BLOOD

Principles & Practice of Hematology

EDITED BY

***Robert I. Handin*, MD**

Professor of Medicine, Harvard Medical School;
Chief, Hematology–Oncology Division,
Brigham and Women's Hospital;
Boston, Massachusetts

***Samuel E. Lux*, MD**

Professor of Pediatrics, Harvard Medical School; Chief, Division of Hematology–Oncology, The Children's Hospital; Associate in Pediatrics, Dana Farber Cancer Institute;
Boston, Massachusetts

***Thomas P. Stossel*, MD**

American Cancer Society Professor of Medicine, Harvard Medical School; Senior Physician, Hematology–Oncology Division;
Chief, Division of Experimental Medicine,
Brigham and Women's Hospital;
Boston, Massachusetts

With 92 Contributors

J.B. LIPPINCOTT COMPANY
Philadelphia

Publisher: Richard H. Lampert
Associate Editor: Paula Callaghan
Associate Managing Editor: Grace R. Caputo
Production Manager: Caren Erlichman
Senior Production Coordinator: Kevin P. Johnson
Designer: Doug Smock
Cover Designer: Tom Jackson
Indexer: Holly Lukens
Compositor: Tapsco, Inc.
Printer/Binder: Courier Book Company/Westford
Color Insert Printer: Walsworth Publishing Company

6 5 4 3 2 1

Library of Congress Cataloging-in-Publication Data

Blood: principles and practice of hematology/edited by Robert I. Handin, Samuel E. Lux, Thomas P. Stossel; with 92 contributors.
p. cm.
Includes bibliographical references and index.
ISBN 0-397-50944-8 (alk. paper)
1. Hematology. 2. Blood—Diseases. I. Handin, Robert I. II. Lux, Samuel E. III. Stossel, Thomas P.
[DNLM: 1. Hematology. WH 100 B65538 1995]
RC636.B575 1995
616.1'5—dc20
DNLM/DLC
for Library of Congress 94-27361
CIP

∞ This paper meets the requirements of ANSI/NISO Z39.48-1992 (permanence of paper).

The authors and publisher have exerted every effort to ensure that drug selection and dosage set forth in this text are in accord with practice at the time of publication. However, in view of ongoing research, changes in government regulations, and the constant flow of information relating to drug therapy and drug reactions, the reader is urged to check the package insert for each drug for any change in indications and dosage and for added warnings and precautions. This is particularly important when the recommended agent is a new or infrequently employed drug.

To Marcia Handin, Kathryn John, and Anne Stossel

CONTRIBUTORS

Peter Agre, MD
Professor of Medicine and Biological Chemistry
Johns Hopkins University School of Medicine
Johns Hopkins Hospital
Baltimore, Maryland

Alan C. Aisenberg, MD, PhD
Professor of Medicine
Harvard Medical School
Massachusetts General Hospital
Boston, Massachusetts

Blanche P. Alter, MD
Professor of Pediatrics
Chief, Division of Pediatric Hematology/Oncology
University of Texas Medical School at Galveston
The Children's Hospital
Galveston, Texas

Joseph H. Antin, MD
Associate Professor of Medicine
Harvard Medical School
Director, Bone Marrow Transplant Program
Brigham and Women's Hospital
Boston, Massachusetts

Robert J. Arceci, MD, PhD
Assistant Professor of Pediatrics
Harvard Medical School
Division of Pediatric Hematology/Oncology
Dana Farber Cancer Institute
The Children's Hospital
Boston, Massachusetts

James O. Armitage, MD
Professor and Chairman
Department of Internal Medicine
University of Nebraska Medical Center
Omaha, Nebraska

Bernard M. Babior, MD
Member and Physician
Division of Hematology/Oncology
Scripps Clinic and Research Foundation
La Jolla, California

Kenneth A. Bauer, MD
Associate Professor of Medicine
Harvard Medical School
Associate Physician
Beth Israel Hospital
Boston, Massachusetts
Chief, Hematology–Oncology Section
Brockton–West Roxbury VA Medical Center
West Roxbury, Massachusetts

Diana Beardsley, MD
Associate Professor of Pediatrics and Internal Medicine
Yale University School of Medicine
Yale–New Haven Hospital
New Haven, Connecticut

Nathan A. Berger, MD
Professor of Medicine, Biochemistry, and Oncology
Case Western Reserve University School of Medicine
Director, Cancer Research Center
University Hospitals of Cleveland
Cleveland, Ohio

Paul D. Berk, MD
Henry and Lillian M. Stratton Professor of Molecular Medicine
Professor of Biochemistry
Chief, Division of Liver Diseases
Mount Sinai School of Medicine of the City University of New York
Mount Sinai Hospital
New York, New York

Kenneth A. Bridges, MD
Assistant Professor of Medicine
Harvard Medical School
Associate Physician
Brigham and Women's Hospital
Boston, Massachusetts

C. Norman Coleman, MD
Alvan T. and Viola D. Fuller–American Cancer Society Professor
Chairman, Joint Center for Radiation Therapy
Boston, Massachusetts

Désire Collen, MD, PhD
Professor of Medicine
University of Leuven
Leuven, Belgium

Harvey R. Colten, MD
Professor of Molecular Microbiology
Washington University School of Medicine
Pediatrician-in-Chief
St Louis Children's Hospital
St Louis, Missouri

Bernard A. Cooper, MD
Louis Lowenstein Professor of Hematology and Oncology
McGill University
Senior Physician
Royal Victoria Hospital
Montreal, Quebec
Canada

Max D. Cooper, MD
Professor of Medicine, Pediatrics, and Microbiology
University of Alabama School of Medicine
University of Alabama Hospital
Birmingham, Alabama

Laurence Corash, MD
Professor of Laboratory Medicine
University of California, San Francisco, School of Medicine
Chief, Hematology Section
Clinical Laboratories
Medical Center at the University of California
San Francisco, California

William M. Crist, MD
Professor of Pediatrics
University of Tennessee, Memphis, College of Medicine
Chairman, Department of Hematology/Oncology
Saint Jude Children's Research Hospital
Memphis, Tennessee

Thomas P. Duffy, MD
Professor of Medicine
Division of Hematology
Yale University Medical School
Yale–New Haven Hospital
New Haven, Connecticut

Cynthia E. Dunbar, MD
Senior Clinical Investigator
Clinical Hematology Branch
National Heart, Lung, and Blood Institute
National Institutes of Health
Bethesda, Maryland

Bruce M. Ewenstein, MD
Assistant Professor of Medicine
Harvard Medical School
Associate Physician
Brigham and Women's Hospital
Boston, Massachusetts

Manlio Ferrarini, MD
Professor of Medical Oncology
University of Genova Medical School
Chief, Division of Clinical Immunology
Isituto Nazionale per la Richerca sul Cancro
Servizio di Immunologia Clinica
Viale Benedetto
Italy

Kenneth A. Foon, MD
Professor and Chief
Division of Hematology and Oncology
Department of Internal Medicine
Director, Lucille Parker Markey Cancer Center
University of Kentucky College of Medicine
Lexington, Kentucky

Bernard G. Forget, MD
Professor of Internal Medicine and Genetics
Chief, Hematology Section
Yale University School of Medicine
Yale–New Haven Hospital
New Haven, Connecticut

Stephen H. Friend, MD, PhD
Assistant Professor of Pediatrics
The Children's Hospital
Boston, Massachusetts
Member, Massachusetts General Hospital Cancer Center
Charlestown, Massachusetts

Steven M. Fruchtman, MD
Assistant Professor of Medicine
Mount Sinai School of Medicine of the City University of New York
Director, Bone Marrow Transplantation
Executive Officer, Polycythemia Vera Study Group
New York, New York

Bruce Furie, MD
Professor of Medicine and Biochemistry
Tufts University School of Medicine
Chief, Division of Hematology–Oncology
New England Medical Center
Boston, Massachusetts

Robert Peter Gale, MD, PhD
Associate Professor of Medicine
University of California, Los Angeles, UCLA School of Medicine
UCLA Medical Center
Los Angeles, California

Stephen J. Galli, MD
Professor of Pathology
Harvard Medical School
Director, Division of Experimental Pathology
Department of Pathology
Beth Israel Hospital
Boston, Massachusetts

Jonathan D. Gitlin, MD
Associate Professor of Pediatrics and Pathology
Washington University School of Medicine
Chief, Division of Immunology and Rheumatology
St Louis Children's Hospital
St Louis, Missouri

Edward J. Goetzl, MD
Robert L. Kroc Professor of Medicine
Professor of Microbiology and Immunology
Director, Immunology and Allergy
University of California, San Francisco, School of Medicine
Director, Immunology and Allergy
Moffitt-Long Hospitals
San Francisco, California

David W. Golde, MD
Professor of Medicine
Cornell University Medical College
Professor of Molecular Pharmacology and Therapeutics
Cornell University Graduate School of Medical Sciences
Head, Division of Hematologic Oncology
Memorial Sloan-Kettering Cancer Center
New York, New York

John M. Goldman, DM, FRCP, FRCPath
Professor of Leukaemia Biology
Royal Postgraduate Medical School
Consultant Physician
Hammersmith Hospital
London, England

James D. Griffin, MD
Professor of Medicine
Harvard Medical School
Division of Tumor Immunology
Dana Farber Cancer Institute
Boston, Massachusetts

Jerome E. Groopman, MD
Dina and Raphael Recanant Professor of Medicine
Harvard Medical School
Chief, Division of Hematology/Oncology
New England Deaconess Hospital
Boston, Massachusetts

Carlo E. Grossi, MD, PhD
Professor
University of Genova School of Medicine
Division of Clinical Pathology
Isituto Nazionale per la Richerca sul Cancro
Genova, Italy

Robert I. Handin, MD
Professor of Medicine
Harvard Medical School
Chief, Hematology–Oncology Division
Brigham and Women's Hospital
Boston, Massachusetts

Laurence A. Harker, MD
Blomeyer Professor of Medicine
Director, Division of Hematology and Oncology
Emory University School of Medicine
Atlanta, Georgia

Elzbieta Kaczmarek, PhD
Instructor
Harvard Medical School
Research Associate
Department of Pathology
Beth Israel Hospital
Boston, Massachusetts

Allen P. Kaplan, MD
Professor and Chairman
Department of Medicine
State University of New York at Stony Brook Health Sciences Center School of Medicine
Service Chief, Department of Medicine
University Hospital at Stony Brook
Stony Brook, New York

Attallah Kappas, MD
Sherman Fairchild Professor
Rockefeller University
Senior Physician and Physician-in-Chief (Emeritus)
Rockefeller University Hospital
New York, New York

John G. Kelton, MD
Professor of Medicine and Pathology
Director, Blood Bank
McMaster University Medical Centre
Hamilton, Ontario
Canada

Stanley J. Korsmeyer, MD
Professor of Medicine and Pathology
Washington University School of Medicine
Associate Investigator
Howard Hughes Medical Institute
Assistant Physician to the Medical Staff
Barnes Hospital
St Louis, Missouri

David J. Kwiatkowski, MD, PhD
Associate Professor of Medicine
Harvard Medical School
Brigham and Women's Hospital
Boston, Massachusetts

Hillard M. Lazarus, MD, FACP
Professor of Medicine
Case Western Reserve University School of Medicine
Director, Bone Marrow Transplant Patient Program
Ireland Cancer Center
Cleveland, Ohio

Myoung Hee Lee, PhD
Instructor
Harvard Medical School
Research Associate
Beth Israel Hospital
Boston, Massachusetts

H.R. Lijnen, MD
Department of Medicine
University of Leuven
Leuven, Belgium

Stuart E. Lind, MD
Associate Professor of Pathology and Medicine
University of Vermont College of Medicine
Director, Coagulation Laboratory
Medical Center Hospital of Vermont
Burlington, Vermont

Samuel E. Lux, MD
Professor of Pediatrics
Harvard Medical School
Chief, Division of Hematology–Oncology
The Children's Hospital
Associate in Pediatrics
Dana Farber Cancer Institute
Boston, Massachusetts

Lucio Luzzatto, MD, FRCP, FRCPath
Professor of Haematology
Royal Postgraduate Medical School of the University of London
Consultant Haematologist
Hammersmith Hospital
London, England

David I. Marks, MD, PhD
Assistant Professor of Medicine
Division of Neoplastic Diseases
Hahnemann University
Philadelphia, Pennsylvania

Peter Mauch, MD
Associate Professor of Radiation Oncology
Joint Center for Radiation Therapy
Harvard Medical School
Boston, Massachusetts

Jeffrey McCullough, MD
Professor, Department of Laboratory Medicine and Pathology
Director, Division of Laboratory Medicine
Director, Section of Transfusion Medicine
University of Minnesota Hospital and Clinic
Minneapolis, Minnesota

Jan McDonagh, PhD
Associate Professor of Pathology
Harvard Medical School
Pathologist
Beth Israel Hospital
Boston, Massachusetts

Kenneth B. Miller, MD
Associate Professor of Medicine
Director, Leukemia and Bone Marrow Transplant Service
Division of Hematology–Oncology
Tufts University School of Medicine
New England Medical Center
Boston, Massachusetts

A. Jacqueline Mitus, MD
Instructor
Harvard Medical School
Associate Physician
Brigham and Women's Hospital
Boston, Massachusetts

Cynthia C. Morton, PhD
Associate Professor of Pathology
Harvard Medical School
Associate Pathologist
Director, Cytogenetics
Brigham and Women's Hospital
Boston, Massachusetts

Scott Murphy, MD
Professor of Medicine
Jefferson Medical College of Thomas Jefferson University
Associate Director for Clinical Programs
Cardeza Foundation for Hematologic Research
Philadelphia, Pennsylvania

Ronald L. Nagel, MD
Professor of Medicine
Head, Division of Hematology
Albert Einstein College of Medicine
Montefiore Medical Center
Bronx, New York

Arthur W. Nienhuis, MD
Director
Saint Jude Children's Research Hospital
Memphis, Tennessee

Stephen D. Nimer, MD
Chief
Hematology Service
Associate Member
Memorial Sloan-Kettering Cancer Center
New York, New York

Stuart H. Orkin, MD
Leland Fikes Professor of Pediatric Medicine
Harvard Medical School
Investigator
Howard Hughes Medical Institute
The Children's Hospital
Boston, Massachusetts

Donald E. Paglia, MD
Professor of Pathology and Laboratory Medicine
University of California, Los Angeles, UCLA School of Medicine
Pathologist
UCLA Center for Health Sciences
Los Angeles, California

Jiri Palek, MD
Professor of Medicine
Tufts University School of Medicine
Chairman, Department of Biomedical Research
Chief, Division of Hematology/Oncology
St Elizabeth's Hospital of Boston
Boston, Massachusetts

Howard A. Pearson
Professor of Pediatrics
Yale University School of Medicine
New Haven, Connecticut

Orah S. Platt, MD
Associate Professor of Pediatrics
Harvard Medical School
Director, Department of Laboratory Medicine
Children's Hospital
Boston, Massachusetts

Sesha R. Reddigari, PhD
Research Assistant Professor
Division of Allergy
Department of Medicine
State University of New York at Stony Brook Health Sciences Center School of Medicine
Stony Brook, New York

Gaston K. Rivera, MD
Professor of Pediatrics
University of Tennessee, Memphis, College of Medicine
Department of Hematology/Oncology
Saint Jude Children's Research Hospital
Memphis, Tennessee

Fred S. Rosen, MD
James L. Gamble Professor of Pediatrics
Harvard Medical School
Senior Associate, Department of Medicine
The Children's Hospital
President, The Center for Blood Research
Boston, Massachusetts

David S. Rosenblatt, MDCM, FCCMG, FRCPC
Professor of Medicine, Pediatrics, and Human Genetics
McGill University Faculty of Medicine
Director, Division of Medical Genetics
Department of Medicine
Montreal General Hospital
Royal Victoria Hospital
Director, The Hess B. and Diane Finestone Laboratory in Memory of Jacob and Jenny Finestone
Montreal, Quebec
Canada

David S. Rosenthal, MD
Henry K. Oliver Professor of Hygiene
Director, Health Services
Harvard University
Associate Professor of Medicine
Harvard Medical School
Brigham and Women's Hospital
Boston, Massachusetts

Wendell F. Rosse, MD
Florence Raynaud McAlister Professor of Medicine
Professor of Immunology
Duke University Medical Center
Durham, North Carolina

Shigeru Sassa, MD, PhD
Associate Professor and Physician
Head, Laboratory of Biochemical Hematology
Rockefeller University
New York, New York

David T. Scadden, MD
Assistant Professor of Medicine
Harvard Medical School
Division of Hematology/Oncology
New England Deaconess Hospital
Boston, Massachusetts

Andrew I. Schafer, MD
W.A. and Deborah Moncrief, Jr., Professor of Medicine
Vice-Chairman, Department of Medicine
Baylor College of Medicine
Chief, Medical Service
Houston VA Medical Center
Houston, Texas

Robert S. Schwartz, MD
Professor of Medicine
Associate Editor
New England Journal of Medicine
Boston, Massachusetts

Paul A. Seligman, MD
Professor of Medicine
Division of Hematology and Oncology
University of Colorado Health Sciences Center
University Hospital
Denver, Colorado

Uri Seligsohn, MD
Professor of Hematology
Sackler School of Medicine
Tel-Aviv University
Chairman, Department of Hematology
Director, Institute of Thrombosis and Hemostasis
Chaim Sheba Medical Center
Tel-Hashomer
Israel

Lawrence N. Shulman, MD
Assistant Professor of Medicine
Harvard Medical School
Clinical Director, Hematology–Oncology Division
Brigham and Women's Hospital
Boston, Massachusetts

Susan Blakely Shurin, MD
Professor of Pediatrics
Case Western Reserve University School of Medicine
Chief, Division of Hematology/Oncology
Rainbow Babies and Children's Hospital
Cleveland, Ohio

Colin A. Sieff, MBBCR
Associate Professor of Pediatrics
Dana Farber Cancer Institute
Harvard Medical School
Senior Associate in Medicine
The Children's Hospital
Boston, Massachusetts

Michael Silverberg, DPhil
Associate Professor of Medicine
State University of New York at Stony Brook Health Sciences Center School of Medicine
Stony Brook, New York

Brian R. Smith, MD
Associate Professor of Internal Medicine, Laboratory Medicine, and Pediatrics
Yale University School of Medicine
Director of Research, Yale Bone Marrow Transplant Unit
Yale–New Haven Hospital
New Haven, Connecticut

Thomas P. Stossel, MD
American Cancer Society Professor of Medicine
Harvard Medical School
Senior Physician, Hematology–Oncology Division
Chief, Division of Experimental Medicine
Brigham and Women's Hospital
Boston, Massachusetts

Marc Verstraete, MD, PhD
Professor of Medicine
Center for Molecular and Vascular Biology
University of Leuven
Leuven, Belgium

Theodore E. Warkentin, MD, FRCPC
Assistant Professor of Pathology and Medicine
McMaster University School of Medicine
Hematologist, Department of Laboratory Medicine
Hamilton Civic Hospitals (General Division)
Hamilton, Ontario
Canada

Howard J. Weinstein, MD
Associate Professor of Pediatrics
Harvard Medical School
Director, Pediatric Bone Marrow Transplant Program
The Children's Hospital
Dana Farber Cancer Institute
Boston, Massachusetts

Leon P. Weiss, MD
Professor of Cell Biology
Chairman, Department of Animal Biology
University of Pennsylvania School of Veterinary Medicine
Philadelphia, Pennsylvania

Alan B. Weitberg, MD
Associate Professor of Medicine
Director, Medical Oncology
Brown University School of Medicine
Chief, Division of Hematology/Oncology
Interim Chairman, Department of Medicine
Roger Williams Medical Center
Providence, Rhode Island

Gilbert C. White II, MD
Professor of Medicine
University of North Carolina at Chapel Hill School of Medicine
University of North Carolina Hospitals
Chapel Hill, North Carolina

David A. Williams, MD
Associate Professor of Pediatrics and Medical and Molecular Genetics
Indiana University School of Medicine
Associate Investigator
Howard Hughes Medical Institute
Indianapolis, Indiana

Lawrence C. Wolfe, MD
Associate Professor of Pediatrics
Tufts University School of Medicine
Chief, Division of Pediatric Hematology–Oncology
New England Medical Center
Boston, Massachusetts

Neal S. Young, MD
Chief
Hematology Branch
National Institutes of Health
National Heart, Lung, and Blood Institute
Bethesda, Maryland

Hagop Youssoufian, MD
Assistant Professor of Medicine
Harvard Medical School
Associate Physician
Brigham and Women's Hospital
Boston, Massachusetts

PREFACE

The editors of *Blood: Principles and Practice of Hematology* have been colleagues and friends at Harvard Medical School for more than 20 years. Our decision to create a new hematology textbook arose primarily from our love of the subject and from our having taught it to medical students, residents, and postdoctoral fellows in the hematology training programs we have directed.

We deliberated at weekly meetings for 6 months to decide what sort of book *Blood* should be, and our desire for contributions that were "just right" was reminiscent of the story "Goldilocks and the Three Bears": The divisions of the field, embodied by the chapters, should not be too long or too short. They should be substantial enough to avoid repetition and fragmentation of material, yet short enough to permit the authors to stay within the bounds of their experience and authority. Each chapter should be complete but not exhaustive. Pathophysiology and clinical lore should be balanced, but one or the other should be emphasized in certain chapters to accommodate anticipated needs of readers and the authority and interests of the authors. Finally, the illustrations had to be new and uniformly executed. To accomplish this end, we commissioned an excellent artist to work with the authors.

The contributors were selected to be a mixture of distinguished scholars and experienced clinicians. Accordingly, they sometimes had their own ideas about what is "just right," and we usually agreed with them. The authors are all busy people who have many more important things to do than write for textbooks, and they are independent spirits. Thus, we were pleasantly surprised by their gracious acquiescence to our sometimes heavy editing. We were even more surprised by and grateful for the forbearance of the authors who completed their chapters in a timely fashion and then revised their work, sometimes more than once, to keep the chapters current. Any success with which this book meets will be due in no small measure to the efforts of our contributing authors.

Readers will decide for themselves how close the textbook comes to being "just right," and we encourage their comments so we can move in that direction with further editions.

Robert I. Handin, MD
Samuel E. Lux, MD
Thomas P. Stossel, MD

ACKNOWLEDGMENTS

We extend our appreciation to Paula Callaghan, Grace Caputo, Richard Lampert, Lisa McAllister, and Richard Winters of J.B. Lippincott for their encouragement as we navigated the not always smooth waters of the voyage to the completed book. We also thank artist Joy Marlowe for her vital contribution.

We acknowledge in particular the support and inspiration of Drs. William Moloney and David Nathan, mentors who introduced us to the marvels of hematology.

CONTENTS

BLOOD

Principles & Practice of Hematology

1

Fundamentals of Hematology: Tools of the Trade

Blood: Principles and Practice of Hematology,
edited by Robert I. Handin, Thomas P. Stossel, and Samuel E. Lux.
J.B. Lippincott Company, Philadelphia © 1995.

1

History and Physical Examination of Relevance to the Hematologist

A. Jacqueline Mitus
David S. Rosenthal

Despite the introduction of sophisticated diagnostic tools, a diligent history and careful physical examination are still of paramount importance in medicine.[1,2] Mandating "observe . . . first the countenance of the patient . . . ," Hippocrates underscored the value of these principles.[3] The eloquent notations of patient complaints and findings by our predecessors serve as the first and often the most accurate descriptions of many hematologic illnesses.

Combe,[4] in 1822, depicted the patient with severe anemia:

> *. . . his face, lips, and the whole extent of the surface, were of a deadly pale colour . . . his motions and speech were languid; he complained of much weakness; his respiration free at rest, became hurried on the slightest exertion; pulse 80 and feeble.*

Craigie[5] colorfully portrayed chronic myelogenous leukemia:

> *. . . listlessness . . . swelling and hardness in the left epigastric region . . . perspiration at night . . . blood vessels filled with grumus and clots containing lymph or purulent matter.*

In 1803, a hemorrhagic disposition existing in certain families was noted by Otto,[6] and probably represents the first reported case of hemophilia:

> *. . . a woman by the name of Smith . . . transmitted the following idiosyncrasy to her descendants. . . . If the least scratch is made on the skin of some of them, as mortal a hemorrhage will eventually ensue as if the largest wound is inflicted . . . generally about a week from the injury, an hemorrhage takes place from the whole surface of the wound, and continues for several days.*

Careful inquiry and meticulous observation remain the most important tools of the physician. In the following sections, aspects of the history and physical examination of particular relevance to the hematologist are highlighted.

HISTORY

Presenting Complaints

Many patients with hematologic disease seek medical attention because of nonspecific complaints such as fatigue, weight loss, fever, and bleeding. Fatigue is one of the most difficult problems to assess in general medical practice, and is ranked fifth among presenting symptoms at a large outpatient clinic.[7,8] Seven percent of those with fatigue had a hematologic abnormality, most frequently iron deficiency anemia. Loss of more than 10% of total body weight during a 6-month period is a worrisome sign of malignancy. Progressive decline in weight despite a good appetite, sweating, and pyrexia characterize the hyperproliferative marrow disorders, especially myeloid metaplasia and chronic myelogenous leukemia. In the setting of lymphoma, these so-called B symptoms signal advanced disease and a poorer prognosis.[9] Bleeding and easy bruising often precipitate hematologic evaluation. Mucocutaneous hemorrhage (epistaxis, menorrhagia, oral and gastrointestinal bleeding), occurring either spontaneously or immediately after mild trauma, suggests a defect in primary hemostasis (platelet plug formation), whereas delayed deep-seated bleeding into joints or muscle indicates an abnormality within the coagulation cascade. For convenience, symptoms of hematologic disease relating to specific organ systems are addressed in conjunction with the physical examination.

Medical History

In a patient with bleeding complaints, details of past hemorrhagic events may prove as predictive as laboratory investigations.[10] Excessive bleeding at circumcision or after tonsillectomy points to a congenital coagulopathy, whereas maternal hemorrhage several weeks after delivery raises the suspicion of an acquired inhibitor to factor VIII.

Recurrent spontaneous abortions may be the first presentation for the woman with α-thalassemia or with the lupus anticoagulant, an acquired thrombotic diathesis noted for fetal wastage, placental infarction, and other signs of thrombosis.[11]

Unusual or repeated infections suggest an immune deficiency state. Children with Wiskott-Aldrich syndrome typically contract opportunistic infections within the first months of life. Patients afflicted with Kostman's congenital agranulocytosis may suffer the first of many bouts of serous skin abscesses at only a few weeks of age. Certain organisms have strong associations with specific ailments. *Salmonella* accounts for about half of culture-positive cases of osteomyelitis in children with sickle cell anemia (SCA),[12] whereas *Mycobacterium avium-intracellulare* is frequently seen in hairy-cell leukemia (HCL) and the acquired immunodeficiency syndrome (AIDS).[13–15] Defective immunoglobulin synthesis predisposes to infection by encapsulated organisms and varicella-zoster virus, common pathogens in multiple myeloma, and chronic lymphocytic leukemia (CLL).

A history of an autoimmune disorder like hypothyroidism or vitiligo should heighten the physician's suspicion of pernicious anemia in a patient with macrocytosis.

Ask the patient about blood donation or transfusion.[16] In the absence of prior blood counts, knowledge that the person has successfully donated blood implies an adequate hematocrit. Receipt of blood not only documents the severity of a bleeding episode but may also serve as an important risk factor for AIDS.

Family History

Hematology is rich in heritable diseases. In his original description of hemophilia, Otto[6] astutely defined sex-linked transmission:

> *It is a surprising circumstance that the males only are subject to this strange affection, and that all of them are not liable to it. . . . Although the females are exempt, they are still capable of transmitting it to their male children.*

Patterns of inheritance must be recognized so that asymptomatic affected persons can receive prompt treatment or appropriate genetic counseling. Up to half the children with Fanconi's anemia (autosomal recessive) do not manifest phenotypic findings of skin, skeletal, and renal abnormalities, potentially delaying recognition of the hematologic condition.[17] At times, the patient is not aware of a genetic disease but reports that many family members have undergone identical procedures or suffered similar deaths. Splenectomy or cholecystectomy at an early age are clues to an inherited hemolytic anemia such as hereditary spherocytosis (autosomal dominant), glucose-6-phosphate dehydrogenase (G6PD) deficiency (sex-linked recessive), and pyruvate kinase deficiency (autosomal recessive). Thrombosis occurring in successive generations may unmask a deficiency of antithrombin III, protein C, or protein S. Detailed family trees prove invaluable in these settings. Familial CLL is reported,[18] and the concurrent development of acute lymphoblastic leukemia in monozygotic twins approaches 20%.[19]

Ethnicity is an excellent clue to the patient's gene pool and allows the clinician to tailor the list of differential diagnoses. Blacks have mild leukopenia, which is usually of no clinical significance.[20] Mediterranean, Asian, or African ancestry signal a possible diagnosis of a hemoglobinopathy or thalassemia. Gaucher's disease is more common in families of Jewish heritage from the Baltic Sea region, whereas pernicious anemia appears more frequently in northern Europeans and factor XI deficiency is prevalent among Ashkenazi Jews. On the other hand, CLL is distinctly unusual in the Asian population. Persons from the endemic areas of Japan, Africa, the Caribbean, and southeastern United States are at risk for exposure to the human T-cell leukemia virus I (HTLV-I) virus and development of adult T-cell leukemia–lymphoma (ATL).[21] Remember that the patient's surname may disguise ancestral origins and careful questioning may provide important genomic information.

Social History

The social history of a patient is too often neglected by subspecialists. Alcohol abuse may cause macrocytic anemia, thrombocytopenia, and coagulopathy. Skillful inquiry regarding drug use and sexual practices helps to assess the risks of HIV infection and its protean hematologic manifestations, including immune thrombocytopenia, myelodysplasia, and diffuse lymphadenopathy.[22] Travel to South America, Cape Cod, or India, locales endemic for malaria, babesiosis, and schistosomiasis, respectively, may provide vital clues in the evaluation of a patient with fever, splenomegaly, and hemolysis.

Detailing environmental exposures at home and at the workplace can help unravel confusing hematologic profiles. Old houses with chipped paint serve as potential sources of lead exposure for young children, and may explain neurologic dysfunction, abdominal pain, and anemia with basophilic stippling. Benzene, a solvent frequently used in the manufacture of dyes, rubber, leather goods, varnishes, and solvents is the most widely recognized toxin associated with hematologic disease, especially aplastic anemia and acute leukemia.[23,24] Heavy metals such as arsenic, arsine, and copper (used in smelting, alloy production, fertilizers, and pesticides) as well as lead and zinc (used in making pottery and in producing batteries) have also been implicated in aplastic, sideroblastic, and hemolytic anemias as well as thrombocytopenia and eosinophilia.[25]

Medications, Diet, and Habits

The hematologist must exhaustively inquire about ingestion of all prescription and nonprescription medications including folk remedies. Aspirin, nonsteroidal anti-inflammatory agents, antibiotics, gold, quinine, phenytoin (Dilantin), and heparin are a few of the many drugs that may affect both the function and number of platelets.[10,26–28] More than 400 medications have been associated with neutropenia and several others have been linked to hemolysis.[29] Memorization of these medications is not necessary since a quick glance through the pharmacopoeia will confirm an adverse reaction.

Exploring dietary habits is invaluable in the evaluation of nutritional anemias. Leafy vegetables and legumes are rich in vitamin K and folate. When eliminated from the diet, coagulopathy and megaloblastic anemias can result in a matter of days (vitamin K) to weeks (folate). More than half the patients with iron deficiency (with or without anemia) demonstrate pica (compulsive eating of nonnutritive substances).[30,31] Clay eating by Southern black women "has the legitimacy of folk medicine and social custom,"[30] whereas pagophagia, the consumption of extraordinary amounts of ice, is a more common manifestation in the population at large.[32] Symptoms promptly reverse with administration of iron.

William Crosby[30] best summarized the approach to eliciting a history of pica:

> *Patients rarely volunteer the story of pica. It requires an investigation of tact, sympathy, and time to explain why you inquire about irrational behavior and how the answers can help with the diagnosis of anemia.*

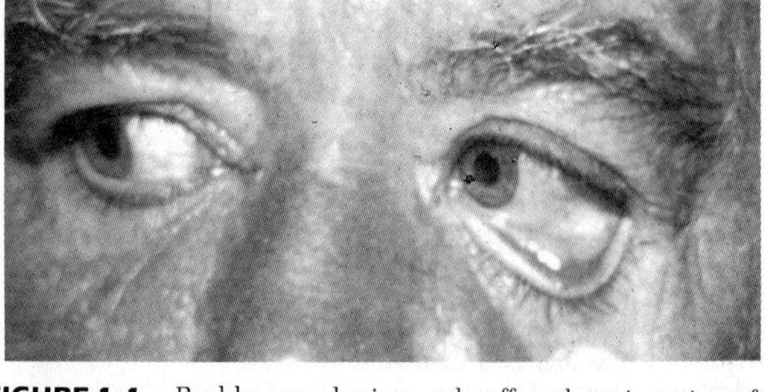

FIGURE 1-1. Ruddy complexion and suffused conjunctiva of a patient with polycythemia vera. (See Color Fig. 1-1.)

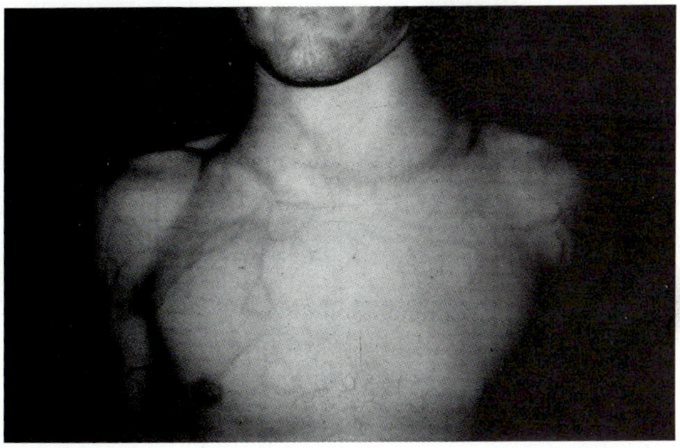

FIGURE 1-2. Venous engorgement secondary to superior vena cava obstruction. (See Color Fig. 1-2.)

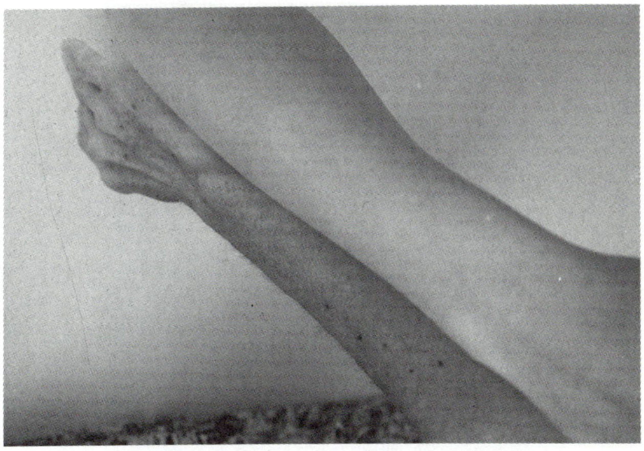

FIGURE 1-3. Slate gray discoloration of the skin of a patient with hemachromatosis compared with normal coloration. (See Color Fig. 1-3.)

Because vitamin B_{12} is plentiful in meat and dairy products, deficiency on a dietary basis is rare, occurring only in strict ovolactovegetarians (vegans) and their children.[33] The anorexic patient may develop profound pancytopenia in association with gelatinous degeneration of the bone marrow.[34]

Common or unusual hobbies are associated with hematologic illness. Exertional hemolysis has been documented in the avid athlete, particularly runners, swimmers, cyclists, and rowers.[35] The builder of model airplanes is at risk for aplastic anemia from serendipitous exposure to glue fumes,[36] whereas storage of winter clothing with mothballs (naphthalene) may provide an oxidant stress for the patient with G6PD deficiency and may precipitate a hemolytic crisis.

PHYSICAL EXAMINATION

Integument

The skin's color and patterns are the first features to strike the examiner. Pallor is best detected by inspection of the normally pink palmar creases, which become pale or silvery white when hemoglobin levels drop below 7 g/dL.[37] By contrast, a ruddy complexion with plethoric facies signifies erythrocytosis (Fig. 1-1). When accompanied by clubbing, perioral, and peripheral cyanosis, a secondary cause is suspect, whereas the presence of acne rosea and eczematoid dermatitis make polycythemia vera more likely. Isolated plethora of the face and upper chest associated with suffused conjunctivae and distended veins (including the sublingual veins) should immediately alert the physician to superior vena cava obstruction, usually by a large mediastinal mass (Fig. 1-2). Up to 4% of patients with non-Hodgkin's lymphomas present with the superior vena cava syndrome.[38] Olive skin in a patient with microcytic anemia suggests possible Mediterranean ancestry and thalassemia, a bronze or slate gray appearance is associated with iron overload (Fig. 1-3), and a lemon yellow hue is characteristic of pernicious anemia. Vitiligo can be seen with pernicious anemia, linking two autoimmune disorders. Café-au-lait spots, patchy brown pigmentations, are found in two thirds of children with Fanconi's anemia.[39]

Abnormal platelet function or number is also reflected in the appearance of the skin. The rare congenital disorder, Hermansky-Pudlak syndrome, is characterized by oculocutaneous albinism, pulmonary fibrosis, inflammatory enteritis, and platelet storage pool deficiency.

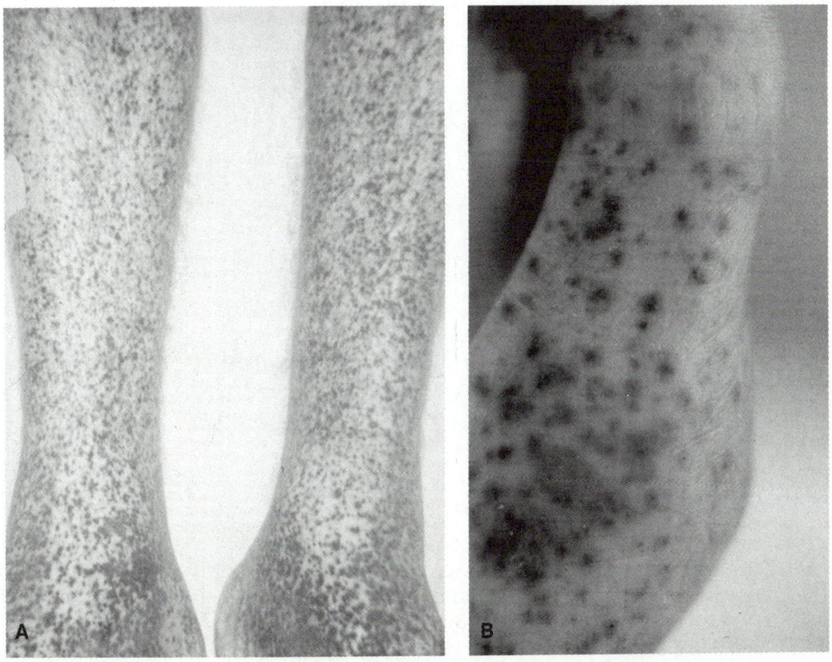

FIGURE 1-4. (**A**) Showers of petechiae and purpura on the legs of a thrombocytopenic patient. (**B**) Close-up of same. (See Color Fig. 1-4.)

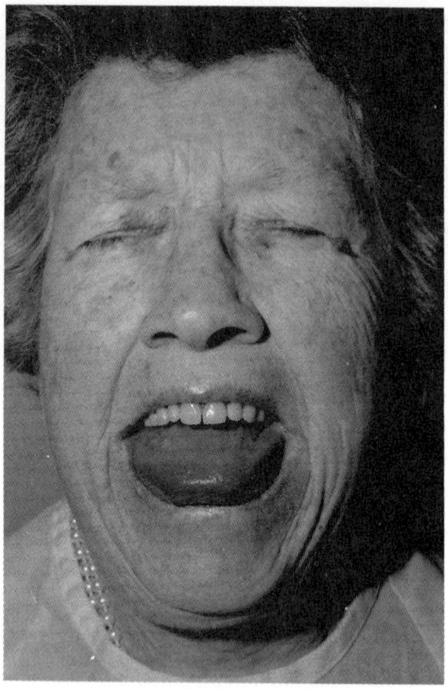

FIGURE 1-5. Periorbital purpura and macroglossia in a patient with amyloidosis. (See Color Fig. 1-5.)

Petechiae, a much more common manifestation of hemostatic abnormalities, are tiny (1- to 3-mm) reddish purple, nonblanching macules that represent small cutaneous hemorrhages. Originally described as flea bitings,[40] petechiae are often found in dependent areas of the body but may be induced by the application of pressure such as with a blood pressure cuff—the tourniquet sign. They arise in the setting of thrombocytopenia or platelet dysfunction or when vascular integrity has been disrupted. Petechiae are hallmark findings in thrombocytopenia of any cause but may also be seen in dysproteinemic states including Waldenström's macroglobulinemia and multiple myeloma. Confluent petechiae or purpura (3 mm to 1 cm) likewise represent sites of hemorrhage into skin and do not blanch with pressure (Fig. 1-4).

Periorbital purpura precipitated by Valsalva maneuver or dependent position of the head is said to be a pathognomonic sign of amyloidosis (AL-type) in the 20% to 40% of

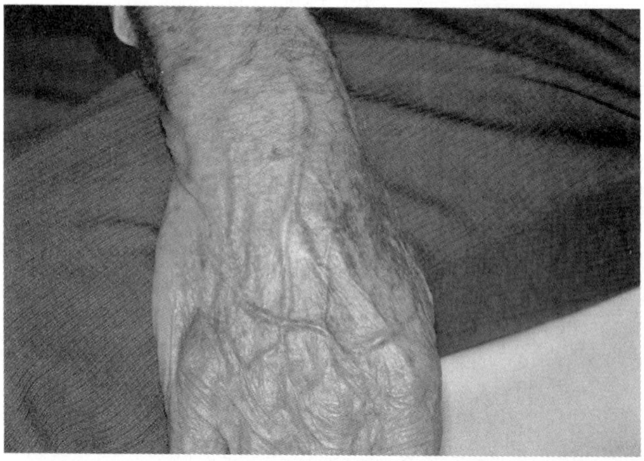

FIGURE 1-6. Senile purpura. Note benign purplish lesions typically found on the dorsum of the hands and the ulnar surface of the forearms. (See Color Fig. 1-6.) (Courtesy of Robert Staszewski, MD)

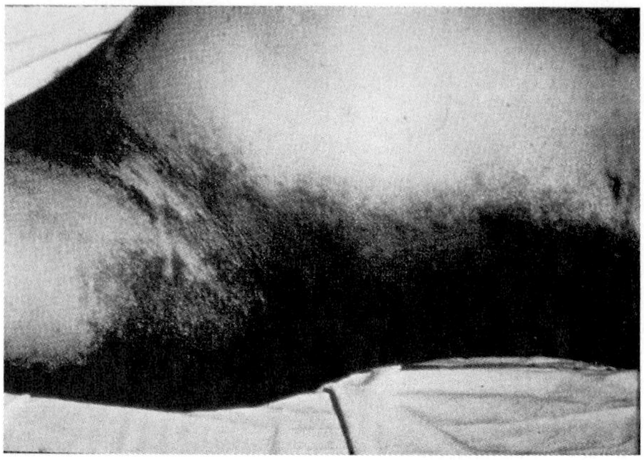

FIGURE 1-7. Grey Turner's sign. Note massive retroperitoneal hemorrhage. (See Color Fig. 1-7.)

these patients who develop cutaneous lesions[41] (Fig. 1-5). Although alarming to the patient, senile purpura are benign and common in the elderly. Resulting from weakened collagen support and ensuing vascular fragility, these large purplish lesions are typically located on the dorsum of the hands and the ulnar surface of the forearm (Fig. 1-6). Vasculitis gives rise to distinct purpura that are palpable. Often urticarial at onset, a reddish brown purpuric eruption of the extremities and buttocks characterizes the rash of the childhood illness, Schönlein-Henoch purpura. The presence of fever, arthralgia, and colicky abdominal pain help clinch the diagnosis.

Ecchymoses larger than 1 cm and hematomas usually predict a defect in secondary hemostasis (coagulation factor deficiency). Grey Turner's sign, a large hematoma at the flanks (Fig. 1-7), and Cullen's sign, blue coloration of the umbilicus, should alert the examiner to massive hemorrhage into the retroperitoneum and peritoneal cavity, respectively. Purpura and hematomas assume a rainbow of colors ranging from red, purple, yellow, and green during the course of resolution (Fig. 1-8).

Telangiectasias, dilations of small cutaneous or mucosal blood vessels that blanch with pressure, are widespread in Rendu-Osler-Weber syndrome (Fig. 1-9). The presence of iron deficiency should raise the suspicion of occult gastrointestinal involvement in patients with this syndrome. Telangiectasias limited to the face are seen in the congenital disorder, Bloom's syndrome. Massive, often disfiguring, capillary hemangiomas or venous malformations can precipitate chronic, low-grade disseminated intravascular coagulation as in the Kasabach-Merritt syndrome (Fig. 1-10).

Kaposi's sarcoma (KS) is a vascular tumor characterized by reddish purple macules or papules. Until recently, KS was an indolent dermal neoplasm afflicting middle-aged men of Mediterranean ancestry or a rare complication of patients with organ transplantation or lymphoma. KS is now recognized as a highly malignant process in the HIV-infected population, affecting up to 46% of homosexual males with this disease.[15] In AIDS, Kaposi's lesions are widespread, and can potentially involve any organ in the body.

Diffuse pruritus heralds a variety of systemic diseases.[42] When exacerbated by hot bathing, it is considered to be pathognomonic of polycythemia vera. Itching can occur without precipitant in this myeloproliferative disorder and often poses a frustrating, refractory clinical problem. Intense pruritus accompanied by skin excoriation has reemerged as an important B symptom of Hodgkin's disease.[43,44] Of 360 patients with this neoplasm, 90 (25%) complained of mild pruritus whereas 20 (6%) experienced

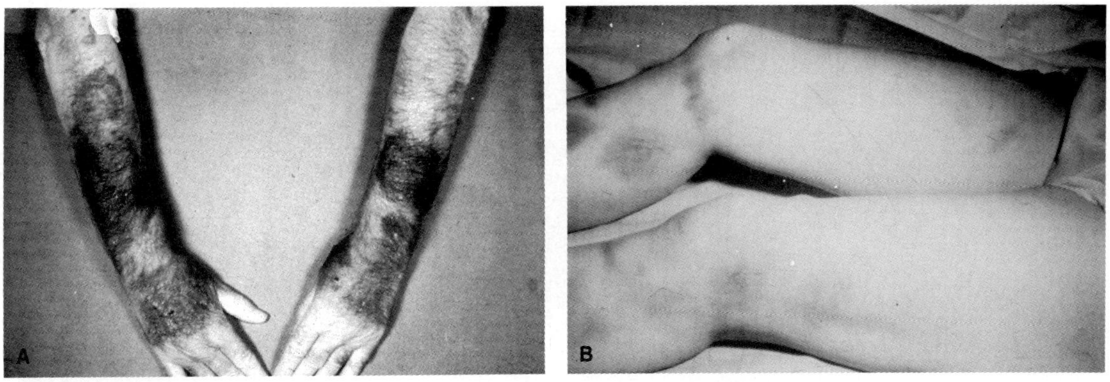

FIGURE 1-8. (**A**) Recent ecchymoses (blue-black). (**B**) Older, resolving ecchymoses (yellow-green). (See Color Fig. 1-8.)

severe symptoms. In the latter group, survival was significantly reduced.[43]

Cutaneous involvement with leukemia or lymphoma takes many forms. The red man syndrome (*l'homme rouge*) is a diffuse, intensely pruritic eczematoid eruption characterizing Sézary's syndrome. In severe conditions, hyperkeratosis with painful fissuring and *leonine facies* are also seen[45] (Fig. 1-11). Subsequent development of serpentine scaling plaques and ulcerated nodules mark the later stages of the T-cell lymphoproliferative process, mycosis fungoides (Fig. 1-12). In contrast, rapidly evolving nonpruritic subcutaneous nodules are typical of HTLV-I associated adult T-cell leukemia- lymphoma[21] (Fig. 1-13).

Of the leukemias, the *monocytic* variants (M4 and M5) have the highest incidence (20% to 30%) of skin infiltration by malignant cells (leukemia cutis).[46] On examination, small, painless, nonpruritic raised nodules of a salmon or pinkish purple color are detected (Fig. 1-14). Overall, leukemia cutis develops in 3% of patients with acute myeloid and lymphoid leukemia.[47,48] Twenty percent of CLL patients have skin findings consisting of macules, nodules, diffuse erythroderma, and bullous pemphigoid.[47,49] Two curious immune phenomena are notable in this lymphoproliferative disease—an exaggerated response to insect bites (especially mosquitoes; Fig. 1-15) and, of greater concern, a potentially fatal necrotizing reaction after live viral vaccination. Xanthomas, café-au-lait spots, and erythematous maculopapules are recognized in over 40% of cases of juvenile chronic myelogenous leukemia.

Chloromas, isolated collections of leukemic myeloblasts, derive their name from the chlorophyll or green color of the myeloperoxidase enzyme present in the cells. Chloromas arise at any site of the body and complicate 2% to 4% of cases of acute and chronic myelogenous leukemia.[51,52] Occasionally, these tumors precede bone marrow involvement.

Cutaneous manifestations of *hairy-cell leukemia* remain underrecognized. Eight percent of patients develop erythematous papules over their extremities, trunk, and palms as a result of infiltration by hairy lymphocytes.[53,54] Cutaneous vasculitis occurs less frequently.[55] The rash of angioimmunoblastic lymphadenopathy with dysproteinemia, seen in 45% of cases, takes many forms such as nonspecific maculopapular eruptions and severe urticaria with excoriation and exfoliation.[56] Intense pruritus, skin nodules, and dermatographism typify *urticaria pigmentosa*, the cutaneous form of systemic mastocytosis (Fig. 1-16).

Among the many nonspecific findings associated with the leukemias and lymphomas, *Sweet's syndrome*, or acute febrile neutrophilic dermatosis, deserves brief mention. In this condition, originally described by Sweet in 1964, intense, focal, perivascular infiltration of the dermis by granulocytes leads to the formation of discrete, small, raised, and tender erythematous plaques on the torso, face, and extremities (Fig. 1-17). Irregular and often studded with

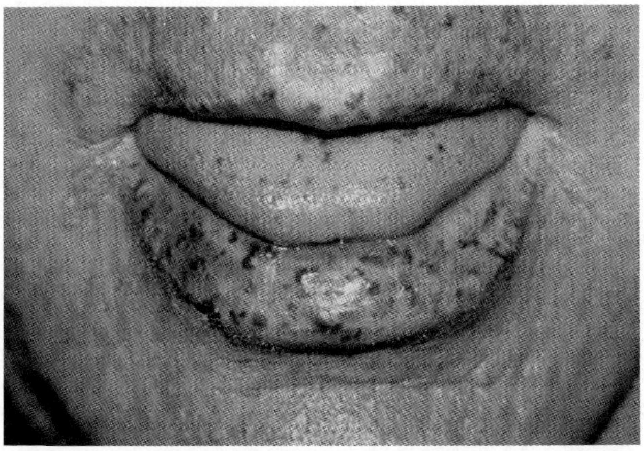

FIGURE 1-9. Mucosal telangiectasias in a patient with Rendu-Osler-Weber syndrome. (See Color Fig. 1-9.)

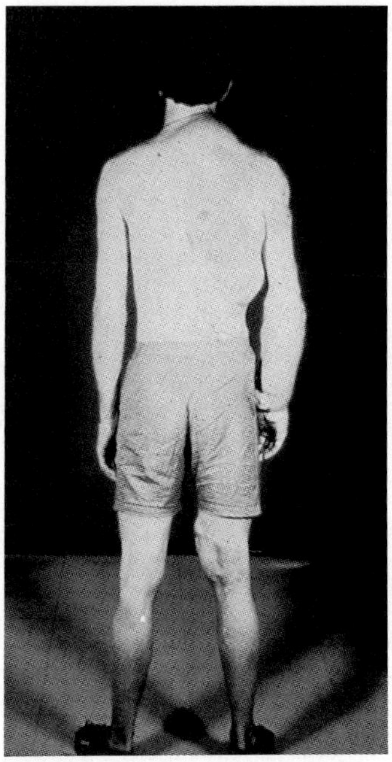

FIGURE 1-10. Massive venous malformation causing chronic disseminated intravascular coagulation.

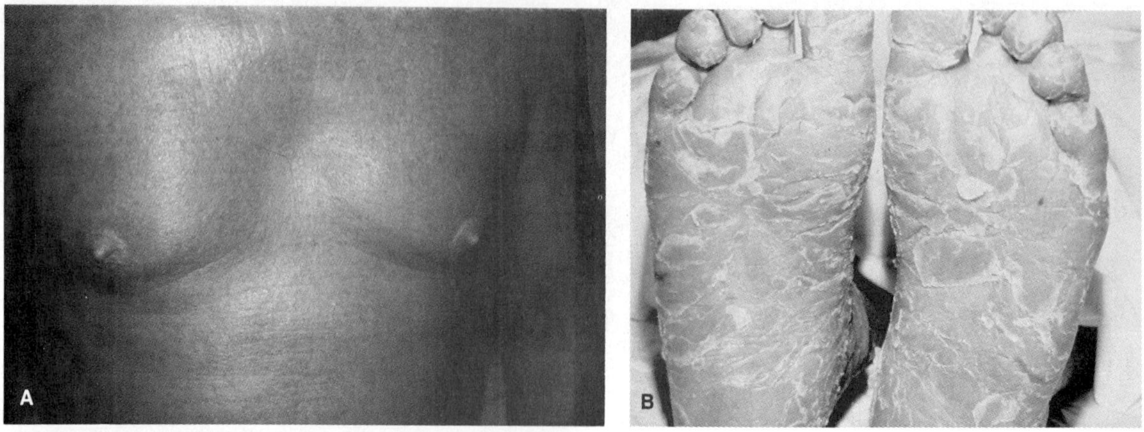

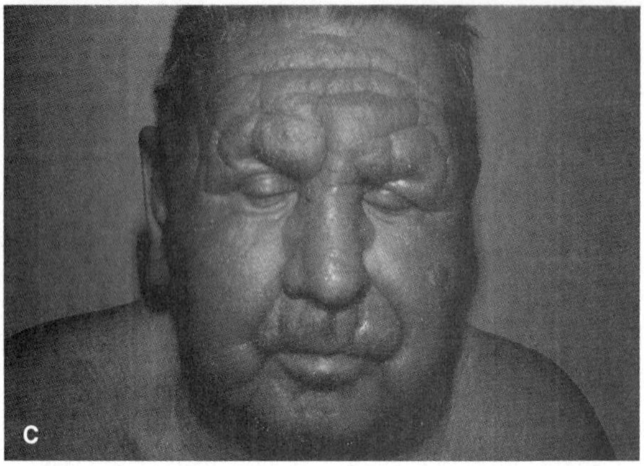

FIGURE 1-11. Sézary's syndrome. (**A**) L'homme rouge. (**B**) Hyperkeratosis with fissuring. (**C**) Leonine facies. (See Color Fig. 1-11.) (Wieselthier JS, Koh HK. Sézary syndrome: diagnosis, prognosis and critical review of treatment options. J Am Acad Dermatol 1990;22:383)

papules, pustules, and crusts, these plaques occur in up to 10% of patients with acute leukemia.[57]

Skin ulceration occurs in several settings, notably in the hemolytic anemias. Herrick[58] first drew attention to this complication in his original description of sickle cell disease:

> *The lesions . . . had been pustular, with formation of ulcers and scabs. . . . The scars . . . were nearly all located on the legs and thighs, some in the former location being as much as 3 cm in diameter. There were perhaps twenty scars in all. They were rounded or oval, sometimes of irregular contour, the edges clean-cut; some were like tissue paper on thin parchment to the touch and were lighter in color than the surrounding skin. (p 517)*

Although rates of leg ulceration higher than 50% have been reported,[59] a large cooperative group study of more than 2000 SCA patients found that only 2.5% demonstrated this complication at entry.[60] The highest incidence occurred in males with SS disease (9.97 per 100,000 patient-years) and S-α-thalassemia (5.73 per 100,000 patient-years), being

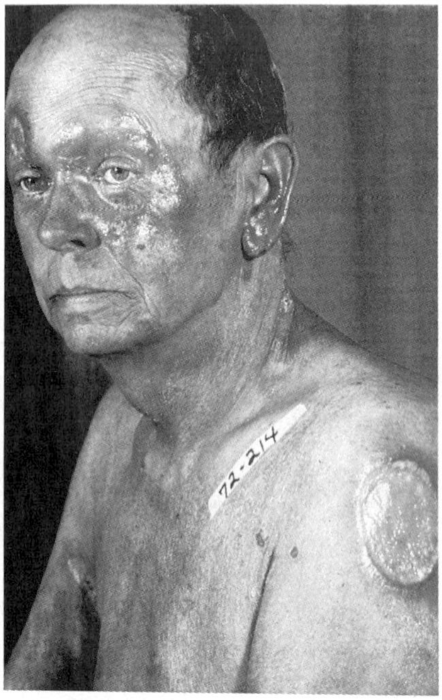

FIGURE 1-12. Mycosis fungoides. Note plaques and ulcerative nodules. (See Color Fig. 1-12.)

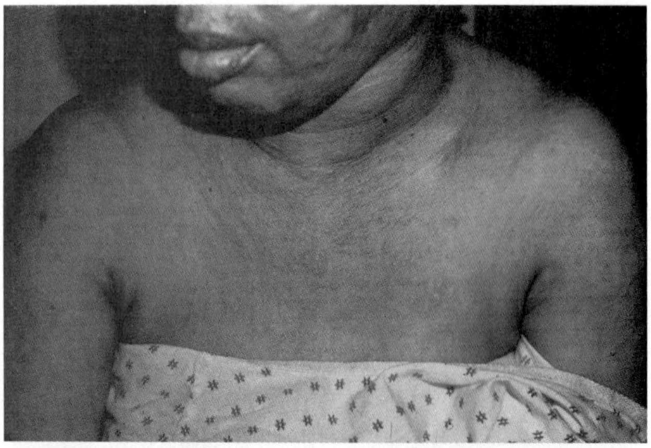

FIGURE 1-13. Erythematous, nonpruritic nodular infiltrate in a patient with adult T-cell leukemia–lymphoma. (See Color Fig. 1-13.)

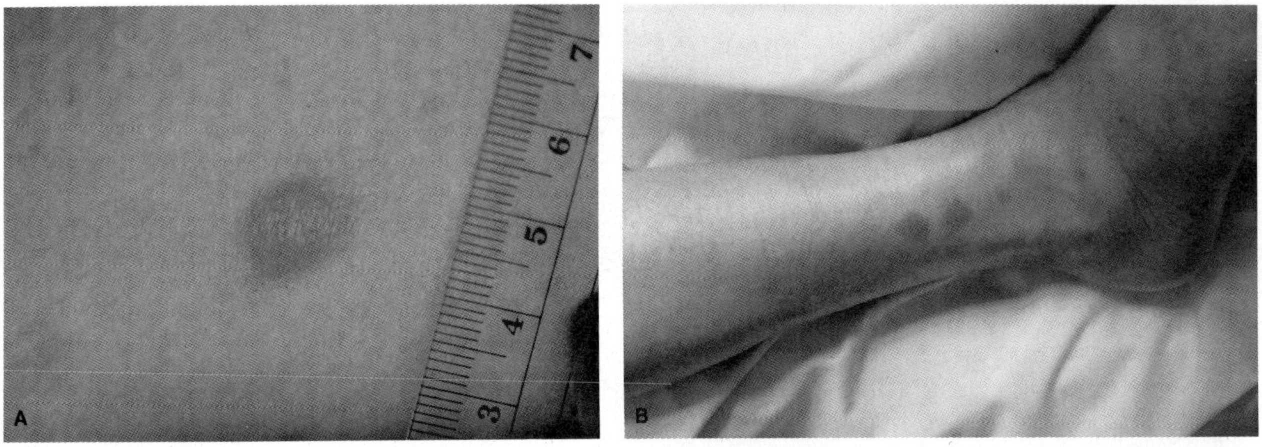

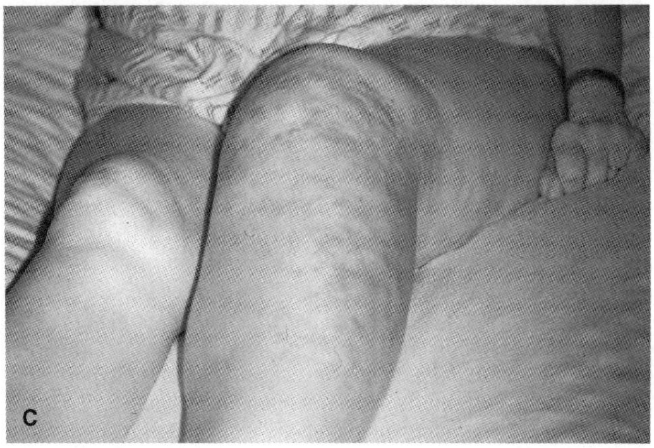

FIGURE 1-14. Leukemia cutis. (**A**) Small salmon-colored nodule. (**B**) Larger purplish subcutaneous lesions. (**C**) Massive cutaneous infiltration by leukemia. (See Color Fig. 1-14.)

distinctly unusual in SC and S-β-thalassemia. Children under the age of 10 years are spared. Ulcers arise spontaneously or after trauma and range in size between 1 and 10 cm. Depressed, irregular scars with hyperpigmented borders (Fig. 1-18), fibrosis and, rarely, distortion of the ankle joint ensue. Photosensitivity, resulting in the formation of cutaneous bullae or vesicles, characterizes certain forms of porphyria. On healing, scars, ulcers, and necrotic lesions may result (Fig. 1-19). The rare disorder, atrophy blanche, is distinguished by recurrent small cutaneous thromboses and microinfarcts. Superficial ulceration, usually involving the distal legs, gives rise to the whitish depressed scars from which this disorder takes its name (Fig. 1-20). The attentive physician searches for protein C or S deficiency in the patient who develops skin necrosis after warfarin (Coumadin) administration (Fig. 1-21).

Eczema is a hallmark finding of the childhood disorders, Wiskott-Aldrich syndrome (immunodeficiency with thrombocytopenia and eczema) and histiocytosis X. The

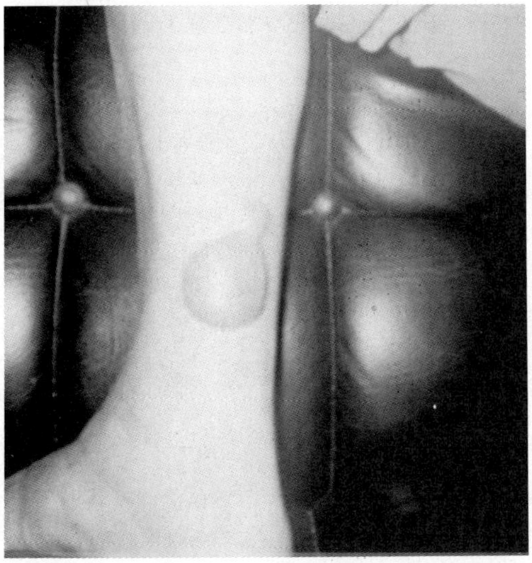

FIGURE 1-15. Exaggerated response to mosquito bite in a patient with chronic lymphocytic leukemia. (See Color Fig. 1-15.)

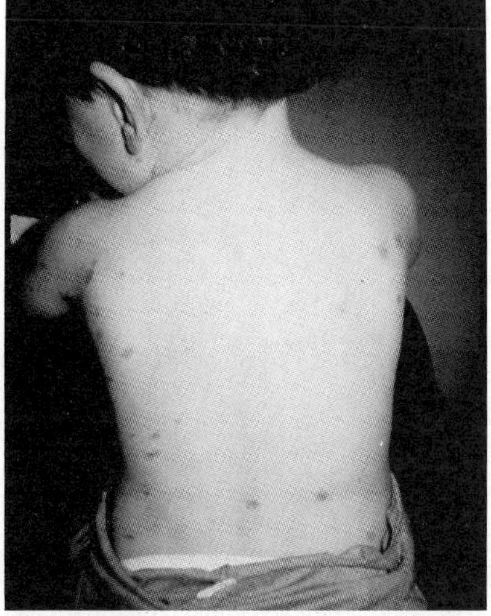

FIGURE 1-16. Multiple reddish brown nodules in a patient with urticaria pigmentosa. (See Color Fig. 1-16.)

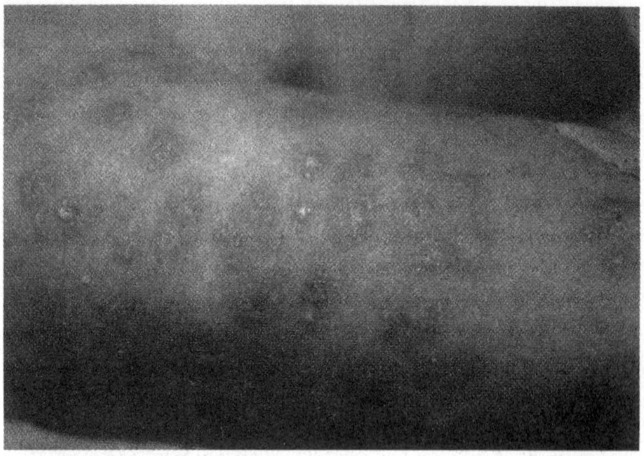

FIGURE 1-17. Patient with Sweet's syndrome. (See Color Fig. 1-17.) (Dover JS. Case records of the Massachusetts General Hospital: a 47-year-old male with a rash, fever and headaches. N Engl J Med 1990;323:255)

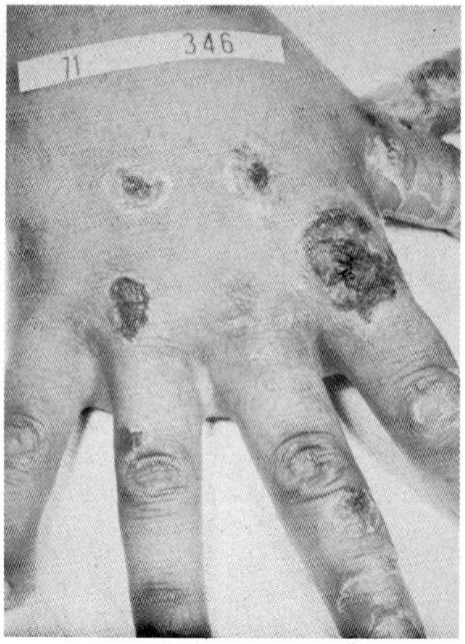

FIGURE 1-19. Necrotic ulcerations in a patient with erythropoietic porphyria. (See Color Fig. 1-19.)

scaling pruritic eruptions may be mistaken for a benign condition, at times delaying diagnosis of the underlying hematologic problem.

The hair and nails are easily overlooked. Although they rarely provide the only clue to diagnosis, they often display characteristic changes in hematologic disease. Koilonychia, brittle, coarsely ridged, and spooned nails, are seen in patients with iron deficiency (Fig. 1-22). Hypertrichosis along with diffuse hyperpigmentation, skin thickening, and edema are skin manifestations of the newly recognized plasmacytic disorder, POEMS syndrome (polyneuropathy, organomegaly, endocrinopathy, m-component, skin change), and occur in 90% of cases.[61,62] Alopecia and thinned and gray hair are notable in patients with pernicious anemia. Originally described in red-haired girls, Job's syndrome is characterized by elevated levels of IgE and chemotactic defects of neutrophils. Job's syndrome is now recognized as a disorder capable of affecting any infant or young child and of giving rise to chronic eczematoid rashes, sterile cutaneous abscesses, and recurrent bacterial infections of the skin and sinopulmonary tract.[63]

Head

In children, the skull serves as a major site of hematopoiesis. Exuberant marrow proliferation in patients with thalassemia results in prominence of frontal and parietal bones (frontal bossing) and in protuberance of the maxilla leading to overbite, protrusion of exposed incisor teeth, and separation of the orbit, a clinical picture called *chipmunk facies* (Fig. 1-23). This disfiguring cephalofacial abnormality correlates with delay in transfusion therapy, less common in the current era of early aggressive treatment.[64] Other skull abnormalities associated with congenital hematologic diseases include microcephaly in Fanconi's anemia, bird-like facies in Bloom's syndrome, and *turmschadel* or tower skull in hereditary spherocytosis. Palpation of the skull can lead to detection of a plasmacytoma in a patient with multiple myeloma or to an osseous lesion in a child with eosinophilic granuloma.

Eyes

The eye can be affected by, or serve as a primary site of, hematologic disease.[65-67] The sclera offers an ideal location for the detection of icterus or plethora by eliminating the confounding problem of skin pigmentation. The normally pink cul-de-sacs of the conjunctivae are pale in the anemic states; in contrast, hyperemia or suffusion typify polycythemia (see Fig. 1-1). Hyperviscosity secondary to erythro-

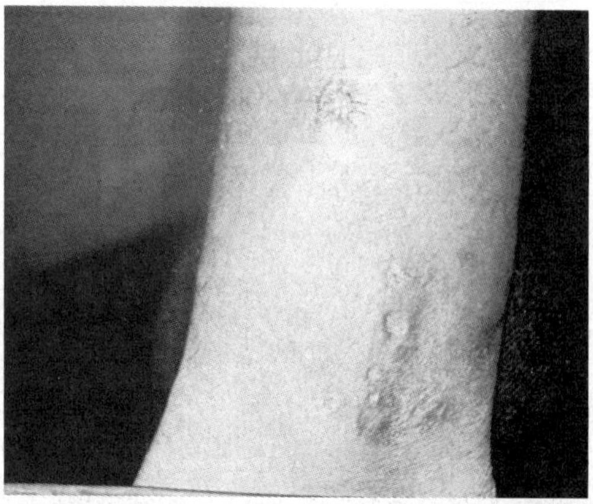

FIGURE 1-18. Scars with hyperpigmented borders due to recurrent ulceration in a patient with sickle cell anemia. (See Color Fig. 1-18.)

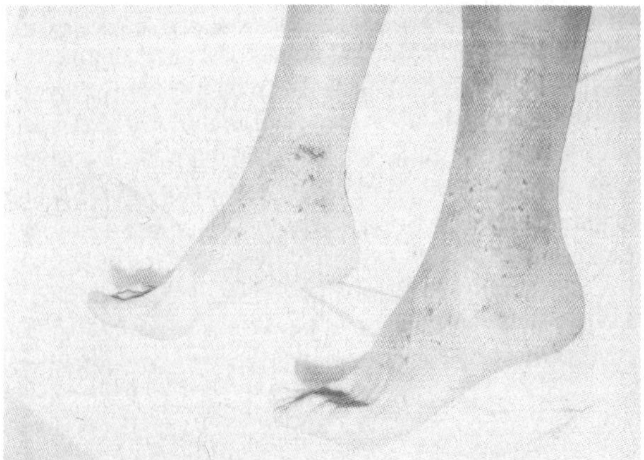

FIGURE 1-20. Small depressed ulcerations on the legs of a patient with atrophie blanche. (See Color Fig. 1-20.)

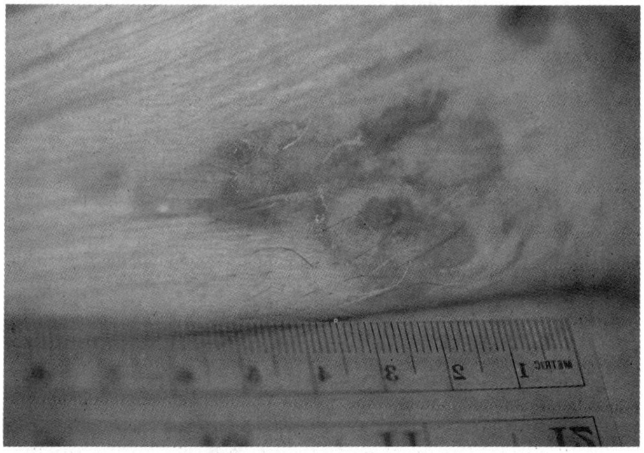

FIGURE 1-21. Necrosis of the skin following warfarin administration in a patient with protein C deficiency. (See Color Fig. 1-21.)

cytosis or hypergammaglobulinemia leads to engorgement, tortuosity, and darkening of conjunctival vessels. Distinctive, asymptomatic, comma-shaped lesions are seen in patients with SCA and result from stasis and ensuing distortion of capillary segments. Pingueculae (brown pterygium) are early findings in patients with Gaucher's disease. Smooth, raised and fleshy, salmon-colored masses on the conjunctivae are likely to represent lymphoma (Fig. 1-24).

Crystalline opacities of the cornea, usually gray or brown, alert the astute examiner to the possibility of an underlying gammopathy. These proteinaceous deposits can precede recognition of Waldenström's macroglobulinemia or multiple myeloma by up to 5 years.[66]

The retina is not spared the pallor of anemia. Rarely, papilledema, hemorrhages, and acute visual loss result when anemia is severe.[67] Visual blurring or darkening and diminished visual acuity are common complaints in disorders in which hyperviscosity can arise. Fifty percent of patients with Waldenström's macroglobulinemia develop fundoscopic changes.[66] Dilatation and tortuosity of the vessels give rise to their description as miniature sausage links or boxcars and may lead to complete central retinal vein occlusion (Fig. 1-25). Left untreated, flame-shaped hemorrhages, microaneurysms, and exudates occur. Cotton-wool spots, vitreous hemorrhage, and papilledema are late sequelae. Truly, the ophthalmoscope can serve as a bedside viscometer.[68]

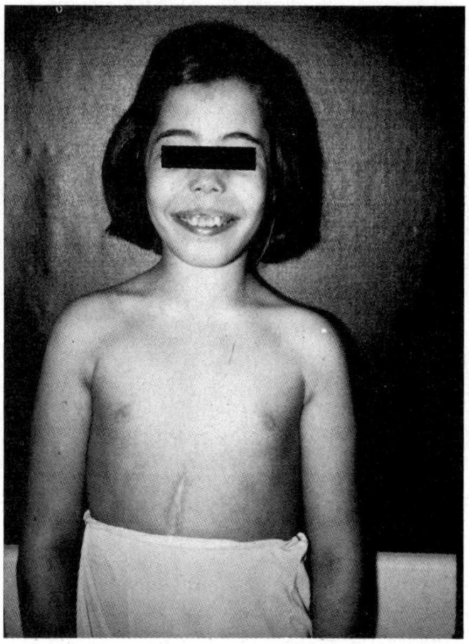

FIGURE 1-23. Chipmunk facies of thalassemia. (See Color Fig. 1-23.)

Routine ophthalmologic examination is an integral component of the care of the patient with SCA and thalassemia. When detected early, asymptomatic neovascularization of the retina may be halted before the development of visual disturbance and blindness, complications of vitreous hemorrhage and retinal detachment. These proliferative changes occur more frequently in persons with SC disease (up to two thirds of all patients) and S-thalassemia (α and β) compared with the homozygous condition (SS) perhaps because of higher hemoglobin levels and viscosity in the former two disorders.[69,70] Other retinal changes found in patients with SCA are overgrowth of retinal pigment giving rise to black sunbursts and salmon-patch hemorrhages arising from peripheral arteriolar occlusion (Fig. 1-26). Angioid streaks are networks of brownish red irregular lines radiating from the optic nerve. Seen in up to 6% patients with SCA, they represent pathologic rupture of Bruch's membrane of the choroid.[67] Hyphema (anterior chamber hemorrhage) may follow blunt trauma to the head. In the child with a sickle hemoglobin, secondary glaucoma and blindness are serious potential complications.

Microembolic events are felt responsible for the retinal

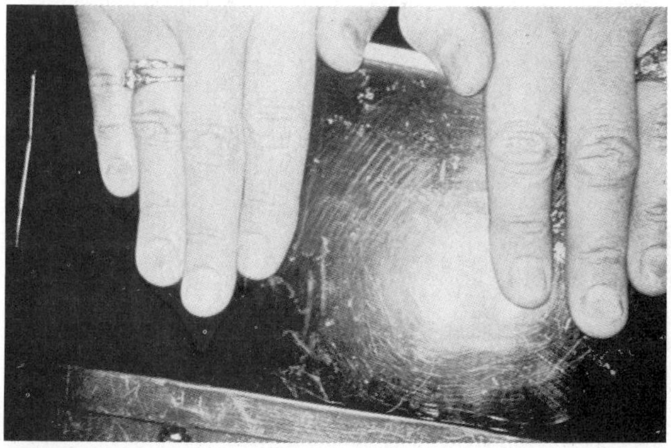

FIGURE 1-22. Koilonychia of iron deficiency. (See Color Fig. 1-22.)

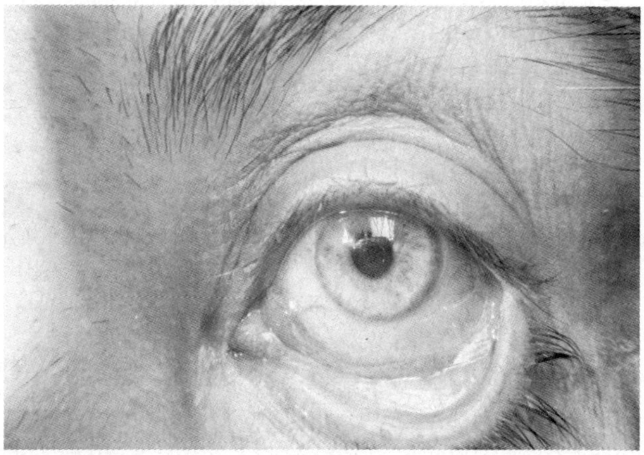

FIGURE 1-24. Smooth fleshy conjunctival mass typical of patient with conjunctival lymphoma. (See Color Fig. 1-24.)

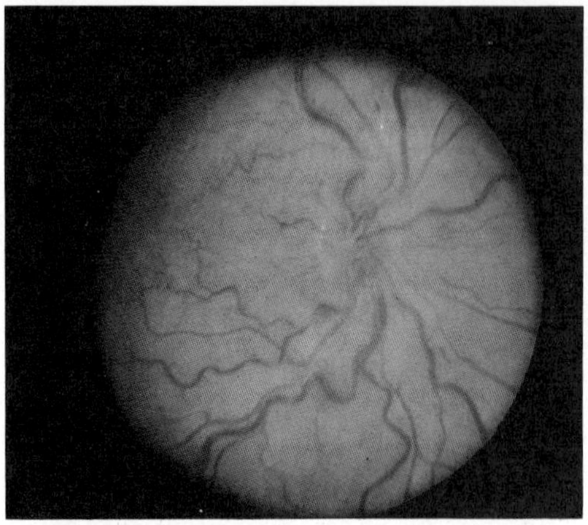

FIGURE 1-25. Hyperviscosity. (See Color Fig. 1-25.) (Courtesy of Rosa Tang, MD; item 0240339, slide no. 22)

and choroidal abnormalities in patients with hypereosinophilic syndrome. Although only a small number of subjects with this disorder have visual complaints, examination reveals abnormalities in up to 92% of patients, such as occlusion of retinal vessels, choroidal infarcts, and patchy or delayed choroidal filling.[71]

Proptosis, periorbital swelling, or masses may bring the patient with an orbital lymphoma or a child with a chloroma or neuroblastoma to the physician's attention. Orbital lymphomas are the most common primary orbital neoplasm in adults.[72] Because orbital involvement occurs in less than 1% of lymphomas and is rarely isolated, other physical findings (adenopathy, splenomegaly) serve to point to a systemic lymphoproliferative disorder.[66,72] Orbital bone infarct in SCA gives rise to frontal headache, proptosis, and lid edema. Persons with hemophilia must be observed closely after trauma to the eye because periorbital hemorrhage, progressive proptosis, and necrosis of surrounding tissue may ensue.

Virtually every tissue of the eye can be affected by leukemia. Thirty-nine percent of prospectively studied children and adults with acute leukemia demonstrate abnormalities on ophthalmologic examination.[73] Despite the number affected, visual loss occurs in only 5% of patients. The choroid is the most common site of leukemic involvement but infiltration of the retina, anterior chamber, and optic nerve is also reported.[66,73,74] Flame-shaped retinal hemorrhages with white leukemic centers (Fig. 1-27), nodular lesions of the iris, and chemosis with papilledema constitute the clinical findings corresponding to these respective anatomic sites of leukemic extension.

Dislocation of the lens and glaucoma are common in the congenital disorder, *homocysteinuria*. Affected persons tend to manifest mental retardation, fair complexion, malar flush, and, of interest to the hematologist, a thromboembolic diathesis. Blue eyes are common in patients with pernicious anemia.[75]

Ears, Nose, and Throat

Rushing, pounding, and ringing in the ears are common complaints in the anemic patient and do not imply pathology in the ears. Although rarely symptomatic, about 12% of children with SCA demonstrate mild high-frequency sensorineural hearing loss on audiometric testing, which probably results from sludging of blood in the cochlea.[76] Epistaxis, the most common mode of presentation for the juvenile with Rendu-Osler-Weber syndrome, is also a central feature of thrombocytopenia and macroglobulinemia.[77] Circulating cryoglobulins or cold agglutinins may lead to necrosis in areas with tenuous blood supply such as the tip of the nose, the ears (Fig. 1-28), and the fingers. Most relevant to the hematologist, the ears, nose, and throat serve as important and at times overlooked sites of lymphoplasmacytic disease. Extraosseous plasmacytomas arise most frequently in the upper respiratory tract, leading to pain, epistaxis, and rhinorrhea. Up to 78% of these tumors are found in the nasopharynx, nasal cavity, paranasal sinuses, tonsils, epiglottis, and other areas in the otolaryngologist's domain.[78,79] Involvement of Waldeyer's ring (lymphoid tissue of the nasopharynx, tonsillar region, base of tongue, and oropharyngeal wall) occurs in about 7% to 10% of non-Hodgkin's lymphoma but is distinctly unusual in Hodgkin's disease.[80]

Oral Cavity

Perhaps because of its rich vascular supply, the oral cavity also serves as a window to hematologic processes. Dentists often have the first opportunity to suspect abnormalities of the blood. Seventeen percent of patients with acute leukemia present solely because of oral symptoms, whereas

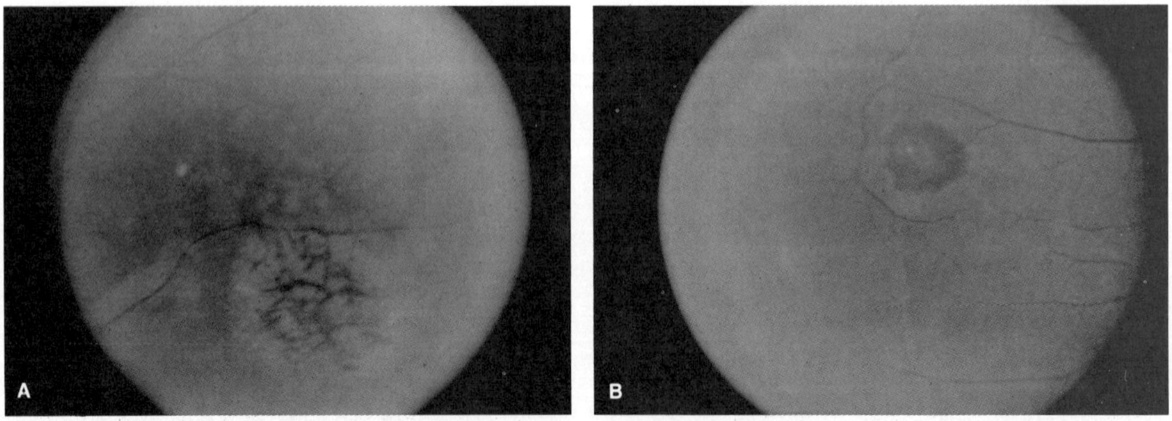

FIGURE 1-26. Retinal changes in a patient with sickle cell anemia. (**A**) Black sun bursts. (**B**) Salmon-colored patch hemorrhages. (See Color Fig. 1-26.) (Bunn HF, Forget BG. Sickle cell disease: clinical and epidemiological aspects. In: Hemoglobin: molecular, genetic and clinical aspects. Philadelphia, WB Saunders, 1986:378)

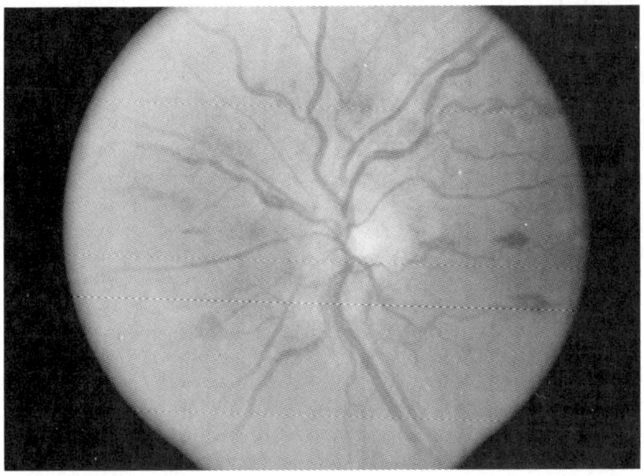

FIGURE 1-27. Retinal hemorrhage with leukemic white centers in a patient with acute monocytic leukemia. (See Color Fig. 1-27.) (Courtesy of Gregory Orloff, MD)

up to 65% have an associated oral problem.[81] Bleeding, pain, and sores are most frequently described and correlate with findings of petechiae, buccal blood blisters, mucosal ulceration, and gingivitis. Uncommon in the leukemias in general (3.6%), gingival infiltration is a notorious development in the monocytic variants, affecting two thirds of patients[46,82–84] (Fig. 1-29). Jaw pain, paresthesias, oral swelling, soft tissue masses, and abnormal mobility or migration of teeth occur in 14% of patients with multiple myeloma. In these instances, lytic bone lesions, osteopenia, or pathologic fractures are likely culprits.[85]

Unsightly and often painful grape-like clusters of hemorrhagic buccal blisters are particularly suggestive of acute idiopathic thrombocytic purpura (ITP). Glossitis arising from vitamin B_{12} and less frequently from folate deficiency, is well described.[86–89] Intense soreness or paresthesias of the tongue with alteration or loss of taste may herald pernicious anemia in which classically the tongue is depapillated, beefy red, and ulcerated on the dorsal and lateral surfaces (Fig. 1-30). The incidence of painful tongue in iron deficiency has been estimated at between 6% and 36% and is frequently accompanied by angular stomatitis.[90] Macroglossia may imply amyloid deposition in someone with multiple myeloma (see Fig. 1-5).

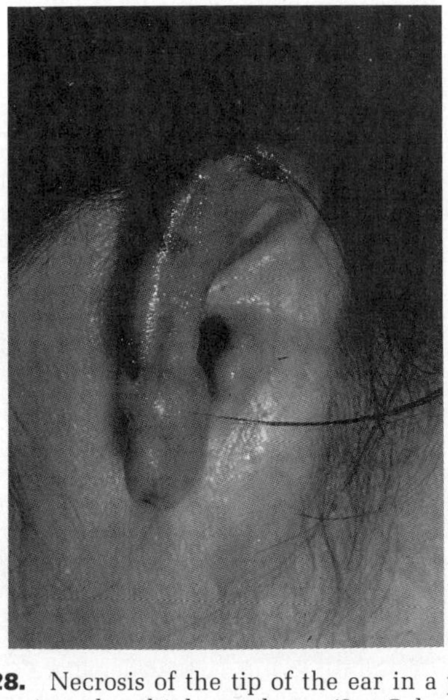

FIGURE 1-28. Necrosis of the tip of the ear in a patient with cryoglobulinemia and multiple myeloma. (See Color Fig. 1-28.)

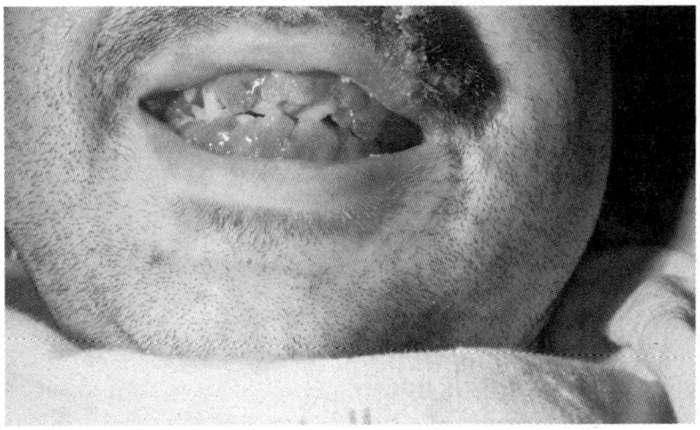

FIGURE 1-29. Gingival infiltration by monoblasts in a patient with M5 leukemia. (See Color Fig. 1-29.)

Lymph Nodes

Examination of the lymph nodes falls mainly in the domain of the hematologist. Although lymphadenopathy serves as the major clinical presentation for non-Hodgkin's lymphomas and Hodgkin's disease, enlarged lymph nodes are more frequently the result of infectious, inflammatory, and other benign disorders[90a] (Table 1-1). Lymph node enlargement in the child often poses a diagnostic problem.[91] It has been said that nodes less than 3 mm in any region or up to 1 cm in the cervical and inguinal areas are normal in the child under 12 years. Palpable adenopathy in the newborn is always pathologic.[92] In a retrospective study of 239 children undergoing peripheral lymph node biopsy, a histologic or microbiologic diagnosis was obtained in only 41% of cases.[93] Reactive hyperplasia (52%), granulomatous disease (32%), and neoplasia (13%) were the most common diagnoses. Anatomic location of the lymph nodes proved an important predictor of pathology (Fig. 1-31). Biopsy of the supraclavicular and lower neck regions had the highest yield: 61% of nodes were abnormal compared with 8% of superior posterior cervical lymph glands.

The incidence of asymptomatic lymphadenopathy in the general adult population is difficult to determine. In a large retrospective chart review of a family practice, the reported incidence of lymphadenopathy was 0.5%, with 45% of these patients having nodes measuring greater than 1 cm.[94] The most common sites of involvement were cervical (44%), inguinal (16%), and submandibular (11%); 24% of patients exhibited lymphadenopathy in more than one location. An infectious cause was suspected in 69% of patients, and cause remained unknown in the rest. No cases of malignancy were diagnosed.

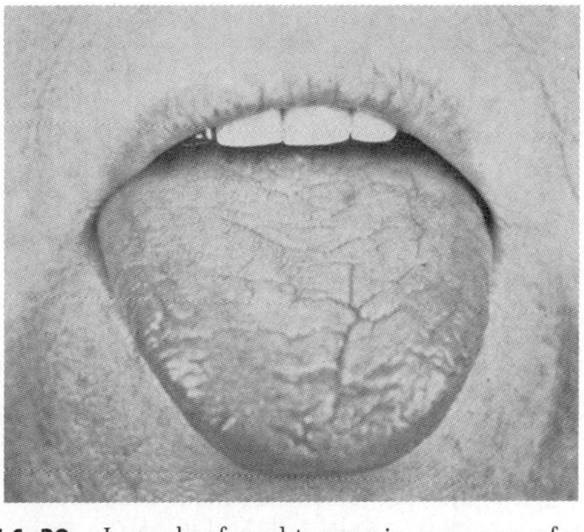

FIGURE 1-30. Large beefy red tongue in a woman of northern European descent with pernicious anemia. (See Color Fig. 1-30.)

TABLE 1-1. **Differential Diagnosis of Lymphadenopathy**

REACTIVE DISEASES

Infectious
- Bacterial: streptococcal, staphylococcal, tuberculosis, chancroid, leprosy, tularemia
- Viral: Epstein-Barr virus, cytomegalovirus, human immunodeficiency virus, measles
- Spirochete: syphilis
- Mycoses: blastomycoses, histoplasmosis
- Other: toxoplasmosis, cat-scratch fever

Dermatopathic

Inflammatory
- Sarcoidosis
- Systemic lupus erythematosus
- Rheumatoid arthritis
- Serum sickness
- Beryliosis

Metabolic
- Hyperthyroidism
- Addison's disease
- Hypopituitarism

Storage diseases
- Gaucher's disease
- Lipidoses

Drugs
- Diphenyhydantoin

Other
- Castleman's disease

MALIGNANT CONDITIONS

Primary hematologic
- Hodgkin's disease
- Non-Hodgkin's lymphoma
- Chronic lymphocytic leukemia
- Acute leukemia (chloroma)

Metastatic disease

It is generally taught that reactive nodes compared with malignant nodes measure less than 2 cm and tend to be soft or tender. The latter are characteristically large, rubbery, painless, matted, and fixed (Table 1-2; Fig. 1-32).

In both child and adult, anatomic localization of lymph node enlargement may point to the probable underlying cause. Hodgkin's disease typically involves axial lymph nodes (cervical, supraclavicular, axillary, mediastinal, and

TABLE 1-2. **Differential Features of Benign Versus Malignant Adenopathy**

Feature	Reactive	Malignant
Size	<2 cm	>2 cm
Texture	Soft, tender, mobile	Firm, rubbery, hard, fixed, nontender, matted
Number	Single	Multiple with satellites

hilar areas) and rarely (5% to 12%) presents in an infradiaphragmatic site.[95] Epitrochlear adenopathy is common in HIV infection, non-Hodgkin's lymphoma, secondary syphilis, and leprosy. Supraclavicular adenopathy is always pathologic. The Valsalva maneuver may aid in examination of the supraclavicular region by bringing deep nodes closer to the surface.

Pain over malignant nodes induced by alcohol consumption is a symptom of considerable interest. This curious phenomenon has been observed in up to 7% of patients with Hodgkin's disease and may be more common in patients with the nodular sclerosis variant.[96] The pace of lymphadenopathy and its duration are also relevant. Waxing and waning adenopathy characterizes angioimmunoblastic lymphadenopathy with dysproteinemia as well as low-grade lymphoma. Isolated rapid growth of a previously stable lymph node group in a patient with chronic lymphocytic leukemia may herald transformation to a large cell lymphoma, know as Richter's syndrome. Enlargement of lymph nodes can occur after administration of phenytoin; although this usually resolves after cessation of the drug, progression to frank lymphoma has been reported.[97] The pathophysiologic mechanisms involved in this process remain to be defined.

Abdomen

Galen first described the spleen as the "*plenum mysterii organon*" (organ full of mystery), but William Crosby most colorfully depicted the special relationship between the hematologist and the spleen, "romancing the spleen has been a pleasure, but marriage was out of the question."[98] An enlarged spleen may give rise to a myriad of local and referred symptoms; left upper quadrant fullness, pain or pulling, early satiety, and left shoulder aching. Visible at times, the spleen expands in an inferomedial direction. When massively enlarged, its most inferior border may be missed unless the examiner begins palpation at the right iliac crest. Dullness over the left upper quadrant (Traube's

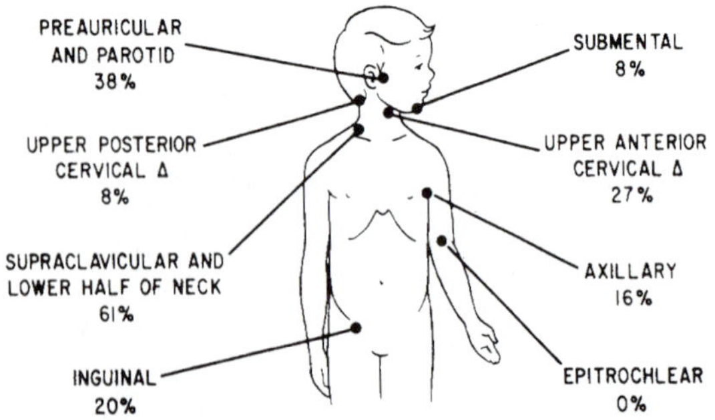

FIGURE 1-31. Lymphadenopathy by site. Percentage at each site of adenopathy is therapeutic yield for that location. High yield from supraclavicular adenopathy was due to Hodgkin's disease, whereas that in upper cervical and preauricular areas was due to atypical mycobacteria. (Knight PJ, Mulne AF, Vassy LE. When is lymph node biopsy indicated in children with enlarged peripheral nodes? Pediatrics 1982;69:394)

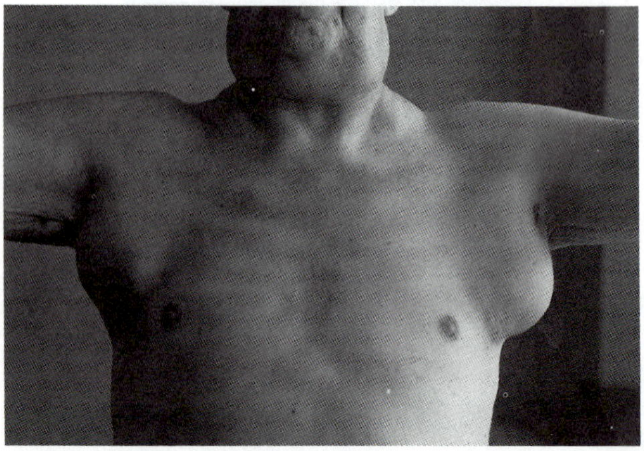

FIGURE 1-32. Malignant adenopathy of lymphoma. Note multiple large, rubbery, nontender lymph nodes. (See Color Fig. 1-32.)

space) on percussion has been considered as an indicator of splenomegaly,[99] but the most reliable method of examination places the patient in the right lateral decubitus position with flexed knees (Fig. 1-33). The presence of a friction rub implies splenic infarction resulting from rapid outgrowth of the blood supply. When this occurs, symptoms of acute, sharp pain and dyspnea may mimic those of a pulmonary embolus.

Splenomegaly, common in many hematologic conditions, may also be detected in healthy persons (Table 1-3). A palpable spleen tip usually represents an increase in size of 1.5 to 3 times normal. A spleen can be appreciated in 5% to 10% of normal children (higher in those with a viral infection)[100] and nearly 3% of college freshman on routine entrance physical examination.[101] During 6 years of follow-up, despite persistence of splenomegaly in a about 30% of students, no increased incidence of disease was found. In general practice, the most common cause of splenomegaly is liver disease whereas among hematology patients, lymphoma, leukemia, myeloproliferative disorders, hemolytic anemias, and storage diseases are more likely. Sixty-five percent of persons with SC disease exhibit splenomegaly with advancing age[102] in contrast to children with homozygous SS disease in whom autoinfarction of the spleen leads to hyposplenism in adolescence.

Right upper quadrant pain, fever, and jaundice in a patient with SCA suggests cholecystitis or hepatic infarction. When associated with massive hepatomegaly and liver failure, intrahepatic cholestasis is likely. Chronic hemolysis leads to bilirubin stone formation in 30% of patients with SCA and 85% of patients with hereditary spherocytosis.[103,104] Relentless accumulation of iron in hemochromatosis accounts for hepatomegaly noted in up to 95% of symptomatic patients.[105] Sudden, painful enlargement of the liver accompanied by ascites is the hallmark of hepatic vein thrombosis (Budd-Chiari syndrome) and should prompt a search for a possible underlying myeloproliferative state.[106] Hepatosplenomegaly and ascites are also detected in about 10% of patients with myeloid metaplasia with myelofibrosis (MMM).[107]

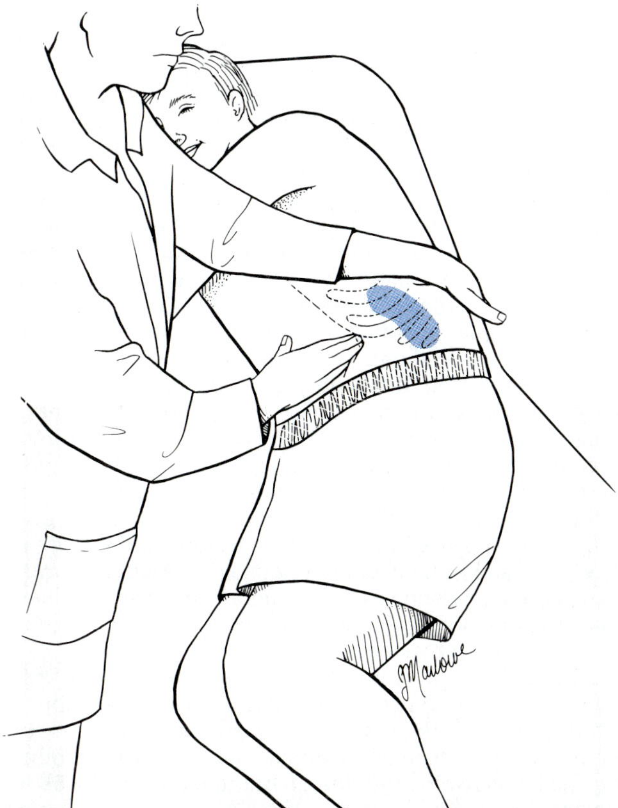

FIGURE 1-33. Drawing of spleen examination.

Dysphagia and pain, typically at the level of the cricoid cartilage, in a patient with iron deficiency, suggest an esophageal web, the Plummer-Vinson or Paterson-Kelly syndrome. Occult involvement of the gastrointestinal tract by non-Hodgkin's lymphoma occurs in 10% to 20% of cases and should be suspected when disease is present in Waldeyer's ring.[108] Infiltration of the stomach and small bowel is most common and may explain diarrhea, abdominal pain, nausea, vomiting, and bleeding. On careful pathologic examination about 5% of all gastric neoplasms are found to be lymphoma[107,110]

Chest

The lymphoproliferative disorders frequently involve the chest and can give rise to a myriad of syndromes including superior vena cava obstruction (secondary to large mediastinal mass), pleural and pericardial effusion, and parenchymal lung infiltration. Most patients with Hodgkin's disease present with mediastinal adenopathy often detected only because of radiographic studies. Likewise, large intrathoracic masses in the child with thalassemia or in the adult with myeloid metaplasia may represent extramedullary hematopoiesis and cause no respiratory difficulties. Conversely, nonproductive cough, dyspnea, and chest pain arise because of pleural effusions, pulmonary infiltrates, or nodules in 10% of patients with Waldenström's macroglobulinemia.[111]

The acute chest syndrome of SCA is caused by infection or pulmonary infarction. Both present with pleuritic chest pain, fever, and cough and their differentiation is not always straightforward. Pneumonia is more common in young children, whereas occlusion of pulmonary vessels by in situ sickling is believed to more of a problem common for adolescents and adults. Pulmonary infarction may also result from emboli of fat or marrow released from infarcted bone. Chronic pulmonary shunting and ventilation–perfusion mismatch can lead to pulmonary hypertension and cor pulmonale heralded clinically by progressive dyspnea, unexplained syncope, and right-sided congestive heart failure.[112]

Shortness of breath, tachypnea, and respiratory failure can develop in myelogenous leukemias when myeloblast counts exceed 50,000 to 100,000/μL. Intravascular leukostasis secondary to plugging of pulmonary vessels with large, sticky, and noncompliant myeloblasts occurs in 17% to 24% of cases of chronic and acute myelocytic leukemia, respectively, and usually responds to prompt antileukemic therapy.[113,114]

The detection of a bruit over the chest may indicate a pulmonary arteriovenous malformation in the person with Rendu-Osler-Weber syndrome. Left uncorrected, this vascular anomaly, found in about 15% of patients, can lead to hemoptysis, hemothorax, large shunting of cardiac output, and congestive heart failure.[115]

Heart

Cardiovascular compromise from anemia depends on the degree of anemia, the rate of its development, and the capacity of the cardiovascular system to compensate for changes in oxygen carrying capacity and volume. With acute blood loss or a sudden drop in hematocrit level, symptoms of hypovolemia including lightheadedness, tachycardia, and postural changes in blood pressure and

TABLE 1-3. Differential Diagnosis of Splenomegaly

INFECTIOUS DISEASES	**PRIMARY HEMATOLOGIC DISEASES**
Infectious mononucleosis	Acquired and hereditary hemolytic disorders; enzymopathies, hemoglobinopathies, autoimmune hemolytic anemia
Cytomegalovirus	Polycythemia vera
Human immunodeficiency virus infection	Myeloid metaplasia with myelofibrosis
Toxoplasmosis	Primary thrombocytosis
Viral hepatitis	Chronic myelogenous leukemia
Salmonellosis	**INFILTRATIVE DISEASES**
Relapsing fever	Leukemia
Tularemia	Lymphoma
Syphilis	Malignant histocytosis
Malaria	Hairy cell leukemia
Subacute bacterial endocarditis	Metastatic cancer
Tuberculosis	Primary tumors: hemangioma, hamartoma, fibroma
Schistosomiasis	**STORAGE DISEASES**
INFLAMMATORY DISEASES	Gaucher's disease
Felty's syndrome	Neimann-Pick disease
Systemic lupus erythematosus	**MISCELLANEOUS CONDITIONS**
Rheumatic fever	Tropical splenomegaly
Serum sickness	Primary splenic hyperplasia
Sarcoid	
CONGESTIVE DISEASES	
Intrahepatic	
Cirrhosis	
Venoocclusive disease	
Congenital hepatic fibrosis	
Portal vein obstruction	
Splenic vein obstruction	
Hepatic vein occlusion (Budd-Chiari syndrome)	
Congestive heart failure	

pulse ensue. In contrast, when anemia develops slowly, symptoms may not become prominent until the hemoglobin falls below 7 g/dL.[116,117] In these cases, compensatory increase in cardiac output at rest and with exertion results from an augmented stroke volume rather than from tachycardia.[116] Dyspnea on exertion, palpitations, and fatigue are common complaints in the patient with anemia. Examination reveals a bounding pulse with a widened pulse pressure, hyperdynamic precordium, gallop rhythm, and systolic flow murmur. In elderly patients, underlying atherosclerotic disease, peripheral edema, unstable angina, and confusion are exacerbated by anemia. Even healthy persons can develop symptoms of congestive heart failure when hemoglobin concentrations fall below 5 g/dL.[116]

Five to 15% of patients with hemochromatosis present with congestive heart failure as the initial manifestation of disease.[105] Reversal of iron overload by phlebotomy generally improves cardiac function.

A benign form of pericarditis with pericardial effusion is frequently seen in children with thalassemia.[118] Spontaneously resolving, it rarely requires therapeutic intervention. Pericardial tamponade can complicate the course of Hodgkin's disease, non-Hodgkin's lymphoma, and the leukemias.[119]

An evaluation of unexplained microangiopathic hemolytic anemia should entail a careful cardiac examination listening for murmurs indicative of valvular abnormalities.

Bones and Joints

Bone pain is a universal complaint in patients with multiple myeloma. This disease often presents with pathologic fractures resulting from osteolytic lesions or severe osteopenia. Tenderness over the sternum, pelvis, and back, bones that are rich in hematopoiesis, is prominent in the patient with leukemia; 50% to 59% of adults and children describe skeletal discomfort as part of their disease.[120] Although pain in children tends to be sharp, intense, and well localized to the peripheral skeleton, pain of adults is generally diffuse, dull, and axial in distribution.

The sickle hemoglobinopathies are perhaps most notorious for painful bone crises. Ten percent of children and adults with SCA develop one or more clinically identified episodes of bone infarction involving the humerus, tibia, and femur, in order of frequency.[121] Localized tenderness, pain, erythema, swelling, and diminished joint motion result and may be difficult to differentiate from the less common complication of osteomyelitis. Occurring equally as frequently in SS and SC disease, avascular necrosis of the femoral head is a dreaded complication, often leading to chronic disability.[122] Fever, irritability, and painful swelling of the hands and feet—the hand–foot syndrome—frequently brings the infant with SCA to medical attention (Fig. 1-34). Impaired growth and development are late sequelae of sickle hemoglobinopathies. Avascular necrosis and pathologic fractures of the femoral and humeral heads may also develop in Gaucher's disease, presumably due to bony expansion by storage cells.[123]

Although less common today because of greater availability of factor replacement, arthropathy is a crippling complication of hemophilia. Hemarthroses—spontaneous or resulting from minor trauma—lead to pain, swelling, erythema, warmth, and flexion of the joint (Fig. 1-35). Synovial thickening, bony ankylosis of larger joints or destruction of smaller joints with associated contractures, and muscle atrophy are consequences of recurrent injury (Fig.

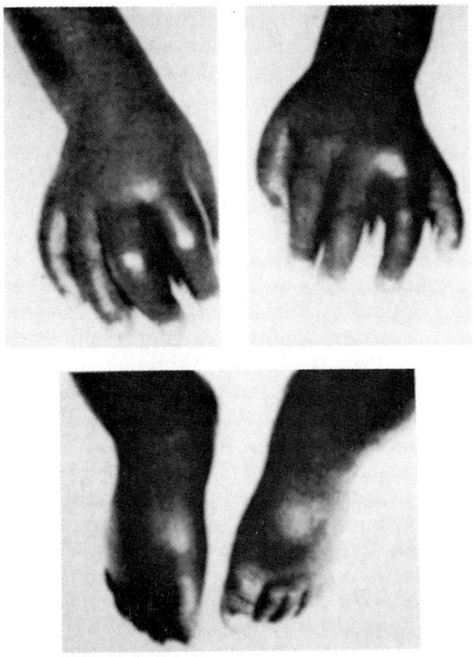

FIGURE 1-34. Hand–foot syndrome. (Konotey-Ahulu FI. The sickle cell disease. Arch Intern Med 1974;133:614)

1-36). In decreasing order of incidence, the knees, elbows, ankles, shoulders, and hips are involved.[124,125]

Acute gout secondary to hyperuricemia develops in several hematologic states characterized by rapid cell turnover—the myeloproliferative disorders, high-grade lymphomas, and acute leukemias. About 14% of leukemic patients develop erythema and swelling of one or more peripheral joints due either to gouty arthropathy or to leukemic infiltration of the synovium and periosteum.[120] The extramedullary hematopoiesis of MMM may extend into joints and give rise to arthritis.[126] Unlike the cardiomyopathy associated with hemochromatosis, the arthropathy present in 20% of these patients does not usually respond to phlebotomy.[105] Rheumatoid arthritis completes the triad (along with splenomegaly and leukopenia) of Felty's syndrome. Sudden onset of joint pain and swelling may be the initial complaints of a child with Schönlein-Henoch purpura, preceeding rash, abdominal pain, and other systemic manifestations.

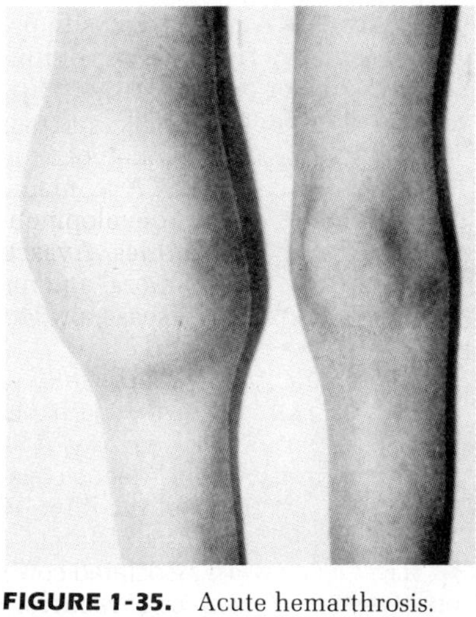

FIGURE 1-35. Acute hemarthrosis.

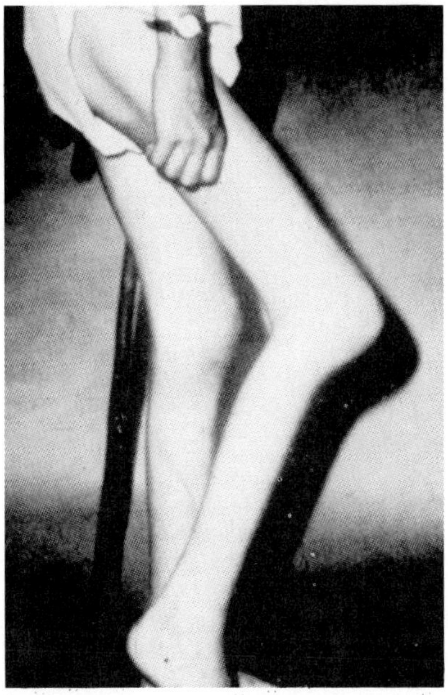

FIGURE 1-36. Joint contracture resulting from chronic hemarthroses in a patient with hemophilia.

The unusual and often disabling syndrome of erythromelalgia deserves special mention. Seen primarily in the chronic myeloproliferative disorders, it serves as the initial complaint in more than half the patients with polycythemia vera and essential thrombocythemia.[127] Mitchell's words and drawings from the late 19th century serve as the most pictorial definition of erythromelalgia[128] (Fig. 1-37):

> *The pain spread from the right toe across the sole beneath the metatarso-phalangeal articulations . . . an intense burning . . . resembling the pain that would be caused by holding the foot very near a red hot stove. . . . pain in the foot or feet; usually it comes in the ball of the foot, or of the great toe, or in the heel; and from these parts it extends so as to involve a large portion of the sole. . . . It is the pain of a burn, the pain of mustard . . . in severer cases, the burning reaches the extreme of torture.* (pp 17–18)

Arteriolar platelet thrombi lead to endothelial swelling fibromuscular intimal proliferation and thrombotic occlusion. Aspirin affords dramatic resolution of symptoms. The observation, one century ago, that erthromelalgia responded to blood letting and cod liver oil may still have clinical implication.

Many bony changes characterize the congenital hematologic diseases. Skeletal abnormalities occur in two thirds of patients with Fanconi's anemia and include short stature as well as absent, hypoplastic, or supernumerary thumbs, sometimes associated with radial hypoplasia.[39] The thrombocytopenia with absent radii (TAR) syndrome derives its name from the isolated bony abnormality. Ten percent of children with Blackfan-Diamond anemia exhibit thumb deformities (triphalangeal, duplicated, subluxated, or hypoplastic digits), and most also have short stature.[129]

Genitourinary Tract

Bouts of gross hematuria occur in both SCA and sickle trait although less frequently seen in patients with the latter disorder. Infarction of renal papillae is presumed to be responsible for most episodes of gross hematuria, but other causes including renal calculi and infection should be routinely excluded. Red or brown-red urine may signal the presence of hemoglobin rather than red blood cells. Only

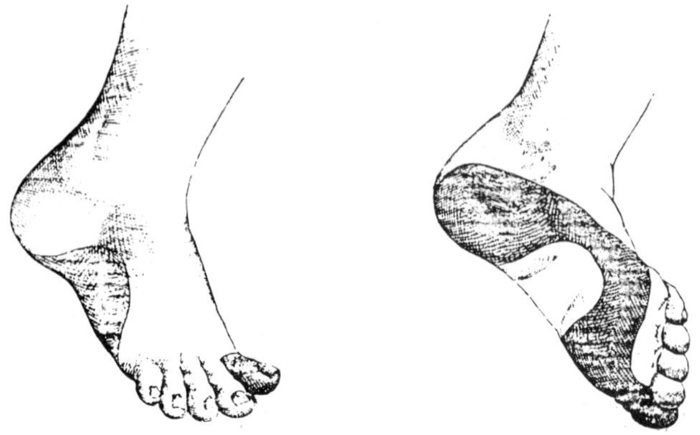

FIGURE 1-37. Erythromelalgia. (Mitchell SW. On a rare vasomotor neurosis of the extremities and on the maladies with which it may be confounded. Am J Med Sci 1878;76:26)

a minority of patients with paroxysmal nocturnal hemoglobinuria develop classic nocturnal exacerbation of hemolysis with ensuing discoloration of the first voided morning urine. Hemoglobinemia occurs during sleep regardless of the time of day and can be avoided by keeping the patient awake. Oliguria heralds renal dysfunction in hyperparaproteinemic states, whereas polyuria may be a clue to hypercalcemia, complicating myeloma, or lymphoma.

Up to 42% of male patients with SCA develop priapism; 25% of these patients subsequently suffer some form of impotence.[130] Priapism is a troubling and painful complication of acute leukemia and is generally a manifestation of leukostasis. Clinically presenting as painless organ enlargement, the testes and ovaries serve as important sanctuary sites in patients with lymphoblastic leukemias and lymphomas and may lead to relapse of disease. Diminished libido and testicular atrophy occur in iron-overload states.

Nervous System

A complete consideration of the nervous system manifestations of hematologic disease is beyond the scope of this chapter. Involvement of the nervous system often occurs as a medical emergency necessitating prompt recognition and treatment. Delays can result in irreversible motor, sensory, and cognitive dysfunction.

Alteration in mentation is an important indicator of hyperviscosity. Headache, sluggishness, visual change, somnolence, and progressive obtundation imply impaired cerebral blood flow in patients with plasma cell disorders, polycythemia, and leukemia. Diminished alertness and cognition, as well as progressive neurologic deterioration, have been shown to correlate with the level of paraprotein, hemoglobin, and WBC count, respectively. Hematocrit counts higher than 45% and leukocrit counts over 3% are associated with increased plasma viscosity, risk of thrombosis, and hemorrhage.[131–135]

Strokes occur in about 7% of children with SCA and usually involve major vessels supplying the brain.[136] Although spontaneous recovery may occur, many children are left with cognitive, motor, and sensory deficits. Transient ischemic attacks probably indicate microvascular occlusion in patients with essential thrombocythemia. Although no doubt more problematic in older patients with underlying cerebrovascular disease, this complication has been reported in 27% of young patients with this myeloproliferative disorder.[137]

Central nervous system (CNS) hemorrhage is the most dreaded complication of thrombocytopenia or coagulopathy. It is less common than might be expected in acute ITP, in which overall mortality rate from cerebral hemorrhage is only about 1%.[138] In contrast, prior to the era of prevalent HIV infection, cerebral hemorrhage was the most common cause of death in patients with hemophilia, carrying a mortality rate of about 35%.[139,140] Symptoms of subdural or subarachnoid bleeding may be delayed in this setting with complaints of headache, nausea, vomiting, blurred vision, and seizures not arising until 4 or more days after head trauma.

Involvement of the CNS is common in non-Hodgkin's lymphoma (about 10%) and less frequent in Hodgkin's disease.[141] Secondary foci of lymphoma may take the form of meningeal infiltration, epidural compression, or intracerebral tumors. Primary CNS lymphoma is rare in persons who are not immunocompromised, occurring in only 1% of such patients. In contrast, in persons with AIDS or in organ transplant recipients, high-grade CNS lymphomas arise in up to 20% of subjects.[142] Meningeal spread of tumor occurs in 2% to 15% of patients with acute leukemia.[143–145] Headache, nausea, and vomiting secondary to increased intracranial pressure as well as isolated cranial neuropathies are common modes of presentation. Nerves III, VI, and VII are most frequently involved (Fig. 1-38), resulting in diplopia, blurred vision, ptosis, and facial droop.

Progressive multifocal leukoencephalopathy is a uniformly fatal complication associated with immunocompromised states (lymphoma, leukemia, AIDS). It manifests clinically by rapid neurologic deterioration secondary to diffuse demyelination. Infection by the JC virus is implicated as etiologic.[146]

Vitamin B_{12} deficiency has protean neurologic manifestations, including irritability, depression, euphoria, agitation, stupor, and coma.[147–149] The classic presentation of combined system disease consists in symmetric paresthesias of the hands and feet, impaired vibratory sensation, and ataxia, particularly at night. Iron deficiency in children may also cause alterations of cognitive function, fatigue, irritability, and lethargy.[150,151]

Neurologic change is a central element of the pentad of thrombotic thrombocytopenic purpura, which also includes fever, microangiopathic anemia, renal insufficiency, and thrombocytopenia. Confusion, headache, delirium, hemiparesis, aphasia, seizures, and altered vision can wax and wane and precede other symptoms and signs.[152]

Spinal cord compression and peripheral neuropathy are important complications of the lymphoplasmacytic disorders. Peripheral nerve involvement is also a key component of the sclerotic variant of myeloma, the POEMS syndrome. Nerve damage may result from compression by a plasmacytoma, direct infiltration by tumor cells, or autoimmune damage from paraprotein. Amyloid deposition in these disorders may in addition give rise to carpal tunnel syndrome. Chloromas in leukemia, or extramedullary hematopoiesis in thalassemia and myeloid metaplasia, can compress cen-

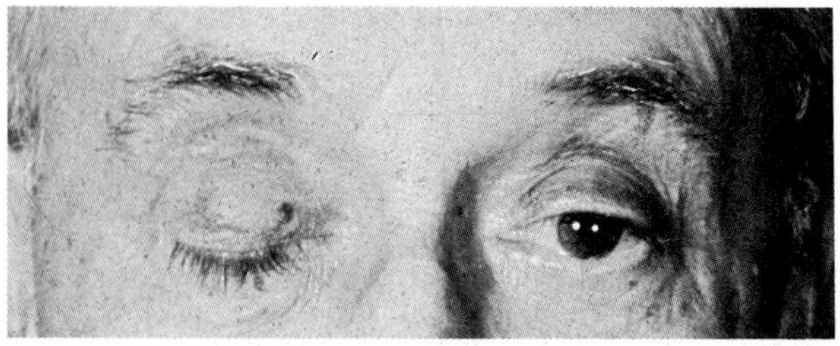

FIGURE 1-38. Third-nerve palsy in a patient with meningeal infiltration by lymphoma.

tral or peripheral nerves causing a variety of neurologic complaints.

SUMMARY

Listening, questioning, and observing provide the physician with information as important as laboratory and x-ray data and are infinitely less expensive. Sleuthful inquiry about the patient's symptoms as well as his or her past history, hobbies, exposures, and social and ethnic background may yield clues vital in unraveling otherwise unexplained hematologic problems. Although more comfortable in the evaluation of splenomegaly or lymphadenopathy, the hematologist must use all aspects of the physical examination. Whereas the clinical and research laboratory in the age of molecular biology herald exciting new advances for hematology, it is well to remember the biddings of Major, "It is noteworthy . . . that chlorosis, pernicious anemia, purpura, and hemophilia were recognized without aid of the microscope or the laboratory."[153]

REFERENCES

1. Major RH. Classic descriptions of disease, ed 3. Springfield, IL, Charles C Thomas, 1955:3.
2. Rich EC, Crowson TW, Harris IB. The diagnostic value of the medical history. Arch Intern Med 1987;147:1957.
3. Hampton JR, Harrison MJG, Mitchell JRA, et al. Relative contributions of history-taking, physical examination, and laboratory investigation to diagnosis and management of medical outpatients. Br Med J 1975;2:486.
4. Combe JS. History of a case of anemia. Trans Med Chir Soc Edinb 1824;1:193.
5. Craigie D. Case of disease of the spleen in which death took place in consequence of the presence of purulent matter in the blood. Edin Med Surg J 1845;64:400.
6. Otto JC. An account of an hemorrhagic disposition existing in certain families. Med Repos 1803;6:1.
7. Gilbert JR, ed. Highlights from a recent seminar on fatigue. Can Med Assoc J 1971;105:309.
8. Spaulding WB. The clinical analysis of fatigue. Appl Therapeutics 1964;6:911.
9. Tubiana M, Attié E, Flamant R, et al. Prognostic factors in 454 cases of Hodgkin's disease. Cancer Res 1971;31:1801.
10. Schafer AI. Bleeding disorders: finding the cause. Hosp Pract 1984;19:88K.
11. Love PE, Santoro SA. Antiphospholipid antibodies: anticardiolipin and the lupus anticoagulant in systemic lupus erythematous (SLE) and in non-SLE disorders. Ann Intern Med 1990;112:682.
12. Barrett-Connor E. Bacterial infection and sickle cell anemia: an analysis of 25 infections in 166 patients and a review of the literature. Medicine 1971;50:97.
13. Maurice PD, Bunker C, Giles F, et al. *Mycobacterium avium-intracellulare* infection associated with hairy cell leukemia. Arch Dermatol 1988;124:1545.
14. Maziarz RT, Tepler I, Antin JH, et al. Reversal of infection with *Mycobacterium avium-intracellulare* by treatment with alpha interferon in a patient with hairy cell leukemia. Ann Intern Med 1988;109:292.
15. Markham PD. Biologic properties and isolation of HTLV-III. Ann Intern Med 1985;102:805.
16. Woolley RJ, Klein HG, Eisenman D. Value of routine inquiry about blood donation. (Letter) N Engl J Med 1990;322:132.
17. Auerbach AD, Sagi M, Adler BA. Fanconi's anemia: prenatal diagnosis in 30 fetuses at risk. Pediatrics 1985;76:794.
18. Gunz JP, Veale AM, et al. Familial leukemia: a study of 909 families. Scand J Hematol 1975;15:117.
19. Pendergrass TW. Epidemiology of acute lymphoblastic leukemia. Semin Oncol 1985;12:80.
20. Mason BA, Lessin L, Schechter GP. Marrow granulocyte reserves in black Americans: hydrocortisone-induced granulocytosis in the "benign" neutropenia of the black. Am J Med 1979;67:201.
21. Kuefler PR, Bunn PA Jr. Adult T cell leukaemia/lymphoma. Clin Haematol 1986;15:695.
22. Scadden DT, Zon LI, Groopman JE. Pathophysiology and management of HIV-associated hematologic disorders. Blood 1989;74:1455.
23. Rinsky RA, Smith AB, Hornung R, et al. Benzene and leukemia: an epidemiologic risk assessment. N Engl J Med 1987;316:1044.
24. Aksoy M, Erdem Ş. Followup study on the mortality and the development of leukemia in 44 pancytopenic patients with chronic exposure to benzene. Blood 1978;52:285.
25. Ringenberg QS, Doll DC, Patterson WP, et al. Hematologic effects of heavy metal poisoning. South Med J 1988;81:1132.
26. Miescher PA, Graf J. Drug-induced thrombocytopenia. Clin Haematol 1980;9:505.
27. King DJ, Kelton JG. Heparin-associated thrombocytopenia. Ann Intern Med 1984;100:535.
28. Lind SE. The prolonged bleeding time. Am J Med 1984;77:305.
29. Jandl JH. Leukocyte anomalies. In: Blood: textbook of hematology. Boston, Little, Brown, 1987:573.
30. Crosby WH. Pica. JAMA 1976;235:2765.
31. Reynolds RD, Binder HJ, Miller MB, et al. Pagophagia and iron deficiency anemia. Ann Intern Med 1968;69:435.
32. Coltman CA Jr. Pagophagia and iron lack. JAMA 1969;207:513.
33. Higginbottom MC, Sweetman L, Nyhan W. A syndrome of methylmalonic aciduria, homocysteinuria, megaloblastic anemia and neurologic abnormalities in a vitamin B_{12}-deficient breast fed infant of a strict vegetarian. N Engl J Med 1978;299:317.
34. Smith RRL, Spivak JL. Marrow cell necrosis in anorexia nervosa and involuntary starvation. Br J Haematol 1985;60:525.
35. Selby GB, Eichner HR. Endurance swimming, intravascular hemolysis, anemia, and iron depletion. Am J Med 1986;81:791.
36. Powars D. Aplastic anemia secondary to glue sniffing. N Engl J Med 1965;273:700.
37. Berry TJ. Hematologic diseases. In: The hand as a mirror of systemic disease. Philadelphia, FA Davis, 1963:135.
38. Jandl JH. Non-Hodgkin's lymphomas in blood. In: Blood: textbook of hematology. Boston, Little, Brown, 1987:935.
39. Alter BP. Bone marrow failure syndromes. In: Nathan DG, Oski FA, eds. Hematology of infancy and childhood, ed 3. Philadelphia, WB Saunders, 1987:177.
40. Major RH. Diseases of the blood. In: Classic descriptions of disease, ed 3. Springfield, IL, Charles C Thomas, 1978:514.
41. Piette WW. Myeloma, paraproteinemias, and the skin. Med Clin North Am 1986;70:155.
42. Kantor GR, Lookingbill DP. Generalized pruritus and systemic disease. J Am Acad Dermatol 1983;9:375.
43. Gobbi PG, Attardo-Parrinello G, Lattanzio G, et al. Severe pruritus should be a B-symptom in Hodgkin's disease. Cancer 1983;51:1934.
44. Gobbi PG, Cavalli C, Gendarini A, et al. Reevaluation of prognostic significance of symptoms in Hodgkin's disease. Cancer 1985;56:2874.
45. Wieselthier JS, Koh HK. Sézary syndrome: diagnosis, prognosis and critical review of treatment options. J Am Acad Dermatol 22:381, 1990.
46. Tobelem G, Jacquillat C, Chastang C, et al. Acute monoblastic leukemia: a clinical and biologic study of 74 cases. Blood 1980;55:71.
47. Dreizen S, McCredie KB, Keating MJ, et al. Leukemia-associated skin infiltrates. Postgrad Med 1989;85:45.
48. Dreizen S, McCredie KB, Keating MJ, Luna MA. Malignant gingival and skin "infiltrates" in adult leukemia. Oral Surg 1983;55:572.
49. Cuni LJ, Grünwald H, Rosner F. Bullous pemphigoid in chronic lymphocytic leukemia with the demonstration of antibasement membrane antibodies. Am J Med 1974;57:987.
50. Castro-Malaspina H, Schaison G, Passe S, et al. Subacute and chronic myelomonocytic leukemia in children (juvenile CML). Cancer 1984;54:675.
51. Muss HG, Moloney WC. Chloroma and other myeloblastic tumors. Blood 1973;42:721.
52. Eshghabadi M, Shojania AM, Carr I. Isolated granulocytic sarcoma: report of a case and review of the literature. J Clin Oncol 1986;4:912.
53. Arai E, Ikeda S, Itoh S, Katayama I. Specific skin lesions as the presenting symptom of hairy cell leukemia. Am J Clin Pathol 1988;90:459.
54. Lawrence DM, Sun NCJ, Mena R, Moss R. Cutaneous lesions in hairy-cell leukemia. Arch Dermatol 1983;119:322.
55. Farcet JP, Weschsler J, Wirquin V, et al. Vasculitis in hairy cell leukemia. Arch Intern Med 1987;147:660.
56. Seldin MF. Clinical description. Ann Intern Med 1988;108:575.
57. Dover JS. Case records of the Massachusetts General Hospital: a 47 year-old man with a rash, fever and headaches. N Engl J Med 1990;323:254.
58. Herrick JB. Peculiar elongation and sickle-shaped red blood corpuscles in a case of severe anemia. Arch Intern Med 1910;6:517.
59. Serjeant GR. Leg ulceration in sickle cell anemia. Arch Intern Med 1974;133:690.
60. Koshy M, Entsuah R, Koranda A. Leg ulcers in patients with sickle cell disease. Blood 74:1403, 1989.
61. Bardwick P. Plasma cell dyscrasia with polyneuropathy, organomegaly, endocrinopathy, M-protein and skin changes: the POEMS syndrome. Medicine 1980;59:311.
62. Takatsuki K. Plasma cell dyscrasia with polyneuropathy and endocrine disorder: clinical and laboratory features of 109 reported cases. Jpn J Clin Oncol 1983;13:543.
63. Donabedian H, Gallin JI. The hyperimmunoglobulin E recurrent-infection (Job's) syndrome: a review of the NIH experience and the literature. Medicine 1983;62:195.
64. Logothetis J, Economidou J, Constantoulakis M, et al. Cephalofacial deformities in thalassemia major (Cooley's anemia). Am J Dis Child 1971;121:300.
65. Shoch D. Blood dyscrasias and the eye. Postgrad Med 1969;45:104.

66. Friedman AH. Ocular manifestations of hematologic disorders. Hosp Pract 1984;19:131.
67. Kolker AE. Ocular manifestations of hematologic disease. Progr Hematol 1966;5:354.
68. Behrman S. Ophthalmoscope as viscosimeter. (Letter) Br Med J 1971;2:399.
69. Bunn HF, Forget BG. Sickle cell disease: clinical and epidemiological aspects. In: Hemoglobin: molecular, genetic and clinical aspects. Philadelphia, WB Saunders, 1986:531.
70. Ballas SK, Lewis CN, Noone AM, et al. Clinical, hematological, and biochemical features of Hb SC disease. Am J Hematol 1982;13:37.
71. Chaine G, Davies J, Kohner EM, et al. Ophthalmologic abnormalities in the hypereosinophilic syndrome. Ophthalmology 1982;89:1348.
72. Reddy EK, Bhatia P, Evans RG. Primary orbital lymphomas. Int J Radiat Oncol Biol Phys 1988;15:1239.
73. Schachat AP, Markowitz JA, Guyer DR, et al. Ophthalmic manifestations of leukemia. Arch Ophthalmol 1989;107:697.
74. Francis IC, Kappagoda MB, Smith JF, et al. Recurrent acute myelomonoblastic leukaemia presenting as a red eye. Med J Aust 1986;145:632.
75. Callender ST, Denborough MA, Sneath J. Blood groups and other inherited characters in pernicious anaemia. Br J Haematol 1957;3:107.
76. Friedman EM, Herer GR, Luban NL, Williams I. Sickle cell anemia and hearing. Ann Otol Rhinol Laryngol 1980;89:342.
77. Stell PM. Epistaxis. Clin Otolaryngol 1977;2:263.
78. Fu Y-S, Perzin KH. Nonepithelial tumors of the nasal cavity, paranasal sinuses and nasopharynx: a clinicopathologic study. IX. Plasmacytomas. Cancer 1978;42:2399.
79. Dolin S, Dewar JP. Extramedullary plasmacytoma. Am J Pathol 1965;32:83.
80. Hoppe RT, Burke JS, Glatstein E, Kaplan HS. Non-Hodgkin's lymphoma: involvement of Waldeyer's ring. Cancer 1978;42:1096.
81. Stafford R, Sonis S, Lockhart P, Sonis A. Oral pathoses as diagnostic indicators in leukemia. Oral Surg 1980;50:134.
82. Brenneise CV, Mattson JS, Commers JR. Acute myelomonocytic leukemia with oral manifestations: report of case. JADA 1988;117:835.
83. Appel BN, Miggantz RJ. Acute nonlymphocytic leukemia, monocytic variant: report of a case. J Periodontol 1987;59:464.
84. Sydney SB, Serio F. Acute monocytic leukemia diagnosed in a patient referred because of gingival pain. JADA 1981;103:886.
85. Epstein JB, Voss NJS, Stevenson-Moore P. Maxillofacial manifestations of multiple myeloma. Oral Surg 1984;57:267.
86. Schmitt RJ, Sheridan PJ, Rogers RS III. Pernicious anemia with associated glossodynia. JADA 1988;117:838.
87. Dayal PK, Mani NJ. Clinical aspects of the tongue in anemia. Ann Dent 1979;38:21.
88. Millard HD, Gobetti JP. Nonspecific stomatitis: a presenting sign in pernicious anemia. Oral Med 1975;39:562.
89. Johnson BE. Glossitis, folic acid and pernicious anemia. (Letter) South Med J 1983;76:1463.
90. Dawson AA, Ogston D, Fullerton HW. Evaluation of diagnostic significance of certain symptoms and physical signs in anaemic patients. Br Med J 1969;3:436.
90a. Libman H. Generalized lymphadenopathy. J Gen Intern Med 1987;2:48.
91. Carithers HA. Lymphadenopathy: a diagnostic enigma. Am J Dis Child 1978;132:353.
92. Barness LA. Manual of pediatric physical diagnosis, ed 4. Chicago, Year Book Medical Pub, 1972:46.
93. Knight PJ, Mulne AF, Vassy LE. When is lymph node biopsy indicated in children with enlarged peripheral nodes? Pediatrics 1982;69:391.
94. Allhiser JN, McKnight TA, Shank JC. Lymphadenopathy in a family practice. J Fam Pract 1981;12:27.
95. Krikorian JG, Portlock CS, Mauch PM. Hodgkin's disease presenting below the diaphragm: a review. J Clin Oncol 1986;4:1551.
96. Atkinson K, Austin DE, McElwain TJ, Peckham MJ. Alcohol pain in Hodgkin's disease. Cancer 1976;37:895.
97. Li FP, Willard DR, Goodman R, Vawter G. Malignant lymphoma after diphenylhydantoin (Dilantin) therapy. Cancer 1975;36:1359.
98. Crosby WC. Foreword. In: Pochedly C, Sills RH, Schwartz D, eds. Disorders of the spleen. New York, Marcel Dekker, 1989:v.
99. Castell DO. The spleen percussion sign: a useful diagnostic technique. Ann Intern Med 1967;67:1265.
100. Vaughan VC, McKay RJ, Behrman RE. Diseases of the blood. In: Nelson WE, ed. Textbook of pediatrics, ed 11. Philadelphia, WB Saunders, 1979:1421.
101. McIntyre OR, Ebaugh FG Jr. Palpable spleens in college freshmen. Ann Intern Med 1967;66:301.
102. Bunn HF, Forget BG. Sickle cell disease: clinical and epidemiological aspects. In: Hemoglobin: molecular, genetic and clinical aspects. Philadelphia, WB Saunders, 1986:533.
103. Bunn HF, Forget BG. Sickle cell disease: clinical and epidemiological aspects. In: Hemoglobin: molecular, genetic and clinical aspects. Philadelphia, WB Saunders, 1986:523.
104. Young LE, Izzo MJ, Platzer RF. Hereditary spherocytosis. I. Clinical, hematologic and genetic features in 28 cases, with particular reference to the osmotic and mechanical fragility of incubated erythrocytes. Blood 1951;6:1073.
105. Halliday JW, Powell LW. Iron overload. Semin Hematol 1982;19:42.
106. Valla D, Casadevall N, LaCombe C. Primary myeloproliferative disorder and hepatic vein thrombosis: a prospective study of erythroid colony formation in vitro in 20 patients with Budd-Chiari syndrome. Ann Intern Med 1985;103:329.
107. Nakai GS, Craddock CG, Figueroa WG. Agnogenic myeloid metaplasia. Ann Intern Med 1962;57:419.
108. Rosenthal DS. Non-Hodgkin's lymphoma: to treat or not to treat? Med Times 1987;115:49.
109. Shimm DS, Dosoretz DE, Anderson T, et al. Primary gastric lymphoma: an analysis with emphasis on prognostic factors and radiation therapy. Cancer 1983;52:2044.
110. Sandler RS. Primary gastric lymphoma: a review. Am J Gastroenterol 1984;79:21.
111. Rausch PG, Herion JC. Pulmonary manifestations of Waldenstrom macroglobulinemia. Am J Hematol 1980;9:201.
112. Collins FS, Orringer EP. Pulmonary hypertension and cor pulmonale in the sickle hemoglobinopathies. Am J Med 1982;73:814.
113. Bloom R, Taveira da Silva AM, Bracey A. Reversible respiratory failure due to intravascular leukostasis in chronic myelogenous leukemia: relationship of oxygen transfer to leukocyte count. Am J Med 1979;67:679.
114. McKee LC Jr, Collins RD. Intravascular leukocyte thrombi and aggregates as a cause of morbidity and mortality in leukemia. Medicine 1974;53:463.
115. Hodgson CH, Burchell HB, Good CA, Clagett OT. Hereditary hemorrhagic telangiectasia and pulmonary arteriovenous fistula: survey of a large family. N Engl J Med 1959;261:632.
116. Varat MA, Adolph RJ, Fowler NO. Cardiovascular effects of anemia. Am Heart J 1972;83:415.
117. Graettinger JS, Parsons RL, Campbell JA. A correlation of clinical and hemodynamic studies in patients with mild and severe anemia with and without congestive failure. Ann Intern Med 1963;58:617.
118. Bunn HF, Forget BG. The thalassemias: clinical manifestations. In: Hemoglobin: molecular, genetic and clinical aspects. Philadelphia, WB Saunders, 1986:335.
119. Shih L-Y, Lin F-C, Kuo T-T. Cutaneous and pericardial extramedullary hematopoiesis with cardiac tamponade in chronic myeloid leukemia. Am J Clin Pathol 1988;89:693.
120. Thomas LB, Forkner CE Jr, Frei E III, et al. The skeletal lesions of acute leukemia. Cancer 1961;14:608.
121. Bunn HF, Forget BG. Sickle cell disease: clinical and epidemiological aspects. In: Hemoglobin: molecular, genetic and clinical aspects. Philadelphia, WB Saunders, 1986:518.
122. Sebes JI, Kraus AP. Avascular necrosis of the hip in sickle hemoglobinopathies. J Can Assoc Radiol 1983;34:136.
123. Amstutz HC, Carey EJ. Skeletal manifestations and treatment of Gaucher's disease. J Bone Joint Surg 1966;48A:670.
124. Epps CH Jr. Painful hematologic conditions affecting the shoulder. Clin Orthop 1983;173:38.
125. Depalma AF. Hemophilic arthropathy. Clin Orthop 1967;52:145.
126. Heinicke MH, Zarrabi MH, Gorevic PD. Arthritis due to synovial involvement by extramedullary haematopoiesis in myelofibrosis with myeloid metaplasia. Ann Rheum Dis 1983;42:196.
127. Michiels JJ, Abels J, Steketee J, et al. Erythromelalgia caused by platelet mediated arteriolar inflammation and thrombosis in thrombocythemia. Ann Intern Med 1985;102:466.
128. Mitchell SW. On a rare vaso-motor neurosis of the extremities and on the maladies with which it may be confounded. Am J Med Sci 1878;76:1.
129. Alter BP. Bone marrow failure syndromes. In: Nathan DG, Oski FA, eds. Hematology of infancy and childhood, ed 3. Philadelphia, WB Saunders, 1987:199.
130. Emond AM, Holman R, Hayes RJ, Serjeant GR. Priapism and impotence in homozygous sickle cell disease. Arch Intern Med 1980;140:1434.
131. Pearson TC, Wetherley-Mein G. Vascular occlusive episodes and venous haematocrit in primary proliferative polycythaemia. Lancet 1978;2:1219.
132. Humphrey PRD, Marshall J, Russell RWR, et al. Cerebral blood-flow and viscosity in relative polycythaemia. Lancet 1979;2:873.
133. Willison JR, du Boulay GH, Paul EA, et al. Effect of high haematocrit on alertness. Lancet 1980;1:846.
134. Lichtman MA, Rowe JM. Hyperleukocytic leukemias: Rheological, clinical, and therapeutic considerations. Blood 1982;60:279.
135. Hild DH, Myers TJ. Hyperviscosity in chronic granulocytic leukemia. Cancer 1980;46:1418.
136. Powars D, Wilson B, Imbus C, et al. The natural history of stroke in sickle cell disease. Am J Med 1978;65:461.
137. Mitus AJ, Schafer AI. Hemostatic complications in young patients with essential thrombocythemia. Am J Med 1990;88:371.
138. Jandl JH. Leukocyte anomalies. In: Blood: textbook of hematology. Boston, Little, Brown, 1987:1056.
139. Biggs R. Haemophilia treatment in the United Kingdom from 1969 to 1974. Br J Haematol 1977;35:487.

140. Eyster ME, Gill FM, Blatt PM, et al. Central nervous system bleeding in hemophiliacs. Blood 1978;51:1179.
141. Levitt LJ, Dawson DM, Rosenthal DS, Moloney WC. CNS involvement in the non-Hodgkin's lymphomas. Cancer 1980;45:545.
142. Lowenthal DA, Straus DJ, Campbell SW, et al. AIDS-related lymphoid neoplasia: the Memorial Hospital experience. Cancer 1988;61:2325.
143. Champlin R, Gale RP. Acute myelogenous leukemia: recent advances in therapy. Blood 1987;69:1551.
144. Clarkson B, Ellis S, Little C, et al. Acute lymphoblastic leukemia in adults. Semin Oncol 1985;12:160.
145. Linker CA, Levitt LJ, O'Donnell M, et al. Improved results of treatment of adult acute lymphoblastic leukemia. Blood 1987;69:1242.
146. Houff SA, Major EO, Katz DA, et al. Involvement of JC virus-infected mononuclear cells from the bone marrow and spleen in the pathogenesis of progressive multifocal leukoencephalopathy. N Engl J Med 1988;318:301.
147. Shulman R. Psychiatric aspects of pernicious anaemia: a prospective controlled investigation. Br Med J 1967;3:266.
148. Rundles RW. Prognosis in the neurologic manifestations of pernicious anemia. Blood 1946;1:209.
149. Victor M, Lear AA. Subacute combined degeneration of the spinal cord. Am J Med 1956;20:896.
150. Dallman PR. Manifestations of iron deficiency. Semin Hematol 1982; 19:19.
151. Oski FA, Honig AS. The effects of therapy on the developmental scores of iron-deficient infants. J Pediatr 1978;92:21.
152. Kwaan HC. Clinicopathologic features of thrombotic thrombocytopenic purpura. Semin Hematol 1987;24:71.
153. Major RH. Diseases of the blood. In: Classic descriptions of disease, ed 3. Springfield, IL, Charles C Thomas, 1978:487.

Blood: Principles and Practice of Hematology,
edited by Robert I. Handin, Thomas P. Stossel, and Samuel E. Lux.
J.B. Lippincott Company, Philadelphia © 1995.

2

Laboratory Hematology: Methods for the Analysis of Blood

Laurence Corash

Enumeration and qualitative classification of the various cell types in blood presents a complicated challenge because of the intrinsic nature of blood. First, blood is a complex suspension of cells in plasma protein. The plasma protein fraction is coagulable, and the process of coagulation may alter the form and quantity of the cellular fraction. Second, blood and its constituents are relatively labile and require immediate processing. Third, some cellular components occur at low frequencies, which presents further problems in achieving adequate measurement precision. Finally, substantial variations among and within individuals exist with respect to sex, age, and ethnicity, which complicate the definition of the normal reference range for interpreting results from single samples. Despite these obstacles, current analytic methods have overcome many of these problems and the analysis of blood is rapid and cost-effective. In fact, this technology has probably led to overuse because it is so cost-effective. The technology of blood analysis continues to evolve at a rapid pace, and physicians, particularly those in the field of hematology, require an ongoing understanding of it to make the best use of the information the technology analysis produces.

SAMPLE COLLECTION AND PREPARATION

Virtually all samples for analysis of blood cells or their constituents, such as hemoglobin, are collected into tubes containing potassium or sodium salts of ethylenediamine tetraacetic acid (EDTA). EDTA, an avid calcium chelator, serves as an effective anticoagulant to inhibit activation of the coagulation system and production of fibrin clots. Samples with clots are not suitable for analysis of cellular components. Usually, these samples are collected in evacuated blood drawing tubes to produce a final EDTA concentration of 4.5 mmol/L. Blood drawn under these conditions is generally stable at room temperature for 24 hours without significant deterioration in the quality or quantity of the different cell classes. Platelet concentrations in EDTA-anticoagulated whole blood are more stable with storage at 4°C, but lower temperatures result in reduction of leukocyte counts and morphologic integrity. In most clinical laboratories, blood samples are retained at room temperatures (20° to 22°C) for 24 hours and discarded.

Under certain circumstances, blood for analysis of cellular constituents may be drawn into sodium citrate or heparin. One volume of sodium citrate (3.2% or 3.8%) is diluted with nine volumes of whole blood; this produces a dilutional error that must be corrected after blood cell enumeration. Citrated samples may be useful for platelet counting when persistent platelet–leukocyte satellitism is observed on peripheral smears prepared from EDTA blood samples. This phenomenon is mediated by agglutinins, either IgG or IgM, which may be calcium-dependent.[1–3] Although platelet–leukocyte satellitism appears to be an in vitro phenomenon, it can result in spurious or pseudothrombocytopenia due to platelet agglutination or leukocyte adherence during sample processing.

Heparin can be used as an anticoagulant without introducing a dilutional error; unfortunately, it causes platelet and leukocyte agglutination, which interferes with accurate cell enumeration. For these reasons, citrate and heparin are not routinely used for blood sample collection. Oxalate, previously used as an anticoagulant, is no longer in common use. Tubes for blood drawing may be prepared (rather than purchased) by placing 0.5 mL of a 100-mmol/L EDTA solution in a dry tube to which 10 mL of whole blood is added.

Red Blood Cell, Platelet, and Leukocyte Morphology

Blood smears can be prepared directly from fingerstick samples or from anticoagulated blood tubes. Either 22-mm square coverslips or standard glass microscope slides (25 × 75 × 1 mm) may be used. Full-sized glass microscope slides offer the advantage that they can be conveniently stained in automated staining devices whereas coverslips can be stained manually only. Blood smears, prepared by either method, should result in a thin blood film with a portion of the smear in which the red blood cells (RBCs) are evenly distributed with adequate preservation of central pallor (Fig. 2-1). The area containing singly distributed RBCs with well-preserved central pallor is the best region to examine RBC, leukocyte, and platelet morphology (Fig. 2-2). Blood smears also may be prepared using automated centrifugal spinner devices that provide excellent morphology.[4] Although the thick portions, or the "feathered edge," of blood smears contain more leukocytes, they gen-

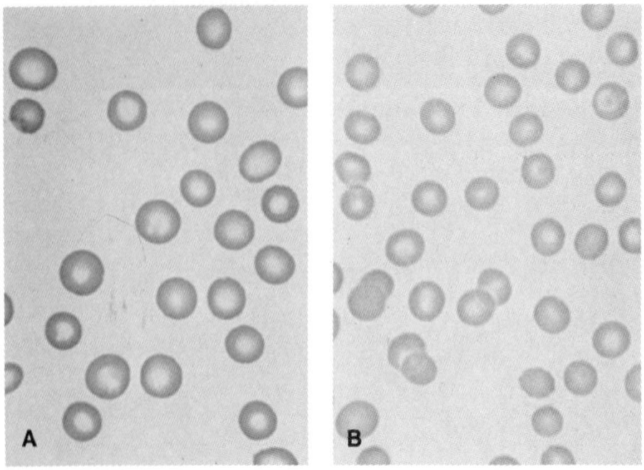

FIGURE 2-1. Thin peripheral blood smear from a newborn infant (**A**) and an adult (**B**). Note the adequate preservation of central pallor. The mean corpuscular volume of the newborn blood is 108 fL, whereas that of the adult blood is 92 fL. This difference is not perceptible on the peripheral smear. (See Color Fig. 2-1.)

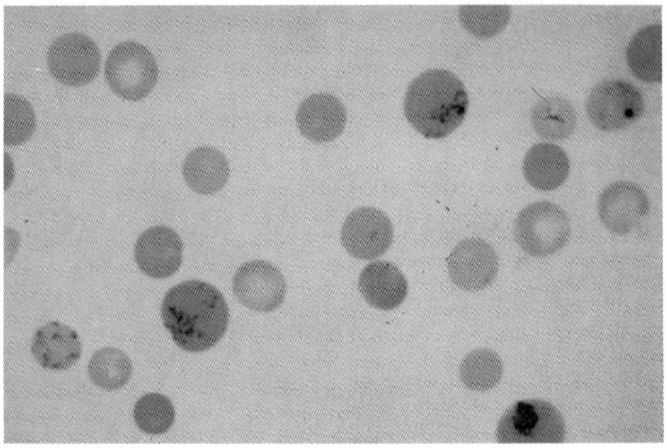

FIGURE 2-3. Reticulocyte preparation using new methylene blue. Precipitated RNA of varying sizes can be seen in the different cells.

erally distort cellular features and can lead to serious errors in interpreting the maturity of nuclear chromatin patterns.

Blood smears should be thoroughly air-dried without heating before staining. Morphologic analysis is best accomplished with polychrome-stained smears using a variety of different stains that are eosin–methylene blue combinations in methyl alcohol—Wright, Giemsa, or Romanowsky.[5] Automated staining devices offer the advantage of greater uniformity of staining conditions with considerable savings in labor.

Reticulocyte Enumeration

Reticulocytes, newly released RBCs containing RNA, also may be enumerated using peripheral smears prepared after RBCs have been incubated with supravital dyes, such as new methylene blue or brilliant cresyl blue. These dyes precipitate intracellular RNA and allow identification of reticulocytes.[6] Reticulocyte counting requires the preparation of thin smears on which reticulocytes containing a blue precipitate can be detected. The amount of reticulum or precipitate varies in reticulocytes of different maturation states (Fig. 2-3). Younger reticulocytes exhibit larger and more dense precipitates.

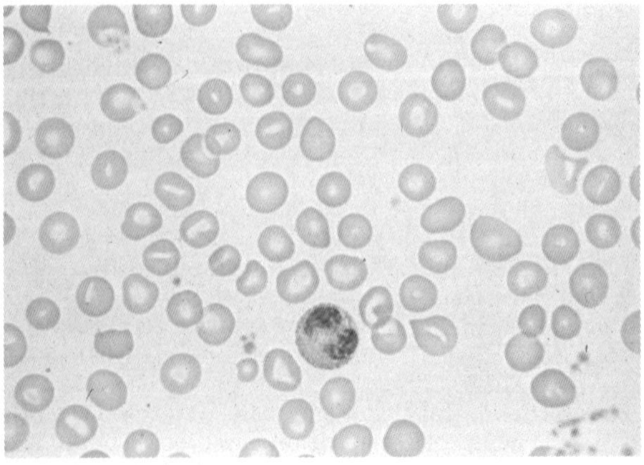

FIGURE 2-2. Peripheral smear with adequate preservation of central pallor. Platelets and a single polymorphonuclear leukocyte are present. RBCs vary in size and shape. (See Color Fig. 2-2.)

Detection of Fetal Hemoglobin

Detection of fetal hemoglobin (hemoglobin F) in individual RBCs is useful to establish the diagnosis of fetal–maternal transfusion and also for the evaluation of hemoglobin F content in patients with hemoglobinopathies. The modified Kleihauer-Betke technique is easily adaptable to the clinical laboratory.[7] Thin blood smears are prepared and fixed with 80% ethanol. The fixed slides are then exposed to an acid–citrate solution at pH 3.3 to elute hemoglobin A followed by hematoxylin counterstain. Cells containing hemoglobin A appear as pale ghosts, whereas cells with hemoglobin F stain pink (Fig. 2-4). Fetal cells demonstrate uniform bright pink staining as do cells from patients that are homozygous for hereditary persistence of hemoglobin F (HPFH). Blood from HPFH heterozygotes demonstrates variation in cell staining intensity, as do samples from heterozygotes for β-thalassemia and $\delta\ \beta$-thalassemia. Alternatively, a commercial kit is available that uses a ferric chloride–hematoxylin eluting solution followed by an erythrosin counterstain to detect hemoglobin F in cells on ethanol fixed air-dried smears (Boehringer Mannheim Diagnostics, Fetal Hemoglobin Elution Method #124249, 1981).

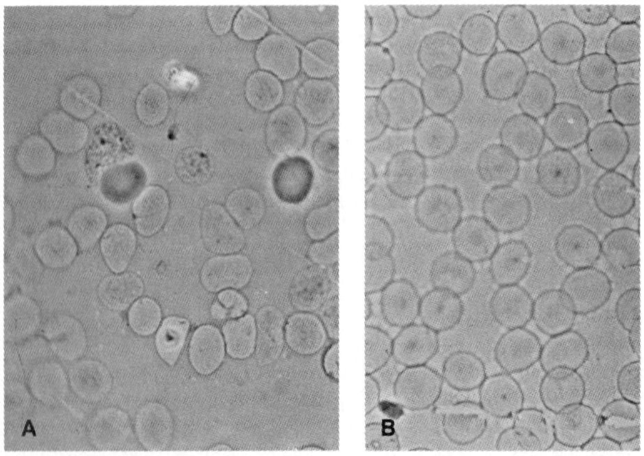

FIGURE 2-4. Detection of fetal hemoglobin using the Kleihauer-Betke acid elution technique. Cells containing fetal hemoglobin are stained pink, and cells containing hemoglobin A appear as pale ghosts. Note the presence of two hemoglobin F cells in a sample of maternal blood (**A**) and the absence of hemoglobin F cells in an adult man's control sample (**B**).

Hemoglobin F also may be detected through the use of monoclonal antibodies to the F specific γ chain.[8,9] Wood and colleagues used a purified anti–hemoglobin F polyclonal antibody conjugated to fluorescein isothiocyanate to measure the incidence of cells containing hemoglobin F in normal whites and blacks. Normal black subjects had an average of 2.8% ± 1.6% standard deviation (SD) F cells, and normal white subjects had an average of 2.6% ± 1% (SD) F cells.[9] The combined average was 2.7% with a range of 0.5% to 7%. Wood and colleagues[9] also concluded that the fluorescence test was much more sensitive than the acid elution technique for the detection of small amounts of hemoglobin F, but they noted that the immunofluorescence technique was less satisfactory than the acid elution technique for samples with higher than 30% fetal cells.

The acid elution technique appears well suited to evaluate samples for fetal–maternal transfusion, but it lacks sensitivity for detection of small amounts of hemoglobin F. Mollison[10] has described the use of a formula to calculate the volume of a fetal–maternal transfusion, for the estimation of Rh_0 (D) immune globulin (RhoGAM) dosage, based on the relative ratio of fetal to maternal cells.

Allen and associates have reported the use of a two-color technique with monoclonal antibodies against the β and γ chains of hemoglobin to establish the absence of β chains in antenatal samples for the diagnosis of β-thalassemia.[11] Fetal blood samples were obtained and cytocentrifuge preparations of the RBCs were fixed and then treated with a combination of anti–β chain and anti–γ chain monoclonal reagents. Monoclonal antibody to γ chain was detected with rhodanine-conjugated goat anti-mouse Ig, and biotin-conjugated anti–β chain was detected with an avidin–fluorescein isothiocyanate conjugate. The dual labeling technique permitted the identification of fetal cells followed by selective examination of these cells for the simultaneous weak expression of β-chain product. Contaminating maternal cells, which stain intensely for β chains, can easily be avoided. Sensitivity was equal to that obtained with radioisotopic β/γ chain ratio synthesis studies.[11]

Flow cytometry should be an ideal method to detect cells containing hemoglobin F to quantitate fetal–maternal bleeding or to diagnose β-thalassemia. A simple flow assay has yet to be described for these purposes. Dover and Boyer[12] reported the use of a monoclonal antibody to hemoglobin F and flow cytometry for the quantitation of mean corpuscular hemoglobin (MCH) content in F and non–F RBCs. Using this technique, they demonstrated that there is a reciprocal relation between hemoglobin F and non–F levels in mature RBCs. Their technique should be adaptable to produce a routine flow cytometric technique.

Detection of Heinz Bodies

Heinz bodies are membrane-bound mixed disulfides of denatured hemoglobin and erythrocyte membrane proteins.[13] They may be seen in association with unstable hemoglobins or in disorders in which the ability of the cell to maintain hemoglobin in a reduced state is impaired, for example, glucose-6-phosphate dehydrogenase deficiency. Spontaneously formed Heinz bodies may be seen on peripheral blood smears after staining with rhodanile blue dye.[14] In contrast to other dyes, such as new methylene blue, rhodanile blue has the advantage of not staining reticulocytes, nor causing oxidative damage. Heinz bodies are not visible in the peripheral blood of most patients with unstable hemoglobin, especially if splenic function is intact.[15] Alternatively, blood samples can be treated with an oxidant agent, acetylphenylhydrazine, then stained and examined for the presence of Heinz bodies. Methyl violet may be used in place of rhodanile blue for the demonstration of Heinz bodies (Fig. 2-5).

The isopropanol solubility test is a sensitive technique to demonstrate the presence of an unstable hemoglobin.[16] A small volume of hemolysate is added to a tube containing a mixture of isopropanol and buffer. If an unstable hemoglobin is present, a flocculent precipitate forms in the presence of an unstable hemoglobin. This simple method appears to have a high level of sensitivity for detecting unstable hemoglobins.

Nomarski Optics

Whole blood may be collected into buffered glutaraldehyde solution and examined using Nomarski optics with an interference phase microscope to visualize the cell surface.[17] As little as 1 drop of fresh blood may be added to 0.5 mL of buffered glutaraldehyde solution, then held for examination at a later time. With intact splenic function, the RBC surface appears uniform and smooth. If splenic function is impaired, the RBC surface contains numerous small craters.[17,18] The incidence of pocked or cratered RBCs can be determined and used as an index of splenic function.[17] Although the presence of Howell-Jolly bodies (Fig. 2-6) also indicates asplenia or splenic hypofunction, their relative sparseness reduces the reliability of the presence or absence of Howell-Jolly bodies as an index of splenic function.[17]

Premature infants frequently have transient functional hyposplenia. One study of 76 full-term and 82 premature infants noted Howell-Jolly bodies transiently in 1 full-term and 4 premature infants.[19] Thus, only a minority of healthy infants have Howell-Jolly bodies.

These RBC inclusions have also been found in patients with megaloblastic anemia, hemolytic anemia, thalassemia, leukemia, idiopathic steatorrhea, nontropical sprue with splenic atrophy, and in circulating late erythroblasts.[19] Examination of the RBC surface using phase contrast microscopy with Nomarski optics had a high degree of sensitivity to detect asplenia and return of splenic function with posttraumatic splenosis.[17] Normal subjects had less than 1% pocked RBCs compared with asplenic children with an average of 20.3% pocked cells. This simple test appears to provide an extremely sensitive means to assess splenic function.

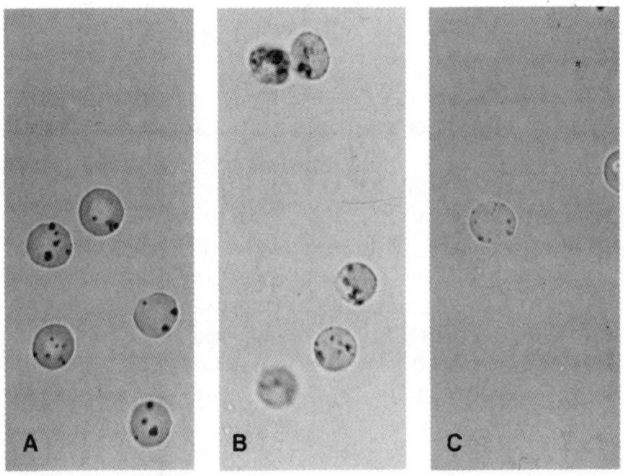

FIGURE 2-5. Heinz body preparation after treatment of normal RBCs (**A** and **C**) and G6PD-deficient RBCs (**B**) with acetylphenhyldrazine and methyl violet stain. Normal RBCs develop a limited number (no more than three) of small Heinz bodies per cell. In contrast, G6PD-deficient cells (**B**) develop more than four Heinz bodies per cell, which are generally large.

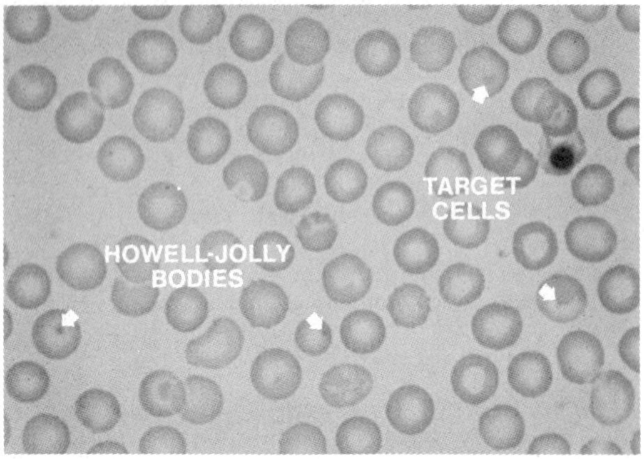

FIGURE 2-6. Peripheral blood smear from an infant with congenital asplenia. Note the presence of increased numbers of target cells and the small round darkly staining cellular inclusions (Howell-Jolly bodies). A nucleated RBC is also present in the field. The Howell-Jolly bodies represent retained nuclear material that has not been removed because of lack of splenic function. (See Color Fig. 2-6.)

Cytochemistry

A number of cytochemical stains may be performed on air-dried peripheral blood smears to aid in the specific identification of abnormal cells and to provide additional diagnostic information about normal-appearing peripheral blood cells.

Leukocyte Alkaline Phosphatase. Leukocyte alkaline phosphatase (LAP) is an enzyme present in the specific granules of myelocytes and more mature cells of the myeloid lineage. The LAP stain of peripheral blood smears is used for evaluation of patients suspected to have chronic myelogenous leukemia or paroxysmal nocturnal hemoglobinuria, and it may be useful in evaluation of granulocytic leukocytosis (leukemoid reactions). This stain is best performed on fresh fingerstick peripheral blood smears without use of EDTA, which inhibits LAP activity. Slides are fixed in citrate–acetone solution and staining is achieved using naphthyl phosphate as a substrate for the enzyme, with formation of an insoluble reaction product using either diazonium salt or fast blue salt as a capture agent.[20,21] Smears are counterstained with hematoxylin to facilitate identification of neutrophils, and positive cells contain either pink or blue granules, depending on the capture agent (Fig. 2-7). After staining, 100 mature neutrophils and band forms are counted and each cell is scored from 0 to 4+ according on the staining intensity.

A total LAP score is obtained by summing the products of the numbers of cells in each staining class times the class intensity score. Although a maximum score of 400 is possible, the normal range is about 11 to 95. Each laboratory should establish its own normal range.

Myeloperoxidase. Myeloperoxidase (MPO) is an enzyme present in the primary granules of myeloid and monocytic lineage cells. Myeloid cells exhibit greater intensity than monocytic cells, eosinophils are intensely positive, basophils are weakly positive, and lymphocytes are negative. Peroxidase staining may be performed on EDTA-anticoagulated specimens after fixation in paraformaldehyde–acetone fixative. Alcohol fixation inhibits peroxidase activity. Hydrogen peroxide is used as the substrate with 3-amino-9 ethyl carbazole as a capture agent for liberated oxygen radicals.[22] Stained smears are counterstained with hematoxylin to facilitate identification of cells. The nuclei are stained pale blue and the peroxidase reaction product is bright red (Fig. 2-8). Although a normal blood

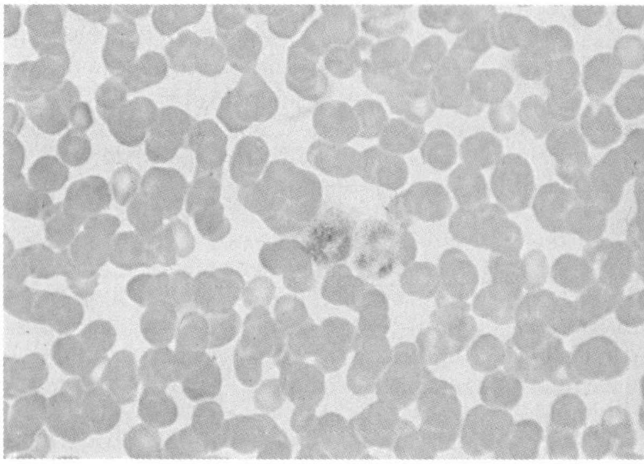

FIGURE 2-7. Leukocyte alkaline phosphatase stain. Note the presence of variable numbers of dark blue granules in the cytoplasm of two mature polymorphonuclear leukocytes. (See Color Fig. 2-7.)

sample is stained in parallel as a control, quality control of the staining procedure is best ensured by identification of a few positive cells in the patient sample. Failure to identify any positive cells should raise questions about the validity of the stain. Congenital or acquired MPO deficiency may be demonstrated by low-intensity staining or by the complete absence of MPO staining in recognizable mature polymorphonuclear cells.

Chloracetate Esterase. Chloracetate esterase is an enzyme present in the primary granules of myeloid cells, but not monocytic cells. It is not present in normal eosinophils or basophils. Chloracetate esterase activity increases with cellular maturation. This stain may be useful to determine the lineage of abnormal or dysplastic cells in the peripheral blood. Acquired chloracetate esterase deficiency may be seen in association with the myelodysplastic syndromes. Eosinophils associated with acute myelomonocytic leukemia with inversion of chromosome 16 demonstrate chloracetate esterase activity in contrast to that seen in normal eosinophils.[23,24] Either α-naphthol chloracetate or naphthol AS-D chloracetate may be used as the substrate for chloracetate esterase with a hematoxylin counterstain.[25] The reaction product is captured with pararosaniline to form a red precipitate (Fig. 2-9). The presence of a positive

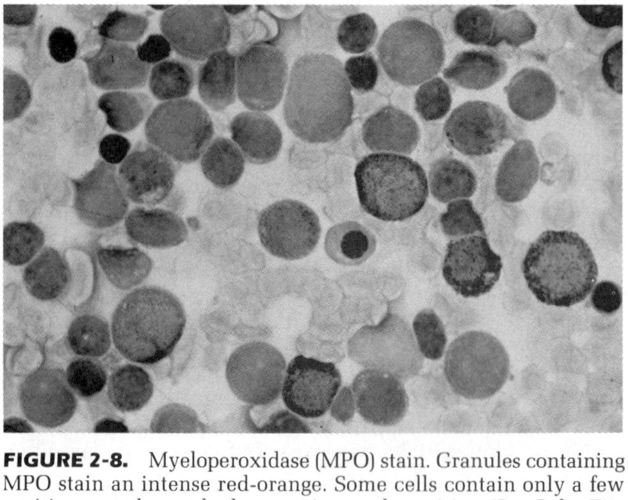

FIGURE 2-8. Myeloperoxidase (MPO) stain. Granules containing MPO stain an intense red-orange. Some cells contain only a few positive granules, and others are intensely positive. (See Color Fig. 2-8.)

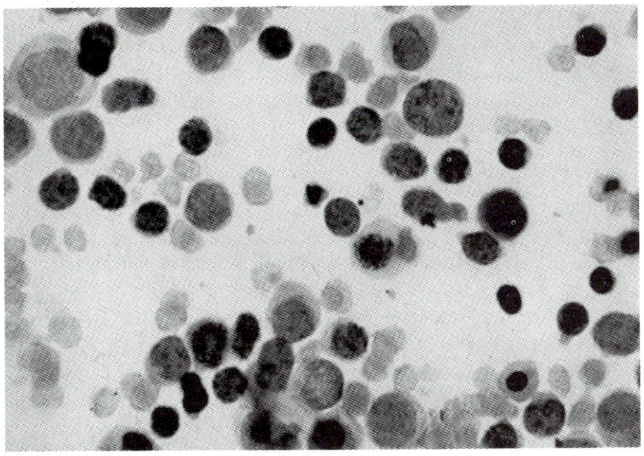

FIGURE 2-9. Chloracetate esterase stain. Two immature band neutrophil cells demonstrate intense cytoplasmic staining. (See Color Fig. 2-9.)

internal control cell confirms that the MPO reaction is working properly.

Nonspecific Esterase. Nonspecific esterase activity may be used as a marker for monocytes, although other cells express variably low levels of activity. Several different substrates may be used for this reaction—α-naphthyl acetate, naphthol AS-D acetate, or α-naphthyl butyrate. The latter produces an intense red after coupling with pararosaniline (Fig. 2-10). The butyrate substrate is less sensitive but more specific than the acetate substrates. Myeloid lineage cells do not contain nonspecific esterase activity; lymphocytes and megakaryocytes may stain weakly, whereas tissue macrophages stain brightly.[26] The nonspecific esterase stain is useful to discriminate monocytes from abnormal T lymphocytes (Sézary cells), both of which have convoluted nuclei.

Tartrate-Resistant Acid Phosphatase. Tartrate-resistant acid phosphatase (TRAP) activity is useful for identification of the abnormal cell of leukemic reticuloendotheliosis (hairy cell leukemia).[27] Lymphoid cells, monocytes, megakaryocytes, macrophages, nucleated erythroid cells, and myeloid cells stain variably for acid phosphatase activity in the absence of tartrate, but only the abnormal cells of leukemic reticuloendotheliosis or other rare lymphomas stain in the presence of tartrate, an inhibitor of most acid phosphatase isoenzymes.[28]

Naphthol AS-BI phosphoric acid is used as the substrate with fast garnet as a capture agent and hematoxylin counterstain. This stain may be difficult to interpret and requires the use of careful controls. Positive cells are identified by the presence of bright red granules (Fig. 2-11). Fresh fingerstick smears are preferred, but peripheral smears made from EDTA-anticoagulated blood may be used. Control slides, obtained from similar specimens, without tartrate should demonstrate platelet and granulocyte staining as well as lymphoid cells. Smears should be freshly prepared, then fixed in citrate–acetone solution, since aged unfixed smears do not stain well. After incubation with tartrate, platelets and granulocytes should be negative. Normal lymphoid cells show a marked reduction in activity, but may not be completely negative. Leukemic reticuloendotheliosis lymphoid cells continue to stain strongly in the presence of tartrate. Examine multiple areas of the smears because staining intensity may vary in different areas of the slide and the counterstain is weak, which makes identification of cells difficult.

A number of other cytochemical stains have been used for identification of abnormal cells, but they are no longer commonly used because of lack of specificity or because they were replaced by better techniques. Sudan black staining for identification of myeloid cells has been largely replaced by MPO staining because of improved counterstaining with the MPO technique. Since the periodic acid–Schiff (PAS) reagent stains glycogen in a wide variety of cells, it has largely been replaced by more specific cytochemical markers to identify abnormal cells. β-Glucuronidase activity also is present in a wide range of lymphoid and myeloid cells and has limited usefulness for evaluation of abnormal cells.

COMPLETE BLOOD COUNT

Red Blood Cell Counting

The complete blood count (CBC), the most commonly ordered test, consists of the following components: leukocyte (white blood cell) count, erythrocyte (RBC) count, hemoglobin concentration, MCH, mean corpuscular volume (MCV), MCH concentration (MCHC), and the hematocrit or packed cell volume. Depending on the methods used, these properties may be either directly measured or calculated from other measured values. Each of these parameters may be measured by manual techniques; except for the hematocrit, manual methods have largely disappeared

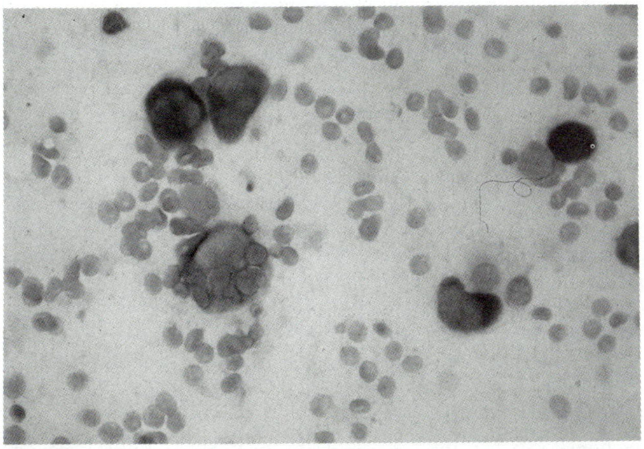

FIGURE 2-10. Nonspecific esterase stain. The butyrate substrate was used to demonstrate a positive reaction in this case of acute monoblastic leukemia (FAB M5a). (See Color Fig. 2-10.)

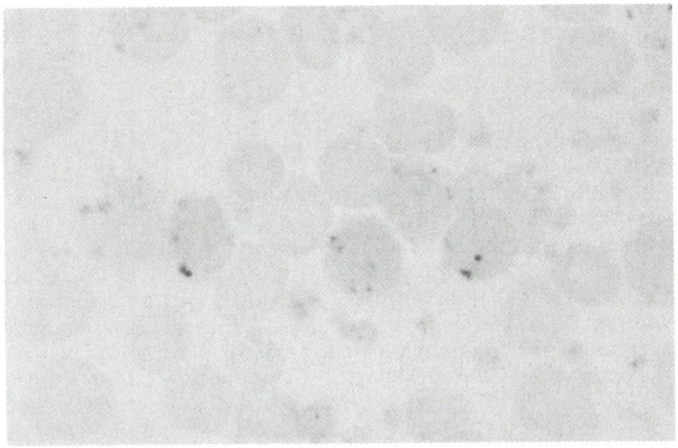

FIGURE 2-11. Tartrate-resistant acid phosphatase stain. Abnormal lymphoid cells from a patient with leukemic reticuloendotheliosis (hairy-cell leukemia) are stained with acid phosphatase in the presence of tartrate. (See Color Fig. 2-11.)

from the routine laboratory. Automated methodology using available instrumentation offers vastly improved precision compared with that provided in the older manual methods, and it has the potential to provide more information than the manual methods do.

As new instrumentation or techniques for performance of laboratory tests are introduced into the clinical laboratory, physicians who use the laboratory may seek guidelines to evaluate the performance of those tests. During the evaluation of new tests, the laboratory carries out comparisons with either existing methods or reference methods. Calibration methods for hemoglobin, hematocrit, and cell counting are described.[29,30] In addition, when new tests or methods are introduced, normal range studies consisting of at least 100 normal subjects should be completed and the reference range for the test established.

Physicians will want to know about the linearity of the test over the dynamic range of patient samples that they may submit. This information should be available from the clinical laboratory before the test is introduced. The most important characteristics of a test are precision and accuracy. Test accuracy is usually assessed through the use of calibrated reference materials, but in the hematology laboratory the only calibrated reference materials available are hemoglobin standards. Commercial cell suspensions may serve as control materials to ensure that instruments are operating within specified limits, but they do not constitute calibrated reference materials that can be used to assess accuracy.

Precision can be assessed by determining the coefficient of variation (CV) for a series of replicate samples, usually 20. The CV equals the standard deviation (SD) divided by the mean for the series of replicate results. As a general rule, a CV of less than 5% for a test is considered acceptable. For many measurements in hematology, CVs of less than 2% can be achieved. For certain tests, such as the reticulocyte count, CVs of 9% to 10% may be the best that can be obtained. Many other quality control procedures are used in the clinical laboratory to ensure correct instrument operation on a daily basis, but this information is rarely of value to the clinical hematologist unless the laboratory indicates that a specific test is out of the normal control range. Knowledge of the reference range for a test and the precision of the test at various levels of measurement provides the clinician with an understanding of the operating characteristics of the test.

In the following sections this information is presented in tabular form for the various tests under discussion.

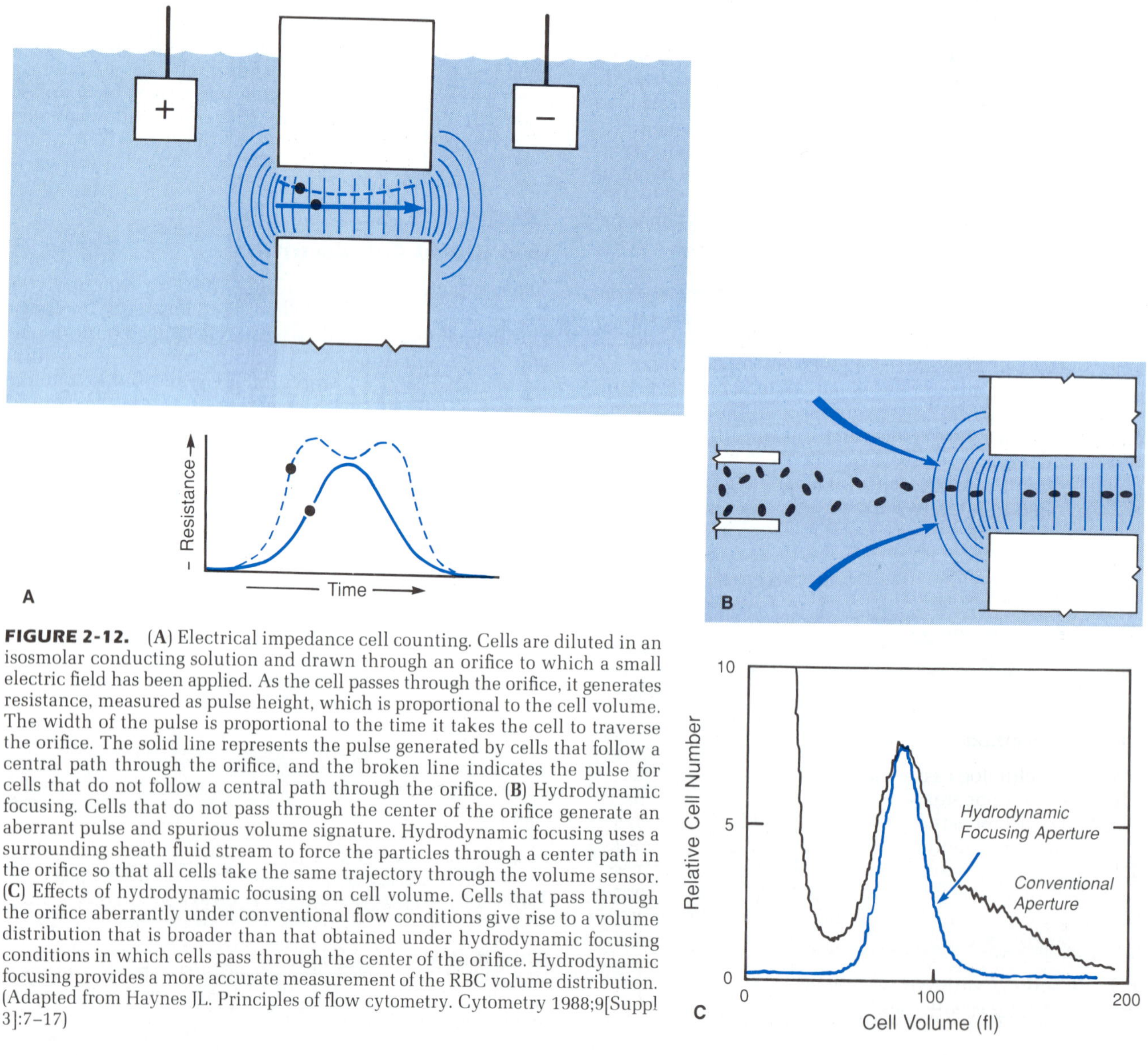

FIGURE 2-12. (A) Electrical impedance cell counting. Cells are diluted in an isosmolar conducting solution and drawn through an orifice to which a small electric field has been applied. As the cell passes through the orifice, it generates resistance, measured as pulse height, which is proportional to the cell volume. The width of the pulse is proportional to the time it takes the cell to traverse the orifice. The solid line represents the pulse generated by cells that follow a central path through the orifice, and the broken line indicates the pulse for cells that do not follow a central path through the orifice. (B) Hydrodynamic focusing. Cells that do not pass through the center of the orifice generate an aberrant pulse and spurious volume signature. Hydrodynamic focusing uses a surrounding sheath fluid stream to force the particles through a center path in the orifice so that all cells take the same trajectory through the volume sensor. (C) Effects of hydrodynamic focusing on cell volume. Cells that pass through the orifice aberrantly under conventional flow conditions give rise to a volume distribution that is broader than that obtained under hydrodynamic focusing conditions in which cells pass through the center of the orifice. Hydrodynamic focusing provides a more accurate measurement of the RBC volume distribution. (Adapted from Haynes JL. Principles of flow cytometry. Cytometry 1988;9[Suppl 3]:7–17)

Manual Red Blood Cell Counting

Manual RBC counting with dilution pipettes, counting chambers, and the microscope has virtually disappeared from the clinical laboratory; descriptions of these methods are available in reference texts.[5] These manual techniques have been replaced by automated flow cytometric instruments, which examine far greater numbers of cells and have improved precision over the entire clinically relevant dynamic range. Modern reference methods for RBC counting rely on the use of single channel or multichannel electrical impedance counting instruments. The only manual methods regularly used in clinical laboratories are hematocrit and hemoglobin measurements.

Manual Hemoglobin and Hematocrit Determinations

Manual hemoglobinometry serves as a reference method for calibration of automated instruments and as an alternative method when interfering substances prevent automated hemoglobinometry. The National Committee for Clinical Laboratory Standards (NCCLS) has published an approved procedure for manual measurement of hemoglobin using the cyanmethemoglobin method.[31] This method depends on the conversion of hemoglobin to a cyanmethemoglobin derivative followed by measurement of the absorbance at 540-nm-wavelength light. The absorbance of this solution is proportional to the hemoglobin concentration according to the Lambert-Beer law. The molar absorption coefficient of cyanmethemoglobin is well characterized, and accurate measurement of hemoglobin concentrations is achievable in the routine hematology laboratory. Hemoglobin concentration is expressed in grams per liter or grams per deciliter and may be converted to millimoles per liter by multiplying the concentration of grams per deciliter by 0.621.

Manual hemoglobinometry is useful when interfering substances, such as lipids or abnormal leukocytes, cause turbidity so that automated optical hemoglobinometry cannot be performed. Excessively high leukocyte counts also may interfere with accurate RBC counting and automated hemoglobinometry, necessitating the use of manually centrifuged hematocrits and manual hemoglobin measurement.

Manual hematocrit determinations, that is, measurement of packed RBC volume, are frequently used to assess the RBC mass. The performance of manual hematocrit requires the use of calibrated centrifuges to ensure uniform cell packing, standard microcapillary tubes, and an acceptable reading device. The NCCLS has published recommended guidelines for the microhematocrit method.[32] The manual hematocrit method is frequently used to provide accurate measurement of the packed cell volume when automated methods give spurious results because of problems with RBC deformability, interfering leukocytes, or plasma proteins.

Automated Methods

Two basic technologies are used for routine measurement of the CBC components—electrical impedance and light scatter. The former is the older technology and has proved its value through many years of usage. With this methodology, blood is aspirated into the system, the sample stream is split, one portion is used for hemoglobinometry, one portion is used for RBC counting, and one portion is used for leukocyte counting. Hemoglobinometry is accomplished after cell lysis and preparation of a cyanmethemoglobin solution with measurement of the hemoglobin concentration by absorbance spectrophotometry. This is a highly precise technique and provides replicate measurements with a CV of replicate samples, within-batch samples, and between-batch samples of 1% or less.[33] Failure of cells to lyse completely, due to abnormal hemoglobin such as hemoglobin AC or to hyperosmolar plasma as in uremia, interferes with hemoglobin measurement.

RBC counting and size analysis are performed by passing the RBCs singly through a small direct current (DC; Fig. 2-12*A*). Passage of the cell through the current generates a small pulse due to a temporary increase in impedance. The height of the pulse is proportional to cell volume and provides information about cell number and cell volume. Pulses that pass through the orifice in a path other than central generate a pulse that is distorted and not a true reflection of cell volume (see Fig. 2-12*B* and *C*). This problem has been resolved by the use of hydrodynamic focusing to force all cells through the central path of the sensing orifice. As for measurement of hemoglobin, the precision of these measurements is excellent with replicate sample CVs of less than 1%.[33]

MCH, MCHC, and hematocrit are not directly measured by electrical impedance systems, but are derived by calculation from the directly measured parameters of hemoglobin, RBC count, and RBC volume. These parameters are calculated from the following formulas:

$$\text{MCH} = \text{Hb(g/L)}/\text{RBC}(10^6/\mu\text{L})$$

$$\text{MCHC} = \text{Hb(g/dL)}/\text{HCT}(\%)$$

$$\text{HCT} = \text{MCV(fL)} \times \text{RBC}(10^6/\mu\text{L})$$

Although precision of the MCV measurement is excellent with replicate samples, abnormalities of membrane deformability or cellular hemoglobin concentration may lead to inaccurate MCV measurements with subsequent inaccuracies of the calculated indices.[33,34]

More recently, new versions of these instruments provide histograms of the RBC volume distribution in addition to the numeric measure of central tendency in the form of the MCV (Fig. 2-13). This format provides information about subpopulations of abnormal cells and also provides a measure of dispersion for the RBC volume distribution, the RBC distribution width (RDW). The RDW is the CV of the RBC volume distribution expressed as a percentage. Combined with the volume distribution, the RDW provides in-

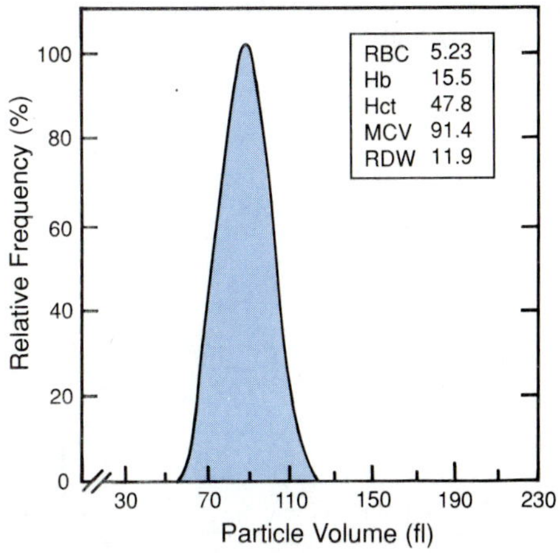

FIGURE 2-13. RBC volume distribution obtained with a Coulter type electrical impedance instrument. Cell number, expressed as relative frequency, is indicated on the Y axis and cell volume is indicated on the X axis. Mean corpuscular volume (MCV) and RBC distribution width (RDW), a measure of the dispersion of the volume distribution curve, are computed and reported. (Adapted from Bessman JD. Automated blood counts and differentials: a practical guide. Baltimore, Johns Hopkins University Press, 1986)

TABLE 2-1. Classification of Anemia Based on Red Cell MCV and RDW

MCV Low RDW Normal	MCV Low RDW High	MCV Normal RDW Normal	MCV Normal RDW High	MCV High RDW Normal	MCV High RDW High
Heterozygous thalassemia	Iron deficiency	Normal	Mixed deficiency	Aplastic anemia	Folate deficiency
Chronic disease	S-β-thalassemia	Chronic disease	Early iron or folate deficiency	Preleukemia	B_{12} deficiency
	Hemoglobin H	Chronic liver disease	Anemic hemoglobinopathy		Immune hemolysis
	Fragmentation	Hemoglobinopathy trait (S, C)	Myelofibrosis, sideroblastic anemia		Cold agglutinins
		Transfusion			CLL*
		Chemotherapy			
		CLL, CML			
		Hemorrhage			
		Hereditary spherocytosis			

MCV, mean corpuscular volume; RDW, red cell distribution width; CLL, chronic lymphocytic leukemia; CML, chronic myelogenous leukemia.
* Due to inclusion of leukocytes in the red cell volume distribution in CLL.
(Data from Bessman JD, et al. Improved classification of anemias by MCV and RDW. Am J Clin Pathol 1983;80:322–326)

formation about variation in cell size (anisocytosis) and is more sensitive than microscopic examination of the smear for detection of abnormal RBC subpopulations. These new parameters have been used to improve the diagnosis of anemia based on a bifunctional algorithm using MCV and RDW.[35] Although this algorithm may not be sensitive for all cases, it does provide a useful approach to the diagnosis of anemia[36] (Table 2-1).

Recently, a newer generation of instrumentation (Technicon H*1, Technicon Instruments, Tarrytown, NY), which offers several improvements for measuring RBC characteristics, has become widely available.[34,37] This instrument measures RBC volume by low-angle forward light scatter after isovolumetric sphering of the RBCs (Fig. 2-14). Under these conditions, using Mie scattering theory, RBC refractive index is directly proportional to the intracellular hemoglobin concentration[38] (Fig. 2-15). Thus, corpuscular hemoglobin concentration (CHC) may now be measured directly, and the distribution of CHC, measures of central tendency of MCHC, and the dispersion of this distribution may be measured (Fig. 2-16). The dispersion of the CHC distribution is termed the *hemoglobin distribution width* and is the CV expressed as a percentage for this distribution. More important, inspection of the CHC distribution (see Fig. 2-16) provides an excellent means of detecting subpopulations of cells with abnormal hemoglobin concentrations, for example, dehydrated cells associated with sickle cell anemia.[34]

The direct measurement of MCHC represents an improvement over earlier electrical impedance systems in which the automated MCHC did not agree well with manual determinations[34] (Fig. 2-17). The lack of agreement was due to poor deformability of RBCs with MCHC levels above 36 g/dL. Sphering of RBCs in the RBC channel resolved this problem and has improved the MCHC measurement as a means of assessing RBC hydration and internal viscosity.[34] The H*1 instrument format now provides direct measurement of four RBC characteristics: hemoglobin, volume, number, and hemoglobin concentration. Because hemoglobin concentration can be precisely measured, calculation of the hematocrit from measured MCV and RBC is of limited value and may gradually be removed from newer instruments. Combined with the histograms for volume and hemoglobin concentration, this information offers

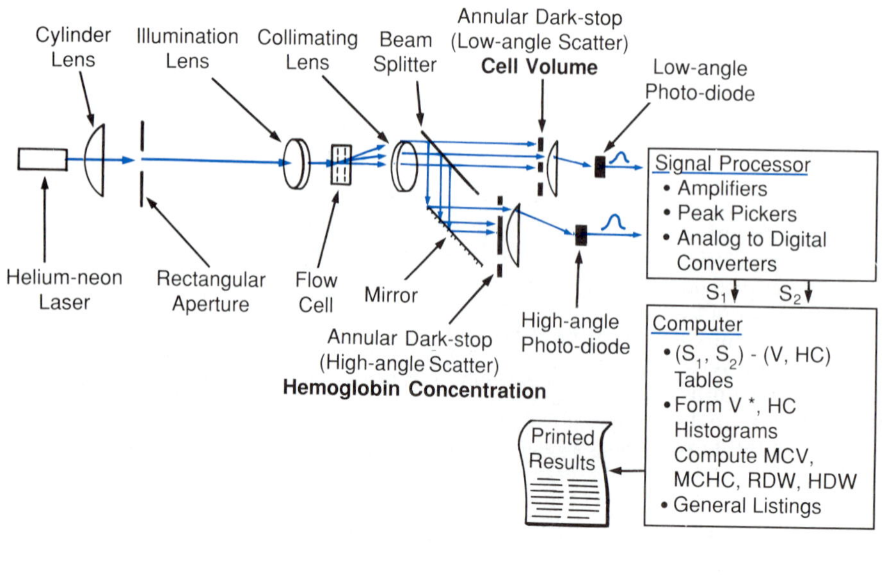

FIGURE 2-14. Schematic representation of the RBC channel of the Technicon H*1 instrument. Five thousand to 10,000 RBCs are sphered and drawn through a flow cell with simultaneous measurement of low-angle (2- to 3-degree) scatter and high-angle (5- to 15-degree) scatter. Low-angle scatter is used as a measure of cell volume and high-angle scatter is used to measure hemoglobin concentration. (Adapted from Mohandas N, et al. Accurate and independent measurement of volume and hemoglobin concentration of individual RBCs by laser light scattering. Blood 1986;68:506–513)

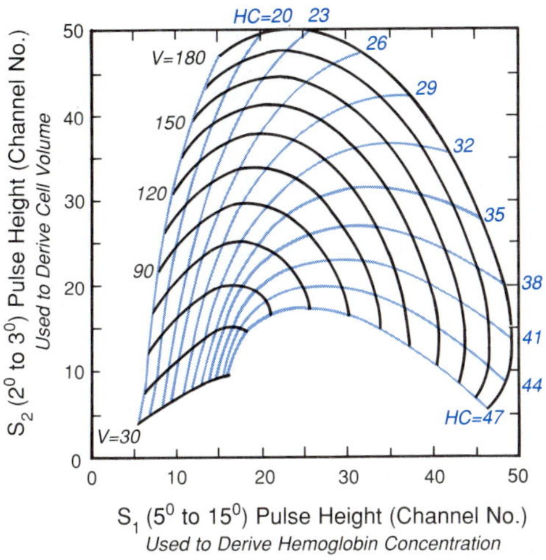

FIGURE 2-15. Bivariant mapping of RBC volume and hemoglobin concentration. The results from the Technicon H*1 RBC channel are represented as a bivariant scatter plot of cell volume (Y axis) and cell hemoglobin concentration (X axis). (Adapted from Mohandas N, et al. Accurate and independent measurement of volume and hemoglobin concentration of individual red cells by laser light scattering. Blood 1986;68:506–513)

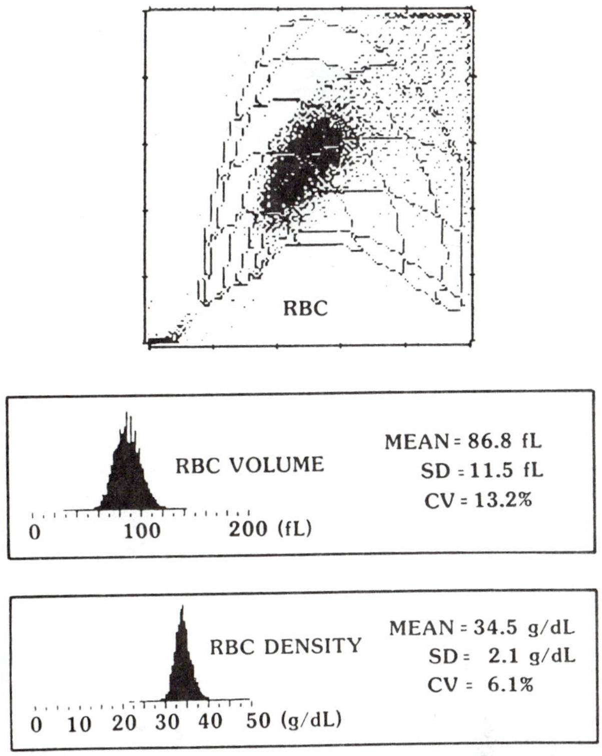

FIGURE 2-16. Analysis of the Technicon H*1 RBC channel. Data from this channel may be presented in three different plots. The bivariant scatter plot is presented and provides a cluster analysis of abnormal cell populations, which may exhibit variation in volume or hemoglobin concentration. The volume distribution is reduced to a single parameter histogram from which mean corpuscular volume (MCV) and the coefficient of variation (CV), a measure of RDW, are computed. The distribution of hemoglobin concentration also is reduced to a single parameter histogram with computation of mean corpuscular hemoglobin concentration and the CV of that distribution which is termed the hemoglobin distribution width. The hemoglobin concentration correlates directly with RBC density and may be presented as a measure of cell density as in this example. The hemoglobin distribution width provides an estimate of the variation in hemoglobin concentration among the RBC population. (Adapted from Mohandas N, et al. Accurate and independent measurement of volume and hemoglobin concentration of individual red cells by laser light scattering. Blood 1986;68:506–513)

an effective means of characterizing RBC disorders and of detecting conditions such as cold agglutinins, which may affect the measurement of RBC properties.[36]

AUTOMATED LEUKOCYTE COUNT

As for RBC counting methods, manual leukocyte counts have virtually disappeared from practice in modern clinical laboratories. Manual leukocyte counts performed with dilution pipettes and calibrated counting chambers exhibited CVs ranging from 10% to 20% for normal leukocyte counts, at lower levels the CV was increased further. Semiautomated or fully automated electrical impedance leukocyte counting offers the advantage of greater precision and efficiency compared with that achieved in older manual methods. Automated leukocyte counting relies on lysis of RBCs in the leukocyte channel with either subsequent electrical impedance or optical detection of intact leukocytes (see Fig. 2-12A).

Leukocyte counts ranging from 2.1 to 26 $\times$ 10^9/L demonstrate CVs from 1.7% to 3.1% for replicate samples, within-batch samples, and between-batch samples using electrical impedance methods.[33] Optical-based instruments exhibit within-run CVs ranging from 6.2% to 0.7% for leukocyte counts ranging from 0.8 to 44 $\times$ 10^9/L.[37]

PLATELET COUNTING

Manual Platelet Counting

The only method of manual platelet counting widely used at this time is the phase microscopic chamber counting method.[39] This method is still the reference method in many laboratories, although its precision limitations are well understood. For platelet counts within the normal range, CVs in the range of 11% to 16.6% have been reported.[39,40] Many laboratories use a peripheral blood smear estimating technique as a rapid means of verifying questionable platelet counts obtained with automated methods.[41,42] With a standard wedge peripheral smear stained with polychrome stain under 1000$\times$ oil magnification, the number of platelets in 10 fields is enumerated in the area of the smear where RBCs are evenly distributed with good preservation of central pallor. The number of platelets per 10 fields is multiplied by 2000 to obtain an estimate of the absolute platelet count per microliter of whole blood.[41] If widefield oculars are used instead of standard oculars, only eight 1000$\times$ fields are counted.[41]

For either optical system, the agreement between the electrical impedance counts and the slide estimates was reasonable (r = .98 to .96). Nosanchuk and colleagues[41] observed a CV of 50% by slide estimate for a platelet count of 27,000/μL established by an automated electrical impedance technique. For automated platelet counts ranging from 65,000 to 100,000/μL, the CV of the slide estimates varied from 20% to 23% and declined to 9% to 15% for platelet counts ranging from 163,000 to 590,000/μL. Thus, slide estimate provides a reliable means to verify the approximate range of automated platelet counts.

The platelet count is frequently used to decide whether to transfuse platelets prophylactically. Most frequently, the transfusion threshold value is 20,000/μL.[43] The uncertainty about whether this is a beneficial practice has led some practitioners to advocate the use of lower thresholds (10,000 to 15,000/μL).[44,45] Pretransfusion and posttransfusion

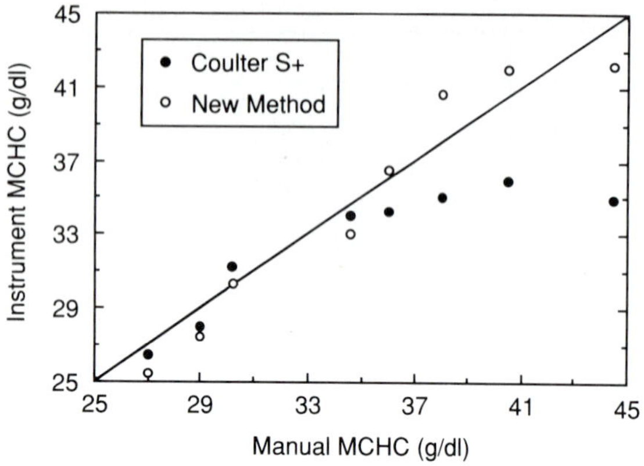

FIGURE 2-17. Comparison of mean corpuscular hemoglobin concentration (MCHC) determined with manual or automated methods. The MCHC of a series of samples was compared using manual methods, the Coulter S Plus, and the Technicon H*1 (new method). Good agreement over the entire range of MCHC values was obtained between the manual and electrooptical Technicon H*1 methods. In contrast, at higher manual MCHC values, the electrical impedance Coulter S Plus MCHC values were lower than the manual values. (Adapted from Mohandas N, et al. Accurate and independent measurement of volume and hemoglobin concentration of individual RBCs by laser light scattering. Blood 1986;68:506–513)

platelet counts should be obtained to determine whether an acceptable increment has been achieved. Thus, the precision of platelet counts in this range and the confidence with which a platelet count of 20,000/μL can be distinguished from a count of 30,000/μL is a relevant issue. Based on the studies of Nosanchuk and colleagues,[41] the slide estimate technique is not sufficiently precise for platelet counts below 65,000/μL.

Automated Platelet Counting

Most current blood counting instruments also offer a whole-blood platelet count using either an electrical impedance or electro-optical detection system.[37,46] The degree of precision for both types of instruments is comparable over a wide range of platelet counts (Table 2-2). The precision of newer instrumentation is superior to that obtained with earlier instruments or phase contrast platelet counts as demonstrated in the study by Wertz and Koepke[47] (Table 2-3). Data from this study provide information about the accuracy of phase contrast platelet counts performed by a group of qualified hematology laboratories.

Information is limited about the ability of automated platelet counting methods to discriminate among varying degrees of severe thrombocytopenia around the critical threshold for platelet transfusion. With the advent of more precise particle counters, the precision of the platelet count at low levels (Table 2-4) has improved so that platelet counts of 10,000/μL can be discriminated from those of 20,000/μL.

TABLE 2-2. Within-Run Precision at Varying Platelet Levels*

Platelet Level†	CV Impedance‡	CV Optical§
13	8.2	7.7
29	4.4	8.9
45	3.0	5.7
100	2.0	2.3
255	1.5	2.2
415	1.5	1.5
700	2.7	1.8

* Comparison of within-run precision for varying platelet counts using two whole blood platelet counting instruments. Twenty replicate counts were performed at each platelet level (×10⁹/L) and the coefficient of variation (CV) expressed as a percentage was determined.

† Random samples ranging from 13 to 700 × 10^9/L were selected and counted using standard automated whole blood platelet counting instruments.

‡ Coulter S-Plus II (Coulter Electronics, Hialeah, FL).

§ Technicon H*1 (Technicon Instruments Corporation, Tarrytown, NY).

(Data from Bollinger PB, et al. The Technicon H*1—an automated hematology analyzer for today and tomorrow. Am J Clin Pathol 1987;87:71–78)

Common Sources of Errors

Errors in measurement of the RBC count, hemoglobin, leukocyte count, platelet count, and RBC indices may arise because of abnormalities that are intrinsic to the sample rather than due to instrument or operator error. Cornbleet[48] has summarized the sources of these errors (Table 2-5).

Measurement of Platelet Volume

Physicians and laboratory technologists have long been cognizant of the variation in platelet size on routine peripheral blood smears. Although the biologic significance of platelet volume heterogeneity remains controversial, effort has continued in the measurement of platelet size as a diagnostic test to evaluate patients with either thrombocytopenia or thrombocytosis.[49,50] Several investigators have reported that microscopic measurement of platelet size on smears may provide useful diagnostic information.[51–53] Microscopic measurement of platelet size has never been widely adopted because of the technical difficulties, labor-intensive methodology, and a time-dependent effect of EDTA anticoagulant on platelet volume.[53] With the advent of electrical impedance measurement of blood cell numbers and volume and the ability to count and size platelets in whole-blood samples, measurement of platelet volume has become a more feasible test. This practice rapidly expanded with the widespread availability of platelet volume measurement on highly automated hematology instruments in clinical laboratories.[54,55] Mean platelet volume (MPV) measurement is routinely available in most clinical laboratories, but controversy as to its diagnostic usefulness persists.

Current laboratory instrumentation measures platelet volume distribution from EDTA-anticoagulated whole-blood samples by either electrical impedance (Coulter S Plus IV, Coulter Electronics, Hialeah, FL) or electro-optical methods (Technicon H*1, Technicon Instruments Corporation, Tarrytown, NY). Both types of instruments measure platelet volume from 2 to 20 fL and use extrapolation and curve fitting techniques with the central portion of the curve to obtain the entire curve. With both techniques, platelet volume has been observed to vary with time of exposure to anticoagulant.[56–59] With electrical impedance instruments, platelet volume in EDTA-anticoagulated whole blood increases over time.[56–58] The greatest increase occurs in the first 2 hours, followed by a progressive increase of up to 50% compared with that found in citrated blood in which platelet volume is stable.[58] In contrast, platelet volume in EDTA-anticoagulated blood may either increase or decrease with time when measured by electro-optical techniques.[59] Although the rate of anticoagulant-induced change in platelet volume may decrease with time, the effect is highly variable over a period of several hours.

TABLE 2-3. **Estimation of Platelet Count Accuracy Using Manual and Automated Methods***

Method	No. of Labs†	Mean Count‡ (×10⁹/L)	SD§	CV‖
LIGHT MICROSCOPY				
Ammonium oxalate	58	104.4	35.2	33.7
Unopette¶	810	82.7	18.2	22.0
Crystal Violet	34	100.6	29.1	28.9
Other#	120	109.6	34.1	31.1
PHASE CONTRAST MICROSCOPY				
Ammonium oxalate	99	104.4	27.7	26.6
Unopette¶	383	84.3	21.6	25.6
AUTOMATED METHODS				
Thrombocounter**	197	77.8	34.4	44.2
Model ZBI**	61	87.4	31.7	36.3
Model FN or F**	109	76.6	39.4	51.5
Autocounter††	52	120.6	26.7	22.2
MK-4HC‡‡	43	95.8	9.7	10.1

CV, coefficient of variation.

* Based on a College of American Pathologists Comprehensive Hematology Survey (1976) in which a calibrated standard platelet suspension was sent to participating laboratories for blinded counting. Results of this survey were reported by Wertz and Koepke.[47] The target value of the prepared standard was 91.52 × 10^9/L with a SD of 1.13 × 10^9/L and a CV of 1.2% based on 56 replicate counts using the Coulter Model Z_f particle counter.

† Within each methodologic class.

‡ For all laboratories within a designated methodologic class.

§ Standard deviation for the designated method.

‖ Coefficient of variation of each method among different laboratories.

¶ Becton-Dickinson.

\# Method not specified.

** Coulter Electronics.

†† Technicon Instruments Corp.

‡‡ J.T. Baker Co.

TABLE 2-4. **Within-Run Precision of Very Low Platelet Counts***

Mean Count†	SD‡	CV§	2-SD Range‖
COULTER S-PLUS IV			
2.0	0.4	20.3	1.2–2.8
8.0	1.8	22.9	4.4–11.6
10.0	0.9	8.5	8.2–11.8
13.0	0.9	6.7	11.2–14.8
16.0	1.8	11.1	12.4–19.6
19.0	1.5	7.7	16.0–22.0
TECHNICON H*1			
6.0	0.6	9.8	4.8–7.2
12.0	0.8	6.9	10.4–13.6
13.0	1.1	8.6	10.8–15.2
14.0	1.6	11.2	10.9–17.1
18.0	1.2	6.4	15.6–20.4
18.0	1.8	9.8	14.4–21.5

* Unpublished observations from the author's laboratory. Random blood samples from patients with severe thrombocytopenia were selected and five replicate counts were performed using two whole blood platelet counting instruments: Coulter S-Plus IV (Coulter Electronics, Hialeah, FL) and Technicon H*1 (Technicon Instruments Corporation, Tarrytown, NY).

† Represents the average platelet (×10^9/L) based on five replicate analyses within a single run.

‡ Standard deviation of the mean platelet count.

§ Coefficient of variation for the five replicate platelet counts.

‖ Indicated for each sample.

Within the confines of the clinical laboratory's operating conditions, it appears impossible to accurately measure platelet volumes on all samples under routine blood collection and sample processing conditions. Lippi and associates[59] have recommended diluting whole-blood samples with Technicon RBC diluent at the time of collection to maintain platelet volume stability. This is feasible for selected specimens so that accurate measurement of platelet volume can theoretically be accomplished.

Levin and Bessman[56] reported an inverse but nonlinear relation between platelet volume and platelet number with EDTA samples from normal subjects. Thompson and colleagues[57] observed an inverse linear relation between platelet volume and number in a second study of normal subjects using citrated blood. The Levin and Bessman study was performed with EDTA-anticoagulated samples in which platelet volumes may not have been adequately stabilized, whereas the Thompson study was performed with stabilized samples. In light of these divergent studies, it is not clear how to define a normal range for the relation between platelet volume and number in the routine clinical laboratory where sample stability and the interval between collection and analysis are highly variable. Both studies were conducted with normal samples for which adequate platelet volume distribution curves could be obtained. When severe thrombocytopenia is present, automated whole-blood measurement of platelet volume distributions may be seriously impaired.

Generally there is greater interest in measurement of mean platelet volume in thrombocytopenic samples. The observation of an increased mean platelet volume in as-

TABLE 2-5. Potential Causes of Erroneous Results With Automated Cell Counters

Parameter	Causes of Spurious Increase	Causes of Spurious Decrease
WBC count	Cryoproteins Heparin Paraproteins Nucleated RBC Platelet clumping Incomplete red cell lysis	Clotting Smudge cells Uremia + immunosuppressants
RBC count	Cryoproteins Giant platelets WBC count > 50,000/μL	Autoagglutination Clotting In vitro hemolysis Microcytic RBC
Hemoglobin	Carboxyhemoglobin > 10% Cryoproteins In vivo hemolysis Heparin WBC count > 50,000/μL Hyperbilirubinemia Lipemia Paraproteins	Clotting Sulfhemoglobin (?)
Hematocrit (automated)	Cryoproteins Giant platelets WBC count > 50,000/μL Hyperglycemia (>600 mg/dL)	Autoagglutination Clotting In vitro hemolysis Microcytic RBCs
Hematocrit (microhematocrit)	Hyponatremia Plasma trapping	Excess EDTA In vitro hemolysis Hypernatremia
MCV	Autoagglutination WBC count > 50,000/μL Hyperglycemia Reduced RBC deformability	Cryoproteins Giant platelets In vitro hemolysis Microcytic RBC Swollen RBC
MCHC	Autoagglutination Clotting In vitro hemolysis Spuriously high hemoglobin Spuriously low hematocrit	WBC count > 50,000/μL Spuriousy low hemoglobin Spuriously high hematocrit
Platelets	Cryoproteins Hemolysis Microcytic RBC RBC inclusions WBC fragments	Clotting Giant platelets Heparin Platelet clumping Platelet satellitosis

(Adapted from Cornbleet J. Spurious results from automated hematology counters. Lab Med 1983;14: 509–514)

sociation with thrombocytopenia is generally interpreted to indicate that thrombopoiesis is stimulated.[51,56,60] When mean platelet volume is normal in the face of thrombocytopenia, thrombopoiesis is assumed to be impaired. Although Bessman and associates[60] have obtained MPV values for thrombocytopenic patients with routine instrumentation, others have been unable to obtain a reliable measurement of platelet volume with routine laboratory instrumentation.[61] This may be partly due to the limited volume measuring range of the automated instruments and to the markedly decreased signal/noise ratio with thrombocytopenic samples. For example, mean platelet volume could not be measured, using routine clinical laboratory automated instrumentation, in a series of patients with the Wiskott-Aldrich syndrome.[62]

Platelet volume measurements in patients with thrombocytosis have been inconsistent and nonreproducible when repeated in different laboratories. Levin and Bessman[56] observed that 16 of 146 patients with thrombocytosis due to benign hematologic disorders had mean platelet volumes higher than the normal range. They also reported that 16 of 18 patients with a myeloproliferative syndrome and thrombocytosis had normal mean platelet volumes, and two patients had elevated platelet volumes. Thus, during either reactive or malignant thrombocytosis, no consistent relation between platelet volume and platelet level exists.

In another study, Bessman and associates[63] described abnormally increased platelet volumes in five of eight patients with CML and elevated platelet levels. Others have not

TABLE 2-6. Reference Ranges for the Differential Leukocyte Count in Adults*

Cell Type	Proportional Count (%)†	Absolute Count (×10⁹/L)‡
Segmented neutrophil	37–80	2.0–6.93
Band neutrophil	0–12	0–0.87
Normal lymphocyte	10–50	0.6–3.44
Variant lymphocyte	0–8.5	0–0.66
Monocyte	0–12	0.03–0.90
Eosinophil	0–9.5	0–0.67
Basophil	0–2.5	0–0.20

* Using the National Committee for Clinical Laboratory Standards (NCCLS) reference method leukocyte differential counts on 114 normal adult subjects with normal complete blood count, normal total leukocyte count and no recent infections.
† Of the total leukocyte population. The central 95th percentile range is indicated.
‡ Calculated from the total leukocyte count (method unspecified). The central 95th percentile for the total leukocyte count was 4.6–10.2 × 10^9/L.

found any deviation from normal in the mean platelet volume of subjects with reactive thrombocytosis or in those in the early phase of myeloproliferative disorders with marked thrombocythemia.[61] Friedhoff and colleagues[64] reported decreased mean platelet volume and increased platelet protein density in six subjects with reactive thrombocytosis. Small and Bettigole[65] measured platelet volume in 20 patients with reactive thrombocytosis and 24 patients with primary myeloproliferative disorders and observed no deviation of mean platelet volume for either group, although the platelet volume distributions associated with myeloproliferative disorders exhibited greater dispersion. Dudley and associates[66] reported a statistically significant increase in platelet volume distribution width (PDW), a measure of dispersion, in myeloproliferative thrombocytosis in comparison to reactive thrombocytosis. The PDW had no diagnostic value when used as an isolated laboratory test.

LEUKOCYTE DIFFERENTIAL

Manual Methods

The microscopic manual differential has been the traditional means of classifying the five basic leukocyte classes: neutrophils, lymphocytes, monocytes, eosinophils, and basophils. In most laboratories, this requires the preparation of a thin, air-dried wedge smear stained with a polychrome stain (see section on red blood cell, platelet, and leukocyte morphology). A reference method for the manual microscopic leukocyte differential has been recommended.[67] Under these guidelines, four technologists perform a 200-cell differential on four different wedge smears prepared from a single venous blood sample anticoagulated with EDTA. The results are calculated from the pooled 800-cell count differential. Normal range reference data are determined by performing 800-cell count differentials on a population of at least 100 normal subjects (adults without evidence of disease).[68]

A typical set of reference data are illustrated from the study of Koepke and associates[68] (Table 2-6). Common practice in the busy routine hematology laboratory is to perform a single 100-cell differential count.[46] Previously, results of leukocyte differentials have been reported as relative frequencies and expressed as percentages. More recently, the calculation of absolute values for each leukocyte class has been encouraged, and most automated instruments now report absolute values expressed as the number of cells per microliter of whole blood. The use of absolute values has made definition of the normal range more precise.

TABLE 2-7. Sensitivity of the Routine Leukocyte Differential in Detecting Distributional and Morphologic Abnormalities*

Referee Finding	n†	Agreement (%)	False-Normals (%)	False-Abnormals (%)
Normal	18	91		9
DISTRIBUTIONAL ABNORMALITIES				
Granulocytosis	9	96	4	
Left shift	19	34	66	
Lymphocytosis	4	100		
Monocytosis	6	80	20	
Eosinophilia	5	72	18	
Agranulocytosis	3	100		
MORPHOLOGIC ABNORMALITIES				
Variant lymphocytosis	10	64	36	
Erythrocyte precursors	15	81	19	
Leukocyte blasts	10	91	2	7

* NCCLS reference method and routine 100-cell leukocyte differentials were performed for a series of slides obtained from patients with the following disorders: acute inflammation, acute allergic reaction, viral infection, acute leukemia, severe anemia or myelophthisic anemia, and aplastic anemia. Five laboratories performed a single routine 100-cell differential on each abnormal slide. The incidences of agreement, false-normal, and false-abnormal results between the routine 100-cell differential and the reference method are expressed as a percentage. Distributional abnormalities indicate differences in the relative proportions of normal cells, and morphologic abnormalities indicate errors in the identification of abnormal cells.
† The number of cases evaluated for each abnormality is indicated.
(Data from Koepke JA, et al. A critical evaluation of the manual/visual differential leukocyte counting method. Blood Cells 1985;11:173–181)

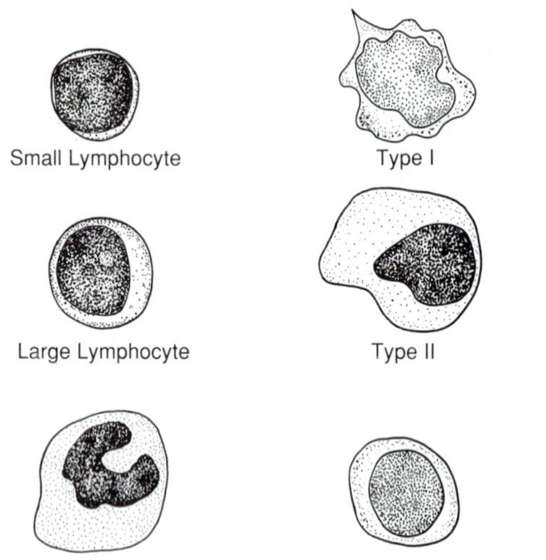

FIGURE 2-18. Schematic representation of the morphology of normal and atypical or variant lymphocytes. (Adapted from Sun NCJ. Hematology: an atlas and diagnostic guide. Philadelphia, WB Saunders, 1983)

Errors in performance of the leukocyte differential have been classified as either distributional or morphologic. Studies to examine the frequency of these types of errors have been conducted and will continue to be carried out and compared with the reference method as new leukocyte differential techniques evolve. Koepke and associates[68] have reported a comparison of the routine 100-cell differential with the NCCLS reference method for detection of a number of diseases in which either distributional or morphologic leukocyte abnormalities exist (Table 2-7).

The sensitivity of the routine differential for detection of a myeloid left shift or monocytosis is low, and specific definitions for the band form and the variant lymphocyte have been published in an effort to improve interlaboratory performance of routine leukocyte differentials.[69] The band cell has been defined as having "a nucleus that could be described as a curve or coiled band, no matter how marked the indentation, if it does not completely segment the nucleus into lobes connected by a filament."[70]

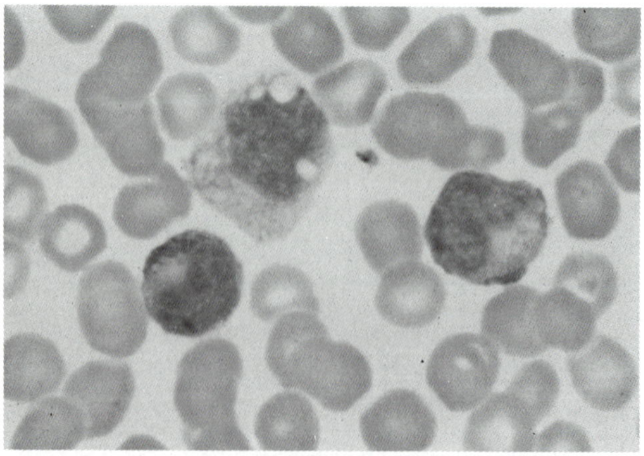

FIGURE 2-19. Examples of variant lymphocytes obtained from the blood of a patient with infectious mononucleosis. Large mononuclear cells with open nuclear chromatin can be seen. (See Color Fig. 2-19.)

TABLE 2-8. Correlation Between the Reference Method and the Routine Differential for Detection of Different Leukocytes*

Cell Type	Slope	*r*
Segmented neurophil	0.88	.87
Band neutrophil	0.53	.67
Normal lymphocyte	0.85	.73
Variant lymphocyte	0.35	.30
Monocyte	0.56	.41
Eosinophil	0.90	.83
Basophil	0.58	.32

* The NCCLS reference method was compared with the routine 100-cell differential for detection of different leukocyte cell classes. (Data from Koepke JA, et al. A critical evaluation of the manual/visual differential leukocyte counting method. Blood Cells 1985;11:173–181)

Identification of atypical or variant lymphocytes has been troublesome because of variation in the morphologic definition of these cells by microscopists. Normal lymphocytes may be small or large, with dense nuclear chromatin and sparse azurophilic cytoplasmic granules. Normal large lymphocytes exhibit more cytoplasm than the small cell, which is typified by a scant rim of cytoplasm. Variant lymphocytes, frequently associated with viral infections, are characterized by increased size, greater cytoplasmic area, basophilia, nuclear convolutions, and nuclear chromatin that is less dense than that of normal cells but not as fine as that found in lymphoblasts (Figs. 2-18 and 2-19). Some variant cells may appear similar to plasma cells; these are referred to as *plasmacytoid lymphocytes*, or stimulated lymphocytes. The latter functional designation is derived from the similarity of these variant lymphocytes to cells in stimulated cultures. Nuclear shape may become kidney bean–like, in contrast to the round configuration of normal lymphocytes. Variant lymphocytes may contain nucleoli. The sensitivity for detection of variant lymphocytes and erythroid precursors is suboptimal, whereas the detection of highly abnormal cells (blasts) is reasonable. The NCCLS standard concluded that new leukocyte differential methods should correlate with the 800-cell reference method and provide the same sensitivity as that achieved in the manual method.

Two critical points in the evaluation process are detection of abnormal proportions of the normal leukocytes (distributional abnormalities) and detection of abnormal cells (morphologic abnormalities). The routine 100-cell manual differential was found to be comparable to the reference method. Thus, new techniques can reliably detect infrequent cell classes such as monocytes, variant lymphocytes, and basophils (Table 2-8).

Electrical Impedance

With improvement in flow cytometric and image analysis technology, a number of automated leukocyte differential cell counters became available to the routine clinical hematology laboratory. A review by Koepke and Ross[71] in 1985 listed 13 different systems that were available at that time. Since that publication, some of these systems have disappeared or have been replaced by newer versions of the same technology. The image analysis pattern recognition systems, which included the Larc, Hematrak 450, Hematrak 450 QP, and Hematrak 590 instruments, are being replaced with less expensive instrumentation that performs a CBC, platelet count, and leukocyte differential. The image analysis systems are not discussed in this chapter and the reader is referred to the excellent study by Wilding and Leboy[72] for an extensive discussion of this technology.

A number of instruments that perform a two-, three-, or five-part automated differential are in common use (Table 2-9). These instruments use a variety of technologies to subclassify leukocytes and have been compared with the manual differential technique using the NCCLS standard.[67] The three-part differential using electrical impedance technology to discriminate granulocytes, lymphocytes, and mononuclear cells has gained widespread acceptance because of its availability in combination with CBC and platelet count capacity in an economical format (Coulter S Plus IV, V, VI series). RBCs are hemolyzed with a reagent system, which leaves leukocytes intact and detectable by electrical impedance. About 20,000 leukocytes are examined, and a single parameter histogram with relative and absolute quantitation of the three cell classes is generated (Fig. 2-20). In addition, region flags (R flags) are generated when the volume distribution of the three regions is abnormal, and if the total leukocyte count is below 1000/μL or above 100,000/μL, no data are computed. Problem samples are also signaled when interference with the small volume portion of the leukocyte distribution (abnormal leukocyte takeoff) or increased numbers of mononuclear cells (more than 1500/μL) is present.

This three-part differential instrument has been evalu-

TABLE 2-9. Automated Leukocyte Differential Instruments

Manufacturer	Model	Method	Result
Clay Adams	QBC	Acridine orange	Granulocytes
		Centrifugation	Nongranulocytes
Coulter	S Plus IV, V, VI	Impedance	Granulocytes*
			Mononuclears†
			Lymphocytes
Ortho	ELT-8ws	Light scatter	Granulocytes
	ELT-800ws		Monocytes
			Lymphocytes
Toa	E-5000	Impedance	Small cell ratio‡
			Middle cell ratio§
			Large cell ratio‖
Technicon	H-6000	Cytochemical	Granulocytes
			Lymphocytes
			Monocytes
			Eosinophils
			Basophils
			Large unstained cells¶
Technicon	H*1	Cytochemical	Granulocytes
		Light scatter	Lymphocytes
			Monocytes
			Eosinophils
			Basophils
			Large unstained cells
Coulter	VCS	Impedance	Granulocytes
		Conductivity	Lymphocytes
		Light scatter	Monocytes
			Eosinophils
			Basophils
Toa	Sysmex NE-8000	Radio frequency	Granulocytes
		Electrical impedance	Lymphocytes
		Selective lysing agents	Monocytes
			Eosinophils
			Basophils
Sequoia Turner	CD 3000	Orthogonal light scatter	Granulocytes
		Depolarized light scatter	Lymphocytes
			Monocytes
			Eosinophils

* Includes eosinophils and basophils.
† Includes monocytes, variant lymphocytes, blasts, progranulocytes, plasma cells, and abnormal lymphocytes.
‡ Lymphocytes.
§ Monocytes, variant lymphocytes, blasts, progranulocytes, eosinophils, basophils, plasma cells, and other abnormal lymphocytes.
‖ Neutrophils (segmented + bands), myelocytes, and metamyelocytes.
¶ Cells that are peroxidase-negative with cell volume greater than that of normal lymphocytes. This class may include variant lymphocytes, peroxidase-negative dysplastic monocytes, peroxidase-negative granulocytes, and peroxidase-negative blast cells.

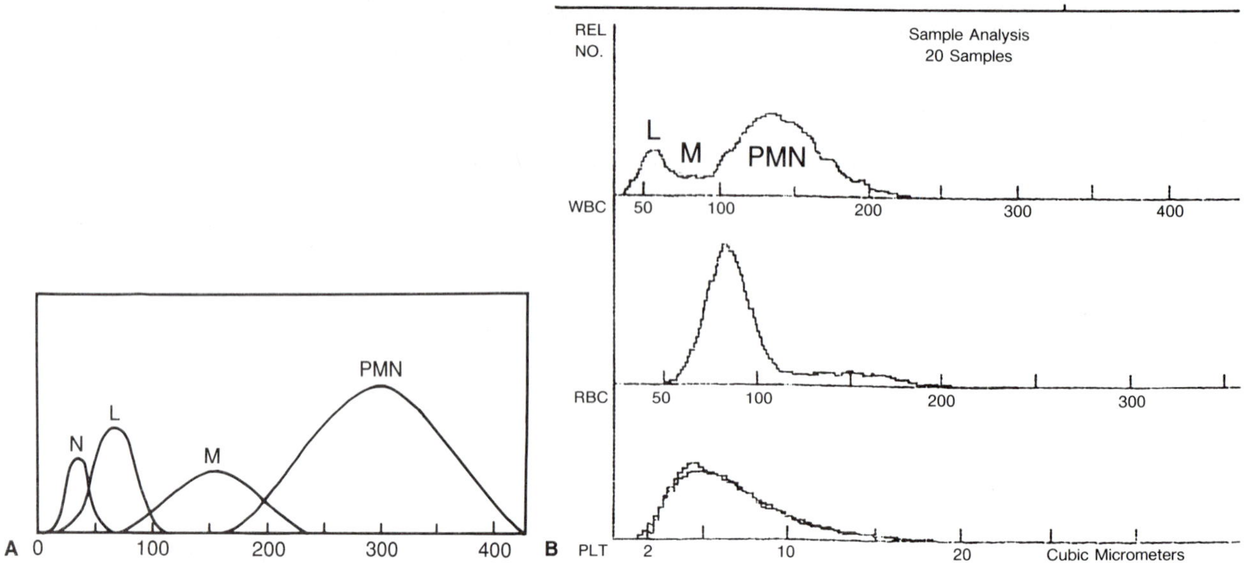

FIGURE 2-20. Electrical impedance RBC volume, platelet volume and leukocyte differential distribution. (**A**) Schematic representation of the volume distribution of nucleated RBCs (N), lymphocytes (L), mononuclear cells (M), and polymorphonuclear leukocytes (PMN). (**B**) An example of the leukocyte differential volume distribution (WBC), RBC volume distribution (RBC), and platelet volume distribution obtained using the Coulter S+IV instrument.

ated using the NCCLS standard and a reference range for the normal three-part differential has been established (Table 2-10).[73] Comparison of precision between the reference method and the S Plus IV demonstrated one order of magnitude improvement in precision using the instrument.[73] The accuracy of the Coulter S Plus IV has been compared with a well-accepted reference method—the 400-cell manual differential. Of 252 patient samples, with a wide range of both distributional and morphologic abnormalities, 188 were abnormal by the reference method. Only 1.6% of those that failed were not detected by the automated technique. Of 185 samples that could be analyzed, 97% were flagged as morphology with either abnormal morphology or distribution and 3% could not be detected. For 64 normal samples, 12.5% were flagged, representing false-positives.

TABLE 2-10. Three-Part Leukocyte Differential Reference Range*

Cell Type	Mean†	Lower‡	Upper‡
144 NORMAL SUBJECTS			
Lymphocyte	2.4	1.2	3.5
Mononuclear	0.4	0.1	0.6
Granulocyte	4.2	1.4	7.0
200 OUTPATIENTS WITHOUT HEMATOLOGIC DISEASE§			
Lymphocyte		1.1	4.6
Mononuclear‖		0.3	0.8
Granulocyte¶		2.3	8.4

* Based on data from a normal range study using 144 adult subjects defined as normal by the NCCLS reference method[73] and 200 outpatients without hematologic disease.[74] Each sample was analyzed four times and the data were averaged.

† Values are expressed as absolute numbers of cells × 10^9/L whole blood.

‡ Lower and upper limits of the normal reference range encompassing 2 standard deviations about the mean are indicated.

§ The lower and upper limits of the central 95% confidence interval determined by nonparametric methods are indicated.

‖ Monocytes, variant lymphocytes, blasts, progranulocytes, plasma cells, and abnormal lymphocytes.

¶ Mature neutrophils, eosinophils, and basophils.

The positive predictive value for this patient population was 95.8%, the negative predictive value was 91.8%, and overall test efficiency was 94.8%.[73] If both distributional and morphologic abnormalities are evaluated in a combined manner, the rates decline slightly, but overall test efficiency remains high (87.6%). The absence of morphologic flags and distributional abnormalities, when compared with the reference range, confirms with a high degree of probability that the specimen is normal. Richardson-Jones and colleagues[73] recognized the limitations of the three-part differential in detecting specific morphologic abnormalities, and outlined a sequential approach that uses a rapid 300- to 400-cell microscopic differential performed under low magnification (Fig. 2-21).

The three-part differential has been evaluated in an acute care hospital setting, which may be a more meaningful test of efficiency.[74] Sixty percent of requested differentials fell within the normal reference range (see Table 2-10) and had no flags. Another 25% were outside the reference range but could be verified on manual review, and 15% did not provide usable results.

The major undetected abnormalities were elevated band counts and eosinophilia. Of specimens with elevated band counts on routine manual differential, 90% were detected by the automated three-part differential method. The false-negative results had no adverse impact on patient care.[74] Overall, the three-part differential combined with a qualitative slide review was successful in analyzing 84% of routine samples.[74]

In another study using a large number of abnormal samples, the precision and efficiency of the S-Plus IV three-part differential were evaluated.[75] Thirty-nine percent of samples generated review flags. The automated counter flagged lymphocyte and monocytic abnormalities more accurately than granulocytic changes. This study emphasized that the mononuclear population should not be equated with the monocyte fraction determined by manual differ-

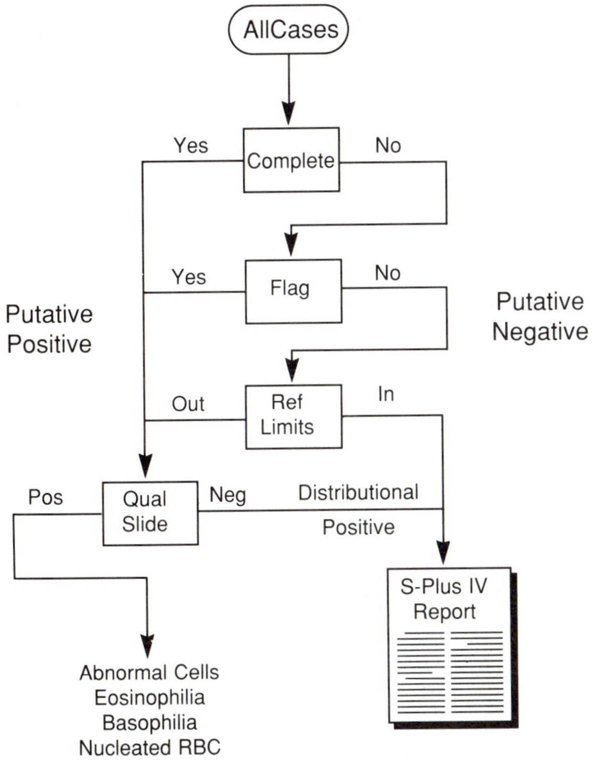

FIGURE 2-21. Work flow algorithm for processing leukocyte differentials using a three-part electrical impedance differential and stained blood smear. If computation by the instrument is incomplete (inc), the smear is automatically reviewed. If computation is complete (comp), the histogram is inspected for regional flags that may indicate distributional abnormalities. If there are no flags, the results are checked against the reference limits. If the data are in limits, the instrument results are reported. If the data are out of limits or there are distributional flags, the slide is reviewed using a high-dry objective to examine 300 to 400 leukocytes to determine whether blasts, immature myeloid cells, nucleated RBCs, variant lymphocytes, increased eosinophils, or basophils are present. (Adapted from Richardson-Jones A, Hellman R, Twedt D. The Coulter Counter leucocyte differential. Blood Cells 1985;11:203–238)

ential.[75] Among the nonflagged samples, 7.6% did not agree with the result obtained from manual differential. The major sources of error were due to leukopenia, monocytosis, and lymphoblastosis (see Table 2-10). The lack of agreement of leukopenic samples may have been due to poor results obtained with the manual method as a result of distributional abnormalities.[75]

The sensitivity and specificity in this large study, in which samples were defined by a routine manual differential, were informative about the relative value of the three-part differential in a clinical laboratory setting (Table 2-11). Both sensitivity and specificity were suboptimal and 39% of samples would have required microscopic review based on morphologic abnormalities without consideration of distributional abnormalities. The precision of the distributional measurements for both granulocytes and lymphocytes was acceptable. Thus, in an inpatient setting the three-part differential would appear to require a high rate of microscopic review with less than optimal sensitivity.

In another study, two three-part differential instruments have been compared with the NCCLS reference method to determine the clinical sensitivity of these methodologies for detection of leukocyte differential abnormalities.[46] The ability to detect both distributional and morphologic abnormalities was examined (Tables 2-12 and 2-13). Sensitivity could be further improved by including criteria other than morphologic flagging to initiate manual review (Table 2-14). When all these algorithms were combined to select samples for manual review, the authors concluded that the sensitivity of the three-part differential was better than that of the routine manual microscopic differential.[46] The major disadvantage of the three-part differential used in this manner is the high false-positive rate, which leads to a large number of manual reviews. This approach is still superior to routine manual differentials on all samples because it results in substantial labor savings and better test completion times.

Alternative strategies, which use a simpler manual microscopic slide review, have been proposed for use along with the three-part differential to improve the usefulness of this automated differential system and to lessen the burden of a high rate of false-positives.[76] For example, the scanning differential uses the following routine: a 15-second general impression at 10× magnification, a 45- to 60-second scan at 20×, and a 15- to 30-second scan at 50×. The authors concluded that this technique was as reliable as the routine manual 100-cell differential for detection of blasts, immature cells, and nucleated erythrocytes, but the ability to detect distributional abnormalities was lower. Thus, the scanning differential technique, used in conjunction with a three-part differential system with distributional and morphologic flags, combined with the limits outlined (see Table 2-14) may be highly efficient.

TABLE 2-11. Specificity and Sensitivity of the Three-Part Differential*

Category	Flagged	Unflagged	Total†
Abnormal‡	81.7%§	18.3%‖	229 (23.9%)¶
Normal	26.3%#	73.7%**	760 (76.1%)††
TOTAL‡‡	387	602	989

* From a study that examined the ability of the three-part differential to detect morphologic abnormalities. Samples were analyzed using the S-Plus IV differential counter and classified as either flagged or unflagged using manufacturer criteria. Whether a sample was flagged or unflagged did not indicate whether it was abnormal or normal. Each sample also was examined with a 100- or 200-cell microscopic differential.

† Total number of samples and relative proportion expressed as a percentage for each category.

‡ Defined by manual 100- or 200-cell microscopic differential as containing detectable nucleated erythrocytes, blasts, promyelocytes, lymphoma cells, more than 5% basophils, more than 5% myelocytes, more than 5% metamyelocytes, more than 10% eosinophils, more than 10% reactive lymphocytes. In contrast, normal samples were defined as all other samples, and distributional abnormalities were not used to define normal and abnormal samples.

§ True positive samples, a measure of sensitivity.

‖ False-negative samples.

¶ Fraction of abnormal samples, a measure of prevalence.

\# False-positive samples for morphologic abnormalities.

** True negative samples, a measure of specificity.

†† Fraction of normal samples.

‡‡ Total number of samples in each category.

(Adapted from Cornbleet J, Kessinger S. Evaluation of Coulter S-Plus three-part differential in population with a high prevalence of abnormalities. Am J Clin Pathol 1985;84:620–626)

Cytochemical Leukocyte Differential

Another leukocyte differential technology that evolved considerably over the past decade is the cytochemical differential. The current version of this approach is used on the Technicon H-6000 and H*1 instruments.[37] These in-

TABLE 2-12. Comparative Reference Ranges for the Routine, Three-Part, and Image Analysis Differential*

Cell Class	Reference†	Routine‡	Hematrak 100 Cell§	S-Plus IV‖	E-5000¶
Lymphocytes	1.0–3.2	0.9–3.1	1.1–3.4	1.3–2.9	1.2–2.8
Mononuclears (S-IV)	0.1–0.8	0.1–0.8	0.1–0.7	0.2–0.8	
Mononuclears (TOA)	0.2–1.0	0.1–1.1	0.1–1.1		0.2–0.9
Granulocytes (S-IV)	2.2–9.1	2.3–9.8	2.1–9.5	2.1–8.7	
Granulocytes (TOA)	2.0–9.1	2.1–9.5	2.0–8.6		1.9–9.0

* From the study in which the routine 100-cell microscopic differential, the Hematrak 100-cell image analysis differential, the Coulter S-Plus IV three-part differential, and the TOA E-500 three-part differential were compared with the NCCLS 800-cell microscopic reference method. The central 95th percentile ranges were determined for 150 normal subjects without disease that alter hematologic values. All results are expressed as absolute values $\times 10^9/L$.

† Values were established using the 800-cell microscopic differential according to the NCCLS standard.[67] The definition of cells included in the granulocyte and mononuclear cell classes were modified for comparison with data from the S-Plus IV and TOA E-5000 instruments. Absolute values were calculated using the total leukocyte count obtained from the S-Plus IV.

‡ 100-cell microscopic differential was performed under routine clinical laboratory conditions. The absolute values were calculated using the total leukocyte count obtained from the S-Plus IV.

§ A 100-cell differential was performed using the image-process analyzer (Geometric Data Hematrak 590, Wayne, PA). The absolute values were calculated using the total leukocyte count obtained from the S-Plus IV.

‖ Three-part leukocyte differential was obtained (Coulter Electronics, Hialeah, FL).

¶ Three-part leukocyte differential was obtained (Toa, Carson, CA). The absolute values were calculated using the total leukocyte count obtained with the E-5000.

(Adapted from Payne BA, Pierre RV, Lee WK. Evaluation of the TOA-E 5000 automated hematology analyzer. Am J Clin Pathol 1987;88:51–57)

struments are based on an earlier five-part cytochemical differential instrument, the Technicon D-90.[77] Both the H-6000 and the H*1 provide a five-part differential based on light scatter and peroxidase cytochemical staining for detection of granulocytes and monocytes.[78] The H-6000 instrument detects immature granulocytes through elevated peroxidase activity, the high peroxidase (HPX) fraction. The H-6000 (Fig. 2-22) contains a discrete cytochemical basophil channel that has been replaced with a noncytochemical technique on the newer H*1 instrument (Fig. 2-23).

Simultaneous measurement of cell size by forward angle light scatter combined with peroxidase staining of individual cells is used to classify cells as lymphocytes, large unstained cells, monocytes, neutrophils, and eosinophils. Basophils are enumerated in a separate channel in which cells are exposed to an acid buffer and lysing reagent, which causes the cytoplasm to be removed from all leukocytes except basophils.[78] In addition, nuclear contour is examined by forward and side light scatter in this channel and a lobularity index (LI) is calculated. It is used to detect im-

TABLE 2-13. Frequency and Type of Errors for Leukocyte Differential Counting*

Correlation and Error Type	E-5000†	S-Plus IV‡	Hematrak 590§	Routine‖
Agreement	69.0%	71.0%	82.7% (85.7%)	85.3% (86.0%)
Distributional false-negative	3.0%	2.3%	5.0% (2.0%)	5.3% (3.7%)
Morphologic false-negative	3.7%	1.7%	5.7% (5.7%)	3.3% (3.3%)
Distributional false-positive	5.0%	3.3%	6.0% (4.7%)	4.7% (5.3%)
Morphologic false-positive	20.3%	21.7%	0.7% (2.0%)	1.3% (1.7%)

* Four different methods of leukocyte differential counting were compared with the NCCLS reference method[67] using 300 patient samples.[46] Correlation with the reference method was based on distribution and morphology using the 95th central percentile of the normal population as the normal range. Samples were classified as follows: complete agreement, morphologic disagreement, or distributional disagreement, where morphologic correlation was given precedence over distributional agreement. The analysis was based on relative distributional values, absolute distributional values, and morphologic flags.

† TOA.

‡ Coulter.

§ Image analysis system. Data are presented using the S-Plus IV three-part differential classification scheme and the TOA E-5000 three-part differential classification scheme (parentheses).

‖ Routine 100-cell microscopic differential. Data are presented using the S-Plus IV three-part differential classification scheme, and the TOA E-5000 three-part differential classification scheme (parentheses).

¶ Agreement indicates that the distributional results were within the 95th percentile of the normal reference range and no morphologic abnormalities were observed. The following morphologic abnormalities were used: variant lymphocytes, fragile cells, blasts, progranulocytes, specific abnormal cells, nucleated erythrocytes, more than 1% myelocytes plus metamyelocytes.[46]

TABLE 2-14. Suggested Criteria for Initiation of Manual Review of the Peripheral Blood Smear*

Variable	Lower Limit	Upper Limit
Lymphocytes (10^9/L)	<1.0	>50.0
Erythrocytes (10^{12}/L)	<2.0	>8.0
Hemoglobin (g/L)	<50	>200
MCV (fL)	<60	>110
MCH (pg)	<20	>37
MCHC (%)	<25	>37
RDW (%)		>20
Platelets (10^9/L)	<40	>1000
Platelet histogram abnormal†		
No platelet results‡		

MCV, mean corpuscular volume; MCH, mean corpuscular hemoglobin; MCHC, mean corpuscular hemoglobin concentration; RDW, red cell distribution width.
* Suggested review criteria to be used in addition to distributional abnormalities and morphologic flags.
† Failure of platelet volume histogram to return to baseline.
‡ Incomplete computation of platelet count.
(Data from Payne BA, et al. Evaluation of the TOA-E 5000 automated hematology analyzer. Am J Clin Pathol 1987;88:51–57)

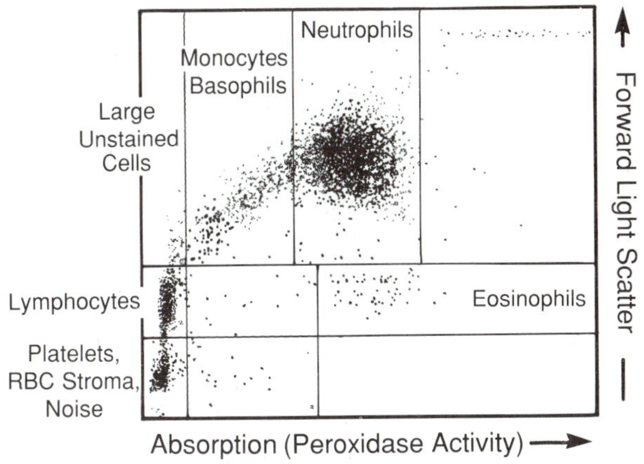

FIGURE 2-22. Bivariant scatter analysis of five-part cytochemical differential using the Technicon H-6000 instrument. The Y axis indicates forward scatter, an index of cell size. The X axis represents peroxidase activity, measured by absorbance. The location of the different cell classes is indicated. Basophils are also counted in a discrete basophil channel, not shown on this diagram. (Adapted from Breakall ES, Marchand A, Marcus R, Simson E. Comparison of performance for leukocyte differential counting of the Technicon H-6000 system with a manual reference method using the NCCLS standard. Blood Cells 1985;11:257–279)

mature cells that have a low LI because of reduced nuclear segmentation.

These instruments offer the advantage of a complete five-part differential with precise monocyte, eosinophil, and basophil measurements. There is a remarkable degree of consistency in the five-part cytochemical differential normal ranges determined in different populations (Table 2-15). The most obvious differences are for the upper limits of the normal ranges for monocytes, eosinophils, and basophils. The ranges for the two most recent studies using the H-6000[79] and the H*1 (UCSF) show good agreement, even for these infrequent cell classes.

Several studies have examined the precision of the H*1 instrument with respect to the total leukocyte count and the leukocyte subclasses (Table 2-16). Precision of the total leukocyte count is excellent even at low levels, and the precision for the infrequent cell classes is superior to that obtainable with manual techniques. The precision in leukopenic patients is important in the management of this group because of the risk associated with profound neutropenia. Kinsey and Watts[80] compared the Technicon H*1 absolute neutrophil count with the routine 100-cell microscopic differential and demonstrated good agreement (r = .9) for absolute counts ranging from less than 100 to 800/μL. The H*1 instrument has limited sensitivity in detecting band neutrophils through the left shift flagging algorithm.[81] For microscopic band counts below 11%, the sensitivity was 76%.[82] Prospective evaluation of a group of patients with documented appendicitis using the H*1 differential demonstrated the following sensitivities: 79% in detecting left shift, 82% in detecting absolute neutrophilia, and 91% in detecting leukocytosis.[82]

An earlier prospective study of patients with acute appendicitis, using the Technicon Hemalog D-90, demonstrated that the total leukocyte count and absolute neutrophil count were more sensitive than the routine microscopic band count, and combinations of the absolute leukocyte count and neutrophil count exhibited high sensitivity (97%).[83] The H*1 differential instrument was more sensitive than an automated image analysis differential performed with the Hematrak 590 system.

Bentley and colleagues[84] examined the sensitivity of the routine 100-cell microscopic band count in comparison with a 200-cell microscopic differential, the H-6000 differential including the HPX flag, and the H*1 differential including the LI and left shift flags in patients with positive blood cultures. The routine microscopic band count had poor sensitivity (30.4%) for detection of bacteremic patients, whereas the automated tests had the following sensitivities: absolute neutrophils (66.1%), HPX (61.6%), LI (49.1%), and left shift flag (71.4%). The diagnostic sensitivity could be further improved by using pairs of these tests. Both the H-6000 and the Hemalog D 90, an earlier version of the five-part cytochemical differential, consistently detected increased numbers of atypical lymphocytes in patients with chronic lymphocytic leukemia and hairy-cell leukemia (HCL).[85]

Volume–Conductivity–Scatter

Recently, a new technology that uses a combination of low-frequency current, high-frequency electromagnetic energy, and light scatter (volume–conductivity–scatter [VCS]) has been introduced to provide a five-part leukocyte differential (Fig. 2-24), the Coulter VCS. Another instrument, the Sysmex NE-8000 (Toa Medical Electronics [USA], Inc, Los Alamitos, CA) uses low-frequency current and high-frequency or radio frequency energy to perform a five-part differential (Fig. 2-25). Preliminary studies with the Coulter VCS system have established a reference range (see Table 2-15) and documented its precision (see Table 2-16). Only the basophil measurements had a high CV in comparison with the H*1 system. The VCS instrument examines 8000 leukocytes during differential analysis. Both precision and accuracy of the VCS system were high. Sensitivity of this system to detect abnormal samples was high (97.3%), and the false-positive VCS rate was acceptable (16.9%), suggesting that the manual microscopic review rate would be tolerable in a busy clinical laboratory.

In addition to the combined use of impedance (low-frequency current) and conductivity (high-frequency current or radio frequency) technology, another system based on light scatter alone has been described and is about to enter the clinical market (Sequoia-Turner CD 3000, Sequoia-Turner Inc, Mountain View, CA).[86] This instrument

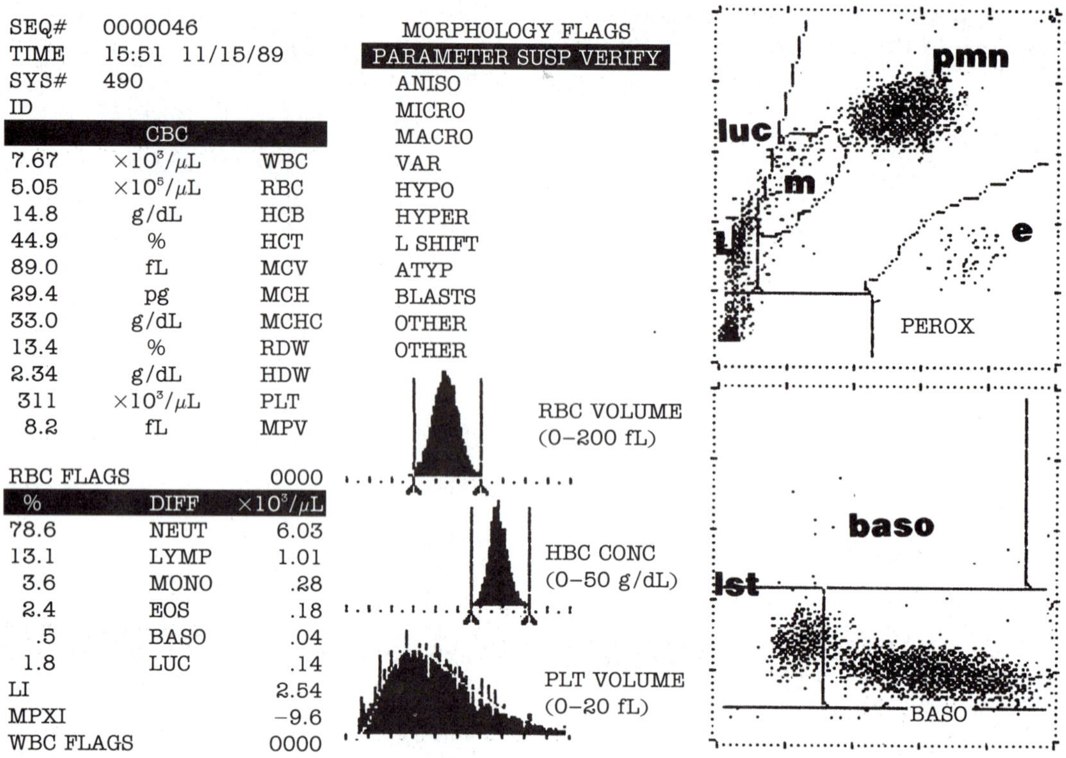

FIGURE 2-23. Results and histogram display for a complete blood count, platelet count, and five-part differential obtained with the Technicon H*1 system. Two channels are used to perform the differential—the peroxidase channel (perox) and the basophil channel (baso). The results from both channels are presented as bivariant scatter plots. In the peroxidase channel (upper panel) the Y axis indicates cell size measured by forward scatter and the X axis represents peroxidase activity measured by absorbance. Respective cell classes are indicated as follows: large unstained cell (luc), monocytes (m), polymorphonuclear leukocytes (pmn), and eosinophils (e). In the basophil channel, the Y axis represents cell size by forward scatter and the Y axis represents nuclear lobularity measured by wide angle light scatter. Cells that exceed the lower scatter threshold (lst) are classified as basophils.

uses a small helium–neon laser with two low-angle scatter detectors (1 to 2.6 degrees and 3 to 11 degrees) combined with depolarized orthogonal light scatter to discriminate lymphocytes, basophils, monocytes, neutrophils, and eosinophils (Fig. 2-26). In comparison with the five-part cytochemical differential methods, this instrument provided excellent correlation for enumeration of neutrophils ($r^2 = .99$), eosinophils ($r^2 = .97$), lymphocytes ($r^2 = .99$), and monocytes ($r^2 = .77$).[86] The lower correlation for monocytes between the two differential counting systems has also been observed when automated H-6000 counts are compared with NCCLS manual reference methods.[87] The developmental instrument described by Terstappen and colleagues[86] has been further modified into the commercial CD3000 system, which is currently being introduced into clinical hematology laboratories. Elimination of the cytochemical channels should improve the efficiency and economy of leukocyte differential counting.

Simplified Two-Part Differential

Another system has been developed for measuring hematocrit, platelet count, and two-part differential, which is easily adaptable to a physician's office.[88] This method is based on centrifugal analysis of a capillary tube of blood (QBC Centrifugal Hematology Analyzer, Clay Adams Division, Becton Dickinson Co, Parsippany, NJ). A special capillary tube coated with acridine orange and oxalate is filled with either venous or capillary blood and a float is inserted into the tube followed by centrifugation. After centrifugation, the RBCs, leukocytes, platelets, and plasma proteins are separated into discrete bands (Fig. 2-27). The processed tube is placed into a reading device that uses blue-violet light to detect the differential fluorescence of the granulocyte and nongranulocyte leukocyte populations. The float device expands the leukocyte layer to provide more efficient separation of the granulocyte and nongranulocyte cells. This device does not provide absolute leukocyte counts but does provide a frequency distribution type of differential.

Sallitt and associates[88] compared the two-part differential system with the NCCLS reference method, with modification of the reference differential to a two-part differential format. They observed a 2.4% bias in measurement of granulocyte and lymphocyte frequencies. A series of abnormal samples produced a false-abnormal distribution rate of 5% and a false-normal distribution rate of 14%. Total agreement between leukocyte distributions using the QBC method and the reference method was 92.5%. The authors concluded that the sensitivity of this test method was comparable to that obtained between reference methods.[88] The QBC system provides a simple method for rapidly performing two-part differentials—a useful screening test.

RETICULOCYTE ENUMERATION

Manual Methods

Enumeration of reticulocytes is the simplest and perhaps best means of evaluating the effectiveness of RBC production. Under conditions of normal hematopoiesis, newly

TABLE 2-15. Leukocyte Differential Reference Range Using Five-Part Differential Instruments*

Study	Neutrophils	Lymphocytes	Monocytes	Eosinophils	Basophils	LUC†
Hemalog D-90‡	1.390–7.880	1.890–4.310	0.110–1.370	0.110–0.740	0.000–0.210	0.000–0.320
H-6000-O§	1.748–9.222	0.440–5.023	0.000–0.920	0.000–0.715	0.000–0.176	0.000–0.440
H-6000-S§	1.677–8.247	0.679–5.772	0.000–1.076	0.000–0.666	0.000–0.155	0.000–0.311
H-6000‖	1.700–6.700^{t}	1.100–3.300^{t}	0.180–0.650^{m}	0.040–0.400^{m}	0.020–0.110^{t}	0.040–0.130^{t}
H*1¶	1.770–6.770	0.900–2.920	0.150–0.570	0.030–0.420	0.010–0.070	0.020–0.020
H*1#	1.200–6.000	0.820–3.260	0.158–0.678	0.000–0.428	0.000–0.052	0.037–0.293
VCS**	1.000–5.600	0.800–3.000	0.200–0.800	0.000–0.500	0.000–0.500	
VCS††	1.400–6.500	1.000–3.600	0.000–0.700	0.000–0.400	0.000–0.100	

LUC, large unstained cells.

* All instruments used in studies perform a five-part differential and some (Hemalog D-90, H-6000, and H*1) include the fraction of LUC. Data are reported as absolute numbers of cells (10^9/L).

† Cells with volume greater than that of small lymphocytes and negative peroxidase staining reaction.

‡ From a study of 64 normal subjects; reference interval definition not specified.

§ From studies by Breakall and colleagues.[87] Absolute values for the ranges were calculated from the reported percentage values for the central 95th percentile and the reported total leukocyte values, thus representing calculated extreme ends of the ranges. These values may not be a precise estimate of the absolute central 95th percentile for absolute leukocyte values. A total of 188 normal subjects were examined in two different studies and are reported separately. H-6000-O indicates the study from Overlook Hospital, Summit, NJ, H-6000-S indicates the study from Stamford Hospital, Stamford, CT. Total leukocyte ranges were 4 to 11.6 and 4.3 to 11.1 × 10^9/L, respectively, for the two populations.

‖ From a study of 42,758 patients in occupational health care practices in which single samples were assumed to indicate absence of hematologic abnormality and the extreme 1% of values were discarded.[79] The normal ranges were derived from the interval between the 2.5th and 97.5th percentiles of the population values after use of a γ distribution fitting function. Data are presented as absolute values × 10^9/L with the following age group limitations: neutrophils 20–49 years, lymphocytes over 10 years, monocytes over 15 years, eosinophils over 15 years, basophils all ages, LUC over 10 years. Data based on both sexes are represented by *t* and where there are sex differences, the larger range is reported and the sex indicated by either *m* or *f*, respectively, for male and female subjects. Comprehensive age- and sex-stratified data were obtained from the same study and are presented in the normal value reference section of this review.

¶ Central 95th percentile values derived from a study of 200 normal blood bank donors from the Irwin Memorial Blood Bank, San Francisco at the University of California, San Francisco. Total leukocyte range was 3.39 to 9.97 × 10^9/L.

From a study of 129 healthy young adults.[152]

** From a study of 210 normal blood donors aged 18 to 65 years.[153] The statistical method by which the normal range determined was not described.

†† From a study of normal subjects, number unspecified.[154]

produced RBCs, *reticulocytes*, constitute 1% to 2% of the peripheral RBC population. The most commonly used test to determine the concentration of reticulocytes in peripheral blood uses supravital stains to precipitate intracellular RNA, the distinguishing feature of reticulocytes. After staining, thin smears are prepared and the percentage of reticulocytes in the RBC population is determined by light microscopy. The NCCLS has published a proposed standard in which a reticulocyte is defined as a RBC containing two or more dots of precipitated RNA.[89] Normal values for the reticulocyte concentration in adults are reported to be 0.5% to 1.5% (24,000 to 84,000/μL).[5]

The raw reticulocyte count may be adjusted for the degree of anemia and the degree of reticulocyte immaturity and expressed as the reticulocyte index.[90] Correction for the level of anemia is derived from an empiric formula in which the raw reticulocyte count is multiplied by the packed cell volume divided by 45 to provide a corrected reticulocyte percentage.[90] This correction may also be performed by determining the absolute number of reticulocytes per microliter of whole blood. This is accomplished by multiplying the reticulocyte percentage by the absolute RBC count. If erythropoiesis is stimulated, the normal reticulocyte maturation time decreases and the corrected reticulocyte count is again adjusted to correct for the prolonged circulation of immature, or shift, reticulocytes.

Hillman and Finch[90] have described an approximate correction factor of 2 based on an assumed halving of the maturation time with stimulated RBC production. This correction may be more precisely calculated using correction factors based on the assumed life-span of the reticulocyte reflected in the degree of anemia as measured by the hematocrit (PCV). For example, with a PCV of 45% the life-span is estimated to be 1 day and no correction is required. With progressive reduction of the PCV, the reticulocyte life-span in the peripheral circulation is prolonged and the corrected count is divided by the appropriate factor to provide a corrected reticulocyte index: if the PCV is 35%, divide by 1.5; if the PCV is 25%, divide by 2; and if the PCV is 15%, divide by 3.

Typically, 1000 RBCs are examined and the number of reticulocytes is determined. Alternative methods using field reduction devices have been introduced to shorten counting time.[91] Both the precision and the accuracy of this manual technique are suboptimal and have been subjects of considerable study.[92,93] The 95% confidence interval (CI) for a reticulocyte count can be expressed as follows:

$$R \pm 2\sqrt{R(100 - R)/N}$$

where:

R = reticulocyte count expressed as a percentage

N = the number of RBCs counted to determine the reticulocyte count

TABLE 2-16. Precision of the Five-Part Cytochemical Leukocyte Differential*

Study	Total	Neutrophils	Lymphocytes	Monocytes	Eosinophils	Basophils	LUC
Kershaw[33] §	(2.1) 3.1%‖						
	(7.4) 2.3%						
	(26.0) 1.3%						
Bollinger[37] ¶	(0.8) 4.9%						
	(1.1) 3.2%						
	(2.2) 3.2%						
	(5.0) 2.1%						
	(8.0) 2.1%						
	(12.0) 1.8%						
	(25.0) 1.5%						
	(44.0) 1.0%						
Wenz[81] #	(12.7) 1.3%	(2.78) 3.7%	(2.12) 1.8%	(0.35) 3.1%	(0.22) 8.2%	(0.05) 16%	(0.15) 11%
Barnard[153] **		[59.3%] 1.2%	[29.1%] 3.3%	[8.9%] 5.7%	[2.4%] 4.3%	[0.3%] 121.5%	
Barnard[153] ††		[59.3%] 1.2%	[29.1%] 3.2%	[8.9%] 5.4%	[2.4%] 2.8%	[0.3%] 120.9%	

LUC, large unstained cells.

* Absolute cell counts ($\times 10^9$/L) are indicated in parentheses and the coefficient of variation is expressed as a percentage.

† Total leukocyte count (10^9/L).

‡ Large unstained cells are defined as peroxidase-negative with cell volume by forward scatter greater than small lymphocytes.

§ From 10 replicate samples within a single run.

‖ Absolute cell counts $\times 10^9$/L are in parentheses.

¶ From 20 replicate determinations within a single run.

\# From within-run studies; number of replicates not indicated.

** From within-run studies on triplicates of 21 separate samples. Cell concentrations are expressed as percentages in brackets.

†† From between-run studies on triplicates of 21 separate samples. Cell concentrations are expressed as percentages in brackets.

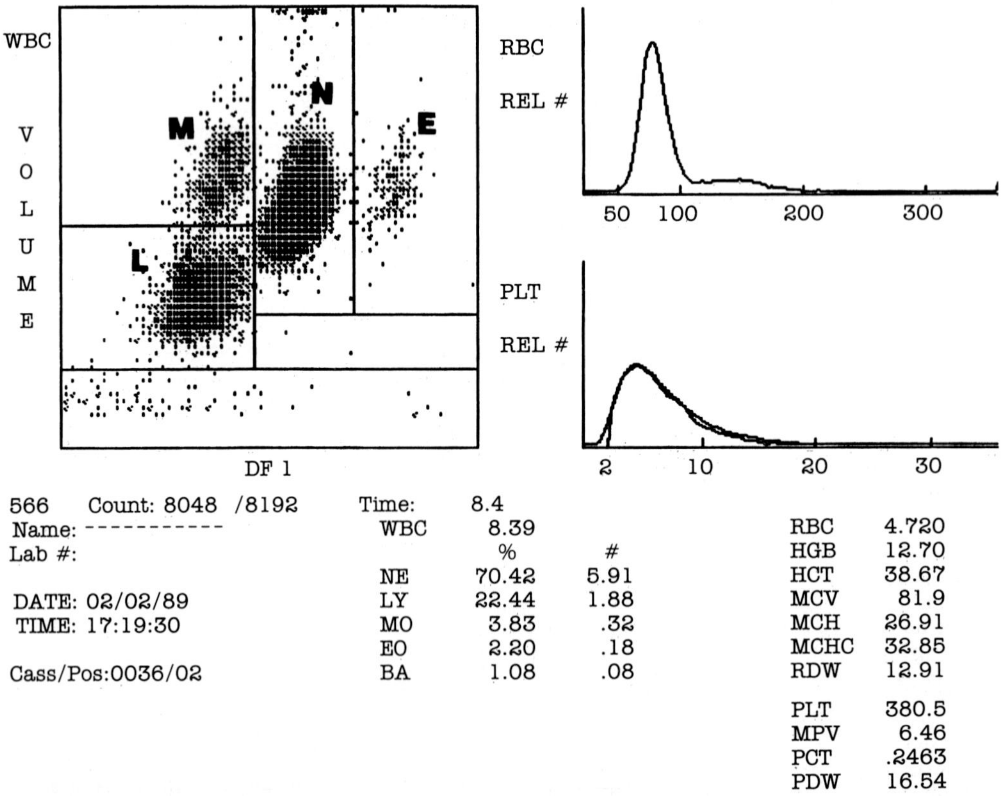

FIGURE 2-24. Coulter VCS instrument display. This system performs a complete blood count, platelet count, and five-part leukocyte differential using a combination of electrical impedance volume sensing, conductivity, and scatter. Conductivity is measured using radio frequency waves. The left panel illustrates the discrimination of four leukocyte cells classes using volume and scatter measurements. L, lymphocytes; M, monocytes; N, neutrophils; E, eosinophils. Basophils are detected using another projection of the data. The right-hand panels illustrate the RBC and platelet volume distribution curves. (Courtesy of Coulter Electronics, Inc, Hialeah, FL)

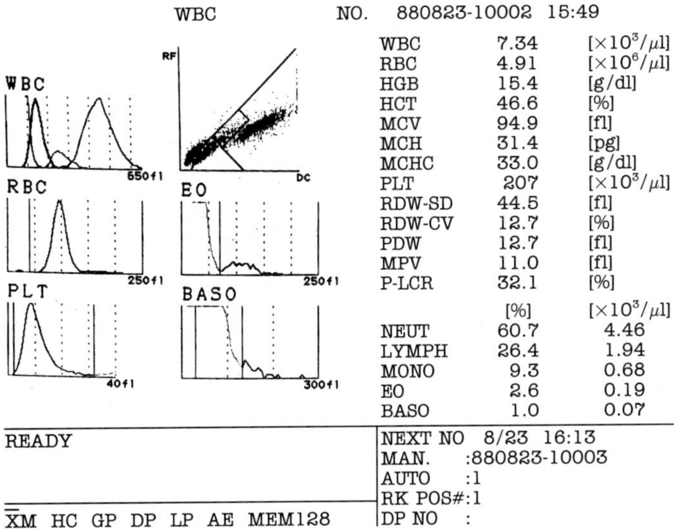

FIGURE 2-25. Sysmex NE-8000 instrument display. This system uses electrical impedance volume sensing, radio frequency conductivity sensing, and selective lysing agents to perform a five-part leukocyte differential. In addition, a complete blood count and platelet count are performed on other channels. (Courtesy of Toa Medical Electronics [USA], Inc, Los Alamitos, CA)

Several specific analytic factors that contribute to the imprecision and inaccuracy of the microscopic reticulocyte count have been identified. The most important factors are interobserver variation in identification of reticulocytes and variation in counting techniques. A recent survey to examine the precision of reticulocyte counting reported CVs as high as 46.05% for manual methods with normal range reticulocyte counts.[92] With respect to accuracy, Savage and associates,[92] in a study of manual reticulocyte counting techniques, concluded that "the degree of imprecision is severe and that inaccuracy is impossible to assess."

Fluorescence-Activated Flow Cytometry

Although standardization of reticulocyte count specimen preparation and counting techniques have been under study, little improvement has been achieved.[94] Recent efforts have focused on developing alternative reticulocyte enumeration techniques. One attractive approach has been the use of fluorescent dyes that selectively bind to intracellular RNA present in reticulocytes, but not in mature RBCs. Under ideal assay conditions, only reticulocytes fluoresce and can be identified using either fluorescence microscopy or fluorescence-activated flow cytometry. The latter technique is advantageous because of greater sample size, easier data collection techniques, and improved analytic methods.

Theoretically, the use of a larger sample size with fluorescence-activated flow cytometric reticulocyte enumeration should result in greater precision than that obtained with the manual technique. The 95% CI around an average reticulocyte count may be calculated. For a count of 1% obtained from a manual 1000-cell count, the CI will be 0.4% to 1.6%; thus with 95% certainty, the true percentage of reticulocytes will lie in this range. For an automated reticulocyte count in which 10,000 cells are counted, the 95% CI will be reduced to 0.8% to 1.2%, with an approximate CV of 20%.

In addition, since the intensity of fluorescence is proportional to the RNA content, the fluorescence technique potentially may provide information on the maturation stages of reticulocytes in the peripheral circulation.[95,96] If the criteria for reticulocyte identification can be based on fluorescence intensity determined by a sensitive photodetector, differences in operator variation for reticulocyte identification should be minimized, which leads to improved accuracy.

Several fluorescent dyes have been described for use in fluorescent reticulocyte enumeration assays and, except for cyanine dye $DiOC_1$ and pyronin Y, have been widely used to develop fluorescence-activated flow cytometric reticulocyte enumeration assays: acridine orange (AO),[97] pyronin Y,[98] thioflavin T (TT),[99–101] cyanine dye $DiOC_1$,[3,102] ethidium bromide (EB),[103] thiazole orange

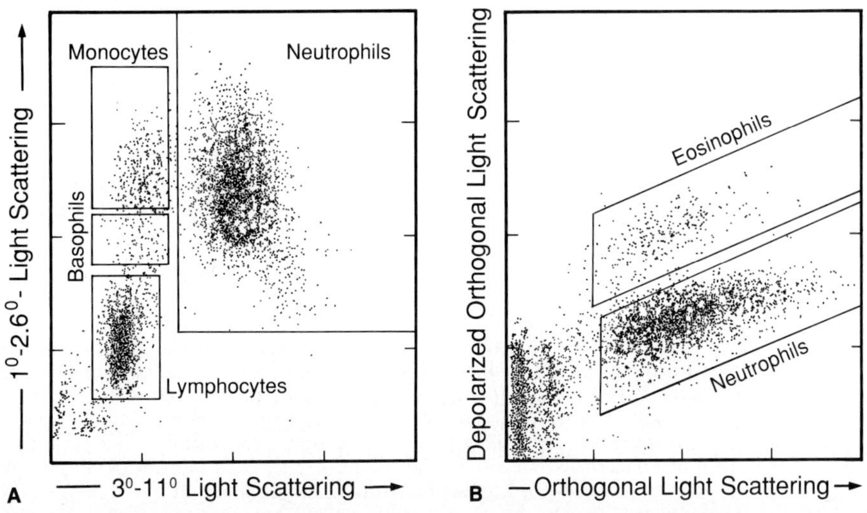

FIGURE 2-26. Sequoia Turner CD 3000 differential system. This instrument uses two low-angle scatter detectors and orthogonal light scatter with depolarized orthogonal light scatter to discriminate leukocyte classes. (**A**) Lymphocytes are detected in box 1, basophils in box 2, monocytes in box 3, and neutrophils in box 4. (**B**) Eosinophils (box 6) are differentiated from neutrophils (box 5) using orthogonal and depolarized orthogonal light scatter. (Adapted from Terstappen LWMM, de Grooth BG, Visscher K, van Kouterik FA, Greve J. Four-parameter white blood cell differential counting based on light scattering measurements. Cytometry 1988;9:39–43)

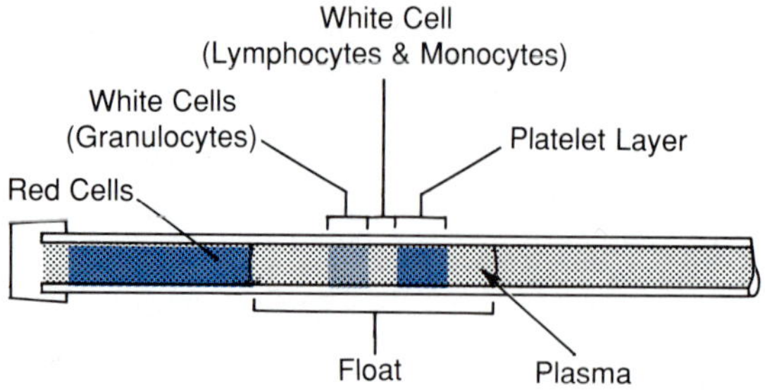

FIGURE 2-27. QBC analyzer differential counter. The system consists of a microcapillary tube coated with acridine orange and oxalate. After filling with either venous or capillary blood, a float is inserted and the tube is centrifuged to separate the various cell classes. After centrifugation, the tube is introduced into a reading device to measure the size of the different cell class bands.

TABLE 2-17. Thioflavin T Fluorescent Reticulocyte Count and Hemoglobin Concentration in Patients With Abnormal Erythropoiesis*

Erythropoiesis	Hgb	Reticulocytes
Decreased	9.3	16.6
range	7.6–13.1	0.4–42.3
Increased	11.1	241.5
range	7.8–15.8	99.8–465.4
Normal	14.0	81.3
range	12.0–16.0	32.5–133.0

* The median value for the hemoglobin concentration (Hgb) in g/dL and the reticulocyte concentration × 1000/μL of whole blood are indicated. Twenty-four subjects with the clinical diagnosis of decreased RBC production and 24 subjects with the clinical diagnosis of increased RBC production were evaluated.

(TO),[6,103,104] and auramine O (AO).[105,106] Only a few of these studies have actually used the fluorescent reticulocyte counting technique in a clinical hematology laboratory setting.[96,100,101,103,106]

Both the normal range for the fluorescent reticulocyte count in adults with normal erythropoiesis and the sensitivity of this technique in patients with abnormal erythropoiesis have been examined.[96,103] Initial studies with this new technique used TT and the FACS Research Analyzer (Becton Dickinson, Mountain View, CA) equipped with a high pressure Hg arc lamp. EDTA-anticoagulated samples were obtained from adult volunteer blood donors who were evaluated by standard procedures at a regional blood bank facility and classified as suitable therapeutic blood donors. Fluorescent reticulocyte counts, expressed as the absolute reticulocyte count per microliter of whole blood, were determined for a population of 246 blood donors of both sexes. The adult normal range was defined as the interval from 2.5% to 97.5% of the reticulocyte concentration cumulative frequency distribution for this population. The reticulocyte count frequency distribution was positively skewed, and the normal range, determined by nonparametric statistics and including all values from percentiles 2.5 to 97.5, was 32,500 to 133,000/μL. The median of this distribution was 81,300/μL. Davis and Bigelow[96] reported a normal range using the TO technique of 2.8% ± 0.6% (SD) with a population of 50 normal adults.

The sensitivity of the fluorescent reticulocyte count in states of abnormal erythropoiesis was determined by examining the reticulocyte concentration in blood from patients with clinical evidence of bone marrow failure and increased RBC destruction with intact bone marrow function (Table 2-17). Patients with bone marrow failure consistently had subnormal reticulocyte levels.[103] In contrast, 20 of 24 patients with documented increased RBC destruction had increased reticulocyte levels and 4 of 20 had levels within the normal range. These patients may have had ineffective erythropoiesis as well as increased RBC destruction.[107]

A comparative study was carried out between the manual reticulocyte count and the TT fluorescent reticulocyte count method using 274 randomly selected patient blood samples submitted to the routine clinical laboratory for reticulocyte enumeration. Manual reticulocyte counts were performed under routine laboratory conditions using the Miller ocular technique.[91] Reticulocyte counts, using either technique, were expressed as the absolute number of reticulocytes per microliter of whole blood. Although there was reasonable agreement between these two techniques ($r = 0.74$), the fluorescent reticulocyte count was consistently greater than the manual reticulocyte count. In another study, there was excellent agreement between the TT reticulocyte count and the 1000-cell manual method.[100]

The precision of the TT fluorescence technique for samples with varying reticulocyte levels was evaluated by performing 30 independent replicate determinations on a series of patient samples with decreased, normal, and increased reticulocyte concentrations. A total of 10,000 cells was examined in each determination, the number of cells identified as reticulocytes was recorded, and the mean values and CVs for each sample were computed.[101] The CVs ranged from 22% for extremely low reticulocyte counts to 6% for elevated counts. Precision was further improved by counting 30,000 RBCs. This did not improve the diagnostic values of the test. Metzger and Charache[100] examined the precision of the TT method at normal, elevated, and markedly elevated reticulocyte levels and observed CVs ranging from 6.4% to 1.3%.

A suitable control material is recommended, which can be independently evaluated with respect to the reticulocyte concentration and used over a period of time to monitor test precision and stability. The ideal control material should have about the same reticulocyte concentration as that of human blood and remain stable for at least 30 days. After evaluation of a series of animal blood samples, rabbit blood was selected. This material exhibited a distribution of reticulocyte fluorescence that was distinct from that of the nonreticulocyte population and contained a reticulocyte concentration and reticulocyte fluorescence intensity distribution that was similar to that found in human blood. Further evaluation of this control material demonstrated that over a 4-month period, although the reticulocyte concentration of individual lots of rabbit blood varied, the overall reticulocyte concentration was consistent and remained in a narrow range (Table 2-18). In comparison, the reticulocyte count was also determined in four lots of rabbit blood by the routine manual technique with the Miller ocular device. The CV for the manual technique was greater for each sample, ranging from 11% to 26%.

TABLE 2-18. Reticulocyte Concentration in Four Lots of Rabbit Blood Evaluated by the Thioflavin T Fluorescent Technique Over a 4-Month Period

Lot	Days	Mean (%)	CV (%)
1198	23	3.1	6.8
0778	27	2.6	8.7
0358	34	3.4	5.5
0078	26	3.0	8.4

CV, coefficient of variation.

TABLE 2-19. Absolute Reticulocyte Concentration Distribution for 176 Normal Newborn Infants Determined by the Thioflavin T Fluorescent Technique

Parameter	Reticulocyte Count*
Minimum value	48.0
Maximum value	358.3
Mean value	131.4
Median value	124.9
Geometric mean	125.5

* Expressed × 1000/μL of whole blood. The interval from 2.5% to 97.5% of the cumulative frequency distribution is 65 to 230 × 10^3/μL.

A study of the normal range of reticulocytes in newborn infants also was performed with the TT method.[101] Previous studies,[108] using manual techniques, demonstrated that newborn infants have a greater reticulocyte concentration than adults. Fluorescent reticulocyte counts were performed on blood samples obtained 2 hours after birth from 176 newborn infants with normal hematocrits, normal birth weights, 5-minute Apgar scores of 7 or higher, and gestational ages of 38 to 42 weeks. The median reticulocyte concentration for this population was greater than that of the normal adult population, and the range was correspondingly shifted (Table 2-19). The fluorescent reticulocyte count levels were consistent with the previously reported manually determined values during the first 5 days of life in normal, full-term infants.[108] The computed range of reticulocytes for normal newborn infants was 65,000 to 230,000/μL of whole blood using the fluorescence technique.

Use of the TT method required precise control of the dye incubation time.[100,101] Other fluorescent dyes, which do not require precise control of incubation times, may be preferable under clinical laboratory conditions. EB is permeable across cell membranes, binds to RNA, and exhibits a quantum yield when bound to RNA about 10-fold greater than that of either TT or the cyanine dye, $DiOC_1$.[3,104] One advantage of EB is that the duration of the incubation of cells with dye does not require precise timing after a minimum 30-minute incubation. The initial EB normal range analysis was performed on the FACS Research Analyzer using 253 samples. The median reticulocyte count for this population was 54,300/μL of whole blood. With the subsequent acquisition of the FACScan instrument, the normal range study with EB was repeated using another population of 104 normal blood donors (Fig. 2-28). The median value for the reticulocyte distribution was 64,000/μL whole blood, which is similar to that obtained with EB and the FACS Research Analyzer and the earlier TT study.

In another study to examine the effect of sex on reticulocyte levels, the median value for males was 56,500/μL and for females 49,100/μL. The 95% CI was similar for both sexes. Comparable sex-biased values also were observed using AO (K. Fujimoto, personal communication, 1990).

Precision studies using EB were carried out using patient samples at several different reticulocyte count levels. The CV for 21 replicate samples at reticulocyte incidences of 2.7%, 4%, and 8.1%, respectively, were 8.1%, 5%, and 4.9% under the described counting conditions using the EB technique and the FACScan instrument.

A third fluorescent dye, TO, which had previously been described by Lee and associates,[104] has become available for fluorescent reticulocyte counting. This dye appeared to be advantageous because it has a higher quantum yield when bound to RNA than other reticulocyte dyes and does not require precise control of incubation times. A normal range study was performed using TO and the FACScan instrument with 115 normal blood donor samples. The median absolute reticulocyte count for this population was 86,800/μL whole blood with a minimum value of 29,000/μL and a maximum value of 225,600/μL. The normal range for this population defined by the 95% CI was from 35,000 to 133,000/μL whole blood. As noted, Davis and Bigelow[96] observed a normal range of 2.8% ± 0.6% SD using this dye, but they did not report their results as absolute numbers of reticulocytes per microliter of whole blood. Compared with the TT and EB normal range studies, the TO normal range and median reticulocyte count values were slightly higher.

A small comparative study using 38 randomly selected patient samples was performed with the TT and TO methods. Correlation coefficient analysis yielded an r of 0.91 between these two techniques.[103] The TO fluorescence technique was compared with the routine methylene blue microscopic technique performed on random patient samples (148 subjects) under routine laboratory conditions. The range of reticulocyte frequencies in this comparative study was from 0.1% to 13%. Under these conditions, a correlation coefficient of 0.85 was observed. The degree of correlation in this study was lower than the value reported by Lee and associates[104] in their more limited study, which contained fewer low reticulocyte count values. Another study compared manual counts with TO flow cytometric counts in 50 patient samples with reticulocyte frequencies ranging from 0.2% to 27%; an excellent correlation coefficient was observed (r = .97).[96]

Davis and Bigelow[96] have described use of the reticulocyte maturation index to detect early recovery of erythropoiesis after bone marrow transplantation. This index should replace the use of the correction for immature reticulocytes, as previously described.[90] Currently, information is insufficient to judge whether the reticulocyte

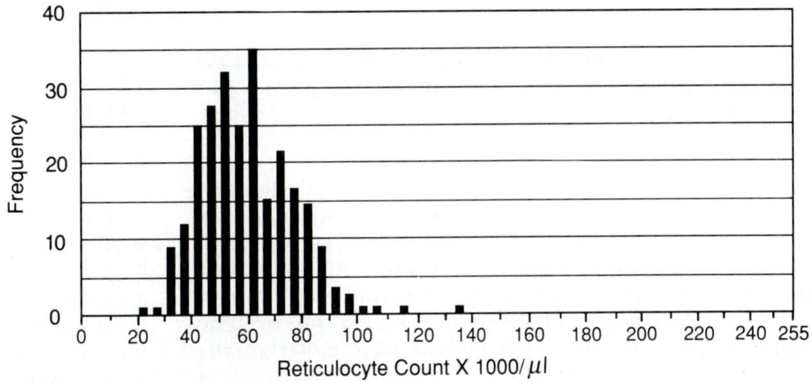

FIGURE 2-28. Reticulocyte count normal range. The reticulocyte count was determined using ethidium bromide and a fluorescence-activated cell analyzer. This study was performed in normal blood bank volunteer donors.

maturation index can be helpful in distinguishing different causes of either stimulated or suppressed erythropoiesis other than recovery from bone marrow transplantation.

The fluorescent reticulocyte technique appears technically feasible for use in the routine hematology laboratory. Comparison of the normal range data for the reticulocyte concentration using the TT method in both adults and newborns demonstrates values that are consistent with those reported with manual reticulocyte counting techniques.[108,109] Collectively, the adult normal range studies carried out with samples from 811 blood bank donors using the TT, EB, or TO methods have yielded comparable data and a well-defined normal range. The fluorescence technique generally yields reticulocyte levels that are slightly higher than those observed with the manual technique. Direct comparison of reticulocyte concentrations, using either normal or abnormal samples, analyzed with the fluorescence technique and the manual technique demonstrated general agreement, but not a high level of correlation between the two techniques. This is not unexpected, since this comparison involves two techniques with substantial differences in precision and the fluorescence technique may detect more reticulocytes than the manual technique when the "two dots of reticulum" rule is rigorously observed for reticulocyte identification with manual methods.[94]

The CV for the fluorescence technique is superior to the previously published values for the manual technique,[92] whether the reticulocyte concentration is low, normal, or high.[96,100,103] The sample size of the fluorescent cytometric technique is much greater than that of the manual technique. Therefore, according to the binomial distribution,[110] the CI for a reticulocyte count, in which the total number of cells enumerated is 10,000 rather than 1000 as in the manual technique, is narrower.

The issue of accuracy in reticulocyte counting is more difficult to assess since there are no well-defined reticulocyte standards with which to compare methodologies. A study of patients with suppressed erythropoiesis demonstrated that the fluorescence technique was able to detect with high sensitivity states of decreased RBC production. When large numbers of replicate determinations were performed on rabbit blood samples, the fluorescent reticulocyte concentrations were in good agreement with manual determinations confirmed by multiple replicate analyses. In addition, the ability of the fluorescence technique to discriminate between the normal ranges for the adult and newborn infant samples suggests that this technique is accurate since the differences in the reticulocyte concentrations of these two populations is well established. The use of rabbit blood as a control material appears to be an acceptable method to ensure quality control for the fluorescence technique. This control material is stable for at least 20 working days and overlapping lots of rabbit blood can be compared to ensure that continuity of the assay system is maintained.

EXAMINATION OF PERIPHERAL BLOOD BY FLUORESCENCE-ACTIVATED CELL ANALYSIS

Rapid progress in the development of accessible fluorescence-activated cell analyzers, fluorochromes, and fluorochrome-conjugated monoclonal antibodies directed against blood cell surface antigens has revolutionized the analysis of peripheral blood. The combined use of these technologies is termed *immunophenotypic analysis*, and it has become commonplace in many hematology laboratories. This technology has been used to improve the identification of abnormal cells and to quantify and assess the function of normal cells. The most widespread use has been in the diagnosis of hematopoietic malignancies and lymphoma and leukemia, and in the analysis of cellular constituents of the immune system. Fluorescence-activated cell analysis also has been used to measure cellular function[111] and to quantify cellular DNA content.[112] The latter application may be useful for identifying neoplastic cells and providing prognostic information about malignant cell populations. These fluorescence-activated techniques are most useful in conjunction with morphologic and functional analytic methods.

Peripheral blood may be examined using fluorescent cytometric methods based on identification of cell surface antigens, internal organelle structure, or DNA content. Greatest use has been made of cell surface antigen analysis with monoclonal antibodies directed against defined surface proteins. The wide array of monoclonal antibodies initially gave rise to a confusing nomenclature, which has been unified under the *cluster designation* or CD system (Table 2-20). Some antibodies are specific for a single cell type or lineage, whereas others may be expressed on several cell types. Combinations of several antibodies may be used to improve specificity.

Instrumentation

The current generation of fluorescence-activated cell analyzers use air-cooled argon ion lasers to generate light at 488 nm for excitation of fluorochromes, measurement of cell size by forward angle light scatter, and measurement of cytoplasmic granularity by wide-angle light scatter (Fig. 2-29). The use of forward scatter and side scatter are important parameters to select cell populations for subsequent fluorescent analysis. The practice of selecting defined cell populations using light scatter is known as *gating* (Fig. 2-30). Within a single cell suspension, multiple populations may be defined by forward and side scatter, with each population examined for expression of selected cell surface proteins using fluorochrome conjugated antibodies. Data from these analyses may be expressed in single parameter format as a frequency histogram. If two properties, such as forward scatter (cell size) and side scatter or fluorescence, are measured simultaneously, the data may be expressed in dual-parameter format using bivariant analysis with a dot plot or contour plot format (Fig. 2-31). After the desired population is selected from a heterogeneous cell suspension using scatter parameters with only a single fluorescent antibody used, the fluorescence intensity of a labeled cell subpopulation may be expressed with a single parameter histogram format. This is the most frequently used format in clinical laboratory applications and is commonly referred to as *single-color flow cytometric analysis* because of the use of one fluorochrome. If the cell suspension is stained with two different antibodies, each conjugated to a different fluorochrome, dual parameter format or bivariant analysis may be used. This is commonly referred to as *two-color flow cytometric analysis*. The use of argon ion lasers is advantageous because multiple fluorochromes with different emission spectra may be excited with 488-nm light.

The fluorescent staining intensity of all cell populations is heterogeneous. An important aspect of this type of cell analysis is to determine where to set the discriminant threshold to divide negative from positive events. This is frequently accomplished by staining one aliquot of the cell suspension with an irrelevant antibody (negatively stained) and the other with the antibody of interest (positively stained; see Fig. 2-30). A threshold is set at the upper end of the fluorescent distribution of the negatively stained suspension, and all events with fluorescent intensity be-

TABLE 2-20. Lymphoid Membrane Antigens Identified by Monoclonal Antibodies

Antigen*	Cell Lineage†	Monoclonal Antibodies‡	Comments
CD1a	Thy, LC	T6, OKT6, Leu-6	
CD1b	Thy		
CD1c	Thy		
CD2	T	T11, OKT11, Leu-5b	SRC receptor
CD3	T	OKT3, Leu-4	TCR complex
CD4	T subset	T4, OKT4, Leu-3a	Helper-inducer
CD5	T	T1, OKT1, Leu-1	B lineage CLL
CD6	T	MBG6, T12	
CD7	T, NK	3A1, Leu-9	FcuR
CD8	T subset	T8, OKT8, Leu-2a	Cytotoxic-suppressor
CD9	Pre-B, P, (M)	J2, BA-2	cALL
CD10	Pre-B	J5, UL-39, CALLA	cALL
CD11a	L		
CD11b	M, G, NK, Tc-s	Mo1, OKM1, Leu-15	C3biR
CD11c	M, (G), NK	Leu-M5, Ki-M1	HCL, AML
CDw12	M, G, P	M67	
CD13	G, M	My7	
CD14	M, (G), FDRC	My4, Leu-M3	
CD15	G, M	My1, Leu-M1	X hapten
CD16	G, NK	Leu-11a, Leu-11b, Leu-11c, VEP13	FcRIII
CD17	G, M, P	T5, A7	Lactosyl ceramide
CD18	L	60.3, MHM23	LFAβ chain
CD19	B	B4, Leu-12	
CD20	B	B1, Leu-16	
CD21	B, FDRC	B2	C3dR
CD22	B	Leu-14, TO15	
CD23	B	PL-13, MHM6	Activation related, FcRII
CD24	B, G	BA-1, HB8	
CD25	Act-T	Tac	IL-2R
CDw26	T	4ELIC7	Activation related
CD27	T, PC, (B)	S152, OKT18A	PC cytoplasm
CD28	T subset	9.3, KOLT2	
CDw29	T subset	4B4	
CD30	Act-T, B	Ki-1	R-S cells
CD31	M, G, P, (T)	SG134, TM3	
CDw32	M, G, P, B	2EI, CIKM5	?FcRII
CD33	BMPC	My9, L4F3	APL
CD34	Myeloid precursor	My10	Leukemia cells
CD35	G, M, FDRC	C3bR, CR1	CR1
CD36	M, P	5F1, CIMegl	
CD37	B, (other)	BL14, HD28	
CD38	PC, (T), (B)	T10, Leu-17	
CD39	B, M	G28-8, G28-10	
CDw40	B, IRC	G28-5	Carcinoma
CDw41	P, Meg	J15, BC5-C4	GPIIb-IIIa
CDw42	P, Meg	HPL14, An51	GPIb
CD43	L		Brain
CD44	L		Brain
CD45	L	4B2, 9.4, HLe-1	T200, LCA
CD45R	B, (T), (M), NK	2H4, Leu-18, HLA-Dr	Restricted T200, B, Act-T, M, G, E

* Defined according to the cluster designation system. Data from Bernard et al,[155] Reinherz et al,[156] McMichael.[157]

† Parentheses indicate a lesser degree of certainty about the presence of the antigen on the indicated lineage or that the reaction is weak.

‡ Commonly available monoclonal antibodies, but not a comprehensive list. Act-B, activated B cells; Act-T, activated T cells; AML, acute myelocytic leukemia; APL, acute promyelocytic leukemia; B, B cells; BMPC, bone marrow precursor cells; cALL, common acute lymphoblastic leukemia, CALLA, common acute lymphoblastic leukemia antigen; C3biR, C3bi receptor; C3dR, C3d receptor; CLL, chronic lymphocytic leukemia; CR1, C3b receptor; E, erythroid; FcR, low affinity receptor for Ig Fc region; FcUR, receptor for Fc region of IgM: FDRC, follicular dendritic reticular cells; G, granulocytes; HCL, hairy-cell leukemia; IL-2R, interleukin 2 receptor; IRC, interdigitating reticulum cells; L, leukocytes, class unspecified; LC, Langerhans' cells; LCA, leukocyte common antigen; M, monocytes; Meg, Megakaryocytes; NK, natural killer cells; P, platelets; PC, plasma cells; ?, questionable association; R, red blood cells; R-S, Reed-Sternberg cells; SRBC, sheep red blood cell; T, T cells; Thy, thymocytes; TCR, T-cell receptor complex.

(Adapted from Deegan MJ. Membrane antigen analysis in the diagnosis of lymphoid leukemias and lymphomas. Arch Pathol Lab Med 1989;113:606–618)

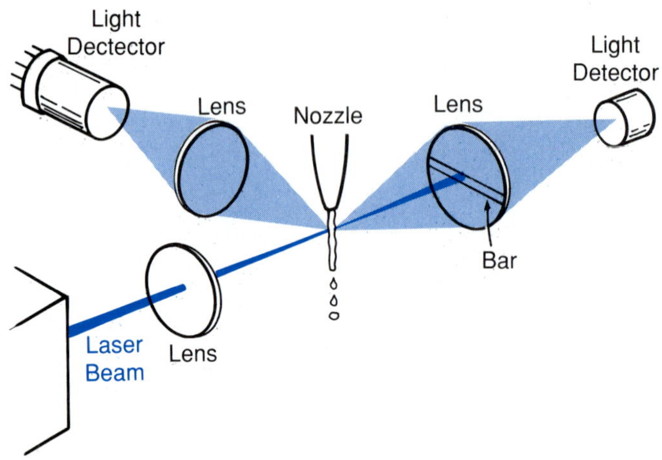

FIGURE 2-29. Diagram of a fluorescence-activated cell analyzer. A laser beam is focused on a particle stream, a forward scatter, a side scatter, and two fluorescence detectors are available to measure two-color emissions and light scatter.

yond that threshold in the positively stained sample are classified as positive events. Under some conditions, only a small fraction of the cell population of interest may stain positively for the selected antigen. This may occur with certain malignant cell populations that may exhibit decreased expression of selected surface antigens. Criteria should be uniform to determine how many cells must be positive to conclude that the designated antigen is significantly expressed by the cell population. No criterion is agreed on and some investigators have used 10% as the critical level,[113] whereas others have chosen 20%.[114,115]

In the evaluation of a series of patients, it is important to use a uniform positive threshold. When antibodies to antigens expressed by normal cells are used to identify a malignant or abnormal cell population, it is important to carefully select the abnormal cell population for analysis.

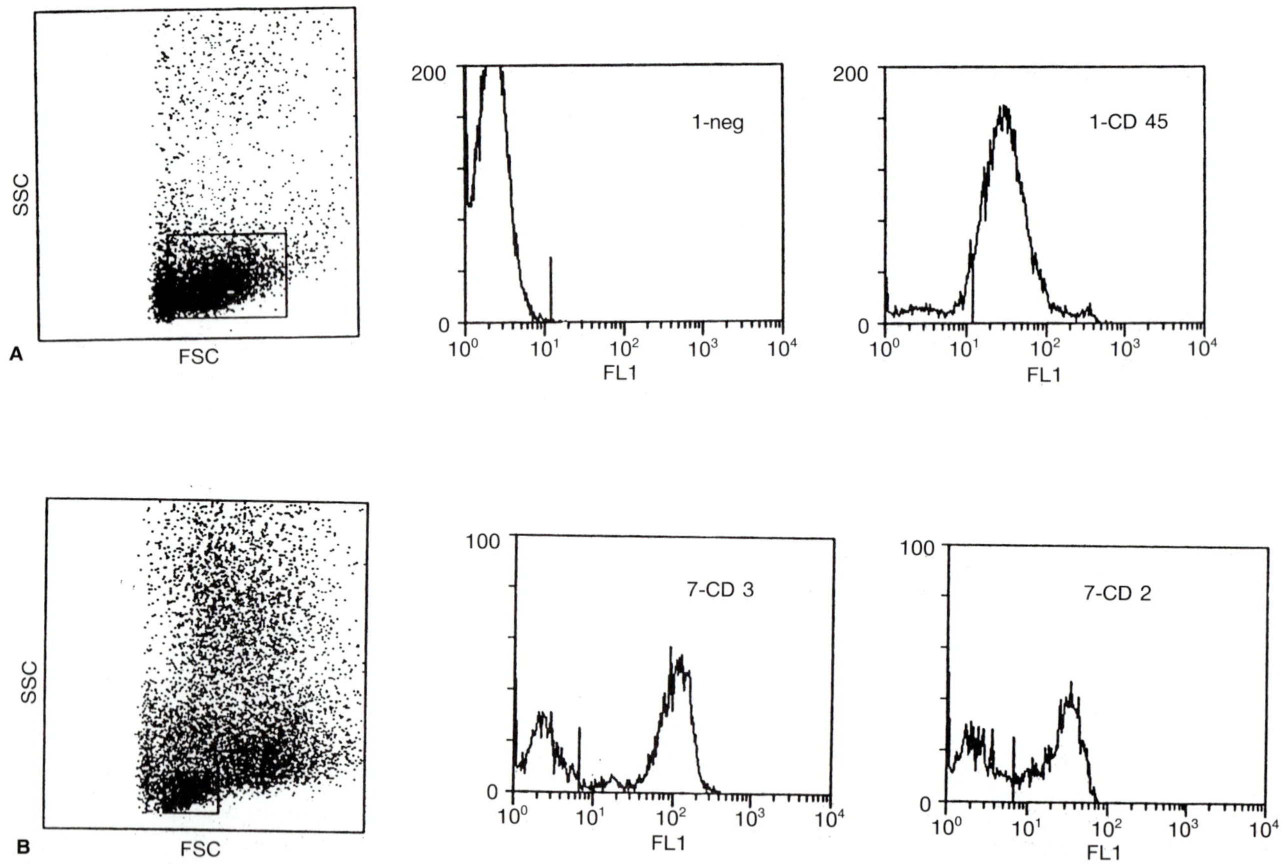

FIGURE 2-30. Data output from a fluorescence-activated analyzer. (**A**) The analysis of peripheral blood from a patient with acute lymphoblastic leukemia. A bivariant dot plot of forward scatter (FSC) versus side scatter (SSC) demonstrates a well-defined blast population outlined by the gating box (*left*). The other panels represent a negatively stained control and a positively stained sample for the CD45 antigen. The vertical line in the negative control sample at the edge of the distribution defines the negative—positive threshold. In the positively stained sample, 95% of the cells lie above the threshold and are defined as positively stained. (**B**) An analysis in which a homogeneous blast population could not be well defined. The gating box was set around a presumed abnormal cell population, but subsequent analysis with CD3 and CD2 demonstrates two cell populations.

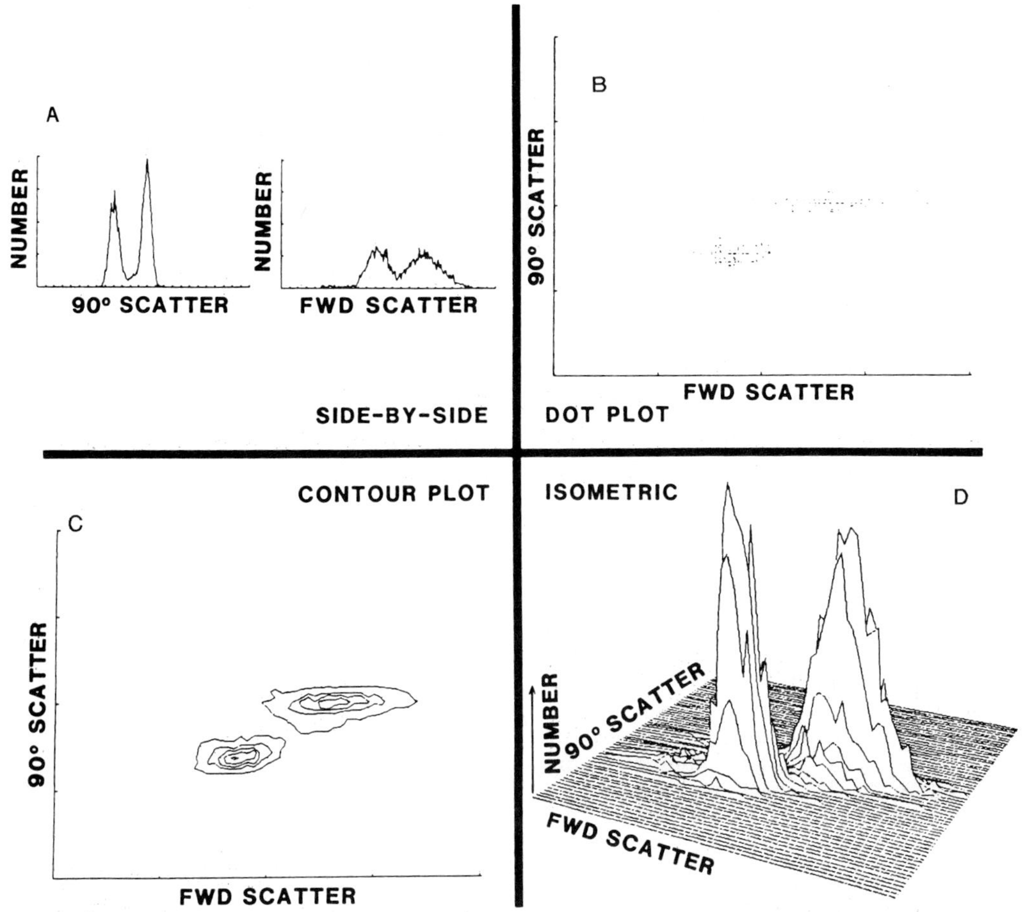

FIGURE 2-31. Data presentation for two different parameters. (**A**) Single-parameter analysis for right angle (90-degree) scatter and forward (FWD) scatter. The data are presented as frequency histograms for each property. (**B**) Bivariant analysis of both 90-degree and FWD scatter presented as a dot or scatter plot. Two cell populations are present; one exhibits greater than 90-degree scatter and FWD scatter. (**C**) Representation of the data from **B** as a contour plot. (**D**) Representation of the data from **B** as an isometric plot so that the cell number in each population can also be examined simultaneously.

If the abnormal cell population cannot be adequately segregated or identified, successful analysis cannot be performed. Immunophenotyping can be achieved with fluorescent microscopy, but most workers think that flow cytometric techniques are superior.[116]

Flow cytometry can examine greater numbers of cells and provide more objective classification criteria than microscopic methods. Flow cytometry is a more sensitive technique to detect infrequent cell subpopulations, since large numbers of cells can be more rapidly examined with flow cytometry than with microscopy. Additionally, the capacity to collect data in list mode for subsequent analysis greatly enhances the value and versatility of this technique. Shapiro[117] has written an excellent text that provides detailed information about instrument configuration, data analysis, and fluorescence techniques.

Sample Preparation

Peripheral blood samples are suitable for immunophenotyping using flow cytometry in conjunction with fluorescent monoclonal antibodies. Blood samples require simple preparatory steps to remove erythrocytes and to stain nucleated cells. Samples may be collected in EDTA or citrate anticoagulants. Heparin may be used, but is less desirable because of increased leukocyte and platelet clumping. In general, cell staining is accomplished with either a single-step direct technique or a two-step indirect method. The direct method uses monoclonal antibodies that are conjugated to fluorochromes. The most commonly used fluorochromes are fluorescein isocyanate and phycoerythrin; the former emits in the green region and the latter emits in the red region. These may be used together to achieve two-color analysis. The two-stage technique uses an unlabeled primary antibody followed by a secondary color developing reagent. This may consist of a heterologous anti-immunoglobulin conjugated to a fluorochrome or biotin. If a biotin conjugate is used, color development is achieved with an avidin conjugated fluorochrome. Biotin conjugates are advantageous since each biotin molecule binds multiple avidin–fluorochrome molecules and primary antibodies can be easily conjugated to biotin to provide greater reagent flexibility.

Several approaches are used for the preparation of peripheral blood samples for fluorescence-activated flow cytometric analysis.[118] Before sample preparation, air-dried smears should be prepared and stained with polychrome stain to provide a morphologic analysis of the cells in the sample. In addition, a leukocyte count should be performed to facilitate calculation of cell recoveries after preparation. At the completion of all preparative and staining procedures, make a cytocentrifuge slide of the final cell suspension so that the morphologic characteristics of the sample can be reviewed.

Whole-blood samples may be directly stained followed by lysis of erythrocytes with buffered ammonium chloride[118] or hypotonic saline. This method is simple and limits the number of tube transfers. If the frequency of abnormal cells is low and large numbers of normal cells remain, data analysis requires highly selective gating to identify the population of interest and to exclude residual normal elements. Excess ammonium chloride must be removed immediately because it produces leukocyte damage with lysis that will affect light scatter and the ability to identify cell subpopulations.

Alternatively, erythrocytes may be lysed first with ammonium chloride followed by washing and antibody staining.[118] The treated sample is then stained with monoclonal antibodies. After staining, samples may be fixed using low concentrations of paraformaldehyde to stabilize the labeled antigens. This permits batch analysis of samples at later times. In addition, this approach allows the use of a prep-and-hold technique in which samples are analyzed only if additional data are required.

A third preparatory method uses partial purification of leukocytes with simple density gradient centrifugation treatment.[118] Whole blood is diluted with buffer, layered over Ficoll-Hypaque solution (1.077 g/mL), and centrifuged (400 g for 30 minutes). During centrifugation, lymphocytes and monocytes collect at the interface, and this leukocyte fraction may be isolated. Some platelet contamination is present and the sample must be washed to remove excess Ficoll-Hypaque solution. Other density gradient media systems such as albumin or the convenient Leuco-Prep system may also be used to isolate leukocyte fractions.

Acute Leukemia

Immunophenotypic analysis of peripheral blood is frequently used in the diagnosis of suspected acute leukemia. Although bone marrow cell suspensions may be a more homogeneous source of abnormal cells, with sufficient numbers of abnormal cells in the peripheral blood, this material may be useful. Griffin and associates[114] compared the results of immunophenotypic analysis on paired samples of peripheral blood and bone marrow from 31 patients with acute myeloblastic leukemia and observed no major differences in diagnostic sensitivity between these two different sources. Peripheral blood is especially useful when an adequate bone marrow sample cannot be obtained. Although immunophenotypic analysis may be of great value, its usefulness is enhanced when used in conjunction with morphology and cytochemistry.

The cytochemical stains of greatest use are MPO, chloracetate esterase, and butyrate or nonspecific esterase. Morphologic analysis of suspected acute leukemias is enhanced by obtaining a plastic-embedded biopsy section on initiation of the work-up.[119] As the diagnostic evaluation evolves, this material can be used to perform multiple cytochemical and immunocytochemical analyses for comparison with the flow cytometric immunophenotypic results. This is especially advantageous since the flow cytometric method does not permit individual cell identification. Identification of individual cells is helpful when abnormal cells may be admixed with reactive normal hematopoietic elements. Final interpretation of flow cytometric data is frequently improved by correlation of morphologic and cytochemical information with immunophenotypic analysis.

Immunophenotypic analysis has been extensively used to classify suspected lymphoid malignancies, primarily acute lymphoblastic leukemia (ALL), and this methodology has further improved with the advent of expanded B-cell lineage reagents.[113,115,116,120–123] If the abnormal cells are peroxidase-negative, the diagnosis of acute lymphoid leukemia should be strongly entertained, although the lack of peroxidase activity is not conclusive proof of lymphoid lineage. A panel of immunophenotypic markers may be used to confirm lymphoid lineage and then to subclassify the abnormal cells as either T-cell or B-cell lineage. This information may be used to determine therapy and to provide a prognosis. Sobol and associates[116] have outlined the antigens of greatest interest (Table 2-21). In addition to the lymphoid antigens, a subset of lymphoid leukemia cells express myeloid antigens (CDw13, CDp16), which may be associated with a poorer prognosis.[115] Some ALL cases lacked lymphoid surface markers, but expressed myeloid antigens and contained either immunoglobulin or T-cell receptor gene rearrangements. Rarely, ALL cells may express surface immunoglobulin as an indicator of mature B-cell lineage. More commonly, ALL cell populations contain intracytoplasmic immunoglobulin indicative of a pre–B-cell lineage. Unfortunately, intracellular immunoglobulin cannot be detected by flow cytometric methods.

Similarly, TdT (terminal deoxynucleotidyl transferase), a useful indicator of lymphoid lineage, is not easily detected by flow cytometric methods. Using an immunophenotypic analysis, Sobol and associates[115] have proposed a classification system for both childhood and adult ALL (Table 2-22). This immunophenotypic classification scheme does not correlate with the Fab classification scheme for lymphoid leukemias.[124]

Immunophenotypic analysis also may be used to classify the myeloid or nonlymphoid leukemias (ANLL). Generally, the use of cytochemical stains such as MPO, chloracetate esterase, and butyrate esterase serve to correctly identify the lineage. In rare circumstances, cytochemical stains may be either negative or inadequate, and immunophenotypic analysis will be of use.

To classify ANLL, a panel of monoclonal antibodies encompassing a relevant series of cell surface antigens has been defined (Table 2-23). Using this panel, Griffin and

TABLE 2-21. Lymphoid Antigens Used for Immunologic Analysis of Acute Lymphoblastic Leukemia

Designation	Identity	Utility
B LINEAGE		
CD19	Pan B	100% of B-ALL
CD20	B subset	<50% of B-ALL
CD24	B and myeloid	Nonspecific
T LINEAGE		
CD1	Thymocytes	Subset of T-ALL
CD2	Pan T	Most T-ALL
CD3	Pan T	Most T-ALL
CD4	Helper-inducer	Subset of T-ALL
CD5	Pan T	Most T-ALL, some CLL
CD7	Pan T	Most T-ALL, few AML
CD8	Suppressor–cytotoxic	Subset of T-ALL
OTHER LYMPHOID MARKERS		
CD10	CALLA, ALL	B- and T-ALL
	TdT	Most ALL, rare AML
	SIg	True B-cell ALL
	Cytoplasmic Ig	Pre–B-ALL

SIg, surface immunoglobulin.
(Adapted from Sobol RE, Bloomfield CD, Royston I. Immunophenotyping in the diagnosis and classification of acute lymphoblastic leukemia. Clin Lab Med 1988;8:151–161)

TABLE 2-22. Immunophenotypic Classification of Childhood and Adult ALL

Classification	Phenotype	Incidence (%)
CHILDHOOD		
Early pre-B	B+cIg−sIg−T−	60–70
Pre B	B+cIg+sIg−T−	15–20
B cell	B+cIg−sIg+T−	1–3
T cell	B−cIg−sIg−T+	15–20
ADULT		
B lineage	B+sIg−T−My−	50–60
T lineage	B−sIg−T+My−	10–15
B-myeloid	B+sIg−T−My+	15–20
T-myeloid	B−sIg−T+My+	5–10
Myeloid*	B−sIg−T−My+	5–10
B cell	B+sIg+T−My−	1–3

* Assigned to lymphoid classification based on germ-line immunoglobulin and T-cell receptor gene configuration.[115]

(Adapted from Sobol RE, Bloomfield CD, Royston I. Immunophenotyping in the diagnosis and classification of acute lymphoblastic leukemia. Clin Lab Med 1988;8:151–161)

TABLE 2-23. Antibodies Used for Immunophenotypic Analysis of ANLL

Designation	Identity
Cp16 (MY9)	Monocytes, promyelocytes, blasts
CDw13 (MY7)	Monocytes, granulocytes, GPC, CFU-GM, BFU-E, CFU-GEMM
CDw15 (MCS-1)	Monocytes, granulocytes, GPC
CD11 (Mo1)	Monocytes, granulocytes, NK cells, GPC
CDw14 (MY4, Mo2)	Monocytes
CD45R (HLA-DR)	Monocytes, B cells, CFU-GM, BFU-E, CFU-GEMM
PM-81	Granulocytes, GPC, CFU-GM
AML-2-23	Monocytes, granulocytes, GPC, CFU-GM
MY8	Monocytes, granulocytes, GPC
MY1	Granulocytes, GPC

ANLL, acute nonlymphocytic leukemia; GPC, granulocyte progenitor cells (promyelocytes, myelocytes, metamyelocytes); CFU-GM, granulocyte-monocyte colony-forming cell; BFU-E, erythroid burst-forming unit; CFU-E, erythroid colony-forming unit; CFU-GEMM, multipotential colony-forming unit.

(Adapted from Griffin JD, Davis R, Nelson D, et al. Use of surface marker analysis to predict outcome of adult myeloblastic leukemia. Blood 1986;68:1232–1241)

associates[114] examined 196 cases of ANLL in which the diagnosis was based on morphology and cytochemical analyses. Most analyses were performed using bone marrow cell suspensions, but in 18% of cases peripheral blood samples also were analyzed. As noted, there was good agreement between bone marrow and peripheral blood samples. Peroxidase activity was present in more than 3% of the blasts in 148 of 164 (90%) of cases examined. Myeloid markers were demonstrated in all but one case and only 2% of the cases expressed lymphoid antigens. Of cases with lymphoid markers, CD10 (CALLA) was weakly expressed on 26% of the cells in one case. The T-cell markers were believed to be expressed on residual or reactive lymphocytes rather than on true blast cells. In three cases, CD19 was expressed on up to 35% of the cells, but multiple myeloid markers were also expressed. A detailed phenotypic analysis of these cases by Fab classification reveals marked heterogeneity and is informative about the relation of the two classification schemes (Table 2-24).

Certain general trends emerged from this complex analysis. Expression of HLA-DR, MY4, MY8, Mo1, AML2–23, MY1, and Mo2 were more common in the Fab M4 and M5 subgroups. My4 and Mo2, late monocyte markers, were not expressed in M3 cells. Immunophenotype did not correlate with patient age, sex, or MPO reactivity of malignant cells. Monocyte markers correlated with esterase-related activity. The absence of MY4 and MY7 was associated with improved remission rates, and the absence of HLA-DR expression was associated with improved remission durability. MY8 and Mo1 were associated with reduced remission duration.

Several studies have examined the diagnostic usefulness of flow cytometric phenotyping to diagnose and classify acute leukemias.[113,122] In 100 patients with acute leukemia, immunophenotypic analysis helped to make the diagnosis in 19% of cases and provided confirmatory support for the diagnosis in the remaining 78%. In a second study of 50 cases, light microscopy with cytochemical stains provided a diagnosis in 86%. The remaining 14% required immunophenotypic analysis to reach a diagnosis. Thus, immunophenotypic analysis is informative in all cases and may be required to arrive at a diagnosis in a minority of cases of acute leukemia. Other studies have shown that it contributes to determining prognosis and management.[114,116] Flow cytometric immunophenotypic analysis has not been helpful in the detection of small amounts of residual disease or in detection of early relapse in marrows with substantial normal hematopoiesis. This is because all the phenotypic antigens, including common acute lymphoblastic leukemia and TdT, are shared by small proportions of normal bone marrow cells; without the presence of a substantial homogeneous population of abnormal cells, it is not possible to detect malignant subpopulations.

Chronic Leukemia and Lymphoma

When sufficient numbers of abnormal cells are present in the peripheral blood, flow cytometric immunophenotypic analysis may be of benefit in diagnosis (Table 2-25). Immunophenotypic analysis is of limited usefulness in providing either a diagnosis or a prognosis for patients with chronic lymphocytic leukemia (CLL). Generally, the diagnosis of CLL is based on the clinical findings and persistent lymphocytosis composed of mature cells. The abnormal lymphocytes of CLL exhibit low-intensity surface IgD or IgM with concomitant anomalous expression of CD5 and B-cell antigens (CD19, CD20, CD24, HLA-DR).[123] Recently, expression of CD5 on subpopulations of peripheral blood cells has been used to facilitate the early diagnosis of CLL.[125] Faguet and Agee[126] have described the cCLLa antigen, which is expressed on B-cell type CLL, prolymphocytic leukemia (PLL), and HCL. This antigen was not present on cells from patients with normal T and B cells, reactive lymphocytosis, or other lymphoid neoplastic conditions. Detection of this antigen with a flow cytometric technique may enhance early detection of CLL. A small proportion of CLL patients have abnormal cells that express T-cell antigens.[127] This observation may be of prognostic value in choosing therapy.[128–130]

These T-cell CLL cases may present with either a helper/inducer (CD4+) phenotype or a suppressor/cytotoxic (CD8+) phenotype. The latter cells frequently have prominent azurophilic cytoplasmic granules, intense acid phosphatase activity, and minimal nonspecific esterase activity.[128] A subset of CD8+ T-cell CLL has been described in which cytoplasmic granules are absent, but with focal cy-

TABLE 2-24. Use of Myeloid Immunophenotypic Analysis in Diagnosis of ANLL*

	FAB Classification Group†								
Antigen	**M-1**	**M-2**	**M-3**	**M-3v‡**	**M-4**	**M-4e‡**	**M-5A**	**M-5B**	**M-6**
CD45R (HLA-DR)	77	83	27	67	95	89	89	92	33
Cp16 (MY9)	68	67	73	67	67	67	100	77	67
PM-81	100	88	62	0	98	100	89	100	50
AML-2-23	62	76	25	0	87	100	78	100	50
CDw13 (MY7)	55	53	64	33	56	78	44	46	67
CDw15 (MCS-1)	28	44	11	0	38	56	44	78	33
MY8	23	41	18	0	62	89	44	100	67
CD11 (Mo1)	19	47	9	0	70	67	78	100	33
CDw14 (MY4)	18	30	0	0	48	78	33	77	0
CDw14 (Mo2)	15	26	0	0	35	78	33	45	0
CD15 (MY1)	33	38	10	0	57	56	67	75	50

* Between 124 and 161 cases were evaluated with respect to each antigen. The relative incidences for each antigen are expressed as a percentage. A reaction was classified as positive if 20% of the abnormal cells reacted with the designated antibody.

† FAB classifications are based on the proposed revised criteria (adapted from Bennett et al[158]).

‡ M-3v indicates the micrograndular variant, and M-4e indicates myelomonocytic leukemia with eosinophilia.

(Adapted from Griffin JD, Davis R, Nelson D, et al. Use of surface marker analysis to predict outcome of adult myeloblastic leukemia. Blood 1986;68:1232–1241)

toplasmic staining using the PAS reagent, acid phosphatase, and nonspecific esterase.[130] The variant CD8+ cases had a more aggressive course than the typical CD8+ T-cell patients. Flow cytometric studies of peripheral blood combined with cytochemical stains help to classify these cases.

In contrast to CLL, PLL is characterized by strong expression of surface immunoglobulin staining (sIg) but weak expression of CD5. The cells in PLL also have a lower nuclear/cytoplasmic ratio with fine nuclear chromatin and frequent prominent nucleoli. As in CLL, a subset of patients with T-cell phenotype has been described.[131] These T-cell phenotypes may be either helper (CD4+) or suppressor (CD8+) subsets and exhibit focal nonspecific esterase activity. Similar to patients B-cell PLL, these T-cell PLL patients appear to have a worse prognosis.[131]

Hairy-cell leukemia cells typically demonstrate strong sIg staining with expression of B-cell antigens (see Table 2-25), Leu-M5 (CD11c), and CD25, the interleukin-2 receptor.[132] Kristensen and colleagues[133] have described a two-color flow cytometric assay for the detection of circulating hairy cells. The assay makes use of a pan B marker CD20 and the SHCL-3/Leu-M5 (CD11c) antibody. The authors did not observe double-labeled cells in samples from patients with CLL, AML, or malignant lymphomas. The sensitivity of detection was about 1%. A few cases of HCL with TRAP-negative cells demonstrated staining with this two-color system; thus, it may enhance diagnostic sensitivity. In rare patients without circulating hairy cells evidenced by light microscopy, this technique may improve diagnostic sensitivity. It may also be useful for monitoring HCL patients after therapeutic intervention. Vokes and colleagues[134] have followed a group of patients with another type of flow cytometric assay to monitor the effects of therapy and assess tumor burden. A cautionary note about the specificity of the CD11c antigen has been raised since cells from patients with splenic lymphoma were positive for this marker.[135] Previous studies have shown that some lymphoma cells may also be TRAP-positive.[136] A double labeling technique was not used in these cases. Caution must be exerted in assuming absolute specificity of any immunologic marker.

Waldenström's macroglobulinemia is a partially differentiated B-cell neoplasm in which the abnormal cells should demonstrate both surface and cytoplasmic monoclonal IgM staining (see Table 2-25). Clonal excess assays have been used to diagnose and to monitor these patients.[137]

TABLE 2-25. Immunophenotypic Analysis of Chronic B-Cell Lymphoproliferative Disorders

Disorder	sIg	cIg	DR	CD5	CD10	CD19	CD20	CD11c	FMC-7	CD38	PCA-1	PC-1	CD25
CLL	IgM ± IgD	(−)*	+	+	−	+	+	−	(−)	−	−	−	−
PLL	IgM ± IgD	−	+	(+)	−	+	+	−	+	−	−	−	−
HCL	IgG, IgM, IgA	(−)	+	−	−	+	+	+	+	−	−	−	+
WM	IgM	+	(−)	−	−	(+)	(+)	−	NA	(+)	+	+	−
MM	—	+	−	−	(−)	−	−	−	NA	+	+	+	−

CLL, chronic lymphocytic leukemia; PLL, prolymphocytic leukemia, HCL, hairy-cell leukemia; WM, Waldenström's macroglobulinemia; MM, multiple myeloma; sIg, surface immunoglobulin; cIg, cytoplasmic immunoglobulin.

* Results in parentheses are the most common presentation, but the opposite has been reported.

(Adapted in part from Deegan MJ. Membrane antigen analysis in the diagnosis of lymphoid leukemias and lymphomas. Arch Pathol Lab Med 1989;113:606–618)

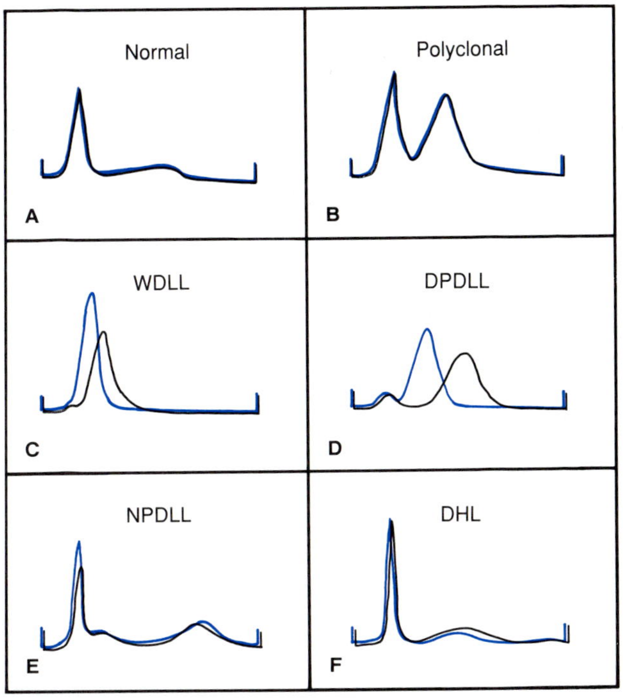

FIGURE 2-32. The clonal excess assay. Samples of peripheral blood have been stained with anti-κ and anti-λ monoclonal antibodies. (**A**) A normal sample with identical distribution of anti-κ and anti-λ stained lymphocytes. (**B**) Polyclonal proliferation of B cells with identical distributions. (**C**) The analysis from a patient with well-differentiated lymphoma (WDLL). There is a second population of cells with increased fluorescence intensity indicative of a clonal excess. (**D**) The analysis from a patient with diffuse poorly differentiated lymphocytic lymphoma (DPDLL). A second more intensely fluorescent cell population indicates clonal excess. (**E**) The analysis from a patient with nodular poorly differentiated lymphocytic lymphoma (NPDLL). The small difference in the two curves indicates clonal excess. (**F**) The analysis from a patient with diffuse histiocytic lymphoma (DHL) with a small difference in fluorescence intensity distribution indicative of clonal excess. (Adapted from Ault KA. Flow cytometric evaluation of normal and neoplastic B cells. In: Rose NR, Friedman H, Fahey JL, eds. Manual of clinical laboratory immunology, ed 3. Washington, DC, American Society for Microbiology, 1986:247–253)

The presence of an excess of cells staining with either anti-κ or anti-λ light chain antibodies indicates a monoclonal population. The abnormal cells of multiple myeloma express cytoplasmic immunoglobulin, but are negative for the common B-cell antigens. Rare cases may express CD10, which is associated with a more aggressive clinical course.[138] Barlogie and colleagues[139] have described the use of a two-color flow cytometric technique to simultaneously examine cytoplasmic immunoglobulin staining, as a means to select myeloma cells, and ploidy as an index of neoplasia. With this technique, myeloma cells with either decreased RNA content or aneuploidy can be identified and used to guide therapy. Although the two-color flow cytometric technique was described with bone marrow cell suspensions, it is amenable to peripheral blood samples with sufficient numbers of circulating plasma cells.

Most attention with respect to immunophenotypic analysis of non-Hodgkin's lymphoma has been directed toward study of lymph node samples. Ault and associates[140–142] have used the clonal excess assay to detect circulating abnormal cells in the peripheral blood of patients with B-cell lymphomas. The clonal excess assay, as described by Ault and associates[140,143] is based on statistical comparison of the distributions of the fluorescence intensity of peripheral blood cells stained with either κ or λ antisera. The presence of a difference in the fluorescence distribution between the two samples indicates the presence of a clonal excess (Fig. 2-32). This assay appears to be highly sensitive and provides a means for detection of small numbers of abnormal cells for diagnosis and therapeutic monitoring.

In addition to T-cell CLL, other T-cell malignancies may be evaluated using immunophenotypic analysis (Table 2-26). These disorders include cutaneous T-cell lymphoma (CTCL or Sézary's syndrome), T-cell leukemia secondary to HTLV-I infection, and the T γ-lymphoproliferative syndrome. Caution must be exerted in concluding that the immunophenotypic pattern for CTCL is necessarily specific in view of the observations by Haynes and associates[144] that the immunophenotypic cellular composition of skin infiltrates of benign reactive lymphoid lesions may be similar to those of CTCL.

The T γ-lymphoproliferative syndrome is generally characterized by neutropenia and peripheral lymphocytosis.[145] The abnormal cell population consists of lymphocytes which carry receptors for the Fc portion of IgG (CD16) and the sheep rosette receptor (CD2). Some of these cells are part of the large granular lymphocyte subpopulation classified as natural killer cells and also antibody-dependent cytotoxicity cells. Other lymphoproliferative disorders in which Tγ cells predominate have been described and include more aggressive lymphomas, T-cell acute leukemia, and T-cell lymphoproliferations without evidence of Fc receptor expression.

During the accelerated and blast crisis phases of chronic myelogenous leukemia, the peripheral blood contains increased numbers of blast cells. If these cells are present in sufficient numbers, they may be classified using immunophenotypic analysis. Adachi and associates[146] examined 20 cases during blastic transformation, of which 9 had only peripheral blood samples studied. Eight cases (40%) were of myeloid lineage, 6 (30%) exhibited lymphoid markers, 3 (15%) exhibited megakaryoblastic antigens, and 3 (15%) did not mark with the antigen panel used in this study. The failure to identify 15% of cases may have been due to the absence of erythroid markers from the study panel. Other workers have shown that chronic myelogenous leukemia cells after transformation may exhibit erythroid markers.[147] Immunophenotypic classification may be helpful in detection of lymphoid blast crisis that appears to be more responsive to therapy than other forms, and, in the

TABLE 2-26. Immunophenotypic Analysis of Chronic T-Cell Lymphoproliferative Disorders

Disorder	sIg	HLA-DR	CD1	CD2	CD3	CD4	CD8	CD16	CD25	CD38	CD57
CTCL	−	−	−	+	+	+	−	−	−	−	−
ATLL	−	−	−	+	+	+	−	−	+	−	−
TγLPD	−	+	−	+	+	−	+	+	−	−	+

CTCL, cutaneous T-cell lymphoma (Sézary syndrome); ATLL, adult T-cell leukemia (HTLV-I); TγLPD, T γ-lymphoproliferative disease; sIg, surface immunoglobulin staining.

TABLE 2-27. Immunophenotypic Analysis of Primary Immunodeficiency Disorders

Disorder	B Cells	T Cells	Natural Killer Cells
SCID	Variable mature B cells (CD19, CD20, CD21)	3 T-cell phenotypes; CD3−, CD4−, CD8−, CD2−, CD3−, CD4−, CD8−, CD38+ Transferrin receptor+, CD3+, CD4+, CD8+, CD38+	Variable CD16, CD56
ADD	Absent	Absent	
Bare lymphocyte syndrome	Normal, ↑ sIgD+, sIgM+	Normal numbers; CD2+, CD3+, CD4+ are CD45R+ (virgin T cells); CD8+ are CD28+ (cytotoxic phenotype)	
X-linked hypogammaglobulinemia	Mature cells absent; immature cells present	Normal numbers; Virgin T-cell phenotype, CD4:CD8 normal	
Common variable immunodeficiency	Normal numbers	Normal numbers; CD2+, CD3+, CD4+5:9+ ↓, CD4: CD8 often ↓	
Selective IgA deficiency	Normal numbers; most sIgA+ are sIgD+ sIgM+	Normal numbers; CD2+, CD3+	
DiGeorge syndrome	Normal numbers	↓ CD3+, CD8+ often ↓	
Wiskott-Aldrich syndrome	Decreased numbers	↓ CD3+, ↓CD2+	

SCID, severe combined immunodeficiency; ADD, adenosine deaminase deficiency; ↑, increased; ↓, decreased.

(Adapted from Nicholson JKA. Use of flow cytometry in the evaluation and diagnosis of primary and secondary immunodeficiency diseases. Arch Pathol Lab Med 1989;113;598–605)

future, this information may be helpful in decisions about bone marrow transplantation.

Immunophenotyping

Flow cytometric immunophenotypic analysis has enhanced the ability of clinicians to evaluate patients with immunodeficiency disorders (Table 2-27); immunophenotype and function may not always be well correlated.[148] Patients with severe combined immunodeficiency (SCID) exhibit several different patterns. According to the classification of Reinherz and associates,[149] one group lacked expression of mature T-cell antigens (CD2, CD3, CD4, CD8) and an immature antigen (CD38). A second group lacked mature T cells but had some immature CD38-bearing cells. The third group had cells that coexpressed mature antigens (CD3, CD4, CD8) and immature antigens as well. SCID patients appear to exhibit variable numbers of B cells with surface immunoglobulin or mature B-cell antigens (CD19, CD20, CD21), but these cells apparently do not synthesize immunoglobulin in a normal manner. Another subset of SCID patients have adenosine deaminase deficiency associated with reduced numbers of either T or B lymphocytes, so that immunologic studies are not informative.[148] Linch and associates[150] have suggested that flow cytometric analysis of fetal blood samples is useful in the prenatal diagnosis of SCID.

Other rare syndromes may also be defined using flow cytometric studies, and the development of new antibodies and direct conjugates with fluorochromes enhances the ability to perform dual-label studies to further define the cell phenotypes associated with these syndromes. A number of the primary immunodeficiency syndromes have been studied with immunophenotypic analysis and the results can best be summarized from the work of Nicholson[148] (see Table 2-27).

Acquired immunodeficiency may be associated with acute viral infections such as cytomegalovirus or chronic viral infections (eg, human immunodeficiency virus). Viral infections generally result in an increased frequency of CD8+ cells in the peripheral blood. Human immunodeficiency virus infection is characterized by coexpression of immature antigens such as CD38 on the CD8+ cells and a decrease in CD4 cells.[148] Precise measurement of CD4 cell concentrations in peripheral blood of patients with acquired immunodeficiency–related syndromes is an important diagnostic step in clinical assessment. Koepke and Landay[151] have emphasized the importance of obtaining precise absolute lymphocyte counts. Use of a combination of an automated total leukocyte count and the relative lymphocyte frequency derived from a 100-cell routine microscopic differential does not provide adequate precision to calculate the absolute lymphocyte count. Automated three-part and five-part leukocyte differential counters are capable of enumerating lymphocytes with a CV of less than 5%, an acceptable level for use in calculating the number of CD4 cells. The absolute lymphocyte concentration may then be used in conjunction with immunophenotypic analysis to estimate absolute concentrations of lymphocyte subsets. Normal range data expressed as absolute concen-

TABLE 2-28. Monoclonal Antibody Panel for Evaluation of Acquired Immunodeficiency Syndrome

Minimal Panel	Expanded Panel
CD3	CD3, CD19
CD4	CD4, CD8
CD8	CD8, Leu-7
CD19 or CD20	CD4, CD45R
CD16 and/or Leu-19	CD4, CDw29
	CD4, class II MHC
	CD8, class II MHC
	CD16 and/or Leu-19
	CD8, CD38

(Adapted from Nicholson JKA. Use of flow cytometry in the evaluation and diagnosis of primary and secondary immunodeficiency diseases. Arch Pathol Lab Med 1989;113:598–605) trations of lymphocyte subsets have been difficult to obtain thus far. Variation in racial and ethnic populations may account for some of these difficulties. Nicholson has recommended the use of monoclonal antibody panels for use in these analyses[148] (Table 2-28).

REFERENCES

1. Kjeldsberg CR, Swanson J. Platelet satellitism. Blood 1974;43:831–836.
2. Greipp P, Gralnick HR. Platelet to leukocyte adherence phenomena associated with thrombocytopenia. Blood 1976;47:513–521.
3. Onder O, Weinstein A, Hoyer LW. Pseudothrombocytopenia caused by platelet agglutinins that are reactive in blood anticoagulated with chelating agents. Blood 1980;56:177–182.
4. Ingram M, Minter FM. Semiautomatic preparations of coverglass blood smears using a centrifugal device. Am J Clin Pathol 1969;51:214.
5. Nelson DA, Morris MW. Basic methodology. In: Henry JB, ed. Clinical diagnosis and management, ed 17. Philadelphia, WB Saunders, 1984: 578–625.
6. Brecher G. New methylene blue as a reticulocyte stain. Am J Clin Pathol 1949;19:895–896.
7. Shepard MK, Weatherall DJ, Conley CL. Semiquantitative estimation of the distribution of fetal hemoglobin in red cell populations. Bull Johns Hopkins Hosp 1962;110:293.
8. Tomoda Y. Demonstration of foetal erythrocytes by immunofluorescent staining. Nature 1964;202:910.
9. Wood WG, Stamatoyannopoulos G, Lim G, Nute PE. F-cells in the adult: normal values and levels in individuals with hereditary and acquired elevations of Hb F. Blood 1975;46:671–682.
10. Mollison PL. Blood transfusion in clinical medicine, ed 7. Oxford, Blackwell Scientific Publications, 1983:367–370, 792–794.
11. Allen C, Weereratne H, Gale R, Beverly PCL, Huehns ER. The use of monoclonal antibodies UCHβ and UCHΓ for the antenatal diagnosis of β-thalassemia. Br J Haematol 1987;65:199–203.
12. Dover GJ, Boyer SH. Fetal hemoglobin-contaning cells have the same mean corpuscular hemoglobin as cells without fetal hemoglobin: a reciprocal relationship between gamma- and beta-globin gene expression in normal subjects and in those with high fetal hemoglobin production. Blood 1987;69:1109–1113.
13. Sears DA, Friedman JM, White DR. Binding of intracellular protein to the erythrocyte membrane during incubation: the production of Heinz bodies. J Lab Clin Med 1975;86:722–732.
14. Simpson CE, Carlisle JW, Mallard L. Rhodanile blue: a rapid selective stain for Heinz bodies. Stain Technol 1970;45:221–223.
15. Zinkham WH, Winslow RM. Unstable hemoglobins: influence of environment on phenotypic expression of a genetic disorder. Medicine 1989;68:309–320.
16. Carrell RW, Kay R. A simple method for the detection of unstable hemoglobins. Br J Haematol 1972;23:615–619.
17. Pearson HA, Johnston D, Smith KA, Touloukian RJ. The born-again spleen: return of splenic function after splenectomy for trauma. N Engl J Med 1978;298:1389–1392.
18. Holroyde CP, Oski FA, Gardner FH. The "pocked" erythrocyte: red-cell surface alterations in reticuloendothelial immaturity of the neonate. N Engl J Med 1969;281:516–520.
19. Padmanabhan J, Risemberg HM, Rowe RD. Howell-Jolly bodies in the peripheral blood of full-term and premature neonates. Johns Hopkins Med J 1973;132:146–150.
20. Kaplow LS. Cytochemistry of leukocyte alkaline phosphatase: use of complex naphthol as phosphatase in azo dye-coupling techniques. Am J Clin Pathol 1963;39:430–449.
21. Kaplow LS. Leukocyte alkaline phosphatase cytochemistry: application and methods. Ann NY Acad Sci 1968;155:911.
22. Kaplow LS. Substitute for benzidine in myeloperoxidase stain. J Clin Pathol 1975;63:451.
23. Liso V, Troccoli G, Specchia G, Magno M. Cytochemical "normal" and "abnormal" eosinophils in acute leukemias. Am J Hematol 1977;2: 123–131.
24. Le Beau MM, Larson RA, Bitter MA, Vardiman JW, Golomb HM, Rowley JD. Association of an inversion of chromosome 16 with abnormal marrow eosinophils in acute myelomonocytic leukemia. N Engl J Med 1983;309:630–636.
25. Yam LT, Li CT, Crosby WH. Cytochemical identification of monocytes and granulocytes. Am J Clin Pathol 1971;55:283–290.
26. Li CY, Lam KW, Yam LT. Esterases in human leukocytes. J Histochem Cytochem 1973;21:1–12.
27. Yam LT, Li CY, Lam KW. Tartrate-resistant acid phosphatase isoenzyme in the reticulum cells of leukemic reticuloendotheliosis. N Engl J Med 1972;284:357–360.
28. Neiman RS, Sullivan AL, Jaffe R. Malignant lymphoma simulating leukemic reticuloendotheliosis: a clinicopathologic study of ten cases. Cancer 1979;43:329–342.
29. Gilmer Jr PR, Williams LJ, Koepke JA, Bull BS. Calibration methods for automated hematology instruments. Am J Clin Pathol 1977;68:185–190.
30. Gilmer PR Jr, Williams LJ. The status of methods of calibration in hematology. Am J Clin Pathol 1980;74:600–605.
31. Reference Procedure for the Quantitative Determination of Hemoglobin in Blood. Villanova, PA, National Committee for Clinical Laboratory Standards, 1984.
32. Procedure for Determining Packed Cell Volume by the Microhematocrit Method. Villanova, PA, National Committee for Clinical Laboratory Standards, 1985.
33. Kershaw GW, Robin H, Kronenberg H. Evaluation of the Technicon H-1 hematology analyser. Pathology 1987;19:305–309.
34. Mohandas N, Kim YR, Tycko DH, Orlik J, Wyatt J, Groner W. Accurate and independent measurement of volume and hemoglobin concentration of individual red cells by laser light scattering. Blood 1986;68: 506–513.
35. Bessman JD, Gilmer PR Jr, Gardner FH. Improved classification of anemias by MCV and RDW. Am J Clin Pathol 1983;80:322–326.
36. Fossat C, David M, Harle JR, et al. New parameters in erythrocyte counting. Arch Pathol Lab Med 1987;111:1150–1154.
37. Bollinger PB, Drewinko B, Brailas CD, Smeeton NA, Trujillo JM. The Technicon H*1®: an automated hematology analyzer for today and tomorrow. Am J Clin Pathol 1987;87:71–78.
38. Tycko DH, Metz MH, Epstein EA, Grinbaum A. Flow-cytometric light scattering measurement of red blood cell volume and hemoglobin concentration. Appl Optics 1985;24:1355–1365.
39. Brecher G, Schneiderman M, Cronkite EP. The reproducibility and constancy of the platelet count. Am J Clin Pathol 1953;23:15–26.
40. Bull BS, Schneiderman MA, Brecher G. Platelet counts with the Coulter counter. Am J Clin Pathol 1965;44:678–688.
41. Nosanchuk J, Chang J, Bennett J. The analytical basis for the use of platelet estimates from peripheral blood smears. Am J Clin Pathol 1978;69:383–387.
42. Abbey A, Belliveau RP. Enumeration of platelets. Am J Clin Pathol 1978;69:55–56.
43. Murphy S, Litwin S, Herring L, et al. Indications for platelet transfusion in children with acute leukemia. Am J Hematol 1982;12:347–356.
44. Patten E. Blood component therapy for cancer patients. Texas Med 1985;81:31–34.
45. Strauss RG. The risks of thrombocytopenia and the standard uses of platelet transfusions. Plasma Ther Transfus Technol 1986;7:279–285.
46. Payne BA, Pierre RV, Lee WK. Evaluation of the TOA-E 5000® automated hematology analyzer. Am J Clin Pathol 1987;88:51–57.
47. Wertz RK, Koepke JA. A critical analysis of platelet counting methods. Am J Clin Pathol 1977;68:195–201.
48. Cornbleet J. Spurious results from automated hematology counters. Lab Med 1983;14:509–514.
49. Corash L. Platelet density heterogeneity. (Letter) Blood 1985;65:779–780.
50. Martin JF, Trowbridge EA. Platelet density heterogeneity. (Letter) Blood 1985;65:779.
51. Garg SK, Amorosi EL, Karpatkin S. Use of the megathrombocyte as an index of megakaryocyte number. N Engl J Med 1971;284:11–17.
52. Kraytman M. Platelet size in thrombocytopenias and thrombocytosis of various origins. Blood 1973;41:587–598.
53. Zeigler Z, Murphy S, Gardner FH. Microscopic platelet size and morphology in various hematologic disorders. Blood 1978;51:479–486.
54. Rowan RM, Fraser C, Gray JH, McDonald GA. The Coulter counter model S-plus: the shape of things to come. Clin Lab Haematol 1979;1: 29–40.
55. Giles C. The platelet count and mean platelet volume. Br J Haematol 1981;48:31–37.
56. Levin J, Bessman JD. The inverse relation between platelet volume and platelet number: abnormalities in hematologic disease and evidence that platelet size does not correlate with platelet age. J Lab Clin Med 1983;101:295–307.
57. Thompson CB, Diaz DD, Quinn PG, Lapins M, Kurtz S, Valeri CR. The role of anticoagulation in measurement of platelet volumes. Am J Clin Pathol 1983;80:327–332.
58. Threatte GA, Adrados C, Ebbe S, Brecher G. Mean platelet volume: the need for a reference method. Am J Clin Pathol 1984;81:769–772.
59. Lippi U, Schinella M, Modena N, Nicoli M. Unpredictable effects of K_3 EDTA on mean platelet volume. Am J Clin Pathol 1987;87:391–393.
60. Bessman JD, Gilmer PR, Gardner FH. Use of mean platelet volume improves detection of platelet disorders. Blood Cells 1985;11:127–135.
61. Corash L. Platelet sizing techniques: biologic significance and clinical applications. Curr Top Hematol 1983;4:99–122.
62. Corash L, Shafer B, Blaese RM. Platelet-associated immunoglobulin, platelet size, and the effects of splenectomy in the Wiskott-Aldrich syndrome. Blood 1985;65:1439–1443.
63. Bessman JD, Williams LJ, Gilmer PR. Platelet size in health and hematologic disease. Am J Clin Pathol 1982;78:150–153.
64. Friedhoff AJ, Miller JC, Karpatkin S. Heterogeneity of human platelets VII. Platelet monoamine oxidase activity in normals and patients with autoimmune thrombocytopenic purpura and reactive thrombocytosis: its relationship to platelet protein density. Blood 1978;51:317–323.
65. Small BM, Bettigole RE. Diagnosis of myeloproliferative disease by analysis of the platelet volume distribution. Am J Clin Pathol 1981;76: 685–691.

66. Dudley JM, Messinezy M, Eridani S, et al. Primary thrombocythaemia: diagnostic criteria and a simple scoring system for positive diagnosis. Br J Haematol 1989;71:331–335.
67. Tentative Standard H20-T: leukocyte differential counting. Villanova, PA, National Committee for Clinical Laboratory Standards, 1984.
68. Koepke JA, Dotson MA, Shifman A. A critical evaluation of the manual/visual differential leukocyte counting method. Blood Cells 1985;11: 173–181.
69. Koepke JA. Standardization of the manual leukocyte differential leukocyte count. Lab Med 1980;11:371–375.
70. Mathay KA, Koepke JA. The clinical usefulness of segmented vs. stab: neutrophil criteria for differential leukocyte counts. Am J Clin Pathol 1974;61:947–958.
71. Koepke JA, Ross DW. White blood cell differential: a call for standards. Blood Cells 1985;11:1–11.
72. Wilding P, Leboy EL. Use of pattern recognition technology for determination of the human differential leukocyte count. Blood Cells 1985;11:187–199.
73. Richardson-Jones A, Hellman R, Twedt D. The Coulter counter® leucocyte differential. Blood Cells 1985;11:203–238.
74. Duncan KL, Gottfried EL. Utility of the three-part leukocyte differential count. Am J Clin Pathol 1987;88:308–313.
75. Cornbleet J, Kessinger S. Evaluation of Coulter® S-Plus three-part differential in population with a high prevalence of abnormalities. Am J Clin Pathol 1985;84:620–626.
76. Arkin CF, Medeiros LJ, Pevzner LZ, et al. The white blood cell differential: evaluation of rapid impression scanning versus the routine manual count. Am J Clin Pathol 1987;87:628–632.
77. Corash L. Automated leukocyte differential analysis by flow cytochemistry. Lab Med 1983;14:503–508.
78. De Cresce R. The Technicon H*1: a discrete, fully automated complete blood count differential analyzer. Lab Med 1986;17:17–21.
79. Swaanenburg JCJM, Rutten WPF, Holdrinet ACJM, van Strik R. The determination of reference values for hematologic parameters using results obtained from patient populations. Am J Clin Pathol 1987;88: 182–191.
80. Kinsey SE, Watts MJ. Accurate automated leucocyte differential counts despite profound leucopenia. J Clin Pathol 1988;41:1236–1239.
81. Wenz B, Ramirez MA, Burns ER. The H*1 hematology analyzer. Arch Pathol Lab Med 1987;111:521–524.
82. Banez E, Bacaling HD. An evaluation of the Technicon H-1 automated hematology analyzer in detecting peripheral blood changes in acute inflammation. Arch Pathol Lab Med 1988;112:885–888.
83. Marchand A, van Lente F, Galen RS. The assessment of laboratory tests in the diagnosis of acute appendicitis. Am J Clin Pathol 1983;80: 369–374.
84. Bentley SA, Pegram MD, Ross DW. Diagnosis of infective and inflammatory disorders by flow cytometric analysis of blood neutrophils. Am J Clin Pathol 1987;88:177–181.
85. Lai AP, Martin PJ, Cawley JC, Richards JDM, Goldstone AH. Automated leucocyte differential counts in chronic lymphocytic and hairy-cell leukemias: a comparison of the Hemalog D, H-6000 and Coulter S Plus IV. Clin Lab Haematol 1987;9:169–174.
86. Terstappen LWMM, de Grooth BG, Visscher K, van Kouterik FA, Greve J. Four-parameter white blood cell differential counting based on light scattering measurements. Cytometry 1988;9:39–43.
87. Breakall ES, Marchand A, Marcus R, Simson E. Comparison of performance for leukocyte differential counting of the Technicon H6000® system with a manual reference method using the NCCLS standard. Blood Cells 1985;11:257–279.
88. Sallitt RL, Ho TT, Rodriquez R. Evaluation of leukocyte differential counts on the QBC(R) centrifugal hematology analyzer according to NCCLS standard H 20-T. Blood Cells 1985;11:281–294.
89. Proposed standard: method for reticulocyte counting. Villanova, PA, National Committee for Clinical Laboratory Standards, 1985.
90. Hillman RS, Finch CA. Annotation: the misused reticulocyte count. Br J Haematol 1969;17:313–315.
91. Brecher G, Schneiderman M. A time-saving device for the counting of reticulocytes. Am J Clin Pathol 1950;20:1079–1083.
92. Savage RA, Skoog DP, Rabinovitch A. Analytic inaccuracy and imprecision in reticulocyte counting: a preliminary report from the College of American Pathologists reticulocyte project. Blood Cells 1985;11:97–112.
93. Peebles DA, Hochberg A. Analysis of manual reticulocyte counting. Am J Clin Pathol 1981;76:713–717.
94. Gilmer PR, Koepke JA. The reticulocyte: an approach to definition. Am J Clin Pathol 1976;66:262–267.
95. Tanke HJ, Rothbarth PH, Vossen JMJJ, Koper GJM, Ploem JS. Flow cytometry of reticulocytes applied to clinical hematology. Blood 1983;61:1091–1097.
96. Davis BH, Bigelow NC. Flow cytometric reticulocyte quantification using thiazole orange provides clinically useful reticulocyte maturity index. Arch Pathol Lab Med 1989;113:684–689.
97. Seligman PA, Allen RH, Kirchanski SJ, Natale PJ. Automated analysis of reticulocytes using fluorescent staining with both acridine orange and an immuno-fluorescence technique. Am J Hematol 1983;14:57–66.
98. Tanke HJ, Nieuwenhuis IAB, Koper GJM, Slats JCM, Ploem JS. Flow cytometry of human reticulocytes based on RNA fluorescence. Cytometry 1980;1:313–320.
99. Sage BH, O'Connell JP, Mercolino TP. A rapid vital staining procedure for flow cytometric analysis of human reticulocytes. Cytometry 1983;4: 222–227.
100. Metzger DK, Charache S. Flow cytometric reticulocyte counting with thioflavin T in a clinical hematology laboratory. Arch Pathol Lab Med 1987;111:540–544.
101. Corash L, Rheinschmidt M, Lieu S, Meers P, Brew E. Fluorescence activated flow cytometry in the hematology clinical laboratory. Cytometry 1988;Suppl 3:60–64.
102. Jaccoberger JW, Horan PK, Hare JD. Flow cytometric analysis of blood cells stained with cyanine dye DiOC-1-[3]: reticulocyte quantification. Cytometry 1984;5:589–600.
103. Corash L, Rheinschmidt M, Lieu S, Meers P, Brew E. Enumeration of reticulocytes using fluorescence-activated flow cytometry. Pathol Immunopathol Res 1988;7:381–394.
104. Lee LG, Chen C, Chiu LA. Thiazole orange: a new dye for reticulocyte analysis. Cytometry 1986;7:508–517.
105. Kojima K, Niri M, Setoguchi K, Tsuda I, Tatsumi N. An automated optoelectronic reticulocyte counter. Am J Clin Pathol 1989;92:57–61.
106. Tichelli A, Gratwohl A, Driessen A, et al. Evaluation of the Sysmex R-1000. 1990;93;70–78.
107. Conley CL, Lippman SM, Ness PM, Petz LD, Branch DR, Gallagher MT. Autoimmune hemolytic anemia with reticulocytopenia and erythroid marrow. N Engl J Med 1982;306:281–286.
108. Matoth Y, Zaizov R, Varsano I. Postnatal changes in some red cell parameters. Acta Paediatr Scand 1971;60:317–323.
109. Deiss A, Kurth D. Circulating reticulocytes in normal adults as determined by the new methylene blue method. Am J Clin Pathol 1970;53: 481–484.
110. Greenberg ER, Beck JR. The effects of sample size on reticulocyte counting and stool examination. Arch Pathol Lab Med 1984;108:396–399.
111. Stelzer GT. Analysis of leukocyte function by flow cytometric techniques. Cytometry 1988;9(Suppl 3):52–59.
112. Coon JS, Landay AL, Weinstein RS. Biology of disease: advances in flow cytometry for diagnostic pathology. Lab Invest 1987;57:453–479.
113. Chan LC, Pegram SM, Greaves MF. Contribution of immunophenotype to the classification and differential diagnosis of acute leukemia. Lancet 1985;1:475–479.
114. Griffin JD, Davis R, Nelson D, et al. Use of surface marker analysis to predict outcome of adult myeloblastic leukemia. Blood 1986;68:1232–1241.
115. Sobol RE, Mick R, Royston I, et al. Clinical importance of myeloid antigen expression in adult acute lymphoblastic leukemia. N Engl J Med 1987;316:1111–1117.
116. Sobol RE, Bloomfield CD, Royston I. Immunophenotyping in the diagnosis and classification of acute lymphoblastic leukemia. Clin Lab Med 1988;8:151–161.
117. Shapiro HM. Practical flow cytometry. New York, Alan R. Liss, 1985.
118. Jackson AL, Warner NL. Preparation, staining, and analysis by flow cytometry of peripheral blood leukocytes. In: Rose NR, Friedman H, Fahey JL, eds. Manual of clinical laboratory immunology, ed 3. Washington, DC, American Society for Microbiology, 1986:226–235.
119. Beckstead JH, Halverson PS, Ries CA, Bainton DF. Enzyme histochemistry and immunohistochemistry on biopsy specimens of pathologic human bone marrow. Blood 1981;57:1088–1097.
120. Foon KA, Todd RF III. Immunologic classification of leukemia and lymphoma. Blood 1986;68:1–31.
121. Foon KA, Gale RP, Todd RF III. Recent advances in the immunologic classification of leukemia. Semin Hematol 1986;23:257–283.
122. Krause JR, Penchansky L, Contis L, Kaplan SS. Flow cytometry in the diagnosis of acute leukemia. Am J Clin Pathol 1988;89:341–346.
123. Deegan MJ. Membrane antigen analysis in the diagnosis of lymphoid leukemias and lymphomas. Arch Pathol Lab Med 1989;113:606–618.
124. Bennett JM, Catovsky D, Daniel MT, Flandrin G, Galton DAG, Gralnick HR, Sultan C. The morphological classification of acute lymphoblastic leukemia: concordance among observers and clinical correlations. Br J Haematol 1981;47:553–561.
125. International Workshop on Chronic Lymphocytic Leukemia. Chronic lymphocytic leukemia: recommendations for diagnosis, staging, and response criteria. Ann Intern Med 1989;110:236–238.
126. Faguet GB, Agee JF. Monoclonal antibodies against chronic lymphocytic leukemia antigen cLLa: characterization and reactivity. Blood 1987;70: 437–443.
127. Brouet J, Flandrin G, Sasportes M, Preud'homme JL, Seligmann M. Chronic lymphocytic leukaemia of T-cell origin: immunological and clinical evaluation in eleven patients. Lancet 1975;2:890–893.
128. Phyliky RL, Li C, Yam LT. T-cell chronic lymphocytic leukemia with morphologic and immunologic characteristics of cytotoxic/suppressor phenotype. Mayo Clin Proc 1983;58:709–720.
129. Huhn D, Thiel E, Rodt H, Schlimok G, Theml H, Rieber P. Subtypes of T-cell chronic lymphatic leukemia. Cancer 1983;51:1434–1447.
130. Hui PK, Feller AC, Pileri S, Gobbi M, Lennert K. New aggressive variant of suppressor/cytotoxic T-CLL. Am J Clin Pathol 1987;87:55–59.

131. Volk JR, Kjeldsberg CR, Eyre HJ, Marty J. T-cell prolymphocytic leukemia: clinical and immunologic characterization. Cancer 1983;52: 2049–2054.
132. Chilosi M, Semenzato G, Cetto G, et al. Soluble interleukin-2 receptors in the sear of patients with hairy cell leukemia: relationship with the effects of recombinant α-interferon therapy on clinical parameters and natural killer in vitro activity. Blood 1987;70:1530–1535.
133. Kristensen JS, Ellegaard J, Hokland P. A two-color flow cytometry assay for detection of hairy cells using monoclonal antibodies. Blood 1987;70: 1063–1068.
134. Vokes E, Bitter MA, Ratain M, Prystowsky MB, Daly K, Golomb HM. Flow cytometry in hairy cell leukemia before and during interferon alfa-2b therapy. Cancer 1987;59:1987–1991.
135. Vardiman JW, Gilewski TA, Ratain MJ, Bitter MA, Bradlow BA, Golomb HM. Evaluation of Leu-M5 (CD11c) in hairy cell leukemia by the alkaline phosphate anti-alkaline phosphatase technique. Am J Clin Pathol 1988;90:250–256.
136. Nieman RS, Sullivan AL, Jaffe R. Malignant lymphoma simulating leukemic reticuloendotheliosis: a clinicopathologic study of ten cases. Cancer 1979;43:329–342.
137. Smith BR, Robert NJ, Ault KA. In Waldenstrom's macroglobulinemia the quantity of detectable circulating monoclonal B lymphocytes correlates with clinical course. Blood 1983;61:911–914.
138. Durie BGM, Grogan TM. CALLA-positive myeloma: an aggressive subtype with poor survival. Blood 1985;66:229–232.
139. Barlogie B, Alexanian R, Pershouse M, Smallwood L, Smith L. Cytoplasmic immunoglobulin content in multiple myeloma. J Clin Invest 1985;76:765–769.
140. Ault KA. Detection of small numbers of monoclonal B lymphocytes in the blood of patients with lymphoma. N Engl J Med 1979;300:1401–1405.
141. Weinberg DS, Pinkus GS, Ault KA. Cytofluorometric detection of B cell clonal excess: a new approach to the diagnosis of B cell lymphoma. Blood 1984;63:1080–1087.
142. Smith BR, Weinberg DS, Robert NJ, et al. Circulating monoclonal B lymphocytes in non-Hodgkin's lymphoma. N Engl J Med 1984;311: 1476–1481.
143. Ault KA. Flow cytometric evaluation of normal and neoplastic B cells. In: Rose NR, Friedman H, Fahey JL, eds. Manual of clinical laboratory immunology, ed 3. Washington, DC, American Society for Microbiology, 1986:247–253.
144. Haynes BF, Hensley LL, Jegasothy BV. Phenotypic characterization of skin infiltrating T cells in cutaneous T-cell lymphoma: comparison with benign cutaneous T-cell infiltrates. Blood 1982;60:463–473.
145. Reynolds CW, Foon KA. T(*$_g$-lymphoproliferative disease and related disorders in humans and experimental animals: a review of clinical, cellular, and functional characteristics. Blood 1984;64:1146–1158.
146. Adachi K, Okumura M, Tanimoto M, Morishima Y, Ohno R, Saito H. Analysis of immunophenotype, genotype, and lineage fidelity in blastic transformation of chronic myelogenous leukemia: a study of 20 cases. J Lab Clin Med 1988;111:125–132.
147. Ekblom M, Borgstrom G, von Willebrand E, Gahmberg CG, Vuopio P, Andersson LC. Erythroid blast crisis in chronic myelogenous leukemia. Blood 1983;62:591–596.
148. Nicholson JKA. Use of flow cytometry in the evaluation and diagnosis of primary and secondary immunodeficiency diseases. Arch Pathol Lab Med 1989;113:598–605.
149. Rheinherz EL, Cooper MD, Schlossman SF, Rosen FS. Abnormalities of T cell maturation and regulation in human beings with immunodeficiency disorders. J Clin Invest 1981;68:699–705.
150. Linch DC, Levinsky RJ, Rodeck CH, MacLennan KA, Simmonds HA. Prenatal diagnosis of three cases of severe combined immunodeficiency: severe T cell deficiency during the first half of gestation in fetuses with adenosine deaminase deficiency. Clin Exp Immunol 1984;56:223–232.
151. Koepke JA, Landay AL. Precision and accuracy of absolute lymphocyte counts. Clin Immunol Immunopathol 1989;52:19–27.
152. Ross DW, Bentley SA. Evaluation of an automated hematology system (Technicon H-1). Arch Pathol Lab Med 1986;110:803–808.
153. Barnard DF, Barnard SA, Carter AB, Patterson KG, Yardumian A, Machin SJ. An evaluation of the Coulter VCS differential counter. Clin Lab Haematol 1989;11:255–266.
154. Richardson-Jones A. Evaluation of the Coulter VCS automated differential counter: a hematology flow cytometer. Hialeah, FL, Coulter Electronics, 1989.
155. Bernard A, Boumsell L, Dausett J, Milstein C, Schlossman SF, eds. Leucocyte typing: human leucocyte differentiation antigens detected by monoclonal antibodies. New York, Springer-Verlag, 1985.
156. Reinherz EL, Haynes BF, Nadler LM, Bernstein ID, eds. Leukocyte typing II. New York, Springer-Verlag, 1986.
157. McMichael J, ed. Leucocyte typing III: white cell differentiation antigens. New York, Oxford University Press, 1987.
158. Bennett JM, Catovsky D, Daniel MT, Flandrin G, Galton DAG, Grainick HR, Sultan C. Proposed revised criteria for the classification of acute myeloid leukemia. Ann Intern Med 1985;103:626–629.

Blood: Principles and Practice of Hematology,
edited by Robert I. Handin, Thomas P. Stossel, and Samuel E. Lux.
J.B. Lippincott Company, Philadelphia © 1995.

3

Study of Bone Marrow

Alan B. Weitberg

Ever since the role of bone marrow in blood cell production was described in 1868, this organ has been examined intensively, particularly by anatomists, pathologists, and hematologists.[1] As techniques to sample the marrow in vivo emerged, observation of the process of blood formation became a reality.[2] Few organs are as accessible to sampling as bone marrow. In concert with review of the peripheral blood smear, bone marrow examination provides the bulk of attainable information regarding the status of the hematopoietic system. Although aspiration and biopsy of the marrow are simple procedures technically, samples can be processed by increasingly sophisticated methods (flow cytometry, immunohistochemistry, cytogenetics, electron microscopy) to yield more information than morphology alone can yield. This chapter reviews these methods and offers a standard methodology to obtain and process bone marrow specimens.

INDICATIONS FOR BONE MARROW EXAMINATION

The decision to perform a bone marrow examination is based on the assumption that relevant data will be obtained and that the attendant risks of the procedure are acceptable. Although the risks of marrow sampling are few, the probability of useful information being garnered for specific cases is difficult to estimate. Retrospective estimates are flawed by sampling bias; specific prospective series are lacking, even for common marrow diseases, except where generated as part of treatment protocols for hematologic and nonhematologic malignancies. As will be discussed in subsequent sections, even these indications are controversial.

Because meaningful pretest probabilities are unavailable, current suggestions represent the collective opinion of hematologists and pathologists, even though complete agreement is lacking.[3–5] Because marrow aspiration is virtually risk-free and biopsy is only minimally invasive, bone marrow examination procedures should be performed when the practitioner can justify a probable benefit of the information obtained.

Situations in which bone marrow examination is regularly performed are listed in Table 3-1. Several of these warrant further mention and will be discussed in more detail in succeeding sections.

Although of low yield, bone marrow sampling in patients with fever of undetermined origin (FUO) is justifiable. In most such cases, abnormalities of peripheral blood counts prompt examination of the marrow, but even when lacking, blind biopsies are worth performing. In about 10% of cases, marrow sampling establishes the diagnosis—most commonly hematologic malignancies or tuberculosis—which represent 21% and 5%, respectively, of the diagnoses in patients presenting with FUO.[6]

Bone marrow culture is useful for the diagnosis of certain infections, particularly histoplasmosis. Most studies reveal a high yield of histoplasmosis on bone marrow culture ranging from 25% to 70%; in 30% to 80% of cases of histoplasmosis not confirmed by marrow fungal stains, the marrow culture is positive.[7–9] The yield of bone marrow culture in patients with miliary tuberculosis is variable (15% to 55%) and is complimentary to the liver biopsy in establishing the diagnosis.[7] In patients with brucellosis, the organism has been cultured from the bone marrow in 40% to 90% of cases.[7,10]

As a test for identifying cancer metastases, bone marrow sampling is diagnostic in 15% to 25% of patients with nonhematologic tumors.[11] It should be reserved for patients with signs of marrow invasion (eg, leukoerythroblastosis), for those in whom a positive finding will significantly alter treatment, and for patients with malignancies commonly metastatic to the bone marrow, such as small cell carcinoma of the lung.

Blind bone marrow biopsy in an attempt to establish a diagnosis in a patient with constitutional symptoms is of low yield unless some objective evidence of disease exists (eg, hypercalcemia, elevated alkaline phosphatase). In a large series of bone marrow biopsies reviewed retrospectively, only 11% were of specific diagnostic value. Of these, 1.7% established the diagnosis of metastatic carcinoma and 2.5% revealed the presence of a hematologic malignancy. Granulomatous disease was identified in 52 of 100 biopsies.[12]

TECHNICAL ASPECTS

Instruments

A variety of needles are available for aspiration or biopsy of the bone marrow. Simple needles with obturators such as the Osgood or Rosenthal needles suffice for aspiration alone. The Illinois sternal puncture needle, although similar in design to the latter, is equipped with a guard to prevent traversing the adult sternum completely (Fig. 3-1).

Percutaneous instruments have been developed as an alternative to open surgical biopsy of the bone marrow. In 1943, the Turkel trephine needle was produced[13] and in

TABLE 3-1. Indications for Bone Marrow Examination

ABSOLUTE INDICATIONS
Anemia, leukopenia, or thrombocytopenia of unknown etiology
Pancytopenia
Macrocytic anemia
Leukoerythroblastosis
Immature forms on peripheral smear suggestive of leukemia
Unexplained teardrop forms on peripheral blood smear
Staging of Hodgkin's and non-Hodgkin's lymphomas
Work-up of myeloproliferative or myelodysplastic disorders
For the purpose of
Evaluation of paraproteinemia or paraproteinuria
Diagnosis of lipid storage diseases
Monitoring the effect of therapy for leukemia
Staging of small cell carcinoma of the lung when clinically indicated
RELATIVE INDICATIONS
Iron-deficiency anemia
Bacteriologic and histologic evaluation of granulomatous diseases
Investigation of fungal, parasitic diseases
Bone marrow culture
Fever of unknown origin

1958, the Vim-Silverman needle, originally designed to obtain a tumor tissue biopsy percutaneously, was adapted for biopsy of the bone marrow.[14] Various adaptations ensued, including the Westerman-Jensen modification[15]; each was designed to avoid the small and often crushed specimens obtained with the earlier models. The Jamshidi-Swaim needle, described in 1971, yields biopsy specimens with well-preserved architecture and can be used for obtaining bone marrow aspirates and biopsies through the same needle.[16] Disposable Jamshidi needles are available and now are in common use (Fig. 3-2). A newer instrument, the Islam needle, is equipped with a core securing device to prevent the biopsy from slipping out of the needle during the process of extraction.[17]

Sites for Aspiration and Biopsy

The choice of a site for bone marrow aspiration or biopsy is dependent on several factors such as age, weight, marrow distribution, patient status, and physician experience. In infants and small children, a variety of sites for aspiration are available, including the tibia and the femur (Table 3-2), whereas the posterior iliac crest is the preferred site for needle biopsy. Biopsy in infants also may be obtained from the anterior iliac crest or the proximal tibia.[18]

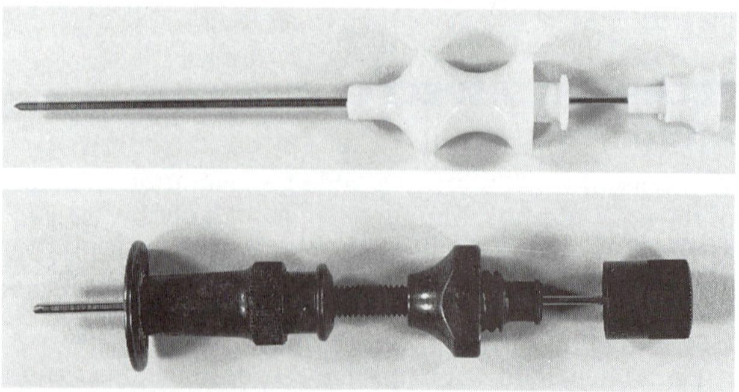

FIGURE 3-1. Aspiration needles. (*Top*) Disposable Rosenthal needle. (*Bottom*) Illinois needle with guard.

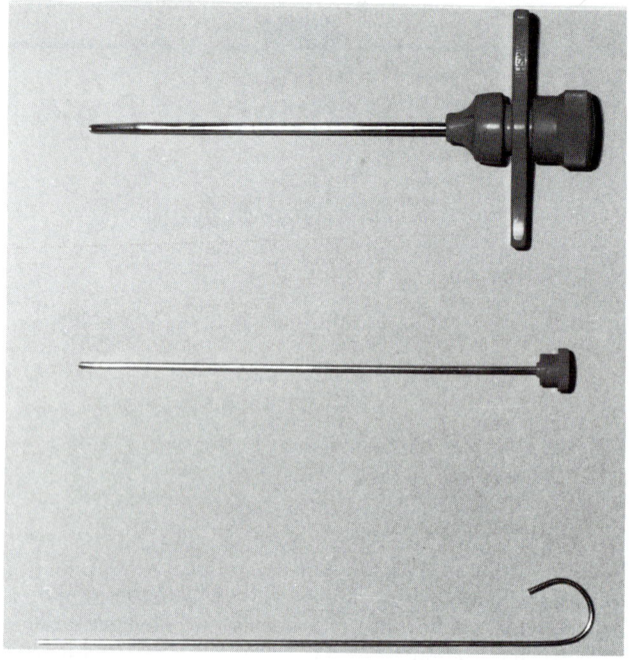

FIGURE 3-2. (*Top*) Disposable Jamshidi needle. (*Middle*) Obturator. (*Bottom*) Stylet.

The normal adult skeleton contains about 1500 g of marrow, 40% of which is concentrated in the pelvis[19] (Table 3-3), since the marrow in long bones is replaced by fat. The once-popular sternal marrow has been abandoned for pelvic sites, primarily for greater safety and convenience. The posterior iliac spine is easily identified and sampled in most patients. When properly biopsies are done, specimens are of good size and quality. In obese patients, whose landmarks are obliterated by flank fat and whose posterior iliac spines lie too deep beneath the skin, the anterior iliac spine may be used. Sampling discordance is not significant between these two sites.[19]

When marrow cannot be aspirated after three or four attempts from one site (dry tap), a biopsy should be obtained, touch preps prepared, and plastic embedding considered. Plastic-embedded marrow biopsy specimens provide better morphologic detail.[20] Not all authorities agree that the increased cost of this technique can be justified.[21] Depending on the urgency for obtaining an aspirate, additional punctures may be made at the anterior iliac spine or the sternum or both. In patients having received radiation therapy or chemotherapy, indium-111 bone marrow scintigraphy demonstrates the distribution of normal mar-

TABLE 3-2. Sites for Bone Marrow Puncture in Infants and Children

Site	Age When Usable
Tibia	Birth to 12 mo
Femur	Birth to 12 mo
Anterior iliac crest	Any age
Posterior iliac crest	Any age
Vertebral spinous process	2 y and older
Sternum	6 mo* and older

* Only when supervised.
(Pochedly C. How to perform bone marrow puncture in small children. Clin Pediatr 1969;8:705)

TABLE 3-3. Marrow Distribution of the Adult

Site	Marrow Weight (g)	Red Marrow Weight (g)	Red Marrow Total (%)
Head	182.2	136.6	13.1
Upper limb girdle	115.5	86.7	8.3
Sternum	39.0	23.4	2.3
Ribs	206.8	82.6	7.9
Vertebrae (cervical)	47.4	35.8	3.4
Vertebrae (thoracic)	197.0	147.9	14.1
Vertebrae (lumbar)	152.2	114.1	10.9
Sacrum	194.0	145.6	13.9
Lower limb girdle	363.6	273.0	26.1
TOTAL	1497.7	1045.7	100.0

(Adapted from Ellis RB. The distribution of active bone marrow in the adult. Phys Med Biol 1961;5:255)

row and guides the physician to a specific site for aspiration or biopsy.[22,23]

Procedure for Bone Marrow Aspiration

The bone marrow aspiration procedure and its possible complications should be explained fully to the patient, and documentation of consent should be entered in the patient's medical record. The following equipment should be assembled and kept easily available:

- One Jamshidi needle
- One aspiration needle (optional)
- Ten to 15 clean glass slides and coverslips
- Zenker's solution
- Ethylenediaminetetraacetic acid (EDTA; lavender top vacutainer)
- Syringes (10 mL)
- Lidocaine hydrochloride
- Gauze pads
- Povidone–iodine solution
- Sterile gloves

As a rule, pretreatment with antianxiety medications is not required. For the extremely anxious patient, 2 to 5 mg of diazepam can be administered parenterally 15 to 20 minutes before the procedure. For the posterior iliac spine approach, the patient should be in the prone position or on one side with legs slightly bent (Fig. 3-3). In either case, the patient should be made comfortable to ensure maximal cooperation.

The posterior iliac spine is located and marked as shown in Figure 3-3. In thinner patients, the posterior iliac spine can be palpated as a bony prominence that is superior and about 3 fingerbreadths lateral to the intergluteal cleft. The skin overlying its upper aspect may be dimpled. The area is cleansed thoroughly with a betadine solution and wiped dry. The overlying skin is anesthetized with intradermal lidocaine hydrochloride using a 25-gauge needle. With a larger needle (19 gauge), the skin is pierced and the needle advanced to the periosteum. An area of about 1 cm in diameter should be injected by withdrawing and redirecting the needle several times. The needle tip should be firmly planted in the bone as the anesthetic is injected under pressure. Allow several minutes for the anesthetic to take effect.

A small skin incision is made with a surgical blade. The bone marrow needle with its obturator fixed in place is pushed through the skin and twisted several times in a clockwise–counterclockwise fashion while forward pressure is exerted until the solid, gritty surface of the periosteum is reached. Because of the curvature of the posterior iliac spine, the needle should be directed cephalad, in the direction of the anterior iliac spine (Fig. 3-4). Again using clockwise–counterclockwise rotations, the needle is advanced through the periosteum and cortex until firmly in place. The operator may sense a sudden lack of resistance as the softer trabecular bone is entered. The stylet is removed and a 10-mL syringe is attached to the anchored needle. By swiftly withdrawing the plunger, negative pressure is created and about 0.5 mL of marrow is collected. The patient experiences a sharp, fleeting pain as the marrow is aspirated, a reliable sign that the marrow cavity was entered successfully.[24]

The liquid marrow is discharged onto the upper end of a slanted glass slide to allow any contaminating peripheral blood to run off. A marrow smear is prepared by laying a

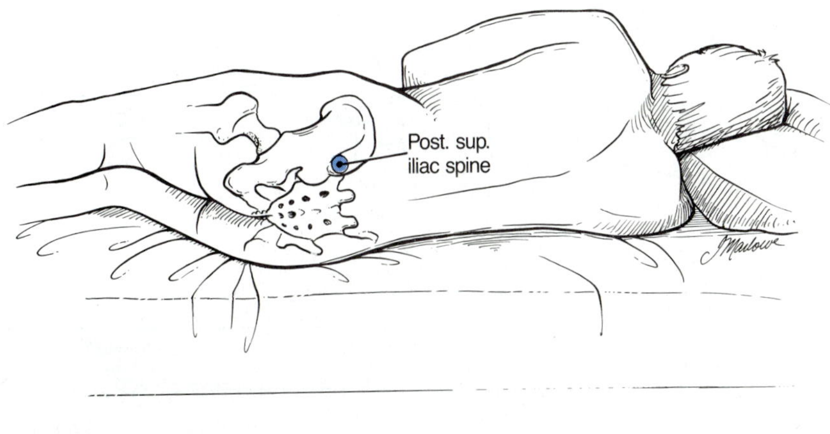

FIGURE 3-3. Positioning of patient and insertion of needle for bone marrow examination.

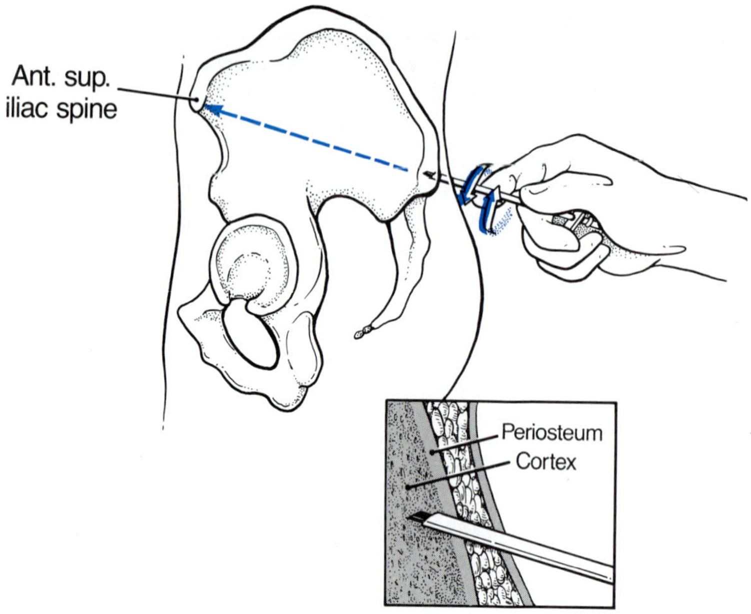

FIGURE 3-4. Direction of bone marrow needle (lateral view).

second slide over the first and gently pulling laterally without exerting direct pressure, the weight of the second slide being sufficient to crush the marrow particles (Fig. 3-5). Alternatively, from the inclined slide, marrow particles are picked up with the corner of a coverslip and smeared across a slide or coverslip held between thumb and index finger while resting firmly on the middle finger. Gentle pressure is applied while smearing the marrow to crush the particles and to avoid undue morphologic distortion. The marrow particles may be distinguished from fat by their smaller size and are easily appreciated when viewed at an angle. Whether or not smears are prepared at the bedside, some marrow promptly should be anticoagulated with ethylenediaminetetraacetic acid (EDTA). This sample is useful for smears to be prepared in the pathology or hematology laboratory. EDTA is superior to heparin as an anticoagulant because the latter may cause considerable morphologic distortion.[25] An additional 5 to 10 mL of marrow is then aspirated and discharged into EDTA for the preparation of histologic sections and for special procedures as will be described. Anticoagulated marrow can be processed in many ways; thus, a sample should be obtained routinely.

Procedure for Bone Marrow Biopsy

Techniques for bone marrow biopsy have evolved considerably over the 30 years since the procedure was popularized by McFarland and Damashek.[14]

Patient preparation for biopsy is the same as aspiration, which usually is performed first to avoid aspirating at a site that had previously undergone biopsy. The needle is removed and directed to an anesthetized area adjacent to the aspiration site to avoid biopsy distortion, although some authors advocate advancing the needle several centimeters after aspiration to obtain a biopsy, noting that hematopoietic cellularity is unaltered.[26] The stylet is locked in place and the needle ensemble is advanced through the cortical bone using a clockwise–counterclockwise rotation until firmly anchored. The stylet is removed and the process continued until a depth of 2 to 3 cm is reached. The length of the core can be approximated by reinserting the obtu-

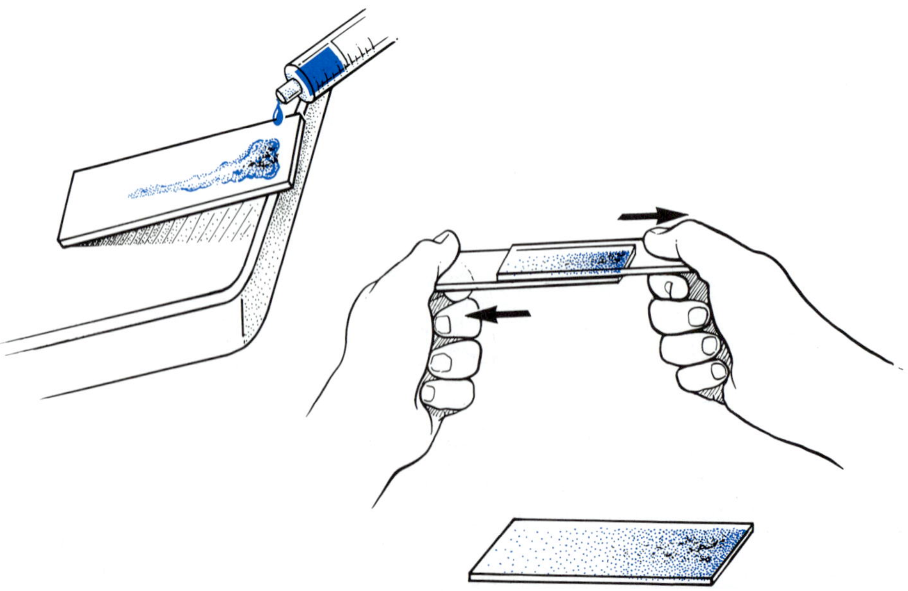

FIGURE 3-5. Preparation of bone marrow smears. The slides are pulled laterally with no downward pressure.

rator and estimating the length that protrudes beyond the proximal end of the shaft of the needle. To loosen the core from its bony moorings, the needle is rotated in place in a counterclockwise–clockwise motion, gently jiggled in several directions, then slowly removed with alternating rotary motions.

The most common reason for failure to obtain a biopsy specimen is that the core has been left in place while the needle was being withdrawn. Care must be taken to dislodge the core completely from the adjacent bone as just described before removing the needle. After the core is obtained, the bone marrow biopsy is dislodged onto a clean glass slide by inserting the probe into the distal, tapered end of the biopsy needle. If the probe is inserted into the proximal end of the needle, the specimen is crushed. Adequate biopsy sections should be at least 2 cm in length and 2 mm in diameter.[16] The incidence of inadequate biopsy specimens is in the range of 5% to 8%.[15,27]

Touch preparations of the biopsy are prepared by applying a second slide to the biopsy along its long axis and making several imprints 1.5 to 2 cm apart. If cultures are desired, small (3- to 5-mm) sections can be cut off using a sterile surgical blade and placed in the appropriate culture containers. The remainder of the biopsy specimen is placed in a container of Zenker's acetic acid solution and submitted for decalcification and preparation of paraffin-embedded sections.

Biopsy Versus Aspiration

Whether bone marrow biopsy augments the diagnostic yield of the aspirate is controversial. An accurate interpretation of published data comparing the two requires attention to the method of aspirate preparation: particle smears, histologic sections or buffy coat preparations, and the most likely diagnoses to be confirmed or excluded.

These caveats notwithstanding, several large series have concluded that the bone marrow biopsy increases the diagnostic accuracy of the aspirate by 10% to 12% (Table 3-4), especially in cases of disseminated granulomas, myelofibrosis, aplastic anemia, metastatic carcinoma, metabolic bone disease, malignant lymphoma, and vasculitis.[15,16,28,29] The procedures tend to be complementary in diagnosing acute leukemia, chronic lymphocytic leukemia, and chronic myelogenous leukemia, whereas all would agree that biopsy is indicated after a dry tap. It is impossible to predict from these data those cases in which the aspirate or the biopsy will be diagnostic.

In experienced hands, procurement of a biopsy should not significantly increase patient discomfort, although the cost of biopsy and aspiration is about twice that of aspiration alone. It may prove to be cost-effective to perform these procedures concurrently rather than sequentially when the aspirate proves nondiagnostic. Furthermore, the biopsy may illuminate important additional pathology (eg, fibrosis, infiltrative processes, vascular lesions) even in instances in which aspiration alone traditionally has been indicated, such as in megaloblastic anemias, microcytic or normocytic anemias, neutropenias, and thrombocytopenias.[30] A cogent argument can be made to aspirate and perform biopsy in all cases even though indications for each have been suggested and clearly overlap.[25,31] Diagnostic yield is increased and a more thorough bone marrow study is obtained at minimal risk to the patient for a modestly increased cost.

TABLE 3-4. Comparison of Positive Yields from Bone Marrow Aspirates and Biopsies

Series	Biopsies	Positive Biopsies	Positive Aspirates
Ellis[4]	1445	253 (10%)	96 (7%)
Grann[27]	238	91 (37%)	63 (27%)
Jamshidi[29]	150	21 (14%)	7 (5%)
Bearden[13]	205	67 (33%)	42 (21%)

(Adapted from Bearden JD, Ratkin GA, Coltman CA. Comparison of the diagnostic value of bone marrow biopsy and bone marrow aspiration in neoplastic disease. J Clin Pathol 1974;27:738)

Complications

Complications of both bone marrow aspiration and biopsy are rare. The infection rate in one large series of bone marrow biopsies was only 0.14% in spite of the fact that most procedures were performed by medical residents and, not infrequently, in neutropenic patients.[22] Although its specific incidence is unknown, hemorrhage is uncommon even in severely thrombocytopenic patients if the procedure is performed carefully and a pressure dressing is applied.[30] Some investigators believe patients with hemophilia and patients with coagulopathies should receive factor replacement before bone marrow examination.[31] Others refute this, simply advising cautious technique in those patients without ill effects. In the absence of hard data, either approach is reasonable, but if the procedure is deemed necessary, the presence of a hemorrhagic disorder is not a contraindication to proceeding as planned. Only two isolated case reports have documented retroperitoneal hemorrhage in patients with osteoporosis after bone marrow biopsy of the ilium.[32,33]

Sternal aspiration is associated with more severe complications. Although the sternum is not a common site for aspiration today, 15 fatalities were reported in the literature prior to 1964; most were due to myocardial or aortic lacerations.[34] Occasional bone marrow embolization to the lung also has been reported.[35]

Although of no clinical importance, a circular, lytic lesion with sclerotic borders can be observed on plain films of the abdomen after biopsy of the posterior iliac spine, and is occasionally accompanied by exostoses.[36,37] Bone scans are normal after bone marrow biopsy.[38]

PROCESSING OF SPECIMENS

Preparation of Samples

In general, the bone marrow aspirate is smeared at the bedside (as described previously) and submitted in an anticoagulant for preparation of histologic sections (particle or clot), additional air-dried smears as needed, and for special procedures (eg, flow cytometry, cytogenetics, electron microscopy, culture, buffy coat preparation). Particle sections differ from clot sections only in that marrow particles are concentrated prior to fixation and sectioning in the former, whereas aspirated marrow is directly deposited into Zenker's solution in the latter. Marrow particles collected in EDTA may be concentrated by one of several filtration methods, embedded in paraffin, and cut into sections 4 μm thick.[39–41] The advantage of histologic sections over smears in increasing diagnostic yields has been well documented.[39,40] Smears preserve cytologic detail, whereas sections reveal the spatial relationships of cells within the marrow particle.

Anticoagulated marrow aspirates may be treated with Ficollpaque or discontinuous Percoll gradients to separate and concentrate bone marrow fractions.[42] Five layers are observed—fat and perivascular cells, plasma, lymphocytes, myeloid layer (buffy coat), and erythrocytes. The fat layer is rich in macrophages, thus particularly suitable for iron staining. Cells from the buffy coat layer may be smeared onto glass slides and stained as required. The buffy coat smear aids in the evaluation of hypoplastic bone marrows as happens when searching for residual blast cells in the bone marrow of patients with acute leukemia in the post-chemotherapy period.

Touch preps of the bone marrow biopsy are prepared routinely prior to fixation in Zenker's solution, and samples may be cut off with a surgical blade for culture or plastic embedding, which allows for thinner sectioning and finer resolution of cytologic detail after staining (as already discussed).

As listed in Tables 3-5 and 3-6, many diagnostic procedures may be performed on the bone marrow biopsy and aspirate. Requirements for submission to the pathology and other special laboratories are noted, but may vary slightly from institution to institution. A complete bone marrow study should include the following:

- Six to eight air-dried particle smears
- Several milliliters of EDTA-anticoagulated marrow
- One bone marrow biopsy
- One or two slides of touch preps
- Samples of the biopsy for culture or special processing
- One peripheral smear

Because anticoagulated marrow is used to prepared histologic sections and is required for many special studies, enough must be submitted to complete the tests requested.

Communicating with a pathologist before obtaining bone marrow samples is important. As the options for processing marrow have increased, the practitioner must be cognizant of how to prepare these specimens to take full advantage of the diagnostic tests available. The expertise of a well-informed pathologist serves as an invaluable aid in this regard.

Staining and Special Procedures

Bone marrow may be examined in many ways, depending on how it is prepared and stained. Know in advance what information is sought and direct the preparation of the marrow specimens accordingly. Although several stains are applied routinely, others must be specially ordered as dictated by the clinical situation.

TABLE 3-5. Processing of Bone Marrow Aspirate

Desired Test*	Requirement
Wright–Giemsa stain	Air-dried smear
Hematoxylin and eosin stain	Histologic sections
Iron stains	Air-dried smear
	Histologic sections
	Fat layer from buffy coat preparation
Histochemical stains	Air-dried smear
	Buffy coat smear
Immunohistochemical stains	Air-dried smear
	Air-dried cytospin smear
Cytogenetics	Anticoagulated sample
Flow cytometry	Anticoagulated sample
DNA/RNA for Southern/Northern blots	Anticoagulated sample
Electron microscopy	Anticoagulated sample
Microbiologic cultures	Anticoagulated sample
Bone marrow cultivation	Anticoagulated sample

* See text for description of each stain or procedure. In general, EDTA-anticoagulated samples are submitted; although 1 to 2 mL of aspirated marrow usually is sufficient for most procedures, this may vary among laboratories.

TABLE 3-6. Processing of Bone Marrow Biopsy

Desired Test	Requirement
Touch prep	Glass slide
Hematoxylin and eosin stain	Paraffin-embedded section
Plastic sections	Karnovsky's fixative
Immunohistochemical stains	Cryostat section
Reticulin stain	Paraffin-embedded section
Microbiologic cultures	Sterile culture tube

Wright-Giemsa Stain. The most commonly used stain, Wright-Giemsa stain, contains a combination of acidic and basic components that produce a variety of color reactions; it is used to stain marrow smears. Acid tissue components such as nuclear DNA and cytoplasmic RNA stain blue with basic stains, whereas acid stains color hemoglobin and eosinophilic granules pink.[43] In well-stained specimens, the nuclei of neutrophils and lymphocytes stain deep blue and those of monocytes, light bluish purple. The cytoplasm of neutrophils stains pink and that of lymphocytes, light blue. Neutrophilic granules stain purple, eosinophilic granules stain orange, and basophilic granules stain deep violet. Erythrocytes appear pink to rose, whereas platelets contain a central reddish purple granule with a light blue halo.

Prussian Blue Stain. Gomori's Prussian blue stain is used to identify nonheme iron in the iron storage compound ferritin and hemosiderin.[44] Acid ferrocyanide reacts with ferric ions in these compounds to yield a characteristic Prussian blue pigment. For best results, the stain is applied to smears or sections of marrow particles, the latter producing more reliable results.[45] The fatty layer obtained from buffy coat preparations is an excellent substrate for iron staining (Fig. 3-6). Particulate iron is observed intracellularly in macrophages, sideroblasts (nucleated red blood cells), and siderocytes (anucleated red blood cells) and should be evaluated for amount, particle size, and distribution within cells. A crude scale designates marrow iron content as absent or markedly decreased, present or increased, and it is prone to observational error.

A more quantitative appraisal of marrow iron can be determined after examining 50 or more oil immersion fields. If no iron is observed, the amount of marrow iron is scored as 0; if only rare intracellular iron granules are identified, the marrow is scored as trace; if iron granules are seen occasionally, but fewer than normal, the marrow is graded as +. A normal amount of iron (iron granules observed in 10% or more of the fields) in the iron marrow is classified as 2+; considerable amounts of iron in every field is scored as 3+; and a considerable degree of iron excess is graded as 4+.[46] Macrophage iron is represented as finely granular particles and, in normal marrows, as many as 40% of normoblasts contain one to four small iron granules.[47] Siderocytes are rarely observed in marrow preparations. In the sideroblastic anemias, iron granules are large and multiple (usually more than six) and they aggregate in a perinuclear arc extending around one third or more of the nucleus, thus forming the ringed sideroblast.

Reticulin Stain. Paraffin-embedded sections of the bone marrow biopsy are treated with silver impregnations to demonstrate reticulin fibers that are increased in myelofibrosis. Using this method, the fibers stain black to deep purple. Collagen fibers are coarser and stain with trichrome stains. Bone marrow reticulin is quantitated as follows[48]:

0 No reticulin fibers demonstrable
N Occasional fine individual fibers only

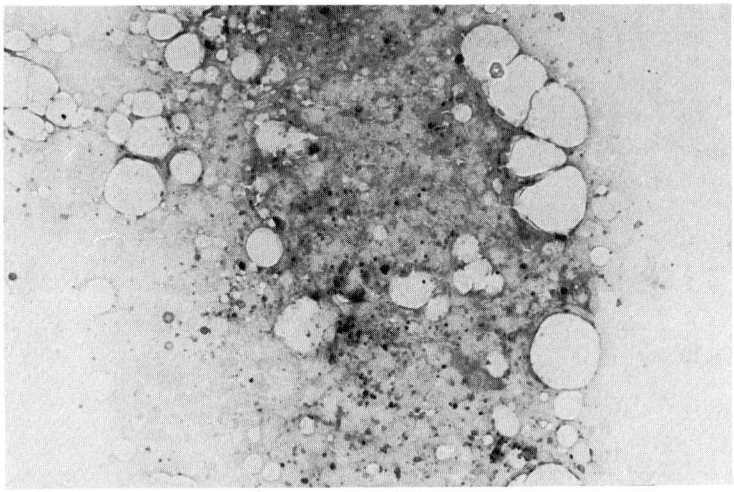

FIGURE 3-6. Iron stain of the fat layer from a buffy coat preparation of a bone marrow aspirate (Prussian blue, ×250). (See Color Fig. 3-6.)

1+ Occasional fine individual fibers, plus foci of fine fiber network
2+ Fine fiber network throughout most of the section; no coarse fibers demonstrated
3+ Diffuse fiber network with scattered thick, coarse fibers but no true collagen (negative trichrome stain)
4+ Diffuse, often coarse, fiber network with areas of collagenization (positive trichrome stain)

Histochemical Stains. Histochemical stains take advantage of the cytochemistry of bone marrow elements of specific lineages and most commonly are used to categorize the leukemias. For this purpose, aspirate smears or buffy coat preparations are stained. The specificities of these stains for identifying individual cell types are demonstrated in Table 3-7.

Immunohistochemical Stains. Advances in understanding of the immunologic changes during the maturation and differentiation of myeloid,[49] lymphoid,[50,51] and erythrocytic cells have resulted in the development of immunohistologic and immunocytologic techniques capable of identifying these changes.[52,53] The production of monoclonal antibodies directed against antigens of normal and neoplastic cells made this technology possible (Table 3-8).

TABLE 3-7. Histochemical Stains

Stain	Targets Positively Stained
Myeloperoxidase	Neutrophils and eosinophils
Sudan black B	Neutrophils and eosinophils
Specific esterase	
Naphthol AS-D chloracetate	Neutrophils
Nonspecific esterases	
α-Naphthyl acetate esterase	Monocytes (inhibited by sodium fluoride)
α-Naphthyl butyrate esterase	Monocytes
Periodic acid–Schiff	Neutrophils (diffuse granular pattern)
	Monocytes (weakly positive)
	Lymphoblasts (in ALL, coarse granular pattern)
	Erythroleukemia (blasts and erythroid precursors)
Muramidase	Neutrophils and monocytes

ALL, acute lymphoblastic leukemia.
(Prepared with J. Khorsand)

Most monoclonal antibodies react against cell surface antigens, which disintegrate after routine fixation and paraffin embedding procedures. For this reason, air-dried aspirate smears, cytospin preparations or cryostat sections of bone marrow biopsies are used when immunoperoxidase staining is applied.

A variety of antibody-conjugated enzymes are used as markers after the marrow preparation has been exposed to a specific monocolonal antibody. The most widely used immunoperoxidase techniques are the peroxidase–antiperoxidase and the avidin–biotin methods[54,55] (Fig. 3-7). In the bone marrow, the presence of endogenous peroxidase in erythrocytes and granulocytes may limit their usefulness. This problem is eliminated by substituting alkaline phosphatase for peroxidase as in the alkaline phosphatase–antialkaline phosphatase method.[56–58] This technique has become an excellent diagnostic tool especially in immunophenotyping leukemias using air-dried smears or cytospin preparations.

Flow Cytometry. The flow cytometer senses electronic and optical signals from cells illuminated by laser or mercury arc light. With this technology, a fluorescent dye, such as fluorescein, is conjugated to a monoclonal antibody, samples of bone marrow cells are stained, and specific cell surface antigens (CSA) are recognized.[59] The fluorescence characteristic of each cell in the sample is measured and displayed as frequency histograms, two-parameter dot plots, or contour maps. Although immunophenotypic analysis of human lymphocytes by flow cytometry is performed routinely, myeloid and megakaryocytic elements may be examined as well, with the major limitation being the availability and quality of appropriate monoclonal antibodies.

A sample of EDTA-anticoagulated bone marrow aspirate is submitted and prepared using a density gradient separation medium to isolate lymphocytes from myeloid cells. A particular cell fraction is stained with fluorescein-conjugated antibody and should be quantitated within 24 hours of obtaining the marrow specimen.

Antibodies directed against the antigens listed in Table 3-8 can be applied to the marrow in differentiating T-cell, B-cell, and myeloid malignancies as is done for leukemia and lymphoma phenotyping. For example, the common acute lymphocytic leukemia antigen (CALLA) recognizes pre–B and early B cells normally and is present in up to 90% of acute lymphocytic leukemias.[60] Although some technical difficulties arise when processing bone marrow specimens by this method, flow cytometry is a powerful adjunct to the evaluation of bone marrow morphology.[61]

TABLE 3-8. Selected Cell Surface Markers

Antigen	CD	Lineage Restriction/ Stage of Differentiation
T LYMPHOCYTES		
T11	CD2	T cells
T3	CD3	T cells
T4	CD4	T cells (helper/inducer)
T8	CD8	T cells (suppressor/cytotoxic)
T10	—	T cells, plasma cells, myeloid progenitors
T6	CD1	T cells, Langerhans' cells
IL2R	CD25	Activated T cells, B cells, monocytes
Ia	—	Activated T cells, B cells, monocytes
B LYMPHOCYTES		
CALLA	CD10	Pre-B cells, granulocytes
B1	CD20	B cells
B2	CD21	B cells
B4	CD19	B cells
sIg	—	B cells
PCA-1	—	Plasma cells, myeloid cells
BA-1	CD24	B cells, granulocytes
MYELOID CELLS		
My7	W13	CFU-GEMM, CFU-GM, granulocytes, monocytes
My9		CFU-GEMM, CFU-GM, promyelocytes, monocytes
My10		CFU-GM, myeloblasts, monoblasts
Mo1, My8	CD11	Myeloblasts, granulocytes, monocytes
Mo2, My4, UCHM1	W14	Promonocytes, monocytes

CD, cluster designation; CALLA, common acute lymphocytic leukemia antigen; CFU-GEMM, colony-forming unit–granulocyte–erythroid–macrophage–megakaryocyte; CFU-GM, colony-forming unit–granulocyte–macrophage; sIg, surface immunoglobulin; IL2R, interleukin-2 receptor.

(Adapted from Freedman A, Nadler LM. Cell surface markers in hematologic malignancies. Semin Oncol 1987;14:193)

EXAMINATION OF BONE MARROW

Evaluation of Specimens

To evaluate bone marrow accurately, its composition in various age groups must be understood. Generally, yellow marrow is composed of fat and red marrow contains hematopoietic cells and adipocytes in addition to plasma, stromal cells, and reticulum.

The marrow of the newborn is devoid of fat. After birth, red marrow is replaced by yellow marrow beginning in the distal extremities and proceeding centripetally (Fig. 3-8). As noted previously, red marrow in the adult is most abundant in the central skeleton, primarily in the skull, sternum, ribs, spine, and pelvis. This distribution has been documented by radionuclide scanning.[62]

Wright-Giemsa–stained marrow smears are scanned at 10× magnification to assess cellularity, megakaryoctyes, and clumps of abnormal (nonhematologic) cells. Cellularity is better assessed on the bone marrow biopsy, but no consensus regarding quantification of cellularity exists. Problems assessing cellularity include sampling error, since only a minor portion of total marrow volume is reviewed, and observer error, which is most dramatically demonstrated in mild or moderate changes in cellularity. Only when marrow hypocellularity is severe (less than 15% to 20% of normal), can cellularity be recognized reproducibly as abnormal.[63] Absolute measurement of marrow cellularity is tedious and not performed routinely.[64]

In general, about 80% of marrow is cellular during the first decade of life, declining to 50% in a 30-year-old and decreasing further after a person reaches 70 years.[65] The mean percent of hematopoietic tissue from the iliac crest by age has been measured and can be used as points of reference as follows: under 10 years, 78.8%; 10 to 19 years, 64.3%; 20 to 29 years, 58%; 30 to 39 years, 47.6%; 40 to 49 years, 48.2%; 50 to 59 years, 46.3%; 60 to 69 years, 45.7%; and 70 to 79 years, 28.9%.[65]

A complication is that the quantity of hematopoietic tissue varies from site to site; therefore, cellularity may vary from particle to particle within the same bone marrow aspirate.[65,66] Conclusions based on isolated bone marrow examinations must be tentative. The bone marrow is too large an organ to be evaluated accurately by the small volumes obtained by aspirates or biopsies.

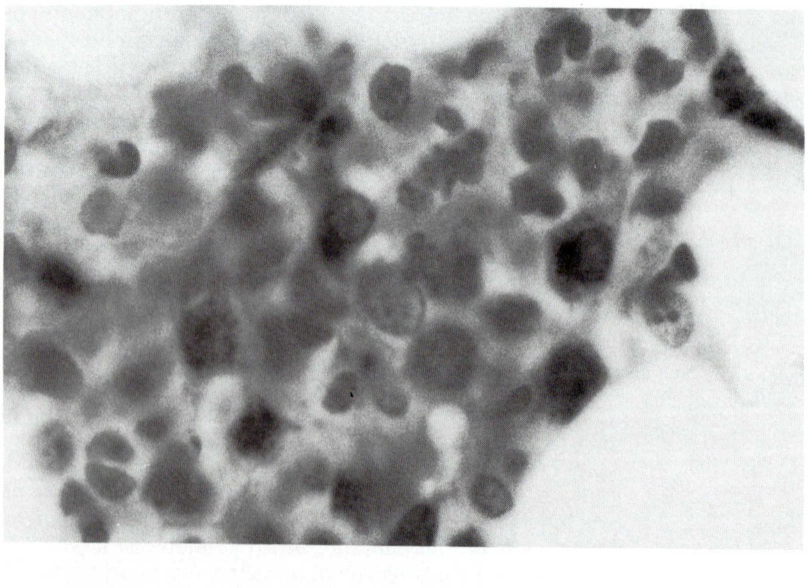

FIGURE 3-7. Immunohistochemical staining of plasma cells with anti-κ antibody using the avidin–biotin complex method. Note the intracytoplasmic staining of antibody (×1000). (See Color Fig. 3-7.) (Courtesy of Dr. Jila Khorsand)

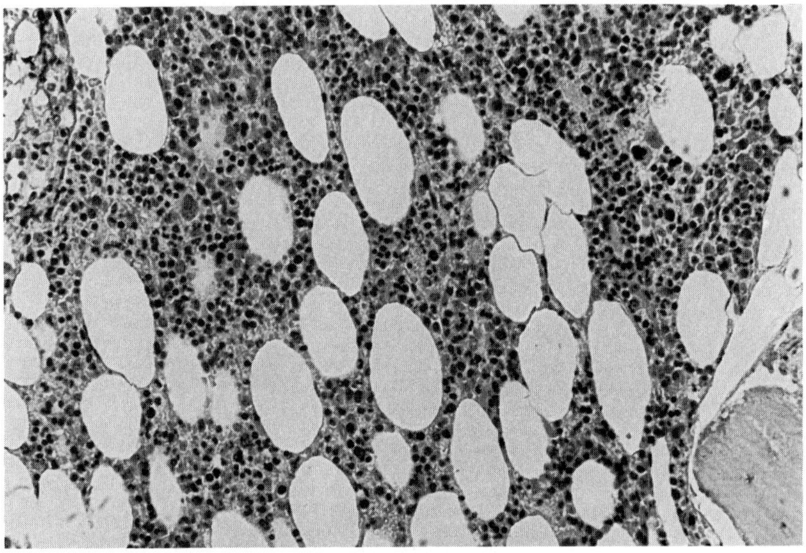

FIGURE 3-8. Normal bone marrow biopsy showing distribution of cells, fat, and trabecular bone (×250). (See Color Fig. 3-8.)

Quantitation of Marrow Elements

Quantitation of hematopoietic cells in the marrow should be performed on aspirate smears at high-power magnification under oil immersion. Normal differential counts for adults are listed in Table 3-9. A total of 300 to 500 cells should be examined in well-stained, evenly spread areas on paired slides after scanning several smears for optimal quality. The percentage of each cell type is calculated and the myeloid/erythroid (M/E) ratio noted. Although normally 2.5:3.1, the ratio is unchanged in cases in which both series are depressed or increased equally. Although a rough guide of normalcy, the M/E ratio is semiquantitative at best. The normal morphology of cells of the myeloid series and the erythroid series is shown in Figures 3-9 through 3-12 and Figures 3-13 and 3-14, respectively.

TABLE 3-9. Differential Counts of Bone Marrow Aspirates From 20 Normal Adults

Cell Type	Mean (%)	Range (%)
Neutrophil series	56.0	45.1–66.5
Myeloblasts	1.0	0.5–1.8
Promyelocytes	3.4	2.6–4.6
Myelocytes	11.9	8.1–16.9
Metamyelocytes	18.0	9.8–25.3
Band forms	11.0	8.5–20.8
Segmented forms	10.7	8.0–16.0
Eosinophil series	3.2	1.2–6.2
Myelocytes	0.9	0.3–1.9
Metamyelocytes	1.4	0.5–2.3
Band forms	1.0	0.3–2.7
Segmented forms	0.9	1.1–1.7
Basophil series	<0.1	0.0–0.2
Erythroid series	21.5	14.2–30.4
Proerythroblasts	0.6	0.2–1.4
Basophilic erythroblasts	2.0	0.7–3.7
Polychromatophilic erythroblasts	12.4	12.2–24.2
Orthochromatic erythroblasts	6.5	2.0–22.7
Lymphocytes	15.8	10.8–22.7
Monocytes	1.8	0.2–2.8
Plasma cells	1.8	0.2–2.2
Reticulum cells	0.3	0.0–0.5
Megakaryocytes	<0.1	0.0–0.2

(Jandl JH. Blood: textbook of hematology. Boston, Little, Brown, 1987:27)

Megakaryocytes are best quantitated at low magnification and recorded as the number viewed per low-power field (Fig. 3-15). No normal value has been calculated, but three or four megakaryocytes per low-power field generally are observed in healthy persons.[67] Complete absence or marked abundance of megakaryocytes are appreciated easily.

Lymphocytes account for about 16% of marrow cells. Lymphoid nodules are aggregates of lymphocytes measuring about 0.3 mm in diameter with an admixture of a few macrophages, plasma cells, and mast cells, and serrated borders fashioned as lymphocytes extend into spaces between fat cells (Fig. 3-16). Up to 47% of older patients (mean age, 71.9 years) without lymphoproliferative disorders, exhibit lymphoid nodules if aspirated particles are concentrated before examination.[68] These nodules are 1.5 to 2 times more common in women. Lower figures have been reported for younger patients evaluated by routine marrow aspiration.

Other elements of normal marrow are macrophages, osteoclasts, osteoblasts, mast cells, fibroblasts, and storage cells. Macrophages, earlier known as reticulum cells or histiocytes, appear in the marrow as large cells (20 to 30 μm) with a round or oval nucleus, pale blue nucleoli, and a cytoplasm composed of fine reticulin fibers (Fig. 3-17). They are often damaged during smearing of the aspirate, making it difficult to identify them. Mast cells or tissue basophils are identified rarely in marrow smears, but are characterized by abundant cytoplasmic blue-black granules that often obscure the nucleus, by their round or polygonal shape, and by their proximity to blood vessels (Fig. 3-18).

Osteoclasts and osteoblasts reside in the marrow to direct the degradation, growth, and remodeling of bone. They are evident rarely in marrow aspirates, surfacing in the course of a variety of rare pathologic conditions. Osteoclasts are huge, outdistancing the diameter of any other marrow resident (100 μm or larger; Fig. 3-19) and multinucleated with indistinct margins, and they contain cytoplasmic azurophilic granules. Their nuclei are composed of moderately fine chromatin filaments and contain at least one nucleolus.

(text continues on page 73)

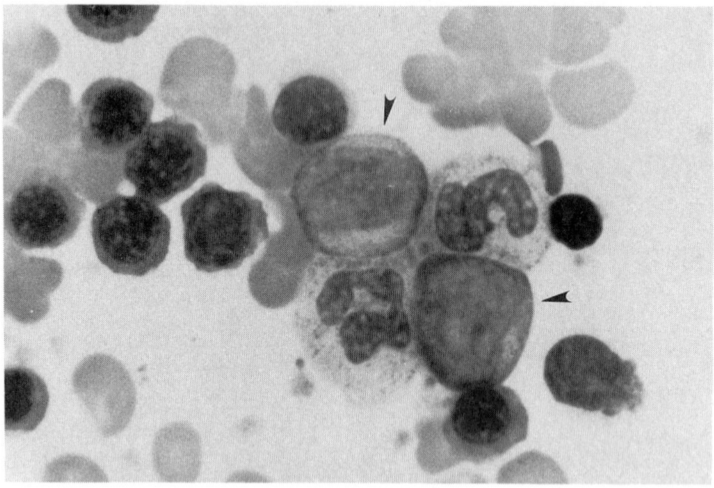

FIGURE 3-9. Myeloblasts (*arrows*; ×1000). (See Color Fig. 3-9.)

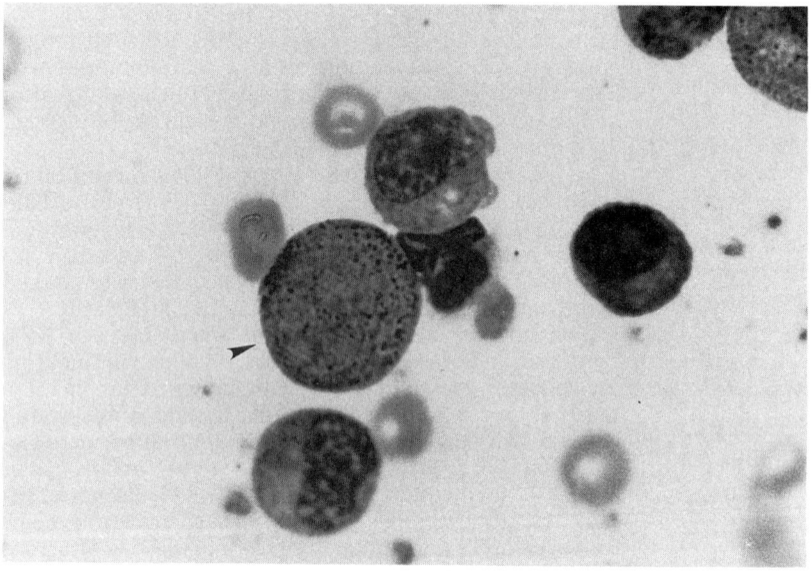

FIGURE 3-10. Promyelocyte (*arrow*; ×1000). (See Color Fig. 3-10.)

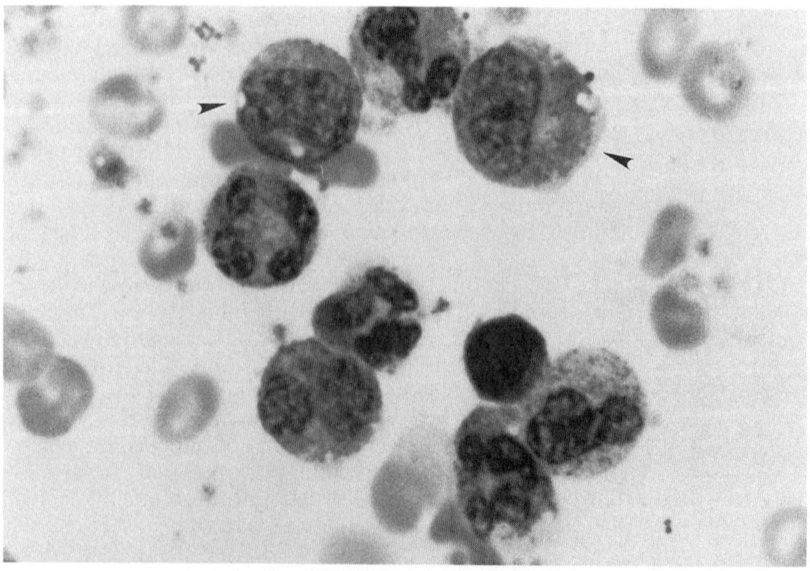

FIGURE 3-11. Myelocytes (*arrows*; ×1000). (See Color Fig. 3-11.)

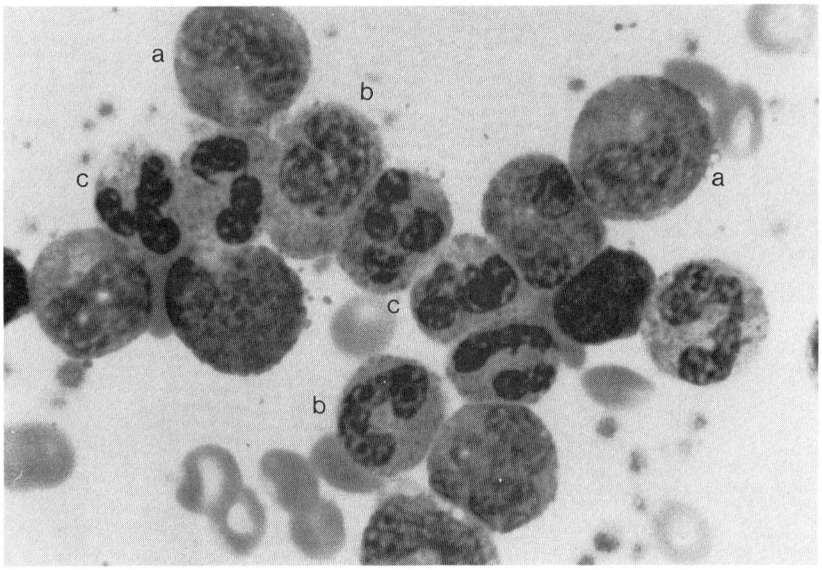

FIGURE 3-12. Metamyelocytes (a), bands (b), and segmented neutrophils (c; ×1000). (See Color Fig. 3-12.) (Courtesy of Dr. Jila Khorsand)

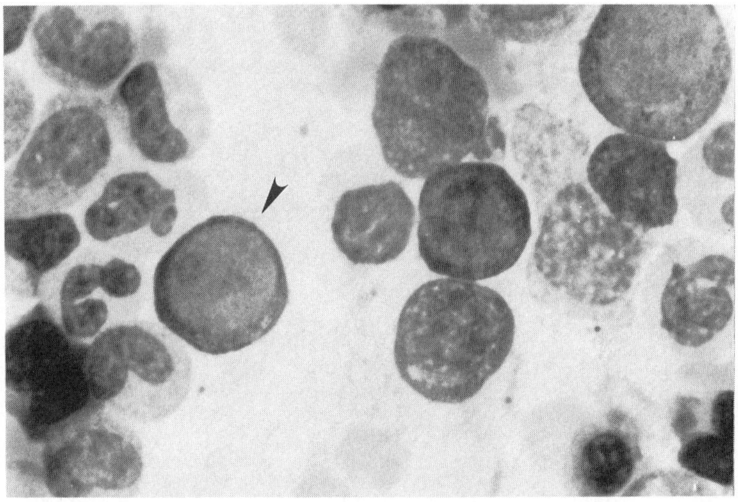

FIGURE 3-13. Proerythroblast (*arrow*; ×1000). (See Color Fig. 3-13.)

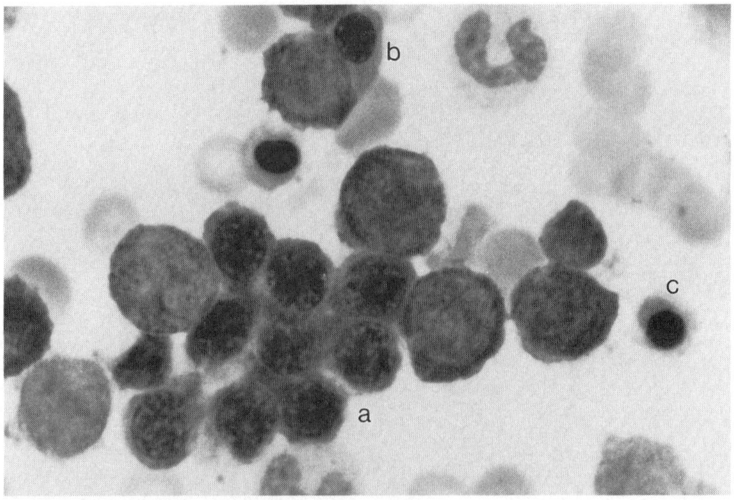

FIGURE 3-14. Basophilic erythroblasts (a), polychromatophilic erythroblasts (b), and orthochromatic erythroblasts (c) (×1000). (See Color Fig. 3-14.) (Courtesy of Dr. Jila Khorsand)

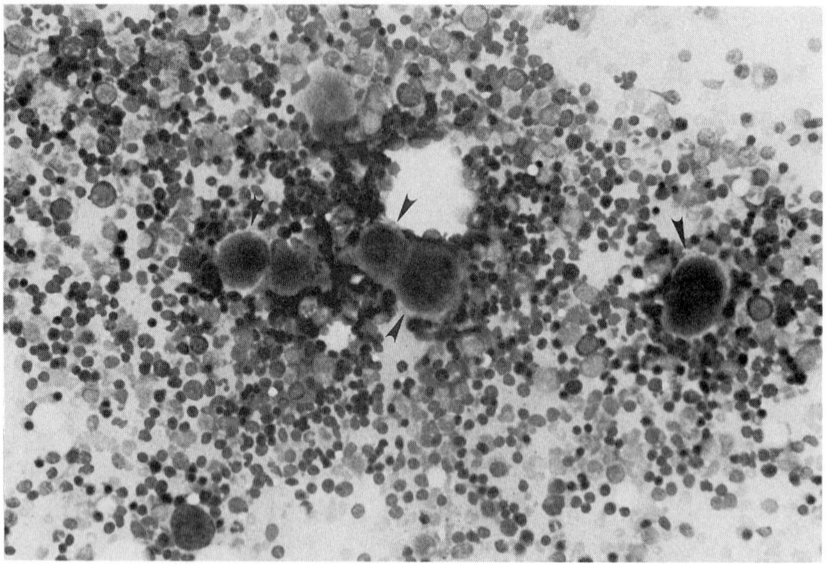

FIGURE 3-15. Megakaryocytes in a bone marrow aspirate (*arrows*; ×250). (See Color Fig. 3-15.)

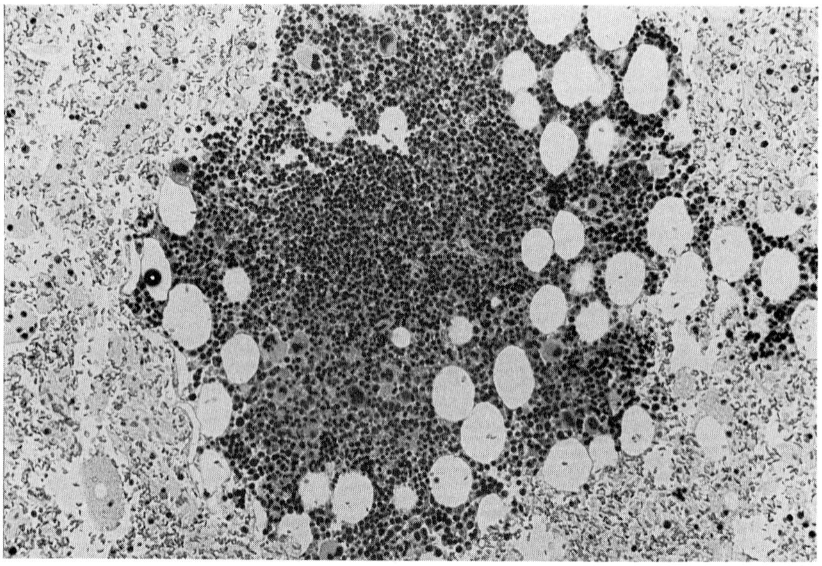

FIGURE 3-16. Lymphoid nodule in a bone marrow aspirate (×160). (See Color Fig. 3-16.) (Courtesy of Dr. Jila Khorsand)

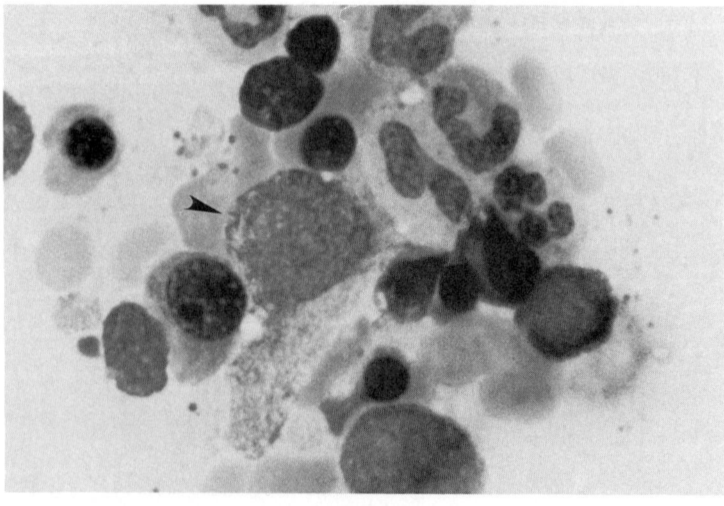

FIGURE 3-17. Reticulum cell (*arrow*; ×1000). (See Color Fig. 3-17.) (Courtesy of Dr. Jila Khorsand)

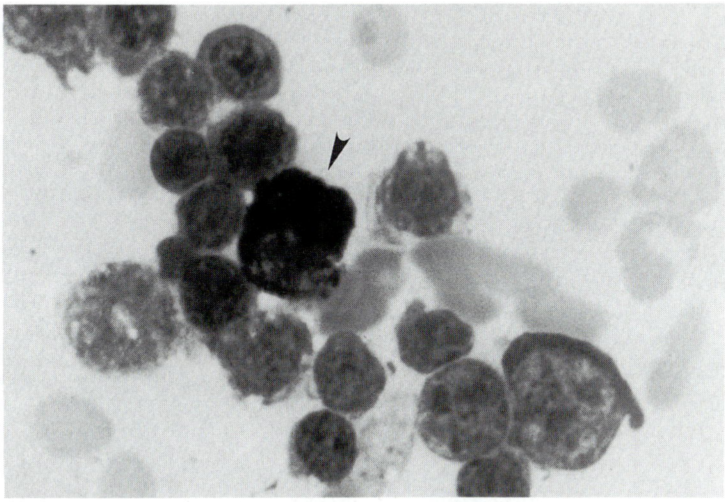

FIGURE 3-18. Mast cell (*arrow*; ×1000). (See Color Fig. 3-18.)

Osteoblasts are smaller cells (up to 30 μm), which tend to be grouped with eccentric nuclei and pale blue nucleoli resembling plasma cells (Fig. 3-20). The cytoplasm is a pale bluish gray, generally devoid of granules.

Gaucher's disease and Niemann-Pick disease are inherited lipidoses in which glucocerebroside accumulates in leukocytes in the former and sphingomyelin accumulates in the latter. During their death, this cellular debris is scavenged by monocytes and macrophages in the marrow resulting in storage cells with characteristic morphologies. Gaucher cells are round to oval with eccentrically placed nuclei and a faintly stained fibrillary appearance of the cytoplasm. Pseudo-Gaucher cells are observed in chronic myelogenous leukemia. Although indistinguishable from true Gaucher cell, methods for differentiating the two have been described[69,70] (Fig. 3-21). Storage cells in Niemann-Pick disease are up to 90 μm in diameter, with a foamy cytoplasm caused by an abundance of lipid-filled droplets that differentiate these cells from the typical Gaucher cell.

Ceroid-containing histiocytes (sea blue histiocytes) are mononuclear cells containing peroxidized fatty acids that appear blue-green after application of Wright-Giemsa stain (Fig. 3-22). They are large (50 to 60 μm) with an eccentric nucleus possessing a single nucleolus and often vacuolated cytoplasm. These histiocytes may be observed in persons with the lipidoses, chronic myelogenous leukemia, acute leukemia, other assorted disorders, and the sea blue histiocyte syndrome, which is characterized by its benign course, splenomegaly, thrombocytopenia, and numerous sea blue histiocytes in the bone marrow.[71,72]

SPECIAL CONDITIONS

Acquired Immunodeficiency Syndrome

Although the bone marrow in patients with acquired immunodeficiency syndrome (AIDS) has been characterized, no pathognomonic feature has been delineated.[73–75] Of marrows studied, 15% to 20% are hypocellular, and over 80% reveal a polyclonal plasmacytosis and iron studies consistent with the anemia of chronic disease. Of patients with *Mycoplasma avium-intracellulare* cultured from bone marrow biopsy specimens (20%), over 50% do not exhibit granulomas in the marrow. Unsuspected B-cell lymphomas and lymphoplasmacytic aggregates progressing to lymphoma rarely are discovered (2% to 3%) if marrows are performed on a series of AIDS patients for heterogeneous indications.

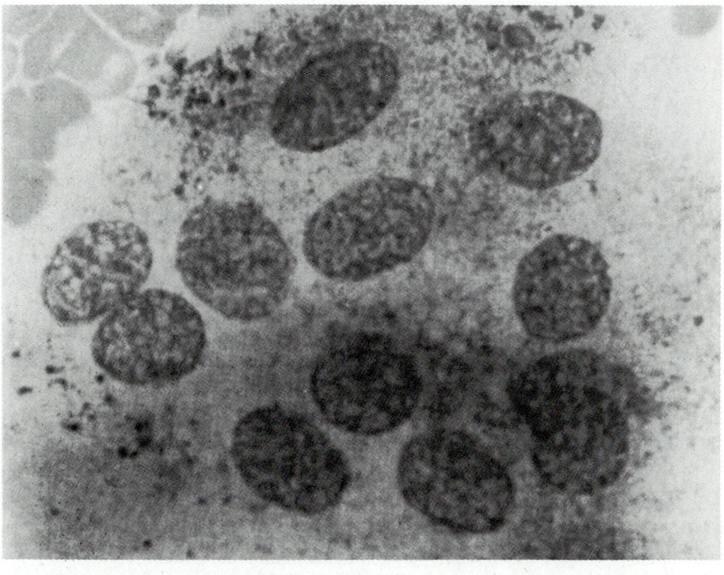

FIGURE 3-19. Osteoclast (×2000). (See Color Fig. 3-19.)

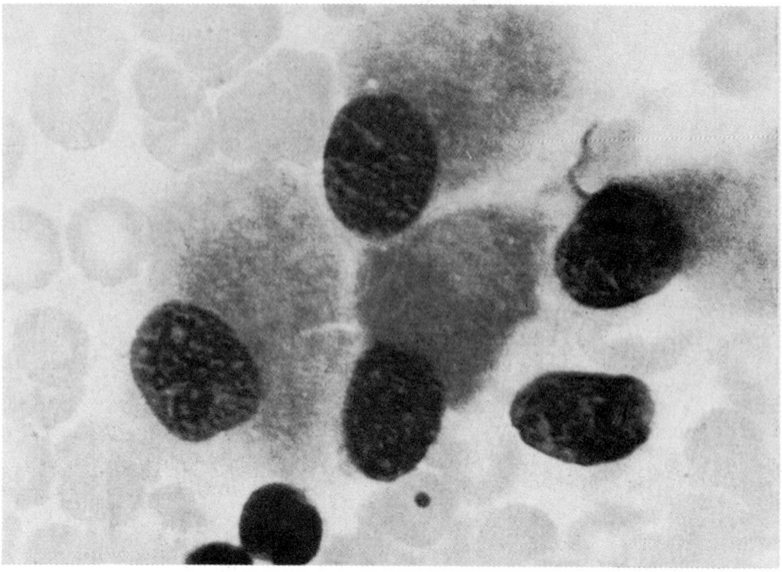

FIGURE 3-20. Osteoblast (×2000). (See Color Fig. 3-20.)

Myelofibrosis

Replacement of hematopoietic tissue and fat in the bone marrow is termed myelofibrosis. Myelofibrosis occurs in a variety of bony diseases, metastatic carcinoma, inflammatory disorders, and hematopoietic diseases, including agnogenic myeloid metaplasia, chronic leukemias, polycythemia vera, megakaryoblastic leukemia, and essential thrombocythemia, and it occurs as a familial syndrome.[76,77] Myelofibrosis may be localized or diffuse and is correlated with age, sex, marrow cellularity, anatomic site, and method of obtaining the bone marrow specimen. The amount of marrow reticulin may vary from particle to particle, but remember that reticulin normally is concentrated around blood vessels and bone spicules.[78]

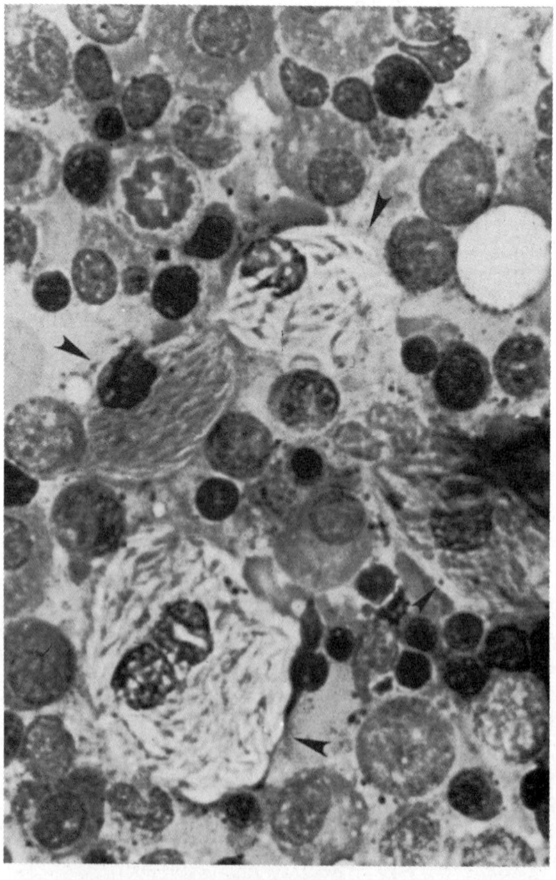

FIGURE 3-21. Pseudo-Gaucher cells (*arrows*; ×600). (See Color Fig. 3-21.) (Kapff CT, Jandl JH. Blood: atlas and sourcebook of hematology. Boston, Little, Brown, 1981:91)

Bone Marrow Necrosis

Bone marrow necrosis with gelatinous transformation has been described in patients with anorexia nervosa and involuntary starvation.[79] Its association with other diseases is not well established. Fat necrosis occurs in infarcts, fracture sites, malignancy, and pancreatitis. Macrophages surround necrotic fat cells and become glutted with their fatty debris, resulting in their designation as *foam cells.*

Granulomas

Granulomas form when mononuclear phagocytes react to inflammation, aggregate into discrete nodules, and sometimes coalesce, resulting in the genesis of multinucleated giant cells. When these cells exhibit eosinophilic cytoplasm and form compact masses activated by T-cell–mediated immune reactions, they are known as epithelioid granulomas, which may necrose centrally as seen in tuberculosis. Nonnecrotic granulomas are characteristic for sarcoidosis. Epithelioid granulomas also are a feature of leprosy, lymphogranuloma venereum, tularemia, cat-scratch fever, syphilis, infectious mononucleosis, brucellosis, histoplasmosis, lymphomas, Hodgkin's disease, and other fungal diseases.[80] Infection (frequently primarily histoplasmosis) and malignancy (primarily lymphoma) account for more than 50% of all diseases associated with bone marrow granulomas.[81]

Lipoid granulomas are composed of fat-laden macrophages, plasma cells, lymphocytes, mast cells, and eosinophils, and they are the most common granulomas encountered in the marrow (9%).[82] Their clinical significance is unclear.

Metastatic Tumor Cells

Metastatic tumor cells to the bone marrow are recognized most easily in histologic sections of aspirated particles or bone marrow biopsy. The two procedures are complementary.[83,84] The preparation should be viewed under low power, because metastatic carcinoma cells are large and

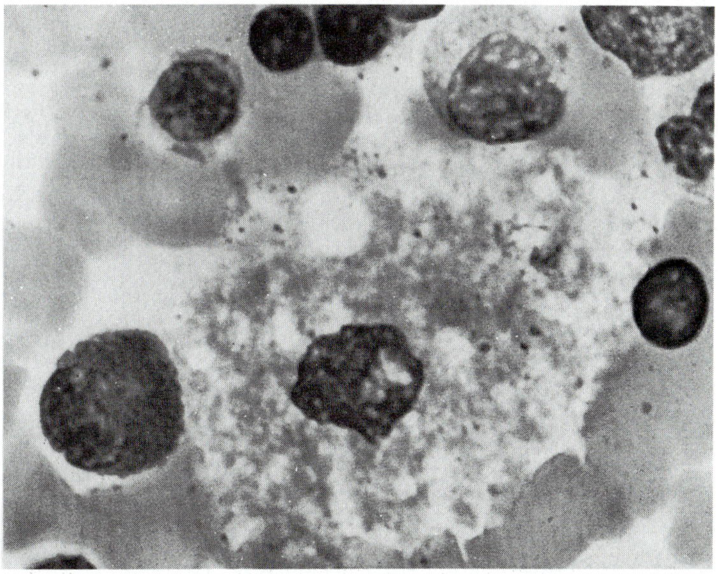

FIGURE 3-22. Sea blue histiocytes (×1260). (See Color Fig. 3-22.) (Kapff CT, Jandl JH. Blood: atlas and sourcebook of hematology. Boston, Little, Brown, 1981:91)

grouped, and may completely replace the marrow elements. They tend to resemble the pattern of the primary neoplasm. In patients with various malignancies, the incidence of a dry tap is 6.6% and in these cases touch preparations are invaluable.[85,86]

Bone marrow examination has been used as a staging procedure in a variety of malignancies. Although routinely performed in patients with small cell carcinoma of the lung in whom the incidence of bone marrow involvement may be as high as 45%, most patients with positive marrows exhibit metastatic disease elsewhere, since only 1.7% had extensive disease based on bone marrow biopsy alone in one series.[87,88] In patients with breast carcinoma, only 1.6% evidenced marrow metastases when radiologic examination of the skeleton was negative. This incidence jumps to 28% when bony metastases are demonstrable.[89]

For prostatic carcinoma, acid phosphatase levels in the bone marrow may be helpful in diagnosing early metastases.[90] Although generally useful in staging patients with nonhematologic malignancies, the use of the bone marrow examination should be individualized based on these and similar data. Common artifacts simulating tumor cells in the marrow include megakaryocytic nuclei, platelet clumping, and clumping of erythroblasts.[91]

Because treatment for the lymphomas has become increasingly sophisticated, accurate staging is of paramount importance. As a staging procedure, bone marrow biopsy is important for patients with non-Hodgkin's lymphoma, regardless of initial stage, and yields positive results nearly twice as often as smears of aspirated marrow.[92] Bilateral sampling increases the yield by about 20% over unilateral biopsies.[93] In patients with Hodgkin's disease, the incidence of positive bone marrow metastases is stage related. From 12% to 25% of patients with stage III disease are upstaged to stage IV after bone marrow biopsy even though the initial aspirates were negative.[94,95] Bilateral biopsies increase the diagnostic yield.[93] The reader should be aware of continued controversy regarding the frequency with which bone marrow biopsy alters patient management in Hodgkin's disease.[96,97]

Pediatric Malignancies

Bone marrow aspiration and biopsy are complimentary procedures in the workup for metastases in children with solid tumors. In one series of children with nonhematologic malignancies, the bone marrow biopsy was positive in 45%, and in slightly more than 50% of these, the aspirate was nondiagnostic. Conversely, the aspirate was positive in 55% of cases when the biopsy was negative and, in 21%, both the biopsy and the aspirate were diagnostic.[98] Neuroblastoma, which frequently metastasizes to the marrow, can be identified in marrow biopsies or aspirates in at least 50% of cases.[99]

REPORTING OF RESULTS

The bone marrow report should be orderly, consistent, and logically organized to provide the optimal amount of information gleaned from the study. The peripheral smear is described after reviewing each cell series under low-power magnification, then under high-power magnification using oil immersion. The quantity and morphology of each cell line are recorded and any foreign cells or parasites are noted. This information is crucial to the accurate interpretation of the findings in the bone marrow.

Descriptions of the bone marrow aspirate and biopsy should be reported separately, but in an orderly fashion. Smears and sections stained routinely and with iron stains are reported first, followed by any special stains or procedures performed on the specimens. For each slide reviewed, the following information should be provided:

- Cellularity
- M/E ratio
- Morphology, quantitation, and maturation of the erythroid, myeloid, and megakaryocytic series
- Description of lymphocytes and plasma cells
- Presence and distribution of hemosiderin
- Stromal reactions
- Bony and vascular lesions
- Presence and description of foreign cells

Additional information provided by special stains, flow cytometry, cytogenetics, electron microscopy, and other specialized procedures should be included at this point if available. A diagnosis, in morphologic terms, is rendered and a section for additional comments is included. The purpose of the latter is to provide the reviewer with an opportunity to correlate the morphologic diagnoses with clinical diagnoses to the extent that the data at hand allow.

NEWER TECHNIQUES: BONE MARROW IMAGING

The bone marrow may be imaged by one of several methods including scintigraphy, computed tomography, and magnetic resonance imaging.

Scintigraphy uses a transferrin-bound isotope to yield a direct physiologic assessment of hematopoiesis or the mononuclear phagocyte system (RES) and an indirect evaluation of total marrow function by surveying surrounding osseous structures. For erythropoietic marrow imaging, radiolabeled iron (^{52}Fe) is the prototypic tracer used,[100] whereas technetium-99m (^{99m}Tc) sulfur colloid is infused for imaging the RES. Although erythropoietic marrow and the RES can be imaged individually, distribution of the isotope in each case is similar. Indirect imaging assesses bone remodeling using the labeled colloid ^{99m}Tc diphosphonate. Radioiron and colloid isotopes provide equally sensitive studies, but lack of anatomic detail and low specificity are drawbacks of scintigraphy in general.[101]

Images produced by computed tomography (CT) occur as an x-ray beam is attenuated by marrow elements of varying electron densities. Fatty marrow generates low-density images, whereas hematopoietic marrow and trabecular bone yield higher-density images with positive Hounsfield values. Thus, the appearance of computed tomograms are location dependent and should be compared with contralateral views. CT provides excellent anatomic detail: trabecular bone is well defined, and some separation of fatty and hematopoietic marrow can be made.[102]

Magnetic resonance imaging (MRI) generates the most detailed evaluation of all bone marrow elements. The biophysical differences of bone marrow tissues resulting in variations in MRI scans include proton density and T1 and T2 relaxation times.[103] Although spin-echo sequences with T1- and T2-weighted images are used frequently, newer approaches are under investigation.[104,105]

Yellow marrow produces a signal similar to that of subcutaneous fat, whereas red marrow is hypodense in comparison.[106] In sites with increased red marrow fractions such as the spine, the signal intensity is lower than in locations predominantly populated with fatty marrow (distal skeleton). As conversion of red to yellow marrow proceeds with age, focal replacement with fat is demonstrated as bright spots on T1 images.[107] Bony trabeculae appear as bands of low-signal intensity on short and long repetition time–echo delay sequences (TR/TE).

MRI reliably can identify infiltrative lesions in the marrow, but is unable to delineate tissue histology, and the appearances of images overlap for benign and malignant processes.[108] Specific patterns for leukemic infiltration as well as marrow alterations after chemotherapy or radiotherapy are being described and thus MRI may evolve as a useful means of monitoring marrow changes in these patients.[109] In conditions resulting in myeloid depletion, the MRI signal pattern is characteristic of fatty marrow although signal intensity varies with the clinical condition. MRI is highly sensitive for demonstrating bone marrow ischemia,[110] and bone marrow edema results in signals on short TR/TE images commensurate with the degree of increase in tissue water.[111]

REFERENCES

1. Neumann E. Ueber die Beduetung des Knochenmarks fur die Blutbildung. Centralblatt Med Wiss 1868;6:689.
2. Damashek W. Biopsy of the sternal bone marrow. Am J Med Sci 1935;190:617.
3. Frankel S, Reitman S, Sonnenwirth AC, eds. Gradwohl's clinical laboratory methods and diagnosis. St Louis, CV Mosby, 1970:652.
4. Miale JB. Laboratory medicine: hematology, 4th ed. St Louis, CV Mosby, 1972:319.
5. Sonnenwirth AC, Jarett L, eds. Gradwohl's clinical laboratory methods and diagnosis. St Louis, CV Mosby, 1980:643.
6. Larson EB, Featherstone HJ, Petersdorf RG. Fever of undetermined origin: diagnosis and follow-up of 105 cases, 1970–1980. Medicine 1982;61:269.
7. Bodem CR, Hamory BH, Taylor HM, Kleopfer L. Granulomatous bone marrow disease. Medicine 1983;62:372.
8. Sarosi GA, Voth DW, Dahl BA, Doto IL, Tosh FE. Disseminated histoplasmosis: results of long-term follow-up. Ann Intern Med 1971;75:511.
9. Smith JW, Utz JP. Progressive disseminated histoplasmosis. Ann Intern Med 1972;76:557.
10. Spink WW. The laboratory in the diagnosis of brucellosis. Am J Clin Pathol 1952;22:201.
11. Garrett TJ, Gee TS, Lieberman PH, McKenzie S, Clarkson BD. The role of bone marrow aspiration and biopsy in detecting marrow involvement by nonhematologic malignancies. Cancer 1976;38:2401.
12. Ellis LD, Wallace NJ, Westerman MP. Needle biopsy of bone and marrow. Arch Intern Med 1964;114:213.
13. Turkel H, Bethell FH. Biopsy of bone marrow performed by a new and simple instrument. J Lab Clin Med 1943;28:1246.
14. McFarland W, Damashek W. Biopsy of the bone marrow with the Vim-Silverman needle. JAMA 1958;166:1464.
15. Ellis LD, Wallace NJ, Westerman MP. Needle biopsy of bone and marrow. Arch Intern Med 1964;114:213.
16. Jamshidi K, Swaim WR. Bone marrow biopsy with unaltered architecture: A new biopsy device. J Lab Clin Med 1971;77:335.
17. Islam A. A new bone marrow biopsy needle with core securing device. J Clin Pathol 1982;35:359.
18. Pochedly C. How to perform marrow puncture in small children. Clin Pediatr (Phila) 1969;8:705.
19. Ellis RB. The distribution of active marrow in the adult. Phys Med Biol 1961;5:255.
20. Moosavi H, Lichtman MA, Donnelly JA, Churukian CJ. Plastic-embedded human marrow biopsy specimens. Arch Pathol Lab Med 1981;105:269.
21. Gatter KC, Heryet A, Brown DC, Mason DY. Is it necessary to embed bone marrow biopsies in plastic for haematological diagnosis? Histopathology 1987;11:1.
22. Gilbert EH, Earle JD, Glatstein E, Goris ML, Kaplan HS, Kriss JP. ^{111}Indium bone marrow scintigraphy as an aid in selecting marrow biopsy sites for the evaluation of marrow elements in patients with lymphoma. Cancer 1976;38:1560.
23. Gilbert EH, Goris ML, Earle JD, Kaplan HS, Kriss JP. The accuracy of $^{111}InCl_3$ as a bone marrow scanning agent. Radiology 1976;119:167.
24. Colvin BT. Practical procedures: how to biopsy the marrow. Br J Hosp Med 1980;24:176.
25. Byrnes RK, McKenna RW, Sundberg RD. Bone marrow aspiration and trephine biopsy: an approach to a thorough study. Am J Clin Pathol 1978;70:753.
26. Wolff SN, Katzanstein AL, Phillips GL, Herzig GP. Aspiration does not influence interpretation of bone marrow biopsy cellularity. Am J Clin Pathol 1983;80:60.
27. Birch CD, Fischer S, Zibell A, Jensen ME. Diagnostic bone marrow studies extended routinely by iliac crest biopsy, using the method of Schaadt-Fischer. Acta Pathol Microbiol Immunol Scand (Sect A) 1982;90:229.
28. Bearden JD, Ratkin GA, Coltman CA. Comparison of the diagnostic value of bone marrow biopsy and bone marrow aspiration in neoplastic disease. J Clin Pathol 1974;27:738.
29. Grann V, Pool JL, Mayer K. Comparative study of bone marrow and biopsy in patients with neoplastic disease. Cancer 1966;19:1898.
30. Bemis EL. Bone marrow examination. Postgrad Med 1970;48:49.
31. Bird AR, Jacobs P. Trephine biopsy of the bone marrow. S Afr Med J 1983;64:271.
32. Fisher WB. Hazard in bone marrow biopsy. N Engl J Med 1971;285:804.
33. McNutt DR, Fudenberg HH. Bone marrow biopsy and osteoporosis. N Engl J Med 1972;286:46.
34. Garnier H, Reynier J, Dimopoulos F. A propos des accidents de la ponction sternale. Ann Chir 1964;18:308.
35. Yoell JH. Bone marrow embolism to lung following sternal puncture. Arch Pathol 1959;67:373.
36. Gilsanz V, Grunebaum M. Radiographic appearance of iliac marrow biopsy sites. AJR 1977;128:597.
37. Murphy WA. Exostosis after iliac bone marrow biopsy. AJR 1977;129:114.
38. Tyler JL, Powers TA. Bone scanning after marrow biopsy. J Nuclear Med 1982;23:1085.
39. Cetto GL, Ianucci A, Perini A, Capitanio A, Alloush N, Fiore-Donati L. Bone marrow evaluation: the relative merits of particle sections and smear preparation. Appl Pathol 1983;1:181.
40. Liao KT. The superiority of histologic sections of aspirated bone marrow in malignant lymphomas. Cancer 1971;27:618.
41. Rywlin AM, Marvan P, Robinson MJ. A simple technic for the preparation of bone marrow smears and sections. Am J Clin Pathol 1970;53:389.
42. Ellis WM, Georgiou GM, Roberton DM, Johnson GR. The use of dis-

continuous percoll gradients to separate populations of cells from human bone marrow and peripheral blood. J Immunol Methods 1984;66:9.
43. Cramer AD, Rogers ER, Parker JW, Lukes RJ. The Giemsa stain for tissue sections: an improved method. Am J Clin Pathol 1973;60:148.
44. Gomori G. Microtechnical demonstration of iron. Am J Pathol 1936;12:655.
45. Lundin P, Persson E, Weinfeld A. Comparison of hemosiderin estimation in bone marrow sections and bone marrow smears. Acta Med Scand 1964;175:383.
46. Beutler E, Robson MJ, Buttenwieser E. A comparison of the plasma iron, iron-binding capacity, sternal marrow iron and other methods in the clinical evaluation of iron stores. Ann Intern Med 1958;48:60.
47. Kaplan E, Zuelzer WW, Mouriquand C. Sideroblasts: a study of stainable nonhemoglobin iron in marrow normoblasts. Blood 1954;9:203.
48. Bauermeister DE. Quantitation of bone marrow reticulin: a normal range. Am J Clin Pathol 1971;56:24.
49. Freedman A, Nadler LM. Cell surface markers in hematologic malignancies. Semin Oncol 1987;14:193.
50. Romain PL. Schlossman SF. Human T lymphocyte subsets. Functional heterogeneity and surface recognition structure. J Clin Invest 1984;74:1559.
51. Volger B. Bone marrow B-cell development. Clin Haematol 1982;11:509.
52. Falini B, Martelli MF, Tarallo F, et al. Immunohistological analysis of human bone marrow trephine biopsies using monoclonal antibodies. Br J Haematol 1984;56:365.
53. Wood GS, Warnke RA. The immunologic phenotyping of bone marrow biopsies and aspirates: frozen section techniques. Blood 1982;59:913.
54. Sternberger LA, Hardy PH Jr, Cuculis JJ, Meyer HG. The unlabeled antibody enzyme method of immunohistochemistry: preparation and properties of soluble antigen-antibody complex (horseradish peroxidase-antiperoxidase) and its use in the identification of spirochetes. J Histochem Cytochem 1970;18:35.
55. Hsu SM, Rain L, Fanger H. A comparative study of the peroxidase-antiperoxidase method and an avidin-biotin complex method for studying polypeptide hormones with radioimmunoassay antibodies. Am J Clin Pathol 1981;75:734.
56. Cordell JL, Falini B, Erber WN, et al. Immunoenzymatic labelling of monoclonal antibodies using immune complexes of alkaline phosphatase and monoclonal antialkaline phosphatase (APAAP complexes). J Histochem Cytochem 1984;32:219–229.
57. Moir DJ, Glosh AR, Abdulaziz Z, Knight PM, Mason DY. Immunoenzymatic staining of hematological samples with monoclonal antibodies. Br J Haematol 1983;55:395.
58. Neumann MP, deSolis I, Parkin JL, et al. Monoclonal antibody study of Philadelphia chromosome positive blastic leukemias using the alkaline phosphatase antialkaline phosphatase (APAAP) technique. Am J Clin Pathol 1986;85:564.
59. Steinkamp JA. Flow cytometry. Rev Sci Instrum 1984;55:1375.
60. Greaves MF. Monoclonal antibodies as probes for leukemic heterogeneity and hematopoetic differentiation. In: Knapp W, ed. Leukemia markers. New York, Academic Press, 1981:19.
61. Giorgi JV. Lymphocyte subset measurements: significance in clinical medicine. In: Rose NR, Friedman H, Fahey JL, eds. Manual of clinical laboratory immunology. Washington, American Society for Microbiology, 1986:245.
62. Dibos PE, Judisch JM, Spaulding MB, Wagner HN, McIntyre PA. Scanning the reticulendothelial system (RES) in hematological disease. Johns Hopkins Med J 1972;130:68.
63. Morley A, Blake J. Observer error in histological assessment of marrow hypocellularity. J Clin Pathol 1975;28:104.
64. Harrison WJ. The total cellularity of the bone marrow in man. J Clin Pathol 1962;15:254.
65. Hartsock RJ, Smith EB, Petty CS. Normal variations with aging of the amount of hematopoietic tissue in bone marrow from the anterior iliac crest. Am J Clin Pathol 1965;43:326.
66. Rywlin AM. Histopathology of the bone marrow. Boston, Little, Brown, 1976:22.
67. Sonnenwirth AC, Jarett L, eds. Gradwohl's clinical laboratory methods and diagnosis. St Louis, CV Mosby, 1980:643.
68. Rywlin AM, Ortega RS, Dominguez CJ. Lymphoid nodules of bone marrow: normal and abnormal. Blood 1974;43:389.
69. Lee RE, Ellis LD. The storage cells of chronic myelogenous leukemia. Lab Invest 1971;24:261.
70. Kapff CT, Jandl JH. Blood: atlas and sourcebook of hematology. Boston, Little, Brown, 1981:91.
71. Dosik H, Rosner F, Sawitsky A. Acquired lipidoses: Gaucher-like cells and "blue cells" in chronic granulocytic leukemia. Semin Hematol 1972;9:299.
72. Silverman MN, Ellefson RD, Ahern EF. The syndrome of the sea-blue histiocyte. N Engl J Med 1970;282:1.
73. Castella A, Croxson TS, Mildvan D, et al. The bone marrow in AIDS: a histologic, hematologic and microbiologic study. Am J Clin Pathol 1985;84:425.
74. Cohen RJ, Samoszuk MH, Busch D, Lagios M. Occult infections with M. intracellulare in bone marrow biopsy specimens from patients with AIDS. N Engl J Med 1983;308:1475.
75. Reichert CM, O'Leary TJ, Levens DL, Simrell CR, Smacher AM. Autopsy pathology in the acquired immunodeficiency syndrome. Am J Pathol 1983;112:357.
76. Bennett JM, Catovsky D, Daniel MT, et al. Criteria for the diagnosis of acute leukemia of megakaryocytic lineage (M7): a report of the French-American-British Cooperative Group. Ann Intern Med 1985;103:460.
77. Patakfalvi B, Csete B, Horvath T. Familial myelofibrosis. Haematologica 1969;3:217.
78. Bauermeister DE. Quantitation of bone marrow reticulin: a normal range. Am J Clin Pathol 1971;56:24.
79. Smith RRL, Spivak JL. Marrow cell necrosis in anorexia nervosa and involuntary starvation. Br J Haematol 1985;60:525.
80. Peace G. Granulomatous lesions in bone marrow. Blood 1956;11:720.
81. Bodem CR, Hamory BH, Taylor HM, Kleopfer L. Granulomatous bone marrow disease. Medicine 1983;62:372.
82. Rywlin AM, Ortega RS. Lipid granulomas of the bone marrow. Am J Clin Pathol 1972;57:457.
83. Garrett TJ, Gee TS, Lieberman PH, McKenzie S, Clarkson BD. The role of bone marrow aspiration and biopsy in detecting marrow involvement by nonhematologic malignancies. Cancer 1976;38:2401.
84. Singh G, Krause JR, Breitfield V. Bone marrow examination for metastatic tumor. Aspirate and biopsy. Cancer 1977;40:2317.
85. Engeset A, Nesheim A, Sokolowski J. Incidence of "dry tap" on bone marrow aspirations in lymphomas and carcinomas. Scand J Haematol 1979;22:417.
86. James LP, Stass SA, Schumacher HR. Value of imprint preparations of bone marrow biopsies in hematologic diagnosis. Cancer 1980;46:173.
87. Hansen HH, Muggia FM, Selawry OS. Bone-marrow examination in 100 consecutive patients with bronchogenic carcinoma. Lancet 1971;2:443.
88. Campling B, Quirt I, DeBoer G, et al. Is bone marrow examination in small-cell lung cancer really necessary? Ann Intern Med 1986;105:508.
89. Ridell B, Landys K. Incidence and histopathology of metastases of mammary carcinoma in biopsies from the posterior iliac crest. Cancer 1979;44:1782.
90. Chua DT, Veenema RJ, Muggia F, Graff A. Acid phosphatase levels in bone marrow: value in detecting early bone metastases from carcinoma of the prostate. J Urol 1970;103:462.
91. Vernon SE. Clumping of erythroblasts simulating a metastatic neoplasm. Arch Pathol Lab Med 1985;109:569.
92. Vinciguerra V, Silver RT. The importance of bone marrow biopsy in the staging of patients with lymphosarcoma. Blood 1973;41:913.
93. Brunning RD, Bloomfield CD, McKenna RW, Peterson L. Bilateral trephine bone marrow biopsies in lymphoma and other neoplastic diseases. Ann Intern Med 1975;82:365.
94. Han T, Stutzman L, Roque AL. Bone marrow biopsy in Hodgkin's disease and other neoplastic diseases. JAMA 1971;217:1239.
95. Webb DI, Ubogy G, Silver RT. Importance of bone marrow biopsy in the clinical staging of Hodgkin's disease. Cancer 1970;26:313.
96. Bennett JM, Gralnick HR, Devita VT. Bone-marrow biopsy in Hodgkin's disease. N Engl J Med 1968;278:1179.
97. Macintyre EA, Hudson BV, Linch DC, Hudson GV, Jelliffe AM. The value of staging bone marrow trephine biopsy in Hodgkin's disease. Eur J Haematol 1987;39:66.
98. Penchansky L. Bone marrow biopsy in the metastatic work-up of solid tumors in children. Cancer 1984;54:1447.
99. Gaffney PC, Hansman CF, Fetterman GH. Experience with smears of aspirates from bone marrow in the diagnosis of neuroblastoma. Am J Clin Pathol 1959;31:213.
100. Fordham EW, Amjad A. Radionuclide imaging of bone marrow. Semin Hematol 1981;18:222.
101. Datz FL, Taylor A Jr. The clinical use of radionuclide bone marrow imaging. Semin Nucl Med 1985;15:239.
102. Genant HK, Wilson JS, Bovill EG, et al. Computed tomography of the musculoskeletal system. J Bone Joint Surg 1980;62A:1088.
103. Mitchell DG, Burk DL Jr, Vinitski S, Rifkin MD. The biophysical basis of tissue contrast in extracranial MR imaging. AJR 1987;149:831.
104. Hendrick RE, Kneeland JB, Stark DD. Maximizing signal-to-noise and contrast-to-noise ratios in FLASH imaging. Magn Reson Imaging 1987;5:117.
105. Winkler ML, Ortendahl DA, Mills TC, et al. Characteristics of partial flip angle and gradient reversal MR imaging. Radiology 1988;166:17.
106. Wismer GL, Rosen BR, Buxton R, Stark DD, Brady TJ. Chemical shift imaging of bone marrow: preliminary experience. AJR 1985;145:1031.
107. Hajek PC, Baker LL, Goobar JE, et al. Focal fat deposition in axial bone marrow: MR characteristics. Radiology 1987;162:245.
108. Nyman R, Rehn S, Glimelius B, et al. Magnetic resonance imaging in diffuse malignant bone marrow disease. Acta Radiol (Diagn) 1987;28:199.
109. McKinstry CS, Steiner RE, Young AT, Jones L, Swirsky D, Aber V. Bone marrow in leukemia and aplastic anemia: MR imaging before, during and after treatment. Radiology 1987;162:701.
110. Beltran J, Herman LJ, Burk JM, et al. Femoral head avascular necrosis: MR imaging with clinical-pathologic and radionuclide correlation. Radiology 1988;166:215.
111. Vogler JB, Murphy WA. Bone marrow imaging. Radiology 1988;168:679.

Blood: Principles and Practice of Hematology,
edited by Robert I. Handin, Thomas P. Stossel, and Samuel E. Lux.
J.B. Lippincott Company, Philadelphia © 1995.

4

A Molecular Genetics Primer for the Hematologist

Hagop Youssoufian
Stuart H. Orkin

Molecular genetic technology provides a highly powerful and efficient means of analyzing cellular function, gene expression, and human disease. Although originally accessible only to laboratories dedicated to molecular biology, recombinant DNA methods are now widely applied to a variety of biomedical problems. The usefulness of recombinant DNA technology to medicine was first evident from the analysis of hematologic disorders. In this chapter, general principles and methodologic aspects of molecular genetics are described, especially those that relate to the general field of hematology. For additional background, refer to basic textbooks on cell and molecular biology.[1,2] In addition, a number of excellent manuals are also available for detailed descriptions of the techniques of recombinant DNA.[3,4]

The essence of genetics is variation. At the molecular or organismic level, variation may be viewed either as normal, termed *polymorphism*, or abnormal and disease related. Whichever the case, the ultimate reservoir of genetic variation is the DNA that constitutes the genome of an organism. Until recently, it was not feasible to establish the precise relationship between observed variation (eg, a trait or disease) and a specific change in cellular DNA. Recombinant DNA technology, largely developed throughout the past 15 years, provides the means by which a direct association between a particular phenotype and genotype can be established. A specific gene and an alteration in that gene can be related to a disease with certainty, rather than by inference. For example, if a structurally abnormal protein is found in association with a clinical disorder, analysis of the gene encoding the mutant protein provides the most fundamental demonstration of the underlying molecular pathology. An amino acid replacement, for example, may be predicted as the basis of the disorder by demonstration of a nucleotide substitution in the DNA sequence and examination of the known genetic code. The crowning glory of this approach was found in sickle cell anemia, in which case the replacement of glutamic acid by valine at the sixth amino acid position of the β-globin chain was accounted for by a single nucleotide substitution in cellular DNA.

With recombinant DNA methods, the products of genes may be produced in virtually unlimited quantities for biochemical, structural, and physiologic studies, as well as for clinical administration. Moreover, in the molecular equivalent of Koch's postulates, the introduction of genes into cells or animals has become a powerful and incisive approach to the study of normal gene function and the consequences of specific mutations. The implications of this revolution in biology and medicine are just becoming fully appreciated. The development of recombinant DNA methods has profoundly advanced our understanding of normal cellular physiology and development, the pathophysiology of inherited disease and cancer, and the design of new approaches to therapy. Hematology has consistently been at the forefront of these developments.

COMPLEXITY AND ORGANIZATION OF THE HUMAN GENOME

The flow of genetic information is primarily from cellular DNA to messenger RNA to protein. DNA is a linear polymer of two interwoven chains (double helix) composed of four monomeric units, the deoxyribonucleotides (also called *nucleotides* or *bases*) adenine (A), cytosine (C), guanine (G), and thymine (T). Because of strict pairing rules of A to T and G to C, the sequence of the two strands of DNA is complementary.

Genetic information is present in both nuclei and mitochondria of eukaryotic cells. Although mitochondrial genes and inheritance are becoming increasingly appreciated, most of our knowledge to date has focused on the nucleus. Nuclear genes are considerably larger than the messenger RNAs (mRNAs) transcribed from them (Fig. 4-1). This was first demonstrated for genes of animal viruses and soon thereafter for mouse β-globin and immunoglobulin genes. The additional sequences, called *intervening sequences* or *introns*, interrupt split genes into two or more units. Although the precise role and function of introns has generated considerable discussion, it has been noted that they often subdivide coding regions, or *exons*, of genes into structural blocks that correspond to functional domains of proteins. Such an arrangement may provide a mechanism by which exons of eukaryotic genes are shuffled during evolution to produce new proteins from smaller units.

Transcription of eukaryotic DNA into RNA is followed by several modifications that result in translatable mRNA found in the cytoplasm. Unlike mature mRNA, the primary transcript of a eukaryotic gene, called *hnRNA*, contains intervening sequences that are removed during RNA proc-

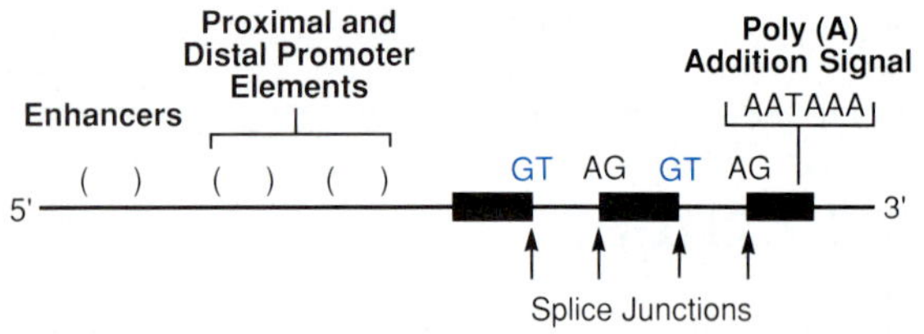

FIGURE 4-1. Schematic diagram of a prototypical eukaryotic gene illustrating the exons (*black boxes*), introns (*solid lines connecting exons*), splice junctions within introns (GT, AG), 5' regulatory elements, and a 3' polyadenylation site.

essing (*splicing*), so that the interrupted exons are joined precisely to assemble the mature mRNA. Short-sequence motifs within genes delineate the beginning and end of intervening sequences. Intervening sequences generally begin with a GT dinucleotide and end with an AG dinucleotide.

Other sequence motifs within the gene near its 3' end direct processing and polyadenylation, whereas sequences within the mRNA itself may influence mRNA stability. Within or nearby genes are additional DNA elements called *cis*-elements, which serve important regulatory functions. Just upstream of the position at which mRNA synthesis is initiated are *promoter elements* required for RNA transcription. Promoters often include short-sequence motifs, which are recognized by sequence-specific DNA-binding proteins located within the nucleus. Through the combined action of many ubiquitous and fewer cell-specific nuclear proteins, the activity of promoter elements is thought to be established.[5] In addition to promoters, *cis*-elements located considerably upstream, downstream, or even within eukaryotic genes may play major roles in regulating gene expression, especially transcription within specialized cell types. Although such DNA elements, called *enhancers*, have no intrinsic promoter function, they often augment transcription from linked promoters.

Finally, DNA regions far removed from a gene may be responsible for activating entire chromosomal domains. The interplay of these *cis*-elements with nuclear proteins generates the exquisite and complex regulation of eukaryotic genes during normal development and differentiation. Given the numerous steps involved in transcription of a gene into mRNA, it should come as no surprise that mutations may interfere with the regulatory process at virtually any stage of gene expression.

In man, cellular DNA is packaged with *nucleoproteins* into chromosomes: 22 autosomes and 2 sex chromosomes (X and Y). (See Chapter 5 for a discussion of chromosomes and cytogenetics.) The astounding complexity of the genome is attributed partly to its large size: the DNA of a single cell contains about 6×10^9 nucleotides, or 6000 megabases (Mb). Although a precise number cannot yet be assigned, it is generally believed that about 10,000 genes are contained in the human genome. Studying a specific gene apart from all others is akin to searching for a needle in a haystack. Therefore, methods have been devised to enrich and to purify individual genes. The extent of purification required to purify a particular gene to homogeneity in amounts suitable for subsequent analysis is far beyond the scope of traditional biochemistry. Gene cloning not only achieves this degree of purification, but also provides an unlimited supply of a specific gene for direct analysis and manipulation.

MOLECULAR CLONING

General Strategies

Cloning is the process by which a DNA molecule is joined to another DNA molecule (vector) that can propagate autonomously in a microbial host, usually a bacterium. An indispensable tool of molecular cloning is the use of *restriction endonucleases* (Fig. 4-2), which are bacterial enzymes that generate predictable cleavages in double-stranded DNA at or near specific recognition sequences. Many of these enzymes have the property of generating staggered DNA ends with short single-stranded regions (sticky ends), which facilitate joining of unrelated, but similarly digested, DNA molecules.

After they are annealed, such molecules may be covalently joined by another enzyme, DNA ligase. Thus, as an initial step in molecular cloning, restriction enzymes provide the essential reagents whereby human or other DNA may be reproducibly cleaved to smaller fragments, then recombined with vector DNA to generate recombinant molecules.

Numerous and often inventive vectors have been developed for gene cloning. (A complete survey of each system is beyond the scope of this chapter.) The choice of vector depends largely on the nature of the DNA clones desired. The sizes of DNA molecules accepted by the various vector systems range from short molecules (a few hundred to several thousand nucleotides) to megabases. To date, most

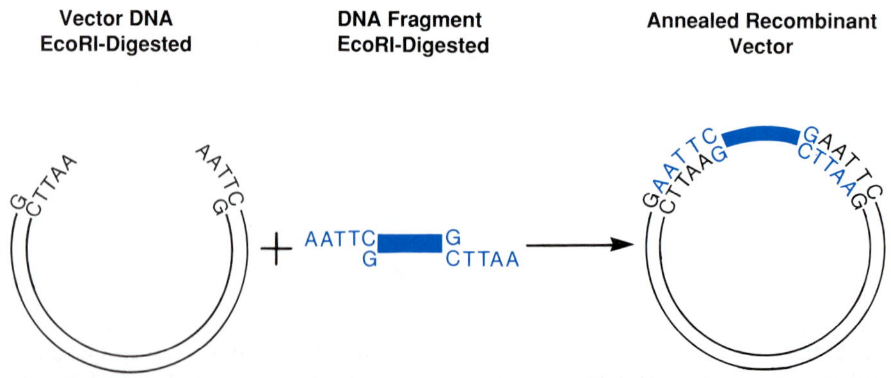

FIGURE 4-2. Cleavage and rejoining of DNA at a restriction site. The restriction enzyme EcoRI recognizes and cleaves the double-stranded oligonucleotide sequence 5'-GAATTC-3', generating single-stranded sticky ends. Cleavage of a hypothetic plasmid or bacteriophage vector at a suitable EcoRI recognition site with this enzyme would allow the annealing of an unrelated DNA fragment that contains complementary, EcoRI-generated sticky ends. The two ends of the annealed DNA fragments can be joined covalently with DNA ligase, resulting in a new recombinant vector.

cloning has been performed in plasmid or bacteriophage vectors.

Because the human genome is complex, the cloning of moderately large genomic DNA segments is experimentally advantageous, since it reduces the number of independent recombinant clones needed to encompass it completely. A collection of independent clones sufficient in number on a statistical basis to include virtually all genes expressed in a particular tissue is often referred to as a *library*. Among the most convenient and widely used vectors for the cloning of mammalian genes has been the *bacteriophage λ*; Fig. 4-3). This bacterial virus, normally about 50 kilobases (kb) in length, infects and propagates efficiently in *Escherichia coli* as a host. Because the central region of the bacteriophage is expendable, foreign DNA sequences can be inserted between the phage arms to generate recombinant DNA, which can then be encapsidated into infectious virions in vitro. After infection of a bacterial lawn, these recombinant phages generate plaques upon lysis of host cells.

Efficient procedures for the screening of large numbers of plaques have been developed, so that entire genome libraries can be examined for specific genes in a matter of days. Most often, this screening process uses radiolabeled DNA fragments, generated either from a previously cloned segment or from chemically synthesized DNA (see text that follows). Phage DNA, transferred by adsorption to filters, is denatured in situ and allowed to anneal (or hybridize) to a complementary DNA strand of the labeled probe. On average, each bacteriophage clone can accommodate about 1 to 20 kb of foreign DNA. Generation of essentially random DNA fragments of this size from genomic DNA permits construction of a total *genomic library*. About 50,000 independent clones in a library are considered to represent the equivalent of a complete genome. In addition, recent advances in the enrichment or isolation of specific chromosomes by microdissection techniques, fluorescence-activated sorting or somatic cell hybrids have made possible the construction of chromosome-specific genomic libraries.[6]

Plasmids are closed circular double-stranded DNA molecules that are most often used for cloning smaller DNA fragments and for the manipulation of cloned DNA segments (Fig. 4-4). Plasmid vectors contain an origin of replication to allow maintenance of the vector at high copy numbers in the bacterial host, a selectable marker (usually an antibiotic-resistance gene) to facilitate identification of bacterial clones harboring the plasmid, and restriction enzyme sites into which DNA fragments may be introduced. In general, DNA fragments of less than 20 kb are conveniently carried and manipulated in these vectors.

For analysis of large stretches of DNA, it is often preferable to use cloning vectors that accept larger DNA fragments. Vectors known as *cosmids*, which share features with both bacteriophage and plasmids, permit propagation of DNA molecules roughly 40 to 50 kb in length.[7] The cloning of much larger DNA fragments often approaching 1 Mb

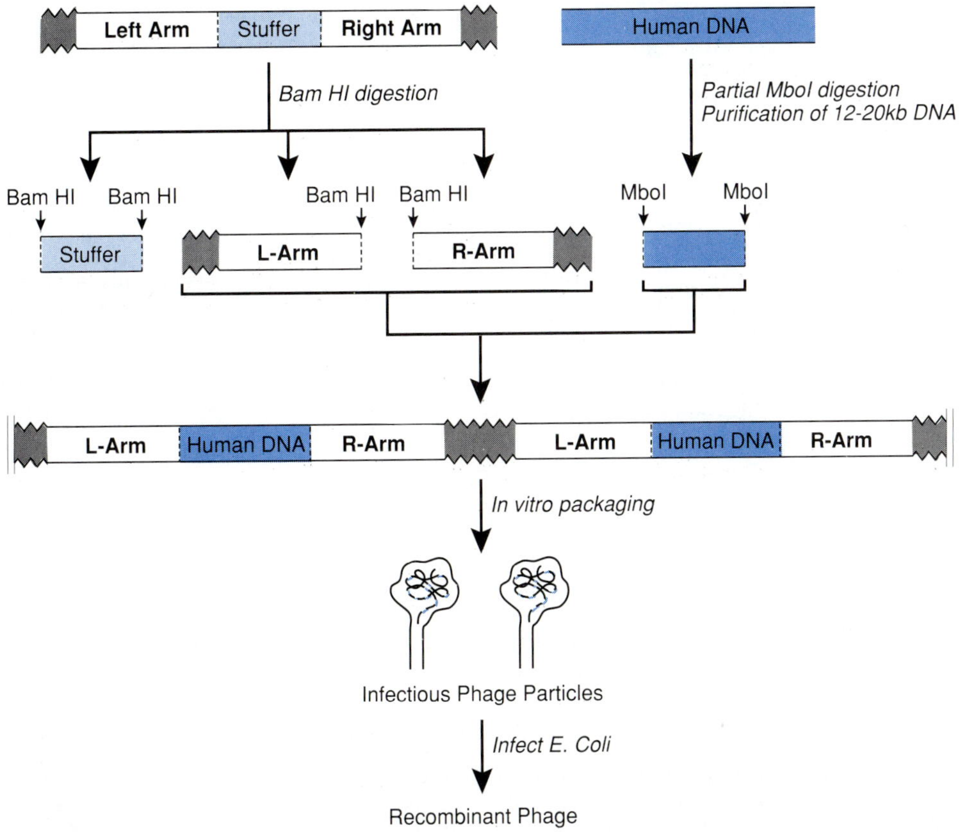

FIGURE 4-3. Cloning of genomic DNA in bacteriophage λ vectors. The cloning of human genomic DNA into bacteriophage λ vectors begins by cleavage of the vector and human DNAs with restriction enzymes that result in compatible sticky ends. In this example, the recognition sequence of MboI (5'-GATC-3') is a subset of the recognition sequence of BamHI (5'-GGATCC-3'). Ligation of the two types of DNA fragments into a recombinant molecule and its packaging into infectious bacteriophage particles are accomplished by the incubation of the DNA ligation mixture with extracts of bacteriophage proteins. The resulting recombinant virions are now capable of infecting suitable bacterial hosts. Typically, the infected bacteria are plated on nutrient agar plates, and plaques are generated in the bacterial lawn after lysis of the bacterial host cells by phage particles.

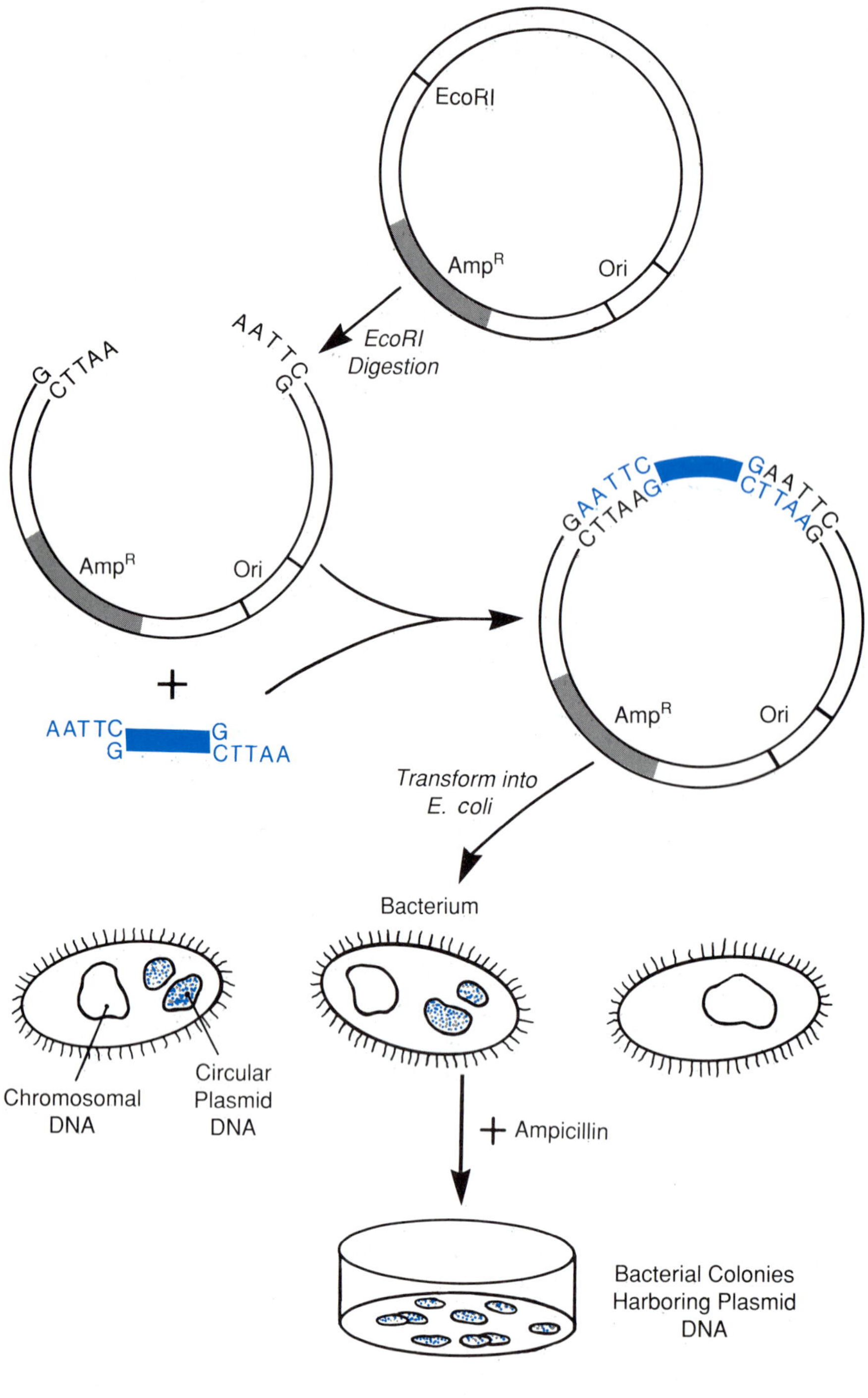

FIGURE 4-4. The closed circular plasmid vector carries a bacterial origin of DNA replication (Ori), and it encodes an ampicillin resistance gene (Amp). The vector also contains an EcoRI site in a nonessential region, which is cleaved to allow the insertion of foreign DNA sequences that have matching EcoRI ends. Suitable strains of bacteria can be rendered competent to accept foreign DNA sequences by pretreating them with calcium chloride or other chemicals. Incubation of plasmid DNA with competent bacteria leads to the transformation of a fraction of the host bacteria. The circular plasmid DNA replicates autonomously, and bacteria-harboring plasmids may be selected for by growth on nutrient agar plates containing ampicillin.

or more is made possible by yeast artificial chromosomes (or YACs).[8] These cloning vehicles are adapted from segments of yeast chromosomes that include centromeric sequences and allow autonomous replication of the recombinant vectors in host yeast cells.

Because only a subset of genomic DNA is ultimately expressed by being transcribed into mRNA, the cloning of mRNA or its complementary copy, known as *cDNA*, offers another strategy by which reagents for, and specific information about, particular genes may be obtained. cDNA may be generated in vitro by copying mRNA with the RNA-dependent DNA polymerase, reverse transcriptase. Subsequent modifications of the cDNA termini facilitates cloning into plasmid or bacteriophage vectors. Thus, depending on the nature of the cloned insert DNA, libraries may be referred to as either genomic libraries or *cDNA libraries*.

Identification of Recombinant Clones

Several different strategies have been developed to identify a specific clone among the numerous recombinant clones in a genomic or cDNA library. In practice, the approach chosen is dictated by the abundance of the clone in the library, the nature of the gene product, and the reagents available to the investigator. If a desired clone is thought to be highly abundant in a cDNA library, it may be sufficient to isolate a few clones at random and subject each to direct DNA sequencing (see text that follows). For example, since the mRNA for β-globin is the major mRNA in a reticulocyte, brute force isolation of cDNA clones from reticulocyte libraries would readily yield β-globin cDNA clones. More commonly, the abundance of a desired clone is far lower and precludes use of this approach. At present, three general strategies are used in the identification of recombinant clones: identification by homology, identification by function, and positional cloning.

Identification by Homology

The most common screening approach employs *nucleic acid hybridization*. If, for example, a cDNA clone for a specific mRNA has been previously isolated and a genomic clone is desired, the cDNA clone may be radiolabeled and used to identify the desired gene within a bacteriophage library.[9] If a gene or cDNA related to a previously isolated sequence is sought, reduced stringency (usually lower temperature or higher salt concentration) of hybridization and washing of filters may permit identification of these homologous members. If a short stretch of polypeptide sequence is known, synthetic oligonucleotides that are designed based on codon degeneracies or a "best guess" can be used as hybridization probes to cloned libraries. The success of this approach relies on the greatly favored stability of perfectly matched versus mismatched hybrid nucleic acids.

Identification by Function

Often no structural data are available on a protein of interest, but antibody reagents or specific functional assays are on hand. In a general strategy referred to as *expression cloning*, a cDNA or genomic clone is isolated by taking advantage of such reagents. In one of the most widely exploited methods, *antisera* are used to screen cDNAs expressed in bacteria as C-terminal fusions to *E coli* β-galactosidase contained within a bacteriophage vector. If an antibody is sufficiently specific and the epitope it recognizes is available in the fusion protein, appropriate clones may be identified with few false-positives.[10] Following isolation of a segment of the desired cDNA with this method, nucleic acid hybridization may be used to recover additional, perhaps complete, cDNA clones.

In another approach that has been successfully exploited in hematology, a cDNA or genomic clone is isolated by transfection (see text in next section) of suitable libraries into mammalian cells, conferring the function of a particular clone on negative cell lines. Thus, if a *biologic assay* exists for a protein, such as a hematopoietic growth factor, assay of the tissue culture media from cells harboring the expressible cDNAs provides a means of identifying the appropriate clone. The success of this method depends on the sensitivity and reliability of a bioassay. Many of the cDNAs encoding hematopoietic growth factors have been recovered in this manner.[11] Similarly, a number of genes encoding receptors for hematopoietic growth factors have also been isolated by expression of appropriate cDNA or genomic libraries in heterologous cells (eg, fibroblasts, COS cells), followed by detection of the receptor on the cell surface by the *binding* of its radioactive ligand.

Introduction of total genomic DNA directly into mammalian cells may also be used to identify DNA fragments that confer *phenotypic alterations* to the host cells. Early examples of this strategy centered on the identification of dominant-acting oncogenes, which can lead to malignant transformation of suitable host cells.[12] Other prominent examples relevant to hematology include cloning of the transferrin receptor gene[13] and the genes that activate V(D)J recombination in B and T cells.[14] Several procedures have been devised to allow recovery of the foreign DNA segment that confers the transformed phenotype to the transfected cell.

Identification by Position

The ability to map chromosomes and subregions by DNA *linkage analysis* and by newly developed gel electrophoresis procedures suitable for large DNA molecules, combined with the availability of naturally occurring alterations in genes that lead to disease states, offers the potential to identify genes responsible for disease without prior protein data, homologous nucleic acid sequences, antisera, or functional assays. This powerful but tedious strategy—commonly referred to as *reverse genetics* or, more properly, *positional cloning*[15]—relies on the fine mapping of a particular disease gene to a chromosomal region by linkage analysis of affected individuals and polymorphic DNA markers. The disease gene locus is narrowed further by identifying contiguous genomic regions using chromosome walking or chromosome jumping techniques. Finally, candidate cDNAs that hybridize with the genomic clones are tested further for any specific role in the disease of interest.

FROM STRUCTURE TO FUNCTION: AN OVERVIEW

Cloning of a cellular gene is merely the first step in the analysis of gene structure and function or in the study of mutations that may affect expression or lead to a disease phenotype. From this perspective, cloned DNA is analogous to a purified protein in traditional biochemistry. Although each cloned gene often presents unique challenges for analysis, in practice a set of core techniques is often used to characterize the molecular structure and function of a DNA clone. These techniques include but are not limited to an analysis of the physical organization, transcriptional activity, protein product (if any), the effect of mutations (both in vitro–generated and in disease states), and chromosomal localization of a gene. A number of the more commonly encountered techniques are reviewed further in the chapter.

As the primary amino acid sequence defines a protein, the nucleotide sequence defines DNA. Two elegant methods, the dideoxy-chain termination procedure[16] and the chemical degradation method,[17] permit rapid and highly accurate determination of *DNA sequence*. In practice, about 10 to 50 kb of sequence can be generated by one laboratory worker in 1 year. With the advent of automated DNA sequencing, it is anticipated that the volume of sequence information already accumulated in computerized databases will expand greatly. The primary nucleotide sequence of a gene or a cDNA provides a substantial database for further analysis. The coding potential of cDNA immediately predicts the amino acid sequence of the encoded protein and may suggest possible functions by identifying relationships to previously described polypeptides. From such comparisons domains of proteins may also be placed into gene families and thereby suggest additional functional and evolutionary relatedness.

If it were not for methods to assess the function of cloned genes and their products, assignment of specific functions to different genetic domains, such as *cis*-acting elements, or the consequences of particular mutations on gene function would remain an inferential exercise. Numerous approaches are now available for the expression of cloned DNA in either prokaryotic or eukaryotic cells, particularly bacteria, yeast, and mammalian cells. Naturally, each system has its advantages and drawbacks. For example, in choosing a bacterial expression system to express the cDNA of a mammalian glycoprotein, although it would be possible to obtain large amounts of the protein, the inability of bacteria to glycosylate must be recognized. If such a modification is deemed important for protein function, an alternative system is then chosen.

Transfection is the introduction of recombinant genes or genomic DNA into mammalian cells. It can be facilitated by various chemical agents (eg, DEAE dextran, calcium phosphate, polyetylene glycol) and liposomes. A special category of transfection that uses viral vectors (eg, retroviruses, vaccinia viruses) is called *transduction*. DNA as well as other macromolecules may also be introduced into individual cells by microinjection. Another versatile strategy used to introduce recombinant DNA into cells is electroporation.[18] This method relies on the formation of transient pores in the cell membrane during the delivery of a high-voltage electrical discharge. For certain cell types in which chemical transfection methods are either ineffective or toxic, electroporation serves as an efficient alternative strategy. In fact, it is currently the method of choice in many laboratories for transferring genes into hematopoietic cells.

By choosing appropriate transfection strategies and cell lines, recombinant genes may be expressed in mammalian cells either over many cell generations in pure cellular clones or for a period of a few days among a pool of positive and negative cells; these two approaches are referred to as *stable* and *transient expression*, respectively. Two mammalian cell culture systems that illustrate some of the differences between stable and transient transfection and allow for *overexpression* of recombinant genes deserve mention. These are Chinese hamster ovary (CHO) and COS cells. For unknown reasons, CHO cells can rapidly amplify stably integrated genes for dihydrofolate reductase (DHFR). CHO cells that are deficient in DHFR can be cotransfected with a DHFR-containing plasmid and a second plasmid containing the gene of interest. Interestingly, the test gene integrates close to the DHFR gene, forming a cointegrant unit, which is subsequently amplified by growing these cells in increasing amounts of methotrexate. Cell lines that carry over 1000 copies of the cointegrant unit can be generated.[19] Stable derivatives of CHO cells that express erythropoietin and coagulation factors have been invaluable for generating large amounts of these recombinant proteins for patient care. COS cells, derived from African green monkey kidney cells, are transformed with a defective mutant of SV40 and express high levels of the SV40 large tumor (large T) antigen. After binding to the sequence-specific origin of replication on the viral genome, the large T antigen initiates high levels of viral DNA replication. This property of the large T antigen has been exploited by cloning the SV40 origin of replication into plasmid vectors. The recombinant plasmids can now be replicated autonomously to very high numbers in COS cells under the influence of the large T antigen. Transfection of COS cells with recombinant plasmid DNA is usually performed with the DEAE-dextran method. Two or 3 days after transfection, 10% or 20% of the cells express the cDNA at sufficiently high levels to allow detection with sensitive bioassays or immunofluorescence. This system has been widely used to clone and transiently express a variety of molecules of importance in hematology.[11]

In recent years there has been an explosion of information on the characterization of regulatory *cis* elements and the proteins, called *trans-acting factors*, that interact with them. In addition to histone and nonhistone proteins, nucleoproteins also include *trans*-acting factors that may play critical roles in determining transcriptional activity.

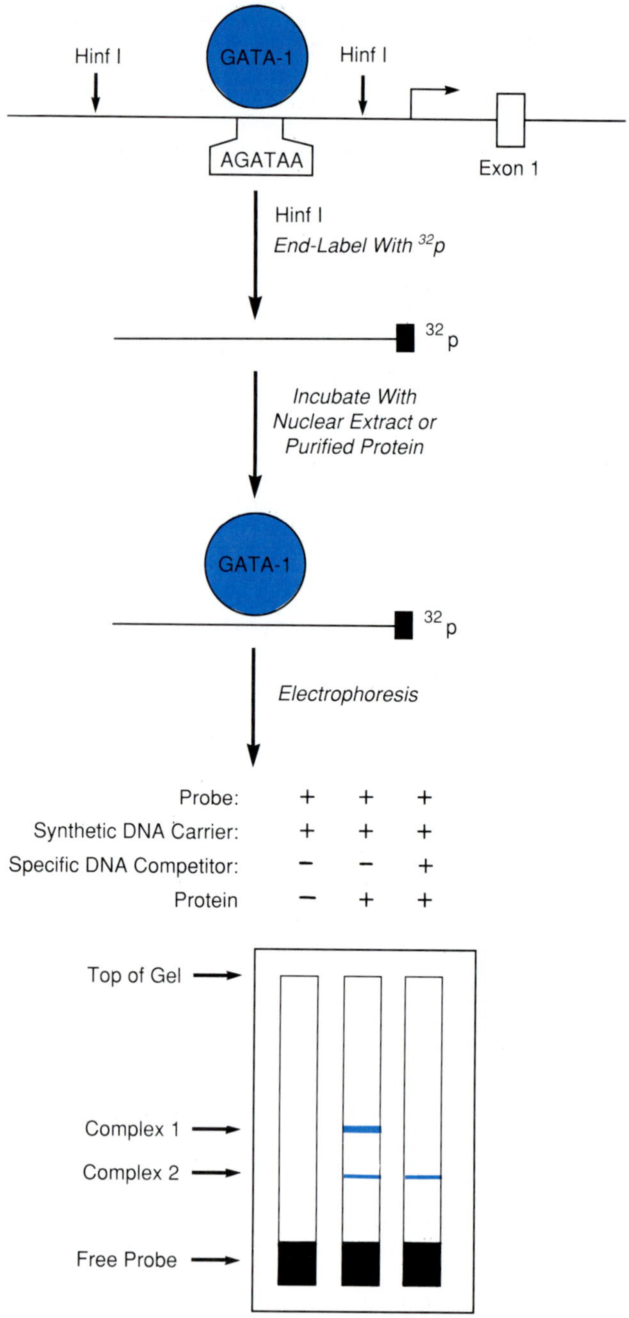

FIGURE 4-5. Schematic diagram of gel mobility retardation assay. A DNA fragment obtained by cleavage of the 5′ regulatory region of an erythroid-specific gene with the restriction enzyme HinfI is used as a probe to identify proteins that bind to this region. This restriction fragment contains the nucleotide sequence AGATAA, which constitutes the binding site for the hematopoietic transcription factor GATA-1. Incubation of the radiolabeled HinfI fragment with a protein source containing GATA-1 allows the formation of a noncovalent complex between GATA-1 and its target sequence on the DNA. Formation of the protein–DNA complex is then detected by electrophoresis of the mixture on relatively porous, nondenaturing acrylamide gels. Migration of the bound complex relative to the free probe is detected as slow-moving bands (complexes 1 and 2) by autoradiography. To ascertain the specificity of interaction between GATA-1 and its target sequence, appropriate competitor DNA fragments are included in the incubation mixture. Addition of a nonradiolabeled HinfI fragment competes for binding of GATA-1 and thus abolishes the complex (complex 1), whereas the addition of an unrelated DNA fragment that lacks the GATA-1 binding site does not disturb the specific complex. Bent arrow indicates the transcriptional start site.

Two complementary approaches are used to delineate such interactions. In the first approach the function of *cis* elements containing candidate promoters or enhancers is assessed by linking them to unrelated (reporter) genes encoding easily detectable proteins, such as chloramphenicol acetyltransferase (CAT) and human growth hormone. The resultant recombinant constructs are transfected into appropriate cell lines, and the presence or absence of *cis* regulatory elements is inferred from the activity or level of the reporter protein. Similarly, this type of analysis can also be performed in the context of the whole animal by generation of transgenic mice bearing reporter constructs (see later discussion). A second approach relies on the physical and biochemical characterization of *trans*-acting factors. Perhaps the most basic method used to characterize *protein–DNA interactions* is the gel mobility retardation assay (also called the "gel shift," "band retardation," and so on). In this assay (Fig. 4-5), a radiolabeled DNA fragment spanning a putative transcriptional regulatory element (eg, a promoter or an enhancer) is incubated with a protein extract from an appropriate tissue source, and the DNA–protein mixture is subjected to electrophoresis. The difference in migration through the gel between the protein–DNA complex versus the unbound DNA can be a clue to specific binding.[20] These protein–DNA interactions can be further refined by footprinting techniques, which delineate specific nucleotide residues that are in contact with the protein, and ultimately by more sophisticated biophysical techniques, including nuclear magnetic resonance.

Methods of *site-directed mutagenesis* allow a more complete analysis of the function of cloned cDNAs. These methods include the introduction of simple deletions and insertions when convenient restriction sites are available in the gene of interest. Other methods of introducing deletions use exonucleases that digest DNA processively from one end. More commonly, such restriction sites are not available, and in any case it is often desirable to insert, delete, or substitute single base pairs at critical regions of a cDNA which are not accessible to DNA-modifying enzymes. Many of these strategies take advantage of mutant synthetic oligonucleotides to create single base mismatches. A popular method uses uracil incorporation into a single-stranded DNA template, use of the uracil-containing template to synthesize a complementary strand in vitro in the presence of a mutant oligonucleotide primer, and selection against the original strand that contains uracil in vivo, leaving only the strand that has incorporated the mutant oligonucleotide for propagation[21] (Fig. 4-6).

Finally, introduction of foreign DNA sequences into the germline of mice and generation of transgenic mouse strains offers another powerful means by which gene structure and function may be correlated[22] (Fig. 4-7). Transgenic mice are particularly useful in delineating *cis* regulatory sequences required for tissue and developmental stage-

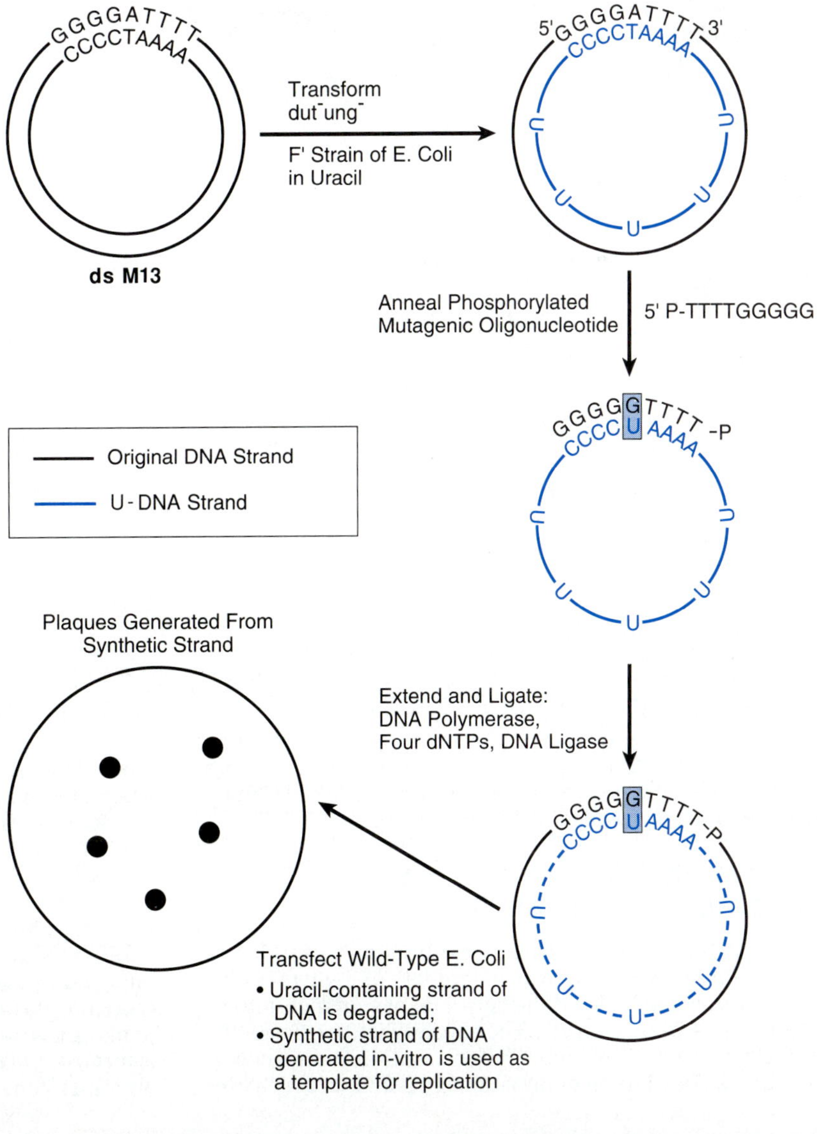

FIGURE 4-6. A strategy of site-directed mutagenesis. A strain of *Escherichia coli* that is deficient in dUTPase and uracil-N-glycosylase, called *dut*- and *ung*-, accumulates dUTP and is unable to remove misincorporated uracil from DNA. When a recombinant M13 bacteriophage is grown in such a strain in the presence of uracil, a fraction of thymine residues are replaced by uracil. Uracil-substituted, single-stranded M13 bacteriophage particles are extruded from the E *coli*, which are used in vitro as templates for DNA synthesis in the presence of mutant oligonucleotides. The nascent DNA chain contains the mutant oligonucleotide and thymine, but no uracil. Transformation of wild-type E *coli* with this DNA results in the replication of the uracil-free strand and destruction of the uracil-containing strand.

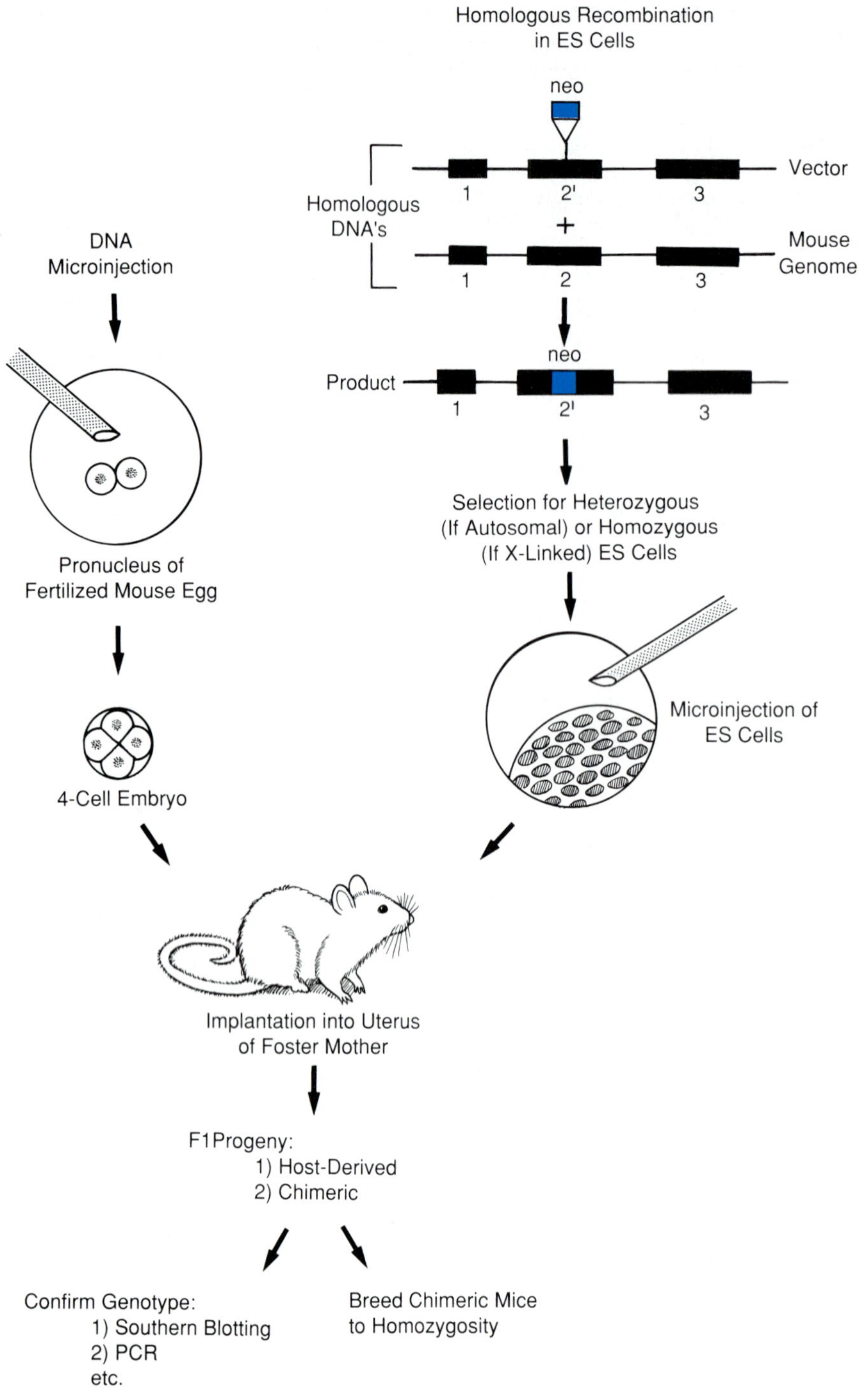

FIGURE 4-7. Manipulation of the mouse genome. The most widely used technique for creating transgenic mice involves the microinjection of cloned DNA into the pronucleus of a one-cell fertilized mouse egg. The DNA integrates randomly in the mouse genome. A second technique initially uses embryonic stem cells as a target for foreign DNA, which is usually introduced by electroporation. The vector contains a selection marker (*neo*) that is inserted in a part of a gene that is otherwise homologous to sequences on the mouse genome. The selection marker disrupts the normal coding region of the gene. Recombination of vector DNA with the homologous mouse genomic locus substitutes the new inactive allele bearing the insertion for the endogenous functional one. Selection for recombinant embryonic stem (ES) cells is accomplished by a variety of strategies conferring drug resistance. The embryo is implanted into the uterus of a foster mother (whose genotype is irrelevant). The foster mother gives birth to either chimeric offspring or those that are host derived. Male chimeras are then mated to breed the new genotype to homozygosity. Polymerase chain reaction (PCR) and Southern analysis are used most frequently to screen for integration of the foreign DNA.

specific gene expression. In addition, the effects of expressing various gene products in a developing animal may be evaluated through introduction of foreign sequences into the mouse germline. As noted below, new models of human disease may be provided by transgenic mice.

SPECTRUM OF MUTATIONS AND POLYMORPHISMS

Much of the clinical impact of analysis of mutations in human disease rests on the development of highly specific and sensitive methods for the detection of subtle mutations in uncloned DNA samples. The capacity to assign specific defects in limited DNA samples permits widespread analysis of the distribution of mutations in populations, carrier detection in families at risk or those possibly at risk, prenatal diagnosis of inherited disease early in pregnancy, and even identification of acquired abnormalities (such as those associated with malignancies) and assessment of minimal residual disease in these latter conditions (see further explanation in text that follows). Prior to describing the technology used to characterize such differences, the more frequently encountered types of polymorphisms and mutations are reviewed here.

Differences in the structure of a particular region of DNA among individuals may reflect either normal variation (polymorphism) or a structural alteration in the gene or its flanking DNA. The most simple form of DNA polymorphism is termed *restriction fragment length polymorphism* (RFLP), which is generated by single nucleotide substitutions at every few hundred base pair intervals in the genome, resulting in the creation or loss of a restriction endonuclease cleavage site. RFLPs have provided invaluable genetic markers within families and populations, and have formed the basis for genetic linkage analysis that has led to the construction of large-scale human gene maps. Repetitive DNA sequences have also been used with great success to construct physical maps or to identify variations among individuals. *Minisatellites*, also called variable number of tandem repeats, are composed of tandem arrays of a core unit that includes 10 nucleotides or more, where the number of units in different alleles is highly variable. The distribution of minisatellites is biased toward the ends of chromosomes. Perhaps the most versatile and informative polymorphisms are *microsatellites*, also called simple repeats, which are composed of tandem repeats of mononucleotides, dinucleotides, trinucleotides, and tetranucleotides (eg, dinucleotide repeat GTGTGT). These markers are being discovered and applied more frequently in DNA fingerprinting. The number of copies of a particular DNA fragment may be estimated by comparison with control DNA samples. For an autosomal gene, the deletion of a single copy would be expected to result in reduction of the hybridization signal by half. Additional copies of a gene, perhaps acquired through *gene amplification* that often is associated with malignancy, are similarly detected by an increase in band intensity.

The structure or expression of a particular gene product may be influenced by alterations in the sequence of the cellular gene. These mutations may take various forms and include deletion or insertion of nucleotide sequences, as well as single base substitutions. Deletion or insertion of larger DNA segments may cause either gross alterations that are detected by cytogenetic techniques or more subtle alterations that are detected principally by sensitive molecular techniques.

Characterizations of mutations in inherited disorders have provided invaluable lessons for the spectrum of mutations that can affect DNA. Almost all mutations that can be predicted to affect gene expression or function have already been observed in inherited disorders. Loss of gene function is readily accomplished by deletion, as seen in α-thalassemias. More frequently, single nucleotide changes are responsible for defective gene or protein function in inherited disorders. Although nucleotide substitutions may occur spontaneously, they appear to arise more frequently at CpG dinucleotides in the DNA.

The effects of single base changes on protein function can be dramatic. A classic example is that of the A-to-T change in the sixth codon of the β-globin gene that results in the substitution of valine for glutamic acid in sickle cell anemia. The altered solubility of sickle hemoglobin ultimately leads to the clinical sequelae. Rather than resulting in an amino acid replacement, a single base change may introduce a stop signal for translation (termed a *nonsense mutation*) and cause production of a truncated polypeptide. This has been documented, for example, in some forms of β-thalassemia. Nucleotide changes in the conserved sequences near the junctions of exons and intervening sequences often lead to deleterious effects on RNA processing, as is also evident in various forms of thalassemia.[23] Finally, single nucleotide mutations may also adversely affect promoter function or 3′ mRNA processing.

ANALYTIC METHODS: STRUCTURE OF DNA AND RNA

Highly sensitive and specific analytic methods have been developed, which form the basis for much of the experimental work required in gene analysis. Two classic procedures, known as Southern blot and Northern blot analyses have been used widely to characterize the molecular structure of DNA and RNA, respectively (Fig. 4-8).

Southern transfer, named after its originator, EM Southern, combines the digestion of DNA by restriction enzymes, electrophoresis of the resulting fragments and their transfer in situ to a solid paper support, and nucleic acid hybridization to identify DNA fragments bearing specific nucleotide sequences among a mixture of fragments. A great strength of the method is its sensitivity: a single gene or a portion thereof can be readily detected within total human DNA. First, the presence or absence of a specific fragment can be ascertained. This may be especially relevant in the analysis of material from a patient who cannot synthesize a given gene product. Second, the size of the detected DNA fragments provides direct information regarding the position of restriction enzyme cleavage sites that flank a DNA segment. With use of a variety of restriction enzyme digests, a physical map of a DNA region may be constructed.

Northern blot analysis is a similar procedure by which RNA, rather than DNA, is examined. This method provides information on the size and abundance of RNA transcripts and is especially useful in revealing the tissue distribution of particular mRNAs in tissue or cell samples and major abnormalities, either structural or quantitative, in samples from patients with a particular disorder.

Additional methods have expanded the analysis of both cellular DNA and RNA. Whereas conventional Southern blot analysis is best suited for study of DNA fragments 20 kb or less in length, long-range mapping methods allow resolution of substantially larger DNA fragments up to 1-Mb range.[24] With these techniques, known as pulsed-field gel electrophoresis, field inversion gels, contour-clamp homogeneous electric field electrophoresis, restriction maps for megabase regions of chromosomes may be constructed. These advances bring the resolution of physical mapping of DNA near to that of contemporary cytogenetics. *RNA structure* may be evaluated more precisely by various nuclease procedures (S1 nuclease and RNase mapping methods) in which a radiolabeled DNA or RNA strand is hybridized to mRNA and mismatched regions are removed by enzymatic digestion.[3,4] Examination of the fragments of these protected probes provides direct information regarding the structural integrity and organization of mRNA.

Within the past few years, an ingenious method developed by Mullis[25] and coworkers has revolutionized gene analysis (Fig. 4-9). This approach, termed *polymerase chain reaction* (PCR), uses in vitro amplification of a DNA region with specific DNA primers and a heat-stable DNA polymerase. With short synthetic primers flanking it, a targeted DNA segment can be amplified more than 1 million times in vitro to provide abundant material for direct analysis either by restriction enzyme digestion, blot hybridization, or DNA sequencing. The method is amazingly versatile and modifications in the basic procedure permit many applications in molecular genetics. Experimental protocols have been refined such that exceedingly small samples of blood or biopsy specimens are required as starting material. In many instances, PCR has replaced the necessity of using molecular cloning to isolate a DNA region of interest.

For the most part, the precise techniques used for detection of a mutation depend on the particular situation at hand. Often, conventional Southern blot analysis can be used, especially if gross structural alterations, such as gene deletions, are anticipated. Increasingly, PCR is being applied for detection of mutations, particularly in the identification and characterization of single or few nucleotide alterations in which Southern blotting is generally insensitive. PCR-generated fragments may be subjected to nucleotide sequence analysis without further manipulations.

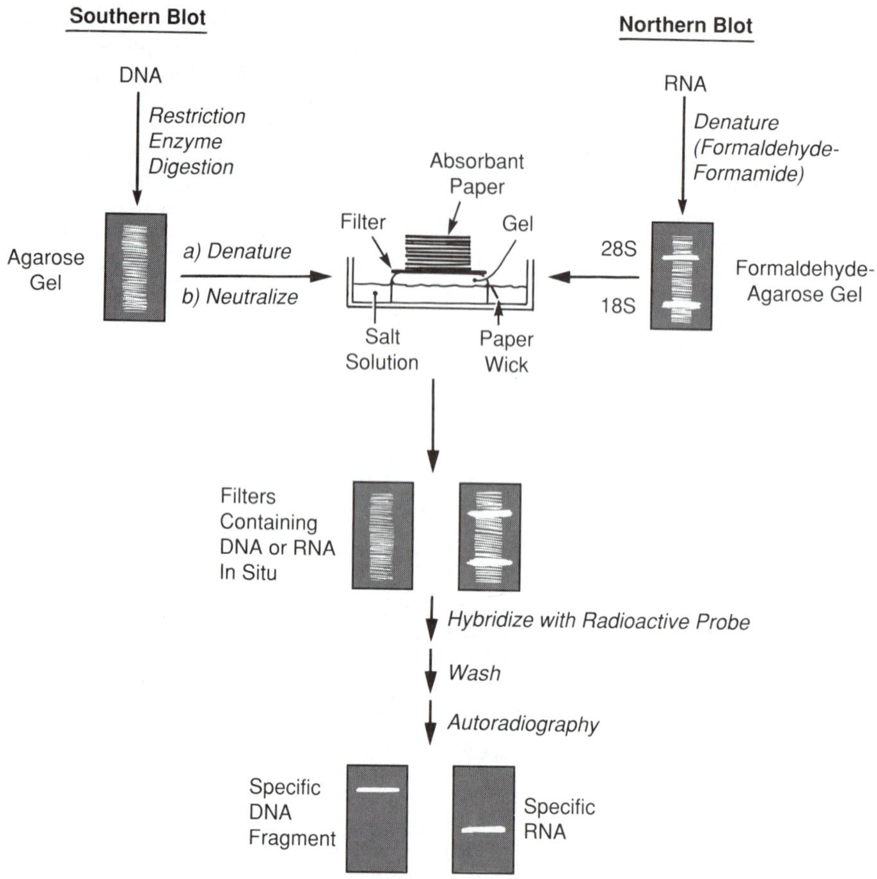

FIGURE 4-8. Schematic illustrations of Southern and Northern blot procedures. In the Southern blot procedure, DNA is cleaved with restriction enzymes, subjected to electrophoresis on agarose gels, and denatured with sodium hydroxide to yield single-stranded fragments in situ. In the Northern blot procedure, strong denaturants are used to disrupt intramolecular secondary structure formation as well as to prevent degradation of RNA. The RNA is subjected to electrophoresis on agarose gels in the presence of formaldehyde. Further transfer and hybridization steps for the two procedures are similar. Binding of denatured DNA or RNA to filters (nitrocellulose or nylon) is generally accomplished by capillary transfer procedures, whereby the nucleic acids are eluted from the gel by the upward movement of buffer. Filters containing immobilized DNA or RNA can now be hybridized with radioactive probes and subjected to autoradiography.

However, it is often desirable to delimit the region of mutation in an otherwise large gene prior to sequencing.

Two of the more effective methods that have been combined with PCR are the denaturing gradient gel electrophoresis (DGGE) and the single-stranded conformational polymorphism (SSCP) methods. In the former, PCR-amplified DNA is tested for heteroduplex formation on denaturing polyacrylamide gel systems, and variant bands are detected at regions of single base mismatches.[26] The latter method is based on the observation that single-stranded DNA fragments assume unique conformations by intramolecular interactions within a particular DNA strand.[27] Thus, migration of a single-stranded DNA fragment on nondenaturing gels are exquisitely sensitive to single nucleotide alterations. These methods have greatly simplified screening for single-base mutations.

CREATING NEW ANIMAL MODELS OF DISEASE

The principal advances in animal models have been made in murine models. The ability to manipulate cloned genes and introduce them into the germline of mice have led to exciting possibilities for the generation of animal models of disease. Without doubt, these developments will have a considerable impact on our understanding of the biology of hematopoietic cells and on potential approaches to management of disease. On the one hand, expression of a gene product may be targeted to a particular tissue to assess its consequences on cell growth, development, and behavior. The major experimental approaches are (1) microinjection of cloned DNA into the pronucleus; (2) infection of embryos with retroviral vectors (insertional mutagens) to create mutant phenotypes; (3) transfer of genetic sequences to hematopoietic stem cells via retroviruses; and (4) transfer of DNA or retroviruses into embryonic stem cells and subsequent injection into blastocysts to generate chimeric mice.

The value of transgenic mice to modern science is no more apparent than in the field of hematology. To date, numerous oncogenes under the transcriptional control of various regulatory elements have been introduced into the mouse germline to generate mice with inherited mammary tumors, insulinomas, and B-cell lymphomas. Such animals with an inherited predisposition to malignancy can be evaluated for the possible role of other oncogenes in facilitating the onset of cancer or factors that might abrogate its development. Through the use of transgenic mice, the expression of different oncogenes in the same tissues may have different consequences for tumor development. Thus, a specific relation exists between the oncogene and target tissues.

In addition to oncogenes, other molecules of importance to hematology have also been introduced into the mouse germline. For example, a line of transgenic mice has been established recently in which the human multidrug resistance gene (MDR1) is expressed in all cell lineages of the bone marrow.[28] This mouse model should be invaluable for assessing the activity of chemotherapeutic agents.

Infection of hematopoietic stem cells by retroviruses followed by adoptive transfer into immunodeficient mice has also been used to create murine models of human disease. For example, to understand the evolution and pathogenesis of chronic myelogenous leukemia (CML), the recombinant retroviruses that encode the hybrid *bcr-abl* gene are used to infect hematopoietic stem cells in vitro, followed by adoptive transfer of these cells into irradiated mice.[29] The observation that the disease may be transferred by transplantation of bone marrow cells to syngeneic recipients makes it an important disease model. Furthermore, human somatic gene therapy based on similar approaches is

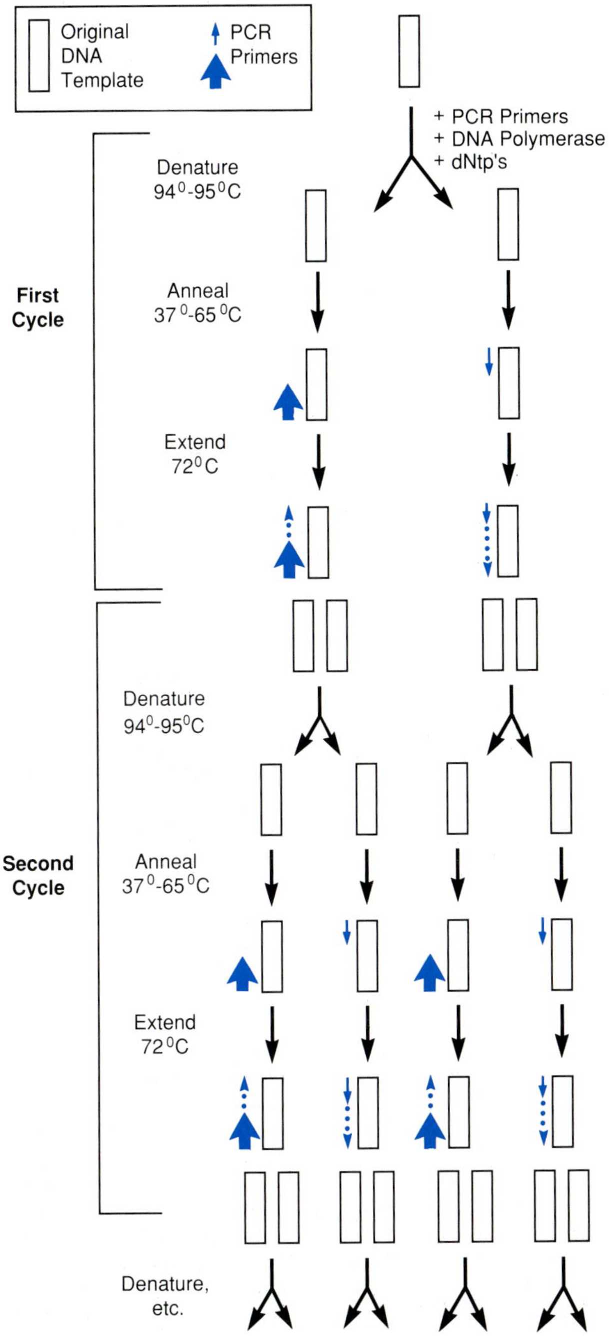

FIGURE 4-9. The principles of the polymerase chain reaction (PCR) technique. The PCR technique involves the successive repetition of three core steps—denaturation, annealing, and extension. In the first step, the double-stranded DNA template is denatured at high temperature. While the temperature is decreased, the denatured strands that have remained free in solution anneal to extension primers, a pair of synthetic oligonucleotides that are complementary to one or the other strand of the template. Because the primers are present in large excess relative to the DNA template, the formation of primer–template complex is favored over the reassociation of the two strands at lower temperatures. Finally, the primer is extended in a 5′-to-3′ direction by DNA polymerase. A set of these three steps is called a *cycle.* Repetition of this cycle 20 or 30 times in an automated apparatus causes an exponential increase in the amount of the nascent product.

now being studied (see section on the potential for gene therapy).

A new and particularly exciting technology is the development of mouse embryonic stem (ES) cells as targets for gene introduction and modification (see Fig. 4-7). ES cells are derived from the inner cell mass of the embryo. With the use of feeder layers, conditioned media, or leukemia inhibitory factor, ES cells may be maintained in tissue culture in an undifferentiated state. Upon injection into blastocysts, ES cells contribute to the host embryo, giving rise ultimately to a chimeric mouse. Under optimal conditions, these cells also contribute to the germline. Breeding of the chimeric mice can lead to germline transmission of genes introduced into the cultured ES cells. As ES cells are susceptible to various methods of gene transfer and also to homologous recombination, directed modifications of endogenous mouse genes may be achieved. Ultimately, mice homozygous for a directed mutation or modification can be produced by matings. The power and potential of this approach are immense. For example, it is now possible in principle to generate animal models for many of the inherited, single-gene disorders of man. As the molecular basis of specific disorders is dissected by molecular genetics, efforts can be made to produce similar conditions in mice. Although the phenotype of a genetic disorder in mice may often be similar to that in man, this may not always be the case. For example, the apparently normal behavior of mice with disruption of the HPRT locus is in stark contrast to Lesch-Nyhan disease in humans as a result of HPRT deficiency. Nonetheless, it is anticipated that for most human gene defects, corresponding mouse phenotypes may be observed.

The animal models of human diseases will be useful in understanding the pathophysiology of various disorders and in evaluating approaches to somatic or pharmacologic gene therapy. A second major area of investigation with ES cells relates to the role of many genes in cell differentiation and development. In many instances, it is currently believed that various oncogenes and transcriptional factors (particularly those expressed in a cell-restricted manner) play major roles in cell commitment during development and differentiation. Disruption of the genes encoding these products provides a genetic means to evaluate their participation in specific cellular programs. The biology of hematopoietic cell differentiation is likely to be addressed through these strategies in the coming years.

APPLICATIONS OF RECOMBINANT DNA TECHNOLOGY TO HEMATOLOGY

The development of recombinant DNA methods in the past decade has profoundly influenced the practice of modern hematology. The identification of specific gene mutations in hematologic disorders such as thalassemia has caused significant reductions in the incidence of births of affected persons, partly because of the successful application of molecular diagnostic techniques. The following selected examples illustrate some of the techniques and strategies discussed in the preceding sections.

Diagnosis of Inherited Hematologic Disorders

At the clinical level, the newer genetic methods have had their greatest impact on the diagnosis of disease states, largely because of their power to detect gene defects in uncloned DNA samples. After a specific mutation is identified and associated with an inherited condition, a diagnostic test for this primary defect can be designed, using conventional Southern blot analysis, synthetic oligonucleotides, or PCR. A classic example of tailoring of a test for a specific mutation is in the molecular analysis of sickle cell anemia. It is fortuitous that the sickle mutation abolishes a recognition site in the β-globin gene for the restriction enzyme Mst II, altering the sizes of genomic fragments generated upon digestion of total DNA. With the Southern blot or PCR methods, carriers of sickle cell disease and sickle homozygotes may be readily and accurately distinguished from normal patients. This approach has been used widely in the prenatal diagnosis of sickle cell anemia. Likewise, specific tests for various forms of thalassemia have been devised and used to examine family members and fetuses at risk for the disorder.

Diagnosis of Acquired Hematologic Disorders

In many hematologic malignancies, specific chromosomal translocations are commonly seen, such as that found in CML, where the *c-abl* proto-oncogene on chromosome 9 is fused to the *bcr* gene on chromosome 22. To the extent that translocations occur within a limited target gene, the chromosomal alterations may be detected with PCR using primers flanking the breakpoints. Besides identifying the translocations at the molecular level, such approaches also provide highly sensitive assays by which a few malignant cells can be detected from a vast population of normal cells. With PCR, a single abnormal cell may be detected among more than 10^6 normal cells. Therefore, PCR provides a new method for the identification and enumeration of residual neoplastic cells. The use of molecular techniques to detect minimal residual disease during chemotherapy for malignant disease will undoubtedly expand greatly in coming years.

A related application of recombinant DNA methods is the assessment of clonality in cell populations. Specific clonal expansion of lymphoid cells, for example, is taken to reflect the proliferation of malignant cells, whereas polyclonal expansion is generally thought to represent nonmalignant states, such as inflammatory conditions. Differentiation of B and T lymphoid cells is accompanied by a stage-specific rearrangement of the immunoglobulin genes and T-cell receptor genes, respectively. As a result, Southern blot analysis of DNA from lymphoid cells with suitable molecular probes can be used to detect clonal expansion of specific cell populations. Together with other findings, such information can help to make clinical diagnoses more secure and precise.

Another related application is the use of RFLPs to establish the origin of cells following allogeneic bone marrow transplantation. Because the cellular DNAs of virtually any two (or more) individuals can be distinguished with RFLPs or other polymorphic sequences, particularly when highly variable fingerprinting probes are used, molecular techniques can rapidly provide the means by which to analyze the relative contribution of host and donor hematopoietic cells in a transplanted individual. Such an approach can provide confirmation for the engraftment of donor marrow, reemergence of host elements, and mixed cell chimerism.

Characterizing the Genetic Basis of Hematologic Disease

Often, the protein product that is altered in an inherited disorder is not apparent from conventional biochemical and cellular studies. With the use of an approach that unites classic genetics and recombinant DNA methods, the gene mutated in a disorder can now be identified without prior knowledge of its protein product. DNA markers that are closely linked to a particular disease locus may be identified by tracking RFLPs within families at risk for an inherited disorder. The chromosomal locus of the relevant gene may be narrowed further by additional linkage mapping or with the use of patient samples bearing DNA deletions or chromosomal translocations. After the region in which the gene is thought to reside is narrowed sufficiently, genomic fragments derived from this region are used as probes to search for expressed sequences. Identification of mRNA transcripts that show either quantitative or qualitative abnormalities in association with the disease state gives strong evidence for the assignment of the gene.

DNA sequence analysis of the gene or its mRNA may provide clues about the nature of the protein product encoded by the gene. Taken together with the pathology seen in the disease, a preliminary model for the role of the protein in cell physiology may then be proposed. Subsequently, for more definitive biochemical and cellular studies, synthetic peptides based on the predicted protein sequence or recombinant proteins derived by overexpression of the cloned gene is used to generate antibodies against the putative protein. As previously cited, this general approach of identifying and characterizing an affected gene and its protein product is referred to as reverse genetics or positional cloning. One of the first examples of this approach involved the characterization of the X-linked form of chronic granulomatous disease, an inherited disorder of phagocyte function.

Molecular Pathology of a Hematologic Disease

For over three decades, it was known that thalassemia syndromes result from a quantitative disturbance of globin chains. As a result of reduced or absent synthesis of specific globin chains, the pathophysiologic basis of thalassemia syndromes was attributed to the unbalanced synthesis of globin polypeptides. With the advent of Northern analysis, deficiencies of specific mRNAs were also correlated with disease states. It was impossible to state a priori whether such deficiencies were secondary to mutations in the globin genes themselves or reflected mutations of regulatory genes that somehow led to reduced mRNA production. This dilemma was resolved with the application of molecular cloning techniques to the analysis of globin genes from patients with thalassemia. Mutant globin genes were cloned, sequenced, and analyzed for expression upon reintroduction into mammalian cell test systems. Rather than representing a single type of mutation, thalassemia syndromes demonstrated a rich spectrum of gene mutations that were predicted to interfere with gene function.[23] Taken together, the thalassemia syndromes were the first genetic disorders to be described in nearly complete molecular detail. They represent a paradigm for the analysis of other genetic conditions.

Impact on Treatment of Hematologic Disorders

Recombinant DNA technology provides new products for direct administration to patients. The availability of hematopoietic growth factors through cDNA cloning and expression is beginning to change the clinical management of several disorders. Among the most dramatic of these examples is the use of erythropoietin to ameliorate the chronic anemia of renal disease. In addition, abnormalities of white cell production, such as the transient neutropenia resulting from cancer chemotherapy, is being more effectively treated with the administration of colony-stimulating factors active on myelomonocytic progenitors. Similarly, the production of blood clotting factors by molecular genetic methods promises to develop as a treatment for the hemophilias.

As more is learned about the precise mechanisms by

which genes are regulated in eukaryotic cells, new strategies for management of disorders are being considered and evaluated. Provocative attempts have been made to influence gene expression in vivo in an effort to correct an inherited deficiency. For example, since the production of fetal hemoglobin appears to reduce the severity of sickle cell anemia or thalassemia, a number of pharmacologic agents have been tested for their ability to stimulate fetal hemoglobin production in adult patients. Based on the association of lower levels of gene activity with methylation of cytosine residues in DNA, 5′-azacytidine, a drug that leads to widespread demethylation, was tested for its effects on fetal hemoglobin production in patients with sickle cell anemia or thalassemia. Although the precise mechanism of action of this drug in vivo is controversial, it often produces a substantial increase in fetal hemoglobin. A variety of other cytotoxic agents, such as hydroxurea, also appear to exert a similar effect on fetal hemoglobin production in vivo. Whatever the basis of these effects, it is gratifying that the observed increase in the level of fetal hemoglobin is often in the range considered to be of clinical benefit.

A related example of modulating gene expression as a means of treating an inherited disorder is the administration of the lymphokine γ-interferon to patients with chronic granulomatous disease. For a number of years, γ-interferon has been known to augment the capacity of phagocytic cells to kill microbes, which may be due to its ability to induce transcription of some of the genes encoding essential components of the superoxide-generating system of phagocytes. Preliminary clinical trials suggested that administration of γ-interferon may appreciably enhance phagocytic function in selected patients with chronic granulomatous disease. From the two examples cited here, it is apparent that knowledge of the molecular biology of specific gene systems will lead to the design and development of novel strategies for the treatment of hematologic disease.

Potential for Genetic Therapy

Methods for the isolation of genes and their reintroduction into cells has suggested the possibility of using gene therapy to achieve permanent correction of a deficiency state in the cells. The primary goal of such an approach is to target the somatic cells of an affected person (somatic gene therapy), rather than the cells of the germline. At present, somatic gene therapy is being contemplated primarily for severe and life-threatening disorders for which current medical management is unsatisfactory. In the course of research efforts, many different methods of introducing a normal version of a gene into cells bearing mutant copies have been considered. Currently, a great deal of effort is being devoted to the use of modified recombinant retroviruses as transduction vehicles, as they have successfully adapted through evolution for efficient cellular infection, gene transfer, integration of their genetic material into the host genome, and stability of the integrated sequences in host cells.

The hematopoietic system represents one of the most attractive and suitable targets for gene therapy, principally because of the self-renewal potential of pluripotent stem cells. Transfer of new genetic material into the most primitive hematopoietic stem cells ensures its presence in more differentiated progenitors. In addition, the extensive clinical experience in the field of bone marrow transplantation provides the necessary tools for reconstitution of the hematopoietic system by infusion of the donor cells and management of the host after transplantation. It is envisioned that in somatic gene therapy experiments involving marrow transplantation, the genetically modified cells of the affected patient, rather than stem cells from a histocompatible donor, would be used for reconstitution. This situation is akin to autologous bone marrow transplantation.

Among the severe disorders for which genetic therapy is being considered, those involving cells of the hematopoietic system are particularly prominent. Appropriate examples are severe combined immunodeficiency due to lack of adenosine deaminase, the hemoglobinopathies (sickle cell anemia and thalassemia), and metabolic storage disorders (such as Gaucher's disease). In addition, plasma deficiencies of coagulation factors, such as factor VIII, might be treated by using hematopoietic cells as in vivo factories for production of normal protein.

In the past few years, considerable progress has been made in the use of retroviruses for gene transfer into pluripotent hematopoietic stem cells of mice. Infection of sufficient numbers of stem cells by recombinant retroviruses and adequate expression of introduced gene sequences in stem cells and their progeny remain formidable technical problems. Attempts are underway to use stronger promoters in an effort to optimize gene expression, and to enrich stem cell preparations for more efficient infection. Until these problems are resolved through further experimentation in mice, successful extension of such methods to larger animals (eg, primates) and their clinical application for correction of disease states are difficult.

Somatic gene therapy is generally regarded as synonymous to gene addition, that is, supplementation of a deficient cell with the normal version of a gene rather than correction of the genetic defect itself. Because precise correction of a mutant gene, in situ, in the chromosome would ensure appropriate regulation of expression throughout cellular differentiation, it would be far more preferable to use targeted methods of gene insertion or modification. Such directed gene mutations have been achieved in mammalian cells through the use of specially designed vector and selection systems (see Fig. 4-7). At present, an estimated 1 per 1000 integration events may be through homologous recombination rather than random integration. This incidence is too low to permit its use in clinical settings. Nonetheless, if site-specific homologous recombination can be made substantially more efficient in mammalian cells, it is likely that greater attention will be paid in the future to more refined strategies for genetic therapy.

CONCLUSION

This brief survey of molecular genetics may provide the reader with general principles that are likely to be common to future investigations of hematologic biology and disease. In the context of this review, it is impossible to communicate the full sense of excitement and promise of molecular genetics in modern hematology. Nevertheless, it is apparent that molecular methods are being assimilated as indispensable tools with which to dissect numerous cellular processes that are directly relevant to hematology. Specific hypotheses may be tested with genetic and molecular approaches, and new experimental strategies for treatment may be evaluated in a logical and systematic manner. For the past decade, hematology has been at the forefront of application of molecular genetics to medical science. Recent developments suggest that this tradition will continue in force in the future.

REFERENCES

1. Darnell J, Lodish H, Baltimore D. Molecular cell biology, 2nd ed. New York, Scientific American Books, 1990.
2. Watson JD, Tooze J, Kurtz DT. Recombinant DNA: a short course. New York, WH Freeman, 1983.
3. Ausubel FM, Brent R, Kingston RE, et al. Current protocols in molecular biology. New York, John Wiley & Sons, 1989.

4. Sambrook J, Fritsch EF, Maniatis T. Molecular cloning: a laboratory manual. Cold Spring Harbor, NY, Cold Spring Harbor Laboratory Press, 1989.
5. Johnson PF, McKnight SL. Eukaryotic transcriptional regulatory proteins. Annu Rev Biochem 1989;58:799.
6. Meltzer PS, Guan X-Y, Burgess A, et al. Rapid generation of region specific probes by chromosome microdissection and their application. Nature Genet 1992;1:24.
7. Collins J, Hohn B. Cosmids: a type of plasmid gene-cloning vector that is packageable *in vitro* in bacteriophage λ heads. Proc Natl Acad Sci USA 1978;75:4242.
8. Burke DT, Carle GF, Olson MV. Cloning of large segments of exogenous DNA into yeast by means of artificial chromosome vectors. Science 1987;236:806.
9. Benton WD, Davis RW. Screening λgt recombinant clones by hybridization to single plaques in situ. Science 1977;196:180.
10. Young RA, Davis RW. Efficient isolation of genes by using antibody probes. Proc Natl Acad Sci USA 1983;80:1194.
11. Wong GG, Witek J, Temple PA. Human GM-CSF: molecular cloning of the complementary DNA and purification of the recombinant protein. Science 1985;228:810.
12. Goldfarb M, Shimizu K, Perucho M, et al. Isolation and preliminary characterization of a human transforming gene from T24 bladder carcinoma cells. Nature 1982;296:404.
13. Kühn LC, McClelland A, Ruddle FH. Gene transfer expression and molecular cloning of the human transferrin receptor gene. Cell 1984;37:95.
14. Schatz DG, Oettinger MA, Baltimore D. The V(D)J recombination activating gene, RAG-1. Cell 1989;59:1035.
15. Collins FS. Positional cloning: let's not call it reverse anymore. Nature Genet 1992;1:3.
16. Sanger F, Nicklen S, Coulson AR. DNA sequencing with chain-terminating inhibitors. Proc Natl Acad Sci USA. 1977;74:5463.
17. Maxam AM, Gilbert W. A new method for sequencing DNA. Proc Natl Acad Sci USA 1977;74:560.
18. Potter H. Review. Electroporation in biology: methods, applications, and instrumentation. Anal Biochem 1988;174:361.
19. Kaufman RJ. Strategies for obtaining high level expression in mammalian cells. Technique 1990;2:221.
20. Gluzman Y. SV40-transformed simian cells support the replication of early SV40 mutants. Cell 1981;23:175.
21. Kunkel TA, Roberts JD, Zakour RA. Rapid and efficient site-specific mutagenesis without phenotypic selection. Methods Enzymol 1987;154:367.
22. Jaenisch R. Transgenic animals. Science 1988;240:1468.
23. Orkin SH, Kazazian HH Jr. The mutation and polymorphism of the human β-globin gene and its surrounding DNA. Annu Rev Genet 1984;18:131.
24. Chu G, Vollrath D, Davis RW. Separation of large DNA molecules by contour-clamped homogeneous electric fields. Science 1986;234:1582.
25. Saiki R, Gelfand D, Stoffel S, et al. Primer-directed enzymatic amplification of DNA with a thermostable DNA polymerase. Science 1988;239:487.
26. Lerman LS, Silverstein K. Computational simulation of DNA melting and its application to denaturing gradient gel electrophoresis. Methods Enzymol 1987;155:482.
27. Orita M, Suzuki Y, Sekiya T, et al. Rapid and sensitive detection of point mutations and DNA polymorphisms using the polymerase chain reaction. Genomics 1989;5:874.
28. Galski H, Sullivan M, Willingham MC, et al. Expression of a human multidrug-resistance cDNA (*MDR1*) in the bone marrow of transgenic mice: resistance to daunomycin-induced leukopenia. Mol Cell Biol 1989;9:4357.
29. Daley GQ, Van Etten RA, Baltimore D. Induction of chronic myelogenous leukemia in mice by the P210$^{bcr/abl}$ gene of the Philadelphia chromosome. Science 1990;247:824.

Blood: Principles and Practice of Hematology,
edited by Robert I. Handin, Thomas P. Stossel, and Samuel E. Lux.
J.B. Lippincott Company, Philadelphia © 1995.

5

Cytogenetics for the Hematologist

Cynthia C. Morton

Cytogenetics is the area of biology that deals with the study of chromosomes. In the past decade, this discipline has witnessed remarkable developments with significant scientific contributions of relevance to the field of hematology. No longer is cytogenetics restricted to its traditional descriptive role in dysmorphology, reproductive medicine, and prenatal diagnosis. It is now an integral part of the clinical practice of hematology. Beyond the clinical relevance of cytogenetic studies in diagnosis, prognosis, and treatment, this science has been used widely in gene mapping and in the identification of genes, and, in some instances, has led to the cloning of genes responsible for specific diseases. Two hematologic disorders, chronic myelogenous leukemia and Burkitt's lymphoma, provide paradigms for interfacing cytogenetics, gene mapping, and molecular cloning to achieve a better understanding of the molecular pathogenesis of disease.

ORGANIZATION OF HUMAN CHROMOSOMES AND METHODS OF STUDY

The human chromosome is a complex structure that consists of DNA and several different proteins. A single helix of DNA is bounded on each end by a structure known as a *telomere*. Each normal human chromosome has one centromere. The *centromere* is the site at which the kinetochore forms for attachment of the mitotic spindle, which is required for proper movement of the chromosome during cell division. The centromere divides the chromosome into two arms. In human chromosomes, the position of the centromere is either central (metacentric), distal (acrocentric), or somewhere in between (submetacentric), providing a useful landmark in the identification of a particular chromosome (Fig. 5-1). The two arms of the human chromosome are identified as p (petite) for the short arm and q for the long arm.

Human chromosomes vary in size, with the largest chromosome designated number 1. In 1956, Tjio and Levan[1] determined that there are a total of 46 chromosomes: 22 pairs of autosomes and one pair of sex chromosomes. With the exception of pairs 21 and 22, the numeric designation reflects the size of the chromosome (eg, chromosome 4 is the fourth largest chromosome). Although chromosome 21 is smaller than chromosome 22, this inconsistency in nomenclature has been perpetuated to avoid confusion due to historical references to Down syndrome as trisomy 21. Prior to development of banding techniques that provide unequivocal identification of each chromosome, the size and position of the centromere were used to place chromosomes into groups. Although infrequently used today to refer to a particular chromosome, the groupings still are useful in instances in which banding may be inadequate to identify precisely the chromosome in question. The groups are as follows: A (1 to 3), B (4 to 5), C (6 to 12,X), D (13 to 15), E (16 to 18), F (19 to 20), and G (21 to 22,Y) (Fig. 5-2).

A karyotype is a display of chromosomes from largest to smallest (with the exception of pairs 21 and 22) with chromosomes oriented so that the p arm is on top. In the human species, the female is the homogametic sex and a normal female karyotype is designated 46,XX; the male is the heterogametic sex and a normal male karyotype is described as 46,XY. Excluding chromosomal abnormalities and variants, karyotypes of two unrelated males or females may appear virtually identical; furthermore, excluding sex chromosomes, karyotypes of males and females are indistinguishable.

Metaphase Preparations of Cultured Cells

Most cytogenetic analyses are performed on chromosomes that are in metaphase of mitosis. At this stage of the cell cycle, condensation of DNA results in distinguishable entities that are characteristic for each species. Special studies to investigate a particular region of a chromosome may require less condensed chromosomes such as those found in prometaphase. The most frequently used tissues for cytogenetic evaluation, due primarily to their accessibility, are peripheral blood lymphocytes, amniotic fluid cells, chorionic villus, skin fibroblasts, and bone marrow. The process of preparing chromosomes for analysis is known as a harvest.

Chromosomes are harvested either after culture of the tissue, or, in the case of bone marrow, some solid tumors, or cord blood, after direct harvest of mitotic cells. Any of a variety of mitogens such as phytohemagglutinin or pokeweed is routinely added to lymphocyte cultures to promote cell growth. Peripheral blood lymphocyte cultures are typically harvested after 48 to 72 hours of culture, a technique introduced by Moorhead and associates[2] in 1960. The addition of mitogen to these cultures synchronizes cells so that several rounds of division will have occurred. Fibroblast and amniotic fluid cell cultures are judged to be mitotically active by the presence of rounded refractile cells, which must be distinguished from dead cells. The harvest

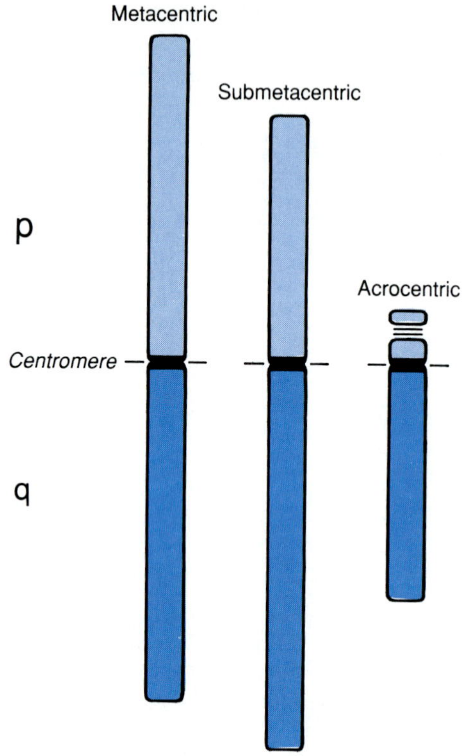

FIGURE 5-1. Schematic diagram of prototypic human chromosomes demonstrating metacentric, submetacentric, and acrocentric chromosomes, p, short arm; q, long arm.

itself may be performed in solution, as is commonly performed for lymphocyte cultures and for other cultures in which attached cells have been released from the tissue culture vessel, or it may be performed in situ, that is, attached to the tissue culture surface.

The in situ procedure is frequently used for amniotic fluid cultures where it may be desirable to evaluate colonies of cells to ascertain chromosomal mosaicism. In all cases, dividing cells must be arrested during mitosis. This is accomplished typically by the addition of colchicine to the culture. Colchicine functions to shorten chromosomes, destroy the mitotic spindle, and arrest the cells in metaphase. After incubation in colchicine, the harvest proceeds with a hypotonic treatment, ordinarily 0.075 mol potassium chloride or 0.8% sodium citrate, which serves to swell the cells. Several rounds of fixation in methanol–acetic acid (3:1) complete the harvest. Depending on the type of harvest that has been performed, metaphases will now either be ready for spreading on a coverslip or slide if harvested in situ or dropped onto slides if they have been harvested in solution.

Preparation of slides or coverslips following the harvest is one of the most critical steps in obtaining quality material for analysis. Factors that influence surface tension such as temperature and humidity are doubtless crucial variables in slide making.

Banding Techniques

Many different banding techniques are used routinely in cytogenetics laboratories. Several of the most popular

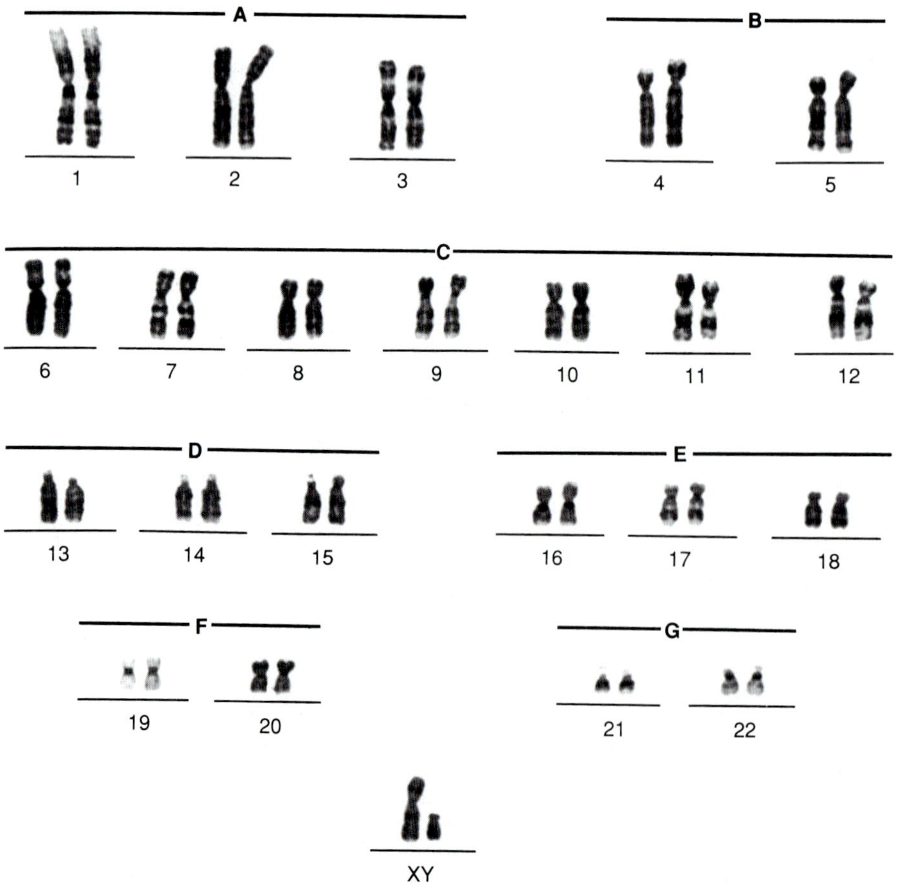

FIGURE 5-2. A representative normal human male GTG-banded karyotype (46,XY).

techniques are G-banding,[3,4] Q-banding,[5] and R-banding[6-8] (Fig. 5-3).

GTG-Banding

Although various methods for producing a G-banded karyotype exist, a popular technique uses proteolytic digestion of chromosomes with trypsin followed by staining in Giemsa. A pattern of alternating light and dark bands are produced enabling identification of each chromosome pair by bright field microscopy. Investigations of chromosome banding patterns with antinucleotide antibodies indicate that light G bands are predominantly GC rich and that dark G bands are AT rich.[9] Light bands are believed to contain more euchromatin, DNA that is replicated early in S phase of the cell cycle and is transcribed. In contrast, dark bands are thought to be composed largely of heterochromatin, DNA that is more condensed and late-replicating.

QFQ-Banding

The Q-banded karyotype is generated by intercalation of quinacrine dihydrochloride or quinacrine mustard dihydrochloride between nucleotide bases of the DNA helix. A pattern of bands similar to those seen in the G-banded karyotype is produced. This is a fluorescent staining method and requires fluorescence microscopy for visualization. In addition, Q-banding permits detection of regions of variable staining known as polymorphisms. Polymorphisms are located at the centromeres of chromosomes 3, 4, 13, and 22, at the short arms and satellites of acrocentric chromosomes (pairs 13 to 15, 21, and 22), and at the distal region of the Y chromosome. Generally, these polymorphisms are stable heritable markers without clinical significance.[10-12] They can be a valuable diagnostic tool because they may permit determination of paternity.[13] These polymorphisms may also mark the parental origin of a particular chromosome[14,15] or indicate maternal cell admixture in a mixed tissue sample.[16]

R-Banding

Reverse banding or R-banding produces a banding pattern that is essentially the opposite of that seen with G- or Q-banding. In other words, a light G band will be a dark R band and vice versa. Terminal regions of many chromosomes tend to be pale by G- or Q-banding, and small deletions or rearrangements in these regions may be difficult to detect. In such cases an R-banded preparation may make such an aberration visible. Protocols exist for both bright field and fluorescent R-banding.

Special Stains and Other Methodologies

Special staining techniques have been developed to assist in analysis of particular chromosomes or regions of particular chromosomes. For example, C-banding or centric banding is particularly useful in analysis of centromeres.[17] This technique involves acid treatment followed by incubation in alkali (eg, barium hydroxide), then staining in Giemsa. The basis of the banding is that a different kind of chromatin, known as *constitutive heterochromatin*, is present in the centromeric regions of all normal chromosomes and the distal portion of the Y chromosome. (Constitutive heterochromatin is a type of heterochromatin consisting of DNA that remains condensed and genetically inactive. A special type of heterochromatin, *facultative heterochromatin*, may decondense and become genetically active.) Chromosomes 1, 9, and 16 tend to have larger amounts of C-banded material in the pericentromeric region, and considerable variation exists in the human population.[18] An inversion in the pericentromeric region of chromosome 9 is another common polymorphism, and C-banding may be used to show that such an inversion is limited to heterochromatin.[19] C-banding is also used to elucidate the structure of unidentified marker chromosomes or derivative chromosomes.

Other special stains are silver staining, also known as NOR-staining,[20] which identifies active nucleolar organizer regions (the sites of the rRNA genes) on acrocentric chromosomes, and DA-DAPI staining,[8] which reacts with centromeres of chromosomes 1, 9, and 16, the short arm of chromosome 15, and the distal end of the Y chromosome. Most recently, banding patterns have been produced with a combination of molecular genetic and cytogenetic techniques. For example, enzymatic digestion of chromosomes with restriction endonucleases[21] and hybridization with repetitive DNA sequences[22] has produced banding patterns reminiscent of G and C bands, and of R bands, respectively.

High-Resolution Banding

In general, clinical laboratories perform banding techniques on chromosomes in mid-metaphase, at which time 350 to 400 bands can be resolved. Other techniques that enrich for chromosomes in earlier stages of metaphase or in prophase provide higher-resolution banding methods and are used when a particular region of a chromosome is being studied. High-resolution methods in practice include amethopterin synchronization of cell cultures with thymidine release[23] and addition of Actinomycin D (dactinomycin)[24,25] or ethidium bromide[26] to the final hours of culture before the harvest.

Idiograms and Chromosome Nomenclature

An idiogram is a schematic standardized karyotype (Fig. 5-4) that is derived from measured band sizes. The idiogram and chromosome nomenclature have been designed by an international committee that has met periodically since 1960 (the Denver Report) to establish uniform language for describing chromosome bands and chromosomal aberrations.[27] Chromosome regions are subdivided into bands and, at higher resolution, into subbands. For example, the designation 14q24 indicates chromosome 14, the long arm, region 2, band 4. On the idiogram, chromosome bands are numbered in an ascending fashion from centromere to telomere on each arm of the chromosome.

A fairly sophisticated set of rules governs the description of chromosomal abnormalities; these rules are set out in the 1985 International System for Human Cytogenetic Nomenclature (ISCN)[28] and a supplement published in 1991 with guidelines for cancer cytogenetics.[29] Basically, the total number of chromosomes is specified first followed by the sex chromosomes (eg, the normal male karyotype is given as 46,XY). Any additions or deletions of entire chromosomes are specified next and are designated by a plus or

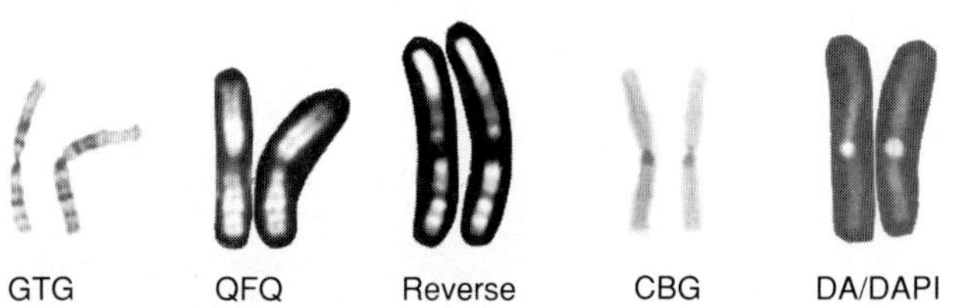

FIGURE 5-3. Chromosome 1 shown after various banding techniques—GTG, QFQ, reverse, CBG, and DA/DAPI.

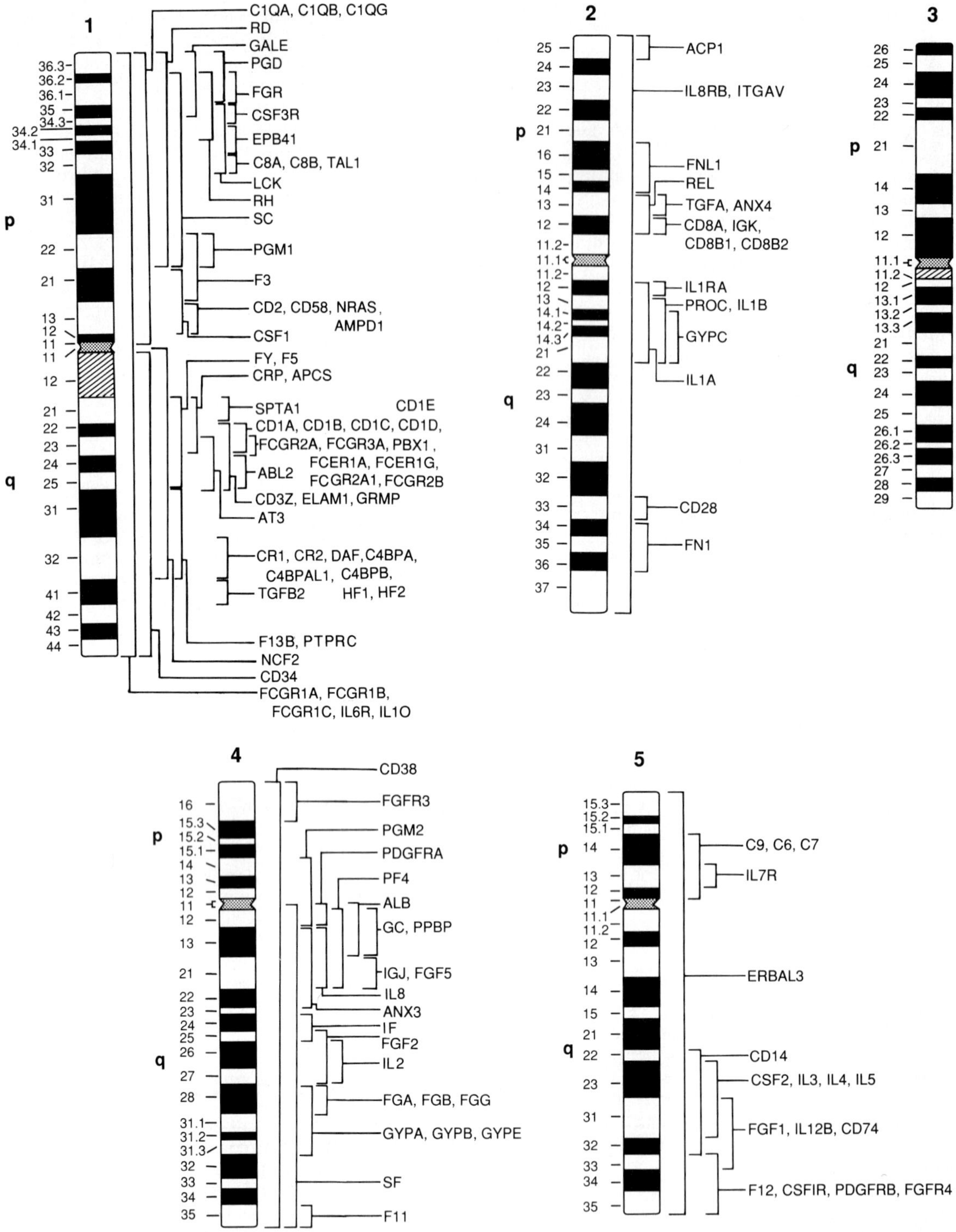

FIGURE 5-4. Location of genes with relevance to hematology displayed on the standardized idiogram of human chromosomes at the 400 band stage.[28]

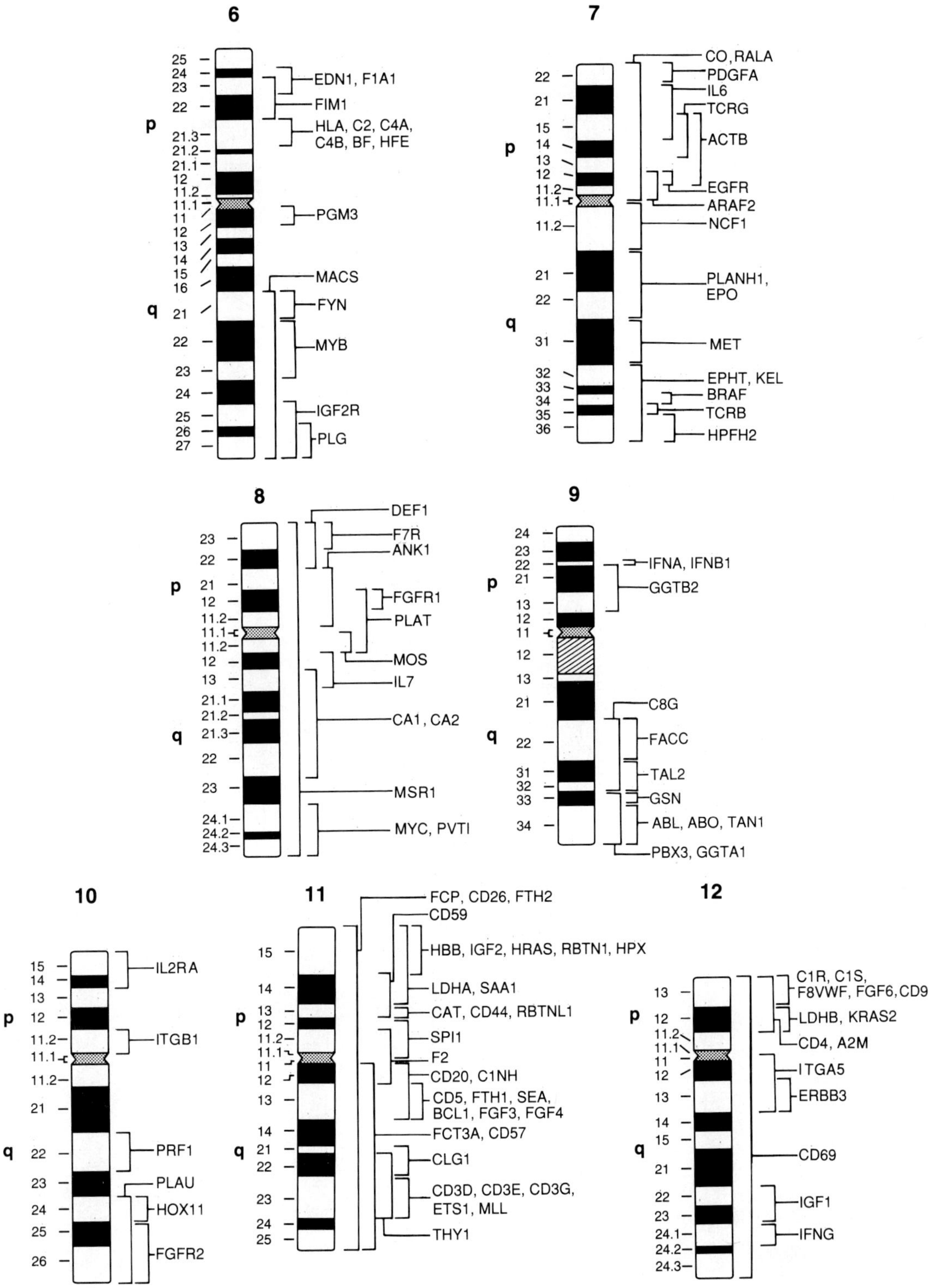

FIGURE 5-4. (Continued)

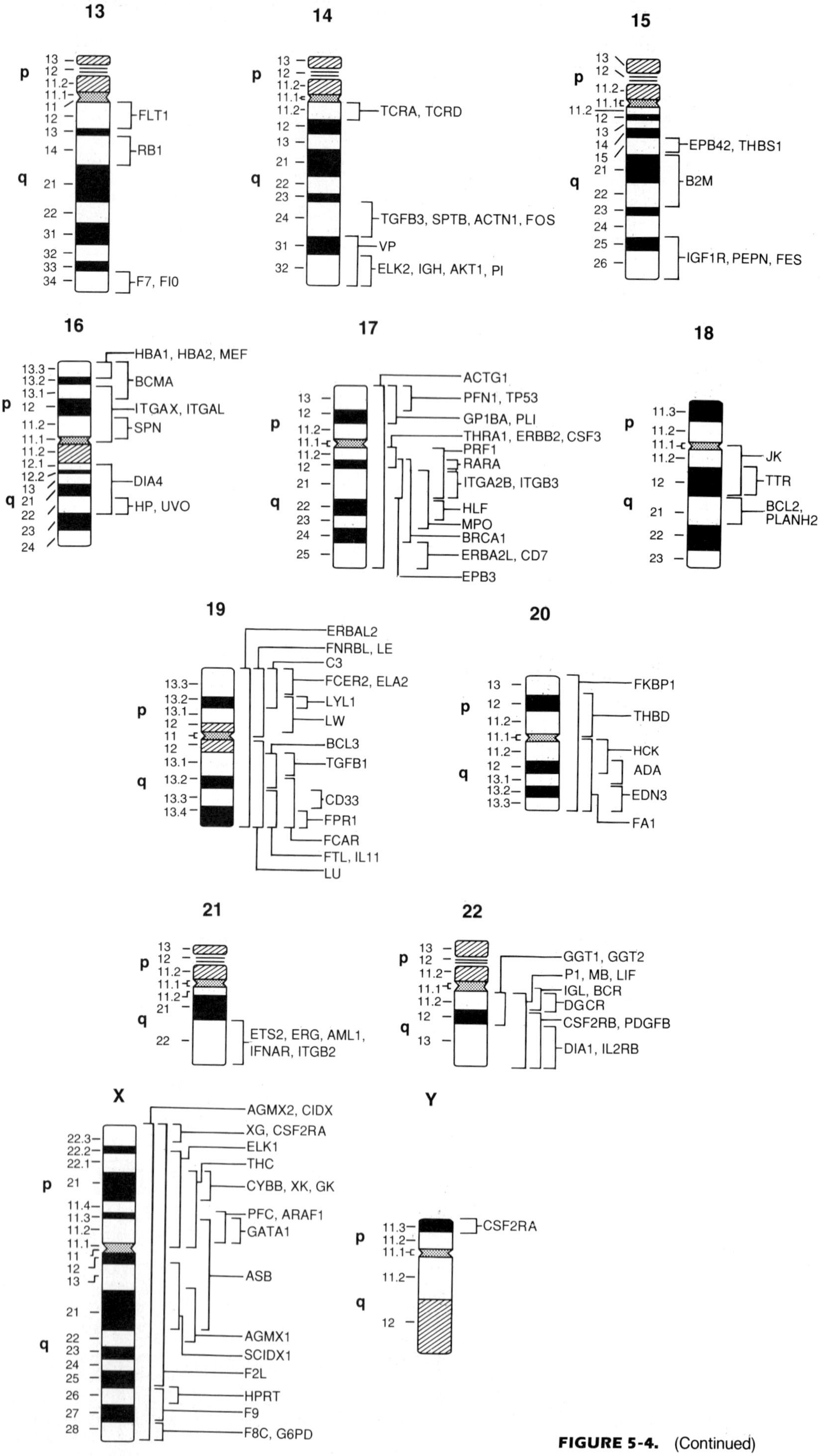

FIGURE 5-4. (Continued)

minus sign preceding the chromosome number (a female with trisomy 21 may be designated as 47,XX,+21). Last, any structural aberration is listed. In the case of translocations, which are common aberrations in leukemias and lymphomas, a t precedes two sets of parentheses. The first set of parentheses contains the numbers of the chromosomes involved, with the lower numbered chromosome listed first except for X or Y, and the second set indicates the corresponding breakpoints (a male with the classic chromosome rearrangement in chronic myelogenous leukemia (CML) may be indicated as 46,XY,t(9;22)(q34;q11)). A frequently used term that is especially useful in describing rearranged chromosomes is the designation *derivative* or *der*. This indicates that a particular rearranged chromosome is generated from a rearrangement involving two or more chromosomes and has the centromere from the indicated chromosome (eg, der[14]).

Somatic Cell Hybrids

Mapping of genes to specific human chromosomes was revolutionized by the development of somatic cell genetics.[30-32] After fusion of rodent and human cells, human chromosomes were lost somewhat randomly and cell lines with a reduced number of human chromosomes could be established. Panels of such cell lines containing various human chromosomes were established. The concordance (and discordance) of a protein from an enzymatic assay on the cell line could be correlated with the constellation of chromosomes present in the hybrid. When cloned genes and anonymous DNA segments became available, DNA was extracted from the hybrids, and Southern blots were prepared. Blots are hybridized with the DNA fragment to be mapped, and presence or absence of a particular restriction fragment scored with respect to chromosomes present in the hybrid. Most recently, polymerase chain reaction (PCR) of hybrid DNAs has been performed with primers specific for the gene under investigation; the advantage of this methodology is that only minute amounts of precious hybrid DNA are required.

In addition to hybrid lines made with intact human chromosomes, hybrid lines have been developed also by fusion of rodent cells with human cell lines that have chromosomal rearrangements. Segregation of derivative products of a translocation in separate hybrid lines permits determination of a gene assignment with respect to the chromosomal breakpoints. In this way, it is possible to make a more precise regional assignment on a chromosome. The development of hybrid lines from patients with rearrangements within a small region of the genome provides an excellent method to map genes with respect to one another.

In Situ Hybridization

The tools of cytogenetics and molecular biology contribute jointly to a powerful new mapping technique, chromosomal in situ hybridization.[33] The advantage of this technique is that a rather precise chromosomal assignment can be determined in a relatively short time frame.

The two different approaches to chromosomal in situ hybridization are isotopic[33,34] and nonisotopic.[35,36] Probes are labeled with radionucleotides in the isotopic method, or with biotin or digoxigenin, typically, in the nonisotopic method, and are then hybridized to slides on which metaphase chromosomes have been prepared and denatured. Following hybridization and washing, slides are dipped in photographic emulsion for detection of radionucleotide signal; alternatively, slides may be incubated with avidin conjugated to a fluorescent dye such as fluorescein, or streptavidin conjugated with peroxidase for detection of biotinylated probes. Metaphases are analyzed and scored for hybridization to a particular chromosome region over the background hybridization to other chromosomes (Fig. 5-5).

A valuable application of in situ hybridization is in the interpretation of chromosome rearrangements. For example, knowledge of the location of a particular gene with respect to a chromosome translocation may aid an effort to clone the translocation breakpoint by providing an orientation for the rearrangement.[37,38] Furthermore, investigation of a cryptic chromosome rearrangement by localization of gene sequences known to be present in a particular chromosome region may elucidate the rearrangement.[39]

THE HUMAN GENOME AND HEMATOLOGY

Mapping the human genome is a task now being approached in a serious fashion by numerous organizations in the United States, including the National Institutes of Health and the Department of Energy, as well as various groups in other countries. Although discussed only in terms of its feasibility in the recent past, this goal has now become a reality. Many valid reasons exist for undertaking such a large project but chief among them is identification of markers or genes for human disease loci. As of the Chromosome Coordinating Meeting (CCM92; Baltimore), 2708 genes had been assigned to chromosomes. Far in excess of gene assignments were localizations of anonymous DNA segments.

Many different perspectives can be used to view the gene map. In this chapter, we consider locations of genes of relevance to the field of hematology (Table 5-1 and Fig. 5-4).

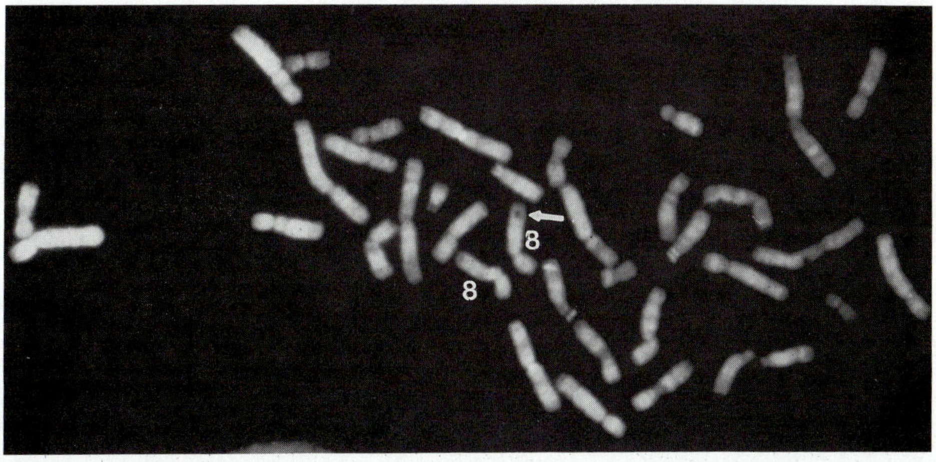

FIGURE 5-5. Chromosome in situ hybridization with a probe for the *myc* gene showing hybridization at 8q24.

TABLE 5-1. Map Locations of Genes with Relevance to Hematology

Marker Name	Gene Symbol	Map Location
RED CELL ENZYMES AND MEMBRANE PROTEINS		
ABO blood group	*ABO*	9q34.1-q34.2
Colton blood group	*CO*	7p
Duffy blood group	*FY*	1q21-q25
Gerbich blood group (glycophorin C)	*GYPC*	2q14-q21
Ii blood group	*II*	linkage group 3
Kell blood group	*KEL*	7q32-qter
Kell blood group precursor (McLeod)	*XK*	Xp21.1
Kidd blood group	*JK*	18q11-q12
Landsteiner-Wiener blood group	*LW*	19p13.2-cen
Lewis blood group	*LE*	19p
Lutheran blood group	*LU*	19q12-q13
MN blood group (glycophorin A)	*GYPA*	4q28-q31
P blood group	*P1*	22q11.2-qter
Radin blood group	*RD*	1p36-p22.1
Rhesus blood group	*RH*	1p36.2-p34
Scianna blood group	*SC*	1p36.2-p22.1
Ss blood group (glycophorin B)	*GYPB*	4q28-q31
Stoltzfus blood group	*SF*	4q
Xg blood group	*XG*	Xp22.3
Acid phosphatase 1, soluble	*ACP1*	2p25
AMP deaminase	*AMPD1*	1p13
Aminolevulinate, δ-, synthase 1	*ALAS1*	3p21
Anemia, sideroblastic/hypochromic	*ASB*	Xp11.21-q21.31
Ankyrin 1, erythrocytic	*ANK1*	8p21.1-p11.2
Antigen CD2 (p50), sheep red blood cell receptor	*CD2*	1p13
Carbonic anhydrase I	*CA1*	8q13-q22.1
Carbonic anhydrase II	*CA2*	8q13-q22.1
Catalase	*CAT*	11p13
Diaphorase (NADH) (cytochrome b-5 reductase)	*DIA1*	22q13.31-qter
Diaphorase (NADH/NADPH) (cyt b-5 reductase)	*DIA4*	16q12-q22
Erythrocyte surface protein band 3	*EPB3*	17q12-q21
Erythrocyte surface protein band 3-like	*EPB3L1*	7q35-q36
Erythrocyte surface protein band 4.1 (elliptocytosis 1, RH-linked)	*EPB41*	1p34.2-p33
Erythrocyte surface protein band 4.2	*EPB42*	15q15
Fanconi anemia 1	*FA1*	20q
Fanconi anemia, complementation group C	*FACC*	9q22.3
Ferritin, heavy polypeptide 1	*FTH1*	11q13
Ferritin, heavy polypeptide 2	*FTH2*	11
Ferritin, light polypeptide	*FTL*	19q13.3-q13.4
UDP-galactose-4-epimerase	*GALE*	1p36-p35
GATA-binding protein 1 (globin transcription factor 1)	*GATA1*	Xp11.23
Glucose-6-phosphate dehydrogenase	*G6PD*	Xq28
Glycerol kinase deficiency	*GK*	Xp21.3
Glycoprotein, α-galactosyltransferase 1	*GGTA1*	9q33-q34
Glycoprotein, 4-β-galactosyltransferase 2	*GGTB2*	9p21-p13
Glycophorin E	*GYPE*	4q28-q31
Haptoglobin	*HP*	16q22.1
Hemoglobin, α 1 and α 2	*HBA1/A2*	16p13.3
Hemoglobin, β, cluster	*HBB*	11p15.5
Hemoglobin F-cell production	*FCP*	11
Hemochromatosis	*HFE*	6p21.3
Hereditary persistence of HbF	*HPFH2*	7q36
Hypoxanthine phosphoribosyltransferase	*HPRT*	Xq26.1
Lactate dehydrogenase A	*LDHA*	11p15.1-p14
Lactate dehydrogeanse B	*LDHB*	12p12.2-p12.1
Myoglobin	*MB*	22q11.2-qter

(continued)

TABLE 5-1. *(Continued)*

Marker Name	Gene Symbol	Map Location
RED CELL ENZYMES AND MEMBRANE PROTEINS (continued)		
Phosphoglucomutase 1	*PGM1*	1p22.1
Phosphoglucomutase 2	*PGM2*	4p14-q12
Phosphoglucomutase 3	*PGM3*	6q12
Phosphogluconate dehydrogenase	*PGD*	1p36.3-p36.13
Spectrin, α, erythrocytic 1 (elliptocytosis 2)	*SPTA1*	1q21
Spectrin, β, erythrocytic (includes spherocytosis, clinical type I)	*SPTB*	14q24.1-q24.2
Variegate porphyria (protoporphyrinogen oxidase)	*VP*	14q31-q32
WHITE CELL AND PLATELET MEMBRANE PROTEINS		
Actin, β	*ACTB*	7p15-p12
Actin, γ1	*ACTG1*	17
Actinin, α1	*ACTN1*	14q24.1-q24.2
Collagenase I, neutrophil	*CLG1*	11q21-q22
Cytochrome b-245, β polypeptide	*CYBB*	Xp21.1
Defensin	*DEF1*	8p23-p22
Elastase 2, neutrophil	*ELA2*	19p13.3
Fc fragment of IgA, receptor	*FCAR*	19q13.2-q13.4
Fc fragment of IgE, high-affinity I receptor, α polypeptide	*FCER1A*	1q23
Fc fragment of IgE, high-affinity I receptor, γ polypeptide	*FCER1G*	1q23
Fc fragment of IgE, low-affinity II receptor (CD23A)	*FCER2*	19p13.3
Fc fragment of IgG, high-affinity Ia receptor	*FCGR1A*	1
Fc fragment of IgG, high-affinity Ib receptor	*FCGR1B*	1
Fc fragment of IgG, high-affinity Ic receptor	*FCGR1C*	1
Fc fragment of IgG, low-affinity IIa receptor (CD32)	*FCGR2A*	1q23
Fc fragment of IgG, low-affinity IIa receptor	*FCGR2A1*	1q23
Fc fragment of IgG, low-affinity IIb receptor	*FCGR2B*	1q23
Fc fragment of IgG, low-affinity III-1 receptor (CD16)	*FCGR3A*	1q23
Fc fragment of IgG, low-affinity III-2 receptor	*FCGR3B*	1q23
Formyl peptide receptor 1	*FPR1*	19q13.4
Gelsolin (amyloidosis, Finnish type)	*GSN*	9q33
Glycoprotein Ib (platelet), α polypeptide	*GP1BA*	17pter-p12
Glycoprotein IX (platelet)	*GP9*	3
Granule membrane protein (140kD, CD62)	*GRMP*	1q22-q25
Integrin, α2b (platelet glycoprotein IIb of IIb/IIIa complex, antigen CD41B)	*ITGA2B*	17q21.32
Integrin, β3 (platelet glycoprotein IIIa, antigen CD61)	*ITGB3*	17q21.32
Macrophage scavenger receptor 1	*MSR1*	8
Macrophage stimulating 1 (hepatocyte growth factor-like)	*MST1*	3p21
Myeloperoxidase	*MPO*	17q21.3-q23
Myristoylated alanine-rich protein kinase C substrate (MARCKS, 80K-L)	*MACS*	6q21-q27
Neutrophil cytosolic factor 1 (chronic granulomatous disease, autosomal 1)	*NCF1*	7q11.23
Neutrophil cytosolic factor 2 (chronic granulomatous disease, autosomal 2)	*NCF2*	1cen-q32
Perforin	*PRF1*	10q22 and 17q11.2-q21.3
Platelet factor 4	*PF4*	4q12-q21
Profilin 1	*PFN1*	17p13.3
Proplatelet basic protein (includes platelet basic protein, β-thromboglobulin, neutrophil-activating peptide-2)	*PPBP*	4q12-q13
Stromelysin 1	*STMY1*	11q22.3-q23
Thrombomodulin	*THBD*	20p12-cen
Thrombospondin	*THBS1*	15q15
Thrombocytopenia I (X-linked)	*THC*	Xp21-p11
LYMPHOCYTE CELL SURFACE PROTEINS AND ANTIGENS		
T-cell receptor, α polypeptide	*TCRA*	14q11.2
T-cell receptor, β polypeptide	*TCRB*	7q35
T-cell receptor, γ polypeptide	*TCRG*	7p15-p14
T-cell receptor, δ polypeptide	*TCRD*	14q11.2

(continued)

TABLE 5-1. *(Continued)*

Marker Name	Gene Symbol	Map Location
LYMPHOCYTE CELL SURFACE PROTEINS AND ANTIGENS (continued)		
Antigen CD1A, a polypeptide	*CD1A*	1q22-q23
Antigen CD1B, b polypeptide	*CD1B*	1q22-q23
Antigen CD1C, c polypeptide	*CD1C*	1q22-q23
Antigen CD1D, d polypeptide	*CD1D*	1q22-q23
Antigen CD1E, e polypeptide	*CD1E*	1q22-q23
Antigen CD3D, δ polypeptide (TiT3)	*CD3D*	11q23
Antigen CD3E, ϵ polypeptide (TiT3)	*CD3E*	11q23
Antigen CD3G, γ polypeptide (TiT3)	*CD3G*	11q23
Antigen CD3Z, ζ polypeptide (TiT3)	*CD3Z*	1q22-q25
Antigen CD4 (p55)	*CD4*	12pter-p12
Antigen CD5 (p56-62)	*CD5*	11q13
Antigen CD7 (p41)	*CD7*	17q25.2-q25.3
Antigen CD8A (p32)	*CD8A*	2p12
Antigen CD8B, β polypeptide 1 (p37)	*CD8B1*	2p12
Antigen CD8B, β polypeptide 2 (p37)	*CD8B2*	2p12
Antigen CD9 (p24)	*CD9*	12p13
Antigen CD10 (membrane metalloendopeptidase)	*MME*	3q21-q27
Antigen CD14	*CD14*	5q22-q32
Antigen CD20	*CD20*	11q12-q13.1
Antigen CD26 (p250)	*CD26*	11
Antigen CD28 (Tp44)	*CD28*	2q33
Antigen CD33 (gp67)	*CD33*	19q13.3
Antigen CD34	*CD34*	1q12-qter
Antigen CD38 (p45)	*CD38*	4
Antigen CD43 (sialophorin, gpL115)	*SPN*	16p11.2
Antigen CD44	*CD44*	11p13
Antigen CD48 (B-cell membrane protein)	*CD48*	1q21.3-q22
Antigen CD57 (LEU7)	*CD57*	11q12-qter
Antigen CD58	*CD58*	1p13
Antigen CD59	*CD59*	11p14-p13
Antigen CD69 (p60, early T-cell activation)	*CD69*	12
Antigen CD74 (invariant polypeptide of MHC class II antigen associated)	*CD74*	5q31-q33
Complement component (3b/4b) receptor 1	*CR1*	1q32
Complement component (3d/Epstein Barr virus receptor)	*CR2*	1q32
Decay accelerating factor for complement	*DAF*	1q32
Fucosyltransferase 3A (antigen CD15)	*FCT3A*	11q12-qter
Integrin, α M (antigen, CD11b (p170), complement component receptor 3)	*ITGAM*	16p11.2
Integrin, α L (antigen CD11A (p180), lymphocyte function-associated antigen 1, α polypeptide)	*ITGAL*	16p13.1-p11
Integrin, β2 (antigen CD18 (p95), lymphocyte function-associated antigen 1; macrophage antigen 1 (mac-1))	*ITGB2*	21q22.3
Peptidase N, amino- (antigen CD13, p150)	*PEPN*	15q25-q26
Protein tyrosine phosphatase (antigen CD45)	*PTPRC*	1q31-q32
Thy-1 cell surface antigen	*THY1*	11q22.3-q23
Uvomorulin	*UVO*	16q22.1
IMMUNE SYSTEM, COMPLEMENT, AND OTHER PLASMA PROTEINS		
Immunoglobulin heavy chain	*IGH*	14q32.3
Immunoglobulin κ chain	*IGK*	2p12
Immunoglobulin λ chain	*IGL*	22q11.1-q11.2
Immunoglobulin J polypeptide	*IGJ*	4q21
Complement component 1 inhibitor	*C1NH*	11q12-q13.1
Complement component 1, q subcomponent, α polypeptide	*C1QA*	1p
Complement component 1, q subcomponent, β polypeptide	*C1QB*	1p
Complement component 1, q subcomponent, γ polypeptide	*C1QG*	1p
Complement component 1, r subcomponent	*C1R*	12p13
Complement component 1, s subcomponent	*C1S*	12p13

(continued)

TABLE 5-1. *(Continued)*

Marker Name	Gene Symbol	Map Location
IMMUNE SYSTEM, COMPLEMENT, AND OTHER PLASMA PROTEINS (continued)		
Complement component 2	*C2*	6p21.3
Complement component 3	*C3*	19p13.3-p13.2
Complement component 4A	*C4A*	6p21.3
Complement component 4B	*C4B*	6p21.3
Complement component 4 binding protein, α	*C4BPA*	1q32
Complement component 4 binding protein, α-like 1	*C4BPAL1*	1q32
Complement component 4 binding protein, β	*C4BPB*	1q32
Complement component 5	*C5*	9q33
Complement component 6	*C6*	5p14-p12
Complement component 7	*C7*	5p14-p12
Complement component 8, α polypeptide	*C8A*	1p32
Complement component 8, β polypeptide	*C8B*	1p32
Complement component 8, γ polypeptide	*C8G*	9q22.3-q32
Complement component 9	*C9*	5p14-p12
H factor 1 (complement)	*HF1*	1q32
H factor 2 (complement)	*HF2*	1q32
Complement component I	*IF*	4q24-q25
Properdin P factor, complement	*PFC*	Xp11.3-p11.23
Interferon, α (leukocyte)	*IFNA*	9p22
Interferon, α and β receptor	*IFNAR*	21p22.1
Interferon, β 1, fibroblast	*IFNB1*	9p22
Interferon, γ	*IFNG*	12q24.1
Interferon regulatory factor 1	*IRF1*	5q23-q31
Interferon regulatory factor 2	*IRF2*	4q34.1-q35.1
β-2-Microglobulin	*B2M*	15q21-q22.2
Major histocompatibility complex, classes I and II	*HLA**	6p21.3
Properdin factor B	*BF*	6p21.3
Adenosine deaminase	*ADA*	20q12-q13.11
Agammaglobulinemia, X-linked 1 (Bruton)	*AGMX1*	Xq21.33-q22
Agammaglobulinemia, X-linked 2	*AGMX2*	X
Albumin	*ALB*	4q11-q13
α-1-Antitrypsin (protease inhibitor)	*PI*	14q32.1
α-2-Macroglobulin	*A2M*	12p13.3-p12.3
Amyloid P component, serum	*APCS*	1q21-q23
B-cell maturation	*BCMA*	16p13
Combined immunodeficiency, X-linked	*CIDX*	X
C-reactive protein	*CRP*	1q21-q23
DiGeorge syndrome chromosome region	*DGCR*	22q11.21-q11.23
FK506-binding protein 1 (12kD)	*FKBP1*	20
Fibronectin 1	*FN1*	2q34-q36
Fibronectin-like 1	*FNL1*	2p16-p14
Group-specific component (vitamin D binding)	*GC*	4q12-q13
Hemopexin	*HPX*	11p15.5-p15.4
Lymphocyte-specific protein tyrosine kinase	*LCK*	1p35-p32
Mediterranean fever	*MEF*	16p13.3
Serum amyloid A1	*SAA1*	11p15.1-p14
Severe combined immunodeficiency, X-linked 1	*SCIDX1*	Xq13-q21.1
Transferrin	*TF*	3q21
Transferrin receptor (p90)	*TFRC*	3q26.2-qter
Transthyretin (prealbumin, amyloidosis type I)	*TTR*	18q12.1
COAGULATION PROTEINS AND RELATED GENES		
Coagulation factor II	*F2*	11p11-q12
Coagulation factor II-like	*F2L*	Xpter-q25
Coagulation factor III	*F3*	1p22-p21
Coagulation factor V	*F5*	1q21-q25

(continued)

TABLE 5-1. *(Continued)*

Marker Name	Gene Symbol	Map Location
COAGULATION PROTEINS AND RELATED GENES (continued)		
Coagulation factor VII	*F7*	13q34
Coagulation factor VII regulator	*F7R*	8p23.2-p23.1
Coagulation factor VIIIc	*F8C*	Xq28
Coagulation factor VIII VWF	*F8VWF*	12p13.3-p13.2
Coagulation factor IX	*F9*	Xq26.3-q27.1
Coagulation factor X	*F10*	13q34
Coagulation factor XI	*F11*	4q35
Coagulation factor XII	*F12*	5q33-qter
Coagulation factor XIII, A1 polypeptide	*F13A1*	6p24.2-p23
Coagulation factor XIII, B polypeptide	*F13B*	1q31-q32.1
Annexin III (placental anticoagulant protein III)	*ANX3*	4q13-q22
Annexin IV (placental anticoagulant protein II)	*ANX4*	2p13
Antithrombin III	*AT3*	1q23-q25.1
γ-Glutamyltransferase 1	*GGT1*	22q11.2-q12.1
γ-Glutamyltransferase 2	*GGT2*	22q11.2-q12.1
Protein C (inactivator of Va and VIIIa)	*PROC*	2q13-q21
Kallikrein 1	*KLK1*	19q13.3
Kallikrein 2	*KLK2*	19q13.3
Kallikrein 3	*KLK3*	4q34-q35
Kininogen	*KNG*	3q26-qter
ONCOGENES, GROWTH FACTORS, AND TUMOR CHROMOSOME BREAKPOINTS		
v-*abl* Abelson murine leukemia homologue 1	*ABL1*	9q34.1
v-*abl* Abelson murine leukemia homologue 2	*ABL2*	1q24-q25
v-*akt* murine thymoma homologue 1	*AKT1*	14q32.32-q32.33
v-*erb*-a avian erythroblastic leukemia homologue 1 (thyroid hormone receptor, α 1)	*THRA1*	17q11.2-q12
v-*erb*-a avian erythroblastic leukemia homologue 2 (thyroid hormone receptor, β)	*THRB*	3p24.1-p22
v-*erb*-a avian erythroblastic leukemia homologue 2-like	*ERBA2L*	17q25
v-*erb*-a avian erythroblastic leukemia homologue-like 2	*ERBAL2*	19
v-*erb*-a avian erythroblastic leukemia homologue-like 3	*ERBAL3*	5
v-*erb*-b avian erythroblastic leukemia homologue (epidermal growth factor receptor)	*EGFR*	7p12
v-*erb*-b2 avian erythroblastic leukemia homologue 2	*ERBB2*	17q11.2-q12
v-*erb*-b2 avian erythroblastic leukemia homologue 3	*ERBB3*	12q13
v-*ets* avian erythroblastosis homologue 1	*ETS1*	11q23.3
v-*ets*-avian erythroblastosis homologue 2	*ETS2*	21p22.3
v-*ets*-related avian erythroblastosis	*ERG*	21q22.3
v-*fes*/v-fps feline sarcoma (Snyder-Theilen)/Fujinami avian sarcoma (PRCII) homologue	*FES*	15q25-qter
v-*fos* FBJ murine osteosarcoma homologue	*FOS*	14q24.3
v-*fgr* Gardner-Rasheed feline sarcoma homologue	*FGR*	1p36.3-p36.1
v-*Ha*-ras Harvey rat sarcoma homologue	*HRAS*	11p15.5
v-*Ki*-ras2 Kirsten rat sarcoma 2 homologue	*KRAS2*	12p12.1
v-*mos* Moloney murine sarcoma homologue	*MOS*	8q11
v-*myb* avian myeloblastosis homologue	*MYB*	6q22-q23
v-*myc* avian myelocytomatosis homologue	*MYC*	8q24.12-q24.13
v-*raf*-1 murine leukemia homologue 1	*RAF1*	3p25
v-*raf* murine sarcoma 3611 oncogene homologue 1	*ARAF1*	Xp11.3-p11.23
v-*raf* murine sarcoma 3611 oncogene homologue 2	*ARAF2*	7p12-cen
v-*raf* murine sarcoma oncogene homologue B1	*BRAF*	7q34
v-*ral* simian leukemia homologue A	*RALA*	7p22-p15
v-*ras* neuroblastoma RAS homologue	*NRAS*	1p13
v-*rel* avian reticuloendotheliosis homologue	*REL*	2p13-p12
Avian lymphoma virus–derived transforming sequence	*BLYM*	1p32
aml 1 (acute myeloid leukemia 1) oncogene	*AML1*	21q22
ELK1, member of ETS oncogene family	*ELK1*	Xp22.1-p11
ELK2, member of ETS oncogen family	*ELK2*	14q32.1-qter
Friend-murine leukemia virus integration site 1 homologue	*FIM1*	6p23-p22.3

(continued)

TABLE 5-1. *(Continued)*

Marker Name	Gene Symbol	Map Location
ONCOGENES, GROWTH FACTORS, AND TUMOR CHROMOSOME BREAKPOINTS (continued)		
Friend-murine leukemia virus integration site 3 homologue	*FIM3*	3q27
FYN oncogene related to SRC, FGR, YES	*FYN*	6q21
met proto-oncogene	*MET*	7q31
pvt-1 murine homologue, *MYC* activator	*PVT1*	8q24
S13 avian erythroblastosis homologue	*SEA*	11q13
Spleen focus forming proviral integration	*SPI1*	11p12-p11.2
Colony-stimulating factor 1 (macrophage)	*CSF1*	1p21-p13
Colony-stimulating factor 1 receptor	*CSF1R*	5q33-q35
Colony-stimulating factor 2	*CSF2*	5q23-q31
Colony-stimulating factor 2 receptor, α	*CSF2RA*	Xp22.32; Yp11.3
Colony-stimulating factor 2 receptor, β	*CSF2RB*	22q12.2-q13.1
Colony-stimulating factor 3	*CSF3*	17q11.2-q12
Colony-stimulating factor 3 receptor	*CSF3R*	1p35-p34.3
Endothelin 1	*EDN1*	6p24.2-p23
Endothelin 2	*EDN2*	1p34
Endothelin 3	*EDN3*	20q13.2-q13.3
Endothelial adhesion molecule 1	*ELAM1*	1q22-q25
Erythropoietin	*EPO*	7q21.3-q22.1
eph tyrosine kinase/erythropoietin producing hepatoma amplified sequence	*EPHT*	7q32-q36
Fibrinogen, A α polypeptide	*FGA*	4q28
Fibrinogen, B β polypeptide	*FGB*	4q28
Fibrinogen, γ polypeptide	*FGG*	4q28
Fibroblast growth factor-1, acidic	*FGF1*	5q31.3-q33.2
Fibroblast growth factor-2, basic	*FGF2*	4q25-q27
Fibroblast growth factor-3 (murine mammary tumor virus integration site (v-int-2))	*FGF3*	11q13
Fibroblast growth factor-4 (heparin secretory transforming protein 1, Kaposi sarcoma)	*FGF4*	11q13.3
Fibroblast growth factor-5	*FGF5*	4q21
Fibroblast growth factor-6	*FGF6*	12p13
Fibroblast growth factor receptor-1 (*fms*-related tyrosine kinase)	*FGFR1*	8p12
fms-related tyrosine kinase (vascular endothelial growth factor/vascular permeability factor receptor)	*FLT1*	13q12
Fibroblast growth factor receptor-2	*FGFR2*	10q25.3-q26
Fibroblast growth factor receptor-3	*FGFR3*	4p16.3
Fibroblast growth factor receptor-4	*FGFR4*	5q33-qter
Insulin-like growth factor 1 (somatomedin C)	*IGF1*	12q22-q23
Insulin-like growth factor 1 receptor	*IGF1R*	15q25-qter
Insulin-like growth factor 2	*IGF2*	11p15.5
Insulin-like growth factor 2 receptor	*IGF2R*	6q25-q27
Interleukin-1, α	*IL1A*	2q12-q21
Interleukin-1, β	*IL1B*	2q12-q21
Interleukin-2	*IL2*	4q26-q27
Interleukin-3	*IL3*	5q23-q31
Interleukin-4	*IL4*	5q23-q31
Interleukin-5 (colony-stimulating factor, eosinophil)	*IL5*	5q23-q31
Interleukin-6 (interferon, β 2)	*IL6*	7p21-p15
Interleukin-7	*IL7*	8q12-q13
Interleukin-8	*IL8*	4q13-q21
Interleukin-9	*IL9*	5q22-q32
Interleukin-10	*IL10*	1
Interleukin-11	*IL11*	19q13.3-q13.4
Interleukin-12A	*IL12A*	3p12-q13.2
Interleukin-12B	*IL12B*	5q31.1-q33.3
Interleukin-1 receptor, α	*IL1RA*	2q12
Interleukin-2 receptor, α	*IL2RA*	10p15-p14
Interleukin-2 receptor, β	*IL2RB*	22q13
Interleukin-4 receptor	*IL4R*	16p12.1-p11.2
Interleukin-5 receptor, α	*IL5RA*	3p26-p24

(continued)

TABLE 5-1. *(Continued)*

Marker Name	Gene Symbol	Map Location
ONCOGENES, GROWTH FACTORS, AND TUMOR CHROMOSOME BREAKPOINTS (continued)		
Interleukin-6 receptor	*IL6R*	1
Interleukin-7 receptor	*IL7R*	5p13
Interleukin-8 receptor, β	*IL8RB*	2
α_2-Plasmin inhibitor	*PLI*	17pter-p12
Plasminogen	*PLG*	6q26-q27
Plasminogen activator, tissue	*PLAT*	8p12-q11.2
Plasminogen activator, urokinase	*PLAU*	10q24-qter
Plasminogen activator inhibitor, type I	*PLANH1*	7q21.3-q22
Plasminogen activator inhibitor, type II	*PLANH2*	18q21.3
Platelet-derived growth factor-α polypeptide	*PDGFA*	7p22
Platelet-derived growth factor-β polypeptide	*PDGFB*	22q12.3-q13.1
Platelet-derived growth factor receptor–α polypeptide	*PDGFRA*	4q11-q12
Platelet-derived growth factor receptor–β polypeptide	*PDGFRB*	5q33-q35
Transforming growth factor-α	*TGFA*	2p13
Transforming growth factor–β1	*TGFB1*	19q13.1
Transforming growth factor–β2	*TGFB2*	1q41
Transforming growth factor–β3	*TGFB3*	14q24
B-cell CLL/lymphoma 1	*BCL1*	11q13.3
B-cell CLL/lymphoma 2	*BCL2*	18q21.3
B-cell CLL/lymphoma 3	*BCL3*	19q13.1-q13.2
B-cell/lymphoma 5	*BCL5*	17q22
Antigen CD30 (Ki-1 antigen)	*CD30*	2q33
Breakpoint cluster region	*BCR*	22q11
Breast cancer 1, early onset	*BRCA1*	17q12-q24
Hemopoietic cell kinase	*HCK*	20q11-q12
Hepatic leukemia factor	*HLF*	17q22
Homeobox 11 (T-cell lymphoma 3–associated breakpoint, Drosophila Notch homologue)	*HOX11*	10q24
Leukemia inhibitory factor (differentiation-stimulating factor)	*LIF*	22q11.2-q13.1
Lymphoblastic leukemia-derived sequence 1	*LYL1*	19p13.2
Myeloid/lymphoid or mixed-lineage leukemia Drosophilia trithorax homologue	*MLL*	11q23
Pre-B-cell leukemia transcription factor 1	*PBX1*	1q23
Pre-B-cell leukemia transcription factor 2	*PBX2*	3q22-q23
Pre-B-cell leukemia transcription factor 3	*PBX3*	9q33-q34
Promyelocytic leukemia	*PML*	15q22
Protein S, α	*PROS1*	3p11-q11.2
Retinoic acid receptor, α	*RARA*	17q12
Retinoblastoma 1 (including osteosarcoma)	*RB1*	13q14.2
Rhombotin 1	*RBTN1*	11p15
Rhombotin-like 1	*RBTNL1*	11p13
T-cell acute lymphocytic leukemia 1	*TAL1*	1p32
T-cell acute lymphocytic leukemia 2	*TAL2*	9q31-q32
Translocation-associated Notch (*Drosophila*) homologue 1	*TAN1*	9q34.3
Tumor protein p53 (Li-Fraumeni syndrome)	*TP53*	17p13.1

* Individual gene symbols are assigned for the different genes within each MHC class.
(Adapted from the 1992 catalog of mapped human genes[318])

Noteworthy are several examples of clusters of functionally related genes. These clusters are located in regions of the genome that are involved nonrandomly in chromosomal rearrangements in various human neoplasms.

Complement Receptor Locus on Chromosome 1

Numerous genes involved in the regulation of complement are located on the long arm of chromosome 1. The C3b/C4b receptor (CR1); the C3d/Epstein-Barr virus receptor (CR2); complement component H factors 1 and 2 (HF1 and HF2); C4-binding protein α, α-like, and β (C4BPA, C4BPAL1, and C4BPB); and decay-accelerating factor for complement (DAF) all reside at 1q32. Also located in this region of chromosome 1 is protein tyrosine phosphatase, receptor-type (PTPRC; previously known as CD45). CR1, CR2, HF1, HF2, C4BPA, C4BPAL1, and C4BPB are related structurally by the presence of a 60–amino acid repeated sequence, which is also found in complement component 2 (C2), properdin factor B (BF), complement component 1, r subcomponent (C1R), the IL2 receptor-α (IL2RA), and the α_1-polypeptide

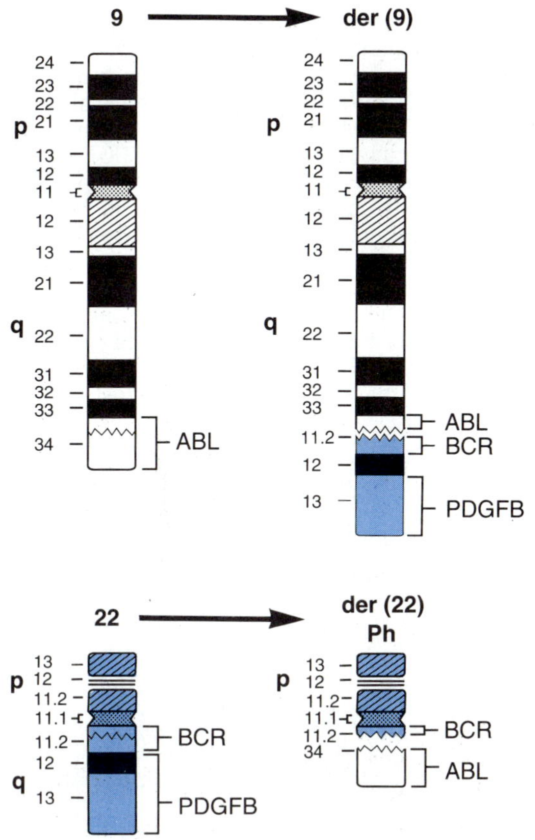

FIGURE 5-6. Ideogram of GTG-banded chromosomes 9 and 22 and derivative chromosomes 9 and 22, demonstrating the t(9;22)(q34;q11) translocation as seen in CML. The distal ends of chromosomes 9 and 22 are exchanged, resulting in the *BCR–ABL1* fusion. PDGFB is relocated from chromosome 22 to chromosome 9 and is distal to the translocation breakpoint.

of coagulation factor XIII (F13A1).[40] A *complement activation* locus including genes encoding proteins that constitute the C3-activating enzymes is present in the major histocompatibility complex at 6p21.3. These genes are C2, complement component 4A (C4A) and 4B (C4B), and BF.

Hematopoietic Growth Factor and Receptor Locus on Chromosome 5

A cluster of hematopoietic growth factors and their receptors have been mapped to the long arm of chromosome 5. Granulocyte/macrophage colony-stimulating factor 2 (CSF2), interleukin-3 (IL3), interleukin-4 (IL4), and interleukin-5 (IL5) are assigned in the region including 5q23-q33.1. Genes for colony-stimulating factor 1 receptor (CSF1R), formerly known as the McDonough feline sarcoma viral (v-*fms*) oncogene homologue, and the β-polypeptide of platelet-derived growth factor receptor (PDGFRB) also reside in this area of chromosome 5. CSF1R and PDGFR are members of the transmembrane protein tyrosine kinase gene family of receptors and probably originate from a gene duplication event.[41,42] In addition, CD14 and an early growth response gene (EGR1) are located in this segment of chromosome 5. A deletion of the long arm of chromosome 5, del(5q) is associated with refractory anemia and therapy-related ANLL, suggesting that loss of function of one or more of these genes may contribute to the pathogenesis of these disorders.[43]

Genes for Cell Proliferation and Differentiation on Chromosome 11

A conserved gene cluster important in cell proliferation and differentiation is located on the long arm of chromosome 11 in band q23.[44] Genes assigned here include δ-, ϵ-, and γ-polypeptides (CD3D, CD3E, and CD3G, respectively) of the T3/T-cell receptor complex, Thy-1 (*THY1*) cell surface antigen, neural cell adhesion molecule (*NCAM*), and the avian erythroblastosis virus E26 (v-*ets*) oncogene (*ETS1*).

Cell Adhesion Cluster on Chromosome 16

A cluster of genes involved in cell adhesion is located on the short arm of chromosome 16. Genes encoding α-subunits of integrins, lymphocyte function-associated antigen 1 (ITGAL; previously known as CD11A), macrophage antigen 1 (ITGAM; previously known as CR3A and CD11B), and p150,95 (ITGAX; previously known as CD11C) are all found within 16p13.1-p11. These α-subunits are transmembrane polypeptides with long extracellular domains containing putative divalent cation-binding sequences. A common evolutionary origin for the three polypeptides is suggested by their structural similarity: ITGAM and ITGAX are 63% identical at the amino acid level, and ITGAL is 35% identical to ITGAM and ITGAX.[45]

CHROMOSOMAL ABERRATIONS AND HEMATOLOGIC DISORDERS

Current understanding of the origin of chromosomal abnormalities is elementary at best. Since discovery of the extra copy of chromosome 21 in Down syndrome in 1959, it has been clear that chromosomal abnormalities are associated with particular phenotypes.[46] Knowledge of gene sequences present in excess and those involved at translocation breakpoints has already resulted in an explosion of new ideas and approaches to the study of chromosome changes in malformation syndromes and malignancy. Despite these advances, little satisfying information exists regarding the cellular mechanism that causes a chromosome to segregate improperly during cell division, or the manner in which two genes, present among 100,000 human genes and located on different chromosomes, become joined together through a translocation.

Constitutional Versus Acquired Chromosome Changes

Chromosomal aberrations are considered to be either constitutional (present in all cells in the body) or acquired (occurring in a particular tissue or stem cell). Whenever aberrations are present in some cells of a particular tissue but not in other cells of the same or a different tissue, the patient is a mosaic or chimera. Aberrations may be divided into two categories, those of number and those of structure. Numeric changes include either gain or loss of chromosomes such as monosomy X or trisomy 21 and gain of an entire set or sets of chromosomes such as triploidy or tetraploidy. Structural changes include translocations, in which chromatin is exchanged between two or more chromosomes; inversion in which chromatin is repositioned within a chromosome arm (paracentric) or between the p and q arms thus involving the centromere (pericentric); deletions, in which there is net loss of chromatin; duplications, in which addition or amplification of chromatin occurs as seen in homogeneously staining regions, or double minute chromosomes; duplication/deficiencies, in which concurrent gain and loss of regions of chromosomes occur;

and breaks, in which a discontinuity in chromatin may lead to an acentric fragment and an abnormal deleted chromosome.

Constitutional abnormalities may be inherited from a parent, who may also have the same rearrangement in all cells or who may be a mosaic with the abnormality having arisen in a single cell sometime after fertilization. Alternatively, a constitutional chromosome rearrangement may occur de novo in a conceptus. In either case, a karyotype of various tissues such as fibroblasts or lymphocytes would reveal the abnormality to be present in all cells. Overall, constitutional rearrangement of chromosomes is a rare event that may not result in any phenotypic abnormality in the individual. Ascertainment of persons with chromosome rearrangements may be only through birth of abnormal offspring or through infertility clinics, since chromosomally unbalanced zygotes are likely to cause first trimester spontaneous abortions. Constitutional rearrangements, although not manifesting themselves in any overt physical changes, may predispose the individual to some neoplastic change in accordance with Knudson's two-hit theory of carcinogenesis.[47] Several examples of such predisposition have now been documented.

Acquired abnormalities are those associated largely with cancer development and tumor progression. Our understanding of the cause of these acquired rearrangements is still limited, but the association of specific rearrangements in particular disorders is well documented. Acquired genomic alterations fall into two groups: those that are considered to be primary changes and are most useful diag-

TABLE 5-2. Chromosomal Abnormalities and Genes in Hematopoietic Disorders

Hematopoietic Disorders	Chromosomal Abnormality	Genes Involved		References
Chronic myeloid leukemia				
	t(9;22)(q34;q11)	*ABL1*	*BCR*	69, 72, 75, 285
Acute myeloid leukemia				
	t(6;9)(p23;q34)	*DEK*	*CAN*	126, 286
	t(8;21)(q22;q22)	*ETO/CDR*	*AML1*	103, 104
	t(9;11)(p22;q23)		*ALL1/MLL/TRX1*	118–120, 287
	t(9;22)(q34;q11)	*ABL1*	*BCR*	97
	t(15;17)(q22;q11-21)	*PML*	*RARA*	113–115, 288–290
	inv(16)(p13q22) or t(16;16)(p13;q22)	*MYH11*	*CBFB*	
B-cell leukemias and lymphomas				
	t(1;19)(q23;p13)	*PBX1/PRL*	*E2A*	208, 209, 281
	t(2;8)(p12;q24)	*IGK*	*MYC, PVT1*	156, 157, 161, 163, 291, 292
	t(2;14)(p13;q32)		*IGH* *IGHG2*	293, 294
	t(4;11)(q21;q23)	*AF4*	*ALL1/MLL/TRX1*	118–120
	t(5;14)(q31;q32)	*IL3*	*IGH*	295, 296
	t(8;12)(q24;q22)	*MYC*	*BTG1*	297
	t(8;14)(q24;q32)	*MYC*	*IGH*	54, 152, 155, 156, 164
	t(8;22)(q24;q11)	*MYC, PVT1*	*IGL*	158, 292, 298
	t(9;14)(p11;q32)		*IGHA*	299
	t(9;14)(p13;q32)		*IGHA*	300
	t(9;22)(q34;q11)	*ABL1*	*BCR*	94, 95, 301
	t(10;14)(q24;q32)	*LYT10*	*IGHA1*	302
	t(11;14)(q13;q32)	*BCL1/PRAD1*	*IGH*	199–201
	t(11;14)(q23;q32)	*RCK*	*IGH*	303–305
	t(11;19)(q23;p13)	*ALL1/MLL/TRX1*		119, 287
	t(14;18)(q32;q21)	*IGH*	*BCL2*	180
	t(14;19)(q32;p13)	*IGH*	*BCL3*	204, 306
	t(17;19)(q22;p13)	*HLF*	*E2A*	307
T-cell leukemias and lymphomas				
	t(1;3)(p34;p21)	*TAL1*		308
	t(1;7)(p32;q35)	*TAL1*	*TCRB*	309
	t(1;7)(p34;q34)	*LCK*	*TCRB*	310, 311
	t(1;14)(p32;q11)	*TAL1*	*TCRD*	197, 269–271
	ins(2;2)(p13;p11-14)	*REL*		312
	t(4;16)(q26;p13)	*IL2*	*BCMA*	313
	inv(7)(p15q35)	*TCRG*	*TCRB*	228
	t(7;9)(q35;q32)	*TCRB*	*TAL2*	314
	t(7;9)(q35;q34.3)	*TCRB*	*TAN1*	284
	t(7;10)(q35;q24)	*TCRB*	*HOX11*	282
	t(7;11)(q35;p13)	*TCRB*	*RBTNL1*	315
	t(7;14)(q35;q32)	*TCRB*		196
	t(7;19)(q35;p13)	*TCRB*	*LYL1*	281
	t(8;14)(q24;q11)	*MYC* *PVT1*	*TCRA* *TCRD*	249, 267, 272, 316
	t(10;14)(q24;q11)	*HOX11*	*TCRD*	280–282
	t(11;14)(p13;q11)	*RBTNL1*	*TCRD*	194, 274, 275
	t(11;14)(p15;q11)	*RBTN1*	*TCRD*	194, 274, 276, 317
	inv(14)(q11q32.1)	*TCRA*	*IGH*	232
	t(14;14)(q11;q32)	*TCRA*		222

(Adapted from the 1992 catalog of mapped human genes[318])

nostically and those that are secondary and likely reflect evolution of the neoplasm. A simple view of the potential biologic implications of primary versus secondary rearrangements is that the primary rearrangement establishes a proliferative advantage for the tumor stem cell, whereas secondary rearrangements may enable the tumor to invade and metastasize in the host.

Nonrandom Chromosomal Aberrations in Neoplasms

The observation of chromosomal changes in human tumors dates to 1914 when Theodor Boveri[48] presented his somatic mutation theory of cancer in his famous book, *Zur Frage der Entstehung Maligner Tumoren.* Not until 1960 was the first specific chromosomal abnormality described by Nowell and Hungerford[49]—the Philadelphia (Ph) chromosome in CML. Today, a growing number of consistent rearrangements have been associated with specific human neoplasms. The Committee on Chromosome Changes in Neoplasia, which is a committee of the Human Gene Mapping Workshops, has made a valiant effort to sort through large numbers of reported chromosomal abnormalities to come up with a list of rearrangements that are consistent within and between laboratories for a particular neoplasm. Because this information is constantly being updated, it is important to refer to the most recent report of this committee. Table 5-2 is adapted from the 1992 report of this committee. Most of these nonrandom changes are translocations, although isochromosomes (chromosomes that are in essence mirror images around a centromere—i [17q]), deletions, insertions, inversions, duplications, and dicentrics (two centromeres present) are also found. Several general statements can be made regarding Table 5-2 and are considered in the following sections.

Cytologically Identical Chromosomal Defects

An interesting finding is that in most instances, chromosomal defects, as characterized by standard cytogenetic methods, are not unique to a specific neoplasm.[50] Molecular technologies are beginning to uncover different sites of chromosome rearrangement at the level of the gene in cytologically indistinguishable rearrangements. Of particular note is the t(9;22)(q34;q11) translocation seen in CML as well as in acute nonlymphocytic leukemia (ANLL) and acute lymphocytic leukemia (ALL). If these three leukemic disorders have the same stem cell,[51] different rearrangements or additional genetic events must account for varying hematologic pictures.[50] Other well-known translocations—such as t(2;8)(p12;q24), t(8;14)(q24;q32), and t(8;22)(q24;q11) of Burkitt's lymphoma–are also characteristic of ALL of the B-lymphocyte type. In this case, the finding of the same chromosomal abnormality in closely related disorders suggests that additional events must be necessary to determine whether the tumor manifests predominantly as a leukemia or as a lymphoma. Similarly, the t(11;14)(q13;q32) translocation found in chronic lymphocytic leukemia (CLL) of the B-cell type is also noted in malignant lymphoma. Alternatively, the t(15;17)(q22;q11-q12) translocation that is characteristic of acute promyelocytic leukemia (APL), M3 and M3 variant, has not been found in any other type of leukemia or in lymphomas or solid tumors.[52]

Hot Spots for Chromosomal Rearrangement

Some chromosomes are involved in rearrangements more frequently than others. In particular, rearrangements of chromosome 14 in band q32 are noted in many lymphoid malignancies. Genes for the immunoglobulin heavy chain reside precisely in this location and have been shown by molecular cloning to be directly involved in rearrangements with the *myc* protooncogene at 8q24 in Burkitt's lymphoma.[53,54] Rearrangements at 14q11 (inv[14] [q11q32]), the locus of the T-cell receptor α chain, are characteristic of T-cell CLL and have been documented by molecular analyses.[55] Besides CLL, rearrangements at 14q11 are also found in ALL (T-cell type). A common site of rearrangement on chromosome 11 involving band q23 is seen in ANLL and in ALL. The q23 band is the site of several genes involved in cell proliferation and differentiation; the reported heterogeneity of chromosomal rearrangements at 11q23 is even greater than that for immunoglobulin and T-cell receptor loci. It was postulated that a gene important in myelomonocytic differentiation, equivalent to the heavy-chain immunoglobulin genes at 14q32, resided at 11q23[50]; molecular cloning revealed a gene that is a homologue of *Drosophila* trithorax involved in homeotic gene regulation.[56]

Translocations

Reciprocal translocations are the most common class of chromosomal rearrangements in leukemias and lymphomas. When other aberrations are seen, such as inversions, deletions, or insertions, they often involve the same chromosome bands as those in translocations.[57] For example, three rearrangements are seen in the M4EO type of ANLL (Table 5-3), all of which involve band q22 of chromosome 16: t(16;16)(p13;q22), inv(16)(p13q22), and del(16)(q22). In the M5 type of ANLL, regions of chromosomes 10 and 11 are consistently rearranged by two different mechanisms: t(10;11)(p15-p11;q23) and ins(10;11)(p11;q23q24). Another nonrandom chromosomal abnormality in ANLL interrupts sequences in two positions on the long arm of chromosome 3 in three different ways: t(3;3)(q21;q26), ins(3;3)(q26;q21q26), and inv(3)(q21q26).

PHYSIOLOGIC CHANGES MEDIATED BY CHROMOSOMAL ABERRATIONS

The significance of structural alterations, which are more common in hematopoietic disorders than are numeric changes of structurally normal chromosomes, is that DNA sequences are brought together that do not normally reside next to each other. Such rearrangements may or may not result in physiologic changes. These changes occur when repositioning produces a novel transcript from the chimeric gene sequence as well as possible deregulation of genes residing at or near the translocation junction. (Both phenomena have been observed and are discussed in the text that follows.) Alternatively, the rearrangement may have

TABLE 5-3. French–American–British Classification of Acute Nonlymphocytic Leukemia

Classification	Definition
M1	Acute myelogenous leukemia without maturation
M2	Acute myelogenous leukemia with maturation
M3	Acute promyelocytic leukemia
M3 variant	Microgranular variant
M4	Acute myelomonocytic leukemia
M4EO	M4 with eosinophilia
M5	Acute monocytic leukemia
M5a	Poorly differentiated (monoblastic) type
M5b	Differentiated type
M6	Acute erythroleukemia
M7	Acute megakaryoblastic leukemia

occurred in a region of noncoding or repetitive DNA sequences, or the alteration, whether it is a novel transcript or deregulation, is not a dominant effect. These silent events are less amenable to study but undoubtedly occur since karyotypes of some tumors demonstrate pronounced genetic instability. This genetic instability is reflected in the occasional finding of rearrangements with no known clinical significance; for example, they may involve moderately repetitive DNA sequences (robertsonian translocations).[58]

Chronic Myelogenous Leukemia and the Philadelphia Chromosome

Cytogenetics and Discovery of the Translocation Breakpoint

Chronic myelogenous leukemia has the distinction of being the first human malignant disease for which a consistent chromosomal rearrangement was identified.[59] In 1960, Nowell and Hungerford[49] reported the observation of an unusually small chromosome in leukemic cells of two males with CML. Originally considered to be a Y chromosome, observation of the same abnormality in leukemic cells of female patients with CML suggested that this chromosome was a member of the G group (either a 21 or a 22).[60] The chromosome was designated the Philadelphia chromosome (Ph) after the location of the laboratory in which it was first discovered, and is now recognized as a diagnostic criterion in CML. Following introduction of banding methods, the Ph chromosome was identified as a deleted chromosome 22 (22q-)[61,62]; this rearrangement was further elucidated by Rowley[59] in 1973 to be a reciprocal translocation between the long arms of chromosomes 9 and 22—t(9;22)(q34;q11) (Fig. 5-7). t(9;22) was shown to be truly a reciprocal chromosome rearrangement (parts of chromatin are exchanged from two or more chromosomes in contrast to loss of material from one only chromosome) when the protooncogene *ABL1*, assigned to 9q34.1, was shown by somatic cell hybrids to reside on the Ph chromosome,[63] and the cellular homologue of the v-*sis* oncogene (known now as PDGFB, the B chain of platelet-derived growth factor) mapped to 22q12.3-q13.1, was found to be translocated to chromosome 9.[64]

Although the t(9;22) is the most common rearrangement producing the Ph chromosome,[65] variant translocations have been described in which three or more different chromosomes are involved[66] (Fig. 5-8*A*). Both chromosomes 9 and 22 are involved in complex rearrangements with the consistent translocation of *ABL1* to a rather limited region on chromosome 22 known as *BCR* for breakpoint cluster region (Fig. 5-9). (The juxtaposition of *ABL1* and *BCR* sequences is sometimes referred to as the Ph gene.) During the blastic or terminal phase of CML, which can be either myeloid (70% of patients) or lymphoid (30% of patients), additional chromosome changes are often seen including an extra Ph chromosome and either an additional chromosome 8, or an extra chromosome 17 or isochromosome for 17q.[67] These additional changes are consistent with the notion of tumor progression. Accordingly, molecular alterations in the tumor suppressor p53 gene, located at 17p13.1 have been noted in 30% of CML patients in blast crisis.[68]

The *BCR* gene was so named because breakpoints of translocations on chromosome 22 were found to be clustered in a small, 5.8-kb region, in contrast to breakpoints on chromosome 9 in the *ABL1* gene, which were found to be spread over a distance of more than 200 kb.[69] The *ABL1* gene spans about 230 kb and has 12 exons including two alternative 5′ exons, 1a and 1b. Exon 1b is located more than 200 kb 5′ to exon 2, requiring a large segment of the nascent transcript to be spliced out to make mature mRNA.[70] As shown in Figure 5-7, rearrangements in *ABL1* occur anywhere within the 200-kb intron 5′ of exon 2, including one breakpoint 5′ of exon 1b. The *BCR* gene spans about 140 kb and has 23 exons. Rearrangements in *BCR* are clustered in the center of the gene between exons 2 and 3 in the *BCR*, although some have been found between exons 3 and 4.

Recently, three additional *BCR*-like (*BCRL*) genes that also map to 22q11 have been discovered.[71] The biologic significance of these sequences (*BCRL2*, *BCRL3*, and *BCRL4*), which retain only the 3′ region of *BCR*, including the last 7 exons and 6 introns, is unknown.

Biologic Significance

Translocation of *ABL1* into *BCR* produces a novel *BCR/ABL1* transcript of 8.5 kb[72] and an abnormal chimeric P210$^{BCR\text{-}ABL1}$ protein with tyrosine kinase activity.[73] The transcript is larger than either the normal *ABL1* mRNAs of 6 kb (exon 1a transcript) and 7 kb (exon 1b transcript) seen in most tissues[74] or the *BCR* mRNAs of 4.5 and 6.7 kb detected in all hematopoietic cell lines and in bone marrow.[72,75] The P210$^{BCR\text{-}ABL1}$ phosphoprotein is also larger than

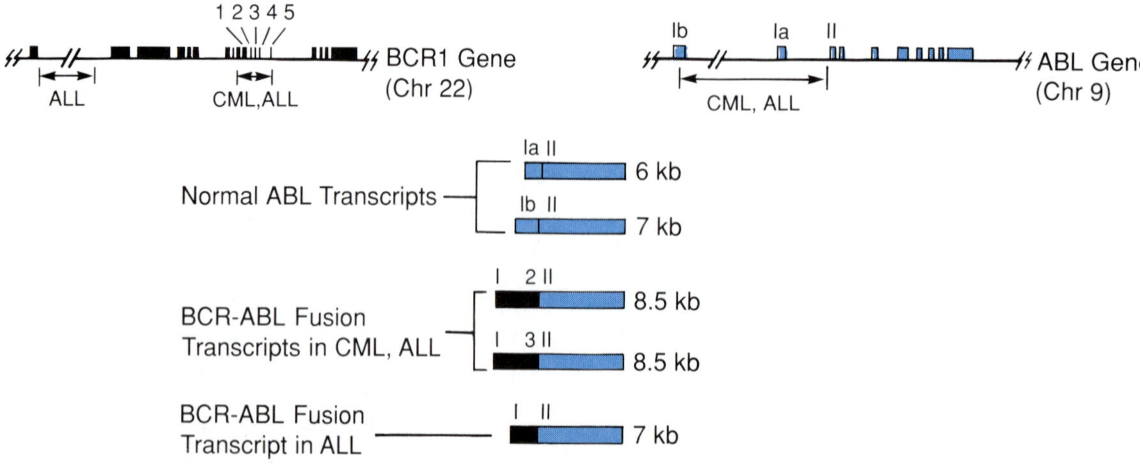

FIGURE 5-7. Schematic diagram of the translocation of *ABL1* into chromosome 22 in the *BCR* gene. (Adapted from Hooberman AL, Carrino JJ, Leibowitz D, et al. Unexpected heterogeneity of BCR-ABL fusion mRNA detected by polymerase chain reaction in Philadelphia chromosome–positive acute lymphoblastic leukemia. Proc Natl Acad Sci USA 1989;86:4259)

the normal *ABL1* protein of 145 kd[76] or the 190-kd *BCR* protein.[73] The function of the *BCR* gene product is unknown although suggested to be a serine kinase that is autophosphorylated, or a substrate for a serine kinase that is not itself evident.[73] The normal *ABL1* gene product shows weak tyrosine kinase activity. This activity is altered upon substitution of 5′ *ABL1* exons with *BCR* sequences and is likely to be fundamental in the pathogenesis of CML. Activation of tyrosine kinase activity by 5′ rearrangement of *ABL1* is analogous to its activation by fusion to gag-encoded sequences in Abelson murine leukemia virus.[77]

Analysis of *BCR–ABL1* transcripts from CML patients in acute phase has demonstrated that 20% of patients have two chimeric RNAs.[78] Furthermore, patients in lymphoid blast crisis usually have a *BCR* exon 2 or *ABL1* exon 2 transcript, whereas patients in chronic phase or myeloid crisis have roughly equal proportions of *BCR* exon 2, *BCR* exon 3, or *ABL1* exon 2 transcripts.[78] Correlation of clinical course and *BCR* breakpoint in one investigation suggests that presence of *BCR* exon 3 portends a shorter survival[79]; other studies have not detected any difference in disease duration with *BCR* breakpoint location.[80,81]

Ph-Negative CML and Ph-Positive ALL

Intense research into the molecular nature of the Ph chromosome has shed light on the nature of Ph-negative CML and Ph-positive ALL. Several different lines of investigation by different groups suggest that, with rare exceptions, Ph-negative CML does not exist. These investigations included a reexamination of bone marrow specimens classified as Ph-negative CML, resulting in reclassification of many of these patients as having chronic myelodysplastic leukemia or refractory anemia.[82,83] Chromosomal in situ hybridization experiments were performed for localization of *ABL1* in some Ph-negative patients and hybridization detected a cytogenetically normal appearing chromosome 22.[84] In these cases, the Ph chromosome is masked; similar-sized pieces of chromatin with banding patterns indistinguishable from the normal chromosome 22 have been exchanged, resulting in a rearranged chromosome 22 that appears cytogenetically normal. Similar analyses by Southern blotting of Ph-negative CML cells have shown translocation of *ABL1* to chromosome 22 with insertion after exon 2 or 3 of the *BCR*.[85] Using PCR followed by hybridization to oligonucleotide probes specific for the Ph gene, several Ph-negative CML patients were shown to express chimeric mRNA.[86]

Although seen in virtually all patients with CML, the Ph chromosome is also present in 10% to 25% of patients with ALL and rarely seen in ANLL.[87] Most ALL and ANLL patients have morphologic features of Fab subtype M1, although M2 and M4 also occur (see later description of Fab classification system).[88] Molecular analyses indicate that t(9;22) breakpoints in CML and ALL may be heterogenous.[89–92] Little or no information is available concerning the Ph chromosome in ANLL patients. DNA analysis of some Ph-positive ALL cells has shown a breakpoint on chromosome 22, at least 50 kb 5′ of the *BCR*, within the large, 70-kb first intron of the *BCR* gene.[93] Thus, the breakpoint on chromosome 22 in ALL may be either within *BCR* or at some distance upstream from it (see Fig. 5-7). The size of the fusion message in ALL cases with more 5′ breakpoints in the *BCR* gene is 7 kb, and it consists of only the 5′-most exon of *BCR* fused to *ABL1* at exon 2. It is translated into a 190-kb *BCR/ABL1* protein.[94,95] Tyrosine kinase activity of the 190-kb protein is greater than that of the 210-kb protein characterizing CML; this may account for a more aggressive leukemia in ALL patients.[96]

The method whereby molecular subtype affects clinical manifestations of Ph-positive leukemia is unknown; more confusing is that the 190-kd protein has been observed in CML as well as ALL cells.[97] Perhaps different *BCR–ABL* fusion messages are manifestations of disease progression. In this light, an investigation of fusion messages in ALL patients using PCR technology noted neither the 7-kb nor 8.5-kb messages in one of six patients with *BCR* rearrangements or in one of five *BCR*-unrearranged patients, and one *BCR*-rearranged patient contained both 7- and 8.5-kb messages.[98]

Acute Nonlymphocytic Leukemia

The acute nonlymphocytic leukemias have been divided into subtypes delineated by the French–American–British classification on the basis of morphology of the predominant cell (see Table 5-3).[88] This classification includes cases of acute myelocytic/myeloblastic leukemia (M1, M2), acute promyelocytic leukemia (M3), and the microgranular variant (M3 variant), acute myelomonocytic leukemia (M4) and M4 with eosinophilia (M4EO), acute monocytic leukemia (M5), erythroleukemia (M6), and acute megakaryoblastic leukemia (M7). Because ANLL is a clinically heterogeneous grouping, specific cytogenetic abnormalities, either alone or in combination with molecular analyses, may aid in the classification and prognosis of patients, as has analysis of the Ph chromosome in CML. Although clonal abnormalities were found originally in only about 50% of patients with ANLL, improved banding and cell culture techniques have resulted in the finding of aberrations in more than 75% of cases studied[52]; some investigators believe that most, if not all, patients with ANLL have chromosomal abnormalities.[99] Overall, the most common karyotypic changes seen in ANLL are trisomy 8 and monosomy 7.[52]

Acute Myeloblastic Leukemia (AML-M2)

In 1973, Rowley[100] identified a specific translocation, t(8;21)(q22;q22) (see Fig. 5-8*B*), that accounts for about 10% of all karyotypically abnormal cases of ANLL.[65,87,101] A median survival time of 11.5 months has been reported for patients with this translocation.[52] Loss of a sex chromosome accompanying t(8;21) is not uncommon, whereas abnormalities of sex chromosomes are otherwise rare in ANLL patients.[102] Initially believed to be specific for M2 subtype, loss of a sex chromosome has been detected also in a small percentage of M4 patients.[101] As in CML patients, where chromosomes 9 and 22 may be involved in complex rearrangements, the same phenomenon is observed in this case permitting the critical translocation junction to be identified as the der(8) chromosome. Thus, physiologic changes mediated by t(8;21) are due to position effect of gene sequences on chromosome 8, proximal to the breakpoint on 8, juxtaposed to DNA sequences distal to the breakpoint on chromosome 21.

The translocation breakpoint has recently been cloned and the genes involved designated ETO (for eight twenty-one) or CDR (for cyclin *D*–related gene), located on chromosome 8, and AML1, located on chromosome 21.[103–105] A fusion transcript results from the translocation. Analysis of the chromosome 21 rearrangement revealed clustering of breakpoints within a limited region in AML1.[103] The AML1 gene has recently been determined to be identical to the α subunit of a mouse heterodimeric transcription factor (CBFα, core-binding factor α), which regulates genes expressed in T cells.[106] It is also homologous to the α subunits of another DNA-binding factor named PEBP2. One of these α subunits shares a 130–amino acid homology with the *Drosophila* segmentation gene runt[107]; an ETO/CDR-AML1 fusion transcript has been characterized, which

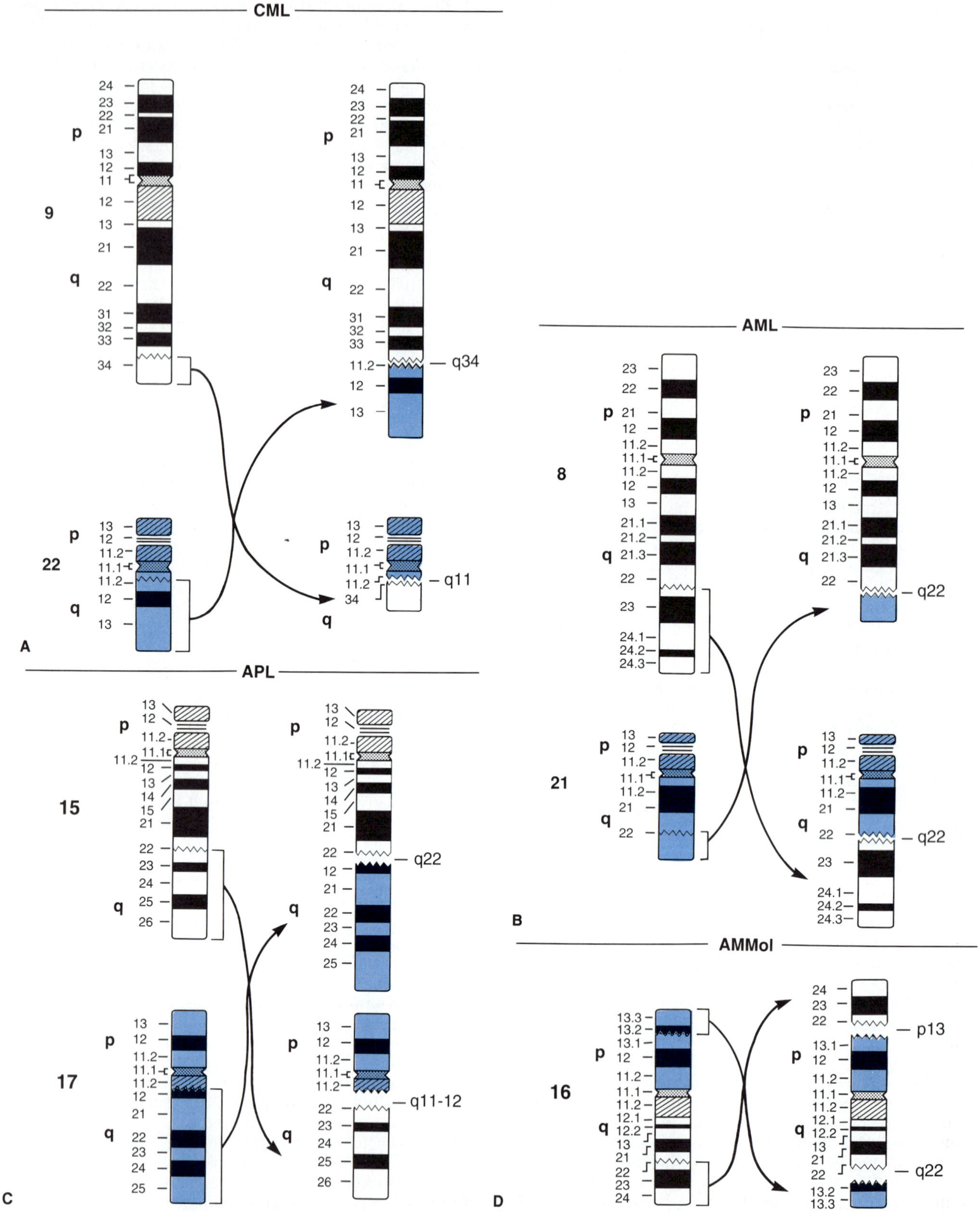

FIGURE 5-8. Critical junction regions in characteristic translocations: (**A**) t(9;22)(q34;q11) in CML, AML, and ALL; (**B**) t(8;21)(q22;q22) in AML-M2; (**C**) t(15;17)(q22;q21) in APL-M3; (**D**) inv(16)(p13q22) in AMMol-M4; and (**E**) t(6;9)(p23;q34) in ANLL with increased basophils. (Adapted from Rowley JD. Identification of a translocation with quinacrine fluorescence in a patient with acute leukemia. Ann Genet 1973;16:109)

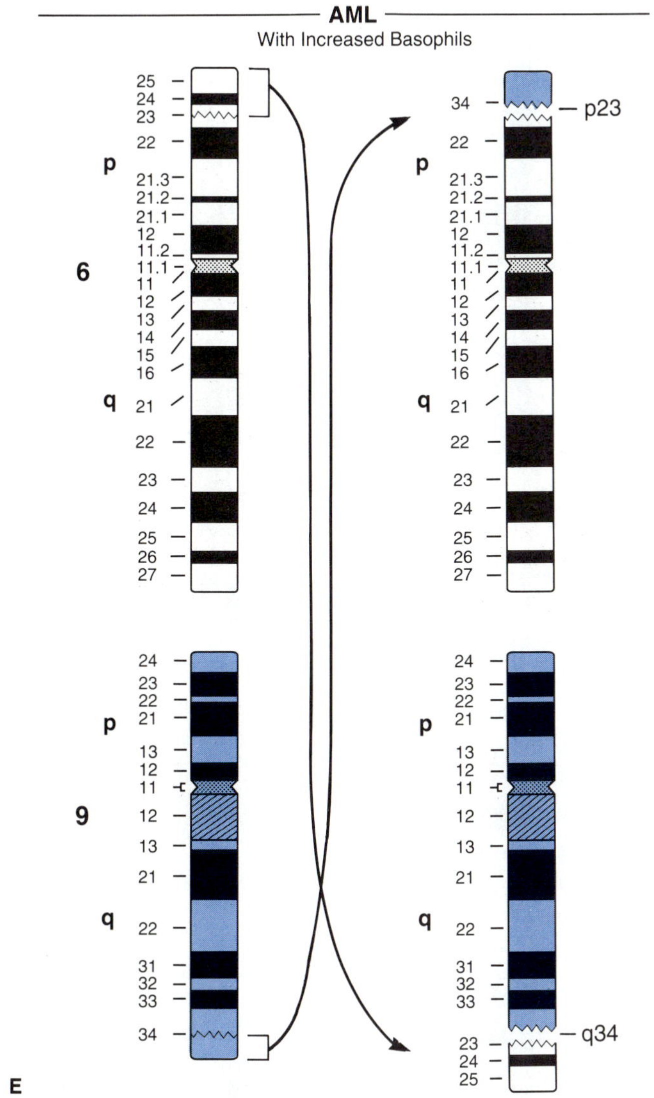

FIGURE 5-8. (Continued)

diverges at the end of the homology to runt.[104] The t(8;21) interrupts a DNA binding basic region in AML1 typical of transcription factors and deletes a glutamine/proline-rich region, which may function as a potential transactivating domain. The site of rearrangement on chromosome 8 resides within a gene (ETO/CDR) that has a region of homology with the cyclin D2 gene[105]; cyclins are involved in control of the mitotic cell cycle, and the D class normally participates in the G1 phase of the cell cycle.

The q22 region of chromosome 21 is intriguing because it is the pathogenetic band for the most common malformation syndrome in humans, trisomy 21, or Down syndrome.[46] One of the features associated with this disorder is an increased incidence of acute leukemias.[108] This increased incidence has been suggested to be directly related to the presence of an extra chromosome 21 as a constitutional abnormality.[109] Furthermore, an extra copy of chromosome 21 is the most common cytogenetic abnormality seen in leukemic blasts of children with ALL who have a normal constitutional karyotype.[110]

Acute Promyelocytic Leukemia (APL-M3)

An APL-specific translocation involving chromosomes 15 and 17, t(15;17)(q22;q21) (see Fig. 5-8C), was first described by Rowley and associates[111] and now appears to be present in every patient with APL-M3.[52] Unlike t(9;22) in CML, ANLL, and ALL and t(8;21) in AML-M2 and AMMol-M4, t(15;17) is specific to APL-M3 and APL-M3 variant (APL patients without coarse granules in the leukemic promyelocytes). As with t(9;22) and t(8;21), complex rearrangements have been noted, which have provided valuable information as to critical translocation junctions. In this instance, the der(15) chromosome has come to be recognized as the pathogenetic unit in leukemogenesis.

Intense efforts by several groups have recently culminated in successful identification of DNA sequences that are involved in t(15;17).[112–114] The retinoic acid receptor α (RARA) on chromosome 17 at q21 is fused to a novel transcribed locus on chromosome 15, designated "PML" for promyelocytic leukemia. PML, a myeloid gene product, may represent either a DNA-binding protein, novel transcription factor, or recombinase. These initial studies indicate that the translocation results in production of a chimeric transcript in which the N-terminal region of RARA has been replaced by PML; a predicted chimeric protein would include most of PML joined to a large part of RARA including DNA and hormone-binding regions.[115] The finding of a rearrangement involving RARA is particularly interesting as it may account for clinical usefulness of retinoic acid in achieving differentiation of APL cells in vivo.

Acute Myelomonocytic Leukemia (AMMoL-M4)

Rearrangement of chromosome 16 involving band q22 (see Fig. 5-8*D*) is associated with AMMoL with abnormal eosinophils, M4EO.[116] This rearrangement occurs through three different structural aberrations. In 25% of patients an inversion of chromosome 16, inv(16)(p13q22), is seen, and, less frequently, either a deletion of 16, del(16)(q22), or a reciprocal translocation, t(16;16)(p13;q22), may be noted. Identification of a patient with a complex translocation has made it possible to identify critical junctions from the inv(16) and the t(16;16) to be distal 16p13 sequences next to proximal 16q22 sequences.[117]

Recently, genes involved in the inv(16) have been identified to be within CBFB (core-binding factor β) on 16q, the human homologue of a mouse subunit of a heterodimeric transcription factor regulating genes expressed in T cells, and MYH11 on 16p, a smooth muscle myosin heavy chain gene.[107] A fusion messenger RNA was identified involving the 5′ region of CBFB and the 3′ portion of MYH11, and elucidation of the role of the fusion protein in leukemogenesis will now be possible. Interestingly, as discussed earlier, the mouse CBFα subunit has been shown to be identical to the AML1 gene.[106]

Acute Monocytic Leukemia (AMoL-M5)

Aberrations of the long arm of chromosome 11 at q23 can be seen in monocytic leukemia blast cells. These abnormalities include translocations, with various chromosomes as the reciprocal partner, deletions, or insertions. Because 11q abnormalities have been reported in patients with acute leukemias other than AMoL, Rowley[52] has pointed out that it will be interesting to learn whether chromosomal abnormalities reveal a spectrum of morphologic features in AMoL not previously recognized.

A gene that is the human homologue of *Drosophila* trithorax located at 11q23 (designated ALL1 or MLL or TRX1)[56,118–120] has been found to be rearranged in acute myeloid and lymphoid leukemias involving a variety of other chromosomes including 1, 2, 4, 6, 9, 10, 17, 19, and X. Based on knowledge of the function of trithorax as a regulator of homeotic genes, it is likely that ALL1/MLL/TRX1 is a transcription factor participating in regulation of human genes involved in development and differentiation.

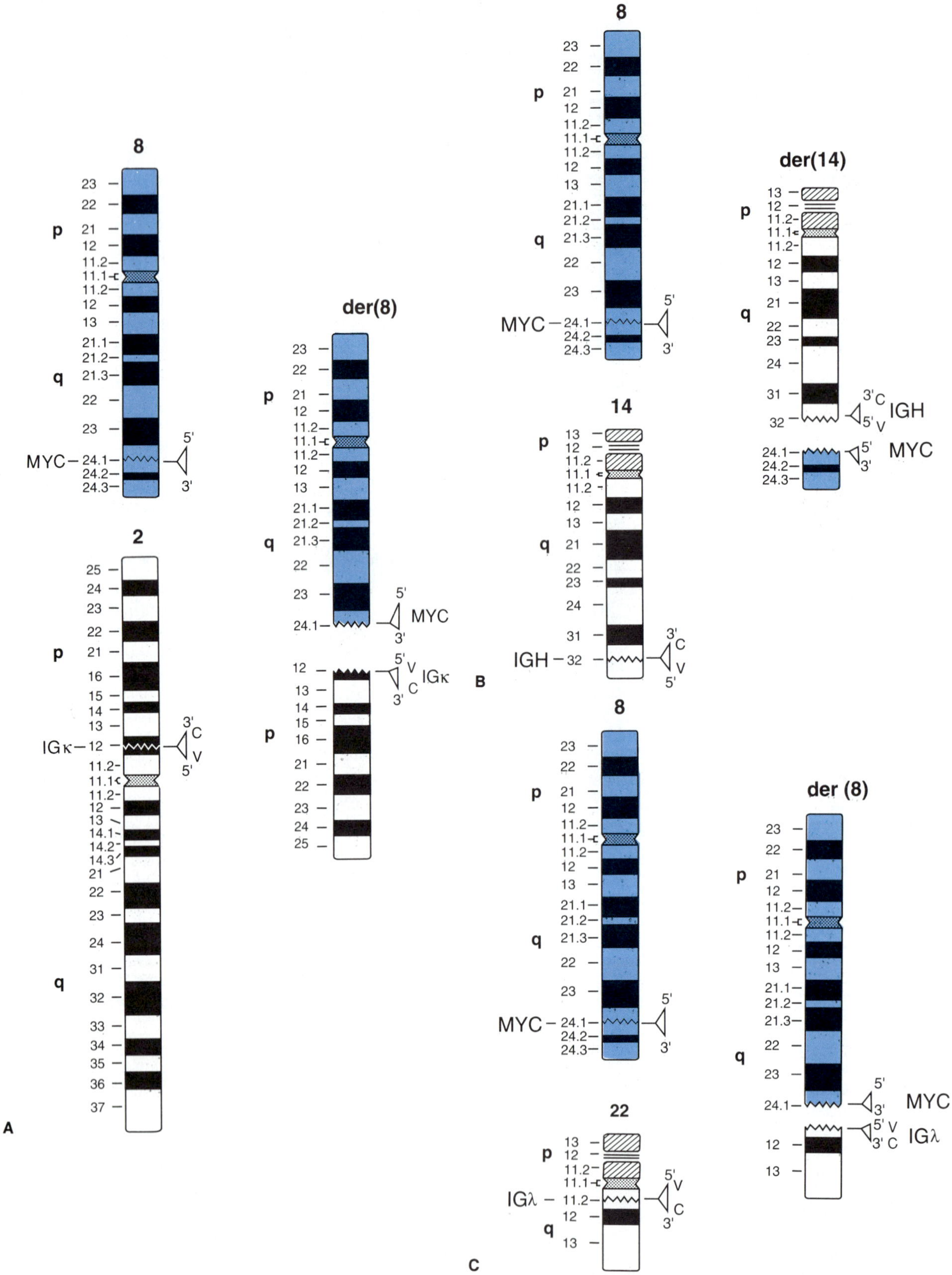

FIGURE 5-9. Characteristic translocations seen in Burkitt's lymphoma: variant, t(2;8)(p11;q24) (**A**), classic, t(8;14)(q24;q32) (**B**), and t(8;22)(q24;q11) (**C**). (Adapted from Rowley JD. Biological implications of consistent chromosome rearrangements in leukemia and lymphoma. Cancer Res 1984;44:3159)

Erythroleukemia (EL-M6)

Little is known concerning chromosomal abnormalities in ANLL-M6 and previous analyses have not suggested any characteristic findings besides hypodiploidy and various unidentified marker chromosomes.[121] Two interesting patients with erythroleukemia have been reported. In one patient, a hypodiploid karyotype with numerous rearranged chromosomes showed a translocation at 11p15, the locus of β-globin, whereas in the other, a relatively simple karyotype had a translocation in the short arm of chromosome 16, the locus of α-globin.[122] Additional cytogenetic and molecular studies of patients with erythroleukemia are needed to determine whether rearrangement in a globin locus might contribute to pathogenesis of this disorder.

Acute Nonlymphocytic Leukemia With Increased Basophils

A translocation involving chromosomes 6 and 9, t(6;9)(p23;q34) (see Fig. 5-8E), characterizes this distinct subtype of ANLL with increased basophils.[123] The translocation breakpoint at 9q34 is at the same cytologic site as that of the breakpoint in the t(9;22) seen in CML. Interestingly, basophilia is also a common finding in CML. One complex chromosome rearrangement in this disorder supported a critical translocation junction of 9q sequences moved onto 6p.[124] Molecular analyses in two patients indicated that the rearrangement did not involve translocation of *ABL1* to chromosome 6; the translocation is 3′ of the *ABL1* gene unlike the rearrangement in CML, which occurs in the 5′ region of *ABL1*.[125] Furthermore, rearrangement does not result in an aberrantly sized *ABL1* fusion protein or in acquisition of in vitro tyrosine kinase activity.[125]

The pathogenetic regions in the t(6;9) have now been cloned; breakpoints on chromosome 6 occur in one intron of the DEK gene and rearrangements in chromosome 9 reside some 360 kb downstream of *ABL1* in a large intron of the CAN gene.[126] An invariant, leukemia-specific, 5.5-kb DEK-CAN transcript results because of translocation within intronic sequences. Comparison of DEK and CAN sequences with the EMBL data base did not reveal homology with any known protein sequences and function of these genes in leukemogenesis remains to be elucidated. However, it has been speculated that CAN may be a transcription factor and that replacement of N-terminal CAN sequences with the DEK protein may activate the transforming potential of CAN.[126]

Refractory Anemia and Therapy-Related ANLL and Myeloblastic Syndromes

Refractory anemia, therapy-related ANLL (t-ANLL), and therapy-related myeloblastic syndromes (t-MDS) are characterized by deletion of a portion of chromosome 5 in refractory anemia, and by a deletion of a portion or the entire chromosome 5 or 7 in the latter two disorders.[127–129] A variety of interstitial deletions of the long arm of chromosome 5 in refractory anemia identify a critical region, band q31, which is deleted in all patients.[43] The chromosome 5 deletion in refractory anemia generally portends a relatively mild clinical course characterized by transfusion-dependent anemia, mild leukopenia, and thrombocytosis that usually does not progress to acute leukemia.[130] In contrast, therapy-related leukemias carry a poor prognosis, and additional chromosomal anomalies usually accompany the deletion or monosomy. The finding of a relatively high incidence of complete or partial monosomy of chromosome 5 or 7 in patients with t-ANLL or t-MDS, and a lower incidence in patients with ANLL or MDS de novo, has led to the suggestion that these abnormalities may be mediated by toxic environmental agents.[131,132]

The region of the long arm of chromosome 5 that is deleted in these disorders is also the location of a cluster of hematopoietic growth factors and receptors. (These genes were discussed previously in the section on human genome and hematology.) In several patients with typical refractory anemia syndrome, it has been shown that CSF1R,[130,133] CSF2,[130] CSF1,[134] IL3,[135] IL4,[43] and IL5[43] are deleted. Studies of additional patients with del(5q) demonstrated deletions of IL3,[135] IL4,[43] and IL5[43] in t-ANLL, and CSF2,[130] CSF1,[133] and IL3[135] in ANLL de novo. Recently, interferon regulatory factor (IRF1) was mapped to 5q31.1 and shown to be deleted consistently at one or both alleles in 13 cases of leukemia or myelodysplasia with aberrations of 5q31.[136] As a transcriptional activator of IFNα, IFNβ, and other IFN-inducible genes, IRF1 manifests growth inhibitory and antioncogenic activity. The significance of deletion of any of these genes in these disorders has yet to be elucidated; the role of these genes in altered hematopoiesis associated with del(5q) is an area of intense investigation. Breakpoints on chromosome 7 indicate a critical region in either 7q32-q33 or 7q34-q35[129]; the identity of the relevant gene is currently unknown.

These disorders highlight the significance of chromosomal deletions in tumorigenesis. Although deletions are not a common aberration in leukemia and lymphoma, their significance in the neoplastic process has been documented in various tumors including retinoblastoma,[137] Wilms' tumor,[138] renal cell carcinoma,[139] meningioma,[140] colorectal carcinoma,[141] osteosarcoma,[142] acoustic neuroma,[143] and small cell lung carcinoma.[144] Several possible mechanisms mediated by chromosomal deletion may contribute to pathogenesis of these disorders. One consideration is reduction in gene product. A 50% decrease in a particular protein may disrupt a delicate stoichiometric balance in hematopoiesis, which could interfere with cellular maturation. Alternatively, deletion of a normal gene may uncover a mutated gene which is then expressed in the hemizygous state. Loss of normal gene product would have a role in neoplasia. Finally, the retinoblastoma-type model is that of functional loss, by deletion or other chromosomal mechanisms, of a tumor suppressor gene. Tumors develop when both alleles are altered by mutations so that no normal gene product is produced.

B-Cell Neoplasms

Burkitt's Lymphoma and the *myc* Gene

Identification of Genes at Translocation Breakpoints. A 14q+ chromosome was identified by Manolov and Manolova[145] in 1972 as the first consistent abnormality in cells from patients with Burkitt's lymphoma. Subsequently, it was determined that the 14q+ was derived from a presumably balanced translocation between chromosomes 8 and 14, t(8;14)(q24;q32).[146] The t(8;14) was present in both EBV-positive as well as EBV-negative lymphomas. Additional variant translocations were identified involving chromosome 2 or 22 with chromosome 8 at band q24, t(2;8)(p13;q24) or t(8;22)(q24;q11)[147–151] (see Fig. 5-9). Whether the variant translocations have prognostic implications that differ from those of the more common t(8;14) is not known. As discussed previously, these translocations are seen also in B-cell ALL, and t(8;14) has been observed in other lymphomas, particularly in the large cell immunoblastic type or small cell lymphocytic varieties.

Ten years after identification of the 14q+ abnormality, molecular genetic analyses revealed that these translocations occurred largely between a cellular protooncogene, *myc*, at 8q24, and immunoglobulin (Ig) gene sequences located at the breakpoints of the translocations on chromosomes 2 (κ light chain, Igκ), 14 (heavy chain, IgH), and 22 (λ light chain, Igλ).[152–155] Unlike the finding in CML, a chimeric mRNA and protein do not result from the translocation. Thus, the physiologic significance of the chromosomal aberration to the disease must be considered to be by a different mechanism. In fact, the t(8;14) translocation has occurred so the direction of transcription of IgH and *myc* genes is away from each other. That is, they are positioned in a head-to-head array. In contrast to the t(8;14), in which the *myc* gene is translocated to chromosome 14, the variant translocations are arranged such that *myc* remains on chromosome 8 and the direction of transcription of both Ig and *myc* is in a 5′ to 3′ orientation (head-to-tail) away from the centromere of chromosome 8 (Fig. 5-10).[156–158]

Molecular[157,159] and cytogenetic[160] analyses of some variant translocations have identified a breakpoint on chromosome 8 that appears to be at a substantial distance 3′ of *myc*. Cloned human chromosome 8 DNA from this region is equivalent, although the degree of homology is limited to murine chromosome 15 DNA (known as the *PVT1* locus) isolated from a plasmacytoma with a t(6;15).[161] In addition, this region of chromosome 8 is the site where an interstitial deletion occurs in an HTLV-1+ adult T-cell leukemia and where three *myc* amplicons terminate in amplified tumors.[162] Cytogenetic analysis of several t(8;22) Burkitt's lymphoma cell lines indicates that the site of rearrangement is on chromosome 8 in subband 24.22, whereas subband 24.1 is rearranged in cell lines with t(8;14).[160] The significance of this distant site of rearrangement to tumorigenesis is an active area of investigation that will likely contribute to a better understanding of the pathobiology of chromosome translocations in these disorders.

Origin of the Translocations. Genomic rearrangement is part of the process whereby a mature Ig molecule is produced. During this process discrete units encoding variable (V), joining (J), and diversity (D; IgH only) regions must be spliced together.[163] The cause of the Burkitt trans-

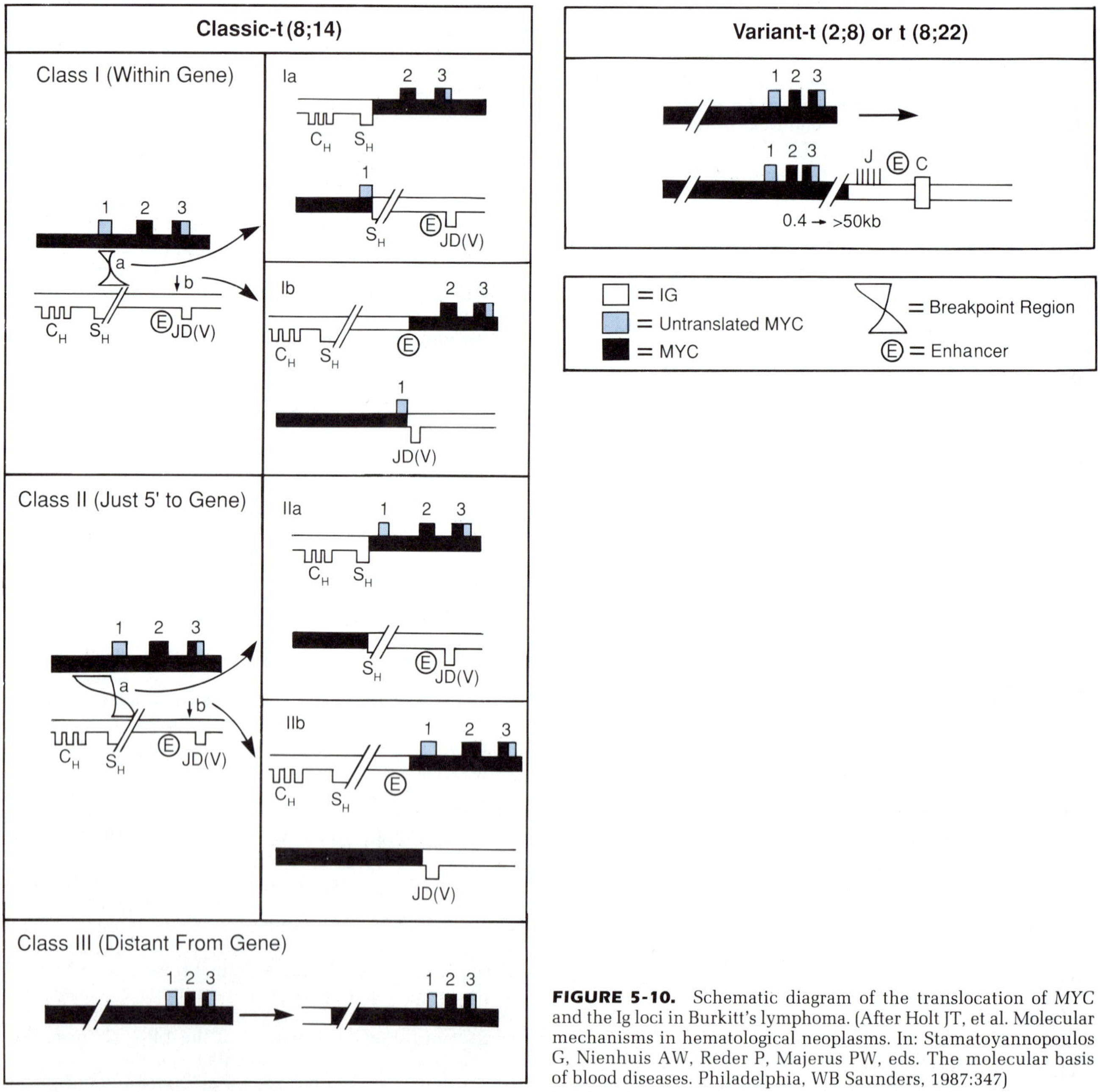

FIGURE 5-10. Schematic diagram of the translocation of *MYC* and the Ig loci in Burkitt's lymphoma. (After Holt JT, et al. Molecular mechanisms in hematological neoplasms. In: Stamatoyannopoulos G, Nienhuis AW, Reder P, Majerus PW, eds. The molecular basis of blood diseases. Philadelphia, WB Saunders, 1987:347)

locations remains elusive although, in this example and those rearrangements involving the T-cell receptor molecules that also undergo genomic rearrangement as a part of their normal maturation, it is possible to postulate a form of illegitimate recombination occurring within a locus that normally undergoes recombination. Whether a region of homology to Ig in DNA at or around 8q24 might promote such a rearrangement remains to be determined. Alternatively, the translocation might be viewed in the context of the cell in which it is occurring; that is, a B-cell tumor has arisen from an aberrant rearrangement involving a gene or genes that are known to be actively transcribed in the mature B cell with genes intimately involved in regulating growth.[122,164]

Deregulation of the *myc* Gene. Prior to actual discovery of the gene partners involved in the translocations in Burkitt's lymphoma, Klein[165] and Rowley[166] suggested that translocations might alter the expression of a cellular transforming gene by placing it under control of a new promoter. Although much still remains to be learned about the role of *myc* in normal cellular processes, extensive investigation into its expression and regulation in both normal and tumor cells has shown that a correlation exists between neoplasia and altered *myc* expression.[156,167,168] Through chromosomal rearrangement in Burkitt's lymphoma, deregulation of *myc* results from a variety of molecular breakpoints in addition to point mutations and insertions.[169–171] Besides quantitative change in levels of *myc* mRNA and protein, the rearranged allele is unable to respond to normal cellular regulatory processes.

A primary mechanism whereby *myc* is deregulated is through the decapitation of the first exon and 5′ regulatory regions from the remainder of the gene by translocation within exon 1 or intron 1. The first *myc* exon is untranslated and contains two promoters, P1 and P2, from which transcription of mRNAs of 2.4 and 2.2 kb, respectively, is initiated. Because a significant degree of homology exists between murine and human *myc* genes, which includes not only the translated portion of the gene (exons 2 and 3) but also exon 1 and regions upstream from the promoters, the decapitation releases *myc* from crucial regulatory sequences. Furthermore, stability or translation of the mRNA may be altered without the presence of an untranslated sequence from exon 1.

Other factors to consider in deregulation of *myc* are potential effect of an Ig enhancer sequence on *myc* expression and, somatic mutations in *myc*. An Ig enhancer may be brought into close proximity to *myc* depending on the particular molecular breakpoint, and its ability to confer tissue-specific expression on various promoters is well established.[172–174] With regard to somatic mutations, DNA sequence analysis of rearranged *myc* genes has uncovered point mutations in the promoter region, 5′ untranslated exon, intron 1, and within coding exons 2 and 3.[168–170,175,176] Both of these alterations may contribute to deregulation of rearranged *myc* genes.

Follicular Lymphoma

IgH at 14q32, which is rearranged in Burkitt's lymphoma, is consistently involved in a translocation, t(14;18)(q32;q21), seen in another B-cell neoplasm. In this case, the gene partner in the translocation was a previously uncharacterized DNA sequence, which has come to be known as the *BCL2* gene (B-cell lymphoma). The t(14;18) translocation is found in 85% of follicular, small, cleaved B-cell lymphomas and about 20% of diffuse lymphomas.[177–179] Molecular cloning has shown that *BCL2*, located at 18q21, moves into the IgH locus at the 5′ end of J_H regions,[180–182] and that this rearrangement occurs early in pre–B-cell development during attempted Ig gene rearrangement.[183] In 60% to 70% of t(14;18) lymphomas, the translocation site on chromosome 18 occurs in a 2.8-kb major breakpoint region (MBR) within the 3′ noncoding region of the third exon.[183,184] This rearrangement does not interrupt the protein coding region of *BCL2*, although somatic mutation, resulting in coding-region changes have been found.[185] A *BCL2*–Ig fusion gene from the MBR translocation on the der(14) produces heterogenous chimeric mRNAs encoding alternative *BCL2* 5′ exons and various Ig 3′ untranslated regions.[185,186] In addition to MBR, a minor breakpoint cluster region (mBR) has been identified in which breakpoints in the remaining t(14;18) cluster near the 5′ end of *BCL2*.[184]

The pathogenetic defect in t(14;18) in follicular lymphoma appears to be inappropriate *BCL2* expression. The *BCL2* gene is normally expressed in pre–B cells and proliferating B cells, is down-regulated in differentiated B cells, and is quiescent in resting B cells.[187–189] Despite the mature B-cell phenotype of t(14;18) lymphomas, *BCL2*–Ig fusion (and expression) represents an early stage of pre–B-cell development. Thus, inappropriately elevated levels of *BCL2*–Ig fusion mRNA are likely to be the pathologically significant result of chromosome translocation.

In at least some cases of t(14;18), as well as other translocations involving IgH (and T-cell receptor genes discussed later), there is evidence to suggest that chromosomal breakage and reunion are due to mistakes in VDJ joining by the lymphocyte recombinase.[190–198] The recombinase recognizes heptamer-nonamer–like recognition sequences near a breakpoint. Such sequences are known to signal sites of breakage during normal VDJ gene rearrangement. At the same time it is important to note that not all translocations analyzed demonstrate this motif and that recombinase-catalyzed recognition cannot be the only mechanism for chromosomal rearrangement.[183,195]

Chronic Lymphocytic Leukemia

B-cell CLL is characterized by trisomy for chromosome 12 and rearrangements at 14q32. Once again, IgH is involved in a critical rearrangement.[199] A t(11;14)(q13;q32) translocation is detected in about 10% of patients with B-cell CLL, and the translocation breakpoint has been cloned using Ig probes to isolate an aberrantly rearranged Ig gene.[200] As in the t(14;18) described earlier, the translocation did not identify a known gene. The site of rearrangement on chromosome 11 has subsequently been named *BCL1/PRAD1*.[201] An expressed gene for *BCL1* has not yet been identified. Molecular analyses of two cell lines, one from a patient with CLL with a t(11;14) and one from a patient with diffuse large cell lymphoma with a t(11;14), have shown clustered breakpoints on chromosome 11 suggesting that the same gene (*BCL1*) may be involved in these B-cell malignancies.[200] Sequence analysis of the t(11;14) from this CLL patient and the t(11;14) from another patient with CLL revealed the chromosome 11 breakpoints to be within eight nucleotides of each other.[202] Nucleotide sequence at the breakpoint on chromosome 11 has homology to heptamer-nonamer sequences used in VDJ joining, as does the chromosome 14 breakpoint, suggesting that the translocation may have evolved from an aberrant VDJ joining event.[202] Independently, a candidate oncogene (*PRAD1*) located at 11q13 that was found to be clonally rearranged in parathyroid tumors was determined to be the *BCL1* oncogene.[201] *BCL1/PRAD1* corresponds to the cyclin D1 gene, and as mentioned previously in conjunction with the ETO/CRD gene in the t(8;21), the D class of cell cycle genes normally function in G1.

Some cases of B-cell CLL are characterized by a t(14;19)(q32;q13.1) translocation.[203] Cloning of the translocation breakpoint has identified a rearrangement between IgH in a switch region with a newly identified gene, *BCL3*, which also has homology with a number of genes involved in cell cycle control and lineage determination.[204]

Pre–B-Cell Leukemia: The t(1;19) Translocation

In about 30% of a characteristic subset of pediatric pre–B cell ALL, a t(1;19)(q23′3.3) translocation is seen.[205,206] Assignment of the E2A gene, that codes for proteins with the properties of immunoglobulin enhancer binding factors E12/E47 and contains a helix–loop–helix DNA binding motif, to 19p13.2-p13.3, led to an investigation of potential involvement of E2A in the t(1;19).[207] Southern blot analysis of leukemias and cell lines with the t(1;19) revealed rearrangements in most samples tested, implicating the E2A gene in the pathogenesis of leukemia. Molecular cloning of the translocation breakpoint revealed a sequence from chromosome 1, designated *PRL/PBX1* (pre–B-cell leukemia), which contains a putative DNA binding domain of a homeoprotein.[208,209] A fusion transcript was cloned in which the DNA binding domain of E2A was replaced by the putative DNA binding domain of *PRL/PBX1*; the chimeric protein resulting from this translocation may be found to contribute to leukemogenesis by altering expression of genes regulated by the *PRL* homeoprotein.

T-Cell Neoplasms

Rearrangements of T-Cell Receptor Genes

Consistent chromosome rearrangements in T-cell neoplasms frequently involve the T-cell receptor (*TCR*) genes.[210] These genes are analogous in many respects to immunoglobulin genes as they both undergo genomic rearrangement as a normal part of their maturation. TCR genes include α chains[211,212] and δ chains[213] located at 14q11, β chain at 7q35[214,215] and the γ chain at 7p15.[216] The locations of these genes, particularly of α- and δ-chain genes on proximal 14q, are at sites of frequent chromosome rearrangements in T-cell–related disorders including chronic T-cell leukemia or lymphoma,[217,218] childhood T-cell acute lymphoblastic leukemia[206] and adult T-cell leukemia.[219]

Homologous or heterologous rearrangements seen involving chromosomes 7 and 14 at *TCR* loci include inversion of chromosome 14, inv(14)(q11;q32)[217,218,220,221]; tandem 14 to 14 translocation, t(14;14)(q11;q32)[217,221,222]; translocations between chromosomes 7 and 14, t(7;14)(p15;q11) and t(7;14)(q32;q11)[196,223–225]; inversion of chromosome 7, inv(7)(p15q32)[226–228]; and chromosome 7 to 7 translocation, t(7;7)(p15;q32).[226,227] Analyses of the inv(14) have uncovered two different rearrangements. In a T-cell lymphoma cell line (SUP-T1), a productive rearrangement between V_H and J_α results in a hybrid Ig–*TCR* transcript,[55,229,230] whereas in various T-cell tumors with inv(14) or t(14;14), rearrangement in 14q32 occurs 15 to 20 mega–base pairs centromeric to IgH at a locus now known as tcl1.[222,231–234]

Also, metaphase preparations from persons with the rare autosomal recessive disorder ataxia telangiectasia,[226,227,235–238] as well as from normal persons,[239–246] have rearrangements in these regions. A translocation at 14q32 with *TCRB* has been examined in a T-cell leukemia of a patient with ataxia telangiectasia, and like the inv(14) and t(14;14), reveals rearrangement proximal to the IgH locus in 14q32 at the *TCL1* locus.[196] The rare finding of chromosomal rearrangement at sites of *TCR* genes in phytohemagglutinin-stimulated lymphocytes from normal persons has recently been addressed at the molecular level.[247] Chimeric V-(Dδ)-Jδ and Vδ-(Dδ)-J TCR gene rearrangements have been found in several normal tissues including peripheral blood. Whether these rearrangements represent aberrant recombinase-mediated rearrangements, not unlike those proposed for various translocations associated with tumors, or whether they are a normal part of the generation of diversity within the lymphocyte antigen receptor repertoire remains to be known.

Other Translocations in T-Cell Tumors Involving T-Cell Receptor Genes

Additionally, translocations are seen involving 14q11 (*TCRA*) with 1p33,[248] 1p32,[249,250] 8q24,[206,251–256] 10q24,[220,257–259] 11p13,[206,260,261] and 11p15.[262,263] Translocations have been noted involving distal 7q in the *TCRB* region with 1p32, 2p21, 6p21,[264] 9q32,[224] 9q34,[224,265] and 19p13.[266]

Molecular analyses have primarily focused on *TCRA* genes and, following their discovery nested within *TCRA* at 14q11, with *TCRD* genes. Undoubtedly, some early publications in which *TCRA* genes were found to be split between J_α and C_α were actually interruptions in TCRD.[194,262,267,268] Also, the nomenclature of genes involved in rearrangements with *TCR* genes has undergone various revisions that complicate the reading of the literature on this subject. Translocation of 14q11 (*TCRD*) with 1p32–34 in a early T-cell precursor ALL results in a fusion transcript that identifies a previously unknown gene, *TAL1* (for T-cell acute lymphoblastic leukemia), important in hematopoietic development and oncogenesis.[197,269–271] The gene *TAL1* contains sequences that encode an amphipathic helix–loop–helix motif.[270] This motif is a DNA-binding domain found in a variety of proteins that control cell growth and differentiation, including the gene *LYL1* (described subsequently and also implicated in T-cell leukemogenesis).

A familiar theme from the variant translocations studied in Burkitt's lymphomas recurs with the t(8;14)(q24;q11) translocation. Translocation of either *TCRA* or *TCRD* occurs 3′ of *myc* [191,193,256,267,268,272] with deregulation of *myc*. [267] Two rearrangements involve 14q11 and the short arm of chromosome 11 at 11p13[195,255,273] and 11p15.[194,262] In four cases of rearrangement at 11p13, breakpoints were found to be clustered on chromosome 11 within a region of less than 800 bp and involved the *TCRD* gene in most cases.[195] The gene at 11p13 is now identified as rhombotin-like 1 (RHBTNL1)[274,275] and the 11p15 site as rhombotin 1 (RBTN1).[274,275] The rhombotin genes encode proteins with duplicated cysteine-rich regions called LIM domains, which show homology to zinc-binding proteins and iron-sulfur centers of ferredoxins. Probes derived from 11p15 that are translocated to the der(14), and downstream of the Vα locus, detect a 4-kb mRNA in the RPMI 8402 T-cell acute leukemia cell line from which it was cloned, but not in some other T-cell lines tested suggesting that only a small subset of thymus cells express the gene.[194,277] Investigation of the t(10;14)(q24;q11) translocation revealed another previously uncharacterized gene identified as *HOX11*, the first homeobox gene implicated in T-cell neoplasia.[270,282] A cloned DNA fragment from a region distal to the 10q24 breakpoint, expected to be translocated to the der(14), detects a 2.9 kb mRNA in a t(10;14) leukemia. No transcript was detected in a variety of other normal or neoplastic T cells supporting deregulation of *HOX11* by translocation into *TCRD*.[279]

Fewer analyses of rearrangement of *TCRB* have been performed reflecting the more frequent rearrangement at 14q11 of *TCRA* or TCRD genes. Among those that have been analyzed molecularly are t(7;9), with breakpoints on 9q at either q32[192,198] or q34.[192,283] The q32 locus has been designated *TAL2*, another helix–loop–helix gene transcriptionally activated by chromosome rearrangement. Intensive analysis of the 9q34 breakpoint (the band to which

ABL1 is assigned) indicated that there were no rearrangements within 250 kb in either direction of *ABL1* and no apparent alteration in *ABL1* protein.[283] A probe from the 9q34 locus detected multiple abundant transcripts in a T-cell ALL cell line from which it was cloned and small amounts of larger transcripts in T cells without the t(7;9).[192] The locus on chromosome 9 was determined to be a gene highly homologous to the *Drosophila* gene Notch and is designated *TAN1* for translocation-associated Notch homologue.[284] Finally, a t(7;19)(q35;p13) was characterized and a transcriptional unit detected from chromosome 19 designated *LYL1*.[272,282]

Translocation with *TCRB* sequences resulted in production of aberrantly sized RNAs from a head-to-head juxtaposition with *LYL1*. The *LYL1* gene is similar to *TAL1* and *TAL2* (described above) in that it too contains a potential helix–loop–helix DNA binding motif.

PERSPECTIVE

Although much has been learned about the relationship between chromosome rearrangement and human cancer, much remains to be known about how these genomic alterations effect cellular changes that promote altered growth and proliferation. The initiating and subsequent events in chromosome rearrangement have yet to be elucidated.

Molecular cloning has permitted dissection of translocation breakpoints, especially in B- and T-cell neoplasms, in which immunoglobulin and T-cell receptor genes provided a landmark from which to isolate largely unknown genes. The characterization of previously unknown sequences identified in this way has only just begun, and their role in normal growth and development must be studied to interpret alterations that accompany tumorigenesis. The function of known identified cellular proto-oncogenes requires further investigation as their participation in normal cellular processes remains poorly defined.

Ultimately, a more complete understanding of the precise contribution of genes to deregulated cellular growth will doubtless enhance our knowledge of the processes that control normal cellular growth and will contribute to new approaches for the diagnosis and treatment of cancer.

REFERENCES

1. Tjio JH, Levan A. The chromosome number of man. Hereditas 1956;42: 1.
2. Moorhead PS, Nowell PC, Mellman WJ, et al. Chromosome preparations of leukocytes cultured from human peripheral blood. Exp Cell Res 1960;20:613.
3. Seabright M. A rapid banding technique for human chromosomes. Lancet 1971;2:971.
4. Drets ME, Shaw MW. Specific banding patterns of human chromosomes. Proc Natl Acad Sci USA 1971;68:2073.
5. Caspersson T, Lomakka G, Zech L. The 24 fluorescence patterns of the human metaphase chromosomes: distinguishing characters and variability. Hereditas 1971;67:89.
6. Sehested J. A simple method for R banding of human chromosomes showing a pH-dependent connection between R and G bands. Humangenetik 1974;21:55.
7. Sahar E, Latt SA. Enhancement of banding patterns in human metaphase chromosomes by energy transfer. Proc Natl Acad Sci USA 1978;75:5650.
8. Schweizer D. Simultaneous fluorescent staining of R bands and specific heterochromatic regions (DA-DAPI bands) in human chromosomes. Cytogenet Cell Genet 1980;27:190.
9. Schreck RR, Warburton D, Miller OJ, et al. Chromosome structure as revealed by a combined chemical and immunochemical procedure. Proc Natl Acad Sci USA 1973;70:804.
10. Robinson JA, Buckton KE, Sporvart G, et al. The segregation of human chromosome polymorphisms. Ann Hum Genet 1976;40:113.
11. Phillips RB. Inheritance of Q and C band polymorphisms. Can J Genet Cytol 1977;19:405.
12. Morton CC, Corey LA, Nance WE, et al. Quinacrine mustard and nucleolar organizer region heteromorphisms in twins. Acta Genet Med Gemellol 1981;30:39.
13. de la Chapelle A, Fellman J, Unnerus V. Determination of human paternity from the length of the Y chromosome. Ann Genet 1967;10: 60.
14. Robinson JA. Origin of extra chromosome in trisomy 21. Lancet 1973;1: 131.
15. Mikkelsen M, Hallberg A, Poulsen H. Maternal and paternal origin of extra chromosome in trisomy 21. Hum Genet 1976;32:17.
16. Hauge M, Poulsen H, Halberg A, Mikkelsen M. The value of fluorescence markers in the distribution between maternal and fetal chromosomes. Humangenetik 1975;26:187.
17. Arrighi F, Hsu TC. Localization of heterochromatin in human chromosomes. Cytogenetics 1971;10:81.
18. Brown T, Robertson FW, Dawson BM, et al. Individual variation of centric heterochromatin in man. Hum Genet 1980;55:367.
19. de la Chapelle A, Schroder J, Stenstrand K, et al. Pericentric inversions of human chromosomes 9 and 10. Am J Hum Genet 1974;26:746.
20. Bloom SE, Goodpasture C. An improved technique for selective silver staining of nucleolar organizer regions in human chromosomes. Hum Genet 1976;34:199.
21. Miller DA, Choi Y-C, Miller OJ. Chromosome localization of highly repetitive human DNA's and amplified ribosomal DNA with restriction enzymes. Science 1983;219:395.
22. Korenberg JR, Rykowski MC. Human genome organization: alu, lines and the molecular structure of metaphase chromosome bands. Cell 1988;53:391.
23. Yunis JJ. High resolution of human chromosomes. Science 1976;191: 1268.
24. Yu RL, Aronson MM, Nichols WW. High resolution bands in human fibroblast chromosomes induced by actinomycin D. Cytogenet Cell Genet 1981;31:111.
25. Rybak J. A simple reproducible method for prometaphase chromosome analysis. Hum Genet 1982;60:328.
26. Ikeuchi T. Inhibitory effect of ethidium bromide on mitotic chromosome condensation and its application to high-resolution chromosome banding. Cytogenet Cell Genet 1984;38:56.
27. Denver Report. A proposed standard system of nomenclature of human mitotic chromosomes. J Hered 1960;51:221.
28. ISCN. An International System for Human Cytogenetic Nomenclature. In: Harnden DG, Klinger HP, eds. (In collaboration with Cytogenet Cell Genet) Basel, Karger, 1985.
29. ISCN. Guidelines for cancer cytogenetics. In: Mitelman F, ed. Supplement to an International System for Human Cytogenetic Nomenclature. Basel, Karger, 1991.
30. Harris H. Cell fusion. Cambridge, MA, Harvard University Press, 1970.
31. Ephrussi B. Hybridization of somatic cells. Princeton, Princeton University Press, 1972.
32. Ringertz NR, Savage RE. Cell hybrids. New York, Academic Press, 1976.
33. Harper ME, Saunders GF. Localization of single copy DNA sequences on G-banded human chromosomes by in situ hybridization. Chromosoma 1981;83:431.
34. Morton CC, Kirsch IR, Taub RA, et al. Localization of the beta-globin gene by chromosomal *in situ* hybridization. Am J Hum Genet 1984;36: 576.
35. Van Prooijen-Knegt AC, Van Hoek JFM, Bauman JGJ, et al. In situ hybridization of DNA sequences in human metaphase chromosomes visualized by an indirect fluorescent immunocytochemical procedure. Exp Cell Res 1982;141:397.
36. Pinkel D, Straume T, Gray JW. Cytogenetic analysis using quantitative, high-sensitivity, fluorescence hybridization. Proc Natl Acad Sci USA 1986;83:2934.
37. Bartram CR, de Klein A, Hagemeijer A, et al. Translocation of c-*abl* oncogene correlates with the presence of a Philadelphia chromosome in chronic myelocytic leukaemia. Nature 1983;306:277.
38. Diaz MO, Le Beau MM, Pitha P, Rowley JD. Interferon and c-*ets*-1 genes in the translocation (9;11)(p22;q23) in human acute monocytic leukemia. Science 1986;231:265.
39. Phelan MC, Morton CC, Stevenson RE, et al. Molecular and cytogenetic characterization of a *de novo* t(5p;21q) in a patient previously diagnosed as monosomy 21. Am J Hum Genet 1988;43:511.
40. Medof ME, Lublin DM, Holers VM, et al. Cloning and characterization of cDNAs encoding the complete sequence of decay-accelerating factor of human complement. Proc Natl Acad Sci USA 1987;84:2007.
41. Coussens L, Van Beveren C, Smith D, et al. Structural alteration of viral homologue of receptor proto-oncogene fms at carboxy terminus. Nature 1986;320:277.
42. Yarden Y, Escobedo JA, Kuang WJ, et al. Structure of the receptor for platelet-derived growth factor helps define a family of closely related growth factor receptors. Nature 1986;323:226.
43. Le Beau MM, Lemmons RS, Espinosa R, et al. Interleukin-4 and interleukin-5 map to human chromosome 5 in a region encoding growth factors and receptors and are deleted in myeloid leukemias with a del(5q). Blood 1989;73:647.
44. Gold DP, van Dongen JJM, Morton CC, et al. The gene encoding the ϵ subunit of the T3/T-cell receptor complex maps to chromosome 11

in humans and to chromosome 9 in mice. Proc Natl Acad Sci USA 1987;84:1664.
45. Corbi AL, Larson RS, Kishimoto TK, et al. Chromosomal location of the genes encoding the leukocyte adhesion receptors LFA-1, Mac-1 and p150, 95. Identification of a gene cluster involved in cell adhesion. J Exp Med 1988;167:1597.
46. Lejeune J, Gautier M, Turpin R. Étude des chromosomes somatiques de neuf enfants mongoliens. C R Acad Sci (Paris) 1959;248:1721.
47. Knudson AG Jr. Mutation and cancer: statistical study of retinoblastoma. Proc Natl Acad Sci USA 1971;68:820.
48. Boveri T. Zur Frage der Entstehung maligner Tumoren. Jena, Gustav Fisher, 1914.
49. Nowell PC, Hungerford Da. A minute chromosome in human chronic granulocytic leukemia. Science 1960;132:1497.
50. Yunis JJ. The chromosomal basis of human neoplasia. Science 1983;221: 227.
51. Bloomfield CD, Lindquist LL, Brunning RD, et al. The Philadelphia chromosome in acute leukemia. Virchows Arch (B) 1978;29:81.
52. Rowley JD. Biological implications of consistent chromosome rearrangements in leukemia and lymphoma. Cancer Res 1984;44:3159.
53. Kirsch IR, Morton CC, Nakahara K, Leder P. Human immunoglobulin heavy chain genes map to a region of translocations in malignant B lymphocytes. Science 1982;216:301.
54. Battey J, Moulding C, Taub R, et al. The human *c-myc* oncogene: structural consequences of translocation into the IgH locus in Burkitt lymphoma. Cell 1983;34:779.
55. Baer R, Chen KC, Smith SD, Rabbitts TH. Fusion of an immunoglobulin variable gene and a T cell receptor constant gene in the chromosome 14 inversion associated with T cell tumors. Cell 1985;43:705.
56. Tkachuk DC, Kohler S, Cleary ML. Involvement of a homolog of Drosophila trithorax by 11q23 chromosomal translocations in acute leukemias. Cell 1992;71:691.
57. Hecht F. Hematologic malignancy breakpoint update. Cancer Genet Cytogenet 1988;31:132.
58. Therman E. Human chromosomes: structure, behavior, effects, ed 2. New York, Springer-Verlag, 1985:243.
59. Rowley JD. A new consistent chromosomal abnormality in chronic myelogenous leukaemia identified by quinacrine fluorescence and Giemsa staining. Nature 1973;243:290.
60. Baikie AG, Court Brown WM, Jacobs PA. Chromosome studies in leukaemia. Lancet 1960;2:168.
61. Caspersson T, Gahrton G, Lindsten J, Zech L. Identification of the Philadelphia chromosome as a number 22 by quinacrine mustard fluorescence analysis. Exp Cell Res 1970;63:238.
62. O'Riordan ML, Robinson JA, Buckton KE, Evans HJ. Distinguishing between the chromosomes involved in Down's syndrome (trisomy 21) and chronic myeloid leukemia (Ph1) by fluorescence. Nature 1971;230: 167.
63. de Klein A, Geurts van Kessel A, Grosveld G, et al. A cellular oncogene is translocated to the Philadelphia chromosome in chronic myelocytic leukemia. Nature 1982;300:765.
64. Groffen J, Heisterkamp N, Stephenson JR, et al. *c-sis* is translocated from chromosome 22 to chromosome 9 in chronic myelocytic leukemia. J Exp Med 1983;158:9.
65. Rowley JD, Testa JR. Chromosome abnormalities in malignant hematologic diseases. Adv Cancer Res 1983;36:103.
66. Lessard M, Le Prisé P-Y. Cytogenetic studies in 56 cases with Ph-positive hematologic disorders. Cancer Genet Cytogenet 1982;5:37.
67. Rowley JD. Ph-positive leukemia, including chronic myelogenous leukemia. Clin Haematol 1980;9:54.
68. Kelman Z, Prokocimer M, Peller S, et al. Rearrangements in the p53 gene in Philadelphia chromosome positive chronic myelogenous leukemia. Blood 1989;74:2318.
69. Groffen J, Stephenson JR, Heisterkamp N, et al. Philadelphia chromosomal breakpoints are clustered within a limited region, bcr, on chromosome 22. Cell 1984;36:93.
70. Bernards A, Rubin CM, Westbrook CM, et al. The first intron in the human *c-abl* gene is at least 200 kilobases long and is a target for translocations in chronic myelogenous leukemia. Mol Cell Biol 1987;7: 3231.
71. Lifshitz B, Fainstein E, Marcelle C, et al. *bcr* Genes and transcripts. Oncogene 1988;2:113.
72. Shtivelman E, Lifshitz B, Gale RP, Canaani E. Fused transcript of *abl* and *bcr* genes in chronic myelogenous leukaemia. Nature 1985;315: 550.
73. Ben-Neriah Y, Daley GQ, Mes-Masson A-M, et al. The chronic myelogenous leukemia-specific P210 protein is the product of the *bcr/abl* hybrid gene. Science 1986;233:212.
74. Gale RP, Canaani E. An 8-kilobase *abl* RNA transcript in chronic myelogenous leukemia. Proc Natl Acad Sci USA 1984;81:5648.
75. Stam K, Heisterkamp N, Grosveld G, et al. Evidence of a new chimeric *bcr* /*c-abl* mRNA in patients with chronic myelocytic leukemia and the Philadelphia chromosome. N Engl J Med 1985;313:1429.
76. Konopka JB, Watanabe SM, Witte ON. An alteration of the human *c-abl* protein in K562 leukemia cells unmasks associated tyrosine kinase activity. Cell 1984;37:1035.
77. Dreazen O, Canaani E, Gale RP. Molecular biology of chronic myelogenous leukemia. Semin Hematol 1988;25:35.
78. Marcelle C, Gale RP, Prokocimer M, et al. Analysis of *BCR-ABL* mRNA in chronic myelogenous leukemia patients and identification of a new *BCR*-related sequence in human DNA. Genes Chromosomes Cancer 1989;1:172.
79. Grossman A, Silver RT, Arlin Z, et al. Fine mapping of chromosome 22 breakpoints within the breakpoint cluster region (*bcr*) implies a role for bcr exon 3 in determining disease duration in chronic myeloid leukemia. Am J Hum Genet 1989;45:729.
80. Dreazen O, Berman M, Gale RP. Molecular abnormalities of *bcr* and *c-abl* in chronic myelogenous leukemia associated with a long chronic phase. Blood 1988;71:797.
81. Shtalrid M, Talpaz M, Kurzrock R, et al. Analysis of breakpoints within the *bcr* gene and their correlation with the clinical course of Ph-positive chronic myelogenous leukemia. Blood 1988;72:485.
82. Pugh WC, Pearson M, Vardiman JW, Rowley JD. Philadelphia chromosome–negative chronic myelogenous leukaemia: a morphologic reassessment. Br J Haematol 1985;60:457.
83. Travis LB, Pierre RV, Dewald GW. Ph-negative chronic granulocytic leukemia: a nonentity. Am J Clin Pathol 1986;85:186.
84. Morris CM, Reeve AE, Fitzgerald PH, et al. Genomic diversity correlates with clinical variation in Ph-negative chronic myeloid leukaemia. Nature 1986;320:281.
85. Dreazen O, Klisak I, Rassool F, et al. The *bcr* gene is joined to *c-abl* in Ph chromosome negative chronic myelogenous leukemia. Oncogene Res 1988;2:167.
86. van der Plas DC, Hermans AB, Soekarman D, et al. Cytogenetic and molecular analysis in Philadelphia negative CML. Blood 1989;73:1038.
87. First International Workshop on Chromosomes in Leukemia. Br J Haematol 1978;39:311.
88. Bitter MA, LeBeau MM, Rowley JD, et al. Associations between morphology, karyotype, and clinical features in myeloid leukemias. Hum Pathol 1987;18:211.
89. Erikson J, Griffin CA, ar-Rushdi A, et al. Heterogeneity of chromosome 22 breakpoint in Philadelphia-positive (Ph+) acute lymphocytic leukemia. Proc Natl Acad Sci USA 1986;83:1807.
90. Naumovski L, Morgan R, Hecht F, et al. Philadelphia chromosome–positive acute lymphoblastic leukemia cell lines without classical breakpoint cluster region rearrangement. Cancer Res 1988;48:2876.
91. Rubin CM, Carrino JJ, Dickler MN, et al. Heterogeneity of genomic fusion of *BCR* and *ABL* in Philadelphia chromosome–positive acute lymphoblastic leukemia. Proc Natl Acad Sci USA 1988;85:2795.
92. van der Feltz MJ, Shivji MK, Allen PB, et al. Nucleotide sequence of both reciprocal translocation junction regions in a patient with Ph positive acute lymphoblastic leukemia, with a breakpoint within the first intron of the BCR gene. Nucl Acids Res 1989;17:1.
93. Rubin CM, Westbrook CA, Smith SD, et al. Philadelphia chromosome–positive acute lymphoblastic leukemia: detection of a DNA rearrangement 50–250 kilobases proximal to BCR. In: Gale RP, Golde DW, eds. Recent advances in leukemia and lymphoma. UCLA Symposia on Molecular and Cellular Biology: new series, vol 61. New York, Alan R Liss, 1987:125.
94. Clark SS, McLaughlin J, Crist WM, et al. Unique forms of the *abl* tyrosine kinase distinguish Ph-positive CML from Ph-positive ALL. Science 1987;235:85.
95. Chan LC, Karhi KK, Rayter SI, et al. A novel *abl* protein expressed in Philadelphia chromosome positive acute lymphoblastic leukaemia. Nature 1987;325:635.
96. Lugo TG, Pendergast A-M, Muller AJ, Witte ON. Tyrosine kinase activity and transformation potency of *bcr-abl* oncogene products. Science 1990;247:1079.
97. Kurzrock R, Shtalrid M, Talpaz M, et al. Expression of *c-abl* in Philadelphia-positive acute myelogenous leukemia. Blood 1987;70:1584.
98. Hooberman AL, Carrino JJ, Leibowitz D, et al. Unexpected heterogeneity of BCR-ABL fusion mRNA detected by polymerase chain reaction in Philadelphia chromosome–positive acute lymphoblastic leukemia. Proc Natl Acad Sci USA 1989;86:4259.
99. Yunis JJ, Bloomfield CD, Ensrud K. All patients with acute nonlymphocytic leukemia may have a chromosomal defect. N Engl J Med 1981;305:135.
100. Rowley JD. Identification of a translocation with quinacrine fluorescence in a patient with acute leukemia. Ann Genet 1973;16:109.
101. Fourth International Workshop on Chromosomes in Leukemia. Cancer Genet Cytogenet 1984;11:249.
102. Second International Workshop on Chromosomes in Leukemia. Cancer Genet Cytogenet 1980;2:89.
103. Miyoshi H, Shimizu K, Kozu T, et al. t(8;21) breakpoints on chromosome 21 in acute myeloid leukemia are clustered within a limited region of a single gene, *AML* 1. Proc Natl Acad Sci USA 1991;88:10431.
104. Erickson P, Gao J, Chang K-S, et al. Identification of breakpoints in t(8;21) acute myelogenous leukemia and isolation of a fusion transcript, *AML 1/ETO*, with similarity to *Drosophila* segmentation gene, *runt*. Blood 1992;80:1825.
105. Nisson PE, Watkins PC, Sacchi N. Transcriptionally active chimeric gene derived from the fusion of the *AML* 1 gene and a novel gene on

chromosome 8 in t(8;21) leukemic cells. Cancer Genet Cytogenet 1992;63:81.
106. Wang S, Wang Q, Crute BE, et al. Cloning and characterization of subunits of the T-cell receptor and murine leukemia virus enhancer core-binding factor. Mol Cell Biol 1993;13:3324.
107. Liu P, Tarlé SA, Harja A, et al. Fusion between transcription factor CBFβ/PEBP2β and a myosin heavy chain in acute myeloid leukemia. Science 1993;261:1041.
108. Fong C, Brodeur GM. Down's syndrome and leukemia: epidemiology, genetics, cytogenetics and mechanisms of leukemogenesis. Cancer Genet Cytogenet 1987;28:55.
109. Rowley JD. Down syndrome and acute leukemia: increased risk may be due to trisomy 21. Lancet 1981;2:1020.
110. Hecht F, Hecht BK, Morgan R, et al. Chromosome clues to acute leukemia in Down's syndrome. Cancer Genet Cytogenet 1986;21:93.
111. Rowley JD, Golomb HM, Dougherty C. 15/17 translocation, a consistent chromosomal change in acute promyelocytic leukaemia. Lancet 1977;1: 549.
112. Lemmons RS, Eilender D, Waldmann RA, et al. Cloning and characterization of the t(15;17) translocation breakpoint region in acute promyelocytic leukemia. Genes Chrom Cancer 1990;2:79.
113. Borrow J, Goddard AD, Sheer D, Solomon E. Molecular analysis of acute promyelocytic leukemia breakpoint cluster region on chromosome 17. Science 1990;249:1577.
114. de Thé H, Chomienne C, Lanotte M, et al. The t(15;17) translocation of acute promyelocytic leukaemia fuses the retinoic acid receptor α gene to a novel transcribed locus. Nature 1990;347:558.
115. de Thé H, Lavau C, Marchio A, et al. The PML-RARα fusion mRNA generated by the t(15;17) translocation in acute promyelocytic leukemia encodes a functionally altered RAR. Cell 1991;66:675.
116. Le Beau MM, Larson RA, Bitter MA, et al. Association of an inversion of chromosome 16 with abnormal marrow eosinophils in acute myelomonocytic leukemia. N Engl J Med 1983;309:630.
117. de la Chapelle A, Lahtinen R. Chromosome 16 and bone-marrow eosinophilia. N Engl J Med 1983;309:1394.
118. Gu Y, Cimino G, Alder H, et al. The (4;11)(q21;q23) chromosome translocations in acute leukemia involve the VDJ recombinase. Proc Natl Acad Sci USA 1992;89:10464.
119. Ziemin-van der Poel S, McCabe NR, Gill HJ, et al. Identification of a gene, MLL, that spans the breakpoints in 11q23 translocations associated with human leukemias. Proc Natl Acad Sci USA 1991;88:10735.
120. Djabali M, Selleri L, Parry P, et al. A trithorax-like gene is interrupted by chromosome 11q23 translocations in acute leukemias. Nat Genet 1992;2:113.
121. Sandberg AA. Erythroleukemia (EL). In: The chromosomes in human cancer and leukemia. New York, Elsevier North-Holland, 1980:323.
122. Kirsch IR, Brown JA, Lawrence J, et al. Translocations that highlight chromosomal regions of differentiated activity. Cancer Genet Cytogenet 1985;18:159.
123. Rowley JD, Potter D. Chromosomal banding patterns in acute nonlymphocytic leukemia. Blood 1976;47:705.
124. Yunis JJ. Recurrent chromosomal defects are found in most patients with acute nonlymphocytic leukemia. Cancer Genet Cytogenet 1984;11: 125.
125. Westbrook CA, Le Beau MM, Diaz MO, et al. Chromosomal localization and characterization of c-*abl* in the t(6;9) of acute nonlymphocytic leukemia. Proc Natl Acad Sci USA 1985;82:8742.
126. von Lindern M, Fornerod M, van Baal S, et al. The translocation (6;9), associated with a specific subtype of acute myeloid leukemia, results in the fusion of two genes, *dek* and *can*, and the expression of a chimeric, leukemia-specific *dek-can* nRNA. Mol Cell Biol 1992;12:1687.
127. Van den Berghe H, Cassiman J-J, David G, Fryns J-P. Distinct haematological disorder with deletion of long arm of No. 5 chromosome. Nature 1974;251:437.
128. Van den Berghe H, Vermaelen K, Mecucci C, et al. The 5q-anomaly. Cancer Genet Cytogenet 1985;17:189.
129. Le Beau MM, Albain KS, Larson RA, et al. Clinical and cytogenetic correlations in 63 patients with therapy-related myelodysplastic syndromes and acute nonlymphocytic leukemia: further evidence for characteristic abnormalities of chromosomes no. 5 and 7. J Clin Oncol 1986;4:325.
130. Le Beau MM, Westbrook CA, Diaz MO, et al. Evidence for the involvement of *GM-CSF* and *FMS* in the deletion (5q) in myeloid disorders. Science 1986;231:984.
131. Mitelman F, Brandt L, Nilsson PG. Relation among occupational exposure to potential mutagenic/carcinogenic agents, clinical findings, and bone marrow chromosomes in acute nonlymphocytic leukemia. Blood 1978;52:1229.
132. Golomb HM, Alimena G, Rowley JD, et al. Correlation of occupation and karyotype in adults with acute nonlymphocytic leukemia. Blood 1982;60:404.
133. Neinhuis AW, Bunn HF, Turner PH, et al. Expression of the human c-*fms* proto-oncogene in hematopoietic cells and its deletion in the 5q-syndrome. Cell 1985;42:421.
134. Pettenati MJ, Le Beau MM, Lemons RS, et al. Assignment of *CSF-1* to 5q33.1: evidence for clustering of genes regulating hematopoiesis and for their involvement in the deletion of the long arm of chromosome 5 in myeloid disorders. Proc Natl Acad Sci USA 1987;84:2970.
135. Le Beau MM, Epstein ND, O'Brien SJ, et al. The interleukin 3 gene is located on human chromosome 5 and is deleted in myeloid leukemias with a deletion of 5q. Proc Natl Acad Sci USA 1987;84:5913.
136. Willman CL, Sever CE, Pallavicini MG, et al. Deletion of *IRF-1*, mapping to chromosome 5q31.1, in human leukemia following alkeran therapy. Cancer Genet Cytogenet 1985;15:95.
137. Cavenee WK, Dryja TP, Phillips RA, et al. Expression of recessive alleles by chromosomal mechanisms in retinoblastoma. Nature 1983;305:779.
138. Orkin SH, Goldman DS, Sallan SE. Development of homozygosity for chromosome 11p markers in Wilms' tumour. Nature 1984;309:172.
139. Zbar B, Brauch H, Talmadge C, Linehan M. Loss of alleles of loci on the short arm of chromosome 3 in renal cell carcinoma. Nature 1987;327:721.
140. Seizinger BR, de la Monte S, Atkins L, et al. Molecular genetic approach to human meningioma: loss of genes on chromosome 22. Proc Natl Acad Sci USA 1987;84:5419.
141. Solomon E, Voss R, Hall V, et al. Chromosome 5 allele loss in human colorectal carcinomas. Nature 1987;328:616.
142. Hansen MF, Koufos A, Gallie BL, et al. Osteosarcoma and retinoblastoma: a shared chromosomal mechanism revealing recessive predisposition. Proc Natl Acad Sci USA 1985;82:6216.
143. Seizinger BR, Martuza RL, Gusella JF. Loss of genes on chromosome 22 in tumorigenesis of human acoustic neuroma. Nature 1986;322:644.
144. Naylor SL, Johnson BE, Minna JD, Sakaguchi AY. Loss of heterozygosity of chromosome 3p markers in small-cell lung cancer. Nature 1987;329: 451.
145. Manolov G, Manolova Y. Marker band in one chromosome 14 from Burkitt lymphoma. Nature 1972;237:33.
146. Zech L, Haglund U, Nilsson K, Klein G. Characteristic chromosomal abnormalities in biopsies and lymphoid-cell lines from patients with Burkitt and non-Burkitt lymphomas. Int J Cancer 1976;17:47.
147. Miyoshi I, Hiraki S, Kimura I, et al. 2/8 translocation in a Japanese Burkitt's lymphoma. Experientia 1979;36:742.156. Van den Berghe H, Parlior C, Gosseye S, et al. Variant translocation in Burkitt lymphoma. Cancer Genet Cytogenet 1979;1:9.
148. Van den Berghe H, Parlior C, Gosseye S, et al. Variant translocation in Burkitt lymphoma. Cancer Genet Cytogenet 1979;1:9.
149. Berger R, Bernheim A, Weh H-J, et al. A new translocation in Burkitt's tumor cells. Hum Genet 1979;53:111.
150. Bernheim A, Berger R, Lenoir G. Translocations t(2;8) et t(8;22) dans des lignées cellulaires continues de lymphomes de Burkitt africain. C R Acad Sci (Paris) 1980;291:237.
151. Bernheim A, Berger R, Lenoir G. Cytogenetic studies on African Burkitt's lymphoma cell lines: t(8;14), t(2;8) and t(8;22) translocations. Cancer Genet Cytogenet 1981;3:307.
152. Taub R, Kirsch I, Morton C, et al. Translocation of the c-*myc* gene into the immunoglobulin heavy chain locus in human Burkitt lymphoma and murine plasmacytoma cells. Proc Natl Acad Sci USA 1982;79:7837.
153. Adams JM, Gerondakis S, Webb E, et al. Cellular *myc* oncogene is altered by chromosome translocation to an immunoglobulin locus in murine plasmacytomas and is rearranged similarly in human Burkitt lymphomas. Proc Natl Acad Sci USA 1983;80:1982.
154. Dalla-Favera R, Martinotti S, Gallo RC, et al. Translocations and rearrangements of the c-*myc* oncogene locus in human undifferentiated B-cell lymphomas. Science 1983;219:963.
155. Hamlyn PH, Rabbitts TH. Translocation joins c-*myc* and immunoglobulin 1 genes in a Burkitt lymphoma revealing a third exon in the c-*myc* oncogene. Nature 1983;304:135.
156. Erikson J, Nishikura K, ar-Rushdi A, et al. Translocation of an immunoglobulin locus to a region 3′ of an unrearranged c-*myc* oncogene enhances c-*myc* transcription. Proc Natl Acad Sci USA 1983;80:7581.
157. Taub R, Kelly K, Battey J, et al. A novel alteration in the structure of an activated c-*myc* gene in a variant t(2;8) Burkitt lymphoma. Cell 1984;37:511.
158. Hollis GF, Mitchell KF, Battey J, et al. A variant translocation places the immunoglobulin genes 3′ to the c-*myc* oncogene in Burkitt's lymphoma. Nature 1984;307:752.
159. Sun LK, Showe LC, Croce CM. Analysis of the 3′ flanking region of the human c-myc gene in lymphomas with the t(8;22) and t(2;8) chromosomal translocations. Nucl Acids Res 1986;14:4037.
160. Manolov G, Manolova Y, Klein G, et al. Alternative involvement of two cytogenetically distinguishable breakpoints on chromosome 8 in Burkitt's lymphoma associated translocations. Cancer Genet Cytogenet 1986;20:95.
161. Graham M, Adams JM. Chromosome 8 breakpoint far 3′ of the c-*myc* oncogene in a Burkitt's lymphoma 2;8 variant translocation is equivalent to the murine *pvt*-1 locus. EMBO J 1986;5:2845.
162. Mengle-Gaw L, Rabbitts TH. A human chromosome 8 region with abnormalities in B cell, HTLV-1+ T cell and c-*myc* amplified tumours. EMBO J 1987;6:1959.
163. Leder P. The genetics of antibody diversity. Sci Am 1982;246:102.
164. Leder P, Battey J, Lenoir G, et al. Translocations among antibody genes in human cancer. Science 1983;222:765.

165. Klein G. The role of gene dosage and transposition in carcinogenesis. Nature 1981;294:313.
166. Rowley JD. Identification of the constant chromosome regions involved in human hematologic malignant disease. Science 1982;216:749.
167. Alitalo K, Schwab M, Lin CC, et al. Homogeneously staining chromosomal regions contain amplified copies of an abundantly expressed cellular oncogene (c-*myc*) in malignant neuroendocrine cells from a human colon carcinoma. Proc Natl Acad Sci USA 1983;80:1707.
168. Taub R, Moulding C, Battey J, et al. Activation and somatic mutation of the translocated c-*myc* gene in Burkitt lymphoma cells. Cell 1984;36:339.
169. Rabbitts TH, Forster A, Hamlyn P, Baer R. Effect of somatic mutation within translocated c-*myc* genes in Burkitt's lymphoma. Nature 1984;309:592.
170. Murphy W, Sarid J, Taub R, et al. A translocated human c-*myc* oncogene is altered in a conserved coding sequence. Proc Natl Acad Sci USA 1986;83:2939.
171. Pelicci P-G, Knowles DM II, Magrath I, Dalla-Favera R. Chromosomal breakpoints and structural alterations of the c-*myc* locus differ in endemic and sporadic forms of Burkitt lymphoma. Proc Natl Acad Sci USA 1986;83:2984.
172. Queens C, Baltimore D. Immunoglobulin gene transcription is activated by downstream sequence elements. Cell 1983;33:741.
173. Gillies SD, Morrison SL, Oi VT, Tonegawa S. A tissue-specific transcription enhancer element is located in the major intron of a rearranged immunoglobulin heavy chain gene. Cell 1983;33:717.
174. Bergman Y, Rice D, Grosschedl R, Baltimore D. Two regulatory elements for immunoglobulin kappa light chain gene expression. Proc Natl Acad Sci USA 1984;81:7041.
175. Wiman KG, Clarkson B, Hayday AC, et al. Activation of a translocated c-*myc* gene: role of structural alterations in the upstream region. Proc Natl Acad Sci USA 1984;81:6798.
176. Showe LC, Ballantine M, Nishikura K, et al. Cloning and sequencing of a c-*myc* oncogene in a Burkitt's lymphoma cell line that is translocated to a germ line alpha switch region. Mol Cell Biol 1985;5:501.
177. Fukuhara S, Rowley JD, Variakojis D, Golomb HM. Chromosome abnormalities in poorly differentiated lymphocytic lymphoma. Cancer Res 1979;39:3119.
178. Yunis JJ, Frizzera G, Oken MM, et al. Multiple recurrent genomic defects in follicular lymphoma. A possible model for cancer. N Engl J Med 1987;316:79.
179. Levine EG, Arthur DC, Frizzera G et al. There are differences in cytogenetic abnormalities among histologic subtypes of the non-Hodgkin's lymphomas. Blood 1985;66:1414.
180. Tsujimoto Y, Finger LR, Yunis J, et al. Cloning of the chromosome breakpoint of neoplastic B cells with the t(14;18) chromosome translocation. Science 1984;226:1097.
181. Bakhshi A, Jensen JP, Goldman P, et al. Cloning the chromosomal breakpoint of t(14;18) human lymphomas: clustering around J_H on chromosome 14 and near a transcriptional unit on 18. Cell 1985;41:899.
182. Cleary ML, Sklar J. Nucleotide sequence of a t(14;18) chromosomal breakpoint in follicular lymphoma and demonstration of a breakpoint-cluster region near a transcriptionally active locus on chromosome 18. Proc Natl Acad Sci USA 1985;82:7439.
183. Bakhshi A, Wright JJ, Graninger W, et al. Mechanism of the t(14;18) chromosomal translocation: structural analysis of both derivative 14 and 18 reciprocal partners. Proc Natl Acad Sci USA 1987;84:2396.
184. Cleary ML, Galili N, Sklar J. Detection of a second t(14;18) breakpoint cluster region in human follicular lymphomas. J Exp Med 1986;164:315.
185. Seto M, Jaeger U, Hockett RD, et al. Alternative promoters and exons, somatic mutation and deregulation of the *Bcl-2-Ig* fusion gene in lymphoma. EMBO J 1988;7:123.
186. Cleary ML, Smith SD, Sklar J. Cloning and structural analysis of cDNAs for *BCL2* and a hybrid *BCL2*/immunoglobulin transcript resulting from the t(14;18) translocation. Cell 1986;47:19.
187. Graninger WB, Seto M, Boutain B, et al. Expression of Bcl-2 and Bcl-2-Ig fusion transcripts in normal and neoplastic cells. J Clin Invest 1987;80:1512.
188. Reed JC, Tsujimoto Y, Alpers JD, et al. Regulation of *BCL2* proto-oncogene expression during normal human lymphocyte proliferation. Science 1987;236:1295.
189. Gurfinkel N, Unger T, Givol D, Mushinski JF. Expression of the *BCL2* gene in mouse B lymphocytic cell lines is differentiation stage specific. Eur J Immunol 1987;17:567.
190. Tsujimoto Y, Gorham J, Cossman J, et al. The t(14;18) chromosome translocations involved in B-cell neoplasms result from mistakes in VDJ joining. Science 1985;229:1390.
191. Finger LR, Harvey RC, Moore RCA, et al. A common mechanism of chromosomal translocation in T- and B-cell neoplasia. Science 1986;234:982.
192. Reynolds TC, Smith SD, Sklar J. Analysis of DNA surrounding the breakpoints of chromosomal translocations involving the β T cell receptor gene in human lymphoblastic neoplasms. Cell 1987;50:107.
193. Bernard O, Larsen C-J, Hampe A, et al. Molecular mechanisms of a t(8;14)(q24;q11) translocation juxtaposing c-*myc* and TcR-α genes in a T-cell leukaemia: involvement of a Vα internal heptamer. Oncogene 1988;2:195.
194. Boehm T, Baer R, Lavenir I, et al. The mechanism of chromosomal translocation t(11;14) involving the T-cell receptor of Cδ locus on human chromosome 14q11 and a transcribed region of chromosome 11p15. EMBO J 1988;7:385.
195. Boehm T, Buluwela L, Williams D, et al. A cluster of chromosome 11p13 translocations found via distinct D-D and D-D-J rearrangements of the human T cell receptor δ chain gene. EMBO J 1988;7:2011.
196. Russo G, Isobe M, Pegoraro L, et al. Molecular analysis of a t(7;14)(q35;q32) chromosome translocation in a T cell leukemia of a patient with ataxia telangiectasia. Cell 1988;53:137.
197. Begley CG, Aplan PD, Davey MP, et al. Chromosomal translocation in a human leukemic stem-cell line disrupts the T-cell antigen receptor δ-chain diversity region and results in a previously unreported fusion transcript. Proc Natl Acad Sci USA 1989;86:2031.
198. Tycko B, Reynolds TC, Smith SD, Sklar J. Consistent breakage between consensus recombinase heptamers of chromosome 9 DNA in a recurrent chromosomal translocation of human T cell leukemia. J Exp Med 1989;169:369.
199. Erikson J, Finan J, Tsujimoto Y, et al. The chromosome 14 breakpoint in neoplastic B cells with the t(11;14) translocation involves the immunoglobulin heavy chain locus. Proc Natl Acad Sci USA 1984;81:4144.
200. Tsujimoto Y, Yunis J, Onorato-Showe L, et al. Molecular cloning of the chromosomal breakpoint of B-cell lymphomas and leukemias with the t(11;14) chromosome translocation. Science 1984;224:1403.
201. Motokura T, Bloom T, Kim HG, et al. A novel cyclin encoded by a *bcl* 1-linked candidate oncogene. Nature 1991;350:512.
202. Tsujimoto Y, Jaffe E, Cossman J, et al. Clustering of breakpoints on chromosome 11 in human B-cell neoplasms with the t(11;14) chromosome translocation. Nature 1985;315:340.
203. Ueshima Y, Bird ML, Vardiman J, Rowley J. A 14;19 translocation in B-cell chronic lymphocytic leukemia: a new recurring chromosome aberration. Int J Cancer 1985;36:287.
204. Ohno H, Takimoto G, McKeithan TW. The candidate proto-oncogene *bcl-3* is related to genes implicated in cell lineage determination and cell cycle control. Cell 1990;60:991.
205. Carroll AJ, Crist WM, Parmley RT, et al. Pre-B cell leukemia associated with chromosome translocation 1;19. Blood 1984;63:721.
206. Williams DL, Look AT, Melvin SL, et al. New chromosomal translocations correlate with specific immunophenotypes of childhood acute lymphoblastic leukemia. Cell 1984;36:101.
207. Mellentin JD, Murre C, Donlon TA, et al. The gene for enhancer binding proteins E12/E47 lies at the t(1;19) breakpoint in acute leukemias. Science 1989;246:379.
208. Nourse J, Mellentin JD, Galili N, et al. Chromosomal translocation t(1;19) results in synthesis of a homeobox fusion mRNA that codes for a potential chimeric transcription factor. Cell 1990;60:535.
209. Kamps MP, Murre C, Sun X-h, Baltimore D. A new homeobox gene contributes the DNA binding domain of the t(1;19) translocation protein in pre-B ALL. Cell 1990;60:547.
210. Boehm T, Rabbitts TH. The human T cell receptor genes are targets for chromosomal abnormalities in T cell tumors. FASEB J 1989;3:2344.
211. Croce CM, Isobe M, Palumbo A, et al. Gene for α-chain of human T-cell receptor: location on chromosome 14 region involved in T-cell neoplasms. Science 1985;227:1044.
212. Caccia N, Bruns GAP, Kirsch IR, et al. T cell receptor α chain genes are located on chromosome 14 at 14q11–14q12 in humans. J Exp Med 1985;161:1255.
213. Chien Y-h, Iwashima M, Kaplan KB, et al. A new T-cell receptor gene located within the alpha locus and expressed early in T-cell differentiation. Nature 1987;327:677.
214. Morton CC, Duby AD, Eddy RL, et al. Genes for β chain of human T-cell antigen receptor map to regions of chromosomal rearrangement in T cells. Science 1985;228:582.
215. Le Beau MM, Diaz MO, Rowley JD, Mak TW. Chromosomal localization of the human T cell receptor β-chain genes. Cell 1985;41:335.
216. Murre C, Waldmann RA, Morton CC, et al. Human λ-chain genes are rearranged in leukaemic T cells and map to the short arm of chromosome 7. Nature 1985;316:549.
217. Ueshima Y, Rowley JD, Variakojis D, et al. Cytogenetic studies on patients with chronic T-cell leukemia/lymphoma. Blood 1984;63:1028.
218. Zech L, Gahrton G, Hammarström L, et al. Inversion of chromosome 14 marks human T-cell chronic lymphocytic leukaemia. Nature 1984;308:858.
219. Miyamoto K, Tomita N, Ishii A, et al. Chromosome abnormalities of leukemia cells in adult patients with T-cell leukemia. J Natl Cancer Inst 1984;73:353.
220. Hecht F, Morgan R, Hecht BK-M, Smith SD. Common region on chromosome 14 in T-cell leukemia and lymphoma. Science 1984;226:1445.
221. Sadamori N, Kusano M, Nishino K, et al. Abnormalities of chromosome 14 at band 14q11 in Japanese patients with adult T-cell leukemia. Cancer Genet Cytogenet 1985;17:279.
222. Davey MP, Bertness V, Nakahara K, et al. Juxtaposition of the T-cell

receptor α-chain locus (14q11) and a region (14q32) of potential importance in leukemogenesis by a 14;14 translocation in a patient with T-cell chronic lymphocytic leukemia and ataxia-telangiectasia. Proc Natl Acad Sci USA 1988;85:9287.
223. Fukuhara S, Hinuma Y, Gotoh Y-I, Uchino H. Chromosome aberrations in T lymphocytes carrying adult T-cell leukemia-associated antigens (ATLA) from healthy adults. Blood 1983;61:205.
224. Smith SD, Morgan R, Link MP, et al. Cytogenetic and immunophenotypic analysis of cell lines established from patients with T cell leukemia/lymphoma. Blood 1986;67:650.
225. Kaneko, Maseki N, Homma C, et al. Chromosome translocations involving band 7q35 or 7p15 in childhood T-cell leukemia/lymphoma. Blood 1988;72:534.
226. Aurias A, Dutrillaux B, Buriot D, Lejeune J. High frequencies of inversions and translocations of chromosomes 7 and 14 in ataxia telangiectasia. Mutat Res 1980;69:369.
227. O'Conner RD, Brown MG, Francke U. Immunologic and karyotypic studies in ataxia-telangiectasia: specificity of break points on chromosomes 7 and 14 in lymphocytes from patients and relatives. In: Bridges BA, Harnden DG, eds. Ataxia-telangiectasia: a cellular and molecular link between cancer, neuropathology, and immune deficiency. Chichester, UK, John Wiley & Sons, 1982:259.
228. Stern M-H, Lipkowitz S, Aurias A, et al. Inversion of chromosome 7 in ataxia telangiectasia is generated by a rearrangement between T-cell receptor β and T-cell receptor γ genes. Blood 1989;74:2076.
229. Denny CT, Yoshikai Y, Mak TW, et al. A chromosome 14 inversion in a T-cell lymphoma is caused by site-specific recombination between immunoglobulin and T-cell receptor loci. Nature 1986;320:549.
230. Denny CT, Hollis GF, Hecht F, et al. Common mechanism of chromosome inversion in B- and T-cell tumors: relevance to lymphoid development. Science 1986;234:197.
231. Kennaugh AA, Butterworth SV, Hollis R, et al. The chromosome breakpoint at 14q32 in an ataxia telangiectasia t(14;14) T cell clone is different from the 14q32 breakpoint in Burkitts and an inv(14) T cell lymphoma. Hum Genet 1986;73:254.
232. Baer R, Heppell A, Taylor AMR, et al. The breakpoint of an inversion of chromosome 14 in a T-cell leukemia: sequences downstream of the immunoglobulin heavy chain locus are implicated in tumorigenesis. Proc Natl Acad Sci USA 1987;84:9069.
233. Mengle-Gaw L, Willard HF, Smith CIE, et al. Human T-cell tumors containing chromosome 14 inversion or translocation with breakpoints proximal to immunoglobulin joining regions at 14q32. EMBO J 1987;6: 2273.
234. Mengle-Gaw L, Albertson DG, Sherrington PD, Rabbitts TH. Analysis of a T-cell tumor-specific breakpoint cluster at human chromosome 14q32. Proc Natl Acad Sci USA 1988;85:9171.
235. McCaw BK, Hecht F, Harnden DG, Teplitz RL. Somatic rearrangement of chromosome 14 in human lymphocytes. Proc Natl Acad Sci USA 1975;72:2071.
236. Taylor AMR, Oxford JM, Metcalfe JA. Spontaneous cytogeneic abnormalities in lymphocytes from thirteen patients with ataxia telangiectasia. Int J Cancer 1981;27:311.
237. Taylor AMR. Cytogenetics of ataxia-telangiectasia. In: Bridges BA, Harnden DG, eds. Ataxia-telangiectasia: a cellular and molecular link between cancer, neuropathology and immune deficiency. Chichester, UK, John Wiley & Sons, 1982:53.
238. Hecht F, Kaiser-McCaw B. Ataxia-telangiectasia; chromosomes before cancer. In: Bridges BA, Harnden DG, eds. Ataxia-telangiectasia: a cellular and molecular link between cancer, neuropathology, and immune deficiency. Chichester, UK, John Wiley & Sons, 1982:243.
239. Welch JP, Lee CLY. Non-random occurrence of 7–14 translocations in human lymphocyte cultures. Nature 1975;255:241.
240. Beatty-DeSana JW, Hoggard MT, Cooledge JW. Non-random occurrence of 7–14 translocations in human lymphocyte cultures. Nature 1975;255: 242.
241. Hecht F, McCaw BK, Peakman D, Robinson A. Non-random occurrence of 7–14 translocations in human lymphocyte cultures. Nature 1975;255: 243.
242. Zech L, Haglund U. A recurrent structural aberration, t(7;14), in phytohemagglutinin-stimulated lymphocytes. Hereditas 1978;89:69.
243. Mihelick K, McCombs J, Howard-Peebles PN, et al. Translocations involving chromosomes 7 and 14: a non-random occurrence? Am J Hum Genet 1983;35:144A.
244. Wallace C, Bernstein R, Pinto MR. Non-random in vitro 7;14 translocations detected in a routine cytogenetic series: 12 examples and their possible significance. Hum Genet 1984;66:157.
245. Dewald GW, Noonan KJ, Spurbeck JL, Johnson DD. T-lymphocytes with 7;14 translocation: frequency of occurrence, breakpoints, and clinical and biological significance. Am J Hum Genet 1986;38:520.
246. Tawn EJ. The non-random occurrence of exchanges involving chromosomes 7 and 14 in human lymphocytes: a prospective study of control individuals. Mutat Res 1988;199:215.
247. Tycko B, Palmer JD, Sklar J. T-cell receptor gene trans-rearrangements: chimeric λ/δ genes and in normal lymphoid tissues. Science 1989;245: 1242.
248. Kurtzberg J, Bigner SH, Hershfield MS. Establishment of the DU.528 human lymphohematopoietic stem cell line. J Exp Med 1985;162:1561.
249. Mathieu-Mahul D, Bernheim A, Sigaux F, et al. Translocation t(1;14) and rearrangement of the gene for the alpha chain of the T-cell receptor in acute T-lymphoblastic leukemia. C R Acad Sci 1986;302:525.
250. Lampert F, Harbott J, Ritterbach J, et al. T-cell acute childhood lymphoblastic leukemia with chromosome 14q11 anomaly: a morphologic, immunologic, and cytogenetic analysis of 10 patients. Blut 1988;56: 117.
251. Rivière D, Dutel JL, Desfontaines B, et al. Leucemie aigue lymphoblastique de type T avec translocation t(8;14)(q24;q12). Nouv Rev Fr Hematol 1983; 25:175.
252. Mathieu-Mahul D, Sigaux F, Zhu C, et al. A t(8;14)(q24;q11) translocation in a T-cell leukemia (L1-ALL) with c-*myc* and TCR-alpha chain locus rearrangements. Int J Cancer 1986; 38:835.
253. Hayashi Y, Yamamoto K, Kojima S. T-cell acute lymphoblastic leukemias with a t(8;14) possibly involving a c-*myc* locus and T-cell-receptor α-chain genes. N Engl J Med 1986;314:650.
254. Caubet J-F, Mathieu-Mahul D, Bernheim A, et al. Remaniement du locus du proto-oncogène c-*myc* dans une lignée cellulaire d'origine lymphoblastique T. C R Acad Sci 1985;300:171.
255. Erikson J, Williams DL, Finan J, et al. Locus of the α-chain of the T-cell receptor is split by chromosome translocation in T-cell leukemias. Science 1985;229:784.
256. Shima EA, Le Beau MM, McKeithan TW, et al. Gene encoding the α chain of the T-cell receptor is moved immediately downstream of c-*myc* in a chromosomal 8;14 translocation in a cell line from a human T-cell leukemia. Proc Natl Acad Sci USA 1986;83:3439.
257. Dubé ID, Raimondi SC, Pi D, Kalousek DK. A new translocation, t(10;14)(q24;q11), in T cell neoplasia. Blood 1986;67:1181.
258. Dubé ID, Greenberg ML. Phenotypic heterogeneity in three cases of lymphoid malignancy with chromosomal translocations in 14q11. Cytogenet Cell Genet 1986;41:215.
259. Raimondi SC, Behm FG, Roberson PK, et al. Cytogenetics of childhood T-cell leukemia. Blood 1988;72:1560.
260. White L, Meyer PR, Benedict WF. Establishment and characterization of a human T-cell leukemia line (LALW-2) in nude mice. J Natl Cancer Inst 1984;72:1029.
261. Harbott J, Engel R, Gerein V, et al. (11;14) translocation in three boys with acute lymphoblastic leukemia of T-cell immunophenotype. Blut 1986;52:45.
262. Le Beau MM, McKeithan TW, Shima EA, et al. T-cell receptor α-chain gene is split in a human T-cell leukemia cell line with a t(11;14)(p15;q11). Proc Natl Acad Sci USA 1986;83:9744.
263. Takasaki N, Kaneko Y, Maseki N, et al. Hemophagocytic syndrome complicating T-cell acute lymphoblastic leukemia with a novel t(11;14)(p15;q11) chromosome translocation. Cancer 1987;59:424.
264. Raimondi SC, Pui C-H, Behm FG, Williams DL. 7q32-q36 translocations in childhood T cell leukemia: cytogenetic evidence for involvement of the T cell receptor β-chain gene. Blood 1987;69:131.
265. Hecht F, Morgan R, Gemmill RM, et al. Translocations in T-cell leukemia and lymphoma. N Engl J Med 1985;313:758.
266. Cleary ML, Mellentin JD, Spies J, Smith SD. Chromosomal translocation involving the β T cell receptor gene in acute leukemia. J Exp Med 1988;167:682.
267. Erikson J, Finger L, Sun L, et al. Deregulation of c-*myc* by translocation of the α-locus of the T-cell receptor in T-cell leukemias. Science 1986;232:884.
268. Isobe M, Russo G, Haluska FG, Croce CM. Cloning of the gene encoding the δ subunit of the human T-cell receptor reveals its physical organization within the α-subunit locus and its involvement in chromosome translocations in T-cell malignancy. Proc Natl Acad Sci USA 1988;85: 3933.
269. Finger LR, Kagan J, Christopher G, et al. Involvement of the *TCL 5* gene on human chromosome 1 in T-cell leukemia and melanoma. Proc Natl Acad Sci USA 1989;86:5039.
270. Chen Q, Cheng J-T, Tsai L-H, et al. The *tal* gene undergoes chromosome translocation in T cell leukemia and potentially encodes a helix–loop–helix protein. EMBO J 1990;9:415.
271. Bernard O, Guglielmi P, Jonveaux P, et al. Two distinct mechanisms for the *SCL* gene activation in the t(1;14) translocation of T-cell leukemias. Genes Chromosomes Cancer 1990;1:194.
272. McKeithan TW, Shima EA, Le Beau MM, et al. Molecular cloning of the breakpoint junction of a human chromosomal 8;14 translocation involving the T-cell receptor α-chain gene and sequences on the 3′ side of *MYC*. Proc Natl Acad Sci USA 1986;83:6636.
273. Lewis WH, Michalopoulos EE, Williams DL, et al. Breakpoints in the human T-cell antigen receptor α-chain locus in two T-cell leukaemia patients with chromosomal translocations. Nature 1985;317:544.
274. Boehm T, Greenberg JM, Buluwela L, et al. An unusual structure of a putative T cell oncogene which allows production of similar proteins from distinct mRNAs. EMBO J 1990;9:857.
275. Royer-Pokora B, Loos U, Ludwig W-D. TTG-2, a new gene coding a cysteine-rich protein with the LIM motif, is overexpressed in acute T-cell leukaemia with the t(11;14)(p13;q11). Oncogene 1991;6:1887.
276. McGuire EA, Davis AR, Korsmeyer SJ. T-cell translocation gene 1 (*Ttg*-

1) encodes a nuclear protein normally expressed in neural lineage cells. Blood 1991;77:599.
277. Boehm T, Greenberg JM, Buluwela L, et al. An unusual structure of a putative T cell oncogene which allows production of similar proteins from distinct mRNAs. EMBO J 1990;9:857.
278. Kagan J, Finan J, Letofsky J, et al. α-Chain locus of the T-cell antigen receptor is involved in the t(10;14) chromosome translocation of T-cell acute lymphocytic leukemia. Proc Natl Acad Sci USA 1987;84: 4543.
279. Zutter M, Hockett RD, Roberts CWM, et al. The t(10;14)(q24;qave11) of T cell acute lymphoblastic leukemia juxtaposes the δ T cell receptor with a conserved and activated locus, TCL-3 at 10q24. Proc Natl Acad Sci USA 1990;87:3161.
280. Hatano M, Roberts AWM, Minden M, et al. Deregulation of a homeobox gene, *HOX* 11, by the t(10;14) in T cell leukemia. Science 1991;253: 79.
281. Dubé ID, Kamel-Reid S, Yuan CC, et al. A novel human homeobox gene lies at the chromosome 10 breakpoint in lymphoid neoplasias with chromosomal translocation t(10;14). Blood 1991;78:2996.
282. Kennedy MA, Gonzalez-Sarmiento R, Kees UR, et al. *HOX* 11, a homeobox-containing T-cell oncogene on human chromosome 10q24. Proc Natl Acad Sci USA 1991;88:8900.
283. Westbrook CA, Rubin CM, Le Beau MM, et al. Molecular analysis of *TCRB* and *ABL* in a t(7;9)-containing cell line (SUP-T3) from a human T-cell leukemia. Proc Natl Acad Sci USA 1987;84:251.
284. Ellisen LW, Bird J, West DC, et al. *TAN*-1, the human homolog of the Drosophila *Notch* gene, is broken by chromosomal translocations in T lymphoblastic neoplasms. Cell 1991;66:649.
285. Heisterkamp N, Stephenson JR, Groffen J, et al. Localization of the *c-abl* oncogene adjacent to a translocation break point in chronic myelocytic leukaemia. Nature 1983;306:239.
286. von Lindern M, Puotska A, Lerach H, Grosveld G. The (6;9) chromosome translocation, associated with a specific subtype of acute nonlymphocytic leukemia, leads to aberrant transcription of a target gene on 9q34. Mol Cell Biol 1990;10:4016.
287. Cimino G, Moir DT, Canaani O, et al. Cloning of *ALL*-1, the locus involved in leukemias with the t(4;11)(q21;q23), t(9;11)(p22;q23), and t(11;19)(q23′3) chromosome translocations. Cancer Res 1991;51:6712.
288. Goddard AD, Borrow J, Freemont PS, Solomon E. Characterization of a zinc finger gene disrupted by the t(15;17) in acute promyelocytic leukemia. Science 1991;254:137.
289. Kakizuka A, Miller WH Jr, Warrell RP, et al. Chromosomal translocation t(15;17) in human acute promyelocytic leukemia fuses RAR with novel putative transcription factor. Cell 1991;66:663.
290. Pandolfi PP, Grignani F, Alcalay M, et al. Structure and origin of the acute promyelocytic leukemia myl RARα cDNA and characterization of its retinoid-binding and transactivation properties. Oncogene 1991;6: 1285.
291. Emmanuel BS, Selden JR, Chaganti RSK, et al. The 2p breakpoint of a 2;8 translocation in Burkitt lymphoma interrupts the V locus. Proc Natl Acad Sci USA 1984;81:2444.
292. Shtivelman E, Henlein B, Groitl P, et al. Identification of a human transcription unit affected by the variant chromosomal translocations 2;8 and 8;22 of Burkitt's lymphoma. Proc Natl Acad Sci USA 1989;86: 3257.
293. Fell HP, Smith G, Tucker PW. Molecular analysis of the t(2;14) translocation of childhood chronic lymphocytic leukemia. Science 1986;232: 491.
294. Richardson AL, Humphries CG, Tucker PW. Molecular cloning and characterization of t(2;14) translocation associated with childhood chronic lymphocytic leukemia. Oncogene 1992;7:961.
295. Grimaldi JC, Meeker TC. The t(5;14) chromosomal translocation in a case of acute lymphocytic leukemia joins the interleukin-3 gene to the immunoglobulin heavy chain gene. Blood 1989;73:2081.
296. Meeker TC, Hardy D, Willman C, et al. Activation of the interleukin-3 gene by chromosome traslocation in acute lymphocytic leukemia with eosinophilia. Blood 1990;76:285.
297. Rimokh R, Rouault J-P, Wahbi K, et al. A chromosome 12 coding region is juxtaposed to the *MYC* protooncogene locus in a t(8;12)(q24;q22) translocation in a case of B-cell chronic lymphocytic leukemia. Genes Chromosomes Cancer 1991;3:24.
298. Croce CM, Thierfelder W, Erikson J, et al. Transcriptional activation os: an unrearranged and untranslocated *c-myc* oncogene by translocation of a C locus in Burkitt lymphoma. Proc Natl Acad Sci 1983;80: 6922.
299. Pellet P, Berger R, Bernheim A, et al. Molecular analysis of a t(9;14)(p11;q32) translocation occurring in a case of human alpha heavy chain disease. Oncogene 1989;4:653.
300. Ohno H, Furukawa T, Fukuhara S, et al. Molecular analysis of a chromosomal translocation, t(9;14)(p13;q32), in a diffuse large-cell lymphoma cell line expressing the Ki-1 antigen. Proc Natl Acad Sci USA 1990;87:628.
301. Fainstein E, Marcelle C, Rosner A, et al. A new fused transcript in Philadelphia chromosome positive acute lymphocytic leukaemia. Nature 1987;330:386.
302. Neri A, Chang C-C, Lombardi L, et al. B cell lymphoma-associated chromosomal translocation involves candidate oncogene *lyt*-10, homologous to NF-κB p50. Cell 1991;67:1075.
303. Akao Y, Seto M, Takahashi T, et al. Molecular cloning of the chromosomal breakpoint of a B-cell lymphoma with the t(11;14)(q23;q32) translocation. Cancer Res 1991;51:1574.
304. Akao Y, Seto M, Yamamoto K, et al. The RCK gene associated with the t(11;14) translocation is distinct from the *MLL/ALL*-1 gene with t(4;11) and t(11;19) translocations. Cancer Res 1992.
305. Lu D, Yunis JJ. Cloning, expression and localization of an RNA helicase gene from a human lymphoid cell line with chromosomal breakpoint 11q23.3. Nucleic Acids Res 1992;20:1967.
306. McKeithan TW, Rowley JD, Shows TB, Diaz MO. Cloning of the chromosome translocation breakpoint junction of the t(14;19) in chronic lymphoblastic leukemia. Proc Natl Acad Sci USA 1987;84:9257.
307. Inaba T, Roberts WM, Shapiro LH, et al. Fusion of the leucine zipper gene *HLF* to the *E 2A* gene in human acute B-lineage leukemia. Science 1991;257:531.
308. Aplan PD, Raimondi SC, Kirsch IR. Disruption of the SCL gene by a t(1;3) translocation in a patient with T cell acute lymphoblastic leukemia. J Exp Med 1992;176:1303.
309. Fitzgerald TJ, Neale AM, Raimondi SC, Goorha RM. *c-tal*, a helix–loop–helix protein, is juxtaposed to the T-cell receptor–β chain gene by a reciprocal chromosomal translocation: t(1;7)(p32;q35). Blood 1991;78:2686.
310. Burnett RC, David J-C, Harden AM, et al. The *LCK* gene is involved in the t(1;7)(p34;q34) in the T-cell acute lymphoblastic leukemia derived cell line, HSB-2. Genes Chromosomes Cancer 1991;3:461.
311. Tycko B, Smith SD, Sklar J. Chromosomal translocations joining LCK and TCRB loci in human T cell leukemia. J Exp Med 1991;174:867.
312. Lu D, Thompson JD, Gorski GK, et al. Alterations at the *rel* locus in human lymphoma. Oncogene 1991;6:1235.
313. Laâbi Y, Gras MP, Carbonnel F, et al. A new gene, BCM, on chromosome 16 fused to the interleukin 2 gene by a t(4;16)(q26′3) translocation in malignant T cell lymphoma. EMBO J 1992;11:3897.
314. Xia Y, Brown L, Yang CY-C, et al. TAL2, a helix–loop–helix gene activated by the (7;9)(q34;q32) translocation in human T-cell leukemia. Proc Natl Acad Sci USA 1991;88:11416.
315. Sanchez Garcia I, Kaneko Y, Gonzalez-Sarmiento R. et al. A study of chromosome 11p13 translocations involving TCR and TCR in human T cell leukaemia. Oncogene 1991;6:577.
316. Kasai M, Maziarz RT, Aoki K, et al. Molecular involvement of the *pvt*-1 locus in a γ/δ T-cell leukemia bearing a variant t(8;14)(q24;q11) translocation. Mol Cell Biol 1992;12:4751.
317. McGuire EA, Hockett RD, Pollock KM, et al. The t(11;14)(p15;q11) in a T-cell acute lymphoblastic leukemia cell line activates multiple transcripts, including *Ttg*-1, a gene encoding a potential zinc finger protein. Mol Cell Biol 1989;92:124.
318. Cuticchia AJ, Pearson PL, Klinger HP, eds. Genome priority reports, vol 1. Basel, Karger, 1993.

Blood: Principles and Practice of Hematology,
edited by Robert I. Handin, Thomas P. Stossel, and Samuel E. Lux.
J.B. Lippincott Company, Philadelphia © 1995.

6

Molecular Basis of Oncology

David J. Kwiatkowski
Stephen H. Friend

TRANSFORMATION AND CELL GROWTH CONTROL

Criteria for Transformation

Tumors present clinically as a mass or disseminated metastases, or as the secondary effects of an abnormal clonal expansion. Tumors consist of a clonal expansion of cells that have deranged growth properties. Cells can achieve this alteration in growth by means of many mechanisms. Before considering these mechanisms, consider the differences between normal cells and tumor cells. The process by which a normal cell becomes a cancer cell is referred to as *transformation*. Pathologists have developed morphologic criteria for transformation to distinguish benign from malignant growth. They consider the individual cells and their overall pattern of growth. Tumor cells generally have an abundance of DNA, an increased nucleus/cytoplasm ratio, and clumping of chromatin. Bizarre mitotic figures are frequently present. In some tumors such as leukemias, loss of proper differentiation is a major feature. Some differentiation-specific markers are usually retained, and some tumors are well differentiated. The architecture that malignant cells display also reflects the underlying growth deregulation. The lack of ordered growth, referred to as *anaplasia* or *dysplasia*, and the extent of invasiveness are also pathologic hallmarks of transformation.

For obvious reasons, it is difficult to study the mechanism of malignant transformation in vivo. Human studies are unethical and not feasible; animal model systems are rarely faithful to the human situation and are frequently difficult to interpret. Most studies examining the molecular basis of transformation have therefore been performed in vitro. In turn, many of the criteria that apply to the transformed phenotype apply only to cells that can grow in tissue culture. In vitro studies require either the establishment of tumor cell lines or the transformation of primary cell lines. Remember that most of what has been learned about tumorigenesis is potentially distorted by the limitations inherent in studies of growth in vitro.

Transformation of cells in tissue culture typically causes a series of morphologic changes. Transformed cells display altered cytoskeletal features, are less adherent, and appear more refractile when viewed by phase contrast microscopy. These cytoskeletal changes are likely to be important for tumor formation in vivo. Experiments that artificially alter the adhesiveness of cells indicate that cell shape is important for maintenance of normal growth control. For example, the addition of substances that force cells into a more spherical conformation decreases the rate of DNA synthesis and impedes the cell's progress through the cell cycle.[1]

Another characteristic of cell transformation is the acquisition of the ability to grow in soft agar. Soft agar prevents attachment of cells to the tissue culture dish surface; therefore, growth in soft agar must be anchorage independent. *Anchorage independence* is the single in vitro characteristic of transformed cells that best correlates with tumorigenicity. Transformed cells also frequently grow in lower serum concentrations than other cells.[2] These cellular properties combine to allow transformed cells to grow to a higher density than untransformed cells and to pile on top of each other. Normal cells can be grown in tissue culture for a limited number of divisions before they senesce and die. Transformed cells can be passaged indefinitely. This loss of growth limitation is termed *immortalization*. It appears to be a necessary but insufficient step in the process of transformation. Because gene transfer (or transfection) of certain oncogenes into cells in primary culture can permit the cells to be passed indefinitely, they are classified as immortalization genes. Cells immortalized in this manner usually are incapable of tumor formation in nude mice.

At a biochemical level, a wide range of characteristics are associated with the transformed phenotype. For example, changes occur in 2-deoxyglucose uptake, secretion of proteases, and intracellular levels of cyclic nucleotides. Such biochemical observations have failed to provide clear insights into the mechanisms that control these alterations or the means to use them therapeutically. Consequently, recent work on the mechanism of transformation has focused on an understanding of growth control regulation and its derangement in tumor cells at the molecular level. We begin by outlining the normal growth control pathways of mammalian cells.

Normal Growth Control

Many situations occur in which normal cells must alter their growth. For example, for totipotent germ cells to form a complex set of organs, they must be able to greatly expand unique sets of cells with specific lineage determinants. Work on simple organisms, like the nematode, *Caeno-*

rhabditis elegans, has shown that decisions about growth and differentiation can be accomplished by providing each cell with a limited set of options. Cells can either duplicate themselves, creating two new identical daughter cells, or generate one cell with the original phenotype and a daughter cell with a new phenotype.[3] Armed with these limited options, a complex set of interactions and signaling pathways is needed to create an organism with all the necessary cell types in the correctly sized organs.

Each cluster of cells must sense its environment and surrounding cells. Some of the signals that regulate the process of morphogenesis are gradients of morphogens whose effect can be either long- or short-term. In some cases, organ systems are created and then dismantled. For example, müllerian ducts in males are a transient structure. The end of embryogenesis does not eliminate the requirement for dynamic cell–cell interactions. Virtually all organs continually replenish differentiated cells. The epithelial linings of the alimentary tract and skin do this continually, reforming this protective lining every few days. In contrast, cells in the nervous system are replenished much less frequently.

In addition to signals that regulate normal cellular replacement, unique signals modulate cell behavior during the repair of wounds. In many respects, after wound healing, normal cells transiently develop some of the characteristics of transformed cells. The complex nature of the pathways that control cellular growth has become increasingly evident over time. A working knowledge of these pathways is essential to understanding how cells can be transformed.

The growth potential of a cell may be altered in two ways: (1) the developmental potential may be either expanded or limited, and (2) the rate of growth may be modulated by altering the time spent in different phases of the cell cycle.

Regulation of the Cell Cycle

The biochemical stages that a cell passes through leading up to division may be divided into a sequence referred to as the cell cycle. The cell cycle is conveniently divided into several phases (Fig. 6-1). G1 is the phase of the cycle that follows mitosis (M phase) and precedes DNA synthesis (S phase). If cells are placed in media lacking vital nutrients, they become arrested and leave the cell cycle early in G1 phase to enter a quiescent state that has been termed *G0*. This quiescent phase approximates the state in which most differentiated cells remain in vivo. Viable and metabolically active cells remain in G0 until some mitogenic stimulus allows them to reenter the cell cycle. When cells reenter the cell cycle in G1, they pass through a portion of the G1 phase termed *prestart*. Here, they are exposed to factors that control most of the variation in the length of cell cycle. After passing the R point, or start, most cells are committed to complete the cell cycle. S is an 8- to 10-hour phase during which DNA synthesis occurs. S is followed by a 4-hour G2 period, which follows DNA synthesis. Mitosis occurs after G2 and lasts about 1 hour.

Little is known about the genes and their proteins that regulate the mammalian cell cycle. Much more is known about the analogous cell cycle proteins in lower organisms,

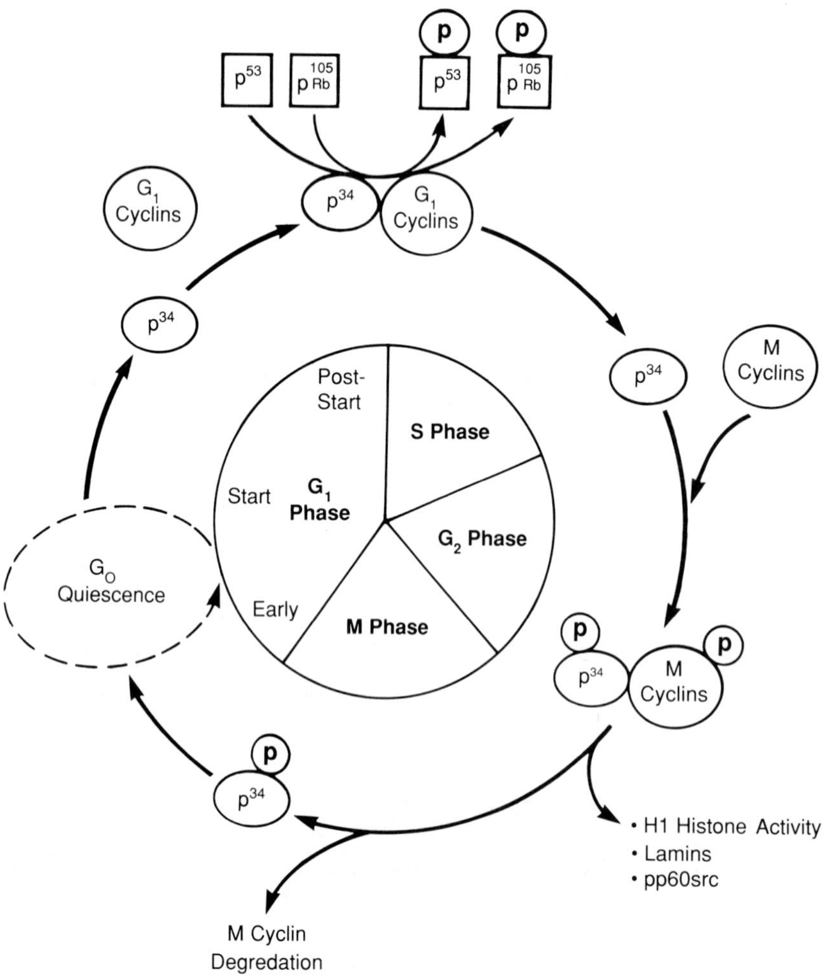

FIGURE 6-1. Mammalian cell cycle. Before the synthesis of DNA during S phase, a G1 phase is divided into early, start, and poststart components. Quiescent cells in G0 enter the cell cycle at the G1 phase. G1 cyclins bind p34, and this complex phosphorylates numerous proteins including p53 and p105 Rb. During S phase, the G1 cyclins are released and p34 is able to bind the M cyclins. The p34/M cyclin complex is then phosphorylated, so that it acquires H1 histone activity. Before reentry into G0, a directed degradation of the M phase cyclins occurs.

particularly yeast. A group of more than 12 yeast proteins have been isolated, which have important roles at specific times in the cell cycle. One of these cell cycle–dependent proteins is a 34-kd serine–threonine kinase called cdc2 in *Schizosaccharomyces pombe* and cdc28 in *Saccharomyces cerevisiae*. This kinase plays a central role in the regulation and functioning of the cell cycle and is the main component of a protein complex known as MPF (maturation-promoting factor). Because it is a kinase, it is able to regulate the function of a large number of other cellular proteins by phosphorylation, and thereby controls progression through the cell cycle. The cdc2 protein phosphorylates distinct proteins at defined times in the cell cycle. This specificity is achieved through regulation of cdc2 kinase activity, by phosphorylation and dephosphorylation of the cdc2 protein itself by different kinases and phosphatases at multiple sites, and through binding of a group of proteins termed *cyclins* to cdc2. Together, the negative and positive regulatory proteins in yeast that modulate cdc2 and the proteins that are phosphorylated by it form the cell cycle regulatory pathway.[4]

Identification of the mammalian homologues of some of these proteins has provided evidence that a similar system regulates the cell cycle in mammalian cells.[5] The homologue of cdc2 in humans has size 34 kd and is termed $p34^{cdc2}$ Many proteins, including the protooncogene pp60 *src* have the ability to phosphorylate $p34^{cdc2}$ and thereby activate it.[6] In turn, p34 phosphorylates numerous proteins including two of the tumor suppressor proteins, p105Rb, and p53 (D. Beach, personal communication). Mitogenic stimulation of cells with a variety of growth factors results in the phosphorylation of p34, which is at the cell cycle hub. This, in turn, leads to the phosphorylation and concomitant inactivation of proteins that restrict cell cycle progression.

As more mammalian proteins are identified within the cell cycle control pathway, insights will be gained into how cells modulate their growth potential. Clearly the cell cycle mechanism does not function autonomously in the cell but interacts with several other physiologic pathways that help to regulate cell growth. It is therefore important to consider how the process of growth is regulated by these pathways and how signals for growth are transmitted within the cell.

Cellular Signaling Pathways Mediate Growth Control

Signaling is a general term used to describe methods by which information is transmitted from one cellular compartment to another. For example, the mechanism by which a growth factor affects a cell and leads to changes in cell behavior, particularly division, can be considered a matter of transducing a signal from the cell exterior to the nucleus. The recognition that an understanding of growth control and differentiation is dependent on an understanding of signaling pathways has led to intensive study of this general phenomenon. Four general signaling pathways are recognized as important in the regulation of cell growth. These are kinase pathways, the phosphoinositide pathway, G proteins, and steroid hormone receptors and their relatives. The first three of these pathways are initiated by cell surface events (growth factor–receptor interactions), which lead to cytoplasmic signaling events, whereas the fourth pathway bypasses the cell surface.

In this chapter, discussion of growth factor–receptor interactions is followed by discussion of these distinct signaling pathways. Although the signaling pathways are discussed separately, they are interconnected in complex ways in most cells, which allow both a high degree of cross-talk and amplification mechanisms for growth control and stimulation.

Growth Factors and Their Receptors

Cells use a vast array of surface molecules to maintain communication with their surroundings. These surface molecules are primarily glycosylated proteins that reside in the cell membrane and may or may not have intracellular extensions. Some of these proteins form the gap junctions and tight junctions commonly seen between cells in epithelia. Other proteins form channels that control the flux of calcium, chloride, sodium, and other ions into and out of cells. A subclass of cell surface proteins, the growth factor receptors, binds growth factors (Fig. 6-2). The discussion here focuses on the nature of these growth factors and their receptors, since these interactions are critical for oncogenesis. This knowledge provides a framework for understanding the various mechanisms by which a cell's growth can be deregulated.

Each cell type displays a different set of growth factor receptors. Some receptors exist at low levels. For example, there are less than 1000 erythropoietin receptors per responsive cell.[7] In contrast, tens of thousands of epidermal growth factor (EGF) receptors are in other cells. The dozens of known growth factors can be divided into two classes: polypeptides and steroid molecules. The steroid growth factors and their receptors use a direct pathway for signaling, which is described in the text that follows. The polypeptide growth factors, their receptors, and signaling pathways are much more diverse and can be subdivided according to their structural and functional similarities. Each of these functional classes defines a different possible mechanism of transformation.

The largest and best-characterized class of growth factor receptors is the receptor kinase family. These growth factor receptors have the ability to phosphorylate themselves and other proteins on tyrosine residues (kinase activity), and they play a major role in the regulation of cellular growth. All these receptors contain both an extracellular domain to which the growth factor binds and an intracellular domain with kinase activity. This structure permits transmission of growth signals from outside the cell to the interior. Many receptor kinases have been identified, including the EGF receptor, the putative c-*neu* receptor, the TGF α-receptor, the insulin and insulin-like growth factor-1 (IGF-1) receptors, and the colony-stimulating factor (CSF-1) and the platelet-derived growth factor (PDGF) receptor. It is not entirely clear how binding of a growth factor to the external domain of a growth receptor leads to changes in the kinase activity of the intracellular domain that is separated from the external domain by the cell membrane. It is known that growth factor binding leads to receptor aggregation, which is followed by endocytosis by means of specialized structures known as coated pits. Aggregation of the receptor appears to be an essential step for activation of the kinase activity. Receptor aggregation also causes autophosphorylation, which enhances the intrinsic kinase activity of the cytoplasmic domain.[8] Cross-modulation of activity occurs between receptor tyrosine kinases. For example, PDGF enhances the mitogenic response of EGF.

Other growth factor receptors use an alternative approach to generate signals, which involve transducing or coupling proteins. The large class of transducing molecules that bind and hydrolyze guanosine triphosphate (GTP) are called *G proteins*. They function to couple many receptors to specific enzyme signaling pathways. The prototype G protein-coupled receptor is the β-adrenergic receptor. Other examples are the rhodopsin, α-adrenergic, muscarinic, vasopressin, and angiotensin receptors.

These receptors share a common structure including seven membrane spanning domains. Each of the seven do-

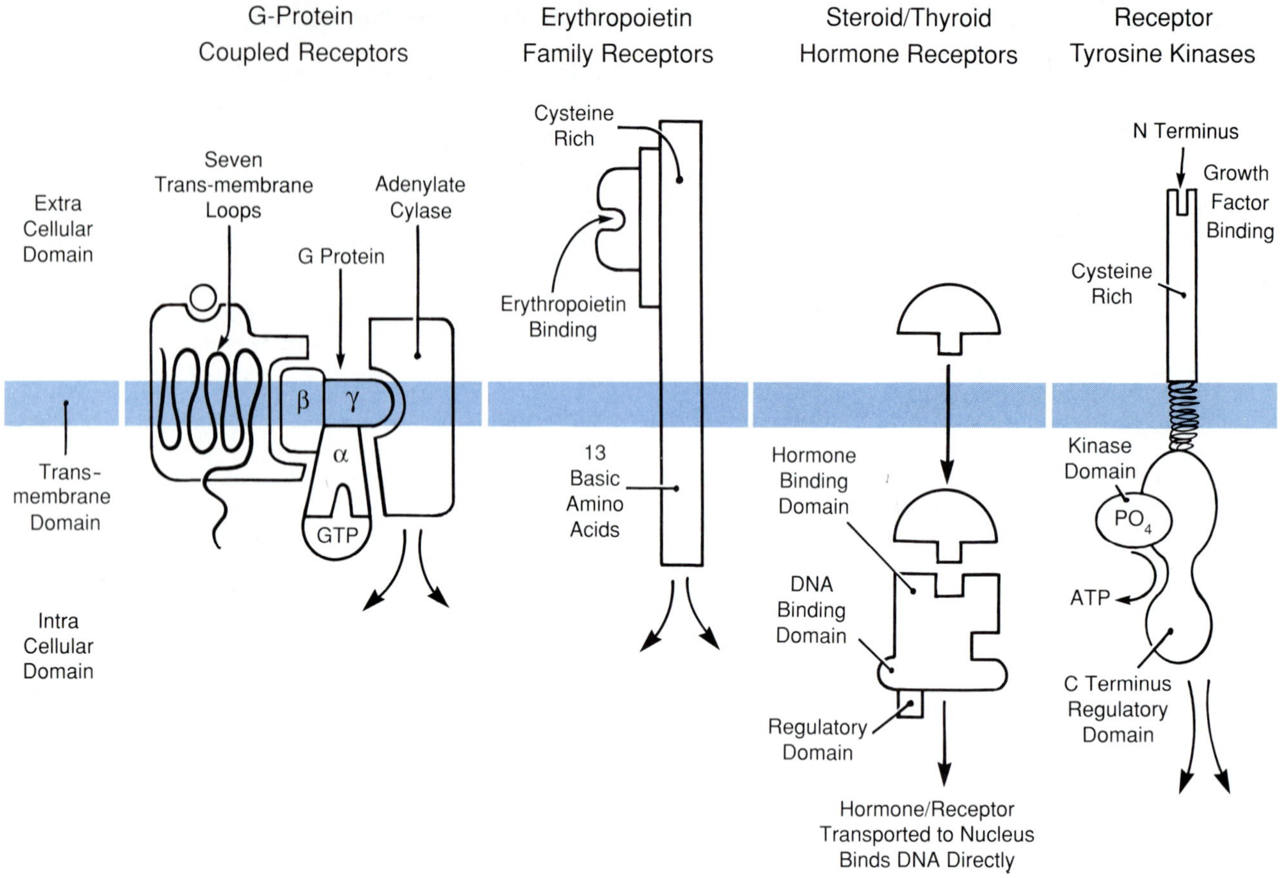

FIGURE 6-2. Cell receptor classes important in growth stimulatory pathways. Component portions of extracellular, transmembrane, and intracellular domains are discussed in the text.

mains has a region rich in serine and threonine, which together form a ligand binding pocket.[9]

The erythropoietin receptor has distinctive features, and consists of a single polypeptide chain. The bulk of the receptor is a cysteine-rich, heavily glycosylated extracellular domain to which erythropoietin binds. A single transmembrane spanning domain is found as well as a short cytoplasmic tail consisting of about 250 amino acids without apparent kinase domain.[10] How the intracellular peptide tail on the erythropoietin receptor is used in cell signaling is unknown. The IL-2 receptor β chain shares structural homology with the erythropoietin receptor. Protein kinase C phosphorylates the IL-2 receptor in response to phorbol myristate acetate, but whether this occurs on the erythropoietin receptor is unknown.[7]

Kinase Signaling

About 100 protein kinases are known to exist, which phosphorylate specific sites on target proteins. They share a highly conserved catalytic domain of 250 to 300 amino acids. Kinases can be classified according to substrate specificities. Some kinases are specific for tyrosine residues, whereas others are specific for serine or threonine residues. Both types of kinase are targets for alterations that produce cellular transformation. The serine–threonine kinases include proteins that are activated by cyclic nucleotides, calcium, phospholipids, and calmodulin. p34^{cdc2}, described earlier, is also a serine–threonine kinase.

Tyrosine kinases may be divided into three families: receptor tyrosine kinases, kinases of the c-*src* protooncogene family, and kinases of the c-*abl* nuclear protooncogene family. Although much is known about the structure of these kinases, little is understood about which particular proteins they activate. This difficulty is easy to appreciate considering that over 100 known kinases are found in the cell, and identification of the direct target of an individual kinase is difficult. Some of the interactions among kinases are shown in Figure 6-3. In most cases, a major target of the kinase is the kinase itself, through autophosphorylation.[11] An activated receptor tyrosine kinase can phosphorylate other kinases that have their own substrates. Thus, a cascade effect of phosphorylation occurs. An example of this cascade effect, as well as the connections among signaling pathways, is that phospholipase C is phosphorylated and activated by several receptor tyrosine kinases. Activated phospholipase C in turn amplifies the signal by its effects on phosphoinositide metabolism, as discussed later.

G Proteins

Many receptors transmit intracellular signals by interaction with a group of signaling proteins that occur as trimers, bind GTP, and are capable of activating other intracellular proteins. These signaling complexes are known as G proteins (see Figs. 6-2 and 6-3). G proteins respond to agonist-mediated receptor stimulation by exchanging guanosine diphosphate (GDP) for GTP, thereby becoming activated and transmitting signals to the cell interior. The activated state of the G protein persists until GTP is hydrolyzed to GDP, a process enhanced by the intrinsic GTPase activity of these proteins. Any process that increases the level of the GTP-bound form leads to increased activity of a G protein. From a growth viewpoint, activating mutations can occur in a G protein by reducing its GTPase activity.

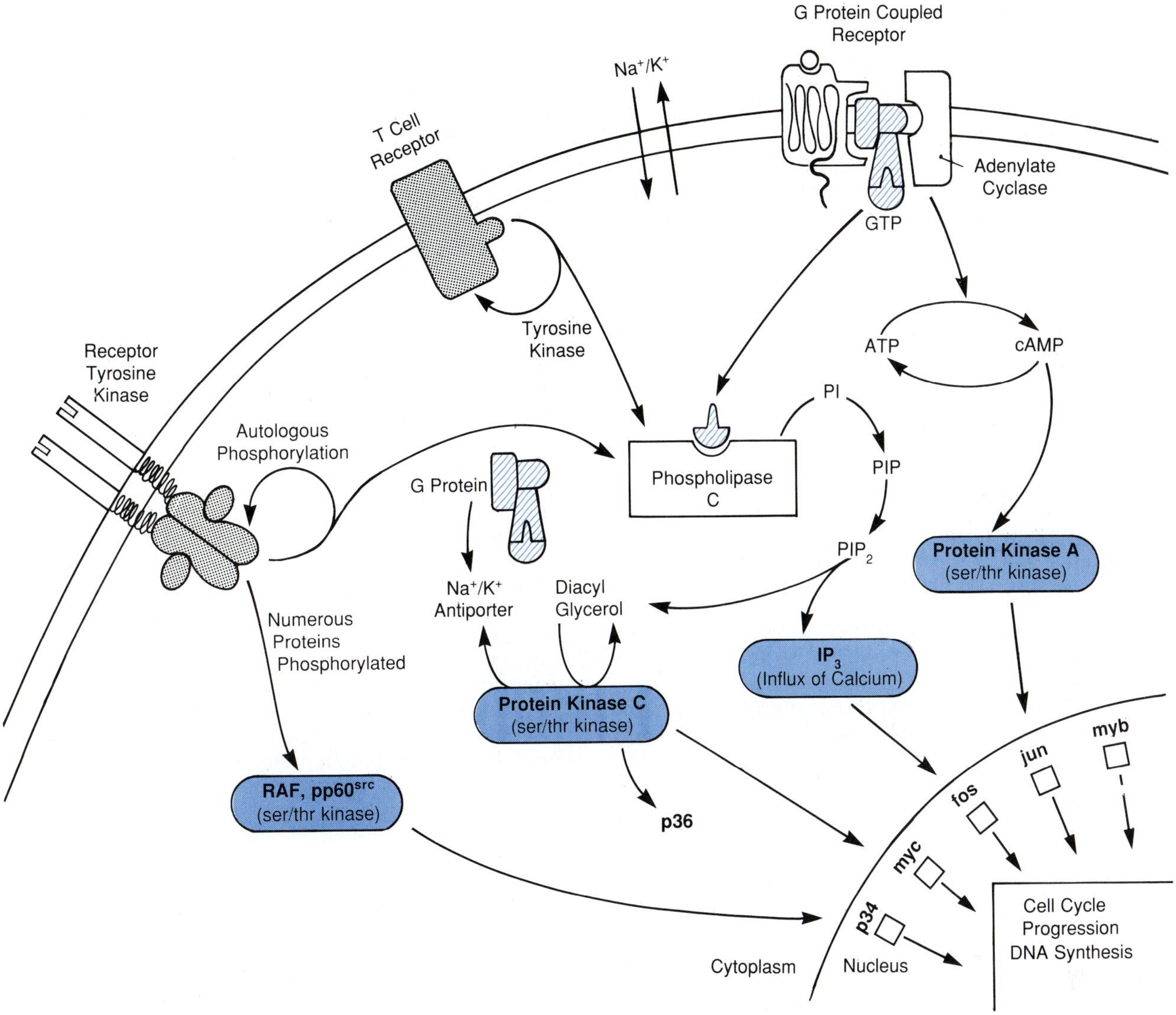

FIGURE 6-3. Intracellular connections of the growth stimulatory pathways. Multiple connections are made between the intermediate components. This cross-talk allows intricate, fine control of DNA synthesis and cell cycle progression.

Some G proteins transmit signals by binding to adenylate cyclase (Gs type), causing the catalytic formation of adenosine 3′,5′-monophosphate (cAMP) molecules, whereas others (Gi type) have inhibitory effects on this pathway, lowering cAMP levels. Other G proteins modulate retinal cell potassium channels and phospholipase C, to name just a few identified functional types.[9] The function of other G proteins are less well understood. *ras* proteins are closely related to G proteins although they occur as monomers and intracellular signaling targets are also unknown (see further discussion later in text).

G proteins typically serve an amplification function in signal transduction. For example, when Gs activates adenylate cyclase, many thousands of molecules of cAMP are generated that may diffuse throughout the cell quickly, and activate a large number of other enzymes. For example, cAMP specifically stimulates the regulatory subunits of certain kinases.[12] This provides another example of the interconnection among signaling pathways. Specificity is achieved by altering the level of expression of these kinases in different cell types. Similar G protein signaling pathways are used by the calcitonin, epinephrine, thyroid-stimulating hormone, and vasopressin receptors. In all these systems, the initial signals result in major growth alterations through the amplification effects of multiple second messengers.

Phosphoinositides

The phosphoinositide pathway uses the phospholipid, phosphatidyl inositol, and its many derivatives as second messengers within the cell. This metabolic pathway is complex, and our understanding of key metabolic and signaling intermediates continues to evolve. We present a brief description of the best understood components of the system. Kinases convert phosphatidyl inositol to phosphatidyl inositol phosphate (PIP), and PIP to phosphatidylinositol biphosphate (PIP_2). Upon cell stimulation, phospholipase C converts PIP_2 to inositol triphosphate (IP_3) and diacylglycerol (DAG). Phospholipase C is regulated by kinases, as well as interactions with G proteins. IP3 and DAG are each important second messengers.[13] DAG activates protein kinase C, a 77-kd serine–threonine kinase, which then phosphorylates a number of proteins. These phosphorylations lead to the synthesis of nuclear factors, including *myc* and *fos*, which in turn increase DNA synthesis and progression through the cell cycle.[13,14] At the same time,

IP_3 causes calcium ion channels to open, causing a transient increase in intracellular calcium ion, an essential cofactor for many intracellular reactions. Molecular analogues of DAG including polycyclic alcohols like phorbol esters are potent tumor promoters because they mimic DAG and activate protein kinase C. Ordinarily within the cell, IP3 and DAG are rapidly converted, through a series of steps, back to PIP_2. Viral and cellular transforming proteins frequently usurp this powerful growth-activating signaling pathway.

Steroid Hormone Receptors

Steroid hormone receptors and their close relatives, the thyroid hormone and retinoic acid receptors, represent one of the best understood signaling pathways used by cells.[15] The ligands or factors bound by these receptors are small and lipid soluble so that they directly traverse the cell membrane to enter the cell cytoplasm, and bind to the receptor (see Fig. 6-2). In the absence of ligand binding, the receptor usually resides in the cytoplasm. Upon ligand binding, the receptor's conformation changes so that nuclear transport occurs. In the nucleus, the ligand–receptor complex binds to a defined set of DNA response elements located in the upstream region of many specific genes. The binding activates (represses, in some cases) transcription of the adjacent gene by affecting RNA polymerase II activity. Members of steroid and thyroid receptor superfamily control vital programs of cellular growth and differentiation. Therefore, it is not surprising that alterations in these receptors can induce transformation.

Nuclear Connections

Although the different signaling pathways within the cytoplasm are understood fairly well, the way in which the signal makes it into the nucleus to signal growth and mitosis is much less clear. The analysis of the nuclear connections of the signaling pathways has been limited to somewhat artificial systems, such as the mitogenic stimulation of quiescent fibroblasts in cell culture. These studies have allowed identification of changes in the level of expression of nuclear proteins that have been recognized as the normal cellular homologues of some viral oncogenes. Much work has focused on identifying the first nuclear proteins to be induced after mitogenic stimulation. This has been done because it is thought that early nuclear events may serve as a switch to lead to all of the changes in gene expression that are necessary for mitosis.

Following growth factor stimulation of quiescent (G0) fibroblasts, the earliest detectable change in the nucleus occurs within the first 5 minutes. For example, PDGF stimulation increases the levels of c-*fos* in less than 5 minutes. This is followed by changes in levels of several other nuclear proteins, including c-*myc*, and numerous other nuclear proteins. Both c-*myc* and c-*fos* appear to regulate numerous other genes. Both exhibit nonspecific binding to DNA, but only c-*fos* has been shown to directly regulate the level of expression of other genes. The c-*myc* gene is a member of a family of *myc* genes that includes L-*myc* and N-*myc*. All three *myc* genes have apparently similar growth regulatory potential.[16,17] A wide variety of proteins are part of the nuclear growth regulatory pathway. Some proteins are kinases such as $p34^{cdc2}$ and phosphatases that modulate the activity of different proteins during the cell cycle. Many other normal nuclear regulatory proteins have been shown to be transcription factors, such as c-*jun* and c-*myb*.[18,19] Interactions among these nuclear factors are poorly understood, but some, particularly c-*fos* and c-*jun*, modulate each other's activity (see also text that follows). These interactions are likely to be part of a complex, tightly regulated growth regulatory pathway present in the nucleus, which rivals the complexity apparent in cytoplasmic signaling pathways. This complexity allows the necessary checks and balances to finely regulate growth and indicates why so many mechanisms exist by which cells can be transformed. This complexity has also prevented a clear understanding of the functional role of any of these nuclear regulatory proteins.

DOMINANT ONCOGENES

In the early 1980s, considerable excitement was generated by the identification of several dominant-acting oncogenes in human cancer specimens. These activated genes have the ability to convert a receptive, untransformed cell into a malignant, transformed cell in a single step. Subsequently, a multitude of dominant oncogenes have been discovered, which have been associated with a diverse spectrum of human malignancies (Table 6-1). Much effort has been invested in determining the normal intracellular function of the protooncogenes, and the deranged functioning of the activated, mutated oncogenes. A detailed understanding of such function would clearly be helpful in strategies aimed at suppressing or controlling oncogene function for use in cancer treatment. In general, the proteins encoded by oncogenes appear to fall into only a few different functional categories with roles in normal growth control: (1) membrane-bound protein tyrosine kinases (including transmembrane growth factor receptors); (2) secreted, extracellular proteins that are growth factors; (3) membrane-bound signal transducing proteins (the *ras* family); and (4) nuclear proteins. In some cases, categorization of an oncogene is based solely on recognized sequence similarity, particularly in the case of the more recently identified and less well-characterized oncogenes. Some other oncogenes do not fit any of these categories, despite extensive study, and functional properties and cellular localization are poorly understood.

In this section, we will discuss mechanisms of dominant oncogene activation and representative members of each group.

Mechanisms of Dominant Oncogene Activation

Dominant-acting oncogenes may be activated from their normal cellular precursor by several different mechanisms—retroviral transduction, proviral insertion, point mutations, chromosomal translocation, and amplification. Several oncogenes have been activated in different instances by more than one of these mechanisms.

Retroviral transduction is the process in which retroviruses accidentally incorporate normal cellular genes into their genome. Retroviruses are small RNA viruses (genomes of less than 10 kb) that infect vertebrate cells and are reverse transcribed into double-stranded DNA (provirus; Fig. 6-4). Human examples of retroviruses are HIV and HTLV-I, II, and III. After the cell is infected, the provirus may be inserted into the host genome and reside there indefinitely, either periodically producing more retrovirus or producing many retroviral copies immediately resulting in rapid cell death. Rarely, after insertion of the provirus into the host genome, a recombination event occurs in which part of the retroviral genome is lost, and a cellular gene or gene fragment is inserted. Most often this process is a lethal event for the provirus, disrupting essential structural features. Occasionally, a complete proviral structure results but with replacement of retroviral genes by hybrid retroviral–cellular genes. Because essential retroviral genes are almost always lost in this process, the retrovirus becomes

TABLE 6-1. Association of Activated Dominant Oncogenes With Human Malignancies*

	Oncogene																		
Malignancy	*abl*	*bcl-1*	*bcl-2*	*erb* B	*fes*	*fos*	*int-2*	*met*	*mos*	*myb*	C-*myc*	N-*myc*	*neu*	*raf*	Ha-*ras*	Ki-*ras*	N-*ras*	*sis*	*src*
Leukemia																			
ALL	26				37	37				37	37					24	24		
AML	26				37	37			28	37	28					37	31		
CML	28	43			37	37				37	37						24	22	37
Lymphoma																			
Non-Hodgkin's		29	26			37				37	37				37				
Burkitt's																	24		
Multiple myeloma		29																	
Carcinoma																			
Bladder															33	39			
Breast		35			37	37	35			37	37		40		37				
Colon						37				40	37				37	33	39		
Head and neck		20					36												
Lung		21			37	37				37	30	32		27	44	33			
Ovary						37					37				37	25			
Pancreas						37										39			
Renal						37					37				37	37			
Stomach													40	27					
Brain tumor				40		41				45	41	41		27				45	41
Melanoma															44				
Neuroblastoma												34					33		
Osteosarcoma						42		40						27					
Rhabdomyosarcoma												37					39	38	45

* Numbers in table indicate references.

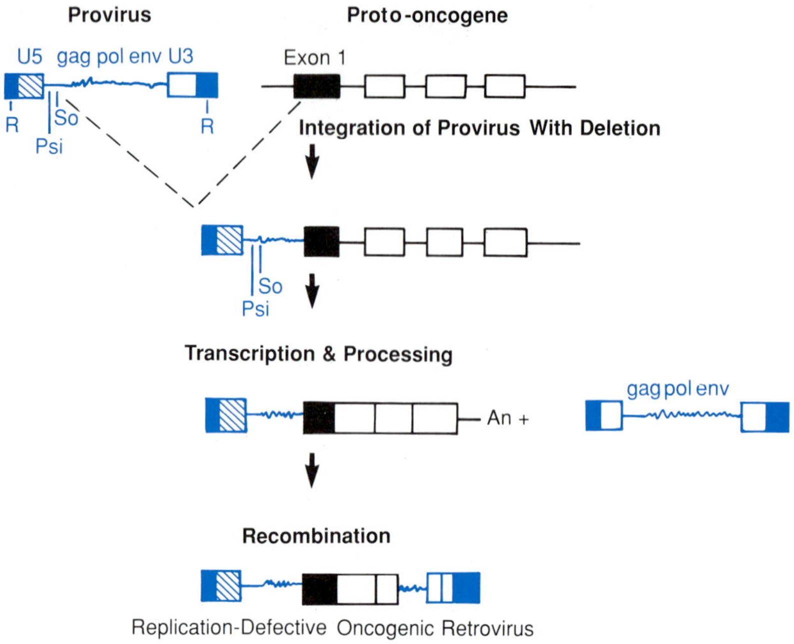

FIGURE 6-4. Retroviral transduction. The retroviral RNA is reverse transcribed into DNA, and inserts into the host genome to create the provirus. Rarely, part of the 3′ region of the provirus is lost and a hybrid, fused retrovirus/cellular gene results. On transcription into RNA, and repair of the 3′ end by attachment of normal 3′ retroviral sequences, a defective oncogenic retrovirus is created.

defective—that is, it is unable to replicate independently in a cell. When such a defective retrovirus coinfects a cell with a normal (helper) retrovirus, it is able to be reproduced, packaged, and released from the cell, thus propagating to a limited extent.

Cellular genes that are acquired by retroviruses in this fashion are usually mutated by single base pair changes (point mutations) or truncation. When a cellular protooncogene is acquired, the gene may be activated to become an oncogene by these mutational events. The oncogenic retrovirus then may have the ability to infect cells and transform them, giving rise to a tumor in the host. This occurrence is also an effective way for a defective oncogenic retrovirus to ensure its own transmission, since the tumor cells all contain the defective retrovirus.

Evidence for oncogenic retroviruses was first described in 1909 by Peyton Rous,[47] who made a cell-free filtrate of a chicken sarcoma and found that it produced similar tumors when injected into normal chickens. More recently, many oncogenic retroviruses have been described, which carry a wide variety of activated oncogenes. No oncogenic retroviruses of this type that infect humans are known. The conversion of a normal cellular protooncogene to an activated oncogene in a retrovirus results from a combination of three different events: mutation of the protooncogene, truncation of the protooncogene, and increased level of expression of the protein due to augmented mRNA transcription driven by retroviral promoter sequences.

Oncogene activation by proviral insertion occurs when a retroviral provirus inserts into the host genome at a site that leads to direct activation of an adjacent endogenous protooncogene. Figure 6-5 illustrates three mechanisms by which retroviral insertion can activate an adjacent oncogene. First, integration of provirus near (but not within) a protooncogene can provide enhancer activity leading to a large increase in the level of transcription and expression

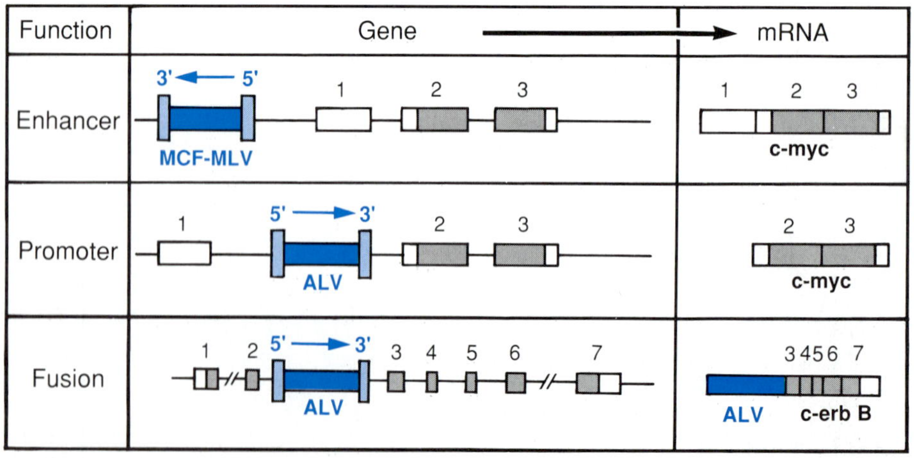

FIGURE 6-5. Proviral insertion. Insertion of provirus leads to oncogene activation by three mechanisms. Enhancer activation occurs when retroviral insertion at some distance from the gene leads to increased mRNA synthesis and expression. Promoter activation occurs when retroviral insertion occurs within the gene, displacing normal promoter sequences and leading to increased mRNA synthesis and expression. Fusion occurs when retroviral insertion occurs within the gene, and a hybrid protein is made, composed of both retrovirally encoded and native (host) sequences.

of the gene. For example, mink cell focus-forming retrovirus frequently integrates upstream of the c-*myc* gene, increasing the expression of the *myc* gene and leading to thymoma formation. Mouse mammary tumor virus activates the *int*-1 gene by inserting near it, causing mammary carcinomas. Avian leukemia virus causes B-cell lymphomas in chickens by integration near the c-*myc* gene.

Second, provirus may insert within a protooncogene leading to replacement of normal, regulated promoter elements by the unregulated retroviral long terminal repeat (LTR) promoter element. This also occurs with avian leukemia virus in some cases. Third, provirus may insert within the coding region of the protooncogene, leading to production of a deregulated, activated fusion protein. This has been demonstrated for avian leukemia virus in erythroblastosis through activation of the c-*erb* B gene, and for Moloney murine leukemia virus in leukemia through activation of the c-*myb* gene. Proviral insertion is a common mechanism that has been important in tumor formation for several different tumors of chickens and rodents. Oncogene activation by proviral insertion has not been described in humans thus far.

Oncogene activation by point mutation, on the other hand, is a common mechanism in human cancer. The *ras* family of oncogenes is invariably activated by point mutations, and tyrosine kinase oncogenes are often activated by both point mutation and truncation.

Chromosomal translocation is the process in which distinct chromosomal regions of the human genome are joined together. The Philadelphia chromosome (Ph) (t9:22;q34:q11) was the first human translocation described, and results from a reciprocal exchange of chromosomal regions on the long arms of chromosomes 9 and 22. The translocation leads to production of a deregulated fusion protein, $p210^{bcr/abl}$, which is an activated form of c-*abl*, as described later. Distinct translocations also result in the activation of c-*myc* and *bcl*-2 oncogenes. Mechanisms of oncogene activation in translocations are similar to those described for proviral insertion and include enhancer or promoter alterations leading to elevated levels of expression and production of deregulated fusion proteins.

Amplification is the process by which a genomic segment is duplicated from 1 up to 50 to 100 times.[46] For an amplified segment containing an oncogene, this is a mechanism for increasing the level of expression of the oncogene. The size of the genomic segment that is amplified, the *amplification unit*, varies from 100 kb to over 1000 kb. Amplification units usually reside either within a single chromosome, where they form tandem arrays with distinct cytogenetic features called a *homogeneously staining region* or in small extrachromosomal fragments called *double minute chromosomes*. In both cases, the amplified material is relatively unstable and tends to be lost by the cell during growth and division in the absence of selection. Consequently, the presence of amplified material indicates that the amplified oncogene must confer a selective growth advantage to the cell, leading to its retention. The increase in level of expression of the gene usually correlates directly with the number of amplified copies, and amplified oncogenes are not commonly affected by concomitant point mutation or translocation.

Oncogene activation by amplification occurs most commonly in the *myc* family of oncogenes but has also been described for several other oncogenes. In some cases amplification has been correlated with a worse prognosis (eg, amplified N-*myc* in childhood neuroblastoma and amplified *neu* in breast cancer). In other cases, variable levels of amplification are seen and do not seem to correlate with clinical virulence, such as the *myc* oncogenes in small cell lung cancer.

Tyrosine Kinase Family

src

The founding member of the tyrosine kinase family of oncogenes, v-*src*, is the protein product of the first described oncogenic retrovirus, the Rous sarcoma virus (RSV), which causes sarcomas in chickens.[47] Antisera derived from rabbits with RSV-induced tumors, permitted the identification of the v-*src* protein as a 60-kd phosphoprotein ($p60^{v\text{-}src}$) that possesses inherent protein kinase activity specific for tyrosine residues. v-*src* is the oncogenic derivative of the intrinsic chicken gene, c-*src*.

After biosynthesis, the v-*src* protein of RSV rapidly associates with 50- and 90-kd cellular proteins to form a multimeric complex.[48,49] In addition, during or just after synthesis, the aminoterminal methionine of v-*src* is removed and the rare, 14-carbon fatty acid, myristic acid, is attached by an amide bond.[50,51] This postbiosynthetic processing, myristoylation, is required for both the membrane localization and the transforming activity of v-*src*. The oncogene c-*src* is also myristoylated, so this modification is clearly not in itself sufficient to cause transformation. v-*src* protein is found predominantly at the inner surface of the plasma membrane and is particularly concentrated in adhesion plaques.[52] Adhesion plaques serve as sites of attachment of the cytoskeleton to the plasma membrane in cultured cells and contain several structural proteins including integrins, talin, vinculin, and α-actinin (Fig. 6-6). PDGF stimulation of cells also leads to an association between c-*src* and the PDGF receptor, which may be important in transmitting growth signals to the cell interior.[53]

The tyrosine kinase activity of v-*src* (and other tyrosine kinase oncogenes) is essential for its transforming ability. All viral isolates of v-*src* have activated kinase activity, whereas the normal cellular c-*src* has more regulated kinase activity. The oncogene c-*src* participates in a control network of phosphorylation–dephosphorylation reactions in the cell whose dysregulation results in disordered cell growth. As discussed previously, the organization and essential elements of this control network are only beginning to be understood. For the v-*src* oncogene, the key question is, which intracellular protein substrate represents the critical substrate for its oncogenic activity?

Whole cell studies have shown that phosphotyrosine labeling is enriched at membrane sites, particularly near adhesion plaques. Numeric abundance of phosphotyrosine residues, however, by no means implies critical importance.

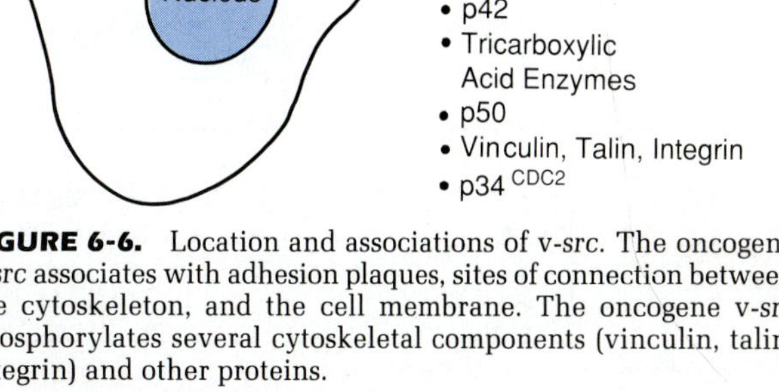

FIGURE 6-6. Location and associations of v-*src*. The oncogene v-*src* associates with adhesion plaques, sites of connection between the cytoskeleton, and the cell membrane. The oncogene v-*src* phosphorylates several cytoskeletal components (vinculin, talin, integrin) and other proteins.

In vitro, a large number of proteins can be phosphorylated on tyrosine residues by v-*src*, such as the immunoglobulins used in immunoprecipitation. In vivo substrates are somewhat more limited but also numerous, including p42, a protein that undergoes M-phase–specific phosphorylation on tyrosine residues in both normal and transformed cells[54]; enzymatic components of the tricarboxylic acid cycle; p50, the protein that rapidly associates with v-*src* after its biosynthesis[55]; and vinculin, talin, and the fibronectin receptor complex (integrin), cytoskeletal components of adhesion plaques. The importance of each of these in the oncogenic activity of v-*src*, as well as the question of whether each protein represents a direct or secondary substrate for c-*src*, remains in doubt. Recently, phosphorylation of $p34^{cdc2}$, the 34-kd serine–threonine protein kinase component of the cell cycle control element MPF (maturation promotion factor), by c-*src* has also been reported.[6]

The oncogenes v-*src* and c-*src* are in turn subject to complex regulation by phosphorylation at serine, threonine, and tyrosine residues (Fig. 6-7). The major site of regulatory phosphorylation in $p60^{c\text{-}src}$ is at tyrosine 527, which decreases its protein kinase activity.[56] $p60^{c\text{-}src}$ is also phosphorylated at ser12 and ser17 by protein kinase C, and cAMP-dependent protein kinase, respectively. Phosphorylation of $p60^{c\text{-}src}$ at thr34, thr46, and ser72 during fibroblast mitosis has also been reported and appears to be due to the kinase activity of $p34^{cdc2}$.[57,58] This observation has led to the hypothesis that $p60^{c\text{-}src}$ may serve an important role during mitosis as an effector kinase, amplifying the signal derived from $p34^{cdc2}$ to induce a variety of cytoskeletal and morphologic changes. This hypothesis is supported by the observation that a fraction of $p60^{c\text{-}src}$ occurs in the perinuclear region where it could well interact with $p34^{cdc2}$. Oncogenic derivatives of c-*src* may act by constitutively stimulating morphologic changes that are part of mitosis and thus short-circuiting cell growth control.

Although the most important pathogenic activity of v-*src* is in cell growth control, c-*src* is likely to serve important roles in nonproliferating cells as well as in dividing cells. For example, c-*src* is found at relatively high levels in platelets and neurons. In neurons, it is associated with nerve growth cones and neurosecretory granules.

Efforts to understand essential primary sequence differences between c-*src* and v-*src* that account for the increased kinase and transforming activity of v-*src* have also given some insight into the mechanism of action of src[59] (see Fig. 6-7). All RSV v-*src* genes have undergone a number of scattered single amino acid changes in residues 1 to 514. In addition, in all strains, residues 515 to 533 have been replaced with sequences resulting in the deletion of tyrosine 527. Studies using hybrid v-*src*/c-*src* proteins have indicated that mutations essential for transforming activity are derived from both the first 514 residues and the C-terminal tail. Single amino acid substitutions at any of four residues in the main portion of the protein result in acquisition of transforming ability,[60] whereas a variety of substitutions of the C-terminal tail that result in loss of tyr527 all produce this property. Similarly, mutagenesis of tyr527 to phenylalanine also results in transforming ability but with subtle differences in comparison with wild-type v-*src*.[61–63] Tyr527 thus is a critical site for mutagenesis in generation of v-*src*, but other sites are also important. These latter sites are likely to represent important regulatory domains within the protein.

More than a dozen protein kinase oncogenes have been identified and have variable sequence similarity to the *src* oncogene.[64] In most cases, these tyrosine kinases are activated by retroviral transduction with production of fusion proteins that have disordered localization or regulation of the kinase activity, generating the oncogenic effect. Most prominent among these from a hematologic standpoint is the *abl* oncogene.

abl

The oncogene v-*abl* is the protein product of the Abelson murine leukemia virus,[65] which causes lymphomas in mice.[66] v-*abl* arose by transduction of the murine cellular *abl* gene, c-*abl*, into the Moloney murine leukemia virus with truncation of both 5′ and 3′ sequences[67] (Fig. 6-8). Translation of the viral RNA produces a chimeric viral/*abl* protein, $p120^{v\text{-}abl}$. A second, entirely different retrovirus (HZ-2) has been described in cats; it also encodes a v-*abl* oncogene.[68] In contrast to Ab-MLV, HZ-2 causes fibrosarcomas in cats. Genetic swap experiments using Ab-MLV and HZ-2 indicate that this difference in clinical biology is due to differences in other components of the retroviruses, particularly the LTR segments and helper virus-derived envelope antigens.[69]

After the c-*abl* gene had been identified, its localization to human chromosome 9 band q34[65,70,71] suggested the possibility that *abl* was involved in the Philadelphia chromosome translocation (Ph) (t9:22;q34:q11)[72,73] that occurs in chronic myelogenous leukemia (CML). Structural studies examining the c-*abl* locus in CML cells indicated that most of c-*abl* is translocated to the middle of a gene on chro-

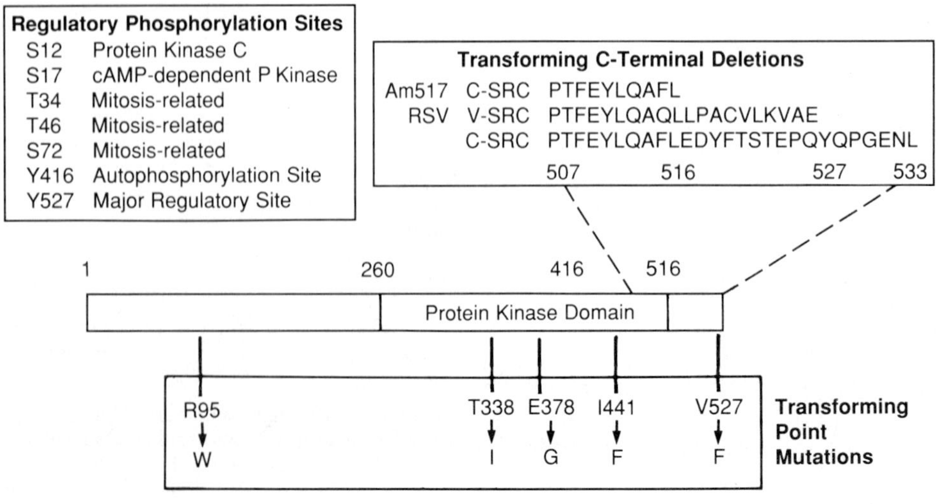

FIGURE 6-7. Structure, regulation, and transforming mutations of *src*. The major site of regulatory phosphorylation in *src* is *tyr*-527, and its loss, by mutation or truncation, activates the protein. Other sites at which mutation leads to activation of the protein (R45, T338, E378, 1441) are also indicated. Sites of regulatory phosphorylation are shown. (After Hunter T. A tail of two *src*'s: mutatis mutandis. Cell 1987;49:1)

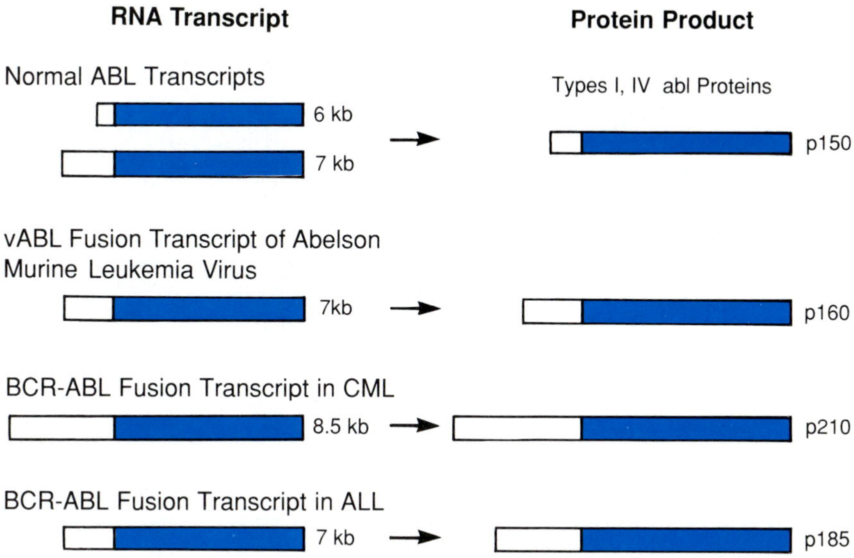

FIGURE 6-8. Structure of normal and oncogenic derivatives of *abl*. At top, the normal c-*abl* mRNA transcripts and protein products are presented schematically. Fusion mRNA and protein products that occur in v-*abl*, chronic myelogenous leukemia (CML), and acute lymphocytic leukemia (ALL) are then shown. Dark boxes are regions of the protein that are common to all four *abl* proteins; light boxes are regions that differ because of gene fusion events.

mosome 22, called *bcr* (for breakpoint cluster region), in a head-to-tail arrangement. This results in the synthesis of a chimeric *bcr/abl* protein, $p210^{bcr/abl}$,[74] that consists of N-terminal *bcr* sequence and almost all of the normal c-*abl* sequence. Thus, structurally the *bcr/abl* protein that occurs in CML is similar to the recombinant *abl* proteins expressed by the murine and feline retroviruses (see Fig. 6-8). The chromosomal translocations in CML are discussed in detail in Chapter 5.

The c-*abl* oncogene is a tyrosine protein kinase and contains three regions of homology to the c-*src* gene, one of which corresponds to the kinase domain.[75] A variety of studies suggest that the tyrosine kinase activity of the v-*abl* and *bcr/abl* oncogenes is essential for their oncogenic activity. For example, mutants of v-*abl* with temperature-sensitive kinase activity have been isolated, which cause mouse fibroblast lines to display morphologic evidence of transformation only at the permissive temperature.[76,77] By itself, a marked increase in the level of expression of c-*abl* is not sufficient for transformation, suggesting that loss of regulation from truncation or mutation is also important in its transforming activity. As for *src*, numerous cellular proteins are phosphorylated on tyrosine in v-*abl* infected murine or in CML cells. Also similar to *src*, several cellular substrates are found at the plasma membrane and at sites of cell–substratum contact.[78] Knowledge of critical substrates for *abl*'s transforming activity is lacking. Recent observations suggest that an alteration in localization of v-*abl* is important in its transforming ability. c-*abl*, expressed at high levels in fibroblasts, has a predominantly nuclear distribution.[79] v-*abl*, on the other hand, as well as other activated *abl* derivatives, has a cytoplasmic distribution.

Mutagenesis experiments performed on v-*abl* and c-*abl* have recently helped clarify which regions of c-*abl* are required for transforming activity and which regions must be eliminated. A series of deletion mutants of c-*abl* have defined a critical region in the N-terminal 139 residues, the deletion of which converts c-*abl* to an oncogene with full transforming activity in fibroblast and lymphoid cells.[80,81] Homologues of this N-terminal domain are also found in *src* and other kinases,[82] and this domain appears to function as a regulatory domain, controlling the kinase activity of the kinase domain. Transforming N-terminal truncated c-*abl* derivatives, as well as v-*abl*, lack this domain, and are themselves tyrosine phosphorylated and have elevated tyrosine kinase activity, in contrast to normal c-*abl*. Phosphorylation of *abl* occurs as a result of its intrinsic autokinase activity. Lack of phosphorylation of c-*abl* is likely because of the presence of the regulatory N-terminal domain.[80,83] Thus, the activation of c-*abl* that occurs during viral transduction is at least partially due to deletion of this N-terminal region and substitution of gag-derived residues in $p120^{v\text{-}abl}$. N-terminal gag sequences also lead to N-terminal myristoylation (similar to *src*), but one of the two normal mouse c-*abl* gene products (c-*abl*[IV]) is also myristoylated on its N-terminal glycine.[81]

The functions of the large C-terminal domain in c-*abl* are less clear. The property of fibroblast transformation is maintained in v-*abl* derivatives that are truncated just past the kinase domain.[84] C-terminal deleted v-*abl* proteins are much less active in lymphoid transformation.[85]

In CML, the translocated Ph chromosome occurs in the pluripotential stem cell as shown by analysis of isozyme markers or restriction fragment length polymorphism markers of blood cells from a variety of lineages.[86] Although the junction sites between chromosomes 9 and 22 in the Ph chromosome are somewhat variable, the fusion *bcr/abl* gene product always has a similar structure, in which N-terminal *bcr* sequences are joined to c-*abl* sequences (starting at exon II) and resulting in the synthesis of a large fusion protein $p210^{bcr/abl}$.[74,86] Although $p210^{bcr/abl}$ does not have transforming activity in fibroblasts, in contrast to v-*abl* products, it has been shown to directly transform an IL-3 dependent murine hematopoietic cell line to growth factor independence.[87] Interestingly, this concatenation of *bcr* and *abl* proteins does nothing to directly alter the regulatory N-terminal region of c-*abl*. This may explain the lack of fibroblast transformation but also begs the question of how the protein transforms hematopoietic cells. Expression of the *bcr/abl* fusion protein in transgenic mice reproduces the essential clinical features of CML. These mice serve as an animal model system for further study of the pathogenesis of and possible therapies in CML.

More than 90% of CML cells contain the Ph chromosome, and an even higher fraction have the translocation when assessed by Southern blot analysis of CML cell DNA using *bcr* and c-*abl* probes. In de novo acute lymphocytic leukemia (ALL), a Ph chromosome is seen in 10% to 20% of all cases. In Ph+ ALL, the junction site between chromosomes 9 and 22 is usually farther upstream in the *bcr* gene, resulting in production of a smaller fusion protein, $p190^{bcr/abl}$[88,89] (Fig. 6-9). The highly consistent appearance

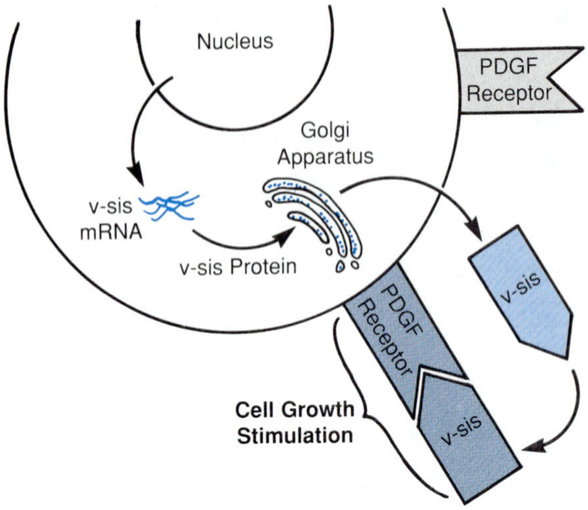

FIGURE 6-9. Oncogenic activity of v-*sis*. Production of v-*sis* by the cell leads to binding to the PDGF receptor intracellularly within the Golgi apparatus and to constitutive growth stimulation.

of the Ph chromosome in CML suggests that it plays an essential role in the pathogenesis of the disease. This chromosomal translocation is usually accompanied by other genetic derangements at the time of progression to blast crisis (see also Chap. 13).

Receptor Tyrosine Kinases and Growth Factors

Receptor tyrosine kinases are transmembrane proteins, which contain an intracellular tyrosine kinase domain and an extracellular domain capable of binding peptide hormones and which participate in cell signaling. They transduce growth (and other) signals from the extracellular space to the cell interior. Receptor tyrosine kinase oncogenes may be constitutively activated by oncogenic processes leading to dysregulation of their intrinsic kinase activity, causing them to behave as if they were continuously receiving a growth factor signal. Alternatively, growth factor oncogenes act by unregulated, constitutive expression, resulting in continuous activation of their corresponding tyrosine kinase receptors. Although these broad mechanisms are correct, the genetic alterations leading to dysregulation of growth factor receptors and their mechanisms of action are inevitably more complex.

The Growth Factor Family: v-*sis*

The growth factor family of oncogenes was identified more recently than *ras* and tyrosine kinase oncogenes but has grown in number rather quickly. Mechanisms of activation include retroviral transduction (v-*sis*),[90] insertional activation (int-2),[91] and mutagenesis of normal human genes (hst),[92] KS3.[93]

The v-*sis* oncogene of simian sarcoma virus (SSV) was the first described growth factor oncogene, and encodes a protein product, p28$^{v\text{-}sis}$, which is derived from the PDGF B chain.[90] SSV causes sarcomas in woolly monkeys, with short latency after infection.

PDGF is a potent growth factor secreted by platelets that is thought to facilitate wound healing at sites of tissue injury. As a constitutively produced variant of c-*sis*, the following mechanisms of action of v-*sis* have been postulated: (1) intracellular activation of the PDGF receptor, (2) extracellular activation of the PDGF receptor on producer cells, or (3) extracellular activation of the PDGF receptor on nonproducer cells.[90] The first two mechanisms represent autocrine models, whereas the third mechanism is a paracrine model for the action of v-*sis*. Much evidence now indicates that the first mechanism is correct. First, the amount of secreted PDGF B chain in the media of cells infected with v-*sis* is extremely low. Second, application of anti–v-*sis* antisera to cells infected with v-*sis* fails to block transformation. More recently, the receptor has been shown to be activated prior to reaching the cell surface.[94]

Expression of a derivative v-*sis* that is completely retained in the endoplasmic reticulum and Golgi of the cell also results in transformation[95] (see Fig. 6-9). Thus, attempts to block transformation by v-*sis*, and more broadly to block the actions of other growth factor oncogenes, must be directed within the cell, rather than at the cell surface. These observations also serve to focus attention on the intracellular effects of activation of the PDGF receptor.

Receptor Tyrosine Kinases

Receptor tyrosine kinases mediate the effects of growth factors and are structurally related to the larger family of tyrosine kinases containing the *src* and *abl* oncogenes.[96] Several dominant oncogenes are derived from growth factor receptors: v-*erb* B from the EGF receptor[8,97]; v-*fms* from the CSF-1 receptor[98]; v-*kit* from the c-*kit* receptor;[99] and activated *neu* from the HER2/*neu* putative receptor.[100] Knowledge of the mechanism of action of these proteins is important both in understanding their own transforming ability, as well as how v-*sis* and other growth factor oncogenes dysregulate cell growth and induce transformation. We will begin by describing general properties of these proteins, and then examine in detail current understanding of the best characterized receptor tyrosine kinase—the PDGF receptor. Finally, we will compare the v-*fms* oncogene with its native receptor, the macrophage colony-stimulating factor receptor, a hematopoietic example of activation of a receptor tyrosine kinase.

Receptor tyrosine kinases have a uniform structure (proceeding from N to C terminus)[96]: an extracellular domain, a transmembrane domain, a juxtamembrane domain, a tyrosine kinase domain, and a carboxy-terminal tail (see Fig. 6-2). The extracellular domain follows a signal peptide and is usually large (500 to 850 amino acids) and heavily glycosylated. Although the primary sequence of this region is not highly conserved, the general features of the extracellular domain may be grouped into two categories: those with highly conserved cysteine residues and those with immunoglobulin-like repetitive domains. These structural features are likely to be important in defining common structural motifs in the extracellular domain among groups of receptors.

The transmembrane domain consists of hydrophobic residues and is followed by a short moderately conserved juxtamembrane sequence that signals stop transfer (to lock the protein in the cell membrane). This juxtamembrane domain is also involved in modulation of receptor function by stimulation of other growth receptors. The tyrosine kinase domain is homologous to similar domains in c-*src*. The PDGF, CSF-1, and c-*kit* receptors contain an additional insertion of 77 to 107 residues in the middle of the kinase domain, the *kinase insert* region (see later in chapter). The C-terminal tail region is highly variable and likely to have important regulatory functions, which at this time are poorly understood.

Platelet-Derived Growth Factor Receptor

By means of its receptor, PDGF stimulates a number of physiologic and morphologic changes in fibroblasts, including increased phosphatidylinositol turnover[101] and activation of phospholipase Cγ, cytoplasmic alkalinization through Na+/H+ exchange, increased intracellular calcium ion,[102] cytoskeletal reorganization,[103] and increases in the transcription of a small family of genes.[104] How the PDGF–PDGF receptor interaction results in this host of cellular responses has been the subject of intense scrutiny. Binding of PDGF by the receptor is known to cause a change in receptor conformation, aggregation of receptors (termed *receptor oligomerization*), internalization of the receptor, and autophosphorylation, as well as phosphorylation of a number of intracellular proteins.[105] Tyrosine kinase activity is essential for mitogenic functions of the PDGF receptor (and transforming activity of oncogenic relatives of the PDGF receptor), but identification of primary critical substrates for phosphorylation by the receptor has been difficult.

Recent results have indicated the importance of the kinase insert domain in the function of the PDGF receptor.[106] The kinase insert region of the PDGF receptor appears to modulate binding of the receptor to intracellular substrates including the serine–threonine kinase *raf*-1 protooncogene (c-*raf*-1),[107] phospholipase Cγ[108,109] (mediates hydrolysis of PIP_2 to IP_3 and DAG, important intracellular second messengers). Direct substrates for the tyrosine kinase of the PDGF receptor include c-*raf*-1, phosphatidylinositol 3-kinase, and the *ras* GTPase-activating protein.[110–112] These multiple components (c-*raf*-1, phospholipase Cγ, phosphoinositol 3-kinase, and GTPase-activating protein) appear to exist as a complex within the cell, ready to interact with activated PDGF (and other) receptors and mediate dissemination of signal to intracellular targets. The full spectrum of proteins involved in this complex and precise details of signal dissemination are not yet clear, but a control pathway is emerging.

v-*fms*

The oncogene v-*fms* is the protein product of the Susan McDonough strain of feline sarcoma virus, which causes fibrosarcomas in domestic cats.[113] The identification and cloning of the v-*fms* oncogene led to the identification of its protooncogene, a receptor expressed exclusively on cells of the mononuclear phagocyte series, which is probably the macrophage colony-stimulating factor CSF-1 (or M-CSF) receptor.[98] Comparison of v-*fms* with the CSF-1 receptor indicates that retroviral transduction resulted in the production of a transmembrane receptor whose major alteration is a 40 amino acid deletion at the C terminus with replacement by 11 amino acids from the retroviral envelope gene.[99] The CSF-1 receptor has closest structural homology to the PDGF receptor and contains a kinase insert domain. The alterations in v-*fms* do not appear to affect its binding to CSF-1.[114] Transformation of cells in culture by v-*fms* does not depend on addition of CSF-1, and antibodies against CSF-1 have no effect on its transforming ability. The precise effects of the COOH-terminal alterations that occur in v-*fms* on the regulation of the receptor's activity are not known, but they are suspected to be critical for its transforming ability. Given the presence of the kinase insert region in the CSF-1 receptor, it is anticipated that it may participate in the same dissemination pathways outlined for the PDGF receptor. Elevated phospholipase Cγ activity has been described in v-*fms* transformed cells,[115] and evidence exists of an association between the CSF-1 receptor and some components of the complex described above, particularly phosphoinositol 3-kinase.[116]

The *ras* Family

Oncogenes in the *ras* family were first identified as the transforming genes of the Harvey and Kirsten strains of rat sarcoma viruses.[117,118] Subsequently, activated versions of these same genes were found to be present in a wide range of human carcinomas and sarcomas. Gene transfer experiments demonstrated that activated *ras* genes have the ability to transform NIH3T3 cells in one step from an immortalized cell line to a malignant cell line. This occurred despite the presence of the normal wild-type gene in the cells, so that these genes are dominant in the genetic sense. The *ras* genes have become the most intensively studied oncogenes because of (1) their involvement in 10% to 15% of all human tumors[119]; (2) their small size, which permits precise molecular dissection of mechanisms of pathogenic activation; and (3) the advent of polymerase chain reaction DNA amplification technology, making it possible to rapidly identify *ras* mutations in any tumor.[120] Although a great deal has been learned regarding the biochemistry and function of *ras* in the cell, significant gaps in our understanding persist.

The *ras* genes are ubiquitous in eukaryotic cells, being found in organisms as diverse as humans, yeasts, and plants, and *ras* protein is expressed in nearly all mammalian cell types.[119] In humans and other mammals, three functional *ras* genes are found: H-*ras*-1, K-*ras*-2, and N-*ras*. H-*ras*-1 and K-*ras*-2 are the oncogenes of the Harvey and Kirsten rat sarcoma viruses, respectively, whereas N-*ras* was first discovered as the oncogene of a human neuroblastoma cell line. The three human ras genes encode proteins of length 189 residues that are similar in amino acid sequence and have identical molecular weight—21 kd. These genes are therefore denoted p21. The human K-*ras* gene undergoes alternative splicing at its COOH-terminus to generate two proteins whose sequence varies in the last 25 residues.

Four domains may be identified within human *ras* proteins based on sequence comparisons.[119] The first domain consists of almost 50% of the protein, beginning at the N terminus, and is identical among all three *ras* genes. The next domain extends from that point until the C terminal 25 residues and displays 85% identity among the different human *ras* genes. A variable domain is then found, extending to the last four residues, which are a constant Cys A-A-X sequence (where A is any hydrophobic residue and X is any residue).

Activating changes in *ras* genes have been well characterized in both human cancers and the v-*ras* genes. Activating mutations occur in codons 12, 13, 59, and 61 within *ras*, thus affecting the primary sequence of the highly conserved N-terminal domain.[121–123] In human cancer, *ras* oncogenes all contain a single activating mutation affecting one of these sites. *ras* gene activation therefore serves as an example of dominant oncogene activation by point mutation. The sites of the activating mutations in the *ras* protein have indicated the probable functional importance of these changes, which will be discussed in further detail later in this chapter. In contrast, all four retroviral *ras* oncogenes contain two activating mutations, affecting one or more of these sites. The *ras* genes of invertebrate eukaryotes are more diverged from the human *ras* genes, but all contain highly conserved N-terminal regions.[119]

Biochemical and Functional Properties

Proteins in the *ras* family are localized to the cytoplasmic surface of the plasma membrane, and this property appears essential for their normal and oncogenic functions.[124,125] The membrane localization of *ras* occurs through a posttranslational modification at the C terminus of the protein, which requires the presence of the CAAX sequence.[126,127] The A-A-X peptide is removed, and a thioether linkage is made between the (now) C-terminal cysteine and the branched-chain, polyunsaturated hydrocarbon alcohol, farnesol. Farnesol is derived from mevalonic acid and is a metabolic intermediate of cholesterol biosynthesis. A second cysteine residue proximal to the C-terminal C-A-A-X sequence (in N-*ras* and H-*ras*) also undergoes reversible attachment to the fatty acid palmitic acid. These covalently bound lipids are thought to mediate the membrane attachment of *ras*. The reversible nature of the palmitoylation reaction suggests that it may provide a means of regulating the protein's function in the cell.[126] The necessity of farnesol attachment at the C terminus of *ras* for its oncogenic function has spurred the thought that sterol biosynthetic inhibitors, such as drugs that block the activity of hydroxymethylglutaryl coenzyme A (HMG CoA) reductase might have beneficial effects in the therapy of human cancer. Such considerations are mitigated by the observation that this same metabolic pathway is used for a number of other proteins, so that nonspecific effects within the body could be serious and limiting.

Activated *ras* oncogenes are the most potent genes known in NIH3T3 cell transformation assays. To understand this property, the functional properties of *ras* proteins have been studied by several techniques.[128] Injection of neutralizing antibodies against *ras* into quiescent fibroblasts blocks growth induction by subsequent application of several different growth factors, indicating the central role of *ras* in cell growth control. In addition, injection of recombinant oncogenic *ras* protein into quiescent fibroblasts stimulates cell division. Protein kinase C activity is increased in *ras*-transformed cells, and antibodies against phospholipase C have the ability to block the growth stimulation of microinjection of *ras*.[129] A direct role for *ras* in stimulation of phosphoinositide turnover has not been found. Consequently, the precise second messengers involved in the growth stimulatory properties of *ras* remain poorly understood but seem likely to be related to their ability to bind to GTP and GDP.

The ability of *ras* proteins to hydrolyze GTP and GDP represents an essential function-related property.[119] Mutant *ras* proteins that cannot bind GTP do not transform NIH3T3 cells in standard gene transfer assays, and moreover the GTPase activity of *ras* genes is markedly reduced in mutagenized oncogenic forms of *ras*. These observations, along with the structural homology between the signal transducing G proteins[130] and ras, suggest that ras proteins participate in the transduction of signals across the cell membrane.

Recent identification of a cellular protein of molecular weight 110, termed *GAP* (for GTPase-activating protein), has led to further insight into regulation of *ras* function.[131] GAP stimulates the hydrolysis of GTP bound by wild-type *ras*, but not that of GTP bound by mutant oncogenic *ras*. Similarly, overexpression of GAP in cells has the ability to prevent transformation through overexpression of wild-type *ras*, but not that caused by mutant oncogenic *ras*.[132] Cell activation, at least in T lymphocytes, results in increased levels of GTP-*ras* with concomitant inhibition of GAP activity.[133] Therefore, GAP appears to be an upstream regular of *ras*, keeping it in the inactivated GDP-bound state, and is ineffective in controlling mutant *ras*. GAP itself is phosphorylated on tyrosine residues after cell stimulation with PDGF or EGF, or in cells transformed by the v-*src* of v-*fps* oncogenes.[111]

Stimulation of cells with PDGF leads to binding between the PDGF receptor and GAP through the kinase insert domain. Thus, GAP may be the critical link between cell stimulation and *ras* activation leading to second messenger production. Other conflicting evidence suggests that GAP may actually lie downstream of *ras* in the network of cell growth control, and further study is required. An understanding of the second messenger pathway by which *ras* microinjection or overexpression leads to cell growth would be helpful in completing the picture of how *ras* works, but such understanding is lacking.

Observations lead to the following model of *ras* function. Under quiescent conditions, *ras* binds GDP. On growth-related (or other) stimulus, *ras* releases GDP, binds GTP, and becomes activated to transmit signals to the cell interior with respect to growth and mitosis. In normal *ras*, the GTP is rapidly hydrolyzed to GDP and signal transmission is turned off. In transforming derivatives of *ras*, GTP hydrolysis is markedly reduced, the mitogenic signal is experienced by the cell much longer, and oncogenesis results.

Because of its relatively small size and efficient, conformationally correct expression in bacterial cells, the three-dimensional structure of *ras* is known in detail[134,135] (Fig. 6-10). *ras* has been crystallized in its inactive form, complexed with GDP, as well as in its activated form, complexed with a nonhydrolyzable analogue of GTP.[136,137] In both these crystal structures the same amino acid groups contribute to binding of the terminal GDP–GTP, which are residues A_{11}–K_{16}, T_{35}, and A_{59}–Q_{61}. Significant differences in conformation occur in residues 30 to 38 and 60 to 76, depending on whether GDP or GTP is bound. The residue 30 to 38 region has also been identified as critical for *ras*

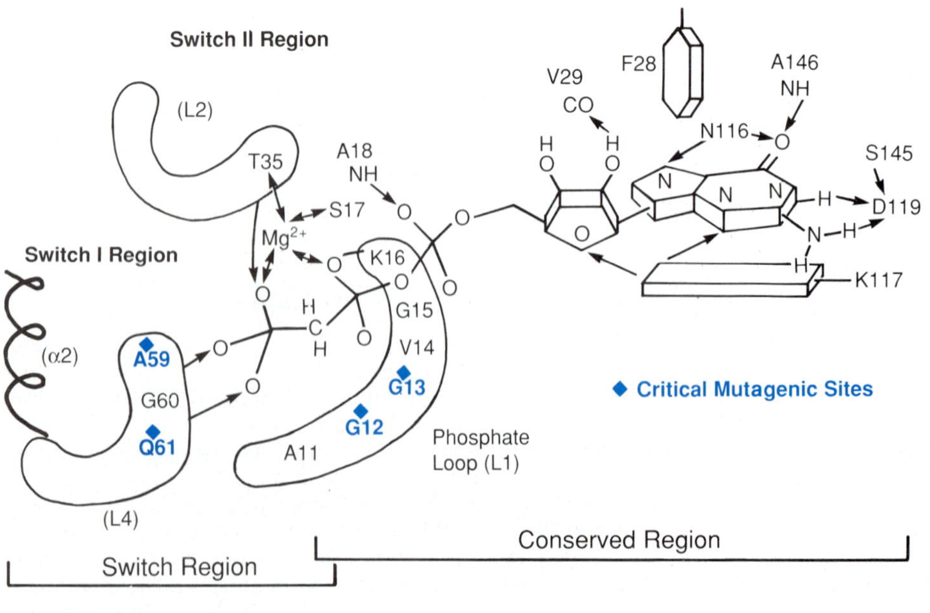

FIGURE 6-10. Binding of GTP by c-H-*ras*. A schematic drawing of the region of the c-H-*ras* protein involved in binding of GDP and GTP is shown. The particular complex drawn involves GDP-CP, a nonhydrolyzable GTP analogue used in crystal formation. Critical sites for mutagenic activation of c-H-*ras* all are directly involved in binding of the gamma-phosphate of GTP. The single amino acid code is used. L1, L2, L4, and α2 represent various peptide chains within the c-H-*ras* protein. (After Milburn, MV, Tong L, deVos AM, et al. Molecular switch for signal transduction: structural differences between active and inactive forms of protooncogenic *ras* proteins. Science 1990;247:939)

function by mutagenesis studies and is likely to interact with other proteins in *ras*-mediated signaling. The most common critical sites of mutation of human *ras* are G_{12} and Q_{61}. *ras* proteins with mutations at these sites have an altered binding pocket for the γ phosphate of GTP and thereby inhibit the normal process of hydrolysis of GTP to $GDP \cdot P_i$.

A large and growing family of proteins with amino acid homology to *ras* has been discovered, including Ral (A and B), Rap1 (A and B), Rap2, R-*ras*, TC21, Rho (A, B, and C), Rab1, Rab2, and Rab3. Most of these proteins interact with cell membranes like *ras*, and some also bind to GAP. Functions of these proteins are poorly understood, but they appear to include signal transduction (Rap1), control of cytoskeletal organization (Rho), and intracellular trafficking of vesicles (Rab family). Oncogenic activation of these proteins has not been described thus far. To the contrary, high level expression of normal Rap1A induces morphologic reversion of a *ras*-transformed cell line.[138]

Mutations in Myelodysplastic Syndromes and Acute Myeloid Leukemia

As noted above, *ras* mutations are probably the most common mutations occurring in human neoplasia and have been found in 30% to 40% of all patients with acute myeloid leukemia (AML) and myelodysplastic syndrome (MDS).[119,139–142] In patients with MDS, the finding of a *ras* mutation appears to confer a poorer prognosis and is associated with subsequent development of AML of M4 and M5 subtypes.[143] In patients with AML, *ras* mutations are also found more commonly in M4 and M5 subtypes but do not appear to have prognostic significance. A significant fraction of patients with MDS who have normal *ras* genes, subsequently develop mutations months or years after their original diagnosis. This suggests that *ras* mutations may serve a secondary or progression factor role rather than being a primary pathogenetic mechanism. On the other hand, in other model systems of carcinogenesis, mutation in *ras* has been shown to occur early in premalignant lesions.[144] The pathogenesis of MDS is discussed in detail in Chapter 10.

bcl-2

The *bcl*-2 oncogene product is also associated with cell membranes but is less well understood than the oncogenes described thus far. *Bcl*-2 was identified by its involvement in follicular lymphomas bearing the t(14;18) (q32;q21) chromosomal translocation.[145,146] It was subsequently recognized to be involved in roughly 85% of all follicular small cleaved B-cell lymphomas[142,147] and 20% of diffuse B-cell lymphomas. It thus represents one of the oncogenes most commonly involved in human hematologic neoplasia. Although *bcl*-2 has never been identified as a retroviral oncogene and lacks direct transforming ability upon introduction into rodent fibroblast cell lines, it appears to play an essential role in lymphomagenesis and is denoted a dominant oncogene.

Translocations t(14;18) occurring in lymphomas result in the juxtaposition of the immunoglobulin heavy-chain gene on chromosome 14 with the *bcl*-2 gene on chromosome 18.[146] Most frequently one of two regions in the 3′ portion of the *bcl*-2 gene serve as breakpoints during the translocation.[147] Much less frequently (less than 5%), translocations occur to the 5′ upstream region of the gene. In all cases, the *bcl*-2 coding region is never disrupted, and the *bcl*-2 gene is expressed at relatively high levels.[148]

The gene encodes two slightly different protein isoforms. Immunolocalization studies have shown that *bcl*-2 protein is associated with membranes in the cell, and a recent report suggests it is found in mitochondria.[149,150] The function of the protein is not known, and this localization is distinct from all other known oncogenes.

The *bcl*-2 gene contains a 370-kb intron, so that the common 3′ translocations occur at considerable distance from the site of transcriptional initiation.[151] Nonetheless, these translocations increase *bcl*-2 transcription, steady state levels of RNA, and protein levels.[152] *bcl*-2 protein levels are uniformly elevated in lymphoma cells containing the translocation. Similar levels of expression are seen only in stimulated normal lymphocytes. By itself, *bcl*-2 does not have classic transforming activity in rodent cell assays but does confer in vivo transforming activity to either rodent fibroblasts[153] or pre–B cells.[154] Conflicting observations regarding the possible function of *bcl*-2 as a signal-transmitting G protein have been made.[155] Based on current understanding, the *bcl*-2 protein confers a relatively weak growth advantage to the cell by unknown mechanisms, consistent with the indolent nature of the B-cell lymphomas in which it is most commonly involved.

Nuclear Oncogenes: *myc, fos, jun*

myc

The *myc* oncogene was first identified as the active element of a group of acute avian leukemia retroviruses known as the *myelocytomatosis viruses*.[156,157] Although the leukemic disorder myelocytomatosis is the most common tumor associated with *myc*-transducing viruses, carcinomas, endotheliomas, and sarcomas, all have been noted in infected animals. Overexpression of c-*myc* alone can immortalize normal rat fibroblasts. When combined with expression of an activated *ras* oncogene, *myc* overexpression transforms primary fibroblasts and renders them tumorigenic in vivo. Two *myc*-related genes, N-*myc* and L-*myc*, have been identified by sequence similarity. These two genes are commonly involved in human neuroblastoma (N-*myc*) and small cell lung cancer (as well as *myc*) but have never been identified as retroviral oncogenes.

The oncogene *myc* is unusual among oncogenes in that activation occurs primarily by elevation of its level of expression, and mutagenesis of its primary sequence appears relatively unimportant. Such increases in the level of expression may occur through mechanisms of retroviral transduction[157]; proviral insertion, as in the case of lymphoid leukosis virus, a slow transforming retrovirus[158]; translocation, as in the characteristic chromosomal translocations of Burkitt's lymphoma[159]; and amplification, as in human small cell lung carcinoma.

The observations that deregulation of *myc* expression alone is sufficient to activate its oncogenic potential and that *myc* is much less often mutagenized have prompted intensive studies of its transcriptional regulation.

Regulation of c-*myc* Expression

The c-*myc* gene is relatively small but has a complex structure and mechanisms for regulation of transcription (Fig. 6-11). Two or three different promoters are used to initiate RNA transcripts at the 5′ end of the gene. Two of these, P1 and P2, are the major sites of transcriptional initiation and are both used in a variety of cell types.[158] Transcription occurs within the c-*myc* gene by RNA polymerase II, which is typically involved in transcription from protein-encoding genes, and by RNA polymerase III, which typically transcribes only short RNA species that are involved in protein synthesis.[160] Thus, multiple transcription initiation sites and polymerases provide a first level of regulation of the c-*myc* locus.

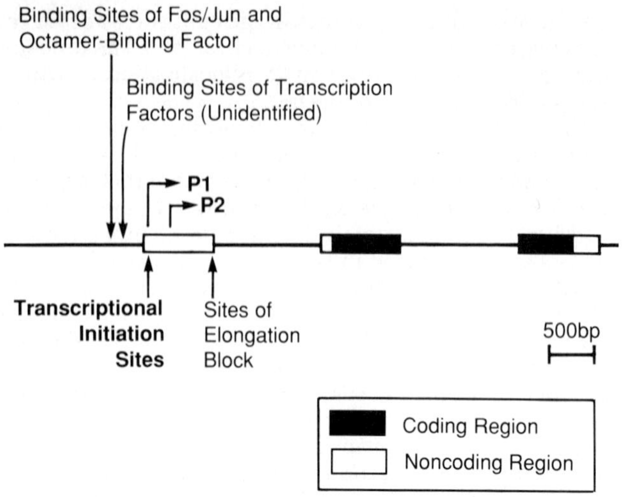

FIGURE 6-11. Regulation of transcription of the c-*myc* gene. Transcriptional initiation sites (P1 and P2), sites of binding by positively and negatively activating factors, and the site of elongation block are indicated.

The c-*myc* gene is also unusual in that its first exon is large (550 nucleotides), highly conserved among mammalian species, and untranslated. The precise role of this unusual first exon is not known, but it is thought to play an important role in regulation of transcription. Analysis of RNA transcripts from the c-*myc* gene have shown that transcription often pauses or terminates in the region near the 3′ border of exon 1.[161] RNA polymerase III, particularly, pauses in this region and may block production of full-length RNA transcripts. Analysis of the DNA sequence of c-*myc* genes that have been translocated, as in Burkitt's lymphoma, has demonstrated that the region 3′ of exon 1 is more frequently mutated than the remainder of the gene.[162] This observation suggests that the increased amounts of c-*myc* RNA expressed in Burkitt's cells may be due to these mutations, which permit synthesis of full-length, functional RNA transcripts.

Enhancer elements are also important in determining the level of expression of the *myc* gene. Regions upstream of the P1 transcriptional initiation site have been defined as important for negative regulation of c-*myc* expression, and several factors have been identified that specifically bind to this region of the gene.[163,164] These include a complex of c-*fos/jun*,[19,165] the octamer-binding factor,[166] and other factors thus far unidentified. In contrast to the usual situation in which these elements serve to increase expression, in c-*myc*, their primary role appears to be to reduce expression, at least under most circumstances. Elevation of c-*myc* expression occurs in normal somatic cells in response to growth stimuli, and this presumably reflects a relaxation of this tonic inhibition of expression. Site-directed mutagenesis of specific residues within this region of the c-*myc* gene in vitro yields enhancement of transcription that is unregulated. Although this mechanism may occur in tumors, this has not yet been directly demonstrated.

Structure and Function of c-*myc*

The c-*myc* protein binds DNA in vitro, is known to be phosphorylated, and has been localized to the cell nucleus. A minor form has been described that has an additional 14 residues at its amino terminus and whose translation initiates at an unusual CTG codon.[167] The functional differences between this slightly larger *myc* protein and the major form, if any, are unknown, but some Burkitt's lymphoma cell lines do not express the larger form. The predominant form of human c-*myc* is a 439–amino acid phosphoprotein. Regions of similarity in the primary amino acid sequence between c-*myc*, N-*myc*, and L-*myc*, as well as mutagenesis studies, have defined four domains (I to IV) within the protein that are important for its transforming ability, nuclear localization, and ability to oligomerize into multimeric complexes. Regions essential for *myc*'s transforming ability depend on the transforming assay used.[168] Domains II and IV are always essential and do not tolerate even small deletions. Deletion of large portions of domain I also affect transforming ability, but small deletions are not important. Domain III is dispensable for transforming activity. The region of the protein essential for nuclear localization has been precisely defined as residues 320 to 328.[169]

The domain required for oligomerization consists of residues 369 to 439, which form an imperfect series of repeating leucines that occur every seventh amino acid.[170] A similar sequence of repeated leucines has been noted in the oncogenes *fos* and *jun* and is thought to be important for dimerization and oligomerization of these proteins into larger aggregates, a process considered essential for their normal physiologic roles in the nucleus.[171]

A clear understanding of the functional role of c-*myc* in normal and malignant cells is not yet available. Studies of a variety of fibroblast and other cell lines in vitro have indicated that *myc* is often expressed transiently at high levels in cells that are making the transition from a quiescent nonreplicative state (G0) to an active growth state, as described earlier.[172] Several other proteins, including *fos*, are expressed at this same time, and these proteins as well as c-*myc* are thought to be important elements in the control of cell proliferation. Furthermore, blockade of c-*myc* expression has been shown to prevent growth factor stimulation of cell growth in vitro in some systems.[173,174] A direct role for *myc* in DNA replication has been proposed based on the ability of antibodies against c-*myc* to inhibit both DNA synthesis and DNA polymerase activity in isolated cell nuclei.[175] Elevated c-*myc* expression has also been reported to facilitate the replication of SV40 DNA in human lymphoma cells.[176] The direct nature of the involvement of c-*myc* in DNA replication has been disputed, however.[177]

c-*myc* Involvement in Burkitt's Lymphoma

The c-*myc* gene is involved in reciprocal translocations with the human immunoglobulin loci in nearly all patients with Burkitt's lymphoma, resulting in the typical cytogenetic findings of t(8;14) (q24;932), t(8;22) (q34;q11), and t(2;8) (p11;q24) in 80%, 15%, and 5% of cases, respectively.[178] A consistent finding in Burkitt's cells is alteration of c-*myc* regulation with overexpression of both RNA and protein. Expression of c-*myc* RNA is derived exclusively from the translocated c-*myc* gene indicating that normal regulatory processes have been disrupted through translocation but remain operational on the nontranslocated c-*myc* gene.[179] Different translocations directly involve several regions of the c-*myc* gene, including within and immediately surrounding exon 1, thereby affecting critical regions for regulation of transcriptional initiation and transcript elongation, as just described.[180] It is more remarkable that translocations also occur at relatively large distances from the c-*myc* gene (more than 50 kb) and still result in upregulation of expression. This may be due to the long-range effects of immunoglobulin gene-derived enhancer elements or to mutagenesis of the translocated c-*myc* locus that occurs as part of the translocation itself.[162,181]

fos and *jun*

The two oncogenes *fos* and *jun* also belong to the family of nuclear oncogenes. The *fos* gene was first identified in the 1960s as the transforming component of two independently isolated osteosarcoma viruses, whereas *jun* was only recently identified.[182] The two proteins are closely related, and recent findings have led to a better understanding of their individual function as well as to greater insights into mechanisms of oncogene action in general.

The story of how recent advances developed also illustrates the often tortuous path of oncogene research.[183] To try to understand *fos*'s normal biochemical function, its tissue-specific expression was investigated. The oncogene *fos* is expressed in a complex pattern in the developing embryo, although in the adult it is expressed in only a few tissues, particularly the bone marrow and other leukocyte-rich tissues. Expression of *fos* is induced in a dramatic way in several in vitro systems.[184] First, *fos* expression increases greatly when quiescent (serum-deprived, G0) fibroblasts are stimulated to grow with serum. Second, *fos* expression increases in several myeloid cell lines when differentiation to macrophage-like cells is induced, particularly with the tumor promoter, phorbol ester. Studies into the regulation of *fos* expression have demonstrated that transcriptional activation occurs in the 5′ region of the gene, but that message stability is also an important control mechanism. Deregulation of *fos* expression occurs in the v-*fos* derivatives analyzed, and this is at least partially due to loss of 3′ untranslated sequences responsible for *fos* message degradation.[185] These observations on the level of expression of *fos* failed to provide any insight into the role of *fos* in normal cellular physiology. The protein *fos* was known to be a nuclear phosphoprotein, but that was all. Immunoprecipitation of *fos* from cells invariably led to the isolation of a second, 39-kd protein whose identity and function were unknown.

The oncogene *jun* was identified in 1987 as the active gene of an avian sarcoma virus. Sequence analysis of the cloned v-*jun* gene indicated that its predicted protein product contained a region whose amino acid sequence was remarkably similar to that of a transcription factor identified in yeast, GCN4. GCN4 is a nuclear protein that binds to a specific sequence in the upstream region of several yeast genes, which are required for amino acid synthesis. Binding of this sequence by GCN4 increases the transcription of these genes. To explore the possibility that *jun* might encode a transcriptional regulatory protein in vertebrate cells, a gene swap experiment was performed. The homologous region of v-*jun* was swapped into the GCN4 gene, and the hybrid protein was shown to bind to the same yeast DNA site as native GCN4 and to functionally replace GCN4 in terms of gene transcription.[186]

A concurrently identified vertebrate transcription factor, AP-1, was known to bind to a sequence that was similar to that bound by GCN4 in yeast. Given the fact that *jun* could functionally substitute for GCN4 in yeast, it was suspected and shown that c-*jun* was a component of the AP-1 complex.[19,187] Even more striking, it was recognized that *jun* binds tightly to *fos* and was the 39-kd protein that had long been observed in close association with *fos* by immunoprecipitation.[188]

At about the same time, a conserved sequence of repeating leucines, occurring every seventh residue, was noted in the COOH-terminal region of GCN4, *fos*, *jun*, *myc*, and other transcriptional enhancing proteins. It was postulated and demonstrated that this "leucine zipper" motif was both necessary and sufficient for the dimerization of *fos* with *jun*, and GCN4 with itself.[189, 190] Dimer formation among these proteins is essential for transcriptional activation.[191] In *fos*, *jun*, and GCN4, the amino acid sequence directly adjacent to the leucine zipper region consists of a cluster of several positively charged residues and is essential for DNA binding and transcriptional activation, although it does not contribute to dimerization.[192] Other regions in both *fos* and *jun* are thought to serve regulatory functions with respect to the transcriptional activation ability of the proteins but this is poorly understood.

Both v-*fos* and v-*jun* contain regions of both single amino acid substitutions and deletions, in comparison with the normal cellular proteins c-*fos* and c-*jun*, respectively, and several of these differences may be important in their oncogenic activation.[193,194] Marked increases in steady state expression of these proteins also occur in v-*fos*/v-*jun*–infected cells so that both mutagenic activation and increased levels of expression may contribute to the transformation process.

Thus, *fos* and *jun* regulate gene transcription and are positioned within the signal transduction pathway in the nucleus. Exactly how the system is regulated (possibly by phosphorylation) is unknown at this point. The transforming activity of the *fos* and *jun* oncogenes is probably the result of their high level and unregulated expression, together with mutagenesis and loss of regulatory domains. At least one *fos*-related protein and two *jun*-related proteins have been identified, and other candidates are under investigation. Heterodimerization among these proteins can greatly augment the repertory of transcriptional factors for precise regulation of gene expression.

TUMOR SUPPRESSOR GENES

Evidence From Somatic Cell Hybrids

During the 1960s, techniques were developed that allowed cells to be fused so that the resulting hybrid contained the combined chromosomal content of both of the original cells. This technique was used to investigate why some tumor cells had a greater malignant potential than others. Henry Harris and coworkers[195] noted that when highly malignant mouse cells were fused with normal mouse embryo cells, the hybrid mouse cells had a low malignant potential. When these hybrid cells were transplanted into mice, in contrast to the original cells that could form tumors, the hybrid cells were nontumorigenic. If, instead, these cells were grown in culture for several passages, they regained their ability to form tumors. To understand why the hybrid cells were only transiently able to suppress the malignant phenotype, chromosome analysis was performed on the tumorigenic segregants. All the tumorigenic segregants were found to have lost many chromosomes compared with the chromosome complement of the original nontumorigenic hybrid. Although formation of the hybrid ablated the tumorigenic phenotype, it was regained as chromosomes were lost. The conclusion was drawn that the presence of certain wild-type genes on the normal chromosomes that had been introduced were able to block the tumorigenic phenotype.[196]

The genes that can block the tumorigenic phenotype are therefore called *tumor suppressor genes*. Since the tumorigenic phenotype could be suppressed by forming somatic cell hybrids, including only a single copy of a normal cellular gene, the phenotype was recessive. Virtually all tumor cells are inhibited by hybrid formation with normal cells, suggesting that the loss of such tumor suppressor genes is an essential pathogenetic feature of nearly all tumors. Hybrids between fibroblasts and cells transformed by DNA tumor viruses represent a notable exception to this general phenomenon because they do not lose their malignant phenotype.[197] As will be discussed, recent evidence suggests that this exception in some ways proves the importance of the suppressor genes because the DNA tumor virus-transforming proteins are thought to functionally inactivate tumor suppressor genes in a transdominant fashion by binding to the tumor suppressor gene protein products.

Analysis of the specific chromosomes that were lost in the intraspecies hybrids that regained tumorigenic properties was aided by use of natural polymorphisms of the centromeric chromosomes to identify the parental origin of the hybrids. Hybrids of malignant mouse cells always appeared to require mouse chromosome 4 to suppress malignancy.[198] A similar suppression of the malignant phenotype could be achieved by introducing human chromosome 1.[199] The fact that human chromosome 1 has a large degree of homology with mouse chromosome 4 suggested that the same tumor suppressor gene could be active in both sets of experiments.[200]

In the 1980s, several different tumors were analyzed for variations in the specific chromosomes that suppressed the tumorigenicity of different tumors. This work indicated that the malignant phenotype of human HeLa cells is suppressed by a gene on chromosome 11. Other potential tumor suppressor genes have been identified on chromosomes 2, 13, 17, and 20 by similar techniques.[201-203] New techniques have further refined this approach by allowing introduction of individual portions of chromosomes by microcell fusion. The overall conclusion from these cell fusion experiments is that malignancy frequently involves inactivation of one or more of a group of cellular genes and that the specific genes inactivated differ for different tumor types.

Familial Tumors as Evidence for Tumor Suppressor Genes

About one third of the United States population will be diagnosed as having cancer during their lifetime. Most of these cancers are not associated with a significantly greater risk of the same malignancy occurring in other family members. For first-degree relatives of cancer patients, the overall risk for most cancers is only two to three times higher than the general population. Rare families carry genes that place them at extremely high risk for specific neoplasms. These families carry gene mutations that can indirectly cause cancer in several distinct ways. Some gene mutations affect the immune system, including the dysgammaglobulinemias, whereas other genes affect DNA repair mechanisms, such as in Bloom's syndrome and xeroderma pigmentosa.[204,205] The discussion here focuses only on the genes that directly alter the propensity of cells to undergo transformation.

When families carry altered genes that directly increase susceptibility for specific tumors, they are referred to as *cancer families*. Over 50 published examples of cancer families exist. In fact, almost all cancers occasionally occur in a familial form.[206] Acute myelogenous leukemia rarely occurs in families, but one such family is shown in Figure 6-12*A*. Other tumors such as retinoblastoma occur in an inherited form almost as often as they occur in a sporadic form (see Fig. 6-12*B*). Familial cancer syndromes also vary in the penetrance of expression of the cancer risk phenotype as well as in the spectrum of tumors that may occur in a given family. An average of three to five retinoblastomas occur in each affected member of a family segregating a high retinoblastoma risk phenotype, and these patients get second tumors, particularly sarcomas, with much higher frequency. On the other hand, entire generations of affected members of families that carry a high Wilms' tumor risk phenotype may not form any tumors but will pass on the high-risk phenotype to their children (see Fig. 6-12*C*). In families with the Li-Fraumeni syndrome, affected members are at greatly increased risk for a wide variety of tumors, including breast cancer and sarcoma (see Fig. 6-12*D*).

Despite these differences, several common features associate the occurrence of tumors in these families. The affected members frequently present with multiple primary tumors. Furthermore, these tumors usually have an early age of onset. Epidemiologic analysis of such families indicates that the difference between the general population and the affected family members may be explained by the fact that the affected members already carry one of the mutational events required for transformation in all their cells.[207] Comings[206] expanded this theory to suggest that the mutation carried by affected family members occurred in tumor release genes capable of coding for transforming factors that could release the cell from normal constraints on growth. The diploid nature of the human genome suggests a model in which a high-risk person has inherited one mutated or deleted gene from his or her parents and also suggests that a second hit occurs in the other normal gene during the pathogenesis of each cancer (Fig. 6-13). The existence of familial forms of most cancers implies that inactivation of growth inhibitory or control genes are important in the genesis of most common tumors. This possibility complements similar indications from cell fusion experiments.

Retinoblastoma: From Hypothesis to Gene

The first tumor suspected to arise from the inactivation of a growth suppressor gene was retinoblastoma. The incidence of retinoblastoma in the general population is less than 1 in 40,000, with a median age of 2 to 4 years. Patients with hereditary retinoblastoma usually have two to five tumors and generally present at a younger age than patients with spontaneous retinoblastoma. In contrast to tumors occurring in adults, which are best modeled as a result of three to seven mutational events leading to cell transformation, Knudsen[207,208] noted that he could model the sporadic retinoblastomas as occurring as a result of two events and the hereditary retinoblastomas as only a single rate limiting event to initiate tumor formation. Using this model, he predicted a difference in age of onset of sporadic versus hereditary retinoblastoma, which the observed data fit well (Fig. 6-14).

The first indication of the possible chromosomal location of the retinoblastoma gene was provided by Yunis, who improved chromosome banding techniques so that more than 1000 bands could be distinguished. He was able to determine that some retinoblastomas contained deletions in the 13q14.1 chromosome region.[209,210] Between 1% and 5% of the retinoblastomas had deletions in one of the two chromosomes 13 detectable by chromosome analysis. Construction of a library of DNA fragments from chromosome 13 permitted the identification of a large set of DNA markers detecting restriction fragment length polymorphisms from the chromosome 13q14 region. One of these markers was able to detect the loss of a region on both copies of chromosome 13 in several retinoblastomas.[211] Chromosome walking techniques were then used to find several DNA fragments nearby that were then analyzed for the possibility that they might encode a gene.

The best candidate DNA fragment within the deleted region was then used to screen a cDNA library produced from mRNA from retinal cells. A 4.7-kb cDNA clone was isolated, which was able to hybridize to mRNA from retinal cells and was missing in some retinoblastomas.[212] This cDNA therefore became a candidate for the gene causing retinoblastoma in these families. The detection of some retinoblastomas that had deletions within the DNA region

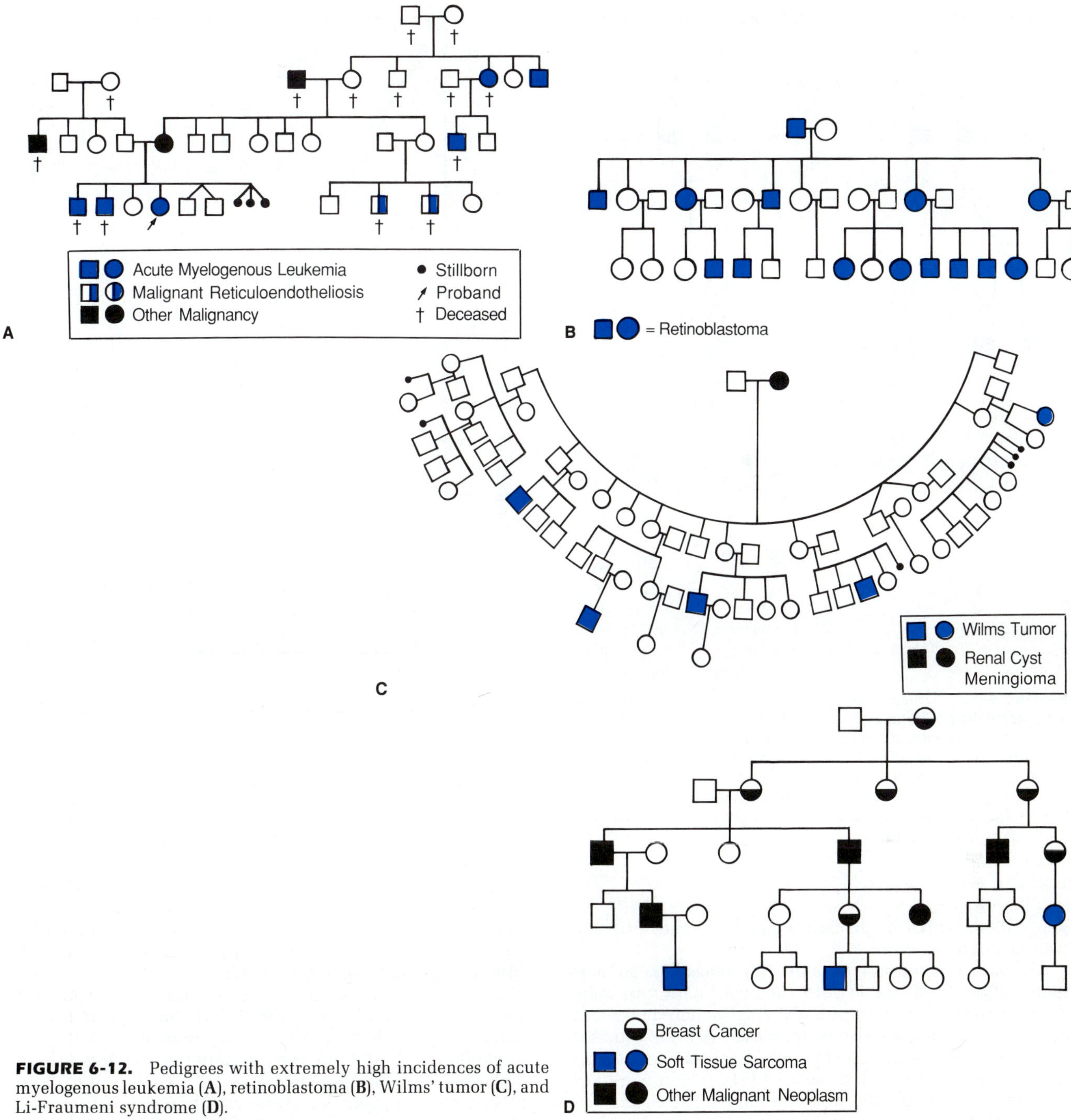

FIGURE 6-12. Pedigrees with extremely high incidences of acute myelogenous leukemia (**A**), retinoblastoma (**B**), Wilms' tumor (**C**), and Li-Fraumeni syndrome (**D**).

encoding this candidate gene provided further evidence that the inactivation of this tumor suppressor gene initiated tumor formation. Since then, extensive studies have documented that about 1 in 10 retinoblastomas has large deletions of this gene detectable by Southern blot analysis.

In addition, antibodies were subsequently made against the protein product of the gene, which was predicted to have length of 105 kd (p105Rb) based on sequence analysis of the cDNA clone. Antibody studies showed an absence of normal p105Rb protein in all retinoblastomas. Further studies have indicated that alterations that inactivate p105Rb range from point mutations that disrupt splice donor and acceptor sites (required for normal processing of mRNA) to large deletions that delete most of the 200 kb containing the exons that encode this protein.[213,214]

Clues about the function of the Rb protein have come from a diverse set of observations. p105Rb expression is not limited to the eye but occurs in all tissues. The mRNA is detectable in embryonic stem cells (T. Jacks, personal communication); by day 11 to 13 of mouse embryo development, it is detectable by Northern blot analysis with the highest level of expression in the liver and brain.[215] The gene is conserved evolutionarily because the human Rb DNA probe has enough homology to hybridize to the Rb gene in sharks and lamprey eels. The antibodies generated against p105Rb show that it is found in the nucleus as a phosphoprotein, which appears to bind nonspecifically to DNA.[213] Sequence analysis indicates that it does not appear to contain a kinase domain or other recognizable active site. It does contain a leucine zipper of the type found in *myc*, *jun*, and *fos*, and it has a nuclear localization signal.[216] p105Rb is therefore considered a ubiquitous nuclear phos-

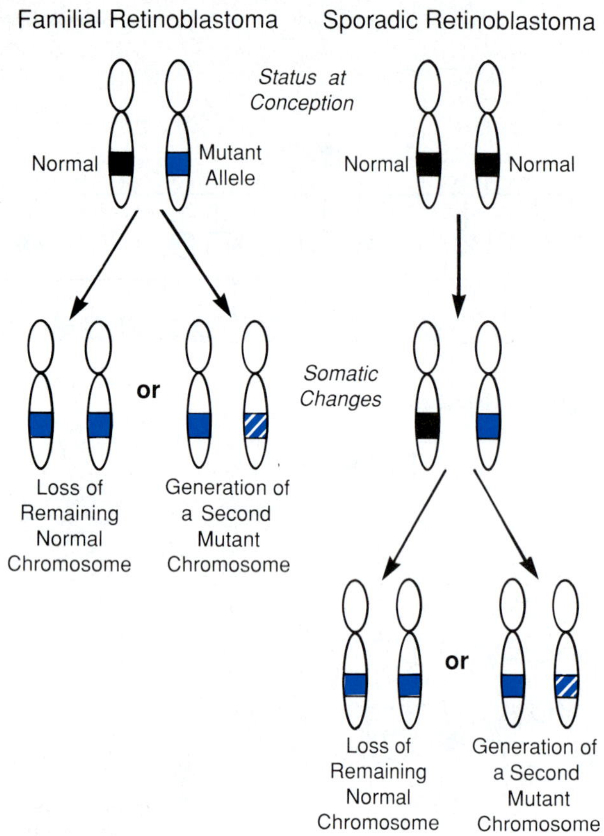

FIGURE 6-13. Differences in the steps required for retinoblastoma formation among patients with the sporadic and familial forms of the disease. Patients with familial retinoblastoma start with one mutant allele and require only one further change. Because patients with sporadic retinoblastoma begin life with two normal copies of the Rb gene, a single retinal cell must undergo two changes, or hits, to inactivate both copies of the Rb gene. (Courtesy of Dr. Fred Li)

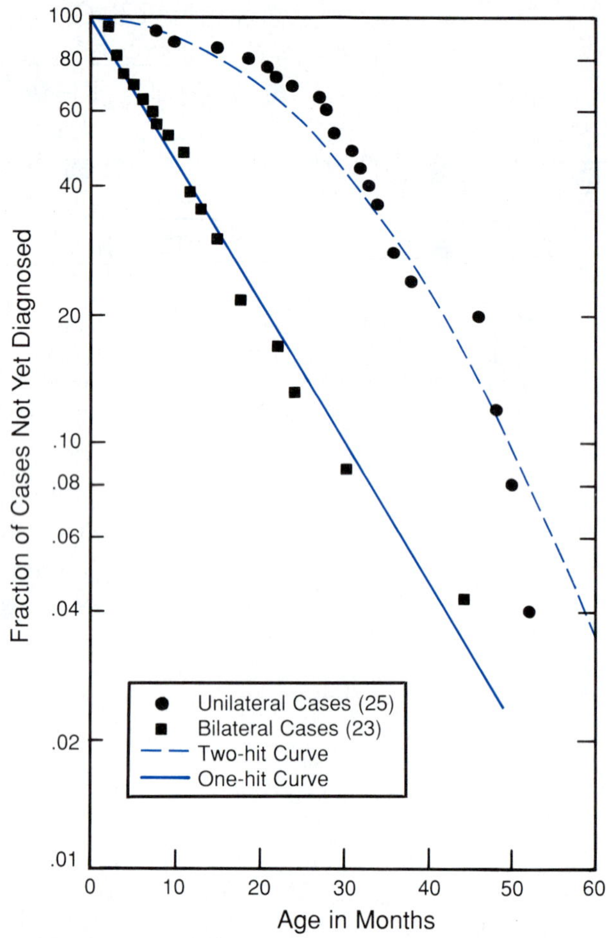

FIGURE 6-14. Comparison between the predicted and actual incidence of retinoblastoma using a two-hit model for unilateral cases and a one-hit model for bilateral cases. (Adapted from Knudsen AG. Mutation and cancer: statistical study of retinoblastoma. Proc Natl Acad Sci USA 1971;68:820)

phoprotein, which might be involved in control of gene transcription.

Although it is referred to as the retinoblastoma gene, its inactivation is associated with tumor formation in many different tissues. Because patients with the hereditary form of retinoblastoma are also at increased risk for osteosarcomas and soft tissue sarcomas, chromosome analysis for loss of alleles in the chromosome 13q14 region were performed on spontaneous osteosarcomas. These analyses were performed by using polymorphic DNA markers from the region of the retinoblastoma gene. These polymorphic DNA markers usually detect two or more distinct alleles in normal persons, based on the presence or absence of a restriction enzyme site (usually in a noncoding region) in the genome. Such markers may be used to examine DNA from a tumor sample and look for the possible loss of one of the two alleles, suggesting that one of two copies of the gene has also been lost. This is referred to as a *loss of heterozygosity* at 13q14. Frequent loss of heterozygosity for the 13q14 alleles in osteosarcomas indicated that retinoblastoma gene inactivation might also be important for formation of spontaneous osteosarcomas.[217] This was confirmed by the presence of internal deletions in the Rb gene in spontaneous osteosarcomas,[212] as well as in spontaneous soft tissue sarcomas.[216]

Other tumors that do not occur more frequently in hereditary retinoblastoma patients also display frequent loss of heterozygosity using these markers near the retinoblastoma gene. Further molecular studies using the cloned Rb gene have shown that, for example, virtually all small cell lung carcinomas have inactivation of p105Rb.[218] On the other hand, several other tumors including carcinomas of the breast, bladder, and prostate have infrequent inactivations in p105Rb.[216] Tumors such as melanomas and colon carcinomas do not appear to undergo inactivation of p105Rb. One model for the observed variation in p105Rb inactivation suggests that tissue variation occurs in the set of genes controlling growth. Despite these possible tissue differences, reintroduction of the normal p105Rb gene severely inhibits the growth of retinoblastoma, osteosarcoma, and prostate carcinoma cells in culture.[219,220]

Some of the first clues about the normal function of the retinoblastoma gene came from studies on the transforming properties of DNA tumor viruses. Although the DNA viruses that cause tumors do not contain dominant oncogenes transduced from the human genome, a subset of the proteins that they encode are able to transform cells. These proteins are therefore termed *DNA tumor virus transforming proteins*. Introduction of random mutations into these proteins results in loss of their ability to transform cells. All these mutations occur in specific conserved domains that control binding to certain normal cellular proteins. For example, the transforming ability of the E1a protein of adenovirus 12 is dependent on its ability to bind to cellular proteins of 105, 107, and 300 kd.[221] A serendipitous examination of the antibodies that recognized the 105-kd cellular protein that binds E1a, and antibodies against the retinoblastoma gene product, revealed that both were recognizing the same protein.[222] Because inactivation of the Rb gene leads to tumor initiation and E1a can complex most of the Rb gene product, the observations suggested that E1a functionally inactivates the growth suppression effects of p105Rb. Therefore, expression of E1a in the cell is equivalent to gene deletion of both copies of p105Rb. p105Rb forms a similar complex with the large T antigen of the SV40 polyoma virus, and with the HPV-16 E7 protein.[223]

The observations in aggregate suggest that many of the DNA tumor viruses functionally inactivate important growth suppressor genes in the process of cell immortalization. The importance of complex formation between DNA virus-transforming proteins and normal cellular proteins such as p105Rb for their pathogenic effects is confirmed by observations in transgenic mice. Transgenic mice, in which expression of the large T antigen of SV40 is driven by a retinal specific promoter, have a high incidence of retinoblastomas.[224]

If p105Rb normally functions as a growth suppressor and is expressed ubiquitously during development, how can cells use p105Rb to turn growth on and off? The answer comes from studies of the posttranslational modifications in p105Rb during the cell cycle. As shown in Figure 6-1, p105Rb is underphosphorylated during the G0, G1, and S phases of the cell cycle. Before the end of the S phase, p105Rb is phosphorylated and remains so throughout the mitotic phase of the cell cycle.[225,226] When cells are quiescent with respect to growth, both in culture and after differentiation, p105Rb is underphosphorylated. The reasonable hypothesis is that phosphorylation probably functionally inactivates p105Rb, so that the cell can progress through mitosis.[225,227] Thus, p105Rb probably serves an important function in DNA synthesis and mitosis. This function is regulated by phosphorylation and dephosphorylation events in the nucleus.

Other Tumor Suppressor Genes

p53

p53 is the second gene recognized to encode a protein that has the properties of a tumor suppressor gene. This gene is a nuclear phosphoprotein initially detected by immunologic methods in transformed cells.[228] Early experiments using what was assumed to be wild-type p53 showed that it could cooperate with the *ras* gene to transform rat embryo fibroblasts.[229] The p53 cDNA clones that were used in those experiments encoded a mutant p53. It is now recognized that p53 forms oligomers. The introduction of mutant p53 therefore was able to complex and functionally inactivate the wild-type p53 present in the cells. The number of human tumors that have mutations in p53 has increased rapidly since the search for alterations has been performed using highly sensitive polymerase chain reaction analysis. The list of tumors includes osteosarcomas, breast, colon, and lung carcinomas, brain tumors, and chronic myelogenous leukemias in blast crisis.[230,231] In all of these tumors, the alterations in p53 represent one of several gene alterations. Therefore, the point during the process of tumor formation that the p53 alterations occur is not clear. The fact that transgenic mice whose cells all express mutant p53 that inactivates normal p53 form a wide range of tumors at high incidences also indicates that p53 inactivation is important in the initiation of many malignancies.[232] Members of families who carry germ line p53 mutations are at significantly higher risk for developing breast cancer, sarcomas, and several other malignancies (the Li-Fraumeni syndrome).[233] This is the first evidence of a mutation in a tumor suppressor gene causing susceptibility to common adult malignancies. It also provides evidence that the inactivation of p53 is a rate-limiting step in the transformation of several tissues.

The little that is known about the biochemical function of p53 reveals many similarities to p105Rb. Both are nuclear phosphoproteins that undergo cell cycle specific phosphorylation and are underphosphorylated in G0 and G1.[234]

DCC

DCC is an acronym for *d*eleted in *c*olon *c*arcinomas. This gene was found by the technique of positional cloning after karyotypic and DNA marker polymorphism analysis of colon carcinomas revealed frequent deletions of the long arm of chromosome 18.[235] The gene was identified in a 370-kb region of 18q21, where deletions in colon carcinomas commonly occur. Expression of the DCC protein product is greatly reduced or absent in most colon carcinomas. Insertions and point deletions within the DNA encoding of this gene are common causes of reduced expression. The importance of the DCC gene loss in tumor initiation is also indicated by the observation that affected members of families with Lynch syndrome, one of the several forms of familial colon carcinoma, have constitutive changes in the DCC gene. The gene is expressed at low levels in most normal tissues and in noncolon tumors. Unlike p105Rb and p53, the DCC gene encodes a cell surface molecule with sequence homology to some neural cell adhesion molecules.[235]

Wilms' Tumor Gene

Wilms' tumor is an embryonal renal tumor of childhood for which the model of sporadic and hereditary components developed for retinoblastoma applies. Important differences are seen in the incidence at which affected members develop tumors. Whereas the number of retinoblastomas in each affected family member is two to five, the penetrance of the Wilms' tumor risk is so low that entire generations of affected members may not form any tumors. This low frequency of tumors suggests that, unlike retinoblastomas, the formation of Wilms' tumors requires multiple initiating events. This appears to be the case since inactivation of at least three candidate genes may be required to alter the normal growth of embryonal renal cells. A gene that is altered in sporadic Wilms' tumors has been cloned from chromosome subregion 11q13.[236,237] This candidate gene is primarily expressed in the kidney and some hematopoietic cell lines. Sequence analysis suggests that it encodes a nuclear transcription factor because it contains four tandem zinc finger motifs (sequences known to be involved in DNA binding in other proteins). This gene is clearly different from one that has been found to be altered among patients with Beckwith-Weidemann syndrome who are at high risk for Wilms' tumors, hyperplasia of many organs, and a predisposition for several other embryonal tumors such as hepatoblastomas and rhabdomyosarcomas. Patients with Beckwith-Weidemann syndrome have alterations in a separate gene that maps to 11p15.5.[238] A third gene is altered in members of families that get Wilms' tumors. This familial Wilms' gene does not map to the short arm of chromosome 11 and gives a higher risk of Wilms' tumor only in affected family members.[239,240] How the products of these three genes interact in the pathogenesis of Wilms' tumor is unknown.

Potential Tumor Suppressor Genes

The genes that have been described represent all the tumor suppressor genes that have been identified to date. Many

TABLE 6-2. Chromosome Deletions Associated With Human Malignancies*

	Chromosome Location											
Pathology	**1p**	**1q**	**2**	**3p**	**5q**	**6q**	**10p**	**11p**	**13q**	**17p**	**18q**	**22**
Adrenocortical carcinoma								266				
Bilateral acoustic neurofibromatosis												273, 202
Bladder carcinoma								203	214 (Rb)			
Breast carcinoma	247	243						241	255, 252 (Rb)		230 (p53)	
Cervical carcinoma				275								
CML blast crisis										231 (p53)		
Colon carcinoma					274					248, 230 (p53)	274 (DCC)	
Gliomas							249			248, 230 (p53)		
Hepatoblastoma								253				
Hepatocellular carcinoma								246		244 (p53)		
Insulinoma								203				
Lung carcinoma (small cell)				262					218 (Rb)	218, 270 (p53)		
Lung carcinoma (NSCLC)				218						230 (p53)		
Melanoma	242					272						
MEN type 1								254				
MEN type 2	256						257, 271					
Meningioma	250					250						267, 245
Myelodysplasia (AML)					251							
Neuroblastoma	258											
Osteosarcoma									212, 217 (Rb)	259 (p53)		
Pheochromocytoma	265											
PNET										264		
Renal cell carcinoma				263, 276								
Retinoblastoma									212 (Rb)			
Rhabdomyosarcoma								253		260		
Soft tissue sarcoma									216 (Rb)			
Thyroid medullary carcinoma	265											
Uveal melanoma			261									
Von Hippel–Lindau disease				268								
Wilms' tumor								269				

CML, chronic myelogenous leukemia; MEN, multiple endocrine neoplasia; PNET, peripheral neuroectodermal tumor.
* Numbers in table indicate references.

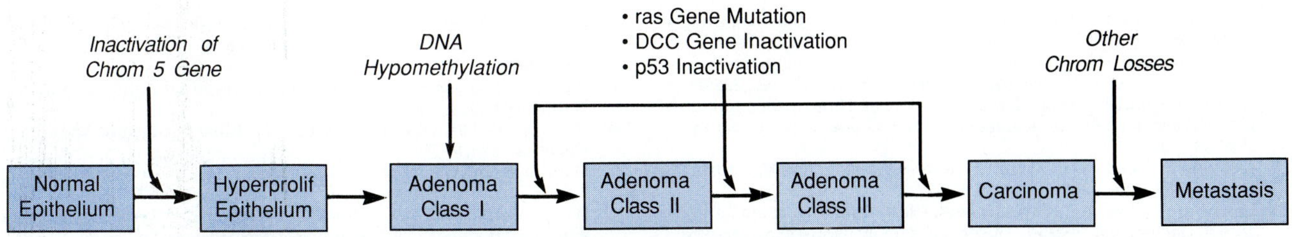

FIGURE 6-15. A model for colorectal carcinogenesis. The multiple steps that result in a carcinoma that is able to metastasize are shown with the series of associated molecular and chromosomal events. (Adapted from Vogelstein B, Fearon ER, Baker SJ, et al. Genetic alterations accumulate during colorectal tumorigenesis. In: Cavenee W, ed. Recessive oncogenes and tumor suppression. Cold Spring Harbor, New York, Cold Spring Harbor Laboratory Press, 1989)

other genomic regions are thought to contain other tumor suppressor genes. Studies looking for evidence of tumor suppressor genes have relied heavily on loss of heterozygosity observations for a large number of polymorphic DNA markers from various regions of the genome. Table 6-2 lists the many sites that may harbor tumor suppressor genes, based on observations of consistent, nonrandom loss of heterozygosity for particular tumors. Because loss of heterozygosity may occur to a certain extent at random, simply as a reflection of the aneuploid state of many tumors, some of the observed losses of heterozygosity may not indicate the location of a potential tumor suppressor gene. The strongest candidate sites have also been found through chromosome analysis to be linked among affected family members. These have been indicated by an asterisk. The list of 31 tumors clearly represents only a partial list that continues to expand as other tumors are examined. In addition, the specific chromosomal regions that have been studied remain a minority of the possible sites, since highly polymorphic DNA probes are not yet available for the entire human genome. Surveying the partial list, several interesting observations can be made. Some tumors have many associated deletions. These tumors are predominantly adult malignancies.

The most coherent attempt at fitting these many changes into a pathogenesis that accounts for all of the steps required from initiation of a malignancy to development of a metastatic cancer has been proposed by Bert Vogelstein for colon carcinoma.[278] As shown in Figure 6-15, colon carcinogenesis occurs as a progressive series of alterations in both dominant oncogenes and tumor suppressor genes. This is an acknowledged simplification of the actual pathway, but it conveys the complexity that is emerging as more of these tumors and genes are studied. Chromosome regions such as 17p, in which the p53 gene is located, are altered in most tumors. This indicates that p53 alterations may result in more general effects than just altering a tissue-specific cell fate. As more complete information is gained about the identities and specific alterations of the tumor suppressor genes that occur in various tumors, our understanding of the process is likely to become less complex as the fundamental rules that govern growth deregulation are discerned.

TABLE 6-3. Major Oncogenes and Tumor Suppressor Genes (Not Comprehensive)

DOMINANT ONCOGENES	TUMOR SUPPRESSOR GENES
Tyrosine kinases	Retinoblastoma gene
src	p53
abl	DCC
Growth factors	Wilms' tumor gene
v-*sis*	
Receptor tyrosine kinases	
v-*fms*	
ras	
Nuclear oncogenes	
myc	
fos	
jun	
bcl-2	

SUMMARY

Two different classes of genes that directly control the proliferation of cells can be defined (Table 6-3). The oncogenes represent activated forms of growth-potentiating genes. They are all members of a signaling cascade from growth factors to the nucleus. The alterations that activate these genes produce either overexpression or inappropriate expression of the protein, or they produce an inappropriate activity of the protein. These activations can sometimes result from observable chromosomal changes. Such changes include gene amplifications (detectable by the presence of homogeneous staining regions or double minutes) and chromosomal translocations. Many dominant oncogenes have been identified by gene transfer studies.

The tumor suppressor genes define a separate class of genes whose normal function is to limit the growth of cells. The inactivation of these genes contributes to the malignant process. Although evidence suggests that tumor suppressor genes exist, only a few genes have been identified. They are likely to define a cell cycle and differentiation control circuit that extends from the cell surface to the nucleus. Observable chromosomal changes associated with the inactivation of tumor suppressor genes are usually the result of translocations or deletions of large portions of a chromosome. Such changes are detectable either by the loss of specific chromosomal markers by cytogenetic analysis. Whereas the gene transfer assay has not been helpful in isolating inactivated tumor suppressor genes, their presence has been detected by cell hybrid fusion assays.

The task of the next decades will be to define the components of the growth-activating and growth-limiting pathways so that the knowledge about the circuits that control cellular growth can suggest rational therapeutic interventions.

REFERENCES

1. Folkman J, Moscona A. Role of cell shape in growth control. Nature 1978;273:345.
2. Pollack R, Chen S, Powess S, et al. Transformation mechanisms at the cellular level. Adv Viral Oncol 1984;4:3.
3. Ruvkin G, Giusho J. The caenorhabditis elegans heterochromic gene lin-14 encodes a nuclear protein but forms a temporal development switch. Nature 1989;338:313.

4. Beach D, Durkacz B, Nurse PM. Functionally homologous cell cycle control genes in budding and fission yeast. Nature 1982;300:706.
5. Lee MG, Nurse P. Complementation used to clone a human homologue of the fission yeast cell cycle control gene cdc 2. Nature 1987;327:51.
6. Draetta G, Piwnica-Worms H, Morrison D, et al. Human cdc2 protein kinase is a major cellcycle regulated tyrosine kinase substrate. Nature 1988;336:738.
7. D'Andrea AD, Lodish HF, Wong GG. Expression cloning of the murine erythropoietin receptor. Cell 1989;57:277.
8. Downward J, Yarden J, Mayes E, et al. Close similarity of epidermal growth factor and v-*erb*-B oncogene protein sequences. Nature 1984;307:521.
9. Gilman AG. G proteins: transducers of receptor-generated signals. Annu Rev Biochem 1987;56:615.
10. D'Andrea AD, Fasman GD, Lodish HF. Erythropoietin receptor and interleukin-2 receptor beta chain: a new receptor family. Cell 1989;58: 1023.
11. Downward J, Parker P, Waterfield MD. Autophosphorylation sites on the epidermal growth factor receptor. Nature 1984;311:483.
12. Stryer L. Biochemistry. New York, WF Freeman, 1988.
13. Parker PJ, Coussens L, Totty N, et al. The complete primary structure of protein kinase c: the major phorbol ester receptor. Science 1986;233: 853.
14. Carpenter D, Jackson T, Hanley MR. Coping with a growing family. Nature 1987;325:107.
15. Evans RM. The steroid and thyroid receptor superfamily. Science 1988;240:889.
16. Kohl NE, Legouy E, DePintro RA, et al. Nature 1986;319:73.
17. Nau M, Brooks BJ, Battey J, et al. L-*myc*, a new *myc*-related gene amplified and expressed in human small cell lung cancer. Nature 1985;318: 69.
18. Turner R, Tjian R. Leucine repeats and an adjacent DNA binding domain mediate the formation of functional cfos-cjun heterodimers. Science 1989;243:1689.
19. Bohmann D, Bos TJ, Admon A, et al. Human proto-oncogene c-*jun* encodes a DNA binding protein with structural and functional properties of transcription factor AP-1. Science 1987;238:1386.
20. Berenson JR, Yang J, Mickel RA. Frequent amplifications of the bcl-1 locus in head and neck squamous cell carcinomas. Oncogene 1989;4: 1111.
21. Berenson JR, Koga H, Yang J. Frequent amplification of the bcl-1 locus in poorly differentiated squamous cell cancer of the lung. Oncogene 1990;5:1343.
22. Brodeur GM. Molecular correlates of cytogenetic abnormalities in human cancer cells. Prog Hematol 1988;14:229.
23. Diaz MO, LeBeau MM, Rowley JD. The role of the c-*mos* gene in the 8:21 translocations in human acute myeloblastic leukemia. Science 1985;229:767.
24. Eva A, Tronick SR. Transforming genes of human hematopoietic tumors: frequent detection of *ras*-related oncogenes whose activation appears to be independent of tumor phenotype. Proc Natl Acad Sci USA 1983;80:4926.
25. Feig LA, Bast RCJ, Knapp RC. Somatic activation of *ras* k gene in a human ovarian carcinoma. Science 1984;223:698.
26. Drucker BJ, J MH, M RT. Oncogenes, growth factors and signal transduction. N Engl J Med 1989;321:1383.
27. Fukui M, Yamamoto T, Kawai S. Detection of a *raf*-related and two other transforming DNA sequences in human tumors maintained in nude mice. Proc Natl Acad Sci USA 1985;82:5954.
28. Heisterkemp N, Stephenson JR, Groffen J. Localization of the c-*abi* oncogene adjacent to a translocation breakpoint in chronic myelogenous leukemia. Nature 1983;306:239.
29. Koduru PRK, Offit K, Filippa DA. Molecular analysis of breaks in bc1-1 proto-oncogene in B-cell lymphomas with abnormalities in 11q13. Oncogene 1989;4:929.
30. Little CD, Nau MM, Carney DN. Amplification and expression of the c-*myc* oncogene in human lung cancer cell lines. Nature 1983;306: 194.
31. Murray MJ, Cunningham JM, Parada L. The Hc-60 transforming sequence: a *ras* oncogene coexisting with altered *myc* genes in hematopoietic tumors. Cell 1983;33:749.
32. Nau MM, Brooks BJ, Carney DN. Human small-cell lung cancers show amplification and expression of the N-*myc* gene. Proc Natl Acad Sci USA 1986;83:1092.
33. Shimizu K, Goldferb M, Suard Y. Three human transformation genes are related to the viral *ras* oncogenes. Proc Natl Acad Sci USA 1983;80: 2112.
34. Schwab M, Alitalo K, Klempnauer KH. Amplified DNA with limited homology to myc cellular oncogene is shared by human neuroblastoma cell lines and a neuroblastoma tumor. Nature 1983;305:245.
35. Theillet C, Adnane J, Szepetowsk P. *bcl*-1 participates in the 11p13 amplification found in breast cancer. Oncogene 1990;5:147.
36. Somers KD, Cartwright SL, Schecter GL. Amplification of the int-2 gene in head and neck squamous cell carcinomas. Oncogene 1990;5: 915.
37. Slamon DJ, deKernion JB, Verma IM. Expression of cellular oncogenes. Science 1984;224:256.
38. Souyri M, Fleissner E. Identification by transfection of transforming sequences in DNA of human T-cell leukemias. Proc Natl Acad Sci USA 1983;80:6676.
39. Pulciani S, Santos E, Laurer AV. Oncogenes in solid human tumors. Nature 1982;300:539.
40. Varmus HE. The molecular genetics of cellular oncogenes. Annu Rev Genetics 1984;18:553.
41. Whittle IR. Oncogenes and neuro-oncology. Br J Neurosurgery 1989;3: 3.
42. Wu JX, Carpenter PM, Gresens GC. The proto-oncogene c-*fos* is over expressed in the majority of human osteosarcomas. Oncogene 1990;5: 989.
43. Yunis JJ. The chromosomal basis of human neoplasia. Science 1983;21: 227.
44. Yuasa Y, L SS, Dunn CY. Acquisition of transforming properties by alternative point mutations within c-*ras-has* human proto-oncogene. Nature 1983;303:775.
45. Israel MA. Molecular cellular biology of pediatric malignancies. In: Pizzo PA, Poplack DG, eds. Principles and practice of pediatric oncology. Philadelphia, JB Lippincott, 1989.
46. Alitalo K, Schwab M. Oncogene amplification in tumor cells: a review. Adv Cancer Res 1986;47:235.
47. Rous P. Transmission of a malignant new growth by means of a cell-free filtrate. JAMA 1911;56:198.
48. Lipsich LA, Cutt JR, Brugge JS. Association of the transforming proteins of Rous, Fujinami and Y73 sarcoma viruses with the same two cellular proteins. Mol Cell Biol 1982;2:875.
49. Brugge J, Erikson E, Erikson RD. The specific interaction of the Rous sarcoma virus transforming protein, pp60*src* with two cellular proteins. Cell 1981;25:362.
50. Buss JE, Sefton BM. Myristic acid, a rare fatty acid, is the lipid attached to the transforming protein of Rous sarcoma virus and its cellular homolog. J Virol 1985;52:7.
51. Garber EA, Cross FR, Hanafusa H. Processing of p60v-*src* to its myristylated membrane-bound form. Mol Cell Biol 1985;5:2781.
52. Rohrschneider LR. Adhesion plaques of Rous sarcoma virus-transformed cells contain the *src* gene product. Proc Natl Acad Sci USA 1980;77:3514.
53. Kypta RM, Goldberg Y, Ulug ET, et al. Association between the PDGF receptor and members of the *src* family of tyrosine kinases. Cell 1990;62: 481.
54. Cooper JA, Bowen-Pope DF, Raines E, et al. Similar effects of platelet-derived growth factor and epidermal growth factor on the phosphorylation of tyrosine in cellular proteins. Cell 1982;31:263.
55. Gilmore TD, Radke K, Martin GS. Tyrosine phosphorylation of a 50K cellular polypeptide associated with the Rous sarcoma virus transforming protein pp60*src*. Mol Cell Biol 1982;2:199.
56. Cooper JA, Gould KL, Cartwright CA, et al. Tyr527 is phosphorylated in pp60c-*src*: implications for regulation. Science 1986;231:1431.
57. Morgan DO, Kaplan JM, Bishop JM, et al. Mitosis-specific phosphorylation of p60c-*src* by p34cdc2-associated protein kinase. Cell 1989;57: 775.
58. Shenoy S, Choi J-K, Bagrodia S, et al. Purified maturation promoting factor phosphorylates pp60c-*src* at the sites phosphorylated during fibroblast mitosis. Cell 1989;57:763.
59. Hunter T. A tail of two *src*'s: mutatis mutandis. Cell 1987;49:1.
60. Levy JB, Iba H, Hanafusa H. Activation of the transforming potential of p60c-*src* by a single amino acid change. Proc Natl Acad Sci USA 1986;83:4228.
61. Cartwright CA, Eckhardt W, Simon S, et al. Cell transformation by pp60c-*src* mutated in the carboxy-terminal regulatory domain. Cell 1987;49:83.
62. Kmiecik TE, Shalloway D. Activation and suppression of pp60c-*src* transforming ability by mutation of its primary sites of tyrosine phosphorylation. Cell 1987;49:65.
63. Piwnica-Worms H, Saunders KB, Roberts TM, et al. Tyrosine phosphorylation regulates the biochemical and biological properties of pp60c-*src*. Cell 1987;49:75.
64. Hanks SK, Quinn AM, Hunter T. The protein kinase family: conserved features and deduced phylogeny of the catalytic domains. Science 1988;241:42.
65. deKlein A, vanKessel AG, Grosveld G, et al. A cellular oncogene is translocated to the Philadelphia chromosome in chronic myelocytic leukaemia. Nature 1982;300:765.
66. Abelson HT, Rabstein LS. Influence of prednisolone on Moloney leukemogenic virus in BALB/c mice. Cancer Res 1970;30:2208.
67. Shields A, Otto G, Goff S, et al. Structure of the Abelson murine leukemia virus genome. Cell 1979;18:955.
68. Besmer P, Hardy WD Jr, Zuckerman EE, et al. The Hardy-Zuckerman 2-FeSV: a new feline retrovirus with oncogene homology to Abelson-MuLV. Nature 1983;303:825.
69. Bergold PJ, Blumenthal JA, D'Andrea E, et al. Nucleic acid sequence and oncogenic properties of the HZ2 feline sarcoma virus v-*abl* insert. J Virol 1987;61:1193.
70. Bartram CR, deKlein A, Hagemeijer A, et al. Translocation of c-*abl* oncogene correlates with the presence of a Philadelphia chromosome in chronic myelocytic leukaemia. Nature 1983;306:277.

71. Heisterkamp N, Groffen J, Stephenson JR, et al. Chromosomal localization of human cellular homologues of two viral oncogenes. Nature 1982;299:747.
72. Nowell PC, Hungerford DA. A minute chromosome in human chronic granulocytic leukemia. Science 1960;132:1497.
73. Rowley JD. A new consistent chromosomal abnormality in chronic myelogenous leukaemia identified by quinacrine fluorescence and Giemsa staining. Nature 1973;243:290.
74. Shtivelman E, Lifshitz B, Gale RP, et al. Alternative splicing of RNAs transcribed from the human abl gene and from the *bcr-abl* fused gene. Cell 1986;47:277.
75. Rosenberg N, Witte ON. The viral and cellular forms of the Ableson (*abl*) oncogene. Adv Virus Res 1988;35:39.
76. Kipreos ET, Lee GJ, Wang JYJ. Isolation of temperature-sensitive tyrosine kinase mutants of v-*abl* oncogene by screening with antibodies for phosphotyrosine. Proc Natl Acad Sci USA 1987;84:1345.
77. Takemori T, Miyazoe I, Shirasawa T, et al. A temperature-sensitive mutant of Abelson murine leukemia virus confers inducibility of IgM expression to transformed lymphoid cells. EMBO J 1987;6:951.
78. Rohrschneider LR, Najita LM. Detection of the v-*abl* gene product at cell-substratum contact sites in Abelson murine leukemia virus–transformed fibroblasts. J Virol 1984;51:547.
79. Van Etten RA, Jackson P, Baltimore D. The mouse type IV c-*abl* gene product is a nuclear protein, and activation of transforming ability is associated with cytoplasmic localization. Cell 1989;58:669.
80. Franz WM, Berger P, Wang JYJ. Deletion of an N-terminal regulatory domain of the c-*abl* tyrosine kinase activates its oncogenic potential. EMBO J 1989;8:137.
81. Jackson P, Baltimore D. N-terminal mutations activate the leukemogenic potential of the myristoylated form of c-*abl*. EMBO J 1989;8:449.
82. Pawson T. Non-catalytic domains of cytoplasmic protein–tyrosine kinases: regulatory elements in signal transduction. Oncogene 1989;3: 491.
83. Wang JY. Negative regulation of c-*abl* tyrosine kinase by its variable N-terminal amino acids. Oncogene Res 1988;3:293.
84. Prywes R, Hoag J, Rosenberg N, et al. Protein stabilization explains the *gag* requirement for transformation of lymphoid cells by Abelson murine leukemia virus. J Virol 1985;54:123.
85. Wantanabe SM, Witte ON. Site-directed deletions of Abelson murine leukemia virus define 3′ sequences essential for transformation and lethality. J Virol 1983;45:1028.
86. Fialkow PJ, Martin PJ, Najfeld V, et al. Evidence for a multistep pathogenesis of chronic myelogenous leukemia. Blood 1981;58:158.
87. Daley GQ, Baltimore D. Transformation of an interleukin 3–dependent hematopoietic cell line by the chronic myelogenous leukemia–specific P210*bcr*/*abl* protein. Proc Natl Acad Sci USA 1988;85:9312.
88. Chan LC, Karhi KK, Rayter SI, et al. A novel abl protein expressed in Philadelphia chromosome positive acute lymphoblastic leukaemia. Nature 1987;325:635.
89. Clark SS, McLaughlin J, Crist WM, et al. Unique forms of the abl tyrosine kinase distinguish Ph1-positive CML from Ph1-positive ALL. Science 1987;235:85.
90. Deuel TF, Jung SH, Huang SS, et al. Expression of a platelet-derived growth factor–like protein in Simian sarcoma virus transformed cells. Science 1983;221:1348.
91. Smith R, Peters G, Dickson C. Multiple RNAs expressed from the int-2 gene in mouse embryonal carcinoma cell lines encode a protein with homology to fibroblast growth factors. EMBO J 1988;7:1013.
92. Yoshida T, Miyagawa K, Odagiri H, et al. Genomic sequence of hst, a transforming gene encoding a protein homologous to fibroblast growth factors and the int-2 encoded protein. Proc Natl Acad Sci USA 1987;84: 7305.
93. Delli Bovi P, Curatola AM, Kern FG, et al. An oncogene isolated by transfection of Kaposi's sarcoma DNA encodes a growth factor that is a member of the FGF family. Cell 1987;50:729.
94. Keating MT, Williams LT. Autocrine stimulation of intracellular PDGF receptors in v-*sis*–transformed cells. Science 1988;239:914.
95. Bejcek BE, Li DY, Deuel TF. Transformation by v-*sis* occurs by an internal autoactivation mechanism. Science 1989;245:1496.
96. Yarden Y, Ullrich A. Growth factor receptor tyrosine kinases. Annu Rev Biochem 1988;57:443.
97. Yamamoto T, Nishida T, Miyajima N, et al. The *erb* B gene of avian erythroblastosis virus is a member of the *src* gene family. Cell 1983;35: 71.
98. Sherr CJ, Rettenmier CW, Sacca R, et al. The c-*fms* proto-oncogene product is related to the receptor for the mononuclear phagocyte growth factor, CSF-1. Cell 1985;41:665.
99. Hampe A, Gobet M, Sherr CJ, et al. Nucleotide sequence of the feline retroviral oncogene v-*fms* shows unexpected homology with oncogenes encoding tyrosine-specific protein kinases. Proc Natl Acad Sci USA 1984;81:85.
100. Bargmann CI, Hung M-C, Weinberg RA. Multiple independent activations of the neu oncogene by a point mutation altering the transmembrane domain of p185. Cell 1986;45:649.
101. Berridge MJ, Heslop JP, Irvine RF, et al. Inositol trisphosphate formation and calcium mobilization in Swiss 3T3 cells in response to platelet-derived growth factor. Biochem J 1984;222:195.
102. Ives HE, Daniel TO. Interrelationship between growth factor–induced pH changes and intracellular calcium. Proc Natl Acad Sci USA 1987;84: 1950.
103. Bockus BJ, Stiles CD. Regulation of cytoskeletal architecture by platelet-derived growth factor, insulin and epidermal growth factor. Exp Cell Res 1984;153:186.
104. Cochran BH, Reffel AC, Stiles CD. Molecular cloning of gene sequences regulated by platelet-derived growth factor. Cell 1983;33:939.
105. Ullrich A, Sclessinger J. Signal transduction by receptors with tyrosine kinase activity. Cell 1990;61:203.
106. Escobedo JA, Williams LT. A PDGF receptor domain essential for mitogenesis but not for many other responses to PDGF. Nature 1988;335: 85.
107. Morrison DK, Kaplan DR, Escobedo JA, et al. Direct activation of the serine/threonine kinase activity of Raf-1 through tyrosine phosphorylation by the PDGF β-receptor. Cell 1989;58:649.
108. Meisenhelder J, Suh P-G, Rhee SG, et al. Phospholipase C-gamma is a substrate for the PDGF and EGF receptor protein-tyrosine kinases in vivo and in vitro. Cell 1989;57:1109.
109. Wahl MI, Daniel TO, Carpenter G. Antiphosphotyrosine recovery of phospholipase C activity after EGF treatment of A-431 cells. Science 1988;241:968.
110. Kaplan DR, Morrison DK, Wong G, et al. PDGF beta-receptor stimulates tyrosine phosphorylation of GAP and association of GAP with a signalling complex. Cell 1990;61:125.
111. Ellis C, Moran M, McCormick F, et al. Phosphorylation of GAP and GAP-associated proteins by transforming and mitogenic tyrosine kinases. Nature 1990;343:377.
112. Kazlauskas A, Ellis C, Pawson T, et al. Binding of GAP to activated PDGF receptors. Science 1990;247:1578.
113. McDonough SK, Larsen S, Brodey RS, et al. A transmissible feline fibrosarcomal of viral origin. Cancer Res 1971;31:953.
114. Sacca R, Stanley ER, Sherr CJ, et al. Specific binding of the mononuclear phagocyte colony-stimulating factor CSF-1 to the product of the v-fms oncogene. Proc Natl Acad Sci USA 1986;83:3331.
115. Jackowski S, Rettenmier CW, Sherr CJ, et al. A guanine nucleotide–dependent phosphatidylinositol 4,5-diphosphate phospholipase C in cells transformed by the v-*fms* and v-*fes* oncogenes. J Biol Chem 1986;261:4978.
116. Varticovski L, Druker B, Morrison D, et al. The colony stimulating factor-1 receptor associates with and activates phosphatidylinositol-3 kinase. Nature 1989;342:699.
117. Harvey JJ. An unidentified virus which causes the rapid production of tumours in mice. Nature 1964;204:1104.
118. Kirsten WH, Mayer LA. Morphologic responses to a murine erythroblastosis virus. J Natl Cancer Inst 1967;39:311.
119. Barbacid M. *Ras* genes. Annu Rev Biochem 1987;56:779.
120. Saiki RK, Scharf S, Faloona F, et al. Enzymatic amplification of β-globin genomic sequences and restriction site analysis for diagnosis of sickle cell anemia. Science 1985;230:1350.
121. Reddy EP, Reynolds RK, Santos E, et al. A point mutation is responsible for the acquisition of transforming properties by the T24 human bladder carcinoma oncogene. Nature 1982;300:149.
122. Tabin CJ, Bradley SM, Bargmann CI, et al. Mechanism of activation of a human oncogene. Nature 1982;300:143.
123. Taparowsky E, Suard Y, Fasano O, et al. Activation of the T24 bladder carcinoma transforming gene is linked to a single amino acid change. Nature 1982;300:762.
124. Willingham MC, Pastan I, Shih TY, et al. Localization of the src gene product of the Harvey strain of MSV to the plasma membrane of transformed cells by electron microscopic immunocytochemistry. Cell 1980;19:1005.
125. Willumsen BM, Christensen A, Hubbert NL, et al. The p21 *ras* C-terminal is required for transformation and membrane association. Nature 1984;310:583.
126. Hancock JF, Magee AI, Childs JE, et al. All *ras* proteins are polyisoprenylated but only some are palmitoylated. Cell 1989;57:1167.
127. Schafer WR, Kim R, Sterne R, et al. Genetic and pharmacologic suppression of oncogenic mutations in RAS genes of yeast and humans. Science 1989;245:379.
128. Hall A. The cellular functions of small GTP-binding proteins. Science 1990;249:635.
129. Smith MR, Liu Y, Kim H, et al. Inhibition of serum- and *ras*-stimulated DNA synthesis by antibodies to phospholipase C. Science 1990;247: 1074.
130. Sigal IS. The *ras* oncogene: structure and some function. Nature 1988;332:485.
131. Trahey M, McCormick F. A cytoplasmic protein stimulates normal N-*ras* p21 GTPase, but does not affect oncogenic mutants. Science 1987;238:542.
132. Zhang K, DeClue JE, Vass WC, et al. Suppression of c-*ras* transformation by GTPase-activating protein. Nature 1990;346:754.
133. Downward J, Graves JD, Warne PH, et al. Stimulation of p21*ras* upon T-cell activation. Nature 1990;346:719.
134. DeVos AM, Tong L, Milburn MV, et al. Three-dimensional structure of an oncogenic protein product catalytic domain of human c-H-*ras* p21. Science 1988;239:888.

135. Pai EF, Kabsch W, Krengel U, et al. Structure of the guanin-nucleotide-binding domain of the Ha-*ras* oncogene product p21 in the triphosphate conformation. Nature 1989;341:209.
136. Krengel U, Schlichting I, Scherer A, et al. Three-dimensional structures of H-*ras* p21 mutants: molecular basis for their inability to function as signal switch molecules. Cell 1990;62:539.
137. Milburn MV, Tong L, deVos AM, et al. Molecular switch for signal transduction: structural differences between active and inactive forms of protooncogenic *ras* proteins. Science 1990;247:939.
138. Kitayama H, Sugimoto Y, Matsuzaki T, et al. A *ras*-related gene with transformation suppressor activity. Cell 1989;56:77.
139. Bos JL, Verlann-de Vries M, van der Eb AJ, et al. Mutations in N-*ras* predominate in acute myeloid leukemia. Blood 1987;69:1237.
140. Hirai H, Kobayashi Y, Mano H, et al. A point mutation at codon 13 of the N-*ras* oncogene in myelodysplastic syndrome. Nature 1987;327:430.
141. Liu E, Hjelle B, Morgan R, et al. Mutations of the Kirsten-*ras* proto-oncogene in human preleukemia. Nature 1987;330:186.
142. Yunis JJ, Frizzera G, Oken MM, et al. Multiple recurrent genomic defects in follicular lymphoma: a possible model for cancer. N Engl J Med 1987;316:79.
143. Yunis J, Boot AJM, Mayer MG, et al. Mechanisms of *ras* mutation in myelodysplastic syndrome. Oncogene 1989;4:609.
144. Kumar R, Sukumar S, Barbacid M. Activation of *ras* oncogenes preceding the onset of neoplasia. Science 1990;248:1101.
145. Fukuhara S, Rowley JD, Variakojis D, et al. Chromosome abnormalities in poorly differentiated lymphocytic lymphoma. Cancer Res 1979;39:3119.
146. Tsujimoto Y, Finger LR, Yunis J, et al. Cloning of the chromosome breakpoint of neoplastic B cells with the t(14;18) chromosome translocation. Science 1984;226:1097.
147. Weiss LM, Warnke RA, Sklar J, et al. Molecular analysis of the t(14;18) chromosomal translocation in malignant lymphomas. N Engl J Med 1987;317:1185.
148. Ngan B, Chen-Levy Z, Weiss LW, et al. Expression in non-Hodgkin's lymphoma of the *bcl*-2 protein associated with the t(14;18) chromosomal translocation. N Engl J Med 1988;318:1638.
149. Chen-Levy Z, Nourse J, Cleary ML. The *bcl*-2 candidate proto-oncogene product is a 24-kilodalton integral-membrane protein highly expressed in lymphoid cell lines and lymphomas carrying the t(14;18) translocation. Mol Cell Biol 1989;9:701.
150. Hockenberry D, Nunez G, Milliman C, et al. *Bcl*-2 is an inner mitochondrial membrane protein that blocks programmed cell death. Nature 1990;348:334.
151. Seto M, Jaeger U, Hockett RD, et al. Alternative promoters and exons, somatic mutation and deregulation of the *Bcl*-2-lg fusion gene in lymphoma. EMBO J 1988;7:123.
152. Reed JC, Tsujimoto Y, Alpers JD, et al. Regulation of *bcl*-2 proto-oncogene expression during normal human lymphocyte proliferation. Science 1987;236:1295.
153. Reed JC, Cuddy M, Slabiak T, et al. Oncogenic potential of *bcl*-2 demonstrated by gene transfer. Nature 1988;336:259.
154. Vaux DL, Cory S, Adams JM. *Bcl*-2 gene promotes haemopoietic cell survival and cooperates with c-myc to immortalize pre-B cells. Nature 1988;335:440.
155. Monica K, Chen-Levy Z, Cleary ML. Small G proteins are expressed ubiquitously in lymphoid cells and do not correspond to *Bcl*-2. Nature 1990;346:189.
156. Beard JW. Avian oncorna viruses: biology. In: Klein G, ed. Viral oncology. New York, Raven Press, 1980.
157. Murray JA, Begg AM. Histology and histogenesis of filtrable endothelioma of fowl. Sci Rep Inv Imp Cancer Res Fund 1930;9:1.
158. Stewart TA, Bellve AR, Leder P. Transcription and promoter usage of the *myc* gene in normal somatic and spermatogenic cells. Science 1984;226:707.
159. Croce CM, Nowell PC. Molecular basis of human B cell neoplasia. Blood 1985;65:1.
160. Chung J, Sussman DJ, Zeller R, et al. The c-*myc* gene encodes superimposed RNA polymerase II and III promoters. Cell 1987;51:1001.
161. Bentley DL, Groudine M. A block to elongation is largely reponsible for decreased transcription of c-*myc* in differentiated HL60 cells. Nature 1986;301:702.
162. Pelicci PG, Knowles DM, Magrath I, et al. Chromosomal breakpoints and structural alterations of the c-*myc* locus differ in endemic and sporadic forms of Burkitt lymphoma. Proc Natl Acad Sci USA 1986;83:2984.
163. Kakkis E, Riggs KJ, Gillespie W, et al. A transcriptional repressor of c-*myc*. Nature 1989;339:718.
164. Takimoto M, Quinn JP, Farina AR, et al. *fos/jun* and ocatmer-binding protein interact with a common site in a negative element of the human c-*myc* gene. J Biol Chem 1989;264:8992.
165. Curran T, Van Beveren C, Ling N, et al. Viral and cellular fos proteins are complexed with a 39,000-dalton cellular protein. Mol Cell Biol 1985;5:167.
166. Singh J, Sen R, Baltimore D, et al. A nuclear factor that binds to a conserved sequence motif in transcriptional control elements of immunoglobulin genes. Nature 1986;319:154.
167. Hann SR, King MW, Bentley DL, et al. A non-AUG translational initiation in c-*myc* exon 1 generates an N-terminally distinct protein whose synthesis is disrupted in Burkitt's lymphoma. Cell 1988;52:185.
168. Morse B, South VJ, Rothberg PG, et al. Somatic mutation and transcriptional deregulation of *myc* in endemic Burkitt's lymphoma disease: heptamer–nonamer recognition mistakes? Mol Cell Biol 1989;9:74.
169. Dang CV, Lee WMF. Identification of the human c-*myc* protein nuclear translocation signal. Mol Cell Biol 1988;8:4048.
170. Dang DV, McGuire M, Buckmire M, et al. Involvement of the "leucine zipper" region in the oligomerization and transforming activity of human c-*myc* protein. Nature 1989;337:664.
171. Landschulz WJ, Johnson PF, McKnight SL. The leucine zipper: a hypothetical structure common to a new class of DNA binding proteins. Science 1988;240:1759.
172. Kelly K, Cochran RH, Stiles CD, et al. Cell-specific regulation of the c-*myc* gene by lymphocyte mitogens and platelet-derived growth factor. Cell 1983;35:603.
173. Heikkila R, Schwab G, Wickstrom E, et al. A c-*myc* antisense oligonucleotide inhibits entry into S phase but not progress from G_0 to G_1. Nature 1987;328:445.
174. Yokoyama K, Imamoto F. Transcriptional control of the endogenous MYC protooncogene by antisense RNA. Proc Natl Acad Sci USA 1987;84:7363.
175. Studzinski GP, Brelvi ZS, Feldman SC, et al. Participation of c-*myc* protein in DNA synthesis of human cells. Science 1986;234:467.
176. Classon M, Henriksson M, Sumegi J, et al. Elevated c-*myc* facilitates the replication of SV 40 DNA in human lymphoma cells. Nature 1987;330:272.
177. Gutierrez C, Guo Z, Burhans W, et al. Is c-*myc* protein directly involved in DNA replication? Science 1988;240:1202.
178. Croce CM, Huebner K, Isobe M, et al. Mapping of four distinct BCR-related loci to chromosome region 22q11: order of BCR loci relative to chronic myelogenous leukemia and acute lymphoblastic leukemia breakpoints. Proc Natl Acad Sci USA 1987;84:7174.
179. Nishikura K, Ar-Rushdi A, Erikson J, Watt R, Rovera G, Croce CM. Differential expression of the normal and of the translocated human c-*myc* oncogenes in B cells. Proc Natl Acad Sci USA 1983;80:4822.
180. Mitchell KF, Battey J, Hollis GF, et al. The effect of translocations on the cellular *myc* gene in Burkitt lymphomas. J Cell Physiol 1984;3(Suppl):171.
181. Kakkis E, Mercola M, Calame K. Strong transcriptional activation of translocated c-*myc* genes occurs without a strong nearby enhancer or promoter. Nucleic Acids Res 1988;16:77.
182. Muller R. Cellular and viral fos genes: structure, regulation of expression and biological properties of their encoded products. Biochim Biophys Acta 1986;823:207.
183. Varmus HE. Oncogenes and transcription control. Science 1987;238:1337.
184. Verma IM, Sassone-Corsi P. Proto-oncogene *fos*: complex but versatile regulation. Cell 1987;51:513.
185. Wilson T, Treisman R. Removal of poly(A) and consequent degradation of c-*fos* mRNA facilitated by 3′ AU-rich sequences. Nature 1988;336:396.
186. Struhl K. The DNA-binding domains of the *jun* oncoprotein and the yeast GCN4 transcriptional activator proteins are functionally homologous. Cell 1987;50:841.
187. Neuberg M, Schuermann M, Hunter JB, et al. Two functionally different regions in fos are required for the sequence-specific DNA interaction of the *fos/jun* protein complex. Nature 1989;338:589.
188. Rauscher FJ, Cohen DR, Curran T, et al. *Fos*-associated protein p39 is the product of the jun proto-oncogene. Science 1988;240:1010.
189. Kouzarides T, Ziff E. The role of the leucine zipper in the fos-jun interaction. Nature 1988;336:646.
190. O'Shea EK, Rutkowski R, Stafford WF, et al. Preferential heterodimer formation by isolated leucine zippers from *fos* and *jun*. Science 1989;245:646.
191. Chiu R, Boyle WJ, Meek J, et al. The c-*fos* protein interacts with c-*jun*/AP-1 to stimulate transcription of AP-1 responsive genes. Cell 1988;54:541.
192. Neuberg M, Adamkiewicz J, Hunter JB, et al. A *fos* protein containing the jun leucine zipper forms a homodimer which binds to the AP1 binding site. Nature 1989;341:243.
193. Bohmann D, Tijian R. Biochemical analysis of transcriptional activation by jun: differential activity of c- and v-*jun*. Cell 1989;59:709.
194. Jenuwein T, Muller R. Structure-function analysis of fos protein: a single amino acid change activates the immortalizing potential of v-*fos*. Cell 1987;48:647.
195. Harris H, Millel OJ, Klein G, et al. Suppression of malignancy by cell fusion. Nature 1969;223:363.
196. Klein G, Bregula U, Wiener F. The analysis of malignancy by cell fusion. J Cell Sci 1974;8:659.
197. Croce DM, Koprowski H. Somatic cell hybrids between peritoneal mouse macrophages and SV40-transformed human cells. J Exp Med 1974;140:1221.
198. Johasson J, Povey S, Harris H. The analysis of malignancy by cell fusion VII. J Cell Science 1977;24:217.

199. Benedict WF, Weissman BE, Mark C, et al. Tumorigenicity of HT 1080 fibrosarcoma x normal fibroblast hybrids. Cancer Res 1984;44:3471.
200. Stoler A, Bouck N. Identification of a single chromosome in the normal human genome essential for suppression of hamster cell transformation. Proc Natl Acad Sci USA 1985;82:570.
201. Stanbridge EJ. Genetic regulation of tumorigenic expression in somatic cell hybrids. Adv Viral Oncol 1987;6:83.
202. Seizinger BR, Martusa RL, Gusella JF. Loss of genes on chromosome 22 in tumorigenesis of human acoustic neuroma. Nature 1986;322: 655.
203. Green AR. Recessive mechanisms of malignancy. Br J Cancer 1988;58: 115.
204. Chan JYH, Becker FF, German J, et al. Altered DNA ligase 1 activity in Bloom's syndrome cells. Nature 1987;325:357.
205. Weeda G, vonHam RCA, Vermeulen W, Bootsma D, et al. A presumed DNA helicase encoded by ERCC-3 involved in the human repair disorders xerodema pigmentosum and cockcaynes syndrome. Cell 1990;62: 777.
206. Comings DE. General theory of carcinogenesis. Proc Natl Acad Sci USA 1973;70:3324.
207. Knudsen AG. Mutation and cancer: statistical study of retinoblastoma. Proc Natl Acad Sci USA 1971;68:820.
208. Knudsen AG. Genetic predisposition to cancer. Cancer Detect Prev 1984;7:1.
209. Sparkes RS, Sparkes ME, Wilson MG, et al. Regional assignment of genes for human esterase D and retinoblastoma to chromosome 13q14. Science 1980;208:1042.
210. Yunis JJ, Ramsey N. Retinoblastoma and sub-band deletion of chromosome 13. Am J Dis Child 1978;132:161.
211. Dryja TD, Rappaport JM, Joyce JM, et al. Molecular detection of deletions involving band q14 of chromosome 13 in retinoblastomas. Proc Natl Acad Sci USA 1986;84:9275.
212. Friend SH, Bernards R, Rogelj S, et al. A human DNA segment with properties of the gene that predisposes to retinoblastoma and osteosarcoma. Nature 1986;323.
213. Lee WH, Bookstein R, Hung F, et al. Human retinoblastoma susceptibility gene. Science 1987;235:1394.
214. Horowitz JM, Yandell DW, Park SH, et al. Point mutational inactivation of the retinoblastoma antioncogene. Science 1989;243:937.
215. Bernards R, Shackleford G, Gerber MR, et al. Structure and expression of the murine retinoblastoma gene and characterization of its encoded protein. Proc Natl Acad Sci USA 1989;86:6474.
216. Friend SH, Horowitz JM, Gerber MR, et al. Deletions of a DNA sequence in retinoblastomas and mesenchymal tumors: organization of the sequence and its encoded protein. Proc Natl Acad Sci USA 1987;84: 9059.
217. Hansen MF, Koufos A, Gallie BL, et al. Osteosarcoma and retinoblastoma: a shared chromosomal mechanism revealing recessive predisposition. Proc Natl Acad Sci USA 1985;82:6216.
218. Harbour JW, Lai SL, Whang-Peng J, et al. Abnormalities in structure and expression of the human retinoblastoma gene in SCLC. Science 1988;241:353.
219. Huang J-JS, Yee JK, Shen JY, et al. Suppression of the neoplastic phenotype by replacement of the RB gene in human cancer cells. Science 1988;242:1541.
220. Bookstein R, Shen J-Y, Chen PL, et al. Suppression of tumorigenicity of human prostate carcinoma calls by replacing a mutated RB gene. Science 1990;247:712.
221. Whyte P, Williamsen NM, Harlow E. Cellular targets for transformation by the adenovirus E1a proteins. Cell 1989;56:67.
222. Whyte P, Buchkovich KJ, Horowitz JM, et al. Association between an oncogene and an anti-oncogene: the adenovirus E1a proteins bind to the retinoblastoma gene product. Nature 1988;334:124.
223. Vousden KH, Jai PS. Functional similarity between HPV16E7,SV40 large T and adenovirus E1a proteins. Oncogene 1989;4:153.
224. Windle JJ, Albert DM, O'Brien JM, et al. Retinoblastoma in transgenic mice. Nature 1990;343:665.
225. Buchkovich K, Duffy LA, Harlow EA. The retinoblastoma protein is phosphorylated during specific phases of the cell cycle. Cell 1989;58: 1097.
226. Chen PL, Scully P, Shew JY, et al. Phosphorylation of the retinoblastoma gene product is modulated during the cell cycle and cellular differentiation. Cell 1989;58:1193.
227. Ludlow JW, Shon J, Pipas JM, et al. The retinoblastoma susceptibility gene product undergoes cell cycle–dependent dephosphorylation and binding to release from SV40 large T. Cell 1990;60:387.
228. Deleo AB, Jay G, Apella E, et al. Detection of a transformation-related antigen in chemically inducted sarcomas and other transformed cells of the mouse. Proc Natl Acad Sci USA 1979;76:2420.
229. Jenkins JR, Rudge K, Curie GA. Cellular immortalization by a cDNA clone encoding the transformation associated phosphoprotein p53. Nature 1984;312:651.
230. Nigro JM, Baker ST, Preisinger AC, et al. Mutations in the p53 gene occur in diverse tumor types. Nature 1989;342:705.
231. Ahuja H, Bar-Eli M, Advani SH, et al. Alterations in the p53 gene and the clonal evolution of the blast crisis of chronic myelocytic leukemia. Proc Natl Acad Sci USA 1989;86:6783.
232. Lavigueur A, Maltby V, Mock D, et al. High incidence of lung, bone, and lymphoid tumors in transgenic mice overexpressing mutant alleles of the p53 oncogene. Mol Cell Biol 1989;9:3982.
233. Malkin D, Lee FP, Strong LC, et al. Germline p53 mutations in a familial syndrome of breast carcinomas, sarcomas, and other neoplasms. Science 1990;250:1233.
234. Diller I, Kessel J, Nelson CE, et al. p53 functions as a cell cycle control protein in osteosarcomas. Mol Cell Biol 1990;10:5772.
235. Fearon ER, Cho KR, Nigro JM, et al. Identification of a chromosome 18q gene that is altered in colorectal cancers. Science 1990;247:49.
236. Gessler M, Poustka A, Cavenee W, et al. Homozygous deletion in Wilm's tumours of a zinc-finger gene identified by chromosome jumping. Nature 1990;343:774.
237. Call KM, Glaser T, Ito CY, et al. Isolation and characterization of a zinc finger polypeptide gene at the human chromosome 11 Wilms' Tumor locus. Cell 1990;60:508.
238. Koufos A, Grundy R, Morgan K, et al. Familial Weidemann Beckwith Syndrome and a second Wilms' tumor locus both map to 11p 1s.s. Am J Hum Genet 1989;44:711.
239. Huff V, Compton DA, Chao LY, et al. Lack of linkage of familial Wilms' tumor to chromosomal band. Nature 1988;336:377.
240. Grundy P, Koufos A, Morgan K, et al. Familial predisposition to Wilms' tumors does not map to the short arm of chromosome 11. Nature 1988;336:374.
241. Ali IV, Lidereau R, Theillet C, et al. Reduction to homozygosity of genes on chromosome 11 in human breast neoplasia. Science 1987;238: 185.
242. Bale SH, Dracopoli NC, Tucker MA, et al. Mapping the gene for hereditary cutaneous malignant melanoma-dysplastic nevus to chromosome 1p. N Engl J Med 1988;320:1367.
243. Chen L-C, Dollbaum D, Smith HS. Loss of heterozygosity on chromosome 12 in human breast cancer. Proc Natl Acad Sci USA 1989;86: 7204.
244. Bressac B, Galvin KM, Liang TJ, et al. Abnormal structure and expression of p53 gene in human hepetocellular carcinoma. Proc Natl Acad Sci USA 1980;87:1973.
245. Dumanski JP, Carlbon E, P CV. Deletions mapping of a locus on human chromosome 22 in the oncogenesis of meningioma. Proc Natl Acad Sci USA 1987;84:9275.
246. Escot C, Theilet C, Lidereau R, et al. Genetic alterations of the c-myc proto-oncogene in primary breast carcinomas. Proc Natl Acad Sci USA 1986;83:4834.
247. Genuerdi M, Tahira H, Anderson DE, et al. Distal deletion of chromosome 1p in ductal carcinoma of the breast. Am J Hum Genet 1989;45: 73.
248. Griffin CA, Hankins AL, Pecker RJ, et al. Chromosome abnormalities in pediatric brain tumors. Cancer Res 1988;48:175.
249. James CD, Caribom E, Dumanski JP, et al. Clonal genomic alterations in glioma malignancy stages. Cancer Res 1988;48:5546.
250. Katsuyama J, Papenhausen PR, Herz F, et al. Chromosome abnormalities in meningiomas. Cancer Genet Cytogenet 1986;22:63.
251. Keneko Y, Rowley JD. Chromosome pattern in childhood acute nonlymphocytic leukemia (ANLL). Biood 1982;60:289.
252. Lee EYHP, To H, Shew JY, et al. Inactivation of the retinoblastoma susceptibility gene in human breast cancers. Science 1988;241:218.
253. Koufos A, Hansen MF, Copeland NG, et al. Loss of heterozygosity in three embryonal tumors supports a common pathogenic mechanism. Nature 1985;316:330.
254. Larsson C, Skogseid B, Oberg D, et al. Multiple endocrine neoplasia type 1 gene maps to chromosome 11 and is lost in insulinoma. Nature 1988;332:85.
255. Lundberg C, Skoog L, C CW, et al. Loss of heterozygosity in human ductal breast tumors indicates a recessive mutation on chromosome 13. Proc Natl Acad Sci USA 1987;84:2372.
256. Matthew CGP, Chin KS, Easton DF, et al. A linked genetic marker for multiple endocrine neoplasia type 2A on chromosome 10. Nature 1986;328:527.
257. Matthew CGP, Smith BA, Thorpe K, et al. Deletion of genes on chromosome 1 in endocrine neoplasia. Nature 1987;328:524.
258. Martinson T, Weith A, Cziepluch, et al. Chromosomal deletions in human neuroblastomas. Genes Chrom Cancer 1989;1:67.
259. Masuda H, Miller C, Battifora H, et al. Rearrangement of the p53 gene in human osteogenic sarcomas. Proc Natl Acad Sci USA 1987;84:7716.
260. Mulligan LM, Matlashewski GJ, Scrabli JH, et al. Mechanism of p53 loss in human sarcomas. Proc Natl Acad Sci USA 1990;87:5863.
261. Mukai S, Dryja T. Loss of alleles at polymorphic loc: on chromosome 2 in uveal melanomas. Cancer Genet Cytogenet 1986;22:45.
262. Naylor SL, Johnson BE, Minna JD, et al. Loss of heterozygosity of chromosome 3p markers in small-cell lung cancers. Nature 1987;329:451.
263. Pathak S, Strong LC, Ferrell RE, et al. Familial renal cell carcinomas with a 3:11 chromosome translocators linked to tumor cells. Science 1982;217:939.
264. Raffel C, Gilles FE, Weinberg KI. Reduction to homozygosity and gene amplification in central nervous system primitive neuroectodermal tumors of childhood. Cancer Res 1990;50:587.
265. Ponder B. Gene losses in human tumors. Nature 1988;335:400.
266. Scrable JH, Sapienza C, Cavenee WK. Genetic and epigenetic losses of

heterozygosity in cancer predisposition and progression. Adv Cancer Res 1990;54:25.
267. Rouleau GA, Wettelecki W, Haines JL, et al. Genetic linkage of bilateral acoustic neurofibromatosis to a DNA marker on chromostome 22. Nature 1987;329:246.
268. Seizinger BR, Rouleau GA, Ozelius LJ, et al. von Hippel- Lindau disease maps to the region of chromosome 3 associated with renal cell carcinoma. Nature 1988;322:268.
269. Rose EA, Glaser T, Jones C, et al. Complete physical map of the WAGR region of 11p13 localizes a candidate Wilms' tumor gene. Cell 1990;60: 495.
270. Takahashi T, Nau MM, Chiba I, et al. p53: a frequent target for genetic abnormalties in lung cancer. Science 1989;246:491.
271. Simpson NE, Kidd KK, Goodfellow PT, et al. Assignment of multiple endocrine neoplasia type 2A to chromosome 10 by linkage. Nature 1987;328:528.
272. Trent JM, Stenbridge EJ, McBridge HL. Tumorigenicity in human melanoma cell lines controlled by introduction of human chromosome 6. Science 1990;247:568.
273. Wertelecki W, Rouleau GA, Supermeau DW, et al. Neurofibromastosis 2: clinical and DNA linkage status of a large kindred. N Engl J Med 1988;319:278.
274. Vogelstein B, Fearon ER, Hamilton ST, et al. Allelotype of colorectal carcinomas. N Engl J Med 1988;319:525.
275. Yokota J, Tsukada Y, Nakayima T, et al. Loss of heterozygosity on the short arm of chromosome 3 in carcinoma of the uterine cervix. Cancer Res 1989;48:3598.
276. Zbar B, Brauch H, Talmadge C, et al. Loss of alleles of loci on the short arm of chromosome 3 in renal cell carcinoma. Nature 1987;327:721.
277. Baker SJ, Fearon ER, Nigro JM, et al. Chromosome 17 deletions and p53 gene mutations in colorectal carcinomas. Science 1989;244:217.
278. Vogelstein B, Fearon ER, Baker SJ, et al. Genetic alterations accumulate during colorectal tumorigenesis. In: Cavenee W, ed. Recessive oncogenes and tumor suppression. New York, Cold Spring Harbor Laboratory Press, 1989.

GLOSSARY

anchorage independence—ability of eukaryotic cells to grow in culture without the need to attach to a surface
cell cycle—biochemical stages that occur during the process of cell division
enhancer—*cis*-acting DNA sequence that increases the synthesis of mRNA from a particular gene independent of location or orientation with respect to the promoter
homogeneous staining regions—tandem array of amplified DNA detectible by karyotypic analysis as staining homogeneously
hormone response elements—DNA sequences that can modulate transcription on binding to a hormone–receptor complex
immortalization—process of conversion of a eukaryotic cell line from limited growth potential (finite number of cell divisions) to unlimited growth potential
kinase—enzyme that phosphorylates proteins on specific hydroxyl groups on serines, threonines, or tyrosine
loss of heterozygosity—deletion of a chromosomal segment that contains a polymorphic marker so that the deletion results in the retention of only one of the two alleles
mitogen—factor that stimulates cell division
oncogene—gene whose product causes malignant transformation of tissue culture cells or tumor formation in vivo
protooncogenes—growth-potentiating genes whose inappropriate activation can render cells malignant; normal cell counterpart to an oncogene
provirus—duplex DNA sequence in an eukaryotic cell corresponding to a reverse-transcribed RNA retrovirus genome
quiescence—portion of the G0 phase of the cell cycle before DNA synthesis that allows a cell to remain viable and metabolically active without cell cycle progression
reverse transcription—synthesis of a DNA template by an enzyme (reverse transcriptase) from an RNA template
second messenger—intracellular molecule that can activate proteins; typically following stimulation of a cell and its surface by an external signal, a second messenger is generated (eg, Ca^{2+}, IP3, cAMP)
transcription factor—protein whose binding to specific DNA sequences modulates synthesis of RNA from a DNA template
transduction—incorporation and transfer of eukaryotic cellular sequences by retroviruses
transformation—conversion of a eukaryotic cell from a normal growth-limited state to one of deregulated growth control that resembles the tumorigenic state
transformation assay—screen for dominant oncogenes by introduction of specific DNA sequences into nontransformed cells followed by analysis of growth potential
tumor suppressor genes—growth-limiting genes whose inactivation can help initiate the deregulated growth that defines tumor cells

2

The Hematopoietic System

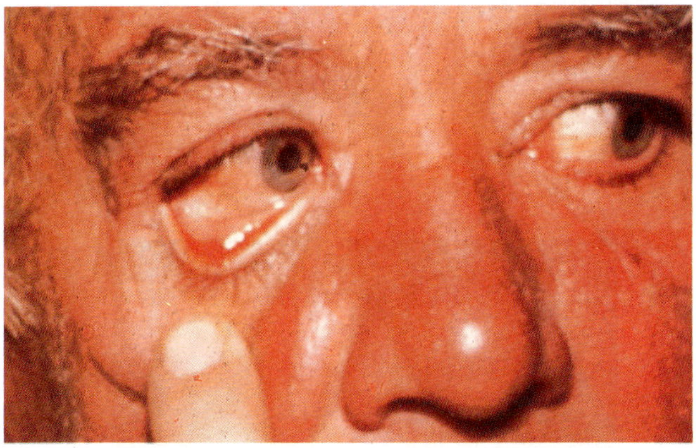

COLOR FIGURE 1-1.

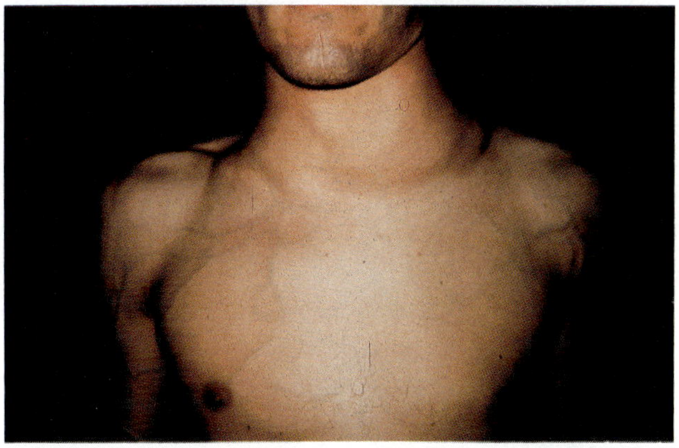

COLOR FIGURE 1-2.

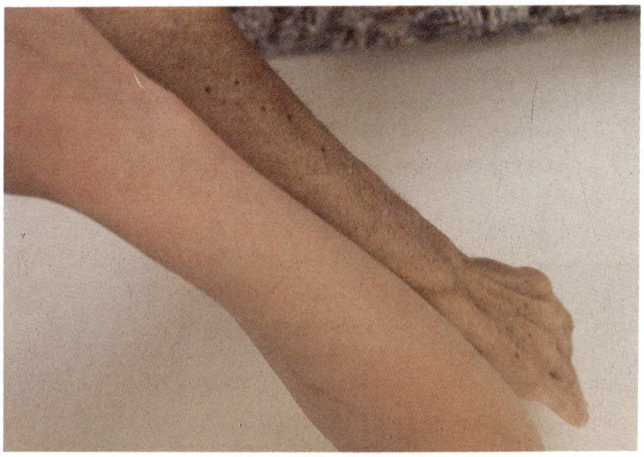

COLOR FIGURE 1-3.

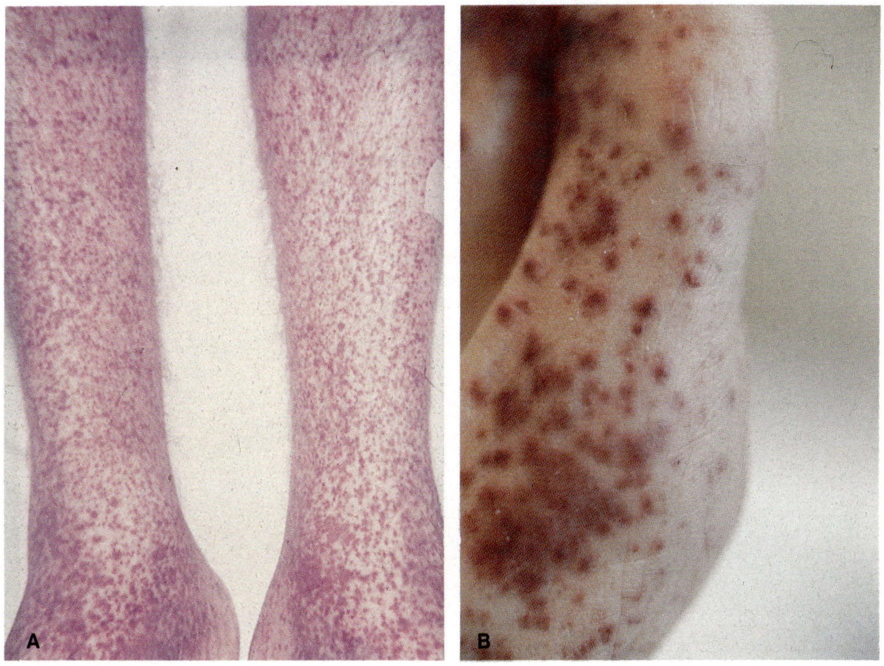

COLOR FIGURE 1-4.

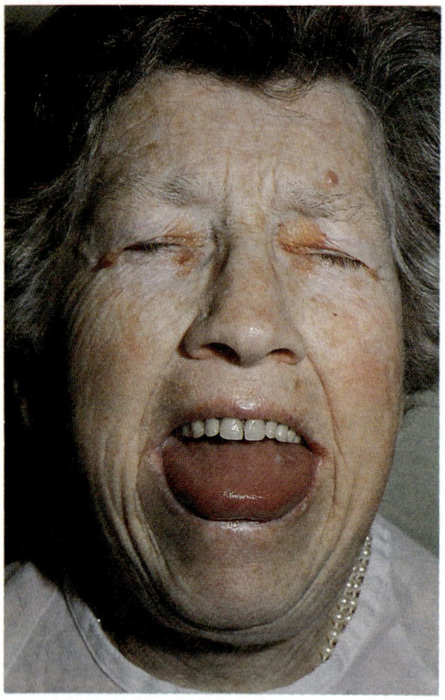

COLOR FIGURE 1-5.

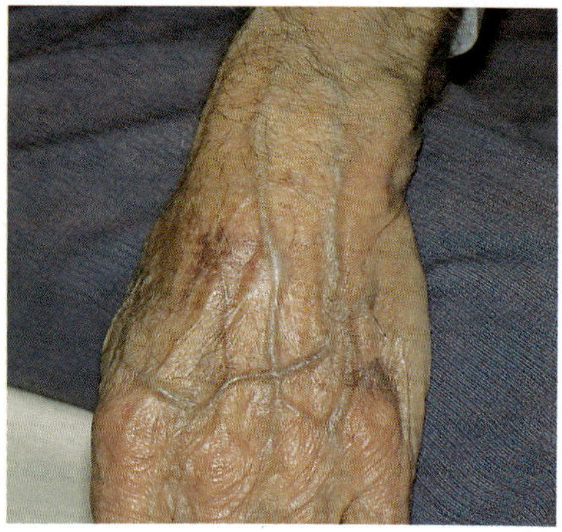

COLOR FIGURE 1-6.

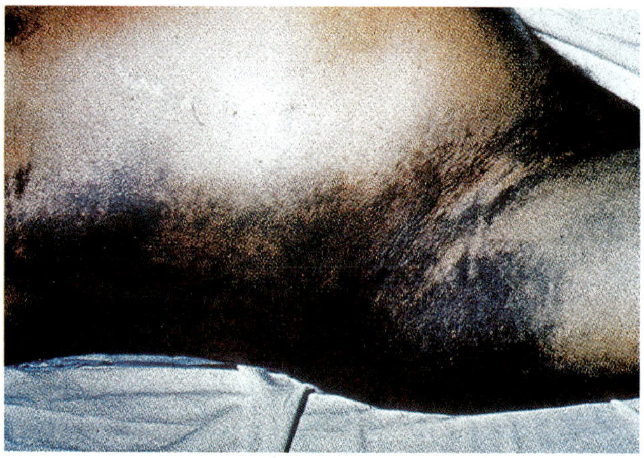

COLOR FIGURE 1-7.

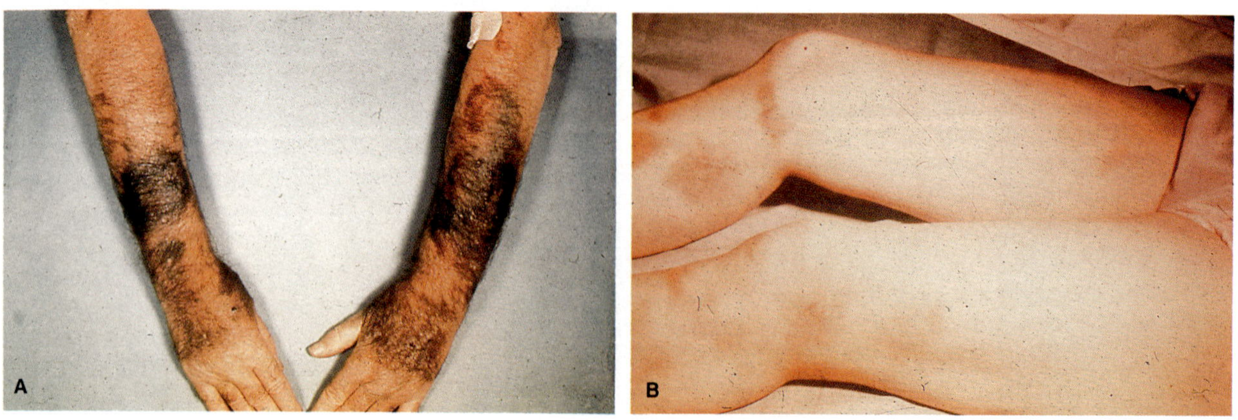

COLOR FIGURE 1-8.

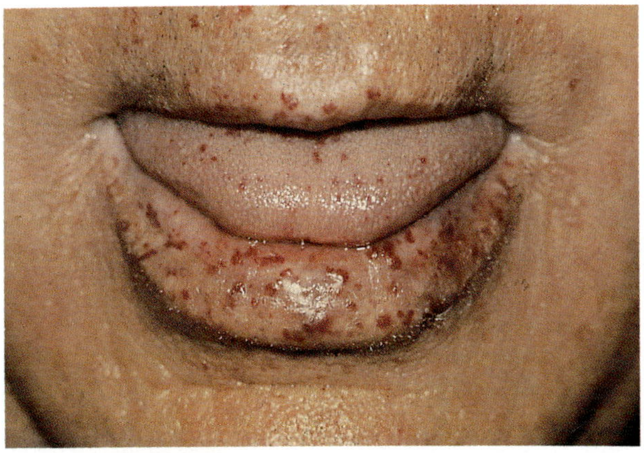

COLOR FIGURE 1-9.

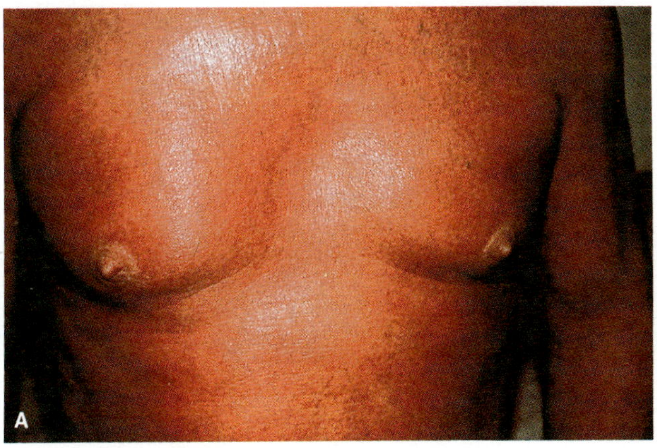

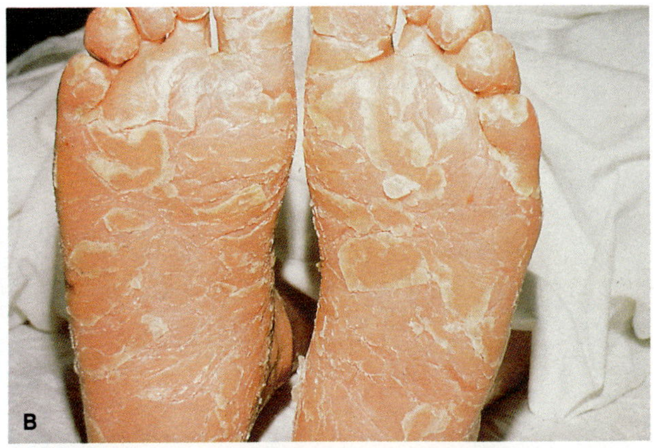

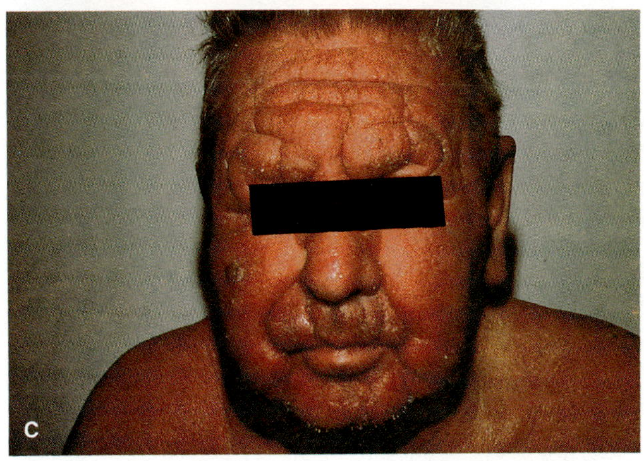

COLOR FIGURE 1-11.

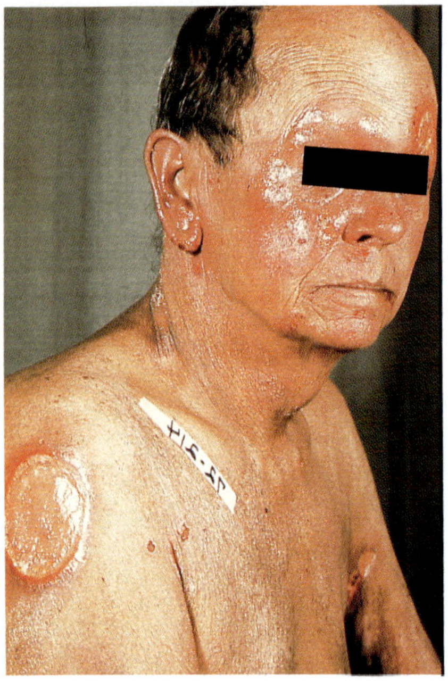

COLOR FIGURE 1-12.

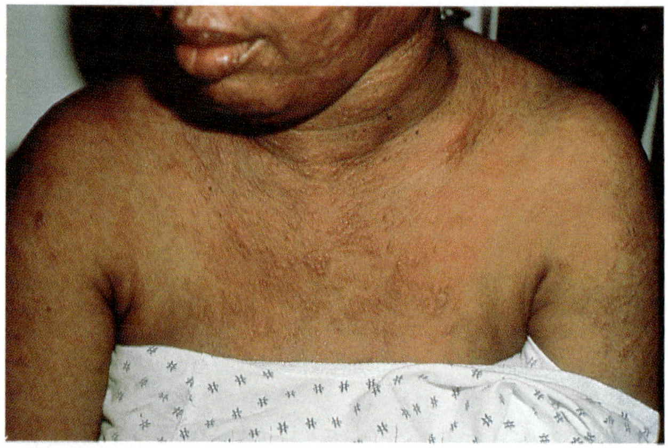

COLOR FIGURE 1-13.

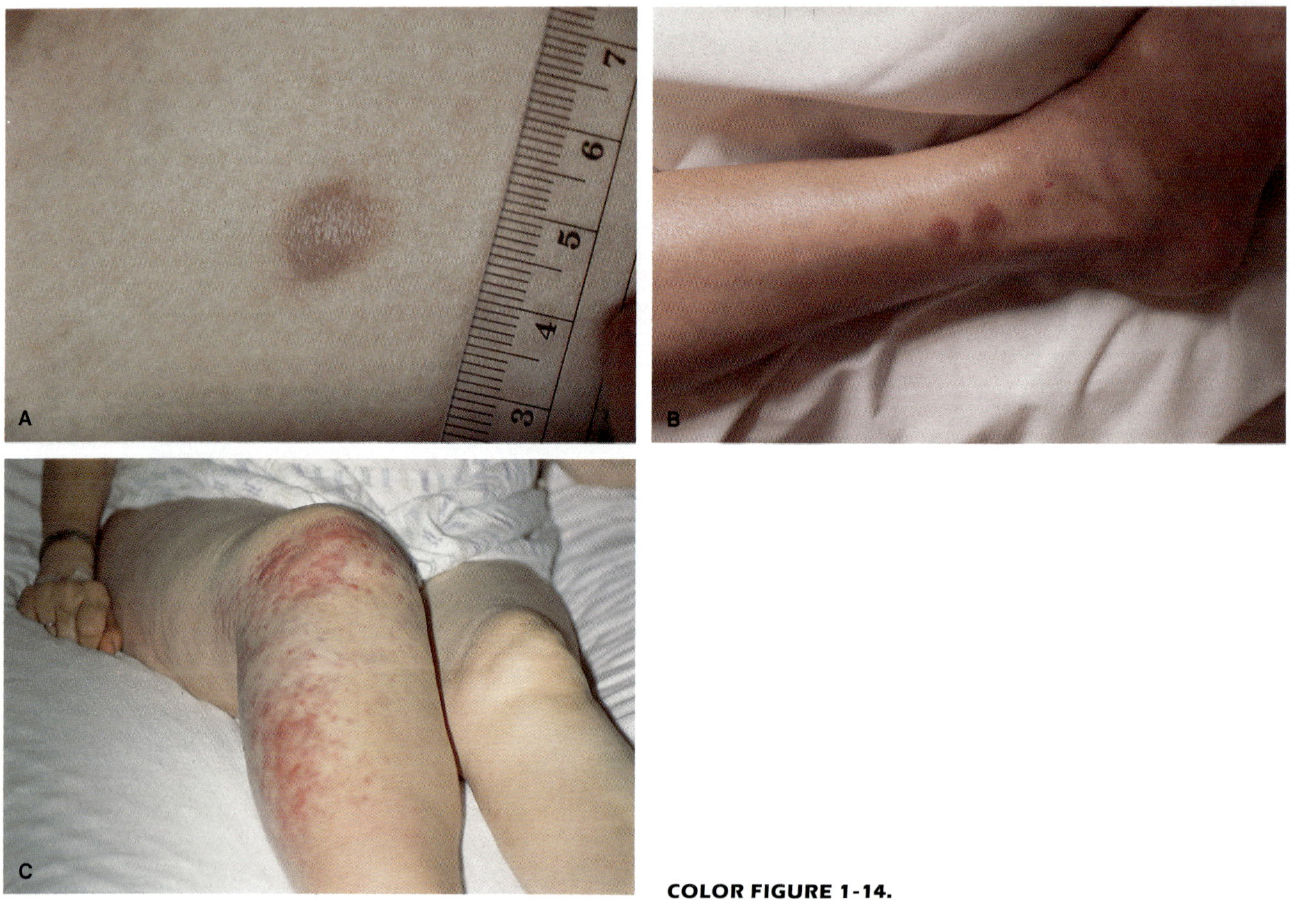

COLOR FIGURE 1-14.

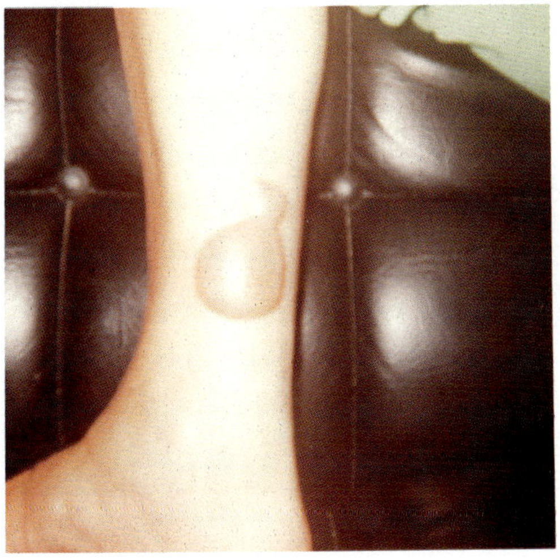

COLOR FIGURE 1-15.

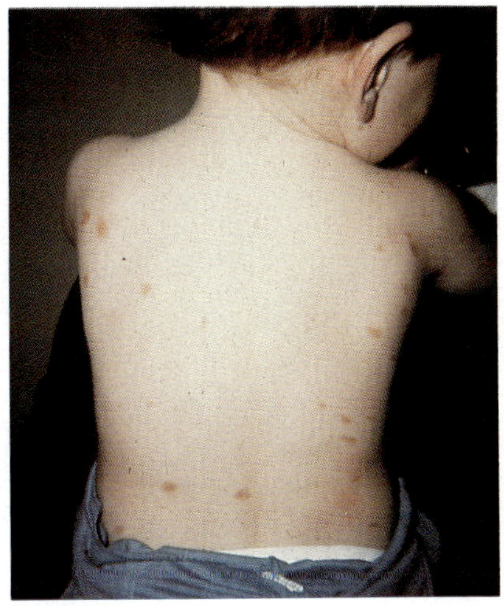

COLOR FIGURE 1-16.

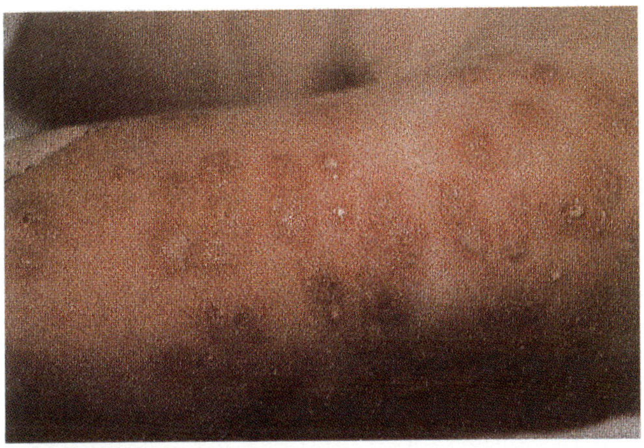

COLOR FIGURE 1-17.

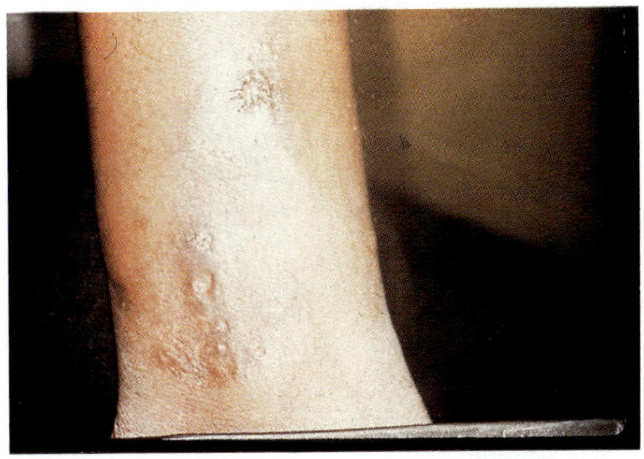

COLOR FIGURE 1-18.

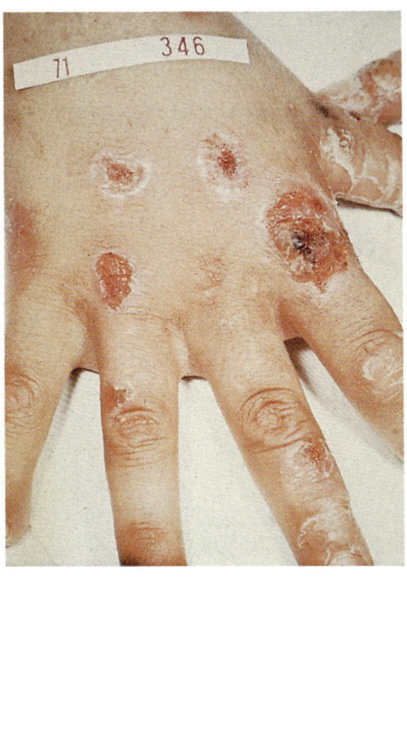

COLOR FIGURE 1-19.

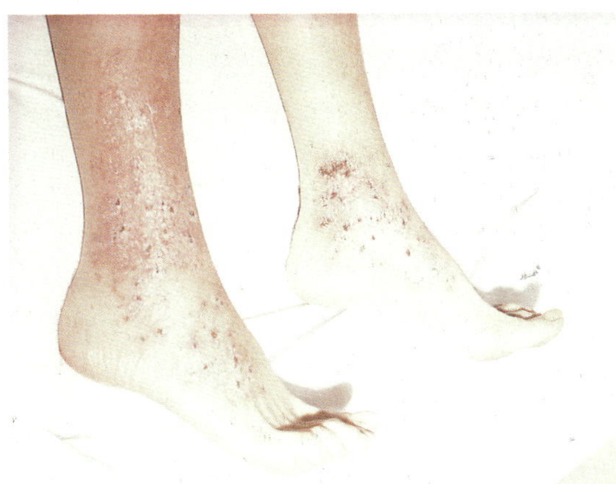

COLOR FIGURE 1-20.

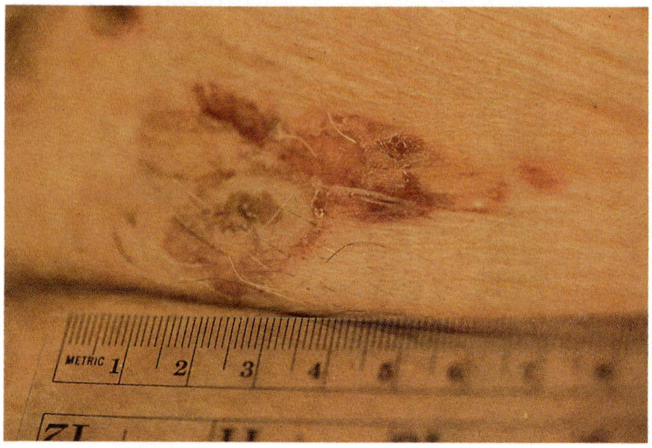

COLOR FIGURE 1-21.

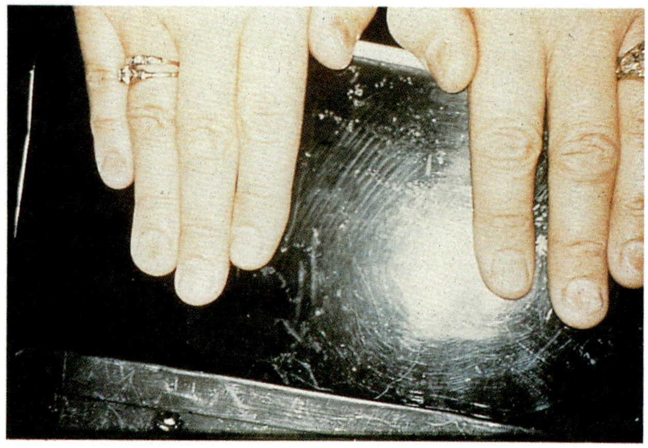

COLOR FIGURE 1-22.

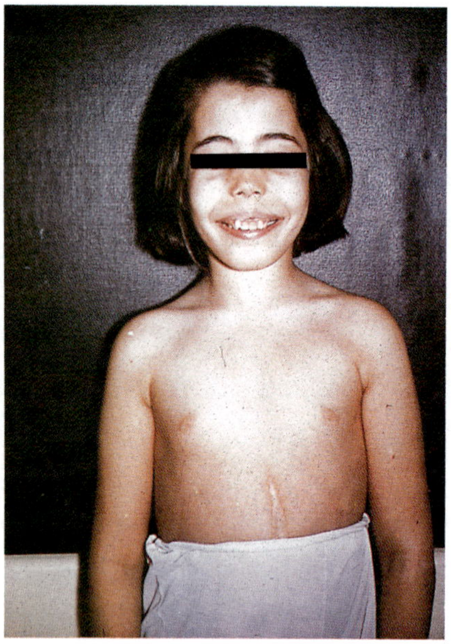

COLOR FIGURE 1-23.

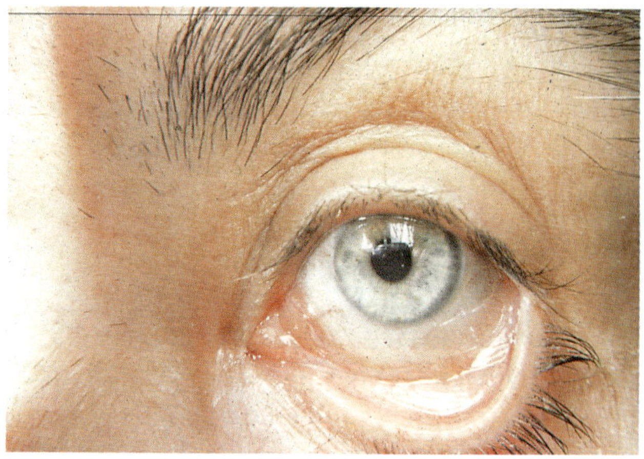

COLOR FIGURE 1-24.

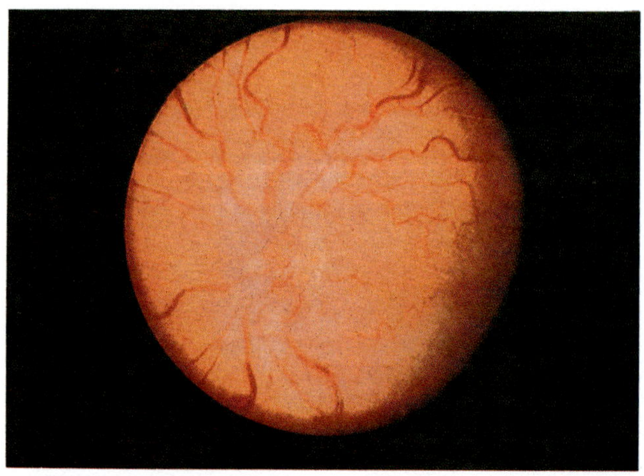

COLOR FIGURE 1-25.

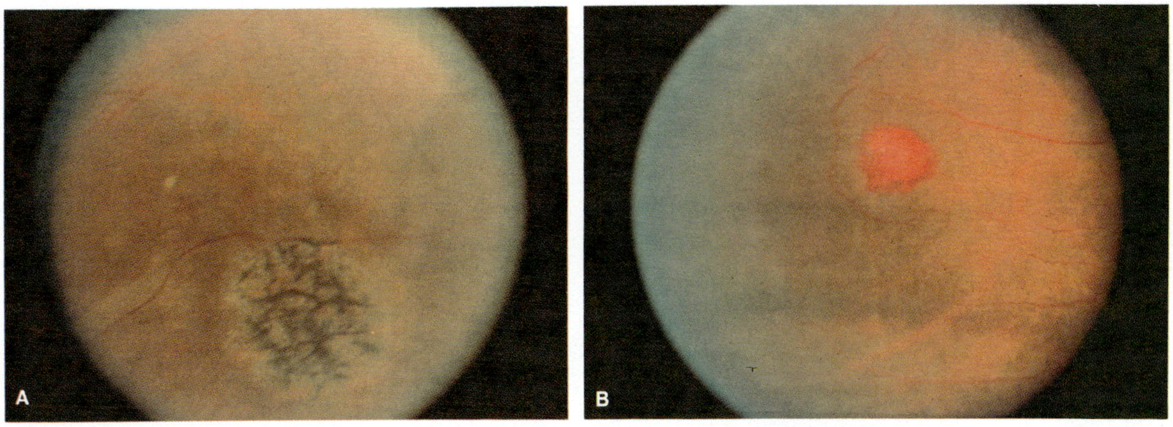

COLOR FIGURE 1-26.

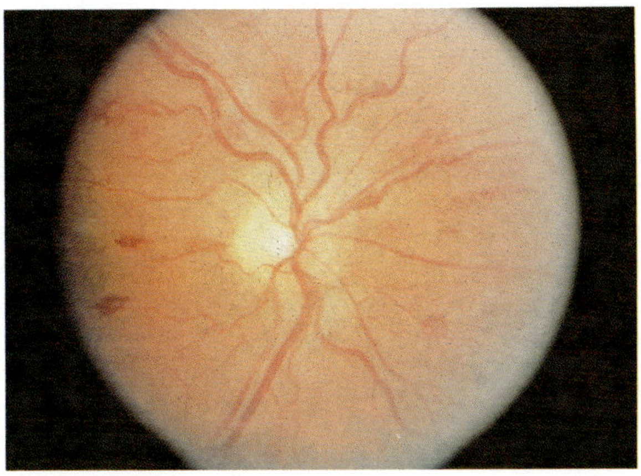

COLOR FIGURE 1-27.

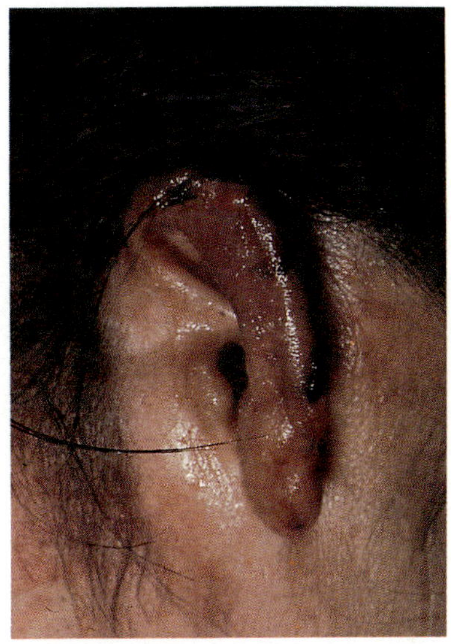

COLOR FIGURE 1-28.

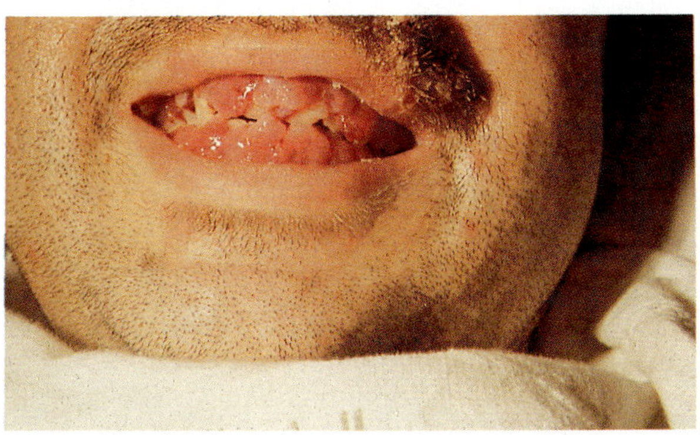

COLOR FIGURE 1-29.

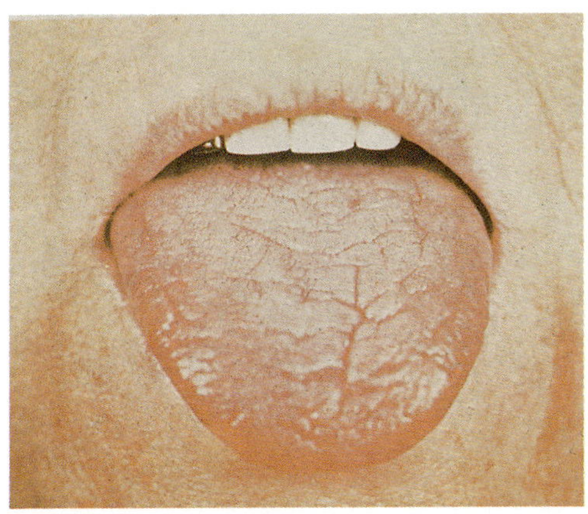

COLOR FIGURE 1-30.

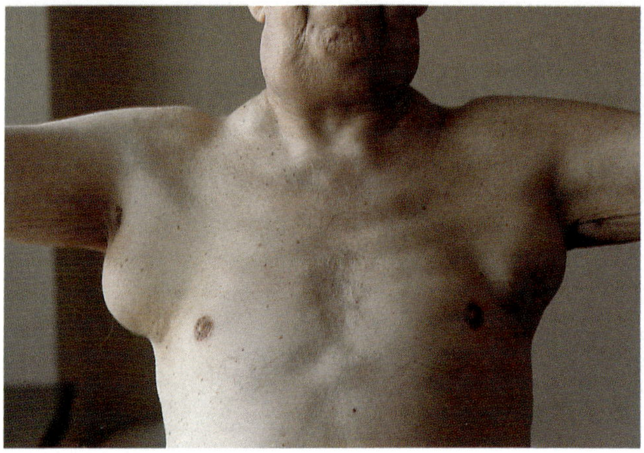

COLOR FIGURE 1-32.

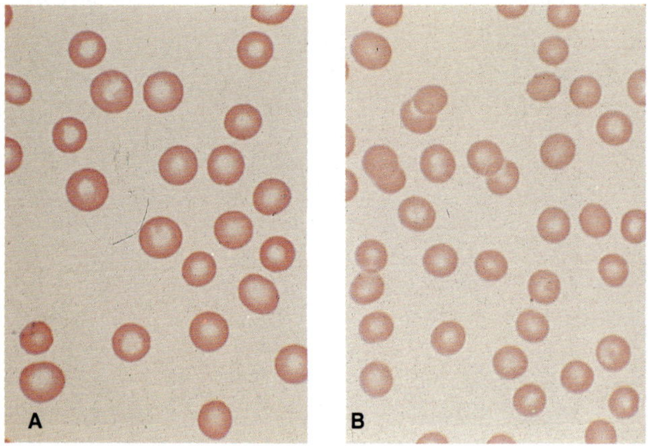

COLOR FIGURE 2-1.

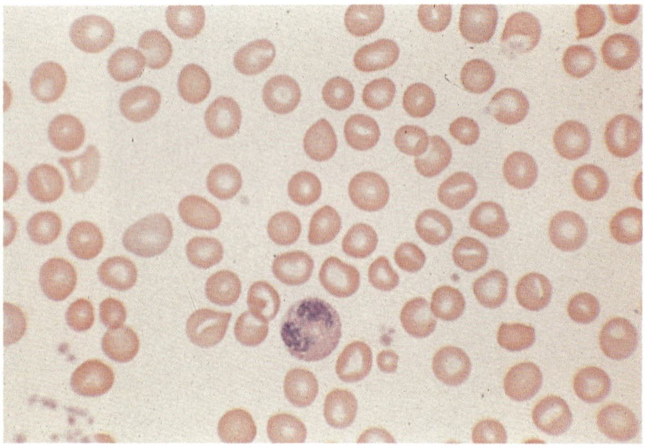

COLOR FIGURE 2-2.

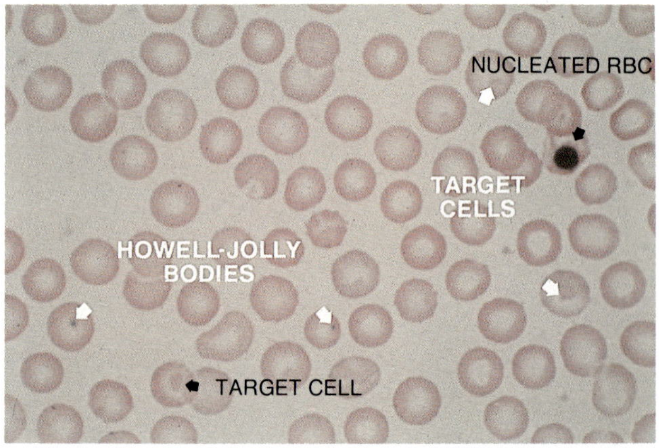

COLOR FIGURE 2-6.

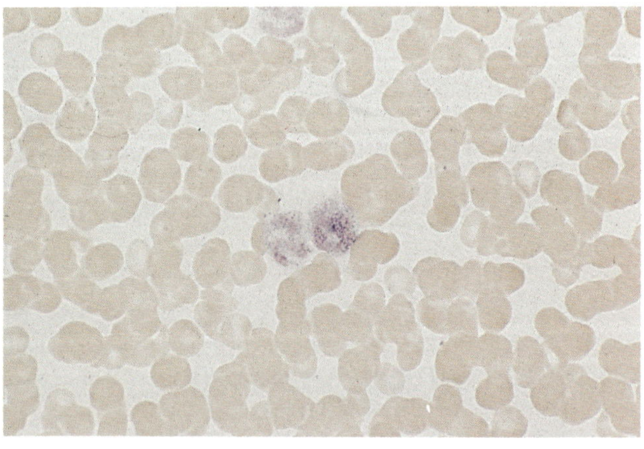

COLOR FIGURE 2-7.

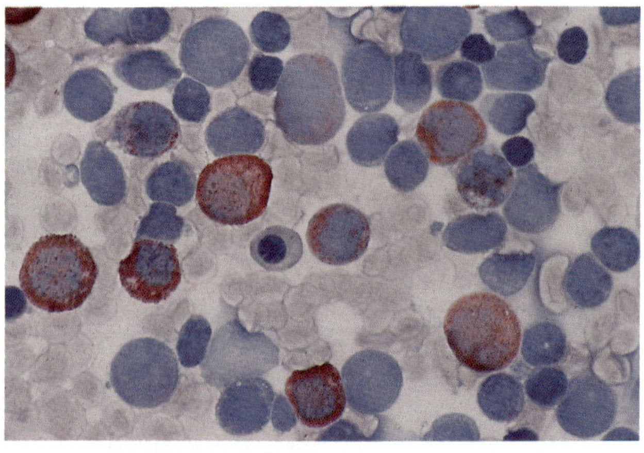

COLOR FIGURE 2-8.

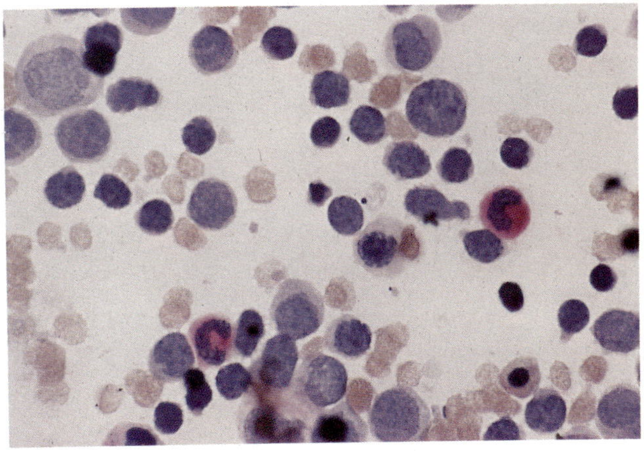

COLOR FIGURE 2-9.

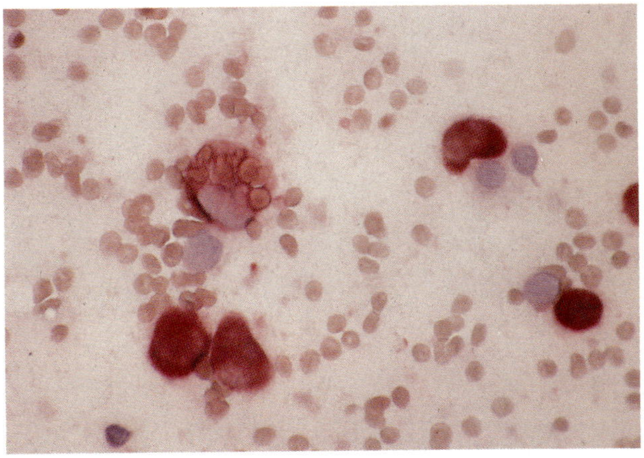

COLOR FIGURE 2-10.

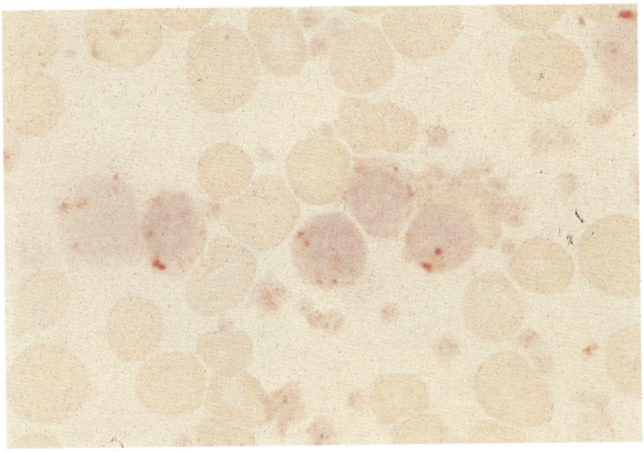

COLOR FIGURE 2-11.

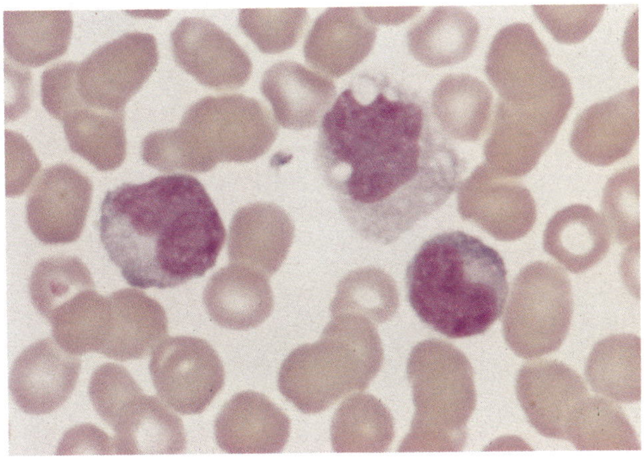

COLOR FIGURE 2-19.

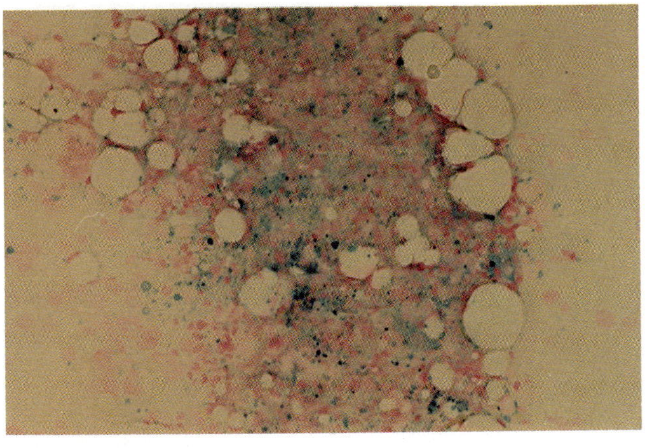

COLOR FIGURE 3-6.

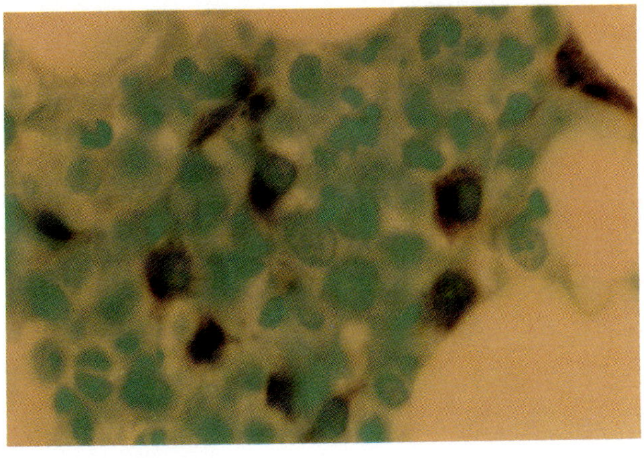

COLOR FIGURE 3-7.

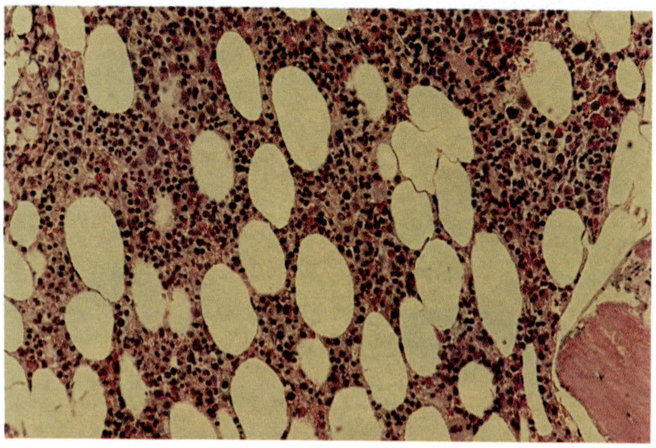

COLOR FIGURE 3-8.

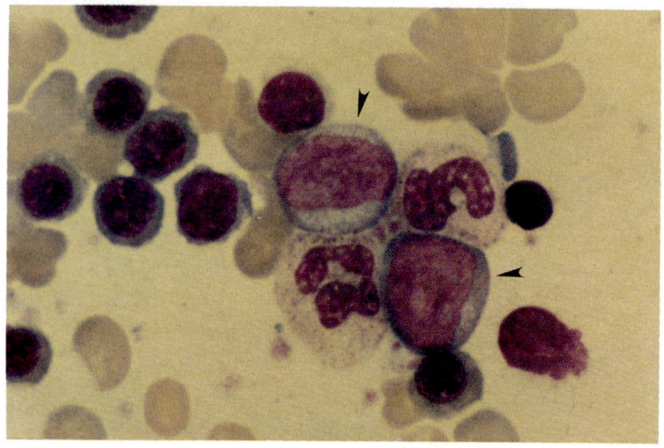

COLOR FIGURE 3-9.

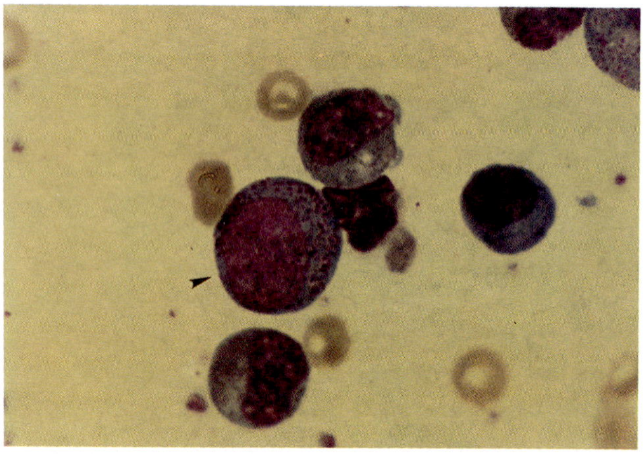

COLOR FIGURE 3-10.

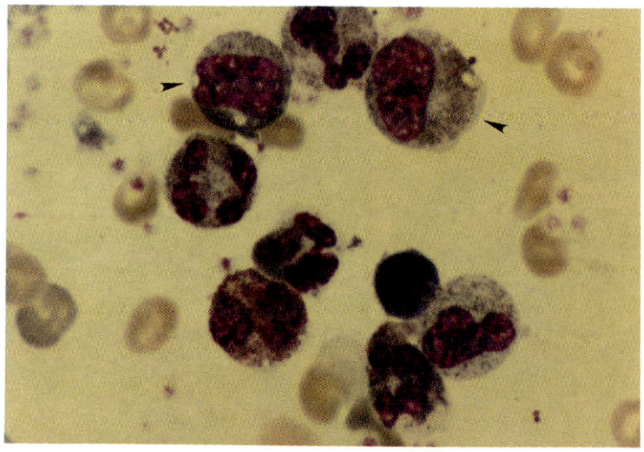

COLOR FIGURE 3-11.

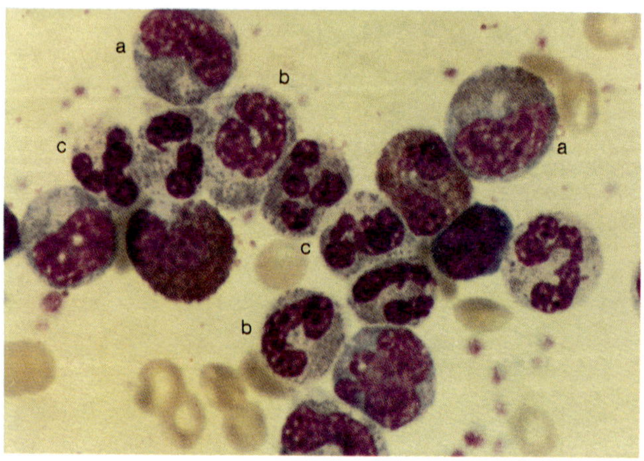

COLOR FIGURE 3-12.

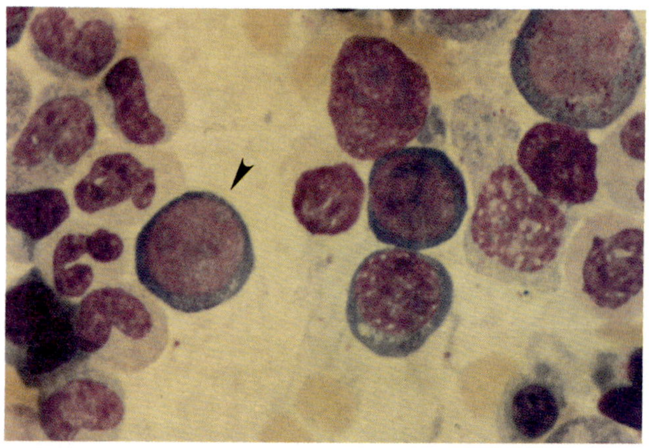

COLOR FIGURE 3-13.

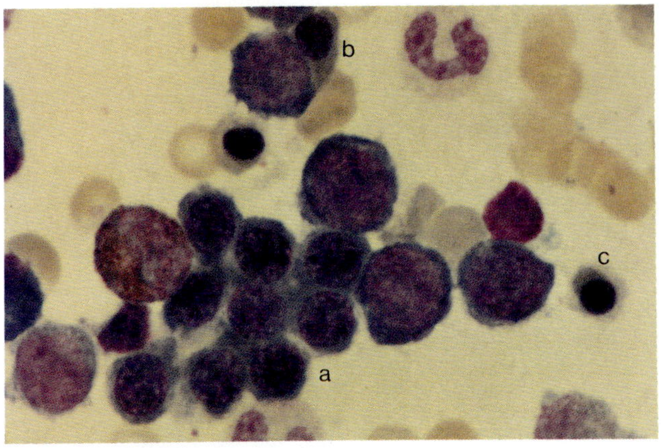

COLOR FIGURE 3-14.

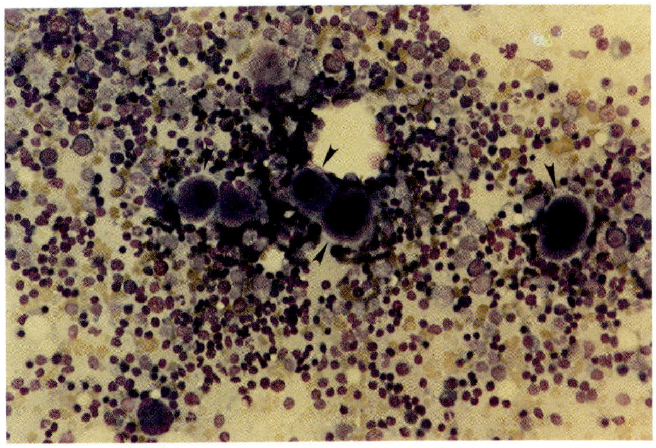

COLOR FIGURE 3-15.

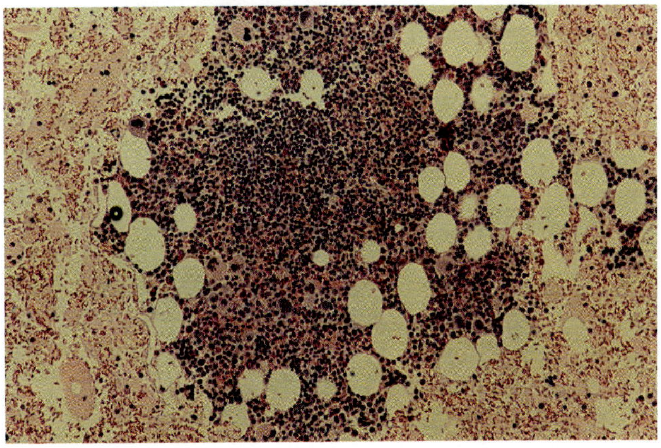

COLOR FIGURE 3-16.

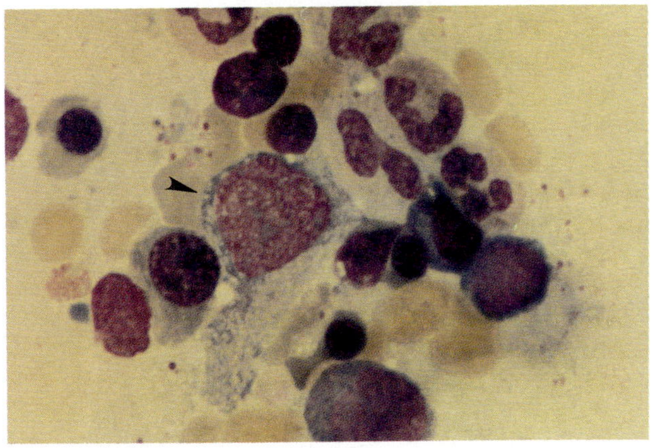

COLOR FIGURE 3-17.

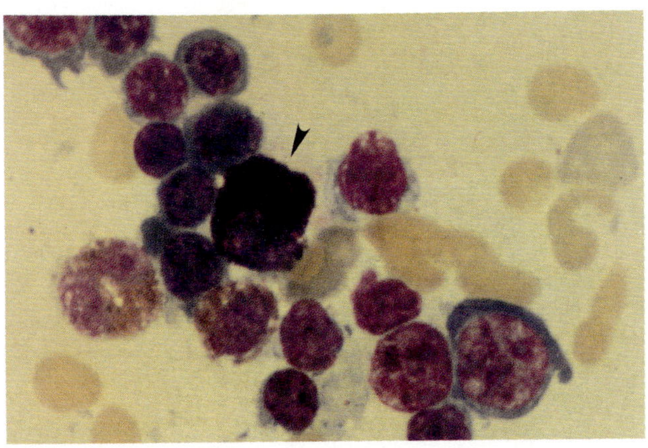

COLOR FIGURE 3-18.

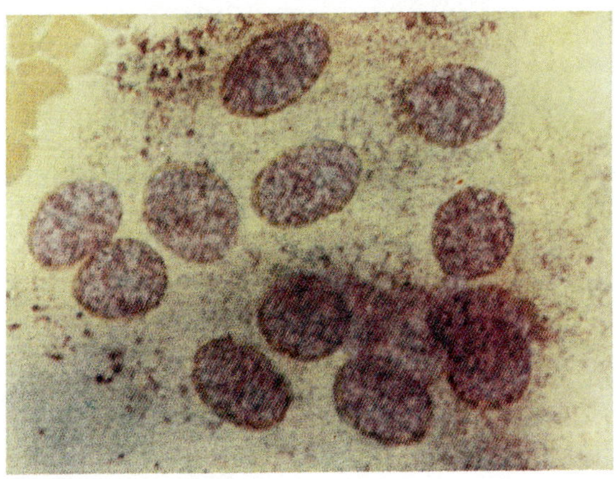

COLOR FIGURE 3-19.

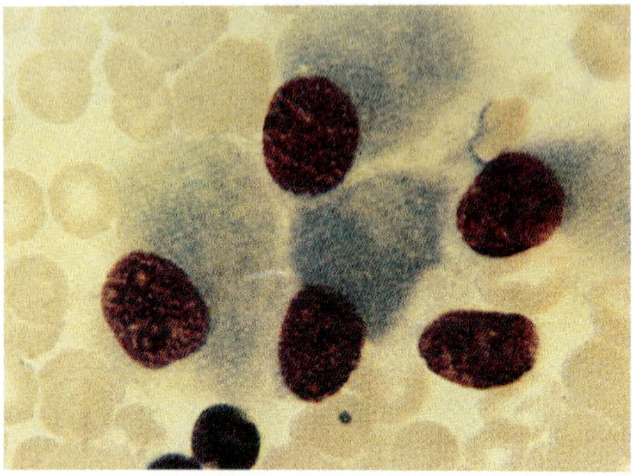

COLOR FIGURE 3-20.

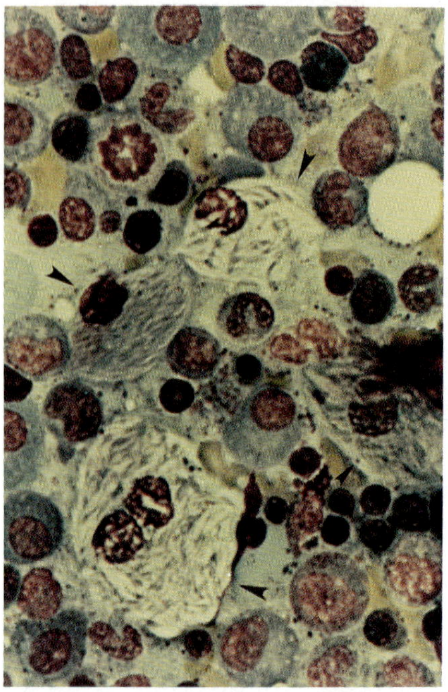

COLOR FIGURE 3-21.

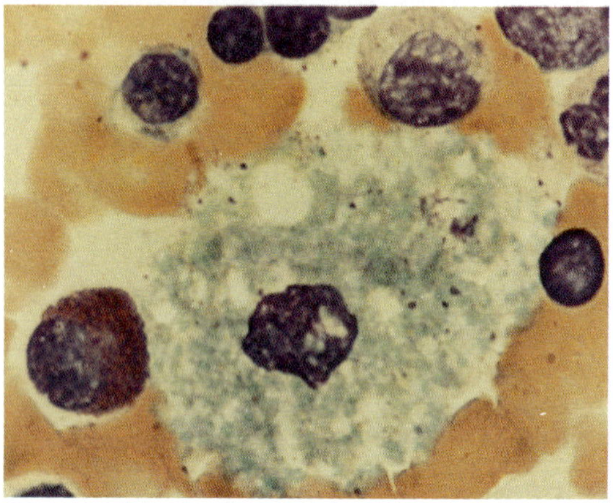

COLOR FIGURE 3-22.

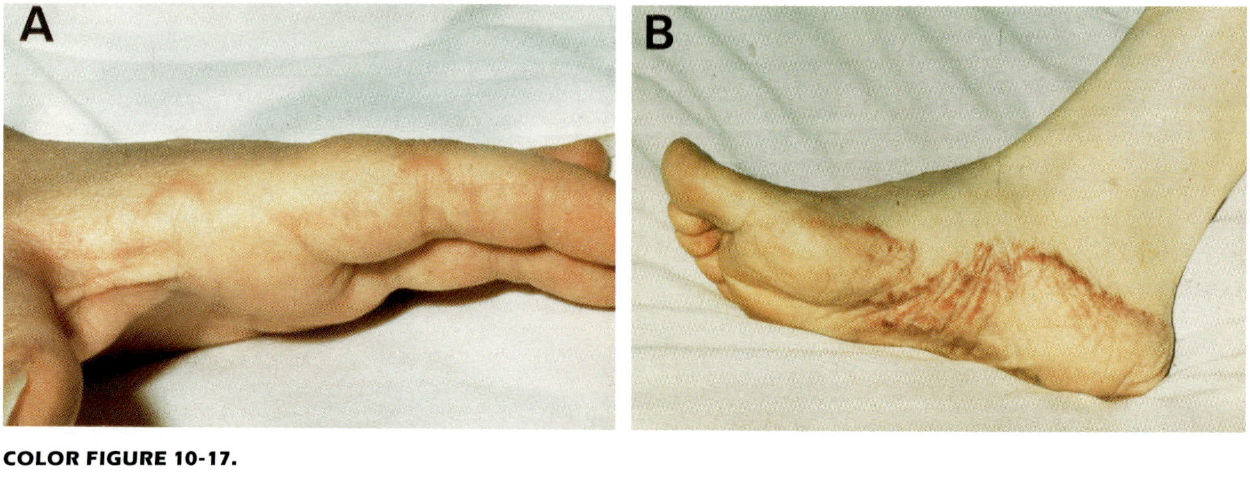

COLOR FIGURE 10-17.

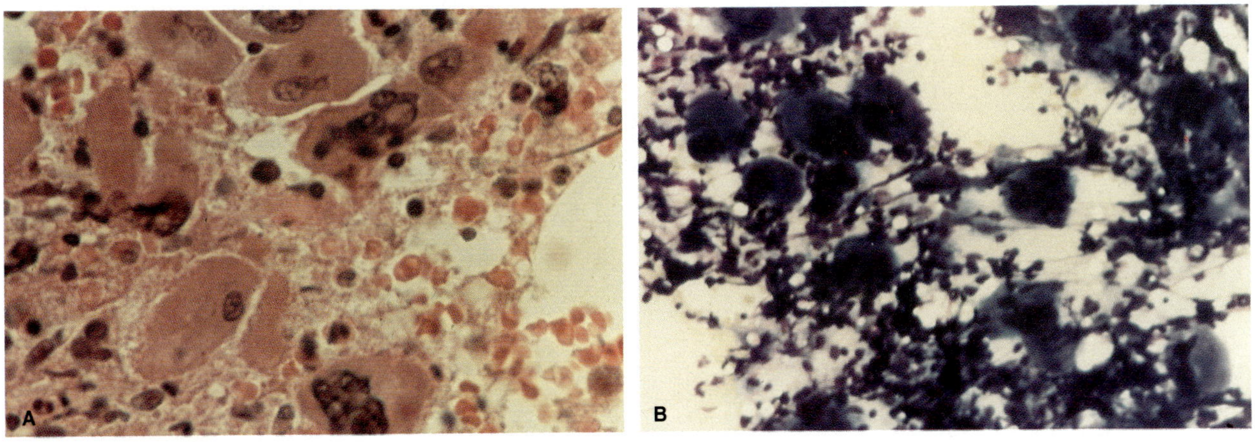

COLOR FIGURE 13-4.

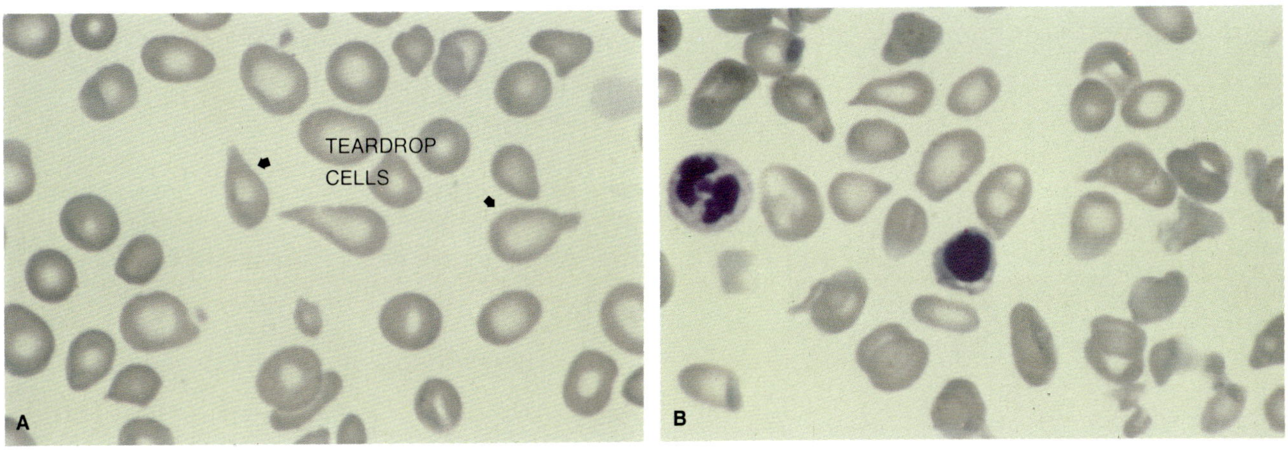

COLOR FIGURE 13-6.

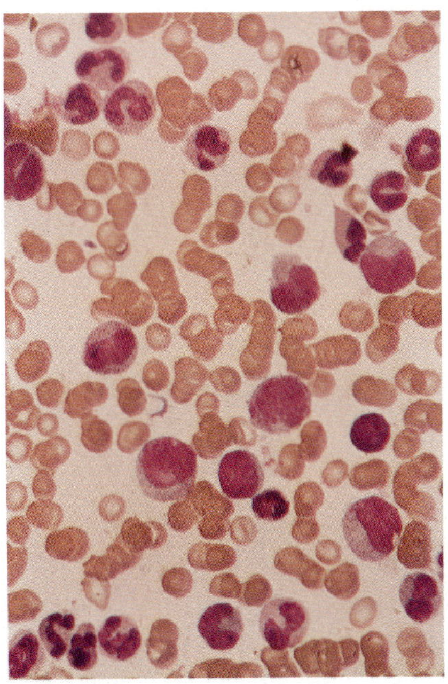

COLOR FIGURE 15-4.

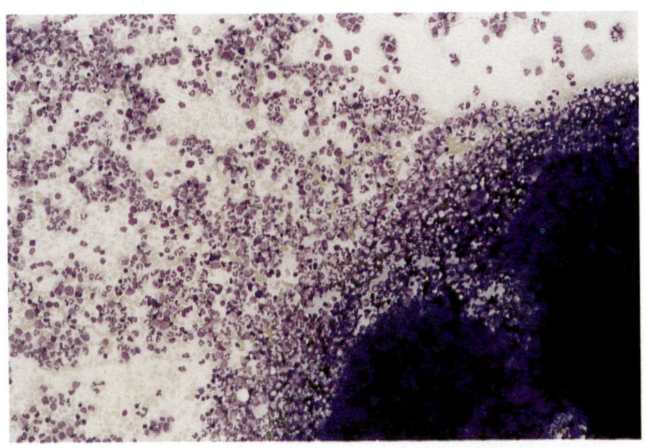

COLOR FIGURE 15-5.

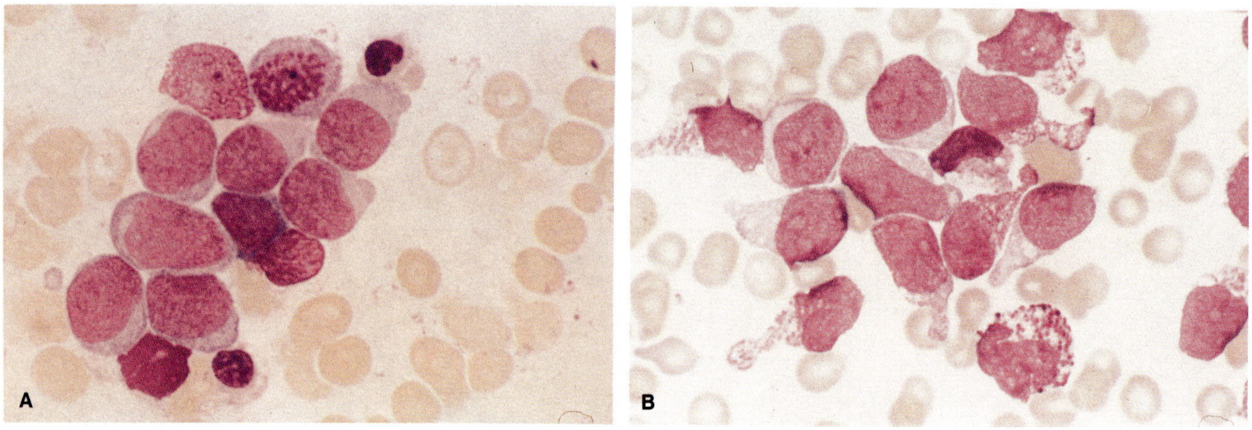

COLOR FIGURE 15-6.

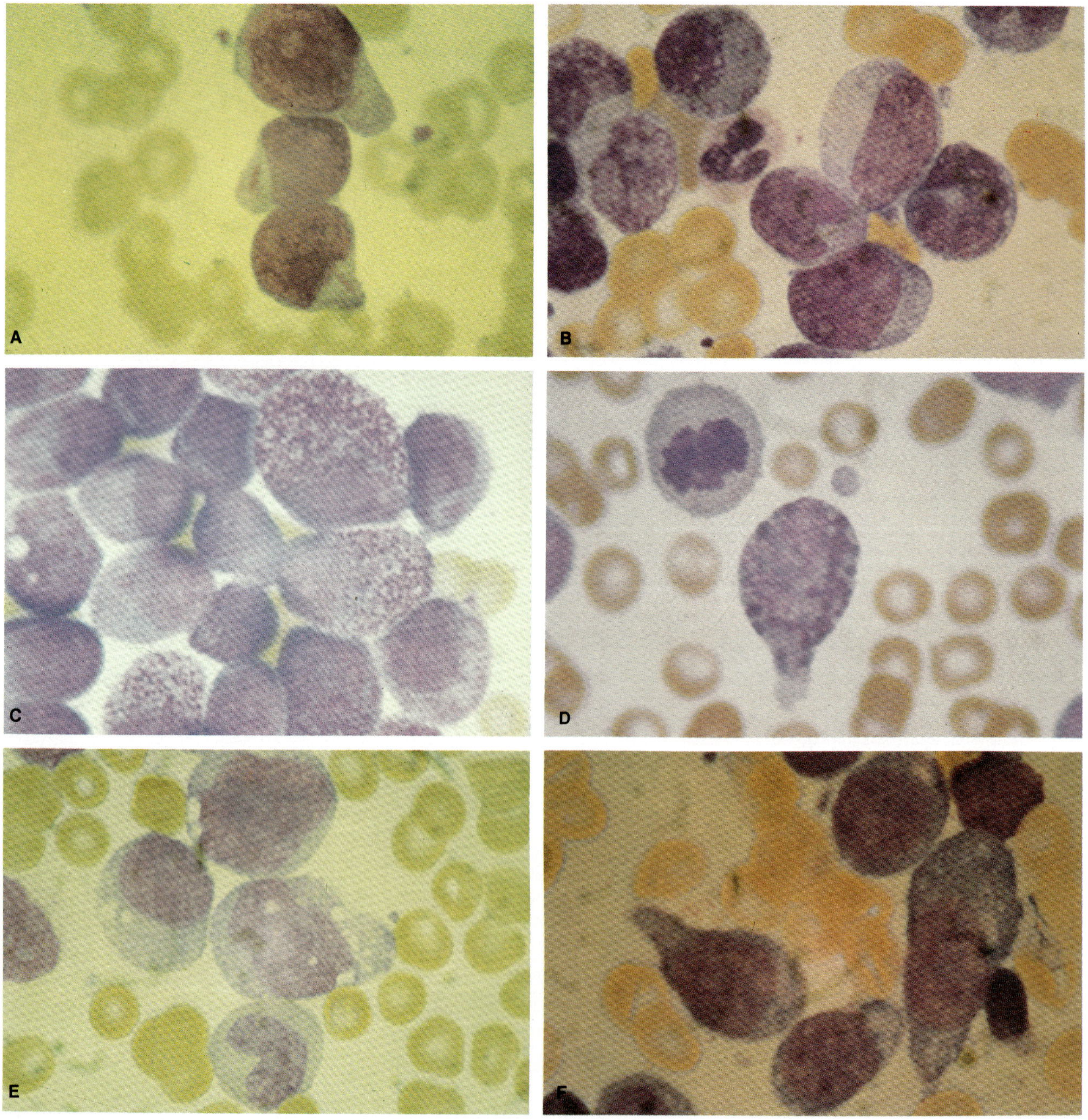

COLOR FIGURE 18-1.

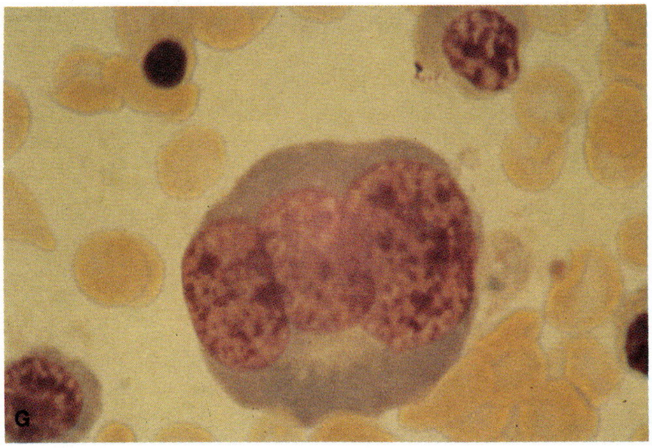

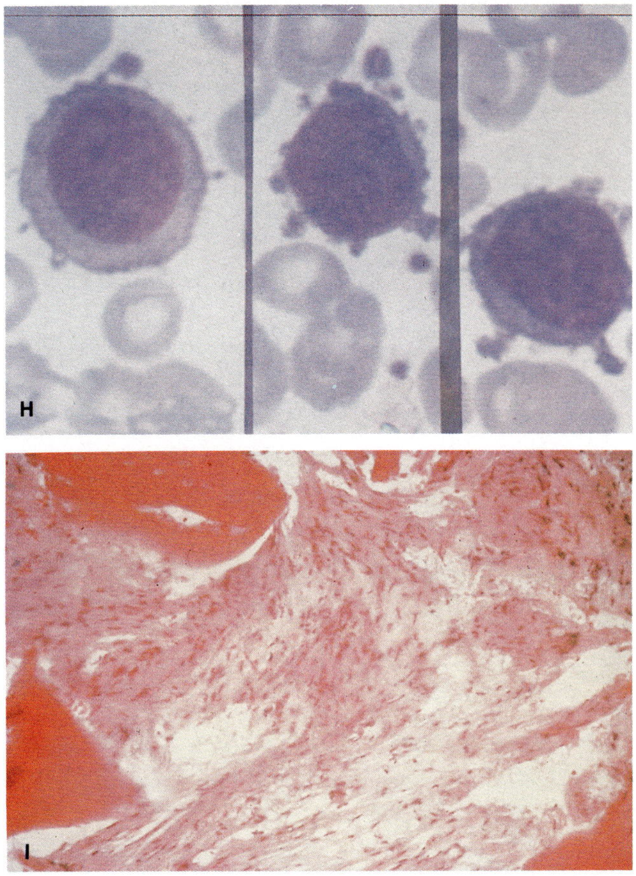

COLOR FIGURE 18-1. (Continued)

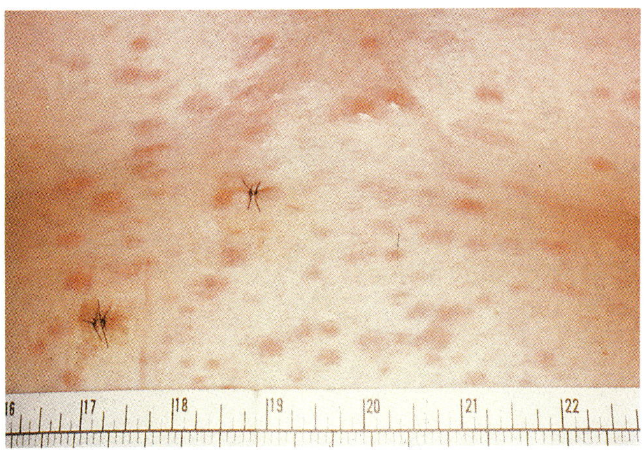

COLOR FIGURE 18-2.

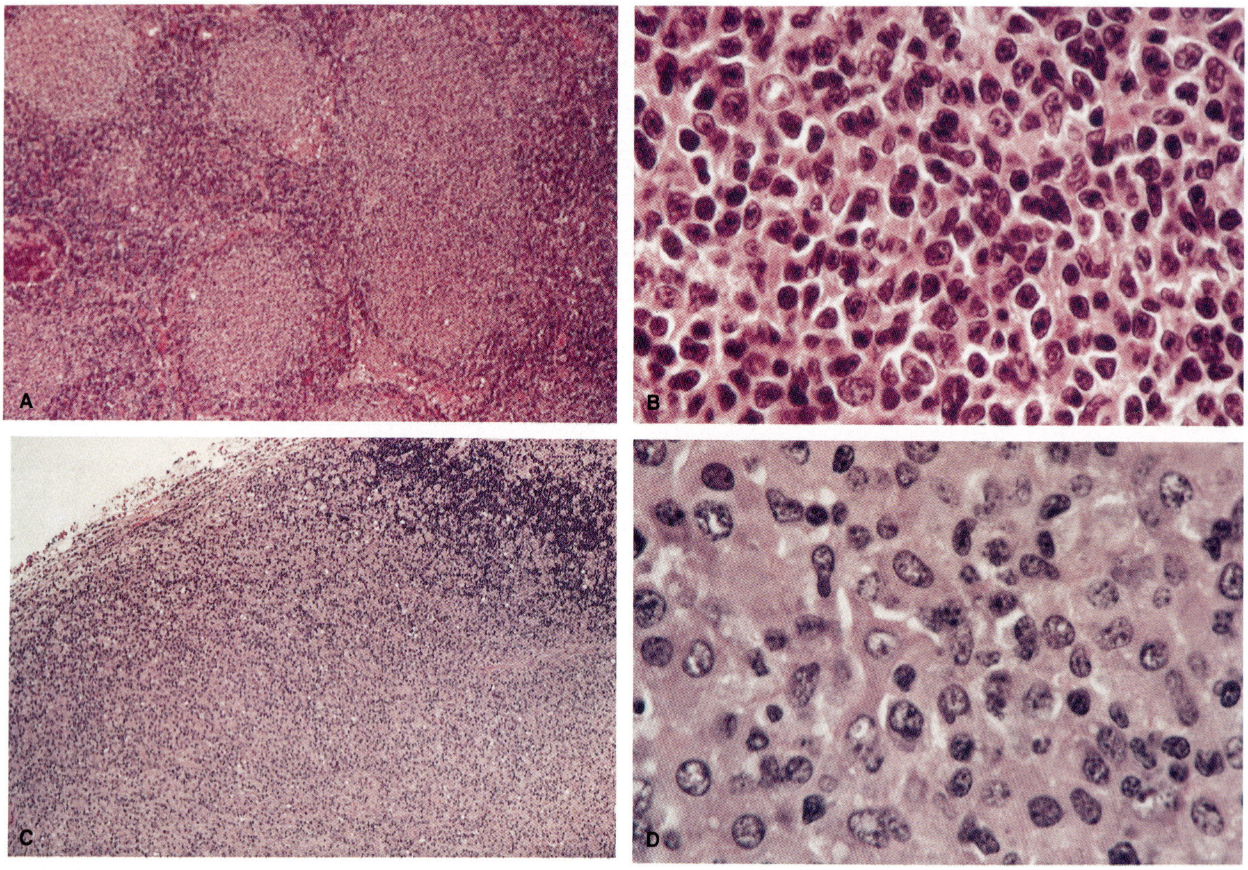

COLOR FIGURE 26-1.

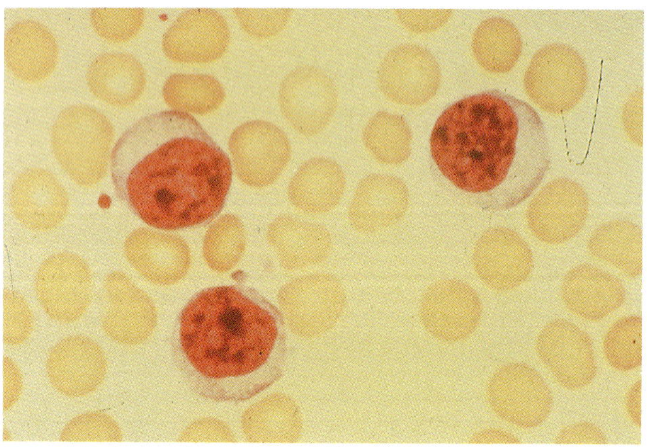

COLOR FIGURE 28-3.

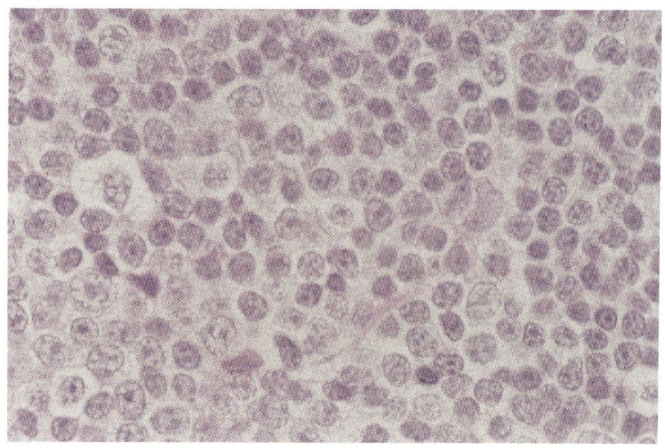

COLOR FIGURE 28-4.

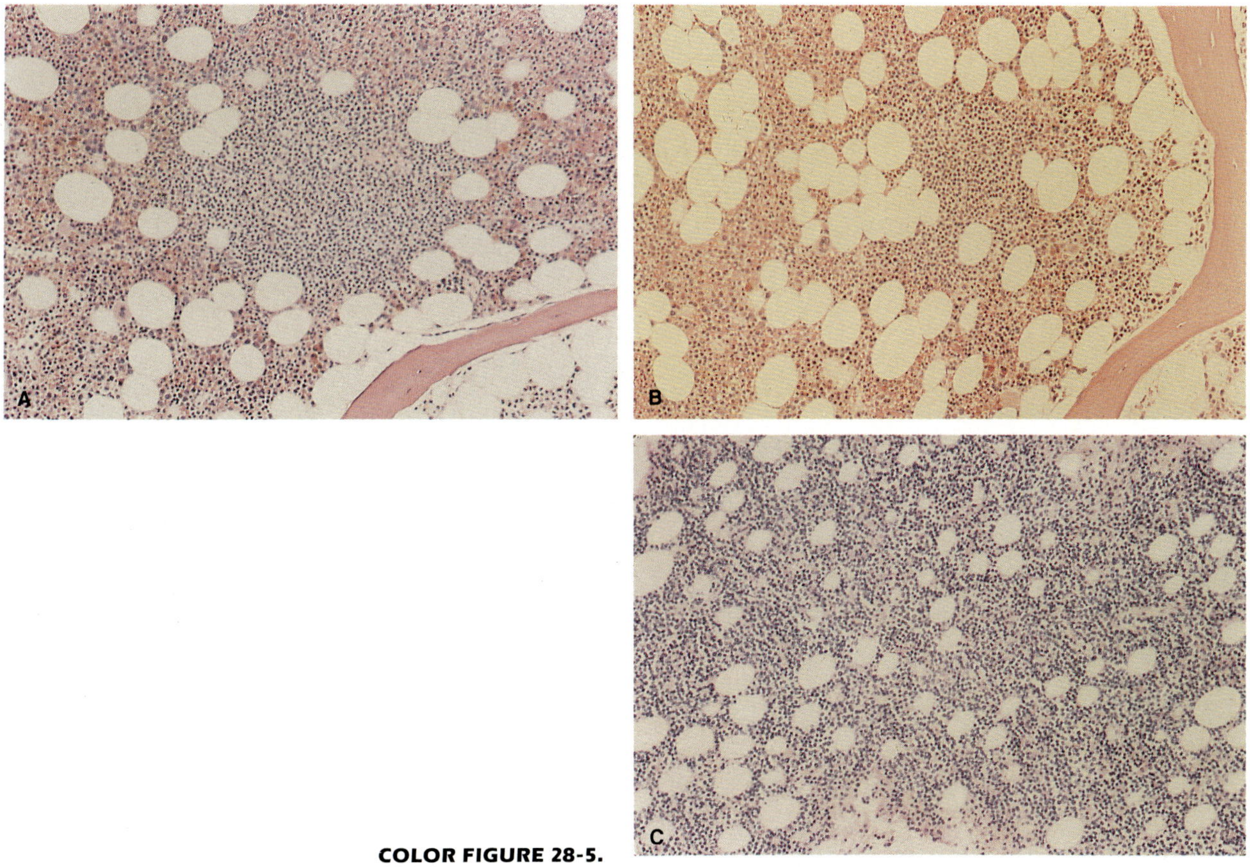

COLOR FIGURE 28-5.

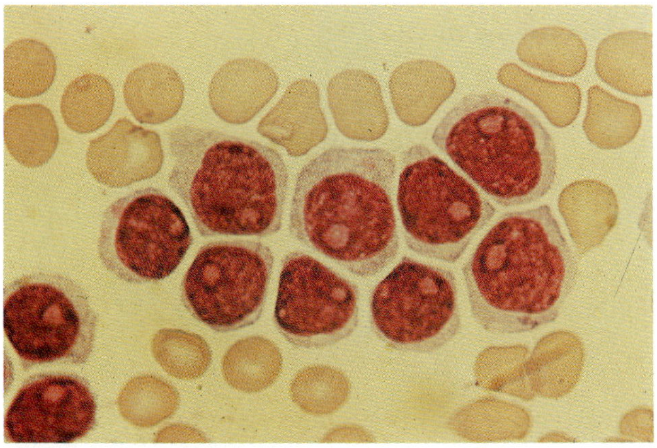

COLOR FIGURE 28-6.

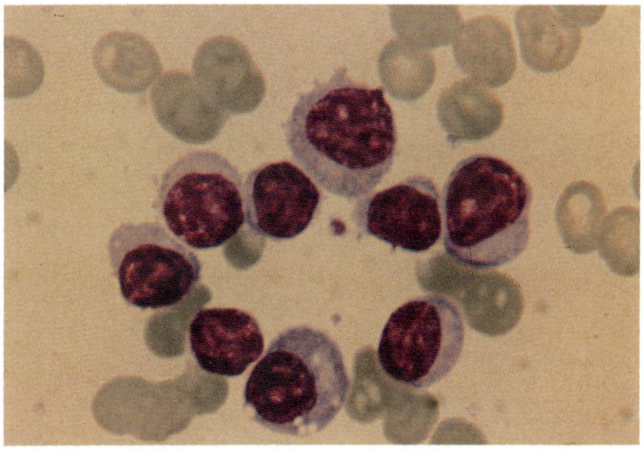

COLOR FIGURE 28-7.

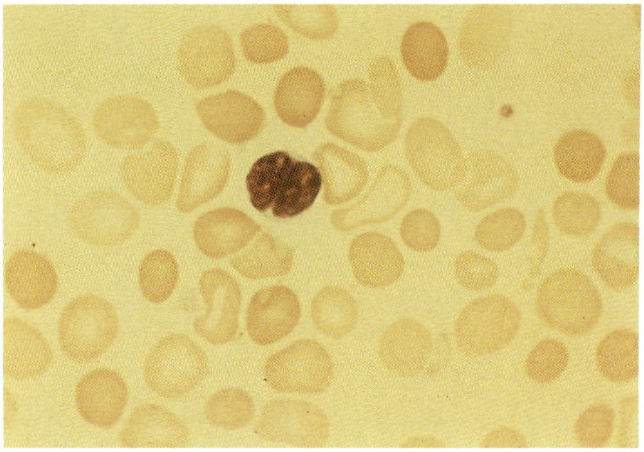

COLOR FIGURE 28-8.

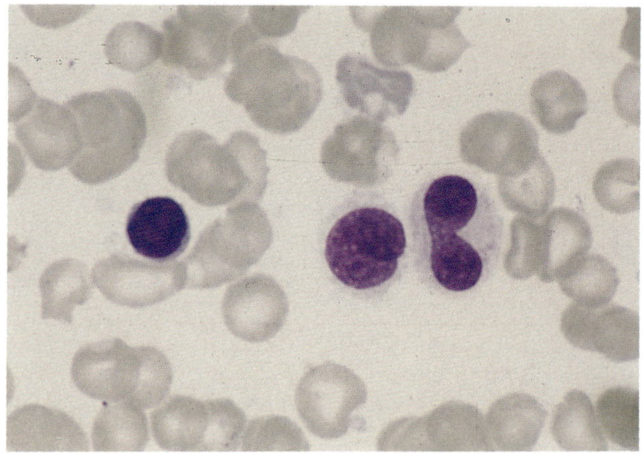

COLOR FIGURE 28-9.

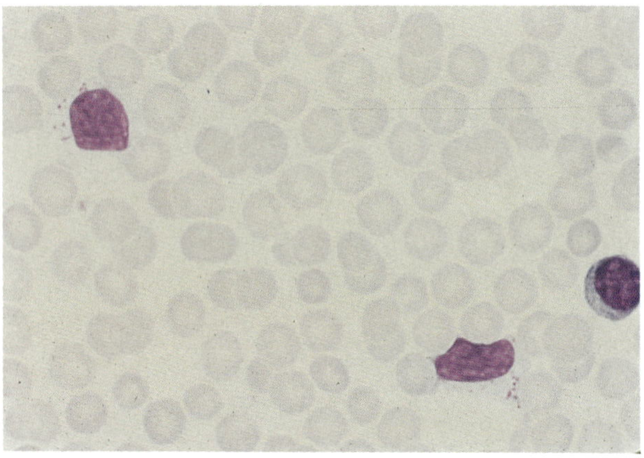

COLOR FIGURE 28-11.

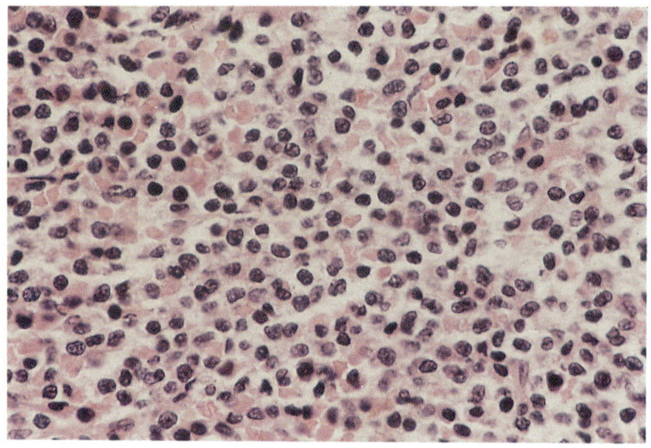

COLOR FIGURE 28-12.

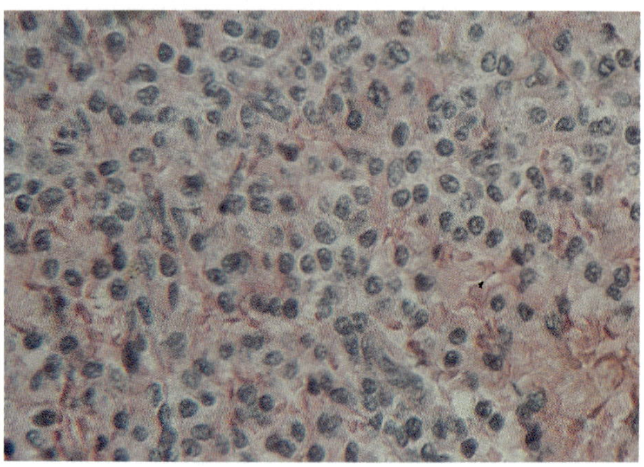

COLOR FIGURE 28-13.

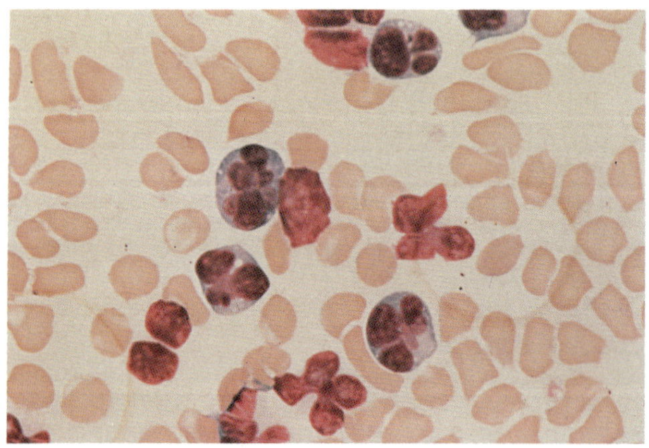

COLOR FIGURE 28-14.

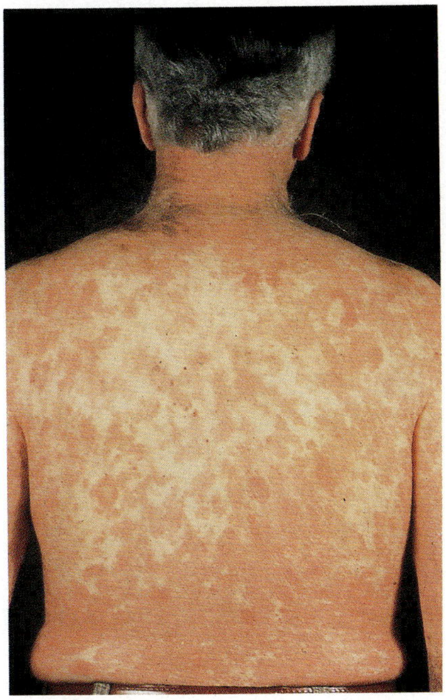

COLOR FIGURE 28-15.

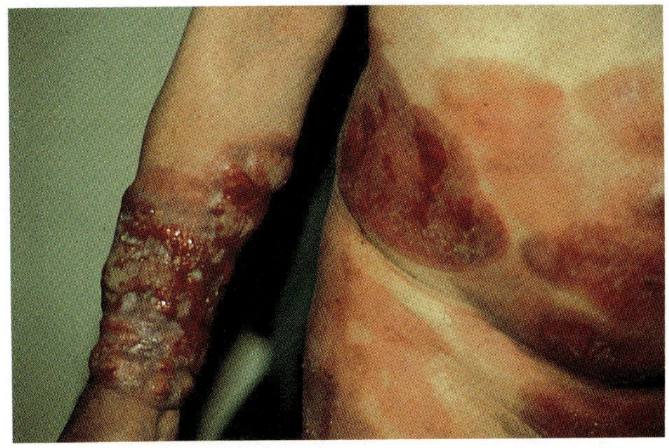

COLOR FIGURE 28-16.

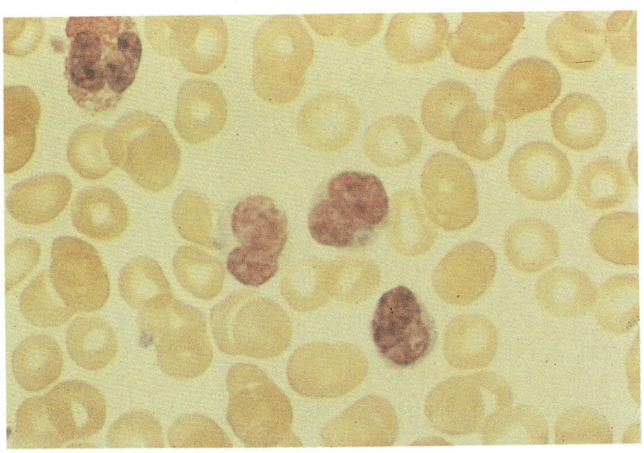

COLOR FIGURE 28-17.

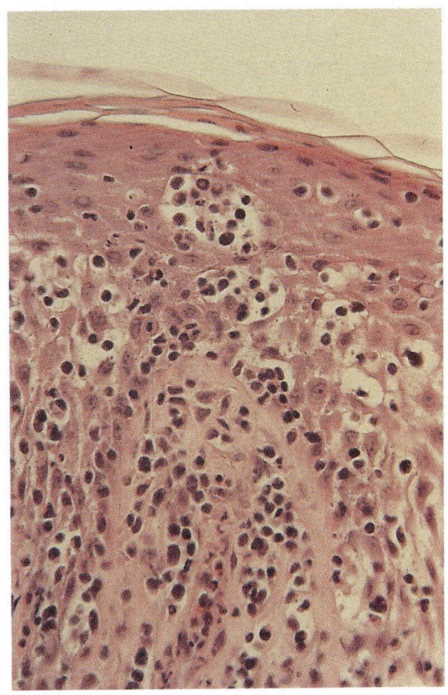

COLOR FIGURE 28-18.

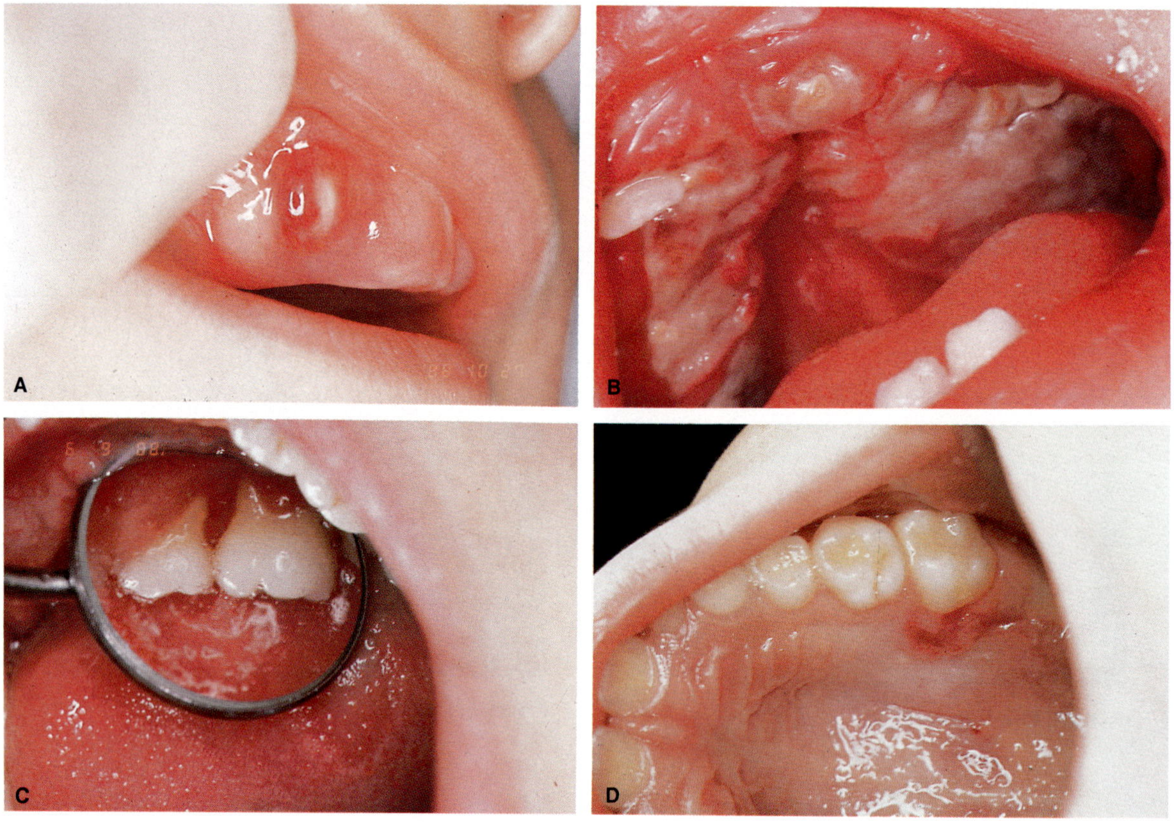

COLOR FIGURE 32-4.

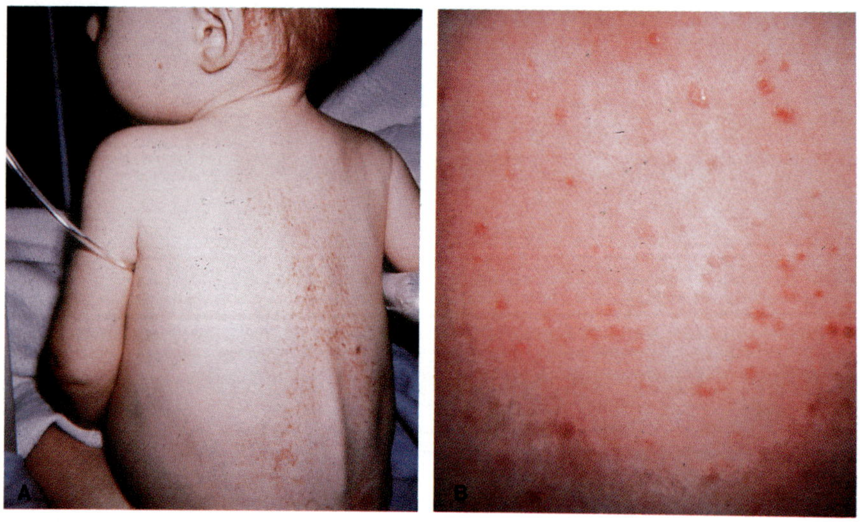

COLOR FIGURE 32-7.

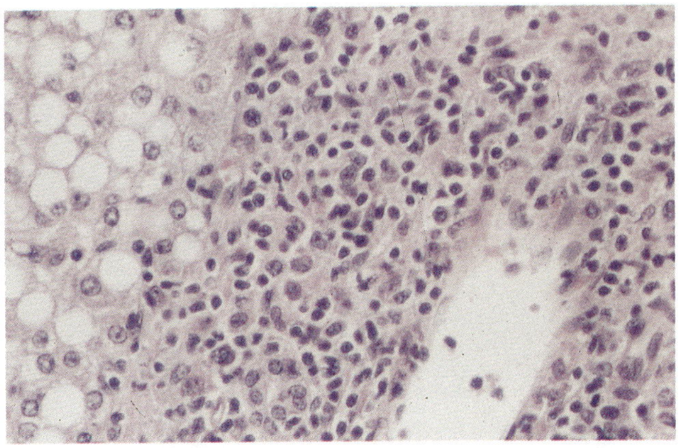

COLOR FIGURE 32-8.

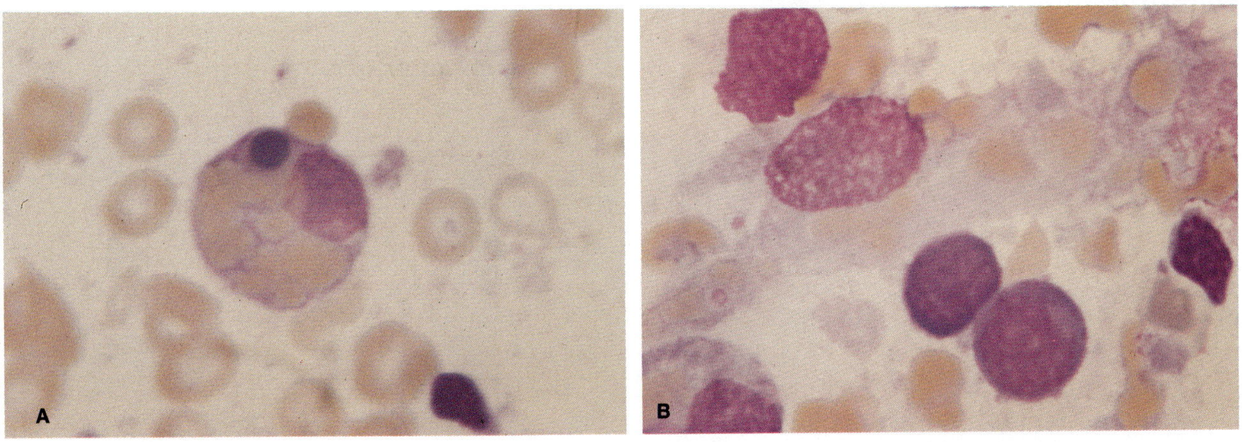

COLOR FIGURE 32-9.

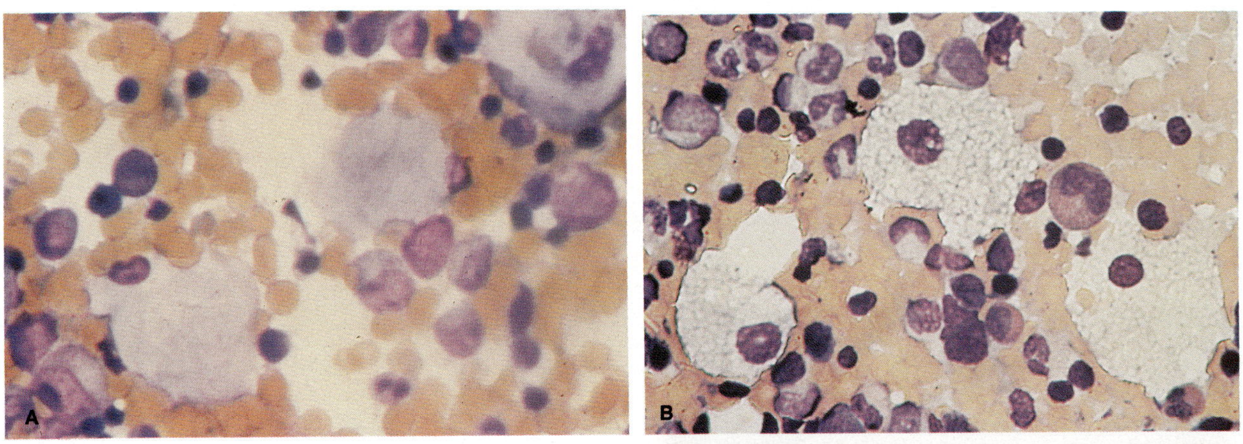

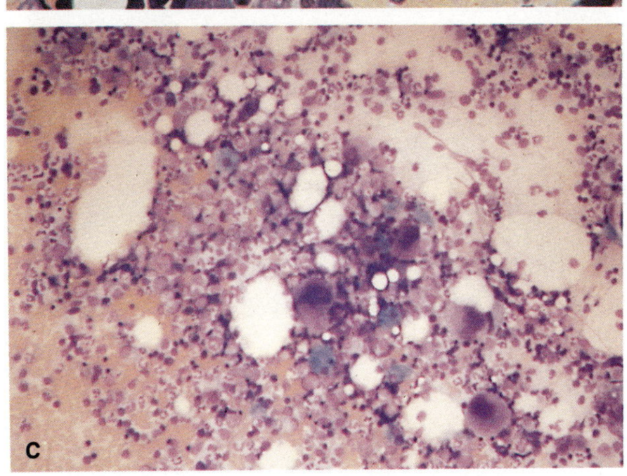

COLOR FIGURE 32-10.

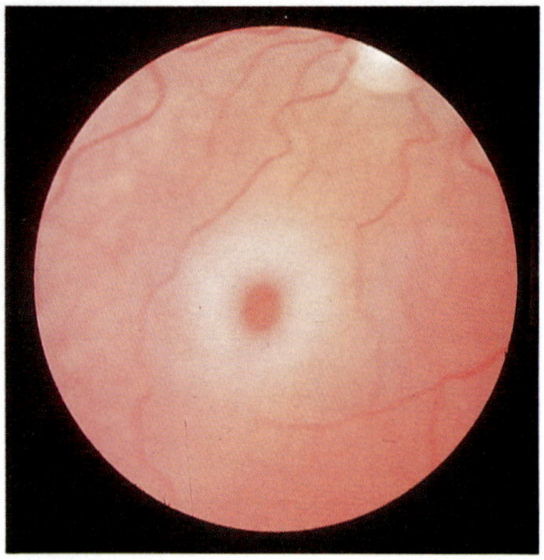

COLOR FIGURE 32-12.

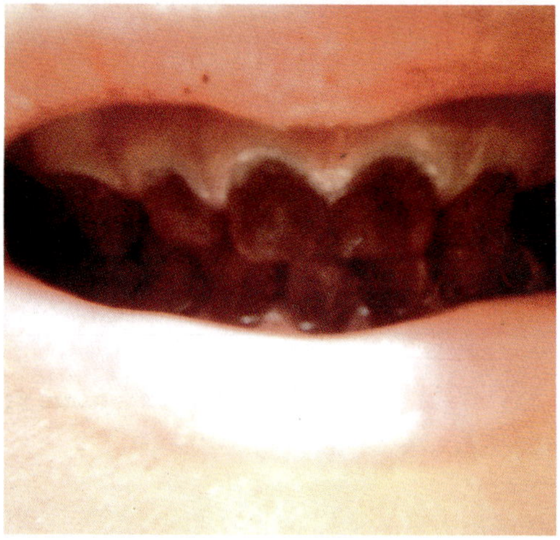

COLOR FIGURE 50-9.

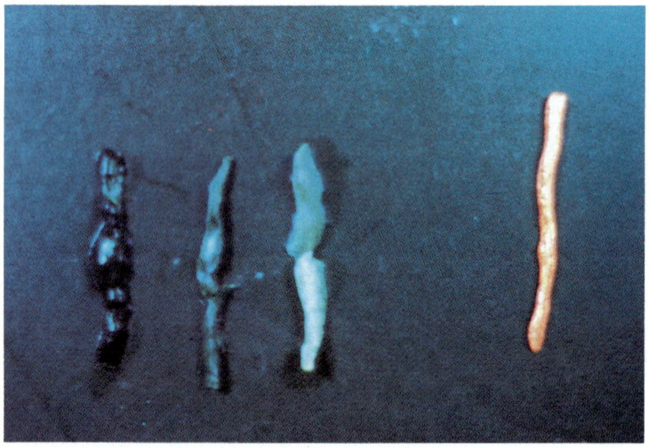

COLOR FIGURE 50-11.

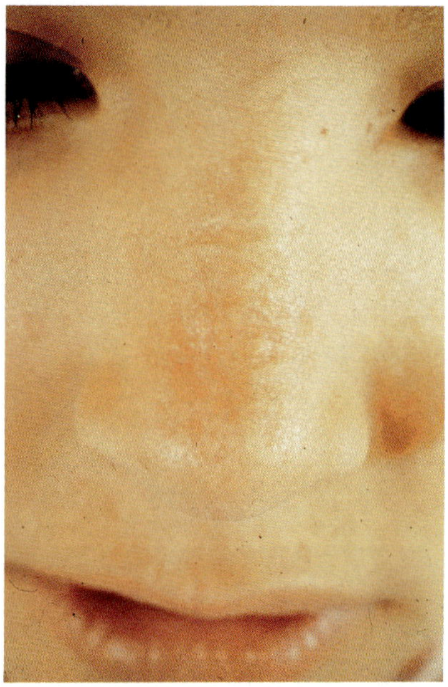

COLOR FIGURE 50-12.

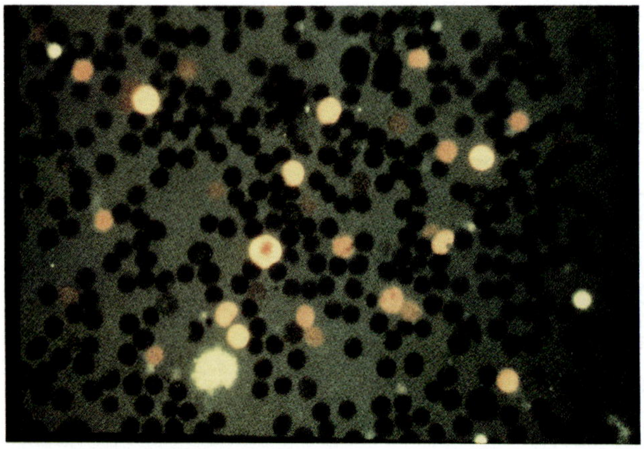

COLOR FIGURE 50-13.

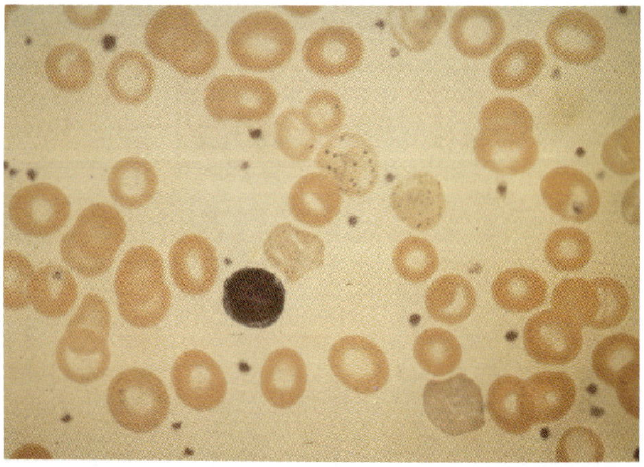

COLOR FIGURE 50-19.

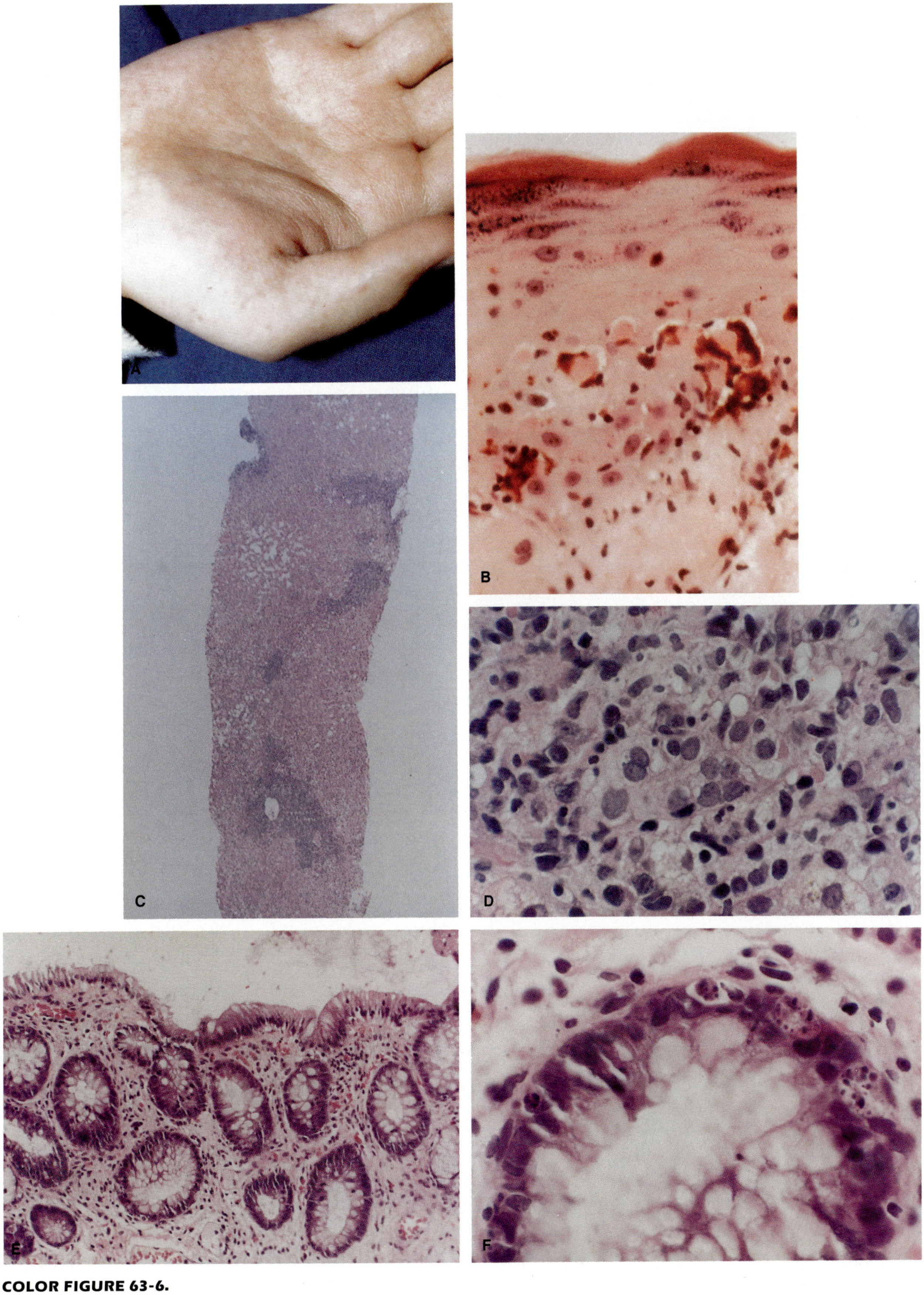

COLOR FIGURE 63-6.

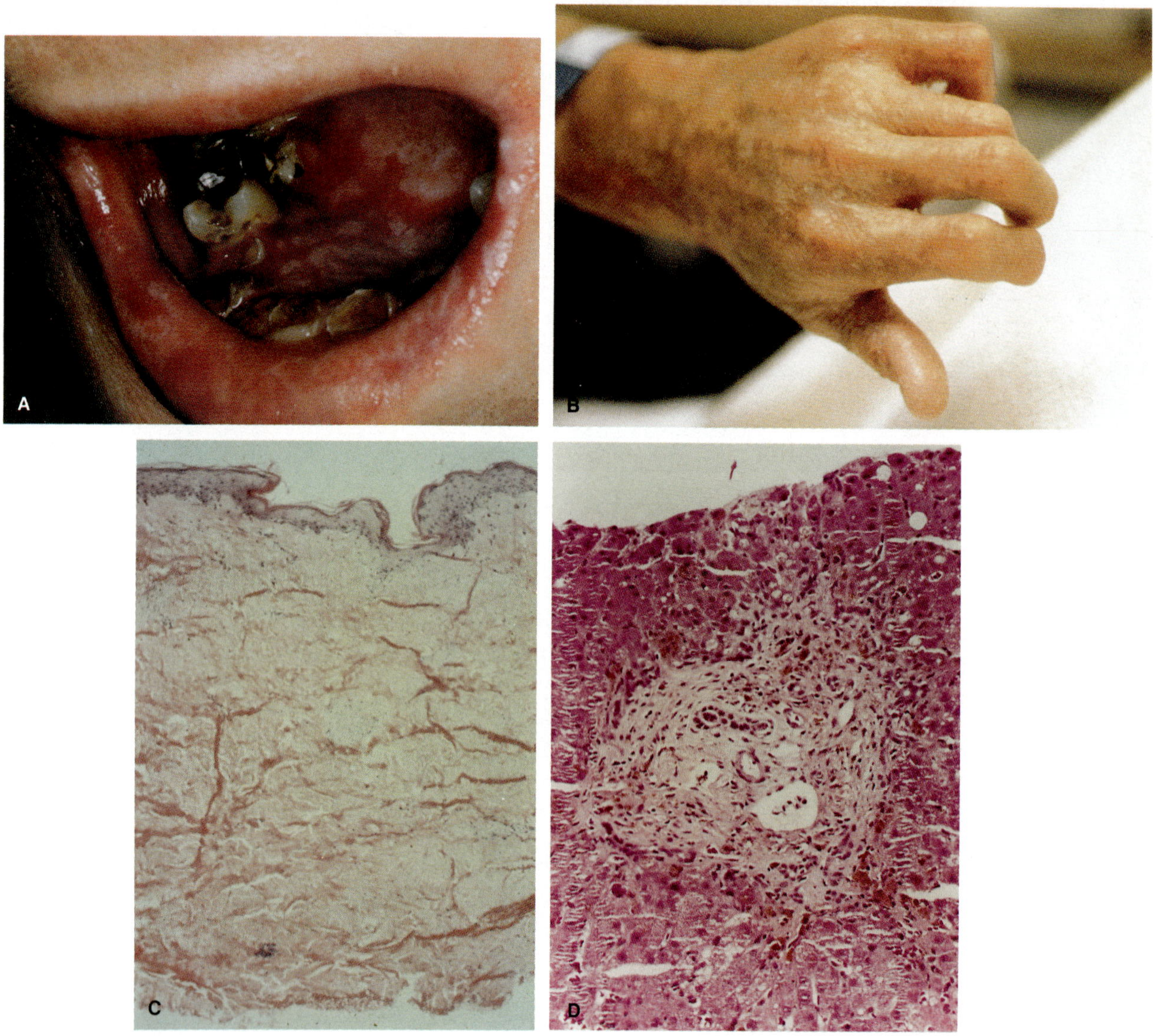

COLOR FIGURE 63-7.

Blood: Principles and Practice of Hematology,
edited by Robert I. Handin, Thomas P. Stossel, and Samuel E. Lux.
J.B. Lippincott Company, Philadelphia © 1995.

7

The Structure of Hematopoietic Tissues

Leon P. Weiss

BLOOD VESSELS

Blood is a highly specialized connective tissue consisting of cells separated by an intercellular fluid, plasma, which allows blood to flow. The friction of flow causes the plasma to layer in concentric laminae. The plasma flowing in the lamina of the central axis moves fast. Moving out to the vessel wall, successive plasma laminae flow slower and slower until, at the wall, the plasma is virtually still. Erythrocytes are relatively dense (specific gravity of 1.069) and flow in the central axial stream. They do have some "wobble" and, as they move from plasma layer to plasma layer or occupy more than one layer, they are subject to shearing forces. These forces may tear apart fragile erythrocytes with unsupported cell membranes such as spectrin-deficient cells. Leukocytes are less dense (specific gravity 1.035) and tend to flow in the middle or peripheral layers. The relatively light leukocytes (such as lymphocytes) are positioned in the most peripheral layer, the very slowly flowing layer of plasma, where they tend to bump along the endothelial surface. This arrangement favors leukocyte–endothelial interactions and, positioned as they are against the endothelium, leukocytes are set for diapedesis (outward passage).

Plasma Skimming

Another consequence of the slow peripheral plasma flow is plasma skimming, favored in arterial vessels with a straight run and right-angled branches. The branches, particularly the more proximal ones, skim off the plasma and leave a high-hematocrit blood to flow on. Perhaps the best-known example of this phenomenon is that of the interlobular renal artery traveling radially from the corticomedullary junction to the outer cortex and giving off right-angled afferent glomerular arterioles as it goes. The juxtamedullary glomeruli receive the lion's share of plasma; the subcortical glomeruli receive high-hematocrit, plasma-poor blood. As a result, more proximal juxtamedullary nephrons make and concentrate a disproportionately large volume of urine. Plasma skimming likely occurs in the spleen into the branches of the central artery as it tunnels through white pulp. Plasma and lymphocytes are preferentially skimmed off to be delivered in and around white pulp, which is the immunologically capable part of the spleen. The red blood cell (RBC)-rich remainder flows out into the red pulp where the RBCs may be stored and conditioned.

Although blood is confined by blood vessels, in different circumstances, elements of the blood escape the vessels, sometimes subtly. As blood circulates through the fine vasculature, a large-scale wash of plasma fluids occurs from the vessels into perivascular tissues and, modified, back into the vessels. Blood cells, too, have extravascular phases, as explained elsewhere in the book. Circulating lymphocytes are part of a recirculating pool of immunologically competent cells, the *recirculating lymphocyte pool* (RLP), which leaves the vasculature at specific sites in lymphatic and related tissues, migrates in a rigorously defined manner through certain tissues, and returns to blood by lymphatic vessels. Leukocytes generally leave the vasculature for the perivascular connective tissues and function there. Monocytes, representing a reserve bank of "professional" phagocytes, may go almost anywhere in the body and quickly differentiate into macrophages.

Although this differentiation may happen within the vasculature where blood flow is slow, and in such specialized intravascular locations as the endothelium of hepatic sinusoids and the lumina of large veins of ear lobes, it ordinarily occurs in the perivascular connective tissues. Macrophages may display a complex life cycle, including vascular phases. They concentrate in such sites as serous cavities and migrate through blood and lymphatic vessels in defined pathways. Macrophages may go on, again in the extracellular tissues, and differentiate into epithelioid cells and fuse into multinuclear giant cells, relatives of osteoclasts and of foreign body giant cells, whose major function is no longer phagocytosis but active transport. Even erythrocytes may leave the vasculature, perhaps through microtrauma, and are picked up by lymphatic vessels and returned to the blood. Lymphatic vessels play a quiet but essential role in hematopoietic tissues. Like lymphatic vessels elsewhere, they carry the fluid lymph and mobile cells in the connective tissues into the venous blood, regularly passing through filtering lymph nodes on the way. In the lymphatic tissues, they constitute a segment in the recirculatory migratory pathway of RLP.

The picture that emerges is that the blood and hematopoietic tissues, the vasculature, and the connective tissues proper are interactive. Nowhere is this interaction better served than in the spleen, an extraordinary hybrid of the vasculature and connective tissues. All the elements of the blood, repeatedly (perhaps 10 to 12 times each hour) interact with one another, with the vasculature, and with the connective tissue in the spleen. The splenic structures that support these interactions are filtration beds, interposed between arteries and veins, fabricated of fibroblastic stromal cells. Yet, these ostensibly extravascular filtration beds may support blood flow as efficiently as conventional blood vessels or may delay elements of the blood and process them as a connective tissue, marshaling all the cells of the connective tissue, including the blood cells, as fully as in inflammation. Because of the unique structure of the spleen, what would be rampant inflammation elsewhere, in the spleen is more structured, more controlled, more confined, and, in many instances, more effective in the control of infectious disease. The spleen allows the full differentiation and the fullest expression of the functional capacities of blood cells and occupies a unique intermediary position between the blood and the connective tissues proper.

SPLEEN

The spleen is both the quintessential filter of the blood and the stage on which the cells and other elements filtered from the blood are stored and modified and on which they function. Weighing about 150 g in adult human beings, the spleen is divided into three zones. The white pulp is the immunologic center; the red pulp is the most versatile filter of the blood and shows the essential structure and functions of the spleen to best advantage; the marginal zone lies between white pulp and red pulp and is a reception center and a major filtration zone.[1]

Open Arterial Circulations

The tissues of the body, with the salient exception of the spleen, have a closed vasculature in which endothelial continuity is found throughout the blood vessels, through the arteries, into and through the microvasculature, into and through the veins.[1-9] In the spleen, arterial vessels, as shown best in red pulp, are not continuous with veins, but are cut off. They may terminate simply, as if sliced across, or they may end with a flare, often with widened interendothelial slits. Blood flows out of terminating vessels through these endings and interendothelial slits.[10] Filtration beds, meshworks fabricated of branched fibroblastic reticular cells and reticular fibers, are interposed between the end of arterial vessels and the vein.

Venous Sinuses

Blood is drained from the spleen by a system of veins. The finest veins form an anastomotic system placed at variable distances from arterial endings. In human beings, these venous vessels are sinusal, termed *venous* or *vascular sinuses*, as in other primates, dogs, armadillos, rabbits, and rats (Figs. 7-1 and 7-2). They are highly specialized vessels that possess rod-like endothelial cells, their long axis parallel with the long axis of vessel, lying tight against one another, side to side. The basal portion of these endothelial cells contain regularly oriented longitudinal fascicles of

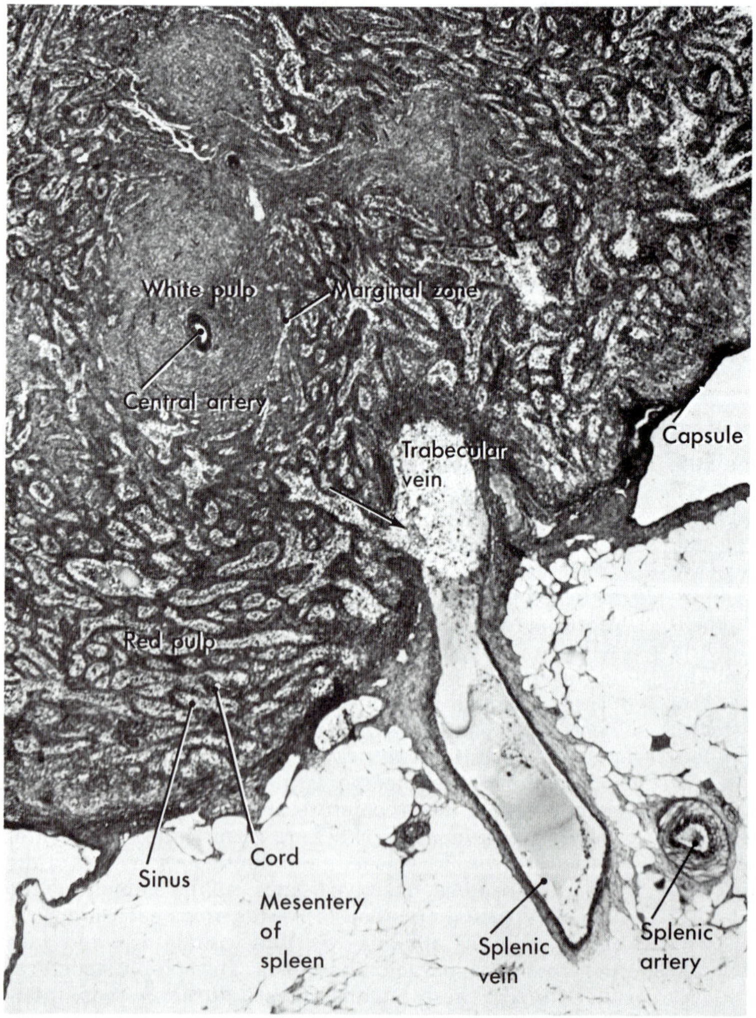

FIGURE 7-1. The spleen of a hedgehog. The white pulp, red pulp, blood outflow tract, and splenic mesentery are shown in this low-power field. The white pulp, occupying a relatively small volume, surrounds a central artery. The red pulp occupies most of the field. It is made up almost entirely of relatively clear spaces, the splenic sinuses, which form an anastomosing system of vessels. The splenic cord (darkly stained tissue lying between the sinuses) consists of reticular meshwork that contains blood cells and macrophages and that receives arterial terminations. Blood is carried out of the spleen through trabecular veins, which drain into the splenic vein. Splenic veins leave the spleen at the hilus and enter the splenic mesentery. The splenic sinuses empty into a pulp vein that drains into a trabecular vein (*arrow*). The marginal zone lies between white pulp and red pulp. The mesentery contains a branch of the splenic artery that will enter the spleen at the hilus (×150).

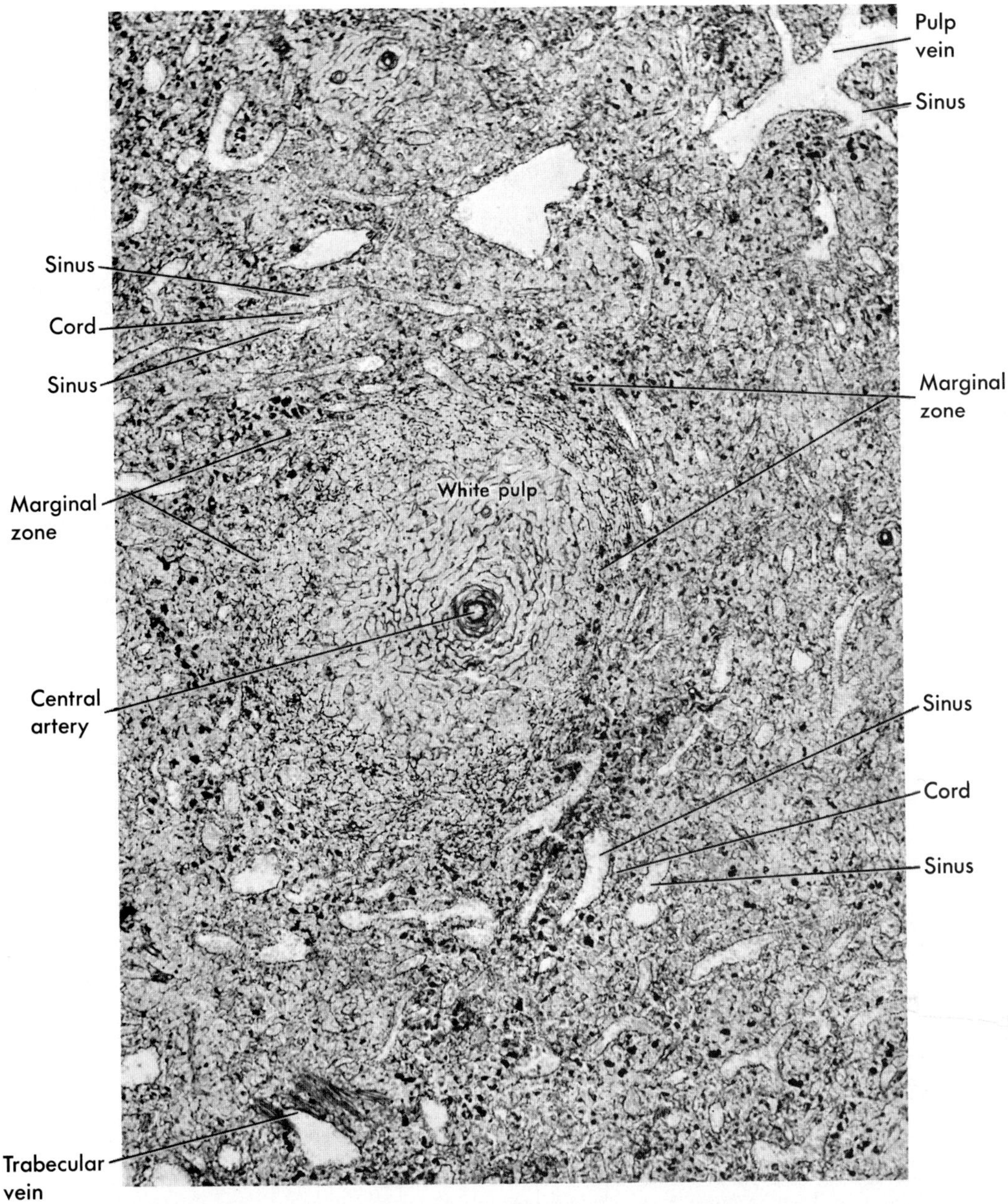

FIGURE 7-2. Spleen of a rat. The extracellular reticulum is stained by the periodic acid–Schiff reaction. The white pulp contains a darkly outlined central artery. Note the circumferential pattern of the reticulum of white pulp. A marginal zone surrounds the white pulp and contains a relatively dense meshwork of the reticulum and many darkly stained cells. Beyond the white pulp and marginal zone lies the red pulp, accounting for most of the splenic sinuses but also pulp veins and trabecular veins. The splenic cords constitute the relatively solid tissue lying between the sinuses (×225). (Weiss L. J Anal 1959;93:465)

contractile intermediate filaments composed of myosin. Microfilaments corresponding to molecules of actin, moreover, have been located by cytochemistry in this region.[11]

The basal surface of endothelial cells lies on a basement membrane. It is not a sleeve-like complete basement membrane as it is in most other locations; it is defective.[1,11] Most of it is missing and the remainder looks like linear strands or fibers, which, as in reticular fibers of the connective tissues, can be selectively stained by silver or by the periodic acid–Schiff (PAS) histochemical reaction. The major components of the basement membrane are arranged as regularly spaced circular bands that encircle the vessel, very much as hoops encircle a barrel, holding the staves (endothelial cells) together. In fact, beneath these circular bands, the endothelial cells may be attached to one another by adherent membranous junctions, and slight, irregular strands of basement membrane run obliquely but predominantly longitudinally, connecting the heavy circular bands. Variations of this pattern exist; human spleen displays it rather well, and in rabbit spleen the basement membrane lacks the heavy circular bands. These details are important in splenic functions because the route that blood cells take in flowing into the veins and out of the spleen is through the bared (uncovered by basement membrane) interendothelial slits of the wall of the venous sinus (Fig. 7-3). Lacking inherent motility, erythrocytes depend

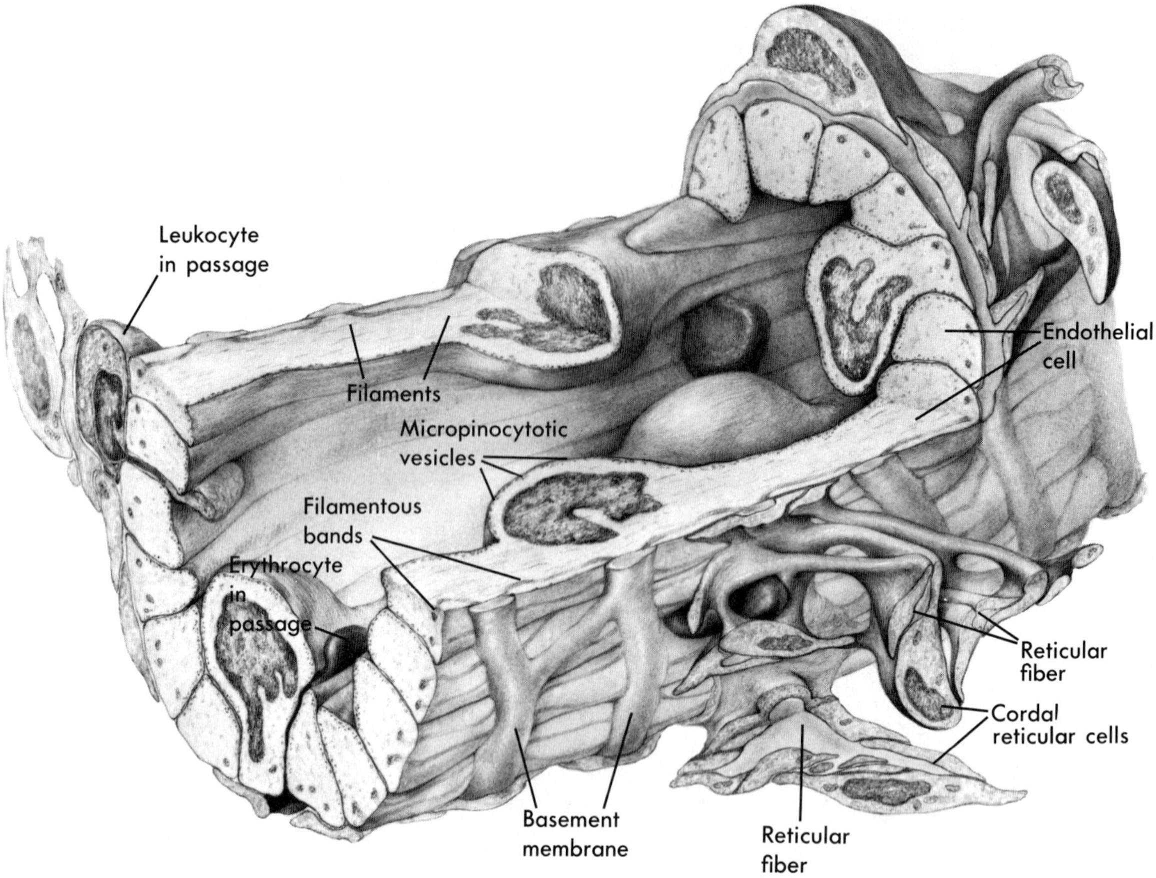

FIGURE 7-3. Schematic depiction of a human splenic sinus in red pulp. The endothelial cells are tapered rods that lie side by side with their long axis parallel to the long axis of the vessel. Virtually all arterial vessels end in the surrounding cords without direct connection to the sinuses. Accordingly, blood entering the vascular sinus must enter from the surrounding cord, squeezing through the slit-like spaces between the sinus endothelial cells. Several blood cells in passage across the sinus wall are shown. The endothelial cells show several distinctive cytologic features. These features include a row of pinocytotic vesicles just beneath the plasma membrane on the luminal and lateral surfaces, and two sets of cytoplasmic filaments. One rather loosely organized set of filaments runs through the cytoplasm. The other set is lightly organized into dense bands in the basal cytoplasm. The bands arch between strands of the basement membrane. They appear to insert into the plasma membrane where it overlies the basement membrane and then to continue through the plasma membrane into the substance of the basement membrane. Those filaments are probably part of the cytoskeletal system, which stiffens the basal cytoplasm and maintains the shape of endothelial cells and the set of filaments, and may be contractile. They play an important role in the spleen's capacity to recognize damaged blood cells and destroy or modify them. The basement membrane is fenestrated, having heavy, strand-like, transverse "ring" components and lighter longitudinal strands joining the rings. The large fenestrae, or apertures, in the basement membrane leave ample unimpeded space for blood cells to pass through the sinus wall. The cordal surface of the basement membrane is covered by cordal reticular cells, which branch into the surrounding cord.

on external forces to squeeze through interendothelial slits. Leukocytes, in contrast, possess a contractile and migratory capacity and can "shoulder" their way through.[1,10]

Blood cells in transendothelial passage can be held or pinched in interendothelial slits, thought to be sites where the "pitting" of an erythrocyte bearing a rigid inclusion, such as an intracellular malarial *Plasmodium* or a Heinz body occurs. Such an inclusion-bearing erythrocyte may be held up as it squeezes through an interendothelial slit. Only the supple, readily deformable, normal part of the erythrocyte easily slips through. The rigid inclusion, enveloped by a portion of erythrocyte plasma membrane, is delayed and may actually snap off, with the plasma membrane "healing" about each part of the severed erythrocyte. The normal, supple portion of the erythrocyte, having navigated the interendothelial slit and gained the venous lumen, flows out of the spleen, whereas the rigid portion lies outside the venous wall. The rigid part is soon phagocytized, but the surviving portion of the erythrocyte is compromised. Shorn of some plasma membrane, it is no longer a supple biconcave disk, but a spherocyte (geometric figure that requires the least amount of plasma membrane). Spherocytes are poorly deformable and are more likely to be retained by the spleen on a subsequent transit.

Sinusal and Nonsinusal Splenic Anatomy

Contractile basal venous endothelial filaments insert into the plasma membrane at the site of the circular hoops of basement membrane, and the plasma membrane is in turn attached to the hoops. Thus, an endothelial cell is marked off into contractile segments by the regularly disposed circular bands of basement membrane. When endothelial segments contract, the effect is to cause side-by-side endothelial cells to separate, converting a closed interendothelial slit into an interendothelial gap, facilitating transendothelial blood cell passage. The rigor and complexity of venous sinusal interendothelial slits are characteristic of the sinusal spleen, of which the human spleen is a good example. In sinusal spleens, therefore, blood flow out of the spleen is regulated by the interendothelial slits of venous sinuses. If these slits become obstructed or do not open, congestion of the spleen occurs.

Fine venous vessels of nonsinusal spleens display a more conventional venous endothelium and are far more likely than sinusal spleens to possess large stable mural apertures and offer little or no impedance to transendothelial blood cell passage. Circulating erythrocytes bearing Heinz bodies are a regular characteristic of feline blood; they form more readily in feline hemoglobin and the feline spleen doesn't pit them.

Spleen as a Filtration and Storage Organ

The distinctive arterial and venous vessels of red pulp are not continuous through a capillary bed. Endothelial continuity typical of the general vasculature is absent. The unique intervascular part of the spleen, interposed between arteries and veins (and lymphatics), serves as filtration beds and supports the spleen's extraordinary capacity to clear the blood, control certain infectious diseases, sustain fetal hematopoiesis, and eliminate damaged erythrocytes, neoplastic cells, and microbes. What are the character and magnitude of splenic clearance? How do the filtration beds provide for splenic clearance and for such derivative activities as phagocytosis and hematopoiesis?

The normal spleen in a normal steady-state adult animal appears to clear the blood of microbes, damaged erythrocytes, platelets, lymphocytes, and other blood cells at effective but modest levels.[1,5,6,12] Limited numbers of T cells and B cells are cleared and, in company with their accessory cells and antigens, are provided a migratory pathway through the two major divisions of white pulp, periarterial lymphatic sheaths (T cells), and lymphatic nodules (B cells) as part of the recirculating lymphocyte pool. Platelets are stored in the filtration beds of all types of spleen. Some animals with a nonsinusal spleen (horse) and some with a sinusal spleen (dog), possess a large spleen with a heavy muscular capsule and trabeculae, a so-called *storage spleen*, which can store large numbers of erythrocytes, granulocytes, and other cells and express them into the circulation as needed. The horse is believed to be able to maintain a sustained running pace because of internal transfusions it can give itself by squeezing out splenic RBC reserves.[7] A splenectomized horse is a poor athlete. The human spleen does not normally have this general storage capacity, although it stores T cells, B cells, macrophages, and platelets.

The clearance capacity of the spleen has been attributed largely to macrophages. Yet, macrophages are not plentiful in normal spleen, and those that are present have few lysosomes, tending not to be activated. They tend to lie along major concourses, surveying cellular traffic, specifically at the orifice of terminating arterial vessels, on the adventitial surface of efferent vessels, and at the interface of splenic zones.

The spleen is involved in the terminal differentiation of blood cells, which are cleared from the circulation after release from bone marrow or thymus.[12] Reticulocytes, for example, are released from bone marrow but do not enter the general circulation until conditioned by the spleen. Eosinophils (at least in the rat) also require some splenic conditioning before joining the general circulation. Mature but "naive" T cells and B cells are released from the thymus and bone marrow, respectively, and travel to the spleen where they may be stabilized and "sophisticated" by small levels of antigen before joining the RLP.

If normal clearance is modest, the spleen is poised to quickly increase its clearance capacities or to decrease them. In many infectious diseases—malaria is the paradigm—the spleen quickly increases its capacity for clearance and often enlarges. The enlargement is due to congestion, to the mobilization and activation of and phagocytosis by macrophages, and to cell proliferation and differentiation, specifically lymphopoiesis and plasmacytopoiesis effecting immune responses, erythropoiesis (in the rodent) in anticipation and compensation for anemia, granulocytopoiesis linked to monocytopoiesis and macrophage production and nonspecific protection against disease. Malaria stresses the spleen extraordinarily. In fact, it has been argued that not only the evolution of hemoglobins, but the character of the spleen, has been driven by vertebrates' ancient and long-term interactions with malaria. In experimental murine malaria, the enlarged spleen changes from functionally asplenic, in the precrisis phase of the disease, to hypersplenic, at crisis.[13,14] It is likely that exaggerated shifts in clearance are characteristic of splenomegaly.

Red Pulp: Reticular Network

The major structural element of the filtration beds is a three-dimensional meshwork, which has been termed a *reticulum* because it is fashioned of reticular cells and reticular fibers.[15] Reticular cells are large, branched, fibroblastic stromal cells, which meet with other reticular cells to form a scaffolding, web, or reticulum.[2,3,16] Reticular cells lie on, ensheathe, and presumably produce delicate reticular fibers that contain a blend of collagens, richest in collagen type IV, and that may be stained selectively with silver or with the PAS histochemical routine. (An older term used to name the substance making up reticular fibers is *reticulin*.) Reticular cells lie on the outside surface of blood vessels, forming an incomplete adventitial coat. From the surface of the vessel, they branch into the perivascular space, their processes meeting those of other reticular cells to form a meshwork or reticulum reinforced by reticular fibers. The interstices of the filtration beds contain blood cells, blood plasma, and cells into which the blood cells differentiate. The specific contents of a filtration bed depend on its location. The mouse spleen readily engages in hematopoiesis, and, even without splenic stress, the subcapsular and peritrabecular filtration beds of red pulp support a balance of megakaryocytopoiesis, granulocytopoiesis, and erythropoiesis.[1,9,13] The human red pulp is far less readily hematopoietic, but similar, if blunted, patterns of splenic hematopoiesis can emerge in hematopoietic stress. This is the structure of the filtration beds in normal spleen, providing basal clearance in a normal steady-state person (Fig. 7-4).

Barrier Cells

The picture changes significantly in splenic stress induced by infection, damaged erythrocytes, or such factors as endotoxin or interleukin-1α. A recently defined, intensely activated, rapidly mobilized, fugitive, fibroblastic stromal cell lineage appears. These stromal cells are generated locally by differentiation from fibroblasts covering the surface of trabeculae and from distantly generated progenitors that circulate into the spleen as mononucleate cells and migrate into the perivascular tissues. Whatever their source, these cells quickly fuse with one another to form extensive syncytial sheets deployed in the filtration beds as diverse barriers, hence termed *barrier cells*.[17]

Barrier cells may quickly degenerate and disappear, re-

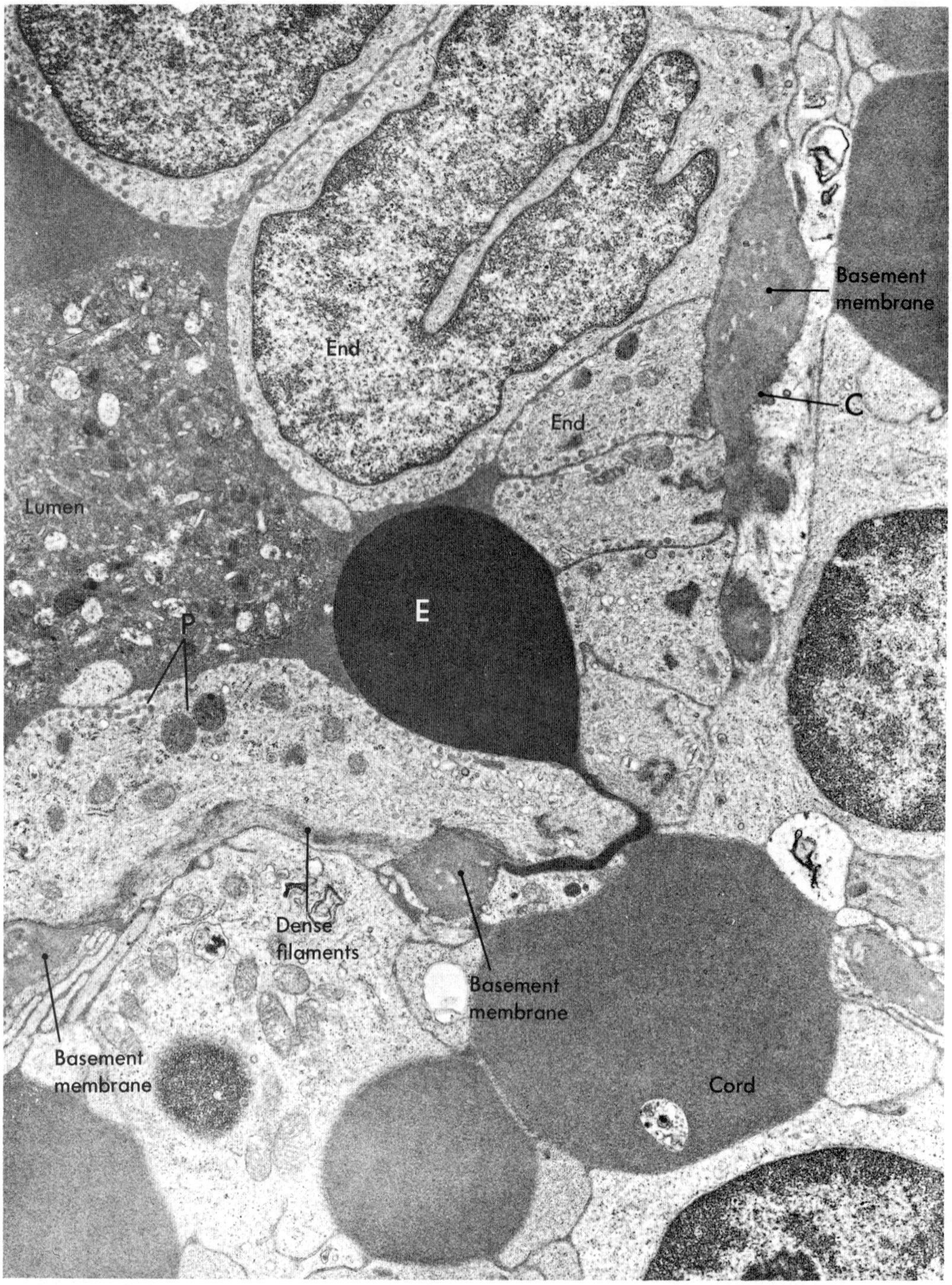

FIGURE 7-4. Human spleen, red pulp. An erythrocyte (E) passes from a cord and through the sinus wall between endothelial cells (End) into the lumen of the sinus. The erythrocyte is drawn into a thin strand as it passes through the mural slit. The endothelial cells contain many pinocytotic vesicles (P) at the luminal surface and dense filaments in the basal cytoplasm, which arches across the fenestrae of the basement membrane. Small portions of cordal reticular cells applied to the abluminal surface of the basement membrane are present. The cord is filled with erythrocytes and free cells (×1000).

vealing a fugitive nature. Barrier cells become intercalated into a basic reticular filtration bed, augmenting its activity, and thereby appear responsible for the increase (and decrease) in splenic clearance above (and below) the basal level supported by the basic reticular cell/fiber filtration bed. Barrier cells ensheathe blood vessels, contributing to blood–spleen barriers. They are aligned to channel blood flow, arrangements that may carry blood into an augmented filtration bed, resulting in heightened clearance, or shunt it past the filtration beds into veins, resulting in a functionally asplenic spleen. Processes of barrier cells extend into channels in which blood cells flow, and entwine platelets, engaging and clustering them, rationalizing the spleen's capacity to clear circulating platelets. Sheets of barrier cells form rafts that float in the moving bloodstream, sometimes tethered by barrier cell processes to a fixed structure as a vascular wall or trabecula. They strip monocytes from the circulation, holding them on their surface and permitting their transformation into macrophages there. Barrier cells enclose hematopoietic colonies. Several consequences follow such enclosure: high concentrations of hematopoietic factors may be maintained within the enclosure; the colony is protected against parasitism, as are the erythroid colonies in murine malaria; and a bone marrow character is conferred on the colony, since the bone marrow offers hematopoietic colonies the protection of an endothelial barrier whereas the filtration beds of the spleen without barrier cells are open to the circulation. Related to the enclosure of hematopoietic colonies is the sealing off of immunologically competent white pulp after the initiation of an immune response. This finding suggests how a segment of white pulp is isolated. The arrangement would concentrate immunoregulatory factors and reduce the diversion of immune resources to new antigens, some of which could stimulate an autoimmune process if responded to.

Barrier cells can be recognized in normal unstressed spleen. They occur inconsistently and in very small numbers. A few ensheathe megakaryocytes in subcapsular murine red pulp. A few are intercalated into the circumferential reticulum that separates white pulp from red pulp. Only when they are induced in large numbers and in characteristic patterns can their significance be readily grasped.

White Pulp

White pulp, an immunologic tissue underlying the spleen's extraordinary capacity to respond to blood-borne antigen, consists of discrete populations of T cells and B cells and their accessory cells (macrophages, interdigitating cells, follicular dendritic cells).[8,18–23] These cell populations are hardly static. In the normal steady state, they maintain nearly constant numbers, because lymphocytes leave, carried away by dedicated efferent lymphatic vessels, and are replaced by immigration of equivalent numbers of like cells from the blood. This significant specialized migratory loop from blood into and through white pulp and out through lymphatic vessels confers on the spleen an important part in the recirculation of the pool of immunologically competent lymphocytes.

The white pulp is organized by a distinctive reticular cell/fiber stroma about arterial and lymphatic vessels. Major splenic arteries pierce the capsule and ramify in the trabecular system. As the arteries branch into trabeculae and become medium- to small-sized arteries, they leave the trabeculae and plunge into the parenchyma or pulp of the spleen. As the arteries leave the trabeculae and enter the pulp, they are surrounded by a dense collection of lymphocytes that make up the white pulp. Two principal portions of white pulp are found. One consists predominantly of T lymphocytes and their accessory cells and forms a sheath symmetrically surrounding the artery. In other words, the artery runs in the central longitudinal axis of the sheath. Appropriately enough, the artery is called the *central artery*, and the sheath is called the *periarterial lymphatic sheath* (PALS).[1] B cells aggregate in nodules—lymphatic nodules (LNs)—lying within the PALS. As the artery branches and tapers, the PALS also tapers, then ends leaving the artery uncovered. The artery, now a metarteriole, emerges from the sheath, leaves the white pulp, and enters the red pulp, where it runs as capillary for some distance and terminates in the filtration beds of the red pulp.

The terminating artery thereby contributes to the filtration unit just described, an arterial terminal carrying blood into a reticular cell–barrier cell filtration bed drained by a system of veins. The lymphocytes and associated mobile cells of the PALS are supported by a fibroblastic stroma of reticular cells and fibers, which tend to assume a circumferential conformation, tracking about the central artery. The circumferential character is especially marked both near the center of the PALS and at the periphery. Indeed, at the periphery of the PALS, the circumferential reticulum is disposed in several layers. Gaps, typically out of register, exist in each of these layers, so that lymphocytes, monocytes, macrophages, interdigitating cells, occasional erythrocytes, and granulocytes move into and out of the white pulp as if through a maze. These maze-like arrangements that bound the PALS thus appear to permit some cellular traffic into and out of the sheath, but offer some restriction to free passage. It is important that as the PALS tapers toward its termination, the circumferential reticulum disappears and no stromal restriction to cellular movement into and out of white pulp occurs. Most of the cellular traffic into white pulp occurs at the attenuated ends of the PALS, particularly that of the recirculating lymphocyte pool.[20,21]

After entering the PALS in its distal, attenuated regions, lymphocytes move proximally in the PALS, sorting themselves out into T-cell and B-cell zones. T cells move about in the PALS, attended by accessory cells, such as macrophages and interdigitating cells, whose diverse functions include antigen presentation. B cells enter the PALS, the traffic being heaviest at the distal PALS as it is for immigrating T cells. These B cells move through the T-cell–rich PALS, heading for compact nodules of lymphocytes (LNs), which lie within the PALS, especially at points of bifurcation. LNs, delimited by stromal reticular cells and fibers, receive B cells and permit them to move about, interacting with other B cells and their accessory cells, macrophages, and follicular dendritic cells. B cells moving through the T-cell–rich PALS toward LNs come in contact with T cells. After they have reached an LN those positioned at the periphery facing the PALS are set to interact with T cells. Thus, the white pulp is efficiently organized to permit T cells and B cells to engage in an antibody response if the proper antigen comes along. If this happens, the white pulp, often at the interface of LN and PALS, becomes the site of antibody formation.

Furthermore, if the antibody response is high level or secondary, antibody-producing cell clusters that consist of B cells differentiating into plasma cells, helper and suppressor T cells, macrophages, and other accessory cells, take up an expanding residence in the center of LN and form germinal centers. These are monoclonal antibody production factories, the lighter zones within the LN. When antibody production wanes, germinal centers show increased numbers of phagocytizing macrophages and at this stage are often termed *reaction centers*. Thereafter, the center disappears, with the whole cycle measured in weeks or months.

The foregoing description is that of an immunologically reactive white pulp. What occurs if the proper antigen fails to meet the proper immunologically competent T cell or B cell? The unengaged lymphocytes leave the white pulp, carried out by a dedicated system of efferent lymphatic vessels. Four to 6 hours after milling about the PALS, as measured in the rodent, T cells move toward the central artery in the central longitudinal axis of the PALS. Taking 6 to 8 hours, B cells move from the lymphatic nodule in the same direction. Girding the artery and its major branches, even arching from one lobule to another, is a system of efferent lymphatic vessels that travel back along the arterial vessels into the trabeculae and back through the capsule, out of the spleen where they become afferent lymphatic vessels, emptying into a cluster of lymph nodes just outside the spleen. From there, they return lymph to the blood through the thoracic duct. The spleen thus provides an important loop in the pathways of the RLP (other loops are in other lymphatic tissues[20,21]) and displays the significance of the pool as a distinct, migratory, immunologically competent tissue rigorously regulated to survey the body, touching important tissues where antigen is efficiently carried, ready to engage in an immune response and to keep circulating and recirculating if not engaged.

Through its reticular cell–barrier cell system the spleen is prepared to wall off the RLP, even shutting it out along with other cells to prevent an immune response. This is an important control under any circumstance, but in the spleen, which is set up to concentrate or even produce damaged self, it may be vital to forestall autoimmune disease, which can be initiated by the pronounced immunogenic proclivity of damaged erythrocytes and other altered cells.[1,13,14]

Note that although the white pulp is the major immune tissue of the spleen, only a small number of lymphocytes entering the spleen take the immunologically significant pathways through the white pulp. Most cross the red pulp and, instead of turning back and entering the distal regions of the PALS, pass through the filtration beds of red pulp and quickly get picked up and carried out by red pulp veins. Clearly, at least several passes through the spleen are needed for all lymphocytes to enjoy the more significant passage through the white pulp. This fits in with the pattern of the spleen. Heinz body–bearing erythrocytes and experimentally heat-damaged erythrocytes are not cleared in one passage through the spleen.

LYMPH NODES

Lymph nodes are organized much like the white pulp of the spleen. The two tissues receive T cells and B cells of the RLP, sort them out into well-organized T-cell and B-cell regions, have a dedicated efferent lymphatic system, and have the capacity to support an immune response. If an immune response is not forthcoming, they can release the T cells and B cells to the RLP. While the spleen clears blood, lymph nodes clear lymph.[1,20,21,24,25]

Lymph nodes occur in clusters at specific regions of the body. Each node is enclosed by a fibrous capsule from whose internal surface a branching system of trabeculae extend into the parenchyma. The parenchyma is dominated by closely packed collections of lymphocytes. A thick dense blanket of lymphocytes lies beneath the capsule. This corresponds to the PALS, the T-cell zone of the spleen. Lymphatic nodules, B-cell zones, lie in the lymphocyte blanket just as the lymphatic nodules of the spleen lie in the PALS. The lymphocytic blanket in which the nodules are embedded is part of the cortex or outer portion of the lymph node. It is divided into two zones, the outer internodular cortex, lying between lymphatic nodules, and the deeper diffuse or tertiary cortex, lying deep to the internodular cortex. These two T-cell portions of the cortex, with the B-cell lymphatic nodules, make up the three components of the cortex.

Deep to the cortex in the center of the node is the medulla. It consists of branched, anastomosing cords of lymphocytes and associated cells, the medullary cords. At one point, the medullary cords displace the cortex and extend to the inner surface of the capsule. Here, the capsule often has an indentation, called the *hilus*, and is perforated, permitting arteries to enter the node and veins and efferent lymphatics to leave it. The capsule is also pierced at many places on its convex surface by afferent lymphatics, which open into the node, carrying lymph into it. If a node is central, the efferent lymphatics from the more distal nodes become its afferent lymphatics, carrying into it lymph released from the more distal nodes. This lymph is discharged into a large bowl-shaped subcapsular sinus. From this intranodal lymphatic vessel, the lymph passes through the cortex, often in the shelter of trabeculae, as radial sinuses. The radial sinuses then enter the medulla, coursing as medullary sinuses between medullary cords (Fig. 7-5). The medullary sinuses coalesce to one or more efferent lymphatic vessels, which pierce the capsule and leave the node, headed toward the thoracic duct to join with the venous system. Depending on the location of their node, efferent vessels may join the thoracic duct directly or become the afferent lymphatics of more proximal nodes.

Lymphatic channels show distinctive modifications. Both afferent and efferent lymphatics are valved, preventing back flow of lymph. Within the nodes, except for a distal segment of radial sinuses, the lymphatic channels are crisscrossed by branches of reticular cells. Lymphatic vessels drain regions of the body and carry regional antigen into lymph nodes. They thus stand in contrast to the spleen,

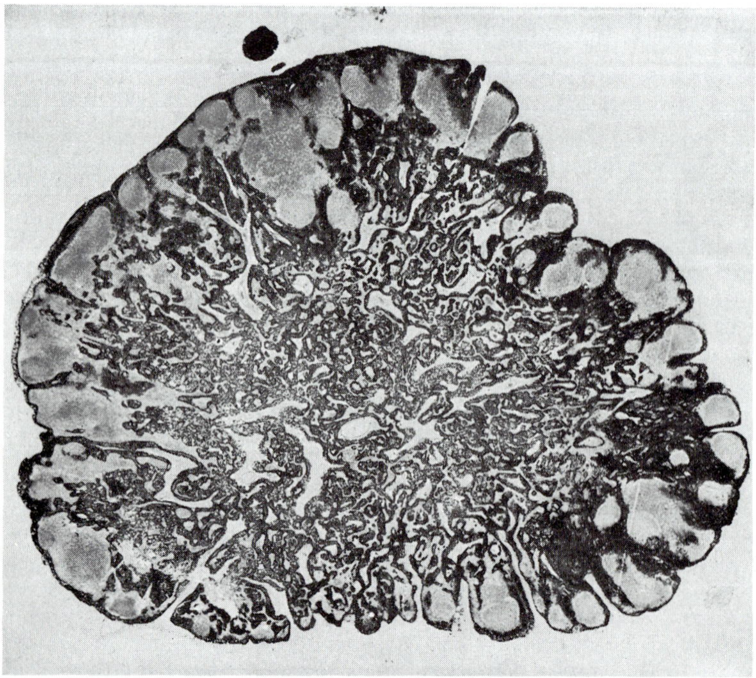

FIGURE 7-5. Lymph node injected with India ink. The sinus system is well outlined (×10).

which receives blood and specializes in the management of systemic antigen. Lymphatics also carry fluids that escaped the fine blood vasculature back to the blood, and this component makes up the largest component of lymph plasma. Lymphatics are important in the migrations of lymphocytes of the RLP, carrying lymphocytes into the node and out of it.

Blood vessels are important both in the nourishment of the tissue and in the migration pathways of the RLP, constituting a major arm carrying lymphocytes into the node. Arteries enter the hilus and branch into a capillary system within the node. Postcapillary venules arch, largely in the deep cortex, and run on into the medulla as veins, exiting the node through the hilus (Fig. 7-6). The postcapillary venule, by a mechanism that depends on the coupling of specific receptors on its endothelium and on the lymphocyte surface, selectively adheres to T cell and B cells in the blood and passes them into the parenchyma.[18] The lymphocytes sort themselves out into T-cell and B-cell zones as in the splenic white pulp, engage in immune responses as in spleen, and, if unengaged, leave the node through efferent lymphatics after a few hours, as in spleen, to rejoin the RLP.[18,20,21]

BONE MARROW

The bone marrow is distinctive among hematopoietic tissues in its capacities to preferentially sequester multipotent hematopoietic stem cells from the circulation and to provide the diverse macroenvironments that induce stem cell differentiation into each of the blood cell lines[1]. The creation of bone marrow obviously depends on the presence and hollowing out of bone, and the presence of bone continues to contribute postnatally to the bone marrow's preeminence as a hematopoietic tissue. The internal surface of bone is covered by a layer of endosteum or bone lining

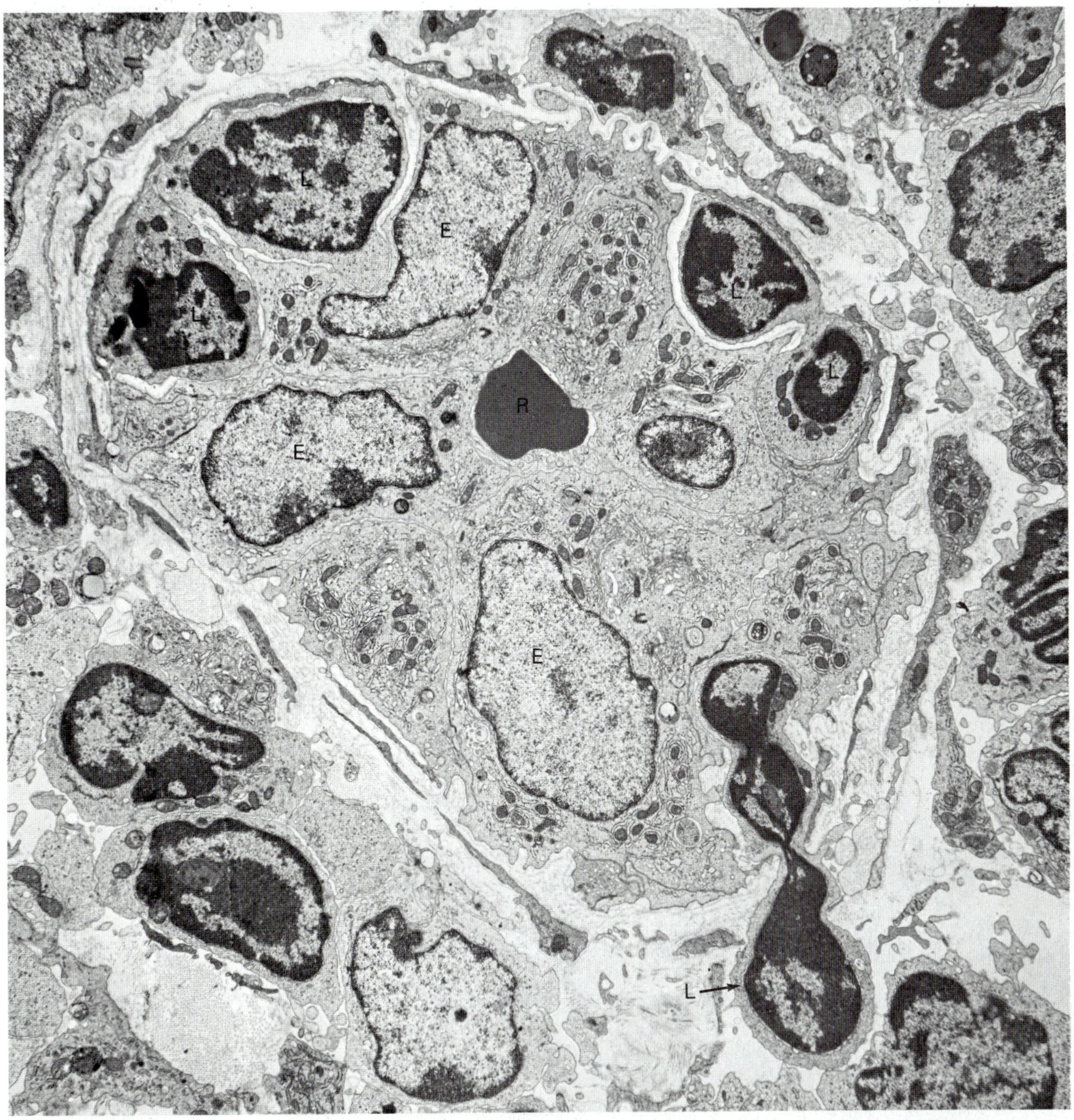

FIGURE 7-6. Postcapillary venules, mouse lymph node. The vessel has a high endothelium containing lightly euchromatic nuclei (E). The lumen is small and contains an erythrocyte (R). The wall of the venule is infiltrated by a number of lymphocytes, the nuclei of which are heterochromatic and thus dense (L). One lymphocyte, its protoplasm beaded as a result of being squeezed by the endothelium, appears to be emerging from the venule and entering the perivascular lymphatic cortex (L; ×1200). (Courtesy of G. D. Levine)

cells that serves as the true capsule of the marrow. The layer is often simple low cuboidal but may be stratified; it is physiologically and sometimes morphologically complex. It contains cells directed toward the regulation of bone, namely, osteoblasts, osteoclasts, and their progenitors. It contains cells directed toward the bone marrow and hematopoiesis, specifically multipotent stem cells, progenitor cells, and stromal cells, notably reticular cells and barrier cells that branch from their subosteal position as bone lining cells into the marrow cavity where they determine the organization of the marrow.[18,19,24,26]

The marrow is organized about its large thin-walled venous sinuses, which, like veins elsewhere, carry blood back toward the heart. In the marrow, they have the additional function of carrying freshly produced blood cells into the general circulation or to other tissues for continued maturation and conditioning before release to the general circulation. The structure of the venous sinus is simple, consisting of an endothelium, a poorly developed basement membrane, and an incomplete outer cover of pericytes or adventitial cells. These adventitial cells are in fact reticular cells, the large fibroblastic stromal cells that branch out from the vascular wall into the perivascular tissue and provide the scaffolding or reticulum that holds and regulates hematopoietic cells (Figs. 7-7 and 7-8). Normally in rodents, they may cover almost 50% of the adventitial surface of the sinuses; in large-scale cell delivery, the cover is considerably reduced. They control access to the wall of the sinus for cells seeking the circulation; they likely also have inductive roles in creating hematopoietic microenvironments. The adventitial cells can accumulate fat droplets and by so doing become marrow adipocytes, which reduce the volume of the perivascular hematopoietic compartment by obtruding on it. Arterial vessels, although not conspicuous, are present in large numbers. They flow into capillaries that join venous sinuses in many places. Endothelial continuity exists from artery to vein so that, unlike the spleen, the circulation is anatomically, as well as physiologically, closed.

The perivenular hematopoietic compartments contain developmental stages of all the blood cell lineages. RBCs tend to be organized as colonies, *erythroblastic islets*, consisting of central macrophages surrounded by differentiating and proliferating erythroblasts (Fig. 7-9). The islet is set at the outside of a vascular sinus. The more mature forms—reticulocytes and normoblasts—lie at the vascular wall, whereas the earlier forms lie at the opposite pole. When reticulocytes are delivered into the sinus lumen, the adventitial reticular cells move away, exposing the outside (adventitial) surface of the endothelium. Reticulocytes penetrate the endothelium, not through interendothelial junctions but through endothelial cytoplasm near an interendothelial junction. Reticulocytes (and other cells crossing into the sinusal lumen) are deeply constricted in passing through a narrow aperture in the endothelial cytoplasm, which heals and disappears after transmural passage is complete. Leukocytes mature away from the sinus wall and move there, entering the sinus lumen where reticulocytes do. Megakaryocytes characteristically lie over apertures in the endothelium, delivering platelets through them.

Normally, there is a close relationship between developing blood cells and fibroblastic stromal cells: adventitial reticular cells on the surface of venous sinuses and other blood vessels within the marrow branch into the perivascular tissue, forming a meshwork supporting differentiating blood cells; reticular cells and, in certain restricted loci, barrier cells, branch into the marrow from the bone lining layer, enveloping differentiating blood cells and blood vessels; adipocytes, derived from reticular cells, are typically closely associated with granulocytes and monocytes and may play a role in their induction. In heightened hematopoiesis, moreover, barrier cells appear throughout the marrow as branched syncytial sheets that enclose hematopoietic cells. Through the production of interleukins and other regulatory factors, these fibroblastic stromal cells are set to not merely support hematopoiesis physically but to regulate blood cell production through paracrine or autochthonous secretion of factors.[1,17,26]

THYMUS

The structure of the thymus is deceptively simple.[1,27] Its central zone, the *medulla*, consists mainly of epithelial cells derived from the third and fourth branchial pouches. The epithelial cells display several conformations. They form a solid epithelial tissue with the cells attached to one another by desmosomes; they layer upon one another in onion-skin pattern, forming large, even multicentric masses with zones of calcification, cystic change, and necrosis. These cellular masses are the thymic or Hassall's corpuscles, which are well developed in human thymus. Epithe-

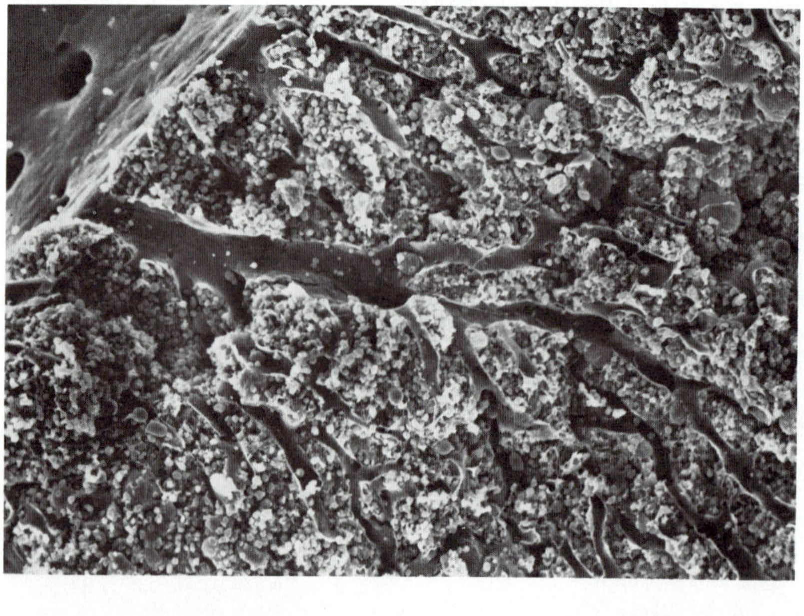

FIGURE 7-7. Rat bone marrow. This is a scanning electron micrograph of the cut surface, showing a system of vascular sinuses originating at the periphery of the marrow (*right side*) and draining into a large vein (*left upper corner*). The large vein has several ruptures in its wall, representing the entry of tributary venous sinuses. Hematopoietic tissue is seen between the vascular sinuses. (Weiss L. Anal Rec 1976;186:161)

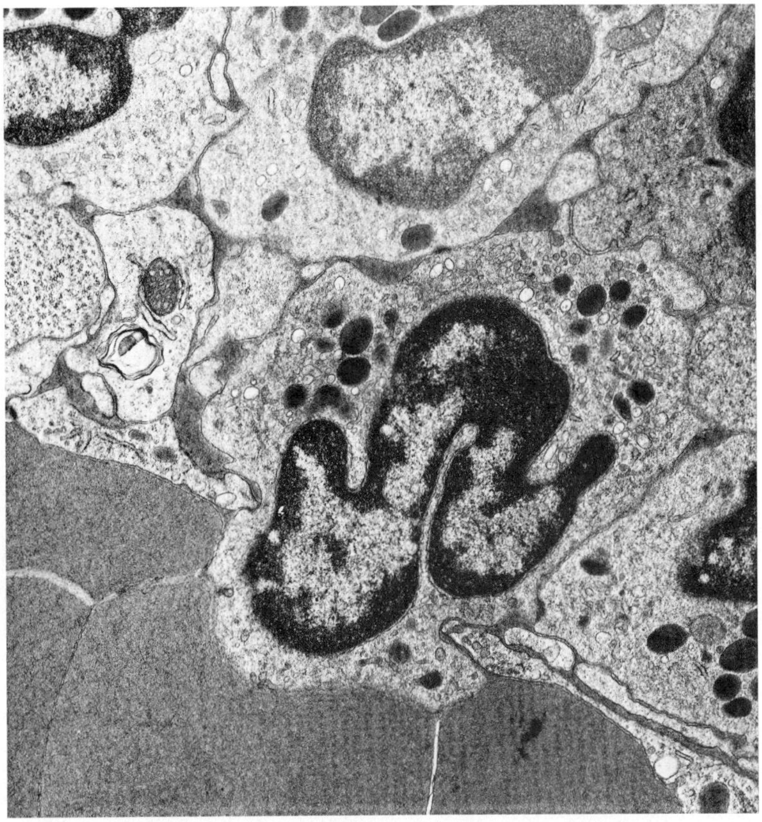

FIGURE 7-8. Mouse bone marrow. An eosinophil is crossing the wall of the vascular sinus, passing from the hematopoietic compartment (*above*) to the blood (*below*; ×9500).

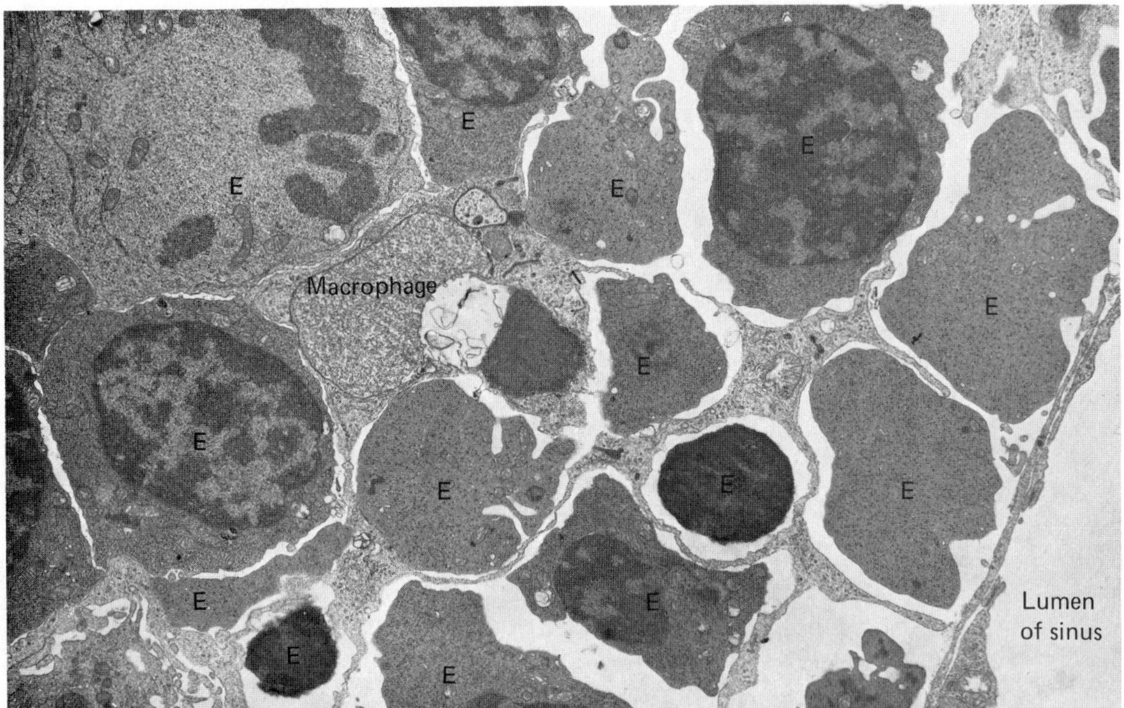

FIGURE 7-9. Rat bone marrow erythroblastic islet. A macrophage lies amid a cluster of red cells and erythroblasts (E). It sends out a system of slender branching cell processes that enclose the surrounding red cells and reach the wall of the vascular sinus on the lower right. (This tissue was perfused; as a result, the cells are separated from one another, thereby revealing the extensive branching of the macrophage clearly.) (×7300.) (Weiss L. Anal Rec 1976;186:161)

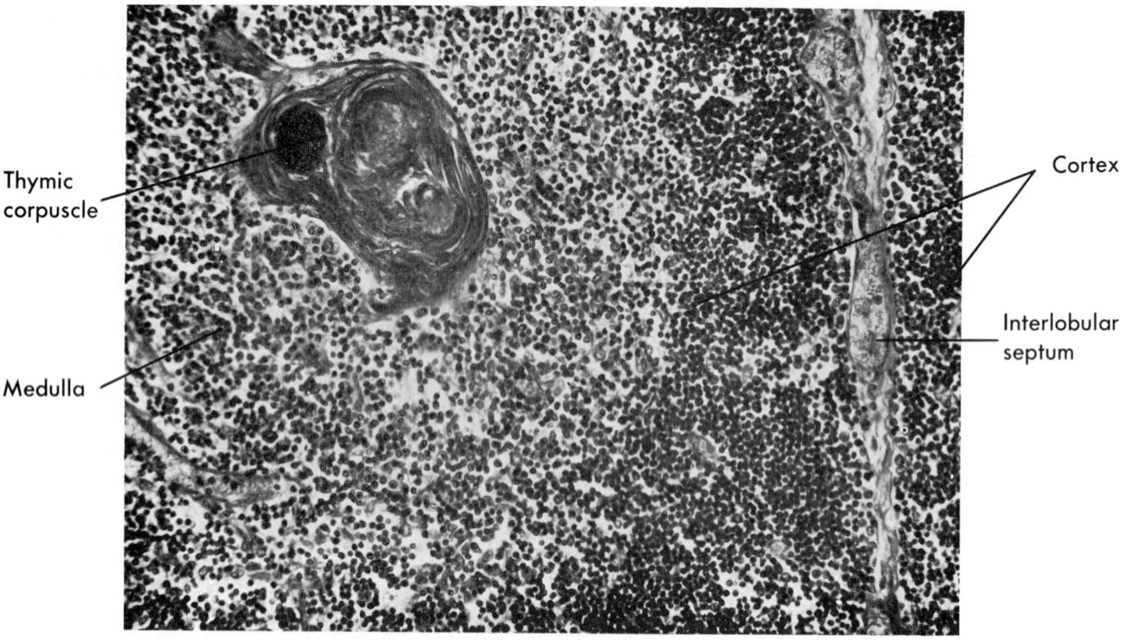

FIGURE 7-10. Thymus of a 20-year-old patient. Lymphocytes are concentrated in the cortex. They are present in the medulla as well but are scattered loosely among epithelial reticular cells. A large, multicentric thymic corpuscle is present in the medulla. The interlobular septum is slender and contains lymphatic vessels, blood vessels, and nerves (×200). (Prepared by B. Castleman)

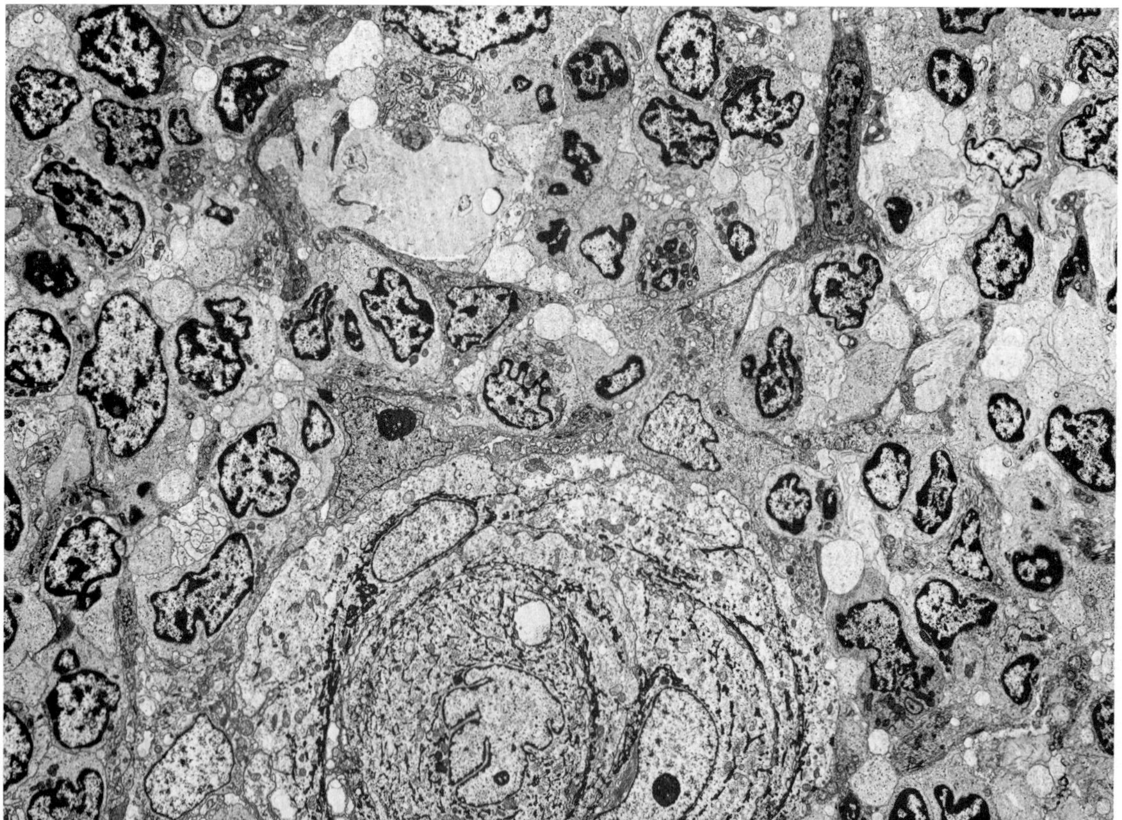

FIGURE 7-11. Human thymus medulla. A large thymic corpuscle is seen along the lower margin. Note the concentric pattern of the epithelial cells and the keratin (dense linear material). The rest of the field consists of branching endothelial cells and lymphocytes and macrophages held within the branches. (Courtesy of Robert Rouse)

lial cells form sheets that ensheathe blood vessels, contributing to a blood–thymus barrier, and enclose thymic lobules, sharply reducing penetration of antigen and other particulate–macromolecule substances into the gland. They form cysts and tubules, expressive of the embryonic tubular prolongations of the branchial pouches from which the epithelial components of the thymus are fashioned. Lymphocytes, which are largely quite mature T cells, some plasma cells, some blood cells, and macrophages, are scattered among the epithelial cells.

The medulla extends thick blunt processes from its central mass. Each of these processes is covered by a layer of densely packed lymphocytes, often continuous from one medullary process to the next. The dense layer of lymphocytes, taken collectively over all the medullary processes, is the cortex of the thymus (Fig. 7-10). In fact, it is structurally much more complex than it appears. It actually consists of epithelial cells with long stretched-out processes, often connected by desmosomes to those of neighboring epithelial cells, with the result that an epithelial meshwork is formed. These epithelial cells are called epithelial–reticular cells. The interstices of their meshwork are packed with developing T cells. These lymphocytes are so dominant in appearance that one must look carefully to find the epithelial cells (Fig. 7-11). The picture is made more complex by the presence of other stromal cells, such as light and dark epithelial cells. Also, "nurse cells" enclose colonies of developing T cells, suggesting that they form brood sacs for the T cells, isolating them and concentrating growth and differentiating factors among them. Barrier cells, reticular cells, interdigitating cells, and macrophages are also present. The important functions of each of these cell types contribute to the thymus.[1,27] The functions contributed by the variants of a given type of cell, such as the varieties of epithelial cells, have not been well sorted out, so that it is difficult to make structural–functional correlates. A few important patterns are worth noting.

With autoradiographic techniques in animals infused with radiolabeled bone marrow cells, it can be shown that immature T cells, or T-cell progenitors, are released from bone marrow and migrate to the subcapsular cortex of the thymus where they proliferate actively and begin a migration, descending through the cortex. In this descent, the developing T cells are attended by epithelial–reticular cells, nurse cells, and other stromal cells. As they migrate, they differentiate through successive stages of T-cell maturation, until at the corticomedullary junction or in the medulla they are picked up by veins or lymphatics. As mature but unsophisticated cells, they then circulate to the spleen for final testing and maturation.

Epithelial cells and possibly other stromal cells secrete thymosin and related factors that may well attract the circulating nascent T cells released from bone marrow into the thymus. After these cells are in the thymus, they are induced to seek appropriate cellular associations, to proliferate, and to differentiate. Furthermore, epithelial cells and possibly other stromal cells appear to "test" the developing T cells by interaction of their major histocompatibility cell surface receptors with the emerging receptors of the differentiating T cells, causing those T cells that would cause autoimmune disease to be suppressed or destroyed. This process likely contributes to the massive cell death of developing T cells: well over 90% die within the thymic cortex.

The cortex holds 90% of thymic lymphocytes. Cortical lymphocytes are not fully mature. For example, they do not survive exposure to cortisone and are not ready to engage in immune responses. The relatively few medullary lymphocytes are a different T-cell population—mature and immunologically competent.

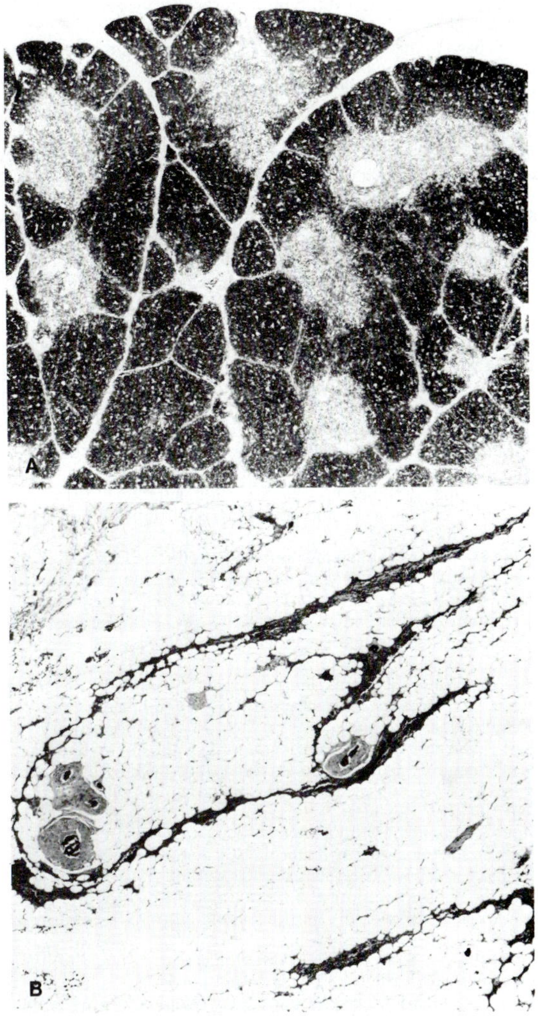

FIGURE 7-12. Human thymus before and after involution: tissue from an infant 3 months old (**A**) and a patient 72 years old (**B**). Note the lobular pattern in **A**. The medella is a branching structure. The cortex surrounds the lobular projections of the medulla. A thin fibrous capsule is present. Involutional changes are evident in **B**. The cortex is markedly diminished, and the organ is fatty. The blood vessels display thickened sclerotic walls (×25). (Courtesy of Robert Rouse)

The thymus is vulnerable to acute large-scale atrophy due to stress (*stress involution*), and it atrophies at puberty and continues to do so on a less dramatic level thereafter ("age involution"; Fig. 7-12). Even an old, withered, fatty, fibrotic thymus, albeit on a reduced level, is capable of generating and exporting T cells.

REFERENCES

1. Weiss L. Cell and tissue biology: a textbook of histology, ed 6. Baltimore, Urban & Schwarzenburg, 1988.
2. Blue J, Weiss L. Vascular pathways in nonsinusal red pulp: an electron microscope study. Am J Anat 1981;161:135–168.
3. Blue J, Weiss L. Electron microscopy of the red pulp of the dog spleen including vascular arrangements, periarterial sheaths (ellipsoids), and the contractile, innervated meshwork. Am J Anat 1981;161:189–218.
4. McCuskey RS, McCuskey RP. In vivo and electron microscopic studies of the splenic microvasculature in mice. Experientia 1985;40:179–192.
5. Schmidt EE, MacDonald IC, Groom AC. Circulatory pathways in the sinusal spleen of the dog, studied by scanning electron microscopy of microcorrosion casts. J Morphol 1983;178:111–123.
6. Groom AC, Schmidt EE, MacDonald IC. Microcirculatory pathways and blood flow in spleen: new insights from washout kinetics, corrosion casts, and quantitative intravital microscopy. 1991;5:159–174.
7. Tablin F, Weiss L. Equine spleen: an electron microscopic analysis. Am J Anat 1983;166:393–416.

8. Tischendorf F. On the evolution of the spleen. Experientia 1985;41: 145–152.
9. Weiss L. New trends in spleen research: conclusions. Experientia 1985;41: 243–248.
10. Weiss L, Powell R, Schiffman FJ. Terminating arterial vessels in red pulp of the spleen: a transmission electron microscopic study. Experientia 1985;41:233–242.
11. Pinkus GS, Warhol MJ, et al. Immunohistochemical localization of smooth muscle myosin in human spleen, lymph node, and other lymphoid tissues. Am J Pathol 1986;123:440–453.
12. MacDonald IC, Schmidt EE, Groom AC. The high splenic hematocrit: a rheological consequence of red cell flow through the reticular meshwork. Microvasc Res 1991;42:60–76.
13. Weiss L. Mechanisms of splenic clearance of blood: a structural overview of the mammalian spleen. In: Bowdler AJ, ed. The spleen: structure, function and clinical significance. London, Chapman & Hall, 1990.
14. Weiss L, Geduldig U, Weidanz WP. Mechanisms of splenic control of malaria: reticular cell activation and the development of a blood-spleen barrier. Am J Anat 1986;176:251–285.
15. Blue J, Weiss L. Periarterial macrophage sheaths (ellipsoids) in cat spleen: an electron microscope study. Am J Anat 1981;161:115–134.
16. Weiss L, Sakai H. The hematopoietic stroma. Am J Anat 1984;170:447–463.
17. Weiss L, Geduldig U. Barrier cells: stromal regulation of hematopoiesis and blood cell release in normal and stressed murine bone marrow. Blood 1991;78:975–990.
18. Butcher EC. The regulation of lymphocyte traffic. In: Clarke A, Compans RW, Cooper M, et al, eds. Current topics in microbiology and immunology. New York, Springer-Verlag, 1986:85–122.
19. Friedenstein AJ, Chailakhan RK, Latsinik NV, et al. Stromal cells responsible for transferring the microenvironment of hematopoietic tissue. Transplantation 1974;17:331–340.
20. Pellas TC, Weiss L. Deep splenic lymphatic vessels in the mouse: a route of splenic exit for recirculating of lymphocytes. Am J Anat 1990;187:347–354.
21. Pellas TC, Weiss L. Lymphocyte migration and recirculation in the mouse: migratory pathways of thoracic duct-derived B cells, L3T4+ and Lyt 2+ T cell subsets in lymphatic and nonlymphatic tissues. Am J Anat 1990;187:347–354.
22. Timens W, Poppema S. Lymphocyte compartments in human spleen: an immunohistologic study in normal spleens and noninvolved spleens in Hodgkin's disease. Am J Pathol 1985;120:443–454.
23. van Ewijk W, Nieuwenhius P. Compartments, domains and migration pathways of lymphoid cells in the splenic pulp. Experientia 1985;41: 199–208.
24. Gowans JL. The recirculation of lymphocytes from blood to lymph in the lymph node in the rat. J Physiol 1959;146:54.
25. Gowans JL, Knight EJ. The recirculation of lymphocytes in the rat. Proc R Soc Lond (Biol) 1964;159:257–284.
26. Grobstein C. Developmental role of the intercellular matrix: retrospective and prospective. In: Slavkin HC, Greulich RC, eds. Extracellular matrix influences on gene expression. New York, Academic Press, 1975:9–16.
27. Ritter MA, Crispe IN. The thymus. New York, IRL Press at Oxford University Press, 1992:9–71.

GLOSSARY

antigen-presenting cell—see *interdigitating cell*

basal lamina—see *basement membrane*

barrier cells—newly recognized connective tissue cell lineage capable of forming barriers or enclosures that may seal or wall off diverse structures. They are branched fibroblastic cells that fuse with one another to form complex multibranched, variegated syncytial sheets. Barrier cells originate locally from archetypical fibroblasts, such as those covering trabeculae, and from circulating progenitors. They ensheathe blood vessels, contributing to blood–tissue barriers. Sealing off segments of white pulp and presumably other immunologically competent tissue after an immune response is initiated, they concentrate regulatory factors and prevent response to additional antigen including those that would initiate an autoimmune process. They enclose hematopoietic colonies, concentrate hematopoietic factors, and offer protection against parasites. Barrier cells work interactively with macrophages and with the immune apparatus in controlling infectious disease.

basement membrane—sheet of extracellular material, made largely of proteoglycans, on which epithelial of various types lie. In addition to providing mechanical support, basement membranes may have roles in controlling transport across the tissues they support and in inducing and regulating the development and functions of vicinal tissues. They may be selectively stained in the PAS histochemical procedure for 1,2-glycol groups and by silver stains. Basement membranes consist of at least two layers: an inner *basal lamina*, itself consisting of dense and light laminae, and an outer layer whose thickness, cell, and fiber content depend on location. The membranes are subject to variations; membrane under the tracheal epithelium is relatively thick, whereas that in the urinary bladder is thin. One of the most extreme variations is that of splenic sinuses in which large, regular defects in the basement membrane cause the remainder of the structure to look like a netting with strong circular components and provide unparalleled freedom for cell crossing.

bone lining cells—see *endosteum*

connective tissues—largely derived from mesenchyme, and consisting of a variety of cell types separated by extracellular matrix and fibers. The two major cell types of the connective tissues are the fibroblast, which produces the extracellular matrix and collagen fibers, and the macrophage, the "professional" phagocyte of the body, which is important in nonphagocytic processes such as regulating hematopoiesis, antigen presentation and immune responses. Mast cells, plasma cells, eosinophils, lymphocytes, and other cells also contribute to the connective tissues. The extracellular connective tissues consist of matrix—largely proteoglycans—and a mixture of collagenous and elastic fibers. In dense connective tissue, such as tendon, heavy bands of collagen are preponderant. The hematopoietic tissues are highly specialized loose connective tissues.

endosteum—lining on the internal surface of bone facing bone on its outside surface and bone marrow on its internal surface. It consists of cells that are concerned with bone—osteoblasts, osteoclasts, and their precursors—and of cells concerned with bone marrow—multipotent hematopoietic stem cells, progenitor cells of the various blood cell lines, reticular cells, other stromal cells, and their progenitors. Another term for endosteum is *bone-lining cells.*

endothelium—specialized simple epithelium that provides an internal lining for blood vessels. It is typically a squamous or flat epithelium, but in significant places in the hematopoietic system it is atypical. In postcapillary venules of lymph nodes supporting traffic of lymphocytes from the blood into the parenchyma of the node, the endothelium is cuboidal or higher. In splenic arterial vessels, the endothelium is pyramidal or cuboidal. Often thought of as mere vessel lining, endothelium is an actively metabolic tissue. Especially in fine vessels, it is beset with small transport vesicles that cross the cell, from basal to luminal surface and from luminal to basal surface (known as *transcytosis*) opening to both luminal and basal surfaces and contributing significantly to vascular permeability. The endothelium secretes factors that maintain blood flow and may regulate blood clotting. Von Willebrand's factor is produced in endothelium, appearing as a characteristic inclusion, the Palade-Weibel body.

epithelioid—see *mononuclear phagocytic system*

follicular dendritic cell—counterpart to the interdigitating cell, presenting antigen to B cells instead of to T cells. Its life cycle has not been as fully worked out as that of the interdigitating cell.

interdigitating cell—found in T-cell areas of lymphatic tissue presenting antigen to T cells. It originates in bone marrow and is released to circulate as a *veiled cell*, so named because it has veil-like processes on its surface, visible by electron microscopy and extending from a round cell that may be mistaken for a monocyte. A distinctive laminar inclusion, a *Birbeck granule*, may be present, and the nucleus tends to have an irregular contour. Veiled cells circulate to stratified squamous epithelia such as the skin, leave the vasculature, and enter the epithelium, extending processes among the keratinocytes. In this guise, the cell type is known as the *Langerhans cell*, named after Paul Langerhans who discovered these cells as a medical student in 1896 by gold toning. The nature of Langerhans cells as antigen-presenting cells remained unclear until the 1970s; they had been thought to be, among other things, effete macrophages, dying keratinocytes, and modified nerve cells. As antigens penetrate the epithelium, they are picked up by the surface of Langerhans cells, which, when replete, migrate out of the epithelium to the vasculature and travel to spleen, lymph node, or other immunologically competent lymphatic tissue. There, the Langerhans cell clusters immunologically competent T cells of the recirculating lymphocyte pool, its processes extending between the T cells; it is now termed an *interdigitating cell.* The interdigitating cell appears to facilitating rosette T cells, their rigorously defined migration through lymphatic tissue and presenting antigen to them. After interdigitating cells present antigen, they may well renew their surface, removing antigen and recirculating as veiled cells. The cells of this system are marked by the high levels of Ia antigen of the major histocompatibility complex on their surface, in addition to Birbeck granules, which are most marked in the Langerhans cell. Antigen presentation may be a widely distributed capacity. Macrophages do it, as do the M cells of the intestinal epithelium and, under stress, endothelial cells.

Langerhans cell—see *interdigitating cell*

macrophage—see *mononuclear phagocyte system*

mononuclear phagocytic system—family of macrophages, including the cell stages in their life cycle: monocytes, macrophages, epithelioid cells, and multinucleate giant cells. Monocytes are produced in bone marrow and enter the circulation as progenitors of macrophages. They leave the vasculature and differentiate into macrophages in the perivascular connective tissues, although in certain parts of the vasculature, such as in the dilated vessels of the earlobe or in blocked-off vessels with still blood, the transformation may occur intravascularly. Macrophages may have a life-span of weeks or months, including movement through blood and lymphatic vessels, and accumulation in certain sites such as the serous cavities and the filtration beds of the spleen. Macrophages may die or may further differentiate into epithelioid cells, which are large polygonal cells showing little evidence of phagocytosis, and which tend to lie next to one another in epithelial-like arrays. Epithelioid cells may then fuse into multinucleate giant cells, which are related to osteoclasts and to the giant cells that may occur pathologically about foreign bodies and in granulomas. Epithelioid cells and giant cells are rich in mitochondria and have few phagosomes; they appear specialized in the active transport of ions rather than phagocytosis.

multinucleate giant cell—see *mononuclear phagocyte system*

recirculating lymphocyte pool (RLP)—distinctive migratory tissue made up of small, immunologically competent, long-lived, as yet not activated T cells and B cells. This tissue migrates in rigorous pathways at rigorous tempos, surveys the body, efficiently bringing together antigen, T cells and B cells, and accessory cells to initiate an immune response. The T cells and B cells circulate in the blood and, on reaching lymph node, spleen, or other peripheral lymphatic tissue, leave the blood, enter the parenchyma of the lymphatic vessel, and sort out into T-cell and B-cell zones. Macrophages, interdigitating cells, follicular dendritic cells, and other accessory cells, together with antigen convene in the lymphatic tissues, with the diverse cells set up to prepare and present antigen and to respond immunologically. The lymphatic tissue is thus organized to house and sustain an immune response. If no immune response occurs, the lymphocytes leave the lymphatic tissue, typically through efferent lymph, pass through proximal lymph nodes (unless engaged by antigen) and lymphatic vessels, and eventually reach the thoracic ducts and thence back to the blood through the great veins in the base of the neck. These long-lived T cells and B cells may circulate and recirculate for years (in the case of T cells) in quest of antigen. Studies of rodent tissues indicate that T cells may remain in a secondary lymphatic tissue for 4 to 6 hours, whereas B cells stay longer, 6 to 8 hours. The RLP thus constitutes a mobile tissue offering vital immunologic protection against microbes and other foreign materials.

reticular cell—branched fibroblastic cell that produces and remains associated with argentophilic reticular fibers. Reticular cells and their fibers produce a three-dimensional meshwork, or *reticulum*, characteristic of the hematopoietic tissues. Such meshworks, which constitute the filtration beds of the spleen, vary in character from place to place, providing different microenvironments, serving different functions. In bone marrow, reticular cells serve as adventitial cells covering the outside surface of blood vessels and branching into the perivascular hematopoietic tissues. They form meshworks that hold hematopoietic tissues and meshworks that hold hematopoietic cells and likely provide distinctive hematopoietic microenvironments. These adventitial cells may modulate into adipocytes, which are large bulky cells that obtrude upon the hematopoietic space, reducing its volume. Adipocytes possess other functions, including the aromatization of estrogen into testosterone and the induction of granulocytopoiesis.

reticuloendothelial system—system of cells having the ability to take up and sequester macrophages and their precursors. Influenced by Metchinokoff's discovery of the amebocyte and phagocytosis, Aschoff, Maximow, Ranvier, Goldmann, Sabin, Downey, and other students of the connective tissues, beginning near the turn of the century, were impressed with the importance of phagocytosis in the control of infectious disease and other activities, such as pigmentation, lipid metabolism, hematopoiesis, and neoplasia. Using vital staining, clearance of particles including microbes from the blood, and selective staining, they identified macrophages in the loose connective tissues and in hematopoietic tissues and characterized them as mobile or free phagocytes. They concluded that reticular cells, the branched fibroblastic cells that produced and remained associated with argentophilic reticular fibers, were phagocytic and that the endothelium of the venous sinuses of hematopoietic and related tissues, was phagocytic as well. Reticular cells and sinusal endothelium, in contrast to the monocyte-derived free macrophage, were fixed macrophages and were widely considered capable of rounding up and differentiating into any of the blood cell lines—in short, as multipotent hematopoietic stem cells. So special was the endothelium of venous sinuses that it was not referred to as endothelium, but its cells were called *littoral* (shore) cells. The evidence for hematopoietic multipotency was morphologic. These cells in hematopoietic stress were observed to round up, come free of their tissue constraints, and become mononuclear cells which in turn developed the granules, pigments, and nuclear changes associated with differentiation into a blood cell type. These inferences were made before the time of labeling cells "innocuously, indubitably, and indelibly," and modern cell biology offers no support to the notion that reticular cells and littoral cells are multipotent. Although they are phagocytic, they are only slightly or moderately so in the presence of heavy phagocytic loads. They are not as phagocytic as the professional phagocyte, the monocyte-derived free macrophage. The reticuloendothelial system was promulgated with the primary view of its being a phagocytic system and the ancillary notion that it is hematopoietically multipotent. Because it was superbly articulated by Aschoff and its other founders, was based on modern, sophisticated, multipronged technology and approach, dealt with important biologic phenomena, and achieved a remarkable synthesis, the idea of the reticuloendothelial system proved compelling. Although it has required revision and has been under attack, it has proved remarkably durable. But there are new, emerging syntheses of the hematopoietic/phagocytic/immune/inflammatory system, integrating regulatory factors, the cells that produce them, the cells that respond to them, the roles of extracellular substances in adhesion and cell induction, and molecular genetic understanding of cell differentiation. The formulation of the reticuloendothelial system is proving irrelevant to these syntheses, and its adaptability is compromised by the accretion of errors and the weakness of intuitive morphology. Scientists are no longer discussing the reticuloendothelial system; as a result, it is slipping, or has slipped, from contemporary science into the history of science. The truly phagocytic component of the reticuloendothelial system has been given its own status in the mononuclear phagocytic system and has been, but should not be, confused with the reticuloendothelial system as a whole.

veiled cell—see *interdigitating cell*

venous sinus—fine venous vessel that receives blood from capillaries in liver, bone marrow, and endocrine organs, as adrenal and pituitary. In spleen, a venous sinus receives blood from filtration beds. It has a relatively large lumen and a thin wall that consists of three layers or tunics: endothelium, basement membrane, and adventitia. The endothelium in spleen may be rod shaped; in long-term, high-level hemolysis, such as in the thalassemias or sickle cell disease, it is slightly to moderately phagocytic. In the venous sinuses within the hepatic lobule, true macrophages or *Kupffer's cells*, are intercalated into the endothelium. In the spleen, the endothelium is reinforced by rods of contractile intermediate filaments, and its interendothelial slits impose a test on erythrocytes, delaying their passage and pitting dense intraerythrocytic particles such as Heinz bodies and malarial plasmodia from them. The basement membrane may be specialized and defective, as in splenic sinuses, and virtually absent, as in bone marrow sinuses. The adventitia consists of reticular cells, which partially cover the outside of the vessel and branch into the perivascular tissue, contributing to meshworks or filtration beds. In addition to the venous function of carrying blood toward the heart, venous sinuses may support the final differentiation of platelets, the recycling of malarial parasites, and cell storage.

Blood: Principles and Practice of Hematology,
edited by Robert I. Handin, Thomas P. Stossel, and Samuel E. Lux.
J.B. Lippincott Company, Philadelphia © 1995.

8

Hematopoiesis

Colin A. Sieff
David A. Williams

The formed elements of the blood together with the stem and progenitor cells that give rise to these functional cells play a vital role in the normal functioning of a healthy person. Certain characteristics of the hematopoietic tissue are clearly different from other vital organs and important in the understanding of normal and abnormal hematopoiesis. These differences include the short life-span of most functional cells of the hematopoietic system, the multiplicity of cell types required for normal hematopoietic functioning, and the wide dispersion of cells performing specific hematopoietic functions throughout the body. Although exceptions exist in the lymphoid compartment, the life-span of most hematopoietic cells is extremely short—from hours to days. The short life-span requires the continuous production of enormous numbers of cells to replace these lost and generally postmitotic cells. Estimates of 10^{10} red blood cells (RBCs) and 10^8 to 10^9 white blood cells produced per hour demonstrate the numbers involved but belie the complexity of the hematopoietic system, since the final number of circulating cells are maintained within strict limits.

The physiologic functioning of the hematopoietic system also requires that the bone marrow be capable of responding quickly to the need for additional cells of any lineage. Finally, despite the requirements for massive production of differentiated cells, stem cells must be maintained in adequate numbers (a process termed *self-renewal*) to constantly provide input progenitor cells throughout the person's lifetime.

Delineation of the relations of different cells in this complex system has been made possible by exemplary research by a number of investigators working in the field of experimental hematology.* Careful study of staining and morphologic characteristics of bone marrow and blood cells by hematologists over the last 50 years has produced a relatively clear idea of the maturational sequence during precursor cell differentiation. Development of an in vivo stem cell assay, the colony-forming unit–spleen (CFU-S) assay (discussed later), by Till and McCulloch[1] in the early 1960s led to an enormous growth of knowledge about stem cell self-renewal and proliferation. Shortly thereafter, the development of in vitro clonogenic culture systems for hematopoietic progenitor cells by Pluznik and Sachs[2] and Bradley and Metcalf[3] led to new understanding of growth factor requirements for hematopoietic cell differentiation. These discoveries ultimately led to the molecular cloning of multiple cytokines that effect hematopoietic cell proliferation and differentiation.[4,5]

Description of an in vitro culture system that allowed continuous proliferation and differentiation of hematopoietic cells in long-term bone marrow cultures by Dexter and coworkers[6] provided new insights into the role of the hematopoietic microenvironment in the physiology of hematopoietic stem cells and the requirement for direct cell–cell contacts in hematopoiesis. Knowledge gained from these and many other studies provides some general concepts with regard to hematopoiesis.

FUNCTIONAL RELATIONS IN HEMATOPOIETIC CELL DIFFERENTIATION

The hematopoietic system can be envisioned as a continuum of functional compartments (Fig. 8-1). In general, the more primitive *stem cell compartment* is made up of rare pluripotent stem cells with high self-renewal capacity, the capacity to give rise to all cell lineages, and a low incidence of mitotically active cells.[7] The self-renewal capacity of the stem cell compartment must be maintained throughout the life-span of the individual and, through a process termed *commitment*, these cells also are constantly capable of providing more differentiated cells into the next compartment.

Transition to the *progenitor compartment* is characterized by some restriction in differentiation and proliferative capacity. This compartment is composed of mostly unipotent progenitor cells, with some bipotent and rare multipotent progenitors. These progenitor cells demonstrate little, if any, self-renewal capacity and are more numerous and mitotically more active than stem cells. In contrast, cells in the most differentiated *precursor compartment* make up most cells in the bone marrow, have no self-renewal capacity, are unipotent, and are mostly in active cell cycle. These precursor cells exhibit well-described nuclear and cytoplasmic morphology during the final steps of differentiation into functional cells. Because of the large quantity of precursor cells, considerable amplification of cell numbers occurs in this compartment.

* For a concise review of previous studies in experimental hematology as they relate to current understanding of hematopoiesis, see Metcalf D. The molecular control of blood cells. Cambridge, MA, Harvard University Press, 1988.

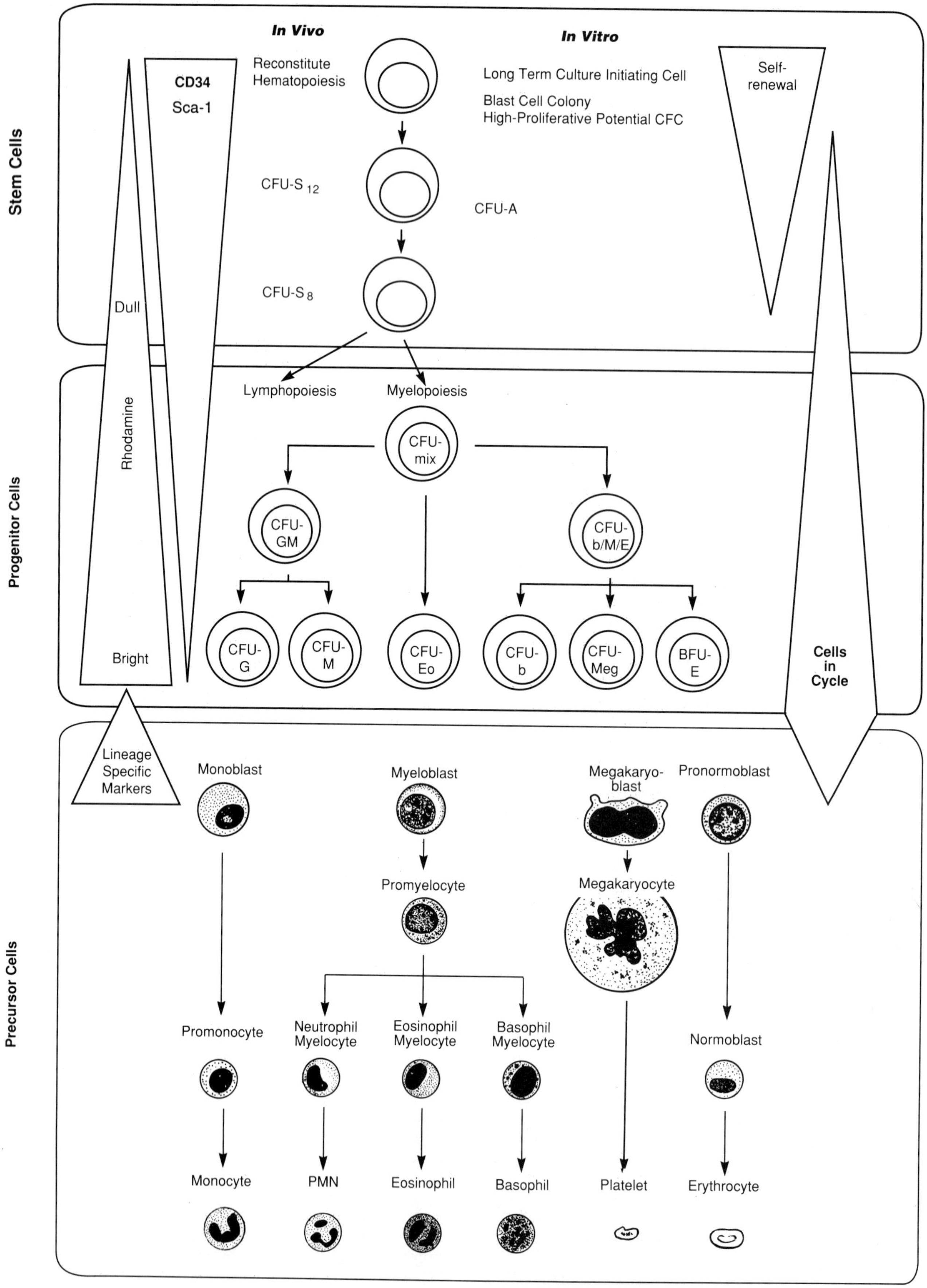
Stem Cells
Progenitor Cells
Precursor Cells
In Vivo
In Vitro
Reconstitute Hematopoiesis
Long Term Culture Initiating Cell
Blast Cell Colony
High-Proliferative Potential CFC
CD34
Sca-1
Self-renewal
CFU-S 12
CFU-A
CFU-S 8
Dull
Rhodamine
Bright
Lymphopoiesis
Myelopoiesis
CFU-mix
CFU-GM
CFU-b/M/E
CFU-G
CFU-M
CFU-Eo
CFU-b
CFU-Meg
BFU-E
Cells in Cycle
Lineage Specific Markers
Monoblast
Myeloblast
Megakaryo-blast
Pronormoblast
Promyelocyte
Megakaryocyte
Promonocyte
Neutrophil Myelocyte
Eosinophil Myelocyte
Basophil Myelocyte
Normoblast
Monocyte
PMN
Eosinophil
Basophil
Platelet
Erythrocyte

In summation, early cells have the capacity to give rise to large numbers of progeny cells on a clonal basis through expansion during differentiation. These principles not only are salient to normal hematopoietic cell biology but also are important concepts when considering the behavior of leukemic cells.

ONTOGENY OF HEMATOPOIESIS

The development of hematopoiesis during gestation is characterized in mammalian systems by sequential change in the major anatomic site of blood cell formation and by multiple changes in the blood cells themselves. Although best studied in relation to globin gene expression (see following text), these changes affect all aspects of hematopoietic cell biology. It is unclear what role programmed changes in hematopoietic cell gene expression compared with local environmental inductive signals play in the progressive developmental differences seen in hematopoietic cells during ontogeny.

Blood cell formation in mammals appears to begin in the fetal yolk sac.[8,9] During early embryogenesis, cells (termed *hemangioblasts*) located in the extraembryonic mesoderm and allantois undergo rapid proliferation at the site of the future blood islands (Fig. 8-2). This induction occurs in response to unknown signals but may require participation of the visceral yolk sac endoderm, a highly secretory cell layer located immediately adjacent to the mesoderm cells[10,11] (Fig. 8-3). These changes occur at days 7.5 through 8.5 postcoitus in mice, the best studied mammalian model of fetal hematopoiesis, and at around 16 days of development in humans.

During further development, hemangioblasts segregate into peripheral cells destined to become vascular endothelial cells and into round mononuclear cells located centrally and destined to become primitive hematopoietic cells[12,13] (see Fig. 8-3, *inset*). The collection of cells, referred to as *blood islands*, subsequently is connected to similar islands and form the circulatory and blood systems of the developing embryo. Although little is known about the yolk sac phase of hematopoiesis, several studies show clear differences between these cells and cells derived later in embryogenesis in the fetal liver or neonatal or adult bone marrow. Differentiation is predominantly (completely in the mouse) limited to erythroid cells,[14–16] although pluripotent cells are present.[9] Yolk sac cells appear to have an altered sensitivity to the hormone, erythropoietin (EPO), since studies in the mouse and sheep suggest an increased sensitivity or lack of dependence on EPO altogether for RBC formation.[17–19]

Yolk sac erythroid cells are macrocytic and most retain nuclei that exhibit a coarse chromatin pattern.[20,21] Yolk sac stem cells exhibit a higher proliferative index when compared with adult stem cells.[19,22,23] Although differentiation is severely restricted to erythroid cells in situ, murine fetal yolk sac stem cells are capable of multilineage differentiation and can effect full reconstitution when injected into lethally irradiated adult recipients.[9] In addition, studies by Micklem and coworkers[24] and Moore and Metcalf[9] show that stem cells located in the yolk sac are capable of extended serial transplantation in irradiated adult syngeneic recipients, data that suggest that these stem cells have higher self-renewal capacity than stem cells derived from adult bone marrow.

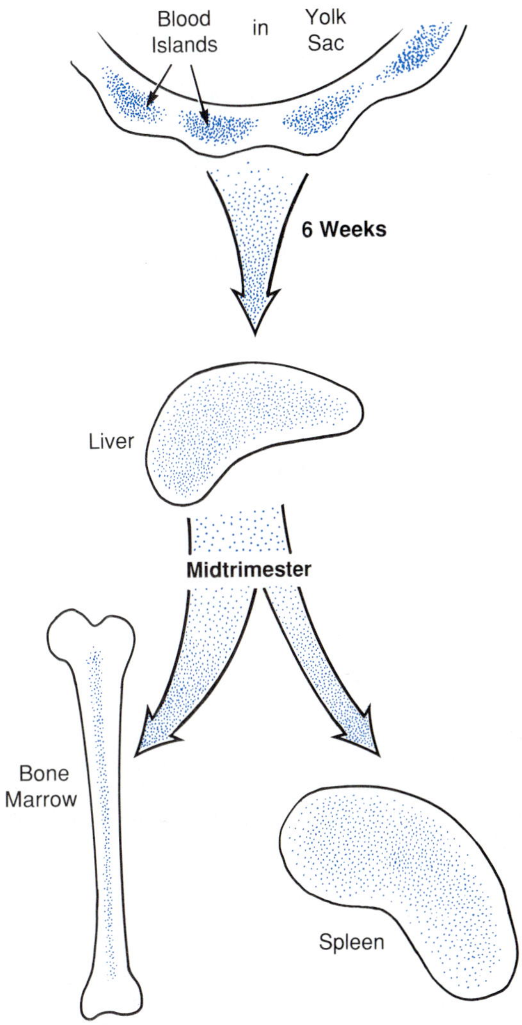

FIGURE 8-2. Ontogeny of hematopoiesis: schematic representation of the anatomic locations of hematopoiesis in the developing fetus. Hematopoiesis begins in blood islands located in extraembryonic tissues (fetal yolk sac) in the first trimester (see Fig. 8-3). At about 6 weeks of gestation, hematopoiesis occurs predominantly in the fetal liver. Beginning at mid-term, the medullary cavity gradually replaces the fetal liver as the main site of hematopoiesis. In some species, such as the mouse, the spleen is a major site of hematopoiesis in the adult.

Definitive adult hematopoiesis appears to arise by seeding of hematopoietic stem cells from the fetal yolk sac to the fetal liver[9,25,26] (see Fig. 8-2). These studies are controversial, since in avian and tadpole embryos a similar migration of fetal stem cells from the yolk sac has not been demonstrated.[27,28] No such observations have been made in humans. One group has recently shown that stem cells derived

◄ **FIGURE 8-1.** Schematic view of some general properties and assays for the heterogeneous cells that make up the stem cell and progenitor cell compartments. As indicated on the diagram, cells capable of permanently reconstituting in vivo hematopoiesis are separable from cells that give rise to day 12 CFU-S, but the precise developmental stage of in vitro long-term culture-initiating cells and blast cell colony progenitors is not established. In the progenitor compartment, mixed colonies of almost all myeloid lineage combinations have been described. The basophil–megakaryocyte–erythroid progenitor (CFU-b/M/E) is inferred from the restricted lineage expression of the transcription factor GATA-1 to cells of these lineages.[716] The precursor cell compartment shows the morphologically recognizable cells of the hematopoietic organs.

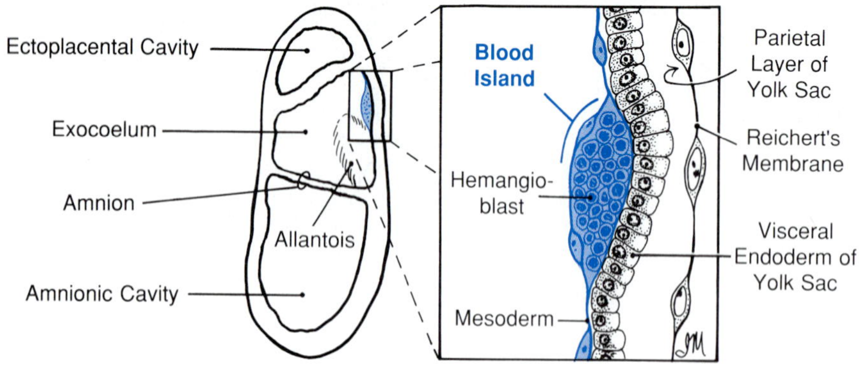

FIGURE 8-3. Schematic view of yolk sac hematopoiesis in the mouse at about 7 days of gestation. Blood islands form in the yolk sac mesoderm and allantois. The yolk sac mesoderm contains multipotent progenitors, termed *hemangioblasts*, that differentiate into endothelial cells lining the blood islands, and primitive hematopoietic stem, and progenitor cells. The visceral endoderm of the yolk sac forms an epithelium directly opposed to the mesoderm.

from human umbilical circulation are capable of hematopoietic reconstitution in an HLA-identical related sibling allogeneic transplant.[29–31]

At about $10\frac{1}{2}$ days postcoitus in mice and 6 weeks in humans, blood islands begin to regress and the major site of hematopoiesis shifts to the fetal liver.[9,32–35] In humans and mice, this change is accompanied by a switch in globin chain production from primitive to fetal globins (fetal to adult in mice; see discussion that follows). Hematopoietic cell differentiation continues to be predominantly restricted to the erythroid lineage[16,36,37] although a large number of myeloid progenitors are present in the fetal liver.[36,38,39] RBCs produced in the fetal liver are smaller than those produced during primitive yolk sac erythropoiesis. Erythroid cell nuclear structure also more closely resembles normoblasts of adult bone marrow, and the site of hematopoiesis is predominantly extravascular.[34,40,41]

Other differences between the hematopoietic cells developing in the fetal liver and the adult cells are expression of i surface antigen (versus I antigen) and low levels of the enzyme carbonic anhydrase, a prominent nonhemoglobin protein of RBCs.[42,43] These fetal characteristics are sometimes seen in adult life during episodes of hematopoietic stress, such as bone marrow failure and posttransplantation reconstitution.

The relation of developing blood cells to stromal or parenchymal hepatic elements during this early phase of hematopoiesis is largely unstudied. Medlock and coworkers[44,45] have reported an orderly morphologic transition from prehepatocytes, apparently secreting reticulum and forming a three-dimensional supporting network for hematopoietic cells, to uniform epithelial cells with evidence of high secretory activity characteristic of the differentiated phenotype of the mature hepatocyte. The full expression of an epithelial cell phenotype coincides with the cessation of hematopoiesis in the fetal liver as the bone marrow medullary cavity becomes the major source of blood cells. Although hematopoietic differentiation in the fetal liver is restricted predominantly to erythroid cells, circulating platelets and granulocytes are seen; evidence suggests, at least in the murine system, that pre–B lymphocytes are present in the liver environment.[45,46] At the time of transition of the anatomic site of hematopoiesis in the mouse from the yolk sac to the fetal liver, an abrupt switch in globin from fetal (EI, EII, EIII) to adult (α_2 and β_2) occurs.[15,47] By the end of the first trimester in human fetuses, the major hemoglobin produced in fetal RBCs is derived from gamma gene expression (hemoglobin F).*[48]

* For an extensive review of hemoglobin switching, see Stamatoyannopoulos G, Neinhuis A. Hemoglobin switching. In: Stamatoyannopoulos G, Neinhuis A, Leder P, Majerus P, eds. The molecular basis of blood diseases. Philadelphia, WB Saunders, 1987.

During the midtrimester, hematopoietic cells are also seen in lymph nodes, thymus, and bone marrow space.[49,50]

The final anatomic site of hematopoiesis during ontogeny is the medullary cavity of bone in humans and the medullary cavity and spleen in mice (see Fig. 8-2). Although human hematopoietic cells can be seen in the medullary cavity space by 8 to 9 weeks, this site becomes the major site of hematopoiesis at about 5 months of gestation.[49] Differentiation occurs along all lineages within the medullary cavity of human fetuses, although little erythropoiesis is observed in the medullary cavity of mice and rats until after birth.[50] By the final trimester, all available medullary space is filled with hematopoietic cells. The medullary cavity of the fetus has little capacity to respond to stress and relies on reactivation of hematopoietic cell production by the liver and cell production in the spleen (extramedullary hematopoiesis) to respond to requirements for additional formed elements during stress.[51,52]

Later in childhood and adult life, the medullary cavity can respond to similar stress by expansion into fatty marrow, and the incidence of extramedullary hematopoiesis is markedly reduced.[52] Thus, blood cell formation proceeds through multiple anatomic sites and displays characteristic changes in gene expression during fetal development. The microenvironment and growth factor requirements for hematopoiesis and specific changes in expression of the major gene studied (globin) during fetal development are described in the text that follows.

Physiologic Changes After Birth

Major changes in erythropoiesis accompany the transition from intrauterine to newborn hematopoiesis. During the last trimester of fetal life, medullary hematopoiesis reaches a stable level with little capacity for expanded cell production without the recruitment of extramedullary sites.[51,52] At the time of birth, erythropoietic activity rapidly declines, as evidenced by decreased reticulocyte counts, falling hemoglobin concentration, and decreased bone marrow cellularity noted in newborn infants.[53–56] The fall in RBC production as well as a shortened half-life of fetal erythrocytes leads to a physiologic hemoglobin nadir at about 2 to 3 months of age in the full-term infant and as early as 4 weeks in the premature infant.[57]

Coincident with the fall in hemoglobin is a gradual shift in the oxygen dissociation curve, which results both from replacement of fetal hemoglobin with adult hemoglobin and from an increase in erythrocyte 2,3-diphosphoglycerate (2,3-DPG).[58–60] This increase in 2,3-DPG increases the oxygen delivery capacity of erythrocytes of newborn infants as the hemoglobin falls and, therefore, the level of hemoglobin must be interpreted in the light of both oxygen delivery and oxygen utilization. The transition from fetal to adult erythropoiesis appears to be a closely regulated multifactorial system allowing replacement of erythroid cells suited for oxygen delivery in the intrauterine environment with erythroid cells suited for oxygen delivery in postnatal life.[61]

The level of fetal hemoglobin gradually falls over the first year after birth, maintaining a low but detectable level in most persons throughout adult life.[62] Conditions associated with erythroid stress as well as mutations around the γ and β gene loci (such as hereditary persistence of fetal hemoglobin [HPFH]) are associated with elevation of fetal hemoglobin levels in childhood and adult life.[63–68] The physiologic nadir of hemoglobin of about 11 g of hemoglobin in the full-term infant is generally attained at about 3 months of age. The nadir is reached earlier in the premature infant and is generally 1 to 2 g less than in full-term infants (9 to 10 g hemoglobin).

Despite the relative hypoplasia of erythroid production during the first months of postnatal life, newborn bone marrow is capable of responding to anemic stress.[69] Infants born after intrauterine hypoxic episodes demonstrate elevated cord blood EPO levels and congenital hemolytic anemias are associated with elevated EPO levels in the amniotic fluid and increased reticulocytes and nucleated RBCs in the peripheral blood.[70,71] Infants with significant ongoing hemolysis occasionally appear to be incapable of sustained compensation during the first 3 to 4 months of life. In addition, some premature infants demonstrate low concentrations of EPO; inadequate production of EPO has been postulated to underlie the anemia seen in these infants.[72–75] Therefore, RBC transfusion requirements for hemolysis and anemia during this period do not predict chronic transfusion dependence. The use of recombinant human EPO for the treatment of anemia in very-low-birthweight infants is under study.[75,76]

THE STEM CELL COMPARTMENT

Pluripotent Stem Cells Retain the Capacity for Self-Renewal and Maintain Hematopoiesis by Clonal Proliferation

The key to sustained hematopoiesis is the pluripotent stem cell. The presence of these stem cells in mice was first indicated by experiments carried out by Jacobson and colleagues.[77] They showed that mice could be protected from the effects of whole-body irradiation if the spleen was exteriorized and excluded from the radiation field. Furthermore, the continued presence of the unirradiated spleen was unnecessary. It could be removed as little as 1 hour after irradiation and still show the effect on improved survival.[78] That this protective effect was cell-mediated rather than noncellular was demonstrated by the observation that injected spleen cells could initiate recovery and reestablish hematopoiesis in irradiated animals.[79] The essential defining characteristic of the most immature stem cells is thus the ability to *repopulate both the immune and hematopoietic lineages* after transfer; in mice, these cells show no decline in repopulating ability with age.[80–82]

Although these repopulation experiments showed the functional importance of stem cells, Till and McCulloch[1] recognized that the colonies that form in the spleens of lethally irradiated mice after injection of bone marrow cells were stem cell–derived, and the following method became available for quantitating stem cells: CFU-S colonies are obtained by injecting a limited number of bone marrow cells intravenously into a heavily irradiated, syngeneic recipient mouse. After 8 to 14 days, the spleens are harvested and can be fixed (for counting or histologic analysis), or the individual spleen colonies can be dissected and analyzed further.

The cells that give rise to these colonies are designated CFU-S. The splenic colonies contain erythroid, phagocytic, or megakaryocyte progenitors and precursors, and spleen colonies that appear late (day 14 or CFU-S_{14}) also contain stem cells that can form additional spleen colonies of differentiated progeny when infused into a second irradiated recipient.[83,84] Analysis of individual CFU-S–derived spleen colonies demonstrates heterogeneity from colony to colony with respect to their content of new CFU-S.[83,85,86] Most colonies contain few CFU-S, whereas some contain large numbers. Experiments with karyotypically marked cells or retroviral-tagged cells have shown that cells that make up CFU-S–derived spleen colonies are of *clonal* origin. Under steady-state conditions, no more than 20% to 30% of CFU-S are in cycle during a 3-hour exposure to high-dose ^{3}H-thymidine or hydroxyurea in suicide experiments, although strain variations have been documented.[87–89]

Many agents are able to increase the proportion of stem cells in cycle, including drugs that stimulate both β-adrenergic and cholinergic receptors and steroids such as testosterone. The physiologic role of such agents is poorly understood. Stem cells are extremely rare. The incidence of reconstituting stem cells is estimated at 1 to 2.5 per 100,000 injected nucleated marrow cells (based on comparative repopulation methods and variabilities using the binomial formula) to 1 per 10,000 transplanted cells (based on limiting dilution analysis).[90–92] Stem cells can repopulate both the myeloid and the lymphoid systems. This has been demonstrated by the use of radiation-induced chromosome markers; by injection of fetal mice with mixtures of cells distinguishable by differences in hemoglobin, isoenzyme, and immunoglobulin types; and by analysis of the progeny of cells marked by unique retroviral integration sites.[93,94]

In summation, the spleen colony technique was used to establish several fundamental properties of hematopoietic stem cells: their ability to generate clonally derived populations of maturing cells; their extensive capacity for self-renewal; their multipotential capacity; and the fact that most of these cells are not in cell cycle.

Purification of Stem Cells

Application of the CFU-S assay and analysis of hematopoietic stem cells generally have been hindered by the low incidence of stem cells in the hematopoietic population and the lack of reagents to identify stem cells. Considerable work by many investigators has led to the ability to enrich stem cells. Murine hematopoietic stem cells can be highly purified by density gradient centrifugation and by labeling with antibodies, lectins, or intracellular dyes (or combinations of these) followed by separation using fluorescence-activated cell sorting (FACS), immunopanning, or immunomagnetic bead separation.[95] Immunologic characteristics that define murine stem cell populations include weak expression of *Thy-1* and expression of antigens defined by Qa-m7, and *Sca-1* (Ly6). Using the combination of lineage depletion and selection of *Thy-1* and *Sca-1* by FACS sorting, Spangrude and coworkers[96] have purified stem cells such that reportedly as few as 30 cells could reconstitute half of lethally irradiated syngeneic recipients.

Bertoncello and coworkers[97,98] used antibodies to the Qa-m7 antigen and immunomagnetic bead separation to purify a primitive murine hematopoietic cell population, termed *high proliferative potential–colony-forming cells* (HPP-CFC). HPP-CFC give rise to macroscopically visible (larger than 5 mm), in vitro colonies considered by some to be the equivalent of the reconstituting stem cell.[99] In these studies, up to 30% of the purified cell populations were HPP-CFC. Visser and coworkers[100,101] used combinations of density gradient centrifugation and labeling with wheat germ agglutinin and rhodamine 123 dye to purify stem cells capable of 30-day radioprotection after transplantation into lethally irradiated syngeneic murine recipients. Studies in humans and nonhuman primates have used similar purification schemes and the CD34 antigen to partially enrich for stem cells.[102–104] Radioprotection of primates with CD34+ selected cells has been achieved, although definitive proof of multilineage reconstitution with these cells has not been shown.[104]

Heterogeneity of Stem Cells

The results of CFU-S and other studies have led to refinements in the assignment of primitive cells in the stem cell compartment and to the realization that the stem cell compartment is heterogeneous[105] (see Fig. 8-1). The stem cell compartment may be observed as a continuum of three broad classes of stem cells with respect to self-renewal and proliferative capacities.[7,106–108] The most primitive stem cell has extensive self-renewal and proliferative capacity and is likely to be responsible for long-term reconstitution of the hematopoietic system after bone marrow transplantation. Less primitive cells, represented by stem cells that give rise to spleen colonies 12 to 14 days after injection into irradiated recipients (CFU-S_{12}) exhibit less self-renewal and proliferative capacity and are generally limited to myeloid differentiation.[83] The least primitive stem cell compartment, represented by stem cells that give rise to spleen colonies 6 to 8 days after transplantation (CFU-S_8), have limited self-renewal and proliferative capacities and may represent cells more restricted to erythroid differentiation.[83,109] The relation between this latter group of stem cells and progenitor cells that give rise to mixed lineage colonies in vitro (CFU-GEMM or CFU-Mix) and colonies of primitive blast cells capable of forming additional colonies after replating (see following text) is at this point unresolved.

Other in vitro assays have been described that measure cells with properties similar to CFU-S_{12}, such as the HPP-CFC,[106] and the type A colony-forming units (CFU-A),[110] which are present at the same frequency, have similar density and cycling characteristics, and respond to growth factors in similar fashion when compared with in vivo CFU-S_{12}. These considerations are of clinical relevance, since any manipulations of human bone marrow before allogeneic or autologous transplantation requires preservation of the most primitive stem cell compartment. Morphologically, stem cells appear to be medium-sized mononuclear cells with large nuclei, prominent nucleoli, and basophilic cytoplasm devoid of granules.

For obvious reasons, examination of human stem cells in vivo has been impossible using the murine techniques previously described. Antin and coworkers[111] have reported microscopic, multilineage hematopoietic colonies in the spleens of humans after bone marrow transplantation. Both human and murine stem cells can form colonies in semisolid media. Several such assays have been established, but the relation of the cells that form in vitro colonies in these assays to pluripotent stem cells with extensive self-renewal capacity is still not clear (see Fig. 8-1).

Multipotent progenitor cells can be assayed by their ability to form colonies of maturing granulocytes, erythrocytes, monocytes, and megakaryocytes when immobilized in a semisolid medium (either methylcellulose or agar) and stimulated with the appropriate hematopoietic growth factors (CFU-GEMM).[112,113] The relation of this cell to the cell or cells detected by the CFU-S assay is not certain; similarities in sedimentation velocities, proliferative state, differentiation potential, and self-renewal properties suggest that they may represent overlapping populations. Reconstitution of hematopoiesis and CFU-S–derived spleen colonies can be obtained after exposure of bone marrow ex vivo to 4-hydroperoxycyclophosphamide, but this treatment renders CFU-GEMM undetectable, and indicates that CFU-GEMM do not contain cells with reconstituting capacity.[114,115] Recent studies have identified a unique type of in vitro colony (CFU-Blast) that contains small numbers of blast cells with higher self-renewal and differentiating capacity than CFU-GEMM.[116] Murine and, to a lesser extent, human stem cells can be cultured for prolonged periods in vitro only in a culture system that provides direct stem cell contact with stromal cells as first described by Dexter and coworkers[6] (see section on hematopoietic microenvironment).

Clonal Succession, or the Continuous Proliferation of Pluripotent Stem Cells

Two stem cells, call them Abraham and Moses
In their first-class compartment, filled with roses
Feeding on royal jelly, one supposes
And ask the question, fateful for each stem
"When should I next divide," says A to M,
"Will both of me become like two of them?"
"These things" said Moses after solemn pause
"Must be determined by almighty cause
And not by chance. We must define our laws."
And swiftly consummating that mitotic burst,
Knowing that two of them must be dispersed,
Two Abrahams were fractionally first
And pushed both Moses through the compartment door
Saying as they did so "What a tedious bore!
Why should they think we need to have a law?"

—*H.E.M. Kay*[117]

The hypothesis that a series of stem cells may contribute clones successively to maintain hematopoiesis throughout the life-span of an individual was first advanced by Kay.[118] Support for this hypothesis comes from transplant studies of recipients of small numbers of bone marrow cells[119,120] and from experiments in which mixtures of fetal liver cells from different inbred mouse strains were introduced into W-mutant fetuses. W-mutants exhibit a genetically determined deficiency of hematopoietic (as well as germ and follicle) stem cells. Long-term monitoring in these mice showed clonal dominance followed by decline of cells of particular genotypes.[121]

Recently, the use of retroviral mediated gene transfer to mark hematopoietic stem cells has lent strong support to this hypothesis. Analysis of the viral integration patterns at intervals after transplantation have documented concurrent contributions of small numbers of stem cells to hematopoiesis, with changing patterns over time.[122–124] These conclusions are not supported by the work of Harrison and coworkers,[91] who measured variances at successive intervals in recipients of marrow mixtures from two congenic donors. The high correlations between congenic contributions observed in these studies suggest that the transplanted stem cells continuously produce descendants.[91] If 10 to 20 clones are contributing to hematopoiesis simultaneously, however, even with clonal succession, variances might be expected to be minimized between two alloenzymes at sequential samplings.

Furthermore, a recent longer-term analysis of viral integration patterns in multiple lineage progeny of stem cells transplanted into mice show that integration patterns are unstable initially, then stabilize and maintain a consistent pattern over many months.[122] Although this consistency does not appear to support the clonal succession hypothesis, the contributory role of unmarked stem cells in these experiments cannot be assessed. Furthermore, it is not possible to determine whether the immediate progeny of the transplanted (and retrovirally marked) stem cells might not all still have self-renewal capacity and subsequently contribute to hematopoiesis successively. Such clones would carry the same integration marker.

The hypothesis of clonal succession remains somewhat controversial, and studies of human transplant recipients suggest that clonal succession is not observed in posttransplantation hematopoiesis.[125]

Influence of Drugs on Cycling of CFU-S

Although the factors that control the decision of CFU-S to undergo either self-renewal or commitment to differentiate down one of the alternate lineage pathways are poorly understood, the cell cycle status of CFU-S can be influenced in a number of ways. Thus, the proportion of CFU-S in cycle can be increased by exposure to agents that act through β-adrenergic or cholinergic mechanisms, suggesting that specific receptors may exist on the surface of these cells; these agents may stimulate proliferation through adenylate cyclase cyclic AMP and cyclic GMP, respectively.[126–128]

Hematopoietic Growth Factors and Stem Cell Function

Hematopoietic growth factors also appear to influence at least some classes of CFU-S. Whereas interleukin-3 (IL-3) is necessary for blast cell colony formation, interleukin-6 (IL-6), granulocyte colony-stimulating factor (G-CSF), and interleukin-11 (IL-11) appear to decrease the time interval until blast cell colonies begin to proliferate in culture.[129–133] In addition, recent studies with retroviral vectors have shown that preincubation of bone marrow cells with IL-3 and IL-6 increase the efficiency of gene transduction of the reconstituting hematopoietic stem cell.[134,135] Such gene insertions require the stem cells to be actively cycling, and these studies provide indirect evidence for the potential roles of IL-3 and IL-6 in stem cell survival.

The recent isolation of the kit ligand, and its receptor, encoded by the c-*kit* protooncogene, has provided a unique insight into genetic factors known for many years to affect stem cell function. Two murine mutations that have been characterized in some detail are the *Steel (Sl)* and *dominant white spotting (W)* mutations (Fig. 8-4). Genetically affected mice defective at these loci have a severe macrocytic anemia associated with increased radiation sensitivity, lack of coat pigmentation, and sterility. Although phenotypically similar, these mutations map to different chromosomes (W to chromosome 5, Sl to chromosome 10) and have distinct hematologic characteristics.[136] Best characterized at the molecular level, the W mutation appears to be a functional deficiency of hematopoietic stem cells. Transplantation of normal bone marrow into compound heterozygote (deficient) W/W^v recipients completely corrects the hematopoietic abnormalities, whereas transplantation of W bone marrow into normal mice fails to reconstitute hematopoiesis.[137]

The W gene has recently been shown to be allelic with the c-*kit* protooncogene, which is known to be a member of the tyrosine kinase receptor family, as is the receptor for CSF-1. Recently, several variants of the W mutation have been shown to be phenotypic expressions of specific molecular mutations of the c-*kit* protooncogene[138,139] and the severity of the phenotypic changes associated with

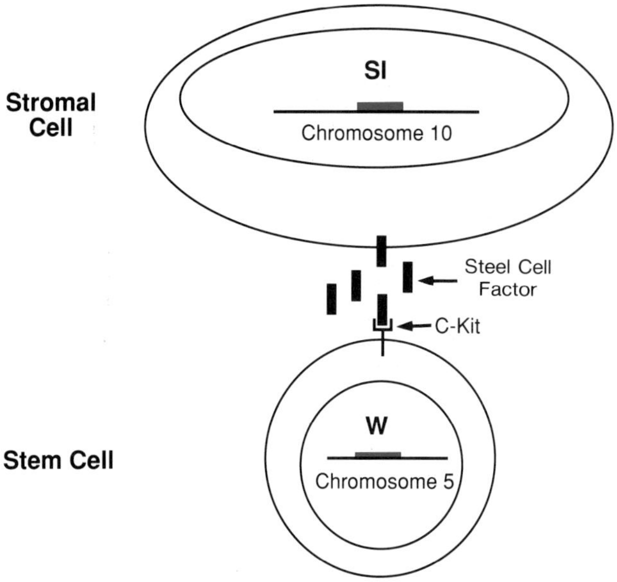

FIGURE 8-4. The White spotting (W) and Steel (S1) gene products. The protooncogene c-*kit* maps to the murine W locus, and its product, a tyrosine–kinase cell surface receptor, is abnormal in numerous mutations of this gene; this leads to abnormalities of hematopoietic stem cells. The S1 gene encodes the ligand for c-*kit*, otherwise known as Steel factor. Mutations at the locus lead to abnormal function of the hematopoietic microenvironment.

specific alleles correlates with the degree of functional impairment of kinase activity.[140]

In contrast, the Steel mutation affects the function of the cells of the microenvironment. Sl/Sl^d bone marrow cells are capable of reconstituting hematopoiesis in irradiated normal mice, whereas transplantation of normal bone marrow into Sl/Sl^d animals fails to cure the defect.[141] A deeper insight into the molecular nature of this defect was recently provided by the purification of a factor that is active on mast cells and on mouse bone marrow treated with 5-fluorouracil (5FU; enriched for primitive stem cells but depleted of mature progenitors).[142,143] This stem cell factor or mast cell growth factor was purified and its cDNA cloned.[144–146] Labeling studies with the purified recombinant protein demonstrate that it is the ligand for c-*kit*.[142,143,146]

Furthermore, administration of the factor to Sl/Sl^d mice corrects their macrocytic anemia and repairs their mast cell deficiency. The *kit* ligand gene maps to the Steel locus on chromosome 10.[147–149] Confirmation for the hypothesis that kit ligand is encoded by the Steel gene comes from Southern analysis of DNA obtained from stromal lines from normal and Sl/Sl homozygotes (the Sl mutation, unlike the commonly studied Steel–Dickie [Sl^d] mutation, is an embryonic lethal). These studies reveal that the coding sequences of the Steel gene locus are completely deleted from the genome of homozygous Steel mice.[149]

Less severe mutations at the Sl locus such as Sl^d are associated with smaller deletions at the Sl locus.[148] The gene encodes a protein that may exist in both transmembrane and secreted forms.[145,150,151] Thus, it is intriguing to speculate that the *kit* ligand may play a role in stromal cell–stem cell interactions. The biologic properties of the *kit* ligand in vitro are characterized by lack of colony-stimulating activity alone but marked synergy with many of the CSFs specific for different cell lineages (a more complete discussion of the Steel gene product is found in the section on hematopoietic microenvironment later in this chapter).

Stochastic Nature of Stem Cell Commitment

Two models have been proposed to explain the mechanisms that influence the choice of stem cells between self-renewal and commitment.[152–154] A stochastic model was proposed by Till and colleagues.[154] In this model, self-renewal or differentiation is considered to occur in a random or stochastic manner, dictated only by a certain probability. Because no extrinsic source of stem cells exists, under steady-state conditions the overall probability of stem cell division resulting in self-renewal must be 0.5; probabilities lesser or greater than this value would lead to progressive stem cell depletion (aplasia) or expansion (leukemia), respectively.

The commitment of stem cells could occur symmetrically, where overall, half of the stem cells divide to produce progeny, both of which enter a differentiation pathway, whereas half of the stem cells generate progeny that are both stem cells. Alternatively, asymmetric division would give rise to one stem cell and one cell committed to differentiate. Analysis of single cells from blast cell colonies has shown that hematopoietic cells can divide asymmetrically; these micromanipulated single cells give rise to colonies that account for almost all possible lineage combinations.[155] These data provide strong support for a stochastic mechanism to explain both commitment and restriction of differentiation potential. Differentiation of single blast cells into mature cells occurs in these methylcellulose cultures in the absence of an intact microenvironment. A source of hematopoietic growth factor is obligatory, as is the case for all colonies grown in semisolid media.

Although these random events occur with a given probability, it must be possible for that probability to be altered. For example, during the regeneration of hematopoietic tissues after injury by radiation or cytotoxic drugs, the probability of generating stem cells must increase. How this probability is altered is one of the outstanding unanswered questions in hematopoiesis.

A contrasting model, proposed by Trentin,[152] postulated that the hematopoietic microenvironment was inductive (HIM) and was based on the observation that domains of a given lineage existed within single spleen colonies.[153] Erythroid HIMs predominate in murine spleen, whereas granulocytic HIMs predominate in bone marrow. Transfer experiments showed that granulocytic cells predominated in the CFU-S–derived spleen colonies arising at junctional regions of bone marrow fragments implanted in spleen, whereas erythroid cells predominate in the splenic portion of the same colony. A major drawback for this model comes from an analysis of progenitors within these colonies. Correlations were not observed between mature cells and their respective committed progenitors.[156]

The preponderance of differentiating cells of one type or other within colonies thus appears to result from later events. The nature of these events has not been established, but possibilities include the release of short-range lineage-specific factors by stromal cells or perhaps the display of such growth factor molecules on the surface of their cell membranes. The Dexter culture system also lends powerful support to an essential role of stromal cells for stem cell survival, since the concentration of stem cells is highest within the adherent stromal layer itself.[157,158] This and other observations related to the morphology of the focal development of hematopoietic islands attached to adherent cells have led to the postulate that hematopoietic stem cells reside within stromal cell "niches" that play a vital role in supporting stem cell survival, perhaps by intimate cell contact.[159]

In summation, it appears likely that two types of control can affect stem cell regulation: at one level is control by stromal cells, perhaps primarily on stem cell survival but also on their response to humoral factors; at a second level are the humoral growth factors, which appear to affect stem cells but probably have a greater effect on committed maturing progenitors and precursors.

THE PROGENITOR CELL COMPARTMENT

The immediate progeny of differentiating stem cells are cells committed to develop into the mature cells of a single lineage. These committed progenitors are characterized by loss of self-renewal capacity and by restriction in differentiating potential. Most of the progenitors that can be analyzed in semisolid cultures are unipotent, and over time can clonally generate colonies composed of 50 to 100,000 mature cells.[2,3] Thus, like stem cells, progenitors show marked heterogeneity within any given lineage. It is convenient to distinguish different progenitor classes based on their proliferative capacity and responsiveness to growth factors. This is probably an artificial classification because a continuum most likely exists in vivo, with the most immature progenitors merging with stem cells and the most mature progenitors merging with recognizable precursors.

Progenitors are assayed by their capacity to form colonies in vitro, and the original technique involved immobilization of a single cell suspension of bone marrow cells in a serum-enriched medium that contained a source of CSF (as conditioned medium) and was rendered semisolid by the addition of agar.[2,3,160] Subsequent modifications to this technique include the use of methylcellulose or agarose in place of agar, the addition of highly purified recombinant CSFs in place of conditioned media, and purification of the progenitor cells. The time required for a progenitor cell to mature into a colony of mature cells depends on both species and stage of differentiation. Mature and immature murine progenitors take about 2 and 7 to 10 days, respectively, whereas the analogous human progenitors require 7 and 14 days. The most mature progenitor-derived colonies are the first to develop into small colonies or clusters in culture, whereas the more immature progenitors take longer to mature and develop into bigger colonies.

Within this continuum, conventional classifications include immature erythroid burst-forming units (BFU-E), large multisubunit colonies of normoblasts that derive their name from their characteristic burst-like morphologic appearance in culture, and more mature single-subunit erythroid colony-forming units (CFU-E); immature granulocyte-macrophage, granulocyte, macrophage, or eosinophil colony-forming units (CFU-GM, CFU-G, CFU-M, CFU-Eo; more than 40 cells) or more mature clusters (less than 40 cells); in some culture systems, progenitors of the basophil–mast cell and megakaryocyte lineages can be identified (CFU-Mast, CFU-MK).

THE PRECURSOR CELL COMPARTMENT

Most cells in the bone marrow of a healthy person are recognizable precursor cells of the myeloid or erythroid cell compartments: 60% to 70% of these cells are myeloid precursors, 20% to 30% are erythroid precursors, and the remaining 10% include lymphocytes, plasma cells, macrophages and the very rare stem and progenitor cells previously discussed. In addition, normally 4 to 5 megakaryocytes are found per 1000 nucleated bone marrow cells. The normal ratio of myeloid to erythroid precursors is 3 to 3.5:1. Alterations in these numbers are difficult to determine with bone marrow aspirate samples because of variations in dilution of peripheral blood. Bone marrow biopsy is the preferred method of quantitation of the relative incidence of precursor types. Specific alterations in the precursor populations are discussed in chapters describing specific pathologic conditions.

As previously discussed, the bone marrow of newborn infants is characteristically very cellular and devoid of fat cells.[51,52] Erythroid precursors make up most marrow cells, and immediately after birth the number of erythroid cells and the total cellularity of the marrow cavity begin to decline.[54] Cellularity may decline by as much as 75% in the first 2 weeks of life but gradually increases thereafter to a maximum at 3 months. (The physiologic nadir of erythroid cells in the newborn was discussed previously.) Thus, in the newborn, the typical myeloid/erythroid ratio is not seen until about 1 month of age, the ratio being 1.2:1 on the first day of life, varying to 4:1 to 6:1 during the next 2 weeks. This dramatic reversal coincides with the diminished erythroid activity typical of the first 3 months of infancy.[53,55] In addition, infant bone marrows are characterized by a large percentage of lymphocytes (the percentage can reach as high as 50% in the first year of life).[56] The relative lymphocytosis generally persists for the first 4 to 5 years and is accompanied by a lymphocytosis in the peripheral blood.

Maturation of the Erythroid Lineage

As seen on standard Wright-Giemsa staining at the light microscope level, the normal differentiation of RBCs occurs in well-defined stages. The first identifiable and also largest precursor of the erythroid lineage is the pronormoblast. The cell diameter is 14 to 19 μm, and the nucleus is large, oval, and homogeneously staining (violet) with indistinct nucleoli. The cytoplasm is darkly basophilic with lighter staining areas (hyaloplasm) usually near the nucleus, reflecting the position of the Golgi and lipid-containing mitochondria. Maturation to the basophilic normoblast is accompanied by reduction in cell size and pronounced changes in the nuclear chromatin structure. The basophilic normoblast is 12 to 17 μm in diameter with basophilic cytoplasm, and the nuclear chromatin shows a coarsening and prominent clumping leading to descriptions of a spoked wheel or cartwheel appearance. Nucleoli are generally not seen. The polychromatic normoblast is nearly the same size as the basophilic normoblast. The accumulation of hemoglobin is now seen by the presence of less basophilic and muddy gray cytoplasm. The nucleus shows further condensation and is nearly black. The last nucleated RBC precursor is the orthochromatic normoblast. The cell now approaches the diameter of a reticulocyte (8 to 12 μm), and the eosinophilic staining cytoplasm contains nearly a full amount of hemoglobin. The nucleus is now fully condensed and pyknotic.

Extrusion of the nucleus results in the *reticulocyte,* a cell slightly larger than a fully mature erythrocyte. The reticulocyte is characterized by the presence of a fine granular or reticular network of ribosomal RNA observed with supravital stains such as cresyl blue or methylene blue. Such cells are present in small quantities in the peripheral blood of normal persons but are increased in response to stress on the erythroid lineage such as hemolysis or blood loss. *Stress reticulocytes* are prematurely released into the peripheral blood, where cellular maturation continues. Stress reticulocytes are larger in diameter than reticulocytes normally found in the peripheral blood, and their cytoplasm is more basophilic.

Other morphologic indications of stress erythropoiesis are polychromatophilia (violet tinting seen with Wright-Giemsa staining) and basophilicstippling (blue or black stippling diffusely distributed throughout the cell). Both are the result of RNA-containing remnants that stain in the cytoplasm of the erythrocyte. The premature destruction of erythroid precursors in the medullary cavity, termed *ineffective erythropoiesis,* is accompanied by elevation of serum lactate dehydrogenase (LDH), decreased levels of haptoglobin, slight elevation of the reticulocyte count (2% to 4%), and the occasional appearance of nucleated erythrocytes in the peripheral blood. The destruction of erythrocyte precursors in the medullary cavity is normally less than 10% of the developing cells, but loss of much larger numbers of cells is seen in hemoglobinopathies and several rare congenital anemias, such as the congenital dyserythropoietic anemias.

The final stage of erythroid maturation is the erythrocyte. The cell is a biconcave, relatively flat, nonnucleated disk of 7 to 8 μm in diameter. The normal survival of the mature erythrocyte is 100 to 120 days.

Leukocyte Differentiation

Leukocytes that circulate in the peripheral blood are divided into those of the myeloid, monocyte–macrophage, and lymphocytic lineages. The differentiation and function of the lymphocytic lineage are discussed elsewhere. Four distinct granule populations are seen in the myeloid and monocyte lineages and distinguish these cells morphologically during differentiation. Azurophilic granules are present in cells of both lineages, stain pink with Romanovsky dyes, and contain myeloperoxidase, acid phosphatase, basic cationic protein, and other hydrolases. Eosinophilic granules are conspicuous reddish orange, and basophilic granules are intensely blue. Specific neutrophilic granules do not stain intensely with standard Wright-Giemsa stains.

Myeloid Differentiation

The earliest identifiable cell of the myeloid lineage is the myeloblast. The cell is about 12 to 14 μm in diameter with a round or oval nucleus and basophilic cytoplasm that lacks granules. Nuclear chromatin is fine and one to five nucleoli are easily visible, with one to five per cell. The nucleus often stains reddish. Promyelocytes are the largest and most common of the primitive myeloid precursors. Promyelocytes are variable in nuclear shape with less prominent nucleoli and chromatin of medium density, which is more coarse than that of the myeloblast. The cytoplasm is deeply basophilic and contains variable numbers of peroxidase-positive granules. These granules can overlie the nucleus and vary in color from deep red to blue and distinguish the promyelocyte from the myeloblast. Myelocytes are characterized by round to oval nuclei with characteristic nuclear indentations, indistinct nucleoli, and unevenly stained, coarse chromatin structure.

The cytoplasm stains pale gray-brown or pink-brown with numerous specific granules covering the nucleus and throughout the cytoplasm except in a clear area near the nuclear indentation (centrosphere), which represents the Golgi apparatus. The myelocyte is also characterized by the first appearance of specific granules and is the last cell capable of cell division during myeloid differentiation. The metamyelocyte, band neutrophil, and segmented neutrophil show progressive condensation and restriction of the nucleus. The metamyelocyte exhibits a characteristic bean-

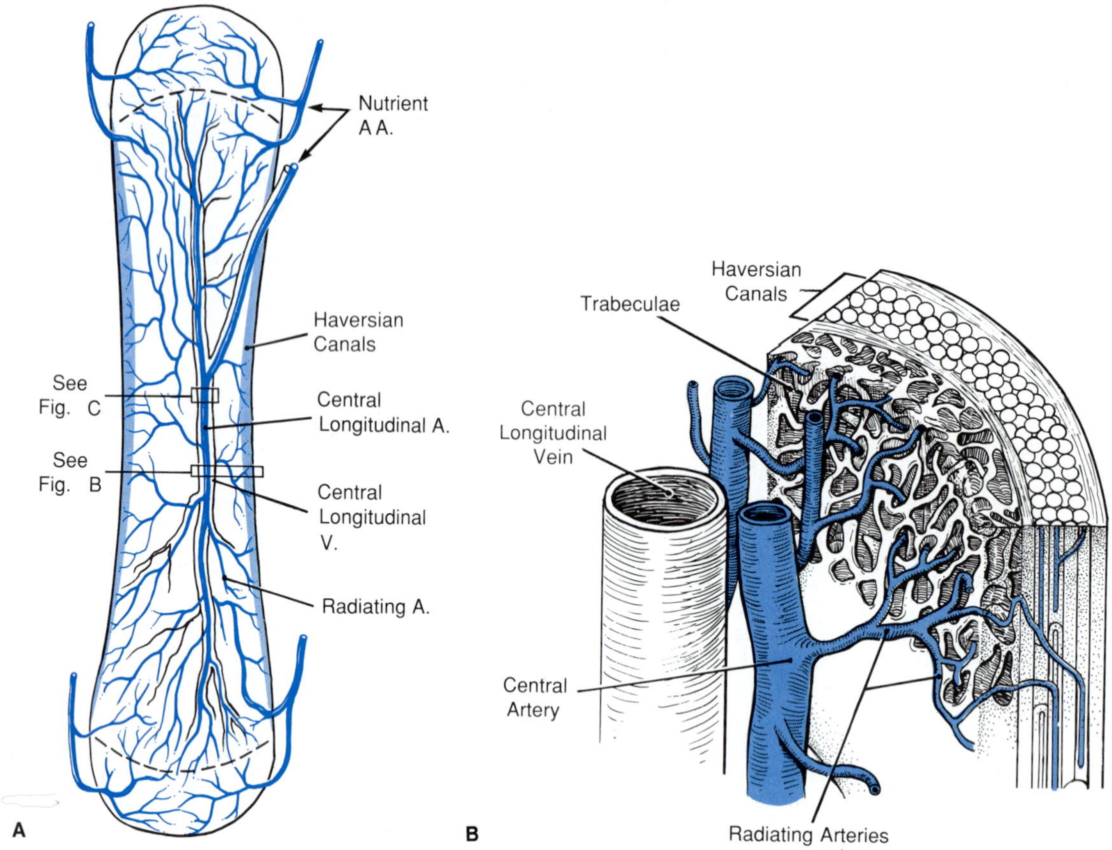

FIGURE 8-5. The hematopoietic microenvironment in the medullary cavity. (**A**) Schematic representation of longitudinal cross section of a long bone. (**B**) Schematic depiction of a sagittal cross section of the medullary cavity. Nutrient arteries feed the bone after entering the medullary space and giving rise to the central longitudinal artery. Progressive branches of this artery (radiating arteries) cross the medullary space toward the outside of the bone, connecting directly with hematopoietic sinuses or indirectly with cords through haversian canals. Hematopoietic cells leaving the medullary cavity collect in venous sinuses, enter the central longitudinal vein, then enter the general circulation. (**C**) Schematic depiction of the hematopoietic compartment of the medullary cavity. Hematopoiesis occurs in cords composed of differentiating hematopoietic cells, stromal cells, adventitial reticular cells, adipocytes (fat cells), and endothelial cells. Megakaryocytes appear to reside in the endothelial cell walls, shedding platelets into the sinus. Erythropoiesis appears to occur, in part, in groups surrounding macrophages, termed *erythroid islands.* Some evidence suggests structured variation in the location of primitive versus differentiated cells, with more primitive cells located nearer the bone surface.

shaped nucleus, the band neutrophil exhibits a horseshoe-shaped or S-shaped nuclear structure without recognizable constrictions, and the segmented neutrophil shows the characteristic nuclear segmentations for which it is named that divide the nucleus into two to five lobes. These myeloid forms exhibit similar cytoplasmic characteristics to the myelocyte without the centrosphere and with progressive reduction in overall cell size. An additional nuclear lobule in the shape of a drumstick is present in 10% to 12% of segmented neutrophils of females.

Maturation of the eosinophil and basophil follows the same morphologic steps as that of the neutrophil until the appearance of specific granules. The eosinophil exhibits a bilobed nucleus with the basophilic cytoplasm filled with prominent orange-red granules. Basophils have less segmentation of the nucleus and cytoplasm that is sparsely filled with deeply staining blue to purple metachromatic granules. The granules often obscure the nucleus and cytoplasm, which stains pink to reddish pink and frequently exhibits vacuoles. The incidence of these latter two cell types in the peripheral blood of normal persons is 1% to 4% and 0% to 0.5%, respectively.

Monocyte Differentiation

The earliest cell of the monocyte/macrophage lineage is difficult to distinguish from the myeloblast. The cell is 12 to 18 μm in diameter, with a round or oval nucleus that is frequently convoluted. The chromatin is fine and nucleoli are variably present. The cytoplasm is basophilic with a grayish cast and, although devoid of granules, may contain vacuoles. Blunt pseudopodia are sometimes present. The naphthol-AS-acetate esterase reaction is positive and inhibited by fluoride. The promonocyte is a large cell with an indented nucleus exhibiting fine chromatin and a single nucleolus. The cytoplasm stains light blue with azurophilic granules and a small centrosphere. The monocyte is the largest cell present in the peripheral blood and measures 13 to 20 μm in diameter. The nucleus is large and lobulated or bean-shaped with coarse nuclear chromatin, lacks nucleoli, and is often eccentric in location. The cytoplasm stains a characteristic smoke blue with azurophilic granules. The chromatin structure of the monocyte is less clumped and the cytoplasm more gray than the lymphocyte—characteristics which, along with nuclear

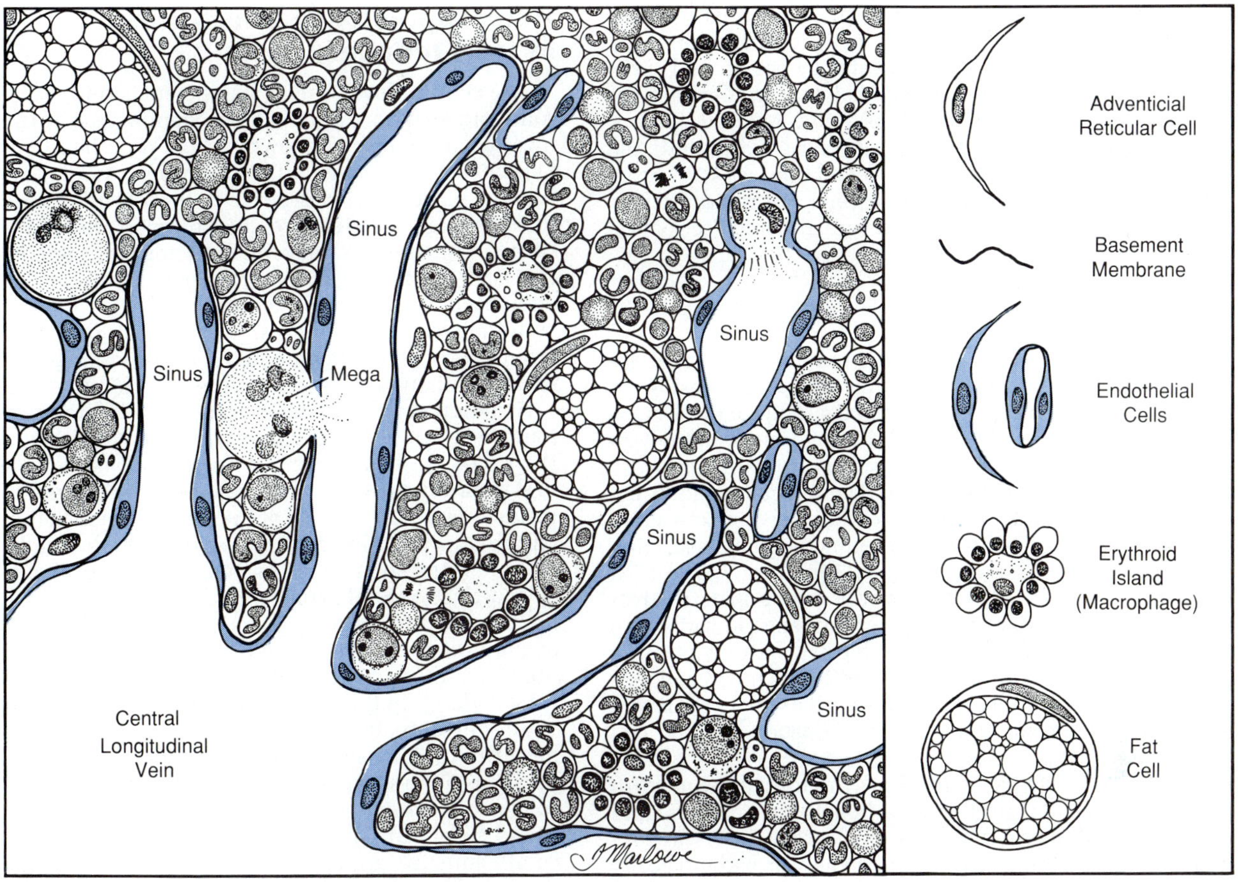

FIGURE 8-5. (Continued)

convolutions, help to distinguish these cells from moderately sized lymphocytes in the peripheral blood.

Blunt pseudopodia provide another helpful distinguishing characteristic. Monocytes usually make up 5% to 10% of the peripheral blood leukocytes. Egress of monocytes from the blood into tissues is associated with increased cell size and larger, lighter-staining nuclei. These cells, termed *macrophages* or *histiocytes*, are phagocytic and mobile, and intracellular debris and pseudopodia are often present.

Megakaryocytes

Morphologic differentiation of platelet-forming cells is different from either erythroid or leukocytic cell lineages. Distinct morphologic maturational steps and divisions do not take place, replaced instead by the process of *polyploidization*. In this process, successive nuclear divisions without concomitant cytoplasmic divisions lead to megakaryocytes with 1 to 32 nuclei representing 2N to 64N nuclear content. The first identifiable cell in this lineage is the megakaryoblast, a distinctly large cell with a high nuclear/cytoplasmic ratio. The nucleus shows variable chromatin coarseness and may contain nucleoli. The nuclear shape varies but the nucleus frequently displays convolutions or deep furrows. The cytoplasm stains basophilic, does not contain granules, and may exhibit fraying at the cytoplasmic membrane. Some megakaryoblasts may contain multiple nuclei. The promegakaryocyte exhibits lobulated nuclear structure without nucleoli and with coarse chromatin structure. The cytoplasm is basophilic with azurophilic granules adjacent to the nucleus and formed platelets are seen on the cytoplasmic cell surface.

Occasionally, the presence of other cells apparently within the cytoplasm (emperipolesis) of the promegakaryocyte is noted, although the mechanism leading to this occurrence is unknown. Mature megakaryocytes are the largest hematopoietic cell of the bone marrow. The nucleus is lobulated and exhibits coarse and clumped chromatin. Nuclear number varies from eight diploid nuclei (65% of marrow megakaryocytes) to four nuclei (10% of marrow megakaryocytes). The cytoplasm is basophilic with numerous azurophilic granules. Platelets can be seen at the periphery of the cytoplasm and attached to the cell membrane. Megakaryocytes constitute 0.1% to 0.5% of cells in the medullary cavity in normal persons.

HEMATOPOIETIC MICROENVIRONMENT

Hematopoiesis occurs within a complex environment in the medullary cavity in mammals.[6,152,161] The spatial arrangements in the medullary cavity are nonrandom and have been studied in some detail in situ and experimentally.[162–164] Branches of the central longitudinal artery traverse the space between the interior of the bone and the cortex, joining either directly to venous sinuses or communicating indirectly by means of the haversian canals in the bony cortex[165] (Fig. 8-5). These vascular connections, now moving toward the interior of the medullary cavity, separate groups of developing hematopoietic cells into so-called hematopoietic cords.166 Within the hematopoietic cords, self-renewal of stem cells and differentiation along all lineages take place. Cells leaving the medullary cavity must traverse the hematopoietic cord and enter the venous sinus by moving through endothelial cells.* This complex series of events involves pores in the endothelial wall, which apparently are located near, but not at, cell junctions.[167] The pores are generally smaller than the diameter of the cells moving into the sinus, and increased deformability appears to be a characteristic of more differentiated cells in both the erythroid and myeloid lineages.[165,168] From the venous sinus, hematopoietic cells are rapidly transported to the central longitudinal vein and into the general circulation.

Cellular Constituents

An important accessory cell of the microenvironment appears to be the adventitial reticular cell, which resides in close approximation to the abluminal surface of the venous endothelium.[169,170] Cells of this type cover most of the vascular adventitial surface and provide a reticular network that supports developing hematopoietic cells. In addition, adventitial cells and preadipocytes may play an active role in hematopoiesis by direct cell contact or local secretion of cytokines or other growth-regulating proteins.[171-177] It appears that such cells also respond to hematopoietic stress by changes in volume. Although adventitial cells and preadipocytes normally contain fat and extend into the hematopoietic cord space, when additional blood cell production is required, these cells become flattened and devoid of fat globules to provide additional space for blood cell production.[169,178]

The marrow cavity of newborn infants, persons with congenital and acquired severe hemolytic anemias, and those exposed to prolonged hypoxia is reduced in fat content.[179,180] In contrast, when hematopoiesis is pathologically impaired, as in aplastic anemia or other bone marrow failure syndromes, the marrow cavity becomes extensively filled with fat leading to the characteristic yellow marrow of hypoplastic marrow syndromes.[179,181] These fatty changes can also be seen in mice after chronic RBC transfusions.[180] A naturally occurring example of cyclical changes in adipocyte content of the medullary cavity is the armadillo. The medullary fat content of armadillo bone marrow increases with decreasing ambient temperatures; these changes correlate with decreased hematopoiesis.[182]

Adipocytes may play additional roles in hematopoiesis as reservoirs for lipids needed in cell metabolism during proliferation.[183,184] Medullary adipocytes demonstrate characteristics similar to both white adipocyte (lipid-containing cells involved in lipid and energy metabolism) and brown adipocyte (lipid-containing cells involved in heat production) tissues.[174] During starvation, white adipocyte tissue is rapidly depleted whereas fat in the bone marrow is spared. Insulin appears to be required for differentiation of white adipocyte cells; these cells exhibit lipogenic responses to insulin treatment. In contrast, bone marrow adipocytes appear to differentiate in response to glucocorticoids and do not respond to insulin.[185] During prolonged starvation, bone marrow fat cells are depleted and the marrow cavity is replaced by a gelatinous tissue.[186,187] Finally, the increasing fat content seen in long bones of older children and adults is associated with decreased limb temperatures compared with that seen in neonates and infants.[51,52] Thus, marrow adipocytes are not clearly classified as either white or brown adipocyte tissue.

* For a complete review of the architecture of the medullary cavity, see Chapter 14, Bone Marrow. In: Weiss L. Cell and tissue biology: a textbook of histology, ed 6. Baltimore, Urban & Schwarzenberg, 1988.

Hematopoietic Organization in the Medullary Sinus

At the cellular level, the hematopoietic sinus also displays some organization, although the significance of this organization remains unknown. Most prominently, megakaryocytes are located adjacent to the vascular endothelium, usually occupying space in the vascular wall. From this location, platelets are shed directly into the venous sinus, reducing any requirements for cell movement on the part of the megakaryocyte. Developing erythrocytes often occur in groups, termed *erythroblastic islands*, around bone marrow macrophages.[169,171,188,189] Studies by several groups show that hematopoietic stem and progenitor cells reside in distinct locations within the medullary cavity.

Hematopoietic stem cells with less proliferative activity tend to reside at the periphery of hematopoietic cords in the subcortical space.[162,163,190] In contrast, stem cells with higher proliferative activity and myeloid progenitor cells reside toward the middle of the hematopoietic sinus. Lord and coworkers[162] have also observed nonrandom localization of erythroid progenitors in murine femoral medullary cavity. Such spatial arrangements may reflect the general flow of cells toward the venous sinus during differentiation or may relate to specific cellular interactions with membrane proteins or extracellular matrix proteins of stromal cells making up the hematopoietic microenvironment.

The hematopoietic microenvironment probably provides more than passive structural support for hematopoietic cells during proliferation and differentiation.† For instance, the spleen environment in the mouse appears particularly suited for erythroid differentiation, whereas the medullary cavity supports granulocytic differentiation.[152] Studies by Wolff and Trentin[153] show effects of specific microenvironments on stem cell differentiation. Femoral shafts placed in spleen pulp give rise to hematopoietic colonies located at the junction of the femur and spleen environments with a geographic distribution of differentiated cells. In these experiments, differentiation within a clonally derived hematopoietic colony was myeloid within the marrow environment and erythroid within the spleen environment. Based on these and other observations, Trentin proposed that specific locations provide an inductive microenvironment for stem cell proliferation and differentiation.[83]

As previously noted, differentiation within the yolk sac and fetal liver microenvironments is severely restricted to the erythroid lineage. The molecular and biochemical bases for the microenvironment regulation of differentiation are not yet known.

In Vitro Cultures Recapitulate the Hematopoietic Microenvironment

The development of an in vitro culture system that mimics the hematopoietic microenvironment has significantly aided the study of hematopoietic stem cell–microenvironment interactions‡ (Fig. 8-6). First described by Dexter and coworkers[6] and later modified by Greenberger,[185] these

† For a wonderful review of the historical background to our understanding of the hematopoietic microenvironment, see Trentin JJ. Hemopoietic microenvironments, historical perspectives, status, and projections. In: Tavassoli M, ed. Handbook of the hemopoietic microenvironment. Clifton, NJ, Humana Press, 1989.

‡ For an extensive review of all aspects of long-term bone marrow cultures and the hematopoietic microenvironment, see Tavassoli M, ed. Handbook of the hemopoietic microenvironment. Clifton, NJ, Humana Press, 1989.

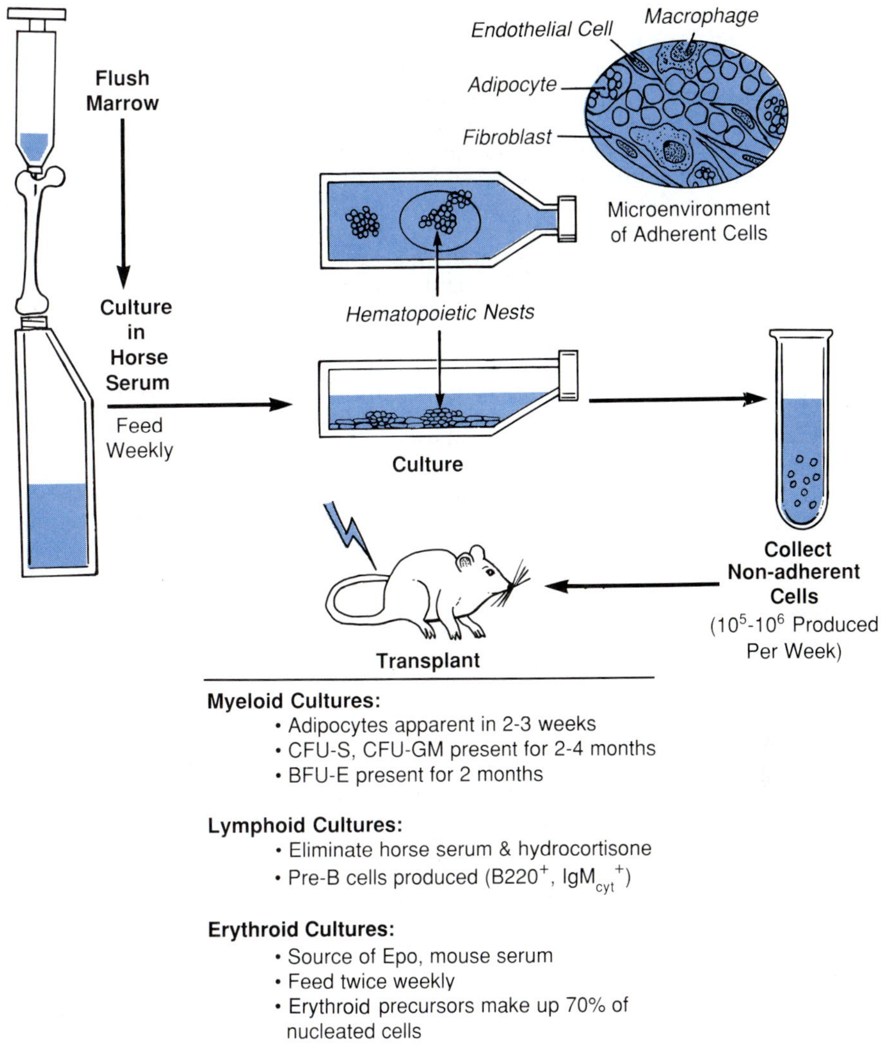

FIGURE 8-6. In vitro analysis of the hematopoietic microenvironment using long-term marrow (Dexter) cultures. Bone marrow is flushed from the marrow cavity and allowed to establish an adherent layer composed of endothelial cells, macrophages, adipocytes, and fibroblasts. Within this stromal layer, hematopoietic nests of actively proliferating stem and progenitor cells enlarge. Hematopoietic cells, including stem and progenitor cells, are shed into the supernatant, which can be harvested and used to rescue lethally irradiated transplant recipients. Such cultures can be modified to yield myeloid, lymphoid, and erythroid elements.

cultures are made up of a complex adherent cell population containing endothelial cells, fibroblasts, macrophages, and preadipocytes. The cultures are created by forcing a large inoculum of medullary cavity cells into flasks with media containing prescreened horse serum (later modified to include hydrocortisone; see Fig. 8-6). Cultures are maintained in high CO_2 at low temperatures (33°C) and depopulated of 50% to 70% of nonadherent cells and media at weekly feedings of fresh media. These culture conditions encourage the growth of the adherent cell population, which matures over about 3 weeks.

Hematopoiesis occurs within the adherent cell population, and on the surface of the adherent cells, hematopoietic cells are continuously shed into the overlying media.[171,191] Large groups of round, refractile cells, termed *hematopoietic islands* or *cobblestone areas*, are present within the adherent cell population and contain stem and progenitor cells.[192] In sharp contrast to other cell culture systems, hematopoietic stem cells are maintained for several months in vitro, and stem cells harvested from such cultures maintain the ability to fully reconstitute the hematopoietic tissues of lethally irradiated recipients.

Maintenance of the stem cell population in such cultures requires direct stem cell–stromal cell contact, since conditioned media from such cultures do not support the survival of stem cells in vitro.[193,194] Hellman and colleagues and other researchers have demonstrated that stem cells present in such cultures exhibit structured variation in self-renewal capacity.[119,157,158,195] Stem cells present in the adherent cell layer demonstrate considerably more self-renewal capacity than stem cells present in the nonadherent media overlying the cultures. These observations support the stem cell "niche" hypothesis proposed by Schofield[159] that direct contact of hematopoietic stem cells with the microenvironment maintains stem cell characteristics.[196] It is proposed that loss of direct stem cell contact with the microenvironment is accompanied by exposure of the stem cell to differentiation pressures with concomitant loss of self-renewal capacity.

The contribution of individual adherent cell types in long-term marrow cultures to the maintenance of stem cells is not known but is the focus of active research. Roles of the hematopoietic microenvironment in hematopoiesis have been proposed to involve direct communication of stromal with stem cells through tight cell-to-cell contact[197]; co-localization of growth factors and stem cells at the point of cell contact or prevention of growth factor degradation by binding of these cytokines to extracellular matrix proteins[198,199]; and secretion of stromal-derived growth-regulating factors,[200,201] including inhibitors of DNA synthesis.[202]

Long-term cultures, as originally described by Dexter,[6] provide an excellent model for myeloid differentiation. Full maturation to granulocytes and macrophages takes place in the cultures, whereas the relative concentration of myeloid compartments (stem, progenitor, precursor, differentiated cell) reflects normal hematopoiesis.[203] Further modification of long-term marrow culture conditions by elimination of horse serum and hydrocortisone leads to proliferation of pre-B lymphocytes as described by Whitlock and Witte.[161,204] Several groups have modified long-term cultures to allow full erythroid differentiation by including a small amount of fetal calf serum, feeding more frequently, and including EPO in the cultures.[205–208]

Long-term cultures have also been useful in the study of human hematopoiesis with several modifications of the techniques used in murine cultures as described.[209] Autologous marrow transplants from long-term cultures have led to successful, but transient, engraftment of normal stem cells in persons with myeloid leukemias.[210,211] Human long-term marrow cultures appear morphologically distinct, lacking the classic cobblestone areas seen in rodent cultures. In addition, stem cells are maintained in vitro for considerably shorter times (usually less than 2 months) in human cultures compared with several months in murine cultures.[212] The basis of these differences in not yet understood.

Stromal Cells Play a Critical Role in Hematopoiesis

The complexity of long-term marrow cultures has hindered some areas of hematopoietic research, specifically the study of stem cell–stromal cell interactions.* Several laboratories have now established immortalized stromal cell lines from long-term marrow cultures.[177,193,194,213–216] Most lines have been established from murine cultures, although a few lines derived from human cultures exist,[217,218] and recently a line from nonhuman primate bone marrow has been established.[200] Such immortalized stromal cell lines are established most frequently by serial trypsinization and passage to select for stromal cells that randomly acquire transformed phenotypes. In addition, Williams and coworkers[193] have used recombinant retroviral vectors that transfer the immortalizing oncogene contained in the simian virus 40 genome (SV40 large T antigen) to efficiently and quickly establish permanent cell lines from murine, primate, and human long-term marrow cultures.[200] Singer and colleagues[217] have used transfection of SV40 large T to establish human stromal cell lines. Immortalized stromal cell lines are generally screened for those that affect some aspect of hematopoiesis; such lines are then studied in detail.

Many stromal cell lines support the maintenance of myeloid and lymphoid progenitors in vitro for several weeks.[177,194,213,214,216–218] In addition, a few lines have been shown to support primitive myeloid stem cells (CFU-S_{12}) for extended periods; these lines effectively replace a complex long-term marrow culture in this regard.[177,193,194] One immortalized stromal cell line has been shown by male–female transplantation to support the maintenance of long-term reconstituting and multipotential stem cells in murine cultures for up to 3 weeks in vitro.[194] Similarly, stromal cell lines have been shown to support the proliferation of pre-B lymphocytes under conditions similar to those established by Whitlock and colleagues[216] and Hunt and coworkers,[213] for long-term lymphocyte cultures.[193] Conditioned media from stromal cell lines contain a variety of known hematopoietic growth factors but cannot support the maintenance of primitive stem cells in culture.[173,176,200,215,219–225] The maintenance of stem and progenitor populations in stromal long-term cultures depends on direct hematopoietic cell–stromal cell contact and therefore closely mimics the stem cell maintenance in traditional long-term marrow cultures.

Established stromal cell lines appear to represent a heterogeneous group of adherent cells.[226]†

Although the appearance of adipocytes in murine long-term marrow cultures is temporally related to increased hematopoietic activity, several stromal cell lines that support progenitor cell proliferation do not appear to be adipocytic. In general, the preadipocyte phenotype appears to correlate with support of myeloid hematopoiesis in vitro.[6,239] In contrast, support of lymphopoiesis appears to be related to the capacity of stromal cell lines to accumulate fat globules.[239] Gimble and coworkers[172,228] have shown that several stromal cell lines respond to inducing agents, such as dexamethasone, hydrocortisone, and methylisobutylxanthine by accumulation of triglycerides and cholesterol esters and increased expression of adipocyte-specific enzymes (adipocyte P2, adipsin, lipoprotein lipase). Stromal cell lines also appear heterogenous with respect to expression of extracellular matrix and intermediate filament proteins.[226]

Many stromal cell lines capable of supporting the proliferation of myeloid progenitor cells are characterized by production of the endothelial proteins laminin and type IV collagen as well as fibronectin.[227,229] Fibroblast-like stromal cell lines appear less capable of supporting hematopoiesis in murine cultures and are characterized by expression of collagens type I and III.[177,226,230–232] A primate stromal cell line recently described expresses collagens type I, III, and V and supports progenitor cells capable of giving rise to both myeloid and mixed colonies for up to 3 weeks in vitro.[200] Therefore, it remains unclear whether key stromal cell types in long-term marrow cultures differ in rodent and other species (including human).

Stromal Cells Produce a Variety of Growth-Regulatory Molecules

Stromal cell lines also differ considerably with respect to production of hematopoietic growth factors.[227,237] Some of these differences may be explained by experimental techniques, since more sensitive assays for growth factor production, such as polymerase chain reaction RNA analysis, have more recently been applied to the analysis of stromal cell lines. Stromal cell lines have been demonstrated to produce IL-6, IL-7, G-CSF, GM-CSF, TGF-β, M-CSF and IL-1, either constitutively or after induction with IL-1 or other inducing agents.[227,233] The induction of growth factor production may play an important role in the microenvironment regulation of hematopoiesis. Cashman and coworkers[221] used IL-1, platelet-derived growth factor (PDGF), transforming growth factor–α (TGF-α), and IL-2; Billips and coworkers[220] used IL-1 and IL-4 to demonstrate induction of stromal cell cytokine production.

In addition, long-term marrow cultures and some stromal cell lines have been shown to inhibit hematopoietic differentiation and stem cell DNA synthesis. Several groups have partially characterized proteins that have apparent negative regulatory roles in hematopoiesis.[234–236]‡ Toksoz and coworkers[202] reported that conditioned media from long-term marrow cultures contain a molecule that pre-

* A summary of stromal cells and hematopoiesis is contained in Singer.[212]

† For a review of stromal cells and hematopoiesis, see Gimble.[174]

‡ For a more complete review of negative regulators in hematopoiesis, see Broxmeyer H. Negative regulators of hematopoiesis. In: Wright D, Greenberger J, eds. Long-term bone marrow culture: present experience and future possibilities. New York, Alan R Liss, 1984.

vents the entry of primitive myeloid hematopoietic stem cells (CFU-S_{12}) into S phase as measured by thymidine suicide. A protein with similar characteristics has recently been defined and molecularly cloned from a macrophage cell line.[237] This protein, termed *stem cell inhibitor*, is identical with a previously characterized cytokine, termed *macrophage inflammatory protein-1-α* (MIP-1-α).[238] Biologic activities of stem cell inhibitor/MIP-1-α suggest that it is an important regulator of stem cell proliferation and may have therapeutic applications in protecting stem cells from cycle-specific chemotherapeutic agents.

Zipori and colleagues[239,240] have demonstrated that hematopoietic cells adherent to stromal cells fail to differentiate into macroscopic colonies of differentiated cell types even in the presence of exogenous CSFs. Thus, it appears that direct cell contact between hematopoietic stem cells and stromal cells can serve to restrict differentiation of stem cells in some culture systems. These same workers have identified a membrane-associated glycoprotein, restrictin-P, which specifically inhibits the growth of the plasmacytoma cell line MPC-11.[241] These studies emphasize the differences between short-term progenitor cultures, in which CSFs are added, hematopoiesis is of short duration, and differentiation predominates, and long-term stromal-associated cultures in which stem cells are maintained for extended periods of time.

A major goal of research is the understanding of these differences. Since the only in vitro system in which stem cells with full reconstitution capacity are maintained involves direct stem cell–stromal cell contact, the hematopoietic microenvironment is likely to play a critical role, either directly or indirectly, in hematopoietic stem cell biology.

The hematopoietic microenvironment may also be important in pathologic conditions affecting hematopoiesis. Murine mutants of bone marrow failure, such as the Steel (Sl) mutants, exhibit characteristics attributable to defective microenvironments, including the hematopoietic microenvironment.[137,242,243] *

Phenotypically, Sl and the better characterized dominant white-spotting (W) mutant are black-eyed white mice with reduced fertility and macrocytic anemia.[136] Careful study has revealed defects in all hematopoietic lineages.[244,245] The hematopoietic abnormalities of the Sl animal are not cured by transplantation of congenic normal marrow, but the anemia can be partially improved by transplantation of intact spleens into the peritoneal cavity, an observation that has led several investigators to postulate that the mutation responsible for the hematologic abnormalities resides in the hematopoietic microenvironment.[141,242,243,246] In support of this view, Dexter and Moore[247] have demonstrated that long-term marrow cultures from Sl mice do not support hematopoietic cells from normal congenic mice in vitro.

Other investigators have postulated that the stromal cells of Sl mice secrete an inhibitor of normal hematopoiesis.[248] The Sl mutation has been mapped to chromosome 10. Several laboratories have recently reported the cloning of the gene product of the Sl mutation and characterized the molecular basis of several of the known Sl mutations.[144,145,147–149,249]

The product of the Sl gene has now been shown to be a 28- to 35-kd growth factor, with a leader sequence, transmembrane domain, and a differentially spliced exon including a proteolytic cleavage site.[142,143,145] The protein product can thus be membrane-bound or secreted, although the physiologic role of these different forms is not clear. Flanagan and coworkers[250] have recently demonstrated that the Steel–Dickie (Sl^d) allele, which is known to be a nonlethal Sl mutation, is encoded by a Sl gene with a deletion of the transmembrane domain. The resulting protein is secreted and biologically active. This observation suggests that the membrane-bound form of the Sl gene product may play an important role in hematopoiesis. The Sl gene product is now known to be the ligand for the c-*kit* protooncogene.[142,147,149] The dominant white spotting mutation is known to be allelic with this tyrosine-kinase receptor family member.[138,139]

Although no congenital human bone marrow failure syndrome has been shown to be due to a microenvironment defect, the failure of bone marrow transplant engraftment in some patients with aplastic anemia suggests that such abnormalities may exist. The use of newer molecular methods, growth-regulatory probes, as well as more powerful genetic approaches to study affected kindreds may define abnormalities in the hematopoietic microenvironment associated with some congenital bone marrow failure syndromes.

FACTORS REGULATING THE EGRESS OF HEMATOPOIETIC CELLS FROM THE BONE MARROW

The movement of cells from the medullary cavity into the bloodstream has been studied in most detail using radiolabeled iron to monitor the development and release of erythroid cells. Classic ferrokinetic studies show that after initial uptake of ^{59}Fe in the bone marrow, newly synthesized erythrocytes are released into the bloodstream in 4 to 6 days.[251] The generation time of proliferating erythroid precursors (pronormoblasts, basophilic and polychromatophilic normoblasts) normally averages about 24 hours at each stage of maturation.[252,253] Nondividing erythroid precursors (orthochromatophilic normoblasts and reticulocytes) reside in the medullary space for about 48 hours each.[254] Normal maturation includes an average of four divisions and the generation of 8 to 16 cells from each pronormoblast. The maturation time can be shortened during stress by one of several mechanisms.

Commonly regarded as a critical mechanism in the erythroid compartment response to stress, erythrocytes can exit the medullary cavity prematurely after having skipped some divisions. These cells maintain primitive characteristics, such as macrocytosis, elevated fetal hemoglobin, and persistence of i (versus I) antigen on the cell surface.[255] In addition, erythrocyte maturation time might be shortened by decreasing the duration of each mitosis or by decreasing the maturation time of nondividing erythrocyte precursors.[256] Finally, RBC mass may be elevated by increasing the number of erythrocytes actually entering the bloodstream.

The last mechanism could result from either less destruction of RBC precursors (*ineffective erythropoiesis*) in the medullary cavity (normally around 10%) or from an expansion in the number of primitive cells entering into the erythroid maturational sequence.[257] The latter appears to be the usual mechanism of expansion of the erythroid compartment during times of increased requirement for RBCs as a result of chronic hemolysis or blood loss.

Recent studies have begun to elucidate the molecular basis for the movement of erythroid cells out of the medullary cavity. Patel and Lodish[258] have demonstrated that an inducible erythroid cell line (murine erythroleukemia cells) binds specifically to the extracellular matrix protein fibronectin and that loss of adhesion to fibronectin occurs during induced differentiation of these cells. Subsequent

* For the most complete review of murine mutations affecting hematopoiesis, see Russell.[136]

studies demonstrated that binding to fibronectin involves a specific peptide in the fibronectin molecule, Arg-Gly-Asp-Ser (RGDS), and this interaction is mediated by a receptor on the surface of erythrocytes, VLA-5, a member of the integrin supergene family of receptors.[259] Loss of adhesion of differentiating erythrocytes is associated with loss of this receptor at the reticulocyte stage of development.[259] It is interesting that the efficiency of enucleation of murine erythroleukemia cells in response to inducers of differentiation is improved dramatically by differentiation on a fibronectin matrix.[260]

Similar molecular studies have not yet elucidated the mechanisms responsible for the release of myeloid cells from the medullary cavity. It is clear that the medullary compartment consists of both a mitotic pool (myeloblasts, promyelocytes, myelocytes) and a storage pool of granulocyte precursors (metamyelocytes and band forms) and granulocytes. Stress and pharmacologic administration of steroids produce a large mobilization of granulocytes into the peripheral blood. The storage pool in the medullary cavity is significantly larger than the peripheral blood pool of granulocytes (estimated at 500,000 and 10,000/μL, respectively, except in newborn infants, in whom marrow reserves of these cells appear to be limited).[261,262]

Tritiated thymidine studies have demonstrated that the maturation time for cells of the neutrophil series is about 8 days. These studies are in good agreement with the response of patients with neutropenia to administration of the late-acting cytokine G-CSF, as well as the recovery of neutrophil counts after administration of cytotoxic chemotherapy.[263–265] The peripheral blood pool of granulocytes is made up of both circulating and marginated compartments of cells with a distribution of about half in each compartment.[266,267] Administration of epinephrine and stress-related endogenous release of cortisol induce rapid demargination of neutrophils with subsequent doubling of the peripheral leukocyte counts within 30 minutes.[266]

Studies have demonstrated at least some of the basic mechanisms involved in the egress of leukocytes from the bloodstream into sites of inflammation. Neutrophils are present in the bloodstream for a relatively short time, probably less than 12 hours. Neutrophils interact with the endothelial wall of blood vessels by means of a group of related leukocyte membrane proteins that belong to the integrin family of heterodimeric receptors. The members of this family include LFA-1(CD11a), Mo1 (also known as Mac-1)(CD11b), and p150,95(CD11c). Persons with congenital absence of these receptors (CD11/CD18 leukocyte glycoprotein deficiency) suffer from recurrent infections because of the inability of neutrophils to egress from the bloodstream into sites of inflammation (among other abnormalities).[268] All three receptors share a common β-subunit (CD18),[269] and the molecular defect in at least some affected kindreds has been described by several investigators to be the lack of expression of this β-subunit with secondary instability of each of the α-subunits.[270–273]

Similar interactions appear to control the movement of lymphocytes between the bloodstream and specific effector organs such as peripheral lymph nodes and Peyer's patches of the gut.[274] Lymphocyte interactions appear to include not only the integrin family of receptors but also receptors related to the immunoglobulin supergene family and lectin interactions.[274]

Although not as well studied, the homing of hematopoietic stem cells to the microenvironment is now partially characterized.[275] Aizawa and Tavassoli[276,277] have shown that adhesion of hematopoietic stem cells to stromal cells of long-term marrow cultures in vitro and homing of stem cells to the spleen in vivo can be blocked by synthetic proteins containing mannosyl and galactosyl (but not fucosyl) lectins. The native proteins and receptors responsible for this interaction are unknown. Williams and coworkers[278] and Verfaillie and colleagues[279] have shown that hematopoietic stem and progenitor cells interact with the C-terminal heparin-binding domain of fibronectin. This interaction appears to involve the VLA-4 integrin receptor and the CS-1 amino acid sequence in fibronectin. Therefore, stem cells are likely to interact through multiple ligands and receptors with the microenvironment, a situation similar to the homing of lymphocytes to specific environments that specialize in immune function.

Several studies have provided insights into the egress of blood cells from the medullary cavity at the descriptive level. To gain entry into the venous sinus, hematopoietic cells must pass through or between the endothelial cells lining the vascular channel. Electron microscopic evidence supports the former mechanism for most cells, although it appears that the point at which hematopoietic cells move through the endothelial cell is frequently near endothelial cell junctions.[167,280]

Pores can be observed in the endothelial lining of the venous sinus, but it is not clear whether these are permanent features of the surface or whether they are present in response to specific signals from departing cells. In addition, areas of marked attenuation of the endothelial cell thickness have also been observed in scanning electron micrographs.[280] Apparently, cells departing the hematopoietic cord must deform to a considerable degree to gain entry into the venous sinus. These observations, along with physical measurements of cell deformability, have led to the theory that increasing deformability associated with differentiation in both the erythroid and myeloid lineages is an important component of the normal physiology of hematopoietic cell egress from the medullary cavity space.[165,281–283]

Two other mechanisms may contribute to the movement of cells from the medullary cavity into the circulation. One group has shown that a factor or factors in neutropenic serum can stimulate the release of neutrophils from the bone marrow.[284,285] This increase in neutrophil release is not endotoxin related and not a reflection of demargination, and the factor appears distinct from molecules that have a proliferative effect on myeloid precursors. Some evidence suggests that attenuation of the adventitial cover over the sinuses is reduced after endotoxin administration, which may allow more rapid egress of hematopoietic cells.[286] Distinct factors may be involved in the release of each cell type from the marrow cavity, but few data are available. Some evidence suggests that EPO may act as a releasing factor for reticulocytes.[287] Finally, the presence of changes in the blood flow to the medullary cavity has been theorized to play a role in blood cell release, but little experimental evidence has been published in support of this theory.[165]

HEMATOPOIETIC GROWTH FACTORS*

The proliferation, differentiation, and survival of immature hematopoietic progenitor cells is sustained by a family of glycoproteins, the hematopoietic growth factors (Table 8-1). In addition to their effect on immature cells, these factors also influence the survival and function of mature cells.

The nomenclature of the hematopoietic growth factors may appear confusing and unsatisfactory to the uninitiated, but remember that the original names were operationally derived, and therefore the current labels are easier to abide.

* Reviewed in Metcalf,[288,306] Sieff,[298] Clark and Kamen,[4] and Nicola.[299]

TABLE 8-1. Human Hematopoietic Growth Factors

				Protein (kd)		Biologic Activities	
Factor	Synonym	Chromosome	RNA (kb)	Core	Glycosylated	Progenitors	Mature Cells
IL-3	Multi-CSF	5q23-31	1.0	15.4	15–30	All CFC	Eosinophil, basophil
GM-CSF	CSF α	5q23-31	0.8	14.4	14–34	All CFC	Neutrophil, monocyte, eosinophil
G-CSF	CSF β	17q 11.2-21	1.6	18.6	20	CFU-G	Neutrophil
M-CSF	CSF-1	1p13-21	4.0	26	70–90 (35–45 dimer)	CFU-M	Monocyte
			1.6	16	40–50 (20–25 dimer)		
EPO	—	7q11-22	1.6	18.4	34–39	BFU-E CFU-E	
IL-5	EDF BCGF-II TRF	5q31	13.2	15.0	46	CFU-Eo	
IL-6	BSF-2, IFN α_2 26-kd protein	7p15	1.3	20.8	26	Synergistic with IL-3 or SF on blast CFC	
IL-1α (pl5)	—	2q13		31.0	17	Induces HGF production	
IL-1β (pl7)	—	2q13-21	1.6	31.0	17		
IL-4	BSF-1	5q23.2-31.2		15	15–19	Synergistic with EPO, G-CSF, M-CSF on progenitors	
IL-8	—	—	—				Neutrophil chemotaxis
IL-9	—	—	—	16	20–30	BFU-E	
IL-10	Mouse cytokine synthesis inhibitory factor	—	—	—	17–21	—	Inhibits synthesis of IFN-γ
IL-11	—	—	—	20	—	Synergistic with IL-3 or SF on blast CFC	
IL-12	—	—	—	—	75 (40 + 35 dimer)	Supports stem cells (with SF and IL-3)	Induces IFN-γ
IL-13	—	5q23-31	—	—	12	—	Increases monocyte and B-cell CD23 and class II antigen expression; increases Ig synthesis
SF	Mast cell growth factor; stem cell factor	12	5.4–6.5 3.5	20	—	Synergistic with IL-3, GM-CSF, G-CSF, EPO on blast CFC and progenitors	

CFC, colony-forming cell; CFU, colony-forming unit; CFU-G, granulocyte CFU; CFU-M, monocyte/macrophage CFU; BFU-E, erythroid burst-forming unit; CFU-E, erythroid CFU; CFU-Eo, eosinophil CFU; IL, interleukin; GM-CSF, granulocyte–macrophage colony-stimulating factor; G-CSF, granulocyte CSF; M-CSF, monocyte CSF; EPO, erythropoietin; SF, Steel factor; HGF, hematopoietic growth factor; IFN-γ; interferon-γ.

The first factors to be described derived their names as CSFs from the in vitro observation that they stimulate progenitor cells to form colonies of recognizable maturing cells; prefixes are used to denote the cell type in the mature colonies, such as G-CSF for granulocyte CSF.

Another large group of factors, the interleukins, derived their names initially from their cellular sources as well as actions on leukocytes. Recent additions to the family have been given a sequential interleukin numeric notation.

During the past 5 years, the genes for several murine and human hematopoietic growth factors have been cloned. This in turn led to the production and purification of the respective recombinant proteins. The advance afforded by molecular methods has allowed intensive investigations of the actions of purified CSFs, their cellular origins, and their regulatory mechanisms, whereas the availability of large quantities of highly purified CSFs such as granulocyte–macrophage CSF (GM-CSF), G-CSF, macrophage CSF (M-CSF), and EPO, has led to preclinical and clinical evaluation of their effectiveness in vivo.

Types of Hematopoietic Growth Factors

The development of semisolid colony-forming assays for progenitor cells of all the hematopoietic lineages provided the means to distinguish several colony-stimulating activities that were present both in media conditioned by different murine and human cell types and in human urine. Separative protein chemistry applied to large volumes of starting material led to the purification of murine M-CSF, GM-CSF, G-CSF, and IL-3.[288] Human urine yielded M-CSF[289] and EPO[290] and a human bladder carcinoma cell line was used to purify human G-CSF.[291]

In general, IL-3 and GM-CSF stimulate the survival, proliferation, and differentiation of a broad range of progenitors, including cells with stem cell properties. Stem cells may also be stimulated by three other interleukins, IL-1, IL-4, and IL-6, but the actions of these factors may be indirect or may require the presence of other cytokines. In contrast, G-CSF, M-CSF, IL-5, and EPO are lineage-restricted and stimulate the proliferation and differentiation of more mature granulocyte, monocyte, eosinophil, and erythroid progenitor cells, respectively. Both sets of factors influence mature cell function, and the pattern of responsive cells for each CSF broadly coincides with the lineages of the less mature cells affected by each factor.

Recent data indicate that several CSFs may have roles outside the hematopoietic system. GM-CSF and G-CSF influence the migration and proliferation of endothelial cells.[292] High-affinity binding sites for both CSFs are present on these cells. M-CSF acts on trophoblasts and production of M-CSF by uterine cells increases markedly during gestation.[293,294] Placental cells express c-*fms*, (the M-CSF receptor)[295] and low-affinity GM-CSF receptors.[296] Finally, murine neurons and astrocytes express IL-3 mRNA by Northern and in situ hybridization analysis.[297]

Several recent reviews have detailed the steps in the isolation of the hematopoietic growth factor genes.[4,5,298,299] Some general comments follow, together with a brief summary. Two approaches were taken to identify complementary DNAs (cDNAs) for these genes. The first was the classic route by which, for example, the human G-CSF, M-CSF, and EPO proteins were purified, part of their amino acid sequence determined, and oligonucleotide probes constructed to screen appropriate cDNA libraries.[300–303] The CSFs are present in minute concentrations in most starting materials, and for several CSFs, purification has been very difficult. The second approach obviated the obstacle of CSF purification in a novel manner: GM-CSF and IL-3 cDNA libraries were constructed from suitable human cell lines; pools of cDNAs from the library were then introduced into "high expression" vectors and directly expressed in mammalian cell lines after transfection. Because of the potency of these CSFs, the gene products of the cDNA pools could be screened in sensitive bioassays, and the single cDNA isolated by sib selection.[304,305]

Hematopoietic Growth Factor Receptors

Membrane receptors for all five murine hematopoietic growth factors have been characterized using iodinated, purified, natural or recombinant preparations.[299,306] Consistent with the lack of structural homology among the growth factors is the existence of distinct receptors for each factor, which range in size from 50 to 160 kd. Distribution of receptors within the hematopoietic system is restricted

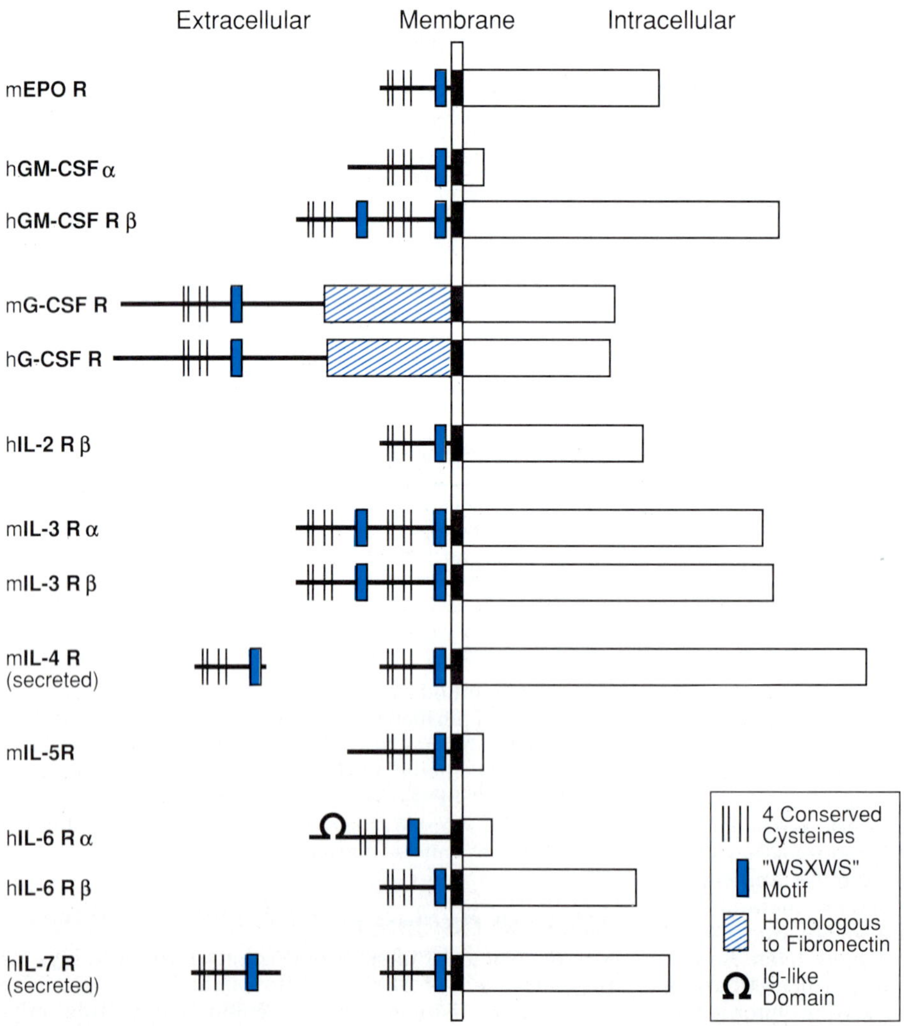

FIGURE 8-7. The hematopoietic growth factor receptor family. Diagram of murine and human hematopoietic growth factor receptors whose genes have been cloned. The extracellular domains are all characterized by one or two regions that contain four conserved cysteines and a tryptophan-serine-x-tryptophan-serine- (WSXWS) motif. Unique features: the IL-6 receptor contains an immunoglobulin-like domain; the G-CSF receptor contains three fibronectin type III–like region repeats (*cross-hatched areas*). The intracellular domains show less homology. Serine and proline residues are enriched in the cytoplasmic domains of several members, such as the IL-2, IL-3, IL-4, IL-7, and erythropoietin receptors.

to undifferentiated and maturing cells of the appropriate target cell lineages. Since progenitor cells respond to more than one factor, overlap in receptor expression occurs. The number of IL-3, GM-CSF, G-CSF, and EPO receptors per cell is strikingly low (1000 sites per cell), whereas M-CSF receptors are present at 10,000 sites per monocyte.

In all cases, affinity of a receptor for its ligand is high, with dissociation constants usually in the picomolar range. Stimulation of target cells can occur at concentrations of factor orders of magnitude lower than the equilibrium constant at which 50% of receptors are occupied; therefore, low receptor occupancy is apparently sufficient to produce biologic effects. Although the four murine CSFs do not cross-compete for binding at 0°, at 21° or 37°C, IL-3 inhibits binding of GM-CSF, G-CSF, and M-CSF to murine bone marrow cells, and GM-CSF inhibits binding of G-CSF and M-CSF.[307] Metcalf and colleagues have suggested that this hierarchical down-modulation results in activation of the modulated receptor without binding ligand, and the model provides an intriguing explanation for the correlation between the pattern of down-regulation and the biologic activity of IL-3 and GM-CSF.

Expression cloning strategies were successfully applied recently to isolate the cDNAs that encode the human or murine IL-1, IL-6, EPO, GM-CSF, IL-3, IL-4, IL-7, and G-CSF receptors have recently been isolated using expression cloning strategies.[296,308–317] Although the IL-1 receptor has three extracellular immunoglobulin-like domains and appears to be a member of the immunoglobulin superfamily, the IL-6, EPO, GM-CSF, IL-3, IL-4, IL-7, and G-CSF receptors are distinct (Fig. 8-7). They show features that are analogous to the (p70 to p75) β chain of the IL-2 receptor[318] and to the prolactin and growth hormone receptors.[319–321] These polypeptides share a number of features as a group and show no apparent homology to other known receptors, but they are all type 1 membrane glycoproteins with extracellular N termini and single transmembrane domains. They contrast with c-*kit* and c-*fms*, which are class III receptor tyrosine kinases (Fig. 8-8).

The major homology lies in the extracellular domain, which is characterized by four conserved cysteine residues in the N-terminal region and a Trp-Ser-X-Trp-Ser (WSXWS, where X is any amino acid) motif just external to the plasma membrane. The IL-6 receptor has both these structural features, but it differs from the other members in that it has one N-terminal immunoglobulin-like domain, and the WSXWS motif is located slightly more proximal.[309] The cytoplasmic regions of the receptor family show much less homology, although there are similarities between the IL-2 β chain and the EPO receptor. The length of the cytoplasmic domains varies from 54 amino acids (GM-CSF receptor) to 568 amino acids (IL-4 receptor). Furthermore, the IL-2, IL-3, IL-4, IL-7, EPO, and a recently isolated isoform of the GM-CSF receptor[324] are rich in serines and prolines. The mechanism by which ligand binding induces a cell signal remains to be determined, but it is interesting that mutational analysis of the IL-2 β chain suggests that the serine-rich region in the cytoplasmic tail is important for signal transduction.

An interesting feature of the cytokine receptor family is that the conserved extracellular structural features are mirrored in conserved structural features of their ligands as well. For example, G-CSF[325] and IL-6 are characterized by four α-helices that fold in a tertiary structure of antiparallel cylinders connected by interhelical loops (Fig. 8-9). This common tertiary structure is based on the radiographic structure of IL-2[326] and of growth hormone–growth hormone receptor complex.[327] Mutational studies of growth hormone receptors suggest that the exposed surface of helix D[328] forms the receptor binding site. The cytokine receptors

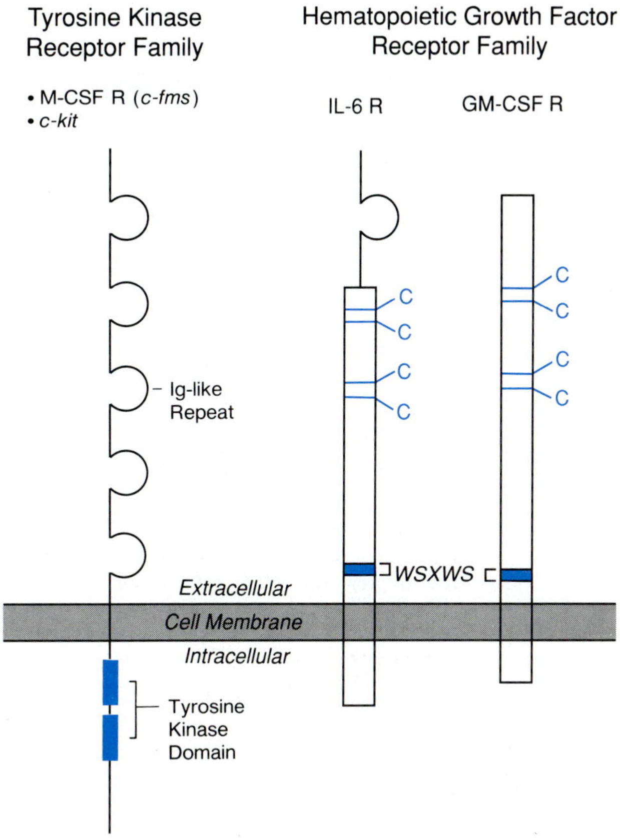

FIGURE 8-8. Hematopoietic growth factor receptors. Two other important hematopoietic growth factor receptors, c-*kit* and the M-CSF receptor c-*fms*, are structurally distinct from the receptor family shown in Figure 8-7, represented here by the GM-CSF and IL-6 receptors. M-CSF (c-*fms*) and c-*kit* are type III tyrosine kinase cell surface receptors; their extracellular domains are characterized by five immunoglobulin-like repeats, whereas the cyptoplasmic regions contain a tyrosine–kinase domain separated by an insert.

in turn share conserved motifs that provide spatial constraints for tertiary folding.[329] The data are consistent with a model in which two clusters of antiparallel β-strands are separated by a V-shaped trough that is formed by a hydrophobic hinge region (the WSXWS loop; Fig. 8-10). This trough may constitute the binding region.

Gene Localization of the Hematopoietic Growth Factors and Their Receptors

The genes for GM-CSF, IL-3, IL-4, IL-5, and the M-CSF receptor c-*fms* have been mapped to the long arm of chromosome 5[330–333] (Fig. 8-11; see also Table 8-1). Both endothelial cell growth factor and the receptor for PDGF have also been mapped to this region. G-CSF and EPO have been mapped to chromosomes 17 and 7, respectively,[334–336] and M-CSF has recently been reassigned to chromosome 1. A proportion of patients with either refractory anemia or acute myeloblastic leukemia have an interstitial deletion of the long arm of chromosome 5 (5q−); these cases appear always to show a critical deletion of bands 5q21 to 32. IL-3 and GM-CSF are deleted in every case, whereas c-*fms* is usually deleted as well. How this deletion bears on the pathogenesis of the myeloproliferative disorder in these patients is unknown. Abnormal function of one of the hematopoietic growth factors or growth factor receptors is one possibility; loss of one allele of an as yet unidentified suppressor gene is also possible.

Several hematopoietic growth factors have recently been

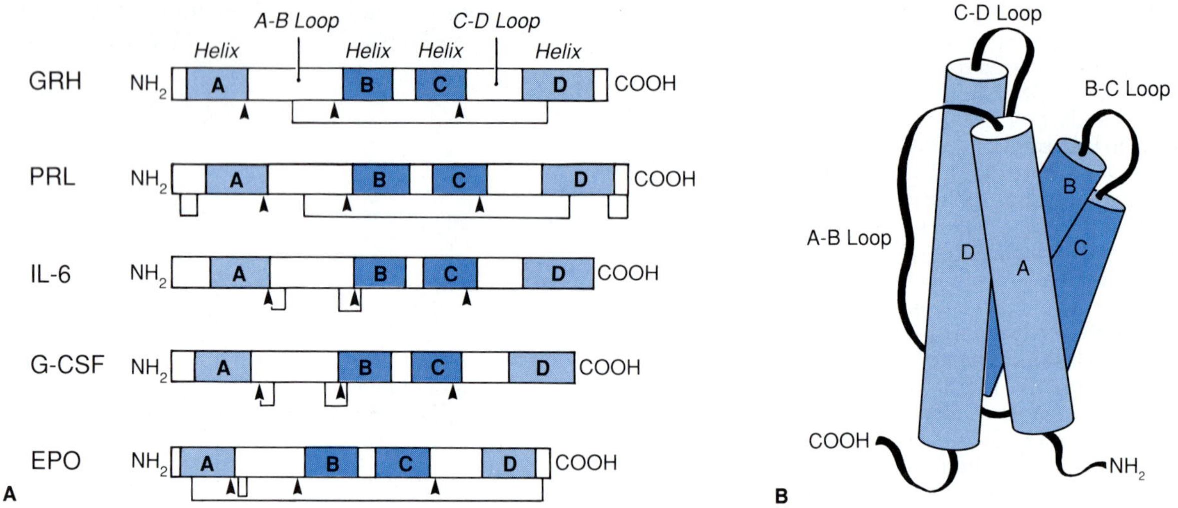

FIGURE 8-9. Secondary and tertiary structure prediction for a group of GRH-like cytokines. (**A**) Location of secondary structural elements in the human sequences for gonadotropin-releasing hormone (GRH), prolactin (PRL), erythropoietin (EPO), IL-6, and G-CSF. The four helices from the GRH x-ray structure[322] are labeled A to D; loops between helices are appropriately named. Known disulfide bridge connections are marked. Gene exon boundaries have been mapped onto the respective protein sequences by arrowheads. An IL-6 variant lacking the amino-terminal 28 residues is bioactive.[323] This deletion would effectively shorten IL-6 helix A but would not affect the overall fold or predicted recognition helix D. (**B**) Drawing of the GRH fold,[322] emphasizing the helix bundle core and loop connectivity. The exposed surface of helix D is thought to play an important role in receptor binding. (Adapted from Bazan JF. Haemopoietic receptors and helical cytokines. Immunol Today 1990;11:350)

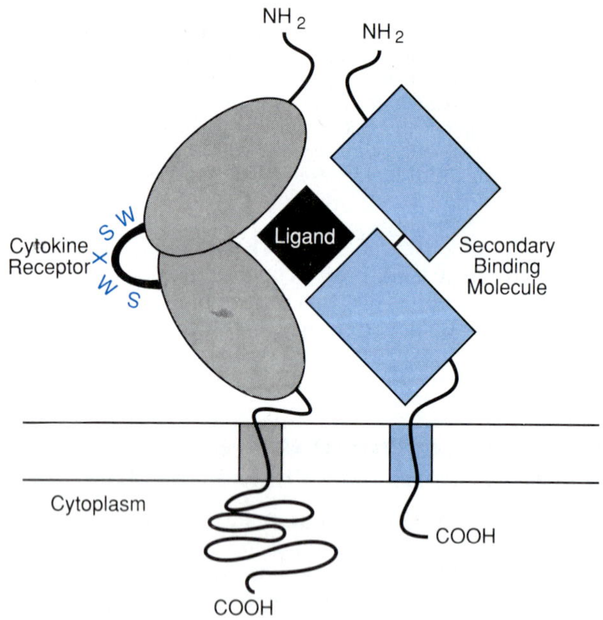

FIGURE 8-10. The tertiary folding of β strands in receptor domains. Predicted configuration of a canonical receptor binding segment on the cell surface. The linked domains pack with barrel axes at an angle so as to create a V-shaped trough lined by β-sheet surfaces; these converge on a hydrophobic hinge region with a proximal WSXWS loop. Linked to a transmembrane helix and a nonspecific cytoplasmic tail, the receptor is shown docked to a cytokine ligand (*black diamond*). In addition, the receptor–cytokine complex interacts with a secondary binding molecule that recognizes the free surface of bound cytokine as well as selected receptor loops distal from the pocket. In this case, the bilobed accessory molecule is analogous to the IL-2 receptor 55-kd chain or the common β chain of the GM-CSF and IL-3 receptors. (Adapted from Bazan JF. Structural design and molecular evolution of a cytokine receptor superfamily. Proc Natl Acad Sci USA 1990;87:6934)

mapped. The EPO receptor gene maps to chromosome 19pter-q12.[337] The GM-CSF receptor α-chain gene maps to the pseudoautosomal region of the X and Y chromosomes,[339] and the IL-5 receptor α gene maps to chromosome 3p24-26.[339] The β common gene maps to chromosome 22q12-2-q13.1.[340]

SPECIFIC GROWTH FACTORS

Interleukin-3

Biochemical Characterization and Molecular Biology

Media conditioned by the murine WEHI-3B myelomonocytic cell line or by activated T lymphocytes contain multiple biologic activities that include mast cell growth factor activity, multipotential colony-stimulating activity, burst-promoting activity, 20α steroid dehydrogenase-inducing activity, and *Thy*-1 antigen-inducing activity. Biochemical purification of a 28-kd glycoprotein from WEHI 3B–conditioned medium[341] or from activated T lymphocytes[342] showed that these activities were all properties of this single protein, named *IL-3*. cDNA clones[343,344] encode a 15.5-kd secreted protein (140 amino acids) after cleavage of the signal peptide. However, native murine IL-3 is considerably larger, a monomer of 23 to 32 kd, as a result of glycosylation.

Four N-glycosylation sites are predicted from the sequence, and variable glycosylation probably accounts for this broad range of molecular weights. Thus, about 30% to 50% of the molecular weight is carbohydrate. However, the carbohydrate is unnecessary for the in vitro or in vivo actions of the protein, since bacterially synthesized IL-3 is fully active.

The cDNA clone for primate IL-3 was isolated by expression screening of a library made from a gibbon T-lymphoblast cell line.[305] This cDNA clone was used to obtain the human gene, and analysis of the gibbon and human recombinant proteins show that they differ in only 11 amino acid positions. The human IL-3 gene encodes a 152–

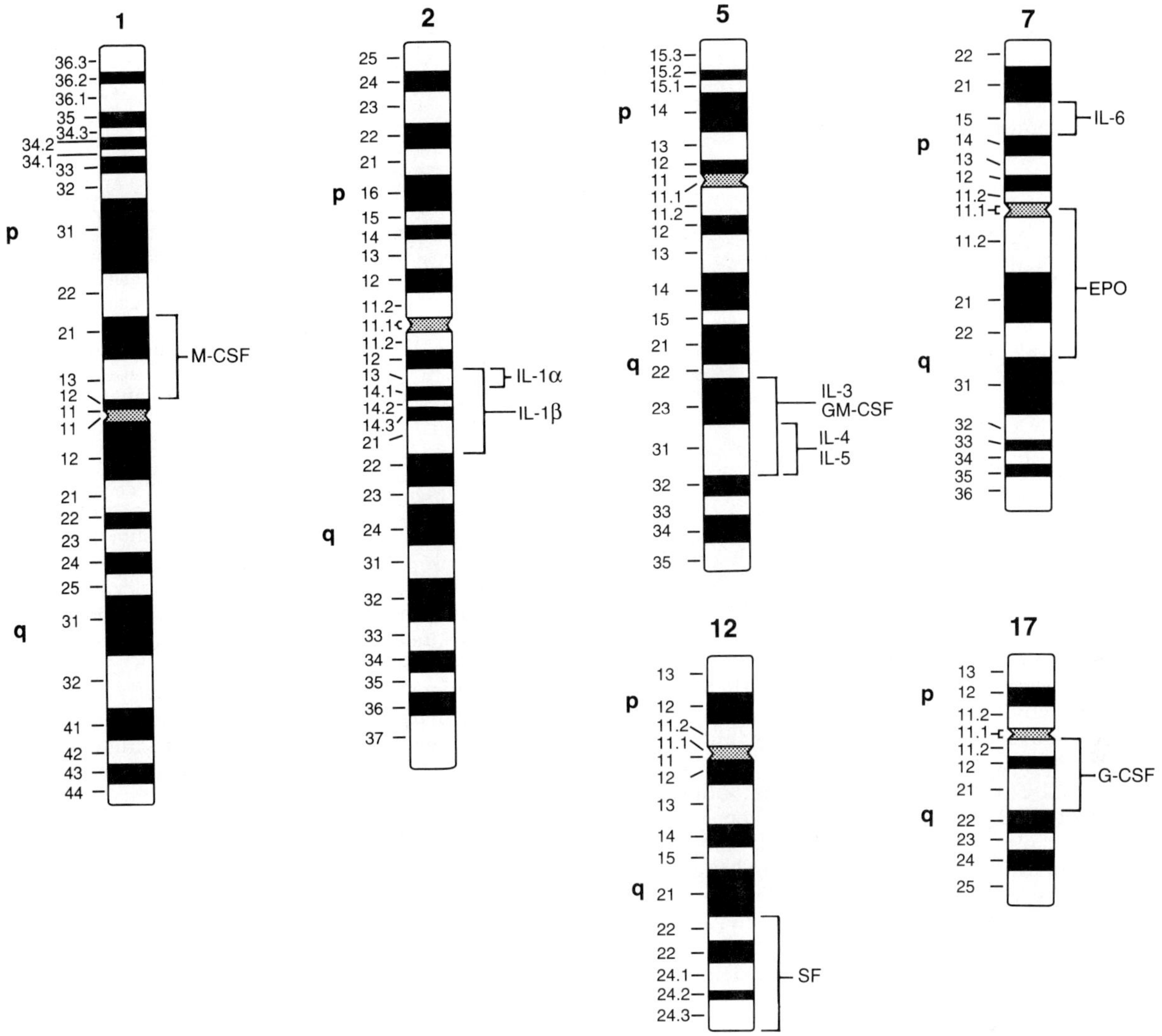

FIGURE 8-11. Chromosome locations of hematopoietic growth factor genes. Schematic representation of the chromosomes on which the hematopoietic growth factor genes have been mapped. In situ hybridization and hybrid analysis were used in most cases to localize the genes to a particular banded region of each chromosome.

amino acid precursor that is N-terminally modified to yield a 133–amino acid mature protein that has one internal disulfide bridge. The human and murine genes have similar structures (5 exons) and show nucleotide homology that is greater in the 5′ and 3′ noncoding regions (59%) than in the coding regions (49%); the proteins are 29% homologous. Biologic activity is not maintained by the human protein on murine cells.

IL-3 and GM-CSF Are Coordinately Regulated in Lymphocytes

Little is known about the levels of production of any of the CSFs or interleukins under steady-state conditions. Levels in normal mice are very low or undetectable, and it has been difficult to detect CSFs in long-term bone marrow cultures. Part of the difficulty may lie in the fact that the hematopoietic growth factors act at picomolar concentrations and thus may function under steady-state conditions at very low concentrations. Another possibility is that GM-CSF and IL-3 may be sequestered by glycosaminoglycans and heparan sulfate in the extracellular matrix.[199]

Injection of bacterial endotoxin into mice results in a rapid but small rise of GM-CSF in the serum.[288] This contrasts with the inability to detect an increase in IL-3 and a marked rise in G-CSF, M-CSF, IL-5, and IL-6. All murine tissues contain extractable growth factors,[288] suggesting that synthesis of the CSFs may occur in cells common to all organs such as fibroblasts, endothelial cells, lymphocytes, and macrophages. Many human organs are capable of synthesizing CSFs, and bioactivity assays on medium conditioned by purified cell populations have documented CSF production by T lymphocytes,[345–347] monocytes,[348–351] endothelial cells,[352,353] and fibroblasts (Fig. 8-12).

Identification of the specific factors produced by these cells has come from mRNA analysis of different purified cell populations, cell lines, or tumors. Phytohemagglutinin-stimulated blood mononuclear cells (made up of monocytes and lymphocytes) contain both GM-CSF and IL-3 mRNAs. Furthermore, phorbol ester–stimulated T-cell clones and T-cell/natural killer (NK) cell fractions isolated from mononuclear cell preparations are the only hematopoietic cell sources that are IL-3 mRNA–positive.[354] In situ hybridization studies of purified lymphocytic subsets indicate that CD4, CD8, and NK fractions are positive for GM-CSF and IL-3 mRNA.[355] Only a small subset of T lymphocytes become GM-CSF– or IL-3–positive after stimulation with phorbol ester and a calcium ionophore ionomycin (10%

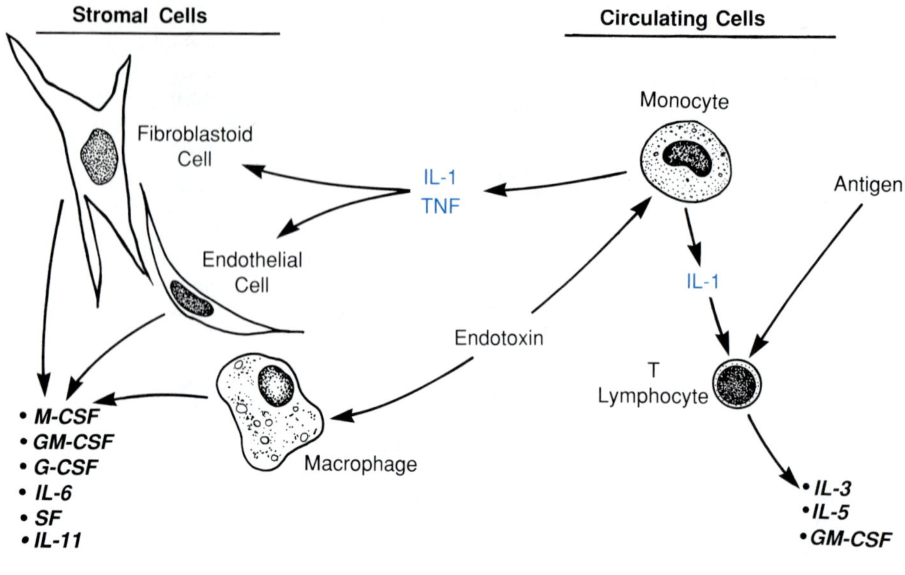

FIGURE 8-12. Major cytokine sources. Cells of the bone marrow microenvironment such as macrophages, endothelial cells, and reticular fibroblastoid cells produce M-CSF, GM-CSF, G-CSF, IL-6, IL-11, and probably Steel factor (SF) after induction with endotoxin or IL-1 or TNF. The cellular sources of SF have not yet been precisely determined, but SF is produced by fibroblasts. T cells produce IL-3, GM-CSF, and IL-5 in response to antigenic and IL-1 stimulation.

and 1%, respectively).[355] This fraction can be increased about five-fold by preincubation with IL-2.

A number of conserved elements in the promoter region of the CSF genes may bind nuclear factors that regulate transcriptional activity. The IL-3 promoter contains several *cis*-acting sequences that play both positive and negative roles in transcription.[356] Although the CK-1 and CK-2 elements of the GM-CSF promoter (see text that follows) are conserved in the IL-3 promoter, they do not appear to play a role in transcription. Two adjacent motifs that are homologous to the cAMP-response element and the "OCT-1" element (in the IL-2 promoter) are important for positive regulation in transient transfection assays in the gibbon T-cell line, MLA-144, as is a more distal AP-1 site. A transcriptional repressor lies between these two elements.[356]

IL-3 Receptors

Murine IL-3 binds to both low- and high-affinity receptors.[357] High-affinity receptors for IL-3 are present on human eosinophils, monocytes, and some cell lines.[358] Cross-linking with human ^{125}I–IL-3 shows at least two bands of net molecular weight 135 and 70 kd,[359] whereas similar murine studies show complexes of 140, 120, and 60 to 70 kd. A murine cDNA clone that encodes an IL-3–binding protein (AIC2A) was recently isolated from an IL-3–dependent mast cell line, MC/9.[311] The mature AIC2A protein has 856 amino acids, with an external domain of 417 amino acids, a transmembrane region of 26 amino acids, and a cytoplasmic domain of 413 amino acids that lacks a tyrosine kinase consensus sequence.

Cross-linking studies with transfected L cells show complexes of 160, 140, and 90 kd, in agreement with the bands seen in the parental MC/9 cell line. Transfected L cells bind IL-3 with low affinity (18 nM) and do not internalize IL-3 in response to ligand binding. The IL-3 receptor belongs to the new family of hematopoietic growth factor receptors but, unlike the other members, has a duplication of the conserved extracellular cysteines and the WSXWS motif. A second cDNA (AIC2B) that encodes an 896 amino acid protein was also isolated from MC/9 cells.[360] It has 91% amino acid homology with AIC2A, but Southern analysis indicates that the proteins are encoded by two genes. After transfection into fibroblasts, AIC2B was expressed at the cell surface as determined by antibody binding, but it did not bind IL-3. Coexpression of both proteins does not alter the affinity of IL-3 binding. The roles of these polypeptides in murine hematopoiesis have been clarified. AIC2A was used to isolate a cDNA (IL-3α) that binds murine IL-3 with low affinity but when coexpressed with either AIC2A or AIC2B confers high-affinity IL-3 binding.[361] AIC2B also acts as a *common β polypeptide* for the murine GM-CSF receptor α and IL-5 receptor α chains and confers high-affinity binding of GM-CSF and IL-5 when coexpressed with those α chains, respectively.[361,362] A human polypeptide whose cDNA was isolated through its homology to these IL-3 receptors plays an important role in high-affinity GM-CSF binding when coexpressed with human GM-CSF receptor α (see section on GM-CSF). This β common cDNA was used to isolate a human cDNA that encodes a low-affinity, IL-3–binding polypeptide (IL-3 receptor α). When β common and IL-3 receptor α are coexpressed, high-affinity IL-3 binding is observed. While serving as the high-affinity converter for the IL-5 receptor α,[363,364] β common but does not itself bind GM-CSF, IL-3, or IL-5.

IL-3 Signal Transduction

Little is known about the precise cascade of intracellular events initiated by the binding of growth factors to their cell surface receptors. IL-3 induces rapid and transient phosphorylation of a variety of cellular substrates in factor-dependent cell lines. These include proteins of 160, 140, 95, 90, 70, 55, and 38 kd in a variety of cell lines.[365–368] The 140-, 90-, 70-, 55-, and 38-kd proteins are phosphorylated on tyrosine. The identity of some of these proteins has been determined. One candidate is phosphatidyl inositol (PI) kinase.[369] Another candidate is c-*raf*, a serine/threonine kinase that is phosphorylated in response to IL-3 in some murine cell lines.[370]

It has recently been shown that the β common component of the IL-3/GM-CSF receptor is tyrosine phosphorylated after IL-3 or GM-CSF stimulation.[371,372] Other proteins that are tyrosine phosphorylated and may be components of a signaling pathway include van,[373] c-*fes*,[374] and mitogen-activated protein kinase (MAPK).[375,376] The tyrosine kinase responsible for ligand-induced receptor phosphorylation could be lyn,[377,378] fyn,[378] of c-*fes*. Evidence has also strongly implicated Jak2 in IL-3 signaling.[379] There are three known members of the Jak kinase family—Jak1, Jak2, and Tyk2. All are 130- to 134-kd, structurally related proteins that share the unusal feature of having two kinase domains. They are particularly well studied in relation to interferon action.[380] Jak1 and Tyk2 are required for interferon α (INF-

α) signaling.[381] It is thought that one or both of these kinases are activated after IFN-α binding and that they phosphorylate cytoplasmic proteins of 113, 91, and 84 kd. The latter two are splice variants of the same gene, whereas p113, although derived from a separate gene, is structurally related to p91 and p84. The three phosphorylated proteins migrate into the nucleus and assemble into a complex—the interferon-stimulated gene factor 3α (ISGF3α) complex—with the forth component, a 48-kd, sequence-specific DNA-binding protein. As a consequence, the affinity of p48 for the IFN-α response elements in IFN-α–induced genes is significantly enhanced, resulting in increased gene expression.[382,383] Signal transduction by interferon-γ (IFN-γ) occurs by a similar mechanism. The 91-kd component of ISGF3α is tyrosine phosphorylated after IFN-γ binds to the IFN-γ receptor, and this event is associated with tyrosine phosphorylation of Jak1 and Jak2.[384] The 91-kd protein then translocates to the nucleus and binds to the IFN-γ response element, thereby transcriptionally activating genes that contain this sequence in their promoters. Although IL-3 has not yet been shown to activate a transcription factor, it has been shown that ligand-induced activation of gp130—the signal-transducing component of the IL-6, LIF, IL-11, oncostatin M, and ciliary neurotropic factor family of hematopoietic growth factor receptors (see discussion that follows)—leads to tyrosine phosphorylation of the Jak-Tyk family and activation of DNA binding of acute-phase response factor, an 89-kd phosphoprotein antigenically related to the 91-kd protein of ISGF3α.[385,386]

Evidence that tyrosine phosphorylation is important for cell proliferation comes from the observation that the introduction of the EGF receptor, a known tyrosine kinase, into an IL-3–dependent cell line can convert it to EGF dependence.[387] Oncogenes such as v-*fms* or v-*src* that encode tyrosine kinases can convert factor-dependent cell lines to factor independence.[388–390]

Ras is a 21-kd, membrane-associated protein that cycles between active GTP-bound and inactive GDP-bound forms in response to extracellular signals from various growth factor receptors, including IL-3 and GM-CSF.[391,392] Excitement has greeted the observation that vav has Ras GDP/GTP nucleotide exchange activity[393] analogous to the *Drosophila* and murine SOS proteins,[394,395] and that Ras GTP can associate with Raf-1 and MAPK kinase.[396] Thus, a possible IL-3/GM-CSF–mediated signaling cascade involves phosphorylation of the β common subunit as well as tyrosine kinases such as vav, with subsequent increased Ras GTP and activation of Raf-1, MAKPK kinase, and MAPK, followed by induction of c-*fos*. Other protooncogenes induced by IL-3 and GM-CSF are c-*myc*[397,398] and *pim*-1,[399,400] although the pathways by which this occurs have not been established.

Some growth factors and receptors can activate phosphatidyl inositol-specific phospholipase C with subsequent diacylglycerol-mediated protein kinase C (PKC) activation and increased inositol triphosphate–mediated intracellular calcium. Activation of PKC has been reported in response to IL-3 in factor-dependent cell lines and in macrophages, whereas other studies have failed to document enhanced enzyme activity.[401–403]

GM-CSF

Biochemical Characterization and Molecular Biology

Complementary cDNA clones for murine GM-CSF were isolated after amino acid sequence was obtained from partial purification of the murine protein.[404] Clones containing cDNAs for human GM-CSF were isolated by constructing a cDNA library from the M-07 leukemia cell line in an expression vector and by directly screening transfected monkey COS cells for transient expression of GM-CSF.[304] The human DNA sequence contains a single open reading frame encoding a 144–amino acid precursor protein. In an analogous fashion to other secreted proteins, 17 amino acids are cleaved from the N-terminal sequence to yield a mature protein of 127 amino acids. Murine and human GM-CSF are only 56% homologous, and the proteins do not cross-react. Purification of both natural and recombinant human GM-CSF (rhGM-CSF) to homogeneity yields identical proteins, which are heterogeneous when analyzed by sodium dodecyl sulfate–polyacrylamide gel electrophoresis (SDS-PAGE), migrating with an apparent molecular mass of 14 to 35 kd.[304] This is due to variable glycosylation; the sequence contains two potential N-linked (asparagine) glycosylation sites, and 0, 1, or 2 asparagines may be occupied by oligosaccharides.[405]

The degree of occupancy appears to affect function. The most heavily glycosylated form of the molecule is not as active in vitro but is cleared much more slowly in vivo from the circulation than the nonglycosylated form. This may have important implications in the choice of bacteria (nonglycosylated) or mammalian/yeast cells (glycosylated) as expression systems for producing recombinant GM-CSF for therapy. The explanation for the difference in bioactivity of the two forms may be related to affinity of the ligand for its cell surface receptor. The glycosylated form of GM-CSF has a lower affinity than the nonglycosylated molecule, and this is accounted for by differences in the kinetic association rate.[406]

The amino acid sequence of murine GM-CSF predicts two α helices close to the N terminus (positions 13 to 27 and 31 to 46). These appear to be required for biologic activity since introduction of a helix-breaking glycine residue markedly reduces the activity of the molecule.[407] The receptor-binding site of human GM-CSF has been mapped to regions between residues 38 and 48 as well as 94 to 111 by chimeric mouse–human hybrid analysis and by mapping with monoclonal antibodies.[408,409] These two regions may lie adjacent to each other in the tertiary structure of the molecule.

Although human IL-3 and GM-CSF are distinct at the gene sequence level, these molecules demonstrate a number of similarities. Like GM-CSF, IL-3 has two potential N-linked glycosylation sites, and polyacrylamide gel analysis of the recombinant protein expressed in mammalian cells shows a similar range of molecular weights (14 to 28 kd). More intriguing are the in situ hybridization and somatic cell hybrid analyses that map the IL-3 and GM-CSF genes within 10 kb of each other on the long arm of chromosome 5 (5q23-q32[410,411]; see Fig. 8-11). The 5′ noncoding regions contain similar eukaryotic promoter elements,[412–414] and the 3′ noncoding regions both contain a sequence rich in adenine–thymidine base pairs that is an important determinant of RNA instability.[415] Finally, the genes appear to be coordinately regulated in T lymphocytes. Despite these similarities, only T lymphocytes produce both CSFs; other mesenchymal cells that produce GM-CSF do not produce IL-3 (see later discussion).

Regulation of GM-CSF Production

Endothelial cells[416–418] and lung, skin, and fetal liver fibroblasts[417,419] accumulate GM-CSF mRNA after induction with IL-1 or TNF, whereas monocytes accumulate GM-CSF mRNA after stimulation with endotoxin[418] (see Fig. 8-12).

Because monocytes produce IL-1 in response to endotoxin,[420] this cell type may perform a central role in inducing increased hematopoiesis during stress, both by producing growth factors, and perhaps more important, by producing IL-1 and tumor necrosis factor (TNF). Together with antigen, IL-1 may induce circulating T lymphocytes to produce both GM-CSF and IL-3. Removal of T lymphocytes from bone marrow before allogeneic bone marrow transplantation to prevent graft-versus-host disease therefore could deplete the marrow of a cell critical for proliferation of the transplanted pluripotent stem cells. Monocyte-derived IL-1 or TNF or both may also induce bone marrow stromal cell populations to produce GM-CSF.[421] This is consistent with published evidence demonstrating the ability of "monokines" present in monocyte-conditioned medium to induce endothelial,[422,423] fibroblast,[424] and T-lymphocyte[425] production of burst-promoting and colony-stimulating activities.

The mechanism by which mesenchymal cells accumulate GM-CSF mRNA is poorly understood. Studies on lung fibroblasts suggest several different mechanisms. Messenger RNA accumulation after exposure to sodium fluoride indicates that a G protein may be involved.[426] The response to tumor promoters such as 12-O-tetradecanoylphorbol-13-acetate (TPA) suggest that PKC is also a stimulatory signal. Another potent stimulator of GM-CSF mRNA accumulation is ouabain, which blocks the Na^+-K^+-ATPase pump and results in elevation of Na^+ and Ca^{2+}. Further studies with Ca ionophores suggest that the increased Ca^{2+} is important for GM-CSF mRNA accumulation. Finally, TNF-stimulated increases of GM-CSF mRNA appear to require neither PKC nor Ca^{2+}; therefore, this potential physiologic regulator operates through an as yet undefined mechanism.

The induction of expression in fibroblasts and endothelial cells is mediated by increased mRNA stability[427] and increased transcriptional activity.[427,428] In contrast, the accumulation of GM-CSF mRNA in murine peritoneal macrophages after exposure to endotoxin is not associated with increased transcription but results from message stabilization.[429] This stabilization requires the synthesis of new protein that prevents RNA degradation, possibly by interaction with an AU-rich sequence that is present in the 3′ untranslated region of many transiently expressed genes, including GM-CSF, IL-1, IL-2, IL-3, G-CSF, α- β-, and γ-IFN, TNF, and protooncogenes such as c-*fos*, c-*myc*, c-*sis* and c-*myb*.[415] Murine macrophages also accumulate GM-CSF mRNA after other events that may occur during inflammation such as phagocytosis and adherence in the presence of fibronectin.[429]

Different elements identified in the GM-CSF promoter may play a tissue- or inducer-specific role. For example, two elements termed CK-1 and CK-2 (−96 to −75) were found to bind two distinct nuclear factors (NF-GMa and NF-GMb).[412] Although gel shift assays show that NF-GMb is induced by phorbol esters in the bladder carcinoma cell line 5637, NF-GMa is constitutively produced in these cells. In contrast, NF-GMa is inducible by TNFα in embryonic fibroblasts, and the CK-1 sequence acts as a TNF-responsive element in transient transfection experiments.[413] T-cell lines show another pattern, with binding of proteins associated with inducible expression localized to a 90-base pair region close to the mRNA cap site (−53 to +37).[414]

GM-CSF Receptors and Cross-Competition With IL-3

Low numbers of high-affinity GM-CSF receptors are expressed by mature polymorphonuclear neutrophils, by eosinophils, and by the myeloid leukemic cell lines, KG1 and HL60.[430–432] Reported affinity constants range from 15 to 1000 pmol/L. Although some investigators note only high-affinity binding sites on human monocytes,[432] other evidence shows that monocytes also express low-affinity receptors.[433] At 4°C, human GM-CSF competes partially for IL-3 binding, and vice versa.[358,434] This contrasts with the murine cross-competition, which occurs only at 37°C. Cross-linking studies with radiolabeled GM-CSF have shown either a single 85-kd receptor[432] or several bands of net 135, 100, and 80 kd.[435] Low-affinity GM-CSF receptors are present on several nonhematopoietic cell lines.[436,437] These include non–small cell carcinoma, adenocarcinoma, and squamous lung carcinoma, gastrointestinal carcinoma, osteosarcoma, and choriocarcinoma lines.

Cross-linking evidence shows that the low-affinity receptor has a net molecular weight of 80 kd[438]; this is in good agreement with expression studies with the receptor whose cDNA was recently isolated from human placenta.[296] This cDNA encodes a 400–amino acid (45-kd) precursor protein. The mature 378–amino acid polypeptide has a 297–amino acid extracellular domain that is heavily glycosylated on 11 potential N-linkage sites. A single transmembrane region (27 amino acids) is followed by a 54–amino acid cytoplasmic domain. The transfected receptor binds GM-CSF with low affinity (K_d 2 to 8 nmol/L) and binds only GM-CSF; IL-3 does not cross-compete. After introduction into the murine factor-dependent cell line FDC-P1, the receptor confers human GM-CSF dependence.[439]

Recently, a second isoform of the human GM-CSF receptor (α_2) was isolated from the factor-dependent cell line M-07.[440] This cDNA encodes a polypeptide that is identical with the placental form (GM-CSF receptor α_1) in its extracellular and transmembrane domains. The intracellular domain is slightly longer (64 versus 54 amino acids) and is identical with GM-CSF receptor α_1 in its proximal portion. An alternate splice results in a polypeptide that diverges completely from GM-CSF receptor α_1 in the distal cytoplasmic region. The divergent sequence is rich in serine, a residue that has been implicated in the function of the IL-2 receptor β. Both isoforms are expressed in bone marrow and placental cells, but expression of GM-CSF receptor α_2 is about 20 times lower. Like GM-CSF receptor α_1, GM-CSF receptor α_2 also binds GM-CSF with low affinity (K_d less than 4 nmol/L) and confers human GM-CSF dependence to FDC-P1 cells.

High-affinity binding may be restricted to hematopoietic cells, and only on hematopoietic cells is the 135-kd band seen.[438] Recently, a human cDNA that is homologous to the murine AIC2B was isolated.[441] It encodes a cell surface protein that binds neither IL-3 nor GM-CSF, but when cotransfected into COS cells with GM-CSF receptor α_1, high-affinity binding is observed. These data suggest that at least two GM-CSF cell surface-binding proteinsexist—an α chain of 80 kd that may be expressed as more than one isoform, and a β chain (β common) of approximately 135 kd. Recent data also suggest the existence of a secreted form of the low-affinity receptor that lacks the transmembrane region.[442] Furthermore, a cDNA clone was recently isolated that encodes a low-affinity IL-3 receptor.[363] When this gene was coexpressed with β common, high-affinity IL-3 binding was observed. These results indicate that the human GM-CSF and IL-3 low-affinity receptors share a common β subunit that confers high-affinity binding on both low-affinity subunits (Fig. 8-13).

FIGURE 8-13. Major cytokine actions. The predominant actions of the different cytokines are indicated schematically. IL-3 and GM-CSF act broadly on most progenitor cells. IL-3, together with SF and IL-6, acts on more primitive cells than GM-CSF. The other cytokines are shown on the lineage pathways to which their actions are restricted.

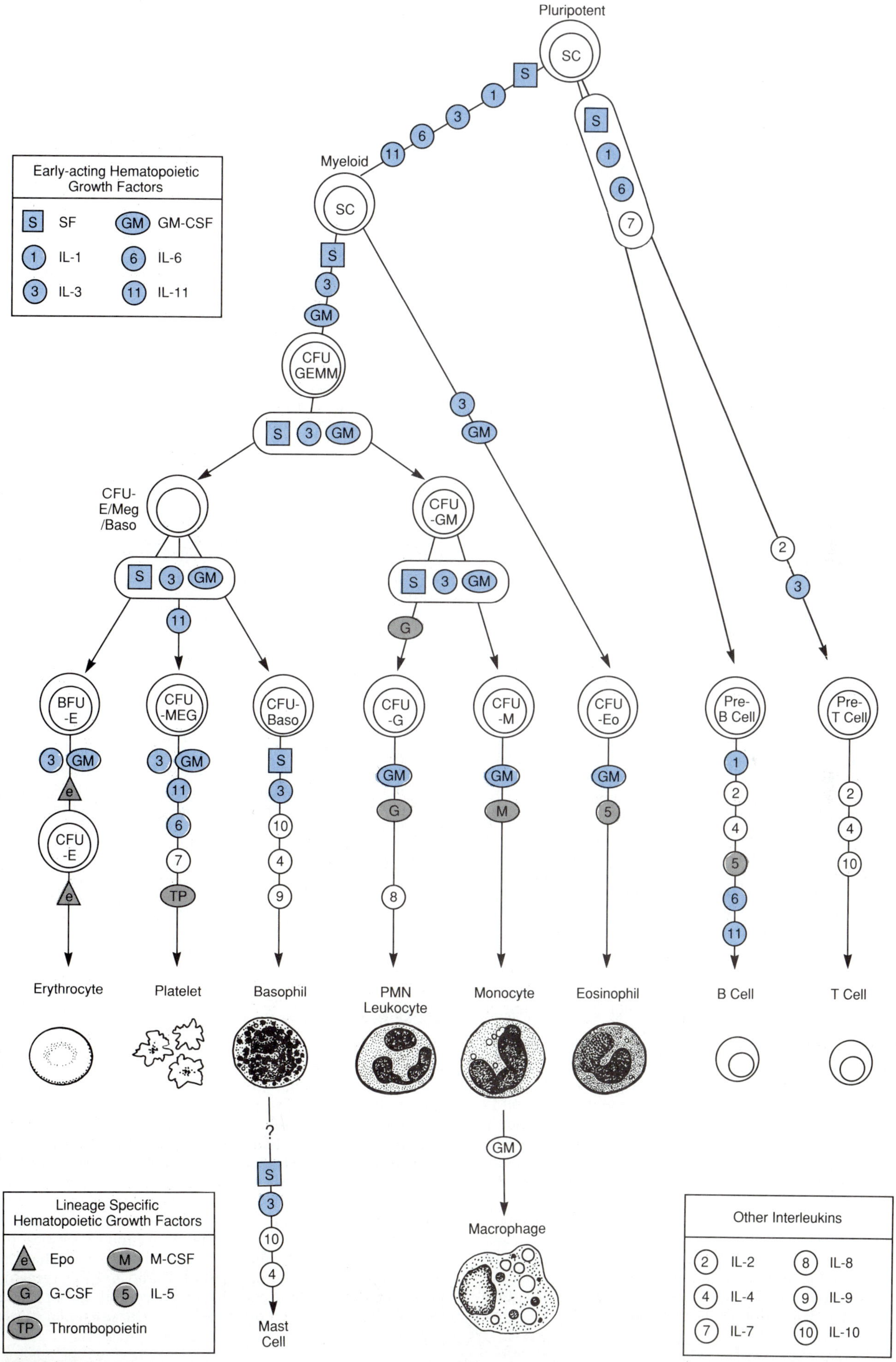
Pluripotent
SC
S
1
3
6
11
Myeloid
SC
S
1
6
7
Early-acting Hematopoietic Growth Factors
S SF
GM GM-CSF
1 IL-1
6 IL-6
3 IL-3
11 IL-11
S
3
GM
CFU GEMM
S 3 GM
3
GM
CFU- E/Meg /Baso
CFU -GM
S 3 GM
S 3 GM
11
G
2
3
BFU -E
CFU -MEG
CFU- Baso
CFU -G
CFU -M
CFU -Eo
Pre- B Cell
Pre- T Cell
3 GM
e
CFU -E
e
3 GM
11
6
7
TP
S
3
10
4
9
GM
G
8
GM
M
GM
5
1
2
4
5
6
11
2
4
10
Erythrocyte
Platelet
Basophil
PMN Leukocyte
Monocyte
Eosinophil
B Cell
T Cell
?
S
3
10
4
Mast Cell
GM
Macrophage
Lineage Specific Hematopoietic Growth Factors
e Epo
M M-CSF
G G-CSF
5 IL-5
TP Thrombopoietin
Other Interleukins
2 IL-2
8 IL-8
4 IL-4
9 IL-9
7 IL-7
10 IL-10

FIGURE 8-13.

GM-CSF Signal Transduction

In contrast to the results with IL-3, GM-CSF induces the tyrosine phosphorylation of only the 90-kd band in B6SUtA1 cells[368] and has a minimal effect on the IC-2.9 cell line. Incubation of human neutrophils with GM-CSF results in increased tyrosine phosphorylation of proteins of 118, 92, 78, and 40 kd,[443] whereas a 75-kd protein that is phosphorylated on tyrosine is present in the HL60 cell line.[444] Exposure of the human GM-CSF– and IL-3–dependent cell line M-07 to either ligand results in the rapid tyrosine phosphorylation of identical 93- and 70-kd proteins.[445] There is considerable overlap in the signaling pathways induced by these two factors.

In neutrophils, preincubation with GM-CSF enhances superoxide production after induction with agents such as f-MLP. This priming does not result from alteration in calcium flux or PKC activity. The effect is inhibited by pertussis toxin, which suggests the involvement of a G-protein, and increased release of arachidonic acid with generation of lipoxygenase products such as leukotriene B4 has been documented.[443,446–449] Murine peritoneal macrophage adenylate cyclase activity is increased rapidly after exposure to GM-CSF, suggesting that cAMP may be involved in transmitting an intracellular signal in macrophages.[450] This contrasts with the decrease in adenylate cyclase and increase in guanylate cyclase activity observed after GM-CSF treatment of neutrophils.[451]

G-CSF

Two G-CSF cDNA clones were isolated from different tumor cell lines. The first clone encodes a 207–amino acid protein, of which 177 amino acids comprise mature G-CSF, whereas 30 hydrophobic amino acids determine the probable leader sequence.[300] The second clone is identical apart from a deletion of 3 amino acids at positions 36 to 38, which results in a 174–amino acid protein.[301] Sequence analysis of a genomic clone that expresses both proteins indicates that alternative use of 2 donor splice sites 9 nucleotides apart at the 5′ end of intron 2 is responsible for the production of the 2 mRNAs.[452] The predicted molecular masses of the two proteins are 19 and 18.6 kd, respectively, whereas purified native G-CSF has a molecular mass of 19.6 kd. This difference is due to O-glycosylation; no N-glycosylation sites exist. Differences in bioactivity of the two proteins may exist, but it is not known whether two analogous forms of native G-CSF are produced.

G-CSF mRNA accumulation in fibroblasts and endothelial cells appears to be coordinately regulated with GM-CSF after exposure to IL-1 or TNFα.[416–419] In endothelial cells, this is mediated by an increase in transcriptional rate.[428] Monocyte synthesis of G-CSF appears to depend on induction with endotoxin[418] (see Fig. 8-12).

Murine and human G-CSF receptor cDNA clones were recently isolated that bind G-CSF with high affinity, similar to the native receptor (K_d 100 to 500 pmol/L).[453,454] The murine receptor is an 812–amino acid polypeptide (90,814 daltons) with an extracellular domain of 601 amino acids, 24 hydrophobic transmembrane amino acids, and a cytoplasmic domain of 187 amino acids. One part (amino acids 95 to 317) of the extracellular domain of the G-CSF receptor is homologous to other members of the hematopoietic growth factor family. Another part (amino acids 375 to 601) is homologous to chicken contactin, a neuronal cell surface glycoprotein that plays a role in cellular communication between neural cells.[455] Contactin is homologous to fibronectin type III, and it is possible that this part of G-CSF receptor acts as a cell adhesion protein.

M-CSF

Because of two alternative splice sites and extensive post-translational modification, the biosynthesis of M-CSF is much more complex (Fig. 8-14). The M-CSF gene is 21 kb in length and comprises 10 exons.[456] Exons 1 to 8 contain the coding sequence, and exons 9 and 10 contain 3′ untranslated sequence. The first reported cDNA, isolated from a library made from a phorbol myristate acetate–stimulated pancreatic tumor cell line, encodes a 1.6-kb mRNA.[457] This is translated into a 26-kd precursor that undergoes N-terminal (32 residue leader sequence) and C-terminal processing to yield a mature subunit of approximately 145 amino acids (16 kd). Analysis of a cDNA that represents the more common 4-kb mRNA shows that this form of message results from alternative splicing during transcription; this leads to an in-frame insertion of 894 nucleotides.[458] The transcript also has a larger 3′ noncoding region that, unlike the untranslated region of the shorter mRNA, contains an AU-rich region that is associated with RNA instability.[415] This mRNA produces a primary translation product of 61-kd that contains an extra 298 residues. Identical N-terminal processing (32 amino acids) and more extensive C-terminal processing (294 residues) yield a mature protein of 223 amino acids (26 kd). Both the 16- and 26-kd forms of M-CSF are N-glycosylated to yield monomers of 20 to 25 kd and 35 to 45 kd, respectively. M-CSF exists as a dimer, and the monomers thus yield two forms of CSF, 40- to 50-kd and 70- to 90-kd glycoproteins, respectively. Native M-CSF of both sizes have been purified.[459–461] However, it is not yet clear whether the smaller protein, purified from human urine, results from biosynthesis of the 1.6-kb mRNA or from proteolysis of the large molecule. The common 75–amino acid C terminal sequence contains a 23–amino acid hydrophobic region, which suggests transmembrane insertion. This is consistent with evidence that membrane and secretory forms of M-CSF may exist.[462–464] The membrane-bound form may be derived from the 1.6-kb cDNA since the latter lacks an intracellular proleolytic cleavage site encoded in the 5′ portion of exon 6. This is present in the 4-kb cDNA and leads to rapid secretion after cleavage within the Golgi apparatus.

Evidence suggests that uninduced monocytes, fibroblasts, and endothelial cells contain M-CSF mRNA.[418] Other investigators report, however, that phorbol myristate acetate, γ-interferon, and GM-CSF induce M-CSF accumulation in monocytes,[465–467] whereas IL-1 and TNF have the same effect in endothelial cells.[428] Fetal calf serum can induce M-CSF mRNA accumulation in monocytes, and it is therefore possible that this led to "constitutive" production in this cell type.

M-CSF Receptor

The interaction of M-CSF with its receptor on bone marrow macrophages has been studied. At 37°C, bone marrow macrophages internalize labeled CSF.[468] Recent evidence shows that the major mechanism of clearance of M-CSF in mice occurs through binding and internalization of circulating M-CSF by liver and splenic macrophages.[469] In contrast to the family of hematopoietic growth factor receptors outlined above, the M-CSF or CSF-1 receptor, encoded by the c-*fms* protooncogene, is a member of the family of receptors that exhibits ligand-induced tyrosine phosphorylation.[470] Evidence that c-*fms* and the M-CSF receptors are identical comes from the observations that the proteins are of similar size (165 kd) and exhibit tyrosine kinase activity; an antibody to c-*fms* precipitates a protein that is phosphorylated on tyrosine in the presence of pu-

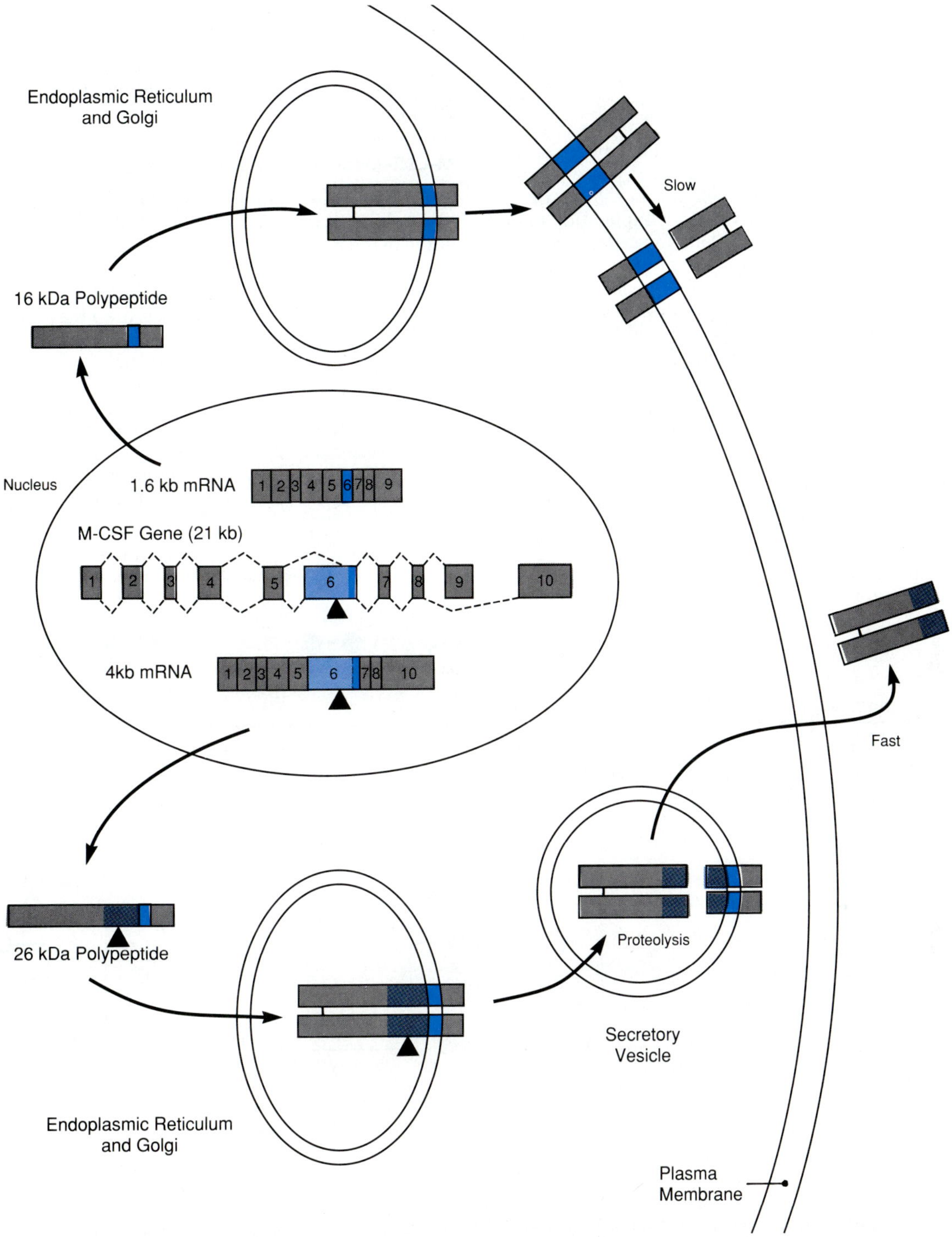

FIGURE 8-14. Biosynthesis of M-CSF. Four M-CSF cDNAs have been isolated. Two are illustrated here to show biosynthesis of the cell surface and soluble forms of M-CSF (see text for explanation). The genome comprises 10 exons. The 4-kb mRNA is encoded by exons 1 to 8 and 10, whereas the 1.6-kb mRNA is encoded by exons 1 to 9, with differential splicing of exon 6 that includes the loss of a sequence that encodes an intracellular proteolytic cleavage site (*arrowhead in exon 6*). The protein product of the 4-kb mRNA is cleaved at this intracellular proteolytic cleavage site in the secretory vesicle, which results in rapid secretion of M-CSF. The 1.6-kb mRNA is expressed on the cell surface and slowly released by extracellular proteolytic cleavage.

rified M-CSF, and [^{125}I] M-CSF can be recovered from immunoprecipitates of receptor-membrane extracts.[471] This family of receptors includes the PDGF, insulin, EGF and c-*kit* receptors (see Fig. 8-8). The PDGF-β isoform shares a high degree of amino acid sequence homology with the M-CSF receptor,[472] and analysis of genomic clones shows that the two genes are juxtaposed in a head-to-tail tandem array, with less than 0.5 kb between the polyadenylation signal of the PDGF receptor β gene and exon 1 of c-*fms*.[473] Presumably, the two genes were divided by duplication of an ancestral gene and subsequent divergence. Each gene is approximately 60 kb long, and transcription is initiated in a tissue-specific manner. Exon 1, which specifies untranslated sequence, is transcribed in placental trophoblasts. In contrast, monocyte transcription is initiated from exon 2, which encodes the signal peptide and is separated by a 26-kb intron from exon 1. The mature human M-CSF receptor is an integral transmembrane glycoprotein 972 amino acids long.[481] The 512–amino acid extracellular domain is organized into 5 immunoglobulin-like regions, and a 25–amino acid transmembrane region separates it from the 435–amino acid intracellular domain that contains the tyrosine kinase activity. The latter is separated into two regions by a 72–amino acid "kinase insert." During biosynthesis of the M-CSF receptor, asparagine-linked glycosylation of a 105-kd precursor protein results in a mature glycoprotein of 150 kd.

M-CSF–Mediated Signal Transduction

M-CSF binding rapidly up-regulates receptor protein tyrosine kinase activity, probably through transphosphorylation of the receptor itself by aggregation of M-CSF receptor subunits (Fig. 8-15). Tyrosine (denoted by the letter Y in the single amino acid code letter) phosphorylation has been mapped to three sites, two within the kinase insert (Y699 and Y708) and one in the C-terminal kinase consensus sequence (Y809). Evidence suggests that the M-CSF receptor is linked through a pertussis toxin–sensitive G protein to activation of PKC.[474] PDGF-β binds to and phosphorylates phospholipase C–γ, an enzyme that cleaves phosphatidyl inositol 4,5-bisphosphate to yield inositol 1,4,5-trisphosphate and 1,2-diacylglycerol, which in turn mobilize calcium and activate PKC, respectively. Phos-

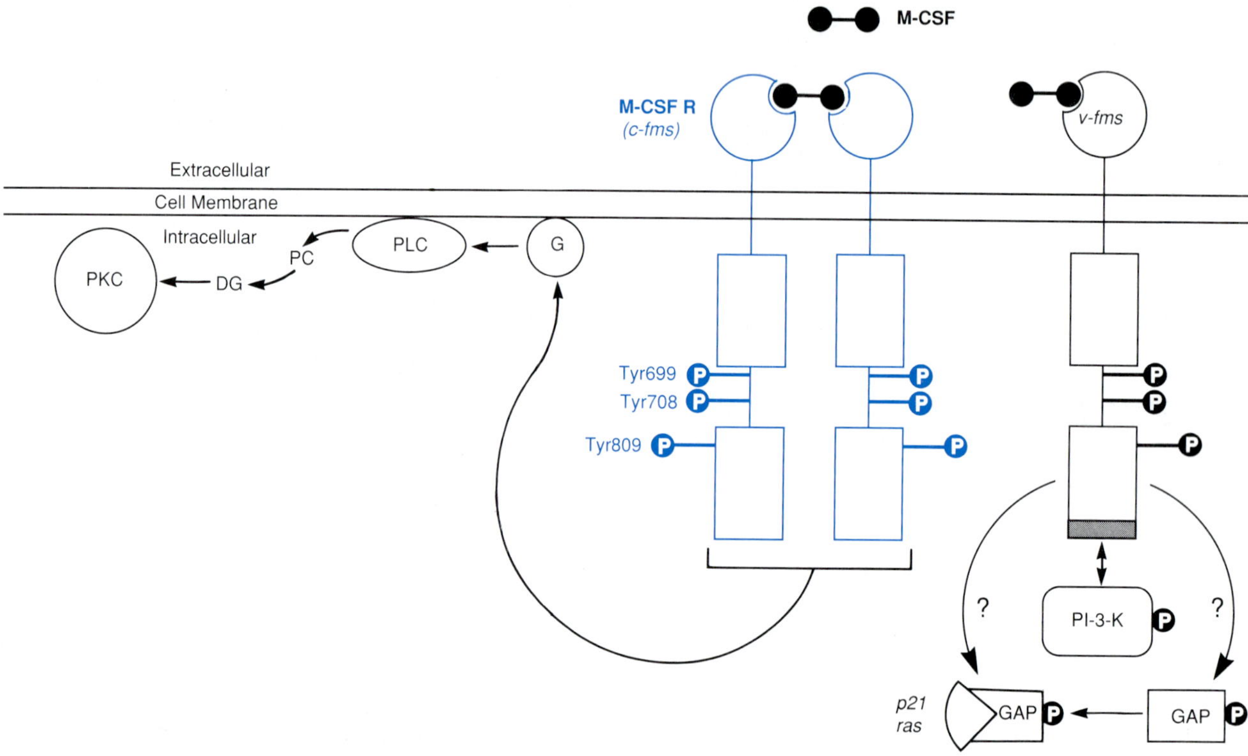

FIGURE 8-15. Signal transduction by M-CSF. M-CSF binds to its receptor and up-regulates receptor protein tyrosine kinase (PTK) activity. By analogy with other receptors of this class, dimerization probably occurs, followed by autophosphorylation or transphosphorylation of the receptor at tyrosines 699, 708, and 809. Activation of receptor PTK activity leads to phosphorylation of heterologous substrates within seconds of M-CSF stimulation. This leads to membrane ruffling and vacuolization, increased Na^+/H^+ exchange resulting in cytoplasmic alkalization, increased hexose transport, and induction of genes such as c-*fos*. The pathways involved in these effects and the protein substrates activated by receptor PTK activity have not yet been identified, but some clues exist. The oncogene v-*fms* has a number of potent mutations and is distinct in its C terminus from c-*fms*. Transformation of cells by v-*fms* induces phosphorylation of the c-*raf* protooncogene, itself a serine–threonine protein kinase. Also, antibodies to the c-*ras* gene product (p21 *ras*) inhibit growth of v-*fms*–transformed cells by an unknown mechanism. p21 *ras* requires bound GTP for its activity. v-*fms* could therefore inhibit GTPase-accelerating protein (GAP), a protein that accelerates the p21 *ras*-mediated hydrolysis of GTP to GDP, and thus decreases p21 *ras* activity. Alternatively, the receptor might increase p21 *ras* activity by another mechanism. A novel phosphatidyl inositol–3′ kinase (PI-3-K) physically associates with v-*fms*. Lastly, activation of protein kinase C (PKC) may occur through receptor-mediated activation of a G protein (G) specific for phosphatidylcholine (PC). M-CSF stimulation of monocytes is associated with hydrolysis of PC to phosphorylcholine and diacylglycerol (DG) by phospholipase C (PLC). DG, in turn, stimulates PKC.

pholipase C–γ does not appear to be a substrate of the activated M-CSF receptor.[482] However, recent evidence shows that M-CSF activation of PKC is mediated by a phosphatidylcholine-specific phospholipase C that catalyses the formation of 1,2-diacylglycerol and phosphoryl choline.[474] After stimulation with M-CSF, the M-CSF receptor also binds to a novel phosphatidylinositol-3-kinase. The association requires tyrosine kinase activity and is triggered by receptor phosphorylation on tyrosine; mutants that lack kinase function show reduced phosphatidylinositol-3-kinase activity.[475]

Several tyrosine-phosphorylated proteins can be detected in macrophages after M-CSF treatment, but none of these polypeptides has been characterized in detail. A possible role for the c-*ras* gene product, p21 ras, is suggested by the observation that microinjected monoclonal antibodies to this protein inhibit the proliferation of fibroblasts transformed by v-*fms*, the M-CSF receptor.[478] Another protooncogene product, c-*raf*, is a serine/threonine kinase and is also phosphorylated after stimulation of fibroblasts by PDGF or their transformation by v-*fms*.[477]

Transformation by v-*fms*

v-*fms* is the oncogene of the McDonough strain of feline sarcoma virus, and expression at the cell surface is required for transformation.[478] The virus was first isolated from a feline fibrosarcoma,[479] and fibroblast cell lines are transformed with the highest efficiency.[470] Since fibroblasts secrete M-CSF[480] and the v-*fms* product appears to contain an almost complete extracellular domain, it is possible that transformation of fibroblasts depends on ligand binding and transduction of a signal through a functional receptor in a cell that does not normally require M-CSF for growth. However, simian virus 40–immortalized macrophages that are CSF-1 dependent do not secrete or express CSF-1. They can be rendered CSF-1 independent after introduction of the v-*fms* gene.[388] The C-terminal end of v-*fms* differs from c-*fms* in that 40 amino acids of c-*fms* are replaced by 11 unrelated residues in the v-*fms* product.[481] This change results in constitutive autophosphorylation of v-*fms*; this is in contrast to c-*fms*, in which autophosphorylation is enhanced by CSF-1. This suggests that the factor independence induced by v-*fms* expression in macrophages is due to unregulated kinase activity that provides growth stimulation in the absence of ligand. v-*fms* has not been implicated in naturally occurring hematopoietic neoplasms in vivo. However, bone marrow infected with helper-free virus containing v-*fms* can be engrafted into irradiated mice. Spleen cells that contain the integrated provirus can be transplanted into irradiated secondary recipients, some of which develop erythroleukemias or B-cell lymphomas.[483] These data are of considerable interest and provide more evidence linking oncogenes and growth factors. Other examples include v-*erb* B, which encodes a protein that is a truncated form of the epidermal growth factor receptor,[484] and c-*sis*, which encodes for a polypeptide chain of PDGF.[485]

Erythropoietin

The EPO molecule was first purified to apparent homogeneity from the urine of patients with aplastic anemia.[290] Analysis of cDNA clones isolated from a fetal liver cDNA library show that a reading frame of 579 nucleotides encodes a 27–amino acid hydrophobic leader sequence followed by the 166–amino acid mature protein.[303] The N terminal of the mature protein was identified by comparison with the sequence of purified human urinary EPO originally determined by Goldwasser and his colleagues.[486] The molecular weight of natural EPO is 34 to 39 kd and the deduced molecular weight of the recombinant polypeptide backbone is 18.4 kd; the difference in molecular weight is due to glycosylation. There are three sites of N-linked glycosylation—at amino acids 24, 38, and 83—and the molecule is also O-glycosylated. There are four cysteine residues, and at least two must be involved in disulphide bonds since biologic activity is lost on reduction.

Cellular Sources

Erythropoietin is produced by fetal liver and adult kidney in response to hypoxia. In situ hybridization studies of anemic murine kidneys have localized production of EPO mRNA to cortical cells that lie in the interstitium between the tubules.[487] Morphologically, these cells resemble peritubular endothelial cells, and immunofluorescent studies show that cells with the same topography are factor VIII–related antigen–positive.[488] Combined immunofluorescent and in situ studies have not been reported, however. Further in situ hybridization studies in mice with varying severities of acute anemia show that serum EPO levels correlate with an alteration in the number of EPO-producing cells and not with degree of positivity, which remains consistent.[489]

Regulation of the Erythropoietin Gene

Two EPO-producing hepatoma cell lines, Hep G2 and Hep 3B, can be induced to produce large amounts of EPO in response to hypoxia or cobalt (II) chloride, a known in vivo inducer of EPO.[490] Further experiments showed that the accumulation of EPO mRNA in response to hypoxia, cobalt, or nickel requires synthesis of new protein in Hep 3B cells.[491] The increase in mRNA levels is due to an increase in transcription,[492] suggesting that the newly synthesized protein could be a *trans*-acting transcription factor. Many proteins that react with molecular oxygen do so through a heme moiety. The classic example is hemoglobin, with oxygen binding reversibly to the ferrous iron atom in the center of the heme porphyrin ring. Oxygen binding alters the conformation of the molecule. Cobalt and nickel can substitute for ferrous iron. The poor binding of oxygen to cobalt and lack of binding to nickel lock the hemoglobin molecule in the deoxy state. An hypothesis for the regulation of EPO production postulates that an unidentified heme protein is sensitive to oxygen tension and triggers EPO mRNA accumulation in renal or hepatic cells when it is in the deoxy conformation.[491] Cobalt and nickel might exert their effects through a common pathway by substituting for the metal in the heme protein and fixing it in a deoxy (active) conformation. Indeed, hypoxia either alone or combined with cobalt or nickel has the same effect, suggesting that they operate through the same pathway. Further support for this hypothesis comes from the observation that carbon monoxide, which substitutes for oxygen and maintains heme in its oxy configuration, reduces EPO production by Hep 3B cells. Also, inhibition of heme synthesis causes a five-fold reduction in hypoxia-induced EPO production. Thus, these results are consistent with the hypothesis that the EPO response is mediated by a heme protein. The new protein that is synthesized after exposure of these cells to hypoxia could be the hypothesized heme protein, the implication being that the promoter of this protein is sensitive to hypoxia. A number of glycolytic enzymes have been shown to be transcriptionally regulated by oxygen availability.[493]

Erythropoietin Signal Transduction

Single cell analysis of erythroblasts derived from cord blood BFU-E, loaded with the Ca^{2+}-sensitive dye fura-2, and analyzed by fluorescence microscopy coupled to digital video imaging showed that EPO or GM-CSF induces a dose-related transient increase in intracellular free calcium concentration [Ca_i].[494] These results were not confirmed in a flow cytometric study of purified murine CFU-E.[495] A resolution to these conflicting data comes from the observation that late erythroblasts (day 10 BFU-E) show a [Ca_i] increase, whereas less mature cells plucked at day 7 do not.[496] The [Ca_i] response to EPO may therefore be linked to later events in maturation rather than to proliferation of immature progenitors.

EPO has also been shown to reduce the serine phosphorylation of a 43-kd membrane phosphoprotein in normal and Rauscher's erythroleukemia cells.[497]. Finally, EPO activates adenylate cyclase and increases cAMP levels in rabbit bone marrow.[498]

Erythropoietin Receptor

About 200 EPO receptors are present on normal erythroid progenitors, with both high-affinity (less than 0.1 nmol/L) and low-affinity (0.5- to 0.8-nmol/L) binding. Cross-linking studies reveal two bands of net 105 and 85 kd, or one of less than 70 kd.[499] Murine erythroleukemia cells express only low-affinity receptors and were used to clone an EPO receptor cDNA.[310] It is surprising that transfection of COS cells with the EPO receptor cDNA revealed both high- and low-affinity binding. The COS transfectants also show two cross-linked complexes similar in size to the complexes observed on normal cells. These data suggest that the low-affinity receptor encoded by the isolated murine EPO receptor cDNA interacts with an endogenous COS cell polypeptide. Among the family of hematopoietic growth factor receptors, the EPO receptor has greatest homology to the IL-2 β chain (35% amino acid identity in the cytoplasmic region). The IL-2 receptor β chain binds IL-2 with intermediate affinity but shows high-affinity binding when complexed with the p55 IL-2 receptor α chain (Tac). Both the IL-2 receptor β chain and the EPO receptor are rich in serines, prolines, and acidic residues in the cytoplasmic region adjacent to the transmembrane domain, and analysis of mutations of the IL-2 receptor β chain shows that the serine-rich region is important for signal transduction.[500] A similar region of the EPO receptor is sufficient for EPO-mediated signal transduction[501] (Fig. 8-16). EPO induces the rapid tyrosine phosphorylation of a number of substrates,[502–505] one of which is Jak2. This leads to activation of the tyrosine kinase function of Jak2, which may mediate the biologic response to EPO.

Deeper insight into a role for the EPO receptor in oncogenesis comes from the recent observation that it interacts with and is activated by the membrane glycoprotein, gp55, of the Friend spleen focus-forming virus (SFFV).[506] SFFV is a defective C-type retrovirus and gp55, encoded by the viral *env* gene, is essential for the induction of erythroleukemia in mice.[507,508] Cotransfection of both EPO receptor and gp55 into an IL-3–dependent cell line results in autocrine cell growth, and immunoprecipitation studies demonstrate physical association between the two proteins. This association could occur in several different subcellular compartments, and direct binding of gp55 may activate the EPO receptor, thus bypassing the normal requirement for EPO. The interaction of gp55 with the EPO receptor is also observed in MEL cells and may account for the absence of high-affinity EPO binding and for the EPO independence of these cells.

Interleukin-1

Interleukin-1 is a monocyte–macrophage product that comprises two distinct polypeptides, IL-1α and IL-1β. The two forms have identical biologic properties, mediated by binding to the same receptor.[509,510]

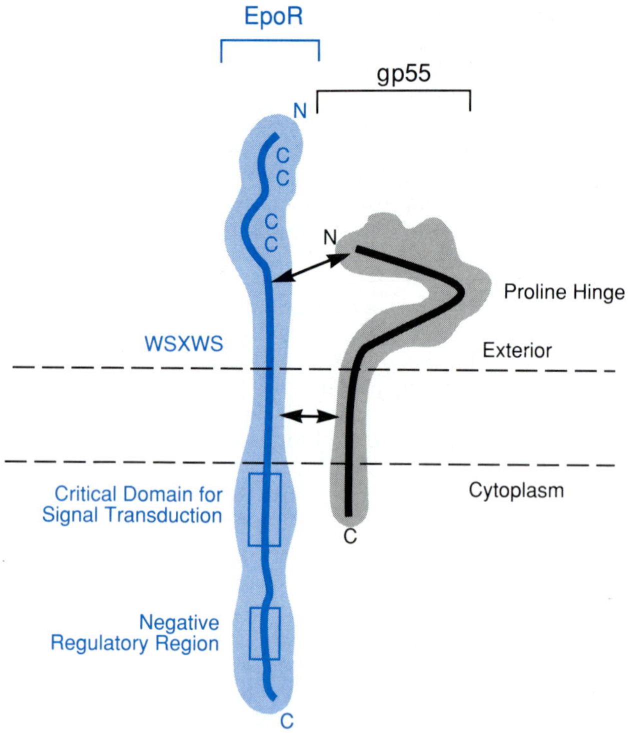

FIGURE 8-16. Functional domains of the erythropoietin receptor (EpoR) and binding to the gp55 envelope protein of the Friend spleen focus-forming virus. Carboxy-terminal truncation mutants of the EPO receptor indicate that the binding site between gp55 and the EPO receptor occurs either in the membrane-spanning region or in the extracellular region of the EPO receptor. These mutants were also used to map the negative regulatory region and the domain critical for signal transduction.

Molecular Structure and Biosynthesis

Both forms of IL-1 have been cloned and are encoded by seven exons that share 45% nucleotide homology.[511–514] Both proteins are synthesized as 31-kd precursors. They lack signal peptides, and the precursor forms, which are found in the cytosolic and liposomal fractions, are released from lysosomes by the action of serine proteases.[515] Forms of 31 and 22 kd remain associated with the monocyte cell membrane, whereas 31- and 17-kd forms, as well as several small polypeptides of 11, 4, and 2 kd, are secreted.[516] Evidence exists that in human monocytes the precursor forms of IL-1α remain primarily cell-associated, whereas both the precursor forms and the mature 17-kd form of IL-1β are released.[517] Furthermore, the IL-1 receptor binds the precursor form of IL-1α but not IL-1β, suggesting that the biologic activity associated with the larger 31-kd form is due to the IL-1α precursor.[518]

IL-1α is produced by blood monocytes and a wide variety of tissue macrophages, including pulmonary alveolar, splenic, and peritoneal macrophages and Kupffer cells. It is also produced by nonphagocytic cells such as fibroblasts, endothelial cells, smooth muscle cells, astrocytes, and epithelial cells from skin, cornea, gingiva, and thymus. A prime stimulus for production is endotoxin, but other microbial products, plant lectins, immune complexes, complement components, and antigens also induce IL-1. Regulation by IL-1 itself and positive and negative regulation by other cytokines is complex and may also be important. IL-1 induces IL-1 production by monocytes, smooth muscle cells, and endothelial cells.[519,520] IL-1 also induces γ-interferon production, which suppresses IL-1–induced IL-1 production but augments production induced by endotoxin.[521] Prostaglandin E_2 and IL-6 also suppress IL-1 production, whereas TNF acts as a positive stimulus.

IL-1 Receptor

The murine IL-1 receptor was cloned from T cells and the cDNA product binds IL-1α and IL-1β in a manner indistinguishable from the native low-affinity (more than 500 pmol/L) receptor.[308] The 319–amino acid extracellular domain of the receptor contains 7 potential N-linked glycosylation sites. Treatment of the IL-1 receptor with N-glycanase removes the carbohydrate chain and reduces the size of the receptor from 80 to 62 kd, close to the predicted size of 64.6 kd. The extracellular region is followed by a 21–amino acid hydrophobic transmembrane region, then a 217–amino acid intracellular domain. The IL-1 receptor belongs to the immunoglobulin (Ig) gene super family, and the extracellular portion is organized in three Ig domains. This is similar to the extracellular domain of some tyrosine kinase receptor family members such as the FGF receptor (3 Ig-like domains and the M-CSF and PDGF receptors (5 Ig-like domains) but is distinct in that the intracellular region does not contain sequences typical of tyrosine kinases or of tyrosine kinase acceptor sites. The sequence His-His-Ser-Arg-Arg (amino acids 429 to 433) resembles a PKC acceptor site.

Other polypeptide(s) may be involved in IL-1 binding. High-affinity binding (K_d 5 to 15 pmol/L) occurs on a variety of cells, and bands distinct from the predicted 80-kd binding protein have been seen in cross-linking studies.[522–524] In view of the unknown mechanism by which the IL-1 receptor transduces its signal, it is likely that, similar to the IL-6 and IL-2 receptors, other polypeptides are involved in both high-affinity binding and signal transmission.

Biologic Activities

IL-1α has been shown to be identical with a factor called hemopoietin 1, which was purified from HBT 5637 cell line–conditioned medium.[525,526] This protein, termed *synergistic factor*,[99] does not stimulate colony formation alone; it acts synergistically with M-CSF to induce the formation of large macrophage colonies from primitive colony-forming cells with high proliferative potential, which are enriched in bone marrow obtained from 5FU-treated mice (HPP-CFC). The data suggest that primitive cells responsive to IL-1 and M-CSF proliferate and differentiate into cells responsive to IL-3 and M-CSF and subsequently to cells responsive to M-CSF alone.[527,528] The synergistic effects of IL-1 are evident when bone marrow cells are plated at low density (500 cells per 35-mm plate), suggesting that its action is direct. IL-1α and IL-1β are now known to be potent inducers of GM-CSF, G-CSF, and IL-6 production by mesenchymal cells, and it is possible that the IL-1 effects are mediated indirectly by induction of known or as yet unidentified hematopoietic growth factors.

IL-1 given in vivo to mice before lethal whole-body irradiation has a marked radioprotective effect, which results from accelerated hematopoietic recovery.[529] Suboptimal doses that are nonradioprotective achieve optimal radioprotection when combined with GM-CSF.[530] These results have been extended to protection from the myelosuppressive effects of 5FU, where IL-1α acts synergistically with G-CSF,[531] and cyclophosphamide.[532] Administration of IL-1β for short periods of time (2 and 7 days) to primates after 5FU is myelostimulatory. In contrast, IL-1 given for longer periods (14 days) is ineffective, partly because of the release of TNFα.[533]

Interleukin-4

Several other interleukins may act synergistically with the CSFs on hematopoietic progenitors. Interleukin-4 (B-cell stimulatory factor 1) is a B-lymphocyte proliferation and activation factor that is also a growth factor for mast cells and T lymphocytes. Complementary DNAs for murine and human IL-4 were isolated.[344,534,535] The human factor is a glycoprotein of 290 amino acids. Its effects are mediated by binding to a single class of high-affinity specific cell surface receptors. Complementary DNA clones for murine and human IL-4 receptor were recently isolated, and encode a 140-kd membrane glycoprotein.[312,313] Two independent clones isolated from two murine cDNA libraries encode a soluble form of the IL-4 receptor.[313] The expressed cDNA is secreted, and the soluble receptor binds IL-4. Although a native secreted receptor has not been identified, a cDNA that encodes a soluble form of the IL-7 receptor has also been found,[314] and soluble IL-6 receptor has been identified in urine.[536] These results raise the possibility that secreted forms of growth factor receptors may play a physiologic role in the regulation of factor action.

Evidence suggests that IL-4 may act as a costimulant with EPO, G-CSF, and possibly M-CSF to increase erythroid, granulocyte, and macrophage colony numbers; paradoxically, it may inhibit IL-3 effects on less mature progenitors.[537,538]

Interleukin-5

IL-5 (eosinophil differentiation factor or B-cell growth factor II) is a 46-kd glycoprotein that, like M-CSF, exists as a dimer of two identical subunits. It was identified as a factor with biologic activities both on eosinophils and their precursors[539] and on B lymphocytes. Complementary DNA clones for both murine[540] and human IL-5[541] have been isolated.

Murine IL-5 induces eosinophil differentiation and acts as a proliferative and differentiating stimulus for B cells. It enhances IgA synthesis in lipopolysaccharide-stimulated B cells. Human recombinant IL-5 stimulates the development of eosinophil colonies from human bone marrow. The effect of IL-5 is lineage specific, and it does not produce as many eosinophil colonies as IL-3 or GM-CSF when tested on unenriched bone marrow mononuclear cells in serum-replete cultures.[542] IL-5 has an additive, not synergistic, effect on eosinophil colonies and appears to stimulate a more mature subset of progenitors than IL-3 or GM-CSF.[542] The appearance of eosinophils in the blood of rodents infected with the nematode *Nippostrongylus brasiliensis* is completely blocked by injection of monoclonal antibody to IL-5,[543] indicating that IL-5 is important for eosinophilia in vivo. In contrast, the IgE response in these animals is unaffected by antibody to IL-5 but is prevented by antibodies to IL-4.[544]

Interleukin-6

Molecular Cloning and Protein Structure

The isolation of cDNA clones for interleukin-6 (IL-6) illustrates the power of the molecular approach to the study of growth factors with broad spectra of biologic activities. A factor that stimulates antibody production by B cells (BSF2) and the differentiation of B cells into antibody-producing cells (BCDF) was purified and its cDNA cloned.[545] The sequence of this cDNA was identical with that of three others cloned at about the same time, interferon-β2,[546] 26-kd protein,[547] and hybridoma/plasmacytoma growth factor activity.[548]

The protein consists of 184 amino acids with two potential N-glycosylation sites, and four cysteine residues that are completely conserved between mouse and human proteins. IL-6 has significant homology to G-CSF, both at the amino acid level (four conserved cysteines) and at the level of gene organization.[545]

Regulation of IL-6 Production

IL-6 is produced by a variety of mesenchymal cells of hematopoietic origin (T cells, B cells, monocytes) and nonhematopoietic origin (fibroblasts, endothelial cells, bone marrow stroma, keratinocytes, astrocytes, mesangial cells). T-cell production is induced by mitogens or by antigen in the presence of macrophages.[549] Lipopolysaccharide enhances IL-6 production by monocytes, whereas lipopolysaccharide, IL-1, TNF, and PDGF induce fibroblast mRNA accumulation (see Fig. 8-12).[548]

IL-6 Receptor

The cDNA for the IL-6 receptor was cloned using high-level COS expression.[309] In contrast to other members of the hematopoietic growth factor receptor family, the 468 amino acid IL-6 receptor is characterized by a 90–amino acid N-terminal immunoglobin-like domain which, like the IL-1, PDGF, and M-CSF receptors, belongs to the C2 set of the immunoglobulin superfamily. The molecular weight of the receptor is 80 kd, and ligand binding induces the association of this polypeptide with a 130-kd membrane protein that is responsible for signal transduction.[550]

IL-6 and Lymphocytic Proliferative Disease

IL-6 has been implicated in the pathogenesis of several diseases. It appears to be an autocrine growth factor for human myeloma cells.[551] Myeloma cells produce and respond in vitro to IL-6, and growth in vitro can be inhibited by antibodies to IL-6. Responsiveness to IL-6 is characteristic of early- but not late-stage myeloma, suggesting that autocrine stimulation of these cells may be an early event.

Castleman's disease is characterized by fever, anemia, hypergammaglobulinemia, and increased acute-phase proteins in association with benign hyperplastic lymphadenopathy.[552] Germinal center B cells produce large amounts of IL-6, and dramatic clinical improvement occurs after surgical excision of involved nodes. Thus, abnormal regulation of IL-6 expression could be important in the pathogenesis of this disease.

Biologic Activities

IL-6 induces B cells to mature into antibody-secreting cells. Like IL-3, it acts as a permissive factor for blast cell colony proliferation in cultures of marrow from 5FU–treated mice, and in human enriched progenitor cell cultures as well. In combination with IL-3, IL-6 reduces the time period during which the blast cells begin to divide to form colonies, suggesting that it influences stem cell cycling.[553]

Interleukin-7

Interleukin-7 is a 25-kd glycoprotein, which was originally defined by its ability to stimulate the proliferation of murine pre–B lymphocytes (B220+, sIg−) in long-term cultures.[554] The murine[201] and human[555] cDNAs have been cloned. The factor binds to two classes of cell surface receptors with low and high affinity. Both murine and human cDNAs for the IL-7 receptor were isolated,[314] and when expressed in COS cells encode a polypeptide that binds IL-7 with low and high affinity. Several human cDNA clones were isolated that encode a secreted form of the receptor.[314]

Interleukin-8

Interleukin-8 was first identified as a small peptide (72 amino acids), which is secreted by monocytes in response to lipopolysaccharide and both activates and attracts polymorphonuclear neutrophils.[556] Recombinant human IL-8 increases expression of CD11b/CD18 and CD11c/CD18 on human polymorphonuclear neutrophils and stimulates CD11b/CD18 binding activity, suggesting that IL-8 may promote leukocyte adhesion and recruit polymorphonuclear neutrophils to sites of tissue inflammation.[557,558] Endothelial cells secrete IL-8 in response to IL-1, TNF, or lipopolysaccharide, and at nanomolar concentrations, IL-8 inhibits neutrophil adhesion to cytokine-activated endothelial cells.[559]

Interleukin-9

Interleukin-9 is a novel growth factor that was cloned from a human T-cell leukemia virus–transformed cell line.[560] The cDNA encodes a 144 amino acid protein (predicted size, 16 kd) with four potential sites for asparagine-linked glycosylation. The secreted protein is variably glycosylated and ranges from 20 to 30 kd. The sequence is homologous with a newly identified murine growth factor for helper T-cell clones designated T-cell growth factor P40.[561]

Recombinant human IL-9 acts selectively on BFU-E in cultures of enriched blood progenitors supplemented with EPO.[562] Large, diffuse, late-maturing BFU-E were observed, suggesting an action on an early immature progenitor. IL-9 is not as effective as IL-3 or GM-CSF in inducing BFU-E in the presence of EPO but appears to be more selective.

Interleukin-10

Interleukin-10 (mouse cytokine synthesis inhibitory factor) is a 17- to 21-kd protein that inhibits the synthesis of IFN-γ and other cytokines produced by stimulated murine T helper 1 (T_H1) clones. The cDNA was isolated for am murine T_H2 clone and contains a 178–amino acid open reading frame with an 18–amino acid hydrophobic signal sequence.[563] IL-10 is closely related to a gene, BCRFI, in the Epstein-Barr virus (EBV) genome, and it is likely that at some time the virus captured with cytokine gene. Because T_H1 clones secrete both IL-2 and IFN-γ and preferentially induce delayed-type hypersensitivity and macrophage activation, it is possible that the EBV exploits the biologic activity of the IL-10 to suppress the immune response in the host.

Interleukin-11

Interleukin-11 is a novel cytokine that was cloned by expression of a plasmacytoma stimulatory factor from an immortalized primate stromal cell line.[564] The cDNA contains a 597-nucleotide open reading frame that encodes a 199–amino acid polypeptide. The first 17 to 20 amino acids are hydrophobic and resemble a leader sequence. SDS-PAGE analysis of transfected COS cell supernatants shows a 20-kd species, consistent with the molecular mass expected for a 180–amino acid secreted protein. The protein lacks cysteine residues and a consensus sequence for asparagine-linked carbohydrate. The primate sequence shares 97% nucleotide identity with the human cDNA.[564]

IL-11 enhances the formation of immunoglobulin-secreting B cells, and enhances IL-3 stimulated megakaryocyte colony formation. Its actions are therefore similar to those of IL-6 and IL-7 though there is no sequence homology to either gene. Evidence indicates that it also acts synergistically with IL-3 to shorten the G_0 period of blast cell colony progenitors.[131]

Interleukin-12

Interleukin-12 is a 75-kd protein that comprises two subunits of 40 and 35 kd (p40 and p35) that are encoded by distinct genes on two different chromosomes. The p40 subunit is related to the extracellular domain of the IL-6 receptor, whereas p35 is distantly related to IL-6 itself. The complex does not signal through gp130. The p40 subunit is expressed mainly by monocytes, macrophages, and B cells, whereas p35 is more widely expressed. IL-12 induces interferon-γ expression in T and NK cells. The recombinant protein also supports hematopoietic stem cell development in combination with SF and IL-3 and is an important regulator of T_H1 cell development.[565]

Interleukin-13

Interleukin-13 is a 12-kd, 113–amino acid protein that was recently cloned from murine T_H2 and human helper T cells.[566–568] The gene maps to human chromosome 5q23-31 close to the IL-4 gene,[569] and the protein has limited homology (20% to 25%) to IL-4. IL-13 acts on monocytes and B cells in a manner somewhat similiar to IL-4. On human monocytes, it increases adherence by inducing expression of CD23 and MHC class II antigens[568] and inhibits antibody-dependent cytotoxicity and lipopolysaccharide-induced cytokine release.[570] Both alone and synergistically with IL-2, it increases large granular lymphocytic IFN-γ synthesis.[570] On human B cells, it increases CD23, MHC class II, CD72, and surface IgM expression and increases B-cell proliferation and synthesis of IgE, IgG, and IgM.[568,571] It competes weakly with IL-4 for binding to its receptor, suggesting that the two receptors share a common β subunit.

HEMATOPOIETIC GROWTH FACTORS IN VITRO

In view of the overlap in activities of the major hematopoietic growth factors, their combined actions on progenitors of the myeloid, erythroid, and megakaryocytic lineages are considered here. In recent years, the availability of pure recombinant growth factors, the enrichment of target progenitor cells, and the use of defined serum-free culture conditions have provided insights into the role of these factors during hematopoiesis. Although much of the fundamental biology has been learned from traditional culture systems using fetal calf serum, conditioned medium, and unfractionated cells, the focus will be on more recently obtained data.

Myelopoiesis

Murine IL-3 stimulates a broad spectrum of myeloid progenitor cells including pluripotent stem cells, granulocyte or macrophage colony-forming cells or units (CFU-GM, CFU-G, CFU-M), BFU-E, eosinophil CFUs (CFU-Eo), megakaryocyte CFUs (CFU-MK), and mast cells. As its name implies, GM-CSF was initially shown to be more restricted as a stimulus of the proliferation and development of CFU-GM. Murine studies with purified or recombinant factor have shown that it also stimulates the initial proliferation of other progenitors such as BFU-E as well.[288] The other murine factors, G-CSF and M-CSF, are more restricted and predominantly stimulate granulocyte and monocyte colony-forming units (CFU-G and CFU-M), respectively.[573,574]

With the possible exception of GM-CSF, the activities of the human CSFs are similar to those of the corresponding murine factors. Because of the lack of an assay for human pluripotent stem cells that is analogous to the murine CFU-S spleen colony assay, it is difficult to compare results in the two species. Both IL-3 and GM-CSF affect a similar broad spectrum of human myeloid progenitor cells. This includes CFU-GEMM, CFU-GM, CFU-G, CFU-M, and CFU-Eo. In full serum cultures, IL-3 and GM-CSF alone stimulate the formation of colonies derived from CFU-GM, CFU-G, CFU-M, and CFU-Eo. Data from serum-free cultures suggest that in the presence of IL-3 or GM-CSF alone, myeloid colony formation is much reduced and that optimal CFU-G or CFU-M proliferation requires the addition of G-CSF or M-CSF, respectively, to the cultures.[575–576] Even in serum-replete conditions, IL-3 acts additively or synergistically with G-CSF to induce more granulocyte colony formation than is observed with either factor alone.[577] The serum-free studies may have important implications for the use of combinations of CSFs in vivo, and it is apparent that the use of such culture conditions may provide further insight into the in vitro activities of the different factors.

In addition to their effects on progenitor differentiation, the CSFs also induce a variety of functional changes in mature cells. GM-CSF inhibits polymorphonuclear neutrophil migration under agarose,[578] induces antibody-dependent cytotoxicity (ADCC) for human target cells,[579] and increases neutrophil phagocytic activity.[580] Some of these functional changes may be related to a GM-CSF–induced increase in the cell surface expression of a family of antigens that function as cell adhesion molecules.[581] The increase in antigen expression is rapid and is associated with increased aggregation of neutrophils; both are maximal at the migration inhibitory concentration of 500 pmol/L, and granulocyte–granulocyte adhesion can be inhibited by an antigen-specific monoclonal antibody. GM-CSF also acts as a potent stimulus of eosinophil ADCC, superoxide production, and phagocytosis.[582]

G-CSF acts as a potent stimulus of neutrophil superoxide production, ADCC, and phagocytosis,[583] whereas M-CSF activates mature macrophages[584] and enhances macrophage cytotoxicity.

The actions of the CSFs on mature cells apparently parallels their spectrum of activity on immature progenitors. Murine IL-3, in contrast to human IL-3, activates neutrophil function. The explanation for this difference lies in the observation that murine IL-3 neutrophils express the IL-3 receptor,[585] whereas it is undetectable on the surface of human neutrophils.

Erythropoiesis

The regulation of the proliferation and maturation of erythroid progenitors depends on interaction with a number of growth factors. EPO is essential for the terminal maturation of erythroid cells. Its major effect appears to be at the level of the CFU-E during adult erythropoiesis, and recombinant preparations[586] are as effective as the natural hormone.[587,588] These progenitors do not require burst-promoting activity (BPA)[214,589] in the form of IL-3 or GM-CSF, and their dependence on EPO is emphasized by the observation that they will not survive in vitro in the absence of EPO. Because most CFU-E are in cycle, their survival in the presence of EPO is probably tightly linked to their proliferation and differentiation to mature erythrocytes. EPO also acts on a subset of presumptive mature BFU-E, which also require EPO for survival and terminal maturation.

A second subset of BFU-E, presumably less mature, survives EPO deprivation if BPA is present, either as IL-3 or GM-CSF. When EPO is added to these cultures on day 3, these BFU-E form typical colonies.[586] Similar results are obtained in serum-deprived methylcellulose cultures in which the usual 30% fetal calf serum is substituted by BSA-adsorbed cholesterol, iron-saturated transferrin, and insulin.[576] Under serum-deprived culture conditions, the combination of IL-3 and GM-CSF results in more BFU-E than either factor alone when EPO is added on day 3.

The *kit* ligand—also termed *Steel factor* (SF), *stem cell factor* (SCF), or *mast cell growth factor*—has been shown to have marked synergistic effects on BFU-E cultured in the presence of EPO.[144] Alone, it has no colony-forming ability. Progenitors obtained from human fetal liver and cultured in serum-free conditions differ in their requirements for BPA and EPO.[37,590] Whereas adult BFU-E require IL-3 or GM-CSF and EPO for the development of maximal BFU-E colony number and size, embryonic BFU-E require only EPO for maximal BFU-E cloning efficiency; the addition of IL-3 or GM-CSF increases BFU-E size but not number. These results suggest that EPO receptors are expressed at an earlier stage of erythroid maturation in fetal cells and that, during ontogeny, expression of the EPO receptor becomes restricted to a subset of mature BFU-E and CFU-E. During fetal development, the EPO receptor may be expressed by even more immature myeloid–erythroid progenitors such as CFU-Mix.

Newborn infants with severe Rh hemolytic disease and very high EPO levels are born with neutropenia and thrombocytopenia.[591] In vitro, high concentrations of EPO reduce the number of CFU-GM colonies and decrease the number of granulocytes per colony, with newborn cells more sensitive to this effect than progenitors from adults.[592] The effect does not appear to result from crowding in the culture dishes, since cord blood cells are plated at low density.

In summation, the data are consistent with the hypothesis that the fetal EPO receptor is expressed on bipotent progenitor cells and can influence the subsequent maturation of these cells.

Factors distinct from the classic CSFs may positively regulate erythropoiesis, either directly or indirectly. Limiting dilution studies of highly purified CFU-E in serum-free culture show that insulin and insulin-like growth factor I act directly on these cells.[593] The presence of EPO is essential in these studies, which contrast with earlier murine studies of unfractionated cells in which CFU-E respond to IGF-1 or insulin in the absence of EPO.[594] Another factor that enhances both BFU-E and CFU-E colony formation is activin. This protein dimer, also known as *follicle-stimulating hormone-releasing protein,* appears to have a lineage-specific effect on erythropoiesis that is indirect, since removal of monocytes or T lymphocytes abrogates its effect.[595] Activin has been identified as the factor produced by vegetal cells during blastogenesis that induces animal ectodermal cells to form primary mesoderm.[596]

Negative Regulation of Erythropoiesis

Observations that subsets of lymphocytes with an immunologic suppressor phenotype isolated from normal subjects can inhibit erythroid activity in vitro[347,597,598] correlate with reports of patients with a variety of disorders in whom anemia or granulocytopenia is associated with an expansion of certain T-lymphocyte populations.[599–603] In the rare disorder, T lymphocytosis with cytopenia,[604] in vitro suppression of erythropoiesis has been correlated with the expansion of a T-lymphocyte population that may be the counterpart of the hematopoietic suppressor cells isolated from normal peripheral blood.

The phenotype of these cells has been described in detail.[598,604] The cell is a large granular lymphocyte that is both E rosette–positive and T8 (classic suppressor phenotype)–positive. Suppressor T cells may also be inhvolved in some cases of aplastic anemia[605,606] or neutropenia[607] without an underlying immunologic disorder or an overt T-cell proliferation. Exactly how such suppressor T cells interact with hematopoietic progenitors and what surface antigens are "seen" by the suppressors is uncertain. Evidence supports the concept that suppression of erythroid colony expression in vitro is regulated by T cells and may be genetically restricted.[598,608] Cell–cell interactions in immunologic systems have been well characterized with regard to surface determinants that allow for cellular recognition. That certain phenotypes of T cells "recognize" distinct classes of histocompatibility antigens on immunologic cell surfaces has been well described.[609] Thus, the observation that hematopoietic progenitors have a unique distribution of class II histocompatibility antigens on their cell surface suggests a role for these antigens in the cell–cell interactions that regulate hematopoietic differentiation.[610–613]

T cells may also inhibit erythropoiesis in a non-HLA–restricted fashion by the production of inhibitory cytokines. Some lymphokines may inhibit erythropoiesis in vitro by a complex lymphokine cascade. Activation of T cells by the T-cell antigen receptor CD3 results in cell surface expression of the IL-2 receptor α chain (p55) and the acquisition of IL-2 responsiveness.[614] IL-2 inhibits BFU-E in the presence of these IL-2 receptor–positive cells, possibly by inducing their release of IFN-γ. CD2 can serve as an alternative pathway of T-cell activation and may do so through binding to its ligand LFA-3 on antigen presenting cells. Blockade of CD2 with monoclonal antibody leads to abrogation of IL-2/IFN-γ–mediated BFU-E suppression.[615] These data are difficult to reconcile with the observation that IL-2 incubation of PMA/calcium ionophore–activated CD4+ T cells leads to marked expansion of IL-3 and GM-CSF mRNA–positive cells by in situ hybridization.[355] Most CD4+ T cells express CD28 as well, and evidence suggests that IL-3 production is restricted to CD28+ T cells.[616] It is thus paradoxical that both potent stimulating and inhibitory lymphokines can be produced by activating T cells through the same pathway.

TNF also suppresses erythropoiesis in vitro.[617,618] The injection of peritoneal macrophages into Friend murine leukemia virus–infected animals results in rapid but transient resolution of the massive erythroid hyperplasia associated with this disease. This may be due to elaboration by macrophages of IL-1α, which does not suppress erythropoiesis itself but acts by the induction of TNF. This effect is reversed by EPO.[619]

Megakaryopoiesis

The regulation of megakaryocyte progenitors, their development into acetylcholinesterase-positive (ACHE+) cells or megakaryoblasts, and their subsequent progressive maturation into platelet-shedding multinucleated cells all are influenced by growth factors. The fundamental system is similar to that observed in erythropoiesis, in that at least two and perhaps four factors interact synergistically for optimal function. Furthermore, strong evidence of positive feedback control exists.

It is well established that megakaryocyte progenitor-derived colonies are best produced in short-term cultures that contain the plasma of patients rendered thrombogenic by aplasia. The activity is usually described as meg-CSA, and the search is on to define the factor or factors that contribute to the activity.[620] The plasma of patients with aplasia due to chemotherapy or marrow transplant conditioning also supports the long-term culture of CFU-MK.[621] Although normal human plasma contains little if any meg-CSA, the activity begins to rise immediately after ablative conditioning for marrow transplantation and peaks 3 weeks after the transplantation.[622] By the 30th day after transplantation, the activity has declined to baseline levels. Furthermore, the level of activity correlates with engraftment. Those with higher plasma activity have slower rates of engraftment, presumably because of persistent thrombocytopenia. Thus, growth factors (some of which circulate) undoubtedly must play an important role in the regulation of thrombopoiesis, and much effort has been directed toward their molecular identity.

As is true of erythrocyte colony formation, the conditioned medium derived from T cells can contribute important growth factor support to megakaryocyte colony formation.[623,624] It is well established that T cells are excellent sources of both GM-CSF and IL-3. Furthermore, recombinant murine GM-CSF promotes megakaryocyte colony formation, enhances the proliferation of megakaryocyte progenitors, and increases the size of megakaryocytes isolated from developing megakaryocyte colonies.[625] In this latter respect, GM-CSF has the functional characteristics of the so-called thrombopoiesis-stimulating factor, or TSF.[626] Yet, GM-CSF itself has no effect on circulating platelets in mice in vivo.[625] In addition to GM-CSF, IL-3 has also recently been shown to support megakaryocyte colony formation,[627,628] and human serum contains at least one other factor with meg-CSA.[629]

Long and coworkers,[628] who have demonstrated a role of either GM-CSF or IL-3 as meg-CSAs in human megakaryocyte colony formation, have evidence that a second synergistic factor is necessary to induce colony formation in concert with IL-3 or GM-CSF but that this second synergistic factor cannot act alone. This is exactly analogous to the requirement for either GM-CSF or IL-3 and EPO in in vitro erythropoiesis. Although Long and coworkers[628] did not examine possible synergy of IL-3 and GM-CSF in vitro, this synergy was detected in vivo; pretreatment of simians with IL-3 followed by a course of low-dose GM-CSF had a pronounced stimulating effect on platelet production.[630]

Erythropoietin and Megakaryopoiesis

For obvious clinical reasons, the second so-called synergistic factor might be EPO, because in situations in which EPO is elevated, thrombocytosis is frequently observed. The thrombocytosis regularly observed in Blackfan-Diamond anemia is an excellent example. Experimental attempts to find a physiologic role for EPO in platelet production have been in vain. High-affinity binding sites for EPO have been found on megakaryocytes (not on platelets)[631] and high concentrations of recombinant EPO promote both an increase in ACHE+ cells in serum-free cultures as well as an increase in megakaryocyte size[632] and megakaryocyte colony formation.[624,633]

The effect of EPO on megakaryocyte colony formation has been disputed,[634] and in vivo studies clearly demonstrate that only enormous doses of EPO actually stimulate platelet production in rodents.[635–637] In fact, physiologic doses of EPO induced by hypoxia have actually decreased the incidence of megakaryocyte colony-forming cells in the spleens and marrows of mice.[638] The latter experiment suggests an element of stem cell competition, but the evidence for that effect is also very weak. The best explanation for the role of EPO in platelet production probably lies in a weak interaction of EPO with the receptor for the second and more specific synergistic factor.

Thrombopoietin

If EPO is not the second synergistic factor (most would agree that it is not), thrombopoietin is certainly the leading candidate. It is believed that either GM-CSF or IL-3 (or another meg-CSF) drive the progenitor differentiation to the ACHE+ stage and beyond. This is exactly analogous to the relation between GM-CSF and IL-3 and EPO in the erythroid system.

Thrombopoietin has been a proposed factor for more than 30 years. Its biology, semipurification, and characterization have recently been reviewed by one of its leading investigators, McDonald.[639,640] A convenient assay of its activity was developed by Greenberg and associates[641] and Tayrien and Rosenberg,[642] who showed that megakaryocyte-stimulating factor (a protein with a molecular mass very close to that described by McDonald for thrombopoietin) markedly stimulates the incorporation of labeled amino acids into megakaryocyte-borne platelet factor 4.

Thrombopoietin enhances megakaryocyte ploidy in vitro,[643] and thrombopoietin is released by stimulated epidermal cells,[644] suggesting a mechanism by which inflammation causes thrombocytosis. Despite all this work (much of which is reviewed elsewhere[599,645,646]), the nature of thrombopoietin has remained elusive. Recently, it has been convincingly demonstrated that IL-6 has thrombopoietin-like activity and that this activity is enhanced by IL-1. IL-6 increases the activity of ACHE and, in the presence of IL-3, the number of megakaryocyte colonies in marrow cultures.[647] Furthermore, the sequence of the first 14 amino acids of IL-6 exactly matches the sequence of a thrombopoietin-like material released by a human lung fibroblast line. Lotem and coworkers[648] have developed a culture system in which they believe that IL-6 induces the formation of megakaryocyte colonies. In serum-free cultures, IL-6 together with IL-3 induces murine megakaryocyte colony formation, but neither is active alone.[649]

Finally, IL-6 or IL-11 administered to normal mice in vivo definitely (if transiently) stimulates platelet production.[650–652] Further studies of the effects of IL-3, IL-6, and Il-11 on simians with chemotherapy-induced thrombocytopenia are now needed to determine whether specific combinations may be useful in some of the persistent hemorrhagic states associated with depressed platelet production. But whether or not such preclinical trials are encouraging, interacting cytokines are clearly involved in megakaryocyte development.[653] None of them are megakaryocyte-specific. They are produced either by stromal cells themselves (GM-CSF, IL-6, and IL-11) or by the T cells embedded in stromal cells (IL-3), and they are aided and abetted by macrophage production of IL-1. If there is a megakaryocyte-specific growth factor, it is yet to be found.

Down-Regulation of Megakaryocytes

Great uncertainty exists about possible down-regulation of megakaryocytes. Platelet factor 4 seems to down-regulate colony formation in vitro, which, if active in vivo, would provide an interesting feedback loop.[654] Transforming growth factor β is also a potent inhibitor in vitro.[655] NK cells, thought by some (but not many) to be general suppressors of hematopoiesis in vitro, actually enhance megakaryocyte colony formation in vitro.[656] When an antibody to NK cells is given intraperitoneally in massive doses to mice, it abolishes the formation of colonies of megakaryocytes that can be grown in culture from murine marrow. This suggests that NK cells may actually play a stimulating role in vivo.[657] These interesting studies are subject to varying interpretations.

HEMATOPOIETIC GROWTH FACTORS IN VIVO

Correction or amelioration of marrow failure syndromes by administration of hematopoietic growth factor has been and continues to be the major goal of research in hematopoiesis. The goal could not be achieved until recombinant DNA technology provided sufficient amounts of the hormones to permit interpretable investigations.

Animal Studies

The discovery, cloning, and expression of the gene for murine multi-CSF or IL-3 presented the first opportunity to evaluate hematopoietic growth factors in an unambiguous fashion.[343,344] Sublethally irradiated mice were infused for 7 days with recombinant multi-CSF or with control protein.[658] The spleens of the multi-CSF–treated marrow recipients were much larger than those of the controls, were more cellular, and contained more progenitors. The increase in progenitor cells affected erythroid and myeloid lineages. In contrast, bone marrow cellularity was unaffected and progenitor content was reduced. Metcalf and colleagues[659] injected mice with purified bacterially synthesized IL-3 by the intraperitoneal route and obtained similar results. In addition, 10-fold increases in blood eosinophil and 2- to 3-fold increases in neutrophil and monocyte levels were observed. The intraperitoneal injections also resulted in 6- to 15-fold increases in peritoneal phagocytes with an increase in macrophage phagocytic activity.

These experiments clearly demonstrate that murine IL-3 influences the replication and growth potential of primitive hematopoietic progenitors and strongly suggest that whatever effect such hormones have on blood counts are related to their influences on progenitor function rather than to their effects on peripheral blood cell kinetics. They also suggest that the function of mature cells can be altered in vivo, an effect that would be expected to decrease rather than increase numbers of circulating phagocytes.

The first indications that human GM-CSF could broadly stimulate hematopoiesis in vivo resulted from studies of the infusion of COS cell–produced GM-CSF into cynomolgus macaques.[660] rhGM-CSF acts on simian progenitors. The disappearance curve of intravenously injected metabolically labeled factor was complex, suggesting a multicompartment turnover model, but the overall initial half-time of 15 to 20 minutes clearly demonstrated that infusion of the hormone at a concentration sufficient to maintain a functional blood level could be achieved.[660] The effects of such infusions into normal *Macaca fasicularis* were striking.

Large increments in all classes of leukocytes, including eosinophils and lymphocytes as well as reticulocytes, were observed during the hormone infusion. When the hormone treatment was terminated, blood counts rapidly fell toward normal. A particularly striking reticulocytosis was observed in an animal with an acquired retroviral infection that was associated with secondary pancytopenia and an elevated EPO level. This "preclinical" trial in a severely ill monkey encouraged the conclusion that GM-CSF plays an important therapeutic role in various cytopenias such as those observed in viral infections, including AIDS, or in autologous or allogeneic marrow transplantation.

The potential role of human recombinant GM-CSF in marrow transplantation was evaluated by the infusion of autologous marrow into rhesus monkeys (*Macaca mulatta*) 2 hours after lethal whole-body irradiation.[661] rhGM-CSF was administered at a daily dosage of 50 IU/min/kg continuously from 10 to 19 days before irradiation or from 9 to 17 days beginning 2 or 3 days after irradiation. Both dosage schedules produced the same final results, although the blood counts of the animals that received the hormone before radiation were much higher at the onset of radiation than those who received the hormone only after radiation. In five separate studies, granulocytes recovered to a level greater than 1000/μL in 9 days rather than the minimum of 17 days observed in two untreated control patients. In four of the five experiments, platelets recovered more rapidly as well.

Human G-CSF has also undergone simian preclinical trials. Cynomolgus monkeys treated with two daily subcutaneous injections of purified G-CSF for 14 to 28 days showed a dose-related increase in polymorphonuclear neutrophils, the plateau being reached after 1 week.[662] At the intermediate dose of 10 μg/kg/d, total white blood cell counts of 40,000 to 50,000/μL were observed. Neutrophil function was also enhanced. Encouraging results were also achieved in two cyclophosphamide-treated animals that received G-CSF either from 6 days before until 21 days after the cyclophosphamide treatment, or for 14 days from the third day after cyclophosphamide. In both monkeys, the neutrophil count increased dramatically by the 6th or 7th day after cyclophosphamide treatment, reaching levels of 50,000/μL by the 10th day. The control animal remained pancytopenic for 3 to 4 weeks after treatment.

Clinical Studies

Several recombinant hematopoietic growth factors are under evaluation in a variety of clinical settings. Largely because of availability, initial studies focused on GM-CSF and G-CSF in both transient and long-standing bone marrow failure syndromes, and EPO in the anemia of chronic renal failure. More recently, other hematopoietic growth factors such as M-CSF and, especially, IL-3 are coming under scrutiny. The availability of recombinant growth factors that stimulate myeloid progenitors raised several possibilities. For instance, they might shorten or prevent the hypoplasia that follows chemotherapy and make more intensive myeloablative chemotherapy regimens possible. Because GM-CSF and IL-3 receptors are expressed by several nonhematopoietic cell types, malignancies of these cell lineages might also respond to growth factor therapy. Table 8-2 summarizes results of several major published studies.

Malignant Disease

G-CSF

In the I/II clinical studies in patients with malignant disease, administration of G-CSF by bolus or continuous intravenous infusion for 5 to 6 days before chemotherapy led to a dose-related increase in polymorphonuclear neutrophils.[663] Rapid increases in neutrophil counts were observed, with maximal counts of 80,000 to 100,000/μL at doses of 10 to 30 mg/kg/d. A transient depression in neutrophil counts was noted to precede this increase in one study.[264] In another study, rhG-CSF was given for 14 days after alternate cycles of intensive chemotherapy.[664] The period of neutropenia was reduced by a median of 80% (52% to 100%) in the chemotherapy/G-CSF cycles, with a return to normal neutrophil counts within 2 weeks after chemotherapy. Infective episodes were observed during the cycles with chemotherapy that did not include G-CSF, whereas no infective episode occurred in those that did.[664] G-CSF treatment after chemotherapy results in a significant reduction in the number of days per patient in which the neutrophil count is less than 1000/μL.[663]

Antibiotic used for fever and neutropenia was also reduced, and all patients could receive their next course of chemotherapy on schedule (compared with 29% of patients who did not receive G-CSF). The mature neutrophils that were produced in response to G-CSF have normal mobility and bactericidal capacity.[665]

The effect of G-CSF on progenitor cells is interesting. After melphalan and G-CSF, the absolute number of *circulating* progenitor cells of the granulocyte-macrophage, erythroid, mixed, and megakaryocyte lineages showed a dose-related increase up to 100-fold after 4 days of treatment with recombinant human G-CSF (rhG-CSF),[666] confirming earlier animal studies.[667,668] The relative proportion of the early and late granulocyte progenitors and of early progenitors of different lineages remained unchanged; CFU-E, normally undetectable in blood, were markedly increased.

In most patients, a slight reduction in number of bone marrow progenitors was found, although this is difficult to interpret in view of the possibility of variable blood cell contamination of bone marrow samples. The mechanism for the increase in all progenitors in the blood is not clear. G-CSF has been shown to affect immature blast colony-forming cells, and stem cells are possibly stimulated in vivo to produce increased progenitors of all classes; alternatively, G-CSF may indirectly stimulate progenitors by induction of hematopoietic growth factor production or by release into the circulation of bone marrow progenitor cells.

GM-CSF

Recombinat human GM-CSF has been administered in phase I/II studies to several groups of patients with advanced malignancy both before and after chemotherapy.[669–671] Glycosylated GM-CSF produced in either mammalian (Chinese hamster ovary [CHO]) cells or yeast, and *Escherichia coli*–derived nonglycosylated GM-CSF have been evaluated with comparable results. A rapid, dose-related increase in polymorphonuclear neutrophils, monocytes, and eosinophils is observed in patients treated before chemotherapy. Neutrophils peak at around 20,000 to 30,000/μL at doses from 4 to 32 mg/kg/d and is well tolerated at doses up to this level. A capillary leak syndrome and venous thrombi are observed at higher doses (64 mg/kg/d).[671] GM-CSF given after chemotherapy is associated with shorter periods of neutropenia (3.5 versus 7.4 days) and higher leukocyte nadirs.

Like G-CSF, GM-CSF also produces an increase in blood progenitor cells of both erythroid and myeloid lineages. Before chemotherapy, an 18-fold increase in blood CFU-GM and an 8-fold increase in BFU-E was noted; after chemotherapy, GM-CSF produced a much greater increase of progenitors (60-fold) when given during the recovery period.[672]

IL-3

A phase I/II study of the effect of recombinant human IL-3 in patients with nonhematopoietic malignancies with normal marrow function, as well as lymphomas and bone marrow failure, has been reported.[673] Doses that ranged from 30 to 500 mg/m^2 were given for 15 days by daily subcutaneous injection. In the patients with normal hematopoiesis, a dose-dependent increase (1.4- to 3-fold) in neutrophils was observed, with the major increase during the second week. This contrasts with the rapid neutrophil response that has been the experience with GM-CSF or G-CSF. Platelets and eosinophils also increased in a dose-dependent fashion up to the dose of 250 mg/m^2 (1.3- to 1.9-fold), and increases in basophil and lymphocytes were noted. Increases in reticulocytes that did not appear to be dose-related were also observed in 70% of the patients. Similar results were observed in the patients with bone marrow failure but stimulation of malignant B cells was seen in two patients with lymphoma. Examination of the bone marrow showed increases in cycling of CFU-GEMM, BFU-E, and CFU-GM, with increased bone marrow cellularity.[674] An increase also occurred in circulating CFU-GEMM and CFU-GM, but a reduction in BFU-E was seen. In conclusion, results from this initial human IL-3 study indicate that IL-3 can induce a multilineage hematopoietic response.

M-CSF

Partially purified urinary M-CSF has been evaluated in patients with different malignancies who received myelotoxic chemotherapy. After treatment, patients received M-CSF for 5 days, and a modest increase in neutrophils was observed. Monocytes and other hematopoietic lineages were unaffected.[675]

Bone Marrow Transplantation

Patients with nonhematopoietic malignancies were treated with high-dose combination chemotherapy, autologous bone marrow transplantation, and rhGM-CSF given by continuous intravenous infusion for 14 days beginning 3 hours after bone marrow infusion. A dose-related increase in the neutrophil count was seen on the 14th day.[676] Although not statistically significant, an improved neutrophil response was found in patients who had not received previous chemotherapy compared with that of those who had (1832 versus 833/mL). Lower morbidity and mortality rates were also noted among the patients who received the GM-CSF; bacteremia occurred in 16% of treated patients compared with 35% of evaluable controls. Comparable results were reported in a study of patients with lymphoid malignancies who received rhGM-CSF as a 2-hour infusion daily for 14 days after chemotherapy, radiotherapy, and autologous bone marrow transplantation.[677] Neutrophil and platelet counts recovered more rapidly, fever lasted for fewer days, and the extent of hospitalization was reduced compared with an historical control group.

The response to GM-CSF after myelosuppression may be dependent on the infusion of sufficient progenitor cells. In an autotransplantation study of patients with acute lymphoblastic leukemia, bone marrows were purged with 4-hydroperoxycyclophosphamide and anti–T-cell or anti–B-cell lineage-specific antibodies before transplantation. Thirty percent of patients who received more than 64 μg/m^2/d achieved an absolute neutrophil count of more than 1000/μL by day 21, whereas none of the nonresponders reached this level by day 27 after transplantation. The responders required only one third as many platelet transfusions and showed a trend to fewer RBC transfusions, higher myeloid/erythroid ratio, and earlier day of discharge in the responder group as well. Although bone marrow cell dose did not differ among the two groups, the number of CFU-GM progenitors infused per kilogram was significantly higher in the responders compared with the nonresponders (17,500/kg [12,000 to 27,000/kg] compared with 2000/kg [0 to 7200/kg]). Although it is possible that this accounts for the more rapid recovery rather than the rhGM-CSF infusion, the responder group showed a rapid decrease in absolute neutrophil count within 48 to 72 hours of discontinuation of GM-CSF. This is consistent with a stimulatory effect on bone marrow. It can be concluded that GM-CSF is effective in this context, provided that sufficient progenitor cells are present.

rhG-CSF was evaluated in patients with hematopoietic and nonhematopoietic malignancies after intensive chemotherapy and reinfusion of cryopreserved autologous bone marrow.[679] The rhG-CSF was given by continuous intravenous infusion from 24 hours after marrow infusion for a maximum of 28 days, beginning at 20 μg/kg/d and reducing the dosage after the neutrophil count persistently exceeded 1000/μL. The mean time to neutrophil recovery (more than 500/μL) occurred by the 11th day, 9 days earlier than in historical controls. This led to significantly fewer days of parenteral antibiotic therapy, but no effect was seen on RBC or platelet recovery.

Although the rate of recovery from neutropenia was

TABLE 8-2. **Recombinant Human Hematopoietic Growth Factors In Vivo**

Factor	Patients	Administration	Response	Toxicity	Reference
CHEMOTHERAPY/MALIGNANCY					
GM-CSF	16 (sarcoma)	4–64 μg/kg/d before and after 1st cycle of chemotherapy	Increase in WBCs and PMNs; decrease in period of neutropenia (after chemotherapy) and higher nadirs	Well tolerated (occasional rash, fever) at 4–32 μg/kg/d; fluid retention, thrombi at 64 μg/kg/d	671
	30 (advanced carcinoma)	120–1000 $\mu g/m^2/d$ bolus or 24-h continuous IV infusion for 5–14 d	Rapid, sustained, dose-related increase in PMNs (2–17×); increased eosinophils and monocytes	Mild—myalgia, fever, nausea, bone pain	669
	20 (advanced carcinoma)	0.3–60 μg/kg/d, 30 min IV for 10 d (2 courses)	Dose-related increase in WBCs (up to 4×); increase in PMNs and eosinophils at ≥10 μg	Severe—capillary leaks, pulmonary embolus at 60 μg/kg/d	670
G-CSF	27	1–60 μg/kg/d IV before or during chemotherapy	Dose-related increase in PMNs (up to 10×); no or shorter period of neutropenia	Bone pain at time of administration	663
	15	1–60 μg/kg/d IV before or after melphalan, 5 d	Dose-dependent increase in PMNs (before chemotherapy); dose-dependent decrease in neutropenia (after chemotherapy)		264
	12	1–40 μg/kg/d, continuous IV infusion	Rapid dose-dependent increase in PMNs; decrease in period of neutropenia		664
M-CSF	24	$2–4 \times 10^6$ U/d, 5 d	Modest increase in PMNs		675
BONE MARROW TRANSPLANTATION (BMT)					
GM-CSF	19 (breast cancer or melanoma; combination chemotherapy → autologous BMT)	2–32 μg/kg/d, continuous IV infusion for 14 d	Total WBCs and PMNs higher at 14 d compared with historical controls	Mild up to 16 μg/kg/d; fluid retention and myalgia at 32 μg/kg/d; decrease in migration of PMNs	676
	15 (lymphoma; chemotherapy → autologous or syngeneic BMT)	15–240 $\mu g/m^2/d$, 2-h IV infusions for 14 d	More rapid recovery of PMNs and decreased period of neutropenia at ≥60 $\mu g/m^2/d$ compared with historical controls	Minimal—cramps, fever	677
	25 (ALL; autologous purged BMT)	16–256 $\mu g/m^2/d$, 1–2 h IV infusions for 14–21 d → autologous purged BMT	More rapid recovery of PMNs at ≥64 $\mu g/m^2/d$; correlated with CFU-GM content infused	Mild—nausea, cramps, fever, deep vein thromboses	678
G-CSF	15 (nonhematopoietic malignancies; chemotherapy → autologous BMT)	20 μg/kg/d; continuous SC infusion up to 28 d; dose adjusted to PMN response	>500/μL PMNs at 11 d (vs 20 d for controls); fewer days on antibiotics		679
M-CSF	51 (allogeneic and autologous BMT)		Slight decrease in time to PMN recovery		681

(continued)

TABLE 8-2. *(Continued)*

Factor	Patients	Administration	Response	Toxicity	Reference
MYELODYSPLASIA					
GM-CSF	8	30–500 μg/m²/d, continuous IV infusion for 14 d (2 courses)	Increase in WBCs (5–70×), PMNs (5–373×), platelets (3 of 8), reticulocytes, lymphocytes, monocytes, eosinophils; decrease in blasts	Mild bone pain, fever, myalgia	682
	7	15–480 μg/m²/d, bolus IV	Increase (5 of 7) in PMNs, monocytes, and reticulocytes	Increase in blasts during treatment	683
	11	15–150 μg/m²/d, continuous IV infusion for 7–14 d (2 courses)	Dose-dependent increase in WBCs (10 of 11; 1.3–18×); increase in monocytes, eosinophils, and lymphocytes; no increase in platelets or reticulocytes	Increase in blasts in RAEB (4 of 5); proliferation and differentiation of leukemic clone	684
	16	0.3–10 μg/kg/d SC	Dose-related increase in PMNs, monocytes, eosinophils	RAEB-T; 1 of 16 progressed to refractory ANLL	685
G-CSF	5 (4 MDS, 1 SMML)	5–1600 μg/m²/d, IV infusion for 6 d	Increase in PMNs		686
	12	Twice-weekly dose escalation 0.1–3 μg/kg/d SC for 8 wk	Increase in WBCs (10 of 12; 2–10×), PMNs (5–40×), reticulocytes (5 of 12); decrease in transfusion requirement (5 of 12)	Minimal—nausea, anorexia, worsening of psoriasis (1 of 12)	687
APLASTIC ANEMIA					
GM-CSF	8	15–480 μg/m²/d for 7 or 14 d	Modest increase (6 of 8) in PMNs, monocytes, and reticulocytes	Minimal—bone pain, anorexia, myalgia	683
	11	4–64 μg/kg/d, continuous IV for 28 d; dose-escalating cohort study	Partial or complete increase (10 of 11) in PMNs, eosinophils, and monocytes; increase (1 of 11) in RBCs and platelets	Minimal—fatigue, myalgia	688
	9	8–32 μg/kg/d continuous IV for 28 d; dose-escalating cohort study	Increase in PMNs (6 of 8; 2.5–31×); trilineage response (1 of 8)	Minimal—fever, rash	690

CSF; colony-stimulating factor; GM-CSF, granulocyte-macrophage CSF; G-CSF, granulocyte CSF; M-CSF, monocyte CSF; IV, intravenous; SC, subcutaneous; WBC, white blood cell; RBC, red blood cell; PMN, polymorphonuclear neutrophil; RAEB, refractory anemia with an excess of blasts; RAEB-T, RAEB in transformation; MDS, myelodysplastic syndrome; SMML, subacute myelomonocytic leukemia; ALL, acute lymphocytic leukemia; ANLL, acute nonlymphocytic leukemia.

faster than that reported for rhGM-CSF, the latter studies were phase I dose-escalation evaluations, and many patients did not receive an optimal dose of GM-CSF. A recent study compared G-CSF with GM-CSF in exactly the same autologous bone marrow transplantation protocol, and a major difference was observed with respect to neutrophil migration to an inflammatory site during CSF infusion after hematopoietic reconstitution.[680] Neutrophils did not migrate to skin chambers filled with autologous serum during GM-CSF treatment, a defect not encountered during the administration of G-CSF. A similar reduction occurred in the incidence of bacteremia with both GM-CSF and G-CSF (18% and 19%, respectively) compared with the historical controls (35%).

In conclusion, if neutrophil recovery is the goal after bone marrow transplantation, G-CSF appears to be the factor of choice. It preserves neutrophil function and is well tolerated. The inability to hasten platelet recovery is still the major challenge.

Human urinary M-CSF has been evaluated in a phase II study of patients with different malignancies who received cyclophosphamide, whole-body irradiation, and either allogeneic or autologous bone marrow.[681] Human urinary CSF was given for 14 days by 2-hour intravenous infusion daily starting at the first, fourth, or fourteenth day. In patients who received CSF early, a significant reduction occurred in the time to a neutrophil count more of than 1000/μL when compared with a control group (16.7 versus 25.4 days). The time to recovery of the control group is somewhat delayed compared with that found in other reports (17 to 21 days).

Myelodysplasia

GM-CSF

Despite the theoretical risks of treating patients with myeloid stem cell clonal diseases with the CSFs, the factors have been evaluated in patients with refractory anemia (RA), RA with an excess of blasts (RAEB), RAEB in transformation (RAEBIT), and chronic myelomonocytic leukemia.[682–684] In an early study, GM-CSF was given by continuous infusion for 14 days, and repeated after a 2-week rest period.[682] Five of the eight patients had received chemotherapy up to 4 weeks before study. Doses of 30 to 500 μg/m^2 were used. Blood leukocytes rose 5- to 70-fold and neutrophils 5- to 373-fold, and an absolute increase in monocytes, eosinophils, and lymphocytes was also observed. Three of the eight patients also had a 2- to 10-fold increase in platelet count and improvement in erythropoiesis, and two of the three became transfusion-independent. Marrow cellularity increased and a reduction in the proportion of blasts occurred, although there was a transient and dose-related increase in the absolute number of circulating blasts. No patient developed overt leukemia during the period of follow-up (up to 32 weeks). No cytogenetic evidence was found for a reduction in abnormal clones, and it is likely that the stimulatory effect on hematopoiesis affects both normal and abnormal cells.

A dose-related increase in neutrophils, monocytes, eosinophils, and lymphocytes was also noted in studies of 11 and 16 patients with myelodysplasia.[685] Four patients who presented with more than 14% of blasts in the bone marrow showed an increase in blasts after therapy, whereas an additional three patients showed an increase in blasts in the blood. Five patients progressed to acute leukemia either during or within 4 weeks after treatment.[684] Unlike the earlier report, none of these patients had received previous chemotherapy.[682] In the other study,[685] one patient with RAEBIT progressed to refractory acute nonlymphoblastic leukemia. Furthermore, the response to GM-CSF was not sustained in four of five patients who went on to maintenance treatment.

G-CSF

A few patients have also been treated with G-CSF.[686] Neutrophil responses were seen in five patients with myelodysplasia who received 50 to 1600 μg/m^2/d by 30-minute infusion daily for 6 days. At the higher doses (400 μg/m^2/d), the increase was sustained and associated with an increase in bone marrow cellularity. No reticulocyte or platelet increases were observed, and no patient progressed to an acute phase. Similar results were reported in a study of 12 patients given G-CSF by daily subcutaneous injection, with dose escalation from 0.1 to 3 μg/kg/d over an 8-week period.[687] Although 10 of the 12 patients showed elevations in neutrophils (5- to 40-fold), an increase in reticulocytes occurred in five patients with reduction in transfusion requirement in two. No response in other cell lineages and no conversion to acute leukemia was seen.

Aplastic Anemia

Establishing a role for the CSFs in aplastic anemia will provide investigators with more of a challenge. Severe aplastic anemia is a heterogeneous disease, which may result from either absent or defective stem cells, from microenvironmental defects or from immunologically mediated suppression. Mortality rate is high and therapeutic options are limited to bone marrow transplantation if an appropriate donor is available, or to immunosuppression (see Chaps. 9 and 10). Although bone marrow transplantation can be curative, treatment with antithymocyte globulin (ATG) is sometimes effective but generally not curative. Other modalities such as administration of cyclosporin A and androgens may be partially effective in some patients. For these reasons, rhGM-CSF has been evaluated in a number of phase I/II studies. Administration of rhGM-CSF by bolus or continuous intravenous infusion for 7 or 14 days resulted in increased granulocytes, monocytes, and reticulocytes in six of eight patients.[688]

In another small study, rhGM-CSF was given to cohorts of patients in escalating doses from 4 to 64 μg/kg/d by continuous intravenous infusion for 14 days.[689] Although a dose-related effect was not observed, 10 of 11 evaluable patients had partial or complete responses in neutrophils, monocytes, and eosinophils, with increases in bone marrow cellularity. It is important that the greatest increments occurred in patients with higher pretreatment neutrophil counts and more cellular marrows. Only 10% to 20% of patients show an increase in hemoglobin concentration and platelet count, and in all cases counts return to baseline after cessation of treatment.[688,689] In the first report of rhGM-CSF treatment in childhood, 75% of evaluable patients responded with a significant rise in neutrophil count during the 28-day induction period.[690] Although neutrophil counts returned to baseline after cessation of treatment in all the responders with severe aplastic anemia, one patient with moderate aplasia maintained a trilineage response off therapy for more than 1 year. One cannot extrapolate from such a small experience, but the data underscore the point that responses are more likely in less severely affected patients.

In summation, it appears that rhGM-CSF is palliative in patients with aplastic anemia, with greater neutrophil responses evident in less severely affected patients. The most severely affected patients respond poorly.[691] No infections were observed during the study period in several reports, whereas infections were observed in others. Longer-term prospective comparative studies are necessary to investigate morbidity rate.

Human Immunodeficiency Virus Infection

Human immunodeficiency virus (HIV) infection is associated with several hematologic abnormalities including neutropenia. Anemia and neutropenia can be exacerbated by treatment with zidovudine, and rhGM-CSF has been evaluated in an effort to enhance immunologic and hematopoietic function and to improve tolerance to therapeutic agents. In the first report of the use of rhGM-CSF in humans, cohorts of AIDS patients were treated with increasing doses of factor given by continuous intravenous infusion for 14 days.[692] This resulted in a rapid, dose-related increase in neutrophils, bands, and eosinophils, with a slight increase in monocytes. A follow-up study with subcutaneous administration showed that these effects could be sustained for up to 6 months without evidence of tachyphylaxis.[693]

A concern with the use of GM-CSF in AIDS is possible enhancement of HIV replication. In one study of zidovudine given on an alternate-week schedule with GM-CSF, some patients showed increased viral p24 levels during therapy with GM-CSF. Evidence exists that GM-CSF may in fact augment zidovudine levels in monocytes, which suggests that the combination of zidovudine and GM-CSF might be advantageous.[694]

Neutropenia

Severe congenital neutropenia or Kostmann's syndrome (see also Chap. 17) is a disorder of myelopoiesis characterized by impaired neutrophil differentiation and absolute neutrophil counts of less than 200/μL. In contrast, monocytes and eosinophil are normal or increased. The bone marrow shows maturation arrest at the promyelocyte stage, and these cells are often atypical with abnormal nuclei and vacuolated cytoplasm. The pathophysiology is uncertain. Reduced production or abnormal G-CSF is possible but unlikely in view of recent data that show that serum from these patients contains normal or elevated levels of G-CSF, as determined by Western blot and bioassay.[695] A progenitor defect is more likely, since in vitro cultures show normal CFU-Ms and CFU-Eos but impaired differentiation of CFU-Gs in the presence of either GM-CSF or G-CSF. Another possibility is that the GM-CSF or G-CSF receptor is abnormal. The responses of these patients to exogenous G-CSF and GM-CSF are therefore of great interest.

One study has compared the effects of GM-CSF and G-CSF in a small number of patients, and G-CSF alone was evaluated in an earlier study.[696,697] In both investigations *G-CSF produced a remarkable increase in neutrophils in all patients.* The dose necessary to maintain a neutrophil count of more than 1000/μL varied, and ranged from 3 to 15 μg/kg/d. The monocyte count was also increased. In contrast, rhGM-CSF produced an increase in neutrophils in only one patient, whereas the other patients showed an increase in eosinophils and monocytes. Although the period on study was short, no new episodes of severe bacterial infection occurred during either GM-CSF or G-CSF treatment; this contrasts with the recurrent bacterial and fungal infections that occurred before treatment.

Cyclic neutropenia (see also Chap. 17) is a rare hematopoietic stem cell disease characterized by regular 21-day cyclic fluctuations in numbers of neutrophils, monocytes, eosinophils, lymphocytes, platelets, and reticulocytes. Patients typically have recurrent episodes of fever, malaise, mucosal ulceration, and, occasionally, life-threatening infection during periods of neutropenia. Six patients were treated with intravenous or subcutaneous rhG-CSF for 3 to 15 months at doses ranging from 3 to 10 μg/kg/d.[698] The median neutrophil count increased from 700 to 9800/μL. In five patients, cycling of blood counts continued, but the length of cycles decreased from 21 to 14 days. The number of days of severe neutropenia (less than 200/μL) was reduced from a mean of 12.7 per month to less than one per month and the nadir counts increased; neutrophil turnover increased almost 4-fold; and migration to a skin window was normal. Average counts of other cells did not increase. One patient with disease of adult onset had a qualitatively different response with an increase in neutrophils and disappearance of the cyclic fluctuations in count. Therapy reduced the incidence of oropharyngeal inflammation, fever, and infections, demonstrating that treatment with recombinat human G-CSF is effective management for such patients.

Chronic idiopathic neutropenia is a disorder of myelopoiesis characterized by maturation arrest of neutrophil precursors in the bone marrow, neutrophil counts of fewer than 1500/μL, and normal other cell lineages. Patients have mucosal ulcers, periodontal disease, and recurrent infections. The pathophysiology is uncertain; in vitro bone marrow culture shows normal numbers of myeloid progenitors; and antineutrophil antibodies are absent. A single patient who received 1 to 3 μg/kg/d rhG-CSF by subcutaneous injection showed normalization of the absolute neutrophil count with healing of chronic oral ulceration, reduction of episodes of recurrent infection, and minimal side effects.[699] Cycling of neutrophils, monocytes, and platelets was induced with a 40-day periodicity. This contrasts with the normal 21-day cycle and out-of-phase fluctuation of neutrophils and monocytes seen in cyclic neutropenia.

Toxicity

The CSFs tested in all these clinical trials have in general been well tolerated. Both GM-CSF and G-CSF induce a transient leukopenia in the first 30 minutes after administration by intravenous bolus injection. GM-CSF rapidly induces surface expression of the leukocyte adhesion protein CD11b (Mo1) in vitro, and this is accompanied by an increase in neutrophil aggregation.[581] CD11a (LFA-1) and CD11c (gp 150, 95), two other members of this family of cell surface adhesion glycoproteins that have distinct α chains but share a common β chain (CD18) with CD11b, are unaffected by GM-CSF. These results have been corroborated by in vivo studies of sarcoma patients who received 32 or 64 g/kg/d GM-CSF. A marked increase of CD11b was evident by 30 minutes after administration and persisted for 12 to 24 hours after treatment was terminated.[700] Radionuclide-labeled leukocytes are sequestered in the lungs after GM-CSF treatment, probably because of the aggregability and adhesiveness induced by increased CD11b expression.[701] Breathlessness and hypoxia have been observed in some patients, particularly after short-duration intravenous administration. CD11b is not modulated by G-CSF, and the reason for the transient leukopenia after treatment with G-CSF is not clear.

Both GM-CSF and G-CSF have been associated with bone pain coincident with or shortly after administration. Occasional increases in leukocyte alkaline phosphatase or lactate dehydrogenase have been noted. GM-CSF has also induced flu-like symptoms, including fever, flushing, malaise, myalgia, arthralgia, anorexia, and headache. Mild elevations of transaminase levels and rash are also reported. These effects are usually mild, are alleviated by antipyretics, and usually disappear with continued drug administration. More serious GM-CSF toxicity has been observed at higher dose levels (more than 32 μg/kg/d intravenously or more than 15 μg/kg/d subcutaneously). These include a capillary leak syndrome with weight gain due to fluid retention, manifested as pericardial or pleural effusions, ascites, or edema.[671,676] Phlebitis was noted in initial studies when the GM-CSF was infused into small veins, and large-vessel thrombosis has occurred with infusion of high doses into central veins.[671]

Antibodies to Recombinant Factors

Recombinant human GM-CSF that is produced in mammalian cells (CHO cells) is variably glycosylated on both O- and N-linked sites. Production in *E coli* results in nonglycosylated GM-CSF, and the yeast product is glycosylated at N-linked sites. All three products appear to be equally effective, but antibodies have been reported in 4 of 13 patients given the yeast-derived product in phase I/II studies.[702] These IgG antibodies developed by 7 days after infusion in all four patients, three of whom had received a bolus test dose. The antibodies were nonneutralizing as judged by bone marrow colony-forming assay and were directed at sites on the protein backbone of the GM-CSF molecule that are normally protected by O-linked glycosylation but are exposed in the yeast and *E coli*–derived products. No dose-limiting toxicity has been observed with G-CSF.

One case of pathogenic neutrophil infiltration (acute febrile neutrophilic dermatosis or Sweet's syndrome) has been reported.[703] One patient with Kostmann's syndrome developed cutaneous necrotizing vasculitis (leukoclastic vasculitis) while on G-CSF treatment.[696]

Fever is the most common side effect associated with

administration of human urinary M-CSF.[675,681] Malaise and headache and slight depression of blood pressure have also been observed.

Erythropoietin

Anemia is a major complication of end-stage renal failure and is primarily caused by a reduction in EPO production. Other mechanisms that may be involved are shortened RBC survival, iron deficiency, hypersplenism, possible circulating inhibitors of erythropoiesis, and aluminum-induced microcytosis. Several phase I, II, and III studies have documented that rhEPO can induce a dose-dependent increase in effective erythropoiesis.[704–706]

In a phase III study, patients received 150 or 300 IU rhEPO three times per week after hemodialysis and reached a target hematocrit of 35% by 8 to 12 weeks.[705] Most patients required 50 to 125 IU/kg intravenously three times per week after dialysis to maintain a hematocrit of less than 35%. The increase in erythropoiesis required to normalize the hemoglobin requires mobilization of a considerable amount of iron; patients who improve, especially those who improve rapidly, can develop absolute or relative iron deficiency. If iron is not given, the response to rhEPO becomes blunted; the standard corrective measure is intravenous administration of iron dextran or oral iron supplementation. Regular measurements of ferritin and transferrin saturation are necessary to ensure that iron stores are adequate.

EPO has been well tolerated, has resulted in elimination of transfusion dependency, and has not led to antibody formation. Hypertension, occasionally with encephalopathy, has been observed, particularly with rapid rises in hematocrit that lead to an increase in peripheral vascular resistance; induction with doses not to exceed 150 IU/kg is recommended to produce a gradual increase in hemoglobin levels. Some patients require either the initiation of antihypertensive medication or an adjustment of dose.

The effect of rhEPO in most studies appears to be restricted to the erythroid lineage. A phase III study of 303 patients showed a significant increase in mean platelet count (224,000 to 241,000/μL at 6 months), which is not biologically meaningful.[705] Also, slight increases occur in blood urea nitrogen, creatinine, and serum potassium levels. The bone marrow progenitors from patients with end-stage renal failure were studied before and 2 weeks after rhEPO treatment. The concentration of BFU-E, CFU-E, and CFU-MK increased after therapy. It is surprising that an increment in CFU-GM also occurred, and the number of progenitors of all classes in the cell cycle almost doubled.[707] Subjective improvement in appetite, energy, sleep pattern, and libido is also noted. A Canadian double-blind placebo-controlled study of rhEPO treatment has provided objective evidence of benefit.[708]

Extending this treatment to patients who do not yet require dialysis has met with similar success.[709] An issue that has yet to be resolved is financial; rhEPO is not inexpensive, and the National Kidney Foundation in the United States has issued guidelines for the use of rhEPO in which all patients with hematocrits of less than 30% are eligible. rhEPO is more effective when administered by the subcutaneous route. This is more convenient for patients and also allows a dose reduction. In predialysis patients, 100 IU/kg administered subcutaneously provided a similar response to 150 IU/kg given intravenously.[710,711] Evidence suggests that the bioavailability of subcutaneous EPO is seven times greater than that of the intravenously administered drug.

Preliminary data suggest that rhEPO may be useful in the treatment of patients with the anemia of chronic disease associated with rheumatoid arthritis,[712] the anemia that complicates zidovudine treatment in patients with AIDS,[713] and possibly the anemia of prematurity.[75,76]

In simian studies, hemoglobin F levels can be increased by administration of EPO.[714] If similar changes occur in humans, EPO may have a role in the management of sickle cell anemia and thalassemia. Finally, EPO can be used to increase the number of units of blood that can be obtained preoperatively in the context of autologous blood donation.[715]

REFERENCES

1. Till JE, McCulloch EA. A direct measurement of the radiation sensitivity of normal mouse bone marrow cells. Rad Res 1961;14:213.
2. Pluznik DH, Sachs L. The cloning of normal "mast" cells in tissue cultures. J Cell Comp Physiol 1965;66:319.
3. Bradley TR, Metcalf D. The growth of mouse bone marrow cells *in vitro*. Aust J Exp Biol Med Sci 1966;44:287.
4. Clark SC, Kamen R. The human hematopoietic colony-stimulating factors. Science 1987;236:1229.
5. Metcalf D. The molecular biology and functions of the granulocyte-macrophage colony-stimulating factors. Blood 1986;67:257.
6. Dexter TM, Allen TD, Lajtha LG. Conditions controlling the proliferation of haemopoietic stem cells *in vitro*. J Cell Physiol 1977;91:335.
7. Botnick LE, Hannon EC, Hellman S. Nature of the hematopoietic stem cell compartment and its proliferative potential. Blood Cells 1979;5:195.
8. Tyan ML. Studies on the ontogeny of the mouse immune system. I. Cell bound immunity. J Immunol 1968;100:535.
9. Moore MAS, Metcalf D. Ontogeny of the haemopoietic system: yolk sac origin of *in vivo* and *in vitro* colony forming cells in the developing mouse embryo. Br J Haematol 1970;18:279.
10. Miura Y, Wilt FH. Tissue interaction and the formation of the first erythroblasts of the chick embryo. Devel Biol 1969:19:201.
11. Haar JL, Ackerman GA. A phase and electron microscopic study of vasculogenesis and erythropoiesis in the yolk sac of the mouse. Anatom Rec 1970;170:199.
12. Edmonds RH. Areas of attachment between developing blood cells. J Ultrastruct Res 1964;11:577.
13. Edmunds RH. Electron microscopy of erythropoiesis in the avian yolk sac. Anat Rec 1966;154:785.
14. Russel ES, Bernstein SE. Blood and blood formation. In: Green EL, ed. Biology of the laboratory mouse. New York, McGraw-Hill, 1966:351.
15. Barker JE. Development of the mouse hematopoietic system. I. Types of hemoglobin produced in embryonic yolk sac and liver. Dev Biol 1968;18:14.
16. Kelemen E, Calvo W, Fliedner TM. Atlas of human hematopoietic development. Berlin, Springer-Verlag, 1979.
17. Roodman GD, Zanjani ED. Endogenous erythroid colony forming cells in fetal and newborn sheep. J Lab Clin Med 1979;94:699.
18. Rich IN, Kubanek B. The autogeny of erythropoiesis in mouse detected by the erythroid colony-forming technique. II. Transition on erythropoietin sensitivity during development. J Embryol Exp Morphol 1980;58:143.
19. Peschel C, Migliaccio AR, Migliaccio G, et al. Identification and characterization of three classes of erythroid progenitors in human fetal liver. Blood 1981;58:565.
20. Block M. An experimental analysis of hematopoiesis in the rat yolk sac. Anat Rec 1946;96:289.
21. Bethlenfalvay NC, Block M. Fetal erythropoiesis: maturation in megaloblastic (yolk sac) erythropoiesis in the C57Bl/6J mouse. Acta Haematol 1970;44:240.
22. Weinberg S, Stohlman F Jr. Growth of mouse yolk sac cells cultured *in vitro*. Br J Haematol 1976;32:543.
23. Weinberg SR, Stohlman F Jr. Factors regulating yolk sac hematopoiesis in diffusion chambers: various types of sera, cyclophosphamide, irradiation and long-term culture. Exp Hematol 1977;5:374.
24. Micklem HS, Ford CE, Evans EP, Ogden DA, Papworth DS. Competitive *in vivo* proliferation of fetal and adult hematopoietic cells in lethally irradiated mice. J Cell Physiol 1972;79:293.
25. Weissman I, Papaioannou V, Gardner R. Fetal hematopoietic origins of the adult hematolymphoid system. In: Differentiation of normal and neoplastic hematopoietic cells. Cold Spring Harbor, NY, Cold Spring Harbor Laboratory, 1978:33.
26. Moore, MAS, Owen JJT. Hypothesis: stem-cell migration in developing myeloid and lymphoid systems. Lancet 1967;1:658.
27. Dieterlen-lievre F. On the origin of haemopoietic stem cells in the avian embryo: an experimental approach. J Embryol Exp Morphol 1975;33:607.
28. Hollyfield JG. The origin of erythroblasts in *Rana pipiens* tadpoles. Dev Biol 1966;14:461.
29. Linch DC, Brent L. Marrow transplantation: can cord blood be used? Nature 1989;340:676.

30. Gluckman E, Broxmeyer HA, Auerbach AD, et al. Hematopoietic reconstitution in a patient with Fanconi's anemia by means of umbilical-cord blood from an HLA-identical sibling. N Engl J Med 1989;321:1174.
31. Broxmeyer HE, Douglas GW, Hangoc G, et al. Human umbilical cord blood as a potential source of transplantable hematopoietic stem/progenitor cells. Proc Natl Acad Sci USA 1989;86:3828.
32. Thomas DB, Yoffey JM. Human foetal haematopoiesis. Br J Haematol 1964;10:193.
33. Rifkind RA, Chui D, Epler H. An ultrastructural study of early morphogenetic events during the establishment of foetal hepatic erythropoiesis. J Cell Biol 1969;40:343.
34. Jones RO. Ultrastructursal analysis of hepatic haematopoiesis in the foetal mouse. J Anat 1970;107:301.
35. Hahn IM, Bodger MP, Hoffbrand AV. Development of pluripotent hematopoietic progenitor cells in the human fetus. Blood 1983;62:118.
36. Slaper-Cortenback I, Ploemacher R, Lowenberg B. Different stimulative effects of human bone marrow and fetal liver stromal cells on erythropoiesis in long-term culture. Blood 1987;69:135.
37. Migliaccio AR, Migliaccio G. Human embryonic hemopoiesis: control mechanisms underlying progenitor differentiation *in vitro*. Dev Biol 1988;125:127.
38. Barak Y, Karov Y, Levin S, et al. Granulocyte-macrophage colonies in cultures of human fetal liver cells: morphologic and ultrastructural analysis of proliferation and differentiation. Exp Hematol 1980;8:837.
39. Symann M, Quesenberry P, Fontebuoni A, Stohlman F Jr. Fetal hemopoiesis in diffusion chamber cultures. II. Cell proliferation and differentiation. Nouv Rev Fr Hematol 1976;16:321.
40. Ackerman GA, Grasso JA, Knouff RA. Erythropoiesis in the mammalian embryonic liver as revealed by electron microscopy. Lab Invest 1961;10:787.
41. Grasso JA, Swift H, Ackerman GA. Observations on the development of erythrocytes in mammalian fetal liver. J Cell Biol 1962;14:235.
42. Marsh WL. Anti-i: a cold antibody defining the Ii relationship in human red cells. Br J Haematol 1961;7:200.
43. Weatherall DJ, McIntyre PA. Developmental and acquired variations in erythrocyte carbonic anhydrase isozymes. Br J Haematol 1967;13:106.
44. Medlock ES, Haar JL. The liver hemopoietic environment. I. Developing hepatocytes and their role in fetal hemopoiesis. Anat Rec 1983;207:31.
45. Medlock ES, Landreth KS, Kincade PW. Putative B lymphocyte lineage precursor cells in early murine embryos. Dev Comp Immunol 1984;8:887.
46. Denis KA, Treiman LJ, St Claire JI, Witte ON. Long-term cultures of murine fetal liver retain very early B lymphoid phenotype. J Exp Med 1984;160:1087.
47. Craig ML, Russell EL. A developmental change in hemoglobins correlated with an embroyonic red cell population in the mouse. Dev Biol 1964;10:191.
48. Karlsson S, Nienhuis AW. Developmental regulation of human globin genes. Ann Rev Biochem 1985;54:1071.
49. Rosenberg M. Fetal hematopoiesis: case report. Blood 1969;33:66.
50. Metcalf D, Moore MAS. Embryonic aspects of haemopoiesis. In: Neuberger A, Tatum EL, eds. Frontiers of biology. Amsterdam, North Holland, 1971:172.
51. Hudson G. Bone-marrow volume in the human foetus and newborn. Br J Haematol 1965;11:446.
52. Custer RP, Ahlfeldt FE. Studies on the structure and function of bone marrow. II. Variations in cellularity in various bones with advancing years of life and their relative response to stimuli. J Lab Clin Med 1932;17:960.
53. Garby L, Sjolin S, Viulle JC. Studies on erythrokinetics in infancy. III. Disappearance from plasma and red cell uptake of radioactive iron injected intravenously. Acta Paediatr 1963;52:537.
54. Glaser K, Limarzi LR, Poncher HG. Cellular composition of the bone marrow in normal infants and children. Pediatrie 1950;6:789.
55. Siep M. The reticulocyte level and the erythrocyte production judged from reticulocyte studies in newborn infants during the first week of life. Acta Paediatr 1955;44:355.
56. Sturgeon P. Volumetric and microscopic pattern of bone marrow in normal infants and children. II. Cytologic pattern. Pediatrie 1951;7:642.
57. Pearson HA. Life-span of the fetal red blood cell. J Pediatr 1967;70:166.
58. Delivoria-Papadopoulos M, Roncevic NP, Oski FA. Postnatal changes in oxygen transport of term, premature, and sick infants: the role of red cell 2,3-diphosphoglycerate and adult hemoglobin. Pediatr Res 1971;5:235.
59. Bunn HF, Kitchen H. Hemoglobin function in the horse. The role of 2,3-diphosphoglycerate in modifying the oxygen affinity of maternal and fetal blood. Blood 1973;42:471.
60. Dhindsa DA, Hoversland AS, Templeton JW. Postnatal changes in oxygen affinity and concentrations of 2,3-diphosphoglycerate in dog blood. Biol Neonate 1972;20:226.
61. Bunn BG, Forget HF. Animal hemoglobins. In: Dyson J, ed. Hemoglobin: molecular, genetic and clinical aspects. Philadelphia, WB Saunders, 1986:126.
62. Huehns ER, Beaven GH. Developmental changes in human hemoglobins. Clin Dev Med 1971;37:175.
63. Dover GJ, Boyer SH, Bell WR. Microscopic method for assaying F cell production: illustrative changes during infancy and in aplastic anemia. Blood 1978;52:664.
64. Collins FS, Boehm CD, Waber PG, et al. Concordance of a point mutation 5′ to the ^{G}gamma globin gene with ^{G}gamma β^{+} hereditary persistence of fetal hemoglobin in the black population. Blood 1984;64:1292.
65. Gilman JG, Huisman THJ. DNA sequence variation associated with elevated fetal ^{G}gamma-globin production. Blood 1985;66:783.
66. Collins FS, Metherall JE, Yamakawa M, Pan J, Weissman SM, Forget BG. A point mutation in the ^{A}gamma-globin gene promoter in Greek hereditary persistence of fetal haemoglobin. Nature 1985;313:325.
67. Gelinas R, Endlich B, Pfeiffer C, Yagi M, Stamatoyannopoulos G. G to A substitution at the distal CCAAT box of the ^{A}gamma-globin gene in Greek hereditary persistence of foetal haemoglobin. Nature 1985;313:323.
68. Giglioni B, Casini C, Mantovani R, et al. A molecular study of a family with Greek hereditary persistence of fetal hemoglogin and β-thalassemia. EMBO 1984;3:2641.
69. Oski FA. Clinical implications of the oxyhemoglobin dissociation curve in the neonatal period. Crit Care Med 1979;7:412.
70. Halvorsen S. Plasma erythropoietic levels in cord blood and in blood during the first week of life. Acta Paediatr Scand 1963;52:425.
71. Gilmour JR. Erythroblastosis fetalis. Arch Dis Child 1944;19:1.
72. Ross MP, Christensen RD, Rothstein G, et al. A randomized trial to develop criteria for administering erythrocyte transfusions to anemic preterm infants 1 to 3 months of age. J Perinatol 1989;9:246.
73. Stockman JA III, Graeber JE, Clark DA, McClellam K, Garcia JF, Kavey REW. Anemia of prematurity: determinants of the erythropoietin response. J Pediatr 1984;105:786.
74. Brown MS, Garcia JF, Phibbs RH, Dallman PR. Decreased response of plasma immunoreactive erythropoietin to "available oxygen" in anemia of prematurity. J Pediatr 1984;105:793.
75. Christensen RD. Recombinant erythropoietic growth factors as an alternative to erythrocyte transfusion for patients with "anemia of prematurity." Pediatrie 1989;83:793.
76. Halperin DS, et al. Effects of recombinant human erythropoietin in infants with the anemia of prematurity: a pilot study. J Pediatr 1990;116:779.
77. Jacobson LO, Marks EK, Gaston EO, Robson MJ, Zirkle RE. Role of the spleen in radiation injury. Proc Soc Exp Biol Med 1949;70:7440.
78. Jacobson LO, Simmons EL, Marks EK, Gaston EO, Robson MJ, Eldredge JH. Further studies on recovery from radiation injury. J Lab Clin Med 1951;37:683.
79. Ford CE, Hamerton JL, Barnes DWH, Loutis JF. Cytological identification of radiation chimeras. Nature 1956;177:452.
80. Ogden DA, Micklem HS. The fate of serially transplanted bone marrow cell populations from young and old donors. Transplantation 1976;22:287.
81. Harrison DE, Astle CM, Delaittre JA. Loss of proliferative capacity in immunohemopoietic stem cells caused by serial transplantation rather than aging. J Exp Med 1978;147:1526.
82. Harrison DE, Astle CM. Loss of stem cell repopulating ability upon transplantation: effects of donor age, cell number, and transplantation procedure. J Exp Med 1982;156:1767.
83. Curry JL, Trentin JJ. Hemopoietic spleen colony studies. I. Growth and differentiation. Dev Biol 1967;15:395.
84. Juraskova V, Tkadlecek L. Character of primary and secondary colonies of haematopoiesis in the spleen of irradiated mice. Nature 1965;206:951.
85. Siminovitch L, Till JE, McCulloch EA. The distribution of colony-forming cells among spleen colonies. J Cell Comp Physiol 1963;62:327.
86. Lewis JP, Trobaugh FE. Haematopoietic stem cells. Nature 1964;204:589.
87. Becker AJ, McCulloch EA, Siminovitch L, Till JE. The effect of differing demands for blood cell production on DNA synthesis by hemopoietic colony-forming cells of mice. Blood 1965;26:296.
88. VanZant G, Eldridge PW, Behringer RR, Dewey MJ. Genetic control of hematopoietic kinetics revealed by analyses of allophenic mice and stem cell suicide. Cell 1983;35:639.
89. Necas E, Znojil V, Frindel E. Thymidine suicide and hydroxyurea kill ratios accurately reflect and proliferative status of stem cells (CFU-S). Exp Hematol 1989;17:53.
90. Micklem HS, Lennon JE, Ansell JD, Gray RA. Numbers and dispersion of repopulating chimeras as functions of cell dose. Exp Hematol 1987;15:251.
91. Harrison DE, Astle CM, Lerner C. Number and continuous proliferative pattern of transplanted primitive immunohematopoietic stem cells. Proc Natl Acad Sci USA 1988;85:822.
92. Boggs DR, Boggs SS, Saxe DR, Cress KA, Confield DR. Hematopoietic stem cells with high proliferative potential. J Clin Invest 1982;70:242.
93. Lemischka IR, Paulet DH, Mulligan RC. Developmental potential and dynamic behavior of hematopoietic stem cells. Cell 1986:917.
94. Wu AM, Till JE, Siminovitch L, McCulloch EA. A cytological study of the capacity for differentiation of normal hematopoietic colony-forming cells. J Cell Physiol 1967;69:177.

95. Visser JWM, VanBekkum DW. Purification of pluripotent hemopoietic stem cells: past and present. Exp Hematol 1990;18:248.
96. Spangrude GJ, Heimfeld S, Weissman IL. Purification and characterization of mouse hematopoietic stem cells. Science 1988;241:58.
97. Bertoncello I, Bartelmez SH, Bradley TR, Hodgson GS. Increased Qa-m7 antigen expression is characteristic of primitive hemopoietic progenitors in regenerating marrow. J Immunol 1987;139:1096.
98. Bertoncello I, Bartelmez SH, Bradley TR, Stanley ER, Harris A, Sandrin MS, Kriegler AB, McNiece IK, Hunter SD, Hodgson GS. Isolation and analysis of primitive hemopoietic progenitor cells on the basis of differential expression of Qa-m7 antigen. J Immunol 1986;136:3219.
99. Bradley TR, Hodgson GS. Detection of primitive macrophage progenitor cells in mouse bone marrow. Blood 1979;54:1446.
100. Visser JWM, Bauman JGJ, Mulder AH, Eliason JF, deLeeuw AM. Isolation of murine pluripotent hemopoietic stem cells. J Exp Med 1984;59: 1576.
101. Visser JWM, deVries P. Isolation of spleen-colony forming cells (CFU-S) using wheat germ agglutinin and rhodamine 123 labeling. Blood Cells 1988;14:369.
102. Civin CI, Strauss LC, Brovall C, Fackler MJ, Schwartz JF, Shaper JH. Antigenic analysis of hematopoiesis. III. A hematopoietic progenitor cell surface antigen defined by a monoclonal antibody raised against KG-la cells. J Immunol 1984;133:157.
103. Tindle RW, Nichols RAB, Chan L, Campana D, Catovsky D, Birnie GD. A novel monoclonal antibody BI-3C5 recognizes myeloblasts and non-B non-T lymphoblasts in acute leukemias and CGL blast crises, and reacts with immature cells in normal bone marrow. Leuk Res 1985;9:1.
104. Berenson RJ, Andrews RG, Bensinger WI, Kalamasz D, Knitter G. Antigen CD 34+ marrow cells engraft lethally irradiated baboons. J Clin Invest 1988;81:951.
105. Lajtha LG. Stem cell concepts. Differentiation 1979;14:23.
106. Hodgson GS, Bradley TR. Properties of haematopoietic stem cells surviving 5-fluorouracil treatment: evidence for a pre-CFU-S cell? Nature 1979;281:381.
107. Botnick LE, Hannon EC, Obbagy J, Hellman S. The variation of hematopoietic stem cell self-renewal capacity as a function of age: further evidence for heterogenicity of the stem cell compartment. Blood 1982;60:268.
108. Mauch P, Botnick LE, Hannon EC, Obbagy J, Hellman S. Decline in bone marrow proliferative capacity as a function of age. Blood 1982;60: 245.
109. Magli MC, Iscove NN, Odartchenko N. Transient nature of early haematopoietic spleen colonies. Nature 1982;295:527.
110. Eckmann L, Freshney M, Wright EG, Sproul A, Wilkie N, Pragnell IB. A novel *in vitro* assay for murine haematopoietic stem cells. Br J Cancer 1988;58:36.
111. Antin JH, Weinberg DS, Rappeport JM. Evidence that pluripotential stem cells form splenic colonies in humans after marrow transplantation. Transplantation 1985;39:102.
112. Fauser AA, Messner HA. Proliferative state of human pluripotent hemopoietic progenitors (CFU-GEMM) in normal individuals and under regenerative conditions after bone marrow transplantation. Blood 1979;54:1197.
113. Fauser AA, Messner HA. Granuloerythropoietic colonies in human bone marrow, peripheral blood, and cord blood. Blood 1978;52:1243.
114. Porcellini A, Manna A, Talevi N, et al. Effect of two cyclophosphamide derivatives on hemopoietic progenitor cells and pluripotential stem cells. Exp Hematol 1984;12:863.
115. Yeager AM, Kaizer H, Santos GW, et al. Autologous bone marrow transplantation in patients with acute nonlymphocytic leukemia, using ex vivo marrow treatment with 4-hydroperoxycyclophosphamide. N Engl J Med 1986;315:141.
116. Hara H, Ogawa M. Murine hemopoietic colonies in culture containing normoblasts, macrophages, and megakaryocytes. Am J Hematol 1978;4: 23.
117. Kay HEM. Stem-cells: a poem. Blut 1983;46:183.
118. Kay HEM. Hypothesis: how many cell-generations? Lancet 1965;1:418.
119. Hellman S, Botnick LE, Hannon EC, Vignuelle RM. Proliferative capacity of murine hematopoietic stem cells. Proc Natl Acad Sci USA 1978;75:490.
120. Micklem HS, Ansell JD, Wayman JER, Forrester L. The clonal organization of hematopoiesis in the mouse. Prog Immunol 1983;5:633.
121. Mintz B, Anthony K, Litwin S. Monoclonal derivation of mouse myeloid and lymphoid lineages from totipotent hematopoietic stem cells experimentally transplanted in fetal hosts. Proc Natl Acad Sci USA 1984;81:7835.
122. Lemischka IR, Raulet DH, Mulligan RC. Developmental potential and dynamic behavior of hematopoietic stem cells. Cell 1986;45:917.
123. Chapel B, Hawley R, Covarrubias L, Hawley T, Mintz B. Clonal contributions of small numbers of retrovirally marked hematopoietic stem cells engrafted in unirradiated neonatal W/W^v mice. Proc Natl Acad Sci USA 1989;86:4564.
124. Keller G, Snodgrass R. Life span of multipotential hematopoietic stem cells *in vivo*. J Exp Med 1990;171:1407.
125. Nash R, Storb R, Neiman P. Polyclonal reconstitution of human marrow after allogeneic bone marrow transplantation. Blood 1988;72:2031.
126. Byron JW. Comparison of the action of $_3$H-leucine and hydroxyurea on testosterone-treated hematopoietic stem cells. Blood 1972;40:198.
127. Byron JW. Manipulation of the cell cycle of the hematopoietic stem cell Exp Hematol 1975;3:44.
128. Byron JW. Drug receptors and the haematopoietic stem cell. Nature 1973;241:152.
129. Ikebuchi K, Wong GG, Clark SC, et al. Interleukin-6 enhancement of interleukin-3–dependent proliferation of multipotential hematopoietic progenitors. Proc Natl Acad Sci USA 1987;85:9035.
130. Ikebuchi K, Clark SC, Ihle JW, et al. Granulocyte colony-stimulating factor enhances interleukin-3–dependent proliferation of multipotential hematopoietic progenitors. Proc Natl Acad Sci USA 1988;85:3445.
131. Musashi M, Yang Y-C, Paul SC, et al. Direct and synergistic effects of interleukin 11 on murine hematopoiesis in culture. Proc Natl Acad Sci USA 1991;88:765.
132. Leary AG, Ikebuchi K, Hirai Y, et al. Synergism between interleukin-6 and interleukin-3 in supporting proliferations of human hematopoietic stem cells: comparison with interleukin-1a. Blood 1988;71:1759.
133. Tsuji K, Lyman SD, Sudo T, et al. Enhancement of murine hematopoiesis by synergistic interactions between Steel factor (ligand for c-*kit*), interleukin-11, and other early acting factors in culture. Blood 1992;11:2855.
134. Lim B, Apperley JF, Orkin SH, Williams DA. Long-term expression of human adenosine deaminase in mice transplanted with retrovirus-infected hematopoietic stem cells. Proc Natl Acad Sci USA 1989;86: 8892.
135. Bodine DM, Karlsson S, Nienhuis AW. Combination of interleukins 3 and 6 preserves stem cell function in culture and enhances retrovirus-mediated gene transfer into hematopoietic stem cells. Proc Natl Acad Sci USA 1989;86:8897.
136. Russell ES. Hereditary anemias of the mouse: a review for geneticists. Adv Genet 1979;20:357.
137. Bernstein SE, Russell ES, Keighley G. Two hereditary mouse anemias (Sl/Sl^d and W/W^v) deficient in response to erythropoietin. Ann NY Acad Sci 1968;149:475.
138. Chabot B, Stephenson DA, Chapman VM, Besmer P, Bernstein A. The proto-oncogenic *c-kit* encoding a transmembrane tyrosine kinase receptor maps to the mouse W locus. Nature 1988;335:88.
139. Geissler EN, Ryan MA, Housman DE. The dominant-white spotting (W) locus of the mouse encodes the c-kit proto-oncogene. Cell 1988;55: 185.
140. Reith AD, Rottapel R, Giddens E, Brady C, Forrester L, Bernstein A. *W* mutant mice with mild or severe developmental defects contain distinct point mutations in the kinase domain of the *c-kit* receptor. Genes Dev 1990;4:390.
141. McCulloch EA, Siminovitch L, Till JE, Russel ES, Bernstein SE. The cellular basis of the genetically determined hemopoietic defect in anemic mice of genotype Sl/Sl^d. Blood 1965;26:399.
142. Williams DE, Eisenman J, Baird A, et al. Identification of a ligand for the *c-kit* proto-oncogene. Cell 1990;63:167.
143. Zsebo KM, Wypych J, McNeice IK, et al. Identification, purification, and biological characterization of hematopoietic stem cell factor from buffalo rat liver–conditioned medium. Cell 1990;63:195.
144. Martin FH, Suggs SV, Langley KE, et al. Primary structure and functional expression of rat and human stem cell factor DNAs. Cell 1990;63:203.
145. Anderson DM, Lyman SD, Baird A, et al. Molecular cloning of mast cell growth factor: a hematopoietin that is active in both membrane bound and soluble forms. Cell 1990;63:235.
146. Nocka K, Buck J, Levi E, Besmer P. Candidate ligand for the *c-kit* transmembrane kinase receptor: KL, a fibroblast derived growth factor stimulates mast cells and erythroid progenitors. EMBO J 1990;9:3287.
147. Huang E, Nocka K, Beier DR, et al. The hematopoietic growth factor KL is encoded at the Sl locus and is the ligand of the *c-kit* receptor, the gene product of the *W* locus. Cell 1990;63:225.
148. Copeland NG, Gilbert DJ, Cho BC, et al. Mast cell growth factor maps near the steel locus on mouse chromosome 10 and is deleted in a number of steel alleles. Cell 1990;63:175.
149. Zsebo KM, Williams DA, Geissler EN, et al. Stem cell factor (SFC) is encoded at the Sl locus of the mouse and is the ligand for the *c-kit* tyrosine kinase receptor. Cell 1990;63:213.
150. Flanagan JG, Leder P. The *kit* ligand: a cell surface molecule altered in steel mutant fibroblasts. Cell 1990;63:185.
151. Flanagan JG, Chan DC, Leder P. Transmembrane form of the *kit* ligand growth factor is determined by alternative splicing and is missing in the $S1^d$ mutant. Cell 1991;64:1025.
152. Trentin JJ, Curry JC, Wolf N, Cheng V. Factors controlling stem cell differentiation and proliferation: the hematopoietic inductive microenvironment (HIM). In: The proliferation and spread of neoplastic cells. MD Anderson Hospital 21st Annual Symposium on Fundamental Cancer Research. Baltimore, Williams & Wilkins, 1967:713.
153. Wolff NS, Trentin JJ. Hemopoietic colony studies. V. Effect of hemopoietic organ stroma on differentiation of pluripotent stem cells. J Exp Med 1968;127:205.
154. Till JE, McCulloch EA, Siminovich L. A stochastic model of stem cell proliferation based on growth of spleen colony-forming cells. Proc Natl Acad Sci USA 1964;51:29.
155. Suda T, Suda J, Ogawa M. Disparate differentiation in mouse hemo-

poietic colonies derived from paired progenitors. Proc Natl Acad Sci USA 1984;81:2520.
156. Gregory CJ, McCulloch EA, Till JE. Repressed growth of C57BL marrow in hybrid hosts reversed by antisera directed against non-H-2 alloantigens. Transplantation 1972; 13:138.
157. Coulombel L, Eaves AC, Eaves CJ. Enzymatic treatment of long-term human marrow cultures reveals the preferential location of primitive hemopoietic progenitors in the adherent layer. Blood 1983;62:291.
158. Mauch P, Greenberger JS, Botnick L, Hannon E, Hellman S. Evidence for structured variation in self renewal capacity within long term bone marrow cultures. Proc Natl Acad Sci USA 1980;77:2927.
159. Schofield R. The relationship between the spleen colony-forming cell and the haemopoietic stem cell: a hypothesis. Blood Cells 1978;4:7.
160. Metcalf D, Moore MAS. Colony-stimulating factor (CSF). In: Neuberger A, Tatum EL, eds. Frontiers of biology: haemopoietic cells. Amsterdam, North Holland, 1971:399.
161. Whitlock CA, Witte ON. Long term culture of B lymphocytes and their precursors from murine marrow. Proc Natl Acad Sci USA 1982;79: 3608.
162. Lord BI, Testa AG, Hendry JH. The relative spatial distributions of BFUs and CFUs in the normal mouse femur. Blood 1975;46:65.
163. Lambertsen RH, Weiss LA. A model of intramedullary hematopoietic microenvironments based on stereologic study of the distribution of endocloned marrow colonies. Blood 1984;63:287.
164. Frassoni F, Testa NG, Lord BI. The relative spatial distribution of erythroid progenitor cells (BFUe and CFUe) in the normal mouse femur. Cell Tissue Kinet 1982;15:447.
165. Lichtman MA, Chamberlain JK, Weed RI, Pincus A, Santillo PA. The regulation of the release of granulocytes from normal marrow. In: Greenwalt TJ, Jamieson GA, eds. The granulocyte: function and clinical utilization. New York, Alan R. Liss, 1977:53.
166. Weiss L, Chen L-T. The organization of hematopoietic cords and vascular sinuses in bone marrow. Blood Cells 1975;1:617.
167. Campbell FR. Ultrastructural studies of transmural migration of blood cells in the bone marrow of rats, mice and guinea pigs. Am J Anat 1972;135:521.
168. Lichtman MA. The ultrastructure of the hemopoietic environment of the marrow: a review. Exp Hematol 1981;9:391.
169. Weiss L. The hematopoietic microenvironment of the bone marrow: an ultrastructural study of the stroma in rats. Anat Rec 1976;186:161.
170. Shaklai M, Tavassoli M. Cellular relationship in the rat bone marrow studied by freeze fracture and lanthanum impregnation thin-sectioning electron microscopy. J Ultrastruct Res 1979;69:343.
171. Allen TD, Dexter TM. Long-term bone marrow cultures: an ultrastructural review. Scan Electron Microsc 1983;4:1851.
172. Gimble JM, Dorheim M-A, Cheng Q, et al. Response of bone marrow stromal cells to adipogenic antagonists. Mol Cell Biol 1989;57:4587.
173. Iscove NN, Fagg B, Keller G. A soluble activity from adherent marrow cells cooperates with IL-3 in stimulating growth of pluripotential hematopoietic precursors. Blood 1988;71:953.
174. Gimble JM. The function of adipocytes in the bone marrow stroma. New Biologist 1990;2:304.
175. Tavassoli M. Marrow adipose cells and hemopoiesis: an interpretative review. Exp Hematol 1984;12:139.
176. Hines DL. Lipid accumulation and production of colony-stimulating activity by the 266AD cell line derived from mouse bone marrow. Blood 1983;61:397.
177. Kodama H-A, Sudo H, Koyama H, Kasai S, Yamamoto S. *In vitro* hemopoiesis with a microenvironment created by MC3T3-G2/PA6 preadipocytes. J Cell Physiol 1984;118:233.
178. Tavassoli M. Marrow adipose cells: histochemical identification of labile and stable components. Arch Pathol Lab Med 1976;100:16.
179. Weiss L. The structure of bone marrow: functional interrelationships of vascular hematopoietic compartments in experimental hemolytic anemia. J Morphol 1965;117:467.
180. Brookoff D, Weiss L. Adipocyte development and the loss of erythropoietic capacity in the bone marrow of mice after sustained hypertransfusion. Blood 1982;60:1337.
181. Islam A. Do bone marrow fat cells or their precursors have a pathogenic role in idiopathic anaemia? Med Hypotheses 1988;25:209.
182. Weiss LP, Wislocki GB. Seasonal variations in hematopoiesis in the dermal bones of the nine-banded armadillo. Anat Rec 1956;126:143.
183. Hussian MM, Mahley RW, Boyles JK, Fainaru M, Brecht WJ, Lindquist PA. Chylomicron-chylomicron remnant clearance by liver and bone marrow in rabbits. J Biol Chem 1989;264:9571.
184. Hussian MM, Mahley RW, Boyles JK, Lindquist PA, Brecht WJ, Innerarity TL. Chylomicron metabolism: chylomicron uptake by bone marrow in different animal species. J Biol Chem 1989;264:17931.
185. Greenberger JS. Sensitivity of corticosteroid-dependent, insulin-resistant lipogenesis in marrow preadipocytes of mutation diabetic-obese mice. Nature 1978;275:752.
186. Bathija A, Davis S, Trubowitz S. Bone marrow adipose tissue: response to acute starvation. Am J Hematol 1979;6:191.
187. Tavassoli M, Eastlund DT, Yam LT, Neiman RS, Finkel H. Gelatinous transformation of bone marrow in prolonged self-induced starvation. Scand J Haematol 1976;16:311.
188. Besis M, Breton-Gorius J. Rev Hematol 1959;14:165.
189. Crocker PR, Gordon S. Isolation and characterization of resident stromal macrophages and hematopoietic cell clusters from mouse bone marrow. J Exp Med 1985;162:993.
190. Lord BI, Hendry JH. The distribution of haemopoietic colony-forming units in the mouse femur and its modification by x-rays. Br J Radiol 1972;45:110.
191. Roberts RA, Spooncer E, Parkinson EK, Lord BI, Allen TD, Dexter TM. Metabolically inactive 3T3 cells can substitute for marrow stromal cells to promote the proliferation and development of multipotent haemopoietic stem cells. J Cell Physiol 1987;132:203.
192. Dexter TM, Spooncer F, Simmons P, Allen TD. Long-term marrow culture: an overview of techniques and experience. In: Wright DG, Greenberger JS, eds. Long-term bone marrow culture. Kroc Foundation Series. New York, Alan R Liss, 1984:57.
193. Williams DA, Rosenblatt MF, Beier DR, Cone RD. Generation of murine stromal cell lines supporting hematopoietic stem cell proliferation by use of recombinant retrovirus vectors encoding simian virus 40 large T antigen. Mol Cell Biol 1988;8:3864.
194. Rios M, Williams DA. Systematic analysis of the ability of stromal cell lines derived from different murine adult tissues to support maintenance of hematopoietic stem cells *in vitro*. J Cell Physiol 1990;145:434.
195. Goodman R, Grate H, Hannon E, Hellman S. Hematopoietic stem cells: effect of preirradiation, bleeding, and erythropoietin on thrombopoietic differentiation. Blood 1977;49:253.
196. Gordon MY, Greaves MF. Physiological mechanisms of stem cell regulation in bone marrow transplantation and haemopoiesis. Bone Marrow Transplant 1989;4:335.
197. Dexter TM, Spooncer E, Varga J, Allen TD, Lanotte M. Stromal cells and diffusible factors in the regulation of haemopoietic cell development. In: Killman S-A, Cronkite EP, Muller-Berat CN, eds. Haemopoietic stem cells. Copenhagen, Munksgaard, 1983:303.
198. Gordon MY, Riley GP, Watt SM, Greaves MF. Compartmentalization of a haematopoietic growth factor. Nature 1987;326:403.
199. Roberts R, Gallagher J, Spooncer E, Allen TD, Bloomfield F, Dexter TM. Heparin sulphate bound growth factors: a mechanism for stromal cell mediated haemopoiesis. Nature 1988;332:376.
200. Paul SR, Yang Y-C, Donahue RE, Goldring S, Williams DA. Stromal cell-associated hematopoiesis: immortalization and characterization of a primate bone marrow–derived stromal cell line. Blood 1991;77: 1723.
201. Namen AE, Lupton S, Hjerrild K, et al. Stimulation of B-cell progenitors by cloned murine interleukin-7. Nature 1988;333:571.
202. Toksoz D, Dexter TM, Lord BI, Wright EG, Lajtha LG. The regulation of hematopoiesis in long-term bone marrow cultures. II. Stimulation and inhibition of stem cell proliferation. Blood 1980;55:931.
203. Allen TD, Dexter TM. Cellular interelationships during *in vitro* granulopoiesis. Differentiation 1976;6:191.
204. Whitlock CA, Robertson D, Witte ON. Murine B cell lymphopoiesis in long term cultures. J Immunol Methods 1984;67:353.
205. Dexter TM, Testa NG, Allen TD, Rutherford T, Scolnick E. Molecular and cell biologic aspects of erythropoiesis in long-term bone marrow cultures. Blood 1981;58:699.
206. Eliason JF, Testa NG, Dexter TM. Erythropoietin-stimulated erythropoiesis in long term bone marrow culture. Nature 1979;281:382.
207. Corey CA, DeSilva A, Williams DA. Erythropoiesis in murine long term marrow cultures following transfer of the erythropoietic cDNA into marrow stromal cells. Exp Hematol 1990;18:201.
208. Oddos T, Nacol-Lizard S, Blanchet JP. Erythropoiesis in murine long-term bone-marrow cell cultures: dependence on erythropoietin and endogenous production of an erythropoietic stimulating activity. J Cell Physiol. 1987;133:72.
209. Gartner S, Kaplan HS. Long-term culture of human bone marrow cells. Proc Natl Acad Sci, USA 1980;77:4756.
210. Chang J, Coutino L, Morgenster G, et al. Reconstitution of haematopoietic system with autologous marrow taken during relapse of acute myeloblastic leukemia and grown in long-term culture. Lancet 1986;1: 294.
211. Coulombel L, Kalousek DK, Eaves CJ, Gupta CM, Eaves AC. Long-term marrow culture reveals chromosomally normal hematopoietic progenitor cells in patients with Philadelphia chromosome positive chronic myelogenous leukemia. N Engl J Med 1983;308:1493.
212. Singer JW. Studies with human long-term marrow cultures. In: Wright DG, Greenberger JS, eds. Long-term bone marrow culture. New York, Alan R Liss, 1984:235.
213. Hunt P, Robertson D, Weiss D, Rennick D, Lee F, Witte ON. A single bone marrow–derived stromal cell type supports the *in vitro* growth of early lymphoid and myeloid cells. Cell 1987;48:997.
214. Li CL, Johnson GR. Stimulation of multipotential erythroid and other murine haematopoietic progenitor cells by adherent cell lines in the absence of detectable multi-CSF (IL3). Nature 1985;316:633.
215. Rennick D, Yang G, Gemmell L, Lee F. Control of hemopoiesis by a bone marrow stromal cell clone: lipopolysaccharide-and interleukin-1-inducible production of colony-stimulating factors. Blood 1987;69: 682.
216. Whitlock CA, Tidmarsh GF, Muller-Sieburg C, Weissman IL. Bone marrow stromal cell lines with lymphopoietic activity express high levels of a pre-B neoplasia-associated molecule. Cell 1987;48:1009.

217. Singer JW, Charbord P, Keating A, et al. Simian virus 40-transformed adherent cells from human long-term marrow cultures: cloned cell lines produce cells with stromal and hematopoietic characteristics. Blood 1987;70:464.
218. Harigaya K, Handa H. Generation of functional clonal cell lines from human bone marrow stroma. Proc Natl Acad Sci USA 1985;82:3477.
219. Slack JL, Nemunaitis J, Andrew DF III, Singer JW. Regulation of cytokine and growth factor gene expression in human bone marrow stromal cells transformed with simian virus 40. Blood 1990;75:2319.
220. Billips LG, Petitte D, Landreth S. Bone marrow stromal cell regulation of B lymphopoiesis: interleukin-1 (IL-1) and IL-4 regulate stromal cell support of pre-B cell production *in vitro*. Blood 1990;75:611.
221. Cashman JD, Eaves AC, Raines EW, Ross R, Eaves CJ. Mechanisms that regulate the cell cycle status of very primitive hematopoietic cells in long term human marrow culture. I. Stimulatory role of a variety of mesenchymal cell activities and inhibitory role of TGF-β. Blood 1990;75:96.
222. Godard CM, Augery YL, Ginsbourg M, Jasmin C. Established cell lines of mouse marrow adherent cells producing differentiation factor(s) for the granulocyte-macrophage lineage. In Vitro 1983;19:897.
223. Song ZX, Shadduck RK, Innes DJ Jr, Waheed A, Quesenberry PJ. Hematopoietic factor production by a cell line (TC-1) derived from adherent murine marrow cells. Blood 1989;66:273.
224. Harigaya K, Cronkite EP, Miller ME, Shadduck RK. Murine bone marrow cell line producing colony-stimulating factor. Proc Natl Acad Sci USA 1981;6963.
225. Lanotte M, Metcalf D, Dexter TM. Production of monocyte-macrophage colony-stimulating factor by preadipocyte cell lines derived from murine stroma. J Cell Physiol 1982;112:123.
226. Zipori D, Duksin D, Tamir M, Argaman A, Toledo J, Malik Z. Cultured mouse marrow stromal cell lines. II. Distinct subtypes differing in morphology, collagen types, myelopoietic factors, and leukemic cell growth modulating activities. J Cell Physiol 1985;122:81.
227. Zipori D. Cultured stromal cell lines from hemopoietic tissues. In: Tavassoli M, ed. Handbook of the hematopoietic microenvironment. Clifton, NJ, Humana Press, 1989;287.
228. Gimble JM, Dorheim M-A, Cheng Q, et al. Adipogenesis in a murine bone marrow stromal cell line capable of supporting B lineage lymphocyte growth and proliferation: biochemical and molecular characterization. Eur J Immunol 1990;20:379.
229. Perkins S, Fleischman RA. Stromal cell progeny of murine bone marrow fibroblast colony-forming units are clonal endothelial-like cells that express collagen IV and laminin. Blood 1990;75:620.
230. Zipori D, Toledo J, von der Mark K. Phenotypic heterogeneity among stromal cell lines from mouse bone marrow disclosed in their extracellular matrix composition and interactions with normal and leukemic cells. Blood 1985;66:447.
231. Zipori D, Friedman A, Tamir M, Silverberg D, Malik Z. Cultured mouse marrow cell lines: interactions between fibroblastoid cells and monocytes. J Cell Physiol 1984;118:143.
232. Garnett HM, Harigaya K, Cronkite EP. Influence of a fibroblastoid cell line derived from murine bone marrow (H-1 cells) on stem cell proliferation. Proc Soc Exp Biol Med 1984;175:70.
233. Gimble JM, Pietrangeli C, Henley A, et al. Characterization of murine bone marrow and spleen-derived stromal cells: analysis of leukocyte marker and growth factor mRNA transcript levels. Blood 1989;74: 303.
234. Pojda Z, Dexter TM, Lord BI. Production of a multipotential cell (CFU-S) proliferation inhibitor by various populations of mouse and human macrophages. Br J Haematol 1988;68:153.
235. Lenfant M, Wdzieczak-Bakala J, Guittet E, Prome J-C, Sotty D, Frindel E. Inhibitor of hematopoietic pluripotent stem cell proliferation: purification and determination of its structure. Proc Natl Acad Sci USA 1989;86:799.
236. Pragnell IB, Wright EG, Lorimore SA, et al. The effect of stem cell proliferation regulators demonstrated with an in vitro assay. Blood 1988;72:196.
237. Graham GJ, Wright EG, Hewick R, et al. Identification and characterization of an inhibitor of haemopoietic stem cell proliferation. Nature 1990;344:442.
238. Wolpe SD, Cerami A. Macrophage inflammatory proteins 1 and 2: members of a novel superfamily of cytokines. FASEB 1989;3:2565.
239. Zipori D, Kalai M, Tamir M. Restrictins: stromal cell associated factors that control cell organization in hemopoietic tissues. Nat Immun Cell Growth Regul 1988;7:185.
240. Zipori D. Stromal cells from the bone marrow: evidence for a restrictive role in regulation of hemopoiesis. Eur J Haematol 1989;42:225.
241. Zipori D, Tamir M, Toledo J, Oren T. Differentiation stage and lineage-specific inhibitor from the stroma of mouse bone marrow that restricts lymphoma cell growth. Proc Natl Acad Sci USA 1986;83:4547.
242. Altus MS, Bernstein SE, Russell ES, Casten AL, Upton AC. Defect extrinsic to stem cells in spleens of Steel anemic mice. Proc Soc Exp Biol Med 1971;138:985.
243. Fried W, Chamberlin W, Knospe WH, Husseini S, Trobaugh FE Jr. Studies on the defective haematopoietic microenvironment. Br J Haematol 1973;24:643.
244. Ruscetti FW, Boggs DR, Torok BJ, Boggs SS. Reduced blood and marrow neutrophils and granulocytic colony-forming cells in Sl/Sl^d mice. Proc Soc Exp Biol Med 1976;152:398.
245. Ebbe S, Phalen E, Stohlman F Jr. Abnormalities of megakaryocytes in Sl/Sl^d mice. Blood 1973;42:865.
246. Bernstein SE. Tissue transplantation as an analytic and therapeutic tool in hereditary anemias. Am J Surg 1969;119:448.
247. Dexter TM, Moore MAS. *In vitro* duplication and cure of haemopoietic defects in genetically anaemic mice. Nature 1977;269:412.
248. Zuckerman KS, Prince CW, Ribadeneira M. Sl/Sl^d mouse bone marrow stroma in vitro contains an active radiation-sensitive inhibitor of normal hemopoiesis. Blood 1986;68:1201.
249. Witte ON. Steel locus defines new multipotent growth factor. Cell 1990;63:5.
250. Flanagan JG, Chan DC, Leder P. Transmembrane form of the kit ligand growth factor is determined by alternative splicing and is missing in the Sl^d mutant. Cell 1991;64:1025.
251. Botwell TH, Callender S, Mallett B, Witts LT. Study of erythropoiesis using tracer quantities of radioactive iron. Br J Haematol 1956;2:1.
252. Donohoe DM, Reiff RH, Hanson ML, Betson Y, Finch CA. Quantitative measurement of the erythrocytic and granulocytic cells of the marrow and blood. J Clin Invest 1958;37:1571.
253. Lajtha LG, Gilbert CW, Guzman EE. Kinetics of haematopoietic colony growth. Br J Haematol 1971;20:343.
254. Hillman RS, Finch CA. Erythropoiesis: normal and abnormal. Semin Hematol 1967;4:327.
255. Hillman RS, Giblett ER. Red cell membrane alteration associated with "marrow stress." J Clin Invest 1965;44:1730.
256. Hanna IRA, Spicer SS, Green WB, Horn RG. Shortening of the cell-cycle time of erythroid precursors in response to anaemia. Br J Haematol 1969;16:381.
257. Eaves CJ, Eaves AC. Erythroid progenitor cell numbers in human marrow-implications for regulation. Exp Hematol 1979;7:54.
258. Patel VP, Lodish HF. Loss of adhesion of murine erythroleukemia cells to fibronectin during erythroid differentiation. Science 1984;224:996.
259. Patel VP, Losich HF. The fibronectin receptor on mammalian erythroid precursor cells: characterization and developmental regulation. J Cell Biol 1986;102:449.
260. Patel VP, Lodish HF. A fibronectin matrix is required for differentiation of murine erythroleukemia cells into reticulocytes. J Cell Biol 1987;105: 3105.
261. Baehner RL. Disorders of leukocytes leading to recurrent infection. Pediatr Clin North Am 1972;19:935.
262. Cartwright GE, Athens JW, Wintrobe MM. The kinetics of granulopoiesis in normal man. Blood 1964;24:780.
263. Cronkite EP, Fliedner TM. Granulocytopoiesis. N Engl J Med 1964;270: 1347.
264. Morstyn G, Campbell L, Souza LM, et al. Effect of granulocyte colony stimulating factor on neutropenia induced by cytotoxic chemotherapy. Lancet 1988;1:667.
265. Glaspy JA, Golde DW. Clinical applications of the myeloid growth factors. Semin Hematol 1989;26:14.
266. Athens JW, Raab SO, Haab OP, et al. Leukokinetic studies. III. The distribution of granulocytes in the blood of normal subjects. J Clin Invest 1961;40:159.
267. Craddock GG Jr, Perry S, Ventzke LE, Lawrence JS. Evaluation of marrow granulocyte reserves in normal and disease states. Blood 1960;15: 840.
268. Todd RF, Freyer DR. The CD11/CD18 leukocyte glycoprotein deficiency. Hematol Oncol Clin North Am 1988;2:13.
269. Sanchez-Madrid F, Nagy JA, Robbins E, Simon P, Springer TA. A human leukocyte differentiation antigen family with distinct α-subunits and a common β-subunit: the lymphocyte function–associated antigen (LFA-1), the C3bi complement receptor (OKM1/Mac-1), and the p150,95 molecule. J Exp Med 1983;158:1785.
270. Dana N, Todd RF III, Pitt J, Springer TA, Arnaout MA. Deficiency of a surface membrane glycoprotein (Mo1) in man. J Clin Invest 1984;73: 153.
271. Arnaout MA, Spits H, Terhorst C, Pitt J, Todd RF III. Deficiency of a leukocyte surface glycoprotein (LFA-1) in two patients with Mo1 deficiency: effects of cell activation on Mo1/LFA-1 surface expression in normal and deficient leukocytes. J Clin Invest 1984;74:1291.
272. Beatty PG, Ochs HD, Harlan JM, et al. Absence of monoclonal-antibody defined protein complex in a boy with abnormal leukocyte function. Lancet 1984;1:535.
273. Springer TA, Thompson WS, Miller LJ, et al. Inherited deficiency of the Mac-1, LFA-1, p150 glycoprotein family and its molecular basis. J Exp Med 1986;160:1901.
274. Gallatin M, St John TP, Siegelman M, Reichert R, Butcher EC, Weissman IL. Lymphocyte homing receptors. Cell 1986;44:673.
275. Gordon MY. Annotation: adhesive properties of haemopoietic stem cells. Br J Haematol 1988;68:149.
276. Aizawa S, Tavassoli M. Marrow uptake of galactosyl-containing neoglycoproteins: implications in stem cell homing. Exp Hematol 1988;16: 811.
277. Aizawa S, Tavassoli M. Interaction of murine granulocyte-macrophage progenitors and supporting stroma involves a recognition mechanism with galactosyl and mannosyl specificities. J Clin Invest 1987;80:1698.

278. Williams DA, Rios M, Stephens C. Fibronectin and VLA-4 in hematopoietic stem cells: microenvironment interactions. Nature 1991;352:438.
279. Verfaillie C, McCarthy J, McGlave P. Differentiation of primitive human lin-34+ DR− hematopoietic progenitors is accompanied by transition of adhesion from the heparin-binding domain to the cell-binding domain of fibronectin (FN). (Abstract) Blood 1990;76:10.
280. De Bruyn, PP, Michelson S, Thomas TB. The migration of blood cells of the bone marrow through the sinusoidal wall. J Morphol 1971;133:417.
281. Litchman MA. Cellular deformability during maturation of the myeloblast: possible role in marrow egress. N Engl J Med 1970;283:943.
282. Litchman MA, Weed RI. Alteration of the cell periphery during granulocyte maturation: relationship to cell function. Blood 1972;39:301.
283. Litchman MA, Weed RI. Peripheral cytoplasmic characteristics of leukocytes in monocytic leukemia: relationship to clinical manifestations. Blood 1972;40:52.
284. Boggs DR, Cartwright GE, Wintrobe MM. Neutrophilia-inducing activity in plasma of dogs recovering from drug induced myelotoxicity. Am J Physiol 1966;211:51.
285. Boggs DR, Marsh JC, Chevernick PA, Cartwright GE, Wintrobe MM. Neutrophil releasing activity in plasma of normal human subjects injected with endotoxin. Proc Soc Exp Biol Med 1968;127:689.
286. Weiss L. Transmural cellular passage in vascular sinuses of rat bone marrow. Blood 1970;36:189.
287. Chamberlain JK, Leblond PF, Weed RI. Reduction of adventitial cell cover: an early direct effect of erythropoietin on bone marrow ultrastructure. Blood Cells 1975;1:655.
288. Metcalf D. The hemopoietic growth factors. Amsterdam, Elsevier, 1984.
289. Das SK, Stanley ER, Guilbert LJ, Forman LW. Human colony-stimulating factor (CSF-1) radioimmunoassay: resolution of three subclasses of human colony-stimulating factors. Blood 1981;58:630.
290. Mikake T, Kung CK-H, Goldwasser E. Purification of human erythropoietin. J Biol Chem 1977;252:5558.
291. Welte K, Platzer E, Lu L, Gabrilove JL, Levi E, Mertelsmann R, Moore MAS. Purification and biochemical characterization of human pluripotent hematopoietic colony-stimulating factor. Proc Natl Acad Sci USA 1985;82:1526.
292. Bussolino F, Wang JM, Defilippi P, et al. Granulocyte- and granulocyte-macrophage-colony stimulating factors induce human endothelial cells to migrate and proliferate. Nature 1989;337:471.
293. Athanassakis I, Bleackley RC, Paetkau V, Guilbert L, Barr PJ, Wegmann TG. The immunostimulatory effect of T cells and T cell lymphokines on murine fetally derived placental cells. J Immunol 1987;138:37.
294. Pollard JW, Bartocci A, Arceci R, Orlofsky A, Ladner MB, Stanley ER. Apparent role of the macrophage growth factor, CSF-1, in placental development. Nature 1987;330:484.
295. Arceci RJ, Shanahan F, Stanley ER, Pollard JW. Temporal expression and location of colony-stimulating factor 1 (SFC-1) and its receptor in the female reproductive tract are consistent with CSF-1–regulated placental development. Proc Natl Acad Sci USA 1989;86:8818.
296. Gearing DP, King JA, Gough NM, Nicola NA. Expression cloning of a receptor for human granulocyte-macrophage colony-stimulating factor. EMBO 1989;8:3667.
297. Farrar WL, Vinocour M, Hill JM. In situ hybridization histochemistry localization of interleukin-3 mRNA in mouse brain. Blood 1989;73:137.
298. Sieff CA. Hematopoietic growth factors. J Clin Invest 1987;79:1549.
299. Nicola NA. Hemopoietic cell growth factors and their receptors. Annu Rev Biochem 1989;58:45.
300. Nagata S, Tsuchiya M, Asano S, et al. Molecular cloning and expression of cDNA for human granulocyte colony-stimulating factor. Nature 1986;319:415.
301. Souza LM, Boone TC, Gabrilove JL, et al. Recombinant human granulocyte colony-stimulating factor: effects on normal and leukemic myeloid cells. Science 1986;232:61.
302. Kawaski ES, Lander MB, Wang AM, et al. Molecular cloning of a complimentary DNA encoding human macrophage-specific colony-stimulating factor (CFS-1). Science 1985;230:291.
303. Jacobs KC, Shoemaker C, Rudersdorf R, et al. Isolation and characterization of genomic and cDNA clones of human erythropoietin. Nature 1985;313:806.
304. Wong GG, Witek JS, Temple PA, et al. Human GM-CSF: molecular cloning of the complementary DNA and purification of the natural and recombinant proteins. Science 1985;228:810.
305. Yang Y-C, Ciarletta AB, Temple PA, et al. Human IL-3 (multi-CSF): identification by expression cloning of a novel hematopoietic growth factor related to murine IL-3. Cell 1986;47:3.
306. Metcalf D. The molecular contol of blood cells. Cambridge, MA, Harvard University Press, 1988.
307. Walker F, Nicola NA, Metcalf D, Burgess AW. Hierarchical down-modulation of hemopoietic growth factor receptors. Cell 1985;43:269.
308. Sims JE, March CJ, Cosman D, et al. cDNA expression cloning of the IL-1 receptor, a member of the immunoglobulin superfamily. Science 1988;241:585.
309. Yamasaki K, Taga T, Hirata Y, et al. Expression of the human interleukin-6 (BSF-2/IFNbeta 2) receptor. Science 1988;241:825.
310. D'Andrea AD, Lodish HF, Wong GG. Expression cloning of the murine erythropoietin receptor. Cell 1989;57:277.
311. Itoh N, Yonehara S, Schreurs J, et al. Cloning of an interleukin-3 receptor gene: a member of a distinct receptor gene family. Science 1990;247:324.
312. Idzerda RL, March CL, Mosley B, et al. Human interleukin 4 receptor confers biological responsiveness and defines a novel receptor superfamily. J Exp Med 1990;171:861.
313. Mosley B, Beckmann MP, March CJ, et al. The murine interleukin-4 receptor: molecular cloning and characterization of secreted and membrane bound forms. Cell 1989;59:335.
314. Goodwin R, Friend D, Ziegler SF, et al. Cloning of the human and murine interleukin-7 receptors: demonstration of a soluble form and homology to a new receptor superfamily. Cell 1990;60:941.
315. Fukunaga R, Ishizaka-Ikeda E, Seto Y, Nagata S. Expression cloning of a receptor for murine granulocyte colony-stimulating factor. Cell 1990;61:341.
316. Fukunaga R, Seto Y, Mizushima S, Nagata S. Three different mRNAs encoding human granulocyte colony-stimulating factor receptor. Proc Natl Acad Sci USA 1990;87:8702.
317. Cosman D, Lyman SD, Idzerda RL, et al. A new cytokine receptor superfamily. TIBS 1990;15:265.
318. Hatakeyama M, Tsudo M, Minamoto S, et al. Interleukin-2 receptor beta chain gene: generation of three receptor forms by cloned human alpha and beta chain cDNAs. Science 1989;244:551.
319. Leung DW, Spencer SA, Cachianes G, et al. Growth hormone receptor and serum binding protein: purification, cloning and expression. Nature 1987;330:537.
320. Boutin J-M, Jolicoeur C, Okamura H, et al. Cloning and expression of the rat prolactin receptor, a member of the growth hormone/prolactin receptor gene family. Cell 1988;53:69.
321. Edery M, Jolicoeur C, Levi-Meyrueis C, et al. Identification and sequence analysis of a second form of prolactin receptor by molecular cloning of complementary DNA from rabbit mammary gland. Proc Natl Acad Sci USA 1989;86:2112.
322. Abdel-Meguid SS, Shieh H-S, Smith WW, et al. Three-dimensional structure of a genetically engineered variant of porcine growth hormone. Proc Natl Acad Sci USA 1987;84:6434.
323. Brankenhoff JPJ, Hart M, Aarden LA. Analysis of human IL-6 mutants expressed in *Escherichia coli*: biologic activities are not affected by deletion of amino acids 1-28. J Immunol 1989;143:1175.
324. Crosier KE, Wong GG, Mathey-Prevot B, Nathan DG, Sieff CA. A functional isoform of the human granulocyte-macrophage colony-stimulating factor receptor contains a unique cytoplasmic domain. Proc Natl Acad Sci USA 1991;88:7744.
325. Lu HS, Boone TC, Souza LM, Lai P-H. Disulfide and secondary structures of recombinant human granulocyte colony stimulating factor. Arch Biochem Biophys 1989;268:81.
326. Brandhuber BJ, Boone T, Kenney WC, McKay DB. Three-dimensional structure of interleukin-2. Science 1987;238:1707.
327. deVos AM, Ultsch M, Kossiakoff AA. Human growth hormone and extracellular domain of its receptor: crystal structure of the complex. Science 1992;255:306.
328. Cunningham BC, Wells JA. High resolution epitope mapping of hGH-receptor interactions by alanine-scanning mutagenesis. Science 1989;244:1081.
329. Bazan JF. Structural design and molecular evolution of a cytokine receptor superfamily. Proc Natl Acad Sci USA 1990;87:6934.
330. Huebner K, Isobe M, Croce CM, Golde DW, Kaufman SE, Gasson JC. The human gene encoding GM-CSF is at 5q 21-q32, the chromosome region deleted in the 5q− anomaly. Science 1985;230:1282.
331. LeBeau MM, Epstein ND, O'Brien SJ, et al. The interleukin 3 gene is located on human chromosome 5 and is deleted in myeloid leukaemias with a deletion of 5q. Proc Natl Acad Sci USA 1987;84:5913.
332. Pettenati MJ, LeBeau MM, Lemons RS, et al. Assignment of CSF-1 to 5q33.1: evidence for clustering of genes regulating hematopoiesis and for their involvement in the deletion of the long arm of chromosome 5 in myeloid disorders. Proc Natl Acad Sci USA 1987;84:2970.
333. LeBeau MM, Westbrook CA, Diaz MO, et al. Evidence for the involvement of GM-CSF and FMS in the deletion (5q) in myeloid disorders. Science 1987;231:984.
334. Watkins PC, Eddy R, Hoffman N, et al. Regional assignment of the erythropoietin gene to human chromosome region 7pter-q22. Cytol Cell Genet 1986;42:214.
335. Law ML, Cai G-Y, Lin F-K. Chromosomal assignment of the human erythropoietin gene and its DNA polymorphism. Proc Natl Acad Sci USA 1986;83:6920.
336. Simmers RN, Webber LM, Shannon MF, et al. Localization of the G-CSF gene on chromosome 17 proximal to the breakpoint in the t (15;17) in acute promyelocytic leukemia. Blood 1987;70:330.
337. Budarf M, Huebner K, Emanuel B, et al. Assignment of the erythropoietin receptor (EPOR) gene to mouse chromosome 9 and human chromosome 19. Genomics 1990;8:575.
338. Gough NM, Gearing DP, Nicola NA, et al. Localization of the human GM-CSF receptor gene to the X-Y pseudoautosomal region. Nature 1990;345:734.
339. Isobe M, Kumura Y, Murata Y, et al. Localization of the gene encoding

the alpha subunit of human interleukin-5 receptor (IL5RA) to chromosome region 3p24-3p26. Genomics 1992;14:755.
340. Shen Y, Baker E, Callen DF, et al. Localization of the human GM-CSF receptor beta chain gene (CSF2RB) to chromosome 22q12.2→q13.1. Cytol Cell Genet 1992;61:175.
341. Ihle JN, Keller J, Henderson L, Klein F, Palaszynski E. Procedures for the purification of interleukin 3 to homogeneity. J Immunol 1982;129:2431.
342. Cutler RL, Metcalf D, Nicola NA, Johnson GR. Purification of a multipotential colony-stimulating factor from pokeweed mitogen-stimulated mouse spleen cell conditioned medium. J Biol Chem 1985;260:6579.
343. Fung MC, Hapel AJ, Yuner S, et al. Molecular cloning for cDNA for murine interleukin-3. Nature 1984;307:238.
344. Yokota T, Lee T, Rennick D, et al. Isolation and characterization of a mouse cDNA clone that expresses mast-cell growth factor activity in monkey cells. Proc Natl Acad Sci USA 1984;81:1070.
345. Cline MJ, Golde DW. Production of colony stimulating activity by human lymphocytes. Nature 1974;248:703.
346. Nathan DG, Chess L, Hillman DG, et al. Human erythroid burst-forming unit: T-cell requirement for proliferation in vitro. J Exp Med 1978;147:324.
347. Mangan KF, Chikkappa G, Sieler LZ, Scharfman WB, Parkingson DR. Regulation of human blood erythroid burst-forming unit (BFU-E) proliferation by T lymphocyte subpopulations defined by Fc receptors and monoclonal antibodies. Blood 1982;59:990.
348. Chervenick PA, LoBuglio AF. Human blood monocytes: stimulation of granulocyte and mononuclear colony formation in vitro. Science 1972;178:164.
349. Golde DW, Cline MJ. Identification of colony-stimulating cells in human peripheral blood. J Clin Invest 1972;51:2981.
350. Zuckerman KS. Human erythroid burst-forming unit growth in vitro is dependent on monocytes but not T lymphocytes. J Clin Invest 1981;67:702.
351. Reid CPL, Batista LC, Chanarin I. Erythroid colony growth in vitro from human peripheral blood null cells: evidence for regulation by T lymphocytes and monocytes. Br J Haematol 1981;48:155.
352. Knudson S, Mortenson BT. Growth stimulation of human bone marrow cells in agar culture by vascular cells. Blood 1975;46:937.
353. Quesenberry PJ, Gimbrone MA. Vascular endothelium as a regulator of granulopoiesis: production of colony stimulating activity by cultured human endothelial cells. Blood 1990;76:1060.
354. Niemeyer CM, Sieff CA, Mathey-Prevot B, Bierer BE, Clark SC, Nathan DG. Interleukin 3 (IL-3) is produced only by activated human T-lymphpocytes. Blood 1987;73:945.
355. Wimperis JZ, Niemeyer CM, Sieff CA, Mathey-Prevot B, Nathan DG, Arceci RJ. Granulocyte-macrophage colony-stimulating factor and interleukin 3 mRNAs are produced by a small fraction of blood mononuclear cells. Blood 1989;74:1525.
356. Mathey-Prevot B, Andrews NC, Murphy HS, Kreissman SG, Nathan DG. Positive and negative elements regulate human interleukin 3 expression. Proc Natl Acad Sci USA 1990;87:5046.
357. Schreurs J, Arai K, Miyajima A. Evidence for a low-affinity interleukin-3 receptor. Growth Factors 1990;2:221.
358. Park LW, Friend D, Price V, et al. Heterogeneity in human interleukin-3 receptors. J Biol Chem 1989;264:5420.
359. Kuwaki T, Kitamura T, Tojo A, et al. Characterization of human interleukin-3 receptors on a multi-factor–dependent cell line. Biochem Biophys Res Comm 1989;161:16.
360. Gorman DM, Itoh N, Kitamura T, et al. Cloning and expression of a gene encoding an interleukin 3 receptor-like protein: identification of another member of the cytokine receptor gene family. Proc Natl Acad Sci USA 1990;87:5459.
361. Hara T, Miyajima A. Two distinct functional high affinity receptors for mouse interleukin-3 (IL-3). EMBO J 1992;11:1875.
362. Devos R. Plaetinck G, Van der Hayden J, et al. Molecular basis of a high affinity murine interleukin-5 receptor. EMBO J 1991;10:2133.
363. Kitamura T, Sato N, Arai K, Miyajima A. Expression cloning of the human IL-3 receptor cDNA reveals a shared beta subunit for the human Il-3 and GM-CSF receptors. Cell 1991;66:1165.
364. Tavernier J, Devos R, Cornelis S, et al. A human high affinity interleukin-5 receptor (IL5R) is composed of an IL5-specific alpha chain and a beta chain shared with the receptor for GM-CSF. Cell 1991;66:1175.
365. Morla AO, Schreurs J, Miyajima A, Wang JYJ. Hematopoietic growth factors activate the tyrosine phosphorylation of distinct sets of proteins in interleukin-3–dependent murine cell lines. Mol Cell Biol 1988;8:2214.
366. Isfort RJ, Stevens D, May WS, Ihle JN. Interleukin 3 binds to a 140-kDa phosphotyrisine-containing cell surface protein. Proc Natl Acad Sci USA 1988;85:7982.
367. Isfort R, Huhn RD, Frackelton AR, Ihle JN. Stimulation of factor-dependent myeloid cell lines with interleukin 3 induces tyrosine phosphorylation of several cellular substrates. J Biol Chem 1988;263:19203.
368. Sorensen PHB, Mui AL-F, Murphy SC, Krystal G. Interleukin-3, GM-CSF, and TPA induce distinct phosphorylation events in an interleukin-3-dependent multipotential cell line. Blood 1989;73:406.
369. Kaplan DR, Whitman M, Schaffhausen B, et al. Common elements in growth factor stimulation and oncogenic transformation: 85 kd phosphoprotein and phosphatidylinositol kinase activity. Cell 1987;50:1021.
370. Carroll, MP, Clark-Lewis I, Rapp UR, May WS. Interleukin-3 and granulocyte-macrophage colony-stimulating factor mediate rapid phosphorylation and activation of cytosolic c-*raf*. J Biol Chem 1990;265:19812.
371. Sakamaki K, Miyajima I, Kitamura T, Miyajima A. Critical cytoplasmic domains of the common beta subunit of the human GM-CSF, IL-3 and IL-5 receptors for the growth signal transduction and tyrosine phosphorylation. EMBO J 1992;11:3541.
372. Duronio V, Clark-Lewis I, Federspiel B, et al. Tyrosine phosphorylation of receptor beta subunits and common substrates in response to interleukin-3 and granulocyte-macrophage colony stimulating factor. J Biol Chem 1992;267:21856.
373. Mui AL-F, Cutler R, Alai M, et al. Steel factor and interleukin-3 stimulate the tyrosine phosphorylation of $p95^{vav}$ in hematopoietic cell lines. (Abstract) Exp Hematol 1992;20:752.
374. Hanazono Y, Chiba S, Sasaki K, et al. c-*fos*/fes protein-tyrosine is implicated in a signalling pathway triggered by granulocyte-macrophage colony-stimulating factor and interleukin-3. EMBO J 1993;12:1641.
375. Okuda K, Sanghera JS, Pelech SL, et al. Granulocyte-macrophage colony-stimulating factor, interleukin-3 and Steel factor induce rapid tyrosine phosphorylation of p42 and p44 MAP kinase. Blood 1992;79:2880.
376. Welham MJ, Duronio V, Sanghera JS, et al. Multiple hematopoietic growth factors stimulate activation of mitogen-activated protein kinase family members. J Immunol 1992;149:1683.
377. Torigoe T, O'Connor R, Santoli D, Reed JC. Interleukin-3 regulates the activity of the LYN protein-tyrosine kinase in myeloid-committed leukemic cell lines. Blood 1992;80:617.
378. Kobayashi N, Kono T, Hatakeyama M, et al. Functional coupling of the *src*-family protein tyrosine kinases $p59^{fyn}$ and $p53/56^{lyn}$ with the interleukin 2 receptor: implications for redundancy and pleiotopism in cytokine signal transduction. Proc Natl Acad Sci USA 1993;90:4201.
379. Silvennoinen O, Wittuhn BA, Quelle FW, et al. Structure of the murine Jak2 protein tyrosine kinase and its role in IL-3 signal transduction. Proc Natl Acad Sci USA 1993.
380. Hunter T. Cytokine connections. Nature 1993;366:114.
381. Valasquez L, Fellous LM, Stark GR, Pellegrini S. A protein tyrosine kinase in the interferon a/b signalling pathway. Cell 1992;70:313.
382. Fu X-Y. A transcription factor with SH2 and SH3 domains is directly activated by and interferon α–induced cytoplasmic protein tyrosine kinase(s). Cell 1992;70:323.
383. Fu X-Y, Schindler C, Improta T, Aebersold R, Darnell JE. The proteins of ISGF-3, the interferon α–induced transciptional activator, define a gene family involved in signal transduction. Proc Natl Acad Sci USA 1992;89:7840.
384. Watling D, Guschin D, Muller M, et al. Complementation by the protein tyrosine kinase Jak2 of a mutant cell line defective in the interferon-g signal transduction pathway. Nature 1993;366:166.
385. Lütticken C, Wegenka UM, Yaun J, et al. Association of transcription factor APRF and protein kinase Jak1 with the interleukin-6 signal transducer gp130. Science 1994;263:89.
386. Stahl N, Boulton TG, Farruggella T, et al. Association and activation of Jak-Tyk kinases by CNTF–LIF–OSM–IL-6b receptor components. Science 1994;263:92.
387. Pierce JH, Ruggiero M, Fleming TP, et al. Signal transduction through the EGF receptor transfected in IL-3–dependent hematopoietic cells. Science 1988;239:628.
388. Wheeler EF, Rettenmeier CW, Look AT, Sherr CJ. The v-*fms* oncogene induces factor independence and tumorigenicity in CSF-1 dependent macrophage cell line. Nature 1986;324:377.
389. Wheeler EF, Askew D, May S, Ihle JN, Sherr CJ. The v-*fms* oncogene induces factor-independent growth and transformation of the interleukin-3-dependent myeloid cell line FDC-P1. Mol Cell Biol 1987;7:1673.
390. Watson JD, Jenkins DR, Eszes M, Leung E. Effect of granulocyte-macrophage colony-stimulating factor and interleukin 3 on the v-*src* oncogene. J Immunol 1988;140:501.
391. Satoh T, Nakafuku M, Miyajima A, Kaziro Y. Involvement of ras p21 protein in signal-transduction pathways from interleukin 2, interleukin 3, and granulocyte/macrophage colony-stimulating factor, but not from interleukin 4. Proc Natl Acad Sci USA 1991;88:3314.
392. Duronio V, Welham MJ, Abrahams S, et al. $p21^{ras}$ activation via hemapoietin receptors and c-*kit* requires tyrosine kinase activity but not phosphorylation of $p21^{ras}$ GTPase-activating protein. Proc Natl Acad Sci USA 1993;89:1587.
393. Gulbins E, Coggeshall KM, Baier G, et al. Tyrosine kinase–stimulated guanine nucleotide exchange activity of vav in T cell activation. Science 1993;260:822.
394. McCormick F. How receptors turn Ras on. Nature 1993;363:15
395. Feig L. The many roads that lead to Ras. Science 1993;260:767.
396. Moodie SA, Willumsen BM, Weber MJ, Wolfman A. Complexes of Ras-

GTP with Raf-1 and mitogen-activated protein kinase. Science 1993;260: 1658.

397. McColl SR, DiPersio JF, Caon AC, et al. Involvement of tyrosine kinases in the activation of human peripheral blood neutrophils by granulocyte-macrophage colony-stimulating factor. Blood 1991;78:1842.
398. Schwartz EL, Chamberlain H, Brechbuhl AB. Regulation of c-*myc* expression by granulocyte-macrophage colony-stimulating factor in human leukemia cells. Blood 1991;77:2716.
399. Berns A. Tumorigenesis in transgenic mice: identification and characterization of synergizing oncogenes. J Cell Biochem 1991;47:130.
400. Lilly M, Le T, Holland P, Hendrickson S. Sustained expression of the *pim-1* kinase is specifically induced in myeloid cells by cytokines whose receptors are structurally related. Oncogene 1992;7:727.
401. Farrar WL, Thomas TP, Anderson WB. Altered cytosol/membrane enzyme redistribution on interleukin-3 activation of protein kinase C. Nature 1985;315:235.
402. Whetton AD, Monk PN, Consalvey SD, Huang SJ, Dexter TM, Downes CP. Interleukin 3 stimulates proliferation via protein kinase C activation without increasing inositol lipid turnover. Proc Natl Acad Sci USA 1988;85:3284.
403. Whetton AD, Monk PN, Consalvey SD, Downes CP. The haematopoietic growth factors interleukin 3 and colony stimulating factor-1 stimulate proliferation but do not induce inositol lipid breakdown in murine bone-marrow–derived macrophages. EMBO J 1986;5:3281.
404. Gough N, Gough J, Metcalf D, et al. Molecular cloning of cDNA encoding a murine haematopoietic growth regulator, granulocyte-macrophage colony stimulating factor. Nature 1984;309:763.
405. Donahue RE, Wang EA, Kaufman RJ, et al. Effects of N-linked carbohydrate on the in vivo properties of human GM-CSF: Cold Spring Harbor symposium. Quant Biol 1986;51:685.
406. Cebon J, Nicola N, Ward M, Gardner I, et al. Granulocyte-macrophage colony stimulating factor from human lymphocytes. J. Biol. Chem. 1990; 265:4483.
407. Gough NM, Grail D, Gearing DP, Metcalf D. Mutagenesis of murine granulocyte/macrophage colony-stimulating factors reveals critical residues near the N terminus. Eur J Biochem 1987;169:353.
408. Kaushansky K, Shoemaker SG, Alfaro S, Brown C. Hematopoietic activity of granulocyte/macrophage colony-stimulating factor is dependent upon two distinct regions of the molecule: functional analysis based upon the activities of interspecies hybrid growth factors. Proc Natl Acad Sci USA 1989;86:1213.
409. Brown CB, Hart CE, Curtis DM, Bailey MC, Kaushansky K. Two neutralizing monoclonal antibodies against human granulocyte-macrophage colony-stimulating factor recognize the receptor binding domain of the molecule. J Immunol 1990;144:2184.
410. Yang Y-C, Kovacic S, Kriz R, et al. The human genes for GM-CSF and IL 3 are closely linked in tandem on chromosome 5. Blood 1988;71: 958.
411. Yang Y-C, Clark SC. Molecular cloning for interleukin 3. Lymphokines 1991;15:375.
412. Shannon MF, Gamble JR, Vadas MA. Nuclear proteins interacting with the promoter region of the human granulocyte/macrophage colony-stimulating factor gene. Proc Natl Acad Sci USA 1988;85:674.
413. Shannon MF, Pell LM, Lenardo MJ, et al. A novel tumor necrosis factor–responsive transcription factor which recognized a regulatory element in hemopoietic growth factor genes. Mol Cell Biol 1990;10:2950.
414. Nimer SD, Morita EA, Martis MJ, Wachsman W, Gasson J. Characterization of the human granulocyte-macrophage colony-stimulating factor promoter region by genetic analysis: correlation with DNase I footprinting. Mol Cell Biol 1988;8:1979.
415. Shaw G, Kamen R. A conserved AU sequence from the 3′ untranslated region of GM-CSF mRNA mediates selective mRNA degradation. Cell 1986;46:659.
416. Broudy VC, Kaushansky K, Segal GM, Harland JM, Adamson JW. Tumor necrosis factor type alpha stimulates human endothelial cells to produce granulocyte/macrophage colony-stimulating factor. Proc Natl Acad Sci USA 1986;83:7467.
417. Munker R, Gasson J, Ogawa M, Koeffler HP. Recombinant human TNF induces production of granulocyte-monocyte colony-stimulating factor. Nature 1986;323:79.
418. Sieff CA, Tsai S, Faller DV. Interleukin 1 induces cultured human endothelial cell production of granulocyte-macrophage colony stimulating factor. J Clin Invest 1987;79:48.
419. Yang Y-C, Tsai S, Wong GG, Clark SC. Production of colony-stimulating factors by interleukin-1–induced human stromal cells. J Cell Physiol 1988;134:292.
420. Dinarello CA. Interleukin 1 and the pathogenesis of the acute-phase response. N Engl J Med 1984;311:1413.
421. Broudy VC, Zuckerman KS, Jetmalani S, Fitchen JH, Bagby GC. Monocytes stimulate fibroblastoid bone marrow stromal cells to produce multilineage hematopoietic growth factors. Blood 1986;68:530.
422. Bagby GC, McCall E, Bergstrom KA, Burger D. A monokine regulates colony-stimulating activity production by vascular endothelial cells. Blood 1983;62:663.
423. Zuckerman KS, Bagby GC, McCall E, et al. A monokine stimulates the production of human erythroid burst-promoting activity by endothelial cells in vitro. J Clin Invest 1985;75:722.
424. Bagby GC, McCall E, Layman DL. Regulation of colony stimulating activity production: interactions of fibroblasts, mononuclear phagocytes, and lactoferrin. J Clin Invest 1983;71:340.
425. Bagby GC, Rigas VD, Bennett RM, Vandenbark AA, Garewal HS. Interaction of lactoferrin, monocytes, and T lymphocyte subsets in the regulation of steady-state granulopoiesis in vitro. J Clin Invest 1981;68: 56.
426. Yamato K, El-Hajjaoui Z, Kuo JF, Koeffler HP. Granulocyte-macrophage colony-stimulating factor: signals for its mRNA accumulation. Blood 1989;74:1314.
427. Koeffler HP, Gasson J, Tobler A. Transcriptional and posttranscriptional modulation of myeloid colony-stimulating factor expression by tumor necrosis factor and other agents. Mol Cell Biol 1988;8:3432.
428. Seelentag WK, Mermod J-J, Montesano R, Vassalli P. Additive effects of interleukin 1 and tumor necrosis factor alpha on the accumulation of the three granulocyte and macrophage colony-stimulating factor mRNAs in human endothelial cells. EMBO 1987;6:2261.
429. Thorens B, Mermod J-J, Vassalli P. Phagocytosis and inflammatory stimuli induce GM-CSF mRNA in macrophages through posttranscriptional regulation. Cell 1987;48:671.
430. Gasson JC, Kaufman SE, Weisbart RH, Tomonaga M, Golde DW. High-affinity binding of granulocyte-macrophage colony-stimulating factor to normal and leukemic human myeloid cells. Proc Natl Acad Sci USA 1986;83:669.
431. Park LW, Friend D, Gillis S, Urdal DL. Characterization of the cell surface receptor for human granulocyte/macrophage colony-stimulating factor. J Exp Med 1986;164:251.
432. DiPersio J, Billing P, Kaufman S, Eghtesady P, Williams RE, Gasson J. Characterization of the human granulocyte-macrophage colony-stimulating factor receptor. J Biol Chem 1988;263:1834.
433. Sieff CA, Kannourakis G. Interleukin-3 and granulocyte-macrophage colony-stimulating factor are synergistic and interact at the cell surface. In: Abraham NG, Kowalinka G, Sachs L, Wiedermann CJ, eds. Molecular biology of hematopoiesis. Andover, MA, Intercept, 1991.
434. Gesner TG, Mufson RA, Norton CR, Turner KJ, Yang Y-C, Clark SC. Specific binding, internalization, and degradation of human recombinant interleukin-3 by cells of the acute myelogenous, leukemia line KG-1. J Cell Physiol 1988;136:493.
435. Chiba S, Tojo A, Kitamura T, Urabe A, Miyazono K, Takaku F. Characterization and molecular features of the cell surface receptor for human granulocyte-macrophage colony-stimulating factor. Leukemia 1990;4:29.
436. Baldwin GC, Gasson JC, Kaufman SE, et al. Nonhematopoietic tumor cells express functional GM-CSF receptors. Blood 1989;73:1033.
437. Miyagawa KS, Chiba S, Shibuya K, et al. Frequent expression of receptors for granulocyte-macrophage colony-stimulating factor on human nonhematopoietic tumor cell lines. J Cell Physiol 1990;143: 483.
438. Chiba S, Shibuya K, Piao Y-F, et al. Identification and cellular distribution of distinct proteins forming human GM-CSF receptor. Cell Regula 1990;1:327.
439. Metcalf D, Nicola NA, Gearing DP, Gough NM. Low-affinity placenta-derived receptors for human granulocyte-macrophage colony-stimulating factor can deliver a proliferative signal to murine hematopoietic cells. Proc Natl Acad Sci USA 1990;87:4670.
440. Croiser KE, Wong GG, Mathey-Prevot B, Nathan DG, Sieff CA. A functional isoform of the human granulocyte-macrophage colony-stimulating factor receptor. Proc Natl Acad Sci USA 1991;88:7744.
441. Hayashida K, Kitamura T, Gorman DM, Ken-Ichi A, Takashi T, Miyajima A. Molecular cloning of a second subunit of the receptor for human granulocyte-macrophage colony-stimulating factor (GM-CSF): reconstitution of a high-affinity GM-CSF receptor. Proc Natl Acad Sci USA 1990;87:9655.
442. Ashworth A, Kraft A. Cloning of a potentially soluble receptor for human GM-CSF. Nucleic Acids Res 1990;18:7178.
443. Gomez-Cambronero J, Yamazaki M, Metwally F, et al. Granulocyte-macrophage colony-stimulating factor and human neutrophils: role of guanine nucleotide regulatory proteins. Proc Natl Acad Sci USA 1989;86:3569.
444. Evans JPM, Mire-Sluis AR, Hoffbrand AV, Wickremasinghe RG. Binding of G-CSF, GM-CSF, tumor necrosis factor-alpha, and gamma-interferon to cell surface receptors on human myeloid leukemia cells triggers rapid tyrosine and serine phosphorylation of a 75-Kd protein. Blood 1990;75:88.
445. Kanakura Y, Druker B, Cannistra SA, Furukawa Y, Torimoto Y, Griffin JD. Signal transduction of the human granulocyte-macrophage colony-stimulating factor and interleukin-3 receptors involves tyrosine phosphorylation of a common set of cytoplasmic proteins. Blood 1990;76: 706.
446. Sullivan R, Griffin JD, Simons ER, et al. Effects of recombinant human granulocyte and macrophage colony-stimulating factors on signal transduction pathways in human granulocytes. J Immunol 1987;139: 3422.
447. Sullivan R, Griffin JD, Wright J, et al. Effects of recombinant human

granulocyte-macrophage colony-stimulating factor on intracellular pH in mature granulocytes. Blood 1988;72:1665.
448. Dahinden CA, Zingg J, Maly FE, De Weck AL. Leukotriene production in human neutrophils primed by recombinant human granulocyte/macrophage colony-stimulating factor and stimulated with the complement component C5A and FMLP as second signals. J Exp Med 1988;167:1281.
449. Corey SJ, Rosoff PM. Granulocyte-macrophage colony-stimulating factor primes neutrophils by activating a pertussis toxin-sensitive G protein not associated with phosphatidylinositol turnover. J Biol Chem 1989;264:14165.
450. Coleman DL, Liu J, Bartiss AH. Recombinant granulocyte-macrophage colony-stimulating factor increases adenylate cyclase activity in murine peritoneal macrophages. J Immunol 1989;143:4134.
451. Coffey RG, Davis JS, Djeu JY. Stimulation of guanlyate cyclase activity and reduction of adenylate cyclase activity by granulocyte-macrophage colony stimulating factor in human blood neutrophils. J Immunol 1988;140:2695.
452. Nagata S, Tsuchiya M, Asano S, et al. The chromosomal gene structure and two mRNAs for human granulocyte colony-stimulating factor. EMBO 1986;5:575.
453. Fukunaga R, Ishizaka-Ikeda E, Seto Y, Nagata S. Expression cloning of a receptor for murine granulocyte colony-stimulating factor. Cell 1990;61:341.
454. Fukunaga R, Seto Y, Mizushima S, Nagata S. Three different mRNAs encoding human granulocyte colony-stimulating factor receptor. Proc Natl Acad Sci USA 1990;87:8702.
455. Ranscht B, Dours MT. Sequence of contactin, a 130-kD glycoprotein concentrated in areas of interneuronal contact, defines a new member of the immunoglobulin supergene family in the nervous system. J Cell Biol 1988;107:1561.
456. Ladner MB, Martin GA, Noble JA, et al. Human CSF-1: gene structure and alternative splicing of mRNA precursors. EMBO 1987;6:2693.
457. Kawaski ES, Lander MB, Wang AM, Van Arsdell J, et al. Molecular cloning of a complimentary DNA encoding human macrophage–specific colony-stimulating factor (CSF-1). Science 1985; 230:291.
458. Wong GG, Temple PA, Leary AC, et al. Human CSF-1: molecular cloning and expression of a 4kb cDNA encoding the human urinary protein. Science 1987;235:1504.
459. Stanley ER, Heard PM. Factors regulating macrophage production and growth: purification and some properties of the colony stimulating factor from medium conditioned by mouse L-cells. J Biol Chem 1977;252:4305.
460. Stanley ER, Hansen G, Woodcock J, Metcalf D. Colony stimulating factor and the regulation of granulopoiesis and macrophage production. Fed Proc 1975;34:2272.
461. Motoyoshi K, Suda T, Kusumoto K, Takaku F, Miura Y. Granulocyte-macrophage colony-stimulating and binding activities of purified human urinary colony-stimulating factor to murine and human bone marrow cells. Blood 1982;60:1378.
462. Cifone M, Defendi V. Cyclic expression of a growth conditioning factor (MGF) on the cell surface. Nature 1974;252:151.
463. Stanley ER, Cifone M, Heard PM, Defendi V. Factors regulating macrophage production and growth: identity of colony-stimulating factor and macrophage growth factor. J Exp Med 1976;143:631.
464. Rettenmier CW, Roussel MF, Ashman RA, Ralph P, Price K, Sherr CJ. Synthesis of membrane-bound colony-stimulating factor 1 (CSF-1) and down modulation of CSF-1 receptors in NIH 3T3 cells transformed by cotransfection of the human CSF-1 and c-frms (CSF-1 receptor) genes. Mol Cell Biol 1987;7:2378.
465. Horiguchi J, Warren MK, Ralph P, Kufe D. Expression of the macrophage specific colony-stimulating factor (CSF-1) during human monocyte differentiation. Biochem Biophys Res Comm 1986;141:924.
466. Rambaldi A, Young DG, Griffin JD. Expression of the M-CSF (CSF-1) gene by human monocytes. Blood 1987;69:1409.
467. Ralph R, Warren MK, Lee MT, et al. Inducible production of human macrophage growth factor, CSF-1. Blood 1986;68:633.
468. Guilbert LJ, Stanley ER. The interaction of ^{125}I-colony-stimulating factor-1 with bone marrow-derived macrophages. J Biol Chem 1986;261:4024.
469. Bartocci A, Mastrogiannis DS, Migliorati G, Stockert RJ, Wolkoff AW. Macrophages specifically regulate the concentration of their own growth factor in the circulation. Proc Natl Acad Sci USA 1987;84:6179.
470. Sherr CJ. Colony-stimulating factor-1 receptor. Blood 1990;75:1.
471. Sherr CJ, Rettenmier CW, Sacca R, et al. The *c-fms* proto-oncogene product is related to the receptor for the mononuclear phagocytic growth factor CSF-1. Cell 1985;41:665.
472. Yarden Y, Escobedo JA, Kuang W-J, et al. Structure of the receptor for platelet-derived growth factor helps define a family of closely related growth factor receptors. Nature 1986;323:226.
473. Roberts WM, Look AT, Moussel MF, Sherr CJ. Tandem linkage of human CSF-1 receptor (c-fms) and PDGF receptor genes. Cell 1988;55: 655.
474. Imamura K, Dianoux A, Nakamura T, Kufe D. Colony-stimulating factor 1 activates protein kinase C in human monocytes. EMBO J 1990; 2423.
475. Shurtleff SA, Downing JR, Rock CO, Hawkins SA, Roussel MF, Sherr CJ. Structural features of the colony-stimulating factor 1 receptor that affects its association with phosphatidylinositol 3-kinase. EMBO J 1990;2415.
476. Smith MR, DeGudicubus SJ, Stacey DW. Requirement for c-ras proteins during viral oncogene transformation. Nature 1986;320:540.
477. Morrison DK, Kaplan DR, Rapp U, Roberts TM. Signal transduction from membrane to cytoplasm: growth factors and membrane-bound oncogene products increase Raf-1 phosphorylation and associated protein kinase activity. Proc Natl Acad Sci USA 1988;85:8855.
478. Roussel MF, Rettenmier CW, Look AT, Sherr CJ. Cell surface expression of v-fms–coded glycoproteins is required for transformation. Mol Cell Biol 1984;4:1999.
479. McDonough SK, Larsen S, Brodey RS, Stock ND, Hardy WDJ. A transmissible feline fibrosarcoma of viral origin. Cancer Res 1971;31:953.
480. Tushinski RJ, Oliver IT, Guilbert LJ, Tynan PW, Warner JR, Stanley ER. Survival of mononuclear phagocytes depends on a lineage-specific growth factor that the differentiated cells selectively destroy. Cell 1982;28:71.
481. Coussens L, Van Beveren C, Smith D, et al. Structural alteration of viral homologue of receptor proto-oncogene fms at carboxy terminus. Nature 1986;320:277.
482. Downing JR, Margolis BL, Zilberstein A, Ashmun RA, et al. Phospholipase C-gamma, a substrate for PDGF receptor kinase, is not phosphorylated on tyrosine during the mitogenic response to CSF-1. EMBO J 1989;8:3345.
483. Heard J-M, Roussel MF, Rettenmier CW, Sherr CJ. Multilineage hematopoietic disorders induced by transplantation of bone marrow cells expressing the v-fms oncogene. Cell 1987;51:663.
484. Downward J, Yarden Y, Mayes E, et al. Close similarity of epidermal growth factor receptor and v-erb-B oncogene protein sequences. Nature 1984;307:521.
485. Waterfield MD, Scrace GT, Whittle N, et al. Platelet-derived growth factor is structurally related to the putative transforming protein P28^{sis} of simian sarcoma virus. Nature 1983;304:35.
486. Lai P-H, Everett R, Wang F-F, Arakawa T, Goldwasser E. Structural characterization of human erythropoietin. J Biol Chem 1986;261:3116.
487. Koury ST, Bondurant MC, Koury MJ. Localization of erythropoietin synthesizing cells in murine kidneys by *in situ* hybridization. Blood 1988;71:524.
488. Lacombe C, DaSilva J-L, Bruneval P, et al. Peritubular cells are the site of erythropoietin synthesis in the murine hypoxic kidney. J Clin Invest 1988;81:620.
489. Koury ST, Koury MJ, Bondurant MC, Caro J, Graber SE. Quantitation of erythropoietin-producing cells in kidneys of mice by *in situ* hybridization: correlation with hematocrit, renal erythropoietin mRNA, and serum erythropoietin concentration. Blood 1989;74:645.
490. Goldberg MA, Glass GA, Cunningham JM, Bunn HF. The regulated expression of erythropoietin by two human hepatoma cell lines. Proc Natl Acad Sci USA 1987;84:7972.
491. Goldberg MA, Dunning SP, Bunn HF. Regulation of the erythropoietin gene: evidence that the oxygen sensor is a heme protein. Science 1988;242:1412.
492. Schuster SJ, Badiavas EV, Costa-Giomi P, Weinmann R, Erslev AJ, Caro J. Stimulation of erythropoietin gene transcription during hypoxia and cobalt exposure. Blood 1989;73:13.
493. Webster KA. Regulation of glycolytic enzyme RNA transcriptional rates by oxygen availablity in skeletal muscle cells. Mol Cell Biochem 1987;77:19.
494. Miller BA, Scaduto RC, Tillotson DL Jr, Botti JJ, Cheung JY. Erythropoietin stimulates a rise in intracellular free calcium concentration in single early human erythroid precursors. J Clin Invest 1988;82:309.
495. Imagawa S, Smith BR, Palmer-Crocker R, Bunn HF. The effect of recombinant erythropoietin on intracellular free calcium in erythropoietin-responsive cells. Blood 1989;73:1452.
496. Miller BA, Cheung JY, Tillotson DL, Hope SM, Scaduto RC Jr. Erythropoietin stimulates a rise in intracellular-free calcium concentration in single BFU-E derived erythroblasts at specific stages of differentiation. Blood 1989;73:1188.
497. Choi H-Y, Wojchowski DM, Sytkowski AJ. Erythropoietin rapidly alters phosphorylation of pp43, an erythroid membrane protein. J Biol Chem 1987;262:2933.
498. Bonanou-Tzedaki SA, Setchenska MS, Arnstein HRV. Stimulation of the adenylate cyclase activity of rabbit bone marrow immature erythroblasts by erythropoietin and haemin. Eur J Biochem 1986;155:363.
499. D'Andrea AD, Zon LI. Erythropoietin receptor subunit structure and activation. J Clin Invest 1990;86:681.
500. Hatakeyama M, Mori H, Doi T, Taniguchi T. A restricted cytoplasmic region of IL-2 receptor beta chain is essential for growth signal transduction but not for ligand binding and internalization. Cell 1989;59: 837.
501. D'Andrea AD, Yoshimura A, Youssoufian H, Zon LI, et al. The cytoplasmic region of the erythropoietin receptor contains nonoverlapping positive and negative growth-regulatory domains. Mol Cell Biol 1991;11: 1980.
502. Linnekin D, Evans GA, D'Andrea A, Farrar WL. Association of the erythropoietin receptor with protein tyrosine kinase activity. Proc Natl Acad Sci USA 1992;89:6237.
503. Miura O, D'Andrea A, Kabat D, Ihle JN. Induction of tyrosine phos-

phorylation by the erythropoietin receptor correlates with mitogenisis. Mol Cell Biol 1991;11:4895.
504. Yoshimura A, Lodish HF. In vitro phosphorylation of the erythropoietin receptor and an associated protein, pp130. Mol Cell Biol 1992;12:706.
505. Witthun BA, Quelle FW, Silvennoinen O, et al. Jak2 associates with the erythropoietin receptor and is tyrosine phosphorylated and activated following stimulation with erythropoietin. Cell 1993;74:227.
506. Li J-P, D'Andrea AD, Lodish HF, Baltimore D. Activation of cell growth by binding of Friend spleen focus–forming virus gp55 glycoprotein to the erythropoietin receptor. Nature 1990;343:762.
507. Friend C. Cell-free transmission in adult Swiss mice of a disease having the character of a leukemia. J Exp Med 1957;105:307.
508. Wolff L, Ruscetti S. Malignant transformation of erythroid cells in vivo by introduction of a nonreplicating retrovirus vector. Science 1985;228: 1549.
509. Dinarello CA, Cannon JG, Mier JW, et al. Multiple biological activities of human recombinant interleukin 1. J Clin Invest 1986;77:1734.
510. Schindler R, Dinarello CA. Interleukin 1. In: Habenicht A, ed. Growth factors, differentiation factors, and cytokines. Berlin, Springer-Verlag, 1990;85.
511. Lomedico PT, Gubler U, Hellman CP, et al. Cloning and expression of murine interleukin-1 cDNA in *Escherichia coli*. Nature 1984;312:458.
512. Furitani Y, Notake M, Fukui T, et al. Complete nucleotide sequence of the gene for human interleukin-1 alpha. Nucl Acid Res 1986;14: 3167.
513. Auron PE, Webb AC, Rosenwasser LJ, Mucci SF, Rich A, Wolff SM, Dinarello CA. Nucleotide sequence of human monocyte interleukin 1 precursor cDNA. Proc Natl Acad Sci USA 1984;81:7907.
514. Clark BD, Collins KL, Gandy MS, Webb AC, Auron PE. Genomic sequence for human prointerleukin 1 beta: possible evolution from a reverse transcribed prointerleukin 1 alpha gene. Nucl Acids Res 1986;14:7897.
515. Bakouche O, Brown DC, Lachman L. Subcellular localization of human monocyte interleukin 1: evidence for an inactive precursor molecule and a possible mechanism for IL 1 release. J Immunol 1987;138:4249.
516. Auron PE, Warner SJC, Webb AC, et al. Studies on the molecular nature of human interleukin 1. J Immunol 1987;138:1447.
517. Hazuda DJ, Lee JC, Young PR. The kinetics of interleukin 1 secretion from activated monocytes: differences between interleukin 1-alpha and interleukin 1-beta. J Biol Chem 1988;263:8473.
518. Mosley B, Urdal DL, Prickett KS, et al. The interleukin-1 receptor binds the human interleukin-1-alpha precursor but not the interleukin-1-beta precursor. J Biol Chem 1987;262:2941.
519. Warner SJC, Auger KR, Libby P. Human interleukin 1 induces interleukin 1 gene expression in human vascular smooth muscle cells. J Exp Med 1987;165:1316.
520. Warner SJC, Auger KR, Libby P. Interleukin 1 induces interleukin 1. II. Recombinant human interleukin 1 induces interleukin 1 production by adult human vascular endothelial cells. J Immunol 1987;139:1911.
521. Ghezzi P, Dinarello CA. IL-1 induces IL-1. III. Specific inhibition of IL-1 production by IFN-gamma. J Immunol 1988;140:4238.
522. Bird TA, Gearing AJH, Saklatvala J. Murine interleukin-1 receptor: differences in binding properties between fibroblastic and thymoma cells and evidence for a two- chain receptor model. FEBS 1987;225: 21.
523. Bird TA, Saklatvala J. Identification of a common class of high affinity receptors for both types of porcine interleukin-1 on connective tissue cells. Nature 1986;324:263.
524. Kroggel R, Martin M, Pingoud V, Dayer JM, Resch K. Two-chain structure of the interleukin 1 receptor. FEBS 1988;229:59.
525. Mochizuki DY, Eisenman JR, Conlon PJ, Larsen AD, Tushinski RJ. Interleukin 1 regulates hematopoetic activity, a role previously ascribed to hemopoietin 1. Proc Natl Acad Sci USA 1987;84:5267.
526. Jubinsky PT, Stanley ER. Purification of hemapoietin-1, a multilineage hemapoietic growth factor. Proc Natl Acad Sci USA 1985;82:2764.
527. Bartelmez SH, Stanley ER. Synergism between hemopoietic growth factors (HGF) detected by their effects on cells bearing receptors for a lineage specific HGF: assay of hemopoietin-1. J Cell Physiol 1985;122: 370.
528. McNiece IK, Bradley TR, Kriegler AB, Hodgson GS. Subpopulations of mouse bone marrow high-proliferative-potential colony-forming cells. Exp Hematol 1986;14:856.
529. Neta R, Douches S, Oppenheim JJ. Interleukin-1 is a radioprotector. J Immunol 1986;136:2483.
530. Neta R, Oppenheim JJ, Douches SD. Interdependence of the radioprotective effects of human recombinant interleukin 1-alpha, tumor necrosis factor alpha, granulocyte colony-stimulating factor, and murine recombinant granulocyte-macrophage colony-stimulating factor. J Immunol 1988;140:108.
531. Moore MAS, Warren DJ. Synergy of interleukin 1 and granulocyte colony-stimulating factor: *in vivo* stimulating of stem-cell recovery and hematopoietic regeneration following 5-fluorouracil treatment of mice. Proc Natl Acad Sci USA 1987;84:7134.
532. Stork L, Barczuk L, Kissinger M, Robinson W. Interleukin-1 accelerates murine granulocyte recovery following treatment with cyclophosphamide. Blood 1989;73:938.
533. Gasparetto C, Laver J, Abboud M, et al. Effects of interleukin-1 on hematopoietic progenitors: evidence of stimulatory and inhibitory activities in a primate model. Blood 1989;74:547.
534. Noma Y, Sideras P, Naito T, et al. Cloning of cDNA encoding the murine IgGl induction factor by a novel strategy using SP6 promoter. Nature 1986;319:640.
535. Yokoto T, Otsuka T, Mossman T. Isolation and characterization of a human interleukin cDNA clone, homologous to mouse B-cell-stimulatory factor 1, that expresses B-cell and T-cell-stimulating activities. Proc Natl Acad Sci USA 1986;83:5894.
536. Novick D, Engelmann H, Wallach D, Rubinstein M. Soluble cytokine receptors are present in normal human urine. J Exp Med 1989;170: 1409.
537. Peschel C, Paul WE, Ohara J, Green I. Effects of B cell stimulatory factor-1/interleukin 4 on hematopoietic progenitor cells. Blood 1987;70: 254.
538. Broxmeyer HE, Lu L, Cooper S, Tushinski R, et al. Synergistic effects of purified recombinant human and murine B cell growth factor-1/IL-4 on colony formation in vitro by hematopoietic progenitor cells: multiple actions. J Immunol 1988;141:3852.
539. Sanderson CJ, Warren DJ, Strath M. Identification of a lymphokine that stimulates eosinophil differentiation in vitro. J Exp Med 1985;162: 60.
540. Kinashi T, Harada N, Severinson E, et al. Cloning of complementary DNA encoding T cell replacing factor and identity with B-cell growth factor II. Nature 1986; 324:70.
541. Azuma C, Tanabe T, Konishi M, et al. Cloning of cDNA for human T-cell replacing factor (interleukin-5) and comparison with the murine homologue. Nucleic Acids Res 1986; 14:9149.
542. Clutterbuck EJ, Hirst EMA, Sanderson CJ. Human interleukin-5 (IL-5) regulates the production of eosinophils in human bone marrow cultures: comparison and interaction with IL-1, IL-3, IL-6, and GMCSF. Blood 1989;73:1504.
543. Coffman RL, Seymour BWP, Hudak S, Jackson J, Rennick D. Antibody to interleukin-5 inhibits helminth-induced eosinophilia in mice. Science 1989;245:308.
544. Sieff CA, Emerson SG, Donahue RE, et al. Human recombinant granulocyte-macrophage colony-stimulating factor: a multilineage hematopoietin. Science 1985;230:1171.
545. Hirano T, Yasukawa K, Harada H, et al. Complementary DNA for a novel human interleukin (BSF-2) that induces B lymphocytes to produce immunoglobulin. Nature 1986;324:73.
546. Zilberstein A, Ruggieri R, Korn JH, Revel M. Structure and expression of cDNA and genes for human interferon-beta-2, a distinct species inducible by growth-stimulatory cytokines. EMBO J 1986;5:2529.
547. Haegeman G, Content J, Volkaert G, Derynck R, Tavernier J, Fiers W. Structural analysis of the sequence coding for an inducible 26 kDa protein in human fibroblasts. Eur J Biochem 1986;159:625.
548. Van Damme J, Opdenakker G, Simpson RJ, et al. Identification of the human 26-kD protein, interferon-beta2 (IFN-beta2), as a B cell hybridoma/plasmocytoma growth factor induced by interleukin 1 and tumor necrosis factor. J Exp Med 1987;165:914.
549. Horii Y, Muraguchi A, Suematsu S, et al. Regulation of BSF-2/IL-6 production by human mononuclear cells: macrophage-dependent synthesis of BSF-2/IL-6 by T cells. J Immunol 1988;141:1529.
550. Taga T, Masahiko H, Hirata Y, et al. Interleukin-6 triggers the association of its receptor with a possible signal transducer, gp130. Cell 1989;58: 573.
551. Kawano M, Hirano T, Matsuda T, et al. Autocrine generation and requirement of BSF-2/IL-6 for human multiple myelomas. Nature 1988;332:83.
552. Castleman B, Iverson L, Menendez VP. Localized mediastinal lymph node hyperplasia resembling thymoma. Cancer 1956;9:822.
553. Ikebuchi K, Wong GG, Clark SC, Ihle JN, Hirai Y, Ogawa M. Interleukin-6 enhancement of interleukin-3–dependent proliferation of multipotential hemopoietic progenitors. Proc Natl Acad Sci USA 1987;84:9035.
554. Namen AE, Schmierer AE, March CJ, et al. B cell precursor growth-promoting activity. J Exp Med 1988;167:988.
555. Goodwin RG, Lupton S, Schmierer A, et al. Human interleukin 7: molecular cloning and growth factor activity on human and murine B-lineage cells. Proc Natl Acad Sci USA 1989;86:302.
556. Baggiolini M, Walz A, Kunkel SL. Neutrophil-activating peptide-1/interleukin 8: a novel cytokine that activates neutrophils. J Clin Invest 1989;84:1045.
557. Schmid J, Weissmann C. Induction of mRNA for a serine protease and a beta-thromboglobulin–like protein in mitogen-stimulated human leukocytes. J Immunol 1987;139:250.
558. Detmers PA, Lo SK, Olsen-Egbert E, Walz A, Baggiolini M, Cohn ZA. Neutrophil-activating protein 1/interleukin 8 stimulates the binding activity of the leukocyte adhesion receptor CD11b/CD18 on human neutrophils. J Exp Med 1990;171:1155.
559. Gimbrone MA, Obin MS, Brock AF, et al. Endothelial interleukin-8: a novel inhibitor of leukocyte-endothelial interactions. Science 1989;246:1601.
560. Yang Y-C, Ricciardi S, Ciarletta A, et al. Expression cloning of a cDNA encoding novel human hematopoietic growth factor: human homologue of murine T-cell growth factor P40. Blood 1989;74:1880.
561. Van Snick J, Goethals A, Renauld J-C, et al. Cloning and characterization

of a cDNA for a new mouse T cell growth factor (P40). J Exp Med 1989;169:363.
562. Donahue RE, Yang Y-C, Clark SC. Human P40 T-cell growth factor (interleukin-9) supports erythroid colony formation. Blood 1990;75: 2271.
563. Moore KW, Vieira P, Fiorentino DF, et al. Homology of cytokine synthesis inhibitory factor (IL-10) to the Epstein-Barr virus gene BCRFI. Science 1990;248:1230.
564. Paul SR, Bennett F, Calvetti JA, et al. Molecular cloning of a cDNA encoding interleukin 11: a stromal cell–derived lymphopoietic and hematopoietic cytokine. Proc Natl Acad Sci USA 1990;87:7512.
565. Clark S. Interleukin-12: a heterodimeric cytokine with multiple biologic activities. Molecular Biology of Hematopoiesis, 8th Symposium, Basel, Switzerland, July 9–13, 1993.
566. Cherwinski HM, Schumacher JH, Brown KD, Mosmann TR. Two types of mouse helper T cell clone. III. Further differences in lymphokine synthesis between Th1 and Th2 clones revealed by RNA hybridization, functionally monospecific bioassays, and monoclonal antibodies. J Exp Med 1987;166:1229.
567. Brown KD, Zurawski SM, Mosmann TR, Zurawski G. A family of small inducible proteins secreted by leukocytes are members of a new superfamily that includes leukocyte- and fibroblast-derived inflammatory agents, growth factors, and indicators of various activation processes. J Immunol 1989;142:679.
568. McKenzie ANJ, Culpepper JA, de Waal Malefyt R, et al. Interleukin 13, a T-cell–derived cytokine that regulates human monocyte and B-cell function. Proc Natl Acad Sci USA 1993;90:3735.
569. Morgan JG, Dolganov GM, Robbins SE, et al. The selective isolation of novel cDNAs encoded by the regions surrounding the human interleukin 4 and 5 genes. Nucleic Acids Res 1992;20:5173.
570. Minty A, Chalon P, Derocq J-M, et al. Interleukin 12 is a new human lymphokine regulating inflammatory and immune responses. Nature 1993;362:248.
571. Punnonen J, Aversa G, Cocks BG, et al. Interleukin 13 induces interleukin 4–independent IgG4 and IgE synthesis and CD23 expression by human B cells. Proc Natl Acad Sci USA 1993;90:3730.
572. Zurawski SM, Vega F Jr, Huyghe B, Zurawski G. Receptors for interleukin-13 and interleukin-4 are complex and share a novel component that functions in signal transduction. EMBO J 1993;12:2663.
573. Metcalf D, Stanley ER. Haematological effects in mice of partially purified colony stimulating factor (CSF) prepared from human urine. Br J Haematol 1971;21:481.
574. Metcalf D, Nicola NA. Proliferative effects of purified granulocyte colony-stimulating factor (G-CSF) on normal mouse hemopoietic cells. J Cell Physiol 1983;116:198.
575. Sonoda Y, Yang Y-C, Wong GG, Clark SC, Ogawa M. Analysis in serum-free culture of the targets of recombinant human hemopoietic growth factors: interleukin 3 and granulocyte-macrophage colony-stimulating factor are specific for early developmental stages. Proc Natl Acad Sci USA 1988;85:4360.
576. Sieff CA, Ekern SC, Nathan DG, et al. Combinations of recombinant colony stimulating factors are required for optimal hematopoietic differentiation in serum-deprived culture. Blood 1989;73:688.
577. Sieff CA, Niemeyer CM, Nathan DG, et al. Stimulation of human hematopoietic colony formation by recombinant gibbon multi-colony–stimulating factor or interleukin-3. J Clin Invest 1987;80:818.
578. Gasson JC, Weisbart RH, Kaufman SE, Clark SC, et al. Purified human granulocyte-macrophage colony-stimulating factor: direct action on neutrophils. Science 1984;226:1339.
579. Weisbart RH, Golde DW, Clark SC, Wong GG, et al. Human granulocyte-macrophage colony-stimulating factor is a neutrophil activator. Nature 1985;314:361.
580. Metcalf D, Begley CG, Johnson GR. Biologic properties *in vitro* of a recombinant human granulocyte-macrophage colony-stimulating factor. Blood 1986;67:37.
581. Arnaout MA, Wang EA, Clark SC, Sieff CA. Human recombinant granulocyte macrophage colony-stimulating factor increases cell to cell adhesion and surface expression of adhesion promoting surface glycoproteins on mature granulocytes. J Clin Invest 1986;78:597.
582. Lopez AF, To LB, Yang Y-C, Gamble JR, et al. Stimulation of proliferation, differentiation, and function of human cells by primate interleukin 3. Proc Natl Acad Sci USA 1987;84:2761.
583. Lopez AF, Nicola NA, Burgess AW, et al. Activation of granulocyte cytotoxic function by purified mouse colony stimulating factors. J Immunol 1983;131:2983.
584. Hamilton JA, Stanley ER, Burgess AW, Shadduck RK. Stimulation of macrophage plasminogen activator activity by colony-stimulating factors. J Cell Physiol 1980;103:435.
585. Nicola NA, Metcalf D. Binding of iodinated multipotential colony-stimulating factor (interleukin-3) to murine bone marrow cells. J Cell Physiol 1986;128:180.
586. Sieff CA, Emerson SG, Mufson A, Gesner TG, et al. Dependence of highly enriched human bone marrow progenitors on hemopoietic growth factors and their response to recombinant erythropoietin. J Clin Invest 1986;77:74.
587. Eaves CJ, Eaves AC. Erythropoietin (Ep) dose-response curves for three classes of erythroid progenitors in normal human marrow and in patients with polycythemia vera. Blood 1978;52:1196.
588. Eaves AC, Eaves CJ. Erythropoiesis in culture. Clin Haematol 1984;13: 371.
589. Iscove NN. Erythropoietin-dependent stimulation of early erythropoiesis in adult bone marrow cultures by conditioned media from lectin stimulated mouse spleen cells. In: Golde DW, Cline MJ, Metcalf D, Fox CF, eds. Hematopoietic cell differentiation. New York, Academic Press, 1978:37.
590. Valtieri M, Gabbianelli M, Pelosi E, Bassano E, et al. Erythropoietin alone induces erythroid burst formation by human embryonic but not adult BFU-E in unicellular serum-free culture. Blood 1989;74:460.
591. Koenig JM, Christensen RD. Neutropenia and thrombocytopenia in infants with Rh hemolytic disease. J Pediatr 1989;114:625.
592. Christensen RD, Koenig JM, Viskochil DH, Rothstein G. Down-modulation of neutrophil production by erythropoietin in human hematopoietic clones. Blood 1989;74:817.
593. Sawada K, Krantz SB, Dessypris EN, Koury ST, et al. Human colony-forming units–erythroid do not require accessory cells, but do require direct interaction with insulin-like growth factor I and/or insulin for erythroid development. J Clin Invest 1989;83:1701.
594. Kurtz A, Jelkmann W. Insulin stimulates erythroid colony formation independently of erythropoietin. Br J Haematol 1983;53:311.
595. Yu J, Shao L, Vaughan J, Vale W, et al. Characterization of the potentiation effect of activin on human erythroid colony formation in vitro. Blood 1989;73:952.
596. Smith JC, Price BM, van Nimmen K, Huylebroeck D. Identification of a potent xenopus mesoderm–inducing factor as a homologue of activin A. Nature 1990;345:729.
597. Torok-Storb BJ, Martin PJ, Hansen JA. Regulation of in vitro erythropoiesis by normal T cells: evidence for two T cell subsets with opposing functions. Blood 1981;58:171.
598. Lipton JM, Nadler LM, Canellos GP, Kudisch M, Reiss CS, Nathan DG. Evidence for genetic restriction in the suppression of erythropoiesis by a unique subset of T lymphocytes in man. J Clin Invest 1983;72: 694.
599. Hoffman R, Kopel SD, Hsu SD, Dainiak N, Esmail Zanjani. T cell chronic lymphocytic leukemia: presence in bone marrow and peripheral blood of cells that suppress erythropoiesis in vitro. Blood 1978;52:255.
600. Bagby GC Jr. T lymphocytes involved in inhibition of granulopoiesis in two neutropenic patients are of the cytotoxic/suppressor ($T3^+T8^+$) subset. J Clin Invest 1981;68:1597.
601. Abdou JI, NaPombejara C, Balentine L, Abdou NL. Suppressor cell-mediated neutropenia in Felty's syndrome. J Clin Invest 1978;61:738.
602. Sugimoto M, Wakabayashi Y, Shiokawa Y, Takaku F. Effect of peripheral blood lymphocytes from systemic lupus erythematosus patients on human bone marrow granulocyte precursor cells (colony-forming units in culture). Stem Cells 1982;2:164.
603. Bom-van Noorloos AA, Pegels JG, van Oers RHJ, et al. Proliferation of T-gamma cells with killer-cell activity in two patients with neutropenia and recurrent infections. N Engl J Med 1980;302:933.
604. Linch DC, Cawley JC, MacDonald SM, et al. Acquired pure red cell aplasia associated with an increase of T cells bearing receptors for the Fc of IgG. Acta Haematol 1981;65:270.
605. Torok-Storb BJ, Sieff C, Storb R, Adamson J, Thomas ED. In vitro tests for distinguishing possible immune-mediated aplastic anemia from transfusion-induced sensitization. Blood 1980;55:211.
606. Bacigalupo A, Podesta M, Mingari MC, Moretta L, van Lint MT, Marmont A. Immune suppression of hematopoiesis in aplastic anemia: activity of T lymphocytes. J Immunol 1980;125:1449.
607. Linch DC, Cawley JC, Worman CP, et al. Abnormalities of T-cell subsets in patients with neutropenia and an excess of lymphocytes in the bone marrow. Br J Haematol 1981;48:137.
608. Torok-Storb BJ, Hansen JA. Modulation of in vitro BFU-E growth by normal Ia-positive T cells is restricted by HLA-DR. Nature 1982;298: 473.
609. Krensky AM, Reiss CS, Mier JW, Strominger JJ, Burakoff SJ. Long-term human cytolytic T-cell lines allospecific for HLA-DR6 antigen are OKT4+. Proc Natl Acad Sci USA 1982;79:2365.
610. Falkenburg JHF, Jansen J, van der Vaart-Duinkerken N, et al. Polymorphic and monomorphic HLA-DR determinants on human hematopoietic progenitor cells. Blood 1984;63:1125.
611. Sieff C, Bicknell D, Caine G, Robinson J, Lam G, Greaves MF. Changes in cell surface antigen expression during hemopoietic differentiation. Blood 1982;60:703.
612. Greaves MF, Katz FE, Myers CD, Davies L, Sieff C. Selective expression of cell surface antigens on human haematopoietic progenitor cells. In: Palek J, ed. Hematopoietic stem cell physiology. New York, Alan R Liss, 1985;301.
613. Sparrow RL, Williams N. The pattern of HLA-DR and HLA-DQ antigen expression on clonable subpopulations of human myeloid progenitor cells. Blood 1986;67:379.
614. Burdach SEG, Levitt LJ. Receptor-specific inhibition of bone marrow erythropoiesis by recombinant DNA-derived interleukin-2. Blood 1987; 69:1368.
615. Burdach S, Shatsky M, Wagenhorst B, Levitt L. The T-cell CD2 deter-

minant mediates inhibition of erythropoiesis by the lymphokine cascade. Blood 1988;72:770.
616. Guba SC, Stella G, Turka LA, et al. Regulation of interleukin 3 gene induction in normal human T cells. J Clin Invest 1989;84:1701.
617. Roodman DC, Bird A, Hutzler D, Montgomery W. Tumor necrosis factor-alpha and hematopoietic progenitors: effects of tumor necrosis factor on the growth of erythroid progenitors CFU-E and BFU-E and the hematopoietic cell lines K562, HL60, and HEL cells. Exp Hematol 1987;15:928.
618. Broxmeyer HE, Williams DE, Lu L, et al. The suppressive influences of human tumor necrosis factor on bone marrow hematopoietic progenitor cells from normal donors and patients with leukemia: synergism of tumor necrosis factor and interferon-gamma. J Immunol 1986;136: 4487.
619. Furmanski P, Johnson CS. Macrophage control of normal and leukemic erythropoiesis: identification of the macrophage-derived erythroid suppressing activity as interleukin-1 and the mediator of its in vivo action as tumor necrosis factor. Blood 1990;75:2328.
620. Hoffman R. Regulation of megakaryocytopoiesis. Blood 1989;74:1196.
621. Chauvet M, Leger J, Molina L, Chabannon C, Hollard D. Study of megakaryocytic progenitors (CFU-MK) in human long-term bone marrow cultures (LTBMC): adjuvant effect of plasma from aplastic patients. Exp Hematol 1990;18:61.
622. Yamasaki K, Solberg LA Jr, Jamal N, et al. Hemopoietic colony growth-promoting activities in the plasma of bone marrow transplant recipients. J Clin Invest 1988;82:255.
623. Kanz L, Lohr GW, Fauser AA. Lymphokine(s) from isolated T lymphocyte subpopulations support multilineage hematopoietic colony and megakaryocytic colony formation. Blood 1986;68:991.
624. Geissler D, Konwalinka G, Peschel C, Braunsteiner H. The role of erythropoietin, megakaryocyte colony-stimulating factor, and T-cell–derived factors on human megakayrocyte colony formation: evidence for T-cell–mediated and T-cell–independent stem cell proliferation. Exp Hematol 1987;15:845.
625. Ishibashi T, Kimura H, Shikama Y, Uchida T, Kariyone S, Maruyama Y. Effect of recombinant granulocyte-macrophage colony-stimulating factor on murine thrombocytopoiesis in vitro and in vivo. Blood 1990;75: 1433.
626. Straneva JE, Briddell RA, McDonald TP, Yang HH, Hoffman R. Effects of thrombocytopoiesis-stimulating factor on terminal cytoplasmic maturation of human megakaryocytes. Exp Hematol 1989;17:1122.
627. Bruno E, Briddell R, Hoffman R. Effect of recombinant and purified hematopoietic growth factors on human megakaryocyte colony formation. Exp Hematol 1988;16:371.
628. Long MW, Hutchinson RJ, Gragowski LL, Heffner CH, Emerson SG. Synergistic regulation of human megakaryocyte development. J Clin Invest 1988;82:1779.
629. Mazur EM, Cohen JL, Bogart L. Human serum megakaryocyte colony-stimulating activity appears to be distinct from interleukin-3, granulocyte-macrophage colony-stimulating factor, and lymphocyte-conditioned medium. Blood 1990;76:290.
630. Donahue RE, Seehra J, Metzger M, et al. Human interleukin-3 and GM-SCF act synergistically in stimulating hematopoiesis in primates. Science 1988;241:1820.
631. Fraser JK, Tan AS, Lin F-U, Berridge MV. Expression of specific high-affinity binding sites for erythropoietin on rat and mouse megakaryocytes. Exp Hematol 1989;17:10.
632. Ishibashi T, Koziol JA, Burstein SA. Human recombinant erythropoietin promotes differentiation of murine megakaryocytes in vitro. J Clin Invest 1987;79:286.
633. Clark DA, Dessypris EN. Effects of recombinant erythropoietin on murine megakaryocytic colony formation in vitro. J Lab Clin Med 1986;108: 423.
634. Lu L, Briddell RA, Graham CD, Brandt JE, Bruno E, Hoffman R. Effect of recombinant and purified human haematopoietic growth factors on in vitro colony formation by enriched populations of human megakaryocyte progenitor cells. Br J Haematol 1988;70:149.
635. McDonald TP, Cottrell MB, Clift RE, Cullen WC, Lin F-K. High doses of recombinant erythropoietin stimulate platelet production in mice. Exp Hematol 1987;15:719.
636. Berridge MV, Fraser JK, Carter JM, Lin F-K. Effects of recombinant human erythropoietin on megakaryocytes and on platelet production in the rat. Blood 1988;72:970.
637. Grossi A, Vannucchi AM, Rafanelli T, Ferrini PR. Recombinant human erythropoietin has little influence on megakaryocytopoiesis in mice. Br J Haematol 1989;71:463.
638. Cullen WC, McDonald TP. Effects of isobaric hypoxia on murine medullary and splenic megakaryocytopoiesis. Exp Hematol 1989;17:246.
639. McDonald TP. Thrombopoietin: its biology, purification, and characterization. Exp Hematol 1988;16:201.
640. McDonald TP, Clift RE, Cottrell MB. A four-step procedure for the purification of thrombopoietin. Exp Hematol 1989;17:865.
641. Greenberg SM, Kuter DJ, Rosenberg RD. In vitro stimulation of megakaryocyte maturation by megakaryocyte stimulatory factor. J Biol Chem 1987;262:3269.
642. Tayrien G, Rosenberg RD. Purification and properties of a megakaryocyte stimulatory factor present both in the serum-free conditioned medium of human embryonic kidney cells and in thrombocytopenic plasma. J Biol Chem 1987;262:3262.
643. Hill RJ, Leven RM, Levin FC, Levin J. The effect of partially purified thrombopoietin on guinea pig megakaryocyte ploidy in vitro. Exp Hematol 1989;17:903.
644. Clark DA, Dessypris EN, Koury MJ. Induction of megakaryocytic colony-stimulating activity in mouse skin by inflammatory agents and tumor promoters (42474). Proc Soc Exp Biol & Med 1987;184:245.
645. Murphy MJ. Megakaryocyte colony-stimulating factor and thrombopoiesis. Hematol Oncol Clin North Am 1989;3:465.
646. McDonald TP. The regulation of megakaryocyte and platelet production. Int J Cell Cloning 1989;7:139.
647. Yamamoto R, Lin LS, Lowe R, Warren MK, White TJ. The human lung fibroblast cell line, MRC-5, produces multiple factors involved with megakaryocytopoiesis. J Immunol 1989;144:1808.
648. Lotem J, Shabo Y, Sachs L. Regulation of megakaryocyte development by interleukin-6. Blood 1989;74:1545.
649. Koike K, Nakahata T, Kubo T, et al. Interleukin-6 enhances murine megakaryocytopoiesis in serum-free culture. Blood 1990;75:2286.
650. Ishibashi T, Kimura H, Shikama Y, et al. Interleukin-6 is a potent thrombopoietic factor in vivo in mice. Blood 1989;74:1241.
651. Hill RJ, Warren MK, Levin J. Stimulation of thrombopoiesis in mice by human recombinant interleukin-6. J Clin Invest 1990;85:671.
652. Neben T, Loebelenz J, Hayes L. Recombinant human interleukin-11 stimulates megakaryocytopoiesis and increases peripheral platelets in normal and splenectomized mice. Blood 1992;81:901.
653. Bruno E, Miller ME, Hoffman R. Interacting cytokines regulate in vitro human megakaryocytopoiesis. Blood 1989;73:671.
654. Gewirtz AM, Calabretta B, Rucinksi B, Niewiarowski S, Xu WY. Inhibition of human megakaryocytopoiesis in vitro by platelet factor 4 (PF4) and a synthetic COOH-terminal PF4 peptide. J Clin Invest 1989;83: 1477.
655. Ishibashi T, Miller SL, Burstein SA. Type beta transforming growth factor is a potent inhibitor of murine megakaryocytopoiesis in vitro. Blood 1987;69:1737.
656. Gewirtz AM, Zu WY, Mangan KF. Role of natural killer cells, in comparison with T lymphocytes and monocytes, in the regulation of normal human megakaryocytopoiesis in vitro. J Immunol 1987;139:2915.
657. Pantel K, Nakeff A. Differential effect of natural killer cells on modulating CFU-meg and BFU-E proliferation in situ. Exp Hematol 1989;17: 1017.
658. Kindler J, Thorens B, De Kossodo S, et al. Stimulation of hematopoiesis *in vivo* by recombinant bacterial murine interleukin 3. Proc Natl Acad Sci USA 1986;83:1001.
659. Metcalf D, Begley CG, Johnson GR, Nicola NA, Lopez AF, Williamson DJ. Effects of purified bacterially synthesized murine multi-CSF (IL-3) on hematopoiesis in normal adult mice. Blood 1986;68:46.
660. Donahue RE, Wang EA, Stone DK, et al. Stimulation of hematopoiesis in primates by continuous infusion of recombinant human GM-CSF. Nature 1986;321:872.
661. Nienhuis AW, Donahue RE, Karlsson S, et al. Recombinant human granulocyte-macrophage colony stimulating factor (GM-CSF) shortens the period of neutropenia after autologous bone marrow transplantation in a primate model. J Clin Invest 1987;80:573.
662. Welte K, Bonilla MA, Gillio AP, et al. Recombinant human granulocyte-colony-stimulating factor: effects on hematopoiesis in normal and cyclophosphamide treated primates. J Exp Med 1987;165:941.
663. Gabrilove J, Jakubowski A, Scher H, et al. Effect of granulocyte colony-stimulating factor on neutropenia and associated morbidity due to chemotherapy for transitional-cell carcinoma of the urothelium. N Engl J Med 1988;318:1414.
664. Bronchud MH, Scarffe JH, Thatcher N, et al. Phase I/II study of recombinant human granulocyte colony-stimulating factor in patients receiving intensive chemotherapy for small cell lung cancer. Br J Cancer 1987;56:809.
665. Kodo H, Tajika K, Takahashi S, Ozawa K, Asano S, Takaku F. Acceleration of neutrophilic granulocyte recovery after bone-marrow transplantation by the administration of recombinant human granulocyte colony-stimulating factor. Lancet 1988;2:38.
666. Duhrsen U, Villeval JL, Boyd J, Kannourakis G, Morstyn G, Metcalf D. Effects of recombinant human granulocyte colony-stimulating factor on hematopoietic progenitor cells in cancer patients. Blood 1988;72: 2074.
667. Tamura M, Hattori K, Nomura H, et al. Induction of neutrophilic granulocytes in mice by administration of purified human native granulocyte colony-stimulating factor (G-CSF). Biochem Biophys Res Comm 1987;142:454.
668. Shimaura M, Kobayashi Y, Yuo A, et al. Effect of human recombinant granulocyte colony-stimulating factor on hematopoietic injury in mice induced by 5-fluorouracil. Blood 1987;69:353.
669. Herrmann F, Schulz G, Lindemann A, et al. Hematopoietic responses in patients with advanced malignancy treated with recombinant human granulocyte-macrophage colony-stimulating factor. J Clin Oncol 1989;7: 159.
670. Steward WP, Scarffe JH, Austin R, et al. Recombinant human granu-

locyte macrophage colony stimulating factor (rhGM-CSF) given as daily short infusions: a phase I dose-toxicity study. Br J Cancer 1989;59: 142.
671. Antman KS, Griffin JD, Elias A, et al. Effect of recombinant human granulocyte-macrophage colony-stimulating factor on chemotherapy-induced myelosuppression. N Engl J Med 1988;319:593.
672. Socinski MA, Cannistra SA, Elias A, Antman KH, Schnipper L, Griffin JD. Granulocyte-macrophage colony stimulating factor expands the circulating haemopoietic progenitor cell compartment in man. Lancet 1988;1:1194.
673. Ganser A, Lindemann A, Seipelt G, et al. Effects of recombinant human interleukin-3 in patients with normal hematopoiesis and in patients with bone marrow failure. Blood 1990;76:666.
674. Ottmann OG, Ganser A, Seipelt G, Eder M, Schulz G, Hoelzer D. Effects of recombinant human interleukin-3 on human hematopoietic progenitor and precursor cells in vivo. Blood 1990;76:1494.
675. Motoyoshi K, Takaku F, Maekawa T, et al. Protective effect of partially purified human urinary colony-stimulating factor on granulocytopenia after antitumor chemotherapy. Exp Hematol 1986;14:1069.
676. Brandt SJ, Peters WP, Atwater SK, et al. Effect of recombinant human granulocyte-macrophage colony-stimulating factor of hematopoietic reconstitution after high-dose chemotherapy and autologous bone marrow transplantation. N Engl J Med 1988;318:869.
677. Nemunaitis J, Singer JW, Buckner CD, et al. Use of recombinant human granulocyte-macrophage colony-stimulating factor in autologous marrow transplantation for lymphoid malignancies. Blood 1988;72:834.
678. Blazar BR, Kersey JH, McGlave PB, et al. In vivo administration of recombinant human granulocyte/macrophage colony-stimulating factor in acute lymphoblastic leukemia patients receiving purged autografts. Blood 1989;73:849.
679. Sheridan WP, Morstyn G, Wolf M, et al. Granulocyte colony-stimulating factor and neutrophil recovery after high-dose chemotherapy and autologous bone marrow transplantation. Lancet 1989;1:891.
680. Peters WP, Stuart A, Affronti ML, Kim CS, Coleman RE. Neutrophil migration is defective during recombinant human granulocyte-macrophage colony-stimulating factor infusion after autologous bone marrow transplantation in humans. Blood 1988;72:1310.
681. Masaoka T, Motoyoshi K, Takaku F, et al. Administration of human urinary colony-stimulating factor after bone marrow transplantation. Bone Marrow Transplant 1988;3:121.
682. Vadhan-Raj S, Keating M, LeMaistre A, et al. Effects of recombinant human granulocyte-macrophage colony-stimulating factor in patients with myelodysplastic syndromes. N Engl J Med 1987;317:1545.
683. Antin JH, Smith BR, Holmes W, Rosenthal DS. Phase I/II study of recombinant human granulocyte-macrophage colony-stimulating factor in aplastic anemia and myelodysplastic syndrome. Blood 1988;72:705.
684. Ganser A, Volkers B, Greher J, et al. Recombinant human granulocyte-macrophage colony-stimulating factor in patients with myelodysplastic syndromes: a phase I/II trial. Blood 1989;73:31.
685. Thompson JA, Lee DJ, Kidd P, et al. Subcutaneous granulocyte-macrophage colony-stimulating factor in patients with myelodysplastic syndrome: toxicity, pharmacokinetics, and hematological effects. J Clin Oncol 1989;7:629.
686. Kobayashi Y, Okabe T, Ozawa K, et al. Treatment of myelodysplastic syndromes with recombinant human granulocyte colony-stimulating factor: a preliminary report. Am J Med 1989;86:178.
687. Negrin RS, Haeuber D, Nagler A, et al. Treatment of myelodysplastic syndromes with recombinant human granulocyte colony-stimulating factor: a phase I/II trial. Ann Intern Med 1989;110:976.
688. Champlin RE, Nimer SD, Ireland P, Oette DH, Golde DW. Treatment of refractory aplastic anemia with recombinant human granulocyte-macrophage colony-stimulating factor. Blood 1989;73:694.
689. Vadhan-Raj S, Buescher S, Broxmeyer HE, et al. Stimulation of myelopoiesis in patients with aplastic anemia by recombinant human granulocyte-macrophage colony-stimulating factor. N Engl J Med 1988;319:1628.
690. Guinan E, Sieff C, Oette D, Nathan DG. Recombinant granulocyte macrophage colony stimulating factor in severe aplastic anemia of childhood. Blood 1989;74.
691. Nissen C, Tichelli A, Gratwohl A, et al. Failure of recombinant human granulocyte-macrophage colony-stimulating factor therapy in aplastic anemia patients with very severe neutropenia. Blood 1988;72:2045.
692. Groopman JE, Mitsuyasu RT, DeLeo MJ, Oette DH, Golde DW. Effects of recombinant human granulocyte-macrophage colony-stimulating factor on myelopoiesis in the acquired immunodeficiency syndrome. N Engl J Med 1987;317:593.
693. Groopman JE, Molina JM, Scadden DT. Hematopoietic growth factors: biology and clinical applications. N Engl J Med 1989;321:1449.
694. Perno CF, Yarchian R, Conney DA, et al. Replication of human immunodeficiency virus in monocytes: granulocyte/macrophage colony-stimulating factor (GM-CSF) potentiates viral production yet enhances the antiviral effect mediated by 3′-azido-2′,3′-dideoxythymidine (AZT) and other dideoxynucleoside congeners of thymidine. J Exp Med 1989;169:933.
695. Pietsch T, Buhrer C, Mempel K, et al. Blood mononuclear cells from patients with severe congenital neutrophenia are capable of producing a granulocyte colony-stimulating factor. Blood 1991;77:1234.
696. Welte K, Zeidler C, Reiter A, et al. Differential effects of granulocyte-macrophage colony-stimulating factor and granulocyte-stimulating factor in children with severe congenital neutropenia. Blood 1990;75: 1056.
697. Bonilla MA, Gillio AP, Ruggiero M, et al. Effects of recombinant human granulocyte colony-stimulating factor on neutropenia in patients with congenital agranulocytosis. N Engl J Med 1989;320:1574.
698. Hammond WP, Price TH, Souza LM, Dale DC. Treatment of cyclic neutropenia with granulocyte colony-stimulating factor. N Engl J Med 1989;320:1306
699. Jakubowski AA, Souza L, Kelly F, et al. Effects of human granulocyte colony-stimulating factor in a patient with idiopathic neutropenia. N Engl J Med 1989;320:38.
700. Socinski MA, Cannistra SA, Sullivan R, et al. Granulocyte-macrophage colony-stimulating factor induces the expression of the CD11b surface adhesion molecule on human granulocytes in vivo. Blood 1988;72:691.
701. Devereaux S, Linch DC, Campos-Costa D, Spittle MF, Jelliffe AM. Transient leukopenia induced by granulocyte-macrophage colony-stimulating factor. Lancet 1987;2:1523.
702. Gribben JG, Devereux S, Thomas NSB, et al. Development of antibodies to unprotected glycosylation sites on recombinant human GM-CSF. Lancet 1990;335:434.
703. Glaspy JA, Baldwin GC, Robertson PA, et al. Therapy for neutropenia in hairy cell leukemia with recombinant human granulocyte colony-stimulating factor. Ann Intern Med 1988;109:789.
704. Winearls CG, Oliver DO, Pippard MJ, Reid C, Downing MR, Cotes PM. Effect of human erythropoietin derived from recombinant DNA on the anemia of patients maintained by chronic haemodialysis. Lancet 1986;2:1175.
705. Eschbach JW, Abdulhadi MH, Browne JK, et al. Recombinant human erythropoietin in anemic patients with end-stage renal disease. Ann Intern Med 1989;111:992.
706. Adamson JW. The promise of recombinant human erythropoietin. Semin Hematol 1989;26(Suppl 2):5.
707. Dessypris EN, Graber SE, Krantz SB, Stone WJ. Effects of recombinant erythropoietin on the concentration and cycling status of human marrow hematopoietic progenitor cells in vivo. Blood 1988;72:2060.
708. Laupacis A. Changes in quality of life and functional capacity in hemodialysis patients treated with recombinant human erythropoietin. Semin Nephrol 1990;10(Suppl 1):11.
709. Eschbach JW, Kelly MR, Haley NR, Abels RI, Adamson JW. Treatment of the anemia of progressive renal failure with recombinant human erythropoietin. N Engl J Med 1989;321:158.
710. MacDougall IC, Roberts DE, Neubert P, Dharmasena AD, Coles GA, Williams JD. Pharmacokinetics of recombinant human erythropoietin in patients on continuous ambulatory peritoneal dialysis. Lancet 1989;1: 425.
711. Bommer J, Ritz E, Weinrich T, Bommer G, Ziegler T. Subcutaneous erythropoietin. Lancet 1988;2:406.
712. Means RT, Olsen NJ, Krantz SB, et al. Treatment of the anemia of rheumatoid arthritis with recombinant human erythropoietin: clinical and in vitro studies. Arthritis Rheum 1989;32:638.
713. Fischl M, Galpin JE, Levine JD, et al. Recombinant human erythropoietin for patients with AIDS treated with zidovudine. N Engl J Med 1990;322:1488.
714. Umemura T, al-Khatti A, Donahue RE, Papayannopoulou TH. Stamatoyannopoulos G. Effects of interleukin-3 and erythropoietin on in vivo erythropoiesis and F-cell formation in primates. Blood 1989;74: 1571.
715. Goodnough LT, Rudnick S, Price TH, et al. Increased preoperative collection of autologous blood with recombinant human erythropoietin therapy. N Engl J Med 1989;321:1163.
716. Martin DIK, Zon LI, Mutter G, Orkin SH. Expression of an erythroid transciption factor in megakaryocytic and mast cell lineages. Nature 1990;344:444.

3

Stem Cell Disorders

Blood: Principles and Practice of Hematology,
edited by Robert I. Handin, Thomas P. Stossel, and Samuel E. Lux.
J.B. Lippincott Company, Philadelphia © 1995.

9

Inherited Bone Marrow Failure Syndromes

Blanche P. Alter

Constitutional aplastic anemia was defined by O'Gorman Hughes[1] as "chronic bone marrow failure associated with other features, such as congenital anomalies, a familial incidence, or thrombocytopenia at birth." In fact, he was referring to inherited aplastic anemia. Patients with constitutional aplastic anemia are genetically at risk for bone marrow failure, which may be expressed at birth (and therefore congenital), but often develops later. O'Gorman Hughes further divided constitutional aplastic anemia into three types using terminology that is confusing and no longer relevant. We will refer to each disorder by its eponym until more specific information becomes available and to the entire group as the *inherited bone marrow failure syndromes* (see section on acquired aplastic anemia).

One hypothesis regarding "acquired" aplastic anemia is that it develops in patients whose genotype predisposes them to the marrow-suppressant effects of detrimental environmental factors. We can sometimes identify homozygotes for autosomal recessive types of inherited bone marrow failure syndromes (or hemizygotes for X-linked disorders) by phenotype, but we cannot yet identify heterozygotes except by inference from family studies. The tools of molecular biology are being applied to these disorders, and our hypothesis may soon be testable.[2] Inherited bone marrow failure is probably more common than published reports indicate, since the phenotype may range from severely abnormal to entirely normal (see following text). In this section, we discuss the classic phenotypes in the major inherited bone marrow failure syndromes and emphasize the variation within each category. Some of this variation may result from the inadvertent inclusion of patients with congenital but not inherited phenotypes that resemble the genetic conditions, since for most disorders there is no specific diagnostic test.

The incidence of inherited marrow failure is difficult to ascertain from the literature. Among 134 patients with all types of aplastic anemia seen at the Children's Hospital Medical Center in Boston from 1958 to 1977, 40 had inherited disorders[3] (Fig. 9-1). Twenty-six patients had Fanconi's anemia (all diagnosed in the era before definitive testing of chromosome breakage after clastogenic stress), 4 developed aplastic anemia after amegakaryocytic thrombocytopenia, and 10 had familial aplastic anemia without physical or cytogenetic evidence for Fanconi's anemia. In 21 years at the Prince of Wales Hospital in Australia (1964 to 1984), 12 of 34 were found to have inherited syndromes, including 8 patients with Fanconi's anemia.[4]

In our previous analysis of the literature, we found that approximately 25% of childhood aplastic anemia was diagnosed as inherited, which is probably an underestimate.[5] The genetic syndromes must be considered carefully in patients of any age with aplastic anemia because the prognosis, treatment, and approach to bone marrow transplantation are different when the hematologic disorder is inherited rather than acquired.

PANCYTOPENIAS

Fanconi's Anemia

Fanconi's anemia was first described by Fanconi[6] in 1927 in three brothers with pancytopenia combined with physical abnormalities. The anemia was macrocytic and thus called pernizioisiforme, despite no further evidence for megaloblastic anemia. Uehlinger[7] then reported a similar patient with aplastic anemia and abnormalities of the thumb and kidney, and Fanconi[8] indicated that Naegeli suggested in 1931 that familial aplastic anemia plus congenital anomalies be called Fanconi's anemia.

Fanconi's anemia is defined by the finding of characteristic chromosomal breaks after clastogenic stress. The patient's physical appearance may or may not be normal, and he or she may or may not have aplastic anemia.[9] A recent review of Fanconi's anemia and current research can be found in a book edited by Schroeder-Kurth and coworkers.[10]

More than 700 cases of Fanconi's anemia have been mentioned in the literature with sufficient detail provided in many for the analyses described in this section.[5,11] For some of our analyses, cases were separated according to the intervals in which they were reported (1927 to 1960; 1961 to 1970; 1971 to 1980; 1981 to 1989) to determine whether any trends are present (Table 9-1).

In the total group of 688, the male/female ratio is 1.3:1. Figure 9-2 shows the distribution of ages at diagnosis for males and females. Although diagnoses were initially made most often when aplastic anemia was detected, the diagnosis was made occasionally in the nonanemic sibling of an affected patient. More recently, diagnoses have also been made after cytogenetic studies in patients with physical anomalies and normal hematologic status. The mean age at diagnosis in males was 7.9 years; in females, it was 8.8 years.

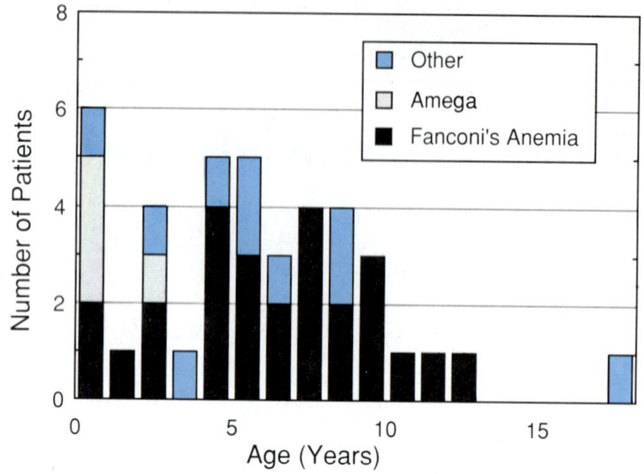

FIGURE 9-1. Age at diagnosis of inherited aplastic anemia in 40 patients seen at the Children's Hospital Medical Center, Boston, 1958 to 1970. Twenty-six patients had Fanconi's anemia; 4 patients had amegakaryocytic thrombocytopenia and developed aplastic anemia; and 10 patients (in 6 families) had other familial bone marrow failure syndromes. (Adapted from Alter BP, Potter NU, Li FP. Classification and aetiology of the aplastic anaemias. Clin Haematol 1978;7:431)

Although 75% of patients were between 3 and 14 years of age at the time of diagnosis of Fanconi's anemia, it is interesting to examine the extremes. Four percent were diagnosed between birth and 1 year of age[12–35]; only 10 of the 27 had hematologic manifestations at the time of diagnosis. Eighteen were males; 9 were females. Thus, Fanconi's anemia can be responsible for aplastic anemia in the first year of life and cannot be excluded because the patient is too young. At the other end of the age spectrum, 10% were diagnosed at 16 years of age or older.[21,32,36–78] Thirty-eight were male and 28 were female. The proportion of Fanconi's anemia patients who are adults is undoubtedly underestimated, both in the literature and in reality. Particularly when a patient lacks characteristic physical findings and is beyond childhood, inherited aplastic anemia is not usually considered. In the case of Fanconi's anemia, testing for chromosome breakage can provide a specific diagnosis.

Physical Examination

Initially, patients were diagnosed with Fanconi's anemia because of the combination of aplastic anemia and physical anomalies or other family members with aplastic anemia, anomalies, or both. This bias in the literature may have contributed to the perception that patients must have physical anomalies for the diagnosis of Fanconi's anemia to be made. The availability of the specific chromosome test in the last decade may have changed the pattern of diagnosis. In fact, the distribution and incidence of anomalies did not differ in those without and those with breakage analyses (Table 9-2). Because many patients had multiple anomalies even within one system, the number of patients with each category of abnormality is less than the number of abnormalities reported. Overall, only 7% had an absolutely normal appearance, whereas a similar percentage (9%) demonstrated only short stature, pigment abnormalities, or both (Table 9-3). These proportions were not affected by the availability of chromosome studies nor by the age of the patients. Figure 9-3 shows a boy with almost all the classic anomalies seen in those with Fanconi's anemia (to be described). The breadth of anomalies is wide, and some patients clearly have none.

The types of abnormalities seen in patients with Fanconi's anemia are listed in detail in Table 9-4. The most common anomaly is skin hyperpigmentation, a generalized brown melanin-like darkening, which is most prominent on the trunk, neck, and intertriginous areas and which becomes more obvious with age. Affected children are often thought to have a permanent suntan. Café-au-lait spots are common, alone or combined with hyperpigmentation, and hypopigmented areas are also seen. The number and size of these pigment changes also increases with the person's age.[79] Café-au-lait spots may actually be more common than hyperpigmentation, but many case reports probably did not differentiate between them.[80]

Microsomia, manifested by short stature and small delicate features, was often the presenting complaint in patients with Fanconi's anemia before the development of hematologic problems. Many patients did not eat or grow well in the early years. Upper limb abnormalities were reported in more than half. The thumbs were involved most frequently, with absence or hypoplasia in 22%. Absent or hypoplastic radii were always associated with absent or hypoplastic thumbs (unlike thrombocytopenia with absent radii (TAR) syndrome, in which the thumbs are always present despite the absence of the radii). Supernumerary, bifid thumbs and thumbs attached only by threads are also common. Flattening of the thenar eminence was reported in only 20 of all approximately 700 patients reported on, but it probably occurs much more frequently, as does weakness of one radial pulse, which are both subtle but common findings in our own experience.

TABLE 9-1. Fanconi's Anemia Literature

	1927–1960	1961–1970	1971–1980	1981–1989	Total
No. of patients	116	107	256	209	688
Male/female	1.4:1	1.7:1	1.5:1	1.1:1	1.3:1
Mean age at diagnosis, male (y)	7.5	7.8	7.6	8.7	7.9
Median	6	7	6.3	7	6.5
Range	2–30	0.6–21	0–27	0.2–24	0–30
Mean age at diagnosis, female (y)	7.7	9.6	9.0	9.0	8.8
Median	7	8.7	7.5	8	8
Range	1–14	0–35	0–48	0–32	0–48
Males ≤1	1	1	9	7	18
Females ≤1	2	1	3	3	9
Males ≥16	5	5	14	14	38
Females ≥16	0	5	11	12	28

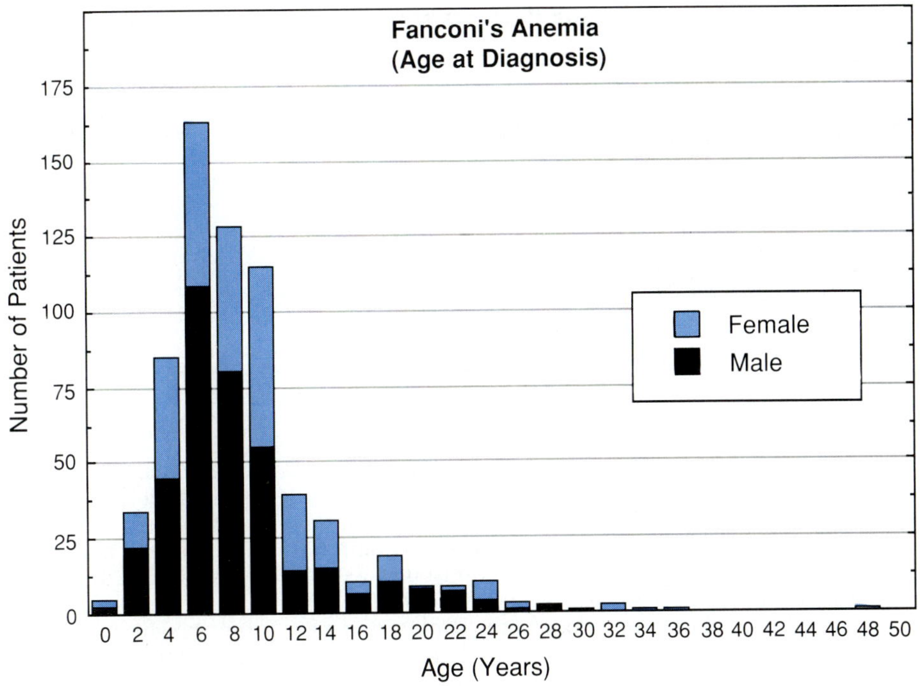

FIGURE 9-2. Age at diagnosis in nearly 700 published cases of Fanconi's anemia.

The next most common physical problem seen in patients with Fanconi's anemia involves the genitalia in close to 40% of males, with underdevelopment in 50% and undescended testes in 25%. Gonadal development in females was commented on in only eight cases, although abnormalities in menses and early menopause were mentioned in a few instances.

Abnormally shaped heads were reported in 30% of patients with Fanconi's anemia, with most having microcephaly. The facies are often characteristic (see Fig. 9-3). Neck anomalies lead to the perception of short or webbed necks, and spine anomalies also occur. The most common abnormalities of the eyes (in over 30%) are microphthalmia and strabismus, as well as epicanthal folds, hypertelorism, and ptosis. Ear problems occur in over 10%, with deafness as well as structural abnormalities of the external or middle ear being found.

Renal defects are found in more than 25% of Fanconi's anemia patients, with ectopic, pelvic, or horseshoe kidneys seen most frequently, as well as absent or hypoplastic kid-

TABLE 9-2. Physical Abnormalities in Fanconi's Anemia*

Abnormality	All Patients	No Cytogenetics	Breaks		Age	
			Spontaneous	Induced	<1 Year	≥16 Years
Skin	62	60	68	43	37	70
Short stature	59	53	65	65	63	67
Upper limbs	49	43	56	42	78	47
Hypogonads, male	39	39	39	33	33	61
Hypogonads, female	3	5	0	3	11	4
Head	26	29	25	17	22	18
Eyes	25	24	27	20	26	24
Renal	24	24	25	18	33	23
Birth weight ≤2500 g	14	12	15	18	52	9
Retardation	13	15	12	8	7	8
Lower limb	10	10	11	8	11	9
Ears	10	9	11	8	19	14
Reflexes increased	8	8	9	0	4	5
Other skeletal	6	4	9	3	4	14
Cardiopulmonary	7	5	8	7	19	5
Gastrointestinal	4	3	4	8	19	0
Other	4	4	4	7	4	2
No anomalies	7	8	6	12	8	7
Short stature and/or skin only	9	5	10	16	4	12
TOTAL PATIENTS	682	331	297	60	27	66

* Data are percentages of patients with the abnormality. The proportions are underestimates, since some reports did not provide physical descriptions.

TABLE 9-3. Fanconi's Anemia Patients Without Major Anomalies* (Estren-Dameshek Type)

Description	All Patients	No Cytogenetics	Breaks		Age	
			Spontaneous	Induced	<1 Year	≥16 Years
Café-au-lait spots	4	0	2	2	0	1
Pigmented areas	17	5	11	1	0	3
Short stature	8	4	2	2	0	1
Short stature + café-au-lait spots	5	1	2	2	1	0
Short stature + pigmented areas	18	5	10	3	0	3
Totally normal	43	22	15	6	2	4
TOTAL	95	37	42	16	3	12

* Data are numbers of patients with each characteristic.

neys. Most of the renal problems are structural, although functional defects resulting in reflux or infections can occur. The incidence of renal structural abnormalities may actually be higher than cited here, since many patients did not have intravenous pyelograms or ultrasound examinations. The incidence of some of the more overt anomalies such as those involving the upper limbs, kidney and gastrointestinal tract, as well as low birthweight, was higher in patients diagnosed as infants, in whom surgery was sometimes required, than it was in older patients.

Several abnormalities were described in fewer than 100 patients. These included low birthweight in at least 90 patients (particularly those diagnosed in infancy), developmental delay in 80, and defects involving the lower limbs in more than 60. Congenital heart disease was reported in 40 patients, and gastrointestinal anomalies in 20. Some of the feeding difficulties of infants with Fanconi's anemia might be due to gastrointestinal abnormalities that were not sought by radiographic studies. More than 50 patients had hyperreflexia, which may be more common than that number indicates, because hematologists often neglect to check reflexes. The incidence and types of anomalies are similar in both sexes.

Auerbach and colleagues[10,81] used a stepwise multivariate

TABLE 9-4. Specific Types of Anomalies in Fanconi's Anemia Patients*

SKIN

Generalized hyperpigmentation, on trunk, neck, and intertriginous areas; café-au-lait spots, hypopigmented areas

BODY

Short stature, delicate features

UPPER LIMBS

Thumbs—absent or hypoplastic, supernumerary, bifid, rudimentary, short, low-set, attached by a thread, triphalangeal, tubular, stiff, hyperextensible

Radii—absent or hypoplastic (only with abnormal thumbs), absent or weak pulse

Hands—clinodactyly, hypoplastic thenar eminence, 6 fingers, absent first metacarpal, enlarged, abnormal fingers, short fingers

Ulnae—dysplastic

GONADS

Males—hypogenitalia, undescended testes, hypospadias, abnormal, absent testis, atrophic testes, azospermia, phimosis, abnormal urethra, micropenis, delayed development

Females—hypogenitalia, bicornuate uterus, abnormal, aplasia of uterus and vagina; atresia of uterus, vagina, ovary

OTHER SKELETAL ANOMALIES

Head and face—microcephaly, hydrocephalus, micrognathia, peculiar face, bird face, flat head, frontal bossing, scaphocephaly, sloped forehead, choanal atresia

Neck—Sprengel's, short, low hairline, webbed

Spine—spina bifida (thoracic, lumbar, cervical, occult sacral), scoliosis, abnormal ribs, sacrococcygeal sinus, Klippel-Feil, vertebral anomalies, extra vertebrae

EYES

Small, strabismus, epicanthal folds, hypertelorism, ptosis, slanted, cataracts, astigmatism, blindness, epiphora, nystagmus, proptosis, small iris

EARS

Deaf (usually conductive), abnormal shape, atresia, dysplasia, low-set, large, small, infections, abnormal middle ear, absent drum, dimples, rotated, canal stenosis

KIDNEYS

Ectopic or pelvic, abnormal, horseshoe, hypoplastic or dysplastic, absent, hydronephrosis or hydroureter, infections, duplicated, rotated, reflux, hyperplasia, no function, abnormal artery

GASTROINTESTINAL SYSTEM

High arch palate, atresia (esophagus, duodenum, jejunum), imperforate anus, tracheoesophageal fistula, Meckel's diverticulum, umbilical hernia, hypoplastic uvula, abnormal biliary ducts, megacolon, abdominal diastasis, Budd-Chiari syndrome

LOWER LIMBS

Feet—toe syndactyly, abnormal toes, flat feet, short toes, clubfoot, 6 toes, supernumerary toe

Legs—congenital hip dislocation, Perthes, coxa vara, abnormal femur, thigh osteoma, abnormal legs

CARDIOPULMONARY SYSTEM

Patent ductus arteriosus, ventricular septal defect, abnormal, peripheral pulmonic stenosis, aortic stenosis, coarctation, absent lung lobes, vascular malformation, aortic atheromas, atrial septal defect, tetralogy of Fallot, pseudotruncus, hypoplastic aorta, abnormal pulmonary drainage, double aortic arch, cardiac myopathy

OTHER ANOMALIES

Slow development, hyperreflexia, Bell's palsy, CNS arterial malformation, stenosis of the internal carotid, small pituitary

* Abnormalities are listed in approximate order of occurrence within each category.

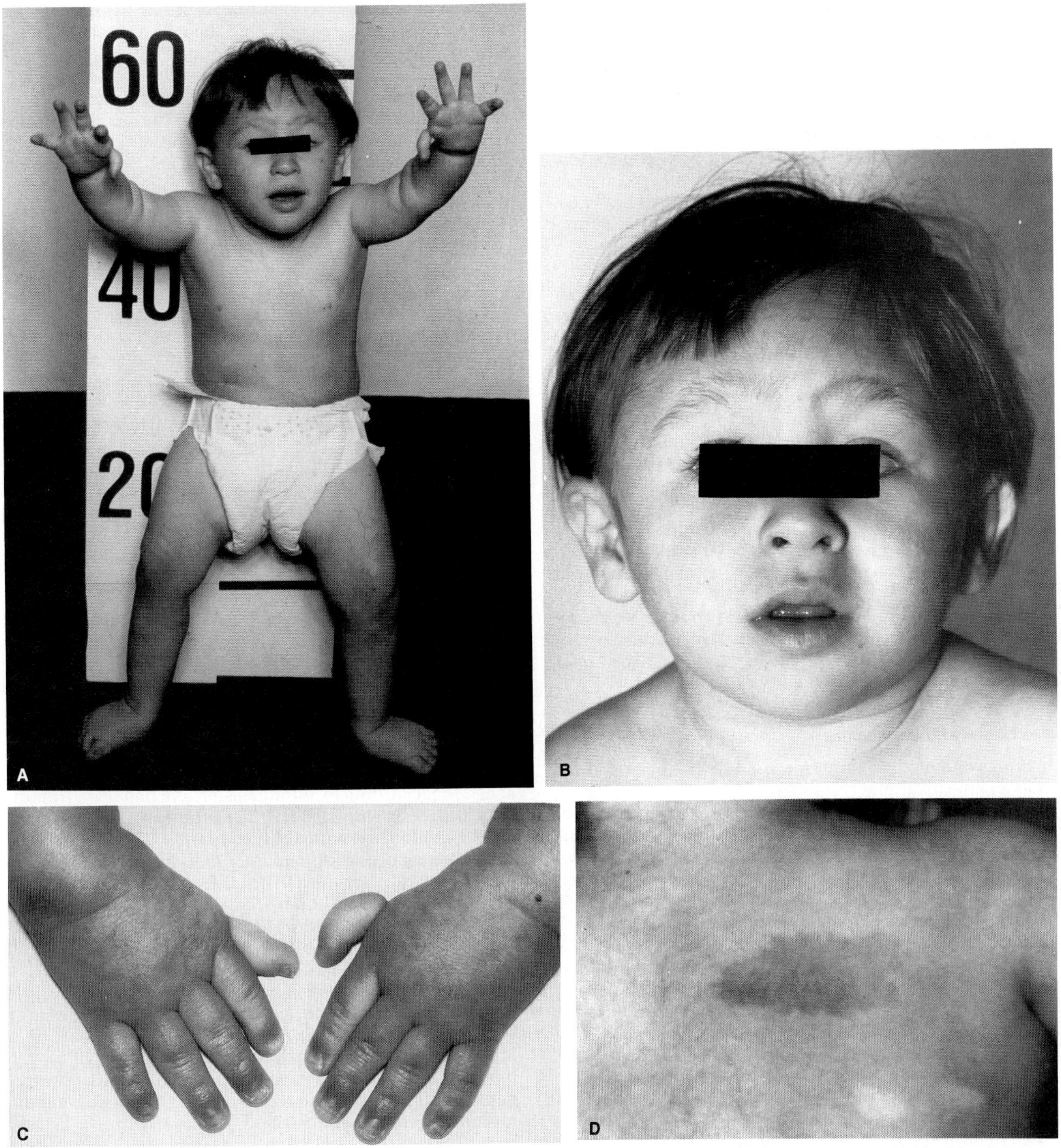

FIGURE 9-3. Three-year-old boy with Fanconi's anemia, with several phenotypic features. (**A**) Front view. (**B**) Face. (**C**) Hands. (**D**) Back of the right shoulder. Features to be noted are short stature, thumbs attached by threads, microcephaly, broad nasal base, epicanthal folds, micrognathia, and café-au-lait spot with hypopigmented areas beneath.

analysis of the first 162 patients in the International Fanconi Anemia Registry (IFAR) to identify eight variables that best discriminated patients with clastogenic stress-induced chromosome breakage (using diepoxybutane [DEB]) and those without chromosome breakage, and suggested a scoring system. One point each is added for microphthalmia, birthmarks, genitourinary abnormalities, growth retardation, absence of radius or thumb or both, and thrombocytopenia. One point is subtracted for learning disabilities and one for other skeletal abnormalities. Higher scores mean that the probability of Fanconi's anemia is increased.

The terms *constitutional aplastic anemia type II* and *Estren-Dameshek aplastic anemia* were used to describe patients with familial aplastic anemia but lacking anomalies. The original paper by Estren and Dameshek[82] described two such families. In fact, two of the patients did have undescended testes. Li and Potter[83] reinvestigated one of these families and discovered that a second cousin, whose parents were both cousins of the original parents, had typical Fanconi's anemia. Now that chromosome testing is available, patients whose anemia might have been called Estren-Dameshek can be correctly diagnosed as having Fanconi's anemia (see Table 9-3).

In the literature survey, 43 patients were entirely normal, and 52 had short stature, skin pigment changes, or both. The proportion of patients without anomalies was higher in the older group and in those studied by the more sensitive cytogenetic methods. Other than a recent increase in awareness of this diagnosis, this subset of patients does not differ from the overall group, and it is not a distinct syndrome.

Further evidence that the Estren-Dameshek patients are just part of the Fanconi's anemia spectrum is provided by the IFAR data[9] (Table 9-5). The diagnosis of Fanconi's anemia was made only when clastogenic stress-induced chromosome breaks were found, independent of physical appearance and family history (although many of the physically and hematologically normal children were tested only because of a positive family history). Thirty percent of the Fanconi's anemia group had aplastic anemia without anomalies, and 7% had neither. These proportions may be inflated, because the conclusion of no physical abnormalities was based on reporting by the referring physician, and not always by thorough examination by the IFAR organizers themselves. Two smaller studies in which the siblings of affected patients were examined also showed that at least 25% of those affected lacked anomalies.[84,85] Until analyses of the Fanconi's anemia gene or genes are available, Fanconi's anemia is considered to consist of a spectrum of physical findings, ranging from totally normal to the extreme of all the problems listed above.

Inheritance and Environment

Fanconi's anemia is clearly inherited in an autosomal recessive pattern, despite the apparent slight preponderance of males in the literature (see Table 9-1). In a large study, 30% of families had two affected children, and consanguinity was found in 10%.[21] In our literature review, we found 52 families with consanguinity, 160 with affected siblings, and 10 with affected cousins. Mothers of Fanconi's anemia patients appear to have an unusual number of miscarriages (22 noted in our survey); in some cases, the fetuses were examined and found to have significant physical anomalies. Rogatko and Auerbach[86] confirmed a monogenic autosomal recessive pattern by segregation analysis of the 86 cases in the report of Schroeder and coworkers[21] and of 88 affected persons in the IFAR. Patients have been reported from more than 40 countries, representing all ethnic and racial groups, including whites, blacks, Asians, Native Americans, and persons from India.

The heterozygote incidence may be 1 in 300 persons in the United States and 1 in 100 Afrikaans in South Africa; this is due to a founder effect.[21,87,88] Physical abnormalities were reported in a few parents.[89,90] It has been suggested that relatives of persons with Fanconi's anemia (possible heterozygotes) have an increased incidence of congenital malformations, particularly genitourinary and hand.[91] Some siblings had characteristic physical abnormalities without hematologic disease.[19,43,92,93] (These children may have developed aplastic anemia subsequently.) Some families have children with pancytopenia and normal physical examinations in addition to those with classic malformations.[94–96] A family was described in 1944 with one child with typical Fanconi's anemia, and his brother with paroxysmal nocturnal hemoglobinuria, who developed lung cancer and was proved to have Fanconi's anemia in 1987 by DEB-induced chromosome breakage[97] (Gordon-Smith EC, personal communication). A cousin, related both maternally and paternally, died of leukemia. These variations may reflect incomplete expression of the homozygous state or may occur in heterozygotes. Most of the reports antedated stress-induced chromosome breakage studies. The varied expression may indicate allelic but different genetic mutations, interacting mutant genes, or the influence of the environment on the Fanconi's anemia phenotype.

Patients with Fanconi's anemia can now be diagnosed by chromosome breakage studies before the onset of hematologic or malignant complications (preanemic phase[15,24,26,57,98]). The advantages of presymptomatic diagnoses are several. Patients can be told to avoid drugs and other agents that have been implicated in the development of acquired aplastic anemia. Prospective analysis in such venues as the IFAR will lead to a determination of the actual incidences of aplastic anemia, leukemia, and other malignancies. Factors that lead to the development of these complications (second hits) may be identified.

The environment has been invoked to explain the aplastic anemia in some cases. In one family with three Fanconi's anemia homozygotes,[99] one sister died of aplastic anemia at age 16 (according to another sister, she had been treating skin infections with coal tar). The other two sisters, proved to be Fanconi's anemia homozygotes by DEB-induced chromosome breakage, had only mild hypoplastic anemia more than 20 years later (Alter BP, Auerbach AD, unpublished data). Aplastic anemia developed in some Fanconi's anemia patients after viral illnesses, hepatitis, and tuberculosis.[95,96,100,101] Cases of Fanconi's anemia have been reported in which the patient received chloramphenicol before the onset of aplastic anemia.[89,102–105] These infectious or drug-related cases suggest a role for the environment in the development of bone marrow failure. The reporting of other families in whom siblings had the onset of pancytopenia at the same age suggest a genetic component.[21,100,106,107] Thus, the relative roles of genetics and environment are not yet clarified.

TABLE 9-5. International Fanconi's Anemia Registry

	FA	Non-FA
Aplastic anemia + anomalies	39%	10%
Aplastic anemia only	30%	65%
Anomalies only	24%	25%
Neither	7%	0%
TOTAL PATIENTS	202	108

(Adapted from Auerbach A, Rogatko A, Schroeder-Kurth TM. International Fanconi Anemia Registry: relation of clinical symptoms to diepoxybutane sensitivity. Blood 1989;73:391)

Laboratory Findings

The blood counts of patients often show thrombocytopenia or leukopenia before pancytopenia, which is usually mild or moderate initially; severe aplasia eventually develops in most cases. Even in the Fanconi's anemia patient with normal blood counts (the preanemic, or the treatment-responsive patient), erythrocytes are macrocytic, with mean cell volumes (MCVs) usually above 100 fl. The blood smear shows large red blood cells (RBCs) with mild poikilocytosis and anisocytosis, as well as a paucity of platelets and leukocytes if the numbers of these components are reduced (Fig. 9-4). Eventually, all three cell lines may fail.

The Fanconi's anemia patient may have larger RBCs with higher levels of fetal hemoglobin (Hb F) than a patient with severe acquired aplastic anemia, but these features are not diagnostic. At the aplastic stage, the bone marrow is hy-

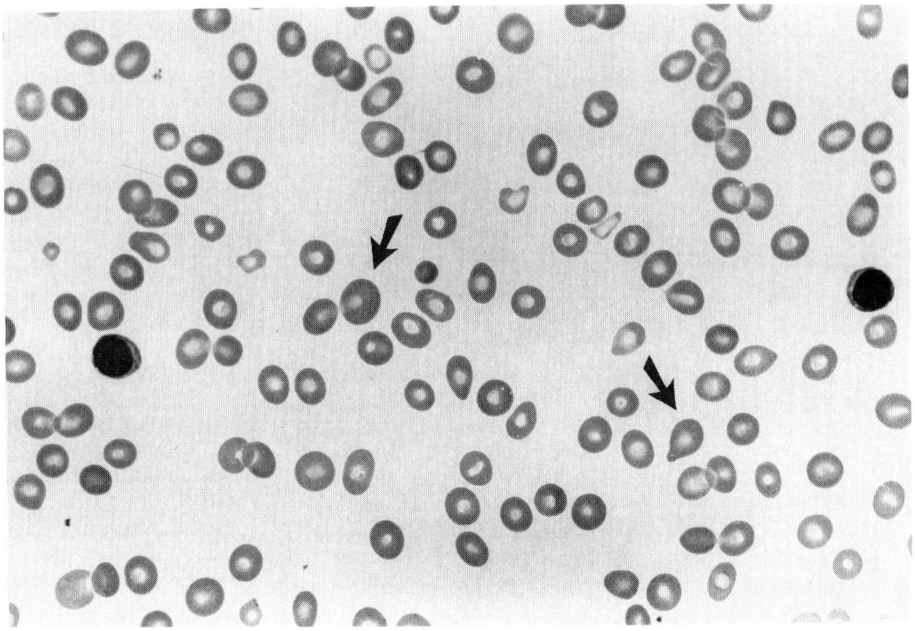

FIGURE 9-4. Peripheral blood from a patient with Fanconi's anemia. Note anisocytosis, macrocytes (*arrows*), thrombocytopenia, and neutropenia. (Courtesy of Dr. Gail Wolfe. Alter BP. The bone marrow failure syndromes. In: Nathan DG, Oski FA, eds. Hematology of infancy and childhood, ed 3. Philadelphia, WB Saunders, 1987:159)

pocellular and fatty, with few hematopoietic elements and a relative increase in lymphocytes, reticulum cells, mast cells, and plasma cells, identical with that found in the marrow in patients with acquired aplasia. In early Fanconi's anemia, areas of hypercellular marrow may be evident, but these disappear as aplasia progresses.[8]

Erythropoiesis in the Fanconi's anemia patient is characterized as stress erythropoiesis and is associated with the production of erythrocytes with fetal characteristics, as in patients with acquired aplastic anemia during recovery—either spontaneous or after marrow transplantation.[108,109] The features of this fetal-like erythropoiesis, which occurs during stress and is present in preanemic, anemic, and remission stage Fanconi's anemia patients, include macrocytosis, increased Hb F (by both alkali denaturation and Kleihauer-Betke acid elution), and presence of the i antigen. These features have also helped to identify nonanemic affected siblings of known patients. The Hb F is distributed unevenly, not clonally, and no concordance of the various fetal-like features exists at the level of single cells.[110] The level of Hb F or degree of macrocytosis does not provide any prognostic information.

Erythrokinetic studies were reported in a few patients.[56,89,96,111,112] RBC life-span was found to be slightly short, but hemolysis is not a major component of the anemia. Some patients with apparently short RBC life-span may have had blood loss associated with thrombocytopenia. Ferrokinetic studies suggest that most patients have a component of ineffective erythropoiesis in addition to relative marrow failure. Dyserythropoiesis was noted in the marrow erythroblasts in some cases, with fragmentation and multinuclearity.[89,101,113] Bone marrow imaging with technetium-99m sulfur colloid showed paradoxic and irregular tracer distribution in Fanconi's anemia, distinct from the uniform reduction seen in acquired aplastic anemia.[114] This may be related to the varied and irregular onset of aplasia in Fanconi's anemia patients. RBC enzymes have been decreased, increased, or normal in several contradictory studies[49,98,115,116]; the variable results may reflect the heterogeneity of Fanconi's anemia.

The small stature of Fanconi's anemia patients was ascribed to growth hormone (GH) deficiency in 14 of 19 patients in whom GH was reported to be measured,[117–130] whereas five were found not to be GH deficient.[66,122,131] Treatment with GH led to documented increased growth in only 5 of 11 patients,[118,119,122,128,130] and lack of growth in three.[121,124,127] No hematologic improvement was found with GH. In some families, GH deficiency and Fanconi's anemia segregated independently.[126,127] Because recombinant GH is available, its role in growth as well as hematopoiesis in Fanconi's anemia needs to be reexamined.[132] Reports suggest a possible association between GH therapy and leukemia, and thus its use in Fanconi's anemia must be considered carefully.[133]

Chromosome Breakage. The characteristic laboratory finding is the abnormal chromosome pattern, seen most easily in metaphase preparations of phytohemagglutinin-stimulated cultured peripheral blood lymphocytes. These reveal breaks, gaps, rearrangements, exchanges, and endoreduplications (Fig. 9-5), which are seen in less than 10% of the cells from normal persons, but in much higher proportions in cells from Fanconi's anemia homozygotes.[39,41,134–138] These features are seen infrequently in direct preparations of bone marrow cells, perhaps because cells with significant abnormalities may divide slowly, or may not survive in vivo.[135,139–141] Cultured skin fibroblasts also have abnormal chromosomes.[41,134,136] It is thought that the spontaneous aberrations seen in cultured blood lymphocytes or fibroblasts may be artifacts of culture, induced by unknown factors in the medium. Because marrow studies are direct, not cultured, these artifacts would not appear. The abnormal lymphocyte chromosomes have no relation to any hematologic findings, and variations in the proportions of abnormal cells or in the number of breaks per cell do not correlate with the clinical course. Furthermore, spontaneous breaks are sometimes absent in bona fide Fanconi's anemia cases.[9] Similar chromosomal changes have been reported in Bloom's syndrome and ataxia-telangiectasia[142] (also, see following text).

Cells from Fanconi's anemia patients are sensitive to oncogenic agents, such as SV40 viral transformation,[143] ionizing radiation,[144] and alkylating agents.[145] These agents damage DNA and produce significantly increased numbers of chromosomal aberrations in Fanconi's anemia cells. The chemicals used in several laboratories include DEB, nitrogen mustard, mitomycin C (MMC), cyclophosphamide, and platinum compounds.[31,145–149] Homozygotes are diagnosed based on an amplification of several times the rate of chro-

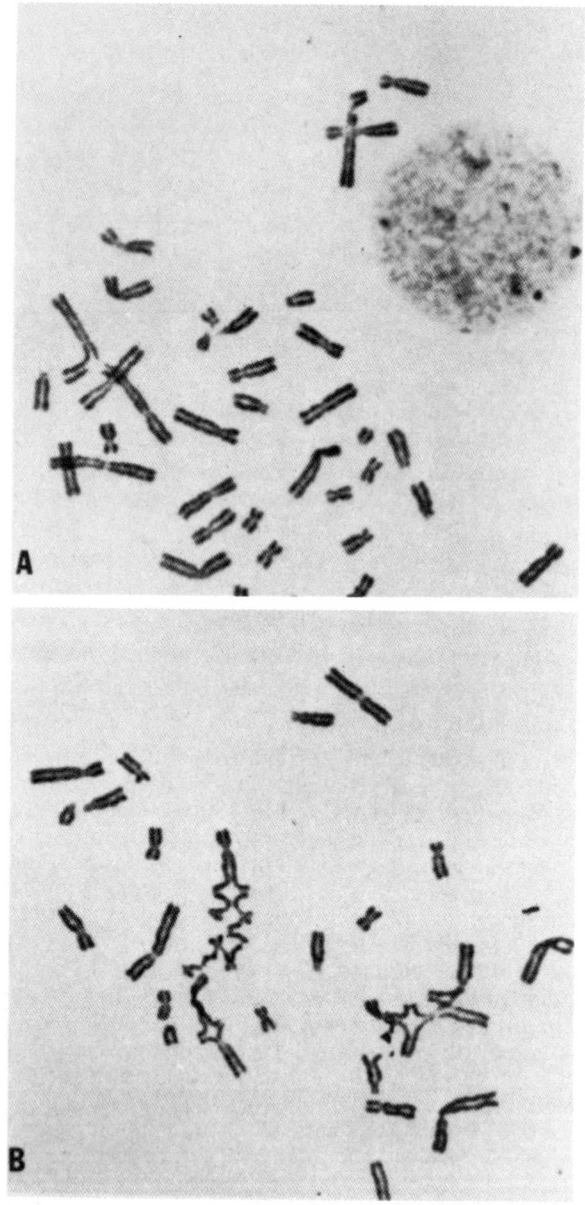

FIGURE 9-5. Cytogenetic findings in a patient with Fanconi's anemia. (**A**) No elastogen. (**B**) After culture with diepoxybutane. (Auerbach AD, Adler B, Chaganti RSK. Prenatal and postnatal diagnosis and carrier detection of Fanconi anemia by a cytogenetic method. Pediatrics 1981;67:128.

mosomal aberrations compared with the baseline spontaneous rate. The agents just cited do not result in increased breakage in the cells of patients with non-Fanconi's anemia chromosome breakage syndromes. In addition, although cells of patients with Bloom's syndrome show increased sister chromatid exchange after treatment with 5-bromodeoxyuridine (BUDR), Fanconi's anemia patients' cells do not.[150] Fanconi's anemia heterozygotes may also be detected, although in most studies an overlap occurs with the normal range.[28,65,147,151–153] Another approach to the diagnosis of Fanconi's anemia by means of alkylating agents involves flow cytometry rather than the counting of chromosomal aberrations. Cells so treated fail to divide, but undergo DNA replication and accumulate in the G2 phase of the cell cycle, where they are detected because of the increased amount of DNA per cell.[154]

The IFAR definition of Fanconi's anemia involves increased numbers of chromosome breaks per cell after culture with DEB, with a mean of 0.06 (range 0 to 0.36) in normal controls and 8.96 (1.3 to 23.9) in Fanconi's anemia patients.[9] Details of the technique are provided elsewhere.[155,156] Although most patients had multiple chromatid breaks and exchanges in most of their peripheral blood lymphocytes, 10% of the patients reported by Auerbach[156] had breaks in 10% to 40% of their DEB-treated lymphocytes. Clonal results have been reported by others as well.[157] These patients can be diagnosed, since the number of breaks per cell with breaks is still high. In addition, fibroblasts show breaks in a consistent and nonclonal manner.

A potentially simpler diagnostic test has been described by German and colleagues[158] and Arwert and Kwee,[157] involving coculture of equal numbers of sex-mismatched normal and patient lymphocytes in the presence of MMC, with the expectation that MMC will decrease growth of the Fanconi's anemia cells and lead to an unbalanced sex ratio. This test may result in false-negative diagnoses in those cases with clonal expression of Fanconi's anemia in their lymphocytes.

Prenatal diagnosis can be performed by examination of fetal amniotic fluid cells obtained at 16 weeks' gestation, or chorionic villus specimens (CVS) at 9 to 12 weeks.[28,103,155,156,159–166] Approximately 75 fetuses have been examined for risk of Fanconi's anemia. In the largest series, 14 samples were obtained by CVS, three of which had increased spontaneous and DEB-induced breaks.[156] In the same series, 7 of 46 fetuses studied by amniocentesis also had increased breaks by both assays. Of the total 10 affected, 8 pregnancies were terminated and 2 continued. One false-negative was obtained by CVS, with no confirmatory amniocentesis sample. In the positive cases, the cultured cells also grew more slowly. Three cases were also examined using fetal blood obtained prenatally, either primarily,[164] or to confirm an abnormal CVS or amniotic fluid result.[159,162] Of the affected cases, only 3 had physical anomalies, further supporting the suggestion that a large proportion of Fanconi's anemia homozygotes do not have malformations. The spontaneous and the clastogenic stress tests also suggested Fanconi's anemia prenatally in two cases in which the fetuses were not known to be at risk for Fanconi's anemia but in which cytogenetic studies were being performed for other reasons.[159,165]

The laboratory evaluation of patients in whom Fanconi's anemia is suspected should include complete blood counts, RBC size analysis, and Hb F measurement. Skeletal radiographs and intravenous pyelography or renal ultrasonography can be used for those with physical anomalies, or after the diagnosis has been proved by analysis of chromosomes. The specific diagnostic test is for chromosome breakage rates, both spontaneous and after clastogenic stress. Such tests have identified Fanconi's anemia homozygosity as the reason for physical anomalies in patients who were not anemic at the time,[15,24,26] and have diagnosed Fanconi's anemia in patients with aplastic anemia who lack malformations.[166,167]

Pathophysiology

The underlying defect in Fanconi's anemia is unknown. The relation among birth defects, hematopoietic failure, increased risk of malignancies, chromosome breakage, and DNA repair remains elusive. In utero, development of hematopoiesis and the organs that are most frequently abnormal in Fanconi's anemia occurs at approximately the same time (at 25 to 34 days of gestation), and a common toxic insult has been invoked.[107] The Fanconi's anemia genotype may make homozygotes more susceptible to the agents that can cause acquired aplastic anemia in normal persons (see acquired aplastic anemia section; Table 9-6). The oncogenic compounds that damage DNA in vitro may also be toxic in vivo.

Several types of agents are toxic to Fanconi's anemia cells in vitro, including the broad categories of alkylating agents and DNA cross-linkers.[29,31,144–147,149,168–173] Assays for the effects of these agents include cell growth kinetics and survival curves, DNA size, synthesis and repair, micronucleus formation, and chromosome breakage.

Many analyses have focused on DNA biochemistry. Excision repair of DNA damaged by ultraviolet (UV) radiation was reported to be impaired by some laboratories but not by others.[169,170,174–176] Decreased DNA repair after UV or γ-radiation was noted by one laboratory, whereas another laboratory reported normal excision repair using MMC, x-rays, or UV radiation.[177,178] Decreased DNA ligase was observed[165] whereas DNA topoisomerase was found to be increased in the cytoplasm and decreased in the nuclei of three Fanconi's anemia placentas and four Fanconi's anemia fibroblast lines.[179,180] Fanconi's anemia cells in culture grow more slowly than normal cells, without or with the addition of clastogenic agents.[181–186] They accumulate in G2.[154]

A theory regarding Fanconi's anemia is that cells are unable to remove oxygen free radicals and are damaged by these molecules. Thirty percent reduction of RBC superoxide dismutase (SOD) was reported by several groups,[55,187–190] and both RBCs and white cells were found to have low SOD by another group.[191] Normal RBC SOD, catalase, and glutathione peroxidase were reported, although glutathione transferase was increased.[192] Normal levels of SOD were found in Fanconi's anemia fibroblasts, which were also reported to have increased Mn-SOD, catalase, and glutathione peroxidase.[193,194] Thus, the suggestion was made that antioxidant effects in Fanconi's anemia cells may be restricted to the hematopoietic system.[195] The addition of SOD and catalase to Fanconi's anemia lymphocyte cultures decreased the numbers of breaks.[196]

In another study, SOD, catalase, or cysteine decreased MMC-induced breaks, but in similar proportions in normal as in Fanconi's anemia fibroblasts.[197] Culture of lymphocytes in increased oxygen tension resulted in increased spontaneous breaks in some Fanconi's anemia and not in normal cells, and in all Fanconi's anemia cells after MMC.[198,199] SOD increased the survival of Fanconi's anemia fibroblasts cultured with MMC.[200] Antioxidants were used to decrease spontaneous and DEB-induced chromosome breaks in Fanconi's anemia lymphocytes.[192] Two Fanconi's anemia patients were treated with SOD, with transient decreases in the number of spontaneous chromosome breaks.[201]

Sister chromatid exchanges (SCEs) are increased in some chromosome breakage syndromes. SCEs were found to be *not* increased in Fanconi's anemia lymphocytes, and actually decreased after culture with MMC[148,202] Some groups found that Fanconi's anemia and normal fibroblasts had similar levels of SCEs,[125,153,202–204] whereas others reported that MMC increased SCEs in both normal and Fanconi's anemia lymphocytes,[205,206] and that nitrogen mustard also increased SCEs.[153]

Diffusible clastogenic and normal factors were suggested by studies in which coculture of Fanconi's anemia with normal or Chinese hamster ovary (CHO) cells led to decreased chromosome breakage in the Fanconi's anemia and increased breakage in the non-Fanconi's anemia cells[207,208]; others were unable to demonstrate such an effect in coculture.[209] In fact, the coculture assay for the diagnosis of Fanconi's anemia just discussed would not work if there were diffusible factors.[157,210]

Hybrid cells formed from Fanconi's anemia and normal cells resulted in correction of the Fanconi's anemia breakage.[211–215] Other cell fusion studies using cell lines from a variety of Fanconi's anemia patients led to the demonstration of at least two complementation groups, involving at least nine patients,[213–215] although only a single group was found in five Japanese patients.[216] Duckworth-Rysiecki and coworkers[212] also found two complementation groups. The identification of distinct complementation groups has led to efforts to reconcile previously contradictory results, by either prospective studies or retrospective analysis of previous experiments.[217] Several laboratories in fact had examined group A cells.[165,174,218,219] Where both group A and group B were evaluated, group A cells had a more severe in vitro defect than did group B.[175,217,220–224] The complementation group does not appear to correlate with clinical status.

Efforts are underway to identify the specific molecular defect in Fanconi's anemia. Transfection of a Fanconi's anemia fibroblast cell line with normal high molecular weight DNA was reported to lead to cells with improved survival in the presence of MMC.[225] Buchwald and colleagues[226] were unable to demonstrate any foreign DNA in similar experiments, suggesting that the resistant cells might be revertants. Microinjection of fibroblasts of complementation group A with normal cell extracts improved the defect after 8-MOP/UVA.[227] Transfection of Fanconi's anemia fibroblasts with CHO DNA cured the growth inhibition and chromosome breakage of DEB; CHO DNA was shown to be present.[228] Auerbach and coworkers[229] fused Fanconi's anemia and normal, heterozygote, or homozygote lymphoblastoid cell lines, and improved survival in MMC. They emphasized that since any of the manipulations discussed here involve cloning of cells, a more normal Fanconi's anemia clone or a revertant might be selected. Direct attempts to identify the Fanconi's anemia gene with molecular techniques are being attempted by Auerbach and coworkers,[2] who have so far probably eliminated most of the chromosome 7q region by genetic linkage analysis. This group has suggested that group A patients have a mutation on 20q,[230] whereas Buchwald and colleagues have recently cloned the gene for Fanconi's anemia group C and have shown that it is on 9q.[231,232]

The hematopoietic defect in Fanconi's anemia patients is evident at the progenitor cell level in both bone marrow and peripheral blood. The numbers of hematopoietic pro-

TABLE 9-6. Agents Toxic to Fanconi's Anemia Cells in Vitro

AGENTS
γ-Irradiation
Ultraviolet irradiation
8-Methoxypsoralen + ultraviolet irradiation
DRUGS
Tetrametansulfonil-d-mannit
Nitrogen mustard
Mitomycin C
Diepoxybutane
Ethylmethanesulfonate
Isonicotinyl hydrazide
Cisplatin
Cyclophosphamide (Cytoxan) or its activation products

genitor cells (CFU-GM, CFU-E, BFU-E) were reduced in several patients, most of whom had aplastic anemia at the time of study,[121,233–240] as well as in a few who were not aplastic.[27] Only one patient had even close to normal progenitor cell numbers.[241] Prospective studies of nonanemic Fanconi's anemia patients may help to predict their hematologic status. Failure to grow in vitro, combined with the fact that cures can be obtained with bone marrow transplantation, suggest that the pluripotent stem cell is defective. Because the DNA repair defect is in all cells, the hematopoietic system just happens to be the one that fails most frequently.

Prognosis

In the past, when patients were diagnosed because they had already developed aplastic anemia and when the only treatment was red blood cell transfusions, 80% were reported to die within 2 years.[111] Almost all died within 4 years, with only rare long-term survivals.[242,243] Because diagnoses can be made before the onset of clinically significant hematologic or malignant symptoms, survival from the time of diagnosis is longer. More reliable information will eventually emerge from the prospective IFAR data, in which a large proportion of patients are entered who have no symptoms.

The cumulative survival of the Fanconi's anemia patients in the literature is shown in Figure 9-6 and Table 9-7. Fifty percent of the patients are predicted to die by the time they reach age 16, and only 25% are expected to live beyond age 26. Preliminary data from the IFAR and literature data for the most recent decade indicate a median survival of 25 years of age.[244] The expected median survival age for the more than 400 patients who did not receive androgens was 16 years, or 4 years from diagnosis, and for the more than 200 who did receive androgens was only age 17, or 7 years after the diagnosis of Fanconi's anemia. The androgen responders were distinguished by slightly better numbers: the projected median survival was age 20, or 9 years from diagnosis. Those who were either 1 year or less or 16 or more years of age when Fanconi's anemia was diagnosed fared slightly worse than the entire group, with an expected survival of only 3 years after diagnosis.

Older Patients. The older Fanconi's anemia males are often small, with underdeveloped genitalia, and abnormalities in spermatogenesis.[245] There is one report of a Fanconi's anemia male who fathered a child.[21]

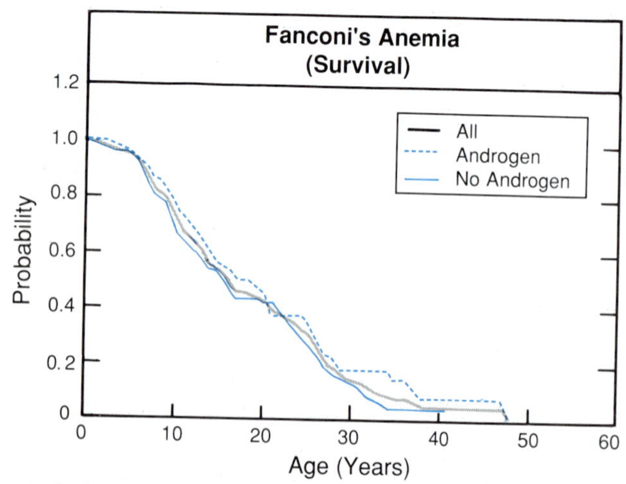

FIGURE 9-6. Kaplan-Meier plot of cumulative survival in Fanconi's anemia patients. Time is shown as years since diagnosis. Of 677 cases published from 1927 to 1989, 440 patients apparently did not receive androgens and 237 received androgens.

TABLE 9-7. Projected Survivals of Fanconi's Anemia Patients*

Group	Age (y)		Interval From Diagnosis (y)	
	50%	25%	50%	25%
All	16	26	6	14
Male	16	26	6	12
Female	16	27	5	14
No androgens	16	26	4	11
Androgens	17	26	7	17
No response	17	26	6	12
Response	20	28	9	17
Leukemia	15	21	5	9
Cancer	27	33	16	18
Liver disease	13	23	6	10
Diagnosis ≤1 y	3	11	3	10
Diagnosis ≥16 y	27	32	3	8
ED, totally normal	21	24	5	11
ED, short stature or skin abnormalities	24	28	11	17

ED, Estren-Dameshek.
* Survivals are determined from Kaplan-Meier estimates. Interval is from diagnosis of Fanconi's anemia.

The older females have irregular menses and early menopause.[41,66,246] Eleven Fanconi's anemia patients have been reported to have pregnancies and four more are known to us, resulting in nine infants.[41,42,57,59,67,70,246–250] Transfusions were often necessary because of worsening of maternal anemia, and cesarian sections were performed in at least four cases because of cephalopelvic disproportion between normal size infants and small Fanconi's anemia mothers. The incidence of miscarriages was high.

Androgen Therapy

Shahidi and Diamond[251] reported the use of androgens in 1959, with improvement in the first six patients. The response rate was noted to be 75% in the series by Sanchez-Medal[252] and Najean.[253] As with any new therapy, initial enthusiasm must give way to reality, and the response rate is now closer to 50%. The first sign of response is a rise in the reticulocyte count, followed by a rise in hemoglobin within 1 to 2 months. The white blood cell count is somewhat slower, and the platelet response, usually incomplete, may take 6 to 12 months.

Only a few patients were reported to be able to discontinue androgen therapy (often at the time of puberty) and maintain their blood counts.[22,27,98,248,254–260] Androgens have added about 2 years to actual (not actuarial) reported survivals (mean of 3.1 without and 5.2 years with androgens). The mean interval to death in those who did not respond to androgens was 3.3 years, similar to the interval in those who never received androgens. The interval to death was extended by more than 4 years to 6.9 years in those who showed some response to androgen treatment. Most patients eventually become refractory to the androgen with which they are treated, and changing to another only occasionally succeeds in buying more time. Some of the complications to be described in the following text develop in older patients, in whom androgens may have prolonged life sufficiently for these complications to appear, or they may have contributed to these developments.

Although some reports suggest that androgens alone are as effective as androgens combined with corticosteroids, the general recommendation is for a combination of the two.[253] The growth acceleration of androgens may be counterbalanced by the growth retardation of the corticosteroids.[261] In addition, corticosteroids may decrease bleeding at a given platelet count, perhaps by promoting vascular stability.[262] The most frequently used androgen is oxymetholone, an oral 17-α alkylated androgen, at 2 to 5 mg/kg/d. Prednisone is also given, at 5 to 10 mg every other day. If an injectable androgen is desired because of decreased risk of hepatotoxicity, the usual form is nandrolone decanoate, 1 to 2 mg/kg/wk, injected intramuscularly, with ice packs and pressure applied to prevent hematomas.

Etiocholanolone has been used with success in an otherwise refractory patient (Gardner FH, unpublished data, 1984). The first sign of response in this patient was the appearance of macrocytic RBCs (Fig. 9-7), as well as an increase in the proportion of RBCs containing Hb F. Potential side effects of androgens are obstructive liver disease, peliosis hepatis, and liver tumors. Patients receiving androgens should be monitored frequently with liver chemistries and ultrasonography. If a response occurs, the drug should be tapered slowly but probably not discontinued entirely. The only group of patients in whom discontinuation might routinely be considered are those from South Africa, who may be a genetically distinct Fanconi's anemia variant.[263] In most experiences elsewhere, relapses ensue when androgens are stopped, and subsequent remissions on the same or different preparations are sometimes elusive.

Bone Marrow Transplantation

Reconstitution of Fanconi's anemia patients with allogeneic hematopoietic stem cells offers the potential of a cure for the aplastic anemia and perhaps cure or prevention of leukemia. It does not prevent and may even accelerate the appearance of other malignancies (see later in text). Close to 100 transplantations have been performed worldwide, with the survival curves shown in Figure 9-8. Twenty-three were transplanted from HLA-matched siblings or matched parents, using the standard aplastic anemia cyclophosphamide regimen of 100 to 200 mg/kg given over 3 to 4 days.[264–274] Eleven (48%) of the 23 survived. Several studies

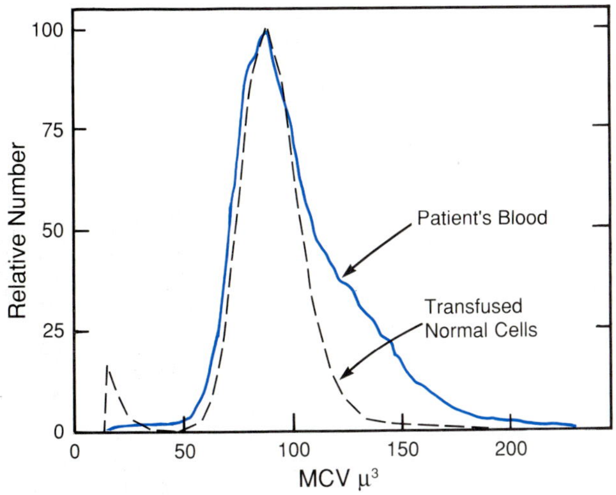

FIGURE 9-7. Red cell size distribution analysis in a patient with Fanconi's anemia treated with etiocholanolone. Note the positive skew and macrocytic shoulder, which indicate the beginning of a response to treatment. (Courtesy of Dr. Frank Gardner. Alter BP. The bone marrow failure syndromes. In: Nathan DG, Oski FA, eds. Hematology of infancy and childhood, ed 3. Philadelphia, WB Saunders, 1987:159)

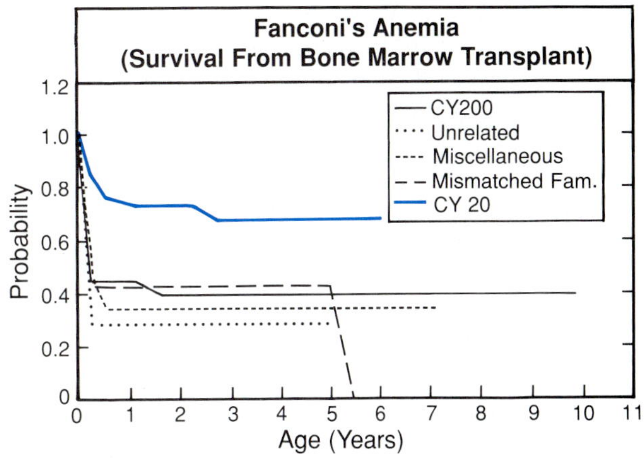

FIGURE 9-8. Kaplan-Meier plot of cumulative survival following bone marrow transplantation for patients with Fanconi's anemia. Time is shown as days from transplantation. Thirty-seven patients were treated with modified cyclophosphamide and TAI (CY20); 20 were treated with standard cyclophosphamide (CY200); 11 were treated with a variety of nonstandard preparations (miscellaneous); 7 had unrelated donors; and 7 had partially mismatched family donors.

have shown that a metabolite of cyclophosphamide is toxic to DNA, which explains the clinical symptoms of severe mucositis with intestinal malabsorption and hemorrhages, fluid retention, cardiac failure, and hemorrhagic cystitis.[31,173,275] Several modifications were then attempted, primarily involving the addition of procarbazine and antithymocyte globulin in 11 patients, as well as in three using thoracoabdominal radiation and T-cell depletion of donor marrow.[31,264,266,270,276–279] Of these 14 patients, only 5 (36%) were reported to be alive.

Gluckman introduced a modified protocol, using a total cyclophosphamide dose of 20 mg/kg, divided over 4 days, plus 5 Gy of thoracoabdominal radiation.[280] This protocol has been reported in a total of 37 patients, with 26 survivors, or 71%.[271,279–286] Problems of graft rejection and of graft-versus-host disease were no more frequent than in transplantations for acquired aplastic anemia.

In many instances, no HLA-compatible sibling is found who can be a marrow donor. Partially mismatched family members were used in seven reported cases, using the modified cyclophosphamide–thoracoabdominal radiation preparation.[279,287] Two survivors (29%) were reported. Unrelated computer-matched donors were also recorded in seven cases, with two survivors.[287–290] Persons with such transplants are particularly at risk for rejection or graft-verus-host disease.

The preferred donors for Fanconi's anemia transplantations are HLA-matched siblings who themselves need to be screened with thorough physical examinations, complete blood counts (including examination of the RBC, MCV, and Hb F), and cytogenetic studies for chromosome breakage, both baseline and after culture with a clastogenic stress agent such as DEB. In one case, the donor turned out to have Fanconi's anemia that had not been diagnosed before transplantation.[269] Parents have an unexpectedly high rate of HLA identity with Fanconi's anemia patients, only partly related to consanguinity, and may serve as marrow donors.[291,292]

Because umbilical cord blood apparently contains hematopoietic progenitor cells, some investigators have proposed cryopreservation of these cells from a non-Fanconi's anemia sibling diagnosed in utero, to use for later transplantation.[293] Two such cases were reconstituted at later than 6 months[294] (Gluckman E, unpublished data). Finally, the use of mismatched family members or unrelated donors should be reserved for the courageous.

The incidence of malignancies is increased in Fanconi's anemia patients (see section on complications). It is clear that bone marrow transplantation does not reduce this (except for hematologic malignancies); in fact, the cytoreductive therapy and radiation may increase this risk. Cancer of the tongue has been reported in two patients among almost 50 Fanconi's anemia long-term transplantation survivors, which is within the expected frequency so far.[295,296]

Other Treatment

Supportive care must be provided as for any patient with aplastic anemia. ϵ-Aminocaproic acid may be used for symptomatic bleeding, at a dose of 0.1 g/kg every 6 hours orally.[297] No family member should be used as a blood product donor until it is decided that a transplantation will not be done (even from an unrelated donor) to decrease the chance of sensitization. Washed or filtered RBCs should be used to reduce the risk of reactions and of HLA sensitization from white cells. The possibility of marrow transplantation must be considered early in the course of the patient's anemia. Although the use of androgens and transfusions does not preclude transplantation, the best results are seen in those whose medical complications are minimal. Drugs and chemicals that may be implicated as causal in acquired aplastic anemia should be avoided. In addition, medications or substances that interfere with platelet function (such as aspirin, antihistamines, nonsteroidal antiinflammatory drugs, glycerol guaiacolate, vitamin E, and cod liver oil) should not be given to thrombocytopenic patients. If a severe allergic reaction occurs during a blood transfusion, diphenhydramine (Benadryl) can be used acutely.

Splenectomy has no apparent role in the management of Fanconi's anemia. Thirty-eight cases were reported to have had this procedure, with no apparent long-term benefit. In some patients, transient improvement of pancytopenia occurred, but at a time when their bone marrow was not yet hypocellular.

Immunotherapy has no theoretical or factual basis. Although the use of high-dose methylprednisolone[298] and antithymocyte globulin[299] have been reported rarely in Fanconi's anemia, there are unreported instances of many patients in whom these modalities as well as cyclosporin A were used without success. In fact, approximately 10% of adults who failed to respond to any of these approaches were shown subsequently by clastogenic stress-induced chromosome breakage studies to have previously undiagnosed Fanconi's anemia (Auerbach AD, Young NS, unpublished data).

Lithium was reported to improve the blood counts in two of five Fanconi's anemia patients, presumably those whose marrow reserve was still present.[301]

Hematopoietic growth factors may have a role in the future management of Fanconi's anemia patients, but this area is awaiting investigation. Factors such as GM-CSF are beginning to be investigated in patients with acquired aplastic anemia, with some limited but encouraging responses.[302] One Fanconi's anemia patient was treated briefly with GM-CSF, with an increase in neutrophil count.[303] Although such factors may also predispose to leukemia,[304] these and others such as interleukin-3 (IL-3) still need to be tested for their role in the aplastic anemia of Fanconi's anemia.

Complications

The in vitro data regarding defects in DNA repair and cellular damage in Fanconi's anemia suggest that it might be a premalignant condition, which is borne out by the in vivo observations. More than 100 cases have been reported with leukemia or tumors, an overall incidence of close to 20%. Because this incidence reflects the biased reporting of interesting cases, the true figure must await long-term prospective analysis by the IFAR. More than 60 patients were reported with leukemia, and approximately 30 were reported with liver tumors and 30 with other cancers (Table 9-8). German[305] observed that cancer in Fanconi's anemia patients has been reported only since the mid-1960s and suggested that androgen therapy, which began in the early 1960s, allowed patients to survive long enough to develop the malignancy for which they were at risk. He also suggested that androgens might be implicated in causing these malignancies. Several patients who never received androgens developed leukemia or cancer; thus, the role of these drugs is unproved.

The finding of a single gene for Fanconi's anemia was thought to be sufficient to confer a risk of malignancy. Garriga and Crosby[306] reported an increased incidence of leukemia in Fanconi's anemia families, and Swift[307,308] found a predisposition to cancer in heterozygotes. Subsequently, these analyses were extended from the original eight fam-

TABLE 9-8. Complications in Fanconi's Anemia

	All Cases	Leukemia	Other Cancer	Liver Disease
No. of cases	688	63	32	30
Percentage of total	100	9.2	4.7	4.4
Male/female	1.3:1	1.5:1	0.4:1	1.5:1
Age at diagnosis (y)				
Mean	8	10	13	10
Median	7	8	12	7
Range	0–48	0.1–28	0.3–32	1–48
≥16	10%	22%	32%	25%
Age at complication (y)				
Mean		14	23	16
Median		14	23	13
Range		0.1–29	0.3–38	3–48
No. without pancytopenia	24 (3.5%)	11 (17.5%)	4 (12.5%)	1 (3.3%)
No. without androgens	447 (65%)	28 (44%)	11 (34%)	1 (3.3%)
No. reported deceased	290 (42%)	51 (81%)	19 (59%)	27 (90%)

ilies to 25 by Swift and colleagues,[309] and to nine families by Potter and coworkers[310]; neither study found an increase in cancer in Fanconi's anemia families. (Another disorder thought to be present at increased incidence in Fanconi's anemia heterozygotes is diabetes mellitus[311,312]). The earlier erroneous conclusions regarding cancer were attributed to small numbers, incorrect assignment of Fanconi's anemia heterozygotes, and biased selection.

Leukemia. Leukemia was reported in more than 60 cases, representing close to 10% of Fanconi's anemia patients in the literature. In a single series of 44 patients, 9 developed leukemia (20%), and 5 more were preleukemic.[32] Eleven of those with leukemia never had a preceding aplastic anemia, and the diagnosis of Fanconi's anemia was made only during the evaluation for leukemia. These 11 patients plus an additional 14 apparently never received androgens. Thus, androgens had no possible role in the development of leukemia in almost half of the patients. A recent communication[313] cites 2 additional patients who presented with acute myelomonocytic leukemia in whom

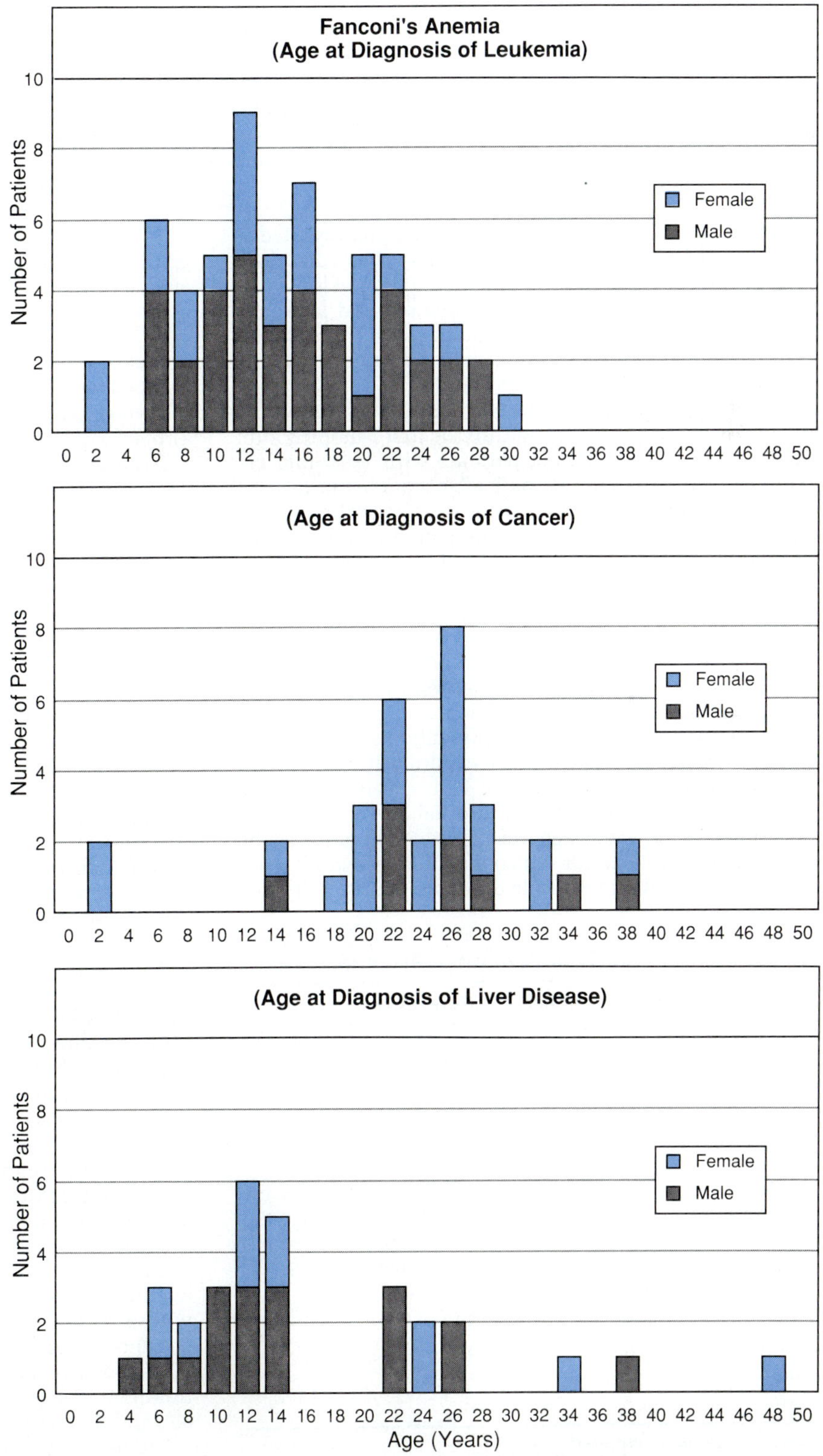

FIGURE 9-9. Age at diagnosis of complications of Fanconi's anemia in patients with leukemia, cancer, or liver disease.

the diagnosis of Fanconi's anemia was not made until after bone marrow transplantation; they developed toxicity from the preparation. These patients were found retrospectively to have chromosome breakage.

The characteristics of patients with Fanconi's anemia and leukemia are compared with those of the total group and those with other malignancies in Table 9-8 and Figure 9-9. The male/female ratio is 1.5:1. The diagnosis of Fanconi's anemia was made at a mean age of 10 years in those who eventually developed leukemia, and leukemia itself was diagnosed at a mean age of 14 years. The proportion of patients over 16 at diagnosis was higher in the leukemia group (13 patients) and includes four patients in their 20s whose Fanconi's anemia was first diagnosed when they presented with leukemia.

Because the most common leukemia in children is lymphocytic, it is noteworthy that until 1989 all leukemias reported in Fanconi's anemia were myeloid. Two cases of acute lymphocytic leukemia (ALL) have been reported, and two others mentioned, although it is not clear from the reports that these patients in fact had ALL.[129,263,314,315]

Table 9-9 lists the specific types of leukemia reported in Fanconi's anemia. At least six patients have been discussed in more than one publication, and the number of literature reports of patients with Fanconi's anemia and leukemia probably exceeds the actual number of cases. Four patients with leukemia had coincidental hepatic tumors, usually discovered at postmortem examination.[316–319]

Treatment of the leukemia was less than satisfactory, and deaths were on average within the first 2 months after diagnosis. Fanconi's anemia patients with leukemia are exquisitely sensitive to the toxic effects of chemotherapy, as predicted by the previous discussion regarding agents that increase damage to DNA. The combination of forms of leukemia that are difficult to treat in anyone (eg, myeloid), abnormal DNA repair, and lack of marrow reserve does not afford a good prognosis. The only apparent long-term remission reported was one of 9 years[30,330,339] (Roozendaal KJ, personal communication, 1989). One 2-year survivor after reduced-dosage chemotherapy subsequently succumbed to varicella[31] (Auerbach AD, personal communication). Bone marrow transplantation from an unrelated donor was attempted unsuccessfully in one patient (Lux S, unpublished data, 1984). Figure 9-10 shows the Kaplan-Meier plots for survival interval after diagnosis of Fanconi's anemia. Although the 50% survival rate was the same for leukemia as for Fanconi's anemia overall, subsequently those with leukemia did more poorly. Fifty-one

TABLE 9-9. Leukemia in Fanconi's Anemia

Type	Number*	References
Acute myeloblastic	22	22, 32, 54, 58, 72, 89, 237, 239, 260, 317, 318, 320–324, F.H. Gardner (unpublished)
Acute myelomonocytic	17	21, 30, 37, 52, 61, 65, 135, 138, 316, 325–330
Acute monocytic	7	71, 74, 101, 135, 331–334
Erythroleukemia	6	22, 63, 74, 121, 141, 245, 335–337
Acute (unspecified)	5	21, 32, 104, 329, 338
Acute nonlymphocytic	1	71
Acute megakaryoblastic	1	339
Chronic myelomonocytic	1	319
Acute lymphocytic	2	129, 315
TOTAL	63	

* Several cases were reported more than once.

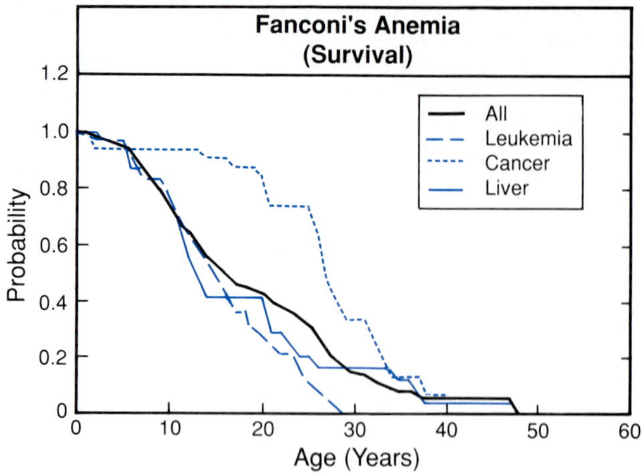

FIGURE 9-10. Kaplan-Meier plot of cumulative survival in patients with Fanconi's anemia with complications. Sixty patients had leukemia, 32 had cancer, and 30 had liver disease.

of the 63 patients (81%) had died at the time of the reports, and follow-up was not available for most of the other patients.

Will all patients develop leukemia if they do not succumb to aplastic anemia first? Probably not, since the older patients have the additional risk of other malignancies. Only long-term prospective studies can answer this question properly.

Preleukemia. Patients with Fanconi's anemia may develop syndromes that are variably called myelodysplastic, refractory anemia, or preleukemia. Some conditions evolve into full-blown leukemia, and other patients die in their preleukemic phase or are reported before further developments ensue.[32,34,57,71,76,141,237,322,340–344] Eighteen patients were reported with clonal cytogenetic abnormalities in bone marrow who did not yet have leukemia.[32,34,48,54,71,76,101,130,257,322,340,344,345] No consistent pattern was found in the involved chromosomes, although 1 and 7 were more common than others; partial or complete deletions, translocations, and marker chromosomes were found. Details of the cytogenetic findings can be found in the cited articles, and in a summary by Berger and Le Coniat,[341] Four patients (22%) went on to develop leukemia within 2 years and died at 7 months to 2 years (mean, 1.1 years), whereas seven died at 2 months to 6 years (mean, 1.4 years) without leukemia and seven were alive at up to 5 years (mean, 1.9 years) also without leukemia.

Three Fanconi's anemia patients were reported with Sweet's syndrome (acute neutrophilic infiltration of skin, associated 20% of the time with malignancy[345]). All had myelodysplastic bone marrow, and two had clonal chromosomal abnormalities. The skin infiltrates responded to prednisone, but sustained treatment was required. This differs from responses in non-Fanconi's anemia patients, where permanent resolution of symptoms occurs.

Cancers. Thirty-two patients (5%) were reported with cancers other than leukemia or liver. The group with cancer is different from the entire Fanconi's anemia population (see Table 9-8 and Fig. 9-9). The preponderance of females (male/female ratio is 1:0.4) was due to the prevalence of gynecologic malignancies. The age at diagnosis of Fanconi's anemia was an average of 13 years in the cancer group, with 32% being 16 years or older when diagnosed. Four patients never had aplastic anemia, and those plus seven more never received androgen therapy. All but two of the tumors developed in patients who were at least 13 years old, and the average age was 23. The younger patients were a 4-month-old who had a bone marrow lymphoma, and a

1½-year-old who had a Wilms' tumor and a medulloblastoma, both unusual tumors in Fanconi's anemia patients.[35,346] The types of tumors are listed in Table 9-10. Most tumors were gastrointestinal, from oropharynx to anus. The next most common tumors were gynecologic (vulva or cervix). Many of the gynecologic cancers had also extended into the anus and gastrointestinal tract, and some of the tumors that are listed separately but in the same patient could be local extension or metastasis. Most of the tumors were squamous cell carcinomas.

The survival curves in Figure 9-10 suggest that survival is longer from diagnosis of Fanconi's anemia in those with cancer. This can be interpreted to indicate that cancer is clearly a disease of the older Fanconi's anemia patient. Thus, if they do not die from aplastic anemia, or leukemia, or liver disease, they are at a high risk for another cancer. The expected 50% survival age for those who will have cancer is 27 years, at which age 80% of the original group of Fanconi's anemia patients have already died. This is 15 years from diagnosis of Fanconi's anemia, again a point at which 80% have died. Of particular concern is the older female Fanconi's anemia patient.

After the diagnosis of a malignancy is made, survival is on average less than 8 months. In one patient, a bronchogenic carcinoma was not detected until death from bleeding.[363] Another patient developed breast cancer at age 26 and died from metastatic disease 3 years later.[258] Treatment of these tumors is difficult, because of increased toxicity from chemotherapy or radiation therapy. Surgery is performed whenever possible. More than half of the patients had died at the time that they were reported.

Liver Disease. Liver disease, consisting mostly of hepatic tumors, was reported in 30 patients (5%). The male/female ratio of 1.5:1 and mean age of diagnosis of Fanconi's anemia of 10 years (see Table 9-8) indicate that this group is not different from the general group. The age at which liver complications was detected averaged 16 years, although the range was wide and encompassed the oldest patients (see Fig. 9-9). Only one patient did not have antecedent androgen treatment; thus, it might be argued that androgen treatment increases the risk of liver disease in Fanconi's anemia patients. The most common liver tumors were hepatocellular carcinomas, hepatomas, and adenomas (Table 9-11). One patient also had tongue cancer,[348] and four had leukemia.[316–319] In two, the liver tumors were found only at postmortem examination.[53,364]

TABLE 9-10. Cancer in Fanconi's Anemia

Type	Number*	References
GASTROINTESTINAL	25	
Gingiva	6	44, 46, 60, 316, 347
Tongue	6	67, 316, 348–351
Esophagus	7	42, 60, 62, 73, 105, 352, 353
Pharynx	1	354
Stomach	1	355
Colon	1	326
Anus	3	41, 46, 326
GYNECOLOGIC	11	
Vulva	9	41, 46, 326, 350, 356–359
Cervix	1	356
Breast	1	258
OTHER	6	
Bronchial	1	21
Mandible	1	360
Lymphoma	1	35
Medulloblastoma	1	361
Skin	1	362
Wilms' tumor	1	361
TOTAL	42	

* Number of tumors (42) exceeds number of patients (32) because some patients had two primary sites. Combinations include Wilms' plus medulloblastoma, two with anus plus vulva in situ, gingiva plus tongue, colon plus anus plus vulva, gingiva plus esophagus, cervix plus vulva, anus plus vulva, and tongue plus vulva. Some of these may have been local extension or metastasis.

TABLE 9-11. Liver Disease in Fanconi's Anemia

Type	Number	References
Hepatocellular cancer	10	248, 319, 348, 365–371
Hepatoma	7	45, 316–318, 364, 372–374
Adenoma	5	53, 375–378
Tumor	1	378
Coma	1	21
Peliosis alone (4 with tumor)	6	23, 25, 45, 50, 248, 318, 369, 372, BP Alter (unpublished)
TOTAL	30	

In three patients, discontinuation of androgens, alone or combined with bone marrow transplantation, led to resolution of the tumors.[248,378] Peliosis hepatis also reverses when androgens are stopped. Surgical removal of tumors was undertaken occasionally. The prognosis is poor with liver tumors. Twenty-seven of the 30 patients had died at the time of the reports. The projected survival rates shown in Figure 9-10 indicate that the patients with liver disease are again indistinguishable from the total Fanconi's anemia group. The average survival was under 4 months, with only a single patient who lived more than 6 months after the diagnosis of liver tumor.[365,366]

Summary of Malignancy in Fanconi's Anemia. The risk of developing leukemia, liver tumor, or another cancer in Fanconi's anemia patients totals at least 20% in the literature, although the true incidence may be obscured by overreporting. It is an important risk, particularly in older patients, since the average age at which malignancies are diagnosed is beyond the age of survival of half of Fanconi's anemia patients. Prolongation of survival by a combination of androgens, better supportive care, and bone marrow transplantation may lead to more time for malignancies to appear. In addition, Fanconi's anemia may be diagnosed in patients with malignancies but without any other stigmata of Fanconi's anemia, using chromosome breakage analysis. Concerns about the development of malignancies in older patients cannot be used as contraindications for aggressive management such as bone marrow transplantation. Cytoreductive chemotherapy and irradiation may themselves increase the risk of malignancies. To some degree, aplastic anemia may be considered to be the least of the problems of the Fanconi's anemia patient.

Dyskeratosis Congenita

Dyskeratosis congenita, also known as Zinsser-Cole-Engman syndrome, named after the first physicians who described these patients, is a rare form of ectodermal dysplasia, with approximately a 50% incidence of aplastic anemia and a 10% incidence of cancer. Dermatologic manifestations and nail dystrophies usually begin in the first decade, and leukoplakia in the second decade; all of these become more extreme with increasing age. These systems represent the diagnostic triad. Aplastic anemia usually develops in the second decade, and cancer in the third and fourth decades.

Inheritance and Environment

More than 160 cases have been reported, many of which are summarized elsewhere.[5,379,380] All ethnic groups are involved. Although the impression is that dyskeratosis congenita is an X-linked disorder, the male/female ratio is 4.7:1 in the literature[5] (Table 9-12).

Several categories of patients have what has been called dyskeratosis congenita:

Presumed X-linked recessive. More than 100 males have been reported as single cases or from families with males only. Nineteen were in sibships, with an additional three families with uncles and nephews, and three with maternal cousins.

Possible autosomal recessive. Two of the males and two brother–sister pairs were the products of consanguineous marriages.[381–383] Three more sets of brothers and sisters were found.[384–386] Ten females were reported as sporadic cases.[387–396]

Possible autosomal dominant. Four families were reported with apparent dyskeratosis congenita in males and females in two or three generations.[397–400] One family also had consanguinity.[400]

The possibly autosomal recessive or dominant families might be X-linked with inactivation of the normal chromosome, and variable levels of expression, but it is more likely that the dyskeratosis congenita phenotype may be due to more than one gene. Similarly, the presumably X-linked male group may contain autosomal recessive patients who happen to be male, as well as new mutation dominants. These possibilities may explain the apparent preponderance of females in the autosomal groups. The X-linked recessive group can be defined more specifically using Xq28 restriction fragment length polymorphisms.[401] No ethnic and sex association was found, since the X-linked male group included four black and six Asian families, the autosomal recessive group two black and one Asian, and the dominant group one black family.

The data in Tables 9-12 and 9-13 are separated by category, in an effort to determine whether the clinical conditions differ. The autosomal dominant group appears to be milder, with a lower incidence of all the findings in the diagnostic triad, and a lower rate of complications. The autosomal recessive group, albeit small, appears to have more physical abnormalities and a higher incidence of cancer and aplastic anemia.

The age at diagnosis of dyskeratosis congenita in the three groups is depicted in Figure 9-11. These data are skewed to the high side because in many cases the only age available was at the time of the report. The mean age for X-linked males was 19 years, autosomal recessives 15, and autosomal dominants 32, again distinguishing the latter group. The ages at development of the components of the diagnostic triad are summarized in Table 9-12. Nail and skin changes were noted at similar ages in the first decade in X-linked and autosomal recessive cases of dyskeratosis congenita, and leukoplakia was noticed earlier in recessives. Over 65% of the X-linked and autosomal recessive patients had all of the diagnostic triad, whereas this was true of less than 20% of the dominant cases.

Physical Examination

The major skin finding in patients with dyskeratosis congenita is reticulated hyperpigmentation, with dark, grayish macules on an atrophic and sometimes hypopigmented background, involving the face, neck, shoulders, and trunk. These changes become more dramatic with increasing age.

TABLE 9-12. Dyskeratosis Congenita Literature

Characteristic	X-linked Male	Autosomal Recessive	Autosomal Dominant
No. of cases	121	20	23
Male/female	121:0	6:14	8:15
Age at diagnosis (or report)			
Mean	19 y	15 y	32 y
Range	0.3–47 y	4–42 y	7–50
Median	16 y	15 y	28 y
Nail changes			
No.	111 (92%)	18 (90%)	7 (30%)
Mean age	9 y	7 y	NA
Skin pigmentation			
No.	115 (95%)	17 (85%)	13 (57%)
Mean age	10 y	6 y	NA
Oral leukoplakia			
No.	83 (69%)	13 (65%)	4 (17%)
Mean age	12 y	8 y	NA
Cancer			
No.	9 (7%)	4 (20%)	1 (4%)
Mean age	30 y	30 y	43 y
Aplastic anemia			
No.	57 (47%)	14 (70%)	2 (9%)
Mean age	15 y	13 y	22 y
Deceased			
No.	34 (28%)	4 (20%)	0 (0%)
Mean age	20 y	19 y	NA
Projected 50% survival age	32 y	33 y	>50 y

NA, not available.

TABLE 9-13. Physical Abnormalities in Dyskeratosis Congenita

Characteristic	X-Linked Males (%)	Autosomal Recessive Males (%)	Autosomal Recessive Females (%)	Autosomal Dominant Males (%)	Autosomal Dominant Females (%)
No. of cases	121	6	14	8	15
Skin pigmentation	95	83	86	38	67
Dystrophic nails	92	100	86	25	33
Leukoplakia	69	67	64	13	20
Eye abnormalities	44	67	43	13	7
Teeth anomalies	22	67	36	13	7
Developmental delay	18	33	21	0	0
Skeletal anomalies	16	17	43	13	7
Short stature	14	33	29	0	7
Hyperhidrosis	16	17	7	13	7
Hair loss	12	33	21	25	20
Urinary tract abnormalities	12	0	7	0	7
Gastrointestinal	8	50	7	0	7
Other conditions	8	17	21	0	7
Gonadal anomalies	5	17	14	0	7
Leg ulcers	2	0	0	0	0

The nail changes (hands and feet) include small nail plates, which may develop longitudinal ridging, then may become hypoplastic and eventually disappear. Leukoplakia involves the oral and other mucous membrane surfaces. The incidences of these and other physical findings are compared for both sexes in all groups in Tables 9-12 and 9-13. Several other systems are also involved.

The eyes are affected in half of the patients, most often with epiphora (excessive tearing) due to blocked lacrimal ducts, or blepharitis, as well as cataracts, no eyelashes, conjunctivitis, ectropion, abnormal fundi, glaucoma, strabismus, and ulcers. Many patients have poor dentition, with caries and early loss of all teeth. Skeletal abnormalities include osteoporosis, frequent fractures, aseptic necroses (all but one of the latter eight patients had received prednisone), and scoliosis. Seven patients had intracranial calcifications. Several patients were short, slender, delicate, or asthenic in appearance. Hyperhidrosis of palms and soles is common. Early hair thinning or loss and premature graying have also been reported. Urinary tract involvement is primarily mucosal, with meatal and urethral stenosis, phimosis, hypospadias, pyelonephritis, penile leukoplakia, and one horseshoe kidney reported. Gastrointestinal problems include esophageal stenosis, diverticula, spasm, duodenal ulcer, anal leukoplakia, bifid uvula, and umbilical hernia. Male hypogonadism with hypoplastic testes was reported in five cases, as in Fanconi's anemia. One female had a vaginal constriction, one had vulvar leukoplakia, and one had a hysterectomy. Four females apparently had successful pregnancies. Other rare reports include deafness, absent eardrum, bird face, cardiac disease, Dandy-Walker deformity, cholesteatoma, and five cases of microcephaly.

Because of the coincidence of skin abnormalities, aplastic anemia, and malignancies, dyskeratosis congenita has sometimes been confused or compared with Fanconi's anemia.[379,402–406] In fact, in one series of five Fanconi's anemia patients, one probably had dyskeratosis congenita and not Fanconi's anemia.[243] The genetics and physical abnormalities of patients with Fanconi's anemia and dyskeratosis congenita are actually different (Table 9-14); although the same systems may be involved, the types of anomalies are characteristic. In addition, aplastic anemia usually occurs earlier in Fanconi's anemia than in dyskeratosis congenita. These disorders should not be confused clinically and can be definitively distinguished by analysis of chromosome breakage after clastogenic stress.

Aplastic Anemia

Fifty-seven (50%) of the X-linked male dyskeratosis congenita patients and 14 (70%) of the autosomal recessive patients were reported to develop aplastic anemia at a mean age of 15 and 13 years, respectively (see Table 9-12). Aplastic anemia occurred in only 2 of the autosomal dominant patients. The distribution of ages at the diagnosis of hematologic disease is shown in Figure 9-12. In many cases, hematologic symptoms preceded the diagnosis of dyskeratosis congenita, although in retrospect the physical abnormalities of dyskeratosis congenita had been present for several years. In the younger patients, hematologic changes may have occurred before the appearance of the dyskeratosis congenita triad.

Laboratory Findings

Blood Counts. Thrombocytopenia or anemia or both are the initial signs in most patients who ultimately develop aplastic anemia. Macrocytosis and elevated Hb F are common (manifestations of stress erythropoiesis), even in patients without pancytopenia. Bone marrow aspirates may be hypercellular at first, and several patients were initially thought to have hypersplenism. Decreased megakaryocytes, hypocellularity, and aplasia eventually ensue. Ferrokinetic studies are consistent with aplastic anemia.[403,404,407] A few patients had decreased immunoglobulins, or decreased cellular immunity, but this has been inconsistent.[408]

Chromosome breakage was studied in several patients. In 12 patients, baseline breakage was apparently increased, but the data from patients and particularly from controls were often not cited. Breakage studies were normal in more than 25 patients, including 12 who were examined with DEB, MMC, or nitrogen mustard.[341,399,406,409] Patients with dyskeratosis congenita probably do not have increased

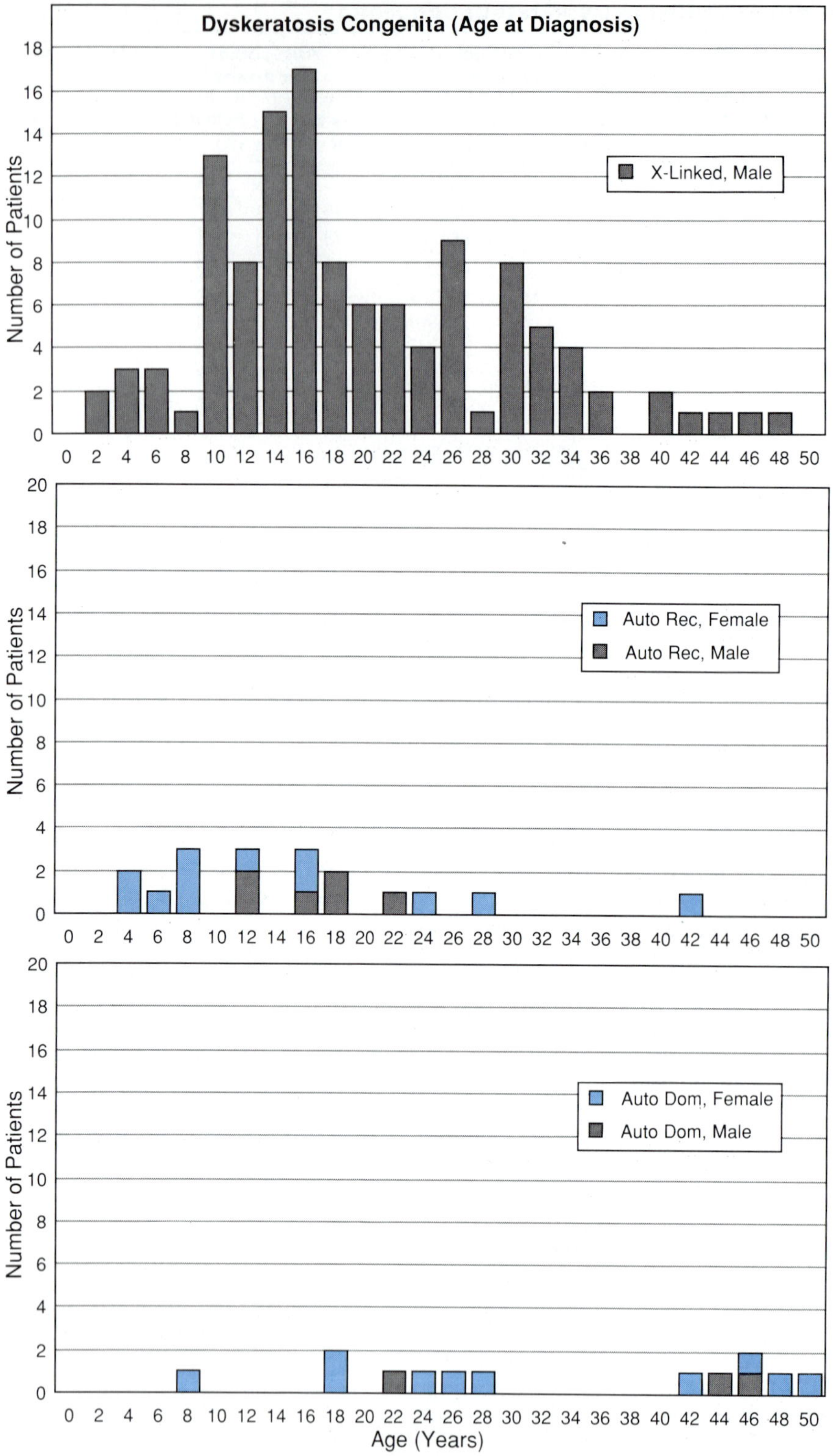

FIGURE 9-11. Age at diagnosis of dyskeratosis congenita in published cases from 1910 to 1989.

breakage, particularly with clastogenic stress, and can be differentiated from those with Fanconi's anemia on this basis.

Hematopoietic cultures have been performed in a few instances of patients with dyskeratosis congenita. In all patients, the numbers of progenitors were reduced or there were none. All these patients were studied when they already had hematologic symptoms.[234,386,410–415] In one report, GM-CSF was added to the culture and increased the number of colonies.[414]

Pathophysiology

Dyskeratosis congenita is inherited in a predominantly X-linked pattern, but there are families with apparently autosomal recessive as well as others with dominant inheritance. The autosomal recessives might have X-linked inheritance with lyonization, and variable expression in males and females. The more compelling explanation is that there are three dyskeratosis congenita genes. The X-linked gene has been localized to Xq28 with restriction

TABLE 9-14. Comparison of Dyskeratosis Congenita and Fanconi's Anemia

Feature	Dyskeratosis Congenita*	Fanconi's Anemia
Predominant inheritance	X-linked	Autosomal recessive
Male/female	4.7:1	1.3:1
Physical features		
Low birthweight	12%	14%
Skin pigmentation	95%	62%
Nail dystrophy	92%	None
Leukoplakia	69%	None
Eye abnormalities	44%	25%
Teeth abnormalities	22%	None
Developmental delay	18%	13%
Skeletal (includes hands)	16%	64%
Short stature	14%	59%
Hyperhidrosis	16%	None
Hair loss	12%	None
Renal anomalies	12%	24%
Gastrointestinal problems	8%	4%
Gonadal anomalies in males	5%	39%
Head abnormalities	3%	26%
Ear abnormalities	3%	10%
Hyperreflexia	None	8%
Cardiopulmonary	1%	7%
Onset of aplastic anemia (mean age)	15 y	8 y
Malignancy		
Tumors of all types	7%	9%
Leukemia	None	9%
Chromosome breaks	10%†	100%

* Dyskeratosis congenita data include only the possible X-linked males.
† Probably not abnormal.

fragment length polymorphisms.[401] This type of analysis can be used for *prenatal diagnosis,* although its usefulness is limited because the diagnosis of dyskeratosis congenita is usually not made until adolescence or later. Whatever the gene, all germ layers are involved: ectoderm, with dyskeratosis; endoderm, with leukoplakia; and mesoderm, with aplastic anemia. Dyskeratosis congenita, like Fanconi's anemia, is also a premalignant condition (see section on cancer).

Dyskeratosis congenita is probably not a chromosome breakage syndrome, since the data showing that breakage is increased are far from convincing. The suggestion of Carter and coworkers[416] that there was a defect in DNA cross-linkage repair was not confirmed by others.[417–419] A report of increased sister chromatid exchange also was not supported by others.[399,417,420] In contrast to that seen in Fanconi's anemia, no increase in transformation by SV40 was seen.[421] Dyskeratosis congenita fibroblasts did resemble those of Fanconi's anemia in showing a decreased plating efficiency, increased sensitivity to MMC, and improvement when SOD was added.[200]

Patients with dyskeratosis congenita have a genetic risk for bone marrow failure, but an environmental factor may be required for its manifestation. At least one patient received chloramphenicol before the development of pancytopenia.[388] The risk of aplastic anemia appears to be higher in the autosomal recessive than in the X-linked recessive patients.

Prognosis

The prognosis is not good in dyskeratosis congenita. One third of the X-linked male dyskeratosis congenita patients and one fifth of the autosomal recessive patients had died by the time of the reports, with a mean age at death of 20 and 19 years, respectively (see Table 9-12). The projected median survival age for males is 32 years; for the autosomal recessive group it was 33 years, whereas none of the autosomal dominant patients had died when the report was made (Fig. 9-13). The reported death rate in those with *aplastic anemia* was 25% in the males and 21% in the autosomal recessive patients. Neither of the two dominant patients with aplastic anemia had died when the report was made. The deaths were at an average of 4 years after the diagnosis of aplastic anemia, similar to that found in patients with Fanconi's anemia. The predicted median survival ages are 28 for X-linked males and 33 for autosomal recessive patients with aplastic anemia. In those with cancer (see following section), deaths were reported in five of eight males, at a mean age of 33, and in two of four autosomal recessive patients, at ages 24 and 34. Four of the six patients with both aplastic anemia and cancer were reported to have died.[385,387,407,422,423] Subtraction of the deaths due to aplastic anemia and those due to cancer from the total number who died leaves 13 X-linked males, for a proportion of 11% dying from other causes (infection or not defined). In the autosomal recessive group, one death (5%) occurred that was not defined.

Cancer

Cancers were reported in nine X-linked males with dyskeratosis congenita, four autosomal recessive patients (one male, three females), and one male in the autosomal dominant group (Table 9-15). Two patients had two or more tumors. Eight of the total of 15 tumors were squamous cell carcinomas, and two were adenocarcinomas; the rest were all unique. The sites were similar to those reported in those with Fanconi's anemia (see Table 9-10) and involve areas known to be abnormal in dyskeratosis congenita, such as mucous membranes and the gastrointestinal tract. Six patients (four X-linked and two autosomal recessive) had both cancer and aplastic anemia. Among those who developed cancer, the predicted median survival is age 35 (see Fig. 9-13). Of interest and unlike Fanconi's anemia patients, only a rare patient with dyskeratosis congenita has yet been reported to have leukemia.

Treatment

Treatment for the aplastic anemia of dyskeratosis congenita is similar to that for Fanconi's anemia. Overall, 23 patients were reported to receive *androgens,* usually combined with prednisone, as described earlier for Fanconi's anemia. Fifty-two percent responded, a similar response rate to that seen in Fanconi's anemia. The interval from diagnosis of aplastic anemia to reported death was 3 years in those who did not receive androgens and 5 years in those who did. As in Fanconi's anemia, responses are not cures, and androgens must be maintained; subsequent failures do ensue. *Splenectomies* were reported in at least eight patients, with only temporary improvements. *Supportive care* with RBC and platelet transfusions, antibiotics, and ε-aminocaproic acid[430] should all be provided when indicated clinically. There are no reports on the use of antilymphocyte globulin or cyclosporin A, but these agents would not be expected to work (one of our patients received these at another institution without response).[396]

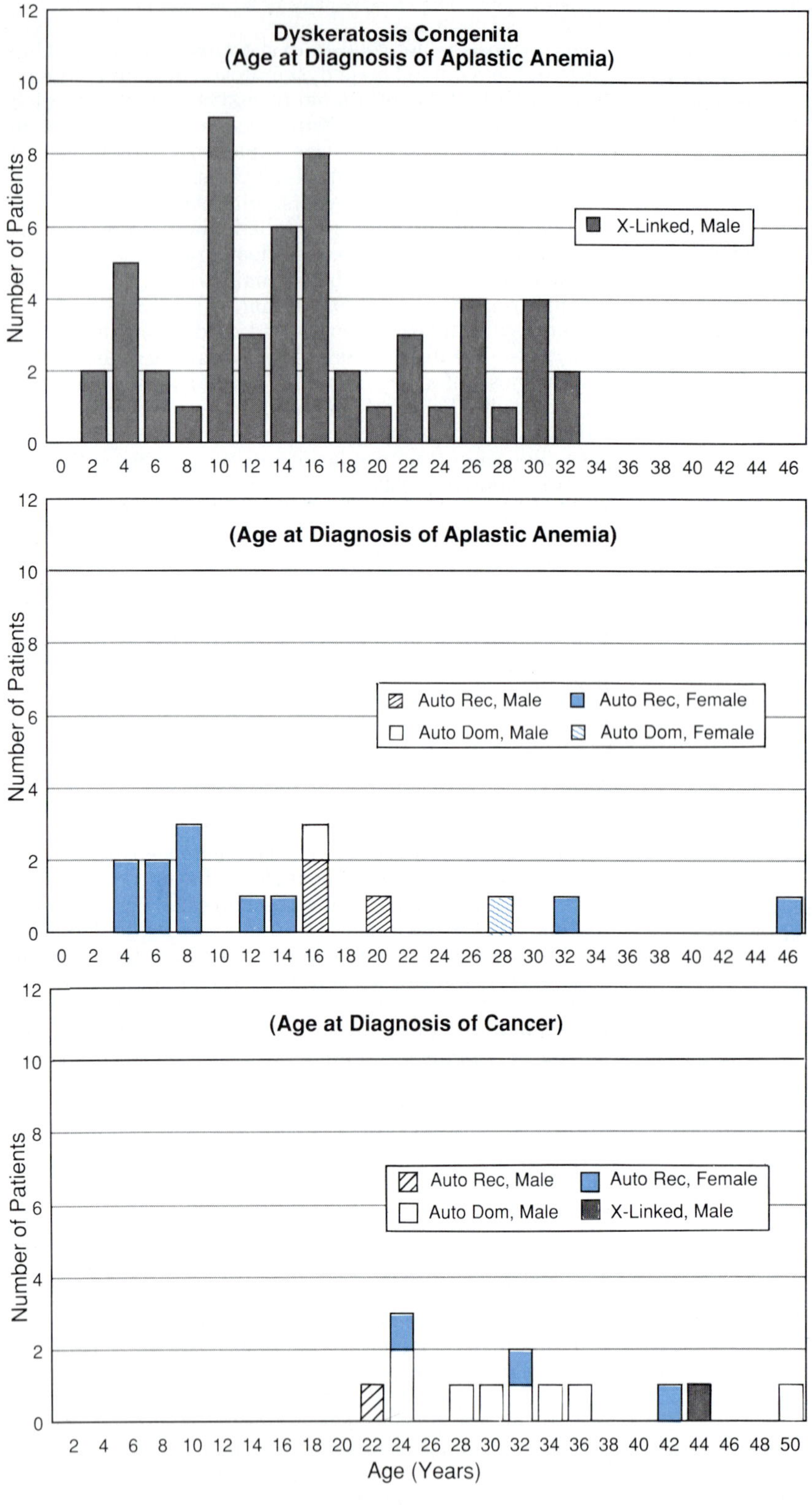

FIGURE 9-12. Age at diagnosis of aplastic anemia or cancer in dyskeratosis congenita.

Bone marrow transplantation has been reported in five patients, with only one survivor.[392,395,431–433] Two died with acute graft- versus-host disease, whereas two patients developed diffuse vasculitis at 2 and 7 years after transplantation. The fourth developed a mucositis syndrome similar to that seen in Fanconi's anemia patients who received standard levels of cyclophosphamide preparation, as did this patient. Thus, transplantation in dyskeratosis congenita patients must be approached with caution. In addition, since the physical features of dyskeratosis congenita may appear late or may be subtle, potential donors who may in fact be affected with dyskeratosis congenita may be difficult to detect. Finally, as in Fanconi's anemia, marrow transplantation does not reduce (and may increase) the risk of development of tumors. *Hematopoietic growth factors* such as GM-CSF or IL-3 may have a role in the future treatment of dyskeratosis congenita.

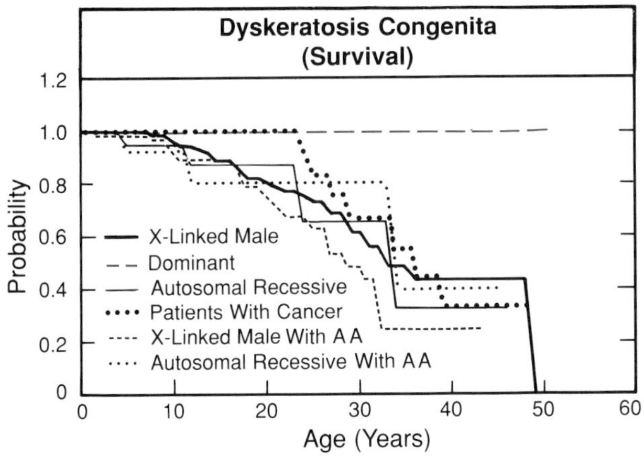

FIGURE 9-13. Kaplan-Meier plot of cumulative survival in dyskeratosis congenita. Time is shown as age in years, since the time of diagnosis is not always clear.

Shwachman-Diamond Syndrome

The Shwachman-Diamond (Bodian Shwachman) syndrome consists of exocrine pancreatic insufficiency plus neutropenia.[434–436] More than 150 cases have been reported[436–439] (Table 9-16). Signs of pancreatic insufficiency, usually apparent in infancy, are diarrhea, malabsorption, steatorrhea, and failure to thrive. Neutropenia is identified early, as part of the general work-up or because of skin infections or pneumonia. Additional hematologic problems develop in more than 40% of patients, with anemia in 15%, thrombocytopenia in 7%, and pancytopenia in 20%. Occasionally, anemia or thrombocytopenia is the initial hematologic problem. The ratio of males to females is 1.8:1 overall and 1.2:1 in those with pancytopenia. More than 20 families were reported with at least two affected children, and the inheritance is thought to be autosomal recessive, although no reports of consanguinity exist. Shwachman-Diamond syndrome has been reported in all racial groups, with no ethnic propensity. Pregnancies and birth histories are uneventful, although 15% had low birthweight.

TABLE 9-15. **Malignancies in Dyskeratosis Congenita**

Type of Cancer	Reference
Nasopharynx, tongue (both squamous cell), rectum (adenocarcinoma)	417
Rectum (adenocarcinoma), cheek (epidermoid)	418
Mouth (basal squamous cell epithelioma)	419
Mouth (squamous cell)	420
Hodgkin's disease	421
Pancreatic adenoma	421
Stomach	402
Tongue	410
Plantar skin	422
Cervix and vagina (squamous cell)	383
Mouth (squamous cell)	380
Nose (squamous cell)	381
Hand (squamous cell epithelioma)	423
Skin (carcinoma in situ)	28

TABLE 9-16. **Shwachman-Diamond Syndrome Literature***

	Total	Pancytopenia
No. of cases	165	33
Male/female	1.8:1	1.2:1
No. with metaphyseal dysostosis	66 (40%)	11 (33%)
Age at malabsorption		
Mean	9 mo	6 mo
Median	4 mo	2 mo
Range	0–15 y	0–9 y
No. with leukemia	9 (5%)	4 (12%)
No. of deaths	27 (16%)	12 (36%)
Age at death		
Mean	6 y	8.9 y
Median	3 y	8 y
Range	0.4–35 y	1.7–35 y
Projected 50% survival (y)	35	14

* All patients had pancreatic insufficiency and neutropenia.

The most prominent physical findings are related to malnourishment, including short stature in more than half, protuberant abdomen, and low weight. Forty percent had radiographic evidence for metaphyseal dysostosis. Fifteen percent had mental retardation, and 2% had microcephaly. Several had an ichthyotic skin rash. Rare physical anomalies include hypertelorism, retinitis pigmentosa, toe or finger syndactyly, cleft palate, dental dysplasia, ptosis, strabismus, short neck, coxa valga, and skin pigmentation.

The combination of pancreatic dysfunction plus bone marrow failure was noted by Ozsoylu and Argun,[440] who found decreased duodenal trypsin in patients with acquired aplastic anemia or Fanconi's anemia. Those patients did not have symptomatic malabsorption. In addition, patients with Shwachman-Diamond syndrome have decreased amylase and lipase as well as trypsin.

Six cases were reported who had exocrine pancreatic insufficiency and who had *refractory sideroblastic anemia with vacuolization of bone marrow precursors* (Pearson's syndrome).[441–443] Anemia was more significant than neutropenia, myeloid and erythroid precursors had vacuoles, and there were ringed sideroblasts. Three of the six patients with Pearson's syndrome died at less than 3 years of age, two from sepsis and one from acidosis and liver failure, whereas the other three improved. At autopsy, pancreatic fibrosis was found, and not the liposis seen in patients with Shwachman-Diamond syndrome. Pearson's syndrome has been shown recently to be due to a deficiency in mitochondrial DNA.[444]

Patients with *cartilage hair hypoplasia* have metaphyseal dysostosis, short stature, and characteristic fine hair.[445] Although lymphopenia and immunodeficiencies were observed in 25% of patients with cartilage hair hypoplasia,[446,447] neutropenia and pancreatic insufficiency were rare[448,449] Shwachman-Diamond syndrome and cartilage hair hypoplasia are probably distinct conditions.

Laboratory Findings

By definition, all patients with Shwachman-Diamond syndrome have neutropenia (neutrophils below 1500/μL on at least one occasion). It may be chronic, intermittent, or cyclic, and is usually noted early in childhood. Anemia occurs in more than one third, but is not usually sufficient to require transfusion. Thrombocytopenia below 100,000/μL is seen in 20% of Shwachman-Diamond syndrome patients. The bicytopenic combination of neutropenia with anemia was reported in 15% of patients, and with thrombocytopenia in 7%. Pancytopenia occurred in 33 patients (20%), at a mean age of 6 years, median of 3 years, and range of 1 to 35 years.

The neutrophils that are produced in Shwachman-Diamond syndrome may not be totally normal. There may be a defect in neutrophil mobility,[450–452] which may explain infections even when the neutrophil count is not extremely low.

Bone marrow examination shows myeloid hypocellularity or maturation arrest. The erythroid series is normal or hyperplastic. Hb F levels are often elevated, even without anemia, suggesting hematopoietic stress.[438] Immunoglobulins are occasionally decreased. Hepatic dysfunction and fibrosis have also been noted. Pancreatic insufficiency is documented as low or absent duodenal trypsin, amylase, and lipase. Patients do not have cystic fibrosis, and sweat chloride levels are normal. Radiographs show metaphyseal dysostosis in 37% of patients. Chromosomes are normal, and no increased breakage is found after clastogenic stress.

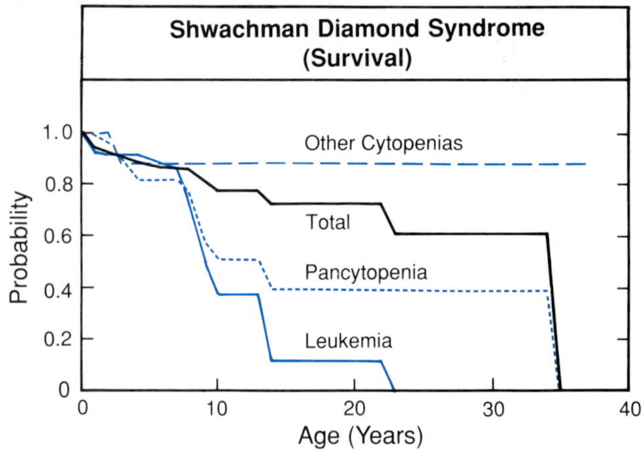

FIGURE 9-14. Kaplan-Meier plot of cumulative survival in Shwachman-Diamond syndrome.

Pathophysiology

The inheritance of Shwachman-Diamond syndrome appears to be autosomal recessive, despite the preponderance of males. Although the exocrine pancreas and bone marrow hematopoiesis develop at about the same time during gestation, familial cases as well as Shwachman-Diamond syndrome in only one of a pair of twins argue against an intrauterine insult as the cause.[453] Culture of bone marrow progenitors shows decreased CFU-GM and CFU-E in most patients, suggesting a stem cell deficit.[454–458] No evidence is found for humoral or cellular inhibitors of granulopoieis. Shwachman-Diamond syndrome thus resembles other forms of inherited bone marrow failure disorders, with reduced numbers of hematopoietic progenitor cells.

Therapy and Outcome

Malabsorption responds to treatment with oral pancreatic enzymes. Infections are treated with the appropriate antibiotics and may decrease with age. Supportive care should be provided, with transfusions for anemia and platelets for thrombocytopenia. Less than 12 patients were treated with corticosteroids, with hematologic improvement in 6. Even fewer received androgens plus steroids (see section on Fanconi's anemia), with some improvement. Two patients recently received G-CSF with an elevation of their neutrophil counts.[459]

Pancytopenia developed in 20% of the patients, at between 1 and 6 years of age. Leukemia (see next section) was reported in nine cases. Deaths were reported in 16% of the total Shwachman-Diamond syndrome group, 36% of those with pancytopenia, 90% of those with leukemia, and 9% of those with neutropenia alone or combined with anemia or thrombocytopenia (see Table 9-16). The projected median survival age for the entire group is 35 years, 14 years for those with aplastic anemia, and 9 for those with leukemia; those without these complications reach a plateau of almost 90% survival by age 6 years (Fig. 9-14). The reported deaths were usually due to infection or bleeding. One patient received a bone marrow transplant, but died from complications due to cyclophosphamide cardiotoxicity.[460] As with other inherited bone marrow failure disorders, cases may have been reported because of severity or complications (eg, leukemia), and Shwachman-Diamond syndrome may be milder than it would appear from the literature.

Leukemia. Nine patients (eight males) developed leukemia (5%) at a mean of 10 years (range 2 to 23). Two had Shwachman-Diamond syndrome siblings. Three had acute lymphoblastic leukemia, two had acute myeloblastic leukemia, and one each had acute myelomonocytic leukemia, monocytic leukemia, erythroleukemia, and juvenile chronic myelocytic leukemia.[436,456,457,461–465] Only one patient had received prednisone plus androgen treatment for aplastic anemia. One of those with ALL was still alive after 1 year, whereas the others succumbed at 1 month to 2 years after diagnosis of leukemia. Three patients had cytogenetic abnormalities, two with additional G group chromosomes, and one with monosomy 7 plus a marker. One patient had an apparent 8-month preleukemic phase. Shwachman-Diamond syndrome thus resembles many of the other inherited bone marrow failure syndromes in that it has a malignant propensity.

Reticular Dysgenesis

Reticular dysgenesis (thymic alymphoplasia with aleukocytosis) refers to infants with congenital agranulocytosis, lymphopenia, and absent cellular and humoral immunity. Since the first description by de Vaal and Gitlin[466] in 1959, 12 cases have been reported, including 10 males and 2 females, with one set of twins, and two sets of brothers.[467–475] Thus, there is a preponderance of males, although the numbers are too low to define an X-linked disorder. The observation of this condition in two sets of brothers and one family with consanguinity is also compatible with an autosomal recessive inheritance. One case in which the mother received azathioprine for renal disease is also included because the phenotype is similar, although this may be acquired rather than inherited.[467,468]

The typical presentation of Shwachman-Diamond syndrome is with signs of infection at birth or early in infancy. The mean age was 14, the median 2, and the range 0 to 105 days. Eight infants had birthweights below 2500 g. Physical examinations reveal no lymph nodes or tonsils, Radiographs have no thymic shadow, and pathologic examinations indicate that thymuses are extremely small, that lymph nodes are absent, and that spleens lack follicles. All patients have severe lymphopenia and granulocytopenia. Anemia was reported in seven patients, and thrombocytopenia in only one. Bone marrow is hypocellular, with no myeloid or lymphoid precursors, and often a reduction in erythropoiesis as well.

All but one patient died—eight in the first month, and the other three before 4 months, at a mean of 34 days, a median of 2 weeks, and a range of 3 days to 17 weeks. The patient who lived the longest was maintained in a gnotobiotic environment.[473] One patient was apparently cured by a bone marrow transplant[475]; another was transplanted but died of sepsis before engraftment ensued.[469]

The successfully transplanted patient was not prepared with immunosuppression, but became a complete chimera, with donor erythrocytes, unlike the situation with patients with severe combined immunodeficiency, in whom only the lymphocytes become donor. This suggests that the defect is in the pluripotent hematopoietic stem cell. This theory is supported by bone marrow culture data from three patients, in whom hematopoietic colonies were zero or extremely low.[469,473,475] Although most of the patients did not have complete aplastic anemia, they are certainly examples of multicytopenia.

Amegakaryocytic Thrombocytopenia

A small number of patients present with thrombocytopenia, usually in infancy, and subsequently develop aplastic anemia. This was called type III constitutional aplastic anemia by O'Gorman Hughes,[52] but the term *amegakaryocytic thrombocytopenia* is more descriptive. Although the differential diagnosis of neonatal thrombocytopenia is lengthy, the entity to be discussed here excludes those with increased bone marrow megakaryocytes as well those due to congenital infection (particularly viral, such as rubella). Immune thrombocytopenias are also not included, despite the occasional development of amegakaryocytosis, which is presumably due to the reactivity of antiplatelet antibodies with megakaryocytes.[476] In addition, the syndrome of TAR is discussed separately below, since it represents a pure single cytopenia. Fanconi's anemia, which can begin with thrombocytopenia, was already discussed. Finally, children with associated trisomies, such as trisomy 13 and 18, have also been excluded. The accepted cases are summarized in Table 9-17, with separate analyses of those with normal appearances and those with congenital anomalies.

Sixteen reports of thrombocytopenia occurred in the first year (12 in the first week), and five with onset at 2 to 9 years, all of whom had no physical anomalies, but who did have absent or reduced bone marrow megakaryocytes.[1,3,52,135,234,477–486] The male/female ratio was 2.3:1.

Fifteen children were described with amegakaryocytic thrombocytopenia in the first year (11 in the first week), who did have physical abnormalities that fit no other specific syndrome.[1,52,486,487–495] The male/female ratio was 2.8:1. Cerebellar and cerebral atrophy was reported in two brothers by Høyeraal and colleagues,[493] as well as one male by Hreidarsson and colleagues,[494] and another child by Saracco and coworkers.[490] Additional patients with neurologic findings were described by Eisenstein[492] and by Gardner and coworkers.[487] Other common abnormalities were cardiac disease in five patients, abnormal facies in two, microcephaly in five, retarded development in five, abnormal hips or feet in four, kidney abnormalities in two, eye anomalies in two, and cleft or high arched palate in two. The physical findings in some resembled those seen in Fanconi's anemia, and the diagnosis of Fanconi's anemia cannot be excluded retrospectively from the reports.

The male preponderance in both groups suggests that some cases might be X-linked and that others may be autosomal recessive. In those with no physical abnormalities, 10 families could be X-linked (males only), and 5 autosomal recessive (including females). Two affected male sibs, a set of fraternal twins, a sibship with 1 male and 2 females, and 1 boy with a brother and a cousin with thrombocytopenia and physical abnormalities were seen.[3,477,480,486] In addition to the 4 families with thrombocytopenic sibs, 1 family each had an anencephalic sibling, relatives with missing fingers,[52] and a male sibling who died of leukemia.[483]

TABLE 9-17. Amegakaryocytic Thrombocytopenia Literature

	No Anomalies	Anomalies
No. of cases	21	15
Male/female	2.3:1	2.8:1
Age at thrombocytopenia		
Mean	1 y	2 mo
Median	7 d	5 d
Range	0–9 y	0–1 y
No. with aplastic anemia*	12	4
Age at aplastic anemia		
Mean	3.9 y	2.3 y
Median	3.5 y	2.3 y
Range	0.4–12.5 y	1.1–3.5 y
No. with leukemia/preleukemia	2	0
No. of deaths, thrombocytopenia	6	9
Age at death		
Mean	1.9 y	0.5 y
Median	2 wk	10 wk
Range	4 d–7 y	0–1.9 y
No. of deaths, aplastic anemia	9	4
Age at death		
Mean	8 y	2.7 y
Median	6 y	2.8 y
Range	7 mo–21 y	1.9–3.5 y
Total projected 50% survival age	6 y	2 y

* Patients with aplastic anemia include the two with leukemia and preleukemia.

In those with anomalies, six families could be X-linked and two autosomal recessive. Sibships included one with one male and two females, one with two brothers, and the thrombocytopenic brother and cousin of a normal-appearing male.[486,487,493] Clearly, separation of cases according to physical appearance may be arbitrary. One family had parental consanguinity.[494]

In both groups, the pregnancies and deliveries were essentially unremarkable, although the incidence of spontaneous abortions was increased (reported in seven families). Three with low-birthweight infants were seen in each group.

The presentation was usually due to bleeding in the skin, mucous membranes, or gastrointestinal tract. Evolution to aplastic anemia was reported in 12 of those with no anomalies, and 4 of those with anomalies (57% and 27%, respectively).

Laboratory Findings

The initial abnormality is thrombocytopenia, with normal white blood counts and hemoglobin levels. Reported platelet counts ranged from 0 to 80,000/μL at diagnosis, white blood counts were normal, and hemoglobins were low only after bleeding had occurred. Macrocytosis, as well as increased Hb F and i antigen, suggested a broader level of marrow failure. One 5-year-old boy with amegakaryocytic thrombocytopenia had increased MCV and Hb F but had not yet developed aplastic anemia.[484] Bone marrow cellularity is normal until aplastic anemia appears, except for markedly decreased or absent megakaryocytes; those that are present are small and apparently inactive. Homologous platelet survival is normal, since the defect is underproduction, not increased destruction.[483] Peripheral blood chromosomes do not show the increased breaks characteristic of Fanconi's anemia.[135,484,486,493,494] In one patient who was clinically preleukemic, abnormalities involved chromosome 19, with absence, partial deletion, or trisomy in 11 of 50 marrow cells (Harris MB, Najfeld V, Weiner MA, Shah L, Alter BP, Hirschhorn K, unpublished data, 1984).

Prenatal diagnosis is possible by means of platelet counts in fetal blood obtained during the midtrimester. Mibashan and Millar[496] examined three fetuses at risk and detected thrombocytopenia in one fetus.

Pathophysiology

The familial occurrence of amegakaryocytic thrombocytopenia in some cases suggests that it is inherited, and the preponderance of males suggests that some are X-linked. The thrombocytopenia is apparently due to a defect in production, since megakaryocytes are decreased or absent, although no studies of megakaryocyte colony-forming units (CFU-Meg) have been reported. After pancytopenia develops, hematopoietic progenitor cells are decreased or absent.[234,485,486] Thrombocytopenia may be the first sign of aplastic anemia in many conditions, although this group is distinguished by the relatively long duration before pancytopenia.

Outcome

Thrombocytopenia Alone. Among the 21 patients with thrombocytopenia without anomalies, 9 did not develop aplastic anemia. One was alive at the time of the report, with macrocytosis and elevated Hb F.[484] Four died at 4 days to 2 weeks after birth from bleeding or infection. Three others died from bleeding at ages 4, 7, and 9. No information was available about 1 patient. In the 15 with anomalies, 11 did not evolve to pancytopenia. One died at birth, 3 in the first 2 weeks, 3 in 2 to 6 months, and 2 before 2 years of age. Only 2 were alive at 1.6 and 2 years, 1 of whom was stated to have improved by 10 months. The few reported causes of death were hemorrhage or infection; many of these babies had complex cardiovascular or cerebral problems. Most cases were described before 1980, and systematic platelet support was not reported.

Aplastic Anemia. Twelve of the 21 thrombocytopenic patients with normal physical examinations developed aplastic anemia at a mean of 3.9 years, range of 5 months to 12.5 years, and median of 3.5 years. The only long-term survivor is a boy who received a bone marrow transplant from his sister[485] (Gelfand E, personal communication); a brother had died at age 10 after evolution to androgen-unresponsive aplastic anemia. Deaths occurred at 7 months to 21 years, usually a result of bleeding or sepsis. Four of those with physical anomalies also developed aplastic anemia, at 1.1 to 3.5 years (mean and median, 2.3 years). They died at 1.9 to 3.5 years, also from hemorrhage or infection or both.

Leukemia. One male with normal physical appearance had amegakaryocytic thrombocytopenia from day 1, developed aplastic anemia at age 5 years, responded poorly to androgens plus steroids, and evolved further into acute myelomonocytic leukemia at age 16, with death at age 17[52] (Potter N, Alter BP, unpublished data). A female had thrombocytopenia at age 2 months, pancytopenia at 5 months, and a preleukemic picture with abnormalities involving chromosome 19 (Harris MB, Najfeld V, Weiner MA, Shah L, Alter BP, Hirschhorn K, unpublished data, 1984). Thus, amegakaryocytic thrombocytopenia may also be one of the marrow failure syndromes with a propensity to malignancy.

Treatment

Steroids alone were used in one third of the cases, with no apparent efficacy. Steroids plus androgens were given to five of those with normal physical appearance and aplastic anemia, with temporary or partial responses in three of these, all of whom subsequently died. Four of those with anomalies received steroids (three had pancytopenia) with no responses. Splenectomies were performed in four patients in all, without effect.

Figure 9-15 shows the survival curves for those without and those with anomalies. The projected median survivals are 6 and 2 years, respectively, and the average ages at reported deaths were 5 and 1.2 years. For those who had aplastic anemia, the mean ages at death were 8 and 2.7 years. Those with thrombocytopenia only died at mean ages of 1.9 and 0.5 years. We can speculate that platelet support might prevent early deaths from thrombocytopenia, but the rate of evolution to aplastic anemia might then be higher. Bone marrow transplantation seems to offer the only possibility for cure at this time, although hematopoietic growth factors should be considered when they become available.

Familial Marrow Dysfunction

Several families have been reported with various combinations of physical and immunologic abnormalities, in which hematopoietic defects and often leukemia have occurred. The ages at the development of hematologic manifestations vary from childhood to adulthood, and the inheritance patterns have been of all types. Table 9-18 summarizes some of these conditions, which are discussed briefly. Some of the families have anomalies that resemble but in fact differ from those described in Fanconi's anemia. One group, the Estren-Dameshek familial aplastic patients, has been reclassified as Fanconi's anemia. Another group of patients has anomalies resembling those seen in Fanconi's anemia patients but does not have Fanconi's anemia. Other patients fit into known genetic syndromes, such as Dubowitz's, Seckel's, and Down's syndromes, and are discussed separately. Several patients with physical anomalies and aplasia are sporadic and are listed in Table 9-19.

Some patients inherited their disease in an autosomal dominant manner. The *IVIC syndrome*, named for the initials of the institution that first reported it (Instituto Ve-

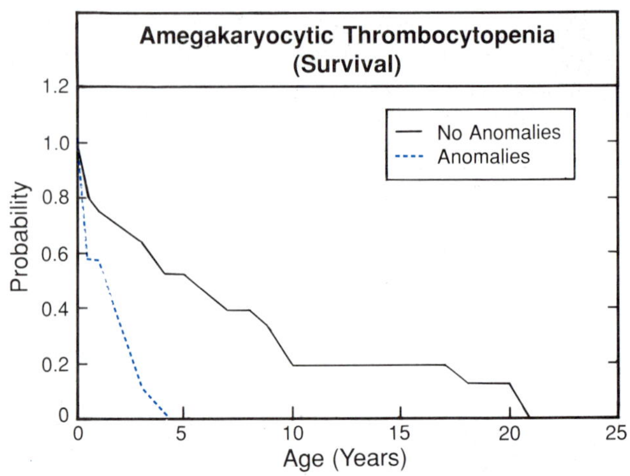

FIGURE 9-15. Kaplan-Meier plot of cumulative survival in amegakaryocytic thrombocytopenia. Patients with only thrombocytopenia and those with aplastic anemia are pooled, since the numbers are small.

TABLE 9-18. Familial Aplastic Anemia

Disorder	Age Group	No. Affected	No. of Generations	References
AUTOSOMAL DOMINANT				
IVIC: Radial hypoplasia, deaf, thrombocytopenia	Children and adults	24	5	491–493
		3	2	
		2	2	
WT: Hand anomalies, leukemia	Children and adults	4	3	494
		8	5	
Aplasia, leukemia, pigmentation, immune deficiency	Adults	4	2	495
Vascular occlusions	Adults	14	5	496
Fused radius and ulna	Adults	6	4	497
		10	2	
Neutropenia	Adults	2	2	498
Ataxis, ANLL, monosomy 7, immune deficiency	Children	4 M, 1 F	1	499–501
		3	2	
Acquired aplastic anemia	Adults, 4 families	9	2	502
AUTOSOMAL RECESSIVE				
Immune deficiency, cutaneous malignancies	Children	2 M	1	503
Immune deficiency	Adults	1 M, 3 F	1	504
ANLL, monosomy 7	Adults	2 M, 6 F	1	505
Acquired aplastic anemia	Adults, 4 families	8 M, 2 F	1	502
X-LINKED RECESSIVE				
Leukemia, light-chain disease	Adults	8 M	3	506
X-linked lymphoproliferative syndrome	Children, 25 families	17 M	4	507

M, male; F, female; IVIC, IVIC syndrome; WT, Wilms' tumor; ANLL, acute nonlymphocytic leukemia.

nezolano de Investigaçiones Cientificas), is characterized by radial ray hypoplasia, with absent thumbs or hypoplastic radial carpal bones, hearing impairment, strabismus, imperforate anus, and thrombocytopenia. The physical anomalies were noted in 24 members of five generations in the first family, two children and their father in the second family, and a mother and son in the third family reported.[497–499] Mild thrombocytopenia and leukocytosis appeared before the age of 50 years in 13 persons in the first family. The incidence of hematologic abnormalities is unknown, since many patients are still young. Baseline chromosome breakage was normal. Despite the lack of complete aplastic anemia, the physical findings resemble those seen in Fanconi's anemia. It has been suggested that this syndrome be renamed *oculootoradial syndrome*.[517]

The *WT syndrome* was named after the initials of the first (and so far the only) two families reported.[500] Twelve patients were described—three generations in one family and five in the other family. They had radial–ulnar hypoplasia, abnormal thumbs, short fingers, fifth finger clinodactyly, pancytopenia or thrombocytopenia, and leukemia. Baseline chromosomes were normal without increased breakage. As in the IVIC syndrome, the physical findings in the WT syndrome were subtly different from those in Fanconi's anemia. The authors suggested that several cases of atypical Fanconi's anemia might be WT syndrome instead. Chromosome studies after clastogenic stress should help to sort out this confusion.

A family was recently described with dominant bone marrow failure, acute nonlymphocytic leukemia, hyperpigmented skin, warts, immune dysfunction, and multiple spontaneous abortions.[501] DEB-induced chromosome breakage was not increased. This disorder resembles Fanconi's anemia clinically but not genetically.

Aufderheide[502] reported a five-generation family with 14 members who developed mild to profound single cytopenias or pancytopenia by the third decade. Vascular occlusions were also present in 9 members of this family. One patient had chromosome breaks in 20% of his cells, but his father, who also had aplastic anemia, had normal chromosomes. Dokal and colleagues[503] recently reported two families with dominantly inherited proximal fusion of

TABLE 9-19. Aplastic Anemia With Anomalies*

Disorder	Age Group	No. Affected	Reference
Friedreich's ataxia, short stature, hypogonadism	Child	1 M	514
Short stature, web neck, epicanthi, proximal thumbs	Child	1 F	515
Short, abnormal thumbs	Children	Twins, F	516
Various anomalies, reported to the IFAR	Children	11	9

M, male; F, female.
* All cases are sporadic.

the radius and ulna. Among the 16 cases with this anomaly, 4 had adult onset aplastic anemia or leukemia. Kato and coworkers[504] reported a mother with aplastic anemia and her son with adult onset neutropenia and thrombocytopenia.

Li and colleagues[505,506] described a family with cerebellar atrophy and ataxia in four brothers and the father, as well as ataxia and mild unexplained anemia in the only sister. Two brothers died from aplastic anemia, a third from acute myelogenous leukemia, and the fourth brother was followed through hypoplastic anemia, immune deficiency, preleukemia, and monosomy 7 until his death from acute myelomonocytic leukemia. A second family with similar features was described recently by Daghistani and coworkers.[507] One brother died at age 5 with monosomy 7 acute nonlymphocytic leukemia, which had been preceded by pancytopenia, and the sister and mother have cerebellar ataxia. The inheritance appears to be autosomal dominant with variable expression.

In a report on 19 members of 8 families with acquired aplastic anemia, 4 families with 9 patients had a vertical pattern, with a parent or aunt or uncle who also had aplasia.[508] These could be due to common environmental factors or to a genetic propensity for bone marrow failure.

Autosomal recessive inheritance is the apparent pattern in several other families. Abels and Reed[509] reported two brothers who had short stature and macrocytosis, and who developed pancytopenia at approximately 10 years of age. One brother had immune deficiency and multiple cutaneous squamous and basal cell carcinomas. He also had oral telangiectasias, and neck and chest poikilodermia, but insufficient to diagnose dyskeratosis congenita. Because the patients were both male, the inheritance might also be X-linked recessive. Another family with associated immune disorders and hematopoietic failures was described by Linsk and colleagues.[510] Four of six siblings from a consanguineous marriage had pure red cell aplasia, neutropenia, or both, as well as unusual crystalloid structures demonstrated in the neutrophils by electron microscopy. Chitambar and coworkers[511] described 8 members of 14 in one generation of a large maternal kindred in which aplastic anemia, acute nonlymphocytic leukemia, and monosomy 7 were found. This association of aplasia and leukemia was also noted in families with possible X-linked recessive inheritance. In the Scandinavian report on acquired aplastic anemia with multiple family members,[508] 10 patients in four families belonged to sibships.

Monosomy 7 was also a feature in the family just discussed by Chitambar and coworkers.[511] A sporadic patient with ataxia and hypoplastic anemia was described by Samad and colleagues.[514] This 16-year-old male had Friedreich's ataxia, short stature, hypogonadism, and hyperreflexia. His macrocytic anemia responded to testosterone. Peripheral blood but not marrow chromosomes showed baseline increased breakage.

A clearly X-linked family was presented by Li and coworkers,[512] in which eight males in three generations had adult onset pancytopenia, acute myelogenous leukemia, light chain disease, or ALL (one).

Another X-linked syndrome with hematopoietic complications is the *X-linked lymphoproliferative syndrome*, to which more than 25 kindreds belong.[513] At least 17 of these boys developed fatal aplastic anemia during or before malignant infectious mononucleosis. Other components of this syndrome include hypoproliferative disorders, agranulocytosis, and hypogammaglobulinemia, as well as proliferative disorders associated with the Epstein-Barr virus, including American Burkitt's lymphoma, immunoblastic B-cell sarcoma, plasmacytoma, and fatal mononucleosis. DNA mapping with restriction fragment length polymorphisms has localized this gene to the region of Xq24-q27.[518]

Sporadic cases with aplastic anemia and physical abnormalities are summarized in Table 9-19. One patient and a set of twins had anomalies similar to those seen in those with Fanconi's anemia, and increased baseline chromosome breaks were seen in one patient.[515,516] This case did not have increased breakage after clastogenic stress (Auerbach AD, personal communication). In a larger series of cases reported to the IFAR, 11 children had aplastic anemia and anomalies, whose chromosome breakage was not increased by DEB.[9] It is probable that many cases that were called Fanconi's anemia in the older literature and are included in our own analyses did not have Fanconi's anemia. Only modern testing with DEB or MMC will help to properly categorize all of these cases.

Also, there are cases that do not fit into any categories. Two adult siblings had thrombocytopenia (not pancytopenia) and a robertsonian translocation (t13;14), although 6 others with the translocation did not have hematologic problems.[519] In 3 of the 8 families with 19 members with aplastic anemia previously cited,[508] anemia might have been related to drugs. In other reports, 4 families had more than 1 patient with chloramphenicol-related aplastic anemia.[520–523] Two families had siblings with aplastic anemia after hepatitis.[524,525] Gold, methyprylon (piperidine), and idiopathic aplastic anemia also have each been reported in sets of siblings.[526–528] A mother and child pair with idiopathic aplastic anemia was also reported.[529]

Thus, aplastic anemia might be associated with familial (genetic) predisposition to specific adverse environments. In some cases, physical abnormalities may call attention to the possibly inherited nature of the condition. The familial and inherited marrow failure syndromes are clearly heterogeneous, with a large variety of phenotypes and all the possible inheritance patterns. It remains for future investigations to elucidate the relevant genetic and environmental factors.

Laboratory Findings

The patients in this heterogeneous group with familial marrow dysfunction have variable degrees of pancytopenia, macrocytosis, elevated Hb F, and hypocellular bone marrow. Families with additional findings, such as immune deficiencies, novel chromosomes, or monosomy 7, may be distinguishable from those with nonfamilial disorders, but those with familial disease without characteristic findings are more difficult to diagnose. Baseline chromosome breakage is usually normal in the non-Fanconi's anemia familial cases, but examination with clastogenic agents is required for definitive distinction. The numbers of hematopoietic stem cells are also reduced, but this, too, is nondiagnostic.[485]

Pathophysiology

The combination of genetic and environmental factors is essentially unique to each of the types of cases outlined in this section of familial marrow dysfunctions. The inheritance patterns are autosomal dominant, autosomal recessive, X-linked recessive, and multifactorial. We can only speculate that some of the genes are allelic with Fanconi's anemia, based on similarities of the physical findings. Even at the hematopoietic level, the defects may be multiple because some of the patients have only single cytopenias. Thus, the pluripotent or committed progenitor cells may be defective.

Therapy and Outcome

Several of the patients just described were treated with transfusions, antilymphocyte globulin, or androgens, with some limited success. Because each case is practically unique, no guidelines can be established, except to suggest that androgens might be more effective than immunosuppression. Because immune dysfunction is part of some of the syndromes, even that statement is overly simplistic. In general, the drug and supportive care should be the same as described previously for patients with Fanconi's anemia or acquired aplastic anemia. Although bone marrow transplantation cannot be dismissed out of hand, it is risky because related donor may have the same condition. In several families, aplastic anemia is just the first step to preleukemia and leukemia. Overall, the prognosis for familial bone marrow failure is not good.

Down's Syndrome

Trisomy 21, or Down's syndrome, is often associated with a neonatal transient myeloproliferative syndrome, and later with an increased risk of leukemia.[530] A few patients have been reported with aplastic anemia. A 17-year-old boy had idiopathic aplastic anemia and trisomy 21 and apparently responded to androgen treatment.[531] Vetrella and colleagues[532] described a newborn with trisomy 21, cystic fibrosis, and amegakaryocytic thrombocytopenia who died at 49 days with pancytopenia shortly before death. A 12-year-old boy developed aplastic anemia that was unresponsive to androgens and died within 10 weeks,[533] and another patient was mentioned with aplastic anemia at 19 months, who appeared to respond to androgens.[534] A fifth case was published recently in which a patient developed aplastic anemia at 9 months and died at 26 months with gastroenteritis.[535] Although bone marrow was generally hypocellular in these patients, the last case had increased numbers of CFU-GM, apparently with both cellular and serum inhibitors of hematopoiesis. The few patients with trisomy 21 who developed aplastic anemia raises the question of whether this is a true association or merely coincidence.

Dubowitz's Syndrome

A rare, apparently autosomal recessive condition in which aplastic anemia has occurred is Dubowitz's syndrome. Approximately 40 cases have been reported, with hematologic abnormalities noted in three. The major features are intrauterine and postnatal growth retardation, microcephaly, moderate mental retardation, hyperactivity, eczema, and facial anomalies such as hypertelorism, epicanthal folds, blepharophimosis, broad nose, and abnormal ears. The most recent summary of the literature included 17 males and 21 females, with one set of twins and four sibling pairs, as well as one family with consanguinity; all these suggest autosomal recessive inheritance.[536] Three patients had bone marrow failure. Walters and Desposito[537] described a girl with pancytopenia beginning at age 10, who had a hypoplastic bone marrow, macrocytosis, and elevated Hb F. Chromosome breakage studies were normal, including a study with DEB, ruling out Fanconi's anemia. She responded to treatment with oxymetholone and is now 17 years old. Her brother, 2 years older, has a macrocytic hypoplastic anemia, with increased Hb F, but no need yet for treatment. The third patient with Dubowitz's syndrome, reported on by Berthold and coworkers,[538] developed fatal aplastic anemia at age 3. Thus, approximately 10% of the patients with Dubowitz's syndrome have had hematopoietic problems. An additional three patients were reported with malignancies, namely, lymphoma, acute lymphoblastic leukemia, and neuroblastoma.[539,540] This syndrome is another with growth defects associated with hematopoietic disorders and malignancies.

Seckel's Syndrome

Another rare autosomal recessive condition in which aplastic anemia has been reported is Seckel's syndrome. Although more than 60 patients have been published as having this syndrome, it may be an overused term, applied to a heterogeneous group of microcephalic dwarfs; thus, the true number is not clear. The stringent definition includes severe intrauterine and postnatal growth retardation, severe microcephaly, severe mental retardation, typical face with receding forehead and chin, antimongoloid slant of palpebral fissures, prominently curved nose, relatively large eyes and teeth, highly arched palate, hirsutism, and clinodactyly.[541]

Among the group with Seckel's syndrome, at least six (10%) developed aplastic anemia,[542–545] although two also had hypersplenism.[543] There were three boys and three girls, aged 4 to 11 at the time of presentation with anemia. Three were reported to have died from sepsis (or causes not reported) at 7, 9, and 12 years of age, 2 to 5 years after diagnosis. All received transfusions, and androgen treatment was tried in two without response. One died 2 weeks after bone marrow transplantation. Fanconi's anemia was considered in all cases, because they were small, microcephalic, and retarded, and had pancytopenia. In fact, the patients with Seckel's syndrome are much smaller and more severely microcephalic and retarded than those with Fanconi's anemia. Chromosome studies were normal in two of the patients with aplastic anemia. Endogenous breakage was increased in one patient and further increased with MMC in the sibling of that patient, but the diagnosis of Fanconi's anemia could not be firmly established. By contrast, two patients with Seckel's syndrome who did not have aplastic anemia had normal chromosomes, by the criteria of endogenous breakage, as well as SCEs.[546] Seckel's syndrome is another autosomal recessive syndrome with growth retardation, occasional aplastic anemia, and probably no association with increased chromosome breakage.

SINGLE CYTOPENIAS: RED BLOOD CELLS

Diamond-Blackfan Anemia

The first descriptions of red cell aplasia in infancy consisted of two cases reported by Josephs[547] in 1936 and four cases by Diamond and Blackfan[548] in 1938. A variety of synonyms and eponyms have been used—congenital hypoplastic anemia (CHA), chronic congenital aregenerative anemia, erythrogenesis imperfecta, chronic idiopathic erythroblastopenia with aplastic anemia (type Josephs-Diamond-Blackfan), and Diamond-Blackfan anemia (DBA). Diamond and Blackfan used the term *congenital hypoplastic anemia* because they thought the disorder differed from complete aplastic anemia only in degree. The term *hypoplastic* is now used when marrow depression (pancytopenia) is only partial; thus, the term is not appropriate for a single cytopenia. Erythrogenesis imperfecta is probably the most descriptive appellation, but the commonly used term now is *Diamond-Blackfan anemia.*

The following are diagnostic criteria for DBA:

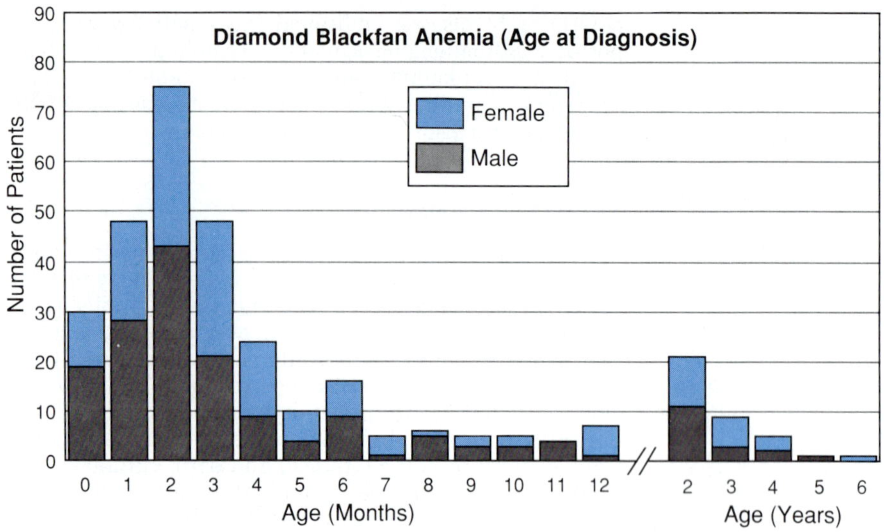

FIGURE 9-16. Age at onset of anemia in close to 400 published cases with Diamond-Blackfan anemia. Note the change in the scale on the abscissa.

- Normochromic, usually macrocytic, but occasionally normocytic anemia developing early in childhood
- Reticulocytopenia
- Normocellular bone marrow with selective deficiency of red cell precursors
- Normal or slightly decreased leukocyte counts
- Normal or often increased platelet counts.

These criteria clearly differentiate DBA from aplastic anemia, but may not always distinguish it from transient erythroblastopenia of childhood (TEC; see section later in text).

About 400 cases of DBA have been reported, and many of the references are cited in previous reviews.[5,549–551] The ages at which DBA was diagnosed (or the first transfusion or treatment initiated) are shown in Figure 9-16 and summarized by decade intervals in Table 9-20. Boys were slightly younger than girls (mean 5.2 compared with 6.6 months). Ten percent were severely anemic at birth, 25% by 1 month, 50% by 2 months, 80% by 6 months, and 90% by 1 year of age. Five percent were diagnosed between 1 and 2 years, and the remaining 5% before age 6. The males/females ratio is 1.1:1. Most of the reports are of whites, but DBA has been described in more than 20 blacks,[552–565] more than 12 Japanese,[566–571] 2 Indians,[572,573] and 1 Navajo.[574]

Very rare cases have presented at an older age. A 34-year-old man with anemia had an anemic daughter and subsequently a grandson with classic DBA.[575,576] Two adults with long-standing anemia responded to prednisone, were short-statured, and had findings typical of DBA, including webbed necks and thenar atrophy.[577]

Inheritance and Environment

The inheritance of DBA appears to have more than a single pattern. There were 13 families with *dominant* disease. The father was the link among affected stepchildren in 3 families, and the mother in 1.[564,578–581] The carrier parent had increased Hb F and macrocytosis without significant anemia. The other dominant families included four affected fathers and five mothers. One parent had childhood anemia, requiring transfusions or steroids, and one or more children had classic DBA.[550,555,558,582–588] In one family, the maternal grandfather, the mother, and one son all were involved.[575,576] In another family with two affected DBA children, the grandfather had refractory sideroblastic anemia.[582,589] There were two reports of three-generation families with seven and six patients, respectively.[581,590] The ratio of males to females in the dominant group was 1.1:1. The incidence of physical abnormalities was less, and the clinical course was generally milder than in the overall DBA population.

Another 30 families might be construed as *recessive*, since apparently there were affected siblings and normal parents, or consanguinity[566,573,591–594] (in 7 of the 30 families). Details were provided for 43 cases, and the sex of the affected sibs for 8 more. Twice as many males as females were in this small group.[555,559,561,582,595–610] Twelve sets of siblings are male only, eight male and female or female only, and in three families the sex of the sibs was not reported. In addition to one set of male twins in a sibship with three affected males,[607] a set of affected identical twins has also been reported.[611] The incidence of anomalies was actually slightly

TABLE 9-20. Diamond-Blackfan Anemia Literature

	1936–1960	1961–1970	1971–1980	1981–1989	Total
No. of patients*	79	110	91	99	379
Male/female	0.8	1.2	1.1	1.4	1.1
Age at diagnosis, male (mo)	3.6	5.4	7.6	3.0	5.2
Median	2	2	2	2	2
Range	0–24	0–48	0–54	0–18	0–54
Age at diagnosis, female (mo)	6.2	5.4	8.2	6.9	6.6
Median	3	3	3	3	3
Range	0–28	0–46	0–48	0–72	0–72
No. of males >1 y	1	7	8	1	17
No. of females >1 y	6	4	7	3	20

* Total of males plus females is less than the total because sex was not always stated.

higher in the recessives than in the overall group, but the anemia was milder and more responsive.

The recessive cases are probably autosomal, although X-linked inheritance cannot be ruled out for the families with only males. The inheritance in the recessive families might also be dominant with variable expression, but that is less likely since there are several families with consanguinity. Removal of all of the patients in families leaves more than 300 cases that are apparently sporadic, suggesting that DBA occurs as a new mutation, or as an acquired disease, or that penetrance is extremely variable.

Several patients were the products of problem pregnancies, suggesting that they had congenitally acquired marrow failure. The problems include preeclampsia, toxemia, rashes, premature placental separation, hemorrhage, spotting, and positive tests for syphilis. Exposures during pregnancy include diethylstilbestrol, x-rays, chlorothiazide, reserpine, thyroid hormone, prednisone, phenylbutazone, chloramphenicol, and anagyrine. A few mothers had previous spontaneous abortions or miscarriages. More than 30 patients weighed 2500 g or less at birth, but only 12 of these were premature; thus, most were small for gestational age (intrauterine growth retardation). The low birthweight might reflect pregnancy problems or poor growth intrinsic to DBA itself.

The anemia in patients with DBA was often noted at birth or during infancy. Jaundice due to hemolytic disease of the newborn from Rh or ABO incompatibility occurred occasionally, leading to prolonged anemia that became chronic[608] or that sometimes resolved after a few months.[612] A few patients had antecedent illnesses such as diarrhea, respiratory infections, urinary tract infections, measles, or mumps, or a smallpox vaccination. One child was treated with chloramphenicol.[613] In most patients, the illness was more likely to be due to the anemia or unrelated, rather than to be the cause of the anemia. The signs of anemia were usually pallor, lethargy, irritability, and heart failure.

TABLE 9-21. Physical Abnormalities in Patients With Diamond-Blackfan Anemia*

Abnormality	Males (%)	Females (%)	Total (%)
Birthweight ≤ 2500 g	7	14	10
Head, face, palate	9	16	13
Upper limbs	8	12	10
Short	4	10	7
Eyes	8	6	7
Renal	4	4	4
Neck	2	6	3
Hypogonads	5	1	3
Retardation	2	4	3
Lower limbs	1	4	2
Cardiopulmonary	2	2	2
Nose	1	1	1
Other skeletal	1	1	1
Other	3	5	4
At least one anomaly	25	34	49
TOTAL PATIENTS	182	164	379

* The totals exceed male + female, since the sex was not always stated. Severeal patients had more than one anomaly. Category, "at least one anomaly," excludes low birthweight as the only finding.

Physical Examination

Physical abnormalities were described in more than 100 patients (29%) with DBA, more frequently in females (25% and 34% of males and females, respectively; Table 9-21). Abnormalities of the head and face were most common. The typical face was described by Cathie[614] as "tow-coloured hair, snub noses, thick upper lips, rather wide set eyes, and an intelligent expression" (p 314), and was observed in many of the children, who resemble each other more than they do their own family members. Cleft lip and palate occurred in 3%. Other findings include micrognathia, microcephaly or macrocephaly, macroglossia, wide fontanelle, and dysmorphic features.

Upper limbs, particularly thumbs, are often abnormal. In our experience, the most common features are subtle flattening of the thenar eminences and weakness of radial pulses. Other radial hand anomalies are also common. Triphalangeal thumbs were noted in 15 patients (bilateral in 9 and unilateral in 6) who were otherwise similar to the total group of patients.[582,587,602,615–625] Although this association has been separated by some into the *Aase syndrome*, it is probably an inappropriate example of splitting rather than lumping.[626] Other thumb anomalies are bifid, supernumerary, absent, or subluxed thumbs,[582,597,599,604,608,625,627–632] which are either unilateral or bilateral. The presence of abnormal thumbs does not predict the course of the anemia.

Another common finding in DBA patients is short stature. Because many have received corticosteroids, it is often difficult to identify genetic short stature, but it was seen in at least 25 patients. There were four reports of dwarfism, including achondroplasia,[591,633] metaphyseal dysostosis,[634] and cartilage hair hypoplasia.[634] Short or webbed necks were reported in more than 12 cases, including both Klippel-Feil syndrome (fused cervical vertebrae) and Sprengel's deformity (elevation of the scapula). A Turner-like phenotype was sometimes mentioned.

Twenty-five patients had eye anomalies, most frequently hypertelorism, as well as blue sclerae, glaucoma, epicanthal folds, microphthalmos, cataracts, and strabismus. Kidney abnormalities including horseshoe, duplicated, and absent kidney were also noted in a few patients. Ten patients had hypogonadism, and 10 were retarded. Lower limb problems included dislocated hips, achondroplasia, and clubfoot. Congenital heart disease of all kinds was seen occasionally. The presence of anomalies serves more to confirm the diagnosis of DBA than to provide any prognosis regarding the course of the disease.

Laboratory Findings

All patients with DBA are by definition anemic. Hemoglobin levels at birth show a range of 2.6 to 14.8 g/dL, with a median of 7. In approximately 60 infants diagnosed with DBA between birth and 2 months, the median hemoglobin was 4 g/dL, with a range from 1.5 to 10. In those diagnosed later, the hemoglobin was also usually in the 4 g/dL range. Macrocytosis was almost uniform, and reticulocytes were usually absent. Figure 9-17 shows a representative blood film, with anisocytosis, macrocytosis, and an occasional teardrop.

White cell counts are generally normal in DBA patients, although counts sometimes decrease with the person's age. Values of 5000/μL or less were found at some time in 20% of patients, and below 3000/μL in 5%. Two heavily transfused older patients developed significant neutropenia (Young NS, unpublished data). Platelet counts are also usually normal, although 25% of patients had at least one count below 150,000/μL and 20% had one count above 400,000/μL. Buchanan and coworkers[635] noted elevated platelets in 50% of 38 patients and decreased platelets in 25% on at least one occasion. They found that platelet function was normal.

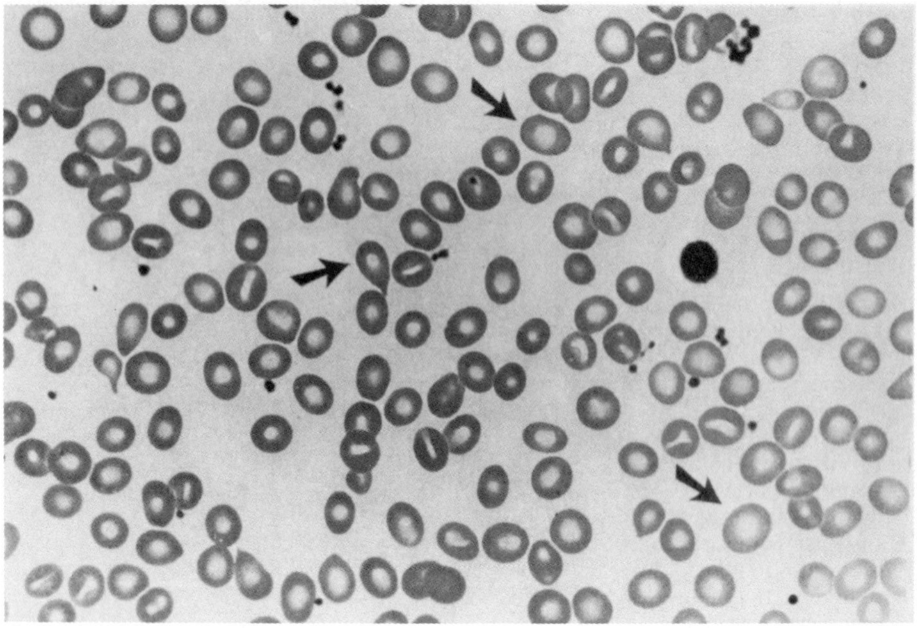

FIGURE 9-17. Peripheral blood from a patient with Diamond-Blackfan anemia. Note anisocytosis with both microcytosis and macrocytosis, as well as teardrop erythrocytes (*arrows*). (Courtesy of Dr. Gail Wolfe. Alter BP. The bone marrow failure syndromes. In: Nathan DG, Oski FA, eds. Hematology of infancy and childhood, ed 3. Philadelphia, WB Saunders, 1987:159)

Hb F is usually increased and is distributed heterogeneously (Fig. 9-18), indicating that the patients do not have a single clone of completely fetal cells. The proportion of $G\gamma$ to $A\gamma$ plus $G\gamma$ is over 50%, similar to that found in fetal RBCs. The titer of red cell membrane i antigen is also increased, as in fetuses, whereas the adult counterpart, I antigen, remains at adult levels. These fetal-like erythrocyte features are seen in newly diagnosed patients, patients responding to corticosteroids, and those in spontaneous remissions. They are not unique to those affected with DBA, but are characteristic of the stress erythropoiesis seen in any type of bone marrow failure.[108,109]

Bone marrow examination by aspiration or biopsy shows normal cellularity, myeloid cells, and megakaryocytes. Lymphocytes are often increased (seen even in normal infants; most of the marrow tests are done in infants with DBA) and were initially thought to be hematogones.[636] Eosinophilia is occasional.[637] Three patterns of erythroid development were described by Bernard and colleagues[597]:

1. Erythroid hypoplasia or total aplasia is seen in 90% of patients with DBA (Fig. 9-19). The only erythroid precursors in some patients are immature proerythroblasts.
2. Five percent of cases have normal numbers and maturation of erythroblasts.
3. The remaining 5% have erythroid hyperplasia, but with a maturation arrest, with increased numbers of immature precursors.

Despite the variable bone marrow picture, all DBA patients have reticulocytopenia. Thus, a few patients must have ineffective erythropoiesis. Dyserythropoietic morphology has been seen occasionally (see section on congenital dyserythropoietic anemia). Ringed sideroblasts were

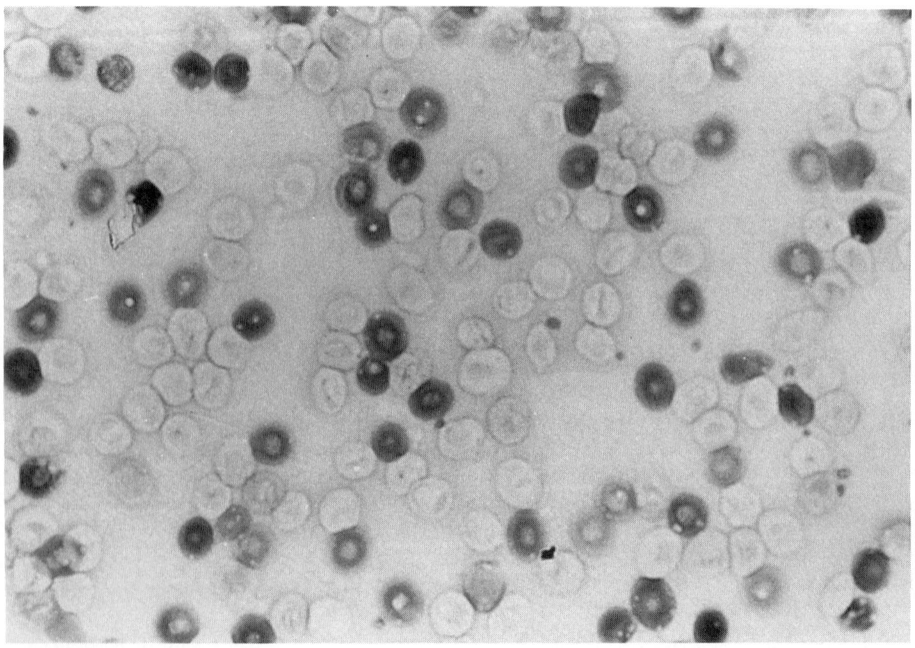

FIGURE 9-18. Kleihauer-Betke acid elution study of blood from a patient with Diamond-Blackfan anemia, showing the heterogeneous distribution of the fetal hemoglobin. (Courtesy of Dr. Gail Wolfe. Alter BP. The bone marrow failure syndromes. In: Nathan DG, Oski FA, eds. Hematology of infancy and childhood, ed 3. Philadelphia, WB Saunders, 1987:159)

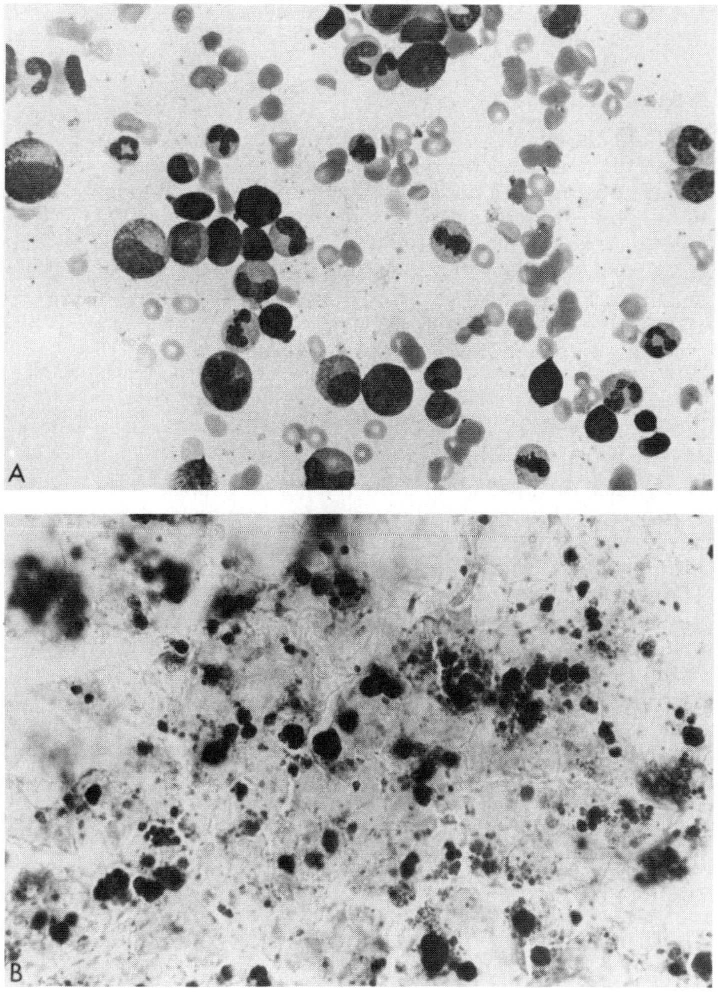

FIGURE 9-19. (**A**) Bone marrow aspirate from a patient with Diamond-Blackfan anemia, showing normal cellularity with erythroid hypoplasia. (**B**) Iron stain of bone marrow aspirate from a 2-year-old child with transfusion-dependent DBA. (Courtesy of Dr. Gail Wolfe. Alter BP. The bone marrow failure syndromes. In: Nathan DG, Oski FA, eds. Hematology of infancy and childhood, ed 3. Philadelphia, WB Saunders, 1987:159)

noted rarely, then disappeared.[638,639] Patients who receive many transfusions accumulate iron in the marrow (see Fig. 9-19) and other organs.

Serum levels of iron, ferritin, folic acid, vitamin B_{12}, and erythropoietin (EPO) all are elevated, and DBA is not due to deficiency of any of the normal hematinic agents.[640] DBA patients do not have antibodies to EPO. Routine urinalysis is normal. It was once thought that an abnormality in tryptophan metabolism occurs,[641,642] but other investigators failed to confirm this.[643] Hypocalcemia was reported only once,[600] and mild hypogammaglobulinemia was noted in several patients.[549,569,597,644] These parameters are normal in many other patients. Low numbers of T lymphocytes, and a reduction in the ratio of helper to suppressor T cells, were reported by Finlay and coworkers,[645] but abnormalities of T-cell function were not observed. Ferrokinetic studies showed the delay in plasma iron clearance and low RBC utilization expected in aplastic anemia.[597,600,629] Autologous RBC survival times were slightly shortened,[549,646] and haptoglobins were low in three patients,[549,647] suggesting a mild hemolytic anemia.

Patients with DBA have negative direct antiglobulin (Coombs') tests, and their disease is not due to RBC autoantibodies, although alloantibodies may develop after many transfusions. Results of bone marrow cultures and erythropoietic inhibitor assays are described below in the section on pathophysiology.

Abnormalities were observed in RBC enzymes involving purine or pyrimidine metabolism. Giblett and colleagues[592] described a patient with atypical DBA who also had lymphopenia and nucleoside phosphorylase deficiency; other patients had normal nucleoside phosphorylase levels.[648,649]Increased levels of the pyrimidine enzymes orotate phosphoribosyl transferase and orotidine monophosphate decarboxylase (ODC) were reported in 5 patients in one study,[649] and increased ODC was reported in 5 of 10 patients in another study.[650] ODC is an age-dependent enzyme that is increased in cord blood cells, and the elevation is consistent with the presence of young, fetal-like erythrocytes.

Glader and associates have observed increased RBC adenosine deaminase (ADA) in 26 of 29 DBA patients.[648,650,651] ADA, a critical enzyme in the purine salvage pathway, is not elevated in erythrocytes from cord blood or patients with hemolytic or other aplastic anemias. ADA was also elevated in 2 of 12 DBA parents.[648] Whitehouse and coworkers[652] found an increase in ADA in 9 of 19 patients and 2 of 15 relatives. The significance of ADA is not clear, since it is also increased in some children with acute lymphoblastic leukemia, and thus may indicate disordered erythropoiesis distinct from fetal-like erythropoiesis.[651] Increased ADA may distinguish DBA from TEC.

Chromosomes are normal in most patients with DBA.[549] Rare abnormalities include an achromatic area in a chromosome 1,[600] a pericentric inversion in one patient,[653] enlargement of chromosome 16 in three of six patients,[630] and breaks and endoreduplication of chromosome 16.[654] One patient had increased spontaneous and x-ray–induced chromosome breakage, without increased breakage due to MMC.[606] Others showed no increased breakage to DEB.[587,622] Sister chromatid exchange is normal. Chromosome studies are not informative, except to distinguish DBA from Fanconi's anemia.

Prenatal Diagnosis

One fetus in a family with two DBA children had an apparent high output cardiac failure when studied with two-dimensional fetal Doppler echocardiography,[610] although its reliability has been questioned.[655] Erythrocyte ADA might be increased in a fetus with DBA, but this has not yet been tested. DBA fetal blood BFU-E might be decreased, but this also has not been examined. Because only about 10% of the DBA cases are familial, the opportunities for prenatal testing are limited.

Pathophysiology

Diamond-Blackfan anemia may have more than a single basis, since the genetics and the phenotypes appear to be multiple. Most in vitro studies of the erythropoietic defect have been limited to small numbers of patients. Differing results may be related to true variability of the disease. The general consensus is that the erythroid progenitor cell is intrinsically abnormal, although a few studies suggested that there may be extrinsic abnormalities in accessory cells or in the serum.

The major erythropoietic hormone, erythropoietin (EPO), is increased in DBA patients to levels higher than expected for a given degree of anemia.[640] A few patients appeared to improve when treated with plasma,[640,656] but the mechanism of this response is unknown and the observation has not generally been substantiated. The mechanism was probably not the replacement of EPO, since the plasmas were from normal, not anemic, persons.

A few of the early patients appeared to have RBC alloantibodies.[608,612,657,658] These patients had neonatal jaundice and ABO or Rh incompatibility, in whom anemia persisted longer than expected or in whom bona fide DBA was eventually diagnosed. Antibody specificity may have extended to erythroblasts or progenitors, or blood group sensitization may have been a real but unrelated episode. Blood group incompatibility was not found to be significant in a large number of patients.[550]

One group reported that DBA serum was inhibitory to EPO stimulation of heme synthesis by suspension cultures of both autologous and allogeneic bone marrow, and that patient marrow had a decreased response to EPO.[659] Two other groups could not confirm these findings.[605,660] Treatment of patient serum with an antibody to EPO failed to unmask an inhibitor. In later studies using erythroid progenitor cultures in semisolid media, only one patient had a serum erythroid-blocking factor, evident only in allogeneic and not in autologous cultures.[563]

Cellular inhibitors have also been proposed. Hoffman and coworkers[661] found that peripheral blood lymphocytes from six multiply transfused DBA patients inhibited normal bone marrow colony-forming units—erythroid (CFU-E). One of those patients was later studied by Nathan and coworkers,[662] who were unable to detect inhibitory lymphocytes when HLA-identical marrow was used as the target population. Another was found to have normal erythroid progenitors and no cellular inhibitors.[663] Steinberg and colleagues[563] also reported suppressor T cells in the blood of two adults who had been transfused as children, which they proposed was overcome by an immunoglobulin blocking factor.[664] One patient out of five studied by Finlay and coworkers[645] was found to have T-cell suppression of normal erythroid colony growth. Inhibitory monocytes were suggested by Zanjani and Rinehart.[665] One adult had normal bone marrow colonies, but heme synthesis was inhibited by bone fragments, implying a microenvironmental defect.[666]

Nathan and associates[667] found no inhibition of normal or autologous marrow CFU-E by the lymphocytes from four transfusion-dependent patients and no inhibition of normal or patient blood burst-forming units erythroid (BFU-E) by the lymphocytes of eight patients, ranging from transfusion-dependent to steroid-independent remissions. They demonstrated that patient T cells were actually stimulatory to normal blood null cell BFU-E, as are normal T cells.[668] The occasional cellular suppression may relate to transfusion sensitization, rather than the pathophysiology of the disease.

Cumulative evidence indicates that the erythroid stem cell is abnormal in DBA. Cultures of bone marrow and blood mononuclear cells in plasma clot or methylcellulose showed reduced numbers of CFU-E or BFU-E in more than 50 patients, and normal numbers in about 12.[241,563,570,571,624,625,645,660,667,669–675] Those with normal quantities of progenitors may have been younger, untreated patients. It was suggested that those patients who subsequently responded to prednisone had better erythroid growth in vitro.[670,672,676] Addition of steroids in vitro was also found to increase erythropoiesis in a few studies.[241,677]

Several studies suggested that DBA erythroid progenitor cells required unusually high concentrations of EPO. Nathan and colleagues[667] demonstrated right-shifted EPO dose–response curves in two relapsed patients, with improvement in one after a prednisone-induced clinical remission. An increased EPO requirement was also noted by others.[625,670,672,676] These EPO studies used crude EPO, which may have contained other erythroid growth-promoting factors. Lipton and colleagues[672] demonstrated increased erythroid growth as well as increased EPO sensitivity in DBA bone marrow cultures to which a source of burst-promoting activity (BPA) was added. They recently found that enrichment of erythroid progenitor cells by removal of monocytes and lymphocytes produced a population of cells in which the BPA effect was more pronounced, suggesting that BPA might act directly on the progenitor cell and not through accessory cell mediation.[676] The identity of BPA is not known, but specific growth factors with in vitro erythroid activity such as granulocyte macrophage colony-stimulating factor (GM-CSF) and IL-3 are available through recombinant DNA methodology. Halpérin and coworkers[625] found that IL-3 increased the size and number of marrow BFU-E. The earlier suggestion that DBA erythroid progenitor cells were insensitive to EPO may have reflected an insensitivity to BPA or to IL-3 specifically. This has important therapeutic considerations, since GM-CSF is already in clinical trials for hematopoietic disorders, and IL-3 soon will be.

Therapy and Outcome

Transfusions. The only treatment initially available for DBA patients was transfusions, without which affected children died of anemia.[547] This remains the mainstay of the steroid-resistant patient. Packed RBCs are given every 3 to 6 weeks as needed to keep the hemoglobin above 6 g/dL. If transfusion reactions develop, white cell-free preparations are provided with either washed or filtered RBCs. Frozen and washed RBCs may be necessary to further reduce the incidence of reactions as well as the risk of viral transmissions. Careful cross-matching for minor blood groups is necessary only when alloantibodies develop from sensitization.

The major complication from transfusions is hemosiderosis. This was the cause of death in at least 20% of the more than 50 patients for whom the cause of death was stated. The side effects of iron overload in DBA are identical with those seen in thalassemia major, including diabetes, cardiac failure, liver disease, growth failure, and failure to enter puberty. These complications do not develop as rapidly in DBA patients as they do in thalassemia patients, in whom there is the added complication of a hemolytic rather than an aplastic anemia. Chelation of iron with subcutaneous desferrioxamine should begin as soon after the patients have begun a chronic transfusion program as they are shown to have increased iron stores.

Splenectomy was reported in almost 24 patients, with no apparent benefit except in those who had hypersplenism related to transfusions. Fifty percent of the splenectomized patients were reported to have died, and at least half of those deaths were due to infections. Splenectomy is not usually recommended today.

Corticosteroids. Gasser first proposed treatment of DBA patients with steroids, based on his observations of transient erythroblastopenia in patients with transient allergic disorders and of eosinophils in the bone marrow of DBA patients.[637,678] The first drugs were cortisone or adrenocorticotropic hormone (ACTH),[679] but prednisone and prednisolone have become the drugs of choice. Twelve of 22 patients responded in the first series by Allen and Diamond.[680]

The current recommendation is prednisone, 2 mg/kg/d, in three or four divided doses. Reticulocytes usually appear within 1 to 2 weeks. Some of the erythropoiesis is apparently ineffective because a sustained rise in hemoglobin may not occur for several weeks, although it usually appears within 1 month. The high divided-dose protocol is maintained until the hemoglobin reaches 10 g/dL. It is then tapered slowly, by sequential removal of the divided doses, until the patient is on a single daily dose that maintains the hemoglobin. This dose is then doubled and administered on alternate days, followed by a slow reduction in the amount. Treatment on alternate days reduces the side effects of the steroids. One group used prednisone daily for a week, followed by 1 to 2 weeks without any drug, to permit better growth.[629] This protocol did not work in our hands. The alternate day dose depends on the patient and varies from as low as 1 mg to more than 40 mg; some patients are sensitive to small doses, as well as to small changes in dose. Steroid side effects include growth retardation in more than half the patients,[550] and osteoporosis, weight gain, cushingoid appearance, hypertension, diabetes, fluid retention, gastric ulcers, and cataracts and glaucoma.

The following are patterns of response to steroids:

- Rapid response, followed by steroid-independent remission (less than 5%)
- Intermittent response (approximately 5%)
- Response, followed by steroid dependence (60%). Up to 20% of these patients may eventually be able to maintain their hemoglobin levels without steroids.
- Steroid response and dependence, followed by later failure to respond to the same or higher doses (5%)
- Requirement for large daily doses, which usually means resuming transfusions because of the steroid side effects (less than 5%)
- No response (30% to 40%). Overall, steroid nonresponders, high-dose responders, or subsequent failures make up almost 50% of cases.

In the total group, 15% to 20% of patients may eventually have a spontaneous remission, unrelated to their treatment response. The steroid or spontaneous remission literature data are summarized in Table 9-22.

Failure to remit with the above prednisone protocol is an indication for a trial of 4 to 6 mg/kg/d, or a trial of prednisolone or dexamethasone. Any medications that might be marrow-suppressive or affect the metabolism of prednisone, such as phenytoin or phenobarbital, should be discontinued. Allen and Diamond[680] found that the response was better when the interval between diagnosis and steroid treatment was short, but this may have been due to the development of hemosiderosis when the interval was long. In fact, steroid remissions have occurred in patients after 10 years of transfusions[549,613,681]; thus, a history of transfusions should not preclude an adequate trial of steroids combined with iron chelation as needed.

Several other therapeutic approaches also have been attempted. Androgens (see section on Fanconi's anemia) were reported in more than 50 patients, with apparent response in only three. Immunosuppressive drugs were given to a few patients. 6-Mercaptopurine was used successfully in one patient[682] and unsuccessfully in another.[605] Two patients had transient reticulocytosis after administration of cyclophosphamide and antilymphocyte globulin[683] (Young NS, unpublished data), whereas others had no response to cyclophosphamide.[564,605,684] Vincristine has also been ineffective.[683–685] Ozsoylu[686] suggested that high doses of intravenous methylprednisolone are effective, as previously described for severe acquired aplastic anemia. Cyclosporin A permitted the reduction but not elimination of prednisone in some patients, but only transiently in others.[609,687–690] Responses to immunosuppressive agents suggest that DBA is an autoimmune disease, but in vitro data are inconclusive.

Bone Marrow Transplantation. Bone marrow transplantation is a potential option for those who do not respond to reasonable doses of steroids. At least 13 patients have been transplanted from HLA-matched sibling donors, with 10 survivors.[674,685,691–693] Their ages at transplantation ranged from 1 to 16 years, and they were all steroid nonresponders or had relapsed on steroids. All had received transfusions. Deaths were related to posttransplantation infection in a

TABLE 9-22. Steroid Therapy in Patients With Diamond-Blackfan Anemia

	1936–1960	1961–1970	1971–1980	1981–1989	Total
No. of patients	79	110	91	99	379
No. treated	26	86	73	74	259
No. responding	18	58	38	48	162
Percentage of treated responding	69	67	53	65	63
No. with SR	13	19	19	9	60
Percentage of total with SR	16	17	21	9	16
No. of treated with SR	1	12	16	7	36
Percentage of treated with SR	4	14	22	9	14

SR, spontaneous remission.

patient with hemochromatosis and a patient with graft-verus-host disease. Transplantation preparations included combinations of antilymphocyte globulin, procarbazine, total lymphoid irradiation, busulfan, and cyclophosphamide. All donors were HLA-identical siblings. The decision for bone marrow transplantation in DBA is not easy, since perhaps 20% of patients may eventually have a spontaneous remission. Marrow transplantations are generally more successful in young, relatively untransfused (and unsensitized) patients; thus, the decision sometimes must be made before the outcome is entirely clear. Most DBA patients who were successfully transplanted did have multiple transfusions, including a minimum of 4 years in a series of four patients.[674]

Survival Data. The *survival data* on almost 400 patients reported in the literature are shown in Figure 9-20. Those who did not receive steroid treatment had a worse outcome than those who did; the best prognosis is for those who do respond to steroids. The projected median survival age for all is 31 years. No substantial differences were seen when the patients were separated by sex or when those with thumb or other abnormalities were analyzed separately.

Fifty-five patients were reported to have died (15%) at a mean age of 10 years in the entire group, 6 years in the 38 who died before 1970, and 17 years in the 17 who died after 1970 (Table 9-23). Seventeen percent of the males and 13% of the females had died. Steroids made a substantial difference in life expectancy. Three of those with dominant DBA had died (10%) at ages 9, 10, and 39, and none of the 43 with recessive disease had died, suggesting that the latter is a milder disorder. Two of 27 with thumb anomalies, including 1 of 15 with triphalangeal thumbs, died at ages 2 and 31. The most common causes of death were complications of iron overload and pneumonia or sepsis. Other deaths were due to bone marrow transplantation complications, leukemia, renal disease, anesthesia, pulmonary emboli, and undefined central nervous system disorders.

The long-term prognosis remains uncertain. On the survival curves shown in Figure 9-20, the only group that seems to reach a plateau is the group that responds to corticosteroids, approximately half the patients. The approaches for the other half include transfusions and chelation, bone marrow transplantation if there is a donor, and perhaps new agents such as hematopoietic growth factors (see section on pathophysiology).

The quality of life is good for most. The spontaneous remitters and the steroid responders who can be maintained on low doses live essentially normal lives. Those who must be transfused can receive chelation therapy, as do patients with thalassemia major. Many DBA patients have grown to adulthood and have had normal children. Temporary worsening of anemia has been noted during pregnancy in some patients, perhaps due to marrow suppression by estrogens'.

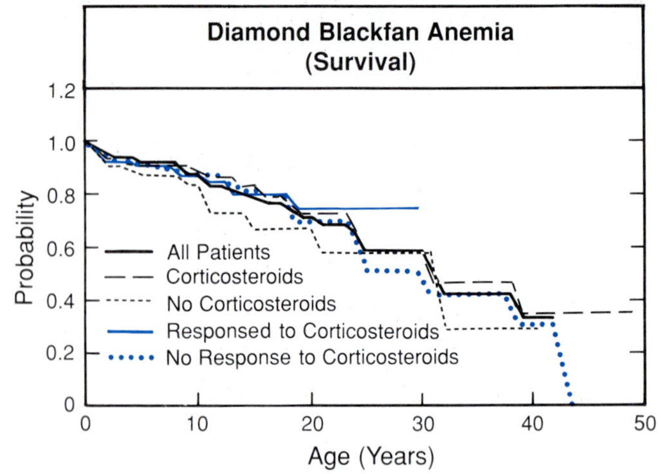

FIGURE 9-20. Kaplan-Meier plot of cumulative survival in Diamond-Blackfan anemia. Time is shown as age in years, since most cases are diagnosed in infancy. From 1938 to 1989, 358 cases were published, and 99 patients apparently did not receive steroids. Of 259 patients who received steroids, 97 did not respond to them, and 162 responded at least transiently.

Leukemia developed in at least five patients. One girl developed ALL at age 13, having had a spontaneous remission of DBA at age 5.[694] A complete remission of the ALL occurred, and she was free from both conditions at age 17 (Schaison G, personal communication). A female and a male from Diamond and coworkers' original series[582] had intermittent remissions of DBA, but died of acute myeloblastic leukemia at ages 31 and 43[695] (Gardner FH, unpublished data, 1984). The male had received radiation to his thymus and long bones to stimulate the bone marrow. One girl whose DBA treatment had included cyclophosphamide died of acute promyelocytic leukemia at age 13.[684] A boy developed acute megakaryoblastic leukemia at age 14 months; it is possible that his anemia from 2 months of age was really a long preleukemic phase.[696] Finally, one patient died at age 25 from metastatic hepatocellular carcinoma, which developed in a hemosiderotic liver.[697] The incidence of malignancies is not high in DBA patients, but is probably above normal.

Evolution to complete aplastic anemia has not been documented in DBA patients, although it was mentioned once without details by Najean.[698] Pancytopenia has occurred owing to severe iron overload or terminal sepsis. In general, DBA remains a single cytopenia, and the prognosis is better than in many of the other marrow failure disorders.

TABLE 9-23. **Age at Death in Patients With Diamond-Blackfan Anemia**

	1936–1960	1961–1970	1971–1980	1981–1989	Total
Total group					
No.	10	28	11	6	55
Years	1.7	8.6	17.5	16.6	9.7
No steroids					
No.	10	8	2	0	20
Years	1.7	9.2	21.5		6.4
Steroids					
No.	0	20	9	6	35
Years		8.3	16.6	16.6	11.9

Transient Erythroblastopenia of Childhood

Acute erythroblastopenia in previously hematologically normal children was first described by Gasser[678] in 1949 in 12 children in whom erythroblastopenia followed toxic, allergic, or infectious episodes. These children did not develop anemia because of their rapid recovery. Baar[699] then studied RBC life-span in an 8-year-old with "complete transient aplasia of the erythropoietic tissue" (p 22). The term *erythroblastopenia of childhood* was first used by Wranne[700] in 1970 to describe four cases with temporary red cell aplasia. Almost 400 cases have been reported since 1970, half as detailed case reports and half as series of cases without individual data.[701–719] TEC is defined as peripheral blood reticulocytopenia, usually with anemia and usually with bone marrow erythroblastopenia, with normal white blood cell and platelet counts, and of temporary duration. Some of the younger patients with TEC were sometimes initially thought to have DBA; Table 9-24 lists some of the features that distinguish the two conditions.

The male/female ratio is 1.3:1 among those with TEC. It is an acquired condition, occurring at a mean age of 26 months in males and 29 months in females, and a median age of 23 months in both (Fig. 9-21). Almost 90% of patients studied were older than 1 year, compared with 10% of those with DBA (compare Figs. 9-16 and 9-21). Only 10% of TEC patients were over 3 years of age, with the oldest male being 10 years and the oldest female 16 years of age.

TABLE 9-24. Comparison of Diamond-Blackfan Anemia and Transient Erythroblastopenia of Childhood

	DBA	TEC
No. of reported cases*	379	394
Male/female	1.1	1.3
Age at diagnosis, male		
Mean	5.2 mo	26 mo
Range	0–54 mo	1–120 mo
Age at diagnosis, female		
Mean	6.6 mo	28 mo
Range	0–72 mo	2–192 mo
Males > 1 y	9%	87%
Females > 1 y	12%	86%
Etiology	? Inherited	Acquired
Antecedent history	None	Viral illness
Physical examination abnormal	30%	0%
Laboratory		
Hemoglobin	1.5–10 g/dL	2.4–11 g/dL
WBCs < 5000/μL	20%	20%
Platelets ≥ 400,000/μL	20%	20%
Adenosine deaminase	Increased	Normal
MCV increased at diagnosis	80%	5%
During recovery	100%	90%
In remission	100%	0%
Hb F increased at diagnosis	100%	20%
During recovery	100%	100%
In remission	85%	0%
i Antigen increased	100%	20%
During recovery	100%	60%
In remission	90%	0%

MCV, mean cell volume.
* No. of males + females is less than the total, because sex not always stated.
(Adapted from Alter[5,543])

The presentation of TEC was that of pallor in a previously normal child, in whom prior normal blood counts were sometimes available. More than half gave a history of a preceding illness (mean, 1 month; range, 0 to 4 months), which was usually viral, either upper respiratory or gastrointestinal. Because these illnesses are common in young children, their relevance is difficult to ascertain, although a viral cause of the aplasia is appealing (see section on pathophysiology). Five children had neurologic manifestations of anemia, either seizures or transient ischemic attacks.[720–722] Drug or toxin exposure included piperazine, aspirin, sulfonamides, valproic acid, phenytoin, and phenobarbital.[704,707,712,723,724]

Familial TEC has been recorded only three times. One set of identical twins and a set of fraternal twins had simultaneous onset of anemia.[707,717] A pair of siblings had TEC at similar ages, 21 and 19 months, but 2 years apart.[725] In these familial cases, TEC might have been caused by the same viral or environmental factor combined with a genetic propensity. All ethnic groups have been represented, including blacks and Japanese.[726,727] Most of the reports have been from temperate climates.

Several series suggested that TEC is seasonal, with apparent clusters from June to October in several cases,[707,716–718,728] and from November to March in one.[713] All but one of these groups was in North America.[716] No statistically significant temporal clustering has been found. The average is 10.6 cases in each month, with a standard deviation of 3.9; the number of cases is sufficiently small that the reported monthly variations may be due to chance alone. At a given center, clusters may be due to specific local viral epidemics. Until the putative etiologic virus is identified, the cause remains speculative.

Physical examinations in TEC patients are normal except for pallor and findings related to anemia such as tachycardia. The anemia is of gradual onset; thus, the pallor often is not noticed by parents until the anemia is profound.

Laboratory Findings

Hemoglobin levels ranged from 2.4 to 10.9 g/dL, with a mean of 5.8 and a median of 5.7 g/dL. Reticulocytes were below 1% in 90% of the children. White blood cell counts were generally normal, but the absolute neutrophil count was below 1000/μL in 34 of 339 patients for which data are available (10%).[711,712,717–719,722,726,729–733] In two series of reasonable size, neutrophil counts below 1000/μL were noted in 5 of 24, and 12 of 64 children. Thrombocytopenia below 100,000/μL was reported in only 5 children (2%), 3 of whom were also neutropenic.[704,706,733] It is possible that whatever suppresses the erythroid series affects all cell lines in a few patients. Twenty-one children had white blood counts higher than 10,000/μL, perhaps associated with intercurrent infections. Platelet counts over 400,000/μL were noted in 65 patients (25%), similar to the proportion of DBA children with increased platelet counts. The MCVs were usually normal for age, with mean and median of 80 fl, although the range was from 63 to 112 fl. Hb F levels also were usually normal, although the range was from 0.2% to 9.2%. A suggestion from one small study that blood group A patients predominate[703] was not borne out in another small study.[708] Bone marrow examinations showed significant to profound erythroblastopenia in more than 90% of patients. In those in whom erythroblasts were seen, a maturation arrest was often present. Marrow lymphocytes were frequently elevated and led to the incorrect diagnosis of acute leukemia in at least one case.[734] The 5% to 10% of patients with reticulocytosis or erythroid hyperplasia at

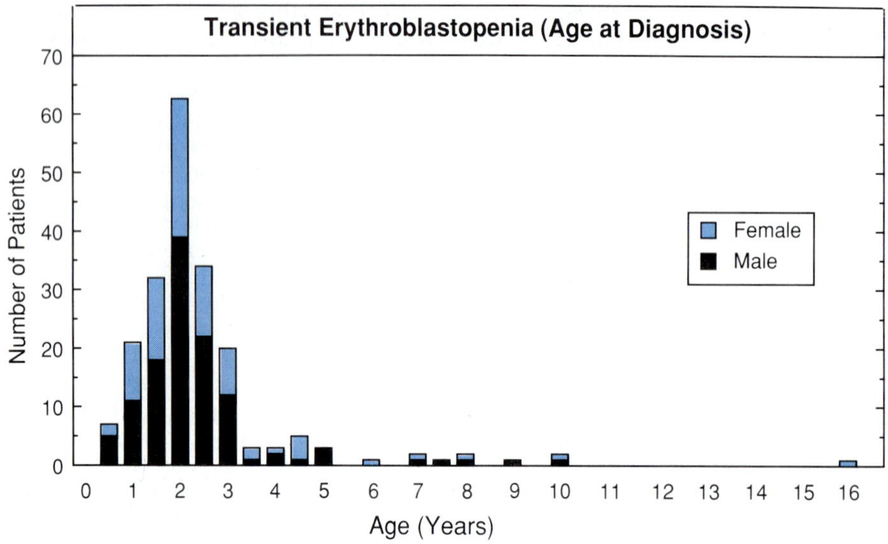

FIGURE 9-21. Age at diagnosis in more than 200 published cases with transient erythroblastopenia of childhood. Compare this with Figure 9-16 for Diamond-Blackfan anemia.

presentation presumably began to recover without the benefit of medical attention.[702–704,706,713,714,735,736]

Several erythrocyte characteristics may distinguish TEC from DBA. Wang and Mentzer[715] pointed out that the RBCs in TEC were "adult" or normal for age in MCV, Hb F, i antigen, and RBC enzyme levels. In DBA, these parameters were more fetal-like. This distinction based on normal versus fetal-like features is only relevant to the reticulocytopenic patient at the time of diagnosis. During the patient's recovery from TEC, the RBCs have the features of stress erythropoiesis, identical with those seen during any bone marrow recovery. This transient cohort of fetal-like erythrocytes[108,109,702,704,708,711] can be detected as soon as the first reticulocytes appear, using a sensitive immunologic assay for F-reticulocytes.[705,737] As Link and Alter[708] documented, this cohort of fetal-like erythrocytes then evolves again into normal RBCs. Thus, interpretation of fetal-like features depends on the stage of the disorder, and the ultimate distinction between TEC and DBA may be clear only from the outcome. Macrocytosis, elevated Hb F, and reticulocytopenia as well as marrow erythroblastopenia in a child under 1 year of age most likely indicates DBA. RBC ADA may also be useful, since it is elevated in most cases of DBA, and normal in TEC.[651]

Pathophysiology

A viral cause for TEC is most likely. The history of an antecedent (usually viral) illness 2 months before TEC is intriguing. Suppression of erythropoiesis in a normal person would require 1 to 2 months to be manifest as symptomatic anemia. It is not clear why recovery would then occur within another month. If the cause is viral, the time course of the development of specific antibodies would be relevant. The prime suspect is parvovirus. Almost 50 cases have been analyzed for parvovirus antibody individually or by one laboratory, and only 2 were found to be positive.[733,738] Because parvovirus inhibits the growth of CFU-E, it is logical that this particular virus leads to aplasia in patients with shortened RBC survival due to hemolytic anemia. Its role in those with previously normal erythropoiesis has not yet been proved and requires sensitive assays for antigen or for parvoviral DNA.[738–740] (See more-detailed discussion of viruses and aplastic anemia in Chapter 10.)

Several groups have investigated the erythropoietic defect in TEC. Levels of EPO are high.[701] Erythroid progenitor cell cultures were performed in close to 50 patients by more than 12 laboratories; the results are summarized in Table 9-25. Among the more than 30 patients whose own bone marrow erythroid progenitors were assayed, 15 (50%) had decreased CFU-E and 9 (30%) had decreased BFU-E, suggesting that the defect might be in CFU-E.[709,710,712,729,732,733,741–745] Koenig and coworkers[746] identified serum or IgG inhibitors of normal progenitors in 4 patients and showed autologous inhibition as well in 1 patient. Serum inhibitors were examined in more than 30 other patients and were observed in both autologous and allogeneic assays.[709,710,712,732,733,742,744,745] Cellular inhibitors were also reported in both types of assays.[710,729,732,733,743,745,747]

A consensus of all of these culture studies is difficult to reach, since not all parameters were examined in all patients. Probably half of all cases of TEC have reduced erythroid progenitor cell numbers. More than half have serum inhibitors in autologous or allogeneic cultures, usually IgG. Inhibitory mononuclear cells may be present in one fourth of cases. No patients had both serum and cellular inhibitors, but only nine were examined for both. TEC may be due to an as yet unknown virus, which may infect CFU-E and not be cleared until specific antibodies develop to the virus. In some cases, a specific IgG may be directed against epitopes on erythroid progenitors themselves, thus inhibiting growth of autologous or allogeneic erythroid colonies. Recovery in these cases might require anti-idiotype antibodies.

Therapy and Outcome

As indicated by the name of this disorder, TEC is transient, and all patients recover. Recurrent TEC was observed only twice and occurred within 1 year.[701,749] Most patients show signs of recovery within the first month after diagnosis, and 5% to 10% have already begun to recover when first seen. The longest interval to recovery without recurrence was 8 months, and only 6 patients took more than 4 months. No treatment was necessary for 144 of 353 patients for whom the clinical course was described (40%). In most patients, the nadir hemoglobin was reached by the time they were seen. Transfusions were given to 209 children (60%), with more than one transfusion in less than 10%. Prednisone was administered to more than 60 patients (20%); reticulocytes appeared within 1 day in many, almost certainly unrelated to the treatment.

Our recommendation for TEC is watchful waiting, with transfusion only when anemia leads to cardiovascular

TABLE 9-25. **Erythroid Cultures in Transient Erythroblastopenia of Childhood***

Assay	No. Studied	Result	No.	Percentage	References
Progenitor cell assays	34				710, 712, 733, 741–743
BM CFU-E	32	Decreased	17	53	709, 729, 732, 744, 745
BM BFU-E	27	Decreased	8	30	
Both	25	Both decreased	8	32	
		CFU-E decreased	4	16	
Serum inhibitors	37				709, 710, 712, 733, 742
Autologous serum	21	Inhibitory IgG 9, IgM 1	13	62	732, 744, 745, 747, 748
Allogeneic serum	26	Inhibitory IgG 9	16	62	
Both	10	Inhibit both IgG 2	5	50	
		Inhibit autologous	1	10	
Cellular inhibitors	16				710, 729, 732, 733, 743, 745, 747
Autologous MNC	8	Inhibitory	2	25	
Allogeneic MNC	6	Inhibitory	2	33	
Both MNC	4	Inhibitory	1	25	
Autologous T cells	8	Inhibitory	1	13	
Allogeneic T cells	2	Inhibitory	0	0	

* A total of 46 patients had cultures performed using some or all of the following: bone marrow cells, serum, IgG, IgM, peripheral blood mononuclear cells (MNC), T cells.

compromise. These children tolerate their anemia extremely well because it has developed gradually, and it is often the cardiovascular status of the physician rather than the patient that leads to transfusion. Prednisone, anabolic steroids, and other immunosuppressive therapies have no apparent role in the management of TEC. The prognosis is excellent, and the distinction from DBA is simple in retrospect (see Table 9-24).

Congenital Dyserythropoietic Anemia

Dyserythropoiesis refers to ineffective, morphologically abnormal erythroid production. *Dysplastic* indicates qualitative abnormalities of the stem cell or the microenvironment. *Aplastic* refers to quantitative abnormalities of the same compartments. Although these congenital conditions are not, strictly speaking, bone marrow failure syndromes, they are inherited marrow disorders, which may result in anemia without reticulocytosis. Erythropoiesis is ineffective because a discrepancy exists between erythroid output from marrow to circulation (anemia) and erythroid marrow content (erythroid hyperplasia), implying intramedullary destruction.

In normal persons, approximately 1 in 1000 bone marrow erythroblasts is abnormal.[750] Multinucleated erythroblasts and karyorrhexis are occasionally seen in megaloblastic anemia, iron deficiency, leukemia, and hemolytic anemia—indicative of bone marrow stress. The incidence of dyserythropoietic erythroblasts may be substantial in acquired or inherited aplastic anemia. In one study of aplastic anemia, 5% to 90% of erythroblasts were megaloblastic or showed nuclear–cytoplasmic asynchrony, 1% to 3% were binucleate, and up to 5% had cytoplasmic connections or chromatin bridges.[751] During recovery from bone marrow transplantation, all patients transiently had up to 30% dyserythropoietic erythroblasts.[752] These morphologic abnormalities are more extreme in congenital dyserythropoietic anemia (CDA) than in aplastic anemia or in marrow transplantation recovery.

All patients with CDA have anemia with insufficient reticulocytosis and ineffective erythropoiesis, and all ethnic groups are affected. The major types of CDA were described in detail in a book by Lewis and Verwilghen[753] in 1977. Table 9-26 outlines the major types:

Type I—macrocytosis, with bone marrow megaloblastoid changes and internuclear chromatin bridges between cells

Type II—normocytosis or macrocytosis, with binucleated and multinucleated erythroblasts, pluripolar mitoses, and karyorrhexis

Type III—macrocytosis, with erythroblastic multinuclearity of up to 12 nuclei (gigantoblasts)

Types I and III are diagnosed primarily due to bone marrow morphology. Type II is characterized by positive reaction to some acidified normal sera (called HEMPAS, or hereditary erythroblastic multinuclearity with a positive acidified serum test[754]). More than 30 additional cases have been reported that do not clearly fit into types I to III.

Type I

About 60 cases of type I CDA have been reported (the first 20 by Heimpel[755,756]). The onset of anemia, jaundice, or both ranges from infancy to old age, with a mean of 15 years. The male/female ratio is 1.25:1, and the inheritance is autosomal recessive. Consanguinity was reported in 8 families, and affected siblings or cousins in 10. Physical examination may show icterus and splenomegaly, as well as brown skin pigmentation; a few patients had toe syndactyly or abnormal fingers.

The anemia is often mild, with a mean Hb of 9 g/dL and a range of 3 to 12 g/dL. Reticulocytes range from 1% to 7%. RBCs are macrocytic, with a MCV of 100 fL and a range of 70 to 120 fL. The blood film shows anisocytosis, poikilocytosis, punctuate basophilia, and occasional Cabot's rings. White blood cells and platelets are normal. Indirect bilirubin is elevated (1 to 4 mg/dL), as is serum lactate

TABLE 9-26. Types of Congenital Dyserythropoietic Anemias

Feature	Type 1	Type II	Type III
Reported cases	60	121	30
Anemia	Mild to moderate	Mild to severe	Mild to moderate
Red cell size	Macrocytic	Normo- to macrocytic	Macrocytic
Bone marrow erythroblasts	Megaloblastoid, binucleated (2–5%) chromatin bridges	Bi- and multi-nucleated (10–40%) karyorrhexis	Gigantoblasts (10–40%)
Inheritance	Recessive	Recessive	Dominant
Acid serum hemolysis	Negative	Positive	Negative
Reaction			
Anti–i antibody	Slight	Strong	Slight
Anti–i antibody	Slight	Strong	Slight

(Modified from Alter BP. The bone marrow failure syndromes. In: Nathan DG, Oski FA, eds. Hematology of infancy and childhood, ed 3. Philadelphia, WB Saunders, 1987:159)

dehydrogenase, whereas haptoglobin is low and transferrin is saturated. Plasma iron turnover is as much as 10 times the normal, and RBC utilization is reduced to below 30%. RBC survival is slightly shortened, with chromium-51 (^{51}Cr) half-life of 15 to 28 days (mean 21 days). Globin synthesis studies usually show non-α/α ratios of 1, although imbalance of 0.5 to 0.7 was observed occasionally.[757,758] Negative reactions are seen in the acidified serum test, and i antigen titer is usually in the adult low range, in contrast to that seen in type II CDA.

Bone marrow examination shows marked erythroid hyperplasia.[759] The abnormalities are confined to the more mature erythroblasts, the polychromatophilic and orthochromatic series (Fig. 9-22). Nuclear maturation and cytoplasmic maturation are dissociated, and nuclei are immature and megaloblastoid. Up to 2% of erythroblasts are large cells with incomplete nuclear division, often with double nuclei in which one component is more mature than the other. Up to 2% of cells show thin chromatin bridges connecting the nuclei of two cells. Electron microscopy demonstrates widening of nuclear membrane pores in mature erythroblasts, with condensation, vacuolization, and disintegration of nuclear chromatin, with cytoplasmic penetrance. Structural changes are found of the nucleolus, microtubules, and siderotic material in the cytoplasm.[759–761]

The defect in CDA is at the stem cell level. The numbers

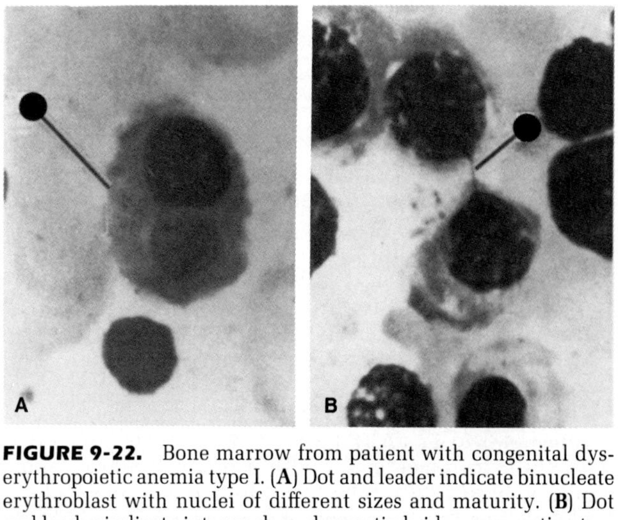

FIGURE 9-22. Bone marrow from patient with congenital dyserythropoietic anemia type I. (**A**) Dot and leader indicate binucleate erythroblast with nuclei of different sizes and maturity. (**B**) Dot and leader indicate internuclear chromatin bridges connecting two erythroblasts. (Lewis SM, Verwilghen RL, eds. Dyserythropoiesis. London, Academic Press, 1977)

of CFU-E and BFU-E are normal, but the colonies contain a mixture of normal and abnormal cells when examined by electron microscopy.[762] This suggests that the abnormality is expressed variably in the mature progeny of each stem cell.

Treatment with the usual hematinics, such as vitamins, metals, and steroids, is without effect. A few transfusions were required in 15% of patients. Splenomegaly is common, but splenectomy (reported in 10 cases) does not improve the anemia. Some patients develop gallstones from the hemolytic anemia. Hemosiderosis is the most important long-term complication because of increased intestinal absorption of iron, ineffective erythropoiesis, and mild hemolysis; phlebotomy or iron chelation with deferroxamine warrants consideration. Two of the 60 patients were reported to have died, 1 at age 10 from complications of splenectomy, and the other at age 84 from old age.

Type II

Type II CDA, also known as HEMPAS, has been reported in approximately 120 patients. Many of the early cases were summarized by Verwilghen.[763,764] Twenty-five were in sibships, and six were in families with consanguinity. The male/female ratio is 1:1, and the inheritance is autosomal recessive. Anemia is noted between infancy and adulthood, at an average of 15 years of age and varies from mild to requiring regular transfusions. Jaundice, hepatosplenomegaly, and gallstones are more common in patients with type II than in those with type I CDA.

Although anemia may be severe in patients with type II CDA, reticulocytosis is inadequate, averaging 4%. RBCs are usually normochromic and normocytic, although macrocytosis has been observed; the average MCV is 93 fL, and the range 77 to 114 fL. The smear shows anisocytosis, poikilocytosis, teardrops, and basophilic stippling, all nonspecific findings. The anemia and the RBC life-span are worse in type II than in type I patients; the ^{51}Cr half-life averages 17 days (range, 7 to 31).

Electron microscopy shows an excess of endoplasmic reticulum parallel with the cell membrane, leading to the appearance of a characteristic double membrane, or cistern, in late erythroblasts and some erythrocytes.[760,761] Many patients with type II CDA also have bone marrow reticuloendothelial cells that resemble Gaucher cells, with birefringent, PAS-positive (paraaminosalicylic acid) needle-like inclusions. These inclusions may be the products of catabolism from the rapidly turning-over marrow erythroblasts. The marrow shows erythroid hyperplasia, with binucleated and multinucleated mature erythroblasts in 10% to 40% of the erythyroid precursors (Fig. 9-23). The internuclear

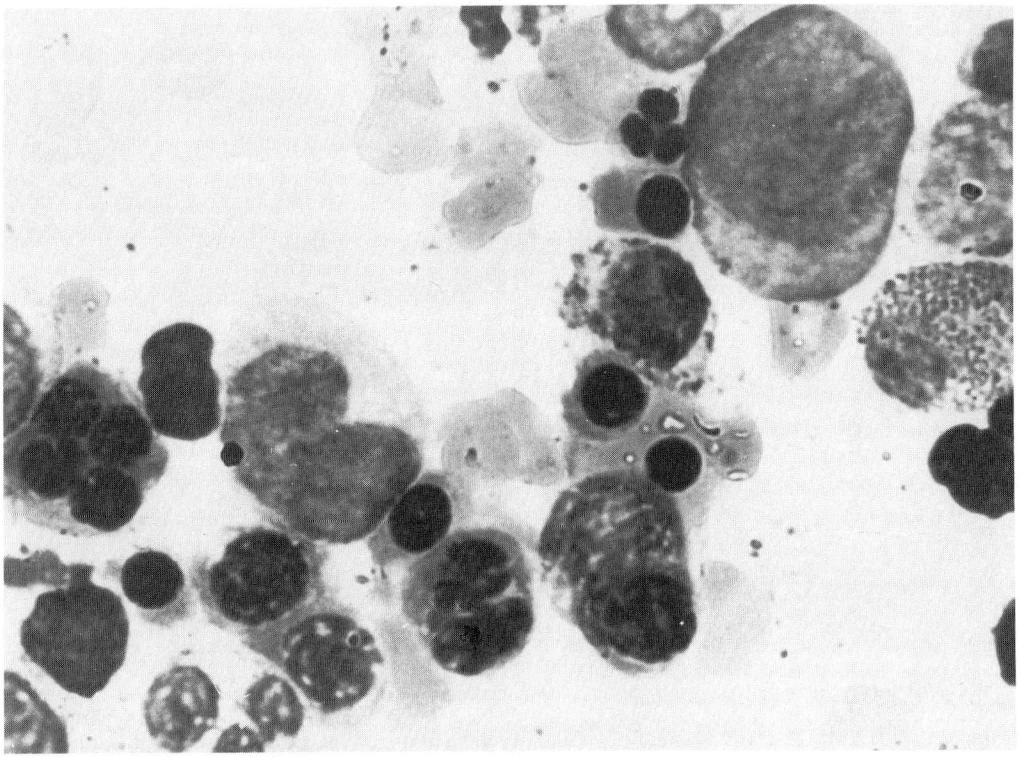

FIGURE 9-23. Bone marrow from patient with congenital dyserythropoietic anemia type II, showing binucleated and multinucleated erythroblasts. (Courtesy of Dr. Gail Wolfe. Alter BP. The bone marrow failure syndromes. In: Nathan DG, Oski FA, eds. Hematology of infancy and childhood, ed 3. Philadelphia, WB Saunders, 1987:159)

chromatin bridges of type I CDA are not seen, nor is the multinuclearity as extreme as is seen in type III.

The pathognomonic findings in HEMPAS are serologic.[754,765,766] HEMPAS RBCs are lysed by approximately 30% of acidified sera from normal persons, but not by the patient's own serum. In contrast, in paroxysmal nocturnal hemoglobinuria, patient cells are lysed by acidified patient serum. In CDA type II, the RBCs have a specific HEMPAS antigen, and many normal sera contain an anti-HEMPAS IgM antibody. In some cases of type II CDA, up to 30 normal sera must be examined until a positive acidified test results; some were thought not to be type II until this was obtained.[767] HEMPAS erythrocytes are also distinct in being more strongly agglutinated with anti-i antibody than cells of newborn infants or of patients with stress erythropoiesis.[768] Fluorescent labels demonstrated i antigen on all RBCs in HEMPAS. Heterozygotes also have increased expression of i antigen.[754,769] HEMPAS RBCs also express increased amounts of I antigen. HEMPAS erythrocytes were shown by Rosse and associates[770] to bind a normal amount of complement (C1), but more antibody and less C4 than normals. This causes binding of an excess of C3 and hemolysis. The RBC plasma membrane abnormality in HEMPAS is related to decreased *N*-acetylglucosaminylphosphotransferase II. Bands 3 and 4.5 lack glycosylation with lactosaminoglycans.[771]

The number of erythroid progenitors is probably normal in marrow and blood. Although one study found only normal morphology of the erythroblasts produced in culture,[772] other studies reported multinuclearity similar to that seen in the bone marrow.[773,774] As in type I CDA, the defect in type II CDA is in the erythroid stem cell and is expressed variably in more mature erythroblasts.

Patients whose anemia is severe are supported by blood transfusions. Unlike in type I, splenectomy is effective in type II, leading to an increase in RBC life-span and abrogation of transfusions. Iron accumulation is a major complication, both from transfusions and from increased intestinal absorption, even in untransfused patients. Phlebotomy and iron chelation have a definite role in the management of patients with type II CDA.[775] Two of the 120 patients with this disease died of hemochromatosis at ages 25 and 30.

Type III

Approximately 30 patients have been reported on with type III CDA.[776,777] Three families had apparently dominant CDA, involving members of two generations, and an additional set of brothers. The male/female ratio was 1.9:1. The average age at diagnosis was 22 years, with a range from birth to old age, similar to that in types I and II. Anemia is mild to moderate, and MCVs may be normal or increased. The bone marrow shows erythroid hyperplasia, with multinuclearity in 10% to 40% of erythroblasts, including some large gigantoblasts with up to 12 nuclei (Fig. 9-24). Hemolysis does not occur with acidified sera, and reactions with anti-i antigen are similar to those seen in stress erythropoiesis. RBC survival is slightly shortened, with ^{51}Cr survival half-life of 21 days. The defect is in the stem cell, and in vitro culture results in colonies containing both normal and abnormal erythroblasts.[778]

The need for transfusions or splenectomy is rare. As in the other CDAs, hemosiderosis is the major problem and resulted in one death at age 42.

Variants

More than 30 patients have been reported with apparent CDA that does not conform to the types just described.

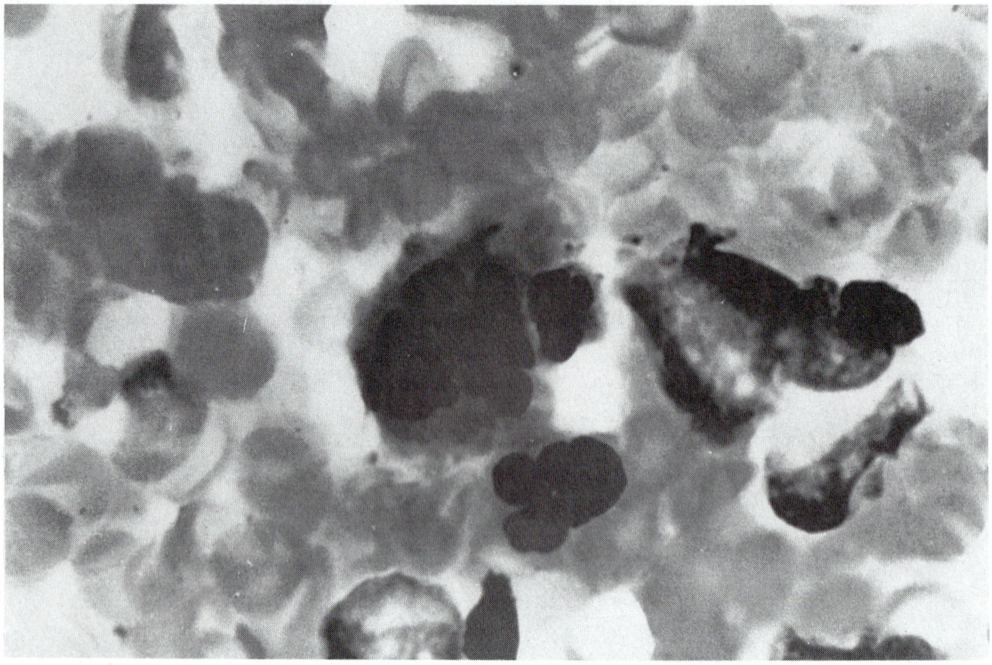

FIGURE 9-24. Bone marrow from patient with congenital dyserythropoietic anemia type III, showing multinucleated erythroblast. (Courtesy of Dr. Gail Wolfe. Alter BP. The bone marrow failure syndromes. In: Nathan DG, Oski FA, eds. Hematology of infancy and childhood, ed 3. Philadelphia, WB Saunders, 1987:159)

Others have attempted to classify them into discrete categories.[779,780]

In four reports, the bone marrow morphology resembled type II; the cases were classified as type IV. The acidified serum tests were negative, which might indicate only that an insufficient number of sera were examined. The level of i antigen was not increased. The inheritance was apparently dominant in one family; thus, at least some of these cases might indeed belong to a different type.[781–784] Anemia was mild in all but one case and was diagnosed from infancy to adulthood. Binucleated erythroblasts made up 10% to 40% of the marrow erythroblasts. The clinical course was relatively benign in the seven cases reported, with splenectomy in only one.

Another group of 10 patients in three families has been termed *CDA with thalassemia*. One family had dominant inheritance, and one family had three affected siblings.[785–787] The age at diagnosis ranged from infancy to old age, the anemia was mild to moderate, MCVs ranged from microcytic to macrocytic, and multinuclearity was present in 25% to 35% of the erythroblasts. Tests with acidified sera were negative, and i antigen was positive in two of the three families. Globin chain synthesis was imbalanced, with β/α ratios of 0.5, similar to those seen in β-thalassemia trait. There may have been coincidence of thalassemia trait and CDA, but two families were from ethnic groups without a high incidence of thalassemia.

More than a dozen additional families have been reported with CDAs that are even harder to classify. Two families had an affected parent and child, two had consanguinity, and three had affected siblings. These cases all may represent different disorders. The proportion of binucleated or multinucleated erythroblasts was always low, under 4%. In some, the morphology resembled type I, with rare internuclear bridges, as well as type II, with symmetric binuclearity, karyorrhexis, and even double membranes by electron microscopy. The ages at diagnosis of anemia ranged from birth to adulthood, and the anemia from mild to severe. MCVs encompassed the entire spectrum. Acidified serum testing was usually negative, i antigen was variable, and RBC ^{51}Cr half-life was from 5 to 29 days. Splenectomy was reported in 6 of 18 patients, with some usefulness. Erythroid cultures from one case demonstrated that multinuclearity was present in some cells in each colony, indicating a stem cell disorder as in the other CDAs.[788] The clinical variability suggests that these cases may represent several types of CDA. Perhaps these patients are double heterozygotes, instead of homozygotes, for recessive CDA genes.

SINGLE CYTOPENIAS: WHITE BLOOD CELLS

Kostmann's Syndrome

Inherited isolated neutropenia was first recognized as a distinct entity by Kostmann[789,790] in 1956, who called it infantile genetic agranulocytosis. Another name for this condition is severe chronic neutropenia, but this fails to differentiate it adequately from other the neutropenias of childhood (see Chap. 17 for a complete discussion of neutropenia). We use the term *Kostmann's syndrome* (KS) to describe the disorder in infants with extreme neutropenia, severe pyogenic infections, and early deaths. More than 100 cases in the literature fit this description (Table 9-27). The male/female ratio is 0.8:1, and the inheritance is autosomal recessive. Most of Kostmann's original 14 and subsequent 10 cases were members of a large intermarried kinship in northern Sweden, and a founder effect is clearly relevant.[791] Cases have been reported in all ethnic groups, including blacks, Native Americans, and Asians. At least 10 were in families with parental consanguinity, and more than 20 had affected siblings.

Age at presentation is very young, with 50% of the patients symptomatic within the first month after birth and 90% by 6 months. In fact, the few who were diagnosed

TABLE 9-27. Kostmann's Syndrome Literature

No. of cases	121
Male/female	0.8:1
Age at diagnosis	
Mean	2.6 mo
Median	3 wk
Range	0–48 mo
No. with leukemia	2 (2%)
Age at leukemia	14 y
No. of deaths	63 (52%)
Age at death	
Mean	2 y
Median	7 mo
Range	2 wk–20 y
Projected 50% survival	3 y

later may not have had KS. Birthweights are generally normal, as are physical examinations, except for signs of infection such as skin abscesses. Short stature was noted in four patients, mental retardation in four, cataracts in three, and microcephaly in two.

Laboratory Findings

Neutropenia is extreme in KS patients, although several infants had almost normal absolute neutrophil counts in the first week or two, which declined rapidly. The average absolute neutrophil count is under 200/μL; many patients have total neutropenia. Eosinophils and monocytes are frequently high (up to 50% monocytes in some patients), but these are not as effective as phagocytes as are neutrophils. Immunoglobulin levels are also frequently increased. KS is a single cytopenia because the hemoglobins are usually normal (mean, 10 g/dL), and platelet counts are normal or even high. Bone marrow is cellular, with absent or markedly decreased myeloid precursors. When precursors are present, there is an arrest at the myelocyte or promyelocyte stage.

Pathophysiology

Kostmann's syndrome is inherited as an autosomal recessive and primarily affects the neutrophil series. Bone marrow cultures have decreased, increased, or, most often, normal numbers of colony-forming units (CFU-C). The colonies that do grow in semisolid media, which contain neutrophils in normal persons, have been reported rarely to contain neutrophils,[792] or more frequently to contain eosinophils, monocytes, and abnormal or arrested myeloid precursors.[793] A block in myeloid differentiation was also seen in long-term cultures from some patients.[792] Thus, in some patients the in vivo defect in myeloid differentiation is apparent in vitro.

Therapy and Outcome

The prognosis for patients with KS has been poor, with more than half reported to have died at a mean age of 2 years, a median of 7 months, and a range of 2 weeks to 20 years. The Kaplan-Meier survival plot (Fig. 9-25) indicates a projected median survival of 3 years, and only 10% long-term survivors. Most of the deaths were from sepsis or pneumonia. No cases have evolved into aplastic anemia, showing that KS is a true single cytopenia.

Infections are treated with antibiotics, and many patients receive prophylactic treatment. Lithium therapy was suggested because of its ability to raise white counts in hematologically normal persons. Lithium was relatively ineffective in KS patients.[794,795] Bone marrow transplantation cured one patient,[796] but the graft was lost in another.[797]

The most exciting therapeutic advance is the use of recombinant growth factors. Subcutaneous G-CSF (granulocyte colony-stimulating factor) in a dose-related manner is effective at raising neutrophil counts in children with KS. The factor must be administered chronically, but seems to be without major side effects.[798]

Prenatal diagnosis has been considered for KS, using fetal blood obtained in the mid-trimester.[799] The absolute neutrophil count is less than 200/μL in normal fetuses.[800] Therefore, absolute neutropenia would be required to diagnose KS in utero.

Leukemia. Two patients developed acute monocytic leukemia, both at age 14, and died at 4 and 6 months.[801,802] One family was reported to have one child with KS and a sibling with ALL.[803] Thus, a propensity for malignancy is seen in KS as in many other bone marrow failure syndromes.

SINGLE CYTOPENIAS: PLATELETS

Syndrome of Thrombocytopenia With Absent Radii

Thrombocytopenia with absent radii represents a true single cytopenia, with no reports of evolution to pancytopenia or malignancy. Comprehensive reviews are provided by Hall and associates[804,805] and by Hedberg and Lipton.[806] The patients are often diagnosed at birth, due to the combination of the characteristic physical appearance plus thrombocytopenia. The pathognomonic physical finding is bilateral absence of the radii, with thumbs present (Fig. 9-26). The presence of thumbs differentiates TAR from Fanconi's anemia (and from trisomy 18), in which thumbs are absent if radii are absent. Hemorrhagic manifestations in TAR patients are often also present at birth, with petechiae, bloody diarrhea, or both apparent in 60% within the first week and in over 95% by 4 months.

Table 9-28 compares several features of TAR with Fanconi's anemia. The inheritance pattern in TAR is autosomal recessive, with more than 20 families reported with affected siblings; having an affected child increases the chances of having another to one in four. The preponderance of females reported as having TAR is similar to the preponderance of males in Fanconi's anemia. A set of identical twins

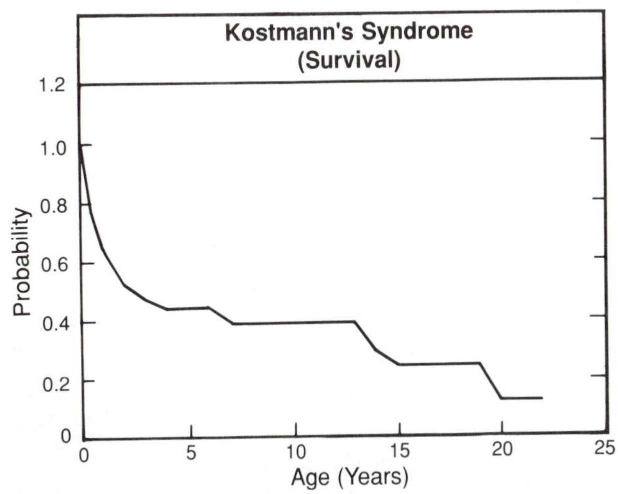

FIGURE 9-25. Kaplan-Meier plot of cumulative survival in Kostmann's syndrome.

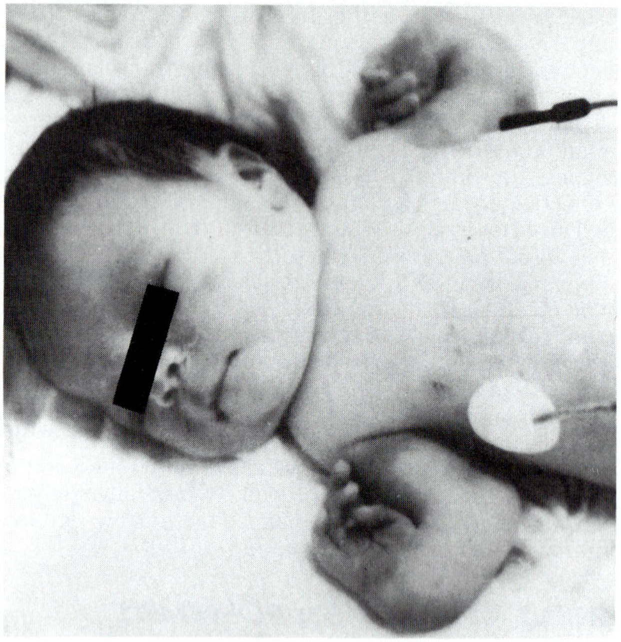

FIGURE 9-26. Newborn infant with thrombocytopenia with absent radius syndrome. Note that thumbs are present. (Courtesy of Dr. Jeffrey Lipton. Alter BP. The bone marrow failure syndromes. In: Nathan DG, Oski FA, eds. Hematology of infancy and childhood, ed 3. Philadelphia, WB Saunders, 1987:159)

had TAR,[807] whereas only one of a pair of fraternal twins was affected.[808] This finding is consistent with the cause being genetic rather acquired. Only two cases of TAR were reported with consanguinity,[809,810] suggesting that TAR patients may be double heterozygotes for genes with similar effects rather than true homozygotes. In most cases, parents of TAR patients are normal, and four normal offspring of affected mothers have been reported.[804,811] At least four families involved more than one generation (aunts or uncles and nephews or nieces, with one example of parent–child transmission), four others included cousins[804,811–817] and one family had two affected half-sibs,[818] suggesting that dominant (or perhaps pseudodominant) inheritance might be relevant in a few families. Although all ethnic groups are affected, including blacks,[233,817,819–821] reports of Asians are rare, but this may reflect a reporting rather than a genetic bias.[822]

All TAR patients have absent radii, with thumbs present (see Fig. 9-26). Most are affected bilaterally, with only three apparently bona fide cases in which the absent radius was unilateral and the hematologic picture was typical.[821,823,824] Short stature is common in both TAR and Fanconi's anemia patients, but those with Fanconi's anemia are often smaller. The other hand abnormalities in TAR are shortening of the middle phalanx of the fifth finger, clinodactyly, occasional finger syndactyly, and sometimes hypoplasia of the thumbs. Almost 50% of patients have additional abnormalities of the forearms, with absent ulnae in more than 15%, and 30% with ulnar shortening or bowing. About 30% have abnormal upper arms, with either short (15%) or absent (10%) humeri. Over 90% of the time the ulnar or humeral lesions are bilateral. Scapular hypoplasia and web necks in approximately 10% further account for abnormal upper body appearances, along with micrognathia and occasional brachycephaly or microcephaly. Hypertelorism, epicanthal folds, strabismus, and low-set ears are also seen. Facial hemangiomas occur in 10%.

The lower limbs are abnormal in 40%. Abnormalities include deformed, subluxed, or hypoplastic knees[825]; dislocated hips or patellae; and varus or valgus rotation at hips, knees, or feet. Short legs and absent tibiae or fibulae have been observed. Congenital heart disease (in 10%) includes atrial or ventricular septal defects, tetralogy of Fallot, dextrocardia, and ectopia cordis. Five patients had gonadal anomalies, such as undescended testes, hypoplasia, unicornuate uterus, and vaginal atresia. Low birthweight was observed at term in 15% of the babies.

TABLE 9-28. **Comparison of Thrombocytopenia With Absent Radii and Fanconi's Anemia**

Feature	TAR	FA
No. of reported cases	160	688
Age at diagnosis	0 y	8 y
Male/female	0.7:1	1.3:1
Inheritance	Recessive	Recessive
Low birthweight	8%	14%
Stature	Short	Short
Skeletal deformities		
Absent radii, thumbs present	100%	0%
Hand anomalies	49%	49%
Shoulders, neck	14%	7%
Lower limbs	39%	10%
Cardiac anomalies	9%	7%
Skin		
Hemangiomas	9%	0%
Pigmentation	0%	62%
Blood	Thrombocytopenia	Pancytopenia
Marrow	Absent megakaryocytes	Aplastic
Marrow colonies decreased	CFU-Mega	CFU-GM, CFU-E
Hb F	Normal	Increased
Chromosome breaks	Absent	Present
Malignancies	0%	20%
Reported deaths	24%	43%

A major distinction of TAR from Fanconi's anemia is that in Fanconi's anemia thumbs are absent when radii are normal. In additon, TAR involves only thrombocytopenia, whereas Fanconi's anemia eventually develops panycytopenia. There are four reports of trisomy 18 with absent or hypoplastic radii, thrombocytopenia, or both,[826–829] but they are distinguished by other characteristic anomalies as well as the cytogenetic abnormality. Roberts' syndrome and SC phocomelia may have a similar phenotype.[830,831] Other syndromes with radial anomalies are beyond the scope of this analysis.

Close to 20% of patients were reported to have bloody diarrhea in infancy, which was ascribed specifically to allergy to cow's milk.[804,824] Removal of milk from the diet alleviates that symptom and may perhaps lead to improvement of the thrombocytopenia.

Laboratory Findings

Platelet counts are less than 50,000/μL at the time of diagnosis in almost 90% of patients. Anemia is probably secondary to bleeding, and reticulocytosis is usually associated. Leukocytosis is a common finding, with white blood counts higher than 15,000/μL in more than 75% of those reported, over 20,000 in two thirds, and over 40,000 in one third of infants (Fig. 9-27). Levels of 100,000 to 133,000/μL were reported in at least four patients. More than 12 patients had immature myeloid precursors in the circulation, but none had true leukoerythroblastosis. This leukemoid reaction has been mistaken for congenital leukemia, but it is in fact transient and usually subsides during infancy. Splenomegaly may occur due to extramedullary hematopoiesis, and eosinophilia is not uncommon. Bone marrow examinations show normal cellularity and normal or increased myeloid and erythroid cell lines, with absence of megakaryocytes in most, and decreased, hypoplastic, or immature megakaryocytes in the rest.

Laboratory tests with normal results include MCV, Hb F, and studies of chromosome breakage, both spontaneous and with clastogenic stress, distinguishing TAR from Fanconi's anemia. Karyotypic analysis also distinguishes TAR from trisomy 18. Hypogammaglobulinemia was reported in one group of patients from Nigeria but has not been a general problem.[821] Platelet size is normal except in one report[832] and platelet function is generally normal,[833–835] although abnormalities of platelet aggregation and storage pool defects were reported.[832,836,837] Clinical symptoms are likely related to be due to quantitative rather than qualitative defects.

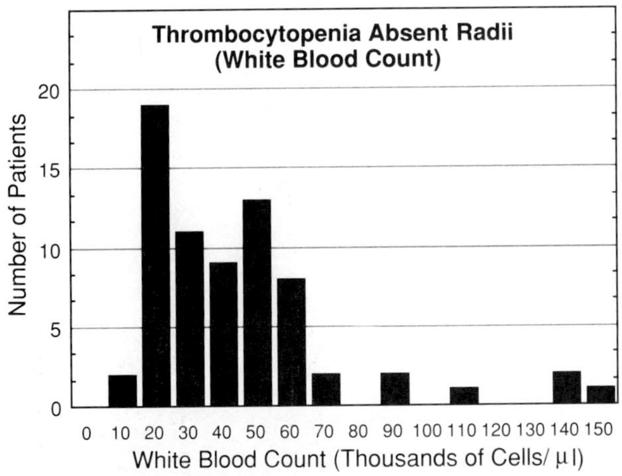

FIGURE 9-27. White blood cell counts in infants with thrombocytopenia with absent radii syndrome.

Pathophysiology

The inheritance pattern is most likely autosomal recessive, for a single or for more than one genetic defect, with a recurrence risk of one in four. TAR is one of several inherited hematologic conditions associated with radial ray anomalies (the others are Fanconi's anemia and DBA). In the case of TAR, only the platelet lineage is significantly affected. Cultures of hematopoietic progenitor cells indicate that the myeloid and erythroid lineages are normal.[233,838–841] Although some studies found no growth of megakaryocytic progenitors,[839–842] others found essentially normal numbers[843] (Hoffman R, personal communication). A unique megakaryocyte colony-stimulating factor was increased in the plasma of one patient.[842] Because TAR is a true single cytopenia, without evolution to aplastic anemia or leukemia, the defect presumably involves only the megakaryocytic lineage.

Therapy and Outcome

Most infants with TAR have hemorrhagic manifestations, which they may outgrow after the first year. Close to 40 deaths were reported (25%), 29 in the first year, 9 in the second, and 1 at 44 months. The projected survival curve is shown in Figure 9-28 and has a plateau of 70% survival at 44 months. Most deaths were from intracranial or gastrointestinal bleeding. The data cited here encompass 40 years of reports of TAR cases, most of whom received limited treatment. Those who survive the perilous first year demonstrate an increase in platelet count to above 100,000/μL, adequate for the orthopedic surgical procedures needed for their arms and legs. Thrombocytopenia may recur during illnesses, but it usually is not severe. Dietary change may be helpful for those with milk allergy.

The most important therapy is platelet transfusions. These are provided during bleeding episodes or operations and are clearly indicated as prophylaxis for infants with severe symptomatic thrombocytopenia. Single donors should be used to reduce the risk of sensitization, and HLA-matched platelets can be obtained, if necessary. The platelet count should be maintained at over 10,000 to 15,000/μL. The prediction is that the duration of this support is finite and short (less than 1 year). Other approaches have included splenectomy, corticosteroids, and androgens, all without apparent benefit. One adult showed a transient elevation of the platelet count after splenectomy.[833] A small dose of prednisone might decrease the bleeding tendency at a given platelet count, and ε-aminocaproic acid may also be useful during bleeding episodes (see section on treatment of Fanconi's anemia for details).

The leukemoid reaction and eosinophilia disappear during the first year in patients with TAR, and aplastic anemia and leukemia have not been reported, although the high white count has led to some infants being diagnosed with *congenital leukemia*. Heroic treatments such as myelotoxic drugs or bone marrow transplantation are generally contraindicated, since spontaneous improvement occurs. One patient who had a life-threatening central nervous system hemorrhage was treated successfully by bone marrow transplantation.[844] In general, this approach is excessive, and the prognosis for TAR patients is good.

Prenatal diagnosis has been reported in more than 12 cases. Absent radii may be diagnosed using radiography[845,846] or ultrasonography.[496,810,811,847–851] Because a few patients were reported with unilateral radial aplasia, both forearms must be examined. In one case, micrognathia was detected by ultrasonography.[810] The diagnosis can then be confirmed by a platelet count in fetal blood obtained by fetoscopy or cordocentesis.[496,849,851] Nine of the 16 fetuses studied so far were affected.

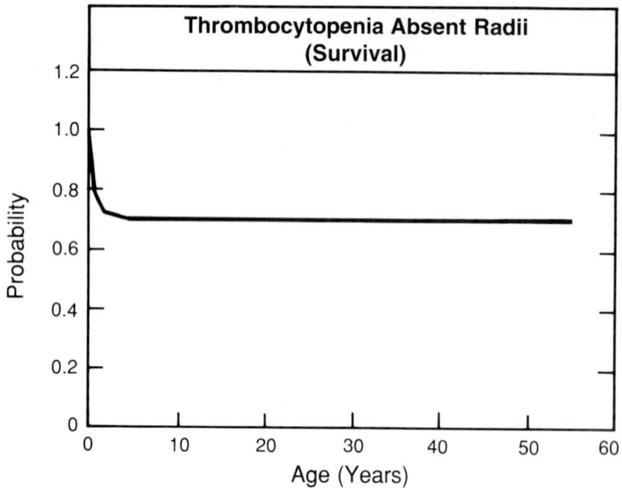

FIGURE 9-28. Kaplan-Meier plot of cumulative survival in thrombocytopenia with absent radii syndrome. The plateau is above 70%, with no deaths reported beyond age 4 years.

LEUKOERYTHROBLASTOSIS

Leukoerythroblastosis is the term suggested by Vaughan[852] in 1936 to describe "an anemia charaterised by the presence in the peripheral blood of immature red cells and a few immature white cells of the myeloid series" (p 541), that is, erythroblasts and leukoblasts. The RBCs are usually normochromic and normocytic, with poikilocytes, fragments, target cells, and teardrops. Giant platelets may also be seen. Leukoerythroblastosis must be distinguished from a *leukemoid reaction*, which is a reactive leukocytosis with an orderly progression of immature through mature myeloid cells. Another related term, *leukemic hiatus*, applies when the myeloid cells are immature and mature but without intermediate forms; thus, there is a gap or hiatus.

The disorders in which leukoerythroblastosis has been seen are outlined in Table 9-29, a composite of several large adult and pediatric series.[853,854] The initial descriptions focused on the association with bone marrow invasion, particularly from metastatic solid tumors, hematologic malignancies, infections, or other marrow components, in which cells might be crowded out of the marrow prematurely (myelophthisis). Hypoxia from nonhematologic or hematologic causes might also stimulate premature release. In myeloproliferative disorders, the premature release of nucleated cells might be related to the intrinsic abnormality of the cells.

Diseases in which leukoerythroblastosis occurs are discussed in many other chapters in this book; this section is restricted to osteopetrosis.

Osteopetrosis

Osteopetrosis, marble bone disease, or Albers-Schönberg disease, was first described in 1904.[855] It is seen in a benign autosomal dominant and a malignant autosomal recessive form.[856] The latter, which is diagnosed in infancy and early childhood, is characterized by dense bones that fracture easily because of a defect in bone resorption. The patients have large heads, sclerotic bones, and hepatosplenomegaly; they experience blindness, deafness, cranial nerve palsies, and pancytopenia. Many cases are familial, with a high degree of consanguinity. The disease may be severe in utero, since there is often a history of stillbirths and spontaneous abortions.

Laboratory Findings

The hematologic complications of osteopetrosis are severe, with macrocytic anemia, reticulocytosis, teardrop RBCs, circulating erythroblasts, and leukocytosis with immature myeloid elements, all components of leukoerythroblastosis. One manifestation of the stress erythropoiesis that occurs is an increase in Hb F.[857] The marrow cavity is gradually narrowed by bone, and the diploic spaces are small. Bone marrow aspiration is difficult, and needles often break in attempts to penetrate the sclerotic bone. The marrow that remains is hypocellular and fibrotic. Osteoblasts as well as osteoclasts are increased.[858] Hepatosplenomegaly develops because of extramedullary hematopoiesis. Hypersplenism ensues, leading to thrombocytopenia, leukopenia, and hemolytic anemia due to extracorpuscular destruction of intrinsically normal erythrocytes.[859]

Pathophysiology

The osteoclasts are apparently abnormal in osteopetrosis, unable to resorb bone and produce the remodeling that

TABLE 9-29. Conditions Associated With Leukoerythroblastosis

MARROW INVASION
Tumor
Solid tumor with bone marrow metastases
Lymphoma
Hodgkin's disease
Multiple myeloma
Leukemia
Neuroblastoma
Preleukemia
Infection
Osteomyelitis
Sepsis
Tuberculosis
Congenital
Marrow Components
Osteopetrosis
Storage disease
Histiocytosis
Vasculitis, including rheumatoid arthritis
MYELOPROLIFERATIVE DISORDERS
Polycythemia vera
Myelofibrosis, myeloid metaplasia
Down's syndrome, transient myeloproliferative disease
Chronic myelogenous leukemia
Erythroleukemia
Thrombocythemia
HEMATOLOGIC DISEASE
Erythroblastosis fetalis
Pernicious anemia
Thalassemia major
Other hemolytic anemias
HYPOXIA
Cyanotic congenital heart disease
Congestive heart failure
Respiratory disease

occurs in normal bone. In experiments using osteopetrotic mice, Walker[860,861] showed that bone marrow or spleen cells from normal mice led to bone remodeling in osteopetrotic litter mates, and spleen cells from affected mice led to osteopetrosis in normal mice. Marrow transplantations that cured osteopetrosis and contained a cytoplasmic marker (giant lysosomes in Chediak-Higashi mice) replaced recipient with donor osteoclasts.[861] Similar studies using donors with defective erythropoiesis (W^e/W^v) indicated that the stem cell that gives rise to osteoclasts may be more primordial than the CFU-S.[862] Although osteopetrosis was cured and donor leukocytes and platelets were sustained, the defective donor erythrocytosis was replaced by the normal erythropoiesis of the recipient. Several laboratories have used in vitro studies to suggest that osteoclasts are derived from hematopoietic stem cells that are in the mononuclear light density fraction.[863]

Hematopoiesis is intrinsically normal in osteopetrosis. The peripheral blood contains increased numbers of CFU-GM, BFU-E, and even CFU-E (normally found only in marrow), which may migrate from the crowded bone marrow cavity to sites of extramedullary hematopoiesis.[864,865] Osteoclasts are numerically normal, morphologically normal or abnormal, and functionally abnormal.

Therapy and Outcome

Death usually occurs in infancy or early childhood in osteopetrosis patients; no patients have survived beyond 20 years of age. Most deaths are from the complications of bone marrow failure, infection, and hemorrhage. Circulating phagocytes, which may be derived from the same lineage as the osteoclasts, may function abnormally, leading to reduced host resistance to infection.[866,867]

Symptomatic anemia and thrombocytopenia can be treated with transfusions of RBCs and platelets, although hypersplenism decreases the efficacy of such treatment. Splenectomy offers temporary improvement, but the rest of the reticuloendothelial system remains active and the primary bone disorder is not cured. Prednisone therapy was used in several patients, again with transient improvement, from decreased hypersplenism and reticuloendothelial suppression.[866,868]

The only possible cure for osteopetrosis at this time is offered by bone marrow transplantation, which has been reported in more than 12 patients.[797,869–873] In those situations in which a sex marker was found, the osteoclasts were of donor origin, whereas the osteoblasts remained host. Short-term follow-up indicated restoration of normal hematopoiesis, improvement of radiographic findings, and stabilization of physical changes.

Prenatal diagnosis by radiography was first performed in 1943,[874] although it was not always successful.[875] More recently, increased bone density, fractures, macrocephaly, and hydrocephaly were detected by ultrasonography and confirmed by radiography.[876]

PRELEUKEMIA

Most bone marrow failure disorders (both acquired and inherited) are associated with the subsequent appearance of leukemia in at least a few patients[877] (Table 9-30). Several examples were discussed already, and many are presented elsewhere in this book. In this section, we discuss a few of the conditions in which pancytopenia is followed by leukemia, as well as specific genetic syndromes that may superficially resemble Fanconi's anemia and in which leukemia may occur.

TABLE 9-30. Preleukemic Bone Marrow Disorders

ACQUIRED	INHERITED
Aplastic anemia	Fanconi's anemia
Irradiation	Shwachman-Diamond syndrome
Drugs	Kostmann's agranulocytosis
Toxins	Diamond-Blackfan anemia
Pure red cell aplasia	Amegakaryocytic thrombocytopenia
Thrombocytopenia	Familial marrow failure
Neutropenia	Familial myeloproliferative disease
Paroxysmal nocturnal hemoglobinuria	Trisomy 21
Refractory sideroblastic anemia	Bloom's syndrome
Preacute lymphocytic leukemia	Ataxia telangiectasia
Myelodysplastic syndromes	Poland's syndrome
Myeloproliferative disorders	

Bloom's Syndrome

Bloom's syndrome is a chromosome breakage syndrome, which may resemble Fanconi's anemia at the physical and cytogenetic levels and is associated with the development of leukemia and other malignancies. The Bloom's Syndrome Registry is maintained by Dr. James German; the most recent update was published in 1989.[878] Bloom's syndrome is inherited as an autosomal recessive trait, has a male/female ratio of 1.5:1 in the 130 cases, and is found predominantly in Ashkenazi Jews, although it has been reported in all ethnic groups. Homozygotes are born at term, but are substantially below normal weight and length. They feed poorly and grow slowly, developing into short delicate persons with fine-featured bird-like faces, and small heads. The diagnostic triad, which may not be apparent in infancy, includes stunted growth, telangiectatic facial erythema, and sun sensitivity. Café-au-lait spots are common. Additional physical findings are hypertrichosis, toe syndactyly, absent toes, supernumerary digits, clinodactyly, prominent ears, hypospadias, and cryptorchidism. Some of the physical findings are reminiscent of those seen in Fanconi's anemia.

Mild anemia has been reported occasionally, and one patient had macrocytosis, dyserythropoietic features, 6% multinucleated erythroblasts, and an elevated Hb F.[879] Several patients had low immunoglobulin levels. Chromosomes are abnormal, with breaks, rearrangements, and quadriradii. The specific diagnostic test is an elevation of sister chromatid exchange,[204] which is not increased in Fanconi's anemia. There is apparently a single complementation group, even among diverse ethnic origins.[880]

Long-term follow-up has identified 44 patients at a mean age of 25 years with a total of 57 cancers: 14 leukemias, both lymphocytic and myelocytic; 5 lymphomas; 1 reticulum cell sarcoma; 2 Hodgkin's disease; 2 breast; 3 tongue; 3 cervical; and 2 esophageal cancers. Other tumors were basal cell, skin, colon, larynx, osteogenic sarcoma, rectum, eyelid, sigmoid, Wilms' tumor, meningioma, and an unknown primary cancer metastatic to liver. Aplastic anemia has not been reported. The mortality rate is 34 of 130, or 26%.

Prenatal diagnosis should be possible for Bloom's syndrome by detection of chromosomal breaks and increased SCEs in amniocytes or chorionic villi. In those monitored to date, only normal results and infants were found.[363]

Ataxia-Telangiectasia

The third of the chromosome breakage syndromes associated with hematologic malignancy is ataxia-telangiectasia (Fanconi's anemia and Bloom's syndrome are more common). Ataxia-telangiectasia is inherited as a autosomal recessive trait and is manifest in childhood by progressive cerebellar ataxia, along with telangiectases and multiple infections.[881,882] T cells, particularly helper T cells, are decreased, as are levels of IgA. Chromosome breaks are seen in T cells and fibroblasts but not in B cells, and the cells that show breakage are also sensitive to γ-radiation. Breakpoints in ataxia-telangiectasia are nonrandom and involve rearrangements of chromosome 14 and others in the areas of genes of the immune system. Several complementation groups are seen in ataxia-telangiectasia; the gene for one has been localized to 11q22-23.[883]

Nearly 300 US patients with ataxia-telangiectasia were summarized by Morrell and coworkers[884] in 1986. Over 50% had died by the time of their report. Approximately 20% had cancer, with lymphoma in 60% of those and lymphocytic leukemia in 27%. Other tumors included epithelial carcinomas, such as stomach, brain, ovary, skin, liver, larynx, parotid, breast, and uterus. The median age at death was less than 19 years.

Poland's Syndrome

Poland's syndrome consists of the absence of one pectoralis major muscle (75% on the right), syndactyly or brachydactyly of the ipsilateral hand, and hypoplasia of the ipsilateral arm. More than 150 cases have been reported, with a male/female ratio of 3:1. The condition is thought to be sporadic and perhaps not genetic, with an incidence of 1 in 32,000.[885,886] Absence of the pectoralis major muscle alone occurs much more frequently. Eleven patients were reported with Poland's syndrome who had leukemia (seven acute lymphocytic, two acute myeloblastic) and three with lymphoma, although five of these only had absence of a pectoralis major muscle. The ages were between 3 and 15 years, except for one who was 25 and one who was 28 years old. The association of malignancy with Poland's syndrome may not be more than that due to chance alone.[887]

Aplastic Anemia Preceding Acute Leukemia in Adults

The term *preleukemia* usually refers to patients with refractory anemia and myelodysplasia, more than half of whom go on to develop leukemia. This specific disorder is discussed briefly in the text that follows and in depth in Chapter 12. A small number of both children and adults who eventually develop leukemia appear to have aplastic anemia without myelodysplastic features. In several series of adults with aplastic anemia, 5% to 10% developed leukemia—usually acute nonlymphocytic.[888–899] From the perspective of leukemia, 1% to 2% of those ultimately diagnosed as leukemia began with a hypoplastic phase.[898]

The initial diagnosis is classic aplastic anemia, with pancytopenia and hypocellular marrow. In approximately 50 adult cases (Table 9-31), the male/female ratio was 1.5:1. The age at the first hematologic diagnosis was slightly younger than seen in those with aplastic anemia in general (Fig. 9-29). The interval between aplasia and leukemia was an average of 3 years.

Laboratory Findings

Patients with aplastic anemia usually have pancytopenia, although they may present with a single cytopenia such as thrombocytopenia. Bone marrow examinations demonstrate decreased cellularity, usually of all lineages. Neither dysmyelopoiesis nor fibrosis are featured, and increased proportions of blasts are not seen until later when leukemia is diagnosed. The few reports of bone marrow chromosomes include monosomy 7 in three patients, deletion of Y in one, 21+ in one, and one with C+, G+ clones.

Pathophysiology

Half the adults with aplastic anemia had been exposed to a potential marrow toxin, including seven who had taken chloramphenicol; five, phenylbutazone; and one each, benzene, cyclophosphamide, sulfonamides, chloroquine, chlorthalidone, antibiotics, herbicides, and cobalt-60. Most of these agents appear on lists of drugs that may cause aplastic anemia or leukemia; in these patients, they caused both. Dameshek[900] many years ago suggested that aplasia and leukemia may have a common etiology.

Leukemia may begin with a pancytopenic phase, and the proportion of blasts in the marrow may be low or unevenly represented (hence, not seen on a random aspirate); thus, some of the patients may have had leukemia from the onset of symptoms. In 50% of the patients, there was more than a 1-year interval until leukemia could be diagnosed; in 20%, the gap was 5 years or more. Therefore,

TABLE 9-31. Comparison of the Cytopenic Preleukemias

	Hypoplastic		Myelodysplastic Children			
Feature	**Adults**	**Children**	**Total**	**Chromosomal 7/C**	**Other**	**Normal**
No. of cases	54	70	120	59	22	39
Male/female	1.5:1	0.9:1	1.9:1	2.3:1	2.1:1	1.3:1
Age at diagnosis (y)						
Mean	53	6.3	6.6	5.3	9.1	7.1
Median	58	5	5	3	11	5
Range	19–75	0.5–19	0.3–19	0.3–19	1.3–16	0.4–18
Interval to leukemia (y)						
Mean	3.3	0.75	1.7	1.9	1.8	1.3
Median	1.1	0.33	1	1.9	2.2	0.8
Range	0.1–23	0.04–6	0–14	0–14	0–4	0–8
Reported dead	76%	49%	71%	81%	68%	56%
Projected 50% survival (y)	2	4	3	2	3	3
5-year survival	39%	39%	22%	18%	13%	37%

Chromosomal 7/C, clonality involving 7 or a C chromosome; other, other clonal cytogenetic abnormality; normal, normal chromosomes or not reported.

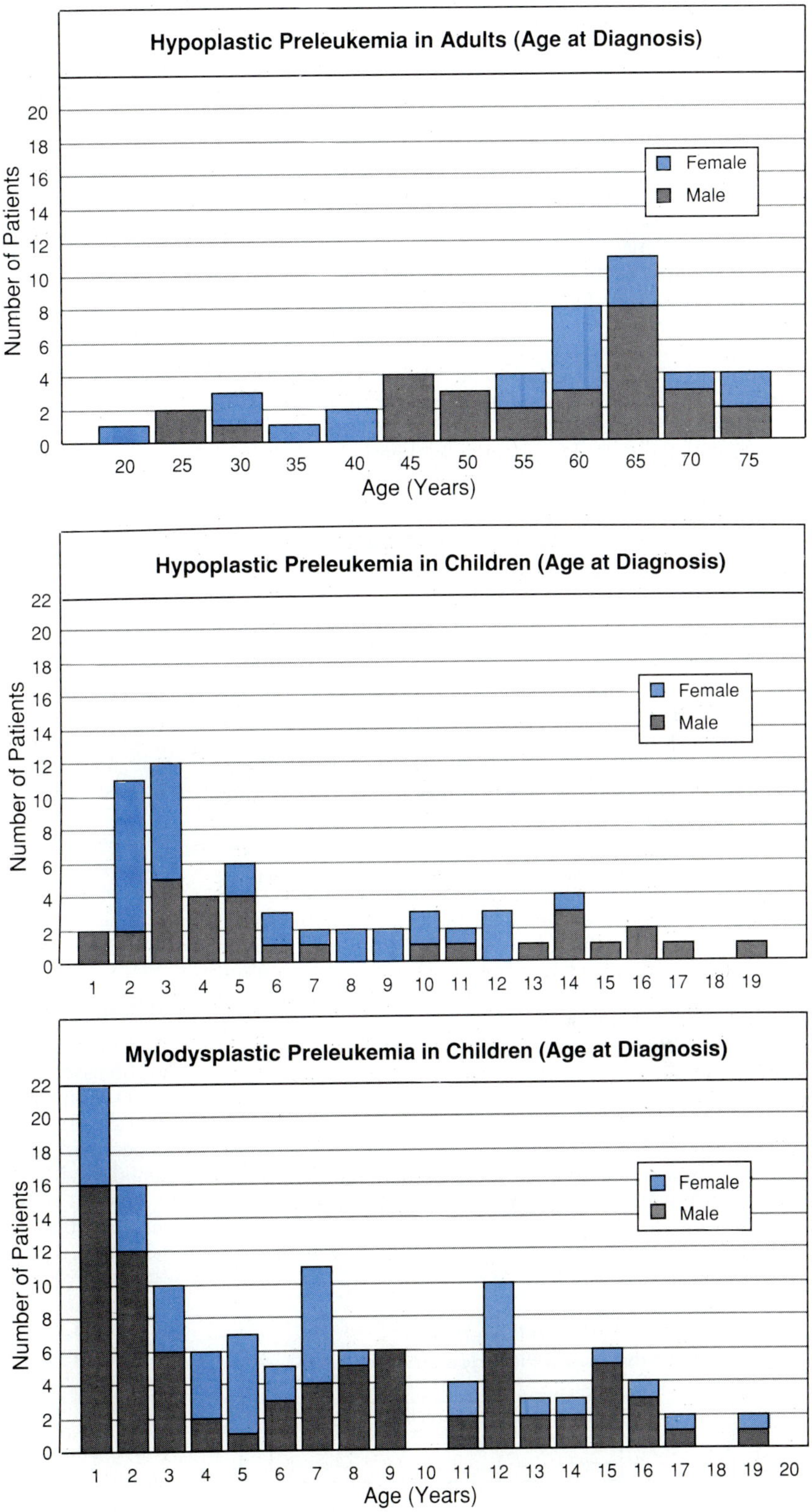

FIGURE 9-29. Age at diagnosis of first hematologic problem in cases with cytopenias followed by leukemia.

some patients may have leukemia as the outcome of the stem cell aberration that led to aplastic anemia initially. The first step in malignant transformation of the stem cell could have led to hypoproliferation, whereas further evolution of changes then resulted in hyperproliferation. This is consistent with the observation that most of the leukemias were myeloid, which is thought to be from a clonal stem cell.

Therapy and Outcome

More than half of the reports precede 1980, and the aplastic anemia was treated by the conventional approaches of the time. Half received corticosteroids plus androgens, with only one third of these responding. Antithymocyte globulin was used in five patients, without good responses, but with survival. In general, pancytopenia appeared to improve in many of the patients only to present later with leukemia. Most patients also received supportive care such as transfusions.

The leukemias were diagnosed at 0.1 to 23 years later. Four patients had acute lymphoblastic leukemia, 32 had acute nonlymphocytic leukemia, 3 had erythroleukemia, 7 had hairy-cell leukemia, 1 had chronic myelogenous leukemia, and the rest evolved into preleukemic myelodysplasia followed by leukemia. These types of leukemia are in the proportions expected in adults.

Seventy-six percent of the patients had died at the time of the reports at an average of 4.6 years (range, 0 to 24; median, 2 years) from the initial hematologic sign. The analysis of projected survivals is shown in Figure 9-30; the median survival is predicted to be 2 years and the 5-year survival 39%. In most cases, the interval from leukemia to death was short, reflecting the difficulties in successful treatment of acute nonlymphocytic leukemia in adults (see Chap. 18).

Aplastic Anemia Preceding Acute Leukemia in Children

As described for adults, approximately 5% of children with aplastic anemia (hypoplastic anemia) progress to leukemia, and 2% of those with acute lymphoblastic leukemia began with a hypoplastic phase.[1,901–905] The largest series was that of Bernard and Schaison,[903] in which 13 of 200 children with aplastic anemia and 2000 with ALL showed this transition. Approximately 70 cases were reported in detail (see Table 9-31). The male/female ratio is 0.9:1. The average age at diagnosis of aplastic anemia was 6.3 years, with a median of 5 and range of 6 months to 19 years. These patients are slightly younger than all children with acquired aplastic anemia. In particular, a peak occurs at ages 2 and 3, similar to the age at diagnosis of children with classic ALL. In contrast to the adults with aplastic anemia who develop leukemia (discussed previously), the children develop leukemia more quickly, with an average interval of 9 months, but a median of only 4 months. The range is 2 weeks to 6 years, but only 15% of patients had an interval of more than 1 year.

Laboratory Findings

Most children with aplastic anemia had pancytopenia. Three had pure red cell aplasia,[903,906,907] one had neutropenia,[908] and four had bicytopenias.[903] Bone marrow was hypocellular. Unlike classic acquired aplastic anemia, megakaryocytes were normal in 15% of cases. Bone marrow karyotypes were normal when examined.

Shackelford and colleagues[907] pointed out that radiographic studies might contribute to the distinction of aplastic anemia and leukemia. Patients with leukemia may have generalized bony rarefaction, transverse metaphyseal radiolucent lines at the ends of the long bones, osteolytic lesions, subperiosteal new bone formation, or osteosclerosis. Rheumatoid arthritis, another great pretender among the pancytopenias, may also have distinctive radiologic findings.

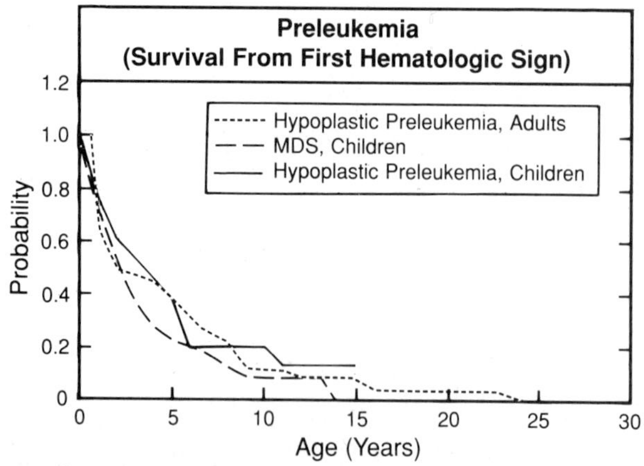

FIGURE 9-30. Kaplan-Meier plot of cumulative survival in preleukemias. Time is shown as years from the first hematologic problem (aplastic anemia or myelodysplasia).

Pathophysiology

In hypoplastic preleukemia, the leukemia may have been present at the outset, but not detected in the randomly sampled bone marrow aspirate. At the least, biopsies would provide a better assessment of overall cellularity. Because bone marrow from young children, as well as from patients with aplastic anemia, may have increased proportions of lymphocytes, lymphoblasts may have been overlooked. Because patients with ALL often respond initially to corticosteroid treatment, the rapid apparent recoveries from aplastic anemia may really have been early remissions in ALL. All of these possibilities are consistent with the short interval from the hypoplastic phase to frank leukemia in children.

The explanations just provided in the section on adult aplastic anemia–leukemia may apply to children as well. Exposure to drugs or toxins that might cause aplasia or leukemia was less common in children. Four children had received chloramphenicol; one had paroxysmal nocturnal hemoglobinuria, and one had hepatitis. In general, the pediatric and adult conditions differ in the interval to leukemia and the type of leukemia and may also differ in their pathophysiology.

Therapy and Outcome

As in the cases of adult hypoplastic leukemia, almost half of the cases were studied before 1980. Treatment consisted of transfusions as needed, as well as the administration of corticosteroids to half of the patients (combined with androgens in 10 cases). Remissions were frequent and rapid, usually within 1 month. Leukemia was then diagnosed by a median of 4 months, much more quickly than in the adults. Almost 80% of patients were diagnosed with ALL—55 with ALL, 10 with acute myeloblastic leukemia, and the rest with myelodysplasia or lymphoma. Perhaps because ALL has a better prognosis than acute myeloblastic leukemia, only 50% of the children were reported to have died, compared with 75% of the adults. The average age reported at death was 9 years—2 years after the diagnosis of leukemia—and the projected median survival is 4 years from the first hematologic problem (see Fig. 9-30). The 5-year survival rate is predicted to be 39%. The survival curve continues down; thus, the only possibility of a cure might be through bone marrow transplantation during leukemic remission.

Myelodysplastic Preleukemia

More than 100 pediatric patients have been studied who resembled adults with preleukemia,[877] and the pediatric perspective has been summarized several times.[909–912] The working definition for myelodysplastic preleukemia is peripheral blood cytopenias with usually hypercellular bone marrow, that is, ineffective hematopoiesis. The literature regarding adult patients uses the terms *myelodysplasia* and *refractory anemia*, and the evolution of that syndrome was classified in 1982 by Bennett[913] for the French-American-British (Fanconi's anemia B) Co-Operative Group. A detailed discussion is provided in Chapter 12. Briefly, the classification is the following:

- Refractory anemia (RA), anemia and reticulocytopenia, with normal or hypercellular marrow, erythroid hyperplasia, or dyserythropoiesis, and less than 5% blast cells
- Refractory anemia with ringed sideroblasts (RARS) constituting more than 15%
- Refractory anemia with excess blasts (RAEB), hypercellular marrow with dysgranulopoiesis, dyserythropoiesis, or dysmegakaryocytopoiesis, plus 5% to 20% marrow blasts and below 5% circulating blasts
- Chronic myelomonocytic leukemia, absolute monocytosis, increased marrow monocytes, less than 5% circulating blasts
- Refractory anemia in transformation (RAEBIT), with more than 5% blasts in the blood, 20% to 30% blasts in marrow, Auer rods, and not yet fitting any of the acute myeloblastic leukemia types M1 to M6 (see Chap. 18 for details)

The abbreviation for myelodysplastic syndromes, MDS, is often used generically and is used in this section as well. The incidence of MDS resulting in acute nonlymphocytic leukemia in children was estimated as 17%, within the 5% to 20% range in adult series.[910,914] The hypercellularity of the marrow, along with dysmyelopoietic changes, serves to differentiate the myelodysplastic preleukemia patients from the hypoplastic preleukemia patients discussed in the previous section. More than 100 cases have been cited in the literature (see Table 9-31). Of these, half had clonal abnormalities involving chromosome 7, usually described as a C-deletion, or monosomy 7. Because this may be a distinct syndrome, with some resemblance to chronic myelogenous leukemia, it is analyzed separately in Table 9-31.[915-917] Those with other clonal abnormalities and those with normal chromosomes are also summarized separately.

The age at diagnosis of MDS is shown in Figure 9-29. A larger proportion was symptomatic within the first year, compared with the hypoplastic preleukemic patients. The mean, median, and ranges were similar in the two groups. Within the MDS patients, those with monosomy 7 presented at a younger age than the others (means of 5.3 for monosomy 7, 9.1 for other clones, and 7.1 years for normal chromosomes). Unlike in the hypoplastic preleukemic group, there were several cases of familial MDS: nine siblings or cousins reported by Randall and coworkers,[918] four sets of siblings reported by Smith and coworkers,[919] Luddy and colleagues,[920] Carroll and coworkers,[921] and Paul and colleagues,[922] one set of monozygotic twins,[923] and a case with parental consanguinity.[924] In the entire group with MDS, the male/female ratio is 1.9:1, the ratio being highest among those with a clonal abnormality and lowest among those with normal chromosomes. Thus, there is a male preponderance in the MDS group, unlike in the hypoplastic preleukemic group.

Diagnosis of MDS is based on symptoms of cytopenias, combined with a cellular bone marrow. Many patients have hepatosplenomegaly with some extramedullary hematopoiesis. In the cases summarized here, all did not develop frank leukemia, but those who resembled those who did were included.

Laboratory Findings

The peripheral blood findings in MDS patients range from single to bicytopenias to pancytopenias. Signs of leukoerythroblastosis are seen, with a few nucleated RBCs, and left-shifted myeloid cells. Stress erythropoiesis is present in MDS patients, manifested by increased levels of Hb F, i antigen, and fetal RBC enzyme patterns.[925,926] Bone marrow shows varying degrees of the manifestations outlined above for the various types of MDS, but it is basically hypercellular and dyshematopoietic. Bone marrow chromosomes were abnormal in 70% of MDS patients. Deletion or abnormality of a C chromosome, shown later to be 7, was reported in 50% of cases. The other clonal abnormalities included six cases with +8, four with abnormalities of 21, and 12 with a variety of other deletions, inversions, or markers. Two families discussed earlier in this chapter with familial aplastic anemia or leukemia as well as other anomalies (cerebellar atrophy or immunologic abnormalities) had monosomy 7[505,511]). Chromosomes were not described in most of the familial cases of MDS, but monosomy 7 was seen in two families.[921,927]

Pathophysiology

Adult preleukemia is a clonal hemopathy, according to glucose-6-phosphate dehydrogenase isoenzymes.[928] Similar studies have not been done in children. When clonal cytogenetic abnormalities are present in the preleukemic phase, they persist in the leukemia, indicating a direct evolution. Hogge and coworkers[916] showed that the same clonal abnormality was present in myeloid and erythroid progenitors. Hematopoiesis is ineffective in vivo, and in vitro assays show decreased CFU-GM as well as blood and marrow BFU-E.[929,930] Thus, presumably a single stem cell mutation occurs, leading to myelodysplasia and evolving into leukemia. There is a familial propensity to MDS in some families, leading to a predicted recurrence risk of 25%.

Therapy and Outcome

The interval from the onset of cytopenias to frank leukemia was longer in children with MDS–leukemia than those with hypoplastic preleukemia (see Table 9-31). The mean was 1.7 years, the median 1 year, and the range 0 to 14 years. Those without clonality may have evolved faster (or their MDS was not diagnosed as early because of the lack of a chromosomal marker). No remissions of MDS occurred. The diagnoses included 1 ALL, 30 acute myeloblastic leukemia, 10 myelomonocytic or monocytic leukemia, 9 acute nonlymphocytic leukemia not further described, 6 chronic myelomonocytic leukemia, 3 erythroleukemia, 1 juvenile chronic myelogenous leukemia, 7 RAEB, and 23 RAEBIT. About 10% had not evolved further when reported, but follow-up may not have been long enough. Over 70% had died when they were reported, at an average of 8.7 years, or 1 year after progression to leukemia. The projected median survival (see Fig. 9-30) is 3 years; the 5-year survival rate would be 22%.

Treatment for childhood myelodysplasia is less than satisfactory, and basically involves supportive transfusions. Splenectomy was performed in 14 patients, with claims to its efficacy in raising blood counts, although usually temporarily. Steroids were used in 14 cases, with improvement in five (35%), perhaps as a result of chemical shrinkage of the reticuloendothelial system. Cytoreductive agents such as 6-mercaptopurine or cytosine arabinoside have been tried without success.[931] Experimental protocols such as those used in adults involving low-dose cytosine arabinoside or 5-azacytidine have not been used in children.

Because of the high risk of leukemia in MDS, bone marrow transplantation is proposed as the treatment of choice for those patients who have a donor. In a series of eight

TABLE 9-32. Inherited Bone Marrow Failure Syndromes

Feature	Fanconi's Anemia	Dyskeratosis Congenita	Shwachman-Diamond Syndrome	Amegakaryocytic Thrombocytopenia	Diamond-Blackfan Anemia	Kostmann's Syndrome	Thrombocytopenia–Absent Radius
No. of cases	700	150	175	36	400	120	160
Male/female	1.3:1	4.7:1	1.8:1	2.6:1	1.1:1	0.8:1	0.7:1
Genetics	Autosomal recessive	X-linked, autosomal recessive, dominant	Autosomal recessive	X-linked or autosomal recessive	Autosomal recessive, dominant, or sporadic	Autosomal recessive	Autosomal recessive
Physical abnormalities	50%–75%	100%	40%	40%	30%	0%	100%
Hand/arm anomalies	50%	15%	<2%	0%	10%	0%	100%
Median age at diagnosis, initial hematologic disease	8 y	16 y	<1 y	<1 wk	2 mo	1 mo	<1 wk
First hematologic manifestation	Pancytopenia	Pancytopenia	Neutropenia	Thrombocytopenia	Anemia	Neutropenia	Thrombocytopenia
Bone marrow	Aplastic	Aplastic	Hypocellular or myeloid arrest	Absent or small megakaryocytes	Erythroid hypoplasia	Myeloid hypoplasia	Megakaryocytes absent or immature
Aplastic anemia	>90%	50%	20%	45%	0%	0%	0%
Leukemia	9%	0%	5%	6%	1%	2%	0%
Liver disease	4%	0%	0%	0%	0.3%	0%	0%
Cancer	5%	7%	0%	0%	0%	0%	0%
Hb F	Increased	Increased	Increased	Increased	Increased	Normal	Normal
Chromosomes	Breaks increased with clastogens	Normal	Normal	Normal	Normal	Normal	Normal
Spontaneous remissions	Very rare	None	Very rare	None	15%	0%	70%
Treatment, responses	Androgens, 50%, transient	Androgens, 50%, transient	Steroids or androgens, 50%, transient	None	Steroids, 60%	G-CSF, excellent	Platelets, needed < 1 y
Prognosis	Poor	Poor	Fair	Poor	Good	Poor	Good
Prenatal diagnosis	Chromosomes	Xq28 RFLP	Neutropenia	Thrombocytopenia	?Anemia, ADA ?BFU-E	Neutropenia	Absent radii, thrombocytopenia
Long-term survival after hematologic disease	<10%	<30%	40%	0%	40%	<20%	70%
Median survival age	16 y	32 y	35 y	4 y	30 y	3 y	>50 y

patients, four are long-term cures.[932] This may be the only cure for this otherwise fatal condition. Trials of recombinant human growth factors are currently in progress in adults with MDS but not yet in children. Both GM-CSF and G-CSF may lead to dose-dependent increases in neutrophils in almost all patients, but changes in platelet counts and transfusion requirements are the exception rather than the rule, and the proportion of blasts may increase in some patients.[933,934] There is some concern that use of these factors may accelerate the transformation to leukemia.

SUMMARY

The major inherited bone marrow failure disorders are summarized in Table 9-32. The diagnosis of acquired aplastic anemia should be made only after serious consideration of these conditions. Physical anomalies may be absent, but family histories or specific tests (chromosome breakage) may provide clues. The number of patients with each condition and the proportions with the cited complications *cannot* be construed as prevalence figures, since they are based on literature reports, not epidemiologic studies. Despite underreporting and underdiagnosis, the numbers do provide some perspective on these entities.

Most of the conditions discussed in this chapter and summarized in Table 9-32 are expressed in probable homozygotes (for autosomal recessives) or hemizygotes (X-linked). Because heterozygotes cannot yet be identified (except as parents), patients with multiple bone marrow failure genes or those with acquired diseases that may in fact be inherited cannot be defined at this time.

Treatment depends on diagnosis. Patients with pancytopenia due to Fanconi's anemia, dyskeratosis congenita, amegakaryocytic thrombocytopenia, or Shwachman-Diamond syndrome may respond to androgens. Those with DBA should receive corticosteroids, patients with Kostmann's syndrome should receive G-CSF, and patients with TAR should receive platelets. Bone marrow transplantation for those with Fanconi's anemia requires modification of the preparative protocols, patients with dyskeratosis congenita and Shwachman-Diamond syndrome need protocols that have yet to be developed, and DBA and TAR, which, respectively, might and will improve spontaneously, may not need transplantation at all.

In all cases in which transplantation is used, the donor must prove to be unaffected by the disease. Immunotherapy and growth factor treatment must be tailored for specific diseases. Risks of evolution of leukemia or other malignancies must be considered for all treatments, and those therapies with higher risk considered carefully in patients whose underlying condition is premalignant. Treatment of malignant complications is also difficult in these inherited disorders in which abnormalities may extend beyond hematopoietic tissues.

Prenatal diagnosis is possible for many of the inherited marrow failure disorders. Families at risk are usually identified through a propositus, after which subsequent pregnancies may be monitored. Early diagnosis of an affected fetus may eventually permit treatment in utero or at birth. Diagnosis of a fetus that is not affected and is HLA matched to the patient may provide placental blood for treatment of the patient.

Much remains to be understood about the genetics, pathophysiology, and treatment of both inherited and acquired aplastic anemia. This requires correct diagnoses, proper treatment, and careful follow-up. The prognoses for most of these disorders have improved with recent therapeutic advances, and it is anticipated that this improvement will accelerate with more knowledge of the specific molecular and cellular defects.

REFERENCES

1. O'Gorman Hughes DW. The varied pattern of aplastic anaemia in childhood. Aust Paediatr J 1966;2:228.
2. Auerbach AD, Venkatraj VS, Mann WR, et al. Genetic linkage studies in Fanconi anemia. J Cell Biochem Suppl 1989;13D:49.
3. Alter BP, Potter NU, Li FP. Classification and aetiology of the aplastic anaemias. Clin Haematol 1978;7:431.
4. Windass B, Vowels MR, O'Gorman Hughes D, White L. Aplastic anaemia in childhood: prognosis and approach to therapy. Med J Aust 1987;146: 15.
5. Alter BP. The bone marrow failure syndromes. In: Nathan DG, Oski FA, eds. Hematology of infancy and childhood, ed 3. Philadelphia, WB Saunders, 1987:159.
6. Fanconi G. Familiäre infantile perniziosaartige Anämie (perniziöses Blutbild und Konstitution). Jahrbuch Kinder 1927;117:257.
7. Uehlinger E. Konstitutionelle infantile (perniziosaartige) Anämie Klin Wochenschr 1929;32:1501.
8. Fanconi G. Familial constitional panmyelocytopathy, Fanconi's anemia (F.A.). I. Clinical aspects. Semin Hematol 1967;4:233.
9. Auerbach AD, Rogatko A, Schroeder-Kurth TM. International Fanconi Anemia Registry: relation of clinical symptoms to diepoxybutane sensitivity. Blood 1989;73:391.
10. Schroeder-Kurth TM, Auerbach AD, Obe G. Fanconi anemia. Clinical, cytogenetic and experimental aspects. Berlin, Springer-Verlag, 1989: 264.
11. Alter BP, Potter NU. Long-term outcome in Fanconi's anemia: description of 26 cases and review of the literature. In: German J, ed. Chromosome mutation and neoplasia. New York, Alan R Liss, 1983:43.
12. Baumann T. Konstitutionelle Panmyelophthise mit multiplen Abartungen (Fanconi-Syndrom). Ann Paediatr 1951;177:142.
13. Genz H. Klinische Beobachtungen and Untersuchungen bei einem Fall von Fanconi-anamie. Arch Kinderheilkd 1952;145:237.
14. Lorenz K. Beitrag zum Krankheitsbild des sog: "Fanconi-Syndroms." Kinderarztl Prax 1957;25:11.
15. Varela MA, Sternberg WH. Preanaemic state in Fanconi's anaemia. Lancet 1967;2:566.
16. Bacigalupo A, Van Lint MT, Cerri R, et al. Treatment of severe aplastic anemia with bolus 6-methylprednisolone and antilymphocytic globulin. Blut 1980;41:168.
17. Coutinho V, Falcao RP, Bottura C. Cytogenetic observations in congenital familial panmyelopathy (Fanconi's syndrome). Nouv Rev Fr Hematol 1971;11:781.
18. Farkas EE, Hadnagy C, Pap-Tuka P. Fanconi: Panmyelopathie. Arch Kinderheilkd 1971;183:306.
19. Gershanik JJ, Morgan SK, Akers R. Fanconi's anemia in a neonate. Acta Paediatr Scand 1972;61:623.
20. Prindull G, Stubbe P, Kratzer W. Fanconi's anemia. Z Kinderheilkd 1975;120:37.
21. Schroeder TM, Tilgen D, Kruger J, Vogel F. Formal genetics of Fanconi's anemia. Hum Genet 1976;32:257.
22. Meisner LF, Taher A, Shahidi NT. Chromosome changes and leukemic transformation in Fanconi's anemia. In: Hibino S, Takaku F, Shahidi NT, eds. Aplastic anemia. Tokyo, University of Tokyo Press, 1976:253.
23. Nadell J, Kosek J. Peliosis hepatis: twelve cases associated with oral androgen therapy. Arch Pathol Lab Med 1977;101:405.
24. Pignatti CB, Bianchi E, Polito E. Fanconi's anaemia in infancy: report of a case diagnosed in the pre-anaemic stage. Helv Paediatr Acta 1977;32:413.
25. Bank JI, Lykkebo D, Hägerstrand I. Peliosis hepatis in a child. Acta Paediatr Scand 1978;67:105.
26. McIntosh S, Breg WR, Lubiniecki AS. Fanconi's anemia: the pre-anemic phase. Am J Pediatr Hematol Oncol 1979;1:107.
27. Daneshbod-Skibba G, Martin J, Shahidi NT. Myeloid and erythroid colony growth in non-anemic patients with Fanconi's anaemia. Br J Haematol 1980;44:33.
28. Auerbach AD, Adler B, Chaganti RSK. Prenatal and postnatal diagnosis and carrier detection of Fanconi anemia by a cytogenetic method. Pediatrics 1981;67:128.
29. Wunder E, Fleischer-Reischmann B. Response of lymphocytes from Fanconi's anemia patients and their heterozygous relatives to 8-methoxy-psoralene in a cloning survival test system. Hum Genet 1983;64:167.
30. Kwee ML, Poll EHA, Van De Kamp JJP, De Koning H, Eriksson AW, Joenje H. Unusual response to bifunctional alkylating agents in a case of Fanconi anaemia. Hum Genet 1983;64:384.
31. Auerbach AD, Adler B, O'Reilly RJ, Kirkpatrick D, Chaganti RSK. Effect of procarbazine and cyclophosphamide on chromosome breakage in Fanconi anemia cells: relevance to bone marrow transplantation. Cancer Genet Cytogenet 1983;9:25.
32. Schaison G, Leverger G, Yildiz C, Berger R, Bernheim A, Gluckman E. L'anémie de Fanconi: fréquence de l'évolution vers la leucémie. Presse Med 1983;12:1269.
33. Gebhart E, Kysela D, Matthee H, Nikol M. Cytogenetic analyses utilizing various clastogens in two sibs with Fanconi anemia, their relatives, and control individuals. Hum Genet 1985;69:309.
34. Schindler D, Kubbies M, Hoehn H, Schinzel A, Rabinovitch PS. Con-

firmation of Fanconi's anemia and detection of a chromosomal aberration (1Q12-32 triplication) via BRDU/Hoechst flow cytometry. Am J Pediatr Hematol Oncol 1987;9:172.
35. Van Niekerk CH, Jordan C, Badenhorst PN. Pancytopenia secondary to primary malignant lymphoma of bone marrow as the first hematologic manifestation of the Estren-Dameshek variant of Fanconi's anemia. Am J Pediatr Hematol Oncol 1987;9:344.
36. Rohr K. Familial panmyelophthisis: Fanconi syndrome in adults. Blood 1949;4:130.
37. Cowdell RH, Phizackerley PJR, Pyke DA. Constitutional anemia (Fanconi's syndrome) and leukemia in two brothers. Blood 1955;10:788.
38. Killmann S-A. A case of pancytopenia in hypopituitarism: with a review of the hematological changes in clinical and experimental pituitary insufficiency. Acta Haematol 1956;15:34.
39. Schroeder TM, Anschütz F, Knopp A. Spontane Chromosomenaberrationen bei familiärer Panmyelopathie. Humangenetik 1964;1:194.
40. Lohr GW, Waller HD, Anschutz F, Knopp A. Biochemische Defekte in den Blutzellen bei familiarer Panmyelopathie (Typ Fanconi). Humangenetik 1965.383.
41. Swift MR, Hirschhorn K. Fanconi's anemia: inherited susceptibility to chromosome breakage in various tissues. Ann Intern Med 1966;65: 496.
42. Esparza A, Thompson WR. Familial hypoplastic anemia with multiple congenital anomalies (Fanconi's syndrome): report of three cases. RI Med J 1966;49:103.
43. Perkins J, Timson J, Emery AEH. Clinical and chromosome studies in Fanconi's aplastic anaemia. J Med Genet 1969;6:28.
44. McDonough ER. Fanconi anemia syndrome. Arch Otolaryngol 1970;92: 284.
45. Port RB, Petasnick JP, Ranniger K. Angiographic demonstration of hepatoma in association with Fanconi's anemia. AJR 1971;113:82.
46. Swift M, Zimmerman D, McDonough ER. Squamous cell carcinomas in Fanconi's anemia. JAMA 1971;216:325.
47. Lieber E, Hsu L, Spitler L, Fudenberg HH. Cytogenetic findings in a parent of a patient with Fanconi's anemia. Clin Genet 1972;3:357.
48. Crossen PE, Mellor JEL, Adams AC, Gunz FW. Chromosome studies in Fanconi's anaemia before and after treatment with oxymetholone. Pathology 1972;4:27.
49. De Grouchy J, De Nava C, Marchand JC, Feingold J, Turleau C. Etudes cytogénetique et biochimique de huit cas d'anémie de Fanconi. Ann Genet 1972;15:29.
50. Naeim F, Copper PH, Semion AA. Peliosis hepatis: possible etiologic role of anabolic steroids. Arch Pathol 1973;95:284.
51. Schuller A, Jelavic D, De La Fuente AG, Betancor P, Ramirez J, Valdivieso L. Peculiaridades de un caso de panmielopatia familiar de Fanconi. Sangre 1974;19:320.
52. O'Gorman Hughes DW. Aplastic anaemia in childhood. III. Constitutional aplastic anaemia and related cytopenias. Med J Aust 1974;1:519.
53. Farrell GC. Fanconi's familial hypoplastic anaemia with some unusual features. Med J Aust 1976;1:116.
54. Perona G, Cetto GL, Bernardi F, Todeschini G, D'Andrea F. Fanconi's anaemia in adults: study of three families. Haematologica 1977;62:615.
55. Joenje H, Eriksson AW, Frants RR, Arwert F, Houwen B. Erythrocyte superoxide-dismutase deficiency in Fanconi's anaemia. Lancet 1978;1: 204.
56. Barosi G, Cazzola M, Marchi A, et al. Iron kinetics and erythropoiesis in Fanconi's anaemia. Scand J Haematol 1978;21:29.
57. Schroeder TM, Pohler E, Hufnagl HD, Stahl-Mauge C. Fanconi's anemia: terminal leukemia and "forme fruste" in one family. Clin Genet 1979;16:260.
58. Eldar M, Shoenfeld Y, Zaizov R, et al. Pulmonary alveolar proteinosis associated with Fanconi's anemia. Respiration 1979;38:177.
59. Dosik H, Steier W, Lubiniecki. Inherited aplastic anaemia with increased endoreduplications: a new syndrome or Fanconi's anaemia variant? Br J Haematol 1979;41:77.
60. Nara N, Miyamoto T, Kurisu A, et al. Two siblings with Fanconi's anemia developing squamous cell carcinomas. Rinsho Ketsueki 1980;21: 1944.
61. Stein AC, Blanck DM, Bennett AJ, Gold BD, Berger J. Acute myelomonocytic leukemia in a patient with Fanconi's anemia. J Oral Surg 1981;39:624.
62. Kozarek RA, Sanowski RA. Carcinoma of the esophagus associated with Fanconi's anemia. J Clin Gastroenterol 1981;3:171.
63. Rotzak R, Kaplinsky N, Chaki R, et al. Giant marker chromosome in Fanconi's anemia transforming into erythroleukemia in an adult. Acta Haematol 1982;67:214.
64. Cervenka J, Hirsch BA. Cytogenetic differentiation of Fanconi anemia, "idiopathic" aplastic anemia, and Fanconi anemia heterozygotes. Am J Med Genet 1983;15:211.
65. Alimena G, Avvisati G, De Cuia MR, Gallo E, Novelli G, Dallapiccola B. Retrospective diagnosis of a Fanconi's anemia patient by dyepoxybutane (DEB) test results in parents. Haematologica 1983;68:97.
66. Berkovitz GD, Zinkham WH, Migeon CJ. Gonadal function in two siblings with Fanconi's anemia. Hormone Res 1984;19:137.
67. Helmerhorst FM, Heaton DC, Crossen PE, Von Dem Borne AEGK, Engelfriet CP, Natarajan AT. Familial thrombocytopenia associated with platelet autoantibodies and chromosome breakage. Hum Genet 1984;65: 252.
68. Saini RK, Sharma SK, Sharma SK. Fanconi's anaemia with psoriasis and polycolonal gammopathy. J Indian Med Assoc 1984;82:327.
69. Duckworth-Rysiecki G, Hulten M, Mann J, Taylor AMR. Clinical and cytogenetic diversity in Fanconi's anaemia. J Med Genet 1984;21:197.
70. Carbone P, Barbata G, Mirto S, Granata G. Inherited aplastic anemia with abnormal clones in bone marrow and increased endoreduplication in peripheral lymphocytes. Cancer Genet Cytogenet 1986;13:259.
71. Stivrins TJ, Davis RB, Sanger W, Fritz J, Purtilo DT. Transformation of Fanconi's anemia to acute nonlymphocytic leukemia associated with emergence of monosomy 7. Blood 1984;64:173.
72. Submoke S, Kessacorn W. Fanconi's syndrome: presentation of a case of acute myeloblastic leukemia. J Med Assoc Thailand 1985;68:480.
73. Rockelein G, Ulmer R, Kniewald A, Wagner H. Osophaguskarzinom bei Fanconi-Syndrom. Pathologe 1986;7:343.
74. Meddeb B, Azzouz MM, Hafsia R, Boussen M. Transformation en leucémie aigue de l'anémie de Fanconi: à propos de 2 cas dans une série de 21 malades. Tunis Med 1986;64:755.
75. Benitez J, Paz y Mino MC, Escudero A, Lapuente L, Ruiz Moreno M. Diagnostico citogenetico de pacientes con anemia de Fanconi utilizando metabolitos de ciclofosfamida como agente clastogenico. Sangre 1986;31: 513.
76. Huret JL, Tanzer J, Guilhot F, Frocain-Herchkovitch C, Savage JRK. Karyotype evolution in the bone marrow of a patient with Fanconi anemia: breakpoints in clonal anomalies of this disease. Cytogenet Cell Genet 1988;48:224.
77. Opinya GN, Kaimenyi JT, Meme JS. Oral findings in Fanconi's anemia. J Periodontol 1988;50:461.
78. Villamor N, Ribera JM, Ballesta F, Rozman C. Abnormal drainage of the pulmonary vessels in a patient with Fanconi's aplasia. Sangre 1988;33:318.
79. Shahidi NT. Fanconi anemia, dyskeratosis congenita, and WT syndrome. Am J Med Genet Suppl 1987;3:263.
80. Akar N, Gozdasoglu S. Spectrum of anomalies in Fanconi anaemia. J Med Genet 1984;21:75.
81. Auerbach A, Schroeder T. First announcement of the Fanconi Anemia International Registry. Blood 1982;60:1054.
82. Estren S, Dameshek W. Familial hypoplastic anemia of childhood: report of eight cases in two families with beneficial effect of splenectomy in one case. Am J Dis Child 1947;73:671.
83. Li FP, Potter NU. Classical Fanconi anemia in a family with hypoplastic anemia. J Pediatr 1978;92:943.
84. Glanz A, Fraser FC. Spectrum of anomalies in Fanconi anaemia. J Med Genet 1982;19:412.
85. Riley E, Caldwell R, Swift M. Comparison of clinical features in Fanconi anemia probands and their subsequently diagnosed siblings. Am J Hum Genet 1979;31:82A.
86. Rogatko A, Auerbach AD. Segregation analysis with uncertain ascertainment: application to Fanconi anemia. Am J Hum Genet 1988;42: 889.
87. Swift M. Fanconi anaemia: cellular abnormalities and clinical predisposition to malignant disease. In: Congenital disorders of erythropoiesis. CIBA Foundation Symposium 37. Amsterdam, Elsevier, 1976:115.
88. Rosendorff J, Bernstein R, Macdougall L, Jenkins T. Fanconi anemia: another disease of unusually high prevalence in the Afrikaans population of South Africa. Am J Med Genet 1987;27:793.
89. Skikne BS, Lynch SR, Bezwoda WR, et al. Fanconi's anaemia, with special reference to erythrokinetic features. S Afr Med J 1978;53:43.
90. Altay C, Sevgi Y, Pirnar T. Fanconi's anemia in offspring of patient with congenital radial and carpal hypoplasia. N Engl J Med 1975;293: 151.
91. Welshimer K, Swift M. Congenital malformations and developmental disabilities in ataxia-telangiectasia, Fanconi anemia, and xeroderma pigmentosum families. Am J Hum Genet 1982;34:781.
92. Reinhold JDL, Neumark E, Lightwood R, Carter CO. Familial hypoplastic anemia with congenital abnormalities (Fanconi's syndrome). Blood 1952;7:915.
93. O'Neill EM, Varadi S. Neonatal aplastic anaemia and Fanconi's anaemia. Arch Dis Child 1963;38:92.
94. Nilsson LR. Chronic pancytopenia with multiple congenital abnormalities (Fanconi's anaemia). Acta Paediatr 1960;49:518.
95. Cassimos C, Zannos L. Congenital hypoplastic anemia associated with multiple developmental defects (Fanconi's syndrome). Am J Dis Child 1952;84:347.
96. Beard MEJ, Young DE, Bateman CJT, et al. Fanconi's anaemia. Q J Med 1973;42:403.
97. Dacie JV, Gilpin A. Refractory anaemia (Fanconi type): its incidence in three members of one family, with in one case a relationship to chronic haemolytic anaemia with nocturnal haemoglobinuria (Marchiafava-Micheli disease or "nocturnal haemoglobinuria"). Arch Dis Child 1944;19:155.
98. Jalbert PP, Leger J, Bost M, Bachelot C, Mouriquand C, Sele B, Frappat P. L'anémie de Fanconi: aspects cytogéenétiques et biochimiques—a propos d'une famille. Nouv Rev Fr Hematol 1975;15:551.
99. Shahidi NT, Gerald PS, Diamond LK. Alkali-resistant hemoglobin in aplastic anemia of both acquired and congenital types. N Engl J Med 1962;266:117.
100. Jones R. Fanconi anemia: simultaneous onset of symptoms in two siblings. J Pediatr 1976;88:152.

101. De Vroede M, Feremans W, De Maertelaere-Laurent E, et al. Fanconi's anaemia: simultaneous onset in 2 siblings and unusual cytological findings. Scand J Haematol 1982;28:431.
102. Silver HK, Blair WC, Kempe CH. Fanconi syndrome: multiple congenital anomalies with hypoplastic anemia. Am J Dis Child 1952;83:14.
103. Voss R, Kohn G, Shaham M, et al. Prenatal diagnosis of Fanconi anemia. Clin Genet 1981;20:185.
104. Götz M, Pichler E. Zur Panmyelopathie im Kindesalter. Klin Pädiatr 1972;148:377.
105. Romero MG, Ortiz HC. Anemia de Fanconi: respuesta a dosis bajas de anabolicos y asociation con carcinoma de esofago. Rev Invest Clin 1984;36:353.
106. Schroeder TM, Drings P, Beilner P, Buchinger G. Clinical and cytogenetic observations during a six-year period in an adult with Fanconi's anaemia. Blut 1976;34:119.
107. Althoff H. Zur Panmyelopathie Fanconi als Zustandsbild multipler Abartungen. Z Kinderheilkd 1953;72:267.
108. Alter BP. Fetal erythropoiesis in stress hematopoiesis. Exp Hematol 1979;7:200.
109. Alter BP. Fetal erythropoiesis in bone marrow failure syndromes. In: Stamatoyannopoulos G, Neinhuis AW, eds. Cellular and molecular regulation of hemoglobin switching. New York, Grune & Stratton, 1979:87.
110. Shepard MK, Weatherall DJ, Conley CL. Semi-quantitative estimation of the distribution of fetal hemoglobin in red cell populations. Bull Johns Hopkins Hosp 1962;110:293.
111. Bernard J, Mathé G, Najean Y. Contribution à l'étude clinique et physiopathologique de la maladie de Fanconi. Rev Franc Etudes Clin Biol 1958;3:599.
112. Sjölin S, Wranne L. Erythropoietic dysfunction in a case of Fanconi's anaemia. Acta Haematol 1962;28:230.
113. Dell'Orbo C, Arico M, Podesta A, Bianchi E. Fanconi's anemia: ultrastructural observations on erythroblasts. Ultrastruct Pathol 1983;4:145.
114. Chu J-Y, Ho JE, Monteleone PL, O'Connor DM. Technetium colloid bone marrow imaging in Fanconi's anemia. Pediatrics 1979;64:635.
115. Löhr GW, Waller HD, Anschütz F, Knopp A. Hexokinasemangel in Blutzellen bei einer Sippe mit familiärer Panmyelopathie (Typ Fanconi). Klin Wochenschr 1965;43:870.
116. Magnani M, Novelli G, Stocchi V, Alimena G, Dallapiccola B. Red blood cell hexokinase in Fanconi's anemia. Acta Haematol 1984;71:341.
117. Pochedly C, Colipp PJ, Wolman SR, Suwansirikul S, Rezvani I. Fanconi's anemia with growth hormone deficiency. J Pediatr 1971;79:93.
118. Costin G, Kogut MD, Hyman CB, Ortega J. Fanconi's anemia associated with isolated growth hormone (GH) deficiency. Clin Res 1972;20:253A.
119. Schonberg D. Plasma growth hormone in cerebral gigantism, Laurence-Moon-Bardet-Biedl syndrome, Bloom syndrome and Fanconi anemia. Acta Paediatr Scand 1973;62:111A.
120. Schettini P, Cavallo L. Deficit di ormone somatotropo nell'anemia di Fanconi. Haematologica 1988;58:800.
121. Prindull G, Jentsch E, Hansmann I. Fanconi's anaemia developing erythroleukaemia. Scand J Haematol 1979;23:59.
122. Zachmann M, Illig R, Prader A. Fanconi's anemia with isolated growth hormone deficiency. J Pediatr 1972;80:159.
123. Clarke WL, Weldon VV. Growth hormone deficiency and Fanconi anemia. J Pediatr 1975;86:814.
124. Gleadhill V, Bridges JM, Hadden DR. Fanconi's aplastic anaemia with short stature: absence of response to human growth hormone. Arch Dis Child 1975;50:318.
125. Hayashi K, Schmid W. The rate of sister chromatid exchanges parallel to spontaneous chromosome breakage in Fanconi's anemia and to Trenimon-induced aberrations in human lymphocytes and fibroblasts. Hum Genet 1975;29:201.
126. Stubbe P, Prindull G. Fanconi's anemia. II. Are multiple endocrine insufficiencies a substantial part of the disease? Acta Paediatr Scand 1975;64:790.
127. Aynsley-Green A, Zachmann M, Werder EA, Illig R, Prader A. Endocrine studies in Fanconi's anaemia: report of 4 cases. Arch Dis Child 1978;53:126.
128. Nordan UZ, Humbert JR, MacGillivray MH, Fitzpatrick JE. Fanconi's anemia with growth hormone deficiency. Am J Dis Child 1979;133:291.
129. Wada E, Murata M, Watanabe S. Acute lymphoblastic leukemia following treatment by human growth hormone in a boy with possible preanemic Fanconi's anemia. Jpn J Clin Oncol 1989;19:36.
130. Standen GR, Hughes IA, Geddes AD, Jones BM, Wardrop CAJ. Myelodysplastic syndrome with trisomy 8 in an adolescent with Fanconi anaemia and selective IgA deficiency. Am J Hematol 1989;31:280.
131. Scharer K, Baumann T. Die Behandlung der idiopathischen Panmyelopathien mit Steroiden und hypophysarem Wachstumshormon. Schweiz Med Wochenschr 1964;38:1322.
132. Golde DW, Herschman HR, Lusis AJ, Groopman JE. Growth factors. Ann Intern Med 1980;92:650.
133. Fisher DA, Job J-C, Preece M, Underwood LE. Leukaemia in patients treated with growth hormone. Lancet 1988;1:1159.
134. Schmid W, Schärer K, Baumann T, Fanconi G. Chromosomenbrüchigkeit bei der familiären Panmyelopathie (Typus Fanconi). Schweiz Med Wochenschr 1965;43:1461.
135. Bloom GE, Warner S, Gerald PS, Diamond LK. Chromosome abnormalities in constitutional aplastic anemia. N Engl J Med 1966;274:8.
136. German J, Pugliatti Crippa L. Chromosomal breakage in diploid cell lines from Bloom's syndrome and Fanconi's anemia. Ann Genet 1966;9:143.
137. Bloom GE. Disorders of bone marrow production. Pediatr Clin North Am 1972;19:983.
138. Gmyrek D, Witkowski R, Syllm-Rapoport I, Jacobasch G. Chromosomal aberrations and abnormalities of red-cell metabolism in a case of Fanconi's anaemia before and after development of leukaemia. German Med Mon 1968;13:105.
139. Wolman SR, Swift M. Bone marrow chromosomes in Fanconi's anemia. J Med Genet 1972;9:473.
140. Shahid MJ, Khouri FP, Ballas SK. Fanconi's anaemia: report of a patient with significant chromosomal abnormalities in bone marrow cells. J Med Genet 1972;9:474.
141. Berger R, Bernheim A, Le Coniat M, Vecchione D, Schaison G. Chromosomal studies of leukemic and preleukemic Fanconi's anemia patients: examples of acquired "chromosomal amplification." Hum Genet 1980;56:59.
142. Schroeder TM, Kurth R. Spontaneous chromosomal breakage and high incidence of leukemia in inherited disease. Blood 1971;37:96.
143. Todaro GJ, Green H, Swift MR. Susceptibility of human diploid fibroblast strains to transformation by SV40 virus. Science 1966;153:1252.
144. Higurashi M, Conen PE. In vitro chromosomal radiosensitivity in Fanconi's anemia. Blood 1971;38:336.
145. Sasaki MS, Tonomura A. A high susceptibility of Fanconi's anemia to chromosome breakage by DNA cross-linking agents. Cancer 1973;33:1829.
146. Auerbach AD, Wolman SR. Susceptibility of Fanconi's anaemia fibroblasts to chromosome damage by carcinogens. Nature 1976;261:494.
147. Berger R, Bernheim A, Le Coniat M, Vecchione D, Schaison G. Nitrogen mustard-induced chromosome breakage: a tool for Fanconi's anemia diagnosis. Cancer Genet Cytogenet 1980;2:269.
148. Cervenka J, Arthur D, Yasis C. Mitomycin C test for diagnostic differentiation of idiopathic aplastic anemia and Fanconi anemia. Pediatrics 1981;67:119.
149. Poll EHA, Arwert F, Joenje H, Eriksson AW. Cytogenetic toxicity of antitumor platinum compound in Fanconi's anemia. Hum Genet 1982;61:228.
150. Chaganti RSK, Schonberg S, German J. A many fold increase in sister chromatid exchanges in Bloom's syndrome lymphocytes. Proc Natl Acad Sci USA 1974;71:4508.
151. Auerbach AD, Wolman SR. Carcinogen-induced chromosome breakage in Fanconi's anaemia heterozygous cells. Nature 1978;271:69.
152. Marx MP, Smith S, Heynes ADP, Van Tonder IZ. Fanconi's anemia: a cytogenetic study on lymphocyte and bone marrow cultures utilizing 1,2:3,4-diepoxybutane. Cancer Genet Cytogenet 1983;9:51.
153. Berger R, Bernheim A, Le Coniat M, Vecchione D, Schaison G. Sister chromatid exchanges induced by nitrogen mustard in Fanconi's anemia: application to the detection of heterozygotes and interpretation of the results. Cancer Genet Cytogenet 1980;2:259.
154. Kaiser TN, Lojewski A, Dougherty C, Juergens L, Sahar E, Latt SA. Flow cytometric characterization of the response of Fanconi's anemia cells to mitomycin C treatment. Cytometry 1982;2:291.
155. Auerbach AD, Ghosh R, Pollio PC, Zhang M. Diepoxybutane test for prenatal and postnatal diagnosis of Fanconi anemia. In: Schroeder-Kurth, TM, Auerbach AD, Obe G, eds. Fanconi anemia: clinical, cytogenetic and experimental aspects. Berlin, Springer-Verlag, 1989:71.
156. Auerbach AD, Alter BP. Prenatal and postnatal diagnosis of aplastic anemia. In: Alter BP, ed. Methods in hematology: perinatal hematology. Edinburgh, Churchill Livingstone, 1989:225.
157. Arwert F, Kwee ML. Chromosomal breakage in response to cross-linking agents in the diagnosis of Fanconi anemia. In: Schroeder-Kurth, TM, Auerbach AD, Obe G, eds. Fanconi anemia: clinical, cytogenetic and experimental aspects. Berlin, Springer-Verlag, 1989:83.
158. German J, Schonberg S, Caskie S, Warburton D, Falk C, Ray JH. A test for Fanconi's anemia. Blood 1987;69:1637.
159. Trunca C, Watson M, Auerbach A, Kaplan C, Mahoney M, Baker D. Prenatal diagnosis of Fanconi anemia in a fetus not known to be at risk. Am J Hum Genet 1984;36:198S.
160. Bonnet-Gajdos M, Vasmant D, Baruchel S, Mamou JF, Boue J, Lasfargues G. Diagnostic antenatal de l'anemie de Fanconi. Presse Med 1985;14:1612.
161. Auerbach AD, Zhang M, Ghosh R, et al. Clastogen-induced chromosomal breakage as a marker for first trimester prenatal diagnosis of Fanconi anemia. Hum Genet 1986;73:86.
162. Boue PJ, Deluchat C, Nicolas H, Oury JF, Dumez Y. Diagnostic prénatal des maladies géniques sur villosités choriales. J Genet Hum 1986;34:221.
163. Dallapiccola B, Carbone LD L, Ferranti G, Cristiani ML, Bricarelli FD. Monitoring of pregnancies at risk for Fanconi's anemia by chorionic villi sampling. Acta Haematol 1985;73:157.
164. Shipley J, Rodeck CH, Garrett C, Galbraith J, Giannelli F. Mitomycin C–induced chromosome damage in fetal blood cultures and prenatal diagnosis of Fanconi's anaemia. Prenat Diagn 1984;4:217.
165. Hirsch-Kauffmann M, Schweiger M, Wagner EF, Sperling K. Deficiency of DNA ligase activity in Fanconi's anemia. Hum Genet 1978;45:25.

166. Auerbach AD, Sagi M, Adler B. Fanconi anemia: prenatal diagnosis in 30 fetuses at risk. Pediatrics 1985;76:794.
167. Cohen MM, Simpson SJ, Honig GR, Maurer HS, Nicklas JW, Martin AO. The identification of Fanconi anemia genotypes by clastogenic stress. Am J Hum Genet 1982;34:794.
168. Bigelow SB, Rary JM, Bender MA. G2 chromosomal radiosensitivity in Fanconi's anemia. Mutat Res 1979;63:189.
169. Remsen JF, Cerutti PA. Deficiency of gamma-ray excision repair in skin fibroblasts from patients with Fanconi's anemia. Proc Natl Acad Sci USA 1976;73:2419.
170. Poon PK, O'Brien RL, Parker JW. Defective DNA repair in Fanconi's anaemia. Nature 1974;250:223.
171. Schroeder TM, Stahl-Maugé C. Mutagenic effects of isonicotinic acid hydracide in Fanconi's anemia. Hum Genet 1979;52:309.
172. Joenje H, Oostra AB. Clastogenicity of cyclophosphamide in Fanconi's anemia lymphocytes without exogenous metabolic activation. Cancer Genet Cytogenet 1986;22:339.
173. Berger R, Bernheim A, Gluckman E, Gisselbrecht C. In vitro effect of cyclophosphamide metabolites on chromosomes of Fanconi anaemia patients. Br J Haematol 1980;45:565.
174. Klocker H, Burtscher HJ, Auer B, Hirsch-Kauffmann M, Schweiger M. Fibroblasts from patients with Fanconi's anemia are not deficient in excision of thymine dimer. Eur J Cell Biol 1985;37:240.
175. Kaye J, Smith CA, Hanawalt PC. DNA repair in human cells containing photoadducts of 8-methoxypsoralen or angelicin. Cancer Res 1980;40:696.
176. Fujiwara Y, Tatsumi M, Sasaki MS. Cross-link repair in human cells and its possible defect in Fanconi's anemia cells. J Mol Biol 1977;113:635.
177. Rainbow AJ, Howes M. Defective repair of ultraviolet- and gamma-ray–damaged DNA in Fanconi's anaemia. Int J Radiat Biol 1977;31:191.
178. Fornace AJ Jr, Little JB, Weichselbaum RR. DNA repair in a Fanconi's anemia fibroblast cell strain. Biochim Biophys Acta 1979;561:99.
179. Wunder E, Burghardt U, Lang B, Hamilton L. Fanconi's anemia: anomaly of enzyme passage through the nuclear membrane? Hum Genet 1981;58:149.
180. Wunder E. Further studies on compartmentalisation of DNA-topoisomerase I in Fanconi anemia tissue. Hum Genet 1984;68:276.
181. Sasaki MS. Is Fanconi's anaemia defective in a process essential to the repair of DNA cross links? Nature 1975;257:501.
182. Fujiwara Y, Tatsumi M. Repair of mitomycin C damage to DNA in mammalian cells and its impairment in Fanconi's anemia cells. Biochem Biophys Res Commun 1975;66:592.
183. Elmore E, Swift M. Growth of cultured cells from patients with Fanconi anemia. J Cell Physiol 1976;87:229.
184. Weksberg R, Buchwald M, Sargent P, Thompson MW, Siminovitch L. Specific cellular defects in patients with Fanconi anemia. J Cell Physiol 1979;101:311.
185. Dutrillaux B, Aurias A, Dutrillaux A-M, Buriot D, Prieur M. The cell cycle of lymphocytes in Fanconi anemia. Hum Genet 1982;62:327.
186. Auerbach AD, Sagi M, Adler B. Fanconi anemia: prenatal diagnosis in 30 fetuses at risk. Pediatrics 1985;76:794.
187. Joenje H, Frants RR, Arwert F, et al. Erythrocyte superoxide dismutase deficiency in Fanconi's anaemia established by two independent methods of assay. Scand J Clin Lab Invest 1979;39:759.
188. Okahata S, Kobayashi Y, Usui T. Erythrocyte superoxide dismutase activity in Fanconi's anaemia. Clin Sci 1980;58:173.
189. Mavelli I, Ciriolo MR, Rotilio G, De Sole P, Castorino M, Stabile A. Superoxide dismutase, glutathione peroxidase and catalase in oxidative hemolysis: a study of Fanconi's anemia erythrocytes. Biochem Biophys Res Commun 1982;106:286.
190. Scarpa M, Rigo A, Momo F, Isacchi G, Novelli G, Dallapiccola B. Increased rate of superoxide ion generation in Fanconi anemia erythrocytes. Biochem Biophys Res Commun 1985;130:127.
191. Yoshimitsu K, Kobayashi Y, Usui T. Decreased superoxide dismutase activity of erythrocytes and leukocytes in Fanconi's anemia. Acta Haematol 1984;72:208.
192. Dallapiccola B, Porfirio B, Mokini V, Alimena G, Isacchi G, Gandini E. Effect of oxidants and antioxidants on chromosomal breakage in Fanconi anemia lymphocytes. Hum Genet 1985;69:62.
193. Brown KW, Harnden DG. Erythrocyte superoxide dismutase in ataxia telangiectasia and Fanconi's anaemia. Lancet 1978;2:1260.
194. Abeliovich D, Cohen MM. Normal activity of nucleoside phosphorylase, superoxide dismutase and catalase in skin fibroblasts cultured from ataxiatelangiectasia patients. Isr J Med Sci 1978;14:284.
195. Gille JJP, Wortelboer HM, Joenje H. Antioxidant status of Fanconi anemia fibroblasts. Hum Genet 1987;77:28.
196. Nordenson I. Effect of superoxide dismutase and catalase on spontaneously occurring chromosome breaks in patients with Fanconi's anemia. Hereditas 1977;86:147.
197. Raj AS, Heddle JA. The effect of superoxide dismutase, catalase and L-cysteine on spontaneous and on mitomycin c–induced chromosomal breakage in Fanconi's anemia and normal fibroblasts as measured by the micronucleus method. Mutat Res 1980;78:59.
198. Joenje H, Arwert F, Eriksson AW, De Koning H, Oostra AB. Oxygen-dependence of chromosomal aberrations in Fanconi's anaemia. Nature 1981;290:142.
199. Joenje H, Oostra AB. Effect of oxygen tension on chromosomal aberrations in Fanconi anaemia. Hum Genet 1983;65:99.
200. Nagasawa H, Little JB. Suppression of cytotoxic effect of mitomycin-C by superoxide dismutase in Fanconi's anemia and dyskeratosis congenita fibroblasts. Carcinogenesis 1983;4:795.
201. Izakovic V, Strbakova E, Kaiserova E, Krizan P. Bovine superoxide dismutase in Fanconi anaemia: therapeutic trial in two patients. Hum Genet 1985;70:181.
202. Latt SA, Stetten G, Juergens LA, Buchanan GR, Gerald PS. Induction by alkylating agents of sister chromatid exchanges and chromatid breaks in Fanconi's anemia. Proc Natl Acad Sci USA 1975;72:4066.
203. Sperling K, Wegner RD, Riehm H, Obe G. Frequency and distribution of sister-chromatid exchanges in a case of Fanconi's anemia. Humangenetik 1975;27:227.
204. Chaganti RSK, Schonberg S, German J. A manyfold increase in sister chromatid exchanges in Bloom's syndrome lymphocytes. Proc Natl Acad Sci USA 1974;71:4508.
205. Novotna B, Goetz P, Surkova NI. Effects of alkylating agents on lymphocytes from controls and from patients with Fanconi's anemia. Hum Genet 1979;49:41.
206. Miura K, Morimoto K, Koizumi A. Proliferative kinetics and mitomycin C–induced chromosome damage in Fanconi's anemia lymphocytes. Hum Genet 1983;63:19.
207. Zakrzewski S, Sperling K. Antagonistic effect of cocultivation on mitomycin C–induced aberration rate in cells of a patient with Fanconi's anemia and in chinese hamster ovary cells. Hum Genet 1980;56:85.
208. Nordenson I, Björksten B, Lundh B. Prevention of chromosomal breakage in Fanconi's anemia by cocultivation with normal cells. Hum Genet 1980;56:169.
209. Shaham M, Adler B. Chromosome breakage in Fanconi's anemia and normal cells following in vitro and in vivo cocultivation. Cancer Genet Cytogenet 1986;23:315.
210. Arwert F. Cocultivation of Fanconi's anemia and normal lymphocytes in response to mitomycin C. Clin Genet 1984;25:210.
211. Yoshida MC. Suppression of spontaneous and mitomycin C–induced chromosome aberrations in Fanconi's anemia by cell fusion with human fibroblasts. Hum Genet 1980;55:223.
212. Duckworth-Rysiecki G, Cornish K, Clarke CA, Buchwald M. Identification of two complementation groups in Fanconi anemia. Somatic Cell Mol Genet 1985;11:35.
213. Zakrzewski S, Sperling K. Genetic heterogeneity of Fanconi's anemia demonstrated by somatic cell hybrids. Hum Genet 1980;56:81.
214. Zakrzewski S, Sperling K. Analysis of heterogeneity in Fanconi's anemia patients of different ethnic origin. Hum Genet 1982;62:321.
215. Zakrzewski S, Koch M, Sperling K. Complementation studies between Fanconi's anemia cells with different DNA repair characteristics. Hum Genet 1983;64:55.
216. Yoshida MC. The absence of genetic heterogeneity in Fanconi's anemia in five patients demonstrated by somatic cell hybridization. Cytogenet Cell Genet 1982;32:329.
217. Digweed M, Zakrzewski-Ludcke S, Sperling K. Fanconi's anaemia: correlation of genetic complementation group with psoralen/UVA response. Hum Genet 1988;78:51.
218. Klocker H, Auer B, Hirsch-Kauffmann M, Altmann H, Burtscher HJ, Schweiger M. DNA repair dependent NAD+ metabolism is impaired in cells from patients with Fanconi's anemia. EMBO J 1983;2:303.
219. Gruenert DC, Cleaver JE. Repair of psoralen-induced cross-links and monoadducts in normal and repair-deficient human fibroblasts. Cancer Res 1985;45:5399.
220. Papadopoulo D, Averbeck D, Moustacchi E. The fate of 8-methoxypsoralenphotoinduced DNA intrastrand crosslinks in Fanconi's anemia cells of defined genetic complementation groups. Mutat Res 1987;184:271.
221. Moustacchi E, Papadopoulo D, Diatloff-Zito C, Buchwald M. Two complementation groups of Fanconi's anemia differ in their phenotypic response to a DNA-crosslinking treatment. Hum Genet 1987;75:45.
222. Coquerelle TM, Weibezahn KF. Rejoining of DNA double-strand breaks in human fibroblasts and its impairment in one ataxia telangiectasia and two Fanconi strains. J Supramolec Struct Cell Biochem 1981;17:369.
223. Digweed M, Zakrzewski-Ludcke S, Sperling. Complementation studies in Fanconi anemia using cell fusion and microinjection of mRNA. In: Schroeder-Kurth TM, Auerbach AD, Obe G, eds. Fanconi anemia: clinical, cytogenetic and experimental aspects. Berlin, Springer-Verlag, 1989:236.
224. Matsumoto A, Vos J-M, Hanawalt PC. Repair analysis of mitomycin C–induced DNA crosslinking in ribosomal RNA genes in lymphoblastoid cells from Fanconi's anemia patients. Mutat Res 1989;217:1985.
225. Diatloff-Zito C, Papadopoulo D, Averbeck D, Moustacchi E. Abnormal response to DNA crosslinking agents of Fanconi anemia fibroblasts can be corrected by transfection with normal human DNA. Proc Natl Acad Sci USA 1986;83:7034.
226. Buchwald M, Ng J, Clarke C, Duckworth-Rysiecki G. Studies of gene transfer and reversion to mitomycin C resistance in Fanconi anemia cells. Mutat Res 1987;184:153.
227. Gök MM, Wunder E. Microinjection of normal cell extracts into Fanconi anemia fibroblasts corrects defective scheduled DNA synthesis recovery after 8-methoxypsoralen plus UVa treatment. Hum Genet 1987;75:350.

228. Shaham M, Adler B, Ganguly S, Chaganti RSK. Transfection of normal human and Chinese hamster DNA corrects diepoxybutane-induced chromosomal hypersensitivity of Fanconi anemia fibroblasts. Proc Natl Acad Sci USA 1987;84:5853.
229. Auerbach AD, Koorse RE, Ghosh R, Venkatraj VS, Zhang M. Complementation studies in Fanconi anemia. In: Schroeder-Kurth TM, Auerbach AD, Obe G, eds. Fanconi anemia: clinical, cytogenetic and experimental aspects. Berlin, Springer-Verlag, 1989:213.
230. Mann WR, Ventatraj VS, Allen RG, et al. Fanconi anemia: evidence for likage heterogeneity on chromosome 20q. Genomics 1991;9:329.
231. Strathdee CA, Gavish H, Shannon WR, Buchwald M. Cloning of cDNAs for Fanconi's anaemia by functional complementation. Nature 1992;356:763.
232. Strathdee CA, Duncan AMV, Buchwald M. Evidence for at least four Fanconi anemia genes including FACC on chromosome 9. Nature Genetics 1992;1:196.
233. Lui VK, Ragab AH, Findley HS, Frauen BJ. Bone marrow cultures in children with Fanconi anemia and the TAR syndrome. J Pediatr 1977;91:952.
234. Saunders EF, Freedman MH. Constitutional aplastic anaemia: defective haematopoietic stem cell growth in vitro. Br J Haematol 1978;40:277.
235. Chu JY. Granulopoiesis in Fanconi's aplastic anemia. Proc Soc Exp Biol Med 1979;161:609.
236. Greenberg BR, Wilson FD, Woo L, Knox S, Jenks H, Taplett J. Cytogenetics and granulopoietic effects of bone marrow fibroblastic cells in Fanconi's anaemia. Br J Haematol 1981;48:85.
237. Auerbach AD, Weiner M, Warburton D, Yeboa K, Lu L, Broxmeyer HE. Acute myeloid leukemia as the first hematologic manifestation of Fanconi anemia. Am J Hematol 1982;12:289.
238. Mera CL, Freedman ML. Clostridium abscess and massive hemolysis: unique demise in Fanconi's aplastic anemia. Clin Pediatr 1984;23:126.
239. Barton JC, Parmley RT, Carroll AJ, Huang ST, Goodnough LT, Findley HW Jr. Preleukemia in Fanconi's anemia: hematopoietic cell multinuclearity, membrane duplication, and dysgranulogenesis. J Submicrosc Cytol 1987;19:355.
240. Shihab-El-Deen A, Guevara C, Prchal JF. Bone marrow cultures in dysmyelopoietic syndrome: diagnostic and prognostic evaluation. Acta Haematol 1987;78:17.
241. Claustres M, Margueritte G, Sultan C. In vitro CFU-E and BFU-E responses to androgen in bone marrow from children with primary hypoproliferative anaemia: a possible therapeutic assay. Eur J Pediatr 1986;144:467.
242. Dawson JP. Congenital pancytopenia associated with multiple congenital anomalies (Fanconi type). Pediatrics 1955;15:325.
243. McDonald R, Goldschmidt B. Pancytopenia with congenital defects (Fanconi's anaemia). Arch Dis Child 1960;35:367.
244. Auerbach AD, Frissora CL, Rogatko A. International Fanconi anemia registry (IFAR): survival and prognostic factors. Blood 1989;74:43a.
245. Bargman GJ, Shahidi NT, Gilbert EF, Opitz JM. Studies of malformation syndromes of man. XLVII. Disappearance of spermatogonia in the Fanconi anemia syndrome. Eur J Pediatr 1977;125:163.
246. Van Buchem FSP, Samson N, Nieweg HO. Familial pancytopenia with congenital abnormalities (Fanconi's syndrome). Acta Med Scand 1954;149:19.
247. Alter BP, Frissora CL, Halpérin DS, et al. Fanconi's anemia and pregancy. Br J Haematol 1991;77:410.
248. Kew MC, Van Coller B, Prowse CM, et al. Occurrence of primary hepatocellular cancer and peliosis hepatis after treatment with androgenic steroids. S Afr Med J 1976;50:1233.
249. Bauters F, Jouet JP, Lacroix D, Lai JL, Deminatti M. Maladie de Fanconi de révélation tardive en cours de grossesse: etude cytogénétique. Presse Med 1984;13:2519.
250. Zakut H, Lotan M, Virag I. Pregnancy in Fanconi's anemia. Harefuah 1984;107:238.
251. Shahidi NT, Diamond LK. Testosterone-induced remission in aplastic anemia. Am J Dis Child 1959;98:293.
252. Sanchez-Medal L. The hemopoietic action of androstanes. Prog Hematol 1971;7:111.
253. Najean Y. Androgen therapy in aplastic anaemia in childhood. In: Congenital disorders of erythropoiesis. CIBA Foundation Symposium 37. Amsterdam, Elsevier, 1976:354.
254. Desposito F, Akatsuka J, Thatcher LG, Smith NJ. Bone marrow failure in pediatric patients. I. Cortisone and testosterone treatment. J Pediatr 1964;64:683.
255. McDonald R, Mibashan RS. Prolonged remission in Fanconi type anemia. Helv Paediatr Acta 1968;23:566.
256. Wasserman HP, Fry R, Cohn HJ. Fanconi's anaemia: cytogenetic studies in a family. S Afr Med J 1968;42:1162.
257. Hirschman RJ, Schulman NR, Abuelo JG, Whang-Peng J. Chromosomal aberrations in two cases of inherited aplastic anemia with unusual clinical features. Ann Intern Med 1969;71:107.
258. Jacobs P, Karabus C. Fanconi's anemia: a family study with 20-year follow-up including associated breast pathology. Cancer 1984;54:1850.
259. Rogers PCJ, Desai F, Karabus CD, Hartley PS, Fisther RM. Presentation and outcome of 25 cases of Fanconi's anemia. Am J Pediatr Hematol Oncol 1989;11:141.
260. El Mauhoub M, Sudarshan G, Banerjee G, Aggarwal VP, Shembish N. Fanconi's anemia with associated acute nonlymphocytic leukemia. Indian Pediatr 1988;25:1124.
261. Shahidi NT, Crigler JF Jr. Evaluation of growth and of endocrine systems in testosterone-corticosteroid–treated patients with aplastic anemia. J Pediatr 1967;70:233.
262. Kitchens CS. Amelioration of endothelial abnormalities by prednisone in experimental thrombocytopenia in the rabbit. J Clin Invest 1977;60: 1129.
263. Smith S, Marx MP, Jordaan CJ, Van Niekerk CH. Clinical aspects of a cluster of 42 patients in South Africa with Fanconi anemia. In: Schroeder-Kurth TM, Auerbach AD, Obe G, eds. Fanconi anemia: clinical, cytogenetic and experimental aspects. Berlin, Springer-Verlag, 1989: 34.
264. Dooren LJ, Kamphuis RP, De Koning J, Vossen JM. Bone marrow transplantation in children. Semin Hematol 1974;11:369.
265. Storb R, Thomas ED, Buckner CD, et al. Allogeneic marrow grafting for treatment of aplastic anemia. Blood 1974;43:157.
266. Gluckman E, Devergie A, Schaison G, et al. Bone marrow transplantation in Fanconi Anaemia. Br J Haematol 1980;45:557.
267. Ramsay NKC, Kim TH, McGlave PB, et al. Bone marrow transplantation from severe aplastic anemia using the conditioning regimen of cyclophosphamide and total lymphoid irradiation. Exp Hematol 1982;12: 139.
268. Kallenberg CGM, Mulder NH, The TH, Speck B. Defective stimulating capacity of leukocytes in mixed leukocyte culture in constitutional aplastic anemia caused by suppressor T cells. Acta Haematol 1980;63: 181.
269. Deeg HJ, Storb R, Thomas ED, et al. Fanconi's anemia treated by allogeneic marrow transplantation. Blood 1983;61:954.
270. Barrett AJ, Brigden WD, Hobbs JR, et al. Successful bone marrow transplant for Fanconi's anaemia. Br Med J 1977:420.
271. Gluckman E, Berger R, Dutreix J. Bone marrow transplantation for Fanconi anemia. Semin Hematol 1984;21:20.
272. Stuart RK, Sensenbrenner LL, Zinkham WH, Santos GW, Saral R. Successful elective bone marrow transplant (BMT) in an untransfused patient with Fanconi's anemia. Blood 1985;66:255a.
273. Hinterberger W, Gadner H, Hocker P, et al. Survival and quality of life in 23 patients with severe aplastic anemia treated with bone marrow transplantation (BMT). Blut 1987;54:137.
274. Appelbaum FR, Storb R, Ramberg RE, et al. Treatment of preleukemic syndromes with marrow transplantation. Blood 1987;69:92.
275. Gluckman E, Devergie A, Dutreix J. Bone marrow transplantation for Fanconi anemia. In: Schroeder-Kurth TM, Auerbach AD, Obe G, eds. Fanconi anemia: clinical, cytogenetic and experimental aspects. Berlin, Springer-Verlag, 1989:60.
276. Storb R, Thomas ED, Weiden PL, et al. Aplastic anemia treated by allogeneic bone marrow transplantation: a report on 49 new cases from Seattle. Blood 1976;48:817.
277. Camitta BM. Aplastic anemia. In: Hibino S, Takaku F, Shahidi NT, eds. Aplastic anemia. Tokyo, University of Tokyo Press, 1976:428.
278. Holl RA, Dooren LJ, Vossen JMJJ, Roos MTL, Schelleken PTA. Bone marrow transplantation in children with severe aplastic anemia: reconstitution of cellular immunity. Transplantation 1981;32:418.
279. Ebell W, Friedrich W, Kohne E. Therapeutic aspects of Fanconi anemia. In: Schroeder-Kurth TM, Auerbach AD, Obe G, eds. Fanconi anemia: clinical, cytogenetic and experimental aspects. Berlin, Springer-Verlag, 1989:47.
280. Gluckman E, Devergie A, Dutreix J. Radiosensitivity in Fanconi anaemia: application to the conditioning regimen for bone marrow transplantation. Br J Haematol 1983;54:431.
281. Gluckman E. Bone marrow transplantation for Fanconi's anaemia. Bailliere's Clin Haematol 1989;2:153.
282. Gluckman E, Devergie A, Dutreix J. Bone marrow transplantation for Fanconi anemia. In: Schroeder-Kurth TM, Auerbach AD, Obe G, eds. Fanconi anemia: clinical, cytogenetic and experimental aspects. Berlin, Springer-Verlag, 1989:60.
283. Miale TD, Ahmed I, Gould RC, Rao S, Rosenthal IM. Increased chromosome fragility of donor cells in Fanconi's anemia after bone marrow transplantation. Pediatr Res 1984;18:245A.
284. Ash RC, Geil J, Serwint M, Greenwood M, Coffey C, Maruyama Y. Successful marrow transplantation for Fanconi's aplastic anemia with low-dose cyclophosphamide and fractionated total lymphoid irradiation. Blood 1984;64:208a.
285. Hows J, Durrant S, Swirsky D, Yin J, Worsley A, Gordon-Smith E. Fanconi's anaemia treated by allogeneic marrow transplantation. Exp Hematol 1987;15:566.
286. Hows JM, Chapple M, Marsh JCW, Durrant S, Yin JL, Swirsky D, Gordon-Smith EC. Bone marrow transplantation for Fanconi's anaemia: the Hammersmith experience 1977–89. Bone Marrow Transplant 1989;4: 629.
287. Hows JM, Yin JL, Swirsky D, et al. Histocompatible unrelated volunteer donors compared with HLA nonidentical family donors in marrow transplantation for aplastic anemia and leukemia. Blood 1986;68:1322.
288. Sokal E, Michel M, Ninane J, Latinne D, Debruyere M, Cornu G. Bone marrow transplantation from an unrelated donor for Fanconi's anaemia: two unusual complications. Bone Marrow Transplant 1987;2:99.
289. Gingrich RD, Ginder GD, Goeken NE, et al. Allogeneic marrow grafting

with partially mismatched, unrelated marrow donors. Blood 1988;71:1375.
290. Hows J, Chapple M, Marsh J, et al. Unrelated donor bone marrow transplantation (BMT) for Fanconi's anemia (FA). Blood 1989;74:282a.
291. Hansen JA, Good RA, Dupont B. HLA-D compatibility between parent and child. Transplantation 1977;23:366.
292. O'Reilly RJ, Pollack MS, Auerbach AD, et al. HLA histocompatibility between parent and affected child in Fanconi's anemia. Pediatr Res 1982;16:210A.
293. Broxmeyer HE, Douglas GW, Hangoc G, et al. Human umbilical cord blood as a potential source of transplantable hematopoietic stem/progenitor cells. Proc Natl Acad Sci USA 1989;86:3828.
294. Gluckman E, Broxmeyer HE, Auerbach AD, et al. Hematopoietic reconstitution in a patient with Fanconi's anemia by means of umbilical-cord blood from an HLA-identical sibling. N Engl J Med 1989;321:1174.
295. Witherspoon RP, Fisher L, Martin P, et al. Secondary malignancies following bone marrow transplantation for aplastic anemia or hematologic malignancy. Blood 1988;72:413a.
296. Hamre MR, Kirkpatrick DV, Humbert JR. Squamous cell carcinoma of the tongue in a patient with Fanconi anemia post bone marrow transplant. Pediatr Res 1989;25:151A.
297. Gardner FH, Helmer RE III. Aminocaproic acid: use in control of hemorrhage in patients with amegakaryocytic thrombocytopenia. JAMA 1980;243:35.
298. Ozsoylu S. Treatment of aplastic anemia. J Pediatr 1983;102:484.
299. Speck B, Gratwohl A, Nissen C, et al. Treatment of severe aplastic anaemia with antilymphocyte globulin or bone-marrow transplantation. Br Med J 1981;282:860.
300. Liu JM, Auerbach AD, Young NS. Fanconi anemia presenting unexpectedly in an adult kindred with no dysmorphic features. Am J Med 1991;91:555.
301. Boggs DR, Joyce RA. The hematopoietic effects of lithium. Semin Hematol 1983;20:129.
302. Guinan EC, Sieff CA, Oette DH, Nathan DG. Granulocyte macrophage colony stimulating factor (GM-CSF) in aplastic anemia (AA). Pediatr Res 1989;25:151A.
303. Ferguson L, Hoots K, Beran M, Jeha S, Vedhan-Raj S, Gutterman J. Long-term bone marrow (BM) cultures with recombinant human granulocyte-macrophage colony stimulating factor (rhGM-CSF) in children with cytopenias: a correlation with clinical response. Blood 1988;72:115a.
304. Nathan DG. Hope for hematopoietic hormones. N Engl J Med 1987;317:626.
305. German J. Patterns of neoplasia associated with the chromosome-breakage syndromes. In: German J, ed. Chromosome mutation and neoplasia. New York, Alan R Liss, 1983:97.
306. Garriga S, Crosby WH. The incidence of leukemia in families of patients with hypoplasia of the marrow. Blood 1959;24:1008.
307. Swift M. Fanconi's anaemia in the genetics of neoplasia. Nature 1971;230:370.
308. Swift M. Malignant disease in heterozygous carriers. Birth Defects 1976;12:133.
309. Swift M, Caldwell RJ, Chase C. Reassessment of cancer predisposition of Fanconi anemia heterozygotes. J Natl Cancer Inst 1980;65:863.
310. Potter NU, Sarmousakis C, Li FP. Cancer in relatives of patients with aplastic anemia. Cancer Genet Cytogenet 1983;9:61.
311. Swift M, Sholman L, Gilmour D. Diabetes mellitus and the gene for Fanconi's anemia. Science 1972;178:308.
312. Morrell D, Chase CI, Kupper LL, Swift M. Diabetes mellitus in ataxia-telangiectasia, Fanconi anemia, xeroderma pigmentosum, common variable immune deficiency, and severe combined immune deficiency families. Diabetes 1986;35:143.
313. Gyger M, Perrault C, Belanger R, Bonny Y, Forest L, Lussier P. Unsuspected Fanconi's anemia and bone marrow transplantation in cases of acute myelomonocytic leukemia. N Engl J Med 1989;321:120.
314. Kwee ML, Kuyt LP. Fanconi anemia in the Netherlands. In: Schroeder-Kurth TM, Auerbach AD, Obe G, eds. Fanconi anemia: clinical, cytogenetic and experimental aspects. Berlin, Springer-Verlag, 1989:18.
315. Ahmed OA, Al-Rimawi HS, Al-Rashid AA, et al. Fanconi's anemia with acute lymphoblastic leukaemia in a Bedouin girl. Am Soc Hum Genet Suppl 1989;45:A14.
316. Sarna G, Tomasulo P, Lotz MJ, Bubinak JF, Shulman NR. Multiple neoplasia in two siblings with a variant form of Fanconi's anemia. Cancer 1975;36:1029.
317. Perrimond H, Juhan-Vague I, Thenieau D, Bayle J, Muratore R, Orsini A. Evolution medullaire et hépatique après androgénotherapie prolongée d'une anémie de Fanconi. Nouv Rev Fr Hematol 1977;18:228.
318. Obeid A, Hill FGH, Harnden D, Mann JR, Wood BSB. Fanconi anemia: oxymetholone hepatic tumors, and chromosome aberrations associated with leukemic transition. Cancer 1980;46:1401.
319. Bessho F, Mizutani S, Hayashi Y, Moriwaki K, Yokota S, Inaba T. Chronic myelomonocytic leukemia with chromosomal changes involving lp36 and hepatocellular carcinoma in a case of Fanconi's anemia. Eur J Haematol 1989;42:492.
320. Zawartka M, Restorff-Libiszowska H, Kowalski R, Litwiniszyn-Krzewicka K, Schejbal J. Bialaczka szpikowa w prezebiegu anemii Fanconiego (AF). Wiad Lek 1976;29:145.
321. Berger R, Bussel A, Schenmetzler C. Somatic segregation and Fanconi anemia. Clin Genet 1977;11:409.
322. Nowell P, Bergman G, Besa E, Wilmoth D, Emanuel B. Progressive preleukemia with a chromosomally abnormal clone in a kindred with the Estren-Dameshek variant of Fanconi's anemia. Blood 1984;64:1135.
323. Woods WG, Nesbit ME, Buckley J, et al. Correlation of chromosome abnormalities with patient characteristics, histologic subtype, and induction success in children with acute nonlymphocytic leukemia. J Clin Oncol 1985;3:3.
324. Van Gils JE, Mandel C, Van Weel-Sipman MH, De Koning J, Van'T Veer-Korthof ET. Acute leukemie bij Fanconi anemie. Tijdschr Kindergeneeskd 1987;55:68.
325. Dosik H, Hsu LY, Todaro GJ, Lee SL, Hirschhorn K, Selirio ES, Alter AA. Leukemia in Fanconi's anemia: cytogenetic and tumor virus susceptibility studies. Blood 1970;36:341.
326. Dosik H, Verma RS, Wilson C, Miotti AB. Fanconi's anemia and a familial stable chromosome abnormality in a family with multiple malignancies. Blood 1977;50:190a.
327. Bourgeois CA, Hill FGH. Fanconi anemia leading to acute myelomonocytic leukemia: cytogenetic studies. Cancer 1977;39:1163.
328. Kunze J. Estren-Dameshek-Anämie mit myelomonocytärer Leukämie (Subtyp der Fanconi-Anämie?). In: Spranger J, Tolksdorf M, eds. Klinische Genetik in der Pádiatrie. Stuttgart, Georg Thieme, 1980:213.
329. Gozdasoglu S, Cavdar AO, Arcasoy A, Babacan E, Sanal O. Fanconi's aplastic anemia: analysis of 18 cases. Acta Haematol 1980;64:131.
330. Roozendaal KJ, Nelis KOAH. Leukaemia in a case of Fanconi's anaemia. Clin Genet 1981;25:208.
331. Levy JM, Stoll C, Korn R. Sur un cas de leucémie aigue chez une fillette atteinte d'anémie de Fanconi: revue de la littérature. Nouv Rev Fr Hematol 1974;14:713.
332. Gastearena J, Giralt M, Orue MT, Oyarzabal FJ, Perez-Equiza E, Uriz MJ. Fanconi's anemia: clinical study of six cases. Am J Pediatr Hematol Oncol 1986;8:173.
333. Gastearena J, Orue MT, Perez Equiza E, et al. Eritroleucemia "transitoria" en la evolucion a leucemia monocitica aguda de una anemia de Fanconi. Sangre 1982;27:967.
334. Ahuja HG, Advani SH, Gopal R, Nair CN, Saikia T. Acute nonlymphoblastic leukemia in the first of three siblings affected with Fanconi's syndrome. Am J Pediatr Hematol Oncol 1986;8:347.
335. Aboin J, Villegas A, Suarez J, Gilsanz V. Eritroleucemia como fase final de anemia constitucional de Fanconi. Sangre 1973;28:416.
336. Taher A, Gilbert E, Shahidi NT. Erythroblastic islands in erythroleukemia. Am J Ped Hematol Oncol 1981;3:121.
337. Villegas A, Aboin J, Alvarez-Sala JL, Espinos D. Eritroleucemia en la evolucion de una anemia constitucional de Fanconi. Sangre 1983;28:225.
338. Götz M, Handel H, Pichler E, Weippl G. Fanconi-anämie: Ubergang in Leukämie und Erythrozytenstoffwechselbefunde. Kinderarztl Prax 1974;2:69.
339. Dharmasena F, Catchpole M, Erber W, Mason D, Gordon-Smith EC. Megakaryoblastic leukaemia and myelofibrosis complicating Fanconi anaemia. Scand J Haematol 1986;36:309.
340. Lisker R, De Gutierrez AC. Cytogenetic studies in Fanconi's anemia: description of a case with bone marrow clonal evolution. Clin Genet 1974;5:72.
341. Berger R, Le Coniat M. Cytogenetic studies in Fanconi anemia induced chromosomal breakage and cytogenetics. In: Schroeder-Kurth TM, Auerbach AD, Obe G, eds. Fanconi anemia: clinical, cytogenetic and experimental aspects. Berlin, Springer-Verlag, 1989:93.
342. Tanzer J, Frocrain C, Desmarest MC, Potiron M. Fragilité chromosomique revelée suelement par culture en presence de moutarde à l'azote dans 2 cas de maladie de Fanconi. Nouv Rev Fr Hematol 1981;23:XVI.
343. Schaison G, Jacquillat C, Bernard J. Les états preleucémiques existentils chez l'enfant? Arch Fr Pediatr 1979;36:643.
344. Huret JL, Benz E, Guilhot F, Brizard A, Tanzer J. Fluctuation of a clone 46,XX,i(7q) in bone marrow in a Fanconi anaemia. Hum Genet 1986;74:98.
345. Baron F, Sybert VP, Andrews RG. Cutaneous and extracutaneous neutrophilic infiltrates (Sweet syndrome) in three patients with Fanconi anemia. J Pediatr 1989;115:726.
346. Francis RC, Moir RA, Swift PN. The value of splenectomy in Fanconi's anaemia. Arch Dis Child 1955;30:439.
347. Kozhevnikov BA, Khodorenko CA. Cancer of the mucous membrane of the left side of the mouth associated with congenital hypoplastic Fanconi's anemia in a 14-year-old boy. Vestn Khir 1986;136:105.
348. Guy JT, Auslander MO. Androgenic steroids and hepatocellular carcinoma. Lancet 1973;1:148.
349. Schofield IDF, Worth AT. Malignant mucosal change in Fanconi's anemia. J Oral Surg 1980;38:619.
350. Kennedy AW, Hart WR. Multiple squamous-cell carcinomas in Fanconi's anemia. Cancer 1982;50:811.
351. Kaplan MJ, Sabio H, Wanebo HJ, Cantrell RW. Squamous cell carcinoma in the immunosuppressed patient: Fanconi's anemia. Laryngoscope 1985;95:771.
352. Aho S. Clinical conferences: case of Fanconi's anemia. Kyobu Geka 1980;33:397.
353. Gendal ES, Mendelson DS, Janus CL, Schlossberg I, Vogel JM. Squamous

cell carcinoma of the esophagus in Fanconi's anemia. Dysphagia 1988;2: 178.
354. Reed K, Ravikumar TS, Gifford RRM, Grage TB. The association of Fanconi's anemia and squamous cell carcinoma. Cancer 1983;52: 926.
355. Hill LS, Dennis PM, Fairham SA. Adenocarcinoma of the stomach and Fanconi's anaemia. Postgrad Med J 1981;57:404.
356. Arnold WJ, King CR, Magrina J, Masterson BJ. Squamous cell carcinoma of the vulva and Fanconi anemia. Int J Gynaecol Obstet 1980;18:395.
357. Ortonne JP, Jeune R, Coiffet J, Thivolet J. Squamous cell carcinomas in Fanconi's anemia. Arch Dermatol 1981;117:443.
358. Hersey P, Edwards A, Lewis R, Kemp A, McInnes J. Deficient natural killer cell activity in a patient with Fanconi's anaemia and squamous cell carcinoma: association with defect in interferon release. Clin Exp Immunol 1982;48:205.
359. Wilkinson EJ, Morgan LS, Friedrich EG Jr. Association of Fanconi's anemia and squamous-cell carcinoma of the lower female genital tract with condyloma acuminatum: a report of two cases. J Reprod Med 1984;29:447.
360. Vaitiekaitis AS, Grau WH. Squamous cell carcinoma of the mandible in Fanconi anemia: report of case. J Oral Surg 1980;38:372.
361. De Chadarevian J-P, Vekemans M, Bernstein M. Fanconi's anemia, medulloblastoma, Wilms' tumor, horseshoe kidney, and gonadal dysgenesis. Arch Pathol Lab Med 1985;109:367.
362. Puligandla B, Stass SA, Schumacher HR, Keneklis TP, Bollum FJ. Terminal deoxynucleotidyl transferase in Fanconi's anaemia. Lancet 1978;2:1263.
363. Schroeder TM. Genetically determined chromosome instability syndromes. Cytogenet Cell Genet 1982;33:119.
364. Evans DIK. Aplastic anaemia in childhood. In: Geary CG, ed. Aplastic anaemia. London, Bailliere Tindall, 1979:161.
365. Recant L, Lacy P. Fanconi's anemia and hepatic cirrhosis. Am J Med 1965;39:464.
366. Johnson FL, Feagler JR, Lerner KG, et al. Association of androgenic-anabolic steroid therapy with development of hepatocellular carcinoma. Lancet 1972;2:1273.
367. Cattan D, Kalifat R, Wautier J-L, Meignan S, Vesin P, Piet R. Maladie de Fanconi et cancer du foie. Arch Fr Mal App Dig 1974;63:41.
368. Mokrohisky ST, Ambruso DR, Hathaway WE. Fulminant hepatic neoplasia after androgen therapy. N Engl J Med 1977;296:1411.
369. Shapiro P, Ikeda RM, Ruebner BH, Connors MH, Halsted CC, Abildgaard CF. Multiple hepatic tumors and peliosis hepatis in Fanconi's anemia treated with androgens. Am J Dis Child 1977;131:1104.
370. Cap J, Ondrus B, Danihel L. Focal nodular hyperplasia of the liver and hepatocellular carcinoma in children with Fanconi's anemia after long-term treatment with androgens. Bratisl Lek Listy 1983;79:73.
371. Abbondanzo SL, Manz HJ, Klappenbach RS, Gootenberg JE. Hepatocellular carcinoma in an 11-year-old girl with Fanconi's anemia: report of a case and review of the literature. Am J Pediatr Hematol Oncol 1986;8:334.
372. Bernstein MS, Hunter RL, Yachnin S. Hepatoma and peliosis hepatis developing in a patient with Fanconi's anemia. N Engl J Med 1971;284: 1135.
373. Holder LE, Gnarra DJ, Lampkin BC, Nishiyama H, Perkins P. Hepatoma associated with anabolic steroid therapy. AJR 1975;124:638.
374. Sweeney EC, Evans DJ. Hepatic lesions in patients treated with synthetic anabolic steroids. J Clin Pathol 1976;29:626.
375. Corberand J, Pris J, Dutau G, Rumeau J-L, Regnier C. Association d'une maladie de Fanconi et d'une tumeur hépatique: chez une malade soumise à un traitement androgenique au long cours. Arch Fr Pediatr 1975;32:275.
376. Mulvihill JJ, Ridolfi RL, Schultz FR, Borzy MS, Haughton PBT. Hepatic adenoma in Fanconi anemia treated with oxymetholone. J Pediatr 1975;87:122.
377. Garel L, Kalifa G, Buriot D, Sauvegrain J. Multiple adenomas of the liver and Fanconi's anaemia. Ann Radiol 1980;24:53.
378. Schmidt E, Deeg HJ, Storb R. Regression of androgen-related hepatic tumors in patients with Fanconi's anemia following marrow transplantation. Transplantation 1984;37:452.
379. Sirinavin C, Trowbridge AA. Dyskeratosis congenita: clinical features and genetic aspects: report of a family and review of the literature. J Med Genet 1975;12:339.
380. Trowbridge AA, Sirinavin C, Linman JW. Dyskeratosis congenita: hematologic evaluation of a sibship and review of the literature. Am J Hematol 1977;3:143.
381. Costello MJ, Buncke CM. Dyskeratosis congenita. Arch Dermatol 1956;73:123.
382. Fudenberg HH, Goust JM, Vesole DH, Salinas CF. Active and suppressor T cells: diminution in a patient with dyskeratosis congenita and in first-degree relatives. Gerontology 1979;25:231.
383. Singh K, Kolalapudi S. Dyskeratosis congenita: report of the first case from India. J Dermatol 1986;13:54.
384. Addison M, Rice MS. The association of dyskeratosis congenita and Fanconi's anaemia. Med J Aust 1965;1:797.
385. Llistosella E, Moreno A, De Moragas JM. Dyskeratosis congenita with macular cutaneous amyloid deposits. Arch Dermatol 1984;120:1381.
386. Juneja HS, Elder FFB, Gardner FH. Abnormality of platelet size and T-lymphocyte proliferation in an autosomal recessive form of dyskeratosis congenita. Eur J Haematol 1987;39:306.
387. Sorrow JMJ, Hitch JM. Dyskeratosis congenita. Arch Dermatol 1963;88: 340.
388. Georgouras K. Dyskeratosis congenita. Aust J Dermatol 1965;8:36.
389. Rollier MR, Rollier M, Prost MA. Sur un cas de syndrome de Zinsser-Engman-Cole. Bull Soc Franc Dermatol Syphiligr 1966;73:383.
390. La Grutta A, Lo Curto M, Cammarata M, Villardita S. Dykeratosis congenita and panmyelopathy: report of a case (Fanconi-Zinsser). Haematologica (Pavia) 1980;65:481.
391. Javier G, Ortega JJ, Tuset M, Velazquez LE. Aplastic anemia associated with congenital dyskeratosis (Zinsser-Fanconi syndrome). Sangre 1981;26:367.
392. Ling NS, Fenske NA, Julius RL, Espinoza CG, Drake LA. Dyskeratosis congenita in a girl simulating chronic graft-vs-host disease. Arch Dermatol 1985;121:1424.
393. Duprey PA, Steger JW. An unusual case of dyskeratosis congenita with intracranial calcifications. J Am Acad Dermatol 1988;19:760.
394. Pai GS, Morgan S, Whetsell C. Etiologic heterogeneity in dyskeratosis congenita. Am J Med Genet 1989;32:63.
395. Conter V, Johnson FL, Paolucci P, Ruggiero M, Janco RL. Bone marrow transplantation for aplastic anemia associated with dyskeratosis congenita. Am J Pediatr Hematol Oncol 1988;10:99.
396. Drachtman R, Alter BP. Dyskeratosis congenita: clinical and genetic heterogeneity—report of a new case and review of the literature. Am J Pediatr Hematol Oncol 1992;14:297.
397. Degos MMR, Bernard J, Belaich S, Flandrin G, Varet B. Syndrome de Zinsser-Cole-Engman (Zinsser-Fanconi). Bull Soc Franc Dermatol Syphiligr 1969;76:15.
398. Scoggins RB, Prescott KJ, Asher GH, Blaylock WK, Bright RW. Dyskeratosis congenita with Fanconi-type anemia: investigations of immunologic and other defects. Clin Res 1971;19:409.
399. Auerbach AD, Lieblich LM, Ehrenbard L, Auerbach R, Chaganti FSK. Dyskeratosis congenita: cytogenetic studies in a family with an unusual pattern of inheritance. Am J Hum Genet 1979;31:87A.
400. Tchou P-K, Kohn T. Dyskeratosis congenita: an autosomal dominant disorder. J Am Acad Dermatol 1982;6:1034.
401. Connor JM, Gatherer D, Gray FC, Pirrit LA, Affara NA. Assignment of the gene for dyskeratosis congenita to Xq28. Hum Genet 1987;72:348.
402. Texier L, Maleville J. La symptomatologie cutanée de l'anémie perniciosiforme de Fanconi: rapports avec la dyskératose congénitale de Zinsser-Cole-Engman. Ann Dermatol Syphiligr 1963;90:553.
403. Steier W, Van Voolen GA, Selmanowitz VJ. Dyskeratosis congenita: relationship to Fanconi's anemia. Blood 1972;39:510.
404. Inoue S, Mekanik G, Mahallati M, Zuelzer WWA. Dyskeratosis congenita with pancytopenia: another constitutional anemia. Am J Dis Child 1973;126:389.
405. Korz R, Wienert V, Knechten H. Dyskeratosis congenita (Zinsser-Engman-Cole-Syndrom) und Fanconi-Anamie. Hautarzt 1982;33:112.
406. Schneider A, Mayer U, Gebhart E, Harms D, Gromball J, Glockel U, Beck JD. Clastogen-induced fragility may differentiate pancytopenia of congenital dyskeratosis from Fanconi anaemia. Eur J Pediatr 1988;145:37.
407. Jacobs P, Saxe N, Gordon W, Nelson M. Dyskeratosis congenita. Haematologic, cytogenetic, and dermatologic studies. Scand J Haematol 1984;32:461.
408. Ortega JA, Swanson VL, Landing BH, Hammond GD. Congenital dyskeratosis. Zinsser-Engman-Cole syndrome with thymic dysplasia and aplastic anemia. Am J Dis Child 1972;124:701.
409. Pai GS, Morgan S, Tennyson R. Etiologic heterogeneity in dyskeratosis congenita. Clin Res 1988;36:60A.
410. Smith CM, II, Ramsay NKC, Branda R, Nesbit ME, Krivit W. Response to androgens in the constitutional aplastic anemia of dyskeratosis congenita (DC). Pediatr Res 1979;13:441.
411. Hanada T, Abe T, Nakazawa M, Aoki Y, Uyeno K. Bone marrow failure in dyskeratosis congenita. Scand J Haematol 1984;32:496.
412. Colvin BT, Baker H, Hibbin JA, Gordon-Smith MC, Gordon MY. Haemopoietic progenitor cells in dyskeratosis congenita. Br J Haematol 1984;56:513.
413. Friedland M, Lutton JD, Spitzer R, Levere RD. Dyskeratosis congenita with hypoplastic anemia: a stem cell defect. Am J Hematol 1985;20: 85.
414. Michalevicz R, Baron S, Nordan U, Rahmani R. Granulocytic macrophage colony stimulating factor restores in vitro growth of granulocyte-macrophage bone marrow hematopoietic progenitors in dyskeratosis congenita. Isr J Med Sci 1989;25:193.
415. Misawa M, Haku Y, Ifuku H, et al. Pancytopenia. Dyskeratosis congenita: a case report of dyskeratosis congenita with pancytopenia in special reference to hemopoietic stem cells. Rinsho Ketsueki 1982;23:1222.
416. Carter DM, Pan M, Gaynor A, Mcguire JS, Sibrack L. Psoralen-DNA cross-linking photoadducts in dyskeratosis congenita: delay in excision and promotion of sister chromatid exchange. J Invest Dermatol 1979;73: 97.
417. Kano Y, Fujiwara Y. Dyskeratosis congenita: survival, sister-chromatid exchange and repair following treatments with crosslinking agents. Mutat Res 1982;103:327.
418. Lam LH, Reynolds RJ. Repair of closely opposed cyclobutyl pyrimidine

dimers in UV-sensitive human diploid fibroblasts. Mutat Res 1986;166: 199.
419. Vuksanovic L, Cleaver JE. Unique cross-link and monoadduct repair characteristics of a xeroderma pigmentosum revertant cell line. Mutat Res 1987;184:255.
420. Burgdorf W, Kurvink K, Cervenka J. Sister chromatid exchange in dyskeratosis congenita lymphocytes. J Med Genet 1977;14:256.
421. Gutman A, Frumkin A, Adam A, Bloch-Shtacher H, Rozenszajn LA. X-linked dyskeratosis congenita with pancytopenia. Arch Dermatol 1976;114:1667.
422. Cole HN, Cole HNJ, Lascheid WP. Dyskeratosis congenita. Arch Dermatol 1957;76:712.
423. Garb J. Dyskeratosis congenita with pigmentation, dystrophia unguium, and leukoplakia oris: a follow-up report of two brothers. Arch Dermatol 1958;77:704.
424. Kubicz J. Syndroma Zinsser-Engman-Cole cum dyschromia extensiva corporis. Pezegl Derm 1970;57:239.
425. Cannell H. Dyskeratosis congenita. Br J Oral Surg 1971;9:8.
426. Connor JM, Teague RH. Dyskeratosis congenita: report of a large kindred. Br J Dermatol 1981;105:321.
427. Kopysc Z, Jankowska-Skrzypek A, Bielniak J, Sokolowska B, Grochowina T. Zinsser-Engman-Cole syndrome (dyskeratosis congenita) in a 13-year-old boy. Wiad Lek 1988;41:525.
428. Costello MJ. Dyskeratosis congenita with superimposed prickle-cell epithelioma on the dorsal aspect of the left hand. Arch Dermatol 1957;75:451.
429. Marsh JCW, Will AJ, Hows JM, et al. "Stem cell" origin of the hematopoietic defect in dyskeratosis congenita. Blood 1992;79:3138.
430. Woog JJ, Dortzbach RK, Wexler SA, Shahidi NT. The role of aminocaproic acid in lacrimal surgery in dyskeratosis congenita. Am J Ophthalmol 1985;100:728.
431. Mahmoud HK, Schaefer UW, Schmidt CG, Becher R, Götz GF, Richter HJ. Marrow transplantation for pancytopenia in dyskeratosis congenita. Blut 1985;51:57.
432. Lemarchand-Venencie F, Gluckman E, Devergie A, Civatte J. Syndrome de Zinsser-Cole-Engmann. Ann Dermatol Venereol (Paris) 1982;109: 783.
433. Gluckman E, Esperou H, Devergie A, Traineau R, Leverger G, Schaison G. Pediatric bone marrow transplantation for leukemia and aplastic anemia: report of 222 cases transplanted in a single center. Nouv Rev Fr Hematol 1989;31:111.
434. Shwachman H, Diamond LK, Oski FA, Khaw K-T. The syndrome of pancreatic insufficiency and bone marrow dysfunction. J Pediatr 1964;65:645.
435. Bodian M, Sheldon W, Lightwood R. Congenital hypoplasia of the exocrine pancreas. Acta Paediatr 1964;53:282.
436. Aggett PJ, Cavanagh NPC, Matthew DJ, Pincott JR, Sutcliffe J, Harries JT. Shwachman's syndrome: a review of 21 cases. Arch Dis Child 1980;55:331.
437. Burke V, Colebatch JH, Anderson CM, Simons MJ. Association of pancreatic insufficiency and chronic neutropenia in childhood. Arch Dis Child 1967;42:147.
438. Shwachman H, Holsclaw D. Some clinical observations on the Shwachman syndrome (pancreatic insufficiency and bone marrow hypoplasia). Birth Defects 1972;8(3):46.
439. Hill RE, Durie PR, Gaskin KJ, Davidson GP, Forstner GG. Steatorrhea and pancreatic insufficiency in Shwachman syndrome. Gastroenterology 1982;83:22.
440. Ozsoylu S, Argun G. Tryptic activity of the duodenal juice in aplastic anemia. J Pediatr 1967;70:60.
441. Pearson HA, Lobel JS, Kocoshis SA, et al. A new syndrome of refractory sideroblastic anemia with vacuolization of marrow precursors and exocrine pancreatic dysfunction. J Pediatr 1979;95:976.
442. Stoddard RA, McCurnin DC, Shultenover SJ, Wright JE, DeLemos RA. Syndrome of refractory sideroblastic anemia with vacuolization of marrow precursors and exocrine pancreatic dysfunction presenting in the neonate. J Pediatr 1981;99:259.
443. Demeocq F, Storme G, Schaison G, Bezou MJ, Bourges M, Chassagne J. Anémie réfractaire sidéroblastique avec vacuolisation des précurseurs médullaires et déficit de la fonction exocrine du pancreas: étude d'une nouvelle observation. Arch Fr Pediatr 1983;40:631.
444. Rotig A, Cormier V, Blanche S, et al. Pearson's marrow–pancreas syndrome: a multisystem mitochondrial disorder in infancy. J Clin Invest 1990;86:1601.
445. McKusick VA, Eldridge R, Hostetler JA, Ruangwit U, Egeland JA. Dwarfism in the Amish. II. Cartilage-hair hypoplasia. Bull Johns Hopkins Hosp 1965;116:285.
446. Virolainen M, Savilahti E, Kaitila I, Perheentupa J. Cellular and humoral immunity in cartilage-hair hypoplasia. Pediatr Res 1978;12:961.
447. Trojak JE, Polmar SH, Winkelstein JA, et al. Immunologic studies of cartilage-hair hypoplasia in the Amish. Johns Hopkins Med J 1981;148: 157.
448. Lux SE, Johnston RB Jr, August CS, et al. Chronic neutropenia and abnormal cellular immunity in cartilage-hair hypoplasia. N Engl J Med 1970;282:231.
449. Burgert EO, Dower JC, Tauxe WN. A new syndrome: a regenerative anemia, malabsorption (celiac), dyschondroplasia and hypophosphatemia. J Pediatr 1965;67:711.
450. Thong YH. Impaired neutrophil kinesis in a patient with the Shwachman-Diamond syndrome. Aust Paediatr J 1978;14:34.
451. Aggett PJ, Harries JT, Harvey BAM, Soothill JF. An inherited defect of neutrophil mobility in Shwachman syndrome. J Pediatr 1979;94:391.
452. Ruutu P, Savilahati E, Repo H, Kosunen TU. Constant defect in neutrophil locomotion but with age decreasing susceptibility to infection in Shwachman syndrome. Br J Haematol 1984;70:502.
453. Hudson E, Aldor T. Pancreatic insufficiency and neutropenia with associated immunoglobulin deficit. Arch Intern Med 1970;125:314.
454. Saunders EF, Gall G, Freedman MH. Granulopoiesis in Shwachman's syndrome (pancreatic insufficiency and bone marrow dysfunction). Pediatrics 1979;64:515.
455. Ikuta K, Sasaki H, Koiso Y, et al. A case of Shwachman's syndrome (pancreatic insufficiency and bone marrow dysfunction): evaluation of hemopoietic disorder by in vitro culture technique. Jpn J Clin Hematol 1980;21:1989.
456. Woods WG, Krivit W, Lubin BH, Ramsay NKC. Aplastic anemia associated with the Shwachman syndrome: in vivo and in vitro observations. Am J Pediatr Hematol Oncol 1981;3:347.
457. Woods WG, Roloff JS, Lukens JN, Krivit W. The occurrence of leukemia in patients with the Shwachman syndrome. J Pediatr 1981;99:425.
458. Suda T, Ikuta K, Mizoguchi H, et al. Hemopoietic colony-forming cells in Shwachman's syndrome. Am J Pediatr Hematol Oncol 1982;4:129.
459. Bonilla MA, Gilmore B, Gillio AP, et al. In vivo administration of recombinant human G-CSF corrects the neutropenia associated with Schwachman-Diamond syndrome. Blood 1989;74:324a.
460. Tsai PH, Sahdev I, Herry A, Lipton JM. Fatal cyclophosphamide-induced congestive heart failure in a 10-year-old boy with Shwachman-Diamond syndrome and severe bone marrow failure treated with allogeneic bone marrow transplantation. Am J Pediatr Hematol Oncol 1989;12:472.
461. Nezeloff C, Watchi M. L'hypoplasie congénitale lipomateuse du pancreas exocrine chez l'enfant (deux observations et revue de la littérature). Arch Fr Pediatr 1961;18:1135.
462. Huijgens PC, Van Der Veen EA, Meijer S, Muntinghe OG. Syndrome of Shwachman and leukaemia. Scand J Haematol 1977;18:20.
463. Strevens MJ, Lilleyman JS, Williams RB. Shwachman's syndrome and acute lymphoblastic leukaemia. Br Med J 1978;2:18.
464. Caselitz J, Klöppel G, Delling G, Grüttner R, Holdhoff U, Stern M. Shwachman's syndrome and leukaemia. Virchows Arch [A] 1979;385: 109.
465. Gretillat F, Delepine N, Taillard F, Desbois JC, Misset JL. Shwachman's syndrome transformed into leukaemia. Presse Med 1985;14:45.
466. De Vaal OM, Seynhaeve V. Reticular dysgenesia. Lancet 1959;2:1123.
467. DeWitte DB, Buick MK, Cyran SE, Maisels MJ. Neonatal pancytopenia and severe combined immunodeficiency associated with antenatal administration of azathioprine and prednisone. J Pediatr 1984;105:625.
468. Alter BP. Neonatal pancytopenia after maternal azathioprine therapy. J Pediatr 1985;106:691.
469. Roper M, Parmley RT, Crist WM, Kelly DR, Cooper MD. Severe congenital leukopenia (reticular dysgenesis). Am J Dis Child 1985;139:832.
470. Gitlin D, Vawter G, Craig JM. Thymic alymphoplasia and congenital aleukocytosis. Pediatrics 1964;33:184.
471. Alonso K, Dew JM, Starke WR. Thymic alymphoplasia and congenital aleukocytosis (reticular dysgenesia). Arch Pathol 1972;94:179.
472. Ownby DR, Pizzo S, Blackmon L, Gall SA, Buckley RH. Severe combined immunodeficiency with leukopenia (reticular dysgenesis) in siblings: immunologic and histopathologic findings. J Pediatr 1976;89:382.
473. Haas RJ, Niethammer D, Goldmann SF, Heit W, Bienzle U, Kleihauer E. Congenital immunodeficiency and agranulocytosis (reticular dysgenesia). Acta Paediatr Scand 1977;66:279.
474. Espanol T, Compte J, Alvarez C, Tallada N, Laverde R, Peguero G. Reticular dysgenesis: report of two brothers. Clin Exp Immunol 1979;38: 615.
475. Levinsky RJ, Tiedeman K. Successful bone-marrow transplantation for reticular dysgenesis. Lancet 1983;1:671.
476. Bizzaro N, Dianese G. Neonatal alloimmune amegakaryocytosis. Vox Sang 1988;54:112.
477. Roberts MH, Smith MH. Thrombopenic purpura. Am J Dis Child 1950;79:820.
478. Matoth Y, Mundel G. Isolated megakaryocytopenia. Acta Haematol 1954;12:209.
479. Bernard J, Boivin P, Caen J. Les cytopénies hypoplastiques congénitales dissociées: purpura thrombopénique congénital avec mégacaryocytopénie—neutropénie congénitale. Sem Hop Paris 1956;28:1597.
480. Bernheim M, Monnet P, Germain D. La thrombopénie hypoplastique amégacaryocytic congénitale. Pediatrie 1963;28:367.
481. Smith CH. Aplastic anemia with onset as congenital thrombocytopenic purpura: blood diseases of infancy and childhood. St Louis, CV Mosby, 1966:714.
482. Berry AM, Agarwal KN, Bajaj G. Congenital amegakaryocytic thrombocytopenia. J Indian Med Assoc 1968;50:209.
483. Buchanan GR, Scher CS, Button LN, Nathan DG. Use of homologous platelet survival in the differential diagnosis of chronic thrombocytopenia in childhood. Pediatrics 1977;59:49.
484. Van Oostrom CG, Wilms RHH. Congenital thrombocytopenia, associated with raised concentrations of haemoglobin F. Helv Paediatr Acta 1978;33:59.

485. Freedman MH. Congenital failure of hematopoiesis in the newborn infant. Clin Perinatol 1984;11:417.
486. Griffiths AD. Constitutional aplastic anaemia: a family with a new X linked variety of amegakaryocytic thrombocytopenia. J Med Genet 1983;20:361.
487. Gardner RJM, Morrison PS, Abbott GD. A syndrome of congenital thrombocytopenia with multiple malformations and neurologic dysfunction. J Pediatr 1983;102:600.
488. Greenwald HM, Sherman I. Congenital essential thrombocytopenia. Am J Dis Child 1929;38:1245.
489. Zetterstrom R, Strindberg B. Sporadic congenital spherocytosis associated with congenital hypoplastic thrombocytopenia and malformations. Acta Paediatr 1958;47:14.
490. Saracco P, Martano C, Bracco G, Fabris C, Miniero R. A case report of congenital amegacaryocytic thrombocytopenia. Panminerva Med 1983;25:23.
491. Landolt RF. Kongenitale (neonatale) Thrombopenien. Helv Paed Acta 1948;3:3.
492. Eisenstein EM. Congenital amegakaryocytic thrombocytopenic purpura. Clin Pediatr 1966;5:143.
493. Høyeraal HM, Lamvik J, Moe PJ. Congenital hypoplastic thrombocytopenia and cerebral malformations in two brothers. Acta Paediatr Scand 1970;59:185.
494. Hreidarsson S, Kristjansson K, Johannesson G, Johannsson JH. A syndrome of progressive pancytopenia with microcephaly, cerebellar hypoplasia and growth failure. Acta Paediatr Scand 1988;77:773.
495. Akerren Y, Reinard T. Thrombocytopenia in the new-born period. Acta Med Scand 1950(ppl.246:281.
496. Mibashan RS, Millar DS. Fetal haemophilia and allied bleeding disorders. Br Med Bull 1983;39:392.
497. Arias S, Penchaszadeh VB, Pinto-Cisternas J, Larrauri S. The IVIC syndrome: a new autosomal dominant complex pleiotropic syndrome with radial ray hypoplasia, hearing impairment, external ophthalmoplegia, and thrombocytopenia. Am J Med Genet 1980;6:25.
498. Sammito V, Motta D, Capodieci G, Sanfilippo S, Neri G. IVIC syndrome: report of a second family. Am J Med Genet 1988;29:875.
499. Czeizel A, Goblyos P, Kodaj I. IVIC Syndrome: report of a third family. Am J Med Genet 1989;32:282.
500. Gonzalez CH, Durkin-Stamm MV, Geimer NF, et al. The WT syndrome: a "new" autosomal dominant pleiotropic trait of radial/ulnar hypoplasia with high risk of bone marrow failure and/or leukemia. Birth Defects 1977;13(3B):31.
501. Alter CL, Levine PH, Bennett J, et al. Dominantly transmitted hematologic dysfunction clinically similar to Fanconi's anemia. Am J Hematol 1989;32:241.
502. Aufderheide AC. Familial cytopenia and vascular disease: a newly recognized autosomal dominant condition. Birth Defects 1972;8(3): 63.
503. Dokal I, Ganly P, Riebero I, et al. Late onset bone marrow failure associated with proximal fusion of radius and ulna: a new syndrome. Br J Haematol 1989;71:277.
504. Kato J, Niitsu Y, Ishigaki S, et al. Chronic hypoplastic neutropenia: a case of familial occurrence of chronic hypoplastic neutropenia and aplastic anemia. Rinsho Ketsueki 1986;27:407.
505. Li FP, Potter NU, Buchanan GR, Vawter G, Whang-Peng J, Rosen RB. A family with acute leukemia, hypoplastic anemia and cerebellar ataxia: association with bone marrow C-monosomy. Am J Med 1978;65: 933.
506. Li FP, Hecht F, Kaiser-McCaw B, Baranko PV, Potter NU. Ataxia-pancytopenia: syndrome of cerebellar ataxia, hypoplastic anemia, monosomy 7, and acute myelogenous leukemia. Cancer Genet Cytogenet 1981;4:189.
507. Daghistani D, Curless R, Toledano SR, Ayyar DR. Ataxia-pancytopenia and monosomy 7 syndrome. J Pediatr 1989;115:108.
508. Sleijfer DT, Mulder NH, Niewig HO, Anders GJPA, Gouw W-L. Acquired pancytopenia in relatives of patients with aplastic anaemia. Acta Med Scand 1980;207:397.
509. Abels D, Reed WB. Fanconi-like syndrome: immunologic deficiency, pancytopenia, and cutaneous malignancies. Arch Dermatol 1973;107: 419.
510. Linsk JA, Khoory MS, Meyers KR. Myeloid, erythroid, and immune system defects in a family: a new stem-cell disorder? Ann Intern Med 1975;82:659.
511. Chitambar CR, Robinson WA, Globe LM. Familial leukemia and aplastic anemia associated with monosomy 7. Am J Med 1983;75:756.
512. Li FP, Marchetto DJ, Vawter GR. Acute leukemia and preleukemia in eight males in a family: an X-linked disorder? Am J Hematol 1979;6: 61.
513. Purtilo DT, Sakamoto K, Barnabei V, Seeley J, Bechtold T, Rogers G, Yetz J, Harada S. Epstein-Barr virus–induced diseases in boys with the X-linked lymphoproliferative syndrome (XLP): update on studies of the registry. Am J Med 1982;73:49.
514. Samad FU, Engel E, Hartmann RC. Hypoplastic anemia, Friedreich's ataxia and chromosomal breakage: case report and review of similar disorders. South Med J 1973;66:135.
515. Sackey K, Sakati N, Aur RJA, Shebib S, Sabbah RS, Rifai S. Multiple dysmorphic features and pancytopenia: a new syndrome? Clin Genet 1985;27:606.
516. Poole S, Smith ACM, Hays T, Clemmens M, McGavran L. Fanconi anemia in monozygotic twin females. Am J Hum Genet 1988;43:A65.
517. Neri G, Sammito V. Re: IVIC syndrome report by Czeizel et al. Am J Med Genet 1989;33:284.
518. Skare JC, Milunsky A, Byron KS, Sullivan JL. Mapping the X-linked lymphoproliferative syndrome. Proc Natl Acad Sci USA 1987;84: 2015.
519. Nowell P, Besa E, Emanuel B, Pathak S, Finan J. Two adult siblings with thrombocytopenia and a familial 13;14 translocation. Cancer Genet Cytogenet 1984;11:169.
520. Rosenthal RL, Blackman A. Bone-marrow hypoplasia following use of chloramphenicol eye drops. JAMA 1965;191:148.
521. Nora AH, Fernbach DJ. Acquired aplastic anemia in children. Texas Med 1969;65:38.
522. Nagao T, Mauer AM. Concordance for drug-induced aplastic anemia in identical twins. N Engl J Med 1969;281:7.
523. Polak BCP, Wesseling H, Schut D, Herxheimer A, Meyler L. Blood dyscrasias attributed to chloramphenicol: a review of 576 published and unpublished cases. Acta Med Scand 1972;192:409.
524. Boga M, Szemere PA. Infectious hepatitis and aplastic anaemia: in two sisters. Lancet 1971;2:708.
525. Sears DA, George JN, Gold MS. Transient red blood cell aplasia in association with viral hepatitis: occurrence four years apart in siblings. Arch Intern Med 1975;135:1585.
526. Davidson LSP, Davis LJ, Innes J. Studies in refractory anaemia. Edinb Med J 1943;50:355.
527. McLaren GD, Doukas MA, Muir WA. Methyprylon-induced bone marrow suppression in siblings. JAMA 1978;240:1744.
528. Stolte JB. Familiäre aplastische Anämie. Ned Tijdschr Geneeskd 1948;92:4053.
529. Keiser G. Erworbene Panmyelopathien. Schweiz Med Wochenschr 1970;100:1938.
530. Weinstein HJ. Congenital leukemia and the neonatal myeloproliferative disorders associated with Down's syndrome. Clin Haematol 1978;7: 147.
531. Erdogan G, Aksoy M, Dincol K. A case of idiopathic aplastic anemia associated with trisomy-21 and partial endoreduplication. Acta Haematol 1967;37:137.
532. Vetrella M, Barthelmai W, Matsuda H. Kongenitale amegakaryocytare Thrombocytopenie mit finaler Pancytopenie bei Trisomie 21 mit cystischer Pankreasfibrose. Z Kinderheilkd 1969;107:210.
533. Weinblatt ME, Higgins G, Ortega JA. Aplastic anemia in Down's syndrome. Pediatrics 1981;67:896.
534. McWilliams NB, Dunn NL. Aplastic anemia and Down's syndrome. Pediatrics 1982;69:501.
535. Hanukoglu A, Meytes D, Fried A, Rosen N, Shacked N. Fatal aplastic anemia in a child with Down's syndrome. Acta Paediatr Scand 1987;76: 539.
536. Kuster W, Majewski F. The Dubowitz syndrome. Eur J Pediatr 1986;144: 574.
537. Walters TR, Desposito F. Aplastic anemia in Dubowitz syndrome. J Pediatr 1985;106:622.
538. Berthold F, Fuhrmann W, Lampert F. Fatal aplastic anaemia in a child with features of Dubowitz syndrome. Eur J Pediatr 1987;146:605.
539. Grobe H. Dubowitz syndrome and acute lymphatic leukemia. Monatsschr Kinderheilkd 1983;131:467.
540. Sauer O, Spelger G. Dubowitz syndrome with immunodeficiency and solid malignant tumor in two siblings. Monatsschr Kinderheilkd 1977;125:885.
541. Majewski F, Goecke T. Studies of microcephalic primordial dwarfism. I. Approach to a delineation of the Seckel syndrome. Am J Med Genet 1982;12:7.
542. Upjohn C. Familial dwarfism associated with microcephaly, mental retardation and anemia. Proc Soc Med 1955;48:334.
543. Seckel HPG. Bird-headed dwarfs. Basel, S Karger, 1960.
544. Lilleyman JS. Constitutional hypoplastic anemia associated with familial "bird-headed" dwarfism (Seckel syndrome). Am J Pediatr Hematol Oncol 1984;6:207.
545. Butler MG, Hall BD, Maclean RN, Lozzio CB. Do some patients with Seckel syndrome have hematological problems and/or chromosome breakage? Am J Med Genet 1987;27:645.
546. Cervenka J, Tsuchiya H, Ishiki T, Suzuki M, Mori H. Seckel's dwarfism: analysis of chromosome breakage and sister chromatid exchanges. Am J Dis Child 1979;133:555.
547. Josephs HW. Anaemia of infancy and early childhood. Medicine 1936;15:307.
548. Diamond LK, Blackfan KD. Hypoplastic anemia. Am J Dis Child 1938;56: 464.
549. Alter BP. Childhood red cell aplasia. Am J Pediatr Hematol Oncol 1980;2:121.
550. Diamond LK, Wang WC, Alter BP. Congenital hypoplastic anemia. Adv Pediatr 1976;22:349.
551. Alter BP, Nathan DG. Red cell aplasia in children. Arch Dis Child 1979;54:263.
552. Davel JGA, Cronje RE. Congenital hypoplastic anaemia with aminoaciduria in a Bantu infant. S Afr Med J 1962;36:226.
553. Shapiro H, White W, Diseker M, Bentley HPJ. Congenital (erythroid) hypoplastic anemia. Am J Dis Child 1964;108:674.

554. Ibrahim JM, Rawstron J, Booth J. A case of red cell aplasia in a Negro child. Arch Dis Child 1966;41:213.
555. Starling KA, Fernbach DJ. Congenital hypoplastic anemia: review of eight cases. Texas Med 1967;63:63.
556. Hankes LV, Brown RR, Schiffer L, Schmaeler M. Tryptophan metabolism in humans with various types of anemias. Blood 1968;32:649.
557. Chitiyo ME, Maar SA, Pritchard J. A case of congenital erythroid hypoplasia in an African infant (Diamond-Blackfan syndrome). Cent Afr J Med 1969;15:226.
558. Falter ML, Robinson MG. Autosomal dominant inheritance and amino aciduria in Blackfan-Diamond anaemia. J Med Genet 1972;9:64.
559. Starling KA, Fernbach DJ. Hypoplastic anemia. J Pediatr 1973;82:735.
560. Akinyanju O, Johnson A. Congenital red cell aplasia with splenic and other abnormalities in an African child. Niger Med J 1975;5:381.
561. Guillozet N, Mbantankhu JF. Congenital hypoplastic red cell anaemia of childhood (the Blackfan-Diamond syndrome): case report, diagnosis and management. East Afr Med J 1977;54:345.
562. Kinoti SN, Kasili EG, Bwibo NO. Congenital pure red cell aplasia (case reports from Kenya). East Afr Med J 1978;55:530.
563. Steinberg MH, Coleman MF, Pennebaker JB. Diamond-Blackfan syndrome: evidence for T-cell mediated suppression of erythroid development and a serum blocking factor associated with remission. Br J Haematol 1979;41:57.
564. Altman AC, Gross S. Severe congenital hypoplastic anemia: transmission from a healthy female to opposite sex step-siblings. Am J Pediatr Hematol Oncol 1983;5:99.
565. Knutsen AP, O'Connor DM. Antibody deficiency with normal immunoglobulins in a child with hypoplastic anemia. Clin Immunol Immunopathol 1985;36:330.
566. Tada K, Kudo T, Nakagawa I, et al. Anémie congénitale hypoplastique. Arch Fr Pediatr 1958;15:183.
567. Fujiwara K, Matsumura T, Tanaka T, et al. Congenital pure red cell anemia: a case of congenital pure red cell anemia, accompanied by thenar defect, syndactyly, and cardiovascular anomalies. Rinsho Ketsueki 1981;22:1948.
568. Sawada K. Studies on the pathogenesis of congenital hypoplastic anemia (Diamond-Blackfan syndrome). Hokkaido Igaku Zasshi 1986;72:61.
569. Ogasawara T, Kasahara H, Watanabe T, Izawa M, Takagi S, Hirose I. A case report of constitutional erythroid hypoplasia (Josephs-Blackfan-Diamond type) with immunodeficiency. Jpn J Pedodontics 1987;25:174.
570. Kojima S, Matsuyama K. Congenital hypoplastic (Diamond-Blackfan) anemia: a possible role of natural killer cells in erythropoietic suppression. Acta Haematol Jpn 1988;51:698.
571. Horita S, Koizumi S, Miura M, Nakarai T, Katayama Y, Taniguchi N. Impaired ability of T4+ lymphocytes in the active stage of congenital hypoplastic anemia to promote in vitro growth of blood erythroid burst-forming units (BFU-E). Acta Haematol Jpn 1988;51:985.
572. Khatua SP. Congenital hypoplastic anaemia (pure red cell type). Indian Pediatr 1964;1:276.
573. Sharda DC, Seif Eldin SA, Qattawi S. Congenital (erythroid) hypoplastic anemia (Diamond-Blackfan syndrome). Indian Pediatr 1982;19:803.
574. Ambruso DR, Mahony BS, Githens JH, Rhoades ED. Effect of subcutaneous deferoxamine and oral vitamin C on iron excretion in congenital hypoplastic anemia and refractory anemia associated with the 5q− syndrome. Am J Pediatr Hematol Oncol 1982;4:115.
575. Wallman IS. Hereditary red cell aplasia. Med J Aust 1956;2:488.
576. Gray PH. Pure red-cell aplasia: occurrence in three generations. Med J Aust 1982;1:519.
577. Balaban EP, Buchanan GR, Graham. M., Frenkel EP. Diamond-Blackfan syndrome in adult patients. Am J Med 1985;78:533.
578. Förare S-A. Pure red cell anaemia in step siblings. Acta Paediatr 1963;52:159.
579. Mott MG, Apley J, Raper AB. Congenital (erythroid) hypoplastic anaemia: modified expression in males. Arch Dis Child 1969;44:757.
580. Hunter RE, Hakami N. The occurrence of congenital hypoplastic anemia in half brothers. J Pediatr 1972;81:346.
581. Viskochil DH, Carey JC, Glader BE, Rothstein G, Christensen RD. Congenital hypoplastic (Diamond-Blackfan) anemia in seven members of one kindred. Am J Med Genet 1990;35:251.
582. Diamond LK, Allen DM, Magill FB. Congenital (erythroid) hypoplastic anemia. Am J Dis Child 1961;102:403.
583. Wang WC, Mentzer W, Alter B. Congenital hypoplastic anemia—Diamond-Blackfan syndrome: comments and additional data on clinical aspects of Diamond-Blackfan syndrome. Blood Cells 1978;4:215.
584. Hamilton PJ, Dawson AA, Galloway WH. Congenital erythroid hypoplastic anaemia in mother and daughter. Arch Dis Child 1974;49:71.
585. Lawton JWM, Aldrich JE, Turner TL. Congenital erythroid hypoplastic anaemia: autosomal dominant transmission. Scand J Haematol 1974;13:276.
586. Brody J. Diamond-Blackfan syndrome in father and son. Aust Paediatr J 1982;18:128.
587. McFarland G, Say B, Carpenter NJ, Plunket DC. A condition resembling congenital hypoplastic anemia occurring in a mother and son. Clin Pediatr 1982;12:755.
588. Michelson AD. Inheritance of Diamond-Blackfan anaemia. Med J Aust 1982;2:409.
589. Gardner FH, Nathan DG. Hypochromic anemia and hemochromatosis: response to combined testosterone, pyridoxine, and liver extract therapy. Trans Am Clin Climatol Assoc 1961;73:121.
590. Krivit W, Nelson E, Sundberg D. Erythrogenesis imperfecta in seven individuals in three generations. Pediatr Res 1978;12:467.
591. Sacrez R, Levy J-M, Godar G, Castanier J. Anémie de Blackfan-Diamond associée a des malformations multiples. Med Infant 1965;72:493.
592. Giblett ER, Ammann AJ, Wara DW, Sandman R, Diamond LK. Nucleoside-phosphorylase deficiency in a child with severely defective T-cell immunity and normal B-cell immunity. Lancet 1975;1:1010.
593. Ramavat LG. Diamond Blackfan syndrome with congenital dislocation of right hip. Indian Pediatr 1978;15:179.
594. Lubani MM, Sharda DC, Qattawi SA, A1-Shab T, Hassanein AA. Congenital hypoplastic anaemia in Arab children (Diamond-Blackfan syndrome). Ann Trop Paediatr 1987;7:227.
595. Burgert EO Jr, Kennedy RLJ, Pease GL. Congenital hypoplastic anemia. Pediatrics 1954;13:218.
596. Gordon RR, Varadi S. Congenital hypoplastic anaemia (pure red-cell anaemia) with periodic erythroblastopenia. Lancet 1962;1:296.
597. Bernard J, Seligmann M, Chassigneux J, Dresch C. Anémie de Blackfan-Diamond. Nouv Rev Fr Hematol 1962;2:721.
598. Seligmann M, Bernard J, Chassigneux J, Dresch C. Anemia hypoplastique familiale. Nouv Rev Fr Hematol 1963;3:209.
599. Ravaille C, Ravaille-Mauer ML. Deux cas de maladie de Blackfan-Diamond dans la meme famille, avec bifidite du pouce et résultat favorable du traitement hormonal chez l'ainé. Pediatrie 1965;20:51.
600. Tartaglia AP, Propp S, Amarose AP, Propp RP, Hall CA. Chromosome abnormality and hypocalcemia in congenital erythroid hypoplasia (Blackfan-Diamond syndrome). Am J Med 1966;41:990.
601. Hildner FJ, Monto RW, Rebuck JW. Congenital erythroblastic hypoplasia: treatment of transfusion hemosiderosis with desferrioxamine B. Henry Ford Hosp Med J 1968;16:147.
602. Aase JM, Smith DW. Congenital anemia and triphalangeal thumbs: a new syndrome. J Pediatr 1969;74:471.
603. Sensenbrenner JA. Congenital hypoplastic anemia of Blackfan and Diamond in sibs. In: Bergsma D, ed. The clinical delineation of birth defects. XIV. Blood. Baltimore, Williams & Wilkins, 1972:166.
604. Rafinska J, Bernatowska E. Multiple developmental anomalies in Blackfan-Diamond anaemia of familial occurrence. Pol Tyg Lek 1974;29:61.
605. Geller G, Krivit W, Zalusky R, Zanjani ED. Lack of erythropoietic inhibitory effect of serum from patients with congenital pure red cell aplasia. J Pediatr 1975;86:198.
606. Iskandar O, Jager MJ, Willenze R, Natarajan AT. A case of pure red cell aplasia with high incidence of spontaneous chromosome breakage: a possible x-ray sensitive syndrome. Hum Genet 1980;55:337.
607. Bello A, Dorantes S, Alvarez-Amaya C. La anemia hipoplastica en la edad pediatrica. Bol Med Hosp Infant Mex 1983;40:718.
608. Freedman MH. Diamond-Blackfan anemia. Am J Pediatr Hematol Oncol 1985;7:327.
609. Seip M, Zanussi GF. Cyclosporine in steroid-resistant Diamond-Blackfan anaemia. Acta Paediatr Scand 1988;77:464.
610. Visser GHA, Desmedt MCH, Meijboom EJ. Altered fetal cardiac flow patterns in pure red cell anaemia (the Blackfan-Diamond syndrome). Prenat Diagn 1988;8:525.
611. Waterkotte GW, McElfresh AE. Congenital pure red cell hypoplasia in identical twins. Pediatrics 1974;54:646.
612. Giblett ER, Varela JE, Finch CA. Damage of the bone marrow due to Rh antibody. Pediatrics 1956;17:37.
613. Schorr JB, Cohen ES, Schwarz A, Wallerstein H. Hypoplastic anemia in childhood. Jewish Mem Hosp Bull 1962;6/7:126.
614. Cathie IAB. Erythrogenesis imperfecta. Arch Dis Child 1950;25:313.
615. Harvey DR. Congenital hypoplastic anaemia. Proc R Soc Med 1966;59:490.
616. Murphy S, Lubin B. Triphalangeal thumbs and congenital erythroid hypoplasia: report of a case with unusual features. J Pediatr 1972;81:987.
617. Jones B, Thompson H. Triphalangeal thumbs associated with hypoplastic anemia. Pediatrics 1973;52:609.
618. Paradis D, Simard H. Erythroblastopénie congénitale, phalange surnuméraire au pouce et luxation de la hanche. Union Med Can 1974;103:1599.
619. Terheggen HG. Hypoplastische Anämie mit dreigliedrigem Daumen. Z Kinderheilkd 1974;118:71.
620. Van Weel-Sipman M, Van De Kamp JJP, De Koning J. A female patient with "Aase syndrome." J Pediatr 1977;91:753.
621. Higginbottom MC, Jones KL, Kung FH, Koch TK, Boyer JL. The Aase syndrome in a female infant. J Med Genet 1978;15:484.
622. Pfeiffer RA, Ambs E. The Aase syndrome: autosomal-recessive hereditary, connatal erythroid hypoplasia and triphalangeal thumbs. Monatsschr Kinderheilkd 1983;131:235.
623. Muis N, Beemer FA, Vandijken P, Klepdepater JM. The Aase syndrome: case report and review of the literature. Eur J Pediatr 1986;145:153.
624. D'Avanzo M, Pistoia V, Tolone C, Toraldo R, Santinelli R, Iafusco F. Aase-Smith syndrome: report of a new case. Br J Haematol 1988;70:125.
625. Halperin DS, Estrov Z, Freedman MH. Diamond-Blackfan anemia:

promotion of marrow erythropoiesis in vitro by recombinant interleukin-3. Blood 1989;73:1168.
626. Alter BP. Thumbs and anemia. Pediatrics 1978;62:613.
627. Marver HS. Studies on tryptophan metabolism. I. Urinary tryptophan metabolites in hypoplastic anemias and other hematologic disorders. J Lab Clin Med 1961;58:425.
628. Lundmark KM. Congenital hypoplastic anaemia. Acta Paediatr Scand 1966;162(Suppl):54.
629. Sjölin S, Wranne L. Treatment of congenital hypoplastic anaemia with prednisone. Scand J Haematol 1970;7:63.
630. Philippe N, Requin Ch, Germain D. Etudes chromosomiques dans 6 cas d'anémie de Blackfan-Diamond. Pediatrie 1971;26:47.
631. Zito GE, Lynch EC. Prednisone-responsive congenital erythroid hypoplasia. JAMA 1977;237:991.
632. Ortega JA, Lazerson J. Anagyrine-induced red cell aplasia, vascular anomaly, and skeletal dysplasia. J Pediatr 1987;111:87.
633. O'Gorman Hughes DW. Hypoplastic anaemia in infancy and childhood: erythroid hypoplasia. Arch Dis Child 1961;36:349.
634. Harris RE, Baehner RL, Gleiser S, Weaver DD, Hodes ME. Cartilage-hair hypoplasia, defective T-cell function, and Diamond-Blackfan anemia in an Amish child. Am J Med Genet 1981;8:291.
635. Buchanan GR, Alter BP, Holtkamp CA, Walsh EG. Platelet number and function in Diamond-Blackfan anemia. Pediatrics 1981;68:238.
636. Vogel P, Bassen FA. Sternal marrow of children in normal and in pathologic states. Am J Dis Child 1939;57:245.
637. Gasser C. Aplastische Anämie (chronische Erythroblastophthise) und Cortison. Schweiz Med Wochenschr 1951;81:1241.
638. Boxer LA, Hussey L, Clarke TL. Sideroblastic anemia following congenital erythroid hypoplasia. J Pediatr 1971;79:681.
639. Girot R, Griscelli C. Erythroblastopénie à rechutes: à propos d'un cas suivi pendant 22 ans. Nouv Rev Fr Hematol 1977;18:555.
640. Hammond D, Shore N, Movassaghi N. Production, utilization and excretion of erythropoietin. I. Chronic anemias. II. Aplastic crisis. III. Erythropoietic effects of normal plasma. Ann NY Acad Sci 1968;149: 516.
641. Altman KI, Miller G. A disturbance in tryptophan metabolism in congenital hypoplastic anaemia. Nature 1953;172:868.
642. Pearson HA, Cone TE Jr. Congenital hypoplastic anemia. Pediatrics 1957;19:192
643. Price JM, Brown RR, Pfaffenbach EC, Smith NJ. Excretion of urinary tryptophan metabolites by patients with congenital hypoplastic anemia (Diamond-Blackfan syndrome). J Lab Clin Med 1970;75:316.
644. Brookfield EG, Singh P. Congenital hypoplastic anemia associated with hypogammaglobulinemia. J Pediatr 1974;82:529.
645. Finlay JL, Shahidi NT, Horowitz S, Borcherding W, Hong R. Lymphocyte dysfunction in congenital hypoplastic anemia. J Clin Invest 1982;70: 619.
646. Feldges D, Schmidt R. Erythrogenesis imperfecta (Blackfan-Diamond-Anämie). Schweiz Med Wochenschr 1971;101:1813.
647. Fondu P, Mandelbaum IM, Stryckmans PA, Delalieux G, Heyder-Bruckner C, Loeb H. Un cas d'érythroblastopénie de l'enfant à début tardif. Nouv Rev Fr Hematol 1972;12:5.
648. Glader BE, Backer K, Diamond LK. Elevated erythrocyte adenosine deaminase activity in congenital hypoplastic anemia. N Engl J Med 1983;309:1486.
649. Zielke HR, Ozand PT, Luddy RE, Zinkham W, Schwartz AD, Sevdalian DA. Elevation of pyrimidine enzyme activities in the RBC of patients with congenital hypoplastic anaemia and their parents. Br J Haematol 1979;42:381.
650. Glader BE, Backer K. Comparative activity of erythrocyte adenosine deaminase and orotidine decarboxylase in Diamond-Blackfan anemia. Am J Hematol 1986;23:135.
651. Glader BE, Backer K. Elevated red cell adenosine deaminase activity: a marker of disordered erythropoiesis in Diamond-Blackfan anaemia and other haematologic diseases. Br J Haematol 1988;68:165.
652. Whitehouse DB, Hopkinson DA, Pilz AJ, Arredondo FX. Adenosine deaminase activity in a series of 19 patients with the Diamond-Blackfan syndrome. Adv Exp Med Biol 1986;195(A):85.
653. Heyn R, Kurczynski E, Schmickel R. The association of Blackfan-Diamond syndrome, physical abnormalities, and an abnormality of chromosome 1. J Pediatr 1974;85:531.
654. Brizard CP, Fayard C, Fraisse J, Le Petit JC, Gannat B, Hermouet Y. Anemie par anerythroblastose (type Blackfan-Diamond) chez une enfant porteuse d'anomalies chromosomiques constitutionnelles. Pediatrie 1971;26:305.
655. Van Der Mooren K. Fetal anemia. Pren Diag 1989;9:450.
656. Gurney CW, Pierce MI, Schreier SE, Carson PE, Jacobson LO. The stimulatory effect of "anemic plasma" in congenital hypoplastic anemia. J Lab Clin Med 1957;50:821.
657. Smith CH. Chronic congenital aregenerative anemia (pure red-cell anemia) associated with isoimmunization by the blood group factor "A." Blood 1949;4:697.
658. Moody EA. Hypoplastic anemia following exchange transfusion for erythroblastosis fetalis associated with isoimmunization to blood group factor "A." J Pediatr 1954;44:244.
659. Ortega JA, Shore NA, Dukes PP, Hammond D. Congenital hypoplastic anemia inhibition of erythropoiesis by sera from patients with congenital hypoplastic anemia. Blood 1975;45:83.
660. Freedman MH, Amato D, Saunders EF. Haem synthesis in the Diamond-Blackfan syndrome. Br J Haematol 1975;31:515.
661. Hoffman R, Zanjani ED, Vila J, Zalusky R, Lutton JD, Wasserman LR. Diamond-Blackfan syndrome: lymphocyte-mediated suppression of erythropoiesis. Science 1976;193:899.
662. Nathan DG, Hillman DG, Breard J. The influence of T cells on erythropoiesis. In: Stamatoyannopoulos G, Nienhuis AW, eds. Cellular and molecular regulation of hemoglobin switching. New York, Grune & Stratton, 1979:291.
663. Harris RE, Baehner RL, Gleiser S, Weaver DD, Hodes ME. Cartilage-hair hypoplasia, defective T-cell function, and Diamond-Blackfan anemia in an Amish child. Am J Med Genet 1981;8:291.
664. Steinberg MH, Coleman MB, Pennebaker JB. Diamond-Blackfan anemia: the role of immunoglobulin blocking factor in remission. Am J Hematol 1980;8:213.
665. Zanjani EM, Rinehart JJ. Role of cell–cell interaction in normal and abnormal erythropoiesis. Am J Pediatr Hematol Oncol 1980;2:233.
666. Ershler WB, Ross J, Finlay JL, Shahidi NT. Bone-marrow microenvironment defect in congenital hypoplastic anemia. N Engl J Med 1980;302:1321.
667. Nathan DG, Clarke BJ, Hillman DG, Alter BP, Housman DE. Erythroid precursors in congenital hypoplastic (Diamond-Blackfan) anemia. J Clin Invest 1978;61:489.
668. Nathan DG, Hillman DG, Chess L, et al. Normal erythropoietic helper T cells in congenital hypoplastic (Diamond-Blackfan) anemia. N Engl J Med 1978;298:1049.
669. Cornaglia-Ferraris P, Ghio R, Mori P, et al. T-gamma lymphocytes in a case of congenital hypoplastic anemia (Diamond-Blackfan syndrome). Haematologica 1981;66:269.
670. Chan HSL, Saunders EF, Freedman MH. Diamond-Blackfan syndrome. I. Erythropoiesis in prednisone responsive and resistant disease. Pediatr Res 1982;16:474.
671. Sawada K-I, Koyanagawa Y, Sakurama S, Nakagawa S, Konno T. Diamond-Blackfan syndrome: a possible role of cellular factors for erythropoietic suppression. Scand J Haematol 1985;35:158.
672. Lipton JM, Kudisch M, Gross R, Nathan DG. Defective erythroid progenitor differentiation system in congenital hypoplastic (Diamond-Blackfan) anemia. Blood 1986;67:962.
673. Scimeca PG, Weinblatt ME, Slepowitz G, Harper RG, Kochen JA. Diamond-Blackfan syndrome: an unusual cause of hydrops fetalis. Am J Pediatr Hematol Oncol 1988;10:241.
674. Lenarsky C, Weinberg K, Guinan E, et al. Bone marrow transplantation for constitutional pure red cell aplasia. Blood 1988;71:226.
675. Willis TB, Seale NS. Oral manifestations in congenital hypoplastic anemia (Diamond-Blackfan anemia): clinical report. Pediatr Dent 1984;6:162.
676. Tsai PH, Arkin S, Lipton JM. An intrinsic progenitor defect in Diamond-Blackfan anemia. Br J Haematol 1989;73:112.
677. Chan HSL, Saunders EF, Freedman MH. Diamond-Blackfan syndrome. II. In vitro corticosteroid effect on erythropoiesis. Pediatr Res 1982;16: 477.
678. Gasser C. Akute erythroblastopenie. Schweiz Med Wochenschr 1949;79: 838.
679. Hill JM, Hunter RB. ACTH therapy in refractory anemias. In: Mote JR, ed. Proceedings of the Second Clinical ACTH Conference, vol II. Therapeutics. New York, Blakiston & Son, 1951:181.
680. Allen DM, Diamond LK. Congenital (erythroid) hypoplastic anemia. Am J Dis Child 1961;102:416.
681. Seaman AJ. Cobalt and cortisone therapy of chronic erythrocytic hypoplasia. Am J Med 1952;13:99.
682. Siegler J, Bognar I, Keleman K. Genesung einer isolierten chronischen Erythrozytenaplasie während einer Behandlung mit 6-Merkaptopurin. Kinderaztl Prax 1970;38:145.
683. Marmont AM. Congenital hypoplastic anaemia refractory to corticosteroids but responding to cyclophosphamide and antilymphocytic globulin: report of a case having responded with a transitory wave of dyserythropoiesis. Acta Haematol 1978;60:90.
684. Krishnan EU, Wegner K, Garg SK. Congenital hypoplastic anemia terminating in acute promyelocytic leukemia. Pediatrics 1978;61:898.
685. August CS, King E, Githens JH, et al. Establishment of erythropoiesis following bone marrow transplantation in a patient with congenital hypoplastic anemia (Diamond-Blackfan syndrome). Blood 1976;48:491.
686. Ozsoylu S. High-dose intravenous corticosteroid treatment for patients with Diamond-Blackfan syndrome resistant or refractory to conventional treatment. Am J Pediatr Hematol Oncol 1988;10:217.
687. Tötterman TH, Nisell J, Killander A, Gahrton G, Lönnqvist B. Successful treatment of pure red-cell aplasia with cyclosporin. Lancet 1984;2: 693.
688. Finlay JL, Shahidi NT. Cyclosporine A (CyA)–induced remission in Diamond-Blackfan anemia (DBA). Blood 1984;64:104A.
689. Peters C, Dover GJ, Casella JE, Zinkham WH. Cyclosporine A (CSA) induces transient remissions in red cell aplasias. Pediatr Res 1986;20: 285A.
690. Leonard EM, Raefsky E, Griffith P, Kimball J, Nienhuis AW, Young NS. Cyclosporine therapy of aplastic anaemia, congenital and acquired red cell aplasia. Br J Haematol 1989;72:278.

691. Iriondo A, Garijo J, Conde E, et al. Complete recovery of hemopoiesis following bone marrow transplant in a patient with unresponsive congenital hypoplastic anemia (Blackfan-Diamond syndrome). Blood 1984;64:348.
692. Ash RC, Montgomery T, Moreno H, Geil J, Greenwood M. Cure of steroid-refractory congenital hypoplastic anemia (Diamond Blackfan syndrome) by marrow ablation and allogeneic marrow transplantation: pre- and posttransplant hematopoietic progenitor cell studies and pathogenetic implications. Clin Res 1985;33:334A.
693. Wiktor-Jedrzejczak W, Szczylik C, Pojda Z, et al. Success of bone marrow transplantation in congenital Diamond-Blackfan anaemia: a case report. Eur J Haematol 1987;38:204.
694. D'Oelsnitz M, Vincent L, De Swarte M, Albertini M, Boutte P. A propos d'un cas de leucémie aigue lymphoblastique survenue après guérison d'une maladie de Blackfan-Diamond. Arch Fr Pediatr 1975;32:582.
695. Wasser JS, Yolken R, Miller DR, Diamond LK. Congenital hypoplastic anemia (Diamond-Blackfan syndrome) terminating in acute myelogenous leukemia. Blood 1978;51:991.
696. Basso G, Cocito MG, Rebuffi L, Donzelli F, Milanesi C, Zanesco L. Congenital hypoplastic anaemia developed in acute megakarioblastic leukaemia. Helv Paediatr Acta 1981;36:267.
697. Steinherz PG, Canale VC, Miller DR. Hepatocellular carcinoma, transfusion-induced hemochromatosis and congenital hypoplastic anemia (Blackfan-Diamond syndrome). Am J Med 1976;60:1032.
698. Hardisty RM. Diamond-Blackfan anaemia. In: Congenital disorders of erythropoiesis. CIBA Foundation Symposium 37. Amsterdam, Elsevier, 1976:89.
699. Baar HS. The life span of red blood corpuscles in erythronophthisis. Acta Haematol 1952;7:17.
700. Wranne L. Transient erythroblastopenia in infancy and childhood. Scand J Haematol 1970;7:76.
701. Lovric VA. Anaemia and temporary erythroblastopenia in children: a syndrome. Aust Ann Med 1970;1:34.
702. Tillman W, Prindull G, Schröter W. Severe anemia due to transient pure red cell aplasia in early childhood: arrest at the level of the committed stem cells? Eur J Pediatr 1976;123:51.
703. Wegelius R, Weber TH. Transient erythroblastopenia in childhood: a study of 15 cases. Acta Paediatr Scand 1978;67:513.
704. Toogood IRG, Speed IE, Cheney KC, Rice MS. Idiopathic transient normocytic, normochromic anaemia of childhood. Aust Paediatr J 1978;14:28.
705. Papayannopoulou T, Vichinsky E, Stamatoyannopoulos G. Fetal Hb production during acute erythroid expansion. I. Observations in patients with transient erythroblastopenia and post-phlebotomy. Br J Haematol 1980;44:535.
706. Corrigan JJ. Transient erythroblastopenia of childhood. Arizona Med 1981;38:436.
707. Labotka RJ, Maurer HS, Honig GR. Transient erythroblastopenia of childhood. Review of 17 cases, including a pair of identical twins. Am J Dis Child 1981;135:937.
708. Link MP, Alter BP. Fetal erythropoiesis during recovery from transient erythroblastopenia of childhood (TEC). Pediatr Res 1981;15:1036.
709. Dessypris EN, Krantz SB, Roloff JS, Lukens JN. Mode of action of the IgG inhibitor of erythropoiesis in transient erythroblastopenia of childhood. Blood 1982;59:114.
710. Freedman MH, Saunders EF. Transient erythroblastopenia of childhood: varied pathogenesis. Am J Hematol 1983;14:247.
711. Gerrits GPJM, Van Oostrom CG, De Vaan GAM, Bakkeren JAJM. Transient erythroblastopenia of childhood: a review of 22 cases. Eur J Pediatr 1984;142:266.
712. Ritchey AK, Dainiak N, Hoffman R. Variable in vitro erythropoiesis in patients with transient erythroblastopenia of childhood. Yale J Biol Med 1985;58:1.
713. Bhambhani K, Inoue S, Sarnaik SA. Seasonal clustering of transient erythroblastopenia of childhood. Am J Dis Child 1988;142:175.
714. Hirt A, Luthy A, Muller B, Gugler E, Wagner HP. Transient erythroblastopenia of children. Schweiz Med Wochenschr 1988;118:703.
715. Wang WC, Mentzer WC. Differentiation of transient erythroblastopenia of childhood from congenital hypoplastic anemia. J Pediatr 1976;88:784.
716. Sorva R, Wegelius R, Weber TH, Siimes MA. Transient erythroblastopenia of childhood: a retrospective study of 57 cases with a review of the literature. Eur Paediatr Haematol Oncol 1984;1:189.
717. Glader BE. Diagnosis and management of red cell aplasia in children. Hematol Oncol Clin North Am 1987;1:431.
718. Hays T, Lane PA, Shafer F. Transient erythroblastopenia of childhood: a review of 26 cases and reassessment of indications for bone marrow aspiration. Am J Dis Child 1989;143:605.
719. Rogers ZR, Bergstrom SK, Amylon MD, Buchanan GR, Glader BE. Reduced neutrophil counts in children with transient erythroblastopenia of childhood. J Pediatr 1989;115:746.
720. Young RSK, Rannels E, Hilmo A, Gerson JM, Goodrich D. Severe anemia in childhood presenting as transient ischemic attacks. Stroke 1983;14:622.
721. Michelson AD, Marshall PC. Transient neurological disorder associated with transient erythroblastopenia of childhood. Am J Pediatr Hematol Oncol 1987;9:161.
722. Beresford CH, Macfarlane SD. Temporal clustering of transient erythroblastopenia (cytopenia) of childhood. Aust Paediatr J 1987;23:351.
723. Schroder H. Transient erythroblastopenia in children. Ugeskr Laeger 1983;145:2140.
724. Douchain F, Leborgne JM, Robin M, Macart M, Kremp L. Erythroblastopénie aigue par l'intolérance au dipropyl acétate de sodium: première observation. Nouv Press Med 1980;9:1715.
725. Seip M. Transient erythroblastopenia in siblings. Acta Paediatr Scand 1982;71:689.
726. Bhambani K, Inoue S. Natural history of transient erythroblastopenia of childhood (TEC). Blood 1982;60:33a.
727. McLaughlin OE, Kinney TR, Falletta JM, Holbrook CT, McMillan CW. Survey of transient erythroblastopenia of childhood (TEC) in North Carolina. Pediatr Res 1983;17:238A.
728. Kubic PT, Warkentin PI, Levitt CJ, Coccia PF. Transient erythroblastopenia of childhood (TEC) occurring in clusters. Pediatr Res 1979;13:435.
729. Inoue S, Ravindranath Y, Lusher JM, Ito T. Absence of inhibitory cells from patients with aplastic anemia or transient erythroblastopenia of childhood on the in vitro growth of erythroid colonies. Acta Haematol Jpn 1980;43:76.
730. Dickerman JD. Transient erythroblastopenia of childhood presenting with reticulocytosis and erythroid hyperplasia in the bone marrow. Pediatrics 1981;67:562.
731. Ross JM. Transient erythroblastopenia of childhood. Nurs Times 1981;77:358.
732. Hanada T, Ehara T, Nakahara S, Suzuki T, Nagasawa T, Takita H. Simultaneous transient erythroblastopenia and agranulocytosis: IgG-mediated inhibition of erythrogranulopoiesis. Eur J Haematol 1987;38:200.
733. Hanada T, Koike K, Hirano C, Takeya T, Suzuki T, Matsunaga Y, Takita H. Childhood transient erythroblastopenia complicated by thrombocytopenia and neutropenia. Eur J Haematol 1989;42:77.
734. Gerrits GPJM, Van Oostrom CG, De Vaan GAM. Severe anemia caused by transient erythroblastopenia in children (TEC). Tijdschr Kindergeneeskd 1982;50:97.
735. Davis D, Gordon J. Transient erythroblastopenia. Pediatrics 1982;69:250.
736. Muntean W. What is your diagnosis? Padiatr Padol 1982;17:713.
737. Dover GJ, Boyer SH, Zinkham WH. Production of erythrocytes that contain fetal hemoglobin in anemia: transient in vivo changes. J Clin Invest 1979;63:173.
738. Young NS, Mortimer PP, Moore JG, Humphries RK. Characterization of a virus that causes transient aplastic crisis. J Clin Invest 1984;73:224.
739. Mortimer PP, Humphries RK, Moore JG, Purcell RH, Young NS. A human parvovirus–like virus inhibits haematopoietic colony formation in vitro. Nature 1983;302:426.
740. Mortimer PP. A virological perspective on bone marrow failure. In: Young NS, Levine AS, Humphries RK, eds. Aplastic anemia: stem cell biology and advances in treatment. New York, Alan R Liss, 1984:121.
741. Lipton JM, Kudisch M, Gross R, Nathan DG. Defective erythroid progenitor differentiation system in congenital hypoplastic (Diamond-Blackfan) anemia. Blood 1986;67:962.
742. Iwai A, Iwai T, Ninomiya T, Miyao M. A case of transient erythroblastopenia of childhood: serum inhibitor of BFU-E development. Jpn J Clin Hematol 1986;27:1688.
743. Hanada T, Abe T, Takita H. T-cell mediated inhibition of erythropoiesis in transient erythroblastopenia of childhood. Br J Haematol 1985;59:391.
744. De Montalembert M, Girot R, Cheron G, Picot C, Lenoir G, Casadevall N. Transient erythroblastopenia of childhood. Arch Fr Pediatr 1986;43:127.
745. Sheridan BL, Rockwell AJ, Pyesmany A. Transient erythroblastopenia of childhood (TEC): a study of cellular interaction upon erythropoiesis. Exp Hematol 1981;9:180.
746. Koenig HM, Lightsey AL, Nelson DP, Diamond LK. Immune suppression of erythropoiesis in transient erythroblastopenia of childhood. Blood 1979;54:742.
747. Zwerdling T, Finlay J, Glader BE. Transient erythroblastopenia of adolescence. Clin Pediatr 1986;25:563.
748. Tachibana N, Onodera N, Ikeda Y, et al. Transient erythroblastopenia of childhood: immune suppression of erythroid progenitor cells in the presence of the patient's serum. Jpn J Clin Hematol 1985;26:1486.
749. Freedman MH. "Recurrent" erythroblastopenia of childhood: an IgM-mediated RBC aplasia. Am J Dis Child 1983;137:458.
750. Lewis SM, Verwilghen RL. Dyserythropoiesis: definition, diagnosis and assessment. In: Lewis SM, Verwilghen RL, eds. Dyserythropoiesis. London, Academic Press, 1977:3.
751. Frisch B, Lewis SM. The bone marrow in aplastic anaemia: diagnostic and prognostic features. J Clin Pathol 1974;27:231.
752. Rozman C, Feliu E, Granena A, Brugues R, Woessner S, Vives Corrons JL. Transient dyserythropoiesis in repopulated human bone marrow following transplantation: an ultrastructural study. Br J Haematol 1982;50:63.
753. Lewis SM, Verwilghen RL, eds. Dyserythropoiesis. London, Academic Press, 1977.

754. Crookston JH, Crookston MC, Burnie KL, Francombe WH, Dacie JV, Davis JA, Lewis SM. Hereditary erythroblastic multinuclearity associated with a positive acidified-serum test: a type of congenital dyserythropoietic anaemia. Br J Haematol 1969;17:11.
755. Heimpel H. Congenital dyserythropoietic anaemia type I: clinical and experimental aspects. In: Congenital disorders of erythropoiesis. CIBA Foundation Symposium 37. Amsterdam, Elsevier, 1976;135.
756. Heimpel H. Congenital dyserythropoietic anaemia, type I. In: Lewis SM, Verwilghen RL, eds. Dyserythropoiesis. London, Academic Press, 1977:55.
757. Alloisio N, Jaccoud P, Dorleac E, et al. Alterations of globin chain synthesis and of red cell membrane proteins in congenital dyserythropoietic anemia I and II. Pediatr Res 1982;16:1016.
758. Wickramasinghe SN, Pippard MJ. Studies of erythroblast function in congenital dyserythropoietic anaemia, type I: evidence of impaired DNA, RNA, and protein synthesis and unbalanced globin chain synthesis in ultrastructurally abnormal cells. J Clin Pathol 1986;39:881.
759. Heimpel H, Forteza-Vila J, Queisser W, Spiertz E. Electron and light microscopic study of the erythroblasts of patients with congenital dyserythropoietic anemia. Blood 1971;37:299.
760. Lewis SM, Frisch B. Congenital dyserythropoietic anaemias: electron microscopy. In: Congenital disorders of erythropoiesis. CIBA Foundation Symposium 37. Amsterdam, Elsevier, 1976:171.
761. Breton-Gorius J, Daniel MT, Clauvel JP, Dreyfus B. Anomalies ultrastructurales des érythroblastes et des érythrocytes dans six cas de dysérythropoiése congénitale. Nouv Rev Fr Hematol 1973;13:23.
762. Vainchenker W, Guichard J, Bouguet J, Breton-Gorius J. Congenital dyserythropoietic anaemia type I: absence of clonal expression in the nuclear abnormalities of cultured erythroblasts. Br J Haematol 1980;46:33.
763. Verwilghen RL, Lewis SM, Dacie JV, Crookston JH, Crookston MC. HEMPAS: congenital dyserythropoietic anaemia (type II). Q J Med 1973;42:257.
764. Verwilghen RL. Congenital dyserythropoietic anaemia type II (Hempas). In: Congenital disorders of erythropoiesis. CIBA Foundation Symposium 37. Amsterdam, Elsevier, 1976:151.
765. Crookston JH, Crookston M. Hereditary anemia with multinuclear erythroblasts (HEMPAS). Birth Defects 1972;8(3):15.
766. Crookston JH, Crookston MC, Rosse WF. Red-cell abnormalities in HEMPAS (Hereditary erythroblastic multinuclearity with a positive acidified-serum test). Br J Haematol 1972;23:83.
767. Seip M, Skrede S, Bjerve K, Hovig T, Gaarder PI, Stavem P. A case of variant congenital dyserythropoietic anemia revisited. Scand J Haematol 1982;28:278.
768. Giblett ER, Crookston MC. Agglutinability of red cells by anti-i in patients with thalassaemia major and other haematological disorders. Nature 1964;201:1138.
769. Enquist RW, Gockerman JP, Jenis EH, Warkel RL, Dillon DE. Type II congenital dyserythropoietic anemia. Ann Intern Med 1972;77:371.
770. Rosse WF, Logue GL, Adams J, Crookston JH. Mechanisms of immune lysis of the red cells in hereditary erythroblastic multinuclearity with a positive acidified serum test and paroxysmal nocturnal hemoglobinuria. J Clin Invest 1974;53:31.
771. Fukuda MN, Dell A, Scartezzini P. Primary defect of congenital dyserythropoietic anemia type II. Failure in glycosylation of erythrocyte lactosaminoglycan proteins caused by lowered N-acetylglucosaminyltransferase II. J Biol Chem 1987;262:7195.
772. Tebbi K, Gross S. Absence of morphological abnormalities in marrow erythrocyte colonies (CFU-E) from a patient with HEMPAS-II. J Lab Clin Med 1978;91:797.
773. Vainchenker W, Guichard J, Breton-Gorius J. Morphological abnormalities in cultured erythroid colonies (BFU-E) from the blood of two patients with HEMPAS. Br J Haematol 1979;42:363.
774. Roodman GD, Clare CN, Mills G. Congenital dyserythropoietic anaemia type II (CDA-II): chromosomal banding studies and adherent cell effects on erythroid colony (CFU-E) and burst (BFU-E) formation. Br J Haematol 1982;50:499.
775. Cazzola M, Barosi G, Bergamaschi G, et al. Iron loading in congenital dyserythropoietic anaemias and congenital sideroblastic anaemias. Br J Haematol 1983;54:649.
776. Wolff JA, Von Hofe FH. Familial erythroid multinuclearity. Blood 1951;6:1274.
777. Goudsmit R. Congenital dyserythropoietic anaemia, type III. In: Lewis SM, Verwilghen RL, eds. Dyserythropoiesis. London, Academic Press, 1977:83.
778. Vainchenker W, Breton-Gorius J, Guichard J, Bouguet J, Henri A, Rochant H, Goudsmit R. Congenital dyserythropoietic anemia type III. Studies on erythroid differentiation of blood erythroid progenitor cells (BFU_E) in vitro. Exp Hematol 1980;8:1057.
779. David G, Van Dorpe A. Aberrant congenital dyserythropoietic anaemias. In: Lewis SM, Verwilghen RL, eds. Dyserythropoiesis. London, Academic Press, 1977:93.
780. Boogaerts MA, Verwilghen RL. Variants of congenital dyserythropoietic anaemia: an update. Haematologia 1982;15:211.
781. McBride JA, Wilson WEC, Baillie N. Congenital dyserythropoietic anaemia: type IV. Blood 1971;38:837.
782. Weatherly TL, Flannery EP, Doyle WF, Shohet SB, Garratty G. Congenital dyserythropoietic anemia (CDA) with increased red cell lipids. Am J Med 1974;57:912.
783. Benjamin JT, Rosse WF, Dalldorf FC, McMillan CW. Congenital dyserythropoietic anemia: type IV. J Pediatr 1975;87:210.
784. Bird AR, Karabus CD, Hartley PS. Type IV congenital dyserythropoietic anemia with an unusual response to splenectomy. Am J Pediatr Hematol Oncol 1985;7:196.
785. Weatherall DH, Clegg JB, Knox-Macaulay HHM, Bunch C, Hopkins CR, Temperley IJ. A genetically determined disorder with features both of thalassaemia and congenital dyserythropoietic anaemia. Br J Haematol 1973;24:681.
786. Hruby MA, Mason RG, Honig GR. Unbalanced globin chain synthesis in congenital dyserythropoietic anemia. Blood 1973;42:843.
787. Eldor A, Matzner Y, Kahane I, Levene C, Polliack A. Aberrant congenital dyserythropoietic anemia with negative acidified serum tests and features of thalassemia in a Kurdish family. Isr J Med Sci 1978;14:1138.
788. Brochstein JA, Siena S, Weinberg RS, Bianchi E, Alter BP. Congenital dyserythropoietic anemia (CDA) with karyorrhexis. Pediatr Res 1985;19:258A.
789. Kostmann R. Infantile genetic agranulocytosis: a new recessive lethal disease in man. Acta Paediatr Scand 1956;45:1.
790. Kostmann R. Infantile genetic agranulocytosis. A review with presentation of ten new cases. Acta Paediatr Scand 1975;64:362.
791. Iselius L, Gustavson KH. Spatial distribution of the gene for infantile genetic agranulocytosis. Hum Hered 1984;34:358.
792. Coulombel L, Morardet N, Veber F, Leroy C, Mielot F, Fisher A, Teillet-Thiebaud F, Tchernia G, Griscelli C, Paramentier C. Granulopoietic differentiation in long-term bone marrow cultures from children with congenital neutropenia. Am J Hematol 1988;27:93.
793. Zucker-Franklin D, L'Esperance P, Good RA. Congenital neutropenia: an intrinsic cell defect demonstrated by electron microscopy of soft agar colonies. Blood 1977;49:425.
794. Barrett AJ. Clinical experience with lithium in aplastic anemia and congenital neutropenia. Adv Exp Med Biol 1980;127:305.
795. Chan HSL, Freedman MH, Saunders EF. Lithium therapy of children with chronic neutropenia. Am J Med 1981;70:1073.
796. Rappeport JM, Parkman R, Newburger P, Camitta BM, Chusid MJ. Correction of infantile agranulocytosis (Kostmann's syndrome) by allogeneic bone marrow transplantation. Am J Med 1980;68:605.
797. O'Reilly RJ, Brochstein J, Dinsmore R, Kirkpatrick D. Marrowtransplantation for congenital disorders. Semin Hematol 1984;21:188.
798. Bonilla MA, Gillio AP, Ruggeiro M, et al. Effects of recombinant human granulocyte colony-stimulating factor on neutropenia in patients with congenital agranulocytosis. N Engl J Med 1989;320:1574.
799. Cividalli G, Yarkoni S, Dar H, Kohn G. Can infantile hereditary agranulocytosis be diagnosed prenatally? Prenat Diagn 1983;3:157.
800. Millar DS, Davis LR, Rodeck CH, Nicolaides KH, Mibashan RS. Normal blood cell values in the early mid-trimester fetus. Prenat Diagn 1985;5:367.
801. Gilman PA, Jackson DP, Guild HG. Congenital agranulocytosis: prolonged survival and terminal acute leukemia. Blood 1970;36:576.
802. Rosen RB, Kang S-J. Congenital agranulocytosis terminating in acute myelomonocytic leukemia. J Pediatr 1979;94:406.
803. Lui V, Ragab AH, Findley H, Frauen B. Infantile genetic agranulocytosis and acute lymphocytic leukemia in two sibs. J Pediatr 1978;92:1028.
804. Hall JG, Levin J, Kuhn JP, Ottenheimer EJ, Van Berkum KAP, McKusick VA. Thrombocytopenia with absent radius (TAR). Medicine 1969;48:411.
805. Hall JG. Thrombocytopenia and absent radius (TAR) syndrome. J Med Genet 1987;24:79.
806. Hedberg VA, Lipton JM. Thrombocytopenia with absent radii: a review of 100 cases. Am J Pediatr Hematol Oncol 1988;10:51.
807. Messen S, Vargas L, Garcia H, Miranda P. Congenital thrombocytopenia and absent radius syndrome in identical twins. Rev Clin Pediatr 1986;57:559.
808. Dodesini G, Frigerio G, Cocco E. La trombocitopenia congenita ipoplastica con aplasia bilaterale del radio. Minerva Pediatr 1979;31:1023.
809. Teufel M, Enders H, Dopfer R. Consanguinity in a Turkish family with thrombocytopenia with absent radii (TAR) syndrome. Hum Genet 1983;64:94.
810. Shalev E, Weiner E, Feldman E, Cohen H, Zuckerman H. Micrognathia: prenatal ultrasonographic diagnosis. Int J Gynaecol Obstet 1983;21:343.
811. Turner RJ, Spencer RA, Miyazawa K. Successful cesarean section in a gravida with the thrombocytopenia with absent radius syndrome: a case report. J Reprod Med 1986;31:260.
812. Gross H, Groh C, Weippl G. Kongenitale hypoplastische Thrombopenie mit Radiusaplasie: ein Syndrom multipler Abartungen. Neue Oesterr Z Kinderheilkd 1956;1:574.
813. Edelberg SB, Cohn J, Brandt NJ. Congenital hypomegakaryocytic thrombocytopenia associated with bilateral absence of the radius: the TAR syndrome: intra-family variation of the clinical picture. Hum Hered 1977;27:147.
814. Temtamy SA, McKusick VA. Radial defects with blood dyscrasias. In: Bergsma D, ed. The genetics of hand malformations. Birth Defects 1978;14(3):101.

815. Hays RM, Bartoshesky LE, Feingold M. New features of thrombocytopenia and absent radius syndrome. Birth Defects 1982;18(3B):115.
816. Ward RE, Bixler D, Provisor AJ, Bader P. Parent to child transmission of the thrombocytopenia absent radius (TAR) syndrome. Am J Med Genet Suppl 1986;2:207.
817. Schnur RE, Eunpu DL, Zackai EH. Thrombocytopenia with absent radius in a boy and his uncle. Am J Med Genet 1987;28:117.
818. Haarmann M, Lenz W, Petersen D. Radiusaplasie mit Thrombocytopenie. Ergeb Inn Med Kinderkeilkd 1975;37:57.
819. Rubin SL. A case of congenital amegakaryocytic thrombocytopenia with leukemoid blood picture and congenital deformities. Arch Pediatr 1959;76:251.
820. Ray R, Zorn E, Kelly T, Hall JG, Sommer A. Lower limb anomalies in the thrombocytopenia absent-radius (TAR) syndrome. Am J Med Genet 1980;7:523.
821. Adeyokunnu AA. Radial aplasia and amegakaryocytic thrombocytopenia (TAR syndrome) among Nigerian children. Am J Dis Child 1984;138:346.
822. Akatsuka J. Fanconi's anemia and radial aplasia–thrombocytopenia. Nippon Rinsho 1978;Suppl:1488.
823. Nilsson LR, Lundholm G. Congenital thrombocytopenia associated with aplasia of the radius. Acta Paediatr 1960;49:291.
824. Whitfield MF, Barr DGD. Cow's milk allergy in the syndrome of thrombocytopenia with absent radius. Arch Dis Child 1976;51:337.
825. Schoenecker PL, Cohn AK, Sedgwick WG, Manske PR, Salafsky I, Millar EA. Dysplasia of the knee associated with the syndrome of thrombocytopenia and absent radius. J Bone Joint Surg 1984;66A:421.
826. Rabinowitz JG, Moseley JE, Mitty HA, Hirschhorn K. Trisomy 18, esophageal atresia, anomalies of the radius, and congenital hypoplastic thrombocytopenia. Radiology 1967;89:488.
827. Stoll C, Sacrez R, Willard D, Freysz H. Un cas de trisomie 18 avec aplasie bilatérale du radius et thrombopénie. Pediatrie 1972;27:537.
828. Juif J-G, Stoll C, Korn R. Thrombopénie hypoplasique congénitale avec aplasie du radius. Arch Franc Ped 1972;29:513.
829. Christodoulou CBW. A girl with 18-trisomy and thrombocytopenia. Acta Genet 1967;17:77.
830. Waldenmaier C, Aldenhoff P, Klemm T. The Robert's syndrome. Hum Genet 1978;40:345.
831. Lenz W. Phenocopies. J Med Genet 1973;10:34.
832. Bessman JD, Harrison RL, Howard LC, Peterson D. The megakaryocyte abnormality in thrombocytopenia–absent radius syndrome. Blood 1983;62:143.
833. Armitage JO, Hoak JC, Elliott TE, Fry GL. Syndrome of thrombocytopenia and absent radii: qualitatively normal platelets with remission following splenectomy. Scand J Haematol 1978;20:25.
834. Thevenieau D, Mattei JF, Juhan I, et al. Anomalies du membre supérieur, thrombopénie et thrombopathie: a propos de trois observations. Arch Franc Ped 1978;35:631.
835. Giuffre L, Cammarata M, Corsello G, Vitaliti SM. Two new cases of thrombocytopenia absent radius (TAR) syndrome: clinical, genetic and nosologic features. Klin Padiatr 1988;200:10.
836. Sultan Y, Scrobohaci ML, Jeanneau C, Rendu F, Caen JP. Anomalies de la lignée plaquettaire au cours du syndrome d'aplasie radiale avec thrombocytopénie. Nouv Rev Fr Hematol 1973;13:573.
837. Day HJ, Holmsen H. Platelet adenine nucleotide "storage pool deficiency" in thrombocytopenic absent radii syndrome. JAMA 1972;221:1053.
838. Linch DC, Stewart JW, West C. Blood and bone marrow cultures in a case of thrombocytopenia with absent radii. Clin Lab Haematol 1982;4:313.
839. Homans AC, Cohen JL, Mazur EM. Defective megakaryocytopoiesis in the syndrome of thrombocytopenia with absent radii. Br J Haematol 1988;70:205.
840. Michalevicz R, Baron S, Burstein Y. Osteoclast-like cells grow in cultures of multipotent hematopoietic progenitors in thrombocytopenia and absent radii (TAR) syndrome. Isr J Med Sci 1988;24:42.
841. Akabutu J, Vergidis D, Poololak-Doiwidziak M, Janowska-Wieczorek A. Studies of hematopoietic progenitor cells in thrombocytopenia with absent radii (TAR) syndrome. Blood 1988;72:78a.
842. Kanz L, Kostjelniak E, Welte K. Colony-stimulating activity (CSA) unique for the megakaryocytic hemopoietic cell lineage, present in the plasma of a patient with the syndrome of thrombocytopenia with absent radii (TAR). Blood 1989;74:248a.
843. De Alarcon PA, Graeve JLA, Levine RF, McDonald TP, Schmieder JA. Thrombocytopenia and absent radii syndrome: a defect in megakaryocyte maturation. Blood 1988;72:321a.
844. Brochstein J, Shank B, Kernan NA, Terwilliger JW, O'Reilly RJ. Marrow transplantation for thrombocytopenia–absent radii syndrome. J Paediatr 1992;121:587.
845. Omenn GS, Figley MM, Graham CB, Heinrichs WL. Prospects for radiographic intrauterine diagnosis: the syndrome of thrombocytopenia with absent radii. N Engl J Med 1973;288:777.
846. Luthy DA, Hall JG, Graham CB. Prenatal diagnosis of thrombocytopenia with absent radii. Clin Genet 1979;15:495.
847. Luthy DA, Mack L, Hirsch J, Cheng E. Prenatal ultrasound diagnosis of thrombocytopenia with absent radii. Am J Obstet Gynecol 1981;141:350.
848. Hobbins JC, Bracken MB, Mahoney MJ. Diagnosis of fetal skeletal dysplasias with ultrasound. Am J Obstet Gynecol 1982;142:306.
849. Filkins K, Russo J, Bilinki I, Diamond N, Searle B. Prenatal diagnosis of thrombocytopenia absent radius syndrome using ultrasound and fetoscopy. Prenat Diagn 1984;4:139.
850. Seemanova E, Spicakova V, Kulovany E, Salichova J, Veprek P, Zwinger A. TAR syndrome in three unrelated children. Cesk Pediatr 1985;40:511.
851. Daffos F, Forestier F, Kaplan C, Cox W. Prenatal diagnosis and management of bleeding disorders with fetal blood sampling. Am J Obstet Gynecol 1988;158:939.
852. Vaughan JM. Leuco-erythroblastic anaemia. J Pathol Bacteriol 1936;42:541.
853. Weick JK, Hagedorn AB, Linman JW. Leukoerythroblastosis. Diagnostic and prognostic significance. Mayo Clin Proc 1974;49:110.
854. Sills RH, Hadley RAR. The significance of nucleated red blood cells in the peripheral blood of children. Am J Pediatr Hematol Oncol 1983;5:173.
855. Albers-Schonberg H. Roentgenbilder einer seltenen Knochenerkrankung. Munchen Med Wochensschr 1904;51:365.
856. Johnston CC Jr, Lavy N, Lord T, Vellios F, Merritt AD, Deiss WP Jr. Osteopetrosis: a clinical, genetic, metabolic, and morphologic study of the dominantly inherited, benign form. Medicine 1968;47:149.
857. Schiliro G, Musumeci S, Pizzarelli G, et al. Fetal haemoglobin in early malignant osteopetrosis. Br J Haematol 1978;38:339.
858. Farber S, Vawter GF. Clinical pathological conference. J Pediatr 1965;67:133.
859. Sjölin S. Studies on osteopetrosis. II. Investigations concerning the nature of the anaemia. Acta Paediatr 1959;48:529.
860. Walker DG. Spleen cells transmit osteopetrosis in mice. Science 1975;190:785.
861. Ash P, Loutit JF, Townsend KMS. Osteoclasts derived from haematopoietic stem cells. Nature 1980;283:669.
862. Marshall MJ, Nisbet NW, Menage J, Loutit JF. Tissue repopulation during cure of osteopetrotic (mi/mi) mice using normal and defective (W^e/W^v) bone marrow. Exp Hematol 1982;10:600.
863. Scheven BAA, Visser JWM, Nijweide PJ. In vitro osteoclast generation from different bone marrow fractions, including a highly enriched haematopoietic stem cell population. Nature 1986;321:79.
864. Ragab AH, Ducos R, Crist WM, Duck SC. Granulopoiesis in osteopetrosis. J Pediatr 1975;87:422.
865. Marcus JR, Fibach E, Akrer M. Circulating myeloid and erythroid progenitor cells in malignant osteopetrosis. Acta Haemat 1982;67:185.
866. Reeves J, Huffer W, August CS, Hathaway WE, Koerper M, Walters CE. The hematopoietic effects of prednisone therapy in four infants with osteopetrosis. J Pediatr 1979;94:210.
867. Beard CJ, Key L, Newburger PE, et al. Neutrophil defect associated with malignant infantile osteopetrosis. J Lab Clin Med 1986;108:498.
868. Moe PJ, Skjaeveland A. Therapeutic studies in osteopetrosis: report of 4 cases. Acta Paediatr Scand 1969;58:593.
869. Ballet JJ, Griscelli C, Coutris C, Milhaud G, Maroteaux P. Bone-marrow transplantation in osteopetrosis. Lancet 1977;2:1137.
870. Coccia PF, Krivit W, Cervenka J, et al. Successful bone-marrow transplantation for infantile malignant osteopetrosis. N Engl J Med 1980;302:701.
871. Sorrell M, Kapoor N, Kirkpatrick D, et al. Marrow transplantation for juvenile osteopetrosis. Am J Med 1981;70:1280.
872. Sieff CA, Chessells JM, Levinsky RJ, et al. Allogeneic bone-marrow transplantation in infantile malignant osteopetrosis. Lancet 1983;1:437.
873. Fischer A, Friedrich W, Levinsky R, et al. Bone-marrow transplantation for immunodeficiencies and osteopetrosis: European survey, 1968–1985. Lancet 1986;2:1080.
874. Jenkinson EL, Pfisterer WH, Latteier KK, Martin M. A prenatal diagnosis of osteopetrosis. AJR 1943;49:455.
875. Golbus MS, Koerper MA, Hall BD. Failure to diagnose osteopetrosis in utero. Lancet 1976;2:1246.
876. Khazen NE, Faverly D, Vamos E, et al. Lethal osteopetrosis with multiple factures in utero. Am J Med Genet 1986;23:811.
877. Pierre RV. Preleukemic states. Semin Hematol 1974;11:73.
878. German J, Passarge E. Bloom's syndrome. XII. Report from the registry for 1987. Clin Genet 1989;35:57.
879. Freeman AI, Edwards JA, Cohen M, Sinks LF. Morphologic studies in a recently described dyserythropoietic state. Blood 1972;40:473.
880. Weksberg R, Smith C, Anson-Cartwright L, Maloney K. Bloom syndrome: a single complementation group defines patients of diverse ethnic origin. Am J Hum Genet 1988;42:816.
881. Gatti RA, Hall K. Ataxia-telangiectasia: search for a central hypothesis. In: German J, ed. Chromosome mutation and neoplasia. New York, Alan R Liss, 1983:23.
882. Waldmann TA, Misiti J, Nelson DL, Kraemer KH. Ataxia-telangiectasia: a multisystem hereditary disease with immunodeficiency, impaired organ maturation, x-ray hypersensitivity, and a high incidence of neoplasia. Ann Intern Med 1983;99:367.
883. Gatti RA, Berkel I, Boder E, et al. Localization of an ataxia telangiectasia gene to chromosome 11q22–23. Nature 1988;336:577.
884. Morrell D, Cromartie E, Swift M. Mortality and cancer incidence in 263 patients with ataxia-telangiectasia. J Natl Cancer Inst 1986;77:89.

885. David TJ. Nature and etiology of the Poland anomaly. N Engl J Med 1972;287:487.
886. McGillivray BC, Lowry RB. Poland syndrome in British Columbia: incidence and reproductive experience of affected persons. Am J Med Genet 1977;1:65.
887. Gilman PA, Miller RW. No link between Poland syndrome and leukemia? Am J Dis Child 1982;136:176.
888. Adams EB. Aplastic anaemia: review of twenty-seven cases. Lancet 1951;1:657.
889. Mohler DN, Leavell BS. Aplastic anemia: an analysis of 50 cases. Ann Intern Med 1958;49:326.
890. Lewis S. Course and prognosis in aplastic anaemia. Br Med J 1965;1: 1027.
891. Aksoy M, Erdem S. Followup study on the mortality and the development of leukemia in 44 pancytopenic patients with chronic exposure to benzene. Blood 1978;52:285.
892. Koeppen KM, Paulisch R, Schneider D, Gerhartz H. Panmyelopathie: ein praleukamisches Stadium? Klin Wochensschr 1975;53:581.
893. Mir MA, Delamore IW. Oxymetholone in aplastic anaemia. Postgrad Med J 1974;50:166.
894. Najean Y. Long-term follow-up in patients with aplastic anemia: a study of 137 androgen-treated patients surviving more than two years. Am J Med 1981;71:543.
895. Garewal G, Mohanty D, Das KC. A study of hypoplastic anaemia. Indian J Med Res 1981;73:558.
896. Fohlmeister I, Fischer R, Modder B, Rister M, Schaefer H-E. Aplastic anaemia and the hypocellular myelodysplastic syndrome: histomorphological, diagnostic, and prognostic features. J Clin Pathol 1985;38: 1218.
897. Appelbaum FR, Barrall J, Storb R, et al. Clonal cytogenetic abnormalities in patients with otherwise typical aplastic anemia. Exp Hematol 1987;15:1134.
898. Orlandi E, Alessandrino EP, Caldera D, Bernasconi C. Adult leukemia developing after aplastic anemia: report of 8 cases. Acta Haematol 1988;79:174.
899. De Planque MM, Kluin-Nelemans HC, Van Krieken HJM, et al. Evolution of acquired severe aplastic anaemia to myelodysplasia and subsequent leukaemia in adults. Br J Haematol 1988;70:55.
900. Dameshek W. Riddle: what do aplastic anemia, paroxysmal nocturnal hemoglobinuria (PNH) and "hypoplastic" leukemia have in common? Blood 1967;30:251.
901. Li FP, Nathan DG. Therapy-linked leukaemia. Br Med J 1971;ii:765.
902. Rokicka-Milewska R, Derulska D. Aplastic anemia in the early period of acute leukemia in children. Mater Med Pol 1974;6:24.
903. Bernard J, Schaison G. Transitory bone marrow failure: a series of 13 preleukemic cases in children. Am J Pediatr Hematol Oncol 1980;2: 141.
904. Breatnach F, Chessells JM, Greaves MF. The aplastic presentation of childhood leukaemia: a feature of common-ALL. Br J Haematol 1981;49: 387.
905. Revesz T, Kardos G, Kajtar P, Schuler D. The adverse effect of prolonged prednisolone pretreatment in children with acute lymphoblastic leukemia. Cancer 1985;55:1637.
906. De Alarcon PA, Miller ML, Stuart MJ. Erythroid hypoplasia. An unusual presentation of childhood acute lymphocytic leukemia. Am J Dis Child 1978;132:763.
907. Shackelford GD, Bloomberg G, McAlister WH. The value of roentgenography in differentiating aplastic anemia from leukemia masquerading as aplastic anemia. AJR 1972;116:651.
908. Toledano SR. Preleukemic phase in childhood acute lymphoblastic leukemia. J Pediatr 1977;91:507.
909. Kleihauer E. The preleukemic syndromes (hematopoietic dysplasia) in childhood. Eur J Pediatr 1980;133:5.
910. Blank J, Lange B. Preleukemia in children. J Pediatr 1981;98:565.
911. Saarinen UM, Wegelius R. Preleukemic syndrome in children. Report of four cases and review of literature. Am J Pediatr Hematol Oncol 1984;6:137.
912. Wegelius R. Preleukaemic states in children. Scand J Haematol 1986;36(Suppl 45):133.
913. Bennett JM, Catovsky D, Daniel MT, et al. Proposals for the classification of the myelodysplastic syndromes. Br J Haematol 1982;51:189.
914. Niebrugge DJ. Preleukemia in children. J Pediatr 1982;100:507.
915. Merrick MV, Gordon-Smith EC, Lavender JP, Szur L. A comparison of ^{111}In with ^{52}Fe and ^{99m}Tc-sulfur colloid for bone marrow scanning. J Nucl Med 1975;16:66.
916. Hogge DE, Shannon KM, Kalousek DK, et al. Juvenile monosomy 7 syndrome: evidence that the disease originates in a pluripotent hemopoietic stem cell. Leuk Res 1987;11:705.
917. Evans JPM, Czepulkowski B, Gibbons B, Swansbury GJ, Chessells JM. Childhood monosomy 7 revisited. Br J Haematol 1988;69:41.
918. Randall DL, Reiquam CW, Githens JH, Robinson A. Familial myeloproliferative disease: a new syndrome closely simulating myelogenous leukemia in childhood. Am J Dis Child 1965;110:479.
919. Smith WB, Ablin A, Goodman JR, Brecher G. Atypical megakaryocytes in preleukemic phase of acute myeloid leukemia. Blood 1973;42: 535.
920. Luddy RE, Champion LAA, Schwartz AD. A fatal myeloproliferative syndrome in a family with thrombocytopenia and platelet dysfunction. Cancer 1978;41:1959.
921. Carroll WL, Morgan R, Glader BE. Childhood bone marrow monosomy 7 syndrome: a familial disorder? J Pediatr 1985;107:578.
922. Paul B, Reid MM, Davison EV, Abela M, Hamilton PJ. Familial myelodysplasia: progressive disease associated with emergence of monosomy 7. Br J Haematol 1987;65:321.
923. Svarch E, De La Torres E. Myelomonocytic leukaemia with a preleukaemic syndrome and Ph1 chromosome in monozygotic twins. Arch Dis Child 1977;52:72.
924. Sheffer R, Cividalli G, Zaharan Y, Tamari H, Okon E. Disturbed patterns of globin chain synthesis in childhood monosomy 7 myeloproliferative syndrome. Br J Haematol 1988;68:357.
925. Rochant H, Dreyfus B, Bouguerra M, Tont-Hat H. Refractory anemias, preleukemic conditions, and fetal erythropoiesis. Blood 1972;39: 721.
926. Valentine WN, Konrad PN, Paglia DE. Dyserythropoiesis, refractory anemia, and "preleukemia": metabolic features of the erythrocytes. Blood 1973;41:857.
927. Nowell P, Wilmoth D, Lange B. Cytogenetics of childhood preleukemia. Cancer Genet Cytogenet 1983;10:261.
928. Raskind WH, Tirumali N, Jacobson R, Singer J, Fialkow PJ. Evidence for a multistep pathogenesis of a myelodysplastic syndrome. Blood 1984;63:1318.
929. Koeffler HP, Golde D. Human preleukemia. Ann Intern Med 1980;93: 347.
930. Chui DHK, Clarke BJ. Abnormal erythroid progenitor cells in human preleukemia. Blood 1982;60:362.
931. Creutzig U, Cantu-Rajnoldi A, Ritter J, et al. Myelodysplastic syndromes in childhood. Am J Pediatr Hematol Oncol 1987;9:324.
932. Guinan EC, Tarbell NJ, Tantravahi R, Weinstein HJ. Bone marrow transplantation for children with myelodysplastic syndromes. Blood 1989;73:619.
933. Vadhan-Raj S, Keating M, LeMaistre A, et al. Effects of recombinant human granulocyte-macrophage colony-stimulating factor in patients with myelodysplastic syndromes. N Engl J Med 1987;317:1545.
934. Negrin RS, Haeuber DH, Nagler A, et al. Treatment of myelodysplastic syndromes with recombinant human granulocyte colony-stimulating factor. Ann Intern Med 1989;110:976.

Blood: Principles and Practice of Hematology,
edited by Robert I. Handin, Thomas P. Stossel, and Samuel E. Lux.
J.B. Lippincott Company, Philadelphia © 1995.

10

Acquired Bone Marrow Failure

Neal S. Young

HISTORICAL BACKGROUND

The medical study of bone marrow failure dates to 1888, when Paul Ehrlich[1] described a young woman with an explosive fatal illness marked by severe anemia, bleeding into the skin and retina, and high fever. The empty bone marrow and its devastating consequences for the patient have rightfully fascinated hematologists for a century, provoking an interest far out of proportion to the incidence of the disease. What other medical specialty is faced with the apparent disappearance of its organ of interest? The study of this disease has not lost its luster. Effective therapy is now available for most patients, but the implementation of curative regimens and the supportive care of the patient require high levels of technical competence and physician responsibility. In more recent times, we may be approaching understanding of the basic mechanisms of marrow failure through the application of such disciplines as cell biology, immunology, virology, and toxicology.

Nosology

As a pathologist, Ehrlich stressed the complete replacement of the patient's bone marrow tissue with fat at autopsy, and he inferred from the morphologic appearance of the marrow only a failure of blood cell regeneration. The combination of low blood cell counts and absent marrow precursor cells remains the essential feature of aplastic anemia and its relatives, pure red cell aplasia (PRCA), agranulocytosis, and amegakaryocytic thrombocytopenia. Unfortunately, the clarity of Ehrlich's discovery was soon lost, and some of the early assumptions had enduring deleterious effects on the medical and experimental approaches to aplastic anemia. Two major problems beset the early literature and to some extent current practice: first, the too-facile identification of depressed blood counts with aplastic anemia; second, unwarranted inferences concerning pathogenesis from bone marrow appearance.

Chauffard[2] introduced the term *aplastic anemia*, which is derived from the Greek verb πλάϑω, "to create and give shape to" (άπλάστκή, the adjective "unformed"). It emphasized the then easily determined low red blood cell (RBC) count rather than the deficiency of cells of all three hematopoietic lineages. More important, the name stressed an apparent functional abnormality rather than the structural characteristic of the empty bone marrow. In fact, Chauffard's original article was entitled, "A case of pernicious aplastic anemia." Ehrlich had distinguished his case from the cellular morphology of pernicious anemia, but well into the 20th century aplastic anemia appeared in medical textbooks as a subheading of pernicious anemia.[3] Unfortunately, inaccuracy and imprecision continue, with consequences for the individual misdiagnosed patient and for the interpretation of group data in clinical studies.

The pernicious anemia that was once a clinical cousin to aplasia is now recognized as a vitamin deficiency disorder with predominantly hematologic manifestations; the sequence of biochemical events that produce megaloblastic cells and the origins of deficiency of B_{12} or folate are well understood. Improvements in pathologic examination and, more recently, in cytogenetics and the molecular analysis of individual chromosomes have led to other bone marrow failure states being classified by such dominant morphologic features as the pattern of myelodysplasia (sideroblastic anemia) or the absence of genetic material (the 5q− syndrome). As a final example, deficient marrow function is a feature of many of the leukemias and may be out of proportion to apparent marrow replacement, but these diseases are obviously classified by their malignant aspect. Conversely, the conception of aplastic anemia as an intrinsic marrow disease,[4,5] certainly useful in the differential diagnosis, is far more applicable to inherited marrow failure than to acquired disease in the adult.

Differential Diagnosis of Pancytopenia

An empty bone marrow is usually obvious (Fig. 10-1). The most important and difficult choice of diagnoses in the pancytopenic patients rests among primary bone marrow diseases (Table 10-1). Several complicating factors should be recognized. In moderate aplastic anemia, only modest depression of marrow cellularity may be present. Bone marrow cellularity is imprecisely quantitated, sampling error is large, and "hot spots" of hematopoietic activity in an otherwise acellular specimen indicate heterogeneity in the pattern of cell loss. Chronic aplastic anemia can evolve into other diseases (including acute myeloblastic leukemia,[6] hairy-cell leukemia,[7] multiple myeloma,[8] and myelodysplasia[9,10]). Leukemia, dysplasia, and aplasia share etiologic risk factors (radiation, chemicals, congenital chromosomal abnormalities). In some cases, separate pathophysiologic processes may be operating in a single patient who manifests more than a single disease (aplastic anemia and myelofibrosis,[11] RBC hypoplasia, myelodysplasia,[12] and others) or show a mixture of pathologic features on bone marrow examination.

Occasional patients with aplastic anemia do not have

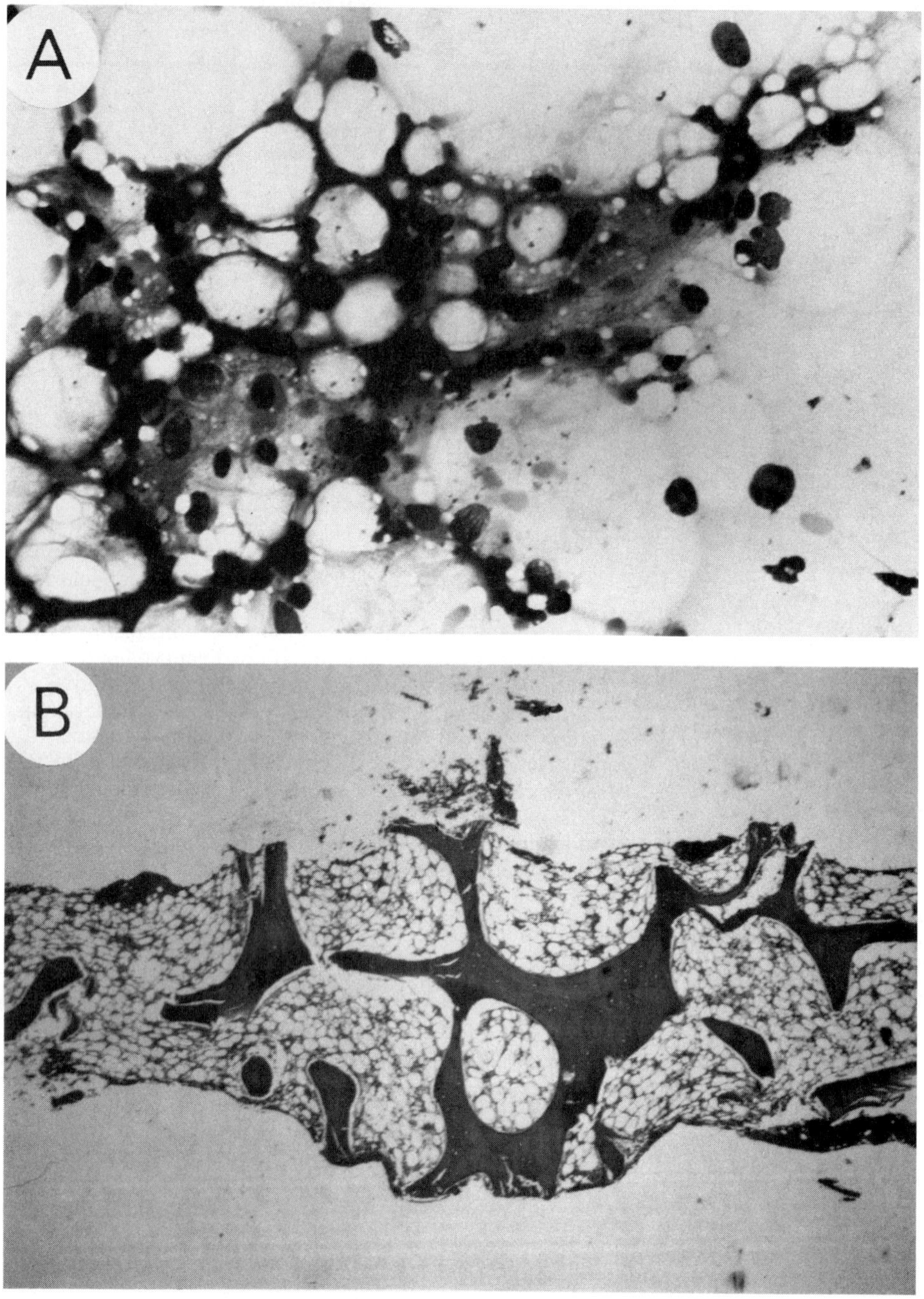

FIGURE 10-1. Bone marrow in aplastic anemia. Core biopsy (**A**) and aspirate smear (**B**) from a patient with severe aplastic anemia show residual stromal and lymphoid elements.

pancytopenia, and they do not have uniform depression of RBC, white blood cell (WBC), and platelet production, despite an empty bone marrow. Their clinical course is dominated by failure in two or even a single hematopoietic lineage. Related aplastic conditions such as PRCA, amegakaryocytic thrombocytopenia, and agranulocytosis, although usually distinctive in their clinical presentation, may unfold into more generalized marrow failure. In the absence of better markers, sometimes the only accurate diagnosis of pancytopenia is a description of the clinical features and specific marrow morphology.

The acute leukemias and myelodysplastic syndromes can atypically be associated with marrow hypocellularity and confused with aplastic anemia. The syndrome of hypoplastic or hypocellular acute leukemia has been estimated to account for 5% to 8% of acute nonlymphocytic leukemia.[13–15] Acute lymphoblastic leukemia also can present as aplastic anemia in children[16,17] and adults.[18] Some patients with myelodysplasia also have hypocellular bone marrows, and aplastic anemia and myelodysplasia are probably most often confused. In a series of 183 patients referred to the University of Washington with a diagnosis of aplastic anemia, only 4% had myelodysplasia.[10] A higher percentage of cases with cellular atypia has been found by other investigators. In a German study of 111 bone marrow specimens labeled aplastic, 21 showed megakaryocytic atypia, 12 showed dyserythropoiesis, 8 showed dysmyelopoiesis, and 43 showed fibrosis; the presence of dysmorphic changes highly correlated with the risk of developing acute nonlymphocytic leukemia.[19]

A high rate of evolution was documented in a Dutch longitudinal study. Of 38 patients with successfully treated aplastic anemia with normal cytogenetics who had survived more than 2 years, 5 evolved to myelodysplasia (3 had monosomy 7), and 3 of these 5 ultimately developed acute myelogenous leukemia.[9] A diagnosis of myelodys-

TABLE 10-1. Differential Diagnosis of Pancytopenia

PANCYTOPENIA WITH HYPOCELLULAR BONE MARROW
Acquired aplastic anemia
Inherited aplastic anemia (Fanconi's anemia)
Some myelodysplasia syndromes
Rare aleukemic leukemia (acute myelogenous or lymphoblastic leukemia)
Some acute lymphoblastic leukemia
Some lymphomas of bone marrow
PANCYTOPENIA WITH CELLULAR BONE MARROW
Primary Bone Marrow Diseases
Myelodysplasia syndromes
Paroxysmal nocturnal hemoglobinuria
Myelofibrosis
Some aleukemic leukemia
Myelophthisis
Bone marrow lymphoma
Hairy cell leukemia
Secondary to Systemic Diseases
Systemic lupus erythematosus[1334]
Hypersplenism
Vitamin B_{12}, folate deficiency (familial defect[1335])
Overwhelming infection
Alcohol
Brucellosis[1336]
Sarcoidosis
Tuberculosis[1337–1339]
HYPOCELLULAR BONE MARROW WITH OR WITHOUT CYTOPENIA
Q fever[1340]
Legionnaire's disease[1341]
Anorexia nervosa,[1342–1344] starvation[1343,1345]
Mycobacteria[1346]

plasia or hypoplastic leukemia carries a worse prognosis than moderate aplastic anemia.[20] Bone marrow aplasia has been observed during the evolution of refractory anemia to leukemia and has been associated with progressive karyotypic changes,[21] and a case of myelomonocytic leukemia with an abnormal karyotype evolved from aplastic anemia.[22]

Pancytopenia can result from peripheral blood processes with relatively normal bone marrow function, but such syndromes usually occur in an obvious clinical context as complications of nonhematologic primary disease. Pancytopenia is unlikely to be the presenting feature of hypersplenism in cirrhosis or of Evans' syndrome in systemic lupus erythematosus. Findings on physical examination may point strongly toward another diagnosis; for example, the patient with myelofibrosis usually has splenomegaly, whereas a patient with aplastic anemia rarely has a large spleen. Although B_{12} and folate deficiency have been reported to be associated with erythroid hypoplasia,[23] it is rare. In general, the likelihood of confusion with other intrinsic bone marrow processes is not equal for all conditions. Therefore, before a bone marrow examination is performed, the list of possible diagnoses should be shortened by analyzing the patient's history and physical examination and by judging the probability of the alternative disorders.

The bone marrow examination is the ultimate basis for the diagnosis of most primary hematologic causes of pancytopenia. Both the aspirate smear and the biopsy must be examined to arrive at an accurate diagnosis. Observation during the procedure itself may be helpful in the differential diagnosis; a fatty specimen can usually be aspirated without difficulty from a patient with aplastic anemia, and a true dry tap is more typical of the packed bone marrow seen in patients with chronic lymphocytic leukemia, hairy-cell leukemia, and acute leukemia or the fibrotic marrow of myelofibrosis. The morphology of individual cells is best displayed on Wright-Giemsa stain of the aspirate smear, the architecture of the marrow, on the biopsy section. A stained smear can be prepared within minutes of the procedure and should be examined within hours of its preparation for the presence of characteristic individual cells or patterns of differentiation that point toward a specific diagnosis. Examination of the cells close to the spicules of a sparse aspirate smear may disclose a distinct population of leukemic blasts; or, the dysmorphic appearance of residual erythroid cells may more strongly suggest dysplasia than aplasia.

Cytogenetic analysis is also useful because chromosomal analysis is usually normal in aplastic anemia patients and frequently abnormal in myelodysplasia patients.[10] Lymphoid aggregates, nests of tumor cells, granulomas, and infectious particles may be visible only on the fixed biopsy specimen. An uncertain diagnosis jeopardizes not only the patient, who may be directed to an improper treatment, but also the integrity of clinical trials; in older hematologic studies, because of inadequate sampling and interpretation, diverse processes are often treated together, and inferences concerning natural history and therapeutic effects should be treated by the modern reader with caution.

APLASTIC ANEMIA

Aplastic anemia is the paradigm of bone marrow failure.[24–30] The name encompasses heterogeneous disorders: the Chernobyl fireman with severe radiation damage, the child with infectious mononucleosis-associated aplasia who responds to immunosuppression, the adolescent presenting late with Fanconi's anemia. All affected persons exhibit the same pathology but suffer different disease processes. Patients with aplastic anemia are united by practical management considerations and also by apparently similar pathophysiologic mechanisms. These common features are stressed in this chapter.

Epidemiology

Recent studies in Europe and the United States suggest an annual incidence of aplastic anemia of 2 to 6 cases per 1 million population[31–35] (Table 10-2). By comparison, the incidences of acute myelogenous leukemia and multiple myeloma are about 35 and 27 cases per 1 million people, respectively. Although an apparent increase in the incidence of aplastic anemia during the 1950s and 1960s was reported by some authors,[36,37] more recent surveys show that the incidence has probably been stable in the past 20 years.[31,34,35] Earlier studies may have been in error by inclusion of cases of pancytopenia secondary to cytostatic drug therapy or resulting from other diseases such as myelodysplasia. Figures of occurrence of aplastic anemia may be heavily influenced by the method of ascertainment and exclusion criteria[35,38]. Few studies have included rigorous confirmation of the diagnosis by a hematologist's review of the chart and tissue. Until recently, chromosome analysis was infrequently performed in adults, and some cases of apparently acquired aplastic anemia almost certainly were misdiagnosed inherited aplastic anemia.

The incidence of aplastic anemia varies significantly with

TABLE 10-2. Epidemiology of Aplastic Anemia*

Study	Dates	Method, Data Base	Population Size (Millions)	Total No. of Cases	Incidence per Million People
US Army[57]	1942–1945	Retrospective, marrow tissue	—	57	0.4–1.8 6.6–28.4†
California[140]	1960	Retrospective, death certificates	15.7	81	5.2
California[141]	1963–1964	Death certificates	2.4	93	7.8
Uppsala, Sweden[1347]	1964–1968	Retrospective, discharge diagnosis	1.3	13	
Uppsala[1220]	1973–1977	Retrospective, medical records	1.3	90	14.0
Israel[1331]	1961–1965	Retrospective, hospital/clinic records	17.5	93	7.8
Japan[42]	1970–1973	Prospective, nationwide hospital survey	—	471	13.9
Japan[51]	1970–1973	Prospective, industry survey	11.3	166	14.7
Baltimore[31]	1970–1978	Retrospective, medical records and death certificates	2.1	118	6.1
Northern Region, UK[35]	1971–1978	Hospital records	3.3	174	6.8
South Carolina[56]	1970–1981	Retrospective, medical records and death certificates	3.1	27	8.7
United Kingdom[33]	1985	Prospective survey of hematologists	21.0	49	2.3
Denmark[34]	1967–1982	Retrospective registry (children only)	1.1	39	2.2
Europe[32]	1980–1984	Population-based case control survey	22.3	168	2.2
Buenos Aires[1348]	1966–1977	Retrospective, medical records	0.5	35	6.0
France[1349]	1984–1987	Prospective, medical records	—	250	1.4

* Studies are listed in order of their date of publication.
† Pacific theater.

age. The incidence curve shows two peaks, with patients mainly presenting at 15 to 25 years or over 60 years of age, and with a trough in middle life[35,39] (Figs. 10-2 and 10-3). (If inherited disease is included, a third peak appears in the first decade.) American mortality figures indicate a major peak in deaths in late middle age.[40]

The most remarkable feature of the epidemiology of aplastic anemia is an apparently large and unexplained geographic variation in its incidence.[41,42] For years, physicians in the Orient and their foreign visitors have believed that aplastic anemia (and the related paroxysmal nocturnal hemoglobinuria [PNH]) is far more common there than in the West.[39,43,44] Certainly, the *prevalence* (total number of cases in a population at a single time) of aplastic anemia is high in the Far East. Hospitals in China (Y. Hao, Institute of Hematology, Tianjin, personal communication), Korea,[45,46] and Thailand (S. Issaragrasil, Sirriraj Hospital, Bangkok, personal communication) may see hundreds of cases of aplastic anemia annually, making it nearly as common as acute myelogenous leukemia as an admitting diagnosis; in most American hospitals, acute myelogenous leukemia is 5 to 10 times more common than aplastic anemia as an admitting diagnosis. A nationwide survey in Japan in 1972 led to an estimate of prevalence of aplastic anemia

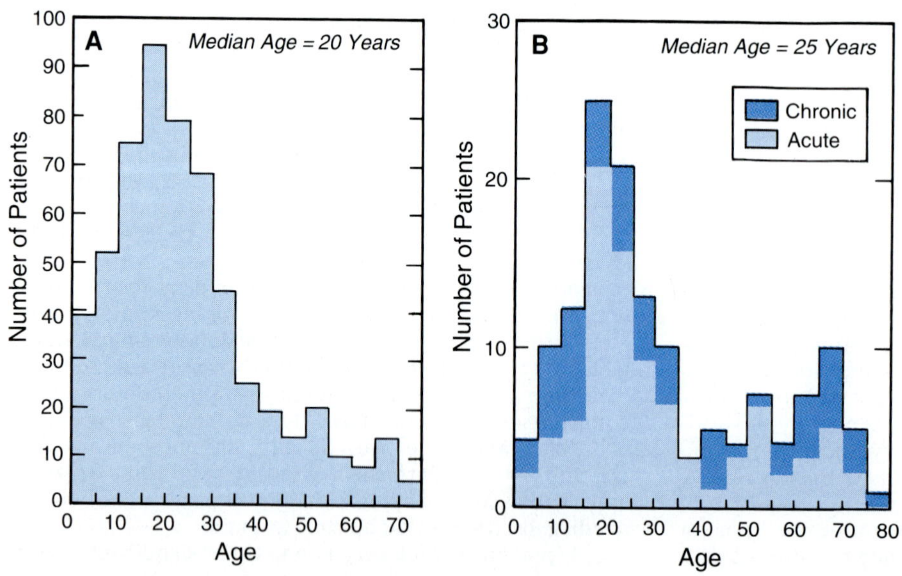

FIGURE 10-2. Incidence of aplastic anemia by age. (**A**) Age at first treatment for patients referred to the University of Washington, mainly for bone marrow transplantation. (**B**) Age at diagnostic bone marrow biopsy for patients referred to the NIH (1983 to 1989), where bone marrow transplantation is not performed. Acute, less than 3 months between diagnosis and presentation at NIH; chronic, more than 3 months.

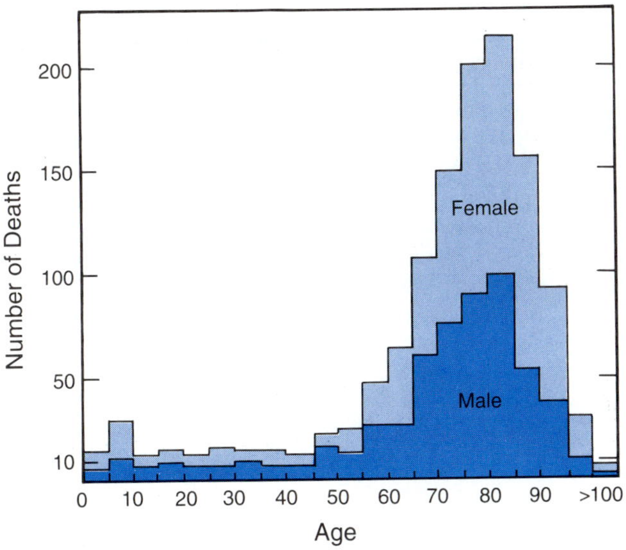

FIGURE 10-3. Mortality from aplastic anemia by age. In this year (1986), a total of 1254 deaths occurred from all aplastic anemia, 27 of which were listed as constitutional aplastic anemia, 366 as other aplastic anemia, and 861 as unspecified aplastic anemia. (Data from US Department of Health and Human Services. Mortality. In: Vital statistics of the United States, ed 2. Washington, DC, 1986: 122)

of 31 to 48 per 1 million population.[47] Two large population surveys in China arrived at similar estimates of 19 to 21 per 1 million people [48,49]; for comparison, the prevalence of acute myelogenous leukemia was 37 per 1 million people (Wang, Peoples' Hospital, Beijing, personal communication).

Incidence, a rate figure defined as the number of new cases in a population per year, is more difficult to determine. An autopsy series suggested that the incidence of aplastic anemia might be at least three times higher in the East than in the West.[50] Comparison of age-adjusted mortality statistics from 1968 to 1971 showed mortality rates in Japan (9.2 per 1 million people) to be about two to three times higher than those in the United States and Europe (3 to 6 per 1 million people).[41] Accurate incidence figures for most of Asia are lacking, and the true ratio may be higher. In Japan, for example, an industry-based national survey found an incidence of 14.4 per 1 million workers aged 19 to 61 years old.[51] Marked and unexplained degrees of variation in the incidence of aplastic anemia have also been observed in European cities, although at rates generally much lower than in the Far East (ranging from 0.6 per 1 million people in Budapest to 3.1 per 1 million people in Milan).[32]

The incidence of aplastic anemia in other parts of the world is unknown. The disease may be particularly prevalent in Mexico and perhaps also in other parts of Latin America.[52] Aplastic anemia occurs frequently in Africa but is probably underdiagnosed,[53-55] and a relatively high incidence was reported among American blacks in a small area of South Carolina.[56]

The explanation for the geographic variation in aplastic anemia is probably mainly environmental rather than genetic, since Japanese in Hawaii seem to have aplastic anemia at the same rate as Americans.[41] (Conversely, American soldiers in the Pacific theater during World War II had a high incidence of aplastic anemia, attributed to use of quinacrine.[57]) Chloramphenicol is a popular antibiotic in much of Asia, because of its efficacy and low cost, but reductions in its use have not been correlated with changes in incidence of aplastic anemia in Japan[58,59] or elsewhere[31,60,61]; chloramphenicol sales are high in Hong Kong, where the rate of aplastic anemia is about the same as that in England.[62] A case control study has shown relations to chemical exposures and exposures to viruses through blood transfusions, hepatitis, and occupation.[63] As noted, a cluster of cases of aplastic anemia, also suggestive of an environmental pathogen, has been reported in South Carolina.[56,64] An environmental influence is also suggested by a trend toward seasonal variation in the onset of aplastic anemia, with peak occurrence in spring and fall.[33,34,65]

Clinical Associations and Pathogenesis

The importance of a classification scheme (Tables 10-3 and 10-4) is to assist in determining prognosis, therapy, and common features that can be related to pathogenesis. A too-strict division into categories can obscure important relations, the genetic basis for susceptibility to drugs or viruses, and common interactions with the immune system. Most patients have idiopathic disease, really meaning cause unknown, but for most clinical associations the inductive mechanisms are uncertain. The determination of clinical association has generally been imprecise, and the basis for assigning patients in practice is the history: How closely is the patient questioned? How biased and repetitive are the inquiries? How conscientiously sought is a significant distant toxic exposure or how exaggerated is a brief episode? Patients with idiopathic and secondary disease require similar support and definitive therapies; with few exceptions, little basis exists for major differences in their clinical management.

Genetic Factors

Inherited forms of aplastic anemia are described in greater detail in Chapter 9. Patients with inherited aplastic anemia may present as adults. The expansion of diagnostic cytogenetic testing has revealed that many patients with Fanconi's anemia lack physical signs and, most important, may become pancytopenic well beyond childhood. The diagnosis of Fanconi's anemia, defined cytogenetically, should be pursued by chromosome analysis of peripheral blood cells in patients in middle life as well as in childhood. About half of the patients with reported cases of dyskeratosis congenita have had aplastic anemia; typically, pancytopenia in this congenital disease does not appear until the third decade of life. Because of its rarity, the association between the skin and blood disorders may be overlooked.

Familial aplastic anemia that is not Fanconi's anemia must be extremely rare. Occasional patients with acquired aplastic anemia describe aplastic anemia in relatives. Pancytopenia in relatives was found in 8 of 55 adult patients,[66] but some of these families probably represented inherited aplastic anemia with presentation late in life. Case reports of idiopathic aplastic anemia in siblings[67] and parent and child[68] are subject to the same reservation.

Genetic factors likely predispose rather than predetermine aplasia. Clinical evidence of pancytopenia in Fanconi's anemia patients commonly appears after a chemical exposure, although the chromosomal abnormalities are present from birth. Other, as yet undefined, genetic variability in DNA repair enzymes, drug metabolizing enzymes, and the immune response may underlie susceptibility to inciting drugs and viruses. Perhaps the reportedly abnormal susceptibility of lymphocyte DNA to bleomycin,[69,70] a strand breaker, and ultraviolet light[71] in adult acquired aplastic anemia reflects a Fanconi's-like defect, but prospective studies cannot easily be performed in these patients. Aplastic anemia has occurred among siblings in six families

TABLE 10-3. Classification of Aplastic Anemia

Acquired Aplastic Anemia	Inherited Aplastic Anemia
SECONDARY APLASTIC ANEMIA	Fanconi's anemia
Radiation	Dyskeratosis congenita
Drugs and chemicals	Shwachman-Diamond syndrome
Regular effects	Reticular dysgenesis
Cytotoxic agents	Amegakaryocytic thrombocytopenia
Benzene	Other (familial aplastic anemias)
Idiosyncratic reactions	Preleukemia (monosomy 7 and others)
Chloramphenicol	Nonhematologic syndromes
Nonsteroidal antiinflammatories	Down's, Dubowitz, Seckel syndromes
Antiepileptics	
Gold	
Other drugs and chemicals	
Viruses	
Epstein-Barr virus (infectious mononucleosis)	
Hepatitis C virus (non–A, non–B hepatitis)	
Parvovirus (transient aplastic crisis, pure red cell aplasia)	
Human immunodeficiency virus	
Immune diseases	
Eosinophilic fasciitis	
Hypoimmunoglobulinemia	
Thymoma and thymic carcinoma	
Graft-versus-host disease in immunodeficiency	
Paroxysmal nocturnal hemoglobinuria	
Pregnancy	
IDIOPATHIC APLASTIC ANEMIA	

exposed to chloramphenicol,[72–75] in occasional families exposed to other drugs,[76,77] and in siblings of two families after hepatitis.[78,79] One form of genetic susceptibility is dramatically exemplified by the high frequency of aplastic anemia in boys with the X-linked lymphoproliferative syndrome, which is characterized by an abnormal immune response to Epstein-Barr virus (EBV).[80]

A model of experimental aplastic anemia in mice, which is mediated by transplantation of lymph node cells into HLA-matched irradiated recipients, is dependent on narrow differences in nonhistocompatibility loci.[81] Increased representation of some class I (HLA A2) and class II (HLA DR2, HLA DR4, HLA DPw3) antigens among patients with acquired aplastic anemia has been reported.[82–85]

Ionizing Radiation

Acute Exposure. Marrow aplasia is a major result of acute toxicity of radiation, [86–89] from nuclear bomb explosions, fallout, reactor accidents, and accidental exposure to radiation sources in medicine and industry. Radiation is widely used not only for medical research and therapy (as radioisotopes and x-rays or particles generated from high-energy accelerators) but also for seed sterilization, food preservation, and industrial radiography of metals. A scale of radiation doses is shown in Figure 10-4. Large radioactive sources have fallen off trucks, been retrieved from junkyards and abandoned medical clinics, and been used in murder and suicide attempts. Although radiation injuries are relatively unusual and often dramatic, in major catastrophes such as the atomic bomb explosions over Hiroshima and Nagasaki, radiation accounted directly for only about 15% of the total casualties, with burn and blast injuries predominating[90]; even in more restricted episodes such as the Chernobyl reactor accident, most fatalities were the result of skin burns and damage to the gastrointestinal and pulmonary systems.[91] Collateral local injuries, especially burns, also greatly complicate the management of pancytopenia.

Precisely how radiant energy damages cells is uncertain.[92,93] Radiant energy generates ions, peroxides, and free radicals, and radiation doses are defined in terms of ionization in tissue (1 gray [Gy] = absorbed energy equivalent to 1 joule/kg unit mass; 1 Gy = 100 rad). Large macromolecules, especially DNA, can be damaged (1) directly by large amounts of radiant energy that can rupture covalent bonds or (2) indirectly by interaction with highly charged

TABLE 10-4. Classification of the Single Cytopenias

Acquired Cytopenias	Inherited Cytopenias
Pure red cell aplasia	
Idiopathic	Diamond-Blackfan anemia
Drugs, toxins	
Immune	
Thymoma	
Transient erythroblastopenia of childhood	
Neutropenia	
Idiopathic	Kostmann's syndrome
Drugs, toxins	Shwachman-Diamond syndrome
	Reticular dysgenesis
Thrombocytopenia	
Idiopathic amegakaryocytic	Amegakaryocytic thrombocytopenia with absent radii
Drugs, toxins	

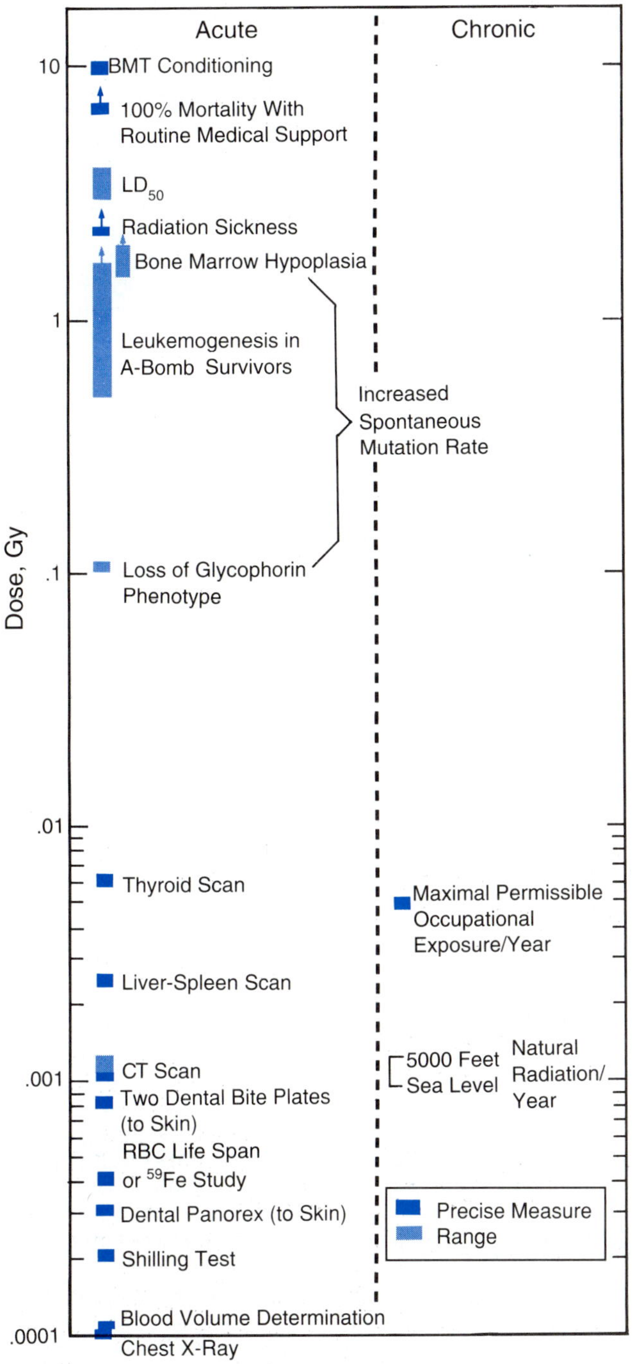

FIGURE 10-4. Scale of whole-body radiation doses.

and reactive small molecules resulting from ionization or free radical formation occurring in solution. With the singular exception of lymphocytes, a round of replication is required for radiation damage to become manifest. Mitotically active hematopoietic tissue is exquisitely sensitive to almost all types of radiation. In atomic bomb explosions, γ radiation has been the major effector of tissue damage, whereas α, β, γ, and neutron emissions all figure to variable degrees in civilian accidents. Bone marrow cells are probably most affected by high-energy γ rays, which penetrate the viscera, and secondarily by ingested or absorbed α and β particles (low-energy β particles burn but do not penetrate beyond the skin).

Cytotoxicity and bone marrow hypoplasia occur with radiation doses higher than 1.5 to 2 Gy to the whole body. The median lethal dose (LD_{50}) is dependent on the quality of medical care applied; at intermediate radiation doses around the LD_{50}, bone marrow toxicity is limiting to survival. For the Hiroshima atomic bomb explosion, which effectively destroyed the medical support system, the LD_{50} was estimated at 2.2 to 3 Gy.[28] From assessment of the outcome of radiation accidents and the high-dose radiation of patients with Ewing's sarcoma (in total, a small number of cases), all of whom have received fuller medical support, the LD_{50} has been estimated at about 4.5 Gy.[28,94,95] Of course, the LD_{50} for bone marrow transplant recipients conditioned by total body irradiation is about 10 Gy. The capacity for mitosis is much more sensitive than the viability functions of a cell to the effects of radiation, and the dose-related occurrence of pancytopenia 2 to 4 weeks after a single large exposure is due to injury to the actively replicating pool of marrow progenitor and precursor cells. (An exception is the lymphocyte, which is extremely sensitive to radiation and is directly lysed by relatively low doses, independent of proliferation.) The ability to recover hematopoietic function after even massive single-radiation exposure is considerable, reflecting the resistance of the quiescent stem cell to damage and the enormous marrow repopulating potential of even a greatly reduced stem cell pool.

Autopsies of atomic bomb victims in Japan showed acellular bone marrows in persons dying within the first 2 weeks of the explosion, but frequently bone marrow was regenerating in those who survived to 6 weeks.[96] Physical structures and the body itself can create complicated patterns of shielding. Because of the heterogeneous pattern of exposure in accidental compared with experimental irradiation, some areas of bone marrow may escape with relatively light radiation damage.

The hematologist is required to care for the patient who has received a sufficient dose to suppress the bone marrow but not such an overwhelming dose that death from other causes is inevitable.[86,89,97,98] Although the principles of management of pancytopenia after a single large dose of radiation are similar to those for aplastic anemia in general, some exceptional points should be made concerning immediate evaluation and long-term prognosis. The type and intensity of the source of radiation and the distance and shielding of the subject are the major determinants of radiation injury; given the nature of the exposure, these factors are often difficult to assess either immediately or retrospectively. Early recognition of the nature of the accident provides the best opportunity for dosimetry by accident reconstruction and the collection of biologic specimens; full characterization of the event may also allow the use of blocking, displacing, or chelating agents and avoid the inadvertent exposure of other persons, including medical personnel.[99,100]

Serial monitoring of blood counts also can provide a good measure of radiation dose.[86,101,102] For atomic bomb victims, exposure correlated well with the degree of pancytopenia.[103] Lymphocytes are particularly sensitive to radiation, with rapid changes in number and morphology. The rate of fall of lymphocytes is a dose-related function up to about 3 Gy of total body exposure[87,103]; at higher doses, the fall in granulocytes and the severity of thrombocytopenia and reticulocytopenia can be used to estimate dose.[89]

Patients with severe pancytopenia who do not die immediately of acute radiation sickness often survive a radiation accident. Bone marrow and fetal liver transplantation were used in the Chernobyl nuclear reactor accident but with uncertain benefit (almost all the patients with transplants died).[104,105] Thirty years earlier, Mathé[106] had performed unmatched bone marrow transplants after a Yugoslav reactor accident; the survival of his patients (and others who were not transplanted) suggests in retrospect that autologous marrow reconstitution occurs in most who survive the immediate consequences of radiation.[107] On the other hand, a radiation accident patient with a mean whole-body exposure of 6 Gy showed reversal of the typical pancytopenia in 15 to 19 days, rather than in the usual 28 to 32 days, after receiving a marrow transplant from an identical twin.[108]

Hematopoietic growth factor administration may be helpful. Direct destruction of lymphocytes by radiation could result in deficiency of growth factors,[109] and hematopoietic growth factors can shorten the period of neutropenia after acute radiation exposure and prolong survival in rodent models; IL-1,[110,111] GM-CSF,[112] and G-CSF[113] have all been effective. In clinical use, GM-CSF increased granulocyte counts in seven of eight patients (three of whom died) who had been exposed to a cesium-137 (^{137}Cs) source discarded from a radiation therapy clinic in Brazil.[114]

Aplastic anemia, in contrast to acute leukemia, is not a late consequence of atomic bomb exposure or fallout.[115–117] Both single large doses and chronic radiation exposure result in prolonged depression of amount of progenitor and the self-renewing capacity of the stem cell compartment as a whole[118]; experiments with long-term bone marrow culture suggest that stem cells that survive radiation damage behave normally.[119] As observed after other insults to the bone marrow, normal blood counts and normal marrow morphology can be maintained from a limited stem cell pool (see section on pathophysiology). Experiments with irradiation of single limbs in animals and with long-term tissue culture have suggested that the degree of injury to stromal cells, which are much less sensitive to radiation (of more than 40 Gy), ultimately may determine recovery in a localized region of marrow. "Second" waves of aplasia in irradiated limbs are presumably due to stromal failure. Late aplasia may not occur in whole-body exposures because the high doses required to ablate the stroma invariably produce acute and fatal cutaneous, gastrointestinal, and neurologic damage.

Chronic Exposure. Chronic radiation is associated with many bone marrow diseases. Repeated exposures to low doses are less damaging to stromal cells, which may tolerate 40 to 50 Gy of fractionated radiation with some repair.[88] Continuous low-dose γ radiation produces aplasia in about half of exposed dogs after a total dose of 20 Gy, with the survivors dying of granulocytic leukemia.[120] Repeated low doses of radiation can damage human bone marrow and have been associated with aplastic anemia. Some of the workers in the luminous watch industry died of aplastic anemia, including not only the unfortunate young women who pointed their radium-tinged brushes with their tongues but also the company's technical director who had formulated the paint.[121] Mesothorium that was injected rather than ingested as the contrast material, Thorotrast, produced iatrogenic aplasia, as well as acute leukemia and myelofibrosis, often decades after the injection caused by the relentless destruction of marrow cells by slowly disintegrating isotope.[122,123]

Excessive deaths from aplastic anemia (and acute leukemia) have occurred after therapeutic irradiation of the spine for ankylosing spondylitis.[124] Excessive deaths from aplastic anemia, and to a lesser degree from acute leukemia and multiple myeloma, occurred among American radiologists who died between 1948 and 1961, presumably the victims of γ scatter.[125] The bone marrow of Hodgkin's disease patients who have been irradiated is much less tolerant of chemotherapy,[126] but aplastic anemia was not found in unexpected numbers in a large population of cancer patients who had received therapeutic radiation.[127] Although the distinction of aplastic anemia from myelodysplasia in some of the older reports is not reliable and a cellular, or "regenerative," phase may occur before the development of frank aplasia, chronic radiation exposure probably can cause accumulated stem cell injury, depletion of stem cells through continued recruitment from a quiescent reserve, or stromal injury.

Drugs and Chemicals

Drug or chemical exposure is the most frequently cited specific cause of aplastic anemia in both clinical series of patients and epidemiologic surveys[128–133] (Figs. 10-5 and 10-6). The agents cited vary with place and over time: benzene and chloramphenicol have been replaced by hydantoin and phenylbutazone with changing patterns of industrial exposure and choice of medications[134] (Tables 10-5 and 10-6). Remarkably, aplastic anemia patients with a history of drug or toxin exposure have demographic and clinical characteristics, a similar prognosis, and equivalent responses to therapy that are identical with those of patients with idiopathic disease.[133] Drug histories may be inadequate or chemical exposures unrecognized in patients with "idiopathic" disease, who may be genetically predisposed to exquisite drug susceptibility. On the other hand, the high percentage of patients in the clinical series with aplastic anemia from a chemical cause may be a biased overestimate. Although about one third of aplastic anemia patients studied by the European cooperative group had significant exposures, twice the percentage of control patients with other hematologic diseases had a similar history of drug exposure.[134] Drug use or chemical exposure also did not figure significantly in a case control study of aplastic anemia.[63]

Clear causal relations between drugs or chemicals and bone marrow failure have been established in only rare instances. The literature on idiosyncratic reactions is best approached with some skepticism. Many studies suffer from the lapses in scientific standards pointed out by Feinstein[135] in his criticism of epidemiologic studies of the "menace of daily life": lack of specific hypotheses, poor quality data, absence of mechanism, and, especially, detection bias. In general, the link between drugs and adverse reactions is more often conditional or dubious than definitive or even probable.[136] Case reports beget case reports, and patients with aplastic anemia are undoubtedly more closely questioned about potentially toxic exposures than patients with most other diseases. Interpretation of case reports is often confounded because many drugs are used in combination. The onset of marrow failure is notoriously difficult to accurately date and therefore to place temporally in relation to drug use; the delay in marrow disease after benzene use may be years or decades. Conversely, trivial case reports of drug use are virtually coincident with the onset of marrow failure.

Authors are often explicit in incriminating an exposure only because there is no other blameworthy preceding event. Aplastic anemia has been ascribed to traditional herbal medicines in Africa.[137] Even the large, thorough, and expensive International Agranulocytosis and Aplastic Anemia Study has been faulted for biases in susceptibility, recall and interviewer, diagnostic suspicion, and choice of control group and exclusion.[138]

Even confirmed associations do not establish causality. Some drugs may be preferentially used in a patient population that has an inherently high risk of marrow failure. Antibiotics may be prescribed for the first symptom of neutropenia or for the preceding causal viral infection. The platelet inhibitory effect of nonsteroidal antiinflammatory drugs may precipitate bleeding in an already thrombocytopenic patient. Some associations, especially with drugs or chemicals in common use, are simply misconstrued. An example of error that is obvious in retrospect decades later is the association of aplastic anemia with glue sniffing; five of the six patients described in the initial report had sickle cell disease with transient aplastic crisis,[139] now recognized as resulting from parvovirus infection.

Aplastic anemia has been called "the most disabling, most frequently fatal, and, next to agranulocytosis, the most frequently reported of adverse reactions to drugs."[140] Quantitative estimates of risk are only approximate. In most retrospective studies, cases have been collected, drug use ascertained, and calculations based on the amount of drug produced and an average dose; each of these procedures is subject to error. The risk of aplastic anemia from a course of chloramphenicol has been estimated at 1 in 20,000 to 60,000, based on an average therapeutic course of 4 g and the assumption of causality with every association (some of the original cases used chloramphenicol after the onset of disease[140,141]; other estimates have been far lower[61]).

A course of chloramphenicol was estimated to increase the risk of aplastic anemia 13-fold. For quinacrine, the risk has been estimated at 1 in 40,000 (a 10-fold increase over the control population)[57]; for phenylbutazone, 1 to 6 in 100,000 (a 5-fold increase).[142] Other estimates have ranged from 1 in 100,000 to 1 in 1,000,000 treatment courses,[143] the uncertainty as usual due to the denominator in the equation). The incidence of aplastic anemia secondary to

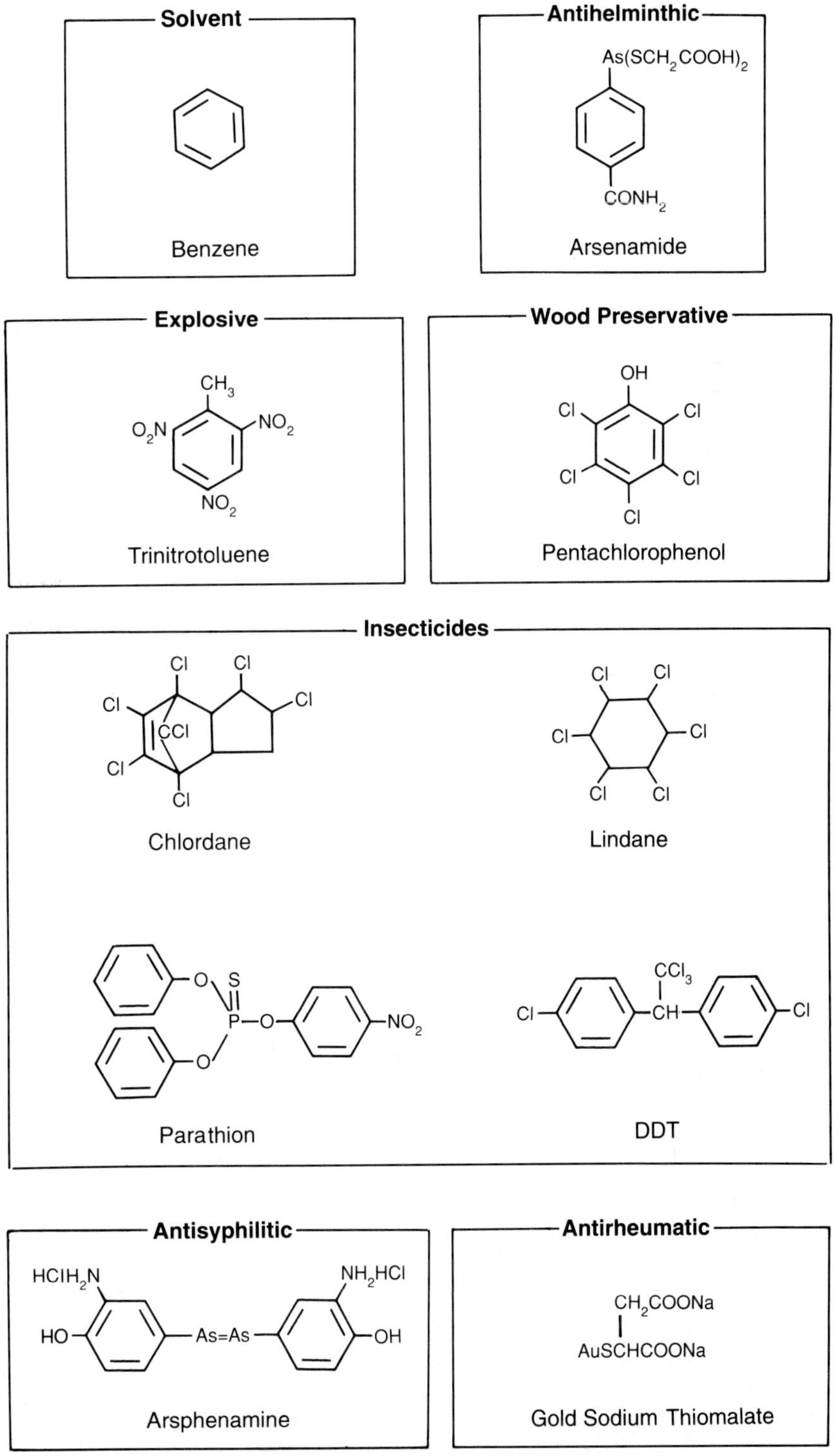

FIGURE 10-5. Structure of some chemicals associated with aplastic anemia.

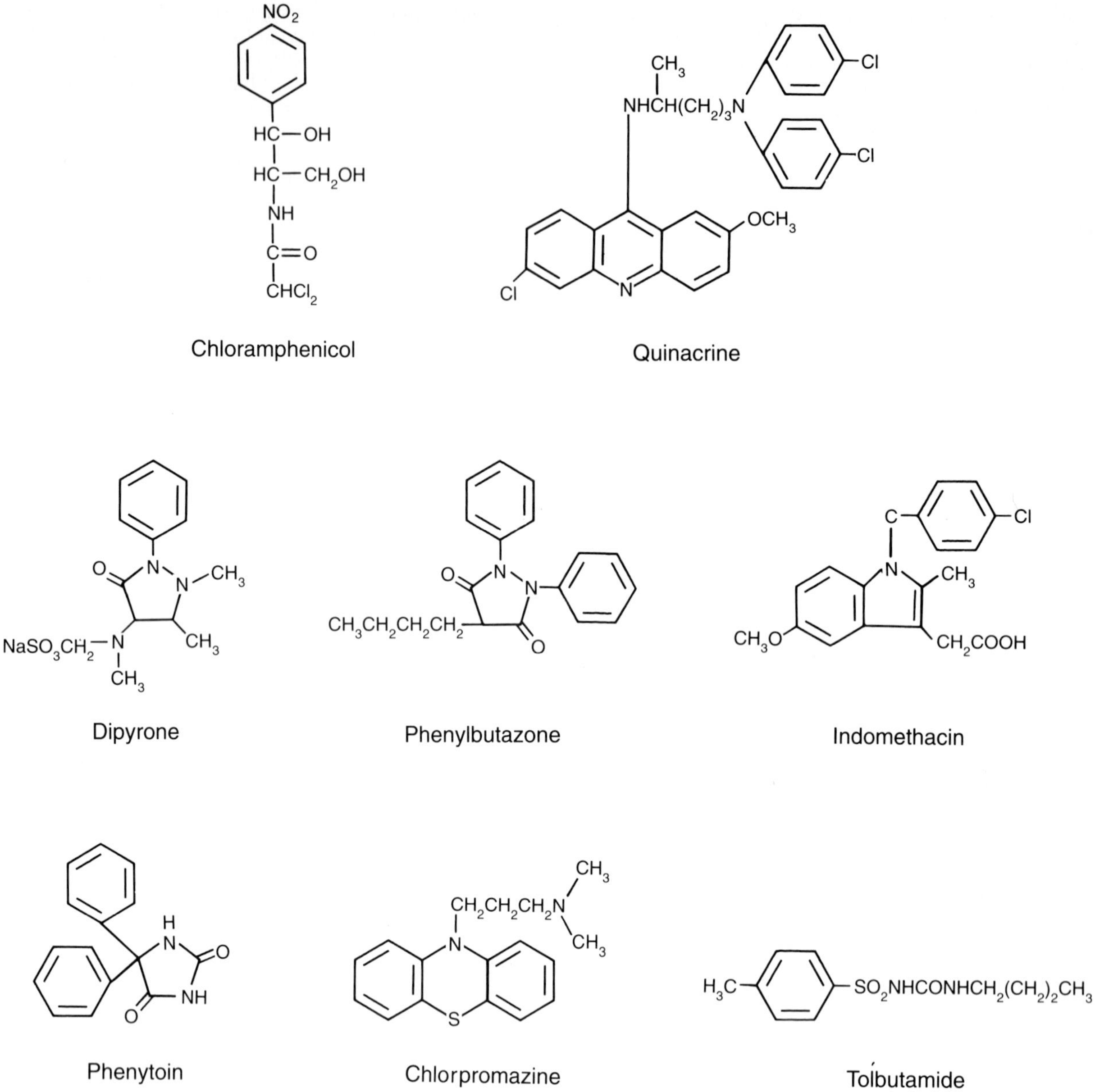

FIGURE 10-6. Structure of some drugs associated with aplastic anemia.

the H_2-receptor antagonist, cimetidine, has been estimated at 1 in 350,000 patients treated,[144] with the incidence of aplasia secondary to carbamazepine at 0.5 in 100,000.[145] Considering the nature of the studies, these numbers are probably not significantly different. Additional more stringent prospective case control studies often lead to reduced risk estimates (for dipyrone, for example, from about 0.8% to 0.0003% of patients who use it for 14 days or more[32]). For many drugs, risk has been estimated solely by enumeration of case reports; these numbers have little meaning in the absence of accurate denominators (eg, drug use, population exposed, average dose).

The distinction between regular and idiosyncratic reactions is useful but not absolute. Many drugs associated idiosyncratically with aplastic anemia are linked more frequently with other forms of marrow suppression, such as agranulocytosis with phenylbutazone or gold, moderate neutropenia with antieleptics, and reticulocytopenia with chloramphenicol. A low incidence of aplastic anemia may be a function of the doses commonly used in clinical practice; at very high doses, chloramphenicol, phenytoin, chlorpromazine, thiouracil, and methicillin all have been reported to occasionally produce reversible marrow depression in human subjects. In vitro, toxic drug effects can be demonstrated at high concentrations, which may be achieved in the rare patient with decreased renal or hepatic clearance or a specific drug metabolism defect. Presumably, many agents could be shown to affect marrow function at high doses if these were attainable without toxicity to other organ systems. Although it is a difficult point to prove, some dose–response relation probably exists even for idiosyncratic occurrences. Exquisitely small doses of drugs—a whiff of insecticide, an eyedrop of chloramphenicol—are unlikely to play a role in aplastic anemia,[132] and, conversely, many case reports document administration of very large doses of drugs for use in the setting of hepatic or renal failure.

Dose-related and idiosyncratic marrow depression have been reported only rarely in the same person, but it is reasonable to assume that at least one mechanism responsible

TABLE 10-5. **Drug and Chemical Associations With Aplastic Anemia***

CLINICAL SERIES Agent	1950–1959	1960–1969	1970–1979	1980–1989	1970–1979 (Far East)
Chloramphenicol	227 (30%)	90 (27%)	194 (17%)	28 (3%)	626 (19%)
Phenylbutazone	1 (<1%)	30 (9%)	67 (6%)	22 (3%)	81 (2%)
Sulfonamides	27 (4%)	3 (1%)	13 (1%)	5 (1%)	42 (1%)
Anticonvulsants	15 (2%)	8 (2%)	16 (2%)	4 (<1%)	35 (1%)
Gold	0 (0%)	3 (1%)	12 (1%)	12 (2%)	11 (<1%)
Benzene, solvents	24 (6%)	14 (4%)	37 (3%)	21 (3%)	95 (3%)
Insecticides	9 (1%)	29 (9%)	15 (1%)	11 (1%)	122 (4%)
Other drugs	118 (16%)	26 (8%)	169 (13%)	60 (7%)	451 (12%)
Total drug cases	427 (57%)	203 (60%)	523 (45%)	163 (20%)	1469 (43%)
Total cases	756	339	1292	811	3391

EPIDEMIOLOGIC SURVEYS Country	Dates	Design	No.	% Drug Cases
Israel	1961–1965	Nationwide, retrospective hospital survey	93	45[1331]
Sweden	1964–1968	Provincial retrospective survey	80	28[1347]
Japan	1970–1973	Nationwide survey	1594	17[42]
England	1971–1978	Provincial retrospective survey	174	36[35]

* Data are derived from published collected series of adult patients in the United States and Europe and from Asia; dates indicate publication period.

(Adapted from reference 1350 with additional material from reference 133 and, for Asian data, from Japan,[1351] Korea,[45] and Thailand).

TABLE 10-6. **Classification of Drugs and Chemicals Associated With Aplastic Anemia***

AGENTS THAT REGULARLY PRODUCE MARROW DEPRESSION AS MAJOR TOXICITY IN COMMONLY USED DOSES OR NORMAL EXPOSURES

Cytotoxic drugs used in cancer chemotherapy, alkylating agents (busulfan, melphalan, cyclophosphamide), antimetabolites (antifolic compounds, nucleotide analogues), antimitotics (vincristine, vinblastine, colchicine,[1352,1353] some antibiotics (daunorubicin, adriamycin)

Benzene (less often benzene-containing chemicals): kerosene,[1354–1356] carbon tetrachloride,[1357] Stoddard's solvent,[1360] chlorophenols[227,228]

AGENTS PROBABLY ASSOCIATED WITH APLASTIC ANEMIA BUT WITH A RELATIVELY LOW PROBABILITY RELATIVE TO THEIR USE

Chloramphenicol

Insecticides

Antiprotozoals: quinacrine and chloroquine[1361–1365]

Nonsteroidal antiinflammatory drugs: phenylbutazone (see text), indomethacin,[1366–1369] ibuprofen,[1370] sulindac,[1371,1372] aspirin,[1373,1374]

Anticonvulsants[1375,1376]: hydantoins,[1377–1381] carbamazepine,[1382–1388] phenacemide[1389]

Gold and arsenic (and other heavy metals, like bismuth,[1390–1392] mercury[1393–1395])

Sulfonamides as a class: some antibiotics,[1395–1399] antithyroid drugs (methimazole,[1400–1402] methylthiouracil,[1403] propylthiouracil[1404]), antidiabetes drugs (tolbutamide,[1405–1407] chlorpropamide),[1408,1409] carbonic anhydrase inhibitors (acetazolamide, methazolamide[1410–1414])

D-Penicillamine[1415–1420]

Estrogens (in pregnancy and in high doses in animals; see text)

AGENTS MORE RARELY ASSOCIATED WITH APLASTIC ANEMIA

Antibiotics: streptomycin,[1421–1423] tetracycline,[1424] methicillin,[1425] mebendazole,[1426] sulfonamides,[1427–1430] trimethoprim/sulfamethoxazole,[1431,1432] flucytosine[1433–1435]

Antihistamines[1436]: cimetidine,[1031,1437,1438] ranitidine,[144] chlorpheniramine[1439,1440]

Sedatives and tranquilizers: chlorpromazine,[1038,1441–1443] prochlorperazine,[1444] piperacetazine,[1445] chlordiazepoxide,[1446] meprobamate,[1447–1449] methyprylon[77]

Allopurinol (may potentiate marrow suppression by cytotoxic drugs[1450–1452])

Methyldopa[1453]

Quinidine[1454,1455]

Lithium[1456,1457]

Guanidine[1458]

Potassium perchlorate[1459–1461]

Thiocyanate[1462]

Carbimazole[1463]

* In the absence of references, see extended discussion in text. Citations are provided for archival interest and do not imply acceptance by the authors of a causal relation.

for rare drug reactions is a metabolic pathway that reproduces in the unusual individual the condition of excess drug administration.[146] Similarly, the probability of developing aplastic anemia with a course of drugs may be a quantitative reflection of the number of genes for metabolic enzymes or histocompatibility types in the human population.

Cytotoxic Chemotherapy. Aplastic anemia is regularly produced by a chemically diverse group of drugs—the chemotherapeutic agents used in the treatment of cancer.[147] Acute myelosuppression resulting from their use is usually dose dependent and predictable. These drugs have been selected for their antiproliferative effects on tumors, and their activity can be measured in tissue culture and animal models. Although virtually all chemotherapeutic drugs exert dose-dependent myelotoxicity, higher doses are not well correlated with late or irreversible damage to stem cells. Some agents, such as busulfan, at doses that cause relatively limited immediate reductions in colony-forming unit–spleen (CFU-S) and self-renewal capacity, can cause profound late depression of bone marrow and reduce marrow regenerative capacity as measured in repopulation assays. In contrast, 5-fluorouracil and cyclophosphamide appear to spare the regenerating cell population, and long-term administration of cyclophosphamide in animals does not reduce CFU-S or repopulating ability.

Late effects of chemotherapeutic agents are well documented in animal models of bone marrow failure such as the busulfan-treated mouse. The marrow of patients who have been subjected to chemotherapy is similarly damaged. Frank marrow failure in patients with chronic myelogenous leukemia, an uncommon occurrence, has been interpreted as a late effect of busulfan therapy.[148–150]

Benzene. Benzene is the chemical most convincingly linked to aplastic anemia by clinical and epidemiologic studies, with animal and in vitro data.[130,151] Benzene myelotoxicity can be placed between the regular effects of chemotherapeutic agents and idiosyncratic drug reactions. Benzene is efficient enough at decreasing the WBC count to have been used briefly in the early treatment of leukemia; on the other hand, many workers have tolerated high doses in industry without developing aplastic anemia.

Enormous quantities of benzene are produced, used in industry, released into the atmosphere, and found in the household[130,151–153] (Table 10-7). In the United States alone, benzene production was estimated at 11 to 12 billion pounds in 1983. The highest exposures occur to workers in the large number of industries that use benzene, estimated in the United States at 2 million.[152] The American chemical industry was initiated to benzene during World War I, when German imports ceased; during the 1920s, voluntary efforts established a ceiling of 100 parts per million (ppm; 100 ppm = 32 μg/L),[154] but application of these standards was erratic and inconsistent. The limit of benzene exposure was further decreased to 10 ppm in the 1950s, which was the level adopted in the 1970s in the first government standard. The Occupational Safety and Health Administration has advocated 1 ppm as being safer yet.

The concentrations of benzene set for industry in other countries, if subject to regulation at all, can be far higher[152,155,156] and are comparable to concentrations found in American factories in the 1920s and 1930s.[154,157] Reports have been made of workers continuously exposed to levels of 200 to 500 ppm in Italian factories[158] and up to 650 ppm in Turkish shoe artisans working at home.[159] Reduced industrial benzene exposure clearly resulted in a decrease in hematologic disease among workers.[160–162]

Benzene is ubiquitous. Its low boiling point (80.1°C) and high vapor pressure ensure rapid evaporation, and fugitive industrial emissions add greatly to the biologic sources of ambient benzene.[152] Present in crude oil and generated with refining, benzene can account for 0.8% (average American) to 5% (average European) of the volume of gasoline,[152] and the proportion of benzene has increased with reductions in leaded antiknock additives. Benzene exposure can occur outside of industry.[152,163,164] Benzene has been measured in pristine Antarctic air and at higher levels in the urban environment near refineries, chemical plants, and roadways.[165] We have treated patients whose benzene exposure was mundane, for example, a 50-year-old man who used benzene product as a wig cleaner in an unventilated bathroom and a 12-year-old girl who cleaned brushes in her family's housepainting project. The concentrations of benzene to which consumers are exposed are much lower in magnitude than those in industry; the effect on a population of chronic exposure to low doses of benzene, as with most threshold phenomena, is unknown.[166]

Inhaled benzene is rapidly absorbed into the body[167]; uptake through mucous membranes and skin is relatively minor. Because of its low partition coefficient, benzene is

TABLE 10-7. Sources of Benzene Exposure

INDUSTRIAL SOURCES*

Made as a Byproduct

Petrochemical plants
Petroleum refineries

Used in Manufacture

Drugs
Chemicals (nitrobenzene, aniline, styrene, cumene, maleic anhydride, monochlorobenzene, dichlorobenzene, and phenol)
Explosives
Cements and adhesives
Dyes
Leathers and shoes
Enamel
Rubber and waterproof fabrics
Lacquers, shellac, and paint thinners
Bronzing, silvering, and gilding liquids
Batteries, electroplating, lithography and photography
Dry cleaning
Feather preparation
Lineoleum and celluloid

Solvent

Rubber
Gum
Resins
Fats
Alkaloids
Grease

HOUSEHOLD SOURCES

Solvent and Solvent Component

Rubber solvent (1.5% benzene)
Varnish maker and naphtha (0.1%), mineral spirits
Stoddard solvent (0.1–0.7%)

Gasoline Storage and Dispensing

Cigarette Smoke

* Listed are industries in which workers have been exposed or continue to be exposed to benzene and likely sources of benzene outside of industry.[154] Exposure is likely to be greater in open industries in which benzene is used for some secondary purpose than in closed-system industry in which benzene is produced.

concentrated in the fat of the bone marrow.[168] Although the primary site of benzene metabolism is the liver, active metabolism also occurs in bone marrow.[169,170] Water-soluble intermediate products such as phenols, hydroquinones, and catechols probably mediate toxicity.[151,152,171–173] Benzene and its intermediate metabolites covalently and irreversibly bind to bone marrow DNA,[169,173–175] inhibit DNA synthesis,[176,177] and introduce DNA strand breaks.[178] Chromosomal abnormalities are produced by chronic administration in animals[177,179] and are present in benzene workers.[180,181] The decrease in cell proliferation frequently measured in vitro could result from any number of indirect effects on cell function such as irreversible protein binding,[182,183] as well as from a direct action on DNA.

Administration of benzene to animals produces bone marrow depression.[130,151] Practical difficulties are encountered in reproducing typical industrial exposure in route (inhalation rather than injection) and in duration (years rather than weeks), and the metabolism of benzene varies among animal species[184,185] and tissues.[170,184] Benzene administration in animals decreases marrow cell proliferation. In acute exposures, the more mature actively cycling marrow precursor cells are preferentially damaged compared with more primitive progenitors, but marked depression of colony-forming unit–erythroid (CFU-E), granulocyte-macrophage colony-forming unit (CFU-GM), and burst-forming unit–erythroid (BFU-E) progenitors. CFU-S can be measured within days.[186–190] Intermittent exposure is more damaging to stem cell count than continuous exposure.[188,191] The stroma is also damaged by benzene, and marrow from chronically exposed mice does not support long-term bone marrow cultures.[192,193] In benzene-treated mice, CFU-S–derived colonies fail to implant[188] and physically extirpated marrow does not regenerate.[194] Benzene also has diverse effects on the immune system, reducing lymphocyte count and suppressing lymphocyte function.[195,196] In vitro, low concentrations of benzene are mildly stimulatory of myeloid colony number, whereas benzene metabolites are strongly inhibitory.[197] These results also are consistent with the leukocytosis and marrow hypercellularity seen in the early stages of human benzene poisoning.

Hamilton described the typical clinical picture of human benzene poisoning: "progressive anemia with malaise, epistaxis, then rapid decline, petechiae, hemorrhage [from many organs] . . . fever more or less intense, sometimes chills . . . and death."[160] In fact, the range of hematologic disease attributable to benzene is broad, from relatively common alterations in blood counts to aplastic anemia or hematologic malignancy.[198–203] The early American studies suggested that the risk of aplastic anemia was 3% to 4% in workers exposed to concentrations higher than 300 ppm, and that half of the persons exposed to 100 ppm showed some blood count depression. The prevalence of some form of marrow suppression in heavily exposed workers can still be astonishingly high. Over 10% of workers surveyed in China in the 1950s showed leukopenia; with improved hygiene, the figure was lowered to 0.5%, a percentage that still represented more than 2000 cases in half a million workers.[155] The incidence of aplastic anemia in one group of Chinese shoemakers was estimated to be increased sixfold (a 2% incidence of aplastic anemia occurred in a single factory).[155] In 217 apparently healthy Turkish shoe factory workers, 25% had some combination of leukopenia, thrombocytopenia, or pancytopenia.[203]

Leukopenia,[203] thrombocytopenia,[204] and anemia[201] each have been cited as the most common hematologic consequences of benzene; lymphocytopenia is also common. Other manifestations are macrocytosis, acquired Pelger-Huët anomaly, eosinophilia, basophilia, elevated fetal hemoglobin, and, less commonly, polycythemia, leukocytosis, thrombocytosis, and splenomegaly.[156,202,203,205] The marrow of healthy workers is usually normocellular but may show moderate hypocellularity or hypercellularity[203]; a hypercellular phase may precede complete aplasia in the course of benzene toxicity. The predictive value of abnormal blood counts is uncertain. Most workers with borderline values in one large clinic returned to normal, despite continued exposure to benzene[202]; most workers with severe hematologic benzene poisoning completely recover.[159,206] Chronic benzene exposure clearly increases the risk of acute myelogenous leukemia[207–209] and a variety of lymphohematopoietic malignancies, including multiple myeloma.[207,210–212] Aplastic anemia and acute leukemia have occurred in the same person.[213] Both aplastic anemia and acute leukemia in benzene workers can manifest decades after exposure, but similar to the effects of radiation, malignancy may be the more common late consequence. Cumulative benzene exposure has been statistically correlated with the risk of acute leukemia[207] and probably is an important variable for marrow failure (even short exposure to high doses can provoke blood changes).[214]

Other Aromatic Hydrocarbons. The common perception that other molecules resembling benzene in structure or containing a benzene ring also cause marrow suppression is not well supported by facts. Not all aromatic hydrocarbons share biologic activities. In contrast to benzene, neither the closely related alkylbenzenes[215] nor pure toluene and xylene[216–218] are marrow toxins. Often, an aromatic hydrocarbon has been implicated clinically only because no other apparent cause of aplastic anemia was found. For some substances, toxicity may be due to the presence of benzene itself, either as a contaminant in the synthesis of the molecule (as with benzene hydrochloride, xylene, toluene) or in the petroleum distillates used to dissolve the product (Stoddard's solvent and organic arsenicals contain benzene). Nevertheless the total number of bone marrow failure cases reported is small considering the large populations exposed to this heterogeneous group of chemicals.

In the case of insecticides, for example, surveys of aplastic anemia patients directed toward causes have found 2%,[134,219] 6%,[42,129] and 9%[45] of cases associated with exposure. The significance of a handful of case reports in the context of vast use is questionable.[220] Perhaps the fatal effect of insecticides on insects has created a bias; it is worth recalling that insecticides were associated with far fewer cases of pancytopenia reported to the American Medical Association Drug Registry than tetracyclines and penicillins.[221] The extensiveness of aromatic hydrocarbons in daily life would greatly amplify even a small individual risk for aplasia. Insecticides and herbicides are used not only in gardening but also are present as residues in food from their massive use in agriculture; aromatic hydrocarbons are present in the atmosphere,[222] in body fat,[223,224] and in the bone marrow[225] of normal persons.

Case reports greatly outnumber series of patients, and only a few rigorous epidemiologic surveys have been performed. Twenty-four cases of aplastic anemia in the British explosives industry in two world wars were credited to trinitrotoluene.[226] Dinitrophenol used to effect weight reduction,[227] pentachlorophenol used as a wood preservative,[227,228] and substituted aromatic hydrocarbons used in the wood pulp industry[229] have also been associated with a few cases of aplasia. Only 14 cases of aplasia related to hair dyes could be collected in 1985, despite their abundant use.[230] Heavy insecticide exposure was implicated in 16 of 20 cases of aplastic anemia and in the high incidence of the disease in general in Mexico[52] and blamed for aplasia in 6 children in California,[231] 6 heavily exposed professional users in Germany,[232] and 4 agricultural workers in Brazil.[233] Forty-four cases could be collected from the literature in 1967.[232] The most frequently cited insecticides are chlordane[234–236] and lindane[232,237–240] or these products in combination with DDT.[240–244]

The results of systematic epidemiologic surveys of users of aromatic hydrocarbons are mixed. British Columbia farmers had a statistically significant proportional mortality ratio (observed number of deaths divided by expected number of deaths, usually age adjusted, multiplied by 100) of 174 from 1950 to 1978, with most of the increase in a single 10-year period.[245] In a special study, the United States Bureau of the Census coded the usual occupation and industry from 1975 death certificates for four rare diseases, including aplastic anemia. Job exposure matrices, which allow cross-classification of persons employed with agents found in industries, were then used to measure chemical exposure as a variable for disease.[246] Significant excesses of aplastic anemia were found in those employed in printing and publishing industries (odds ratio [OR] of 6.2), lumber and wood products manufacture (OR of 3.7), agriculture (OR of 2.4), and construction (OR of 2).

Other surveys of pesticide makers or users[247–251] and farmers[252–255] have failed to show an increased mortality rate from aplastic anemia, even though some of these workers have detectable blood levels of pesticide.[256] Neutropenia was correlated with insecticide exposure among Canadian apple pickers and exposed residents.[257] Bone marrow hypocellularity was discovered in a large percentage of apparently healthy printers exposed to a range of glycol ethers and organic solvents.[258]

Some organophosphate insecticides depress rodent blood counts and inhibit hematopoietic colony formation in vitro.[259,260]

Chloramphenicol. Chloramphenicol was isolated from a Venezuelan *Streptomyces* sp in 1947; the crystalline antibiotic was named chloromycetin because it contained chlorine and came from an actinomycete. The chemical structure of chloramphenicol contains a nitrobenzene ring, a unique property for a natural compound; its similarity to the structure of amidopyrine, a drug known to cause agranulocytosis, led to an early prediction of blood dyscrasias.[261,262] Chloramphenicol was introduced into practice in 1949 and rapidly gained popularity because of its broad spectrum of antimicrobial activity and minimal gastrointestinal toxicity. The first published case of aplastic anemia associated with chloramphenicol appeared in 1950, followed by such an explosion of reports that the Food and Drug Administration was able to collect several hundred reports within a few years.[263,264] A still remarkable feature of chloramphenicol was that, in contrast to most other agents associated with marrow suppression, pancytopenia, which is frequently fatal, was by far the most common hematologic toxicity encountered (Table 10-8).

During the period of unrestrained use of chloramphenicol, it was considered the most common cause of aplastic anemia in the United States.[219] Most affected patients died; a few survivors developed acute leukemia.[265,266] Chloramphenicol use has been associated with leukemia independent of the occurrence of aplastic anemia.[267] From 1949 to 1952, 47% of the 296 patients of aplastic anemia collected were associated with prior chloramphenicol use[264]; from 1952 to 1954, after deservedly adverse publicity, 15% of 607 patients had prior exposure.[263] Chloramphenicol use rebounded and continued to be the drug most frequently associated with aplastic anemia for several decades. In clinical series, chloramphenicol usually accounted for 20% to 30% of the total cases of aplastic anemia and half of the drug-associated cases; in epidemiologic surveys in California done in the early 1960s, chloramphenicol was associated with most of the drug-related cases of aplastic anemia.[140,141]

In a small Japanese case control study, 14 of 28 patients with aplastic anemia reported chloramphenicol ingestion during the previous year compared with 1 of 16 patients with leukemia.[41] With narrowing indications for the use of chloramphenicol, aplastic anemia associated with its use has almost disappeared. In 160 patients with acquired aplastic anemia admitted to the National Institutes of Health from 1978 to 1989, none had a history of chloramphenicol use. The International Agranulocytosis and Aplastic Anemia Study failed to find chloramphenicol use in any of 135 patients with aplastic anemia.[268]

The perception that the introduction of chloramphenicol into the American market increased the number of cases of bone marrow failure[219,269] was only weakly supported by epidemiologic data.[140] The decline in chloramphenicol use in Japan and Sweden has not been associated with a decrease in the incidence of aplastic anemia, and in regions where chloramphenicol continues to be widely used, aplastic anemia associated with its use is either infrequent (Hong Kong,[62] Israel[270]) or may even have declined since its introduction (Colombia[271]). An inference from these data is that chloramphenicol affected a subpopulation prone to drug effects on the bone marrow, with only the rapid introduction and popularity of the antibiotic leading to its recognition as a dramatic destructive agent. Genetic susceptibility is supported by the appearance of aplasia in family members treated with chloramphenicol.[74,272] Although its medical use has substantially diminished, it has not disappeared, especially in surgical service.[273] Chloramphenicol continues to be in wide but illegal use in food-producing animals, and, occasionally, high concentrations are found in the muscle tissue of animals brought to slaughter.[274]

The dose–response relation of chloramphenicol and aplastic anemia has never been satisfactorily resolved. The early case collections and epidemiologic surveys stressed excessive dosage, often given in repeated or intermittent courses, and a high proportion of cases occurred among children.[140,141,263,264,275] In a later collection of nearly 600 cases, most patients had received a dose of less than 10 g.[75]

Whether the first series underestimated the extent of toxicity or the later ones exaggerated the relation is not

TABLE 10-8. Epidemiologic Studies of Chloramphenicol and Aplastic Anemia

Area	Years	Percentage of Drug Cases	Percentage of Total Cases	Data Base
California	1957–1961	78	29	Death certificates[140]
California	1963–1964	59	17	Death certificates[141]
Sweden	1966–1971	17	6	Hospital discharges[1347]
Israel	1961–1965	56	25	Hospital survey[1331]
Japan	1958–1974	30	3	Autopsies[1464]
Japan	1973	45	8	Hospital survey[42]
Europe and Israel	1980–1986	0	0	Case control[268]

clear. Certainly, chloramphenicol's notoriety prompted unusual case reports: aplastic anemia in a shepherd who used a chloramphenicol sheep dip,[276] in a child treated for only 2 days,[277] and in persons after using chloramphenicol ophthalmic drops.[278,279] Such trivial exposures have been cited as convincing evidence of chloramphenicol's marrow toxicity[280] or have been dismissed as coincidental.[132] The culpability of chloramphenicol administered years prior to the appearance of aplastic anemia appears to be slight, and in most cases, the duration between exposure and onset of symptoms was relatively brief, around 2 months.[75]

A dose–response relation is also suggested by the occurrence of anemia, leukopenia, or pancytopenia with the therapeutic,[281] accidental,[282] or experimental[283,284] administration of extremely high doses of chloramphenicol, usually more than 40 g. These blood changes are reversible but have been fatal.[146] Hematologic toxicity has been associated with high blood levels[284] and delayed clearance of chloramphenicol in patients with hepatic or renal disease, presumably because chloramphenicol is conjugated in the liver and excreted in the urine.[285] The rarity of cases that result after intravenous chloramphenicol therapy may be attributed to its relatively infrequent parenteral use.[286] The bioavailability of chloramphenicol is higher after administration of the palmitate form (as in oral suspensions given to children) than in the free-base formulation of pills and lowest after parenteral injection of the succinate salt.[287,288] Chloramphenicol can also inhibit the metabolism of other drugs that have been implicated in bone marrow failure, including sulfonamides and hydantoins.[289]

At the usual therapeutic doses, a stereotypical pattern of reversible alterations in erythropoiesis occurs in virtually every patient treated with chloramphenicol[290] (Table 10-9). Suppression of erythropoiesis is probably secondary to drug inhibition of mitochondrial protein synthesis, especially of heme synthesis enzymes such as ferrochelatase, which catalyzes the insertion of iron into protoporphyrin.[291] Other enzymes inhibited include cytochrome oxidase, cytochrome b, and an ATPase.[292] Vacuolization of erythroblasts represents mitochondria with condensed and fragmented matrix.[293] Decreased iron utilization and reticulocytopenia may occur earlier in patients than in normal volunteers because of their increased erythropoietic activity.[292,294] Suppression of erythropoiesis has not been correlated with the later occurrence of aplastic anemia.[295] Chloramphenicol can inhibit hematopoietic colony formation, especially early erythroid,[296–299] or diminish colony size,[300] but usually at doses greater than that achieved in patients. Inhibition of marrow stromal cell proliferation[301] and production of growth factors[298] have also been reported. No consistent evidence shows abnormal marrow cell sensitivity to the drug in affected persons.[302,303] Low chloramphenicol[300] and thiamphenicol[304] doses may actually stimulate CFU-GM–derived colony formation; in the mouse, these doses may increase hematopoietic colony-forming and stem cell counts, either directly or in response to alterations in more mature marrow compartments. These results may account for the paradoxical stimulation of myelopoiesis observed in a single neutropenic patient.[305] Chloramphenicol also suppresses some lymphocyte functions,[306,307] and karyotype abnormalities involving C chromosomes have been described in a few cases of chloramphenicol-associated aplasia.[308] The explanation for chloramphenicol's idiosyncratic effect probably lies in its metabolism, described later.

Nonsteroidal Antiinflammatory Drugs. It took far longer to associate phenylbutazone with aplastic anemia than it did for chloramphenicol.[309] These drugs have been most frequently used in the treatment of rheumatic syndromes, and other therapies (gold and penicillamine) have also been associated with aplastic anemia in this group of patients. Neutropenia is far more common than pancytopenia as a hematologic toxicity of phenylbutazone.[310] Fatal aplasia has occurred with butazone treatment of a child with juvenile rheumatoid arthritis[311] and a jockey who used his horse's tablets.[312]

Other nonsteroidal antiinflammatory drugs have been associated by occasional case reports with aplastic anemia, including aspirin, indomethacin, and ibuprofen (see Table 10-6). The large case control investigation conducted by the International Agranulocytosis and Aplastic Anemia Study not only confirmed the risk of aplastic anemia with phenylbutazone but identified even higher probabilities with some of the other nonsteroidal antiinflammatory drugs.[32] Risk ratio estimates (based on any exposure in the 5-month period before onset of disease) were 12.7 for indomethacin, 8.8 for diclofenac sodium, and 8.7 for the butazones (equivalent to excess risks of 10.1, 6.8, and 6.6 per 1 million, respectively, for these exposures). Increased use of salicylates was also observed but did not reach statistical significance.

In the International Study, an increased risk was suggested for taking drugs regularly for a prolonged period.[32] Many patients with the early cases of butazone-associated aplasia had been treated with very high doses of butazone.[310] Large doses of phenylbutazone consistently produce neutropenia in horses.[313] As with chloramphenicol, hematologic toxicity has been associated with decreased clearance rates.[314] Hematopoietic colony formation in vitro by patients with drug-associated neutropenia was shown to be abnormally sensitive to phenylbutazone,[315] but these studies suffer from the common defect of poor controls for patently abnormal bone marrow.

Gold and Other Heavy Metals. Gold salts cause an extraordinarily high incidence of fatal adverse reactions, estimated at 1.6 in 10,000 prescriptions. Dose-dependent

TABLE 10-9. Hematologic Toxicity From Chloramphenicol

	Reversible Toxicity	Aplastic Anemia
Incidence	Common	Rare
Blood	Reticulocytopenia progressing to anemia if treatment is prolonged; increased serum iron; occasional moderate leukopenia, thrombocytopenia	Pancytopenia, usually severe
Bone marrow appearance	Normal cellularity; decreased late erythroid cells, erythroblast nuclear/cytoplasmic vacuolization	Aplastic
Dose relation	Dose dependent	Either dose independent or greater drug sensitivity
Onset	With drug therapy	Several months after treatment
Symptoms	None (pallor with anemia)	Bleeding, infection, etc.
Outcome	Recovery	Usually fatal

neutropenia is common, but several dozen cases of aplastic anemia have been reported.[316,317] Gold was demonstrated in the bone marrow by electron microscopy in one case of aplastic anemia.[318] Chelation therapy has not been helpful,[319] but patients have been successfully treated with bone marrow transplantation[320] and immunosuppression.[321–323] High concentrations of gold salts inhibit hematopoietic colony formation in vitro[324]; some evidence suggests a dose–response relation in patients, since high doses of gold have been associated with the development of blood dyscrasias in general and fatal pancytopenia, as opposed to transient neutropenia or thrombocytopenia.[325]

The consistent leukopenic effect of inorganic arsenic once led to the use of potassium arsenite in the treatment of leukemia. Arsenic poisoning can result in neutropenia, anemia, and thrombocytopenia,[326,327] with characteristic basophilic stippling as seen in lead poisoning. Organic arsenicals, originally used in the treatment of syphilis (Arsphenamine) and now as anthelmintics (Arseneamide), have also been associated with aplastic anemia,[328] possibly because of the combined effect of the arsenic and benzene moieties. Bone marrow depression has been associated with other heavy metals, including bismuth and mercury.

Drug Metabolism and Toxic-Reactive Intermediate Compounds

Many drugs and chemicals, especially if they have limited water solubility, must be enzymatically degraded before conjugation and excretion[130] (Fig. 10-7; see Table 10-6). Degradative pathways for xenobiotics as for most drugs and chemicals are complex, specific, redundant, and interrelated. For some aromatic hydrocarbons, polar groups are added by phase I enzymes, which are part of the cytochrome P-450 mitochondrial system. These metabolites become the substrate for phase II enzyme systems that add glucuronide, sulfate, acetate, and glycine moieties to increase solubility and permit excretion. Other xenobiotics are directly metabolized by addition of methyl or acetyl groups. Intermediate compounds, especially arene oxides, are often highly electrophilic and therefore highly reactive with macromolecules, especially DNA.[329]

Toxic intermediate molecules are difficult to study because they may be produced in relatively small concentrations through a minor metabolic pathway and because they are intrinsically unstable. Metabolic pathways in other species, especially rodents, are often different from those of humans. The rarity of idiosyncratic responses requires the study of large numbers of animals or normal persons to detect a metabolic defect. The four examples of detoxifying enzyme systems described in the following text are chosen because they are directly applicable to bone marrow failure and because they also demonstrate genetic variability.

Arylhydrocarbon Hydroxylase. Cyclical aromatic hydrocarbons are metabolized by the P-450 enzyme system, a microsomal catalytic group of monooxygenases that are inducible by specific substrates.[330] Arylhydrocarbon hydroxylase can be induced by polycyclic aromatic hydrocarbons in wild mice who bear the Ah^b locus, encoding a cytosolic receptor for the hydrocarbon. Unresponsive Ah^d animals develop aplastic anemia when they ingest benzo[*a*]pyrene. Animals can be protected against marrow failure by phenobarbital, which induces drug-conjugating enzymes, and α-naphthoflavone, which inhibits P-450 metabolism. In vitro, Ah^b/Ah^b myeloid cells are paradoxically more sensitive than Ah^d/Ah^d cells, probably because they generate toxic metabolites more efficiently. In the intact animal, the marrow is protected by first-pass detoxification of metabolites in the intestine and liver, whereas large quantities of unaltered hydrocarbon reach the marrow of Ah^b/Ah^b animals. Phenobarbital, which induces P-450 microsomal oxidases, can protect animals against benzene myelotoxicity.[331]

Epoxide Hydrolase. A mechanism of detoxification of arene oxides is conversion of epoxides to phenols, a function of a large and poorly defined system of epoxide hydroxylases. These enzymes are substrate-specific, and their activity varies widely among individuals and ethnic groups. Epoxide hydroxylase activity has been measured indirectly by generating reactive intermediates from a test compound with rat hepatic microsomes, then by monitoring their cytotoxicity for patient lymphocytes in vitro. The cells serve as a source of the enzyme and a marker for the effect of the toxic intermediates. This system has identified persons susceptible to phenytoin hepatotoxicity and to birth defects. In a patient who had recovered from phenytoin-associated aplastic anemia, dose-dependent killing of the patient's lymphocytes, no toxicity for normal donors' cells, and intermediate killing of cells of the patient's mother occurred in vitro.[332] The patient's cells were unaffected by phenytoin alone or by the metabolites generated from closely related compounds.

***S*-Methylation.** Methylation is an important step in the metabolism of many drugs, chemicals, and neurotransmitters.[333] Thiopurine methyltransferase catalyzes the S-methylation of 6-mercaptopurine, 6-thioguanine, and azathioprine. The activity of this enzyme can be measured in erythrocytes, and population and family studies have shown a pattern of inheritance of a single genetic locus, with estimated gene frequencies of 94% for high-enzyme activity ($TPMT^H$) and 6% for low-enzyme activity ($TPMT^L$). Most persons have high (89%) or intermediate (11%) levels of activity, but those who are homozygous for $TPMT^L$—only 0.03% of the population—have undetectable enzyme. These homozygous persons, on treatment with azathioprine or 6-mercaptopurine, accumulate intracellular 6-thioguanine, which is a purine analogue that can be incorporated into DNA. 6-Thioguanine levels were elevated in the RBCs of patients with thiopurine-induced myelosuppression[334,335]; in three patients with hematologic complications of azathioprine, an enzyme level was undetectable in two and intermediate in the other.[336]

***N*-Acetylation.** N-Acetyltransferase activity is a polymorphic activity inherited as an autosomal recessive trait.[337] Acetylation rates vary greatly among the races, with fast acetylation far more frequent among Orientals than among whites. Acetylation phenotypes have been associated with isoniazid failure in persons with tuberculosis (fast), drug-induced lupus erythematosus, leprosy, and bladder cancer (slow). Sulfonamide toxic reactions are strongly associated with the slow acetylation phenotype.[338] Under these circumstances, sulfa may be shunted away from the acetylation detoxification pathway to a cytochrome P-450 pathway, with generation of a toxic intermediate such as an hydroxylamine. N-Acetylation is also a major pathway for procainamide metabolism.

Chloramphenicol Metabolism. Chloramphenicol is relatively nontoxic in tissue culture of mammalian cells, and it is not concentrated in the bone marrow. Thiamphenicol, in which the paranitro group is substituted by a methylsulfonyl group, was originally thought to be an innocent relative of chloramphenicol, but it has been associated with at least six cases of irreversible aplastic anemia,[339–342] a frequency of serious marrow failure that may be proportional to its use. Both chloramphenicol and thiamphenicol cause dose-related reversible suppression of erythropoiesis in patients and similarly inhibit hematopoietic colony formation.[296]

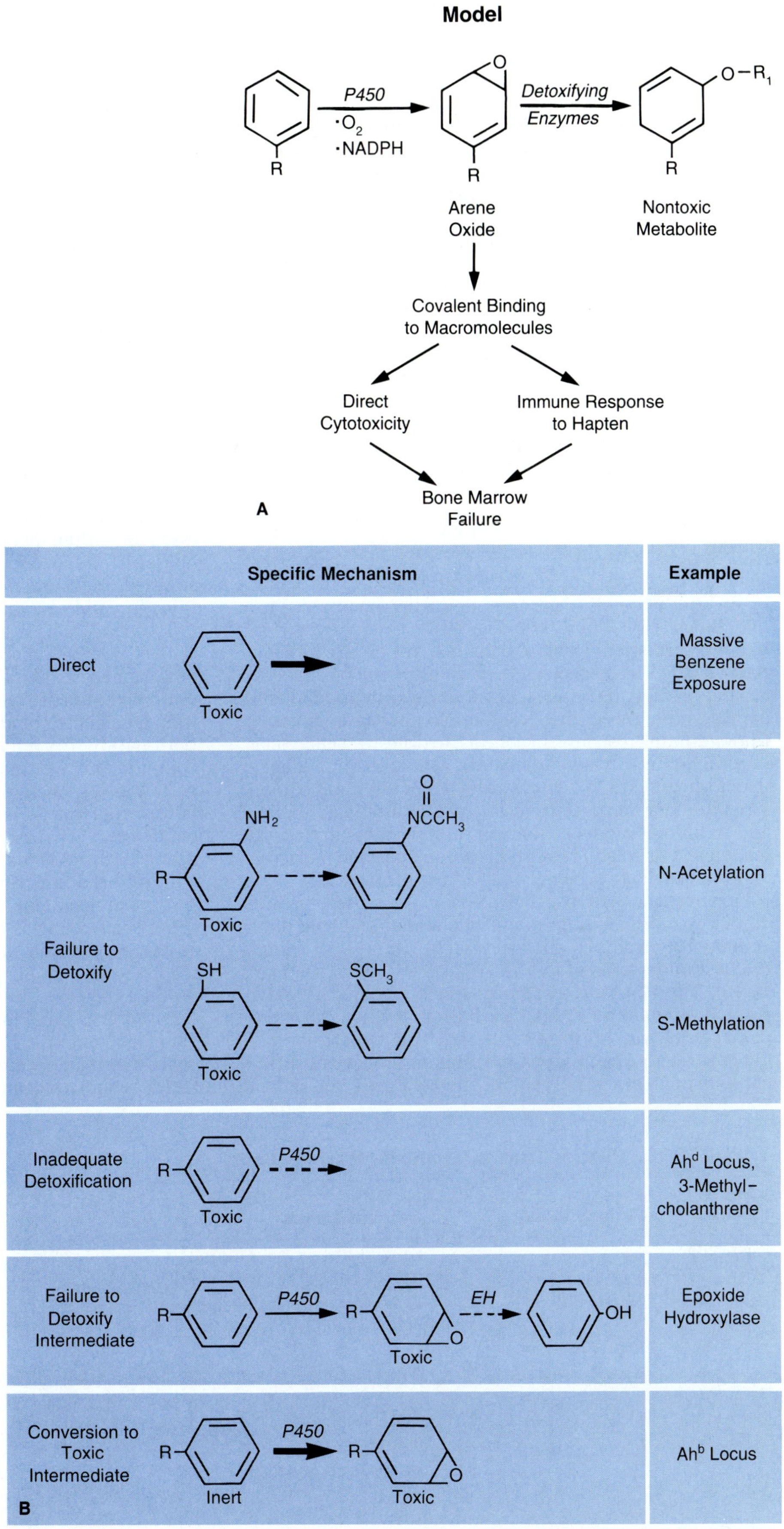

FIGURE 10-7. General model for the generation of toxic intermediate metabolites (**A**) and some specific mechanisms of chemical or drug-mediated toxicity (**B**).

The cellular uptake and metabolism of chloramphenicol and thiamphenicol differ, but no clear comprehensive theory exists as to the precise toxic intermediates involved, the mechanisms of cellular damage, or the basis of rare individual susceptibility. Yunis[343] has shown that nitrosochloramphenicol (in which the paranitro group [$-NO_2$] has been reduced to the nitroso [$-NO$] form), can efficiently degrade isolated[344] and cellular DNA.[345] However, the nitroso derivative is not made in the bone marrow and has a brief half-life.

Dehydrochloramphenicol, another toxic metabolite in culture and strand scission assays, is produced by gut bacteria[346]; individual susceptibility is hypothesized to be caused by differences in intestinal bacteria, clearance of toxic metabolites, or hematopoietic cell sensitivity.[343,346] Others have proposed that chloramphenicol toxicity is the result of covalent binding to cellular proteins of reactive oxidative metabolites, an oxalic acid derivative produced by cytochrome P-450–mediated oxidative dehalogenation or reduction to produce a chloramphenicol free radical and hydroxylamine intermediate, all capable of acylating proteins.[347,348]

Viruses

Temporary depression of blood counts, especially leukocytes and platelets, is frequent during common virus infections[349–351] (Table 10-10; Fig. 10-8). The role of viruses in more permanent forms of bone marrow failure has been recognized. Virus species of many different families are capable of infecting human bone marrow cells and inducing damage either by causing direct cytotoxicity or by invoking a host immune response. In contrast to drugs and chemicals, in which clinical associations are numerous but mechanisms are difficult to demonstrate in an individual patient, virus interactions with cells are readily produced in vitro and in animal models, whereas the presence of virus infection and its role in the patient require specific molecular and immunologic probes.

Parvovirus. B19 parvovirus is more closely related clinically to PRCA than to aplastic anemia, but its interaction with hematopoietic cells and the immune system is the best understood of all the viruses[352–354] (Figs. 10-9 and 10-10). The *Parvoviridae*, small single-stranded DNA viruses, are common animal pathogens. Feline panleukopenia virus was the first virus that was experimentally demonstrated to cause disease in animals; this virus infects cat hematopoietic and lymphocytic cells and causes fatal neutropenia.[355] The first parvovirus shown to cause human disease was only discovered in 1975.[356] Acute infection with B19 parvovirus (named from the blood bank code for the donor from whom the virus was isolated) causes the childhood exanthem fifth disease (erythema infectiosum).[357–359] Children with fifth disease are usually not very ill, but the characteristic rash—the "slapped cheek" facial erythema and a lacy, reticular, evanescent maculopapular eruption over the trunk and proximal extremities—combined with extreme contagion allow recognition of parvovirus infection in the individual patient and of the epidemic in the community. Adults with fifth disease suffer joint pains or frank arthritis more frequntly than a rash; symptoms that mimic rheumatoid arthritis can occasionally persist for months and even years[360,361]

Transient Aplastic Crisis. In persons with underlying hemolysis, acute parvovirus infection causes transient aplastic crisis (TAC), an abrupt cessation of erythropoiesis characterized by reticulocytopenia, absent erythroid precursors in the bone marrow, and precipitous worsening of anemia. The aregenerative quality of anemic crisis was recognized early from observations on hereditary spherocytosis in large Scandinavian kindreds,[362] later appreciated also for other persons with underlying hemolysis.[363] Owren[364] introduced the term *aplastic crisis*, and he stressed the relation between anemic crisis and previous infection and also the temporary quality of RBC failure.

TAC occurs as a unique event in the lives of patients with sickle cell disease, erythrocyte membrane defects, enzymopathies, thalassemias, and in those who are under circumstances of erythroid stress, such as hemorrhage and iron deficiency,[353] and after bone marrow transplantation.[365] Both parvovirus infection and stressed bone marrows are common; in retrospect, parvovirus infection was almost certainly responsible for cases of transient erythropoietic failure that were blamed on kwashiorkor,[366,367] folic acid deficiency,[368,369] some drugs (especially immunosuppressive agents or drugs given to immunocompromised patients),[370] and bacterial infections.[371,372]

It is not accidental that many reported cases of aplastic crisis occurred in hospitalized patients, since the virus is easily transmitted nosocomially among patients,[373,374] as well as among hospital personnel[375] and from blood products.[376]

Parvovirus infection was probably responsible for cases of aplastic anemia that were imputed to glue sniffing (five of six of which occurred in sickle cell patients, who really had TAC not aplastic anemia).[139]

TABLE 10-10. Viruses That Infect Bone Marrow Cells

Virus Family	Animal Model	In Vitro Target	Human Disease
Parvovirus	FePV	FePV: hematopoietic progenitors, lymphocyte[355] B19: CFU-E, BFU-E (human)[410,1466]	Transient aplastic crisis, pure red cell aplasia, nonimmune hydrops fetalis
Herpesvirus	Murine CMV[488]	CMV: fibroblast, hematopoietic progenitors (?)[491,492] EBV: lymphocytes, macrophage, BFU-E (?)	Post-BMT graft failure Infectious mononucleosis, aplastic anemia
Flavivirus	Bovine viral diarrhea[1467]	Dengue: macrophage, hematopoietic progenitors[449]	Hematodepressive diseases; hepatitis C, aplastic anemia
Retrovirus	FeLV[517] FV	FeLV: BFU-E[520,523] FV: CFU-E HIV: macrophage/monocyte,[954,1468–1472] megakaryocyte,[508] marrow stroma cells,[1473] CFU-GM (?)	Acquired immunodeficiency syndrome

BFU, burst-forming unit—erythroid; CFU-E, colony-forming unit—erythroid; CFU-GM, granulocyte-macrophage colony-forming unit; EBV, Epstein-Barr virus; BMT, bone marrow transplantation; FePV, feline panleukopenia virus; CMV, cytomegalovirus, FeLV, feline leukemia virus; FV, Friend virus.

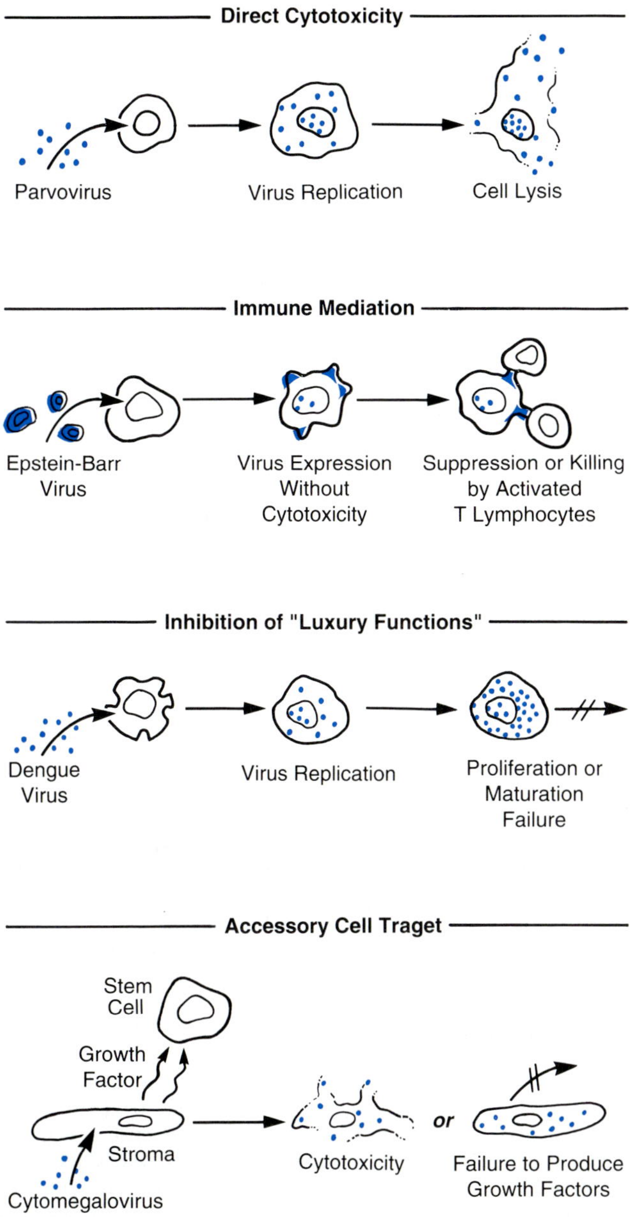

FIGURE 10-8. Mechanisms of virus-induced bone marrow failure.

Although suffering from a self-limited illness, the patient with an aplastic crisis may be profoundly ill; symptoms may include not only the usual dyspnea and fatigue but also extreme lassitude, confusion, and congestive heart failure. Death can occur. An aplastic crisis may be the first evidence of hereditary spherocytosis in a patient with compensated hemolysis.[377,378] TAC is readily treated by blood transfusion but can be fatal. TAC,[379–381] as well as experimental parvovirus infection in humans,[382] is often associated with variable degrees of neutropenia and thrombocytopenia; some cases of idiopathic thrombocytopenic purpura and Henoch-Schönlein purpura[383,384] have apparently followed acute parvovirus infection. Rarely, TAC may be complicated by bone marrow necrosis.[385,386] Transient pancytopenia[387–389] and a case of typical severe aplastic anemia[390] have been reported to follow acute parvovirus infection.

Community-acquired TAC is almost always caused by parvovirus infection.[391–393] B19 parvovirus should be the presumptive diagnosis in TAC and sought in any patient with anemia due to an abrupt cessation of erythropoiesis. Patients with TAC are often viremic at presentation, with concentrations of viral genomes as high as 10^{14}/mL as determined by DNA dot blot hybridization of serum.[394,395] IgM antibody appears during the first week of convalescence and is a specific indicator of recent infection.[392] IgG to parvovirus is present in about half the adult population. Both IgG and IgM antibody to parvovirus can be measured in capture immunoassays, but these tests have not been generally available because of the limited amounts of antigen

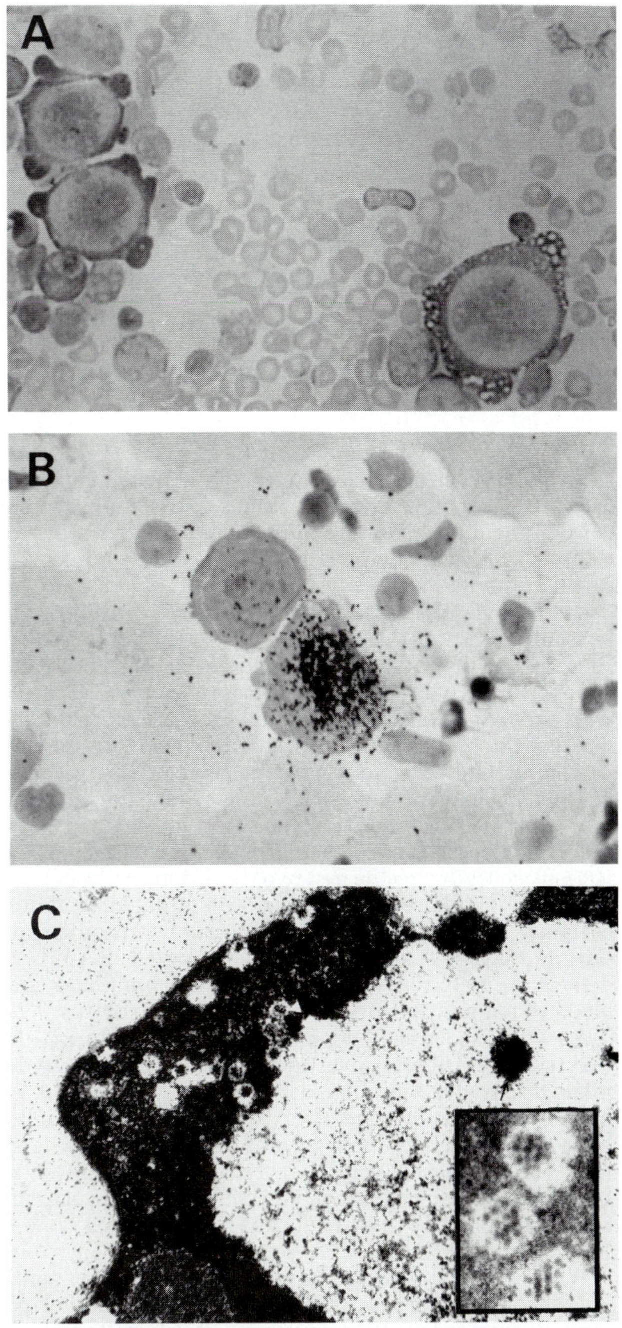

FIGURE 10-9. B19 parvovirus infection of bone marrow cells. (**A**) Giant pronormoblasts in the bone marrow of a patient with chronic anemia due to persistent infection. (**B**) Electron micrograph of a human late erythroid progenitor infected in vitro with B19 parvovirus. Inset shows viral particles in the marginated chromatin of the cell's nucleus. (**C**) Viral protein detected by immunoperoxidase staining with a specific anti–B19 parvovirus capsid antibody in the bone marrow cells of a patient with acquired immunodeficiency syndrome and persistent parvovirus infection.

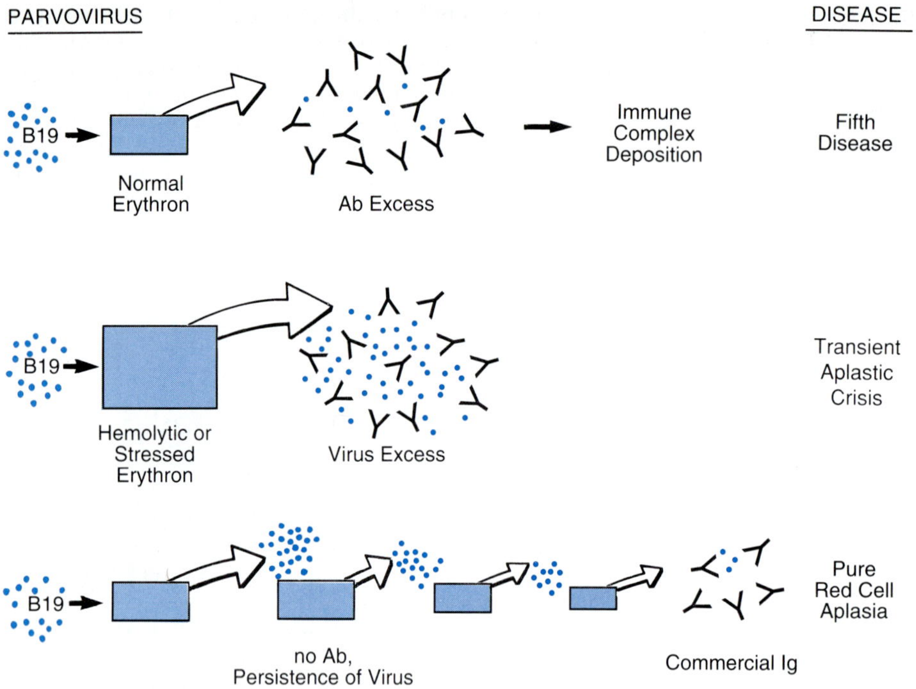

FIGURE 10-10. Pathogenesis of parvovirus disease in humans.

recoverable from infected sera.[396] The development of a cell line by genetic engineering that expresses empty viral capsids should remedy the antigen shortage.[397] Immunoglobulin assays are not useful in cases of persistent infection (see text that follows).

Hydrops Fetalis Due to B19 Parvovirus. In utero infection with B19 parvovirus is a cause of nonimmune hydrops fetalis, in which death occurs as a result of severe anemia.[398,399] Hydropic infants born of mothers infected with parvovirus have similar pathologic features, including leukoerythroblastosis, iron deposition in the liver, and viral cytopathic alterations of erythroblasts in the liver. Virus has been demonstrated by DNA hybridization and immunofluorescence for protein, mainly in the liver.[400,401] The risk of a fatal fetal outcome is probably greatest when infection occurs during the first two trimesters. Although the probably of stillbirth has not been quantitated, it almost certainly is low; of 170 reported cases of seroconversion during pregnancy, only a few have resulted in stillborn deliveries, including some in which the umbilical cord blood tested positive for IgM antibody to parvovirus.[398]

An increased risk of spontaneous abortion during the first trimester is being investigated in several large epidemiologic surveys; a preliminary estimate is that about 5% of infected women aborted.[398] No congenital anomalies have been associated with intrauterine parvovirus infection, either prospectively or in retrospective analysis of banked fetal tissue, although viral infection of myocardial cells was shown by in situ hybridization at autopsy of one hydropic infant.[402]

While the overall risk of a poor outcome to pregnancy is probably low, the concern of the pregnant mother potentially exposed to B19 parvovirus is not low. Parvovirus is extremely contagious. Pregnant women are commonly exposed to fifth disease through other children in the household, at schools and day care centers, and through nursing and medical personnel who are caring for persistently infected patients. About half the pregnant population has acquired protective immunity, as determined by assay for IgG antibody to parvovirus. Evidence of seroconversion should be sought in seronegative women. Hydrops can be detected by ultrasonography, and treatment of a suspected hydropic infant with intrauterine RBC transfusion has been reported.[403] The usefulness of this type of intervention, or of the administration of commercial immunoglobulins containing antiparvovirus antibodies as prophylaxis or treatment, needs to be determined.

B19 parvovirus can persist in children and adults who fail to produce an adequate immune response (see section on PRCA).

Pathogenesis of Parvovirus Infection. The pattern of disease that follows parvovirus infection is the result of balance among virus, marrow target cell, and immune response. Bone marrow depression in parvovirus infection occurs during the early viremic phase, and under normal conditions it is terminated by a neutralizing antibody response. The immune response produces the clinical manifestations of fifth disease—in children a rash illness, in adults a rheumatic syndrome—which occur during the period of antibody formation and are immune-complex–mediated (fifth disease symptoms can be precipitated by treatment of persistent infection with immunoglobulin).

In patients with hyperactive erythropoiesis, large amounts of virus are produced and the immune response may be weak, resulting in relatively greater quantities of antigen to antibody and little immune complex formation; rash and joint pains are rare in patients with TAC.[379] In persistent infection in children and adults and in in utero infection, failure to mount a neutralizing antibody response allows parvovirus to persist and cause chronic anemia.[404] In acute infection, the period of viremia is brief, usually 1 to 3 days, and virus titers are extremely high (10^{11} to 10^{14} genome copies per milliliter). In persistent infection, virus can be demonstrated in serum samples obtained months apart; the viral titer is often lower (10^6), although AIDS patients may have serum concentrations equal to those seen in acute infection.

B19 parvovirus is extraordinarily tropic for human erythroid progenitor cells. The virus binds to erythroid progenitors on the P blood group antigen [404a] (a glycosphingolipid called a *globoside*). Erythrocytes lacking P antigen are not agglutinate by the virus and purified P antigen blocks binding of the virus to erythroid cells and infectivity of erythroid progenitors.[404a] Replication of B19 parvovirus occurs only in erythroid bone marrow cells,[405] and replicative double-stranded DNA forms can be detected in the bone marrow of infected patients.[380,406,407] In tissue culture, B19 parvovirus has been propagated only in the erythroid cells of human bone marrow[408] and fetal liver.[409] Erythroid colony formation by CFU-E and BFU-E, but not by CFU-GM, is strongly inhibited by virus.[410] Parvovirus is directly cytotoxic and induces characteristic light[408] and electron[411] microscopic morphologic changes in erythroid precursors (see Fig. 10-8). The virus cytopathic effect is manifest as giant pronormoblasts, first recognized by Owren[364] in 1948 in the bone marrow of patients with TAC and reproduced by tissue culture infection.[408] Virus toxicity is the result of expression of the single nonstructural protein of the virus, and limited expression of this gene may explain inhibition of myelopoiesis and megakaryocytopoiesis in patients in the absence of virus replication in these cells.[412]

Hepatitis and Flaviviruses. Aplastic anemia may follow an episode of acute hepatitis.[413–418] The association of hepatitis and aplastic anemia is not rare, and almost 200 cases could be collected in the literature to 1972.[416] As an identifiable clinical event, a prior episode of hepatitis is recognized in 2% to 5% of aplastic anemia patients in western series[419] and about twice this percentage in the Far East.[44] A previous episode of hepatitis was a significant risk factor in a case control study of aplastic anemia.[63] In a much greater number of patients, antecedent hepatitis may be subclinical, since about half of patients may have abnormally elevated hepatic transaminases on presentation before their first transfusion.[24]

Hepatitis is frequently associated with mild blood count depression, but aplasia is a rare sequela, estimated to occur in less than 0.07% of total pediatric hepatitis cases[420] and less than 2% of non-A, non-B hepatitis cases.[421–423] In patients with hepatic failure after non-A, non-B hepatitis, an astonishing 28% (9 of 32) developed aplastic anemia after liver transplantation.[424–426]

Hepatitis-associated aplastic anemia has several peculiar features.[415,416,418,427] Bone marrow depression usually occurs just when the patient is recovering from acute liver inflammation, as judged by serum hepatic transaminase elevation, generally about 2 months from the episode of hepatitis. A large percentage of patients are male and young. Hepatitis confers a particularly poor prognosis on aplastic anemia patients. In Hagler's series of 174 cases, over 90% of patients had died within 1 year of diagnosis, and the average duration of survival was only 11 weeks from onset of pancytopenia.[416] A history of hepatitis has been considered an indication for early bone marrow transplantation[427]; patients have been successfully transplanted,[427–429] but some have also responded to antithymocyte globulin (ATG)[424] or androgen therapy.[430] Aplastic anemia has occurred in some family members affected with hepatitis[78,79] and not in others[414]; a genetic predisposition is suggested by the presence of HLA-B8 antigen in 6 of 11 cases (also associated with autoimmune hepatitis).[431] Blood count depression during the course of hepatitis is common, and the leukopenia, atypical lymphocytosis, erythroid macrocytosis, and thrombocytopenia mimic in milder form the hematologic changes of aplastic anemia. Much rarer sequelae than severe aplastic anemia are reports of transient pancytopenia,[432,433] PRCA,[79,434] agranulocytosis,[435] and hypoplastic acute lymphocytic leukemia.[436]

Inconsistent immune system changes have been reported. Hepatitis-associated aplastic anemia has been associated with generally diminished immune responsiveness, including decreased T-cell count and function and lower serum immunoglobulins, compared with idiopathic disease.[437,438] Comparison with patients with hepatitis alone was not carried out. In contrast, others have reported heightened immune responsiveness, with more circulating activated suppressor T lymphocytes in children with hepatitis-associated aplasia,[439,440] likely reflecting a cytotoxic lymphocyte response to the viral infection (see section on immune suppression of hematopoiesis). A serum sickness–like illness can occur during the course of hepatitis-associated aplastic anemia.[423]

Aplastic anemia is probably most frequently associated with non-A, non-B hepatitis. In one series of 16 patients, hepatitis types A and B could be confidently excluded in 13 patients and was considered doubtful as a preceding illness in the remaining 3 patients[417]; subsequently other serologically well-defined cases have been reported.[421–423,441] Non-A, non-B hepatitis has, until recently, been a diagnosis of exclusion, but in 1989 the etiologic agent of non-A, non-B hepatitis was molecularly cloned.

Hepatitis C is a small, enveloped, positive-stranded RNA virus[442]; these properties allow its classification as flavivirus-like. Flaviviruses are the etiologic agents of the arbovirus hemorrhagic fevers, dengue (Thai hematodepressive disease),[443,444] Russian spring-summer fever,[445] South American hemorrhagic fever,[446] Omsk hemorrhagic fever, and many others.[447] These are acute infectious hematodepressive syndromes; in dengue, the neutrophil and platelet counts fall, often to very low levels, during the early viremic phase of illness, whereas immune events, probably secondary to cytokine release and reflected in atypical lymphocytosis, predominate during the second, shock phase of the disease. The bone marrow in dengue is hypocellular with abnormal megakaryocyte appearance. Experimental inoculation of flaviviruses into human volunteers produced pancytopenia and marrow aplasia.[448] Flaviviruses propagate efficiently in human bone marrow cultures and hematopoietic cell lines.[449] Although not directly cytotoxic to marrow cells,[449] dengue infection in vitro induces lymphocyte activation and release of cytokines such as γ-interferon (γ-IFN) that suppress hematopoiesis[450] (see section on pathophysiology).

In a large study of histocompatibility phenotypes, 6 of 11 patients with hepatitis-associated aplasia expressed the HLA-B8 antigen,[431] and aplasia has occurred in family members with hepatitis,[79] both observations suggesting a genetic basis for the immune response. Patients with hepatitis-associated aplastic anemia can successfully undergo transplantation,[427,433] although a syngeneic transplant required prior conditioning.[451] These clinical findings are more consistent with a dominant immune pathophysiologic mechanism than with direct viral destruction of cells.

Occasional case reports of aplasia after hepatitis B[452,453] and hepatitis A[454–456] have not been supported by epidemiologic evidence.[457] These are common pathogens, and perhaps some of the patients were coinfected with hepatitis C, which may travel with hepatitis B.[458] Hematopoietic colony formation in vitro can be inhibited (modestly) by hepatitis B,[459,460] hepatitis A,[461] and perhaps hepatitis C.[462] Hepatitis B surface antigen has been detected in the nuclei of immature myeloid cells[459] and hepatitis B DNA in circulating WBCs.[463] Murine hepatitis virus, a coronavirus, also causes pancytopenia and bone marrow necrosis associated with acute liver inflammation.[464,465]

Epstein-Barr Virus. Herpesviruses are large, genetically complex DNA viruses; two herpesviruses have been associated clinically and experimentally with bone marrow failure. Acute infection with EBV causes infectious mononucleosis, which has been rarely complicated by severe bone marrow failure. Agranulocytosis[466–468] and PRCA[469,470] have also been associated with EBV infection. Only nine cases of pancytopenia occuring shortly after infectious mononucleosis could be collected in 1981, and bone marrow hypocellularity was not documented in all. Agranulocytosis[466–468] and PRCA[469,470] also have been associated with EBV infection. Some aplastic patients had spontaneous recoveries, others recovered with corticosteroid therapy, and some died.[471] In our study, EBV was demonstrated by immunologic and molecular techniques in bone marrow cells of six patients with aplastic anemia.[472] All patients had serologic evidence of recent infection or reactivation, but only two had a previous history of typical infectious mononucleosis, suggesting that the virus may be involved more frequently than inferred from the history alone, especially since a large number of primary EBV infections are unrecognized.[472,473] After our observation of a sustained remission after acyclovir therapy in a young woman with aplastic anemia and herpes simplex infections, other patients with aplastic anemia have apparently responded to acyclovir therapy.[474,475]

Suppressor T cells are activated during infectious mononucleosis[476] and may mediate hematopoietic failure (Fig. 10-11). Lymphocyte suppression of hematopoiesis was shown in one patient with postmononucleosis aplastic anemia who responded to ATG therapy.[477] An aberrant genetically determined immune response to the virus is suggested by the frequent mortality from bone marrow failure in boys with X-linked lymphoproliferative syndrome, a familial syndrome characterized by various combinations of hypogammaglobulinemia, chronic or fatal acute infectious mononucleosis, B-cell lymphomas, and aplastic anemia.[80]

Aplastic anemia has occurred in both sexes of a German Mennonite family in which a high frequency of nasopharyngeal carcinoma and high antibody titers to EBV were also present.[478] Hematopoietic cells may be targets of EBV infection. Although the B lymphocyte is the most obvious target, EBV has also been detected in T lymphocytes in some patients with lymphoma[479] and in nasopharyngeal epithelial cells infected in vitro[480] and in vivo.[481] The virus is present in monocyte-macrophage cell lines established from children with a variety of clinical defects in hematopoiesis.[482]

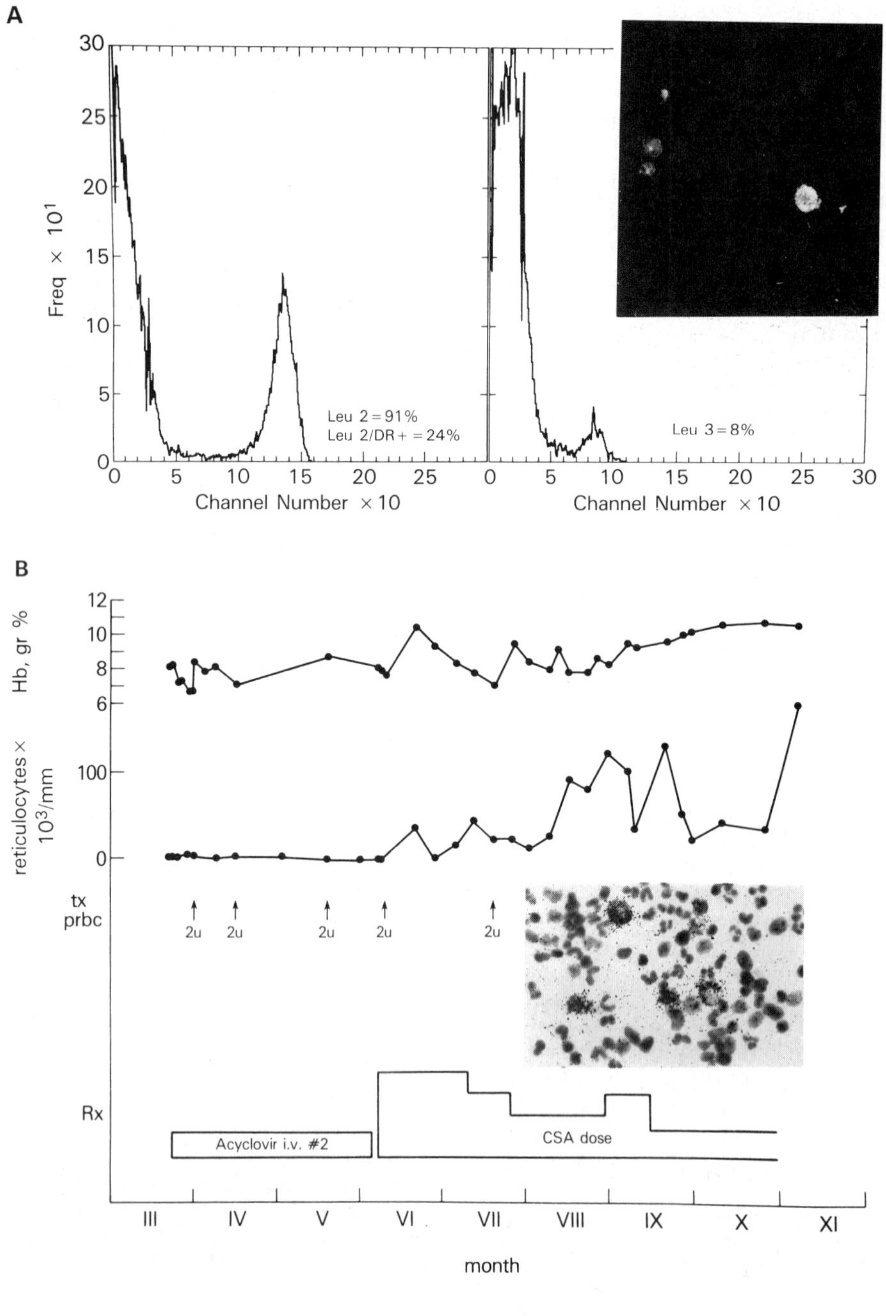

FIGURE 10-11. Clinical findings in patients with EBV-associated aplastic anemia. (**A**) A 16-year-old girl who developed severe and ultimately fatal pancytopenia 1 month after an episode of infectious mononucleosis. Essentially all her circulating leukocytes were suppressor/cytotoxic lymphocytes, as shown in the flow cytometry profiles, and a large proportion of these cells were activated. (HLA-DR normally is expressed on less than 1% of T cells.) EBV was detected in the bone marrow by immunofluorescence for nuclear antigen, shown in the inset. Low concentrations of γ-interferon were present in the circulation. (**B**) A 12-year-old girl with hereditary pure red cell aplasia suffered an atypical relapse (RBCs were not macrocytic) after infectious mononucleosis. She developed a slight reticulocytosis with parenteral acyclovir therapy (not shown) and a complete, sustained remission with cyclosporine treatment. EBV was easily detected in the bone marrow by in situ hybridization, as shown in the inset.

The rare virus-associated hemophagocytic syndrome is a related but clinically distinct syndrome also associated mainly with EBV infection.[483] Here, the bone marrow is characterized by histiocytic hyperplasia and erythrocyte phagocytosis (although hematopoietic cell hypoplasia is also present), and the peripheral blood count depression is often associated with abnormalities of other organ systems, especially hepatosplenomegaly, lymphadenopathy, cutaneous eruptions, and pulmonary infiltrates.[483–485] Hemophagocytosis is often observed on supravital stains of the marrow of patients with idiopathic aplastic anemia.[486]

Cytomegalovirus. Like EBV, cytomegalovirus (CMV) infection is common and usually benign in its effects. Even in immunosuppressed patients, CMV infection, as a result of either reactivation or new exposure, is not associated with a characteristic clinical syndrome.[487] In the immunosuppressed bone marrow transplant patient, a second episode of marrow failure may follow CMV infection. In immunodeficient mice, murine CMV prevented bone marrow reconstitution despite the presence of stem cells, and cytotoxic (CD8+) lymphocytes protected animals against this lethal effect[488,489]; virus can be demonstrated in thrombocytopenic mouse megakaryocytes.[490] CMV promiscuously infects fibroblasts of many tissues, and its infection of bone marrow stromal cells is the probable mechanism of marrow failure.[491] Some clinical isolates of CMV inhibited colony formation (both CFU-GM– and BFU-E–derived), but no good correlation exists between these in vitro effects and the presence of neutropenia in the patient donor.[492] As in EBV infection, CMV infection is associated with reversal of the helper/suppressor T-lymphocyte ratio, but in contrast to that seen in EBV, T-cell function is diminished.[493]

Human Immunodeficiency Virus. Hematologic changes are common in patients with the acquired immunodeficiency syndrome (AIDS).[494–497] Although most patients have anemia and granulocytopenia and one third have thrombocytopenia, many of these abnormalities may be secondary to opportunistic infections, medications, and neoplasms. Pancytopenia and marrow hypocellularity can occur.[498] Marrow hypocellularity may be present in up to 20% of bone marrow biopsies performed in patients with AIDS,[495,499,500] but need not be associated with pancytopenia.[501] Hypocellularity almost always has been reported in patients with concomitant infections and suppressive drug therapy[502,503]; one patient had PNH.[504] Much more frequently, blood count depression is associated with normal cellularity or hypercellularity,[494,501–503] which is often dysplastic.[502,503,505–507] Atypical lymphocytosis and lymphocytic infiltration of the bone marrow are common features.

Thrombocytopenia in patients with AIDS has been partly explained by the presence of platelet antibodies or immune complexes, but retroviral particles are visible in megakaryocytes from thrombocytopenic patients.[508] A similar mechanism for neutrophils is supported by in vitro experiments, in which CFU-GM–derived colony formation by patients' bone marrow was inhibited by serum-containing antibodies to envelope glycoprotein.[509] The numbers of hematopoietic colonies recovered from patients with AIDS have been variable, reported as both normal[509] and decreased.[510] These differences may be a function of the balance between virus and antibody response in different patient populations or may reflect hematopoietic suppression by marrow infected with opportunistic organisms.[511] An immune mechanism of hematopoietic suppression has been inferred from in vitro studies of another pathogenic human retrovirus, HTLV-1 or the adult T-cell leukemia–lymphoma virus. In a case of PRCA associated with HTLV-1 infection, T lymphocytes that suppressed BFU-E–derived progenitor growth were detected in colony culture experiments.[512] A nonviral glycoprotein inhibitor of myelopoiesis was partially purified from supernatants of the bone marrow of patients with AIDS in one study.[513]

Human T-cell leukemia virus type II has been isolated from a patient with pancytopenia and hemophilia,[514] and HIV has been found in the brain of a patient with aplastic anemia.[515] Efforts by ourselves and others[516] to expand these observations have failed to detect a retrovirus in aplastic anemia bone marrow and blood cells, using reverse transcriptase assays and electron microscopy.

Animal retroviruses can infect hematopoietic cells and offer useful models of bone marrow failure secondary to virus infection; leukemia viruses of cats[517] and mice[518] are the best examples. Feline leukemia virus is a clinically important pathogen that causes more marrow failure, usually myelodysplastic in morphology, than leukemia.[517,519] Infection of laboratory animals with a strain of the C group of feline leukemia virus produces PRCA. Primitive erythroid progenitor cells (BFU-E) are not detectable in kittens infected with this virus,[520] and CFU-E are absent in adult animals.[521] Feline leukemia virus can persist as a latent infection of marrow cells, with virus undetectable except by in vitro culture of bone marrow cells; it can be reactivated by corticosteroid treatment.[522] Progenitor cells from group C–infected animals bear viral glycoprotein, and erythroid cells acquire sensitivity to complement that resembles PNH.[523] The determinants for erythroid pathology have been matched to limited regions of the viral genome.[524]

Other Viruses. As an organ of actively proliferating cells accessible to the circulation, the bone marrow undoubtedly provides an attractive milieu for many types of viruses. Infection of human megakaryocytes has been inferred in congenital and acquired rubella,[525–527] measles,[528] and mumps,[529] and has been found after live attenuated measles vaccination[530] and demonstrated in varicella (chickenpox)[531] and in animals infected with CMV,[490] Newcastle disease virus,[532] encephalomyocarditis virus,[533] and retrovirus-associated lymphomas.[534] Aplastic anemia has been reported after influenza A infection.[535]

Paroxysmal Nocturnal Hemoglobinuria

Aplastic anemia and PNH are clinically related syndromes.[536–540] During the course of PNH, pancytopenia is common, and about one third of patients die of bone marrow failure. Some patients have a positive sucrose hemolysis test and a negative acid lysis test on presentation with pancytopenia, later evolving into a fully typical laboratory pattern.[536,538] A fairly high percentage of patients with pancytopenia and marrow hypocellularity have either a positive sucrose hemolysis test (10%)[538] or an acidified serum hemolysis test (15%).[536] Other patients with aplastic anemia evolve to PNH, or, possibly, the diagnosis was initially undetermined or mistaken.[540] The acid or sucrose hemolysis test can be positive in patients on presentation or during the course of otherwise typical idiopathic aplastic anemia, and in patients with drug-[541] or benzene-associated[542] aplastic anemia. PNH, aplastic anemia, and acute myelogenous leukemia all have occurred in a single patient.[543]

Hematopoietic progenitor count is severely decreased in patients with cytopenias and PNH, even when the marrow is cellular.[544,545] Studies with fractionated erythrocytes[546] and progenitor cell cultures[547] have suggested that complement-sensitive cells are relatively frequent in aplastic anemia. Aplastic patients with positive Ham tests can respond to immunosuppressive therapy. PNH, like aplastic anemia, is also relatively common in the Far East, where it is more frequently associated with aplastic anemia and less often with thromboses.[548] The origin of complement-sensitive cells is an acquired genetic defect in PIG-A, an enzyme on the X chromosome that catalyzes an early step in the biosynthesis of the glycosylphosphatidylinositol (GPI) moiety that anchors some proteins to membranes.[548a,548b] Several GPI-linked proteins protect cells from complement damage. Presumably, lack of these proteins or others related to growth and proliferation can cause aplastic anemia.

The concept of PNH as a clonal disorder is based on the observation of a single glucose-6-phosphate dehydrogenase (G6PD) type in the affected erythrocytes of two female patients heterozygous at this locus.[539] Both normal and sensitive erythrocytes circulate, and identification of distinct populations of complement-sensitive and normal progenitors has been reported by some[549,550] but not other investigators.[545,551,552] The coexistence with normal cells of a clone with deficient growth properties is paradoxical. Clonal hematopoiesis in a single patient with moderate aplastic anemia (and multiple physical anomalies but negative cytogenetic studies[553]) may represent a similar development in the presumed absence of markers for PNH; alternatively, reduction of number of stem cells in aplasia may favor the generation of circulating cells from limited numbers of stem cells, as occurs after experimental chemotherapy or virus infection.

Immunologic Abnormalities

Aplastic anemia commonly occurs during the course of the rare syndrome eosinophilic fasciitis, a collagen vascular disease similar to scleroderma.[554,555] Of the first 100 cases reported in the literature, nearly 10% had bone marrow failure. The rheumatologic symptoms of fasciitis respond to corticosteroids, but the associated aplastic anemia has a poor prognosis[554]; some patients have responded to immunosuppression.[556]

Aplastic anemia occasionally occurs in persons with hypogammaglobulinemia[557,558] or in association with thymoma, thymic hyperplasia,[559] or thymic carcinoma.[560] In one case, suppressor T cells, already implicated in B-cell inhibition, were shown to suppress erythropoietic colony formation.[561]

Iatrogenic fatal aplastic anemia has been produced by the transfusion of competent lymphocytes into immunodeficient hosts,[562–566] and runt disease in some animal species may also be accompanied by aplasia with a histiocytic, phagocytic cell infiltrate.

Other than the specific and possibly pathophysiologic immunologic abnormalities to be described in the text that follows, immune system function is not severely impaired in most cases of aplastic anemia. Patients with aplastic anemia generally have normal immunoglobulin levels and normal antibody titers to common viral antigens.[558,567–569] About half of patients show skin test anergy to a common panel of antigens, but in vitro lymphocyte proliferation is normal.[567] Monocytopenia and lymphocytopenia are responsible for reported specific abnormalities such as deficient differentiation of B cells on lectin stimulation[558] or lymphocyte proliferation that requires monocyte help.[569] Aplastic patients do not behave clinically as if they were immunodeficient, and susceptibility to virus and protozoan organisms is related to immunosuppressive therapy.

Pregnancy

The first patient with aplastic anemia described by Ehrlich[1] was pregnant. Pregnancy is common in the age groups most susceptible to marrow failure, and in many cases its association is probably only coincidental. Etiology is suggested by the temporal relation between the onset of pancytopenia and pregnancy and remissions with normal,[570] forceps,[571] or cesarean delivery[572] at term or spontaneously[573] or by therapeutic abortion.[574,575] Occasional patients have developed aplastic anemia during pregnancy and remitted after each delivery.[576] The paucity of cases is apparent from periodic literature reviews,[577,578] and only 43 could be collected in 1975. Several larger series have come from the Orient,[580,581] and in the largest literature survey half the cases were reported originally in Japanese.[579] In the latter review, many cases were dismissed because of inadequate documentation.[579] Of the 43 well-described cases, aplasia was diagnosed during the pregnancy in 30 patients. Bone marrow hypoplasia may be relatively common during pregnancy, as it was detected in 8 of 101 anemic pregnant women without overt iron deficiency.[582]

Survival rates for aplastic anemia in pregnancy in recent years have been relatively high for mother (83%) and baby (75%), with most pregnancies (69%) being successful.[579] Death during pregnancy or delivery is usually caused by hemorrhage. The published data are insufficient to guide the management of the pregnant aplastic woman, especially since aplastic anemia in some cases is clearly serendipitously diagnosed and can persist beyond parturition. On the one hand, pregnancy complicates the problems of pancytopenia; on the other hand, most patients can be successfully supported.[575,576,578–581] A woman who desires a child can be maintained with transfusions, with the understanding that clinical deterioration is a criterion for interruption or termination of the pregnancy. Bleeding can be better controlled with surgical intervention than during a vaginal delivery.

That estrogens are related to the aplasia of pregnancy is suggested by the effect of large doses of these hormones on hematopoiesis in animals. Estrus-associated aplastic anemia occurs in ferrets,[583] and administration of large doses of estrogens can produce blood count depression in ferrets[584] and dogs,[585–587] although the bone marrow is more usually hyperplastic than acellular.[588] Estrogens can blunt the erythrokinetic response to erythropoietin in rats.[589] Estrogen administration has decreased the number of CFU-S in the spleen and bone marrow of mice, in association with thrombocytopenia and neutropenia.[590] The positive action of androgens on hematopoiesis is discussed later in this chapter.

Pathophysiology

Hematopoietic Stem Cells

The most consistent laboratory finding in aplastic anemia is very low numbers of blood and bone marrow hematopoietic progenitor cells, including myeloid CFU-GM,[591–598] BFU-E, CFU-E,[599–601] and pluripotent CFU-GEMM.[602] Some preservation of numbers of progenitors, such as residual hematopoiesis on bone marrow specimens, has been associated with an improved prognosis.[594,598,601] Decreased progenitors persist in patients long after successful treatment with bone marrow transplantation[603] or immunosuppression.[597,604] Blast colonies, a stem cell equivalent in semisolid medium, are also undetectable. Nevertheless, an absence of stem cells was reasonably inferred from an inability to detect progenitors and seemingly confirmed by the dramatic efficacy of stem cell replacement in the form of bone marrow transplantation. The success of nonreplacement immunosuppressive therapies in aplastic anemia, however, has made a simple thesis of quantitative deficiency of stem cells untenable.

The W/W^v mouse is an animal model of stem cell-based bone marrow failure; these heterozygotes have a macrocytic anemia that is curable by transplantation, but their own cells form microscopic rather than macroscopic spleen colonies in normal host animals.[605,606] The anemia, out of proportion to depression of other blood counts, and the CFU-S assay itself, reflect a mainly erythropoietic lesion.[607] The W/W^v phenotype results from mutations in the c-*kit* locus. This gene is a transmembrane tyrosine kinase, expressed primarily in erythroid cells, and is the cell surface receptor for stem cell factor (SCF; kit ligand), a hematopoietic growth factor[608–609g] (see Chap. 8). Mutations in SCR are responsible for steel disease, an inherited aplastic anemia in mice.[609d–609g] The relevance of the W/W^v model to acquired aplastic anemia is dubious because a somatic mutation that confers a growth disadvantage suffers negative selective pressure in the marrow. On the other hand, mutations in genes for growth factor receptors must be responsible for some hereditary cytopenias such as congenital red cell aplasia (Diamond-Blackfan anemia) and congenital neutropenia (Kostmann's syndrome).

The stem cell compartment is not homogeneous but organized in a hierarchy of cells according to generational age[610,611] (Fig. 10-12). If a mouse is treated with a cell-cycle–active drug such as hydroxyurea[612,613] or 5-fluorouracil,[614] the remaining hematopoietic stem cells have increased capacities to proliferate, differentiate, and renew themselves. Similar results can be seen in long-term bone marrow cultures, in which the initial phase of establishing the culture leaves a population in the adherent cell layer that has a high proliferative capacity.[615] Stem cells of different properties can be physically separated, so that highly purified CFU-S are not effective in repopulating an irradiated mouse.[616] The hierarchical model predicts that as stem cells age by undergoing repeated cell divisions, they would increase their probability of entering another division and of being recruited to leave the stem cell compartment and differentiate. The behavior of the compartment best fits a model of clonal succession, in which stem cell entry into the more active part of the compartment and ultimately to terminal differentiation is orderly but random.

The quantity of extremely primitive, repopulating cells, the true stem cells, is limited, and only a small percentage of primitive stem cells is likely to be in mitotic cycle at any time. By inference from the distribution of G6PD phenotype in heterozygous persons, 10 to 24 cells were estimated to be actively maintaining hematopoiesis.[617] Primitive repopulating cells are about 10-fold less common than the CFU-S; clonal analysis has shown that a single pluripotent stem cell repopulates.[618,619] Nevertheless, normal hematopoiesis is maintained from these few cells for the life-span of the animal, and little evidence exists for aging of hematopoiesis. Elderly mice make as good bone marrow donors as young mice, and serially transplanted stem cells can maintain normal blood counts in animals through several life-spans.[620]

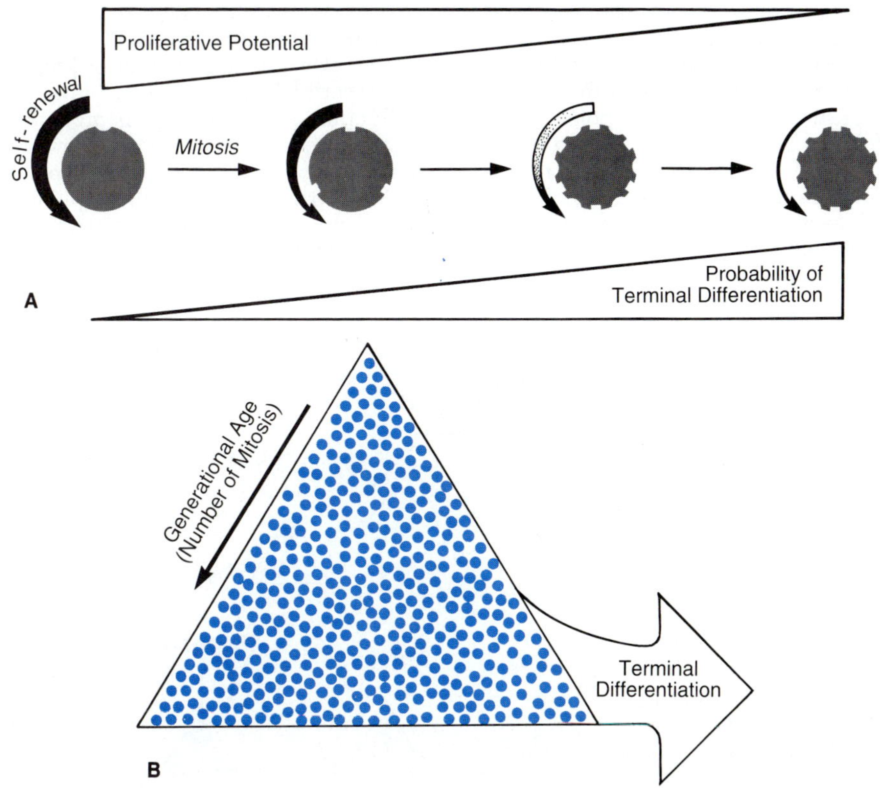

FIGURE 10-12. Stem cell aging and a model of stem cell hierarchical organization by generational age. (**A**) Functional changes in an individual cell are followed through several mitotic cycles. With each cell cycle, the cell's proliferative potential for expansion or self-renewal decreases, and its likelihood of entering a pathway of terminal differentiation increases. Proliferation, self-renewal, and differentiation are regulated by a combination of internal cell mechanisms (genetic) and environmental influences (cell–cell interactions, growth factors, hormones). For example, increasing cell surface receptors is one way to increase the probability of a response to a specific proliferative or differentiative stimulus, such as a constant concentration of hematopoietic growth factor molecules in the environment. Each mitosis also increases the number of cells. (**B**) The organization of the entire compartment is diagrammed. The stochastic or random nature of regulatory events can be envisioned from this model. As the cell number increases because of mitosis, the number of cells available to a signaling event is much higher among the mitotically older members of the population. Cell numbers also increase during terminal differentiation.

Given this enormous capacity, it is paradoxical that the stem cell compartment should suffer drastic loss in quantity and especially in self-renewal capacity in a wide variety of experimental situations. That relatively late CFU-S should decline in colony-forming ability with serial transplantation is perhaps not surprising,[621] but the same occurs when repopulation is the endpoint,[622] as in the shielded limb of an irradiated animal[623] and after a single bone marrow transplantation.[624] Stem cell loss and deterioration of stem cell function are observed with parabiosis instead of physical removal of donor cells in W/W^v mice (which are only mildly anemic) as in the irradiated host.[625] Similar permanent loss of self-renewal capacity can be observed at the stressful initiation of a long-term bone marrow culture[626] and after cell irradiation in vitro.[119] Deregulation of hematopoiesis results not only in reduction in the size of the stem cell compartment but also in alteration of its most important functional properties. Recent experiments with purified pluripotent hematopoietic stem cells can be interpreted as showing that monoclonal succession of stem cell differentiation is operative and limiting when stem cell count is low.[627,628]

In contrast to the effect of hydroxyurea in improving the quantity and quality of the hematopoietic stem cell compartment, treatment with busulfan produces latent bone marrow failure.[629–631] Similar bone marrow damage can be produced by other alkylating agents[632] and frequent small doses of γ radiation.[633] At an appropriate dose, the busulfan-treated mouse maintains normal or near-normal blood counts and bone marrow cellularity, near-normal or only moderately reduced progenitor cell and stem cell counts for 1 year, until CFU-S counts decrease and the animals develop frank aplasia. Estimates that hematopoiesis failed when the percentage of CFU-S fell to 10%, based on the effects of busulfan or split-dose irradiation,[633] can now be reinterpreted as disappearance of the less common repopulating cell. A self-renewal deficit in busulfan-treated animals can be demonstrated in vitro,[632,634] and normal cell transplants largely ameliorate busulfan-induced marrow failure, two results that implicate the stem cell directly (although there may be concomitant damage by drug to the stroma[629,635,636]).

Two different pathways of bone marrow damage are seen, based on the paradigms of animals treated with busulfan and hydroxyurea (Fig. 10-13). Common to both pathways is the crucial position of the most primitive hematopoietic stem cells at the top of the hierarchy. These primitive cells are mitotically quiescent. Quiescence must serve to prevent stem cell compartment depletion. Quiescence would protect the most primitive stem cell from a variety of environmental toxins, which would be expected to be most injurious to metabolically active cells, and from viruses, which favor replication in mitotically active or differentiated cells. Severe or continuing damage in both pathways would result in a similar appearance of total acellularity, but the mechanism of progression and recovery would be different. In pathway I, damage to the hematopoietic compartment is random, striking all cells with an equal probability. Pathway I is the likely mechanism of direct injury to cellular DNA; examples of exogenous agents are radiation, alkylating drugs, reactive benzene metabolites, and possibly chloramphenicol. Although the likelihood of injury would be the same for all cells, the effect would be selective for more primitive cells, because primitive cells require many mitoses to mature and because late cells have accomplished most of their mitotic life and need only a few divisions to reach terminal maturation.

Recovery would occur from throughout the stem cell compartment, but a severe defect in stem cell quantity and self-renewal capacity would be the permanent result, as just described, of busulfan or radiation treatment. The introduction of DNA defects is probably rare outside of iatrogenic or experimental drug and x-ray exposure. In nature, the genetic defects that make up Fanconi's anemia, in which repair of DNA is inadequate, would be the most common examples of bone marrow failure by pathway I.

In contrast, most environmental damage to the stem cell compartment is probably directed at mitotically and met-

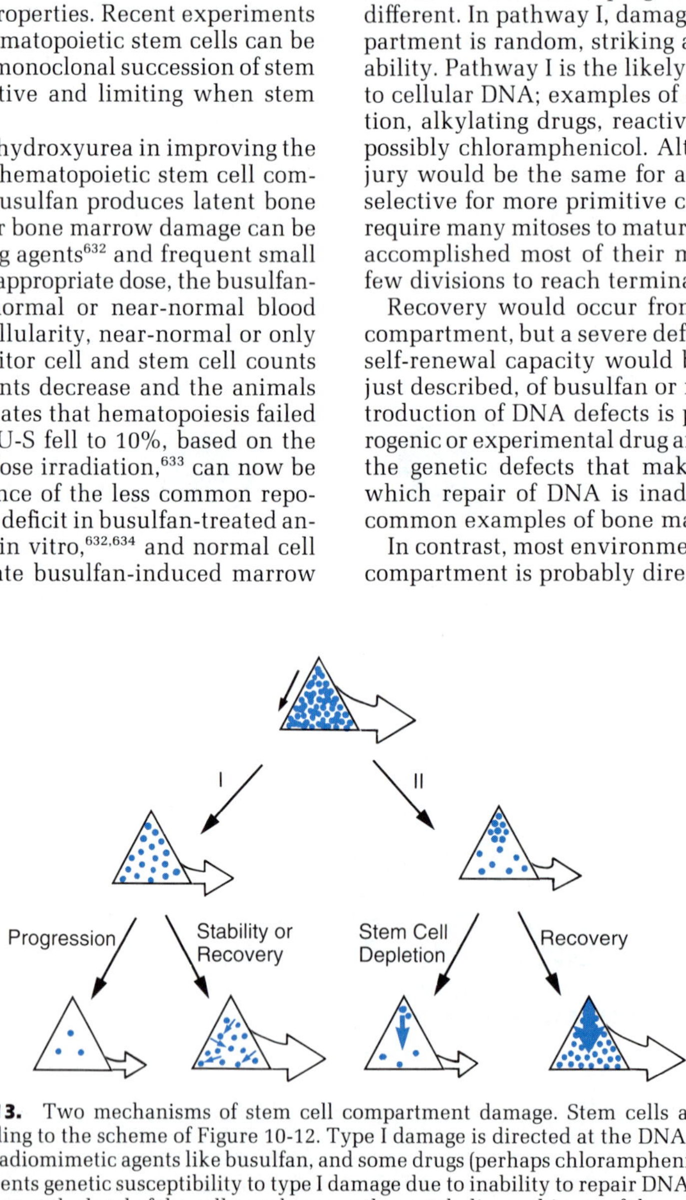

FIGURE 10-13. Two mechanisms of stem cell compartment damage. Stem cells are depicted in outline according to the scheme of Figure 10-12. Type I damage is directed at the DNA and is typified by radiation, radiomimetic agents like busulfan, and some drugs (perhaps chloramphenicol). Fanconi's anemia represents genetic susceptibility to type I damage due to inability to repair DNA damage. Type II damage occurs at the level of the cell membrane or the metabolic machinery of the cell and includes most drugs, viruses, and immune-mediated marrow failure. Of course, the diagram is a simplification. Some exogenous agents may act to injure a late cell's metabolic machinery and also to introduce genetic damage (benzene may be an example), and genetic susceptibility, as in Fanconi's anemia, implies an external precipitating event. Primitive stem cells feed recovery when loss has occurred to actively cycling cells, as shown on the right, whereas later stem cells are needed to repair random damage as shown on the left. At some point in either scheme, qualitative alterations in the compartment can become an absolute quantitative loss of stem cells. Nonetheless, hematopoietic recovery should be easier with type II damage, in which the repopulating cells are preserved.

abolically active cells. Differentiating cells acquire a distinct phenotype as they express antigens absent on immature cells; differentiating, metabolically dynamic, and mitotically active cells are the preferred targets of most viruses. In pathway II, damage occurs to the proliferating stem cells and progenitors, spares the primitive cells, and is probably mediated at the cell surface or through the cell's metabolic machinery. The response to continuous removal or suppression of late cells, by viral infection or immune response, is movement from the most primitive stem cells at the top of the pyramid. Depletion of stem cells has been suggested by some experiments, for example, decreased CFU-S self-renewal after prolonged severe hemolysis in the mouse.[626] On the other hand, the most primitive stem cells, even when not depleted, may be too quiescent, too unresponsive to positive stimuli, although the probability of response would increase with time in a stochastic model. The high rate of response in aplastic anemia to immunosuppressive therapy implies that most patients suffer from type II damage to the stem cell compartment.

The different pathways to bone marrow failure also help to clarify the confusing relation of aplastic anemia to other diseases (Fig. 10-14). Aplasia caused by genetic damage may resemble clinically and share pathophysiology with the myelodysplasias and leukemias, whereas the aplasia that results from immune, drug, and virus damage is related to less complicated diseases of the immune system: the single cytopenias and acute viral infections.

Hematopoietic Stroma and Growth Factors

The hypothesis that bone marrow failure is a lesion of "soil" rather than "seed"[637] was based on several experimental observations: regeneration in isolated limbs after irradiation (discussed previously); defects of the sinusoidal vasculature in animals rejecting allogeneic bone marrow grafts; intrinsic differences in the ability of red and yellow, or predominantly fatty, marrow to support hematopoiesis after transplantation to extramedullary sites.[638] Abnormal adipocyte proliferation, based on morphologic characteristics of fatty marrow in patients and controls, has even been proposed as the primary lesion in aplastic anemia.[639] Direct evidence for a microenvironmental defect in aplastic patients has not been found in biochemical analysis of the composition

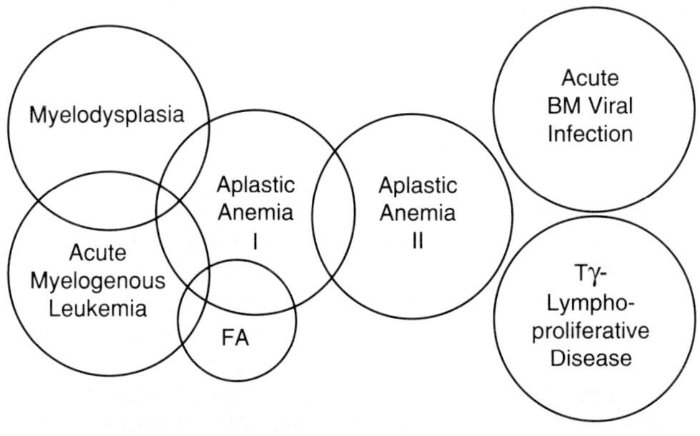

FIGURE 10-14. Venn diagram that relates type I and II aplastic anemia to other hematologic diseases. Real overlap exists between type I aplastic anemia and myelodysplastic and leukemic syndromes because of the commonality of DNA damage in these diseases. The fact that only some patients with ordinary viral infections develop aplasia is probably a function of the immune response. Monoclonal (if not malignant) proliferation of similar cytotoxic lymphocytes, as are detected in some cases of type II aplastic anemia, results in Tγ-lymphoproliferative disease. BM, bone marrow; FA, Fanconi's anemia.

of fat cells[640] or in ultrastructural studies of marrow microvasculature.[641]

Bone marrow failure due to a stromal defect occurs in the Sl/Sl^d mouse.[605,606] In this disorder, a genetic defect of the Sl^d allele results in an anemia that is not corrected by stem cell infusion but is cured by spleen transplantation. The product of the Sl allele is SCF, the ligand for c-kit.[609d–609g] The presence of normal stem cells in Sl/Sl^d mice is shown by the ability of their spleen or bone marrow to cure W/W^v animals. Parallel results occur in long-term bone marrow cultures: stroma of Sl/Sl^d animals does not support hematopoiesis by W/W^v cells, whereas W/W^v stroma supports hematopoiesis from Sl/Sl^d mice.[642]

In contrast to the stem cell, the human marrow microenvironment has resisted quantitative assessment, but important qualitative conclusions have been inferred from in vitro studies. First, in long-term bone marrow cultures the stroma is composed of morphologically diverse components, including cells resembling macrophages, fibroblasts, and fat cells.[644,645] Second, analyses of patients with clonal disorders of hematopoiesis[646] and virus-transformed cell lines[647] have shown that at least some of the cell types in the stroma share a common origin with stem cells. Third, the stroma after human bone marrow transplantation is of host and not of donor origin, with the exception of macrophages, as demonstrated by chromosomal analysis with Y-specific markers in sex-mismatched transplants.[648,649]

Studies of the bone marrow of aplastic anemia patients must be interpreted in the context of the aforementioned findings. Long-term bone marrow cultures with recognizable cobblestone stromal layers can be established from most patients with aplastic anemia,[650–652] although their capacity to support colony formation in the nonadherent layer may be deficient.[653] These culture systems are inherently unstable and difficult to quantitate, and their failure can be a secondary phenomenon or a technical artifact as well as evidence of a primary stromal defect. Numbers of bone marrow fibroblast colonies (CFU-F) in aplastic anemia has occasionally been low[654] but more often normal,[655,656] although their growth characteristics may be abnormal.[650] Functional abnormalities of aplastic marrow stromal cells have been described. Their decreased capacity to generate colony-stimulating factors[655–657] may be related to the profound inability of monocytes from aplastic patients to generate IL-1, a cytokine that releases a variety of growth factors from fibroblast-like cells.[658–662]

A deficiency of colony-stimulating activity release in the presence of autologous serum, which has been correlated with a poor prognosis, may also reflect monocyte function.[663] (Monocytes are the one element of the stroma that is transplanted; see previous text.) Conversely, adherent cell activity that inhibits hematopoiesis has been reported by some investigators using aplastic bone marrow[664,665] or peripheral blood[665,666] (these results have not been duplicated by others[666] and may not be specific to aplastic anemia).[667] Bone marrow stromal cells can produce β-IFN (IL-6),[668,669] and the monocyte is the main producer of interferons after some viral infections.[670] Production of an inhibitor by S1/S1^d stroma has been reported.[671,672]

Factors that stimulate hematopoiesis are almost always abundant in patients with aplastic anemia. The urine of these patients has been a favorite source of erythropoietin for purification, and high levels of this hormone circulate.[673] Other hematopoietic colony activities have, until recently, been difficult to measure except in cumbersome and semiquantitative double-layer culture systems. Production of burst-promoting activity by aplastic anemia patients' mononuclear cells in vitro is high,[674,675] and high activity levels have been measured in these patients' sera.[676–678] Similarly, elevated levels of colony-stimulating activities for granulocyte-macrophage colonies have usually[593,679–681] if not always been observed.[682] Megakaryocyte-stimulating activities are also increased in aplastic sera patients.[683–687] Undefined serum activities that release growth factors or enhance colony formation are also high[685,688,689] and may correlate with response to treatment.[689] Determination of stimulatory activities in sera is muddied by the concomitant presence of serum inhibitors.[690] When directly measured by radioimmunoassay, granulocyte colony-stimulating activity was elevated in 9 of 11 patients with aplastic anemia and inversely related to the absolute neutrophil count (ANC).[691]

A case of congenital hypoplastic anemia was imputed to a microenvironmental defect because erythroid colony formation was normal, whereas erythropoiesis by marrow fragments was depressed.[692] Deficient burst-promoting activity by T lymphocytes in Diamond-Blackfan syndrome is also consistent with an accessory cell defect.[693,694] In contrast, virtually all patients with aplastic anemia have markedly depressed hematopoietic colony formation with appropriate hematopoietic growth factor production. Although stromal cell function may be damaged or affected by viral pathogens or chemical toxins, it probably occurs in combination with effects on marrow stem cells, and marrow failure as a result of a specific stromal defect in acquired aplastic anemia probably occurs rarely if at all.

Immune Suppression of Hematopoiesis

Clinical observations provide a powerful impetus to the development of an immune theory of aplastic anemia. Mathé[695] first suggested an immune mechanism when he observed improvement in autologous bone marrow function after failed, mismatched bone marrow transplantation. His patients had been conditioned with antilymphocyte sera. Other cases were reported after cyclophosphamide conditioning.[696–698] Systematically applied protocols using antilymphocyte globulins have a high rate of success, averaging about 50% hematopoietic recovery[699] and in some series over 75%.[700,701] About half of bone marrow transplantations between syngeneic twins fail unless the host receives cytotoxic conditioning treatment,[702] and marrow graft failure can occur even with adequate preparation.[703] The laboratory data marshalled in support of an immune pathophysiology on the whole are persuasive of a lymphocyte-mediated process, but this is a controversial area and conflicting findings have been reported by reputable centers.

Lymphocytes. In mixing and depletion experiments, T cells were first implicated by in vitro studies of an aplastic patient's bone marrow, who was studied at Memorial Sloan-Kettering Hospital in 1973.[704,705] Hematopoietic colony formation occurred only after physical separation of myeloid cells from lymphocytes; colony formation was improved by addition of antilymphocyte serum; and the patient's bone marrow cells inhibited normal bone marrow colony formation. Confirmatory case reports followed,[561,706–709] and in several larger series, inhibition was detected in most patients[710–713] or in a substantial minority.[714–716] In other studies, only a minority of cases showed cellular suppression of hematopoiesis,[717–719] and some efforts to identify inhibitory cells were completely unrewarding.[720] In some patients, suppressor cell activity disappeared with successful therapy,[721] but in others it was present after hematologic improvement.[712,722]

Major criticism of these studies came from workers in Seattle, who argued that prior transfusion of patients affected lymphocyte function measured in vitro. Small numbers of blood transfusions in dogs sensitized the recipients' lymphocytes, so that they failed to stimulate or actively decrease colonies in coculture experiments.[723] In humans, coculture inhibition was observed much more frequently in cells from patients who had been transfused and in coculture with histoincompatible marrow; only 3 of 16 untransfused patients inhibited HLA-compatible hematopoietic progenitors.[724,725] Use of T-cell depletion was proposed to distinguish the transfusion effect; marrow BFU-E–derived colony formation was increased by this maneuver in 8 of 32 patients.[726] Although other studies had used heavily transfused patients with diverse hematologic diseases as controls[704,711] or were based on the T-cell depletion assay,[712,714] the Seattle results tempered enthusiasm for the immune mediation hypothesis.

Analysis of Cell Surface Phenotype and Cytokines. A new approach to the problem of immune cell suppression of hematopoiesis was initiated by Bacigalupo and colleagues.[727] They generated suppressor cells from normal bone marrow by in vitro lectin stimulation; in comparison, the bone marrow cells of aplastic patients were spontaneously inhibitory and their lymphocytes required only mild activation.[728] In addition, the inhibitory activity was found in the supernatants of cultured cells.[727] In studies performed at the NIH, this soluble inhibitor was identified as γ-IFN.[729] The interferons as a class were known to be potent inhibitors of hematopoietic colony formation in vitro,[729–733] in treated patients,[734] and in animals.[735] γ-IFN acts both directly on progenitors[736] and through accessory immune system cells.[731] It also induces HLA-DR expression[737] (therefore target cell recognition) and production of other inhibitors, such as tumor necrosis factor[738,739] and lymphotoxin,[740] and it increases the susceptibility of target cells to cytotoxic lymphocytes and natural killer cells.[741] Coexpression of lymphokines is common,[742] and subsequently lectin stimulation was shown to also release lymphotoxin,[743] a molecule that acts synergistically with interferons to suppress hematopoiesis.[744–748]

Lymphokine production in vitro was associated with acquisition of activation markers on the stimulated lymphocytes, with the receptor for interleukin-2 (IL-2R) appearing early and HLA-DR appearing late.[729] In vitro inhibitory activity usually has been found in Fc γ-receptor–bearing cells[749] (CD8+)[750–752] or nonhelper cells,[753] and much less frequently localized to the subset of normal helper–inducer lymphocytes (CD4+).[754,755] The ability of normal activated lymphocytes to inhibit hematopoiesis can be demonstrated by other methods of activation, such as exposure to alloantigens in mixed lymphocyte culture[751,754] and in allogeneic spleen organ cultures,[756] or by triggering of the CD3 antigen receptor complex with antibody.[755] CD3 receptor activation leads to acquisition of the IL-2 receptor, dependence for proliferation on IL-2, and γ-IFN mediation, at least in part, of BFU-E inhibition.[757,758]

Potentially pathophysiologic immune system abnormalities were observed in aplastic anemia patients analogous to those seen with stimulated normal lymphocytes in vitro. The Italian group[604,759] had localized inhibitory activity to a specific subset of radiation-sensitive lymphocyte-bearing receptors for IgG (T_G+, also termed $T\gamma$+, the subpopulation containing cells that functionally suppress B-lymphocyte immunoglobulin production), which were present in seven of seven aplastic patients tested but not in patients with normal bone marrow. In measurements of specific lymphokines, γ-IFN was much overproduced by mononuclear cells from aplastic patients,[760] and production of IL-2[761] and tumor necrosis factor[762] was also excessive in vitro.[761] γ-IFN activity was present in sera, and antibodies to γ-IFN enhanced aplastic marrow progenitor growth.[760] Many patients showed inverted helper–inducer/suppressor–cytotoxic lymphocyte ratios in blood[763,764]; a distinctive population of circulating activated lymphocytes was detected by the presence of CD8, HLA-DR, and the receptor for IL-2 on the cell surface using two-color flow cytometry.[765] This population mediated suppression of hematopoiesis in vitro through lymphokine production. The expanded T-cell population in aplastic anemia was polyclonal by T-cell receptor rearrangement studies[766] (Kurtzman and Young, unpublished data). These studies extended earlier reports implicating T8+ cells as mediators of myelopoietic suppression in isolated cases of neutropenia to aplastic anemia in general.[106]

The functional importance of immunologic dysfunction has been suggested by the reduction in activated lymphocytes that followed successful immunosuppressive therapy with ATG[767] or cyclosporine.[762] In a parallel investigation, CD8+ T-cell, γ-IFN–mediated immune suppression in nine patients disappeared after ATG treatment, and the presence of this cell population was correlated with the probability of improvement with immunosuppression.[768] Lymphokine overproduction and lymphocyte activation are not related to prior blood transfusion.[760,762,765] Findings of lymphocyte activation and lymphokine overproduction have been broadly if not uniformly confirmed (Table 10-11). γ-IFN was easier to detect by bioassay than was the molecule itself by immunoassays, but tumor necrosis overproduction by aplastic cells,[769] the synergy among inhibitors, and the instability of γ-IFN may explain this discrepancy.[447] Elevated neopterin levels in blood have been proposed as a surrogate for γ-IFN.[447,769,770] Most patients with aplastic anemia also have elevated serum levels of the soluble form of CD8[771] and the IL-2 receptor (Maron, Young, and Nelson, unpublished data).

Natural Killer Cells. In their lymphocyte origin, the presence of CD8 antigen on the cell surface and the ability to produce γ-IFN, IL-2, and colony-stimulating activities,[772,773] natural killer cells share important properties with suppressor–cytotoxic lymphocytes, and more distinction has been made between natural killer cells and cytotoxic lymphocytes than may be justified. For example, some unstimulated cytotoxic lymphocytes appear as large granular lymphocytes, and natural killer cell activity can be generated from cloned murine cytotoxic T cells.[774]

Like suppressor–cytotoxic lymphocytes, natural killer cells can inhibit hematopoiesis in vitro. Human natural killer cells inhibit in vitro myelopoietic[775–778] and erythropoietic[777–779] colony formation. Analysis of individual human natural killer cell clones has suggested that some cells may preferentially affect CFU-E or CFU-GM.[778] Murine natural killer cells have been reported to particularly inhibit either differentiating marrow cells[780] or more primitive spleen colony-forming cells.[781,782] Usually, inhibition requires intimate cell contact between effector and target and increases with time; soluble inhibitors, including γ-IFN, can be effectors[776,778] as well as increasing natural killer activity[780] and possibly HLA-DR expression on target cells. In some cases, natural killer cell activity may behave as if it were HLA-DR restricted,[777] a property of suppressor lymphocytes. Natural killer cell activity may be dominant in hematopoietic suppression by IL-2–stimulated lymphocytes (so-called *lymphokine-activated cells*).[783]

Natural killer cells are pathogenic in at least one bone marrow failure condition, Tγ-lymphoproliferative disease, which is large granular lymphocytosis in which neutropenia and other single cell cytopenias are common manifestations.[784–786] Tγ-lymphoproliferative disease is marked by a relatively benign monoclonal proliferation of natural killer cells, which may regress with a brief course of corticosteroids or even spontaneously.[787,788] Little evidence exists for a role for natural killer cells in aplastic anemia. Natural killer cell activity in the blood[789–791] and bone marrow[789,792] is uniformly low in aplastic patients, HNK-1+ cells are deficient in the peripheral blood,[789] and both activity and phenotypically identifiable cells return with hematopoietic recovery.[789]

Stimuli for T-Cell Activation. In some series, immunologic abnormalities have clustered in a subset of patients with virus-associated (usually hepatitis) aplastic anemia, as, for example, low helper–inducer/suppressor–cytotoxic lymphocyte ratios and elevated activated suppressor–cytotoxic cells.[439,440] Cell lines with the activated suppressor–cytotoxic cell phenotype have been isolated from the blood of a patient with non-A, non-B hepatitis–associated aplastic anemia[793] and from a patient with EBV-associated aplastic anemia (Baranski and Young, unpublished data); both cell lines made γ-IFN and suppressed hematopoiesis in vitro. The development of a CD8+ adult T-cell leukemia in a recovered aplastic anemia patient has also been reported.[766]

The CD8+ cells implicated in bone marrow failure are probably cytotoxic lymphocytes. Activation of cytotoxic lymphocytes is a feature of the immune response to some of the viruses implicated in aplastic anemia, such as flaviviruses[450,794] and herpesviruses.[489,795] Cytotoxic lymphocytes can recognize hematopoietic cells, since class I antigens are expressed on all hematopoietic cells and class II antigens are present on hematopoietic progenitors.[796,797] The lymphocyte response itself may be more destructive than the original viral infection; murine lymphocytic choriomeningitis virus is the paradigm of cytotoxic lymphocyte-mediated pathology.[798] The amount of virus may be low and still provoke a cytopathic immune response; cytotoxic lymphocytes may be targeted to cells by nonstructural viral

TABLE 10-11. Summary of Studies of Immune Pathophysiology in Aplastic Anemia

Phenomenon	Positive Studies	Negative Studies
Activated T cells	CD8+, DR+, IL-2R+ in 10/12[765]; IL-2R+ pre–BMT;[1474] T8+ mediate suppression[768]; DR+ in 4/21[440]	Normal mean[759,769,1475]
High γ-IFN production	Spontaneous and stimulated,[760,769,1476] stimulated only[768]	Normal 7/7[1477]
Serum γ-IFN	Bioassay,[760] RIA[447]	RIA[769,1476]
High IL-2 production	12/17,[761] 18/34[681]	
$CD4^+/CD8^+ < 1$	15/28,[763] 8/31,[764] 12/22,[1478] 10/21,[440] low mean,[1474] 11/18[1479]	3/18,[439] 3/18,[1480] 6/27,[1475] normal mean,[768] 2/19,[759] 2/7[1477]
Clinical correlation	Decreased IL-2R+ T cells with recovery;[767] CD4+/CD8+ with recovery;[1478] falling IL-2R+ cells with ATG;[956] CD8+ number, activation with BMT;[1474] γ-IFN production with ATG[768]	γ-IFN production with ATG,[1469] CD4+/CD8+ with ATG,[1479] CD4+/CD8+ with therapy[1475]

ATG, antithymocyte globulin; BMT, bone marrow transplantation; IFN, interferon; IL-2R, interleukin-2 receptor; RIA, radioimmunoassay.

proteins synthesized in latently infected cells or by viral peptides passively attached to the MHC antigens on the cell surface. Viruses differ in the pattern of host response that they provoke, with great variation in experimental infection in the relative importance of CD8+, CD4+, natural killer, and antibody responses.

Finally, the presence and magnitude of the host immune response is genetically regulated.[799] In humans, permissivity for persistent parvovirus infection appears as a restricted immunodeficiency syndrome, and susceptibility to EBV's malignant and destructive complications is an X-linked trait. Genetic differences among viruses or genetic differences among people offer ample explanation for the variability in the consequences of bone marrow infection.

The complexity of interactions among immune cells and hematopoietic targets should not be underestimated. T cells also have positive effects on hematopoiesis, mediated by the production of hematopoietic growth factors such as IL-3 and GM-CSF.[125,758,800,801] In culture, addition of an excess of hematopoietic growth factors can overcome and mask inhibition of colony formation by negative regulators such as interferon.[736] Opposing activities for cell proliferation are present in the culture supernatants of cloned murine cytotoxic lymphocytes, which produce IL-3, GM-CSF, and γ-IFN.[802] Hematopoietic growth factors can also influence cells of the immune system, leading to lymphocyte activation in vitro[803] and in vivo.[804] Inhibitory molecules can, in turn, stimulate production of colony-stimulating activities.[805,806] IL-2 has been reported to enhance T-cell release of colony stimulating[807] and burst-promoting[808] activities as well as to suppress hematopoiesis.[758] (The therapeutic use of IL-2 is associated with lymphocyte activation in vivo, release of γ-IFN and tumor necrosis factor, and hematopoietic suppression.[809,810]) Although immune system activation is most likely pathophysiologic in aplastic anemia, either secondary activation of cellular immunity by hematopoietins or concurrent stimulation of the immune system as a response to pancytopenia cannot be rigorously excluded.

Antibodies. Immunoglobulin inhibition of hematopoiesis is a less important mechanism in aplastic anemia than in the single cell cytopenias (PRCA, transient erythroblastopenia of childhood, and drug-induced agranuocytosis). A convincing demonstration of antibody-mediated disease includes isolation and identification of an immunoglobulin fraction, determination of complement dependence, and some clinical correlation with the presence of the inhibitor in the patient. Well-characterized antibody inhibitors have been described in patients with two types of disease, atypical bone marrow failure (rare) and drug-associated aplastic anemia (occasional). In the former category are single patients with unusual patterns of disease: episodic panleukopenia,[811] aplasia with normal in vitro colony formation,[812] pure WBC aplasia,[813] transient agranulocytosis and erythroblastopenia,[814] and, most often, aplastic anemia associated with systemic lupus erythematosus.[815–818] (Systemic lupus erythematosus is also associated with antibody-mediated RBC and WBC aplasia, immune-mediated neutropenia, thrombocytopenia, and autoimmune hemolytic anemia.) Some of these patients have recovered with plasmapheresis or immunosuppressive drug therapy.[811,815,816,818–820]

Antibody inhibitors have been defined by their ability to inhibit hematopoietic colony formation in vitro. Antibody activity is usually complement dependent,[815,817,818,821] but may be independent of complement.[813,815] In some cases, both humoral and cellular inhibition of in vitro hematopoiesis has been detected in the same patient.[812,816] Cellular inhibition has been localized to the B-cell fraction by some experimenters.[712]

Antibodies to progenitor cells have also been demonstrated in drug-associated bone marrow failure, but much more rarely in pancytopenia compared with those found in agranulocytosis and PRCA. In one patient with aplastic anemia after quinidine administration, acute phase serum plus drug (but not either alone or convalescent phase serum plus drug) inhibited normal bone marrow colony formation, analogous to the mechanism of quinidine-induced peripheral blood destruction.[822] In contrast, drug-dependent antibody inhibition of colony formation has been reported for agranulocytosis due to diphenylhydantoin,[823] quinidine,[824] amidopyrine,[825] chlorpropamide,[826] propylthiouracil,[827] and ibuprofen,[828] and for PRCA due to diphenylhydantoin.[829] In most cases, progenitor cells act as innocent bystanders that bind antibody–drug complexes.[830] For metamizole and diclofenac agranulocytosis, putative drug metabolites present in urine, rather than the parent compound, have been antigenic.[830] Detection of antibodies is greatly complicated by the specificity of the antibody response for an intermediate metabolite. Autoantibodies are also present in the sera of some patients with drug-associated agranulocytosis,[823,830] but whether they are pathogenic or whether they represent an immune response to a damaged cell membrane or lysed cell constituent is unknown.

In most cases of aplastic anemia, the clinical significance and specificity of serum inhibitors are uncertain. In an early study, inhibition of CFU-GM–derived colonies was a property of sera from seven of eight aplastic patients[819]; serum inhibitor activity has been reported in a substantial minority of cases in subsequent series.[595,820,821,831] Serum inhibitory activity in most cases is associated with transfusions, often directed against HLA antigens, and frequently not directed at the patient's own cells.[820,821] Serum inhibitors may be present in multiparous women, in multiply transfused patients with other hematologic diseases, and occasionally in normal persons.[595,832,833]

History and Physical Examination

Most patients with aplastic anemia seek medical attention for symptoms, which may occur as a result of depression of any or all of the hematopoietic cell lines. Bleeding is the most alarming manifestation of pancytopenia and most frequently brings the patient to a doctor. Thrombocytopenia is usually not associated with massive bleeding. Instead, the patient reports easy bruising (ecchymoses) and red spots (petechiae) usually over dependent surfaces, bleeding gums with tooth brushing, and nosebleeds (epistaxis). Heavy menstrual flow or menorrhagia is common in menstruating women. In classic cases of PNH, dark red urine is reported, but visible bleeding from the genitourinary and gastrointestinal tracts is rare on presentation in patients with aplastic anemia. Massive hemorrhage from any organ does occur in aplastic anemia, but late in the course of the disease and almost always in association with infections (especially invasive fungi), drug therapy (ulcerogenic corticosteroids), or traumatic therapeutic procedures (intravenous line placements).

The physiologic adaptation to a gradual reduction in hemoglobin concentration is usually good. The patient with the insidious onset of anemia may report fatigue, lassitude, shortness of breath, or ringing in the ears, but some persons can tolerate astonishingly low hemoglobins without effect. Angina precipitated by anemia may be a presenting symptom in the older patient. Even abrupt cessation of erythropoiesis leads only to a slow decline in hemoglobin (about 1 g/dL/wk), but the presence, absence, or severity of anemia is not useful in judging the onset of disease since blood counts do not necessarily fall (or rise) concurrently.

Infection is not common in patients presenting with aplastic anemia. The sore throat and fever of agranulocytosis are not observed frequently, presumably because other symptoms have appeared earlier in the patient with pancytopenia.

Except for specific complaints referable to the blood counts, most patients have no systemic symptoms; their sense of well-being is belied by the blood counts. Weight loss, persistent fever, and loss of appetite point to another diagnosis. Pain is unusual.[834] A careful, persistent, and reiterative history often reveals exposure to implicated drugs or chemicals or a preceding viral infection, but for purposes of management, a history of blood diseases in other family members is most important.

Laboratory Features

Peripheral Blood

In typical cases of aplastic anemia, all the blood cell counts are uniformly decreased. This simple finding indicates that cessation of bone marrow function is probably neither abrupt nor uniform among the hematopoietic cell lineages. (The presence of even small amounts of circulating blood elements also implies some degree of bone marrow function.) From the half-life in the circulation of granulocytes (about 6 to 12 hours), platelets (5 days), and erythrocytes (60 days), most patients would be expected to show neutropenia and thrombocytopenia, but anemia is common and the granulocyte count often decreases during the first weeks of observation. The blood smear usually shows an obvious paucity of platelets and leukocytes but normal RBC morphology; toxic granulations may be present in the neutrophils. Automated cell counting frequently shows erythrocyte macrocytosis and a normal RBC distribution width, indicating little variation in RBC size.[835,836]

Platelet size is normal and not increased, as it is in immune peripheral destruction, but the low platelet count may cause greater heterogeneity of size.[835] The absolute reticulocyte count is inaccurate in the lower range but is greatly diminished. Prior transfusions obviously alter platelet, reticulocyte, and hemoglobin values. Most patients show a decrease in monocyte and lymphocyte counts as well as neutrophil numbers.[837]

There is no characteristic pattern for other routine hematologic and clinical chemistry tests. Increased fetal hemoglobin concentrations[838] and i antigen (fetal) expression on erythrocytes,[839] decreased erythrocyte membrane sialic acid content,[840] and macrocytosis all may be evidence of stress erythrocytosis. The Ham test or sucrose hemolysis test may be positive. (A negative Ham test may not be valid if the patients' RBCs have been replaced by transfusion.) Folate, vitamin B_{12}, and erythropoietin levels are usually increased. Serum transaminases may be mildly elevated in patients with hepatitis-associated aplastic anemia.

Bone Marrow

The marrow must be assessed quantitatively and qualitatively for cellularity and morphology of residual cells. The invention of the Jamshidi bone marrow needle has allowed withdrawal of an undistorted biopsy with little more effort than with aspiration[841]; both samples should always be obtained. The bone marrow biopsy should be at least 1 cm long. Although the cellularity of aspirate smear and biopsy is correlated,[842,843] dilution by sinusoidal blood often occurs, and the aspirate can be especially misleadingly hypocellular when the biopsy is hypercellular[844] or shows local areas of active hematopoiesis.[843] No compromise should be made over inadequate specimens and no hesitation should be made in requesting and performing second biopsies or sternal aspirations. Biopsy point counting (determination of numbers of cells in small grids) is the most accurate method of determining cellularity, but visual estimation is more frequently used.[842] The lower limit of normal marrow cellularity is about 30%. In most aplastic patients, cellularity approaches 0%; in some, significant residual cellularity is present because of lymphocytosis; "hot pockets" of hematopoiesis may be present in a minority of patients.[845] The marrow tends to contract centripetally with age and pathology, so in adults the sternal bone marrow is often more cellular than iliac crest sites.[846]

The appearance of individual cells is best appreciated on Wright-Giemsa stain of the aspirate smear. In acellular specimens, the only cells visible usually are lymphocytes, plasma cells, and stromal elements, and fibroblastoid and histiocytic cells. Dyserythropoiesis is common, usually the "megaloblastoid" features of macrocytosis and some nuclear–cytoplasmic maturation asynchrony, but sometimes more complex degenerative changes in nuclei and cytoplasm can be observed by light[847] and electron microscopy.[848] These features are common to aplastic anemia and myelodysplasia, which may be difficult to distinguish prospectively.[10] An increase in myeloblast count is not seen in patients with aplastic anemia and, if not evidence of aleukemic leukemia, may herald the evolution of leukemia from pancytopenia.[849]

Clinical Measures of Bone Marrow Function

Bone marrow activity can be assessed in patients by radiographic methods. In ferrokinetic studies of aplastic anemia, plasma iron concentrations are increased, transferrin is saturated, and the clearance of radioactively labeled iron is prolonged[850]; binding of labeled ^{59}Fe to transferrin before injection more specifically distinguishes iron uptake by erythroid cells.[850,851] Indium-111 (^{111}In), which also binds to transferrin, has been used for bone marrow scintigraphy; aplastic anemia patients almost always show markedly decreased ^{111}In uptake.[852–855] Generally, good correlation has existed with marrow imaging, ferrokinetic measurements, and bone marrow morphologic estimates of erythroid activity. The technique has been limited by the poor ability to quantitate differences at the low end of the scale and the unavailability of the indium isotope. ^{111}In scanning also measures only erythropoiesis, and the correlation with blood counts has been imperfect.[855]

Despite suggestions that increased uptake,[852,856] such as morphologically identified "hot pockets," might be associated with an improved prognosis, scanning has not been widely applied. Bone marrow fat and marrow cells differ in their density, and measurement of these different signal intensities by spin-echo magnetic resonance imaging has been used to observe aplastic and recovering bone marrow.[857,858] Positron emission tomography, which measures tissue metabolism using radioactively labeled oxygen, might also be adapted to measure the reduced cellular activity of hypoplastic bone marrow.

Treatment

Severe aplastic anemia is a medical emergency. Severity is determined by the peripheral blood counts, the most common criteria being greatly reduced counts in two of three lineages: ANC less than 500/μL, platelet count less than 20,000/μL, and corrected reticulocyte count less than 1%.[859] The patient with severe aplastic anemia is at immediate risk for catastrophe if neutropenia and thrombocytopenia are carelessly regarded. In addition, there are advantages to rapid institution of definitive therapy. For example, early arrangement of histocompatibility testing can speed the appropriate patient to bone marrow transplantation, and tissue typing becomes more difficult if the leukocyte count later falls. Patients not seriously considered transplant candidates may receive unnecessary blood products, even transfusions from family members, which increase the risk of marrow graft rejection. Because of the delay in the hematologic response to immunosuppressive therapy, its institution before the complications of pancytopenia develop is also worthwhile.

Bone Marrow Transplantation

Bone marrow was infused into an aplastic anemia patient as early as 1939,[865] and in the 1960s several identical twins were successfully treated by infusion of syngeneic bone marrow.[866] Sixty-six other allogeneic bone marrow transplants that were performed between 1959 and 1962 failed.[867] Application of bone marrow transplantation beyond twins required the definition of the human histocompatibility gene complex, the development of immunosuppressive regimens, and the supporting systems needed to maintain severely pancytopenic patients, especially with blood bank products and broad-spectrum antibiotics.[860] Early trials of histocompatible sibling marrow transplantations conclusively demonstrated their value compared with conventional supportive therapy; in a controlled trial of the International Aplastic Anemia Study Group, patients with severe disease who had early transplantation had actuarial survival rates of more than 60% compared with about 20% in patients who received androgens and blood transfusions only.[868] With current conditioning regimens, immunosuppressive therapies for graft-versus-host disease, and transplant unit support, long-term survival rates in most severe aplastic anemia patients of 60% to 70%[860,863,864,869] and more than 80% survival rate in the most favorable subgroups have been achieved[861] (Table 10-12; Fig. 10-15).

Bone marrow transplantation is curative therapy for most aplastic patients, but the general applicability of marrow transplantation to marrow failure has remained limited. The major problems are designing conditioning regimens that balance the risks of rejection and graft-versus-host disease, particularly in patients receiving transfusions; the continuing independent problem of complications in the older patient; and transplantation across major histocompatibility barriers.

Graft Rejection. Graft rejection is a greater problem for aplastic anemia patients than for patients with any other disease, and it remains the major predictor of posttransplantation survival.[870] The more intensive conditioning regimens used to eradicate malignant disease may also more fully ablate the host immune system. Graft rejection may be underestimated because failure to engraft, which may have a similar mechanism, usually leads to an early death from infection. That graft rejection might be intrinsic to the pathophysiology of aplastic anemia has been suggested by the unexpectedly high percentage of failure in unprepared syngeneic transplants,[702,871,872] even with adequate preconditioning.[703] Mixed hematologic chimerism occurs commonly after transplantation in aplastic anemia, and persistence of donor lymphocytes is highly associated with graft rejection (30% versus 5% in complete chimeras).[873] More rapid regeneration of bone marrow grafts has been observed in the presence of cyclosporine,[874] and second grafts have been successful when ATG has been added to the conditioning regimen.[875] Conversely, graft rejection can occur when cyclosporine is discontinued.[876]

Successful engraftment requires that sufficient numbers of hematopoietic stem cells be transplanted. An early study from the major transplant center at the University of Washington showed a correlation between the quantity of infused donor cells and graft acceptance.[877] Hematopoietic stem cells circulate and can reconstitute hematopoietic function after ablation,[878] and the addition of peripheral blood buffy coat cell infusion increased graft acceptance, but at the cost of increased graft-versus-host disease, so that survival rate was not improved.[879] In more recent retrospective analyses, addition of buffy coat cells has correlated with improved graft acceptance in the Seattle series[870] but not among patients in the International Bone

TABLE 10-12. Mismatched or Unrelated Bone Marrow Transplant in Aplastic Anemia

			Graft-Versus-Host Disease		
Study	**No.**	**Alive**	**No.**	**Survivors (%)**	**Early Death or Graft Failure**
PARTIALLY MISMATCHED RELATED DONOR					
O'Reilly[1481]	7	2*	2	0	4
Seattle[1482]	24	8	9	69	10
UCLA[1483]	4	0	1		3
Minnesota[1484]	6	1	2	100	3
Royal Marsden[1485]	7	2	1	0	4
EGBMT[904]	35	8	—		—
Milwaukee[906]	11	4	0		3
MATCHED UNRELATED DONOR					
O'Reilly[1481]	3	0	—		3
Iowa[1486]	4	1	1	100	3
Royal Marsden[1485]	11	2*	3	0	5
EGBMT[904] †	11	4	—		—
Milwaukee[906]	4	3	1	33	0

EGBMT, European Group for Bone Marrow Transplantation.
* Autologous reconstitution.
† Some of the patients reported in Hows and coworkers[1485] are duplicated in the EGBMT results.[904]

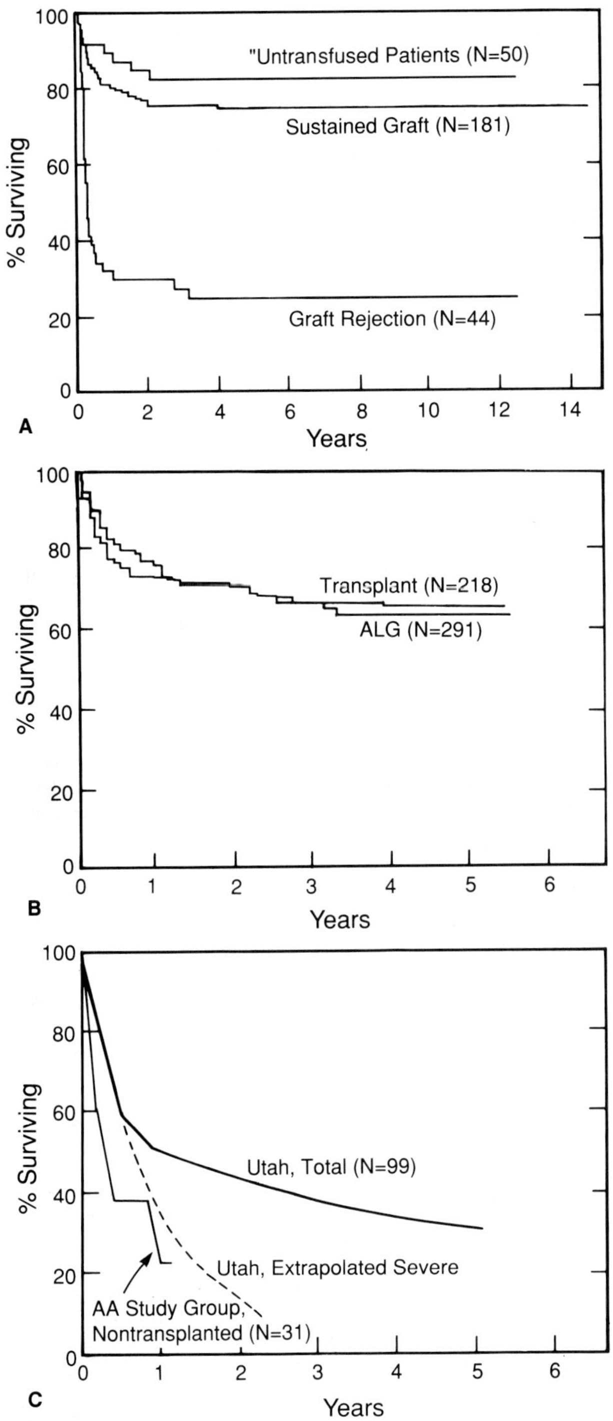

FIGURE 10-15. Survival rate (actuarial) in aplastic anemia patients. (**A**) Severe aplastic anemia patients treated with bone marrow transplantation, demonstrating the critical role of graft acceptance in determining outcome (data from the University of Washington[870]). (**B**) Bone marrow transplantation versus immunosuppression with antilymphocyte globulin (ALG) (data from the European Group for Bone Marrow Transplantation[862]). (**C**) Natural history of aplastic anemia. University of Utah data are for all patients, with the extrapolation based on retrospective analysis of the cases with the poorest outcome[1025]; the control group for the Aplastic Anemia Study was prospectively assigned to not receive a bone marrow transplantation.[868] In both cases, some patients were treated with androgens.

Marrow Transplant Registry[880]; in the European Bone Marrow Transplant Group studies, survival rate has correlated with marrow cell dose (41% for 0.9 to 1.9 $\times$ 10^8 cells/kg to 60% for more than 4 $\times$ 10^8 cells/kg.[881] Infusions of about 3 $\times$ 10^8 cells/kg can routinely be accomplished with aggressive harvesting.[880,881]

Transfusion sensitization as a mechanism of graft failure was predicted from dog experiments, in which animals given as few as three transfusions rejected marrow from litter mates and transfusion sensitization of donor lymphocytes was predictive of graft acceptance.[882,883] Graft rejection was observed in the first large trials of marrow transplantation in aplasia.[877,884] Actuarial survival rate of 82% achieved in untransfused patients approximated that of identical twin transplants, with an incidence of graft rejection of only 10%.[885] Better survival in patients without transfusions could also reflect the influence of other dependent variables, especially the absence of hemorrhage and infection in the patient who receives a transplant soon after diagnosis.[881] Despite the fact that about 80% of recipients receive transfusions before transplantation, the risk of graft rejection has progressively decreased since 1970.[870,886] This improvement in outcome has been credited in part to changes in blood product preparation, especially the routine use of leukocyte-free platelet and RBC transfusions and the strict avoidance of family members as donors.[870] The influence of transfusion on graft rejection is relative and not absolute. In the International Bone Marrow Transplant registry analysis, while untransfused patients had a low risk of rejection of about 5% and heavily transfused patients (more than 40 units) had a risk of over 25%, patients who received 1 to 40 units had an intermediate risk of about 15% for graft rejection[880]; in the Seattle retrospective analysis, increased graft rejection was observed in patients who had received more than 10 units of erythrocytes or 40 or more units of platelets.[870]

The influence of intensification of the immunosuppressive conditioning regimens on graft rejection in patients without transfusions is more of a problem. Graft rejection on the one hand and GVHD on the other behave as counterbalancing adverse consequences in protocol design. Frequently, protocols that are successful in improving graft acceptance result in greater GVHD. A neat sample from a single institution is one early study in which addition of irradiation to cyclophosphamide decreased the rejection rate from 42% to 0% but increased chronic GVHD from 17% to 48%. Combination conditioning chemotherapy,[887,888] total body irradiation,[889] and total lymphoid irradiation[890,891] all have improved graft acceptance in single-center studies, but they have not been shown to influence long-term survival in large retrospective analyses.[863,880,881]

Graft-Versus-Host Disease. Donor mature T cells that recognize minor histocompatibility antigens mediate GVHD. Age is a major risk factor for GVHD, possibly because defective thymic function and lymphocyte maturation in older persons leads to inappropriate immune responses such as increased nonspecific suppressor activity and a deficiency of specific suppressor T cells. Corticosteroid therapy previous to transplantation also increases the risk of GVHD[892] (as it increases the risk of graft rejection[880]). Untreated chronic GVHD has a high mortality but has been successfully treated with immunosuppression.[893] However, some posttransplantation therapy that reduces GVHD has a deleterious effect on the incidence of fungal infections and interstitial pneumonitis.[894]

Although centers agree that age is correlated with GVHD and generally with a lower survival, there is less agreement as to an upper age limit for transplantation. The incidence of GVHD in the Seattle series showed a progressive increase with age (19% for patients 0 to 10 years old, 46% at 11 to

30 years, and 90% in patients over 31 years old).[895] Several studies have suggested that the major difference in survival figures occurs at about 20 years of age. In the European Bone Marrow Transplant Group, a significant difference was observed in survival for those less than 20 years old (65%) compared with patients over 20 years old (56%), and there was no difference in survival for patients between 21 and 30 and those 31 to 55 years old.[881] Young adults have fared better in other series. At UCLA, the actuarial survival rate was 79% in patients under 20 years old, 41% for those 21 to 35 years old, and 20% for those over 35 years old.[896] At Minnesota, survival of adults (median age, 27 years) was equivalent to children (median age, 10 years), although morbidity from severe GVHD was far more prevalent in the older patients (43% versus 10%).[897]

While efforts to reduce GVHD, like complete T-cell depletion, have had disastrous effects on graft acceptance,[898] more limited or specific efforts to modulate the immune system at the time of transplantation may be more effective. Mixed hematologic chimeras have a significantly lower incidence of acute GVHD,[873] a major risk factor for development of chronic GVHD. Dramatic prevention of GVHD in transplantation for malignancy occurred using partial T-cell depletion that left 5% of the donor cells in the infusion.[899] In a swine model, mixing of T-cell–depleted syngeneic bone marrow with allogeneic marrow prevents GVHD, an effect thought to be secondary to generation of suppressor lymphocytes from the syngeneic component.[900] Specific manipulations of the marrow inoculum by removal of lymphocyte subsets is a promising approach to this problem.[901]

Nonsibling and Nonhistocompatible Donors. About 70% of patients with aplastic anemia do not have histocompatible sibling donors (see Table 10-12). Recent clinical experience suggests the feasibility of alternative donors, especially in young patients, with intense conditioning regimens (to prevent graft rejection) and aggressive prophylaxis with cyclosporine (for GVHD). Alternative potential donors include phenotypically matched relatives, partially matched (mismatched) relatives, and histocompatible but unrelated volunteers. Haplotype sharing between parents occasionally has allowed successful transplantation between phenotypically matched (but genotypically mismatched) siblings,[902,903] although long-term survival appears to be inferior to genotypically matched transplantations.[904] A successful mismatched marrow transplantation into an 18-month-old was first performed a decade ago,[905] but the general experience with these alternative donors until recently has been dismal, with about half the patients dying early, usually as a result of graft failure, and severe GVHD in the few survivors. In the European Bone Marrow Transplant Group, 46 patients received marrow from mismatched relatives or unrelated matched donors.[904] Actuarial survival was 45% for phenotypically identical matches, 25% for patients with a single locus mismatch, 11% for two or three loci mismatch. More intense conditioning to prevent rejection and added cyclosporine for GVHD were associated with the most favorable outcomes. At the Royal Marsden Hospital, 1 of 5 antigenically mismatched family transplantations, that in a 33-year-old woman, was successful,[903] and 2 of 10 transplantations between unrelated donors resulted in engraftment without severe GVHD. The best results have been obtained in young children, who received intensive conditioning with various combinations of cyclophosphamide, irradiation, cytosine arabinoside, corticosteroids, and T-cell depletion: 10 of 13 transplantations resulted in engraftment (including all patients who received closely matched bone marrow from either relatives or unrelated donors), 7 of 10 survived, and severe GVHD occurred in only 1 case.[906]

Transplantation between closely matched HLA types is feasible using either family or unrelated donors; if long-term survival validates preliminary results, an alternative donor transplantation could be considered early in the course of children with severe disease. Perhaps in anticipation that the major problems related to alternative transplantation may be solved, a national donor registry of more than 20,000 volunteers has been established.[907] A file of this size has been calculated to provide four antigen matches for 75% and six antigen matches for 25% of patients; a donor pool of 100,000 to 200,000 would be required to match 80% to 90% of all patients.[908] A much smaller donor number would serve patients with common haplotypes, but an even larger donor population is required for unusual haplotypes and for nonwhite patients.[909]

Fetal liver infusion has apparently been effective in some patients[910,911] but, for practical and political reasons, has not been widely practiced.

Antilymphocyte Sera

Clinical Trials. Antithymoctye globulin (ATG) and antithoracic duct lymphocyte globulin (ALG) are the most important definitive therapies for aplastic anemia patients who do not receive bone marrow transplantations[698] (Fig. 10-16; Table 10-13). In a study of ALG as a conditioning regimen for bone marrow transplantation, Mathé[694] noted clinical improvement in two aplastic anemia patients, at least one of whom was genotypically mismatched with the donor; other cases followed of autologous marrow reconstitution after infusion of incompatible bone marrow and

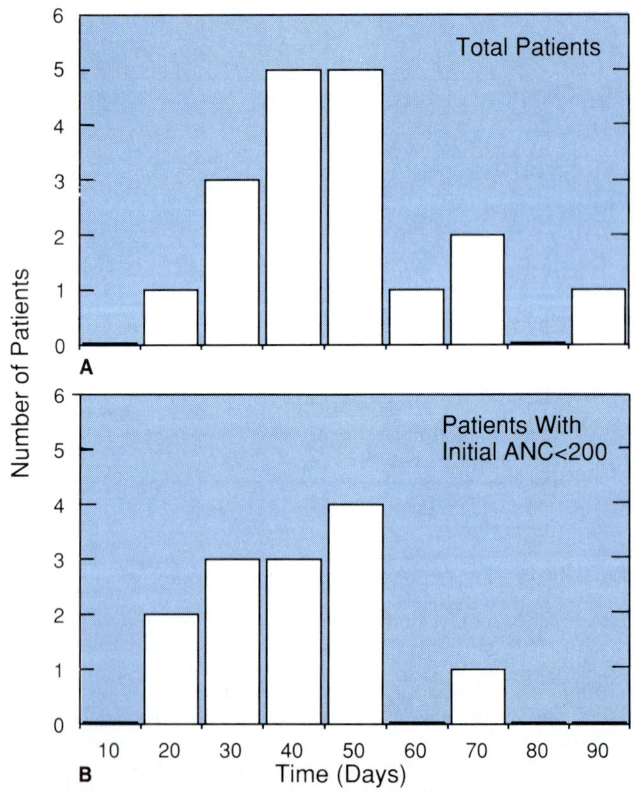

FIGURE 10-16. Time to response after treatment with antithymocyte globulin (ATG). (**A**) Distribution of patients with severe aplastic anemia by time to achieve an increase in the ANC (absolute neutrophil count) of 1000/μL. (**B**) Distribution of those patients with an initial ANC of less than 200/μL by time to achieve an ANC of 1000/μL. (After Young N, Griffith P, Brittain E, Elfenbein G, et al. A multicenter trial of anti-thymocyte globulin in aplastic anemia and related diseases. Blood 1988;72:1861)

TABLE 10-13. Large Trials of ATG/ALG in Aplastic Anemia Patients*

Center	Other Treatment	No.	Severe	Hematologic Improvement	Survival
EGBMT[930]	BMT ± androgens	125	100%	41/125 (33%)	50% (1 y)
Leiden[931]	±BMT	20	100%	7/20 (35%)	55% (5 y)
Cleveland[967]	CS only	11	100%	6/11 (54%)	50% (3 y)
UCLA[920]	CS only	33	67%	17/32 (53%)	62% (2 y)
Aplastic Anemia Study Group[919]	BMT, androgens	29	100%	20/29 (69%)	76% (2 y)
Minnesota[1487]	CS only	19	100%	10/16 (63%)	71% (1 y)
Base[700]	Androgens ± BMT	72	100%	44/72 (61%)	75% (>1.5 y)
Austria[924]	High-dose CS	15	100%	11/14 (79%)	12/15 (1 y)
Seattle[938]	CS, androgens	46	34%	19/46 (41%)	65% (3 y)
NHLBI Multicenter Trial[921]	CS only	77	100%	36/75 (48%)	58% (1 y)
Postgraduate Medical School[926]	CS only	64	47%	25/64† (40%)	53% (6 y)
Vanderbilt[934]	±Androgens	22	78%	10/22† (44%)	62% (2 y)
Mexico[1488]	Prednisone only	22	100%	10/22 (42%)	51% (1.5 y)

EGBMT, European Group for Bone Marrow Transplantation; ALG, antilymphocyte globulin; ATG, antithymocyte globulin; BMT, bone marrow transplantation; CS, corticosteroids.

* Only studies enrolling more than 10 patients are shown; earlier reports from the same institution are excluded if overlap of patients appeared likely. When early deaths (usually within 1 month of initiation of therapy) are specified, the denominator for hematologic response has been adjusted. Criteria for hematologic response are variable but are usually equivalent to transfusion independence. Moderate doses of corticosteriods were almost invariably administered; their use is noted only when they were the sole concomitant therapy. For individual center and other reports see references 80, 923, 1004, 1489 and text.

† Includes some patients who received two courses of ALG.

preconditioning with ALG[912] or cyclophosphamide,[695,696,913] or with ALG alone[914] or cyclophosphamide alone.[697,915,916] In a collection of European patients treated with different antilymphocyte sera in a variety of dose regimens, sustained hematologic improvement occurred in 12 of 29 patients with severe aplastic anemia (41%) and the 1-year survival rate of the entire group was 55%.[917] Skepticism greeted Mathé's original report and the early European studies,[918] but the effectiveness of antilymphocyte sera has been repeatedly confirmed. Two important controlled trials were performed in the United States. In a combined center study, Swiss ALG was clearly superior to androgen treatment in a concurrent population and in historical controls; nearly 70% (20 of 29) ALG-treated patients responded, compared with 18% (7 of 38) androgen-treated patients, and the 1-year survival rate was 76% versus 22% for the combined control groups.[919] At UCLA, patients were randomly assigned to receive ATG or supportive care only; 11 of 12 treated patients (52%) responded hematologically, whereas there was no improvement over 3 months in an equal number of patients given supportive care (6 of 12 control patients later responded to ATG).[920] Patients with aplastic anemia of many suspected causes—including hepatitis-associated bone marrow failure[881,921] and gold-associated aplasia[318-320]—have responded to ATG.

Variability in patient populations, differences in the definition of hematologic response and the time at which a response is measured, and duplication of case material in the literature make an overall response rate difficult to approximate. The choice of specific criteria for improvement in aplastic anemia can include transfusion independence (which may be subjective and does not measure neutrophil improvement), blood counts (which are altered by transfusion and affected by error at the low rate range of reticulocyte and platelet determinations), and clinical assessments of improvement.[921] Although the average time to improvement in neutrophil number (the only objective measure unaffected by transfusion) is 1 to 2 months[921] and to transfusion independence is about 2 to 3 months,[922,923] continued improvement without further therapy commonly occurs after 3 months, and some patients may be true late responders (10%,[920] 19%,[922] and 35%[923] of responses occurred at 3 to 9 months). Some improvement in clinical status by 3 months is strongly correlated with long-term survival.[918,921] Although the true response rate probably lies between 40% and 60%, reported remission rates for ATG and ALG have varied greatly, from low values of about 24% in severe disease[922] to extraordinarily high success rates approximating 85%.[699,924] There is little statistical evidence for "inactive" lots of ATG or ALG or for variation in lymphocytotoxicity.[925] Patient selection is important, since the likelihood of response to ALG has been correlated to disease severity,[926] and, in particular, poor response rates have been measured in patients with "supersevere" disease, defined by an absolute neutrophil count of less than 200/μL.[881] If they can survive the first month of therapy, severely neutropenic patients respond to ATG with the same probability as patients with higher neutrophil counts.[921] Some centers or protocols may intentionally exclude patients who are too sick to tolerate treatment or who require an observation period that selects for the better prognosis cases.

Regimens that include androgens appear to work well in some institutions[699,924] but not in others.[18,926] Androgens are often administered concomitantly in Europe but seldom in the United States. In a randomized controlled trial in Los Angeles, no difference was noted in response rate between patients treated with ATG alone (12 of 27) and those treated with ATG and oxymetholone (11 of 26).[927] In contrast, a German study[928] that used longer follow-up and a different androgen, methenolone acetate, showed a significant difference in response rate (11 of 15 versus 4 of 15) and a large but not significant difference in survival at more than 2 years (87% versus 43%). In European cooperative trials, androgen addition was associated with improved survival, although the advantage in severely neutropenic patients was not statistically significant.[929,930] Mismatched bone marrow was originally combined with ALG for historical reasons, but marrow infusion plays no role in ALG's effect.[917,918,923,931]

The intensity of immunosuppression may be an important variable. In the NHLBI trial that compared 10 days versus 28 days of ATG, a trend toward more rapid, frequent, and complete remissions was seen with the 28-day regimen, although there was no statistical difference in response rates.[921] Horse serum administered beyond 10 days is given in the face of the host's immune response and rapid clearance of heterologous protein by the immune system; ATG's average half-time of 5.7 days is much shorter in the presence of anti–horse immunoglobulin.[932] It is more rational to administer equivalent doses of ATG or ALG by the schedule originally used in Europe, 40 mg/kg/d for 4 days; horse immunoglobulin, both free and cell-bound, will then have reached low levels in the circulation[933] by the time host IgG is circulating. A 4- to 5-day regimen is easier to administer, associated with less serum sickness, and is equally as effective as a more prolonged course. Whether higher doses acutely administered would be more effective is a moot point that is unlikely to be tested. Patients have responded to repeated courses of immunosuppression, either repeated ALG (22%[926], 25%[699], 45%[934] response rate among refractory patients to the second course) or high-dose corticosteroids and ALG (27% response to the second therapy),[935] and patients treated with sequential immunosuppression may have better prospects of survival.[936]

Corticosteroids are usually administered in moderate doses (1 mg/kg of prednisone or methylprednisolone) during the first 2 weeks to ameliorate serum sickness; they would not be expected to affect host antibody production[937] but may blunt the inflammatory response. The addition of high-dose methylprednisolone (see later discussion) to ALG has been associated with high response rates in some European trials (68%[699], 73%[924]) but not in other studies.[938] Survival in the European Group for Bone Marrow Transplantation was the same for low- and high-dose methylprednisolone,[881] nor has a retrospective analysis of published series shown any advantage for the high-dose regimen.[698] Very high doses of corticosteroids can be associated with serious toxicity. ALG has been successfully combined with cyclosporine to produce a high response rate in a German cooperative study (see later discussion).

ATG also has been effective in patients with pancytopenia and cellular bone marrow morphology,[921,939] PRCA[940–942] (transitory responses have been observed also in hereditary PRCA[943]), pure white cell aplasia,[944] and amegakaryocytic thrombocytopenia.[945,946] The platelet refractory state may be improved by ATG therapy.[947]

Toxicity. Antilymphocyte sera have three major toxicities: immediate allergic phenomena, serum sickness, and transient blood count depression.

Immediate Allergic Phenomena. Fever, rigors, and urticaria are common on the first day or two of therapy and respond to antihistamines and meperidine. Anaphylaxis is rare, but its occurrence has been fatal even in the prepared medical setting.[948] A positive immediate wheal and flare reaction to the epicutaneous application of the 50-mg/mL stock solution of ATG may be predictive of massive histamine release on systemic infusion, and desensitization with gradually increasing doses of ATG administered intradermally, subcutaneously, and then intravenously has permitted ATG use in allergic individuals.[948] Skin tests only occasionally convert to positive after ATG therapy, and patients have been treated with a second course of IgG of the same animal species.

Serum Sickness. The consequence of host production of antibody to horse protein, serum sickness occurs in almost all patients treated with ATG for 10 days or longer.[949,950] Serum sickness usually begins 5 to 11 days after the first dose of horse immunoglobulin, and although usually a brief illness, symptoms can persist for weeks. Serum sickness is a pleomorphic syndrome, with prominent symptoms of fever, lassitude, a cutaneous maculopapular eruption, arthralgia and myalgia, and, less commonly, gastrointestinal and neurologic complaints. A serpiginous rash at the volardorsal border of the hands and feet is pathognomonic and precedes the full syndrome by about a day (Fig. 10-17). Although the urine sediment and creatinine clearance may become transiently abnormal, frank azotemia is unusual. Severe serum sickness may include rhabdomyolysis and myocarditis. Corticosteroids are usually prescribed with ATG to prevent serum sickness, and their dose is increased to ameliorate its manifestations, but there is little evidence that they are effective in either role since the illness is self-limited. Serum sickness is much less frequent and less severe when horse immunoglobulin is administered over a shorter period of 4 or 5 days. Serum sickness correlates with the formation of circulating immune complexes and complement fixation; horse immunoglobulin can be demonstrated by immunofluorescence in affected skin, and immune complexes presumably are deposited in many organs.[949] Hematologic recovery does not require the occurrence of serum sickness.[951]

Contaminating Antibodies. Neither ATG nor ALG is an immunologically specific reagent. The immunogen for ATG is normal human thymocytes, collected at pediatric cardiac surgery, and for ALG it is thoracic duct lymphocytes, collected during therapeutic cannulation. The immunized animals respond with production of antibodies that recognize a variety of human cell surface antigens. Removal of antierythrocyte antibodies is a major limitation on commercial processing of horse sera, since the sera must be absorbed with erythrocyte stroma, derived from outdated human blood, and often residual human hemoglobin must be physically separated from the IgG fraction. Some batches of ALGs have been associated with positive antiglobulin tests in patients and, rarely, frank immune hemolytic anemia.[491,952] ATG reacts with lymphocytes of all classes and also with cell surface antigens present on granulocytes, platelets, thymocytes, and testicular cells, as well as with intracellular antigens of many human types.[953] Decreased granulocyte and platelet number are common during the immediate period of ATG use.

Mechanism of Action. Immunosuppression is almost certainly the major mechanism of action of antilymphocyte sera in aplastic anemia. ATG and ALG contain a heterogeneous mix of antibody specificities for lymphocytes, and direct binding and blocking studies have shown reactivity with antigens such as CD2, CD3, CD4, CD5, CD8, CD25 (the receptor for IL-2), and HLA-DR.[925,954,955] Horse sera fix human complement efficiently, and all preparations are equally cytotoxic in vitro, with little difference between ATG and ALG or among lots for lymphocyte killing in vitro.[925] Administration of ATG and ALG in patients results in rapid reduction in the number of circulating lymphocytes, usually to below 10% of staring values, and lymphocytopenia persists for several days after the last infusion. When lymphocyte numbers have returned to pretreatment values at 3 months, reductions in activated lymphocyte numbers in recovered patients persist.[766,956] Although ATG and monoclonal antibodies compete for the same antigenic binding sites in vitro, monoclonal antibodies directed to pan–T-cell specificities (as single agents[896] or in combination[957]) or a monoclonal antibody to the IL-2 receptor (anti-Tac; Waldmann and Young, unpublished data) have not been effective in aplastic anemia, probably because they are inadequately immunosuppressive. Naked antibody preparations have not found wide use in clinical practice, and even toxin-conjugated monoclonal antibodies that are

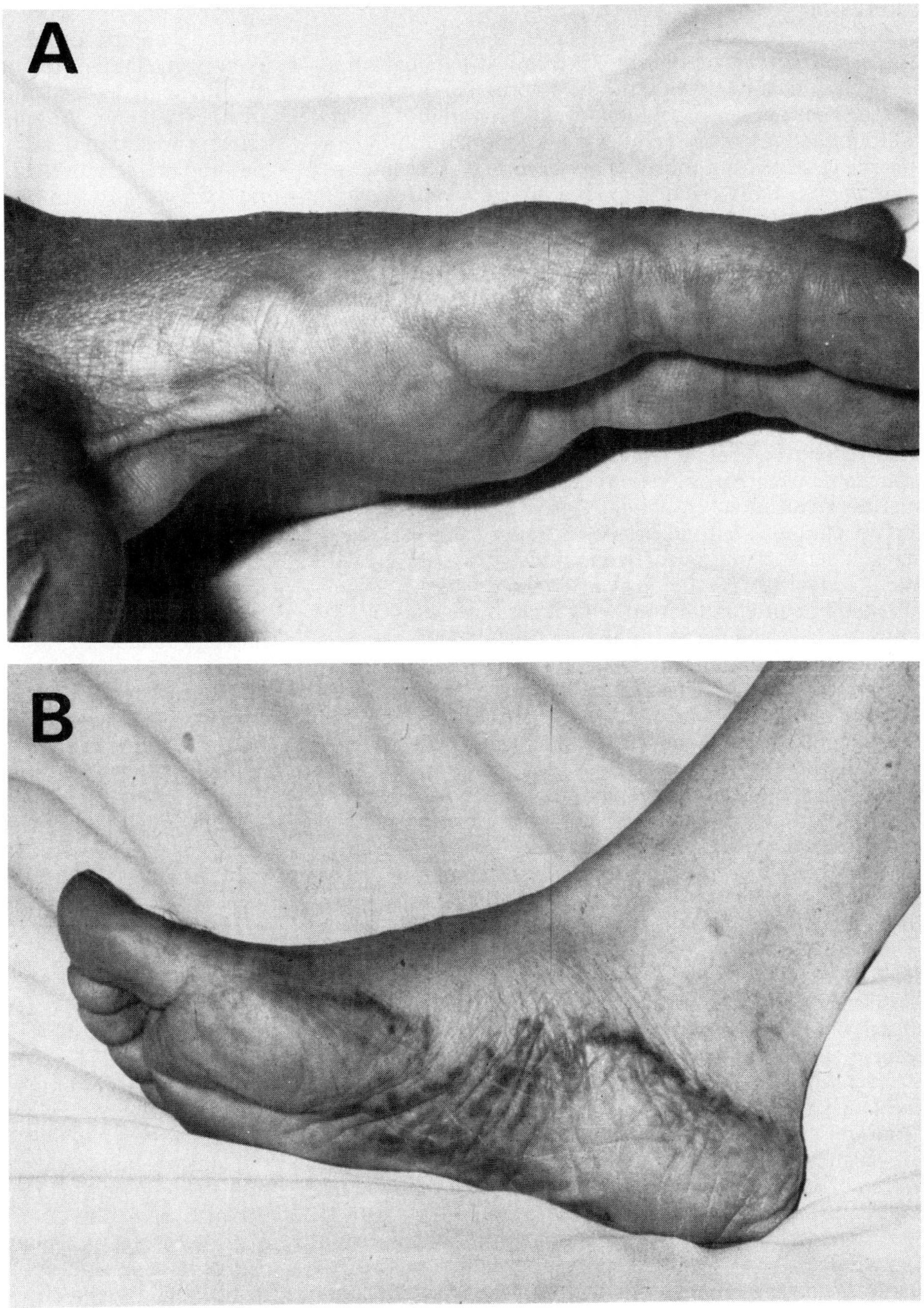

FIGURE 10-17. Serum sickness rash of the hand (**A**) and foot (**B**). If the patient has severe thrombocytopenia, petechiae may etch the serpiginous margin between volar and dorsal surfaces. (See Color Fig. 10-17.)

potent in vitro may be without visible effect when injected into an animal.

In the absence of complement to effect lysis in vitro, ATG and ALG can stimulate lymphocyte function, suggesting the possibility that stimulations of hematopoiesis might be important in the therapeutic effect. ATG acts as a mitogen to stimulate lymphocyte proliferation, and it provokes both IL-2 and hematopoietic growth factor production by peripheral blood mononuclear cells; these effects are exaggerated for the cells of patients with aplastic anemia, perhaps reflecting their already activated status.[760] T cells cloned after ALG stimulation produce GM-CSF or IL-3, and, less frequently, IL-2 and γ-interferon.[958] Variation in stimulatory activity measured in vitro has been correlated with clinical response rates by some[959] but not others.[760] In a mouse model, ATG increased circulating levels of colony-stimulating activity.[960] ATG also binds directly to bone marrow precursor[953] and progenitor[961] cells. In normal marrow progenitor assays, ATG can stimulate erythroid colony formation[962] and growth of a peculiar, unusually mature type of myeloid colon, effects mediated at least partly through accessory T lymphocytes; direct action on myeloid precursor cells has been inferred by analogy from ATG induction of HL-60 leukemic cell differentiation.[962]

Manipulation of bone marrow cultures in vitro before therapy might be expected to predict a response to therapy. In occasional cases, lymphocyte inhibitory activity disappeared after successful ATG therapy.[963,964] Good correlations were reported between clinical response to immunosuppression and pretreatment improvement in hematopoietic colony formation after T-cell depletion,[713] incubation of marrow with ALG,[965] or in co-culture assays,[966] but these promising findings have not been confirmed in other studies.[918,931,967,968]

Cyclosporine

Cyclosporine (or cyclosporin A), a fungal cyclical undecapeptide, is an effective immunosuppressive drug.[969] Cyclosporine is not lymphocytotoxic, but it has highly specific inhibitory effects on T-lymphocyte function, inhibiting inducible gene transcription and preferentially affecting production of IL-2 and γ-interferon but not colony-stimulating factors.[970,971] Cytotoxic T-cell activation of IL-2 receptors in response to lectins and alloantigens is prevented by cyclosporine. Cyclosporine has been successfully used in a number of diseases in which autoimmune pathology has been suspected, such as noninfectious uveitis, type I diabetes, and rheumatoid arthritis.

Shahidi and others[972–977] had success with cyclosporine in individual patients with aplastic anemia, many of whom had failed with other therapies. These results were clouded by the frequent concomitant use of androgens. In a larger trial from South Africa,[978] there was no response to cyclosporine given alone (6 patients) or in combination with ALG (6 patients); in other trials,[979,980] only 2 of 9 refractory aplastic patients improved. In one study,[981] 22 patients who had failed with ATG therapy were treated with cyclosporine alone or in combination with moderate doses of corticosteroids; 8 patients responded, 6 to sustained transfusion independence and 1 who appeared to require continued cyclosporine maintenance. Of the patients able to complete 3 months of treatment, more than half responded. Most patients showed some blood count increase during the first 3 months, but maximal effects were not seen until 6 months of cyclosporine therapy or even after discontinuation of the drug in some cases. No patients with absolute neutrophil counts of under 200/μL responded. A major difference between the NIH protocol and previous regimens was the higher dose, 12 mg/kg/d for adults and 16 mg/kg/d, with adjustment after 1 month to maintain blood levels by immunoassay between 200 and 400 ng/mL. In this study, none of 5 patients treated for briefer periods before ATG therapy responded to cyclosporine, but a French cooperative study[982,983] randomly assigned severely aplastic patients to receive either ALG or cyclosporine as initial therapy, with apparently equivalent (but low) remission rates and survival. A striking increase in the response rate to immunosuppression has been observed in a cooperative German trial[700] in which patients treated initially with a combination of ALG and cyclosporine showed an 85% hematologic remission rate at 6 months compared with a rate of 50% in those treated with ALG alone, and cyclosporine appeared to increase the rapidity and extent of the responses. The combination of lymphocytotoxicity and lymphocyte blocking is rational but may expose some patients unnecessarily to the serious toxicity of cyclosporine.

In most case, remissions have continued even after discontinuation of cyclosporine therapy. Some patients clearly experienced relapse when cyclosporine administration was discontinued and responded to its reinstitution[979,984] or require maintenance cyclosporine treatment.[976,981] Optimal therapy requires periodic measurement of blood levels both to ensure adequately immunosuppressive levels and to avoid toxicity; trough serum levels of 100 to 250 ng/mL are desirable (when cyclosporine and its metabolites are assayed together nonselectively).[969] Variability in cyclosporine metabolism, especially in children, may require serum levels to be determined every 2 weeks for dose adjustments.[985] Cyclosporine toxicity is not minor. Hypertension, azotemia, hirsutism, and gingival hypertrophy are common, and increasing serum creatinine levels are an indication to lower the dose.[969] Chronic, irreversible nephrotoxicity can occur with long-term exposure. Cyclosporine, especially in combination with corticosteroids, converts patients with aplastic anemia to temporary immunodeficiency and new susceptibility to unusual infectious agents; tuberculous pericarditis has been reported,[986] and *Pneumocystis carinii* pneumonia, otherwise not seen in aplasia, can occur and be fatal. Unfortunately, and similar to the situation with ATG, clinical responses cannot be predicted by in vitro tests because cyclosporine does not increase progenitor growth in vitro.[987] The efficacy of cyclosporine, a far more specific agent than the antilymphocyte sera, is a strong argument for T-cell mediation of disease in some patients.

Corticosteroids

Corticosteroids were used in the 1950s and 1960s in the treatment of aplastic anemia. These uncontrolled observations are now difficult to evaluate for many reasons: lack of objective criteria for classification and response, frequent combination of corticosteroids and androgens, an acknowledged preference to treat the most affected patients, and the limited availability of transfusion support. Bias is introduced because of the high proportion of patients with moderate disease and the mixing of acquired and inherited cases. Sporadically observed apparent remissions[988,989] were not reproduced in more systematic surveys,[217,267,990] and the general impression among experienced hematologists was that corticosteroids were without utility in aplastic anemia[217,991–993] and might even be harmful.[606,994] Despite the devaluation of corticosteroids in acquired bone marrow failure, patients continue to undergo therapeutic trials as initial treatment, probably to their detriment.

More recently, large amounts of corticosteroids have been administered, as intravenous boluses of 6-methylprednisolone (20/mg/kg/d on days 1 to 3, 10 mg/kg/d on days 4 to 7, 5 mg/kg/d on days 8 to 11, 2 mg/kg/d on days 12 to 20, and 1 mg/kg/d until day 30, followed by maintenance at 0.1 to 0.2 mg/kg/d).[995] In a series of patients treated by the originators of this program, 15 of 39 patients (38%) responded.[491,935,995] At first treatment, there was no difference on retrospective analysis in survival between patients treated with ALG and those treated with bolus methylprednisolone.[930] There are several reasons, however, to prefer ATG or ALG as initial therapy. First, a high proportion of patients who failed with corticosteroid therapy subsequently remitted with ALG treatment.[491,935] Second, these industrial doses of corticosteroids have great toxicity, especially metabolic (hypertension, hyperglycemia, volume overload, potassium wasting), infectious (an apparent increase in susceptibility to fungal disease and masking of fever), and psychiatric (psychosis); late aseptic necrosis of femoral and humeral heads also has occurred. Unfortunately, achievement of a complete response has been correlated with recent diagnosis (under 4 weeks), limiting the usefulness of the regimen to salvage ATG failures (cyclosporine is preferable). High-dose corticosteroids have been substituted for ATG in countries where the cost of antilymphocyte sera is prohibitively high (Thailand[968] and Turkey[996]). As with antilymphocyte sera, in vitro progenitor assays have not predicted clinical responses.[997]

Immunosuppression Versus Bone Marrow Transplantation

Antilymphocyte sera and bone marrow transplantation are alternative effective therapies for aplastic anemia (see Fig. 10-15). In Basel, patients treated with ALG continue to have superior probability of survival (65% versus 46%) compared with those treated with bone marrow transplantation from a histocompatible sibling.[699,923] One-year survival figures are similar from the European Group for Bone Marrow Transplantation (69% for immunosuppression, 65% for bone marrow transplantation).[936] and long-term survival curves are superimposable (52% for either treatment).[881] In Seattle, a similar long-term survival figure (65%)[938] would be compared with a better outcome from transplantation (see earlier discussion). Survival is not the only criterion for judgment, however. Bone marrow transplantation is more expensive and riskier in the short term, but it is capable of restoring permanently normal hematopoiesis. Immunosuppression is cheaper, much less toxic, but more often results in partial remission[698] or in gradual recovery[998] than prompt reconstitution of entirely normal blood counts. Five to 10% of patients who respond to ATG experience relapse. Myelodysplasia, acute leukemia, and PNH may evolve from the "cured" aplastic bone marrow[9,999,1000]; in the large European series, 31 of 223 patients who survived for more than 2 years developed clonal disorders, including 12 with acute leukemia.[998] Bone marrow transplantation is also not without its late problems. A small number of patients may show late graft loss[895]; 10% in one series had graft failure when cyclosporine, administered for GVHD, was stopped.[903] Chronic thrombocytopenia occurred in 23% of patients who underwent transplants for diverse hematologic diseases.[1001] Acute leukemia has been reported to follow shortly on bone marrow transplantation for aplastic anemia.[1002] The conditioning drugs and radiation of the transplantation procedure produce their own delayed complications, including pulmonary disease, endocrine dysfunction and infertility, leukoencephalopathy, cataracts, and secondary malignancies.[895]

Two circumstances dictate immunosuppressive therapy: lack of money and lack of a histocompatible sibling donor. Even for children, transplantation across major HLA barriers must be considered experimental. In other circumstances, factors weigh less absolutely. Although children appear to respond to immunosuppression at the same rate as adults (12 of 13 collected cases responded with a 48% 1-year survival[1003]; 8 of 9 responded to ATG followed by cyclosporine),[977] the outcome with bone marrow transplantation is far better in younger patients.[1004,1005] In a direct comparison of patients under age 25 years, 2-year survival after transplantation was 72% and only 45% after ATG.[1004] How old is too old for a marrow transplantation? The high risk of GVHD in older patients makes transplantation less attractive even with a histocompatible donor, especially if the patient has undergone transfusion, whereas extreme neutropenia tips the balance toward bone marrow transplantation.[881] Even its enthusiasts do not recommend transplantation as first-line therapy in patients over 50 years old,[1006] and it works best in those "older" patients, beyond 20 to 25 years, who have had minimal transfusions with a fully compatible sibling donor. The difficulty, expense, and glamour of bone marrow transplantation have made it a holy grail for patients and practitioners, and its hazards should not be undertaken lightly, but it is equally unsatisfactory to deny a suitable patient the possibility of cure because of ignorance, carelessness, or logistical inertia. In any event, recommendations concerning the choice of definitive therapy must be considered conditional in light of the likely improvements to be made in intensifying immunosuppression on the one hand and preventing chronic GVHD in the older marrow recipient on the other.

Androgens[1007-1009]

Clinical Experience. Testosterone was first successfully used by Shahidi and Diamond, who reported hematologic remissions in 9 of 17 children with acquired aplastic anemia and 6 of 7 with hereditary aplasia.[1010] The Boston investigators noted the often prolonged duration of therapy required to response, the predictive value of residual marrow hematopoiesis, and occasional dependence of hematopoietic recovery on androgens.[1010,1011] At that time, androgens represented the only effective therapy directed at underlying bone marrow failure in aplastic anemia, and they were widely employed with good response rates in clinics in Mexico,[1012] Boston,[1013] Chile,[1014] Hong Kong,[1015] Korea,[45] Sweden,[1016,1017] Holland,[1018] and Japan[1019]). Some centers, however, reported low numbers of remissions and no improvement in survival[1020-1024]; one major retrospective analysis actually found poorer survival in androgen-treated patients.[1025]

The early androgen studies were uncontrolled, used different androgen preparations in different doses, lacked clearly defined endpoints, and described different measures of success, from hematologic normalization to improvement in survival. An important flaw was selection bias. Although the clinical data are often inadequate for an accurate retrospective analysis, many series were composed of a large proportion of patients with moderate or chronic disease who could tolerate and survive a 3-month or longer treatment regimen and who constituted a disproportionate fraction of the androgen responders. The response rate to androgens has in general been lower in severe than in moderate disease (8% versus 56% in one comparison[1026]), and, in a large cooperative study of multiple androgens, only 20% of surviving patients had severe disease compared with 58% in the initial group.[1027] In a randomized American trial that compared androgen therapy to bone marrow transplantation in patients with severe aplastic anemia,[859] there was no difference in survival between patients without transplants who were treated with androgens (administered as oxymetholone, 3 to 5 mg/kg/d orally, or nandrolone decanoate, 3 to 5 mg/kg/wk intramuscularly) and those who did not receive androgens. Three of 13 "untreated" patients (23%) appeared to go into remission, a figure no different from 11 of 50 patients (22%) treated with androgens who showed some degree of improvement.

Nevertheless, it would be unwise to discount androgen therapy in aplastic anemia, for several reasons. First, 30% to 50% response rates,[1027] even if restricted to moderate or chronic disease, may represent the difference between transfusions and independence from continuous medical care. Second, some cases that would be classified retrospectively as severe have apparently responded to androgens, such as most of Shahidi's original series.[1010] Third, androgen dependence of hematologic recovery in some patients is strong evidence of a role of these agents in improving hematopoiesis.[1027-1029] Fourth, androgen dose and type may be important variables. Some patients who had failed with conventional androgen therapy apparently responded to etiocholanolone, a 5β-metabolite androstane metabolite,[1030] and in European cooperative trials significant differences in remission quality and survival were measured among androgens (fluoxymesterone greater than norethandrolone) and between high- and low-dose regimens.[1031] In some hands, treatment with etiocholanolone metabolites has resulted in remission and survival rates comparable to those with immunosuppression.[1032] More Japanese patients may respond to androgens than to immunosuppressive therapy,[1033] but in a randomized multicenter trial, the response rate in patients with moderate or severe disease was higher with ATG (28%) than with high-dose nandrolone decanoate (0%).[921]

If they are used, androgens should be administered to patients who have failed immunosuppressive therapy. It should be anticipated that the hemoglobin response will be more impressive than improvement in granulocytes and, particularly, in platelets.[1010,1027] An adequate trial is at least 3 months and possibly as long as 6 months at full doses. Androgen therapy has multiple toxic effects, especially virilization, hirsutism and acne, fluid retention, and psychological alterations. Hepatotoxicity can occur with all preparations but is less frequent with parenteral preparations.[1034] The cholestatic pattern of liver function test abnormalities is usually reversible when androgens are discontinued, but the rare syndrome peliosis hepatis has been associated with androgen therapy.[1035] Children can tolerate high doses of androgens for more than a year without lasting effects on growth or maturation.[1036] Scintigraphy[856,1008] and in vitro progenitor cultures have been proposed as predictors of clinical improvement.[1037]

Androgen Effects on Experimental Hematopoiesis. Androgens have a wide variety of biologic effects,[1038,1039] including several actions on hematopoiesis.[1008,1009,1040,1041] High endogenous testosterone and the administration of testosterone correlate with higher hemoglobin levels and RBC mass as a result of androgenic stimulation of erythropoietin production by the kidney,[1042–1045] and experiments with plethoric mice have suggested that the major erythropoietic effect of testosterone is exerted through this hormone.[1046–1048] This is unlikely to be a major mechanism of action in aplastic patients who produce abundant amounts of erythropoietin. Androgens have direct effects on hematopoietic cells independent of their effect on erythropoietin secretion. Injection of mice with a variety of testosterone derivatives has increased granulocyte[1049,1059] and platelet[1051] numbers as well as hemoglobin[1042,1052] and accelerated recovery from irradiation[1053] and chemotherapy.[1054,1055] Androgens stimulate hematopoiesis in marrow suspension cultures,[1056] in recovery of progenitor cells from treated animals[1049,1055,1059] or suspension cultures,[1058] and when directly added to semisolid colony cultures.[1057,1059–1062] In general, steroids with an angular, 5β-configuration (oxymetholone, fluoxymesterone, etiocholanolone) are more active than planar 5α-steroids (testosterone) in stimulating colony formation.[1009,1057,1059,1060] Testosterone is incorporated into the nuclei of rat bone marrow cells[1063] and stimulates RNA metabolism,[1064] and an increase in the proportion of CFU-S in mitotic cycle has been observed with testosterone[1065] and its 5β-metabolites.[1066,1067] In a few experiments, androgens have also been implicated in increasing production of colony-stimulating factors by normal blood adherent cells[1050] and in treated mice.[1068] Androgens have diverse, generally suppressive effects on the immune system,[1008] hypothesized to be an explanation for the heightened immune response and prevalence of autoimmune disease in female mice.[1069] Androgens were without effect in experimental busulfan marrow failure[1070] but increased colony numbers in the immune cell–mediated model.[1071]

Hematopoietic Growth Factors

These factors have some promise in aplastic anemia, for even if patients with aplasia probably do not suffer a deficiency of hematopoietins, pharmacologic stimulation, especially of neutrophil production, might permit patients to survive long enough to respond to definitive therapy. Clinical experience remains limited to a few patients treated with granulocyte-macrophage colony stimulating factor (GM-CSF). GM-CSF has been given by continuous intravenous infusion for 2 weeks to two groups of patients (21 cases) with chronic refractory aplastic anemia; almost all patients showed increased granulocyte, monocyte, and eosinophil numbers; increased bone marrow cellularity; and higher proportions of recognizable myeloid cells in the marrow,[1072,1073] although without increased myeloid progenitor cells.[1073] Responses almost always have been restricted to the myeloid series, dependent on continuous administration of factor, and, at least in one series,[1072] proportionate to the initial granulocyte blood counts. In comparison to its effect in patients with myelodysplasia, GM-CSF blood count improvements are restricted in lineage, often modest, and can occur late, after 2 weeks of therapy.[1074] Most treated patients have had more than 500 neutrophils/μL; in some cases, the clinical significance of two- to three-fold increases may be marginal. We have treated six patients with severe aplastic anemia at diagnosis; of these, two responded with significant, factor-dependent granulocytosis, and both later responded satisfactorily to ATG (Young, unpublished data). GM-CSF has not been successful in the treatment of severely neutropenic and infected patients[1075] (Young, unpublished data). Current clinical trials will establish the ability of GM-CSF to protect patients from infection and to improve survival. Other factors, especially those acting early on hematopoietic cells like IL-1 (which may be deficient in severe aplasia) and IL-3 and growth factors given in combination may broaden the hematologic response in bone marrow failure.

Other Therapies

Antiviral Therapy. Occasional patients treated by ourselves and subsequently by others[472,473] improve after therapy with acyclovir, although the responses are temporary in most cases. Immunoglobulin therapy is curative in patients with persistent B19 parvovirus infection (see later discussion).

Plasmapheresis. To effectively remove immunoglobulins, plasmapheresis must be intensive and frequent (at least three times weekly); lymphocytopheresis that removes both soluble inhibitory factors and circulating lymphocytes should be most efficient in combination with cytotoxic chemotherapy to inhibit generation of new active cells. Lymphocytopheresis has only occasionally been successful in producing remissions in patients with aplastic anemia, although improvement was sustained in two cases in which it was combined with either prednisone or cyclophosphamide.[1076,1077]

Splenectomy. A splenectomy was first done for aplastic anemia in 1913. In a literature review to 1957, 35 had been performed with benefit in 20; in 12 patients with marrow hypoplasia operated on at Walter Reed Army Hospital, 6 improved.[1078] Favorable results in individual patients were reported subsequently,[217,988,991] and the operation has been employed most recently in 26 patients in Basel to facilitate supportive care.[699] Postoperative deaths can occur, usually from intraperitoneal hemorrhage or infection. Improvement is often slow and incomplete and therefore difficult to confidently accredit to the procedure. Some eminent hematologists have been skeptical of the usefulness of splenectomy in patients with severe depression of neutrophils and platelets.[217,921] Although a modest decrease in RBC survival is seen in aplastic anemia, there is little other rationale for splenectomy, and the organs removed have almost invariably been normal in size and histology. Thus, despite some promising data, splenectomy has not been popular and, with many noninvasive medical alternatives available, is infrequently used.

Lithium. Psychiatric patients treated with lithium may have neutrophilia and increased neutrophil mass and production,[1079,1080] an effect reproduced in rat[1081] and dog models.[1082] The in vitro myelopoietic effect of lithium has been credited to augmentation of colony-stimulating activity[1083,1084] and an indirect action independent of hematopoietins.[1085] Lithium can correct canine cyclic hematopoiesis,[1086] a disease curable also by growth factor administration. Long-term bone marrow cultures were depleted more rapidly in the presence of lithium.[1087] Modest and transient improvement in two cases[1088] and rapid complete remission in another[1089] are the published experience with lithium in aplastic anemia. Initial reports of lithium abbreviating postchemotherapy neutropenia[1090] have not been confirmed in controlled trials.[1091]

Unusual Anecdotal Responses. A patient with moderate aplastic anemia that had responded to androgens in the past apparently also improved hematologically with repeated low does of anti-Rh immunoglobulin.[1092] The plant lectin phytohemagglutinin has been administered intravenously to six patients with aplastic anemia (one appeared to have aleukemic chronic myelogenous leukemia, others had postirradiation or postchemotherapy aplasia) with improvement in the bone marrow appearance and variable and temporary increases in blood counts,[1093] perhaps as a result of stimulation of growth factor production by lymphocytes.

Management of Bleeding

Bleeding is a common and disturbing symptom in aplastic anemia, and death due to hemorrhage was frequent in the premodern era. Platelet transfusions can prevent and effectively treat bleeding during the period of definitive treatment with marrow transplantation or immunosuppression, and they can sustain a large minority of chronically thrombocytopenic patients for months or years; the effective use of platelet transfusions has been credited with a substantial improvement in survival in this disease.[1094] In autopsy studies of patients with leukemia, the introduction of routine platelet transfusions had dramatically lowered hemorrhage as a cause of death but had not altered the proportion of death in which hemorrhage complicated infection.[1095] The older literature on aplastic anemia also indicates that death from bleeding was relatively common. In contrast, in our own series of more than 150 patients with aplastic anemia treated at the Clinical Center, death due to bleeding alone occurred in only three cases, one of which was associated with intravenous line placement. However, bleeding continues to complicate the management of serious infection, especially invasive fungal processes.

Platelets can be collected from individual units of blood or by apheresis; the latter method is preferred because it reduces antigenic exposure of the recipient. As defined by the American Association of Blood Banks,[1096] one platelet unit (from a single unit of blood) contains a minimum of 5.5×10^{10} platelets; an apheresis pack must contain at least 3×10^{11}, but efficient harvesting technique can net up to 6×10^{11}. A single unit of platelets should increase the platelet count in the recipient by 5000 to 10,000/μL. In patients with bone marrow failure, 56% of the platelets calculated to have been transfused can be recovered, and transfused platelets have survival of 5.2 ± 1.1 days. The slightly lower values in patients with marrow failure compared to normal recipients (65% recovery with 9.6 ± 0.6 days survival) have been thought to be secondary to vascular consumption, an obligatory interaction of platelets with endothelium, that removes a higher proportion of cells from the circulation of thrombocytopenic than normal persons.[1098]

Few studies of platelet therapy in aplastic anemia patients are available to guide transfusion practice, and transfusion principles have usually been extrapolated from studies in acute leukemia, often childhood populations. Specific problems in aplastic anemia—the chronicity of disease, the absence of repeated intensive chemotherapy, and differences in immune system function—have not been addressed. Certain aspects of platelet transfusion therapy remain controversial, especially relating to prophylaxis and alloimmunization, and some common practices that are assumed to (and may well) be effective owe less to clinical trials than to the availability of large technologically advanced blood banks.

The bleeding time, the most realistic measure of a thrombocytopenic hemorrhagic diathesis, is linearly related to the platelet count below 100,000/μL. In patients with bone marrow failure, performance of a bleeding time is unnecessary and may be hazardous. The efficacy of platelet transfusions is related to the platelet count 1 hour after transfusion,[1009] and this is as effective and practical a method, and far simpler, as many other more cumbersome assays of platelet effectiveness.[1095,1100] Correction of thrombocytopenia by transfusion can end hemorrhage. Major bleeding episodes (melena, epistaxis, hematuria, hematemesis) in one study of leukemic patients[1101] were controlled 83% of the time with increments over 40,000/μL but only 33% of the time if the increments were below 20,000/μL. Rapid bleeding is usually not due to thrombocytopenia alone, and other reasons for massive hemorrhage should always be sought. Platelet recovery falls with fever and probably even more so with frank sepsis[1102] and disseminated intravascular coagulation; exacerbation of thrombocytopenia may be an early indication of gram-negative bacteremia.[1103,1104] Amphotericin therapy has been associated with a poor response to platelet transfusions.[1105] Although splenomegaly is not a feature of aplastic anemia, occasional patients recover bone marrow function, yet remain thrombocytopenic despite the presence of megakaryocytes in the bone marrow, and functionally demonstrate splenic sequestration. Conversely, bleeding may persist, despite good increments, if platelet function is inhibited by aspirin, other nonsteroidal antiinflammatory agents, and some penicillins.

Alloimmunization. By far the most common reason for a poor response to platelet therapy is alloimmunization.[1106] The circulatory life span of the transfused platelet is dramatically shortened by host antibodies, almost always directed to HLA A and B antigens present on the platelet surface and much less frequently to immunogenic public histocompatibility antigens (Bw4/Bw6) or platelet antigens. Alloimmunization is suggested by poor recovery at the 1-hour posttransfusion platelet count and is confirmed by finding specific HLA antibodies in the patient's serums by lymphotoxicity testing.[1095,1100,1106,1107] Although the reactivity of anti-HLA antibodies is quantitatively correlated with clinical refractoriness in retrospective analysis,[1105,1108] the ability to predict a platelet increment in an individual patient by cross-matching tests is only around 50%,[398,1109] probably because of the formation of non-HLA–reactive antibodies.[1110] Refractoriness to platelets can be overcome in many cases by selection of HLA-matched donors,[1108,1111] but 6% to 39% of perfect HLA-matched transfusions fail.[1106] The size of donor pools and rare haplotypes represents practical limitations. One or two antigen mismatches are often acceptable; some histocompatibility proteins appear to be more antigenic than others,[1112,1113] and trial and error of near-matches may uncover suitable donors.

In the era that preceded easy histocompatibility typing, some patients appeared to benefit from splenectomy[1114] and corticosteroids.[1115] More recent short-term therapies include plasma exchange[1116] and high-dose intravenous immunoglobulins. The latter therapy was given at a dose of 400 to 800 mg/kg/d for 5 days and led to good increments in 6 of 10 alloimmunized patients in one study[1117] but was without effect in another study.[1118] Platelets should not be administered prophylactically to alloimmunized patients, and there is only a weak experimental rationale for their use in the bleeding patient.[1119]

The use of single donor platelets rather than pooled platelets significantly reduces the rate of alloimmunization,[1120–1122] and collection of platelets by apheresis rather than centrifugation of whole blood is now routine practice at many centers. Leukocyte depletion also would be expected to decrease alloimmunization because the class II HLA antigens, which are necessary to initiate sensitization, are not present on platelets (presentation of class I antigens in the absence of class II antigens does not result in alloimmunization). Leukocyte depletion by centrifugation of platelet packs appeared to be useful in some studies[1123] but not in others.[1124] Filtration is more efficient in removing WBCs, wastes fewer platelets, and is cheaper; it has resulted in a lower rate of anti-HLA antibodies and less frequent clinical refractoriness.[1125] The threshold for sensitization appears to be about 10^7 leukocytes. Centrifugation does not achieve this level of depletion, whereas filtration commonly results in a product with 10^6 WBCs and only 10% platelet loss. A consensus is growing that newer filters that reduce leukocytes by 99.9% (three logs) can prevent alloimmunization.[1126,1127] Avoidance of platelet transfusions, except in the presence of active bleeding, is another alternative, but the dose–response between administered platelets and the probability of alloimmunization is controversial.[1106]

Early reports suggested that alloimmunization increased with time,[1128] but in other studies, about half of patients with leukemia did not become alloimmunized, regardless of the number of transfusions.[1129,1130] Aplastic patients, who do not receive repetitive courses of chemotherapy and whose immune system is often activated, would be expected to be less tolerant of repeated antigen infusions than patients with leukemia receiving chemotherapy. In serial analyses of bone marrow failure patients receiving platelet transfusions, high percentages became immunized (66%[1131] to 88%[1132]). In a retrospective analysis of aplastic anemia patients, clinical refractoriness was correlated with the number of previous platelet transfusions, but the percentage of refractory patients increased sharply only at more than 40 units and was not different in groups receiving 0 to 9 and 10 to 39 units.[1108]

Prophylaxis. Since thrombocytopenic bleeding is not massive and most bleeding episodes are not serious, the major indication for platelet prophylaxis is to reduce the risk of intracranial hemorrhage. In children with leukemia, prophylactic platelet transfusions, usually to maintain counts at more than 20,000/μL, clearly decreases the number of bleeding episodes,[1133–1135] but no evidence suggests that prophylaxis alters survival.[1095,1107,1135–1138] Because most patients with leukemia die as a result of progressive malignancy and not during induction chemotherapy, these studies are difficult to extrapolate to aplastic anemia, and a controlled trial to assess benefit would require a large number of subjects.[1095] Aplastic anemia patients probably continue to receive platelets to relieve relatively minor discomfort from hemorrhage rather than to prevent death or serious morbidity. Although no data support this, it is probably prudent to administer platelets before performing a lumbar puncture because of the consequences of local subarachnoid bleeding. Bone marrow can be obtained without prior platelet transfusions.

The level at which the risk of hemorrhage greatly increases has also been debated. Because bleeding and serious hemorrhage in a leukemia population increase with lower platelet counts and are infrequent at levels higher than 20,000/μL,[1139] this value has been adopted as a threshold to trigger intervention. Other studies in similar patient populations suggest increased risks associated with platelet counts of 10,000/μL[1133] to 25,000/μL.[1140] Reanalysis of the original data suggests that little difference exists in the risk of bleeding between 5000 and 100,000/μL and that only one of eight patients suffers intracranial hemorrhage at a platelet count of more than 5000/μL (and less than 10,000/μL).[1095,1102,1137] Quantitative determination of stool blood loss in thrombocytopenic patients also has shown a sharp breakpoint at a platelet count of 5000/μL.[1141] Certainly, many patients with chronic aplastic anemia and thrombocytopenia have little bleeding at platelet counts between 5000 and 20,000/μL. Any prophylaxis program must be modified to the individual patient, but a goal of maintaining platelet counts higher than 5000/μL is reasonable and usually can be achieved with transfusion of 1 to 2 pheresis packs per week.

Other Measures. Common sense measures to prevent bleeding include maintenance of dental hygiene to decrease gingival inflammation, avoidance of trauma, control of hypertension, and avoidance of vasoconstrictive drugs (from pseudoephedrine to cocaine). Intramuscular injections can be administered to patients with thrombocytopenia if followed by 15 minutes of firm pressure. Topical Gelfoam, collagen, or thrombin may be useful to treat local oozing. Anterior nasal packing should be avoided because of the risk of infection. Antifibrinolytic agents such as aminocaproic acid and tranexamic acid may decrease bleeding episodes and the need for platelet and RBC transfusions.[1142,1143] Amicar is inconvenient to administer because of the need for frequent dosing, variability in the optimal dosage, and gastrointestinal discomfort; we usually start with 5 g/d, given every 3 to 6 hours, and adjust upward to 30 g to control hemorrhagic symptoms. The administration of low doses of prednisone (10 to 15 mg/d) to ameliorate bleeding has a very weak experimental basis. Improvement in endothelial cell thinning in rabbits[1144] and humans[1145] was observed, but the doses used in these studies were high (1 mg/kg); a change in the electron micrographic appearance of vessels has not been correlated with less bleeding, and the animal studies have not been reproducible.[1146]

Management of Infections[1147–1150]

As with platelet transfusion therapy, most recommendations are based on studies of neutropenia from chemotherapy, studies that have themselves been criticized for inconsistent measures of outcome[1151] and statistical naiveté.[1152] Few specific studies of infections in patients with aplastic anemia are available.[837,1153] Duration is the major difference between the neutropenia of bone marrow failure and that induced by cytotoxic chemotherapy; severe granulocytopenia can persist for months and even years in patients with aplastic anemia. A second major dissimilarity is that neutropenia is part of a complex of problems in malignant disease. Immunosuppression is often an intrinsic feature of specific tumors or leukemias, and malignant tissue invasion, radical surgery, radiation therapy, and cytotoxic drug effects on mucosa and gut can directly compromise organ integrity. In aplastic anemia, in contrast, the immune system is activated and, with the exception of intravenous catheter placement, the integument is preserved. In patients with cancer, malignant progression remains a dominant cause of death; in our experience, most patients with aplastic anemia who do not respond to definitive therapy for their marrow failure die of infection. Studies of cancer patients have usually identified a "low-risk" category, determined by the relatively brief period of neutropenia; by this criteria, almost all unresponsive patients with aplastic anemia are "high risk."

Neutropenia increases susceptibility to bacterial infections. (In one study of a small number of aplastic anemia patients, monocytopenia was also correlated with infectious episodes.[1153]) In general, the number of infectious episodes correlates with the degree and duration of neutropenia. In an early classic study at the National Cancer Institute, 9% to 10% of days at granulocyte levels higher than 1500/μL were associated with proven infection, but this rose to 20%

at granulocyte counts of 500 to 1000/μL, to 36% at 100 to 500/μL, and to 53% at less than 100 neutrophils/μL.[1154] Levels of extreme neutropenia, less than 100 neutrophils/μL, were associated with the most serious infections and high mortality rate.[1155] Susceptibility is so extremely high if the ANC is less than 200/μL that this value has been used to define a category of "supersevere" disease.

As severe granulocytopenia becomes prolonged, infection is inevitable.[1156] Neutropenia itself greatly complicates the diagnosis of infection, since patients usually are unable to mount an inflammatory response. Minimal local inflammation around a catheter insertion site, mild tenderness and erythema rather than an obvious abscess in the perianal area, absence of a pulmonary infiltrate or sputum, and scanty WBCs in the urine all represent the most subtle indicators of infection, if there are any signs at all.[1157] Bacteremia is present in only 20% of febrile neutropenic episodes, and in only about 40% can a microbiologic cause or localizing physical findings be identified.[1158] The ability to document sepsis or to locate the site of infection decreases with subsequent febrile episodes.[1159] There is no reliable method of distinguishing fever due to infection from a noninfectious cause.

Infection in neutropenia is caused by a relatively small number of common bacterial species: the gram-negative bacilli, *Escherichia coli, Klebsiella pneumoniae,* and *Pseudomonas aeruginosa,* and the gram-positive cocci, *Staphylococcus aureus* and *Staphylococcus epidermidis,* and some *Streptococcus* sp.[1148] Twenty years ago, gram-negative bacteremia and pneumonia had a fearsome reputation,[1160] whereas infections due to gram-positive organisms, which were generally extremely sensitive to the penicillin derivatives then available, were considered less serious. In the intervening decades, entirely new antibiotics and their aggressive and early use have greatly reduced the mortality of gram-negative infections, whereas the general prevalence of antibiotics and the use of indwelling catheters have caused a striking increase in gram-positive bacteria compared with gram-negative bacteria cultured from neutropenic patients[1161–1164] (Possibly gram-negative bacteremia was especially prevalent during the 1970s.[1150])

In the individual patient, repeated treatment with antibiotics is associated with the emergence of resistant organisms, especially among the gram-negative bacteria,[1159] to cephalothins and some of the semisynthetic penicillins[1158] and to fungal disease, presumably because of the altered microbial microenvironment of the host. The organisms that cause serious infection are almost always endogenous, originating from the patient's own gut, skin, oropharynx, and upper respiratory tract; this bacterial microenvironment is radically altered by illness and hospitalization.[1165] The rate of decrease of neutrophils may also be an important variable, and patients with chronic neutropenia may eventually tolerate their low WBCs surprisingly well. Global immunosuppression, produced by conditioning for bone marrow transplantation in the treatment of graft-versus-host disease, and with ATG and cyclosporine, is associated with unusual bacterial and fungal pathogens and with serious viral and protozoan infections.[1166]

Fever in the Neutropenic Patient. Fever is the cardinal symptom of sepsis in the neutropenic patient; even after thorough assessment, fever commonly is the only evidence of infection.[1167] Afebrile patients who have vague symptoms of sepsis (malaise, a sense of impending doom, mental disorientation) should also be seriously evaluated, especially if they are receiving corticosteroids.[1168] A patient with sepsis from a Hickman catheter may be asymptomatic. Initial assessment should include a pertinent history and physical examination, with special attention to the oral mucosa and perianal areas and to indwelling catheter sites. Microbial cultures of blood (including specimens obtained through catheters), urine, and sputum need to be obtained. The results of these investigations may be helpful in prescribing antibiotic therapy, but the decision to treat is not dependent on the results of any diagnostic tests. *If the ANC is less than 500/μL and infection is suspected, immediately begin broad-spectrum, parenteral antibacterial therapy.* Adherence to this principle usually prevents fatal overwhelming sepsis and seeding of organisms to tissues. Adoption of empirical antibiotic therapy has reduced the mortality rate from 80% (mainly because of gram-negative bacteria) to 10% to 40% overall.[1147,1169]

The exact choice of antibiotics is often determined by the epidemiology of hospital flora and the preference of the infectious disease consulting service, but the use of an adequate regimen is the responsibility of the attending hematologist. A combination of a semisynthetic penicillin, cephalosporin, and aminoglycoside is standard; monotherapy with ceftazidime, a third-generation cephalosporin, may be equally effective.[1170] Either regimen may require modification based on results of cultures or the clinical course (Table 10-14), but generally broad-spectrum antibiotics buy time for the later addition of more specific agents such as vancomycin.[1158,1171] Specific organisms are isolated during only a minority of putative infectious episodes, but early discontinuation of antibiotics in persistently neutropenic patients is unwise.

In general, we continue antibiotics for a full 14-day course[1172]; briefer therapy of 4 to 7 days for afebrile, clinically stable patients whose cultures are negative has also been advocated, provided that antibiotics are promptly reinstituted on recrudescence.[1173] Even when an organism is successfully cultured, narrowing of the antibiotic spectrum in continuing neutropenia often results in recrudescence due to polymicrobial or secondary infection. Persistently neutropenic patients often remain on antibiotics for many weeks or months because of recurrent fever or sepsis.

Fungemia during an initial febrile episode is rare,[1158] but fungal infection becomes more likely with repeated courses of antibiotics. The frequency and rapidity of appearance of fungemia may be increasing because of the success of conventional antibiotic regimens and the prolongation of neutropenia from days to months.[1174,1175]

Candida and *Aspergillus* sp account for almost all fungal disease in aplastic anemia patients. Colonization of the oropharynx and upper respiratory tract with fungus is common in patients receiving antibiotics. Fungal infection should be suspected when a neutropenic patient develops sinusitis, and routine nasal cultures may be helpful in predicting aspergillosis. *Candida* tends to disseminate and may be associated with septic cutaneous emboli[1176] or a hepa-

TABLE 10-14. Common Modifications of Antibiotic Regimens in Neutropenic Fever

Clinical Event	Modification
Breakthrough bacteremia	Vancomycin for gram-positive
	New regimen for resistant gram-negative
Catheter infection	Vancomycin
Perianal or oropharyngeal localization	Anaerobic coverage (clindamycin, metronidazole)
Pneumonia	Trimethoprim–sulfamethoxazole and erythromycin
Persistent fever after 1 wk	Antifungal therapy with amphotericin B

tosplenic syndrome with abdominal pain and rise in alkaline phosphatase level[1177]; *Candida* esophagitis also occurs.[1178] Aspergillosis usually localizes to the lungs.[1175,1179]

Distinguishing colonization from tissue invasion in documenting fungal infection may require invasive techniques,[1180] and biopsies are often impossible in the severely thrombocytopenic patient. Antifungal therapy is often unavoidably empiric, and the data supporting the efficacy of treatments are often indirect. Early aggressive treatment of neutropenic patients who remain febrile for more than 7 days despite adequate antibacterial therapy can reverse fungal disease, as demonstrated in individual cases[1179] and comparison of autopsy series.[1181] Patients with documented fungal infection should receive a total dose of 2 g of amphotericin B; alternatives to amphotericin B have not conclusively proved its equal, although the addition of flucytosine was useful in an animal model of candidiasis.[1182]

Granulocyte Transfusions. Polymorphonuclear cells have a relatively brief life in the circulation, with their major activity being in infected tissue. No simple measures of therapeutic efficacy are known (ANC is not measurably increased by standard transfusions). Nonetheless, several controlled trials performed in the 1970s demonstrated significant improvement in survival in patients who received granulocyte transfusions, particularly when the neutropenia was prolonged for 10 days or more. The negative studies were criticized because of the relatively low numbers of granulocytes transfused (less than $10^{10}/m^2/d$),[1183–1187] since a dose effect is readily demonstrated in animal models with gram-negative infection.[1188] The development of more effective antibiotic regimens independently has greatly reduced mortality in patients with neutropenic infections, especially for gram-negative bacilli. Granulocyte transfusions are expensive and associated with serious toxicity: severe febrile reactions, pulmonary capillary leak syndrome when amphotericin is concurrently administered, increased risk of CMV, and inevitable alloimmunization. Not only does alloimmunization create a refractory state for platelet transfusions, but infused granulocytes fail to localize to sites of infection in the alloimmunized host.[1189] Unfortunately, when granulocyte transfusions are not routinely offered, they tend to be used in situations of last resort.

Prevention. About simple measures for prevention of infection, there is little dispute. Most important is hand washing, by the patient and by all medical personnel, since transmission of bacteria usually requires a human vector.[1147] The physical surroundings of a hospital ward should be well maintained to reduce nosocomial infection (two examples are the "miniepidemics" of legionellosis from water sources[1190] and of aspergillosis from local construction activity).[1191] Dental hygiene should be maintained and sources of infection removed with antibiotic and platelet prophylaxis.[1192] Nystatin oral rinses prevent thrush.[1193] In general, early attention to the signs of infection and good communication between patient and physician, especially after hospital discharge, can avert many of the catastrophic complications of initially minor infectious episodes.

Granulocytopenic mice do not become infected in a germ-free environment. Sterilization of the patient and his or her surroundings has been applied successfully in occasional immunosuppressed or neutropenic humans. Occasional patients have been maintained for years in protective bubbles that include not only barrier isolation but sterilization of the patient's internal milieu, food, and the objects with which he or she comes in contact. Total protective environments,[1194–1196] nonabsorbable antibiotics or selective gut decontamination to preserve some anaerobic bacteria,[1197] and prophylactic antibiosis with trimethoprim–sulfamethoxazole[1198–1200] or quinolones[1201] all have had their advocates. Serious arguments can be made against such regimens on psychological, economic, and ethical grounds—they are almost always expensive, unpleasant, and poorly tolerated, and often are of unproven efficacy in improving survival (as opposed to reducing bacterial contamination or colonization).[1147] Laminar flow rooms with gut sterilization are not obviously superior to simpler methods of isolation,[1195] but simple reverse isolation accomplishes little more than compulsive hand washing[1202]; all isolation methods severely reduce personal interaction of medical personnel with the patient. Long-term treatment with oral antibiotics for gut sterilization is poorly tolerated by most patients, and lack of compliance greatly reduces the effectiveness of the regimen.[1203] Furthermore, resistant organisms emerge,[1204] and other portals of bacterial entry are unprotected.

Surveillance cultures can help document the acquisition of new gut bacteria and predict the species responsible for bacteremia,[1205,1206] but their cost is high and their general value is controversial.[1207] Most neutropenic patients receive broad-spectrum antibiotic therapy, regardless of the results of surveillance cultures. One exception is routine nasal culture for aspergillosis.[1208] Sterile diets, avoidance of fresh fruits and vegetables, and no flowers in the room are easy proscriptions but of similarly unproven practical value.[1209–1211]

Red Blood Cell Transfusions and Hemochromatosis

Complete replacement of erythrocytes requires transfusion of about 1 unit of packed RBCs per week, usually given as 2 units every 2 weeks. (There is no rationale for allowing a patient to suffer symptoms of anemia.) After equilibrium is achieved, a constant amount of blood is required to maintain any hemoglobin concentration. With acclimation, fit individuals are usually not symptomatic at hemoglobin concentrations of more than 7 g/dL; patients with underlying cardiovascular disease should be maintained at a higher concentration, around 9 g/dL or more. In patients with anemia who are likely to remain dependent on erythrocyte transfusions, deferoxamine therapy is effective in chelating iron.[1212] Iron accumulation in critical organs, especially the heart, liver, and endocrine glands, can be prevented and sometimes reversed in the compliant patient who self-administers deferoxamine by subcutaneous infusion[1212] or more aggressively by intravenous infusion[1213] of 1.5 to 2.5 g/d. Iron chelation should be used in patients with unresponsive chronic anemia. As hemochromatotic damage to viscera begins after about 100 units of transfusion, a convenient starting time is after 50 to 100 units have been transfused or when the serum ferritin exceeds 500 ng/mL (usually 1 to 2 years after diagnosis) in a patient refractory to definitive therapy of aplastic anemia.

Spontaneous Recovery

Even minimal intervention, by modern standards, alters the natural history of bone marrow failure; a reading of the medical literature of the 1950s reveals the enormous impact of simple blood transfusions on the prospects of the patient with aplastic anemia. Certainly, spontaneous recovery was reported by physicians in the era predating even corticosteroid usage: a 9-year-old boy with severe symptoms of aplasia who was comatose for 2 weeks before recovery,[1214] a 47-year-old woman with chloramphenicol-associated aplastic anemia whose severe pancytopenia persisted for 22 months before recovery.[1215] In most of the early clinical series, a small proportion of patients appeared to improve, sometimes to completely normal hematologic values, when supported only by RBC transfusions,[1216,1217] and after the introduction of corticosteroids.[219,988,989,993,1218] In a series of pediatric patients treated mainly with transfusions, 14 of 33 achieved remission.[1219] These historical data are obscured by uncertainties in diagnosis, especially by the confounding influence of Fanconi's anemia and transient pancytopenias due to drug or toxin exposure, and by the inclusion of cases of myelodysplasia.

In those series in which blood counts of individual patients were published, it is clear that recovery usually occurred among patients who would now be classified as having moderate disease (at least 22 of 31 patients by the most conservative estimate in three series).[219,993,1217] In a more recent study that randomized 21 patients to supportive care only, none improved during 3 months of observation.[920] The fact that rare patients with aplastic anemia may recover even after years of severe pancytopenia is not an argument against therapy—rather, it is the opposite. Even in an era in which blood transfusions, corticosteroids, and penicillin constituted the entire armamentarium, the consensus of an eminent expert panel was "Never give up—at least almost never."[991]

Our time offers powerful broad-spectrum antibiotics, facile use of platelet transfusions, effective immunosuppression, bone marrow transplantation over histocompatibility barriers, a multiplicity of newly cloned hematopoietic growth factors, and every expectation of future therapeutic successes. Patients should be determinedly sustained, aggressively treated. Although good clinical judgment dictates when the only effect of treatment is to prolong suffering, an important consolation for the family and the physician is that all effective measures had been used to cure the disease.

Prognosis

Blood counts are the most important indicators of prognosis in aplastic anemia. The most popular Camitta criteria define severe disease as the presence of two of three greatly diminished blood counts: ANC below 500/μL; platelet count below 20,000/μL; corrected reticulocyte count of less than 1% (fewer than 40,000/μL).[868] Other criteria and algorithms have been proposed: a low initial reticulocyte count (below 10,000/μL)[1220]; a low reticulocyte count combined with progressive neutropenia[1221]; the Camitta criteria with a lower reticulocyte figure[1222]; the lowest individual blood counts during the course of disease[1223,1224]; and rapid progression with low neutrophil and platelet numbers.[1015]

More complex formulas[179,1225] have incorporated features of the clinical history and bone marrow examination. Some of these parameters reiterate the clinical manifestation of low blood counts (presence of bleeding[1225] or infection[179] or mean RBC volume),[836,1223] or mask logically circular arguments concerning survival (length of time from symptoms to presentation[1223,1225] or improvement or worsening in the first 6 weeks of observation[179]). These quantitate what experienced clinicians intuit—that patients who tolerate low blood counts without symptoms do better than those who bleed or become infected, that patients who do well continue to do well, at least for a time, and those who do not do well "go steadily down from bad to worse," in Cabot's phrase.[1226] This was the conclusion of a comparative study of prognostic indices, in which decreasing blood counts during the first 3 months of therapy were found to be uniformly associated with death before 5 years, whereas stable or increased counts correctly predicted long-term survival in 75% of patients.[1227] Of the prognostic indices, the Camitta criteria were most accurate at 6 months, correctly predicting poor survival in 85% of patients with 100% sensitivity. Fifteen percent of patients were incorrectly predicted to have a limited survival, and the errors were even higher for other scoring systems. All the indices are much less accurate when applied to cohorts different from the one used for their generation.[1228]

Other investigators have proposed the morphology of the bone marrow as a component of their prognostic formulas (as the percentage of nonmyeloid cells in the bone marrow[179,1225,1229] or stromal disorganization).[179] Predominance of lymphoid cells in the bone marrow has been associated with a bad prognosis in some studies[847,1229,1230] and not in others[843,1231,1232]; whether marrow lymphocyte predominance represents a pathologic process or the residua of severe hypocellularity remains unclear. Conversely, the presence of residual hematopoiesis, particularly erythropoiesis, in the bone marrow has been associated with a good outlook in some studies.[843,1015,1229,1233] In China, acute disease and chronic disease are separated by the overall cellularity on marrow aspirations from as many as six separate sites (anterior and posterior iliac crests, sternum, and vertebrae).[846]

Other tests to predict marrow recovery have been proposed. The detection of a peculiar subset of erythroid cells that bound an antibody to T cells and monocytes was highly correlated to recovery with immunosuppressive therapy.[1234]

Many of the prognostic scoring systems evolved prior to the widespread use of prophylactic and therapeutic platelet transfusions and effective immunosuppressive therapy. Control of bleeding has had a major impact on survival. Platelet transfusion, not antibiotic therapy, is credited with a significant improvement in the mortality of aplastic anemia in Japan in the 1970s.[1094] Bleeding was a major cause of death in the early large series, whereas infection kills the most patients now. In our own series of NIH patients, bleeding alone was responsible for death in only 4 of 75 deaths. In the large European cooperative trials, the category of "supersevere" aplastic anemia has recently been defined solely by an ANC below 200/μL.[881]

A modern algorithm would probably score neutrophil count much more heavily than platelet count, subtract heavily for established infection at time of diagnosis, and add a negative factor for the development of refractoriness to platelet transfusion. Finally, the traditional prognostic systems were developed specifically to define a patient category to subject to the travail of bone marrow transplantation. Now marrow transplantation is a much safer, almost routine procedure, especially in the younger patient, and effective alternative medical treatments also exist. The choice for one or the other treatment need not be exclusive nor based too heavily on prognostic criteria.

PURE RED CELL APLASIA

Pure red cell aplasia is a rare disease; only a few hundred cases have been reported.[1236] PRCA shares many clinical associations and pathophysiologic mechanisms with aplastic anemia. In particular, a variety of inciting causes that activate a common immune response may result in identical pathology (Table 10-15). Although many cases of PRCA are idiopathic, a large proportion is associated with clinical immunologic abnormalities, and erythropoiesis may be suppressed by either humoral or cellular immune effectors or both. A variant of PRCA, transient erythroblastopenia of childhood (TEC), is discussed in detail in Chapter 9.

Clinical Features

Women are more commonly affected with PRCA than men, especially within the large subcategory of immune-mediated disease. For PRCA associated with thymoma, male/female ratios are 2:1[1237,1238] or higher[372]; males may

TABLE 10-15. Clinical Classification of Pure Red Blood Cell Aplasia

SELF-LIMITED

Transient erythroblastopenia of childhood
Transient aplastic crisis of hemolysis (B19 parvovirus infection)

FETAL RED BLOOD CELL APLASIA

Nonimmune hydrops fetalis (in utero B19 parvovirus infection)

HEREDITARY PURE RED CELL APLASIA

Congenital pure red cell aplasia (Diamond-Blackfan syndrome)

ACQUIRED PURE RED CELL APLASIA

Thymoma[1237,1238,1248,1250]

Lymphoid Malignancies

Chronic lymphocytic leukemia (see text)
Malignant lymphoma[1312,1313,1490]
Malignant histiocytosis[1491]
Kaposi's sarcoma[1492]
Acute lymphocytic leukemia[1493]
Hodgkin's disease[1494]
Multiple myeloma[1495]

Other Hematologic Diseases

Myelodysplasia[12]
Chronic myelogenous leukemia[1496]
Myelofibrosis[1497]

Paraneoplastic to Solid Tumors[1236,1259]

Carcinoma of the bronchus, breast, stomach, thyroid, bile duct, and skin[1236,1498,1499]

Collagen Vascular Disease

Systemic lupus erythematosus[1500–1502]
Juvenile rheumatoid arthritis[1503]
Rheumatoid arthritis[1504]
Multiple endocrine gland insufficiency[1505]

Virus

B19 parvovirus[353]
Hepatitis[79,434,1506]
Adult T-cell leukemia virus[512]
Epstein-Barr virus[469,470]

Pregnancy[1507–1509]

Drugs

Probably causative associations
- Antiepileptics (diphenylhydantoin,[829,1260,1510–1515] carbamazepine,[1516] sodium dipropylacetate,[1517] sodium valproate[1518])
- Azathioprine[1519–1522]
- Chloramphenicol (see text) and thiamphenicol[1523,1524]
- Sulfonamides (salicylazosulfapyridine,[1272] sulfathalazine,[1525] methazolamide [with hepatitis],[1506] chlorpropamide,[1409,1526–1528] sulfathiazole,[1529,1530] cotrimoxazole[1531])
- Isoniazid[1510,1532–1534]
- Procaineamide[147,1535]

Possibly coincidental associations*
- Nonsteroidal antiinflammatory drugs (aminopyrine,[1536] phenylbutazone,[1537] fenoprofen,[1538,1539] sulindac[1372])
- Allopurinol[1540]
- Halothane (and hepatitis[1541])
- D-penicillamine[1542]
- Maloprim (dapsone and pyrimethamine)[1543]
- Metalozone[1544]
- Quinidine[824,1454] and quinacrine[1545]
- Gold[1546]
- Benzene[1530] and benzene-containing compounds (pentachlorophenol,[1547] arsenicals,[1548] and insecticides[1239,1549])

Idiopathic

* Some drugs have been linked to PRCA in patients with diseases that may be predisposed to PRCA (sulfonamides for ulcerative colitis, nonsteroidal antiinflammatories for rheumatoid arthritis). Some of the more dubious cases cited by Dessypris[1236] have been omitted, especially when bone marrow giant pronormoblasts were described or pictured and there was a history typical of transient aplastic crisis.[139,363,370] These cases more likely represent acute parvovirus infection.

also predominate in series in which PRCA is mainly associated with drugs or toxins[1239] or with chronic lymphocytic leukemia.[1240] The mean age of onset in immune-mediated disease is about 60 years.[1237,1238] There is no racial predisposition, and the disease is not apparently more common in Asia. Anemia, reticulocytopenia, and absent erythroid precursor cells define PRCA.[1241–1244] The erythrocytes are usually normocytic or occasionally macrocytic. Neutrophil and platelet counts are normal, but neutropenia, thrombocytopenia, or full pancytopenia can develop. The bone marrow cellularity is normal and remarkable for the lack or paucity of recognizable erythroid cells. Marrow erythropoiesis can be monitored with ^{111}In scintigraphy.[1245] Cytogenetics are usually normal, and abnormal results of chromosome analysis suggest the possibility of myelodysplasia,[1246] including the 5q− syndrome.[1247] In children, PRCA may be acute and self-limited (TEC); in contrast, acquired disease in adults is almost always chronic. The clinical associations and probably the pathogenesis of the two diseases are different. Unless otherwise noted, the discussion here focuses on adult PRCA. TEC is covered in Chapter 9.

Clinical Associations

Most cases of PRCA are idiopathic, but a large number are associated with illnesses. The most interesting association is with thymoma, but the often quoted 50% incidence of associated thymoma has almost certainly been greatly exaggerated because of the propensity to report an unusual combination. The true percentage is probably closer to 10%.[1236,1238,1248] Conversely, about 5% of thymomas have been estimated to be associated with RBC aplasia.[1236] Thymoma can precede the onset of PRCA by many years, and PRCA may have its onset after removal of the tumor.[1249] The thymic mass is commonly composed of spindle cells and is usually benign (contained within the capsule), but the tumors can be malignant and metastatic.[1237,1238,1248,1250,1251] In one large survey of published cases, 46 of 56 were well encapsulated.[1238] PRCA can complicate thymoma associated with several other autoimmune diseases such as myasthenia gravis,[1252,1253] collagen vascular syndromes, and endocrine failure states.[1254] PRCA can occur with these syndromes individually or with associated thymoma. The association of thymoma and PRCA is most common in older women; its occurrence in childhood is extremely rare. The possibility of a mediastinal mass should be excluded in adult patients by computed tomography of the chest, which is far more sensitive than routine thoracic radiography.[1255]

PRCA in adults is also associated with other immunologic abnormalities, including hypoimmunoglobulinemia,[469,1241,1256] monoclonal gammopathy,[1257,1258] anergy, antinuclear antibodies, and autoimmune hemolysis.[1244]

PRCA can accompany a wide variety of other neoplasms,[1259] most frequently lymphoid.[1240] The incidence of PRCA in chronic lymphocytic leukemia was estimated at 6% in one large series; PRCA may be present initially but more commonly appears several years after diagnosis.[1240] PRCA also can complicate other hematologic malignancies and nonthymic solid tumors. T-cell inhibition has been implicated in the pathophysiology of PRCA in lymphoproliferative disease; many of these same illnesses—or their therapy—are immunosuppressive and would be permissive for persistent parvovirus infection.

A large number of drugs has been associated with PRCA,[1236] most of which are included in the black list for aplastic anemia treatment. For only a few agents is there more than a single case report. Diphenylhydantoin is causally related to PRCA: patients have developed marrow failure on drug rechallenge,[1260,1261] and one patient has demonstrated a drug-dependent antibody that inhibited in vitro erythropoiesis.[829]

Practically, it is most important to distinguish among PRCA that is (1) immunologically mediated (most idiopathic cases and those associated with thymoma, systemic lupus erythematosus, and chronic lymphocytic leukemia), (2) caused by primary bone marrow failure (myelodysplasia, myeloproliferative disease, cytogenetic abnormalities, and others), (3) secondary to persistent parvovirus infection, and (4) hereditary and presents in adulthood.[1262]

Pathogenesis and Pathophysiology

Antibodies to Erythroid Precursor Cells

A marrow-suppressing factor was first identified in a patient with PRCA, thymoma, and Hodgkin's disease.[1263] Antibody mediation of PRCA was proposed by Krantz and associates on the basis of observations in several patients: their plasma contained an IgG that inhibited heme synthesis in suspension cultures of normal bone marrow cells[1264,1265] and in the presence of complement, lysed erythroblasts.[1266] Immunoglobulin preparations from some patients were later shown to inhibit CFU-E–derived erythroid colony formation but not myeloid colony formation in the presence[1267–1270] or absence[1271] of complement. The prevalence of antibody to erythroid precursor cells in PRCA is difficult to assess because of the limited number of patients and because of reporting bias; in a cooperative study, an antibody that inhibited erythropoiesis was found in 13 of 16 patients,[1272] but antibody generally has not been detected in patients with RBC aplasia secondary to lymphoma and other malignancies.[1240] A remarkable feature of the cytotoxic antibody in PRCA is its cross-species reactivity, including release of ^{59}Fe from murine cells in vitro, inhibition of RBC production after injection into mice, and depletion of CFU-E in treated animals (although some inhibitors have been species specific).[1272] The target antigen on erythroid precursor cells has not been identified. In two cases, erythropoiesis was inhibited by an antibody that bound directly to erythropoietin,[941,1273] but in all others antibody has bound to precursor cells and erythropoietin levels are high.[1272]

The strongest evidence of a pathogenic role for cytotoxic antibodies is their disappearance from the circulation of patients who respond to therapy, including antilymphocyte sera and immunosuppressive drugs,[941] thymectomy,[1274] and plasmapheresis.[1275,1276] In contrast, an immunoglobulin that specifically stained erythroblast nuclei, which was also found in patient plasma, often persisted despite effective therapy and hematologic improvement.[1275,1277] It may represent a secondary antibody formed to the contents of lysed erythroblasts. Alloimmunized patients may have other antibodies directed to antigens on mature erythrocyte surfaces that can be distinguished from the characteristic inhibitor of erythropoiesis.[1269] In one case of PRCA and thymoma, a serum inhibitor of antigen-induced lymphocyte transformation was present[1249]; such an activity might account for defective production of erythropoietic factors by lymphocytes in some patients with PRCA.[1270]

IgG inhibitors of erythropoiesis have also been documented in children with transient erythroblastopenia of childhood.[1278]

Cytotoxic Lymphocytes. T-cell inhibition of erythropoiesis is probably a more common mechanism of depression of RBC production than antibody formation.[1279] Lymphocyte inhibition may be particularly common in PRCA associated with chronic lymphocytic leukemia.[1240,1280] T-cell inhibition of either CFU-E– or BFU-E–derived colony formation was present in eight of eight cases, whereas none showed a serum inhibitor of erythropoiesis[1240]; cells with the suppressor phenotype and function in erythropoietic colony culture were present in early, nonanemic stages of disease in a high percentage of patients.[1281] As in aplastic anemia, there may be increased numbers of lymphocytes with receptors for IgG (Tγ cells) [1282–1284] or with the suppressor cell phenotype (CD8+),[1283–1286] which inhibit erythroid colony formation by CFU-E and BFU-E. Genetic restriction of lymphocytic suppression of erythropoiesis by CD8+, HLA-DR+ lymphocytes was shown in one well-studied case.[1287] Clinical remission has been correlated with the disappearance of the suppressive population after immunosuppressive therapy or chemotherapy-induced remission of chronic lymphocytic leukemia.[1283–1286,1288] In some cases, the implicated population was a true suppressor cell, capable of inhibiting in vitro immunoglobulin synthesis as well as erythropoiesis.[1289,1290]

Persistent Parvovirus Infection. Patients with persistent B19 parvovirus infection have PRCA. Persistence is possible because patients fail to mount a neutralizing antibody response to the virus. Such patients lack the immune complex–mediated symptoms of fifth disease—fever, rash, and polyarthralgia or polyarthritis. Persistent parvovirus infection and PRCA have been documented in three patient populations: patients with congenital immunodeficiency (Nezelof's syndrome),[406,1291] children with lymphoblastic leukemia in remission on chemotherapy,[407] and patients with AIDS.[1292] Defective antibody production occurs also in other diseases associated with PRCA, such as chronic lymphocytic leukemia and malignancies treated with cytotoxic drugs. Some of these cases may have represented occult viral infection (parvovirus infection likely was unrecognized previously as a cause of PRCA in AIDS[1293,1294] and leukemia,[1295] in reticulocytopenic episodes associated with hemolytic disease,[1296] and in starvation and severe protein deficiency[366,1297]).

Clinically, the anemia is severe and infected patients depend on erythrocyte transfusions; neutropenia may be an associated condition. The bone marrow should contain some giant pronormoblasts, which are the cytopathic sign of parvovirus infection, although these are usually infrequent. The anemia may be intermittent, with periods of relapse associated with viremia and periods of remission with spontaneous disappearance of virus from the circulation, possibly caused by depletion of the erythroid target cell population. The diagnosis is established by detection of B19 parvovirus genome in the serum, blood, or bone marrow cells by dot blot hybridization; polymerase chain reaction amplification of viral DNA may be necessary in rare cases.[404] Antibodies to parvovirus, as determined in capture immunoassays or ELISA, are not present in most patients, but a pattern of antibody response suggestive of early infection (IgM antibody and IgG antibody directed to the major capsid protein) may be found in patients with congenital immunodeficiency.[1298] A poor reaction on immunoblot testing is a consistent finding and correlates with poor neutralizing activity for the virus in erythroid colony assays.[1298] Persistent parvovirus infection may be the dominant manifestation of some inherited immunodeficient states.

Effective therapy consists of infusion of commercial immunoglobulin preparations, which are a good source of neutralizing antibodies because most of the adult population has been exposed to the virus. The best treatment regimen has not been established. One patient with congenital immunodeficiency was cured by a 10-day course followed by intermittent immunoglobulin injections until virus had disappeared from his serum.[1291] Patients with AIDS respond to a 5- to 10-day course of immunoglobulin but may relapse months later, and they can respond to a second course.[1292] Patients with AIDS have had extremely high virus serum concentrations, comparable to levels found in TAC patients, and much higher than found in other patients with chronic parvovirus infection.[1292] Measurement of serum virus is helpful in predicting relapse and may assist in determining optimal treatment regimens.

Treatment

About two thirds of patients with PRCA respond to some form of immunosuppression, although trials of alternative forms of therapy may be necessary.[1299–1301] Prednisone can induce remission in about 45% of cases, and the addition of a cytotoxic agent may improve the remission rate and lower the corticosteroid dose.[1300] Cytotoxic drug regimens include azathioprine, cyclophosphamide, and 6-mercaptopurine with titration to leukopenia; a 3- to 4-month trial is adequate. Relapse occurs in about half of the treated cases and chronic cytotoxic chemotherapy may be required to maintain transfusion independence.[1302] Patients have responded to ATG[940–942,1279] and cyclosporine,[980,981,1303,1304] including cases refractory to conventional immunosuppression.

Plasmapheresis[1275,1276,1305] and lymphocytopheresis[1305] have been successful in inducing sustained remissions; in some patients, the clinical response has been correlated with removal of an antibody inhibitory to erythropoiesis in vitro.[1275,1276] Splenectomy may sometimes be helpful.[1243,1300] Some patients have responded to androgens,[1306] including three of three patients who responded to Danazol in one small series.[1307] Apparent responses have also been noted after high doses of intravenous immunoglobulin.[1304,1308–1310] A small percentage of patients (about 15%) may have apparently spontaneous remissions.[1300] Patients with PRCA secondary to malignant disease can also respond to specific immunosuppressive therapy or cytotoxic chemotherapy.[1240,1300,1311–1313] A thymoma is necessarily removed for diagnosis and treatment of a possibly malignant chest mass, but the procedure probably benefits only a minority of patients. The percentage commonly quoted for remission of anemia after thymectomy is 30%, based on an analysis of the 9 of 26 patients who showed improvement[1238]; in three of these patients remission occurred only with the postoperative addition of corticosteroids, and in three others no benefit was sustained. (It also is worth remembering that PRCA can occur years after removal of a thymoma.)

PRCA may be one of the few diseases in which hematopoietic colony cultures have clinical value in predicting response to treatment. In general, patients whose marrow contains CFU-E progenitors have a high probability of response to immunosuppression, whereas patients without detectable CFU-E–often cases secondary to myeloproliferative or malignant disease—have not responded.[1279,1314] These results confirm the earlier observation that a proliferative response in suspension culture to added erythropoietin predicts clinical improvement with therapy.[1264,1265] In contrast, the presence of an antibody to erythroid progenitors in coculture does not correlate with responsiveness to immunosuppressive treatment, and antibodies are often undetectable in patients who behave clinically as if they have an autoimmune process.[1252,1314]

The obvious mainstay of therapy is RBC transfusion, and the same principles as were described earlier for the support of the patient with aplastic anemia should be applied here.

AMEGAKARYOCYTIC THROMBOCYTOPENIC PURPURA

Amegakaryocytic thrombocytopenic purpura is a rare disorder. It exists in adult and pediatric forms; the latter is discussed in Chapter 9. Only 30 adult patients have been reported. As in PRCA, females predominate (2.6:1) and half the patients are older than 55 years.[1315] Patients present with easy bruising, gingival bleeding, epistaxis, menorrhagia, or other symptoms of a thrombocytopenic bleeding diathesis. The bone marrow examination, which shows reduced or absent megakaryocytes, differentiates amegakaryocytic thrombocytopenia from thrombocytopenia due to peripheral destruction. About 20% of the reported 30 cases have progressed to aplastic anemia.[1315] Other cases have been diagnosed as myelodysplasia[1316] or preleukemia,[1317] and cytogenetic abnormalities include the 5q− lesion[1316] and partial duplication of chromosome 3.[1318] The presence of a single cytogenetic (XO) cell type in the bone marrow of a sex chromosome mosaic with amegakaryocytic thrombocytopenia suggested clonality in one case.[1319]

Familial amegakaryocytic thrombocytopenia presenting in adulthood has been associated with hemochromatosis.[1320] A number of parallels can be found between amegakaryocytic thrombocytopenia and more generalized bone marrow failure. Like aplastic anemia, amegakaryocytic thrombocytopenia is associated with systemic lupus erythematosus[1321] and other collagen vascular diseases,[1322] with hepatitis[1323,1324] and other viral infections,[1315] and with drug use (oxyphenbutazone).[1325] Many patients have shown peripheral RBC macrocytosis.[1326]

In vitro studies suggest diverse pathophysiologic mechanisms. Megakaryocyte colony formation (but not formation of myeloid colonies) is usually low or absent.[1326,1327] Megakaryocyte colony-stimulating factor and thrombopoietic activities also have usually been normal or increased,[1326] but in some patients defective growth factor production has been documented.[1328] In one patient, it is associated with the 5q− abnormality,[1316] and in another patient with cyclical thrombocytopenia, it is associated with an immunoglobulin that blocked the action of granulocyte-macrophage colony-stimulating factor.[1329] T-lymphocyte–mediated suppression of megakaryocytopoiesis[1321,1330,1331] and serum inhibitors[1323,1326] has been described in several patients. Patients have responded to ATG,[945,946] cyclophosphamide,[1332] lithium,[1317] androgens,[1333] and prednisone.[945,1315]

Acknowledgments

I am grateful to many critical readers of the manuscript, especially to members of my laboratory (Dr. Johnson Liu and Dr. Norbert Frickhofen), Dr. David Bodine of the Clinical Hematology Branch (stem cell section), Dr. Niel Wald of the University of Pittsburgh, Dr. Eli Glatstein of the National Cancer Institute (radiation section), Dr. Paul Leaverton of Florida State University at Tampa, Dr. Samuel Shapiro of Boston University (epidemiology), Dr. Susan Leitman of the Clinical Center Blood Bank (management of bleeding), and Dr. Phillip Pizzo of the National Cancer Institute (management of infection). Ms. Nysa Sanders provided excellent secretarial assistance.

REFERENCES

1. Ehrlich P. Ueber einen Fall von Anämie mit Bemerkungen über regenerative Veranderungen des Knochenmarks. Charit-Annalen 1888;13:300.
2. Chauffard M. Un cas d'anaemie pernicieuse aplastique. Bull Med Soc Hôp Paris 1904;21:313.
3. Cabot RC. The general pathology of the blood-forming organs. In: Osler W, ed. System of medicine, ed 2. London, Froude, 1908:595.
4. Frank E. Aleukia hemorrhagica: aplastische (aregenerative) anämie-panmyelophthise. Berl Klin Wochenschr 1915;37:961.
5. Minot GR. Diminished blood platelets and marrow insufficiency. Arch Intern Med 1917;19:1062.
6. Delamore IW, Geary CG. Aplastic anaemia, acute myeloblastic leukaemia, and oxymetholone. Br J Haematol 1971;2:743.
7. Krause JR. Aplastic anemia terminating in hairy cell leukemia. Cancer 1984;53:1533.
8. Beyer GS, Glant MD, Hoffman R. Development of IgA multiple myeloma in a patient with aplastic anemia treated with antithymocyte globulin. N Engl J Med 1986;314:247.
9. de Planque MM, Kluin-Nelemans HC, van Krieken HJM, et al. Evolution of acquired severe aplastic anaemia to myelodysplasia and subsequent leukaemia in adults. Br J Haematol 1988;70:55.
10. Appelbaum FR, Barrall J, Storb R, et al. Clonal cytogenetic abnormalities in patients with otherwise typical aplastic anemia. Exp Hematol 1987;15:1134.
11. Antonucci R, Walker R, Herion J. Myelofibrosis and aplastic anemia: first report of the two disorders occurring sequentially in the same person. Am J Med 1989;86:352.
12. Craig A, Geary CG, Love EM, Liu-Yin J. Red cell hypoplasia, thrombocytosis, and leucocytosis: myelodysplastic and proliferative syndrome. J Clin Pathol 1988;41:1168.
13. Geary CG. Myelodysplasia. In: Whittaker JA, Delamore IW, eds. Leukaemia. Oxford, Blackwell, 1987:420.
14. Needleman SW, Burns CP, Dick FR, Armitage JO. Hypoplastic acute leukemia. Cancer 1981;48:1410.
15. Block M, Jacobson LO, Bethard WF. Preleukemic acute human leukemia. JAMA 1953;152:1018.
16. Cheng PNM, Ng CS, Brearley RL. Acute lymphoblastic leukaemia presenting as aplastic anaemia. J R Soc Med 1987;80:116.
17. Klingemann H-G, Storb R, Sanders J, et al. Acute lymphoblastic leukaemia after bone marrow transplantation for aplastic anaemia. Br J Haematol 1986;63:47.
18. Nakamori Y, Takahashi M, Moriyama Y, et al. The aplastic presentation of adult acute lymphoblastic leukaemia. (Letter) Br J Haematol 1986;62:782.
19. Fohlmeister I, Fischer R, Modder B, et al. Aplastic anaemia and the hypocellular myelodysplastic syndrome: histomorphological, diagnostic, and prognostic features. J Clin Pathol 1985;38:1218.
20. Riccardi A, Giordano M, Girino M, et al. Refractory cytopenias: clinical course according to bone marrow cytology and cellularity. Blut 1987;54:153.
21. Tomonaga M, Tomonaga Y, Kusano M, Ichimaru M. Sequential karyotypic evolutions and bone marrow aplasia preceding acute myelomonocytic transformation from myelodysplastic syndrome. Br J Haematol 1984;58:53.
22. Aso T, Okamura T, Shibuya T, et al. A case of hybrid phenotypic chronic myelomonocytic leukemia transformed from aplastic anemia. Jpn J Med 1989;28:385.
23. Pezzimenti JF, Lindenbaum JF. Megaloblastic anemia associated with erythroid hypoplasia. Am J Med 1972;53:748.
24. Camitta BM, Storb R, Thomas ED. Aplastic anemia: pathogenesis, diagnosis, treatment, and prognosis. N Engl J Med 1982;306:645–652.
25. Young N. Aplastic anemia: research themes, clinical issues. Prog Hematol 1981;12:227.
26. Young NS, Levine AS, Humphries RK, eds. Aplastic anemia: stem cell biology and advances in treatment. New York, Alan R Liss, 1984.
27. Geary CG, ed. Aplastic anaemia. London, Ballière Tindall, 1979.
28. Gavirtz AM, Hoffman R. Current considerations of the etiology of aplastic anemia. Crit Rev Oncol Hematol 1985;4:1.
29. Hibino S, Takaku F, Shahidi NT, EDS. Aplastic anemia. Baltimore, University Park Press, 1978.
30. Marmont AM, Bacigalupo A. Aplastic anemia: pathogenesis and treatment. Haematologica 1988;73:133.
31. Szklo M, Sensenbrenner L, Markowitz J, et al. Incidence of aplastic anemia in metropolitan Baltimore: a population-based study. Blood 1985;66:115.
32. Risks of agranulocytosis and aplastic anemia: a first report of their relation to drug use with special reference to analgesics. JAMA 1986;256:1749.
33. Cartwright RA, McKinney PA, Williams L, et al. Aplastic anaemic incidence in parts of the United Kingdom in 1985. Leuk Res 1988;12:459.
34. Clausen N. A population study of severe aplastic anemia in children: incidence, etiology and course. Acta Paediatr Scand 1986;75:58.
35. Davies SM, Walker DJ. Aplastic anaemia in the Northern Region 1971–1978 and follow-up of long-term survivors. Clin Lab Haematol 1986;8:307.
36. Donski S, Bucher U. Increase of the number of pancytopenias between 1954 and 1964. Helv Med Acta 34:337.
37. Kletter G. Aplastiche anämien im Obduktionsgut. Wien Klïn Wochenschr 1972;84:145.
38. Levy M, Slone D, Shapiro S, et al. Incidence of aplastic anemia: the relevance of diagnostic criteria. Blood 1987;70:1718.
39. Bottiger LE. Epidemiology and aetiology of aplastic anemia. In: Heimpel H, Gordon-Smith EC, Heit W, Kubanek B, eds. Aplastic anemia: pathophysiology and aproaches to therapy. Berlin, Springer-Verlag, 1979:27.
40. US Department of Health and Human Services. Mortality. In: Vital statistics of the United States, ed 2. Washington, DC, 1986:122.
41. Aoki K, Fujiki N, Shimizu H, Ohno Y. Geographic and ethnic differences of aplastic anemia in humans. In: Najean Y, ed. Medullary aplasia. New York, Masson, 1980:79.
42. Aoki K, Ohtani M, Shimizu H. Epidemiological approach to the etiology of aplastic anemia. In: Hibino S, Takaku F, Shahidi NT, eds. Aplastic anemia. Baltimore, University Park Press, 1978:155.
43. Dameshek W. Riddle: what do aplastic anemia, paroxysmal nocturnal hemoglobinuria (PNH) and "hypoplastic" leukemia have in common? Blood 1967;30:251.
44. Young NS, Issaragrasil S, Ch'en WC, Takaku F. Aplastic anemia in the Orient. Br J Haematol 1986;62:1.
45. Whang KS. Aplastic anemia in Korea: a clinical study of 309 cases. In: Hibino S, Takaku F, Shahidi NT, eds. Aplastic anemia. Baltimore, University Park Press, 1978:225.
46. Lee CM, Hong CY, Choi KW, et al. Aplastic anemia in Korea (an analysis of 862 cases). Korean J Hematol 1975;10:3.
47. Aoki K. Comments on epidemiology. In: Hibino S, Takaku F, eds. Aplastic anemia. Tokyo, Igaku-Shoin, 1979:1.
48. Yin D, Wu Y, Lin Z, et al. Epidemiological and etiological studies on aplastic anemia in the Mudanjiang area. Chin J Hematol 1980;1:33.
49. Aplastic anemia. In: Deng J, Yang CL, Yang TY, eds. Clinical hematology. Shanghai, China, Science and Technology Publishing Company, 1985.
50. Corrigan GE. An autopsy survey of aplastic anemia. Am J Clin Pathol 1974;62:488.
51. Shima S, Kato Y. Incidence of aplastic anemia among workers in major industries in Japan and suspected causal factors. In: Aoki K, Hosoda Y, Yanagawa H, et al, eds. Epidemiology of intractable diseases in Japan. Nagoya, Department of Preventive Medicine, Nagoya University School of Medicine, 1986:53.
52. Sánchez-Medal L, Castanedo JP, Garcia-Rojas F. Insecticides and aplastic anemia. N Engl J Med 1963;269:1365.
53. Mukiibi J, Paul B, Nkrumah F. Aplastic anaemia in Zimbabweans. Cent Afr J Med 1987;33:1.
54. Esan GJF. Aplastic anaemia in Nigerians. W Afr Med J 1973;22:534.
55. Mabin TA, Gelfand M. Aplastic anaemia in Africans. Trop Geogr Med 1974;26:423.
56. Linet MS, McCaffrey LD, Morgan WF, et al. Incidence of aplastic anemia in a three county area in South Carolina. Cancer Res 1986;46:426.
57. Custer RP. Aplastic anemia in soldiers treated with atabrine. Am J Med Sci 1946;212:211.
58. Shimizu H, Kuroishi T, Tominaga S, et al. Production amount of

chloramphenicol and mortality rate of aplastic anemia in Japan. Acta Haematol Jpn 1979;42:689.
59. Mizuno S, Aoki K, Ohno Y, et al. Time series analysis of age-sex specific death rates from aplastic anemia and the trend in production amount of chloramphenicol. Nagoya J Med Sci 1982;44:103.
60. Bottiger LE, Furhoff AK, Holmberg L. Drug-induced blood dyscrasias. Acta Med Scand 1979;205:457.
61. Bottiger LE. Drug-induced aplastic anemia in Sweden with special reference to chloramphenicol. J Postgrad Med 1974;50:127.
62. Kumana CR, Li KY, Chau PY. Worldwide variation in chloramphenicol utilization: should it cause concern? J Clin Pharmacol 1988;28:1071.
63. Linet MS, Markowitz JA, Sensenbrenner LL, et al. A case-control study of aplastic anemia. Leuk Res 1989;13:3.
64. Linet MS, Tielsch JM, Markowitz JA, et al. An apparent cluster of aplastic anemia in a small population of teenagers. Arch Intern Med 1985;145:635.
65. de Gramont A, Najean Y, Beaune R. Does the monthly frequency of medullary aplasia vary throughout the year? Acta Haematol 1982;68:71.
66. Sleifer DT, Mulder NH, Nieweg HO, et al. Acquired pancytopenia in relatives of patients with aplastic anaemia. Acta Med Scand 1980;207:397.
67. Stolte JB. Familiäre aplastische anämie. Ned Tijdschr Geneeskd 1948;92:4053.
68. Keiser G. Erworbene panmyelopathien. Schweiz Med Wochenschr 1970;100:1938.
69. Morley A, Trainor K, Seshadri R, Sorrell J. Is aplastic anaemia due to abnormality of DNA? Lancet 1978;2:9.
70. Turner DR, Morley AA, Seshadri RS. Lymphocyte DNA in aplastic anaemia. Br J Haematol 1981;48:207.
71. Kovacs E, Nissen C, Speck B, Signer E. Repair of UV-induced DNA damage in aplastic anaemia: changes after treatment with antilymphocyte globulin (ALG). Eur J Haematol 1988;40:430.
72. Rosenthal RL, Blackman A. Bone-marrow hypoplasia following use of chloramphenicol eye drops. JAMA 1965;191:136.
73. Nora AH, Fernbach DJ. Acquired aplastic anemia in children. Tex Med 1969;65:38.
74. Nagao T, Mauer AM. Concordance for drug induced aplastic anemia in identical twins. N Engl J Med 1969;281:7.
75. Meyler L, Polak BCP, Wesseling H, et al. Blood dyscrasias attributed to chloramphenicol. Acta Med Scand 1972;192:409.
76. Davidson LSP, Davis LJ, Innes J. Studies in refractory anaemia. Edinb Med J 1943;50:355.
77. McLaren GD, Doukas MA, Muir WA. Methyprylon-induced bone marrow suppression in siblings. JAMA 1978;240:1744.
78. Boga M, Szemere PA. Infectious hepatitis and aplastic anaemia—in two sisters. (Letter) Lancet 1971;2:703.
79. Sears DA, George JN, Gold MS. Transient red blood cell aplasia in association with viral hepatitis: occurrence four years apart in siblings. Arch Intern Med 1975;135:1585.
80. Purtilo DT, Sakamoto K, Barnabei V, et al. Epstein-Barr virus-induced diseases in boys with the X-linked lymphoproliferative syndrome (XLP): update on studies of the registry. Am J Med 1982;73:49.
81. Chiu KM, Knospe WH. Immunologically mediated aplastic anemia in mice: effects of varying the source and composition of donor cells. Exp Hematol 1987;15:269.
82. Dausset J, Gluckman E, Lemarchand F, et al. Exces d'HLA-A2 et d'homozygotes HLA-A2 parmi les malades atteints d'aplasie medullaire et maladie de fanconi. Nouv Rev Fr Hematol 1977;18:315.
83. Chapuis B, Von Fliedner VE, Jeannet M, Merica H, et al. Increased frequency of DR2 in patients with aplastic anaemia and increased DR sharing in their parents. Br J Haematol 1986;63:51.
84. Aaron S, Davis P, Bertouch J. HLA-DR antigens in gold-induced neutropenia. Arthritis Rheum 1986;29:1515.
85. Odum N, Platz P, Morling N, Jacobsen N, et al. Increased frequency of HLA-DPw3 in severe aplastic anemia (AA). Tissue Antigens 1987;29:184.
86. Champlin R. Bone marrow aplasia due to radiation accidents: pathophysiology, assessment and treatment. In: Hinton K, Tindall B, eds. Clinical haematology. London, Bailliere Tindall, 1989:69.
87. Warren S, Dunlap CE. Effects of radiation on normal tissues. III. Effects of radiation on the blood and the hemopoietic tissues, including the spleen, the thymus and the lymph nodes. Arch Pathol 1942;34:562.
88. Knospe WH. Long-term bone marrow damage after irradiation. In: Testa NG, Gale RP, eds. Hematopoiesis: long-term effects of chemotherapy and radiation. New York, Marcel Dekker, 1988:93.
89. Wald N, Thoma GE, Broun G Jr. Hematological manifestations of radiation exposure in man. Prog Hematol 1962;3:1.
90. Bruegge CFV. Radiation injury following an A-bomb explosion. Ann Intern Med 1952;36:1444.
91. Gale RP. Immediate medical consequences of nuclear accidents: lessons from Chernobyl. JAMA 1987;258:625.
92. Pollard EC. The biological action of ionizing radiation. Am Scientist 1969;57:206.
93. Puck TT. The effect of radiation on mammalian cells. Am Naturalist 1960;94:95.
94. Adams GE. Lethality from acute and protracted radiation exposure in man. Int J Radiat Biol 1984;46:209.
95. Mole RH. The LD50 for uniform low LET irradiation of man. Br J Radiol 1984;57:355.
96. Liebow AA, Warren S, DeCoursey E. Pathology of atomic bomb casualties. Am J Pathol 1949;25:853.
97. Wald N. Diagnosis and therapy of radiation injuries. Bull NY Acad Med 1983;59:1129.
98. Cronkite EP. Hematology, diagnosis and therapy of radiation injury. US Armed Forces Med J 1951;56:661.
99. Andrews GA. The medical management of accidental total-body irradiation. In: Hübner KF, Fry SA, eds. The medical basis for radiation accident preparedness. New York, Elsevier/North Holland, 1980:297.
100. Langweiler M, Cockerell GL, deNoronha F. Role of suppressor cells in feline leukemia virus-associated immunosuppression. Cancer Res 1983;43:1957.
101. Adelstein SJ, Dealy JB Jr. Hematologic responses to human whole body irradiation: analytical approaches to biologic dosimetry. AJR 1965;93:927.
102. Lawrence JS, Dowdy AH, Valentine WN. Effects of radiation on hemopoiesis. Radiology 1948;51:400.
103. LeRoy GV. Hematology of atomic bomb casualties. Arch Intern Med 1950;86:691.
104. Gale RP, Reisner Y. The role of bone-marrow transplants after nuclear accidents. Lancet 1988;1:923.
105. Gale RP. Dose injury assessment and medical effects at Chernobyl. In: Bond VP, Cronkite EP, eds. Workshop on short-term health effects of reactor accidents: Chernobyl, August 8–9, 1986. Upton, Brookhaven National Laboratory, 1989:12.
106. Hübner KF, Fry SA. The medical basis for radiation accident preparedness. New York, Elsevier/North Holland, 1980.
107. Mathé G, Jammet H, Pendic B, Schwarzenberg L, et al. Transfusions et greffes de moelle osseuse homologue chez des humaines irradiés à haute dose accidentellement. Rev Fr Études Clin Biol 1959;4:226.
108. Gilberti MV. The 1967 radiation accident near Pittsburgh, Pennsylvania, and a follow-up report. In: Hubner KF, Fry SA, eds. The medical basis for radiation accident preparedness. New York, Elsevier/North Holland, 1980:131.
109. Cronkite EP. Regulation of hemopoiesis, its perturbation by ionizing radiation and new therapeutic approaches involving recombinant molecular regulators. In: Bond VP, Cronkite EP, eds. Workshop on short-term health effects of reactor accidents: Chernobyl, August 8–9, 1986. Upton, Brookhaven National Laboratory, 1986:33.
110. Neta R, Douches SD, Oppenheim JJ. Interleukin 1 is a radioprotector. J Immunol 1986;136:2483.
111. Morrissey P, Charrier K, Bressler L, Alpert A. The influence of IL-1 treatment on the reconstitution of the hemopoietic and immune systems after sublethal radiation. J Immunol 1988;140:4204.
112. Monroy RL, Skelly RR, Taylor P, et al. Recovery from severe hematopoietic suppression using recombinant human granulocyte-macrophage colony-stimulating factor. Exp Hematol 1988;16:344.
113. Schuening FG, Storb R, Goehle S, et al. Effect of recombinant human granulocyte colony-stimulating factor on hematopoiesis of normal dogs and on hematopoietic recovery after otherwise lethal total body irradiation. Blood 1989;74:1308.
114. Butturini A, Gale RP, Lopes DM, et al. Use of recombinant granulocyte-macrophage colony stimulating factor in the Brazil radiation accident. Lancet 1988;2:471.
115. Kirshbaum JD, Matsuo T, Sato K, et al. A study of aplastic anemia in an autopsy series with special reference to atomic bomb survivors in Hiroshima and Nagasaki. Blood 1971;38:17.
116. Lange RD, Wright SW, Tomonaga M, et al. Refractory anemia occurring in survivors of the atomic bombing in Nagasaki, Japan. Blood 1955;10:312.
117. Conrad RA, Cronkite EP, Bond VP, et al. Fallout radiation: effects on Marshallese people. In: Behrens CF, King ER, Carpender JWJ, eds. Atomic medicine, ed 5. Baltimore, Williams & Wilkins, 1969: 308.
118. Fliedner TM, Nothdurft W, Calvo W. The development of radiation late effects to the bone marrow after single and chronic exposure. Int J Radiat Biol 1986;49:35.
119. Reincke U, Hannon EC, Hellman S. Residual radiation injury exhibited in long-term bone marrow cultures. J Cell Physiol 1982;112: 345.
120. Seed TM, Cullen SM, Kaspar LV, et al. Hemopathologic consequences of protracted gamma irradiation: alterations in granulocyte reserves and granulocyte mobilization. Blood 1980;56:42.
121. Martland HS. Occupational poisoning in manufacture of luminous watch dials. JAMA 1929;92:466.
122. Spier J, Cluff LE, Urry WD. Aplastic anemia following administration of thorotrast. J Lab Clin Med 1947;32:147.
123. Duane GW. Aplastic anemia fourteen years following administration of thorotrast. Am J Med 1957;23:499.
124. Court-Brown WM, Doll R. Leukemia and aplastic anaemia in patients irradiated for ankylosing spondylitis. In: Medical Research Council (Brit). Special Report Series No. 295. London, HM Stationery Office, 1957.

125. Lewis EB. Leukemia, multiple myeloma, and aplastic anemia in American radiologists. Science 1963;142:1492.
126. Curran RE, Johnson RE. Tolerance to chemotherapy after prior irradiation for Hodgkin's disease. Ann Intern Med 1970;72:505.
127. Kitabatake T, Sakai K, Saito A. Expectation of aplastic anemia following radiotherapy for malignancy. Radiology 1978;129:169.
128. Bithell TC, Wintrobe MM. Drug-induced aplastic anemia. Semin Hematol 1967;4:194.
129. Williams DM, Lynch RE, Cartwright GE. Drug-induced aplastic anemia. Semin Hematol 1973;10:195.
130. Young N. Drugs and chemicals as agents of bone marrow failure. In: Testa N, Gale RC, eds. Hematopoiesis: long-term effects of chemotherapy and radiation. New York, Marcel Dekker, 1988:131.
131. Vincent PC. Drug-induced aplastic anemia and agranulocytosis: incidence and mechanisms. Drugs 1986;31:52.
132. Gordon-Smith EC. Aplastic anaemia: aetiology and clinical features. In: Hinton K, Tindall B, eds. Clinical haematology. London, Baillere Tindall, 1989:1.
133. Heimpel H, Heit W. Drug-induced aplastic anaemia: clinical aspects. Clin Haematol 1980;9:641.
134. Aksoy M, Erdem S. Dincol G, et al. Aplastic anemia due to chemicals and drugs: a study of 108 patients. Sex Trans Dis 1984;11:347.
135. Feinstein AR. Scientific standards in epidemiologic studies of the menace of daily life. Science 1988;242:1257.
136. Karch FE, Lasagna L. Adverse drug reactions: a critical review. JAMA 1975;234:1236.
137. Lowenthal MN, Jones IG, Desai M. Aplastic anaemia and optic fundus haemorrhages due to traditional herbal remedies. J Trop Med Hyg 1978;81:177.
138. Imperiale TF, Horwitz RI. Scientific standards and the design of case-control research. Biomed Pharmacother 1989;43:187.
139. Powars D. Aplastic anemia secondary to glue sniffing. N Engl J Med 1965;273:700.
140. Smick KM, Condit PK, Proctor RL, Sutcher V. Fatal aplastic anemia: an epidemiological study of its relationship to the drug chloramphenicol. J Chron Dis 1964;17:899.
141. Wallerstein RO, Condit PK, Kasper CK, et al. Statewide study of chloramphenicol therapy and fatal aplastic anemia. JAMA 1969;208: 2045.
142. Inman WHW. Study of fatal bone marrow depression with special reference to phenylbutazone and oxyphenbutazone. Br Med J 1977;1: 1500.
143. Chaplin S. Bone marrow depression due to mianserin, phenylbutazone, oxyphenbutazone, and chloramphenicol. I. Adverse Drug React Acute Poisoning Rev 1986;5:97.
144. Aymard J-P, Aymard B, Netter P, et al. Haematological adverse effects of histamine H2-receptor antagonists. Med Toxicol 1988;3:430.
145. Hart RG, Easton JD. Carbamazepine and hematological monitoring. Ann Neurol 1982;11:309.
146. Daum RS, Cohen DL, Smith AL. Fatal aplastic anemia following apparent "dose-related" chloramphenicol toxicity. J Pediatr 1979;94: 403.
147. Testa NG, Hendry JH, Molineux G. Long-term bone marrow damage after cytotoxic treatment: stem cells and microenvironment. In: Testa NG, Gale RP, eds. Hematopoiesis, ed 8. New York, Marcel Dekker, 1988:75.
148. Bowcock SJ, Galton DAG, Goldman JG. Marrow aplasia developing 3 years after treatment with busulphan for chronic myeloid leukemia. Eur J Hematol 1989;42:496.
149. Krug K, Stenzel L. Verlaufsvarianten von panzytopenien nach busulfanbehandlung der chronischen myeloischen leukämie (CML). Folia Haematol 1978;2:181.
150. Furuse N, Hayasaka S, Yamamoto Y, Setogawa T. Retinal microaneurysms in a patient with drug-induced aplastic anemia. Ophthalmologica 1987;195:188.
151. Snyder R, Kocsis JJ. Current concepts of chronic benzene toxicity. CRC Crit Rev Toxicol 1975;3:265.
152. Fishbein L. An overview of environmental and toxicological aspects of aromatic hydrocarbons. I. Benzene. Sci Total Environ 1984;40: 189.
153. Brief RS, Lynch J, Bernath T, Scala RA. Benzene in the workplace. Am Ind Hyg Assoc J 1980;41:616.
154. Winslow C-EA. Summary of the national safety council study of benzol poisoning. J Ind Hyg 1927;9:61.
155. Yin S-N, Li Q, Liu Y, et al. Occupational exposure to benzene in China. Br J Ind Med 1987;44:192.
156. Moszczynski P, Lisiewicz J. Hematological indices of peripheral blood in workers occupationally exposed to benzene, toluene and xylene. Zentralbl Bakt Hyg I Abt Orig B 178 1983.
157. Bowditch M, Elkins HB. Chronic exposure to benzene (benzol). I. The industrial aspects. J Ind Hyg Toxicol 1939;21:321.
158. Vigliani EC, Saita G. Benzene and leukemia. N Engl J Med 1964;271: 872.
159. Aksoy M, Erdem S. Followup study on the mortality and the development of leukemia in 44 pancytopenic patients with chronic exposure to benzene. Blood 1978;52:285.
160. Hamilton A. Benzene (benzol) poisoning. Arch Pathol 1931;11:434, 601.
161. Rejsek K, Rejsková M. Long term observation of chronic benzene poisoning. Acta Med Scand 1955;152:71.
162. Vigliani EC, Forni A. Benzene and leukemia. Environ Res 1976;11: 122.
163. Wester RC, Maibach HI, Gruenke LD, Craig JC. Benzene levels in ambient air and breath of smokers and nonsmokers in urban and pristine environments. J Toxicol Environ Health 1986;18:567.
164. Brandi L, Nilsson PG, Mitelman F. Non-industrial exposure to benzene as leukæmogenic risk factor. Lancet 1977;2:1074.
165. Wallace L, Pellizzari ED, Hartwell T, et al. Concentrations of 20 volatile organic compounds in the air and drinking water of 350 residents of New Jersey compared to concentrations in their exhaled breath. Environ Res 1984;35:293.
166. Cronkite EP. Benzene hematotoxicity and leukemogenesis. Blood Cells 1986;12:129.
167. Srbová J, Teisinger J, Skramovsky S. Absorption and elimination of inhaled benzene in man. Arch Ind Hyg Occ Med 1950;2:1.
168. Sato A, Nakajima T, Fujiwara Y, Hirosawa K. Pharmacokinetics of benzene and toluene. Int Arch Arbeitsmed 1974;33:169.
169. Irons RD, Dent JG, Baker TS, Rickert DE. Benzene is metabolized and covalently bound in bone marrow in situ. Chem Biol Interact 1980;30:241.
170. Andrews LS, Sasame HA, Gillette JR. 3H-benzene metabolism in rabbit bone marrow. Life Sci 1979;25:567.
171. Kalf GF, Post GB, Snyder R. Solvent toxicology: recent advances in the toxicology of benzene, the glycol ethers, and carbon tetrachloride. Annu Rev Pharmacol Toxicol 1987;27:399.
172. Sawahata T, Rickert DE, Greenlee WF. Metabolism of benzene and its metabolites in bone marrow. In: Irons RD, ed. Toxicology of the blood and bone marrow. New York, Raven Press, 1985:141.
173. Greenlee WF, Sun JD, Bus JS. A proposed mechanism of benzene toxicity: formation of reactive intermediates from polyphenol metabolites. Toxicol Appl Pharmacol 1981;59:187.
174. Lutz WK, Schlatter Ch. Mechanism of the carcinogenic action of benzene: irreversible binding to rat liver DNA. Chem Biol Interact 1977;18:241.
175. Dipple A, Pigott MA, Agarwal SK, et al. Optically active benzo [c] phenanthrene diol epoxides bind extensively to adenine in DNA. Nature 1987;327:535.
176. Lee EW, Garner CD, Johnson JT. A proposed role played by benzene itself in the induction of acute cytopenia: inhibition of DNA synthesis. Res Comm Chem Pathol Pharmacol 1988;60:27.
177. Kissling M, Speck B. Further studies on experimental benzene induced aplastic anemia. Blut 1972;25:97.
178. Pellack-Walker P, Blumer JL. DNA damage in L5178YS cells following exposure to benzene metabolites. Mol Pharmacol 1986;30:42.
179. Rithidech K, Au WW, Ramanujam VMS, et al. Induction of chromosome aberrations in lymphocytes of mice after subchronic exposure to benzene. Mutat Res 1987;188:135.
180. Tough IM, Brown WMC. Chromosome aberrations and exposure to ambient benzene. Lancet 1965;1:684.
181. Jablonická A, Vargová M, Karelová J. Cytogenetic analysis of peripheral blood lymphocytes in workers exposed to benzene. J Hyg Epidemiol Microbiol Immunol 1987;31:127.
182. Snyder R, Lee EW, Kocsis JJ. Binding of labeled benzene metabolites to mouse liver and bone marrow. Res Comm Chem Pathol Pharmacol 1978;20:191.
183. Tunek A, Platt KL, Bentley P, Oesch F. Microsomal metabolism of benzene to species irreversibly binding to microsomal protein and effects of modifications of this metabolism. Mol Pharmacol 1978;14: 920.
184. Harper C, Drew RT, Fouts JR. Species differences in benzene hydroxylation to phenol by pulmonary and hepatic microsomes. Drug Metabol Disposition 1975;3:381.
185. Sabourin PJ, Bechtold WE, Birnbaum LS, et al. Differences in metabolism and disposition of inhaled [3H] benzene by F344/N rats and B6C3F1 mice. Toxicol Appl Pharmacol 1988;94:128.
186. Moeschlin S, Speck B. Experimental studies on the mechanism of action of benzene on the bone marrow (radioautographic studies using H-thymidine). Acta Haematol 1967;38:104.
187. Uyeki EM, Ashkar AE, Shoeman DW, Bisel TU. Acute toxicity of benzene inhalation to hemopoietic precursor cells. Toxicol Appl Pharmacol 1977;40:49.
188. Gill DP, Jenkins VK, Kempen RR, Ellis S. The importance of pluripotential stem cells in benzene toxicity. Toxicology 1980;16:163.
189. Hilderbrand RL, Murphy MJ. The effects of benzene inhalation on murine hematopoietic precursor cells (CFU-e, BFU-e and CFU-gm). Int J Cell Cloning 1983;1:240.
190. Seidel HJ, Barthel E, Zinser D. The hematopoietic stem cell compartments in mice during and after long-term inhalation of three doses of benzene. Exp Hematol 1989;17:300.
191. Green JD, Snyder CA, LoBue J, et al. Acute and chronic dose/ response effects of inhaled benzene on multipotential hematopoietic stem (CFU-S) and granulocyte/macrophage progenitor. Toxicol Appl Pharmacol 1981;58:492.
192. Garnett HM, Cronkite EP, Drew RT. Effect of in vivo exposure to benzene on the characteristics of bone marrow adherent cells. Leuk Res 1983;7:803.

193. Gaido K, Wierda D. In vitro effects of benzene metabolites on mouse bone marrow stromal cells. Toxicol App Pharmacol 1984;76:45.
194. Steinberg B. Bone marrow regeneration in experimental benzene intoxication. Blood 1949;4:550.
195. Aoyama K. Effects of benzene inhalation on lymphocyte subpopulations and immune response in mice. Toxicol Appl Pharmacol 1986;85:92.
196. Hsieh GC, Sharma RP, Parker RDR. Subclinical effects of groundwater contaminants. I. Alteration of humoral and cellular immunity by benzene in CD-1 mice. Arch Environ Contam Toxicol 1988;17:151.
197. Bostrom B, Smith K, Ramsay N. Low concentrations of benzene stimulate CFU/GM. Blood 1985;66:119a.
198. Jacobs RH, Cornbleet MA, Vardiman JW, et al. Prognostic implications of morphology and karyotype in primary myelodysplastic syndromes. Blood 1986;67:1765.
199. Hunter FT. Chronic exposure to benzene (benzol). II. The clinical effects. J Ind Hyg Toxicol 1939;21:331.
200. Erf LA, Rhoads CP. The hematological effects of benzene (benzol) poisoning. J Ind Hyg Toxicol 1939;21:421.
201. Goldwater LJ. Disturbances in the blood following exposure to benzol. J Lab Clin Med 1941;26:957.
202. Oldfeldt CO. Benzene poisoning: clinical considerations. Acta Med Scand 1944;119:380.
203. Aksoy M, Koray D, Akgun T, Erdem S, et al. Haematological effects of chronic benzene poisoning in 217 workers. Br J Ind Med 1971;28:296.
204. Savilhati M. Mehr also 100 Vergiftungsfälle durch Benzol in einer Schufabrik. Arch Gwerberpath Gewerbehyg 1956;15:147.
205. Aksoy M, Dincol K, Erdem S, et al. Details of blood changes in 32 patients with pancytopenia associated with long-term exposure to benzene. Br J Ind Med 1972;29:56.
206. Hernberg S, Savilahti M, Ahlman K, Asp S. Prognostic aspects of benzene poisoning. Br J Indust Med 1966;23:204.
207. Rinsky RA, Smith AB, Hornung R, et al. Benzene and leukemia: an epidemiologic risk assessment. N Engl J Med 1987;316:1044.
208. Austin H, Delzell E, Cole P. Benzene and leukemia: a review of the literature and a risk assessment. Am J Epidemiol 1988;127:419.
209. Jacobs A. Benzene and leukaemia. Br J Haematol 1989;72:119.
210. Arp EW, Wolf PH, Checkoway H. Lymphocytic leukemia and exposures to benzene and other solvents in the rubber industry. J Occup Med 1983;25:598.
211. Decoufle P, Blattner WA, Blair A. Mortality among chemical workers exposed to benzene and other agents. Environ Res 1983;30:16.
212. Aksoy M. Chronic lymphoid leukaemia and hairy cell leukaemia due to chronic exposure to benzene: report of three cases. Br J Haematol 1987;66:209.
213. DeGowin RL. Benzene exposure and aplastic anemia followed by leukemia 15 years later. JAMA 1963;185:748.
214. Stewart RD, Dodd HC, Baretta ED, et al. Chronic overexposure to benzene vapor. Toxicol Appl Pharmacol 1967;10:381. Abstract.
215. Gerarde HW. Toxicological studies on hydrocarbons. II. A comparative study of the effect of benzene and certain mono-n-alklybenzenes on hemopoiesis and bone marrow metabolism in rats. AMA Arch Ind Health 1956;13:468.
216. Wolf MA, Rowe VK, McCollister DD, et al. Toxicological studies of certain alkylated benzenes and benzene. AMA Arch Ind Health 1956;14:387.
217. Speck B, Moeschlin S. Die Wirkung von Toluol, Xylol, Chloramphenicol und Thiouracil auf das Knochenmark: experimentelle autoradiographische Studien mit H3-Thymidin. Schweiz Med Wochenschr 1968;98:1684.
218. Jenkins LJ Jr, Jones RA, Siegel J. Long-term inhalation screening studies of benzene, toluene, o-xylene, and cumene on experimental animals. Toxicol App Pharmacol 1970;16:818.
219. Scott JL, Cartwright GE, Wintrobe MM. Acquired aplastic anemia: an analysis of thirty-nine cases and review of the pertinent literature. Medicine 1958;38:119.
220. Mastromatteo E. Hematological disorders following exposure to insecticides. Can Med Assoc J 1964;90:1166.
221. Erslev AJ, Wintrobe MM. Detection and prevention of drug-induced blood dyscrasias. JAMA 1962;181:114.
222. Richards RP, Kramer JW, Baker DB, Krieger KA. Pesticides in rainwater in the northeastern United States. Nature 1987;327:129.
223. Dale WE, Quinby GE. Chlorinated insecticides in the body fat of people in the United States. Science 1963;142:593.
224. Hoffman WS, Adler H, Fishbein WI, Bauer FC. Relation of pesticide concentrations in fat to pathological changes in tissues. Arch Environ Health 1967;15:758.
225. Anselstetter V, Ballschmiter K, Dmochewitz S, Heimpel H. Aplastic anaemia: residue analysis of chlorinated hydrocarbons in human bone marrow biopsy specimens by high resolution gas chromatography. Acta Haematol 1985;73:6.
226. Crawford MAD. Aplastic anaemia due to trinitrotoluene intoxication. Br Med J 1954.
227. Imerman SW, Imerman CP. Dinitrophenol poisoning with thrombocytopenia, granulopenia, anemia and purpura complicated by lung abscess. JAMA 1936;106:1085.
228. Roberts HJ. Aplastic anemia due to pentachlorophenol and tetrachlorophenol. South Med J 1963;56:632.
229. Carlson GW. Aplastic anemia following exposure to products of the sulfite pulp industry. Ann Intern Med 1946;24:277.
230. Hopkins JE, Manoharan A. Severe aplastic anaemia following the use of hair dye: report of two cases and review of literature. Postgrad Med J 1985;61:1003.
231. Reeves JD, Driggers DA, Kiley VA. Household insecticide associated aplastic anaemia and acute leukaemia in children. Lancet 1981;2:368.
232. Stieglitz R, Stobbe H, Schüttmann W. Knochenmarkschäden nach beruflicher Einwirkung des Insektizids gamma-hexachlorcyclohexan (Lindan). Acta Haematol 1967;38:337.
233. Lorand IC, Souza CA, Costa FF. Haematological toxicity associated with agricultural chemicals in Brazil. (Letter) Lancet 1984;1:404.
234. Infante PF, Epstein SS, Newton WA. Blood dyscrasias and childhood tumors and exposure to chlordane and heptachlor. Scand J Work Environ Health 1978;4:137.
235. Epstein SS, Ozonoff D. Leukemias and blood dyscrasias following exposure to chlordane and heptachlor. Mutagenesis 1987;7:527.
236. Stormont RT. The present status of chlordane. JAMA 1955;158:1364.
237. Loge JP. Aplastic anemia following exposure to benzene hexachloride (lindane). JAMA 1965;193:104.
238. West I. Lindane and hematologic reactions. Arch Environ Health 1967;15:97.
239. Stormont RT. Toxic effects of technical benzene hexachloride and its principal isomers. JAMA 1951;147:571.
240. Woodliff HJ, Connor PM, Scopa J. Aplastic anæmia associated with insecticides. Med J Aust 1966;1:628.
241. Jenkyn LR, Budd RC, Fein SH, Cornell CJ. Insecticide/herbicide exposure, aplastic anaemia, and pseudotumor cerebri. Lancet 1979.
242. Stormont RT. Pharmacologic and toxicologic aspects of DDT (chlorophenothane U.S.P.). JAMA 1951;135:728.
243. Friberg L, Martensson J. Case of panmyelophthisis after exposure to chlorophenothane and benzene hydrochloride. AMA Arch Ind Hyg 1953;8:166.
244. Clinico-Pathologic Conference. Exposure to insecticides, bone marrow failure, gastrointestinal bleeding, and uncontrollable infections. Am J Med 1955;19:274.
245. Gallagher RP, Threlfall WJ, Jeffries E, et al. Cancer and aplastic anemia in British Columbia farmers. J Natl Cancer Inst 1984;72:1311.
246. Spirtas R, Hoar SK, Kaminski R, Rosenberg H. Aplastic anemia mortality and occupational exposures. In: Proceedings of the 1985 Public Health Conference on Records and Statistics. Health and Human Services Publication No. PHS 86-1214. Washington, DC, Department of Health and Human Services, 1986:53.
247. Blair A, Grauman DJ, Lubin JH, Fraumeni JF. Lung cancer and other causes of death among licensed pesticide applicators. J Natl Cancer Inst 1983;71:31.
248. Stein WJ, Hayes WJ. Health survey of pest control operators. Ind Med Surg 1964;33:549.
249. Frinci F, Spurbeck GH. A study of workers exposed to the insecticides chlordan, aldrin, dieldrin. Arch Ind Hyg Occup Med 1951;3:64.
250. Ditraglia D, Brown DP, Namekata T, Iverson N. Mortality study of workers employed at organochlorine pesticide manufacturing plants. Scand J Work Environ Health 1981;7:140.
251. Samuels AJ, Milby TH. Human exposure to lindane: clinical, hematological and biochemical effects. J Occup Med 1971;13:147.
252. Wang HH, Grufferman S. Aplastic anemia and occupational pesticide exposure: a case-control study. J Occup Med 1981;23:364.
253. Burmeister LF, Everett GD, Van Lier SF, Isacson P. Selected cancer mortality and farm practices in Iowa. Am J Epidemiol 1983;118:72.
254. Blair A, Thomas TL. Leukemia among Nebraska farmers: a death certificate study. Am J Epidemiol 1979;110:264.
255. Linos A, Kyle RA, O'Fallon WM, Kurland LT. A case-control study of occupational exposures and leukaemia. Int J Epidemiol 1980;9:131.
256. Milby TH, Samuels AJ, Ottoboni F. Humane exposure to lindane: blood lindane levels as a function of exposure. J Occup Med 1968;10:584.
257. Davignon LF, St-Pierre J, Charest G, Tourangeau FJ. A study of the chronic effects of insecticides in man. Can Med Assoc J 1965;92:597.
258. Cullen MR, Rado T, Waldron JA, et al. Bone marrow injury in lithographers exposed to glycol ethers and organic solvents used in multicolor offset and ultraviolet curing printing processes. Arch Environ Health 1983;38:247.
259. Gallichio VS, Casale GP, Bartholomew PW, Watts TD. Altered colony-forming activities of bone marrow hematopoietic stem cells in mice following short-term in vivo exposure to parathion. Int J Cell Cloning 1987;5:231.
260. Gallicchio VS, Casale GP, Watts T. Inhibition of human bone marrow-derived stem cell colony formation (CFU-E, BFU-E, and CFU-GM) following in vitro exposure to organophosphates. Exp Hematol 1987;15:1099.
261. Smadel JE, Jackson EB. Chloromycetin, an antibiotic with chemotherapeutic activity in experimental and viral infections. Science 1944;106:418.

262. Smadel JE. Chloramphenicol (chloromycetin) in the treatment of infectious diseases. Am J Med 1949;7:671.
263. Lewis CN, Putnam LE, Hendricks FD, et al. Chloramphenicol (chloromycetin) in relation to blood dyscrasias with observations on other drugs: a special study. Antibiot Chemother 1952;2:601.
264. Welch H, Lewis CN, Kerlan I. Blood dyscrasias: a nationwide survey. Antibiot Chemother 1954;4:607.
265. Hellriegel KP, Gross R. Follow-up studies in chloramphenicol-induced aplastic anaemia. Postgrad Med J 1974;50:136.
266. Brauer MJ, Dameshek W. Hypoplastic anemia and myeloblastic leukemia following chloramphenicol therapy. N Engl J Med 1967;277:1003.
267. Xiao OS, Yu TG, Linet MS, et al. Chloramphenicol use and childhood leukaemia in Shanghai. Lancet 1987;2:934.
268. Kelly JP, Kaufman DW. Anti-infective drug use in relation to the risk of agranulocytosis and aplastic anemia. Arch Intern Med 1989;149:1036.
269. Wolff JA. Anemias caused by infections and toxins, idiopathic aplastic anemia and anemia caused by renal disease. Pediatr Clin North Am 1957;469.
270. Weiner H. Less drug reactions in Jews? (Letter) N Engl J Med 1969;281:740.
271. Ghitis J. Chloramphenicol in South America. (Letter) N Engl J Med 1970;282:813.
272. Yunis AA. Chloramphenicol-induced bone marrow suppression. Semin Hematol 1973;10:225.
273. Fink TJ, Gump DW. Chloramphenicol: an inpatient study of use and abuse. J Infect Dis 1978;138:690.
274. Settepani JA. The hazard of using chloramphenicol in food animals. J Am Vet Med Assoc 1984;184:930.
275. Hodgkinson R. Blood dyscrasias associated with chloramphenicol. Lancet 1954;1:285.
276. Plaut ME, Best WR. Aplastic anemia after parenteral chloramphenicol: warning renewed. (Letter) N Engl J Med 1982;306:1486.
277. Cone TE Jr, Abelson SM. Aplastic anemia following two days of chloramphenicol therapy: case report of a fatality in a 6-year old girl. J Pediatr 1952;41:340.
278. Fraunfelder FT, Bagby GC, Kelly DJ. Aplastic anemia and chloramphenicol. Am J Ophthalmol 1982;94:268.
279. Brodsky E, Zeidan Z, Biger Y, Schneider M. Topical application of chloramphenicol eye ointment followed by fatal bone marrow aplasia. Israel J Med Sci 1989;25:54.
280. Jandl JH. Aplastic anemias. In: Jandl JH, ed. Blood: textbook of hematology. Boston, Little, Brown, 1987:115.
281. Volini IF, Greenspan I, Ehrlich L, et al. Hemopoietic changes during administration of chloramphenicol (chloromycetin). JAMA 1950;142:1333.
282. Ozer FL, Truax WE, Levin WC. Erythroid hypoplasia associated with chloramphenicol therapy. Blood 1960;16:997.
283. Krakoff IH, Karnofsky DA, Burchenal JH. Effects of large doses of chloramphenicol on human subjects. N Engl J Med 1950;253:7.
284. Scott JL, Finegold SM, Belkin GA, Lawrence JS. A controlled double-blind study of the hematologic toxicity of chloramphenicol. N Engl J Med 1965;272:1137.
285. Suhrland LG, Weisberger AS. Delayed clearance of chloramphenicol from serum in patients with hematologic toxicity. Blood 1969;34:466.
286. Alavi JB. Aplastic anemia associated with intravenous chloramphenicol. Am J Hematol 1983;15:375.
287. Kauffman RE, Thirumoorthi MC, Buckley JA, et al. Relative bioavailability of intravenous chloramphenicol succinate and oral chloramphenicol palmitate in infants and children. J Pediatr 1981;99:963.
288. Kramer WG, Rensimer ER, Ericsson CD, Pickering LK. Comparative bioavailability of intravenous and oral chloramphenicol in adults. J Clin Pharmacol 1984;24:181.
289. Christensen LK, Skovsted L. Inhibition of drug metabolism by chloramphenicol. Lancet 1969;2:1397.
290. Gussoff BD, Lee SL. Chloramphenicol-induced hematopoietic depression: a controlled comparison with tetracycline. Am J Med Sci 1966;251:8.
291. Abou-Khalil S, Salem Z, Yunis AA. Mitochondrial metabolism in normal, myeloid, and erythroid hyperplastic rabbit bone marrow: effect of chloramphenicol. Am J Hematol 1980;8:71.
292. Smith AL, Weber A. Pharmacology of chloramphenicol. Pediatr Clin North Am 1983;30:209.
293. Rosenbach LM, Caviles AP, Mitus WJ. Chloramphenicol toxicity: reversible vacuolization of erythroid cells. N Engl J Med 1960;263:724.
294. Rubin D, Weisberger AS, Botti RE, Storaasli JP. Changes in iron metabolism in early chloramphenicol toxicity. J Clin Invest 1958;37:1286.
295. Oski FA. Hematologic consequences of chloramphenicol therapy. J Pediatr 1979;94:515.
296. Ratzan RJ, Moore MAS, Yunis AA. Effect of chloramphenicol and thiamphenicol on the in vitro colony-forming cell. Blood 1974;43:363.
297. Bostrom B, Smith K, Ramsay NKC. Stimulation of human committed bone marrow stem cells (CFU-GM) by chloramphenicol. Exp Hematol 1986;14:156.
298. Sawada H, Tezuka H, Kamamoto T, et al. Effects of chloramphenicol on hemopoietic cells and their microenvironment in vitro. Acta Haematol 1985;48:1323.
299. Hara H, Kohsaki M, Noguchi K, Nagai K. Effect of chloramphenicol on colony formation from erythrocytic precursors. Am J Hematol 1978;5:123.
300. Firkin FC, Sumner MA, Bradley TR. The influence of chloramphenicol on the bone marrow haemopoietic stem cell compartment. Exp Hematol 1974;2:264.
301. Nara N, Bessho M, Hirashima K, Momoi H. Effects of chloramphenicol on hematopoietic inductive microenvironment. Exp Hematol 1982;10:20.
302. Yunis AA. Mechanisms underlying marrow toxicity from chloramphenicol and thiamphenicol. In: Silber R, LoBue J, Gordon AS, eds. The year in hematology. New York, Plenum, 1978:143.
303. Howell A, Andrews TM, Watts RWE. Bone marrow cells resistant to chloramphenicol in chloramphenicol-induced aplastic anæmia. Lancet 1975;1:65.
304. Goris H, Loeffler M, Bungart B, et al. Hemopoiesis during thiamphenicol treatment. I. Stimulation of stem cells during eradication of intermediate cell stages. Exp Hematol 1989;17:957.
305. Adams GR, Pearson H. Chloramphenicol-responsive chronic neutropenia. N Engl J Med 1983;309:1039.
306. Pazdernik TL, Corbett MD. Role of chloramphenicol reduction products in aplastic anemia. Pharmacology 1980;20:87.
307. Couderc J, Perrodon Y, Ventura M, et al. Specification of the immune response: its suppression induced by chloramphenicol in vitro. Bioscience Rep 1983;3:19.
308. Rowley JD, Blaisdell RK. Abnormal marrow karyotype in chloramphenicol associated aplastic anemia. Clin Res 1967;15:287. Abstract.
309. Venning GR. Identification of adverse reactions to new drugs. II. How were 18 important adverse reactions discovered and with what delays? Br Med J 1983;286:365.
310. McCarthy DD, Chalmers TM. Hematological complications of phenylbutazone therapy: review of the literature and report of two cases. Can Med Assoc J 1964;90:1061.
311. Gaisfort W. Fatality after oxyphenbutazone in Still's disease. Br Med J 1962;2:1517.
312. Ramsey R, Golde DW. Aplastic anemia from veterinary phenylbutazone. JAMA 1976;236:1049.
313. MacKay RJ, French TW, Nguyen HT, Mayhew IG. Effects of large doses of phenylbutazone administration to horses. Am J Vet Res 1983;44:774.
314. Cunningham JL, Leyland MJ, Delamore IW, Price Evans DA. Acetanilide oxidation in phenylbutazone-associated hypoplastic anaemia. Br Med J 1974;3:313.
315. Smith CS, Chinn S, Watts RWE. The sensitivity of human bone marrow granulocyte/monocyte precursor cells to phenylbutazone, oxyphenbutazone and gamma-hydroxyphenylbutazone in vitro, with observations on the bone marrow colony formation in phenylbutazone-induced granulocytopoenia. Biochem Pharmacol 1977;26:847.
316. MacCarty DJ, Brill JM, Harrop DH. Aplastic anemia secondary to gold-salt therapy: report of fatal case and a review of literature. JAMA 1962;179:655.
317. Shearer CA, Parker WA. Chrysotherapy-induced aplastic anemia: a case report. Am J Hosp Pharm 1978;35:1095.
318. Cheson BD, Clegg DO, Moatamed F. Ultrastructural evidence for persistent gold in the bone marrow of a patient with aplastic anemia. Arthritis Rheum 1986;29:128.
319. Bower JS. Aplastic anemia due to gold therapy unsuccessfully treated with BAL. NC Med J 1952;13:340.
320. Baldwin JL, Storb R, Thomas ED, Mannik M. Bone marrow transplantation in patients with gold-induced marrow aplasia. Arthritis Rheum 1977;20:1043.
321. Mant MJ, Russell AS, Percy JS, et al. Immunosuppression as initial treatment for gold induced aplastic anemia. J Rheumatol 1987;14:1026.
322. Alvaro-Gracia JM, Castañeda-Sanz S, Arranz R, et al. Antithymocyte globulin in the treatment of gold induced severe aplastic anemia. J Rheumatol 1988;15:43.
323. Doney K, Storb R, Buckner CD, Thomas ED. Treatment of gold-induced aplastic anaemia with immunosuppressive therapy. Br J Haematol 1988;68:469.
324. Howell A, Gumpel JM, Watts RWE. Depression of bone marrow colony formation in gold-induced neutropenia. Br Med J 1975;1:432.
325. Kay AGL. Myelotoxicity of gold. Br Med J 1976;1:1266.
326. Lawson GB, Jackson WP, Cattanach GS. Arsenic poisoning. Report of twenty-eight cases. JAMA 1925;85:24.
327. Kyle RA, Prase GL. Hematologic aspects of arsenic intoxication. N Engl J Med 1965;273:18.
328. Loveman AB. Toxic granulocytopenia, purpura hemorrhagica and aplastic anemia following the arsphenamines. Ann Intern Med 1932;5:1238.

329. Jerina DM, Daly JW. Arene oxides: a new aspect of drug metabolism. Science 1974;185:573.
330. Nebert DW, Gonzalez FJ. P450 genes: structure, evolution and regulation. Annu Rev Biochem 1987;56:945.
331. Gill DP, Kempen RR, Nash JB, Ellis S. Modifications of benzene myelotoxicity and metabolism by phenobarbital, SKF-525A and 3-methylcholanthrene. Life Sci 1979;25:1633.
332. Gerson WT, Fine DG, Spielberg SP, Sensenbrenner LL. Anticonvulsant-induced aplastic anemia: increased susceptibility to toxic drug metabolites in vitro. Blood 1983;61:889.
333. Weinshilboum R. Pharmacogenetics of methyl conjugation and thiopurine drug toxicity. Prog Clin Biol Res 1983;135:167.
334. Lennard L, Rees CA, Lilleyman JS, Maddocks JL. Childhood leukaemia: a relationship between intracellular 6-mercaptopurine metabolites and neutropenia. Br J Clin Pharmacol 1983;16:359.
335. Lennard L, Murphy MF, Maddocks JL. Severe megaloblastic anaemia associated with abnormal azathioprine metabolism. Br J Clin Pharmacol 1984;17:171.
336. Lennard L, VanLoon JA, Lilleyman JS, Weinshilboum RM. Thiopurine pharmacogenetics in leukemia: correlation of erythrocyte thiopurine methyltransferase activity and 6-thioguanine nucleotide concentrations. Clin Pharmacol Ther 1987;41:18.
337. Price DA. Acetylation. In: Kalow W, Goedde HW, Agarwal DP, eds. Ethnic differences in reactions to drugs and xenobiotics. New York, Alan R Liss, 1986:209.
338. Shear NH, Spielberg SP, Grant DM, et al. Differences in metabolism of sulfonamides predisposing to idiosyncratic toxicity. Ann Intern Med 1986;105:179.
339. DeRenzo A, Formisano S, Rotoli B. Bone marrow aplasia and thiamphenicol. Haematology 1981;66:98.
340. Roussy P, Reiffers J, Broustet A, et al. Insuffisance medullaire au thiamphenicol: deux observations. Nouv Presse Med 1978;7:2073.
341. Ferrari V. Introductory address: salient features of thiamphenicol: review of clinical pharmacokinetics and toxicity. Sex Transm Dis 1984;11:336.
342. Bernard J. Note on thiamphenicol. In: Hibino S, Takaku F, Shahidi NT, eds. Aplastic anemia. Baltimore, University Park Press, 1978: 355.
343. Yunis AA. Chloramphenicol toxicity: 25 years of research. Am J Med 1989;87:3–44N.
344. Murray TR, Downey KM, Yunis AA. Chloramphenicol-mediated DNA damage and its possible role in the inhibitory effects of chloramphenicol on DNA synthesis. J Lab Clin Med 1983;102:926.
345. Yunis AA, Arimura GK, Isildar M. DNA damage induced by chloramphenicol and its nitroso derivative: damage in intact cells. Am J Hematol 1987;24:77.
346. Jimenez JJ, Arimura GK, Abou-Khalil WH, Isildar M, et al. Chloramphenicol-induced bone marrow injury: possible role of bacterial metabolites of chloramphenicol. Blood 1987;70:1180.
347. Krishna G, Aykac I, Siegel D. Recent studies on the mechanisms of chloramphenicol activation responsible for aplastic anemia. In: Najean Y, ed. Safety problems related to chloramphenicol and thiamphenicol therapy. New York, Raven Press, 1981:5.
348. Pohl LR, Reddy GB, Krishna G. A new pathway of metabolism of chloramphenicol which influences the interpretation of its irreversible binding to protein in vivo. Biochem Pharmacol 1979;28: 2433.
349. Camitta BM. The role of viral infections in aplastic anemia. Haematol Blood Transfus 1979;24:39.
350. Kurtzman G, Young N. Virus-associated bone marrow failure. Clin Haematol 1989;2:51.
351. Baranski B, Young N. Hematologic manifestations of viral illness. Hematol Oncol Clin North Am 1987;1:167.
352. Young N, Mortimer PP. Viruses and bone marrow failure. Blood 1984;63:729.
353. Young N. Hematologic and hematopoietic consequences of B19 parvovirus infection. Semin Hematol 1988;25:159.
354. Young NS. Human parvoviruses. In: Gorbach SL, Bartlett JG, Blacklow NR, eds. Infectious diseases in medicine and surgery. Philadelphia, WB Saunders, 1992.
355. Kurtzman GJ, Platanias L, Lustig L, Frickhofen N, et al. Feline parvovirus propagates in cat bone marrow cultures and inhibits hematopoietic colony formation in vitro. Blood 1989;74:71.
356. Cossart YE, Field AM, Cant B, et al. Parvovirus-like particles in human sera. Lancet 1975;1:72.
357. Ager EA, Chin TDY, Poland JD. Epidemic erythema infectiosum. N Engl J Med 1966;275:1326.
358. Balfour Jr HH. Erythema infectiosum (fifth disease): clinical review and description of 91 cases seen in an epidemic. Clin Pediatr 1969;8: 721.
359. Chorba TL, Coccia P, Holman RC, et al. Role of parvovirus B19 in aplastic crisis and erythema infectiosum (fifth disease). J Infect Dis 1986;154:383.
360. Reid DM, Reid TMS, Rennie JAN, et al. Human parvovirus-associated arthritis: a clinical and laboratory description. Lancet 1985;1:419.
361. White DG, Woolf AD, Mortimer PP, et al. Human parvovirus arthropathy. Lancet 1985;1:422.
362. Lyngar E. Samtidig optreden av anemisk kriser hos 3 barn i en familie med hemolytisk ikterus. Nord Med 1942;14:1246.
363. Gasser C. Akute erythroblastopenie: 10 falle aplastischer erythroblastenkrisen mit riesenproerythroblasten bei allergisch-taxischen Zustandsbildern. Helv Paediatr Acta 1949;4:107.
364. Owren PA. Congenital hemolytic jaundice: the pathogenesis of the "hemolytic crisis." Blood 1948;3:231.
365. Weiland HT, Salimans MMM, Fibbe WE, et al. Prolonged parvovirus B19 infection with severe anaemia in a bone marrow transplant recipient. (Letter) Br J Haematol 1989;710:300.
366. Lien-Keng K. Erythroblastopenia with giant pro-erythroblasts in kwashiorkor. Blood 1957;12:171.
367. Zucker JM, Tchernia G, Vuylsteke P, et al. Acute and transitory erythroblastopenia in kwashiorkor under treatment. Nouv Rev Fr Hematol Blood Cells 1971;11:131.
368. Pierce LE, Rath CE. Evidence for folic acid deficiency in the genesis of anemic sickle cell crisis. Blood 1962;20:19.
369. Alperin JB. Folic acid deficiency complicating sickle cell anemia. Arch Intern Med 1967;120:398.
370. Broccia G, Dessalvi P. Acute pure red cell aplasia following bromosulphophthalein injection in a patient with non-Hodgkin lymphoma. Haematologica 1983;68:680.
371. Choremis CB, Megas HA, Liaromati AA, Michael SC. Aplastic crisis in the course of infectious diseases: report of 10 cases. Helv Paediatr Acta 1961;2:134.
372. Jootar S, Srichaikul R, Atichartakaran V. Pure red cell aplasia in Thailand: report of twenty four cases. Southeast Asian J Trop Med Public Health 1985;16:291.
373. Evans JPM, Rossiter MA, Kumaran TO, et al. Human parvovirus aplasia: case due to cross infection in a ward. (Letter) Br Med J 1984;288:681.
374. Shneerson JM, Mortimer PP, Vandervelde EM. Febrile illness due to a parvovirus. Br Med J 1980;280:1580.
375. Bell LM, Naides SJ, Stoffman P, et al. Human parvovirus B19 infection among hospital staff members after contact with infected patients. N Engl J Med 1989;321:485.
376. Mortimer PP, Luban NLC, Kelleher JF, Cohen BJ. Transmission of serum parvovirus-like virus by clotting-factor concentrates. Lancet 1983;2:482.
377. Lefrère J, Courouc A, Bertrand Y, et al. Human parvovirus and aplastic crisis in chronic hemolytic anemias: a study of 24 observations. Am J Hematol 1986;23:271.
378. McLellan NJ, Rutter N. Hereditary spherocytosis in sisters unmasked by parvovirus infection. Postgrad Med J 1987;63:49.
379. Nunoue T, Koike T, Koike R, et al. Infection with human parvovirus (B19), aplasia of the bone marrow and a rash in hereditary spherocytosis. J Infect 1987;14:67.
380. Kurtzman G, Gascon P, Caras M, et al. B19 parvovirus replicates in circulating cells of acutely infected patients. Blood 1988;71:1448.
381. Doran HM, Teall AJ. Neutropenia accompanying erythroid aplasia in human parvovirus infection. (Letter) Br J Haematol 1988;69:287.
382. Anderson MJ, Higgins PG, Davis LR, et al. Experimental parvoviral infection in humans. J Infect Dis 1985;152:257.
383. Lefrere JJ. Peripheral thrombocytopenia in human parvovirus infection. (Letter) J Clin Pathol 1987;40:469.
384. Lefrère JJ, Courouc AM, Kaplan C. Parvovirus and idiopathic thrombocytopenic purpura. (Letter) Lancet 1989;1:279.
385. Conrad ME, Studdard H, Anderson LJ. Case report: aplastic crisis in sickle cell disorders—bone marrow necrosis and human parvovirus infection. Am J Med Sci 1988;295:212.
386. Pardoll DM, Rodeheffer RJ, Smith RRL, Charache S. Aplastic crisis due to extensive bone marrow necrosis in sickle cell disease. Arch Intern Med 1982;142:2223.
387. Frickhofen N, Raghavachar A, Heit W, et al. Human parvovirus infection. (Letter) N Engl J Med 1986;314:646.
388. Saunders PWG, Reid MM, Cohen BJ. Human parvovirus induced cytopenias: a report of five cases. (Letter) Br J Haematol 1986;63: 407.
389. Hanada T, Koike K, Takeya T, et al. Human parvovirus B19-induced transient pancytopenia in a child with hereditary spherocytosis. Br J Haematol 1988;70:113.
390. Hamon MD, Newland AC, Anderson MJ. Severe aplastic anaemia after parvovirus infection in the absence of underlying haemolytic anaemia. (Letter) J Clin Pathol 1988;41:1242.
391. Serjeant GR, Topley JM, Mason K, et al. Outbreak of aplastic crises in sickle cell anaemia associated with parvovirus-like agent. Lancet 1981;2:595.
392. Saarinen UM, Chorba TL, Tattersall P, et al. Human parvovirus B19-induced epidemic acute red cell aplasia in patients with hereditary hemolytic anemia. Blood 1986;67:1411.
393. Lefrère JJ, Courouc A-M, Bertrand Y, et al. Human parvovirus and aplastic crisis in chronic hemolytic anemias: a study of 24 observations. Am J Hematol 1986;23:271.
394. Anderson MJ, Jones SE, Minson AC. Diagnosis of human parvovirus infection by dot-blot hybridization using cloned viral DNA. J Med Virol 1985;15:163.

395. Clewley JP. Detection of human parvovirus using a molecularly cloned probe. J Med Virol 1985;15:173.
396. Cohen BJ, Mortimer PP, Pereira MS. Diagnostic assays with monoclonal antibodies for the human serum parvovirus-like virus (SPLV). J Hyg Camb 1983;91:113.
397. Kajigaya S, Shimada T, Fujita S, Young NS. A genetically engineered cell line that produces empty capsids of B19 (human) parvovirus. Proc Natl Acad Sci USA 1989;86:7601.
398. Anderson LJ, Hurwitz ES. Human parvovirus B19 and pregnancy. Clin Perinatol 1988;15:273.
399. Leads from the MMWR: risks associated with human parvovirus B19 infection. JAMA 1989;261:1406.
400. Anand A, Gray ES, Brown T, et al. Human parvovirus infection in pregnancy and hydrops fetalis. N Engl J Med 1987;316:183.
401. Cotmore SF, McKie VC, Anderson LJ, et al. Identification of the major structural and nonstructural proteins encoded by human parvovirus B19 and mapping of their genes by procaryotic expression of isolated genomic fragments. J Virol 1989;60:548.
402. Porter HJ, Quantrill AM, Fleming KA. B19 parvovirus infection of myocardial cells. (Letter) Lancet 1988;1:535.
403. Schwarz TF, Roggendorf M, Hottentrager B, et al. Human parvovirus B19 infection in pregnancy. (Letter) Lancet 1988;2:566.
404. Frickhofen N, Young NS. Persistent parvovirus B19 infections in humans. Microbial Pathogen 1989;7:319.
404a. Brown KE, Anderson SM, Young NS. Erythrocyte P antigen: cellular receptor for B19 parvovirus. Science 1993;262:114.
405. Ozawa K, Kurtzman G, Young NS. Replication of the B19 parvovirus in human bone marrow cultures. Science 1986;233:883.
406. Kurtzman G, Ozawa K, Hanson GR, et al. Chronic bone marrow failure due to persistent B19 parvovirus infection. N Engl J Med 1987;317:287.
407. Kurtzman G, Cohen B, Myers P, et al. Persistent B19 parvovirus infection as a cause of severe anemia in children with acute lymphocytic leukemia in remission. Lancet 1988;2:1159.
408. Ozawa K, Kurtzman G, Young N. Productive infection by B19 parvovirus of human erythroid bone marrow cells in vitro. Blood 1987;70:384.
409. Yaegashi N, Shiraishi H, Takeshita T, et al. Propagation of human parvovirus B19 in primary culture of erythroid lineage cells derived from fetal liver. J Virol 1989;63:2422.
410. Mortimer PP, Humphries RK, Moore JG, et al. A human parvovirus-like virus inhibits hematopoietic colony formation in vitro. Nature 1983;302:426.
411. Young NS, Harrison M, Moore HG, et al. Direct demonstration of the human parvovirus in erythroid progenitor cells infected in vitro. J Clin Invest 1984;74:2024.
412. Ozawa K, Ayub J, Kajigaya S, et al. The gene encoding the nonstructural protein of B19 (human) parvovirus may be lethal in transfected cells. J Virol 1962;62:2884.
413. Rubin E, Gottlieb C, Vogel P. Syndrome of hepatitis and aplastic anemia. Am J Med 1968;45:88.
414. Levy RN, Sawitsky A, Florman AL, Rubin E. Fatal aplastic anemia after hepatitis. N Engl J Med 1965;273:1118.
415. Ajlouni K, Doeblin TD. The syndrome of hepatitis and aplastic anaemia. Br J Haematol 1974;27:345.
416. Hagler L, Pastore RA, Bergin JJ, Wrensch MR. Aplastic anemia following viral hepatitis: report of two fatal cases and literature review. Medicine 1975;54:139.
417. Zeldis JB, Dienstag JL, Gale RP. Aplastic anemia and non-A, non-B hepatitis. Am J Med 1983;74:64.
418. Viala J-J, Bryon P-A, Cordel J-C, et al. Discussions du role des hépatitis virales dans le déclenchement des insuffisances médullaires chroniques. Lyons Méd 1970;223:1019.
419. Böttiger LE, Westerholm B. Aplastic anemia. III. Aplastic anaemia and infectious hepatitis. Acta Med Scand 1972;192:323.
420. Pikis A, Kavaliotis J, Manios S. Incidence of aplastic anemia in viral hepatitis in children. Scand J Infect Dis 1988;20:109.
421. Cargnel A, Vigano P, Davoli C, et al. Sporadic acute non-A non-B hepatitis complicated by aplastic anemia. Am J Gastroenterol 1983;78: 245.
422. Sandberg T, Lindquist O, Norkrans G. Fatal aplastic anaemia associated with non-A, non-B hepatitis. Scand J Infect Dis 1984;16:403.
423. Perrillo RP, Pohl DA, Roodman ST, Tsai CC. Acute non-A, non-B hepatitis with serum sickness-like syndrome and aplastic anemia. JAMA 1981;245:494.
424. Tzakis AG, Arditi M, Whitington PF, et al. Aplastic anemia complicating orthotopic liver transplantation for non-A, non-B hepatitis. N Engl J Med 1988;319:393.
425. Stock PG, Steiner ME, Freese D, et al. Hepatitis-associated aplastic anemia after liver transplantation. Transplantation 1987;43:595.
426. Forbes G, O'Grady HG, Williams R. Aplastic anemia after liver transplantation for non-A, non-B hepatitis. N Engl J Med 1989;320: 122.
427. Camitta BM, Nathan DG, Forman EN, et al. Posthepatic severe aplastic anemia: an indication for early bone marrow transplantation. Blood 1974;43:473.
428. Kojima S, Matsuyama K, Kodera Y. Bone marrow transplantation for hepatitis-associated aplastic anemia. Acta Haematol 1988;79:7.
429. Witherspoon RP, Storb R, Shulman H, et al. Marrow transplantation in hepatitis-associated aplastic anemia. Am J Hematol 1984;17:269.
430. Linares M, Jarque I, Pallares P, Tuset T. Recovery from aplastic anemia after non-A, non-B posttranfusion hepatitis. (Letter) Ann Intern Med 1988;109:513.
431. Albert E, Thomas ED, Nisperos B, Storb R. HLA antigens and haplotypes in 200 patients with aplastic anemia. Transplantation 1976;22: 528.
432. Dhingra K, Michels SD, Winton EF, Gordon DS. Transient bone marrow aplasia associated with non-A, non-B hepatitis. Am J Hematol 1988;29:168.
433. Firkin FC, Nicholls K, Whelan G. Transient myeloid and erythroid aplasia associated with infectious hepatitis. Br Med J 1978;4:1534.
434. Wilson HA, McLaren GD, Dworken HJ, Tebbi K. Transient pure red-cell aplasia: cell-mediated suppression of erythropoiesis associated with hepatitis. Ann Intern Med 1980;92:196.
435. Nagaraju M, Weitzman S, Baumann G. Viral hepatitis and agranulocytosis. Digest Dis 1973;18:247.
436. Ireland R, Gillett D, Mieli-Vergani G, Mufti G. Pre-ALL and non-A, non-B hepatitis infection. Leuk Res 1988;12:795.
437. Foon KA, Mitsuyasu RT, Schroff RW, et al. Immunologic defects in young male patients with hepatitis-associated aplastic anemia. Ann Intern Med 1984;100:657.
438. Strauss RG, Bove KE, Lake A, Kisker CT. Acquired immunodeficiency in hepatitis-associated aplastic anemia. J Pediatr 1975;86:910.
439. Wang WC, Herrod HG, Presbury GJ. Lymphocyte subsets in children with aplastic anemia. Am J Med Sci 1986;291:304.
440. Kojima S, Matsuyama K, Kodera Y, Okada J. Circulating activated suppressor T lymphocytes in hepatitis-associated aplastic anaemia. Br J Haematol 1989;71:147.
441. Bannister P, Miloszewski K, Barnard D, Losowsky MS. Fatal marrow aplasia associated with non-A, non-B hepatitis. Br Med J 1983;286: 1314.
442. Choo QL, Kuo G, Weiner AJ, LR, et al. Isolation of cDNA clone derived from a blood-borne non-A, non-B viral hepatitis genome. Science 1989;244:359.
443. Bierman HR, Nelson ER. Hematodepressive diseases of Thailand. Ann Intern Med 1965;62:867.
444. Halstead SB. Dengue: hematologic aspects. Semin Hematol 1982;19: 116.
445. Casals J, Hoogstraal H, Johnson KM, et al. A current appraisal of hemorrhagic fevers in the U.S.S.R. Am J Trop Med Hyg 1966;15:751.
446. Johnson KM, Halstead SB, Cohen SM. Hemorrhagic fevers of Southeast Asia and South America: a comparative appraisal. Prog Med Virol 1967;9:106.
447. Young NS. Flaviviruses and bone marrow failure. JAMA 1990;263: 3065.
448. Tigertt WD, Crosby WH, Berge TO, et al. The virus of Venezuelan equine encephalomyelitis as an antineoplastic agent in man. Cancer 1962;15:628.
449. Nakao S, Lai C-J, Young NS. Dengue virus, a flavivirus, propagates in human bone marrow progenitors and hematopoietic cell lines. Blood 1989;74:1235.
450. Kurane I, Innis BL, Nisalak A, et al. Human T cell responses to dengue virus antigens: proliferative responses and interferon gamma production. J Clin Invest 1989;83:506.
451. Royal Marsden Hospital Bone Marrow Transplant Team. Failure of syngeneic bone marrow graft without preconditioning in post-hepatitis marrow aplasia. Lancet 1977;2:742.
452. Nakamura S, Sato T, Maeda T, Sato Y. Viral hepatitis B and aplastic anemia. Tohoku J Exp Med 1975;116:101.
453. Casciato DA, Klein CA, Kaplowitz N, Scott JL. Aplastic anemia associated with type B viral hepatitis. Arch Intern Med 1978;138:1557.
454. Aoyagi K, Ohhara N, Okamura S, et al. Aplastic anemia associated with type A viral hepatitis: possible role of T lymphocytes. Jpn J Med 1987;26:348.
455. Domenech P, Palomeque A, Martinez-Gutiérrez A, et al. Severe aplastic anaemia following hepatitis A. Acta Haematol 1986;76:227.
456. Smith D, Gribble TJ, Yeager AS, et al. Spontaneous resolution of severe aplastic anemia associated with viral hepatitis A in a 6-year-old child. Am J Hematol 1978;5:247.
457. Lin CK, Gau JP. Aplastic anaemia is not aetiologically associated with hepatitis-B in Taiwan. (Letter) Eur J Hematol 1989;42:505.
458. Koziol DE, Holland PV, Alling DW, et al. Antibody to hepatitis B core antigen as a paradoxical marker for non-A, non-B hepatitis agents in donated blood. Ann Intern Med 1986;104:488.
459. Zeldis JB, Mugishima H, Steinberg HN, et al. In vitro hepatitis B infection of human bone marrow cells. J Clin Invest 1986;78:411.
460. Zeldis JB, Farraye FA, Steinberg HN. In vitro hepatitis B virus suppression of erythropoiesis is dependent on the multiplicity of infection and is reversible with anti-HBs antibodies. Hepatology 1988;8:755.
461. Busch FW, deVos S, Flehmig B, et al. Inhibition of in vitro hematopoiesis by hepatitis A virus. Exp Hematol 1987;15:978.
462. Zeldis JB, Boender PJ, Hellings JA, Steinberg H. Inhibition of human

hemopoiesis by non-A, non-B hepatitis virus. J Med Virol 1989;27: 34.
463. Lie-Injo LE, Balasagaram M, Lopez CG, Herrera AR. Hepatitis B virus DNA in liver and white blood cells of patients with hepatoma. DNA 1983;2:301.
464. Piazza M, Piccinino F, Matano F. Haematological changes in viral (MHV-3) murine hepatitis. Nature 1965;205:1034.
465. Hunstein W, Perings E, Eggeling B, Uhl N. Panmyelophthise und Virushepatitis: Experimentelle untersuchungen mit dem Mäuse-hepatitis-virus MHV3. Acta Haematol 1969;42:336.
466. Koziner B, Hadler N, Parrillo J, Ellman L. Agranulocytosis following infectious mononucleosis. JAMA 1973;225:1235.
467. Neel EU. Infectious mononucleosis: death due to agranulocytosis and pneumonia. JAMA 1976;236:1493.
468. Eriksson KF, Holmberg L, Bergstrand CG. Infectious mononucleosis and agranulocytosis. Scand J Infect Dis 1979;11:307.
469. Purtilo DT, Zelkowitz L, Harada S, et al. Delayed onset of infectious mononucleosis associated with acquired agammaglobulinemia and red cell aplasia. Ann Intern Med 1984;101:180.
470. Bruyn GAW, Schelfhout LJDM. Transient syndrome of inappropriate antidiuretic hormone secretion in a patient with infectious mononucleosis and pure red cell aplasia. Neth J Med 1986;29:167.
471. Lazarus KH, Baehner RL. Aplastic anemia complicating infectious mononucleosis: a case report and review of the literature. Pediatrics 1981;67:907.
472. Baranski B, Armstrong G, Truman JT, et al. Epstein-Barr virus in the bone marrow of patients with aplastic anemia. Ann Intern Med 1988;109:695.
473. Ahronheim GA, Auger F, Ghibu F, et al. Primary infection by Epstein-Barr virus presenting as aplastic anemia. (Letter) N Engl J Med 1983;309:313.
474. Bacigalupo A, Frassoni F, van Lint MT. Acyclovir for the treatment of severe aplastic anemia. (Letter) N Engl J Med 1984;310:1606.
475. Gomez-Almaguer D, Marfil-Rivera J, Kudish-Wersh A. Acyclovir in the treatment of aplastic anemia. Am J Hematol 1988;29:172.
476. Tosato G, Magrath I, Koski I, et al. Activation of suppressor T cells during Epstein-Barr-virus–induced infectious mononucleosis. N Engl J Med 1979;301:1133.
477. Shadduck RK, Winkelstein A, Zeigler Z, et al. Aplastic anemia following infectious mononucleosis: possible immune etiology. Exp Hematol 1979;7:264.
478. Schimke RN, Collins D, Cross D. Nasopharyngeal carcinoma, aplastic anemia, and various malignancies in a family: possible role of Epstein-Barr virus. Am J Med Genet 1987;27:195.
479. Jones JF, Shurin S, Abramowsky C, et al. T-cell lymphomas containing Epstein-Barr viral DNA in patients with chronic Epstein-Barr virus infections. N Engl J Med 1988;318:733.
480. Sixbey JW, Vesterinen EH, Nedrud JG, et al. Replication of Epstein-Barr virus in human epithelial cells infected in vitro. Nature 1983;306:480.
481. Sixbey JW, Nedrud JG, Raab-Traub N, et al. Epstein-Barr virus replication in oropharyngeal epithelial cells. N Engl J Med 1983;310: 1225.
482. Revoltella RP, Vigneti E, Fruscalzo A, et al. Epstein-Barr virus DNA sequences in precursor monocyte-macrophage cell lines established from the bone marrow of children with maturation defects of haematopoiesis. J Gen Virol 1989;70:1203.
483. Reiner AP, Spivak JL. Hematophagocytic histiocytosis: a report of 23 new patients and a review of the literature. Medicine 1988;67: 19203.
484. Risdall RJ, McKenna RW, Nesbit ME, et al. Virus-associated hemophagocytic syndrome: a benign histiocytic proliferation distinct from malignant histiocytosis. Cancer 1979;44:993.
485. Tomomasa T, Fukushima N, Kuribayashi T, et al. A case of virus-associated haemophagocytic syndrome with hypoplastic anaemia. Pediatrics 1986;145:550.
486. Marmont AM, Bacigalupo A, van Lint MT, et al. Treatment of severe aplastic anemia with high-dose methylprednisolone and antilymphocyte globulin. In: Young NS, Levine AS, Humphries RK, eds. Aplastic anemia: stem cell biology and advances in treatment. New York, Alan R Liss, 1984:271.
487. Craighead JE, Hanshaw JB, Carpenter CB. Cytomegalovirus infection after renal allotransplantation. JAMA 1967;201:725.
488. Mutter W, Reddehase MJ, Busch FW, et al. Failure in generating hemopoietic cells is the primary cause of death from cytomegalovirus disease in the immunocompromised host. J Exp Med 1988;167:1645.
489. Reddehase MJ, Mutter W, Münch K, et al. CD8-positive T lymphocytes specific for murine cytomegalovirus immediate-early antigens mediate protective immunity. J Virol 1987;61:3102.
490. Osborn JE, Shahidi NT. Thrombocytopenia in murine cytomegalovirus infection. J Lab Clin Med 1973;81:53.
491. Apperley JF, Dowding C, Hibbin J, Buiter J, et al. The effect of cytomegalovirus on hemopoiesis: in vitro evidence for selective infection of marrow stromal cells. Exp Hematol 1989;17:38.
492. Rakusan TA, Juneja HS, Fleischmann WR Jr. Inhibition of hemopoietic colony formation by human cytomegalovirus in vitro. J Infect Dis 1989;159:127.
493. Carney WP, Rubin RH, Hoffman RA, Hansen WP, et al. Analysis of T lymphocyte subsets in cytomegalovirus mononucleosis. J Immunol 1981;126:2114.
494. Scadden DT, Zon LI, Groopman JE. Pathophysiology and management of HIV-associated hematologic disorders. Blood 1989;74:1455.
495. Costello C. Haematological abnormalities in human immunodeficiency virus (HIV) disease. J Clin Pathol 1988;41:711.
496. Ganser A. Abnormalities of hematopoesis in the acquired immunodeficiency syndrome. Blut 1988;56:49.
497. Zon LI, Groopman JE. Hematologic manifestations of the human immune deficiency virus (HIV). Semin Hematol 1988;25:208.
498. Spivak JL, Selonick SE, Quinn TC. Acquired immune deficiency syndrome and pancytopenia. JAMA 1983;250:3084.
499. Castella A, Croxson TS, Mildvan D, et al. The bone marrow in AIDS: a histologic, hematologic, and microbiologic study. Am J Clin Pathol 1985;84:425.
500. Namiki TS, Boone DC, Meyer PR. A comparison of bone marrow findings in patients with acquired immunodeficiency syndrome (AIDS) and AIDS related conditions. Hematol Oncol 1987;5:99.
501. Spivak JL, Bender BS, Quinn TC. Hematologic abnormalities in the acquired immune deficiency syndrome. Am J Med 1984;77:224.
502. Treacy M, Lai L, Costello C, Clark A. Peripheral blood and bone marrow abnormalities in patients with HIV related disease. Br J Haematol 1987;65:289.
503. Zon LI, Arkin C, Groopman JE. Haematologic manifestations of the human immune deficiency virus (HIV). Br J Haematol 1987;66:251.
504. Baumann MA, Pacheco J, Paul CC, et al. Paroxysmal nocturnal hemoglobinuria associated with the acquired immunodeficiency syndrome. Arch Intern Med 1988;148:212.
505. Schneider DR, Picker LJ. Myelodysplasia in the acquired immune deficiency syndrome. Am J Clin Pathol 1985;84:144.
506. Geller SA, Muller R, Greenberg ML, Siegal FP. Acquired immunodeficiency syndrome: distinctive features of bone marrow biopsies. Arch Pathol Lab Med 1985;109:138.
507. Osborne BM, Guarda LA, Butler JJ. Bone marrow biopsies in patients with the acquired immunodeficiency syndrome. Hum Pathol 1984;15:1048.
508. Zucker-Franklin D, Cao Y. Megakaryocytes of human immunodeficiency virus-infected individuals express viral RNA. Proc Natl Acad Sci USA 1989;86:5595.
509. Donahue RE, Johnson MM, Zon LI, et al. Suppression of in vitro haematopoiesis following human immunodeficiency virus infection. Nature 1987;326:200.
510. Carlo-Stella C, Ganser A, Hoelzer D. Defective in vitro growth of the hemopoietic progenitor cells in the acquired immunodeficiency syndrome. J Clin Invest 1987;80:286.
511. Gascon P, Rameshwar P, Sathe S. Studies on the mechanism of AIDS associated anemia. (Abstract) Blood 1988;72(Suppl 1):351a.
512. Levitt LJ, Reyes GR, Moonka DK, et al. Human T cell leukemia virus-I-associated T-suppressor cell inhibition of erythropoiesis in a patient with pure red cell aplasia and chronic T-gamma-lymphoproliferative disease. J Clin Invest 1988;81:538.
513. Leiderman IZ, Greenberg ML, Adelsberg BR, Siegel FP. A glycoprotein inhibitor of in vitro granulopoiesis associated with AIDS. Blood 1987;70:1267.
514. Kalyanaraman VS, Narayanan R, Feorino P, et al. Isolation and characterization of a human T cell leukemia virus type II from a hemophilia-A patient with pancytopenia. EMBO J 1985;4:1455.
515. Vinters HV, Mah V, Mohrmann R, Wiley CA. Evidence for human immunodeficiency virus (HIV) infection of the brain in a patient with aplastic anemia. Acta Neuropathol 1988;76:321.
516. Nissen-Druey C. Pathophysiology of aplastic anaemia. In: Hinton K, Tindall B, eds. Clinical haematology. London, Bailliere Tindall, 1989: 37.
517. Hardy WD Jr, Essex M, McClelland AJ. Feline leukemia virus. New York, Elsevier/North Holland, 1980.
518. Tambourin PE, Wendling F, Jasmin C, Smadja-Joffe F. The physiopathology of Friend leukemia. Leuk Res 1979;3:117.
519. Cotter SM, Essex M. Acute lymphoblastic leukemia, aplastic anemia. Am J Pathol 1977;87:265.
520. Onions D, Jarrett O, Testa N, et al. Selective effect of feline leukemia virus on early erythroid precursors. Nature 1982;296:156.
521. Abkowitz JL, Holly RD, Adamson JW. Retrovirus-induced feline pure red cell aplasia: the kinetics of erythroid marrow failure. J Cell Physiol 1987;132:571.
522. Rojko JL, Hoover EA, Quackenbush SL, Olsen RG. Reactivation of latent feline leukaemia virus infection. Nature 1982;298:385.
523. Abkowitz JL, Holly RD, Grant CK. Retrovirus-induced feline pure red cell aplasia. J Clin Invest 1987;80:1056.
524. Riedel N, Hoover EA, Dornsife RE, Mullins JI. Pathogenic and host range determinants of the feline aplastic anemia retrovirus. Proc Natl Acad Sci USA 1988;85:2758.
525. Rausen AR, Richter P, Tallal L, Cooper LZ. Hematologic effects of intrauterine rubella. JAMA 1967;199:75.
526. Zinkham WH, Medearis DN, Osborn JE. Blood and bone-marrow findings in congenital rubella. J Pediatr 1967;71:512.

527. Bayer WL, Sherman FE, Michaels RH, et al. Purpura in congenital and acquired rubella. N Engl J Med 1965;273:1362.
528. Gresser I, Chany C. Isolation of measles virus from the washed leucocytic fraction of blood. Proc Soc Exp Biol Med 1963;113:695.
529. Fehr J, Hofmann V, Kappeler U. Transient reversal of thrombocytopenia in idiopathic thrombocytopenic purpura by high-dose intravenous gamma globulin. N Engl J Med 1982;306:1254.
530. Oski FA, Naiman JL. Effect of live measles vaccine on the platelet count. N Engl J Med 1966;275:352.
531. Espinoza C, Kuhn C. Viral infection in megakaryocytes in varicella with purpura. Am J Clin Pathol 1974;61:203.
532. Jerushalmy Z, Kaminski E, Kohn A, DeVries A. Interaction of Newcastle disease virus with megakaryocytes in cell cultures of guinea pig bone marrow. Proc Soc Exp Biol Med 1963;114:687.
533. Modai Y, Oren R, de Vries A, Kohn A. Thrombocytopenia in guinea pigs infected by encephalomyocarditis virus (EMC). Thromb Diath Haemorrh 1967;18:686.
534. Dalton AJ, Law LW, Moloney JB, Manaker RA. An electron microscopic study of a series of murine lymphoid neoplasms. J Natl Cancer Inst 1961;27:747.
535. Curzon PGD, Muers MF, Rajah SM. Aplastic anemia associated with influenza A infection. Scand J Haematol 1983;30:232.
536. Lewis SM, Dacie JV. The aplastic anaemia: paroxysmal nocturnal haemoglobinuria syndrome. Br J Haematol 1967;13:236.
537. Gardner FH. Aplastic anemia syndrome in paroxysmal nocturnal hemoglobinuria (PNH). In: Hibino S, Takaku F, Shahidi NT, eds. Aplastic anemia. Baltimore, University Park Press, 1978:273.
538. Conrad ME, Barton JC. The aplastic anemia-paroxysmal nocturnal hemoglobinuria syndrome. Am J Hematol 1979;7:61.
539. Rotoli B, Luzzatto L. Paroxysmal nocturnal hemoglobinuria. Semin Hematol 1989;26:201.
540. Yang T-Y, Yang H-Y, Chu H-T, et al. Differential diagnosis of aplastic anemia and paroxysmal nocturnal hemoglobinuria. Chin Med J 1963;82:740.
541. Quagliana JM, Cartwright GE, Wintrobe MM. Paroxysmal nocturnal hemoglobinuria following drug-induced aplastic anemias. Ann Intern Med 1964;61:1045.
542. Aksoy M. Different types of malignancies due to occupational exposure to benzene: a review of recent observations in Turkey. Environ Res 1980;23:181.
543. Wasi P, Kruetrachue M, Na-Nakorn S. Aplastic anemia–paroxysmal nocturnal hemoglobinuria syndrome-acute leukemia in the same patient: the first record of such occurrence. J Med Assoc Thailand 1970;53:656.
544. Rotoli B, Robledo R, Luzzatto L. Decreased number of circulating BFU-Es in paroxysmal nocturnal hemoglobinuria. Blood 1982;60: 157.
545. Moore JG, Humphries RK, Frank MM, Young N. Characterization of the hematopoietic defect in paroxysmal nocturnal hemoglobinuria. Exp Hematol 1986;14:222.
546. Ben-Bassat I, Brok-Simoni F, Ramot B. Complement-sensitive red cells in aplastic anemia. Blood 1975;46:357.
547. Nissen C, Gratwohl A, Speck B, et al. Acquired aplastic anaemia: a PNH-like disease? Br J Haematol 1986;64:355.
548. Kruatrachue M, Wasi P, Na-Nakorn S. Paroxysmal nocturnal haemoglobinuria in Thailand with special reference to an association with aplastic anaemia. Br J Haematol 1978;39:267.
548a. Takeda J, Miyata T, Kawagoe K, et al. Deficiency of the GPI anchor caused by a somatic mutation of the PIG-A gene in paroxysmal nocturnal hemoglobinuria. Cell 1993;73:703.
548b. Miyata T, Yamada N, Iida Y, et al. Abnormalities of *PIG-A* transcripts in granulocytes from patients with paroxysmal nocturnal hemoglobinuria. N Engl J Med 1994;330:249.
549. Dessypris EN, Clark DA, McKee LC Jr, Krantz SB. Increased sensitivity to complement of erythroid and myeloid progenitors in paroxysmal nocturnal hemoglobinuria. N Engl J Med 1983;309:690.
550. Rotoli B, Robledo R, Scarpato N, Luzzatto L. Two populations of erythroid cell progenitors in paroxysmal nocturnal hemoglobinuria. Blood 1984;64:847.
551. Moore JG, Frank MM, Muller-Eberhard HJ, Young NS. Decay accelerating factor is present on PNH hematopoietic progenitors and lost during in vitro erythropoiesis. J Exp Med 1985;162:1182.
552. Shichishima T, Terasawa T, Uchida T, Kariyone S. Complement sensitivity of erythroblasts and erythropoietic precursors in paroxysmal nocturnal haemoglobinuria (PNH). Br J Haematol 1989;72: 578.
553. Abkowitz JL, Fialkow PJ, Niebrugge DJ, et al. Pancytopenia as a clonal disorder of a multipotent hematopoietic stem cell. J Clin Invest 1984;73:258.
554. Hoffman R, Young N, Ershler WB, et al. Diffuse fasciitis and aplastic anemia: a report of four cases revealing an unusual association between rheumatologic and hematologic disorders. Medicine 1982;61: 373.
555. Moore TL, Zuckner J. Eosinophilic fasciitis. Semin Arthritis Rheum 1980;9:228.
556. Debusscher L, Bitar N, De Maubeuge J, et al. Eosinophilic fasciitis and severe aplastic anemia: favorable response to either antithymocyte globulin or cyclosporine A in blood and skin disorders. Transplant Proc 1988;10:310.
557. Mir MA, Geary CG, Delamore IW. Hypoimmunoglobulinaemia and aplastic anaemia. Scand J Haematol 1977;19:225.
558. Uchiyama T, Nagai K, Yamagishi M, et al. Pokeweed mitogen-induced B cell differentiation in idiopathic aplastic anemia associated with hypogammaglobulinemia. Blood 1978;52:77.
559. Josse JW, Zacks SI. Thymoma and pancytopenia. N Engl J Med 1958;259:113.
560. Thomas CV, Manivel JC. Thymic carcinoma and aplastic anemia: report of a previously undocumented association. Am J Hematol 1987;25:333.
561. Littman BH, Cooke CL, Hoffman R. Hypogammaglobulinemia followed by aplastic anemia with suppressor lymphocytes: a case report. Clin Immunol Immunopathol 1978;10:344.
562. Miller ME. Thymic dysplasia ("Swiss agammaglobulinemia"). I. Graft versus host reaction following bone-marrow transfusion. J Pediatr 1967;70:730.
563. Hathaway WE, Fulginiti VA, Pierce CW, et al. Graft-vs-host reaction following a single blood transfusion. JAMA 1967;201:1015.
564. Hathaway WE, Githens JH, Blackburn WR, et al. Aplastic anemia histiocytosis and erythrodermia in immunologically deficient children: probable human runt disease. N Engl J Med 1965;273:953.
565. Naiman JL, Punnett HH, Lischner HW, et al. Possible graft-versus-host reaction after intrauterine transfusion for Rh erythroblastosis fetalis. N Engl J Med 1969;281:697.
566. Parkman R, Mosier D, Umansky I, et al. Graft-versus-host disease after intrauterine and exchange transfusions for hemolytic disease of the newborn. N Engl J Med 1974;290:359.
567. Elfenbien GJ, Kallman CH, Tutschka PJ, et al. The immune system in 40 aplastic anemia patients receiving conventional therapy. Blood 1989;53:652.
568. Falcao RP, Voltarelli JC, Bottura C. Some immunological studies in aplastic anaemia. J Clin Lab Immunol 1983;10:25.
569. Sabbe LJM, Haak HL, Te Velde J, et al. Immunological investigations in aplastic anemia patients. Acta Haematol 1984;71:178.
570. Goldstein IM, Coller BS. Aplastic anemia in pregnancy: recovery after normal spontaneous delivery. (Letter) Ann Intern Med 1975;82: 537.
571. Maizels G. Aplastic anaemia of pregnancy with recovery. S Afr Med J 1951;25:973.
572. Collins DJ, Rosenthal DS, Goldstein DP, Moloney F. Aplastic anemia in pregnancy. Obstet Gynecol 1972;39:884.
573. Evans IL. Aplastic anaemia in pregnancy remitting after abortion. (Letter) Br Med J 1968;3:166.
574. Crisp AJ. Remission of pregnancy hypoplastic anaemia and "malignant" pre-eclampsia after delivery: a case report and discussion. Br J Clin Pract 1900;34:304.
575. Aitchison RGM, Marsh JCW, Hows JM, et al. Pregnancy associated aplastic anaemia: a report of five cases and review of current management. Br J Haematol 1989;73:541.
576. Fleming AF. Hypoplastic anaemia in pregnancy. J Obstet Gynaec Br Commonw 1968;75:138.
577. Rovinsky JJ. Primary refractory anemia complicating pregnancy and delivery. Obstet Gynecol Survey 1959;14:149.
578. Knispel JW, Lynch VA, Viele BD. Aplastic anemia in pregnancy: a case report, review of the literature, and a re-evaluation of management. Obstet Gynecol Survey 1976;31:523.
579. Suda T, Omine M, Tsuchiya J, Maekawa T. Prognostic aspects of aplastic anemia in pregnancy: experience in six cases and review of literature. Blut 1978;36:285.
580. Issaragrisil S, Vanachivanavin V, Piankijagum A, Kruatrachue M. Aplastic anemia with pregnancy. J Med Assoc Thailand 1982;65: 111.
581. Hsu MC, Ho HN, Lee TY, et al. Aplastic anemia and pregnancy. J Formosan Med Assoc 1984;83:1128.
582. Holly RG. Hypoplastic anemia in pregnancy. Obstet Gynecol 1953;1: 535.
583. Kociba GJ, Caputo CA. Aplastic anemia associated with estrus in pet ferrets. J Am Vet Med Assoc 1981;178:1293.
584. Bernard SL, Leathers CW, Brobst DF, Gorham JR. Estrogen-induced bone marrow depression in ferrets. Am J Vet Res 1983;44:657.
585. Tyslowitz R, Dingemanse E. Effect of large doses of estrogens on the blood picture of dogs. Endocrinology 1941;29:817.
586. Crafts RC. The effects of estrogens on the bone marrow of adult female dogs. Blood 1948;3:276.
587. Van Kruiningen HJ, Friedland TB. Responsive estrogen-induced aplastic anemia in a dog. Clin Rep 1987;191:91.
588. Castrodale D, Bierbaum O, Helwig EB, MacBryde CM. Comparative studies of the effects of estradiol and stilbestrol upon the blood, liver, and bone marrow. Endocrinology 1941;29:363.
589. Dukes PP, Goldwasser E. Inhibition of erythropoiesis by estrogens. Endocrinology 1961;69:21.
590. Fried W, Tichler T, Dennenberg I, et al. Effects of estrogens on hematopoietic stem cells and on hematopoiesis of mice. J Lab Clin Med 1974;83:807.
591. Kurnick JE, Robinson WA, Dickey CA. In vitro granulocytic colony-

forming potential of bone marrow from patients with granulocytopenia and aplastic anemia. Proc Soc Exp Biol Med 1971;137:917.
592. Ragab AH, Gilkerson E, Crist WM, Phelan E. Granulopoiesis in childhood aplastic anemia. J Pediatr 1976;88:790.
593. Kern P, Heimpel H, Heit W, Kubanek B. Granulocytic progenitor cells in aplastic anaemia. Br J Haematol 1977;35:613.
594. Haak HL, Goselink HM, Veenhof W, et al. Acquired aplastic anemia in adults. IV. Histological and CFU studies in transplanted and non-transplanted patients. Scand J Haematol 1977;19:159.
595. Barrett AJ, Faille A, Balitrand N, et al. Bone marrow culture in aplastic anaemia. J Clin Pathol 1979;32:660.
596. Rickard KA, Brown RD, Wilkinson T, Kronenberg H. The colony forming cell in the myeloproliferative disorders and aplastic anaemia. Scand J Haematol 1979;22:121.
597. Yoshida K, Miura I, Takahashi T, et al. Quantitative and qualitative analysis of stem cells of patients with aplastic anemia. Scand J Haematol 1983;30:317.
598. Hinterberger W, Geissler K, Fischer M, et al. Aplastic anemia: assessment of myeloid progenitor cells in the bone marrow and blood provides prognostic information. Acta Haematol 1985;73:1.
599. Hansi W, Rich I, Heimpel H, et al. Erythroid colony forming cells in aplastic anaemia. Br J Haematol 1977;37:483.
600. Moriyama Y, Sato M, Kinoshita Y. Studies on hematopoietic stem cells. XI. Lack of erythroid burst-forming units (BFU-E) in patients with aplastic anemia. Am J Hematol 1979;6:11.
601. Umemura T, Takeichi N, Kaneko S, et al. Significance of abnormally high endogenous CFU-E numbers in aplastic anemia. Acta Haematol Jpn 1985;49:837.
602. Hara H, Kai S, Fushimi M, et al. Pluripotent hemopoietic precursors in vitro (CFU_{mix}) in aplastic anemia. Exp Hematol 1980;8:1165.
603. Li S, Champlin R, Fitchen JH, Gale RP. Abnormalities of myeloid progenitor cells after "successful" bone marrow transplantation. J Clin Invest 1985;75:234.
604. Bacigalupo A, Podesta M, Mingari MC, et al. Immune suppression of hematopoiesis in aplastic anemia: activity of T-gamma lymphocytes. J Immunol 1981;125:1449.
605. Harrison DE. Use of genetic anaemias in mice as tools for haematological research. Clin Haematol 1979;8:239.
606. Russell ES. Hereditary anemias of the mouse: a review for geneticists. Adv Genet 1979;200:357.
607. Lewis JP, O'Grady LF, Bernstein SE, et al. Growth and differentiation of transplanted W/Wv marrow. Blood 1967;30:601.
608. Chabot B, Stephenson DA, Chapman VW, et al. The proto-oncogene c-kit encoding a transmembrane tyrosine kinase receptor maps to the mouse W locus. Nature 1988;335:88.
609. Geissler EN, Ryan MA, Housman DE. The dominant-white spotting (W) locus of the mouse encodes the c-kit proto-oncogene. Cell 1988;55:185.
609a. Williams DE, Ersenman J, Baird A, et al. Identification of a ligand for the c-kit proto-oncogene. Cell 1990;63:167.
609b. Zsebo KM, Wypych J, McNeice IK, et al. Identification, purification, and biological characterization of hematopoietic stem cell factor from buffalo rat liver–conditioned medium. Cell 1990;63:195.
609c. Anderson DM, Lyman SD, Baird A, et al. Molecular cloning of mast cell growth factor, a hematopoietin that is active in both membrane bound and soluble forms. Cell 1990;63:235.
609d. Huang E, Nocka K, Beier DR, et al. The hematopoietic growth factor KL is encoded at the Sl locus and is the ligand of the c-kit receptor, the gene product of the W locus. Cell 1990;63:225.
609e. Copeland NG, Gilbert DJ, Cho BG, et al. Mast cell growth factor maps near the steel locus on mouse chromosome 10 and is deleted in a number of steel alleles. Cell 1990;63:175.
609f. Zsebo KM, Williams DA, Geissler EN, et al. Stem cell factor (SCF) is encoded at the Sl locus of the mouse and is the ligand for the c-kit tyrosine kinase receptor. Cell 1990;63:213.
609g. Flanagan JG, Leder P. The *kit* ligand: a cell surface molecule altered in steel mutant fibroblasts. Cell 1990;63:185.
610. Spangrude G. Enrichment of murine haemopoietic stem cells: diverging roads. Immunol Today 1989;10:344.
611. Ogawa M, Porter PN, Nakahata T. Renewal and commitment to differentiation of hemopoietic stem cells (an interpretive review). Blood 1983;61:823.
612. Rosendaal M, Hodgson GS, Bradley TR. Haemopoietic stem cells are organized for use on the basis of their generation-age. Nature 1976;264:68.
613. Sinclair WK. Hydroxyurea: differential lethal effects on cultured mammalian cells during the cell cycle. Science 1965;150:1729.
614. Hodgson GS, Bradley TR. Properties of haematopoietic stem cells surviving 5-fluorouracil treatment: evidence for a pre-CFU-S cell? Nature 1979;281:381.
615. Mauch PM, Greenberger JS, Botnick LE, et al. Evidence for structured variation in self-renewal capacity in long-term bone marrow cultures. Proc Natl Acad Sci USA 1980;77:2927.
616. Spooncer E, Lord BI, Dexter TM. Defective ability to self-renew in vitro of highly purified primitive haematopoietic cells. Nature 1985;316:62.
617. Fialkow P. Primordial cell pool size and lineage relationships of five human cell types. Ann Hum Genet 1973;37:39.
618. Nakano T, Waki N, Asai H, Kitamura Y. Long-term monoclonal reconstitution of erythropoiesis in genetically anemic W/Wv mice by injection of 5-fluorouracil-treated bone marrow cells of Pgk-1b/Pgk-la mice. Blood 1987;70:1758.
619. Mintz B, Anthony K, Litwin S. Monoclonal derivation of mouse myeloid and lymphoid lineages from totipotent hematopoietic stem cells experimentally engrafted in fetal hosts. Proc Natl Acad Sci USA 1984;81:7835.
620. Harrison DE. Normal production of erythrocytes by mouse marrow continuous for 73 months. Proc Natl Acad Sci USA 1973;70:3184.
621. Siminovitch L, Till JE, McCulloch EA. Decline in colony-forming ability of marrow cells subjected to serial transplantation into irradiated mice. Cell Comp Physiol 1964;64:23.
622. Ross EAM, Anderson N, Micklem HS. Serial depletion and regeneration of the murine hematopoietic system: implications for hematopoietic organization and the study of cellular aging. J Exp Med 1982;155:432.
623. Mauch P, Rosenblatt M, Hellman S. Permanent loss in stem cell self renewal capacity following stress to the marrow. Blood 1988;72:1193.
624. Mauch P, Hellman S. Loss of hematopoietic stem cell self-renewal after bone marrow transplantation. Blood 1989;74:872.
625. Harrison DE, Astle CM. Loss of stem cell repopulating ability upon transplantation: effects of donor age, cell number, and transplantation procedure. J Exp Med 1982;156:1767.
626. MacMillan JR, Wolf NS. Depletion of reserve in the hemopoietic system. II. Decline in CFU-S self-renewal capacity following prolonged cell cycling. Stem Cells 1982;2:45.
627. Lemischka IR, Raulet DH, Mulligan RC. Developmental potential and dynamic behavior of hematopoietic stem cells. Cell 1986;45:917.
628. Spangrude GJ, Heimfeld S, Weissman IL. Purification and characterization of mouse hematopoietic stem cells. Science 1988;241:58.
629. Morley A, Trainor K, Blake J. A primary stem cell lesion in experimental chronic hypoplastic marrow failure. Blood 1975;45:681.
630. Morley A, Blake J. An animal model of chronic aplastic marrow failure. I. Late marrow failure after busulfan. Blood 1974;44:49.
631. Fitchen JH, Cline MJ. The effect of granulopoietic stress in mice with "latent" bone marrow failure. Exp Hematol 1980;8:788.
632. Botnick LE, Hannon EC, Hellman S. Limited proliferation of stem cells surviving alkylating agents. Nature 1976;262:68.
633. Chervenick PA, Boggs DR. Patterns of proliferation and differentiation of hematopoietic stem cells after compartment depletion. Blood 1971;37:568.
634. Fitchen JH, Deregnaucourt J, Cline MJ. An in vitro model of hematopoietic injury in chronic hypoplastic anemia. Cell Tissue Kinet 1981;14:85.
635. McManus PM, Weiss L. Busulfan-induced chronic bone marrow failure: changes in cortical bone, marrow stromal cells, and adherent cell colonies. Blood 1984;64:1036.
636. Fried W, Kedo A, Barone J. Effects of cyclophosphamide and of busulfan on spleen colony-forming units and on hematopoietic stroma. Cancer Res 1977;37:1205.
637. Knospe WH, Crosby WH. Aplastic anaemia: a disorder of the bone-marrow sinusoidal microcirculation rather than stem-cell failure? Lancet 1971;1:20.
638. Tavassoli M, Maniatis A, Crosby WH. Induction of sustained hemopoiesis in fatty marrow. Blood 1974;43:33.
639. Islam A. Do bone marrow fat cells or their precursors have a pathogenic role in idiopathic aplastic anaemia? Med Hypoth 1988;25:209.
640. Malik F, Gordon MY, Goldman JM, Gordon-Smith EC. Comparisons of the composition of fat cells obtained from the marrow of normal individuals or of subjects with aplastic anemia and from bone marrow cultures. Exp Hematol 1984;12:191.
641. Samson JP, Hulstaert CE, Molenaar I, Nieweg HO. Fine structure of the bone marrow sinusoidal wall in idiopathic and drug-induced panmyelopathy. Acta Haematol 1972;48:218.
642. Dexter TM, Moore MAS. In vitro duplication and "cure" of haemopoietic defects in genetically anaemic mice. Nature 1977;269:412.
643. Knospe WH, Hinrichs B, Fried W, et al. Normal colony stimulating factor (CSF) production by bone marrow stromal cells and abnormal granulopoiesis with decreased CFUc in S1/S1d mice. Exp Hematol 1976;4:125.
644. Wright DG, Greenberger JS. Long-term bone marrow culture. New York, Alan R Liss, 1984.
645. Cashman J, Eaves AC, Eaves CJ. Regulated proliferation of primitive hematopoietic progenitor cells in long-term human marrow cultures. Blood 1985;66:1002.
646. Singer JW, Keating A, Cuttner J, et al. Evidence for a stem cell common to hematopoiesis and its in vitro microenvironment: studies of patients with clonal hematopoietic neoplasia. Leuk Res 1984;8:535.
647. Singer JW, Charbord P, Keating A, et al. Simian virus 40-transformed adherent cells from human long-term marrow cultures: cloned cell lines produce cells with stromal and hematopoietic characteristics. Blood 1987;70:464.
648. Simmons PJ, Przepiorka D, Thomas ED, Torok-Storb B. Host origin of marrow stromal cells following allogeneic bone marrow transplantation. Nature 1987;328:429.

649. Laver J, Jhanwar SC, O'Reilly RJ, Castro-Malaspina H. Host origin of the human hematopoietic microenvironment following allogeneic bone marrow transplantation. Blood 1987;70:1966.
650. Juneja HS, Gardner FH, Minguell JJ, Helmer RE III. Abnormal marrow fibroblasts in aplastic anemia. Exp Hematol 1984;12:221.
651. Hotta T, Kato T, Maeda H, et al. Functional changes in marrow stromal cells in aplastic anaemia. Acta Haematol 1985;74:65.
652. Yoshida K, Takatsu H, Miura I, et al. Long-term liquid culture of marrow CFU-C from normal subjects and patients with aplastic anemia. Acta Haematol Jpn 1986;49:829.
653. Juneja HS, Lee S, Gardner FH. Human long-term bone marrow cultures in aplastic anemia. Int J Cell Cloning 1989;7:129.
654. Wiktor-Jedrzejczak W, Siekierzynski M, Szczylik C, et al. Aplastic anaemia with marrow defective in formation of fibroblastoid cell colonies in vitro. Scand J Haematol 1982;28:82.
655. Juneja HS, Gardner FH. Functionally abnormal marrow stromal cells in aplastic anemia. Exp Hematol 1985;13:194.
656. Hirata J, Umemura T, Kaneko S, et al. Difference of bone marrow adipocyte colony-forming capacity between aplastic anemia and iron deficiency anemia. Leuk Res 1988;12:179.
657. Gordon MY, Gordon-Smith EC. Bone marrow fibroblast function in relation to granulopoiesis in aplastic anemia. Br J Haematol 1983;53: 483.
658. Nakao S, Matsushima K, Young N. Deficient interleukin 1 production by aplastic anemia monocytes. Br J Haematol 1989;71:431.
659. Broudy VC, Zuckerman KS, Jetmalani S, et al. Monocytes stimulate fibroblastoid bone marrow stromal cells to produce multilineage hematopoietic growth factors. Blood 1986;68:530.
660. Zsebo KM, Yuschenkoff VN, Schiffer S, et al. Vascular endothelial cells and granulopoiesis: interleukin-1 stimulates release of G-CSF and GM-CSF. Blood 1988;71:99.
661. Lee M, Segal GM, Bagby GC. Interleukin-1 induces human bone marrow-derived fibroblasts to produce multilineage hematopoietic growth factors. Exp Hematol 1987;15:983.
662. Fibbe WE, van Damme J, Billiau A, et al. Interleukin 1 induces human marrow stromal cells in long-term culture to produce granulocyte colony-stimulating factor and macrophage colony-stimulating factor. Blood 1988;71:430.
663. Nissen C, Moser Y, dalle Carbonare V, et al. Complete recovery of marrow function after treatment with anti-lymphocyte globulin is associated with high, whereas early failure and development of paroxysmal nocturnal haemoglobinuria are associated with low endogenous G-CSA-release. Br J Haematol 1989;72:573.
664. Merchav S, Tatarsky I, Sharon R. Aplastic anemia associated with in vitro inhibition of erythropoiesis by bone marrow-adherent cells. Eur J Haematol 1988;41:429.
665. Suda T, Mizoguchi H, Miura Y, et al. Suppression of *in vitro* granulocyte-macrophage colony formation by the peripheral mononuclear phagocytic cells of patients with idiopathic aplastic anaemia. Br J Haematol 1981;47:433.
666. Hanada T, Abe T. The effect of peripheral blood adherent cells from patients with aplastic anemia on in vitro hematopoiesis. Exp Hematol 1983;11:298.
667. Roodman GD, Horadam VW, Wright TL. Inhibition of erythroid colony formation by autologous bone marrow adherent cells from patients with the anemia of chronic disease. Blood 1983;62:406.
668. Shah G, Dexter TM, Lanotte M. Interferon production by human marrow stomal cells. Br J Haematol 1983;54:365.
669. Resnitzky D, Yarden A, Zipori D, Kimchi A. Autocrine β-related interferon controls c-myc suppression and growth arrest during hematopoietic cell differentiation. Cell 1986;46:31.
670. Saksela E, Virtanen I, Hovi T, et al. Monocyte is the main producer of human leukocyte alpha interferons following Sendai virus induction. Prog Med Virol 1984;30:78.
671. Zuckerman KS, Prince CW, Ribadeneira M. S1/S1d mouse bone marrow stroma in vitro contains an active radiation-sensitive inhibitor of normal hemopoiesis. Blood 1986;68:1201.
672. Onoue H, Ebi Y, Nakayama H, et al. Suppressive effect of S1/S1d mouse embryo-derived fibroblast cell lines on diffusible factor-dependent proliferation of mast cells. Blood 1989;74:1557.
673. Alexanian R. Erythropoietin excretion in bone marrow failure and hemolytic anemia. J Lab Clin Med 1973;82:438.
674. Takeichi N, Umemura T, Nishimura J, et al. Regulation of erythropoietin and burst-promoting activity production in patients with aplastic anemia and iron deficiency anemia. Acta Haematol 1988;80: 145.
675. Fukamachi H, Urabe A, Saito T, et al. Burst-promoting activity in anemia and polycythemia. Int J Cell Cloning 1986;4:74.
676. Hara H, Okamoto T, Ohe Y, Kanamaru A. Mixed colony inducing activity in sera from patients with acquired aplastic anemia. Acta Haematol 1983;46:35.
677. Okamoto T, Kanamaru A, Hara H, Nagai K. Burst-promoting activity (BPA) without erythropoietin (Ep) activity in sera of aplastic anemia patients fractionated by chromatofocusing column. Exp Hematol 1982;10:844.
678. Yen YP, Zabala P, Doney K, et al. Hematopoietic growth factors in human serum: erythroid burst-promoting activity in normal subjects and in patients with severe aplastic anemia. J Lab Clin Med 1985;106: 384.
679. Dicke KA, Lowenberg B. In vitro analysis of pancytopenia: its possible relevance to the clinical course and to the preleukemic state in the aplastics. In: Lindahl-Kiessling K, Osoba D, eds. Proceedings of the 8th Leukocyte Culture Conference. London, Academic Press, 1974: 417.
680. Entringer MA, Robinson WA, Dreging CJ. Colony stimulating activity in normal human serum tested against human bone marrow. Exp Hematol 1980;8:1232.
681. Nissen C, Moser Y, Weis J, et al. The release of interleukin-2 (IL-2) and colony stimulating activity (CSA) in aplastic anemia patients: opposite behaviour with improvement of bone marrow function. Blut 1986;52:221.
682. Weatherly TL, Fleisher TA, Strong DM. Reduced granulocyte-macrophage colony-stimulating activity by mitogen-stimulated lymphocytes from patients with aplastic anaemia. Br J Haematol 1979;43:335.
683. Enomoto K, Kawakita M, Kishimoto S, Katayama N, Miyake T. Thrombopoiesis and megakaryocyte colony stimulating factor in the urine of patients with aplastic anaemia. Br J Haematol 1980;45:551.
684. Hoffman R, Mazur E, Bruno E, Floyd V. Assay of an activity in the serum of patients with disorders of thrombopoiesis that stimulates formation of megakaryocytic colonies. N Engl J Med 1981;305:533.
685. Adams JA, Barrett AJ. Haematopoietic stimulators in the serum of patients with severe aplastic anaemia. Br J Haematol 1982;52:327.
686. Miyake T, Kawakita M, Enomoto K, Murphy MJ. Partial purification and biological properties of thrombopoietin extracted from the urine of aplastic anemia patients. Stem Cells 1982;2:129.
687. Ogata K, Kuriya S, Dan K, Nomura T. Partial purification of human urinary megakaryocyte colony-stimulating factor. Exp Cell Biol 1989;57:19.
688. Nissen C, Moser Y, Weis J, Speck B. Stimulatory serum factors in aplastic anaemia. I. Serum "releaser" activity for haemopoietic growth factors, a regulator? Br J Haematol 1985;61:491.
689. Nissen C, Moser Y, Speck B, et al. Stimulatory serum factors in aplastic anaemia. II. Prognostic significance for patients treated with high dose immunosuppression. Br J Haematol 1985;61:499.
690. Nissen C, Moser Y, Speck B, Bendy J. Haemopoietic stimulators and inhibitors in aplastic anaemia serum. Br J Haematol 1983;54:519.
691. Watari K, Asano S, Shirafuji N, et al. Serum granulocyte colony-stimulating factor levels in healthy volunteers and patients with various disorders as estimated by enzyme immunoassay. Blood 1989;73:117.
692. Ershler WB, Ross J, Finlay JL, Shahidi NT. Bone-marrow microenvironment defect in congenital hypoplastic anemia. N Engl J Med 1980;302:1321.
693. Horita S, Koizumi S, Miura M, et al. Impaired ability of T4+ lymphocytes in the active stage of congenital hypoplastic anemia to promote in vitro growth of blood erythroid burst-forming units (BFU-E). Acta Haematol Jpn 1988;51:985.
694. Lipton JM, Kudisch M, Gross R, Nathan DG. Defective erythroid progenitor differentiation system in congenital hypoplastic (Diamond-Blackfan) anemia. Blood 1986;67:962.
695. Mathé G, Amiel JL, Schwarzenberg L, et al. Bone marrow graft in man after conditioning by antilymphocytic serum. Br Med J 1970;2: 131.
696. Thomas ED, Storb R, Giblett ER, et al. Recovery from aplastic anemia following attempted marrow transplantation. Exp Hematol 1976;4: 97.
697. Territo MC. Autologous bone marrow repopulation following high dose cyclophosphamide and allogeneic marrow transplantation in aplastic anemia. Br J Haematol 1977;36:305.
698. Bussel A, Dumont J, Schenmetzler C, et al. Long-term complete autologous reconstitution following cyclophosphamide and allogeneic marrow infusion in a case of severe aplastic anemia. Nouv Rev Fr Hematol 1985;27:15.
699. Young N, Speck B. Antithymocyte and antilymphocyte globulins: clinical trials and mechanism of action. In: Young NS, Levine A, Humphries RK, eds. Aplastic anemia: stem cell biology and advances in treatment. New York, Alan R Liss, 1984:221.
700. Speck B, Gratwhol A, Nissen C, et al. Treatment of severe aplastic anemia. Exp Hematol 1986;14:126.
701. Frickhofen N, Kaltwasser JP. Immunosuppressive treatment of aplastic anemia: a prospective, randomized multicenter trial evaluating antilymphocyte globulin (ALG) versus ALG and cyclosporin A. Blut 1988;56:191.
702. Champlin RE, Feig SA, Sparkes RS, Gale RP. Bone marrow transplantation from identical twins in the treatment of aplastic anaemia: implication for the pathogenesis of the disease. Br J Haematol 1984;56: 455.
703. Appelbaum FR, Cheever MA, Fefer A, et al. Recurrence of aplastic anemia following cyclophosphamide and syngeneic bone marrow transplantation: evidence for two mechanisms of graft failure. Blood 1985;65:553.
704. Kagan WA, Ascensao JA, Pahwa RN, et al. Aplastic anemia: presence in human bone marrow of cells that suppress myelopoiesis. Proc Natl Acad Sci USA 1976;73:2890.

705. Ascensao J, Kagan W, Moore M, et al. Aplastic anaemia: evidence for an immunological mechanism. Lancet 1976;1:669.
706. Bagby GC Jr, Goodnight SH, Mooney WM, Richert-Boe K. Prednisone-responsive aplastic anemia: a mechanism of glucocorticoid action. Blood 1979;54:322.
707. Gorski A, Rowinska D, Skopinska E, Orlowski T. Circulating suppressor cells in aplastic anemia. Vox Sang 1979;36:356.
708. Roodman GD, Ascensao JL, Banisadre M, et al. Autoimmune pancytopenia: lymphocyte inhibition of autologous but not allogenic bone marrow growth in vitro. Am J Med 1980;69:325.
709. Saitoh H, Yagi Y, Nakahata T, et al. A case of severe childhood aplastic anemia associated with lymphocyte mediated hemopoietic suppression: recovery following cyclophosphamide treatment. Acta Haematol Jpn 1983;46:808.
710. Hoffman RA, Zanjani ED, Lutton JD, et al. Suppression of erythroid-colony formation by lymphocytes from patients with aplastic anemia. N Engl J Med 1977;296:10.
711. Hoffman R, Zanjani ED, Lutton JD, et al. Suppression of erythroid-colony formation by lymphocytes from patients with aplastic anemia. N Engl J Med 1977;296:10.
712. Nissen C, Cornu P, Gratwohl A, Speck B. Peripheral blood cells from patients with aplastic anaemia in partial remission suppress growth of their own bone marrow precursors in culture. Br J Haematol 1980;45:233.
713. Shionoya S, Motoyoshi K, Saito M, et al. Immunosuppressive therapy in aplastic anemia based on in vitro culture studies. Acta Haematol Jpn 1986;49:1282.
714. Bacigalupo A, Podesta M, van Lint MT, et al. Severe aplastic anaemia: correlation of *in vitro* tests with clinical response to immunosuppression in 20 patients. Br J Haematol 1981;47:423.
715. Takaku F, Suda T, Mizoguchi H, et al. Effect of peripheral blood mononuclear cells from aplastic anemia patients on the granulocyte-macrophage and erythroid colony formation in samples from normal human bone marrow in vitro: a cooperative work. Blood 1980;55: 937.
716. Da WM. In vitro studies on the pathogenesis of aplastic anemia in Chinese patients. Exp Hematol 1988;16:336.
717. Abdou NI, Verdirame JD, Amare M, Abdou NL. Heterogeneity of pathogenetic mechanisms in aplastic anemia. Ann Intern Med 1981;95:43.
718. Morris TCM, Vincent PC, Young GAR, et al. CFU-C inhibitors in aplastic anaemia. Blut 1984;48:61.
719. Nagasawa T, Abe T, Hanada T. Inhibitory effects of T cells on in vitro granulopoiesis, erythropoiesis, and immunoglobulin production in patients with aplastic anemia. Scand J Haematol 1982;28:389.
720. Sullivan R, Quesenberry PJ, Parkman R, et al. Aplastic anemia: lack of inhibitory effect of bone marrow lymphocytes on in vitro granulopoiesis. Blood 1980;56:625.
721. Hanada T, Aoki Y, Ninomiya H, Abe T. T cell-mediated inhibition of haematopoiesis in aplastic anemia: serial assay of inhibitory activities of T cells to autologous CFU-E during immunosuppressive therapy. Br J Haematol 1986;63:69.
722. Bacigalupo A, Podesta M, Raffo MR, et al. Lack of in vitro colony (CFU_c) formation and myelosuppressive activity in patients with severe aplastic anemia after autologous hematologic reconstitution. Exp Hematol 1980;8:795.
723. Torok-Storb BJ, Storb R, Graham TC, et al. Erythropoiesis in vitro: effect of normal versus "transfusion-sensitized" mononuclear cells. Blood 1978;52:706.
724. Singer JW, Brown JE, James MC, et al. Effect of peripheral blood lymphocytes from patients with aplastic anemia on granulocytic colony growth from HLA-matched and -mismatched marrows: effect of transfusion sensitization. Blood 1978;52:37.
725. Singer JW, Doney KC, Thomas ED. Coculture studies of 16 untransfused patients with aplastic anemia. Blood 1979;54:180.
726. Torok-Storb BJ, Sieff C, Storb R, et al. In vitro tests for distinguishing possible immune-mediated aplastic anemia from transfusion-induced sensitization. Blood 1980;55:211.
727. Bacigalupo A, Podesta M, Mingari MC, et al. Generation of CFU-C/suppressor T cells in vitro: an experimental model for immune-mediated marrow failure. Blood 1981;57:491.
728. Bacigalupo A, Podesta M, Frassoni F, et al. Generation of CFU-C suppressor T cells *in vitro*. V. A multistep process. Br J Haematol 1982;52:421.
729. Zoumbos NC, Djeu JY, Young NS. Interferon is the suppressor of hematopoiesis generated by stimulated lymphocytes in vitro. J Immunol 1984;133:769.
730. Rigby WFC, Ball ED, Guyre PM, Fanger MW. The effects of recombinant-DNA-derived interferons on the growth of myeloid progenitor cells. Blood 1985;65:858.
731. Mamus SW, Beck-Schroeder S, Zanjani ED. Suppression of normal human erythropoiesis by gamma interferon in vitro: role of monocytes and T lymphocytes. J Clin Invest 1985;75:1496.
732. Broxmeyer HE, Cooper S, Rubin BY, Taylor MW. The synergistic influence of human interferon-gamma and interferon-α on suppression of hematopoietic progenitor cells is additive with the enhanced sensitivity of these cells to inhibition by interferons at low oxygen tension in vitro. J Immunol 1985;135:2502.
733. Ganser A, Carlo-Stella C, Greher J, et al. Effect of recombinant interferons alpha and gamma on human bone marrow-derived megakaryocytic progenitor cells. Blood 1987;70:1173.
734. Talpaz M, Spitzer G, Hittelman W, et al. Changes in granulocyte-monocyte colony-forming cells among leukocyte-interferon-treated chronic myelogenous leukemia patients. Exp Hematol 1986;14:668.
735. Koren S, Klimpel GR, Fleischmann WR Jr. Treatment of mice with macrophage colony stimulating factor (CSF-1) prevents the in vivo myelosuppression induced by murine alpha, beta, and gamma interferons. J Biol Response Mod 1986;5:481.
736. Raefsky E, Platanias L, Zoumbos N, Young NS. Studies of interferon as a regulator of hematopoietic proliferation. J Immunol 1985;135: 2507.
737. Basham TY, Merigan TC. Recombinant interferon-gamma increases HLA-DR synthesis and expression. J Immunol 1983;130:1492.
738. Collart MA, Belin D, Vassalli J-D, et al. Gamma interferon enhances macrophage transcription of the tumor necrosis factor/cachectin, interleukin 1, and urokinase genes, which are controlled by short-lived repressors. J Exp Med 1986;164:2113.
739. Cannistra SA, Groshek P, Griffin JD. Monocytes enhance gamma-interferon-induced inhibition of myeloid progenitor cell growth through secretion of tumor necrosis factor. Exp Hematol 1988;16: 865.
740. Wallach D, Hahn T. Enhanced release of lymphotoxins by interferon-treated cells. Cell Immunol 1983;76:390.
741. Stötter H, Wiebke EA, Tomita S, et al. Cytokines alter target cell susceptibility to lysis. II. Evaluation of tumor infiltrating lymphocytes. J Immunol 1989;142:1767.
742. Conta BS, Powell MB, Ruddle NH. Production of lymphotoxin, IFN-gamma and IFN-α,β by murine T cell lines and clones. J Immunol 1983;130:2231.
743. Murphy M, Loudon R, Kobayashi M, Trinchieri G. Gamma-interferon and lymphotoxin released by activated T cells synergize to inhibit granulocyte/monocyte colony formation. J Exp Med 1986;164:263.
744. Williams TW, Bellanti JA. In vitro synergism between interferons and human lymphotoxin: enhancement of lymphotoxin-induced target cell killing. J Immunol 1983;130:518.
745. Lee SH, Aggarwal BB, Rinderknecht E, et al. The synergistic anti-proliferative effect of gamma-interferon and human lymphotoxin. J Immunol 1984;133:1083.
746. Czarniecki CW, Fennie CW, Powers DB, Estell DA. Synergistic antiviral and antiproliferative activities of Escherichia coli-derived human, alpha, beta, and gamma interferons. J Virol 1984;49:490.
747. Fleischmann WR Jr, Fleischmann CM. Potentiating effect of murine interferon-gamma-containing lymphokine preparations on the antiviral and antiproliferative effects of murine interferon-α/β: identification of the potentiation factor as murine interferon-gamma itself. Antiviral Res 1984;4:221.
748. Broxmeyer HE, Williams DE, Lu L, et al. The suppressive influences of human tumor necrosis factors on bone marrow hematopoietic progenitor cells from normal donors and patients with leukemia: synergism of tumor necrosis factor and interferon-gamma. J Immunol 1986;136:4487.
749. Spitzer G, Verma DS, Abramowitz S, Tomasovic B. Cells with Fc gamma receptors from normal donors suppress granulocytic macrophage colony formation. Blood 1982;60:758.
750. Broxmeyer HE, Lu L, Bognacki J. Transferrin, derived from an OKT8-positive subpopulation of T lymphocytes, suppresses the production of granulocyte-macrophage colony-stimulatory factors from mitogen-activated T lymphocytes. Blood 1983;62:37.
751. Nakao S, Harada M, Kondo K, et al. Effect of activated lymphocytes on the regulation of hematopoiesis: suppression of *in vitro* granulopoiesis by $OKT8^+Ia^+T$ cells induced by alloantigen stimulation. J Immunol 1984;132:160.
752. Verma DS, Johnston DA, McCredie KB. Evidence for the separate human T-lymphocyte subpopulations that collaborate with autologous monocyte/macrophages in the elaboration of colony-stimulating activity and those that suppress this collaboration. Blood 1983;62:1088.
753. Torok-Storb B, Martin PJ, Hansen JA. Regulation of in vitro erythropoiesis by normal T cells: evidence for two T-cell subsets with opposing function. Blood 1981;58:171.
754. Harada M, Nakao S, Kondo K, et al. Effect of activated lymphocytes on the regulation of hematopoiesis: enhancement and suppression of in vitro BFU-E growth by T cells stimulated by autologous non-T cells. Blood 1986;67:1143.
755. Burdach S, Shatsky M, Wagenhorst B, Levitt L. The T-cell CD2 determinant mediates inhibition of erythropoiesis by the lymphokine cascade. Blood 1988;72:770.
756. von Melchner H, Bartlett PF. The influence of T lymphocytes and their products on hemopoietic precursor cell regeneration in spleen organ cultures. Blood 1983;61:200.
757. Burdach SEG, Levitt LJ. Receptor-specific inhibition of bone marrow erythropoiesis by recombinant DNA-derived interleukin-2. Blood 1987;69:1368.
758. Burdach S, Shatsky M, Wagenhorst B, Levitt L. Receptor-specific modulation of myelopoiesis by recombinant DNA-derived interleukin 2. J Immunol 1987;139:452.

759. Koller U, Hinterberger W, Geschwandtler L, et al. Identification of activated T cells and the suppressor/inducer subset in patients suffering from severe aplastic anemia. Blut 1989;58:21.
760. Zoumbos N, Gascon P, Djeu J, Young NS. Interferon is a mediator of hematopoietic suppression in aplastic anemia in vitro and possibly in vivo. Proc Natl Acad Sci USA 1985;82:188.
761. Gascon P, Zoumbos N, Djeu J, et al. Lymphokine abnormalities in aplastic anemia: implications for the mechanism of action of ATG. Blood 1985;65:407.
762. Hinterberger W, Adolf G, Bettelheim P, et al. Lymphokine overproduction in severe aplastic anemia is not related to blood transfusions. Blood 1989;74:2713.
763. Zoumbos NC, Ferris WO, Hsu S-M, et al. Analysis of lymphocyte subsets in patients with aplastic anemia. Br J Haematol 1984;58:95.
764. Ruiz-Argüelles GJ, Katzmann JA, Greipp PR, et al. Lymphocyte subsets in patients with aplastic anemia. Am J Hematol 1984;16:267.
765. Zoumbos N, Gascon P, Trost S, et al. Circulating activated suppressor T lymphocytes in aplastic anemia. N Engl J Med 1985;312:257.
766. Mehta AB, Chiu E, Harhalakis N, et al. A T-cell lymphoma of suppressor phenotype arising in a patient with severe aplastic anaemia. (Letter) Br J Haematol 1989;72:287.
767. Platanias L, Gascon P, Bielory L, et al. Lymphocyte subsets and lymphokines following anti-thymocyte globulin therapy in patients with aplastic anaemia. Br J Haematol 1987;66:433.
768. Laver J, Castro-Malaspina H, Kernan NA, et al. In vitro interferon-gamma production by cultured T-cells in severe aplastic anaemia: correlation with granulomonopoietic inhibition in patients who respond to anti-thymocyte globulin. Br J Haematol 1988;69:545.
769. Hinterberger W, Adolf G, Aichinger G, et al. Further evidence for lymphokine overproduction in severe aplastic anemia. Blood 1988;72:266.
770. Fuchs D, Hausen A, Reibnegger G, et al. Neopterin as a marker for activated cell-mediated immunity: application in HIV infection. Immunol Today 1988;9:150.
771. Raghavachar A, Frickhofen N, Taniguchi Y, et al. Soluble interleukin-2 receptors and CD8 like molecules in the sera of patients with aplastic anemia. Blut 1988;57:240. Abstract.
772. Kasahara T, Djeu JY, Dougherty SF, Oppenheim JJ. Capacity of human large granular lymphocytes (LGL) to produce multiple lymphokines: interleukin 2, interferon, and colony stimulating factor. J Immunol 1983;131:2379.
773. Pistoia V, Ghio R, Nocera A, et al. Large granular lymphocytes have a promoting activity on human peripheral blood erythroid burst-forming units. Blood 1985;65:464.
774. Brooks CG. Reversible induction of natural killer cell activity in cloned murine cytotoxic T lymphocytes. Nature 1983;305:155.
775. Hansson M, Beran M, Andersson B, Kiessling R. Inhibition of *in vitro* granulopoiesis by autologous allogeneic human NK cells. J Immunol 1982;129:126.
776. Degliantoni G, Perussia B, Mangoni L, Trinchieri G. Inhibition of bone marrow colony formation by human natural killer cells and by natural killer cell-derived colony-inhibiting activity. J Exp Med 1985;161:1152.
777. Vinci G, Vernant JP, Nakazawa M, et al. In vitro inhibition of normal human hematopoiesis by marrow CD3$^+$, CD8$^+$, HLA-DR$^+$, HNK$^1_+$ lymphocytes. Blood 1988;72:1616.
778. Herrmann F, Schmidt RE, Ritz J, Griffin JD. In vitro regulation of human hematopoiesis by natural killer cells: analysis at a clonal level. Blood 1987;69:246.
779. Mangan KF, Hartnett ME, Matis SA, et al. Natural killer cells suppress human erythroid stem cell proliferation in vitro. Blood 1984;63:260.
780. O'Brien T, Kendra J, Stephens H, et al. Recognition and regulation of progenitor marrow elements by NK cells in the mouse. Immunology 1983;49:717.
781. Holmberg LA, Miller BA, Ault KA. The effect of natural killer cells on the development of syngeneic hematopoietic progenitors. J Immunol 1984;133:2933.
782. Barlozzari T, Herberman RB, Reynolds CW. Inhibition of pluripotent hematopoietic stem cells of bone marrow by large granular lymphocytes. Proc Natl Acad Sci USA 1987;84:7691.
783. Takahashi M, Oshimi K, Saito H, Mizoguchi H. Inhibition of human granulocyte-macrophage colony formation by interleukin 2-treated lymphocytes. Exp Hematol 1988;16:226.
784. Reynolds CW, Foon KA. T-gamma-lymphoproliferative disease and related disorders in humans and experimental animals: a review of the clinical, cellular, and functional characteristics. Blood 1984;64:1146.
785. Newland AC, Catovsky D, Linch D, et al. Chronic T cell lymphocytosis: a review of 21 cases. Br J Haematol 1984;58:433.
786. Catovsky D, Linch DC, Beverley PCL. T cell disorders in haematological diseases. Clin Haematol 1982;11:661.
787. McKenna RW, Arthur DC, Gajl-Peczalska KJ, et al. Granulated T cell lymphocytosis with neutropenia: malignant or benign chronic lymphoproliferative disorder? Blood 1985;66:259.
788. Winton EF, Chan WC, Check I, et al. Spontaneous regression of a monoclonal proliferation of large granular lymphocytes associated with reversal of anemia and neutropenia. Blood 1986;67:1427.
789. Gascon P, Zoumbos N, Young NS. An analysis of natural killer cells in aplastic anemia. Blood 1986;67:1349.
790. Porwit A, Hast R, Stenke L, et al. Decreased blood natural killer cell activity and immunoglobulin synthesis in vitro in aplastic anemia. Acta Med Scand 1988;224:391.
791. Voltarelli JC, Falcao RP, Carvalho IF, Bottura C. K-cell activity in aplastic anaemia. Scand J Haematol 1983;30:451.
792. Yoda Y, Kawakami Z, Abe T. Decreased frequency of bone marrow NK progenitors in aplastic anemia. Br J Haematol 1989;71:545.
793. Herrmann F, Griffin JD, Meuer SG, Zum Buschenfelde K-HM. Establishment of an interleukin 2-dependent T cell line derived from a patient with severe aplastic anemia, which inhibits in vitro hematopoiesis. J Immunol 1986;136:1629.
794. Kurane I, Meager A, Ennis FA. Dengue virus-specific human T cell clones: serotype crossreactive proliferation, interferon gamma production, and cytotoxic activity. J Exp Med 1989;170:763.
795. Lotz M, Tsoukas CD, Fong S, et al. Release of lymphokines after Epstein Barr virus infection in vitro. I. Sources of and kinetics of production of interferons and interleukins in normal humans. J Immunol 1986;136:3636.
796. Winchester RJ, Meyers PA, Broxmeyer HE, et al. Inhibition of human erythropoietic colony formation in culture by treatment with Ia antisera. J Exp Med 1978;148:613.
797. Fitchen JH, Le Fèvre C, Ferrone S, Cline MJ. Expression of Ia-like and HLA-A, B antigens on human multipotential hematopoietic progenitor cells. Blood 1982;59:188.
798. Ahmed R, Oldstone MBA. Mechanisms and biological implications of virus-induced polyclonal B-cell activation. In: Notkins AL, Oldstone MBA, eds. Concepts in viral pathogenesis. New York, Springer-Verlag, 1984.
799. Brinton MA, Nathanson N. Genetic determinants of virus susceptibility: epidemiologic implications in murine models. Epidemiol Rev 1981;3:115.
800. Wisniewski D, Strife A, Wachter M, Clarkson B. Regulation of human peripheral blood erythroid burst-forming unit growth by T lymphocytes and T lymphocyte subpopulations defined by OKT_4 and OKT_8 monoclonal antibodies. Blood 1985;65:456.
801. Haq AU, Rinehart JJ, Balcerzak SP. T-cell subset modulation of blood erythroid burst-forming unit proliferation. J Lab Clin Med 1983;101:53.
802. Gajewski TF, Fitch FW. Anti-proliferative effect of IFN-gamma in immune regulation. IV. Murine CTL clones produce IL-3 and GM-CSF, the activity of which is masked by the inhibitory action of secreted IFN-gamma. J Immunol 1990;144:548.
803. Santoli D, Clark SC, Kreider BL, et al. Amplification of IL-2 driven T cell proliferation by recombinant human IL-3 and granulocyte-macrophage colony-stimulating factor. J Immunol 1988;141:519.
804. Ho AD, Hass R, Wulf G, et al. Activation of lymphocytes induced by recombinant human granulocyte-macrophage colony-stimulating factor in patients with malignant lymphoma. Blood 1990;75:203.
805. Piacibello W, Lu L, Williams D, et al. Human gamma interferon enhances release from phytohemagglutinin-stimulated T4$^+$ lymphocytes of activities that stimulate colony formation by granulocyte-macrophage, erythroid, and multipotential progenitor cells. Blood 1986;68:1339.
806. Koeffler HP, Gasson J, Ranyard J, et al. Recombinant human TNFα stimulates production of granulocyte colony-stimulating factor. Blood 1987;70:55.
807. Estrov Z, Roifman C, Mills G, et al. The regulatory role of interleukin 2-responsive T lymphocytes on human marrow granulopoiesis. Blood 1987;69:1161.
808. Skettino S, Phillips J, Lanier L, et al. Selective generation of erythroid burst-promoting activity by recombinant interleukin 2-stimulated human T lymphocytes and natural killer cells. Blood 1988;71:907.
809. Ettinghausen SB, Moore JG, Platanias L, et al. Hematologic toxicity of lymphokine activated killer (LAK) cells and recombinant interleukin 2 in cancer patients. Blood 1987;69:1654.
810. Heslop HE, Gottlieb DJ, Bianchi ACM, et al. In vivo induction of gamma interferon and tumor necrosis factor by interleukin-2 infusion following intensive chemotherapy or autologous marrow transplantation. Blood 1989;74:1374.
811. Cline MJ, Opelz G, Saxon A, et al. Autoimmune panleukopenia. N Engl J Med 1976;295:1489.
812. Freedman MH, Gelfand EW, Saunders EF. Acquired aplastic anemia: antibody-mediated hematopoietic failure. Am J Hematol 1979;6:135.
813. Levitt LJ, Ries CA, Greenberg PL. Pure white-cell aplasia. Antibody-mediated autoimmune inhibition of granulopoiesis. N Engl J Med 1983;308:1141.
814. Hanada T, Ehara T, Nakahara S, et al. Simultaneous transient erythroblastopenia and agranulocytosis: IgG-mediated inhibition of erythrogranulopoiesis. Eur J Haematol 1987;38:200.
815. Fitchen JJ, Cline MJ, Saxon A, Golde DW. Serum inhibitors of hematopoiesis in a patient with aplastic anemia and systemic lupus erythematosus. Am J Med 1979;66:537.
816. Dainiak N, Hardin J, Floyd V, et al. Humoral suppression of erythropoiesis in systemic lupus erythematosus (SLE) and rheumatoid arthritis. Am J Med 1980;69:537.
817. Brooks BJ Jr, Broxmeyer HE, Bryan CF, Leech SH. Serum inhibitor

in systemic lupus erythematosus associated with aplastic anemia. Arch Intern Med 1984;144:1474.
818. Bailey FA, Lilly M, Bertoli LF, Ball GV. An antibody that inhibits in vitro bone marrow proliferation in a patient with systemic lupus erythematosus and aplastic anemia. Arthritis Rheum 1989;32:901.
819. Gordon MY. Circulating inhibitors of granulopoiesis in patients with aplastic anaemia. Br J Haematol 1978;39:491.
820. Fitchen JH, Cline MJ. Serum inhibitors of myelopoiesis. Br J Haematol 1980;44:7.
821. Takahashi M. Complement-dependent hematopoietic inhibitors in the sera of patients with aplastic anemia and paroxysmal nocturnal hemoglobinuria. Int J Cell Cloning 1987;5:242.
822. Kelton HG, Huang AT, Mold N, et al. The use of in vitro technics to study drug-induced pancytopenia. N Engl J Med 1979;301:621.
823. Taetle R, Lane TA, Mendelsohn J. Drug-induced agranulocytosis: in vitro evidence for immune suppression of granulopoiesis and a cross-reacting lymphocyte antibody. Blood 1979;54:501.
824. Ascensao JL, Flynn PJ, Slungaard A, et al. Quinidine-induced neutropenia: report of a case with drug-dependent inhibition of granulocyte colony generation. Acta Haematol 1984;72:349.
825. Barrett AJ, Weller E, Rozengurt N, et al. Amidopyrine agranulocytosis: drug inhibition of granulocyte colonies in the presence of patient's serum. Br Med J 1976;2:850.
826. Levitt LJ. Chlorpropamide-induced pure white cell aplasia. Blood 1987;69:394.
827. Fibbe WE, Claas FHJ, van der Star-Dijkstra W, et al. Agranulocytosis induced by propylthiouracil: evidence of a drug dependent antibody reacting with granulocytes, monocytes and haematopoietic progenitor cells. Br J Haematol 1986;64:363.
828. Mamus SW, Burton JD, Groat JD, et al. Ibuprofen-associated pure white-cell aplasia. N Engl J Med 1986;314:624.
829. Dessypris EN, Redline S, Harris JW, Krantz SB. Diphenylhydantoin-induced pure red cell aplasia. Blood 1985;65:789.
830. Salama A, Schütz B, Kiefel V, et al. Immune-mediated agranulocytosis related to drugs and their metabolites: mode of sensitization and heterogeneity of antibodies. Br J Haematol 1989;72:127.
831. Chudomel V, Rerábková E, Cinátl J, et al. Progenitor white cells and serum inhibitors in patients with bone marrow aplasia. Folia Haematol 1979;106:358.
832. Chan SH, Metcalf D. Inhibition of bone marrow colony formation by normal and leukemic human serum. Nature 1980;227:845.
833. Vincent PC, Sutherland R, Morris TCM, Chapman GV. Inhibitor of in-vitro granulopoiesis in plasma of patients with renal failure. Lancet 1978;2:864.
834. Bharucha C, Crosbie J, Bharucha H, Mayne EE. Intractable pain in aplastic anaemia. Br Med J 1981;282:1834.
835. Bessman JD. Automated blood counts and differentials. Baltimore, Johns Hopkins University Press, 1986.
836. Bessman JD, Gardner FH. Persistence of abnormal RBC and platelet phenotype during recovery from aplastic anemia. Arch Intern Med 1985;145:293.
837. Twomey JJ, Douglass CC, Sharkey O Jr. The monocytopenia of aplastic anemia. Blood 1973;41:187.
838. Rao ANR, Brown AK, Rieder RF, et al. Aplastic anemia with fetallike erythropoiesis following androgen therapy. Blood 1978;51:711.
839. Alter BP, Rappeport JM, Huisman THJ, et al. Fetal erythropoiesis following bone marrow transplantation. Blood 1976;48:843.
840. Yoshida M, Takaku F, Nojiri H, et al. Decreased sialic acid content of erythrocytes in patients with aplastic anaemia. Br J Haematol 1987;65:351.
841. Jamshidi K, Swaim WR. Bone marrow biopsy with unaltered architecture: a new biopsy device. J Lab Clin Med 1971;77:335.
842. Fong TP, Okafor LA, Schmitz TH, Thomas W, et al. An evaluation of cellularity in various types of bone marrow specimens. Am J Clin Pathol 1979;72:812.
843. Najean Y. Diagnostic and prognostic value of bone marrow biopsy in aplastic anemia. Nouv Rev Fr Hematol 1986;28:281.
844. Gruppo RA, Lampkin BC, Granger S. Bone marrow cellularity determination: comparison of the biopsy, aspirate, and buffy coat. Blood 1977;49:29.
845. Kansu E, Erslev AJ. Aplastic anaemia with "hot pockets." Scand J Haematol 1976;17:326.
846. Yang C, Wang Z, Li L, et al. Studies of bone marrow of aplastic anemia: preliminary classification study. J Chin Intern Med 1962;12:757.
847. Frisch B, Lewis SM. The bone marrow in aplastic anaemia: diagnostic and prognostic features. J Clin Pathol 1974;27:231.
848. Frisch B, Lewis SM, Sherman D. The ultrastructure of dyserythropoiesis in aplastic anaemia. Br J Haematol 1975;29:545.
849. Clemmesen L, Hansen MM, Mortensen L, et al. The applicability of simple blood and bone marrow variables in prediction of acute leukaemia in patients with acquired bi- or pancytopenia. Scand J Haematol 1981;27:193.
850. Cazzola M, Pootrakul P, Huebers HA, et al. Erythroid marrow function in anemic patients. Blood 1987;69:296.
851. Cazzola M, Bergamaschi G, Huebers HA, Finch CA. Pathophysiological classification of acquired bone marrow failure based on quantitative assessment of erythroid function. Eur J Haematol 1987;38:426.
852. McNeil BJ, Rappeport JM, Nathan DG. Indium chloride scintigraphy: an index of severity in patients with aplastic anemia. Br J Haematol 1976;34:599.
853. Pauwels EKJ, TeVelde J, Hermans J, et al. Indium-chloride bone marrow scintigraphy in aplastic anemia. Scand J Haematol 1981;26:81.
854. Horn NL, Bennett LR, Marciano D. Evaluation of aplastic anemia with indium chloride In 111 scanning. Arch Intern Med 1980;140:1299.
855. Sayle BA, Helmer RE III, Birdsong BA, et al. Bone marrow imaging with indium-111 chloride in aplastic anemia and myelofibrosis: concise communication. J Nucl Med 1982;23:121.
856. Najean Y, Le Danvic M, Le Mercier N, et al. Significance of bone-marrow scintigraphy in aplastic anemia: concise communication. J Nucl Med 1980;21:213.
857. Rosen BR, Fleming DM, Kushner DC, et al. Hematologic bone marrow disorders: quantitative chemical shift MR imaging. Radiology 1988;169:799.
858. McKinstry CS, Steiner RE, Young AT, et al. Bone marrow in leukemia and aplastic anemia: MR imaging before, during, and after treatment. Radiology 1987;162:701.
859. Camitta BM, Thomas D, Nathan DG, et al. A prospective study of androgens and bone marrow transplantation for treatment of severe aplastic anemia. Blood 1979;53:504.
860. O'Reilly RJ. Allogeneic bone marrow transplantation: current status and future directions. Blood 1983;62:941.
861. Kanfer EJ. Bone marrow transplantation: current controversies. Bone Marrow Transplant 1988;3:501.
862. Gordon-Smith EC. Treatment of severe aplastic anemia by bone marrow transplantation. Hematol Oncol 1987;5:255.
863. Sullivan KM, Witherspoon RP, Storb R, et al. Long-term results of allogeneic bone marrow transplantation. Transplant Proc 1988;21:2926.
864. Deeg HJ, Klingemann H-G, Phillips GL. A guide to bone marrow transplantation. Berlin, Springer-Verlag, 1988.
865. Osgood EE, Riddle MC, Mathews TJ. Aplastic anemia treated with daily transfusions and intravenous marrow: case report. Ann Intern Med 1939;13:357.
866. Pillow RP, Epstein RB, Buckner CD, et al. Treatment of bone-marrow failure by isogeneic marrow infusion. N Engl J Med 1966;275:94.
867. Bortin MM. A compendium of reported human bone marrow transplants. Transplantation 1970;9:571.
868. Camitta BM, Thomas ED, Nathan DG, et al. Severe aplastic anemia: a prospective study of the effect of early marrow transplantation on acute mortality. Blood 1976;48:63.
869. Gluckman E, Esperou H, Devergie A, et al. Pediatric bone marrow transplantation for leukemia and aplastic anemia. Nouv Rev Fr Hematol 1989;31:111.
870. Deeg HJ, Self S, Storb R, et al. Decreased incidence of marrow graft rejection in patients with severe aplastic anemia: changing impact of risk factors. Blood 1986;68:1363.
871. Appelbaum FR, Fefer A, Cheever MA, et al. Treatment of aplastic anemia by bone marrow transplantation in identical twins. Blood 1980;55:1033.
872. Lu DP. Syngeneic bone marrow transplantation for treatment of aplastic anemia: report of a case and review of the literature. Exp Hematol 1981;9:257.
873. Hill RS, Petersen FB, Storb R, et al. Mixed hematologic chimerism after allogeneic marrow transplantation for severe aplastic anemia is associated with a higher risk of graft rejection and a lessened incidence of acute graft-versus-host disease. Blood 1986;67:811.
874. Hows JM, Kaffaf S, Palmer S, et al. Regeneration of peripheral blood cells following allogeneic bone marrow transplantation for severe aplastic anaemia. Br J Haematol 1982;52:551.
875. Storb R, Weiden PL, Sullivan KM, et al. Second marrow transplants in patients with aplastic anemia rejecting the first graft: use of a conditioning regimen including cyclophosphamide and antithymocyte globulin. Blood 1987;70:116.
876. Hows J, Palmer S, Gordon-Smith EC. Cyclosporine and graft failure following bone marrow transplantation for severe aplastic anemia. Br J Haematol 1985;60:611.
877. Storb R, Prentice RL, Thomas ED. Marrow transplantation for treatment of aplastic anemia. N Engl J Med 1977;296:61.
878. Kessinger A, Armitage JO, Landmark JD, et al. Autologous peripheral hematopoietic stem cell transplantation restores hematopoietic function following marrow ablative therapy. Blood 1988;71:723.
879. Storb R, Doney KC, Thomas ED, et al. Marrow transplantation with or without donor buffy coat cells for 65 transfused aplastic anemia patients. Blood 1982;59:236.
880. Champlin RE, Horowitz MM, vanBekkum DW, et al. Graft failure following bone marrow transplantation for severe aplastic anemia: risk factors and treatment results. Blood 1989;73:606.
881. Bacigalupo A. Treatment of severe aplastic anaemia. In: Hinton K, Tindall B, eds. Clinical haematology. London, Bailliere Tindall, 1989:19.

882. Storb R, Weiden PL, Deeg HJ, et al. Rejection of marrow from DLA-identical canine littermates given transfusions before grafting: antigens involved are expressed on leukocytes and skin epithelial cells but not on platelets and red blood cells. Blood 1979;54:477.
883. Torok-Storb BJ, Storb R, Deeg HJ, et al. Growth in vitro of donor marrow cultured with recipient lymphocytes predicts the fate of marrow grafts in transfused DLA-identical dogs. Blood 1979;53:104.
884. van Bekkum DW, Bach FH, Bergan JJ, et al. Bone marrow transplantation from donors with aplastic anemia. JAMA 1976;236:1131.
885. Anasetti C, Doney KC, Storb R, et al. Marrow transplantation for severe aplastic anemia. Ann Intern Med 1986;104:461.
886. Gluckman E. Current status of bone marrow transplantation for severe aplastic anemia: a preliminary report from the international bone marrow transplant registry. Transplant Proc 1987;19:2597.
887. Parkman R, Rappeport J, Camitta B, et al. Successful use of multiagent immunosuppression in the bone marrow transplantation of sensitized patients. Blood 1978;52:1163.
888. Gluckman E, Devergie A, Gerotta I, et al. Bone marrow transplantation in 65 patients with severe aplastic anemia. Bull Cancer 1981;68: 74.
889. Feig SA, Champlin R, Arenson E, et al. Improved survival following bone marrow transplantation for aplastic anaemia. Br J Haematol 1983;54:509.
890. Ramsay NKC, Kim TH, McGlave P, et al. Total lymphoid irradiation and cyclophosphamide conditioning prior to bone marrow transplantation for patients with severe aplastic anemia. Blood 1983;62: 622.
891. Miyamura K, Kojima S, Takeyama K, et al. Use of cyclophosphamide and total lymphoid irradiation combined with cyclosporine in bone marrow transplantation for transfused severe aplastic anemia. Bone Marrow Transplant 1988;3:457.
892. Niederwieser D, Pepe M, Storb R, et al. Factors predicting chronic graft-versus-host disease and survival after marrow transplantation for aplastic anemia. Bone Marrow Transplant 1989;4:151.
893. Sullivan KM, Shulman HM, Storb R, et al. Chronic graft-versus-host disease in 52 patients: adverse natural course and successful treatment with combination immunosuppression. Blood 1981;57:267.
894. Weiner RS, Horowitz MM, Gale RP, et al. Risk factors for interstitial pneumonitis following bone marrow transplantation for severe aplastic anaemia. Br J Haematol 1989;71:535.
895. Deeg HJ, Storb R, Thomas ED. Bone marrow transplantation: a review of delayed complications. Br J Haematol 1984;57:185.
896. Champlin R, Ho W, Bayever E, et al. Treatment of aplastic anemia: results with bone marrow transplantation, antithymocyte globulin, and a monoclonal anti-T cell antibody. In: Young NS, Levine AS, Humphries RK, eds. Aplastic anemia: stem cell biology and advances in treatment. New York, Alan R Liss, 1984:227.
897. McGlave PB, Haake R, Miller W, et al. Therapy of severe aplastic anemia in young adults and children with allogeneic bone marrow transplantation. Blood 1987;70:1325.
898. Butturini A, Gale RP. Clinical trials of T-cell depletion: current controversies, future directions. In: Gale RP, Champlin RE, eds. Bone marrow transplantation: current controversies. New York, Alan R Liss, 1989:495.
899. Herve P, Cahn JY, Flesch M, et al. Successful graft-versus-host disease prevention without graft failure in 32 HLA-identical allogeneic bone marrow transplantations with marrow depleted of T cells by monoclonal antibodies and complement. Blood 1987;69:388.
900. Sachs DH, Suzuki T, Sundt TM, Sykes M. A new approach to bone marrow transplantation across MHC barriers. In: Gale RP, Champlin RE, eds. Bone marrow transplantation: current controversies. New York, Alan R Liss, 1989:433.
901. O'Reilly RJ, Kernan NA, Cunningham I, et al. T cell depleted marrow transplants for the treatment of leukemia. In: Gale RP, Champlin RE, eds. Bone marrow transplantation: current controversies. New York, Alan R Liss, 1989:477.
902. Beatty PG, DiBartolomeo P, Storb R, et al. Treatment of aplastic anemia with marrow grafts from related donors other than HLA genotypically-matched siblings. Clin Transplant 1987;1:117.
903. Hows JM, Kaminski E, Brookes P, et al. Unrelated and mismatched transplants for aplastic anaemia. In: Gale RP, Champlin RE, eds. Bone marrow transplantation: current controversies. New York, Alan R Liss, 1989:9.
904. Bacigalupo A, Hows J, Gordon-Smith EC, et al. Bone marrow transplantation for severe aplastic anemia from donors other than HLA identical siblings: a report of the BMT working party. Bone Marrow Transplant 1988;3:531.
905. O'Reilly RJ, Pahwa R, Kirkpatrick D, et al. Successful transplantation of marrow from an HLA-A, -B, -D mismatched heterozygous sibling donor into an HLA-D-homozygous patient with aplastic anemia. Transplant Proc 1978;10:957.
906. Camitta B, Ash R, Menitove J, et al. Bone marrow transplantation for children with severe aplastic anemia: use of donors other than HLA-identical siblings. Blood 1989;74:1852.
907. McCullough J, Hansen J, Perkins H, et al. The national marrow donor program: how it works, accomplishments to date. Oncology 1989;3: 63.
908. Mickey MR. Donor pool size for bone marrow transplantation. In: NIH, ed. Donor registries for bone marrow transplantation: NIH Technology Assessment Meeting, 1985:54.
909. Hansen JA. Donor selection for marrow transplantation. HLA polymorphism and matching. In: Gale RP, Champlin RE, eds. Bone marrow transplantation: current controversies. New York, Alan R Liss, 1989:607.
910. Kelemen E. Recovery from chronic idiopathic bone marrow aplasia of a young mother after intravenous injection of unprocessed cells from the liver (and yolk sac) of her 22 mm CR-length embryo: a preliminary report. Scand J Haematol 1973;10:305.
911. Kochupillai V, Sharma S, Francis S, et al. Fetal liver infusion in aplastic anaemia. Thymus 1987;10:95.
912. Jeannet M, Speck B, Rubinstein A, et al. Autologous marrow reconstitutions in severe aplastic anaemia after ALG pretreatment and HL-A semi-incompatible bone marrow cell transfusion. Acta Haematol 1976;55:129.
913. Sensenbrenner LL, Steele AA, Santos GW. Recovery of hematologic competence without engraftment following attempted bone marrow transplantation for aplastic anemia: report of a case with diffusion chamber studies. Exp Hematol 1977;5:51.
914. Silingardi V, Torelli U. Recovery from aplastic anemia after treatment with antilymphocyte globulin. Arch Intern Med 1979;130:582.
915. Griner PF. A survey of the effectiveness of cyclophosphamide in patients with severe aplastic anemia. Am J Hematol 1980;8:55.
916. Pizzuto J, Conte G, Ambríz R, et al. Cyclophosphamide for aplastic anemia. (Letter) N Engl J Med 1978;298:164.
917. Speck B, Gluckman E, Haak HL, van Rood JJ. Treatment of aplastic anaemia by antilymphocyte globulin with and without allogeneic bone-marrow infusions. Lancet 1977;1145.
918. Doney KC, Weiden PL, Buckner CD, et al. Treatment of severe aplastic anemia using antithymocyte globulin with or without an infusion of HLA haploidentical marrow. Exp Hematol 1981;9:829.
919. Camitta B, O'Reilly RJ, Sensenbrenner L, et al. Antithoracic duct lymphocyte globulin therapy of severe aplastic anemia. Blood 1983;62:883.
920. Champlin R, Ho W, Gale RP. Antithymocyte globulin treatment in patients with aplastic anemia. N Engl J Med 1983;308:113.
921. Young N, Griffith P, Brittain E, et al. A multicenter trial of antithymocyte globulin in aplastic anemia and related diseases. Blood 1988;72:1861.
922. Fairhead SM, Chipping PM, Gordon-Smith EC. Treatment of aplastic anaemia with antilymphocyte globulin (ALG). Br J Haematol 1983;55: 7.
923. Speck B, Gratwohl A, Nissen C, et al. Treatment of severe aplastic anaemia with antilymphocyte globulin or bone-marrow transplantation. Br Med J 1981;282:860.
924. Hinterberger-Fischer M, Hinterberger W, Hockern P, et al. Treatment of severe aplastic anemia with combined immunosuppression (antithymocyte globulin and high dose methylprednisolone). Acta Haematol 1986;76:196.
925. Raefsky E, Gascon P, Gratwohl A, et al. Biological and biochemical characterization of anti-thymocyte globulins (ATG) and antilymphocyte globulins (ALG). Blood 1986;68:712.
926. Marsh JCW, Hows JM, Bryett KA, et al. Survival after antilymphocyte globulin therapy for aplastic anemia depends on disease severity. Blood 1987;70:1046.
927. Champlin RE, Ho WG, Feig SA, et al. Do androgens enhance the response to antithymocyte globulin in patients with aplastic anemia? A prospective randomized trial. Blood 1985;66:184.
928. Kaltwasser JP, Dix U, Schalk KP, Vogt H. Effect of androgens on the response to antithymocyte globulin in patients with hematopoietic progenitor cells from normal donors and patients with leukemia: synergism of tumor necrosis factor and interferon-gamma. Eur J Haematol 1988;40:111.
929. Bacigalupo A, van Lint MT, Congiu M, et al. Treatment of SAA in Europe 1970–1985: a report of the SAA working party. Bone Marrow Transplant 1986;1(Suppl 1):19.
930. Gluckman E, Devergie A, Poros A, Degoulet P. Results of immunosuppression in 170 cases of severe aplastic anaemia. Br J Haematol 1982;51:541.
931. Jansen J, Zwaan FE, Haak HL, et al. Anti-thymocyte globulin treatment for aplastic anemia. Scand J Haematol 1982;28:341.
932. Satoh PS, Davis JW, Fleming WF, et al. Horse IgG, anti-horse IgG, and circulating immune complexes in the plasma of renal transplant patients receiving ATGAM. Upjohn Technical Report 7244/79/7244/35, 1979.
933. Heyworth MF. Effects of anti-lymphocytic globulin in human subjects. J Immunol 1981;43:793.
934. Means RT, Krantz SB, Dessypris EN, et al. Re-treatment of aplastic anemia with antithymocyte globulin or antilymphocyte serum. Am J Med 1988;84:678.
935. Marmont AM, Bacigalupo A, van Lint MT, et al. Treatment of severe aplastic anemia with sequential immunosuppression. Exp Hematol 1983;11:856.
936. Gluckman E, Marmont A, Speck B, Gordon-Smith EC. Immunosup-

pressive treatment of aplastic anemia as an alternative treatment for bone marrow transplantation. Semin Hematol 1984;21:11.
937. Butler WT. Corticosteroids and immunoglobulin synthesis. Transplant Proc 1975;7:49.
938. Doney K, Storb R, Buckner CD, et al. Treatment of aplastic anemia with antithymocyte globulin, high-dose corticosteroids, and androgens. Exp Hematol 1987;15:239.
939. Sulecki M, Shadduck RK, Zeigler Z. Anti-thymocyte globulin for hypoplastic myelodysplastic syndrome. Blood 1988;72(Suppl 1):229a.
940. Krantz SB. Studies on red cell aplasia. III. Treatment with horse antihuman thymocyte gamma globulin. Blood 1972;39:347.
941. Marmont A, Peschle C, Sanguineti M, Condorelli M. Pure red cell aplasia (PRCA): response of three patients to cyclophosphamide and/or anti-lymphocyte globulin (ALG) and demonstration of two types of serum IgG inhibitors to erythropoiesis. Blood 1975;45:247.
942. Harris SI, Weinberg JB. Treatment of red cell aplasia with antithymocyte globulin: repeated inductions of complete remissions in two patients. Am J Hematol 1985;20:183.
943. Marmont AM. Congenital hypoplastic anaemia refractory to corticosteriods but responding to cyclophosphamide and antilymphocytic globulin. Acta Haematol 1978;60:90.
944. Firkin FC, Prewett EJ, Nicholls K, Moran J. Antithymocyte globulin therapy for pure white cell aplasia. Am J Hematol 1987;25:101.
945. Khelif A, French MF, Follea G, et al. Amegakaryocytic thrombocytopenic purpura treated with antithymocyte globulin. (Letter) Ann Intern Med 1985;102:720.
946. Fäldt R. Remission of amegakaryocytic thrombocytopenia induced by antilymphocyte globulin (ALG). (Letter) Br J Haematol 1986;63:205.
947. Sabbe LJM, Claas FHJ, Haak HL, et al. Anti-thymocyte globulin (ATG) can eliminate platelet refractoriness. Blut 1981;42:331.
948. Bielory L, Wright R, Nienhuis AW, et al. Antithymocyte globulin hypersensitivity in bone marrow failure patients. JAMA 1988;260:3164.
949. Lawley TJ, Bielory L, Gascon P, et al. A prospective clinical and immunological analysis of serum sickness in man. N Engl J Med 1984;311:1407.
950. Bielory L, Lawley T, Gascon P, et al. Human serum sickness after equine antithymocyte globulin in patients with bone marrow failure. Medicine 1988;67:40.
951. Bielory L, Gascon P, Lawley TJ, et al. Serum sickness and haematopoietic recovery with antithymocyte globulin in bone marrow failure patients. Br J Haematol 1986;63:729.
952. Marmont AM, Cerri R, Lercari G, et al. Positive direct antiglobulin tests and heteroimmune hemolysis in patients with severe aplastic anemia and pure red cell anemia treated with antilymphocytic globulin. Acta Haematol 1985;74:14.
953. Greco B, Bielory L, Stephany D, et al. Antithymocyte globulin reacts with many normal human cell types. Blood 1983;62:1047.
954. Smith AG, O'Reilly RJ, Hansen JA, Martin PJ. Specific antibody-blocking activities in antilymphocyte globulin as correlates of efficacy for the treatment of aplastic anemia. Blood 1985;66:721.
955. Neudorf S, Jones M. The effects of antithymocyte globulin on natural killer cells. Exp Hematol 1988;16:831.
956. López-Karpovitch X, Zarzosa ME, Cárdenas MR, Piedras J. Changes in peripheral blood mononuclear cell subpopulations during antithymocyte globulin therapy for severe aplastic anemia. Acta Haematol 1989;81:176.
957. Doney K, Martin P, Storb R, et al. A randomized trial of antihuman thymocyte globulin versus murine monoclonal antihuman T-cell antibodies as immunosuppressive therapy for aplastic anemia. Exp Hematol 1985;13:520.
958. Barbano GC, Schenone A, Roncella S, et al. Anti-lymphocyte globulin stimulates normal human T cells to proliferate and to release lymphokines in vitro: a study at the clonal level. Blood 1988;72:56.
959. Kawano Y, Nissen C, Gratwohl A, Speck B. Immunostimulatory effects of different antilymphocyte globulin preparations: a possible clue to their clinical effect. Br J Haematol 1988;68:115.
960. Mookerjee BK, Azzolina L, Poultar L. Interaction of anti-thymocyte serum with hematopoietic stem cells. I. Effects in vitro and in vivo. J Immunol 1974;112:822.
961. Barrett AJ, Longhurst P, Rosengurt N, et al. Crossreaction of antilymphocyte globulin with human granulocyte colony forming cells. J Clin Pathol 1978;31:129.
962. Hunter RF, Mold NG, Mitchell B, Huang AT. Differentiation of normal marrow and HL60 cells induced by antithymocyte globulin. Proc Natl Acad Sci USA 1985;82:4823.
963. Amare, Abdou NL, Robinson MG, Abdou NI. Aplastic anemia associated with bone marrow suppressor T-cell hyperactivity: successful treatment with antithymocyte globulin. Am J Hematol 1978;5:25.
964. Hanada T, Abe T, Fukao K, et al. Severe aplastic anaemia treated with anti-lymphocyte globulin. Scand J Haematol 1982;29:128.
965. Faille A, Barrett AJ, Balitrand N, et al. Effect of antilymphocyte globulin on granulocyte precursors in aplastic anaemia. Br J Haematol 1979;42:371.
966. Blasetti A, Faille A, Balitrand N, et al. Inhibitory effects of peripheral blood cells on in vitro colony formation by autologous bone marrow in aplastic anemia: relation with response to immunosuppressive therapy. J Clin Pathol 1982;35:1316.
967. Rothmann SA, Streeter RR, Bukowski RM, Hewlett JS. Treatment of severe aplastic anemia with antithymocyte globulin. Exp Hematol 1982;10:809.
968. Issaragrisil S, Tangnai-Trisorana Y, Siriseriwan T, et al. Methylprednisolone therapy in aplastic anaemia: correlation of in vitro tests and lymphocyte subsets with clinical response. Eur J Haematol 1988;40:343.
969. Kahan BD. Cyclosporine. N Engl J Med 1989;321:1725.
970. Orosz GG, Roopenian DC, Widmer MB, Bach FH. Analysis of cloned T cell function. II. Differential blockade of various cloned T cell functions by cyclosporine. Transplantation 1983;36:706.
971. Bickel M, Tsuda H, Amstad P, et al. Differential regulation of colony-stimulating factors and interleukin 2 production by cyclosporin A. Proc Natl Acad Sci USA 1987;84:3274.
972. Finlay JL, Toretsky J, Hoffman R, et al. Cyclosporine A (CyA) in refractory severe aplastic anemia (AA). Blood 1984;64(Suppl 1):104a. Abstract.
973. Stryckmans PA, Dumont JP, Velu T, Debusscher L. Cyclosporine in refractory severe aplastic anemia. (Letter) N Engl J Med 1984;310:655.
974. Seip M, Vidnes J. Cyclosporine A in a case of refractory severe aplastic anemia. Scand J Haematol 1985;34:228.
975. Wisloff F, Godal HC. Cyclosporine in refractory severe aplastic anemia. (Letter) N Engl J Med 1985;312:1193.
976. Bridges R, Pineo G, Blahey W. Cyclosporin A for the treatment of aplastic anemia refractory to antithymocyte globulin. Am J Hematol 1987;26:83.
977. Werner EJ, Stout RD, Valdez LP, Harris RE. Immunosuppressive therapy versus bone marrow transplantation for children with aplastic anemia. Pediatrics 1989;83:61.
978. Jacobs P, Wood L, Martell RW. Cyclosporin A in the treatment of severe acute aplastic anemia. Br J Haematol 1985;61:267.
979. Porwit A, Panayotides P, Mansson E, et al. Cyclosporine A treatment in four cases of aplastic anemia. Blut 1987;54:73.
980. Tötterman TH, Höglund M, Bengtsson M, et al. Treatment of pure red-cell aplasia and aplastic anaemia with cyclosporin: long-term clinical effects. Eur J Haematol 1989;42:126.
981. Leonard EM, Raefsky E, Griffith P, et al. Cyclosporine therapy of aplastic anaemia, congenital and acquired red cell aplasia. Br J Haematol 1989;72:278.
982. Gluckman E, Esperous H, Devergie A. Comparison of cyclosporine A (CyA) and horse antithymocyte globulin (H.ATG) for treatment of severe aplastic anemia. Blood 1988;72(Suppl 1):42a. Abstract.
983. Esperou H, Devergie A, Lehn P, et al. A randomized study comparing ciclosporin A and antithymocyte globulin for treatment of severe aplastic anemia. Nouv Rev Fr Hematol 1989;31:65.
984. Bern MM, Roberts MS, Yoburn D. Cyclosporin treatment for aplastic anemia: a case report demonstrating a second response to second exposure to cyclosporin. Am J Hematol 1987;24:307.
985. Kahan BD. Individualization of cyclosporine therapy using pharmacokinetic and pharmacodynamic parameters. Transplantation 1985;40:457.
986. Pogliani EM, Cortellaro M, Foa P, et al. Cyclosporin A in the treatment of severe aplastic anemia: description of a case complicated by the development of tubercular pericarditis during treatment. Am J Hematol 1989;30:257.
987. Bacigalupo A, Frassoni F, Podesta M, et al. Cyclosporin A (CyA) does not enhance CFU-c growth in patients with severe aplastic anaemia. Scand J Haematol 1985;34:133.
988. Mohler DN, Leavell BS. Aplastic anemia: an analysis of 50 cases. Ann Intern Med 1958;49:326.
989. Vincent PC, De Gruchy GC. Complications and treatment of acquired aplastic anemia. Br J Haematol 1967;13:977.
990. Erslev AJ, Iverson CK, Lawrason FD. Cortisone and ACTH in hypoplastic anemia. Yale J Biol Med 1952;25:44.
991. Crosby WH, Feinstein FE, Heilmeyer L, et al. XII. Hypoplastic-aplastic anemia. Blood 1957;12:193.
992. Moore CV. The treatment of refractory anemia or bone marrow failure. J Chron Dis 1957;6:324.
993. Israëls MCG, Wilkinson JF. Idiopathic aplastic anaemia. Lancet 1961;1:63.
994. Najean Y, Pecking A, Le Danvic M. Androgen therapy of aplastic anaemia: a prospective study of 352 cases. Scand J Haematol 1979;22:343.
995. Bacigalupo A, van Lint MT, Cerri R, et al. Treatment of severe aplastic anemia with bolus 6-methylprenisolone and antilymphocytic globulin. Blut 1980;41:168.
996. Ozsoylu S, Coskun T, Minassazi S. High dose intravenous glucocorticoid in the treatment of childhood acquired aplastic anaemia. Scand J Haematol 1984;33:309.
997. Yoshida Y, Sakota H, Taniguchi Y, et al. Lack of correlation between in vitro corticosteroid effect on hemopoietic colony formation and response to corticosteroid therapy in aplastic anemia. (Abstract) Int J Cell Cloning 1986;4:82.

998. de Planque MM, Bacigalupo A, Würsch A, et al. Long-term follow-up of severe aplastic anaemia patients treated with antithymocyte globulin. Br J Haematol 1989;73:121.
999. Tichelli A, Gratwohl A, Würsch A, et al. Secondary leukemia after severe aplastic anemia. Blut 1988;56:79.
1000. Orlandi E, Alessandrino EP, Caldera D, Bernasconi C. Adult leukemia developing after aplastic anemia: report of 8 cases. Acta Haematol 1988;79:174.
1001. First LR, Smith BR, Lipton J, et al. Isolated thrombocytopenia after allogeneic bone marrow transplantation: existence of transient and chronic thrombocytopenic syndromes. Blood 1985;65:368.
1002. Hughes RT, Milligan DW, Smith GM, et al. A second bone marrow transplant for acute myeloid leukaemia after transplantation for aplastic anaemia. (Letter) Br J Haematol 1988;68:391.
1003. Cairo MS, Baehner RL. The use of antithymocyte globulin in the treatment of severe aplastic anemia in children. J Pediatr 1982;100: 307.
1004. Bayever E, Champlin R, Ho W, et al. Comparison between bone marrow transplantation and antithymocyte globulin in treatment of young patients with severe aplastic anemia. J Pediatr 1984;105: 920.
1005. Kojima S, Fukuda M, Horibe K, et al. Comparison between bone marrow transplantation and immunosuppressive therapy in treatment of patients younger than 20 years with severe aplastic anemia. Acta Haematol Jpn 1988;51:28.
1006. Klingemann H-G, Storb R, Fefer A, et al. Bone marrow transplantation in patients aged 45 years and older. Blood 1986;67:770.
1007. Ammus SS. The role of androgens in the treatment of hematologic disorders. Adv Intern Med 1989;34:191.
1008. Gardner FH. Androgen therapy of aplastic anaemia. Clin Haematol 1978;7:571.
1009. Adamson JW. Pharmacological stimulation of marrow function. Clin Haematol 1978;7:555.
1010. Shahidi NT, Diamond LK. Testosterone-induced remission in aplastic anemia of both acquired and congenital types: further observations in 24 cases. N Engl J Med 1961;264:953.
1011. Li F, Alter BP, Nathan DG. The mortality of acquired aplastic anemia in children. Blood 1972;40:153.
1012. Sanchez-Medal L, Gomez-Leal A, Duarte L, Rico MG. Anabolic androgenic steroids in the treatment of acquired aplastic anemia. Blood 1969;34:283.
1013. Allen DM, Fine MH, Necheles TF. Oxymetholone therapy in aplastic anemia. Blood 1968;32:83.
1014. Daiber A, Herve L, Con I, Donoso A. Treatment of aplastic anemia with nandrolone decanoate. Blood 1970;36:748.
1015. Tso SC, Chan TK, Todd D. Aplastic anaemia: a study of prognosis and the effect of androgen therapy. Q J Med 1977;406:513.
1016. Hast R, Skårberg KO, Engstedt L, et al. Oxymetholone treatment in aregenerative anaemia. II. Remission and survival: a prospective study. Scand J Haematol 1976;16:90.
1017. Gustafsson G, Kreuger A, Sjölin S. Acquired aplastic anaemia in children treated with corticosteroids and anabolic steroids. Scand J Haematol 1981;26:195.
1018. Van Hengstum M, Steenbergen J, Haanen C. Clinical course in 28 unselected patients with aplastic anaemia treated with anabolic steroids. Br J Haematol 1979;41:323.
1019. Hirota Y. Effects of androstanes on aplastic anemia: a prospective study. Acta Haematol Jpn 1981;44:1341.
1020. Davis S, Rubin AD. Treatment and prognosis in aplastic anæmia. Lancet 1972;1:871.
1021. Alexanian R, Nadell J, Alfrey C. Oxymetholone treatment for the anemia of bone marrow failure. Blood 1972;40:353.
1022. Haak HL, Hartgrink-Groeneveld CA, Guoit HFL, et al. Acquired aplastic anaemia in adults. Acta Haematol 1977;58:339.
1023. Branda RF, Amsden TW, Jacob HS. Randomized study of nandrolone therapy for anemias due to bone marrow failure. Arch Intern Med 1977;137:65.
1024. Gordon-Smith EC. Treatment of aplastic anaemia; I. Conservative management. In: Geary CG, ed. Aplastic anaemia. London, Bailliere Tindall, 1979:108.
1025. Lynch RE, Williams DM, Reading JC, Cartwright GE. The prognosis in aplastic anemia. Blood 1975;45:517.
1026. Pizzuto J, Conte G, Sinco A, et al. Use of androgens in acquired aplastic anaemia: relation of response to aetiology and severity. Acta Haematol 1980;64:18.
1027. Najean Y. Long-term follow-up in patients with aplastic anemia: a study of 137 androgen-treated patients surviving more than two years. Am J Med 1981;71:543.
1028. Azen EA, Shahidi NT. Androgen dependency in acquired aplastic anemia. Am J Med 1977;63:320.
1029. Yoshida Y, Yamagishi M, Uchino H. Problems in androgen treatment in aplastic anemia with reference to androgen dependency and acquisition of refractoriness. Acta Haematol Jpn 1981;44:1360.
1030. Besa EC, Wolff SM, Dale DC, Gardner FH. Etiocholanolone and prednisolone therapy in patients with severe bone-marrow failure. Lancet 1977;10:728.
1031. Najean Y. Androgen therapy in aplastic anaemia: a comparative study of high and low-doses and of 4 different androgens. Scand J Haematol 1986;36:346.
1032. Gardner FH, Juneja HS. Androstane therapy to treat aplastic anaemia in adults: an uncontrolled pilot study. Br J Haematol 1987;65:295.
1033. Urabe A, Takaku F, Akatsuka J, et al. Immunosuppression or androgen therapy for aplastic anemia: a cooperative study. Jpn J Clin Hematol 1984;25:554.
1034. Peking A, Girot R, Najean Y, Le Joly JM. Liver damage during androgenic anabolic therapy. In: Najean Y, ed. Medullary aplasia. New York, Masson, 1980:189.
1035. McGiven AR. Peliosis hepatis: case report and review of pathogenesis. J Pathol 1970;101:283.
1036. Bourliere B, Najean Y. Influence of long-term androgen therapy on growth: an analysis of 18 cases of aplastic anemia in children. Pediatr Forum 1987;141:718.
1037. Kamamoto T, Ohkubo T, Yamagishi M, et al. Correlation between in vitro and in vivo response to androgens in patients with aplastic anemia. Int J Cell Cloning 1984;2:173.
1038. Mooradian AD, Morley JE, Korenman SG. Biological actions of androgens. Endocr Rev 1987;8:1.
1039. Minguell JJ, Sierralta WD. Molecular mechanism of action of the male sex hormones. J Endocrinol 1975;65:287.
1040. Naets JP, Wittek M. Mechanism of action of androgens on erythropoiesis. Ann NY Acad Sci 1968;149:315.
1041. Viala JJ, Hadjian AJ. Androgens and hematopoiesis: current concepts of mode of action. In: Najean Y, ed. Medullary aplasia. New York, Masson, 1980:177.
1042. Gardner FH, Nathan DG, Piomelli S, Cummins JF. The erythrocythaemic effects of androgen. Br J Haematol 1968;14:611.
1043. Rishpon-Meyerstein N, Kilbridge T, Simone J, Fried W. The effect of testosterone on erythropoietin levels in anemic patients. Blood 1968;31:453.
1044. Alexanian R. Erythropoietin and erythropoiesis in anemic man following androgens. Blood 1969;33:564.
1045. Fisher JW, Samuels AI, Malgor LA. Androgens and erythropoiesis. Israel J Med Sci 1971;7:892.
1046. Schooley JC. Inhibition of erythropoietic stimulation by testosterone in polycythemic mice receiving anti-erythropoietin. Proc Soc Exp Biol Med 1966;122:402.
1047. Fisher JW, Roh BL, Halvorsen S. Inhibition of erythropoietic effects of hormones by erythropoietin antisera in mildly plethoric mice. Proc Soc Exp Biol Med 1967;126:97.
1048. Rencricca NJ, Solomon J, Fimian WJ Jr, et al. The effect of testosterone on erythropoiesis. Scand J Haematol 1969;6:431.
1049. Udupa KB, Reissmann KR. Stimulation of granulopoiesis by androgens without concomitant increase in the serum level of colony stimulating factor. Exp Hematol 1975;3:26.
1050. Francis GE, Berney JJ, Bateman SM, Hoffbrand AV. The effect of androstanes on granulopoiesis in vitro and in vivo. Br J Haematol 1977;36:501.
1051. D'Alessandro N, Gibbia N, Biondo F, et al. Haemopoietic effects of 7 alpha, 17 beta dimethyltestosterone. Pharmacol Res Commun 1979;11:81.
1052. Evens RP, Amerson AB. Androgens and erythropoiesis. J Clin Pathol 1974;94.
1053. Horn Y, Price DC. The effect of androgens on erythroid and granulocytic marrow recovery in the irradiated rat. Acta Haematol 1972;48:300.
1054. Horn Y. The effect of androgenic hormones on bone marrow of rats receiving chemotherapy. Oncology 1971;25:512.
1055. Reissmann KR, Udupa KB, Kawada K. Effects of erythropoietin and androgens on erythroid stem cells after their selective suppression by BCNU. Blood 1974;44:649.
1056. Reisener EH Jr. Tissue culture of bone marrow. II. Effect of steroid hormones on hematopoiesis in vitro. Blood 1966;27:460.
1057. Modder B, Foley JE, Fisher JW. The in vitro and in vivo effect of testosterone and steroid metabolites on erythroid colony forming cells (CFU-E). J Pharmacol Exp Ther 1978;207:1004.
1058. Beran M, Spitzer G, Verma DS. Testosterone and synthetic androgens improve the in vitro survival of human marrow progenitor cells in serum-free suspension cultures. J Lab Clin Med 1982;99:247.
1059. Urabe A, Sassa S, Kappas A. The influence of steroid hormone metabolites on the in vitro development of erythroid colonies derived from human bone marrow. J Exp Med 1979;149:1314.
1060. Singer JW, Adamson JW. Steroids and hematopoiesis. II. The effect of steroids on in vitro erythroid colony growth: evidence for different target cells for different classes of steroids. J Cell Physiol 1976;88: 135.
1061. Ohno Y, Fisher JW. Effects of androgens on burst forming units (BFU-E) in normal rabbit bone marrows. Life Sci 1978;22:2031.
1062. Rosenblum AL, Carbone PP. Androgenic hormones and human granulopoiesis in vitro. Blood 1974;43:351.
1063. Minguell J, Valladares L. Molecular aspects on the mechanism of action of testosterone in rat bone marrow cells. J Steroid Biochem 1974;5:649.
1064. Sierralta W, Gonzalez MC, Minguell J. The effect of testosterone on

rat bone marrow nuclear ribonucleic acid metabolism. J Steroid Biochem 1974;5:645.
1065. Byron JW. Comparison of the action of 3H-thymidine and hydroxyurea on testosterone-treated hemopoietic stem cells. Blood 1972;40:198.
1066. Byron JW. Effect of steroids on the cycling of haemopoietic stem cells. Nature 1970;228:1204.
1067. Jepson JH, Leonard RA, Gorshein D, et al. Review of the induction of cycling of erythropoietin sensitive cells by androgens and their 5 β-H-metabolites. Biomedicine 1974;20:262.
1068. Shimizu M, Sato J, Ishii T, et al. Androgen-induced production of colony-stimulating factor (CSF) and colony-inhibitory factor (CIF) in the submandibular gland in female mice. J Pharmacobiodyn 1989;12:352.
1069. Weinstein Y, Berkovich Z. Testosterone effect on bone marrow, thymus, and suppressor T cells in the (NZB x NZW)F1 mice: its relevance to autoimmunity. J Immunol 1981;126:998.
1070. Morley A, Remes J, Trainor K. A controlled trial of androgen therapy in experimental chronic hypoplastic marrow failure. Br J Haematol 1976;32:533.
1071. Najean Y, Chedeville A, Eberlin A, Balitrand N. A study of the efficacy of 5α- and 5β-androstanes in chronic experimental aplastic anemia in mice. Nouv Rev Fr Hematol 1984;26:391.
1072. Champlin RE, Nimer SD, Ireland P, et al. Treatment of refractory aplastic anemia with recombinant human granulocyte-macrophage-colony-stimulating factor. Blood 1989;73:694.
1073. Vadhan-Raj S, Buescher S, Broxmeyer HE, et al. Stimulation of myelopoiesis in patients with aplastic anemia by recombinant human granulocyte-macrophage colony-stimulating factor. N Engl J Med 1988;319:1628.
1074. Antin JH, Smith BR, Homes W, Rosenthal DS. Phase I/II study of recombinant human granulocyte-macrophage colony-stimulating factor in aplastic anemia and myelodysplastic syndrome. Blood 1988;72:705.
1075. Nissen C, Tichelli A, Gratwohl A, et al. Failure of recombinant human granulocyte-macrophage colony-stimulating factor therapy in aplastic anemia patients with very severe neutropenia. Blood 1988;72:2045.
1076. Young NS, Klein HG, Griffith P, Nienhuis AW. A trial of immunotherapy in aplastic anemia and pure red cell aplasia. J Clin Apheresis 1983;1:95.
1077. Ito T, Hiraiwa M, Ishikawa Y, et al. Lymphocytapheresis in a patient with severe aplastic anemia. Acta Haematol 1988;80:167.
1078. Heaton LD, Crosby WH, Cohen A. Splenectomy in the treatment of hypoplasia of the bone marrow. With a report of twelve cases. Ann Surg 1957;146:637.
1079. Bille PE, Jensen MK, Jensen JPK, Poulsen JC. Studies on the haematologic and cytogenetic effect of lithium. Acta Med Scand 1975;198:281.
1080. Rothstein G, Clarkson DR, Larsen W, et al. Effect of lithium on neutrophil mass and production. N Engl J Med 1978;298:178.
1081. Gallicchio VS, Chen MG. Modulation of murine pluripotential stem cell proliferation in vivo by lithium carbonate. Blood 1980;56:1150.
1082. Rossof AH, Fehir KM. Lithium carbonate increases marrow granulocyte-committed colony-forming units and peripheral blood granulocytes in a canine model. Exp Hematol 1979;7:255.
1083. Harker WG, Rothstein G, Clarkson D, et al. Enhancement of colony-stimulating activity production by lithium. Blood 1977;49:263.
1084. Spitzer G, Verma DS, Barlogie B, et al. Possible mechanisms of action of lithium on augmentation of in vitro spontaneous myeloid colony formation. Cancer Res 1979;39:3215.
1085. Doukas MA, Niskanen EO, Quesenberry PJ. Lithium stimulation of granulopoiesis in diffusion chambers: a model of a humoral, indirect stimulation of stem cell proliferation. Blood 1985;65:163.
1086. Hammond WP, Dale DC. Cyclic hematopoiesis: Effects of lithium on colony-forming cells and colony-stimulating activity in grey collie dogs. Blood 1982;59:179.
1087. Levitt LJ, Quesenberry PJ. The effect of lithium on murine hematopoiesis in a liquid culture system. N Engl J Med 1980;302:713.
1088. Barrett AJ, Faille A. Clinical studies with lithium. In: Najean Y, ed. Medullary Aplasia. New York: Masson, 1980:241.
1089. Blum SF. Lithium therapy of aplastic anemia. (Letter) N Engl J Med 1979;300:677.
1090. Stein RS, Beaman C, Ali MY, Hansen R, et al. Lithium carbonate attenuation of chemotherapy-induced neutropenia. N Engl J Med 1977;297:430.
1091. Scarffe JH, Chang J. Failure of lithium to reduce period of neutropenia during induction therapy of acute myeloid leukemia. Hematol Oncol 1989;7:69.
1092. Rewald E. Repeated low doses of anti-rhesus gammaglobulin in aplastic anaemia. (Letter) Lancet 1987;2:795.
1093. Humble JG. The treatment of aplastic anæmia with phytohæmagglutinin. Lancet 1964;1:1345.
1094. Hamajima N, Sasaki R, Aoki K, Shibata A. A notable change in mortality of aplastic anemia observed during the 1970s in Japan. Blood 1988;72:995.
1095. Kelton JG, Ali AM. Platelet transfusions: a critical appraisal. Clin Oncol 1983;2:549.
1096. Holland PV, ed. Standards for blood banks and transfusion services, ed 13. Arlington, American Association of Blood Banks, 1989.
1097. Freireich EJ. Effectiveness of platelet transfusion in leukemia and aplastic anemia. Transfusion 1966;6:50.
1098. Mustard JF, Rowsell HC, Murphy EA. Platelet economy (platelet survival and turnover). Br J Haematol 1966;12:1.
1099. Daly PA, Schiffer CA, Aisner J, Wiernik PH. Platelet transfusion therapy: one-hour posttransfusion increments are valuable in predicting the need for HLA-matched preparations. JAMA 1980;243:435.
1100. Tomasulo PA, Petz LD. Platelet transfusions. In: Petz LD, Swisher SN, eds. Clinical practice of transfusion medicine, ed 2. New York, Churchill Livingstone, 1989:427.
1101. Djerassi I, Farber S, Evans AE. Transfusions of fresh platelet concentrates to patients with secondary thrombocytopenia. N Engl J Med 1963;268:221.
1102. Slichter SJ. Controversies in platelet transfusion therapy. Annu Rev Med 1980;31:509.
1103. Cohen P, Gardner FH. Thrombocytopenia as a laboratory sign and complication of gram-negative bacteremic infection. Arch Intern Med 1966;117:113.
1104. Poskitt TR, Poskitt PKF. Thrombocytopenia of sepsis: the role of circulating IgG-containing immune complexes. Arch Intern Med 1985;145:891.
1105. Bishop JF, McGrath K, Wolf MM, Matthews JP, et al. Clinical factors influencing the efficacy of pooled platelet transfusions. Blood 1988;71:383.
1106. Menitove JE. Platelet transfusion for alloimmunized patients. Clin Oncol 1983;2:587.
1107. Platelet transfusion therapy: consensus conference. JAMA 1987;257:1777.
1108. Klingemann H-G, Self S, Banaji M, et al. Refractoriness to random donor platelet transfusions in patients with aplastic anaemia: a multivariate analysis of data from 264 cases. Br J Haematol 1987;66:115.
1109. Tosato G, Appelbaum F, Deisseroth AB. HLA-matched platelet transfusion therapy of severe aplastic anemia. Blood 1978;52:846.
1110. Wu KK, Thompson JS, Koepke JA, et al. Heterogeneity of antibody response to human platelet transfusion. J Clin Invest 1976;58:432.
1111. Yankee RA, Grumet FC, Rogentine GN. Platelet transfusion therapy: the selection of compatible platelet donors for refractory patients by lymphocyte HL-A typing. N Engl J Med 1969;281:1208.
1112. Duquesnoy RJ, Filip DJ, Aster RH. Influence of HLA-A2 on the effectiveness of platelet transfusions in alloimmunized thrombocytopenia patients. Blood 1977;50:407.
1113. Dahlke MB, Weiss KL. Platelet transfusion from donors mismatched for crossreactive HLA antigens. Transfusion 1984;24:299.
1114. Flatow FA, Freireich EJ. Effect of splenectomy on the response to platelet transfusion in three patients with aplastic anemia. N Engl J Med 1966;274:242.
1115. Grumet FC, Yankee RA. Long-term platelet support of patients with aplastic anemia. Effect of splenectomy and steroid therapy. Ann Intern Med 1970;73:1.
1116. Bensinger WI, Buckner CD, Clift RA, et al. Plasma exchange for platelet alloimmunization. Transplantation 1986;41:602.
1117. Zeigler ZR, Shadduck RK, Rosenfeld CS, et al. High-dose intravenous gamma globulin improves responses to single-donor platelets in patients refractory to platelet transfusion. Blood 1987;70:1433.
1118. Lee EJ, Norris D, Schiffer CA. Intravenous immune globulin for patients alloimmunized to random donor platelet transfusion. Transfusion 1987;27:245.
1119. Roy AJ, Djerassi I. Effects of platelet transfusions: plug formation and maintenance of vascular integrity. Proc Soc Exp Biol Med 1972;139:137.
1120. Sintnicolaas K, Sizoo W, Haije WG, et al. Delayed alloimmunisation by random single donor platelet transfusions: a randomised study to compare single donor and multiple donor platelet transfusions in cancer patients with severe thrombocytopenia. Lancet 1981;1:750.
1121. Schiffer CA. Management of patients refractory to platelet transfusion: an evaluation of methods of donor selection. Prog Hematol 1987;15:91.
1122. Gmür J, von Felten A, Osterwalder B, et al. Delayed alloimmunization using random single donor platelet transfusions: a prospective study in thrombocytopenic patients with acute leukemia. Blood 1983;62:473.
1123. Eernisse JG, Brand A. Prevention of platelet refractoriness due to HLA antibodies by administration of leukocyte-poor blood components. Exp Hematol 1981;9:77.
1124. Schiffer CA, Dutcher JP, Aisner J, et al. A randomized trial of leukocyte-depleted platelet transfusion to modify alloimmunization in patients with leukemia. Blood 1983;62:815.
1125. Sniecinski I, O'Donnell MR, Nowicki B, Hill LR. Prevention of refractoriness and HLA-alloimmunization using filtered blood products. Blood 1988;71:1402.
1126. Kickler TS, Bell W, Ness PM, et al. Depletion of white cells from platelet concentrates with a new absorption filter. Transfusion 1989;29:411.
1127. Bertholf MF, Mintz PD. Comparison of plateletpheresis using two cell separators and identical donors. Transfusion 1989;29:521.

1128. Howard JE, Perkins HA. The natural history of alloimmunization to platelets. Transfusion 1978;18:496.
1129. Dutcher JP, Schiffer CA, Aisner J, Wiernik PH. Alloimmunization following platelet transfusion: the absence of a dose-response relationship. Blood 1981;57:395.
1130. Dutcher JP, Schiffer CA, Aisner J, Wiernik PH. Long-term follow-up of patients with leukemia receiving platelet transfusions: identification of a large group of patients who do not become alloimmunized. Blood 1981;58:1007.
1131. Pegels JG, Bruynes ECE, Engelriet CP, von dem Borne AEGKR. Serological studies in patients on platelet- and granulocyte-substitution therapy. Br J Haematol 1982;52:59.
1132. Holohan TV, Terasaki PI, Deisseroth AB. Suppression of transfusion-related alloimmunization in intensively treated cancer patients. Blood 1981;58:122.
1133. Roy AJ, Jaffe N, Djerassi I. Prophylactic platelet transfusions in children: a dose response study. Transfusion 1973;13:283.
1134. Highby DJ, Cohen E, Holland JF, Sinks L. The prophylactic treatment of thrombocytopenic leukemic patients with platelets: a double blind study. Transfusion 1974;14:440.
1135. Murphy S, Litwin S, Herring LM, et al. Indications for platelet transfusion in children with acute leukemia. Am J Hematol 1982;12:347.
1136. Solomon J, Bofenkamp T, Fahey JL, et al. Platelet prophylaxis in acute non-lymphoblastic leukemia. (Letter) Lancet 1978;1:267.
1137. Buchanan GR. Hematologic supportive care. In: Pizzo PA, Poplack DG, eds. Principles and practice of pediatric oncology. Philadelphia, JB Lippincott, 1989:823.
1138. Aderka D, Praff G, Santo M, et al. Bleeding due to thrombocytopenia in acute leukemias and reevaluation of the prophylactic platelet transfusion policy. Am J Med Sci 1986;291:147.
1139. Gaydos LA, Freireich EJ, Mantel N. The quantitative relation between platelet count and hemorrhage in patients with acute leukemia. N Engl J Med 1962;266:905.
1140. Cavins JA, Farber S, Roy AJ. Transfusion of fresh platelet concentrates to adult patients with thrombocytopenia. Transfusion 1968;8:24.
1141. Slichter SJ, Harker LA. Thrombocytopenia: Mechanisms and management of defects in platelet production. Clin Haematol 1978;7:523.
1142. Gardner FH, Helmer RE III. Aminocaproic acid: use in control of hemorrhage in patients with amegakaryocytic thrombocytopenia. JAMA 1980;243:35.
1143. Bartholomew JR, Salgia R, Bell WR. Control of bleeding in patients with immune and nonimmune thrombocytopenia with aminocaproic acid. Arch Intern Med 1989;149:1959.
1144. Kitchens CS. Amelioration of endothelial abnormalities by prednisone in experimental thrombocytopenia in the rabbit. J Clin Invest 1977;60:1129.
1145. Kitchens CS, Pendergast JF. Human thrombocytopenia is associated with structural abnormalities of the endothelium that are ameliorated by glucocorticosteroid administration. Blood 1986;67:203.
1146. Shepro D, Sweetman HE, Hechtman HB. Experimental thrombocytopenia and capillary ultrastructure. Blood 1980;56:937.
1147. Hathorn JW, Pizzo PA. Infectious complications in the pediatric cancer patient. In: Pizzo PA, Poplack DG, eds. Principles and practice of pediatric oncology. Philadelphia, JB Lippincott, 1989:837.
1148. Joshi JH, Schimpff SC. Therapy of infection in granulocytopenic patients with cancer. Clin Oncol 1983;2:611.
1149. Marcus RE, Goldman JM. Management of infection in the neutropenic patient. Br Med J 1986;295:406.
1150. Boogaerts M. Empiric antibiotic therapy in the neutropenic patient. (Symposium) Br J Clin Pract 1988;Suppl 57:85.
1151. Elliott CR, Pater JL. The effect of different measures of outcome on the results of studies of empiric antibiotic therapy in febrile neutropenic patients. Clin Invest Med 1988;11:327.
1152. Pater JL, Weir L. Reporting the results of randomized trials of empiric antibiotics in febrile neutropenic patients: a critical survey. J Clin Oncol 1986;4:346.
1153. Keidan AJ, Tsatalas C, Cohen J, et al. Infective complications of aplastic anaemia. Br J Haematol 1986;63:503.
1154. Bodey GP, Buckley M, Sathe YS, Freireich EJ. Quantitative relationships between circulating leukocytes and infection in patients with acute leukemia. Ann Intern Med 1966;64:328.
1155. van der Meer JWM. Infectious episodes in severely granulopenic patients. Infection 7:171,1979.
1156. Gurwith MJ, Brunton JL, Lank BA, et al. Granulocytopenia in hospitalized patients. I. Prognostic factors and etiology of fever. Am J Med 1978;64:121.
1157. Sickles EA, Greene WH, Wiernik PH. Clinical presentation of infection in granulocytopenia patients. Arch Intern Med 1975;135:715.
1158. Klastersky J. Empiric antimicrobial therapy for febrile granulocytopenic cancer patients. Acta Oncol 1988.
1159. Wingard JR, Santos GW, Saral R. Differences between first and subsequent fevers during prolonged neutropenia. Cancer 1987;59:844.
1160. McCabe WR, Jackson GG. Gram-negative bacteremia. I. Etiology and ecology. Arch Intern Med 1962;110:847.
1161. Viscoli C, Van der Auwera P, Meunier F. Gram-positive infections in granulocytopenic patients: an important issue? J Antimicrob Chemother 1988;21(Suppl C):149.
1162. Langley J, Gold R. Sepsis in febrile neutropenic children with cancer. Pediatr Infect Dis J 1988;7:34.
1163. Rubin M, Hathorn JW, Pizzo PA. Controversies in the management of febrile neutropenic cancer patients. Cancer Invest 1988;6:167.
1164. Barnes RA, Rogers TR. An evaluation of empirical antibiotic therapy in febrile neutropenic patients. Br J Haematol 1987;66:137.
1165. Schimpff SC, Young VM, Greene WH, et al. Origin of infection in acute non-lymphocytic leukemia: significance of hospital acquisition of potential pathogens. Ann Intern Med 1972;77:707.
1166. Winston DJ, Gale RP, Meyer DV, et al. Infectious complications of human bone marrow transplantation. Medicine 1979;58:1.
1167. Pizzo PA, Robichaud KJ, Wesley R, Commers JA. Fever in the pediatric and young adult patient with cancer: a prospective study of 1001 episodes. Medicine 1982;61:153.
1168. Dale DC, Petersdorf RG. Corticosteroids and infectious diseases. Med Clin North Am 1973;57:1277.
1169. Love LJ, Schimpff SC, Schiffer CA, Wiernik PH. Improved prognosis for granulocytopenic patients with gram-negative bacteremia. Am J Med 1980;68:643.
1170. Pizzo PA, Hathorn JW, Hiemenz J, et al. A randomized trial comparing ceftazidime alone with combination antibiotic therapy in cancer patients with fever and neutropenia. N Engl J Med 1986;315:552.
1171. Rubin M, Hathron JW, Marshall D, et al. Gram-positive infections and the use of vancomycin in 550 episodes of fever and neutropenia. Ann Intern Med 1988;108:30.
1172. Pizzo PA, Robichaud KJ, Gill FA, Witebsky FG. Empiric antibiotic and antifungal therapy for cancer patients with prolonged fever and granulocytopenia. Am J Med 1982;72:101.
1173. DiNubile MJ. Stopping antibiotic therapy in neutropenic patients. Ann Intern Med 1988;108:289.
1174. Horn R, Wong B, Kiehn TE, Armstrong D. Fungemia in a cancer hospital: changing frequency, earlier onset, and results of therapy. Rev Infect Dis 1985;7:646.
1175. Gerson SL, Talbot GH, Hurwitz S, et al. Prolonged granulocytopenia: the major risk factor for invasive pulmonary aspergillosis in patients with acute leukemia. Ann Intern Med 1984;100:345.
1176. Wingard JR, Merz WG, Saral R. *Candida tropicalis*: a major pathogen in immunocompromised patients. Ann Intern Med 1979;91:539.
1177. Thaler M, Pastakia B, Shawker TH, et al. Hepatic candidiasis in cancer patients: the evolving picture of the syndrome. Ann Intern Med 1988;108:88.
1178. Walsh TJ, Hamilton SR, Belitsos N. Esophageal candidiasis. Managing an increasingly prevalent infection. Postgrad Med J 1988;84:193.
1179. Degregorio MW, Lee WMF, Linker CA, et al. Fungal infections in patients with acute leukemia. Am J Med 1982;73:543.
1180. Albelda SM, Talbot GH, Gerson SL, et al. Role of fiberoptic bronchoscopy in the diagnosis of invasive pulmonary aspergillosis in patients with acute leukemia. Am J Med 1984;76:1027.
1181. Sculier JP, Weerts D, Klastersky J. Causes of death in febrile granulocytopenic cancer patients receiving empiric antibiotic therapy. Eur J Cancer Clin Oncol 1984;20:55.
1182. Thaler M, Bacher J, O'Leary T, Pizzo PA. Evaluation of single-drug and combination antifungal therapy in an experimental model of candidiasis in rabbits with prolonged neutropenia. J Infect Dis 1988;158:80.
1183. McCullough J. Granulocyte transfusion. In: Petz LD, Swisher SN, eds. Clinical practice of transfusion medicine, ed 2. New York, Churchill Livingstone, 1989:469.
1184. Dutcher JP. Platelet and granulocyte transfusions in cancer patients. Adv Immun Cancer Ther 1986;2:211.
1185. Strauss RG. Granulocyte transfusion therapy. Clin Oncol 1983;2:635.
1186. DiNubile MJ. Therapeutic role of granulocyte transfusions. Rev Infect Dis 1985;7:232.
1187. Menitove JE, Abrams RA. Granulocyte transfusions in neutropenic patients. CRC Crit Rev Oncol Hematol 1987;7:89.
1188. Appelbaum FR, Bowles CA, Makuch RW, Deisseroth AB. Granulocyte transfusion therapy of experimental Pseudomonas septicemia: study of dose and collection techniques. Blood 1978;52:323.
1189. Dutcher JP, Schiffer CA, Johnston GS, et al. Alloimmunization prevents the migration of transfused indium-111–labeled granulocytes to sites of infection. Blood 1983;62:354.
1190. Kirby BD, Snyder KM, Meyer RD, Feingold SM. Legionnaires' disease: report of sixty-five nosocomially acquired cases and review of the literature. Medicine 1980;59:188.
1191. Weems JJ Jr, Davis BJ. Construction activity: an independent risk factor for invasive aspergillosis and zygomycosis in patients with hematologic malignancy. Infect Control 1987;8:71.
1192. Lasser SD, Camitta BM, Needleman HL. Dental management of patients undergoing bone marrow transplantation for aplastic anemia. Oral Surg 1989;43:181.
1193. Vogler WR, Malcom LG, Winton EF. A randomized trial comparing ketoconazole and nystatin prophylactic therapy in neutropenic patients. Cancer Invest 1987;5:267.
1194. Schimpff SC, Greene WH, Young VM, et al. Infection prevention in

acute nonlymphocytic leukemia: laminar air flow room reverse isolation with oral, nonabsorbable antibiotic prophylaxis. Ann Intern Med 1975;82:351.
1195. Dietrich M, Gaus W, Vossen J, et al. Protective isolation and antimicrobial decontamination in patients with high susceptibility to infection: a prospective cooperative study of gnotobiotic care in acute leukemia patients. I. Clinical results. Infection 1977;5:107.
1196. van den Broek PJ. Infection control during neutropenia. J Hosp Infect 1988;11(Suppl A):7.
1197. Van Saene HKF, Stoutenbeek CP. Selective decontamination. J Antimicrob Chemother 1987;20:462.
1198. Dekker AW, Rozenberg-Arska M, Sixma JJ, Verhoef J. Prevention of infection by trimethoprim-sulfamethoxazole plus amphotericin B in patients with acute nonlymphocytic leukaemia. Ann Intern Med 1981;95:555.
1199. Bow EJ, Rayner E, Scott BA, Louie TJ. Selective gut decontamination with nalidixic acid or trimethoprim-sulfamethoxazole for infection prophylaxis in neutropenic cancer patients: relationship of efficacy to antimicrobial spectrum and timing of administration. Antimicrob Agents Chemother 1987;31:551.
1200. Young LS. Antimicrobial prophylaxis in the neutropenic host: lessons of the past and perspectives for the future. Eur J Clin Microbiol Infect Dis 1988;7:93.
1201. Karp JE, Merz WG, Hendricksen C, et al. Infection management during antileukemia treatment-induced granulocytopenia: the role for oral norfloxacin prophylaxis against infections arising from the gastrointestinal tract. Scand J Infect Dis 1986;48(Suppl):66.
1202. Nauseef WM, Maki DG. A study of the value of simple protective isolation in patients with granulocytopenia. N Engl J Med 1981;304:448.
1203. Pizzo PA, Robichaud KJ, Edwards BK, et al. Oral antibiotic prophylaxis in patients with cancer: a double-blind randomized placebo-controlled trial. J Pediatr 1983;102:125.
1204. Wilson JM, Guinery DG. Failure of oral trimethoprim-sulfamethoxazole prophylaxis in acute leukemia: isolation of resistant plasmids from strains of Enterobacteriaceae causing bacteremia. N Engl J Med 1982;306:16.
1205. Schimpff SC. Surveillance cultures. J Infect Dis 1981;144:81.
1206. Daw MA, Munnelly P, McCann SR, et al. Value of surveillance cultures in the management of neutropenic patients. Eur J Clin Microbiol Infect Dis 1988;7:742.
1207. Surveillance cultures in neutropenia. Lancet 1989;1:1238.
1208. Aisner J, Murillo J, Schimpff SC, Steere AC. Invasive aspergillosis in acute leukemia: correlation with nose cultures and antibiotic use. Ann Intern Med 1979;90:4.
1209. Aker SN, Cheney CL. The use of sterile and low microbial diets in ultraisolation environments. JPEN 1983;7:390.
1210. Somerville ET. Special diets for neutropenic patients: do they make a difference? Semin Oncol Nurs 1986;2:55.
1211. Pizzo PA, Purvis DS, Waters C. Microbiological evaluation of food items. J Am Diet Assoc 1982;81:272.
1212. Schafer AI, Rabinowe S, Le Boff MS, et al. Long-term efficacy of deferoxamine iron chelation therapy in adult with acquired transfusional iron overload. Arch Intern Med 1985;145:1217.
1213. Cohen AR, Mizanin J, Schwartz E. Rapid removal of excessive iron with daily, high-dose intravenous chelation therapy. J Pediatr 1989;115:151.
1214. Parkinson JP. A case of aplastic anæmia. Br J Child Dis 1919;16:1.
1215. Björkman SE. Case of aplastic anemia caused by chloramphenicol with recovery after 22 months. Acta Haematol 1962;27:124.
1216. Adams EB. Aplastic anaemia: review of twenty-seven cases. Lancet 1951;1:657.
1217. Boon TH, Walton JN. Aplastic anaemia. Q J Med 1951;20:75.
1218. Lewis SM. Course and prognosis in aplastic anemia. Br Med J 1965;1:1027.
1219. Heyn RM, Ertel IJ, Tubergen DG. Course of acquired aplastic anemia in children treated with supportive care. JAMA 1969;208:1372.
1220. Lohrmann H-P, Kern P, Niethammer D, Heimpel H. Identification of high-risk patients with aplastic anaemia in selection for allogeneic bone-marrow transplantation. Lancet 1976;2:647.
1221. Haak HL, Hartgrink-Groenveld CA, Ernisse JG, et al. Acquired aplastic anaemia in adults. I. A retrospective study of 40 cases: single factors influencing prognosis. Acta Haematol 1977;58:257.
1222. Rozman C, Martin P, Nomdedu B, Monteserrat E. Criteria for severe aplastic anaemia. Lancet 1987;2:955.
1223. Rozman C, Marin P, Grañena A, et al. Prognosis in acquired aplastic anaemia: a multivariate statistical analysis of 80 cases. Scand J Haematol 1981;26:321.
1224. Hörmann A, Berchthold W, Rhyner K, et al. Prognosis in acquired aplastic anemia. Acta Haematol 1984;71:81.
1225. Retief FP, Heyns ADP. Pansiopenie en aplastiese anemie 'n retropektiewe beoordeling. S Afr Med J 1976;50:1318.
1226. Cabot RC. Case 13321: bleeding from the gums. Boston Med Surg J 1927;197:236.
1227. Najean Y, Pecking A. Prognostic factors in acquired aplastic anemia: a study of 352 cases. Am J Med 1979;67:564.
1228. Williams DM, Lynch RE, Cartwright GE. Prognostic factors in aplastic anaemia. Clin Haematol 1978;7:467.
1229. Clemmesen L, Hansen MM, Mortensen L, et al. Prediction of survival in adults with acquired bi- or pancytopenia. Scand J Haematol 1984;32:119.
1230. Te Velde J, Haak HL. Aplastic anaemia: histological investigation of methacrylate embedded bone marrow biopsy specimens—correlation with survival after conventional treatment in 15 adult patients. Br J Haematol 1977;35:61.
1231. Sale GE, Rajantie J, Doney K, et al. Does histologic grading of inflammation in bone marrow predict the response of aplastic anaemia patients to antithymocyte globulin therapy? Br J Haematol 1987;67:261.
1232. de Planque MM, van Krieken JHJM, Kluin-Nelemans HC, et al. Bone marrow histopathology of patients with severe aplastic anaemia before treatment and at follow-up. Br J Haematol 1989;72:439.
1233. Bomford RR, Rhoads CP. Refractory anemia. Q J Med 1941;10:175.
1234. Torok-Storb B, Doney K, Sale G, et al. Subsets of patients with aplastic anemia identified by flow microfluorometry. N Engl J Med 1985;312:1015.
1235. Torok-Storb B, Doney K, Brown SL, Prentice RL. Correlation of two in vitro tests with clinical response to immunosuppressive therapy in 54 patients with severe aplastic anemia. Blood 1984;63:349.
1236. Dessypris EN. Pure red cell aplasia. Baltimore, Johns Hopkins University Press, 1988.
1237. Roland AS. The syndrome of benign thymoma and primary aregenerative anemia. Am J Med Sci 1964;247:719.
1238. Hirst E, Robertson TI. The syndrome of thymoma and erythroblastopenic anemia. Medicine 1967;46:225.
1239. Schmid JR, Kiely JM, Pease GL, Hargraves MM. Acquired pure red cell agenesis. Acta Haematol 1963;30:255.
1240. Chikkappa G, Zarrabi MH, Tsan MF. Pure red-cell aplasia in patients with chronic lymphocytic leukemia. Medicine 1986;65:339.
1241. Ammus SS, Yunis AA. Acquired pure red cell aplasia. Am J Hematol 1987;24:311.
1242. Sieff C. Pure red cell aplasia. Br J Haematol 1983;54:331.
1243. Beard MEJ, Krantz SB, Johnson SAN, et al. Pure red cell aplasia. Q J Med 1978;187:339.
1244. Krantz SB. Diagnosis and treatment of pure red cell aplasia. Med Clin North Am 1976;60:945.
1245. Bunn HF, McNeil BJ, Rosenthal DS, Krantz SB. Bone-marrow imaging in pure red blood cell aplasia. Arch Intern Med 1976;136:1169.
1246. Dessypris EN, Gogo A, Russell M, et al. Studies on pure red cell aplasia. X. Association with acute leukemia and significance of bone marrow karyotype abnormalities. Blood 1980;56:421.
1247. DiBenedetto J Jr, Padre-Mendoza T, Albala MM. Pure red cell hypoplasia associated with long-arm deletion of chromosome 5. Hum Genet 1979;46:345.
1248. Schmid JR, Kiely JM, Harrison EG Jr, et al. Thymoma associated with pure red-cell agenesis. Cancer 1965;18:216.
1249. Geary CG, Byron PR, Taylor G, et al. Thymoma associated with pure red cell aplasia, immunoglobulin deficiency and an inhibitor of antigen-induced lymphocyte transformation. Br J Haematol 1975;29:479.
1250. Jacobs EM, Hutter RVP. Benign thymoma and selective erythroid aplasia of the bone marrow. Cancer 1959;12:47.
1251. DeSevilla E, Forrest JV, Zivnuska FR, Sagel SS. Metastatic thymoma with myasthenia gravis and pure red cell aplasia. Cancer 1975;36:1154.
1252. Guillan RA, Zelman S, Smalley RL, Iglesias PA. Malignant thymoma associated with myasthenia gravis, and evidence of extrathoracic metastases: an analysis of published cases and report of a case. Cancer 1971;27:823.
1253. Socinski MA, Ershler WB, Frankel J, et al. Pure RBC aplasia and myasthenia gravis. Arch Intern Med 1983;143:543.
1254. Souadjian JV, Enriquez P, Silverstein MN, Pepin J-M. The spectrum of diseases associated with thymoma. Arch Intern Med 1974;134:374.
1255. Baron RL, Lee JKT, Sagel SS, Levitt RG. Computed tomography of the abnormal thymus. Radiology 1982;142:127.
1256. Linsk JA, Murray CK. Erythrocyte aplasia and hypogammaglobulinemia. Response to steroids in a young adult. Ann Intern Med 1961;55:831.
1257. Resegotti L, Dolci C, Palestro G, Peschle C. Paraproteinemic variety of pure red cell aplasia. Acta Haematol 1978;60:227.
1258. Prasad AS, Berman L, Tranchida L, Poulik MD. Red cell hyploplasia, cold hemoglobinuria and M-type gamma G serum paraprotein and Bence Jones proteinuria in a patient with lymphoproliferative disorder. Blood 1968;31:151.
1259. Doll DC, Weiss RB. Neoplasia and the erythron. J Clin Oncol 1985;3:429.
1260. Brittingham TE, Lutcher CL, Murphy DI. Reversible erythroid aplasia induced by diphenylhydantoin. Arch Intern Med 1964;113:764.
1261. Yunis AA, Arimura GK, Lutcher CL, et al. Biochemical lesion in dilantin-induced erythroid aplasia. Blood 1967;30:587.
1262. Balaban EP, Buchanan GR, Graham M, Frenkel EP. Diamond-Blackfan syndrome in adult patients. Am J Med 1985;78:533.
1263. Field EO, Caughi MN, Blackett NM, Smithers DW. Marrow-suppressing factors in the blood in pure red-cell aplasia, thymoma and Hodgkin's disease. Br J Haematol 1968;15:101.

1264. Krantz SB, Kao V. Studies on red cell aplasia. I. Demonstration of a plasma inhibitor to heme synthesis and an antibody to erythroblast nuclei. Proc Natl Acad Sci USA 1967;58:493.
1265. Krantz SB, Kao V. Studies on red cell aplasia. II. Report of a second patient with an antibody to erythroblast nuclei and a remission after immunosuppressive therapy. Blood 1969;34:1.
1266. Krantz SB, Moore WH, Zaentz SD. Studies on red cell aplasia. V. Presence of erythroblast cytotoxicity in gamma G-globulin fraction of plasma. J Clin Invest 1973;52:324.
1267. Lowenberg B, Ghio R. An assay for serum cytotoxicity against erythroid precursor cells in pure red cell aplasia. Biomedicine 1977;27:285.
1268. Meyer RJ, Hoffman R, Zanjani ED. Autoimmune hemolytic anemia and periodic pure red cell aplasia in systemic lupus erythematosus. Am J Med 1978;65:342.
1269. Mangan KF, Besa EC, Shadduck RK, et al. Demonstration of two distinct antibodies in autoimmune hemolytic anemia with reticulocytopenia and red cell aplasia. Exp Hematol 1984;12:788.
1270. Mangan KF, Chikkappa G, Scharfman WB, Desforges JF. Evidence for reduced erythroid burst (BFUE) promoting function of T lymphocytes in the pure red cell aplasia of chronic lymphocytic leukemia. Exp Hematol 1981;9:489.
1271. Brownman GP, Freedman MH, Blajchman MA, McBride JA. A complement independent erythropoietic inhibitor acting on the progenitor cell in refractory anemia. Am J Med 1976;61:572.
1272. Peschle C, Marmont A, Perugini S, et al. Physiopathology and therapy of adult pure red cell aplasia (PRCA): a cooperative study. In: Hibino S, Takaku F, Shahidi NT, eds. Aplastic anemia. Baltimore, University Park Press, 1978:285.
1273. Jepson JH, Lowenstein L. Panhypoplasia of the bone marrow. I. Demonstration of a plasma factor with anti-erythropoietin-like activity. Can Med Assoc J 1968;99:99.
1274. Al-Mondhiry H, Zanjani ED, Spivack M, et al. Pure red cell aplasia and thymoma: loss of serum inhibitor of erythropoiesis following thymectomy. Blood 1971;38:576.
1275. Messner HA, Fauser AA, Curtis JE, Dotten D. Control of antibody-mediated pure red-cell aplasia by plasmapheresis. N Engl J Med 1981;304:1334.
1276. Freund LG, Hippe E, Strandgaard S, et al. Complete remission in pure red cell aplasia after plasmapheresis. Scand J Haematol 1985;35:315.
1277. Barnes RD. Refractory anaemia with thymoma. (Letter) Lancet 1966;2:1464.
1278. Dessypris EN, Krantz SB, Roloff JS, Lukens JN. Mode of action of the IgG inhibitor of erythropoiesis in transient erythroblastopenia of childhood. Blood 1982;59:114.
1279. Abkowitz JL, Powell JS, Nakamura JM, et al. Pure red cell aplasia: response to therapy with anti-thymocyte globulin. Am J Hematol 1986;23:363.
1280. Hoffman R, Kopel S, Hsu SD, et al. T cell chronic lymphocytic leukemia: presence in bone marrow and peripheral blood of cells that suppress erythropoiesis in vitro. Blood 1978;52:255.
1281. Mangan KF, D'Alessandro L. Hypoplastic anemia in B cell chronic lymphocytic leukemia: evolution of T cell–mediated suppression of erythropoiesis in early-stage and late-stage disease. Blood 1985;66:533.
1282. Linch DC, Cawley JC, MacDonald SM, et al. Acquired pure red-cell aplasia associated with an increase of T cells bearing receptors for the Fc of IgG. Acta Haematol 1981;65:270.
1283. Mangan KF, Chikkappa G, Farley PC. T gamma cells suppress growth of erythroid colony-forming units in vitro in the pure red cell aplasia of B-cell chronic lymphocytic leukemia. J Clin Invest 1982;70:1148.
1284. Abkowitz JL, Kadin ME, Powell JS, Adamson JW. Pure red cell aplasia: lymphocyte inhibition of erythropoiesis. Br J Haematol 1986;63:59.
1285. Mangan KF, Volkin R, Winkelstein A. Autoreactive erythroid progenitor-T suppressor cells in the pure red cell aplasia associated with thymoma and panhypogammaglobulinemia. Am J Hematol 1986;23:167.
1286. Akard LP, Brandt J, Lu Li, et al. Chronic T cell lymphoproliferative disorder and pure red cell aplasia. Am J Med 1987;83:1069.
1287. Lipton JM, Nadler LM, Canellos GP, Kudisch M. Evidence for genetic restriction in the suppression of erythropoiesis by a unique subset of T lymphocytes in man. J Clin Invest 1983;72:694.
1288. Hanada T, Abe T, Nakamura H, Aoki Y. Pure red cell aplasia: relationship between inhibitory activity of T cells to CFU-E and erythropoiesis. Br J Haematol 1984;58:107.
1289. Nagasawa T, Abe T, Nakagawa T. Pure red cell aplasia and hypogammaglobulinemia associated with Tγ-cell chronic lymphocytic leukemia. Blood 1981;57:1025.
1290. Shionoya S, Amano M, Imamura Y, et al. Suppressor T cell chronic lymphocytic leukaemia associated with red cell hypoplasia. Scand J Haematol 1984;33:231.
1291. Kurtzman G, Frickhofen N, Kimball J, et al. Pure red-cell aplasia of 10 years' duration due to persistent parvovirus B19 infection and its cure with immunoglobulin therapy. N Engl J Med 1989;321:519.
1292. Frickhofen N, Abkowitz J, Safford M, et al. Persistent parvovirus infection in patients with human immunodeficiency virus-1: a treatable cause of anemia in AIDS. Ann Intern Med 1990;113:926.
1293. Frickhofen N, Cohen B, Young NS, et al. Parvovirus B19 as a cause of acquired pure red cell aplasia. (Abstract) Blood 1991;78(Suppl 1):336a.
1294. Berner YN, Green L, Handzel ZT. Erythroblastopenia in acquired immunodeficiency syndrome (AIDS). (Letter) Acta Haematol 1983;70:273.
1295. Sallan SE, Buchanan GR. Selective erythroid aplasia during therapy for acute lymphoblastic leukemia. Pediatrics 1977;59:895.
1296. Conley CL, Lippman SM, Ness PM, et al. Autoimmune hemolytic amemia with reticulocytopenia and erythroid marrow. N Engl J Med 1982;306:281.
1297. Foy H, Kondi A, MacDougall L. Pure red-cell aplasia in marasmus and kwashiorkor treated with riboflavine. Br Med J 1961;937.
1298. Kurtzman G, Cohen R, Field AM, et al. The immune response to B19 parvovirus infection and an antibody defect in persistent viral infection. J Clin Invest 1989;84:1114.
1299. Gill PJ, Amare M, Larsen WE. Pure red cell aplasia: three cases responding to immunosuppression. Am J Med Sci 1977;273:213.
1300. Clark DA, Dessypris EN, Krantz SB. Studies on pure red cell aplasia. XI. Results of immunosuppressive treatment of 37 patients. Blood 1984;63:277.
1301. Firkin FC, Maher D. Cytotoxic immunosuppressive drug treatment strategy in pure red cell aplasia. Eur J Haematol 1988;41:212.
1302. Zaentz SD, Krantz SB, Brown EB. Studies on pure red cell aplasia. VIII. Maintenance therapy with immunosuppressive drugs. Br J Haematol 1976;32:47.
1303. Tötterman TH, Nisell J, Killander A, et al. Successful treatment of pure red-cell aplasia with cyclosporin. (Letter) Lancet 1984;2:693.
1304. Katakkar SB. Cyclosporine and pure red cell aplasia. Transplant Proc 1988;10:314.
1305. Berlin G, Liedén G. Long-term remission of pure red cell aplasia after plasma exchange and lymphocytapheresis. Scand J Haematol 1986;36:121.
1306. Chang JC, Slutzker B, Lindsay N. Remission of pure red cell aplasia following oxymetholone therapy. Am J Med Sci 1978;275:345.
1307. Lippman SM, Durie BGM, Garewal HS, et al. Efficacy of danazol in pure red cell aplasia. Am J Hematol 1986;23:373.
1308. Needleman SW. Durable remission of pure red cell aplasia after treatment with high-dose intravenous gammaglobulin and prednisone. Am J Hematol 1989;32:150.
1309. Etzioni A, Atias D, Pollack S, et al. Complete recovery of pure red cell aplasia by intramuscular gammaglobulin therapy in a child with hypoparathyroidism. Am J Hematol 1986;22:409.
1310. Katakkar SB. Pure red blood cell aplasia: response to intravenous immunoglobulins, a blocking antibody. (Letter) Arch Intern Med 1986;146:2288.
1311. Battle JD Jr, Hewlett JS, Hoffman GC. Prolonged erythroid aplasia in chronic lymphocytic leukemia: favorable response to adrenocortical steroids in four cases. (Letter) Ann Intern Med 1963;58:731.
1312. Slater LM, Schlutz MJ, Armentrout SA. Remission of pure red cell aplasia associated with nonthymic malignancy. Cancer 1979;44:1879.
1313. Hunt FA, Lander CM. Successful use of combination chemotherapy in pure red cell aplasia associated with malignant lymphoma, histiocytic type. Aust NZ J Med 1975; 5:469.
1314. Lacombe C, Casadevall N, Muller O, Varet B. Erythroid progenitors in adult chronic pure red cell aplasia: relationship of in vitro erythroid colonies to therapeutic response. Blood 1984; 64:71.
1315. Manoharan A, Williams NT, Sparrow R. Acquired amegakaryocytic thrombocytopenia: report of a case and review of literature. Q J Med 1989; 70:243.
1316. Geissler D, Thaler J, Konwalinka G, Peschel C. Progressive preleukemia presenting amegakaryocytic thrombocytopenic purpura: association of the 5q-syndrome with a decreased megakaryocytic colony formation and a defective production of Meg-CSF. Leuk Res 1987;11:731.
1317. Stoll DB, Blum S, Pasquale D, Murphy S. Thrombocytopenia with decreased megakaryocytes. Ann Intern Med 1981;94:170.
1318. Hallett JM, Martell RW, Sher C, Jacobs P. Amegakaryocytic thrombocytopenia with duplication of part of the long arm of chromosome 3. (Letter) Br J Haematol 1989;71:291.
1319. Nieneltow M, Cooper M, Breg WR, Hoffman R. Evidence for the clonal origin of acquired hypomegakaryocytic thrombocytopenic purpura from a sex chromosome mosaic. Cancer Genet Cytogenet 1984;12:261.
1320. Milnes JP, Schofield KP, Low-Beer TS. Genetic haemochromatosis and thrombocytopenia. (Letter) Lancet 1986;2:1336.
1321. Nagasawa T, Sakurai T, Kashiwagi H, Abe T. Cell-mediated amegakaryocytic thrombocytopenia associated with systemic lupus erythematosus. Blood 1986;67:479.
1322. Subramanian VP. Thrombocytopenia and decreased megakaryocytes. (Letter) Ann Intern Med 1981;94:711.
1323. Slater LM, Katz J, Walter B, Armentrout SA. Aplastic anemia occurring as amegakaryocytic thrombocytopenia with and without an inhibitor of granulopoiesis. Am J Hematol 1985;18:251.
1324. Iannelli S, Petrini MT. Acquired pure megakaryocytic aplasia in course of hepatitis in a patient with immune thrombocytopenic purpura. Acta Haematol 1984;72:355.
1325. Font J, Nomdedeu B, Martinez-Orozco F, et al. Amegakaryocytic

thrombocytopenia and an analgesic. (Letter) Ann Intern Med 1981;95:783.
1326. Hoffman R, Bruno E, Elwell J, et al. Acquired amegakaryocytic thrombocytopenic purpura: a syndrome of diverse etiologies. Blood 1982;60:1173.
1327. Gewirtz AM, Sacchetti MK, Bien R, Barry WE. Cell-mediated suppression of megakaryocytopoiesis in acquired amegakaryocytic thrombocytopenic purpura. Blood 1986;68:619.
1328. Hirsh EH, Vogler WR, McDonald TP, Stein SF. Acquired hypomegakaryocytic thrombocytopenic purpura: occurrence in a patient with absent thrombopoietic stimulating factor. Arch Intern Med 1980;140:721.
1329. Hoffman R, Briddell RA, van Besien K, et al. Acquired cyclic amegakaryocytic thrombocytopenia associated with an immunoglobulin blocking the action of granulocyte-macrophage colony-stimulating factor. N Engl J Med 1989;321:97.
1330. Worman CP, Mills KHG, Linch DC, et al. Amegakaryocytic thrombocytopenia associated with an excess of leu 2a+ suppressor cells. Scand J Haematol 1982;28:215.
1331. Dharmasena F, Galton DAG. Remission of amegakaryocytic thrombocytopenia induced by antilymphocyte globulin. Br J Haematol 1986;63:205.
1332. El Saghir NS, Geltman RL. Treatment of acquired amegakaryocytic thrombocytopenic purpura with cyclophosphamide. Am J Med 1986;81:139.
1333. Kayser W, Euler HH, Schmitz N, et al. Danazol in acquired amegakaryocytic thrombocytopenic purpura: a case report. Blut 1985;51:401.
1334. Michael SR, Vural L, Bassen FA, Schaefer L. The hematologic aspects of disseminated (systemic) lupus erythematosus. Blood 1951;6:1059.
1335. Branda RF, Moldow CF, MacArthur JR, et al. Folate-induced remission in aplastic anemia with a familial defect of cellular folate uptake. N Engl J Med 1978;298:469.
1336. Lynch EC, McKechnie JC, Alfrey CP Jr. Brucellosis with pancytopenia. Ann Intern Med 1968;69:319.
1337. Evans TS, DeLuca VA, Waters LL. The association of miliary tuberculosis of the bone marrow and pancytopenia. Ann Intern Med 1952;37:1044.
1338. Fountain JR. Blood changes associated with disseminated tuberculosis. Br Med J 1954;2:76.
1339. Glasser RM, Walker RI, Herion JC. The significance of hematologic abnormalities in patients with tuberculosis. Arch Intern Med 1970;125:691.
1340. Hitchins R, Cobcroft RG, Hocker G. Transient severe hypoplastic anemia in Q fever. Pathology 1986;18:254.
1341. Hajiroussou VJ, Joshi RC. Hypoplastic anaemia associated with legionnaires' disease. Br Med J 1980;280:366.
1342. Pearson HA. Marrow hypoplasia in anorexia nervosa. J Pediatr 1967;71:211.
1343. Smith RRL, Spivak JL. Marrow cell necrosis in anorexia nervosa and involuntary starvation. Br J Haematol 1985;60:525.
1344. Tavassoli M, Eastlund DT, Yam LT, et al. Gelatinous transformation of bone marrow in prolonged self-induced starvation. Scand J Haematol 1976;16:311.
1345. Drenick EJ, Swendseid ME, Blahd WH, Tuttle SG. Prolonged starvation as treatment for severe obesity. JAMA 1964;187:100.
1346. Engstrom PF, Dewey GC, Barrett O Jr. Disseminated Mycobacterium kansasii infection. Am J Med 1972;52:533.
1347. Bottiger LE, Westerholm B. Aplastic anaemia. I. Incidence and aetiology. Acta Med Scand 1972;192:315.
1348. Aggio MC, Alvarez RV, Bartomioli MA, Maguitman O. Incidence and etiology of aplastic anemia in a defined population of Argentina (1966–1977). Medicina 1988;48:231.
1349. Mary JY, Baumelou E, Guiguet M. Epidemiology of aplastic anemia in France: a prospective multicenter study. Blood 1990;75.
1350. Alter BP, Potter NU, Li FP. Classification and aetiology of the aplastic anaemias. Clin Haematol 1978;7:431.
1351. Abe T, Komiya M. Some clinical aspects of aplastic anemia. In: Hibino S, Takaku F, Shahidi NT, eds. Aplastic anemia. Baltimore, University Park Press, 1978:197.
1352. Boruchow IB. Bone marrow depression associated with acute colchicine toxicity in the presence of hepatic dysfunction. Cancer 1966;19:541.
1353. Liu YK, Hymowitz R, Carroll MG. Marrow aplasia induced by colchicine. Arthritis Rheum 1978;21:731.
1354. Hiebel J, Gant HL, Schwartz SO, Friedman IA. Bone marrow depression following exposure to kerosene: a report of 3 cases. Am J Med Sci 1963;246:185.
1355. Cavanaugh JR, Wilner PR. Aplastic anemia due to kerosene. Med Ann DC 1939;8:140.
1356. Johnson DE. Hypoplastic anemia following chronic exposure to kerosene. J Am Med Wom Assoc 1955;10:421.
1357. Straus B. Aplastic anemia following exposure to carbon tetrachloride. JAMA 1954;155:737.
1360. Prager D, Peters C. Development of aplastic anemia and the exposure to Stoddard solvent. Blood 1970;35:286.
1361. Nagaratnam N, Chetiyawardana AD. Aplasia and leukaemia following chloroquine therapy. J Postgrad Med 1978;54:108.
1362. Biro L, Leone N. Aplastic anemia induced by quinacrine. Arch Dermatol 1945;92:574.
1363. Fishman AP, Kinsman JM. Hypoplastic anemia due to atabrine. Blood 1949;4:970.
1364. Parmer LG, Sawitsky A. Fatal aplastic anemia following quanacrine therapy in chronic discoid lupus erythematosus. JAMA 1953;153:1172.
1365. Paton MD, Riddell MJ, Strong JA. Aplastic anaemia following mepacrine treatment of lupus erythematosus. Lancet 1955;1:281.
1366. Menkes E, Kutas GJ. Fatal aplastic anemia following indomethacin ingestion. (Letter) Can Med Assoc J 1977;117:118.
1367. Shearer CA. Indomethacin and aplastic anemia. (Letter) Can Med Assoc J 1978;118:18.
1368. Canada AT, Burka ER. Aplastic anemia after indomethacin. (Letter) N Engl J Med 1968;278:743.
1369. Fredrick GR, Tanaka KR. Indomethacin and aplastic anemia. (Letter) N Engl J Med 1968;279:1290.
1370. Gryfe CI, Rubenzahl S. Agranulocytosis and aplastic anemia possibly due to ibuprofen. Can Med Assoc J 1976;114:878.
1371. Miller JL. Marrow aplasia and sulindac. (Letter) Ann Intern Med 1980;92:129.
1372. Sanz MA, Martinez JA, Gomis F, Garcia-Borras JJ. Sulindac-induced bone marrow toxicity. Lancet 1980;2:802.
1373. Wijnja L, Snijder JAM, Nieweg HO. Acetylsalicylic acid as a cause of pancytopenia from bone-marrow damage. Lancet 1966;2:768.
1374. Eldar M, Aderka D, Shoenfeld Y, et al. Aspirin-induced aplastic anemia. (Letter) S Afr Med J 1979;55:318.
1375. Robins MM. Aplastic anemia secondary to anticonvulsants. Am J Dis Child 1962;104:614.
1376. Abbott JA, Schwab RS. The serious side effects of the new antiepileptic drugs: their control and prevention. N Engl J Med 1950;242:944.
1377. Sparbert M. Diagnostically confusing complications of diphenylhydantoin therapy. Ann Intern Med 1963;59:914.
1378. Weiss HA, Hawley WD. Pancytopenia following the use of mesantoin and thiantoin. US Armed Forces Med J 1951;2:83.
1379. Witkind E, Waid ME. Aplasia of the bone marrow during Mesantoin therapy. Report of a fatal case. JAMA 1951;147:757.
1380. Pearson PH, Peck JL, Livingston S. Fatal pancytopenia following therapy with nuvarone (3-methyl, 5-phenylhydantoin). Bull Johns Hopkins Hosp 1952;91:341.
1381. Isaacson S, Gold JA, Ginsberg V. Fatal aplastic anemia after therapy with nuvarone (3-methyl-5-phenylhydantoin). JAMA 1956;160:1311.
1382. Donaldson GWK, Graham JG. Aplastic anemia following the administration of tegretol. Br J Clin Pract 1965;19:699.
1383. Dyer NH, Hughes DTD, Jenking GC. Aplastic anemia after carbamazepine. (Letter) Br Med J 1966;1:108.
1384. Pisciotta AV. Hematologic toxicity of carbamazepine. In: Penry JK, Daly DD, eds. Advances in neurology. New York, Raven Press, 1975:355.
1385. Gayford JJ, Redpath TH. The side effects of carbamazepine. Proc R Soc Med 1969;61:615.
1386. Pellock JM. Carbamazepine side effects in children and adults. Epilepsia 1987;28(Suppl 3):S64.
1387. Moore NC, Lerer B, Meyendorff E, Gershon S. Three cases of carbamazepine toxicity. Am J Psychiatry 1985;142:974.
1388. Franceschi M, Ciboddo G, Truci G, et al. Fatal aplastic anemia in a patient treated with carbamazepine. Epilepsia 1988;29:582.
1389. Simpson TW, Wilson EB Jr, Zimmerman SL. Fatal aplastic anemia occurring during anticonvulsant therapy: probable idiosyncrasy to phenurone. Ann Intern Med 1950;32:1224.
1390. Merskey C. A case of aplastic anaemia following the use of mapharside and bismuth for syphilis. Clin Proc 1946;5:256.
1391. Bismuth C, Gaultier M, Conso F. Aplasie médullaire après intoxication aigue à la colchinine: 20 cas. Nouv Presse Med 1977;6:1625.
1392. Dassen R, Rey JC. Intoxicación aguda por el bismuto (estomatitis gangrenosa, púrpura, netritis asuda). Semana Méd 1930;37:1152.
1393. Wilson DR. Mercurial poisoning and aplastic anemia. (Letter) Br Med J 1966;2:1534.
1394. Ryrie DR, Toghill PJ, Tanna MK, Galan GN. Marrow suppression from mercury poisoning? Br Med J 1970;1:499.
1395. Slee PHTHJ, den Ottolander GJ, de Wolff FA. A case of merbromin (mercurochrome) intoxication possibly resulting in aplastic anemia. Acta Med Scand 1979;205:463.
1396. Kutscher AH, Lane SL, Segall R. The clinical toxicity of antibiotics and sulfonamides: a comparative review of the literature based on 104, 672 cases treated systemically. J Allergy 1954;25:135.
1397. Holsinger DR, Hanlon DG, Welch JS. Fatal aplastic anemia following sulfamethoxypyridazine therapy. Mayo Clin Proc 1958;33:679.
1398. Tulloch AL. Pancytopenia in an infant associated with sulfamethoxazole-trimethoprim therapy. J Pediatr 1976;88:499.
1399. Spracklen F. Fatal aplastic anaemia following sulphaphenazole (orisulf=+) therapy. Postgrad Med J 1963;39:488.
1400. Levine B, Rosenberg DV. Aplastic anemia during the treatment of hyperthyroidism with tapazole. Ann Intern Med 1954;41:844.
1401. Edell SL, Bartuska DG. Aplastic anemia secondary to methimazole: case report and review of hematologic side effects. J Am Med Wom Assoc 1975;30:412.

1402. Rosenberg AH. Methimazol-induced aplastic anemia. Conn Med 1970;34:32.
1403. Kurata N, Murakami T, Hojo K, et al. An autopsy case of panmyelophthisis after treatment with methylthiouracil. Acta Haematol Jpn 1964;27:580.
1404. Aksoy M, Erdem S. Aplastic anaemia after propylthiouracil. (Letter) Lancet 1968;1:1379.
1405. Jost F. Blood dyscrasias associated with tolbutamide therapy. Br Med J 1959;169:1468.
1406. Chapman I, Cheung WH. Pancytopenia associated with tolbutamide therapy. JAMA 1963;186:595.
1407. Traumann KJ, Grom E, Schwarzkopf H. Panzytopenie bei Diabetes-Mellitus-Therapie mit Tolbutamid? Deutsch Med Wochenschr 1975;100:250.
1408. White LLR. Fatal marrow aplasia during chlorpropamide therapy. (Letter) Br Med J 1962;1:691.
1409. Recker RR, Hynes HE. Pure red blood cell aplasia associated with chlorpropamide therapy. Arch Intern Med 1969;123:445.
1410. Gangitano JL, Foster SH, Contro RM. Nonfatal methazolamide-induced aplastic anemia. Am J Ophthalmol 1978;86:138.
1411. Werblin TP, Pollack IP, Liss RA. Aplastic anemia and agranulocytosis in patients using methazolamide for glaucoma. JAMA 1979;241:2817.
1412. Underwood LC. Fatal bone marrow depression after the treatment with acetozolamide (Diamox). JAMA 1956;161:1477.
1413. Lubeck MJ. Aplastic anemia following acetazolamide therapy. Am J Ophthalmol 1970;69:684.
1414. Wisch N, Fischbein FI, Siegel R, Glass JL, et al. Aplastic anemia resulting from the use of carbonic anhydrase inhibitors. Am J Ophthalmol 1973;75:130.
1415. Bourke B, Maini RN, Griffith ID, Scott JT. Fatal marrow aplasia in a patient on penicillamine. (Letter) Lancet 1976;2:515.
1416. MacAllister WAC, Vale JA. Fatal marrow aplasia in patient on penicillamine. (Letter) Lancet 1976;2:631.
1417. Barnett AJ, Whiteside MG. Marrow aplasia and penicillamine. Lancet 1976;2:682.
1418. Jones S, Corringham RET, Jain S. Erythro-myeloid aplasia following D-penicillamine treatment in primary biliary cirrhosis. J Postgrad Med 1978;54:834.
1419. Weiss AS, Markenson JA, Weiss MS, Kammerer WH. Toxicity of D-penicillamine in rheumatoid arthritis: a report of 63 patients including two with aplastic anemia and one with the nephrotic syndrome. Am J Med 1978;64:114.
1420. Fishel B, Tishler M, Caspi D, Yaron M. Fatal aplastic anaemia and liver toxicity caused by D-penicillamine treatment of rheumatoid arthritis. Ann Rheum Dis 1989;48:609.
1421. Deyke VF, Wallace JB. Development of aplastic anemia during the use of streptomycin. JAMA 1948;136:1098.
1422. Womack CR, Reiner CB. Fatal aplastic anemia due to streptomycin: case report and brief review of pertinent literature. Ann Intern Med 1951;34:759.
1423. Sacks MS, Bradford GT, Spurling CL. Aplastic anemia complicating streptomycin treatment of pulmonary tuberculosis. JAMA 1951;147:308.
1424. Lehrner LM, Cooke JH, Enck RE. Tetracycline-induced aplastic anemia. South Med J 1979;72:358.
1425. Levitt BH, Gottlieb AJ, Rosenberg IR, Klein JJ. Bone marrow depression due to methicillin, a semisynthetic penicillin. Clin Pharmacol Ther 1964;5:301.
1426. Fernández-Bañares F, González-Huix F, Xiol X, et al. Marrow aplasia during high dose mebendazole treatment. Am J Trop Med Hyg 1986;35:350.
1427. Meyer LM, Perlmutter M. Aplastic anemia due to sulfathiazole. JAMA 1942;119:558.
1428. Johnson FD, Korst DR. Pancytopenia associated with sulfamethoxypyridazine administration. The occurrence of leukopenia suggests an accumulative effect: constant awareness is essential to prevent serious marrow damage. JAMA 1961;175:967.
1429. Sparcklen F. Fatal aplastic anemia following sulphaphenazole (Orisulf=+) therapy. Postgrad Med J 1963;39:488.
1430. Dunning AM. Blood and bone marrow changes following the use of sulfadimethoxine (madribon). Ned Tijdschr Geneeskd 1962;106:1729.
1431. Salter AJ. The toxicity profile of trimethoprim/sulfamethoxazole after four years of widespread use. Med J Aust 1973;1(Suppl 2):70.
1432. Golde DW, Bersh N, Quan SG. Trimethoprim and sulfamethoxazole inhibition of haematopoiesis in vitro. Br J Haematol 1978;40:363.
1433. Meyer R, Axelrod JL. Fatal aplastic anemia resulting from flucytosine. JAMA 1942;119:558.
1434. Meyer R, Axelrod JL. Fatal aplastic anemia resulting from flucytosine. JAMA 1974;228:1573.
1435. Bryan CS, McFarland JA. Cryptococal meningitis. Fatal marrow aplasia from combined therapy. JAMA 1978;239:1068.
1436. Glassmire CR. Fatal pancytopenia following anti-histamine administration. J Maine Med Assoc 1951;42:83.
1437. Chang HK, Morrison SL. Bone-marrow suppression associated with cimetidine. Ann Intern Med 1979;91:580.
1438. Tonkonow B, Hoffman R. Aplastic anemia and cimetidine. (Letter) Arch Intern Med 1980;140:1123.
1439. Spry CJF. Chlorpheniramine-induced bone-marrow suppression. (Letter) Lancet 1976;1:545.
1440. Kanoh T, Jingami H, Uchino H. Aplastic anaemia after prolonged treatment with chlorpheniramine. (Letter) Lancet 1977;1:546.
1441. McKinney WT Jr, Kane FJ Jr. Pancytopenia due to chlorpromazine. Am J Psychiatry 1967;123:879.
1442. Mansour N, Broun GO Jr. Depression of erythropoiesis associated with chlorpromazine therapy. Arch Intern Med 1967;119:113.
1443. Shelton JG, Kingston WR, McRae C. Aplastic anæmia and agranulocytosis following chlorpromazine therapy. Med J Aust 1960;1:130.
1444. Bhaskaran K, Subrahmanyan P, Nand DS. Fatal bone-marrow aplasia complicating prochlorperazine therapy. Am J Psychiatry 1962;119:373.
1445. Yeung KY, Corn M. Fatal aplastic anemia with piperacetazine therapy. (Letter) Ann Intern Med 1974;81:411.
1446. Menon GN. Hypoplastic anaemia: an unusual complication of chlordiazepoxide hydrochloride therapy. J Postgrad Med 1965;41:282.
1447. Meyer LM, Heever WL, Bertscher RW. Aplastic anemia after meprobamate [(methyl) 2-N-propyl-1, 3-propanediol dicarbamate] therapy. N Engl J Med 1957;256:1232.
1448. Cromie BW. Meprobamate and aplastic anaemia. (Letter) Br Med J 1964;1:562.
1449. Anastassiades C. Pancytopenia and meprobamate. (Letter) Br Med J 1971;1:349.
1450. Shapiro S. Allopurinol and bone-marrow depression. Lancet 1974;2:412.
1451. Wilkinson DG. Allopurinol and agranulocytosis. Lancet 1977;2:1282.
1452. Greenberg MS, Zambrano SS. Aplastic agranulocytosis after allopurinol therapy. Arthritis Rheum 1972;15:413.
1453. Durg NG, Vyas HD, Ward RL. Marrow aplasia and methyldopa. (Letter) Lancet 1968;1:695.
1454. Barzel US. Quinine sulfate induced hypoplastic anemia and agranulocytosis. JAMA 1967;201:325.
1455. Kelton JC, Mold N, Huang A. Quinidine-associated pancytopenia and marrow aplasia as demonstrated in marrow cultures. (Letter) Blood 1977;50(Suppl 1):151.
1456. Hussain MZ, Khan AG, Chaudhry ZA. Aplastic anemia associated with lithium therapy. Can Med Assoc J 1973;108:724.
1457. Jefferson JW. Aplastic anemia associated with lithium. (Letter) Lancet 1975;1:413.
1458. Norris FH, Eaton JM, Mielke CH. Depression of bone marrow by guanidine. Arch Neurol 1974;30:184.
1459. Krevans JR, Asper SP Jr, Reinhoff WF Jr. Fatal aplastic anemia following use of potassium perchlorate in thyrotoxicosis. JAMA 1962;181:162.
1460. Gjemdal N. Fatal aplastic anaemia following use of potassium perchlorate in thyrotoxicosis. Acta Med Scand 1963;174:129.
1461. Barzilai D, Sheinfeld M. Fatal complications following use of potassium perchlorate in thyrotoxicosis: report of two cases and a review of the literature. Israel J Med Sci 1966;2:453.
1462. Frohmam LA, Klocke FJ. Recurrent thiocyanate intoxication with pancytopenia, hypothyroidism and psychosis. N Engl J Med 1963;268:701.
1463. Richardson JS, Sarkany I, Campbell CD. Fatal case of marrow aplasia after treatment with carbimazole. Br Med J 1954;1:364.
1464. Shimamine T, Ishihara K, Imamura T. Pathological findings in aplastic anemia. In: Hibino S, Takaku F, Shahidi NT, eds. Aplastic anemia. Baltimore, University Park Press, 1976:3.
1466. Young NS, Mortimer PP, Moore JG, Humphries RK. Characterization of a virus that causes transient aplastic crisis. J Clin Invest 1984;73:224.
1467. Corapi WV, French TW, Dubovi EJ. Severe thrombocytopenia in young calves experimentally infected with noncytopathic bovine viral diarrhea virus. J Virol 1989;63:3934.
1468. Gartner S, Markovits P, Markovitz DM, et al. The role of mononuclear phagocytes in HTLV-III/LAV infection. Science 1986;233:215.
1469. Kunicka JE, Platsoucas CD. Defective helper function of purified T4 cells and excessive suppressor activity of purified T8 cells in patients with B-cell chronic lymphocytic leukemia: T4 suppressor effector cells are present in certain patients. Blood 1988;71:1551.
1470. Nicholson JK, Cross GD, Callaway CS, McDougal JS. In vitro infection of human monocytes with human T lymphotropic virus type III/lymphadenopathy virus (HTLV-III/LAV). J Immunol 1986;137:323.
1471. Folks TM, Kessler SW, Orenstein JM, et al. Infection and replication of HIV-1 in purified progenitor cells of normal human bone marrow. Science 1988;242:919.
1472. Potts B, Hogan D, Lamperth L, et al. Replication of human immunodeficiency viruses 1 and 2 in human bone marrow cultures. (Abstract) Blood 1989;74(Suppl 1):206a.
1473. Zeira M, Scadden DT, Lim B, et al. Human immunodeficiency virus (HIV) infection of human bone marrow stromal cells. (Abstract) Blood 1989;74(Suppl 1):205a.
1474. Mangan KF, Mullaney MT, Rosenfeld CS, Shadduck RK. In vitro evidence for disappearance of erythroid progenitor T suppressor cells following allogenic bone marrow transplantation for severe aplastic anemia. Blood 1988;71:144.
1475. de Planque MM, Brand A, Kluin-Nelemans HC, et al. Haematopoietic

and immunologic abnomalities in severe aplastic anaemia patients treated with anti-thymocyte globulin. Br J Haematol 1989;71:421.
1476. Torok-Storb B, Johnson G, Bowden R, Storb R. Gamma-interferon in aplastic anemia: inability to detect significant levels in sera or demonstrate hematopoietic suppressing activity. Blood 1987;69:629.
1477. Hanada T, Yamamura H, Ehara T, et al. Inhibitory activity of T cells on hematopoiesis and gamma-IFN production by T cells from peripheral blood in patients with aplastic anemia. Acta Haematol Jpn 1988;51:571.
1478. Kuriyama K, Tomonaga M, Jinnai I, et al. Reduced helper (OKT4+): suppressor (OKT8+) T ratios in aplastic anaemia: relation to immunosuppressive therapy. Br J Haematol 1984;57:329.
1479. Lumm LG, Seigneuret MC, Doney KC, Storb R. In vitro immunoglobulin production, proliferation, and cell markers before and after antithymocyte globulin therapy in patients with aplastic anemia. Am J Hematol 1987;26:1.
1480. Falcao RP, Voltarelli JC, Bottura C. T-lymphocyte subpopulations in the peripheral blood and bone marrow of patients with aplastic anemia. Blut 1985;50:103.
1481. Dupont B, O'Reilly RJ, Pollack MS, Good RA. Use of HLA genotypically different donors in bone marrow transplantation. Transplant Proc 1979;11:219.
1482. Clift RA, Storb R. Histoincompatible bone marrow transplants in humans. Annu Rev Immunol 1987;5:43.
1483. Storch S, Gale RP, Champlin R, et al. Partially mismatched marrow transplantation for acute leukemia and aplastic anemia. In: Gale RP, ed. Recent advances in bone marrow transplantation. New York, Alan R Liss, 1983:785.
1484. Filipovich AH, Ramsay NKC, McGlave P, et al. Mismatched bone marrow transplantation at the University of Minnesota: use of related donors other than HLA MLC identical siblings and T-cell depletion. In: Gale RP, ed. Recent advances in bone marrow transplantation. New York, Alan R Liss, 1983:769.
1485. Hows JM, Yin JL, Marsh J, et al. Histocompatible unrelated volunteer donors compared with HLA nonidentical family donors in marrow transplantation for aplastic anemia and leukemia. Blood 1986;68:1322.
1486. Gingrich RD, Ginder GD, Goeken NE, et al. Allogeneic marrow grafting with partially mismatched, unrelated marrow donors. Blood 1988;71:1375.
1487. Miller WJ, Branda RF, Flynn PJ, et al. Antithymocyte globulin treatment of severe aplastic anaemia. Br J Haematol 1983;55:17.
1488. Delgado-Lamas JL, Lopez-Karpovitch X, Marin-Lopez A, et al. Low doses of high-potency antithymocyte globulin (ATG) in severe aplastic anemia: experience with the Mexican ATG. Acta Haematol 1989;81:70.
1489. Cosimi AB, Peters C, Harmon D, Ellman L. Treatment of severe aplastic anemia with a prolonged course of anti-thymocyte globulin. Transplant Proc 1982;14:761.
1490. Carloss HW, Saab GA, Tavassoli M. Pure red cell aplasia and lymphoma. JAMA 1979;242:67.
1491. Hanada T, Yamamura H, Isobe T, et al. Pure red cell aplasia in association with malignant histiocytosis. Cancer 1986;57:2325.
1492. Shimm DS, Logue GL, Rohlfing MB, Gaede JT. Primary amyloidosis, pure red cell aplasia, and Kaposi's sarcoma in a single patient. Cancer 1979;44:1501.
1493. de Alarcon PA, Miller ML, Stuart MJ. Erythroid hypoplasia; an unusual presentation of childhood acute lymphocytic leukemia. Am J Dis Child 1978;132:763.
1494. Morgan E, Pang KM, Goldwasser E. Hodgkin disease and red cell aplasia. Am J Hematol 1978;5:71.
1495. Gilbert EF, Harley JB, Anido V, et al. Thymoma, plasma cell myeloma, red cell aplasia and malabsorption syndrome. Am J Med 1968;44:820.
1496. Kitahara M. Pure RBC aplasia associated with chronic granulocytic leukemia. JAMA 1978;240:376.
1497. Barosi G, Baraldi A, Cazzola M, et al. Red cell aplasia in myelofibrosis with myeloid metaplasia: a distinct functional and clinical entity. Cancer 1983;52:1290.
1498. Entwistle CC, Fentem PH, Jacobs A. Red-cell aplasia with carcinoma of the bronchus. Br Med J 1964;2:1504.
1499. Mitchell ABS, Pinn G, Pegrum GD. Pure red cell aplasia and carcinoma. Blood 1971;37:594.
1500. Nossent JC, Swaak AJG. Pure red-cell aplasia in systemic lupus erythematosus. Clin Rheumatol 1988;7:527.
1501. Cassileth PA, Myers AR. Erythroid aplasia in systemic lupus erythematosus. Am J Med 1973;55:706.
1502. Cavalcant J, Shadduck RK, Winkelstein A, et al. Red-cell hypoplasia and increased bone marrow reticulin in systemic lupus erythematosis: reversal with corticosteroid therapy. Am J Hematol 1978;5:253.
1503. Kimura N, Yamasaki K, Niho Y, et al. Pure red cell aplasia associated with juvenile rheumatoid arthritis: effects of T-lymphocytes on hemopoietic progenitor cells. Acta Haematol Jpn 1982;45:129.
1504. Rodrigues JF, Harth M, Barr RM. Pure red cell aplasia in rheumatoid arthritis. J Rheumatol 1988;15:1159.
1505. Myers TJ, Bower BF, Hild DH. Pure red cell aplasia and the syndrome of multiple endocrine gland insufficiency. Am J Med Sci 1980;280:29.
1506. Krivoy N, Ben-Arieh Y, Carter A, Alroy G. Methazolamide-induced hepatitis and pure RBC aplasia. Arch Intern Med 1981;141:1229.
1507. Miyoshi I, Hikita T, Koi B, Kimura I. Reversible pure red-cell aplasia in pregnancy. (Letter) N Engl J Med 1978;299:177.
1508. Lehman G, Alcoff J. Reversible pure red cell hypoplasia in pregnancy. JAMA 1982;247:1170.
1509. Picot C, Triadou P, Lacombe C, et al. Relapsing pure red-cell aplasia during pregnancy. (Letter) N Engl J Med 1984;311:196.
1510. Hoffman R, McPhedran P, Benz EJ Jr, Duffy TP. Isoniazid-induced pure red cell aplasia. Am J Med Sci 1983;286:2.
1511. Jeong YG, Yung Y, River GL. Pure red blood cell aplasia and diphenylhydantoin. JAMA 1974;229:314.
1512. Hujigens PC, Thijs LG, den Ottolander GJ. Pure red cell aplasia, toxic dermatitis and lymphadenopathy in a patient taking diphenylhydantoin. Acta Haematol 1978;59:31.
1513. Lee CH, Firkin FC, Grace CS, Rozenberg MC. Pure red cell aplasia: a report on three cases with studies on circulating toxic factors against erythroid precursors. Aust NZ J Med 1978;8:75.
1514. Hotta T, Hirabayashi N, Kobayashi T, et al. Five cases showing hemoglobinuria and aplastic crisis following administration of diphenylhydantoin after craniotomy. Jpn J Clin Hematol 1980;21:536.
1515. Sugimoto M, Wakabayashi Y, Shiokawa Y, Takaku F. A case of pure red cell aplasia whose bone marrow heme synthesis was suppressed by diphenylhydantoin in vitro. Jpn J Clin Hematol 1982;23:1446.
1516. Hirai H. Two cases of erythroid hypoplasia caused by carbamazepine. Jpn J Clin Hematol 1977;18:33.
1517. Douchain F, Leborgne JM, Robin M, et al. Erythroblastop nie aiguë par intolerance au dipropyl-acetate de sodium: premiere observation. Nouv Presse Med 1980;9:1715.
1518. MacDougall-Lorna G. Pure red cell aplasia associated with sodium valproate therapy. JAMA 1982;247:53.
1519. McGrath BP, Ibels LS, Raik E, et al. Erythroid toxicity of azathioprine: macrocytosis and selective marrow hypoplasia. Q J Med 1975;44:57.
1520. Old CW, Flannery EP, Grogan TM, et al. Azathioprine-induced pure red cell aplasia. JAMA 1978;240:552.
1521. DeClerk YA, Ettenger RB, Ortega JA, Pennisi AJ. Macrocytosis and pure RBC anemia caused by azathioprine. Am J Dis Child 1980;134:377.
1522. Flury W, Montandon A. Isolierte erythroide Aplasie unter immnosuppressive Therapie mit Azathioprin nach Nierentransplantation. Schweiz Med Wochenschr 1980;110:1614.
1523. Cornet A, Cornu P, Barbier JP, et al. Un cas d'érythroblastophie réversible due au thiamphenicol. Semin Hôp Paris 1974;50:1567.
1524. Estavoyer JM, Singer P, Broda C, Baufle GH. Toxicit hématologique du thiamphenicol: à propos de deux observations d' érythroblastop nie aiguë. Semin Hôp Paris 1981;57:1970.
1525. Dunn AM, Kerr GD. Pure red cell aplasia associated with sulphasalazine. Lancet 1981;2:1288.
1526. Teoh PC, Tan DKS, Da Costa JL, Chew BK. Acquired pure red cell aplasia in adults. Med J Aust 1973;2:373.
1527. Planas AT, Kranwinkel RN, Soletsky HB, Pezzimenti JF. Chlorpropamide-induced pure RBC aplasia. Arch Intern Med 1980;140:707.
1528. Gill MJ, Ratliff DA, Harding LK. Hypoglycemic coma, jaundice, and pure RBC aplasia following chlorpropamide therapy. Arch Intern Med 1980;140:714.
1529. Strauss AM. Erythrocyte aplasia following sulfathiazole. Am J Clin Pathol 1943;13:249.
1530. Tsai SY, Levin WC. Chronic erythrocytic hypoplasia in adults: review of literature and report of a case. Am J Med 1957;22:322.
1531. Stephens ME. Transient erythroid hypoplasia in a patient on long-term co-trimoxazole therapy. Postgrad Med J 1974;50:235.
1532. Mielke HG. Aplastische Anämie (Erythroblastophthise) nach INH-behandlung. Folia Haematol 1958;2:1.
1533. Goodman SB, Block MH. A case of red cell aplasia occurring as a result of antituberculous therapy. Blood 1964;24:616.
1534. Claiborne RA, Dutt AK. Isoniazid-induced pure red cell aplasia. Am Rev Respir Dis 1985;131:947.
1535. Giannone L, Kugler JW, Krantz SB. Pure red cell aplasia associated with administration of sustained-release procainamide. Arch Intern Med 1987;147:1179.
1536. Gasser C. Aplasia of erythropoiesis. Pediatr Clin North Am 1957;4:445.
1537. Swineford O Jr, Curry JC, Cumbia JW. Phenylbutazone toxicity: depression of erythropoiesis. Arthritis Rheum 1958;1:174.
1538. Weinberger KA. Fenoprofen and red cell aplasia. (Letter) J Rheumatol 1979;6:475.
1539. Reitz CL, Bottomley SS. Pure red cell aplasia associated with fenopren. Am J Med Sci 1984;287:62.
1540. Vohra RM, Sturm RE, Patel AR. Pure red cell aplasia in association with allopurinol. Blood 1983;62(Suppl 1):51a.
1541. Jurgensen JC, Abraham JP, Hardy WW. Erythroid aplasia after halothane hepatitis. Am J Digest Dis 1970;15:577.
1542. Gollan JL, Hussein S, Hoffbrand AV, Sherlock S. Red cell aplasia

following prolonged D-penicillamine therapy. J Clin Pathol 1976;29: 135.
1543. Nicholls MD, Concannon AJ. Maloprim-induced agranulocytosis and red cell aplasia. Med J Aust 1982;2:564.
1544. Suh K, Sood R. Hypoplastic anemia associated with metolazone. (Letter) JAMA 1979;242:139.
1545. Foy H, Kondi A. A case of true red cell aplastic anemia successfully treated with riboflavin. J Pathol Bacteriol 1953;65:559.
1546. Reid G, Patterson AC. Pure red cell aplasia after gold treatment. Br Med J 1977;2:1457.
1547. Roberts HJ. Aplastic anemia and red cell aplasia due to pentachlorophenol. South Med J 1983;76:45.
1548. Sharff O, Neumann H. Über eine seltene Form von Knochenmarkschadidung durch Salvarsan. Med Klin 1944;40:500.
1549. Vodopick H. Cherchez la chienne. I. Erythropoietic hypoplasia after exposure to gamma-benzene hexachloride. JAMA 1975;234:850.
1550. Storb R, Thomas ED, Buckner CD, et al. Marrow transplantation in thirty "untransfused" patients with severe aplastic anemia. Ann Intern Med 1980;92:30.

Blood: Principles and Practice of Hematology,
edited by Robert I. Handin, Thomas P. Stossel, and Samuel E. Lux.
J.B. Lippincott Company, Philadelphia © 1995.

11

Paroxysmal Nocturnal Hemoglobinuria

Wendell F. Rosse

Paroxysmal nocturnal hemoglobinuria (PNH) was first described in 1864 in a young tanner who had episodes of "hematinuria," worse in the morning and occurring in episodes lasting a few days.[1] The classic description was that of Paul Strubing,[2] which detailed many of the clinical manifestations of hemolysis, including hemolytic anemia, hemoglobinuria, and hemosiderinuria. With the introduction of the acidified serum lysis test for the diagnosis of the syndrome,[3] other manifestations not apparently related to the hemoglobinuria were described, including unusual venous thromboses,[4] hypoplastic or aplastic hematopoiesis,[5] thrombocytopenia and granulocytopenia,[6] and frequent infections. From these findings, it became apparent that the syndrome is far more complex than simple hemolytic anemia and that it is actually a stem cell disorder that involves all the cells of the marrow.

CLINICAL SYNDROME

The clinical syndrome of PNH is complex and involves primarily three sets of symptoms:

- Hemolytic anemia due to the susceptibility of the red blood cells (RBCs) to the hemolytic action of complement
- Thrombosis that tends to occur in unusual veins such as hepatic and abdominal, cerebral, and subdermal veins
- A deficient hematopoiesis whose manifestations may be minimal or may result in an aplastic anemia-like state

In addition, several less prominent symptoms and signs are seen in some patients, such as increased infections, esophageal spasm, impotence, and malaise. Each symptom is treated in detail in the text that follows.

PNH may occur at any age from children as young as 2 years to adults up to 83 years. PNH is seen most frequently in young adults.[7-9] The clinical manifestations do not vary in any consistent way with differences in age; all of the complications known for adults have occurred in children.

Hemolytic Anemia

The defining characteristic of PNH is hemolytic anemia due to the intravascular destruction of RBCs by complement. The amount of hemolysis and the degree of anemia are highly variable from patient to patient.[7-9] The classic manifestation is the appearance of hemoglobin in the urine formed during the night, with partial or complete clearing during the day. This may occur nearly every day in the most severely affected patient. More frequently, the hemolysis occurs in episodes lasting 3 to 10 days, often preceded or accompanied by an infection. Many patients experience this symptom rarely or not at all.

Both direct and indirect evidence of hemolysis is often present. The reticulocyte count is usually elevated and the erythropoiesis in the bone marrow is active (see explanation later in text). The plasma hemoglobin level is usually elevated, sometimes markedly. Serum haptoglobin is low. Serum lactic acid dehydrogenase is elevated, but the serum alanine aminotransferase (ALT), or SGOT, is usually elevated only minimally.

Hemoglobin may be in the urine only during a hemolytic episode, but hemosiderin is nearly always present if carefully sought.[10] Hemosiderinuria of the kidneys can be detected by computed tomography or magnetic resonance imaging (MRI).[11,12] The hemosiderosis of the kidneys may be so great that airport iron detectors are triggered.

During an acute bout of hemoglobinuria, the patient may experience renal failure as a result of overload of the renal tubules with hemoglobin.[13] This usually occurs when the patient does not drink enough fluids and becomes dehydrated.

For many years, it was thought that the chronic hemoglobinuria of PNH did not affect the kidneys. This apparently is not the case since renal damage ranging from subtle changes (including proximal tubular dysfunction)[14] to marked diminution in renal function occur in this disorder.[15,16] In about 5% of patients, renal failure is the cause of death. At autopsy, little is seen except the marked hemosiderosis of the kidneys with evidence of fibrosis.

Thrombosis

For unknown reasons, thrombosis in PNH almost always involves the venous system.

Hepatic Vein Thrombosis

Many patients with PNH suffer from unusual thrombotic syndromes. The most common syndrome is thrombosis of the hepatic veins, resulting in a variation of the Budd-Chiari syndrome.[17-19] Thrombosis of the veins may be sudden and catastrophic; when this occurs, it is usually in the setting of a hemolytic crisis. The patient has severe abdominal pain, a rapidly enlarging liver, and rapidly accumulating ascites. If sufficiently severe, thrombosis may lead to vascular collapse and death.

More frequently, the onset of thrombosis is insidious, with dull, aching pain in the right upper quadrant, slow accumulation of ascites, and splenomegaly. If the condition continues chronically, diversion of the portal blood through esophageal varices and other anastomoses become apparent; if sufficiently prolonged and severe, hepatic failure may supervene.

The diagnosis of hepatic vein thrombosis can be made by radiographic means.[20,21] A routine technetium-99m colloid scan of liver and spleen often shows diminished function in all portions of the liver except the caudate lobe. This lobe is spared because its venous effluent goes directly to the inferior vena cava rather than through the hepatic veins. This is manifested by a bright caudate lobe in such a scan. Careful analysis of blood flow by MRI or ultrasound can also demonstrate the cessation of flow through the hepatic veins. Finally, an injection contrast study of the inferior vena cava and hepatic veins definitively demonstrates the blockage of the veins; this should be reserved for equivocal cases since the injection of the dye may increase the degree of thrombosis.

Abdominal Vein Thrombosis

Patients with PNH may experience episodes of severe abdominal pain. This pain is frequently in the upper abdomen but may occur in any area. The episode may last from 1 to 6 days and often occurs during a severe hemolytic episode. During the episode, bowel sounds are usually active and direct and rebound tenderness may be present. Often, the pain is so severe that analgesic medications are required for relief.

Until the availability of improved diagnostic methods, the cause of the pain was not clear. In some cases, thrombosis of the splanchnic vessels resulting in infarction of the bowel was demonstrated[22]; the cause is seldom found, even on exploratory celeotomy. When the portal or splenic vein is involved, splenomegaly is usually seen. Often, the problem is manifested only by the pain that ensues. In other cases, the amount of thrombosis may be sufficient to cause severe infarction of the bowel, which may result in death.

Cerebral Vein Thrombosis

The cerebral veins appear to be particularly subject to thrombosis in patients with PNH.[23,24] In its mildest form, thrombosis of these veins is manifest as severe headaches. In more severe cases, neurologic symptoms are common, depending on which veins have thrombosed. The sagittal vein is commonly affected; this results in papilledema, and a syndrome sometimes mistaken for pseudotumor cerebri. Thrombosis of the parietal veins results, when on the dominant side, in Gerstmann's syndrome (agraphia, right–left disorientation, acalculia, and finger agnosia). Veins of the brain stem are seldom affected.

Again, the diagnosis is most effectively made by MRI analysis. Contrast studies can be performed but are not always accurate and may cause further thrombosis. Analysis of the cerebral spinal fluid often shows xanthochromia and a high protein, but this is not specific.

Dermal Vein Thrombosis

Thrombosis of the dermal veins is manifested by the appearance of painful, red, raised areas in any part of the body.[25,26] The nodules, if small, usually subside within a few weeks without necrosis of the skin. The process may spread to involve large areas such as the entire back; in this case, necrosis of the skin often occurs and grafting may be necessary.

Patients with PNH are prone to purpura fulminans, as are other patients with a tendency to thrombosis. This occurs in the setting of fever and infection and results in widespread necrosis of the skin. In rare instances, the involvement may be so extensive as to be fatal.

Thrombosis of Other Veins

Occasionally, the epididymal veins may thrombose, resulting in a syndrome much like orchitis or torsion of the testis. Thrombosis may occur in peripheral limb veins, with resultant pulmonary embolism. Renal vein thrombosis and atrial thrombosis have also been observed.

Arterial thrombosis is not notable in PNH.

Deficient Hematopoiesis

Many patients with PNH have evidence of deficient hematopoiesis.[5,27–29] This may be as little as a suboptimal reticulocyte count even with an actively erythropoietic marrow to as much as nearly complete aplasia of the bone marrow.

The deficit affects the other cell lines as well. More than two thirds of patients have thrombocytopenia or granulocytopenia or both.[6] This was first thought to be caused by excessive destruction of these cells, as with the RBCs. The survival in the circulation of both platelets[30,31] and neutrophils[32] is normal; thus, the low counts must be caused by diminished production.

The relation of PNH to aplastic anemia has been recognized for some time. Ten to 20% of patients with PNH have histories of aplastic anemia. About 5% of all patients with aplastic anemia eventually have PNH. In some instances, the proliferation defect remains predominant and the hemolytic manifestations are minimal; in others, the hemolysis is as great as in patients without previous aplastic anemia.

Aplastic episodes may occur during the course of PNH, often heralded by increasing thrombocytopenia and neutropenia; these episodes may be fatal.

Other Symptoms

Esophageal Spasm

Many patients with severe hemoglobinuria experience tightness of the esophagus. This occurs in the morning and usually, like the dark urine, disappears during the day. It is caused by esophageal spasms in which the peristaltic waves are normally propagated but are 10 to 15 times the strength of normal waves. The cause for this symptom is not known.

Impotence

Many men are unable to obtain or maintain a penile erection during periods of hemoglobinuria. When tested, the neurologic responses have been found to be normal. The cause for this symptom is likewise unknown.

PAROXYSMAL NOCTURNAL HEMOGLOBINURIA IN CHILDHOOD AND ADOLESCENCE

Paroxysmal nocturnal hemoglobinuria occurs in childhood and adolescence but is uncommon. Ware and colleagues[33] collected data on 26 patients who had the onset of the disorder in this age group. They found that a higher percentage of these patients presented with the primary features of aplastic anemia than that of the normal adult population. Other complications (infection, thrombosis) occurred about as frequently. Eight of 20 patients had died of the complications of the disorder, and the median duration of survival from the time of diagnosis was 10.3 years.

DIAGNOSIS

Paroxysmal nocturnal hemoglobinuria is defined as the demonstration of RBCs that are exceptionally sensitive to the hemolytic action of complement. This was originally demonstrated by Hijmans van den Bergh[34] in 1913 by testing the patient's cells in normal and autologous serum under conditions of acidification. He noted that heating the serum (known to destroy complement) abrogated the reaction, but he was not able to restore hemolysis by replacement of complement with more normal serum; he probably used too little fresh serum.

Thomas Hale Ham showed that the RBCs in PNH were lysed by complement when normal serum was acidified or was activated by alloantibodies.[3,35,36] This resulted in the acidified serum lysis or *Ham test*, still a reliable way to diagnose PNH if done properly. In this case, the alternative pathway of complement is activated in a manner not entirely understood.[37–39]

To achieve maximum sensitivity, the pH of the serum is lowered to about 6.2 and the Mg^{2+} level is adjusted to 0.005 mol/L Mg^{2+}.[40] The only known false-positive is seen in congenital dyserythropoietic anemia, type II (hereditary erythroblastic multinuclearity with a positive acidified serum test [HEMPAS])[41]; the lysis in this case is due to the presence of naturally occurring alloantibodies that react with the abnormal cells.[42] The remainder of the syndrome is so different from PNH that little confusion results.

Ham noted that only part of the cells were lysed in this test and that the residual cells would not lyse no matter how many times they were treated with acidified serum. With the advent of more precise tests, it became evident that the cells in PNH consist of two or more populations differing in their sensitivity to complement.[43]

The more precise method for the elucidation of the abnormality in PNH is the *complement lysis sensitivity test* of Rosse and Dacie.[43] In this test, the RBCs are sensitized with a potent lytic anti–i antigen and hemolysed with limiting amounts of normal human serum as a source of complement. Normal cells consist of a single population that is highly resistant to the hemolytic action of complement. Variable proportions of PNH cells are lysed by small concentrations of serum, and it has been possible to denote three types of cells[44,45] (Fig. 11-1):

1. PNH I cells that are virtually normal in their sensitivity to complement
2. PNH II cells that are moderately more sensitive than normal cells
3. PNH III cells that are markedly more sensitive than normal, requiring $\frac{1}{15}$ to $\frac{1}{20}$ the amount of complement for an equal degree of lysis

Patients may have various combinations of these populations. It was long thought that most patients had PNH I and PNH III cells only; careful analysis by other methods has revealed that often a small PNH II population is present.[46] In other patients, the PNH II cells predominate. The differences in these cells is discussed in the text that follows.

The percentage of each population varies greatly from patient to patient; as few as 1% to 2% to as many as 95% abnormal cells may be seen. In a given patient, the percentage of the abnormal cells remains fairly stable for long periods, although it may be found to increase during the onset of the disease and to decrease as the disease ameliorates. Because the PNH III cells are preferentially lysed during a hemolytic episode, their percentage may decrease at that time.

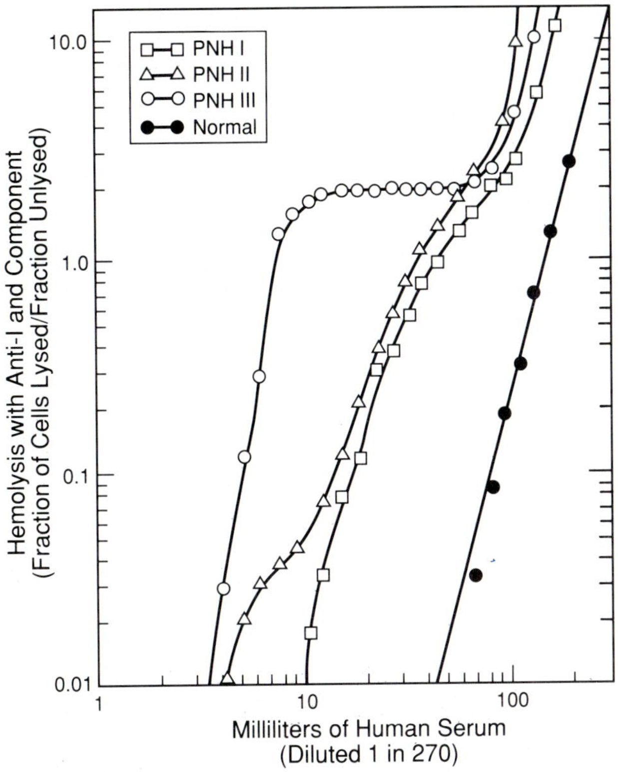

FIGURE 11-1. Demonstration of the populations of differing sensitivity to complement lysis by the complement lysis sensitivity test of Rosse and Dacie.[43] The RBCs are sensitized with large amounts of hemolytic anti–i antibody and lysed with incremental amounts of normal human serum as a source of complement. A function of the amount of lysis (fraction of cells lysed divided by the fraction unlysed) is plotted on logarithmic paper against the amount of serum used. The relative sensitivity of the cells can be determined by estimating the amount of complement needed to lyse half of the population. The proportion of cells in each population can be determined by inspection of the curves. Normal and PNH I RBCs require large amounts of complement, whereas the markedly sensitive PNH III RBCs are lysed by small amounts. The cells of intermediate sensitivity (PNH II cells) require somewhat less complement than normal but much more than PNH III cells.

The PNH III cells are the most sensitive to lysis in vivo as well as in vitro; the mean life-span of these cells is about 10 to 15 days.[47] Therefore, the amount of hemolysis in vivo is roughly proportional to the number of these cells present. PNH II cells are lysed somewhat more readily than normal cells but much less readily than PNH III cells[47]; patients with a large percentage of PNH II cells often have little hemolysis.

Other Tests for Paroxysmal Nocturnal Hemoglobinuria

Other tests for the complement sensitive cells in PNH have been devised. One of the most popular is the so-called sugar water, or sucrose lysis test, in which the ionic strength of serum is reduced by dilution in an isoosmotic solution of sucrose.[48,49] Complement is activated by the classic pathway and the complement-sensitive cells are lysed. Unfortunately, the test is somewhat less specific than the Ham's test as cells of patients with autoimmune hemolytic anemia as well as other disorders (leukemia, aplastic anemia) are sometimes hemolyzed, although usually to a minor degree. The sucrose lysis test is suggested to be more sensitive than Ham's test; this is not the case if the latter is performed correctly with magnesium supplementation.[40]

A factor in the venom of the cobra *Naja naja* is able to activate the terminal portion of the complement sequence resulting in reactive lysis.[37,50] Normal human serum activated in this way is able to hemolyze PNH cells, which has been suggested as a test for the disease. Unfortunately, complement activated in this way hemolyzes PNH III and not PNH II cells[51]; thus, it does not accurately identify those patients who have PNH II but not PNH III cells.

A number of other ways of activating complement have been devised but none of the tests have been shown to be superior to those described. In the future, tests based on the detection of the lack of certain membrane proteins (see following section) may be devised but they are not standard.

PATHOGENESIS

Although PNH is defined by the abnormality of the RBCs, it was recognized as a stem cell disorder and may be classified as a myelodysplastic syndrome. The platelets, granulocytes, and, in some cases, lymphocytes can be demonstrated to have defects in relation to complement and in other respects. Thus, the acquired defect affects the stem cell, and the defect is transmitted to the descendant hematopoietic cells.

The nature of the defect was not understood for many years. It had been known that two enzymes were missing; acetylcholinesterase from the RBCs[52,53] and alkaline phosphatase from the granulocytes[54,55]; neither of these defects appeared to have any effect on the activation of complement. With the finding of the deficiency of a third protein that *did* affect the activation of complement, the decay-accelerating factor (DAF),[56,57] a pattern of selective membrane protein deficiency began to appear. At least nine proteins are known to be missing on the cells of patients with PNH (Table 11-1). Undoubtedly, other proteins will be found that share the common characteristic of these nine.

The Biochemical Defect

All the proteins missing in PNH are bound to the membrane by a glycosyl-phosphatidylinositol (GPI) anchor.[58–63] This anchor (Fig. 11-2) consists of a phosphatidylinositol moiety affixed to four sugars and connected to the protein through an ethanolamine molecule. In addition, an extra lipid entity (usually palmitate) may be attached to the inositol, and other side chains may be attached to the first two mannoses.[63]

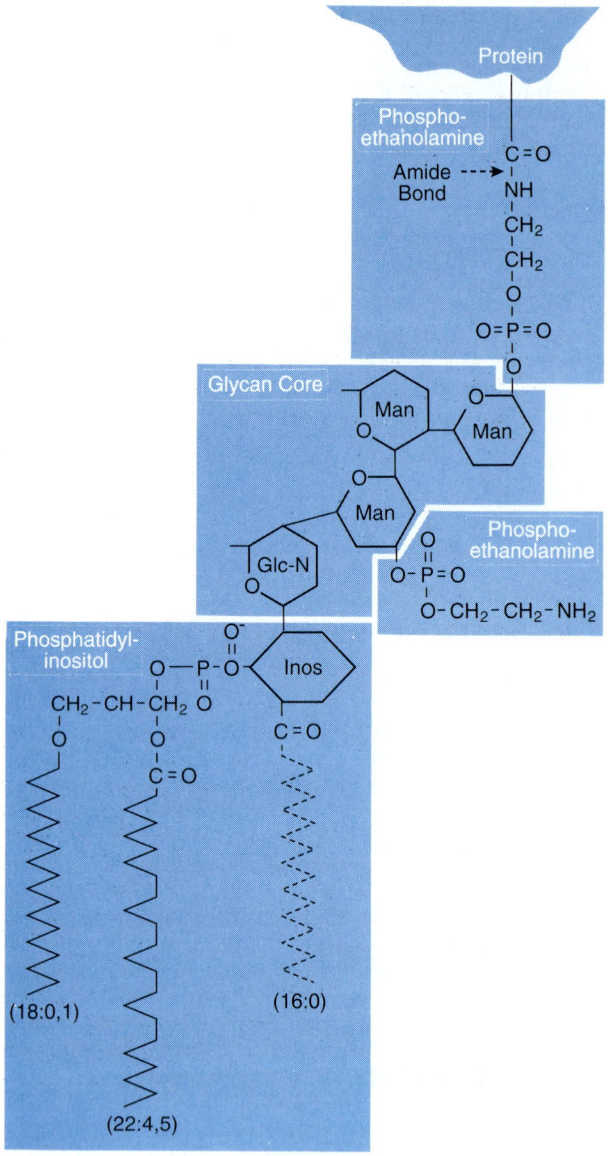

FIGURE 11-2. The phosphatidylinositol-containing glycolipid anchor common to all proteins lacking in PNH cells. The glycan core, consisting of four sugar moieties, is attached to the phosphatidylinositol molecule. A palmityl group (*dashed side chain*) may be attached to the inositol of this core. Ethanolamine is added to the terminal mannose of the core, and the protein is attached by an amide linkage. An additional ethanolamine may be added to the first mannose of the core.

TABLE 11-1. Membrane Proteins Known to Be Missing From Hematopoietic Cells in Paroxysmal Nocturnal Hemoglobinuria

COMPLEMENT-REGULATING PROTEINS
Decay-accelerating factor (CD55) from erythrocytes,[56] granulocytes, and platelets[75,76]
Membrane inhibitor of reactive lysis (protectin or CD59) from PNH III RBCs[76,131]
C8 binding protein or homologous restriction factor[87,88]
MEMBRANE ENZYMES
Erythrocyte acetylcholinesterase[52,53]
Leukocyte alkaline phosphatase[54,55]
Lymphocyte 5′ ectonucleotidase
IMMUNE FUNCTION PROTEINS
Lymphocyte function antigen 3[91]
Neutrophil Fc_γ III receptor (CD16)[90]
Monocyte CD14[92]

Such an anchor was first described for the variable surface glycoproteins of trypanosomes,[64,65] who use them to fool the immune system of the host. The trypanosome changes this coat about every 5 days, substituting an immunologically unrelated protein that does not react with the antibodies produced against preceding coats. The old coat is removed by an enzyme, phosphatidyl inositol-specific phospholipase C that cleaves the phospholipid link.[66]

In the trypanosome, the synthesis of these proteins is fairly well understood.[67] The protein is made with a hydrophobic section that interacts with the lipid bilayer of the endoplasmic reticulum. In the cisterna of the endoplasmic reticulum, the anchor is independently synthesized. An enzyme present in the cisterna cleaves the protein and binds it to the ethanolamine of the anchor (Fig. 11-3). The protein is then processed and finally appears on the external cell membrane.

This sort of anchor is well known for mammalian organisms as well. The advantage of such an anchor resides both in the readiness with which the protein may be enzymatically removed from the membrane and the lateral mobility in the plane of the membrane of proteins anchored in this way; since the insertion molecule is much like the other phospholipids of the membrane, these molecules are thought to have the same mobility as those phospholipids.

The fundamental defect in PNH appears to be an inability to synthesize this GPI anchor. The defect is at the same step in all patients: the first sugar moiety (*N*-acetylglucosamine) cannot be affixed to the phosphatidylinositol molecule.[68–70] The cDNA of the protein that is lacking has been cloned,[70a] but the exact function of the protein is not yet clear. The corresponding gene, called *PIG-A* (for phosphatidylinositol glycan class A), resides on the X chromosome.[70b] This explains how a single recessive somatic mutation in a hematopoietic stem cell can cause PNA, since only a single X chromosome is active in each cell. Twenty-six patients with PNH have been tested, and all have defects in PIG-A protein.[70b,70c] These range from deletions to point mutations. Functionally, the defect appears to be partial in many patients; thus, small amounts of the anchor are made and some of the cells may have small amounts of the GPI proteins on their surface. These are the PNH II cells of intermediate sensitivity to complement.

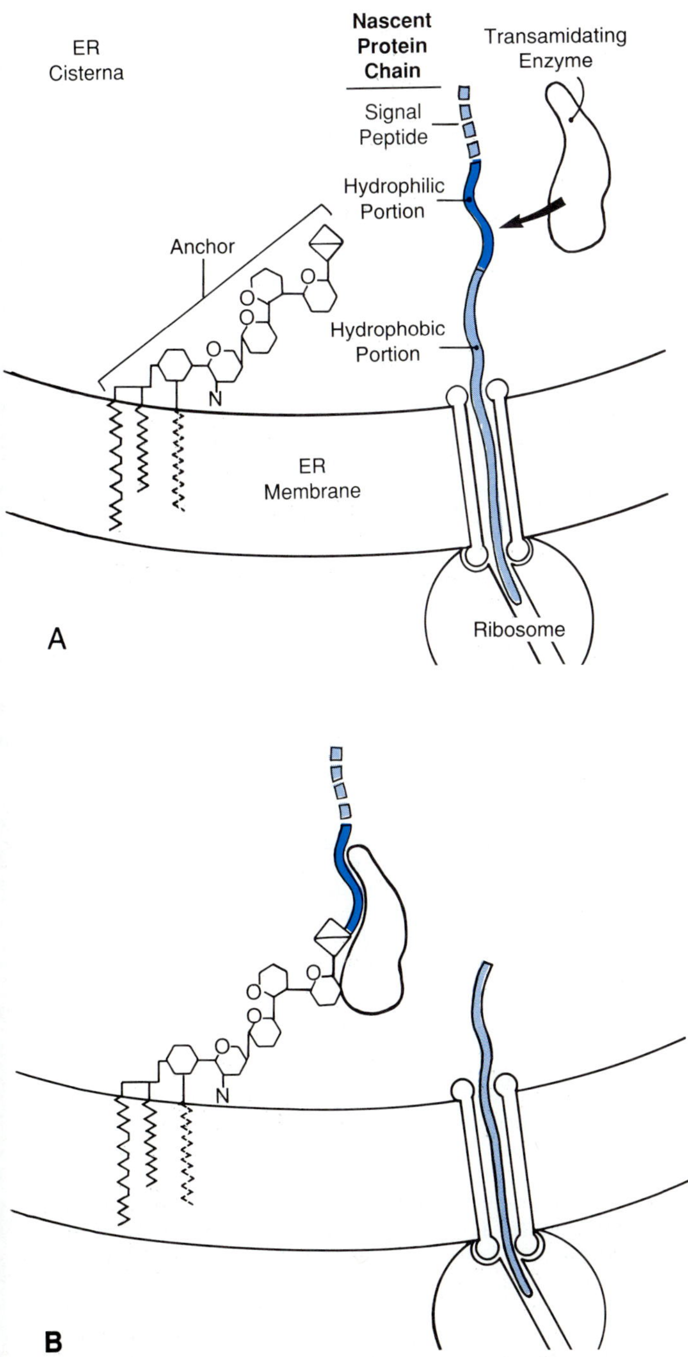

FIGURE 11-3. Attachment of the phosphatidylinositol-glycan anchor to the nascent protein in the endoplasmic reticulum (ER). (**A**) The ribosome attached to the membrane of the ER translates the nascent protein, which is extruded into the cisterna of the ER. There, it encounters the anchor that has been preformed on the inner leaflet of the ER membrane. (**B**) The transamidating enzyme then cleaves the nascent protein and affixes it to the anchor.

Effects of the Biochemical Defect

Modulation of Complement Activation

The defining characteristic of PNH is the diminished modulation of complement activation that results in the excessive sensitivity to its hemolytic action. This is caused by the lack of at least three proteins: DAF, membrane inhibitor of reactive lysis (MIRL), and perhaps C8-binding protein or homologous restriction factor. Each of these proteins normally plays a role in the inactivation of reactions of homologous complement at the membrane surface.

Decay-Accelerating Factor

The first of these to be defined was DAF,[56] a glycoprotein of the complement regulating group coded on chromosome 1.[71] All these proteins contain a 62-unit short consensus repeat that apparently permits them to interact with complement proteins, particularly C3b and C4b.[72] DAF has four of these and apparently acts to dissociate the convertase complexes of the classic and alternative pathways (C4b2a and C3bBb, respectively).[73] In this way, the amplification of the activation of complement is halted.

The absence of DAF explains why a given number of convertase complexes generated on PNH cells and on normal cells results in markedly greater fixation of C3b to the PNH cells, since the function of the convertase complex is the activation of C3 to C3b and C5 to C5b.[74]

The platelets, granulocytes, and, in some cases, the lymphocytes as well as the RBCs in PNH lack DAF.[75,76] The platelets are able to counteract this deficiency in part because their α granules contain protein H (a protein with analogous actions), another member of the complement restriction group of proteins.[77] When the release reaction occurs, factor H is released from the granules locally and inhibits the activation of the convertase complex. Because of this and the fact that the lack of DAF is not greatly injurious to the survival of cells, PNH platelets survive normally.[31]

Membrane Inhibitor of Reactive Lysis

Parker and associates[78] described a protein on normal erythrocyte membranes that appears to regulate the effectiveness of the membrane attack complex (C5b-9). Parker named this protein *membrane inhibitor of reactive lysis*, since he first demonstrated its ability to inhibit lysis generated by activation by cobra venom factor. This name is not entirely correct because the protein also appears to inhibit lysis when generated by the alternative and classic pathways as well. The action of this protein, also called *CD59* or *protectin*, is, at least in part, to prevent the polymerization of C9 in the formation of the membrane attack complex.[79,80]

The membrane attack is initiated by the partial insertion of the complex C5b-7 into the membrane, whereupon it affixes C8. C9 in the plasma reacts with C8 in this complex and is converted into an amphipathic molecule that can span the lipid bilayer. Altered C9 accumulates in polymers of 3 to 12 molecules, and these are responsible for the lysis of the cell. CD59 disrupts this process by preventing the reaction of C9 with C8. When CD59 is missing, as in PNH, more polymeric C9 complexes accumulate and lysis occurs more readily.

MIRL (CD59) has a molecular weight of about 18 kd and is linked to the membrane by the GPI anchor.[81] The cDNA for the protein has been isolated.[82,83] It is a complex protein that is related to the snake toxin bungarotoxin as well as to the urokinase receptor and to Ly6 proteins, a series of murine immunologic signal proteins.

The importance of MIRL is demonstrated by the fact that inhibition of the molecule on normal RBCs by antibody renders them much like PNH III cells in the complement lysis sensitivity test (Fig. 11-4*A*). Furthermore, introduction of the molecule into the membrane of PNH III cells renders them nearly normal with respect to complement sensitivity (see Fig. 11-4*B*). From these studies, it is clear that the lack of MIRL is the most important abnormality with respect to the abnormal down-regulation of complement in PNH cells.

The lack of regulation of the formation of polymeric C9 in the membrane of the platelet because of the lack of CD59 is also probably at least partially responsible for the thrombotic tendency in PNH. When polymeric C9 complexes are generated in the membrane of a normal or PNH platelet, they are gathered into a vesicle that is then removed by budding. These vesicles are highly thrombogenic since they bear sites for the formation of prothrombinase complexes, which in turn generate thrombin.[83a] In addition, PNH platelets are more susceptible to the aggregogenic effects of thrombin. The result of these abnormalities is a marked tendency of the blood to clot, particularly in the venous circulation.

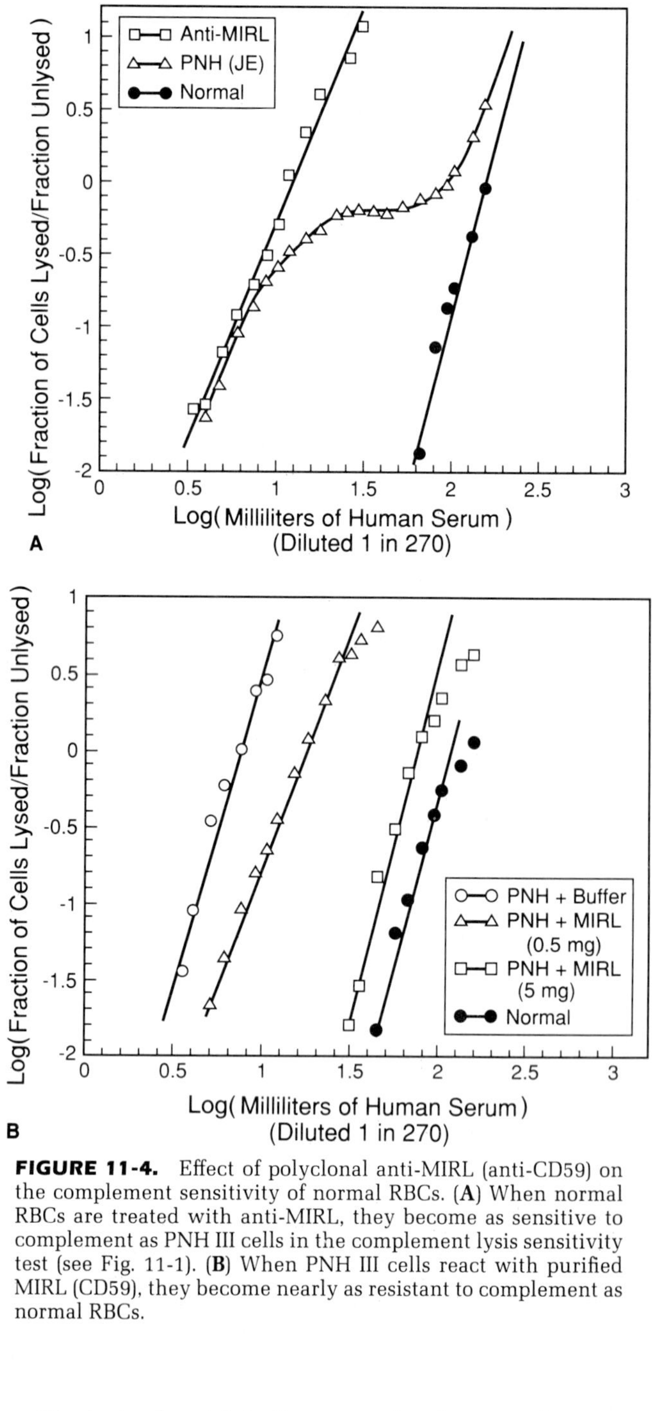

FIGURE 11-4. Effect of polyclonal anti-MIRL (anti-CD59) on the complement sensitivity of normal RBCs. (**A**) When normal RBCs are treated with anti-MIRL, they become as sensitive to complement as PNH III cells in the complement lysis sensitivity test (see Fig. 11-1). (**B**) When PNH III cells react with purified MIRL (CD59), they become nearly as resistant to complement as normal RBCs.

C8-Binding Protein

A third protein that may regulate the activation of the terminal complex of complement has been described. It was purified by its ability to bind to C8 and is thought to interfere with the role of C8 in organizing the polymerized C9 complexes that penetrate the cell membrane.[84,85] The protein has a molecular weight of about 79 kd and is apparently PI linked. It is not well characterized, and its importance in the regulation of complement is in question. C8-binding protein is said to be missing in PNH III but not in PNH II cells.[86,87] This protein and MIRL are possibly the same, but the characteristics of each appear to be different.

Enzymes

Three enzymes are missing on PNH cells: acetylcholinesterase from RBCs,[52,53] alkaline phosphatase from neutrophils,[54,55] and 5′ *ectonucleotidase* from lymphocytes (Devine and Rosse, unpublished). These enzymes serve as markers of the abnormal population but to date no functional abnormality has been ascribed to explain their absence.

The lack of acetylcholinesterase has been used to separate the abnormal population from the PNH I cells, which bear the enzyme.[88] The cells are reacted with monoclonal antibody to acetylcholinesterase, then with a rabbit antibody to mouse IgG. They are then passed through a column of staphylococcal protein A affixed to sepharose. The cells bearing acetylcholinesterase are retained and the abnormal cells are eluted.

Lack of alkaline phosphatase has been used as a marker of the abnormal population as well. In a patient with PNH who had acquired acute myelocytic leukemia (see following text), the blasts were found to lack alkaline phosphatase, whereas the blasts from patients in whom the leukemia was not preceded by PNH bore the enzyme, suggesting that the leukemic population had arisen from the abnormal PNH stem cells.[89]

Immunologic Functional Proteins

The effect of the lack of the three known missing immunologic proteins—neutrophil Fc γ-III receptor, lymphocyte functional antigen-3, and CD14—in PNH is not entirely clear.[90–92] The neutrophils bear other Fc receptors, and no distinct defect of phagocytosis has been demonstrated. The alloantigens NA1 and NA2 are resident on Fc γ-III and are thus missing on the abnormal population of PNH neutrophils.[93]

The lymphocyte functional antigen-3 is missing from the abnormal RBCs in patients with PNH and is partially missing from the nucleated blood cells.[94] It apparently has a phosphatidylinositol-containing, glycolipid-linked form as well as a membrane-anchored form; the latter form is not lacking. The effect of the lack is under investigation. It may have a role in the diminished hematopoiesis seen in PNH.

CD14 is the receptor for the endotoxin-binding protein of plasma.[95] Its gene is located on chromosome 5 (5q23 to q33), the site of the genes of a number of myeloid growth factors and growth factor receptors.[96] The effect of its absence has not been fully described.

Leukemia

An unusual complication of PNH that cannot be explained at the present time by the loss of PI-linked proteins is acute leukemia.[97–100] Patients with PNH have a probability of acquiring leukemia that is much above the general population; the incidence of this complication may be about 1% to 3%. The leukemia occurs about 5 to 8 years after the onset of PNH and is usually preceded by a preleukemic phase. The leukemia is nearly always acute myelogenous leukemia, although erythroleukemia,[101–103] myelomonocytic leukemia,[104] and terminal deoxynucleotidyl transferase–positive acute lymphocytic leukemia[105] have been reported. The leukemia cells appear to arise from the abnormal population of stem cells[89] (see previous text). No specific chromosomal abnormalities have been reported in patients with leukemia arising from PNH.

When leukemia supervenes, the abnormal RBCs usually disappear; this may simply be a reflection of the markedly diminished erythropoiesis in this setting. If remission is obtained (a difficult task in these patients), the abnormal RBCs may return.[104] No patient with leukemia occurring after PNH has been cured by chemotherapy.

TREATMENT

The ideal treatment for PNH is replacement of the abnormal stem cells or correction of the defect. These are not routinely practicable. The abnormal stem cells may be replaced by transplantation and this is successful in treating the disease.[106–108] This requires histocompatible donors, and, even so, appreciable morbidity and mortality rates due to graft-versus-host disease occur. For this reason, replacement has been restricted to those patients with the most serious complications, particularly aplastic anemia. Bone marrow transplantation has not been used in patients in transition to leukemia but might be useful.

Although much is known about the defect and its effects on the cells, this information has not been translated into practical treatment for the disorder. Thus, the treatment of PNH is largely based on symptoms.

Anemia

The treatment for anemia in PNH takes four forms, depending in part on the major causes and the severity.

Modulation of Complement

Because the hemolysis in PNH depends on the activation of complement, it could theoretically be abrogated if complement activation could be controlled. Unfortunately, despite detailed knowledge about the activation of complement, little is known about pharmacologic means for its control. *Glucocorticoids* in large doses apparently diminish the activation of complement by means that are not entirely clear and their use in PNH has been established.[109,110] In most patients, a moderate to marked diminution in hemolysis can be seen with the administration of 20 to 40 mg/d of prednisone for adults (0.3 to 0.6 mg/kg/d); the dose can be given once, preferably in the early evening. The effect is immediate and short lasting; the nocturnal hemoglobinuria for a night can be abrogated by the administration of prednisone in the evening but will return the following evening if the treatment is not repeated (Fig. 11-5).

Because the dose required is high, usually above 20 mg/d (0.3 mg/kg/d) in adults, and since the treatment is by necessity chronic, *prednisone should be given on alternate days except during episodes of hemolysis*, when it is given on a daily basis for periods up to 10 days. On this regimen, about 70% of adult patients with a significant degree of hemolysis experience improvement in the level of hemoglobin.

Replacement of Nutrients

Patients with PNH often lose large amounts of iron either as hemoglobin or as hemosiderin; 200 times the normal daily urinary excretion, which is about 0.1 mg/d,[111] may occur without overt hemoglobinuria. This loss increases the probability of iron deficiency, demonstrated by a diminished hematopoiesis and reduction in the mean corpuscular volume. Iron replacement by oral medication is usually effective in treating or preventing this deficiency.[112]

Sometimes, when iron is given to an iron-deficient patient with PNH, marked exacerbation of hemolysis begins about 5 days after inception of treatment.[113] This was at one time thought to be caused by a toxic effect of iron but is now known to be caused by increased hematopoiesis resulting from iron replenishment, which causes a sudden

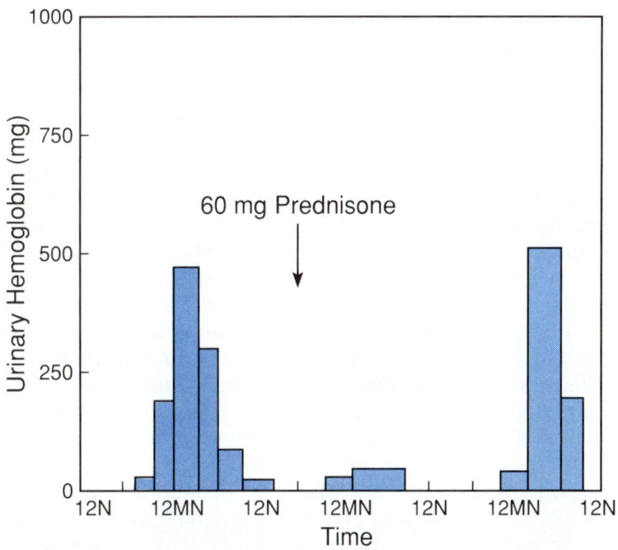

FIGURE 11-5. Effect of prednisone on the excretion of hemoglobin in the urine.

outpouring of complement-sensitive cells.[114] These cells are then subject to lysis with the result that hemoglobinuria may result. This complication can be prevented by administering prednisone (see previous text) or by giving the patient transfusions so that the stimulus to increased hematopoiesis is diminished.

Folic acid deficiency can occur in any patient with hemolytic anemia because of the greater need of the hyperactive bone marrow for this nutrient, which is in limited supply in the diet.[115] This may occur in patients with PNH but is possibly less common since the intracellular folate from RBCs is released into the plasma and can probably be reutilized; in most cases of hemolytic anemia, however, in which the destruction is intracellular, folate cannot be recycled. Nevertheless, most patients with hemolysis are advised to take 1 mg/d of folic acid.

Stimulation of Erythropoiesis

Androgenic hormones stimulate erythropoiesis, probably by increasing the production of erythropoietin.[116] They have been used successfully in the treatment of PNH, particularly in those patients with moderate reduction in erythropoiesis.[112] Any of a number of preparations can be used, usually in moderate dosage: oxymethalone, 10 to 30 mg/d; fluoxymesterone, 10 to 30 mg/d; stanozolol, 2 to 6 mg/d; danazol, 200 to 600 mg/d. All seem effective, but some (danazol, stanozolol) have less androgenizing effects, a property valued by women.

The incidence of hepatic vein thrombosis is thought to be increased in patients taking androgenic hormones. These compounds are also known to have toxic effects on the liver.[117–119] Statistical proof of this relation is lacking.

Transfusion

Transfusion of patients with PNH is generally not attended with special problems. Cases of hemolysis of the patient's RBCs have been recorded[120–122]; this most likely occurs in circumstances in which complement may be activated, as in the transfusion of alloantibodies or the presence of antibodies in the patient's plasma reacting with transfused platelets or neutrophils.[123] The reaction can be prevented by washing the RBCs before transfusion.[124]

Thrombosis

The treatment of thrombosis in a patient with PNH follows principles of treatment of thrombosis in any patient. Acute thrombosis is treated with heparin, and the treatment is switched to coumarin as soon as possible.[18] Thrombolytic agents have been used as well.[125] The administration of heparin has been reported to cause exacerbations of hemolysis[126] and worsening of subdermal thromboses. This may be because heparin in low doses activates complement; in higher doses, it inhibits complement activity.[127] Care must be taken to observe carefully the patient being heparinized to be certain that these complications do not occur.

Because the thrombosis may be due to the sensitivity of the platelets to thrombin activation, the ideal preventive agent might be a drug inhibiting thrombin directly. Hirudin would be useful if it were available.

The activation of the platelet by thrombin can be prevented by inhibition of the cyclooxygenase system.[128] For this reason, powerful inhibitors of this system (such as aspirin, ibuprofen, or sulfinpyrazone) may be useful in preventing thrombosis; statistical evidence for this is lacking.

Stimulation of Hematopoiesis

Bone marrow hypoplasia seen in PNH is a serious cause of morbidity and mortality. It is most effectively treated with bone marrow transplantation; this procedure is often not available because no suitable donor can be found.

Antithymocyte globulin, an antiserum to human T cells prepared in horses, has been used in the treatment of aplastic anemia with considerable success.[129] We have used this treatment in patients with PNH, with evidence of hematopoietic deficit ranging from thrombocytopenia alone to overt aplastic marrow. The treatment has been successful in 11 of 14 patients and has resulted in improvement or complete normalization of blood counts (Huang et al, unpublished data). The disadvantage of this treatment is that the abnormal cells are still made, but the correction of the thrombocytopenia and neutropenia is extraordinarily useful in treating PNH with a hypoplastic component. The mechanism by which antithymocytic globulin stimulates a hypoplastic marrow in either aplastic anemia or PNH is not known. Complications resulting from this treatment in patients with PNH have been no greater than those accompanying its use in aplastic anemia.

PROGNOSIS

The prognosis in PNH is highly variable, so mean survival figures have little meaning. Patients with chronic anemia alone, without thrombotic or hematopoietic complications, can often live relatively normal lives for many years. Clearly, this prognosis is shortened if one of the complications supervenes.

In many patients, the abnormal population of hematopoietic cells tends to disappear. This usually takes at least 5 years and often as long as 15 to 20 years to occur. In about half of long-term patients, marked amelioration or disappearance of hemolysis occurs with time.[130]

REFERENCES

1. Gull WW. A case of intermittent haematinuria, with remarks. Guy's Hosp Rep 1866;12:381.
2. Strubing P. Paroxysmale haemoglobinurie. Deutsch Med Wochenschr 1882;8:1.
3. Ham TH. Chronic hemolytic anemia with paroxysmal nocturnal hemoglobinuria: a study of the mechanism of hemolysis in relation to acid-base equilibrium. N Engl J Med 1937;217:915.
4. Crosby WH. Paroxysmal nocturnal hemoglobinuria: relation of the clinical manifestations to underlying pathogenic mechanisms. Blood 1972;8:769.
5. Dacie JV, Lewis SM. Paroxysmal nocturnal hemoglobinuria: variation in clinical severity and association with bone-marrow hypoplasia. Br J Haematol 1961;7:442.
6. Dacie JV. Paroxysmal nocturnal haemoglobinuria. Proc R Soc Med 1963;56:587.
7. Dacie JV. The haemolytic anaemias: congenital and acquired, part IV, ed 2. New York, Grune & Stratton, 1967:1128.
8. Sirchia G, Lewis SM. Paroxysmal nocturnal haemoglobinuria. Clin Haematol 1975;4:199.
9. Dacie JV, Lewis SM. Paroxysmal nocturnal hemoglobinuria, clinical manifestations, hematology and nature of the disease. Semin Haematol 1972;5:3.
10. Sears DA, Anderson PR, Foy AL, et al. Urinary iron excretion and renal metabolism of hemoglobin in hemolytic diseases. Blood 1966;28:708.
11. Mulopulos GP, Turner DA, Schwartz MM, et al. MRI of the kidneys in paroxysmal nocturnal hemoglobinuria. AJR 1986;146:51.
12. Lupetin AR. Magnetic resonance appearance of the kidneys in paroxysmal nocturnal hemoglobinuria. Urol Radiol 1986;8:101.
13. Rubin H. Paroxysmal nocturnal hemoglobinuria with renal failure. JAMA 1971;215:433.
14. Riley AL, Ryan LM, Roth DA. Renal proximal tubular dysfunction and paroxysmal nocturnal hemoglobinuria. Am J Med 1977;62:125.
15. Clark DA, Butler SA, Braren V, et al. The kidneys in paroxysmal nocturnal hemoglobinuria. Blood 1981;57:83.
16. Hamilton DV, Pryor JS. Paroxysmal nocturnal haemoglobinuria and chronic renal failure. Practitioner 1979;223:381.

17. Petremann R, Rhodes RS, Hartmann RC. Thrombosis in paroxysmal nocturnal hemoglobinuria (PNH) with particular reference to progressive diffuse hepatic venous thrombosis. Semin Haematol 1972;5:115.
18. Hartmann RC, Luther AB, Jenkins DE Jr, et al. Fulminant hepatic venous thrombosis (Budd-Chiari syndrome) in paroxysmal nocturnal hemoglobinuria: definition of a medical emergency. Johns Hopkins Med J 1980;146:247.
19. Horler AR, Shaw MT, Thompson RB. Budd-Chiari syndrome as a complication of paroxysmal nocturnal hemoglobinuria. Postgrad Med J 1970;46:618.
20. Staab EV, Hartmann RC, Parrott JA. Liver imaging in the diagnosis of hepatic venous thrombosis in paroxysmal nocturnal hemoglobinuria. Radiology 1975;117:341.
21. Tavill AS, Wood EJ, Kreel L, et al. The Budd-Chiari syndrome: correlation between hepatic scintography and the clinical, radiological and pathological findings. Gastroenterology 1975;68:509.
22. Blum SF, Gardner FH. Intestinal infarction in paroxysmal nocturnal hemoglobinuria. N Engl J Med 1966;274:1137.
23. Stirling ML, Lenton RJ, Summerling MD. Cerebral vein thrombosis and the contraceptive pill in paroxysmal nocturnal hemoglobinuria. Scott Med J 1980;25:243.
24. Johnson RV, Kaplan SR, Blailock ZR. Cerebral venous thrombosis in paroxysmal nocturnal hemoglobinuria (Marchiafava-Micheli syndrome). Neurology 1970;20:681.
25. Rietschel RL, Lewis CW, Simmons RA, Phyliky RL. Skin lesion in paroxysmal nocturnal hemoglobinuria. Arch Dermatol 1978;114:560.
26. Hansen NE, Killmann SA. Paroxysmal nocturnal hemoglobinuria: a clinical study. Acta Med Scand 1968;184:525.
27. Lewis SM, Dacie JV. The aplastic anaemic-paroxysmal nocturnal haemoglobinuria syndrome. Br J Haematol 1967;13:236.
28. Rosse WF. Paroxysmal nocturnal hemoglobinuria in aplastic anemia. Clin Haematol 1985;14:105.
29. Ben Bassat I, Brok-Simoni F, Ramot B. Complement-sensitive red cells in aplastic anemia. Blood 1975;46:357.
30. Cohen P, Gardner FH, Barnett GO. Reclassification of the thrombocytopenias by the Cr^{51}-labeling method for measuring platelet life span. N Engl J Med 1961;264:1264.
31. Devine DV, Siegel RS, Rosse WF. Interactions of the platelets in paroxysmal nocturnal hemoglobinuria with complement. J Clin Invest 1987;79:131.
32. Brubaker L, Essig LJ, Mangel CE. Neutrophil life span in paroxysmal nocturnal hemoglobinuria. Blood 1977;50:657.
33. Ware RE, Hall SE, Rosse WF. Paroxysmal nocturnal hemoglobinuria with onset in childhood and adolescence. N Engl J Med 1991;325:991.
34. Hijmans van den Bergh AA. Ictère hémolytique avec crises hémoglobinuriques. Fragilité globulaire. Rev Med 1911;31:63.
35. Ham TH. Studies on the destruction of red blood cells. I. Chronic hemolytic anemia with paroxysmal nocturnal hemoglobinuria: an investigation of the mechanism of hemolysis with observations on five cases. Arch Intern Med 1939;64:1271.
36. Ham TH, Dingle JH. Studies on destruction of red blood cells. II. Chronic hemolytic anemia with paroxysmal nocturnal hemoglobinuria: certain immunological aspects of the hemolytic mechanism with special reference to serum complement. J Clin Invest 1939;18:657.
37. Gotze O, Muller-Eberhard HJ. Paroxysmal nocturnal hemoglobinuria: hemolysis initiated by the C3 activator system. N Engl J Med 1972;286:180.
38. Hinz CJ Jr, Jordan WS Jr, Pillemer L. The properdin system and immunity. IV. The hemolysis of erythrocytes from patients with paroxysmal nocturnal hemoglobinuria. J Clin Invest 1956;35:453.
39. Logue GL, Rosse WF, Adams JP. Mechanism of immune lysis of red blood cells in vitro. I. Paroxysmal nocturnal hemoglobinuria. cells. J Clin Invest 1973;42:1129.
40. May, JE, Frank MM, Rosse WF. Alternate complement-pathway-mediated lysis induced by magnesium. N Engl J Med 1973;298:705.
41. Crookston JH, Crookston MC, Burnie KL, et al. Hereditary erythroblastic multinuclearity associated with a positive acidified serum test: a type of congenital dyserythropoietic anaemia. Br J Haematol 1969;17:11.
42. Crookston JH, Crookston MC, Rosse WF. Red cell abnormalities in HEMPAS (hereditary erythroblastic multinuclearity with a positive acidified-serum) test. Br J Haematol 1973;23(Suppl):83.
43. Rosse WF, Dacie JV. Immune lysis of normal human and paroxysmal nocturnal hemoglobinuria red blood cells. I. The sensitivity of PNH red cells to lysis by complement and specific antibody. J Clin Invest 1966;45:736.
44. Rosse WF, Adams JP, Thorpe AM. The population of cells in paroxysmal nocturnal hemoglobinuria of intermediate sensitivity to complement lysis: significance and mechanism of increased immune lysis. Br J Haematol 1974;28:181.
45. Rosse WF. Complement sensitivity of paroxysmal nocturnal hemoglobinuria cells. Semin Haematol 1972;5:101.
46. Rosse WF, Hall S, Campbell M, Borowitz M, Moore JO, Parker CJ. The erythrocytes of paroxysmal nocturnal hemoglobinuria of intermediate sensitivity to complement lysis. Br J Haematol 1991;79:99.
47. Rosse WF. The life-span of complement-sensitive and -insensitive red cells in paroxysmal nocturnal hemoglobinuria. Blood 1971;37:556.
48. Hartmann RC, Jenkins, DE Jr. The "sugar water" test for paroxysmal nocturnal hemoglobinuria. N Engl J Med 1966;275:155.
49. Hartmann RC. Diagnostic specificity of the sucrose hemolysis test for paroxysmal nocturnal hemoglobinuria. Blood 1970;35:462.
50. Kabaci R, Rosse WF, Logue GL. The lysis of paroxysmal nocturnal haemoglobinuria red cells by serum and cobra factor. Br J Haematol 1972;23:693.
51. Parker CJ, Wiedmer T, Sims PJ, Rosse WF. Characterization of the complement sensitivity of paroxysmal nocturnal hemoglobinuria erythrocytes. J Clin Invest 1985;75:2074.
52. Auditore JV, Hartmann RC, Flexner JM, Balchum OJ. The erythrocyte acetylcholinesterase enzyme in paroxysmal nocturnal hemoglobinuria. Arch Pathol 1960;69:534.
53. Kunstling TR, Rosse WF. Erythrocyte acetylcholinesterase deficiency in paroxysmal nocturnal hemoglobinuria (PNH): a comparison of the complement-sensitive and -insensitive populations. Blood 1969;33:607.
54. Lewis SM, Dacie JV. Neutrophil (leucocyte) alkaline phosphatase in paroxysmal nocturnal hemoglobinuria. Br J Haematol 1965;11:549.
55. Beck WS, Valentine WN. Biochemical studies on leucocytes. II. Phosphatase activity in chronic lymphatic leukemia, acute leukemia, and miscellaneous hematologic conditions. J Lab Clin Med 1951;38:245.
56. Nicholson-Weller A, March JP, Rosenfeld SI, Austen KF. Affected erythrocytes of patients with paroxysmal nocturnal hemoglobinuria are deficient in the complement regulatory protein, decay accelerating factor. Proc Natl Acad Sci USA 1983;80:5066.
57. Pangburn MK, Schreiber RD, Muller-Eberhard HJ. Deficiency of an erythrocyte membrane protein with complement regulatory activity in paroxysmal nocturnal hemoglobinuria. Proc Natl Acad Sci USA 1983;80:5430.
58. Davitz MA, Low MG, Nussenzweig V. Release of decay-accelerating factor (DAF) from the cell membrane by phosphatidylinositol specific phospholipase C (PIPLC) J Exp Med 1986;163:1150.
59. Hansch GM, Weller PF, Nicholson-Weller A. Release of C8 binding protein (C8bp) from the cell membrane by phosphatidylinositol-specific phospholipase C. Blood 1988;72:1089.
60. Taguchi R, Suzuke K, Nakabayashi T, Ikezawa H. Acetylcholinesterase release from mammalian erythrocytes by phosphatidyl inositol specific phospholipase C of *Bacillus thuringiensis* and characterization of the released enzyme. J Biochem (Tokyo) 1984;96:437.
61. Low MG, Finean JB. Release of alkaline phosphatase from membranes by a phosphatidylinositol-specific phospholipase C. Biochem J 1977;167:281.
62. Low MG, Finean JB. Specific release of plasma membrane enzymes by a phosphatidylinositol-specific phospholipase C. Biochim Biophys Acta 1978;508:565.
63. Roberts WL, Santikarn S, Reinhold VN, Rosenberry TL. Structural characterization of the glycoinositol phospholipid membrane anchor of human erythrocyte acetylcholinesterase by fast atom bombardment mass spectrometry. J Biol Chem 1988;263:18776.
64. Cardoso de Almeida ML, Turner MJ. The membrane form of variant surface glycoproteins of *Trypanosoma brucei*. Nature 1983;302:349.
65. Ferguson MAH, Low MG, Cross GAM. Glycosyl-*sn*-1,2-dimyristylphosphatidylinositol is covalently linked to *Trypanosoma brucei* variant surface glycoprotein. J Biol Chem 1985;260:14547.
66. Hereld D, Krakow JL, Bangs JD, et al. A phospholipase C from *Trypanosoma brucei* which selectively cleaves the glycolipid on the variant surface glycoprotein. J Biol Chem 1986;261:13813.
67. Bangs JD, Andrews NW, Hart GW, Englund PT. Posttranslational modification and intracellular transport of a trypanosome variant surface glycoprotein. J Cell Biol 1986;103:255.
68. Mahoney JF, Urakaze M, Hall S, et al. Defective glycosylphosphatidylinositol anchor synthesis in paroxysmal nocturnal hemoglobinuria (PNH) granulocytes. Blood 1992;79:1400.
69. Hirose S, Rav L, Prince GM, et al. Synthesis of mannosylglucosaminylinositol phospholipids in normal but not paroxusmal nocturnal hemoglobinuria cells. Proc Natl Acad Sci USA 1992;89:6025.
70. Armstrong C, Schubert J, Ueda E, et al. Affected paroxysmal nocturnal hemoglobinuria T lymphocytes harbor a common defect in assembly of *N*-acetyl-D-glucosamine inositol phospholipid corresponding to that in class A Thy-1-murine lymphoma mutants. J Biol Chem 1992;267:25347.
70a. Miyata T, Takada J, Iida Y, et al. The cloning of PIG-A, a component in the early step of GPI-anchor biosynthesis. Science 1993;259:1318.
70b. Takeda J, Miyata T, Kawagoe K, et al. Deficiency of the GPI anchor caused by a somatic mutation of the PIG-A gene in paroxysmal nocturnal hemoglobinuria. Cell 1993;73:703.
70c. Miyata T, Yamada N, Iida Y, et al. Abnormalties of *PIG-A* transcripts in granulocytes from patients with paroxysmal nocturnal hemoglobinuria. N Engl J Med 1994;330:249.
71. Rodriguez de Cordoba S, Lublin DM, Rubinstein P, Atkinson JP. Human genes for three complement components that regulate the activation of C3 are tightly linked. J Exp Med 1985;161:1189.
72. Kristensen T, D'Eustachio P, Ogata RT, et al. The superfamily of C3b/C4b-binding proteins. Fed Proc 1987;46:2463.

73. Medof ME, Lublin DM, Holers VM, et al. Cloning and characterization of cDNAs encoding the complete sequence of decay-accelerating factor of human complement. Proc Natl Acad Sci (Wash) 1987;84:2007.
74. Parker CJ, Baker PJ, Rosse WF. Increased enzymatic activity in the alternative pathway convertase when bound to the erythrocytes of paroxysmal nocturnal hemoglobinuria. J Clin Invest 1982;69:337.
75. Nicholson-Weller A, Spicer DB, Austen KF. Deficiency of the complement regulatory protein "decay accelerating factor," on membranes of granulocytes, monocytes, and platelets in paroxysmal nocturnal hemoglobinuria. N Engl J Med 1983;312:1091.
76. Kinoshita T, Medof ME, Silbor R, Nussenzweig V. Distribution of decay accelerating factor in the peripheral blood of normal individuals and patients with paroxysmal nocturnal hemoglobinuria. J Exp Med 1985;162:75.
77. Devine DV, Rosse, WF. Regulation of the activity of platelet-bound alternative pathway C3 convertase by intracellular Factor H. Proc Natl Acad Sci 1987;84:5673.
78. Holguin MH, Fredrick LR, Bernshaw NJ, Parker CJ. Isolation and characterization of a membrane protein from normal human erythrocytes that inhibits reactive lysis of the erythrocytes of paroxysmal nocturnal hemoglobinuria. J Clin Invest 1989;84:77.
79. Rollins SA, Sims PJ. The complement-inhibitory activity of CD59 resides in its capacity to block incorporation of C9 into membrane C5b-9. J Immunol 1990;144:3478.
80. Meri S, Morgan BP, Davies A, et al. Human protectin (CD59), an 18,000–20,000 MW complement lysis restricting factor, inhibits C5b-8 catalyzed insertion of C9 into lipid bilayers. Immunology 1990;71:1.
81. Holguin MH, Wilcox LA, Bernshaw NJ et al. Erythrocyte membrane inhibitor of reactive lysis: effects of phosphatidylinositol-specific phospholipase C on the isolated and cell-associated protein. Blood 1990;75:284.
82. Davies A, Simmons DL, Hale G, et al. CD59, an Ly-6 like protein expressed in human lymphoid cells, regulates the action of the complement membrane attack complex on homologous cells. J Exp Med 1989;170:637.
83. Philbrick WM, Palfree RGE, Maher SE, et al. The CD59 antigen is a structural homologue of murine Ly-6 antigens but lacks interferon inducibility. Eur J Immunol 1990;20;87.
83a. Weidmer T, Hall SE, Ortel TL, Kane WH, Rosse WT, Sims PJ. Complement-induced vesiculation and exposure of membrane prothrombinase sites in platelets of paroxysmal nocturnal hemoglobinuria. Blood 1993;82:1192.
84. Schonermark S, Rauterberg EW, Shin ML, et al. Homologous species restriction in lysis of human erythrocytes: a membrane-derived protein with C8-binding capacity functions as an inhibitor. J Immunol 1986;136: 1772.
85. Zalman LS, Wood LM, Muller-Eberhard HJ. Isolation of a human erythrocyte membrane protein capable of inhibition of expression of homologous complement transmembrane channels. Proc Natl Acad Sci USA 1986;83:6975.
86. Zalman LS, Wood LM, Frank MM, Muller-Eberhard HJ. Deficiency of the homologous restriction factor in paroxysmal nocturnal hemoglobinuria. J Exp Med 1987;165:572.
87. Hansch GM, Schonermark S, Roelcke D. Paroxysmal nocturnal hemoglobinuria type III. Lack of an erythrocyte membrane protein restricting the lysis of C5b-9. J Clin Invest 1987;80:7.
88. Chow F-L, Telen MT, Rosse WF. The separation of the populations of red cells in paroxysmal nocturnal hemoglobinuria by monoclonal antibody to acetylcholinesterase Blood 1986;67:893.
89. Devine DV, Gluck WL, Rosse WF, Weinberg JB. Acute myeloblastic leukemia in paroxysmal nocturnal hemoglobinuria: evidence of evolution for the abnormal PNH clone. J Clin Invest 1987;79:314.
90. Selvaraj P, Rosse WF, Silber R, Springer TA. The major Fc receptor in blood has a phosphotidylinositol anchor and is deficient in paroxysmal nocturnal hemoglobinuria. Nature 1988;333:565.
91. Selvaraj P, Dustin ML, Silber R, et al. Deficiency of lymphocyte function-associated antigens 3 (LFA-3) in paroxysmal nocturnal hemoglobinuria: functional correlates and evidence for a phosphatidylinositol membrane anchor. J Exp Med 1987;166:1011.
92. Simmons DL, Tan S, Tenen DG, Nicholson-Weller A, Seed B. Monocyte antigen CD 14 is a phospholipid anchored membrane protein. Blood 1989;73:284.
93. Werner G, von dem Borne AEG, Bos MJE, et al. Localization of NA1 alloantigen on neutrophil Fc (gamma) receptors. In: Reinherz EF, Haynes BF, Nadler LM, Bernstein ID, ed. Leukocyte typing II. New York, Springer-Verlag, 1986:109.
94. Dustin MI, Selvaraj P, Mattaliano RJ, Springer TA. Anchoring mechanisms for LFA-3 cell adhesion glycoprotein at membrane surface. Nature 1987;3290:846.
95. Ulevitch RJ, Mathison JC, Schumann RR, Tobias PS. A new model of macrophage stimulation by bacterial lipopolysaccharide. J Trauma 1990;30:S189.
96. Goyert SM, Ferrero I, Rettig JW, et al. The CD14 monocyte differentiation antigen maps to a region encoding growth factors and receptors. Science 1988;239:497.
97. Holden D, Lichtman H. Paroxysmal nocturnal hemoglobinuria with acute leukemia. Blood 1969;33:283.
98. Jenkins DE Jr, Hartmann RC. Paroxysmal nocturnal hemoglobinuria terminating in acute myeloblastic leukemia. Blood 1969;33:274.
99. Kaufmann RW, Schechter GP, McFarland W. Paroxysmal nocturnal hemoglobinuria terminating in acute granulocytic leukemia. Blood 1969;22:287.
100. Krause JR. Paroxysmal nocturnal hemoglobinuria and acute non-lymphocytic leukemia: a report of three cases exhibiting different cytologic types. Cancer 1983;51:2078.
101. Carmel R, Coltman CA, Yatteau RF, Costanzi JJ. Association of paroxysmal nocturnal hemoglobinuria with erythroleukemia. N Engl J Med 1970;283:1329.
102. Luzzato L, Familusi JB, Williams CKO, et al. The PNH abnormality in myeloproliferative disorders: association of PNH and acute erythremic myelosis in two children. Br J Haematol 1979;64:13.
103. Cowall DE, Pasquale DN, Dekker P. Paroxysmal nocturnal hemoglobinuria terminating as erythroleukemia. Cancer 1979;43:1915.
104. Hirsch VJ, Neubach PA, Parker DM, et al. Paroxysmal nocturnal hemoglobinuria: termination in acute myelomonocytic leukemia and reappearance after leukemic remission. Arch Intern Med 1981;141: 525.
105. Katahira J, Masako A, Oshimi K, et al. Paroxysmal nocturnal hemoglobinuria terminating in TdT-positive acute leukemia. Am J Hematol 1983;14:79.
106. Storb R, Thomas ED, Weiden PL, et al. Aplastic anemia treated by allogeneic bone marrow transplantation: a report of 49 new cases from Seattle. Blood 1976;49:817.
107. Antin JH, Ginsburg D, Smith BR, et al. Bone marrow transplantation for paroxysmal nocturnal hemoglobinuria: eradication of the PNH clone and documentation of complete lymphohematopoietic engraftment. Blood 1985;66:1247.
108. Fefer A, Freeman H, Storb R, et al. Paroxysmal nocturnal hemoglobinuria and marrow failure treated by infusion of marrow from an identical twin. Ann Intern Med 1976;84:692.
109. Firkin F, Goldberg H, Firkin BG. Glucocorticoid management of paroxysmal nocturnal hemoglobinuria. Aust Ann Med 1968;17:127.
110. Rosse WF. The treatment of PNH. Blood 1982;60:20.
111. Roesser HP, Powell LW. Urinary iron excretion in valvular heart disease and after heart valve replacement. Blood 1970;56:785.
112. Hartmann RC, Jenkins DE Jr, McKee LC, Heyssel RM. Paroxysmal nocturnal hemoglobinuria: clinical and laboratory studies relating to iron metabolism and therapy with androgens and iron. Medicine 1966;45: 331.
113. Mengel CE, Kann HE Jr, O'Malley BW. Increased hemolysis after intramuscular iron administration in patients with paroxysmal nocturnal hemoglobinuria. Blood 1965;26:74.
114. Rosse WF, Gutterman LA. The effect of iron therapy in paroxysmal nocturnal hemoglobinuria. Blood 1970;36:559.
115. Chanarin I, Dacie JV, Mollin DL. Folic-acid deficiency in haemolytic anaemia. Br J Haematol 1959;5:245.
116. Alexanian R. Erythropoietin and erythropoiesis in anemic man following androgens. Blood 1969;33:564.
117. Sanchez-Medal L, Gomez-Leal A, Duarte L, et al. Anabolic androgenic steroids in the treatment of acquired aplastic anemia. Blood 1969;34: 283.
118. Nadell J, Kosek J. Peliosis hepatis. Twelve cases associated with oral androgen therapy. Arch Pathol Lab Med 1977;101:405.
119. Nuzzo JL, Marz HJ, Maxted WC. Pelosis hepatis after long-term androgen therapy. Urology 1985;25:518.
120. Dacie JV, Firth D. Blood transfusion in nocturnal hemoglobinuria. Br Med J 1943;1:626.
121. Gockerman JP, Brouillard RP. RBC transfusions in paroxysmal nocturnal hemoglobinuria. Arch Intern Med 1977;137:538.
122. Brecher ME, Taswell HF. Paroxysmal nocturnal hemoglobinuria and the transfusion of washed red blood cells: a myth revisited. Transfusion 1989;29:681.
123. Rosse WF. Transfusion in paroxysmal nocturnal hemoglobinuria: to wash or not to wash? (Editorial) Transfusion 1989;29:663.
124. Dacie JV. Transfusion of saline-washed red cells in nocturnal haemoglobinuria (Marchifava-Micheli disease). Clin Sci 1943;7:65.
125. Sholar PW, Bell WR. Thrombolytic therapy for inferior vena cava thrombosis in paroxysmal nocturnal hemoglobinuria. Ann Intern Med 1985;103:539.
126. Fritzche W, Martin H. Properdin und Hemolyse. Zur Hemmung der Hemolyse der Erythrocyten von Kranken mit paroxymaler Nachtalicher Hemoglobinurie durch Heparin. Klin Wochenschr 1957;35:1166.
127. Logue GL. Effect of heparin on complement activation and lysis of paroxysmal nocturnal hemoglobinuria red cells. Blood 1977;50:239.
128. Marcus AJ. The role of lipids in platelet functions: with particular reference to the arachidonic acid pathway. J Lipid Res 1978;19:793.
129. Young N, Griffith P, Brittain E, et al. A multicenter trial of antithymocyte globulin in aplastic anemia and related diseases. Blood 1988;72: 1861.
130. Charache S. Prolonged survival in paroxysmal nocturnal hemoglobinuria. Blood 1969;33:877.
131. Holguin MH, Wilcox LA, Bernshaw NJ, et al. Relationship between membrane inhibitor of reactive lysis and the erythrocyte phenotypes of paroxysmal nocturnal hematuria. J Clin Invest 1989;84:1387.

Blood: Principles and Practice of Hematology,
edited by Robert I. Handin, Thomas P. Stossel, and Samuel E. Lux.
J.B. Lippincott Company, Philadelphia © 1995.

12

Myelodysplastic Syndromes

Cynthia E. Dunbar
Arthur W. Nienhuis

The myelodysplastic syndromes (MDSs) are a heterogeneous group of disorders characterized by inadequate and dysmorphic hematopoiesis. Varying degrees of reticulocytopenia, leukopenia, or thrombocytopenia may render patients dependent on red blood cell (RBC) transfusions and susceptible to infection or hemorrhage. Persons with MDS are also at high risk for evolution to acute leukemia. Central to consideration of these syndromes is the fact that they are clonal hematopoietic disorders. The progeny of a single myelodysplastic stem cell are able to dominate the bone marrow to the exclusion of their normal counterparts, despite an inability to maintain effective circulating cell populations. This property of clonality, along with demonstrations of cytogenetic abnormalities and mutations in cellular protooncogenes, has stimulated investigation of the myelodysplasias as prototypical premalignant processes.

Overlap of both clinical manifestations and biologic behavior of MDS with other hematologic disorders causes diagnostic confusion and invites errors in interpretation of pathophysiology (Fig. 12-1). Nutritional deficiencies are part of the differential diagnosis and must be excluded by clinical testing. Cytopenias are common to both aplastic anemia and MDS, and a minority of patients with MDS have hypocellular bone marrow. Dysmorphic features may be evident in the few residual bone marrow cells found in patients with aplastic anemia. Diagnostic distinction may be extremely difficult in the absence of a cytogenetic abnormality. In some patients with dysplastic marrow characteristics, monocytosis, neutrophilia, or thrombocytosis bring to mind a myeloproliferative syndrome.

Finally, the aforementioned frequent evolution to leukemia and the clonal nature of MDS emphasize the close relation of these disorders to acute myelogenous leukemia (AML). Despite this, MDSs have emerged as distinct clinical and morphologic entities deserving of clinical and laboratory investigation.

Our purpose in this chapter is to present a full account of the accumulating knowledge about MDSs.[1–11] Their extensive array of clinical, morphologic, biochemical, and genetic abnormalities provides a rich but often confusing tableau for the clinical investigator and the practicing physician. It may not be clear whether a morphologic or laboratory abnormality is an essential element in the pathogenesis of MDS or an inconsequential result of a genetically unstable cellular environment. Furthermore, the clinician must balance a desire for therapy directed at an underlying pathogenetic mechanism with the realization that patients with MDS may be stable for long periods of time with only supportive care. Advances in understanding the regulation of hematopoiesis and the molecular genetics of DNA damage and repair should improve our ability to diagnose, treat, and even prevent these disorders in the future.

HISTORY

The present conceptual framework for MDSs evolved gradually from two historically distinct areas of clinical investigation. During the 1920s and 1930s, a recognition of the nutritional requirements of hematopoietic cells emerged. Iron deficiency, pernicious anemia, and folate deficiency were identified and effectively treated, but many patients with chronic anemia failed to respond to these nutritional interventions. As assays were developed for quantitating iron, B_{12}, and folate, these refractory patients were found to have adequate levels of these substances. In 1938, Rhoads and Barker[12] described 60 patients with refractory anemia (RA), one third of whom would have met the diagnostic criteria for MDS. Neutropenia and thrombocytopenia were noted in some of the patients, but progression to leukemia was not described. Subsequently, those with RA were better characterized with descriptions of specific dyserythropoietic features such as ringed sideroblasts by Bjorkman,[13] and the morphology of hypercellular bone marrows by Vilter and colleagues.[14]

Investigators studying the acute leukemias noted that some patients had a chronic preleukemic phase characterized by cytopenias that preceded overt AML. In his 1949 paper, Hamilton-Paterson[15] suggested that the same dyshematopoietic factor was responsible for both the preceding cytopenias and the development of leukemia. Subsequent series contained descriptions of dysplastic bone marrow abnormalities in patients with preleukemia.[16–19] Between 5% and 31% of patients with AML were found to have had a discernible preleukemic phase.[19,20] By definition, the diagnosis of preleukemia was retrospective, made only after progression to acute leukemia. With the introduction of remission-inducing chemotherapy for AML, prospective identification of patients who would develop acute leukemia became of more than theoretical interest.

These two paths converged as investigators discussed and debated whether RA and preleukemic states were related.[21,22] Dameshek[22] proposed that RA states were neoplastic because they lacked a consistent metabolic defect and were irreversibly progressive, with eventual replace-

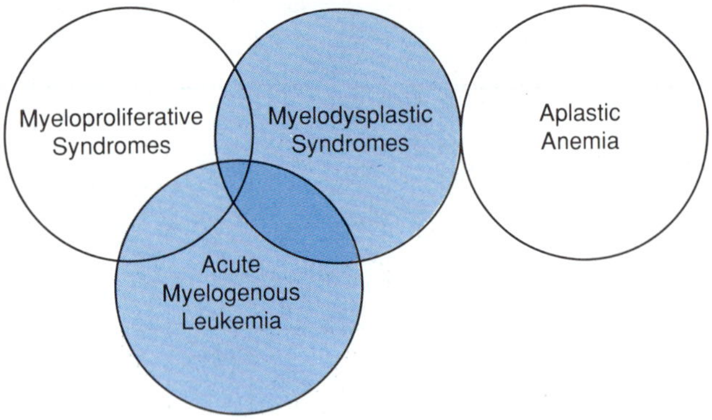

FIGURE 12-1. Venn diagram illustrating the interrelations among the myelodysplastic syndromes (MDSs) and several other hematologic disorders. Differentiation between hypocellular MDSs and aplastic anemia may be difficult, but generally these disorders can be considered separately with distinct epidemiology and pathogenesis. MDSs can progress to acute myelogenous leukemia, and the transition may be indistinct (*overlapping areas*). Patients with chronic myelomonocytic leukemia, the monosomy 7 syndrome, or the 5q− syndrome share characteristics of both MDSs and myeloproliferative syndromes, indicated by the overlap in the diagram.

ment of normal marrow elements. Dreyfus and coworkers,[23,24] Linman and Bagby,[20] and Saarni and Linman[25] made the connection explicit in their careful descriptive studies.

The nomenclature and classifications applied to patients with RA and preleukemia became increasingly confusing. In an effort to provide uniform criteria for diagnosis and for clinical investigation, the French-American-British (FAB) Cooperative Group initially developed guidelines to separate patients with what they termed *myelodysplastic syndromes* from patients with leukemia as part of their classification system for AML.[26] In 1982, the same group focused on MDS more specifically and set forth a classification, defined nomenclature, and catalogued diagnostic morphologic features.[27] By these criteria, most patients who had previously been given diagnoses of RA, idiopathic sideroblastic anemia, marrow dysplasia, preleukemia, oligoleukemia, smoldering leukemia, or chronic myelomonocytic leukemia could be included in the MDS classification system.

The ability, gained during the past two decades, to cure or induce sustained remissions in several types of malignancies with aggressive chemotherapy or radiation therapy has also produced a new category of MDS.[28–30] Long-term survivors of effectively treated neoplasms have an appreciable risk of developing cytopenias with trilineage marrow dysplasia. This hematologic disorder has been termed *therapy-related MDS* (t-MDS). Despite sharing many characteristics with primary MDS, t-MDS differs in many important respects and carries a more dismal prognosis with a higher risk of early progression to leukemia (t-AML).

BONE MARROW MORPHOLOGY

The diagnosis of MDS in a patient with anemia, neutropenia, or thrombocytopenia or all three depends on demonstrating characteristic dysmorphic features in the bone marrow. Indeed, the FAB classification is based almost entirely on abnormalities found on the bone marrow aspirate.[7,27] Although often considered a diagnosis of exclusion, MDS can usually be recognized and differentiated from other hematologic disorders by thorough assessment of bone marrow morphology. Several comprehensive reviews of the bone marrow in MDS have been published, and the characteristic features are summarized in Table 12-1.[31–34]

TABLE 12-1. Morphologic Abnormalities of the Bone Marrow in Myelodysplasia

Abnormality	Incidence (%)
LINEAGE	
Dyserythropoiesis	73–100
Multinuclearity	
Intranuclear bridging	
Nuclear fragments and budding	
Megaloblastic changes	
Vacuolation	
Ringed sideroblasts	
Maturation arrest	
Dysmyelopoiesis	37–88
Giant primary granules	
Decreased primary granules	
Auer rods	
Decreased secondary granules	
Fragmented nuclei	
Maturation arrest	
Abnormal localization of immature myeloid precursors	
Dysmegakaryocytopoiesis	50–87
Micromegakaryocytes	
Decreased nuclear polyploidization	
Separated nuclei ("pawn ball")	
GENERAL FEATURES	
Cellularity	
Increased or normal	81–100
Decreased	0–19
Fibrosis	20–25

(Data from references 5, 27, 58, 67, 74, 137, 568)

Both a bone marrow aspirate and a biopsy should be obtained; cellular morphology and quantitation of myeloblasts can be done on an aspirate, but accurate assessment of cellularity and localization of immature precursors require biopsy sections.[33,35,36] Definitive diagnostic evaluation of patients with MDS may require several separate samples because affected bone marrow may be distributed unevenly.[37] If a bone marrow biopsy from the posterior iliac crest is hypocellular, adequate cells may often be obtained from a sternal aspirate.

Dyserythropoietic abnormalities include a dissociation between nuclear and cytoplasmic maturation and other megaloblastic characteristics[38] and bizarre nuclear configurations including binuclearity, nuclear bridging, and nuclear budding.[39] Ringed sideroblasts, erythroblasts with at least five Prussian blue–staining iron granules encircling more than one third of the nucleus, are an important morphologic characteristic in MDS[40] (Fig. 12-2*A*). These cells were first described in 1956 by Bjorkman in the marrow of a patient with RA[13] and have been historically central to discussions on the nature and classification of MDS.[21,22,27]

Thirty to 50% of normoblasts in the normal bone marrow contain iron granules detectable by light microscopy. These granules are small, located in the cytoplasm, and by electron microscopy are ferritin–iron aggregates.[12,41,42] The number of these granules increases with either ineffective erythropoiesis or iron overload, as in thalassemia or pernicious anemia. In contrast, pathologic ringed sideroblasts contain large perinuclear granules that have been shown, by electron microscopy, to be mitochondria enlarged and

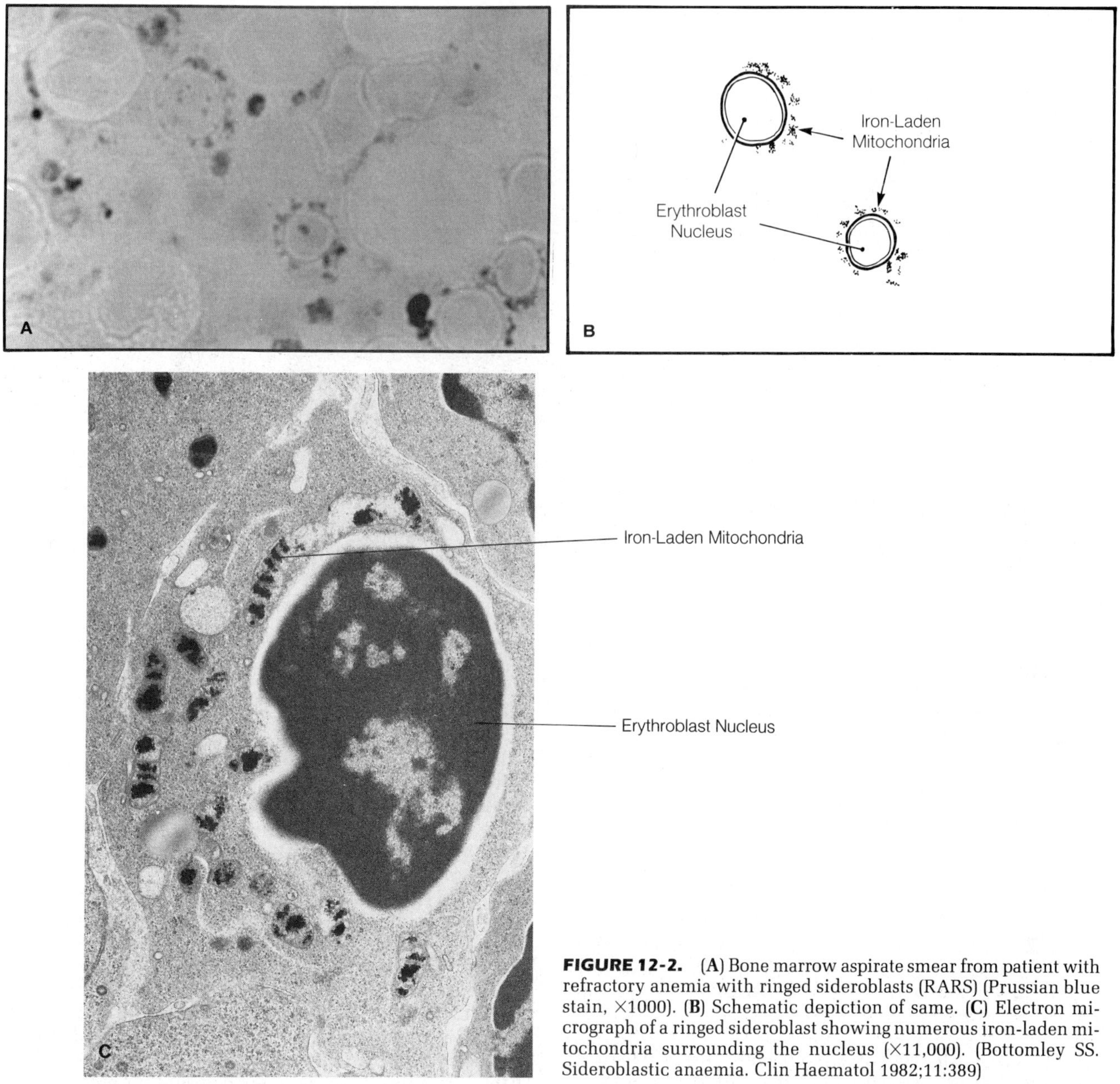

FIGURE 12-2. (**A**) Bone marrow aspirate smear from patient with refractory anemia with ringed sideroblasts (RARS) (Prussian blue stain, ×1000). (**B**) Schematic depiction of same. (**C**) Electron micrograph of a ringed sideroblast showing numerous iron-laden mitochondria surrounding the nucleus (×11,000). (Bottomley SS. Sideroblastic anaemia. Clin Haematol 1982;11:389)

distorted by abnormal nonferritin iron deposition[43,44] (see Fig. 12-2B). More than half of patients with all subtypes of MDS have an appreciable number of ringed sideroblasts.[40]

Megakaryocytes have characteristic abnormalities in MDS.[45] Absolute numbers of megakaryocytes may be increased, normal, or decreased, but individual cells often have defects in nuclear polyploidization and increased nuclear separation ("pawn ball" nuclei).[46] The most unusual megakaryocytes are small, with one or two round and widely separated nuclei and aberrant granulation (Fig. 12-3). These cells are most common in patients with the 5q− syndrome but can also be found in other patients with MDS.[47] Anti–von Willebrand factor antibodies may be used to stain biopsy sections to assist in the identification of megakaryocytes.[48]

Abnormalities of myeloid maturation may be striking or subtle. A left shift toward more immature forms may be seen even without an actual excess of myeloblasts. Specific monoclonal antibodies may be useful in identifying immature myeloid cells that lack the typical morphologic characteristics.[49] Both primary and secondary granulation are often decreased and distributed abnormally within the cell. A lack of synchronization between nuclear and cellular maturation and granule formation is also observed. Some myeloid precursors stain with both specific and nonspecific esterases, suggesting infidelity between granulocytic and monocytic lineages.[50]

The morphology and identification of myeloblasts is particularly pertinent to the FAB classification.[27] Two types of myeloblasts are described on a Wright-Giemsa–stained aspirate; these differ primarily in their cytoplasmic characteristics.[27] Type I myeloblasts are typical myeloblasts with high nuclear/cytoplasmic ratios, distinct nucleoli, uncondensed chromatin, and no cytoplasmic granules. Type II blasts may have a few primary azurophilic granules and lower nuclear/cytoplasmic ratios. Auer rods, elongated azurophilic inclusions resulting from fusion of primary granules, are found in the cells of 20% of patients with certain subtypes of MDS.[51] Cells with eccentric nuclei, a well-developed Golgi apparatus (perinuclear clear zone), condensed chromatin, numerous granules, or a low nuclear/cytoplasmic ratio should be scored as promyelocytes

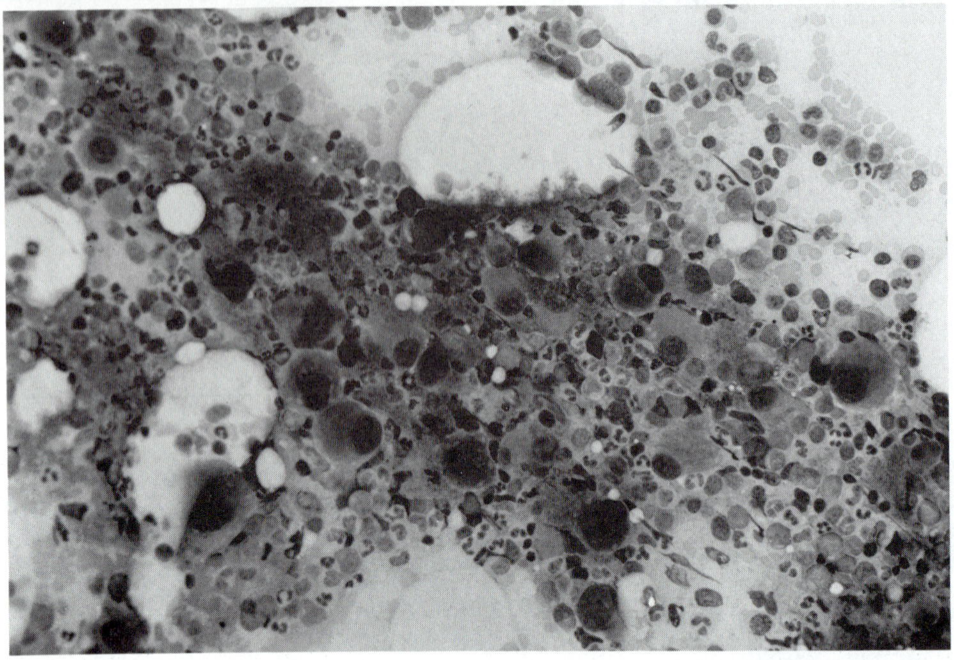

FIGURE 12-3. Bone marrow aspirate from a patient with refractory anemia and the 5q− syndrome. A large number of strikingly abnormal small and uninuclear megakaryocytes are characteristic of both the 5q− syndrome in particular and myelodysplastic syndromes in general (Wright's stain, ×900).

instead of myeloblasts. The bone marrow blasts of most patients with MDS have immunochemical and cytochemical characteristics typical of myeloid or monocytoid blasts.[52] Occasionally, the blasts exhibit features of the megakaryocytic or lymphoid lineage, supporting the concept that the basic defect in MDS is expressed at the level of the pluripotent stem cell.[53,54]

Most characteristically, bone marrow cellularity is either increased or normal in patients with MDS (see Table 12-1), but many studies have included patients with hypocellular bone marrows who have the typical morphologic and clinical characteristics of MDS. Recent reviews comparing patients with a hypocellular bone marrow with those with a hypercellular or normocellular bone marrow report similar biologic characteristics and prognosis.[55–57] Myeloid/erythroid ratios are extremely heterogeneous but typically increased except in RARS, FAB subtype.

A significant increase in reticulin is seen in the bone marrow biopsies of 20% of patients with MDS.[58,59] Patients with bone marrow fibrosis and MDS do not have significant splenomegaly or other clinical features of myelofibrosis with myeloid metaplasia, but rather they have trilineage dysplasia and a prognosis similar to typical patients with MDS.[60] Most such patients exhibit increased numbers of megakaryocytes, leading to speculation that excess fibrosis is due to release of fibroblast mitogens such as platelet-derived growth factor (PDGF) or transforming growth factor-β (TGFβ).[60–62] Elevated levels of PDGF have been reported in the serum of patients with primary myelofibrosis.[63] This is discussed in more detail in Chapter 13.

The anatomic interrelations between hematopoietic precursors and the bone marrow stroma, particularly the interface between marrow and bone, may be disordered in patients with MDS. Such relations may be central to the regulation of normal hematopoiesis. First, stromal cells are an important source of various growth and inhibitory factors. Second, specific binding to stromal matrix proteins may also control the local concentration of growth factors.[64–66] Tricot[36,67] was the first to call attention to abnormally localized immature precursors (ALIPs) in MDS patients. Myeloblasts and other immature forms are normally localized along the endosteal surface, but in many patients they form clusters (ALIPs) that are not contiguous with bony trabeculae.

CLASSIFICATION

The diagnostic criteria and classification system for MDS proposed by the FAB Cooperative Group[7,27] has become widely adopted despite controversy over its morphologic emphasis and skepticism regarding its prognostic usefulness.[10,68–71] The group reviewed morphologic features of bone marrow aspirates from 50 patients as well as clinical data, and they used the observations to define five subtypes of MDS (Table 12-2). (The qualitative morphologic abnormalities were summarized in Table 12-1.) The percentages of bone marrow and peripheral blood myeloblasts used to define categories are arbitrary and are not meant to imply separate biologic entities but to provide information that may be useful in assessing severity of disease and prognosis. The cutoff of 5% marrow myeloblasts used in FAB and other classification schemes derives from a study in which 1827 consecutive unselected bone marrow examinations were reviewed and a myeloblast percentage with respect to total nucleated marrow cells calculated. Patients (127 of 129) with more than 5% myeloblasts either had or later developed leukemia, and 127 of 136 patients who subsequently developed leukemia had previous marrows with greater than 5% myeloblasts.[72]

The original FAB classification scheme defined subtypes by the percentage of myeloblasts in both bone marrow and peripheral blood[27] (see Table 12-2). It has become clear that even patients with RA or RARS can have occasional circulating blasts that are not prognostically ominous.[73,74] When a discrepancy exists between bone marrow and peripheral blood blast percentage FAB class, the marrow percentage should determine assignment. This problem rarely arises.

One difficulty in using the FAB classification scheme has been in calculating the myeloblast percentage in bone marrow specimens with an increased nucleated erythroid cell count. Some have suggested that the denominator should be total cells if the percentage of erythroid cells is less than 50% but that total myeloid cells should serve as the denominator if the erythroid component of the marrow

TABLE 12-2. FAB Classification Criteria

Subtype	Abbreviation	Peripheral Blood	Bone Marrow
Refractory anemia	RA	Blasts < 1%	Blasts < 5%
Refractory anemia with ringed sideroblasts	RARS	Blasts < 1%	Blasts < 5%
Refractory anemia with excess of blasts	RAEB	Blasts 5%	Blasts 5%–20%
Refractory anemia with excess of blasts in transformation	RAEBT	Blasts > 5%	Blasts 20%–30% or Auer rods
Chronic monomyelocytic leukemia	CMML	Monocytes 1 × 10⁹/L	Any of the above
Acute myeloid leukemia	AML		Blasts > 30%

(Bennett JM, Catovsky D, Daniel MT, Flandien G, et al. Proposals for the classification of the myelodysplastic syndromes. Br J Haematol 1982;51:189)

exceeds 50%.[7,75] For example, a marrow specimen with 80% erythroblasts and 20% myeloid cells including 10% myeloblasts would be classified as acute leukemia because the myeloblasts make up 50% of the myeloid component. This scheme gives some weight to the relative size of the erythroid component as an independent prognostic factor. More reasonable would be a consistent practice of expressing the percentage of myeloblasts with reference only to the total number of nonerythroid nucleated hematopoietic cells. Fortunately, this issue arises in few patients with MDS. Most patients with erythroid hyperplasia have RARS and few myeloblasts.[74,76–78] Conversely, patients with prognostically unfavorable subtypes of MDS generally have a smaller marrow erythroid compartment.

In the original FAB classification system, patients with t-MDS were not placed in a separate category but into one of the five subtypes based on the usual criteria. It has become increasingly apparent that these patients behave differently from patients with primary MDS with respect to leukemic transformation and overall prognosis.[7,68,79] Even patients presenting with a low percentage of bone marrow myeloblasts often have severe cytopenias and trilineage dysplasia and rapidly evolve into t-AML.[80] The use of the FAB system in clinical investigation of prognosis or treatment is more meaningful if patients with t-MDS are not simply subsumed into the standard five subtypes but are considered as a separate entity.

Since the introduction of the FAB system, most literature on MDS has incorporated it. Despite the admittedly arbitrary delineations among subtypes, the common language and criteria for diagnosis improve communication among investigators so that cases with similar characteristics can be compared.

Table 12-3 collates data on distribution among FAB subtypes pooled from 12 large published cohorts. These studies classified different percentages of their patient populations into each subtype, leading some to argue that the classification criteria are unreliable.[34] The patient populations in these studies varied widely: some included patients with t-MDS, and some were collected at specialized, tertiary medical centers where only the most clinically severe cases were referred and treated. Also, these studies were not uniform in the assignment of patients who fit into more than one FAB subtype.

Most investigators have found the FAB classification system to have good prognostic applicability, with significantly longer survivals for patients with RA and RARS than for those with RA with excess of blasts (RAEB), RA with excess of blasts in transformation (RAEBT), or chronic myelomonocytic leukemia (CMML).[73,81–84]

Another positive aspect of the FAB classification system for MDS is its functional continuity with the widely used FAB leukemia classification system.[26] The FAB MDS nomenclature also allows for progression from one subtype to another over time. Several longitudinal studies found frequent progression from RA or RARS to RAEB, RAEBT, or CMML, then to AML.[74,85–87] In many ways, the subtypes can be considered as stages of disease rather than distinct entities.

The FAB classification system has also been the focus of criticism and controversy.[10,34,68–71] One problem has been semantic. Patients who present with isolated thrombocytopenia or neutropenia but with unambiguous morphologic or cytogenetic evidence for myelodysplasia fall into the subtype *refractory anemia*.[87] It has been suggested that *refractory cytopenia* might be a preferable term.[7] Another issue has been the classification of patients who fit criteria for more than one subtype, such as a patient with 20% ringed sideroblasts and 10% myeloblasts in the marrow. Prognostic predictions are more accurate in these cases when the patient is assigned to the subtype based on bone marrow myeloblast percentage (RAEB or RAEBT).[73,84] This interpretation of the FAB guidelines has become standard.

The FAB recommendation to include any patient with marrow or circulating Auer rod-laden myeloblasts in RAEBT has also been controversial. In several small groups of patients, Auer rods were not associated with a worse prognosis or a higher risk of leukemic transformation than predicted by the overall myeloblast percentage.[51,83,88] The issue deserves further investigation, but most investigators do not classify patients with Auer rods in RAEBT unless they also have greater than 20% marrow myeloblasts.

TABLE 12-3. Distribution of Myelodysplastic Syndrome Patients at Presentation by FAB Subtype

Subtype	Percentage of Total	Percentage Range*
RA	27	8–43
RARS	20	2–37
RAEB	26	13–38
RAEBT	13	4–27
CMML	14	1–32
t-MDS†		2–15
TOTAL (1709 patients)	100	

* Range of individual study percentages of patients in each subtype or t-MDS.

† Patients with t-MDS were excluded from some studies (references 73, 74, 83, 237, 444, 449, 568). Studies including t-MDS patients assigned them to subclasses through normal FAB criteria.

(Pooled data from references 58, 73, 74, 82, 83, 89, 137, 165, 237, 444, 449, 568).

The inclusion of the CMML subtype in the FAB system has also been criticized. Historically, patients with chronic disorders of the monocytoid lineage have been difficult to classify and characterize. Some investigators have argued that CMML should be considered as a completely separate entity or should be included in the myeloproliferative syndromes.[34,70] Most of these patients clearly have classic trilineage dysplastic marrows and other characteristic features of MDS. CMML patients frequently progress in and out of the CMML subtype to and from other FAB subtypes, supporting their inclusion into the MDS.[74,86] Some confusion exists in the classification of patients with increased circulating monocytes and greater than 5% marrow myeloblasts. For prognostic purposes, inclusion of these patients in RAEB or RAEBT is preferred to inclusion in CMML.[73,83,84,89]

Alternative classification systems have been proposed and adopted by some investigators. Bagby[10,69] introduced a system based on bone marrow myeloblast percentages but separated MDS into only two categories: the *preleukemic syndrome* (marrow blasts less than 5%) and *oligoblastic leukemia* (marrow blasts between 5% and 40%). Separation into two instead of five subtypes may be justified in terms of predicting prognosis, but this nomenclature implies inevitable progression to a proliferative leukemic process in all patients.[73,81] Because less than half of patients with MDS progress to acute leukemia, these terms seem both inaccurate and unnecessarily ominous. Also, the term *preleukemic* has been applied to conditions such as Fanconi's anemia, Bloom's syndrome, or Down's syndrome, which are not myelodysplastic by any other criteria but are associated with a statistically increased risk of leukemia. Other investigators have tried to improve the FAB classification by including clinical as well as morphologic features in simple or complicated scoring systems; these are discussed later in this chapter.

The ability to place patients with MDS into categories with some etiologic or pathophysiologic basis is desirable but impossible based on current knowledge. The situation should improve as investigators progress toward a better understanding of MDS. For the near future, the FAB system can continue to serve as a practical and useful basis for communication and data collection. There is one cautionary note. A recent study pointed out that morphologic features of MDS in the marrow samples of patients presenting with acute leukemia did not affect their prognoses and responses to chemotherapy.[81a] Thus, in some patients, it may be difficult to differentiate antecedent MDS that has progressed to AML from de novo AML.

CLINICAL PRESENTATION

The myelodysplastic syndromes are not common disorders in the general population, but most hematologists follow several such cases. The actual incidence of MDS is unknown. In 1976, Linman and Bagby[20] estimated 1500 new cases per year in the United States, but only patients with less than 5% myeloblasts were included in their calculations. A retrospective review of all bone marrow specimens submitted for interpretation at one institution revealed diagnostic features of myelodysplasia in 1.43% of specimens.[34] After the introduction of the FAB classification system in 1982, the published literature on myelodysplasia has expanded significantly, although no evidence shows that the actual incidence has increased. An exception is t-MDS; since more patients enjoy extended survival after chemotherapy and radiation, this unfortunate complication is being encountered more frequently.

Epidemiologic Characteristics

Table 12-4 summarizes data from several large studies on presenting characteristics of patients with MDS. MDS is primarily a disorder of the elderly,[90,91] with a median onset in the seventh decade, although the syndrome may occur in any age group including in the pediatric population.[92–94] Five to 17% of children experience a myelodysplastic phase before the onset of AML, and similar or higher figures have been estimated for adults.[19,92,95,96] There is a slight male predominance in all age groups. Few reports have been made of the familial occurrence of MDS.[97–100] Initial clinical presentation as children or young adults in these families has been typical, but Fanconi's anemia has not been rigorously excluded in every case.

Chronic exposure to low-dose radiation, especially radiopharmaceuticals that are taken up by the reticuloendothelial system, may increase the risk of MDS or AML.[101–103] A recent pilot case control study reviewed the association between environmental and occupational exposures and MDS. They found that significantly more patients than controls had worked with ammonia, diesel fuel, or other petrochemicals.[104] Significant benzene exposure may also be a risk factor.[105] The development of MDS as a delayed complication of intensive chemotherapy or radiation (t-MDS) is discussed in detail later in this chapter.

Several long-term follow-up studies of patients with aplastic anemia treated with antithymocyte globulin suggest an increased risk of subsequent MDS or AML.[106–110] This increased risk has not been observed in bone marrow

TABLE 12-4. Clinical Characteristics of Myelodysplastic Syndrome Patients at Presentation

Study	Mean Age (y)	Male/Female Ratio	Incidence: Splenomegaly	Anemia*	Thrombocytopenia†	Neutropenia‡
Weisdorf[83]	70	100:0	25	83	28	36
Varela[447]	72	—	18	93	25	31
Mufti[89]	73	51:49	—	67	38	39
Oguma[458]	59	65:35	—	—	—	—
Sanz[136]	68	53:47	12	82	45	24
Tricot[442]	62	58:42	—	45	32	24
Kerkhofs[73]	73	50:50	—	85	—	—
Foucar[82]	68	52:48	12	—	—	—
Coiffier[58]	—	54:46	21	—	—	—

* Anemia: percentage of patients with hemoglobin below 12 g/dL.
† Thrombocytopenia: percentage of patients with platelet counts below 100,000/μL.
‡ Neutropenia: percentage of patients with neutrophil counts below 1500/μL.

transplant recipients. In one study, the initial diagnosis of aplastic anemia may have been erroneous in some patients, since retrospective review of bone marrows obtained at initial presentation revealed trilineage dyplasia, fibrosis, and megakaryocytic hyperplasia.[110] It is also possible that patients with recovered aplastic anemia are left with a greatly reduced number of stem cells, increasing the mutational stress on each stem cell and thus increasing the risk of developing MDS.[111] Abnormal cells that can escape immune surveillance may be selected for in the context of an abnormally active autoimmunue response against hematopoietic cells in aplastic anemia.[111] Several reports have also been cited of MDS in patients who had been in remission from AML.[112,113] The patients had not received alkylating agents, making MDS secondary to chemotherapy unlikely. Perhaps a residual abnormal stem cell clone survived chemotherapy and gradually became dominant, with subsequent emergence of MDS.

The coincident occurrence of myeloma or other lymphoproliferative disorders and MDS has been described more frequently.[114–116] This may be due to the chance occurrence of two diseases that are more common in elderly patients, although some authors have made statistical arguments for a nonrandom association.[114] No clonal markers were shown to be shared by both the dysplastic and the abnormal lymphoid clones in these patients. Perhaps impaired immune function associated with MDS, particularly decreased natural killer (NK) cell activity, could predispose to lymphoproliferative disorders.[117,118]

Symptoms and Signs

Initial symptoms of MDSs are weakness or pallor secondary to anemia and, less frequently, bleeding or infection. Occasionally, patients complain of diffuse arthralgias. Intermittent fevers of unknown origin have also been reported.[119] About half of patients have no symptoms, MDS being discovered during investigation of unrelated complaints or on a routine visit. Macrocytosis or mild anemia may be present for years before the development of more severe cytopenias that precipitate the diagnosis of MDS. Splenomegaly is found in about 20% of patients, most frequently in patients with CMML; hepatomegaly and lymphadenopathy are found less frequently. Physical examination rarely reveals any specific abnormalities. Several unusual dermatologic syndromes have been reported in association with MDS, including acute febrile neutrophilic dermatosis (Sweet's syndrome),[120,121] urticaria pigmentosa,[122] and granulocytic sarcoma.[123]

Hematologic Characteristics

The incidence of anemia, thrombocytopenia, and neutropenia in several large studies is shown in Table 12-4. Pancytopenia or bicytopenia is present in 20% to 35% of patients with MDS. Anemia is the most common isolated abnormality (30% to 35%), and isolated thrombocytopenia or neutropenia can occur in 1% to 9% of cases.[37,58,124–126] Except in patients with CMML, a specific subtype of MDS, the total white count is usually normal or decreased. The granulocytic lineage is primarily affected, but reductions in total lymphocyte count can also occur. Patients with the 5q− syndrome can have thrombocytosis and, more rarely, neutrophilia.[127]

Abnormalities of peripheral blood cell morphology are summarized in Table 12-5. Macrocytosis is common in patients with MDS but not universal.[128,129] A distinctive dimorphic smear is often seen in patients with RARS, with both a hypochromic and microcytic population of cells, as well as a second macrocytic population. Decreased heme synthesis reduces hemoglobin production, and hypochromia results.[130] Teardrops, RBC fragments, and nucleated RBCs are seen, especially in patients with increased marrow reticulin. Giant platelets are characteristic, and platelet granules may be sparse or increased in size. These platelet anomalies are most readily appreciated by electron microscopy.[131,132] Granulocytes may manifest striking abnormalities, including a spectrum of nuclear variants such as hyposegmentation with a Pelger-Huët anomaly,[133] unusual chromatin clumping and myelokathexis-like hypersegmentation,[134–136] and abnormal granulation.

TABLE 12-5. Morphologic Abnormalities in the Peripheral Blood in Myelodysplastic Syndromes

RED CELLS	PLATELETS
Macrocytosis	Giant forms
Dimorphism	Hypogranulation
Anisopoikilocytosis	Megakaryocyte fragments
Punctate basophilia	
Nucleated red blood cells	
Polychromasia	
Erythroblasts	
WHITE CELLS	
Hypogranulation	
Pelgeroid nuclei	
Hyposegmented or hypersegmented nuclei	
Ringed-shaped nuclei	
Dohle bodies	
Myeloblasts or other immature forms	

Occasional circulating myeloblasts can be detected in a large number of patients with MDS,[73] and up to 10% of the differential count in RAEBT patients can be myeloblasts without signaling progression to AML. A sudden increase in circulating myeloblasts should prompt a reexamination of the bone marrow. Generally, peripheral blast percentage changes in tandem with bone marrow blast percentage and is not an independent predictor of prognosis.[74,137]

Laboratory Abnormalities

Blood chemistry analysis is often abnormal but the findings are nonspecific. Ten to 40% of patients have elevated levels of lactate dehydrogenase, alkaline phosphatase, hepatic transaminases, uric acid, or bilirubin, but these abnormalities rarely help make the diagnosis. Vitamin B_{12} levels are usually normal but may be elevated in patients with an expanded myeloid compartment. Serum and urine lysozyme (muramidase) may also be elevated in MDS, especially in CMML patients, presumably because of increased monocyte turnover.[138] Because lysozyme levels may be elevated in many conditions, this test has little routine diagnostic usefulness.[139,140]

Iron Metabolism

The finding of ringed sideroblasts is a characteristic feature of MDS. (What is known about metabolic abnormalities leading to iron deposition within mitochondria is summarized in the section on ringed sideroblast formation.) Directly relevant to clinical evaluation and care of patients with MDS is their predisposition to iron overload. They may have increased total body iron stores on presentation. Measurement of the serum iron, total iron-binding capacity and ferritin is an essential part of the initial evaluation.

Often, patients with MDS have received iron as empiric therapy for RA prior to accurate diagnosis. Furthermore, patients with a large but ineffective erythroid component in their bone marrow are predisposed to excess iron absorption. A strong positive correlation exists between the rate of iron turnover within the erythron and iron absorption independent of total-body iron stores.[141] The mechanism of this relation has not been established. The total iron absorbed, particularly in patients given empiric iron therapy, may be significant. Estimates suggest that 6% to 10% of the population may be heterozygous for primary hemochromatosis. The presence of such an abnormal gene in a patient with MDS undoubtedly enhances excess iron absorption. A possible nonrandom association has been suggested between the HLA A3 allele, which is closely linked to the primary hemochromatosis allele, and RARS, but this remains controversial.[142–146]

The importance of evaluating iron stores on presentation is underscored by the fact that many patients require chronic transfusion therapy. Among those with the best prognoses are patients with ineffective erythropoiesis, who may present with high iron stores. Early institution of chelation therapy may be indicated to help avoid unnecessary morbidity and mortality.

SPECIFIC CLINICAL SYNDROMES

Lack of knowledge about the causes of MDS means that many of the clinical and morphologic delineations are arbitrary and may actually deter insight into pathogenesis and pathophysiology. In general, we have chosen to discuss MDSs collectively with respect to clinical features, pathophysiology, prognosis, and treatment. A large body of literature containing many important observations on several specific clinical syndromes exists and is summarized in this section.

Chronic Myelomonocytic Leukemia

Classification of patients with abnormal proliferation or differentiation of the monocytoid lineage has always been confusing. In their 1956 description of monocytic leukemias, Sinn and Dick[147] noted that a subset of patients with increased circulating monocytoid cell counts had a chronic course without inevitable progression to acute leukemia. Subsequent investigators reported that all hematopoietic lineages were frequently abnormal in these patients.[148,149] In the 1970s, several carefully documented series of patients with these characteristics were described, and their disorder was termed *chronic myelomonocytic leukemia*.[138,150,151]

Usually, such patients were elderly (median age 65) and presented with nonspecific symptoms. Sixty percent of patients had anemia or thrombocytopenia or both in addition to the characteristic peripheral blood monocytosis. Both circulating monocytes and granulocytes were found to have morphologic and functional abnormalities.[152] The bone marrow exhibited trilineage dysplasia, with dyserythropoietic and dysmegakaryocytic features similar to those found in patients with preleukemic syndromes. Their bone marrows were uniformly hypercellular, with increased myeloid/erythroid ratios. Serum lysozyme concentration was almost always significantly elevated.[139,153] Up to 60% of patients had polyclonal hypergammaglobulinemia, perhaps because of hyperstimulation of B cells by increased circulating, activated monocytes.[139]

The 1982 FAB classification system for myelodysplasia included CMML as a subclass.[27] Some controversy has existed about classification of CMML as a myelodysplastic instead of as a myeloproliferative syndrome or as a separate entity.[34,70] The trilineage dysplastic changes seen in these patients and the frequent evolution between CMML and other FAB subtypes seem to justify its inclusion in MDS.[86,149,150] Diagnostic features that distinguish CMML from CML and AML are the lack of a Philadelphia chromosome, trilineage marrow dysplasia, and a less aggressive clinical course.

5q− Syndrome

In 1974 and 1975, van den Berghe and coworkers[154,155] described five patients with an acquired interstitial deletion of the long arm of chromosome 5 (5q−) and RA. The patients had severe macrocytic anemia, leukopenia, and normal or elevated platelet counts. Their bone marrows were hypercellular, with increased myeloblasts in some cases, and characteristic dysplastic, small, and uninuclear megakaryocytes. None of the original patients progressed to leukemia or had short survival times; thus, the authors suggested that these clinical findings portend a relatively good prognosis. They felt the association was specific and termed this constellation the *5q− syndrome*. Since that time, a great deal of interest has been generated in patients with this karyotypic abnormality and hematologic disease, especially after the discovery that the genes for several hematopoietic growth factors and their receptors were localized to the missing area of chromosome 5.[156–160] Several genes located in the deleted area of the 5q−, including IRF1, a putative tumor suppressor gene, have been proposed as candidate genes in the pathogenesis of MDS. One recent study refutes the role of IRF1 and points out that few patients have the requisite loss of *both* alleles needed for IRF1 to play a role in MDS.[160a] The role of candidate genes is discussed later in this chapter.

The syndrome present in patients with the 5q− chromosome is similar to that found in other patients with primary MDS. Several larger studies have reported that many 5q− patients present with thrombocytopenia, along with anemia and neutropenia, and progression to AML has now been documented in many cases, even without evolution of additional cytogenetic abnormalities.[161–163] The distinctive uninuclear or binuclear megakaryocytes, described by some authors as unique to patients with 5q−,[47] can clearly be found in patients with dysplastic megakaryocytes and apparently normal chromosome 5.[157] The 5q− chromosomal abnormality has also been found in patients with a wide variety of other hematologic diseases, including AML, myeloproliferative syndromes, and t-MDS.

Therapy-Related Myelodysplasia

The increased risk of acute leukemia in patients previously treated with cytotoxic chemotherapy for other conditions has been recognized for two decades. After investigators observed that therapy-related AML (t-AML) was a panmyelosis accompanied by trilineage abnormalities, patients who had received chemotherapy began to be followed more closely and evaluated as soon as cytopenia, macrocytosis, or abnormal bone marrow morphology was detected.[29] Most patients who develop t-AML have a detectable t-MDS phase.[28,30] This realization has made risk assessment for these secondary hematologic syndromes more meaningful, because patients dying from complications of the cytopenias prior to developing actual t-AML are now generally included in epidemiologic surveys.[164]

In recent large studies, patients with t-MDS account for up to 15% of total patients with MDS.[58,82,165] The incidence of t-MDS and t-AML has increased because of the prolonged survivals (even cures) now attainable after aggressive chemotherapy and radiation therapy of tumors that were previously rapidly fatal. This unfortunate by-product of aggressive treatment, especially in young patients with curable tumors such as Hodgkin's lymphoma, has stimulated a reexamination of chemotherapy regimens in hopes of designing and implementing less mutagenic or carcinogenic combinations.[166–168]

The primary tumors most frequently reported as preceding t-MDS or t-AML are Hodgkin's and non-Hodgkin's lymphomas, ovarian carcinoma, small cell lung cancer, multiple myeloma, breast cancer, and gastrointestinal tumors treated with adjuvant chemotherapy.[28,164,169–175] Patients given alkylating agents for nonmalignant conditions such as rheumatoid arthritis or scleroderma are also at risk.[176]

The risks of developing t-MDS or t-AML are disturbingly high: up to 13% at 10 years after aggressive Hodgkin's disease chemotherapy[177] and up to 14% at 4 years in one smaller study of patients treated intensively for small cell lung cancer.[172] A 12-fold higher risk has been found in ovarian cancer patients treated with chemotherapy compared with that found in patients treated with surgery alone.[174] The risk increases nonlinearly with duration and intensity of treatment. The highest risk occurs within the first 4 to 5 years after institution of chemotherapy or radiation therapy and reaches a plateau at 8 to 10 years (Fig. 12-4). The mean time to presentation with symptoms of t-MDS or t-AML from initial chemotherapy is 48 to 68 months.[169,173,178–180]

Alkylating agents are strongly implicated, since aggressive chemotherapy regimens without an alkylating agent such as those used for germ cell tumors or acute leukemias do not increase the risk of t-MDS or t-AML.[113,173,178,181,182] Alkylating agents are mutagenic and carcinogenic in vitro and in animal models.[183] They interact directly and covalently with DNA, forming reactive intermediates that cross-link, break, and cause misreading of DNA strands. Agents such as methotrexate and vincristine, which do not directly interact with DNA, have not been shown to increase the risk of secondary neoplasms. It is not understood why agents such as cisplatin or daunorubicin, which do interact with DNA and cause strand breaks or conformational shifts, have not been associated with an appreciable rate of secondary tumors.

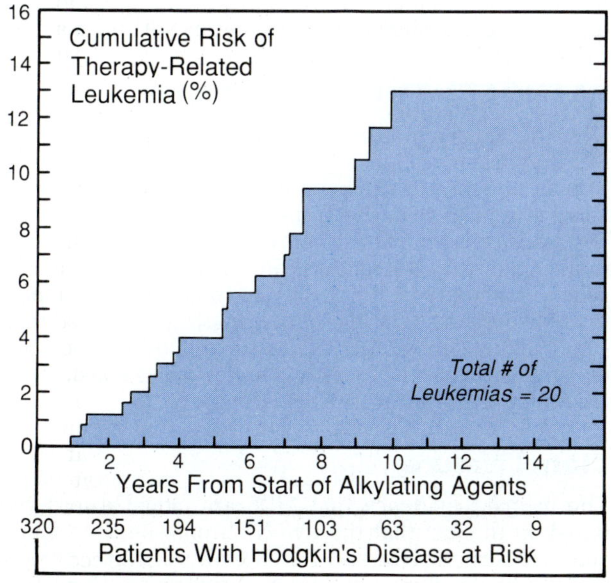

FIGURE 12-4. Kaplan-Meier plot of the cumulative risk of therapy-related myelodysplastic syndrome and acute myelogenous leukemia in a cohort of 320 patients up to 15 years after the start of alkylating agent chemotherapy for Hodgkin's disease. (After Pedersen-Bjergaard J, Larsen SO, Struck J, et al. Risk of therapy-related leukaemia and preleukaemia after Hodgkin's disease: relation to age, cumulative dose of alkylating agents, and time from chemotherapy. Lancet 1987;2:85)

The link between external-beam radiation therapy and a higher risk of t-MDS or t-AML has been less clearly established. Some studies have failed to identify cases in patients treated with external-beam radiation therapy alone.[28,170] Another reported a lower risk and a longer latency than after chemotherapy,[179] whereas at least one other described several patients who had received external-beam radiation therapy alone and soon thereafter developed t-MDS. These patients had received extremely high radiation doses to the spine and pelvis.[173] Chemotherapy, given in conjunction with external-beam radiation therapy, does not result in a higher risk than the same regimen of chemotherapy given alone.[28,164,170,174,175]

Several clinical features of t-MDS should be emphasized. The mean age at presentation is about 10 years earlier than that seen in primary MDS.[30,179] Occurrence of t-MDS in children is more common than primary MDS in this age group.[184] Peripheral blood counts and cell morphology are similar to those found in primary MDS, except that severe pancytopenia is more common and increased numbers of basophils have been noted.[29,169,179] Bone marrow cellularity is generally normal or increased, but 10% to 25% of patients have hypocellular bone marrows.[178,179] The degree of trilineage dysplasia is often striking. Ringed sideroblasts can be found in appreciable numbers in up to 60% of t-MDS bone marrow samples.[29,179]

The FAB classification of patients with t-MDS is much less meaningful than in primary MDS. Even patients with less than 5% myeloblasts or large numbers of sideroblasts (RA or RARS) progress rapidly to AML or succumb to complications of severe cytopenias.[80] Patients with t-MDS should always be separated from those with primary MDS in natural history studies and therapeutic trials, because their clinical course and prognosis are significantly different. Otherwise, results may be distorted, depending on the relative number of patients with t-MDS included. Specific prognostic information and treatment options for t-MDS are discussed in later sections of this chapter.

DIFFERENTIAL DIAGNOSIS

Few if any pathognomonic features are seen in myelodysplasia patients. Many patients must be followed for several months to determine whether their cytopenias have reversible or nonprogressive causes. Table 12-6 lists other possible causes of chronic cytopenias with an adequately cellular marrow, which should be excluded before making the diagnosis of MDS. The impressive macrocytosis and megaloblastic changes that often occur in MDS can strongly suggest B_{12} or folate deficiency, but serum levels or a Schilling test should be obtained before embarking on empiric vitamin replacement. During the regenerating, recovery phase after marrow damage due to chemotherapy, alcohol, or benzene, many of the morphologic changes used to define MDS may be seen. Diagnosis of t-MDS should be made only when cytopenia and marrow dysplasia are persistent or follow an initial period of full bone marrow recovery. Viral infection of erythroid presursors, such as with B19 parvovirus, can also produce bizarre erythroid dysplasia. Parvovirus infections should be excluded, especially in children or adults with immune deficiencies.[185]

Ringed sideroblasts are not specific to MDS, and do not by themselves imply that diagnosis. Table 12-7 gives a differential diagnosis of ringed sideroblasts. Several comprehensive review articles can be consulted for more detail.[12,41] Reversible causes, such as drug- or alcohol-related marrow damage, should be ruled out and treated. A careful family history and hematologic workup are required to rule out

TABLE 12-6. Differential Diagnosis of Chronic Cytopenias With Cellular Marrows

NUTRITIONAL CONDITIONS
Vitamin B_{12} deficiency
Folate deficiency
Iron deficiency

REVERSIBLE MARROW TOXICITY
Alcohol
Recovery phase from chemotherapy or irradiation
Toxins or drugs

ANEMIA OF CHRONIC DISEASE
Renal failure
Collagen vascular disease
Chronic infection

VIRAL INFECTION OF MARROW
B19 parvovirus
Human immunodeficiency virus

NEOPLASTIC CONDITIONS
Leukemia
Nonleukemic tumor infiltration of marrow
Paraneoplastic marrow suppression

CONGENITAL OR HEREDITARY CONDITIONS
Hereditary sideroblastic anemias
Congenital dyserythropoietic anemias
Fanconi's anemia
Diamond-Blackfan syndrome
Down's syndrome
Shwachman's syndrome
Kostmann's syndrome

MYELOPROLIFERATIVE SYNDROMES
Polycythemia vera
Essential thrombocythemia
Chronic myelogenous leukemia
Myelofibrosis with myeloid metaplasia
Monosomy 7 syndrome
Juvenile chronic myelogenous leukemia

PAROXYSMAL NOCTURNAL HEMOGLOBINURIA

HYPERSPLENISM

MYELODYSPLASTIC SYNDROMES
Primary idiopathic
Therapy related

hereditary sideroblastic anemia, especially in children presenting with isolated anemia and no dysplasia of nonerythroid lineages. Monomorphic, microcytic RBCs are also suggestive of hereditary rather than idiopathic acquired sideroblastic anemia.

In our experience, differentiation between aplastic anemia and MDS can be difficult in patients with a hypocellular bone marrow. A judgment regarding the degree of bone marrow dysplasia may be required. The finding of activated suppressor T lymphocytes in peripheral blood may support the diagnosis of aplastic anemia. Conversely, cytogenetic abnormalities of a clonal nature provide evidence that MDS is the correct diagnosis. Care should also be taken to identify patients with aleukemic leukemia who have a hypocellular bone marrow. If the myeloblast percentage is greater than 30%, such persons should be treated aggressively with chemotherapy.[186]

Acquired or congenital hematologic diseases such as paroxysmal nocturnal hemoglobinuria, the myeloproliferative syndromes, Kostmann's syndrome, and Fanconi's anemia should not be classified as MDSs, even though statistically they carry an increased risk of leukemia and in that sense are preleukemic. This also applies to Down's syndrome and Bloom's syndrome. These disorders are not necessarily associated with hematologic abnormalities but are indeed associated with an increased risk of leukemia. MDS is rare in children who have not received chemotherapy; thus, careful family histories, chromosomal studies and bone marrow examinations are required to exclude Diamond-Blackfan syndrome (pure RBC aplasia), congenital dyserythropoietic anemia, Fanconi's anemia, hereditary sideroblastic anemia, Schwachman's syndrome, and other constitutive disorders in young patients with cytopenias.

TABLE 12-7. Differential Diagnosis of Ringed Sideroblasts

CONGENITAL
Hereditary sideroblastic anemias
- X-linked[410–415]
- Autosomal[411,412,569–572]

ACQUIRED
Idiopathic (refractory anemia with ringed sideroblasts)
Drug induced[398]
- Isoniazid[399]
- Other antituberculous drugs[399]
- Chloramphenicol[44]
- Zinc[573]

Ethanol induced[398]

PATHOGENETIC MECHANISMS

Of special consideration in the pathogenesis of MDSs is the fact that these are clonal disorders. Progeny of a single cell gain ascendancy in the bone marrow. Their selective advantage appears to derive from genetic mutations that free dysplastic cells from normal growth constraints and perturb their capacity for full maturation. An acquired or inherent genetic instability within the myelodysplastic clone appears to predispose to additional mutations, leading to the emergence of subclones and progressive evolution of the myelodysplastic process, initially manifesting as bone marrow dysfunction and ultimately as leukemia.

Clonal Nature

The primary evidence that MDS are clonal disorders is based on the fact that the two X chromosomes in female cells are structurally and functionally distinct. Early in embryonic development, one X chromosome in each somatic cell is randomly inactivated by mechanisms that include methylation of specific cytosine residues in DNA. If a female is heterozygous at a specific X-chromosome locus, each of the tissues is composed of cells expressing one or the other allele but not both. The best-known example is glucose-6-phosphate dehydrogenase (G6PD). In heterozygous women, the A and B isozymes of G6PD are present in roughly equal proportions in all tissues. Because X-chromosome inactivation occurs early in embryogenesis, the number of cells expressing either allele are about equal. If a population of cells in such a heterozygous individual is clonal, that is, they derive from a single somatic cell, it is composed of cells that are all producing the same isozyme.[187]

In 1978, Prchal and coworkers[188] reported that a G6PD heterozygous woman with classic RARS expressed only one isozyme in platelets, RBCs, granulocytes, macrophages, B cells, and T cells. In this patient, RARS was shown to be a clonal disorder affecting a hematopoietic stem cell that became ascendant in all myeloid and lymphoid lineages. The observations of these researchers provided the first evidence of a common hematopoietic progenitor for myeloid and lymphoid cells in humans. Several other patients with MDS have since been shown to have clonal expression of G6PD, with a single isozyme present in all myeloid lineages, B cells, and EBV-immortalized B-cell lines, but not in T cells.[189,190] This discrepancy in T-cell involvement among patients suggests that the myelodysplastic process could begin in progenitors or stem cells with varying T-lymphoid repopulating ability. Perhaps polyclonal, unaffected T cells persist for long periods in some patients.

Heterozygosity for G6PD is rare, limiting analysis of clonality in MDS to just a few patients. Recently, more general methods have been developed to investigate clonality. Many cytosine residues on the inactive X chromosome are methylated, whereas the corresponding residues on the active chromosome remain unmethylated. Several X-chromosome probes for restriction fragment length polymorphisms (RFLPs) have been identified. Using these probes, sequential digestion with two restriction enzymes can first identify female heterozygotes, then distinguish the activated from the inactivated X chromosome.[191–193] This procedure is diagrammed in Figure 12-5. The first restriction enzyme distinguishes the maternally and paternally derived copies of the X-chromosome gene via an RFLP. The second enzyme is methylation-sensitive and distinguishes the active from the inactive copy of the gene via differential digestion patterns. Between 30% and 60% of women are heterozygotes for at least one of the presently available RFLP probes. This technique has already been used to demonstrate the monoclonal derivation of bone marrow and peripheral blood nucleated cells in seven of eight patients with MDS.[194]

Cytogenetic studies have also supported the concept of MDS as a clonal disorder of the pluripotent stem cell. The same specific chromosomal abnormalities have been identified in cells derived from either erythroid or myeloid colony-forming units (CFUs) grown in vitro from patients with MDS.[195,196] EBV-immortalized B cells, but not T cells, from one patient had the same interstitial chromosomal deletion as bone marrow myeloid progenitor cells.[197] One recent study provides some convincing evidence that, at least in patients with the 5q− syndrome, the defect is not present in lymphoid cells.[197a]

Besides the documentation of clonal markers in cells of multiple lineages, the transformation of MDS into several different phenotypic varieties of acute leukemia is evidence that the primary defect is at the level of the hematopoietic stem cell. Most patients with MDS who develop acute leukemia have typical AML that can be classified in the FAB scheme as M1 or M2; several instances of transformation to acute megakaryocytic leukemia (M7)[53,61] and several case reports documenting conversion to acute lymphocytic leukemia have been seen.[53,198–201] One patient developed acute leukemia with two distinct populations of blast cells—one myeloid and one lymphoid[202]—and other patients have leukemic populations with lineage infidelity, the coexpression of markers or phenotypic characteristics normally not found coexisting in one cell.[201]

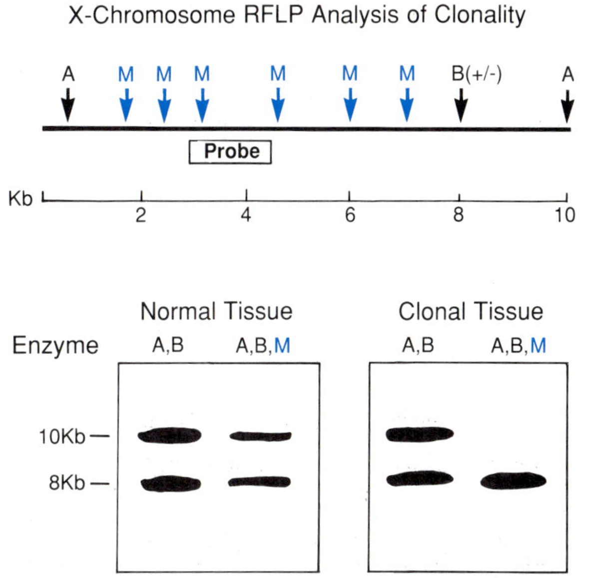

FIGURE 12-5. *(Top)* Representation of a restriction enzyme map of an X-chromosome region that contains a restriction fragment length polymorphism (RFLP). Enzyme A cuts at nonpolymorphic sites present in all X chromosomes. Enzyme B cuts at a polymorphic site present only in some X chromosomes. Enzyme M is methylation sensitive and cuts at sites in the active (undermethylated) X chromosome only. *(Bottom)* Diagrams of expected Southern blot results using normal or neoplastic clonal tissue DNA from a woman heterozygous for this X-chromosome RFLP (enzyme B restriction site). When digested with enzymes A and B, two bands can be detected, corresponding to the two X chromosomes. When the same DNA is further digested with enzyme M, DNA from active X chromosomes is cut into multiple smaller pieces not detectable on the blots. Because in normal, nonclonal tissue, about half of the cells have each X chromosome randomly inactivated, both bands persist, but are of lower intensity. In neoplastic clonal tissue, all cells are derived from the same single progenitor cell and have the same X chromosome inactivated. Thus, when enzyme M is used to digest the clonal DNA from a woman heterozygous for the RFLP, one band disappears (from the active X chromosomes), and the other remains at the same intensity (from the inactive X chromosomes).

Cytogenetic Abnormalities

Patients with MDS have frequently been found to have bone marrow cells with chromosomal abnormalities that are clonal, nonrandom, and prognostically informative,[203–205a] although the exact role of these chromosomal changes in the pathogenesis of MDS is still uncertain. Using standard cytogenetic techniques (see Chap. 5) Thirty-three to 64% of patients with primary MDS have detectable abnormalities.[206–217] Using higher-resolution techniques, Yunis and coworkers[218,219] found chromosomal abnormalities in 79% of patients with primary MDS. Specific abnormalities are not random: the most common are deletion of the long arm of chromosome 5 (5q−), monosomy 7 (7−), and trisomy 8 (+8). The incidences of each karyotype in one large study is reproduced in Figure 12-6.[217] A similar incidence (50%) and distribution of chromosomal changes have been reported in a small group of pediatric patients with MDS,[220] except that abnormalities of chromosome 5 are much less common than in adults.

Deletion of the long arm of chromosome 5 (5q−) has been the most intensely studied chromosomal change associated with MDS for three reasons: (1) it is the most common

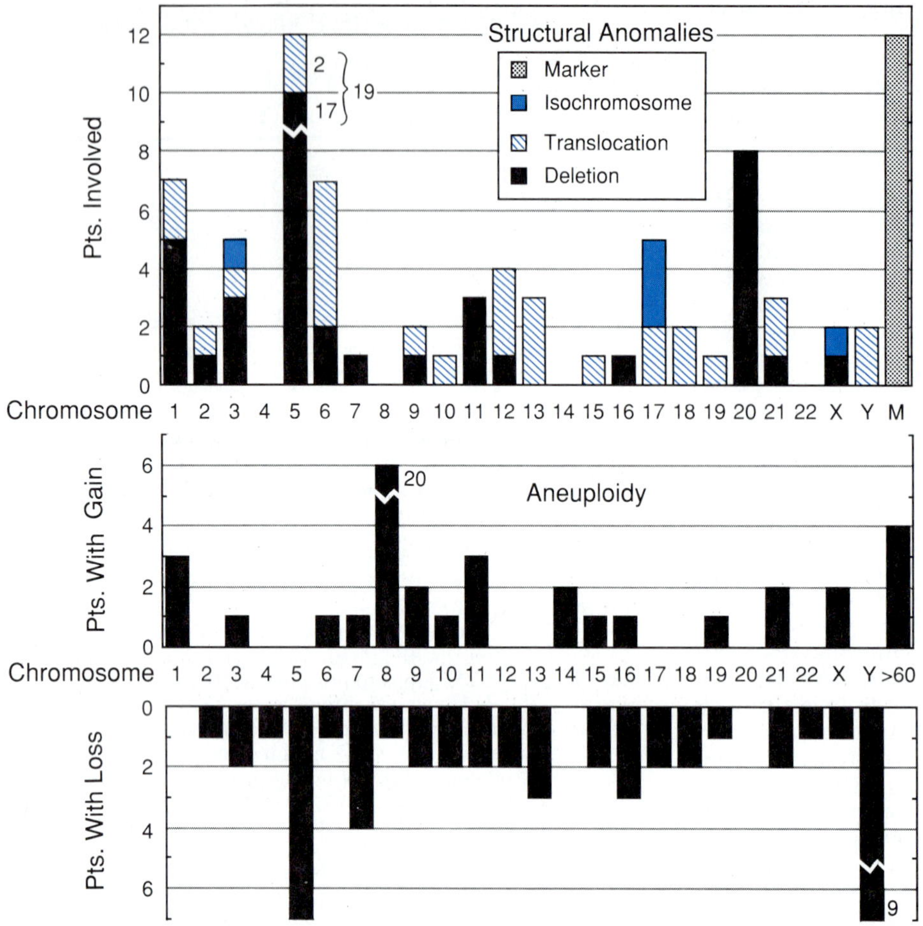

FIGURE 12-6. Chart showing data on the specific chromosome affected in 69 patients with myelodysplastic syndromes and an identifiable chromosomally abnormal clone. (*Top*) The number of patients (pts) with structural abnormalities. (*Middle*) The number of patients with chromosomal gain. (*Bottom*) The number of patients with chromosomal loss. Marker chromosomes are abnormal extra chromosomes that cannot be assigned an identity. (After Knapp RC, Dewald GW, Pierre RV, et al. Cytogenetic studies in 174 consecutive patients with preleukemic or myelodysplastic syndromes. Mayo Clin Proc 1985;60:510)

chromosomal alteration found in association with MDS (3% to 10% of all patients with MDS)[218,221]; (2) a 5q− syndrome, consisting of RA, thrombocytosis, and abnormal megakaryocyte morphology with a relatively good prognosis has been reported; and (3) the genes for several hematopoietic growth factors and receptors have been mapped to the deleted region on chromosome 5. The 5q deletion is an acquired mutation, present in multipotent progenitor cells giving rise to both erythroid and granulocytic lineages,[222] but not to fibroblasts or circulating T lymphocytes.[154] The deletion is almost universely interstitial, with loss rather than translocation of the missing segment.[127,223,224] The 5q− abnormality is also frequently reported in association with other hematologic disorders, including de novo and t-AML, acute lymphoblastic leukemia, polycythemia vera and other myeloproliferative syndromes, and pure RBC aplasia.[127,163,225–228]

Several of the commonly detected abnormalities in MDS are also see in patients with de novo AML, especially the elderly.[229] This suggests a true biologic continuum between MDS and at least some types of AML. On the other hand, several of the translocations that are specifically associated with certain types of leukemia, including 8;21 with M2 AML, 15;17 with M3 (promyelocytic) AML, and 9;22 with chronic myelogenous leukemia (CML), have virtually never been identified in patients with MDS. No consistent associations between FAB subtypes of MDS and specific chromosomal abnormalities have yet been reported, although chromosomal changes are more common in patients with RAEB, RAEBT, and CMML than in those with RARS or RA.[212,217,230]

The incidence of detectable cytogenetic abnormalities in patients with t-MDS is higher than in those with primary MDS—80% to 100% in several studies.[29,173,178–180,231–233] Compared with that seen in other chromosomes, abnormalities of chromosome 5, chromosome 7, or both are relatively more common (50% to 95%) than in primary MDS. Changes in chromosomes 1, 3, 4, 12, 14, 17, 18, 19, and 21 have also been reported as being nonrandomly associated with t-MDS.[173,178,232,234,235] Patients treated with chemotherapy but without active hematologic disease do not have these cytogenetic changes detectable in their marrows.[231] Thus, detection of karyotypic changes may be of value for early diagnosis of t-MDS and could help distinguish t-MDS from other causes of cytopenias in cancer patients, including relapse of the primary tumor with marrow suppression or infiltration.

Many investigators have performed serial karyotypes and have noted an association between progression of MDS, from RA or RARS to RAEB, RAEBT, or frank AML, and new or additional chromosomal changes. In some cases, clonal evolution occurs as an initially abnormal clone acquires additional cytogenetic abnormalities[236–242]; in others, several subclones with independent abnormalities have been shown to arise, coexist, and eventually either disappear or dominate.[243–246] Even stronger correlations between new cytogenetic abnormalities and disease progression have been observed in t-MDS.[173,178,180]

Adequate cytogenetic analysis of bone marrow or peripheral blood in MDS may be difficult because of low proliferation rates or absence of evaluable metaphases.[203,212] Most investigators have cultured marrow cells for 12 to 72 hours in an attempt to increase yield; some have advocated synchronization procedures.[218] Results may be skewed if an abnormal clone has a selective growth advantage or disadvantage in culture. Several studies have documented a difference in the number of or even presence of abnormal clones when bone marrow cells are assayed immediately after harvesting rather than after a period of in vitro culture.[247–249]

Several other methods have been devised for assessing karyotype that do not depend on microscopic analysis of condensed chromosomes. The DNA content of cells can be measured by flow cytometry, which has been used to show that half of patients with MDS have aneuploidy of marrow cells.[250] The advantages of this method are that large numbers of cells can be analyzed easily and rapidly, without requiring in vitro proliferation. A disadvantage is an inability to detect balanced translocations and other pseudodiploid states. Direct DNA image cytometry on fixed cells shares with flow cytometry the advantage of not requiring mitotic cells, while allowing analysis of individual fixed cells on a slide and detection of small populations of abnormal cells.[251] DNA probes specific for frequently altered chromosomal fragments can be used to assess cytogenetic changes in DNA harvested from fractionated MDS cell populations.[252,253] DNA probes isolated from known chromosomal regions have also been useful for mapping breakpoints by pulsed field gel electrophoresis.[254]

Mutations in Specific Genes

Because of the clonal nature of MDS and the frequent cytogenetic abnormalities and mutations in specific oncogenes associated with it, we prefer to consider the pathogenesis of these syndromes in the context of mechanisms operative in neoplastic processes in general. We realize fully that no specific cytogenetic abnormality or gene mutation has been linked causally to MDS and that many of the observed abnormalities may be mechanistically irrelevant, reflecting DNA damage by exogenous agents or inherent genetic instability. The evolving knowledge of oncogenic mechanisms provides several paradigms for considering the pathogenesis of MDS, including dominant-acting oncogenes, recessive oncogenes, and multistep pathogenesis.

An explosion of knowledge about dominant-acting oncogenes has occurred, as detailed in Chapters 5 and 6. Normal cellular genes, the so-called protooncogenes, can be rendered transforming by several possible mechanisms. For example, a point mutation in a *ras* gene results in a single amino acid substitution in the protein product that diminishes its capacity to hydrolyze GTP and dysregulates its role in signal transduction.[255,256] Chromosomal breakpoints characteristic of specific malignancies often pinpoint the location of oncogenes. The translocation between chromosomes 9 and 22 characteristic of CML gives rise to a chimeric *BCR-ABL* gene, the product of which is a dysregulated protein tyrosine kinase.[257] Finally, overexpression of a protooncogene due to a regulatory mutation may contribute to cell transformation. For example, expression of the *myc* protooncogene in Burkitt's lymphoma is increased after its relocation into an immunoglobulin locus.[258–260] Each of these oncogenic mutations can be characterized as dominant because the gene product perturbs cell growth despite an unaltered normal gene on the homologous chromosome.

Recessive oncogenes (classic tumor suppressor genes) are operative only when a normal gene product is dysfunctional, diminished in amount, or absent because of mutations affecting both alleles at a specific locus.[261] The best-studied example is the retinoblastoma (Rb) gene. The Rb gene product undergoes reversible phosphorylation on initiation of S phase and is dephosphorylated as the cell returns to the G1 phase of the cell cycle or a resting state.[262] Retinoblastoma cells lack any of the Rb gene product and are fully neoplastic; introduction and expression of the Rb gene into such cells by recombinant DNA methods markedly reduce their transformed phenotype in vitro and decrease their capacity for tumor formation in vivo.[263] Loss of Rb gene function in retinoblastoma cells occurs by complex mutational mechanisms, which include congenital interstitial deletion, exchange of genetic information among homologous chromosomes, and either deletions or point mutations in the structural gene.[261,264] Several other recessive oncogenes have been described: a gene on chromosome 11 that has been implicated in Wilms' tumor, the p53 gene on chromosome 17 that has been implicated in many malignancies including leukemia and colon cancer, and a recently described gene on chromosome 18 that has been associated with colon cancer.[261,265–268]

Inherent in the concept of neoplastic mechanisms is the notion that a normal cell becomes fully malignant by a series of mutations, each of which represents a single step out of many.[269,270] This hypothesis is best supported in colon cancer: specific chromosomal deletions, chromosomal loss and point mutations in protooncogenes, or recessive oncogenes have been linked with transitions from normal to hyperplastic epithelium, the development of adenomas, and the emergence of carcinomas.[271] The evolution of normal bone marrow to MDS and then to leukemia invites a similar application of the concepts of multistep genetic pathogenesis.

Oncogene Activation

The search for mutations of protooncogenes in the cells of patients with MDS has been focused thus far on the *ras* gene family, Ha-, Ki- and N-*ras*. These genes encode 21-kd GTP-binding proteins that localize to the inner surface of the plasma membrane and play an as-yet-undefined role in the transduction of signals from the cell surface.[256] Overexpression of normal p21 protein can result in transformation of immortalized fibroblast cell lines, but transformation occurs with much lower levels of an altered activated p21 protein produced by *ras* genes mutated at codons 12, 13, or 61. These abnormal p21 proteins have less intrinsic GTPase activity and may be locked in an activated, GTP-bound state.

An activated *ras* gene was first found in DNA isolated from a human bladder tumor.[255,272] Activated *ras* genes have now been found in DNA isolated from many human tumors in up to 40% to 50% in AML, colon cancer, and adenocarcinoma of the lung.[272] The high incidence of *ras* mutations found in AML samples prompted investigators to screen bone marrow cells of patients with MDS with the hope of learning whether *ras* mutations were an early event in the apparent multistep progression toward leukemia or a later event associated with actual leukemic transformation.

Activated *ras* genes have been found in bone marrow or peripheral blood samples of from 8% to 50% of patients with MDS.[194,273–281] Mutations in the N-*ras* gene are most common, but activation of either of the other *ras* genes has also been reported. No consistent association of *ras* mutations with any one FAB subtype has been found, except that these mutations may be more common in patients with CMML.[273,275] Mice that develop T-cell lymphomas secondary to alkylating agents have an extremely high incidence of activating *ras* gene mutations in tumor DNA,[282] but only one of nine patients with t-MDS secondary to chemotherapy was found to have these mutations.[283] In several, a clear relation existed between *ras* gene mutations and progression of MDS to leukemia. Such mutations are found in patients with indolent RA or RARS, and some investigators have not found them to predict more rapid progression to AML.[273,274] However, in one recent study, N-*ras* mutations were associated with a poor prognosis and an increased risk of progression to leukemia in patients with MDS.[274a] Two patients in whom only a small percentage of bone marrow cells initially tested positive for a *ras* mutation developed coincident increases in the percentage of cells with abnormal *ras* genes and bone marrow myeloblasts.[284] Another study reported significantly shorter survivals for patients with MDS with *ras* mutations.[281]

Increased levels of expression from nonactivated *ras* genes has also been explored in relation to the pathogenesis of MDS. Krontiris and coworkers[285] suggested an association between the presence of rare DNA polymorphisms just downstream of the Ha-*ras* coding sequence and a high risk of MDS or AML. This region was hypothesized to function as a modulator of *ras* gene expression, and the rare polymorphisms were thought to be associated with increased levels of p21 production. Two larger studies have failed to verify any association.[286,287] An MDS patient with a chromosomal translocation (5;12) was found to have six times more Ki-*ras*-2 mRNA in bone marrow cells than normal.[288] The Ki-*ras*-2 gene is on the region of chromosome 12 that was translocated in this patient. No structural alterations in the Ki-*ras* gene itself, or in genes on chromosome 5 such as c-*fms* or macrophage colony-stimulating factor (M-CSF), were found. A similar increase in expression from a cellular protooncogene was reported in three patients with (1;7) translocations; mRNA for the *erb* B protooncogene product was elevated 10 to 30 times over that of control levels.[289]

Skeptics have argued that *ras* gene mutations do not have a primary pathogenic role in MDS or other neoplastic processes.[276,290] In patients with AML, *ras* gene mutations in myeloblast cells on presentation were not always detected on relapse.[291] In MDS or AML, only a minority of cells in the total bone marrow population may harbor *ras* mutations. Drawing on the knowledge that mutant *ras* gene products have incontestable transforming properties in vivo and in vitro, we prefer to believe that mutant p21 protein in MDS cells contributes to abnormal growth properties. Such mutations are certainly not an obligatory step in the pathogenesis of MDS. As is discussed in a later section, the multitude of subclones in the bone marrow of patients with MDS may derive their abnormal growth properties from differing constellations of any of a number of different types of mutations.

The *fms* gene encodes the receptor for M-CSF.[292] Activating mutations shown to contribute to the conversion of the *fms* protooncogene to its transforming viral counterpart, v-*fms*, have been localized to codon 301 in the external ligand binding domain and to codon 969, a tyrosine residue in the C-terminal region of the protein that may be involved in kinase control.[293] Using the polymerase chain reaction, Jacobs and colleagues[294] have found mutations in these codons in bone marrow cells of patients with MDS, most frequently with CMML. Twenty percent of the patients had mutations; most were in codon 969. Such mutations would be likely to enhance the ligand-independent protein kinase activity of the receptor, diminishing the dependence on growth factor for cell proliferation. The observed spontaneous growth of myeloid progenitors in cultures of bone marrow from patients with CMML is particularly intriguing in this regard.[295,296] There is a report of three patients with p53 mutations who had MDS.[296a] Two had RAEB and one had RAEBT. Although the number is small, it raises the possibility that this important tumor suppressor gene, involved in the pathogenesis of a number of other malignancies, may also play a role in MDS.

5q Deletion

Several models have been proposed to account for the association of acquired somatic cytogenetic changes with disordered hematopoiesis and increased risk of leukemia. These models are deletion of specific genes necessary for normal growth and differentiation with a resultant gene dosage effect, deletion of a tumor suppressor gene with unmasking of a recessive abnormal allele on the homologous chromosome, and dysregulation of a protooncogene or alteration of its gene product due to abnormal juxtaposition of genetic information at the breakpoint. These hypotheses are discussed in the context of the acquired 5q− chromosomal abnormality; similar considerations apply to the loss of other chromosomal regions or to chromosomal translocations that occur in MDS. As described earlier, the 5q− chromosome is associated with a characteristic hematologic syndrome in which anemia, diminished erythroid activity, thrombocytosis, and abnormal megakaryocyte maturation are seen. The 5q− chromosome is also found in more typical MDSs, t-MDS and t-AML, and in other hematologic disorders.[127,163,225–228] The search for a pathogenetic link between the 5q deletion and hematopoietic abnormalities has not yet been successful. The difficulties encountered are typical of the obstacles in trying to associate any specific chromosomal aberration with a hematologic disease.

Mapping the boundaries of the 5q deletion has generated conflicting results. High-resolution banding techniques localized the proximal breakpoint to q13.3 and the distal breakpoint to q33.1 in 15 of 15 patients with 5q− and MDS.[224] Other reports have described patients with MDS with variations in both proximal and distal breakpoints.[127,223,297] The breakpoints seem to be more variable in t-MDS and t-AML, but the critical shared deleted region is smaller (5q31).[173,297] Figure 12-7 shows the breakpoints compiled by one group of investigators on a large series of MDS, AML, t-MDS, t-AML, and 5q− syndrome patients. The variation in 5q deletion breakpoints has fostered the hypothesis that clinical abnormalities are caused by the loss of genes from a critical region rather than by the abnormal juxtaposition of genes at translocation junctions.

The long arm of chromosome 5 contains several genes relevant to hematopoiesis. Cells containing the 5q deletion are hemizygous for these genes. In 1985, the granulocyte-macrophage colony-stimulating factor (GM-CSF) gene and the *fms* protooncogene, which encodes the M-CSF receptor, were localized to within the deleted region.[298–300] Over the last few years, other hematopoietic growth factors and their receptors have been mapped to this same region. These include M-CSF,[301] interleukin-3 (IL-3),[302,303] interleukin-5 (IL-5),[297,304] and interleukin-4 (IL-4),[297,305,306] as well as the PDGF receptor,[307,308] the β_2-adrenergic receptor,[309] acidic fibroblast growth factor,[310] a glucocorticoid receptor,[311] CD14 (a myeloid membrane antigen),[312] and a zinc-finger protein coregulated with the *fos* protooncogene.[313] Figure 12-7 diagrams the localization of these genes and the critical region deleted in patients with the 5q− syndrome, as well as patients with 5q deletions and other types of MDS or AML. Nature would seem to have perpetrated a cruel hoax indeed if the deletion of these genes were not relevant to disorders in which such evident derangement of hematopoietic cell differentiation occurs.

Possibly, the single copies of growth factor and other genes present on the homologous region of the nonaffected chromosome 5 cannot direct synthesis of sufficient gene product to support normal hematopoiesis. This gene dosage hypothesis seems logical but thus far has been difficult to prove. Monocytes and macrophages can synthesize M-CSF and GM-CSF, so that cells carrying a 5q− chromosome might produce reduced quantities of these growth factors during normal hematopoiesis. Most evidence implicates lymphocytes, fibroblasts, and endothelial cells, which do not carry the 5q deletion, as the primary sites of synthesis for most growth factors involved in hematopoiesis.[314–316]

The M-CSF receptor (*fms* gene product) could also be susceptible to a gene dosage effect. The *fms* gene product influences the pattern of differentiation of hematopoietic cells when it is introduced into cultured cells by DNA

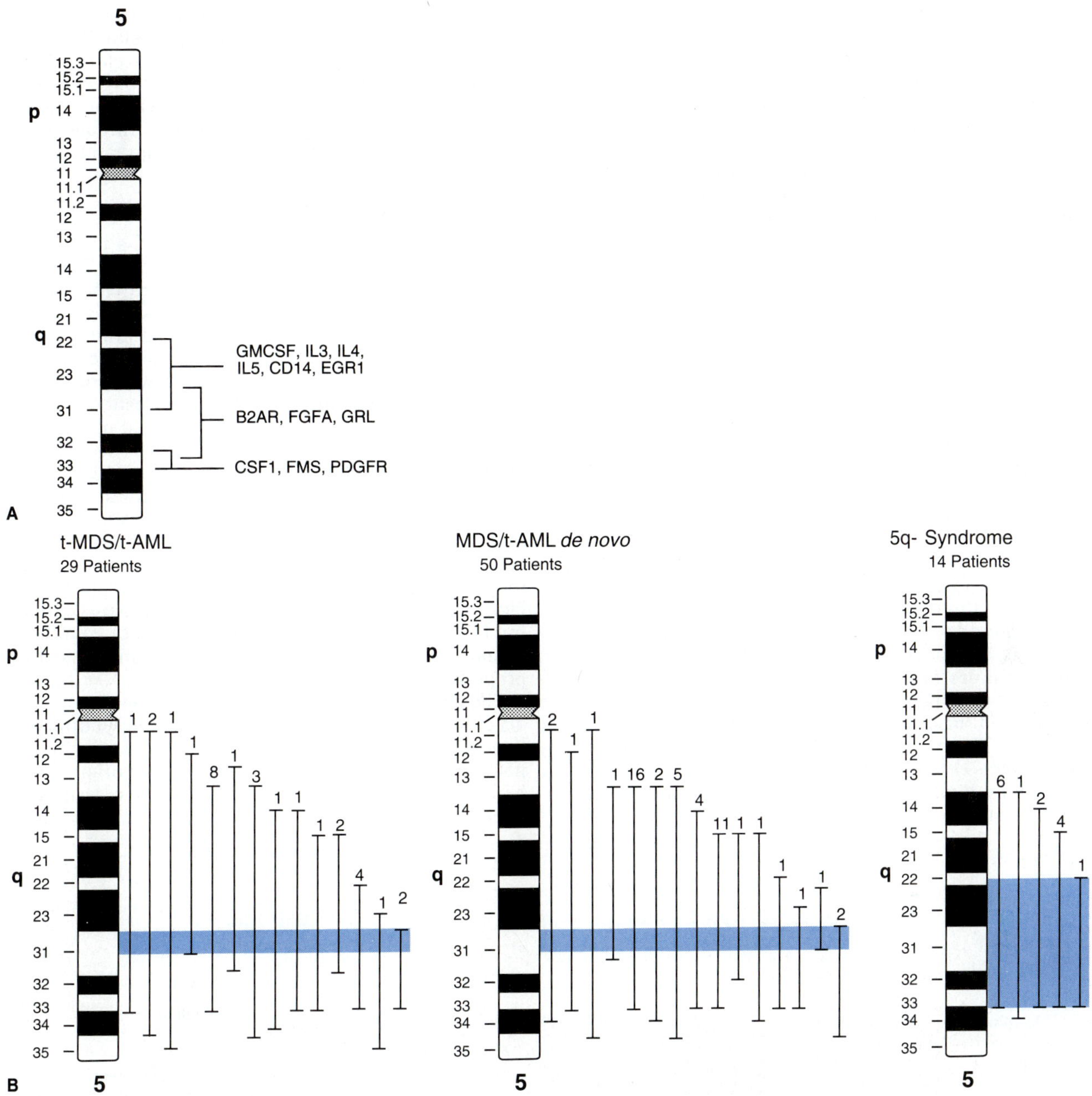

FIGURE 12-7. (A) Map of the normal human chromosome 5, showing assignments on the long arm (g) for granulocyte-macrophage colony-stimulating factor (GM-CSF),[298] interleukin-3 (IL3),[302,303] interleukin-4 (IL4),[297,305,306] interleukin-5 (IL5),[297,304] the myeloid membrane antigen CD14,[312] a DNA-binding zinc finger protein (EGR1),[313] the β-adrenergic receptor (B2AR),[309] acidic fibroblast growth factor,[310] colony-stimulating factor 1 (CSF1) or macrophage colony-stimulating factor,[301] the CSF1 receptor (FMS),[299] and the platelet-derived growth factor receptor (PDGFR).[307,308] (B) Diagram of chromosome 5 illustrating the breakpoints of the interstitial deletions found in patients with therapy-related myelodysplastic syndrome or acute myelogenous leukemia (t-MDS/t-AML), de novo MDS or AML, and the 5q− syndrome. The vertical lines represent the regions that were deleted, and the numbers above these lines indicate the numbers of patients with each deletion. The horizontal lines indicate the critical region in each group, that is, the smallest overlapping region that was deleted in each of the patients. (Courtesy of M. M. Le Beau, University of Chicago)

transfection techniques.[317] Both myeloid progenitors and pre-B lymphocytes exhibit monocytic differentiation under appropriate experimental conditions. Limited production of the M-CSF receptor could influence the pattern of differentiation during a crucial phase of myelopoiesis in patients with MDS.

Several other hypotheses can explain the relation between a chromosomal deletion and dysregulated hematopoiesis. Perhaps loss of one normal allele unmasks a mutated, silent, or dysfunctional allele on the partner chromosome. As yet, no data are available for either specific mutations in or absent expression from the known genes on the grossly normal homologous chromosome 5 in patients with the 5q− abnormality.

The relevant gene might be currently unassociated with hematopoiesis or as yet undiscovered. The gene that is presumably mutated in autosomal dominant familial adenomatous polyposis has been localized to the q21 to q22 region of chromosome 5, a region typically deleted in 5q− MDS.[261,318] Even a heterozygous abnormality of this gene seems to allow the development of colonic polyps. Inactivation of the remaining normal allele by acquired somatic mutation may predispose patients to colon cancer by mechanisms analogous to those that occur in retinoblastoma. A gene important in intestinal cell differentiation can undoubtedly simultaneously have a crucial role in hematopoiesis.

These speculations should convince the reader that there are no definitive insights into the role of the 5q deletion in MDS. This deletion, although relevant in the cells in which it is found, may not be an obligatory element for evolution of the dysplastic process or the development of leukemia. Several patients have been reported with classic clinical features of the 5q− syndrome whose karyotype was normal until years after presentation, when a 5q− chromosome was finally detected.[319–321] This could indicate that the 5q− change itself is not primarily causal or could simply point out the insensitivity of present detection methods. A normal hematopoietic stem cell may give rise to a dysplastic or malignant clone by any one of several multistep pathways, one or more of which might include the 5q− chromosome.

Other Genetic Abnormalities

Figure 12-6 emphasizes the complexity of the cytogenetic abnormalities found in patients with MDS. These changes are the tip of the iceberg, since many deletions and translocations may be too small to be detectable by current techniques and populations of cells with chromosomal changes that are rare or nonviable in culture must often be missed. Many point mutations in specific genes, as yet undiscovered, may be relevant to the evolution of these syndromes. The frequent translocations could create new gene products that contribute to dyshematopoiesis or leukemogenesis. Finally, chromosome loss may influence cellular differentiation either by gene dosage effects or by unmasking recessive oncogenes as described above in our consideration of the 5q− chromosome. It may also be that many of these changes are completely irrelevant to the pathogenesis of MDS but occur as a result of genetic instability produced by the primary mutational event. The interested investigator may be forced to sift through genetic debris in an effort to identify important mutations.

Model for Evolution

A model that addresses many facets of the pathogenesis and biology of MDS is outlined in Figure 12-8. This model is based on a selection-driven process of carcinogenesis as outlined by Temin[269] and first suggested to us in the context of MDS by Dr. Alan Jacobs (personal communication). Implicit within this model is the infrequent occurrence of mutations that subtly enhance the growth properties of cells without rendering them fully neoplastic. Over time, gradual overgrowth occurs within the total population of cells possessing even a modest proliferative advantage. The occurrence of additional mutations is more likely within this expanding population, and gradually a mixture of competing subclones emerges within the population. This process of mutation and selective proliferation of an increasingly complex mixture of subclones and sub-subclones may go on indefinitely until the whole population of cells lacks sufficient maturational capacity to produce circulating blood elements in adequate numbers or until a subclonal population finally arises with frankly leukemic properties.

The model is supported by several of the biologic features of MDS. At any point in the evolution of the syndrome, the bone marrow may contain from one to several distinct subpopulations of cells each derived from the original single hematopoietic stem cell, as well as ever-decreasing numbers of unaffected stem cells. Cytogenetic studies of MDS

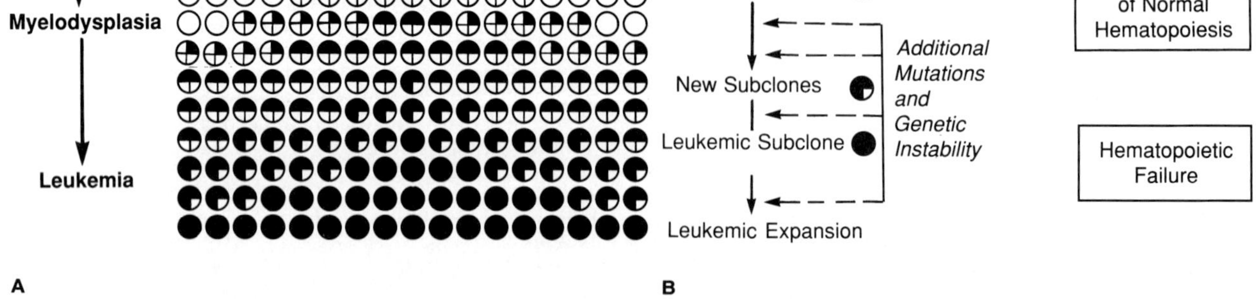

FIGURE 12-8. A model for the pathogenesis of the myelodysplastic syndromes. (**A**) Representation of a selection-driven process of neoplasia. A cohort of cells is shown moving through time (for clarity, no increase in the total number of cells is shown). Each mutation is represented by a filled-in quadrant. A transformed, leukemic cell is completely filled in. Each mutated cell has a growth advantage over less mutated cells. Thus, mutant cells increase in relative quantity and are more likely to suffer further mutations. (**B**) Representation of the possible corresponding events occurring in the development and progression of the myelodysplastic syndromes from an initial genetic insult to death from hematopoietic failure or leukemia. (**A** after Temin HM. Evolution of cancer genes as a mutation-driven process. Cancer Res 1988;48:1698; **B** after Jacobs A, Clark RE. Pathogenesis and clinical variations in the myelodysplastic syndromes. Clin Haematol 1986;15:928)

have documented the coexistence of subclones with unrelated karyotypic abnormalities,[246,322] the accumulation over time of additional cytogenetic or point mutations in an already marked clone,[216,236,237,239,240,284] and gradual replacement of one karyotypically marked subclone by another.[243–245] Each subclone may contain an overlapping but distinct set of mutations that provide it with a selective growth advantage.

Emergence or loss of specific cytogenetic abnormalities or gene mutations may be caused by spontaneous competitive or therapy-induced shifts in subpopulations and need not call into question the relevance of a specific genetic change to the pathogenesis of MDS. Conversely, the disappearance of a specific cytogenetic abnormality need not reflect elimination of the entire dysplastic population of cells from the bone marrow but only that of the most actively proliferating and thus therapy-sensitive subclone. Therapy-induced remissions may be particularly difficult to achieve if the entire stem cell pool is occupied by dysplastic cells. This hypothesis is consistent with the fact that remissions are more difficult to obtain in patients with AML evolving from MDS than in patients with de novo AML, who may have some remaining normal stem cells.

The pathogenetic model contrasts with the genetic mechanisms that induce CML. The chimeric *BCR-ABL* gene arising from the chromosome 9:22 translocation is virtually always present in CML cells.[323] Recent experiments in mice have shown that expression of the *BCR-ABL* gene in normal hematopoietic cells creates a syndrome resembling CML.[324] The *BCR-ABL* gene appears to be a dominant-acting oncogene, providing hematopoietic cells with a potent proliferative advantage and leading to the emergence of a homogeneous, proliferating population of cells with nearly normal maturation. Certainly, the genetic mechanisms in CML are more complex, but the *BCR-ABL* gene appears to have a major pathogenetic role and is specific for the clinical CML syndrome. In contrast, our model of MDS implies the operation of many mutations, each of which has subtle effects on both proliferation and maturation evolving to a mixed population of dysplastic cells.

Damage to DNA must be a common feature of MDS. The multiplicity of cytogenetic abnormalities obvious in MDS supports the notion of inherent genetic instability. As already mentioned, both alkylating agents and irradiation, known to damage DNA, are implicated in t-MDS. The frequent occurrence of identical cytogenetic abnormalities in primary MDS and in t-MDS and t-AML suggests that a search should be made for exposure to mutagens for patients with the primary syndromes and abnormalities of chromosomes 5 and 7. Mitelman and colleagues[325] and Golumb and associates[326] have found that patients with AML and histories of significant exposure to pesticides, industrial metals, petroleum solvents, and other chemicals had significantly higher incidences of karyotypic changes of chromosomes 5 or 7.

Only limited direct experimental data support genetic instability or aberrant DNA repair as causal mechanisms in MDS. MDS shares with Fanconi's syndrome, Bloom's syndrome, and ataxia telangiectasia a predisposition to leukemia or other hematologic malignancies. Patients with these disorders have been shown to have increased chromosomal breakage in response to ultraviolet (UV) light or chemical mutagens. Progress is being made toward identifying specific DNA repair defects in these disorders that produce an inability to withstand environmental mutagenic pressure.[327–329] Preliminary reports of abnormalities of heterochromatin structure, sister chromatid exchange, and DNA repair after UV light mutagenesis in bone marrow cells from patients with MDS have been published.[330–332] As more components of eukaryotic DNA repair pathways are defined, their function can be tested in patients with MDS and specific questions regarding underlying defects addressed.

PATHOPHYSIOLOGY

Much effort has been devoted to characterizing the biologic and biochemical abnormalities of myelodysplastic hematopoietic cells. Recent advances in in vitro culture methodology and the isolation and characterization of hematopoietic growth factors and their receptors have stimulated attempts to define derangements in cellular proliferation and maturation. The myriad functional and biochemical abnormalities that presumably result from damage to the genome and disordered hematopoietic cell maturation are catalogued and their significance to the clinical manifestations of MDS is assessed.

Hematopoiesis

Techniques for growth of bone marrow progenitor cells in semisolid culture media have been developed over the past two decades and have proven invaluable to hematologic research (see Chap. 8).[333] Figure 12-9 is a simplified diagram of hematopoiesis and summarizes the nomenclature used to identify the various hematopoietic progenitors according to their growth requirements and colony morphology.

Several facets of the pathophysiology of MDS can be analyzed with existing culture methodology. An understanding of the properties of hematopoietic progenitors that cause failure of blood cell formation is desired. Relevant parameters are number of progenitors, their capacity for maturation, their interaction with stromal elements and response to growth factors, and the existence of pathologic inhibitory mechanisms. Experiments have been performed to address each of these issues without yet providing simple answers.

Progenitor Growth

Granulocyte-macrophage CFUs (CFU-GM) are usually decreased in blood or bone marrow of patients with MDS.[334–339] In addition, blocks in the differentiation of myeloid cells may be present.[340–343] No strict correlations between colony growth patterns and FAB subclass exist,[344] although patients in a transition phase to acute leukemia often develop increasingly abnormal colony growth characteristics. These patients have even fewer normal colonies with more small clusters and blast cell colonies than are characteristically found in cultures of leukemic marrow.[345–347] Abnormally high cluster/colony ratios are also common in those with t-MDS.[30]

Patients with CMML are an exception, since they often have increased or normal numbers of CFU-GM in their marrow.[337] Additionally, GM colonies can be grown from many CMML patients without addition of the exogenous hematopoietic growth factors that are necessary to grow colonies from normal marrow.[295,296]

Erythroid and megakaryocytic colony formation are also often abnormal in patients with MDS. The number of CFU-erythroid (CFU-E) progenitor can be normal or increased, but the number of less mature burst-forming units–erythroid (BFU-E) progenitor cell is generally profoundly decreased.[334,335,337,348,349] Low numbers of CFU-megakaryocyte (CFU-Meg) usually parallel decreased erythroid colony growth.[348,350,351] Mixed colonies arising from multilineage progenitors (CFU-GEMM) were also decreased in one study.[337] Patients with the 5q− abnormality and RA

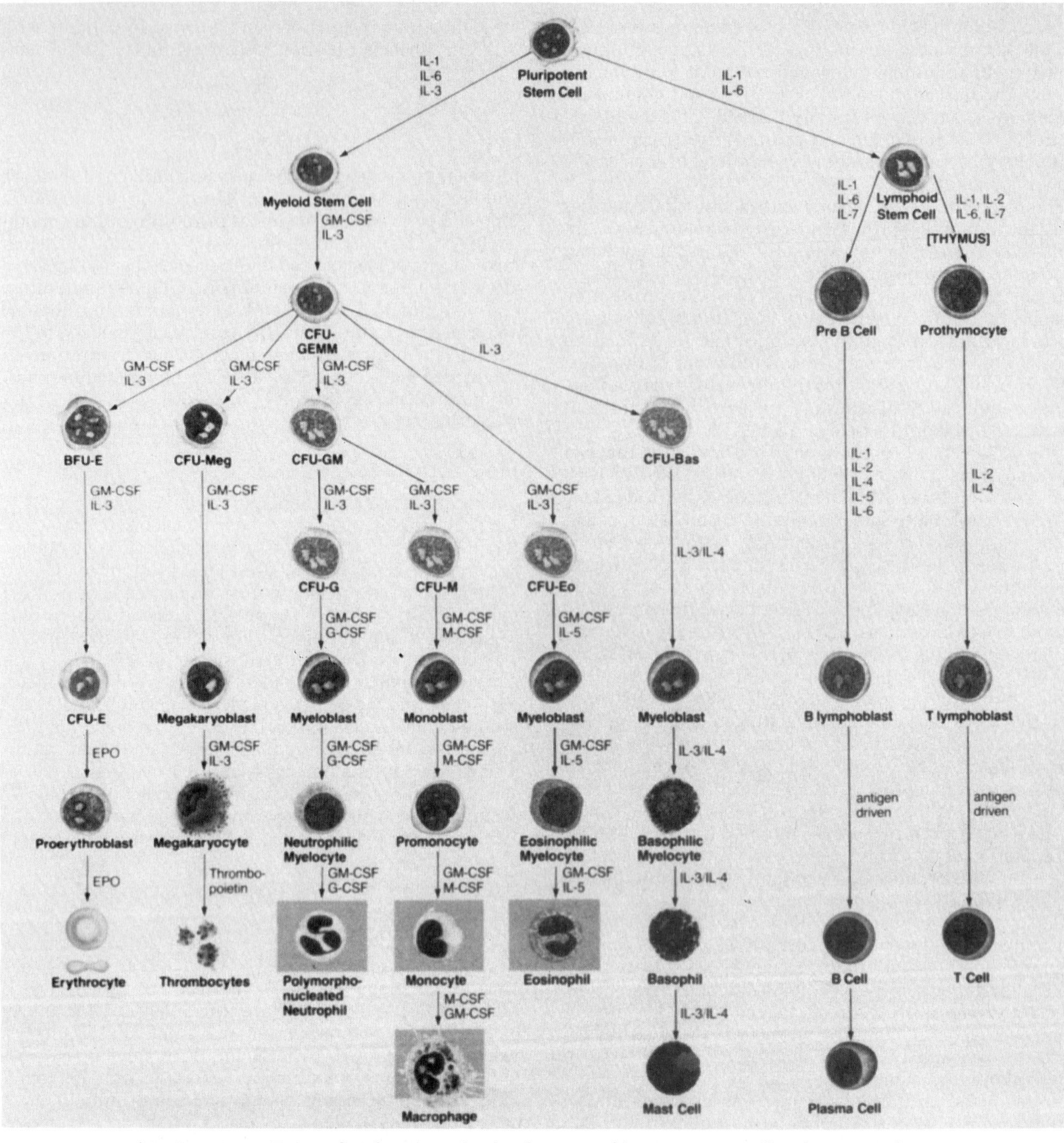

FIGURE 12-9. Proposed pathways in the development of hematopoietic cells. The nomenclature for each cell type is given in bold print below each cell diagram. The growth factors thought to be involved in each step are also indicated. CFU, colony-forming unit; BFU, burst-forming unit; E, erythroid; M, macrophage; G, granulocyte; GM, granulocyte-macrophage; Eo, eosinophil; Bas, basophil; Meg, megakaryocyte; GEMM, mixed; IL, interleukin; CSF, colony-stimulating factor; EPO, erythropoietin. (Courtesy of the Sandoz Pharmaceutical Corporation, East Hanover, NJ)

often have normal numbers of CFU-GM but profoundly decreased BFU-E.[160,352]

The in vitro culture results may not fully reflect disordered hematopoiesis in vivo. Patients with absent CFU-GM growth may maintain adequate neutrophil counts,[33] whereas cytogenetically abnormal progenitors can form both myeloid and erythroid colonies in culture.[196,352,353] The proliferative capability of bone marrow precursors from all lineages as assessed in vitro by DNA synthesis or progression into S phase from G1 is reduced.[354–356] The ability of MDS progenitors to compete with normal progenitors in vivo also may not correlate with their in vitro behavior.[247,249] Colony analysis of hematopoietic progenitors can help predict prognosis and plan therapy in some patients.[30,339,346]

The response of MDS hematopoietic cells to growth factors may also be abnormal. In semisolid culture, CFU numbers can be increased or even normalized by the addition of higher than standard concentrations of growth factors.[357–359] This increased requirement might result from down-regulated or poorly transducing receptors, or from a relative deficiency of accessory cell-derived growth factors in cultures of MDS bone marrow.[359] Most studies examining growth factor production by T cells or stromal cells from patients with MDS have shown normal production of hematopoietic growth factors.[336,360,361]

Even less evidence is available for cell-mediated or humoral inhibition of normal hematopoiesis in patients with MDS. Both murine and human leukemic cells have been shown to secrete substances inhibitory to normal hematopoietic proliferation in vitro.[362,363] Conflicting data exist regarding the presence of humoral factors that inhibit megakaryocytopoiesis in patients with MDS.[350,364,365] One study reported NK cell inhibition of autologous CFU-GM in a small number of patients with MDS.[366] Further investigation is required before the importance of inhibitory activities can be assessed.

Growth Factors

The possibility has been raised that patients with MDS do not respond to cytopenias in vivo by producing appropriately high concentrations of stimulatory hematopoietic growth factors. Several studies have reported much lower levels of megakaryocyte colony-stimulating activity than expected in the serum of patients with MDS and thrombocytopenia compared with that of patients with other causes for thrombocytopenia such as aplastic anemia.[350,364,365] In general, serum erythropoietin (EPO) levels are elevated in patients with MDS, but not always to the extent predicted by the blood hemoglobin level.[367] As in other situations in which the EPO response seems inappropriately blunted, such as in sickle cell anemia, anemia of chronic disease, or megaloblastic anemias, EPO production may be regulated by overall erythroid cellularity in the marrow as well as by blood oxygen carrying capacity.[368–371] Treatment with hematopoietic growth factors including EPO may have some rational basis if an impaired capacity for growth factor production is convincingly demonstrated.

Autocrine Mechanisms

Another intriguing possibility is that release from growth factor requirements allows affected MDS clones to gain dominance in the marrow. This mechanism seems potentially applicable when a dominant proliferative component is present, as in CMML patients, or during evolution to acute leukemia. CFU-GM, CFU-E, and clusters that grow in culture without the addition of exogenous growth factors have been detected in the bone marrow of a small number of patients with MDS,[334,350,361,372] with autonomous CFU-GM especially common in patients with CMML.[295,296] Perhaps hyperresponsive progenitor cells can be stimulated by small amounts of growth factors present in the serum component of the culture media or secreted by accessory cells. Another possible explanation is that some MDS hematopoietic cells have dysregulated growth factor production. They may be able to abnormally produce and then respond to a particular factor (autocrine effects) or to stimulate or inhibit neighboring cells (paracrine effects).

The possibility that release from normal growth constraints by autocrine stimulation could be an important step in the development of neoplasia has been the focus of intense recent interest and experimentation.[373,374] Blast cells from some patients with AML have been found to contain growth factor mRNA and to secrete a variety of factors. Several studies have demonstrated that antibodies that neutralize the secreted growth factors inhibit colony formation by these cells.[374,375] A similar mechanism may contribute to dominance by abnormal clones or initiate progression to leukemia.[376,377] Evidence is thus far lacking, except for a recent study that reported autocrine production of GM-CSF and interleukin-6 (IL-6) from cultured CMML marrow cells, with inhibition of colony formation by neutralizing antibodies to GM-CSF and IL-6.[295] The presence on bone marrow biopsy of ALIPs separated from the bony trabecular surface has suggested to some authors that these cells have become autonomous and are no longer dependent on stromally supplied growth factors.[377]

It is unlikely that autocrine stimulation could be the sole or primary mechanism in MDS. Dysregulated production of several growth factors by hematopoietic progenitors has been shown in several animal models to lead to myeloproliferative states with *preserved* maturation.[378–380] The defective maturation that is the hallmark of MDS probably results from another type of mutation.

Disordered Maturation of Hematopoietic Cells

Normal committed hematopoietic progenitors in each lineage experience a pathway of differentiation that culminates in mature, functional, nonmitotic cells. A myriad of biochemical and functional abnormalities within the cells of all lineages has been described in patients with MDS. An understanding of their incidence and functional consequences is an important goal because many patients with MDS die from infections or bleeding resulting at least partially from dysfunction of circulating cells. Damage to one or a few involved genes may result in disordered patterns of gene expression and thus cellular maturation and function. Observations of lineage infidelity and reversion to fetal cellular characteristics support this hypothesis. Specific biochemical defects might also arise if a mutation affected a normal allele at a locus that already harbored a defect on the opposite chromosome.

Abnormalities in Erythroid Cells

Erythroid activity in MDS bone marrow can vary widely from hypoplasia to hyperplasia with massively ineffective erythropoiesis.[77] Many qualitative abnormalities have also been described, in some instances leading to hemolysis and worsening of anemia. Often, decreased activity is seen of RBC enzymes, including pyruvate kinase, phosphofructokinase, adenylate kinase, and diphosphoglycerate mutase or increases in the activities of 6-phosphogluconate dehydrogenase, and G6PD, hexokinase, aldolase, adenosine deaminase, and enolase.[381–383] The patterns of enzyme alteration may vary among patients. Increased dihydrofolate reductase activity has been shown to persist to an abnormally late stage of erythroid development.[384] Clinically significant hemolysis has been reported in association with a reduction in pyruvate kinase or an increase in adenosine deaminase activities.[385–388]

Decreased expression of blood group antigens within the ABO group has been reported, probably resulting from decreased activity of the galactosyltransferases that add carbohydrate side chains to proteins on the RBC surface.[383,389,390] In some cases, the i antigen (fetal) is expressed rather than the I antigen (adult). Fetal hemoglobin levels are elevated up to 5% to 37% of the total hemoglobin in RBCs from patients with MDS.[391] In a few patients, acquired hemoglobin H (unstable tetramers of β-globin chains) has been detected.[392–394] Decreased α-globin gene transcription can be shown in erythroid cells from these patients. The four α genes are intact, suggesting operation of a transacting mechanism.

Ringed Sideroblast Formation

Ringed sideroblasts are common in patients with MDS and can be detected in various quantities in all FAB subtypes.[40] Over the past three decades, numerous attempts have been made to define the mechanism of ringed sideroblast formation and the connection between the presence of these cells and the underlying primary defects in MDS.[12,41,42,142,395–398] An understanding of the pathogenesis of ringed sideroblasts in patients with MDS has been hampered in many investigations by the grouping together of the several different underlying conditions associated with ringed sideroblasts (see Table 12-7).

Figure 12-10 shows diagrams of some of the steps iron takes between its arrival at an early erythroid cell and its incorporation into hemoglobin (these pathways are discussed in detail elsewhere). Heme synthesis intermediates are transported through the mitochondrial membrane at least twice, and several enzymatic steps occur within the mitochondria. Any hypothesis must account for normal or increased iron uptake into erythroid progenitors and abnormal accumulation within mitochondria, but decreased incorporation into heme, and thus into hemoglobin. At least three mechanisms for abnormal mitochondrial iron deposition in ringed sideroblasts and associated disordered erythropoiesis have been considered: defects in the enzymes or cofactors of the heme synthetic pathway; defects in the transport or processing of iron before it is incorporated into heme; and generalized mitochondrial defects.

Interest in defects of the heme synthetic pathway enzymes or cofactors was generated by several observations. Pyridoxine after phosphorylation to pyridoxal phosphate, is a cofactor for the enzyme δ-aminolevulinic acid synthase (ALA-S), which combines glycine and succinyl coenzyme A into ALA. In hepatic cells and less clearly in erythroid cells, this step is rate-limiting in heme synthesis. In some experimental animals, pyridoxine deficiency produces anemia and ringed sideroblast formation.[398] Patients on isoniazid and other antituberculous drugs occasionally develop anemia and ringed sideroblasts (RARS), which disappear when the drugs are discontinued; the drug interferes with the transport of pyridoxine to the cells.[41,398,399] At least a small percentage of patients with both acquired and hereditary sideroblastic anemia improve while on pharmacologic doses of pyridoxine.[400,401]

ALA-S activity is decreased in bone marrow cells of some patients with either acquired or hereditary types of sideroblastic anemia.[402–405] In several hereditary pyridoxine-responsive patients, the actual amount of ALA-S mRNA is low[406]; in others, the ALA-S protein itself is abnormally sensitive to degradation by a mitochondrial protease.[407,408] Further interest in this enzyme has been generated by the finding that although the hepatic isozyme gene is on chromosome 3,[409] the erythroid ALA-S gene may be on the X chromosome.[406] Most families with hereditary sideroblastic anemia exhibit an X-linked inheritance pattern.[410–415] Other enzymatic steps in the pathway—most frequently that of ferrochelatase (heme synthase)—have also been reported to be affected in at least some patients.[403] Elevated levels

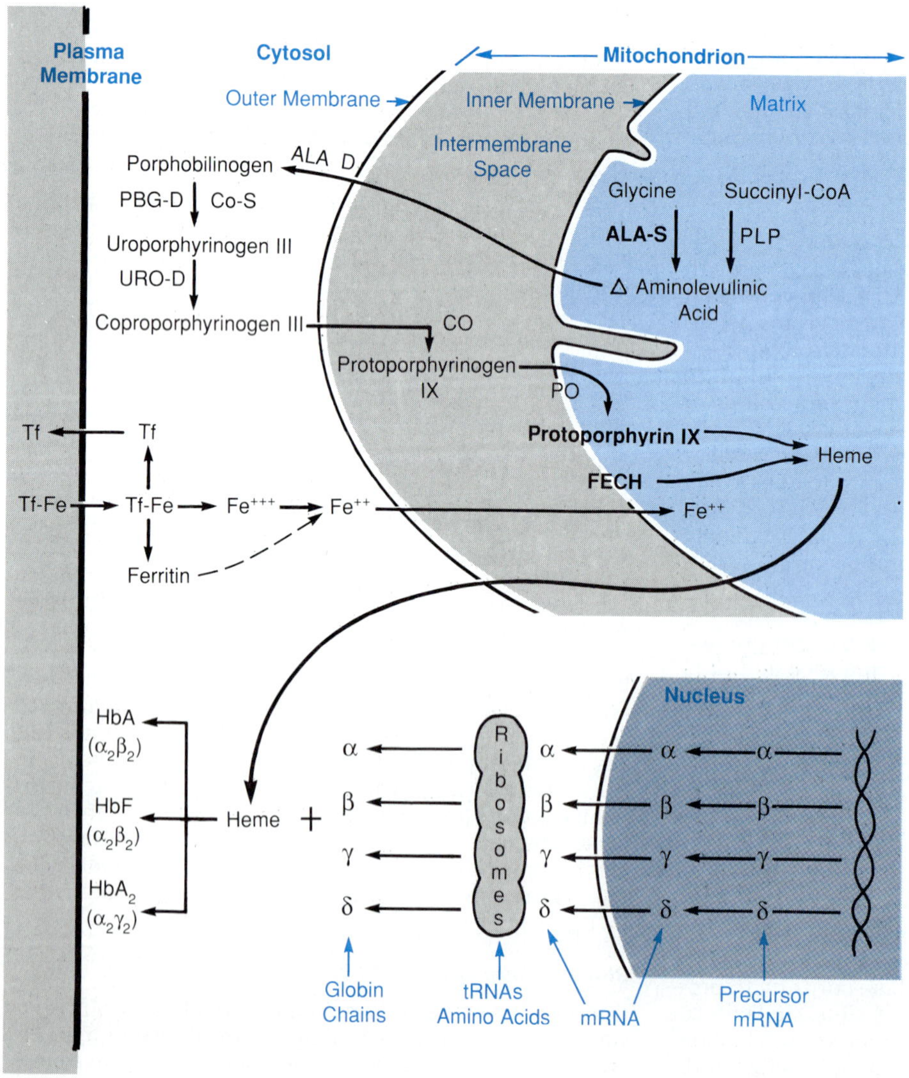

FIGURE 12-10. Pathways of heme synthesis. ALA-S, δ-aminolevulinic acid synthase; PLP, pyridoxal phosphate; ALA-D, δ-aminolevulinic acid dehydratase; PBG-D, porphobilinogen deaminase; CoS, uroporphyrinogen cosynthase; URO-D, uroporphyrinogen decarboxylase; CO, coproporphyrinogen oxidase; PO, protoporphyrinogen oxidase; FECH, ferrochelatase; Tf, transferrin; Hb, hemoglobin. (Courtesy of S.S. Bottomley, MD, University of Oklahoma)

of free erythrocyte protoporphyrin (FEP) result from blockage of the heme synthetic pathway at the ferrochelatase step.[416,417]

Other evidence suggests that these enzyme defects are not the primary mechanisms for ringed sideroblast formation in RARS or in patients with MDS. In these patients, abnormal mitochondrial iron deposition can be detected in early erythroid precursors before initiation of heme synthesis.[418] Lead inhibits heme synthesis enzymes, including ALA-S and ferrochelatase, but ringed sideroblasts are rare or nonexistent in the bone marrow of patients with lead poisoning.[398] No evidence shows actual pyridoxine or PRP deficiency in patients with MDS.[419] In patients with erythropoietic porphyria, a specific defect in ferrochelatase activity is found. These patients have high levels of FEP and urine and stool porphyrins but do not develop ringed sideroblasts.[420] A patient with RARS and high circulating levels of FEP was studied and found to have normal ALA-S and ferrochelatase activities but no photosensitivity or other signs of porphyria.[416] At least two patients with RARS and high levels of FEP developed photosensitivity in conjunction with low ferrochelatase activity.[417,421] Obviously, the situation is complicated and not yet well understood, even when patients with acquired and hereditary forms of sideroblastic anemias are carefully separated.

The second hypothesis involves primary defects of iron uptake or cellular processing. A small study found an association between RARS and the HLA A3 allele, which had previously been strongly linked to hemochromatosis.[143] It was suggested that patients heterozygous for the hemachromatosis allele were in some way predisposed to developing ringed sideroblasts and RARS, but in larger series this association was not borne out.[144–146] Patients with iron overload from primary hemochromatosis or secondary hemosiderosis due to transfusion or ineffective erythropoiesis accumulate iron in normal ferritin storage granules but do not develop ringed sideroblasts.

Others have suggested that there is defective reduction of ferric iron (Fe^{3+}) to ferrous iron (FE^{2+}), which is necessary before incorporation into heme can occur.[41,398,416] An abnormal amount of Fe^{3+} could accumulate, damaging mitochondria via free radical formation, before precipitation as ferric phosphate.[422] Feedback inhibition of iron uptake into cells may normally be controlled by intracellular heme concentration.[398] If heme synthesis decreases, cells may continue to take up iron despite increased intracellular stores. By whatever mechanism, it is likely that abnormal iron deposition in mitochondria further disrupts the heme synthetic pathway and impairs erythropoiesis. Cellular iron deposition inhibits uroporphyrinogen decarboxylase.[423] In fact, some patients with RARS or hereditary sideroblastic anemia have shown hematologic improvement with iron chelation or phlebotomy, presumably by interrupting this vicious cycle of iron deposition and further cellular damage.[423–425,426]

The third hypothesis invokes a generalized mitochondrial defect. Aoki[427] demonstrated that the activities of many mitochondrial enzymes, including nonheme synthetic pathway enzymes, were decreased in patients with RARS, whereas ALA-S activity alone was decreased in patients with pyridoxine-responsive hereditary sideroblastic anemia. These defects were also detected in granulocytes from RARS patients, although not in lymphocytes. Secondary mitochondrial damage from iron deposition could be an explanation of generalized erythroid mitochondrial dysfunction, but the presence of defects in granulocyte mitochondria is difficult to explain except by a primary defect.

We do not yet know which, if any, of these hypotheses will explain the formation of ringed sideroblasts in patients with MDS. As with other functional and morphologic defects found in MDS cells, these abnormalities of the iron metabolic pathway may result from abnormal maturation of hematopoietic precursors. Processes leading to ringed sideroblast formation are probably secondary and not related to the propensity for leukemia seen in these patients. In contrast, hereditary sideroblastic anemias are not preleukemic or trilineage disorders; primary mechanisms in these anemias are much more likely to involve specific genetic defects in the heme synthetic pathway or iron transport.

Abnormalities in Platelets

Abnormalities of platelet function may contribute to the bleeding tendencies sometimes encountered even in patients with MDS with adequate platelet counts. Platelet granules may be sparse or abnormally large. In one study, 15 of 16 patients with MDS had giant dense granules that did not release their contents normally during platelet aggregation. The authors postulated that these granules arose through abnormal fusion of many smaller granules.[131,132] Platelet adenosine diphosphate content and thromboxane A_2 activity are low in some patients with MDS.[428] Responses to collagen and epinephrine can be blunted,[125,428,429] and the bleeding time is increased in as many as half of patients with MDS, even with normal platelet counts.[428] These abnormalities are not unique to patients with MDS, having also been reported in myeloproliferative syndromes.

Abnormalities in Myeloid Cells

As described earlier in this chapter, lineage infidelity of MDS granulocytes and monocytes, as assessed by surface marker and cytochemical phenotyping, is common.[50,430] Tests of neutrophil function yield heterogeneous results, but in the most detailed study, 20 of 20 patients had at least one abnormality of chemotaxis, phagocytosis, adhesion, chemiluminescence, or microbicidal capacity of neutrophil-specific enzyme activity.[431] The myeloperoxidase content of granules in polymorphonuclear leukocytes was low in a number of studies,[432–435] but in vitro killing of *Staphlococcus aureus* or *Candida albicans* was not consistently impaired.[432,433,435,436] Given the high mortality and morbidity rates due to infection in patients with MDS, neutrophil abnormalities may be significant in vivo.

Immune Dysfunction

The involvement of the lymphoid system in both the pathophysiology and the clinical manifestations of MDS has not been extensively investigated but could prove important. As noted previously in some studies, B lymphocytes, and less consistently T lymphocytes, are part of the abnormal affected clone in MDS.[188–190,197,197a] Lymphoid cells are probably the primary source of many of the hematopoietic growth factors in vivo; the lack of normal factor production due to lymphoid dysfunction could be a mechanism for deranged hematopoiesis. It is also possible that disordered immune surveillance permits expansion of abnormal marrow clones. No experimental evidence exists for or against these hypotheses.

Immunophenotyping with monoclonal antibodies to cell surface markers has documented pronounced decreases in T-cell count, specifically helper T4 cells, and a shift in the T4/T8 ratio.[49,437–439] Some authors have suggested that the relative increase in T8 suppressor activity could inhibit both hematopoiesis and antibody production. These changes in T-cell populations might result from the primary disease or may be secondary to the multiple transfusions that most patients with MDS have received.[439]

B-cell numbers are often decreased and antibody-dependent cellular cytotoxicity is impaired in some but not all patients with MDS.[49,118,440] On the other hand, many patients with MDS have hypergammaglobulinemia; one study showed a monoclonal immunoglobulin spike in 12.5%.[73,441] Coombs-positive hemolysis has been documented only rarely in these patients, and other antoantibodies have also been detected.[73,441]

Interest has also focused on NK cell numbers and activity, since NK activity is universally low in MDS because of decreased NK cell counts.[49,117,118,438,442,443] The addition of interferon only partially corrects the defect.[117,118] Because NK cells may be involved in regulation of hematopoiesis and seem to play a role in tumor surveillance, a decrease in NK-cell count could permit toleration of abnormal MDS clones and produce dyshematopoiesis.

CLINICAL COURSE AND PROGNOSIS

The prognosis for most patients with MDS is grim, with overall median durations of survival being only 2 years. Spontaneous complete remission or hematologic improvement rarely if ever occurs. The initial diagnosis of MDS should be critically reevaluated in any patient whose cytopenias or bone marrow dysplasia disappears without intervention. On the other hand, the clinical course is variable in MDS, and some patients live relatively normal lives for many years after diagnosis, with or without treatment. Thus, much effort has been focused on methods for predicting prognosis.

Causes of Morbidity and Mortality

Despite the pervasive application of the term *preleukemia*, transformation to acute leukemia accounts for only 30% of MDS mortality.[58,82,83,165,444] Another 40% of patients die from complications of bone marrow dysfunction, including infection, bleeding, and iron overload. The remaining 30% of patients die from seemingly unrelated conditions, such as cardiovascular disease or nonhematologic malignancies. In fact, survival from the time of diagnosis of MDS is no worse or better in patients who develop leukemia than in those who do not.[84,444,445] One possible explanation for this surprising finding is that patients with severe cytopenias die early from infection or bleeding, whereas those with less severe cytopenias survive longer, increasing the likelihood of progression to leukemia.

The most common infectious complications are bacterial in nature, in the lower respiratory tract, skin, and perineal area. Risk of infection is high even in patients with adequate numbers of neutrophils, presumably because of functional neutrophil impairment or generalized immune dysfunction.[83,114,439] Likewise, bleeding in nonthrombocytopenic patients may occur because of platelet dysfunction so that platelet transfusions may be indicated before major surgery. The surprisingly high percentage of deaths attributed to causes with no known direct relation to MDS most likely reflects the advanced age of the affected population, but the chronic effects of anemia and immune dysfunction may contribute to second malignancies and cardiac mortality.[83]

Parameters Predictive of Prognosis

The FAB classification system has prognostic usefulness.[58,73,74,81,83,84,89,137,165,446,447] Table 12-8 summarizes the median survival after presentation and risk of progression to leukemia by FAB subtype in several large studies. Survival curves are shown in Figure 12-11. The variable results among studies can be accounted for in most cases by exclusion or inclusion of patients with t-MDS, by differences in median age, or by differences due to referral patterns. Variable methods for assignment of patients who seem to fall into two FAB subclasses may also account for some discrepancies; such patients should be assigned to the FAB class with the poorer prognosis, for example, RAEB instead of RARS or CMML, if greater than 5% marrow blasts are present.[7,73] If this is done, RARS patients generally have a somewhat longer median survival than RA patients, followed by CMML, RAEB, and RAEBT, in that order.

TABLE 12-8. Prognosis in Myelodysplastic Syndromes

Study	RA	RARS	RAEB	RAEBT	CMML	Overall
MEDIAN SURVIVAL IN MONTHS FROM PRESENTATION BY FAB SUBTYPE						
Kerkhofs[73]	50	60+	9	6	60+	47
Sanz[137]	26	34	9	5	12	15
Tricot[444]	46	53	28	11	23	15
Varela[449]	38	53	13	3	17	26
Foucar[82]	64	71	7	5	8	10
Coiffer[58]	102	131	26*	26*	28	53
Mufti[89]	32	76	10.5	5	21	23
Teerenhovi[165]	48	41	21	13	16	29
PERCENTAGE LEUKEMIC TRANSFORMATION BY FAB SUBTYPE						
Kerkhofs[73]	25	16	64	60	18	37
Sanz[137]	21	39	57	82	15	—
Tricot[444]	11	11	56	56	56	—
Varela[449]	15	12	41	75	33	29
Foucar[82]	15	0	32	50	27	27
Coiffer[58]	15	20	44*	44*	40	32
Mufti[89]	11	5	28	55	13	—
Teerenhovi[165]	14	17	38	75	28	26.5

* Patients with RAEB and RAEBT were pooled in this study.

Because the range of survival times within each subtype of MDS, especially RA and RARS, may be variable, many investigators have sought additional parameters besides FAB subtype to improve the accuracy of predicting prognosis in patients. Circulating blasts, whether myeloid or erythroid, may be an ominous sign.[58,81] Large numbers of circulating monocytes predict shorter survival in patients with CMML.[153,448] Other studies found trilineage marrow dysplasia prognostically poor in all FAB subtypes.[82,449] Increased erythroid activity, even if ineffective, is more favorable than a predominantly myeloid marrow.[58,341,450,451] A high percentage of ringed sideroblasts is also a good sign and usually occurs in conjunction with a predominantly erythroid marrow.[58,250,452] Paradoxically, a hypocellular marrow is either good or neutral prognostically.[33,56,57,445,447]

Another predictive morphologic abnormality is the presence of ALIPs on bone marrow biopsy, which are clumps of myeloid blast cells or promyelocytes aberrantly localized at a distance from bony trabeculae.[36] Median survival of patients with ALIPs is only 12 months, regardless of FAB subclass, and 50 months without ALIPs.[67,239,444] ALIPs are most useful in identifying RA, RARS, or CMML patients with less favorable prognoses, because almost all patients with RAEB or RAEBT have ALIPs.[76,444,453] Although the presence of Auer rods dictates inclusion in the RAEBT FAB category, these rods have not been clearly shown to herald a higher rate of transformation.[51,82]

In vitro cell culture has also been a source of prognostically useful information. Severely curtailed CFU-GM growth from the bone marrow has been associated with shorter survival in both primary and t-MDS.[30,58,339] For un-

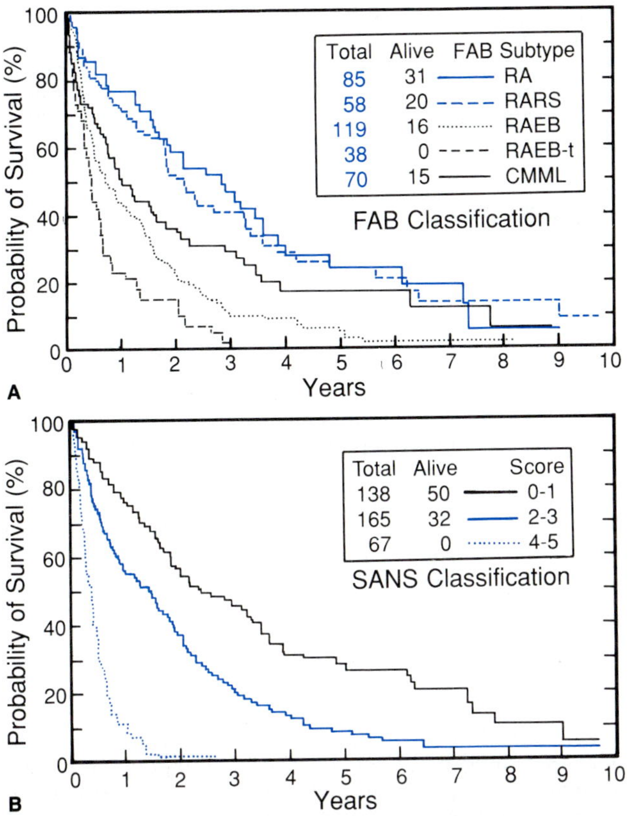

FIGURE 12-11. (A) Survival according to FAB subtype of 370 patients with myelodysplastic syndrome. The Kaplan-Meier product limit was used to estimate probability of survival. RA, refractory anemia; RARS, refractory anemia with ringed sideroblasts; RAEB, refractory anemia with excess of blasts; RAEB-t, refractory with excess of blasts in transformation. (B) Survival according to the Sanz scoring system (see Table 12-9) of the same 370 patients. (After Sanz GF, Sanz MA, Vallespi T, et al. Two regression models and a scoring system for predicting survival and planning treatment in myelodysplastic syndromes: a multivariate analysis of prognostic factors in 370 patients. Blood 1989;74:400)

known reasons, dependence of marrow cells on phytohemagglutinin for growth in vitro is associated with an increased risk for leukemia.[454]

Clinical parameters have also been investigated for their prognostic significance in MDS, both as single variables and by multivariate analysis. As might be expected, most investigators have found pancytopenia,[455] thrombocytopenia,[58,81,165] neutropenia,[58,444] and severe anemia or transfusion dependence[81,84,165,447] to independently predict shorter survival. Several years ago, Mufti and coworkers[89] combined degree of cytopenias and bone marrow blast percentages into the Bournemouth scoring system, shown in Table 12-9. The system is simple and prognostically useful and has been modified to better accommodate CMML,[456] or subdivided based on bone marrow blast percentage for better accuracy[137] (see Table 12-9). Survival curves generated by this scoring system in the largest cohort of patients with MDS studied to date are shown in Figure 12-11.

Most studies have not found sex to be prognostically important, and the predictive value of patient age is limited. Younger patients (defined as from less than 40 years to less than 65 years old, according to the study) have been found by some studies to have longer survival rates,[137,447] but by others to have a worse prognosis, especially due to leukemic transformation.[165,215,444] These discrepancies may stem from the inclusion of younger patients with t-MDS in some cohorts since primary myelodysplasia in patients under 40

TABLE 12-9. Prognostic Scoring Systems

Criteria	Points	Class	Points
BOURNEMOUTH SCORE[89]			
Bone marrow blast > 5%	1	A	0–1
Platelets < 100,000/μL	1	B	2–3
Hemoglobin < 10 g/dL	1	C	4
Neutrophils < 2500/μL	1		
SANZ ET AL[136] MODIFICATION			
Age > 60	1	A	0–1
Platelets			
< 100,000/μL	1	B	2–3
< 50,000/μL	2	C	4–5
Bone marrow blast			
5–10%	1		
> 10%	2		

is extremely rare. There is also a recent report clearly showing that the apparent incidence of MDS is increasing as physicians become more aware of the syndrome and screen their elderly patients.[444a] This increased prevalence may affect the interpretation of previous studies relating age and prognosis.

The few published pediatric studies all define MDS or preleukemia only retrospectively after the onset of acute leukemia.[92–95,220] Refractory cytopenias with dysplastic changes precede 5% to 17% of childhood AML cases.[92,95,220] It is not clear how frequently children with clinical and morphologic characteristics of MDS fail to progress rapidly to AML since an indolent course in children has not been reported. Survivals are brief because resultant leukemias are often refractory to chemotherapy, and a high incidence of serious infections, especially in children with monosomy 7, is seen.[92,95,244,457–459] The incidence of monosomy 5 or 7 in childhood preleukemic disorders has suggested that a potent mutagen is involved in pathogenesis because the same cytogenetic changes are commonly found in t-MDS and in patients with significant chemical exposures.[173]

Complex formulas have been devised for more precise prediction of prognosis based on clinical, morphologic, and biologic variables found to be relevant by multivariate analysis.[460–462] This approach may be useful for research purposes but is too complicated for general clinical usage and offers no significant advantage over the FAB classification tempered with clinical and cytogenetic data.

Cytogenetic Abnormalities and Prognosis

Cytogenetic studies have provided a major source of prognostic information. The occurrence of single nonspecified karyotypic abnormalities is not consistently a poor prognostic sign.[67,209,213,215,463] The presence of complex karyotypic changes, that is, multiple chromosomal abnormalities within one clone or coexisting multiple abnormal clones, accurately predicts a shorter survival.[127,207,209,213,215,218,237] An exception is monosomy 7, which has a prognosis as poor as complex abnormalities.[209,213,215,463] An isolated 5q− abnormality has a more favorable prognosis than any other single karyotype in MDS, including a normal karyotype.[127]

Figure 12-12 shows survival curves for complex, single, and normal karyotypes. Coexistence of cells with both normal and abnormal karyotypes in the bone marrow is less ominous than complete replacement by karyotypically abnormal cells.[73] Sequential determinations may allow assessment of disease extent and pace.[216,242] Cellular DNA content, as measured by flow cytometry, is also prognostically useful; hypodiploidy is associated with shorter survival.[250]

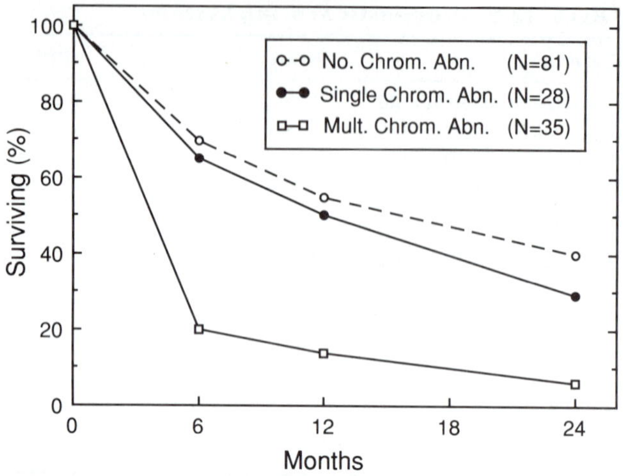

FIGURE 12-12. Survival according to bone marrow karyotype of 144 patients with myelodysplastic syndrome during the 2 years after the initial chromosome study. (After Nowell PC, Besa EC, Stelmach T, Finan JB. Chromosome studies in preleukemic states. Cancer 1986;58:2572)

Complex karyotypic changes are associated not only with lower survival rate but also with a higher rate of transformation to leukemia.[207,211] Many case reports, as well as several larger studies, suggest that acquisition of a new cytogenetic abnormality coincides with transformation to acute leukemia.[161,236,238,239,242,244,464,465] On the other hand, in many cases acute leukemia has developed without a detectable new karyotypic change, and in other cases a new karyotypic change was not accompanied by transformation or any other significant clinical event.[238,239]

Prognosis of Therapy-Related Myelodysplastic Syndromes

Therapy-related MDS almost uniformly has an extremely poor prognosis, with median survival of only 3 to 8 months.[169,171,178,179] The rate of leukemic transformation is higher than in primary MDS (50% to 87%), but length of survival in patients with t-MDS is similar with or without progression to AML.[30,178,179,207] The percentage of myeloblasts at diagnosis, the presence of ringed sideroblasts, and other morphologic criteria seem to have little prognostic meaning in patients with t-MDS; thus, the FAB system has no real usefulness for these patients. Complex chromosomal abnormalities are associated with particularly short survival, but patients with t-MDS and isolated monosomy 7 have relatively good prognoses. This is especially true after leukemic transformation and may result from better responsiveness to chemotherapy.[173,178]

Leukemic Transformation

The central question not yet answered is whether progression to leukemia in patients with MDS results from gradual marrow replacement by the original abnormal clone or from a series of further growth-disruptive mutations. Either pattern might be operative, depending on the nature of the initial genetic event. Longitudinal analyses of patients have revealed clinical patterns of progression toward leukemia that support both models, as discussed in previous sections. Further insight awaits identification of the genes deranged in these disorders.

Most acute leukemias supervening in patients with MDS are myeloid. Relative incidences of FAB leukemia subtypes M1 to M7 are not appreciably different from de novo AML, with the possible exception that a preponderance of CMML patients transform to M5 leukemia.[74,82,83,449] As mentioned in previous sections, coexisting populations of both myeloid and lymphoid blasts,[202,466–468] blast populations exhibiting lineage infidelity,[53,201] and pure lymphoid leukemias[198,199] have been observed occasionally.

TREATMENT

At least three difficulties are inherent in designing and implementing treatment strategies for patients with MDS. First, our lack of basic understanding of the pathogenesis of these syndromes makes the tailoring of specific therapeutic approaches and the prediction of which patients might benefit almost impossible. Second, the heterogeneity of the patient population with respect to manifestations and prognosis means that interpretation of clinical trials is difficult and that results may vary radically depending on types of patients enrolled. For example, inclusion of patients with t-MDS has complicated the interpretation of some clinical trials. In addition, most studies have been small, uncontrolled, and short term. Third, the advanced age of most patients with MDS means that unrelated comorbid conditions are common, complicating survival predictions and often precluding aggressive, potentially toxic therapies.

The results of clinical trials performed thus far are not encouraging. During the past decade, several interventions initially generated excitement but were later shown to have unacceptable side effects or no survival benefit, delay of leukemic transformation, or improvement in cytopenias.[469–471]

Supportive Care

General Measures

Careful supportive care of patients with MDS may allow maintenance of a normal life-style and prevention of necessary morbidity and mortality. Medications that further suppress or damage bone marrow should be avoided, as should excessive amounts of alcohol. Patients need counseling on the importance of obtaining prompt medical evaluation of any symptoms or signs of infection, even if they are not actually neutropenic. Aggressive parenteral antibiotic treatment of documented serious infections or neutropenic fevers is essential, as for any immunocompromised patient. The decision to discontinue antibiotic or antifungal agents is more difficult in patients with MDS than in patients who are neutropenic from chemotherapy, because bone marrow recovery is unlikely. In most patients, platelets should be transfused only when bleeding becomes a clinical problem or in preparation for surgical procedures.

Chelation Therapy

Because most patients with MDS become dependent on RBC transfusions, complications of iron overload are a major cause of mortality and morbidity.[472,473] Even untransfused or minimally transfused patients can sustain clinically significant organ damage, because ineffective erythropoiesis stimulates hyperabsorption of iron.[141,142,145] Elderly patients with underlying cardiac, hepatic, or pancreatic dysfunction may be especially sensitive to further iron-induced organ damage.

The assessment of total body iron stores is not simple in patients with MDS. Serum iron, percentage of iron-binding capacity saturation, and even ferritin values become elevated early in the course of the disease and fluctuate widely, depending on intercurrent illnesses or status of erythropoiesis.[474] Liver biopsy is the best diagnostic test, but an invasive procedure in patients with MDS with thrombocytopenia or platelet dysfunction is impractical and inadvisable. An accurate noninvasive magnetic interference technique for quantitation of liver iron has been developed but is not widely available.[475] The number of units of packed RBCs given is an important determinant of iron stores, but excessive iron absorption also increases the total body iron burden and is harder to quantify.

Daily subcutaneous administration of deferoxamine, 1.5 to 2 g, effectively prevents progressive iron overload in transfusion-dependent patients. Chelation therapy is most effective when used for preventing iron overload than for reversing organ dysfunction such as in diabetes mellitus or cardiac disease after damage is clinically evident. Prophylactic chelation therapy is of little value for a patient with a poor prognosis, such as RAEBT patients, in whom the total transfusion burden is unlikely to reach the level of 100 units of packed RBCs regularly associated with clinical hemochromatosis. Early chelation therapy is most appropriate in patients with RARS. Removal of iron by chelation or phlebotomy can improve erythropoiesis and help to correct anemia in patients with hereditary sideroblastic anemia and possibly those with primary myelodysplasia. Most often, patients with RARS are severely anemic or transfusion dependent before the diagnosis is unequivocally established, rendering phlebotomy impractical. Subcutaneous deferoxamine should be initiated early, since RARS patients are likely to survive long enough to develop complications of iron overload, which are preventable with regular chelation. Patients with RA, CMML, and RAEB may be observed on transfusion with periodic monitoring for endocrine or cardiac dysfunction. If no significant clinical worsening of complications occurs after 12 to 18 months of transfusion (50 to 75 units), chelation should be instituted.

Marrow Stimulation and Immune Suppression

Hematinics

Some physicians have advocated initially treating all patients with MDS with varying combinations of vitamin B_{12}, folate, pyridoxine, riboflavin, and vitamin C.[142] Now that assays for B_{12} and folate are routinely available, this approach can no longer be justified and is not beneficial. A trial of pharmacologic doses of pyridoxine alone may be considered. Before the realization that ringed sideroblasts accompany several different types of anemia (see Table 12-7), all patients with ringed sideroblasts received pyridoxine. Some responded at least partially and became transfusion independent.[400,401,408,410,424,425] No evidence has been found that such patients had pyridoxine deficiency, and pharmacologic doses of 100 mg/d, were required for a response.

Most, if not all, pyridoxine-responsive patients probably had hereditary or drug-induced sideroblastic anemia. Pharmacologic doses of pyridoxine might overcome a functional or absolute deficiency of δ-aminolevulinic acid synthetase (ALA-S) and improve erythropoiesis. Hereditary sideroblastic anemia is the only disorder with evidence for ALA-S deficiency. In recent trials in patients with RARS or RA, after careful exclusion of those with hereditary sideroblastic anemia, pyridoxine had no effect.[142,419] Occasionally, the diagnosis of hereditary sideroblastic anemia is difficult to exclude. Because pyridoxine is a safe drug, a 3-month trial of 100 mg/d orally is warranted in suspected MDS if the patient has isolated anemia and ringed sideroblasts on bone marrow examination.

Heme arginate has been used in 26 patients with MDS.[476] The hemoglobin concentrations of six patients increased significantly, accompanied by a reduction in ringed sideroblast count in the bone marrow. All responders initially had low levels of marrow ferrochelatase activity; heme arginate may allow bypass of this step in heme synthesis. Even though deficiency of this mitochondrial enzyme is unlikely to be the primary cause of the anemia in patients with MDS, secondary ferrochelatase deficiency from mitochondrial iron deposition and damage may contribute to the degree of anemia. Larger cohorts, especially of RARS patients, should be studied using this compound.

Androgens

Androgen treatment has been investigated in several large trials. In an uncontrolled initial study, Najean and Pecking[477] treated 90 RAEB or RAEBT patients with different androgen compounds. Less than 10% showed an increase in hemoglobin concentration or platelet count, and none had significant improvement in neutrophil counts. Side effects were common, including jaundice, muscle cramping, and virilization of female patients. The rate of transformation to leukemia in this androgen-treated cohort was higher than in historical controls. The same investigators then conducted a randomized trial comparing supportive care to androgen therapy, methenolone 2.5 mg/kg/d, or ara-C (cytosine arabinoside), 20 mg/m^2/12 h subcutaneously.[451] Neither modality affected survival or progression to leukemia. Several smaller studies have also reached similar conclusions[478–480]; no evidence suggests that these drugs should be used in most patients with MDS.

Some data suggest that patients with MDS who have hypocellular bone marrows may benefit from androgen therapy. Testosterone enanthate, 7 to 10 mg/wk intramuscularly, was given to 92 patients with either aplastic anemia or MDS.[57] Some patients with MDS responded with clinically significant improvement in peripheral blood counts. Almost all of these responders initially had a hypocellular bone marrow. Those who responded survived longer than nonresponders, but there was no untreated control group. A 3-month trial of androgen therapy would be appropriate for patients with a hypocellular marrow and no other therapeutic options.

Corticosteroids

In most patients with MDS, corticosteroids should be avoided because they are ineffective as well as toxic to already immunocompromised patients.[20,481] Bagby and coworkers[481] found that prednisone improved the peripheral counts of a few patients with MDS and that response could be predicted by the in vitro enhancement of bone marrow CFU-GM by cortisol. These responders did not live demonstrably longer and suffered appreciable toxicity. The potential to improve peripheral blood counts was small and was outweighed by the toxicity of the treatment and the impracticability of performing bone marrow cultures on all patients to identify rare potential responders.

Conventional Chemotherapy

The attainment of complete and often sustained hematologic remissions in most patients with AML given standard antileukemic chemotherapy has prompted clinical trials of this approach in MDS. Several problems with high-dose chemotherapy in these patients could be predicted from the outset. They are on average older and thus less able to tolerate full-scale chemotherapy than patients with de novo AML. The bone marrow may not recover after chemotherapy, because patients with MDA have trilineage marrow replacement with abnormal clonal precursors. No functional repopulating hematopoietic stem cells may remain after chemotherapy-induced aplasia. Finally, it is hard to decide when to initiate chemotherapy, because the clinical course in individual patients varies so widely.

An early retrospective study included 45 patients with RAEB, RAEBT, or CMML treated with one of several antileukemic chemotherapy regimens.[482] Forty-five percent of the patients with RAEB or RAEBT and 64% of the patients with CMML achieved complete remission, but these remissions were brief (median of 8.4 and 6.2 months, respectively). Toxicity and treatment-related mortality rates did not differ from those of patients with de novo AML who were treated during the same period on the same regimens. This cohort of patients with MDS was relatively young (median age of 52 years).

A similar retrospective review of 20 patients with MDS of a more typical median age (69 years) treated with a variety of antileukemic regimens showed a complete remission rate of only 20%. Responding patients were, on average, younger than the rest of the cohort.[483] Nonresponders had a median survival of only 1 month; this was shorter than the survival of five untreated patients from the same cohort and suggested increased mortality from chemotherapy. A more recent study of 29 patients with RAEB or RAEBT, CMML, or AML evolving from MDS showed a higher complete remission rate (48%), but this was significantly less than the 73% complete remission rate that the same investigators found in treating de novo AML with the same regimen.[484] Unfortunately, 35% of the patients died during induction. No difference in complete remission rate or survival time after chemotherapy was found between patients treated in the MDS phase and those who had transformed to AML.

The ability to achieve complete remission in patients with MDS after transformation (t-MDS) to AML supports delaying the use of aggressive chemotherapy until transformation has occurred. Remission rates are not as high as in de novo AML, their duration is shorter, and toxicity is greater, but 22% to 50% of patients obtain complete remission.[482,485–488] Standard regimens of ara-C plus daunorubicin or single agent high-dose ara-C, 3 $g/m^2/12$ h for 12 doses, have been successfully used. For patients under age 50 with RAEB, RAEBT, or life-threatening cytopenias, some researchers have advocated treating with chemotherapy at presentation instead of waiting for progression to AML.[486,489–492] No data from controlled trials support this approach.

In t-MDS, no formal studies of chemotherapy before acute transformation have been published, perhaps because the time until transformation or death from other complications is so brief. Patients with t-MDS treated with standard antileukemic chemotherapy after transformation attained a 41% to 45% complete remission rate, but remissions are short and no evidence of an increase in survival duration has been found.[178,179,490]

Differentiation Therapy

During the 1980s, much attention focused on the treatment of patients with MDS with agents that could, at least theoretically, induce the differentiation of abnormal hematopoietic progenitors.[469,493] This approach seemed promising for several reasons. First, maturation of immature progenitors might increase the number of the functional hematopoietic cells and decrease complications such as infection, bleeding, and iron overload. Second, immature cells might be pushed out of the mitotic compartment into a nonmitotic compartment, from which they might be less likely to overrun remaining normal marrow elements. Finally, toxicity to normal marrow precursors and other rapidly dividing cells might be less from differentiating agents than from cytoreductive regimens. Unfortunately, these agents have not yet fulfilled the promise that they showed in vitro and in early clinical trials; in some instances, their mechanisms of action have been more cytostatic than differentiating.

The initial stimulus to investigation of differentiation induction was the observation that cell lines derived from leukemic mice became more mature by morphologic and functional criteria when exposed to several compounds in vitro.[469,493–495] Lotem[495] and Sachs[493] discovered that only certain leukemic cell lines retain the ability to differentiate, suggesting more than one mechanism for maturation arrest. Clinical interest was generated by demonstration that ara-C, retinoic acid, vitamin D, interferon, dactinomycin, methotrexate, hypoxanthine, 5-azacytidine, and other compounds all induced differentiation of human cells.[469,496–498] In vitro maturation of cells from patients with AML or MDS were less striking than that seen in cell lines, and varied from patient to patient.[499–501] Striking synergism with combinations of different agents, such as retinoic acid and ara-C, has been demonstrated both in cell lines and in primary cells from patients with MDS or AML.[502,503] The mechanism of induction by these compounds is not fully understood and probably varies among inducers. Concentrations of these compounds high enough to produce differentiation also generally inhibit proliferation. No one yet knows whether growth inhibition is a necessary side effect or a consequence of maturation.[493,498]

Several of these above-mentioned agents—alone and in combination—have been tested in clinical trials. Although the clinical trials were based on the hypothesis that these agents would have differentiating ability in vivo, their mechanism of action might involve differential killing of dysplastic cells and hematopoietic repopulation by normal or less severely affected subclones.

Low-Dose Ara-C

Cytosine arabinoside (ara-C) is the arabinoside analogue of deoxycytidine. In its phosphorylated form, ara-C is incorporated into DNA, acting as a chain synthesis terminator. At doses of 100 to 200 $mg/m^2/d$, in combination with daunorubicin, it is part of the standard regimen for remission induction of de novo AML. Low-dose ara-C, 10 to 20 $mg/m^2/d$ by continuous intravenous infusion, or every 12 hours by subcutaneous injection, produces plasma levels high enough to induce differentiation of human promyelocytic (HL-60) cells in vitro without irreversible cytostasis. These concentrations are also high enough to inhibit DNA synthesis.[469,498,504–506] There were initial reports of complete responses in three patients with AML using this low-dose regimen.[507]

Table 12-10 summarizes the results of the larger trials of low-dose ara-C in patients with MDS. Interpretation is made difficult by their small size, intracohort and intercohort heterogeneity, inclusion of patients with frank acute leukemia, lack of untreated controls in all studies but one, differing dose schedules and treatment durations, and differing definitions of response. Najean and Pecking[451] carried out the only controlled trial. They compared supportive care with androgen or low-dose ara-C treatment and found no survival advantage for either therapy. Ara-C was given for only 2 days each month.

More encouraging results were obtained by Griffin and coworkers.[508,509] Eleven of 16 patients had significant improvement in blood counts of one or more lineage, and some became transfusion independent for 2 to 14 months. Other investigators have generally not reported such a high response or complete remission rate. Even among responders, duration of improvement in counts or bone marrow remission has generally been only 2 to 3 months. In some patients, several courses of ara-C were required before a

TABLE 12-10. **Low-Dose ara-C Clinical Trials**

Clinical Study	Daily Dose*	Duration (d)†	CR/PR/Total‡	Median Response (mo)
Wisch et al[508]	20 mg/m²	7–21	2/9/16	3.5
Griffin et al[509]				
Castaigne et al[511]	20 mg/m²	15–21	4/0/5	5.5
Tricot et al[514]	20–50 mg	21–28	3/10/26	5
Jehn et al[512]	20 mg/m²	15–31	3/0/7	2
Winter et al[513]	10–20 mg/m²	10–21	0/5/10	2
Degos et al[574]	20 mg/m²	15–21	9/6/38	—

* Total dose per day shown as milligrams per square meter (mg/m²) or total milligrams. Administration either intravenously or subcutaneously, continuous or every 12 hours.
† Duration in days of ara-C treatment.
‡ Number of patients who obtained a complete remission/number who obtained a partial remission/total number of patients treated in the study.

response occurred.[508,510,511] Significant toxicity was often observed. Even at these low dosages, patients became extremely pancytopenic and required more RBC and platelet transfusions.[506,511–515] Marrow recovery back to pre–ara-C counts did not occur in some cases for up to 1 month after treatment.[508,515] Therapy-related deaths have been reported frequently.[511,514,515]

Some investigators have argued that the mechanism of in vivo response to these dosages of ara-C was mainly differentiation, without significant cytoreduction.[506,507,511] The detection of mature granulocytes with Auer rods in several patients after ara-C treatment and persistent abnormal cytogenetics in patients with complete hematologic remissions support this hypothesis.[506,508] Even in AML prior to treatment, circulating mature granulocytes that originate from the abnormal clone have been detected [191] Many investigators have instead argued that the major mechanism of action of low-dose ara-C must be cytoreductive, with preferential killing or inhibition of the most severely dysregulated immature populations, allowing less severely affected progenitors to restore hematopoiesis.[469,504,516] This hypothesis is supported by the documentation, in many clinical trials, of significant marrow aplasia in patients after ara-C treatment before hematopoietic recovery.[508,512–514,517] In two patients with complete hematologic remissions after ara-C therapy, X-chromosome RFLP (restriction fragment length polymorphism) analysis showed that polyclonal hematopoiesis was restored.

The relatively low response rates, short response durations, and high toxicity and mortality rates associated with low-dose ara-C treatment have not encouraged more general application of these regimens.[469,516] In an attempt to decrease toxicity, a few patients have been treated with very low-dose ara-C, 6 mg/m²/d for 21 days.[518] Marrow suppression was not as severe as at the higher doses, and six of eight patients showed improvement in their counts; three had complete normalization. One study of more than 100 patients found that an adverse outcome after treatment with ara-C could be related to advanced age, low platelet count, the presence of the pseudo-Pelger in leukocytes, and multiple chromosomal abnormalities.[519a] The authors proposed that these parameters be used to develop a predictive model for ara-C therapy. Another small study used low-dose oral 6-thioguanine, but only 4 of 18 patients showed any improvement.[519] We await further investigation of these gentler regimens.

Retinoids

Unlike ara-C, the retinoid class of vitamin A analogues are generally not cytostatic at concentrations sufficient to induce differentiation of HL-60 cells, although their mechanism of action is not completely understood.[496] They are known to regulate the expression of several protooncogenes in vitro. When given to animals before mutagen exposure, they decrease the risk of subsequent development of neoplasms. Retinoids may also increase the sensitivity of hematopoietic precursors to stimulation by growth factors.[496]

In a phase I study of 13-*cis*-retinoic acid, 15 of 45 courses of 25 to 125 mg/m²/d orally were accompanied by some improvement in counts, generally in granulocytes.[520] Similar results were reported in other smaller cohorts.[521,522] Hepatotoxicity was dose limiting, and other side effects included chelosis, hyperkeratosis, stomatitis, and increased serum lipid levels. In another uncontrolled trial, 22% of patients showed appreciable toxicity, including worsening thrombocytopenia.[523]

Two randomized placebo-controlled trials have been published, with conflicting results. In one study, 70 patients with RA or RARS received 13-*cis*-retinoic acid, 20 mg/m²/d, or placebo. Overall survival in the entire cohort was worse than in historical controls, but the 1-year survival rate in RA patients given the drug was 77% compared with 36% in the placebo group, which was statistically significant.[524] Because no significant difference in blood counts or rate of transformation to acute leukemia was found between the two groups, the survival advantage remains unexplained. Sequential bone marrow examinations were not performed. In a second randomized, controlled trial, 68 patients with MDS of all subtypes received 13-*cis*-retinoic acid, 100 mg/m²/d, or placebo for 6 months.[525] Cytopenias were not significantly improved, and the overall course did not improve in the *cis*-retinoic acid–treated group. Over 90% sustained appreciable dermatologic toxicity. The reasons for the discrepancy in results between these two trials are unclear.[526] On balance, the lack of documented hematologic improvement in the patients in the first study and their unusually short overall survival generates skepticism about a beneficial effect of retinoids.

Vitamin D

1,25-Dihydroxyvitamin D_3 effectively differentiates HL-60 cells in vitro at concentrations of 5×10^{-9} mol/L, and AML blasts at 10^{-6} to 10^{-7} mol/L.[2] A clinical trial used 2 μg/d orally in 18 patients with MDS.[2] Minimal transient increases in platelet and white blood cell counts were seen in 8 of 18 patients, but 9 developed clinically significant hypercalcemia. Serum levels of only 2×10^{-10} mol/L were achieved, and higher doses were not practical because of hypercalcemia. Seven of 18 patients developed acute leukemia during treatment.

Interferon

Interferon-α also induces differentiation of leukemic cells in vitro and has been given to a small number of patients with MDS in uncontrolled studies. Besides inducing differentiation, it may stimulate NK cell activity, which was found lacking in patients with MDS. Remarkable sustained responses even after discontinuation of therapy have been reported in two patients.[527,528] Trisomy 8, detectable in most of the marrow metaphases in one patient before treatment, disappeared after interferon-α was given. Only one eighth of patients demonstrated a response in the only clinical trial yet published, which was uncontrolled.[528] Toxicity was minimal.

The possibility that combinations of interferon, vitamin D, retinoic acid, and ara-C could provide in vivo synergy is being investigated. All four given simultaneously are not well tolerated, but the first three given without ara-C produced a 44% response rate in one uncontrolled study.[529]

Hematopoietic Growth Factors

The potent abilities of recently isolated growth factors to support and stimulate hematopoiesis both in vitro and in experimental animals has focused scientific, economic, and clinical attention on their possible usefulness in treating hematologic disease.[315,316,530] The human genes for at least 15 of these factors have been cloned during the past 5 years.[315,333] Recombinant DNA technology allows production of pharmacologic quantities of the proteins in bacteria, yeast, or cultured mammalian cell systems. The lack of normal glycosylation of these recombinant human proteins might affect activity or immunogenicity, although neither has been a problem in clinical trials. Four factors are undergoing active clinical investigation in patients with MDS, and several more are certain to be released for initial studies soon.

A deficiency in production of any particular growth factor has not been shown in MDS, despite the mapping of several growth factor genes to the area deleted from the 5q chromosome. As noted, higher concentrations of these factors may be necessary to stimulate colony formation from MDS marrow than from normal bone marrow.[357,358] Several possible growth factor effects might result in clinical improvement. These include differentiation of abnormal precursors, stimulation of residual normal hematopoietic elements, and enhancement of the function of mature cells. Conversely, adverse effects can also be imagined, such as stimulation of blast cell proliferation without differentiation. At least in culture, hematopoietic growth factors enhance the growth of both leukemic cell lines and primary blasts.[531–533] In the future, combination therapy with two or more growth factors may prove desirable because synergy has already been demonstrated.[534–537] An agent acting early in hematopoietic development, such as interleukin-3, might be more effective in conjunction with a late-acting agent such as EPO.

Granulocyte-Macrophage Colony-Stimulating Factor

More patients with MDS have received granulocyte-macrophage colony-stimulating factor (GM-CSF) than any other growth factor. Vadhan-Raj and coworkers[538] published a phase I/II trial using 30 to 500 $\mu g/m^2/d$ by continuous intravenous infusion for 14 days to eight patients. All had a 5- to 70-fold increase in total leukocyte count, due mainly to increases in granulocytes and eosinophils. Three patients also had an increase in their reticulocyte or platelet counts. The percentage of myeloblasts in the bone marrow decreased in some patients, although small numbers of circulating blasts appeared during extreme leukocytosis. Toxicity was minimal, consisting mainly of nonspecific bone pain and fatigue.

Several small uncontrolled studies have been subsequently published using 7- to 21-day courses of GM-CSF at equivalent doses. An increase in white blood cells occurred in nearly all patients.[539,540] Consistent beneficial effects on platelet count, RBC count, and transfusion requirement have not been observed. Investigators have reported clinically significant decreases in platelet count in some patients receiving GM-CSF, necessitating discontinuation of therapy in several patients.[541] The same study reported similar improvements in neutrophil count using up to 20 times lower doses of GM-CSF, with milder nonhematologic toxicity. One patient with t-MDS experienced a trilineage remission after two courses of GM-CSF, with disappearance of a documented cytogenetic abnormality.[542] Relapse occurred after 1 year. The pathophysiology of this unusual response may have involved terminal differentiation of an abnormal clone precluding further proliferation.

Unfortunately, in one study 5 of 11 treated patients progressed to acute leukemia while on GM-CSF, or within 4 weeks of completing a GM-CSF course.[540] All had bone marrow myeloblast percentages of more than 15% before beginning therapy. It is unclear whether GM-CSF actually accelerated the progression to leukemia or whether the timing of transformation was coincidental.

Most patients do respond to GM-CSF with an increase in their neutrophil count, but the impact of this numeric change on ability to fight infection and on longer-term morbidity and mortality, both from infection and from leukemic progression is unclear. A multicenter, randomized, controlled trial has been carried out, with only preliminary results available.[543] Median neutrophil counts were significantly increased in the treatment arm, but no effect on anemia, transfusion requirements, or platelet counts was seen. Patients on the GM-CSF arm experienced significantly fewer infections during the 3-month treatment period. There was no higher rate of leukemic transformation in the patients given GM-CSF, but follow-up has been brief.

Granulocyte Colony-Stimulating Factor

Fewer patients with MDS have received G-CSF than GM-CSF in formal clinical trials, but less toxicity makes it likely to be used more extensively than GM-CSF in the future. Response rates and patterns in small, uncontrolled trials have been similar to GM-CSF: over 80% of patients significantly increase their neutrophil counts, but only rare responses in erythroid or platelet lineages have been seen. [544–546] G-CSF, 0.1 to 5 $\mu g/kg/d$, has been used for up to 3 months. The first two trials did not report progression to acute leukemia while on therapy,[544,545] but longer follow-up of subsequent patients did reveal progression to AML in several patients with marrow blast percentages of over 10% before therapy.[546] Those patients with abnormal cytogenetics before therapy experienced no change in the percentage of abnormal metaphases detected in bone marrow while on therapy.

Several indices of neutrophil function were shown to be improved in MDS patients on G-CSF, including in vitro phagocytosis and leukocyte alkaline phosphatase levels.[544,547] In patients receiving GM-CSF or G-CSF after autologous bone marrow transplantation for breast cancer, neutrophil migration into skin windows was impaired in the cohort given GM-CSF but not in the G-CSF cohort.[548]

Interleukin-3

Only a limited number of patients in MDS have received IL-3[549]; there is no evidence that IL-3 offers any clinical advantages over GM-CSF or G-CSF. Most patients responded with increases in neutrophil count but to a less pronounced degree than with G-CSF or GM-CSF. Despite increases in reticulocyte counts, only one patient had decreased transfusion requirements. Patients did not show significant responses in the platelet lineage, a particularly disappointing outcome since IL-3 stimulates all lineages in vitro and has increased platelet and reticulocyte counts in primates as well as in humans with normal marrow function.[534,536,550–551a]

Erythropoietin

The blunted EPO response of some MDS patients to severe anemia has encouraged clinicians to treat these patients with recombinant EPO.[367] Most trials have been small and uncontrolled. Overall response rates have been 0% to 25%,[552–556] but the identification of response has varied from minimal increases in hemoglobin concentrations of increased spacing of transfusions to transfusion independence in previously severely anemic patients. Reticulocytosis is often observed, but may not be accompanied by a decrease in transfusion requirements, and may reflect ineffective erythropoiesis. Pretreatment EPO levels do not consistently predict responses, nor do ferrokinetic measurements or transferrin receptor protein levels.[553,554,557] Several of the trials used doses as high as 1000 to 1600 IU/kg/d, and responses were often delayed more than 12 weeks after initiation of treatment.[553,554] Because of the low toxicity and easy availability of EPO, MDS patients are certain to be treated by their physicians with this drug. The low response rate and suggestion of an increased rate of leukemic progression in one study[558] argue for waiting until lager, controlled, multicenter trials are completed.[558a]

Bone Marrow Transplantation

Bone marrow transplantation offers the only real opportunity for cure of MDS. Several early case reports described syngeneic transplantions from identical twins that produced complete hematologic reconstitution and long-term survival without disease recurrence.[321,559] An initial series of patients received marrow from HLA-matched siblings.[560,561] Initially, patients were conditioned with cyclophosphamide alone before transplantation, as is standard in patients undergoing transplantation for aplastic anemia, but the first 3 patients treated in this way had rapid recurrences of MDS. Thus, subsequent patients were conditioned with total body irradiation plus cyclophosphamide as if they had leukemia, and 6 of 7 are alive and well without recurrence 7 to 25 months after transplantation.

The same investigators have recently updated their experience.[562,563] They have performed transplantations for MDS in 59 patients, aged 4 to 54 years, from both HLA-matched and partially matched donors. Twenty-eight are alive and disease-free, with 8 recurrences, 8 deaths from graft-versus-host disease, and 8 deaths from interstitial pneumonitis. Long-term survival was more likely in younger patients with abnormal karyotypes transplanted soon after diagnosis. Similar results have been obtained by other transplant centers both in children and in adults.[564,565] Patients with t-MDS included in these studies generally have not done as well, but several are long-term survivors with normal hematopoiesis.[490,562,563]

These results are encouraging and have led investigators to suggest that bone marrow transplantation from an HLA-matched sibling donor should be first-line therapy for patients with primary or secondary MDS under the age of 40 to 50 years.[470,489,564,565] Optimal timing is not yet clear, but the rapid progression of younger patients with primary or t-MDS to acute leukemia suggests that bone marrow transplantation should be performed early in the course of disease.[563] Tumor burden and tranfusional iron burden are less severe, and the general condition of the patient is usually better. So far, investigators have not given patients conventional antileukemic therapy in an attempt to attain hematologic remission prior to transplant because of the known high mortality rate from induction chemotherapy in these patients.

Recommendations for Treatment

No generally applicable, standard, beneficial therapy for MDS exists, although patients may respond dramatically to any of several available regimens. Our lack of understanding of the basic pathophysiology of these disorders and the heterogeneity of the affected patient population suggest that progress may be difficult. All patients should be enrolled in well-designed clinical trials if they are receiving any form of treatment other than supportive care. Patients with serious complicating medical problems or with good prognostic parameters (such as low bone marrow blast cell counts and normal cytogenetics) may do better with a conservative approach. Patients with t-MDS should be enrolled in separate clinical trials because of the more aggressive course of their disease.

Patients under the age of 50 with a histocompatible donor should be considered for bone marrow transplantation. This is especially true of children and patients with rapidly progressive disease. In the future, histocompatible marrow from unrelated donors, matched through computerized banks, may become more widely available, increasing the number of patients eligible for transplant.

We recommend that patients ineligible for transplant should not receive standard or low-dose chemotherapy until their condition progresses to acute leukemia. The role of hematopoietic growth factors, differentiating agents, and other agents remain uncertain unless long-term, controlled trials can demonstrate a survival advantage for treated patients. Finally, combination therapy, either with several growth factors or with growth factors or differentiating factors plus cytostatic agents, deserves careful clinical study.[566,567]

REFERENCES

1. Yoshida Y. Biology of myelodysplastic syndromes. Intl J Cell Clon 1987;5:356.
2. Koeffler HP. Myelodysplastic syndromes (preleukemia). Semin Hematol 1986;23:284.
3. Hoelzer D. Cytobiology and clinical findings of myelodysplastic syndromes. Recent Results Cancer Res 1988;106:172.
4. Geary CG. Clinical annotation: the diagnosis of preleukaemia. Br J Haematol 1983;55:1.
5. Mufti GJ, Galton DAG. Myelodysplastic syndromes: natural history and features of prognostic importance. Clin Haematol 1986;15:953.
6. Koeffler HP. Preleukaemia. Clin Haematol 1986;15:829.
7. Bennett JM. Classification of the myelodysplastic syndromes. Clin Haematol 1986;15:909.
8. Beris P. Primary clonal myelodysplastic syndromes. Semin Hematol 1989;26:216.
9. Jacobs A, Clark RE. Pathogenesis and clinical variations in the myelodysplastic syndromes. Clin Haematol 1986;15:925.
10. Bagby G. The preleukemic syndrome. Boca Raton, CRC Press, 1985.
11. Galton DAG. The myelodysplastic syndromes. Scand J Haematol 1986;36(Suppl 45):11.
12. Rhoads CP, Barker WH. Refractory anemia. JAMA 1938;110:794.
13. Bjorkman SE. Chronic refractory anemia with sideroblastic bone marrow: a study of four cases. Blood 1956;11:250.
14. Vilter RW, Jarrold T, Will JJ, et al. Refractory anemia with hyperplastic bone marrow. J Haematol 1960;15:1.
15. Hamilton-Paterson JL. Preleukaemic anaemia. Acta Haematol 1949;2:302.
16. Rheingold JJ, Kaufman R, Adelson E, Lear A. Smoldering acute leukemia. N Engl J Med 1963;268:812.
17. Meacham GC, Weisberger AS. Early atypical manifestations of leukemia. Ann Intern Med 1954;41:780.
18. Block M, Jacobson LO, Bethard WF. Preleukemic acute human leukemia. JAMA 1953;152:1018.
19. Boggs DR, Wintrobe MM, Cartwright GE. The acute leukemias. Medicine 1962;41:163.
20. Linman JW, Bagby GC. The preleukemic syndromes (hemopoietic dysplasia). Cancer 1978;42:854.

21. Hayhoe FGJ, Quaglino D. Refractory sideroblastic anaemia and erythraemic myelosis: possible relationship and cytochemical observations. Br J Haematol 1960;6:381.
22. Dameshek W. Sideroblastic anemia: is this a malignancy? Br J Haematol 1965;2:52.
23. Dreyfus B, Rochant H, Salmon C, et al. Anémies réfractaires états préleucemiques et anomalies enzymatiques multiples. C R Acad Sci 1968;266:1627.
24. Dreyfus B, Rochant H, Sultan C, et al. Les anémies réfractaires avec execs de myeloblastes dans la moelle. Étude de onze observations. Presse Med 1970;78:359.
25. Saarni M, Linman J. Preleukemia: hematologic syndrome preceding acute leukemia. Am J Med 1973;55:38.
26. Bennett JM, Catovsky D, Daniel MT, et al. Proposals for the classification of the acute leukemias. Br J Haematol 1976;33:451.
27. Bennett JM, Catovsky D, Daniel MT, et al. Proposals for the classification of the myelodysplastic syndromes. Br J Haematol 1982;51:189.
28. Pedersen-Bjergaard J, Larsen SO. Incidence of acute nonlymphocytic leukemia, preleukemia, and acute myeloproliferative syndrome up to 10 years after treatment of Hodgkin's disease. N Engl J Med 1982;307: 965.
29. Foucar K, McKenna RW, Bloomfield CD, et al. Therapy-related leukemia: a panmyelosis. Cancer 1979;43:1285.
30. Mortensen BT, Pedersen-Bjergaard J, Pedersen NT, et al. Predictive value of bone marrow cultures in 48 patients with acute myeloblastic leukaemia or myelodysplasia both secondary to treatment of other malignant diseases. Scand J Haematol 1985;35:423.
31. Wolf BC, Neiman RS. The bone marrow in myeloproliferative and dysmyelopoietic syndromes. Hematol Oncol Clin North Am 1988;2: 669.
32. Krause JR. An appraisal of the value of the bone marrow biopsy in the assessment of proliferative lesions of the bone marrow. Histopathology 1983;7:627.
33. Frisch B, Bartl R. Bone marrow histology in myelodysplastic syndromes. Scand J Haematol 1986;36(Suppl 45):21.
34. Georgii A, Vykoupil KF, Buhr T. Preleukemia: bone marrow histopathology in myelodysplasia and preleukemic syndrome. Recent Results Cancer Res 1988;106:159.
35. Jacot-Des-Combes E, Beris P, Kapanci Y. Plastic embedded bone marrow biopsy in the evaluation of myelodysplastic syndromes. Pathol Res Pract 1985;180:280.
36. Tricot G, DeWolfe-Peeters C, Hendrick B, Verwilghen RL. Bone marrow histology in myelodysplastic syndromes. Br J Haematol 1984;57: 423.
37. Fohlmeister I, Fischer R, Schaefer H-E. Preleukemic myelodysplastic syndromes (MDS): pathogenetical considerations based on retrospective clinicomorphological sequential studies. Anticancer Res 1985;5: 179.
38. Mitrou PS, Fischer M, Hubner K. Proliferation of ineffective erythropoiesis with nuclear abnormalities and megaloblastoid appearance in preleukaemia. Acta Haematol 1975;54:271.
39. Bethlenfalvey NC, Phaure TAJ, Phyliky RL, Bowman RP. Nuclear bridging of erythroblasts in acquired dyserythropoiesis: an early and transient preleukemic marker. Am J Hematol 1986;21:315.
40. Juneja SK, Imbert M, Sigaux F, et al. Prevalence and distribution of ringed sideroblasts in primary myelodysplastic syndromes. J Clin Pathol 83;36:566.
41. Bottomley SS. Sideroblastic anaemia. Clin Haematol 1982;11:389.
42. Hast R. Sideroblasts in myelodysplasia: their nature and clinical significance. Scand J Haematol 1986;45:53.
43. Caroli J, Bernard J, Bessis M, et al. Hémochromatose avec anémie hypochrome et absence d'hémoglobine anormale. Presse Med 1957;65: 1991.
44. Goodman JR, Hall SG. Accumulation of iron in mitochondria of erythroblasts. Br J Haematol 1967;13:335.
45. Smith WB, Ablin A, Goodman JR, Brecher G. Atypical megakaryocytes in preleukemic phase of acute myeloid leukemia. Blood 1973;42:535.
46. Queisser W, Queisser U, Ansmann M, et al. Megakaryocyte polyploidization in acute leukemia and preleukemia. Br J Haematol 1974;28:261.
47. Thiede T, Engquist L, Billstrom R. Application of megakaryocytic morphology in diagnosing 5q− syndrome. Eur J Haematol 1988;41: 434.
48. Thiele J, Krech R, Wienhold S, et al. The use of the anti–factor VIII method on trephine biopsies of the bone marrow for the identification of immature and atypical megakaryocytes in myeloproliferative diseases and allied disorders: a morphometric study. Virchows Arch 1987;54:89.
49. Hokland P, Kerndrup G, Griffin JD, Ellegaard J. Analysis of leukocyte differentiation antigens in blood and bone marrow from preleukemia (refractory anemia) patients using monoclonal antibodies. Blood 1986;67:898.
50. Scott CS, Cahill A, Bynoe AG, et al. Esterase cytochemistry in primary myelodysplastic syndromes and megaloblastic anaemias: demonstration of abnormal staining patterns associated with dysmyelopoiesis. Br J Haematol 1983;55:411.
51. Seigneurin D, Audhuy B. Auer rods in refractory anemia with excess of blasts: presence and significance. Am J Clin Pathol 1983;80:359.
52. Kass L, Elias JM. Cytochemistry and immunocytochemistry in bone marrow examination: contemporary techniques for the diagnosis of acute leukemia and myelodysplastic syndromes. Hematol Oncol Clin North Am 1988;2:537.
53. San Miguel JF, Gonzalez M, Canizo MC, et al. The nature of blast cells in myelodysplastic syndromes evolving to acute leukaemia. Blut 1986;52:357.
54. Woessner S, Lafuente R, Florensa L, et al. Acquired refractory anaemia with excess of blasts of promegakaryoblastic type. Blut 1986;53:293.
55. Nand S, Godwin JE. Hypoplastic myelodysplastic syndrome. Cancer 1988;62:958.
56. Yoshida Y, Oguma S, Uchino H, Maekawa T. Refractory myelodysplastic anaemias with hypocellular bone marrow. J Clin Pathol 1988;41:763.
57. Riccardi A, Giordano M, Girino M, et al. Refractory cytopenias: clinical course according to bone marrow cytology and cellularity. Blut 1987;54:153.
58. Coiffier B, Adeleine P, Viala JJ, et al. Dysmyelopoietic syndromes: a search for prognostic factors in 193 patients. Cancer 1983;52:83.
59. Sultan C, Sigaux F, Imbert M, Reyes F. Acute myelodysplasia with myelofibrosis: a report of eight cases. Br J Haematol 1981;49:11.
60. Pagliuca A, Layton DM, Manoharan A, et al. Myelofibrosis in primary myelodysplastic syndromes: a clinico-morphological study of 10 cases. Br J Haematol 1989;71:499.
61. Bested AC, Cheng G, Pinkerton PH, et al. Idiopathic acquired sideroblastic anaemia transforming to acute myelosclerosis. J Clin Pathol 1984;37:1032.
62. Assoian RK, Grotendorst GR, Miller DM, Sporn MB. Cellular transformation by coordinated action of three peptide growth factors from human platelets. Nature 1984;309:804.
63. Gersuk GM, Carmel R, Pattengale PK. Platelet-derived growth factor concentrations in platelet-poor plasma and urine from patients with myeloproliferative disorders. Blood 1989;74:2330.
64. Gordon MY. Extracellular matrix of the marrow microenvironment. Br J Haematol 1988;70:1.
65. Gordon MY, Riley GP, Watt SM, Greaves MF. Compartmentalization of a haematopoietic growth factor (GM-CSF) by glycosaminoglycans in the bone marrow microenvironment. Nature 1987;326:403.
66. Islam A, Catovsky D, Goldman JM, Galton DAG. Studies on cellular interactions between stromal and hematopoietic stem cells in normal and leukemic bone marrows. Bibl Haematol 1984;50:17.
67. Tricot G, De Wolf-Peeter C, Vlietinck R, Verwilghen RL. Bone marrow histology in myelodysplastic syndromes. Br J Haematol 1984;58:217.
68. Greenberg P, Bagby G. Biologic rather than morphologic markers in myelodysplastic syndromes. Br J Haematol 1983;52:532.
69. Bagby GC Jr. The concept of preleukemia: clinical and laboratory studies. CRC Crit Rev Oncol Hematol 1980;4:203.
70. Spitzer TR, Goldsmith GH Jr. Myelodysplastic syndromes: is another classification necessary? Br J Haematol 1982;52:343.
71. Greenberg PL. The smoldering myeloid leukemic states: clinical and biologic features. Blood 1983;61:1035.
72. Ibbot JW, Whitelaw DM, Thomas JW. The significant percentage of blast cells in the bone marrow in the diagnosis of acute leukemia. Can Med Assoc J 1960;82:358.
73. Kerkhofs H, Hermans J, Haak HL, Leeksma CHW. Utility of the FAB classification for myelodysplastic syndromes: investigation of prognostic factors in 237 cases. Br J Haematol 1987;65:73.
74. Vallespi T, Torrabadella M, Julia A, et al. Myelodysplastic syndromes: a study of 101 cases according to the FAB classification. Br J Haematol 1985;61:83.
75. Bennett JM, Catovsky D, Daniel MT, et al. Proposed revised criteria for the classification of acute myeloid leukemia. Ann Intern Med 1985;103:620.
76. Kerndrup G, Bendix-Hansen K, Pedersen B. The prognostic significance of cytological, histological and cytogenetic findings in refractory anaemia (RA) and RA with sideroblasts. Blut 1987;54:231.
77. Cazzola M, Bergamaschi G, Huebers HA, Finch CA. Pathophysiological classification of acquired bone marrow failure based on quantitative assessment of erythroid function. Eur J Haematol 1987;38:426.
78. Kushner JP, Lee GR, Wintrobe MM, Cartwright GE. Idiopathic refractory sideroblastic anemia: clinical and laboratory investigation of 17 patients and review of the literature. Medicine 1971;50:139.
79. Bennett JM, Berger R, Brunning RD, et al. Recommendations for a morphologic, immunologic, and cytogenetic (MIC) working classification of the primary and therapy-related myelodysplastic disorders. Cancer Genet Cytogenet 1988;32:1.
80. Khaleeli M, Keane WM, Lee GR. Sideroblastic anemia in multiple myeloma: a preleukemic change. Blood 1973;41:17.
81. Garcia S, Sanz MA, Amigo V, et al. Prognostic factors in chronic myelodysplastic syndromes: a multivariate analysis in 107 cases. Am J Hematol 1988;27:163.
81a. Ballen KK, Gilliland DG, Kalish LA, et al. Bone marrow dysplasia in patients with newly diagnosed acute myelogenous leukemia does not correlate with history of myelodysplasia or with remission rate and survival. Cancer 1994;73:314.
82. Foucar K, Langdon RM II, Armitage JO, et al. Myelodysplastic syndromes: a clinical and pathologic analysis of 109 cases. Cancer 1985;56: 553.

83. WeisdorfDJ, Oken MM, Johnson GJ, Rydell RE. Chronic myelodysplastic syndrome: short survival with or without evolution to acute leukaemia. Br J Haematol 1983;55:691.
84. van der Weide M, Sizoo W, Nauta JJP, et al. Myelodysplastic syndromes: analysis of clinical and prognostic features in 96 patients. Eur J Haematol 1988;41:115.
85. Schmalzl F, Lechleitner M. Disappearance of a sideroblastic cell clone during the chronic phase of a preleukemic myelodysplastic syndrome. Br J Haematol 1986;64:410.
86. Bursztyn B, Douer D, Ramot B. Chronic myelomonocytic leukemia following refractory anemia with sideroblasts: report of two cases. Eur J Haematol 1987;38:197.
87. Fenaux P, Estienne MH, Lepelley P, et al. Refractory anaemia according to the FAB classification: a report on 69 cases. Eur J Haematol 1988;40:318.
88. Weisdorf DJ, Oken MM, Johnson GJ, Rydell RE. Auer rod positive dysmyelopoietic syndrome. Am J Hematol 1981;11:397.
89. Mufti GJ, Stevens JR, Oscier DG, et al. Myelodysplastic syndromes: a scoring system with prognostic significance. Br J Haematol 1985;59:425.
90. Van Dijk JM, Sonnenblick M, Kornberg A, Rosin AJ. Preleukemic syndrome in elderly patients-report of 11 cases. Israel J Med Sci 1985;21:292.
91. Gardner FH. Refractory anemia in the elderly. Adv Intern Med 1987;32:155.
92. Wegelius R. Preleukaemic states in children. Scand J Haematol 1986;36(Suppl 45):133.
93. Blank J, Lange B. Preleukemia in children. J Pediatr 1981;98:565.
94. Saarinen UM, Wegelius R. Preleukemic syndrome in children: report of four cases and review of literature. Am J Pediatr Hematol Oncol Clin North Am 1984;6:137.
95. Blank J, Lange B. Preleukemia in children. J Pediatr 1981;98:565.
96. Niebrugge DJ. Preleukemia in children. J Pediatr 1981;100:507.
97. Paul B, Reid MM, Davison EV, et al. Familial myelodysplasia: progressive disease associated with emergence of monosomy 7. Br J Haematol 1987;65:321.
98. Li FP, Marchetto DJ, Vawter GF. Acute leukemia and preleukemia in eight males in a family: an X-linked disorder? Am J Hematol 1979;6:61.
99. Palmer CG, Heerema NA, Greist A, et al. Cytogenetic findings in siblings with a myelodysplastic syndrome. Cancer Genet Cytogenet 1987;27:241.
100. Shannon KM, Turhan AG, Chang SSY, et al. Familial bone marrow monosomy 7: evidence that the predisposing locus is not on the long arm of chromosome 7. J Clin Invest 1989;84:984.
101. Kamiyama R, Ishikawa Y, Hatakeyama S, et al. Clinicopathological study of hematological disorders after Thorotrast administration in Japan. Blut 1988;56:153.
102. Yoosufani Z, Slavin JD, Hellman RM, et al. Preleukemia following large dose radioiodide therapy for metastatic thyroid carcinoma. J Nuclear Med 1987;28:1348.
103. Kamada N, Uchino H. Preleukemic states in atomic bomb survivors in Japan. Blood Cells 1976;2:57.
104. Farrow A, Jacobs A, West RR. Myelodysplasia, chemical exposure, and other environmental factors. Leukemia 1989;3:33.
105. Van Den Berghe H, Louwagie A, Broeckaert-Van Orshoven A, et al. Chromosome analysis in two unusual malignant blood disorders presumably induced by benzene. Blood 1979;53:558.
106. de Planque MM, Kluin-Nelemans HC, van Krieken HJM, et al. Evolution of acquired severe aplastic anemia to myelodysplasia and subsequent leukemia in adults. Br J Haematol 1988;70:55.
107. Tichelli A, Gratwohl A, Wursch A, et al. Late haematological complications in severe aplastic anaemia. Br J Haematol 1988;69:413.
108. Orlandi E, Alessandrino EP, Caldera D, Bernasconi C. Adult leukemia developing after aplastic anemia: report of 8 cases. Acta Haematol 1988;79:174.
109. Orlandi E, Alessandrino EP, Caldera D, Bernasconi C. Adult leukemia developing after aplastic anemia: report of 8 cases. Acta Haematol 1988;79:174.
110. Fohlmeister I, Fischer R, Modder B, et al. Aplastic anaemia and the hypocellular myelodysplastic syndrome: histomorphological, diagnostic, and prognostic features. J Clin Pathol 1985;38:1218.
111. Young NS. The problem of clonality in aplastic anemia: Dr Dameshek's riddle, restated. Blood 1992;79:1385.
112. Ng J-P, Pati A, Strevens MJ, Swart S. Myelodysplastic relapse of *de novo* acute myeloid leukaemia with trilineage myelodysplasia. Br J Haematol 1988;69:578.
113. Brito-Babapulle F, Catovsky D, Galton DAG. Myelodysplastic relapse of *de novo* acute myeloid leukaemia with trilineage myelodysplasia: a previously unrecognized correlation. Br J Haematol 1988;68:411.
114. Copplestone JA, Mufti GJ, Hamblin TJ, Oscier DG. Immunological abnormalities in myelodysplastic syndromes. Br J Haematol 1986;63:149.
115. Tranchida L, Palutke M, Poulik MD, Prasad AS. Primary acquired sideroblastic anemia preceding monoclonal gammopathy and malignant lymphoma. Am J Med 1973;55:559.
116. Greenberg BR, Miller C, Cardiff RD, et al. Concurrent development of preleukaemic, lymphoproliferative and plasma cell disorders. Br J Haematol 1983;53:125.
117. Takagi S, Kitagawa S, Takeda A, et al. Natural killer-interferon system in patients with preleukaemic states. Br J Haematol 1984;58:71.
118. Kerndrup G, Meyer K, Ellegaard J, Hokland P. Natural killer (NK)-cell activity and antibody-dependent cellular cytotoxicity (ADCC) in primary preleukemic syndrome. Leuk Res 1984;8:239.
119. Zanger B, Dorsey HN. Fever: a manifestation of preleukemia. JAMA 1976;236:1266.
120. Soppi E, Nousiainen T, Seppa A, Lahtinen R. Acute febrile neutrophilic dermatosis (Sweet's syndrome) in association with myelodysplastic syndromes: a report of three cases and a review of the literature. Br J Haematol 1989;73:43.
121. Tikjob G, Kassis V, Thomsen HK, Jensen G. Acute febrile neutrophilic dermatosis and abnormal bone marrow chromosomes as a marker for preleukemia. Acta Derm Venereol 1985;65:177.
122. Vilter RW, Wiltse D. Preleukemia and urticaria pigmentosa followed by acute myelomonoblastic leukemia. Arch Intern Med 1985;145:349.
123. Sadick N, Edlin D, Myskowski PL, et al. Granulocytic sarcoma: a new finding in the setting of preleukemia. Arch Dermatol 1984;120:1341.
124. Stoll DB, Blum S, Pasquale D, Murphy S. Thrombocytopenia with decreased megakaryocytes. Ann Intern Med 1981;94:170.
125. Gardner FH, Bessman JD. Thrombocytopenia due to defective platelet production. Clin Haematol 1983;12:23.
126. Najean Y, Lecompte T. Chronic pure thrombocytopeina in elderly patients. An aspect of the myelodysplastic syndrome. Cancer 1989;64:2506.
127. Dewald GW, Davis MP, Pierre RV, et al. Clinical characteristics and prognosis of 50 patients with a myeloproliferative syndrome and deletion of part of the long arm of chromosome 5. Blood 1985;66:189.
128. Juneja SK, Imbert M, Jouault H, et al. Haematological features of primary myelodysplastic syndromes (PMDS) at initial presentation: a study of 118 cases. J Clin Pathol 1983;36:1129.
129. Tulliez M, Testa U, Rochant H, et al. Reticulocytosis, hypochromia, and microcytosis: an unusual presentation of the preleukemic syndrome. Blood 1982;59:293.
130. White JM, Hoffbrand AV. Haem deficiency and chain synthesis. Nature 1974;248:88.
131. Maldonado J. Platelet granulopathy. Mayo Clin Proc 1976;51:452.
132. Pintado T, Maldonado J. Ultrastructure of platelet aggregation in refractory anemia and myelomonocytic leukemia. Mayo Clin Proc 1976;51:443.
133. Weil SC, Rose VL. A variant myelodysplastic syndrome with multilineage pelgeroid chromatin. Am J Clin Pathol 1986;85:176.
134. Felman P, Bryon P, Gentilhomme O, et al. The syndrome of abnormal chromatin clumping in leucocytes: a myelodysplastic disorder with proliferative features? Br J Haematol 1988;70:49.
135. Varma N, Dash S, Marwaha N, Varma S. A case of myelodysplastic syndrome with abnormal chromatin clumping in leucocytes. Br J Haematol 1989;73:135.
136. Rassam SMB, Roderick P, Al-Hakim I, Hoffbrand AV. A myelokathexis-like variant of myelodysplasia. Eur J Haematol 1989;42:99.
137. Sanz GF, Sanz MA, Vallespi T, et al. Two regression models and a scoring system for predicting survival and planning treatment in myelodysplastic syndromes: a multivariate analysis of prognostic factors in 370 patients. Blood 1989;74:395.
138. Zittoun R. Subacute and chronic myelomonocytic leukaemia: a distinct haematological entity. Br J Haematol 1976;32:1.
139. Solal-Celigny P, Desaint B, Herrera A, et al. Chronic myelomonocytic leukemia according to FAB classification: analysis of 35 cases. Blood 1984;63:634.
140. Youman JD, Saarni M, Linman JW. Diagnostic value of muraminidase (lysozyme) in acute leukemia and preleukemia. Mayo Clin Proc 1970;45:219.
141. Weintraub LR, Conrad ME, Crosby WH. Regulation of intestinal absorption of iron by the rate of cytopoiesis. Br J Haematol 1965;11:432.
142. Beris P, Graf J, Miescher PA. Primary acquired sideroblastic and primary acquired refractory anemia. Semin Hematol 1983;20:101.
143. Cartwright GE, Edwards CQ, Skolnick MH, Amos DB. Association of HLA-linked hemochromatosis with idiopathic refractory sideroblastic anemia. J Clin Invest 1980;65:989.
144. Simon M, Beaumont C, Briere J, et al. Is the HLA-linked haemochromatosis allele implicated in idiopathic refractory sideroblastic anaemia? Br J Haematol 1985;60:75.
145. Peto TEA, Pippard MJ, Weatherall DJ. Iron overload in mild sideroblastic anaemias. Lancet 1983;1:375.
146. Simon M. Secondary iron overload and the haemochromatosis allele. Br J Haematol 1985;60:1.
147. Sinn CM, Dick FW. Monocytic leukemia. Am J Med 1956;20:588.
148. Pretlow TG. Chronic monocytic dyscrasia culminating in acute leukemia. Am J Med 1968;49:130.
149. Saarni MI, Linman JW. Myelomonocytic leukemia: disorderly proliferation of all marrow cells. Cancer 1971;27:1221.
150. Miescher PA, Farquet JJ. Chronic myelomonocytic leukemia in adults. Semin Hematol 1974;11:129.
151. Geary CG, Catovsky D, Wiltshaw E, et al. Chronic myelomonocytic leukemia. Br J Haematol 1975;30:289.
152. Skinnider LF, Card RT, Padmanabh S. Chronic myelomonocytic leukemia: an ultrastructural study by transmission and scanning electron microscopy. Am J Clin Pathol 1977;67:339.

153. Ribera J-M, Cervantes F, Rozman C. A multivariate analysis of prognostic factors in chronic myelomonocytic leukaemia according to the FAB criteria. Br J Haematol 1987;65:307.
154. Van Den Berghe H, Cassiman J-J, David G, Fryns J-P. Distinct haematological disorder with deletion of long arm of No. 5 chromosome. Nature 1974;251:437.
155. Sokal G, Michaux JL, Van Den Berghe H, et al. A new hematologic syndrome with a distinct karyotype: the 5q− chromosome. Blood 1975;46:519.
156. Nimer SD, Golde DW. The 5q− abnormality. Blood 1987;70:1705.
157. Bunn HF. 5q− and disordered haematopoiesis. Clin Haematol 1986;15:1023.
158. Van Den Berghe H. The 5q− syndrome. Scand J Haematol 1986;45:78.
159. Tinegate H, Gaunt L, Hamilton PJ. The 5q−syndrome: an underdiagnosed form of macrocytic anaemia. Br J Haematol 1983;54:103.
160. Mahmood T, Robinson WA, Hamstra RD, Wallner SF. Macrocytic anemia, thrombocytosis and nonlobulated megakaryocytes. Am J Med 1979;66:946.
160a. Boultwood J, Fidler C, Lewis S, et al. Allelicloss of IRF1 in myelodysplasia and acute myeloid leukemia: retention of IRF1 on the 5q− chromosome in some patients with the 5q− syndrome. Blood 1993;82:2611.
161. Donti E, Tabilio A, Donti GV, et al. 5q− syndrome terminating in acute myeloid leukemia: karyotype evolution and immunologic characterization of blast cells. Cancer Genet Cytogenet 1988;32:205.
162. Jume'an HG, Libnoch JA. 5q− myelodysplasia terminating in acute leukemia. Ann Intern Med 1979;91:748.
163. Brusamolino E, Orlandi E, Morra E, et al. Hematologic and clinical features of patients with chromosome 5 monosomy or deletion (5q). Med Pediatr Oncol 1988;16:88.
164. Boice JD, Greene MH, Killen JY, et al. Leukemia and preleukemia after adjuvant treatment of gastrointestinal cancer with semustine (methyl-CCNU). N Engl J Med 1983;309:1079.
165. Teerenhovi L, Lintula R. Natural course of myelodysplastic syndromes-Helsinki experience. Scand J Haematol 1986;36(Suppl 45):102.
166. Calabresi P. Leukemia after cytotoxic chemotherapy-a pyrrhic victory? N Engl J Med 1983;309:1118.
167. Canellos G. Therapy-related leukemia: a necessary complication of successful systemic chemotherapy? J Clin Oncol 1984;2:1077.
168. Coltman CA, Dahlberg S. Treatment-related leukemia. N Engl J Med 1990;322:52.
169. De Gramont A, Louvet C, Krulik M, et al. Preleukemic changes in cases of nonlymphocytic leukemia secondary to cytotoxic therapy. Cancer 1986;58:630.
170. Pedersen-Bjergaard J, Ersboll J, Sorensen HM, et al. Risk of acute nonlymphocytic leukemia and preleukemia in patients treated with cyclophosphamide for non-Hodgkin's lymphomas. Ann Intern Med 1985;103:195.
171. Bennett JM, Moloney WC, Greene MH, Boice JD. Acute myeloid leukemia and other myelopathic disorders following treatment with alkylating agents. Hematol Pathol 1987;1:99.
172. Pedersen-Bjergaard J, Osterlind K, Hansen M, et al. Acute nonlymphocytic leukemia, preleukemia, and solid tumors following intensive chemotherapy of small cell carcinoma of the lung. Blood 1985;66:1393.
173. LeBeau MM, Albain KS, Larson RA, et al. Clinical and cytogenetic correlations in 63 patients with therapy-related myelodysplastic syndromes and acute nonlymphocytic leukemia: further evidence for characteristic abnormalities of chromosomes No. 5 and 7. J Clin Oncol 1986;4:325.
174. Kaldor JM, Day NE, Pettersson F, et al. Leukemia following chemotherapy for ovarian cancer. N Engl J Med 1990;322:1.
175. Kaldor JM, Day NE, Clarke EA, et al. Leukemia following Hodgkin's disease. N Engl J Med 1990;322:7.
176. Tulliez M, Ricard MF, Jan F, Sultan C. Preleukaemic abnormal myelopoiesis induced by chlorambucil: a case study. Scand J Haematol 1974;13:179.
177. Pedersen-Bjergaard J, Larsen SO, Struck J, et al. Risk of therapy-related leukaemia and preleukaemia after Hodgkin's disease: relation to age, cumulative dose of alkylating agents, and time from chemotherapy. Lancet 1987;2:83.
178. Pedersen-Bjergaard J, Philip P, Pedersen NT, et al. Acute nonlymphocytic leukemia, preleukemia, and acute myeloproliferative syndrome secondary to treatment of other malignant diseases. Cancer 1984;54:452.
179. Michels SD, McKenna RW, Arthur DC, Brunning RD. Therapy-related acute myeloid leukemia and myelodysplastic syndrome: a clinical and morphologic study of 65 cases. Blood 1985;65:1364.
180. Rowley JD, Golomb HM, Vardiman JW. Nonrandom chromosome abnormalities in acute leukemia and dysmyelopoietic syndromes in patients with previously treated malignant disease. Blood 1981;58:759.
181. Zarrabi MH, Rosner F, Grunwald HW. Second neoplasms in acute lymphoblastic leukemia. Cancer 1983;52:1712.
182. Rustin GJS, Rustin F, Dent J, et al. No increase in second tumors after cytotoxic therapy for gestational trophoblastic tumors. N Engl J Med 1983;308:473.
183. International Agency for Research on Cancer Overall evaluation of carcinogenicity: an update of IARC monographs volumes 1–42(Suppl 7). Lyons, France, International Agency for Research on Cancer, 1987.
184. Ingram L, Mott MG, Mann JR, et al. Second malignancies in children treated for non-Hodgkin's lymphoma and T-cell leukaemia with the UKCCSG regimens. Br J Haematol 1987;55:463.
185. Kurtzman GJ, Ozawa K, Cohen B, et al. Chronic bone marrow failure due to persistant B19 parvovirus infection. N Engl J Med 1987;317:287.
186. Howe RB, Bloomfield CD, McKenna RW. Hypocellular acute leukemia. Am J Med 1982;72:391.
187. Raskind WH, Fialkow PJ. The use of cell markers in the study of human hematopoietic neoplasia. Adv Cancer Res 1987;49:127.
188. Prchal JT, Throckmorton DW, Carroll AJ, et al. A common progenitor for human myeloid and lymphoid cells. Nature 1978;274:590.
189. Raskind WH, Tirumali N, Jacobson R, et al. Evidence for a multistep pathogenesis of a myelodysplastic syndrome. Blood 1984;63:1318.
190. Abkowitz JL, Fialkow PJ, Niebrugge DJ, et al. Pancytopenia as a clonal disorder of a multipotent hematopoietic stem cell. J Clin Invest 1984;73:258.
191. Fearon ER, Burke PJ, Schiffer CA, et al. Differentiation of leukemia cells to polymorphonuclear leukocytes in patients with acute nonlymphocytic leukemia. N Engl J Med 1986;315:15.
192. Vogelstein B, Fearon ER, Hamilton SR, Feinberg AP. The use of restriction fragment length polymorphisms to determine the clonal origin of human tumors. Science 1985;227:642.
193. Fearon ER, Hamilton SR, Vogelstein B. Clonal analysis of human colorectal tumors. Science 1987;238:193.
194. Janssen JWG, Buschle M, Layton M, et al. Clonal analysis of myelodysplastic syndromes: evidence of multipotent stem cell origin. Blood 1989;73:248.
195. Grier HE, Weinstein HJ, Revesz T, et al. Cytogenetic evidence for involvement of erythroid progenitors in a child with therapy linked myelodysplasia. Br J Haematol 1986;64:513.
196. Amenomori T, Tomonaga M, Jinnai I, et al. Cytogenetic and cytochemical studies on progenitor cells of primary acquired sideroblastic anemia (PASA): involvement of multipotential myeloid stem cells in PASA clone and mosaicism with normal clone. Blood 1987;70:1367.
197. Lawrence HJ, Broudy VC, Magenis RE, et al. Cytogenetic evidence for involvement of B lymphocytes in acquired sideroblastic anemia. Blood 1987;70:1003.
197a. Kroef MJ, Fibbe WE, Mout R. Myeloid but not lymphoid cells carry the 5q deletion: polymerase chain reaction analysis of loss of heterozygosity using mini-repeat sequence on highly purified cell fractions. Blood 1994;81:1849.
198. Inoshita T. Acute lymphoblastic leukemia following myelodysplastic syndrome. Am J Clin Pathol 1985;84:233.
199. Barton JC, Conrad ME, Parmley RT. Acute lymphoblastic leukemia in idiopathic refractory sideroblastic anemia: evidence for a common lymphoid and myeloid progenitor cell. Am J Hematol 1980;9:109.
200. Ariel I, Weiler-Ravell D, Stalnikowicz R. Preleukemia in acute lymphoblastic leukemia. Acta Haematol 1981;66:50.
201. Brusamolino E, Isernia P, Alessandrino EP, et al. Terminal deoxynucleotidyl transferase-positive acute leukemias evolving from a myelodysplastic syndrome. Am J Hematol 1985;20:187.
202. Eridani S, Chan LC, Halil O, Pearson TC. Acute biphenotypic leukaemia (myeloid and null-ALL type) supervening in a myelodysplastic syndrome. Br J Haematol 1985;61:525.
203. Heim S, Mitelman F. Chromosome abnormalities in the myelodysplastic syndromes. Clin Haematol 1986;15:1003.
204. Michels VV, Hoagland HC. Chromosome abnormalities in preleukemic or myelodysplastic syndromes. Mayo Clin Proc 1985;60:555.
205. Nowell PC. Cytogenetics of preleukemia. Cancer Genet Cytogenet 1982;5:265.
205a. Ohyashiki K, Sasao I, Ohyashiki JH, et al. Cytogenetic and clinical findings of myelodysplastic syndromes with a poor prognosis: an experience with 97 cases. Cancer 1992;70:94.
206. Billstrom R, Nilsson PG, Mitelman F. Cytogenetic analysis in 941 consecutive patients with haematologic disorders. Scand J Haematol 1986;37:29.
207. Anderson RL, Bagby GC. The prognostic value of chromosome studies in patients with the preleukemic syndrome (hemopoietic dysplasia). Leuk Res 1982;6:175.
208. Gold EJ, Conjalka M, Pelus LM, et al. Marrow cytogenetic and cell-culture analyses of the myelodysplastic syndromes: insights to pathophysiology and prognosis. J Clin Oncol 1983;1:627.
209. Nowell P, Besa EC, Stelmach T, Finan JB. Chromosome studies in preleukemic states. Cancer 1986;58:2571.
210. Lawler SD, Swansbury GJ. Cytogenetic studies in primary and secondary preleukaemic states. Haematologica (Pavia) 1987;72:49.
211. Jacobs RH, Cornbleet MA, Vardiman JW, et al. Prognostic implications of morphology and karyotype in primary myelodysplastic syndromes. Blood 1986;67:1765.
212. Ayraud N, Donzeau M, Raynaud S, Lambert J-C. Cytogenetic study of 88 cases of refractory anemia. Cancer Genet Cytogenet 1983;8:243.
213. Billstrom R, Thiede T, Hansen S, et al. Bone marrow karyotype and prognosis in primary myelodysplastic syndromes. Eur J Haematol 1988;41:341.

214. Estey EH, Keating MJ, Dixon DO, et al. Karyotype is prognostically more important than the FAB system's distinction between myelodysplastic syndrome and acute myelogenous leukemia. Hematol Pathol 1987;1:203.
215. Musilova J, Michalova K. Chromosome study of 85 patients with myelodysplastic syndrome. Cancer Genet Cytogenet 1988;33:39.
216. Horiike S, Taniwaki M, Misawa S, Abe T. Chromosome abnormalities and karyotypic evolution in 83 patients with myelodysplastic syndrome and predictive value for prognosis. Cancer 1988;62:1129.
217. Knapp RH, Dewald GW, Pierre RV. Cytogenetic studies in 174 consecutive patients with preleukemic or myelodysplastic syndromes. Mayo Clin Proc 1985;60:507.
218. Yunis JJ, Rydell RE, Oken MM, et al. Refined chromosome analysis as an independent prognostic indicator in de novo myelodysplastic syndromes. Blood 1986;67:1721.
219. Yunis JJ. Should refined chromosomal analysis be used routinely in acute leukemias and myelodysplastic syndrome? N Engl J Med 1986;315:322.
220. Nowell P, Wilmoth D, Lange B. Cytogenetics of childhood preleukemia. Cancer Genet Cytogenet 1983;6:261.
221. Nowell PC, Besa EC. Prognostic significance of single chromsomal abnormalities in preleukemic states. Cancer Genet Cytogenet 1989;42:1.
222. Carbonell F, Heimpel H, Kubanek B, Fliedner TM. Growth and cytogenetic characteristics of bone marrow colonies from patients with 5q−syndrome. Blood 1985;66:463.
223. Gyger M, Perreault C, Pichette R, et al. Interstitial deletion of the long arm of chromosome 5 (5q−) in leukemia and other hematological disorders: clinical and biological relevance of variable breakpoint patterns. Leuk Res 1986;10:9.
224. Mitelman F, Manolova Y, Manolov G, et al. High resolution analysis of the 5q− marker chromosome in refractory anemia. Hereditas 1986;105:49.
225. Wisniewski LP, Hirschorn K. Acquired partial deletion of the long arm of chromosome 5 in hematologic disorders. Am J Hematol 1983;15:295.
226. Haas OA, Bettelheim P, Schmidmeier W, et al. 5q− chromosome in acute leukemia with lymphoid morphology and expression of myeloid membrane determinants. Blood 1985;65:1342.
227. Swolin B, Weinfeld A, Ridell B, et al. On the 5q− deletion: clinical and cytogenetic observations in ten patients and review of the literature. Blood 1981;58:986.
228. Kerkhofs H, Hagemeijer A, Leeksma HW, et al. The 5q− chromosome abnormality in haematological disorders: a collaborative study of 34 cases from the Netherlands. Br J Haematol 1982;52:365.
229. Mitelman F. Catalog of chromosome aberrations in cancer, ed 3. New York, Alan R Liss, 1988.
230. Lavezzi AM, Maiolo AT, Chiorboli O, Mozzana R. The bone marrow karyotype in seventeen cases of refractory anemia with excess of blasts (RAEB). Ann Genet 1983;26:220.
231. Gyger M, Forest L, Vuong TE, et al. Therapy-induced preleukaemia in patients treated for Hodgkin's lymphoma: clinical and therapeutic relevance of sequential chromosome banding studies. Br J Haematol 1984;58:61.
232. Pedersen-Bjergaard J, Philip P. Cytogenetic characteristics of therapy-related acute nonlymphocytic leukaemia, preleukaemia and acute myeloproliferative syndrome: correlation with clinical data for 61 consecutive cases. Br J Haematol 1987;66:199.
233. Levin M, Le Coniat M, Bernheim A, Berger R. Complex chromosomal abnormalities in acute nonlymphocytic leukemia. Cancer Genet Cytogenet 1986;22:113.
234. Wilmoth D, Feder M, Finan J, Nowell P. Preleukemia and leukemia with 12p− and 19q+ chromosome alterations following Alkeran therapy. Cancer Genet Cytogenet 1985;15:95.
235. Kledsen N, Philip P, Pedersen-Bjergaard J. Translocations and deletions with breakpoint on 21q are nonrandomly associated with treatment-related acute nonlymphocytic leukemia and preleukemia. Cancer Genet Cytogenet 1987;29:43.
236. Tomonaga M, Tomonaga Y, Kusano M, Ichimaru M. Sequential karyotypic evolutions and bone marrow aplasia preceding acute myelomonocytic transformation from myelodysplastic syndrome. Br J Haematol 1984;58:53.
237. Yunis JJ, Lobell M, Arnesen MA, et al. Refined chromosome study helps define prognostic subgroups in most patients with primary myelodysplastic syndrome and acute myelogenous leukaemia. Br J Haematol 1988;68:189.
238. Pierre RV. Cytogenetic studies in preleukemia: studies before and after transition to acute leukemia in 17 subjects. Blood Cells 1975;1:163.
239. Tricot G, Boogaerts MA, De Wolf-Peeters C, et al. The myelodysplastic syndromes: different evolution patterns based on sequential morphological and cytogenetic investigations. Br J Haematol 1985;59:659.
240. Struli RA, Testa JR, Vardiman JW, et al. Dysmyelopoietic syndrome: sequential clinical and cytogenetic studies. Blood 1980;55:636.
241. Donti E, Tabilio A, Venti Donti G, et al. 5q− syndrome terminating in acute myeloid leukemia: karyotype evolution and immunologic characterization of blast cells. Cancer Genet Cytogenet 1988;32:205.
242. Benitez J, Carbonell F, Sanchez Fayos J, Heimpel H. Karyotypic evolution in patients with myelodysplastic syndromes. Cancer Genet Cytogenet 1985;16:157.
243. Ringressi A, Mecucci C, Grossi A, et al. 6p+ and 9q− in two chromosomally distinct clones occurring in a case of myelodysplastic syndrome evolving to acute nonlymphocytic leukemia. Cancer Genet Cytogenet 1988;35:213.
244. Miller BA, Weinstein HJ, Nell M, et al. Sequential development of distinct clonal chromosome abnormalities in a patient with preleukaemia. Br J Haematol 1985;59:411.
245. Smadja N, Krulik M, De Gramont A, et al. Acquired idiopathic sideroblastic anemia and terminal deletion of chromosome 11. Cancer Genet Cytogenet 1985;16:275.
246. Heim S, Mitelman F. Cytogenetically unrelated clones in hematological neoplasms. Leukemia 1989;3:6.
247. Knuutila S, Vuopio P, Borgstrom GH, De La Chapelle A. Higher frequency of 5q−clone in bone marrow mitoses after culture than by a direct method. Scand J Haematol 1980;25:358.
248. Wang WC, Dow LW, Presbury GJ, et al. Serial cell culture and cytogenetic studies of marrow cells from a patient with monosomy 7 syndrome. Am J Pediatr Hematol Oncol 1985;7:321.
249. Okuda T, Yokota S, Maekawa T, et al. Heterogeneous colony forming ability *in vitro* of the abnormal clone-derived granulocyte-macrophage precursors in myelodysplastic syndromes. Leuk Res 1988;12:687.
250. Clark R, Peters S, Hoy T, et al. Prognostic importance of hypodiploid hemopoietic precursors in myelodysplastic syndromes. N Engl J Med 1986;314:1472.
251. Auffermann W, Fohlmeister I, Bocking A. Diagnostic and prognostic value of DNA image cytometry in myelodysplasia. J Clin Pathol 1988;41:604.
252. Thein SL, Oscier DG, Jeffreys AJ, et al. Detection of chromosomal 7 loss in myelodysplasia using an extremely polymorphic DNA probe. Br J Cancer 1988;57:131.
253. Kere J, Ruutu T, De La Chapelle A. Monosomy 7 in granulocytes and monocytes in myelodysplatic syndrome. N Engl J Med 1987;316:499.
254. Kere J. Chromosome 7 long arm deletion breakpoints in preleukemia: mapping by pulsed field gel electrophoresis. Nucleic Acids Res 1989;17:1511.
255. Tabin CJ, Bradley SM, Bargmann CI, et al. Mechanism of activation of a human oncogene. Nature 1982;300:143.
256. Barbacid M. RAS genes. Ann Rev Biochem 1987;56:779.
257. Davis RL, Konopka JB, Witte ON. Activation of the c-*abl* oncogene by viral transduction or chromosomal translocation generates altered c-*abl* proteins with similar in vitro kinase properties. Mol Cell Biol 1985;5:204.
258. Battey J, Moulding C, Taub R, et al. The human c-*myc* oncogene: structural consequences of translocation into the IgH locus in Burkitt lymphoma. Cell 1983;34:779.
259. Lombardi L, Newcomb EW, Dalla-Favera R. Pathogenesis of Burkitt lymphoma: expression of an activated c-*myc* oncogene causes the tumorigenic conversion of EBV-infected human B lymphoblasts. Cell 1987;49:161.
260. Croce CM, Nowell PC. Molecular basis of B-cell neoplasia. Blood 1985;65:1.
261. Sagar R. Tumor suppressor genes: the puzzle and the promise. Science 1989;246:1406.
262. Cooper JA, Whyte P. RB and the cell cycle: entrance or exit? Cell 1989;58:1009.
263. Huang HJS, Yee JK, Shew JY, et al. Suppression of the neoplastic phenotype by replacement of the RB gene in human cancer cells. Science 1988;242:1563.
264. Cavenee WK, Dryja TP, Phillips RA, et al. Expression of recessive alleles by chromosomal mechanisms in retinoblastoma. Nature 1983;305:779.
265. Baker SJ, Fearon ER, Nigro JM, et al. Chromosome 17 deletions and p53 gene mutations in colorectal carcinomas. Science 1989;244:217.
266. Stanbridge EJ. Identifying tumor suppressor genes in human colorectal cancer. Science 1990;247:12.
267. Fearon ER, Cho KR, Nigro JM, et al. Identification of a chromosome 18q gene that is altered in colorectal cancers. Science 1990;247:49.
268. Solomon E, Voss R, Hall V, et al. Chromosome 5 allele loss in human colorectal carcinomas. Nature 1987;328:616.
269. Temin HM. Evolution of cancer genes as a mutation-driven process. Cancer Res 1988;48:1697.
270. Land H, Parada LF, Weinberg RA. Cellular oncogenes and multistep carcinogenesis. Science 1983;222:771.
271. Vogelstein B, Fearon ER, Hamilton SR, et al. Genetic alterations during colorectal-tumor development. N Engl J Med 1988;319:525.
272. Bos JL. The ras gene family and human carcinogenesis. Mutat Res 1988;195:255.
273. Lyons J, Janssen JWG, Bartram C, et al. Mutation of Ki-RAS and N-RAS oncogenes in myelodysplastic syndromes. Blood 1988;71:1707.
274. Bar-Eli M, Ahuja H, Gonzalez-Cadavid N, et al. Analysis of N-RAS exon-1 mutations in myelodysplastic syndromes by polymerase chain reaction and direct sequencing. Blood 1989;73:281.
274a. Paquette RL, Landaw EM, Pierre RV, et al. N-*ras* mutations are associated with poor prognosis and increased risk of leukemia in myelodysplastic syndrome. Blood 1993;82:590.
275. Padua RA, Carter G, Hughes D, et al. RAS mutations in myelodysplasia

detected by amplification, oligonucleotide hybridization, and transformation. Leukemia 1988;2:503.
276. Toksoz T, Farr CJ, Marshall CJ. RAS genes and acute myeloid leukaemia. Br J Haematol 1989;71:1.
277. Bartram CR. Mutations in ras genes in myelocytic leukemias and myelodysplastic syndromes. Blood Cells 1988;14:533.
278. Janssen JWG, Steenvoorden AGM, Lyons J, et al. RAS gene mutations in acute and chronic myelocytic leukemia, chronic myeloproliferative disorders, and myelodysplastic syndromes. Proc Natl Acad Sci USA 1987;84:9228.
279. Hirai H, Koyabashi Y, Mano H, et al. A point mutation at codon 13 of the N-ras oncogene in myelodysplastic syndrome. Nature 1987;327:430.
280. Liu E, Hjelle B, Morgan R, et al. Mutations of the Kirsten-ras proto-oncogene in human preleukemia. Nature 1987;330:186.
281. Yunis JJ, Boot AJ, Mayer MG, Bos JL. Mechanisms of ras mutation in myelodysplastic syndrome. Oncogene 1989;4:609.
282. Guerrero I, Calzada P, Mayer A, Pellicer A. A molecular approach to leukemogenesis: mouse lymphomas contain an activated c-*ras* oncogene. Proc Natl Acad Sci USA 1984;81:202.
283. Pedersen-Bjergaard J, Janssen JWG, Lyons J, et al. Point mutations of the ras protooncogenes and chromosome aberrations in acute nonlymphocytic leukemia and preleukemia related to therapy with alkylating agents. Cancer Res 1988;48:1812.
284. Hirai H, Okada M, Mizoguchi H, et al. Relationship between an activated N-ras oncogene and chromosomal abnormality during leukemic progression from myelodysplastic syndrome. Blood 1988;71:256.
285. Krontiris TG, DiMartino NA, Colb M, Parkinson DR. Unique allelic restriction fragments of the human Ha-ras locus in leukocyte and tumor DNAs of cancer patients. Nature 1985;313:369.
286. Carter G, Worwood M, Jacobs A. The H-ras polymorphism in myelodysplasia and acute myeloid leukemia. Leuk Res 1988;12:385.
287. Thein SL, Oscier DG, Flint J, Wainscoat JS. Ha-ras hypervariable alleles in myelodysplasia. Nature 1986;321:84.
288. Srivastava A, Boswell HS, Heerema NA, et al. KRAS2 oncogene overexpression in myelodysplastic syndrome with translocation 5;12. Cancer Genet Cytogenet 1988;35:61.
289. Woloschak GE, Dewald GW, Bahn RS, et al. Amplification of RNA and DNA specific for erb B in unbalanced 1;7 chromosomal translocation associated with myelodysplastic syndrome. J Cell Biochem 1986;32:47.
290. Duesberg PH. Activated proto-oncogenes: sufficient or necessary for cancer? Science 1985;228:669.
291. Farr CJ, Saiki RK, Erlich HA, et al. Analysis of RAS gene mutations in acute myeloid leukemia by polymerase chain reaction and oligonucleotide probes. Proc Natl Acad Sci USA 1988;85:1629.
292. Sherr CJ. Colony-stimulating factor-1 receptor. Blood 1990;75:1.
293. Roussel MF, Downing JR, Rettenmier CW, Sherr CJ. A point mutation in the extracellular domain of the human CSF-1 receptor (c-fms proto-oncogene product) activates its transforming potential. Cell 1988;55:979.
294. Jacobs A, Ridge S, Worwood M, Padua RA. Point mutations at codons 301 and 969 in the human c-*fms* gene in myelodysplasia, acute myeloid leukaemia and in normal subjects. Blood 1989;74:245a.
295. Everson MP, Brown CB, Lilly MB. Interleukin-6 and granulocyte-macrophage colony-stimulating factor are candidate growth factors for chronic myelomonocytic leukemia cells. Blood 1989;74:1472.
296. Geissler K, Hinterberger W, Bettelheim P, et al. Colony growth characteristics in chronic myelomonocytic leukemia. Leuk Res 1988;12:373.
296a. Sugimoto K, Hirano N, Toyoshima H. Mutations of the p53 gene in myelodysplastic syndrome (MDS) and MDS-derived leukemia. Blood 1993;81:3022.
297. Le Beau MM, Chandrasekharappa SC, Lemons RS, et al. Molecular and cytogenetic analysis of chromosome 5 abnormalities in myeloid disorders: chromosomal localization and physical mapping of IL-4 and IL-5. In: Cancer cells 7/molecular diagnostics of human cancer. Cold Spring Harbor, New York, Cold Spring Harbor Laboratory, 1989:53.
298. Huebner K, Isobe M, Croce CM, et al. The human gene encoding GM-CSF is at 5q21–q32, the chromosome region deleted in the 5q− anomaly. Science 1985;230:1282.
299. Sherr CJ, Rettenmier CW, Sacca R, et al. The c-*fms* proto-oncogene product is related to the receptor for the mononuclear phagocyte growth factor, CSF-1. Cell 1985;41:665.
300. Nienhuis AW, Bunn HF, Turner PH, et al. Expression of the human c-*fms* proto-oncogene in hematopoietic cells and its deletion in the 5q− syndrome. Cell 1985;42:421.
301. Pettenati MJ, Le Beau MM, Lemons RS, et al. Assignment of CSF-1 to 5q33.1: evidence for clustering of genes regulating hematopoiesis and for their involvement in the deletion of the long arm of chromosome 5 in myeloid disorders. Proc Natl Acad Sci USA 1987;84:2970.
302. Le Beau MM, Epstein ND, O'Brien SJ, et al. The interleukin 3 gene is located on human chromosome 5 and is deleted in myeloid leukemias with a deletion of 5q. Proc Natl Acad Sci USA 1987;84:5913.
303. Yamg YC, Kovacic S, Kriz R, et al. The human genes for GM-CSF and IL-3 are closely linked in tandem on chromosome 5. Blood 1988;71:958.
304. Sutherland GR, Baker E, Callen DF, et al. Interleukin-5 is at 5q31 and is deleted in the 5q− syndrome. Blood 1988;71:1150.
305. Le Beau MM, Lemons RS, Espinosa R III, et al. Interleukin-4 and interleukin-5 map to human chromosome 5 in a region encoding growth factors and receptors and are deleted in myeloid leukemias with a del(5q). Blood 1989;73:647.
306. van Leeuwen BH, Martinson ME, Webb GC, Young IG. Molecular organization of the cytokine gene cluster, involving the human IL-3, IL-4, IL-5, and GM-CSF genes, on human chromosome 5. Blood 1989;73:1142.
307. Yarden Y, Escobedo A, Kuang WJ, et al. Structure of the receptor for platelet-derived growth factor helps define a family of closely related growth factor receptors. Nature 1986;323:226.
308. Roberts WM, Loo AT, Roussel MF, Sherr CJ. Tandem linkage of human CSF-1 receptor (c-fms) and PDGF receptor genes. Cell 1988;55:655.
309. Kolbilka BK, Cison RAF, Frielle T, et al. cDNA for the human beta2-adrenergic receptor: a protein with multiple membrane-spanning domains and encoded by a gene whose chromosomal localization is shared with that of the receptor for platelet-derived growth factor. Proc Natl Acad Sci USA 1987;84:46.
310. Jaye M, Howk R, Burgess W, et al. Human endothelial cell growth factor: cloning, nucleotide sequence and chromosomal localization. Science 1986;233:541.
311. Francke U, Foellmer BE. The glucocorticoid receptor gene is in 5q31–q32. Genomics 1989;4:610.
312. Goyert SM, Ferrero E, Rettig WJ, et al. The CD14 monocyte differentiation antigen maps to a region encoding growth factors and receptors. Science 1988;243:497.
313. Sukhatme VP, Cao X, Chang LC, et al. A zinc finger-encoding gene coregulated with c-*fos* during growth and differentiation and after cellular depolarization. Cell 1988;53:37.
314. Sieff CA. Hematopoietic growth factors. J Clin Invest 1987;79:1549.
315. Groopman JE, Molina J, Scadden DT. Hematopoietic growth factors: biology and clinical applications. N Engl J Med 1989;321:1449.
316. Clark SC, Kamen R. The human hematopoietic colony-stimulating factors. Science 1987;236:1229.
317. Rohrschneider LR, Metcalf D. Induction of macrophage colony-stimulating factor-dependent growth and differentiation after introduction of the murine c-*fms* gene into FDC-P1 cells. Mol Cell Biol 1989;9:5081.
318. Bodmer WF, Bailey CJ, Bodmer J, et al. Localization of the gene for familial adenomatous polyposis on chromosome 5. Nature 1987;328:614.
319. Heim S, Billstrom R, Kristoffersson U, et al. Late appearing 5q− marker in refractory anemia. N Engl J Med 1987;24:159.
320. Baer MR, Dessypris EN. Deletion of the long arm of chromosome 5 (5q−) as a secondary event in the course of refractory anemia. Cancer Genet Cytogenet 1986;22:169.
321. Stuart RK, Mangan KF. Hematologic and cytogenetic remission of 5q− refractory anemia after syngeneic bone marrow transplantation. Am J Med 1986;80:503.
322. Knuutila S, Teerenhovi L, Borgstrom GH. Chromosome instability is associated with hypodiploid clones in myelodysplastic syndromes. Hereditas 1984;101:19.
323. Nowell PC, Hungerford DA. Chromosome studies on normal and leukemic human leukocytes. J Natl Cancer Inst 1960;25:85.
324. Daley GQ, Van Etten RA, Baltimore D. Induction of chronic myelogenous leukemia in mice by the $P210^{bcr/abl}$ gene of the Philadelphia chromosome. Science 1990;247:824.
325. Mitelman F, Brandt L, Nilsson PG. Relation among occupational exposure to potential mutagenic/carcinogenic agents, clinical findings, and bone marrow chromosomes in acute nonlymphocytic leukemia. Blood 1978;52:1229.
326. Golomb HM, Alimena G, Rowley JD, et al. Correlation of occupation and karyotype in adults with acute nonlymphocytic leukemia. Blood 1982;60:404.
327. Arlett CF. Human DNA repair defects. J Inher Metab Dis 1986;9:69.
328. Chaganti RSK, Schonberg S, German J. A manyfold increase in sister chromatid exchanges in Bloom's syndrome lymphocytes. Proc Natl Acad Sci USA 1974;71:4508.
329. Schimke RT, Sherwood SW, Hill AB, Johnston RN. Overreplication and recombination of DNA in higher eukaryotes: potential consequences and biological implications. Proc Natl Acad Sci USA 1986;83:2157.
330. Murthy PB, Kamada N, Kuramoto A. Increased sister chromatid exchange frequency in bone marrow cells of myelodysplastic syndromes. Cancer Genet Cytogenet 1985;15:151.
331. de Vinuesa ML, Larripa I, de Pargament MM, de Salum SB. Heterochromatic variants and their association with neoplasias. II preleukemic states. Cancer Genet Cytogenet 1985;14:31.
332. Murthy PB, Kamada N, Kuramoto A. Defective ultraviolet-induced DNA repair in bone marrow cells and peripheral lymphocytes of patients with refractory anemia with excess of blasts. Jpn J Clin Oncol 1984;14:87.
333. Metcalf D. The hematopoeitic colony stimulating factors. Amsterdam, Elsevier, 1984.

334. Milner GR, Testa NG, Geary CG, et al. Bone marrow culture studies in refractory cytopenia and "smouldering leukaemia." Br J Haematol 1977;35:251.
335. Mizoguchi H, Kubota K, Suda T, et al. Erythroid and granulocyte/macrophage progenitor cells in primary acquired sideroblastic anemia. Intl J Cell Clon 1983;1:15.
336. Baines P, Masters GS, Lush C, Jacobs A. Enrichment of haemopoietic progenitor cells from the marrow of patients with myelodysplasia. Br J Haematol 1988;68:159.
337. Geissler K, Hinterberger W, Jager U, et al. Deficiency of pluripotent hemopoietic progenitor cells in myelodysplastic syndromes. Blut 1988;57:45.
338. Tennant G, Jacobs A, Bailey-Wood R. Peripheral blood granulocyte-macrophage progenitors in patients with the myelodysplastic syndromes. Exp Hematol 1986;14:1063.
339. Greenberg PL, Mara B. The preleukemic syndrome: correlation of in vitro parameters of granulopoiesis with clinical features. Am J Med 1979;66:951.
340. Lidbeck J. In vitro colony and cluster growth in haemopoietic dysplasia (the preleukaemic syndrome). Scand J Haematol 1980;25:113.
341. Rosenthal DS, Moloney WC. Refractory dysmyelopoietic anemia and acute leukemia. Blood 1984;63:314.
342. Elstner E, Schulze E, Ihle R, et al. Proliferation and maturation of hemopoietic cells from patients with preleukemia and aplastic anemia in agar and diffusion chamber cultures. Haematol Blood Transfus 1983;28:358.
343. Zwierzina H, Sepp N, Ringler E, Schmalzl F. Delayed maturation of skin window macrophages in myelodysplastic syndromes. Leuk Res 1989;13:433.
344. May SJ, Smith SA, Jacobs A, et al. The myelodysplastic syndrome: analysis of laboratory characteristics in relation to the FAB classification. Br J Haematol 1985;59:311.
345. Senn JS, Messne HA, Pinkerton PH, et al. Peripheral blood blast cell progenitors in human preleukemia. Blood 1979;54:106.
346. Greenberg P. Clinical relevance of in vitro study of granulocytopoiesis. Scand J Haematol 1980;25:369.
347. Greenberg PL, Nichols WC, Schrier SL. Granulopoiesis in acute myeloid leukemia and preleukemia. N Engl J Med 1971;284:1225.
348. Juvonen E, Partanen S, Knuutila S, Ruutu T. Megakaryocyte colony formation by bone marrow progenitors in myelodysplastic syndromes. Br J Haematol 1986;63:331.
349. Koeffler HP, Cline MJ, Golde DW. Erythropoiesis in preleukemia. Blood 1978;51:1013.
350. Geissler D, Zwierzina H, Pechlaner C, et al. Abnormal megakaryopoiesis in patients with myelodysplastic syndromes: analysis of cellular and humoral defects. Br J Haematol 1989;73:29.
351. Juvonen E, Partanen S, Knuutila S, Ruutu T. Colony formation by megakaryocyte progenitors in myelodysplastic syndromes. Eur J Haematol 1989;42:389.
352. Carbonell F, Heimpel H, Kubanek B, Fleidner TM. Growth and cytogenetic characteristics of bone marrow colonies from patients with 5q− syndrome. Blood 1985;66:463.
353. Koeffler HP, Golde DW. Cellular maturation in human preleukemia. Blood 1978;52:355.
354. Queisser U, Olischlager A, Queisser W, Heimpel H. Cell proliferation in the "preleukaemic" phase of acute leukaemia. Acta Haematol 1972;47:21.
355. Dormer P, Ucci G, Hershko C, Wilmanns W. Cell kinetics in leukemia and preleukemia. Haematol Blood Transfus 1987;30:3.
356. Montecucco C, Riccardi A, Traversi E, et al. Proliferative activity of bone marrow cells in primary dysmyelopoietic (preleukemic) syndromes. Cancer 1983;52:1190.
357. Stella CC, Cazzola M, Bergamaschi G, et al. Growth of human hematopoietic colonies from patients with myelodysplastic syndromes in response to recombinant human granulocyte-macrophage colony-stimulating factor. Leukemia 1989;3:363.
358. Mayani H, Baines P, Bowen DT, Jacobs A. In vitro growth of myeloid and erythroid progenitor cells from myelodysplastic patients in response to recombinant human granulocyte-macrophage colony-stimulating factor. Leukemia 1989;3:29.
359. Merchav S, Nagler A, Fleischer-Kurtz G, Tatarsky I. Regulatory abnormalities in the marrow of patients with myelodysplastic syndromes. Br J Haematol 1989;73:158.
360. Merchav S, Nagler A, Sahar E, Tatarsky I. Production of human pluripotent progenitor cell colony stimulating activity (CFU-GEMM-CSA) in patients with myelodysplastic syndromes. Leuk Res 1987;11:273.
361. Francis GE, Miller EJ, Wonke B, et al. Use of bone-marrow culture in prediction of acute leukaemic transformation in preleukaemia. Lancet 1983;1409.
362. Morris TCM, McNeill TA, Bridges JM. Inhibition of normal in vitro colony forming cells by cells from leukaemic patients. Br J Cancer 1975;31:641.
363. Quesenberry PJ, Rappeport JM, Fountebuoni A, et al. Inhibition of normal murine hematopoiesis by leukemic cells. N Engl J Med 1978;299:71.
364. Geissler D, Thaler J, Konwalinka G, Peschel C. Progressive preleukemia presenting amegakaryocytic thrombocytopenic purpura: association of the 5q− syndrome with a decreased megakaryocytic colony formation and a defective production of Meg-CSF. Leuk Res 1987;11:731.
365. Putintseva E, Garcia-Triana E. Thrombopoietic inhibitory activity in serum of patients with refractory anaemia. Br J Haematol 1987;265.
366. Kerndrup G, Hokland P. Natural-killer cell-mediated inhibition of bone marrow colony formation (CFU-GM) in refractory anemia (preleukaemia): evidence for patient-specific cell populations. Br J Haematol 1988;69:457.
367. Jacobs A, Janowska-Wieczorek A, Caro J, et al. Circulating erythropoietin in patients with myelodysplastic syndromes. Br J Haematol 1989;73:36.
368. Wallner SF, Kurnick JE, Vautrin RM, et al. Levels of erythropoietin in patients with the anemias of chronic diseases and liver failure. Am J Hematol 1977;3:37.
369. Sherwood JB, Goldwasser E, Chilcote R, et al. Sickle cell anemia patients have low erythropoietin levels for their degree of anemia. Blood 1986;67:46.
370. de Klerk G, Rosengarten PCJ, Vet RJWM, Goudsmit R. Serum erythropoietin (ESF) titers in anemia. Blood 1981;58:1164.
371. Ward HP, Kurnick JE, Pisarczyk MJ. Serum level of erythropoietin in anemias associated with chronic infection, malignancy, and primary hematopoietic disease. J Clin Invest 1971;50:332.
372. Lutton JD, Ibraham NG, Hoffman R, et al. Sideroblastic anemia: differences in bone marrow erythroid colony (CFU_E) growth responses to erythropoietin in plasma clot and methylcellulose cultures. Am J Hematol 1984;16:219.
373. Sporn MB, Roberts AB. Autocrine growth factors and cancer. Nature 1985;313:745.
374. Browder TM, Dunbar CE, Nienhuis AW. Private and public autocrine loops in neoplastic cells. Cancer Cells 1989;1:9.
375. Young DC, Griffin JD. Autocrine secretion of GM-CSF in acute myeloblastic leukemia. Blood 1986;68:1178.
376. Griffin JD, Young DC. The role of colony stimulating factors in leukaemogenesis. Clin Haematol 1986;15:995.
377. Russell NH, Reilly AG. Role of autocrine growth factors in the leukemic transformation of the myelodysplastic syndromes. Leukemia 1989;3:83.
378. Chang JM, Metcalf D, Lang RA, et al. Nonneoplastic hematopoietic myeloproliferative syndrome induced by dysregulated multi-CSF (IL-3) expression. Blood 1989;73:1487.
379. Wong PMC, Chung SW, Dunbar CE, et al. Retrovirus-mediated transfer and expression of the interleukin-3 gene in mouse hematopoietic cells result in a myeloproliferative disorder. Mol Cell Biol 1989;9:798.
380. Johnson GR, Gonda TJ, Metcalf D, et al. A lethal myeloproliferative syndrome in mice transplanted with bone marrow cells infected with a retrovirus expressing granulocyte-macrophage colony stimulating factor. EMBO J 1989;8:441.
381. Valentine WN, Konrad PN, Paglia DE. Dyserythropoiesis, refractory anemia, and "preleukemia": metabolic features of the erythrocytes. Blood 1973;41:857.
382. Boivin P, Galand C, Hakim J, Kahn A. Acquired erythroenzymopathies in blood disorders: study of 200 cases. Br J Haematol 1975;31:531.
383. Dreyfus B, Sultan C, Rochant H, et al. Anomalies of blood group antigens and erythrocyte enzymes in two types of chronic refractory anemia. Br J Haematol 1969;16:303.
384. Nano R, Invernizzi R, Rezzani R, Gerzeli G. Qualitative 2nd quantitative study of dihydrofolate reductase in myelodysplastic syndromes. Acta Haematol 1988;79:198.
385. Kanno H, Fujii H, Tani K, et al. Elevated erythrocyte adenosine deaminase activity in a patient with primary acquired sideroblastic anemia. Am J Hematol 1988;27:216.
386. van der Weyden MB, Harrison C, Hallam L, et al. Elevated red cell adenosine deaminase and haemolysis in a patient with a myelodysplastic syndrome. Br J Haematol 1989;73:129.
387. Helmstadter V, Arnold H, Blume KG, et al. Acquired pyruvate kinase deficiency with hemolysis in preleukemia. Acta Haematol 1977;57: 339.
388. Kornberg A, Goldfarb A. Preleukemia manifested by hemolytic anemia with pyruvate-kinase deficiency. Arch Intern Med 1986;146:785.
389. Salmon C. Blood groups changes in preleukemic states. Blood Cells 1976;2:211.
390. Yoshida A, Kumazaki T, Dave V, Dzik WH. Suppressed expression of blood group B antigen and blood group galactosyltransferase in a preleukemic subject. Blood 1985;66:990.
391. Rochant H, Dreyfus B, Bouguerra M, Tont-Hat H. Refractory anemias, preleukemic conditions, and fetal erythropoiesis. Blood 1972;39:721.
392. Abbondanzo SL, Anagnou NP, Sacher RA. Myelodysplastic syndrome with acquired hemoglobin H disease: evolution through megakaryoblastic transformation into myelofibrosis. Am J Clin Pathol 1988;89: 401.
393. Peters RE, May A, Jacobs A. Globin chain synthesis ratios in sideroblastic anaemia. Br J Haematol 1983;53:201.
394. Anagnou NP, Ley TJ, Chesbro B, et al. Acquired alpha-thalassemia in preleukemia is due to decreased expression of all four alpha-globin genes. Proc Natl Acad Sci USA 1983;80:6051.
395. Jacobs A. Primary acquired sideroblastic anemia. Br J Haematol 1986;64:415.

396. Pasanen A, Tenhunen R. Heme synthesis in sideroblastic anaemias. Scand J Haematol 1986;45:60.
397. Hast R, Reizenstein P. Sideroblastic anemia and development of leukemia. Blut 1981;42:203.
398. Bottomley SS. Porphyrin and iron metabolism in sideroblastic anemia. Semin Hematol 1977;14:169.
399. Verwilghen R, Reybrouck G, Callens L, Cosemans J. Antituberculous drugs and sideroblastic anaemia. Br J Haematol 1965;II:92.
400. Horrigan DL, Harris JW. Pyridoxine-responsive anemia: analysis of 62 cases. Adv Intern Med 1989;12:103.
401. Raab SO, Haut A, Cartwright GE, Wintrobe MM. Pyridoxine-responsive anemia. Blood 1961;18:285.
402. Ibraham NG, Lutton JD, Hoffman R, Levere RD. Regulation of heme metabolism in normal and sideroblastic bone marrow cells in culture. J Lab Clin Med 1985;105:593.
403. Konopka L, Hoffbrand AV. Haem synthesis in sideroblastic anaemia. Br J Haematol 1979;42:73.
404. Bottomley SS, Tanaka M, Self J. Delta-aminolevulinic acid synthetase activity in normal human bone marrow and in patients with idiopathic sideroblastic anemia. Enzyme 1973;16:138.
405. Aoki Y, Urata G, Takaku F. Delta-aminolevulinic acid synthetase activity in erythroblasts of patients with primary sideroblastic anemia. Acta Haematol Jpn 1973;36:74.
406. Bottomley SS, Healy HM, May BK. 5-aminolevulinic acid synthetase in sideroblastic anemia revisited. Blood 1989;74:103a.
407. Aoki Y, Muranaka S, Nakabayashi K, Ueda Y. Delta-aminolevulinic acid synthetase in erythroblasts of patients with pyridoxine-responsive anemia. J Clin Invest 1979;64:1196.
408. Meier PJ, Fehr J, Meyer UA. Pyridoxine-responsive primary acquired sideroblastic anaemia. Scand J Haematol 1982;29:421.
409. Sutherland GR, Baker E, Callen DF, et al. 5-Aminolevulinate synthetase is at 3p21 and thus not the primary defect in X-linked sideroblastic anemia. Am J Hum Genet 1988;43:331.
410. Elves MW, Bourne MS, Israels MCG. Pyridoxine-responsive anaemia determined by an X-linked gene. J Med Genet 1966;3:1.
411. Jamel BCJ, Schretlen EDA. Sideroblastic anaemia: a review of seven paediatric cases. Eur J Pediatr 1982;138:130.
412. Pasanen AVO, Eklof M, Tenhunen R. Coproporphyrinogen oxidase activity and porphyrin concentrations in peripheral red blood cells in hereditary sideroblastic anaemia. Scand J Haematol 1985;34:235.
413. Prasad AS, Tranchida L, Konno ET, et al. Hereditary sideroblastic anemia and glucose-6-phosphate dehydrogenase deficiency in a negro family. J Clin Invest 1968;47:1415.
414. Pagon RA, Bird TD, Detter JC, Pierce I. Hereditary sideroblastic anaemia and ataxia: an X linked recessive disorder. J Med Genet 1985;22:267.
415. Partanen S, Pasanen A, Juvonen E, et al. Erythroid colony formation and effect of hemin in vitro in hereditary sideroblastic anemias. Exp Hematol 1988;16:313.
416. Romslo I, Brun A, Sandberg S, et al. Sideroblastic anemia with markedly increased free erythrocyte protoprophyrin without dermal photosensitivity. Blood 1982;59:628.
417. Rothstein G, Lee GR, Cartwright GE. Sideroblastic anemia with dermal photosensitivity and greatly increased erythrocyte protoporphyrin. N Engl J Med 1969;280:587.
418. May A, De Souza P, Barnes K, et al. Erythroblast iron metabolism in sideroblastic marrows. Br J Haematol 1982;52:611.
419. Solomon LR, Hillman RS. Vitamin B6 metabolism in idiopathic sideroblastic anaemia and related disorders. Br J Haematol 1979;42:239.
420. Bottomley SS, Tanaka M, Everett MA. Diminished erythroid ferrochelatase activity in protoporphyria. J Lab Clin Med 1975;86:126.
421. Bottomley SS, Moore MZ. Acquired erythropoietic protoporphyria and sideroblastic anemia. Clin Res 1989;38a.
422. Grasso JA, Myers TJ, Hines JD, Sullivan AL. Energy-dispersive x-ray analysis of the mitochondria of sideroblastic anaemia. Br J Haematol 1980;46:57.
423. Kushner JP, Steinmuller DP, Lee GR. Inhibition of uroporphyrinogen decarboxylase activity by iron. Clin Res 1973;21:266.
424. Hines JD. Effect of pyridoxine plus chronic phlebotomy on the function and morphology of bone marrow and liver in pyridoxine-responsive sideroblastic anemia. Semin Hematol 1976;13:133.
425. Weintraub LR, Conrad ME, Crosby WH. Iron-loading anemia: treatment with repeated phlebotomies and pyridoxine. N Engl J Med 1966;275:169.
426. Jensen PD, Jensen IM, Ellegaard J. Desferrioxamine treatment reduces blood transfusion requirements in patients with myelodysplastic syndrome. Br J Haematol 1992;80:121.
427. Aoki Y. Multiple enzymatic defects in mitochondria in hematological cells of patients with primary sideroblastic anemia. J Clin Invest 1980;66:43.
428. Rasi V, Lintula R. Platelet function in the myelodysplastic syndromes. Scand J Haematol 1986;36(Suppl 45):71.
429. Rao AK, Walsh PN. Acquired qualitative platelet disorders. Clin Haematol 1983;12:201.
430. Clark RE, Hoy TE, Jacobs A. Granulocyte and monocyte surface membrane markers in the myelodysplastic syndromes. J Clin Pathol 1985;38:301.
431. Boogaerts MA, Nelissen V, Roelant C, Goossens W. Blood neutrophil function in primary myelodysplastic syndromes. Br J Haematol 1983;55:217.
432. Cech P, Markert M, Perrin LH. Partial myeloperoxidase deficiency in preleukemia. Blut 1983;47:21.
433. Lehrer RI, Goldberg LS, Apple MA, Rosenthal NP. Refractory megaloblastic anemia with myeloperoxidase-deficient neutrophils. Ann Intern Med 1972;76:447.
434. Breton-Gorius J, Houssay D, Dreyfus B. Partial myeloperoxidase deficiency in a case of preleukemia. Br J Haematol 1975;30:273.
435. Breton-Gorius J, Houssay D, Vilde JL, Dreyfus B. Partial myeloperoxidase deficiency in a case of preleukemia: defects of degranulation and abnormal bactericidal activity of blood neutrophils. Br J Haematol 1975;30:279.
436. Kletter Y, Nagler A. Function of peripheral blood and bone-marrow monocytes in preleukemic patients: normal phagocytosis and intracellular killing of Candida albicans. Acta Haematol 1984;72:379.
437. Bynoe AG, Scott CS, Ford P, Roberts BE. Decreased T helper cells in the myelodysplastic syndromes. Br J Haematol 1983;54:97.
438. Knox SJ, Greenberg BR, Anderson RW, Rosenblatt LS. Studies of T-lymphocytes in preleukemic disorders and acute nonlymphocytic leukemia: in vitro radiosensitivity, mitogenic responsiveness, colony formation, and enumeration of lymphocytic subpopulations. Blood 1983;61:449.
439. Colombat PH, Renoux M, Lamagnere JP, Renoux G. Immunologic indices in myelodysplastic syndromes. Cancer 1988;61:1075.
440. Janowska-Wieczorek A, Jakobisiak M, Dobaczewska H. Decreased antibody-dependent cellular cytotoxicity in preleukemic syndromes. Acta Haematol 1983;69:132.
441. Mufti GJ, Figes A, Hamblin TJ, et al. Immunological abnormalities in myelodysplastic syndromes. I. Serum immunoglobulins and autoantibodies. Br J Haematol 1986;63:143.
442. Anderson RW, Volsky DJ, Greenberg B, et al. Lymphocyte abnormalities in preleukemia. I. Decreased NK activity, anomalous immunoregulatory cell subsets and deficient EBV receptors. Leuk Res 1983;7:389.
443. Oblakowski P. Natural killer activity in preleukemic states. Haematol Blood Transfus 1987;31:132.
444. Tricot G, Vlietinck R, Boogaerts MA, et al. Prognostic factors in the myelodysplastic syndromes: importance of initial data on peripheral blood counts, bone marrow cytology, trephine biopsy and chromosomal analysis. Br J Haematol 1985;60:19.
444a. Aul C, Gattermann N, Schneider W. Age-related incidence and other epidemiologic aspects of myelodysplastic syndromes. J Haematol 1992;82:358.
445. Barlogie B, Johnston DA, Keating M, et al. Evolution of oligoleukemia. Cancer 1984;53:2115.
446. Heimpel H, Drings P, Mitrou P, Queiber W. Verlauf und prognostische kriterien bei patienten mit "praleukamie." Klin Wochenschr 1979;57:21.
447. Riccardi A, Giordano M, Giordano P, et al. Prognostic parameters in myelodysplastic syndromes: a multiple regression analysis. Eur J Haematol 1988;40:158.
448. Jaworkowsky LI, Solovey DY, Rhausova LY, Udris OY. Monocytosis as a sign of subsequent leukemia in patients with cytopenias (preleukemia). Folia Haematol Leipzig 1983;110:395.
449. Varela BL, Chuang C, Woll JE, Bennett JM. Modifications in the classification of primary myelodysplastic syndromes: the addition of a scoring system. Hematol Oncol 1985;3:55.
450. Cazzola M, Barosi G, Gobbi PG, et al. Natural history of idiopathic refractory sideroblastic anemia. Blood 1988;71:305.
451. Najean Y, Pecking A. Refractory anemia with excess of blast cells: prognostic factors and effect of treatment with androgens or cytosine arabinoside. Cancer 1979;44:1976.
452. Vandermolen L, Rice L, Rose MA, Lynch EC. Ringed sideroblasts in primary myelodysplasia. Arch Intern Med 1988;148:653.
453. Kerndrup G, Pedersen B, Ellegaard J, Hokland P. Prognostic significance of some clinical, morphological and cytogenetic findings in refractory anaemia (RA) and RA with sideroblasts. Blut 1986;52:35.
454. Schipperus MR, Hagemeijer A, Ploemacher RE, et al. In myelodysplastic syndromes progression to leukemia is directly related to PHA dependency for colony formation and independent of in vitro maturation capacity. Leukemia 1988;2:433.
455. Greenberg PL, Mara B. The preleukemic syndrome: correlation of in vitro parameters of granulopoiesis with clinical features. Am J Med 1979;66:951.
456. Worsley A, Oscier DG, Stevens J, et al. Prognostic features of chronic myelomonocytic leukaemia: a modified Bournemouth score gives the best prediction of survival. Br J Haematol 1988;68:17.
457. Smith WB, Ablin A, Goodman JR, Brecher G. Atypical megakaryocytes in preleukemic phase of acute myeloid leukemia. Blood 1973;42:535.
458. Weiss K, Stass S, Williams D, et al. Childhood monosomy 7 syndrome: clinical and in vitro studies. Leukemia 1987;1:97.
459. Monosomy 7 in childhood: a preleukemic state. Br J Haematol 1981;49:129.
460. Oguma S, Yoshida Y, Uchino H, Maekawa T. Factors influencing leukemic transformation in refractory anemias with excess of blasts, with ringed sideroblasts, and without ringed sideroblasts. Cancer Res 1986;46:3698.

461. Oguma S, Yoshida Y, Uchino H, Maekawa T. Factors influencing nonleukemic death in refractory anemia, refractory anemia with ringed sideroblasts, and refractory anemia with excess blasts. Cancer Res 1987;47:3599.
462. Jaworkowsky LI, Solovey DY, Rhausova LY, et al. A simple mathematical method revealing the early stage of acute leukemia in patients with cytopenias. Folia Haematol Leipzig 1984;111:701.
463. Nowell PC, Besa EC. Prognostic significance of single chromosomal abnormalities in preleukemic states. Cancer Genet Cytogenet 1989; 42:1.
464. Berghe HVD, David G, Michaux JL, et al. 5q− acute myelogenous leukemia. Blood 1976;48:624.
465. Michiels JJ, Mallios-Zorbala H, Prins MEF, Hahlen K. Simple monosomy 7 and myelodysplastic syndrome in thirteen patients without previous cytostatic treatment. Br J Haematol 1986;64:425.
466. Camba LL, Joyner MV. Refractory anaemia terminating in a combined lymphoproliferative and myeloproliferative disorder. J Clin Pathol 1985;38:297.
467. Hehlmann R, Zonnchen B, Thiel E, Walther B. Idiopathic refractory sideroachrestic anemia (IRSA) progressing to acute mixed lymphoblastic-myelomonoblastic leukemia. Blut 1983;46:11.
468. Bonati A, Delia D, Starcich R. Progression of a myelodysplastic syndrome to pre-B acute lymphoblastic leukaemia with unusual phenotype. Br J Haematol 1986;64:487.
469. Spriggs DR, Stone RM, Kufe DW. The treatment of myelodysplastic syndromes. Clin Haematol 1986;15:1081.
470. Larson RA. Management of myelodysplastic syndromes. Ann Intern Med 1985;103:136.
471. Treatment for pre-leukaemia? Lancet 1984;1:943.
472. Schafer AI, Cheron RG, Dluhy R, et al. Clinical consequences of acquired transfusional iron overload in adults. N Engl J Med 1981;304: 319.
473. Pippard MJ, Callender ST. Clinical annotation: the management of iron chelation therapy. Br J Haematol 1983;54:503.
474. Ley TJ, Griffith P, Nienhuis AW. Transfusion haemosiderosis and chelation therapy. Clin Haematol 1982;11:437.
475. Brittenham GM, Zanzucchi PE, Farrell DE, et al. Non-invasive in vivo measurement of human iron overload by magnetic susceptibility studies. Trans Assoc Am Phys 1980;43:156.
476. Volin L, Tuutu T, Knuutila S, Tenhunen R. Heme arginate treatment for myelodysplastic syndromes. Leuk Res 1988;12:423.
477. Najean Y, Pecking A. Refractory anaemia with excess of myeloblasts in the bone marrow: a clinical trial of androgens in 90 patients. Br J Haematol 1977;37:25.
478. Doll DC, Ringenberg QS, Yarbro JW. Danazol therapy in acquired idiopathic sideroblastic anemia. Acta Haematol 1987;77:170.
479. Aviles A, Rubio E. Danazol in idiopathic sideroblastic anemia. Acta Haematol 1988;79:229.
480. Hupperets P, De Witte T, Haanen CA. Retrospective study of the effect of anabolic steroids on the dyshaematopoietic syndrome (preleukaemic syndrome). Neth J Med 1983;26:181.
481. Bagby GC, Gabourel JD, Linman JW. Gluticocorticoid therapy in the preleukemic syndrome (hemopoietic dysplasia). Ann Intern Med 1980;92:55.
482. Mertelsmann R, Thaler HT, To L, et al. Morphological classification, response to therapy, and survival in 263 adult patients with acute nonlymphoblastic leukemia. Blood 1980;56:773.
483. Armitage JO, Dick FR, Needleman SW, Burns CP. Effect of chemotherapy for the dysmyelopoietic syndrome. Cancer Treat Rep 1981;65: 601.
484. Fenaux P, Lai JL, Jouet JP, et al. Aggressive chemotherapy in adult primary myelodysplastic syndromes. Blut 1988;57:297.
485. Murray C, Cooper B, Kitchens LW Jr. Remission of acute myelogenous leukemia in elderly patients with prior refractory dysmyelopoietic anemia. Cancer 1983;52:967.
486. Tricot G, Boogaerts MA. The role of aggressive chemotherapy in the treatment of the myelodysplastic syndromes. Br J Haematol 1986;63: 477.
487. Preisler HD, Raza A, Barcos M, et al. High-dose cytosine arabinoside in the treatment of preleukemic disorders: a Leukemia Intergroup study. Am J Hematol 1986;23:131.
488. Martiat P, Ferrant A, Michaux JL, Sokal G. Intensive chemotherapy for acute non-lymphoblastic leukemia after primary myelodysplastic syndrome. Hematol Oncol 1988;6:299.
489. Tricot G, Boogaerts MA, Verwilghen RL. Treatment of patients with myelodysplastic syndromes: a review. Scand J Haematol 1986;36(Suppl 45):121.
490. Gyger M, Perreault C, Carnot J, et al. Treatment of therapy-induced preleukemic syndrome. Blut 1984;48:117.
491. Aul C, Schneider W. The role of low-dose cytosine arabinoside and aggressive chemotherapy in advanced myelodysplastic syndromes. Cancer 1989;64:1812.
492. Richard C, Iriondo A, Garijo J, et al. Therapy of advanced myelodysplastic syndrome with aggressive chemotherapy. Oncology 1989; 46:6.
493. Sachs L. Control of normal cell differentiation and the phenotypic reversion of malignancy in myeloid leukaemia. Nature 1978;274:535.
494. Friend C, Scher W, Holland J, Sato T. Hemoglobin synthesis in murine virus-induced leukemic cells in vitro: stimulation of erythroid differentiation by dimethyl sulfoxide. Proc Natl Acad Sci USA 1971;68: 378.
495. Lotem J, Sachs L. Different blocks in the differentiation of myeloid leukemic cells. Proc Natl Acad Sci USA 1974;71:3507.
496. Sporn MB, Roberts AB. Role of retinoids in differentiation and carcinogenesis. Cancer Res 1983;43:3034.
497. Koeffler HP, Hirji K, Itri L, et al. 1, 25-dihydroxyvitamin D_3: in vivo and in vitro effects on human preleukemic and leukemic cells. Cancer Treat Rep 1985;69:1399.
498. Griffin J, Munroe D, Major P, Kufe D. Induction of differentiation of human myeloid leukemia cells by inhibitors of DNA synthesis. Exp Hematol 1982;10:774.
499. Honma Y, Fujita Y, Kasukabe T, et al. Induction of differentiation of human acute non-lymphocytic leukemia cells in primary culture by inducers of differentiation of human myeloid leukemia line HL-60. Eur J Cancer Clin Oncol 1983;19:251.
500. Breitman TR, Collins SJ, Keene BR. Terminal differentiation of human promyelocytic leukemic cells in primary culture in response to retinoic acid. Blood 1981;57:1000.
501. Swanson G, Picozzi V, Morgan R, et al. Responses of hemopoietic precursors to 13-cis retinoic acid and 1, 25-dihydroxyvitamin D_3 in the myelodysplastic syndromes. Blood 1986;67:1154.
502. Gullberg U, Nilsson E, Einhorn S, Olsson I. Combinations of interferon-gamma and retinoic acid or 1-alpha, 25-dihydroxycholecalciferol induce differentiation of the human monoblast leukemia cell line U-937. Exp Hematol 1985;13:675.
503. Francis GE, Guimaraes JETE, Berney JJ, Wing MA. Synergistic interaction between differentiation inducers and DNA synthesis inhibitors: a new approach to differentiation induction in myelodysplasia and acute myeloid leukaemia. Leuk Res 1985;9:573.
504. Kufe DW, Griffin JD, Spriggs DR. Cellular and clinical pharmacology of low-dose Ara-C. Semin Oncol 1985;12:200.
505. Kreis W, Chaudhri F, Chan K, et al. Pharmacokinetics of low-dose 1-beta-D-arabinofuranosylcytosine given by continuous intravenous infusion over twenty-one-days. Cancer Res 1985;45:6498.
506. Ishikura H, Sawada H, Okazaki T, et al. The effect of low dose ara-C in acute nonlymphoblastic leukemias and atypical leukaemia. Br J Haematol 1984;58:9.
507. Housset M, Daniel MT, Degos L. Small doses of ARA-C in the treatment of acute myeloid leukemia: differentiation of myeloid leukemia cells? Br J Haematol 1982;51:125.
508. Wisch JS, Griffin JD, Kufe DW. Response of preleukemic syndromes to continuous infusion of low-dose cytarabine. N Engl J Med 1983;309: 1599.
509. Griffin JD, Spriggs DR, Wisch JS. Treatment of preleukemic syndromes with continuous intravenous infusion of low dose cytosine arabinoside. J Clin Oncol 1985;3:982.
510. Izumi Y, Sawada H, Okazaki T, et al. Favourable remission rate by repeating low dose ARA-C treatment in ANNL and RAEB. Br J Haematol 1985;61:187.
511. Castaigne S, Daniel MT, Tilly H, et al. Does treatment with ARA-C in low dosage cause differentiation of leukemic cells? Blood 1983;62: 85.
512. Jehn U, DeBock R, Haanen C. Clinical trial of low-dose ara-C in the treatment of acute leukemia and myelodysplasia. Blut 1984;48:255.
513. Winter JN, Variakojis D, Gaynor ER, et al. Low-dose cytosine arabinoside (ara-C) therapy in the myelodysplastic syndromes and acute leukemia. Cancer 1985;56:443.
514. Tricot G, de Bock R, Dekker AW, et al. Low dose cytosine arabinoside (Ara C) in myelodysplastic syndromes. Br J Haematol 1984;58:231.
515. Alessandrino EP, Orlandi E, Brusamolino E, et al. Low-dose arabinosyl cytosine in acute leukemia after a myelodysplastic syndrome and in elderly leukemia. Am J Hematol 1985;20:191.
516. Desforges JF. Cytarabine: low-dose, high-dose, no dose? N Engl J Med 1983;309:1637.
517. Baccarani M, Zaccaria A, Bandini G, et al. Low dose arabinosyl cytosine for treatment of myelodysplastic syndromes and subacute myeloid leukemia. Leuk Res 1983;7:539.
518. Worsley A, Mufti GJ, Copplestone JA, et al. Very-low-dose cytarabine for myelodysplastic syndromes and acute myeloid leukaemia in the elderly. Lancet 1986;1:966.
519. Spitzer TR, Lazarus HM, Crum ED, Weisman R. Treatment of myelodysplastic syndromes with low-dose oral 6-thioguanine. Med Pediatr Oncol 1988;16:17.
519a. Hwellstrom-Lindber E, Robert KH, Gahrton G, et al. A predictive model for the clinical response to low dose ara-C: a study of 102 patients with myelodysplastic syndrome or acute leukemia. Br J Haematol 1992;81:503.
520. Gold EJ, Mertelsmann RH, Itri LM, et al. Phase I clinical trial of 13-*cis*-retinoic acid in myelodysplastic syndromes. Cancer Treat Rep 1983;67:981.
521. Kerndrup G, Bendix-Hansen K, Pedersen B, et al. Primary myelodysplastic syndrome: treatment of 6 patients with 13-*cis*-retinoic acid. Scand J Haematol 1986;45:128.
522. Leoni F, Ciolli S, Longo G, et al. 13-cis-retinoic acid treatment in patients with myelodysplastic syndrome. Acta Haematol 1988;80:8.
523. Greenberg BR, Durie BGM, Barnett TC, Meyskens FL Jr. Phase I-II

study of 13-cis-retinoic acid in myelodysplastic syndrome. Cancer Treat Rep 1985;69:1369.
524. Clark RE, Lush CJ, Jacobs A, Smith SA. Effect of 13-cis-retinoic acid on survival of patients with myelodysplastic syndrome. Lancet 1987;1: 763.
525. Koeffler HP, Heitjan D, Mertelsmann R, et al. Randomized study of 13-*cis* retinoic acid *v* placebo in the myelodysplastic disorders. Blood 1988;71:703.
526. Jacobs A, Clark RE. 13-cis-retinoic acid v placebo in myelodysplasia. Br J Haematol 1988.
527. Blok WL, Lowenberg B, Sizoo W. Disappearance of trisomy 8 after alpha-2 interferon in a patient with myelodysplastic syndrome. N Engl J Med 1988;318:787.
528. Galvani DW, Nethersell ABW, Cawley JC. Alpha-interferon in myelodysplasia: clinical observations and effects on NK cells. Leuk Res 1988;12:257.
529. Hellstrom E, Robert K-H, Gahrton G, et al. Therapeutic effects of low-dose cytosine arabinoside, alpha-interferon, 1-alpha-hydroxyvitamin D3 and retinoic acid in acute leukemia and myelodysplastic syndromes. Eur J Haematol 1988;40:449.
530. Nienhuis A. Hematopoietic growth factors: biologic complexity and clinical promise. N Engl J Med 1988;318:916.
531. Delwel R, Salem M, Pellens C, et al. Growth regulation of human acute myeloid leukemia: effects of five recombinant hematopoietic factors in a serum-free culture system. Blood 1988;72:1944.
532. Vellenga E, Ostapovicz D, O'Rourke B, Griffin JD. Effects of recombinant IL-3, GM-CSF and G-CSF on proliferation of leukemic clonogenic cells in short-term and long-term cultures. Leukemia 1987;1: 584.
533. Vellenga E, Young DC, Wagner K, et al. The effects of GM-CSF and G-CSF in promoting growth of clonogenic cells in acute myeloblastic leukemia. Blood 1987;69:1771.
534. Bruno E, Miller ME, Hoffman R. Interacting cytokines regulate in vitro human megakaryocytopoiesis. Blood 1989;73:671.
535. Ikebuchi K, Wong GG, Clark SC, et al. Interleukin 6 enhancement of interleukin 3-dependent proliferation of multipotential hemopoietic progenitors. Proc Natl Acad Sci USA 1987;84:9035.
536. Donahue RE, Seehra J, Metzger M, et al. Human IL-3 and GM-CSF act synergistically in stimulating hematopoiesis in primates. Science 1988;241:1820.
537. Broxmeyer HE, Williams DE, Hangoc G, et al. Synergistic myelopoietic actions in vivo after administration to mice of combinations of purified natural murine colony-stimulating factor 1, recombinant murine interleukin 3, and recombinant murine granulocyte/macrophage colony-stimulating factor. Proc Natl Acad Sci USA 1987;84:3871.
538. Vadhan-Raj S, Keating M, LeMaistre A, et al. Effects of recombinant human granulocyte-macrophage colony-stimulating factor in patients with myelodysplastic syndromes. N Engl J Med 1987;317:1546.
539. Antin JH, Smith BR, Holmes W, Rosenthal DS. Phase I/II study of recombinant human granulocyte-macrophage colony-stimulating factor in aplastic anemia and myelodysplastic syndrome. Blood 1988;72:705.
540. Ganser A, Volkers B, Greher J, et al. Recombinant human granulocyte-macrophage colony-stimulating factor in patients with myelodysplastic syndromes: a phase I/II trial. Blood 1989;73:31.
541. Estey EH, Kurzrock R, Talpaz M, et al. Effects of low doses of recombinant human granulocyte-macrophage colony stimulating factor (GM-CSF) in patients with myelodysplastic syndromes. Br J Haematol 1991;77:291.
542. Vadhan-Raj S, Broxmeyer HE, Spitzer G, et al. Stimulation of nonclonal hematopoiesis and suppression of the neoplastic clone after treatment with recombinant human granulocyte-macrophage colony-stimulating factor in a patient with therapy-related myelodysplastic syndrome. Blood 1989;74:1491.
543. Schuster MW, Larson RA, Thompson JA, Coiffier B, Bennett JM, Israel RJ. Granulocyte-macrophage colony-stimulating factor (GM-CSF) for myelodysplastic syndrome (MDS): results of a multi-center randomized controlled trial. Blood 1990;76:318a.
544. Negrin RS, Haeuber DH, Nagler A, et al. Treatment of myelodysplastic syndromes with recombinant human granulocyte colony-stimulating factor. Ann Intern Med 1989;110:976.
545. Kobayashi Y, Okabe T, Ozawa K, et al. Treatment of myelodysplastic syndromes with recombinant human granulocyte colony-stimulating factor: a preliminary report. Am J Med 1989;86:178.
546. Negrin RS, Haeuber DH, Nagler A, et al. Maintenance therapy of patients with myelodysplastic syndromes using recombinant human granulocyte colony-stimulating factors. Blood 1990;76:36.
547. Yuo A, Kitagawa S, Okabe T, et al. Recombinant human granulocyte colony-stimulating factor repairs the abnormalities of neutrophils in patients with myelodysplastic syndromes and chronic myelogenous leukemia. Blood 1987;70:404.
548. Peters WP, Stuart A, Affronti ML, Kim CS, Coleman RE. Neutrophil migration is defective during recombinant human granulocyte-macrophage colony-stimulating factor infusion after autologous bone marrow transplantation in humans. Blood 1988;72:1310.
549. Ganser A, Seipelt G, Lindemann A, et al. Effects of recombinant human interleukin-3 in patients with myelodysplastic syndromes. Blood 1990;76:455.
550. Ganser A, Bartram CR, Ottman OG, et al. Stimulation of non-clonal hematopoiesis in patients with hematological disorders by recombinant human GM-CSF or interleukin-3. Blood 1990;76:1449.
551. Sonoda Y, Yang Y, Wong GG, et al. Analysis in serum-free culture of the targets of recombinant human hemopoietic growth factors: interleukin 3 and granulocyte/macrophage-colony-stimulating factor are specific for early developmental stages. Proc Natl Acad Sci USA 1988;85:4360.
551a. Nand S, Sosman J, Godwin JE, et al. A phase I/II study of sequential interleukin 3 and granulocyte-macrophage colony-stimulating factor in myelodysplastic syndromes. Blood 1994;83:357.
552. Casadevall N, Belanger C, Goy A, et al. High-dose recombinant human erythropoietin administered intravenously for the treatment of anaemia in myelodysplastic syndromes. Acta Haematol 1992;87(Suppl 1): 25.
553. Adamson JW, Schuster M, Allen S, Haley NR. Effectiveness of recombinant human erythropoietin therapy in myeoldysplastic syndromes. Acta Haematol 1992;87(Suppl 1):20.
554. Hellstrom E, Birgegard G, Lockner D, et al. Treatment of myeoldysplastic syndromes with recombinant human erythropoietin. Eur J Hematol 1991;47:355.
555. Kurzrock R, Talpaz M, Estey E, et al. Erythropoietin treatment in patients with myelodysplastic syndrome and anemia. Leukemia 1991;5:985.
556. Stein RS, Abels RI, Krantz SB. Pharmacologic doses of recombinant human erythropoietin in the treatment of myelodysplastic syndromes. Blood 1991;78:1658.
557. van Kamp H, Prinsze-Postema TC, Kluin PM, et al. Effect of subcutaneously administered human recombinant erythropoietin on erythropoiesis in patients with myelodysplasia. Br J Haematol 1991;78: 488.
558. Schouten HC, Vellenga E, van Rhenen DJ, et al. Recombinant human erythropoietin in patients with myelodysplastic syndromes. Leukemia 1991;5:432.
558a. Negrin RS, Steion R, Vardiman J, et al. Treatment of the anemia of myelodysplastic syndromes using recombinant human granulocyte colony-stimulating factor in combination with erythropoeitin. Blood 1993;82:737.
559. Bhaduri S, Kubanek B, Heit W, et al. A case of preleukemia: reconstitution of normal marrow function after bone marrow transplantation (BMT) from identical twin. Blut 1979;38:145.
560. Appelbaum FR, Storb R, Ramberg RE, et al. Allogeneic marrow transplantation in the treatment of preleukemia. Ann Intern Med 1984;100: 689.
561. Deeg HJ. Marrow transplantation in preleukemia. J Natl Cancer Inst 1986;76:1329.
562. Appelbaum FR, Storb R, Ramberg RE, et al. Treatment of preleukemic syndromes with marrow transplantation. Blood 1987;69:92.
563. Appelbaum FR, Barrall J, Storb R, et al. Treatment of myelodysplasia with marrow transplantation: overall result and effect of pretreatment variables on outcome. Blood 1989;74:52a.
564. Belanger R, Gyger M, Perrault C, et al. Bone marrow transplantation for myelodysplastic syndromes. Br J Haematol 1988;69:29.
565. Guinan EC, Tarbell NJ, Tantravahi R, Weinstein HJ. Bone marrow transplantation for children with myelodysplastic syndromes. Blood 1989;73:619.
565a. Anderson JE, Appelbaum FR, Fisher LD, et al. Allogeneic bone marrow transplantation for 93 patients with myelodysplastic syndrome. Blood 1993;82:677.
566. Hoffken K, Overkamp F, Stirbu J, et al. Recombinant human granulocyte-macrophage colony-stimulating factor and low-dose cytosine-arabinoside in the treatment of patients with myelodysplastic syndromes: a phase II study. Onkologie 1990;13:33.
567. Hoelzer D, Ganser A, Ottman OG, et al. Effect of treatment with rhGM-CSF and low-dose cytosine arabinoside on leukemic blast cells in patients with myelodysplastic syndromes. Haematol Bluttransfus 1990;33:763.
568. van der Weide M, Sizoo W, Krefft J, Langenhuijsen MMAC. Myelodysplastic syndromes: analysis of morphological features related to the FAB-classification. Eur J Haematol 1988;41:58.
569. Weatherall DJ, Pembrey ME, Hall EG, et al. Familial sideroblastic anaemia: problem of Xg and X chromosome inactivation. Lancet 1970;744.
570. Hast R, Miale T, Westin J, et al. Hereditary ring sideroblastic anaemia and Christmas disease in a Swedish family. Scand J Haematol 1983;30: 444.
571. van Waveren Hogervorst GD, van Roermund HPC, Snijders PJ. Hereditary sideroblastic anaemia and autosomal inheritance of erythrocyte dimorphism in a Dutch family. Eur J Haematol 1987;38:405.
572. Claustres M, Vannereau H, Bellet J, et al. A paediatric case of sideroblastic anaemia: ultrastructural studies of erythroblasts cultured from marrow BFU-E in a methylcellulose micromethod. Eur J Pediatr 1986;145:422.
573. Patterson WP, Winkelmann M, Perry MC. Zinc-induced copper deficiency: megamineral sideroblastic anemia. Ann Intern Med 1985;103: 385.
574. Degos L, Castaigne S, Tilly H. Treatment of leukemia with low dose ara-C: a study of 160 cases. Semin Oncol 1985;12(Suppl 3):196.

Blood: Principles and Practice of Hematology,
edited by Robert I. Handin, Thomas P. Stossel, and Samuel E. Lux.
J.B. Lippincott Company, Philadelphia © 1995.

13

Polycythemia Vera and Agnogenic Myeloid Metaplasia

Steven M. Fruchtman
Paul D. Berk

Polycythemia vera (PV) is a primary bone marrow disorder characterized by panhyperplasia of the marrow. The panmyelosis involves the erythroid, myeloid, and megakaryocyte series and causes a rise in peripheral blood counts and an increased red blood cell (RBC) mass.[1] Although the cause has not been established, it is recognized that PV is a clonal disorder of a hematopoietic stem cell with the capacity to differentiate into erythrocytes, granulocytes, platelets, and B lymphocytes.[2] It is not known whether T lymphocytes are part of the abnormal clone.

Polycythemia vera is a subset of a group of related disorders referred to as the *myeloproliferative diseases:* agnogenic myeloid metaplasia or idiopathic myelofibrosis, chronic myeloid leukemia, and essential thrombocythemia (see Chaps. 14 and 15 for discussion of essential thrombocythemia and chronic myelogenous leukemia). In Dameshek's original classification of the myeloproliferative syndrome,[3] erythroleukemia was also included. We believe that the biology and clinical ramifications of acute leukemia are sufficiently different from the other myeloproliferative disorders that this is not warranted.

The myeloproliferative syndromes commonly have increased numbers in the peripheral blood of any of the circulating cellular elements, alone or in combination, although a particular component typically dominates the picture and results in the assignment of a specific diagnosis. Thus, in PV, erythrocytosis is the predominant finding. PV is far more than a pure RBC proliferation. Pancytosis of the peripheral blood is present with combinations of erythrocytosis, leukocytosis, and thrombocytosis. Multilineage hypercellularity in the marrow is often dominated by an extreme increase in megakaryocytes, which may be seen in clusters. The leukocyte count in PV may be normal or may approach the levels found in chronic myelocytic leukemia, with counts of 50,000 cells/μL and sometimes even a shift to immature forms. The platelet count may range from normal to as high as several million per microliter.

Similarly, in many cases of Philadelphia chromosome–positive chronic myelocytic leukemia (CML), which is characterized principally by leukocytosis, there can be profound thrombocytosis. In some cases, megakaryocyte fragments are present in the peripheral circulation, as seen in essential thrombocythemia. Some CML patients may also have an elevated hematocrit early in the disease.

In about 10% to 25% of patients with PV, an increasing anemia gradually develops with a leukoerythroblastic blood picture. The bone marrow may show striking fibrosis, and the spleen and liver may show myeloid metaplasia. Once fully evolved from a more typical case of polycythemia vera, this condition is indistinguishable from an entity referred to as *agnogenic myeloid metaplasia,* in which marrow fibrosis and extramedullary hematopoiesis in the spleen and liver arise de novo and dominate the clinical course. Thus, although the various conditions currently included as myeloproliferative disorders may present differently, they are closely related and are all disorders of a pluripotent marrow stem cell.

PV is a rare disorder. The estimated incidence of PV varies from 4.5 to 16 new cases per million each year.[4,5] The risk of developing PV may be higher among Jews of European extraction.[6] Familial PV is rare; 6% of patients registered with the Polycythemia Vera Study Group (PVSG) have family members with the same disorder, and parents of patients with documented PV have a significant increase in the likelihood of having the disease.[7] This suggests that unknown genetic factors may be important in determining the incidence of PV.

PV is more prevalent in males (about 1.4:1). Various studies report a mean age at diagnosis of between 55 and 60 years[8]; only 20% of patients are under age 50, and the disorder is rarely seen in childhood.[9]

Erythrocytosis in the neonate is a serious clinical entity that occurs primarily in infants of diabetic mothers and in small-for-gestational-age infants; it may be related to a hyperinsulinemic environment in which erythroid progenitors develop.[10] Erythrocytosis must therefore be differentiated from PV, which is uncommon in children, although childhood cases have been reported.[9]

In addition to the diagnostic criteria for PV outlined in Table 13-1, all pediatric patients should first have a normal P_{50} measurement and normal hemoglobin dissociation curve to rule out a hemoglobin with an avid oxygen affinity before the diagnosis of PV is entertained.[11]

Our understanding of PV has a long and interesting course. In 1730, Von Haller[12] recognized the increase in numbers of RBCs. He was perhaps the first to associate thrombosis with gangrene as a frequent occurrence in polycythemia. Since the early 1800s, when Gabriel Andral[13]

TABLE 13-1. Diagnostic Criteria* for Polycythemia Vera (Adapted From Eligibility Criteria of the Polycythemia Vera Study Group)

Category A (Major)	Category B (Minor)
A1. Red cell mass Male ≥36 mL/kg Female ≥32 mL/kg	B1. Thrombocytosis, platelet count >400,000/μL
A2. Normal arterial O_2 saturation ≥92%	B2. Leukocytosis >12,000/μL (no fever or infection)
A3. Splenomegaly	B3. ↑ Leukocyte alkaline phosphatase >100 (no fever or infection) ↑ Serum B_{12} (>900 pg/mL) or unbound B_{12} binding capacity (>2200 pg/mL)

* Diagnosis is acceptable if the following combinations are present: A1 + A2 + A3 or A1 + A2 + any two from category B.

indicated that "true plethoric" was a constitutional disease and not an acquired one, discussion regarding the cause of polycythemia has been heated.

Vaquez's[14] original description of the disease in 1892 noted the typical physical findings and referred to the functional hyperactivity of the hematopoietic organs. He, along with Cabot[15] and Osler[16] at the turn of the century, called the disease *polycythemia vera*. Osler noted the need for careful studies of all forms of chronic cyanosis with polycythemia and mentioned the association of splenomegaly with an increased peripheral count. Turk,[17] a few years later, stressed the leukoerythroblastic blood picture and the association of PV with myeloid metaplasia.

PATHOGENESIS

Although the neoplastic nature of PV has been suspected since Osler's time, it was first confirmed in the mid-1970s by Adamson's and Fialkow's innovative studies of women with PV who were also heterozygotes for isoenzymes of glucose-6-phosphate dehydrogenase (G6PD).[18] This marker system is extremely useful in the study of neoplastic disorders. Early in embryogenesis one of the two X chromosomes in somatic cells of women is randomly inactivated (Fig. 13-1)—a process referred to as *lyonization*, after Mary Lyon, its discoverer. If a woman is a heterozygote for isoenzymes of G6PD, such as the wild type B, and a variant such as A, only one structural gene, Gd^B or Gd^A, remains active in a particular cell. After inactivation occurs, that cell and all its progeny contain the same isoenzyme type. Thus, normal adult women who are G6PD heterozygotes are cellular mosaics; some of the cells of the body contain one isoenzyme, whereas the remaining somatic cells contain the other G6PD isoenzyme. Because X-chromosome inactivation is a random event, heterozygotes have about equal numbers of cells of each isoenzyme type in tissues like the skin, muscle, and blood cells.

Fialkow and associates[19] used this system to study the cellular origins of human neoplasia. In studying neoplasms in G6PD heterozygotes, Fialkow and associates postulated, then confirmed, that if a neoplasm begins in a single cell, then that cell and all the cells involved in the neoplasm have a single G6PD isoenzyme type. If the abnormal proliferation results from stimulation or transformation of several progenitors, the tumor contains a mixture of cells containing two isoenzymes. Chronic myelogenous leukemia was the initial myeloproliferative disorder studied with this technique. Skin from G6PD heterozygotes with chronic myelogenous leukemia showed two isoenzyme types, but only a single isoenzyme was detected in peripheral blood erythrocyte, granulocyte, and platelet preparations.

Similar results were found in patients with PV.[18] Patients treated with myelosuppressive agents whose blood counts normalized, suggesting clinical remission, continued to have clonal hematopoiesis. PV, chronic myelocytic leukemia, agnogenic myeloid metaplasia,[20] and essential thrombocythemia[21] all are clonal hematologic neoplasias in which the peripheral blood abnormalities are the consequence of an abnormal hematopoietic stem cell clone proliferating in the marrow. Remissions induced with myelosuppressive agents are not accompanied by a repopulation of the marrow with normal stem cells; rather, clonal hematopoiesis persists. A clonal origin for PV is also supported by the finding of a cytogenetic abnormality in cells of the erythroid, myeloid, and megakaryocytic hematopoietic lineages, which is lacking in skin fibroblasts (see following text).

In addition to the G6PD and cytogenetic models, evidence of disordered regulation of hematopoiesis is found in patients with PV. Hematopoietic tissues include three cellular compartments: pluripotent stem cells that undergo unlimited self-replication, committed progenitors with restricted potential, and mature precursor cells of each lineage.[22] Progenitor cells retain limited self-renewal potential but are more restricted than the pluripotent stem cell. Precursor cells undergo terminal amplification divisions during maturation but lack potential for self-renewal (Fig. 13-2).

Progenitor cells have been characterized with clonogenic assays that quantitate growth of hematopoietic colonies in semisolid media.[23] Colony growth requires the presence of various hematopoietic factors, added either as components of conditioned media or, more recently, as pure molecules obtained by recombinant DNA techniques. The earliest monopotent erythroid progenitor is called a burst-forming unit–erythroid (BFU-E). The name is derived from the morphology of colonies produced in clonal cultures.[24] Ery-

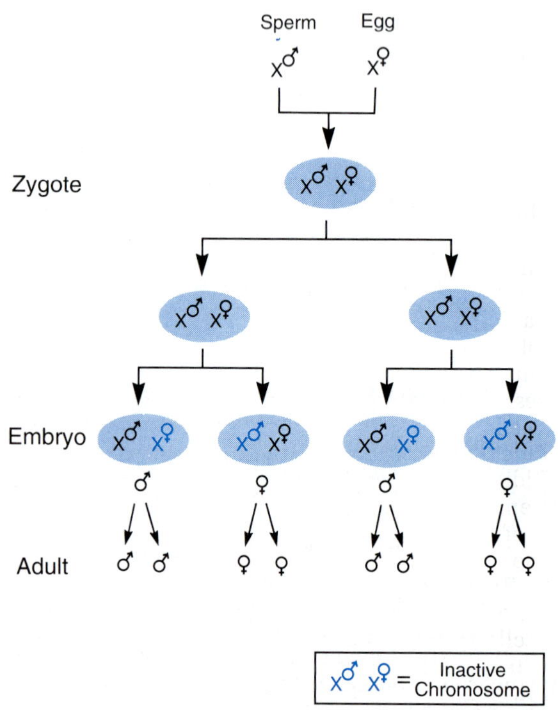

FIGURE 13-1. Diagrammatic representation of X-chromosome inactivation. See text for explanation. (After Fialkow PJ. Clonal and stem cell origin of blood cell neoplasms. Contemp Hematol Oncol 1980;1:1)

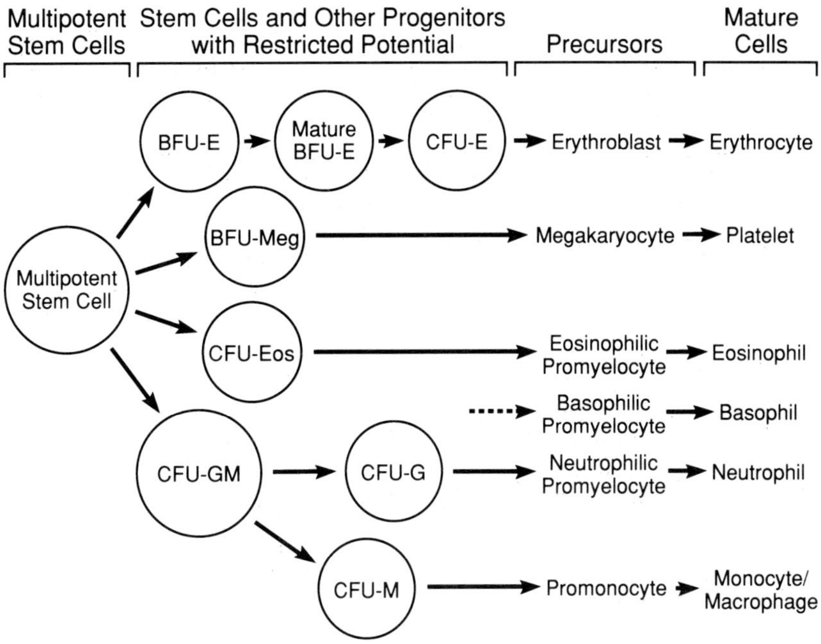

FIGURE 13-2. Current model of the cellular compartments in hematopoiesis. BFU, burst-forming unit; CFU, colony-forming units; CFU-G, colony-forming unit–granulocyte; CFU-GM, colony-forming unit–granulocyte-macrophage. (After Stamatoyannopoulos G, Nienhuis AW. Hemoglobin switching. In: Stamatoyannopoulos G, Nienhuis AW, Leder P, Majerus P, eds. The molecular basis of blood diseases. Philadelphia, WB Saunders, 1987:85)

throid bursts are composed of over 100 and usually of several thousand cells arranged in subclones.

Growth of BFU-E requires burst-promoting activity, usually added in the form of conditioned medium. Such burst-promoting activity may be shared by more than one factor. BFU-E growth is also modulated by cell–cell interactions.[25] BFU-E–T-cell or BFU-E–T-cell–macrophage interactions are believed to result in production of monokines or lymphokines which make erythroid progenitors more sensitive to hematopoietic growth factors.

The progeny of BFU-E are erythropoietin-sensitive cells, the erythroid colony-forming units (CFU-E). These immediate precursors of erythroblasts form colonies of 9 to 64 cells that mature during the first week in culture. Commitment of CFU-E to terminal differentiation initiates an irreversible process, in which proerythroblasts and basophilic, polychromatophilic, and orthochromatophilic erythroblasts develop sequentially. Loss of the nucleus from the orthochromatophilic erythroblasts produces a reticulocyte. Several levels in the erythroid compartment, including more differentiated BFU-E, CFU-E, and proerythroblasts, respond to the erythroid-specific growth hormone, erythropoietin.[26] Erythropoietin stimulates proliferation of committed erythroid progenitors, the formation of erythroblasts, and release of reticulocytes into the circulation. Whole animal studies indicate that erythropoietin increases the number of developing erythroid precursors and accelerates the release of reticulocytes from the marrow without markedly altering the cell cycle length or the number of mitotic divisions involved in the differentiation process.[27] In addition to increasing the pool of maturing erythroblasts, evidence is substantial that erythropoietin increases the pool of cells capable of erythroid differentiation.

The regulation of erythropoietin production in patients with PV is unique. In all other forms of polycythemia, erythropoietin production is either normal or elevated. In PV cells, increased erythropoiesis occurs despite low or undetectable levels of bioassayable erythropoietin in the blood.[28] Urinary levels are also below normal and usually undetectable with the polycythemic mouse assay.[29] These observations have led to the concept that erythropoiesis in this disorder is autonomous and that the increased production of erythrocytes in PV cells results from the proliferation and differentiation of hematopoietic precursor cells that are not under the usual regulatory control.[30] In vitro culture studies of PV bone marrow[31,32] and peripheral blood[33,34] have shown that, in contrast to samples from normal subjects, some erythroid colonies grow without the addition of erythropoietin to the culture system. These so-called endogenous erythroid colonies arise from progenitors that represent a subset of the abnormal clone seen in PV.[32] These colonies are extraordinarily sensitive to low concentrations of erythropoietin in serum constituents added to the culture systems.

The growth of endogenous colonies from patients with PV is reduced or eliminated by adding antierythropoietin antibody to the culture; it is restored by adding minute quantities of the hormone. This suggests that erythroid progenitors in PV cells, rather than being independent of the hormone, may be uniquely sensitive to trace levels of erythropoietin. The reason for the exquisite sensitivity is unclear but may reflect increased numbers of erythropoietin receptors on the membranes of erythroid progenitors.

Other investigators have suggested that the growth of endogenous colonies in cultures from patients with PV may be caused by a peculiar sensitivity of erythropoietic progenitors to growth factors other than erythropoietin.[35] In long-term marrow culture systems, primitive marrow progenitor cells from patients with PV fail to respond to negative signals from the adherent cellular layer, which return their normal counterparts to a quiescent state.[36] This abnormal cycling behavior of PV cells in long-term culture systems mimics what is operative in vivo, where primitive hemopoietic progenitors are also in a continuous state of turnover. This is in contrast to similar primitive progenitor compartments in normal persons, which are more quiescent.[37]

In cases of polycythemia of uncertain etiology, the demonstration of endogenous colonies supports a diagnosis of PV. Endogenous colonies are not observed in all cases of PV at every stage of the disease. When found in other settings, they do not suggest a diagnosis of PV, having been reported by at least some investigators in other myeloproliferative disorders.

In addition to the abnormal clone found in patients with PV, normal erythropoiesis and granulopoiesis can be found.

By using the G6PD model and the differential response to erythropoietin, the progeny of presumed normal stem cells have been shown to persist in marrows of patients with PV.[38] An inhibition of normal erythroid differentiation occurs, and this block appears somewhere between primitive BFU-E and the more mature CFU-E.[38] Also, a steady decline in the proportion of the normal elements occurs as the duration of the illness increases. The observation that presumably normal stem cells are found in patients with PV is similar to the situation in chronic myelogenous leukemia patients, in whom, after ablative chemotherapy, normal stem cells can proliferate and repopulate the marrow.[39] This suggests that the normal stem cells are present with the malignant clone. Because normal committed stem cells from the marrow of these patients can be demonstrated in vitro, their proliferation in vivo appears to be suppressed.

Although all the myeloproliferative disorders are believed to arise from a clonal malignant transformation at the level of a pluripotent hematopoietic stem cell, the following are possible explanations for the histologic differences observed among the various syndromes. First, the transforming event may occur in different stem cell compartments that manifest different degrees of commitment to various cell lineages. Second, differences in the nature of the transforming event per se, at the DNA level, may alter the subsequent behavior of the resulting clone either directly or by modifying the response of clonally derived cells to regulatory factors. Although the major focus has been on erythroid progenitors, there is evidence that granulocyte-macrophage and megakaryocytic precursors are also hypersensitive to the cytokines IL-3 and GM-CSF.[38a,38b] This is in keeping with the stem cell nature of the underlying disorder and the frequent finding of leukocytosis and thrombocytosis along with the predominant finding of erythrocytosis.

DIAGNOSIS

Differential Diagnosis

The diagnosis of PV should be carefully established in every person suspected of having this disorder. In the patient who presents with an elevated hematocrit and hemoglobin concentration or RBC count, a diagnosis of PV can be readily made by the procedures that exclude the various causes of secondary polycythemia. *Polycythemia* is a descriptive term that simply denotes the presence of an elevation of the hemoglobin concentration and hematocrit. Measurements of the hemoglobin concentration, hematocrit, and RBC count are used by clinicians as proxy indicators of the RBC or hemoglobin mass. In fact, these variables are merely measures of the extent to which the RBC mass is diluted in the plasma volume. Both the RBC mass and the plasma volume are regulated by separate and, to a considerable extent, independent physiologic controls. Hence, an elevated hemoglobin, hematocrit, or RBC count may be due to an increased RBC mass (an absolute erythrocytosis), when this more precise determination is performed. These elevations may also be due to a reduction in the plasma volume or to a combination of an RBC mass at the upper end of the normal range and a plasma volume at the lower end of the normal range.

The latter two situations have been termed *relative* or *spurious polycythemia*, since the elevated hemoglobin, hematocrit, and RBC count do not reflect an absolute increase in the mass of circulating erythrocytes. In fact, it would be preferable to use the term *relative* or *spurious erythrocytosis* in these situations, reserving the designation *polycythemia* for conditions associated with increased levels of other formed elements (such as granulocytes and platelets) in addition to erythrocytes.

PV and the secondary polycythemias are accompanied by an absolute increase in the RBC mass. Secondary polycythemia refers to a situation in which the absolute increase in RBC mass is due to and maintained by an increased production of erythropoietin. In the secondary polycythemias, the erythrocytosis disappears when the underlying cause of the increased erythropoietin production can be eliminated.[40]

Accurate separation of patients with absolute erythrocytosis from those with relative erythrocytosis requires direct measurement of both the RBC mass and the plasma volumes, using chromium-51 (^{51}Cr)-labeled erythrocytes and iodine-125 (^{125}I)–albumin, respectively. This is the initial step in evaluating the patient with a persistently elevated hematocrit. It is important because, in the absence of conditions associated with arterial hypoxemia-like cyanotic congenital heart disease or chronic pulmonary disease, cases of relative erythrocytosis are far more common than those with absolute erythrocytosis. These patients need not be subjected to the extensive and expensive investigation that may be required to determine the cause of an absolute increase in the circulating RBC mass. Of all those patients with PV, an estimated three to four patients have spurious polycythemia.[41]

Red blood cell and plasma volumes should be measured when a repeatedly elevated hematocrit is unexplained. The normal RBC mass is 30 ± 3 (SD) mL/kg in men and 27 ± 2 mL/kg in women. Measurements involve injection of autologous ^{51}Cr-labeled RBCs and calculation of the isotope dilution after an appropriate time interval. In patients with severe polycythemia, large amounts of blood remain in distended veins, and mixing is delayed. Blood samples for analysis must be drawn repeatedly until mixing is complete. RBC mass calculated from only the 30- or 60-minute sample may be a gross underestimate of the true value.

In addition, body habitus must be taken into consideration when interpreting the results. A tall muscular person normally has a higher RBC mass than that of a shorter obese person of the same weight, because the blood volume of muscle is much higher than that of fat. This discrepancy can be overcome by the use of a normogram that permits matching of height, weight, and surface area calculations with figures for normal RBC mass on an individual basis. Males with a hematocrit value of 60% or more and females with a hematocrit value of 57% or more virtually always have an increased RBC mass.

Although the radiation dose involved in the previously mentioned techniques is small compared with that of background radiation, it precludes RBC volume measurement in some patients, especially children and pregnant women. A nonradioactive approach using biotin has been described[42]; experience with this method is limited.

If the circulating RBC mass is increased, a systematic consideration of possible causes is in order, with careful evaluation of the history, physical examination, and pertinent laboratory data to determine whether the patient has a secondary polycythemia or PV. As shown in Table 13-2, the cause of the increased mass is one of the following: (1) a physiologically appropriate response to hypoxemia from cardiac or pulmonary disease, smoking, or high-oxygen affinity hemoglobins; (2) a consequence of autonomous erythropoietin production from neoplasms, cysts or renal ischemia, or other causes; or (3) PV.

In the secondary polycythemias, the hematopoietic cellular proliferation results from abnormalities in the erythropoietic regulatory mechanisms extrinsic to the erythroid progenitors themselves. The increased RBC production in these circumstances is driven by increased levels of erythropoietin or by other erythroid stimulator substances, which may be either physiologically appropriate or inappropriate (autonomous). Among the former are cases with

TABLE 13-2. Differential Diagnosis of Polycythemia

ERYTHROCYTOSIS ASSOCIATED WITH A NORMAL OR REDUCED RBC MASS

Acute or chronic hemoconcentration

Spurious polycythemia (stress polycythemia, relative polycythemia, or Gaisböck's syndrome)

ERYTHROCYTOSIS ASSOCIATED WITH AN ELEVATED RBC MASS (ABSOLUTE POLYCYTHEMIA)

Secondary Polycythemia

Increased erythropoietin production (physiologically appropriate)
- High altitude
- Cardiopulmonary disease
- Decreased blood oxygen carrying capacity due to carboxyhemoglobin
- Impaired oxygen delivery, hemoglobin with increased oxygen affinity or congenital decreased red cell 2,3-diphosphoglycerate
- Renal artery stenosis
- Familial elevated erythropoietin with appropriate physiologic response

Autonomous erythropoietin production
- Tumors
  - Hypernephroma
  - Cerebellar hemangioblastoma
  - Hepatoma
  - Uterine fibroids
  - Pheochromocytoma
  - Adrenal cortical adenoma
  - Ovarian carcinoma
- Renal disorders
  - Cysts
  - Hydronephrosis
  - Bartter's syndrome
  - Transplantation
- Familial polycythemia due to autonomous erythropoietin production

Polycythemia Vera

arterial hypoxemia due to diverse causes (see Table 13-2), to genetically determined high-affinity hemoglobins that release oxygen to tissues inadequately, or to reduced tissue perfusion. Determination of the arterial oxygen saturation screens for arterial hypoxemia as a cause of secondary polycythemia. A single normal value does not exclude desaturation at other times. For instance, patients with sleep apnea syndromes may desaturate only during sleep.

Structural differences in the hemoglobin molecule can cause a higher than usual affinity for oxygen. In 1965, hemoglobin Chesapeake was the first such hemoglobin variant to be described; since then, many others have been discovered.[43] In addition, abnormalities in enzymes involved in 2,3-diphosphoglycerate (2,3-DPG) synthesis may result in low RBC 2,3-DPG levels. In this setting, hemoglobin A behaves as a high-affinity hemoglobin. If one of these uncommon situations is suspected, the oxygen–hemoglobin dissociation curve, as reflected by the P_{50}, must be determined. Patients with high-oxygen-affinity hemoglobin have a shift to the left of the dissociation curve; the P_{50} is usually less than 20 mmHg.

Analogous shifts are seen in low 2,3-DPG states. If the P_{50} is reduced, determination of RBC 2,3-DPG indicates whether the defect is in 2,3-DPG metabolism or in the hemoglobin molecule itself. Hemoglobin electrophoresis is less valuable as a screening procedure than a P_{50} determination. Electrophoresis does not identify cases because of low 2,3-DPG, and it also fails to distinguish some of the high-affinity hemoglobins that arise from electrophoretically silent point mutations.

Smokers with an increased RBC mass fall into a special category and may have smoker's polycythemia.[44] The carbon monoxide inhaled in tobacco smoke has a high affinity for hemoglobin, 200 times that of oxygen for heme iron, and it is readily measurable as blood carboxyhemoglobin. The resultant carboxyhemoglobin causes tissue hypoxia and elaboration of erythropoietin. Also, the binding of carbon monoxide to hemoglobin causes a shift in the oxygen dissociation curve of the remaining heme groups, leading to an increased affinity of the hemoglobin for oxygen, a situation akin to high-affinity abnormal hemoglobin states. Smoking is also associated with reduction of plasma volume. Even transient cessation of smoking causes the low plasma volume to increase promptly in most patients, with consequent decline in the hematocrit. More prolonged abstinence causes the RBC volume to return gradually to normal.

If the patient does not have arterial hypoxemia secondary to cardiopulmonary disease, is not smoking, and is not likely to have a high–oxygen affinity hemoglobin variant, autonomous production of erythropoietic stimulatory substances (erythropoietin, androgens, adrenal corticosteroids) must be considered as a cause of polycythemia. Increased autonomous erythropoietin production may occur in certain neoplasms.[45] On a worldwide basis, hepatocellular carcinoma is probably the most common cause. RBC mass may also rise as a result of nonneoplastic lesions in the kidney (hydronephrosis, cysts, vascular lesions, transplantation), which are believed to produce local ischemia and to perturb the renal oxygen sensory mechanism. Cystic renal disease has been associated with polycythemia two to three times more frequently than has renal carcinoma.[46] Because diseases of the kidney are a common cause of secondary polycythemia, either a renal sonogram or renal computed tomography must be obtained in the event that another cause of the polycythemia is not evident. Erythrocytosis may be the presenting sign of renal cell carcinoma at a stage when it is the most amenable to surgical resection and potential cure.

Several rare familial polycythemia syndromes are associated with abnormalities in erythropoietin production. In some families, autonomous, fixed erythropoietin production occurs in the absence of a detectable structural lesion. In others, basal erythropoietin output is increased but appears responsive to physiologic perturbations such as phlebotomy or hypertransfusion.[47,48] Several groups have reported on deletions in the portion of the erythropoietin receptor gene that encodes the cytoplasmic domain of the receptor as a cause of familial polycythemia.[48a] This results in constitutive activation of the receptor.

Polycythemia Vera Study Group Criteria

The PVSG was formed in 1967 and at its inception recognized the need for a simple set of diagnostic criteria to facilitate the accurate diagnosis of PV. The group studied a relatively uniform group of patients over several decades. The resulting criteria, empirically developed from the collective clinical experience of the group, are listed in Table 13-1. In large numbers of patients initially diagnosed on the basis of these widely available studies and subsequently subjected to a more extensive evaluation according to the algorithm indicated in Figure 13-3, the false-positive rate was less than 0.5%. The combination of heavy smoking and excessive alcohol consumption—the former leading to smokers' polycythemia and the latter to alcoholic liver disease with splenomegaly, elevated serum B_{12} levels, and

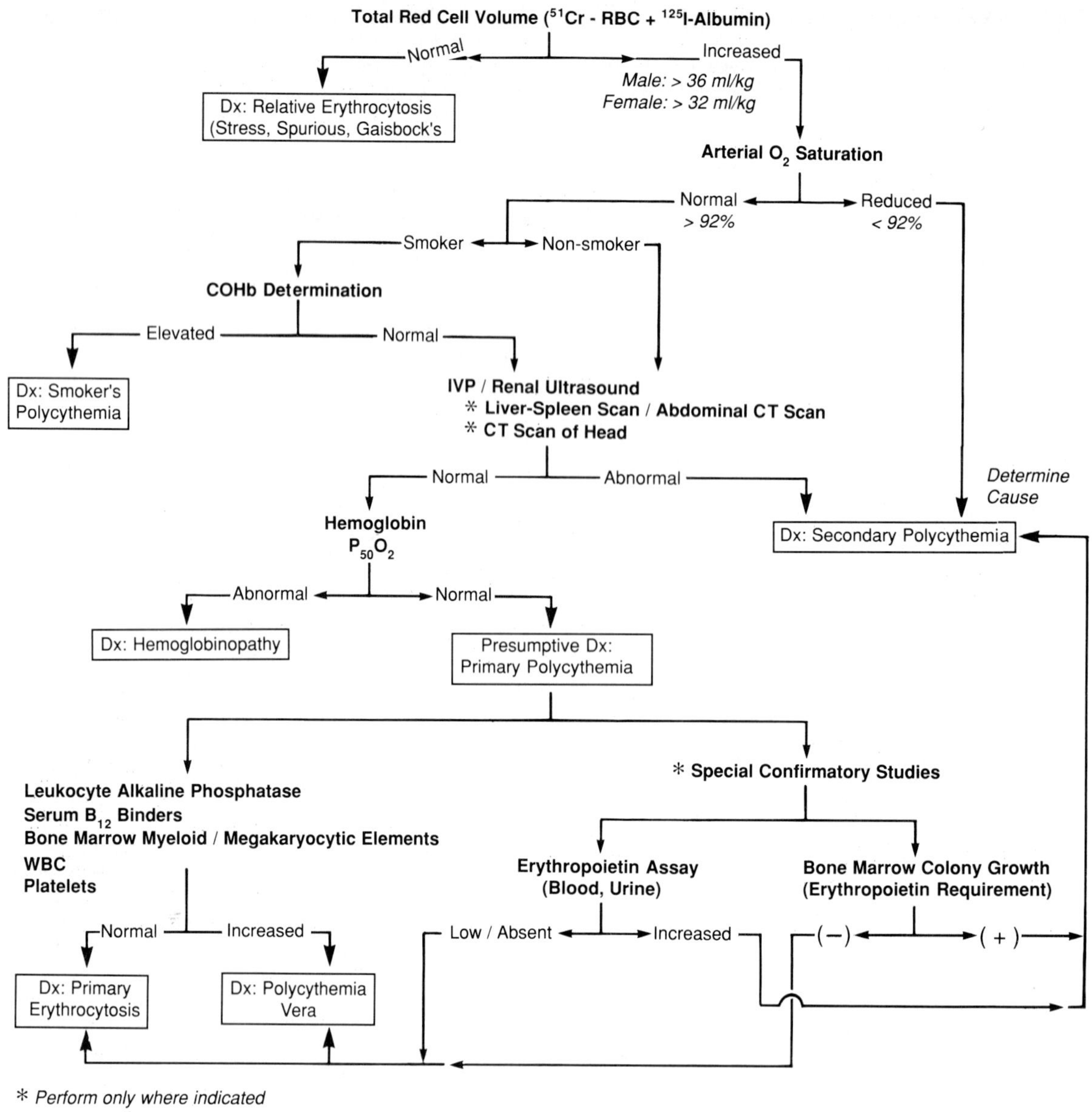

FIGURE 13-3. Algorithm for evaluation of an elevated hematocrit. (After Berlin W. Diagnosis and classification of the polycythemias. Semin Hematol 1975;12:5)

leukocytosis with an elevated leukocyte alkaline phosphatase score—is the patient condition that most often led to a false-positive diagnosis of PV.[49]

The criteria were developed to minimize false-positive results and not necessarily to have a low false-negative rate. Surely, patients early in the course of PV may fail to meet these criteria. In such cases, either continued follow-up or the use of more specialized studies makes it apparent that PV is the correct diagnosis. In patients who are diagnostic dilemmas, the measurement of serum and urinary erythropoietin levels is most helpful in differentiating PV from the secondary polycythemias.

Unfortunately, until recently precise measurement of erythropoietin has been difficult to accomplish. A costly biologic assay system uses the exhypoxic polycythemic mouse.[50] When mice are made polycythemic by either hypertransfusion or temporary exposure to hypoxia (exhypoxic mouse), their endogenous erythropoietin output is suppressed. Subsequent injection of the animals with biologic samples containing exogenous erythropoietin stimulates erythropoiesis and RBC ^{59}Fe (radiolabeled iron) incorporation to a degree that reflects the amount of erythropoietin in the injected material. Depending on the procedures used to concentrate the samples, erythropoietin bioassays have a lower limit of sensitivity of about 5 mIU/mL. Some normal persons have values below this limit of detection. Accordingly, although the presence of measurable serum erythropoietin levels by such assays weighs against a diagnosis of PV, the finding of undetectable levels does not reliably distinguish normal persons from those with PV.

Newer and more sensitive radioimmunoassays for erythropoietin permit its measurement to become more routine.[51] Again, although readily distinguishing normal from elevated erythropoietin levels, several of the available radioimmunoassays cannot distinguish normal serum levels from the reduced values expected in PV, in this case because of the presence of cross-reacting materials and because of the possibility of biologically inactive forms of the hormone in human sera. The presence of an elevated erythropoietin level in a person with a documented increase in RBC mass virtually rules out the diagnosis of PV, suggesting that the disorder is a secondary one.

Specimens for erythropoietin should not be obtained shortly after phlebotomy. Optimally, if these levels are required, they should be obtained at presentation to avoid

the effect of phlebotomy or a lowered hematocrit on the erythropoietin level. Patients with PV may generate increased erythropoietin levels after such a procedure.[52] As indicated in Figure 13-3, erythropoietin assays or studies of in vitro endogenous colony formation may help to distinguish patients with primary erythrocytosis from those with secondary erythrocytosis. In most cases, this distinction can be made with the more conventional diagnostic studies.

Classic laboratory tests important in the evaluation of polycythemia are the leukocyte alkaline phosphatase (LAP) score, B_{12} level, and B_{12}-binding proteins.[53] The principle of the LAP staining method is based on the amount and staining intensity of a precipitated dye at presumed sites of enzyme activity within mature and band-forming neutrophils, which are the only granulocytes with significant LAP activity in the peripheral blood or bone marrow. Usually, peripheral blood is scored semiquantitatively, and 100 neutrophils are graded 0 to 4+. The total score may thus range from 0 to 400. The normal LAP score is considered to be between 25 and 100. A marked increase may be seen in patients with PV; whereas in chronic granulocytic leukemia patients, LAP score is usually below 25. More than 80% of patients with PV have an increase in the alkaline phosphatase of circulating neutrophils.[54] In general, LAP values in uncomplicated secondary polycythemia are normal. Many factors may cause an increase in the LAP score (infection, fever, hemorrhage). Because the LAP may be normal in patients with PV, this test may lose its discriminatory value in the individual case.

Peripheral Blood Findings

The findings in the peripheral blood are often characteristic of patients with PV. In addition to elevation of the hematocrit, 40% of the 431 eligible patients in the initial PVSG study had white blood cell (WBC) counts above 12,000/μL, and 60% had platelet counts higher than 400,000/μL.[55] An increased proportion of basophils and eosinophils may be present. Leukocyte counts of 20,000 to 50,000/μL are common and may accompany erythrocytosis for years. Patients may present with or develop platelet counts exceeding 1,000,000/μL. The RBCs are most often normochromic and normocytic, but they may also be hypochromic and microcytic at presentation, even before therapeutic phlebotomy. This reflects iron-deficient erythropoiesis, which results from a shift of iron stores out of the marrow and into the expanded circulating erythron rather than from true total-body iron deficiency. Immature cells of the myeloid series may be observed in the peripheral blood of 50% of the patients when first seen, and nucleated RBCs are found in about 10% of these patients.

Bone Marrow Histology

Although PV is a disorder of the marrow stem cell, no feature of marrow histopathology is unique by which the diagnosis can be made with confidence. Rather, a constellation of findings may help support the diagnosis. Hypercellularity of the bone marrow is the typical finding in untreated patients with PV.[56] Nevertheless, hypercellularity is not invariable, since cases with a normocellular marrow have been reported with otherwise typical clinical and hematologic findings of PV.[57] Marrow cellularity is proportional to spleen size.[58]

Increase in megakaryocyte number and size in PV has been well documented (Fig. 13-4). The PVSG reported that 95% of patients with documented PV had slight to marked megakaryocyte hyperplasia, which correlated statistically with marrow cellularity. Although at initial review it appears that selective megakaryocyte hyperplasia has outpaced overall marrow hypercellularity, when values for fat-free marrow are calculated, the differences are not significant. Thus, megakaryocytic hyperplasia paralleled overall hyperplasia of other cellular elements. No particular clinical significance can be attached to the occurrence of relatively normal cellularities or of normal concentrations of megakaryocytes in some pretreatment biopsies. In addition to an increase in megakaryocyte numbers, their occurrence in clusters or even in sheets is a feature of all the myeloproliferative diseases, including PV. These large collections of often atypical megakaryocytic cells are best observed in bone marrow biopsies but may often be observed by carefully examining the spicules in marrow aspirate preparations.

Reticulin is a collagen fiber distinguished by its staining characteristics with various silver stains. Of 226 pretreatment biopsies graded for reticulin content, 64% were evaluated as normal, 24% showed only a slight increase in reticulin, and 12% showed a moderate to marked increase in reticulin fibers.[59] The spent phase of PV, discussed in the following text, is often associated with an increase in reticulin, as well as with much denser collagen fibrosis. Patients in the active phase of their disease can also increase the amount of reticulin in their marrow with time. Whether this reflects sampling variability or is of prognostic importance is not obvious. Patients with marrow reticulin fibrosis due to PV have increased circulating levels of the aminoterminal propeptide of type III procollagen,[60] which correlates with histologic assessment of reticulin deposition.

Serum iron concentration is low in most cases of PV in the absence of documented bleeding.[61] An accepted explanation for this phenomenon is that the iron level decreases as a result of both increased hematopoiesis and iron utilization for hemoglobin synthesis. This is reflected in the absence of iron stores in the marrow in most patients with PV. Iron pigment was found by Prussian blue staining in only 17 of 256 pretreatment biopsy specimens (6.6%). Caution should be used in interpretation of iron content of bone marrow based on sections alone, because biopsy sections that are not properly fixed and decalcified may lose appreciable amounts of iron-containing pigment during processing. This is not true of bone marrow aspiration smears, since they are air dried and do not require decalcification. Thus, marrow smears are more accurate than biopsy sections for the determination of marrow iron.

Because of an overlap of features among the various myeloproliferative disorders, study of the bone marrow aspirate and biopsy histology cannot definitively establish the diagnosis of PV, but it can be a valuable diagnostic tool. Hypercellularity is almost always observed in patients with PV. Although the lack of such hypercellularity does not exclude the disease, a normocellular marrow should make the diagnosis suspect, particularly when iron is present and megakaryocytic hyperplasia is absent or unimpressive. Nevertheless, in the setting of an increased RBC mass, the combination of marrow hypercellularity and megakaryocytic hyperplasia, particularly with concomitant reticulin increase, is of diagnostic importance and is strongly suggestive of the disease.

Cytogenetics

Bone marrow examination is also helpful in obtaining specimens for cytogenetic analysis. No single chromosomal defect is associated with PV. It was found that 26% of patients with previously untreated PV showed definite bone marrow chromosome abnormalities, a significant increase over the incidence of cytogenetic abnormalities in the control group studied.[62] Fifty percent of patients with an initial normal karyotype developed an abnormality with further

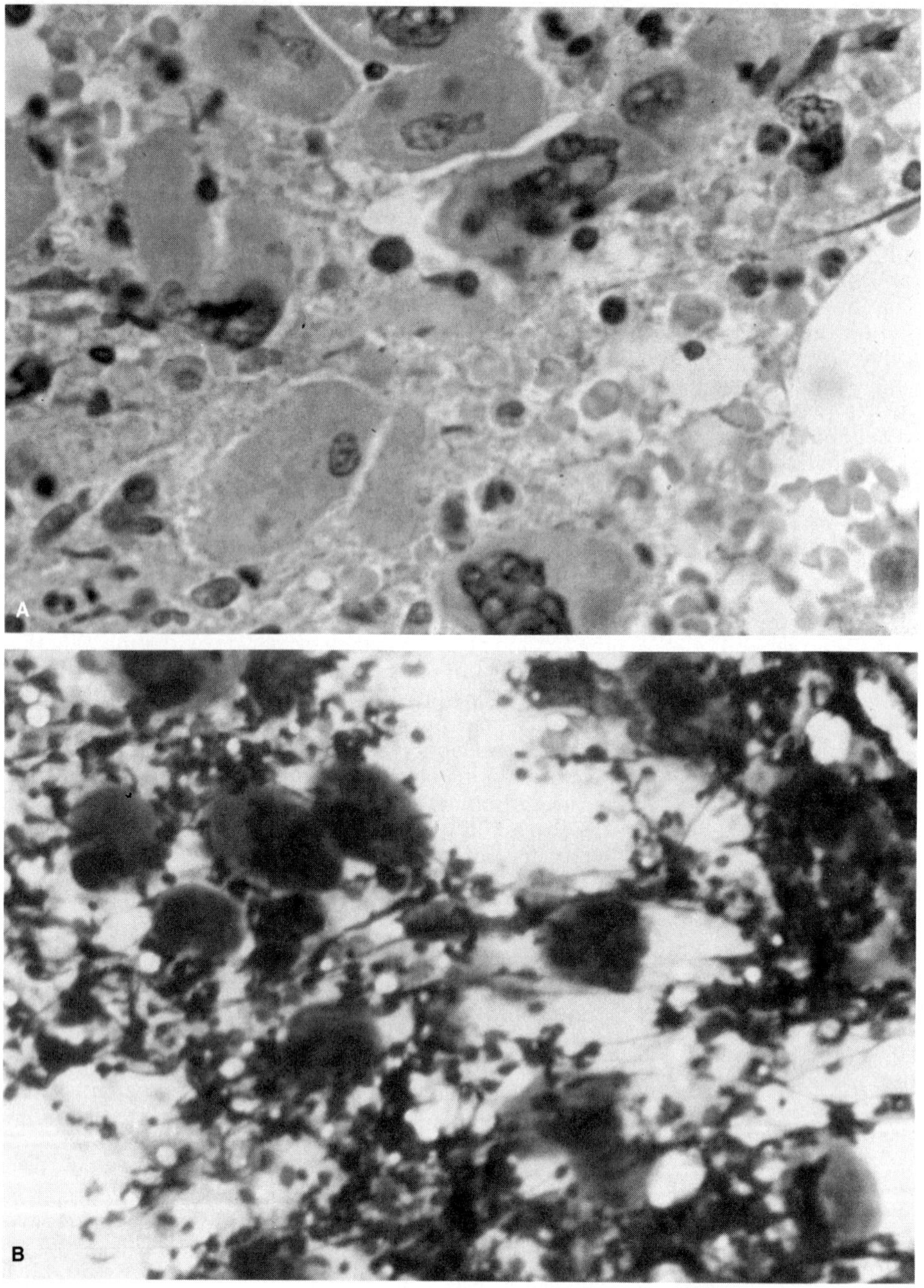

FIGURE 13-4. Photomicrograph showing hypercellular bone marrow biopsy (**A**) due to hyperplasia of erythroid, megakaryocytic, and granulocytic components, and megakaryocyte clumping on bone marrow aspirate (**B**) (hematoxylin–eosin, ×1000). (See Color Fig. 13-4.)

follow-up.[63] Numerical gain of chromosomes 8, 9, or both, and structural abnormalities of chromosome 20 are common in patients with PV. Others report structural abnormalities of chromosomes 13 and 1.[64,65] During the course of the disease, more patients develop abnormalities; in late stages of PV, more than half of the patients have cytogenetically abnormal clones.[66,66a] The prognostic significance of these findings is not clear. In contrast to many other hematopoietic neoplasms, the presence of a cytogenetic abnormality on diagnosis does not predict an aggressive clinical course in PV.

Symptoms and Physical Examination

Headache, weakness, and pruritus are the most common presenting symptoms of patients with PV, being seen in over 40% of patients reported. Dizziness, sweating, visual disturbances, and weight loss are other common nonspecific complaints. Pruritus can be the most persistent of the symptoms, is highly suggestive of PV, and may persist in some patients who are otherwise effectively treated. It is usually aggravated by bathing or showering, particularly with hot water, and by drying off after bathing. The pathogenesis of the pruritus is not known, and it has been reported to precede the development of overt PV.[67] Histamine release from the increased number of basophilic leukocytes has been suggested as being an important factor.[68] This suggestion may be inconsistent with the poor clinical response to antihistamine medications[69] and the absence of pruritus in other myeloproliferative disorders such as chronic myelocytic leukemia, in which basophil counts may be higher than those seen in patients with PV. Others have suggested that skin mast cells,[70] or iron deficiency[71] may play a role, although pruritus is usually not associated with iron deficiency when seen in other disorders.

The presence of splenomegaly is a most useful physical finding in evaluating patients for PV. Seventy percent of patients with PV have an enlarged spleen.[55] Other common findings are facial plethora in 67%, conjunctival plethora in 59%, engorgement of the fundic veins in 46%, and a palpable liver in 40%. These findings are less specific than splenomegaly and may be found in patients with polycythemia from other causes.

The cause of splenomegaly in polycythemia is a source of controversy. Some investigators have suggested that splenic enlargement results primarily from congestion,[72] others state that extramedullary hematopoiesis is responsible for the splenomegaly.[73] A recent morphologic and immunohistologic study showed that spleens from patients in the erythrocytic phase of their disease showed striking congestion of the red pulp sinuses and Billroth's cords with mature erythrocytes and minimal evidence of extramedullary hematopoiesis.[74] In contrast, spleens obtained from patients whose disease had evolved to the spent phase showed prominent extramedullary hematopoiesis. Using RBC pooling studies, it has been shown that RBC pooling occurs in the spleen in patients with PV, whereas with comparable total RBC volumes no significant RBC pooling is found in secondary polycythemia patients.[73] This suggests a unique RBC–splenic structural interaction in patients with PV to explain the splenic pooling and congestive splenomegaly.

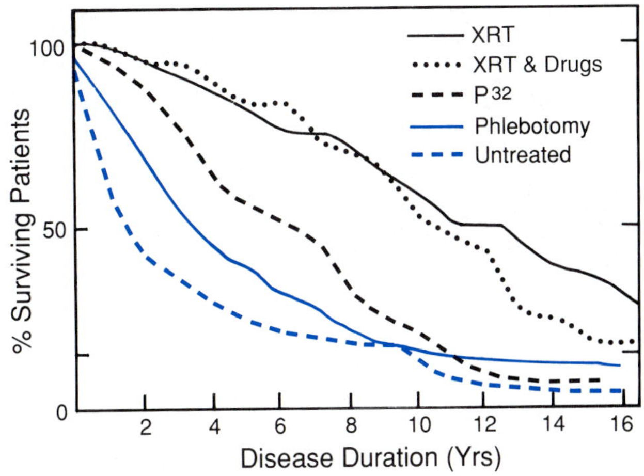

FIGURE 13-5. Percentage survival of patients with polycythemia vera who were left untreated and those who received various therapeutic modalities. (After Chievitz E, Thiede T. Complications and causes of death in polycythemia vera. Acta Med Scand 1962;172:513)

NATURAL HISTORY AND COMPLICATIONS OF POLYCYTHEMIA VERA

Although the onset of PV may be insidious and its course chronic, PV is a hematologic malignancy involving an abnormal clone of the pluripotent marrow stem cell. Clinical observation has helped to confirm the biochemical findings that PV can behave as a malignant process.

Patients with PV who are left untreated do poorly; half are reported to die within 18 months after onset of the first symptom.[75] Untreated patients with PV also have an especially high risk of developing both thrombotic and hemorrhagic complications, with death due to thrombosis of the cerebral, coronary, and pulmonary circulation. Unusual sites for thrombosis, such as the hepatic veins, femoral artery or vein, and mesentery are also seen. In a review of 253 patients with Budd-Chiari syndrome, PV was found to be the cause in over 10%, and other myeloproliferative disorders accounted for an additional 1.2%.[76] In 20 intriguing patients with idiopathic Budd-Chiari syndrome, 16 had endogenous erythroid colonies, only two of whom had an overt myeloproliferative disorder.[77] This suggests that patients with occult, or perhaps early, PV may also be prone to unusual thrombotic complications. This interesting observation requires further study.

Because of the aggressive nature of untreated PV and the broader availability of routine screening blood counts with automated analyzers, it is unusual to see patients with PV who are not diagnosed relatively early in the course of their disease or who are left untreated. Therefore, the natural history of PV can be evaluated only by review of studies prior to the current era.

In 1962, Chievitz and Thiede[75] reported that 50% of untreated patients died within 18 months of the first manifestation of their disease. This compared with $3^1/_2$ years for patients treated with venesection, and between 7 and 13 years for patients treated with various combinations of phosphorus-32 (^{32}P), radiation, and myelosuppressive agents (Fig. 13-5). Sixty-three percent of untreated patients and 40% of all patients died of thrombosis. In more than 20% of patients, the critical presenting sign was thrombosis; in more than 10%, bleeding, especially from the gastrointestinal tract, was the first sign. Cerebral, coronary, pulmonary, and mesenteric thrombosis accounted for 90% of the deaths due to thrombosis. Other causes of death attributable to PV were hemorrhage and leukemia, myelofibrosis, and anemia. The latter three conditions were especially prevalent in patients treated with radiation, although it appeared that these patients lived longer. These findings corroborated those of Wasserman and Bassen,[78] who found thrombosis to be the major cause of death in patients with PV, followed by myeloid metaplasia, leukemia, and hemorrhage.

Myeloid metaplasia with myelofibrosis, or so-called spent polycythemia was the next most common cause of death in Wasserman's series.[79] This phase is the first sign of diminished erythropoietic activity in the marrow. The peripheral blood may show a relatively normal RBC concentration, often with a leukocytosis and perhaps a thrombocytosis. The smear shows a leukoerythroblastic picture, with myelocytes and normoblasts. The RBCs, in particular, show abnormalities characteristic of the evolving myeloid metaplasia, with polychromatophilia and marked anisocytosis and poikilocytosis, including microcytes, elliptic cells, teardrop cells, and other unusual RBC forms (Fig. 13-6). These RBC changes, and the findings in the marrow, are characteristic of either this stage of PV or of the idiopathic type of myeloid metaplasia. The marrow may still appear hyperplastic, but instead of showing a panmyelosis it may show some reduction in the erythropoietic elements with an increase in reticulin and megakaryocytes. Along with the marrow changes, the spleen enlarges and becomes the site of extramedullary blood formation. When splenic punctures were used as a diagnostic tool, they showed a picture similar to that seen in the marrow, with increased reticulin and hematopoietic cell proliferation. At this stage, the anemia may be mild or even absent, and a compensated myelofibrotic state may be seen that may last for months or years.

The marrow eventually becomes almost completely fibrotic with megakaryocytes now especially prominent because of the disappearance of most of the other cellular elements. At this stage, a dry tap on marrow aspiration is seen and the peripheral blood shows anemia, leukopenia, and a variable platelet count, although thrombocytopenia is typical. Others may develop leukocytosis with myeloid immaturity, and some may develop overt acute leukemia.

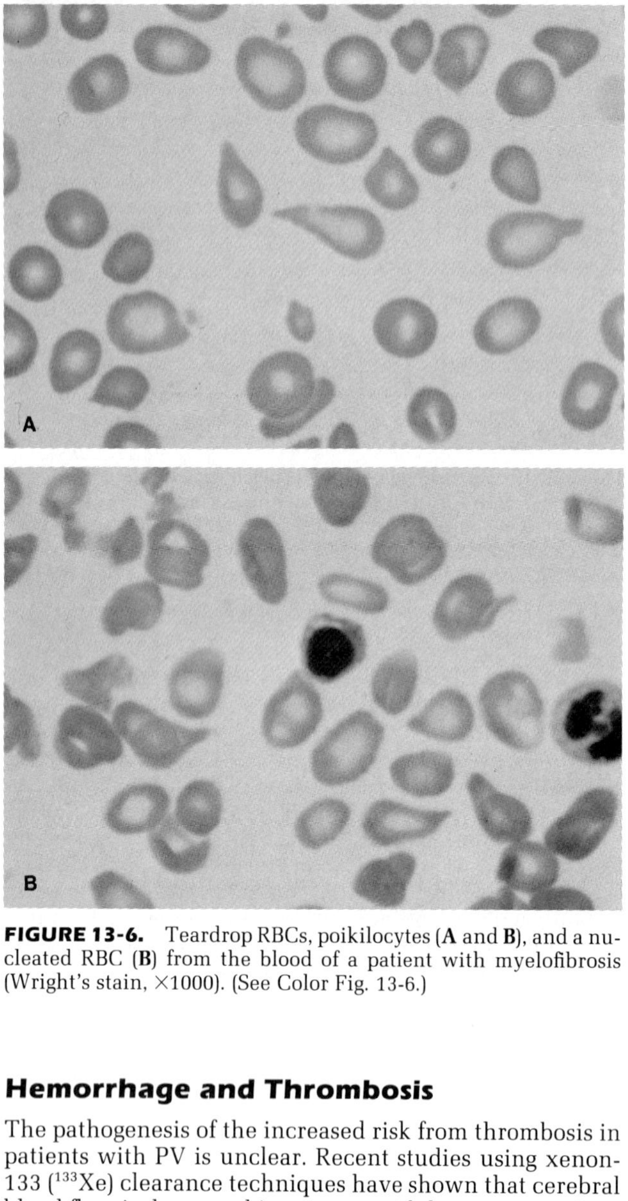

FIGURE 13-6. Teardrop RBCs, poikilocytes (**A** and **B**), and a nucleated RBC (**B**) from the blood of a patient with myelofibrosis (Wright's stain, ×1000). (See Color Fig. 13-6.)

Hemorrhage and Thrombosis

The pathogenesis of the increased risk from thrombosis in patients with PV is unclear. Recent studies using xenon-133 (^{133}Xe) clearance techniques have shown that cerebral blood flow is decreased in persons with hematocrit values above 53% and returns to normal after a reduction in hematocrit to normal levels.[80] Even hematocrit reductions within the normal range, such as from 50% to 45% or less, result in significant augmentation of cerebral blood flow in many patients. Furthermore, cerebral function is impaired by high hematocrit values and improved by reduction of the hematocrit to levels below 45%, the level at which cerebral blood flow is optimally improved.[81] Indeed, the Framingham Study identified the hemoglobin value as an important risk factor for cerebral infarction in the general population.[82] A postmortem study demonstrated a greater incidence of cerebral infarction in patients with packed RBC volume levels over 46% than in those with lower values,[83] and the degree of hematocrit elevation may influence the size of a cerebral infarct in both animals and man.[84] Elevation in hematocrit has been shown to be an important contributory factor toward higher morbidity and mortality rates from cardiovascular disease and myocardial infarction.[85] Thus, the propensity for thrombosis and infarction in polycythemia may be related to a reversible impairment of blood flow.

Hemorrhage is another common cause of early mortality. Epistaxis, ecchymosis, and menorrhagia are also common problems. The gastrointestinal tract is the most common site of severe bleeding, and cerebral hemorrhage may be fatal. Although blood fluidity is important in influencing the thrombotic and hemorrhagic tendencies seen in PV, even when the blood volume is normalized by phlebotomy these patients are prone to thrombotic and hemorrhagic complications. In addition to whole blood viscosity, abnormalities of the circulating elements and the vascular endothelium may play a role. A multitude of platelet abnormalities are found in patients with PV, and the platelet has been incriminated in the thrombohemorrhagic complications of PV with respect to both increased numbers and abnormal function. Typically, patients with PV have elevated platelet counts and a multiplicity of in vitro abnormalities in platelet aggregation; moreover, these platelets may undergo in vivo degranulation.[86,87] Qualitative platelet defects that have been described include lipooxygenase deficiency, loss of response or increased sensitivity to aggregating agents, decreased numbers of adrenergic and prostaglandin D receptors, increased expression of Fc receptors, acquired storage pool disease and abnormal platelet membrane glycoprotein patterns.[88–90a] In addition, there is an intriguing observation that platelets from PV patients synthesize increased quantities of thromboxane A_2 and that this increase is readily suppressed by low-dose aspirin.[90b] This observation may explain the beneficial effect of aspirin in some PV patients. The relation between these platelet defects and clinical bleeding or thrombosis has not been firmly established.

A widespread belief of hematologists has been that an elevated platelet count is a risk factor for thrombotic complications. The PVSG attempted to demonstrate an association between the platelet count or hematocrit and the risk for thrombosis for the 431 patients followed up by this group in its initial long-term study. This effort was confounded by the wide scatter of hematologic values reported, not only among treatment groups, but in the courses of individual patients. To alleviate some of these problems, a retrospective matched-pair analysis was carried out. For each patient who had a thrombotic event, a thrombosis-free control patient of similar age, sex, treatment group, and duration of study was selected. Hematologic parameters measured at the nearest time before the thrombotic event of the index case were then compared with those in the matched control patient at the corresponding time on study. Within this retrospective study of treated patients, neither elevations of the platelet count nor the hematocrit were associated with an increased risk of a thrombotic event, although the number of patients with hematocrits over 52% or with platelet counts of more than 1.5 million was small.[49] Thus, it is not clear that the tendency to thrombosis in these patients is related to platelet number alone.

Leukemia

The occurrence of leukemia in patients with PV as an end result of the natural course of the disease or as a complication of therapy has long been a source of controversy. Acute leukemia is believed to occur as a terminal event in some patients with PV treated only with phlebotomy, and the risk of developing acute leukemia in this setting is several-fold greater than in an age-matched control population.[91] The incidence of acute leukemia in patients with PV receiving various forms of radiation or radiomimetic chemotherapy ranges from 11% to 30%.[92,93] The therapeutic modality chosen was believed to influence the tendency for PV to transform into acute leukemia. A possible role of ^{32}P in the transformation of PV to acute leukemia was first suggested in 1945.[93] Landaw[94] summarized the results of more than 25 large studies that suggested that the treatment of PV with radiation, either in the form of x-rays or ^{32}P, was associated with an increased incidence of acute leu-

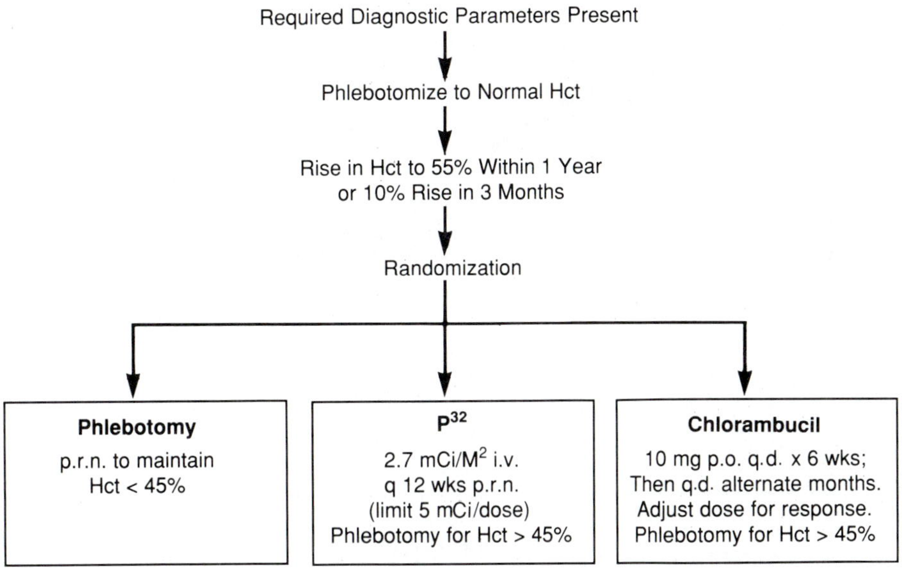

FIGURE 13-7. Protocol of PVSG-01, a long-term randomized controlled trial of three treatment regimens in polycythemia vera patients.

kemia; he suggested that any chemotherapeutic agent capable of suppressing the panmyelosis may increase the inherent tendency to acute leukemia of the untreated disease. Lawrence and coworkers[95] and Osgood[96] have argued that this increased incidence was explained by the longer survival in ^{32}P-treated patients, which permitted fuller expression of the natural history of the disease. That this is not the case was clearly demonstrated in studies by the PVSG, in which both longest survival and lowest incidence of leukemia were observed in patients treated with chronic phlebotomy alone.

THERAPEUTIC STUDIES AND RECOMMENDATIONS OF THE POLYCYTHEMIA VERA STUDY GROUP

Overall Survival

In 1967, in an attempt to clarify the therapeutic dilemma and to determine the optimal treatment for patients with PV, the PVSG began entering patients into a randomized controlled trial, comparing the efficacy of treatment with phlebotomy alone with ^{32}P supplemented by phlebotomy, and with chlorambucil supplemented by phlebotomy. The protocol, designated PVSG-01, is summarized in Figure 13-7. Patients who met the diagnostic criteria for PV as outlined in Table 13-1 were phlebotomized to a normal hematocrit. If the hematocrit level rose to 55% within 1 year or rose 10% above the postphlebotomy value within 3 months, the patient was randomized to one of the three treatment arms. The initial phlebotomies were incorporated into the protocol to ensure that only patients in the active, proliferative stage of the disease were entered into the study.

Between 1967 and 1974, 431 eligible patients were assigned at random to one of the three treatment regimens of PVSG-01. Patients still alive and in the study have been observed for 15 to 22 years. As of the most recent analysis of the data base, 219 patients, representing 51% of the initial cohort, had died while in the study. As indicated in Table 13-3, thrombotic events, acute leukemia and lymphoma, other neoplasias, hemorrhage, and complications of myelofibrosis were the principal causes of death. Together, these five entities accounted for over 75% of all deaths reported among patients on study. Thrombosis and acute leukemia accounted for more than half of all deaths.

Survival curves for the three treatment groups are illustrated in Figure 13-8. Median duration of survival is 9.1 years in chlorambucil-treated patients, 10.9 years in patients treated with ^{32}P, and 12.6 years in patients treated with phlebotomy alone. Thus, a statistically significant difference is seen in long-term survival in these treatment arms (see Fig. 13-8); chlorambucil-treated patients do significantly worse than those treated with phlebotomy or ^{32}P. Note that differences in survival rate, assessed by the Breslow chi-squared test, which emphasizes earlier events, do not achieve statistical significance. When the Logrank test, which emphasizes later events is used, these differences reach statistical significance. Thus, over the first 8 years of study, the three treatment arms were equivalent in terms of overall survival. The late occurrence of malignancies in the two myelosuppressive arms of the protocol, predominantly in the arm using the alkylating agent chlorambucil, contributed to the differences in long-term survival.

Examination of the causes of death by treatment regimen highlights these differences (Table 13-4). Thrombotic events, the most common cause of death in patients with PV in the overall study, accounted for a higher percentage of deaths among phlebotomy-treated patients than among those receiving either of the myelosuppressive regimens. Acute leukemia, the second most prevalent terminal event, was markedly increased in patients treated with chlorambucil. Because of this finding, the PVSG no longer recommends the use of chlorambucil in the treatment of patients with PV.[92] The increase in leukemia in chlorambucil-treated patients was recognized within 4 years after starting therapy. A later but significant increase in acute leukemia

TABLE 13-3. Cause of Death at 10 Years of Study—PVSG-01

Cause of Death*	No.	Percentage Deaths
Thrombosis	64	29
Acute leukemia/lymphoma	51	23
Other neoplasms	35	16
Hemorrhage	15	7
Myelofibrosis	7	3
Miscellaneous	47	22
TOTAL	219	100

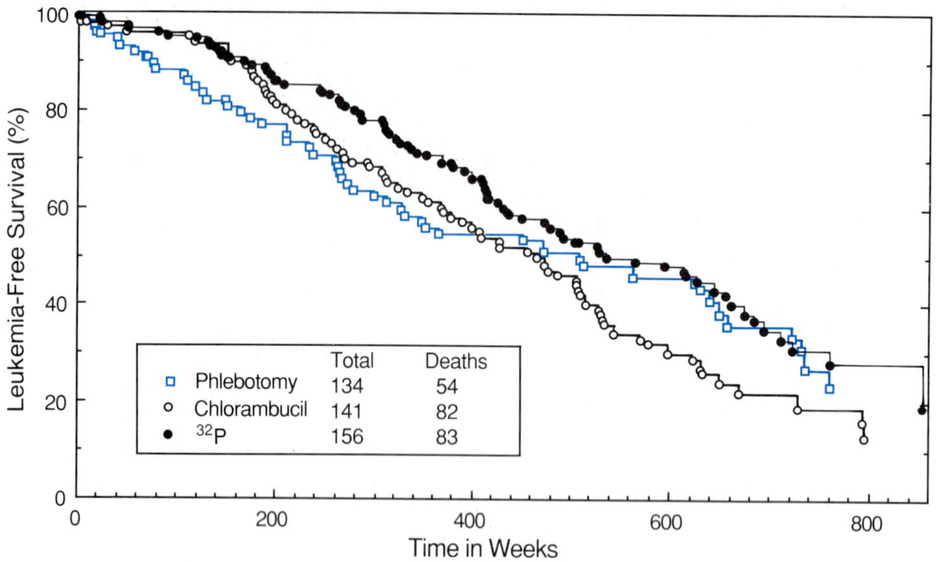

FIGURE 13-8. Cumulative survival of patients with polycythemia vera on three treatment arms of PVSG-01.

was subsequently recognized in patients receiving ^{32}P. The group continues to study the oral, nonalkylating agent hydroxyurea in the management of this disease, as will be discussed later in more detail.

Other malignant diseases, in addition to acute leukemia, also occurred more often in patients with PV treated with either chlorambucil or ^{32}P than in those managed by phlebotomy alone. These malignancies, including both lymphomas and nonhematologic solid tumors, are discussed in detail in the text that follows. A recent European study confirms the PVSG findings and suggests that, with treatment, the mortality of patients with PV does not differ significantly from that of age-matched controls without the disease.[92a]

Thrombotic Events

The 143 initial thrombotic events reported on protocol PVSG-01 are summarized in Table 13-5. Cerebrovascular accidents, myocardial infarctions, peripheral arterial occlusions, pulmonary infarcts, and venous thromboses other than thrombophlebitis accounted for 65% of these initial thrombotic events. Thirty-five percent of the initial thrombotic events in these first five categories were fatal. One third of those who survived the initial thrombotic event have had a second or subsequent thrombosis. The case fatality rate with subsequent thrombosis is also 35%. Figure 13-9 illustrates the thrombosis-free cumulative survival rate in the three treatment arms. Note that differences in the three treatment arms are primarily early, and patients treated with phlebotomy have a higher incidence of thrombotic events only during the first 3 years of study.

In an attempt to determine the factors associated with risk of thrombosis, data from the entire cohort of 431 patients were analyzed using a variety of multivariate methods. Of all the variables examined, treatment with phlebotomy per se was found to be associated with a statistically significant increased risk of early thrombosis. History of prior thrombosis and age over 70 also contributed significantly to the overall risk of thrombosis. Evaluation of other variables, including sex, history of hemorrhage, pretreatment hematocrit, WBC count, platelet count, and RBC indices, individually or jointly, did not contribute significantly to the explanation of the observed data. Among patients treated with phlebotomy alone, the phlebotomy rate was also found to contribute significantly to the incidence of thrombosis. It is not known whether a high phlebotomy rate and an increased risk of thrombosis are causally related or whether both are manifestations of increased disease activity. Hence, treatment with phlebotomy alone, particularly among patients with a high phlebotomy requirement, advanced age, and history of a prior thrombotic event, appear to be major factors contributing to the increased risk of thrombosis.

Iron deficiency with microcytic, hypochromic RBC changes may complicate the management of patients with phlebotomy. Iron should not be given because this may cause the hematocrit and RBC mass values to increase rapidly, thus increasing the phlebotomy requirement. Controversy exists regarding the correlation between whole blood viscosity at a fixed hemoglobin level and mean RBC

TABLE 13-4. Causes of Death by Treatment Group—PVSG-01

	Phlebotomy	Chlorambucil	^{32}P
Number at start	134	141	156
Number of deaths	54	82	83
Percentage of deaths due to:			
Thrombosis	43	23	27
Hemorrhage	0	9	10
Acute leukemia/ lymphoma	4	35	24
Other neoplasms	11	17	18
Myelofibrosis	2	5	2
Miscellaneous and unknown	41	11	19

TABLE 13-5. Initial Thrombotic Events in the First 10 Years of Study—PVSG-01

Type of Event	No.	Percentage Events
Cerebral vascular accident	49	34
Myocardial infarct	18	13
Peripheral arterial occlusion	13	9
Pulmonary infarct	7	5
Venous thrombosis (other than thrombophlebitis)	6	4
Deep vein thrombophlebitis	32	22
Miscellaneous	18	13
TOTAL	143	100

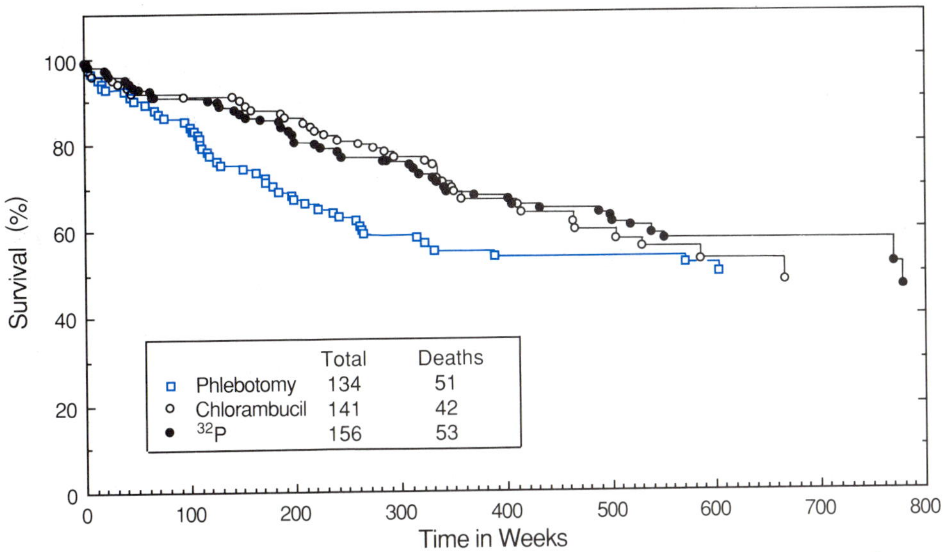

FIGURE 13-9. Incidence of thrombosis in polycythemia vera patients on three treatment arms of PVSG-01.

hemoglobin. It has been reported that iron-deficient RBCs, as indicated by a low MCH (mean corpuscular hemoglobin) value, result in a relative increase in whole blood viscosity, particularly at low shear rates, which may exist with concomitant circulatory disease.[97] These findings contrast with those of other investigators who found no difference in viscosity caused by microcytic, hypochromic RBC changes.[98,99] Debate in the literature on methodologic aspects has not resolved the conflict and requires further investigation.

Whole blood viscosity is also influenced by other factors, including plasma proteins, flow velocity, vessel diameter, and endothelial integrity.[100] Clinically, these factors may play a more important role in the development of thrombosis than do rheologic considerations. In any event, in PVSG-01 no correlation was observed between RBC indices and the incidence of thrombosis. The absence of a strict relationship between red cell count per se and thrombotic events is confirmed by a recent study comparing thromboembolic events in patients with PV "smoker's polycythemia" with equivalent elevations in peripheral blood hemoglobin content.[100a]

Role of Aspirin and Dipyridamole in the Prevention of Thrombosis (PVSG-05)

To determine whether the excess risk of thrombotic complications associated with phlebotomy therapy could be reduced by administration of platelet antiaggregating agents, a randomized controlled trial (PVSG-05) was initiated in 1977.[101] The study consisted of 166 patients who met the diagnostic criteria for PV (see Table 13-1). Eighty-three patients were randomized to receive radioactive phosphorus supplemented by phlebotomy; 83 were treated with phlebotomy plus aspirin, 300 mg by mouth three times daily, and dipyridamole (Persantine), 75 mg orally three times daily. At a median follow-up of 1.5 years, with a maximum period of observation of 3.4 years, seven severe thrombotic complications were found on the phlebotomy–aspirin–persantine regimen and only two on the ^{32}P regimen. Moreover, six patients receiving phlebotomy, aspirin, and dipyridamole had severe gastrointestinal hemorrhages requiring transfusion, compared with none in the patients receiving ^{32}P.

The cumulative 2-year incidence of severe thrombotic complications after treatment with phlebotomy, aspirin, and dipyridamole was similar to that of patients in protocol PVSG-01 who were treated with phlebotomy alone.[101] Hence, aspirin and dipyridamole, in the doses used in this study, did not prevent early thrombotic complications in patients with PV who were treated by phlebotomy without myelosuppression. In addition, these agents were associated with an increased incidence of serious hemorrhage, and the protocol was terminated.

In retrospect, these studies can be criticized for using too high a dose of aspirin. Other investigators continue to study the use of lower doses of aspirin to see whether antiplatelet agents at these doses can prevent thrombosis in patients with PV treated solely with phlebotomy. In other settings, the doses of aspirin and dipyridamole influence the incidence of hemorrhagic side effects. There is no well-documented situation in which these agents failed to reduce thrombotic events at high doses but were efficacious at lower doses. Hence, a significant role for aspirin and dipyridamole in prevention of thrombosis in PV seems highly unlikely.

Hematologic and Nonhematologic Neoplasia (PVSG-01)

The PVSG reported in 1981 that treatment with chlorambucil increased the risk of developing acute leukemia.[92] This is reflected by a predominance of leukemic deaths on this regimen (see Table 13-4). As of January 1987, a total of 20 cases of acute leukemia, confirmed by histopathologic review, have been reported after chlorambucil treatment, 2 after phlebotomy, and 15 among patients treated with ^{32}P. Additionally, 5 cases of large-cell lymphoma, predominantly with an abdominal presentation, have been reported after use of chlorambucil. Nine additional patients with leukemia or lymphoma have been reported, but either death was considered to have another cause or final confirmation of diagnosis was pending.

Figure 13-10 shows the leukemia-free cumulative survival curves for the study. The incidence of hematologic malignancy, that is, of leukemia and non-Hodgkin's lymphoma, is markedly increased in patients treated with either of the two myelosuppressive regimens. The peak incidence of leukemia in ^{32}P-treated patients tends to occur later than among patients treated with chlorambucil. The time interval from the diagnosis of PV to the onset of acute leukemia ranged from 2.1 years to more than 11 years with a median of 4.2 years in the chlorambucil-treated patients. In ^{32}P-treated patients, the interval ranged from 3.2 years to more than 12.5 years with a mean of 7.3 years.[63] Because of the greater incidence of leukemic transformation with myelosuppressive agents, other agents continue to be studied for efficacy and long-term safety.

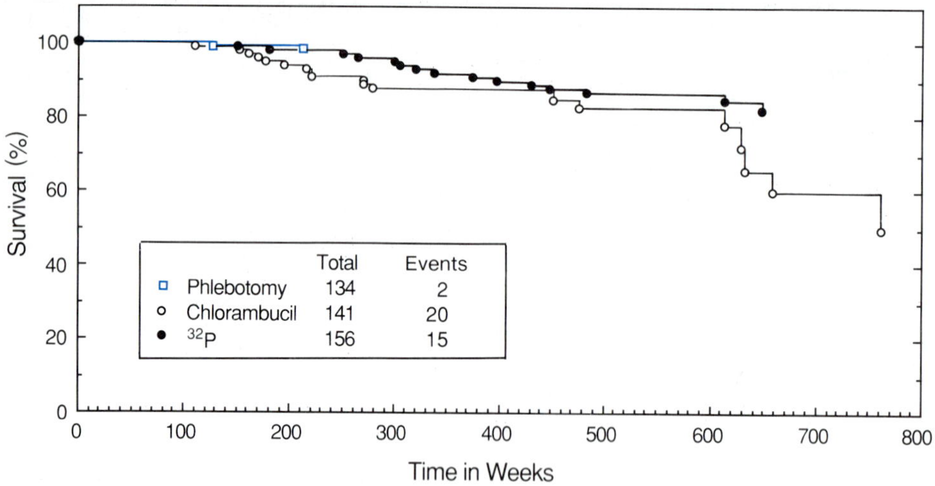

FIGURE 13-10. Incidence of acute leukemia in polycythemia vera patients on three treatment arms of PVSG-01.

Successful treatment of postpolycythemic acute leukemia is difficult. The experience of the PVSG is that postpolycythemic acute leukemia, like the blast crisis of chronic myelogenous leukemia and other secondary acute leukemias, infrequently responds to chemotherapeutic regimens that induce remission in patients with de novo acute leukemia. In addition, the incidence of biphenotypic leukemia is greater in this population than in a population in which acute leukemia does not follow a prior hematologic malignancy. Thirteen patients with postpolycythemic acute leukemia received multiagent combination chemotherapy. Overall median survival among these 13 patients was only 32 days from the time therapy for acute leukemia was initiated; only one complete remission was achieved.[102] By contrast, complete remission rates of 70%, with median survival of more than 1 year, were being widely achieved with similar chemotherapeutic regimens in de novo acute leukemia. Thus, better induction regimens are required for patients with postpolycythemic acute leukemia, who are more refractory to standard treatment strategies. The most important approach must continue to be further study in understanding the pathogenesis of acute leukemia and minimization of the risk of leukemic transformation in patients with PV.

After 20 years of study, 62 nonhematologic neoplasms had been reported among patients in PVSG-01. Fifteen neoplasms were seen in phlebotomy-treated patients, 24 in patients receiving chlorambucil, and 23 in patients treated with ^{32}P. Sixty percent of these tumors were of gastrointestinal or cutaneous origin. When the incidence of reported cancers was compared with that predicted from data for an age- and sex-matched population, the rate of malignancy in chlorambucil-treated patients 14 years after entry in the study was almost 2.5 times over that which was expected. Among patients treated with ^{32}P, it was almost twice that expected. The incidence of nonhematologic malignancy in phlebotomy-treated patients was not significantly increased relative to that in the control group. Differences among the three groups can be attributed to the gastrointestinal and skin cancers. Thus, the malignant transformation may occur in all rapidly proliferating tissues (such as bone marrow, gastrointestinal tract, skin) as a long-term consequence of these types of myelosuppressive agents in patients with PV.[92]

OTHER THERAPEUTIC STRATEGIES

Myelosuppressive Agents

Because patients with PV treated with phlebotomy alone have a significantly higher incidence of serious thrombotic complications earlier in the course of PV than those treated with chlorambucil or ^{32}P, investigators continue to seek myelosuppressive agents that may prove safe for long-term use. Other trials have used melphalan, cyclophosphamide, and busulfan as cytostatic agents. These alkylating agents can control the peripheral blood counts in patients with PV.[103] As has been shown in greatest detail with chlorambucil, no alkylating agent is free of leukemogenic potential, and numerous reports have been made of the association of alkylating agent therapy and leukemia in both hematologic[104,105] and nonhematologic disorders.[106]

Since busulfan's mechanism of action is significantly different from the classic alkylating agents, it may warrant continued study in patients with PV to see whether the tendency to leukemic transformation that is seen with other alkylating agents can be avoided.[107–109] Busulfan has a more marked effect on megakaryocytes than other alkylating agents and may induce long-standing thrombocytopenia. Because of the effect of busulfan on thrombopoiesis, patients must be carefully monitored to detect early any tendency toward thrombocytopenia; failure to do so can lead to severe and potentially life-threatening thrombocytopenia as well as marrow aplasia in sensitive patients. This can make busulfan a difficult agent to manage. Pulmonary fibrosis has also been noted in patients receiving long-term busulfan therapy. Antimetabolites such as 6-thioguanine[110] and azaribine,[111] alkaloids such as harringtonine,[112] and miscellaneous agents such as pipobroman,[113] and dibromomannitol[114] have been used effectively to treat patients with PV. Both long-term efficacy and side effects are unknown, so these agents cannot be recommended as initial therapy. (Recombinant interferon-α is also being studied in the management of myeloproliferative disorders, including PV.) A much greater experience has accumulated with the use of hydroxyurea for patients requiring myelosuppressive therapy.

Hydroxyurea

The need for a safe myelosuppressive agent in patients with PV, in whom phlebotomy is not ideal therapy because of age, history of prior thrombosis, high phlebotomy requirement, or lack of venous access, prompted the study of hydroxyurea.[115] Hydroxyurea had been used primarily in the treatment of patients with chronic granulocytic leukemia and other malignant conditions. It is a nonalkylating, myelosuppressive agent that inhibits cell growth by decreasing DNA synthesis. It does this by inhibiting the enzyme ribonucleoside diphosphate reductase.[116] Because its mechanism of action is different from that of alkylating agents, it was hoped that this easily administered and usually well-tolerated oral agent was safe for long-term use. Hydroxyurea can achieve and maintain good peripheral blood counts in over 80% of patients within 12 weeks of its initiation.[117] When rapid control is deemed important, hydroxyurea should be administered initially at a dose of 15 to 20 mg/kg/d, after normalization of the hematocrit with phlebotomy. The patient is followed up with weekly blood counts. When a steady state is achieved, the interval between blood counts is lengthened to 2 weeks, then to 4 weeks. If the WBC count falls below 3500/μL or the platelet count to less than 100,000/μL, hydroxyurea is withheld and reinstated at 50% of the prior dose when the blood count normalizes. For poorly controlled patients who require frequent phlebotomies or are thrombocythemic (platelet count consistently higher than 600,000/μL), the dose can be increased by 5 mg/kg/d at monthly intervals with frequent monitoring until control is achieved.

Because patient sensitivity to hydroxyurea varies widely, this approach may produce transient leukopenia or thrombocytopenia in a significant minority of cases. In a less urgent circumstance , therapy may be indicated with one 500-mg tablet per day (about 8 to 10 mg/kg/d), with the dose being increased at monthly intervals by one tablet every other day until an effective level is achieved. This requires doses from as little as one 500-mg tablet three times per week to 3 g/d (or rarely, higher); the average maintenance dosage is about 1000 mg/d.

Other than reversible suppression of myelopoiesis and thrombopoiesis, acute toxicity in hydroxyurea therapy is rare. Occasional patients may develop a rash, gastrointestinal complaints, oral ulcerations, or fever. Hydroxyurea therapy, supplemented by phlebotomy, has been shown to diminish the risk of thrombosis associated with phlebotomy alone.[118]

The highest risk of thrombotic complications occurs during the first few years of phlebotomy therapy, and hydroxyurea effectively diminishes this risk. The question of long-term safety of this agent continues to be studied. Analysis of the data at 11 years of maximum follow-up shows that hydroxyurea does not significantly increase the incidence of leukemic transformation when compared with an historical control group of patients treated with phlebotomy on PVSG-01.

Follow-up of these hydroxyurea-treated patients continues, to ensure that hydroxyurea is nonmutagenic. Thus, hydroxyurea may prove to be the drug of choice, particularly for young patients requiring myelosuppression or for the older reliable patient, and for patients who do not have access to ^{32}P. In a recent report, a combination of plateletpheresis and cytotoxic chemotherapy (hydroxyurea or busulfan) was successfully used. The investigators concluded that combined modality treatment would be effective as acute treatment for symptomatic patients with thrombocytosis.[118a]

Adjuvant Therapy and Surgery

Complications of PV, such as a hypermetabolic state or hyperuricemia due to increased nucleoprotein breakdown secondary to accelerated hematopoiesis, can cause acute gout and nephrolithiasis. Hyperuricemia can usually be controlled by effective myelosuppressive therapy. If no other indication for myelosuppression is present and the patient is being managed by phlebotomy alone, allopurinol, 300 mg/d orally, usually controls the hyperuricemia. Colchicine or nonsteroidal antiinflammatory agents are used to manage acute gouty attacks.

Pruritus, present in about half of patients with PV, is usually generalized and may be made worse by bathing or showering and by brisk rubbing with a towel. The skin should be patted gently and not rubbed to dry. During myelosuppressive therapy, when the peripheral blood normalizes, itching frequently subsides. In some patients, pruritus remains a troubling symptom and is difficult to treat.

The pathogenesis of pruritus has not been clearly established. Sixty-six percent of patients with untreated PV have elevated blood and urine histamine levels compared with 7% of treated patients.[68] The water-induced itching seen with patients with PV closely resembles that seen in *aquagenic pruritus*, in which blood histamine[119] and cutaneous fibrinolytic activity[120] are increased after water challenge. Similarly, in patients with PV after water challenge, histamine and cutaneous fibrinolytic activity are also increased.[121] Antihistamines may prove helpful, and both H_1 antagonists, cyproheptadine, 4 mg orally three times daily, or H_2 antagonists, cimetidine, 300 mg orally four times daily, have been used either singly or in combination.[122] Cholestyramine may offer relief to patients with intractable pruritus[123]; the basis for its use is unclear since bile acids are not increased in this disorder.

Because most patients with PV are middle-aged or elderly, surgical and dental intervention are often needed. These procedures are accompanied by excessively high morbidity and mortality rates. The expanded blood volume and platelet abnormalities impair hemostasis. Surgical complication rates of over 30% and a mortality rate of 7% have been reported in patients with PV.[124] In a series of more than 81 operative procedures performed on 68 patients with PV, Wasserman and Gilbert[125] reported a postoperative morbidity rate of almost 50% and a postoperative mortality rate of 16%, compared with an expected mortality rate of 2%. Most of these complications were related to uncontrolled hemorrhage or vascular thrombosis.

The frequency of adverse complications in patients with PV is directly related to hematocrit level. The postoperative mortality rate was seven times greater in patients whose hematocrit was uncontrolled (52% or more) than in those whose hematocrit was normal.[125] In addition, the duration of hematologic control is an important factor in the incidence of postoperative complications. The complication rate when hematologic control was maintained for less than 4 months was more than five times greater than when hematocrit levels of patients were well controlled for more than 4 months. The number of deaths decreased from 15% in patients in whom short-term control was achieved to zero in the group whose disease was controlled for more than 4 months before surgery. The physiologic basis for these latter observations remains unclear[124,125]

Thus, elective surgery should not be contemplated in patients with PV unless hematologic values have been normal for several months. The better the hematologic control and the longer the period of time that control has been achieved, the lower is the incidence of postoperative complications and death. If emergency surgery is required, the patient should be phlebotomized rapidly until a more normal hematocrit is obtained, maintaining the intravascular volume with autologous plasma or intravenous fluids. To minimize thrombotic complications, these patients should be mobilized as soon as possible after surgery.

MANAGEMENT OF HYPOXEMIA-INDUCED POLYCYTHEMIA

An increase in hemoglobin and packed RBC volume is an important adaptation to lowered arterial oxygen saturation, whether the hypoxemia is caused by chronic lung disease, intracardiac right-to-left shunts, or residence at high altitudes where ambient P_{O_2} is less than at sea level. This response may be beneficial because it enhances oxygen carrying capacity. The raised RBC mass increases blood viscosity, thereby decreasing tissue perfusion and possibly predisposing to thrombosis. The development of polycythemia in chronic obstructive airway disease indicates a poor prognosis and increases the risk of cor pulmonale[126]; median survival is 18 to 36 months. In patients with cyanotic congenital heart disease, autopsy studies show a high incidence of thrombosis, especially in the pulmonary and cerebral vessels.[127,128] Some investigators question whether the incidence of stroke is higher in adult patients with cyanotic congenital heart disease.[100]

The balance between improved oxygen carriage provided by the increased hemoglobin concentration and decreased perfusion due to increased viscosity can be studied further by observations before and after reduction in the hematocrit with phlebotomy. In patients with polycythemia secondary to chronic airway obstruction, it appears that pulmonary vascular resistance and right ventricular work, particularly on exercise, are reduced with judicious phlebotomy, although arterial blood gases do not change.[129,130] An improvement in exercise tolerance with phlebotomy has also been demonstrated.[131] The hemodynamic improvements obtained with reduction of the hematocrit to the 50% to 52% range are not enhanced by further reduction. Such further reductions would only reduce oxygen transport and are therefore not recommended in this setting.

The hemodynamic effects of hematocrit reduction in cyanotic congenital heart disease are less well studied; thus, recommendations for management can differ. Reduction of hematocrit from a mean of 73% to 62% and from 66% to 57% decreased peripheral vascular resistance, whereas stroke volume, cardiac output, and systemic blood flow increased.[132,133] Exercise tests repeated 2 weeks after venesection showed an increased oxygen uptake with reduction in oxygen debt. Hyperviscosity symptoms are also improved by venesection. Some investigators suggest that patients with cyanotic congenital heart disease and packed RBC volumes over 60% should have phlebotomy therapy with the aim of reducing the hematocrit to about 55%.[132,133] Others believe that the firmest indications for phlebotomy in adult patients with congenital cyanotic heart disease are significant symptomatic hyperviscosity in patients with hematocrit levels exceeding 65%, or preoperative improvement in hemostasis.[100]

Another characteristic feature of the polycythemia associated with cyanotic congenital heart disease is a deficiency of coagulation factors. Decreased levels of factors II, V, VII, and IX and significant thrombocytopenia have been reported.[134] These deficiencies have been found to be due to hepatic dysfunction and chronic disseminated intravascular coagulation.[135] Although these deficiencies do not usually lead to a clinical bleeding diathesis, defects in hemostasis that accompany the erythrocytosis of cyanotic congenital heart disease warn against incurring the additional risks of anticoagulants that are given to reduce a possible thrombotic predisposition. In patients with hematocrits over 60%, preoperative venesection improves the coagulation abnormalities, and blood loss at surgery is lower than in untreated patients.[136] It must be emphasized that to ensure a proper coagulation evaluation, the correct ratio of anticoagulant to plasma volume must be maintained by increasing the amount of whole blood placed into standard test tubes to compensate for an elevated hematocrit.

MYELOFIBROSIS AND AGNOGENIC MYELOID METAPLASIA

Definition

The clinical presentation of myelofibrosis/myeloid metaplasia can be as variable as the terms used to describe this entity. The condition may arise de novo as a primary myeloproliferative disorder. Alternatively, a similar entity may evolve secondarily in the course of other myeloproliferative disorders, especially PV. Over the years, the former situation has been termed, among other things, *agnogenic myeloid metaplasia, aleukemic myelosis, myelosclerosis, leukoerythroblastic anemia with diffuse osteosclerosis,* and *megakaryocytic splenomegaly.* The constant features are bone marrow fibrosis and extramedullary hematopoiesis in a patient in whom no underlying systemic disorder can be identified. The PVSG defined myelofibrosis as a clinical illness with splenomegaly, fibrosis involving more than one third of the sectional area of a bone marrow biopsy, a leukoerythroblastic blood reaction with significant teardrop poikilocytosis on peripheral smear, and the absence of both an increased RBC mass and the Philadelphia chromosome to exclude PV and chronic myelocytic leukemia, respectively.[137]

After the original description of the disease by Heuck[138] in 1879, an important event in myelofibrosis has been recognized as the fibroblastic proliferation seen within the marrow cavity. Discovering the driving stimulus for this proliferation would help unravel the mysteries of the disease and offer new insights for possible therapeutic intervention.

Pathogenesis and Presentation

Whether agnogenic myeloid metaplasia is truly a hematologic neoplasm, a reactive syndrome, or a combination of both is not clear, although in many cases clones of abnormal hematopoietic stem cells have now been demonstrated. Whatever the underlying cause, fibroblast proliferation, increased collagen deposition, and fibrosis of the bone marrow are present.

Originally, marrow fibrosis was thought to be part of a disordered hematopoietic cell growth. Marrow fibroblasts do not share a common ancestry with the major hematopoietic cell lines, as judged by chromosomal, isoenzyme, and culture studies[139,140] or by analysis of marrow fibroblasts after marrow transplantation.[141] Although the fibroblasts are not part of the neoplastic clone, the collagen they secrete deleteriously influences bone marrow function. Biochemical determination of collagen indicates that the amount found in bone marrow increases with the duration of disease.[142] Increased net collagen deposition is a fundamental and ongoing aspect of the myelofibrotic process.

The clinical syndrome of myelofibrosis has been described in a series of reviews,[143,144] with an excellent and detailed discussion by Ward and Block.[145] These reports emphasize that the diagnosis of myelofibrosis, which requires the demonstration of fibrosis in a bone marrow biopsy, may not always be possible because of the patchy nature of the fibrosis, especially in the early stages. Accordingly, multiple biopsies may be required for diagnosis. A leukoerythroblastic peripheral blood smear and poikilocytic, teardrop-shaped erythrocytes are characteristic features (see Fig. 13-6), but they are not always present nor are they absolutely pathognomonic. Splenomegaly is almost always present, and it may be enormous, encompassing a major portion of the abdomen and interfering with the function of other vital organs such as the intestinal tract. The few patients who present without palpable splenomegaly usually develop it in the course of the disease. Hepatomegaly also occurs in a large percentage of patients.

The triad of leukoerythroblastic anemia, poikilocytosis, and splenomegaly suggests the occurrence of extramedullary hematopoiesis. This may be seen in any site with the potential for blood formation, but the spleen is the principal organ in which this occurs. Morphologic changes may occur in the peripheral blood before the onset of anemia in myelofibrosis, although most patients have modest anemia and a few are profoundly anemic. Modestly reduced hematocrits in the presence of massive splenomegaly may initially reflect dilution by an expanded plasma volume, although an absolute reduction in RBC mass almost invariably develops eventually. A significant number of patients have pancytopenia, and a leukoerythroblastic blood picture is not invariable, although a careful search of the peripheral blood reveals an occasional normoblast.[146] Anisocytosis and poikilocytosis are also the rule, but they may be relatively inconspicuous and the classic teardrop-shaped RBCs may be sparse. The cause of the anisocytosis and poikilocytosis seen in many cases is not clear but may reflect abnormal hematopoiesis in extramedullary sites as well as disorganized bone marrow stroma.

The spleen's role in myelofibrosis is preeminent and complicated, and attempts to better understand it have included the use of radionuclides for determining splenic RBC pooling, splenic RBC sequestration, platelet kinetics, the degree of marrow compared with that of extramedullary erythropoiesis, and the extent of effective compared with ineffective erythropoiesis. These studies may prove helpful when the difficult decision regarding the risks and benefits of splenectomy is under consideration.[147,148] Although the spleen and liver are characteristically involved by myeloid metaplasia in idiopathic myelofibrosis, in advanced cases extramedullary hematopoiesis may occur in any organ that was the site of hematopoiesis in fetal life. Unusual masses of extramedullary hematopoiesis have been reported to occur in lymph nodes, kidneys, lungs, pleura, gastrointestinal tract, peritoneum, dura and central nervous system, skin, and breast.[144] These can lead to diagnostic dilemmas. Their nature often can be elucidated by ^{52}Fe scanning[149]; when required, they can be managed with radiation.

Marrow Collagen

As a result of the application of newer immunologic techniques to the study of collagen metabolism, much knowledge regarding the distribution of collagen in the bone marrow has been obtained; this has caused a reevaluation of the older terminology used in describing bone marrow fibrosis. Classically, pathologists have described two types of marrow fibrosis when studying bone marrow biopsy sections: reticulin and collagen fibrosis. These terms are based on differences in the histochemical staining properties of the fibers causing fibrosis, which were formerly thought to indicate differences in chemical composition. The finer reticulin fiber does not stain with the usual trichrome stains for collagen but rather is argyrophilic, that is, readily impregnable with silver. In contrast, collagen fibers are coarser, stain with the usual trichrome stains such as those of Mallory's triple stain, Masson stain, and Van Gris stain, and are not usually argyrophilic. Nevertheless, some histopathologists reported that it was not possible to distinguish between reticulin and collagen fibers on the basis of their reaction with silver impregnation methods.[150] Variations in staining patterns also depend on the fixative and staining techniques used.

By using more sensitive microscopic and immunologic techniques, both of these fiber types, which are increased in myelofibrosis, are now known to be composed of collagen. Electron microscopy has demonstrated that reticulin is collagen on the basis of its characteristic cross-striations.[151,152] By using immunohistochemical staining techniques with specific antibodies for the various collagen subtypes, the fine reticulin fibers have been shown to be principally type III collagen and the coarse fibers are predominantly type I collagen. Thus, in both reticulin fibrosis and collagen fibrosis, the fibrous protein deposited in the extracellular marrow space is collagen, formed from a genetically distinct precursor molecule, procollagen.

Collagen is the most abundant protein in the human body.[153] It is found in the extracellular matrix of connective tissues, often in association with proteoglycans, glycoproteins, and elastin. Although once regarded as a passive scaffold serving mainly to provide support for extracellular matrices, collagen is now recognized as having several additional physiologic roles. These include a role in morphogenesis and development, chemotaxis, platelet adhesion and aggregation, and cell attachment. Eleven types of collagens have been recognized in vertebrate tissues; humans have at least five different types of collagen.[154]

Collagens are the product of a family of closely related but structurally distinct genes. The collagen types differ in the amino acid composition of their constitutive polypeptides. They are identified by Roman numerals in the chronologic order of their discovery. Each collagen molecule is composed of three polypeptide chains coiled around each other in a triple helix with glycine in every third position of each chain. Proline, hydroxyproline, and hydroxylysine are other characteristic amino acids found in collagen.

Collagen is synthesized in a precursor form that is substantially larger (about 50%) than the collagen molecule.[155] This procollagen (Fig. 13-11) has globular peptide extensions at both the amino and carboxyl termini. These propeptides are believed to enhance solubility and thus facilitate transport of individual procollagen molecules out of the cell. Removal of these propeptides results in insoluble collagen molecules, which subsequently undergo self-assembly into fibrils, and then cross-link. Procollagen itself is not able to aggregate into fibrils because of the bulky propeptide extensions. The procollagen peptides are cleaved, principally in the extracellular space, by specific proteases. Serum levels of the resulting propeptides, measured by radioimmunoassay, have been shown to reflect the degree of organ fibrosis, including bone marrow fibrosis. Serum procollagen III amino-terminal peptide levels have been reported to correlate with the degree of marrow fibrosis[60] and to increase with disease progression.[156]

The normal histologic structure of bone marrow consists of reticulin fibers arranged in a network, which is most concentrated around blood vessels and bone spicules, with fine, branching filaments extending into the adjacent marrow.[157] Bone is a nonhomogeneous tissue, comprising several components, including bony trabeculae, fat spaces, blood vessels, and hematopoietic tissue. It may be anticipated that different collagen types can be found in these different compartments. By using collagen-type specific antibodies under normal conditions, type I collagen has been shown to be almost exclusively restricted to the bone matrix; few fibrils composed of type I collagen molecules occur in the bone marrow cavity.[158] The reticular stroma of the marrow spaces, as well as the endosteal lining of the bone trabeculae, consists largely of a fine network of thin fibrils composed principally of type III collagen molecules. Cells with positive cytoplasmic staining for collagen types I and III are scattered throughout the marrow but are particularly prominent in two sites: in relation to marrow sinusoids and around the margins of fat spaces.[159]

The histologic characteristics of the myelosclerotic process consist primarily of an apparent increase in the number of fibers, in addition to alterations in the basic fiber morphology, including thickening and the formation of wavy forms that transmit polarized light and demonstrate the staining characteristics of collagen, such as staining with Mallory's triple stain and the trichrome technique.[160] Primary myelofibrosis may be further characterized by a proliferation of other marrow cellular elements, especially atypical megakaryocytes.

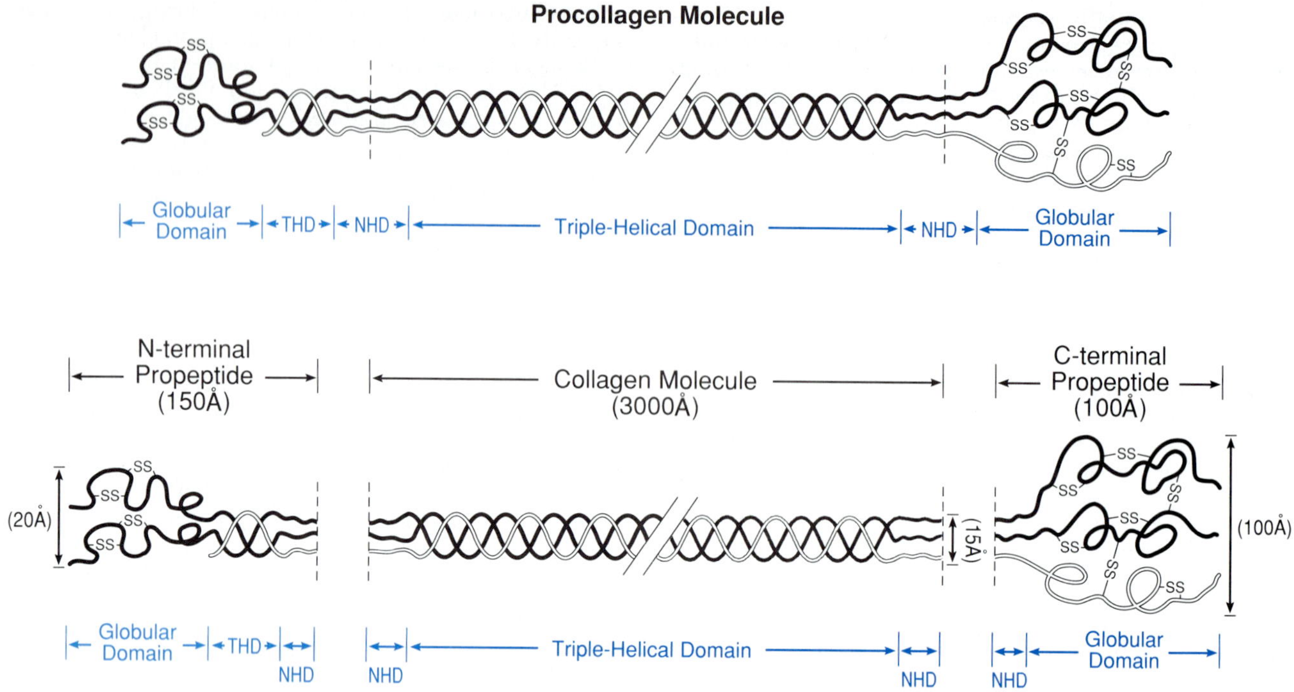

FIGURE 13-11. Schematic representation of the structure of the procollagen molecule. (After Prockop DJ, Kivirikko KI, Tuberman L, et al. The biosynthesis of collagen and its disorders. N Engl J Med 1979;301:13)

Etiology

The range of myeloproliferative disorders in which marrow fibrosis plays an important role is shown in Figure 13-12. It may be found in many myeloproliferative disorders but dominates the histologic picture of primary myelofibrosis. As discussed, evidence from cytogenic and other cell marker studies suggests that marrow fibrosis, although it may dominate the histologic picture, is reactive to the underlying hematopoietic neoplasia and is not part of that process. There are also secondary forms of myelofibrosis, syndromes with similar bone marrow and peripheral blood findings of marrow fibrosis and leukoerythroblastic blood picture. There are found in association with a variety of neoplasms, infections, and other diseases, as well as after toxic exposure to certain chemicals (Table 13-6).

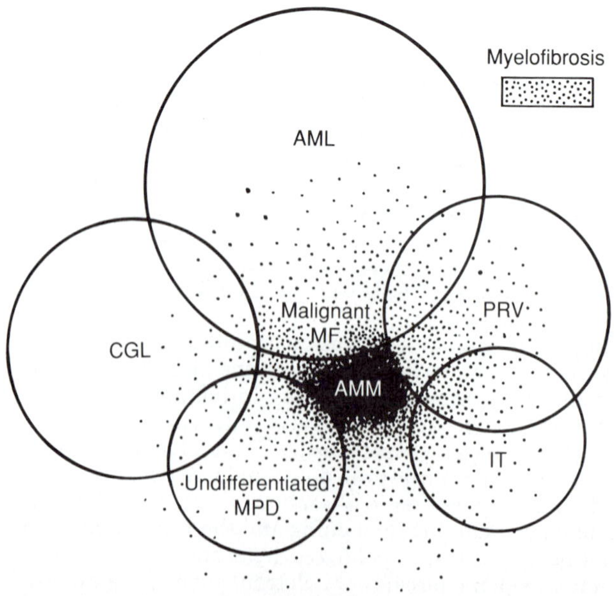

FIGURE 13-12. Myelofibrosis in the myeloproliferative syndromes. (After Geary CG. Clinical and hematological aspects of chronic myelofibrosis in myelofibrosis. In: Lewis SM, ed. Myelofibrosis. New York, Marcel Dekker, 1985:17)

Knowledge about factors that cause fibroblast proliferation and increased collagen synthesis is increasing. Platelet-derived growth factor (PDGF) may be inappropriately released in patients with myeloproliferative disorders, which can then stimulate fibroblasts to divide and secrete collagen.[161] Homogenates of megakaryocytes isolated from normal human bone marrow clearly stimulate fibroblast proliferation,[162] suggesting that abnormal megakaryocytes might release PDGF in vivo and cause fibrosis. Degradation of newly formed collagen may also be inhibited by simultaneous release of platelet factor 4, which can inhibit collagenase.[163] The observation that the numbers of megakaryocytes are frequently increased in patients with idiopathic myelofibrosis, and that fibrosis is an important finding in acute megakaryoblastic leukemia, supports the model of the megakaryocyte and its secretory products playing an important role in these disorders. Ineffective marrow megakaryocytosis, with intramedullary death of these cells, may be the determining factor in the genesis of marrow fibrosis associated with the myeloproliferative disorders.[164]

Further support for the importance of the megakaryocyte and platelet in myeloproliferative disorders comes from the reports of myelofibrosis occurring in the gray platelet syndrome, in which there is excessive release of PDGF.[165,166] In fibrosing disorders of the marrow in which megakaryocytic hyperplasia is not typically found, such as hairy cell leukemia and disseminated carcinoma, mediators of fibrosis are possibly released from these malignant cells or other appropriately stimulated cells, such as the monocyte-macrophage or the T lymphocyte.[167,168]

Malignant or Acute Myelofibrosis

Myelofibrosis with myeloid metaplasia is usually a slowly progressive disorder with a gradually downhill clinical

TABLE 13-6. Conditions Associated With Marrow Fibrosis

HEMATOLOGIC NEOPLASIA
Acute leukemia
Chronic myelocytic leukemia
Polycythemia vera
Essential thrombocythemia
Hairy cell leukemia
Multiple myeloma
Hodgkin's disease and non-Hodgkin's lymphoma
Systemic mastocytosis
SOLID TUMORS
Breast
Prostate
Stomach
Lung
INFECTION
Tuberculosis
Osteomyelitis (focal)
TOXIC EXPOSURE
X-radiation or gamma radiation
Benzene
Fluorine
NONMALIGNANT DISORDERS
Vitamin D deficiency
Gray platelet syndrome
Systemic lupus erythematosus
Hyper- and hypoparathyroidism
Paget's disease (focal)
Marble bone disease

course. The term *malignant myelosclerosis* was introduced in 1963 by Lewis and Szur[169] to differentiate the distinct clinical and laboratory entity of acute myelofibrosis with a rapid clinical demise, similar to that seen in acute leukemia. This syndrome was defined by rapidly developing pancytopenia and the absence of hepatosplenomegaly. The blood smear shows only moderate abnormalities of the RBC, and blasts may be found. Bone marrow aspiration is frequently dry, and the biopsy reveals increased collagen deposition in association with round and oval mononuclear cells (perhaps early reticulin cells) and giant cells similar to megakaryocytes. Cytologic, cytochemical, and electron microscopic investigation of the blast cells of the peripheral blood strongly suggested a megakaryocytic origin.[170] Thus, the common denominators of acute myelofibrosis and acute megakaryocytic leukemia are fibrosis of the marrow and proliferation of the megakaryocytic cell line.

Malignant myelofibrosis is important to recognize because the clinical outcome—thus therapy—is different for acute myelofibrosis than for primary idiopathic myelofibrosis with myeloid metaplasia. Although improved supportive care may have resulted in longer survival, acute myelofibrosis continues to run a rapidly downhill course in most patients. Until recently, the median duration of survival was about 5 months.[171] Pancytopenia usually persists, with increasing blast cell counts. As in acute leukemia, infection and bleeding disorders are the most common causes of death.

Because of the now recognized similarity of acute myelofibrosis to acute leukemia, a more aggressive approach to therapy has been adopted; along with this, the prognosis of the rapidly fatal acute myelofibrosis has improved. Intensive multiagent chemotherapy[172] and bone marrow transplantation[173,174] for appropriate patients have been advocated as therapeutic modalities. If successful, both forms of therapy may result in the interesting phenomenon of gradual disappearance of marrow fibrosis. The mechanisms for resolution of marrow fibrosis require further investigation.

Prognosis and Survival

Primary myelofibrosis is a progressive but usually chronic disorder. The clinical diagnosis may be preceded by a long symptom-free interval lasting many years, which may account for two thirds of the natural history of the disease.[175] During this period, myeloid metaplasia increases gradually with progressive enlargement of the spleen and frequently the liver. The size of the spleen at diagnosis gives some indication of the duration of the disease. On the basis of observations made in untreated patients, Ward and Block[145] estimated that the disease has been present for 1 year for each centimeter that the spleen extends below the costal margin. Many patients are relatively asymptomatic at diagnosis, which is often made incidentally, following a routine blood count, or because the physician detects splenomegaly during routine physical examination. These patients may initially require no therapeutic intervention.

Because of this long asymptomatic period, data for survival from the time of diagnosis are variable. Patients may survive with their disease for decades. Median survival times were estimated to be 10.6 years from onset of disease and 5.2 years from diagnosis.[145] A comparison of survival in primary myelofibrosis with reports of survival for patients with PV and CML is shown in Figure 13-13. When calculated from the date of diagnosis, the survival curve for primary myelofibrosis lies between these two other myeloproliferative diseases. When the duration of disease is calculated from the date of onset, the survival curve is similar to that of PV.

Since the clinical presentation and life expectancy are variable, attempts have been made to identify distinctive features of predictive importance. Many studies, however, are based on small numbers of patients. Most studies do agree that the hemoglobin level at diagnosis, the isotopic measure of total erythroid iron turnover, and the bone marrow histologic finding or red cell aplasia provide independent contributions to poorer prognosis.[176–178] Older patients and a higher value for immature myeloid cells in the peripheral blood are additional indicators for poorer prognosis in some studies.[179] The importance of spleen size, platelet count, and marrow myeloid hyperplasia are more controversial.[176,179–181]

When symptoms of primary myelofibrosis occur, they can be divided into three main groups: those caused by splenic enlargement, those associated with the metabolic consequences of the underlying myeloproliferative disorder, and those caused by bone marrow failure. Clinically, transformation into acute leukemia is relatively uncommon. Bentley and associates,[182] reviewing the literature, estimated the average incidence of acute leukemia to be about 8%, usually within 5 years of the original diagnosis of myelofibrosis. Transformation into acute leukemia may be suspected by any of the following signs or symptoms: rapid increase in spleen size, lymphadenopathy, onset of bone pain, weight loss, or persistent fever. A sudden increase in peripheral blood blastemia should arouse suspicion, although an exaggerated leukoerythroblastic picture and a marked shift to more blastic forms may also occur as a response to infection or hemorrhage.

Common complaints are fullness in the left upper quadrant due to splenomegaly, weakness due to anemia, and gastrointestinal problems due to mechanical pressure from

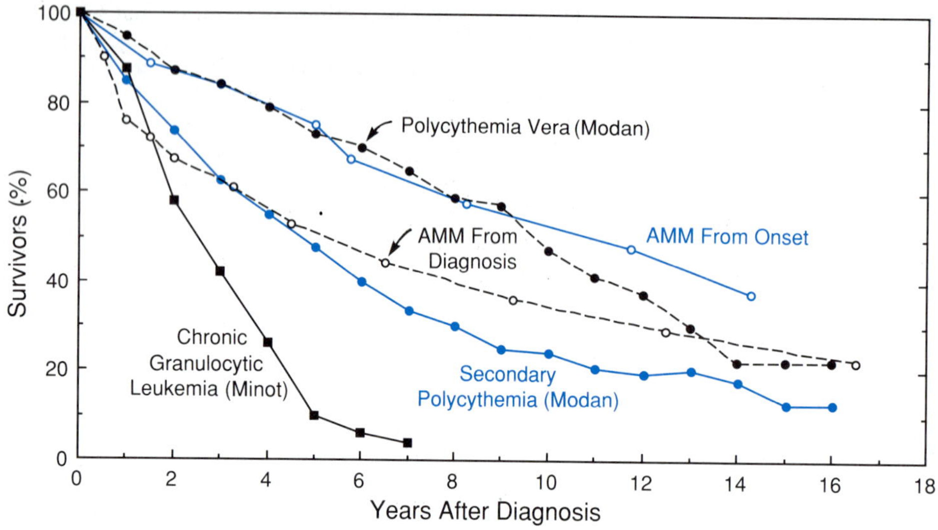

FIGURE 13-13. Survival of patients with idiopathic myelofibrosis compared with that for polycythemia vera, secondary polycythemia, and chronic myelocytic leukemia. (After Ward HP, Block MH. The natural history of agnogenic myeloid metaplasia [MMM] and a critical evaluation of its relationship with the myeloproliferative syndrome. Medicine 1971;50:357)

an enlarged spleen. A minority of patients may have severe pain due to splenic infarction and perisplenitis. Metabolic symptoms of patients with primary myelofibrosis are less conspicuous than in other myeloproliferative disorders, but weight loss is common and occasional patients complain of generalized pruritus, sweating, or fever. Hyperuricemia may lead to acute gout or renal colic. Acute gout is reported in 6% of patients in one series, and 16% of patients in a second series presented with massive splenomegaly.[183,145]

As in other chronic myeloproliferative disorders, fatigue is a common complaint and does not necessarily correlate with the hemoglobin level. Other symptoms due to anemia occur in about 50% of patients and are more common in older subjects. Less than 10% of patients present with a serious bleeding diathesis. This may occur even when the platelet number is normal; in this situation, it is presumably caused by platelet dysfunction. Skin bruising is extremely common.

Therapeutic Modalities

Patients who are asymptomatic at diagnosis require careful observation; therapy is not usually required at this stage. Experimental therapies to prevent the progression of myelofibrosis are being investigated. No definitive therapy to reverse or decrease the ongoing fibrotic process and improve survival is widely accepted, although in appropriate patients, allogeneic bone marrow transplantation has been reported to gradually resolve the fibrosis with normalization of the peripheral blood and bone marrow morphology.[184,185] Bone marrow transplantation is not currently a therapeutic option for most patients with myelofibrosis. Because the risk/benefit ratio has not been clearly established in this setting, it must still be considered experimental.

Besides the possibility of bone marrow transplantation, no therapy for primary myelofibrosis is widely accepted. Colchicine, which appears to ameliorate the excessive collagen deposition in cirrhosis of the liver, has been discussed in relation to myelofibrosis; no data supporting its use in this setting have been developed.[186] The thrust of our therapeutic options remains palliation and improvement in the patient's sense of well-being.

Anemia develops in most patients with myelofibrosis and frequently can be difficult to treat without transfusional support.[183] Deficiencies of iron and vitamins should be sought and corrected. Patients have often been treated with androgen preparations with variable results.[187,188] Since most patients do not benefit from androgen therapy, Gardner and Pringle[187] attempted to develop criteria for selecting those patients who might respond favorably. All eight of their patients who had ^{59}Fe–ferrous citrate incorporation into RBC hemoglobin of more than 50% of the administered dose responded with an increase in circulating hemoglobin level during 3 months of intensive androgen therapy. Typical doses used are oxymetholone, 50 mg by mouth four times per day, or fluoxymesterone, 10 mg orally three times daily. In patients without thrombocytopenia, intramuscular testosterone enanthate, 400 mg every 3 to 4 weeks, is another therapeutic option. Responses to androgen therapy may be delayed for up to 3 to 4 months; thus, these agents should be continued for this period of time before they are considered to be ineffective. Occasional patients who fail on one androgen preparation may respond to another. Careful monitoring of liver function tests is necessary while on androgen therapy. For patients with symptomatic severe anemia, transfusion therapy may have to be initiated. Erythropoietin has also been suggested as a therapy for the severe anemia of myeloid metaplasia. A recent study documents that such patients have an appropriately elevated serum erythropoietin level and that additional exogenous erythropoietin is unlikely to be of benefit.[187a]

Splenomegaly is a common concomitant finding in patients with myelofibrosis. Many patients develop a progressively enlarging, painful spleen, encompassing the entire left side of the abdomen and extending beyond the midline or into the pelvis.[145] The massive splenomegaly can cause disturbances of normal gastrointestinal motility and absorption, with early satiety, diarrhea, hypermetabolism, and weight loss. Severe pain secondary to splenic infarction can also be seen.

Chemotherapeutic agents have been used to shrink the spleen in patients with myelofibrosis. The mainstays of therapy have been busulfan and hydroxyurea. Treatment must be initiated at low doses with frequent monitoring of the peripheral blood (at least weekly) to avoid undue suppression of hematopoiesis; it should be used only by physicians experienced in the use of these agents. Typical doses are busulfan, 2 mg/d orally, or hydroxyurea, 500 mg/d orally, with adjustment of the dose according to peripheral blood counts and shrinkage of the spleen. These drugs can decrease the spleen size and lower the leukocyte and platelet counts, but only rarely does a patient experience an improvement in anemia with this therapeutic approach.[189]

For patients with massive splenomegaly or those with recurrent splenic infarction and painful splenomegaly, low-dose local radiation therapy over the spleen in doses of 25 to 50 rad/d for 4 or 5 days may also be tried with good results.[190] When either chemotherapy or radiation is discontinued, rapid enlargement of the spleen frequently occurs.

Despite attempts at controlling massive splenomegaly in patients with myelofibrosis, it frequently continues to be a problem and splenectomy remains a therapeutic option. It must be emphasized that perioperative morbidity and mortality rates remain high. Older studies cited operative mortality rates of up to 28%,[191] more recent studies of about 10%.[192] Frequently mentioned operative complications are intraabdominal bleeding requiring reoperation, mesenteric thrombosis, septicemia, and subphrenic abscess. Extreme elevations in platelet count may follow splenectomy, even when thrombocytopenia preceded surgery.[144] Hepatic enlargement may also follow splenectomy.

Splenectomy may be required, despite the risks, in a selected group of patients with myelofibrosis. Major considerations are severe anemia and thrombocytopenia refractory to other therapeutic modalities and secondary to splenic pooling, severe portal hypertension secondary to increased portal blood flow, and mechanical bowel syndromes secondary to refractory massive splenomegaly. Shortened intravascular life-span of platelets or RBCs, as well as their localization in the spleen, should be demonstrated by radionuclide studies when splenectomy is contemplated. Estimation of the importance of splenic erythropoiesis, as determined by radioactive iron studies, should also be considered.[193] Difficulties in interpretation of these radionuclide studies and limitations in their ability to predict either a positive or negative clinical outcome after splenectomy have diminished their usefulness.

Experimental Therapies

Evidence suggests that the microskeleton of the fibroblast, the microtubules and microfilaments, is engaged in the transport of procollagen within and outside of the cell. Drugs that interfere with these structures, such as colchicine, inhibit the secretion of collagen in in vitro systems,[194] and have been efficaciously used for the treatment of various fibrosing diseases of man, such as scleroderma[195] and hepatic cirrhosis.[186] D-Penicillamine, a copper chelator, blocks aldehyde groups involved in the intermolecular and intramolecular cross-linkages of mature collagen.[196] It has been used in patients with primary biliary cirrhosis and scleroderma. Lathyrogens, such as β-aminoproprionitrile, block the cross-linking of collagen by inhibiting lysyl oxidase, a copper-dependent enzyme important in collagen cross-linking. The usefulness of these agents in myelofibrosis is under study.[196]

Myelofibrosis can occur in a number of nonmalignant disorders. Cooperberg and Singer[197] describe an infant with rickets and myelofibrosis. The myelofibrosis regressed after treatment with vitamin D. Other investigators also reported bone marrow improvement in children with rickets and myelofibrosis, who were treated with vitamin D.[198] 1,25-dihydroxyvitamin D_3 has been used to treat patients with myelofibrosis in association with hematologic neoplasia with apparent improvement.[199] 1,25-dihydroxyvitamin D_3, the active metabolite of vitamin D_3, inhibits the proliferation of human megakaryocytes in vitro and induces myeloid cells from normal persons and from patients with chronic granulocytic leukemia to mature toward monocytes and macrophages.[200] Because megakaryocytes may promote collagen formation and monocytes promotes its degradation, 1,25-dihydroxyvitamin D_3 may thus indirectly modulate net collagen deposition.[201] Its role in the therapy of myelofibrosis requires further study.

REFERENCES

1. Berk PD. Erythrocytosis and polycythemia. In: Wyngaarden JB, Smith LH, Plum F, eds. Cecil's textbook of medicine, ed 17. Philadelphia, WB Saunders, 1985:963.
2. Raskind WH, Jacobson R, Murphy S, et al. Evidence for the involvement of B lymphoid cells in polycythemia vera and essential thrombocytopenia. J Clin Invest 1985;75:1388.
3. Dameshek W. Some speculations on the myeloproliferative syndromes. Blood 1951;6:372.
4. Modan B. An epidemiological study of polycythemia vera. Blood 1965;26:657.
5. Silverstein MN, Lanier AP. Polycythemia vera, 1935–1969: an epidemiologic survey in Rochester, Minnesota. Mayo Clin Proc 1971;4B: 751.
6. Modan B, Kallner H, Zemer D, et al. A note on the increased risk of polycythemia vera in Jews. Blood 1971;37:172.
7. Brubaker LH, Wasserman LR, Goldberg JD, et al. Increased prevalence of polycythemia vera in parents of patients on PVSG protocols. Am J Hematol 1984;16:367.
8. Osgood E. Polycythemia vera: age relationship and survival. Blood 1965;26:243.
9. Natelson EA, Lynch EC, Britton HA. Polycythemia vera in childhood. Am J Dis Child 1971;122:241.
10. Perrine SP, Greene MF, Lee PD. Insulin stimulates cord blood erythroid progenitor growth: evidence for an etiological role in neonatal polycythemia. Br J Haematol 1986;64:503.
11. Golde DW, Hockwing WG, et al. Polycythemia: mechanisms and management. Ann Intern Med 1971;95:71.
12. Von Haller A. Elementa, physiologie corporis humani, vol 2. Lausanne, 1757:34.
13. Andral G. Essai d'hematologie pathologique. Paris, Fortin, Masson et Cie, 1843.
14. Vaquez H. Sur une forme speciale de cyanose s'accompanant d'hyperglobulie excessive et persistente. Compt Rend Soc Biol 1892;44: 384.
15. Cabot RC. A case of chronic cyanosis without discovering cause, ending in cerebral hemorrhage. Boston Med Surg J 1899;141:574.
16. Osler W. Chronic cyanosis with polycythemia and enlarged spleen: a new clinical entity. Am J Med Sci 1903;126:187.
17. Turk W. Beitrage zur Kenntnis des Symptom-enbildes Polyzythame mit Milztumor and Zyanose. Wien Klin Wochenschr 1904;17:153,189.
18. Adamson JW, Fialkow PJ, Murphy S, et al. Polycythemia vera: stem cell and probable clonal origin of the disease. N Engl J Med 1976;295: 913.
19. Fialkow PJ, Gartler SM, Yoshida A. Clonal origin of chronic myelocytic leukemia in man. Proc Natl Acad Sci USA 1976;58:1468.
20. Jacobson RJ, Salo A, Fialkow PJ. Agnogenic myeloid metaplasia: a clonal proliferation of hematopoietic stem cells with secondary myelofibrosis. Blood 1978;51:189.
21. Fialkow PJ, Faguet G, Jacobson R, et al. Evidence that essential thrombocythemia is a clonal disorder with origin in a multipotent stem cell. Blood 1981;58:916.
22. Ogawa M, Porter PN, Nakahata T. Renewal and commitment to differentiation of hemopoietic stem cells: an interpretative review. Blood 1983;61:823.
23. Metcalf D. The hemopoietic colony stimulating factors. Amsterdam, Elsevier, 1984.
24. Gregory CJ, Eaves AC. Human marrow cells capable of erythropoietic differentiation in vitro: definition of three erythroid colony responses. Blood 1977;49:855.
25. Wagemaker G. Cellular and soluble factors influencing the differentiation of primitive erythroid progenitor cells (BFU-e) in vitro. In: Murphy MJ Jr, ed. In vitro aspects of erythropoiesis. New York, Springer-Verlag, 1978:44.
26. Goldwasser E. The action of erythropoietin as the inducer of erythroid differentiation. In: Cronkite EP, Dainiak N, McCaffrey RP, Palek J, Quesenberry PJ, eds. Hematopoietic stem cell physiology. New York, Alan R Liss, 1985:77.
27. Papayannopoulou T, Finch CA. On the in vivo action of erythropoietin: a quantitative analysis. J Clin Invest 1972;51:1179.
28. Erslev AJ, Caro J, Kansu E, et al. Plasma erythropoietin in polycythemia. Am J Med 1979;66:243.
29. Adamson JW. The erythropoietin-hematocrit relationship in normal and polycythemia man: implications of marrow regulation. Blood 1968;32:597.
30. Gurney CW. Pathogenesis of the polycythemias. In: Klein H, ed. Polycythemia: theory and management. Springfield, IL, Charles C Thomas, 1973:42.
31. Eaves CJ, Eaves AC. Erythropoietin (Epo) dose–response curves for three classes of erythroid progenitors in normal human marrow and in patients with polycythemia. Blood 1978;52:1196.
32. Zanjani ED, Lutton JD, Hoffman R, et al. Erythroid colony formation by polycythemia vera bone marrow in vitro. J Clin Invest 1977;59: 841.
33. Horland A, Ludman S, Murphy MJ, et al. Proliferation of erythroid colonies in semi-solid agar. Br J Haematol 1977;36:495.
34. Lutton JD, Levere RD. Endogenous erythroid colony formation by

peripheral blood mononuclear cells from patients with myeolofibrosis and polycythemia vera. Acta Haematol 1979;62:94.
35. Eridani S, Dudley JM, Sawyer BM, et al. Erythropoietic colonies in a serum-free system: results in primary proliferative polycythemia and thrombocytopenia. Br J Haematol 1987;67:387.
36. Cashman JD, Eaves CJ, Eaves AC. Unregulated proliferation of primitive neoplastic cells in long term polycythemia vera marrow cultures. J Clin Invest 1988;81:87.
37. Fauser AA, Messner HA. Pluripotent hemopoietic progenitors CFU-GEMM in polycythemia vera: analysis of erythropoietin requirements and proliferative activity. Blood 1981;58:1224.
38. Prchal JF, Adamson JW, Murphy S, et al. Polycythemia vera: the in vitro response of normal and abnormal sten cell lines to erythropoietin. J Clin Invest 1978;61:1044.
38a. Dai CH, Dessypris EN, Means RT Jr, et al. Polycythemia veras. II. Hypersensitivity of bone marrow erythroid, granulocyte-macrophage, and megakaryocytic progenitor cells to interleukin 3 and granulocyte-macrophage colony stimulating factor. Blood 1992;80:891.
38b. Kobayashi S, Teramura M, Hoshino S, et al. Circulating megakaryocyte progenitors in myeloproliferative disorders are hypersensitive to interleukin-3. 1993. Br. J. Haematol. 83:539.
39. Singer JW, Arlin ZA, Najfeld V, et al. Restoration of nonclonal hematopoiesis in chronic myelogenous leukemia (CML) following a chemotherapy-induced loss of the Ph[1] chromosome. Blood 1987;56:356.
40. Balcerzak SP, Bromberg PA. Secondary polycythemia. Semin Hematol 1975;12:353.
41. Weinstein IM. Clinical manifestations. In: Klein H, ed. Polycythemia: theory and management. Springfield, IL, Charles C Thomas, 1973.
42. Cavill I, Trevett D, Fisher J, et al. The measurement of the total volume of red cells in man: a non-radioactive approach using biotin. Br J Haematol 1988;70:491.
43. Weatherall DJ. Polycythemia resulting from abnormal hemoglobins. N Engl J Med 1969;280:604.
44. Smith JR, Landaw SA. Smokers' polycythemia. N Engl J Med 1978; 298:6.
45. McFadzean AJS, Todd D, Tsang KC. Polycythemia in primary carcinoma of the liver. Blood 1958;13:427.
46. Jones NF, Payne RW, Hyde RD, et al. Renal polycythemia. Lancet 1960;1:299.
47. Adamson JW, Stamatoyannopoulous G, Kontrass, et al. Recessive familial erythrocytosis: aspects of marrow regulation in two families. Blood 1973;4:641.
48. Adamson JW. Familial polycythemia. Semin Hematol 1975;12:49.
48a. Prchal JT, Prchal JF. Evolving understanding of the cellular defect in polycythemia vera: implications for its clinical diagnosis and molecular pathophysiology. Blood 1994;83:1.
49. Berk PD, Goldberg JD, Donovan PB, et al. Therapeutic recommendations in polycythemia vera based on polycythemia vera study group protocols. Semin Hematol 1986;23:132.
50. Camiscolle JF, Weintraub AH, Gordon AS. Comparative assay of erythropoietin standards. Ann NY Acad Sci 1968;149:40.
51. Egrie JC, Cotes PM, Lane J, et al. Development of radioimmunoassays for human erythropoietin using recombinant erythropoietin as tracer and immunogen. J Immunol Methods 1987;99:235.
52. Bomchil G, Carinena AD, Segade A, et al. Studies on the response to hypoxia and relative hyperoxia in two polycythemia vera patients. Indian J Med Res 1967;55:543.
53. Gilbert HS, Kraus S, Pasternack B, et al. Serum vitamin B12 content and unsaturated vitamin B12-binding capacity in myeloproliferative disease. Ann Intern Med 1969;71:71.
54. Adamson JW. The polycythemias: diagnosis and treatment. Hosp Pract 1983;12:49.
55. Berlin W. Diagnosis and classification of the polycythemias. Semin Hematol 1975;12:5.
56. Kurnick JE, Ward HP, Block MH. Bone marrow sections in the differential diagnosis of polycythemia. Arch Pathol 1972;94:489.
57. Lundin PM, Ridell B, Weinfeld A. The significance of bone marrow morphology for the diagnosis of polycythemia vera. Scand J Haematol 1972;9:271.
58. Roberts BE, Miles DW, Woods CG. Polycythemia vera and myelosclerosis: a bone marrow study. Br J Haematol 1969;16:75.
59. Ellis TJ, Silver RT, Coleman M, et al. The bone marrow in polycythemia vera. Semin Hematol 1975;12:99
60. Hochweiss S, Fruchtman S, Hahn EG, et al. Increased serum procollagen III aminoterminal peptide in myelofibrosis. Am J Hematol 1983;15:343.
61. Schachner E, Ronen M, Pinkhas J, et al. Iron absorption in patients with polycythemia vera. Eur J Nucl Med 1978;3:125.
62. Wurster-Hill D, Whang-Peng J, McIntyre OR, et al. Cytogenetic studies in polycythemia vera. Semin Hematol 1976;13:13.
63. Minutes of the PVSG Meeting, New York, November 14, 1987:31.
64. Rege-Cambien G, Mecucci C, Tricot G, et al. A chromosomal profile of polycythemia. Cancer Genet Cytogenet 1987;25:233.
65. Swolin B, Weinfeld A, Westin J. Trisomy 1q in polycythemia vera and its relation to disease transition. Am J Hematol 1986;22:155.
66. Testa JR, Kanofsky JR, Rowley JD, et al. Karyotypic patterns and their clinical significance in polycythemia vera. Am J Hematol 1981;11:29.
66a. Dies-Martin JL, Graham DI, Petitt RM, et al. Chromosome studies in 104 patients with polycythemia vera. Mayo Clinic Proc 1991;66:287.
67. Reid CD. Pruritus preceding the development of polycythemia vera. Lancet 1988;2:964.
68. Gilbert HS, Warner RP, Wasserman LR. A study of histamine in myeloproliferative disease. Blood 1966;28:795.
69. Harrison AR, Littenberg G, Goldstein L, et al. Pruritus, cimetidine and polycythemia. N Engl J Med 1979;300:433.
70. Jackson N, Burt D, Crocker J, et al. Skin mast cells in polycythemia vera: relationship to the pathogenesis and treatment of pruritus. Br J Dermatol 1987;116:21.
71. Vickers CF. Nutrition and the skin. In: Ledingham JGG, ed. Proceedings of the 10th Symposium on Advanced Medicine. London, Royal College of Physicians, 1974:311.
72. Rappaport H. Tumors of the hematopoietic system, atlas of tumor pathology, section 3, fascicle 8. Washington, DC, US Armed Forces Institute of Pathology, 1966:303.
73. Westin J, Lanner L-O, Larsson A, et al. Spleen size in polycythemia: a clinical and scintigraphic study. Acta Med Scand 1972;191:263.
74. Wolf BC, Banks PM, Mann RB, et al. Splenic hematopoiesis in polycythemia vera: a morphologic and immunohistologic study. Am J Clin Pathol 1988;89:69.
75. Chievitz E, Thiede T. Complications and causes of death in polycythemia vera. Acta Med Scand 1962;172:513.
76. Mitchell MC, Biotnott JK, Kaufman S, et al. Budd-Chiari syndrome: etiology, diagnosis and management. Medicine 1982;61:199.
77. Valla D, Casadevall N, Lacombe C, et al. Primary myeloproliferative disorder and hepatic vein thrombosis: a prospective study of erythroid colony formation in vitro in 20 patients with Budd-Chiari syndrome. Ann Intern Med 1985;103:329.
78. Wasserman LR, Bassen F. Polycythemia vera. J Mt Sinai Hosp 1959; 26:1.
79. Wasserman LR. Polycythemia vera: its course and treatment—relation to myeloid metaplasia and leukemia. Bull NY Acad Med 1954;3:343.
80. Thomas DJ, BuBoulay GH, Marshall J, et al. Cerebral blood flow in polycythemia. Lancet 1977;2:1161.
81. Willison JR, Thomas DJ, Boulay GH, et al. Effect of high hematocrit on alertness. Lancet 1980;1:846.
82. Kannel WB, Gordon T, Wolf PA, et al. Hemoglobin and the risk of cerebral infarction: the Framingham study. Stroke 1972;3:409.
83. Tohgi H, Yamanouchi H, Murakami M, et al. Importance of the hematocrit as a risk factor in cerebral infarction. Stroke 1978;9:369.
84. Harrison MJG, Pollock S, Kendall BE, et al. Effect of haematocrit on carotid stenosis and cerebral infarction. Lancet 1981;2:114.
85. Burch GE, DePasquale NP. Hematocrit, blood viscosity and myocardial infarction. Am J Med 1962;32:161.
86. Berger S, Aledort LM, Gilbert HS, et al. Abnormalities of platelet function in patients with polycythemia vera. Cancer Res 1973;33: 2683.
87. Viero P, Cortelazzo S, Bassan R, et al. Effect of aspirin on platelet 5-hydroxytryptamine and β-thromboglobulin plasma levels in patients with myeloproliferative disease. Thromb Haemostas 1982;48:125.
88. Schafer AJ. Deficiency of platelet lipoxygenase activity in myeloproliferative disorders. N Engl J Med 1982;306:381.
89. Zucher S, Mielke CH. Classification of thrombocytosis based on platelet function tests: correlation with hemorrhagic and thrombotic complications. J Lab Clin Med 1972;80:385.
90. Cooper B, Schafer AJ, Puchelsky D, et al. Platelet resistance to prostaglandin D2 in patients with myeloproliferative disorders. Blood 1978;52:618.
90a. Stenke L, Edenius C, Samuelsson J, et al. Deficient lipoxin synthesis: a novel platelet dysfunction in myeloproliferative disorders with special reference to blastic crisis of chronic myelogenous leukemia. Blood 1991;78:2989.
90b. Landolfi R, Ciabattoni G, Patrignani P, et al. Increased thromboxane biosynthesis in patients with polycythemia vera: evidence for aspirin-suppressible platelet activation in vivo. Blood 1992;88:1965.
91. Wasserman LR, Balcerzak S, Berk PD, et al. Influence of therapy on causes of death in polycythemia vera. Trans Assoc Am Phys 1981;154: 30.
92. Berk PD, Goldberg JD, Silverstein MN, et al. Increased incidence of acute leukemia in polycythemia vera associated with chlorambucil therapy. N Engl J Med 1981;304:441.
92a. Rozman C, Giralt M, Feliu E. Life expectancy of patients with chronic nonleukemic myeloproliferative disorders. Cancer 1991;67:2658.
93. Wiseman BK, Rohn RJ, Bouroncle, et al. The treatment of polycythemia vera with radioactive phosphorus. Ann Intern Med 1951;64:311.
94. Landaw SA. Acute leukemia in polycythemia vera. Semin Hematol 1976;13:38.
95. Lawrence JH, Winchell HS, Donald WG. Leukemia in polycythemia vera: relationship to splenic myeloid metaplasia and therapeutic radiation dose. Ann Intern Med 1969;70:763.
96. Osgood EE. Contrasting incidence of acute monocytic and granulocytic leukemia in P^{32} treated patients with polycythemia vera and chronic lymphocytic leukemia. J Lab Clin Med 1964;64:560.
97. Milligan DW, MacNamee R, Roberts BE, et al. The influence of iron deficient indices on whole blood viscosity in polycythemia. Br J Haematol 1982;50:467.

98. Pearson TC, Ring CP, Wetherley-Mein G. Plasma and whole blood viscosity in treated primary polycythemia. Clin Lab Haematol 1980;2: 73.
99. Birgegard G, Carlsson M, Sandhagen B, et al. Does iron deficiency in treated polycythemia vera affect whole blood viscosity? Acta Med Scand 1984;216:165.
100. Perloff JK, Rosove MH, Child JS, et al. Adults with cyanotic congenital heart disease, hematologic management. Ann Intern Med 1988;109: 406.
100a. Schwarcz TH, Hogan LA, Endean ED, et al. Thromboembolic complications of polycythemia: polycythemia vera versus smokers' polycythemia. J Vasc Surg 1993;17:518.
101. Tartaglia AP, Goldberg JD, Berk PD, et al. Adverse effects of antiaggregating platelet therapy in the treatment of polycythemia vera. Semin Hematol 1986;23:177.
102. Donovan PB, Landaw SA, Dresch C, et al. Resistance to therapy of acute leukemia developing in the course of polycythemia vera. Nouv Rev Fr Hematol 1981;23:187.
103. Gilbert HS. Problems relating to control of polycythemia vera: the use of alkylating agents. Blood 1968;32:500.
104. Weinfeld A, Westin J, Ridell B, et al. Poloycythemia vera terminating in acute leukemia: a clinical, cytogenetic and morphologic study in 8 patients treated with alkylating agents. Scand Haematol 1977;19: 255.
105. Casciato DA, Scott JL. Acute leukemia following prolonged cytotoxic ageant therapy. Medicine 1979;58:32.
106. Reimer RR, Hoover R, Fraumeri J, et al. Acute leukemia after alkylating agent therapy of ovarian cancer. N Engl J Med 1977;297:177.
107. Brodsky I. Busulphan treatment of polycythemia vera. Br J Haematol 1982;52:1.
108. Haanan L, Mathe G, Hayat M. Treatment of polycythemia vera by radiophosphorous or busulphan: a randomized trial. Br J Cancer 1981;44:75.
109. Messinezy M, Pearson TC, Prochayke A, et al. Treatment of primary proliferative polycythemia by venesection and low dose busulphan: retrospective study from one centre. Br J Haematol 1985;01:657.
110. Milligan DW, Thein SL, Roberts BE. Secondary treatment of polycythemia vera with 6-thioguanine. Cancer 1982;50:836.
111. Deconti RC, Calabresi P. Treatment of polycythemia vera with azauridine and azarabine. Ann Intern Med 1970;73:575.
112. Lian-Huang Lu, Shu-ping L, Yu-ying L. Harringtonine in treatment of polycythemia vera. Chin Med J 1989;96:533.
113. Brusamolino E, Salvaneschi L, Canevari A, et al. Efficacy trial of pipobroman in polycythemia vera and incidence of acute leukemia. J Clin Oncol 1874;2:558.
114. Keleman E, Tura S. Mitobronitol: an alkylating agent that does not induce extra leukemia cases if applied as pulse therapy for polycythemia vera. Ann NY Acad Sci 1985;459:335.
115. Wet Wo, Rff DJ, Yarbo JW. Response of polycythemia to treatment with a new agent: hydroxyurea. J Lab Clin Med 1968;74:1002.
116. Krakoff IH, Brown NC, Reichard P. Inhibition of ribonucleoside diphophatase reductase by hydroxyurea. Cancer Res 1968;28:1559.
117. Donovan PB, Kaplan ME, Goldberg JD. Treatment of polycythemia vera with hydroxyurea. Am J Hematol 1984;17:329.
118. Kaplan ME, Mack K, Goldberg JD, et al. Long-term management of polycythemia vera with hydroxyurea: a progress report. Semin Hematol 1986;23:167.
118a. Baron BW, Micka R, Baron JM. Combined plateletpheresis and cytotoxic chemotherapy for symptomatic thrombocytosis in myeloproliferative disorders. Cancer 1993;72:1209.
119. Greaves MW, Black AK, Eady RAJ, et al. Aquagenic pruritus. Br Med J 1981;282:2007.
120. Lotti T, Cappugi P, Lattari P, et al. Increased cutaneous fibrinolytic activity in a case of aquagenic pruritus. Int J Dermatol 1984;23:61.
121. Steinman HK, Kobza-Black A, Lotti TM, et al. Polycythemia rubra vera and water-induced pruritus: blood histamine levels and cutaneous fibrinolytic activity before and after water challenge. Br J Dermatol 1987;116:329.
122. Easton P, Galbraith PR. Cimetidine treatment of pruritus in polycythemia vera. (Letter) N Engl J Med 1978;299:1234 .
123. Chavarian I, Szur L. Relief of intractable pruritus in polycythemia rubra vera with cholestyramine. Br J Haematol 1975;29:669.
124. Rigby PB, Leavell BS. Polycythemia vera. Arch Intern Med 1960;106: 622.
125. Wasserman LR, Gilbert HS. Surgical bleeding in polycythemia vera. Ann NY Acad Sci 1964;115:122.
126. Renzetti AD, McClement JH, Litt BD. The Veterans Administration cooperative study of pulmonary infarction III: mortality in relation to respiratory function in chronic obstructive pulmonary disease. Am J Med 1966;44:115.
127. Bethrong M, Sabiston DC. Cerebral lesions in congenital heart disease. Bull Johns Hopkins Hosp 1951;89:384.
128. Ferenz C. The pulmonary vascular bed in tetralogy of Fallot. Bull Johns Hopkins Hosp 1960;106:81.
129. Segel N, Bishop JM. The circulation in patients with chronic bronchitis and emphysema at rest and during exercise with special reference to the influence of changes in blood viscosity and blood volume on the pulmonary circulation. J Clin Invest 1966;45:1555.
130. Weisse AB, Moschos CB, Frank MJ, et al. Hemodynamic effects of staged hematocrit reduction in patients with stable cor pulmonale and severely elevated hematocrit levels. Am J Med 1975;58:92.
131. Hart G, Strokes TC, Harrison BDW, et al. Erythrapheresis in patients with polycythemia secondary to hypoxic lung disease. Br Med J 1983;286:1284.
132. Rosenthal A, Nathan DG, Marty TL, et al. Acute hemodynamic effects of red cell volume reduction in polycythemia of cyanotic congenital heart disease. Circulation 1970;42:297.
133. Oldershaw PJ, St John Sutton MG. Hemodynamic effects of haematocrit reduction in patients with polycythemia secondary to cyanotic congenital heart disease. Br Heart J 1980;44:584.
134. Henriksson D, Varendh G, Lundrstrom N-R. Hemostatic defects in cyanotic congenital heart disease. Br Heart J 1979;41:23.
135. Rosve MH, Hocking WG, Harwig SS, et al. Studies of betathromboglobulin, platelet factor 4, and fibrinopeptide A in erythrocytosis due to cyanotic congenital heart disease. Thromb Res 1983;29:225.
136. Wedemeyer AL, Lewis JH. Improvement in hemostasis following phlebotomy in cyanotic patients with heart disease. J Pediatr 1973;83: 46.
137. Lazlo J. Myeloproliferative disorders (MPD): myelofibrosis, myelosclerosis, extramedullary hematopoiesis, undifferentiated MPD, and hemorrhagic thrombocythaemia. Semin Hematol 1975;12:75.
138. Heuck G. Zivei falle von leukamie mit eigenthumlichen blutresp knochenmarksbefund. Virchows Arch [A] 1879;78:475.
139. Nowell P, Jensen J, Gardner F, et al. Chromosome studies in "preleukemia." III. Myelofibrosis. Cancer 1976;38:1873.
140. Van Slyck EJ, Weiss L, Dully M. Chromosomal evidence for the secondary role of fibroblastic proliferation with acute myelofibrosis. Blood 1970;36:729.
141. Golde DW, Howking WG, Quan SG, et al. Origin of human bone marrow fibroblasts. Br J Haematol 1980;44:183.
142. Charron D, Robert L, Couty M-C, et al. Biochemical and histologic analysis of bone marrow collagen in myelofibrosis. Br J Haematol 1979;41:151.
143. Wyatt JP, Somers SC. Chronic marrow failure, myelosclerosis and extramedullary hematopoiesis. Blood 1950;5:329.
144. Bouroncle BA, Doan CA. Myelofibrosis: clinical, hematologic and pathologic study of 110 patients. Am J Med Sci 1962;243:697.
145. Ward HP, Block MH. The natural history of agnogenic myeloid metaplasia (AMM) and a critical evaluation of its relationship with the myeloproliferative syndrome. Medicine 1971;50:357.
146. Njoku OS, Lewis SM, Catovsky D, et al. Anemia in myelofibrosis: its value in prognosis. Br J Haematol 1983;54:79.
147. Lewis SM. The spleen: mysteries solved and unresolved. Clin Haematol 1983;12:363.
148. Goldman JM, Nolasco I. The spleen in myeloproliferative disorders. Clin Haematol 1983;12:505.
149. Cornfield DB, Shipkin P, Alavi A, et al. Intracranial myeloid metaplasia: diagnosis by CT and Fe^{52} scans and treatment by cranial irradiation. Am J Hematol 1983;15:273.
150. Puchtler H, Waldrop FS. Silver impregnation methods for reticulin fibers and reticulin: a re-investigation of their origins and specificity. Histochemistry 1978;57:177.
151. Irving EA, Tomlin SG. Collagen reticulin and their argyrophilic properties. Proc R Soc Lond (Biol) 1954;142:113.
152. Kramer H, Little K. Nature of reticulin. In: Randall JT, Jackson SF, eds. Nature and structure of collagen. New York, Academic Press, 1990.
153. Pinnell SR, Murad S. Disorders of collagen. In: Stanbury JB, Wyngaarden JB, Fredrickson DS, Goldstein J, eds. Metabolic basis of inherited disease, ed 5. New York, McGraw-Hill, 1983.
154. Mayne R, Burgeson RE, eds. Structure and function of collagen types. New York, Academic Press, 1987.
155. Fessler JH, Fessler LI. Biosynthesis of procollagen. Annu Rev Biochem 1978;47:129.
156. Barosi G, Costa A, Liberato LN, et al. Serum procollagen III peptide level correlates with disease activity in myelofibrosis with myeloid metaplasia. Br J Haematol 1989;72:16.
157. Sabin F, Miller FR. Normal bone marrow v. bone marrow in the adult. In: Downey H, ed. Handbook of hematology, vol 3. New York, Paul B Hoeber, 1938;1821.
158. Gay S, Gay R, Prchal JT. Immunohistological studies of bone marrow in collagen. Progr Clin Biol Res 1984;154:291.
159. Bentley SA, Alabester O, Foidart J. Collagen heterogeneity in normal bone marrow. Br J Haematol 1981;48:287.
160. Roberts BE, Miles DW, Woods CG. Polycythemia and myelosclerosis: a bone marrow study. Br J Haematol 1969;16:75.
161. Groopman JE. The pathogenesis of myelofibrosis in myeloproliferative disorders. Ann Intern Med 1980;92:857.
162. Castro-Malaspina H, Rabellino EM, Yen A, et al. Human megakaryocyte stimulation of proliferation of bone marrow fibroblasts. Blood 1981;57:781.
163. Hiti-Harper, Wohl E, Harper E. Platelet factor 4: an inhibitor of collagenase. Science 1978;199:991
164. Castro-Malaspina H, Moore MAS. Pathophysiological mechanisms operating in the development of myelofibrosis: role of megakaryocytes. Nouv Rev Fr Hematol 1982;24:221.

165. Drouet L, Praloran V, Cywirer-Golenzer C, et al. Deficit congenital en alpha granules plaquettaires et fibrose reticulinique medullaire: hypotheses physiopathogenique. Nouv Rev Fr Hematol 1981;23:95.
166. Coller BS, Haltin MB, Nurden AT, et al. Isolated alpha granule deficiency (gray platelet syndrome) with slight increase in bone marrow reticulin and possible glycoprotein and/or protease defect. Thromb Haemost 1983;50:211.
167. Aalto M, Potila M, Kubonen E. The effect of silica-treated macrophages on the synthesis of collagen and other proteins in vitro. Exper Cell Res 1976;97:193.
168. Leibovich SJ, Ross R. A macrophage dependent factor that stimulates the proliferation of fibroblasts in vitro. Am J Pathol 1976;84:501.
169. Lewis SM, Szur L. Malignant myelosclerosis. Br Med J 1963;2:472.
170. Bain BJ, Catovsky D, O'Brien M, et al. Megakaryoblastic leukemia presenting as acute myelofibrosis: a study of four cases with the platelet peroxidase reaction. Blood 1981;58:206.
171. Bearman RM, Pangalis GA, Rappaport H. Acute ("malignant") myelosclerosis. Cancer 1979;43:279.
172. Chan WC, Brynes RK, Kim, et al. Acute megakaryoblastic leukemia in early childhood. Blood 1983;62:92.
173. Smith JW, Shulman HM, Thomas ED, et al. Bone marrow transplantation for acute myelofibrosis. Cancer 1981;48:2198.
174. Wolf JL, Spruce WE, Bearman, et al. Reversal of acute ("malignant") myelosclerosis by allogeneic bone marrow transplantation. Blood 1982;59:191.
175. Block M. Phylogenetic and embryological basis of myeloid metaplasia. In: Burkhardt R, Conley CL, eds. "Dahlem" workshop on myelofibrosis–osteosclerosis syndrome. 1975.
176. Barosi G, Berzuini C, Liberato L, et al. A prognostic classification of myelofibrosis with myeloid metaplasia. Br J Haematol 1988;70:397.
177. Njoku OS, Lewis SM, Catovsky D, et al. Anemia in myelofibrosis: its value in prognosis. Br J Haematol 1983;54:79.
178. Najean Y, Cacchione R, Castro-Malaspina H, et al. Erythrokinetic studies in myelofibrosis: their significance for prognosis. Br J Haematol 1978;40:205.
179. Chelloul N, Briere J, Leval-Jeantet M, et al. Prognosis of myeloid metaplasia with myelofibrosis. Biomedicine 1976;24:272.
180. Varki A, Lottenberg R, Griffith R, et al. The syndrome of idiopathic myelofibrosis: a clinical review with emphasis on the prognostic variables predicting survival. Medicine (Baltimore). 1983;62:353.
181. Manoharan A, Smart RC, Pitney WR. Prognostic factors in myelofibrosis. Pathology 1982;14:455.
182. Bentley SA, Murray KH and Lewis SM, et al. Erythroid hypoplasia in myelofibrosis: a feature associated with blastic transformation. Br J Haematol 1977;36:41.
183. Silverstein MN. Agnogenic myeloid metaplasia. Acton, MA, Massachusetts Publishing Science Group, 1975.
184. Fruchtman SM. Therapeutic implications of collagen metabolism in myelofibrosis. In: Berk PD, Castro-Malaspina H, Wasserman LR, eds. Myelofibrisis and the biology of connective tissue. Progress in clinical and biological research. 1984;154:467.
185. Dokel I, Jones L, Deenmamode M, et al. Allogeneic bone marrow transplantation for primary myelofibrosis. Br J Haematol 1989;71:158.
186. Kershenobich D, Vargas F, Garcia-Tsao G, et al. Colchicine in the treatment of cirrhosis of the liver. N Engl J Med 1988;318:1709.
187. Gardner FH, Pringle JC. Androgens and erythropoiesis. II. Treatment of myeloid metaplasia. N Engl J Med 1961;264:103.
187a. Barosi G, Liberato LN, Guarnone R. Serum erythropoietin in patients with myelofibrosis with myeloid metaplasia. Br J Haematol 1993;83: 365.
188. Hast R, Engstedt L, Jameson S, et al. Oxymetholone treatment in myelofibrosis. Blut 1978;37:19.
189. Silver RT. Use of testosterone and busulfan in the treatment of myelofibrosis with myeloid metaplasia. Blood 1964;23:341.
190. Silverstein MN. Control of hypersplenism and painful splenomegaly in myeloid metaplasia by irradiation. Int J Radiat Oncol Biol Phys 1977;2:1221.
191. Benbassat J, et al. Splenectomy in patients with agnogenic myeloid metaplasia: an analysis of 321 published cases. Br J Haematol 1979;42: 207.
192. Silverstein MN, Remine WH. Splenectomy in myeloid metaplasia. Blood 1979;53:515.
193. Pettit JE, et al. Quantitative studies of splenic erythropoiesis in polycythemia and myelofibrosis. Br J Haematol 1976;34:465.
194. Bornstein P. The biosynthesis of collagen. Annu Rev Biochem 1974;43: 567.
195. Alacon-Segovia D, Ramos-Niembro F, Shaney de Kasep G, et al. Long-term evaluation of colchicine in the treatment of scleroderma. J Rheumatol 1979;6:705.
196. Silverstein MN. Treatment of myelofibrosis in Myelofibrosis: pathophysiology and clinical management. In: Lewis SM, ed. New York, Marcel Dekker, 1985.
197. Cooperberg AA, Singer OP. Reversible myelofibrosis due to Vitamin D deficiency rickets. Can Med Assoc J 1966;94:392.
198. Vetgin S, Ozsoylu S. Myeloid metaplasia in vitamin D deficiency rickets. Scand J Haematol 1982;28:180.
199. Arlet PH, Nicodeme R, Adoue D, et al. Clinical evidence for 1,25 hydroxycholecaliferol action in myelofibrosis. Lancet 1984;1:1013.
200. McCarthy DM, Hibbin JA, San Miguel JF, et al. The effect of vitamin D_3 metabolites on normal and leukemic bone marrow cells in vitro. Int J Cell Clon 1984;2:227.
201. McCarthy DM, Hibbin JA, Goldman JM. A role for 1,25 hydroxyvitamin D_3 in control of bone marrow collagen deposition. Lancet 1984;1: 78.
202. Fialkow PJ. Clonal and stem cell origin of blood cell neoplasms. Contemp Hematol Oncol 1980;1:1.
203. Stamatoyannopoulos G, Nienhuis AW. Hemoglobin switching. In: Stamatoyannopoulos G, Nienhuis AW, Leder P, Majerus P, eds. The molecular basis of blood diseases. Philadelphia, WB Saunders, 1987: 85.
204. Prockop DJ, Kivirikkoki KI, Tuberman L, et al. The biosynthesis of collagen and its disorders. N Engl J Med 1979;301:13.
205. Geary CG. Clinical and hematological aspects of chronic myelofibrosis. In: Lewis SM, ed. Myelofibrosis. New York, Marcel Dekker, 1985: 17.

Blood: Principles and Practice of Hematology,
edited by Robert I. Handin, Thomas P. Stossel, and Samuel E. Lux.
J.B. Lippincott Company, Philadelphia © 1995.

14

Thrombocytosis

David S. Rosenthal
Scott Murphy

Thrombocytosis, like erythrocytosis, may be a primary marrow disorder or a secondary phenomenon. The primary disorder is a well-recognized type of myeloproliferative disorder[1,2] that was first described in 1934 as *hemorrhagic thrombocythemia*.[3] Various other names have been given to the disorder, including *thrombocythemia, idiopathic thrombocythemia, primary hemorrhagic thrombocythemia*, and *primary thrombocythemia*.[2–11] The preferred term is *essential thrombocythemia* (ET). This distinct entity is closely related to the other chronic myeloproliferative disorders: polycythemia vera (PV), myeloid metaplasia with myelofibrosis (MMM), and chronic myelogenous leukemia (CML). Each of the four chronic myeloproliferative disorders has clear diagnostic criteria based on cytogenetics, bone marrow biopsy, red blood cell (RBC) mass, and iron studies. In most instances, ET can be differentiated from the thrombocytosis of PV, MMM, CML, and reactive thrombocytosis (RT). Occasionally, patients are seen in whom clear distinctions cannot be made.

Thrombocytosis is simply defined as an elevation in the platelet count and may be due to a number of causes other than ET. With the routine use of automated counters, thrombocytosis has become a more common clinical finding. This chapter attempts to differentiate reactive from essential thrombocytosis, discusses the clinical problems associated with both disorders, describes the diagnostic approach, and recommends whom to treat and when. The relationships between platelet function, membrane defects, light and electron microscopic changes, and clinical symptoms also are presented. The major complications of ET are the paradoxical problems of thrombosis and bleeding. As in other myeloproliferative disorders, there is a well-recognized risk of transformation to acute leukemia.

PATHOGENESIS

Clonality

Essential thrombocythemia presumably is a clonal disorder and originates in a pluripotent stem cell. Since there is no specific cytogenetic marker for ET, like the Philadelphia (Ph) chromosome in CML, chromosomal analysis has not helped to document the pluripotential stem cell compartment as the source of the malignant clone.[12–15] Chromosomal studies are important, however, to exclude CML. The sporadic finding of a 21q− or a marker chromosome in euploid or polyploid cells is not helpful in determining clonality. The Polycythemia Vera Study Group (PVSG) did not find any cytogenetic abnormalities specific for the disease. By studying the X-linked glucose-6-phosphate dehydrogenase (G6PD) locus as a cell marker, it was shown that heterozygous female patients with chronic myeloproliferative disorders such as ET, who have types A and B of G6PD in nonhematopoietic tissue, have only a single enzyme type in granulocytes, RBCs, and platelets.[16–18] Clonality can be shown in subjects heterozygous for other G6PD variants, such as Gd^{Mediterranean}.[19] Use of the polymerase chain reaction in heterozygous females may further document that the adult marrow cells are clonal.[20–22] This strategy involves amplification of a segment of a gene located on the X chromosome, such as the phosphoglycerate kinase (pgk) gene, from small numbers of peripheral blood cells. The *pgk* gene locus was chosen because it contains a methylation-sensitive restriction fragment length polymorphism for the enzyme BSTX1 and because the site is fully methylated on the inactive X chromosome. In a female who is heterozygous for the BSTX1 polymorphic site, clonality can be determined by electrophoretic analysis of amplified and restriction-digested DNA from peripheral blood cells. With this technique, in contrast to earlier studies using G6PD isoenzyme markers, monocytes, T lymphocytes, and non-T lymphocytes were not involved in the clonal proliferation in ET patients. Techniques such as the polymerase chain reaction may be the best test for clonality and may aid in distinguishing ET from secondary causes.

Platelet Megakaryocyte Morphology and Function

Under the light microscope, ET platelets are heterogeneous, with a mixture of normal and abnormal forms. Although they are usually discoid in shape, platelets may either be granular or agranular, and they range from small to giant forms, with considerable variation in size.[23,24] Platelet size can be measured directly on Wright-stained blood smears or by using the platelet volume (MPV) or platelet distribution width (PDW; an index of heterogeneity of cell volume), which is available with the automated counters.[23–26] With the Coulter S Plus II and IV counters, ET platelets have a normal MPV, while the MPV of RT platelets is slightly less than normal. The PDW is increased significantly in ET, suggesting an increased number of both large and small forms. The PDW is greater in blood samples from patients with myeloproliferative disease compared with samples from RT patients.[27] Thus, the PDW may help differentiate ET from RT (Fig. 14-1). In one study,[27] mean PDW was 17.29 in ET, compared with 16.48 in RT ($P < .01$). The discrepancy in size between direct and automated measurements most likely is due to the artificial spreading of the cell when in contact with glass. Spectophotometric measurements of the optical density of platelets correlates well with cell density (Fig. 14-2). In ET, the decreased mean cell density correlates with increased dispersion, a measurement reflecting heterogeneity of cell volume.[28–30]

Electron microscopy demonstrates some minor differences in size, number, and distribution of the organelles and, in ET platelets, demonstrates some features of immaturity.[31,32] Platelets are generally larger than normal, with frequent diameters of 10 μm or greater. There is either disorganization or scarcity of microtubules, and membranous hypertrophy is observed. Electron microscopy studies confirm the absence of granulation and, in some specimens, document a proliferation of interwoven membranes of the open canalicular and dense tubular systems.

ET megakaryocytes are markedly increased in the marrow and usually mature normally. The megakaryocyte is large, measuring 15 to 120 μm in diameter.[33–35] Dwarf forms are not seen and are more characteristic of myelofibrosis, the myelodysplastic syndromes, and CML. The nuclei may be multilobulated and have variable chromatin, irregular margins, and an elongated appearance without a clear cytoplasmic demarcation.[36] The megakaryocytes are found dispersed diffusely throughout marrow sinusoids and in clusters. This is a useful feature since clusters of megakaryocytes are not seen in normal people or in those with RT. Overall marrow cellularity may be normal or increased, with accompanying granulocytic hyperplasia.

Studies of megakaryocyte volume and nuclear lobe counts suggest that the platelet count in ET is elevated autonomously.[28,37] *Total megakaryocyte volume*, which is the total volume occupied by cells in a marrow biopsy, is increased, and there is a roughly linear relation between the space occupied by megakaryocytes and platelet production, indicating increased platelet production rather than ineffective thrombopoiesis (Fig. 14-3). In patients with RT, some, but not all, studies have shown that the mean megakaryocyte volume may be decreased, suggesting that

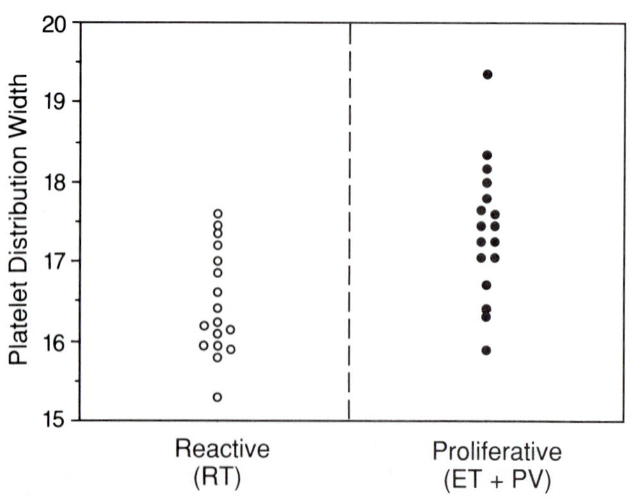

FIGURE 14-1. Distribution of platelet distribution width in reactive and proliferative groups. (After Dudley JM, Messinezy M, Eridani S, et al. Primary thrombocythaemia: diagnostic criteria and a simple scoring system for positive diagnosis. Br J Haematol 1989;71:331)

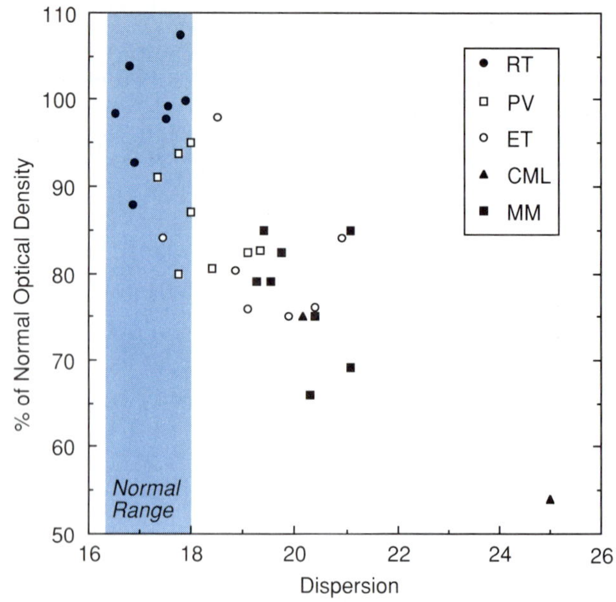

FIGURE 14-2. Correlation between two measurements that reflect platelet morphology in patients with myeloproliferative disease. Percentage of normal optical density is a spectrophotometric measurement[24] that correlates with cell density (weight/volume). The dispersion is a reflection of the breadth (degree of anisocytosis) of the platelet size distribution as measured by Coulter counter. The measurements correlate with each other ($r = -.81$) and are normal in reactive thrombocytosis (RT), modestly abnormal in polycythemia vera (PV) and essential thrombocytopenia (ET), and highly abnormal in myeloid metaplasia (MM) and in two patients with the accelerated phase of CML. (After Murphy S. Thrombocytosis and thrombocythaemia. Clin Hematol 1983;12:89)

the increased platelet count is due to increased numbers of megakaryocytes.[28,38–40] Nuclear lobes and nuclear number are also increased in these patients. Nuclear lobes can be counted directly on smears or estimated by DNA quantitation.[37,41] Normal modal megakaryocyte ploidy value is 32N, with less than 10% of cells having 2N and 4N and with few cells having 64N and 128N. No normal preparations had a ploidy greater than 128N[37] (Fig. 14-4). In patients with ET, high ploidy values are frequent, with 10% of cells having 256N and with some as high as 512N. These findings are unique for ET and may help in the differential diagnosis of thrombocytosis.

Growth Characteristics in Culture Studies

Cell lines derived from marrow precursors have been useful in studying some aspects of megakaryocyte proliferation and differentiation, but most studies of megakaryocyte kinetics have used short-term in vitro cultures.[42–53] In addition, the putative humoral regulators of megakaryocyte development have not been well characterized. These studies are technically difficult because megakaryocytes are relatively rare and constitute only 0.03% to 0.06% of the marrow nucleated cells. Theories of the pathogenesis of ET include the following: (1) an inappropriate expansion in the number of megakaryocyte progenitor cells resulting from an increased input from the pluripotent hematopoietic stem cell pool[48]; (2) an increase in the number of megakaryocyte progenitors secondary to accelerated self-renewal at the committed stem cell level; (3) presence of a normal regulatory system with excessive mitotic or endomitotic megakaryocyte development; and (4) autonomous production and proliferation of megakaryocytes.[49,50]

Culture studies of megakaryocytes derived from periph-

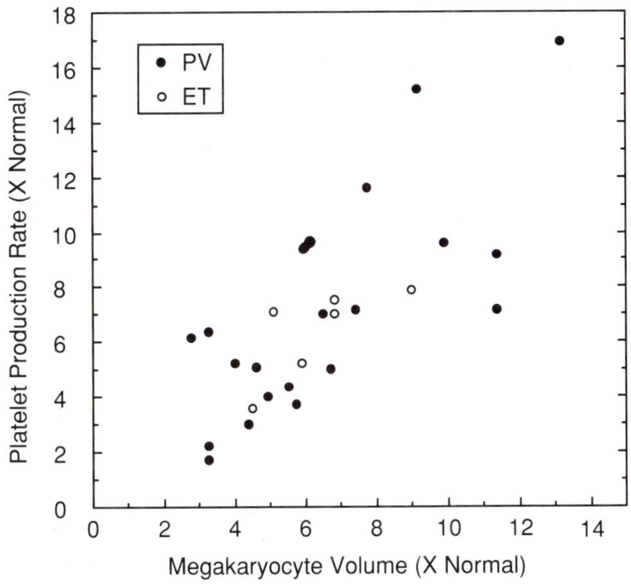

FIGURE 14-3. Rate of platelet production and megakaryocyte volume in polycythemia vera (PV) and essential thrombocytopenia (ET). Megakaryocyte volume is an estimate of the total volume occupied by megakaryocyte throughout the marrow. There is equal increase in both measurements, suggesting an increase in platelet production without evidence for ineffective thrombopoiesis. (After Kutti J, Ridell B, Weinfeld A, Westin J. The relation of thrombokinetics to bone marrow megakaryocytes and to the size of the spleen in polycythaemia vera. Scand J Haematol 1973;10:88; and Branehög I, Ridell B, Swolin B, Weinfeld A. Megakaryocyte quantifications in relation to thrombokinetics in primary thrombocythaemia and allied diseases. Scand J Haematol 1975;15:321)

eral blood and marrow have given conflicting results and have yet to confirm the pathogenesis of the thrombocytosis. In short-term cultures, some patients with thrombocytosis secondary to myeloproliferative disorders produce a substance with thrombopoietin-like properties that may cause thrombocytosis in ET.[53] More likely, ET results from the growth of an abnormal clone of colony-forming unit megakaryocyte (CFU-M) cells that is ultrasensitive to the megakaryocyte colony-stimulating activity present in normal plasma. The finding of an increased number of megakaryocyte colonies would certainly support this mechanism and would be similar to the mechanism proposed for erythrocytosis in PV. In one study,[42] when mononuclear cells from ET patients were assayed for CFU-M in the presence of normal AB serum, they gave rise to many more megakaryocytes than normal. The number of cells per colony was also increased. This is most likely due to autonomous growth and proliferation. Using a method for cloning human CFU-M in plasma clot cultures, Gerwitz and colleagues[45] described a putative megakaryocyte colony-stimulating activity in patients with amegakaryocytic thrombocytopenia, which stimulates CFU-M growth. This factor, however, does not increase CFU-M in patients with RT or ET. Using a megakaryocyte colony assay in methyl cellulose–containing plasma and medium conditioned by phytohemagglutinin-stimulated leukocytes, platelet-released materials and platelet-derived growth factor, as well as serum from both normal subjects and patients with thrombocytosis, decrease megakaryocytic colony formation.[46] These studies imply that platelet-derived factors in the *serum* are inhibitory, whereas *plasma* from ET patients, when compared with normal plasma, is more efficient in supporting megakaryocyte colony formation by normal or ET marrow cells.[46]

In short-term assays, there may be spontaneous growth of megakaryocyte progenitors under minimal or even suboptimal conditions, for example, using only normal human plasma.[49] However, recent evidence indicates that circulating megakaryocyte progenitors are hypersensitive to interleukin-3 and that this increased sensitivity may account for the "autonomous" growth of megakaryocyte colonies in ET patients.[49a] In addition, most patients with ET develop spontaneous erythroid colonies without the addition of erythropoietin.[50] Since no patients with secondary thrombocytosis or RT developed spontaneous erythroid colonies, this pattern of growth may be helpful in differential diagnosis. In ET patients, the concentration of circulating megakaryocyte progenitors is increased, but the CFU-M developed abnormally.[51] The endomitotic component of megakaryocyte growth was disordered in all patients. The finding of abnormal endoreduplication after almost 2 weeks in culture might explain the abnormally high-ploidy megakaryocytes.[52]

Megakaryocyte differentiation and maturation may be more appropriately studied in long-term culture. Despite many attempts, there are relatively few permanent cell lines that uniformly express the megakaryocytic phenotype. Several human megakaryocytic cell lines (MEG-01, T-33, EST-IU, CMK, MEG-1S, and DAMI) have been established.[54–59] The study of these cells should produce useful information regarding megakaryocytopoiesis and the various control mechanism involved. For example, in 1986, a human megakaryocytic cell line (DAMI) was established from a patient with thrombocytosis secondary to MMM.[54] The cultured cells achieved ploidy levels greater than 4N and have maintained the initial megakaryocytic-like phenotype, expressing GpIb/II and GpIIb/IIIa complexes. The HLA class I antigens, as well as MY9 (an early myeloid antigen), are also expressed. Transmission electron microscopy shows these cells to contain a lobulated nucleus with multiple prominent nucleoli and a high nuclear/cytoplasmic volume ratio. Cytoplasmic budding was frequently observed, but no demarcation membranes were

FIGURE 14-4. Combined ploidy distribution histograms from 13 patients with normal platelet counts (Nl), 7 patients with idiopathic thrombocytopenic purpura (ITP), and 5 patients with essential thrombocytopenia (ET). Error bars represent 1 standard deviation. Significant rightward ploidy shifts relative to control population are seen both for patients with ITP ($P < .01$) and for those with ET ($P < .001$). (After Mazur EM, Lindquist DL, de Alarcon PA, et al. Evaluation of bone marrow megakaryocyte ploidy distributions in persons with normal and abnormal platelet counts. J Lab Clin Med 1988;11:194)

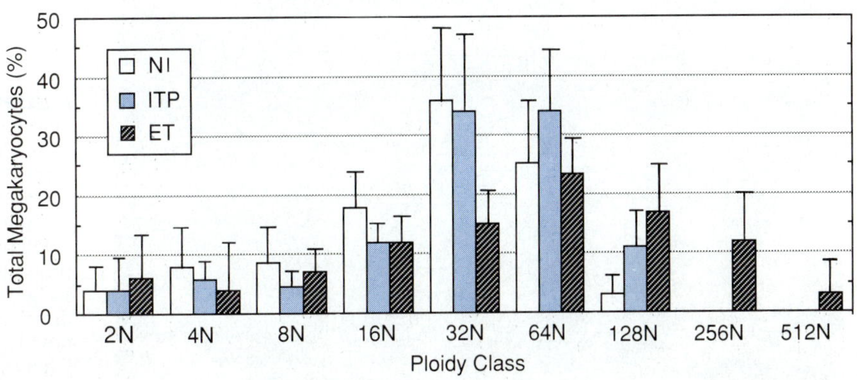

noted. Morphologic and biochemical studies performed after 1 year of continuous culture were unchanged. These cells are polyploid with budding cytoplasm and occur in conjunction with smaller blast forms with similar nuclear and membrane features (Fig. 14-5). DAMI cells, in the presence of PMA or DMSO, secrete vWF antigen and other platelet proteins and undergo differentiation and endomitosis (after PMA). Study of these or other cell lines may improve our understanding of megakaryocytic proliferation and differentiation.

ESSENTIAL THROMBOCYTHEMIA: A MYELOPROLIFERATIVE DISORDER

Essential thrombocythemia, PV, and MMM constitute the nonleukemic chronic myeloproliferative disorders. As discussed, the use of G6PD isoenzymes in heterozygous patients as markers suggests that a clonal stem cell defect is responsible for increased production of RBCs, granulocytes, and platelets in the marrow.[16,17] ET has a well-recognized presentation but shares many similarities with PV, CML, and MMM. ET, the rarest of the chronic myeloproliferative disorders, increased in incidence as the platelet count became a more routine laboratory study.

The presenting symptoms of ET are not too dissimilar from those of PV. Many patients may present with a masked PV, with the initial striking feature being thrombocytosis. Thrombocytosis secondary to CML is also a common phenomenon, and many patients may have preexistent thrombocytosis for some time, with only minimal leukocyte elevation; these patients are recognized by finding the Ph chromosome. Patients with myelofibrosis may also present with signs and symptoms related to significant thrombocytosis. ET has remained the least well defined of the chronic myeloproliferative disorders. The following is the list of strict diagnostic criteria established by the PVSG[10]:

- Persistent platelet count higher than $600 \times 10^9/L$
- Hemoglobin 13 g/dL or less, or normal RBC mass

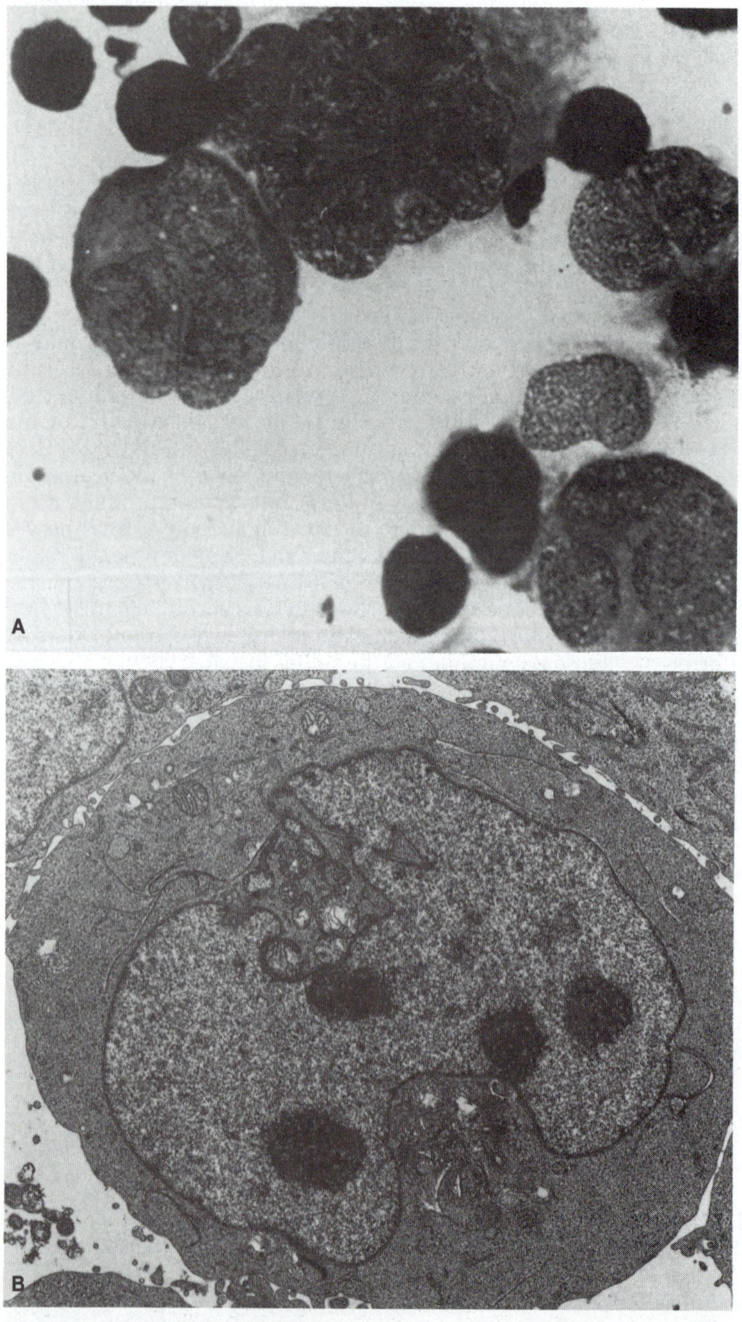

FIGURE 14-5. (**A**) DAMI culture cell smears prepared after 1 year of continuous culture. Shown are polyploid cells with budding cytoplasm as well as smaller blast forms with similar nuclear and membrane features (×630). (**B**) Transmission electron micrograph of DAMI cell after 8 months in culture. Multiple prominent nucleoli in a lobulated nucleus. The cytoplasm contained prominent smooth endoplasmic reticulum, extensive Golgi complexes, and numerous enlarged mitochondria; no granules or demarcation membranes were noted (×9555). (After Greenberg SM, Rosenthal DS, Greeley TA, et al. Characterization of a new megakaryocytic cell line: the Dami cell. Blood 1988;72:1968)

- Stainable iron in marrow or failure of iron trial (less than 1-g/dL rise in hemoglobin after 1 month of trial)
- No Ph chromosome, no *bcr/abl* gene rearrangement, or both
- Absent marrow fibrosis (or less than one third marrow fibrosis without splenomegaly and leukoerythroblastic blood smear)
- No known cause for RT

In one series of patients thought to have ET, application of rigid diagnostic criteria often revealed a mistaken cause of thrombocytosis, such as PV, CML, or MMM.[10,27,60,61] For example, of 50 patients studied with presumed ET at the Mayo Clinic from the years 1965 to 1975, 2 transformed into a state indistinguishable from PV, 2 evolved into a clinical situation indistinguishable from CML, and 2 evolved into a state similar to MMM (MN Silverstein, unpublished data, 1980). In addition, the states of 2 of the 50 patients transformed directly into acute nonlymphocytic leukemia.

The ultimate complication of all myeloproliferative disorders is transformation to acute leukemia or a blastic transformation. Most patients develop anemia, splenomegaly, leukocytosis, and thrombocytopenia as they enter the blast phase. As with PV, the transformation is not always related to previous chemotherapy.[62] The numbers of ET-related leukemia cases reported are few, and there is insufficient follow-up time of prospective studies of ET to make any definite conclusions regarding risk factors.[63–67] The leukemic transformation is primarily of myeloblastic, myelomonoblastic, or megakaryoblastic phenotypes. There was one report of combined myeloblastic and lymphoblastic transformation.[65] Once the blast transformation occurs, death follows within months. Occasional complete remissions can be obtained with aggressive chemotherapy, but they are brief.

DIFFERENTIAL DIAGNOSES

Although thrombocytosis is a necessary requirement for the diagnosis of ET, an elevated platelet count frequently accompanies the chronic myeloproliferative disorders as well as a number of acute and chronic diseases. Diagnostic requirements have varied in the literature and have included the presence of a spleen, the absence of the Ph chromosome, the presence or absence of thrombotic or hemorrhagic complications, and the absence of erythrocytosis and marrow fibrosis.[7,8–11] The diagnosis of ET should be considered when there is a persistent elevation of platelet count in excess of $600 \times 10^9/L$, splenomegaly, marrow megakaryocytic hyperplasia, absence of the Ph chromosome, absence of an increased RBC mass, presence of abnormal platelet function studies, and presence of thrombohemorrhagic disease. Many patients who have ET, however, have platelet counts under $1000 \times 10^9/L$; and some patients with RT have platelet counts of $1000 \times 10^9/L$ or greater. A schema of clinical findings and laboratory tests was devised to aid in the diagnosis of the disorder causing the thrombocytosis[60] (see Fig. 14-6).

Table 14-1 lists the differential diagnosis of thrombocytosis, subclassifying the laboratory abnormality into those disorders that are associated with a reactive or secondary thrombocytosis and those disorders, such as ET, that are part of the myeloproliferative or myelodysplastic syndromes. Thrombocytosis is commonly found in patients with many acute and chronic inflammatory diseases.[28–69] Chronic infections, such as tuberculosis, osteomyelitis, and subacute bacterial endocarditis, frequently raise the platelet count to 500 to $700 \times 10^9/L$. In addition, many other acute or chronic bacterial and fungal infections raise the platelet count. Rheumatic diseases, such as rheumatoid arthritis, ankylosing spondylitis, and polyarteritis nodosa, commonly cause thrombocytosis. Gastrointestinal inflammatory disease, such as regional enteritis, ulcerative colitis, Crohn's disease, Whipple's disease, tropical sprue, and dermatitis herpetiformis, may result in persistent thrombocytosis.[70]

The platelet count is increased in patients with acute and chronic bleeding, iron deficiency, hemolytic anemia, and many types of malignancy, such as Hodgkin's and non-Hodgkin's lymphoma. In addition, thrombocytosis occurs after splenectomy, postpartum, and postoperatively.[71–74] The platelet count rarely exceeds $1000 \times 10^9/L$ in reactive states, and the platelet count gradually decreases toward

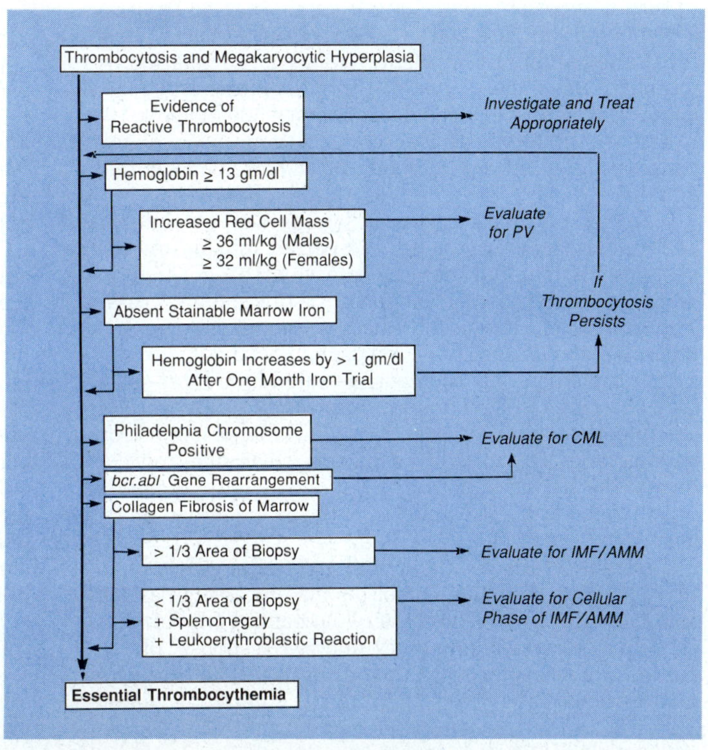

FIGURE 14-6. Schematic approach to the diagnosis of essential thrombocytosis. PV, polycythemia vera, CML, chronic myelogenous leukemia, IMF/AMM, idiopathic myelofibrinosis/agnogenic myeloid metaplasia. (After Iland HJ, Laszlo J, Peterson P, et al. Essential thrombocythemia: clinical and laboratory characteristics at presentation. Trans Assoc Am Physicians 1983;96:165)

TABLE 14-1. Differential Diagnosis of Thrombocytosis

REACTIVE THROMBOCYTOSIS
Persistent
Accompanies many acute and chronic inflammatory diseases
Rheumatoid arthritis
Polyarteritis nodosa
Regional enteritis
Ulcerative colitis
Tuberculosis
Malignancies
Polymyalgia rheumatica
Chronic pneumonia
Transient
Acute and chronic hemorrhages
Hemolytic anemia
Iron deficiency
Postsplenectomy disease
Postpartem disease
MYELOPROLIFERATIVE AND MYELODYSPLASTIC THROMBOCYTOSIS
Essential thrombocythemia
Chronic myelogenous leukemia
Polycythemia vera
Myeloid metaplasia with myelofibrosis
Refractory anemia with ringed sideroblasts
5q− syndrome

normal or remains mildly elevated. Two myelodysplastic disorders, the 5q− syndrome and refractory anemia with ringed sideroblasts, may produce platelet counts greater than 1000 × 10^9/L at presentation and during the course of the disease.[75–77]

The cause of thrombocytosis in acute and chronic inflammatory states is not well explained.[78–81] There is no consistently measurable increase in thrombopoietic activity in serum of patients with RT, although existing bioassays are not well standardized and are relatively insensitive. In the limited number of available studies, no correlation was found between the degree of thrombocytosis and serum activity; patients with platelets counts of 500 to 600 × 10^9/L had stimulatory activity, while patients with platelet counts as high as 1000 to 2000 × 10^9/L had no measurable activity.

Many patients with chronic inflammatory bowel disease and autoimmune disease have impaired splenic function, and it is possible that immune complexes are formed that result in microvascular occlusion of the splenic vessels. The finding of Howell-Jolly bodies, target cells, and increased platelets suggests a hyposplenic state. Hyposplenism or asplenism has been corroborated by a liver-spleen scan showing reduced or absent uptake of test material in the spleen. In addition, chromium-51–labeled heated RBC studies have shown delayed plasma clearance and confirmed the hypofunction of the spleen. Many of the disorders listed as RT in Table 14-1 may be explained on this basis.

Thrombocytosis occurs immediately after splenectomy in all patients, and platelet counts may be as high as 1000 to 2000 × 10^9/L.[82–88] There are two potential explanations: (1) as part of an inflammatory marrow response, platelet counts increase after many operations; or (2) with removal of the spleen, about one third of the total-body platelet mass is released into the circulation from the splenic pool. After splenectomy, however, patients with previously normal platelet counts develop counts that are far in excess of what can be explained on the basis of these two considerations. Some have proposed that the spleen produces a circulating factor that suppresses platelet production. Postsplenectomy thrombocytosis, even with platelet counts as high as 1000 to 2000 × 10^9/L, usually subsides over weeks to several months and levels off at high-normal or just above normal range. In patients who have chronic myeloproliferative disorders, elevated platelet counts may persist indefinitely after splenectomy. In patients with no primary marrow disorder, the high platelet counts cause no increased incidence in thrombotic or bleeding complications. A recognized exception to this generalization is the situation in which severe anemia coexists with thrombocytosis. Anemia related to hemolysis, ineffective erythropoiesis, or iron deficiency has been associated rarely with thrombotic complications.[73] For most patients with postsplenectomy thrombocytosis, however, no therapy is indicated unless there was a prior thrombotic complication, an underlying myeloproliferative disorder, or persistent significant anemia.

Iron-deficiency anemia has been associated with platelet counts over 2000 × 10^9/L. Rarely, a thromboembolic complication has been reported in this situation, but the relation may be coincidental. The thrombocytosis responds dramatically to iron replacement even before there is any recognizable improvement in the RBC values.[73] In the postpartum period, the increased number of platelets has been attributed to the bleeding associated with delivery and to the postoperative state.

The following is a list of major variables that help differentiate RT from ET:

- Platelet count: less than 5% of RT patients have counts greater than 1000 × 10^9/L
- Platelet distribution width
- Platelet aggregation studies
- Platelet adenosine triphosphate (ATP)/adenosine diphosphate (ADP) ratio
- Response of marrow cultures to exogenous erythropoietin
- Size of the spleen
- Clinical evidence of thromboses or bleeding
- Other abnormal cell lines

The finding of myelodysplasia is suggested by significant anemia (hemoglobin less than 10 g/dL) and a marrow revealing ineffective erythropoiesis, ringed sideroblasts, and an abnormal karyotype. Most patients with RT who have platelet counts over 600 × 10^9/L cannot be separated from ET patients on the basis of age, sex, or presenting platelet count. The PDW is increased significantly in most patients with ET and is relatively normal in the reactive group. Platelet aggregation studies in RT are occasionally abnormal with epinephrine, but as many as 10% of normal subjects have absence of platelet aggregation to epinephrine. There are no reports of spontaneous aggregation. The platelet ATP/ADP ratio is significantly higher in thrombocytosis patients with myeloproliferative disease. Cell cultures analyzing burst-forming unit–erythroid (BFU-E) product, when increased above normal spontaneous colonies without erythropoietin (EPO), always indicate a myeloproliferative cause. This study has never been abnormal in RT. A scoring system[27] was developed based on splenic enlargement (two points), unstimulated BFU-E–derived colonies (two points), elevated ATP/ADP ratio (one point), elevated PDW (one point), and presence of clinical ischemia (one point; Table 14-2). A score of three or higher indicates

TABLE 14-2. Diagnostic Scoring System: Reactive Versus Proliferative Thrombocytosis

Diagnostic Test	Points*
Abnormal platelet distribution width	1
ATP/ADP ratio	1
Unstimulated BFU-E—derived colony formation	2
Spleen scan	2

* A score of 3 points or more indicates proliferative thrombocytosis; less than 3 points indicates reactive thrombocytosis.

a proliferative thrombocytosis such as ET; a score below three indicates RT. This scoring system yielded no false predictions of ET, and the overall predictive value was 87%.

The routine schema of evaluating thrombocytosis in everyday practice should consist of a complete history and physical examination and examination of the blood smear to rule out iron deficiency, hemolysis, leukoerythroblastosis, ineffective erythropoiesis, and the postsplenectomy state or hyposplenism. In addition, sedimentation rate, antinuclear antibodies, protein electrophoresis (noting changes of chronic inflammation), serum iron, total iron-binding capacity, and ferritin should be measured, all of which should be normal in ET. If there is no evidence for RT, a marrow examination to look for megakaryocyte clustering and cytogenetics should complete the evaluation.

Thrombocytosis Secondary to Other Myeloproliferative Disorders

Essential thrombocythemia is generally considered a diagnosis of exclusion, and by convention, many patients are classified as having PV if thrombocytosis is associated with an increased RBC mass.[10,11,28,61] About one third of patients with PV have thrombocytosis (platelet counts higher than 400 × 10^9/L), and in about 5%, the platelet count exceeds 1000 × 10^9/L.[8,10,27,60] From 1974 to 1982, the PVSG enrolled 151 patients in a clinical trial of the management of thrombocytosis secondary to myeloproliferative disorders.[10] Of the 151 patients with platelet counts greater than 1000 × 10^9/L, only 50 satisfied the rigid diagnostic criteria for ET. Of the remaining 101 patients, 19 satisfied all the criteria for ET, with the exception that masked PV had not been adequately excluded. These patients either had no RBC mass study (despite a hemoglobin of 13 g/dL or more), or they were iron-deficient at presentation and had not been given an adequate trial of iron replacement before myelosuppressive therapy. Of the remaining 82 patients, 25 had MMM with secondary thrombocytosis, some had classic PV, and 6 were later shown to have CML identified by the finding of the Ph chromosome.

In a univariate comparison of a group of strictly defined ET patients with a series of PV patients who had platelet counts greater than 1000 × 10^9/L, patients with PV had significantly higher leukocyte counts and a higher incidence and degree of splenomegaly.[10] The hematocrit value was helpful in differentiation only at the extreme levels since almost half of the patients with thrombocytosis secondary to PV or ET had hematocrits of 43% to 57%, a considerable overlap (Fig. 14-7). Differentiating ET from PV is important because patients with ET have a better overall prognosis. Median total survival for the PV patients is 8 years, compared with an 83% survival at 8 years for the ET patients in the same cohort. In differentiating PV from ET, the RBC mass or the response to an oral iron trial are the most helpful diagnostic tests. If it is not possible to perform either of these studies, an algorithm based on measurement of the hematocrit, leukocyte count, and palpable spleen size has been shown to be helpful in differentiating the two disorders.[61] The model used specifies the probability of a diagnosis of ET or PV with thrombocytosis (P_{ET}/P_{VT}). This algorithm can be used to derive a simple computer program. To calculate the probability of the diagnosis, one only needs to know the hematocrit (percentage), the leukocyte count (10^9/L), and the spleen size (in centimeters):

$$\text{final probability} = \frac{a}{(1 + a)}$$

where:
$a = 23.0188 - (0.374255 \times \text{hematocrit}) - (0.227586 \times \text{leukocyte count}) - (0.833028 \times \text{spleen size})$

The closer the final probability (*P* value) is to unity, the greater is the likelihood that a patient with a given set of values has a diagnosis of ET; whereas, as the *P* value approaches 0, the more likely the patient is to have PV. For example, if the probability is greater than 0.65, then the most likely diagnosis is ET (Fig. 14-8). If the probability is less than 0.35, then PV is most likely. With these calculations, it was shown that the correct diagnosis could be made with 92% accuracy, compared with only 52% when the hematocrit was used alone.

The interrelation of the myleoproliferative diseases has been suspected since Dameshek[1] and others[89–91] reported suspected ET patients who later developed CML. In a series of PVSG patients referred with platelet counts greater than 1000 × 10^9/L, six patients, all female, had the Ph chromosome.[89] Each patient presented without anemia, marked splenomegaly, and the extreme leukocytosis characteristic of CML. The leukocyte counts were 8000 to 32,000 × 10^9/L, and the differential showed only a small percentage of immature cells and rare nucleated RBCs; whereas the platelet counts ranged from 1700 to 2900 × 10^9/L. The leukocyte alkaline phosphatase (LAP) score was not helpful in diagnosis since it was normal in five of the six patients. In another retrospective analysis of six adults presenting with the classic clinical features of ET, five had a Ph chromosome.[90] A sixth patient developed leukemic blast crisis 4 years after diagnosis, and although the cells were Ph chromosome–negative by cytogenetic examination, Southern blots of leukemic DNA showed that the *abl* oncogene had been translocated to the breakpoint cluster region on chromosome 22, the same molecular gene change as occurs in cases of Ph-positive CML. The clinical impor-

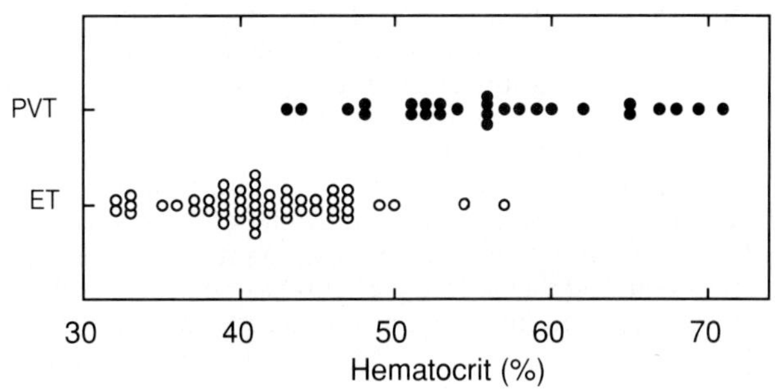

FIGURE 14-7. Distributions of presenting hematocrits in patients with essential thrombocythemia (ET) and polycythemia vera with thrombocytosis (PVT), that is, platelet counts over 1000 × 10^9/L. A hematocrit in the range 40% to 60% is consistent with either diagnosis. (After Murphy S, Iland H, Rosenthal D, Laszlo J. Essential thrombocythemia: an interim report from the Polycythemia Vera Study Group. Semin Hematol 1986;23:177)

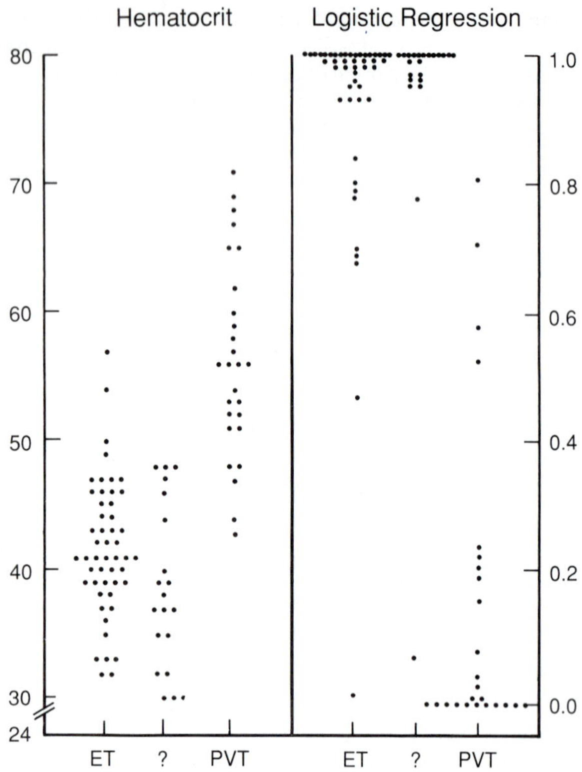

FIGURE 14-8. Distribution of hematocrits (*left*) and P_{ET}/P_{VT} values obtained with the logistical regression algorithm (*right*) in PVSG patients with essential thrombocytopenia (ET), polycythemia vera with thrombocytosis (PVT), and myeoloproliferative-related thrombocytosis. (After Iland HJ, Laszlo J, Case DC, et al. Differentiation between essential thrombocythemia and polycythemia vera with marked thrombocytosis. Am J Hematol 1987;25:191)

tance of finding the Ph chromosome in an otherwise classic case of ET is most important in predicting prognosis. Most of these patients with the Ph chromosome develop an accelerated phase of CML or blast crisis and have a much shorter survival than ET patients without the Ph chromosome.[91]

CLINICAL DATA

Presentation at diagnosis is variable, and a large percentage of ET patients are totally asymptomatic.[8,9,11] Symptoms do not correlate well with platelet count. The male/female incidence ratio is about 1.2:1. This is based on an analysis of older patients. Several series of patients under age 45 years were predominantly female. From PVSG data, about 85% of the patients were over the age of 50 years.[10] The actual age distribution is still unclear since most age curves were constructed from patients admitted to protocol studies, and many investigators may not have enrolled younger patients for the chemotherapy or radiation trials.[28] Occasional patients may present with thrombotic manifestations or hemorrhage prior to the development of thrombocytosis.[28a] Good evidence also suggest that the risk of thrombosis and arterial ischemic events is increased in patients with additional cardiovascular risk factors.[28b] Series of younger patients have since been reported.[92–95] In 1978, Hoagland and Silverstein[92] described nine patients under the age of 30 years who were evaluated because of platelet counts exceeding 1000×10^9/L. These patients fit the criteria for diagnosis of ET but, despite a long follow-up, did not develop the complications usually associated with ET. In fact, two patients had normal pregnancies without significant bleeding or thrombosis. In another series of 44 patients under the age of 45 years, there was a 39% incidence of hemorrhage or thrombosis, and two patients died of thrombotic complications.[95] Other case reports have been published of serious and fatal episodes of hemorrhage and thrombosis complicating the course of ET in young patients.[93,94,96–103] Cardiac ischemia and infarction, superior sagittal sinus thrombosis, brachial and mesenteric arterial thrombosis, and placental infarcts leading to termination of pregnancy have been documented. With the advent of automated platelet counting, increasing numbers of asymptomatic adults with ET are being found. Follow-up of these patients should resolve this discrepancy in the literature.

As with the other chronic myeloproliferative disorders, the major clinical symptoms are related to bleeding or thrombosis. Of 50 patients initially evaluated at the Mayo Clinic in the years 1965 to 1975, 30% were asymptomatic and were discovered because of an unexplained increase in the platelet count. Under the age of 45 years, over 70% of patients were asymptomatic at diagnosis.[95] The clinical presentations of symptomatic patients in the younger age group were hemorrhage and microvascular thrombotic occlusions. Patients may also have easy bruising, epistaxis, unexplained gastrointestinal hemorrhage, and postoperative hemorrhage. The latter complication explains the labeling of ET as *hemorrhagic thrombocythemia*. Thrombotic complications are also frequent and include microvascular occlusions of the extremities, central nervous system, and coronary circulation.[104,105] The most frequent complications include digital ischemia, erythromelalgia, cerebrovascular ischemia, Budd-Chiari syndrome, recurrent spontaneous abortions, and gastrointestinal hemorrhage. In a PVSG study,[10] the most frequent symptoms were weakness, hemorrhage, headache, paresthesia, and dizziness. Although the headaches and weakness were generally nonspecific, there were several instances of classic migraine accompanied by contralateral weakness and paresthesia. Bleeding was usually mild. Epistaxis, ecchymosis, and uterine, buccal, and urinary tract hemorrhage occurred. Only a minority of patients had severe bleeding or massive postoperative blood loss.[51]

Microvascular occlusive lesions are frequent in ET. They may lead to peripheral gangrene and may be the sole clinical manifestation of the disease.[104,106] Distal gangrene of the toes may be the presenting feature, and the skin's purple, mottled appearance resembles lesions of livedo reticularis.[107] Patients with distal gangrene generally do not have any bleeding or hemorrhagic symptoms, and the symptoms and signs can often be alleviated by ingestion of aspirin. About one third of patients develop localized paresthesia, described as tingling, burning, or numbness.[108–113] Involvement of the hands or feet, simulating a diabetic neuropathy, is most common (see Fig. 14-9).

Mitchell first described erythromelalgia in 1878:

> *Usually it comes in the ball of foot, or of the great toe, or in the heel; and from these parts it extends so as to involve a large portion or all of the sole and to reach the dorsum and even the leg. . . . The pain is of a burning character: it is the pain of a burn, the pain of mustard, of intense sunburn . . . is throbbing, aching and burning.*[108]

The sensations are accompanied by redness and increased skin temperature. The symptoms may be exacerbated by increasing temperatures or diminished by cooling the skin. In some instances, erythromelalgia may precede the diagnosis of thrombocytosis for as long as 10 to 16 years.[110] The warm congestion in the extremities can be accurately documented with thermography.[113] Skin-punch biopsy specimens taken from affected areas demonstrate arteriolar inflammation and thrombotic occlusions.[111,113] There is no

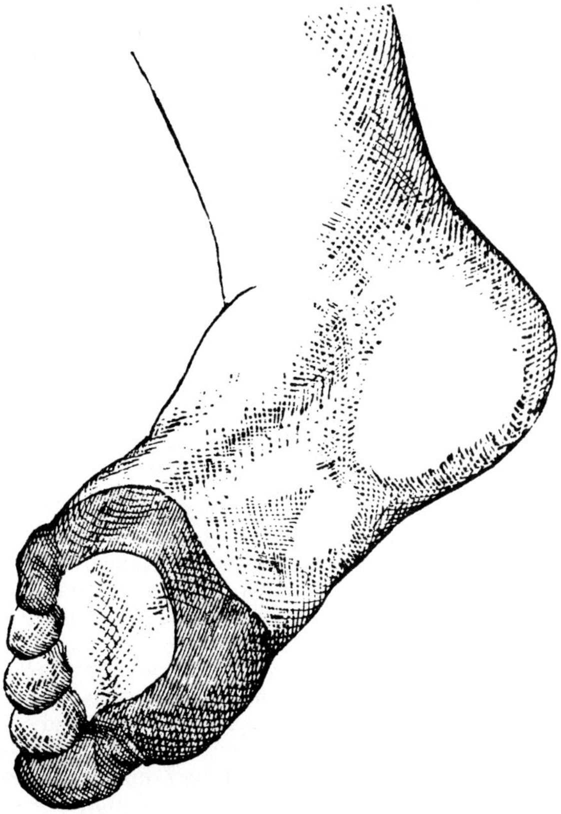

FIGURE 14-9. Area of pain in the foot. (Am J Med Sci 1878; 76:2)

involvement of venules, capillaries, or nerves. The inner layer of the vessel wall is thickened by proliferation of cells, with vascularization and swelling of the cytoplasm and deposition of intercellular material (Fig. 14-10).

Many patients obtain relief from aspirin therapy—an important diagnostic test for erythromelalgia. It is thought that the thrombus occluding the arteriole is composed of platelet aggregates,[111] and concomitant with the symptoms, platelet consumption is significantly increased. The relation between platelet number and erythromelalgia is unclear. Two studies have come to different conclusions.[110,113] Migraine, confused states, transient ischemic attacks, amaurosis fugax, dizziness, lightheadedness, syncope, visual disturbances, and epileptic seizures have all been described.[105] The pathophysiology is presumed to be similar to that of digital ischemia, that is, obstruction in the microvasculature of the cerebral circulation.[104] Antiplatelet agents such as aspirin often reduce or eliminate these symptoms.[107,114]

The Budd-Chiari syndrome, or hepatic vein thrombosis, is frequently observed in patients with an underlying myeloproliferative disorder such as PV or ET.[115,116] Although more common in PV, this complication has occurred in several documented cases of ET.[116] The increased incidence of spontaneous abortions may be secondary to placental insufficiency from the multiple thromboses in the placental circulation.[101–103] In one instance, a 29-year-old patient had an intrauterine fetal death at 30 weeks but had a second successful term delivery while being treated throughout the pregnancy with aspirin.[101] In addition, platelet consumption with placental thrombosis has been described as a cause of preeclampsia and fetal growth retardation.[103]

Several reports have been made of fatal coronary heart disease occurring in young patients with ET.[98–100] The presence of thromboemboli in the intramural coronary arteries and in peripheral, splenic, pulmonary, and renal arteries supports the view that the arterial narrowings are due to thrombocytosis.[117] Sudden catastrophic events of massive arterial thrombosis in the cerebral and coronary arteries can occur.[95,98–100]

Bleeding complications in primary thrombocytosis are characteristic of platelet and vascular disorders, as opposed to a clotting factor deficiency.[118,119] Bruising, epistaxis, and superficial mucosal hemorrhages in gastrointestinal, genitourinary, or gingival areas are most common, whereas deep tissue and muscle bleeding is uncommon. Excessive local bleeding after surgery has also been frequent in ET, as it has in PV.

Physical examination generally is unremarkable other than signs of bleeding or thrombosis. The median Karnofsky performance status was 90% in one study,[10] indicating a limited clinical effect of the disease. Splenomegaly is seen in about 38% of patients and liver enlargement in only 16%. The degree of splenomegaly is usually minimal, with the lower border rarely extending more than 3 cm below the left costal margin.[10]

Routine Laboratory Studies

Tables 14-3 through 14-5 list the blood and marrow findings in 37 patients who satisfied the strict ET criteria of the PVSG and who had platelet counts over 1000×10^9/L.[60] Six (16%) of 37 patients had hemoglobin levels less than 12 g/dL despite the absence of iron deficiency. No patient had a hemoglobin level less than 10 g/dL. The RBC mass correlated fairly well with hemoglobin levels, although there was considerable variation. The leukocyte counts ranged from 6000 to 41,100/μL, with 16 patients (43%) having counts greater than 12,000/μL but only 8% of patients having leukocyte counts higher than 20,000/μL. There was only mild basophilia and mild eosinophilia, with a rare nucleated RBC and immature leukocyte in the blood.

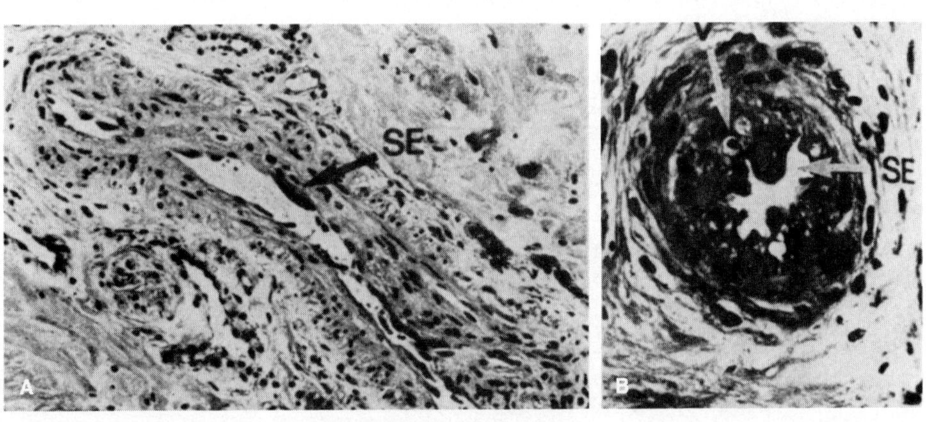

FIGURE 14-10. Arterioles with swollen endothelial cells (SE) and cell proliferation of the inner part of the media with associated degenerative vascular cytoplasmic swelling (V) (hematoxylin–azophyloxine; **A**, ×120, **B**, ×300). (After Michiels JJ, Ten Kate FWJ, Vuzevski VD, Abels J. Histopathology of erythromelalgia in thrombocythaemia. Histopathology 1984;8: 669)

TABLE 14-3. Clinical Features of Essential Thrombocythemia in 37 Patients

Symptom	Affected Patients
Splenomegaly	14 (38%)
Weakness	14 (38%)
Hemorrhage	13 (35%)
Headache	13 (35%)
Paresthesia	11 (30%)
Dizziness	9 (24%)
Weight loss	9 (24%)
Sweating	8 (22%)
Visual phenomena	7 (19%)
Hepatomegaly	6 (16%)
Fever	6 (16%)
Peripheral vascular insufficiency	5 (14%)
Pruritus	5 (14%)
Venous thrombosis	4 (11%)
Myocardial ischemia	4 (11%)
Gout	4 (11%)
Epilepsy	2 (5%)
Stroke	1 (3%)
Peptic ulcer	1 (3%)
Transient drooping of eyelid	1 (3%)

(Iland HJ, Laszlo J, Peterson P, et al. Essential thrombocythemia: clinical and laboratory characteristics at presentation. Trans Assoc Am Physicians 1983;96:165)

TABLE 14-4. Peripheral Blood Findings in 37 Patients With Essential Thrombocythemia

Parameter	Median	Range
Platelet count (per μL)	1,300,000	1,000,000–2,650,000
Hemoglobin (gm/dL)	13.8	10–18.8
Hematocrit (%)	41	32–57
Red cell mass (mL/kg)	25	15–34
Reticulocyte count (per μL)	61,600	17,000–555,700
Leukocyte count (per μL)	11,500	6000–41,100
Basophil count (per μL)	0	0–346
Eosinophil count (per μL)	242	0–1780
Leukocyte alkaline phosphatase score	79	0–171

(Iland HJ, Laszlo J, Peterson P, et al. Essential thrombocythemia: clinical and laboratory characteristics at presentation. Trans Assoc Am Physicians 1983;96:165)

One third of patients had a slightly increased reticulocyte count. LAP scores ranged from zero to 171, with a median of 79; only three patients had scores less than 20. One patient had a LAP score of zero, but no other features suggestive of CML. RBC morphology was normal, and no patient had changes in RBC morphology suggestive of splenic atrophy.

All 37 patients studied had marrow aspirates and biopsies. The reticulin content was only slightly increased in 20% of patients. Cellularity was moderately increased, whereas megakaryocyte number was moderately to markedly increased. The megakaryocytes were abnormal and had varying degrees of cellular atypia, including hyperlobulated nuclei and irregular chromatin. Clustering of megakaryocytes was seen frequently. Erythroid and myeloid precursors were also increased, but not as significantly as those of the megakaryocyte line. Iron stains revealed adequate iron stores, and ringed sideroblasts were rarely seen.

Marrow cytogenetic studies do not show a characteristic abnormality. Of the 37 PVSG patients studied, 29 had acceptable karyotypes for review. In 23, the karyotypes were totally normal. Four patients with aneuploidy had random abnormalities. There was only one karyotype with a definite abnormal clone, which included a 20q− cell and one or more of the following cell types: 1p−, 2p−, 8p−, or −7. Two patients had a lesser degree of aneuploidy and were classified as possibly being abnormal. By definition, none of the patients had the Ph chromosome. In one study,[13] five consecutive untreated patients with ET had a nonrandom clone of 21q− cells. In another study,[120] however, 12 of 14 patients were totally normal, with one patient showing a translocation between chromosomes 2 and 9 (t:2q+;9p−), and the other a 16q− cell. The 21q− abnormality has not been a consistent finding.

Uric acid was elevated in 22% of males and 28% of females.[10,60] Serum B_{12} levels were elevated in 29% of the patients, with the unbound vitamin B_{12}–binding capacity at a median of 1400 pg/mL. Only one patient had a value over 2200 pg/mL. Serum vitamin B_{12}– and unbound B_{12}–binding capacity levels are similar to those seen in PV but are less markedly elevated than has been reported in CML. Lactate dehydrogenase (LDH) levels are also increased, with a mean in one study of 342 IU. Plasma LDH levels are similar to serum levels, indicating that platelets were probably not the source of the elevation of the enzyme. LDH levels are also increased in PV and all the other chronic myeloproliverative disorders; the highest levels are seen in MMM. Elevated serum potassium levels and low blood sugar levels may be in vitro artifacts caused by the excessive number of platelets.

Bleeding times vary but are usually normal in ET.[28,121,119] There is no observable relation between the bleeding times and the degree of thrombocytosis (Fig. 14-11). Despite the relatively normal bleeding times, a number of qualitative platelet defects have been defined.[28,30,97,118,119,122] Abnormal

TABLE 14-5. Bone Marrow Findings in 37 Patients With Essential Thrombocythemia

Parameter	Normal	Slightly Increased	Moderately Increased	Markedly Increased
Cellularity	4	7	22	4
Megakaryocyte number	0	3	10	24
Erythroid elements	6	12	15	4
Myeloid elements	7	11	17	2
Reticulin content	29	7	1	0

(Iland HJ, Laszlo J, Peterson P, et al. Essential thrombocythemia: clinical and laboratory characteristics at presentation. Trans Assoc Am Physicians 1983;96:165)

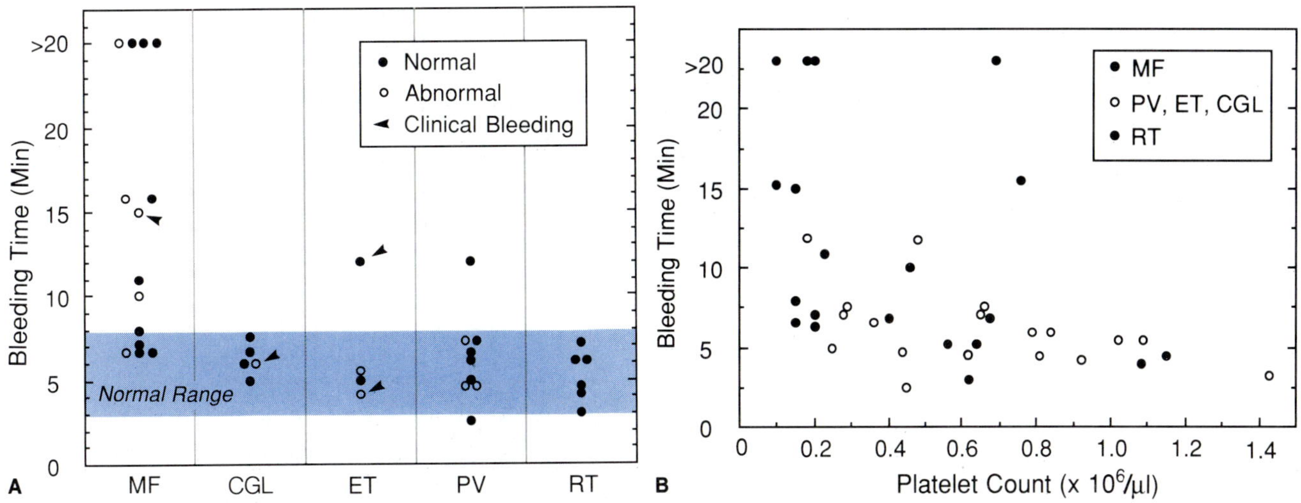

FIGURE 14-11. (**A**) Template bleeding time in myeloproliferative disease (MPD). Subclassifications are myelofibrosis (MF), chronic granulocytic leukemia (CGL), essential thrombocytopenia (ET), polycythemia vera (PV), and reactive thrombocytosis (RT). Bleeding time commonly was elevated in MF but rarely in other diseases. (**B**) Template bleeding times compared with platelet count in MPD. Prolonged bleeding times were seen at all levels of platelet count in MF. Thrombocytosis per se did not result in prolongation of bleeding time. (After Murphy S, Davis JL, Walsh PN, Gardner FH. Template bleeding time and clinical hemorrhage in myeoloproliferative disease. Arch Intern Med 1978;138:1252)

platelet aggregation to epinephrine, collagen, and ADP is frequent. In addition, defects characteristic of acquired storage pool disease, as well as abnormalities in the platelet membrane and within the platelet itself, have been described (Table 14-6). Unfortunately, there is no single specific qualitative abnormality that helps define a patient as having ET or that helps predict bleeding or thrombosis. Although a number of abnormalities have been found in platelet aggregation studies, the most characteristic defect is loss of both the primary and secondary wave of aggregation with epinephrine. In more than 325 studies of platelet aggregation in myeloproliferative disorders, including ET, 57% of the patients had abnormal aggregation with epinephrine, 37% with collagen, and 39% with ADP.[97] In the same study, only 17% had abnormal bleeding times. Figure 14-12 demonstrates the comparative analysis of platelet aggregation in patients with ET, PV, CML, and RT. The patterns in PV and ET are similar. There is no correlation between aggregation abnormalities and clinical

TABLE 14-6. Qualitative Platelet Abnormalities

Bleeding time
Abnormal platelet aggregation
Epinephrine
Collagen
ADP
Acquired storage-pool disease
Abnormal platelet membrane
Glycoprotein abnormalities
Receptor abnormalities:
α_2-Adrenergic receptors reduced
Fc receptors increased
Prostaglandin D_2 receptors reduced
Decreased procoagulant activity
Acquired von Willebrand's disease
Abnormal arachidonic acid metabolism
Reduced lipoxygenase activity

events. Six of 14 patients studied had no symptoms, 5 had thrombotic complications, and 3 had bleeding tendency. These studies revealed a clear difference between MPD thrombocytosis and RT, with consistently normal studies in the latter.

The epinephrine aggregation defect is in contrast to the absence of only the second wave of aggregation seen in storage pool disease and aspirin-like defects. Epinephrine-induced aggregation is initiated by the binding of epinephrine to α_2-adrenergic receptors on the platelet surface membrane. A 50% to 60% reduction in the number of α_2-adrenergic receptors is associated with a diminished aggregation response and serotonin release. A similar defect has also been found in a family whose members have impaired platelet aggregation and secretion responses to epinephrine with normal responses to ADP and collagen.[123] This familial disorder was associated with a mild bleeding diathesis.

Spontaneous platelet aggregation at either 23° or 37°C is seen in a significant number of patients with thrombocytosis secondary to myeloproliferative disorders.[124] The supernatant derived from ET patients' platelet-rich plasma after spontaneous aggregation can induce aggregation of normal platelet-rich plasma. Aspirin administration can abolish spontaneous aggregation in practically all cases. Circulating platelet aggregates may be estimated by a formalin fixation method described by Wu and Hoak.[125] Aliquots of blood are collected into formalin or ethylenediaminetetraacetic acid (EDTA). Formalin fixes circulating platelet aggregates while EDTA breaks up the aggregates. Therefore, the ratio of the platelet count in a formalin solution to that of an EDTA solution is referred to as the *platelet aggregate index*. With this method, circulating platelet aggregates were significantly increased in ET patients, and their number correlated with the clinical occurrence of thrombosis[126] (Table 14-7). Circulating platelet aggregates were also increased in PV but did not always correlate with clinical complications.[124] Whether the thromboses are actually caused by circulating platelet aggregates or the aggregates form as a result of the thrombosis remains unclear.

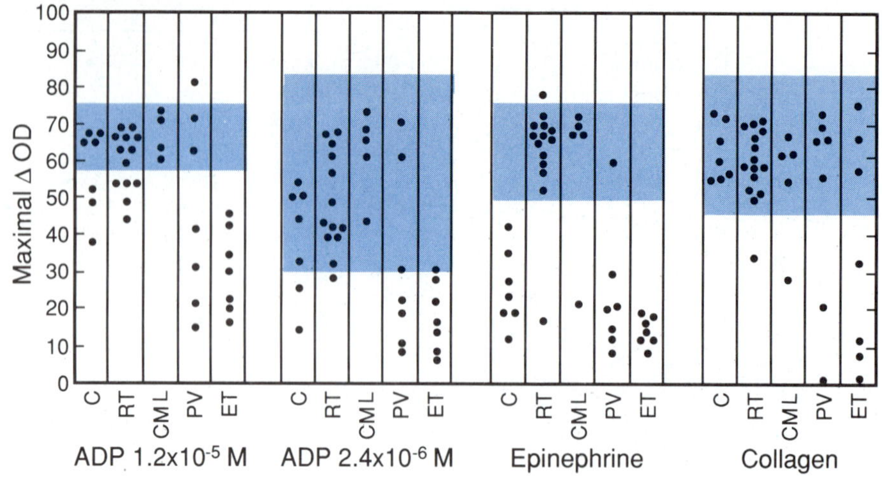

FIGURE 14-12. Platelet aggregation in thrombocytosis. Each dot represents the maximal change in optical density (OD) of platelet-rich plasma from a single individual after aggregation with the varying aggregating agents shown. The columns group patients in the different diagnostic categories. The shaded areas represent 2 standard deviations on either side of the mean calculated from maximum optical densities noted in 48 normal subjects. The columns showing abnormal controls refer to 7 subjects arbitrarily excluded from these calculations because of impaired adrenaline (epinephrine) aggregation. ADP, adenosine diphosphate; C, abnormal controls; RT, reactive thrombocytosis; CML, chronic myeloid leukemia; PV, polycythemia vera; ET, essential thrombocytopenia. (After Ginsburg AD. Platelet function in patients with high platelet counts. Ann Intern Med 1975;82:506)

Boughton and colleagues[127] theorized that the platelets produced in ET are normal but acquire abnormalities in the circulation (Fig. 14-13). This theory would help explain the many conflicting reports on platelet function in thrombocytosis of myeloproliferative disorders. Functionally viable platelets are released into the circulation and are then injured by various factors that cause diffuse intravascular platelet aggregation. Platelet aggregates could result in (1) large vessel thromboembolism followed by hemorrhagic infarction and bleeding; (2) platelet functional injury and impaired hemostasis; or (3) microvascular symptoms such as erythromelalgia, and distal gangrene. Supporting this theory are the observations that platelet survival is shortened and that damaged, or "spent," platelets are seen in circulating blood.[40] In addition, elevated levels of β-thromboglobulin, a platelet-specific protein, are found in the plasma of ET patients and reflect platelet activation.[128] The appearance of "disseminated intravascular platelet aggregation" leading to thrombosis or bleeding, or both, may be due to an acquired storage-pool disease. This theory is supported by the observed depletion of serotonin and α-granule proteins like platelet factor 4 and β-thromboglobulin.[128–131] The combination of shortened platelet survival, depletion of platelet-specific proteins, and the increased plasma levels of these same proteins supports the theory that storage-pool disease in ET is acquired as platelets are activated and degranulate in the circulation. This theory conflicts with the concept that platelet changes originate in an abnormal megakaryocyte clone and suggests that both abnormal production and aberrant degranulation may take place.

Platelet Membrane and Receptor Abnormalities

Various abnormalities in membrane glycoproteins have been described.[132–135] There is a reduction in glycoproteins Ib, IIb, and IIIa, with a simultaneous increase in glycoprotein IV. No correlation has been made between bleeding or thrombosis and these glycoprotein abnormalities. Abnormalities in prostaglandin D_2 receptor and Fc receptor have also been described.[136–139] A decrease in prostaglandin D_2 receptors is not a unique finding for ET since it is also found in patients with acute venous thrombosis who have

TABLE 14-7. Summary of Platelet Hyperaggregability Studies

Group	Total No. of Patients	Circulating Platelet Aggregate Index	Spontaneous Platelet Aggregation (%)
Essential thrombocythemia	14	0.72 ± 0.05*	13.5 ± 7.5*
Polycythemia vera	7	0.76 ± 0.08†	12.6 ± 5*
Chronic myelocytic leukemia	3	0.92 ± 0.02	1
Myeloid metaplasia with myelofibrosis	4	0.82 ± 0.08	1.3
Reactive thrombocytosis	11	0.82 ± 0.06	2.1 ± 0.5
Normal subjects	32	0.91 ± 0.03	1.3 ± 1

* Denotes statistical significance with a *P* value < .01.
† Denotes statistical significance with a *P* value < .05.
(Wu KK. Platelet hyperaggregability and thrombosis in patients with thrombocythemia. Ann Intern Med 1978;88:7–11)

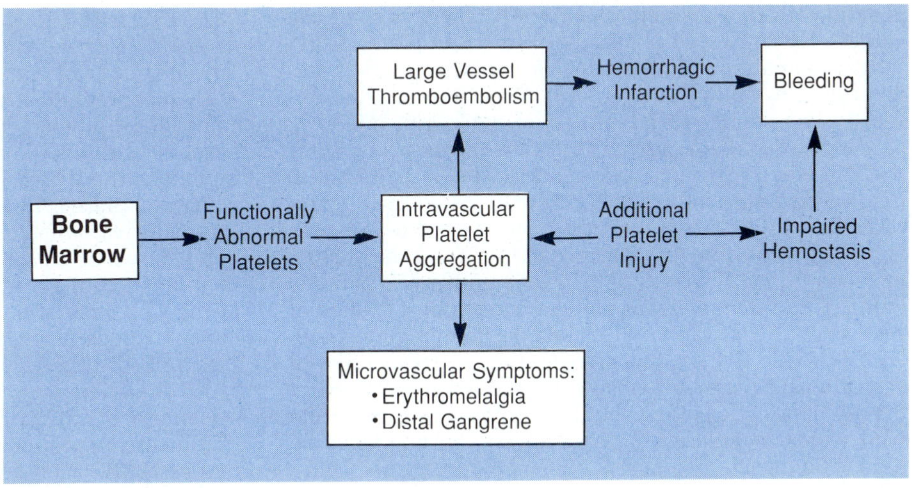

FIGURE 14-13. Schematic drawing showing the events surrounding diffuse intravascular platelet aggregation. (After Boughton BJ, Corbett WEN, Ginsburg AD. Myeloproliferative disorders: a paradox of in-vivo and in-vitro platelet function. J Clin Pathol 1977;30:228)

no evidence of a myeloproliferative disorder. The loss of these receptors, however, could lead to the platelet becoming more resistant to the antiaggregating activity of this prostaglandin. The increase in Fc receptors correlates with an increased release response to immunoglobulin aggregates, but there is no clinical correlation with the increased number of Fc receptors.

Platelet membrane abnormalities may also be characterized by abnormal platelet coagulant activity. Coagulation in plasma proceeds more rapidly in the presence of platelets. This procoagulant (factor X–activating) activity is decreased in ET.[129,140] One would expect increased bleeding associated with this abnormality, but there is no clinical correlation between decreased factor Xa activity and clinical symptoms.

Plasma Defects

An association has been reported between ET and acquired von Willebrand's disease.[141–145] A reduction in the large multimer forms of the vWF protein was first described in 1984.[141] There is a disproportionate reduction in the level of ristocetin cofactor activity, and the laboratory findings resemble the type II form of von Willebrand's disease. The mechanism underlying this phenomenon is unknown, and no anti-vWF antibodies or other inhibitory factors have been described. Both clinical bleeding and the laboratory abnormality have been corrected with reduction of the platelet count or infusion of the vasopressin analogue, DDAVP. The platelet receptor for vWF, glycoprotein Ib, and ristocetin-dependent vWF binding to platelets are normal in ET patients with acquired von Willebrand's syndrome.[146] The etiology of the acquired von Willebrand's syndrome in patients with ET is not completely understood. Leukocyte enzymes, possibly elastase, may degrade plasma vWF multimers. A recent study reports a close relation between platelet count and loss of high-molecular-weight multimers and suggests that vWF multimers are adsorbed to the platelet surface in ET and related myeloproliferative disorders.[146a]

Abnormal Arachidonic Acid Metabolism

A significant number of patients with myeloproliferative disorders, including ET, have abnormalities in platelet arachidonic acid metabolism.[147–152] Stimulated platelets release arachidonic acid from membrane phospholipids, which is then metabolized either by cyclooxygenase to PGG2 and then to thromboxane or by 12-lipoxygenase to 12-HPETE and then to 12-HETE. In one study,[150] most patients with myeloproliferative disease and ET had selective deficiency of platelet lipoxygenase with a compensatory increase in cyclooxygenase activity that resulted in increased thromboxane A_2 formation. It would have been anticipated that the clinical result of increased thromboxane production would be an increased incidence of thrombosis. Paradoxically, the risk of bleeding was significantly greater than the thrombotic risk in patients with lipoxygenase deficiency.

In summary, there are multiple platelet abnormalities in this disorder (see Table 14-6). The thrombotic and bleeding complications, however, cannot be directly correlated with the degree of thrombocytosis, prolongation of the bleeding time, or abnormalities of platelet aggregation.[122] In myeloproliferative disease with thrombocytosis, prolonged bleeding times were seen at all levels of platelet count. In addition, there is no correlation between bleeding time and aggregation abnormalities because a normal bleeding time did not rule out the possibility of clinical bleeding or a platelet aggregation abnormality. In addition, a prolonged bleeding time could be associated with both normal platelet aggregation and clinical bleeding. None of these findings has consistently correlated with clinical outcome. Although there are some associations, none has been definitive. Some abnormalities may be inherent to the platelet as it leaves the marrow or acquired as it travels through the circulation. Although controlling platelet count has significantly reduced the complications of bleeding and thrombosis, it has not eliminated them and raises the possibility of other etiologic factors.

THERAPY

The two most difficult clinical problems in ET are making the diagnosis and deciding whether to treat the patient. The PVSG has clearly shown that lowering the red count and hematocrit in PV reduces the risk, in asymptomatic patients, of a major complication.[153] The importance of lowering the platelet count in asymptomatic patients with ET has not been well demonstrated. The first step in evaluating patients for therapy is to determine whether the patient is symptomatic. The symptomatic patient is defined as one who is either in the midst of or has a history of acute thrombosis or hemorrhage. As was described earlier, there is no clearcut correlation between the degree of thrombocytosis and the risk of these complications. Therefore, in the asymptomatic patient, there is no convincing evidence that lowering the platelet count, even when the platelet count is 1000 to 2000 $\times$ 10^9/L, is warranted. No study of ET patients has demonstrated risk factors for complications in this asymptomatic group. There is some argument for considering therapy in the asymptomatic geriatric population, but it is not clear whether there is any difference in complications with respect to age. A prospective randomized trial of platelet reduction in elderly patients has not been carried out, nor is the natural history of ET in elderly patients well defined. The decision not to treat the asymptomatic patient is complicated by the concern that the first complication may be severe and irreversible. In addition, the concern of increased thrombosis in the perioperative setting may be amplified in patients with ET and may warrant platelet control or antiplatelet agents or anticoagulants in that setting. If immediate platelet suppression is needed preoperatively, irrespective of age, intensive plateletpheresis can be considered. Whether the asymptomatic patient should be further defined as one who has normal platelet aggregation and normal bleeding time is not clear.

Little controversy exists over the need to treat patients with prior or current thrombotic or hemorrhagic complications; however, the best therapy is unclear. Treatments that have been employed include plateletpheresis, alkylating agents (busulfan, melphalan (Alkeran), chlorambucil, uracil mustard), radiation therapy in the form of P^{32}, hydroxyurea, interferon, anagrelide, and antiplatelet agents. Dramatic reduction of the platelet count can be achieved safely and swiftly by plateletpheresis.[154–158] With each procedure, about 2 to 9 trillion platelets can be removed. Most patients have also been given myelosuppressive agents to maintain the therapeutic response initiated by plateletpheresis. In one study,[156] long-term suppression of platelet count was attempted with continued plateletpheresis. Although intensive pheresis at the rate of four to five procedures per week produced rapid lowering of the patient's platelet count, continued therapy at the rate of two or three procedures per week failed to maintain a normal or reduced platelet level, and the platelet count gradually increased to pretreatment levels. Thus, long-term plateletpheresis, a difficult procedure, is not cost-effective and is inadequate for long-term control. It should be reserved for rapid reduction of platelets in patients who have life-threatening thrombotic or hemorrhagic complications.

The platelet count can be lowered rapidly by administering an intravenous alkylating agent such as nitrogen mustard or thiotepa.[159] Both act rapidly, with the median platelet count falling from 1700 to to 1000 $\times$ 10^9/L within 3 weeks, and below 400 $\times$ 10^9/L by 6 weeks. Neither of these methods of intravenous chemotherapy produces unmaintained responses. Busulfan (Myleran), melphalan, uracil mustard, and radioactive phosphorous all cause a more gradual reduction in platelets.[160–162] The only randomized trial conducted in ET compared melphalan with radioactive phosphorous.[162] The initial dose for melphalan-treated patients was 10 mg/d for 5 consecutive days, with the dose then reduced to 2 mg/d for the next 3 weeks. The subsequent dose of melphalan was adjusted to maintain the platelet count between 200 and 400 $\times$ 10^9/L. The initial dose of P^{32} was 2.9 MCi/m^2, not to exceed 5 MCi per dose. Radioactive phosphorous was administered at 3-month intervals, if needed, to maintain the platelet count under 450 $\times$ 10^9/L. With melphalan, 11 of 13 patients had platelet counts under 450 $\times$ 10^9/L at both 3 and 6 months. This response rate was significantly better than the response to radioactive phosphorous at these early evaluation intervals. After 12 months, the response rates were similar. Thus, the response to P^{32} was gradual and would certainly be unsatisfactory for treating symptomatically acute patients, but it may provide a good means for long-term control. Pipobroman, another alkylating agent, resulted in a complete platelet response in 22 of 24 previously untreated patients.[163] The median time to a complete response was 12 weeks, with a range of 2 to 22 weeks. Unfortunately, 13 of the 22 patients who achieved a complete remission relapsed in spite of continued therapy. Despite good control with pipobroman, major thrombocythemia-related complications occurred, including gastrointestinal bleeding, cerebral thrombosis, retinal thrombosis, and progressive anemia without bleeding. With both alkylating agents and radiation, there is little difficulty in lowering the platelets, the major variable being the speed with which this is accomplished. Of great concern is the potential for long-term complication of a malignancy secondary to the alkylating agents and irradiation. From the experience with ovarian cancer, Hodgkin's disease, and PV, both forms of therapy may increase the incidence of acute leukemia and other types of malignancy.[164–166]

Concern about using mutagenic agents in patients with chronic myeloproliferative diseases has led to a search for other effective agents. Hydroxyurea and anagrelide are two such drugs. Hydroxyurea is an inhibitor of ribonucleoside reductase and does not induce mutations in vitro.[167] This agent, however, does cause chromosome breaks and is teratogenic in several species of animals. The PVSG tested hydroxyurea at 15 mg/kg/d by mouth in the therapy of thrombocytosis.[10] Initial reports suggested a response rate of over 80%. It is still too early to assess long-term side effects. In 51 patients with PV treated with hydroxyurea in a similar fashion, there have been three leukemic patients (P = 0.11 to 0.18) and an incidence of 15.7% for all thrombotic events.[168,168a] Discontinuation of the drug is associated with the rapid return of high levels of platelets, indicating that continued maintenance therapy is necessary.

Anagrelide (imidazole-2,1-b,quinazolin-2-1), while undergoing testing as a potential anticoagulant, was found to have a side effect of thrombocytopenia. In a phase I trial, Silverstein[169] treated 17 patients with ET, and 15 had a complete response. Anagrelide did not change marrow cellularity, morphology, or number of megakaryocytes, and the agent had no effect on short-term megakaryocyte cultures or production of CFU-M.[170,171] The method of action is unknown, although decreased platelet release from the marrow may be its mechanism.[171] Induction was best achieved with doses of 1.5 to 2.5 mg every 6 hours orally. Once a platelet level of under 400 $\times$ 10^9/L was achieved, the patient was given maintenance dose of 0.5 mg twice a day. Side effects included nausea, headache, and mild hypotension. Anagrelide inhibits platelet function and may cause bleeding complications. This agent is undergoing phase II and phase III studies in the treatment of myeloproliferative disease thrombocytosis.

Recombinant α-interferon has shown promising results when given subcutaneously at 3 million units three times a week.[172–175] In several studies, there was a greater than 50% decrease in the platelet count by day 28, and symptoms related to thrombocytosis resolved within 1 week. Maintenance therapy was required for continued control. The complications of α-interferon are well known, and about 20% of patients had to withdraw from therapy because of influenza-like symptoms. In addition, the leukocyte count fell during the treatment period. When added in vitro at initiation of culture, α-interferon inhibited the CFU-M growth of marrows from both normal subjects and patients with ET.[176] The obvious drawbacks of this form of therapy are the expense and the need to continue α-interferon on a maintenance schedule indefinitely.

Antiplatelet agents such as aspirin are efficient in alleviating the symptoms of erythromelalgia and transient central nervous system ischemia.[107,114] These agents have been used alone or in combination with a myelosuppressive agent, such as P^{32}, or an alkylating agent. It is likely that the risk of serious bleeding complications is increased with aspirin. Schafer[119] suggested an approach to the use of aspirin in patients with thrombocytosis. With the presence of digital ischemia or cerebral vascular ischemia in patients who have normal bleeding times and normal or spontaneous aggregation, antiplatelet agents are indicated. In a patient with a history of bleeding or a prolonged bleeding time, antiplatelet agents are contraindicated. The decision is more difficult when a patient gives a history of both thrombosis and bleeding, and empiric, individualized decisions are necessary.

A number of questions about aspirin therapy remain unanswered. First, the use of aspirin by asymptomatic patients may increase their risk of bleeding. For example, in the Physician's Aspirin Trial for Prevention of Myocardial Infarction,[177] there was a modest increase in the number of intracerebral bleeds in the aspirin-treated patients. The PVSG, which used older patients and higher doses of aspirin than are generally employed, showed that antiplatelet agents, even when given to patients who had a normal bleeding time and no history of bleeding, frequently caused hemorrhage that required hospitalization and transfusion.[178] We think that the risk/benefit ratio, particularly for patients over 45 years of age, is low enough that low-dose (eg, 80 to 325 mg/d) aspirin can be recommended. A second unanswered question is whether aspirin or other antiplatelet agents should be given to symptomatic patients without concomitant myelosuppression.

REFERENCES

1. Damashek W. Some speculations on the myeloproliferative syndromes. Blood 1951;6:372.
2. Laszlo J. Myeloproliferative disorders (MPD): myelofibrosis, myelosclerosis, extramedullary hematopoiesis, undifferentiated MPD, and hemorrhagic thrombocythemia. Semin Hematol 1975;12:409.
3. Epstein E, Goedel A. Hämorrhagische Thrombocythämie bei vasculärer Schrumfmilz. Virchows Arch [A] 1934;292:233.
4. di Guglielmo G. Eritroleucemia e plastrinemia. Folia Med 1920;1:36.
5. Fanger H, Cella LJ Jr, Lichtman H. Thrombocythemia: report of three cases and review of literature. N Engl J Med 1954;250:456.
6. McCabe WR, Bird RM, McLaughlin RA. Is primary hemorrhagic thrombocythemia a clinical myth? Ann Intern Med 1955;43:182.
7. Ozer FL, Truax WE, Miesch DC, Levin WC. Primary hemorrhagic thrombocythemia. Am J Med 1960;28:807.
8. Gunz FW. Hemorrhagic thrombocythemia: a critical review. Blood 1960;15:706.
9. Silverstein MN. Primary or hemorrhagic thrombocythemia. Arch Intern Med 1968;122:18.
10. Murphy S, Iland H, Rosenthal D, Laszlo J. Essential thrombocythemia: an interim report from the Polycythemia Vera Study Group. Semin Hematol 1986;23:177.
11. Bellucci S, Janvier M, Tobelem G, et al. Essential thrombocythemias: clinical evolutionary and biological data. Cancer 1986;58:2440.
12. Frick PG. Primary thrombocythemia: clinical, hematological, and chromosomal studies of 13 patients. Helv Med Acta 1969;35:20.
13. Zaccaria A, Tura S. A chromosomal abnormality in primary thrombocythemia. N Engl J Med 1978;298:1422.
14. Third International Workship on Chromosomes in Leukemia, 1980. Report of essential thrombocythemia. Cancer Genet Cytogenet 1981;4:138.
15. Knuutila S, Ruutu T, Partanen S, Vuopio P. Chromosome 1q+ in erythroid and granulocyte-monocyte precursors in a patient with essential thrombocythemia. Cancer Genet Cytogenet 1983;9:245.
16. Adamson JW, Fialkow PJ. The pathogenesis of myeloproliferative syndromes. Br J Haematol 1978;38:299.
17. Fialkow PJ, Faguet GB, Jacobson RJ, et al. Evidence that essential thrombocythemia is a clonal disorder with origin in a multipotent stem cell. Blood 1981;58:916.
18. Singal U, Prasad AS, Halton DM, Bishop C. Essential thrombocythemia: a clonal disorder of hematopoietic stem cell. Am J Hematol 1983;14:193.
19. Gaetani GF, Ferraris AM, Galiano S, et al. Primary thrombocythemia: clonal origin of platelets, erythrocytes, and granulocytes in a $Gd^{B}/Gd^{Mediterranean}$ subject. Blood 1982;59:76.
20. Gilliland G, Levy J, Perrin S, et al. Determination of clonality in myeloproliferative diseases using polymerase chain reaction. Clin Res 1989;37:601A.
21. Tefferi A, Thibodeau SN, Solberg LA. Clonal studies in the myelodysplastic syndrome using X-linked restriction fragment length polymorphisms. Blood 1990;75:1770.
22. Vogelstein B, Fearon ER, Hamilton SR, Feinberg AP. Use of restriction fragment length polymorphisms to determine the clonal origin of human timers. Science 1985;8:642.
23. Ts'ao CH, Rossi EC, Lestina FC. Abnormalities in platelet function and morphology in a case of thrombocythaemia. Arch Pathol Lab Med 1977;101:526.
24. Zeigler Z, Murphy S, Gardner FH. Microscopic platelet size and morphology in various hematologic disorders. Blood 1978;51:479.
25. Holme S, Simmonds M, Ballek R, Murphy S. Comparative measurements of platelet size by Coulter counter, microscopy of blood smears and light transmission studies. J Lab Clin Med 1981;97:610.
26. Small BM, Bettigole RE. Diagnosis of myeloproliferative disease by analysis of the platelet volume distribution. Am J Soc Clin Pathol 1981;76:685.
27. Dudley JM, Messinezy M, Eridani S, et al. Primary thrombocythaemia: diagnostic criteria and a simple scoring system for positive diagnosis. Br J Haematol 1989;71:331.
28. Murphy S. Thrombocytosis and thrombocythaemia. Clin Hematol 1983;12:89.
28a. Vadher BD, Machin SJ, Patterson KG, et al. Life-threatening thrombotic and haemorrhagic problems associated with silent myeloproliferative disorders. Br J Haematol 1993;85:213.
28b. Watson KV, Key N. Vascular complications of essential thrombocythaemia: a link to cardiovascular risk factors. Br J Haematol 1993;83:198.
29. Holme S, Murphy S. Studies of the platelet density abnormality in myeloproliferative disease. J Lab Clin Med 1984;103:373.
30. Boneu B, Nouvel C, Sie P, et al. Platelets in myeloproliferative disorders. I. A comparative evaluation with certain platelet function tests. Scand J Haematol 1980;25:214.
31. Maldonado JE, Pintads T, Pierre RV. Dysplastic platelets and circulating megakaryocytes in chronic myeloproliferative diseases. I. The platelets: ultrastructure and peroxidase reaction. Blood 1974;43:797.
32. Boughton BJ, Jerrome DW, Rychetnik M. Chronic myeloproliferative disorders: a quantitative assessment of platelet ultrastructure. Acta Haematol 1980;64:319.
33. Branehög I, Ridell B, Swolin B, Weinfeld A. Megakaryocyte quantifications in relation to thrombokinetics in primary thrombocythaemia and allied diseases. Scand J Haematol 1975;15:321.
34. Burkhardt R, Bartl R, Jager K, et al. Working classification of chronic myeloproliferative disorders based on histological, haematological, and clinical findings. J Clin Pathol 1986;39:237.
35. Thiele J, Schneider G, Hoeppnedr B, et al. Histomorphometry of bone marrow biopsies in chronic myeloproliferative disorders with associated thrombocytosis: features of significance for the diagnosis of primary (essential) thrombocythaemia. Virchows Arch [A] 1988;413:407.
36. Thiele J, Jansen B, Orth K-H, et al. Ultrastructure of megakaryocytes in the human bone marrow of patients with primary (essential) thrombocythemia. J Submicrosc Cytol Pathol 1988;20:671.
37. Mazur EM, Lindquist DL, de Alarcon PA, et al. Evaluation of bone marrow megakaryocyte ploidy distributions in persons with normal and abnormal platelet counts. J Lab Clin Med 1988;11:194.
38. Kutti J, Ridell B, Weinfeld A, Westin J. The relation of thrombokinetics to bone marrow megakaryocytes and to the size of the spleen in polycythaemia vera. Scand J Haematol 1973;10:88.
39. Branehög I, Ridell B, Swolin B, Weinfeld A. Megakaryocyte quantifications in relation to thrombokinetics in primary thrombocythaemia and allied diseases. Scand J Haematol 1975;15:321.
40. Harker LA, Finch CA. Thrombokinetics in man. J Clin Invest 1969;48:963.
41. Tomer A, Friese P, Conklin R, et al. Flow cytometric analysis of megakaryocytes from patients with abnormal platelet counts. Blood 1989;74:594.
42. Mazur EM, Hoffman R, Bruno E. Regulation of human megakaryocytopoiesis: an in vitro analysis. J Clin Invest 1981;68:733.
43. Hoffman R, Mazur E, Bruno E, Floyd V. Assay of an activity in the serum of patients with disorders of thrombopoiesis that stimulates formation of megakaryocyte colonies. N Engl J Med 1981;305:533.
44. Messner HA, Jamal N, Izaguirre C. The growth of large human megakaryocyte colonies from bone marrow. J Cell Physiol 1982;1:45.
45. Gerwitz AM, Bruno E, Elwell J. In vitro studies of megakaryocytopoiesis in thrombocytotic disorders of man. Blood 1983;61:384.
46. Komatsu N, Suda T, Eguchi M, et al. Megakaryocytopoiesis in vitro of patients with essential thrombocythaemia: effect of plasma and serum on megakaryocytic colony formation. Br J Haematol 1986;64:241.
47. Kimura H, Ishibashi T, Sato T, et al. Megakaryocytic colony formation (CFU-Meg) in essential thrombocythemia: quantitative and qualitative abnormalities of bone marrow CFU-Meg. Am J Hematol 1987;24:23.
48. Juvonen E, Partanen S, Ruutu T. Colony formation by megakaryocytic progenitors in essential thrombocythaemia. Br J Haematol 1987;66:161.
49. Han ZC, Briere J, Abgrall JF, et al. Spontaneous formation of megakaryocyte progenitors (CFU-MK) in primary thrombocythaemia. Acta Haematol 1987;78:51.
49a. Kobayashi S, Teramura M, Hoshino S, et al. Circulating megakaryocyte progenitors in myeloproliferative disorders are hypersensitive to interleukin-3. Br J Haematol 1993;83:539.
50. Eridani S, Sawyer B, Pearson TC. Patterns of in vitro BFU-E prolif-

eration in different forms of polycythaemia and thrombocythaemia. Eur J Haematol 1987;38:363.
51. Mazur EM, Cohen JL, Bogart L. Growth characteristics of circulating hematopoietic progenitor cells from patients with essential thrombocythemia. Blood 1988;71:1544.
52. Han ZC, Briere J, Abgrall JF, et al. Characteristics of megakaryocyte colony formation in normal individuals and in primary thrombocythemia: studies using an optimal cloning system. Exp Hematol 1989;17:46.
53. Shreiner DP, Weinberg J, Enoch D. Plasma thrombopoietic activity in humans with normal and abnormal platelet counts. Blood 1980;56:183.
54. Greenberg SM, Rosenthal DS, Greeley TA, et al. Characterization of a new megakaryocytic cell line: the Dami cell. Blood 1988;72:1968.
55. Ogura M, Morishima Y, Ohno R, et al. Establishment of leukemia cell line MEG-01 with positive Philadelphia chromosome. Blood 1985;66:1384.
56. Tange T, Nakahara K, Mitani K, et al. Establishment of a human megakaryoblastic cell line (T-33) from chronic myelogenous leukemia in megakaryoblastic crisis. Cancer Res 1988;48:6137.
57. Sledge G, Glant M, Jansen J, et al. Establishment in long term culture of megakaryocytic leukemia cells (EST-IU) from the marrow of a patient with leukemia and a mediastinal germ cell neoplasm. Cancer Res 1986;46:2155.
58. Komatsu N, Suda T, Morui M, et al. Growth and differentiation of a human megakaryoblastic cell line, CMK. Blood 1989;74:42.
59. Ogura M, Morishima Y, Okumura M, et al. Functional and morphological differentiation induction of a human megakaryoblastic leukemia cell line (MEG-01S) by phorbol diesters. Blood 1988;72:49.
60. Iland HJ, Laszlo J, Peterson P, et al. Essential thrombocythemia: clinical and laboratory characteristics at presentation. Trans Assoc Am Physicians 1983;96:165.
61. Iland HJ, Laszlo J, Case DC, et al. Differentiation between essential thrombocythemia and polycythemia vera with marked thrombocytosis. Am J Hematol 1987;25:191.
62. Berk PD, Goldberg JD, Silverstein MN, et al. Increased incidence of acute leukemia in PV associated with chlorambucil therapy. N Engl J Med 1981;304:441.
63. Rosenthal DS, Moloney WC. Occurrence of acute leukaemia in myeloproliferative disorders. Br J Haematol 1977;36:373.
64. Fickers M, Speck B. Thrombocythaemia: familial occurrence and transition into blast crisis. Acta Haematol 1974;51:257.
65. Geller SA, Shapiro E. Acute leukemia as a natural sequel to primary thrombocythemia. Am J Clin Pathol 1982;77:353.
66. Frei-Lahr D, Barton JC, Hoffman R, et al. Blastic transformation of essential thrombocythemia: dual expression of myelomonoblastic/megakaryoblastic phenotypes. Blood 1984;63:866.
67. Sedlacek SM, Curtis JL, Weintraub J, Levin J. Essential thrombocythemia and leukemic transformation. Medicine 1986;65:353.
68. Ginsburg AD. Thrombocytosis and thrombocythaemia. In: Root WS, Berliner RW, eds. Physiological pharmacology, vol 5. New York, Academic Press, 1974:199.
69. Iland H, Laszlo J. Thrombocytosis. Med Grand Rounds 1984;3:225.
70. Morowitz DA, Allen LW, Kirsner JB. Thrombocytosis in chronic inflammatory bowel disease. Ann Intern Med 1968;68:1013.
71. Levin J, Conley CL. Thrombocytosis associated with malignant disease. Arch Intern Med 1964;114:497.
72. Silvis SE, Turkbas N, Doscherholmen A. Thrombocytosis in patients with lung cancer. JAMA 1970;211:1852.
73. Knizley H Jr, Noyes WD. Iron deficiency anemia, papilledema, thrombocytosis, and transient hemiparesis. Arch Intern Med 1972;129:483.
74. Desforges JF, Bigelow FS, Chalmers TC. The effects of massive gastrointestinal hemorrhage on hemostasis. I. The blood platelets. J Lab Clin Med 1954;43:501.
75. Bunn HF. 5q− and disordered haematopoiesis. Clin Hematol 1986;15:1023.
76. Swolin B, Weinfeld A, Ridell B, et al. On the 5q− deletion: clinical and cytogenetic observations in ten patients and review of literature. Blood 1981;58:986.
77. Streeter RR, Presant CA, Reinhard E. Prognostic significance of thrombocytosis in idiopathic sideroblastic anemia. Blood 1977;50:427.
78. Ghosh P. Thrombocytosis in rheumatoid arthritis. Br J Clin Pract 1986;40:388.
79. Marchasin S, Wallerstein RD, Aggeler PM. Variation of the platelet count in disease. Calif Med 1964;101:95.
80. Baynes RD, Bothwell TH, Flax H, et al. Reactive thrombocytosis in pulmonary tuberculosis. J Clin Pathol 1987;40:676.
81. Thomas GA, O'Brien RT. Thrombocytosis in children with hemophilus influenzae meningitis. Clin Pediatr 1986;25:610.
82. Lipson RL, Bayrd ED, Watkins CH. The postsplenectomy blood picture. Am J Clin Pathol 1959;32:526.
83. Hirsh J, Dacie JC. Persistent post-splenectomy thrombocytosis and thrombo-embolism: a consequence of continuing anaemia. Br J Haematol 1966;12:44.
84. Bensinger TA, Logue GL, Rundles RW. Hemorrhagic thrombocythemia: control of postsplenectomy thrombocytosis with melphalan. Blood 1970;36:61.
85. Starksen NF, Day AT, Gazzaniga AB. Does splenectomy result in a higher incidence of limb deep venous thrombosis? Am J Surg 1978;135:202.
86. Coon WW, Penner J, Clagett GP. Deep venous thrombosis and postsplenectomy thrombocytosis. Arch Surg 1978;113:429.
87. Boxer MA, Braun J, Ellman L. Thromboembolic risk of post-splenectomy thrombocytosis. Arch Surg 1978;113:808.
88. Gordon DH, Schaffner D, Bennett JM, Schwartz SI. Postsplenectomy thrombocytosis. Arch Surg 1978;113:713.
89. Stoll DB, Peterson P, Exten R, et al. Clinical presentation and natural history of patients with essential thrombocythemia and the Philadelphia chromosome. Am J Hematol 1988;27:77.
90. Morris CM, Fitzgerald PH, Hollings PE, et al. Essential thrombocythaemia and the Philadelphia chromosome. Br J Haematol 1988;70:13.
91. Michiels JJ, Prins ME, Hagermeijer A, et al. Philadelphia chromosome-positive thrombocythemia and megakaryoblast leukemia. Am J Clin Pathol 1987;88:645.
92. Hoagland HC, Silverstein MN. Primary thrombocythemia in the young patients. Mayo Clin Proc 1978;53:578.
93. Davis RB. Acute thrombotic complications of myeloproliferative disorders in young adults. Am J Clin Pathol 1985;84:180.
94. Eyster ME, Saletan SL, Rabellino EM, et al. Familial essential thrombocythemia. Am J Med 1986;80:497.
95. Mitus AJ, Barbui T, Shulman LN, et al. Hemostatic complications in young patients with essential thrombocythemia. Blood 1989;74:274a.
96. Murphy MF, Clarke CRA, Brearley BL. Superior sagittal sinus thrombosis and essential thrombocythaemia. Br Med J 1983;287:1344.
97. Ginsburg AD. Platelet function in patients with high platelet counts. Ann Intern Med 1975;82:506.
98. Virmani R, Popovsky MA, Roberts WC. Thrombocytosis, coronary thrombosis and acute myocardial infarction. Am J Med 1979;67:498.
99. Pick RA, Glover MU, Nanfro JJ, et al. Acute myocardial infarction with essential thrombocythemia in a young man. Am Heart J 1983;106:406.
100. Saffitz JE, Phillips ER, Temesy-Armos PN, et al. Thrombocytosis and fatal coronary heart disease. Am J Cardiol 1983;52:651.
101. Kaibara M, Kubayashi T, Matsumoto S. Idiopathic thrombocythemia and pregnancy: report of a case. Obstet Gynecol 1985;65:185.
102. Mercer B, Drouin J, Jolly E, D'Anjou G. Primary thrombocythemia in pregnancy: a report of two cases. Am J Obstet Gynecol 1988;159:127.
103. Falconer J, Pineo G, Blahey W, et al. Essential thrombocythemia associated with recurrent abortions and fetal growth retardation. Am J Hematol 1987;25:345.
104. Singh AK, Wetherley-Mein G. Microvascular occlusive lesions in primary thrombocythaemia. Br J Haematol 1977;36:553.
105. Jabaily J, Iland HJ, Laszlo J, et al. Neurologic manifestations of essential thrombocythemia. Ann Intern Med 1983;99:513.
106. Lahuerta-Palacios JJ, Bornstein R, Fernandez-Debora FJ, et al. Controlled and uncontrolled thrombocytosis: its clinical role in essential thrombocythemia. Cancer 1988;61:1207.
107. Preston FE, Emmanuel IG, Winfield DA, Malia RG. Essential thrombocythaemia and peripheral gangrene. Br Med J 1974;3:548.
108. Mitchell SW. On a rare vaso-motor neurosis of the extremities, and on the maladies with which it may be confounded. Am J Med Sci 1878;76:2.
109. Babb RR, Alarcon-Segovia D, Fairbairn JF II. Erythermalgia: review of 51 cases. Circulation 1964;29:136.
110. Alarcon-Segovia D, Babb RR, Fairbairn JF II. Erythermalgia: a clue to the early diagnosis of myeloproliferative disorders. Arch Intern Med 1966;117:511.
111. Redding KG. Thrombocythemia as a cause of erythermalgia. Arch Dermatol 1977;113:468.
112. Michiels JJ, Ten Kate FWJ, Vuzevski VD, Abels J. Histopathology of erythromelalgia in thrombocythaemia. Histopathology 1984;8:669.
113. Michiels JJ, Abels J, Steketee J, et al. Erythromelalgia caused by platelet-mediated arteriolar inflammation and thrombosis in thrombocythemia. Ann Intern Med 1985;102:466.
114. Vera JC. Antiplatelet agents in the treatment of thrombotic complications of primary thrombocythemia. Can Med Assoc J 1979;120:60.
115. Alexandridis K, Cocovinis C, Tsigalidou V. Syndrome de Budd-Chiari et polythémie vraie. Rev Int Hepatol 1959;9:293.
116. Valla D, Casdevall N, Lacombe C, et al. Primary myeloproliferative disorder and hepatic vein thrombosis: a prospective study of erythroid colony formation in vitro in 20 patients with Budd-Chiari syndrome. Ann Intern Med 1985;103:329.
117. Bello Nicolau I, Conde Zurita JM, Barrientos Guzman A, et al. Essential thrombocytosis with acute renal failure due to bilateral thrombosis of the renal arteries and veins. Nephron 1982;32:73.
118. Colman RW, Hirsh J, Marder V, Salzman E. Platelet production and destruction. In: Hemostasis and thrombosis, ed 2. Philadelphia, JB Lippincott, 1982:752.
119. Schafer AI. Bleeding and thrombosis in the myeloproliferative disorders. Blood 1984;64:1.
120. Köpf I, Swolin B, Weinfeld A. Cytogenetic studies on primary thrombocythaemia. Heriditas 1982;97:217.
121. Murphy S, Davis JL, Walsh PN, Gardner FH. Template bleeding time

and clinical hemorrhage in myeloproliferative disorders. Arch Intern Med 1978;138:1251.
122. Schafer AI. Pathophysiology of bleeding and thrombosis in myeloproliferative disorders. In: Barbui T, Cortelazzo S, Viero P, et al, eds. Cellular blood components in haemostasis and thrombosis. Paris, John Libbey Eurotext, 1988:1.
123. Rao AK, Willis J, Kowalska MA, et al. Differential requirements for platelet aggregation and inhibition of adenylate cyclase by epinephrine: studies of a familial platelet alpha$_2$-adrenergic receptor defect. Blood 1988;71:494.
124. Barbui T, Battista R, Dini E. Spontaneous platelet aggregation in myeloproliferative disorders. Acta Haematol 1973;50:25.
125. Wu KK, Hoak JC. A new method for the quantitative detection of platelet aggregates in patients with arterial insufficiency. Lancet 1974;2:924.
126. Wu KK. Platelet hyperaggregability and thrombosis in patients with thrombocythemia. Ann Intern Med 1978;88:7.
127. Boughton BJ, Corbett WEN, Ginsburg AD. Myeloproliferative disorders: a paradox of in-vivo and in-vitro platelet function. J Clin Pathol 1977;30:228.
128. Boughton BJ, Allington MJ, King A. Platelet and plasma β thromboglobulin in myeloproliferative syndromes and secondary thrombocytosis. Br J Haematol 1978;40:125.
129. Walsh PN, Murphy S, Barry WE. The role of platelets in the pathogenesis of thrombosis and hemorrhage in patients with thrombocytosis. Thromb Haemost 1977;38:1085.
130. Martinez J, Shapiro SS, Holburn R, et al. Metabolism of human prothrombin and fibrinogen in patients with thrombocytosis secondary to myeloproliferative states. Blood 1973;42:35.
131. Luzzatto G, Fabris F, Mazzucato M, Girolami A. PF$_4$ versus βTG as evidence of platelet activation in myeloproliferative disorders. Scand J Haematol 1985;35:299.
132. Bolin RB, Okumura T, Jamieson GA. Changes in distribution of platelet membrane glycoproteins in patients with myeloproliferative disorders. Am J Hematol 1977;3:63.
133. Eche N, Sie P, Caranobe C, et al. Platelets in myeloproliferative disorders. III. Glycoprotein profile in relation to platelet function and platelet density. Scand J Haematol 1981;26:123.
134. Clezardin P, McGregor JL, Dechavanne M, Clemetson KJ. Platelet membrane glycoprotein abnormalities in patients with myeloproliferative disorders and secondary thrombocytosis. Br J Haematol 1985;60:331.
135. Booth WJ, Berndt MC, Castaldi PA. An altered platelet granule glycoprotein in patients with essential thrombocythemia. J Clin Invest 1984;73:291.
136. Cooper B, Schafer AI, Puchalsky D, Handin RI. Platelet resistance to prostaglandin D_2 in patients with myeloproliferative disorders. Blood 1978;52:618.
137. Schafer AI, Cooper B, O'Hara D, Handin RI. Identification of platelet receptors for prostaglandin I_2 and D_2. J Biol Chem 1979;254:2914.
138. Cooper B, Ahern D. Characterization of the platelet prostaglandin D_2 receptors in platelets of patients with myeloproliferative disorders. J Clin Invest 1979;64:586.
139. Moore A, Nachman RL. Platelet F_c receptor: increased expression in myeloproliferative disease. J Clin Invest 1981;67:1064.
140. Semeraro N, Cortellazzo S, Colucci M, Barbui T. A hitherto undescribed defect of platelet coagulant activity in polycythaemia vera and essential thrombocythaemia. Thromb Res 1979;16:795.
141. Budde U, Schaefer G, Mueller N, et al. Acquired von Willebrand's disease in the myeloproliferative syndrome. Blood 1984;64:981.
142. Sato K. Plasma von Willebrand factor abnormalities in patients with essential thrombocythemia. Keio J Med 1988;37:54.
143. Raman BKS, Sawdyk M, Saeed M. Essential thrombocythemia with acquired von Willebrand's disease. Am J Clin Pathol 1987;88:102.
144. Fabris F, Casonato A, Del Ben MG, et al. Abnormalities of von Willebrand factor in myeloproliferative disease: a relationship with bleeding diathesis. Br J Haematol 1986;63:75.
145. Meschengieser S, Blanco A, Woods A, et al. Intraplatelet levels of vWF:Ag and fibrinogen in myeloproliferative disorders. Thromb Res 1987;48:311.
146. Budde U, Dent JA, Berkowitz SD, et al. Subunit composition of plasma von Willebrand factor in patients with the myeloproliferative syndrome. Blood 1986;68:1213.
146a. Budde U, Scharf RE, Franke P, et al. Elevated platelet count as a cause of abnormal von Willebrand factor multimer distribution in plasma. Blood 1993;82:1749.
147. Okuma M, Uchino H. Altered arachidonate metabolism by platelets in patients with myeloproliferative disorders. Blood 1979;54:1258.
148. Nishimura J, Okamoto S, Ibayashi H. Abnormalities of platelet adenine nucleotides in patients with myeloproliferative disorders. Thromb Haemost 1979;41:787.
149. Russell NH, Salmon J, Keenan JP, Bellingham AJ. Platelet adenine nucleotides and arachidonic acid metabolism in the myeloproliferative disorders. Thromb Res 1981;22:389.
150. Schafer AI. Deficiency of platelet lipoxygenase activity in myeloproliferative disorders. N Engl J Med 1982;306:381.
151. Okuma M. Platelet function and arachidonate metabolism in patients with myeloproliferative disorders. Acta Haematol Jpn 1980;43:1139.
152. Colombi M, Manfreda M, Radaelli F, et al. Platelet thromboxane synthesis in thrombocythemia patients. In: Barbui T, Cortelazzo S, Viero P, et al, eds. Cellular blood components in haemostasis and thrombosis. Paris, John Libbey Eurotext, 1988:175.
153. Berk PD, Goldberg JD, Donovan PB, et al. Therapeutic recommendations in polycythemia vera based on Polycythemia Vera Study Group protocols. Semin Hematol 1986;23:132.
154. Taft EG, Babcock RB, Scharfman WB, Tartaglia AP. Plateletpheresis in the management of thrombocytosis. Blood 1977;50:927.
155. Younger J, Umlas J. Rapid reduction of platelet count in essential hemorrhagic thrombocythemia by discontinuous flow plateletpheresis. Am J Med 1978;64:659.
156. Goldfinger D, Thompson R, Lowe C, et al. Long-term plateletpheresis in the management of primary thrombocytosis. Transfusion 1979;19: 336.
157. Orlin JB, Berkman EM. Improvement of platelet function following plateletpheresis in patients with myeloproliferative diseases. Transfusion 1980;20:540.
158. Greenberg BR, Watson-Williams EJ. Successful control of life-threatening thrombocytosis with a blood processor. Transfusion 1975;15: 620.
159. Case DC. Therapy of essential thrombocythemia with thiotepa and chlorambucil. Blood 1984;63:51.
160. Fountain JR, Losowsky MS. Haemorrhagic thrombocythaemia and its treatment with radioactive phosphorus. Q J Med 1962;31:207.
161. Van de Pette JEW, Prochazka AV, Pearson TC, et al. Primary thrombocythemia treated with busulphan. Br J Haematol 1986;62:229.
162. Murphy S, Rosenthal DS, Weinfeld A, et al. Essential thrombocythemia: response during first year of therapy with melphalan and radioactive phosphorus: a Polycythemia Vera Study Group report. Cancer Treat Rep 1982;66:1495.
163. Brusamolino E, Canevari A, Salvaneschi L, et al. Efficacy trial of pipobroman in essential thrombocythemia: a study of 24 patients. Cancer Treat Rep 1984;68:1339.
164. Berk PD, Goldberg JD, Silverstein MN, et al. Increased incidence of acute leukemia in polycythemia vera associated with chlorambucil therapy. N Engl J Med 1981;304:441.
165. Kaldor JM, Day NE, Pettersson F, et al. Leukemia following chemotherapy for ovarian cancer. N Engl J Med 1990;322:1.
166. Kaldor JM, Day NE, Clarke EA, et al. Leukemia following Hodgkin's disease. N Engl J Med 1990;322:7.
167. Lofvenberg E, Wahlin A. Management of polycythaemia vera, essential thrombocythaemia and myelofibrosis with hydroxyurea. Eur J Haematol 1988;41:375.
168. Kaplan ME, Mack K, Goldberg JD, et al. Long-term management of polycythemia vera with hydroxyurea: a progress report. Semin Hematol 1986;23:167.
168a. Fruchtman SM, Kaplan ME, Peterson P, et al. Hydroxyurea in the management of polycythemia vera (PV): analysis of long-term leukemia gene potential. Clin Res 1992.
169. Silverstein MN, Petitt RM, Solberg LA Jr, et al. Anagrelide: a new drug for treating thrombocytosis. N Engl J Med 1988;318:1292.
170. Solberg LA Jr, Oles KJ, Tarach J, et al. The effects of anagrelide on human megakaryocytopoiesis. Blood 1989;74:20a.
171. Mazur EM, Sohl P, Newton J, Narendron A. Mechanism of anagrelide induced thrombocytopenia. Blood 1989;74:32a.
172. Giles FJ, Singer CRJ, Gray AG, et al. Alpha-interferon therapy for essential thrombocythaemia. Lancet 1988;2:70.
173. Gisslinger H, Ludwig H, Linkesch W, et al. Long-term interferon therapy for thrombocytosis in myeloproliferative diseases. Lancet 1989;1: 634.
174. Talpaz M, Kurzrock R, Kantarjian H, et al. Recombinant interferon-alpha therapy of Philadelphia chromosome-negative myeloproliferative disorders with thrombocytosis. Am J Med 1989;86:554.
175. Tichelli A, Gratwohl A, Berger C, et al. Treatment of thrombocytosis in myeloproliferative disorders with interferon alpha-2a. Blut 1989;58: 15.
176. Gugliotta L, Bagnara GP, Catani L, et al. In vivo and in vitro inhibitory effect of alpha-interferon on megakaryocyte colony growth in essential thrombocythaemia. Br J Haematol 1989;71:177.
177. Manson JE, Grobbee DE, Stampfer MJ, et al. Aspirin in the primary prevention of angina pectoris in a randomized trial of United States physicians. Am J Med 1990;89:772.
178. Barbui T, Buelli M, Cortelazzo S, et al. Aspirin and risk of bleeding in patients with thrombocythemia. Am J Med 1987;83:265.

Blood: Principles and Practice of Hematology,
edited by Robert I. Handin, Thomas P. Stossel, and Samuel E. Lux.
J.B. Lippincott Company, Philadelphia © 1995.

15

Chronic Myelogenous Leukemia

John M. Goldman
David I. Marks

HISTORY AND DEFINITIONS

Chronic myelogenous leukemia (CML), a term used interchangeably with chronic myeloid leukemia, chronic myelocytic leukemia, and chronic granulocytic leukemia, is a well-characterized disease that runs a biphasic or triphasic clinical course. Most patients are diagnosed in the stable or chronic phase, which usually persists for 2 to 6 years. The disease then transforms abruptly to a phase of blast cell transformation (also called blast crisis) or more insidiously to an intermediate phase of acceleration that then proceeds after some months (or sometimes years) to blast transformation.

CML was probably first defined as a discrete entity in 1848.[1] Various reports of leukemias that would today be recognized as CML were published in the second half of the last century. Radiation as a means of treatment was introduced in 1902.[2] The first comprehensive description of CML appeared in 1924.[3] An important landmark in the treatment of CML was the introduction of busulfan in 1953.[4] Of great importance was the discovery in 1960 of the G-group chromosomal abnormality[5] that was later named the Philadelphia (Ph) chromosome. The 1980s were a decade of substantial further progress. The Ph chromosome was found to carry a unique chimeric gene, the *bcr/abl* gene, which is expressed as a protein with pronounced kinase activity and is likely to play a fundamental role in the pathogenesis of the chronic phase of CML.[6,7] At the beginning of the 1980s, CML was generally regarded as an incurable disease; today, the fact that appreciable numbers of patients transplanted with bone marrow from HLA-identical siblings have survived for 10 or more years without evidence of relapse can be interpreted as evidence that CML is indeed curable. The challenges for the current decade are to elucidate further the molecular mechanisms underlying CML and to extend curative treatment to more patients.

One of the first sizable series of cases that could today reasonably be accepted as CML was published by Ward in 1917.[8] The peak age incidence was in the fifth decade, and males were affected more than females. In 1924, Minot and colleagues[3] reviewed 166 typical cases of CML. The greatest number of cases occurred in patients between the ages of 30 and 50 years; 56% of these patients were male and 44% were female. The delay between onset of symptoms and diagnosis was 1.4 years. Of 130 evaluable patients, the duration of disease for those treated by irradiation was 3.5 years, whereas for those not treated by irradiation, it was 3.04 years.

Since that time, a considerable number of patient series have been reported from the United States, Europe, and other countries,[9–13] and the picture is reasonably consistent worldwide. CML is diagnosed in all decades of life but has a peak incidence between the ages of 30 and 50 years. The slight predominance in males compared with females was confirmed. The median duration of survival from diagnosis ranged from 3 to 4.5 years in different series.

Although the morphologic appearances of blood and marrow were reasonably well characterized in the 1950s, nothing whatever was known of the pathogenesis of CML, and little was known about the degree of involvement of different hematopoietic lineages. A new era opened with the discovery of the Ph chromosome in 1960.[5,14] In 1973, Rowley[15] showed that the Ph chromosome was due to a reciprocal translocation involving chromosomes 9 and 22, termed t(9;22) (Fig. 15-1). In 1982, Heisterkamp and colleagues[16] reported that the Abelson (*abl*) protooncogene normally located on the long arm of chromosome 9 was involved in the Ph translocation, and the same group showed in 1984 that the breakpoints on chromosome 22 in different patients were clustered in a relatively small sequence of DNA, which was termed the *breakpoint cluster region* (*bcr*).[17] In 1984, Konopka and colleagues[18] identified an abnormal protein of 210 kd with tyrosine kinase activity. Thereafter, the *bcr/abl* chimeric gene was defined,[19] and an mRNA with *abl* determinants was characterized.[20] The most recent link in the chain connecting the *bcr/abl* gene and the P210-*bcr/abl* with the pathogenesis of CML is the demonstration that retroviral constructs containing *bcr/abl* sequences can be used to transfect murine hematopoietic stem cells and produce a disease closely resembling human CML in mice.[21]

It is commonly believed that CML is a clonal disease derived from a single hematopoietic stem cell, the progeny of which expand to displace at different rates all normal hematopoietic lineages.[22–24] The evidence in support of this belief is circumstantial but convincing. Thus, study of the marrow of a newly diagnosed patient shows the Ph chromosome in all (or almost all) dividing cells. Specialized methods confirm that not only do neutrophil granulocyte progenitors carry a Ph chromosome but so do cells of eosinophilic, basophilic, erythroid, megakaryocytic, and monocytic lineages.[25–29] A proportion of B cells carry the Ph chromosome,[30,31] and probably a small minority of T

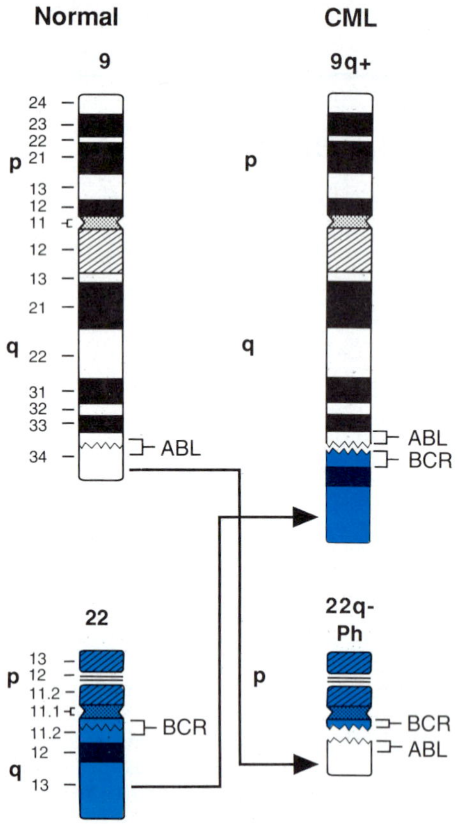

FIGURE 15-1. Diagramatic representation of the formation of the Philadelphia (Ph) chromosome. Note the formation of the *bcr/abl* gene on chromosome 22q− (Ph) and the reciprocal *abl/bcr* gene on chromosome 9q+. The *abl/bcr* gene is expressed in 70% of CML patients but its relevance to CML is unknown.

cells do also.[32,33] Study of female patients with CML who are heterozygotes for the two isoenzymes of glucose-6-phosphate dehydrogenase (G6PD) has revealed that leukemic cells are all of type A or type B but never both.[34,35] This is best interpreted as consistent with the idea that the Ph chromosome translocation occurred originally in a single hematopoietic stem cell of the same isoenzyme type as the bulk of the leukemia. The possibility that the leukemia originates simultaneously in a cohort of stem cells of a single isoenzyme type was involved in the same leukemogenic process is not formally excluded.

The possibility that hematopoiesis may be clonal (and therefore by implication neoplastic or preneoplastic) before the acquisition of the Ph chromosome has been considered by some investigators. Fialkow and colleagues[35] demonstrated a series of acquired chromosomal changes in Ph-negative B-lymphoid lines established from a female G6PD heterozygote with Ph-positive CML. The fact that these changes were found predominantly in cell lines with the same G6PD isoenzyme type as the Ph-positive leukemia cells was interpreted as evidence for the existence of an unstable hematopoietic clone with predisposition to acquire a Ph chromosome. The occasional observation of patients with a Ph-negative CML at diagnosis whose disease proved subsequently to have a Ph chromosome provides further support for this hypothesis.[36,37] It is unknown whether clonal hematopoiesis preceding Ph-positive leukemia is a routine occurrence or merely a curiosity.

The classification of chronic myelogenous or chronic myeloid leukemia is not entirely straightforward. Nevertheless, most patients have a reasonably well-defined disease characterized by splenomegaly, leukocytosis, and the finding of a Ph chromosome in marrow metaphases. Some workers choose to reserve the term *chronic granulocytic leukemia* for these patients and use *chronic myeloid leukemia* as a more comprehensive generic term.[38] This distinction is not widely accepted. A small proportion (5% to 7%) of those with a disease closely resembling CML have normal marrow karyotypes or abnormalities other than 22q−. These patients are usually classified as having Ph-negative CML,[39–42] and closer study may reveal that some do while others do not differ from classic CML on clinical or hematologic grounds. Other rarer forms of CML include juvenile CML,[43,44] chronic myelomonocytic leukemia,[45] and the rare chronic neutrophilic leukemia.[46,47]

CLASSIFICATION OF CML

- Chronic myelogenous leukemia
  - Ph-positive
  - Ph-negative, hematologically typical
  - Ph-negative, hematologically atypical
- Juvenile chronic myeloid leukemia
  - Ph-negative
- Chronic myelomonocytic leukemia
  - Ph-negative, also included in the classification of the myelodysplastic syndromes
- Chronic neutrophilic leukemia

ETIOLOGY AND PATHOGENESIS

Epidemiologic Factors

Chronic myelogenous leukemia accounts for about 15% of all cases of leukemia. As mentioned, it is slightly more common in males than in females and especially prevalent in young and middle-aged adults. In countries where the data are reliable, it occurs with an annual incidence of about 1 per 100,000 persons, and this figure seems to be consistent in different ethnic populations.[48,49] There is no association with social class or race and, in general, no familial incidence. Rare examples of CML that occur more than once in a family are described.[50] Exposure to ionizing radiation is the only known etiologic factor. The incidence of CML was increased to a minor but significant degree in patients treated with radiation therapy for ankylosing spondylitis[51] or metropathia hemorrhagica.[52] The survivors of the explosions of atomic bombs at Hiroshima and Nagasaki in 1945 also showed a small but significantly increased risk of developing CML.[53,54]

The Philadelphia Chromosome

The Ph chromosome is a chromosome 22 that lacks about half the chromosomal material normally present on its long arm. The observation that one member of the G group of chromosomes was abnormal was made in Philadelphia in 1960.[5,14] The original papers described simply the fact that leukemic cells from patients with CML had partial deletion of the long arm of one member of the G group of chromosomes. This specific chromosomal defect was later termed the *Philadelphia chromosome* and described as 22q− because it involved the G-group chromosome other than the one involved in Down's syndrome (trisomy 21).[55] The superscript 1 (Ph^1) was chosen to indicate the first of what was thought would be a series of chromosomal anomalies, each specific for a different malignant disease. More recently, it has been proposed that the superscript 1 be dropped.[56] In 1973, the introduction of newer chromosome-banding techniques permitted Rowley[15] to identify the presence of chromosomal material added to the long arm of chromosome 9, from which she deduced that the Ph chromosome was the result of a reciprocal translocation involving chromosomes 9 and 22 (Fig. 15-2). Subsequently, the positions of the breaks have been defined more precisely, and the translocation is designated t(9;22)(q34;q11).[57] The history of the Ph chromosome is summarized in Table 15-1.

About 90% of patients with hematologically acceptable CML have a classic Ph chromosome in all or almost all analyzable marrow metaphases at diagnosis. These Ph-positive cells are mainly dividing cells of the granulocytic lineage, but studies with iron isotopes[25] and studies involving cells with multiple nuclei[27] led to the conclusion that erythroid and megakaryocyte progenitors also carry a Ph chromosome. A proportion of B lymphocytes are also Ph-positive.[30,31] Most studies of T lymphocytes in CML suggest that they are cytogenetically normal, but the observation that occasional colonies of T lymphocytes cultured in vitro are Ph-positive and the observation that the predominating blast cell in lymphoid transformation occasionally has T-cell features must mean that the Ph-positive stem cell can give rise to cells of T lineage.[32,33] In contrast, fibroblasts from the marrow and other sites are uniformly cytogenetically normal, as are cells of all other lineages in the body.[58,59]

Occasional patients have a mixture of Ph-positive and Ph-negative cells in their marrow at presentation.[60] The Ph-negative cells are presumed to reflect the progeny of residual normal stem cells, although they might be merely leukemic cells that have not yet acquired a Ph chromosome. In these cases, the reason that the Ph-positive cells should have failed to express a complete proliferative advantage is unknown. It was thought at one time that prognosis in these patients with Ph-positive and Ph-negative mosaicism was superior to that of patients with 100% Ph chromosomal positivity in the marrow at diagnosis, but this view has not been confirmed.[61,62]

About 5% of patients with CML have variant chromosomal translocations. These are subclassified as simple when chromosome 22 is involved in addition to a single chromosome other than chromosome 9, and as complex when a t(9;22) is present in conjunction with morphologic changes in one or more additional chromosomes.[63] The sequence of cytogenetic events in complex variant translocations in unknown. It is possible that the Ph translocation occurs as a first step and that further changes occur later in the evolution of CML; alternatively, all cytogenetic changes may occur simultaneously. The term *masked Ph chromosome* refers to a rare situation in which the acquisition of additional cytogenetic material on chromosome 22q− produces a chromosome that is superficially normal and so disguises the fact that a t(9;22) has in fact occurred.[64] Patients with variant Ph chromosomes have the same *bcr/abl* chimeric gene as those with the classic Ph chromosome (discussed later). They also appear to have an overall prognosis that is neither better nor worse than those with the classic translocation.[64,65]

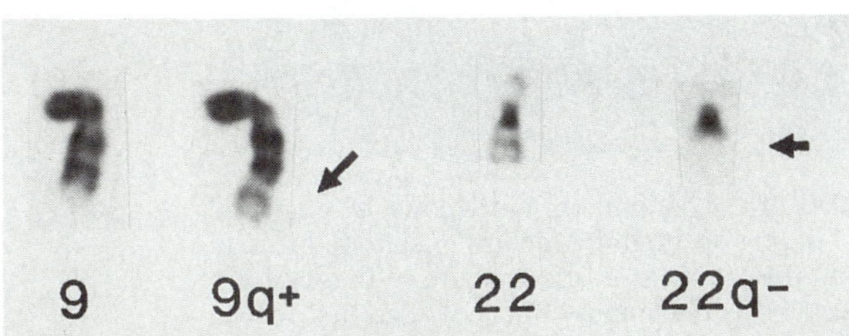

FIGURE 15-2. Photomicrograph of a partial karyotype showing normal chromosomes 9, 9q+, 22, and 22q−. The sites of additional deleted chromosomal material are shown by arrows.

TABLE 15-1. History of the Philadelphia Chromosome and *bcr/abl* Gene

Year	Advance
1960	Discovery of the Philadelphia chromosome
1973	Recognition of translocation t(9;22)
1984	Definition of breakpoint cluster region on chromosome 22q
1985	Discovery of the P210-*bcr/abl* with tyrosine kinase activity
1987	Demonstration of *bcr/abl* chimeric gene in some cases of Ph-negative CML
1990	Mouse model of CML produced with retroviral construct containing human *bcr/abl* gene

A further 5% of patients with more or less typical CML have leukemic cells with a strictly normal karyotype or, less commonly, clonal with cytogenetic changes that involve neither chromosome 9 nor 22. These patients are described as having Ph-negative CML.[39–42,66–68] Some have clinical and hematologic features indistinguishable from patients with Ph-positive disease, while others differ in various ways. The categorization of Ph-negative CML is imprecise, but probably about 40% of patients have the same molecular changes (*bcr/abl* chimeric gene formation and P210 expression) as patients with Ph-positive CML.[69,70] The remainder have no discernible changes involving *bcr/abl* but may be more likely to have *ras* mutations. It was thought at one time that patients with Ph-negative CML had a prognosis distinctly worse than those with Ph-positive disease (1.5 versus 3.5 years),[39,40,66] but this distinction may not apply to Ph-negative patients whose disease resembles Ph-positive CML by hematologic and molecular features.[71]

A summary of the chromosomal classification of CML is given in Table 15-2.

Molecular Changes in Chronic Phase

The Abelson variant of the Moloney murine leukemia virus contains specific RNA sequences capable of transforming target cells in vitro.[72] This viral oncogene is homologous to a human protooncogene located in all normal cells on chromosome 9q34. This oncogene codes for a protein of 140 kd (P140), which is widely expressed in human cells and has weak protein kinase activity.[73] Its normal substrate and thus its normal function are unknown. The human *abl* comprises a number of exons, including one or more that code for the kinase activity. There are two upstream exons (designated Ib and Ia) situated a considerable distance from exon II, which is also known as the *first common exon.* Patients with CML have genomic breakpoints that may be

TABLE 15-2. Chromosomal Classification of CML

Classification	Translocation
Ph-positive CML	
Standard	t(9;22) (q34;q11)
Simple variant	t(?;22)
Complex variant	t(?;9;22)
Masked	Apparently normal chromosome 22
Ph-positive and Ph-negative CML mosaicism	
Ph-negative CML	
With *bcr* rearrangement	
Without *bcr* rearrangement	

located upstream of exon Ib, between exons Ib and Ia, or downstream of exon Ia.[7,74] This means that the precise position of the breakpoint is variable over a distance of perhaps 200 kb.

The situation on chromosome 22 is different. Studies of DNA from different patients with Ph-positive CML showed that breakpoints occur at different points within a relatively restricted genomic region measuring 5.8 kb and containing five coding exons, which was termed the *breakpoint cluster region*.[17] These five exons were designated b1 to b5. Subsequently, it was shown that this small region formed part of a complete gene designated the *bcr* gene.[7] This nomenclature gave rise to some confusion, but the complete gene is now termed the *bcr gene*, and the breakpoint region is referred to as the *major breakpoint cluster region* (M-*bcr*).[7] Most patients with CML have genomic breaks in the introns between exons b2 and b3 or b3 and b4 of the M-*bcr*. Superficially, the *bcr* gene resembles the *abl* gene in that the first exon is situated at some considerable distance from the main body of the gene. Most patients with Ph-positive acute lymphoblastic leukemia have genomic breakpoints in the first intron of the *bcr* gene (some considerable distance upstream of M-*bcr*).[75] These breakpoints occur in the *minor breakpoint cluster regions*, or m-*bcr*.[76] Like the *abl* gene, the normal *bcr* gene product is widely distributed in normal cells, but its function is unknown.

The formation of the Ph chromosome results in every case in juxtaposition of 5′ sequences of the *bcr* gene with 3′ sequences of the *abl* protooncogene, thereby forming a new chimeric or fusion gene on 22q− (Fig. 15-3). The contribution of *abl* sequences to 22q− can be confirmed by studies using in situ hybridization of gene probes to metaphase preparations.[77,78] The *abl* probes hybridize to both the normal 9q and the 22q−. Of considerable interest was the discovery that some patients with Ph-negative CML also had *abl* sequences present on a morphologically normal chromosome 22.[79,80] Furthermore, the *bcr/abl* chimeric gene may on occasion be located on other chromosomes in patients with complex translocations.

The formation of the *bcr/abl* chimeric gene is associated in most cases with production of a unique mRNA measuring 8.5 kb, with *bcr* and *abl* determinants. The mRNA is produced as a result of splicing out of all introns and omission of exons Ib or of Ib plus Ia on the *abl* gene.[81] This mRNA links *bcr* exon b2 or b3 to *abl* exon II (the first common exon). This mRNA can be detected in blast cells from patients in chronic phase and more readily in cells from patients in transformation and in various CML cell lines.[82] It encodes a protein of 210 kd that has the capacity to autophosphorylate and to phosphorylate other proteins on tyrosine residues.[20] Thus, in effect, the replacement of normal upstream sequences on the *abl* protooncogene has unmasked tyrosine kinase activity encoded by downstream exons. This activity can be identified in leukemic cells by a two-stage procedure involving immune precipitation with an *abl* or *bcr* antibody, followed by in vitro assay of kinase activity. It is reasonable to assume that the production of P210-*bcr/abl* is a crucial part of the mechanism by which the function of a normal hematopoietic stem cell is perturbed, but the nature of this action is not defined. The introduction of the *bcr/abl* gene in a retroviral vector into murine hematopoietic stem cells can produce in mice a disease closely mimicking human CML.[21]

The patients with Ph-negative CML referred to previously, who have evidence for translocation of *abl* to the morphologically normal chromosome 22, all have the characteristic mRNA-*bcr/abl* and P210-*bcr/abl*.[69–71] This observation further supports the concept that these molecular changes play a pathogenetic role in CML—even in the absence of a Ph chromosome.

The identification of leukemia-specific transcripts (ie, mRNA-*bcr/abl*) in CML cells relied formerly on Northern analysis or a protection assay, both of which could give false results. The introduction of the polymerase chain reaction (PCR) has greatly simplified the molecular characterization of CML cells.[83,84] Because of the highly variable positions of the breakpoints in *abl* and, to a lesser extent, in *bcr*, it is technically difficult to use DNA for the PCR. However, cDNA reverse-transcribed from the leukemic mRNA reflects the unique *bcr/abl* linkages referred to previously and can be specifically amplified with appropriate oligonucleotide primers in the PCR. This technology is

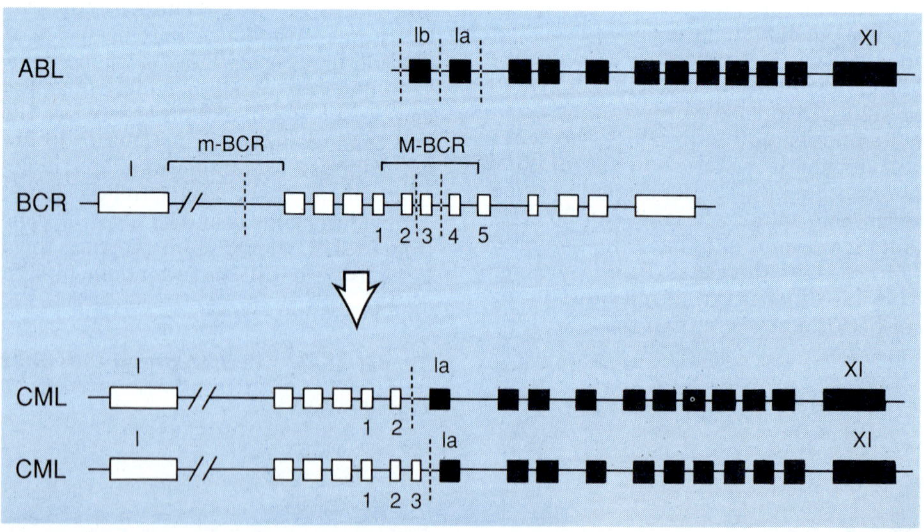

FIGURE 15-3. Schematic representation of the formation of the *bcr/abl* chimeric gene. The normal *abl* and *bcr* genes are shown above. The alternative first exons of the *abl* gene are designated Ib and Ia, respectively. The location of genomic breakpoints in CML and Ph-positive acute leukaemia are shown by vertical dashed lines. The first exon of the *bcr* gene is designated I or (e1). The first intron is designated m-*bcr* (minor breakpoint cluster region). Most breakpoints in CML occur in the region designated M-*bcr* (major breakpoint cluster region). Exons within M-*bcr* are numbered 1 through 5 (also referred to as b1 through b5). The two alternative *bcr/abl* genes—the top one (b2 to a2) excluding exon b3 and the bottom one (b3 to a2) including b3—are shown at the bottom.

TABLE 15-3. Molecular Alterations in Chronic Myeloid and Associated Leukemias

	M-*bcr* Rearranged	*bcr/abl* Transcript	*abl*-Related Protein
Normal	No	No	P145, TPK−
Ph-positive CML (95%)			
M-*bcr*+ (98%)	Yes	8.5	P210, TPK+
M-*bcr*− (2%)	No*	—	—
Ph-negative CML (5%)			
M-*bcr*+ (50%)	Yes	8.5	P210, TPK+
M-*bcr*− (50%)	No	—	None
Ph-positive ALL			
30%	Yes	8.5	P210, TPK+
70%	No†	7.3	P190, TPK+

ALL, acute lymphoblastic leukemia; TPK, tyrosine protein kinase.

* Occasional patients with Ph-positive CML have genomic breakpoints on chromosome 22 outside M-*bcr*.

† Most patients with Ph-positive ALL have breakpoints in the first intron of the *bcr* gene, which is far upstream of M-*bcr*. They have a smaller chimeric *bcr/abl* gene, resulting in a smaller mRNA and protein than those that characterize CML.

useful for characterizing the specific linkage in an individual patient, which may have prognostic relevance (discussed later), and for monitoring minimal residual disease after treatment with interferon-α (IFN-α) or by bone marrow transplantation.[85,86]

A summary of molecular alterations in the chronic myeloid and associated leukemias is given in Table 15-3.

Stem Cell and Progenitor Cell Kinetics

Although there is no assay that measures the number of pluripotential hematopoietic stem cells present in human marrow or blood, much circumstantial evidence suggests that their numbers must be greatly increased in the untreated CML patient.[87] Thus, the numbers of Ph-positive multipotential myeloid progenitor cells (CFU-GEMM or CFU-mix) and the numbers of lineage-committed myeloid progenitor cells, measured as granulocyte-macrophage (CFU-GM), erythroid burst (BFU-E), and megakaryocyte (CFU-Mk) colony-forming cells, are all increased greatly in the marrow and to an even greater extent in the peripheral blood (Figs. 15-4 and 15-5). Such leukemia progenitor cells proliferate almost normally in clonogenic cultures and produce colonies with cells of normal morphology.

One might speculate that the proliferation in vitro of leukemic progenitor cells would proceed autonomously or with greatly increased sensitivity to positive regulatory factors, but there is no evidence to support this. In general, the proliferation in vitro of committed CML progenitor cells requires the presence in the culture of the same hematopoietic growth factors as would be required by their normal counterparts.[87] Some studies have suggested that there may be a subpopulation of progenitor cells with greatly increased sensitivity to certain growth factors,[88] analogous to the increased sensitivity of some erythroid cells to erythropoietin in polycythemia rubra vera, but this has not been confirmed.

Marrow cells from untreated patients with CML can be maintained for some weeks in long-term culture, usually in conjunction with a preformed stromal layer derived from normal marrow cells established in the culture flasks at an earlier date. Assessment of the proportion of myeloid progenitor cells produced in such long-term culture systems has on occasion shown appearance and persistence of Ph-negative cells.[89] Moreover, such putatively normal cells go in and out of proliferative cycle in response to alterations in the culture conditions, while their leukemic counterparts appear to remain permanently in cycle.[90] These experimental observations may have considerable biologic significance. They suggest that untreated patients may have their complete complement of normal stem cells but that

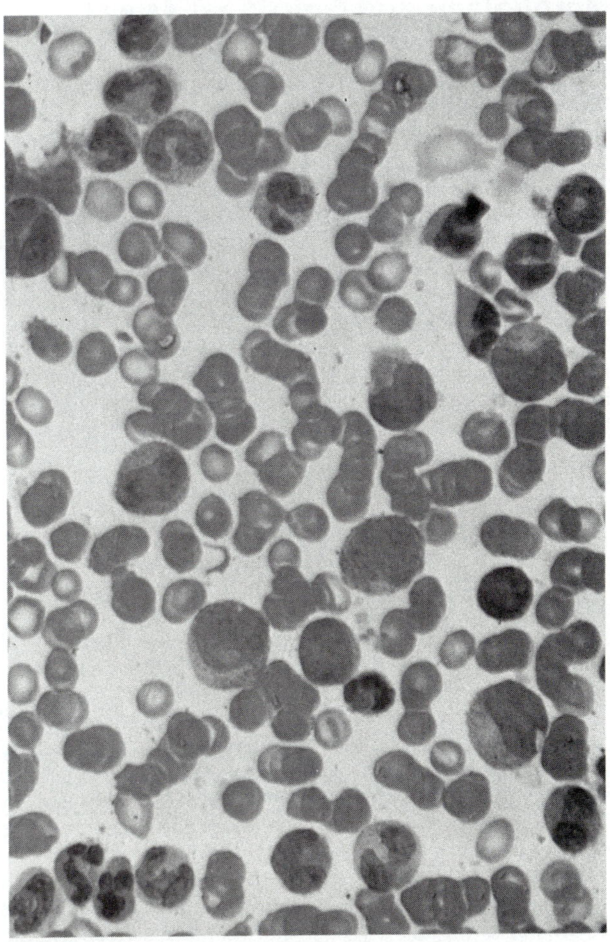

FIGURE 15-4. Appearance of the peripheral blood in CML in chronic phase (May-Grunwald Giemsa stain). (See Color Fig. 15-4.)

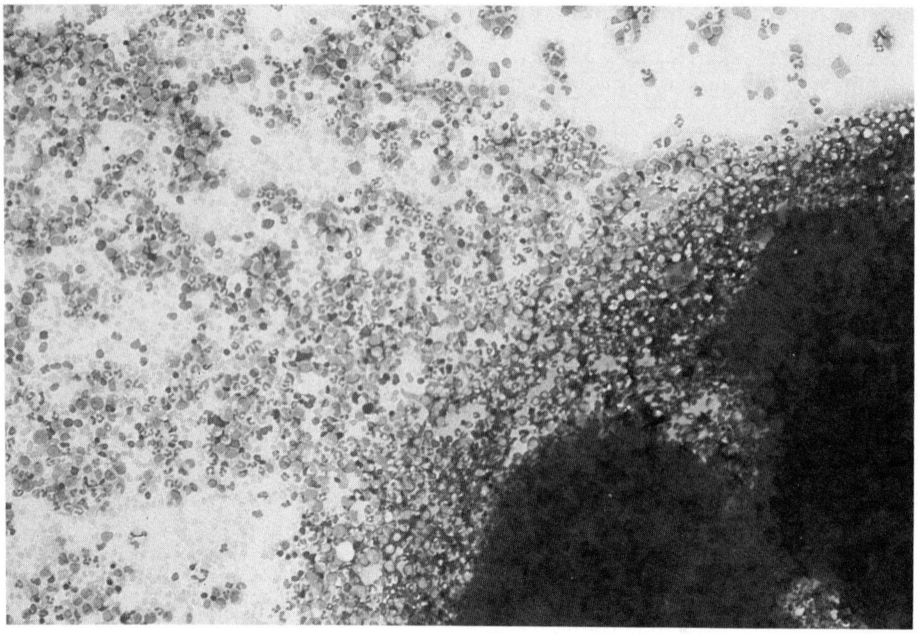

FIGURE 15-5. Appearance of the bone marrow in CML in chronic phase. Note the dense fragment (left) with complete loss of fat spaces. The cell trail is hypercellular (May-Grunwald Giemsa stain). (See Color Fig. 15-5.)

their proliferation is completely suppressed in vivo; they suggest also that there may be a fundamental difference in the manner in which normal and leukemic progenitor cells respond to physiologic inhibitory regulatory mechanisms.[87]

Morphologic and Functional Aspects of Various Lineages

The morphology of the early and mature myeloid cells in the marrow and peripheral blood of patients with CML in chronic phase does not differ greatly from normal.[91] Although the surface antigen characteristics of BFU-E and CFU-GM in the blood of CML patients differ from that of normal people, these changes are not striking.[92] Similarly, although the relative numbers of immature erythroid cells are reduced in the marrow, they appear morphologically unremarkable. A number of studies have been directed at assessment of the phagocytic and microbicidal functions of CML granulocytes. In general, it appears that both these functions are impaired to a minor degree in untreated patients, but the deficiency is more than compensated for by the vast increase in phagocytic cell numbers.[93,94]

Transformation

The existence of the chronic phase of CML appears to predispose a patient to further molecular and cytogenetic evolution, although the speed with which this occurs is largely unpredictable for individual patients. Most patients have a Ph chromosome as the only cytogenetic abnormality in their leukemic cells at diagnosis, although variant translocations are well recognized, and other random clonal changes also occur. Serial cytogenetic studies in individual patients show that the Ph chromosome remains the only abnormality in most cases for a number of years. Additional changes, when they occur, are usually held to presage acceleration of the disease or transformation. They may be random or nonrandom.

About 80% of patients in blast transformation show cytogenetic changes in their leukemic cells in addition to the the Ph chromosome.[95–98] These may comprise an additional Ph chromosome (+Ph), an additional 8 (+8), an additional 19 (+19), or a loss of short arms and replacement by duplicated long arms in chromosome 17 (iso-17q). These new changes may be present in some cells in parallel with other cells that contain only the Ph chromosome, or they may totally replace the chronic phase populations. Complex additional cytogenetic changes are common in which individual cells contain nonrandom changes (listed previously) in conjunction with a wide variety of seemingly random cytogenetic translocations, deletions, and markers chromosomes.

The molecular changes in blast cells from patients with CML in transformation bear little relation to the nonrandom cytogenetic changes (Fig. 15-6). The best characterized molecular changes are clonal rearrangement of immunoglobulin and, less frequently, of T-cell receptor genes that occur in all patients with lymphoid transformation and occasional patients with myeloid transformation.[99–101] These molecular changes are evidence for further evolution in a clone already marked as leukemic by *bcr* rearrangement, but they provide no useful clues about the mechanisms that underlie transformation.

If the *bcr/abl* chimeric gene plays a crucial role in pathogenesis of chronic phase disease, it is reasonable to infer that further genetic changes, presumably involving one or more protooncogenes, underlie disease progression to the accelerated and transformed phases. It is also likely that the molecular route to transformation may differ considerably in different patients. Our knowledge of molecular features underlying transformation is still scanty. There are occasional patients with mutations of *ras* genes identified in transformation but not in chronic phase.[102] One patient has been described with amplification and rearrangement of *myc*.[103] Rare patients have evidence of further changes in the *bcr/abl* rearrangement characteristic of chronic phase disease.[104] Evidence suggests that deletions or point mutations in the *P53* protooncogene located on chromosome 17p may occur in 15% to 20% of patients with blast crisis, predominantly those with myeloid transformation. *P53* is usually regarded as a member of the class of tumor-suppressor or antioncogenes, which are necessary for normal control of cellular growth and whose inactivation or neutralization is associated with tumor progression. One might speculate that acquired alterations in *P53* in chronic phase CML lead to activation of one or more further protooncogenes and thus to blastic transformation. The retinoblastoma gene product, RB, has been found to

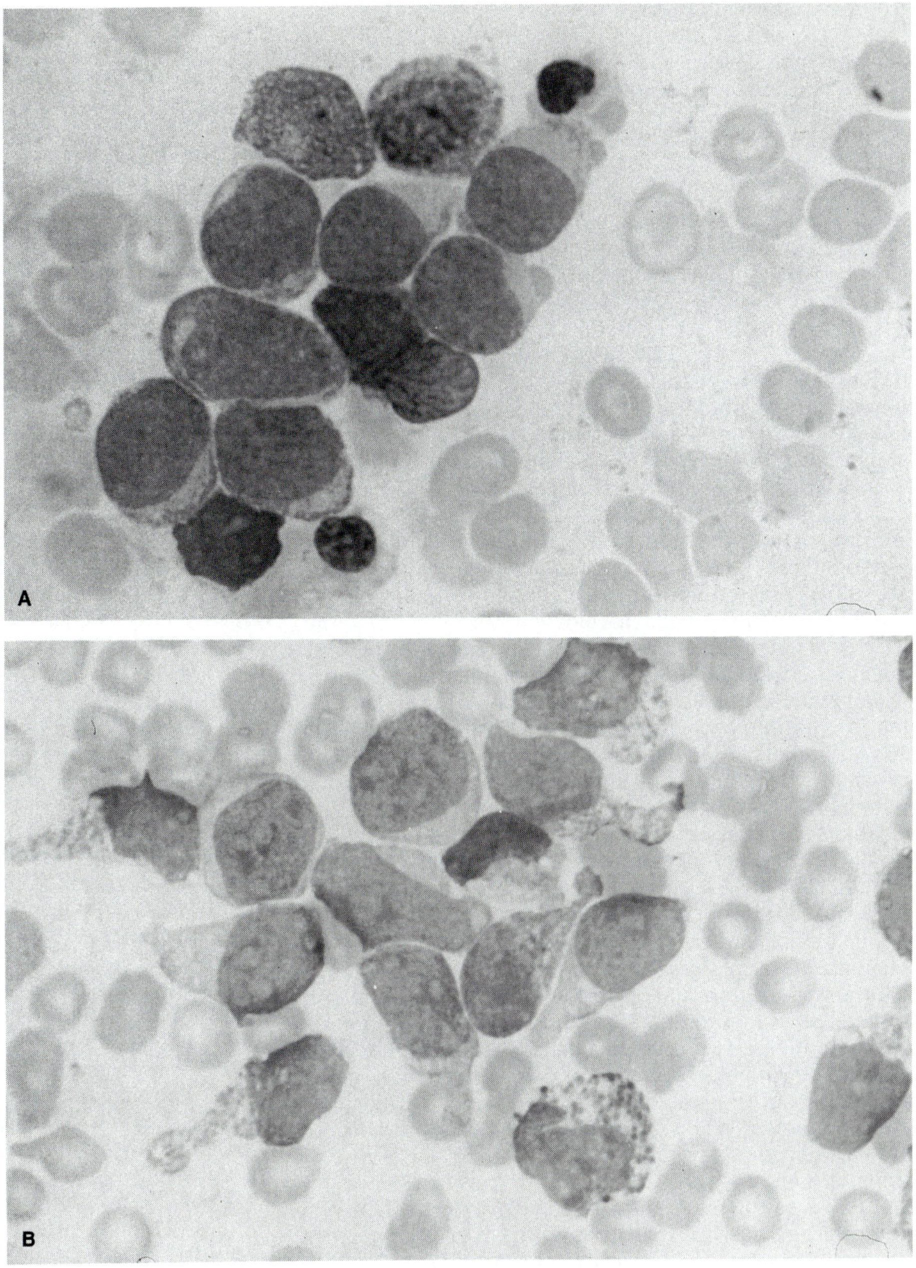

FIGURE 15-6. (**A**) Lymphoid blast cells in chronic myelogenous leukemia in transformation. (**B**) Myeloid blast cells in chronic myelogenous leukemia transformation. (See Color Fig. 15-6.)

be absent from blast crises with a megakaryocytic phenotype and rearranged at a frequency of about 15% in crises of various phenotypes.[105]

CLINICAL PRESENTATION

Symptoms and Signs

Many patients present with symptoms related to the greatly expanded granulocyte mass, to hypermetabolism, or to hemorrhage associated with platelet dysfunction. Thus, patients may have lethargy or weakness due to anemia, a sensation of fullness in the left upper-abdominal quadrant attributable to splenomegaly, or abdominal pain due to splenic infarction.[107–109] Patients may present with ecchymoses or hematoma formation at any site. They may have visual disturbances due to retinal hemorrhages.[110] Other constitutional symptoms include undue sweating and weight loss. Patients occasionally have single or multiple subcutaneous masses of variable size that may be due to small subcutaneous bleeds followed by local proliferation of immature granulocytes. About 1% of males present with priapism, which is usually preceded by some days or weeks of less troublesome intermittent penile erections.[111] An increasing proportion of patients, perhaps as many as 40%, present without symptoms. In these patients, leukocytosis is identified incidentally as a result of a routine blood test performed for a variety of possible reasons, including pregnancy, insurance examinations, blood donation, minor surgery, or other circumstances.

Most patients have few physical signs on examination. Ten to 20% of patients have no palpable splenomegaly, but the spleen may be enlarged to percussion in some. In other patients, the spleen is greatly enlarged and in extreme cases may fill the left iliac fossa and even extend across the midline such as to be palpable in the right hemiabdomen. It is only tender if there is a recent splenic infarct, in which case a splenic rub may be audible. The liver may be modestly enlarged, but the liver edge is usually soft, unlike the firm edge palpable in patients with primary liver disease.

All other physical signs are much rarer. The patient may have ecchymoses or other localized bleeding. Retinal hemorrhages may be present. Retinal veins may be engorged as a consequence of leukostasis.[110,112] Rarely, patients present with features of gout or priapism.

Hematology

Patients with splenomegaly and considerably raised leukocyte counts usually present with anemia (hemoglobin, 6 to 12 g/dL)[91]; however, an appreciable number of patients present with normal hemoglobin values. The leukocyte count is usually raised at diagnosis and ranges between 15 and 500 $\times$ 10^9/L. It is possible to make a diagnosis of CML in patients with leukocyte counts in the normal range if other features, such as the appearance of occasional immature cells or excess of basophils, lead to cytogenetic examination of the marrow. Conversely, rare patients present with leukocyte counts in excess of 700 $\times$ 10^9/L and occasionally even 1000 $\times$ 10^9/L. The blood film is usually characteristic.[91] The morphology of individual leukocytes is normal, but the whole spectrum of immature and mature granulocytes is present in the blood, with relatively high proportions of blast cells, myelocytes, and mature granulocytes. The percentage of blast cells rises with the leukocyte count such that patients with high leukocyte counts may have 10% or even 12% of blasts in the blood. The mature granulocytes are mainly neutrophils, but the relative numbers of eosinophils and basophils are also increased. The percentage of monocytes is reduced, and lymphocyte numbers are relatively low. Occasional nucleated red cells are present in the blood film. Platelet numbers are usually moderately increased, in the range of 300 to 700 $\times$ 10^9/L. Less commonly, platelet numbers are normal and occasionally subnormal.

The cytoplasmic content of alkaline phosphatase (NAP) characteristically is greatly reduced or absent in CML.[113–115] This enzyme appears to be associated with small cytosolic organelles, sometimes referred to as *phosphasomes*,[116] whose function is unknown. The mechanism underlying these reduced NAP levels is unknown, but the enzyme is inducible—NAP levels may rise in pregnancy and infection. Moreover, when granulocytes with low NAP scores from CML patients are transfused to recipients with aplastic anemia, they express normal NAP levels after a few hours.[117] Granulocytes cultured in vitro from CML progenitor cells also have normal amounts of NAP.[118] Some recent evidence suggests that exposure of NAP-deficient cells to granulocyte colony-stimulating factor increases their alkaline phosphatase content.[119] It is possible that ambient levels of granulocyte colony-stimulating factor are low in the marrow and blood of CML patients.

Examination of the bone marrow is not strictly necessary to establish a diagnosis, but it is routinely carried out for a number of reasons. Cytogenetic studies are more likely to be successful on marrow cells. The marrow aspirate is usually densely hypercellular, with multiple small fragments or without identifiable fragments. The distribution of immature leukocytes in the marrow resembles that of the blood. Erythroid precursors are relatively reduced. Megakaryocyte numbers are increased, and some are small and mononuclear. Some marrow specimens contain occasional large mononuclear cells with abundant granular cytoplasm resembling Gaucher cells (designated *pseudo-Gaucher cells*).[120,121] A trephine biopsy specimen is also usually obtained at diagnosis. This characteristically confirms the hypercellularity and shows complete loss of marrow fat spaces. The reticulin content of the marrow is usually normal at diagnosis[122] but may increases insidiously with time.[123] Some patients have moderate or even major increases in marrow reticulin or collagen formation when the marrow is first examined.

Prognostic Features and Disease Progression

The median duration of survival from diagnosis with conventional chemotherapy is about 3.5 years, with a range in different series of 3 to 4.2 years.[124,125] It has been shown in one large series that the chance of dying within 1 year of diagnosis in chronic phase was 10%, the chance of death in the second year was 12%, and the chance in each subsequent year was 22%.[126] If these figures apply to all series of CML patients, the probability of death in any single year does not increase after the third year. Patients with an imperfect understanding of these statistics sometimes believe that their probability of further survival has become significantly shorter once they have survived 3.5 years, the median duration of survival for new patients. This belief is obviously erroneous and must be dispelled.

A considerable number of attempts have been made to define individual features or a constellation of features that predict the duration of chronic phase or of survival in newly diagnosed patients.[127–132] There is general agreement that the size of the spleen (usually measured in centimeters below the left costal margin) is correlated with duration of survival, with patients with small or impalpable spleens having relatively long chronic phases, and vice versa. Other studies have identified the age of the patient, the leukocyte count, the proportion of blast cells in the blood, and the presence of thrombocytopenia or major thrombocytosis as poor prognostic factors. Sokal and colleagues[126,133] studied a large cohort of patients diagnosed in chronic phase and derived an equation (incorporating patient age, spleen size, blast cell percentage, and platelet numbers) from which a prognostic index could be calculated for each patient. When a cohort of patients was divided into three categories in accordance with the prognostic index, the median survivals for each group were 2.5, 4, and 5 years, respectively.

It has been proposed that the precise position of the breakpoint in M-*bcr* correlates with duration of chronic phase and thus with survival.[134,135] Individual patients can be classified as to whether the genomic breakpoint in their leukemic cells occurs either upstream (5′) or downstream (3′) of a Hind III restriction site between exons b3 and b4 of M-*bcr*. Some studies suggest that patients with 5′ breakpoints have significantly better prognoses than those with 3′ breakpoints,[134,135] but this view is not generally accepted.[136]

Occasional patients with CML become long-term survivors (more than 10 years).[137–139] Some of these patients have features at diagnosis that might have marked them as having good prognoses (eg, small spleens, low leukocyte counts), but in general, such long-term survival cannot be predicted. In rare patients, the raised leukocyte count remains relatively low and stable for many years.[140] Spontaneous disappearance of Ph-positive marrow metaphases has been reported.[141]

Complications of Chronic Phase Disease

The patient receiving adequate treatment for CML in chronic phase can expect to have a normal life-style and need anticipate few complications (other than those related to disease progression). Rarely, symptoms of gout develop in the patient undergoing treatment. Most problems are either the result of toxicity of antileukemia drugs (discussed later) or manifestations of disease acceleration, which may in its initial stages be difficult to characterize.

MANAGEMENT OF CHRONIC PHASE

Decisions on treatment strategy, particularly for patients younger than 50 years, have become exceedingly complex in recent years. Undoubtedly, the first obligation for the physician meeting a newly diagnosed patient with CML is to present to the patient an explanation of the nature, natural history, and probable prognosis. The extent to which the physician provides detailed information must depend on how much the physician believes the patient can comprehend, but it is a mistake to underestimate any individual patient. The second question is to decide whether initiation of treatment is in fact indicated. Because there is no convincing evidence that treatment with busulfan or hydroxyurea prolongs the duration of chronic phase, one need not automatically start treatment with one of these agents in an asymptomatic patient. The target should rather be to prevent the onset of symptoms. This means that treatment can reasonably be deferred until the leukocyte count reaches 50 or $100 \times 10^9/L$. Conversely, some patients are happier in the knowledge that their leukocyte counts have in fact been restored to normal soon after diagnosis. For these patients, initiation of treatment is fully justified. If initial treatment with IFN-α is contemplated, or if the patient is a candidate for allogeneic bone marrow transplantation, the decision of when to start treatment is less straightforward.

Conventional Use of Cytotoxic Drugs for Chronic Phase

Busulfan (1,4-dimethanesulfonyloxybutane) has been the mainstay of management of chronic phase CML for nearly 40 years. It is a fat-soluble alkylating agent that is conveniently given by mouth, but the dimethyl derivative can be given intravenously. It acts by damaging or destroying a relatively primitive hematopoietic stem cell; there is no evidence that it acts selectively against CML as opposed to normal stem cells. It was introduced first into clinical practice by Galton in London in 1953.[142,143] In 1968, a formal comparison of clinical results showed that survival was significantly longer in patients treated with busulfan than in those who received radiation therapy,[144] and radiation therapy for chronic phase CML fell largely into disuse. Busulfan may be administered by three different approaches, none of which is obviously best. Patients may be started at a daily dose of 8 mg (more or less regardless of their weight), with early reduction to 4 mg when the leukocyte count has halved and with complete cessation of treatment when the leukocyte count falls to 30 or $20 \times 10^9/L$.[145] The leukocyte count then continues to fall for 2 to 4 weeks and may stabilize in the normal range. Treatment may be recommenced when the leukocyte rises again to 30 or 40 $\times 10^9/L$, but the interval between the first and second course may vary from as little as 6 weeks to more than 1 year. Thereafter, treatment may be continued, with repeated courses lasting 2 to 4 weeks and with each separated by weeks or months. A second approach to treatment involves the attempt to continue busulfan indefinitely at low dosage to maintain the leukocyte count in the normal range. A daily dose ranging between 0.5 and 2 mg usually achieves this objective. The third approach involves administration of relatively large single doses (eg, 50, 100, or 150 mg) on a single occasion at intervals not shorter than 4 weeks.[146] This is convenient for the patient but confers no other discernible advantage.

The toxicity associated with administration of busulfan may be divided into the predictable and the idiosyncratic.[124,147,148] All patients have impaired fertility after treatment with busulfan. Women develop amenorrhea, and ovulation ceases. Men develop azoospermia but not usually loss of libido. These effects develop more rapidly in older patients and are generally irreversible. Patients should be warned of these risks, and cryopreservation of semen should be offered if appropriate. Patients treated with busulfan for some years developed cutaneous pigmentation vaguely suggestive of Addison's syndrome.[149] Overdosage with busulfan, usually consequent on inadequate monitoring of the patient's blood count or confused compliance whereby the drug is inadvertently continued some weeks or months after it should have been stopped, is associated with severe marrow aplasia that may prove fatal.[150,151] Occasional patients recover hematopoiesis after months or years of supportive therapy.[152] Such patients may paradoxically be restored to a Ph-negative status.[153]

Other, much rarer problems associated with administration of busulfan include a syndrome of interstitial and alveolar pulmonary fibrosis, usually referred to as busulfan lung,[154,155] and anecdotally, cataract formation.[156] Moreover, there are occasional patients whose sensitivity to busulfan is such that they become aplastic with standard dosage. This problem must be distinguished from the aplasia associated with true overdosage mentioned previously.

Hydroxyurea is a ribonucleotide reductase inhibitor synthesized originally in Hungary in the 1960s but not introduced into clinical practice until some years later.[125,157–159] It acts more rapidly and at a level of hematopoiesis more differentiated than busulfan. It is usual to start patients at a dosage of 2 g/d by mouth and to continue at this dosage until the leukocyte count reaches normal levels. At that point, the dosage may be reduced in steps of 0.5 g/d, with the intention of maintaining the leukocyte count within the normal range. If the drug is stopped abruptly, as would be appropriate with busulfan treatment, the leukocyte count rebounds rapidly to the consternation of patient and physician alike. Unlike busulfan, treatment with hydroxyurea once initiated must be continued indefinitely. The aim is to titrate the dosage against the leukocyte count, and the maintenance dosage typically ranges between 0.5 and 1.5 g/d.

The toxicity of hydroxyurea is far less than that of busulfan, and mainly for this reason, most hematologists favor hydroxyurea as the initial cytotoxic drug for new patients. It does not impair gonadal function, although it probably is teratogenic if administered in the first trimester of pregnancy. Marrow hypoplasia, if it occurs, is rapidly reversible on stopping the drug. The major toxicity is gastrointestinal disturbance (nausea, vomiting, diarrhea), which is frequently dose-related and reverses on reducing dosage. Occasional patients develop fevers or rashes attributable to hydroxyurea.

A variety of other cytotoxic drugs can be used in the management of CML in chronic phase. Dibromomannitol, 100 to 200 mg/d by mouth, probably acts by alkylation and may sometimes be active in patients who fail to respond to busulfan or hydroxyurea.[160] Cyclophosphamide, melphalan, 6-thioguanine, and other agents have been tested, but none offers advantages over hydroxyurea.

Other Approaches to Chronic Phase Disease

Radiation therapy was used to control CML in chronic phase during the first half of this century.[161] It was administered first as whole-body irradiation from a radium source and subsequently as irradiation to the spleen using kilovoltage apparatus. It was highly effective in inducing clinical remission, but the benefit was relatively short-lived and treatment had to be repeated at frequent intervals. There is little indication for the use of radiation therapy today in the management of patients with uncomplicated chronic phase disease.

The introduction of continuous-flow blood cell separators in the early 1970s led to a number of studies designed to test the merits of mechanical removal of mature leukocytes and incidentally of granulocyte progenitors from the peripheral blood.[162,163] It was considered possible that the commonly used cytotoxic drugs might be mutagenic and that avoiding their use might prolong the duration of chronic phase disease. It rapidly became clear that repeated leukapheresis could indeed reduce the size of the spleen and restore the leukocyte count to normal levels. This effect was maintained for weeks or months after a course of leukapheresis was interrupted. In the small number of patients so treated, transformation was not delayed, and leukapheresis today has no place except in the management of women during the first two trimesters of pregnancy.[164,165]

It also was postulated in the 1970s that splenectomy performed soon after diagnosis might prolong the duration of chronic phase.[166] This postulate was intuitively somewhat naive since successful treatment with cytotoxic drugs reduces spleen size to normal and eliminates most of the myeloid tissue in the previously enlarged spleen. Careful studies failed to show benefit for patients subjected to early elective splenectomy,[129,167–169] and this approach is no longer used.

Newer Approaches to Management of Chronic Phase

The interferons are a group of biologically active glycoproteins originally isolated from hematopoietic cells and fibroblast cell lines that inhibit cell proliferation in vivo. They are now routinely synthesized by recombinant techniques. Early studies showed that natural IFN-α could reduce the splenomegaly and leukocytosis of patients with CML in chronic phase.[170] The same results could be achieved with recombinant molecules.[171,172] This by itself would hold little interest, but cytogenetic studies of marrow cells from patients treated for 6 to 12 or more months have revealed cytogenetic conversion (ie, restoration of partial Ph-negative hematopoiesis) in 20% to 30% of patients. In some cases, this cytogenetic conversion was complete, and on rare occasions, Ph-negative hematopoiesis was maintained for months or even years after the interferon was discontinued.[172] Two patients treated with interferon were described whose marrow showed no evidence of leukemic transcripts when studied by PCR.[173] The mode of action of IFN-α is almost entirely unknown. Myeloid cells have interferon receptors, and the IFN-receptor complex is internalized. How it might act thereafter to suppress myelopoiesis is not known. Similarly, in vitro studies designed to establish the basis for the apparently selective suppression of Ph-positive stem cells are negative or inconclusive.[174,175]

IFN-α must be given by subcutaneous injection. It is usual to start at a low daily dose (eg, 3 MU) and to work gradually up to a maximal dose of 9 MU or 5 MU/m^2/d. The probability of achieving Ph negativity is probably greatest if the leukocyte count can be reduced to normal or subnormal (2 to 4 $\times$ 10^9/L) levels. Unfortunately, the drug has a number of side effects. Most patients experience influenza-like symptoms, such as fevers, sweats, headaches, and lethargy, during the few days or weeks of administration. These symptoms usually subside and do not prevent continued administration. More troublesome is nausea, anorexia, weight loss, and prolonged feelings of lethargy and sleepiness, which sometimes necessitate stopping the drug. Patients who can tolerate the drug and who appear to obtain cytogenetic benefit may be treated with IFN-α for some years. Preliminary studies with IFN-γ alone or in combination with IFN-α suggest that this agent contributes nothing to the management of CML.[176]

Recent data with IFN-α suggest that 70% of patients experience complete hematologic remission and about 20% have complete cytogenetic remission (CCR).[170] The chance of response to IFN-α is higher if the drug is used in the first year after diagnosis; the reason for this observation is not clear. A proportion of patients who achieve CCR are still in remission years later, but 90% are PCR-positive with a two-step PCR. These points notwithstanding, the first randomized study to be reported suggests that patients treated with IFN-α, regardless of whether they achieve cytogenetic remission, may have median survival of 1 to 3 years longer than patients treated with hydroxyurea.[176a] This conclusion needs confirmation from other studies.

Allogeneic Bone Marrow Transplantation

If CML involves a pluripotential hematopoietic stem cell, which may closely resemble a normal stem cell, it is difficult to see how cytotoxic drugs could selectively damage the first population but not the second. The concept therefore of treating CML patients by myeloablative chemotherapy or chemoradiotherapy followed by rescue with stem cells collected from normal donors is attractive. Initial attempts to treat patients with CML in transformation were undertaken in Seattle in the 1970s and were largely unsuccessful.[177] A small number of patients, however, fortunate enough to have hematologically normal identical twins underwent bone marrow transplantation in chronic phase, and some of these patients have become long-term survivors.[178] These preliminary results and the results of allografting for patients with acute myeloid leukemia led a number of specialist centers to begin in the 1980s to treat patients with CML in chronic phase by allogeneic bone marrow transplantation with more promising results.[179–182] It appears that most patients so treated are cured of their leukemia, but the risk of dying of transplantation-related complications is still substantial.

The results of allogeneic bone marrow transplantation for CML in chronic phase can be summarized by reference to an analysis performed by the International Bone Marrow Transplant Registry on 405 patients who underwent transplantation in various countries of Europe and North America[183] (Figs. 15-7 and 15-8). For patients who were

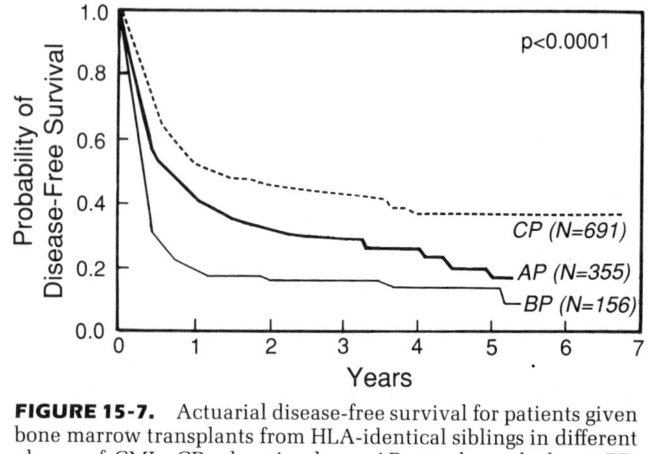

FIGURE 15-7. Actuarial disease-free survival for patients given bone marrow transplants from HLA-identical siblings in different phases of CML. CP, chronic phase; AP, accelerated phase; BP, blastic phase. (Data from the International Bony Marrow Transplant Registry, Milwaukee)

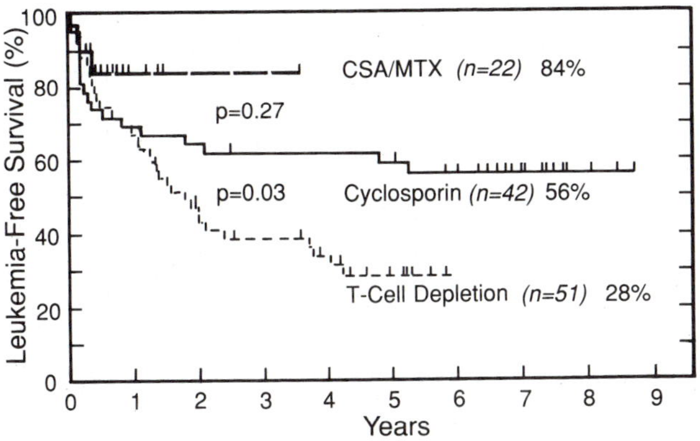

FIGURE 15-8. Actuarial leukemia-free survival for patients with CML in chronic phase given bone marrow transplants from HLA-identical siblings according to method used for prevention of graft-versus-host disease. T-cell depletion involved in vitro incubation of donor marrow with the monoclonal antibody Campath-1M. The patients were treated at the Hammersmith Hospital in London. CSA/MTX, cyclosporin and methotrexate.

mostly under 50 years of age (median, 31.5) and who received conditioning with cyclophosphamide followed by total body irradiation and then transfusion of marrow cells collected from HLA-identical siblings, the actuarial survival at 5 years was 49%, the actuarial leukemia-free survival was 42%, and the actuarial relapse rate was 12%. The principal causes of death for the 169 patients who died were graft-versus-host disease (GVHD), interstitial pneumonitis or a combination of these two complications. The series included 87 patients who had received donor marrow depleted of T cells by various in vitro manipulations to prevent GVHD. It was interesting to note that T-cell depletion in comparison with results in recipients of unmanipulated donor marrow did indeed reduce the incidence and severity of GVHD, but the graft failure rate was increased from 3% to 10% or 12%, and the incidence of relapse increased enormously (from about 12% to 49%).

The observation that the probability of relapse is greatly increased by T-cell depletion of donor marrow cells[183–185] is consistent with the notion that a specific but ill-defined population of cells in the donor marrow (possibly T-lymphocytes or lymphokine-activated killer cells) mediates an antileukemic effect in addition to the more obvious cytotoxic effect of the conditioning regimen. This cell-mediated antileukemic effect has been termed the *graft-versus-leukemia effect.* A comparison of relapse rates in patients who had received unmanipulated donor marrow, T-cell–depleted donor marrow, and syngeneic marrow suggests that the graft-versus-leukemia effect has at least three distinct components, one associated with the occurrence of GVHD, one associated with the presence of allogeneic (but not syngeneic) T cells in donor marrow, and one associated with T cells, allogeneic or syngeneic.[186] The increased risk of relapse resulting from T-cell depletion is smaller in patients with acute leukemia than in CML; this suggests that the graft-versus-leukemia effect in general may be of particular importance in CML.

The recognition and definition of relapse after transplantation for CML is not entirely straightforward. In some cases, patients present again after transplantation with leukocytosis or thrombocytosis in conjunction with Ph-positive hematopoiesis. These patients obviously have hematologic relapse. Other patients may have variable proportions of Ph-positive marrow metaphases without hematologic abnormality. Most patients with these so-called cytogenetic relapses eventually progress to overt hematologic relapse, but there are a number of well-documented instances in which the Ph positivity after transplantation apparently has been reversed on subsequent cytogenetic analysis.[187,188] These patients may be classified as having sustained a *transient cytogenetic relapse.*

More recently, PCR amplification of leukemia-specific transcripts has been able to define patients with minimal residual disease after transplantation.[189–191a] It is common for patients who eventually prove to be cured to be PCR-positive in the first year after bone marrow transplanatation,[190,191] but PCR positivity after this time is associated with an increased risk of relapse. In contrast, nearly all long-term survivors (more than 5 years) are PCR-negative. Quantitative PCR is a refinement that may prove clinically useful.[191a]

Autologous Bone Marrow Transplantation

The marrow and peripheral blood of untreated CML patients both contain hematopoietic stem cells capable of reconstituting autologous hematopoiesis after myeloablative therapy. A number of workers have investigated the possibility that administration of high-dose chemotherapy or chemoradiotherapy followed by transfusion of autologous stem cells might be of clinical benefit. Although the logic of restoring hematopoiesis with leukemic stem cells is not immediately apparent,[192] some patients achieve partial or complete Ph-negative hematopoiesis after autografting, and the procedure could reduce the size of the leukemic stem cell pass and thereby possibly delay the onset of transformation.

Preliminary results of autografting in chronic phase carried out in a number of centers have confirmed that Ph-positive and Ph-negative mosaicism can be identified in the marrow in perhaps half of patients, but this is not usually sustained.[193,194] In a small proportion of patients, Ph-negative hematopoiesis has predominated for more than 3 years.[193] The question of whether it is better to use blood- or marrow-derived stem cells for autografting is unresolved.

The obvious theoretical disadvantage of autografting with leukemic stem cells would be irrelevant if methods could be developed to separate leukemic and normal stem cells in vitro, so that only normal stem cells could be retransfused to the patients. Laboratory studies designed to achieve this objective by incubating marrow cells with cytotoxic drugs or monoclonal antibodies are not promising. Of considerable interest is the observation, mentioned previously, that long-term culture of marrow cells from CML patients may favor the survival of Ph-negative normal myeloid progenitors.[89] This observation formed the basis for clinical studies in which a small number of patients were autografted with marrow cells held in liquid culture for 10 days.[195] Most patients treated by this technique recovered hematopoiesis that was predominantly or exclusively Ph-negative, and the longest follow-up in this series is now 48 months. The clinical contribution to these fascinating results with in vitro marrow culture is not yet established. There is still no formal proof that autografting in chronic phase can prolong a patient's life.

ADVANCED PHASES

After a variable number of years, the chronic phase of CML evolves directly to blastic transformation or may pass more insidiously to a phase intermediate between chronic phase and transformation, usually referred to as the *accelerated phase*[196] (Table 15-4). The definition of transformation is

TABLE 15-4. Proposed Factors for the Recognition of Accelerated Phase CML

FACTORS PROPOSED IN 1983
Persisting splenomegaly after adequate treatment
Increasing leukocyte count resistant to busulphan or hydroxyurea
More than 10% blasts in blood or marrow
More than 20% blasts plus promyelocytes in blood or marrow
Persistent thrombocytosis ($>1.5 \times 10^{12}$/L)
Anemia (<10 g/dL) refractory to treatment
Acquisition of chromosome changes in addition to Ph
More than 20% basophils in blood
More than 20% eosinophils in blood
Increasing marrow fibrosis
FACTORS USED BY THE INTERNATIONAL BONE MARROW TRANSPLANT REGISTRY
Leukocyte count difficult to control with conventional use of bulsulfan or hydroxyurea
Rapid doubling of leukocyte count within 5 days
More than 10% blasts in blood or marrow
More than 20% blasts plus promyelocytes in blood or marrow
More than 20% basophils plus eosinophils in blood
Anemia or thrombocytopenia unresponsive to busulfan or hydroxyurea
Persistent thrombocytosis
Additional chromosomal changes (evolving new clone)
Increasing splenomegaly
Development of chloromas or myelofibrosis
Second chronic phase

somewhat arbitrary, but its identification is straightforward in most cases.[197] Conversely, patients may in some cases pass slowly into an accelerated phase, and some features of acceleration, such as increasing splenomegaly or a rising blast cell count, are probably more ominous than others, such as increasing basophilia or the finding in an otherwise asymptomatic patient of new cytogenetic changes.

Clinical Features

The onset of blastic transformation, sometimes referred to as *blast crisis,* may be entirely silent and revealed only as a result of a routine blood count. More commonly, the patient has nonspecific symptoms, such as fever, weight loss, sweats, or hemorrhagic manifestations, or more localized symptoms, such as bone pain or pain of splenic infarction. Rarely, the patient may have leukemic infiltrates of the skin or develop masses at other sites. Such masses may be designated *granulocytic sarcoma.*[198] The occasional patient in blastic transformation presents with features of neuroleukemia, including headaches, visual disturbances, and focal neurologic signs.

In occasional cases, the first manifestation of blastic transformation is the appearance of localized or generalized lymphadenopathy.[199] The peripheral blood or marrow may at this stage still be compatible with chronic phase disease. A lymph node biopsy reveals obvious infiltration with blast cells (or blast cells plus promyelocytes), which may have myeloid or lymphoid features.

On rare occasions, patients with blastic transformation present with isolated or multiple lytic lesions of bone[200,201] (Fig. 15-9). This presentation superficially may suggest metastatic carcinoma, but knowledge of the preceding CML in chronic phase permits the correct diagnosis. It may be unnecessary to obtain histologic proof of the transformation if biopsy of the lytic lesion is technically hazardous.

In 10% to 15% of patients, the disease progresses to myelofibrosis rather than to overt blastic transformation.[202–204] Such patients may have persistent sweats, with or without low-grade fever; nonspecific pains, especially in the limbs; and sometimes, steadily increasing splenomegaly.

Hematology in Accelerated Phase

In accelerated phase examination, peripheral blood nearly always reveals features no longer consistent with uncomplicated chronic phase CML. The patient may be anemic. The leukocyte differential is no longer typical of chronic phase; instead, there may be an excess of blast forms or promyelocytes. The neutrophils may show morphologic abnormalities, and the NAP score may be normal or raised. The number of eosinophils or basophils may be greatly increased. Nucleated red cells may be abundant. Platelet numbers may be reduced or greatly increased; in the latter case, platelet anisocytosis may be obvious. Examination of the bone marrow may provide little additional information. The finding of blast cells or blasts plus promyelocytes in excess of 30% implies that the patient is already in frank transformation.

In patients with myelofibrotic features, anemia is common. The red cells typically show anisocytosis with nucleated forms present in the blood. Platelet numbers may be increased or reduced. The marrow is difficult or impossible to aspirate, and a trephine biopsy specimen shows increased reticulin and collagen formation. Megakaryocytes may be increased in number and morphologically abnormal.

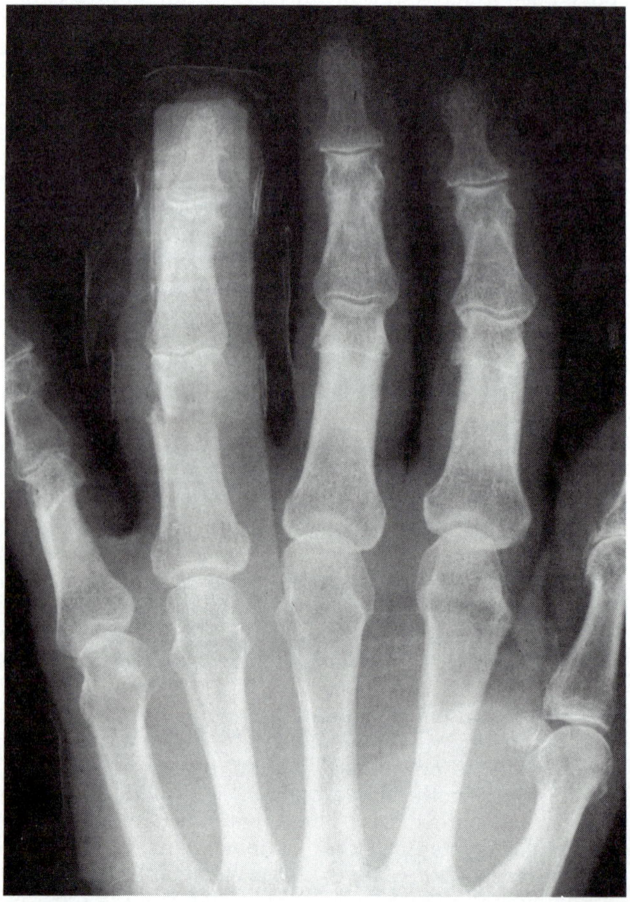

FIGURE 15-9. Radiograph showing lytic lesions in bone due to chronic myelogenous leukemia in transformation.

Hematology in Blastic Transformation

The peripheral blood in blast transformation shows a relatively homogeneous pattern of blasts (or blasts plus promyelocytes) that represent from 30% to nearly 100% of leukocytes. Other, more differentiated granulocytes are relatively reduced. The total leukocyte count is almost always raised. Platelet numbers may be variable. Nucleated red cells may be prominent.

Morphologic and other features reveal that blast cells are myeloid in about 70% of cases, lymphoid in about 20%, and mixed in the remainder.[205-209] The distinction sometimes can be made on Romanowsky-stained preparations. In many cases, the blast cells have features of myeloblasts or promyelocytes. Less frequently, the predominant blast is erythroid, megakaryoblastic, or monoblastic. Rarely, blastic transformation may be predominantly eosinophilic or basophilic. The blast cells cannot usually be classified in accordance with the French-American-British classification[210] (which is intended primarily for use in acute leukemia) but can usually be characterized by ultrastructure, cytochemistry, or study of surface antigen expression. Megakaryoblasts stain positively for platelet peroxidase on the nuclear membrane. Lymphoblasts usually have characteristic morphology by light microscopy. They may show block positivity with periodic acid–Schiff stain. They express common acute lymphoblastic leukemia antigen (CALLA; CD10) and other B-cell antigens on their surface membranes. Their nuclei contain terminal deoxynucleotidyl transferase.[206,208] Their DNA usually shows rearrangement of H-chain immunoglobulin or of both H- and L-chain immunoglobulin genes.[99] The genes for the T-cell receptor may also be rearranged.[100,101] Occasional cases of transformation with T lymphoblasts predominating have been described.[32,33]

When blast cell transformation is obvious from examination of the peripheral blood, examination of the marrow usually serves only as confirmation. As in chronic phase, however, it may be easier to obtain metaphases for cytogenetic studies from marrow cells, and it may be useful to assess the extent of marrow fibrosis.

The increased use of immunophenotyping has shown that morphologic and cytochemical results can be discordant. Occasional cases with apparently myeloid morphology have been shown to have exclusively lymphoid surface antigens. This new technology has also identified the occasional "lymphoid" marker on the surface of cells that have an otherwise myeloid appearance and immunophenotype. In these cases, it may be better to give the patients the benefit of the doubt and treat them (at least initially) as if they had lymphoid differentiation.

Complications of Blastic Transformation

Various complications may occur in accelerated or, more commonly, blastic phase that require recognition and specific therapy. The spleen may enlarge considerably, and the patient may sustain splenic infarction on more than one occasion. A large spleen may be associated with progressive anemia and an increasing requirement for blood transfusion.

The high blast cell count in the peripheral blood may produce features of leukostasis with cerebral dysfunction or pulmonary insufficiency.[112,211,212] A serum uric acid level may precipitate gout or urate nephropathy. Patients with one or more lytic bone lesions may develop mild or severe hypercalcemia.[213] Hypercalcemia may also occur in the absence of bone disease and may then be attributable to synthesis of parathormone-like material by leukemic blast cells. Patients with very high platelet counts may have a spurious or pseudohyperkalemia due to release of platelet potassium into the serum or plasma after the blood is drawn.[214]

A proportion of patients with lymphoid transformation in the blood and marrow develop simultaneously or subsequently features of neuroleukemia.[215-217] These typically include headache with nausea and vomiting, but focal neurologic signs may be detected. Some patients have signs of spinal cord compression. Examination of the cerebrospinal fluid reveals increased pressure and leukemic lymphoblasts in variable numbers.

Prognosis in Acceleration and Transformation Phases

Patients with CML in accelerated phase may respond to a variety of different approaches to treatment (discussed later) and may thereby be maintained in reasonable health for some months or even 1 to 2 years. In contrast, most patients in established myeloid transformation respond poorly to treatment, and their median survival is 2 to 3 months.[218-222] Patients in lymphoid transformation, however, may derive benefit from treatment and be restored to what amounts to second chronic phase; the median survival for such patients ranges from 6 to 18 months.

MANAGEMENT OF ADVANCED PHASES

When blast transformation is diagnosed, the first step must be to characterize the blast cells as far as is possible. If they prove to have a myeloid phenotype, treatment may be undertaken with the same cytotoxic drug combinations as are routinely valuable in the management of acute myeloid leukemia, namely cytosine arabinoside, daunorubicin, and perhaps 6-thioguanine administered over 5 or 7 days. This treatment should be accompanied by full doses of allopurinol to prevent accumulation of uric acid. Most patients respond to such treatment with a reduction in the number of blast cells in their blood and marrow. In most cases, a period of hypoplasia or aplasia is followed by gradual regeneration of blast cells, at which point it may be deemed expedient to continue treatment. Some patients remain aplastic and die eventually of infection or hemorrhage. A minority, perhaps 20%, recover with chronic phase–type hematopoiesis, which is almost invariably Ph-positive but usually lacks the additional cytogenetic changes that characterized the transformation. This second chronic phase lasts for some months, but blastic transformation inevitably recurs.

As an alternative approach to the management of myeloid blast transformation, the use of hydroxyurea in conjunction with plicamycin (mithramycin) was suggested in 1986.[223] Although most patients described in the original report were restored to second chronic phase, subsequent experience in other specialist centers has not been as favorable.

Patients whose blast cells manifest a lymphoid phenotype may be treated with drugs appropriate to acute lymphoblastic leukemia (ALL), notably vincristine and steroids with or without L-asparaginase. Treatment must be monitored with care because prolonged marrow hypoplasia is more common in CML in lymphoid transformation than in patients presenting de novo with ALL. With this treatment, most patients with CALLA-positive, TdT-positive blast cells regain chronic phase–type hematopoiesis. It is probably wise in such patients to continue intensive chemotherapy using a consolidation or maintenance schedule appropriate to adult ALL. It is also probably expedient to administer some form of prophylaxis for neuroleukemia—

probably five or six intrathecal injections of methotrexate. The use of cranial irradiation may be unnecessary.

The value of radiation therapy in treating specific problems for the patient in transformation should not be forgotten. Localized bone pain may be due to focal deposits of blast cell proliferation, which may be detected by radiologic or radionuclide scans. Such local lesions usually respond well to irradiation up to 10 to 20 Gy. An enlarged spleen may also reduce in size after irradiation; the radiation field need not encompass the whole of the enlarged spleen.

The spleen may reach vast proportions in the accelerated or transformed phases of CML. If its large size seriously impairs appetite and food ingestion, and if the patient is anemic or thrombocytopenic, splenectomy should be considered.[224] The surgery carries an appreciable risk of mortality, but the short-term benefits of a successful operation probably justify the risk.

Allogeneic bone marrow transplantation may be considered for the patient in transformation who has an HLA-identical sibling donor. Experience from many centers shows that the risks are considerable (Fig. 15-8); death may occur from any recognized complication of transplantation, and the actuarial risk of relapse is 50% to 60%. Nevertheless, 10% to 12% of patients allografted in transformation have become long-term survivors,[225] and this result is clearly better than could be achieved with cytotoxic drugs alone.

A number of patients in transformation have been treated by high-dose chemotherapy or chemoradiotherapy followed by autografting.[226] The procedure is usually successful at a technical level, but evidence of blast transformation recurs at a median of 3 months after autograft, and the median survival is about 6 months. The procedure may be repeated, and occasional patients autografted on two or three occasions have survived in second chronic phase for more than 1 or even 2 years.[222]

FUTURE PROSPECTS

Great progress has been made in the last decade in understanding stem cell kinetics and molecular features underlying the chronic phase of CML. It seems likely that the molecular features of transformation will be revealed in the foreseeable future. Such knowledge may point the way to more specific methods of controlling and possibly eradicating CML without the need for bone marrow transplantation. In the interim, allogeneic bone marrow transplantation should be undertaken in all suitable patients, and efforts must be made to extend the range of patients for whom the procedure is feasible. The role of autografting and the possible benefits of marrow purging before autografting are not yet defined.

REFERENCES

1. Bennett JH. Case of hypertrophy of the spleen and liver in which death took place from suppuration of the blood. Edinb Med Surg J 1845;64:413–422.
2. Pusey WA. Report of cases treated with roentgen rays. JAMA 1902;38: 911–191.
3. Minot GR, Buckman TE, Isaacs R. Chronic myelogenous leukemia: age incidence, duration and benefit derived from irradiation. JAMA 1924;82:1489–1494.
4. Galton DAG. Myleran in chronic myeloid leukaemia. Lancet 1953;1: 208–213.
5. Nowell PC, Hungerford DA. A minute chromosome in human chronic granulocytic leukemia. Science 1960;132:1497.
6. Gale RP, Canaani E. The molecular biology of chronic myelogenous leukaemia. Br J Haematol 1985;66:395–408.
7. Gale RP, Goldman JM. Rapid progress in chronic myeloid leukemia. Leukemia 1988;2:321–324.
8. Ward G. The infective theory of leukaemia. Br J Child Dis 1917;14: 10–20.
9. Shimkin MB, Mettier SR, Bierman HR. Myelocytic leukemia: an analysis of incidence, distribution and fatality, 1910–1948. Ann Intern Med 1951;35:194–212.
10. Tivey H. The prognosis for survival in chronic granulocytic leukemia and lymphocytic leukemia. Ann Intern Med 1953;72:68–93.
11. Canellos GP. Chronic granulocytic leukemia. Med Clin North Am 1976;60:1001–1018.
12. Kardinal CG, Bateman JR, Weiner J. Chronic granulocytic leukemia: review of 536 cases. Arch Intern Med 1976;136:305–313.
13. Baikie AG. Chronic granulocytic leukaemia. Med J Aust 1974;2:12–17.
14. Nowell PC, Hungerford DA. A minute chromosome in human chronic granulocytic leukemia. J Natl Cancer Inst 1960;25:85–109.
15. Rowley JD. A new consistent chromosomal abnormality in chronic myelogenous leukaemia identified by quinacrine fluorescence and Giemsa staining. Nature 1973;243:290–293.
16. Heisterkamp N, Stephenson JR, Groffen J, et al. Localization of the c-*abl* oncogene adjacent to a translocation breakpoint in chronic myelocytic leukaemia. Nature 1983;306:239–242.
17. Groffen J, Stephenson JR, Heisterkamp N, et al. Philadelphia chromosome breakpoints are clustered within a limited region, *bcr*, on chromosome 22. Cell 1984;36:93–99.
18. Konopka JB, Watanabe SM, Witte O. An alteration of the human c-abl protein in K562 leukemia cells unmasks associated tyrosine kinase activity. Cell 1984;37:1035–1042.
19. Heisterkamp N, Stam K, Groffen J, de Klein A, Grosveld G. Structural organization of the *bcr* gene and its role in the Ph translocation. Nature 1985;315:758–761.
20. Gale RP, Canaani E. An 8-kilobase abl RNA transcript in chronic myelogenous leukemia. Proc Natl Acad Sci USA 1984;81:5648–5652.
21. Daley GQ, van Etten RA, Baltimore D. Induction of chronic myelogenous leukemia in mice by the P210 *bcr/abl* gene of the Philadelphia chromosome. Science 1990;247:824–830.
22. Greaves MF. "Target cells," differentiation and clonal evolution in chronic granulocytic leukaemia: a "model" for understanding the biology of malignancy. In: Shaw MT, ed. Chronic granulocytic leukaemia. New York, Praeger, 1982:15–47.
23. Fialkow PJ, Gartler SM, Yoshida A. Clonal origin of chronic myelocytic leukemia in man. Proc Natl Acad Sci USA 1967;58:1468–1471.
24. Fialkow PJ Jacobson RJ, Papayannopoulou T. Chronic myelocytic leukemia: clonal origin in a stem cell common to the granulocyte, erythrocyte, platelet and monocyte/macrophage. Am J Med 1977;63: 125.
25. Rastrick JM, Fitzgerald PH, Gunz FW. Direct evidence for presence of Ph chromosome in erythroid cells. Br Med J 1974;1:96.
26. Denegri JF, Naiman SC, Gilken J, Thomas JW. In vitro growth of basophils containing the Philadelphia chromosome in the acute phase of chronic myelogenous leukaemia. Br J Haematol 1978;40:351.
27. Whang J, Frei E, Tjio JHY, Carbone PP, Brecher G. The distribution of the Philadelphia chromosome in patients with chronic myelogenous leukemia. Blood 1963;22:664–673.
28. Koeffler HP, Levine AM, Sparkes M, Sparkes RS. Chronic myelocytic leukemia: eosinophils involved in the malignant clone. Blood 1980;55: 1063–1064.
29. Golde DW, Burgaleta C, Sparkes RS, Cline MJ. The Philadelphia chromosome in human macrophages. Blood 1977;49:367.
30. Martin PJ, Najfeld V, Hansen JA, Penfold GK, Jacobson RJ, Fialkow PJ. Involvement of the B-lymphoid system in chronic myelogenous leukaemia. Nature 1980;287:49–50.
31. Bernheim A, Preud'homme JL, Labaume S, Bussel A, Barot-Ciorbaru R. Philadelphia chromosome positive blood B lymphocytes in chronic myelocytic leukemia. Leuk Res 1981;5:331–339.
32. Hernandez P, Carnot J, Cruz C. Chronic myeloid leukaemia blast crisis with T-cell features. Br J Haematol 1982;51:175.
33. Griffin JD, Tautravahi R, Canellos GP, et al. T-cell surface antigens in a patient with blast crisis of chronic myeloid leukemia. Blood 1983;61:640.
34. Yoffe G, Chinault AC, Talpaz M, et al. Clonal nature of Philadelphia chromosome positive and negative chronic myelogenous leukemia by DNA hybridization analysis. Exp Hematol 1987;15:725–728.
35. Fialkow PJ, Martin PJ, Najfeld V, Penfold GK, Jacobson RJ, Hansen JA. Evidence for a multistep pathogenesis of chronic myelogenous leukemia. Blood 1981;58:158–163.
36. Lisker R, Casas L, Mutchinick O, Perez-Chavez F, Labordini J. Late appearing Philadelphia chromosome in two patients with chronic myelogenous leukemia. Blood 1980;56:812–814.
37. Goldman JM, Lu Dao Pei. New approaches in chronic granulocytic leukemia: origin, prognosis and treatment. Semin Hematol 1982;19: 241–256.
38. Shepherd PCA, Ganesan TS, Galton DAG. Haematological classification of the chronic myeloid leukaemias. Baillières Clin Haematol 1987;1:887–906.
39. Ezdinli EZ, Sokal JE, Crosswhite JE. Philadelphia-chromosome-positive and -negative chronic myelocytic leukemia. Ann Intern Med 1970;72:175–183.

40. Canellos GP, Whang-Peng J, De Vita VT. Chronic granulocytic leukemia without the Philadelphia chromosome. Am J Clin Pathol 1976;65:467–470.
41. Pugh WC, Pearson M, Vardiman JW, Rowley JD. Philadelphia chromosome negative chronic myeloid leukaemia: a morphological reassessment. Br J Haematol 1985;60:456–467.
42. Kantarjian HM, Keating MJ, Walters RS, et al. Clinical and prognostic features of Philadelphia chromosome–negative chronic myelogenous leukemia. Cancer 1986;58:2023–2030.
43. Reisman LE, Trujillo JM. Chronic granulocytic leukaemia in childhood. J Pediatr 1963;62:710–723.
44. Hardisty RM, Speed DE, Till R. Granulocytic leukaemia in childhood. Br J Haematol 1964;10:551–556.
45. Bennett JM, Catovsky D, Flandrin G, Galton DAG, Gralnick HR, Sultan C. The French-American-British Cooperative Group: proposals for the classification of the myelodysplastic syndromes. Br J Haematol 1982;51:189–199.
46. Rubin H. Chronic neutrophilic leukemia. Ann Intern Med 1966;65: 93.
47. You W, Weisbrot IM. Chronic neutrophilic leukemia: report of 2 cases and a review of the literature. Am J Clin Pathol 1979;72:233–242.
48. Gunz FW. The epidemiology and genetics of the chronic leukaemias. Clin Haematol 1977;6:3–20.
49. Muir CS, Waterhouse J, Mack T, Powell J, Whelan S. Cancer incidence in 5 continents, vol 5. IARC Scientific Publication no. 88. Lyon: International Agency for Research on Cancer, 1987.
50. Eglin RP, Swann RA, Isaacs D, Moxon ER. Chronic leukaemia in siblings. Lancet 1984;2:984.
51. Court Brown W, Abbatt J. Mortality from cancer and other causes after radiotherapy for ankylosing spondylitis. Br Med J 1965;2:1327–1329.
52. Doll R, Smith PG. The long term effects of X-irradiation in patients treated for metropathia haemorrhagica. Br J Radiol 1968;41:362–368.
53. Lange R, Moloney W, Yamawaki T. Leukemia in atomic bomb survivors. 1. General observations. Blood 1954;9:574–585.
54. Heyssel R, Brill B, Woodbury L. Leukemia in Hiroshima atomic bomb survivors. Blood 1960;15:313–331.
55. Caspersson T, Gahrton G, Lindsten J, Zech L. Identification of the Philadelphia chromosome as a number 22 by quinacrine mustard fluorescence analysis. Exp Cell Res 1970;63:238.
56. Sandberg AA. Nomenclature: the Philadelphia chromosome—Ph[1] or Ph without the superscript. Cancer Genet Cytogenet 1985;14:1.
57. Whang-Peng J, Lee EC, Khutsen TA. The genesis of the Ph[1] chromosome. J Natl Cancer Inst 1974;52:1035.
58. Maniatis AK, Amsels S, Mitus WJ, Colman N. Chromosome pattern of bone marrow fibroblasts in patients with chronic granulocytic leukaemia. Nature 1969;222:1278.
59. Greenberg B, Wilson F, Woo L, Jenks H. Cytogenetics of fibroblastic colonies in Ph-positive chronic myelogenous leukemia. Blood 1978;51: 1039.
60. Brandt L, Mitelman F, Panani A, Lenner HC. Extremely long duration of chronic myeloid leukaemia with Ph[1] negative and Ph[1] positive bone marrow cells. Scand J Haematol 1976;16:321–325.
61. Sokal JE. Significance of Ph-negative marrow cells in Ph-positive chronic granulocytic leukemia. Blood 1980;56:1072–1076.
62. Golde DW, Bersh NL, Sparkes RS. Chromosomal mosaicism associated with prolonged remission in chronic myelogenous leukemia. Cancer 1976;37:1849–1852.
63. de Braekeleer M. Variant Philadelphia translocations in chronic myeloid leukemia. Cytogenet Cell Genet 1987;44:215–222.
64. Hagemeijer A. Chromosome abnormalities in CML. Baillieres Clin Haematol 1987;1:963–981.
65. Hagemeijer A, de Klein A, Godde-Salz E, et al. Translocation of c-abl to "masked" Ph in chronic myeloid leukemia. Cancer Genet Cytogenet 1985;18:95–104.
66. Theologides A. Unfavorable signs in patients with chronic myelocytic leukemia. Ann Intern Med 1972;76:95–99.
67. Travis LB, Pearson M, Vardiman JW, Rowley JD. Ph[1]-negative chronic granulocytic leukemia: a nonentity. Am J Clin Pathol 1986;85:186–193.
68. Pugh WC, Pearson M, Vardiman JW, Rowley JD. Philadelphia-chromosome–negative chronic myelogenous leukaemia: a morphological reassessment. Br J Haematol 1985;60:457–467.
69. Morris CM, Reeve AE, Fitzgerald PH, Hollings, Beard MEJ, Heaton DC. Genomic diversity correlates with clinical diversity in Ph-negative chronic myeloid leukaemia. Nature 1986;320:281–283.
70. Dreazen O, Klisak I, Rassool F, Goldman JM, Sparkes RS, Gale RP. Do oncogenes determine the clinical features in chronic myeloid leukaemia? Lancet 1987;1:1402–1405.
71. Weidemann LM, Karhi KK, Shivji MKK, et al. The correlation of bcr rearrangement and p210phl/abl expression with morphological analysis of Ph-negative CML and other myeloproliferative diseases. Blood 1988;71:349–355.
72. Abelson HT, Rabstein LS. Lymphosarcoma: virus-induced thymic independent disease in mice. Cancer Res 1970;30:2213–2222.
73. Heisterkamp N, Groffen J, Stephenson JR. The human v-*abl* cellular homologue. J Mol Appl Genet 1983:57–68.
74. Groffen J, Heisterkamp N. The BCR/ABL hybrid gene. Baillieres Clin Haematol 1987;1:983–999.
75. Hermans A, Heisterkamp N, von Lindern M, et al. Unique fusion of *bcr* and c-*abl* genes in Philadelphia positive acute lymphoblastic leukemia. Cell 1987;51:333–340.
76. Goldman JM, Grosveld G, Baltimore D, Gale RP. Chronic myelogenous leukemia: the unfolding saga. Leukemia 1990;4:163–167.
77. Bartram CR, De Klein A, Hagemeijer A, et al. Translocation of c-*abl* oncogene correlates with the presence of a Philadelphia chromosome. Nature 1983;306:277–280.
78. Hagemeijer A, Bartram CJ, Smit EME, van Agthoven AJ, Bootsma D. Is the chromosomal region 9q34 always involved in variants of the Ph[1] translocation? Cancer Genet Cytogenet 1984;13:1–16.
79. Morris CM, Reeve AE, Fitzgerald PH, Hollings PE, Beard MEJ, Heaton DC. Genomic diversity correlates with clinical variation in Ph[1]-negative chronic myeloid leukaemia. Nature 1986;320:281–283.
80. Bartram CR, Kleihauer E, de Klein A, et al. c-abl and bcr are rearranged in a Ph[1]-negative CML patient. EMBO J 1985;4:683–686.
81. Shtivelman E, Gale RP, Dreazen O, et al. *bcr-abl* RNA in patients with chronic myelogenous leukemia. Blood 1987;69:971–973.
82. Collins SJ, Groudine MT. Chronic myelogenous leukemia: amplification of a rearranged c-*abl* oncogene in both chronic phase and blast crisis. Blood 1987;69:893–898.
83. Kawasaki ES, Clark SS, Coyne MY, et al. Diagnosis of chronic myeloid and acute lymphocytic leukemias by detection of leukemia-specific mRNA sequences amplified in vitro. Proc Natl Acad Sci USA 1988;85: 5698–5702.
84. Lee MS, Lemaistre A, Kantarjian HM, et al. Detection of two alternative *bcr/abl* mRNA junctions and minimal residual disease in Philadelphia chromosome positive chronic myelogenous leukemia by polymerase chain reaction. Blood 1989;73:2165–2170.
85. Sawyers CL, Timson L, Kawasaki ES, et al. Molecular relapse in chronic myelogenous leukemia patients after bone marrow transplantation detected by polymerase chain reaction. Proc Natl Acad Sci 1990;87:563.
86. Hughes TP, Martiat P, Morgan G, Sawyers C, Witte ON, Goldman JM. Significance of residual leukaemia transcripts after bone marrow transplant for CML. Lancet 1990;1:50.
87. Eaves CJ, Eaves AC. Cell culture studies in CML. Baillieres Clin Haematol 1987;1:931–961.
88. Wognum AW, Krystal G, Eaves CJ, Eaves AC, Lansdorp PM. Increased erythropoietic-receptor expression on CD34-positive bone marrow cells from patients with chronic myeloid leukemia. Blood 1992;79: 642–649.
89. Coulombel L, Kalousek DK, Eaves CJ, et al. Long term marrow culture reveals chromosomally normal hematopoietic progenitor cells in patients with Philadelphia-positive chronic myelogenous leukemia. N Engl J Med 1983;308:1493–1498.
90. Eaves AC, Cashman JD, Gaboury LA, Kalousek DK, Eaves CJ. Unregulated proliferation of primitive chronic myeloid leukemia progenitors in the presence of normal marrow adherent cells. Proc Natl Acad Sci USA 1986;83:5306.
91. Spiers ASD, Bain BJ, Turner JE. The peripheral blood in chronic granulocytic leukaemia: study of 50 untreated Philadelphia-positive cases. Scand J Haematol 1977;18:25.
92. Robak T, Nolasco I, Hibbin JA, Goldman JM. Antigenic characteristics of circulating CFU-GM in chronic granulocytic leukemia resemble those of CFU-GM in normal marrow and differ from those in normal blood. Leuk Res 1985;9:1023–1029.
93. Odeberg H, Olofsson T, Olsson I. Granulocyte function in chronic granulocytic leukaemia. I. Bactericidal and metabolic capabilities during phagocytosis in isolated granulocytes. Br J Haematol 1975;29: 427.
94. Goldman JM, Th'ng KH. Phagocytic function of leucocytes from patients with acute myeloid and chronic granulocytic leukaemia. Br J Haematol 1973;25:299.
95. Lawler SD. The cytogenetics of chronic granulocytic leukaemia. Clin Haematol 1977;6:55–75.
96. Hagemeijer A, Stenfert-Kroese WF, Abels J. Cytogenetic follow-up of patients with non-lymphocytic leukemia. I. Philadelphia chromosome positive chronic myeloid leukemia. Cancer Genet Cytogenet 1980;2: 317–326.
97. Alimena G, Dallapiccola B, Gastaldi R, et al. Chromosomal, morphological and clinical correlations in blastic crisis of chronic myeloid leukaemia: a study of 69 cases. Scand J Haematol 1982;28:103–117.
98. Rowley JD, Testa JR. Chromosome abnormalities in malignant hematologic diseases. Adv Cancer Res 1982;36:103–148.
99. Bakshi A, Minowada J, Arnold A, et al. Lymphoid blast crisis of chronic myelogenous leukemia represent stages in the development of B-cell precursors. N Engl J Med 1983;309:826–831.
100. Chan LC, Furley AJ, Ford AM, Yardumian DA, Greaves MF. Clonal rearrangement and expression of the T-cell receptor β-gene and involvement of the breakpoint cluster region in blast crisis of CGL. Blood 1986;67:533–536.
101. Uike N, Takeichi N, Kimura N, Takahira H, Kozuru M. Dual rearrangement of immunoglobulin and T-cell receptor genes in blast crisis of CML. Eur J Haematol 1989;42:460–465.

102. Liu E, Hjelle B, Bishop JM. Transforming genes in chronic myelogenous leukaemia. Proc Natl Acad Sci USA 1988;85:1952–1956.
103. McCarthy DM, Rassool FV, Goldman JM, Graham SV, Birnie GD. Genomic alterations involving the *c-myc* protooncogene locus during evolution of a case of chronic granulocytic leukaemia. Lancet 1984;1: 1362–1365.
104. Bartram CR, De Klein A, Hagemeier A, Carbonell F, Kleihauer E, Grosveld G. Additional *c-abl/bcr* rearrangements in a CML patient exhibiting two Ph[1] chromosomes during blast crisis. Leuk Res 1986;10: 221–225.
105. Ahuja H, Bar-Eli M, Advani SH, Benchimol S, Cline MJ. Alterations in the p53 gene and the clonal evolution of the blast crisis of chronic myelocytic leukemia. Proc Natl Acad Sci USA 1989;86:6783–6787.
106. Kelman Z, Prokocimer M, Peller S, et al. Rearrangements in the p53 gene in Philadelphia chromosome positive chronic myelogenous leukemia. Blood 1989;74:2318.
107. Spiers ASD. The clinical features of chronic granulocytic leukaemia. Clin Haematol 1977;6:77–95.
108. Bergsagel DE. The chronic leukemias: a review of disease manifestations and the aims of therapy. Can Med Assoc J 1967;96:1615–1620.
109. Kamada N, Urchino H. Chronologic sequence in appearance of clinical and laboratory findings characeristic of chronic myelocytic leukemia. Blood 1978;51:843–850.
110. Mehta AB, Goldman JM, Kohner E. Hyperleucocytic retinopathy in chronic granulocytic leukaemia: the role of intensive leucapheresis. Br J Haematol 1984;56:661–667.
111. Suri R, Goldman JM, Catovsky D, Johnson SA, Wiltshaw E, Galton DAG. Priapism complicating chronic granulocytic leukemia. Am J Hematol 1980;2:295–299.
112. Thompson DS, Goldstone AH, Parry HF, Richards JDM. Leukostasis in chronic myeloid leukaemia. Br Med J 1978;2:202.
113. Wachstein M. Alkaline phosphatase activity in normal and abnormal human blood and bone marrow cells. J Lab Clin Med 1946;31:1–17.
114. Wiltshaw E, Moloney WC. Histochemical and biochemical studies on leukocyte alkaline phosphatase activity. Blood 1955;10:1120–1123.
115. Mitus WJ, Bergna LJ, Mednikoff IB, Dameshek W. Alkaline phosphatase of mature neutrophils in chronic forms of the myeloproliferative syndrome. Blood 1958;30:285–294.
116. Rustin GJS, Peters TJ. Studies on the subcellular organelles of neutrophils in chronic granulocytic leukaemia with special reference to alkaline phosphatase. Br J Haematol 1979;41:533.
117. Rustin GJS, Goldman JM, McCarthy DM, Mees S, Peters TJ. An extrinsic factor controls neutrophil alkaline phosphatase in chronic granulocytic leukaemia. Br J Haematol 1980;45:381–387.
118. Hellmann A, Goldman JM. Alkaline phosphatase activity of chronic granulocytic leukaemia neutrophils in agar culture. Scand J Haematol 1980;24:237–242.
119. Chikkappa G, Wang GJ, Santella D, et al. Granulocyte colony-stimulating factor (G-CSF) induces synthesis of alkaline phosphatase in neutrophilic granulocytes of chronic myelogenous leukemia patients. Leuk Res 1988;12:491–498.
120. De Marsh QB, Kautz J. Pseudo-Gaucher cells in chronic myelocytic leukemia. Blood 1957;12:324.
121. Kelsey PR, Geary CG. Sea-blue histiocytes and Gaucher cells in bone marrow of patients with chronic myeloid leukaemia. J Clin Pathol 1988;41:960–962.
122. Gralnick HR, Harbor J, Vogel C. Myelofibrosis in chronic granulocytic leukemia. 1971;37:152–162.
123. Clough V, Geary CG, Hashmi K, Davson G, Knowlsen T. Myelofibrosis in chronic granulocytic leukaemia. Br J Haematol 1979;42:515–526.
124. Bolin R, Robinson W, Sutherland J, Hamman R. Busulfan versus hydroxyurea in long-term therapy of chronic myelogenous leukemia. Cancer 1982;50:1683.
125. Kennedy BJ. Hydroxyurea in chronic myelogenous leukemia. Ann Intern Med 1969;70:1084.
126. Sokal JE, Cox EB, Baccarani M. Prognostic discrimination in "good risk" chronic granulocytic leukemia. Blood 1984;63:789–799.
127. Sokal JE, Baccarani M, Tura S, et al. Prognostic discrimination among younger patients with chronic granulocytic leukemia: relevance to bone marrow transplantation. Blood 1985;66:1352–1357.
128. Tura S, Baccarani M, Corbelli G, and the Italian Cooperative Study Group on Chronic Myeloid Leukaemia. Staging of chronic myeloid leukaemia. Br J Haematol 1981;47:105–119.
129. Medical Research Council's Working Party of Therapeutic Trials in Leukaemia. Randomized trial of splenectomy in Ph-positive chronic granulocytic leukaemia, including an analysis of prognostic features. Br J Haematol 1983;54:415–430.
130. Cervantes F, Rozman C. A multivariate analysis of prognostic factors in chronic myeloid leukemia. Blood 1982;60:1298–1304.
131. Oguma S, Takatsuki K, Uchino H, Kamada N, Oguma N, Kuramoto A. Factors influencing survival in Philadelphia-chromosome positive chronic myelocytic leukemia. Cancer 1982;50:2928–2934.
132. Kantarjian HM, Smith TL, McCredie KB, et al. Chronic myelogenous leukemia: a multivariate analysis of the associations of patient characteristics and therapy with survival. Blood 1985;66:1326–1335.
133. Sokal JE. Prognosis in CML. Baillieres Clin Haematol 1987;1:907–929.
134. Schaefer-Rego K, Dudek H, Popenoe D, et al. CML patients in blast crisis have breakpoints localized to a specific region of the BCR. Blood 1987;70:448–455.
135. Mills KI, MacKenzie ED, Birnie GD. The site of the breakpoint within the *bcr* is a prognostic factor in Philadelphia-positive CML patients. Blood 1988;72:1237–1241.
136. Jaubert J, Martiat P, Dowding C, Ifrah N, Goldman JM. The position of the M-*BCR* breakpoint does not predict the duration of chronic phase or survival in chronic myeloid leukaemia. Br J Haematol 1989;74:30–35.
137. Wolf DJ, Silver RT, Coleman M. Factors associated with prolonged survival in chronic myeloid leukemia. Cancer 1978;42:1957–1963.
138. Singer CRJ, McDonald GA, Douglas AS. Twenty-five year survival of chronic granulocytic leukaemia with spontaneous karyotype conversion. Br J Haematol 1984;57:309–314.
139. Nowell PC, Jackson L, Weiss A, Kurzrock R. Historical communication: Philadelphia-positive chronic myelogenous leukemia followed for 27 years. Cancer Genet Cytogenet 1988;34:57–61.
140. Brandt L, Mitelman F, Panani A, Lenner HC. Extremely long duration of chronic myeloid leukaemia with Ph[1] negative and Ph[1] positive bone marrow cells. Scand J Haematol 1976;16:321–325.
141. Provan AB, Majer RV, Herbert A, Smith AG. Spontaneous remission of chronic myeloid leukaemia with loss of Philadelphia chromosome. Br J Haematol 1991;78:578–579.
142. Galton DAG. Myleran in chronic myeloid leukaemia. Lancet 1953;1: 208–213.
143. Galton DAG, Till M, Wiltshaw E. Busulfan (1,4-dimethanesulphonyloxybutane): summary of clinical results. Ann NY Acad Sci 1958;68: 967–973.
144. Medical Research Council's Working Party for Therapeutic Trials in Leukaemia. Chronic granulocytic leukaemia: comparison of radiotherapy and busulphan therapy. Br Med J 1968;1:201–208.
145. Galton DAG. Treatment of the chronic leukaemias. Br Med Bull 1959;15:79–86.
146. Vicariot M, Goldman JM, Catovsky D, Galton DAG. Treatment of chronic granulocytic leukaemia with repeated single doses of busulphan. Eur J Cancer 1979;15:559–563.
147. Weatherall DJ, Galton DAG, Kay HEM. Busulphan and bone marrow depression. Br Med J 1969;1:638.
148. Dunn CD. The chemical and biological properties of busulfan. Exp Hematol 1974;2:101–117.
149. Kyle RA, Schwartz RD, Oliner HL, Dameshek W. A syndrome resembling adrenal cortical insufficiency associated with long-term busulfan (Myleran) therapy. Blood 1961;18:497–510.
150. Finney R, McDonald GA, Baikie AG, Douglas AS. Chronic granulocytic leukaemia with Ph[1] negative cells in bone marrow and a ten year remission after busulphan hypoplasia. Br J Haematol 1972;23:283–288.
151. Speed DE, Lawler SD. Chronic granulocytic leukaemia: the chromosomes and the disease. Lancet 1964;1:403–407.
152. Greig HBW. Myleran in the treatment of chronic granulocytic leukaemia. Acta Haematol 1956;16:171–180.
153. Finney R, McDonald GA, Baikie AG, et al. Chronic granulocytic leukaemia with Ph[1] negative cells in bone marrow and a ten year remission after busulphan hypoplasia. Br J Haematol 1972;23:283.
154. Oliner HL, Schwartz RS, Rubio F, Dameshek W. Interstitial pulmonary fibrosis following busulfan therapy. Am J Med 1961;31:134–139.
155. Kirschner RH, Esterly JR. Pulmonary lesions associated with busulfan therapy for chronic myelogenous leukemia. Cancer 1971;27:1074–1080.
156. Podos SM, Canellos GP. Lens changes in chronic granulocytic leukemia: possible relationship to chemotherapy. Am J Opthalmol 1969;68:500–504.
157. Kennedy BJ, Yarbro JW. Metabolic and therapeutic effects of hydroxyurea in chronic myeloid leukemia. J Am Med Assoc 1966;195: 1038.
158. Kennedy BJ. Hydroxyurea therapy in chronic myelogenous leukemia. Cancer 1972;29:1052–1056.
159. Bolin RW, Robinson WA, Sutherland J, et al. Busulphan versus hydroxyurea in long-term therapy of chronic myelogenous leukemia. Cancer 1982;50:1683–1686.
160. Silver RT, Mick R, Cooper R, et al. A comparative study of dibromomannitol and busulfan in the treatment of chronic myeloid leukemia. Blood 1987;60:1442–1448.
161. Renon L, Dreyfus L. Radium therapie de la leucemie myeloide. Arch Elec Med 1933;23:366.
162. Morse EE, Carbone PP, Freireich EJ, Bronson W, Kliman A. Repeated leukapheresis of patients with chronic myelocytic leukemia. Transfusion 1966;6:175–182.
163. Lowenthal RM, Buskard NA, Goldman JM, et al. Intensive leukapheresis as initial therapy for chronic granulocytic leukemia. Blood 1975;46:835–844.
164. Caplan SN, Coco FV, Berkman EM. Management of chronic myelocytic leukemia in pregnancy by cell pheresis. Transfusion 1978;18:120–124.
165. Fitzgerald D, Rowe JM, Heal J. Leukapheresis for control of chronic myelogenous leukemia during pregnancy. Am J Hematol 1986;22: 213–218.

166. Spiers ASD, Baikie AG, Galton DAG. Chronic granulocytic leukaemia: effect of elective splenectomy on the course of the disease. Br Med J 1975;1:175–179.
167. Gomez GA, Sokal JE, Mittelman A, Aungst CW. Splenectomy for palliation of chronic myelocytic leukemia. Am J Med 1976;61:14–22.
168. Ihde DC, Canellos GP, Schwartz JH, De Vita VT. Splenectomy in the chronic phase of chronic granulocytic leukemia. Ann Intern Med 1976;84:17–21.
169. Italian Cooperative Study Group on Chronic Myeloid Leukaemia. Effect of early splenectomy and cyclic acute leukemia-like chemotherapy on the course of chronic myeloid leukemia. Boll Ist Sieroter Milan 1978;57:360.
170. Talpaz M, McCredie KB, Mavligit GM, Gutterman J. Leukocyte interferon-induced myeloid cytoreduction in chronic myelogenous leukemia. Blood 1983;62:689–692.
171. Talpaz M, Kantarjian HM, McCredie K, et al. Hematologic remission and cytogenetic improvement induced by recombinant human interferon alpha A in chronic myelogenous leukemia. N Engl J Med 1986;314:1065–1069.
172. Talpaz M, Kantarjan HM, McCredie KB, Keating MI, Trujillo, Gutterman J. Clinical investigation of human alpha interferon in chronic myelogenous leukemia. Blood 1987;69:1280–1288.
173. Lee M, Kantarjian H, Deisseroth A, Freireich E, Trujillo J, Stass S. Clinical usage of polymerase chain reaction (PCR) to analyze the BCR/ABL splicing patterns and minimal residual disease (MRD) in Philadelphia chromosome positive chronic myelogenous leukemia. Blood 1989;74:199a.
174. Galvani DW, Cawley JC. Mechanism of action of alpha interferon in chronic granulocytic leukaemia: evidence of preferential inhibition of late progenitors. Br J Haematol 1989;73:475–479.
175. Oladipupo-Williams CK, Svet-Moldavskaya I, Vilcek J, Ohnuma T, Holland JF. Inhibitory effects of human leukocyte and fibroblast interferons on normal and chronic myelogenous leukemia granulocytic progenitor cells. Oncology 1981;38:356.
176. Kurzrock R, Quesada JR, Talpaz M, et al. Phase I study of multiple-dose intramuscularly administered recombinant gamma interferon. J Clin Oncol 1986;4:1101.
176a. Italian Cooperative Study Group on Chronic Myeloid Leukemia. Progress in treatment of chronic myeloid leukemia: interferon versus conventional chemotherapy. N Engl J Med (in press).
177. Doney K, Buckner CD, Thomas ED, et al. Allogeneic bone marrow transplantation for chronic granulocytic leukemia. Exp Hematol 1981;9:966–971.
178. Fefer A, Cheever MA, Thomas ED, et al. Disappearance of Ph-positive cells in four patients with chronic granulocytic leukemia after chemotherapy, irradiation and marrow transplantation from an identical twin. N Engl J Med 1979;300:333–337.
179. Clift RA, Thomas ED, Buckner CD, et al. Treatment of chronic granulocytic leukaemia in chronic phase by bone marrow transplantation. Lancet 1982;2:623–625.
180. Goldman JM, Baughan ASJ, McCarthy DM, et al. Marrow transplantation for patients in chronic phase of chronic granulocytic leukaemia. Lancet 1982;2:623–625.
181. Thomas ED, Clift RA, Fefer A, et al. Marrow transplantation for the treatment of chronic myelogenous leukemia. Ann Intern Med 1986;104:155–163.
182. Goldman JM, Apperley JF, Jones L, et al. Bone marrow transplantation for patients with chronic myeloid leukemia. N Engl J Med 1986;314:202–207.
183. Goldman JM, Gale RP, Horowitz MM, et al. Bone marrow transplantation for chronic myelogenous leukemia in chronic phase: increased risk of relapse associated with T-cell depletion. Ann Intern Med 1988;108:806–814.
184. Apperley JF, Mauro F, Goldman JM, et al. Bone marrow transplantation for chronic myeloid leukaemia in chronic phase: importance of a graft-versus-leukaemia effect. Br J Haematol 1988;69:239–245.
185. Maraninchi D, Gluckman E, Blaise D, et al. Impact of T-cell depletion on outcome of allogeneic bone marrow transplantation for standard-risk leukaemias. Lancet 1987;2:175–178.
186. Horowitz MM, Gale RP, Sondel PM, Goldman JM, et al. Graft-versus-leukemia reactions after bone marrow transplantation. Blood 1990;75:555–562.
187. Arthur CK, Apperley JF, Guo AP, et al. Cytogenetic events after bone marrow transplantation for chronic myeloid leukemia in chronic phase. Blood 1988;71:1179–1186.
188. Zaccaria A, Rosti G, Sassarego M, et al. Relapse after allogeneic bone marrow transplantation for chronic myeloid leukemia: cytogenetic analysis of 24 patients. Bone Marrow Transplant 1988;3:413–424.
189. Bartram CR, Janssen JWG, Schmidberger M, et al. Minimal residual leukaemia in chronic myeloid leukaemia patients after T-cell depleted bone marrow transplantation. Lancet 1989;1:1260.
190. Roth MS, Antin JH, Bingham EL, Ginsburg D. Detection of Philadelphia chromosome positive cells by the polymerase chain reaction following bone marrow transplant for chronic myelogenous leukemia. Blood 1989;74:882.
191. Morgan GJ, Hughes T, Janssen JWG, et al. Polymerase chain reaction for the detection of residual leukaemia. Lancet 1989;1:928–929.
191a. Cross NCP, Feng Lin, Chase A, et al. Competitive PCR to estimate the number of BCR-ABL transcripts in chronic myeloid leukemia patients after bone marrow transplantation. Blood 1993;82:1929–1936.
192. Butturini A, Keating A, Goldman JM, Gale RP. Autotransplants in chronic myelogenous leukaemia: strategies and results. Lancet 1990;1:1255–1258.
193. Brito-Babapulle F, Bowcock S, Marcus RE, et al. Autografting for patients with chronic myeloid leukaemia in chronic phase: peripheral blood stem cells may have a finite capacity for maintaining haemopoiesis. Br J Haematol 1989;73:76–81.
194. McGlave PB, Arthur D, Miller WJ, Lasky L, Kersey J. Autologous transplantation for CML using marrow treated ex vivo with recombinant human interferon gamma. Bone Marrow Transplant 1990;6:115–120.
195. Barnett MJ, Eaves CJ, Phillips GL, et al. Successful autografting in chronic myeloid leukaemia after maintenance of marrow in culture. Bone Marrow Transplant 1989;4:345–351.
196. Kantarjian HM, Dixon D, Keating MJ, et al. Characteristics of accelerated disease in chronic myelogenous leukemia. Cancer 1988;61:1441–1446.
197. Karanas A, Silver RT. Characteristics of the terminal phase of chronic granulocytic leukemia. Blood 1968;32:445–459.
198. Neiman RS, Barcos M, Berard C, et al. Granulocytic sarcoma: a clinicopathologic study of 61 biopsied cases. Cancer 1981;48:1426–1437.
199. Jacknow G, Frizzera G, Gajl-Paczaslska K, et al. Extramedullary presentation of the blast crisis of chronic myelogenous leukaemia. Br J Haematol 1985;61:225–236.
200. Chabner BA, Hasell CM, Canellos GP. Destructive bone lesions in chronic granulocytic leukemia. Medicine 1969;48:401–410.
201. Longo DL, Whang-Peng J, Jaffe E, Triche TJ, Young RC. Myeloproliferative syndromes: a unique presentation of chronic myelogenous leukemia (CML) as a primary tumor of bone. Blood 1978;52:793–801.
202. Lazzarini M, Mora E, Castello A, et al. Myelofibrosis in chronic granulocytic leukaemia: clinicopathologic correlations and prognostic significance. Br J Haematol 1986;64:227–240.
203. Moloney WC. Natural history of chronic granulocytic leukaemia. Clin Haematol 1971;6:41.
204. Gralnick HR, Harbor J, Vogel C. Myelofibrosis in chronic granulocytic leukemia. Blood 1971;37:152.
205. Janossy G, Greaves MF, Revesz T, et al. Blast crisis of chronic myeloid leukaemia (CML). II. Cell surface marker analysis of "lymphoid" and myeloid cases. Br J Haematol 1976;34:179–192.
206. Marks SM, Baltimore D, McCaffrey R. Terminal transferase as a predictor of initial responsiveness to vincristine and prednisone in blastic chronic myelogenous leukemia. N Engl J Med 1978;298:812–814.
207. Janossy G, Woodruff RK, Pippard MJ, et al. Relation of "lymphoid" phenotype and response to chemotherapy incorporating vincristine-prednisone in the acute phase of Ph positive leukemia. Cancer 1979;43:426–434.
208. Tanaka M, Kaneda T, Hirota Y, Yoshida S, Kitajima K. Terminal deoxynucleotidyl transferase in the blastic phase of chronic myelogenous leukemia: an indicator of response to vincristine and prednisone therapy. Am J Hematol 1980;9:287–293.
209. San Miguel JF, Tavares De Castro J, Matutes E, et al. Characterization of blast cells in chronic granulocytic leukaemia in transformation, acute myelofibrosis and differentiated leukaemia. II. Studies with monoclonal antibodies and terminal transferase. Br J Haematol 1985;59:297–309.
210. Bennett JM, Catovsky D, Daniel MT, et al. Proposals for the classification of the acute leukaemias. Br J Haematol 1976;33:451–458.
211. Lichtman MA, Rowe JM. Hyperleukocytic leukaemia: rheological, clinical and therapeutic considerations. Blood 1982;60:279.
212. Stirling ML, et al. Leukapheresis for papilloedemia in chronic granulocytic leukaemia. Br Med J 1971;2:676.
213. Haskell CM, de Vita VT, Canellos GP. Hypercalcemia in chronic granulocytic leukemia. Cancer 1971;27:872–880.
214. Wulkan RW, Michiels JJ. Pseudohyperkalaemia in thrombocythaemia. J Clin Chem Biochem 1990;28:489–491.
215. Kwaan HC, Pierre RV, Long DL. Meningeal involvement as first manifestation of acute myeloblastic transformation of chronic granulocytic leukemia. Blood 1969;33:348–352.
216. Atkinson K, Kay HEM, Lawler SD, Wells DG, McElwain TJ. Meningeal leukemia after blastic transformation of chronic myeloid leukemia. Cancer 1975;35:529–533.
217. Woodruff RK, Malpas JS, Wrigley PFM, Lister TA, Paxton AM, Janossy G. Meningeal leukaemia in lymphoid blast crisis of chronic myeloid leukaemia. Br Med J 1977;2:1325–1326.
218. Canellos GP. The treatment of chronic granulocytic leukaemia. Clin Haematol 1977;6:113–128.
219. Vallejos CS, Trujillo JM, Cork A, et al. Blastic crisis in chronic granulocytic leukemia: experience in 39 patients. Cancer 1974;34:1806–1812.
220. Spiers ASD, Costello C, Catovsky D, Galton DAG, Goldman JM. Chronic granulocytic leukaemia: multiple drug chemotherapy for acute transformation. Br Med J 1974;2:77–80.

221. Coleman M, Silver R, Pajak T, et al. Combination chemotherapy for terminal phase chronic myelocytic leukemia. Blood 1980;55:29–36.
222. Kantarjian HM, Keating MJ, Talpaz M, et al. Chronic myelogenous leukemia in blast crisis: analysis of 242 patients. Am J Med 1987;83: 445–454.
223. Koller CA, Miller DM. Preliminary observations in the therapy of myeloid blast phase of chronic granulocytic leukemia with plicamycin and hydroxyurea. N Engl J Med 1986;315:1433–1438.
224. Spiers ASD, Baikie AG, Galton DAG, et al. Splenectomy for complications of chronic granulocytic leukaemia. Lancet 1975;2:627.
225. Speck B, Bortin MM, Champlin R, et al. Allogeneic marrow transplantation for chronic myelogenous leukaemia. Lancet 1984;1:665–668.
226. Haines ME, Goldman JM, Worsley AM, et al. Chemotherapy and autografting for patients with chronic granulocytic leukemia in transformation: probable prolongation of life for some patients. Br J Haematol 1984;58:711–722.
227. Reiffers J, Trouette R, Marit G, et al. Autologous blood stem cell transplantation for chronic granulocytic leukaemia in transformation: a report of 47 cases. Br J Haematol 1991;77:339–345.

4

White Blood Cells

Blood: Principles and Practice of Hematology,
edited by Robert I. Handin, Thomas P. Stossel, and Samuel E. Lux.
J.B. Lippincott Company, Philadelphia © 1995.

16

Immunoproteins

Harvey R. Colten
Jonathan D. Gitlin

The discovery and application of the principles of specific immunity in 1796 antedated by about 200 years concepts pertaining to the mechanisms involved. That is, Jenner's recognition of the value of vaccination for protection against smallpox and the eventual acceptance of this as an effective prophylaxis were pure empiricism. In the late 19th century, however, the field of immunology emerged in tandem with studies of microbes and microbial pathogenesis. These developments permitted formulation of hypotheses to describe well-recognized phenomena and to make predictions about host defenses against infectious agents. Indeed, many of the theoretic formulations of Erhlich, Metchnikoff, Pasteur, Bordet, and others were surprisingly close to our current concepts of molecular and cellular immunologic mechanisms. It was soon obvious to these investigators that specific immunity required prior encounter with the infectious agent but that nonspecific factors were important in host defenses as well. The full complexity of the systems serving these functions was appreciated only as methods for fractionating plasma and cellular subsets were developed. However, the broad outline of the sequential interactions of humoral and cellular elements in immune function was recognized almost from the beginning.

In this chapter, we review our current knowledge of the structure and function of immunoglobulin and complement proteins. We recognize that these proteins interact with many other systems, but we limit the scope of our discussion to the interface among immunoglobulins, the complement proteins, and their specific receptors.

IMMUNOGLOBULINS

In 1937, Tiselius[1] developed a method to separate the proteins of plasma by electrophoresis, and soon after, Kabat and Tiselius[2] demonstrated that the antibody activity of plasma was confined to the slow migrating γ-globulin fraction. The onset of World War II created an urgent need for preservable plasma fractions, providing further impetus to the isolation and purification of the human plasma proteins. Salt fractionation of plasma was used by Cohn and others to purify the globulin proteins. Antisera to these globulins were used in the study of children with undue susceptibility to infection, revealing that the antibodies of the plasma consisted of three antigenically distinct groups (IgG, IgM, IgA).[3] Each antigenic group was found to have a different electrophoretic mobility, and thus the more general term *immunoglobulin* was introduced. By the mid-1960s, analysis of myeloma proteins revealed two additional antigenic groups, termed IgD and IgE, which were shown to be present in normal sera in amounts below the usual methods of detection.[4,5] We define the immunoglobulins as a heterogeneous group of proteins found in the blood plasma and body fluids and on the cell surface of B lymphocytes. These proteins are all related in structure and biologic function and are considered to be a family of proteins that possess the unique capacity to function as antibodies, that is, to recognize and bind specifically to antigen. Although all antibodies are immunoglobulins, we include in this group immunoglobulins with no known antibody activity; these proteins are structurally and antigenically related to antibodies but are more often found in pathologic states (eg, Bence Jones proteins, heavy-chain fragments). Immunoglobulins are found in the sera of all vertebrate species and as such represent the cumulative output of the immunologic memory of each individual. Originally identified as proteins capable of preventing infection, the immunoglobulins are now regarded, along with the T-cell receptor and the major histocompatibility complex (MHC) surface molecules, as integral components of the host immune recognition system. Produced solely by lymphocytes of the B-cell lineage, immunoglobulins serve both as membrane-bound, cell-surface antigen receptors and as secreted antigen-recognition molecules available to interact with a variety of other cell types and soluble components of the immune system. We are concerned here primarily with immunoglobulins as secreted antibody molecules.

Structure

The discovery that papain proteolysis of rabbit IgG results in two identical nonprecipitating fragments with antibody-binding activity (Fab) and a third crystallizable fragment devoid of antibody activity (Fc) permitted the elucidation of the structure of antibody molecules.[6] Biochemical analysis of these proteolytic fragments of IgG provided a structural model of the immunoglobulins. Subsequently, chemical reduction and acid gel chromatography of intact IgG demonstrated the presence of multiple peptide chains in each molecule.[7] We now recognize that all immunoglobulin molecules consist of a pair of identical polypeptide chains linked by disulfide bonds and electrostatic forces. The prototype molecule consists of a pair of identical heavy chains, which determine the immunoglobulin class, found in combination with a pair of identical light chains (Fig.

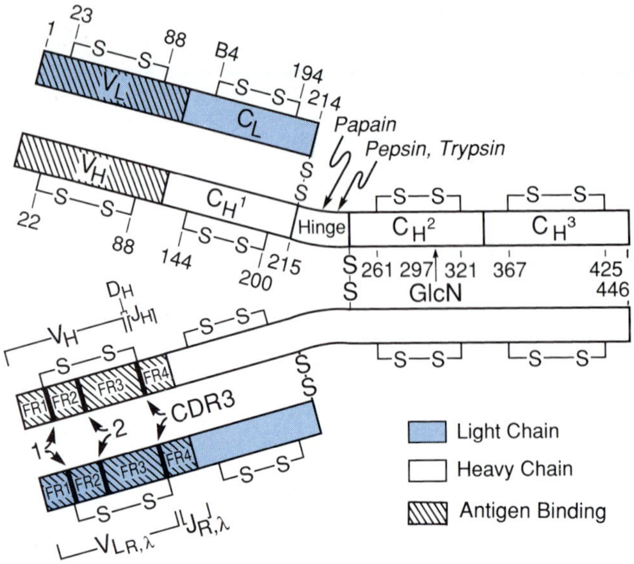

FIGURE 16-1. Structural schematic depiction of prototypic immunoglobulin molecule (monomer). The identical light (L) and heavy (H) chains are shown linked by interchain disulfide bonds. The unique amino acid sequences of the complementarity-determining regions (CDR) and the framework regions (FR) of the antibody-binding site of the H and L chains are illustrated in one of two identical halves of the molecule. N-linked oligosaccharide sites are located on each H chain within the C_H2 domain (GlcN).

16-1). Each immunoglobulin-synthesizing cell secretes only one type of heavy and light chain, so that each immunoglobulin molecule consists of identical halves of heavy and light chains. Each immunoglobulin molecule (monomer) has two antigen-combining sites, which are contained within the Fab fragment and involve regions on both the heavy and light chains. Sequences in the Fc region of the heavy chain are involved in mediating immunoglobulin effector functions.

Amino acid sequence analysis reveals that the heavy and light chains are composed of a series of distinct repeating homology units termed the *immunoglobulin domains.*[8] These domains consist of regions of 100 to 120 amino acids linked by an intrachain disulfide bond. X-ray crystallography indicates that each immunoglobulin domain consists of two β sheets of 3 or 4 antiparallel β strands that contain 5 to 10 amino acids each (Fig. 16-2). The domain structures are stabilized by the interior hydrophobic region between each sheet and by an intrachain disulfide bond. The immunoglobulin domains function as independent structural determinants that permit a variety of interactions through the accessible surfaces of the immunoglobulin molecule. Interactions between domains occur on the face of the β sheets, while interactions with other molecules (eg, antigens, complement) occur on contact residues near the ends of the domains. X-ray crystallography of an entire immunoglobulin molecule reveals that each pair of homologous domains compacts together to form a globular unit[9,10] (Fig. 16-3). In this model, molecular flexibility is provided by the sequences in the interdomain regions.

Recent studies have revealed that a considerable number of mammalian cell-surface molecules are constructed of similar immunoglobulin-like domains. Collectively, these proteins are members of the immunoglobulin superfamily, which includes receptors and adhesion molecules within the immune system (eg, the MHC class 1 molecules, T-cell receptor) and beyond (eg, neural cell adhesion molecule, carcinoembryonic antigen, platelet-derived growth factor receptor).[8] In each case, the known functions of these molecules appear to involve binding to and subsequent triggering of events at the cell surface, supporting the concept that the immunoglobulin domain functions as a protein framework for displaying determinants that permit molecular recognition of other molecules and transduction of biologic effects.[11]

The systematic analysis of the amino acid sequence of light and heavy chains revealed an enormous diversity of sequences in the N-terminal half of each chain. This region on each chain is termed the *variable* (V_L and V_H) *region*, and the antigen-binding sites are determined by the amino acid sequence of this region (see Fig. 16-1). On careful analysis, the V_L and V_H region sequence variation can be localized to three regions, termed the *hypervariable* or *complementarity-determining regions* (CDR1, CDR2, and CDR3).[12] The remainder of the V region is more conserved throughout all light and heavy chains and is termed the *framework region*, which consists of four clusters of framework segments (FR1 through FR4; see Fig. 16-1). In all, about one third of the amino acid sequences in the V region are hypervariable, the remaining two thirds consisting of framework regions. The heavy-chain CDR3 is slightly longer and more variable in amino acid sequence than in light chains. X-ray crystallographic studies reveal that the framework-region amino acids are organized as the β strands of the V region domain, while the amino acids constituting the hypervariable regions loop out of the domain structure[13] (see Fig. 16-2). This arrangement

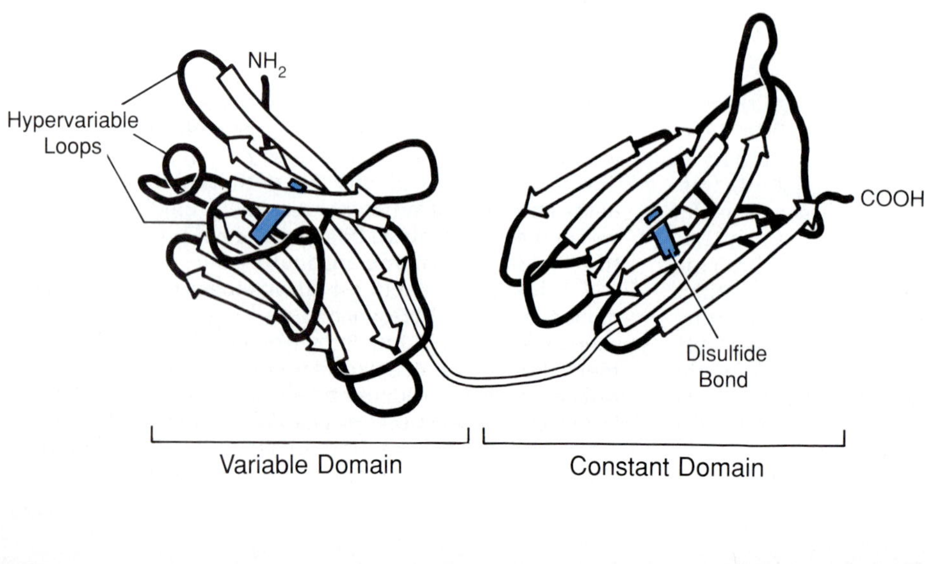

FIGURE 16-2. Tertiary structure of immunoglobulin light chain. The characteristic immunoglobulin fold is seen in both the V_L and C_L domains as two β-pleated sheets connected by an intrachain disulfide bond. In the V_L, the hypervariable amino acid regions (CDR1 to CDR3) are seen as loops independent of the fold, which, together with the V_H CDRs, determine the three-dimensional structure of the antibody-binding site. (After Schiffer M, Girling RL, Ely KR, Edmunson AB. Structure of the lambda-type Bence Jones protein at 3.5Å resolution. Biochemistry 1970;12:4620)

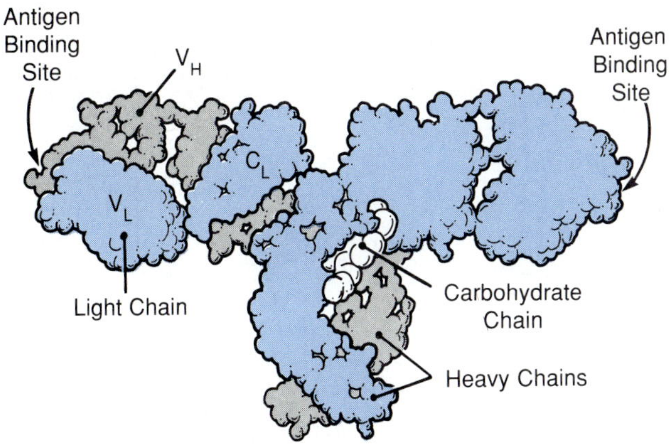

FIGURE 16-3. Quaternary structure of IgG molecule. The interactions among H- and L-chain components are displayed at the level of individual amino acids. Stabilizing carbohydrate structure on C_H2 is shown as occurring between each C_H2 chain. (After Silverton EW, Navia MA, Davis DR. The dimensional structure of an intact human immunoglobulin. Proc Natl Acad Sci USA 1977; 74:5140)

allows considerable variability in the sequence of the complementarity-determining regions without disturbing the framework of the antibody-binding site. The constraints on amino acids necessary to stabilize the hydrophobic β-sheet interior provide the stringent requirements that produce sequence conservation. The antibody-binding site is thus viewed as a concave pocket lined by the six complementarity-determining regions and built on the framework region scaffold. Proof of this molecular model was elegantly demonstrated in experiments in which a synthetic hybrid antibody was constructed by placing the heavy-chain framework regions of a human myeloma protein with the complementarity-determining regions from a murine-specific antibody. The hybrid antibody molecule retained the specificity determined by the murine complementarity-determining regions, verifying the precise role of these regions in determining the antigen-binding characteristics.[14,15]

The immunoglobulin molecule is encoded in a series of three unlinked gene families in the human genome: the κ or λ light-chain genes and the heavy-chain genes. The amino-terminal half of each light chain is encoded by a series of germ-line V κ or λ genes. These V-region genes encode the enormous diversity of the V-region sequence. The carboxy-terminal half of each light chain is encoded by germ-line C κ or λ genes, which determine the light-chain class. In humans, the κ light chain is encoded at a single locus, whereas the λ light chain is encoded by at least six separate loci.[16] In the heavy chain, the amino-terminal 110 amino acids constitute a single V-region domain (V_H). As is the case with the light-chain V region, the heavy-chain V region is encoded by a series of germ-line genes. Distinct from the light chain, however, the same V_H region is shared by each heavy-chain constant (C) region.[17,18] The heavy-chain C region is encoded in a series of germ-line genes (γ_1, γ_2, γ_3, γ_4, μ, α_1, α_2, ϵ, δ), which determine the heavy-chain class. The C region of the heavy chain is subdivided into three (IgG, IgA, IgD) or four (IgM, IgE) C-region domains[19] ($C\mu_H1$, $C\mu_H2$, $C\mu_H3$, and $C\mu_H4$; Fig. 16-4). The C region of each heavy-chain class is different, and it is the sequence of this region that confers the biologic functions unique to each immunoglobulin class (eg, cell-binding, complement activation). An additional segment, termed the *hinge region*, is unique to each immunoglobulin class and is not related by amino acid sequence to any other portion of the immunoglobulin gene locus. This hinge region is essential for both the antibody-binding and effector functions of certain immunoglobulin classes.

Like most plasma proteins, immunoglobulins contain oligosaccharides. Each immunoglobulin class varies in the amount and structure of the attached carbohydrate. In IgG, the oligosaccharides are found in the Fc region linked to asparagine-297 in C_H2 and to a more variable degree in the Fab region (depending on the presence of oligosaccharide consensus sequences in the hypervariable region).[21] X-ray crystallographic analysis of IgG reveals a direct interaction between the C_H2-linked oligosaccharides, suggesting a role for these structures in stabilizing the immunoglobulin molecule.[22] The oligosaccharide structures of each IgG molecule show a large degree of heterogeneity, resulting in many "glycoforms" of each polypeptide. This heterogeneity is found in each molecule and is not the result of polyclonality because similar results are seen in myeloma and hybridoma (monoclonal) derived immunoglobulins.[23] The occurrence of oligosaccharides in the Fab region further increases the diversity of antibodies and has been implicated in IgG aggregation and cryoprecipitation.[24,25] More recently, site-directed mutagenesis has been used to explore the role of carbohydrate in IgG function. These studies suggest that the carbohydrate on the heavy chain of IgG serves to provide a structural conformation essential in complement binding and activation. The biologic functions of IgG carbohydrate have also been explored using aglycosyl monoclonal IgG. These studies suggest that carbohydrate is essential for Fc-receptor binding and immune clearance.[26,27]

Diversity

Immunoglobulin diversity is entirely genetically determined, but the nomenclature of this diversity is based on differences in structure identified by specific antiglobulin antibodies before the genetic basis of this diversity was understood. Diversity in the C region is limited and results in the immunoglobulin classes (isotypes) and the genetic polymorphisms of these classes (allotypes). Diversity in the V region is much greater and forms the basis of the immunologic repertoire (idiotypes).

Isotypic Diversity

Immunoglobulin determinants recognized by antisera prepared in a different (iso) species are termed *isotypes*. Each C-region gene encodes a specific immunoglobulin isotype. The heavy-chain isotypes define the immunoglobulin classes and the subclasses of IgG and IgA. Nine heavy-chain isotypes have been identified in humans (Table 16-1). The isotype differences in subclasses are antigenically related more to each other than to the class isotypes, and it is therefore speculated that subclasses represent a relatively late evolutionary diversification in mammals.[28] Diversity of the light-chain isotypes are confined to the λ chain in humans.[29] Four distinct λ isotypes have been characterized, but DNA analysis suggests that many more exist in the λ gene complex. Because the isotypes each represent distinct gene products, every individual has the capacity to produce each isotypic variant. In addition to determining the unique functions of each antibody class or subclass, isotypes may play a role in immune regulation. Isotypic determinants on membrane-bound antibody molecules may interact directly with T lymphocytes and thus regulate antibody responses during antigenic challenge.[30] Consistent with this possibility, isotype-restricted antibody expression has been observed in humans in response to specific bacterial and viral infections. Antiisotypic antibodies (C-region auto-

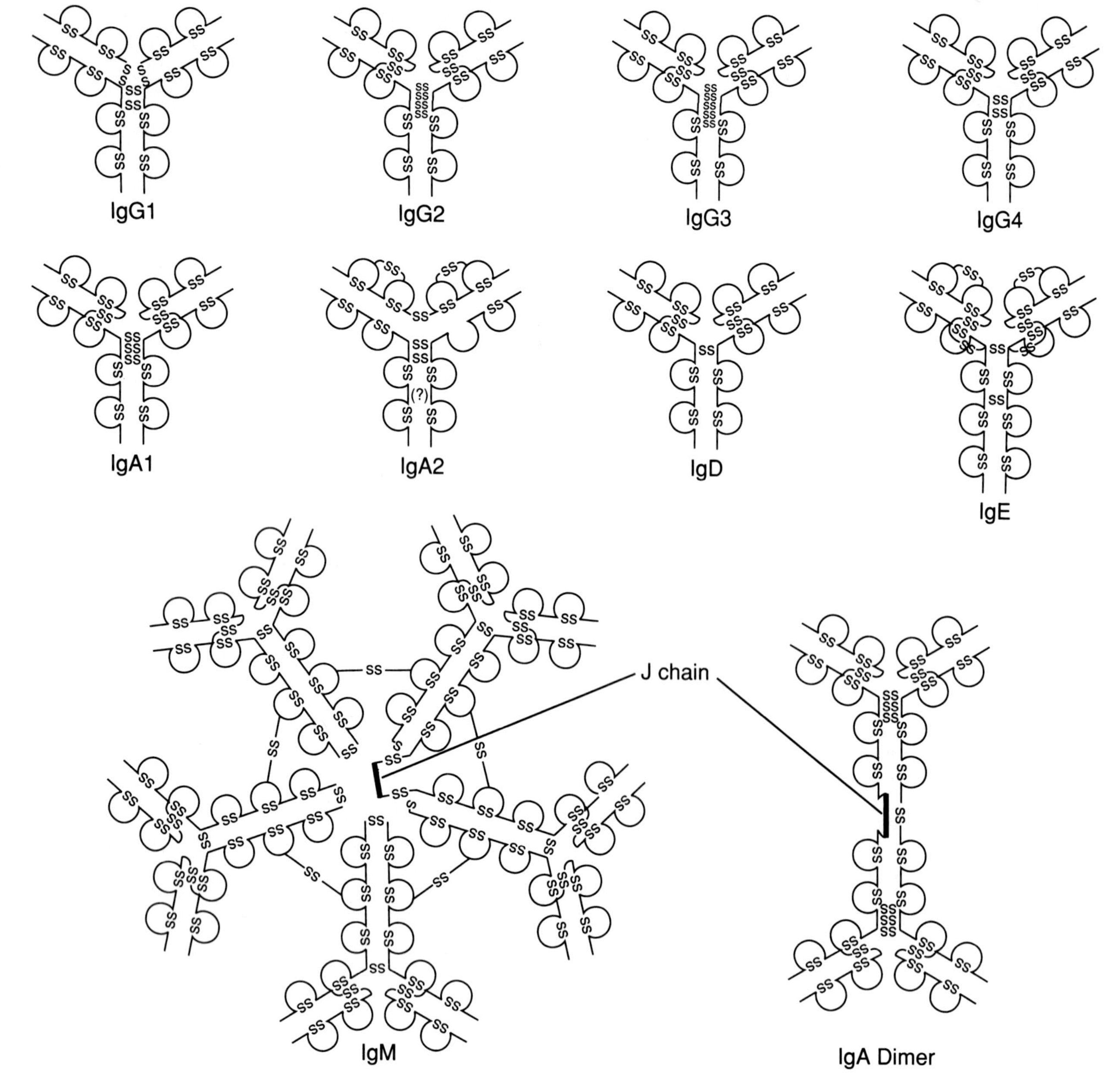

FIGURE 16-4. Structural characteristics of individual immunoglobulin isotypes. Dimeric structure of serum IgA and pentameric structure of IgM are illustrated linked by unique J-chain component. Variations in isotype structure are noted among isotype subclasses and each isotype in terms of both disulfide bond structure and number of domains. (After Gally J. Structure of immunoglobulins. In: Sela M, ed. The antigens. New York, Academic Press, 1973)

antibodies) are found in low abundance in the sera of most normal people and in increased amounts in patients with certain autoimmune disorders. The best characterized of these antiisotypic antibodies are the rheumatoid factors, which are IgM (and to a lesser degree IgG) antibodies directed against IgG subclass isotypes.[31] The structure and function of these autoantibodies are discussed in detail later.

Allotypic Diversity

Genetically determined allelic differences in antibody structure are termed *allotypes*. These determinants are recognized by antisera prepared from the same species (allo) in which they occur. Antibody allotypes represent individual genetic alternatives and thus occur only in certain members in a given population. Allotypic diversity was first discovered by Grubb[32] using sera containing rheumatoid factors that were found to be directed against specific allotypes of the IgG heavy-chain isotype. Due to the lack of specificity of most rheumatoid factors, allotypes are now generally characterized using the sera of multiply-transfused patients. The detection system involves inhibition of red cell agglutination, and the antiallotypic IgG antibodies found in the transfusion sera are termed *serum normal agglutinins*. In addition, because allotypes represent inherited differences in immunoglobulin amino acid sequence, these differences can be identified directly by DNA analysis using specific probes.

Gm Group. The Gm allotypes are found on the heavy chain of the IgG isotype, and most are localized in the Fc domain.[33] The nomenclature for these allotypes denotes

TABLE 16-1. Biochemical and Genetic Features of Human Immunoglobulins

Biochemical Properties	IgG						IgA				
	IgG1	IgG2		IgG3	IgG4	IgM	IgA1		IgA2	IgE	IgD
Structure											
Heavy chain	$\gamma 1$	$\gamma 2$		$\gamma 3$	$\gamma 4$	μ	$\alpha 1$		$\alpha 2$	ϵ	δ
Light chain	κ or λ	κ or λ		κ or λ	κ or λ	κ or λ	κ or λ		κ or λ	κ or λ	κ or λ
Molecular formula	$(\gamma 1)_2, \kappa_2$ $(\gamma 1)_2, \lambda_2$	$(\gamma 2)_2, \kappa_2$ $(\gamma 1)_2, \lambda_2$		$(\gamma 3)_2, \kappa_2$ $(\gamma 3)_2, \lambda_2$	$(\gamma 4)_2, \kappa_2$ $(\gamma 4)_2, \lambda_2$	$(\mu_2, \kappa_2)5$ $(\mu_2, \lambda_2)5$	$((\alpha 1)_2, \kappa_2)$ 1 or 2 $((\alpha 1)_2, \lambda_2)$ 1 or 2		$([\alpha 2]_2, \kappa_2)$ 1 or 2 $([\alpha 2]_2, \lambda_2)$ 1 or 2	ϵ_2, κ_2 ϵ_2, λ_2	δ_2, κ_2 δ_2, λ_2
Interchain S–S bonds	4	6		14	4	26	4		3 (or 4)	4	3
Molecular mass (kd)	146	146	155	165	146	900 —		160–385 —		190 —	180 —
Sedimentation coefficient (Svedberg units)			6.6			19		7, 11		8	7
Electrophoretic mobility (serum)			2			1		β		β	—
Carbohydrate content (%)			2.8			10.2		10		12	10
Allotypes	G1m1, 2, 3, 17	G2m2, 3	Gm; Km1, 2, 3	G3m5, 6, 10, 11, 13, 14, 15, 16, 21, 24, 26, 27	G4m4a, 4b	Km1, 2, 3 —	—	Am; Km1, 2, 3	A2m1, 2	Km1, 2, 3	Km1, 2, 3

the occurrence on each of the IgG subclasses (see Table 16-1). In some cases, the amino acid determinants of the Gm allotypes have been characterized; in others, the molecular bases of Gm allotypy have been inferred from genetic study. All the Gm allotypes are serologically defined, and the antigenic recognition of some Gm groups appears to require the combination of heavy and light chains, suggesting that tertiary structure is necessary in determining certain antigenic characteristics.[34] Analysis of immunoglobulin allotypia at the DNA level obviates these problems and expands the number of allotypes detected. Some Gm groups, termed *isoallotypes*, are allotypic only for a given IgG subclass and are always present on the other subclasses. Serologic studies reveal that certain Gm groups are inherited together as haplotypes, making these useful tools for population genetics.[35]

Am Group. This group is confined to the α_2 heavy-chain subclass isotype. The variant allele (Am1) encodes for an IgA molecule with a distinct disulfide bridge pattern in which the heavy and light chains are linked only by electrostatic forces. The amino acid difference in these allotypes also results in a differential sensitivity of these proteins to certain clostridial proteases, although the relevance of this to host immunity is unclear.[36,37]

Km Group. The three allotypes of the Km group are defined by two amino acid substitutions on the κ light chain.[38,39] The presence of allotypic diversity in a light chain implies that this can be represented in all the immunoglobulin isotypes.

The biologic role of allotypic diversity is unclear. There are no clearly identified associations between immunologic disorders and allotypic haplotypes. In some cases, specific Gm alleles are associated with a two-fold variation in the serum level of specific IgG subclasses, but the significance of this variation appears minimal to host defense.[40] The antibody response to certain polysaccharide antigens may also be related to allotypic diversity. In one study,[41] the response to *Haemophilus influenzae* vaccination was 10-fold greater in children lacking the Km1 allotype. The anti-Gm antibodies seen after exogenous γ-globulin administration or exposure of pregnant women to paternally derived Gm allotypes do not appear to influence IgG synthesis, suggesting that allotypic diversity plays a small role in the network of immunologic regulation.[42,43]

Idiotypic Diversity

The enormous diversity of antibodies was first appreciated independently by Kunkel[44] and Oudin,[45] who demonstrated by experimental immunization that each purified myeloma protein (immunoglobulin) had different antigenic characteristics. These antigenic differences among all antibodies are due to differences in the amino acid sequences found in the V regions of the immunoglobulin molecule. The V-region sequence determines the unique specificity of each antibody molecule, and the unique structure created by this sequence is termed an *idiotype*. The determinants of idiotypes are recognized by antisera from the same individual in which they occur. The individual antigenic components that determine a given idiotype are called *idiotopes*. Every antibody molecule contains idiotopes, which can be further defined as (1) α idiotopes, which are outside the antigen-binding site; (2) β idiotopes, which are not in the antigen-binding site but are close enough to affect antigen binding; and (3) γ idiotopes, which are directly in the antigen-combining site.[46] Although some idiotopes can be localized to light- or heavy-chain V regions, most require an intact region of both chains for antigenic recognition.

All idiotypes are capable of generating an antibody response in an appropriate host, and these elicited antibodies are termed *antiidiotypic*. Because the V-region idiotypes generated in response to any antigenic challenge are foreign to the host, antiidiotypic antibodies arise during the normal course of an immune response.[47] Antiidiotypic antibodies that develop under these circumstances are autoantibodies directed against immunoglobulin molecules. These autoantibodies are directed only against the V regions and are distinct from rheumatoid factors directed against C-region isotypes. Antiidiotypic antibodies also have unique idiotopes, resulting in multiple generations of antiidiotypic responses. The recurrent nature of the idiotype response prompted Jerne[48] to propose a fundamental role for these antibodies in a network of immune regulation linking antibodies and lymphocytes in the modulation of the immune response. Although the details of this network are still poorly understood, there is evidence that idiotypes may profoundly regulate the immune humoral response in humans both in health and disease states.[49,50]

Although idiotypes represent unique individual components, some are present in many individuals in a given population and indeed appear to follow distinct patterns of inheritance. These antigenically similar cross-reactive idiotypes probably result from idiotypes in the framework domains of the V-region locus (α or β idiotopes) and are thus inherited in the germ-line DNA common to related individuals.[51] In addition, some cross-reactive idiotypes may result from natural constraints on the antibody response to a given antigen, resulting in common idiotypes.[52] Idiotypes that are antigenically similar among individuals can also occur in certain autoimmune disorders, suggesting that selection of the V-region repertoire may be limited under certain pathologic circumstances.

Function

The dual function of all antibody molecules is to recognize antigen and to communicate with host effector systems (humoral and cellular). Although the V-region structural diversity determines the antigenic specificity of each antibody molecule, it is the C-region diversity that determines the range of biologic functions of these molecules. Indeed, the evolution of C-region diversity has resulted in an expanded range of functions for each antibody molecule. These functions are different but overlapping for each immunoglobulin class.

IgG

IgG is the most abundant immunoglobulin class in human serum, accounting for more than 75% of all the antibody activity found in this compartment. This protein circulates as a 155-kd monomer in the plasma; normally, about 45% of the total body IgG is in the extravascular compartment. The abundance and distribution of IgG, along with the long half-life relative to most plasma proteins, allows for its functions in immune defense. The production of IgG after antigenic challenge is associated with the development of immunologic memory such that further antibody production remains in this isotype class. The essential nature of IgG in host defense is best illustrated by patients deficient in IgG production—these patients suffer recurrent infections and eventually succumb if not treated with exogenous immunoglobulin.[53,54] IgG is the sole isotype transported in any significant amount across the placenta, providing the human newborn with adequate passive immunity for the first 3 to 4 months of life.[55] The human fetus is able to mount an effective humoral response in utero, and IgG synthesis has been detected in the human conceptus by 11 weeks of gestation, but under normal conditions, fetal IgG synthesis contributes little to total IgG in the newborn.[56]

IgG mediates host defense in several ways (Table 16-2). IgG can bind directly to a variety of toxins, resulting in neutralization in the plasma. After antigen binding, IgG is effective at activating the complement system. This activation is the result of direct protein interaction with the initial components of the complement pathway and is determined by unique sequences in the heavy-chain C region of this isotype[57] (discussed later). The activation of complement results in mononuclear phagocyte uptake of antigen–antibody complexes and the enzymatic production of anaphylotoxins, which promote inflammatory cell chemotaxis, migration, phagocytosis, and target cell lysis (discussed later). In addition, IgG can interact directly with receptors on the surface of cells by means of determinants in the Fc region (Fc receptors).[58] The presence of these receptors on mononuclear phagocytes and neutrophils promotes immune complex uptake and phagocytosis of particulate antigens. These interactions also mediate a variety of other cell functions essential to host survival during inflammation and tissue injury. Finally, the presence of IgG on defined target cell antigens such as tumors or allogeneic transplant tissue mediates the processes of antibody-dependent cellular cytotoxicity whereby lymphocyte cell populations are directed to lyse cells recognized as foreign.[59]

IgG is also the predominant isotype involved in antibody-mediated tissue injury, such as immune complex renal and pulmonary disease. IgG antibodies to the cellular elements of the blood may arise in the course of infection, passive immunization, or disorders of immunologic regulation. These antibodies may result in a variety of hematologic disorders, including idiopathic thrombocytopenic purpura, Rh hemolytic disease, autoimmune hemolytic anemia, red cell aplasia, and agranulocytosis. The passive administration of specific IgG antibodies can be of therapeutic value in abrogating certain antibody-mediated diseases, perhaps best exemplified clinically in the near absolute effectiveness of anti-Rh antibody in preventing Rh hemolytic disease of the newborn.[60] Immunization with specific allergens (antigens) can result in the acquisition of IgG antibodies, which may be important in interrupting the pathologic consequences of allergen hypersensitivity. A similar IgG response is seen in the case of tumor antigens; in these cases, the "blocking antibodies" are almost always of the IgG isotype and may work to the detriment of the host.[61]

After the recognition of IgG allotypic diversity, a number of investigators noted distinct electrophoretic fractions of IgG with different physicochemical properties. These fractions were characterized and found to be antigenically distinct, leading to the recognition of four IgG subclasses (isotypes) in humans.[62] Various classes of antigens result in marked differences in antibody responses among these subclasses. The reasons for these differences are unclear but may have to do with the selection of the V-region class at the time of an initial response. Differences in IgG–effector protein interactions and IgG–cell-surface binding account for the functional biologic differences seen among IgG isotypes. A striking example is seen in complement activation, where only IgG1 and IgG3 are able to effectively activate the classic complement cascade. The importance of IgG isotype differences in biologic function is further highlighted by the predominance of certain isotypes in immune complex–mediated disorders. Patients have been described with isolated IgG subclass deficiency in association with increased susceptibility to infection. Although some of these patients have deficient antibody responses and additional immunologic deficits, a specific role for IgG isotypes in the regulation of the humoral immune response remains unclear.[63]

IgM

IgM circulates in the serum as a pentamer of disulfide-linked immunoglobulin molecules joined by a single cross-linking peptide[64] (the J chain). Under normal circumstances, the size of this pentameric structure (over 900 kd) limits the distribution of IgM to the vascular compartment. In contrast to IgG, the affinity of monomeric IgM is low. This is balanced, however, by a high-IgM antibody avidity due to the multivalent structure of the molecule. In addition, this multivalent structure provides a flexibility to the IgM antibody molecule that is important in mediating the specific biologic functions of this isotype. IgM antibodies are the first isotype to appear in the plasma after antigenic stimulation. These antibodies usually appear within 3 to 5 days, are transient in nature, and are not associated with the development of immunologic memory. For this reason, the presence of specific IgM antibodies can be indicative of recent antigenic exposure. Active synthesis of IgM has been detected in the human conceptus as early as 10.5 weeks of gestation.[54] Because this isotype is not transported across the placenta, the presence of specific IgM antibodies in the human fetus or newborn can be used as prima facie evidence of intrauterine infection. Certain polysaccharide antigens result in an antibody response that is predominantly IgM. An example is the naturally occurring isohemagglutinins, which are IgM antibodies to erythrocyte blood-group antigens. Isotype-specific autoantibodies, such as rheumatoid factors, are also predominantly IgM antibodies.

IgM antibodies mediate host defense in several important ways. The IgM molecule is more efficient in activating the classic complement cascade than any other immunoglobulin isotype, and many of the biologic effects of IgM are mediated by means of complement activation. The pentameric structure confers multivalency to the IgM molecule, and the molecular structure appears to afford a range of motion (flexibility) that permits conformational changes to accommodate this multivalent ligand binding. The localization of IgM antibodies in the serum, combined with

TABLE 16-2. Biologic Properties of Human Immunoglobulins

	IgG					IgA			
Biologic Properties	**IgG1**	**IgG2**	**IgG3**	**IgG4**	**IgM**	**IgA1**	**IgA2**	**IgE**	**IgD**
Primary antibody response	−				+	−		−	−
Secondary antibody response	+				−	−		−	−
Complement activation									
Classic pathway	+	+	+	−	+	−		−	−
Alternate pathway	−	−	−	−	−	+/−		+/−	+/−
Transplacental transport	+	+	+	+	−	−		−	−
Opsonization	+	+	+	+	++	−		−	−
Reagenic activity	−	−	−	−	−	−		++	−

efficient complement activation, results in a prominent role for this isotype in serum particle clearance by macrophages. Thus, IgM functions as a first line of specific immunologic defense in the serum.

IgM is the first isotype expressed during human lymphoid ontogeny, and under these circumstances, the molecule is found as a monomer on the B-lymphocyte cell surface.[65] IgM monomers can be detected free in the plasma, generally in association with immunodeficiency or autoimmune disorders. These IgM monomers have been found to have antibody activity, and in certain cases, this involves the common blood-group isoantigens.[66] Defects in IgM polymerization or J-chain production can also result in IgM monomer formation. The J chain, a 137–amino acid polypeptide, is synthesized only in immunoglobulin-producing cells and preferentially in those cells producing polymeric (IgM or IgA) immunoglobulin. The amino acid sequence of the J chain is not homologous to the immunoglobulin domains, and the role of this protein in the regulation of IgM biosynthesis is poorly understood.[67,68]

IgA

IgA is by far the most abundant immunoglobulin isotype found in humans.[69] In the serum, IgA exists as a monomer (160 kd), accounting for about 10% of the total amount of immunoglobulin found in this compartment. IgA is also found in abundance in all external secretions (secretory IgA), where it exists as a dimer (500 kd) attached to a J-chain peptide identical to that found in IgM. The IgA found in secretions (S-IgA) is not derived from the serum but rather is produced by plasma cells localized in and around mucosal tissues. S-IgA is generally found in secretions attached to an additional protein termed the *secretory component* (SC). SC is synthesized by epithelial cells of mucosal tissues and hepatocytes and is derived from proteolytic cleavage of the receptor used to facilitate the secretion of polymeric IgA (receptor-mediated transcytosis) into body fluids and bile (discussed later). Although difficult to quantify, the amount of S-IgA produced each day probably exceeds all other immunoglobulin isotypes combined. Two IgA subclasses (isotypes) have been identified (designated IgGA1 and IgGA2; see Table 16-1). Differences in the amino acid sequence of the hinge region of IgA2 (found preferentially in secretions) confer partial resistance to bacterial proteases.[70] As noted previously, allotypic differences in IgA2 further differentiate this protease susceptibly.

Despite the presence of IgA antibodies in the plasma, the primary role of IgA in host defense appears to be localized to mucosal surfaces. After antigenic stimulation, lymphoid tissues associated with specific organs, such as the lung and gastrointestinal tract, mediate the local synthesis and secretion of specific polymeric IgA antibodies. In addition, homing of locally sensitized cells to distant tissue sites results in an elaborate system of mucosal defense in which specific IgA antibodies are present at all potential portals of entry.[71] IgA antibodies do not activate the classic complement pathway and are not particularly effective in promoting phagocytosis. The overall importance of IgA in host defense is not known.[72]

IgE

The concentration of IgE in normal plasma is below the limits of conventional immunochemical detection. Nevertheless, Ishizaka and colleagues[73] were able to identify IgE in the plasma, and subsequent characterization of serum from a patient with IgE myeloma permitted detailed analysis of this isotype, which normally accounts for less than 0.0001 of the immunoglobulin concentration in serum.[74] IgE circulates in the plasma in monomeric form (190 kd). As noted previously, this isotype lacks a hinge region and contains four C-region heavy-chain domains. IgE is synthesized in most lymphoid tissues in the body but probably in greatest abundance in the lung and gastrointestinal tract. Unlike IgA, this isotype is not secreted and appears in increased concentrations in certain body fluids only during inflammatory exudation.

The primary biologic function of IgE appears to be the mediation of immediate hypersensitivity reactions. Antigen-specific IgE interacts with tissue mast cells by means of a receptor specific for the IgE Fc region. On antigenic stimulation, Fc-bound IgE mediates mast cell degranulation, with resultant bronchoconstriction, tissue edema, and urticaria.[75] Although these responses may be beneficial to the host, the presence of IgE-mediated allergic reactions are at best a nuisance and at times life-threatening. The presence of elevated serum IgE in patients with certain parasitic infections suggests that this isotype may play a role in host defense to parasitic infection and that encounter with parasites may be the evolutionary driving force for the persistence of an otherwise disadvantageous immunoglobulin.[76] IgE antibodies cannot activate complement and are not effective opsonins. These data lend support to the suggestion that under certain circumstances an immediate hypersensitivity reaction may benefit the host by increasing access of other immunologic defenses at local sites of inflammation. The serum levels of IgE are regulated by T-cell–dependent lymphokines (IgE-binding factors), which can either induce or suppress B-lymphocyte IgE synthesis. In this regard, IgE-binding factors from non-atopic patients can actively suppress endogenous IgE synthesis in the lymphocytes of certain atopic patients with markedly elevated serum IgE (ie, hyper-IgE syndrome).[77,78]

IgD

IgD is found in trace quantities in human plasma and appears to have no direct role as a soluble antibody molecule. IgD antibody does not activate the complement cascade and does not interact directly with effector cells. The membrane-bound form of IgD is widely distributed on immunoglobulin-synthesizing cells, suggesting a possible regulatory role in primary antigen recognition.[79]

Metabolism

Static Measurements

The concentration of immunoglobulins in the plasma can be qualitatively assessed by serum protein electrophoresis. For example, in most cases of hypogammaglobulinemia, the γ-globulin fraction is reduced or absent, while the other separated protein fractions appear normal (Fig. 16-5). Serum protein electrophoresis is also useful in differentiating cases of secondary immunoglobulin deficiency (eg, generalized protein loss) because, in these cases, the level of other protein fractions also is decreased. Finally, in cases of monoclonal and oligoclonal gammopathies, when the total concentration of immunoglobulins may be normal or even elevated, the monoclonal nature of the immunoglobulin can be appreciated on serum electrophoresis as a well-focused band (or series of bands) distinct from the normal diffuse pattern (see Fig. 16-5). Quantitative immunoglobulin determination should always accompany serum protein electrophoresis. Enzyme-linked immunoassays using antisera specific to a given immunoglobulin isotype are sensitive and specific and can be readily adapted to the clinical laboratory. Immunoglobulin subclasses and genetic variants can be similarly quantitated providing the appropriate

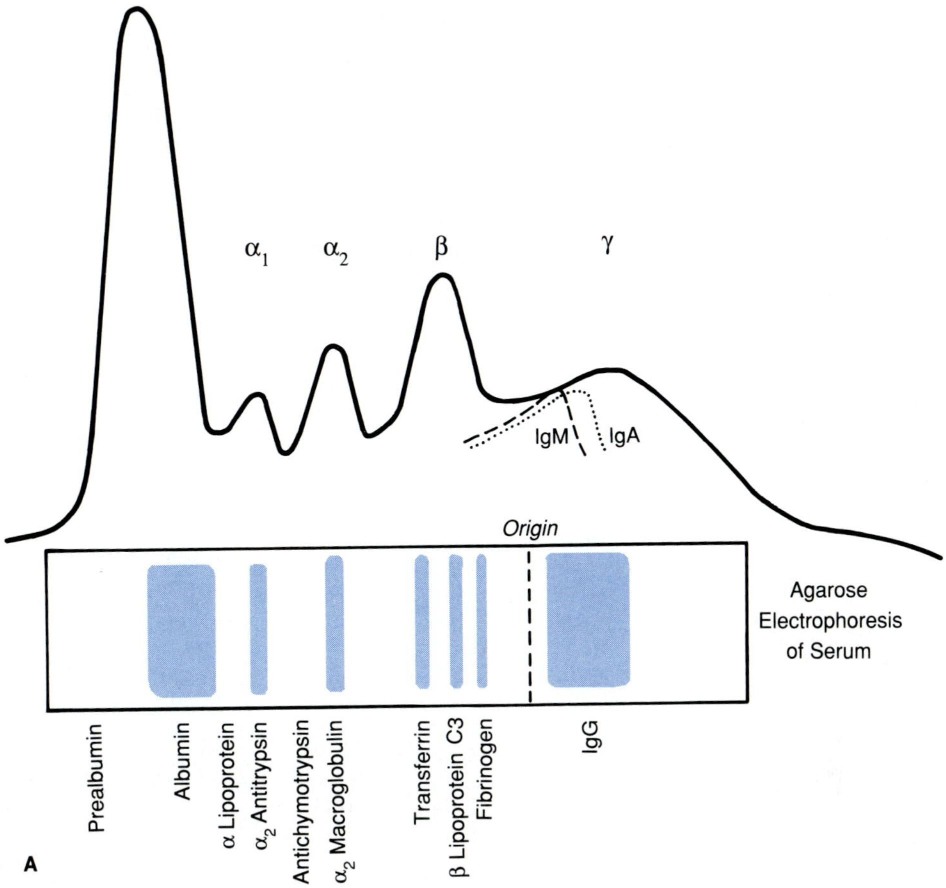

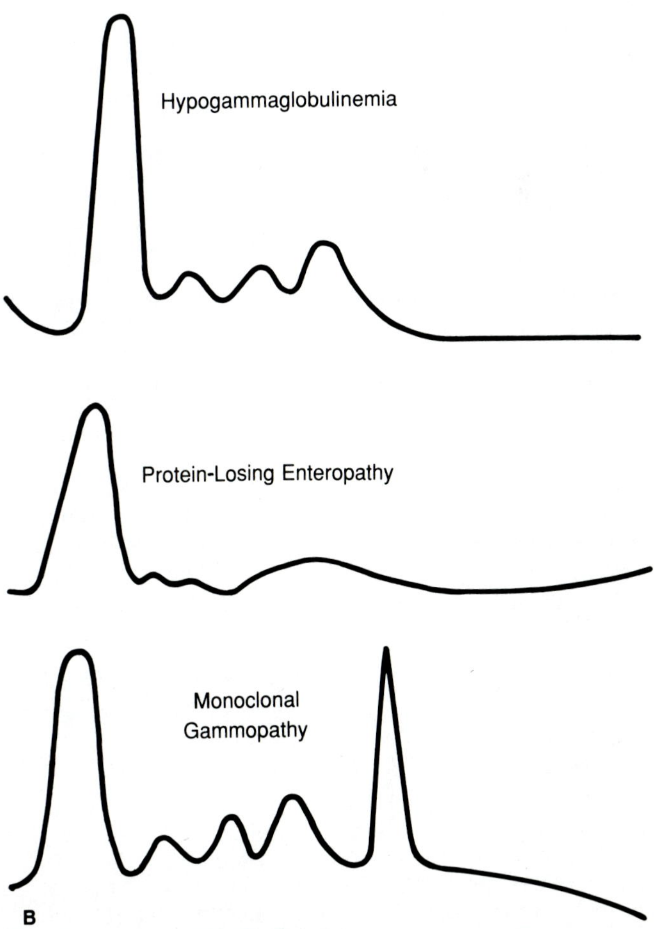

FIGURE 16-5. (*A*) Agarose gel electrophoresis of serum with notation of major protein components and the fractions (α_1, α_2, β, γ) obtained by densitometry. The immunoglobulins (IgM and IgA) are contained within the β fractions as well as the predominant γ (IgG) fraction. (*B*) Illustrative patterns of serum protein electrophoresis in various disorders of immunoglobulin metabolism. There is a selective loss of fraction in hypogammaglobulinemia as opposed by the general decrease in all fractions in protein-losing enteropathy. A single homogenous spike is illustrated in monoclonal gammopathy.

specific antisera are available. A caveat in all methods for quantitation of immunoglobulins is that each antiserum and each immunoglobulin standard used for quantitation will be heterogeneous. Thus, variation in sample measurements between and even within laboratories can result. Fortunately, the normal biologic variation in immunoglobulin metabolism is much broader than the usual degree of uncertainty in these determinations, so that these measurements are useful in the clinical setting.

Several important limitations in the interpretation of serum immunoglobulin measurements should be noted. First, all values must be interpreted in light of the changes that occur during development and aging. Although the variations in immunoglobulin levels are considerable under such circumstances, these have been carefully defined, and reference values allow adequate interpretation (Table 16-3). Second, the assessment of immunoglobulin levels provides no information regarding antibody activity. Such information is important because some patients with normal immunoglobulin levels have marked deficiency in antibody production after antigen exposure. The diagnostic approach in such cases is a part of the overall evaluation of immunologic competence and is discussed elsewhere. Finally, the static measurement of immunoglobulin concentration in the plasma provides no information about immunoglobulin flux, synthesis rates, body fluid distribution, or catabolism. Such metabolic data are essential to the interpretation of static measurements of immunoglobulin levels, helping to define the pathogenesis of disorders associated with variations in immunoglobulin concentration. For these reasons, it is important to understand the principles and methods used in making such metabolic measurements and the resulting data regarding immunoglobulin metabolism.

Dynamic Measurements

The plasma concentration of any protein is a reflection of the balance between the rate of protein synthesis, the distribution in the body fluids, and the rate of protein catabolism.[80] For each protein, the synthetic and catabolic rate and the factors determining these rates are different. During adult life, the concentrations of proteins in the plasma remain relatively constant, reflecting a steady state in which the amount of new protein synthesized each day is equivalent to that which is degraded. Plasma protein degradation depends directly on the total body pool of protein (P). The rate of degradation of a given protein (D) is defined as

$$D = \frac{0.693\ P}{t½}$$

where:
t½ (the half-life of the protein) = time required for degradation of half the molecules present in P at any given time

It follows that:

$$D/P = \frac{0.693}{t½}$$

where:
D/P = fractional rate of degradation of the protein or the fractional catabolic rate (FCR)

The FCR is the fraction of the total-body pool of protein degraded per day and in a steady state is equal to the fraction synthesized in this same period. It is apparent from this that the half-life of a given protein is inversely proportional to the FCR.

Most of the data concerning immunoglobulin metabolism have been obtained using passively administered (intravenous) radioiodinated purified proteins. These studies have revealed that each immunoglobulin isotype has a characteristic synthesis, transport, distribution, and catabolism[81] (see Table 16-3). It is apparent from these data that differences in the rates of catabolism are as important as changes in the rates of synthesis in determining serum immunoglobulin concentration for each isotype. For some, including IgM and IgA, the FCR remains constant over a wide range of plasma concentrations, implying that short-term changes in the rate of synthesis have little or no effect on plasma concentration. On the other hand, the mean half-life of IgG is inversely proportional to the plasma IgG concentration.[82] A decrease in the IgG synthetic rate re-

TABLE 16-3. Metabolic Parameters of Human Immunoglobulins

	IgG					IgA			
	IgG1	IgG2	IgG3	IgG4	IgM	IgA1	IgA2	IgE	IgD
Serum concentration (mg/dL)									
Adult		600–1500			75–150	200–300		0.02–0.06	0.01–3
Range		1200			97	250		0.04	2.2
Mean	840	240	80	40	—	220	30	—	—
Fetus (6 months; mean)		300			20	ND		0.003	0.05
Newborn		1200 (all maternal)			30	ND		0.003	0.1
6-Month-old		400			40	25		0.006	0.1
1-Year-old		800			60	60		0.01	0.3
Fraction of total serum immunoglobulin (%)		75–80			10	10–15		<0.01	<1
Fraction of total serum IgG (%)	70	18	8	4	—	—		—	—
Fraction of body pool intravascular (%)		45			80	42		50	75
Time (days)		23			5.1	5.8		2.5	2.6
	23	23	9	23	—	—		—	—
Fractional catabolic rate (plasma pool catabolized/d)		6.7			25	18		91	37
Metabolic rate (mg/kg/d)		33			6.9	24		0.003	0.4

ND, not determined.

sulting in a decrease in serum IgG will thus result in an increase in the IgG half-life. This serves to diminish the impact of decreased IgG synthesis on the plasma IgG concentration. Thus, although the mean half-life of IgG is 23 days, in patients with agammaglobulinemia, this value may be prolonged to 30 days.[83] The plasma levels of other immunoglobulin isotypes do not affect the half-life of IgG. In some cases, the metabolic data must be interpreted with additional caveats. For example, for IgE, which has a short-half life and a large FCR in serum, a fraction of the body pool bound to tissue mast cells turns over much more slowly.

During development of the human fetus, the plasma concentration of an immunoglobulin is a reflection not only of net fetal synthesis and degradation but also of net exchange of protein between the mother and fetus.[79] Providing that the half-lives of a given protein are similar in the mother and the fetus, it is possible to use the methods described previously to study immunoglobulin metabolism in the fetus. The transfer of immunoglobulins to the fetus takes place directly through the placenta and indirectly through the amniotic fluid.[55,84] All immunoglobulin isotypes are exchanged from mother to fetus and from fetus to mother by both these routes, albeit in small amounts. Nevertheless, the placental transfer of IgG from mother to fetus in the later portion of gestation is much more efficient than is the maternofetal or fetomaternal transfer of any other immunoglobulin. Indeed, this process is so efficient that by term, the human infant is born with an IgG concentration equal to or greater than that of the mother. The kinetics of IgG transport across the placenta have been carefully studied and are consistent with both passive and active transport mechanisms. Analogous to the effects of plasma IgG levels on IgG half-life, active transport is most efficient at low maternal IgG concentrations and is inhibitable at high levels. Presumably, this process tends to stabilize the fetal levels of IgG over a wide range of maternal plasma IgG concentrations and serves to enhance fetal survival regardless of the maternal level.[85] Because the transport process begins at about 20 weeks of gestation, premature infants are born with lower IgG levels, but it is unclear if this contributes to the increased susceptibility to infection seen in these patients. Under certain circumstances, the markedly limited transfer of some immunoglobulin isotypes may be advantageous to the fetus, such as in the prevention of immediate hypersensitivity reactions (IgE).

Many of the physiologic factors that regulate the rates of immunoglobulin synthesis, transport, and catabolism are unknown. In certain disorders, such as Wiskott-Aldrich syndrome and primary idiopathic nephrotic syndrome, these factors are apparently altered, resulting in marked increases in immunoglobulin turnover.[86]

Effector Functions

The biologic effects of antibody molecules are mediated by the highly conserved molecular framework of the Fc region. The mechanisms determining these biologic effects involve interaction of this Fc domain with either fluid-phase (complement activation) or cell-surface–bound (Fc receptor) molecules.

Fc Receptors. Cellular receptors for IgG were first recognized on the surface of macrophages containing cytophilic antibody.[87] These receptors specifically bind the Fc region of the immunoglobulin molecule and are found on a variety of cells that participate in the immune response (Table 16-4). Fc receptors mediate phagocytosis of antigen–antibody complexes, acquisition of passive immunity during development, stimulation of mediator release during inflammation, immunoglobulin clearance and catabolism, and antibody-dependent cell-mediated cytotoxicity. In addition, these receptors mediate the proliferation of lymphocytes and thereby influence the synthesis and secretion of immunoglobulins.[88] The molecular analysis of Fc receptors indicates that these receptors are part of the immunoglobulin superfamily differing in ligand affinity and primary structure. The diversity of the cytoplasmic regions of each receptor determines the unique signals transmitted and the distinct cellular function.

Fe Receptors Mediating Transcytosis. The polyimmunoglobulin receptor (PIgR) is expressed only in epithelial cells and appears to transport both IgA and IgM across the epithelial cell surface.[89] The pIgR was the first immunoglobulin receptor to be cloned. Sequencing of the pIgR cDNA revealed five extracellular domains homologous to each other and to the immunoglobulin V regions.[90] The sequence of the pIgR cDNA also demonstrated that the secretory component found in association with IgA is derived from proteolytic cleavage of the pIgR. Although the precise recognition sequences involved in IgA binding have not been determined, computer modeling suggests that the receptor binds to the hydrophobic faces of the domains in the Fc region of IgA.

The acquisition of passive immunity in utero occurs by transmission of maternal IgG across the placenta (humans) or the placenta and suckling intestine (rodents). High-affinity receptors for the Fc region of IgG have been purified from rat intestine and have been shown to consist of two proteins, p51 (52 kd) and p14 (14 kd).[91] The protein p14 has been identified as β_2-microglobulin and most recently a cDNA clone for p51 has been isolated.[92] Sequence of this cDNA reveals that the p51 molecule has three extracellular domains and a transmembrane region highly homologous to MHC class I antigens. The cytoplasmic tail of p51 is unique and probably subserves the intracellular transport and recycling of the receptor. The relation of the FcγRn to the putative trophoblastic Fc receptor involved in placental IgG transfer in rodents and humans is not known.[93]

Feγ Receptors. The molecular cloning of the Feγ receptors revealed that the diversity of biologic responses mediated by antibody molecules is due to the cell-specific expression and structural heterogeneity of these receptors. Three classes of Fcγ receptors are recognized, each of which is encoded by genes located on chromosome 1[88] (see Table 16-4). Leukocytes have an IgG receptor found predominately on the surface of monocytes and macrophages that binds monomeric IgG with high avidity. This Fc receptor is a glycoprotein of 72 kd, and monoclonal antibodies interacting with receptor suggest a role in antibody-dependent cellular cytotoxicity and immune complex clearance. In accord with this, cytokines such as γ-interferon, which regulate these biologic functions, also regulate expression of FcγRI on the surface of monocytes. cDNA clones for FcγRI were isolated using a ligand-affinity cloning system.[94] The extracellular region of FcγRI contains three IgG-like domains, two of which are homologous to the domains of FcγRII and FcγRIII (discussed later). The third domain is unique, and site-directed mutagenesis suggests that this region may be essential for high-affinity binding of IgG. Binding of IgG to FcγRI is localized to the C_H2 domain. Site-directed mutagenesis of residue$_{235}$ in IgG_3 completely abrogates FcγRI binding, and conversion of glutamine$_{235}$ to leucine in a non-FcγRI–binding murine isotype results in high-affinity IgG binding.[95] Peptide sequences from this region can also inhibit IgG binding. As noted previously, carbohydrate chains on C_H2 also play a role in determining IgG binding to FcγRI presumably by stabilizing molecular interaction between the two C_H2 domains. Current data suggest that distinct FeγRI transcripts are derived from a single gene, some of which represent

TABLE 16-4. Human Fc Receptors

Receptor Nomenclature	Biochemical Features	Biologic Characteristics
Transcytosis receptors; FcαR, FcμR	Single chain; 92 kd Cleaved extracellular domain forms secretary component of S-IgA Ig-like domains	Found on glandular epithelia and hepatocytes Binds polymeric IgA and IgM—transports these immunoglobulins into secretions (including bile)
FcγRn (data from rat)	Dimer P14; 14 kd (β_2-microglobulin) P51; 51 kd P51—Ig-like domains; homology to MHC class I antigens	Found on proximal intestine of suckling rodent High-affinity binding of IgG Transports maternal IgG intact across gut into serum of newborn
IgG/IgE Fe receptors		
FcγRI	Single chain; 72 kd Three extracellular domains, each Ig-like in structure Two domains homologous to FcγRII and FcγRIII, one unique domain	Found on monocytes and macrophages High-affinity binding of monomenic IgG ($K_a \sim 10^8$ M^{-1}) cDNA sequence and RNA blot analysis suggest multiple transcripts Expression modulated by IFN-γ; may play role in antibody-dependent cell-mediated cytotoxicity
FcγRII	Single chain; 45 kd CDW32 Multiple forms by cDNA sequence Ig-like domains	Found on most leukocytes—predominant on platelets Low-affinity binding of aggregated IgG ($K_a \sim 10^6$ M^{-1}) Highly polymorphic Gene located on chromosome 1—linked to FcγRIII gene May regulate oxidative metabolism in polymorphonuclear leukocytes
FcγRIII	Single chain; 46 kd (50–70 kd) Phosphoinositol membrane linkage forms CD16	Found on neutrophils, macrophages, and T lymphocytes Low-affinity binding of IgG in immune complex ($K_a \sim 5 \times 10^5$ M^{-1}) May interact with C3 receptors; may be family of receptors Promotes immune complex clearance; phagocytosis; natural killer cell function
FcεRI	Tetramer (α, β, γ2) α chain; 50 kd; Ig-like domains β chain; 32 kd γ chain; 7 kd All chains needed for expression of activity	Found on mast cells and basophils High-affinity IgE binding Mediates mast cell activation and degranulation
FcεRII	Single chain; 45 kd CD23; 25 kd fragment is IgEbF in serum Lectin-like homology (mannose-binding protein; asialoglycoprotein receptor) No Ig-like domains	Found on most leukocytes Low-affinity binding of monomeric IgE Potential role in B-lymphocyte activation and growth

polymorphisms.[96] The precise role of various isoforms is unclear.

FcγRII is a low-affinity receptor responsible for the binding of aggregated IgG molecules.[97] The FeγRII receptors are encoded by three closely linked genes, resulting in the generation of at least six distinct transcripts.[48,99] Although each receptor is characterized by two homologous extracellular Ig-like domains, diversity is generated by cell-specific expression and divergent cytoplasmic domains.[100,101] All cell types except large granular lymphocytes (natural killer cells) have been observed to have FcγRII receptors.[102] Transfection of these cDNA molecules indicates that each can combine with ligand at the expected affinity, and, therefore, each represents a form of FcγRII. In addition to this molecular heterogeneity, the FcγRII receptor is apparently highly polymorphic with multiple alleles, which are functionally as well as electrophoretically distinct.[103]

A low-affinity Fc receptor (FcγRIII) is found on macrophages, neutrophils, and natural killer cells.[104,105] FcγRIII appears to play a role in the clearance of immune complexes, and studies with monoclonal antibodies indicate that this is the receptor responsible for the clearance of IgG-sensitized erythrocytes in experimental studies.[106] The FeγRIII receptor is encoded by two separate genes, resulting in two forms of the receptor. Thus, the FcγRIII is distinct in that it appears to be anchored to the cell surface in both phosphotidylinositol (PI) linkage and polypeptide-anchor forms.[107–109] cDNA cloning suggests that the PI linkage form is differentially expressed on neutrophils, while the polypeptide-anchor occurs only in natural killer cells and macrophages. The PI anchor in neutrophils may promote receptor mobility through lateral membrane diffusion, although the role of this process in facilitating immune complex clearance is not known. Biosynthesis and assembly of the polypeptide anchor FeγRIII requires expression of accessory molecules shared with other lymphocyte receptors.

Fcε Receptors. Multiple receptors for the IgE isotype have been characterized. A high-affinity receptor (FcεRI) is found only on mast cells and basophils and consists of a tetramer of α, β, and γ chains.[110] cDNA cloning has revealed that the α chain is homologous to the other Fc receptors and contains immunoglobulin-like domains; however, the β and γ chains are not part of the immunoglobulin superfamily.[111] Expression of a functional FcεRI requires the presence of all these chains.[111] A recombinant-generated three-domain IgE fragment, $C_H2,3,4$, is able to totally inhibit passive cutaneous anaphylaxis in vivo by blocking IgE binding to the mast cell FcεRI.[112] Synthetic peptides that can block binding of radiolabeled IgE to mast cells should be useful to more precisely localize the IgE Fc binding sites.

The Fc receptor for IgE on lymphocytes, Langerhans cells, and monocytes (FcεRII) is recognized by a monoclonal antibody termed CD23.[113,114] Isolation of the cDNA for this receptor indicates that it is homologous to lectins such as the mannose-binding protein, surfactant protein A, and the asialogylcoprotein receptor.[115–117] Expression of the FcεRII (CD23 molecule) in fibroblasts indicates that this molecule alone is sufficient to bind IgE. Recombinant-generated IgE lacking carbohydrate is able to bind to FcεRII, suggesting that despite the homology to lectin-like proteins, at least some of the interactions between IgE and FcεRII occur through protein–protein interactions.[117] Treatment of lymphocytes with interleukin-4 or Epstein-Barr virus (EBV) infection increases cell-surface expression of FcεRII in parallel with the interleukin-2 receptor.[118] A proteolytic fragment of this FcεRII has been shown to be identical to a soluble IgE-binding factor that was previously characterized as a B-cell growth factor.[115] Taken together, these results suggest that FcεRII may be involved in mediating B-cell proliferation.

In addition to the FcεRI and FcεRII receptors, multiple other IgE receptors have been identified. Both FeγRII and FeγRIII bind IgE immune complexes.[119] A second lectin-like receptor, moc-z, has also been characterized, which, like FeεRII, is expressed on multiple hematopoietic cell lines.[120] To determine the unique role of each of these receptors in IgE-mediated anaphylactic reactions, the FcεRI-specific α chain was deleted from the germline of mice by homologous recombination.[121] The results of this experiment revealed that the high-affinity FeεRI receptor is essential for IgE-dependent anaphylaxis. The serum clearance of IgE is normal in these animals, implicating other IgE receptors in the sequestration of IgE. In an analogous study, the subunit of Fe receptors was also deleted by homologous recombination.[122] This subunit associates with FeγRIII and FcεRI, where it is essential for expression and signal transduction. Mice with this subunit deleted were immunocompromised and somewhat surprisingly displayed dysfunction of all three Fcγ receptors, as well as lack of expression of the FcεRI receptor and resistance to anaphylaxis as observed in the α-chain–delted mice. These studies establish the essential role of Fc receptors in immune complex clearance, cell-mediated cytotoxicity, and allergic responses mediated by mast cell degeneration.

The role of Fe receptors in B-cell functions, including proliferation and cytokine production, has recently been identified and, as with the effector functions, is determined by structural diversity and molecular heterogeneity of each receptor.[123]

In addition to these Fc receptors, other Fc-binding proteins can affect the phagocytic capacity of cells toward opsonized particles. Complement acts synergistically with IgG to promote macrophage phagocytosis, and C1q has been shown to function as an Fc receptor on monocytes and macrophages. In the case of C1q, the collagenous domain of the molecule mediates this phagocytic enhancement, which appears to enhance the IgG-mediated uptake and killing of certain microorganisms.[124]

Paraproteins

The immunoglobulins are synthesized and secreted by terminally differentiated B lymphocytes termed *plasma cells*. Each plasma cell secretes only one light-chain and one heavy-chain isotype, and thus all antibody molecules originating from a single plasma cell are identical. Under normal circumstances, the heterogeneity of circulating antibody molecules reflects the diversity of B-cell clones synthesizing immunoglobulin. Despite the well-orchestrated series of events that results in antibody synthesis and secretion, there occurs at times a striking imbalance in immunoglobulin production. Complete absence of single or multiple immunoglobulin isotypes is seen in the immune deficiency disorders. Although the details of many immunopathologic disorders are presented elsewhere, we review in this chapter some specific examples in which the contribution of abnormal immunoglobulin production to tissue pathology has provided insight into immunoglobulin structure and function.

Monoclonal Gammopathies

Monoclonal immunoglobulins (M components) are seen as sharp, well-focused bands on electrophoretic separation of serum or urine (see Fig. 16-5). Immunofixation with antibody specific to light-chain or heavy-chain isotypes is used to identify a particular M component. The presence of an M component generally reflects a dyscrasia of the plasma cells with selected expression of a single clone of cells (monoclonal gammopathy; Table 16-5). Immunoglobulin synthesis and assembly in these plasma cells is often abnormal, frequently resulting in secretion of excess light chains. Free serum light chains are small enough to permit glomerular filtration and urinary excretion. In addition to plasma cell dyscrasia, M components may occur transiently after antigenic challenge in normal people, and they may also occur after immunologic reconstitution of bone marrow.[125] M components have also been described in children with immunologic deficiency.[126]

The incidence of monoclonal gammopathy in the population increases with advancing age. In an analysis at the Mayo Clinic[127] of more than 50,000 serum samples, about 900 new cases of monoclonal gammopathy were recognized. In most (over 70%) of these cases, no disease process was associated with the presence of the M component. Ten percent of patients had multiple myeloma, 8% primary amyloidosis, 6% lymphoma, 2% chronic lymphocytic leu-

TABLE 16-5. Monoclonal Gammopathies

Syndrome	M Component	Prominent Clinical Features
Multiple myeloma	IgG; IgA; (to a lesser degree: IgD, IgE)	Osteolysis and fractures
	Free L chain	Renal failure
		Recurrent infections
		Amyloidosis
Waldenström's disease	IgM	Hyperviscosity
	Free L chain	Cryoglobulinemia
		Bleeding diathesis
H-chain diseases	H-chain fragment	Organ infiltration
		Recurrent infections

kemia, 2% macroglobulinemia, and the 1% a variety of disease processes, including chronic liver and hematologic disorders.

Monoclonal Gammopathy of Undetermined Significance

This classification signifies all patients with an M component but no detectible findings of an underlying plasma cell neoplasia. The presence of a detectable serum M component increases with age, occurring in about 1% of the population above 50 years of age and in more than 3% by age 70 years.[128] Most of these patients never develop plasma cell neoplasia. In almost all cases, quantitation of the M component in plasma indicates relatively small amounts of protein (usually less than 3 g/dL), and bone marrow aspiration reveals less than 5% plasma cells. These patients are healthy and have normal serum albumin and serum immunoglobulin levels. An increase in the M component by more than 50% often heralds progression to neoplasia.[129]

Multiple Myeloma

Multiple myeloma results from the neoplastic proliferation of a single clone of plasma cells within the bone marrow, resulting in disruption of normal marrow architecture and function. The neoplastic plasma cells usually produce an M component in amounts proportional to the burden of tumor cells present. The cause of this disorder is unknown, but cases occur most commonly in the elderly. The pathophysiology of the disorder is related not only to the tumor burden but also to the secreted products (predominantly the M component) and the host response to these products. The M component of multiple myeloma is most often IgG, IgA, or light chain. The secreted light chains are generally dimers and are rapidly catabolized, precluding detection in the serum. The plasma concentration of these light chains can exceed the renal threshold, with subsequent excretion in the urine. Thus, the presence of a serum M component composed entirely of light chains identical to those seen in the urine often indicates renal failure.[130]

M components contribute to the pathophysiology of multiple myeloma in several ways. Intrinsic antibody activity of an M component can result in hemolytic anemia or a bleeding diathesis.[131] Patients with multiple myeloma are often hypogammaglobulinemic and may have an increased susceptibility to infection. The hypogammaglobulinemia may result either from an increase in the FCR of IgG secondary to the increase in plasma IgG concentration from the M component or from suppression of normal B-cell growth and differentiation by abnormal B-cell clones.[132]

Waldenström's Macroglobulinemia

In this neoplastic disorder, the uncontrolled proliferation of "lymphocytoid" plasma cells in the bone marrow, spleen, and lymphoid tissue results in weakness, fatigue, and recurrent infections.[133] The proliferation of the lymphocytoid cells is associated with secretion of an IgM M component (macroglobulin), which often results directly in disease symptomatology. Waldenström's macroglobulinemia is more common in male patients and is frequently seen in patients over 60 years of age. The circulating M component is frequently associated with free light-chain dimers in the urine (over 75% of which are κ), reflecting imbalanced immunoglobulin chain production in the lymphocytoid cells. The presence of a significant concentration of the IgM M component in the serum (more than 3 g/dL) can result in hyperviscosity syndrome, with mucosal bleeding, gastrointestinal tract hemorrhage, retinal hemorrhages with blurring and loss of vision, and a variety of neurologic syndromes, including dizziness, paresthesia, and coma.[134]

Heavy-Chain Diseases

These disorders represent an uncommon group of plasma cell neoplasias associated with secretion of a heavy-chain M component. The heavy-chain disorders are classified according to the isotype of the circulating M component, and the clinical syndromes are similar to that described for multiple myeloma. The first heavy-chain disorder to be recognized was γ-chain disease. These patients have a characteristic infiltrative edema of Waldeyer's ring in addition to a generalized lymphadenopathy and splenomegaly.[135] Free γ-heavy chains are detectable in the serum and urine, and in all cases, amino acid deletions in the heavy-chain V region are observed.[136] These heavy chains arise from aberrant immunoglobulin gene rearrangement and not from secondary degradation of monoclonal immunoglobulin in the plasma.

α-Chain disease occurs predominantly among young people in the Mediterranean region of the Middle East. Plasma cell infiltration of the gastrointestinal tract is found in association with malabsorption, weight loss, and diarrhea.[137] μ-Chain disease is a rare plasma cell neoplasia found in some patients with chronic lymphocytic leukemia.[138] These patients have abnormal-appearing plasma cells, hypogammaglobulinemia, and detectable monomeric serum μ chains. The presence of urinary κ light chains suggests that the disorder results from aberrant immunoglobulin assembly similar to Waldenström's macroglobulinemia. δ-Heavy chain disease has been reported in a patient with multiple myeloma-like features but with an abnormal tetrameric δ chain present in the serum.[139] The abnormal δ heavy chain is most likely the result of aberrant rearrangements of δ-immunoglobulin genes rather than degradation of a normal monoclonal heavy-chain component.

Amyloidosis

The amyloid disorders are a diverse group of syndromes all associated with the deposition of insoluble fibrillar protein at various tissue sites (Table 16-6). The syndromes are classified clinically according to the particular proteins isolated from these deposits. In all cases, the fibrillar amyloid protein is identified by a characteristic green birefringence under polarized light after staining of the deposits with Congo red dye.[140] The symptomatology of amyloidosis is related both to the underlying disease process and to the direct effects of the deposited amyloid on organ function.

Primary (immunoglobulin-type) amyloidosis is the most common form of the systemic amyloidoses. In primary amyloidosis, the amyloid protein fibrils are homogeneous and contain a protein identical to the V region of immunoglobulin κ or λ light chains.[141] Primary amyloidosis is therefore a systemic illness of unknown cause that is associated with the deposition of immunoglobulin light-chain fragments in various tissues. Patients with primary amyloidosis have organ enlargement secondary to amyloid deposition, including hepatosplenomegaly, skin plaques and nodules, and cardiac infiltration. A urinary M component of light-chain dimers is detected in over 90% of these patients. About 15% of patients have associated multiple myeloma, often with a serum M component. The prognosis in primary amyloidosis is poor, and death usually results from cardiac or renal failure. There is a direct relation between the circulating M component and the amyloid fibrils. Amino acid sequence analysis of the light-chain component of amyloid deposits in patients with primary amyloidosis indicates that the deposited light chains are identical in N-terminal sequence to light chains in immunoglobulin molecules isolated from normal people.[142] Although x-ray crystallographic analysis has demonstrated that the light chains from these plaques are arranged in a β-pleated sheet, the

TABLE 16-6. Systemic Amyloidoses

Syndrome	Biochemistry	Features
Primary amyloidosis (immunoglobulin-type)	L-chain deposits (N terminal)	Organ infiltration with renal, cardiac failure 15% associated multiple myeloma
Secondary amyloidosis	AA protein deposit (derived from serum SAA)	Associated with multiple chronic diseases GI, CNS symptoms common Secondary organ infiltration
Hereditofamilial forms (and miscellaneous examples)	AF prealbumin	Familial amyloid Polyneuropathy
	Calcitonin peptide	Medullary carcinoma of the thyroid
	Protein (SAP)	Found in most systemic forms of amyloidosis

structural features of light chains that result in deposition in amyloid fibrils are unknown. A similar β-pleated sheet can be produced in vitro by limited proteolysis of certain light chain dimers (Bence Jones proteins), but the significance of this finding is unclear.[143] Because there appears to be a preponderance of certain λ light chains found in amyloid fibrils, it has been speculated that certain amino acid sequences in light chains may predispose to the formation of amyloid deposits.[144] Not all light-chain tissue deposition occurs as amyloid fibrils. Patients with clinical features similar or identical to those seen in primary amyloidosis have been described with so called nonamyloid light-chain deposition.[145]

Immunoglobulin molecules are not found in the amyloid plaques of other forms of amyloidosis. In secondary amyloidosis, the predominant protein, amyloid A (AA) protein, is derived from a plasma precursor serum amyloid A protein (SAA). In patients with secondary amyloidosis, SAA degradation may be abnormal, contributing to AA deposition.[146] Serum amyloid protein (SAP), a member of the pentraxin family of serum proteins, is found as a nonfibrillar component of most forms of amyloid deposits apparently derived directly from the plasma without proteolytic cleavage. The role of SAP in amyloidogenesis is not known.[147]

In the hereditary forms of amyloidosis, SAA or other plasma proteins (eg, prealbumin) are found in the amyloid plaques.[148]

Cryoglobulinemia

The term *cryoglobulin* identifies a group of serum proteins that reversibly precipitate on exposure of plasma to the cold.[149] C- tain cryoglobulins are present normally in small amounts in the serum, and in some cases, these proteins can be concentrated and purified by cold precipitation (eg, factor VIII). Cryoglobulins can appear in the plasma in association with the onset of disease states and may contribute directly to organ pathology. Although cryoglobulins can include plasma proteins, such as fibrinogen and C-reactive protein, most cryoglobulins are immunoglobulins. The presence of naturally occurring cryoimmunoglobulins was first appreciated in studies on the reaction of pneumococcal type-specific antibody with capsular polysaccharide, in which it was noted that, at certain antibody concentrations, an insoluble precipitate was reversibly formed in the cold.[150] Clinically, cryoimmunoglobulins were first recognized in patients with myeloma with reversible cold-induced precipitation of plasma in association with the presence of a significant concentration of circulating M components.[151] Detection of cryoimmunoglobulins in the serum requires that blood collection and clotting be carried out at 37°C before analysis of serum at 4°C. Cryoimmunoglobulins can be quantitated by immunologic methods and the isotype identified by specific antisera. The overall incidence of cryoimmunoglobulinemia increases with age, occurring in 2% to 3% of healthy patients over 60 years of age.[152]

The physiochemical basis for cryoprecipitation has been studied using monoclonal cryoimmunoglobulins. Polymerization of individual components appears to be both temperature and concentration dependent, suggesting that the solubility of cryoimmunoglobulins in the plasma may play a role in determining the initiation of precipitation.[153] Amino acid sequences of monoclonal cryoimmunoglobulins and noncryoimmunoglobulins are identical, and no specific sequences have been discovered that can be related to cryoprecipitation. Differences in carbohydrate quantity and quality have been found between cryoimmunoglobulins and noncryoimmunoglobulins, suggesting that these determinants may contribute to the structural alterations determining cold precipitation.[154] The physiochemical basis for cryoprecipitation remains largely unknown.

Analysis of cryoimmunoglobulins in a variety of disease states has led to the following classification:

1. Cryoimmunoglobulins occurring as M components in individuals with an underlying monoclonal gammopathy
2. Cryoimmunoglobulins that are M components directed against an immunoglobulin isotype (generally IgM). These cryoimmunoglobulins are generally found bound to the specific immunoglobulin and are termed *mixed cryoglobulins* because of the nature of the isolated complex.
3. Polyclonal cryoimmunoglobulins, which are often found in association with other immunoglobulins or proteins as immune complexes. The mixed polyclonal cryoimmunoglobulins are the most commonly seen (about half the total) but occur in low concentrations and are the most difficult to accurately characterize.

The precise relation of cryoimmunoglobulins to various disease states is not well defined. Certain cryoimmunoglobulins (particularly M components) have been shown to have antibody activities that may contribute to pathology. The mixed cryoglobulins found in patients with immune complex disease frequently demonstrate antibody activity against single- or double-stranded DNA or RNA, suggesting a role for these proteins in autoimmune disease.[155] Recent studies have demonstrated a clear association between hepatitis C virus infection and type II mixed cryoglobulinemia, although the pathogenesis of cryoglobulinemia in these circumstances remains unclear.[155a,155b] The relation between the immunochemical properties of the cryoglobulins and symptoms in patients with underlying disorders remains unclear. Although many patients have symptoms that could be related to cold-precipitating globulins, the underlying disease processes, such as vasculitis and glomerulonephritis, make it difficult to differentiate the causality of these symptoms. In the absence of any underlying disorder, the presence of polyclonal mixed cryoimmunoglobulins is termed *essential cryoglobulinemia*. The incidence of this disorder is unknown, but recent studies suggest that it may be more common than previously appreciated. In patients with symptomatology that can be demonstrated to be due to cryoimmunoglobulins (Raynaud's phenomenon), minimalization of cold precipitation is the most important therapeutic approach. In addition, plasmapheresis has been used with limited success to remove the cryoglobulins from the circulation.[156]

Rheumatoid Factors

Rheumatoid factors are autoantibodies that react predominately with antigenic determinants in the Fc region of IgG isotype. Most rheumatoid factors are of the μ isotype (IgM) and frequently occur as M components and cryoglobulins. Rheumatoid factors were originally isolated from the sera of patients with chronic rheumatoid arthritis. Evidence has accumulated indicating that rheumatoid factors are synthesized transiently after a secondary immune response in most normal people.[157] The presence of rheumatoid factors in normal people suggests that these immunoglobulins may play a role in regulation of the immune network.[158]

Rheumatoid factors produced after antigenic stimulation are IgM M components. After the production of an anti-idiotypic antibody to a rheumatoid factor M component (anti-Wa), it was noted that this antiserum recognized more than half of the monoclonal rheumatoid factors isolated from unrelated people.[159] The presence of cross-reactive idiotypes among these rheumatoid factors suggested that the V-region sequences of each of the rheumatoid factor antibodies were similar or identical. Analysis of a large series of rheumatoid factor M components and subsequent cloning of rheumatoid factor light-chain gene determinants has confirmed this V-region identity.[160,161] These data indicate that the genes encoding rheumatoid factor light chains are both conserved and widely distributed in the human population. Antiidiotypic antibodies prepared from synthetic peptides derived from the hypervariable regions of rheumatoid factor light chains also identify the cross-reactive rheumatoid factor idiotypes supporting the concept of conservation of genetic structure.[162] In this regard, the V regions of several distinct autoantibodies from patients with autoimmune disorders have been found to be identical to germ-line–encoded genes.[163] These results extend the observations with rheumatoid factors and support the concept that the autoantibodies that arise in health and disease states may be structurally identical.

Rheumatoid factor is associated with immunopathology in a variety of circumstances. In Waldenström's macroglobulinemia, many of the IgM M components are rheumatoid factors. In addition, many of these are cryoimmunoglobulins that can precipitate in serum, causing symptoms under circumstances of increased protein concentration. These monoclonal IgM proteins also share cross-reactive idiotypic determinants, suggesting conserved V-region gene usage during production of M components in this disorder. IgM rheumatoid factors are also seen in patients with chronic lymphocytic leukemia and other lymphoproliferative disorders. Under these circumstances, the light chain of the IgM M component appears to arise from conserved κ-region genes, suggesting expression of a restricted set of idiotypic antigens during neoplastic transformation. The rheumatoid factors found in patients with rheumatoid arthritis are diverse and polyclonal, although the antigens involved in inducing rheumatoid factor in rheumatoid arthritis have not been identified. These IgM rheumatoid factors are often localized as antigen–antibody complexes in the synovia of patients with rheumatoid arthritis, suggesting a direct role for rheumatoid factor in tissue pathology.[164]

THE COMPLEMENT PROTEINS

The complement system, now known to comprise about two dozen plasma and cell membrane proteins, was first recognized nearly 100 years ago as a cofactor in specific immune defenses against pathogenic bacteria. The complexity of the complement cascade and its role in many other biologic functions have only been appreciated within the last two decades, following advances in protein chemistry, molecular genetics, and cell biology. The recognition of genetic deficiencies of these complement components and their phenotypic expression provided insights into the physiologic role of the complement system and validation of the relative importance of the vast array of complement-mediated phenomena observed in vitro. We devote the balance of this chapter to the complement genes, proteins, and activities.

Interaction of antigens with antibodies of several immunoglobulin classes and subclasses initiates binding and activation of the classic complement pathway. Specificity of the classic pathway reaction is imposed by antibody. In a few instances, such as viral agents,[165–168] DNA, C-reactive protein,[169,170] and mitochondrial membranes,[171,172] activation of classic pathway can apparently proceed in the absence of antibody. Activation of the alternative complement pathway always involves antibody-independent recognition of structures, such as repeating polysaccharides, endotoxin, and so forth, that are highly represented among pathogenic microorganisms. This activation therefore involves relatively nonspecific binding; localization of the alternative pathway reaction is accomplished by permissive propagation of the cascade under conditions when control of protein inactivation of the effector proteins is limited. Amplification is an important feature of both pathways since deposition of one or few molecules (immunoglobulin or C3b fragment) can yield enzymatic cleavage of thousands of later components in the cascade and the consequent generation of complement-dependent biologic activities. A positive activation loop involving the proteins of the alternative pathway further augments the biologic amplification caused by the complement system. The bases for these conclusions are summarized in several recent reviews.[173,174] With cleavage of the complement protein C5, a polypeptide (C5b) is generated that serves as a nidus for assembly of the terminal complement proteins, also known as the *membrane attack complex* (MAC).[175] When the target of antibody-dependent or -independent complement activation is on a cell surface, the membrane lesions are clustered about the initial recognition site. In the course of this reaction, however, numerous biologically active complement-derived polypeptides are released in the fluid phase. The effects of these may be exerted at great distance and, in most instances, through interaction with specific cell-surface receptors. Modulation of the complement cascade is accomplished by fluid-phase and membrane proteins (inhibitors/cofactors) as well as intrinsic decay or instability of several of the complement activities. Figure 16-6 shows the complement pathways.

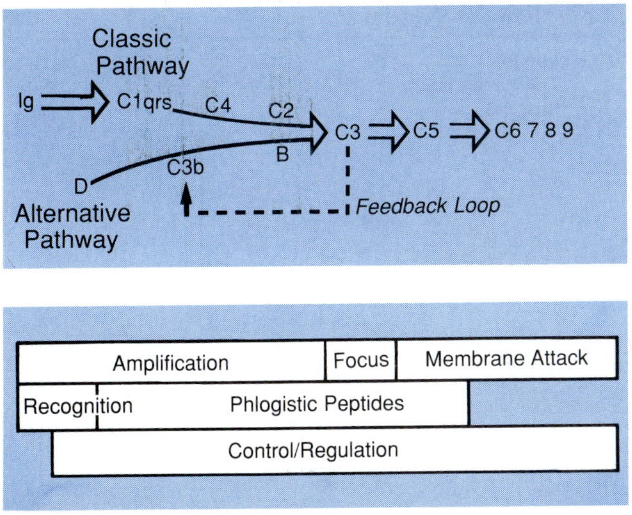

FIGURE 16-6. Classic and alternative complement activation pathways leading to assembly of the membrane attack complex.

Nomenclature

The first[176] and subsequent attempts to reach agreement on nomenclature of the complement system have resulted in a standard for describing the complement proteins and their cleavage products. The soluble proteins are designated numerically (eg, C1 through C9) or by upper-case letters (eg, factor B, factor D); their cleavage products by lower-case letters (eg, C2a, C3b); and the polypeptide subunits of the multichain proteins by lower-case Greek letters (eg, C4α, β, γ). A common system has not yet been agreed on for all the membrane-bound complement receptors and control proteins, but in this chapter, we use the most current accepted terminology. Table 16-7 outlines several physicochemical properties of the complement proteins, approximate serum concentrations, sizes of the mRNA, and genes encoding the complement proteins.

Classic Activation Pathway

First Component (C1)

The C1 complement component is a Ca^{2+}-dependent metalloprotein complex of a collagen-like recognition molecule C1q (410 kd) and dimers of the serine proteinases C1r and C1s, each 85 to 95 kd.[177] The C1q is composed of six globular domains connected by triple helical regions to a central fibril.[178,179] The globular heads interact with the Cγ2 domain of IgG[180] and Cμ3 or Cμ4 of IgM immunoglobulins.[181] Two dimeric structures consisting of zymogen C1r and C1s are thought to reside in a cone formed by the C1q fibrils (Fig. 16-7). Binding to immunoglobulin leads to distortion of the C1q cone, and the resulting activation of C1r leads to cleavage and activation of the C1s serine proteinase.[182,183] C1q is present in normal human serum at a concentration of about 70 μg/mL, mostly in the complex $C1qr_2s_2$, but up to 20% to 30% may be found as free C1q and $C1r_2s_2$.[184] Binding of C1q to immunoglobulin increases the affinity of $C1r_2s_2$ for C1q by an order of magnitude. On cell surfaces, a single IgM or an IgG doublet (30 to 50 nm or less from each other) in complex with antigen is capable of binding a single C1 molecule and initiating the complement cascade.[185]

C1 is synthesized in epithelial cells, mononuclear phagocytes, and fibroblasts in tissue culture[186]; and C1r and C1s synthesis has been demonstrated in a hepatocellular cell line.[187] C1q is the product of three distinct mRNA species. The gene encoding the β chain (2.6 kb) has been characterized, and cDNA clones corresponding to the C1q β[188] and α[189] chains have been identified.

The C1r and C1s primary translation products are programmed by mRNA species varying in size from 2.9 to 3.1 kb and encoded by closely linked genes on chromosome 12p. For C1r and possibly C1s, the multiple mRNA sizes are generated from single genes but differ due to differences in 3′ untranslated region.[190–193] Details of the synthesis and postsynthetic processing and assembly of the C1 protein have not yet been elucidated, but it is likely that the synthesis of each subunit is under independent control.

Fourth Component (C4)

C4, the natural substrate of the C1s enzyme, is a disulfide-linked heterotrimer (200 kd) consisting of α (93 kd), β (78 kd), and γ (33 kd) chains.[194] Cleavage of a 9-kd amino-terminal fragment of C4 (C4a) from α chain between residues 74 and 75 exposes a reactive thiolester, the binding site for the C4b fragment to immunoglobulin, antigen, or cell surfaces.[195] Two isotypes of C4, products of the separate genes C4A and C4B,[196,197] are found in human serum. The previously identified red cell antigens Rodgers and Chido are, in fact, cleavage fragments of C4A and C4B proteins, respectively.[198] The two forms differ by only four residues, but these differences account for a profound difference in affinity for hydroxyl (C4B) or amino group (C4A) acceptor sites.[199,200] Both forms of C4b serve as binding sites for the cleavage product of C2 activation (C2a), thus generating the classic pathway C3 convertase enzyme.

The C4A and C4B genes are polymorphic in overall size (16 and 22 kb) and in fine structure.[196] C4 protein polymorphisms are readily detected in agarose gel electrophoresis (Fig. 16-8). In addition, deletions and duplications of the C4 genes are frequently observed.[201,202] Each gene programs transcription of C4 mRNA, which is processed to a 5.5-kb template for translation of prepro-C4, the single-chain precursor of the mature protein.[203] Cosynthetic and postsynthetic processing of prepro-C4 involves cleavage of signal peptide, excision of two interchain-linking peptides, sulfation, modification of residues to produce the thiol ester reactive site, glycosylation of α and β chain, and a carboxy-terminal modification of α chain by an extracellular metalloenzyme.[204]

Second Component (C2)

C2 is a single-chain glycoprotein that binds to C4b in the presence of Mg^{2+} and is cleaved into an amino-terminal, 223–amino acid polypeptide, C2b, and into a carboxy-terminal, 509–amino acid fragment, C2a. The latter bears the active site and thus is unusual among serine proteinases since the active polypeptide site is the larger of the two fragments generated during activation and cleavage.[205] The C3-cleaving enzyme C4b2a is unstable. First order decay of the C4b2a complex[206] represents an intrinsic control mechanism in the classic pathway (Fig. 16-9), but decay is accelerated by cell-surface control proteins as described in detail later. On the cell membrane, a single C1 molecule can generate a cluster of C4b2a molecules that function to generate membrane lesions at or near the recognition site.[207]

C2 is the product of a 14-kb gene within the MHC class III region on chromosome 6p.[208] Several C2 primary translation products (84, 79, and 70 kd)[209] programmed by one or few C2 mRNA species (2.8 kb) are synthesized in liver, mononuclear phagocytes, fibroblasts, and perhaps in other cells.[210] The largest is glycosylated and secreted in about 60 minutes, but the other two forms remain cell-associated. The function of these cell-associated C2 proteins has not been determined.

TABLE 16-7. Proteins, Regulators, and Receptors of the Complement System

	Molecular Mass (kd)	Subunit Structure	Serum Concentration (μg/mL)	mRNA Size*† (kb)	Gene Size* (kb)
COMPLEMENT PROTEIN					
C1q	410	6A: 24 kd 6B: 23 kd 6C: 22 kd	70	A: ND B: 1.5 C: ND	A: ND B: 2.6 C: ND
C1r	95	Single chain	35	2	ND
C1s	87	Single chain	35	2	ND
C2	110	Single chain	25	2.9	18
B	93	Single chain	200	2.6	6
D	24	Single chain	1	1	ND
C3	185	α: 110 kd β: 75 kd	1500	5.2	24
C4	200	α: 93 kd β: 78 kd γ: 33 kd	400–600	5.3	A: 22 B: 16/2
C5	190	α: 115 kd β: 75 kd	75	5.5	>70
C6	115	Single chain	75	ND	ND
C7	115	Single chain	65	3.9	ND
C8	163	α: 64 kd β: 64 kd γ: 22 kd	55	α: 2.5 β: 2.6 γ: 1	α: ND β: ND γ: ND
C9	71	Single chain	60	2.4	80
C1 inhibitor	104 (34% CHO)	Single chain	150	1.8	17
P	~224	6: 56,000	25	1.6	ND
C4bp	500	7: 70,000 (6α: 70,000) (1β: 45,000)	~150	2.5	20
I	88	46,000 39,000	35	2.4	ND
H	155	Single chain	500	4.4	>100‡
S	~80	Single chain	500	1.6	ND
MEMBRANE RECEPTORS AND REGULATORS					
DAF	70	Single chain	—	3.1 2.7 2	ND
MCP	58–63	Single chain	—	4.2	ND
HRF	20	Single chain	—		
CR1	A: 190§ B: 220 C: 160 D: 250	Single chain	—	A: 8.6 B: 11.6 C: 7.3 D: 12.8	ND
CR2	140	Single chain	—	5	ND
CR3	260	α: 165,000 β: 95,000	—	α: 6 β: 3	α: ND β: 32
C5aR	~45	Single chain	—	ND	ND
C1qR	~70	ND	—	ND	ND

ND, not determined.
* Approximate values.
† Only major mRNAs are shown.
‡ Murine gene (human unknown).
§ Allotypes.

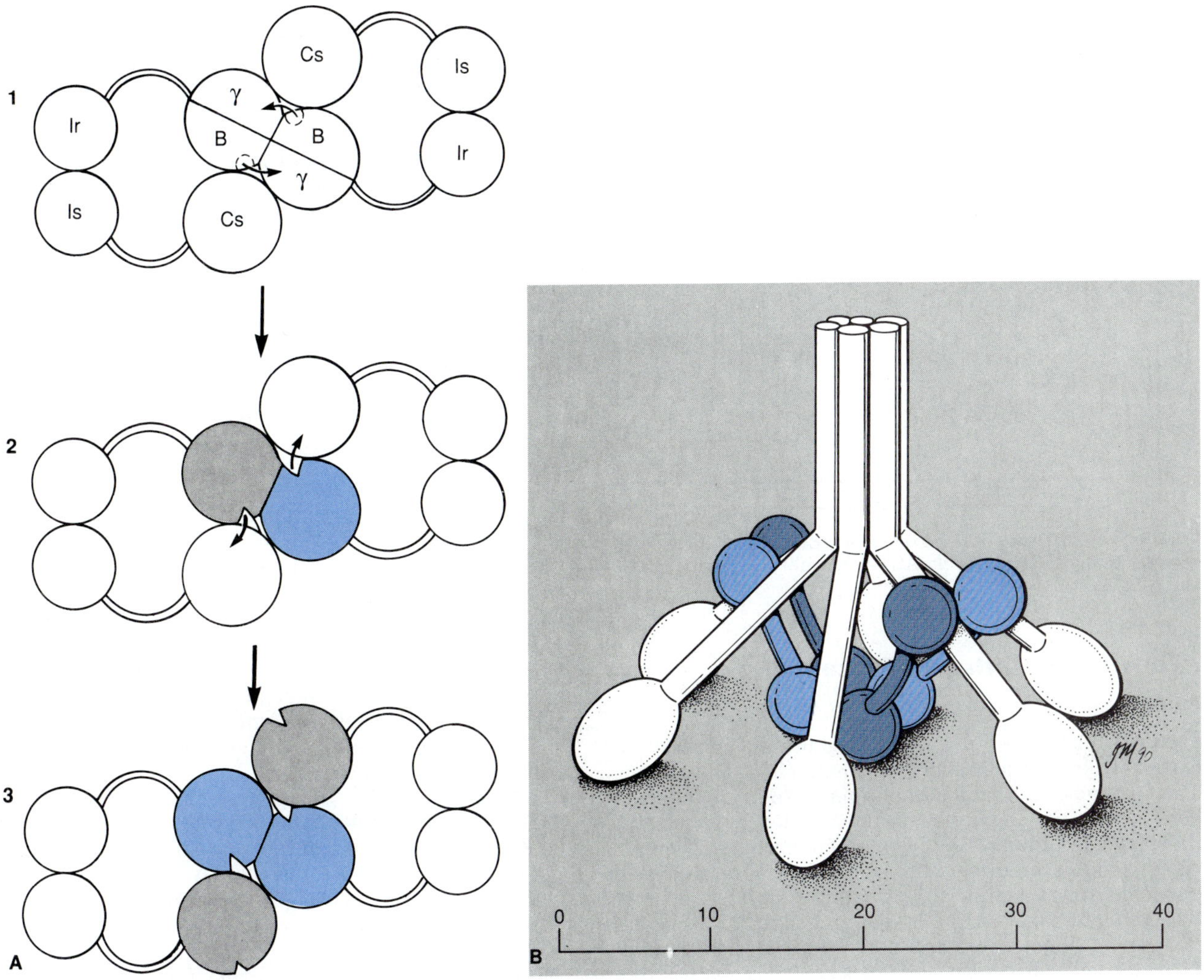

FIGURE 16-7. (*A*) Schematic representation of the C1r-C1s catalytic subunit of the first component of complement. The diagram shows the autoactivation of C1r (1), C1s activation by C1r (2), leading to full activation of C1s-C1r-C1r-C1s macromolecular complex (3). Dotted circles represent active sites in zymogen form, nicks represent true active sites, and curved arrows represent proteolytic cleavage sites. Cs, catalytic domain of C1s; Ir and Is, interaction domains of C1r and C1s. (After Arlaud GJ, et al. Molecular characterization of the catalytic domains of human complement serine protease Clr. Biochemistry 1986;25:5177) (*B*) Model of C1r-C1s with C1q. C1q is white, and C1r2-C1s2 is dark. The ruler is in nanometers. (After Colomb MG, Arlaud GJ, Viliers CL. Activation of Cl. Trans R Soc Lond [Biol] 1984;306:283)

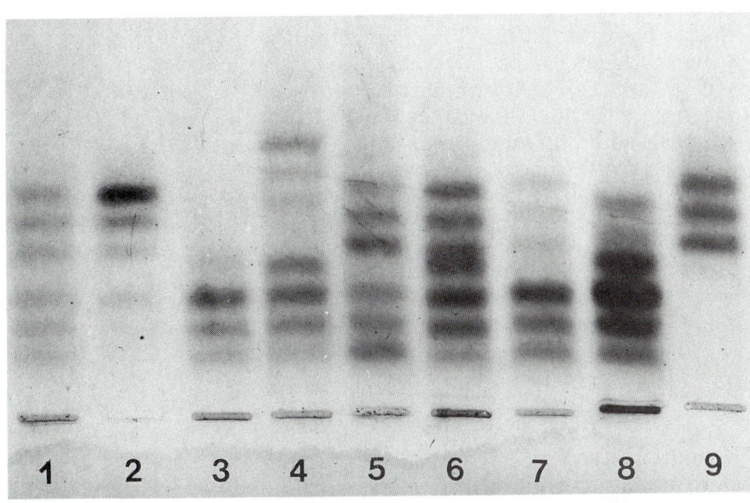

FIGURE 16-8. C4 patterns produced by immunofixation with antiserum to C4 after agarose gel electrophoresis of neuraminidase-treated ethylenediaminetetraacetic acid plasma samples from selected patients. Patients 1, 2, 3, 4, 7, 8, and 9 bear C4-null alleles. (Hauptmann G, Tappeiner G, Schifferli JA. Inherited deficiency of the fourth component of human complement. Immunodefic Rev 1988;1:9)

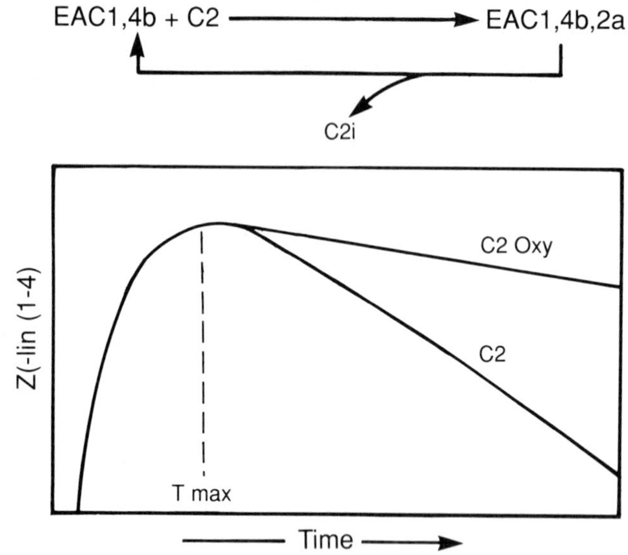

FIGURE 16-9. Decay of classic pathway convertase. Lower panel shows a plot of the kinetics of EAC142 assembly and decay for C2 and oxidized C2.

Alternative Pathway Proteins

Factor D

Factor D, a 24-kd serine proteinase is present in serum at extremely low concentrations, apparently in its active form. The enzyme can circulate in plasma as an active enzyme because it is not susceptible to inactivation by the serine proteinase inhibitor (SERPIN) family of proteins. Factor D shows a high degree of substrate specificity for cleavage of a specific Arg-Lys amino acid bond in factor B when factor B is bound to C3b. Factor D is synthesized in mononuclear phagocytes,[211] fat cells, and peripheral nerves (perhaps Schwann cells). In the fat cell, it has been designated *adipsin*,[212,213] and its expression has been shown to alter markedly in obese mice as a function of nutritional status.

Factor B

Factor B is the structural and functional alternative pathway homologue of the C2 protein of the classic pathway. The gene for factor B (6 kb), is about 400 base pair 5′ of the terminus of the C2 gene on chromosome 6P.[214,215] From mature factor B mRNA (2.5 kb), an 83-kd primary product is synthesized, processed, and secreted with kinetics similar to that observed for C2.[216,217] The factor B protein is activated by factor D–mediated cleavage of the zymogen to yield Bb, the carboxy-terminal fragment that bears the serine proteinase site. The Bb fragment in an Mg^{2+}-dependent complex with C3b forms an unstable C3-cleaving enzyme analogous to the classic pathway C4b2a complex.[218] In addition to its role in alternative pathway complement activation, factor B also serves as a cofactor in antibody-independent monocyte-mediated cytotoxicity,[219] macrophage spreading,[220] activation of plasminogen,[221] and as a growth factor for clonal expansion of antigen-stimulated B lymphocytes.[222]

Properdin

Properdin is isolated as a polydisperse mixture of noncovalently bound multimers of a 56-kd subunit.[223] The principal function of properdin is to stabilize the alternative pathway C3 convertase (C3bBb) by decreasing the rate of decay dissociation and by interfering with binding of the cofactor protein factor H to the C3 convertase (discussed later). Isolation of murine properdin cDNA and comparison with the partial amino acid sequence of human properdin reveals greater than 75% identity.[224] An interesting 60-residue repeating motif homologous to many other complement and clotting proteins, cell-surface receptors, the circumsporozoite, and the thrombospondin-related anonymous protein (proteins of malaria), is found in properdin.[224,225] These proteins represent examples of molecular mimicry, one among several microbial strategies that subvert complement-mediated defenses (others are discussed later). Recent studies have established that the properdin gene is on chromosome Xp11.23 to 21.1, near the retinitis pigmentosa locus. In the mouse, the 1.6-kb properdin mRNA is expressed in spleen, lung, and activated macrophages but is not detectable under resting conditions in liver (K.B.M. Reid, personal communication). The tissue sites of human properdin synthesis have not yet been established.

Third Component (C3)

Convergence of the classic and alternative pathways of complement activation on C3 results in the generation of most of the biologic activities associated with the complement system. The C3 protein (185 kd) is a disulfide-linked heterodimer of α (110 kd) and β (75 kd) chains.[226] It is the most abundant of the complement proteins in serum (1 to 1.5 mg/mL). Genetically determined polymorphic variants of C3 have been identified,[227] each with about the same biologic-specific activity.[228]

Cleavage of C3 at Arg_{77}-Ser_{78} of α chain liberates the C3a fragment, a potent anaphylatoxin that elicits histamine release, smooth muscle contraction, and noncytotoxic liberation of arachidonate metabolites.[229] These effects are mediated by specific receptors for C3a on mast cells, smooth muscle cells, and leukocytes. Covalent binding of C3b to a carboxyl- or amino-acceptor site is accomplished by its labile thiolester.[230,231] Deposition of C3 on a cell is relatively inefficient (less than 5% to 10% is bound under optimal conditions), so that much of the metastable C3b reacts with water and cannot bind to target cell or immune complex. Nevertheless, C3b, whether surface-bound or hydrolyzed, can bind C5, factors B and H, properdin, and the C3b receptor, CR1.

Binding and activation of factor B to C3b generates the alternative pathway amplification loop (Fig. 16-10), the flux of which is controlled by intrinsic decay of the enzyme C3bBb and control and cofactor protein dissociation of the

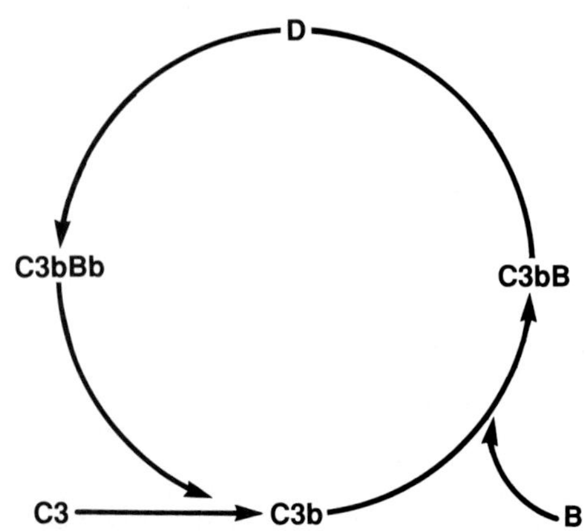

FIGURE 16-10. Amplification loop of the complement cascade. Regulation of this loop is due primarily to the C3b inactivator (factor I).

complex and cleavage of the C3b.[218] Both fluid-phase and cell-surface proteins participate in the regulation of the complement cascade at this point in the sequence. Interestingly, some microorganisms, such as EBV and various bacteria, have evolved strategies for control of C3b activity that mimic the physiologic regulatory mechanisms (discussed later). A second C3b bound to the C3bBb complex results in generation of a C5-cleaving enzyme and generation of the MAC.[173,175] This is but one of the several pathways for further generation of active complement proteins since many of the products of C3b cleavage have important biologic activity (Fig. 16-11).

Cleavage of C3b by one of the natural control proteins, factor I, is facilitated by the fluid-phase component factor H and on erythrocytes, lymphocytes, granulocytes, mononuclear phagocytes, and other cells by the C3b receptor, CR1. C3b α chain is cleaved by factor I at two sites to generate C3bi, consisting of disulfide-linked α-chain fragments of 62.5 kd and 39.5 kd, bound to β chain, and a 2-kd fragment (C3f) of uncertain function. A member of the integrin family of proteins is found on phagocytes. CR3 is a specific receptor for C3bi (discussed later). The C3bi undergoes further cleavage by factor I, dissociating a 62.5-kd amino-terminal fragment to generate C3dg, a 40-kd C3 product that remains covalently bound to the target of complement activation. Further cleavage of a 5-kd fragment, C3g, from the amino terminus by plasmin generates C3d (35-kd), for which a specific receptor CR2 is found on B lymphocytes. The balance of the C3 molecule, C3c, is released from the site. The sequential reactions in which C3 serves as substrate are summarized in Figure 16-11.[231]

The C3 gene (24 kb)[232] localized to chromosome 19p[233] programs synthesis of the 5.2-kb mature C3 mRNA, from which prepro-C3 is synthesized. As for C4 and C5, C3 is synthesized as a single-chain precursor that is modified postsynthetically and secreted within about 2 hours.[234] The source of most of the plasma C3 is liver, but extrahepatic synthesis of C3 is important in host defenses and immunopathophysiology.[235] This is also true for many other components of the two activation pathways and the complement-regulatory proteins.

Fifth Component (C5)

C5, a 190-kd glycoprotein, is homologous to C3, C4, and α_2-macroglobulin but lacks the characteristic thiolester sites found in the other three proteins.[226] Native C5 binds to the macromolecular complex C5-cleaving enzymes of classic and alternative pathways (C4b2a3b/$[C3b]_2$Bb) by interaction with sites on C4b or C3b, respectively. Cleavage of the α chain yields an 11-kd C5a molecule that shows structural and functional similarity to the corresponding amino-terminal α-chain polypeptides (C3a and C4a) of C3 and C4. C5a has spasmogenic activity, induces chemotaxis, increases adherence and noncytotoxic release of intracellular enzymes, and induces an oxidative burst and arachidonate metabolism in granulocytes. A carboxypeptidase found in plasma cleaves the carboxy-terminal arginine in C5a to generate C5a des-Arg with modification of several of these biologic activities.[236] C5a des-Arg is about 100 times less potent as a chemotaxin than C5a. Complexing of C5a des-Arg with the vitamin D–binding protein Gc globulin specifically enhances the chemotactic effect of the C5 cleavage products but does not affect FMLP- or leukotriene B4–mediated leukocyte migration.[237,238] Both C5a and C5a des-Arg have an amplifying effect on antibody responses and T-cell proliferation. C3a has similar, but less potent, effects. C5b, the remaining portion of the C5 molecule, remains bound to the convertase, where it expresses a binding site for C6 and the assembly of the proteins of the MAC.[239] This C5b6 complex is unstable and decays with a relatively short half-life. C5b6 can remain bound or transfer to other cells generating sites for the phenomenon of reactive lysis[240] and diffusion of the effects of complement activation, but its short half-life limits this phenomenon unless the complex is stabilized (discussed later).

C5 is encoded by a large gene (more than 50 kb) on chromosome 9q,[241] which generates a mature mRNA of 5.5 kb and a pro-C5 translation product that requires postsynthetic processing to yield the heterodimeric native C5 protein.[242] C5 is synthesized in liver, mononuclear phagocytes, and possibly in other cells. Hence, the tissue distribution of C5 gene expression is somewhat more restricted than for proteins of the classic and alternative complement-activation pathways.

Sixth and Seventh Components (C6 and C7)

The single-chain glycoproteins C6 (115 kd) and C7 (115 kd) are considered together because of similarities in function of these two proteins in the MAC. The complete primary structure of C7 has been deduced from cDNA cloning and sequence analysis.[243] The amino-terminal two thirds of C7 is about 30% homologous with C8α and C8β chains and C9. Several other proteins show sequence homology with a cysteine-rich region of the C7 molecule. These include, for example, the low-density lipoprotein receptor, thrombospondin, factors IX and X of the clotting system, and many other proteins. Functional and structural data support the concept that binding of C7 to C5b6 generates from

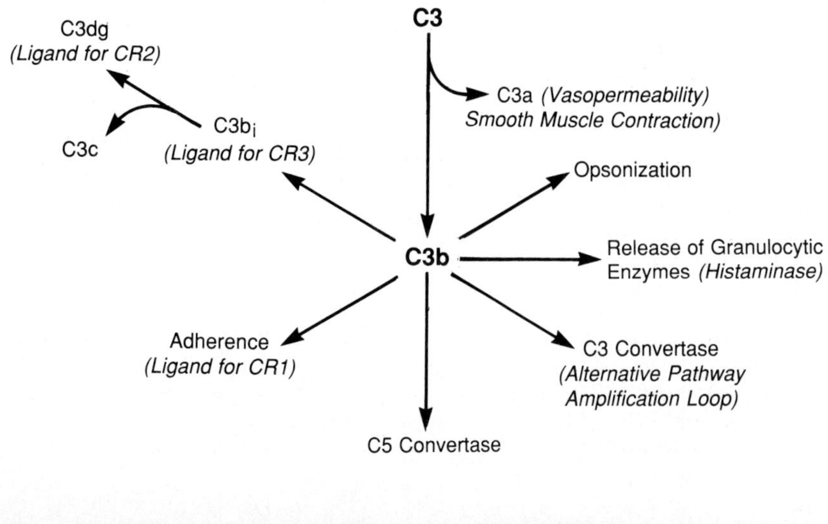

FIGURE 16-11. Biologic functions of C3 cleavage products.

the hydrophilic precursors (C5b6 and C7), an amphiphilic complex that permits insertion of the complex into a lipid bilayer and generation of discrete membrane lesion.

Eighth Component (C8)

The penultimate component in the complement cascade leading to cytolysis, C8 is a complex of three polypeptides: disulfide-linked α (64 kd) and γ (22 kd) chains and a noncovalently associated β chain (64 kd).[244] The polypeptides are translated from three separate mRNA species derived from three genes: two (α and β) on chromosome 1p and γ on 9q.[245,246] As indicated previously, C8β and C8α chains show sequence homology with other MAC and functionally unrelated membrane plasma proteins. On binding of C8 to the 5b67 complex, the α-γ subunit inserts into the membrane, and a functional lesion with an effective pore size of about 10 to 30 nm is generated.[247,248] Thus, slow lysis of a cell can occur in the absence of C9.

Ninth Component (C9)

In plasma, C9 is a soluble glycoprotein (70 kd) with amino-terminal hydrophilic and carboxy-terminal relatively hydrophobic domains.[249] When C9 interacts with a single C5b8 complex, it expresses amphiphilic properties, inserts in the membrane, and polymerizes with 10 to 15 additional C9 molecules to generate an effective lesion of about 100 nm.[250] These pores result in disruption of osmotic integrity of the cell, loss of small intracellular molecular species, and then loss and degradation of macromolecules. Complement-dependent hemolysis is efficient, but lysis of nucleated cells is less so because the latter are capable of repairing these membrane lesions.[251] Perforin, a protein produced by cytolytic T lymphocytes and natural killer cells, is a 70-kd channel-forming protein[252] that bears striking functional and structural homology with C9. That is, the proximate mechanisms of fluid-phase and cell-mediated cytolysis seem to be rather similar.

Regulatory Proteins

The complement cascade is modulated to some extent by (1) the intrinsic decay of multimolecular enzyme complexes (eg, C4b2a and C3bBb); (2) labile reactive sites with microsecond half-lives (eg, the thiolester of C3); and (3) dissociation of incompletely assembled MAC from cell surfaces. Nevertheless, the absence of regulatory proteins of the system results in uncontrolled wasteful activation and consumption of complement. A naturally occurring example of this is the genetic deficiency of a key complement-regulatory protein factor I (discussed later). Many of the regulatory proteins are products of extended gene families, including some with no apparent functional relation to the complement system.

Soluble Regulators

Factor I. Factor I is a disulfide-linked, heterodimeric, 88-kd glycoprotein synthesized in liver and in extrahepatic tissues as a 63-kd single-chain precursor.[253] Factor I, like factor D, circulates in plasma as an active serine proteinase. The active serine esterase site is on the light chain, a polypeptide with extensive primary sequence homology to tissue plasminogen activator. The heavy chain shows homology with low-density lipoprotein and epidermal growth factor receptors as well as the terminal complement components C8 and C9. Factor I displays exquisite substrate specificity for C3b and C4b.[254] The cleavage of these substrates is facilitated in fluid phase by factor H and C4-binding protein (C4bp) and on cell surfaces by the complement C3b/C4b receptor, CR1.[255] As indicated previously, cleavage of C3b and C4b render these proteins hemolytically inactive, but at least for C3b, several new biologic activities are generated by factor I–mediated cleavage. The gene encoding factor I is on chromosome 4, but details about its size and structure are lacking.

Factor H. The complement-regulatory cofactor protein factor H is a 150-kd glycoprotein found in plasma at a concentration of about 500 μg/mL. It is synthesized in liver, macrophages, fibroblasts, and possibly platelets (where it is found in the α granules) from a 4.4-kb mRNA.[256] Liver is also the site of synthesis of a truncated form of H (43 kd), but its function and fate are unknown.[257] Recent studies have identified multiple factor H–related proteins in serum, some of which are derived from distinct genes, but the function of these proteins in complement regulation is unknown.[257a] The gene for factor H is on chromosome 1 within the complement-regulatory gene complex. Studies of the murine factor H gene indicate that it is large (100 kb) and complex.

The primary structure of factor H shows homology to several other proteins displaying a characteristic 60-residue cysteine-rich repeating unit. Based on physicochemical properties, amino acid composition, and electromicroscopic data, the protein is thought to have an unusual higher order structure and elongated shape.[258] Factor H binds to C3b, thereby leading to dissociation and decay of the alternative pathway C3 convertase (C3bBb) and the C5 convertase, $(C3b)_2Bb$. Additional binding sites for heparin have been characterized in factor H, raising the potential for direct interaction with carbohydrate moieties in the extracellular matrix.[257a] This facilitates cleavage of C3b by factor I. The findings of factor H–binding sites on B cells and of H bound to leukocytes and studies suggesting ligand-mediated functional consequences of H binding in several cell types raise the possibility that other physiologic roles for factor H are mediated perhaps by specific receptors.

C4-Binding Protein (C4bp). The functional analogue of factor H, C4bp, that regulates the classic pathway C3 convertase (C4b2a) is structurally unique but does show a repeating homology unit similar to that for many of the complement-regulatory proteins.[258] It is a disulfide-linked multimer of seven identical chains (70 kd each), which appears spider-like when visualized in the electron microscope.[259] In plasma, C4bp is free or noncovalently complexed with protein S, a cofactor in protein C degradation of clotting factors Va and VIIIa.[260] Multiple sites facilitate association of the binding protein with C4b, leading to dissociation of the C4b2a complex. In addition, C4bp acts as cofactor to enhance generation of the products of factor I cleavage and dissociation of C4b to the C4c and C4d fragments.

Vitronectin (S-protein). Vitronectin, or S-protein, is an 80-kd glycoprotein that functions as an inhibitor of the MAC of the complement system[261] and in the heparin-accelerated inactivation of thrombin by antithrombin III.[262] This protein must be distinguished from the vitamin K–dependent protein S, another cofactor in the clotting system alluded to previously. Several distinct structural domains of vitronectin mediate its multiple functional activities.[263] A sequence characteristic of integrins facilitates cell-surface binding and enhancement of Fc-mediated phagocytosis. A basic region, the heparin-binding domain, important for its function in the clotting system, also interacts with a negatively charged region conserved in C9, perforin, C6, C7, and C8.[264] The latter is involved in what is likely the most important role of vitronectin in modulating complement, that is, limiting the extent of reactive lysis and potential innocent bystander damage after complement activation. Vitronectin also contains at the amino terminus a peptide identical to somatomedin B, but the functional meaning of this homology is unknown. Complement MAC activity can also be inhibited in the fluid phase by plasma lipoproteins, but the relative importance of this mechanism compared with vitronectin control of the complement cascade is not certain.

C1 Inhibitor. C1 inhibitor is a highly glycosylated (35% carbohydrate by weight) 104-kd plasma protein member of the SERPIN family. It is the only known inhibitor of the C1r and C1s enzymes, but it also forms 1:1 stoichiometric complexes with factors XII and XI of the clotting cascade, kallikrein, and plasmin.[265] It is encoded by a gene on chromosome 11 that directs synthesis of a mature 2-kb mRNA, from which the 64-kd primary translation product is generated.[266] In primary structure, C1 inhibitor shows homology to other SERPINS, but it also contains a large amino-terminal nonhomologous extension.[267,268] C1 inhibitor is synthesized in liver[187] and at extrahepatic sites in mononuclear phagocytes, fibroblasts, and perhaps megakaryocytes.[269] The importance of C1 inhibitor as a regulator of complement activation is evidenced by the profound life-threatening symptoms associated with genetically determined and acquired deficiencies of the protein (discussed later).

Cell-Associated Regulators

Membrane Cofactor Protein. The membrane cofactor protein (MCP) is one of the several fluid-phase and membrane proteins that inhibit the C3 convertases by facilitating factor I cleavage of C3b/C4b. Unlike the others, MCP does not promote dissociation and decay of the convertase.[270] MCP is encoded by a gene on chromosome 1q within the regulator of complement-activation (RCA) complex. This integral membrane protein is present on all leukocytes, platelets, endothelial and epithelial cells, and fibroblasts.[271] The primary structure of MCP displays the typical 60-residue homologous repeat units shared among the proteins of the RCA. Atkinson and colleagues[272] proposed MCP as an important constituent in limiting complement activation on autologous tissues. Recent observations have revealed that MCP (CD46) is the measles virus receptor and that CD46+ cells are susceptible to measles infection, resulting in synctra and productive infectious measles viral particles.[272a,272b]

Homologous Restriction Factor. Homologous restriction factor (CD59) is a glycophospholipid-anchored membrane protein that restricts lysis of homologous platelets, leukocytes, and erythrocytes.[273] CD59 was shown to be deficient in a patient with symptomatic paroxysmal nocturnal hemoglobinuria,[274] revealing the importance of this protein in limiting complement-induced host cell injury. The CD59 glycolipid anchor apparently permits lateral mobility in the lipid bilayer, facilitating blocking of the randomly distributed MAC on a cell surface by a minimal number of HRF molecules per cell. Only about 9000 HRF molecules per erythrocyte are required for effective blockade of lysis.[275]

Decay-Accelerating Factor. DAF, another member of the supergene family exhibiting the characteristic highly repetitive homology units, is encoded by a gene on chromosome 1p within the RCA complex.[276,277] It is a 70-kd polypeptide anchored to membranes of erythrocytes, leukocytes (T and B lymphocytes, monocytes, neutrophils), platelets, and vascular endothelium by means of a characteristic glycolipid.[278] DAF and proteins such as acetylcholinesterase, 5-nucleotidase, and many others are released from cell surfaces by a phosphatidylinositol-specific phospholipase C (PIPLC). Support has been obtained for the existence of a secreted form of DAF generated by alternative mRNA splicing.[279] Thus, three mechanisms by which fluid-phase DAF can be generated have been described: PIPLC, proteolytic cleavage[280] of DAF from cell surfaces, and secretion. DAF limits association of the constituents and facilitates decay and dissociation of the C3 convertases (C4b2a, C3bBb) and C5 convertases, but it does not serve as cofactor for factor I cleavage of C3b/C4b (the obverse of MCP functions). Recurrent lysis of erythrocytes observed in paroxysmal nocturnal hemoglobinuria in patients with normal DAF but deficient CD59 emphasizes the relative HRF in regulating complement activation in vivo.[281] Recombinant secreted DAF has been shown to decrease inflammation in experimental immune complex disease[281a] and cell-associated MCP, CD59, and DAF can protect heterologous cell types from complement-mediated lysis.[281b] These studies suggest a potential role for this protein and HRF (CD59) in the inhibition of xenotransplant rejection.

Complement Receptors

Complement Receptor Type 1

The receptor for C3b binding (complement receptor type 1 [CR1])[282] is a single-chain integral membrane glycoprotein found on erythrocytes, lymphocytes, monocytes, granulocytes, glomerular podocytes, and dendritic cells. The number of receptors varies among these cell types, but where measured, the affinities for C3b are similar. Erythrocytes bear 50 to 1500 copies per cell, and polymorphonuclear leukocytes have between 3000 to 4000 CR1 receptors under resting conditions. A substantial intracellular pool of CR1 is translocated to the cell surfaces of polymorphonuclear leukocytes[283] after exposure to several stimuli, including C5a, FMLP, tumor necrosis factor, and viral agents such as herpes simplex,[284] a phenomenon potentially important in the pathogenesis of several disorders characterized by neutropenia and sequestration. Phorbol esters induce phosphorylation of CR1 in myelomonocytic cells but not in B lymphocytes.[285] CR1 is detected early in the B-cell lineage, is present in circulating B cells (2000 to 4000 per cell), but expression is down-regulated just before plasma cell differentiation.[286] The protein is encoded by a single-copy gene on chromosome 1q32 within the RCA complex, but four codominantly expressed allelic size variants (160, 190, 220, and 250 kd) have been recognized.[287] These allelic variants arise from intragenic duplications within the C3b-binding portion of CRI, thus varying the number of C3b-binding sites from one to four among each variant.[287a] Another variant, resulting in decreased CR1 expression, with a specific restriction fragment length polymorphism (detected on DNA blot analysis with a CR1 cDNA probe), may be a disease susceptibility marker for systemic lupus erythematosus (SLE).[288] The finding of reduced CR1 on cells of patients with SLE also results from nongenetic factors. Hence, the meaning of relative CR1 deficiency in this disorder remains uncertain.

CR1 exhibits saturable, relatively high-affinity binding of multimeric C3b or C4b.[289] The subsequent cleavage products, C3bi and C4bi, also bind to CR1, but with lower affinity. Binding is through a domain within the C3c fragment of C3α chain, so that further cleavage to generate C3dg releases C3c (Fig. 16-12), and the surface-bound C3 product no longer interacts with CR1. This reaction sequence is facilitated by interaction of C3b with CR1 because the receptor is also a complement-regulatory protein that mediates decay and dissociation of classic and alternative complement-activation pathways and is a cofactor for factor I cleavage of C3b on leukocytes.[282] Because erythrocytes are more abundant than other vascular cells, over 80% of

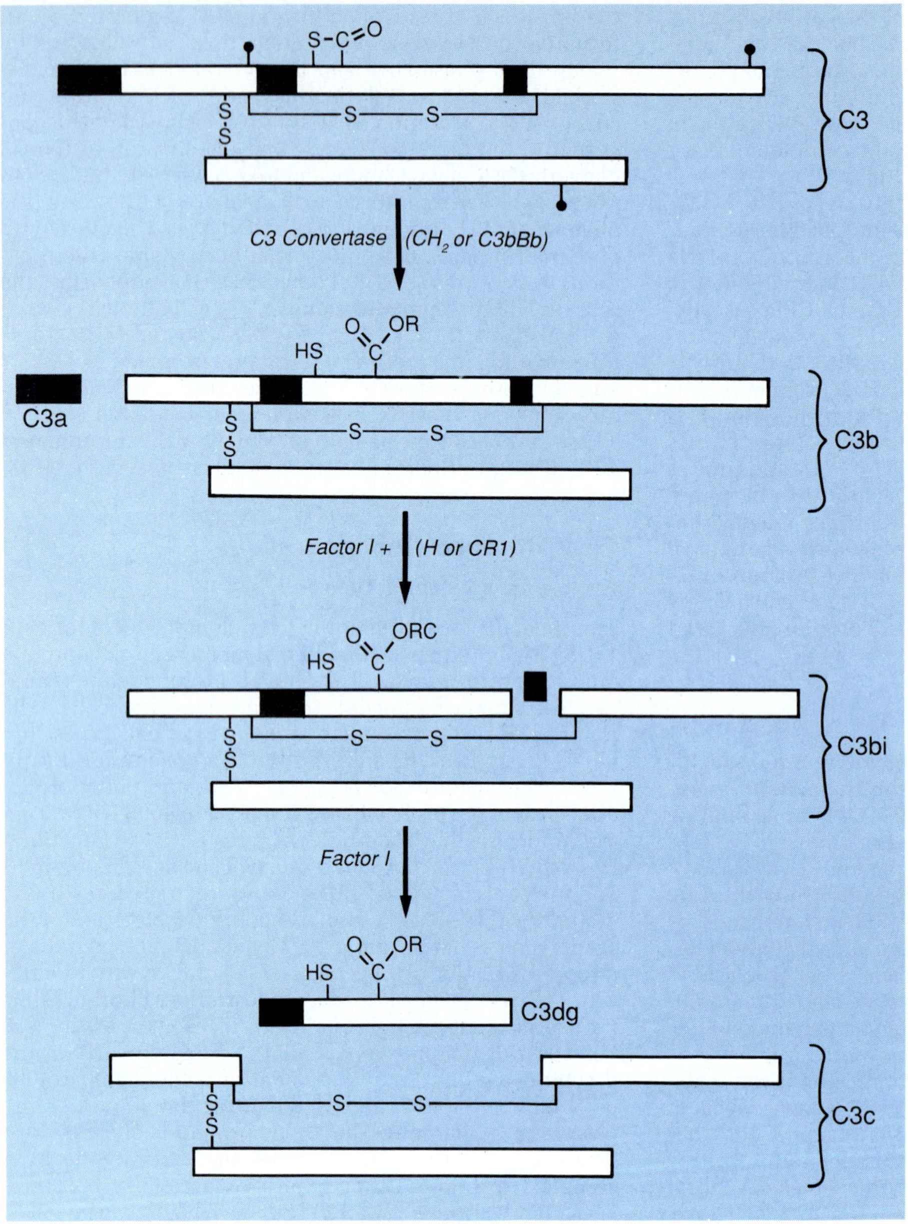

FIGURE 16-12. Diagram of C3 cleavage products.

circulating CRI is erythrocyte bound. As such, erythrocyte CR1 plays an important role as a carrier for complement-fixing immune complexes that are cycled to fixed mononuclear phagocytes for removal.[290] This mechanism reduces the concentration of free soluble immune complexes in plasma (discussed later). CR1, like many other products of the RCA, displays a repeating structural motif of about 60 residues. Multiples of these short consensus repeats are found within larger homologous repeating units. These structural features are thought to be important in the interaction with C3 and C4 cleavage products.

Complement Receptor Type 2

Complement receptor type 2 (CR2) receptor has a more limited cellular distribution than the other complement receptors. That is, CR2 is found primarily on B lymphocytes (later in maturation than CR1) and follicular dendritic cells.[291] The CR2 binds C3 fragments C3bi, C3dg, C3d bearing the C3d domain of C3 and the EBV protein, gp350. The latter, a specific EBV product that mediates binding of the virus to CR2, shows sequence homology with the C3d region.[292] The mature form of CR2 is a 145-kd glycoprotein encoded by a gene within the RCA complex on chromosome 1q32.[293] It also displays the 60- to 75-residue repeating structure, a typical transmembrane region, and a 34–amino acid cytoplasmic tail. Interaction of the C3d domain or EBV with CR2 induces phosphorylation of the receptor[285] and a nuclear ribonucleoprotein[294] and induction or enhancement of B-cell proliferation.[295] The activation of B-cell proliferation has been shown to be linked to the ability of CR2 to associate with B-cell CD19.[296] This CR2–CD19 complex mediates the binding of C3 activation fragments and, when inhibited by soluble CR2, can induce humoral immunosuppression.[296] This is but one mechanism by which complement modulates specific immune responses.

Complement Receptor Type 3

Complement receptor type 3 (CR3) receptor is a heterodimer consisting of one of the three α-chain membrane glycoproteins (CD11/18) that share a common β chain. The specific function of each of the dimeric proteins (LFA-1, CR3, and p150,95) is defined by its α chain. CR3 is distributed on mononuclear phagocytes, polymorphonuclear leukocytes, natural killer cells, and antibody-dependent cell-mediated cytotoxicity effector lymphocytes.[298] This receptor, in the presence of calcium, binds to the C3 cleavage products C3bi (with high affinity) and C3dg (with much lower affinity). The receptor also binds to yeast cell wall constituents and can, by this means, facilitate ingestion of unopsonized microorganisms. Other functions of CR3 include binding to endothelium, phagocytosis, and various activities that depend on the adhesive properties of the receptor. The CR3 α chain is synthesized from a 6-kb mRNA, postsynthetically processed, and transported to specific granules and cell membranes.[299] It contains a 26-residue transmembrane region, a 19-residue cytoplasmic tail, and a large extracellular domain with homologies to complement factor B, the von Willebrand factor, and to other members of the integrin protein family (ie, receptors for vitronectin, fibronectin, and platelet IIb/IIIa). The CR3 α subunit also shows sequence homology with another member of the CD11 group, the α chain of p150,95, a protein perhaps involved in binding to other C3 cleavage products and designated CR4.[300] The third of the α subunits defines LFA-1, a leukocyte adhesion molecule found on monocytes, T and B lymphocytes, and natural killer cells. The β chain is encoded by a gene (about 32 kb) on chromosome 21.[301] It has a structure typical of membrane proteins, with extracellular cysteine-rich transmembrane and cytoplasmic domains. The β chain also shows significant homology with the integrin family of proteins, moieties that interact with extracellular matrix and promote adhesion.

Intercellular adhesion molecule (ICAM)-1 is the counterreceptor for CR3, interacting with the third immunoglobulin-like domain in the ICAM-1 moeity.[302] The activation of CR3 on neutrophils and monocytes by endotoxin promotes leukocyte–endothelial interaction, suggesting that CR3 function is highly regulated by extracellular stimuli and facilitates the accumulation of these cells during an inflammatory response.[303] CR3 is the predominant integrin found on polymorphonuclear leukocytes and, as such, plays a key role in host defense during the initial stages of leukocyte extravasation and phagocytosis. This role is apparent in children with an inherited deficiency of CR3, who are unable to mount an inflammatory response and who have undue susceptibility to infection.[303a]

C5a Receptor

Specific and saturable receptors for C5a have been identified on blood leukocytes and alveolar macrophages as well as on several cell lines of mononuclear origin. The characterization of C5a receptors was accomplished by cDNA cloning.[304,305] The cDNA encodes a 350–amino acid protein that predisects a seven-membrane–spanning domain structure typical of G-protein–linked receptors. Recent studies have revealed that this receptor is a part of a family of related chemotaxis receptors, including the FMLP receptor, which are localized to chromosome 19q13.3.[305a] Functional data support the concept of a distinct C3a receptor, but attempts to isolate and characterize the C3a-binding protein have not been successful.

C1q Receptor

A 70-kd surface glycoprotein with C1q-binding properties appears to be a component of the saturable C1q receptor found on all leukocytes, platelets, endothelial cells, and fibroblasts.[306–308] After activation of C1, interaction of the $C1r_2C1s_2$ tetramer with the C1 inhibitor favors dissociation of the C1 complex, revealing a site on C1q that binds to its receptor. The C1qR satisfies criteria for signal transduction since C1q induces chemotaxis and K^+ conductance in fibroblasts,[309] platelet activation, and enhanced phagocytosis.[310] The C1q receptor may also serve in the transfer of soluble immune complexes to vascular endothelium.[308] Functional C1q binding proteins have been isolated from the surface of phagocytic cells using an affinity matrix of C1q. a monoclonal antibody against these proteins inhibits C1q enhancement of phagocytosis.[310a] These C1q receptors may also function in recognition and binding of an additional family of proteins termed *collections*, which includes serum mannose-binding protein and surfactant proteins A and D. The C1q receptor most likely binds to the C1q-like collagen domain in these proteins, initiating phagocytosis as an innate immune defense.[310b] Partial sequence data of this C1q receptor has revealed homology to calreticulum, the Ro/SSA antigen and a surface antigen of *Onchoceroa volvulus*.[310c]

Clinical Applications

Complement and Infectious Diseases

The complement cascade serves as an important mechanism for defense against microbial agents.[311] For encapsulated pyogenic microorganisms, deposition of C3 fragments on the bacterial surface prepares the bacterium for ingestion by phagocytic cells. When antibody is limited or when alternative pathway activation results in antibody-independent complement deposition, interaction of the C3 fragments with receptors (CR1, CR3) on phagocytes facilitates adherence of the bacteria to the host cell. The state of activation of the phagocyte[312] and the participation of other proteins (fibronectin,[313] small amounts of IgG[314]) determine whether the complement protein serves as a sufficient signal for ingestion. Adherence of microbe to phagocyte by means of C3b interaction with CR1 obviously facilitates generation of the factor I–mediated C3b cleavage products that interact with the CR3 receptor as well. Multiple ligand-receptor interactions therefore characterize the host cell bacterial adherence, that is, a redundancy that favors the host.

Resolution of bacteremia (pyogenic encapsulated organisms) involves complement-dependent clearance in liver and, to a lesser extent, in spleen. Liver is the principal site of sequestration in normal animals, whereas complement depletion results in a shift toward splenic clearance.[315] Some studies[316] suggest that complement also plays a role in the efficiency of intracellular killing of bacteria once ingested by the phagocyte, but the molecular mechanisms accounting for this phenomenon are not clear. Finally, bacteriolysis represents another complement-dependent host defense mechanism (Fig. 16-13). The details of complement-mediated bacteriolysis are beyond the scope of this chapter and are summarized elsewhere.[311] This represents a clinically important mechanism only for a few bacterial species (eg, *Neisseria*).

Molecular Mimicry: Microbial Subversion of Complement-Dependent Host Defenses

The advent of molecular cloning techniques has generated an enormous amount of primary sequence data for complement components and for proteins of microbial origin. As a result, the molecular bases of microbial strategies aimed at subverting complement-dependent host defenses previously only suspected from functional data have been established. Such mechanisms used by viruses, bacteria, yeast, and parasites often involve the production of proteins that are structural and functional homologues of the complement-regulatory proteins. These homologues in-

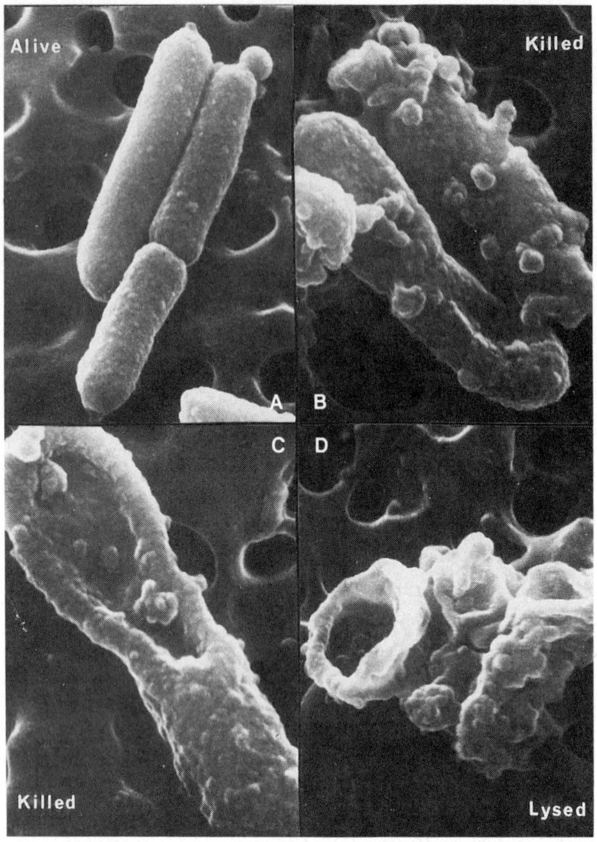

FIGURE 16-13. Scanning electron micrograph of *Escherichia coli* killed or lysed by alternative pathway proteins. (*A*) Heat-inactivated proteins (control). (*B*) Active proteins. (*C*) Active proteins plus lysozyme. (*D*) Active proteins plus C4-depleted serum. Organisms in *B* and *C* were killed but not lysed; organisms in *D* were killed and lysed (×30,000). (Schreiber RD, Morrison DC, Podack ER, Müller-Eberhard HJ. Bactericidal activity of the alternative complement pathway generated from 11 isolated plasma proteins. J Exp Med 1979;149:878)

activate complement or facilitate complement-activation pathways favorable to the pathogen. Herpes simplex virus (HSV) and EBV provide interesting examples of this general phenomenon.

HSV-1– and HSV-2–infected cells express the proteins gC-1 and gC-2, which share sequence homology with each other and with the complement-regulatory proteins.[270] Expression of the viral gC-1 protein generates C3b- and C3bi-binding activities on the infected cells since the human C3b/C4b receptor CR1 is antigenically and functionally similar to gC-1. In addition, gC-1 (and possibly gC-2) promotes decay and dissociation of the alternative pathway C3 convertase, thereby limiting alternative pathway–mediated deposition of C3 fragments on the viral envelope.[317,318] Both gC-1 and gC-2 thus protect against antibody-dependent, complement-mediated viral neutralization by means of several different strategies.

EBV-infected cells produce complement-regulatory activities that serve to accelerate decay of the alternative pathway convertase and produce a cofactor for factor I cleavage of C3b → C3bi → C3c + C3dg.[319] This leads not only to control of the complement cascade but also to generation of the C3 product, C3dg, a fragment that effectively does not interact with CR1 and CR3 on phagocytic cells but does interact with the CR2 receptor on B lymphocytes, facilitating viral adherence and infectivity. EBV does not accelerate classic pathway (C4b2a) dissociation but does function as cofactor for factor I cleavage of C4b and C4bi, so that the virus also limits classic pathway activation.

Vaccinia, a member of the pox virus family, produces a 35-kd polypeptide that reveals the repeating structural motif characteristic of the complement-regulatory proteins.[320] Preliminary data suggest a potential role for this protein in blocking classic pathway activation. Other organisms, such as *Trypanosoma cruzi*, produce a decay-accelerating activity for both complement-activation pathways. This activity is associated with polypeptides of 87 to 93 kd.[321,322] Yeast (*Candida albicans*) also expresses complement receptor-like molecules. For the trypanosomes and for other parasites such as malaria (*Plasmodium falcipalum*) that produce a protein homologous to properdin and thrombospondin, expression of these products is developmentally regulated.[224,225] Hence, at certain stages in its life cycle, when most vulnerable to complement-mediated injury, the organism expresses a counter to the action of complement.

Mechanisms employed by bacteria to limit complement-dependent opsonization include expression by group B streptococci of inhibitors of C5-dependent chemotaxis.[323] Elaboration of surfaces that are nonpermissive for alternative pathway activation and several other less well-defined resistance mechanisms are employed by *Neisseria* sp and *Escherichia coli*.

Immune Complexes

Complement serves several roles in the disposition of immune complexes.[324] As shown in the work of several investigators, complement activation results in solubilization of antigen–antibody precipitates.[325] Perhaps of greater importance, however, is the role of complement in clearance of soluble immune complexes. Complexes composed of complement-fixing antibody and antigen are cleared from the circulation in liver and spleen. Studies in nonhuman primates have established a critical function for CR1 on erythrocytes in mediating this clearance.[290] That is, deposition of C3b on the immune complex allows binding to the erythrocytes, thereby decreasing the fluid-phase concentration of the immune complex in plasma. The complexes are presumably then transferred to Kupffer cells as the erythrocytes traverse liver, possibly by conversion of C3b to C3bi and interaction with the CR3 on Kupffer cells (Fig. 16-14). Whatever the precise mechanism, the erythrocytes emerge from the liver capable of accepting complexes, so that the erythrocyte complement receptor serves as an immune complex buffer system. Clearance of immune complexes in complement-depleted experimental animals bypasses this mechanism and results in rapid deposition of complexes in other tissues, including lung and kidney. Recently, similar studies in normal humans and patients with SLE have established the generality of these conclusions.[326] Consistent with these concepts, soluble CRI is effective in inhibiting inflammation and tissue injury in vivo in several different models of complement-mediated injury.[326a–326c]

Genetic Deficiencies of Complement Proteins

Deficiencies of nearly all the complement components have been reported (Table 16-8). With two exceptions, these complement deficiencies are inherited as autosomal recessive traits (codominant when analyzed at the protein level). The exceptions are deficiency of C1 inhibitor (hereditary angioneurotic edema), which is inherited as an autosomal dominant trait, and properdin deficiency, inherited as an X-linked disorder. All but one of the complement deficiencies are associated with clinical symptoms;

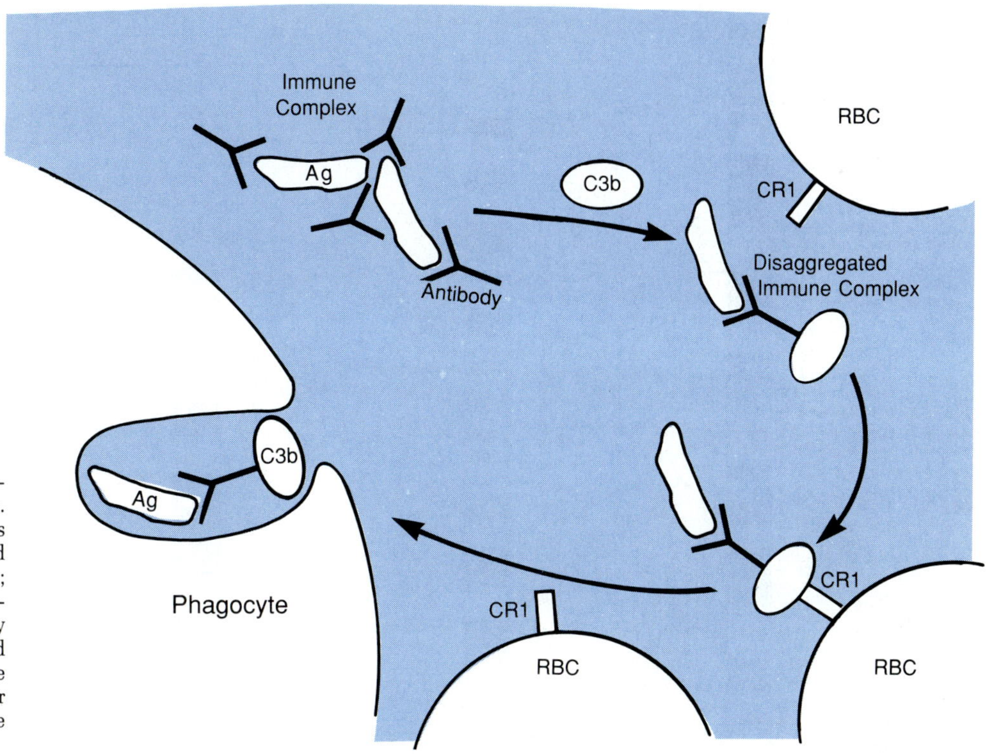

FIGURE 16-14. Immune complex solubilization and transport. C3b binding to Ag-Ab complexes facilitates solubilization and binding to erythrocytes by CR1; release of complexes to liver-fixed macrophages, presumably by C3b to C3bi conversion; and binding to CR3. The erythrocyte CR1 thus serves as a buffer system for soluble immune complexes.

C9-deficient patients are asymptomatic.[327] Chromosomal assignment of most of the complement gene loci has been accomplished by classic genetic linkage and molecular biologic methods (Fig. 16-15).

Deficiencies of the early complement components (C1q, C1r, C1s, C2, and C4) are generally associated with rheumatic disorders.[328] These include discoid lupus, SLE, glomerulonephritis, dermatomyositis, anaphylactoid purpura, and nonspecific vasculitis. The pathophysiologic basis for the association between these disorders and complement deficiencies is unclear, but a number of hypotheses have been proposed:

1. The association is due to an impairment of host defenses against viral or other microbial agents.
2. The MHC class III genes (C2, C4) are in linkage disequilibrium with specific HLA haplotypes,[329] and thus the deficiency may simply be genetically linked to a gene primarily involved in the autoimmune disorder.
3. The role of complement in processing immune complexes may be impaired.
4. A critical function of complement in initiating antibody responses may be altered.

It is impossible to distinguish among these hypotheses.

Important differences between rheumatic diseases seen in complement-deficient patients and non–complement-deficient patients have been recognized. For example, the SLE-like illness found in association with complement deficiencies is characterized by an early onset (often in childhood), prominent annular photosensitive skin lesions resembling discoid lupus, relatively limited renal and pleuropericardial involvement, and an infrequent deposition of immunoglobulin and C3 in the skin.[331–333] In addition, sera from complement-deficient patients with SLE contain low levels of antinuclear antibodies and antinative DNA antibodies. In contrast, anti-Ro antibodies are found more frequently in the complement-deficient patients.

Deficiencies of C3, factor H, and factor I predispose to recurrent infection with encapsulated pyogenic bacteria. Patients who lack the terminal components C5, C6, C7, and C8 display increased susceptibility to recurrent or disseminated neisserial infections.[330] C1-inhibitor deficiency results in angioneurotic edema. Acquired deficiency of C1 inhibitor is also characterized by intermittent episodes of visceral and cutaneous edema. The acquired disease, often found in association with lymphomas, results from complement-fixing antiidiotypic antibody directed against the tumor-derived immunoglobulin or, in some instances, autoantibody to C1 inhibitor.[334,335]

With the advent of molecular biology, it has become possible to examine mechanisms accounting for these deficiencies at the genomic level and to address more comprehensively the reasons for association of disease with the deficiency. Complementary DNA clones have been obtained for nearly all complement proteins, including the complement receptors and regulatory proteins. Several reviews[327,328] detail our current understanding of the mo-

TABLE 16-8. Clinical Conditions Associated With Complement Deficiencies

Clinical Features	Associated Complement Deficiency
Glomerulonephritis	C1q, C3
SLE and SLE-like syndromes	C1q, C1r, C1s, C4, C2
Angioneurotic edema	C1 inhibitor
Increased susceptibility to infection	
Pyogenic encapsulated bacteria (eg, *Streptococcus pneumoniae, Haemophilus influenzae, Staphylococcus aureus*)	C3, I, P, CR3
Neisseria gonorrhoeae, meningitidis	C5, C6, C7, C8
Paroxysmal nocturnal hemoglobinuria	DAF

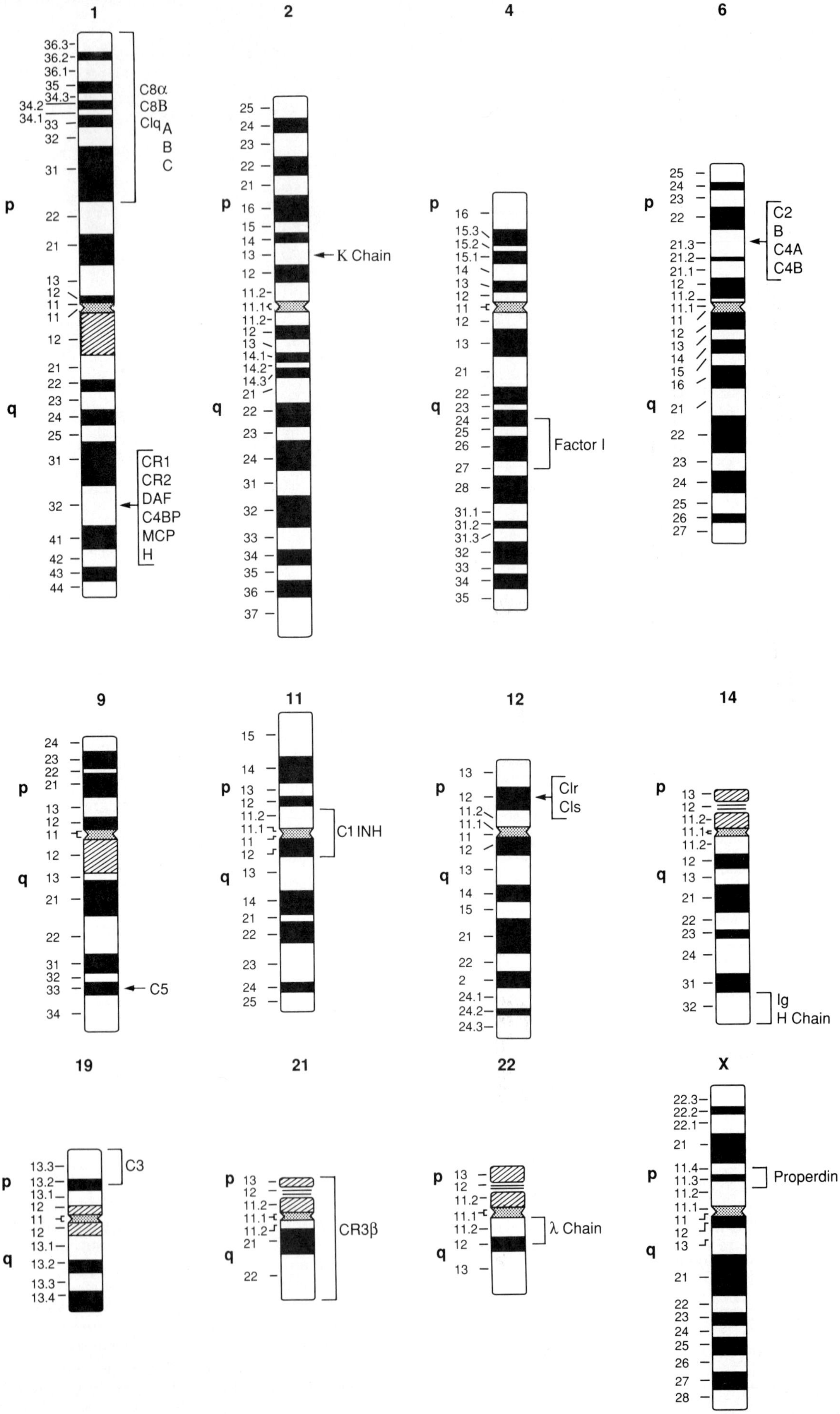

FIGURE 16-15. Complement immunoglobulin and receptor gene localization.

lecular basis for the genetic deficiencies of the complement system.

Polymorphic Variants of the Complement Proteins

Genetically determined electrophoretic variants of the C3 protein were first observed about two decades ago.[336,337] The common C3 variants are found in all major racial groups, and about 20 rare variants have been detected. Genetic variants of the other polymorphic complement proteins, such as factor B, C2, C4, C6, C7, C8, and factor D, have also been revealed.[336] In some instances, the structural basis for this genetic variation has been determined by sequence analysis of cDNA clones.[196] Associations between polymorphic forms of individual components of complement and certain diseases have been recognized,[327,337] but the basis for these associations is not known.

Considerable attention has been given to an analysis of the complement proteins encoded by genes within the MHC. Studies of protein polymorphisms of the C2, factor B, C4A, and C4B loci, together with typing of the class I and class II genes, have generated the concept of *extended haplotypes*,[329] which are defined as chromosomes displaying a decreased frequency of recombinant events extending over a 10-million base-pair region of chromosome 6. The extended haplotypes account for nearly 30% of haplotypes in normal white populations. These observations have relevance for the well-recognized association of a number of diseases (eg, SLE, type I diabetes mellitus, celiac disease, congenital adrenal hyperplasia) with certain extended haplotypes and the remarkable finding that mixed lymphocyte cultures from unrelated patients sharing the same extended haplotypes exhibit low or absent reactivity.[338] The latter has obvious implications for clinically relevant transplantation biology.

Cryoglobulins and Paraproteins

As alluded to previously, either antiidiotypic antibody (eg, acquired C1-inhibitor deficiency), antiimmunoglobulins with other specificities (rheumatoid factor), autoantibodies to complement-regulatory proteins (eg, acquired C1-inhibitor deficiency) to the C3 convertases (nephritic factors), or immunoglobulins with unusual physicochemical properties (eg, cryoglobulinemia) have been implicated in complement-mediated diseases.[339] In the instance of rheumatoid factor or cryoglobulin-induced disease, complement fixation by means of classic pathway activation is thought to be the mechanism leading to inflammation and tissue injury. Considerable uncertainty about this point, however, derives from the difficulty of determining to what extent a reduction in classic pathway component activity and the association of proteins in cryoprecipitates represent in vitro artifacts. That is, to what extent are intravascular temperatures, even in superficial cutaneous vessels, sufficiently low to generate complement-fixing aggregates?

In certain disorders, autoantibodies to complement proteins have been implicated in the pathogenesis of tissue injury. For instance, nephritic factor, an antibody to the alternative pathway (C3bBb) or to classic pathway (C4b2a) C3 convertase is observed in some patients with glomerulonephritis and SLE, respectively.[340] Again, their precise role in the pathogenesis of these disorders is uncertain.

Hemolytic Anemias

Clinical and experimental evidence has established a major role of complement in the pathogenesis of many autoimmune and drug-induced hemolytic anemias whereby antigen–antibody reactions at or near erythrocyte cell membranes lead to deposition of complement proteins on the cell surface. The extent of complement activation is a function of properties of the antibody (Ig class) and distribution of the antigen (cell-bound or fluid-phase). For instance, the pattern and tissue distribution of erythrocyte clearance from the circulation is profoundly influenced by immunoglobulin class and quantity of antibody bound to the erythrocytes.

A series of elegant studies[341–343] established what had been inferred from a larger number of clinical observations. That is, IgM antibody bound to the erythrocytes, even at low multiplicity (about 40 molecules per cell), results in rapid clearance of the sensitized erythrocytes by liver, then release into the circulation, followed by clearance at a rate markedly less than the first phase of hepatic clearance (see Fig. 16-14). This pattern is generated by the efficient activation of classic pathway deposition on the membrane of hundreds to thousands of C3b molecules per IgM molecule and the cleavage of C3b-C3bi in the presence of factor I plus fluid-phase or cell-bound cofactor. The C3 fragments permit binding to fixed mononuclear phagocytes in liver, release, and then clearance by phagocytosis. This latter process is facilitated at higher IgM antibody content per cell, so that if sufficient C3bi is generated, release from liver does not occur. Similar studies in complement-deficient or -depleted animals established that C3 is a necessary component.[344] The necessity for factor I–mediated cleavage of the C3b to generate this pattern is evident from the presence and relatively slow clearance of C3b-coated erythrocytes from the circulation in factor I–deficient patients.[345]

When immune hemolytic anemia is mediated by IgG antibody, the amount of antibody and antigen distribution on the erythrocytes are important determinants because a doublet of IgG is required for C1 binding and activation. If antigen distribution is unfavorable for formation of the C1-fixing doublet (more than 30 nm), the IgG antibody concentration is low or is of a subclass that binds C1 poorly (if at all), and little complement activation occurs. In any event, clearance of IgG-sensitized erythrocytes occurs largely in splenic macrophages and is markedly accelerated but not strictly dependent on complement activation since interaction with Fc receptor, as well as complement receptor, promotes adherence and uptake of the erythrocytes.[340] Cells sensitized with "cold" antibodies of the IgM (eg, anti-I cold agglutinin) or IgG (Donath-Landsteiner antibody directed against P red cell antigen) can undergo intravascular lysis due to activation of the complement cascade even when the antibody has dissociated from the erythrocyte after activation of the classic pathway. At low temperatures, C1 binding by IgG antibody is almost 10 times more than at 37°C,[346] thus narrowing the difference between IgG and IgM antibody efficiency in complement-mediated hemolysis.

Corticosteroids profoundly decrease the clearance of IgG-sensitized erythrocytes irrespective of whether complement has been deposited on the erythrocyte, and except at extremely high concentrations, corticosteroids do not affect clearance of IgM-sensitized erythrocytes.[347] These data suggest that this effect of corticosteroid is primarily mediated by Fc receptor–IgG interaction.

Similar principles apply to drug-induced hemolytic anemias when the hapten (drug) is bound to the erythrocyte and when complement is deposited by an innocent-bystander mechanism, as in C3 deposition due to fluid-phase complement activation. The mechanisms of drug-induced hemolytic anemias are not well explored, but our current understanding of complement activation and control should make further study worthwhile. A similar conclusion can be drawn regarding the participation of complement in immune thrombocytopenias and decrease in other formed elements of the blood. Nevertheless, in most of these instances (eg, idiopathic thrombocytopenic purpura), accelerated clearance is likely Fc-receptor, and not complement-receptor, mediated.

Paroxysmal Nocturnal Hemoglobinemia

This interesting, but relatively rare, condition emphasizes the importance of two membrane-associated complement-regulatory proteins: DAF and HRF. Absence of these glycolipid-anchored proteins in paroxysmal nocturnal hemoglobinemia *leads* to increased deposition of C3b and more efficient lysis of the cells by the MAC, although the reasons for nocturnal attacks or attacks occurring after acute-phase stimuli (eg, surgery, infection, trauma) are not clear. The defect leading to loss of these proteins and others anchored by glycophospholipid is due to molecular defects in the phosphatidylinositol glycan class A (PIG-A) gene, which is involved in the first step of glycophosphoinositol biosynthesis.[348,349]

REFERENCES

1. Tiseluis A. Electrophoretic analysis and the constitution of native fluids. Harvey Lect 1939;35:37.
2. Tiseluis A, Kabat EA. Electrophoresis of immune serum. Science 1938;87:416.
3. Gitlin D, Hitzig WH, Janeway CA. Multiple serum protein deficiencies in congenital and acquired agammaglobulinemia. J Clin Invest 1956;35: 1199.
4. Ishizaka K, Ishizaka T. Physiochemical properties of reaginic antibody. I. Association of reaginic activity with immunoglobulin other than γA or γG globulin. J Allergy 1966;37:169.
5. Rowe DS, Fahey JL. New class of human immunoglobulins. I. Unique myeloma protein. J Exp Med 1965;121:171.
6. Porter RR. The hydrolysis of rabbit γ-globulin and antibodies with crystalline papain. Biochem J 1959;73:119.
7. Edelman GM, Cunningham BA, Gall WE, et al. The covalent structure of an entire γG immunoglobulin molecule. Proc Natl Acad Sci 1969;63: 78.
8. Amzel LM, Poljak RJ. Three dimensional structure of Igs. Annu Rev Biochem 1979;48:961.
9. Silverton EW, Navia MA, Davies DR. Three dimensional structure of an intact human immunoglobulin. Proc Natl Acad Sci 1977;74:5140.
10. Alzari PM, Lascombe MB, Poljak RJ. Three-dimensional structure of antibodies. Annu Rev Immunol 1988;6:555.
11. Williams AF, Barclay AN. The immunoglobulin superfamily: domains for cell surface recognition. Annu Rev Immunol 1988;6:381.
12. Wu TT, Kabat EA. Analysis of the sequences of the variable regions of Bence-Jones proteins and myeloma light chains and their implications for antibody complimentarity. J Exp Med 1970;132:211.
13. Edmundson AB, Ely KR, Abola EE, et al. Rotational allomerism and divergent evolution of domains in immunoglobulin light chains. Biochemistry 1975;14:3953.
14. Jones PT, Dear PH, Foote J, et al. Replacing the complementarity-determining regions in a human antibody with those from a mouse. Nature 1986;321:522.
15. Alzari PM, Lascombe MB, Poljak RJ. Three-dimensional structure of antibodies. Annu Rev Immunol 1988;6:555.
16. Seidman JG, Leder A, Edgell MH, et al. Multiple related immunoglobulin variable-region genes identified by cloning and sequence analysis. Proc Natl Acad Sci 1978;75:3881.
17. Hieter PA, Hollis GF, Korsmeyer SJ, et al. Clustered arrangement of immunoglobulin lambda constant region genes in man. Nature 1981;294:536.
18. Siedman JG, Leder P. The arrangement and rearrangement of antibody genes. Nature 1978;276:790.
19. Honjo T, Kataoka T. Organization of immunoglobulin heavy chain genes. Cell 1978;19:37.
20. Putnam FW, Takahashi N, Tetaert D, et al. Amino acid sequence of the first constant region domain and the hinge region of the δ heavy chain of human IgD. Proc Natl Acad Sci 1981;78:504.
21. Rademacker TW, Dwek RA. Structural, functional and confirmational analysis of immunoglobulin G-derived asparagine-linked oligosaccharides. Prog Immunol 1984;5:95.
22. Sutter BJ, Phillips DC. The three-dimensional structure of the carbohydrate within the Fc fragment of immunoglobulin G. Biochem Soc Trans 1983;11:130.
23. Burton DR. Immunoglobulin G: functional sites. Mol Immunol 1985;22: 161.
24. Middaugh CR, Litman GW. Atypical glycosylation of an IgG monoclonal cryoimmunoglobulin. J Biol Chem 1987;262:3671.
25. Rademacher TW, Parekh RB, Dwek RA. Glycobiology. Annu Rev Biochem 1988;57:785.
26. Heyman B, Nose M, Weigle WO. Carbohydrate chains on IgG2b: a requirement for efficient feedback in immunosuppression. J Immunol 1985;134:4018.
27. Leatherbarrow RJ, Rademacher TW, Dwek RA. Effector functions of a monoclonal aglycosylated mouse IgG2a: binding and activation of complement component C1 and interaction with human monocyte Fc receptor. Mol Immunol 1985;22:407.
28. Takahashi N, Ueda S, Obata M, et al. Structure of human immunoglobulin gamma genes: implications for evolution of a gene family. Cell 1982;29:671.
29. Solomon A. Bence-Jones proteins and light chains of immunoglobulins. N Engl J Med 1976;294:17.
30. Guercio P. Regulatory structures on the V and C regions of immunoglobulin molecules. Immunol Today 1987;8:304.
31. Welch MJ, Fong S, Vaughan JH, et al. Increased frequency of rheumatoid factor precursor B lymphocytes after immunization of normal adults with tetanus toxoid. Clin Exp Immunol 1983;51:299.
32. Grubb R. Agglutination of erythrocytes coated with "incomplete" anti Rh by certain rheumatoid arthritic sera and some other sera. Acta Pathol Microbiol Scand 1956;35:195.
33. Fudenberg HH. Hereditary human gamma globulin (GM) groups: interpretations and extensions. Prog Allergy 1963;7:1.
34. Natvig JB, Kunkel HG. Human immunoglobulins, classes, subclasses, genetic variants and idiotypes. Adv Immunol 1973;16:1.
35. Steinberg AG. Globulin polymorphisms in man. Annu Rev Genet 1969;3:25.
36. Vyas GN, Fudenberg HH. Am(1), the first genetic marker of human immunoglobulin A. Proc Natl Acad Sci 1969;64:1211.
37. Kunkel HG, Smith WK, Joslin PG, et al. Genetic marker of the gamma-A2 sub group of gamma A immunoglobulins. Nature 1969;223:1247.
38. Baglioni C, Alescio ZL, Cioli A, et al. Chemical basis of the allelic antigenic factor Im^v(2) of light chains of human immunoglobulins. Science 1966;152:1519.
39. Milstein CP, Steinberg AG, McLaughlin CL, Solomon A. Amino acid sequence change associated with genetic marker Imv(2) of human immunoglobulin. Nature 1974;248:160.
40. Yount WJ, Kunkel HG, Litwin SD. Studies of Vi(γ-2c) subgroups of gamma globulin. J Exp Med 1967;125:177.
41. Granoff DM, Pandey JP, Boies E, et al. Response to immunization with Hemophilus influenza type b polysaccharide-pertusis vaccine and the risk of Hemophilus meningitus in children with the Km(1) immunoglobulin allotype. J Clin Invest 1984;74:1708.
42. Allen JC, Kunkel HG. Antibodies against gamma-globulin after repeated blood transfusions in man. J Clin Invest 1966;45.
43. Fudenberg HH, Fudenberg BR. Antibody to hereditary human gamma-globulin (GM) factor resulting from maternal-fetal incompatibility. Science 1964;145;170.
44. Kunkel HG, Mannik M, Williams RC. Individual antigenic specificity of isolated antibodies. Science 1963;140:1218.
45. Oudin J, Michel M. One nouvelle forme d'allotypie des globulines γ du serum de lapin, apparemenment liee a la fraction et ala specificite anticorps. CRHS Acad Sci 1963;257:805.
46. Kieber-Emmons T, Kohler H. Towards a unified theory of immunoglobulin structure-function relations. Immunol Rev 1986;90:29.
47. Geha RS. Presence of auto-anti-idiotypic antibody during the normal response to tetanus toxoid antigen. J Immunol 1982;129:139.
48. Jerne NK. Towards a network theory of the immune system. Ann Immunol 1974;15C:373.
49. Jerne NK. Idiotypic networks and other preconceived ideas. Immunol Rev 1984;79:5.
50. Geha RS. Idiotypic interactions in the treatment of human diseases. Adv Immunol 1986;39:255.
51. Williams R, Kunkel HG, Capra JD. Antigenic specificities related to the cold agglutinin activity of IgM globulins. Science 1968;161:379.
52. Davie JM, Seiden MV, Greenspan NS, et al. Structural correlates of idiotopes. Annu Rev Immunol 1986;4:147.
53. Gitlin D, Janeway CA, Apt L, Craig JM. Agammaglobulinemia. In: Lawrence HS, ed. Cellular and humoral aspects of hypersensitivity states. (Symposium) New York, Hoeber-Harper, 1959:375.
54. Rosen FS, Janeway CA. Immunologic competence of the newborn infant. Pediatrics 1964;33:159.
55. Gitlin D, Kumate J, Urrusti J, Morales C. Selectivity of human placenta in the transfer of plasma proteins from mother to fetus. J Clin Invest 1964;43:1939.
56. Gitlin D, Biasucci A. Development of gamma G, gamma A, gamma M, beta-1c/beta-1a, C'l esterase inhibitor, ceruloplasmin, transferin, hemopexin, haptoglobin, fibrinogen, plasminogen, alpha-1-antitrypsin, orosomucoid, beta-lipoprotein, alpha-2-macroglobulin and prealbumin in the human conceptus. J Clin Invest 1969;48:1433.
57. Burton DR. Immunoglobulin G: functional sites. Mol Immunol 1985;22: 161.

58. Unkeless JC. Function and heterogeneity of human Fc receptors for immunoglobulin G. J Clin Invest 1989;83:355.
59. Moller E. Contact induced cytotoxicity by lymphoid cells containing foreign isoantigens. Science 1965;147:873.
60. Freda VJ, Gorman JG, Pollack W. Successful prevention of experimental Rh sensitization in man with an anti-Rh γ-globulin antibody preparation. Transfusion 1964;4:26.
61. Old LJ, Boyse EA. Current enigmas in cancer research. Harvey Lect 1973;67:273.
62. Schur PH. IgG subclasses: a historical perspective. Monogr Allergy 1988;23:1.
63. Schur PH, Borel H, Gelfand EW, et al. Selective gamma-G globulin deficiencies in patients with recurrent pyogenic infections. N Engl J Med 1970;283:631.
64. Mestecky J, Zikan J, Butler WT. Immunoglobulin M and secretory immunoglobulin A: presence of a common polypeptide chain different from light chain. Science 1971;171:163.
65. Abney ER, Cooper MD, Kearney JF, et al. Sequential expression of immunoglobulin on developing mouse B-lymphocytes. A systematic survey which suggests a model for the generation of immunoglobulin isotype diversity. J Immunol 1978;120:2041.
66. Metzger H. Structure and function of gamma M macroglobulins. Adv Immunol 1970;12:57.
67. Yagi M, D'Eustachio P, Ruddle FH, et al. J chain is encoded by a single gene unlinked to other immunoglobulin structural genes. J Exp Med 1982;155:647.
68. Koshland ME. Structure and function of the J chain. Adv Immunol 1975;20:41.
69. Heremans JF. Immunoglobulin A. In: Seki J, ed. The antigens, vol 2. New York, Academic Press, 1974:365.
70. Tsuzukida Y, Wang CC, Putnam FW. Structure of the A2m(1) allotype of human IgA: a recombinant molecule. Proc Natl Acad Sci 1979;76:1104.
71. Mestecky J, McGhee JR. Immunoglobulin A(IgA): molecular and cellular interactions involved in IgA biosynthesis and the immune response. Adv Immunol 1987;40:153.
72. Bachmann R. Studies in serum γA-globulin level III: frequency of A γ-A globulinemia. J Clin Lab Invest 1965;17:316.
73. Ishizaka K, Ishizaka T, Hornbrook MM. Physiochemical properties of reaginic antibody V: correlation of reaginic activity with gamma-ε-globulin antibody. J Immunol 1961;97:840.
74. Johansson SGO, Bennich H. Immunologic studies of an atypical (myeloma) immunoglobulin. Immunology 1967;13:381.
75. Solley GO, Gleich GJ, Jordan RE, Schroeter AL. The late phase of the immediate wheal and flare skin reaction: its dependence upon IgE antibodies. J Clin Invest 1976;58:408.
76. Capron A, Dessaent JP, Capron M, Bazin H. Specific IgE antibodies in immune adherence of normal macrophages to schistosoma mansoni schisto-somules. Nature 1975;253:474.
77. Sarayan JA, Leung DY, Geha RS. Induction of human IgE synthesis by a factor from T cells of patients with hyper IgE states. J Immunol 1983;130:242.
78. Ishizaka I. IgE binding factors and regulation of the IgE antibody response. Annu Rev Immunol 1988;6:513.
79. Blattner FR, Tucker PW. The molecular biology of immunoglobulin D. Nature 1984;307:417.
80. Gitlin D, Gitlin JD. Fetal and neonatal development of human plasma proteins. In: Putnam FW, ed. The plasma proteins, vol 3. New York, Academic Press, 1975:264.
81. Waldman TA. Methods for the study of the metabolism of immunoglobulin. Methods Enzymol 1985;116:201.
82. Solomon A, Waldmann TA, Fahey JL. Clinical and experimental metabolism of normal 6.6S γ-globulin in normal subjects and in patients with macroglobulinemia and multiple myeloma. J Lab Clin Med 1963;62:1.
83. Janway CA, Rosen FS. The gamma globulins IV: therapeutic uses of human gamma globulin. N Engl J Med 1966;275:826.
84. Gitlin D, Kumate J, Morales C, et al. The turnover of amniotic fluid protein in the human conceptus. Am J Obstet Gynecol 1972;113:632.
85. Gitlin D. Morphis LG. Systems of materno-fetal transport of γG immunoglobulin in the mouse. Nature 1969;223:195.
86. Waldman TA, Strober N. Metabolism of immunoglobulins. Prog Allergy 1969;13:1.
87. Berken A, Benacerraf B. Properties of antibodies cytophilic for macrophages. J Exp Med 1966;123:119.
88. Ravetch JV, Kinet JP. Fe receptors. Annu Rev Immunol 1991;9:457.
89. Mostov KE, Simister NE. Transcytosis. Cell 1985;43:389.
90. Mostov KE, Friedlander M, Blobel G. The receptor for transepithelial transport of IgA and IgM contains multiple immunoglobulin-like domains. Nature 1984;308:37.
91. Simister NE, Rees AR. Isolation and characterization of an Fc receptor from neonatal rat small intestine. Eur J Immunol 1985;15:733.
92. Simister NE, Mostov KE. An Fc receptor structurally related to MHC class I antigens. Nature 1989;337:184.
93. Gitlin JD, Gitlin D. Protein binding by specific receptors on human placenta, murine placenta, and suckling murine intestine in relation to protein transport across these tissues. J Clin Invest 1974;54:1155.
93. Perussia B, Dayton ET, Lazarus R, et al. Immune interferon induces the receptor for monomeric IgG1 on human monocytic and myeloid cells. J Exp Med 1983;158:1092.
94. Allen JM, Seed B. Isolation and expression of functional high-affinity Fc receptor complementary DNAs. Science 1989;243:378.
95. Duncan AR, Woof JM, Partridge LJ, et al. Localization of the binding site for the human high-affinity Fc receptor on IgG. Nature 1988;332:563.
96. Porges AJ, Redecha PB, Doebela R, et al. Novel Fcγ receptor I family gene products in human mononuclear cells. J Clin Invest 1992;90:2102.
97. Anderson CL. Isolation of the receptor for IgG from a human monocyte cell line (U937) and from human peripheral blood monocytes. J Exp Med 1982;156:1794.
98. Brooks DG, Qiu WQ, Luster WQ, Ravetcg JV. Structure and expression of a human IgG FeRII (Cd32): functional heterogeneity is encoded by alternatively spliced products of multiple genes. J Exp Med 1989;170:1369.
99. Qiu WQ, de Bruin D, Brownstein BH, Pearse R, Raveth JV. Organization of the human and mouse low affinity Fe R genes: evidence for duplication and recombination. Science 1990;248:732.
100. Odin JA, Edberg JC, Painter CJ, Kimberly RP, Unkeless JC. Regulation of phagocytosis and [Ca^{2+}]i flux by distinct regions of an Fe receptor. Science 1991;254:1785.
101. Amigorena S, Bonnerot C, Drake J, et al. Cytoplasmic domain heterogeneity and functions of IgG Fe receptors in B lymphocytes. Science 1992;256:1808.
102. Fridman WH. Fe receptors and immunoglobulin binding factors. FASEB J 1991;5:2684.
103. Anderson CL, Ryan DH, Looney RJ, Leary PC. Structural polymorphism of the human monocyte 40 kilodalton Fc receptor for IgG. J Immunol 1987;138:2254.
104. Fleit HB, Wright SD, Unkeless JC. Human neutrophil Fc gamma receptor distribution and structure. Proc Natl Acad Sci 1982;79:3275.
105. Fleit HB, Wright SD, Dime CJ, et al. Ontogeny of Fc receptors and a complement receptor (CR3) during human myeloid differentiation. J Clin Invest 1984;73:516.
106. Clarkson SB, Kimberly RP, Valinsky JE, et al. Blockage of clearance of immune complexes by an anti-Fc gamma receptor monoclonal antibody. J Exp Med 1986;164:474.
107. Simmons D, Seed B. Fcγ receptor of a natural killer cell is a phospholipid-linked membrane protein. Nature 1988;333:568.
108. Peltz GA, Grandy HO, Lebo RV, et al. Human FcγRIII: cloning, expression and identification of the chromosomal locus of two Fc receptors for IgG. Proc Natl Acad Sci 1989;86:1013.
109. Scallon BJ, Scigliano E, Freedman VH, Miedel MC, et al. A human immunoglobulin G receptor exists in both polypeptide-anchored and phosphatidylinositol-glycan-anchored forms. Proc Natl Acad Sci 1989;86:5079.
110. Beaven MA, Metxger H. Signal transduction by Fc receptors: the FcϵRI case. Immunol Today 1993;14:222.
111. Blank U, Ra C, Miller L, et al. Complete structure and expression in transfected cells of high affinity IgE receptor. Nature 1989;337:187.
112. Geha RA, Helm B, Gould H. Inhibition of the Prausnitz-Küstner reaction by an immunoglobulin E-chain fragment synthesized in E coli. Nature 1985;315:577.
113. Yukawa K, Kibutani H, Owaki H, et al. A B-cell specific differentiation antigen CD23 is a receptor for IgE ($Fc_{\epsilon}R$) on lymphocytes. J Immunol 1987;138:2476.
114. Bonnefay JY, Aubry JP, Peronne R, et al. Production and characterization of a monoclonal antibody specific for the human lymphocyte low affinity receptor for IgE: DC23 is a low affinity receptor for IgE. J Immunol 1987;138:2970.
115. Ikuta K, Takami M, Kim L, et al. Human lymphocyte Fc receptor for IgE: sequence homology of its cloned cDNA with animal lectins. Proc Natl Acad Sci 1987;84:819.
116. Kibutani H, Inui S, Sato R, et al. Molecular structure of human lymphocyte receptor for immunoglobulin E. Cell 1986;47:657.
117. Ludin C, Hofstetter H, Sarfati M, et al. Cloning and expression of the cDNA coding for a human lymphocyte IgE receptor. EMBO J 1987;6:109.
118. Defrance T, Aubry JP, Rousset F, et al. Human recombinant interleukin 4 induces Fc_{ϵ} receptors (CD23) on normal human B lymphocytes. J Exp Med 1987;165:1459.
119. Takizawa F, Adamczewski M, Kinet JP. Identification of the low-affinity receptor for immunoglobulin E on moose mast cells and macrophages as FcγRII and FcγRIII. J Exp Med 1992;176:469.
120. Frigeri LG, Liu FT. Surface expression of functional IgE binding protein, an endogenous lectin, on mast cells and macrophages. J Immunol 1992;148:861.
121. Dombrowicz D, Flamaud V, Bingman KK, Koller BH, Kinet JP. Abolition of anaphylaxis by targeted disruption of the high-affinity immunoglobulin E receptor α chain gene cell. 1993;75:969.
122. Takai T, Li M, Syvestre D, Clynes R, Ravetch JV. FcR γ chain deletion results in pleitropic effector cell defects. Cell 1994;76:519.
123. Fridman WH. Regulation of B-cell activation and antigen presentation by Fc receptors. Curr Opin Immunol 1993;5:355.

124. Bobak DA, Gaither TA, Frank MM, Terner AJ. Modulation of FcR function by complement: subcomponent of C1q enhances the phagocytosis of IgG opsonized targets by human monocytes and culture derived macrophages. J Immunol 1987;138:1150.
125. Radl J, Dooren LJ, Eijsvoogel VP, et al. An immunological study during post transplantation follow-up of a case of severe combined immunodeficiency. Clin Exp Immunol 1971;10:367.
126. Geha RS, Schneeberger E, Gaiten J, et al. Synthesis of an M component by circulating B lymphocytes in severe combined immunodeficiency. N Engl J Med 1974;290:726.
127. Kyle RA, Griepp PA. Plasma cell dyscrasias: current status. CRC Crit Rev Oncol Hematol 1988;8:93.
128. Crawford J, Eye MK, Cohen HJ. Evaluation of monoclonal gammopathies in the "well" elderly. Am J Med 1987;82:39.
129. Kyle RA. "Benign" monoclonal gammopathy: a misnomer? JAMA 1984;251:1849.
130. Fong LST. Light-chain nephropathy. Kidney Int 1985;27:582.
131. Fontz E, Ludwig H, Scheithauer W, Sinzinger H. Shortened platelet half life in multiple myeloma. Blood 1986;68:514.
132. Broder S, Waldman TA. The suppressor cell network in cancer. N Engl J Med 1978;299:1281.
133. Waldenström J. Studies in conditions associated with disturbed gamma globulin formation (gammopathies). Harvey Lect 1961;56:211.
134. MacKenzie MR, Fudenberg HH. Macroglobulinemia: an analysis of 40 patients. Blood 1972;39:874.
135. Kyle RA, Griepp PR, Banks PM. The diverse picture of gamma heavy-chain disease: a report of seven cases and review of literature. Mayo Clin Proc 1981;56:439.
136. Franklin EC. Some impacts of clinical investigation on immunology: surface IgD, IgE and heavy-chain variants. N Engl J Med 1976;294:531.
137. Seligman M. Immunochemical, clinical and pathologic features of α-chain disease. Arch Intern Med 1975;135:71.
138. Franklin EC. μ-Chain disease. Arch Intern Med 1975;135:75.
139. Vilpo JA, Irjala K, Viljanen MK, et al. δ-Heavy chain disease: a study of a case. Clin Immunol Immunopathol 1980;17:584.
140. Cohen AS, Connors LH. The pathogenesis and biochemistry of amyloidosis. J Pathol 1987;151:1.
141. Kyle RA, Greipp RA. Amyloidosis (AL) clinical and laboratory features in 229 cases. Mayo Clin Proc 1983;58:665.
142. Glenner GG, Turg W, Harada M, et al. Amyloid fibril proteins: proof of homology with immunoglobulin light chains by sequence analysis. Science 1971;172:1150.
143. Glenner GG, Ein D, Eanes ED, et al. Creation of "amyloid" fibrils from Bence-Jones proteins in vitro. Science 1971;174:712.
144. Solomon A, Frangione B, Franklin EC. Bence-Jones proteins and light chains of immunoglobulins: preferential association of the lambda VI subgroup of human light chains with amyloidosis AL (lambda). J Clin Invest 1982;70:453.
145. Feiner HD. Pathology of dysproteinemia: light chain amyloidosis, non-amyloid immunoglobulin deposition disease, cryoglobulinemia syndromes, and macroglobulinemia of Waldenström. Hum Pathol 1988;19:1255.
146. Lavie G, Zucker-Franklin D, Franklin EC. Degradation of severe amyloid A protein by surface associated enzymes of human blood monocytes. J Exp Med 1978:148:1020.
147. Colten HR, Gitlin JD. Molecular regulation of the acute phase complement proteins. In: Pepys M, ed. Acute phase proteins and the acute phase response. London, Springer Verlag, 1989.
148. Husby G. Amyloidosis. Semin Arthritis Rheum 1992;22:67.
149. Malchesky PS, Clough JD. Cryoimmunoglobulins: properties, prevalence in disease and removal. Cleve Clin Q 1985;52:175.
150. Heidelberger M, Kendal FE. Quantitative study of the precipitin reaction between type III pneumococcus polysaccharide and purified homologous antibody. J Exp Med 1929;50:809.
151. Wintrobe MM, Buell MV. Hyperproteinemia associated with multiple myeloma, with report of a case in which an extraordinary hyperproteinemia was associated with thrombosis of the retinal veins and symptoms suggesting Raynaud's disease. Bull Johns Hopkins Hosp 1933;52:156.
152. Brouet JC, Clauvel JP, Danon F, et al. Biologic and clinical significance of cryoglobulins: a report of 86 cases. Am J Med 1974;57:775.
153. Meltzer M, Franklin EC. Cryoglobulinemia: a study of twenty-nine patients. 1. IgG and IgM cryoglobulins and factors affecting cryoprecipitability. Am J Med 1966;40:828.
154. Middaugh CR, Oshman RG, Litman GW. Localization of a confirmational anomaly to the Fab mu region of a monoclonal IgM cryoglobulin. Clin Exp Immunol 1978;31:126.
155. Davis JS, Godfrey SM, Winfield JB. Direct evidence for circulating DNA/anti-DNA complexes in systemic lupus erythermatosus. Arthritis Rheum 1978;21:17.
155a. Agnello V, Chung RT, Kaplan LM. A role for hepatitis C virus infection in type II cytoglobulinemia. N Engl J Med 1992;327:1490.
155b. Abel G, Zhang QX, Agnello V. Hepatitis C virus infection in type II mixed cryoglobulinemia. Arthritis Rheum 1993;36:1341.
156. McLeod BC, Sassetti RJ. Plasmapheresis with return of cryoglobulin-depleted autologous plasma (cryoglobulinpheresis) in cryoglobulinemia. Blood 1980;55:866.
157. Welch MJ, Fong S, Vaughan JH, Carson DA. Increased frequency of rheumatoid factor precursor B lymphocytes after immunization of normal adults with tetanus toxoid. Clin Exp Immunol 1983;51:299.
158. Carson DA, Chen PP, Fox RI, et al. Rheumatoid factor and immune networks. Annu Rev Immunol 1987;5:109.
159. Kunkel HG, Agnello V, Joslin FG, et al. Cross-idiotypic specificity among monoclonal IgM proteins with anti-gammaglobulin activity. J Exp Med 1973;137:331.
160. Goni F, Chen PP, Pons-Estel B, et al. Sequence similarities and cross-idiotypic specificity of L chains among human monoclonal IgM-κ with antigamma globulin activity. J Immunol 1985;135:4073.
161. Chen PP, Robbins DL, Jirik FR, et al. Isolation and characterization of a light chain variable region gene for human rheumatoid factors. J Exp Med 1987;166:1900.
162. Crowley JJ, Goldfien RD, Schrohenloher RE, et al. Incidence of three cross-reactive idiotypes on human rheumatoid factor paraproteins. J Immunol 1988;140:3411.
163. Sanz I, Capra JD. The genetic origin of human autoantibodies. J Immunol 1988;140:3283.
164. Winchester RJ, Agrello V, Kunkel HG. Gamma globulin complexes in synovial fluids of patients with rheumatoid arthritis: partial characterization and relationship to lowered complement levels. Clin Exp Immunol 1970;6:689.
165. Welsh RM, Cooper NR, Jensen FC, Oldstone MBA. Human serum lyses RNA tumor viruses. Nature 1975;257:612.
166. Cooper NR, Jensen FC, Welsh RM, Oldstone MBA. Lysis of RNA tumor viruses by human serum: direct antibody-independent triggering of the classical complement pathway. J Exp Med 1976;144:970.
167. Bartholomew RM, Esser AF. Mechanism of antibody-independent activation of the first component of complement (C1) on retrovirus membranes. Biochem 1980;19:2847.
168. Bartholomew RM, Esser AF, Muller-Eberhard HJ. Lysis of oncocornaviruses by human serum: isolation of the viral complement (C1) receptor and identification as p15E. J Exp Med 1978;147:844.
169. Kaplan MH, Volanakis JE. Interaction of C-reactive protein complexes with the complement system. I. Consumption of human complement associated with the reaction of C-reactive protein with pneumococcal C-polysaccharide and with choline phosphatides, lecithin and sphingomyelin. J Immunol 1974;112:2135.
170. Richards RL, Gewurz H, Osmand AP, Alving CR. Interactions of C-reactive protein and complement with liposomes. Proc Natl Acad Sci USA 1977;74:5672.
171. Pinckard RN, O'Rourke RA, Crawford MH, et al. Complement localization and mediation of ischemic injury in baboon myocardium. J Clin Invest 1980;66:1050.
172. Storrs SB, Kolb WP, Pinckard RN, Olson MS. Characterization of the binding of purified human C1q to heart mitochondrial membranes. J Biol Chem 1981;256:10924.
173. Muller-Eberhard HJ. Molecular organization and function of the complement system. Annu Rev Biochem 1988;57:321.
174. Pangburn MK, Muller-Eberhard HJ. The alternative pathway of complement. Springer Semin Immunopathol 1984;7:163.
175. Muller-Eberhard HJ. The membrane attack complex of complement. Annu Rev Immunol 1986;4:503.
176. Austen KF, et al. Nomenclature of complement. Bull WHO 1968;39:935.
177. Cooper NR. The classical complement pathway: activation and regulation of the first complement component. Adv Immunol 1985;37:151.
178. Svehag S-E, Manhem L, Bloth B. Ultrastructure of human C1q protein. Nature New Biol 1972;238:117.
179. Reid KBM, Porter RR. Subunit composition and structure of subcomponent C1q of the first component of human complement. Biochem J 1976;155:19.
180. Burton DR, Boyd J, Brampton AD, et al. The C1q receptor site on immunoglobulin G. Nature 1980;288:338.
181. Hurst MM, Volanakis JE, Hester RB, et al. The structural basis for binding of complement by immunoglobulin M. J Exp Med 1974;140:1117.
182. Colomb MG, Arlaud GJ, Villiers CL. Activation of C1. Philos Trans R Soc Lond 306:283.
183. Schumaker VN, Zavodszky P, Poon PH. Activation of the first component of complement. Annu Rev Immunol 1987;5:21.
184. Ziccardi RJ, Cooper NR. Direct demonstration and quantitation of the first complement component in human serum. Science 1978;199:1080.
185. Borsos T, Rapp HJ. Complement fixation on cell surfaces by 19S and 7S antibodies. Science 1965;150:505.
186. Morris KM, Colten HR, Bing DH. The first component of complement (C1): a quantitative comparison of its biosynthesis in culture by human epithelial and mesenchymal cells. J Exp Med 1978;148:1007.
187. Morris KM, Aden DP, Knowles BB, Colten HR. Complement biosynthesis by the human hepatoma derived cell line HepG2. J Clin Invest 1982;70:906.
188. Reid KMB. Molecular cloning and characterization of the cDNA and gene coding for the B-chain of C1q of the human complement system. Biochem J 1985;231:729.

189. Sellar GC, Goundis D, McAdam RA, et al. Cloning and chromosomal localization of human C1q A-chain. Identification of molecular defect in a C1q deficient patient. Complement 1987;4:225.
190. Journet A, Tosi M. Cloning and sequencing of full-length cDNA encoding the precursor of human complement component C1r. Biochem J 1986;240:783.
191. Tosi M, Duponchel C, Meo T, Julier C. Complete cDNA sequence of human complement C1s and close physical linkage of the homologous genes C1s and C1r. Biochemistry 1987;26:8516.
192. Mackinnon CM, Carter PE, Smyth SJ, et al. Molecular cloning of cDNA for human complement component C1s. The complete amino acid sequence. Eur J Biochem 1987;169:547.
193. Nguyen VC, Tosi M, Gross MS, et al. Assignment of the complement serine protease genes C1r and C1s to chromosome 12 region 12p13. Hum Genet 1988;78:363.
194. Schreiber RD, Muller-Eberhard HJ. Fourth component of human complement: description of a three polypeptide chain structure. J Exp Med 1974;140:1324.
195. Campbell RD, Dodds AW, Porter RR. The binding of human complement component C4 to antibody-antigen aggregates. Biochem J 1980;189:67.
196. Yu CY, Belt KT, Giles CM, et al. Structural basis of the polymorphism of human complement components C4A and C4B: gene size, reactivity and antigenicity. EMBO J 1986;5:2873.
197. Belt KT, Carroll MC, Porter RR. The structural basis of the multiple forms of human complement component C4. Cell 1984;36:907.
198. O'Neill GJ, Yang SY, Tegoli J, et al. Chido and Rodgers blood groups are distinct antigenic components of human complement C4. Nature 1978;273:668.
199. Isenman DE, Young JR. The molecular basis for the difference in immune hemolysis activity of the Chido and Rodgers isotypes of human complement component C4. J Immunol 1984;132:3019.
200. Law SKA, Dodds AW, Porter RR. A comparison of the properties of the two classes, C4A and C4B of the human complement component C4. EMBO J 1984;3:1819.
201. Schneider PM, Carroll MC, Alper CA, et al. Polymorphism of human complement C4 and steroid 21-hydroxylase gene: restriction fragment length polymorphism revealing structural deletions, homoduplications, and size variants. J Clin Invest 1986;78:650.
202. Palsdottir A, Fossdal R, Arnason A, et al. Heterogeneity of human C4 gene size. Immunogenetics 1987;25:299.
203. Hall RE, Colten HR. Cell-free synthesis of the fourth component of guinea pig complement (C4): identification of a precursor of serum C4 (pro-C4). Proc Natl Acad Sci USA 1977;74:1707.
204. Perlmutter DH, Colten HR. Structure and expression of the complement genes. Pharmacol Ther 1987;34:247.
205. Cooper NR. Enzymatic activity of the second component of complement. Biochemistry 1975;14:4245.
206. Rapp HJ, Borsos T. Molecular basis of complement action. New York, Appleton-Century Crofts, 1970.
207. Opferkuch W, Rapp HF, Colten HR, Borsos T. Immune hemolysis and the functional properties of the second (C2) and fourth (C4) components of complement. II. Clustering of effective C42 complexes at individual hemolytic sites. J Imunol 1971;106:407.
208. Carroll MC, Campbell DR, Bentley DR, Porter RR. A molecular map of the human major histocompatibility complex class III region linking complement genes C4, C2 and factor B. Nature 1984;307:237.
209. Perlmutter DH, Cole FS, Goldberger G, Colten HR. Distinct primary translation products from human liver mRNA give rise to secreted and cell-associated forms of complement (C2). J Biol Chem 1984;259: 10380.
210. Colten HR. Complement biosynthesis. Clin Immunol Allergy 1985;5: 287.
211. Barnum SR, Volanakis JE. In vitro biosynthesis of complement protein D by U937 cells. J Immunol 1985;134:1799.
212. Rosen BS, Cook KS, Yaglom J, et al. Adipsin and complement factor D activity: an immune related defect in obesity. Science 1989;244: 1483.
213. Flier JS, Cook KS, Usher P, Spiegelman BM. Severely impaired adipsin expression in genetic and acquired obesity. Science 1987;237:405.
214. Campbell RD, Bentley DR, Morley BJ. The factor B and C2 genes. Philos Trans R Soc Lond 1984;306:367.
215. Nonaka M, Gitlin JD, Colten HR. Regulation of human and murine complement: comparison of 5′ structural and functional elements regulating human and murine complement factor B gene expression. Mol Cell Biochem 1989;89:1.
216. Woods DE, Markham A, Ricker A, et al. Isolation of cDNA clones for the human complement protein factor B, a class III major histocompatibility complex gene product. Proc Natl Acad Sci USA 1982;79: 5661.
217. Cole FS, Schneeberger EE, Lichtenberg NA, Colten HR. Complement biosynthesis in human breast milk macrophages and blood monocytes. Immunology 1982;46:429.
218. Pangburn MK. The alternative pathway. In: Ross GD, ed. Immunobiology of the complement system. New York, Academic Press, 1986: 45.
219. Hall RE, Blaese RM, Davis AE III, et al. Cooperative interaction of factor B and other complement components with mononuclear cells in the antibody-independent lysis of xenogeneic erythrocytes. J Exp Med 1982;156:834.
220. Sundsmo JS, Gotze O. Human monocyte spreading induced by factor Bb of the alternative pathway of complement activation. J Exp Med 1981;154:763.
221. Sundsmo JS, Wood LM. Activated factor B (Bb) of the alternative pathway of complement activation cleaves and activates plasminogen. J Immunol 1981;127:877.
222. Peters MG, Ambrus JL, Fauci AS, Brown EJ. The Bb fragment of complement factor B acts as a B cell growth factor. J Exp Med 1988;168: 1225.
223. Smith CA, Pangburn MK, Vogel CW, Muller-Eberhard HJ. Molecular architecture of human properdin, a positive regulator of the alternative pathway of complement. J Biol Chem 1984;259:4582.
224. Goundis D, Reid KBM. Properdin, the terminal complement components, thrombospondin and the circumsporozoite protein of malaria parasites contain similar sequence motifs. Nature 1988;335:82.
225. Robson KJH, Hall JRS, Jennings MW, et al. A highly conserved amino-acid sequence in thrombospondin, properdin and in proteins from sporozoites and blood stages of a human malaria parasite. Nature 1988;335:79.
226. Tack BF, Janatova J, Thomas ML, et al. The third, fourth, and fifth components of human complement: isolation and biochemical properties. Methods Enzymol 1981;80:64.
227. Alper CA, Propp RP. Genetic polymorphism of the third component of human complement. J Clin Invest 1968;47:2181.
228. Colten HR, Alper CA. Hemolytic efficiencies of genetic variants of human C3. J Immunol 1972;108:1184.
229. Hugli TE. Biochemistry and biology of anaphylotoxins. Complement 1986;3:111.
230. Thomas ML, Janatova J, Gray WR, Tack BF. Third component of human complement: localization of the internal thiolester bond. Proc Natl Acad Sci 1982;79:1054.
231. Wetsel RA, Barnum SR. Molecular biology and biochemistry of the third (C3) and fifth (C5) complement components. In: Sim RB, ed. Biochemistry and molecular biology of complement. Lancaster, MTP Press, 1990.
232. Wiebauer K, Domdey H, Diggelmann H, Fey G. Isolation and analysis of genomic DNA clones encoding the third component of mouse complement. Proc Natl Acad Sci USA 1982;79:7077.
233. Whitehead AS, Solomon E, Chambers S, et al. Assignment of the structural gene for the third component of human complement to chromosome 19. Proc Natl Acad Sci USA 1982;79:5021.
234. Morris KM, Goldberger G, Colten HR, et al. Biosynthesis and processing of a human precursor complement protein, pro-C3, in a hepatoma-derived cell line. Science 1982;215:399.
235. Perlmutter DH, Colten HR. Molecular immunobiology of complement biosynthesis: a model of single cell control of effector–inhibitor balance. Annu Rev Immunol 1986;4:231.
236. Bokisch VA, Muller-Eberhard HJ. Anaphylatoxin inactivator of human plasma: its isolation and characterization as a carboxy-peptidase. J Clin Invest 1970;49:2427.
237. Perez HD, Kelly E, Chenoweth D, Elfman F. Identification of the C5a des Arg cochemotaxin: homology with vitamin-D binding protein (group-specific component globulin). J Clin Invest 1988;82:360.
238. Kew RR, Webster RO. Gc-globulin (vitamin-D binding protein) enhances the neutrophil chemotactic activity of C5a and C5a des Arg. J Clin Invest 1988;82:364.
239. Bhakdi S, Tranum-Jensen J. Membrane damage by complement. Biochem Biophys Acta 1983;737:343.
240. Lachmann PJ, Thompson RA. Reactive lysis: the complement-mediated lysis of unsensitized cells. II. The characterization of activated reactor as C56 and the participation of C8 and C9. J Exp Med 1970;131:643.
241. Wetsel RA, Lemons RS, LeBeau MM, et al. Molecular analysis of human complement component C5: localization of the structural gene to chromosome 9. Biochemistry 1988;27:1474.
242. Ooi YM, Colten HR. Biosynthesis and post-synthetic modification of a precursor (pro-C5) of the fifth component of mouse complement (C5). J Immunol 1979;123:2494.
243. DiScipio RG, Chakravarti DN, Muller-Eberhard HJ, Fey GH. The structure of human complement component C7 and the C5b-7 complex. J Biol Chem 1988;263:549.
244. Steckel EW, York RG, Monahan JB, Sodetz JM. The eighth component of human complement: purification and physiochemical characterization of its unusual subunit structure. J Biol Chem 1980;255:11997.
245. Rao AG, Howard OMZ, Ng SC, et al. Complementary DNA and derived amino acid sequence of the alpha subunit of human complement protein C8: evidence for the existence of a separate alpha subunit messenger RNA. Biochemistry 1987;26:3556.
246. Howard OMZ, Rao AG, Sodetz JM. Complementary DNA and derived amino acid sequence of the β subunit of human complement protein C8: identification of a close structural and ancestral relationship to the α subunit and C9. Biochemistry 1987;26:3565.
247. Esser AF, Kolb WP, Podack ER, Muller-Eberhard HJ. Molecular reorganization of lipid bilayers by complement: a possible mechanism for membranolysis. Proc Natl Acad Sci USA 1979;76:1410.
248. Mayer MM. Membrane attack by complement (with comments on

cell-mediated cytotoxicity). In: Clark WR, Golstein P, eds. Mechanisms of cell-mediated cytotoxicity. New York, Plenum, 1982:193.
249. Stanley KK, Kocher HP, Luzio JP, et al. The sequence and topology of human complement component C9. EMBO J 1985;4:375.
250. Podack ER, Biesecker G, Kolb W, Muller-Eberhard HJ. The C5b-6 complex: reaction with C7, C8, C9. J Immunol 1978;121:484.
251. Ohanian SH, Schlager SI, Borsos T. Molecular interaction of cells with antibody and complement: influence of metabolic and physical properties of the target on the outcome of humoral immune attack. In: Reisfeld RA, Inman FP, eds. Contemporary topics in molecular immunology, vol 7. New York, Plenum, 1978:153.
252. Podack ER, Dennert G. Cell-mediated cytolysis: assembly of two types of tubules with putative cytolytic function by cloned natural killer cells. Nature 1983;302:442.
253. Goldberger G, Bruns GAP, Rits M, et al. Human complement factor I: analysis of cDNA-derived primary structure and assignment of its gene to chromosome 4. J Biol Chem 1987;262:10065.
254. Pangburn MK, Schreiber RD, Muller-Eberhard HJ. Human complement C3b inactivator: isolation, characterization and demonstration of an absolute requirement for the serum protein B1H for cleavage of C3b and C4b in solution. J Exp Med 1977;146:257.
255. Pangburn MK. The alternative pathway. In: Ross GD, ed. Immunobiology of the complement system. London, Academic Press, 1986:45.
256. Kristensen T, Ogata RT, Chung P, et al. cDNA structure of murine C4b-binding protein, a regulatory component of the serum complement system. Biochem 1987;26:4668.
257. Schwaeble W, Schulz TF, Zwirner J, et al. Complement factor H: expression of an additional truncated mRNA and corresponding protein in human liver. Complement 1987;4:224a.
257a. Zipfel PF, Skerka C. Complement factor H and related proteins: an expanding family of complement-regulating proteins? Immunol Today 1994;15:121.
258. Kristensen T, D'Eustachio P, Ogata RT, et al. The superfamily of C3b/C4b-binding proteins. Fed Proc 1987;46:2463.
259. Dahlback B, Smith CA, Muller-Eberhard HJ. Visualization of human C4b-binding protein and its complexes with vitamin K–dependent protein S and complement protein C4b. Proc Natl Acad Sci USA 1983;80:3461.
260. Suzuki K, Nishioka J. Binding site for vitamin K–dependent protein S on complement C4b-binding protein. J Biol Chem 1988;263:17034.
261. Podack ER, Muller-Eberhard HJ. Isolation of human S-protein, an inhibitor of the membrane attack complex of complement. J Biol Chem 1979;254:9908.
262. Podack ER, Dahlback B, Griffin JH. Interaction of S-protein of complement with thrombin and antithrombin III during coagulation. J Biol Chem 1986;16:7387.
263. Suzuki S, Oldberg A, Haymann EG, et al. Complete amino acid sequence of human vitronectin deduced from cDNA: similarity of cell attachment sites in vitronectin and fibronectin. EMBO J 1985;10:2519.
264. Tschopp J, Masson D, Schafer S, et al. The heparin binding domain of S-protein/vitronectin binds to complement components C7, C8 and C9 and perforin from cytolytic T-cells and inhibits their lytic activities. Biochemistry 1988;27:4103.
265. Davis AE. C1 inhibitor and hereditary angioneurotic edema. Annu Rev Immunol 1988;6:595.
266. Davis AE, Whitehead AS, Harrison RA, et al. Human inhibitor of the first component of complement, C1: characterization of cDNA clones and localization of the gene to chromosome 11. Proc Natl Acad Sci USA 1986;83:3161.
267. Tosi M, Duponchel C, Bougarel P, et al. Molecular cloning of human C1 inhibitor: sequence homologies with alpha-1-antitrypsin and other members of the serpins superfamily. Gene 1986;42:265.
268. Carter PE, Dunbar B, Fothergill JE. Genomic and cDNA cloning of the human C1 inhibitor: intron–exon junctions and comparison with other serpins. Eur J Biochem 1988;173:163.
269. Schmaier AH, Smith PM, Colman RW. Platelet C1 inhibitor: a secreted alpha-granule protein. J Clin Invest 1985;75:242.
270. Holers VM, Cole JL, Lublin DM, et al. Human C3b- and C4b-regulatory proteins: a new multi-gene family. Immunol Today 1985;6:188.
271. Lublin DM, Liszewski MK, Post TW, et al. Molecular cloning and chromosomal localization of human membrane cofactor protein (MCP): evidence for inclusion in the multigene family of complement-regulatory proteins. J Exp Med 1988;168:181.
272. Atkinson JP, Farries T. Separation of self from non-self in the complement system. Immunol Today 1987;8:212.
272a. Döring RE, Marcil A, Chopne A, Richardson CD. The human CD46 molecule is a receptor for measles virus. Cell 1993;75:295.
272b. Naniche D, Vanor-Krishnau G, Cervoni F, et al. Human membrane cofactor protein (CD46) acts as a cellular receptor for measles virus. J Virol 1994 (in press).
273. Zalman LS, Wood LM, Muller-Eberhard HJ. Isolation of a human erythrocyte membrane protein capable of inhibiting expression of homologous complement transmembrane channels. Proc Natl Acad Sci USA 1986;83:6975.
274. Yamashina M, Ueda E, Kinoshita T, et al. Inherited complete deficiency of 20-kilodalton homologous restriction factor (CD59) as a cause of paroxysmal nocturnal hemoglobinuria. N Engl J Med 1990;323:1184.
275. Schonermark S, Rauterberg EW, Shin ML, et al. Homologous species restriction in lysis of human erythrocytes: a membrane-derived protein with C8-binding capacity functions as an inhibitor. J Immunol 1986;136:1772.
276. Lublin DM, Lemons RS, LeBeau MM, et al. The gene encoding decay-accelerating factor (DAF) is located in the complement regulatory locus on the long arm of chromosome 1. J Exp Med 1987;165:1731.
277. Rey-Campos J, Rubinstein P, de Cordoba SR. Decay-accelerating factor: genetic polymorphism and linkage to the RCA (regulator of complement activation) gene cluster in humans. J Exp Med 1987;166:246.
278. Kinoshita T, Medof ME, Silber R, Nussenzweig V. Distribution of decay-accelerating factor in the peripheral blood of normal individuals and patients with paroxysmal nocturnal hemoglobinuria. J Exp Med 1985;162:75.
279. Caras IW, Davitz MA, Rhee L, et al. Cloning of decay-accelerating factor suggests novel use of splicing to generate two proteins. Nature 1987;325:545.
280. Seya T, Farries T, Nickells M, Atkinson JP. Additional forms of human decay-accelerating factor (DAF). J Immunol 1987;139:1260.
281. Nicholson-Weller A, March JP, Rosenfeld SI, Austen KF. Affected erythrocytes of patients with paroxysmal nocturnal hemoglobinuria are deficient in the complement regulatory protein, decay-accelerating factor. Proc Natl Acad Sci USA 1983;80:5066.
281a. Moran P, Beasly H, Borrel A, et al. Human recombinant decal accelerating factor inhibits complement activation in vitro and in vivo. J Immunol 1992;149:1736.
281b. Tomlinson PS. Complement defense mechanisms. Curr Opin Immunol 1993;5:83.
282. Krych M, Atkinson JP, Holers VM. Complement receptors. Curr Opin Immunol 1992;4:8.
283. Fearon DT, Collins LA. Increased expression of C3b receptors on polymorphonuclear leukocytes induced by chemotactic factors and by purification procedures. J Immunol 1983;130;370.
284. Kubota Y, Gaither TA, Cason J, O'Shea JJ, Lawley TJ. Characterization of the C3 receptor induced by herpes simplex virus type 1 infection of human epidermal, endothelial and A431 cells. J Immunol 1987;138:1137.
285. Changelian PS, Fearon DT. Tissue-specific phosphorylation of complement receptors CR1 and CR2. J Exp Med 1986;163:101.
286. Tedder TF, Clement LT, Cooper MD. Expression of C3d receptors during human B cell differentiation: immunofluorescence analysis with the HB-5 monoclonal antibody. J Immunol 1984;133:678.
287. Holers VM, Chaplin DD, Leykam JF, et al. Human complement C3b/C4b receptor (CR1) mRNA polymorphism that correlates with the CR1 allelic molecular weight polymorphism. Proc Natl Acad Sci USA 1987;84:2459.
287a. Wong WW, Farrell SA. Proposed structure of the F′ allotype of human CRI: loss of a C3b binding site may be associated with altered function. J Immunol 1991;146:656.
288. Dykman TR, Hatch JA, Atkinson JP. Polymorphism of the human C3b/C4b receptor: identification of a third allele and analysis of receptor phenotypes in families and patients with systemic lupus erythematosus. J Exp Med 1983;159:691.
289. Arnaout MA, Dana N, Melamed, J, et al. Low ionic strength or chemical-crosslinking of monomeric C3b increases its binding affinity to the human complement C3b receptor. Immunology 1983;48:229.
290. Cornacoff JB, Hebert LA, Smead WL, et al. Primate erythrocyte-immune complex-clearing mechanism. J Clin Invest 1983;71:236.
291. Ross GD, Medof ME. Membrane complement receptors specific for bound fragments of C3. Adv Immunol 1985;37:217.
292. Moore MD, Cooper NR, Tack BF, Nemerow GR. Molecular cloning of the cDNA encoding the Epstein-Barr virus/C3d receptor (complement receptor type 2) of human B lymphocytes. Proc Natl Acad Sci USA 1987;84:9194.
293. Weis JH, Morton CC, Bruns GAP, et al. A complement receptor locus: genes encoding C3b/C4b receptor and C3d/Epstein-Barr virus receptor map to 1q32. J Immunol 1987;138:312.
294. Delcayre AX, Fiandino A, Barel M, Frade R. gp140, The EBV/C3d receptor (CR2) of human B lymphocytes, is involved in cell-free phosphorylation of p120, a nuclear ribonucleoprotein. Eur J Immunol 1987;17:1827.
295. Melchers F, Erdei A, Schulz T, Dierich M. Growth control of activated, synchronized murine B cells by the C3d fragment of human complement. Nature 1985;317:264.
296. Matsumoto AK, Kopicky-Burd J, Carter RH, et al. Intersection of the complement and immune systems: a signal transduction complex of the B-lymphocytic–containing complement receptor type 2 ans CD19. J Exp Med 1991;173:55.
297. Itebell T, Ahearn JM, Fearn DT. Suppression of the immune response by a soluble complement receptor of B lymphocytes. Science 1991;254:102.
298. Todd RF III, Freyer DR. The CD11/CD18 leukocyte glycoprotein deficiency. Hematol Oncol Clin North Am 1988;2:13.
299. Corbi AL, Kishimoto TK, Miller LJ, Springer TA. The human leukocyte adhesion glycoprotein Mac-1 (complement receptor type 3, CD11b) α subunit: cloning, primary structure, and relation to the integrins, von Willebrand factor and factor B. J Biol Chem 1988;263:12403.
300. Arnaout MA, Gupta SK, Pierce MW, Tenen DG. Amino acid sequence

of the alpha subunit of human leukocyte adhesion receptor Mo1 (complement receptor type 3). J Cell Biol 1988;106:2153.
301. Kishimoto TK, O'Connor K, Lee A, et al. Cloning of the β subunit of the leukocyte adhesion proteins: homology to an extracellular matrix receptor defines a novel supergene family. Cell 1987;48:681.
302. Diamond MS, Staunton DE, Marlin SD, et al. Binding of hte integrin Mac-1 (CD11b/CD18) to the third immunoglobulin-like domain of ICAM-1 (CD54) and its regulation by glycosylation. Cell 1991;65:961.
303. Wright SD, Ramos RA, Hermanowski-Vosatka A, et al. Activation of the adhesive capacity of CR3 on neutrophils by endotoxin: dependence on lipopolysacharide-binding protein and CD14. J Exp Med 1991;173:1281.
303a. Arnost MA. Leukocyte adhesion molecule deficiency: its structural basis, pathophysiology and implications for modulating the inflammatory response. Immunol Res 1990;114;145.
304. Gerard NP, Gerard C. The chemotactic receptor for human C5a anaphylaxotoxin. Nature 1991;349:614.
305. Boulay F, Mery L, Tardif M, et al. Expression cloning of a receptor for human C5a anaphylotoxin on differentiated HL-60 cells. Biochemistry 1991;30:2993.
305a. Gerard NP, Bao L, Xiao-Ping H, Eddy RL Jr, Shous TB, Gerard C. Human chemotaxis receptor genes cluster at 19q13.3–13.4: characterization of the C5a receptor. Biochemistry 1993;32:124.
306. Tenner AJ, Cooper NR. Identification of types of cells in human peripheral blood that bind C1q. J Immunol 1981;126:1174.
307. Peerschke EIB, Ghebrehiwet B. Identification and partial characterization of human platelet C1q binding sites. J Immunol 1988;141: 3505.
308. Daha MR, Miltenburg AMM, Hiemstra PS, et al. The complement subcomponent C1q mediates binding of immune complexes and aggregates to endothelial cells in vitro. Eur J Immunol 1988;18:783.
309. Oiki S, Okada Y. C1q induces chemotaxis and K^+ conductance activation coupled to increased cytosolic Ca^{2+} in mouse fibroblasts. J Immunol 1988;141:3177.
310. Bobak DA, Gaither TA, Frank MM, Tenner AJ. Modulation of FcR function by complement: subcomponent C1q enhances the phagocytosis of IgG-opsonized targets by human monocytes and culture-derived macrophages. J Immunol 1987;138:1150.
310a. Guan E, Burgess WH, Robinson SL, Goodman EB, McTique KJ, Tenner AJ. Phagocytic cell molecules that bind the collagen-like region of C1q. J Biol Chem 1991;266:20345.
310b. Malhorta R, Laursen SB, Willis AC, Sim RB. Localization of the receptor-binding site in the collection family of proteins. Biochem J 1993;293:15.
310c. Malhorta C, Willis AC, Jenserius JC, Jackson J, Sim RB. Structure and homology of the human C1q receptor (collection receptor). Immunology 1993;78:341.
311. Joiner KA, Brown EJ, Frank MM. Complement and bacteria: chemistry and biology in host defense. Annu Rev Immunol 1984;2:461.
312. Bianco C, Griffin FM, Silverstein SC. Studies of the macrophage complement receptor. Alteration of receptor function on macrophage activation. J Exp Med 1975;141:1278.
313. Pommier CG, Inada S, Fries LF, et al. Plasma fibronectin enhances phagocytosis of opsonized particles by human peripheral blood monocytes. J Exp Med 1983;157:1844.
314. Mantovani B, Rabinovitch M, Nussenzweig V. Phagocytosis of immune complexes by macrophages. Different roles of the macrophage receptor sites for complement (C3) and for immunoglobulin IgG. J Exp Med 1972;135:780.
315. Brown EJ, Hosea SW, Frank MM. The role of complement in the localization of pneumococci in the splanchnic reticuloendothelial system during experimental bacteremia. J Immunol 1981;126:2230.
316. Leigh PCJ, van den Burselaar MT, van Zwet TL, et al. Requirement of extracellular complement and immunoglobulin for intracellular killing of microorganisms by human monocytes. J Clin Invest 1979;63: 772.
317. McNearney TA, Odell C, Holers VM, et al. Herpes simplex virus glycoproteins gC-1 and gC-2 bind to the third component of complement and provide protection against complement-mediated neutralization of viral infectivity. J Exp Med 1987;166:1525.
318. Eisenberg RJ, Ponce de Leon M, Friedman HM, et al. Complement component C3b binds directly to purified glycoprotein C of herpes simplex virus types 1 and 2. Microbiol Pathogenesis 1987;3:423.
319. Cohen JHM, Fischer E, Kazatchkine MD, et al. Expression of CR1 and CR2 complement receptors following Epstein-Barr virus infection of Burkitt's lymphoma cell lines. Scand J Immunol 1987;25:587.
320. Kotwal GJ, Moss B. Vaccinia virus encodes a secretory polypeptide structurally related to complement control proteins. Nature 1988;335: 176.
321. Rimoldi MT, Sher A, Heiny S, et al. Developmentally regulated expression by *Trypanosoma cruzi* of molecules that accelerate the decay of complement C3 convertases. Proc Natl Acad Sci USA 1988;85: 193.
322. Joiner KA, daSilva WD, Rimoldi MT, et al. Biochemical characterization of a factor produced by trypomastigotes of Trypanosoma cruzi that accelerates the decay of complement C3 convertases. J Biol Chem 1988;263:11327.
323. Hill HR, Bohnsack JF, Morris EZ, et al. Group B streptococci inhibit the chemotactic activity of the fifth component of complement. J Immunol 1988;141:3551.
324. Schifferli JA, Ng YC, Peters DK. The role of complement and its receptor in the elimination of immune complexes. N Engl J Med 1986;315:488.
325. Miller GW, Nussenzweig V. A new complement function: solubilization of antigen-antibody aggregates. Proc Natl Acad Sci USA 1975;72: 418.
326. Schifferli JA, et al. The clearance of tetanus toxoid/anti-tetanus toxoid immune complexes from the circulation of humans. J Immunol 1988;140:899.
326a. Mulligan MS, Yeh CG, Rudolph AR, Ward PA. Protective effects of soluble CK1 in complement and neutrophil mediated tissue damage. J Immunol 1992;148:1479.
326b. Hill J, Lindsay TF, Orhz F, Yeh CG, Hechtman HB, Moore FD. Soluble complement reception type 1 ameliorates the local and remote organ injury after intestinal ischemia-reperfusion in the rat. J Immunol 1992;149:1723.
326c. Weisman HF, Bartow T, Leppo MK, et al. Soluble human complement receptor type 1: in vivo inhibitor of post-ischemic myocardial inflammation and necrosis. Science 1990;249:146.
327. Winkelstein JA, Colten HR. Genetically determined disorders of the complement system. In: Scriver CR, Beaudet AL, Sly WS, Valle DL, eds. The metabolic basis of inherited disease, ed 6. New York, McGraw-Hill, 1989:2711.
328. Wetsel RA, Colten HR. The molecular biology of complement deficiency syndromes. In: Avner ED, ed. Topics in renal medicine: the genetics of hereditary nephropathies. Boston, Kluwer Academic Publishers, 1990.
329. Awdeh ZL, Raum D, Yunis EJ, Alper CA. Extended HLA/complement allele haplotypes: evidence for the T/t-like complex in man. Proc Natl Acad Sci USA 1983;80:259.
330. Ross SC, Densen P. Complement deficiency states and infection: epidemiology, pathogenesis and consequences of neisserial and other infections in an immune deficiency. Medicine 1984;63:243.
331. Meyer O, Hauptmann G, Tappeiner G, et al. Genetic deficiency of C4, C2 or C1q and lupus syndromes: association with anti-Ro (SS-A) antibodies. Clin Exp Immunol 1985;62:678.
332. Glass D, Raum D, Gibson D, Stillman JS, Schur P. Inherited deficiency of the second component of complement: rheumatic disease associations. J Clin Invest 1976;58:853.
333. Provost TT, Arnett FC, Reichlin M. Homozygous C2 deficiency, lupus erythematosus, and anti-Ro (SSA) antibodies. Arthritis Rheum 1983;26:1279.
334. Geha RS, Quinti I, Austen KF, et al. Acquired C1 inhibitor deficiency associated with anti-idiotypic antibody to monoclonal immunoglobulins. N Engl J Med 1985;312:534.
335. Jackson J, Sim RB, Whelan A, Feighery C. An IgG auto antibody which inactivates C1 inhibitor. Nature 1986;323:722.
336. Raum D, Donaldson VH, Rosen FS, Alper CA. Genetics of complement. Curr Top Hematol 1980;3:111.
337. Schur PH. Inherited complement component abnormalities. Annu Rev Med 1986;37:333.
338. Awdeh ZL, Alper CA, Eynon E, et al. Unrelated individuals matched for MHC extended haplotypes and HLA-identical siblings show comparable responses in mixed lymphocyte culture. Lancet 1985;2:853.
339. Dalmasso AP. Complement in the pathophysiology and diagnosis of human diseases. CRC Crit Rev Clin Lab Sci 1986;24:123.
340. Vallota EH, Forristal J, Davis NC, West CD. The C3 nephritic factor and membranoproliferative nephritis: correlations of serum levels of the nephritic factor with C3 levels, with therapy and with progression of the disease. J Pediatr 1972;80:947.
341. Brown DL, Lachmann PJ, Dacie JV. The in vivo behavior of complement-coated red cells: studies in C6-deficient, C3-depleted, and normal rabbits. Clin Exp Immunol 1970;7:401.
342. Schreiber AD, Frank MM. Role of antibody and complement in the immune clearance and destruction of erythrocytes. I. In vivo effects of IgG and IgM complement-fixing sites. J Clin Invest 1972;51:575.
343. Schreiber AD, Frank MM. The role of antibody and complement in the immune clearance and destruction of erythrocytes. II. Molecular nature of IgG and IgM complement fixing sites and effects of their interaction with serum. J Clin Invest 1972;51:583.
344. Ellman L, Green I, Frank M. Genetically controlled total deficiency of the fourth component of complement in the guinea pig. Science 1970;170:74.
345. Abramson N, Alper CA, Lachmann PJ, et al. Deficiency of C3 inactivator in man. J Immunol 1971;107:19.
346. Colten HR, Borsos T, Rapp HJ. Complement fixation by different classes of immunoglobulins: the effect of temperature. Protides Biol Fluids 1967;15:471.
347. Atkinson JP, Schreiber AD, Frank MM. Effects of corticosteroids and splenectomy on the immune clearance and destruction of erythrocytes. J Clin Invest 1973;52:1509.
348. Miyata T, Yamada N, Iida Y, et al. Abnormalities of PIG-A transcripts in granulocytes from patients with paroxysmal nocturnal hemoglobinuria. N Engl J Med 1994;330:249.
349. Rosse WF. The glycolipid anchor of membrane surface proteins. Semin Hematol 1993;30:219.

Blood: Principles and Practice of Hematology,
edited by Robert I. Handin, Thomas P. Stossel, and Samuel E. Lux.
J.B. Lippincott Company, Philadelphia © 1995.

17

Molecular, Cellular, and Clinical Biology of Phagocytic Cells

Stephen D. Nimer
David W. Golde

As described in Chapter 19, the primary role of the phagocytic system is to kill invading microorganisms; however, mononuclear phagocytes (MNPs) are also important in localizing and eliminating biologic debris, removing effete cells, processing antigen, and producing immune mediators. This chapter addresses historical studies of the life cycle of neutrophils and MNPs.

NEUTROPHIL LIFE CYCLE

The neutrophil plays a critical role in host defense against microbial invasion and is an important mediator of inflammatory responses. About 1×10^9 neutrophils per kilogram are produced in the bone marrow daily[1,2]; the numbers of neutrophils and their state of activation must be tightly regulated to respond appropriately for host defense needs while avoiding self-injury. Production of the mature neutrophil from its precursor cells involves an orderly series of morphologic and functional changes coincident with changes in gene expression.

Morphologic Development

Two primary morphologically characteristic processes occur during the formation of the mature neutrophil (polymorphonuclear neutrophil [PMN]). First, the nuclei of the immature cells become progressively smaller, more dense, more lobulated, and less functionally active. Second, neutrophil precursors acquire cytoplasmic primary granules and then develop specific or secondary granules (Fig. 17-1). The earliest morphologically identifiable neutrophil precursor is the myeloblast, a large (15 to 20 μm) round cell with a large nucleus and scant cytoplasm. Its nucleus contains fine chromatin and several nucleoli, and the cytoplasm is lightly basophilic and generally without granules. The myeloblast matures into the promyelocyte, which is characterized by many azurophilic granules, also referred to as *primary* or *nonspecific* granules (Fig. 17-2). The promyelocyte nucleus is similar to the myeloblast nucleus, but slight chromatin clumping may occur. The next stage of development is the myelocyte, the most differentiated myeloid cell still capable of undergoing mitosis. This cell is considerably smaller than the promyelocyte and has distinct clumping of its nuclear chromatin. The myelocyte nucleus is usually eccentrically placed in the cell and has no visible nucleoli. A cytoplasmic clear zone can be seen representing the Golgi apparatus, which is actively synthesizing specific or secondary neutrophil granules. Myeloblasts, promyelocytes, and myelocytes constitute the proliferative compartment of the bone marrow and normally account for 20% to 30% of the myeloid cells present.[3]

Postmitotic neutrophil forms include metamyelocytes, band neutrophils, and mature segmented neutrophils, which constitute 70% to 80% of the myeloid cells in the bone marrow. The metamyelocyte cytoplasm appears pink with the usual Romanowsky stains and contains numerous small neutrophil-specific granules. The nucleus of the metamyelocyte is indented, with coarsely clumped chromatin. It is incapable of cell division, but matures to form the band or stab form. Metamyelocytes and bands are distinguished from mature segmented neutrophils by the thickness of chromatin connecting the lobes of the neutrophil nucleus. Mature neutrophils (PMNs) have a dark blue segmented nucleus with heavily clumped chromatin. Mature neutrophil cytoplasm contains predominantly secondary (specific) granules, and although primary granules are not visible by light microscopy,[4] about one third of the mature neutrophil granules are azurophilic (primary) granules (Fig. 17-3). Normally, only mature segmented neutrophils and band forms circulate in the blood, but in times of stress, progressively earlier neutrophilic forms can be seen in blood smears.

Concomitant with morphologic development, neutrophil precursors acquire the functional capabilities of mature phagocytic effector cells discussed in Chapter 19. Many neutrophil functional activities require constituents of the neutrophilic granules. Neutrophil granules vary in size, but primary and secondary granules are biochemically and functionally distinct.[4] Neutrophil primary granules are azurophilic (purple- or blue-staining) and rich in myeloperoxidase, an iron-containing enzyme involved in oxidative killing of microorganisms.[5–7] These primary granules are easily identified by a histochemical stain for peroxidase activity. Primary granules also contain lysozyme,[8] β-glucuronidase,[9] acid phosphatase,[4] neutral proteases such as elastase and cathepsin G,[10,11] and a variety of cationic proteins with potent antibacterial and antifungal properties, including defensins,[12] bactericidal permeability–increasing

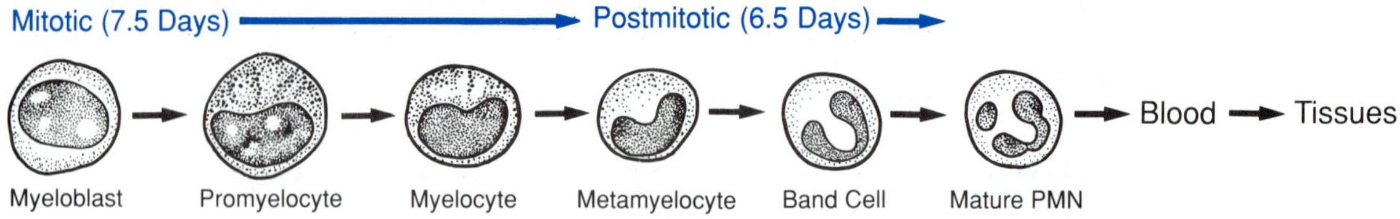

FIGURE 17-1. Development of the neutrophil. (After Bainton DF, Ullyot JL, Farquhar MG. The development of neutrophilic polymorphonuclear leukocytes in human bone marrow. J Exp Med 1971;134:907)

factor,[13] and azurophil-derived bactericidal factor[14] (see Chap. 19).

Neutrophil-specific or secondary granules appear at the myelocyte stage of development.[4] Secondary granules are smaller and less dense than primary granules, and although they lack peroxidase, they are rich in lysozyme, collagenase, plasminogen activator, lactoferrin, and vitamin B_{12}–binding proteins.[8,15] Secondary granules also contain a variety of membrane receptors that can be shuttled to the surface for ligand binding. These include C3b, laminin, and N-formyl-methionyl-leucyl-phenylalanine (f-MLP) receptors,[16–19] which are discussed in Chapter 19. PMNs contain twice as many peroxidase-negative secondary granules as peroxidase-positive primary granules. After neutrophil activation, specific granules can fuse with plasma membrane or endocytic vacuoles (phagosomes) and can deliver their granule contents to the phagosome, to the cell membrane, or externally into the extracellular milieu.[20] Primary granules do not normally release their contents extracellularly, although they fuse with phagosomes, forming secondary phagosomes.[21,22] There appears to be preferential degranulation of secondary granules before primary granules.[23] A third type of granule (*tertiary*) containing gelatinase has been suggested, based on the time course of its release from stimulated neutrophils and subcellular fractionation studies.[24] Recent localization data, however, indicate that gelatinase is present in specific (secondary) granules.[25]

Functional Development

During development, the neutrophil must acquire the full range of cell-surface molecules needed to mediate its major functional activity: to phagocytize and kill invading bacteria. To perform this task, the neutrophil must be attracted to the site of bacterial invasion, move directionally to that location, identify bacteria, engulf, and ultimately kill them.

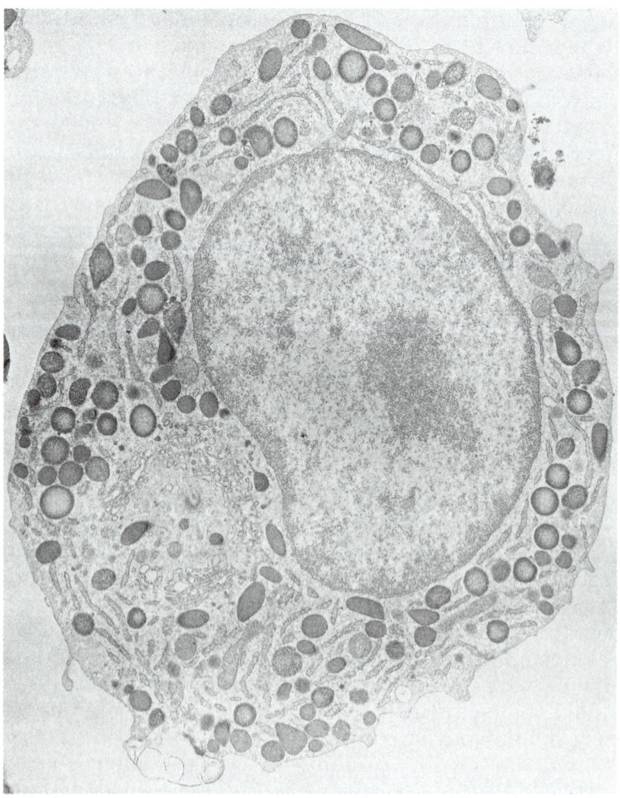

FIGURE 17-2. Promyelocyte stained for peroxidase. A prominent Golgi apparatus and spherical and elliptoid azurophilic granules can be seen. (Bainton DF, Ullyot JL, Farquhar MG. The development of neutrophilic polymorphonuclear leukocytes in human bone marrow: origin and content of azurophil and specific granules. J Exp Med 1971;134:907; copyright 1971 Rockefeller University Press)

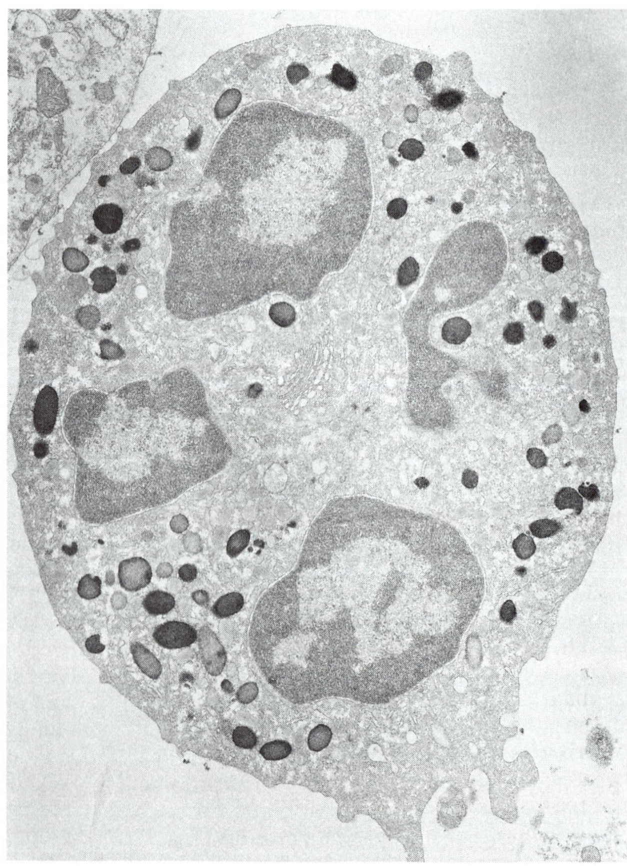

FIGURE 17-3. Normal blood neutrophil as seen under the electron microscope. (Bainton DF, Ullyot JL, Farquhar MG. The development of neutrophilic polymorphonuclear leukocytes in human bone marrow: origin and content of azurophil and specific granules. J Exp Med 1971;134:907; copyright 1971 Rockefeller University Press)

These processes are guided by interactions with specific surface receptors on the neutrophil. Chemoattractant molecules act through cell-surface receptors to direct neutrophils to a site of inflammation where they can also activate neutrophil functions. Receptors for the major physiologic chemoattractants, C5a,[17] platelet-activating factor (PAF),[26] leukotriene B_4,[27] and N-formylated bacterial peptides,[28] have been characterized on mature neutrophils.[29] Bacteria opsonized by immunoglobulins are more rapidly phagocytosed through neutrophil IgG Fc receptors (Fc RII and Fc RIII)[30,31] and C3b receptors.[19,32]

As the neutrophil matures, it becomes more deformable, more adherent to surfaces, more actively mobile, and it more avidly ingests particles.[33] Phagocytic ability appears to be acquired just after expression of IgG Fc receptors at the promyelocyte stage.[34] Next, neutrophils express receptors for complement components (the myelocyte-metamyelocyte stage), and then acquire the ability to kill microbes using oxygen-independent mechanisms and the ability to migrate in response to a variety of chemotactic stimuli.[35] These latter functions are acquired during the terminal stages of maturation of the human neutrophil. Although promyelocytes can phagocytize bacteria, and promyelocyte granules contain a variety of lysosomal enzymes and bactericidal proteins, they have little ability to kill bacteria by either oxidative or oxygen-independent mechanisms. Myelocytes and metamyelocytes can kill bacteria, although neither cell demonstrates a respiratory burst. Thus, oxygen-dependent bacterial killing is a late manifestation of neutrophil maturation.[35] Receptors for f-MLP are not detectable on normal myeloblasts but occur in increasing numbers as myeloid cells mature.[36,37] Morphologically mature marrow neutrophils exist that are still functionally immature, and they have decreased ability to phagocytize and generate an oxidative burst and decreased alkaline phosphatase activity.[38,39]

TABLE 17-1. Cluster Differentiation Antigens on Human Phagocytic Cells of Various Developmental Stages

Cluster	Antibody	Cell Reactivity
CD10	CALLA	Early B cells, granulocytes
CD11a	LFA-1, gp180, 95	Leukocytes
CD11b	Mac-1, Mo-1 C3biR	Monocytes, granulocytes
CD11c	3.9 gp150, 95	Monocytes, granulocytes
CD13	My7	Monocytes, granulocytes
CD14	MO2, UCH M1, My4	Monocytes > granulocytes
CD15	Leu M1, My1	Granulocytes > monocytes
CD16	3G8, Fc RIII	Granulocytes, natural killer cells
CD17	G 035	Granulocytes, monocytes, platelets
CD18	60.3	Leukocytes
CD24	BA-1	B cells, granulocytes
CD25	Tac	Macrophages, T cells, B cells
CD31	SG134	Monocytes, granulocytes, platelets
CDW32	2E1	Monocytes, granulocytes, platelets
CD33	My9	Myeloid progenitors
CD34	My10	Myeloid progenitors
CD35	T05	Granulocytes, monocytes
CD36	4C7	Monocytes, platelets
CD38	OKT10	Multiple lineages
CD39	G28-2	Macrophages, B cells
CD43	G19-1	Leukocytes
CD44	F10-44-2	Leukocytes
CD45	T200	Leukocytes
CD46	J4B	Leukocytes
CDW50	101-1D2	Leukocytes
CD64	Fc RI	Monocytes
CDW65	V1M2	Granulocytes, monocytes
CD66	VTH71.3	Granulocytes
CD67	JML-H16	Granulocytes
CD68	EBM11	Macrophages

Gene Expression During Polymorphonuclear Neutrophil Maturation

Morphologic and functional changes result from specific patterns of gene expression in the maturing neutrophil. Genes encoding a variety of important neutrophil constituents (cytoplasmic and granule components, cell-surface molecules, and nuclear proteins) have been molecularly cloned, making it possible to monitor gene expression at different stages of maturation. Analysis of myeloid cell lines (discussed later) that are arrested at various stages of development have also been helpful in evaluating neutrophil gene expression.

Myeloperoxidase, a bactericidal heme-containing enzyme, is a 130- to 150-kd molecule composed of two heavy and two light chains. The myeloperoxidase cDNA has been cloned[40–42] and the gene encoding myeloperoxidase localized to the long arm of chromosome 17.[42] Expression of the myeloperoxidase gene occurs only during the formation of primary granules at the promyelocyte stage. Differentiation of the promyelocytic HL-60 cell line toward monocytes (by phorbol esters or 1,25-dihydroxyvitamin D_3), or toward granulocytes (by dimethylsulfoxide), results in a drastic decrease in levels of myeloperoxidase mRNA.[43]

The cluster differentiation (CD) system for designation of antigens present on myeloid cells is given in Table 17-1. Expression of CD11b/CD18 (Mo1, Mac1), the C3bi receptor of myeloid cells, has also been studied during myeloid differentiation.[44] The CD11b/CD18 molecule belongs to the family of cell-surface adhesion heterodimers that includes LFA-1 (CD11a/CD18) and p150,95 (CD11c/CD18), all of which share a common β chain (CD18).[45] These molecules are critical to cell–cell interactions involved in the inflammatory process.[46] The genes encoding CD11a, CD11b, and CD11c have all been localized to chromosome 16.[47] Differentiation of HL-60 cells toward monocytes or granulocytes results in an induction of CD11b and CD18 mRNA, commensurate with increased expression of the CD11b/CD18 heterodimer on the differentiated cell surface. These findings are in accordance with functional studies that demonstrate acquisition of cell adhesiveness during neutrophil maturation.

Expression of a protein called p53 has been studied in cells from patients with hematopoietic malignancies and in a variety of human leukemia cell lines. The protein p53 plays a role in regulating cell division and is involved in the transition from a resting to an actively proliferating state.[48,49] Wild-type p53 acts as a tumor-suppressor gene and can bind DNA in a sequence-specific fashion.[50] Mutations in p53 are the most frequent genetic abnormalities observed in human cancers. A variety of gross structural mutations or point mutations have been identified in patients with acute myelogenous leukemia (AML) or chronic myelogenous leukemia (CML).[51,51a] The p53 gene has been localized to the short arm of chromosome 17,[52] and rearrangement of the gene has been reported in patients with CML in blast crisis.[52a]

Expression of the c-*fes*/c-*fps* gene is believed to be involved in differentiation of hematopoietic progenitors toward granulocyte-macrophages. The c-*fes* gene encodes a 92-kd protein that has tyrosine-specific protein kinase activity[53] and may function as a receptor for an unidentified growth factor. The c-*fes* gene is expressed in the human myeloid cell lines HL-60 and KG-1.[54] The c-*src* gene is the cellular homologue of the Rous sarcoma virus–transforming gene and encodes a membrane-associated tyrosine kinase.[55] The levels of PP-60 c-*src* kinase activity are increased when HL-60 cells are induced toward monocyte, macrophage, or granulocyte differentiation by a variety of inducing agents.[56] The function of c-*src* in mature myeloid cells is unknown. Another member of the *src* oncogene family, c-*fgr*, is expressed in mature monocytes and granulocytes, with little expression in B or T lymphocytes.

Neutrophil Kinetics

Bone Marrow

Classic kinetic studies have started with the myeloblast, the first morphologically identifiable myeloid precursor, and have examined proliferation, maturation, and storage pools in the bone marrow (Fig. 17-4). Mathematic formulas used to calculate steady-state kinetics are available in the literature,[57] although formal kinetic studies are seldom conducted clinically.

About five cell divisions occur between the myeloblast and the myelocyte stages.[57,58] There are four times as many myelocytes in the bone marrow as promyelocytes; therefore, myelocytes likely undergo three cycles of cell division, and the major expansion of the neutrophil pool probably occurs through cell division at the myelocyte stage. The myeloblasts, promyelocytes, and myelocytes constitute the mitotic pool, whose size is estimated at 2×10^9 cells/kg.[3] The postmitotic pool (metamyelocytes, bands, and segmented neutrophils) constitutes a maturation-storage compartment of about $6.5 - 13 \times 10^9$ cells/kg.[1,3,59,60] Radionuclide studies[3] suggest that cells spend 135 hours in transit from myeloblast to myelocyte, with 14 hours at the myeloblast stage, 19 hours as a promyelocyte, and 102 hours as a myelocyte. Transit from myelocyte to mature blood neutrophil has been estimated at 131 to 158 hours. Data from one study[3] indicate that the neutrophil spends 30 hours as a metamyelocyte, 50 hours as a band neutrophil, and 72 hours as a segmented neutrophil. Thus, it normally takes about 11 or 12 days for the mature neutrophil to form from the precursor to the myeloblast.[61,62]

Thymidine incorporation studies suggest an orderly progression from metamyelocytes to PMNs, which then leave the storage compartment of bone marrow for the bloodstream. Labeled metamyelocytes may be identified by autoradiography about 3 hours after injection of tritiated thymidine (^{3}H-TdR). Labeled neutrophils appear in the blood 4 to 7 days after administration of ^{3}H-TdR; thus, the transition from myelocyte to circulating PMN takes about 5 to 7 days.[1,57] In the presence of active infection, the myelocyte–PMN transit may require only 48 hours.[63] At any given time, the reserve of mature neutrophils in the bone marrow greatly exceeds the number of neutrophils circulating in the blood. Under stress conditions, the number of myeloid progenitors increases, and maturation times are shortened; however, release of functionally mature neutrophils from the storage compartment is the mechanism used to immediately respond to a need for additional circulating PMNs.[64]

Blood

Once the neutrophil leaves the marrow storage compartment and enters the blood, there is no significant reentry into the marrow.[65] The total blood neutrophil pool consists of cells that circulate freely in vascular spaces, referred to as the *circulating neutrophil pool* (CNP), and neutrophils that adhere to the endothelium of capillaries and postcapillary venules, referred to as the *marginated blood pool* (MBP).[59] Marginated neutrophils are particularly common in the lung, liver, and spleen. When labeled neutrophils are injected into normal subjects, about half remain in the CNP, while the other half enters the MBP, suggesting that these pools are roughly of equal size[60] (estimated at 31×10^7 cells/kg[61]; Table 17-2).

Many factors affect the size of the CNP and MBP. Stress, exercise, and epinephrine injection can lead to movement of neutrophils from the MBP to the CNP.[59] The effects of stress and exercise are probably mediated in part by changes in circulating levels of epinephrine and glucocorticoids. Glucocorticoids increase the total blood neutrophil pool as well as the proportion of neutrophils in the CNP. The increase in blood neutrophils is the result of an increased efflux of neutrophils from marrow storage and a decreased rate of loss of neutrophils from the circulation.[66] Whereas neutrophils normally leave the circulation with a mean disappearance time of 6 to 8 hours,[1,61] in the presence of glucocorticoids, the half-life of circulating neutrophils increases to 10 hours. The disappearance time of neutrophils from the circulation should not be confused with the granulocyte life-span since the granulocyte spends most of its life in the bone marrow and tissue.

Neutrophils that have migrated into tissue do not return to the bloodstream. Although they appear to leave the bone marrow in a first-in, first-out manner,[67] movement of neutrophils from the circulation into tissue is random. Thus, neutrophils newly released from the bone marrow are as

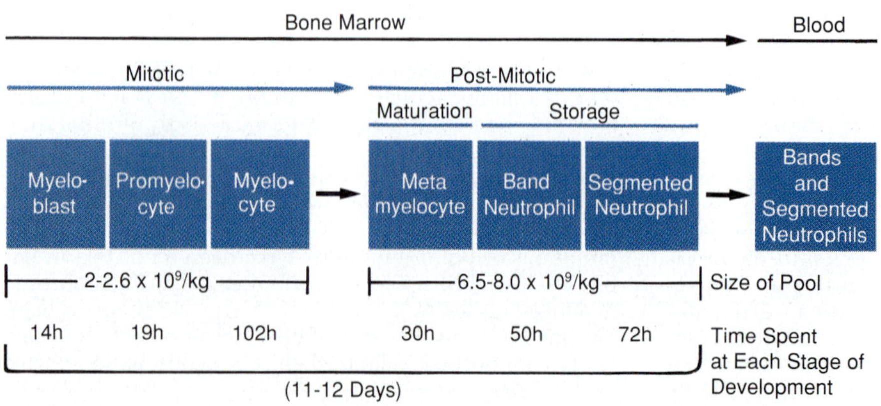

FIGURE 17-4. Neutrophil kinetics.

TABLE 17-2. **Absolute Blood Phagocyte Concentrations**

Population	Concentration (cells/μL; 95% range [mean])			
	Band Forms	Segmented Forms	Band and Segmented Forms	Monocytes
AMERICAN ADULTS*				
White subjects	200–2150 (600)	1500–6050 (3000)		220–950 (460)
Black subjects	60–1650 (300)	1100–6700 (2700)		210–1050 (470)
EUROPEAN ADULTS†				
White subjects			3487–9206	221–843
AMERICAN INFANTS AND CHILDREN‡				
Birth			6000–26000 (11000)	400–3100 (1050)
7 d			1500–10000 (5500)	300–2700 (1100)
4 y			1500–8500 (3800)	0–800 (450)
10 y			1800–8000 (4400)	0–800 (350)

* Orfanakis NG, Ostlund RE, Bishop CR, Athens JW. Normal blood leukocyte concentration values. Am J Clin Pathol 1970;53:647.
† England JM, Bain BJ. Total and differential leukocyte count. Br J Haematol 1976;33:1.
‡ Altman PL, Katz DD. Human health and disease. In: FASEB biology handbooks II. Washington, DC, FASEB, 1977:161.

likely to leave the blood as neutrophils that have been circulating for several hours.[3] In contrast, senescent neutrophils may be removed from the circulation by the MNP network with a different set of kinetics.[63] The fate of neutrophils in tissue is largely unknown. Normally, neutrophils migrate into the lung, oral cavity, gastrointestinal tract, liver, and spleen.[68] They may be lost from mucosal surfaces, die in tissue, or be engulfed by tissue macrophages.[69] The life-span of neutrophils in tissue has not been defined but is likely to be short (1 to 2 days). Factors influencing neutrophil survival in tissue are unknown, but inflammation or infection in tissue leads to neutrophil activation and a decrease in neutrophil survival. Activation of the neutrophil can be seen in response to a variety of cytokines, such as granulocyte-macrophage colony-stimulating factor (GM-CSF), granulocyte colony-stimulating factor (G-CSF),[70] tumor necrosis factor-α (TNF-α),[71,72] PAF,[73] and the chemotactic factors, C5a, f-MLP, and leukotriene B_4.[74–76]

Evaluation

A variety of techniques have been used in assessing neutrophil kinetics. Many of these are of historical interest only[62]; some have provided useful basic information in the past, but because this information rarely affects patient management, only a few techniques are applied clinically today.

^{3}H-Thymidine Labeling and DNA Measurement. Considerable information about the proliferation of bone marrow progenitors has been obtained through measuring the amount or rate of ^{3}H-TdR incorporation into cellular DNA of actively growing cells.[77,78] Tritiated thymidine has been used to label cells in S phase and to follow their progression through the various bone marrow compartments. Labeling studies using tritiated thymidine have several advantages, including selective DNA labeling, rapid degradation of unincorporated material, and a weak β-particle emission that is ideal for radioautography; however, administration of ^{3}H-TdR in vivo is associated with an unacceptable level of radiation exposure for routine human studies, and the kinetics of cell proliferation in vitro may not be equivalent to that in the intact subject. In general, ^{3}H-TdR methodology also is too difficult and time-consuming for routine use.

Mitotic Index. Cell division can be assessed directly by measuring the mitotic index (MI). The MI is the ratio of cells in mitosis to the total number of cells in the population. To be useful, such determinations should be made in morphologically homogeneous cell populations. The clinical utility of the MI alone or in combination with ^{3}H-TdR–labeling studies has been modest at best because identifying mitoses in various cell populations is difficult, and the range of MI in humans is wide (from 7 to 43 per 1000 nucleated marrow cells). MI and ^{3}H-TdR–labeling studies have proved more useful in diseases associated with uniform cell populations, such as multiple myeloma.

Diisopropyl Fluorophosphate and Chromium-51 Labeling. Diisopropyl fluorophosphate (DFP), containing either radioactive phosphate (^{32}P) or tritium, was introduced as a granulocyte marker in the late 1950s.[59,60,79] This radioactively-labeled compound binds to mature granulocytes and monocytes and also binds to erythrocytes, which must be eliminated when the isotope is counted. DFP may be employed as an in vivo or in vitro label and has been used to determine blood neutrophil turnover[61] and the size and compartmentalization of the total blood neutrophil pool.[79,80] Kinetic studies of intravenously administered DFP permit measurement of marrow transit times, neutrophil reserves, and marrow myelocyte turnover rates under steady-state and non–steady-state conditions.[59,60,79,81–83] The major drawbacks to DFP studies are that the DFP may be toxic to tagged leukocytes and that ^{32}P can elute from a labeled cell in vivo and be taken up by unlabeled cells.[1,81]

γ-Ray–emitting chromium-51 (^{51}Cr) has also been used to label leukocytes.[81,84–87] Although its radioactive emission permits surface monitoring to ascertain the distribution of label, it has low labeling efficiency, it labels leukocytes other than neutrophils (lymphocytes and monocytes preferentially), and the label can slowly elute from the cells. Agreement between DFP and ^{51}Cr studies of leukocyte kinetics has been variable,[81,82,86,88] and while DFP and chromium-labeling techniques have given valuable information about normal and abnormal neutrophil kinetics, both are too cumbersome for routine clinical use.

Gallium-67, Technetium-99m, and Indium-111 Labeling. Recently, several newer isotopes have been used to radiolabel leukocytes for in vivo studies, including gallium-67 (^{67}Ga), technetium-99m (^{99m}Tc), and indium-111 (^{111}In). Because of nonspecific accumulation of ^{67}Ga in the liver and gut and binding of ^{67}Ga to serum proteins and tumors, ^{67}Ga has not proved useful as a leukocyte label. ^{99m}Tc has a shorter half-life and has been used to label PMNs[89,90]; however, it too accumulates in the liver. Indium-labeled leukocytes have demonstrated the greatest in vivo and in vitro stability, and the cells retain most of their functional capacities. Unlike the β-emitters ^{32}P-phosphate and ^{3}H-thymidine, ^{111}In emits two γ photons that can be detected externally with commercially available radioactivity detectors. Using an ^{111}In–oxine complex and a leukocyte fraction, about 75% to 90% of the label appears in the polymorphonuclear cells. Recently, ^{111}In–tropolone complexes have been used because of ease of labeling. ^{111}In-labeled leukocytes and whole-body scanning with a γ counter may be useful to identify or localize inflammatory or infectious processes that cannot be identified using other diagnostic studies. This technique has been applied in evaluating fevers of unknown origin, osteomyelitis, and inflammatory bowel disease.[91]

Indium has also been used clinically to measure the half-disappearance time of neutrophils from the circulating blood; the half-disappearance time of radioactivity from the blood was 4 to 5 hours, somewhat shorter than that measured by other techniques. One drawback to the use of ^{111}In as a label for neutrophils is that its half-life (2.8 days) is relatively long compared with the clearance time of neutrophils (6 to 7 hours). Thus, radioactive neutrophils taken up by the MNP system can deliver significant radiation to the liver, spleen, and bone marrow.[1,92,93] Ruthenium-97 may be useful in in vivo studies because it has a low affinity to blood protein, is similar to ^{111}In in its physical characteristics, and delivers less radiation to each cell labeled.

Measurement of Leukocyte Products. Measurement of leukocyte products has been proposed as a simple means to assess blood cell kinetics. Measurement of serum and marrow lysozyme (muramidase), an enzyme contained in neutrophil and monocyte granules, has been used to assess neutrophil production,[94,95] but correlation with cell kinetics is disappointing, and measurement of lysozyme for clinical purposes is not useful in assessing neutrophil production.[96]

Circulating concentrations of transcobalamin I, found in immature neutrophils such as the promyelocytes and more abundantly in mature neutrophils,[94,97] have also been studied as a means of estimating neutrophil production but rarely provide information on neutrophil kinetics.

In Vitro Bone Marrow Culture. The colony-forming unit, granulocyte-macrophage (CFU-GM), usually regarded as the committed progenitor of neutrophils and macrophages, gives rise to colonies of neutrophils and MNPs in semisolid culture. The maximal number of colonies formed in agar from marrow aspirates should be reflective of the number of CFU-GM existing in vivo; however, the technique gives information only about the relative concentration of CFU-GM among all nucleated marrow cells and does not provide information about the total number of these progenitors. Although the total circulating CFU-GM can be quantified in peripheral blood, this determination may be more reflective of the distribution of CFU-GM than of its production in the bone marrow.[98] In vitro culture techniques permit assessment of abnormalities of granulocytic development in various hematologic disorders and have been of particular interest in assessing patients with aplastic anemia, myelodysplasia, and acute leukemia.[99] The CFU-GM assay is useful in determining the viability of cryopreserved bone marrow for transplantation.

In the steady state, the number of neutrophils entering the circulation must equal the number leaving it. The number entering the CNP reflects the rates of neutrophil production and distribution of neutrophils between the CNP and MBP. The absolute neutrophil count is a fair guideline to the balance between neutrophil production and destruction, particularly when evaluated in the context of overall bone marrow biopsy cellularity and the myeloid/erythroid ratio.

Bone Marrow Aspiration and Biopsy. Although gauging neutrophilic granulopoiesis by the appearance of marrow films, clot sections, or biopsies suffers from the limitations of sampling error and relatively poor correlation with kinetics, as measured by other techniques,[100] it does provide a rough estimate of leukocyte production. By combining bone marrow biopsy cellularity data with the myeloid/erythroid ratio, one can determine whether granulocytic hypoplasia or hyperplasia is present and distinguish granulocytic hypoplasia from erythroid hyperplasia. Although more precise information is obtained by performing radioisotopic labeling studies, they are usually too cumbersome to be used in all but rare instances.

Assessment of neutrophil production by bone marrow examination has several limitations. For example, morphologic findings in the marrow of a maturation arrest with diminished neutrophil development beyond the myelocyte stage does not distinguish between a true defect in cellular maturation and rapid mobilization of cells from marrow. Despite these limitations, when absolute neutrophil count and marrow cellularity (ascertained from a bone marrow biopsy) are used together, they provide a practical and useful guide in most clinical settings. An absolute neutrophil count of less than 1000/μL and hypocellular marrow invariably reflect impaired production of neutrophils. Hypercellular marrow generally reflects increased production of neutrophils, although it can be difficult morphologically to distinguish neutropenia due to ineffective neutrophilic granulopoiesis from that caused by peripheral destruction of neutrophils.

Newer techniques of marrow biopsy section preparation and staining allow for more accurate assessment of cellularity and differential cell counts. When an accurate neutrophil/erythroid ratio is obtained, total neutrophil cellularity in marrow may be derived from an estimate of total erythroblasts, based on measurement of erythroid iron incorporation with ^{59}Fe.[1] These studies, in conjunction with ^{3}H-TdR radioautography, provide detailed information on neutrophil kinetics; however, the laborious nature of these investigations limits their clinical utility, except in research settings.

REGULATION OF PHAGOCYTE PRODUCTION (MYELOPOIESIS)

All the cellular elements of blood are derived from stem cells in the bone marrow. There is a hierarchy of stem cells, the earliest of which are multipotent and able to give rise to cells of myeloid, erythroid, lymphoid, and megakaryocyte lineages.[101] Stem cells are not morphologically recognizable, but they have the capacity for extensive self-replication as well as differentiation along several lineages. The earliest stem cells give rise to more restricted stem cells, with the ultimate appearance of committed progenitors, which can proliferate and mature along only a single pathway (Fig. 17-5).

Differentiation in the stem cell compartment is manifested by expression of cellular receptors for various growth factors that allow progenitor cells to respond to hormonal signals in the environment, regulating the body's requirements for blood cell production. For example, expression of erythropoietin receptors is a characteristic of cells committed to erythroid differentiation, whereas expression of GM-CSF receptors is associated with granulocyte and MNP development.

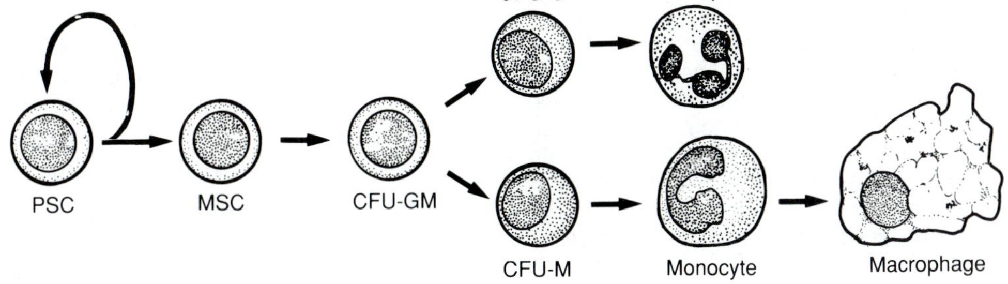

FIGURE 17-5. Stem cell development of neutrophils and macrophages. PSC, totipotent hematopoietic stem cell; MSC, myeloid stem cell; CFU-GM, colony-forming unit, granulocyte-macrophage; CFU-G, colony-forming unit, granulocyte; CFU-M, colony-forming unit, monocyte.

A variety of in vivo and in vitro models have been used to study the multipotent stem cells. The first assay used to identify stem cells was based on their ability to form hematopoietic colonies in the spleens of lethally irradiated mice. This assay, developed by Till and McCulloch,[102] defined the colony-forming unit, spleen (CFU-S), which is capable of forming erythroid, granulocytic, megakaryocytic, and mixed colonies in the spleen. Since then, a number of investigations have shown that the CFU-S has limited self-renewal properties and thus does not represent the true multipotent hematopoietic stem cell.[103]

The initial development of semisolid culture techniques[104,105] provided a system that could be used to study the clonal proliferation of hematopoietic progenitors. In this system, colonies of maturing myeloid cells develop from progenitors in response to the presence of CSF (Fig. 17-6). In humans, a primitive myeloid progenitor cell, the CFU-blast, can be identified in in vitro culture assays,[106] characterized by high in vitro self-renewal capability and complete myeloid potential, but these cells are also probably not the true hematopoietic stem cells. Recently, stem cells have been purified from mouse bone marrow that have properties attributable to a stem cell for all hematopoietic lineages. These stem cells were isolated with monoclonal antibodies; they are weakly *Thy-1*–positive, lineage marker-negative, and *Sca-1*–positive, and they can completely repopulate hematopoiesis in lethally irradiated mice.[107]

Studies in humans and mice (thymidine suicide, 5-fluorouracil resistance of CFU-S) demonstrate that most multipotent stem cells are not actively cycling but are resting in the nonproliferating state of the cell-cycle (G_0).[108,109] Various hormonal signals have been identified that can act to stimulate movement of cells from phase G_0 to G_1; these include interleukin-6 (IL-6),[110] IL-1,[111,112] and G-CSF.[113] Proliferation of primitive hematopoietic progenitors in culture is factor-dependent, and IL-3 is the most effective in supporting proliferation of multipotent progenitors, including CFU blast cells.[114–116]

Recently, a factor variously called Steel factor, stem cell factor, mast cell growth factor, or *kit* ligand has been cloned that has synergistic effects with previously identified growth factors on the growth of very primitive hematopoietic precursor cells.[116a]

Growth Factors

In vitro clonogenic culture systems have permitted the identification and isolation of hormones regulating hematopoietic cell proliferation and maturation. Characterization of these CSFs in mice led to the description of four distinct CSFs named according to type of colonies that resulted from adding the factor to murine bone marrow cultures. They are known as GM-CSF, G-CSF, macrophage colony-stimulating factor (M-CSF, also referred to as CSF-1) and multi-CSF (or IL-3).[117–120] Human analogues of these molecules have now been identified and their cognate cDNAs molecularly cloned.

Granulocyte-Macrophage Colony-Stimulating Factor

Human GM-CSF is a glycoprotein of 19 to 32 kd first purified from a human T-lymphoblastic cell line infected with human T-cell leukemia virus type II.[121] Isolation of GM-CSF cDNA[122–124] permitted generation of large amounts of recombinant GM-CSF protein for characterization of its in vitro and in vivo activities. Cellular sources of GM-CSF are limited; GM-CSF is made by activated but not resting T-lymphocytes and by all T-cell lines infected by human T-cell leukemia virus.[125] GM-CSF is also produced by monocytes,[126] fibroblasts,[127] endothelial cells,[128,129] and

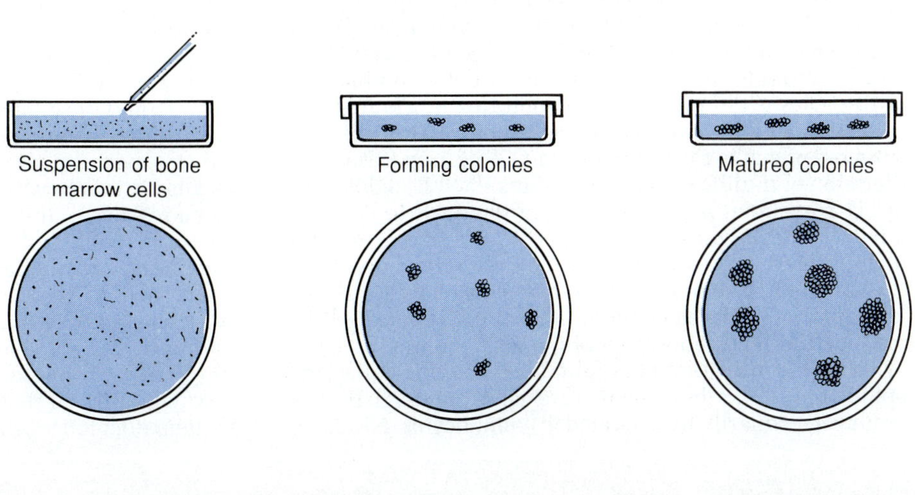

FIGURE 17-6. Colony assay for CFU-GM.

keratinocytes[130] stimulated by cytokines such as IL-1, TNF, or other cellular activators. Although low-level constitutive transcription of the GM-CSF gene can be demonstrated in certain in vitro circumstances, there appears to be little constitutive production of GM-CSF by normal human cells.

Like all CSFs, GM-CSF has activity on bone marrow progenitor cells and mature myeloid effector cells, enhancing their functional activities.[70] Addition of GM-CSF to normal human bone marrow in gel culture results in formation of pure neutrophil, pure eosinophil, mixed neutrophil–monocyte, and pure monocyte colonies.[131–133] In the presence of erythropoietin, GM-CSF can support the growth of erythroid bursts. GM-CSF has weak stimulatory activity on megakaryocyte colony formation[134] and stimulates colony formation of leukemia cell lines, such as KG-1 and HL-60.[133]

The study of the recombinant growth factors and interleukins has demonstrated the wide range of activities present in a single molecule. For example, GM-CSF has a variety of direct (primary) and indirect effects on mature neutrophils, eosinophils, and MNPs.[135–144] Serum concentrations of GM-CSF are very low or undetectable, consistent with a hypothesis that GM-CSF acts in a paracrine fashion locally in bone marrow and at sites of inflammation.[145]

Granulocyte Colony-Stimulating Factor

Granulocyte colony-stimulating factor is a species-nonspecific growth factor with activity on both human and murine cells.[146] Human and mouse G-CSFs are about 75% homologous. Human G-CSF is an 18- to 22-kd glycoprotein originally purified from the CHU-2 squamous carcinoma of the lung cell line,[147] the 5637 human bladder carcinoma cell line,[148] and human placenta–conditioned medium.[146] cDNA clones were isolated,[149,150] and the nonglycosylated bacterially derived G-CSF was used in clinical trials. G-CSF mRNA can be detected in monocytes, endothelial cells, and fibroblasts after cytokine stimulation,[151–153] and the gene encoding G-CSF has been localized to the long arm of chromosome 17 by in situ hybridization.[154] G-CSF has activities similar to GM-CSF on mature neutrophils. Although G-CSF has potent differentiating activity on the murine myelomonocytic leukemia cell line, WEHI-3B,[146,148] it has only weak differentiating activity on the human HL-60 promyelocytic leukemia cell line. G-CSF causes an increase in neutrophil alkaline phosphatase,[155,156] and it is a more potent maturational factor than GM-CSF with regard to neutrophil development.

Interleukin-3

Murine IL-3 was the first of the hematopoietic growth factors to be molecularly cloned.[157] After isolation of a gibbon ape IL-3 cDNA, the human gene for IL-3 was identified and cloned.[158] IL-3 (or multi-CSF) acts at an earlier level of stem cell development than GM-CSF.[114,115,159] Studies in human culture systems show that IL-3 can influence replication of CFU-blasts, the primitive uncommitted progenitors, as well as stimulate growth of committed progenitor cells. IL-3 is more effective than human GM-CSF in supporting proliferation of multipotential progenitors.[114–116] IL-3 does not direct movement of stem cells from phase G_0 to G_1,[115,116] but it synergizes with IL-1α, IL-1β, G-CSF, and IL-6 to stimulate formation of early progenitor cell-derived colonies. Addition of IL-3 to normal human bone marrow results in formation of colonies containing mast cells, neutrophils, monocytes, erythroblasts, eosinophils, and megakaryocytes.[160] IL-3 also stimulates functional activities of eosinophils and MNPs but not mature neutrophils.[161] IL-3 is produced primarily by activated T lymphocytes, NK cells, and mast cells.[162] The genes encoding IL-3 and GM-CSF are located close together on the long arm of chromosome 5,[163–165] separated by only 9 kb.[166] The structure of the genes for IL-3 and GM-CSF is similar, suggesting that they may have evolved from a common ancestral gene.

Macrophage Colony-Stimulating Factor

Macrophage colony-stimulating factor is a lineage-specific hematopoietic growth factor that influences cells committed to the MNP pathway. Human M-CSF was purified from urine[167] and from medium conditioned by the Mia Paca pancreatic cancer cell line.[168] Unlike IL-3, GM-CSF, and G-CSF, which are monomers, M-CSF is a disulfide-joined homodimer of 70 to 90 kd. The structure of M-CSF places it in the family of hormones related to insulin and relaxin. Also unlike G-CSF, GM-CSF, and IL-3, M-CSF is produced by many cell types. M-CSF circulates in plasma and is excreted in urine.[169,170] There are several identified RNA transcripts for M-CSF, and large and small cDNA clones encoding different forms of M-CSF mRNA have been isolated.[171,172] The gene for M-CSF has recently been localized to the short arm chromosome 1, whereas the gene encoding the M-CSF receptor, the product of the c-*fms* protooncogene is on the long arm of chromosome 5.[164,174] Human M-CSF is not species-specific and appears to have more prominent effects on murine MNP proliferation than on human cells. Suboptimal concentrations of GM-CSF are required to observe optimal stimulation of human macrophage colony formation in vitro.[175] M-CSF enhances RNA and protein synthesis in the macrophage and causes an increased release of several monokines, including tissue plasminogen activator, TNF, IL-1, and prostaglandin E_2.[176] M-CSF also induces G-CSF gene expression in macrophages. In vitro studies have also demonstrated prominent synergy between M-CSF and both IL-1α and IL-3.[177,178]

Interleukin-1 and Interleukin-6

Several other factors have shown important effects on the growth and function of myeloid progenitor cells. IL-6, and to some extent, IL-1 and G-CSF, stimulate movement of stem cells from G_0 to G_1.[112] IL-6 is a 26-kd glycoprotein made by IL-1– or TNF-α–stimulated fibroblasts and activated T lymphocytes and monocytes.[179,180] IL-6 has a wide range of biologic activities and is known also as hepatocyte-stimulating factor, hybridoma growth factor, B-cell stimulatory factor 2, and interferon-β_2 (IFN-β_2).[181] Recent studies suggest that several of the activities attributed to IL-1, such as the synergistic activity known as hemopoietin-1,[182–185] may be the result of IL-1–induced expression of IL-6.[112] IL-6 appears to serve as a competence factor in proliferation of progenitor cells, but proliferation of these cells also requires the presence of IL-3.[110,112] In a human blast cell colony assay, addition of IL-6 in combination with IL-3 led to earlier appearance and greater numbers of blast cell colonies than did IL-3 alone.[112] Similarly, IL-6 alone had little or no stimulatory effect on AML blast colony formation, but it synergized with IL-3 or GM-CSF.[186]

IL-1 appears to play an important role in host defense because it is centrally involved in inflammatory and immune responses. IL-1 is an endogenous pyrogen and activates a wide range of cells, including B and T lymphocytes, fibroblasts, endothelial cells, and osteoclasts.[187] When exposed to IL-1, these target cells demonstrate enhanced functional activity and secrete a variety of cytokines, including IL-2, IFN, GM-CSF, G-CSF, IL-3, and IL-6. IL-1 therefore has numerous indirect effects on hematopoiesis, making it difficult to ascertain the direct activities of IL-1 on hematopoietic cell growth. Recently, interleukins 8 through 13 have been molecularly cloned and characterized. All have effects on myeloid cells.

Inhibitors of Hematopoiesis

A variety of inhibitors of hematopoiesis have been identified using in vitro culture techniques. T lymphocytes, capable of suppressing hematopoiesis, have been seen in aplastic anemia and T-cell disorders, such as T-γ disease. A number of T-cell–derived inhibitory substances have been identified, including IFN-γ,[188] lymphotoxin (TNF-β),[189] TNF-α,[190] and several partially characterized activities, such as differentiation-inducing factors,[191] colony-inhibiting lymphokine,[192] and T-cell–derived colony-inhibiting activity.[193] Other factors have been identified using in vitro systems, including transforming growth factor β,[194,195] IFN-α, and prostaglandins. G-CSF causes mature neutrophils to produce IFN-α, which suggests a possible feedback regulation mechanism.[196]

Factors released from neutrophils have also been implicated in negative feedback regulation of neutrophil production.[197] Lineage-specific inhibitors, referred to as chalones,[198] have been described, but their exact nature or role in regulating hematopoiesis is unknown. Lactoferrin, a 79-kd iron-binding glycoprotein[199] and component of neutrophil secondary granules, is a candidate inhibitory substance.[200,201] Although a variety of functions have been postulated for neutrophil lactoferrin,[202,203] patients with congenital lactoferrin deficiency have normal neutrophil counts.[204]

Myeloid Growth Factor Receptors

The process of differentiation of hematopoietic stem cells involves expression of cell-surface receptors that allows the cell to respond to signals in its environment. The CSFs exert their biologic effects by interacting with specific high-affinity receptors present in low numbers on the surface of hematopoietic progenitors and mature effector cells. The hierarchy of receptor expression during the course of differentiation is being characterized for both human and murine hematopoiesis, and down-modulation of growth factor receptor expression by other growth factors has been demonstrated.[205]

Interleukin-3 Receptor

Interleukin-3 interacts with early progenitor cells, and studies in mice have identified a low number (100 to 1000) of high-affinity binding sites on murine bone marrow cells.[206] Other murine IL-3–responsive cells have been reported to have 100 to 13,000 binding sites per cell.[207] The human KG-1 myelogenous leukemia cell line has about 200 IL-3 binding sites per cell, with an apparent dissociation constant (K_d) of 70 to 105 pmol.[208] Receptors for IL-3 have been found on monocytes, eosinophils, and adherence-depleted peripheral blood lymphocytes, but not on mature neutrophils.

Granulocyte-Macrophage Colony-Stimulating Factor Receptor

Granulocyte-macrophage colony-stimulating factor acts on an overlapping but somewhat more mature population of progenitor cells than IL-3. A single class of high-affinity binding sites for GM-CSF has been demonstrated on human bone marrow progenitors, neutrophils, monocytes, and eosinophils.[209] The apparent K_d of 15 to 30 pmol/L is in agreement with the concentrations of GM-CSF that elicit biologic activity in vitro. The HL-60 and KG-1 leukemia cell lines also express high-affinity GM-CSF receptors, and the number of sites increases during differentiation of HL-60 cells toward neutrophils.[210] GM-CSF receptors have also been found on acute and chronic myeloid leukemia cells.

Recently, cloning of the α and β subunits of the IL-3 receptor and GM-CSF receptor have provided the molecular tools for studying receptor physiology. Distinct, low-affinity α subunits for human IL-3, GM-CSF, and IL-5 have been identified. A common β subunit for these three receptors has been identified, which converts the binding of ligand to each receptor from a low-affinity to a high-affinity interaction. Neither the α nor the β subunit of the receptor contains a kinase domain, so the signaling through the receptor complexes requires additional components. The α and β subunits belong to the recently described cytokine receptor superfamily.[210a]

GM-CSF receptors have also been identified on nonhematopoietic cells,[211] and various tumor cell lines can respond to GM-CSF.[212] Normal placental cells have GM-CSF receptors,[213] as do normal endothelial cells, implying that GM-CSF may affect the physiology of nonhematopoietic tissue.[214]

Macrophage Colony-Stimulating Factor Receptor

The c-*fms* protooncogene encodes the receptor for M-CSF. M-CSF receptors are expressed on early cells committed to monocytic differentiation, and the number of M-CSF receptors increases markedly during maturation. Treatment of normal human monocytes with IFN-γ or GM-CSF increases expression of c-*fms*,[215–217] and differentiation of HL-60 cells toward monocytes by either 1,25 dihydroxyvitamin D_3 or TPA increases the levels of c-*fms* RNA. Expression of c-*fms* has also been shown in human AML.[218] The gene encoding c-*fms* is highly complex, contains about 22 exons, and overlaps one of the genes for the platelet-derived growth factor receptor at its 5′ end.[219]

Granulocyte Colony-Stimulating Factor Receptor

Granulocyte colony-stimulating factor stimulates proliferation and maturation of neutrophil progenitors and enhances the functional activity of mature neutrophils by acting through specific high-affinity cell-surface receptors. About 560 receptors (K_d of 250 pmol) have been demonstrated on human neutrophils using a modified human G-CSF ligand. Chemical cross-linking of ligand to its receptor results in a complex of 170 kd, suggesting that the G-CSF receptor is a 150-kd molecule.[220] Studies using radiolabeled mouse G-CSF have demonstrated G-CSF receptors on mouse and human bone marrow, human neutrophils, and a variety of murine myelomonocytic cell lines.[205,206,221,222] These studies demonstrated 600 to 1100 G-CSF receptors per cell, with a K_d of 720 to 880 pmol. G-CSF receptors have also been identified on fresh myeloid leukemia cells.[150] Recently, cDNAs encoding the human G-CSF receptor have been isolated and characterized.[221]

Human Leukemia Cell Lines

The development of immortalized human myeloid leukemia cell lines representing different stages of maturation has provided important tools for analyzing hematopoietic cell differentiation. Cell lines have been established from patients with promyelocytic leukemia (HL-60), erythroleukemia (K562), histiocytic lymphoma (U937), AML (KG-1), acute monocyte leukemia (THP-1).[223] KG-1 cells are myeloblasts, and the KG-1 variant KG-1a cell line is less mature and does not differentiate in response to phorbol esters or other inducers of differentiation.[224] HL-60 cells are promyelocytes and have been studied extensively because of their ability to differentiate toward granulocytes or macrophages. U937 and THP-1 cells are monocytoid lines, and ML-1, ML-2, and ML-3 cells are myelomonoblasts established from a single patient with AML.[225] K562 and HEL differentiate along the erythroid pathway but also show evidence of myeloid maturation.

The HL-60 cell line was derived from the peripheral blood of a patient with the clinical characteristics of acute promyelocytic leukemia.[226,227] Review of the patient's leukemia has led to its classification as the M2 rather than the M3 subtype of AML.[228] HL-60 cells form colonies in semisolid medium and respond to GM-CSF.[133] Treatment with chemical agents, such as dimethyl sulfoxide[229] or dibutyryl cAMP, results in neutrophilic differentiation, while exposure to phorbol esters,[230] retinoic acid,[231] or 1,25 dihydroxyvitamin D_3[232] results in differentiation toward MNPs. The c-*myc* protooncogene is overexpressed in resting HL-60 cells, but with differentiation, c-*myc* mRNA disappears. Enhanced c-*myc* expression is due to gene amplification; about 20 copies of the c-*myc* gene are present at a single chromosomal locus.[233,234] Another nuclear oncogene, c-*myb*, is also transcribed in undifferentiated HL-60 cells, but its transcription is turned off when HL-60 cells undergo terminal neutrophilic differentiation.[235] Recently, an additional gene encoding a serine protease called *myeloblastin* has been shown to be turned off in association with HL-60 differentiation.[236]

HL-60 cells show morphologic features of promyelocytes, and although the cells have several karyotypic abnormalities present in the patients' fresh leukemia cells and contain only 45 chromosomes, they do not have the classic 15: 17 translocation seen in promyelocytic leukemia. HL-60 cells are monosomic for normal chromosome 5 and have a marker chromosome that may include a part of chromosome 5.[163,237,238]

The K562 leukemia cell line was derived from the pleural effusion of a patient with CML in blast crisis.[239] K562 shows capability to differentiate along several myeloid lineages, and although the cells express some myeloid antigens, including MY-1,[240] it is primarily an erythroblast cell line.[239,241,242] K562 cells are used most often to study erythroid differentiation and globin gene expression. Fetal and embryonic hemoglobin are produced when the cells are exposed to butyrate and hemin.[243] The cell line is composed of large, undifferentiated blast cells, with two or more prominent nucleoli and a basophilic cytoplasm containing no granules. The cells stain for erythroid markers such as glycophorin A and spectrin; they do not stain for Sudan black, peroxidase, and ASD-chloroacetate esterase. K562 cells have 70 chromosomes, including the Philadelphia chromosome,[244] and they have amplification of the c-*abl* protooncogene.[233]

HEL cells were established from the peripheral blood of a patient with erythroleukemia.[245] The HEL cells are proerythroblasts and spontaneously synthesize fetal and embryonic hemoglobin. They are positive on periodic acid–Schiff, acid phosphatase, and butyrate esterase stains and negative on myeloid histochemical stains. They contain 66 chromosomes.

KG-1 cells were derived from the bone marrow of a patient with erythroleukemia evolving into AML.[246] More than 90% of the cells stain strongly for ASD-chloroacetate esterase, but only 1% to 2% are peroxidase-positive. Like HL-60 cells, KG-1 cells differentiate into nondividing macrophage-appearing cells when exposed to phorbol esters. KG-1 cells express Ia antigen,[247] i antigen, gp95, and gp105. They have GM-CSF and IL-3 receptors[208,209] and respond to CSF in semisolid medium. The KG-1a cell line arose spontaneously from the KG-1 cell line.[248] The cells are undifferentiated blasts and show no response to CSF.[248] KG-1a cells have acquired several characteristics of T lymphocytes.[224]

The U937 cell line was established from a patient with histiocytic lymphoma and has predominantly monoblastoid characteristics.[249] The cells stain for nonspecific esterase, produce lysozyme, and show some degree of phagocytic activity. U937 cells differentiate toward monocytes in response to IFN-γ, 1,25 dihydroxyvitamin D_3, retinoic acid, or phorbol esters. The activity of differentiated U937 cells can be enhanced by addition of GM-CSF.[250]

The THP-1 cell line was derived from a child with acute monoblastic leukemia.[251] The cells are immature monocytes, stain positively for nonspecific esterase, and stain negatively for myeloid-specific markers. THP-1 cells produce lysozyme; a small number have phagocytic activity.

NEUTROPENIA

Definition

By defining a normal population as being within two standard deviations of the mean, 5% are placed outside the normal range. Therefore, 2.5% of the population have a leukocyte count below the defined lower limits of normal. These people have no hematologic disorder and do not require extensive evaluation of their neutropenia.

The initial evaluation of a patient with a low leukocyte count is to perform a differential count to determine which cellular components are reduced. Normal neutrophil levels vary with age, race,[252] sex,[253] time of day, and other factors, such as exercise, stress, and viral illness. A neutrophil count of less than 2000/μL constitutes neutropenia for adult white persons, whereas the somewhat lower limit of about 1500/μL is normal for African Americans.[254,255]

Profound neutropenia, sometimes called *agranulocytosis*, is usually associated with mucosal ulcerations and a serious risk of bacterial or fungal infections affecting the skin, lungs, and gastrointestinal tract. The exceptions to this rule demonstrate that the peripheral blood neutrophil count is only a crude indicator of neutrophil *turnover*, the determination of which requires sophisticated and rarely performed kinetic measurements described previously. Chronic neutropenia without serious clinical manifestations is often designated *benign neutropenia*.

Causes

Neutropenia can be classified into broad categories of decreased production, increased destruction, or a shift in neutrophil distribution (Table 17-3), although in many cases the kinetic basis of the neutropenic state is unknown. It should be confirmed initially that the number of circulating neutrophils is truly low. Certain paraproteins, for example, cause excessive leukocyte clumping, leading to spurious neutropenia; and abnormally fragile cells can disintegrate after collection, resulting in artificially low leukocyte counts. Factitious neutropenia can also occur if blood counts are performed long after blood has been drawn. Pseudoneutropenia is due to an excessive shift of neutrophils from the CNP to the MBP; the neutrophil production rate is normal. The size of the MBP can be crudely estimated by the epinephrine test,[256] although this procedure is rarely clinically indicated.

Most commonly, neutropenia is caused by decreased production of neutrophils owing to decreased numbers of functional precursor cells or abnormalities in maturation. Although most cases of adult neutropenia are acquired, there are a number of important hereditary and congenital neutropenias (see Table 17-3). Some of these disorders in-

TABLE 17-3. Causes of Neutropenia

DECREASED PRODUCTION
Congenital
Dysgenesis congenita with familial pancytopenia
Reticular dysgenesis with congenital aleukocytosis
Cyclic neutropenia
Kostmann's syndrome
Chronic hypoplastic neutropenia
Schwachman-Diamond syndrome
Familial severe neutropenia
Familial benign neutropenia
Acquired
Aplastic anemia
Infiltrative diseases of the bone marrow (leukemia, myeloma, tumors, tuberculosis, etc)
Suppressor T-cell–associated neutropenia (T-γ disease)
Severe infection
Drug-induced
Predictable
Cytotoxic chemotherapy
Radiation therapy
Idiosyncratic
Chloramphenicol
Semisynthetic penicillins
Cephalosporins
Phenothiazines
Phenylbutazones
Gold
Antithyroid drugs
Quinidine and procainamide
Anticonvulsants
Ineffective Granulopoiesis
Myelodysplastic syndrome
Vitamin B_{12} or folate deficiency
Alcohol
INCREASED DESTRUCTION
Hypersplenism
Idiopathic immune-mediated
Drug-induced
Associated with collagen vascular diseases (Felty's syndrome, systemic lupus erythematosus)
Isoimmune neutropenia
Complement activation neutropenia (hemodialysis, cardiopulmonary bypass)
ALTERED DISTRIBUTION
Pseudoneutropenia
Complement-activation neutropenia

volve the hematopoietic pluripotent stem cell, such as cyclic neutropenia, while other syndromes appear primarily to affect committed stem cells, such as Kostmann's syndrome (infantile genetic agranulocytosis)[257] and neutropenia with exocrine pancreas deficiency (Schwachman-Diamond syndrome).[258] Neutropenia with dysgammaglobulinemia[259] and Chédiak-Higashi syndrome[260] are other hereditary causes of neutropenia that do not involve a defined stem cell abnormality. Chronic benign neutropenia is often discovered in adulthood, and these patients, who are usually women, may have substantial neutropenia without clinical manifestations. This disorder may be familial, and the pathophysiology is unknown. Although the condition can evolve into life-threatening neutropenia, the prognosis is generally good,[261,262] and patients with neutropenia who suffer recurrent infection in infancy and childhood often cease to be affected when older.[263]

Cyclic neutropenia is a stem cell disorder characterized by severe episodes of neutropenia occurring at about 3-week intervals.[264,265] During the time of neutropenia, patients often develop fever, malaise, and oral ulcerations. Some of the cases are clearly inherited as an autosomal dominant, but most appear to arise spontaneously, with manifestations beginning in infancy or early childhood. Cycling of reticulocytes, platelets, and monocytes indicates that the regulatory abnormality occurs at a pluripotent stem cell level. A similar syndrome occurs in gray collie dogs,[266] and these animals may be cured by bone marrow transplantation from a normal litter mate; conversely, the disorder can be induced in a normal dog transplanted with bone marrow from an affected animal.[267,268]

Neutropenia is a common manifestation of acquired intrinsic bone marrow diseases, either neoplastic or nonneoplastic. Acute leukemias, chronic lymphoid leukemia, myelodysplastic disorders, hairy-cell leukemia, multiple myeloma, and malignant histiocytic disorders can cause neutropenia by infiltration of marrow, loss of normal stem cells, and possibly production of inhibitors of hematopoiesis. Disruption of marrow architecture by fibrosis, granulomas, or lipid-laden macrophages can also result in neutropenia. Ineffective granulopoiesis occurs in myelodysplastic syndromes and in megaloblastic anemia caused by folic acid or vitamin B_{12} deficiency.

Although infections most often cause neutrophilia (discussed later), certain infections are sometimes associated with neutropenia. These include viral infections, especially in children; bacterial infections in chronic alcoholics (in which case alcoholic toxicity to the bone marrow and vitamin deficiency may play a contributory role); and some infections caused by *Salmonella* and *Pseudomonas* sp as well as by *Staphylococcus aureus*. In these latter cases, the microorganisms may elaborate toxins, known as leukocidins, that destroy neutrophils or their precursors.[269]

The mechanisms summarized here as underlying many of the neutropenic states described are more or less tentative because it has not been possible to perform detailed kinetic studies. In many instances, mechanisms inferred in the literature based on morphologic appearances of bone marrow aspirates have not been tested by more sophisticated means.[270]

Drug-Induced Neutropenia

Drug-related neutropenia is probably the most common cause of isolated neutropenia. Cytotoxic drugs predictably cause neutropenia, as does extensive bone marrow irradiation. Table 17-4 lists the different classes of drugs associated with idiosyncratic drug-induced neutropenia.

The approach most commonly used with patients who develop neutropenia of unclear cause is to evaluate their medications and determine whether a specific drug could be causing the neutropenia. Issues to be addressed include the indications for use of the drug; how well established the link is between any particular drug and neutropenia; whether host factors that affect drug metabolism are present, such as age or liver or renal disease; and whether alternative effective drugs are available. Thus, if an antibiotic is considered as a possible cause of neutropenia, the prudent approach is to switch to an alternative class of antibiotics. If the medication in question has few alternatives, such as an effective antiseizure medication, it becomes essential that the role of the medication in the patient's neutropenia be accurately assessed.

TABLE 17-4. Drugs Associated With Neutropenia or Agranulocytosis

ANALGESICS
Aminopyrine
Dipyrone

ANTIBIOTICS
Cephalosporins
Chloramphenicol
Clindamycin
Doxycycline
Flucytosine
Gentamicin
Griseofulvin
Isoniazid
Lincomycin
Metronidazole
Nitrofurantoin
Penicillins
Rifampin
Streptomycin
Sulfonamides
Vancomycin

ANTICONVULSANTS
Carbamazepine
Ethosuximide
Mephenytoin
Phenytoin
Primidone
Trimethadione

ANTIHISTAMINES
Brompheniramine
Cimetidine
Pyribenzamine
Rantidine
Thenalidine

ANTIINFLAMMATORY AGENTS
Fenoprofen
Gold salts
Ibuprofen
Indomethacin
Phenylbutazone

ANTIMALARIALS
Amodiaquine
Dapsone
Hydroxychloroquine
Pyrimethamine
Quinine

ANTITHYROID DRUGS
Carbimazole
Methimazole
Methylthiouracil
Potassium perchlorate
Propylthiouracil

CARDIOVASCULAR AGENTS
Captopril
Diazoxide
Hydralazine
Methyldopa
Pindolol
Procainamide
Propanolol
Quinidine

DIURETICS
Acetazolamide
Bumetanide
Chlorothiazide
Hydrochlorothiazide
Hydrochlorthalidone
Methazolamide
Spironolactone

HYPOGLYCEMIC AGENTS
Chlorpropamide
Tolbutamide

PHENOTHIAZINES
Chlorpromazine
Methylpromazine
Prochlorperazine
Promazine
Thioridazane
Trifluoperazine
Trimeprazine

SEDATIVES AND NEUROPHARMACOLOGIC AGENTS
Chlordiazepoxide
Clozapine
Desipramine
Diazepam
Imipramine
Meprobamate
Metoclopramide

MISCELLANEOUS
Allopurinol
Colchicine
Ethanol
Levamisole
Levodopa
D-Penicillamine

(Adapted from Vincent PC. Drug-induced aplastic anemia and agranulocytosis. Drugs 1986;31:52)

Aminopyrine, which was introduced as an analgesic in the 1920s, was probably the first drug to be convincingly associated with neutropenia, often resulting in a total absence of granulocytes (agranulocytosis). Epidemiologic studies clearly implicated aminopyrine as a cause of agranulocytosis, which led to its elimination from medical use.[271–273] Aminopyrine-related agranulocytosis appears to be immunologically mediated.[274,275]

Chloramphenicol was introduced in 1948, but its possible association with aplastic anemia was not suspected until 2 years later, and it was another 2 years before reports indicating its association with aplastic anemia began to appear in the literature.[276] Chloramphenicol can cause a dose-related suppression of hematopoiesis and an idiosyncratic aplastic anemia or severe neutropenia that is often irreversible.[277,278] The variety of hematologic abnormalities seen in patients receiving chloramphenicol are well described.[278]

The Council on Drugs of the American Medical Association Registry on Adverse Reactions no longer tracks drug-related hematologic reactions. The precise incidence of drug-related neutropenia has always been difficult to assess partly because of problems in obtaining reliable information regarding drug usage. During a 5-year period, 215 cases of drug-induced neutropenia were reported in Sweden, an overall incidence of 0.01%. Sulfonamides and antithyroid drugs were most frequently implicated.[279,280]

The most common drugs associated with neutropenia in the United States were the phenothiazine derivatives.[281,282] In these studies, the reported incidence of agranulocytosis was 1 in 1300 patients receiving phenothiazines, although transient milder neutropenia was commonly seen. Women had a higher incidence of agranulocytosis than men, and most patients developing agranulocytosis were over 40 years old. Agranulocytosis due to phenothiazines occurs concomitantly with treatment, usually after a 10- to 20-g cumulative dose (20 to 40 days of therapy). Occasional use of phenothiazines as antiemetics, tranquilizers, or antihistamines is generally not complicated by this reaction. A dose-dependent suppression of neutrophil production may be seen after weeks of continuous phenothiazine therapy, leading to a modest degree of neutropenia, with neutrophil production slowly increasing after withdrawal of the drug or decrease in dosage. Phenothiazines can be readministered in smaller doses to some sensitive patients without recurrence, consistent with a toxic rather than immunologically mediated reaction in most patients.

Clozapine, a dibenzodiazepine antipsychotic drug that is used for the treatment of schizophrenia refractory to phenothiazines, was found when introduced to be associated with a 1% to 2% incidence of potentially fatal agranulocytosis occurring within the first 6 months of treatment. Neutrophil counts usually fell gradually over a 6-week period but occasionally fell precipitously. Recovery took place within 2 to 4 weeks after drug therapy was stopped. The high incidence of blood dyscrasias led the manufacturer to release the drug only as part of a care package in which patients under treatment must have their blood counts monitored.[283] A recent analysis of more than 11,000 patients in the monitoring program revealed a 0.8% incidence of agranulocytosis at 1 year and of 0.9% during 1.5 years of treatment. There were two deaths of infections resulting from the neutropenia. Most cases of agranulocytosis occurred in the first 6 months of treatment and in older patients (average age, 49 yearss).[283a]

The commonly used penicillins and cephalosporins are remarkably nontoxic. Five to 15% of patients receiving high-dose penicillin, penicillin derivative, or cephalosporin therapy for 10 days or more develop varying effects of neutropenia. Nafcillin, oxacillin, cephalothin, and methicillin have been most frequently reported to cause neutropenia in high doses, but probably all β-lactam antibiotics can cause neutropenia. Most patients who develop neutropenia have been given a prolonged course (more than 10 days) of high-dose penicillin therapy,[284] suggesting a direct effect of the penicillin. Toxic effects of penicillin G breakdown products on human bone marrow myeloid cell growth have been demonstrated in vitro.[285] Some patients have had recurrent neutropenia after a single-dose rechallenge, suggesting that both immune and nonimmune mechanisms are involved in β-lactam–associated neutropenia. Drug-dependent antibodies to neutrophils in some patients suggest that occasionally the mechanism of neutropenia is similar to that observed in penicillin-induced immune hemolytic anemia. Given the frequency with which penicillin is prescribed, the risk of significant neutropenia from penicillin therapy is low. In most cases of penicillin-induced neutropenia, neutrophil counts return to normal within 2 weeks of discontinuing therapy. Because a slow, progressive fall in neutrophil counts is common,[286] patients with osteomyelitis or endocarditis who are receiving high-dose chronic β-lactam antibiotics should have their leukocyte counts monitored regularly. Rash, fever, or eosinophilia can be seen in up to 70% of cases of β-lactam–associated neutropenia.[286] The role that chronic high-dose β-lactam therapy may play in prolonging neutropenia in the neutropenic host is difficult to address. Some studies suggest that double β-lactam therapy has less nephrotoxicity than a β-lactam and aminoglycoside combination, patients may have a longer duration of granulocytopenia.

Captopril has been associated with several cases of neutropenia or aplastic anemia. Certain patients are at high risk for developing captopril-induced neutropenia, particularly those with renal insufficiency, who have delayed clearance of the drug, and those with collagen vascular diseases. Of 6000 patients receiving captopril in formal clinical studies, there were 44 cases of captopril-associated neutropenia.[287] The incidence of patients with normal serum creatinine and no collagen vascular disease was 0.2%, but for patients with a creatinine of 2 or greater, the incidence of neutropenia was 0.4%, and for patients with collagen vascular disease and a serum creatinine greater than 2, the incidence was 7.2%. The neutropenia associated with captopril therapy is usually rapidly reversible, with 90% of the cases resolving within 3 weeks. Fatal bone marrow suppression associated with captopril treatment has been reported.[288]

Data identifying subsets of patients susceptible to hematologic toxicity are not available for most drugs. A priority should be to develop such data for drugs that have limited therapeutic alternatives. Drugs such as chloramphenicol or phenylbutazone, which can cause fatal neutropenia, should be used with extreme caution because alternative therapies are available for most of their indications.

Other drugs that can cause severe neutropenia include levamisole,[288a] the sulfonamides and sulfonamide derivatives (chlorpropamide, sulfasalzine, carbonic anhydrase inhibitors)[289–291] and antiinflammatory agents, such as phenylbutazone,[292] indomethacin, ibuprofen,[293] and gold.[294,295] Antithyroid drugs are frequently associated with neutropenia,[296,297] and the commonly used H_2 blockers, cimetidine and ranitidine, rarely but definitely can cause neutropenia.[298,299]

Patients beginning therapy with one of the many drugs associated with neutropenia should be cautioned to contact their physician if they develop unexplained fever, chills, sore throat, or malaise within the first weeks to months after starting treatment. With the reversible drug-induced neutropenias, the leukocyte count usually begins to recover within 1 week of drug discontinuance, and long-term sequelae are uncommon. Patients with more profound neutropenia may require prolonged hospitalization for treatment of infection, yet they usually recover in 3 weeks.

Autoimmune Neutropenia

Humoral and cellular immune responses have been implicated in the pathogenesis of various acquired neutropenic syndromes. Although methods for demonstrating antibodies to red blood cell (RBC) and lymphocyte antigens are well standardized, techniques for assaying antibodies to neutrophils tend to be reliable only at institutions experienced at performing them. Neutrophils are difficult to work with in vitro because of low viability and a tendency to spontaneously agglutinate; also, they tend to adsorb normal immunoglobulins and other plasma proteins. Techniques used for identifying neutrophil antibodies include cytotoxicity and agglutination assays, adherence to staphylococcal protein A, immunofluorescence, and indirect methods whereby serum is tested against fixed target neutrophils using a fluorescent-labeled anti-IgG antibody. Also, direct and indirect antiglobulin tests using ^{125}I-labeled reagents have been developed for assessing neutrophil antibodies. Using serum from cases of alloimmune neonatal neutropenia, as well as from children with autoimmune neutropenia, five neutrophil-specific antigens have been identified (Table 17-5). Some of these antigens are isoforms of the FcγIII receptor (see Chap. 16).

Autoimmune neutropenia due to circulating antibody can occur as an isolated condition or in association with other autoimmune or collagen vascular diseases (eg, systemic lupus erythematosus[300]). The antibodies may be directed at the mature neutrophil, at morphologically identifiable precursors,[301] or at progenitor cells at about the level of the CFU-GM. Autoantibodies against human myeloid progenitors can cause isolated neutropenia or pancytopenia.[301–308] Immune neutropenia may be associated with immune thrombocytopenia purpura[309] or autoimmune hemolytic anemia. Also, a syndrome of autoimmune neutropenia after bone marrow transplantation has been described[310] and is associated with Graves' disease and certain lymphomas.[311,312]

Febrile, nonhemolytic transfusion reactions are frequently caused by antineutrophil antibodies developed in response to repeated transfusions. Some of these antibodies are neutrophil specific. Granulocyte-agglutinating antibodies have been shown to reduce intravascular survival of transfused neutrophils using ^{111}In-labeled leukocyte studies.[313]

TABLE 17-5. Neutrophil-Specific Antigens

Antigen	Gene Frequency	Phenotype Frequency
NA1	0.31	53.9
NA2	0.69	92.7
NB1	0.72	92.1
NC1	0.80	96.2
ND1	0.88	98.5
NE1	0.12	23.0

(Adapted from Minchinton RM, Waters AH. The occurrence and significance of neutrophil antibodies. [Annotation] Br J Haematol 1984;56:521; and Class FHJ, Langerak J, Sabbe LJM, van Rood JJ. NE1: a new neutrophil specific antigen. Tissue Antigens 1979;13: 129)

Alloimmune Neonatal Neutropenia

Alloimmune or isoimmune neutropenia may occur in the newborn because of transplacental passage of maternal antineutrophil IgG antibodies. The estimated frequency of alloimmune neonatal neutropenia is 3% of live births[314]; the most common antibodies involved are anti-NA1 and anti-NB1, while cases involving antibodies to NA2 and NC1 have also been reported. These neutrophil-specific antibodies can cause neutropenia for up to 3 months after birth.[315] Severe cases require exchange-transfusion therapy.

Felty's Syndrome

Felty's syndrome is defined by the clinical picture of rheumatoid arthritis, splenomegaly, and neutropenia.[316–318] The mechanism of neutropenia in Felty's syndrome is not completely understood.[319] Many investigators believe that the primary pathogenesis of the syndrome involves development of antineutrophil antibodies, with subsequent margination and destruction of neutrophils.[320] Other researchers have only infrequently identified neutrophil antibodies in serum from patients with Felty's syndrome.[321] Cell-mediated immune mechanisms in Felty's syndrome have also been defined.[322] A major mechanism of neutropenia in Felty's syndrome appears to be excessive margination of neutrophils, but decreased production also occurs in some of these patients.[323] Similarly, hypersplenism may contribute to the neutropenia directly by neutrophil destruction, as well as indirectly, by being a site of production of neutrophil antibodies.

Most patients with Felty's syndrome do not develop infections unless the neutrophil count drops substantially below 500/μL. A significant association between neutrophil counts and the incidence of infection is seen only at neutrophil counts of less than 100/μL, suggesting that a variety of host factors influence the incidence of infection in patients with Felty's syndrome.[324] Splenectomy generally improves neutrophil counts[325,326] and may reduce neutrophil-bound immunoglobulin.[327]

Neutropenia and Suppressor T-Cell Disease

Cell-mediated suppression of hematopoiesis has been well documented in the literature.[328] Suppressor or cytotoxic T-lymphocyte inhibition of granulopoiesis has been shown to occur in two general situations: as part of a syndrome of connective tissue or autoimmune disease, or, more commonly, in association with the disease now referred to as T-γ disease.[329,330] The former may be related to Felty's syndrome. The neutropenic patients have manifestations of rheumatoid arthritis or related disorders, and the peripheral blood contains numerous large granular lymphocytes.[331,332] The latter disorder is generally due to a clonal expansion of suppressor T cells often associated with neutropenia but also with thrombocytopenia and anemia. The disease is clinically characterized by the presence of large granular lymphocytes in the peripheral blood. Successful treatment of the cytopenia in T-γ disease usually requires direct treatment of the lymphoproliferative disorder.

Complement-Activation Neutropenia

Complement-activation neutropenia is due to activation of complement on filtration membranes during hemodialysis,[333,334] cardiopulmonary bypass,[335] and certain apheresis procedures.[336] The activated complement, normally C5a, causes granulocyte aggregation within a few minutes of institution of the procedure.[337] The clinical syndrome is associated with transient neutropenia, dyspnea, and pulmonary infiltrates. It has been proved that the activated complement leads to expression of adhesion proteins on the neutrophils, which then causes neutrophil aggregation and pulmonary capillary occlusion. The syndrome may be severe and lead to hypoxemia. The pathogenetic role of neutrophils in this syndrome may be only one of many factors.[338]

General Approach to the Neutropenic Patient

Evaluation of a patient with neutropenia begins with a careful history to determine the duration of the patient's neutropenia, whether there are associated medical illnesses, and if there is a family history of neutropenia. A thorough drug history and history of exposure to environmental or other toxins should be undertaken, as well as a careful physical examination looking for splenomegaly, infection, stomatitis, and signs of systemic disease. A bone marrow aspirate and biopsy should be performed to assess cellularity and myeloid maturation and to rule out neoplastic disorders and infiltrative diseases. Testing for the presence of neutrophil antibodies in severe cases of neutropenia can be done by sending serum specimens to referral laboratories that perform these assays. It is not feasible to perform neutrophil half-life studies on a routine basis to document increased peripheral destruction of neutrophils, but neutropenia associated with granulocytic hyperplasia and normal maturation in the bone marrow suggests increased destruction of neutrophils, either in the marrow itself (ineffective granulopoiesis) or in the circulation or tissue. A decreased myeloid/erythroid ratio associated with a normal or hypocellular marrow and peripheral neutropenia implies that marrow neutrophil production is decreased. Once spurious neutropenia has been ruled out, all drugs that may induce neutropenia should be stopped.

The most important concern with regard to treatment of neutropenia is the prevention and control of infection. Generally, infections tend to be more common and more severe when the absolute neutrophil count falls below 500/μL, but in cases of immune-mediated neutropenia or in chronic benign neutropenia, this relation may not hold. A patient with severe neutropenia associated with fever should be hospitalized, and prophylactic antibiotics should be administered after cultures have been obtained. The most likely sources of infection are the lungs, skin, and venous catheters, and infecting organisms are usually endogenous. Severely neutropenic patients requiring hospitalization should be placed in reverse isolation, mainly to remind the medical personnel of the importance of sterile technique when accessing venous catheters. Suppression of endogenous gastrointestinal flora with nonabsorbable antibiotics is usually worthwhile since most infections in the neutropenic host are due to endogenous organisms. Systemic administration of prophylactic antibiotics to neutropenic patients without fever has not been proved useful. Although the current approach to neutropenia leaves much to be desired, a survey of neonates yielded a 6% incidence of neutropenia, defined as less than 2×10^9/L, but a low mortality rate in this affected population.[339]

Stimulation of granulopoiesis is a major new therapeutic modality available for the management of neutropenia, and use of CSFs is discussed later. Corticosteroids or other forms of immunosuppression can increase the neutrophil count in autoimmune neutropenia.[302,303] In alloimmune neutropenia of the newborn, plasma exchange may be necessary. In other situations in which there is antibody-mediated immune destruction of neutrophils, plasmapheresis or high-dose γ-globulin may be of empiric value. Amelioration of cytopenia in T-γ disease usually requires treatment with alkylating agents and prednisone.

The urgency for treatment of neutropenia depends principally on the risk of infection. When the neutropenia is caused by one of the many causes of bone marrow failure in which serious infectious complications are predictable, treatment of the underlying disorder, if possible, is mandatory. Unfortunately, however, the treatments for the common neoplastic forms of bone marrow failure exacerbate neutropenia, rendering the patient at risk for infection until bone marrow recovery occurs. A decade of efforts to replace neutrophils by leukocyte transfusion led to abandonment of this approach in all but a few medical centers, although recently the use of neutrophil transfusions has been reevaluated (see Chap. 60). Previously, the low number of neutrophils obtainable with available technology and the risk of inflicting pulmonary injury on the recipient and of transmitting cytomegalovirus and other viral illnesses led to their falling into disfavor. However, the use of CSFs to prepare donors for the collection of neutrophils has led to their reevaluation. As described in further detail later, it is now possible to stimulate granulopoiesis in some of these conditions with CSF. The risk of infection in other neutropenic disorders varies considerably, and the need for therapy with agents such as CSF is less clear. The ability of these substances to raise the neutrophil count in congenital,[340] cyclic,[341] and idiopathic acquired neutropenia[342–345] is of great interest. Even if the baseline clinical picture does not push the clinician to encourage experimental growth factor therapy of a patient with mild neutropenia or with an unimpressive history of infections, it is reassuring to know that treatment exists should infection occur or if major surgical or other intervention is necessary in such a patient.[346]

Clinical Use of Colony-Stimulating Factors

By virtue of their ability to stimulate production of granulocytes and monocytes and to enhance the functional activities of mature myeloid effector cells, the CSFs have broad applications in clinical medicine. Potential uses include the following:

- Reduction of neutropenia caused by chemotherapy or radiation therapy
- Enhancement of host defense against infection
- Treatment of primary hematologic disorders (aplastic anemia, neutropenia, myelodysplasia)
- Facilitation of recovery from allogeneic and autologous bone marrow transplantation
- Harvesting of peripheral blood stem cells for autologous transplantation
- Enhancement of host in vivo antitumor activity

Granulocyte-Macrophage Colony-Stimulating Factor

Based on studies in monkeys,[347,348] recombinant GM-CSF (rGM-CSF) was first administered to patients with acquired immunodeficiency syndrome (AIDS) and neutropenia in a phase I study.[349] Dose-dependent increases in circulating neutrophils, eosinophils, and monocytes were seen, and toxicity was mild at the doses used (1 to 8 μg/kg/d by continuous intravenous infusion for 14 days). The neutrophils and monocytes elicited by GM-CSF were functional in in vitro assays.[350] Side effects included occasional low-grade fever, myalgia, headache, facial flushing, or faint macular skin rash. Four patients receiving GM-CSF by peripheral vein developed phlebitis, so subsequent patients received GM-CSF through central venous catheter.

Studies of GM-CSF in myelodysplastic syndromes and aplastic anemia[351–354] have demonstrated the ability of GM-CSF to raise peripheral leukocyte counts in patients with primary bone marrow disorders. Nearly all patients treated with GM-CSF have had an increase in circulating neutrophils. Eosinophil and monocyte numbers have also increased, although more variably. In aplastic anemia, the height of the neutrophil response appears to correlate with the severity of the pretreatment neutropenia.[352] GM-CSF has been given by a variety of dosing schedules, and a dose-dependent response is generally seen. In most studies, peripheral blood counts rapidly fell to their pretreatment values when GM-CSF administration was discontinued. In several patients with myelodysplasia, peripheral counts did not return to baseline before the next cycle of GM-CSF commenced.[354] Immediately after administration of GM-CSF (within minutes), an abrupt fall in leukocyte counts is observed, perhaps due to sequestration of neutrophils in the lungs or elsewhere. A subsequent rise in leukocyte counts is then seen, probably reflecting changes in the distribution of neutrophils. After several weeks of therapy, bone marrow cellularity increased in patients with aplastic anemia, reflecting the stimulatory effects of GM-CSF on bone marrow proliferation. Although platelet counts and hemoglobin concentrations increased in one study of myelodysplastic patients,[354] the increase in platelet and erythrocyte numbers has been slight and often of little clinical significance. The most prolonged continuous intravenous administration of GM-CSF in patients with aplastic anemia reported is 3 months.[352] Toxicities reported were not significantly different from those seen after 2 weeks of GM-CSF at comparable doses.

GM-CSF has been administered after chemotherapy for sarcoma, and the period of neutropenia was shortened, allowing more chemotherapy to be administered within a given period.[345] GM-CSF has also been administered after bone marrow autotransplantation in an attempt to speed hematologic recovery.[355,356] Because of the ability of GM-CSF to stimulate AML cells in culture, these studies were performed in patients with lymphoid malignancies or solid tumors. Nineteen patients with breast cancer or melanoma were given a 14-day, continuous infusion of rGM-CSF at doses ranging from 2 to 32 μg/kg/d, beginning 3 hours after bone marrow infusion.[356] Although the time required to achieve a neutrophil count of more than 500/μL was not significantly shortened compared with historical controls, the incidence of bacteremia was reduced from 35% in controls to 16% in the GM-CSF–treated patients. After GM-CSF administration was stopped, neutrophil counts returned to expected posttransplantation levels, usually less than 500/μL at 14 days after transplantation. In a second study,[355] 14 patients undergoing autologous bone marrow transplantation for lymphoid malignancies received intravenous GM-CSF for 14 days at doses from 15 to 240 μg/m^2/d (about 0.4 to 6.4 μg/kg/d). Patients receiving less than 60 μg/m^2/d (ie, less than 1.6 μg/kg/d) had no significant response, whereas patients receiving 60 μg/m^2/d or more achieved an absolute neutrophil count of more than 500/μL earlier than historical controls. Platelet recovery and days of fever higher than 38°C were also improved by GM-CSF administration at doses of 60 μg/m^2/d or more. No consistent effects were seen on platelet or red-cell counts. The average length of hospital stay was markedly shortened by GM-CSF administration (from 41 to 29 days).

Doses of GM-CSF of more than 16 μg/kg/d have not been well tolerated by patients undergoing bone marrow transplantation or by patients with aplastic anemia. Doses of 32 μg/kg/d or more have been associated with pulmonary infiltrates, pleuritis, pericarditis, edema, or debilitating myalgia. The toxicity appears to be directly related to the dose of GM-CSF administered rather than due to increased numbers of activated circulating cells.

Granulocyte Colony-Stimulating Factor

Granulocyte colony-stimulating factor has been given by both subcutaneous and intravenous routes to patients undergoing combination chemotherapy. G-CSF administration results in an increase in the number of circulating neutrophils, although at high doses, a slight increase in monocytes is also seen. G-CSF administration has been well tolerated, with bone pain as the most frequent side effect. Examination of functional properties of the G-CSF–induced neutrophils has shown them to be normal.[357]

A study of G-CSF in patients receiving combination chemotherapy for small cell lung cancer demonstrated the ability of G-CSF to considerably shorten the period of absolute neutropenia.[344] The neutrophil nadir was not altered by G-CSF, but neutrophil recovery was hastened, and patients receiving G-CSF had fewer febrile episodes. Similar to GM-CSF, G-CSF administration is associated with a transient decrease in neutrophil counts, followed by a rise above baseline values, presumably due to release of neutrophils into the CNP. The increase in neutrophil counts after days or weeks of G-CSF administration is associated with increases in bone marrow cellularity and presumably reflects the stimulation of myeloid progenitors.

Other studies using G-CSF to abrogate chemotherapy-induced neutropenia have confirmed its effectiveness.[343,358] G-CSF administration to 27 patients with urothelial malignancies undergoing M-VAC chemotherapy showed significant shortening of the duration of significant neutropenia (less than 1000/μL) and no serious toxicity.[343] The number of patients able to receive their planned doses of chemotherapy increased from 29% to 100%; the incidence of mucositis decreased from 44% to 11%. Before receiving chemotherapy, patients received a 6-day course of G-CSF at 1 to 60 μg/kg/d; all patients receiving 3 μg/kg/d or more of G-CSF had a doubling of neutrophil counts. G-CSF has been administered to patients with a variety of solid tumors, and in all studies, a beneficial effect on neutrophil recovery after chemotherapy has been demonstrated.

G-CSF has also been used to treat neutropenia associated with a primary hematologic disorder. Four patients with hairy-cell leukemia received daily subcutaneous injections of G-CSF at 1 to 6 μg/kg/d for 2 to 6 weeks.[357] One patient developed Sweets's syndrome (acute neutrophilic vasculitis of the skin) during the second week of therapy and was withdrawn from the study. The other patients had an increase in absolute neutrophil counts at 1 μg/kg/d, with an initial rise within 3 days of therapy. After the initial rise in neutrophil counts, a dose-dependent increase in neutrophils was noted. Neutrophil levels fell rapidly after G-CSF was discontinued. Two patients cleared recurrent or resistant infections that were present at the initiation of G-CSF therapy.

G-CSF has been administered to patients with idiopathic neutropenia[342] and cyclic neutropenia.[341] The patient with idiopathic neutropenia had normalization of her absolute neutrophil count and healing of chronic oral ulcerations on 3 μg/kg/d subcutaneous G-CSF. The effectiveness of G-CSF therapy for patients with congenital neutropenia has been well demonstrated.[340] Patients with cyclic neutropenia have continued to display cyclic hematopoiesis, but the numbers of circulating neutrophils at nadir is substantially increased, which may serve to prevent repetitive infection by eliminating or decreasing the period of risk.

M-CSF

A modest effect of purified natural M-CSF on granulocyte counts after cancer chemotherapy has been reported.[359] Purified human M-CSF was given to patients with chronic neutropenia of childhood; in most patients, transient increases in neutrophil counts were seen within 4 weeks.[360] Natural M-CSF has also been given after bone marrow transplantation to enhance hematopoietic recovery. Compared with nonrandomized controls, the time recovery of neutrophil counts, to more than 500/μL and more than 1000/μL, was significantly shorter in the M-CSF–treated patients.[361] Side effects in both these studies were minimal. Phase I studies of recombinant M-CSF indicate low toxicity and stimulation of mononuclear phagocyte production. Clinical trials using M-CSF as an adjunct in the treatment of resistant fungal infections are underway.

From initial clinical trials, it appears that G-CSF elevates neutrophil counts with less accompanying toxicity than GM-CSF, which may be due in part to the absence of stimulatory effects on macrophages and eosinophils. The eosinophilia that frequently accompanies chronic administration of GM-CSF is of unknown significance but may also be responsible for some of the side effects of longer-term GM-CSF administration. As experience accumulates with the use of combinations of CSFs, a specific cocktail of CSFs may prove most efficacious for each clinical indication. With further understanding of the role the macrophage plays in hematopoiesis, host defense, and tumoricidal activity, factors that stimulate the macrophage (GM-CSF or M-CSF) may be applied in a clinically advantageous manner. Enhanced in vitro macrophage tumoricidal activity has been demonstrated in patients receiving GM-CSF.[362] Similarly, both GM-CSF[363] and M-CSF[364] administration are associated with a lowering of serum cholesterol.

NEUTROPHILIA

Neutrophilia is arbitrarily defined as an absolute blood neutrophil count greater than 7500/μL in adults.[365] As shown in Table 17-2, neonates have neutrophilia. For unexplained reasons, newborns of hypertensive mothers have higher average blood neutrophil counts than infants of normotensives.[366] Most commonly, neutrophilia results from increased production or release of cells from the bone marrow, although it may also result from a shift of marginated cells to the CNP. Such a change in distribution of neutrophils is sometimes referred to as *pseudoneutrophilia*. Acute neutrophilia can occur in response to severe pain, exercise, extremes of heat and cold, epileptic seizures, or emotional stress. This neutrophilia results from adrenergic stimulation, which increases the basal neutrophil count from 1.5- to 2-fold for 1 to 2 hours.[367]

Glucocorticoids and etiocholanolone can also cause acute neutrophilia,[368,369] which frequently reflects a shift in neutrophil distribution. Glucocorticoids raise the peripheral blood neutrophil count by increasing neutrophil production and also by diminishing the rate of egress of neutrophils from the circulation.[66] In the clinical setting, neutrophilia can accompany the hyperglucocorticism of adrenal endocrinopathy, specifically Cushing's syndrome or, more commonly, the iatrogenic administration of synthetic corticosteroids for therapeutic purposes. A single dose of hydrocortisone (200 mg) or prednisone (40 mg) elevates the neutrophil count by an average of 4000/μL within 5 to 6 hours.[368] During persistent exposure to corticosteroids, the neutrophil count remains elevated, although it may fall somewhat after 2 weeks of treatment.[369]

The most common reason for neutrophilia in the clinical setting is inflammatory disease due to microbial infection or to ischemic, autoimmune, or traumatic injury causing tissue necrosis. Multiple mechanisms may contribute to the neutrophilia, including release of microbial and host tissue constituents that cause neutrophil mobilization from the bone marrow, adrenergic stimulation, increased corticosteroid release, and enhanced elaboration of cytokines that promote myelopoiesis. When the combination of factors is intense, very high neutrophil counts can be encountered as well as immature myeloid forms in the blood. This picture is designated a *leukemoid reaction*. In chronic inflammatory states, neutrophilia can persist for long periods, indicating an enormous capacity of the bone marrow to produce neutrophils. It has been reported, however, that neonates with sepsis can deplete their neutrophil reserves and thereafter more readily succumb to the infection.[370]

Lithium can produce a neutrophilia in patients with psychiatric disorders[371] and can ameliorate neutropenia in occasional patients with a variety of underlying disorders.[372–374] Lithium acts by stimulating leukocyte production rather than altering the distribution, function, or lifespan of neutrophils.[375] Lithium may cause neutrophilia through enhanced production of CSF,[376] direct stimulation of hematopoietic stem cells, and potentiation of the in vitro effects of CSF on myeloid colony formation.[377] Lithium has considerable neurologic and endocrinologic toxicity and is therefore not routinely recommended to treat neutropenia.

A variety of inflammatory conditions (vasculitis, gout) or tumors can cause neutrophilia. Lung cancer, gastric cancer, and renal carcinoma have all been associated with elevated leukocyte counts.[378,379] Production of CSF has been postulated as the mechanism of the sustained neutrophilia associated with certain tumors. In several instances, production of CSF by tumor cells has been demonstrated.[380] A variety of hereditary conditions associated with neutrophilia have been reported, as has neutrophilia after splenectomy. Neutrophil counts can also be elevated in relation to a primary hematologic disorder, including CML and AML. Other myeloproliferative disorders, such as polycythemia vera, essential thrombocythemia, and agnogenic myeloid metaplasia, are associated with neutrophilia. Pregnancy,[381] rebound from a drug- or therapy-induced agranulocytosis, and metabolic disorders such as acidosis or various poisonings can also lead to neutrophilia.

The major distinction to be made in an elevated leukocyte count consisting of predominantly mature blood neutrophils is whether the patient has a leukemoid reaction, CML, or another myeloproliferative disorder. Absence of eosinophilia, thrombocytosis, nucleated RBCs, splenomegaly, and a normal bone marrow cell karyotype favor the diagnosis of leukemoid reaction. The leukocyte alkaline phosphatase score should be normal or elevated in a leukemoid reaction and markedly decreased in CML (see Chap. 15). Cytogenetic data can be obtained, looking for the Philadelphia chromosome, or molecular studies can be performed to detect the *bcr/abl* rearrangement, to identify the malignant cells of CML. The presence of splenomegaly would also point to diagnosis of a myeloproliferative disorder.

LIFE CYCLE OF MONONUCLEAR PHAGOCYTES

Morphologic Development

Monocytes are derived with neutrophils from a common progenitor cell, the CFU-GM.[382,383] Monoblasts arise from monocyte-committed progenitor cells derived from the CFU-GM.[384] Monoblasts mature into promonocytes, which are the first morphologically identifiable cells in the monocyte–macrophage series[385] (Fig. 17-7). Although the

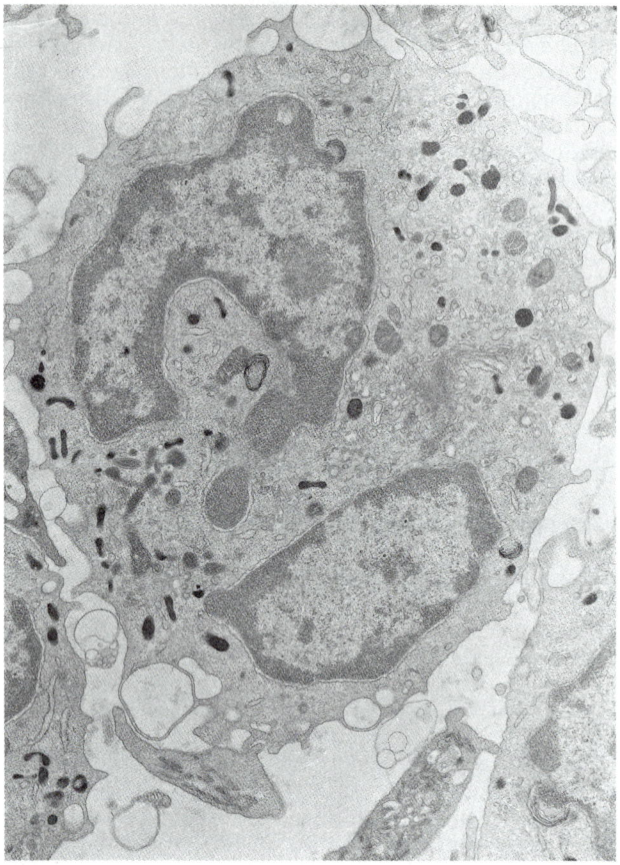

FIGURE 17-7. Development of mononuclear phagocytes. (Cline MJ, Golde DW. A review and reevaluation of the histiocytic disorders. Am J Med 1973;55:49)

decision to differentiate toward monocytes or granulocytes is thought to be made at the level of CFU-GM, differentiation studies with both HL-60 and KG-1 myeloid leukemia cell lines suggest that morphologically identifiable myeloid cells (promyelocytes and myeloblasts, respectively) may still be capable of differentiating along the monocyte–macrophage pathway.

Monoblasts appear identical to myeloblasts at the light microscopic level. They are about 15 μm in diameter and have a clear, deep-blue cytoplasm when stained with Wright Giemsa. There is a large eccentrically placed nucleus, which is indented and contains prominent nucleoli. The promonocyte is larger than the monoblast (up to 18 μm in diameter) and contains a few peroxidase-positive primary granules in a basophilic cytoplasm. The promonocyte nucleus is usually irregularly shaped and indented, containing minimally condensed chromatin and one nucleolus. The monocyte is the largest cell circulating in the blood (12 to 20 μm in diameter) and has a characteristically folded nucleus that is eccentrically placed. Peroxidase-positive and peroxidase-negative granules and many vacuoles are present in the abundant gray-blue cytoplasm.

Electron microscopy demonstrates a progression of ultrastructural features associated with maturation from the monoblast to the monocyte stage. The promonocyte has a well-developed endoplasmic reticulum and an active Golgi apparatus synthesizing peroxidase and other granule components. Promonocytes contain unique bundles of cytoplasmic filaments, which distinguish them from promyelocytes.[386] Peripheral blood monocytes demonstrate surface features consistent with their phagocytic and motile capabilities. Viewed under the scanning electron microscope, the monocyte surface is extensively ruffled, with finger-like microvilli that extend in a polar fashion during cell movement. The monocyte cytoplasm has many microtubules, filament bundles, mitochondria, and an active Golgi apparatus (Fig. 17-8).

The macrophage is a large cell (15 to 80 μm in diameter) with an oval shape and an eccentric nucleus. Its cell membrane is highly ruffled, and there are frequent pseudopodia (arm-like projections). The cytoplasm is clear and often contains ingested particulate matter. There is an extensive endoplasmic reticulum, a prominent Golgi complex, and peroxidase-negative granules. During transformation from the monocyte to the macrophage stage, the cell enlarges 5- to 10-fold, develops vacuoles, begins to spread over surfaces, and loses its peroxidase-positive granules.[387] The nuclear chromatin becomes clumped, and the potential for more active oxidative metabolism is evidenced by an increase in number and activity of mitochondria and more active glycolysis.[388] Activated macrophages are larger than resting cells and have a greater number of cytoplasmic granules, enhanced ability to phagocytize particles, and increased metabolism of glucose through the hexose monophosphate shunt.

Functional Maturation

As MNPs mature from bone marrow precursors to tissue macrophages, they acquire increasing ability to phagocytose microorganisms. Although the promonocyte has few receptors for the Fc portion of IgG and has limited phagocytic capability, mature monocytes express greater numbers of Fc and complement receptors and contain a greater amount of lysozyme. Both promonocytes and monocytes adhere to glass.

Two functionally distinct populations of granules can be detected in bone marrow promonocytes and blood monocytes.[389,390] Monocytes contain a number of hydrolytic enzymes also found in neutrophils, including lysozyme, peroxidase, acid phosphatase, β-glucuronidase, sulfatase, N-acetylglucosaminidase, cathepsins, lipases, elastases, collagenases, plasminogen activator, and nucleases.[391] Monocytes cannot hydrolyze naphthol AS-D chloroacetate, but they hydrolyze esters such as α-naphthyl butyrate and α-naphthyl acetate, which are nonspecific esterase markers

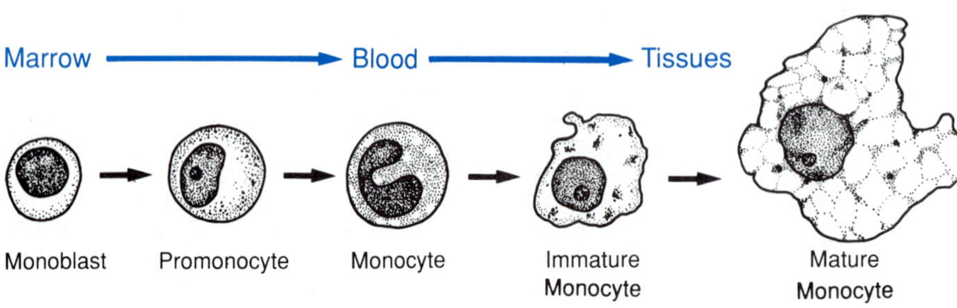

FIGURE 17-8. Mature monocyte. A nucleolus is clearly visible; the abundance of cytoplasmic organelles (Golgi apparatus, rough endoplasmic reticulum, mitochondria) reflects the functional capabilities of the monocyte. (Morris RB, Nichols BA, Bainton DF. Ultrastructure and peroxidase cytochemistry of normal human leukocytes at birth. Dev Biol 1975;44:233)

for MNPs.[392,393] Monocyte esterase is inhibited by sodium fluoride.[394]

Two major subsets of monocytes have been identified, based on functional and morphologic criteria.[395–397] One subset has receptors for the chemoattractant, f-MLP, and receptors for C5a. These monocyte subsets can also be separated by size and density. The slightly larger cells have more intense peroxidase activity and strongly express M1 antigen. The monocyte subset with low peroxidase activity lacks both M1 antigen and a receptor for pokeweed mitogen. The subsets are apparently not a reflection of age of the monocyte.

As described in Chapter 19, monocytes and macrophages play a vital role in multiple host functions, including initiation and regulation of the immune response, phagocytosis and killing of microorganisms, phagocytosis and degradation of aging cells and cellular debris, secretion of various biologically active substances, and antitumor effects. They are "professional" phagocytes. Their ability to phagocytose organisms can be enhanced by a variety of means, including coating of these organisms by complement or immunoglobulin and activation of the macrophage by exposure to bacterial products, adherence to glass, or exposure to various cytokines. Denatured proteins, antigen complexes, activating clotting factors, and aging RBCs are all cleared by macrophages. MNPs are also important in the removal of blood cells coated by antibodies. Thus, in autoimmune hemolytic anemias, thrombocytopenia, or neutropenia, the macrophage plays an important role in reducing the number of circulating cells, a process that may occur by means of the macrophage C3b and IgG-1 and IgG-3 Fc receptors.

Macrophages also respond to C5a, N-formylated bacterial peptides, and hydroxylated derivatives of arachidonic acid. Activated macrophages release a variety of substances (see Chap. 19) that can activate neutrophils (eg, TNF, GM-CSF, neutrophil activating factor) and mesenchymal cells (eg, IL-1, TNF, platelet-derived growth factor). Macrophages and T lymphocytes interact extensively to provide cellular immune function.[398–400] Macrophages present antigen to T cells in the setting of class II major histocompatibility complex compatibility,[401] and macrophage products such as IL-1 are involved in activating T cells to perform effector functions. Activated T cells can release substances, including IFN-γ, GM-CSF, and IL-3, which can enhance various macrophage functions.

Mononuclear Phagocyte Kinetics

It is difficult to measure precisely the behavior of monoblasts because they lack distinctive features separating them from myeloblasts. The mature monocyte is derived from its earliest morphologically identifiable precursor after at least three divisions. The generation time for promonocytes from earlier progenitors is about 30 to 48 hours in humans, and tritiated thymidine-labeling studies suggest that about 80% of promonocytes are in S phase.[402] The time required for a promonocyte to undergo division is about 19.5 hours. After completing their last division, most monocytes leave the bone marrow space within a 24-hour period. Promonocytes constitute about 3% of bone marrow cells, whereas blood monocytes represent 3% to 11% of circulating leukocytes. The total number of monocytes in the bone marrow is estimated at 7.3×10^9 cells.[402] Unlike neutrophils, there is no appreciable bone marrow storage pool of monocytes.[403] The presence of an MBP of peripheral monocytes in humans has been suggested[404] but not definitively shown.[402,405] Circulating monocytes leave the blood randomly; that is, their exit from the blood is independent of their time of entry into the blood from bone marrow. Tritiated thymidine-labeled monocytes are cleared from the circulation with a half-life of about 71 hours (range of 36 to 104 hours), although estimates of the half-life of monocytes in the blood have varied widely depending on the methods used.[402,406] Once monocytes leave the blood, they do not reenter the circulation.

Blood monocytes can enter tissue, where they may participate in inflammatory reactions or die by unknown means. The monocytes can also provide a renewal source for tissue macrophages. Studies in animal and human bone marrow transplantation indicate that the resident tissue macrophages ultimately are derived from bone marrow precursors. Thus, pulmonary alveolar macrophages, Kupffer cells, and dermal Langerhans cells become of donor type after successful bone marrow engraftment.[407,408] It has been estimated that by 100 days after transplantation, all recipient alveolar macrophages are replaced by cells of donor type.[409] Peritoneal and pleural macrophages, osteoclasts,[410] and microglial cells of the brain are also resident macrophages derived from bone marrow precursors. Osteopetrosis, caused by a deficiency in osteoclast activity, can be successfully treated by bone marrow transplantation.[411]

Although tissue macrophage populations derive from the bone marrow, they are not dependent on an influx of marrow-derived cells to maintain their numbers.[412,413] Tissue macrophages have proliferative capability and can sustain their populations by replication in situ. The precise relation between local macrophage replication and mononuclear cell influx from the bone marrow in the maintenance of resident macrophage populations is uncertain. In general, tissue macrophages have a low ^{3}H-thymidine–labeling index,[405] suggesting that a small proportion of the cells are in active cell cycle. Studies using fluorescent dyes for in situ labeling of resident peritoneal macrophages and recruited macrophages demonstrated no replacement of resident macrophages by recruited blood monocytes in the steady state over a 7-week period.[414] Macrophages in inflammatory tissue exudates, however, are largely derived from circulating blood monocytes.[403]

Gene Expression

Protooncogenes are thought to play a critical role in the process of cellular growth and differentiation. Whereas TPA-induced differentiation of HL-60 cells toward macrophages results in decreased expression of c-*myc*[415] and c-*myb*,[416] increased amounts of c-*fos* and c-*fms* accumulate in hematopoietic cells as monocytic maturation proceeds. Expression of these oncogenes may be directly related to the differentiation process.[417–419] Rapid induction of c-*fos* is seen in TPA-induced monocytic differentiation of the HL-60 and U937 cell lines,[420] and high levels of c-*fos* have also been detected in primary cultures of peritoneal macrophages.[421] Low basal levels of c-*fos* transcripts are seen in pure myeloid subtypes of AML, whereas high constitutive c-*fos* expression was detected in the M4 and M5 monocytic subtypes of AML.[422] The levels of c-*fos* RNA correlate with expression of the CD14 (Mo-2) antigen and expression of sodium fluoride–inhibitable α-napthyl acetate esterase. Yet, despite these correlations, studies examining differentiation of HL-60 variants by vitamin D_3 or TPA have demonstrated that c-*fos* expression is not essential for monocyte differentiation.[423]

HL-60 cells can be differentiated toward monocytes by incubation with phorbol diesters,[424,425] 1,25 dihydroxyvitamin D_3,[426,427] or stimulated lymphocyte-conditioned medium (PHA-LCM). These agents can have differential effects on gene expression. Thus, PHA-LCM (which contains IFN-γ[428] and other lymphokines) induces expression of Mo-1 and Mo-2 surface antigens, whereas phorbol diesters such as phorbol-myristate acetate (PMA) induce only Mo-1 expression.[429] Morphologic differentiation of HL-60 cells toward monocytes by vitamin D derivatives is accompanied by increases in secreted lysozyme, nonspecific acid esterase activity, nitroblue tetrazolium (NBT) reduction, phagocytic activity, f-MLP receptor, and Mac-120 surface antigen expression.[430] In contrast, PMA-treated HL-60 cells demonstrate only weak NBT reduction,[431] and although they show a marked increase in OKM-1 positivity, they do not express the monocyte-specific marker, 61D3. Deprivation of a single essential amino acid also results in differentiation of HL-60 cells toward monocytes,[432] defined by OKM-1 or anti-Leu M3 antigen expression. This effect may be the result of a decrease in DNA synthesis since as other interventions that decrease DNA synthesis are also associated with monocytic differentiation of HL-60 cells.

TNF-α can also induce differentiation of myeloid leukemia cells toward monocyte-like cells.[433] Treatment of HL-60 cells with TNF-α had no effect on cell growth or thymidine incorporation but did enhance the nonspecific esterase activity and increase superoxide production, NBT reduction, and acid phosphatase content of the cells. TNF-α synergized with both IFN-γ and 1,25 dihydroxyvitamin D_3 in its effects on the functional activity of these cells and on the expression of monocyte antigens such as Leu M3 (CD14) and OKM-1 (CD11).[434]

HL-60 cells differentiated toward monocytes still display granulocyte-specific markers[435]; thus, they are not fully suitable for studying monocyte differentiation processes. IFN-γ treatment increases antibody-dependent cell-mediated cytotoxicity and surface antigen expression on HL-60 cells.[428] IFN-γ also induces an increase in Fc receptor expression on both HL-60 and U937 cells,[436] which may not be linked to monocytoid differentiation. Additional polypeptide factors capable of inducing monocyte differentiation of HL-60 cells have been characterized and are referred to as *differentiation-inducing factors* (DIFs, also referred to as leukemia inhibitory factors). DIFs were originally described as products of mitogen-stimulated human mononuclear cells[437] but are also produced by T cells[438] and T-cell and monocytic cell lines, such as HUT-102[439] and THP-1,[440] respectively. The DIFs represent a family of polypeptides, and were originally described as a murine factor (D factor) capable of inducing differentiation of murine myeloid leukemia M1 cells. Human macrophage DIF is equivalent to murine leukemia inhibitory factor.[440] Although DIFs have potent differentiation-inducing effects on HL-60 cells, many have little or no effect on U937 cells.

Differentiation of the U937 cell line into monocyte- or macrophage-like cells occurs in response to phorbol diesters, retinoic acid,[441] vitamin D_3,[442] IFN-γ,[443,444] TNF-α, GM-CSF,[445] G-CSF,[446] and a 45- to 55-kd, heat-stable T-cell lymphokine that is distinct from IFN-γ or GM-CSF.[447] U937 cells cannot be induced to differentiate toward granulocytic lineages; thus, they have been useful in studying monocyte and macrophage development. Uninduced U937 cells do not express the c-*fms* gene (which encodes the M-CSF receptor) and therefore do not respond to M-CSF. Exposure of U937 cells to GM-CSF results in induction of c-*fms* expression, allowing the cells to respond to M-CSF, and also leads to expression of C3bi receptors, prominent nonspecific esterase activity, and development of a respiratory burst, as measured by NBT reduction. GM-CSF also induces Mo-1 expression and stimulates TNF-α production, which may have additional effects on monocytes. M-CSF can increase My4 antigen expression (CD14) on peripheral blood monocytes.[446]

Expression of c-*mos* RNA has been observed in U937 cells as they differentiate into macrophages in response to TPA or macrophage differentiation-inducing factor. Inducible expression of the v-*mos* gene in U937 cells results in their differentiation into macrophages.[448] Cell growth was inhibited in proportion to the amount of *mos* mRNA produced, and cells expressing *mos* became adherent and developed the ability to reduce NBT and generate superoxide anions. These cells also became phagocytic and increased their expression of IgG Fc receptors and the Mac-1 surface antigen. Continuous synthesis of a certain amount of *mos* was required for maintenance of the differentiated phenotype, and the quantity of macrophage-associated characteristics corresponded well with the amount of *mos* RNA present. Although *mos* expression by itself does not appear to be sufficient to trigger the differentiation process, expression of *mos* is closely related to activation of a variety of genes involved in macrophage differentiation.

IL-8 is an 8- to 10-kd peptide,[449] also known as monocyte-derived neutrophil chemotactic factor or neutrophil-activating factor (NAF), produced by human monocytes stimulated by lipopolysaccharide, phytohemagglutinin or Con A,[450] lectin-stimulated lymphocytes,[451,452] and stimulated fibroblasts and endothelial cells. NAF is chemotactic for neutrophils and can enhance many of their functional activities. IL-8 induces neutrophil shape change, respiratory burst, and the exocytosis of specific and azurophilic neutrophil granules.[453,454] NAF is partially homologous to β-thromboglobulin and PAF-4.[455]

Regulation of Mononuclear Phagocyte Production

Monocytes and macrophages elaborate a variety of factors that stimulate or inhibit MNP proliferation.[456] These factors include GM-CSF, M-CSF, IL-1, TNF, and IFN.[457] Peripheral blood monocytes stimulated by IFN-γ, PMA, GM-CSF, or TNF[458] produce M-CSF, and mouse peritoneal macrophages produce GM-CSF after cycloheximide treatment or stimulation by adherence or endotoxin.[126,216,217] Production of M-CSF and GM-CSF by MNPs is potentially important in stimulating monocyte production by an autocrine mechanism. Clearance of M-CSF by macrophages has also been implicated in controlling the rate of macrophage production.[459]

Although active in generating murine macrophage colonies, human M-CSF by itself has relatively weak ability to stimulate human macrophage colony formation. However, in combination with IL-1[184] or suboptimal concentrations of GM-CSF,[175] M-CSF is a potent stimulator of macrophage proliferation. M-CSF is present in serum[170] and urine, and in vivo administration of M-CSF results in increased numbers of promonocytes and monocytes. M-CSF appears to be important in the day-to-day regulation of monocyte numbers.

GM-CSF can directly stimulate macrophage colony formation at low concentrations and can prime marrow precursor cells to respond to M-CSF. GM-CSF is produced by stromal cells, such as fibroblasts and endothelial cells, after stimulation by monocyte-derived IL-1 or TNF-α,[127–129] and may also play an important role in controlling macrophage production, particularly during the inflammatory response. Because GM-CSF can stimulate production of TNF by MNPs, several positive feedback loops may exist.[460] The role of the T lymphocyte and its secretory products in the day-to-day control of monocyte proliferation is unknown. Activated T cells produce IL-3 and GM-CSF, suggesting a role for these mediators in stimulating macrophage production and function during immune responses. IL-3 stimulates macrophage colony formation and may act to make macrophage progenitors responsive to more lineage-restricted growth factors, such as GM-CSF and M-CSF.[461]

A variety of factors have been suggested to function as negative regulators of MNP proliferation. Of these, prostaglandin E, lactoferrin, and TNF have all been shown to have inhibitory effects on formation of phagocytic cells in vitro.[462,463] By contrast, TNF-α reportedly supports the viability of skin macrophages (Langerhans cells) in culture but does not affect the maturation of monocytes.[464] Because prostaglandin E is produced by macrophages, it may serve in negative-feedback regulation.[465] Lactoferrin, which is produced by neutrophils, suppresses CSF production by MNPs.[201,466] Tumor growth factor-β (TGF-β), which is secreted by activated macrophages,[467] similarly can inhibit proliferation of macrophages in response to M-CSF.[468]

Monocytosis

In the normal adult, between 1% and 9% of the circulating leukocytes are monocytes. Absolute monocyte counts range from 300 to 700 cells/μL. Monocyte counts of more than 800 cells/μL constitute monocytosis in adults.[469] Monocytosis is normal during the first few weeks of life (see Table 17-2),[470] and children tend to have higher monocyte counts than adults. Increases in monocyte numbers frequently accompany neutrophilia. Because the monocyte plays an important role in immunologic reactions and the host response to neoplasia, a variety of inflammatory, neoplastic, and immune conditions can result in monocytosis.[471] Tuberculosis is associated with a brisk monocytosis,[472] as are chronic infections such as subacute bacterial endocarditis[473] and secondary syphilis.[474] Monocytosis is also seen in response to malignancies,[475] especially lymphomas and Hodgkin's disease,[476,477] and can accompany lipid storage or connective tissue diseases such as rheumatoid arthritis, systemic lupus erythematosus, sarcoidosis, and polyarteritis nodosum. Modest monocytosis is seen in preleukemic conditions.[478] A variety of malignant monocyte disorders have been identified, including acute monocytic leukemia and acute or chronic myelomonocytic leukemia.[479–482]

Monocytosis may also occur after recovery from chemotherapy or drug-induced agranulocytosis or as a compensatory event in association with neutropenic disorders such as cyclic neutropenia. This stem cell disorder is marked by striking periodicity of neutrophil production, often reciprocal to the periodicity affecting monocytes; monocyte numbers change reciprocally to neutrophil numbers and may reach peaks of over 5000 cells/μL.

Monocytopenia

Monocytopenia is observed in patients receiving chronic corticosteroid therapy, even when prednisone is administered on an alternate-day basis.[483,484] Monocytopenia is also seen in conjunction with neutropenia in diseases such as hairy-cell leukemia,[485,486] aplastic anemia,[487] AIDS, and infiltrative diseases of the bone marrow.

REFERENCES

1. Dancey JT, Deubelbeiss KA, Harker LA, Finch CA. Neutrophil kinetics in man. J Clin Invest 1976;58:705.
2. Donohue DM, Reiff RH, Hanson ML, et al. Quantitative measurement of the erythrocytic and granulocytic cells of the marrow and blood. J Clin Invest 1958;37:1511.
3. Cronkite EP, Vincent PC. Granulocytopoiesis. Ser Haematol II 1969;4: 3.
4. Bainton DF, Ullyot JL, Farquhar MG. The development of neutrophilic polymorphonuclear leukocytes in human bone marrow. J Exp Med 1971;134:907.
5. Bainton DF, Farquhar MG. Differences in enzyme content of azurophil and specific granules of polymorphonuclear leukocytes. II. Cytochemistry and electron microscopy of bone marrow cells. J Cell Biol 1968;39:299.
6. Bainton DF, Farquhar MG. Differences in enzyme content of azurophil and specific granules of polymorphonuclear leukocytes. I. Histochemical staining of bone marrow smears. J Cell Biol 1968;39:286.
7. Schultz J, Corlin R, Oddi F, et al. Myeloperoxidase of the leukocyte of normal blood. III. Isolation of the peroxidase granule. Arch Biochem Biophys 1965;111:73.
8. Bretz V, Baggiolini M. Biochemical and morphological characterization of azurophil and specific granules of human neutrophilic polymorphonuclear leukocytes. J Cell Biol 1974;63:251.
9. Olsson I. Isolation of human leukocyte granules using colloidal silica-polysaccharide density gradients. Exp Cell Res 1969;54:325.
10. Dewald B, Rindler-Ludwig R, Bretz U, Baggiolini M. Subcellular localization and heterogeneity of neutral proteases in neutrophilic polymorphonuclear leukocytes. J Exp Med 1975;141:709.
11. Olsson I, Venge P. Cationic proteins of human granulocytes. II. Separation of the cationic proteins of the granules of leukemic myeloid cells. Blood 1974;44:235.
12. Ganz T, Selsted ME, Szklarek D, et al. Defensins: natural peptide antibiotics of human neutrophils. J Clin Invest 1985;76:1427.
13. Elsbach P, Weiss J, Franson RC, et al. Separation and purification of a potent bactericidal/permeability-increasing protein and a closely associated phospholipase A_2 from rabbit polymorphonuclear leukocytes. J Biol Chem 1979;254:11000.
14. Gabay JE, Heiple JM, Cohn ZA, Nathan CF. Subcellular location and properties of bactericidal factors from human neutrophils. J Exp Med 1986;164:1407.
15. Spitznagel JK, Dalldorf FG, Leffell MS, et al. Character of azurophil and specific granules purified from human polymorphonuclear leukocytes. Lab Invest 1974;30:774.
16. Bainton DF, Miller LJ, Kishimoto TK, Springer TA. Leukocyte adhesion receptors are stored in peroxidase-negative granules of human neutrophils. J Exp Med 1987;166:1641.
17. Chenoweth DE, Hugli TE. Demonstration of specific C5a receptor on intact human polymorphonuclear leukocytes. Proc Natl Acad Sci USA 1978;75:3943.
18. Fletcher MP, Gallin JI. Degranulating stimuli increase the availability of receptors on human neutrophils for the chemoattractant f-Met-Leu-Phe. J Immunol 1980;124:1585.
19. O'Shea JJ, Brown EJ, Seligman BE, et al. Evidence for distinct intracellular pools of receptors for C3b and C3bi in human neutrophils. J Immunol 1985;134:2580.
20. Leffell MS, Spitznagel JK. Intracellular and extracellular degranulation of human polymorphonuclear azurophil and specific granules induced by immune complexes. Infect Immunol 1974;10:1241.
21. Gallin JI. Neutrophil specific granules: a fuse that ignites the inflammatory response. Clin Res 1984;32:320.
22. Goldstein IM. Neutrophil degranulation in regulation of leukocyte function. Contemp Top Immunobiol 1984;14:221.
23. Bentwood BJ, Henson PM. The sequential release of granule constituents from human neutrophils. J Immunol 1980;124:855.
24. Dewald B, Bretz U, Baggiolini MR. Release of gelatinase from a novel secretory compartment of human neutrophils. J Clin Invest 1982;70: 518.
25. Hibbs MS, Bainton DF. Human neutrophil gelatinase is a component of specific granules. J Clin Invest 1989;84:1395.
26. O'Flaherty JT, Surles JR, Redman J, et al. Binding and metabolism of platelet-activating factor by human neutrophils. J Clin Invest 1986;78: 381.
27. Goetzl EJ, Pickett CW. The human PMN leukocyte chemotactic activity of complex hydroxy-eicosatetraenoic acids (HETEs). J Immunol 1980;125:1789.
28. Williams LT, Snyderman R, Pike MC, Lefkowitz RJ. Specific receptor sites for chemotactic peptides on human polymorphonuclear leukocytes. Proc Natl Acad Sci USA 1977;74:1204.
29. Gallin J, Seligmann B. Neutrophil chemoattractant fMet-leu-Phe receptor expression and ionic events following activation. In: Synderman R, ed. Regulation of leukocyte function. New York, Plenum, 1984:83.
30. Messner RP, Jelinek J. Receptors for human γG globin on human neutrophils. J Clin Invest 1970;49:2165.
31. Unkeless JC, Scigliano E, Freedman VH. Structure and function of human and murine receptors for IgG. Annu Rev Immunol 1988;6: 251.
32. Berger M, O'Shea J, Cross AS, et al. Human neutrophils increase expression of C3bi as well as C3b receptors upon activation. J Clin Invest 1984;74:1566.
33. Wallace PJ, Packman CH, Lichtman MA. Maturation-associated changes in the peripheral cytoplasm of human neutrophils: a review. Exp Hematol 1987;15:34.
34. Herborn H, Valdimarsson H, Wickramasinghe SN. Development of human granulocyte and monocyte Fc receptors. Scand J Haematol 1979;22:364.
35. Glasser L, Fiederlein RL. Functional differentiation of normal human neutrophils. Blood 1987;69:937.
36. Niedel J, Wilkinson S, Cuatrecasas P. Receptor-mediated uptake and degradation of 125I-chemotactic peptide by human neutrophils. J Biol Chem 1979;254:10700.
37. Sullivan R, Griffin JD, Malech HL. Acquisition of formyl peptide re-

ceptors during normal human myeloid differentiation. Blood 1987;70:1222.
38. Altman AJ, Stossel TP. Functional immaturity of bone marrow bands and polymorphonuclear leucocytes. Br J Haematol 1974;27:241.
39. Berkow RL, Dodson RW. Purification and functional evaluation of mature neutrophils from human bone marrow. Blood 1986;68:853.
40. Johnson KR, Nauseef WM, Care A, et al. Characterization of cDNA clones for human myeloperoxidase: predicted amino acid sequence and evidence for multiple mRNA species. Nucleic Acids Res 1987;15:2013.
41. Morishita K, Kubota N, Asano S, et al. Molecular cloning and characterization of cDNA for human myeloperoxidase. J Biol Chem 1987;262:3844.
42. Weil SC, Rosner GL, Reid MS, et al. Translocation and rearrangement of myeloperoxidase gene in acute promyelocytic leukemia. Science 1988;240:790.
43. Weil SC, Rosner GL, Reid MS, et al. cDNA cloning of human myeloperoxidase: decrease in myeloperoxidase in mRNA upon induction of HL-60 cells. Proc Natl Acad Sci USA 1987;84:2057.
44. Rosmarin AG, Weil SC, Rosner GL, et al. Differential expression of CD11b/CD18 (Mol) and myeloperoxidase genes during myeloid differentiation. Blood 1989;73:131.
45. Sanchez-Madrid F, Nagy JA, Robbins E, et al. A human leukocyte differentiation antigen family with distinct α-subunits and a common α-subunit. J Exp Med 1983;158:1785.
46. Springer TA, Dustin ML, Kishimoto TK, Marlin SD. The lymphocyte function-associated LFA-1, CD2, and LFA-3 molecules: cell adhesion receptors of the immune system. Annu Rev Immunol 1987;5:223.
47. Corbi AL, Larson RS, Kishimoto TK, et al. Chromosomal location of the genes encoding the leukocyte adhesion receptors LFA-1, Mac-1 and p150, 85: identification of a gene cluster involved in cell adhesion. J Exp Med 1988;167:1597.
48. Milner J, Milner S. SV40-53K antigen: a possible role for 53K in normal cells. Virology 1981;112:785.
49. Reich N, Levine AJ. Growth regulation of a cellular tumour antigen, p53, in nontransformed cells. Nature 1984;308:199.
50. Kern SE, Kinzler KW, Bruskin A, et al. Identification of p53 as a sequence-specific DNA-binding protein. Science 1992;252:1708.
51. Koeffler HP, Miller C, Nicolson MA, et al. Increased expression of p53 protein in human leukemia cells. Proc Natl Acad Sci USA 1986;83:4035.
51a. Fenaux P, Preudhomme C, Quiquandon I, et al. Mutations of the P53 gene in acute myeloid leukaemia. Br J Haematol 1992;80:178.
52. McBride OW, Merry D, Givol D. The gene for human p53 cellular tumor antigen is located on chromosome 17 short arm (17p13). Proc Natl Acad Sci USA 1986;83:130.
52a. Ahuja H, Bar-Eli M, Advani SH, Benchimol S, Cline MJ. Alterations in the p53 gene and the clonal evolution of the blast crisis of chronic myelocytic leukemia. Proc Natl Acad Sci USA 1989;86:6783.
53. MacDonald I, Levy J, Pawson T. Expression of the mammalian c-fes protein in hematopoietic cells and identification of a distinct fes-related protein. Mol Cell Biol 1985;5:2543.
54. Koeffler HP. Induction of differentiation of human acute myelogenous leukemia cells: therapeutic implications. Blood 1983;62:709.
55. Bishop JM. Cellular oncogenes and retroviruses. Annu Rev Biochem 1983;52:301.
56. Gee CE, Griffin J, Sastre L, et al. Differentiation of myeloid cells is accompanied by increased levels of pp60c-src protein and kinase activity. Proc Natl Acad Sci USA 1986;83:5131.
57. Vincent PC. Granulocyte kinetics in health and disease. Clin Haematol 1977;6:695.
58. Warner HR, Athens JW. An analysis of granulocyte kinetics in blood and bone marrow. Ann NY Acad Sci 1964;113:523.
59. Athens JW, Haab OP, Raab SO, et al. Leukokinetic studies. IV. The total blood, circulating and marginal granulocyte pools and the granulocyte turnover rate in normal subjects. J Clin Invest 1961;40:989.
60. Athens JW, Raab SO, Haab OP, et al. Leukokinetic studies. III. The distribution of granulocytes in the blood of normal subjects. J Clin Invest 1961;40:159.
61. Cartwright GE, Athens JW, Wintrobe MM. The kinetics of granulopoiesis in normal man. Blood 1964;24:780.
62. Cronkite EP, Fliedner TM. Granulocytopoiesis. N Engl J Med 1964;270:1403.
63. Fliedner TM, Cronkite EP, Robertson JS. Granulocytopoiesis. 1. Senescence and random loss of neutrophilic granulocytes in human beings. Blood 1964;24:402.
64. Boggs DR, Athens JW, Cartwright GE, Wintrobe MM. "Masked" granulocytosis. Proc Soc Exp Biol Med 1965;118:753.
65. Walker RI, Herion JC, Herring WB, Palmer JG. Leukocyte kinetics in hematologic disorders studied by DNA-phosphorus labeling. Blood 1964;23:795.
66. Bishop CR, Athens JW, Boggs DR, et al. Leukokinetic studies. XIII. A non–steady-state kinetic evaluation of the mechanism of cortisone-induced granulocytosis. J Clin Invest 1968;47:249.
67. Maloney M, Patt HM. Granulocyte transit from bone marrow to blood. Blood 1968;31:195.
68. Osgood EE. Number and distribution of human hemic cells. Blood 1954;9:1141.
70. Golde DW, Gasson JC. Cytokines: myeloid growth factors. In: Gallin JI, Goldstein IM, Snyderman R, eds. Inflammation: basic principles and clinical correlates. New York, Raven, 1988:253.
71. Klebanoff SJ, Vadas MA, Harlem JM, et al. Stimulation of neutrophils by tumor necrosis factor. J Immunol 1986;136:4220.
72. Shalaby MR, Aggarwol BB, Rinderknecht E, et al. Activation of human polymorphonuclear neutrophil functions by interferon-γ and tumor necrosis factors. J Immunol 1985;135:2069.
73. Shaw JO, Pinckard RN, Ferrigni KS, et al. Activation of human neutrophils with 1-0-hexadecyl/octadecyl-2-acetyl-sn-glyceryl-3-phosphorylcholine (platelet activating factor). J Immunol 1981;127:1250.
74. Ford-Hutchinson AW, Bray MA, Doig MV, et al. Leukotriene B, a potent chemokinetic and aggregating substance released from polymorphonuclear leukocytes. Nature 1980;286:264.
75. Sanchez-Crespo M, Alonso F, Egido J. Platelet-activating factor in anaphylaxis and phagocytosis. Immunology 1980;40:645.
76. Snyderman R, Goetzl EJ. Molecular and cellular mechanisms of leukocyte chemotaxis. Science 1981;213:830.
77. Cleaver JE. Thymidine metabolism and cell kinetics. Amsterdam, North Holland, 1967.
78. Hughes WL, Bond VP, Brecher G, et al. Cellular proliferation in the mouse as revealed by autoradiography with tritiated thymidine. Proc Natl Acad Sci USA 1958;44:476.
79. Athens JW, Mauer AM, Ashenbrucker H, et al. Leukokinetic studies. I. A method for labeling leukocytes with diisopropylfluorophosphate (DFP32). Blood 1959;14:303.
80. Mauer AM, Athens JW, Ashenbrucker H, Cartwright GE. Leukokinetic studies. II. A method for labeling granulocytes in vitro with radioactive diisopropylfluorophosphate (DFP^{32}). J Clin Invest 1960;39:1481.
81. Dresch C, Najean Y, Bauchet J. Kinetic studies of ^{51}Cr and $DF^{32}P$ labelled granulocytes. Br J Haematol 1975;29:67.
82. Kurth D, Athens JW, Cronkite EP, et al. Leukokinetic studies. V. Uptake of tritiated diisopropylfluorophosphate by leukocytes. Proc Soc Exp Biol Med 1961;107:422.
83. Rothstein G, Bishop CR, Athens JW, Ashenbrucker HE. A method for leukokinetic study in the nonsteady state. Blood 1971;38:302.
84. McCall MS, Sutherland DA, Eisentraut AM, Lanz, H. The tagging of leukemic leukocytes with radioactive chromium and measurement of the in vivo cell survival. J Lab Clin Med 1955;45:717.
85. McMillan R, Scott JL. Leukocyte labeling with ^{51}chromium. I. Technic and results in normal subjects. Blood 1968;32:738.
86. Spivak JL, Perry S. Evaluation of ^{51}Cr as a leukocyte label. Br J Haematol 1973;25:321.
87. Eyre HJ, Rosen PJ, Perry S. Relative labeling of leukocytes, erythrocytes and platelets in human blood by ^{51}chromium. Blood 1970;36:250.
88. Meuret G, Hoffmann G, Fliedner TM, et al. Neutrophil kinetics in man: studies using autotransfusion of ^{3}H-DFP labeled blood cells and autoradiography. Blut 1972;4:10.
89. English D, Anderson BR. Labeling of phagocytes from human blood with ^{99m}Tc-sulfur colloid. J Nucl Med 1975;16:5.
90. Linhart N, Bok B, Gourgerot M, et al. ^{99m}Tc labelled human leukocytes. Acta Haematol 1980;63:71.
91. Froehlich JW, Swanson D. Imaging of inflammatory processes with labeled cells. Semin Nucl Med 1984;14:128.
92. McAfee JG, Thakur ML. Survey of radioactive agents for in vitro labeling of phagocytic leukocytes. I. Soluble agents. J Nucl Med 1976;17:480.
93. McAfee JG, Thakur ML. Survey of radioactive agents for in vitro labeling of phagocytic leukocytes. II. Particles. J Nucl Med 1976;17:488.
94. Catovsky D, Galton DAG, Griffin C, et al. Serum lysozome and vitamin B_{12} binding capacity in myeloproliferative disorders. Br J Haematol 1971;21:661.
95. Hansen NE. The relationship between the turnover rate of neutrophilic granulocytes and plasma lysozome levels. Br J Haematol 1973;25:771.
96. Levi JA, Macqueen A, Vincent PC. Assessment of the value of lysozome assay in neutropenia. Br J Haematol 1973;25:757.
97. Rachmilewitz B, Rachmilewitz M, Moshkowitz B, Gross J. Serum transcobalamin in myeloid leukemia. J Lab Clin Med 1971;78:276.
98. Socinski MA, Cannistra SA, Elias A, et al. Granulocyte-macrophage colony-stimulating factor expands the circulating hematopoietic progenitor cell compartment in man. Lancet 1988.1194.
99. Metcalf D. In-vitro cloning techniques for hemopoietic cells: clinical applications. Ann Intern Med 1977;87:483.
100. Bishop CR, Rothstein G, Ashenbrucker HE, Athens JW. Leukokinetic studies. XIV. Blood neutrophil kinetics in chronic, steady-state neutropenia. J Clin Invest 1971;50:1678.
101. Pharr PP, Ogawa M. Pluripotent stem cells. In: Golde DW, Takaku F, eds. Hematopoietic stem cells. New York, Marcel Dekker, 1985:3.
102. Till JE, McCulloch EA. A direct measurement of the radiation sensitivity of normal mouse bone marrow cells. Radiat Res 1961;14:213.
103. Schofield R. The relationship between spleen colony-forming cells and the haematopoietic stem cell. Blood Cells 1978;4:7.
104. Bradley TR, Metcalf D. The growth of mouse bone marrow cells in vitro. Aust J Exp Biol Med Sci 1966;44:287.
105. Pluznik DH, Sachs L. The cloning of normal "mast" cells in tissue culture. J Cell Comp Physiol 1965;66:319.
106. Nakahata T, Ogawa M. Identification in culture of a class of hematopoietic colony-forming units with extensive capability to self-renew

and generate multipotential colonies. Proc Natl Acad Sci USA 1982;79:3843.

107. Spangrude GJ, Heimfeld S, Weissman IL. Purification and characterization of mouse hematopoietic stem cells. Science 1988;241:58.
108. Vassort F, Winterholer M, Frindel E, Tubiana M. Kinetic parameters of bone marrow stem cells using in vivo suicide by tritiated thymidine or by hydroxyurea. Blood 1973;41:789.
109. Hodgson GS, Bradley TR. Properties of haematopoietic stem cells surviving 5-fluorouracil treatment: evidence for a pre-CFU-S cell? Nature 1979;281:381.
110. Ikebuchi K, Wong GG, Clark SC, et al. Interleukin 6 enhancement of interleukin 3–dependent proliferation of multipotential hematopoietic progenitors. Proc Natl Acad Sci USA 1987;84:9035.
111. Ikebuchi K, Ihle JN, Hirai Y, et al. Synergistic factors for stem cell proliferation: further studies of the target stem cells and the mechanism of stimulation by interleukin-1, interleukin-6, and granulocyte colony-stimulating factor. Blood 1988;72:2007.
112. Leary AG, Ikebuchi K, Hirai Y, et al. Synergism between interleukin-6 and interleukin-3 in supporting proliferation of human hematopoietic stem cells: comparison with interleukin-1α. Blood 1988;71:1759.
113. Ikebuchi K, Clark SC, Ihle JN, et al. Granulocyte colony-stimulating factor enhances interleukin-3–dependent proliferation of multipotential hemopoietic progenitors. Proc Natl Acad Sci USA 1988;85:3445.
114. Leary AG, Ogawa M. Blast cell colony assay for umbilical cord blood and adult bone marrow progenitors. Blood 1987;69:953.
115. Leary AG, Yang YC, Clark S, et al. Recombinant gibbon interleukin 3 supports formation of human multilineage colonies and blast cell colonies in culture: comparison with recombinant human granulocyte-macrophage colony-stimulating factor. Blood 1987;70:1343.
116. Messner HA, Yamasaki K, Jamal N, et al. Growth of human hematopoietic colonies in response to recombinant gibbon interleukin-3: comparison with human recombinant granulocyte-macrophage colony-stimulating factor. Proc Natl Acad Sci USA 1987;84:6765.
116a. Witte OW. Steel locus defines new multipotent growth factor. Cell 1990;63:5.
117. Clark SC, Kamen R. The human hematopoietic colony-stimulating factors. Science 1987;236:1229.
118. Golde DW, Gasson JC. Hormones that regulate blood cell production. Sci Am 1988;259:62.
119. Metcalf D. The molecular biology and functions of the granulocyte-macrophage colony-stimulating factors. Blood 1986;67:257.
120. Sieff CA. Hematopoietic growth factors. J Clin Invest 1987;79:1549.
121. Gasson JC, Weisbart RH, Kaufman SE, et al. Purified human GM-colony-stimulating factor: direct action on neutrophils. Science 1984;226:1339.
122. Kaushansky K, O'Hara PJ, Berkner K, et al. Genomic cloning, characterization and multilineage growth-promoting activity of human granulocyte-macrophage colony-stimulating factor. Proc Natl Acad Sci USA 1986;83:3101.
123. Lee F, Yokota T, Otsuka T, et al. Isolation of a cDNA for a human granulocyte-macrophage colony-stimulating factor by functional expression in mammalian cells. Proc Natl Acad Sci USA 1985;82:4360.
124. Wong GG, Witek JS, Temple PA, et al. Human GM-CSF: molecular cloning of the complementary DNA and purification of the natural and recombinant proteins. Science 1985;228:810.
125. Chan JY, Slamon DJ, Nimer SD, et al. Regulation of expression of human granulocyte-macrophage colony-stimulating factor (GM-CSF). Proc Natl Acad Sci USA 1986;83:8669.
126. Thorens B, Mermod JJ, Vassalli P. Phagocytosis and inflammatory stimuli induce GM-CSF mRNA in macrophages through posttranscriptional regulation. Cell 1987;48:671.
127. Zucali JR, Dinarello CA, Oblon DJ, et al. Interleukin-1 stimulates fibroblasts to produce granulocyte-macrophage colony-stimulating activity and prostaglandin E2. J Clin Invest 1986;77:1857.
128. Munker R, Gasson J, Ogawa M, Koeffler HP. Recombinant human tumor necrosis factor induces production of granulocyte-monocyte colony-stimulating factor mRNA and protein from lung fibroblasts and vascular endothelial cells *in vitro*. Nature 1986;323:79.
129. Broudy VC, Kaushansky K, Segal GM, et al. Tumor necrosis factor type A stimulates human endothelial cells to produce granulocyte/macrophage colony-stimulating factor. Proc Natl Acad Sci USA 1986;83:7467.
130. Kupper TS, Dower S, Birchall N, et al. Interleukin-1 binds to specific receptors on keratinocytes and induces granulocyte/macrophage colony stimulating factor (GM-CSF) mRNA and protein: a potential autocrine role for IL-1 in epidemics. J Clin Invest 1988;82:1787.
131. Metcalf D, Begley CG, Johnson GR, et al. Biologic properties *in vitro* of a recombinant human granulocyte-macrophage colony-stimulating factor. Blood 1986;67:37.
132. Sieff CA, Emerson SG, Donahue RE, et al. Human recombinant granulocyte-macrophage colony-stimulating factor: a multilineage hematopoietin. Science 1985;230:1171.
133. Tomonaga M, Golde DW, Gasson JC. Biosynthetic (recombinant) human granulocyte-macrophage colony-stimulating factor: effect on normal bone marrow and leukemia cell lines. Blood 1986;67:31.
134. Mazur EM, Cohen JL, Wong GG, Clark SC. Modest stimulatory effect of recombinant human GM-CSF on colony growth from peripheral blood human megakaryocyte progenitor cells. Exp Hematol 1987;15:1128.
135. Begley CG, Lopez AF, Nicola NA, et al. Purified colony-stimulating factors enhance the survival of human neutrophils and eosinophils in vitro: a rapid and sensitive microassay for colony-stimulating factors. Blood 1986;68:162.
136. Lopez AF, Williamson J, Gamble JP, et al. Recombinant human granulocyte-macrophage colony-stimulating factor stimulates in vitro mature neutrophil and eosinophil functions, surface receptor expression and survival. J Clin Invest 1986;78:1220.
137. Burgess AW, Begley CG, Johnson GR, et al. Purification and properties of bacterially synthesized human granulocyte-macrophage colony-stimulating factor. Blood 1987;69:43.
138. Fleischmann J, Golde DW, Weisbart RH, Gasson JC. Granulocyte-macrophage colony-stimulating factor enhances phagocytosis of bacteria by human neutrophils. Blood 1986;68:708.
139. Golde DW, Baldwin GC, Weisbart, RH. Responses to neutrophils to myeloid growth factors: CIBA Foundation Symposium 148. In: Molecular control of haemopoiesis. Chichester, NY, Wiley, 1990:62.
140. Grabstein KH, Urdal DL, Tushinski RJ, et al. Introduction of macrophage tumoricidal activity by granulocyte-macrophage colony-stimulating factor. Science 1986;232:506.
141. Silberstein DS, Owen WF, Gasson JC, et al. Regulation of human eosinophil function by granulocyte-macrophage colony-stimulating factor. J Immunol 1986;137:3290.
142. Villalta F, Kierszenbaum F. Effects of human colony-stimulating factor on the uptake and destruction of a pathogenic parasite (*Trypanosoma cruzi*) by human neutrophils. J Immunol 1986;137:1703.
143. Weisbart RH, Golde DW, Clark SC, et al. Human granulocyte-macrophage colony-stimulating factor is a neutrophil activator. Nature 1985;314:361.
144. Weisbart RH, Kwan L, Golde DW, Gasson JC. Human GM-CSF primes neutrophils for enhanced oxidative metabolism in response to the major physiological chemoattractants. Blood 1987;69:18.
145. Gordon MY, Riley GP, Watt SM, Greaves MF. Compartmentalization of a haematopoietic growth factor (GM-CSF) by glycosaminoglycans in the bone marrow microenvironment. Nature 1987;326:403.
146. Nicola NA, Begley CG, Metcalf D. Identification of the human analogue of a regulator that induces differentiation in murine leukaemic cells. Nature 1985;314:625.
147. Nomura H, Imazeki I, Oheda M, et al. Purification and characterization of human granulocyte colony-stimulating factor (G-CSF). EMBO J 1986;5:871.
148. Welte K, Platzer E, Lu L, et al. Purification and biochemical characterization of human pluripotent hematopoietic colony-stimulating factor. Proc Natl Acad Sci USA 1985;82:1526.
149. Nagata S, Tsuchiya M, Asano S, et al. Molecular cloning and expression of cDNA for human granulocyte colony-stimulating factor. Nature 1986;319:415.
150. Souza LM, Boone TC, Gabrilove J, et al. Recombinant human granulocyte colony-stimulating factor: effects on normal and leukemic myeloid cells. Science 1986;232:61.
151. Broudy VC, Kaushansky K, Harlan MJ, Adamson JW. Interleukin 1 stimulates human endothelial cells to produce granulocyte-macrophage colony-stimulating factor and granulocyte colony-stimulating factor. J Immunol 1987;139:464.
152. Kaushansky K, Lin N, Adamson JW. Interleukin 1 stimulates fibroblasts to synthesize granulocyte-macrophage colony-stimulating factors. J Clin Invest 1988;81:92.
153. Vellenga E, Rambaldi A, Ernst TJ, et al. Independent regulation of M-CSF and G-CSF gene expression in human monocytes. Blood 1988;71:1529.
154. Simmers RN, Webber LM, Shannon MR, et al. Localization of the G-CSF gene on chromosome 17 proximal to the breakpoint in the t(15;17) in acute promyelocytic leukemia. Blood 1987;70:330.
155. Chikkappa G, Wang GJ, Santell D, Pasquale D. Granulocyte colony-stimulating factor (G-CSF) induces synthesis of alkaline phosphatase in neutrophilic granulocytes of chronic myelogenous leukemia patients. Leuk Res 1988;12:491.
156. Yuo A, Kitagawa S, Okabe T, et al. Recombinant human granulocyte colony stimulating factor repairs the abnormalities of neutrophils in patients with myelodysplastic syndromes and chronic myelogenous leukemia. Blood 1987;70:404.
157. Fung MC, Hapel AJ, Ymer S, et al. Molecular cloning of cDNA for murine interleukin-3. Nature 1984;307:233.
158. Yang Y-C, Ciarletta AB, Temple PA, et al. Identification by expression cloning of a novel hematopoietic growth factor related to murine IL-3. Cell 1986;47:3.
159. Sonada Y, Yang Y-C, Wong GG, et al. Analysis in serum-free culture of the targets of recombinant human hemopoietic growth factors: interleukin 3 and granulocyte/macrophage colony-stimulating factor are specific for early developmental stages. Proc Natl Acad Sci USA 1988;85:4360.
160. Sieff CA, Niemeyer CM, Nathan DG, et al. Stimulation of human hematopoietic colony formation by recombinant gibbon multi-colony-stimulating factor or interleukin 3. J Clin Invest 1987;80:818.

161. Lopez AF, To LB, Yang Y-C, et al. Stimulation of proliferation, differentiation, and function of human cells by primate interleukin 3. Proc Natl Acad Sci USA 1987;84:2761.
162. Niemeyer CM, Sieff CA, Mathey-Prevot B, et al. Expression of human interleukin-3 (multi-CSF) is restricted to human lymphocytes and T-cell tumor lines. Blood 1989;73:945.
163. Huebner K, Isobe M, Croce CM, Golde DW, Kaufman SE, Gasson JC. The human gene encoding GM-CSF is at 5q21-q32, the chromosome region deleted in the 5q- anomaly. Science 1985;230:1282.
164. Le Beau MM, Westbrook CA, Diaz MO, et al. Evidence for the involvement of GM-CSF and FMS in the deletion (5q) in myeloid disorders. Science 1986;231:984.
165. Le Beau MM, Epstein ND, O'Brien SJ, et al. The interleukin 3 gene is located on human chromosome 5 and is deleted in myeloid leukemias with a deletion of 5q. Proc Natl Acad Sci USA 1987;84:5913.
166. Yang Y-C, Kovacic S, Kriz R, et al. The human genes for GM-CSF and IL 3 are closely linked in tandem on chromosome 5. Blood 1988;71: 958.
167. Stanley ER, Hansen G, Woodcock J, Metcalf D. Colony stimulating factor and the regulation of granulopoiesis and macrophage production. Fed Proc 1975;34:2272.
168. Wu M, Cini JK, Yunis AA. Purification of a colony stimulating factor from cultured pancreatic cells. J Biol Chem 1979;254:6226.
169. Das SK, Stanley ER, Guilbert LJ, Forman LW. Human colony-stimulating factor (CSF-1) radioimmunoassay: resolution of three subclasses of human colony-stimulating factors. Blood 1981;58:630.
170. Hanamura T, Motoyoshi K, Yoshida K, et al. Quantitation and identification of human monocytic colony-stimulating factor in human serum by enzyme-linked immunosorbent assay. Blood 1988;72:886.
171. Wong GG, Temple PA, Leary AC, et al. Human CSF-1: molecular cloning and expression of a 4 kb cDNA encoding the hematopoietin and determination of the complete amino acid sequence of the human urinary protein. Science 1987;235:1504.
172. Kawasaki ES, Ladner MB, Wang AM, et al. Molecular cloning of a complementary DNA encoding human macrophage-specific colony-stimulating factor (CSF-1). Science 1985;230:291.
173. Morris SW, Valentine MB, Shapiro DN, et al. Reassignment of the human *CSF1* gene to chromosome 1p13-p21. Blood 1991;78:2013.
174. Nienhuis AW, Bunn HF, Turner PH, et al. Expression of the human c-*fms* proto-oncogene in hematopoietic cells and its deletion in the 5q-syndrome. Cell 1985;42:421.
175. Caracciolo D, Shirsat N, Wong GG, et al. Recombinant human macrophage colony-stimulating factor (M-CSF) requires subliminal concentrations of granulocyte/macrophage (GM)-CSF for optimal stimulation of human macrophage colony formation in vitro. J Exp Med 1987;166:1851.
176. Warren RK, Ralph P. Macrophage growth factor CSF-1 stimulates human monocyte production of interferon, tumor necrosis factor, and colony-stimulating activity. J Immunol 1986;137:2281.
177. Koike K, Stanley ER, Ihle JN, Ogawa M. Macrophage colony formation supported by purified CSF-1 and/or interleukin 3 in serum-free culture: evidence for hierarchical difference in macrophage colony-forming cells. Blood 1986;67:859.
178. Zhou Y-Q, Stanley R, Clark SC, et al. Interleukin-3 and interleukin-1a allow earlier bone marrow progenitors to respond to human colony-stimulating factor 1. Blood 1988;72:1870.
179. Yasukawa K, Hirano T, Watanabe Y, et al. Structure and expression of human B cell stimulatory factor-2 (BSF-2/IL-6) gene. EMBO J 1987;6: 2939.
180. Zilberstein A, Ruggieri R, Korn JH, Revel M. Structure and expression of cDNA and genes for human interferon-beta-2, a distinct species inducible by growth-stimulatory cytokines. EMBO J 1986;5:2529.
181. Wong GG, Clark SC. Multiple actions of interleukin 6 within a cytokine network. Immunol Today 1988;9:137.
182. Mochizuki DY, Eisenman JR, Conlon PJ, Larsen AD. Interleukin 1 regulates hematopoietic activity, a role previously ascribed to hemopoietin 1. Proc Natl Acad Sci USA 1987;84:5267.
183. Jubinsky PT, Stanley ER. Purification of hemopoietin 1: a multilineage hemopoietic growth factor. Proc Natl Acad Sci USA 1985;82:2764.
184. Stanley ER, Bartocci A, Patinkin D, et al. Regulation of very primitive, multipotent, hematopoietic cells by hemopoietin-1. Cell 1986;45:667.
185. Zsebo KM, Wypych J, Yuschenkoff VN, et al. Effects of hematopoietin-1 and interleukin 1 activities on early hematopoietic cells of the bone marrow. Blood 1988;71:962.
186. Hoang T, Goncalves HO, Wong GG, Clark SC. Interleukin-6 enhances growth factor–dependent proliferation of the blast cells of acute myeloblastic leukemia. Blood 1988;72:823.
187. Dinarello CA. Multiple biological properties of recombinant human interleukin 1 (beta). Immunobiology 1986;172:301.
188. Raefsky EL, Platanias LC, Zoumbos N, Young NS. Studies of interferon as a regulator of hematopoietic cell proliferation. J Immunol 1985;135: 2507.
189. Barber KE, Crosier PS, Watson JD. The differential inhibition of hemopoietic growth factor activity by cytotoxins and interferon-γ^1. J Immunol 1987;139:1108.
190. Murase T, Hotta T, Saito H, Ohno R. Effect of recombinant human tumor necrosis factor on the colony growth of human leukemia progenitor cells and normal hematopoietic progenitor cells. Blood 1987;69: 467.
191. Gullberg U, Peetre K, Olsson E. Differentiation induction in myeloid leukemic cells. (Review) Med Oncol Tumor Pharmacother 1986;3: 55.
192. Trucco M, Rovera G, Ferrero D. A novel human lymphokine that inhibits haematopoietic progenitor cell proliferation. Nature 1984;309: 166.
193. Bacigalupo A, Podesta M, Mingari MC, et al. Immune suppression of hematopoiesis in aplastic anemia: activity of T-γ lymphocytes. J Immunol 1980;125:1449.
194. Hino M, Tojo A, Miyazono K, et al. Effects of type β transforming growth factors on haemopoietic progenitor cells. Br J Haematol 1988;70: 143.
195. Tessier N, Hoang T. Transforming growth factor β inhibits the proliferation of the blast cells of acute myeloblastic leukemia. Blood 1988;72:159.
196. Shirafuji N, Matsuda S, Tani K, et al. Granulocyte colony-stimulating factor stimulates human mature neutrophilic granulocytes to produce interferon-α. Blood 1990;75:17.
197. Lozzio BB. Regulators of cell division: a review. 1. Endogenous mitotic inhibitors of hematopoietic cells. Exp Hematol 1973;1:309.
198. Rytomaa T, Kiviniemi K. Control of granulocyte production. I. Chalone and antichalone, two specific humoral regulators. Cell Tissue Kinet 1986;1:329.
199. Querinjean P, Masson PL, Heremans JF. Molecular weight, single-chain structure and amino acid composition of human lactoferrin. Eur J Biochem 1971;20:420.
200. Broxmeyer HE, DeSousa M, Smithyman A, et al. Specificity and modulation of the action of lactoferrin, a negative feedback regulator of myelopoiesis. Blood 1980;55:324.
201. Broxmeyer HE, Smithyman A, Eger RR, et al. Identification of lactoferrin as the granulocyte-derived inhibitor of colony-stimulating activity production. J Exp Med 1978;148:1052.
202. Boxer LA, Haak RA, Yang HH, et al. Membrane-bound lactoferrin alters the surface properties of polymorphonuclear leukocytes. J Clin Invest 1982;70:1049.
203. Oseas R, Yang HH, Baehner RL, Boxer LA. Lactoferrin: a promoter of polymorphonuclear leukocyte adhesiveness. Blood 1981;57:939.
204. Boxer LA, Coates TD, Haak RA, et al. Lactoferrin deficiency associated with altered granulocyte function. N Engl J Med 1982;307:404.
205. Walker F, Nicola NA, Metcalf D, Burgess AW. Hierarchical down-modulation of hemopoietic growth factor receptors. Cell 1985;43: 269.
206. Nicola NA, Metcalf D. Binding of ^{125}I-labeled granulocyte colony-stimulating factor to normal murine hemopoietic cells. J Cell Physiol 1985;124:313.
207. Palasynski EW, Ihle JN. Evidence for specific receptors for interleukin 3 on lymphokine-dependent cell lines established from long-term bone marrow cultures. J Immunol 1984;132:1872.
208. Gesner TG, Mufson RA, Norton CR, et al. Specific binding, internalization and degradation of human recombinant interleukin-3 by cells of the acute myelogenous leukemia line, KG-1. J Cell Physiol 1988;136: 493.
209. Gasson JC, Kaufman SE, Weisbart RH, et al. High affinity binding of granulocyte-macrophage colony-stimulating factor to normal and leukemic human myeloid cells. Proc Natl Acad Sci USA 1986;83:669.
210. Cosman D, Lyman SD, Idzenda RL, et al. A new cytokine receptor superfamily. Trends Biochem Sci 1990;15:265.
210a. Bazan JF. Haematopoietic receptors and helical cytokines. Immunol Today 1990;11:350.
211. Baldwin GC, Gasson JC, Kaufman SE, et al. Nonhematopoietic tumor cells express functional CSF receptors. Blood 1989;73:1033.
212. Dedhar S, Gaboury L, Galloway P, Eaves C. Human granulocyte-macrophage colony-stimulating factor is a growth factor active on a variety of cell types of nonhematopoietic origin. Proc Natl Acad Sci USA 1988;85:9253.
213. Scheffler JE, Fleissner LC, Seelig GF, et al. Characterization of the human granulocyte-macrophage colony-stimulating factor receptor from placenta. J Cell Biochem 1989;13S:30.
214. Bussolino F, Wang JM, Defilippi P, et al. Granulocyte- and granulocyte-macrophage colony-stimulating factors induce human endothelial cells to migrate and proliferate. Nature 1989;337:471.
215. Horiguchi J, Warren MK, Ralph P, Kufe D. Expression of the macrophage specific colony-stimulating factor (CSF-1) during human monocytic differentiation. Biochem Biophys Res Commun 1986;141: 924.
216. Horiguchi J, Warren MK, Kufe D. Expression of the macrophage-specific colony-stimulating factor in human monocytes treated with a granulocyte-macrophage colony-stimulating factor. Blood 1987;69: 1258.
217. Rambaldi A, Young DC, Griffin JD. Expression of the M-CSF (CSF-1) gene by human monocytes. Blood 1987;69:1409.
218. Rambaldi A, Wakamiya N, Vellenga E, et al. Expression of the macrophage colony-stimulating factor and c-fms genes in human acute myeloblastic leukemia cells. J Clin Invest 1988;81:1030.
219. Yarden Y, Escobedo JA, Kaung WJ, et al. Structure of the receptor for

platelet-derived growth factor helps define a family of closely related growth factor receptors. Nature 1986;323:226.
220. Uzumaki H, Okabe T, Sasaki N, et al. Characterization of receptor for granulocyte colony-stimulating factor on human circulating neutrophils. Biochem Biophys Res Commun 1988;156:1026.
221. Fukunaga R, Seto Y, Mizushima S, Nagata S. Three different mRNAs encoding human granulocyte colony-stimulating factor receptor. Proc Natl Acad Sci USA 1990;87:8702.
222. Nicola NA, Vadas MA, Lopez AF. Down-modulation of receptors for granulocyte colony-stimulating factor on human neutrophils by granulocyte-activating agents. J Cell Physiol 1986;128:501.
223. Ferrero D, Rovera G. Human leukaemic cell lines. Clin Haematol 1984;13:461.
224. Furley AJ, Reeves BR, Mizutani S, et al. Divergent molecular phenotypes of KG1 and KG1a myeloid cell lines. Blood 1986;68:1101.
225. Minowada J. Immunology of leukemic cells. In: Gunz F, Henderson E, eds. Leukemia. New York, Grune & Stratton, 1982:119.
226. Collins SJ, Gallo RC, Gallagher RE. Continuous growth and differentiation of human myeloid leukaemic cells in suspension culture. Nature 1977;270:347.
227. Gallagher R, Collins S, Trujillo T, et al. Characterization of continuous differentiating myeloid cell line (HL-60) from a patient with acute promyelocytic leukemia. Blood 1979;54:713.
228. Dalton WT, Ahearn MJ, McCredie KB, et al. HL-60 Cell line was derived from a patient with FAB-M2 and not FAB-M3. Blood 1988;71: 242.
229. Collins SJ, Ruscetti FW, Gallagher RE, Gallo RC. Terminal differentiation of human promyelocytic leukemia cells induced by dimethyl sulfoxide and other polar compounds. Proc Natl Acad Sci USA 1978;75: 2458.
230. Rovera G, O'Brien TG, Diamond L. Induction of differentiation in human promyelocytic leukemia cells by tumor promoters. Science 1979;204:868.
231. Breitman TR, Selonick SE, Collins SJ. Induction of differentiation of the human promyelocytic leukemia cell line (HL-60) by retinoic acid. Proc Natl Acad Sci USA 1980;77:2936.
232. Shiina Y, Abe E, Miyaura C, et al. Biological activity of 24, 24-difuoro-1α,25-dihydroxyvitamin D_3 and 1a,25-dihydroxyvitamin D_3-26,33-lactone in inducing differentiation of human myeloid leukemia cells. Arch Biochem Biophys 1983;220:90.
233. Collins SJ, Groudine M. Amplification of endogenous *myc*-related DNA sequences in a human leukaemia cell line. Nature 1982;298: 679.
234. Dalla-Favera R, Wong-Staal F, Gallo R. *onc* Gene amplification in promyelocytic leukaemia cell line HL-60 and primary leukaemic cells of the same patient. Nature 1982;299:61.
235. Westin E, Wong-Staal F, Gelmann E, et al. Expression of cellular homologues of retroviral onc genes in human hematopoietic cells. Proc Natl Acad Sci USA 1982;79:2490.
236. Bories, D, M-C Raymal, DH Solomon, Z Darzynkiewicz, and YE Cayre. Down-regulation of a serine protease, myeloblastin, causes growth arrest and differentiation of promyelocytic leukemic cells. Cell 1989;59:959.
237. Mulder A, Alexander S, Engelfreit CP, von dem Borne AEG Kr. Characterization, by immunoprecipitation, of myeloid- and monocyte-specific antigens present on the human promyelocytic cell line (HL-60) in three stages of differentiation. Proc Natl Acad Sci USA 1981;78: 5091.
238. Rovera G, Ferraro D, Pagliardi GL, et al. Induction of differentiation of human myeloid leukemias by phorbol diesters: phenotypic changes and mode of action. Ann NY Acad Sci 1982;397:211.
239. Lozzio CB, Lozzio BB. Human chronic myelogenous leukemia cell-line with positive Philadelphia chromosome. Blood 1975;45:321.
240. Marie JP, Izaguirre CA, Civin CI, et al. The presence within single K-562 cells of erythropoietic and granulopoietic differentiation markers. Blood 1981;58:708.
241. Andersson LC, Nilsson K, Gahmberg CG. K562: a human erythroleukemic cell line. Int J Cancer 1979;23:143.
242. Jokinen M, Gahmberg CG, Andersson LC. Biosynthesis of the major human red cell sialoglycoprotein, glycophorin A, in a continuous cell line. Nature 1979;279:604.
243. Rutherford TR, Clegg JB, Weatherall DJ. K562 Human leukaemic cells synthesize embryonic haemoglobin in response to haemin. Nature 1979;280:164.
244. Klein E, Ben Bassat H, Neumann H, et al. Properties of the K562 cell line, derived from a patient with chronic myeloid leukemia. Int J Cancer 1976;18:421.
245. Martin P, Papayannopoulou T. HEL cells: a new human erythroleukemia cell line with spontaneous and induced globin expression. Science 1982;216:1233.
246. Koeffler HP, Golde DW. Acute myelogenous leukemia: a human cell line responsive to colony-stimulating activity. Science 1978;200:1153.
247. Koeffler HP, Billing R, Sparkes RS, Golde DW. Antigens present on human myeloid leukemia cell lines. Leuk Res 1980;4:69.
248. Koeffler HP, Billing R, Lusis AJ, et al. An undifferentiated variant derived from the human acute myelogenous leukemia cell line (KG-1). Blood 1980;56:265.
249. Sundstrom C, Nilsson K. Establishment and characterization of a human histiocytic lymphoma cell line (U-937). Int J Cancer 1976;17:565.
250. Zuckerman SH, Surprenant YM, Tang J. Synergistic effect of granulocyte-macrophage colony-stimulating factor and 1,25-dihydroxyvitamin D3 on the differentiation of the human monocytic cell line U937. Blood 1988;71:619.
251. Tsuchiya S, Yamabe M, Yamaguchi Y, et al. Establishment and characterization of a human acute monocytic leukemia cell line (THP-1). Int J Cancer 1980;26:171.
252. Shaper AG, Lewis P. Genetic neutropenia in people of African origin. Lancet 1971;2:1021.
253. Bain BJ, England JM. Normal haematological values: sex difference in neutrophil count. Br Med J 1975;1:306.
254. Broun GO, Herbig FK, Hamilton JR. Leukopenia in negroes. N Engl J Med 1966;275:1410.
255. Forbes WH, Johnson RE, Consolazio F. Leukopenia in Negro workmen. Am J M Sci 1941;201:407.
256. Joyce RA, Boggs DR, Hasiba U, Srodes CH. Marginal neutrophil pool size in normal subjects and neutropenic patients as measured by epinephrine infusion. J Lab Clin Med 1976;88:614.
257. Kostmann R. Infantile genetic agranulocytosis. Acta Paediatr 1956;45: 105.
258. Schwachman H, Diamond LK, Oski FA, Khaw KT. The syndrome of pancreatic insufficiency and bone marrow dysfunction. J Pediatr 1964;65:645.
259. Hitzig WH, Schlapfer A. Chronic neutropenia and dysgammaglobulinemia: possible interrelations. X Cong Int Soc Hematol D 1964;23.
260. Blume RS, Bennett JM, Yankee RA, Wolff SM. Defective granulocyte regulation in the Chediak-Higaski syndrome. N Engl J Med 1968;279: 1009.
261. Dale DC, Guerry D, IV, Wewerka JR, et al. Chronic neutropenia. Medicine 1979;58:128.
262. Kyle RA. Natural history of chronic ideopathic neutropenia. N Engl J Med 1980;302:908.
263. Pincus SH, Boxer LA, Stassel TP. Chronic neutropenia in childhood: analysis of 16 cases and a review of the literature. Am J Med. 1976;61: 849–861.
264. Dale DC, Hammond WP IV. Cyclic neutropenia: a clinical review. Blood Rev 1988;2:178.
265. Wright DG, Dale DC, Fauci AS, Wolff SM. Human cyclic neutropenia: clinical review and long-term follow-up of patients. Medicine 1981;60: 1.
266. Lund JE, Padgett GA, Ott RL. Cyclic neutropenia in grey collie dogs. Blood 1967;29:452.
267. Dale DC, Graw RG, Jr. Transplantation of allogeneic bone marrow in canine cyclic neutropenia. Science 1974;183:83.
268. Jones JB, Yang TJ, Dale JB, Lange RD. Canine cyclic haematopoiesis: marrow transplantation between littermates. Br J Haematol 1975;30: 215.
269. Lally ET, Golub ER, Kieba IR, et al. Analysis of the Actinobacillus actinomycetocomitans leukotoxin gene. J Biol Chem 1989;264:15451.
270. Bassan R, Viero P, Minetti B, Commotti B, Barsui T. Myelokathexis: a rare form of chronic benign granulocytopenia. Br J Haematol 1984;58: 115–117.
271. Kracke RR, Parker PP. The relationship of drug therapy to agranulocytosis. JAMA 1935;150:960.
272. Plum P. Clinical and experimental investigations in agranulocytosis. London, HK Lewis, 1937.
273. Squier TL, Madison FW. Drug hypersensitivity as a cause of acute primary granulocytopenia. Wis Med J 1935;34:175.
274. Moeschlin S, Wagner K. Agranulocytosis due to occurrence of leukocyte-agglutinins (pyramidon and cold agglutinins). Acta Haematol 1952;8:29.
275. Barrett AJ, Weller B, Rozengurt H, et al. Amidopyrine agranulocytosis: drug inhibition of granulocyte colonies in the presence of patient's serum. Br Med J 1976;2:850.
276. Smiley RK, Cartwright GE, Wintrobe MM. Fatal aplastic anemia following chloramphenicol (chloromycetin) administration. JAMA 1952;149:914.
277. Polak BC, Wesseling H, Schut D, et al. Blood dyscrasias attributed to chloramphenicol: a review of 576 published and unpublished cases. Acta Med Scand 1972;192:409.
278. Yunis AA. Chloramphenicol-induced bone marrow suppression. Semin Hematol 1973;10:225.
279. Arneborn P, Palmblad J. Drug-induced neutropenia in the Stockholm region 1973–75: frequency and causes. Acta Med Scand 1978;204: 283.
280. Arneborn P, Palmblad J. Drug-induced neutropenias in the Stockholm region 1976–77. Acta Med Scand 1979;206:241.
281. Pisciotta AV. Immune and toxic mechanisms in drug-induced agranulocytosis. Semin Hematol 1973;10:279.
282. Pisciotta V. Drug-induced agranulocytosis. Drugs 1978;15:132.
283. Lieberman JA, Kane JM, Johns CA. Clozapine: guidelines for clinical management. J Clin Psych 1989;50:329.
283a. Alvir J, Lieberman J, Safferman A, Schwimmer J, Schaaf J. Clozapine-induced agranulocytosis: incidence and risk factors in the United States. N Engl J Med 1993;329:162.

284. Walz B, Zupnick J, Uden D, Keating A. Penicillin-induced agranulocytosis. West J Med 1988;149:460.
285. Neftel KA, Muller MR, Walti M, et al. Penicillin G degradation products inhibit in vitro granulopoiesis. Br J Haematol 1983;54:255.
286. Neftel KA, Hauser SP, Muller MR. Inhibition of granulopoiesis in vivo and in vitro by β-lactam antibiotics. J Infect Dis 1985;152:90.
287. Cooper RA. Captopril-associated neutropenia. Arch Intern Med 1983;143:659.
288. El Matri A, Larabi MS, Kechrid C, et al. Fatal bone-marrow suppression associated with captopril. Br Med J 1981;283:277.
288a. Thompson J, Herick J, Klassen L, et al. Studies on levamisole-induced agranulocytosis. Blood 1980;56:388.
289. Fraunfelder FT, Meyer SM, Bagby GC Jr, Dreis MW. Hematologic reactions to carbonic anhydrase inhibitors. Am J Ophthalmol 1985;100: 79.
290. Mitrane MP, Singh A, Seibold JR. Cholestasis and fatal agranulocytosis complicating sulfasalazine therapy. J Rheumatol 1986;13:969.
291. Weitzman SA, Stossel TP. Drug-induced immunological neutropenia. Lancet 1978;1:1068.
292. McCarthy DD, Chalmers MB. Hematologic complications of phenylbutazone therapy: review of the literature and report of 2 cases. Can Med Assoc J 1964;90:1061.
293. Mamus SW, Burton JD, Groat JD, et al. Ibuprofen-associated pure white-cell aplasia. N Engl J Med 1986;314:624.
294. Kay AGL. Myelotoxicity of gold. Br Med J 1976;1:1266.
295. Howell A, Gumpel JM, Watts RWE. Depression of bone marrow colony formation in gold-induced neutropenia. Br Med J 1975;1:432.
296. Cooper DS, Goldminz D, Levin AA, et al. Agranulocytosis associated with antithyroid drugs. Ann Intern Med 1983;98:26.
297. Morton H. Agranulocytosis caused by thiouracil: a review of fifty nine cases in the literature and a report of two additional cases. Am J Med 1947;2:53.
298. Freston JW. Cimetidine and granulocytopenia. Ann Intern Med 1979;90:264.
299. List AF, Beaird DH, Kummet T. Ranitidine-induced granulocytopenia: recurrence with cimetidine. Ann Intern Med 1988;108:566.
300. Budman DR, Steinberg AD. Hematologic aspects of systemic lupus erythematosus: current concepts. Ann Intern Med 1977;86:220.
301. Harmon DC, Weitzman SA, Stossel TP. The severity of immune neutropenia correlates with the maturational specificity of antineutrophil antibodies. Br J Haematol 1984;58:209.
302. Logue G, Shimm DS. Autoimmune granulocytopenia. Annu Rev Med 1980;31:191.
303. Boxer LA, Greenberg MS, Boxer GJ, Stossel TP. Autoimmune neutropenia. N Engl J Med 1975;293:748–754.
304. Levitt LJ. Chlorpropamide-induced pure white cell aplasia. Blood 1987;69:394.
305. Verheugt FWA, von dem Borne AEG Kr, van Noord-Bockhorst JC, Engelfreit CP. Autoimmune granulocytopenia: the detection of granulocyte autoantibodies with the immunofluorescence test. Br J Haematol 1978;39:339–350.
306. Cline MJ, Golde DW. Immune suppression of hematopoiesis. Am J Med 1978;64:301.
307. Cline MJ, Opelz G, Saxon A, et al. Autoimmune panleukopenia. N Engl J Med 1976;295:1489.
308. Fitchen JH, Cline MJ. Serum inhibitors of myelopoiesis. Br J Haematol 1980;44:7.
309. Linker CA, Newcom SR, Nilsson CM, et al. Combined idiopathic neutropenia and thrombocytopenia. Ann Intern Med 1980;93:704.
310. Minchinton RM, Waters AH. The occurrence and significance of neutrophil antibodies. (Annotation) Br J Haematol 1984;56:521.
311. Weitzman SA, Stossel TP, Harmon DC, Daniels G, Maloof F, Ridgeway EC. Antineutrophil antibodies in Grave's disease: implications of thyrotropin binding to neutrophils. J Clin Invest 1985;75:119–123.
312. Kruskall MS, Weitzman SA, Stossel TP, Harris N, Robinson SH. Lymphoma with autoimmune neutropenia and hepatic infiltration: a syndrome. Ann Intern Med 1982;97:202–206.
313. McCullogh J, Weiblen BJ, Clay ME, Forstrom L. Effect of leukocyte antibodies on the fate of in vivo of indium-III–labeled granulocytes. Blood 1981;58:164.
314. Verheugt FWA, van Noord-Bokhorst JC, von dem Borne AEG Kr, Engelfriet CP. A family with allo-immune neonatal neutropenia: group-specific pathogenicity of maternal antibodies. Vox Sang 1979;36: 1.
315. Boxer LA, Yokoyama M, Lalezari P. Isoimmune neonatal neutropenia. J Pediatr 1972;80:783.
316. Felty AR. Chronic arthritis in the adult, associated with splenomegaly and neutropenia. Johns Hopkins Med J 1924;35:16.
317. Sienknecht CW, Urowitz MB, Pruzanski W, Stein HB. Felty's syndrome: clinical and serological analysis of 34 cases. Ann Rheum Dis 1977;36:500.
318. Spivak JL. Felty's syndrome: an analytical review. Johns Hopkins Med J 1977;141:156.
319. Goldberg J, Pinals RS. Felty syndrome. Semin Arthritis Rheum 1980;10: 52.
320. Hashimoto Y, Ziff M, Hurd E. Increased endothelial cell adherence, aggregation and superoxide generation by neutrophils incubated in systemic lupus erythematosus and Felty's syndrome sera. Arthritis Rheum 1982;25:1409.
321. Goldschmeding R, Breedveld FC, Engelfriet CP, von dem Borne AEG Kr. Lack of evidence for the presence of neutrophil autoantibodies in the serum of patients with Felty's syndrome. Br J Haematol 1988;68: 37.
322. Bagby, GC Jr, Lawrence JH, Neerhout RC. T-lymphocyte–mediated granulocytepoietic failure. J Clin Invest 1983;307:1073–1078.
323. Vincent PC, Levi JA, MacQueen A. The mechanisms of neutropenia in Felty's syndrome. Br J Haematol 1974;27:463.
324. Breedveld FC, Fibbe WE, Hermans J, et al. Factors influencing the incidence of infections in Felty's syndrome. Arch Intern Med 1987;147: 915.
325. Laszlo J, Jones R, Silberman HR, Banks PM. Splenectomy for Felty's syndrome: clinicopathological study of 27 patients. Arch Intern Med 1978;138:597.
326. Moore RA, Brunner CM, Sandusky WR, Leavell BS. Felty's syndrome: long-term follow-up after splenectomy. Ann Intern Med 1971;75:381.
327. Blumfelder TM, Logue GL, Shimm DS. Felty's syndrome: effects of splenectomy upon granulocyte count and granulocyte-associated IgG. Ann Intern Med 1981;94:623.
328. Mangan KF. T-cell-mediated suppression of hematopoiesis. N Engl J Med 1985;312:306.
329. Reynolds CW, Foon KA. Tγ-lymphoproliferative disease and related disorders in humans and experimental animals: a review of the clinical, cellular, and functional characteristics. Blood 1984;64:1146.
330. Berliner N, Duby AD, Linch DC, Murre C. T cell receptor gene rearrangements define a monoclonal T cell proliferation in patients with T lymphocytosis and cytopenia. Blood 1986;67:914.
331. Barton JC, Prasthofer EF, Egan ML, Heck LW, Koopman WJ, Grossi CE. Rheumatoid arthritis associated with expanded populations of granular lymphocytes. Ann Intern Med 1986;104:314.
332. Wallis WJ, Loughran TP Jr, Kadin ME, Clark EA, Starkebaum GA. Polyarthritis and neutropenia associated with circulating large granular lymphocytes. Ann Intern Med 1985;103:357.
333. Craddock PR, Fehr J, Dalmasso AP, et al. Hemodialysis leukopenia: pulmonary vascular leukostasis resulting from complement activation by dialyzer cellophane membranes. J Clin Invest 1977;59:879.
334. Craddock PR, Hammerschmidt D, White JG, et al. Complement (C5a)-induced granulocyte aggregation in vitro: a possible mechanism of complement-mediated leukostasis and leukopenia. J Clin Invest 1977;60:260.
335. Chenoweth DE, Cooper SW, Hugli TE, et al. Complement activation during cardiopulmonary bypass: evidence for generation of C3a and C5a anaphylatoxins. N Engl J Med 1981;304:497.
336. Boogaerts ME, Roelant C, Goossens W, Verwilghen RL. Complement activation and adult respiratory distress syndrome during intermittent flow apheresis procedures. Transfusion 1986;26:82.
337. Kaplow LS, Goffinet JA. Profound neutropenia during the early phase of hemodialysis. JAMA 1968;203:1135.
338. Subuk DW, Moore SB. Roles of the neutrophil and other mediators in adult respiratory distress syndrome. Mayo Clin Proc 1989;64:1118.
339. Baley JE, Stork EK, Warkentin PI, Shurin SB. Neonatal neutropenia: clinical manifestations, cause and outcome. Am J Dis Child 1988;142: 1161.
340. Bonilla MA, Gillio AP, Ruggeiro M, et al. Effects of recombinant human granulocyte colony-stimulating factor on neutropenia in patients with congenital neutropenia. N Engl J Med 1989;320:1574.
341. Hammond WP, Price TH, Souza LM, Dale DC. Treatment of cyclic neutropenia with granulocyte colony-stimulating factor. N Engl J Med 1989;320:1306.
342. Jakubowski AA, Souza L, Kelly F, et al. Effects of granulocyte colony-stimulating factor in a patient with idiopathic neutropenia. N Engl J Med 1989;320:38.
343. Gabrilove JL, Jakubowski A, Scher H, et al. Effect of granulocyte colony stimulating factor on neutropenia and associated morbidity due to chemotherapy for transitional cell carcinoma of the urothelium. N Engl J Med 1988;318:1414.
344. Bronchud MH, Scarffe JN, Thatcher N, et al. Phase I/II study of recombinant human granulocyte colony-stimulating factor in patients receiving intensive chemotherapy for small cell lung cancer. Br J Cancer 1987;56:809.
345. Antman KS, Griffin JD, Elias A, et al. Effect of recombinant human granulocyte-macrophage colony-stimulating factor on chemotherapy-induced myelosuppression. N Engl J Med 1988;319:593.
346. Ganser A, Ottmann OG, Erdmann H, Schulz G, Hoelzer D. The effect of recombinant human granulocyte-macrophage colony-stimulating factor on neutropenia and related morbidity in chronic severe neutropenia. Ann Intern Med 1989;111:887.
347. Donahue RE, Wang EA, Stone DK, et al. Stimulation of haematopoiesis in primates by continuous infusion of recombinant human GM-CSF Nature 1986;321:872.
348. Mayer P, Lam C, Obenaus H, et al. Recombinant human GM-CSF induces leukocytosis and activates peripheral blood polymorphonuclear neutrophils in nonhuman primates. Blood 1987;70:206.
349. Groopman JE, Mitsuyasu RT, DeLeo MJ, et al. Phase I/II trial of recombinant granulocyte-macrophage colony-stimulating factor (rGM-

CSF) in the acquired immunodeficiency syndrome. N Engl J Med 1987;317:593.
350. Baldwin GC, Gasson JC, Quan SG, et al. GM-CSF enhances neutrophil function in AIDS patients. Proc Natl Acad Sci USA 1988;85:2763.
351. Antin JH, Smith BR, Holmes W, Rosenthal DS. Phase I/II study of recombinant human granulocyte-macrophage colony-stimulating factor in aplastic anemia and myelodysplastic syndrome. Blood 1988;72:705.
352. Champlin RE, Nimer SD, Ireland P, et al. Treatment of refractory aplastic anemia with recombinant human granulocyte-macrophage colony-stimulating factor. Blood 1989;73:694.
353. Ganser A, Volkers B, Greher J, et al. Recombinant human granulocyte-macrophage colony-stimulating factor in patients with myelodysplastic syndromes: a phase I/II trial. Blood 1989;73:31.
354. Vadhan-Raj S, Keating M, LeMaistre A, et al. Effects of recombinant human granulocyte-macrophage colony-stimulating factor in patients with myelodysplastic syndromes. N Engl J Med 1987;317:1545.
355. Nemunaitis J, Singer JW, Buckner CD, et al. Use of recombinant human granulocyte macrophage colony stimulating factor in autologous marrow transplantation for lymphoid malignancies. Blood 1988;72:834.
356. Brandt SJ, Peters WP, Atwater SK, et al. Effect of recombinant human granulocyte-macrophage colony-stimulating factor on hematopoietic reconstitution after high dose chemotherapy and autologous bone marrow. N Engl J Med 1988;318:869.
357. Glaspy JA, Baldwin GC, Robertson PA, et al. Therapy for neutropenia in hairy cell leukemia with recombinant human granulocyte colony-stimulating factor. Ann Intern Med 1988;109:789.
358. Morstyn G, Souza LM, Keech J, et al. Effect of granulocyte colony-stimulating factor on neutropenia induced by cytotoxic chemotherapy. Lancet 1988;1:667.
359. Motoyoshi K, Takaku F, Maekawa T, et al. Protective effect of partially purified human urinary colony-stimulating factor on granulocytopenia after antitumor chemotherapy. Exp Hematol 1986;14:1069.
360. Komiyama A, Ishiguro A, Kubo T, et al. Increases in neutrophil counts by purified human urinary colony-stimulating factor in chronic neutropenia of childhood. Blood 1988;71:41.
361. Masaoka T, Motoyoshi K, Takaku F, et al. Administration of human urinary colony stimulating factor after bone marrow transplantation. Bone Marrow Transplant 1988;3:121.
362. Wing EJ, Magee DM, Whiteside TL, et al. Recombinant human granulocyte/macrophage colony-stimulating factor enhances monocyte cytotoxicity and secretion of tumor necrosis factor A and interferon in cancer patients. Blood 1989;73:643.
363. Nimer SD, Champlin RE, Golde DW. Serum cholesterol-lowering activity of granulocyte-macrophage colony-stimulating factor. JAMA 1988;260:3297.
364. Motoyoshi K, Takaku F. Serum cholesterol-lowering activity of human monocytic colony-stimulating factor. Lancet 1989;2:326.
365. Altman RL, Dittmer DS. Blood and other body fluids. Washington, DC, FASEB, 1971.
366. Manroe, BL, Weinberg AG, Rosenfeld, CR, Browne R. The neonatal blood count in health and disease. I. Reference values for neutrophilic cells. J Pediatr 1979;95:89.
367. Steel CM, French EB, Atchison WRC. Studies on adrenaline-induced leucocytosis in normal man, I. The role of the spleen and of the thoracic duct. Br J Haematol 1971;21:413.
368. Dale DC, Fauci AS, Guerry D IV, Wolff SM. Comparison of agents producing a neutrophilic leukocytosis in man: hydrocortisone, prednisone, endotoxin and etiocholanolone. J Clin Invest 1975;56:808.
369. Shoeufeld Y, Gurewich Y, Galant LA, Pinkhas J. Prednisone-induced leukocytosis. Am J Med 1981;71:773.
370. Christensen RD, Bradley PP, Rothstein G. The leukocyte left shift in clinical and experimental neonatal sepsis. J Pediatr 1981;98:101–105.
371. O'Connell RA. Leukocytosis during lithium carbonate treatment. Int J Pharmacopsychiatr 1970;4:30.
372. Catane R, Kaufman J, Mittleman A, Murphy GP. Attenuation of myelosuppression with lithium. N Engl J Med 1977;297:452.
373. Gupta RC, Robinson WA, Kurnick JE. Felty's syndrome: effect of lithium on granulopoiesis. Am J Med 1976;61:29.
374. Stein RS, Beaman C, Ali MY, et al. Lithium carbonate attentuation of chemotherapy-induced neutropenia. N Engl J Med 1977;297:430.
375. Rothstein G, Clarkson DR, Larson W, et al. Effect of lithium on neutrophil mass and production. N Engl J Med 1978;178:298.
376. Harker WG, Rothstein G, Clarkson D, et al. Enhancement of colony-stimulating activity production by lithium. Blood 1977;49:263.
377. Barr RD, Koekebakker M, Brown EA, Falbo MC. Putative role for lithium in human hematopoiesis. J Lab Clin Med 1987;109:159.
378. Chen H, Walz DV. Leukemoid reaction in the bone marrow, associated with malignant neoplasms. Am J Clin Pathol 1958;29:345.
379. Meyer LM, Rotter SD. Leukemoid reaction (hyperleukocytosis) in malignancy. Am J Clin Pathol 1942;12:218.
380. Hocking W, Goodman J, Golde D. Granulocytosis associated with tumor cell production of colony-stimulating activity. Blood 1983;61:600.
381. Kuvin SF, Brecher G. Differential neutrophil counts in pregnancy. N Engl J Med 1962;266:877.
382. Van Furth R, Cohn ZA, Hirsch JG, et al. The mononuclear phagocyte system: a new classification of macrophages, monocytes, and their precursor cells. Bull WHO 1972;46:2864.
383. Metcalf D. Hematopoietic colonies: in vitro cloning of normal and leukemic cells. In: Rentchnick P, ed. Recent results in cancer research. Berlin, Springer-Verlag, 1977.
384. Metcalf D. Transformation of granulocytes to macrophages in bone marrow colonies *in vivo*. J Cell Physiol 1971;77:277.
385. Carr I. The biology of macrophages. Clin Invest Med 1978;1:59.
386. De Petris S, Karlsbad G, Pernis B. Filamentous structures in the cytoplasm of normal mononuclear phagocytes. J Ultrastruct Res 1962;7:39.
387. Bainton DF, Golde DW. Differentiation of macrophages from normal human bone marrow in liquid culture: electron microscopy and cytochemistry. J Clin Invest 1978;61:1555.
388. Cohn ZA. Structure and function of monocytes and macrophages. Adv Immunol 1968;9:163.
389. Nichols BA, Bainton DF, Farquhar MG. Differentiation of monocytes: origin, nature and fate of their azurophil granules. J Cell Biol 1971;50:498.
390. Nichols BA, Bainton DF. Differentiation of human monocytes in bone marrow and blood: sequential formation of two granule populations. Lab Invest 1973;29:27.
391. Nathan CF, Murray HW, Cohn ZA. The macrophage as an effector cell. N Engl J Med 1980;303:622.
392. Bozdech MJ, Bainton DF. Identification of α-naphthyl butyrate esterase as a plasma membrane ectoenzyme of monocytes and as a discrete intracellular membrane-bounded organelle in lymphocytes. J Exp Med 1981;153:182.
393. Braunsteiner H, Schmalzl F. Cytochemistry of monocytes and macrophages. In: Van Furth F, ed. Mononuclear phagocytes. Oxford, Blackwell, 1970:62.
394. Li CY, Lam KW, Yam LT. Esterases in human leukocytes. J Histochem Cytochem 1973;21:1.
395. Akiyama Y, et al. Characterization of a human blood monocyte subset with low peroxidase activity. J Clin Invest 1983;71:1093.
396. Figdor CG, Bont WS, Touw I, et al. Isolation of functionally different human monocytes by counterflow centrifugation elutriation. Blood 1982;60:46.
397. Norris DA, Morris RM, Sanderson RJ, Kohler PF. Isolation of functional subsets of human peripheral blood monocytes. J Immunol 1979;123:166.
398. Rosenthal AS. Regulation of the immune response: role of the macrophage. N Engl J Med 1980;303:1153.
399. Unanue ER. Cooperation between mononuclear phagocytes and lymphocytes in immunity. N Engl J Med 1980;303:977.
400. Unanue ER. The regulation of lymphocyte functions by the macrophage. Immunol Rev 1978;40:227.
401. Nossal GVJ. The basic components of the immune system. N Engl J Med 1987;316:1320.
402. Van Furth R, Raeburn JA, van Zwet TL. Characteristics of human mononuclear phagocytes. Blood 1979;54:485.
403. Van Furth R, Diesselhoff-Den Dulk MMC, Mattie H. Quantitative study on the production and kinetics of mononuclear phagocytes during an acute inflammatory reaction. J Exp Med 1973;138:1314.
404. Van Furth R, Sluiter W. Distribution of blood monocytes between a marginating and a circulating pool. J Exp Med 1986;163:474.
405. Van Furth R, Cohn ZA. The origin and kinetics of mononuclear phagocytes. J Exp Med 1968;128:415.
406. Whitelaw DM. Observations on human monocyte kinetics after pulse labeling. Cell Tissue Kinet 1972;5:311.
407. Gale RP, Sparkes RS, Golde DW. Bone marrow origin of hepatic macrophages (Kupffer cells) in humans. Science 1978;201:937.
408. Katz SI, Tamaki K, Sachs DH. Epidermal Langerhans cells are derived from cells orginating in bone marrow. Nature 1979;282:324.
409. Thomas ED, Ramberg RE, Sale GE, et al. Direct evidence for a bone marrow origin of the alveolar macrophage in man. Science 1976;192:1016.
410. Ash P, Loutit JF, Townsend KMS. Osteoclasts derived from haemopoietic stem cells. Nature 1980;283:669.
411. Coccia PF, Krivit W, Cervenka J, et al. Successful bone-marrow transplantation for infantile malignant osteopaetrosis. N Engl J Med 1980;302:701.
412. Golde DW, Byers LA, Finley TN. Proliferative capacity of human alveolar macrophage. Nature 1974;247:373.
413. Golde DW, Finley TN, Cline MJ. The pulmonary macrophage in acute leukemia. N Engl J Med 1974;290:875.
414. Melnicoff MJ, Horan PK, Breslin EW, Morahan PS. Maintenance of peritoneal macrophages in the steady state. J Leukocyte Biol 1988;44:367.
415. Reitsma PH, Rothberg PG, Astrin SM, et al. Regulation of *myc* gene expression in HL-60 leukaemia cells by a vitamin D metabolite. Nature 1983;306:492.
416. Westin EH, Gallo RC, Arya SK, et al. Differential expression of the *amv* gene in human hematopoietic cells. Proc Natl Acad Sci USA 1982;79:2194.
417. Gonda TJ, Metcalf D. Expression of *myb*, *myc* and *fos* proto-oncogenes

during differentiation of murine myeloid leukaemias. Nature 1984;310: 249.
418. Muller R, Curran T, Muller D, Guilbert L. Induction of c-*fos* during myelomonocytic differentiation and macrophage proliferation. Nature 1985;314:546.
419. Sariban E, Mitchell T, Kufe D. Expression of the c-*fms* proto-oncogene during human monocytic differentiation. Nature 1985;316:64.
420. Mitchell RL, Zokas L, Schreiber RD, Verma IM. Rapid induction of expression of proto-oncogene *fos* during human monocytic differentiation. Cell 1985;40:209.
421. Muller R, Muller D, Guilbert L. Differential expression of c-fos in hematopoietic cells: correlation with differentiation of monomyelocytic cells in vitro. EMBO J 1984;3:1887.
422. Pinto A, Colletta G, Vecchio LD, et al. c-*fos* Oncogene expression in human hematopoietic malignancies is restricted to acute leukemias with monocytic phenotype and to subsets of B cell leukemias. Blood 1987;70:1450.
423. Mitchell RL, Henning-Chubb C, Huberman E, Verma IM. c-*fos* Expression is neither sufficient nor obligatory for differentiation of monomyelocytes to macrophages. Cell 1986;45:497.
424. Cooper RA, Braunwald AD, Kuo AL. Phorbol ester induction of leukemic cell differentiation is a membrane-mediated process. Proc Natl Acad Sci USA 1982;79:2865.
425. Koeffler HP, Bar-Eli M, Territo. Phorbol ester effect on differentiation of human myeloid leukemia cell lines blocked at different stages of maturation. Cancer Res 1981;41:919.
426. Bar-Shavit Z, Teitelbaum SL, Reitsma P, et al. Induction of monocytic differentiation and bone resorption by 1,25-dihydroxyvitamin D_3. Proc Natl Acad Sci USA 1983;80:5907.
427. McCarthy DM, San Miguel JF, Freake HC, et al. 1,25-dihydroxyvitamin D_3 inhibits proliferation of human promyelocytic leukaemia (HL60) cells and induces monocyte-macrophage differentiation in HL60 and normal human bone marrow cells. Leuk Res 1983;7:51.
428. Ball ED, Guyre PM, Shen L, et al. Gamma interferon induces monocytoid differentiation in the HL-60 cell line. J Clin Invest 1983;73: 1072.
429. Todd RF III, Griffin JD, Ritz J, et al. Expression of normal monocyte-macrophage differentiation antigens on HL60 promyelocytes undergoing differentiation induced by leukocyte-conditioned medium or phorbol diester. Leuk Res 1981;5:491.
430. Mangelsdorf DJ, Koeffler HP, Donaldson CA, et al. 1,25-dihydroxyvitamin D3-induced differentiation in a human promyelocytic leukemia cell line (HL-60): receptor-mediated maturation to macrophage-like cells. J Cell Biol 1984;98:391.
431. Newburger PE, Baker RD, Hansen SL, et al. Functionally deficient differentiation of HL-60 promyelocytic leukemia cells induced by phorbol myristate acetate. Cancer Res 1981;41:1861.
432. Nichols KE, Weinberg JB. Essential amino acid deprivation induces monocyte differentiation of the human HL-60 myeloid leukemia cell line. Blood 1989;73:1298.
433. Takeda K, Iwamoto S, Sugimoto H, et al. Identity of differentiation inducing factor and tumour necrosis factor. Nature 1986;323:338.
434. Weinberg JB, Larrick JW. Receptor-mediated monocytoid differentiation of human promyelocytic cells by tumor necrosis factor: synergistic actions with interferon-g and 1,25-dihyroxyvitamin D3. Blood 1987;70: 994.
435. Ferrero D, Pessano S, Pagliardi GL, Rovera G. Induction of differentiation of human myeloid leukemias: surface changes probed with monoclonal antibodies. Blood 1983;61:171.
436. Guyre PM, Morganelli PM, Miller R. Recombinant immune interferon increases immunoglobulin G Fc receptors on cultured human mononuclear phagocytes. J Clin Invest 1983;72:393.
437. Olsson I, Olofsson T, Mauritzon N. Characterization of mononuclear blood cell-derived differentiation inducing factors for the human promyelocytic leukemia cell line HL-60. J Natl Cancer Inst 1981;67: 1225.
438. Leung K, Chiao JW. Human leukemia cell maturation induced by a T-cell lymphokine isolated from medium conditioned by normal lymphocytes. Proc Natl Acad Sci USA 1985;82:1209.
439. Olsson IL, Sarngadharan MG, Breitman TR, Gallo RC. Isolation and characterization of a T lymphocyte-derived differentiation inducing factor for the myeloid leukemic cell line HL-60. Blood 1984;63: 510.
440. Abe T, Murakami M, Sato T, et al. Macrophage differentiation inducing factor from human monocytic cells is equivalent to murine leukemia inhibitory factor. J Biol Chem 1989;246:8941.
441. Olsson I, Breitman TR. Induction of differentiation of the human histiocytic lymphoma cell line, U-937, by retinoic acid and cyclic AMP-inducing agents. Cancer Res 1982;42:3924.
442. Dodd RC, Cohen MS, Newman SL, Gray TK. Vitamin D metabolites change the phenotype of monoblastic U937 cells. Proc Natl Acad Sci USA 1983;80:7538.
443. Hattori T, Pack M, Bougnoux P, et al. Interferon-induced differentiation of U937 cells: comparison with other agents that promote differentiation of human myeloid or monocytelike cell lines. J Clin Invest 1983;72:237.
444. Ralph P, Harris PE, Punjabi CJ, et al. Lymphokine inducing "terminal differentiation" of the human monoblast leukemia line U937: a role for γ interferon. Blood 1983;62:1169.
445. Zuckerman SH, Surprenant YM, Tang J. Synergistic effect of granulocyte-macrophage colony-stimulating factor and 1,25-dihyroxyvitamin D3 on the differentiation of the human monocytic cell line U937. Blood 1988;71:619.
446. Geissler K, Harrington M, Srivastava C, Leemhuis T, Tricot G, Broxmeyer HE. Effects of recombinant human colony stimulating factors (CSF) (granulocyte-macrophage CSF, granulocyte CSF, and CSF-1) on human monocyte/macrophage differentiation. J Immunol 1989;143: 140.
447. Clement LT, Roberts RL, Martin AM. Characterization of a monocyte differentiation factor distinct from gamma-interferon, tumor necrosis factor, or G,M-colony-stimulating factor that regulates the growth and function capabilities of the U937 monocytic cell line. J Leukocyte Biol 1988;44:101.
448. Kurata N, Akiyama H, Taniyama T, Marunouchi T. Dose-dependent regulation of macrophage differentiation by mos mRNA in a human monocytic cell line. EMBO J 1989;8:457.
449. Lindley I, Aschauer H, Seifert JM, et al. Synthesis and expression in *Escherichia coli* of the gene encoding monocyte-derived neutrophil-activating factor: biological equivalence between natural and recombinant neutrophil-activating factor. Proc Natl Acad Sci USA 1988;85: 9199.
450. Yoshimura T, Matsushima K, Tanaka S, et al. Purification of a human monocyte-derived neutrophil chemotactic factor that has peptide sequence similarity to other host defense cytokines. Proc Natl Acad Sci USA 1987;84:9233.
451. Gregory H, Young J, Schroder J-M, et al. Structure determination of a human lymphocyte derived neutrophil activating peptide (LYNAP). Biochem Biophys Res Commun 1988;151:883.
452. Van Damme J, van Beeumen J, Opdenakker G, Billiau A. A novel, NH_2-terminal sequence-characterized human monokine possessing neutrophil chemotactic, skin-reactive, and granulocytosis-promoting activity. J Exp Med 1988;167:1364.
453. Peveri P, Walz A, Dewald B, Baggiolini M. A novel neutrophil-activating factor produced by human mononuclear phagocytes. J Exp Med 1988;167:1547.
454. Thelen M, Peveri P, Kernen P, et al. Mechanism of neutrophil activation by NAF, a novel monocyte-derived peptide agonist. FASEB J 1988;2:2702.
455. Schmid J, Weissmann C. Induction of mRNA for a serine protease and a β-thromboglobulin-like protein in mitogen-stimulated human leukocytes. J Immunol 1987;139:250.
456. Stanley ER, Heard PM. Factors regulating macrophage production and growth. J Biol Chem 1977;252:4305.
457. Nathan CF. Secretory products of macrophages. J Clin Invest 1987;79: 319.
458. Oster W, Lindemann A, Horn S, et al. Tumor necrosis factor (TNF)-alpha but not TNF-beta induces secretion of colony-stimulating factor for macrophages (CSF-1) by human monocytes. Blood 1987;70:1700.
459. Bartocci A, Mastrogiannis DS, Migliorati G, et al. Macrophages specifically regulate the concentration of their own growth factor in the circulation. Proc Natl Acad Sci USA 1987;84:6179.
460. Cannistra SA, Rambaldi A, Spriggs DR, et al. Human granulocyte-macrophage colony-stimulating factor induces expression of the tumor necrosis factor gene by the U937 cell line and by normal human monocytes. J Clin Invest 1987;79:1720.
461. Zhou YQ, Stanley ER, Clark SC, et al. Interleukin-3 and interleukin-1α allow earlier bone marrow progenitors to respond to human colony-stimulating factor-1. Blood 1988;72:1870.
462. Kurland JI, Broxmeyer HE, Pelus LM, et al. Role for monocyte-macrophage–derived colony-stimulating factor and prostaglandin E in the positive and negative feedback control of myeloid stem cell proliferation. Blood 1978;52:388.
463. Kurland JI, Bockman RS, Broxmeyer HE, Moore MAS. Limitation of excessive myelopoiesis by the intrinsic modulation of macrophage-derived prostaglandin E. Science 1978;199:552.
464. Koch F, Heufler C, Kämpgen E, Schneeweiss D, Böock G, Schüler G. Tumor necrosis factor α maintains the viability of murine epidermal Langerhans cells in culture, but in contrast to granulocyte/macrophage colony-stimulating factor, without inducing their functional maturation. J Exp Med 1990;171:159.
465. Williams N, Jackson H. Limitation of macrophage production in long term marrow cultures containing prostaglandin E. J Cell Physiol 1980;103:239.
466. Pelus LM, Broxmeyer HE, Kurland JI, Moore MAS. Regulation of macrophage and granulocyte proliferation: specificities of prostaglandin E and lactoferrin. J Exp Med 1979;150:277.
467. Assoian RK, Fleurdelys BE, Stevenson HC, et al. Expression and secretion of type β transforming growth factor by activated human macrophages. Proc Natl Acad Sci USA 1987;84:6020.
468. Strassmann G, Cole MD, Newman W. Regulation of colony-stimulating factor 1-dependent macrophage precursor proliferation by type b transforming growth factor. J Immunol 1988;140:2645.
469. Munan L, Kelly A. Age-dependent changes in blood monocyte populations in man. Clin Exp Immunol 1979;35:161.

470. Kato K. Leukocytes in infancy and childhood. J Pediatr 1935;7:7.
471. Maldonado JE, Hanlon DG. Monocytosis: a current appraisal. Mayo Clin Proc 1965;40:248.
472. Flinn JW. A study of differential blood count in one thousand cases of active pulmonary tuberculosis. Ann Intern Med 1929;2:622.
473. Daland GA, Gottlieb L, Wallerstein RO, et al. Hematologic observations in bacterial endocarditis: especially the prevalence of histiocytes and the elevation and variation of the white cell count in blood from the ear lobe. J Lab Clin Med 1956;48:827.
474. Rosahn PD, Pearce L. The blood cytology in untreated and treated syphilis. Am J Med Sci 1934;187:88.
475. Barrett O Jr. Monocytosis in malignant disease. Ann Intern Med 1970;73:991.
476. Levinson B, Walter BA, Wintrobe MM, Cartwright GE. A clinical study in Hodgkin's disease. Arch Intern Med 1957;99:519.
477. Ultman JE. Clinical features and diagnosis of Hodgkin's disease. Cancer 1966;19:297.
478. Saarni MI, Liman JW. Preleukemia: the hematologic syndrome preceding acute leukemia. Am J Med 1973;55:38.
479. Bearman RM, Kjeldsberg CR, Pangalis GA, Rappaport H. Chronic monocytic leukemia in adults. Cancer 1981;48:2239.
480. Brynes RK, Golomb HM, Desser RK, et al. Acute monocytic leukemia. Am J Clin Pathol 1976;65:471.
481. Geary CG, Catovsky D, Wiltshaw E, et al. Chronic myelomonocytic leukemia. Br J Haematol 1975;30:289.
482. Saarni MI, Liman JW. Myelomonocytic leukemia. Cancer 1971;27:1221.
483. Dale DC, Fauci AS, Wolff SM. Alternate-day prednisone: leukocyte kinetics and susceptibility to infections. N Engl J Med 1974;291:1154.
484. Thompson J, van Furth R. The effect of glucocorticosteroids on the proliferation and kinetics of promonocytes and monocytes of the bone marrow. J Exp Med 1973;137:10.
485. Seshardi RS, Brown EJ, Zipursky A. Leukemic reticuloendotheliosis: a failure of monocyte production. N Engl J Med 1976;295:181.
486. Turner A, Kjeldsberg CR. Hairy cell leukemia. Medicine 1978;57:477.
487. Twomey JJ, Douglass CC, Sharkey O Jr. The monocytopenia of aplastic anemia. Blood 1973;41:187.

Blood: Principles and Practice of Hematology,
edited by Robert I. Handin, Thomas P. Stossel, and Samuel E. Lux.
J.B. Lippincott Company, Philadelphia © 1995.

18

Acute Myelogenous Leukemia

Howard J. Weinstein
James D. Griffin

Acute myelogenous leukemia (AML) is a disorder caused by the malignant transformation of a bone marrow hematopoietic stem cell. This transformed stem cell has an increased rate of self-renewal and is inevitably associated with aberrant or absent differentiation, leading to an accumulation of cells in the marrow with phenotypic features of immature phagocytes, conventionally designated *myeloid cells*. This usurpation of normal bone marrow by leukemic cells ultimately suppresses normal hematopoiesis and produces the clinical signs and symptoms of bone marrow failure. During the past decade, the application of new techniques in molecular biology, cytogenetics, and immunology to the study of AML has greatly improved our understanding of this disease. Further, important advances in the treatment of AML with chemotherapy or bone marrow transplantation have significantly improved the prognosis for most patients with this disease.

Although Virchow[1] recognized leukemia ("white blood") as a clinical entity in 1845, it is likely that most, or all, of Virchow's cases represented chronic lymphocytic or granulocytic leukemias. Leukemia with an acute course was not reported until 1857 by Friedreich.[2] Such cases were considered to be lymphocytic in origin until Naegeli[3] described the myeloblast in 1900 as a precursor of blood neutrophilic granulocytes. It then became evident that many cases of leukemia, both acute and chronic, originated from marrow myeloid cells, and were thus *myelogenous*. Subtypes of AML were recognized as early as 1913, with the reporting of a possible case of acute monocytic leukemia.[4] Later, subsets of monocytic leukemia were described, including myelomonocytic (Naegeli's type) and pure monocytic (Schilling's type) leukemia.[5] In 1946, DiGuglielmo reported an acute disorder that involved primarily the erythroid series.[6] Morphologic subtypes continue to be defined, including acute promyelocytic leukemia (APL) in 1957,[7] acute megakaryoblastic leukemia in 1963,[8] and microgranular APL in 1980.[9] Organization of the various subtypes of AML into a widely accepted classification system has been accomplished in the past decade by a French–American–British (FAB)[10–13] cooperative group, and this has greatly facilitated studies of prognostic features and interpretation of clinical trials in AML.[14]

EPIDEMIOLOGY

Acute myelogenous leukemia accounts for 15% to 20% of the acute leukemias in children and 80% of the acute leukemias in adults. The overall annual incidence of AML in the United States is about 2.3 per 100,000 people.[15] The age-specific incidence of AML increases from fewer than 1 per 100,000 people under age 30 until it reaches about 15 per 100,000 people over age 80. The median age of patients with AML is about 55 years. In contrast to ALL, there is no peak age incidence of AML in childhood.[16] Both ALL and AML are slightly more common in males than females, and the reported incidence is similar in patients of different races. Geographic variations in both incidence and subtypes of leukemia have been observed in children.[17] In Japan and several African countries, in contrast to the United States and Europe, the incidence of childhood AML is greater than childhood ALL. In Turkey, the M4 subtype of AML (discussed later) has been often associated with orbital chloromas and accounts for about 35% of all cases of childhood leukemia.[18]

ETIOLOGY

Although the cause of AML in humans is unknown, several predisposing factors, as well as inciting agents, are well established. Risk factors such as exposure to high-dose radiation, occupational exposure to benzene, and prior chemotherapy for other cancers or benign conditions have been fairly well established, but together these factors probably account for only a small proportion of cases of AML in children and adults.

Radiation

Ionizing radiation remains the most conclusively identified leukemogenic factor in humans.[19] Physicians and scientists exposed to excessive amounts of radiation during the early years of research on medical application of x-rays,[20] patients given low-dose radiation for rheumatoid spondylitis,[21] and Japanese atomic bomb survivors have all been found to have an increased incidence of leukemia.[22] Children and adults exposed to radiation from the atomic bombs in Japan had a 20-fold increased incidence of both AML and chronic myelogenous leukemia (CML) that peaked 5 to 9 years after the explosion, and 20 years later the incidence of acute leukemia remained elevated.[23]

Considerable controversy still surrounds whether the developing fetus is unusually susceptible to radiation-induced carcinogenesis.[19] Studies of atomic bomb survivors have not confirmed an increased risk for leukemia after low-dose intrauterine or preconception irradiation.[24] There are also conflicting reports about whether prenatal exposure to diagnostic x-rays is associated with an increased risk of leukemia and other childhood cancers.[25] An increased risk of leukemia has also been reported to be associated with nuclear power reactors[26] and with occupational or residential exposure to electromagnetic radiation. These reports are controversial and inconclusive.[27,28]

Chemical Agents

Both chemotherapy and occupational chemical exposure have been associated with an increased risk for AML.[29,30] High-dose occupational benzene exposure increases the risk of AML, with bone marrow hypoplasia or pancytopenia often preceding the diagnosis of leukemia. Less convincing reports have implicated chloramphenicol[31] and phenylbutazone[32] as leukemogenic agents. The use of alkylating agents such as nitrogen mustard, chlorambucil, and melphalan, for both neoplastic and benign conditions, has resulted in an increased risk for developing AML or a myelodysplastic syndrome (MDS; see Chap. 12).[33–35] In many cases, these secondary leukemias have developed in the absence of radiation therapy or a predisposing immunodeficiency. From 2% to 10% of patients treated with a regimen of mechlorethamine, Oncovin (vincristine), procarbazine, and prednisone (MOPP) chemotherapy for Hodgkin's disease developed AML within 2 to 12 years after completing chemotherapy, with the peak incidence at 6 years. In several of these Hodgkin's disease studies, splenectomy was an added risk factor for developing AML.[34] Until recently, patients given nonalkylating cytotoxic agents as cancer chemotherapy had not been reported to develop AML as a second neoplasm. Recent reports of children treated for ALL[36] and adults treated for small cell lung cancer[37] suggested that the epipodophyllotoxins (VM 26 or VP 16) may also be leukemogenic.

Viruses

Retroviruses are clearly capable of inducing acute leukemia in mice, domestic cats, cattle, chickens, and gibbon apes.[38,39] With one exception, attempts to identify leukemogenic viruses in humans have been inconclusive. It was only recently demonstrated that any human leukemia was caused by a virus. Clusters of adult T-cell leukemia in Japan and in islands of the Caribbean were independently found to be due to the retrovirus human T-cell leukemia virus type 1.[40,41]

Recent studies have focused on investigating the role of dominant and recessive cellular oncogenes in the pathogenesis of AML rather than continuing the search for leukemogenic viruses in humans. These investigations aim to establish causal relations between altered gene expression and leukemic hematopoiesis.

Oncogenes and Human Leukemogenesis

Many genes involved in the regulation of cell growth and development have been found in mutated forms in retroviruses capable of transforming animal cells.[42] The normal cellular versions of these genes, protooncogenes, are typically involved in stimulating cell proliferation in normal cells and include growth factors, growth factor receptors, and signal-transducing molecules[43–45] (see Chap. 6). In addition to growth-stimulating oncogenes, a growing number of human tumors have been found to have deletions of tumor suppressor genes such as the retinoblastoma gene or p53.[46,47] Such genes are believed to normally regulate cell growth at specific checkpoints in the cell cycle. A third class of oncogene is typified by *bcl*-2, which encodes a protein that reduces programmed cell death, or apoptosis.

Retroviruses that contain mutated versions of growth-stimulating genes such as tyrosine kinases have been shown to effectively transform hematopoietic cells in several non-human animals.[48,49] For example, retroviruses with activated versions of *src*, *abl*, *fgr*, and *yes* readily cause leukemias or other tumors in animals. However, except for *abl*, activating mutations in tyrosine kinase protooncogenes are uncommon in human leukemias. In CML, the activation of *abl* tyrosine kinase activity by the *bcr/abl* rearrangement has been well described.[50,51]

In contrast to tyrosine kinase protooncogenes, mutations are commonly observed (40%) in members of the *ras* family in human AML and MDS.[52–54] The human genome has three *ras* genes, N-*ras* at chromosome 1p11–13, H-*ras* at 11p14.1, and K-*ras* at 12p12.1.[55,56] The three protooncogenes encode proteins of 21-kd molecular mass, which are similar structurally and functionally. The *ras* proteins are guanosine triphosphate (GTP)-binding proteins, have GTPase activity, and have some homology with the α subunit of G proteins involved in transmembrane cellular signal transduction.[55,56] Unlike the classic G proteins, however, human *ras* proteins are not thought to modulate the activity of adenyl cyclase. It is likely, however, that members of this family serve to transduce some type of signal from membrane receptors. For example, some receptors of the hematopoietic growth factor receptor family are known to activate p21 *ras* in normal cells.[57] The *ras* proteins are believed to be activated when GTP is bound and inactivated after hydrolysis of the GTP to guanosine diphosphate (GDP) and Pi.[58] Point mutations that reduce the GTPase activity lead to transformation, presumably by producing a prolonged active state of *ras*. Mutations in *ras* genes have been found to occur primarily in codons 12, 13, 59, and 61.[55,56] These codons all encode for regions of *ras* that are directly involved in GDP–GTP binding.[59] Animal model studies suggest that activation of a *ras* gene is by itself insufficient to cause tumor development. Complementing mutations in other protooncogenes are likely to be required in most tumors. Point mutations have been detected in each of the three *ras* genes in AML but are most common in N-*ras*.[52–54] Mutations in *ras* do not clearly correlate with morphology or prognosis.[60] When relapse samples have been compared with initial diagnostic samples, occasional *ras* mutations are no longer detected.[61] The latter observation suggests that *ras* mutations may be acquired in a subclone of a leukemia and thus may be more important for progression than for initiation of the clone. There is no clinical benefit to the patient in determining the presence or absence of *ras* mutations. If it becomes possible in the future to pharmacologically inhibit *ras* function, this could form the basis for a new strategy of treatment for AML.

Overall, although many oncogenes can be identified that cause leukemias in lower animals, only a small number have been shown to be leukemogenic in humans. In contrast, the cloning of genes at the breakpoints of chromosomal translocations has been used to identify several novel genes that are likely to be involved in causing human myeloid leukemias. These include the PML-RARα fusion gene produced as a result of the t(15;17)(q22;q12-21) translocation in acute promyelocytic leukemia[62–64]; the AML 1/ETO fusion gene produced by the t(8;21) translocation[66–70]; the CBF β/PEBP2 β/myosin heavy-chain fusion protein produced by the inversion 16[71]; the MLL/AF4 fusion gene produced by the t(4;11) translocation[72–76]; and the Dek-Can fusion gene produced as a result of the t(6;9)(p23,q24) translocation.[65] These potential oncogenes are discussed in more detail later in this chapter.

The deletion or mutation of tumor suppresor genes may also play an important role in human myeloid leukemias. Mutations in the retinoblastome gene and decreased expression of the Rb protein have been described in some cases.[77] Similarly, mutations in the p53 gene have been observed in AML and the blast crisis phase of CML.[78] Deletions of the interferon regulatory factor-1 (IRF-1) gene at 5q31 in each of 13 cases of leukemia or myelodysplastic syndrome have been reported.[79] The IRF-1 gene has antioncogenic activity in fibroblasts and may be a tumor suppressor gene.[80]

Host Susceptibility

Clinical observations have identified unusual susceptibility to AML in monozygotic twins[81] and people with certain heritable disorders and genetic syndromes. Hereditary conditions associated with chromosomal instability and a predisposition to AML include Bloom's syndrome and Fanconi's anemia.[82] Congenital bone marrow failure syndromes such as Diamond-Blackfan anemia[83] (see Chap. 10) and Kostmann's syndrome[84] (see Chap. 17) also appear to predispose patients to an increased risk for AML.

Children with Down's syndrome have a 10- to 20-fold increased risk of leukemia during the first decade of life.[85] The types of leukemia follow the usual distribution of acute leukemia in the United States and Europe (ALL/AML ratio is 4:1) in childhood, except during the neonatal period. Neonates with Down's syndrome are more likely to develop AML or MDS than ALL. These data, however, may be biased by inclusion of neonates with trisomy 21 and a disorder called the *transient myeloproliferative syndrome* (TMS).[86] TMS is invariably diagnosed during the first month of life and is clinically and hematologically indistinguishable from congenital AML.[87] In contrast to congenital AML, however, spontaneous regression with normalization of blood counts occurs in most of these infants within weeks to months without specific antileukemia therapy. The blasts associated with this unique syndrome have been shown to have cell-surface antigens that are characteristic of megakaryoblasts[87,88] and data from several cases show that this proliferation is clonal.[89] TMS has also been observed in newborns without the clinical features of Down's syndrome but with a mosaic karyotype and trisomy 21.[90,91] About 20% to 30% of infants with TMS eventually develop AML, often type M7.[92,93]

BIOLOGY

Hematopoietic Stem Cells

Acute myelogenous leukemia cells are derived from immature hematopoietic cells and retain many biologic features of their cell of origin. Understanding the nature of the cellular defects in AML requires an appreciation of normal hematopoiesis, particularly the regulation of granulocyte and monocyte production. Briefly, mature granulocytes, monocytes, and their immediate precursors (myeloid cells) are derived from a small population of pluripotent stem cells that have extensive capacity to self-renew and to differentiate.[94-98] These stem cells reside in and interact with a complex microenvironment composed of endothelial cells, fibroblasts, adipocytes, macrophages, and T lymphocytes, the bone marrow "stroma." Evidence for the existence of self-renewing stem cells first came from the work of Till and McCulloch,[94,97] who noted 30 years ago that injection of syngeneic marrow into lethally irradiated mice resulted in the formation of macroscopic colonies of hematopoietic cells in the spleen. The colonies were shown to be the product of single cells, termed *colony-forming unit–spleen* (CFU-S), through the use of marker chromosomes.[97] Self-renewal of CFU-S was demonstrated by showing that colonies could be excised, homogenized, and reinjected into new irradiated recipients, resulting in the growth of new CFU-S colonies. At about the same time, Pluznick and Sachs,[95] Pike and Robinson,[96] Bradley and Metcalf,[98] and others initiated efforts to define in vitro culture conditions that would support growth of hematopoietic precursor cells. In semisolid media, marrow cells exhibited little spontaneous proliferation, but colonies of single or multiple lineages were readily produced when CSFs were added (initially in the form of media conditioned by exposure to spleen cells, mononuclear blood cells, or certain tumor cell lines).[99-101] The in vitro assays continue to be refined but have made it possible to identify a hierarchy of hematopoietic progenitor cells and determine their individual growth factor requirements. The most primitive and most recently identified clonogenic cell, termed the *CFU–blast cell* by Ogawa and colleagues,[102] gives rise to a small colony composed of blasts with a high secondary plating efficiency. The CFU–blast cell also has some degree of self-renewal. Evidence from murine marrow transplantation studies suggest that blast colony cells are close to true hematopoietic (transplantable) stem cells. The recent efforts of Weissman and colleagues[103] to purify murine hematopoietic stem cells are likely to clarify the relation of CFU-S and CFU–blast to true stem cells.

Several other distinct stages of progenitor cells have been identified that fall between stem cells and mature myeloid elements. The colony-forming unit, granulocyte, erythrocyte, monocyte, megakaryocyte (CFU-GEMM) is a cell that is multipotent by virtue of its ability to give rise to multiple cell lineages (granulocyte, erythrocyte, monocyte, and megakaryocyte) but has a limited capacity for self-renewal.[104] Of particular interest for the study of AML is the existence of several different levels of progenitor cells committed to granulocyte and monocyte differentiation that produce colonies containing only neutrophils, both neutrophils and monocytes, only monocytes, or only eosinophils. These cells, termed *CFU-G, CFU-GM, CFU-M,* or *CFU-Eo,* respectively, have no self-renewal potential, and a high fraction are actively cycling.[105,106] Similarly, clonogenic cells committed to erythroid differentiation can be assayed as burst-forming units (BFU-E) or the more mature CFU-E.[107]

Colony-Stimulating Factors

The factors that regulate the growth of normal stem cells are also important in the growth of AML cells.[108] The conditioned media that were originally used to support the growth of clonogenic cells have been shown to contain several specific factors, including interleukin-3 (IL-3), granulocyte-macrophage colony-stimulating factor (GM-CSF), granulocyte colony-stimulating factor (G-CSF), or macrophage colony-stimulating factor (M-CSF, or CSF-1).[109-114] There is clear evidence that these factors act directly on some progenitor cells to stimulate production of neutrophils or monocytes, and there is evidence to suggest that they are active in vivo as well.[115-122] The cDNAs for all of CSF genes have been cloned and recombinant human and murine factors produced.[109-114] The availability of pure CSFs has allowed precise characterization of their functions and specificity. The cellular and molecular characteristics of IL-3, GM-CSF, G-CSF, and M-CSF are summarized in Table 18-1.

In Vitro Growth of AML Cells

Many advances in our understanding of AML cell biology are a result of studies of the proliferation of leukemic cells in tissue culture.[108] AML cells from the blood or marrow of over 90% of cases grow in semisolid media or liquid suspension culture for periods of 7 days to 6 months or

TABLE 18-1. Biologic Characteristics of Human Colony-Stimulating Factors Affecting AML Cell Growth

Factor	Alternate Name	Major Target Cells	Protein Size (kd)	Chromosome	Effect on AML
IL-3	Multi-CSF	CFU-GEMM, CFU-GM, BFU-E, CFU-meg, CFU-eo, mono	20–26 (133 amino acids)	5q23-31	++++
GM-CSF	CSF-α, pluripoietin-α	CFU-GEMM, CFU-GM, BFU-E, CFU-meg, CFU-Eo, gran, mono	14–30 (127 amino acids)	5q23-31	++++
G-CSF	CSF-β, pluripoietin	CFU-G, neut	18–22 (177 amino acids)	17q11.2-q21	+++
M-CSF	CSF-1	CFU-M, mono	Dimer 40–44 × 2 or 18–26 × 2 (3 different cDNAs; 3 different 1 proteins; 2 different secreted M-CSFs	5q33.1	+

eo, eosinophil; G or gran, granulocyte; E, erythroid; CFU, colony-forming unit; mono, monocyte; BFU-E, erythroid burst-forming unit; meg, megakaryocyte; neut, neutrophil; GEMM, granulocyte, erythrocyte, monocyte, megakaryocyte; GM, granulocyte-macrophage.

more. The assay of leukemic clonogenic cells (CFU-AML) has been particularly informative.[108] Only a small subset of cells (typically 0.1% to 1%) proliferate in agar or methycellulose to form a colony of leukemic blasts.[120] The remaining cells are either nonproliferative or can undergo only one to four cell divisions. The CFU-AML have several properties of leukemic stem cells, including self-renewal capacity[121,122] and the ability to produce daughter cells that have undergone partial differentiation as assessed by analysis of cell-surface antigens.[123] Thus, studies of AML-CFU suggest that production of leukemic leukocytes is similar in some respects to normal myelopoiesis. Small numbers of highly proliferative, self-renewing, leukemic stem cells produce large numbers of partially differentiated but nonfunctional leukemic cells, which fill the marrow and physically suppress normal hematopoiesis. The self-renewal capacity of AML-CFU is limited in culture, and permanent cell lines are only rarely obtained.[124] This suggests that leukemic stem cells may exist that are even earlier than the AML-CFU and that have not been successfully cultured.

The gross appearance of AML colonies in semisolid media is different than normal CFU-GM–derived colonies. The leukemic colonies are smaller and tend not to display the heterogeneity of normal granulocyte and monocyte colonies.[108] Typical AML colony morphology can be seen in preleukemic disorders that may herald the onset of acute leukemia. In remission, colony morphology usually returns to a normal pattern.[125,126] The degree of AML-CFU self-renewal has also been investigated as a prognostic factor in AML. Higher secondary plating efficiency (higher self-renewal) has been associated with a significantly worse treatment outcome.[127] The secondary plating efficiency assay is technically difficult and is not recommended for routine analysis. The sensitivity of AML-CFU to cytotoxic drugs can be readily assessed, and in general, there is a positive correlation between in vitro sensitivity and patient response to induction therapy.[108] Considerable overlap, however, exists between sensitive and resistant cases, and the technique has not found widespread acceptance.

Cell Cycle Analysis and Kinetic Properties of AML Cells

Extensive studies of cell cycle kinetics have been conducted in AML in an effort to better understand the clinical heterogeneity of these patients. Initial studies by Clarkson and colleagues,[128] Killman,[129] and Mauer and colleagues[130] estimated the fraction of cells in S phase by infusing pulses of ^{3}H-thymidine into patients with advanced disease. The labeling indexes were surprisingly low (5% to 7%). More sophisticated studies in which bromodeoxyuridine (BrdU) was infused, followed by detection of labeled cells in marrow biopsy specimens by immunofluorescence, gave a slightly higher value (mean 17%), but this was still lower than the estimates of 35% to 55% labeling index of myeloblasts in normal bone marrow.[131,132] These results suggest that most leukemic cells are not proliferating and thus do not incorporate nucleic acids into DNA. These in vivo results are consistent with in vitro studies of clonogenic AML cells that indicate that only a small fraction of leukemic cells have extensive proliferative capacity and that most leukemic cells rapidly become quiescent.[108]

Limited studies of cell cycle parameters have also been undertaken on clonogenic cells using the technique of "thymidine suicide" or some variation thereof. Marrow or blood cells are briefly (30 to 60 minutes) exposed to high-specific-activity ^{3}H-thymidine. Cells in S phase incorporate a lethal dose of tritium, and the subsequent loss of clonogenic cells (compared with unexposed cells) represents the fraction in S. Such studies have shown that clonogenic cells have a high S phase fraction (30% to 50%). Recent studies suggest that this fraction can be further increased both in vitro and in vivo by exposure of leukemic cells to GM-CSF or other growth factors. This observation has led to the suggestion that it may be possible to augment the effectiveness of S phase–specific chemotherapy drugs, such as cytarabine, by combining such drugs with GM-CSF.[133]

Leukemic cell cycle time has been measured by exposing cells to two separate pulses of labeling agents, such as an in vivo pulse of BrdU followed by an in vitro pulse of ^{3}H-thymidine.[131,132] Cell cycle times have been extremely variable, ranging from about 24 hours to more than 10 days. Such studies are complicated by the heterogeneity of proliferative potential of leukemic cells in each patient. The cell cycle time of clonogenic cells is considerably shorter, with estimates of 9 to 22 hours.

The clinical utility of measuring cell cycle parameters in AML has not been determined. Limited studies have suggested that patients with either very low or very high labeling indexes may have a poorer prognosis. In general, however, technical difficulties with the assays and leukemic cell heterogeneity have limited the clinical usefulness of these studies.

Growth Factors for AML Cells in Tissue Culture

In 20% to 25% of cases, leukemic cells proliferate spontaneously in vitro in fetal calf serum–containing media.[134,135] Such spontaneous proliferation is not observed with normal marrow cells or cells from myelodysplastic patients. In most AML cases, however, proliferation of leukemic cells requires the addition of specific growth factors. With few exceptions, the same factors that support the growth of normal myeloid cells also support the growth of AML cells, including GM-CSF, IL-3, G-CSF, M-CSF, and IL-1.[134–137] The most effective factors to promote growth of AML cells in both semisolid media and in liquid suspension culture are GM-CSF and IL-3 (see Table 18-1). Combinations of CSFs, such as GM-CSF and G-CSF, are more active than single factors.[134] There is no evidence from tissue culture studies that any of these CSFs enhance differentiation of AML cells. In limited clinical trials in myelodysplasia and AML, GM-CSF, G-CSF, and IL-3 were shown to accelerate leukemic cell proliferation in some cases.[138–144] This suggests both that these CSFs are important growth factors in vivo and that supply of CSF may be a limiting factor in the rate of leukemic cell proliferation in patients. However, most patients with MDS receiving CSFs do not progress to AML. Preliminary studies suggest that patients with more advanced disease (refractory anemia with excess blasts in transformation)[RAEB-t] are more likely to convert to AML with CSF stimulation. The rate of transformation may be particularly low with G-CSF.

The response of AML cells in vitro and in vivo to CSFs suggest that a supply of these factors may be critical for progression of AML in patients. Indirect evidence supports this concept in murine leukemias. Several cloned hematopoietic cell lines have been developed, such as FDC-P1, which are immortal but remain dependent on GM-CSF or IL-3 for growth.[145] Such cell lines are not leukemic in syngeneic animals despite an extremely high rate of self-renewal. When FDC-P1 cells are made to secrete GM-CSF or IL-3 after retroviral insertion of a CSF cDNA, these cells rapidly become factor-independent and fully leukemogenic.[146] The autocrine production of CSFs has also been demonstrated in spontaneous and virus-induced murine leukemias.[147,148] In some examples, virus insertion has been shown to occur adjacent to or within a CSF gene.[149] Human leukemias are usually not factor-independent, however, and only about one fifth of cases proliferate spontaneously in culture.[134,135] Some of these spontaneously proliferating cases produce a CSF in culture, usually GM-CSF, IL-1, or G-CSF.[150–154] Evidence that CSFs are being produced in vivo is lacking, although cases have been reported in which serum G-CSF levels have been elevated.[155] Thus, it is possible that autocrine and paracrine stimulation of AML cells occurs in some cases. Excess growth factor supply by itself, however, would not be leukemogenic. The primary transforming event must cause an increase in the rate of self-renewal and a decrease in differentiation. Nonetheless, autonomous proliferation in culture indicates a poor prognosis.[156]

Leukemic Cell Lines

Extensive studies on the growth properties and differentiation of several myeloid leukemia cell lines have been conducted.[124] The most useful cell lines have included the promyelocytic line HL-60,[157] the myeloblast cell line KG-1,[158] the Philadelphia (Ph) chromosome erythroleukemic cell line K562,[159] and the monocytic lines U937[160] and THP-1.[161] These cell lines all have some common features, including that they are all factor-independent for growth and that they can be induced to undergo some degree of differentiation in response to agents such as phorbol ester, tumor necrosis factor, retinoic acid, or 1,25 dihydroxvitamin D_3.[124] HL-60 has been particularly valuable because of the large variety of effective differentiating agents and the finding that it can differentiate to either macrophages or to a neutrophil-like cell in response to different inducing agents.[162] Differentiation of all the cell lines is associated with cessation or diminishment of proliferation. Studies with HL-60, in particular, have been used to identify agents for clinical trials of differentiation therapy. Unfortunately, preliminary clinical studies of such inducers, including interferon-γ, tumor necrosis factor, 13-*cis*-retinoic acid, hexamethylene bisacetamide, and low-dose cytarabine, have produced only modest evidence of either significant in vivo differentiation of AML cells or significant clinical benefit.[163] Many trials are using combinations of differentiating agents with each other or with CSFs. However, all-*trans*-retinoic acid appears to be an effective differentiating agent for patients with acute promyelocytic leukemia with a t(15;17) chromosomal translocation.[164,165]

Although the leukemic cell lines are valuable models of primary AML, there are a number of fundamental biologic differences between the cell lines listed previously and primary AML cells. First, primary AML cells are almost always dependent on CSFs for in vitro growth, while all the commonly used cell lines are factor independent. Also, primary AML cells have a limited life-span in tissue culture, possibly indicating that they may require a stromal cell microenvironment for optimal growth and self-renewal. Improvements in long-term culture of AML cells would solve many of these problems. Finally, many of the cell lines have evolved in culture, acquiring (or losing) new characteristics, including karyotypic changes.

Clonality

In contrast to normal blood cells, myeloid leukemic cells are monoclonal, derived from a single stem cell that has become neoplastic. Evidence for the monoclonal nature of AML comes from three lines of evidence. First, studies of female patients heterozygous for isoenzymes of the X-linked gene encoding glucose-6-phosphate dehydrogenase (G6PD) indicates that while normal cells in heterozygous people are always polyclonal (have about equal amounts of G6PD isoenzymes A and B), AML cells express only a single isoenzyme and are therefore derived from a single cell.[166,167] Second, cytogenetic analysis of AML cells frequently shows specific chromosomal markers that are present in all metaphases.[168–171] Finally, restriction fragment length polymorphism (RFLP) studies of X-chromosomal genes, such as phosphoglycerol kinase, have confirmed the clonality of AML and further indicated that remission cells in occasional patients with AML may also be clonal.[172,173] Although the significance of clonal remissions is not clear, one explanation is that AML in some patients arises in the setting of a clonal blood disorder, such as a myelodysplastic or myeloproliferative syndrome. Successful therapy of the acute leukemia leads to reemergence of the underlying preleukemic disorder.

Cell of Origin

Karyotype, G6PD isoenzyme, and RFLP analyses have been used to investigate clonality of individual lineages in AML to determine at what point in the hierarchy of hematopoietic stem cells the leukemic cells arise. In contrast to CML, in which the cell of origin is always a pluripotent stem cell,[176] similar studies in AML have suggested that as many of two thirds of cases arise at levels more mature

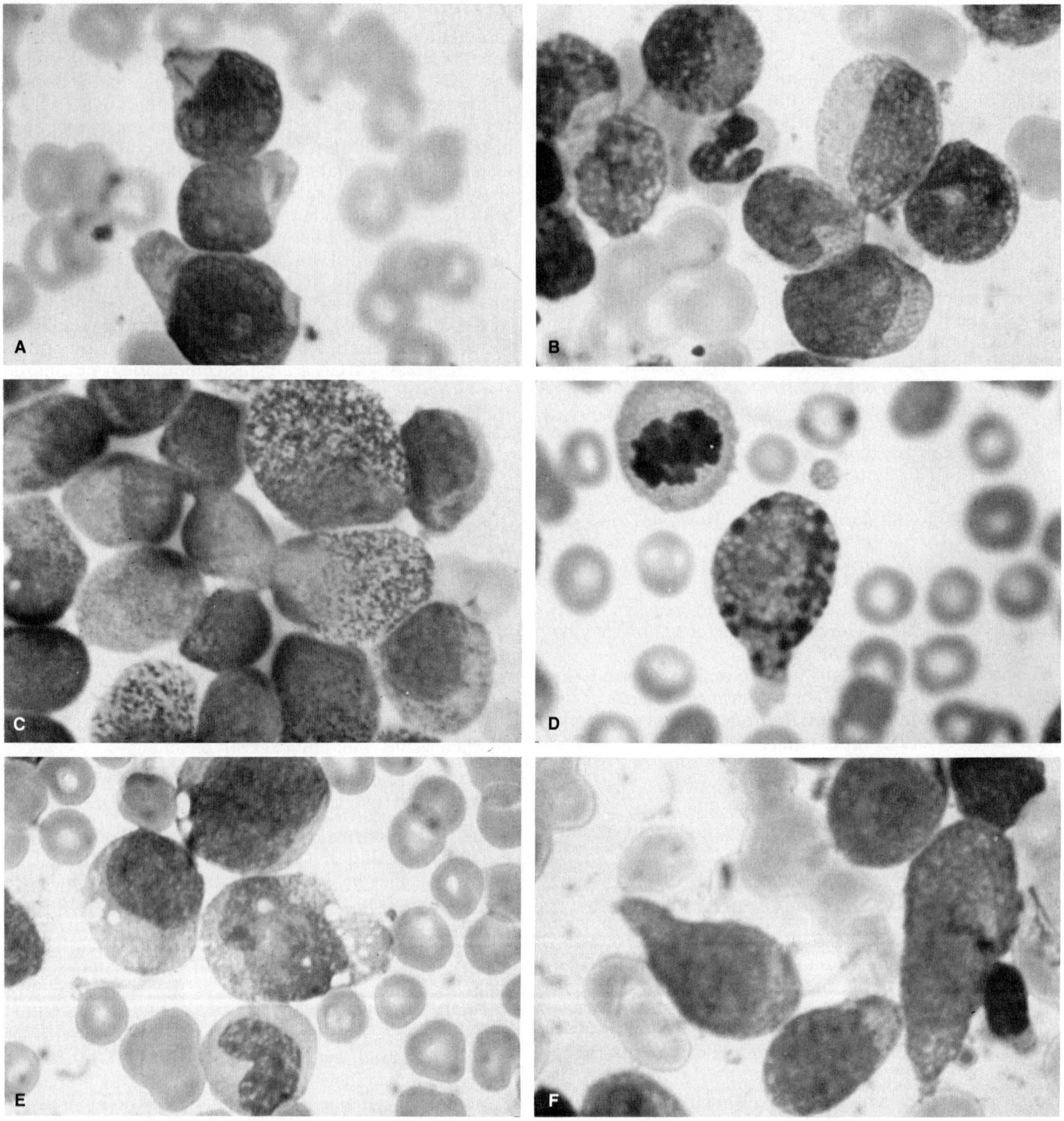

FIGURE 18-1. Morphologic appearance of bone marrow in Wright-Giesma–stained films for each FAB type of acute myelogenous leukemia. (**A**) M1: myeloblastic without maturation; the blasts contain Auer rods. (**B**) M2: myeloblastic with maturation. (**C**) M3: hypergranular promyelocytic. (**D**) M4: myelomonocytic. (**E**) M4Eo: myelomonocytic with abnormal eosinophilic and basophilic granules. (**F**) M5: monocytic. (**G**) M6: erythroleukemic. (**H**) M7: megakaryoblastic. (**I**) M7: myelofibrotic. (See Color Fig. 18-1.) (Courtesy of Pearl Leavitt and Dr. Arthur Skarin, Dana-Farber Cancer Institute, Boston)

than the pluripotent stem cell. Specifically, the erythroid and megakaryocytic lineages are involved in about one third of de novo cases of AML, while in two thirds, only the granulocytic and monocytic lineage is clonal.[166,167] Additional evidence comes from immunophenotype analysis of leukemic clonogenic cells using monoclonal antibodies that identify restricted stages of differentiation of myeloid cells.[177] About one third of cases are found to be related to multipotent progenitor cells and two thirds to committed progenitor cells, such as the CFU-GM. Morphologic abnormalities of erythroid or megakaryocytic cells are observed in up to half of cases. Limited data suggest that patients with AML arising in a multipotent stem cell tend to be older, have secondary (therapy-related) leukemia, or have had MDS.[166,167] These data suggest that AML may arise at any point within the proliferating compartment of the bone marrow, from the pluripotent stem cell to the promyelocyte. This wide variability of the cell of origin of AML is likely to account for some of the striking morphologic, molecular, and clinical heterogeneity of AML.

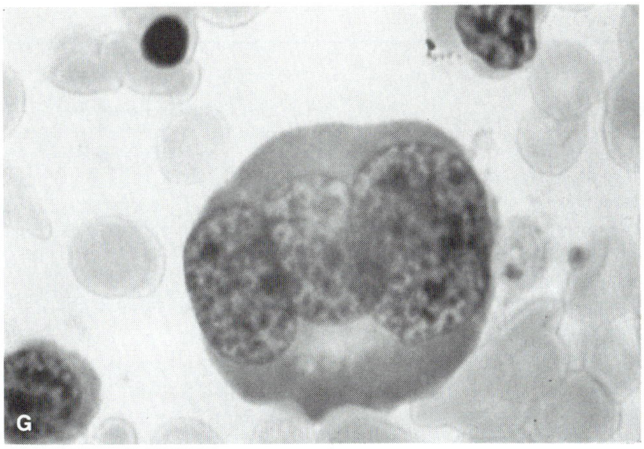

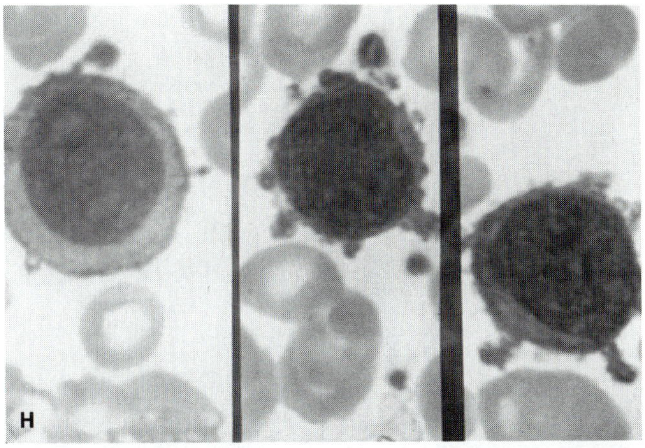

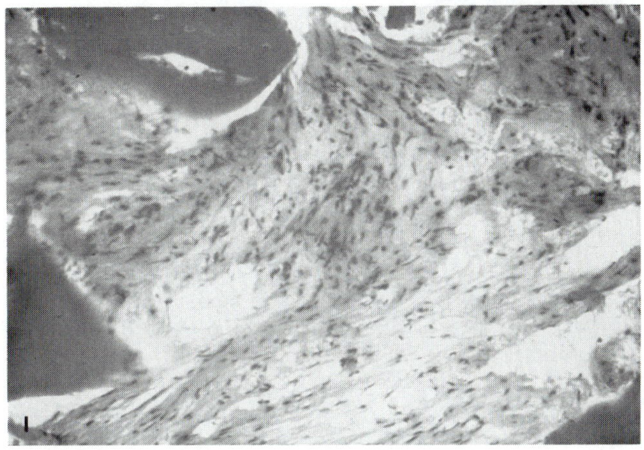

FIGURE 18-1. (Continued)

Clonal Remissions

Studies using RFLP and G6PD techniques have documented clonal hematopoiesis in 1% to as high as 26% of patients with AML in complete remission.[172–174] Discrepancies in these incidence figures of clonal remission can be partly explained by extreme lyonization of polyclonal cells.[175] The significance of this observation has not been determined. It is possible that such patients have an unrecognized underlying clonal stem cell disorder and that, after successful elimination of a frankly leukemic subclone with chemotherapy, morphologically normal but clonal hematopoiesis continues. Alternatively, complete remission induction in these cases may have altered the biologic behavior of AML by selecting out a subclone of leukemic stem cells that can differentiate near-normally. Long-term follow-up of additional cases is warranted.

CLASSIFICATION

French–American–British Classification System

Although all cases of AML share many common biologic features, such as cell of origin, clonality, growth factor requirement, and aberrant differentiation, the morphology is strikingly heterogeneous. The most widely accepted classification scheme, the FAB system, divides AML cases into seven major groups (M1 through M7) and several subgroups[10–13,178] (Fig. 18-1 and Table 18-2). The FAB classification depends on identifying the lineage of the major population of blasts (myeloblast, monoblast, erythroblast, or megakaryoblast) and the degree of differentiation present. Cytochemical identification of myeloperoxidase, specific esterase, nonspecific esterase enzymes, and staining for Sudan black and periodic acid–Schiff (PAS) are used to confirm or extend interpretation of Romanowsky-stained specimens.[11,14]

Five to 20% of specimens are difficult to classify by the FAB system, and this seems to be particularly common in leukemias arising in the setting of preleukemic disorders. Satisfactory classification systems for hybrid or biphenotypic leukemias, hypoplastic leukemias, basophilic leukemias, and primitive erythroblast leukemias have not been devised. Nonetheless, the FAB system is invaluable in providing common ground for comparing patients in different studies and for providing useful prognostic information.

M1: Myeloblastic Leukemia Without Maturation

In this category, marrow cells show minimal evidence of granulocytic maturation, with 3% or more of the blasts being myeloperoxidase- or Sudan black–positive and a varying proportion of the cells expressing a few needle-shaped azurophilic granules (Auer rods), or both. Over 90% of nonerythroid cells are blasts, and the remaining cells are monocytes or maturing granulocytes. Two types of M1 blasts have been defined. Type I blasts are primitive cells that lack granules and usually contain one or more nucleoli. Type II blasts are slightly larger, have a lower nucleus/cytoplasm ratio, and contain one to six azurophilic granules. Unlike promyelocytes, the nucleus of the type II blast is central, the nuclear chromatin is uncondensed, and the Golgi zone is not prominent.

M2: Myeloblastic Leukemic With Maturation

In M2, the sum of type I and II blasts is 30% to 89% of nonerythroid cells, and there is evidence of maturation to

TABLE 18-2. The French–American–British (FAB) Classification System

FAB Type	Blasts		Nucleated Erythroblasts	Morphology	Cytochemistry
	ANC	NEC			
M1	>30	>90	<50	Undifferentiated; <10% promyelocytes or monocytes; acute myeloblastic leukemia	>3% POX or SBB+
M2	>30	30–89	<50	>10% promyelocytes, myelocytes, <20% monocytic cells; AML with partial differentiation	POX+, SBB+, PAS–
M3	>30	30–89	<50	>20% abnormal hypergranular promyelocytes; Auer rods common; acute promyelocytic leukemia	POX+, SBB+, PAS–
M3v	>30	30–89	<50	Microgranular variant, may have folded nucleus	POX+, SBB+, PAS–
M4	>30	30–79	<50	>20% promonocytes and monocytes; >20% granulocytic component; blood monocytes >5 × 10^9/L or lysozyme more than three times normal	POX+, NASDA+
M4Eo	>30	30–79	<50	>5% eosinophils with abnormal eosinophil and basophilic granules	POX+, NASDA+, eosinophils are PAS+
M5a		>80*	<50	>80% of monocytic cells are monoblasts; acute monoblastic leukemia	POX, NASDA+ (inhibited by NaF)
M5b		>80*	<50	<80% of monocytic cells are monoblasts; rest are promonocytes and monocytes	Same as M5a
M6		>30	>50	Megaloblastoid, erythroid, and myeloid blasts; multinucleated; erythroleukemia	PAS+, ringed sideroblasts with iron stain
MDS	<30	<30		Megaloblastoid; nuclear and cytoplasmic dysynchrony; nuclear anomalies; myelodysplastic syndromes	
M7	>30		<50	Large polymorphic blasts, cytoplasmic blebs; gplb or IIb/IIIa+; myelofibrosis; acute magakaryoblastic leukemia	POX–, SBB–, NASDA+; platelet POX+ on electron microsope

ANC, all nucleated cells; MDS, myelodysplastic syndrome; NASDA, napthol-ASD chloroacetate esterase; NEC, nonerythroid cells; PAS, periodic acid–Schiff stain; POX, myeloperoxidase; SBB, Sudan black B stain.

* Includes monoblasts, promonocytes, and monocytes.

the stage of promyelocyte or beyond. Monocytic precursor cells are less than 20%. Nucleoli, azurophilic granules, and Auer rods are common. Myeloblasts with bilobed or reniform nuclei can be distinguished from monocytes by the fine chromatin pattern of the blast.

M3: Hypergranular Promyelocytic Leukemia

Most M3 cells are heavily granulated promyelocytes. The nuclei may be reniform, and the cytoplasmic granules may be coalescent. Auer rods are common, and bundles of Auer rods may be seen.

M3 Variant: Microgranular Promyelocytic Leukemia

The promyelocytes contain large numbers of tiny granules that may be difficult to distinguish by light microscopy.[9] The cytoplasm is usually strikingly myeloperoxidase-positive, however, and the combination of agranular cytoplasm and strong myeloperoxidase staining should suggest this variant. The nuclei may be reniform, and the diagnosis of M4 is initially made in some cases. The diagnosis can be confirmed by cytogenetics, which reveals t(15:17) translocation, or by electron microscopy, which shows multiple dark primary granules and Auer rods.

M4: Myelomonocytic Leukemia

Over 20%, but less than 80%, of the M4 nonerythroid cells are of the monocytic lineage, often *promonocytes*. Greater than 30% of all nonerythroid cells must be blasts. In addition, the blood monocyte concentration should exceed 5 × 10^9/L or the serum (or urine) lysozyme should exceed three times normal. In some cases, the marrow picture may be more consistent with M2, but if there is blood monocytosis or elevated lysozyme, the diagnosis is M4. Esterase stains can be particularly useful to distinguish promonocytes from promyelocytes (see Table 18-2).

M5: Monocytic Leukemia

Two forms are recognized: M5a, in which more than 80% of marrow nonerythroid cells are monoblasts, and M5b, in which less than 80% of nonerythroid cells are monoblasts but more than 80% are monoblasts, promonocytes, and monocytes.

M6: Erythroleukemia

Over 30% of nonerythroid cells are type I or II blasts in M6, but half or more of marrow cells are erythroblasts. Cases in which more than half of marrow cells are erythroblasts but less than 30% of nonerythroid cells are myeloblasts fall into the category of MDS (RAEBIT). In rare cases, there is a monomorphic population of erythroblasts without a significant myeloblast component. These cases are not classifiable within the FAB system but are being recognized more frequently with immunophenotype analysis.

M7: Megakaryoblastic Leukemia

The blast cells are typically polymorphic with round nuclei and finely reticulated nuclear chromatin.[12] Cytoplasmic blebs may be seen, as may bare nuclei surrounded by clusters of platelets. Megakaryocytic fragments may be seen in the blood film. The blasts are peroxidase- and Sudan black–negative but may stain for fluoride-inhibitable nonspecific esterase activity. The PAS and acid phosphatase reactions are frequently positive. Bone marrow fibrosis is a frequent accompaniment of the M7 subtype. The diagnosis should be confirmed with ultrastructural histochemistry, demonstrating platelet peroxidase activity exclusively on the nuclear membrane and the endoplasmic reticulum. Immunophenotype analysis is also useful to confirm the diagnosis of M7.[12] The blasts typically express platelet glycoproteins 11b/11a or 1b.[178] Factor VIII antibodies may also react with cells.

Separation of AML from ALL

Distinguishing AML from ALL is essential for treatment planning and is relatively simple in 80% to 90% of cases. The presence of Auer rods or myeloperoxidase-positive primary granules is pathognomonic of AML. AML cells tend to be larger and are more heterogeneous in size and nuclear morphology than ALL cells. Useful cytochemical stains include myeloperoxidase, Sudan black B, napthol-ASD chloroacetate esterase, and lysozyme. The PAS stain is negative in M1, M2, and M3 but may be positive in M4 and M5 (punctate staining) and M6. The PAS stain may be particularly useful in M6, in which blocks of PAS-positive material are identified in the abnormal erythroid cells of this disease. Terminal deoxynucleotidyl transferase is more commonly expressed by ALL cells than AML cells, but it is not lineage-specific and is consistent with lymphoid differentiation only if other lymphoid specific-markers are present.[178]

In the 10% to 20% of cases in which morphology and cytochemistry are inconclusive or insufficient to distinguish AML and ALL, immunophenotype analysis provides the diagnosis in virtually all cases.[179] A large number of monoclonal antibodies have been generated that recognize antigens expressed on the surface of AML but not ALL cells.[180,181] All the antibodies studied also react with subsets of normal hematopoietic cells, indicating that leukemia-specific antigens in human myeloid leukemias are rare or nonexistent. These antibodies have been grouped into clusters of differentiation (CD) by International Workshops on Leukocyte Differentiation Antigens, and antibodies of several clusters have been shown in extensive studies to be useful in distinguishing myeloid from lymphoid leukemias[179–184] (Table 18-3). Using a combination of antibodies specifically recognizing B-cell, T-cell, and myeloid antigens, it is possible to distinguish AML from ALL in 95% to 99% of cases. Many of the most useful myeloid antigens are expressed by normal cells at specific stages of differentiation, and some investigators have attempted to correlate surface phenotype of AML cells with a normal cell counterpart.[184] There appears to be only a limited utility

TABLE 18-3. Immunophenotype Analysis of AML

CD	Antibodies	M1/M2	M3	M4/M5	M6	M7	B-ALL	T-ALL
MYELOID LINEAGE								
CD11b	Anti-Mo1		+	++	−	−	−	−
CD13	Anti-MY7	+	+	++	+	+	−	−
CD14	Anti-Mo2, MY4	−	−	++	−	−		−
CD15	Anti-My1	+	++	++	−	−	−	−
CD33	Anti-MY9	++	++	++	++	++	−	−
CD34	Anti-MY10	++	+	+	+	+	+	+
T LINEAGE								
CD2	Anti-T11	−	−	−	−	−	−	++
CD3	Anti-T3	−	−	−	−	−	−	+
CD5	Anti-T1	−	−	−	−	−	−	++
CD7	3A1	+	+	+	+	+	+	++
B LINEAGE								
CD10	Anti-CALLA	−	−	−	−	−	+	−
CD19	Anti-B4	−	−	−	−	−	+	−
CD20	Anti-B1	−	−	−	−	−	+	−
ERYTHROID LINEAGE								
	Anti-glycophorin A	−	−	−	++	−	−	−
MEGAKARYOCYTE LINEAGE								
CD41	Anti-gpIIb/IIIa	−	−	−	−	++	−	−
CD42	Anti-gpIb	−	−	−	−	++	−	−

CALLA, common acute lymphoblastic leukemia antigen; CD, cluster differentiation; B-ALL, B lineage acute lymphoblastic leukemia; T-ALL, T lineage acute lymphoblastic leukemia.
+++, expressed by over 20% of blasts in more than 50% of cases; ++, expressed by over 20% of blasts in 20% to 50% of cases; +, expressed by over 20% of blasts in 5% to 20% of cases; −, expressed by less than 5% of cases.

to this type of approach. Cells from AML patients with immature morphology (M1) tend to have an immature phenotype, while cells from patients with M3 or M5 tend to express an immunophenotype typical of the normal promyelocyte or promonocyte.[185–188] Also, limited information may be available from surface antigen phenotype.[185,187,188] Some studies have indicated that expression of CD13, CD14, or CD34 may be associated with a lower than average rate of complete remission.[185,189] Overall, however, the primary value of surface antigen analysis in most cases of AML is in distinguishing AML and ALL.

Hybrid or Biphenotypic Leukemia

About 5% of cases of acute leukemia have morphologic, cytochemical, immunophenotypic, or genetic evidence of more than one hematopoietic lineage.[190–197] This promiscuity may be due to the simultaneous presence of two distinct leukemic populations (bilineage or biclonal) or, more commonly, to the presence of features of more than one lineage in the same cells (hybrid or biphenotypic). This phenomenon has been best studied with immunophenotype analysis, and cases in which there is coexpression of myeloid–T cell, myeloid–B cell, and T cell–B cell phenotypes are commonly reported.[192–196] The pathogenesis of these mixed leukemias has been the subject of much speculation, but it remains poorly understood.[190,197] One popular school of thought is that leukemic cells represent frozen stages of differentiation and that a biphenotypic leukemia represents a clonal expansion of a normal cell that expresses features of more than one lineage. It has been difficult to identify such cells in normal marrow, however, and it is more likely that the molecular events that determine the orderly commitment to one or another lineage in normal hematopoiesis are disrupted in AML. Lineage switching can also be observed in a small fraction of cases.[198] A typical example would be a patient with features of a T-cell phenotype at diagnosis but with a mixed T-cell–myeloid or pure myeloid phenotype at relapse. Hybrid leukemias may be more common in patients with antecedent myelodysplastic disorders; secondary leukemias; translocations involving chromosome 11q23, particularly t(4;11); the Ph chromosome; or age less than 6 months.[189–199] A better understanding of the molecular control of lineage commitment is likely to be required before the precise mechanisms responsible for biphenotypic leukemias are identified.

It is controversial whether patients with hybrid leukemias have a poorer prognosis than patients with classic AML or ALL. Recent pediatric data suggest that the expression of lymphoid-associated cell surface antigens on leukemic cells from children with AML lacks prognostic significance.[194,195] The significance of hybrid acute leukemia in adults may depend on whether the cells are primarily myeloid (AML with lymphoid markers) or lymphoid (ALL with myeloid markers). In a prospective Cancer and Leukemia Group B (CALGB) study of adults with ALL, 31% of patients coexpressed lymphoid and myeloid surface antigens.[200] These hybrid cases had a statistically significant lower complete remission rate than nonhybrid cases (30% versus 73%; $P < .01$) when treated with an aggressive ALL treatment regimen. In contrast, patients whose disease is primarily myeloid but coexpresses lymphoid markers may have a favorable prognosis.[201]

M0: Undifferentiated Myeloid Leukemia

M0 is defined as cases of AML lacking morphologic or cytochemical analyses.[178,202] Evidence of myeloid differentiation can be obtained from immunophenotype analysis with expression of CD13, CD33, or other surface markers[178,203–207] or with demonstration of peroxidase-positive granules by electron microscopy.[208] If platelet peroxidase is positive by electron microscopy, the case should be considered M7.

CYTOGENETIC ABNORMALITIES

Chromosomal analysis has proved to be a valuable aspect of diagnostic, prognostic, and biologic studies of AML[168–171] (see Chap. 5). Nonrandom chromosomal abnormalities have been detected in 50% to 90% of cases of AML using high-resolution banding techniques.[209–214] These abnormalities include internal deletions of single chromosomes, such as 5q− or 7q−; gain or loss of whole chromosomes, +8 or −7); chromosome inversions, inv(3) or inv(16); and specific translocations, such as t(8;21) or t(15:17). Complex chromosomal defects are observed in about 15% of de novo cases (ie, without a preceding myelodysplastic disorder) and constitute a clinical group of patients with particularly poor prognoses. Common cytogenetic abnormalities observed in de novo AML are described in Table 18-4 in relation to FAB classification.[168–170,208–214]

The translocation t(15;17))(q22;q11–12) is uniquely associated with M3, both the hypergranular and hypogranular variants. Several groups showed that the retinoic acid receptor α (RARα) gene on chromosome 17 was rearranged in patients with acute promyelocytic leukemia with a t(15;17)(q22;q12-21) translocation.[62–64] The RARα gene is fused with a gene on chromosome 15 that encodes a putative zinc finger transcription factor, PML.[215–217] Two reciprocal types of fusion RNA species are produced, RARα-PML and PML-RARα. The PML-RARα species contains the zinc finger of PML fused to the DNA- and protein-binding domains of RARα. The aberrent PML-RARα fusion protein may function as a dominant inhibitory oncogene, blocking the normal activities of the RARα receptor.[216] The clinical response of these patients to all-*trans*-retinoic acid may be explained by the ability of this retinoid to bind to the PML-RARα fusion protein and alter its function.[218]

The translocation t(8;21)(q22;q22) is the most frequently occurring translocation in de novo AML, found in 18% of M2 cases. Three-way rearrangements may also be observed, and the t(8;21) is frequently associated with loss of a sex chromosome (−X in females, −Y in males). The t(8;21) produces a fusion protein involving the AML1 gene on chromosome 21 and the ETO gene on chromosome 8.[66–68,70] Remarkably, the AML 1/ETO gene can be deleted in patients in clinical remission for many years.[69]

Structural abnormalities of 11q are associated with myelomonocytic or monocytic leukemias. At the Fourth International Workshop of Chromosomes in Leukemia, 64% of 33 patients with 11q abnormalities were classified as M5, 15% as M4, and 9% as M2.[212] The other chromosome involved in 11q translocations is variable, but 9q23 is common. A gene termed MLL has been shown to span the breakpoint in 11q23.[72–76] Translocation of the c-*ets*-1 protooncogene into the interferon genes has been reported in t(9;11)(q22;q23).[219]

The inv(16)(p12;q22), t(16;16)(p13:q22) and del(16)(q22) have been associated closely with a unique syndrome of M4 with abnormal eosinophils (M4Eo).[220,221] The complete remission rate in this syndrome is high (Table 18-5), and remission durations are favorable. These patients have a higher incidence of relapse in the central nervous system (CNS) than those with other types of AML, except for M5.[222] The inv(16) involves the CBF β gene (a transcritpion factor) and a myosin heavy-chain gene, creating a fusion gene.[71]

Deletions of all or part of chromosomes 5 and 7 and trisomy 8 are generally not associated with a specific FAB

TABLE 18-4. Recurring Chromosome Abnormalities in De Novo AML

Chromosome Defect	Frequency (%)	Main FAB Subtype	Other
inv(3)(q21;q23) or t(3;3)(q21;q26)	1	M7, M4	High platelet count; abnormal megakaryocytes
−5/del(5)(q11-q35)	3–6	All	MDS; older patients; toxic exposure
t(6;9)(p21-22;q34)	<1	M2, M4	Basophilia
−7/del(7)(q22-q36)	9	All	MDS; older patients; toxic exposure
Trisomy 8	13	All	MDS; older patients
t(8;16)(p11;p13)	<1	M5b	Phagocytosis
t(8;21)(q22;q22)	5–7	M2	Auer rods common; myeloblastomas; loss of sex chromosome (−X or −Y)
t(9;11)(q22;q23)*	5–13	M5a, M4	Children, young adults, and most infants; high leukocyte count
del(9)(q11-q32)	1	M2	
t(9;22)(q34;q11)	<1	M1, M2	190-kd *BCR/ABL*
t(15;17)(q22;q21.1)	6	M3, M3v	Coagulopathy
inv(16)(p13;q22), del(16)(q22), t(16;16)(p13;q22)	2–5	M4Eo	Eosinophilia; CNS leukemia
del(11q) or t(11;v)	2–5	M4, M5	Infants, high leukocyte count; CNS leukemia; biphenotypic leukemia t(4;11)

FAB, French–American–British classification system; MDS, myelodysplastic syndrome.
* Other chromosomal bands with 11q23 translocations in AML include 1q21, 2p21, 6q27, 10p11, 17q25, and 19p13.

subtype of AML.[224–226] They are considerably more frequent in older patients, whereas the frequency of the specific translocations and inversions decreases with age. These same abnormalities (+8, −7, −5/5q−) are more common in patients with an antecedent MDS,[169,170] therapy-related AML, and suspected exposure to environmental mutagens.[226] In contrast, specific translocations are relatively uncommon in these patient groups. An exception to this is AML that develops in patients who have received high doses of epipodophyllotoxins (VP 16 or VM 26) for treatment of a previous malignancy.[36,37] Translocations involving 11q23 are commonly observed in this setting.

The frequent involvement of chromosome 5q is of interest because the genes encoding several hematopoietic growth factors are located in this arm, including GM-CSF (5q23-31), IL-3 (5q23-31), and IL-4 (5q23-31).[228] The M-CSF receptor, c-*fms*, is also on this chromosome, at 5q34. The genes for GM-CSF and IL-3 are structurally related and are physically adjacent to each other.[229] The genes for c-*fms* and the platelet-derived growth factor receptor are also physically adjacent.[230] In some 5q− chromosome defects, one or more growth factor genes may be deleted.[228] Rearrangements of genes for both IL-3 and M-CSF have also been reported. The relation of growth factor gene abnormalities to AML or MDS remains undefined. More recent studies have suggested that the 5q deletions always involve the IRF-1.[79] This gene, which maps to 5q31.1, may have the properties of a tumor suppressor gene.[80]

TABLE 18-5. Patient Charactersitics Related to Complete Remission Rate

Characteristics	Favorable Value
Cytogenetics	t(8;21) or inv(16)
Secondary AML	Not present
Age	<60 y
Leukocyte count	<100,000/μL
FAB subtype	M1, M2, M4, M5
Auer rods	Present
Albumin	>3.5 g/dL
Creatinine	<1.1 mg/dL
Leukemia blast self-renewal	Low
Fibrinogen	>250 mg%

FAB, French–American–British classification system.

The Ph chromosome t(9;22)(q34;q11) is observed in about 1% to 2% of all cases of de novo AML and is associated with a poor prognosis.[209–214] The *bcr/abl* rearrangement may be similar either to that seen in classic CML (8.5-kb mRNA, 210-kd *bcr/abl* fusion protein) or to that seen typically in Ph-positive ALL (7-kb *bcr/abl* mRNA, 190-kd *bcr/abl* fusion protein).[231,232] Patients with p210 *bcr/abl* may have CML presenting in a myeloid blast phase, and rare cases develop stable phase CML after treatment. Patients with p190 *bcr/abl* are more likely to have de novo AML.[232] The biologic differences between the p210 *bcr/abl* and p190 *bcr/abl* have not been determined. Molecular studies indicate that different pathogenic mechanisms may be involved in CML and Ph-positive acute leukemia (AML or ALL).

The t(4;11)(q21;q23) may also be observed in AML, particularly in infants and children.[199,233–235] This translocation was originally described in association with ALL, but later studies documented the myeloid or hybrid nature of blasts in some of the patients.[236] The immunophenotype is consistent with a B-cell precursor ALL in patients who have cellular morphology consistent with lymphoblasts. In AML, the t(4;11)(q21;q23) has been associated with M4 or M5.

In summary, specific karyotypic abnormalities are common in AML and may be associated with specific clinical syndromes, such as the association of t(15;17) with promyelocytic leukemia and inv(16) with eosinophilia and M4 AML. Identification of the other new genes involved in AML represents a major challenge for the next decade of research in AML. It is likely that the specific translocations activate or otherwise dysregulate genes controlling proliferation and differentiation of myeloid cells, thus contributing to leukemogenesis.

CLINICAL PRESENTATION

The symptoms of AML may be as nonspecific as weight loss, fatigue, and weakness but more commonly include pallor, fever, and bleeding.[236,237] These symptoms are usually due to anemia, neutropenia, and thrombocytopenia, which are secondary to decreased normal myelopoiesis from leukemic replacement of the bone marrow. Patients rarely have symptoms for more than 6 months before diagnosis and often for only one to several months. AML rarely presents as an incidental finding on a routine blood count in an asymptomatic patient.

About one third of patients have petechiae, bruising, oral bleeding, or epistaxis. Patients with APL often have more extensive bleeding because of disseminated intravascular coagulation (DIC). Another one third of patients present with fever and a serious bacterial infection. Common sites of infection include the respiratory tract, gums, teeth, sinuses, urinary tract, perirectal area, and skin. About 5% of patients present with signs and symptoms that reflect pulmonary or intracerebral leukostasis.[239–241] These may include tachypnea, rales, stupor, coma, or stroke.

The most common sites of clinically overt extramedullary leukemic infiltration include superficial lymph nodes, liver, spleen, gingiva, CNS, and skin. Bulky lymphadenopathy and mediastinal involvement are rare in patients with AML. Leukemic infiltrates in the adenoids, tonsils, or paratracheal area may result in airway obstruction. Splenomegaly is found in about 25% of patients. Bone pain or tenderness and joint pain or swelling may be initial presenting complaints, but these symptoms are more commonly associated with ALL.

Gingival hypertrophy, signs of meningeal leukemia, and leukemia cutis (Fig. 18-2) are much more commonly associated with the monocytic or myelomonocytic subtypes (M4, M5) of AML.[242–244] Interestingly, most neonates with AML have the M5 subtype and present with skin infiltrates that often appear as slate-blue, subcutaneous nodules.[245]

About 2% of patients with AML present with signs and symptoms related to discrete tumors. These tumors are composed of immature myeloid cells and are referred to as *myeloblastomas, chloromas,* or *granulocytic sarcomas.*[246,247] Myeloblastomas may be the initial clinical manifestation of AML or may herald bone marrow and blood involvement by weeks to months.[248,249] They may be found in virtually any location but especially the orbit, paranasal sinuses, brain, spinal cord, bone, breast, skin, and subcutaneous tissues. These tumors were originally called chloromas because of their greenish color secondary to a high myeloperoxidase content. In the past, these tumors were often misdiagnosed as diffuse lymphomas or anaplastic carcinomas. Histochemical and immunoperoxidase studies are helpful in establishing the correct diagnosis.

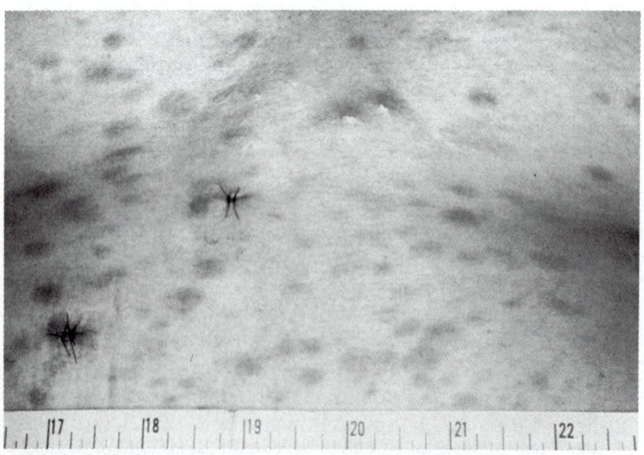

FIGURE 18-2. Leukemia cutis in a patient with M5 (monocytic) acute myelogenous leukemia. (See Color Fig. 18-2.) (Courtesy of Dr. Arthur Skarin, Dana-Farber Cancer Institute, Boston)

Laboratory Findings at Diagnosis

The leukocyte counts at the time of diagnosis in patients with AML can vary from 100 cells/μL to greater than 1,000,000 cells/μL.[250,251] About 15% to 20% of patients present with leukocyte counts greater than 100,000/μL, but most patients present with leukocyte counts less than 50,000/uL. The highest counts have been observed in patients with the M4 and M5 subtypes of AML,[241,252] whereas patients with M3 AML tend to have a low leukocyte count at diagnosis.[253] The differential leukocyte count reveals less than 1000 neutrophils/μL and a variable percentage of blasts in most patients. In about 10% of patients, no peripheral blasts are detectable. Other leukocyte abnormalities may be present, including Pelger-Huët (see Chap. 19) or hypogranular mature neutrophils.[254]

Thrombocytopenia is invariably present at the time of diagnosis.[255] In more than half of patients, the platelet count is less than 50,000/μL, and counts of less than 20,000/μL are common. Giant platelets and poorly granulated platelets with functional abnormalities can occur.[256] Thrombocytopenia is due to either decreased platelet production, reduced megakaryocytes accompanying leukemic infiltration of the bone marrow, or DIC. Hypersplenism as a cause of thrombocytopenia is uncommon in patients with acute leukemia.

Almost all patients have a normocytic, normochromic anemia (hematocrit, 25% to 35%) with occasional nucleated red blood cells (RBCs) and teardrop forms seen on peripheral blood smear.[237,250] The anemia is secondary to either decreased RBC production or blood loss.[257] The rare hemolytic anemia associated with AML is usually not immune-mediated but rather a microangiopathic hemolytic anemia secondary to DIC. The serum uric acid and lactate dehydrogenase (LDH) are usually modestly elevated.[250] Laboratory evidence of DIC (prolonged prothrombin time and partial thromboplastin time, decreased fibrinogen, and increased fibrin degradation products) is commonly associated with the M3 and M5 subtypes of AML.[258–260]

The typical bone marrow findings include a hypercellular biopsy sample and an aspirate showing greater than half leukemic cells (more than 30% being required by FAB criteria for the diagnosis of AML).[237,250] The bone marrow biopsy may be hypocellular, especially in elderly males and in patients with an antecedent hematologic disorder (ie, paroxysmal nocturnal hemoglobinuria, Fanconi's anemia, or MDS) or therapy-related AML.[261,262] A rare patient with AML has fewer than 30% bone marrow blasts but over 30% peripheral blasts.[263] Patients with AML, especially those with M6 or M7 or a preceding MDS, may show morphologic abnormalities in the erythroid, granulocytic, and megakaryocytic lineages.[264,265] These dysplastic changes of multiple lineages are consistent with a malignant transformation of a primitive multipotential progenitor or stem cell.

Differential Diagnosis

Most cases of AML can be readily diagnosed after an examination of the peripheral blood and bone marrow. As previously discussed, AML in infants with Down's syndrome needs to be differentiated from the transient myeloproliferative syndrome.[87] In some situations, it may be difficult to distinguish MDS from AML.[266] This might occur in the setting of a hypoplastic marrow with occasional blasts or M2 AML with marked granulocytic differentiation and a low percentage of typical blasts.[267]

In a small percentage of patients, other diagnoses must be entertained and systematically excluded. For example, bacterial sepsis may either cause a leukemoid reaction or profound neutropenia.[268,269] In this circumstance, the bone marrow aspirate may be confusing. There may be a maturation arrest of the granulocytic precursors at the promyelocyte stage. This morphologic picture has been confused with APL. With resolution of the sepsis, normal granulocytic maturation ensues. Patients with acute infectious mononucleosis may have signs and symptoms similar to those seen in patients with AML. On rare occasions, the atypical lymphocytes have a bizarre mononuclear appearance that may mimic monoblasts, but normal findings on bone marrow examination rule out AML.

Patterns of Spread

Central Nervous System

Central nervous system involvement in patients with AML can be due to meningeal infiltration,[270–272] epidural or brain parenchymal myeloblastomas,[273] or leukostasis.[274] Meningeal leukemia is much more common in patients with ALL than in AML. About 5% to 20% of patients with AML either present with (usually with no symptoms) or develop meningeal leukemia during the course of their disease.[270–272] It has been postulated that leukemic cells reach the meninges by either hematogenous spread or by direct extension from cranial bone marrow.[275] Hematogenous spread may occur either as a result of direct perivascular invasion or deposition from petechial hemorrhages in the pia-arachnoid. The most common signs and symptoms of meningeal leukemia reflect increased intracranial pressure and include nausea, vomiting, lethargy, headache, and papilledema. Other signs and symptoms may include meningism, cranial nerve palsy, root pain, and paresthesia. Symptomatic meningeal leukemia is usually not observed at initial diagnosis.

Clinical or laboratory features at diagnosis that have been strongly associated with the development of CNS leukemia include the M4 and M5 subtypes,[270,271] high leukocyte counts,[240] elevated levels of lysozyme,[276] chromosome abnormality inv(16),[222] high serum LDH levels, and extramedullary involvement at other sites.[264] High blood lysozyme and LDH levels and extramedullary leukemia are associated with M4 and M5 AML, and this probably accounts for their association with meningeal leukemia. The diagnosis of meningeal leukemia is made by examining a cytocentrifuged preparation of cerebrospinal fluid.[277] There is usually an increased number of cells in the CSF, with blast cells present. The cytocentrifuge technique is important because this method may reveal blasts despite a normal routine cell count. On occasion, patients may have clinical evidence of CNS leukemia (ie, cranial nerve palsy) with negative CSF cytology. In this situation, appropriate CNS therapy should be instituted.

CNS disease in patients with AML may also be secondary to intracranial or epidural myeloblastomas.[273] These solid tumors of myeloblasts are believed to arise from hematopoietic tissue and traverse the haversian canals to reach the subperiosteum and dura from and eventually penetrate to the subarachnoid and Virchow-Robin spaces.

Patients with cerebral leukostasis may also develop intraparenchymal brain lesions.[274] These nodular leukemic lesions result from blasts invading and penetrating vessel walls.

Integumentary

Leukemia cutis has been reported to occur in 2% to 13% of cases of AML.[278,279] Skin involvement is associated with M5 AML (especially in neonates) and with extramedullary infiltration at other sites. Such infiltration usually results in small (2- to 5-mm) raised pink or salmon-colored nodules or bluish gray, firm, rubbery nodules. The skin lesions are painless and are most common on the extremities or trunk but may involve the face, scalp, and other areas. These lesions may be difficult to distinguish from infection, hemorrhage, or neutrophilic dermatosis.[280] Biopsy specimens show dense infiltration of the dermis with or without subcutaneous infiltration by myeloblasts or monoblasts, often with eosinophilic myelocytes. Leukemia cutis may antedate bone marrow involvement or be a harbinger of imminent marrow relapse.

Cardiac

Cardiovascular abnormalities due to leukemic infiltration are rarely clinically significant.[281,282] Leukemic infiltration of the pericardium, conduction system, and endocardium have been associated with arrhythmia, heart failure, and death.

Respiratory

Leukemic infiltration or myeloblastomas may lead to laryngeal obstruction, pulmonary parenchymal infiltrates, alveolar septal infiltration, or pleural seeding.[283–285] Pulmonary leukostasis can also lead to respiratory distress with abnormal radiologic findings.[286,287] Pneumonia remains the most common pulmonary lesion associated with AML.

Gastrointestinal

Functional disturbances of the gastrointestinal tract secondary to leukemic infiltration are uncommon. Gingival hypertrophy, secondary to leukemic infiltration, is commonly associated with AML, especially with acute myelomonocytic and monocytic leukemia.[264,288] It is not unusual for the dentist to raise the first suspicion of leukemia after seeing the patient with gingival disease. Esophagitis, enterocolitis, and proctitis usually result from chemotherapy-induced mucosal changes and infection during periods of neutropenia.[289] Leukemic infiltration of the gastrointestinal tract rarely causes significant bleeding, perforation, or other symptoms (ie, obstruction).

Genitourinary

The kidneys may be diffusely enlarged secondary to leukemic infiltration in a small proportion of cases, but functional abnormalities are extremely unusual.[290] Rare cases of bladder neck, prostatic, or testicular involvement with AML have been described.[291] Testicular leukemia has been observed in several young boys with M4 or M5 AML.[292]

Osteoarticular

Osteoarticular symptoms other than bone pain are infrequent in patients with AML.[237,238] Migratory polyarthritis or arthralgia is more common in children with ALL, but these have been observed in patients with AML.[293] The most common radiologic findings of bone seen in children with leukemia are osteoporosis and submetaphyseal lucent lines (growth arrest lines), whereas thinning of the cortex of the long bones is seen in adults.[294] Periosteal elevation or osteolytic lesions are uncommon. Myeloblastomas of bone may give the radiologic appearance of an expanding geographic lesion with well-defined but irregular nonsclerotic margins.

Ocular

About 40% to 50% of patients with AML have ocular manifestations of leukemia at diagnosis.[295,296] Leukemic infiltration of the optic nerve, choroid, and retina is rare, but secondary opthalmic manifestations, including intraretinal hemorrhage, cotton-wool spots, white-centered retinal hemorrhages, central vein obstruction, and vitreous hemorrhage are more commonly observed. Controversy exists concerning the relation between fundus findings in leukemic retinopathy and hematologic parameters, such as platelet count, hematocrit, and leukocyte count.[296] In all studies, patients with retinopathy had significantly lower platelet counts than those without retinopathy. Some studies have found a relation between retinopathy and low hematocrit.

Leukemic infiltration of the eye requires prompt recognition to save vision. Local irradiation combined with intrathecal chemotherapy is recommended in such cases. Leukemic ocular infiltrates are often associated with other evidence of CNS leukemia but may represent the first detectable site of relapse. Anterior chamber involvement is rare but has been reported as the site of first or subsequent relapse in both ALL and AML.[297]

PROGNOSTIC FACTORS

Achieving remission is the prime determinant of survival in patients with AML. The likelihood of achieving remission is age-dependent (see Table 18-5), but it is also related to other clinical and laboratory variables.[298–305] Factors that have been consistently associated with lower remission rates include age greater than 60 years, certain chromosomal abnormalities (−5/5q− or −7/7q−), poor performance status, therapy-related AML, and AML that develops secondary to MDS. In many studies, additional adverse prognostic variables have included leukocyte count higher than 100,000/μL, M6 or M7 AML, low fibrinogen, elevated creatinine, low serum albumin, absence of Auer rods, blasts with low S phase, and a high leukemic blast self-renewal rate.[264,306–310]

Failure to achieve remission may result from early death secondary to infection, hemorrhage, leukostasis, or therapy-resistant leukemia. Several of the previously mentioned prognostic variables, including poor performance status, leukocyte count higher than 100,000/μL, and low albumin, identify patients who are not likely to survive induction owing to complications of leukemia and its treatment. On the other hand, the lower remission rates associated with low labeling index (S phase), unfavorable cytogenetics, and therapy-related AML or AML that develops secondary to MDS are chiefly due to resistant leukemia (ie, persistence of bone marrow blasts after one or two cycles of induction chemotherapy). In addition to having more resistant leukemia, patients with secondary AML or prior MDS have a slow recovery of blood counts after induction chemotherapy, placing them at increased risk for fungal infections and other complications associated with prolonged pancytopenia. The adverse influence of older age on the remission rate is in part due to a greater risk of early death from toxicity but also to disease-related factors, including a higher incidence of prior MDS and unfavorable cytogenetics.[311]

The absence of Auer rods has been shown in some studies to be associated with a low remission rate.[306,312] In a recent pediatric AML report,[313] the absence of Auer rods in the M1 group was correlated with both a low complete remission rate and a short duration of remission. The biologic significance of this association is unknown, but Auer rod–negative M1 AML may represent a less differentiated subtype of AML that is relatively chemotherapy resistant.

The ability to predict durations of remission in patients with AML based on various clinical, laboratory, or therapy-related factors has been difficult and not consistent from one study to another (Table 18-6). For example, there is not a clear relation between age at diagnosis and duration of remission.[300,311,314] In the CALGB studies, however, increasing age had an adverse impact on length of remission (Fig. 18-3). The shortest remissions were observed in patients over 60 years of age. A prior MDS and therapy-related AML are unfavorable factors for both induction response and complete remission duration.[303,304] In several studies, patients (especially children) with M4 and M5 AML and leukocyte counts higher than 30,000/μL have had statistically significant shorter durations of remission compared with those with other FAB subtypes or lower leukocyte counts.[264,315] Other studies have not confirmed these findings. Since many prognostic factors are treatment-dependent, more effective or different therapies will likely influence what emerge as important prognostic variables. It is possible, for example, that the adverse impact of M4 and M5 AML is lost with protocols that include an epipodophyllotoxin.[292,316]

The cytogenetic findings that predict a low remission rate (−5/5q− and −7/7q−) also associate with short durations of response.[300] It appears that patients with inv/del(16)(q22) and t(8;21) have high complete remission rates and relatively favorable durations of remission. In several adult studies,[213,299] patients with rearrangements of band 16q22 had the longest remissions. It has been recognized for many years that patients with M3 AML can have long remissions if they survive the hemorrhagic complications of remission-induction therapy.[317] In a recently reported pediatric AML trial,[318] children with structural abnormalities involving 11q23 were infants (median age, 6 months) with M4 or M5 AML, hyperleukocytosis, and frequent coagulation abnormalities. These infants relapsed early during postremission therapy. This was in contrast to children with M5 AML and t(9;11), who had favorable durations of remission.

The Berlin-Frankfurt-Münster Study Group has identified low- and high-risk groups of children with AML.[313] The low-risk group comprised 37% of the patients who achieved remission and included those with M1 and Auer rods, M2 with leukocyte counts lower than 20,000/μL, M3, and M4 with eosinophilia. The 6-year relapse-free survival

TABLE 18-6. Patient Characteristics Relating to Duration of Remission

Characteristics	Favorable Value
Cytogenetics	t(15;17), inv(16)
Age	<18 y
Secondary AML	Not present
FAB subtype	M1 with Auer rods; M4 with eosinophilia; M3
Marrow blasts and promyelocytes	<80%
Courses to complete remission	1
Leukocyte count	<30,000/μL

FAB, French–American–British classification system.

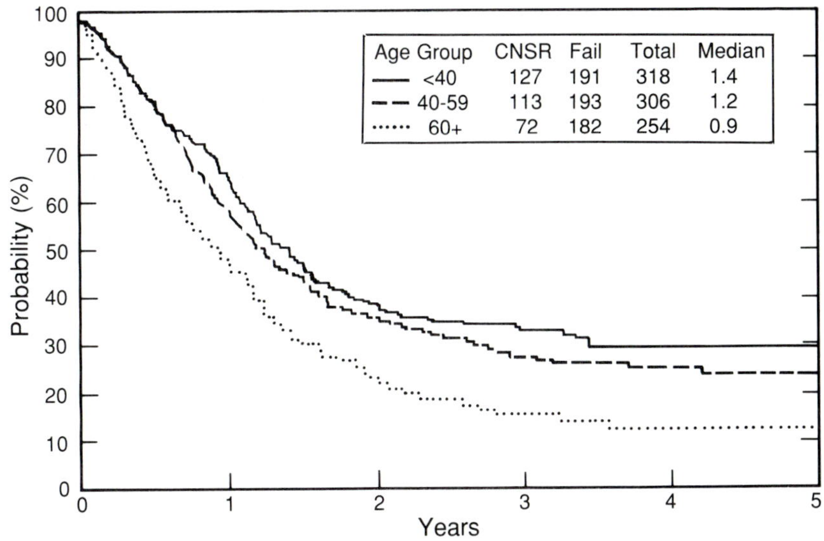

FIGURE 18-3. Kaplan-Meier analysis of disease-free survival for adults with acute myelogenous leukemia who were treated according to CALGB protocols between 1982 and 1985. Outcome by age group is statistically significant ($P < .001$). CNSR, censor. (Data courtesy of Drs. Roger Davis and Charles Schiffer, Cancer and Leukemia Group B)

was 91% for the low-risk children and 42% for those in the high-risk category.

THERAPY

The goal of therapy is to reduce and eventually eradicate the leukemic cell population while preserving normal hematopoiesis (allowing for return of normal bone marrow function). This presupposes that both normal and leukemic cells coexist at diagnosis and that effective therapy will sufficiently reduce the leukemic cell burden to allow regrowth of normal myeloid progenitors. The available data (cytogenetics, G6PD isoenzyme studies, RFLP analyses) suggest that nonneoplastic cells repopulate the marrow after chemotherapy-induced remissions in most patients with AML. AML, if untreated, progresses rapidly in most patients, but it may remain indolent or smolder for many weeks in a small percentage of patients.[319]

Before the late 1940s, there was no treatment available that could reduce the leukemic cell mass and induce a return of normal marrow function. There were rare reports of spontaneous remissions after viral or bacterial infections or transfusions.[320–322] Irradiation with x-rays or gamma emissions was successful in reducing high peripheral blast counts or extramedullary organ infiltration, but complete remission was not achieved.[323,324] It was not until the clinical trials of Farber and colleagues,[325] with the folic acid antagonist, aminopterin, that systemic chemotherapy became the mainstay of therapy for the acute leukemias (Table 18-7). Since 1955, there has been a formal anticancer drug development program supported with public funds at the National Cancer Institute (NCI).[326] The private sector is also active in drug development. During the period from 1970 to 1985, the NCI introduced 83 drugs into clinical trial. Many of these agents, including amsacrine, 5-azacitidine, doxorubicin, etoposide, mitoxantrone, and homoharringtonine, have been shown to be active in AML. During the 1960s, the anthracyclines (doxorubicin, daunorubicin) and cytarabine (ara-C), the two most active agents in the treatment of AML, entered clinical trial.[327,328] New drug development has had a major impact on therapeutic outcome, but improvements in supportive care made

TABLE 18-7. Drugs Commonly Used in the Treatment of AML

Drug (Year Introduced)	Mechanism of Action	Route	Dosage Range
Mercaptopurine or thioguanine (1958)	Inhibits purine synthesis; also incorporated into DNA	PO, IV	50–200 mg/m²/d
Daunorubicin or doxorubicin (1968)	Intercalates between base pairs in DNA; inhibits nucleic acid synthesis	IV	30–60 mg/m²/d
Cytarabine (1962)	Completely inhibits replicative DNA polymerase; also incorporated into DNA	IV, SQ IT	100–200 mg/m²/d (standard) 1000–3000 mg/m²/d (high) 40–60 mg/m² (intrathecal)
Epipodophyllotoxins (1972)	Interact with topoisomerase II to produce protein-associated cross-links; strand breaks DNA	IV	100–200 mg/m²/d
Amsacrine (1978)	Intercalates and interferes with topoisomerase II	IV	450–700 mg/m²/d
Mitoxantrone (1980)	Binds to DNA and has intercalating action	IV	12 mg/m²/d
Azacitidine (1971)	Incorporates into RNA and a lesser extent DNA; inhibits DNA methyltransferase	IV	50–250 mg/m²/d

it safe and feasible to treat patients with myelosuppressive therapies. In addition, carefully designed clinical trials in single institutions and through the cooperative group mechanism, and increasing numbers of physicians trained in the complex medical management of patients with leukemia also contributed to increased survival rates.

Until the 1970s, there were few long-term (more than 5 years) survivors of AML. The first chemotherapy regimens that resulted in long term disease-free survival usually included ara-C and often involved the administration of prolonged courses of maintenance chemotherapy (ara-C and thioguanine) or rotating combinations of drugs with or without concomitant immunotherapy.[329–332] The average remission durations ranged from 6 to 15 months, with about 10% to 15% of complete responders remaining in continuous remission for 5 or more years. Actuarial life-table analyses indicated a decreasing hazard of relapse after 3 to 4 years of remission, suggesting that a small proportion of these patients were cured of their AML.

Supportive Care

The initial hours of treatment are directed toward stabilizing the patient with respect to metabolic parameters, bleeding, fever and infection, and other life-threatening problems, such as a high peripheral blast count or extramedullary leukemic spread (eg, CNS, epidural chloromas). An indwelling central venous catheter (eg, Hickman or Broviac) should be placed by a surgeon early in the treatment course.[333,334] This access facilitates administration of chemotherapy, antibiotics, and blood components and also permits repetitive sampling of blood for diagnostic purposes.

RBC transfusions should be given to a patient with a modest degree of anemia (hemoglobin, 7 to 8 g/dL) who is about to begin remission-induction therapy. During this phase of therapy, there is an expected 3- to 4-week period of complete bone marrow suppression with profound thrombocytopenia and mucosal (skin, mouth, gastrointestinal tract) injury from chemotherapy. In this situation, maintaining a relatively high hemoglobin level provides some reserve in the case of a major bleeding episode. The blood component of choice is packed RBCs.[335] A partial exchange transfusion is sometimes preferred in the severely anemic patient (especially a young infant) with congestive heart failure.[336] Many blood banks are beginning to advocate the use of leukocyte-poor or fresh frozen packed RBCs.[337,338] Their use minimizes exposure to leukocyte antigens and thus reduces the likelihood of allergic and febrile transfusion reactions. These red-cell products have not been known to transmit cytomegalovirus. Several studies also suggest that leukocyte-poor blood products decrease the risk of alloimmunization.[339] A continuing controversy surrounds the issue of whether or not to irradiate blood products to avoid the potentially fatal syndrome of transfusion-associated graft-versus-host disease (GVHD).[340] Although the incidence of transfusion-associated GVHD is exceedingly rare in patients with AML, many investigators recommend irradiation of blood products because it is safe and effective in preventing this disease.

Hemorrhage in the patient with AML is usually secondary to thrombocytopenia. Thrombocytopenia in this setting is nearly always due to decreased production of platelets caused by reduced numbers of megakaryocytes accompanying leukemia cell infiltration of the bone marrow. It may also result from mechanical platelet injury as seen in patients with M3 AML and DIC.[258,259] Bleeding in promyelocytic leukemia may also arise from a fibrinolytic disorder.[341] Severe hemorrhage is uncommon until the platelet count falls below 20,000/μL.[342] Intensive platelet support is required in a patient with AML who has severe thrombocytopenia and is bleeding. Controversies surrounding the use of single-donor or leukocyte-poor platelet units are discussed elsewhere. Prophylactic platelet transfusions have been recommended by many physicians for patients with AML whose platelet counts are less than 20,000/μL because these patients have no marrow compensation for bleeding and are believed to be at risk for diffuse mucosal ulceration and bleeding from the toxicity of chemotherapy. The risk of fatal intracranial hemorrhage can theoretically also be reduced if the platelet count is maintained above 5000/μL. These recommendations notwithstanding, there are no controlled studies to support the efficacy of prophylactic platelet transfusions in the nonbleeding thrombocytopenic patient with AML.[343,344]

DIC is seen primarily in patients with septicemia and with M3 (promyelocytic) and M5 (monocytic) AML.[345,346] The primary therapy for DIC is treatment of the leukemia (effective cytoreductive chemotherapy) or complicating infectious disease. Platelet and fresh frozen plasma transfusions should be given to patients with DIC. The use of heparin remains controversial in patients with APL.[347–349] In several retrospective studies,[347,348] the use of heparin (low dose, 10 to 20 IU/kg/h, or standard dose) has been shown to reduce the likelihood of fatal hemorrhagic complications during remission-induction therapy. This potential benefit of heparin for patients with M3 AML has never been prospectively evaluated in a controlled study.

Most patients with AML are febrile (over 38.5°C) at the time of diagnosis or become febrile within several days after initiation of cytotoxic therapy. Although some of these patients may have fever because of their leukemia, it is probable that most have an overt or occult infection.[350] These patients should be rapidly evaluated and given empiric broad-spectrum antibiotic therapy, even if the site of infection is not defined. The use of empiric antibiotics for the febrile, neutropenic (more than 500 neutrophils/μL) patient has markedly reduced morbidity and mortality rates.[351,352]

Most microbiologically documented infections at diagnosis or early during the course of remission induction in patients with AML are caused by endogenous microflora, and some of the responsible pathogens are nosocomially acquired shortly after admission to the hospital.[352] The neutropenic AML patient with skin disrupted by chemotherapy or by intravenous catheters is especially susceptible to infection. The patient with AML may first come to medical attention because of an infection (respiratory, dental, sinus, perirectal, urinary tract, or skin) that never fully responds to antibiotic therapy.[353] Most pathogens associated with fevers in newly diagnosed patients with AML are bacterial. The antibiotic regimen must cover a broad spectrum to encompass both gram-positive and enteric gram-negative bacteria.[354]

With the increased use of indwelling venous access devices (Broviac catheters, port-a-caths), catheter-associated bacteremia has become more frequent, and most of these infections are caused by gram-positive organisms (coagulase-negative staphylococci or α-hemolytic streptococci).[355] Bacterial pathogens usually predominate as the cause of localized pulmonary infiltrates within the first 2 weeks of induction.

If a period of neutropenia persists to the second to fourth week of induction, patients are more prone to develop a fungal infection, usually *Candida albicans* or *Aspergillus* sp.[352] It is therefore appropriate to institute empiric antifungal treatment for the patient with AML who is febrile for more than 7 days while on antibiotics or who develops a new pulmonary infiltrate. Bronchoalveolar lavage or open-lung biopsy may also be indicated to establish the diagnosis. Localized pneumonia caused by *Legionella* sp must also be considered in the differential diagnosis.[356] It is uncommon for a patient with AML to develop *Pneumocystis carinii* infection, herpes simplex virus, or cytomegalovirus pneumonitis during remission induction.

The most common lesions of the oral cavity during remission induction are superficial infections due to *C albicans*.[357] This infection is easily controlled by nystatin suspension, 1 million IU four times a day, or clotrimazole troches, 10 mg four times a day. Herpes simplex is the most common viral pathogen isolated from mucosal lesions,[358] and intravenous acyclovir, 250 mg/m^2 every 8 hours for 7 to 14 days, is the preferred treatment.[359] Both *C albicans* and herpes simplex may cause clinically significant esophagitis.[360] Chemotherapeutic agents (especially doxorubicin in combination with cytosine arabinoside) are frequently responsible for oral mucositis and esophagitis during remission induction.

The most serious intraabdominal complication observed during remission induction is typhlitis, also called *necrotizing enterocolitis*.[289,361–363] This is an inflammatory cellulitis that involves the distal ileum, cecum, ascending colon, and appendix and occurs in the setting of neutropenia and cytotoxic drug-related mucosal injury. Several of the chemotherapeutic agents commonly associated with typhlitis include daunorubicin, doxorubicin, ara-C, and methotrexate. Typhlitis is characterized by fever, right lower quadrant abdominal pain, and diarrhea. Gram-negative bacillary and occasionally anaerobic organisms are responsible for the bacteremia in this setting. Abdominal radiography may show a lack of gas in the right lower quadrant and minimal distention of the small bowel. An abdominal ultrasound examination may show thickness and edema of the wall of the cecum.[364] The management of typhlitis includes cessation of oral feeding, parenteral nutrition, and administration of broad-spectrum antibiotics. Exploratory laparotomy is reserved for the rare occurrence of perforation, uncontrollable lower gastrointestinal hemorrhage, or abdominal wall fascitis.[361,362]

Metabolic Complications

Metabolic complications of AML may result from both spontaneous and treatment-induced leukemic cell lysis.[250,365] Tumor lysis can lead to hyperuricemia, hyperkalemia, and hyperphosphatemia with concomitant hypocalcemia and hyperphosphaturia.[365–367] The increase in uric acid is from catabolism of purines and may result in precipitation of uric acid in the renal collecting system with subsequent renal failure.[368] Uric acid nephropathy is avoided by prompt attention to intravenous hydration, alkalinization of the urine, and administration of allopurinol, although patients with a massive leukemia burden and a concentrated, acidic urine remain at risk for this complication. Potassium release by leukemic cells during clotting of blood samples may lead to a spurious reporting of hyperkalemia.[369,370] Spurious hypoxia from the effects of a high blast count also can occur.[371] Patients with very high serum lysozyme levels,[250] as happens in M4 or M5 AML, may develop hypokalemia secondary to renal tubular injury from high levels of urinary lysozyme.[276]

Hypercalcemia has been observed on rare occasions in patients with AML.[372,373] The pathogenesis is probably multifactorial, but cases with increased ectopic parathormone-like activity in the plasma have been described.[374] Severe hypernatremia as a consequence of diabetes insipidus can be an initial manifestation,[375] and marked hyponatremia associated with inappropriate antidiuretic hormone secretion has also occurred at presentation.[366]

Leukostasis

Extreme leukocytosis is often associated with early morbidity and mortality among patients with AML.[239,240,286,376–378] Histopathologic studies have revealed leukocyte thrombi and aggregates in the vasculature of AML patients with leukocyte counts greater than 150,000/μL but especially in those with counts over 300,000/μL.[379,380] This phenomenon of leukostasis (white thrombi) affects blood flow in the lung, brain, and other organs and eventually leads to infarction and hemorrhage (Fig. 18-4). The blasts can also compete for oxygen in the microcirculation and invade and damage vessel walls.

Leukostasis can occur in any organ, but the brain and lung appear to be the major target organs. The most common manifestations of leukostasis include stupor, coma, retinal engorgement, acute respiratory distress, and priapism. Chest radiographs may show diffuse pulmonary infiltrates, vascular engorgement, cardiomegaly, and pleural effusions. The immediate goal of therapy is to lower rapidly the peripheral blast count in an attempt to prevent infarction and hemorrhage. This goal may be achieved by the use of a rapidly acting chemotherapeutic agent, such as hydroxyurea, 3 g/m^2/d orally for 2 days,[381] sometimes in conjunction with leukapheresis, once daily. Leukapheresis is recommended for the patient who already has clinical signs and symptoms of leukostasis.[382] In the newly diagnosed patient with AML and a leukocyte count greater than 150,000/μL, it is critical to initiate promptly remission-induction chemotherapy along with intravenous hydration and allopurinol.

Remission Induction

The first step required to provide a significant prolongation of survival for patients with AML is to induce complete remission.[327] For treatment purposes, complete remission has been defined as the reduction of leukemic blasts to less than 5% in the bone marrow and restoration of normal marrow function. Peripheral blood counts should approach normal values and any organomegaly, lymphadenopathy, or other extramedullary evidence of leukemic infiltration should resolve. The patient should also have returned to a normal performance status.

It has been estimated that the leukemic cell burden is reduced by at least 2 to 3 logs (10^9 to 10^{12} cells) during the remission-induction period.[383] Additional therapy therefore is required to eradicate the residual leukemic cell mass. Therapy administered to patients after the induction of complete remission has been referred to as either *intensification, consolidation*, or *maintenance treatment*.

The remission-induction phase of therapy for patients with AML is more toxic than ALL induction. This is due to several factors, including the toxicities of the active drugs in AML and greater impairment of normal marrow reserve in the AML patient.

The induction of complete remission is successful in 70% to 80% of children and adults who are under 60 years of age with AML.[384,385] Lower remission rates are seen in elderly adults and in patients with therapy-related AML or certain cytogenetic findings.[300,304,311]

A bone marrow aspirate and biopsy specimen should be assessed within 1 to 2 weeks after completion of the first cycle of induction chemotherapy. A period of profound marrow hypoplasia and pancytopenia usually precedes a remission marrow. Patients with M3 AML or those receiving low-dose ara-C (20 mg/m^2 for 10 to 20 days) may achieve complete remission after only modest decreases in bone marrow cellularity.[386,387] Posttreatment marrow biopsy specimens in M3 AML are often cellular and contain residual dysplastic promyelocytes. Follow-up marrow aspirates in the absence of additional chemotherapy may show complete remission. If it is difficult to distinguish leukemic blasts or promyelocytes from a recovering myeloid picture, a bone marrow sample should be obtained again in several days. If the repeat marrow shows persistence of blasts, a second induction cycle should commence.

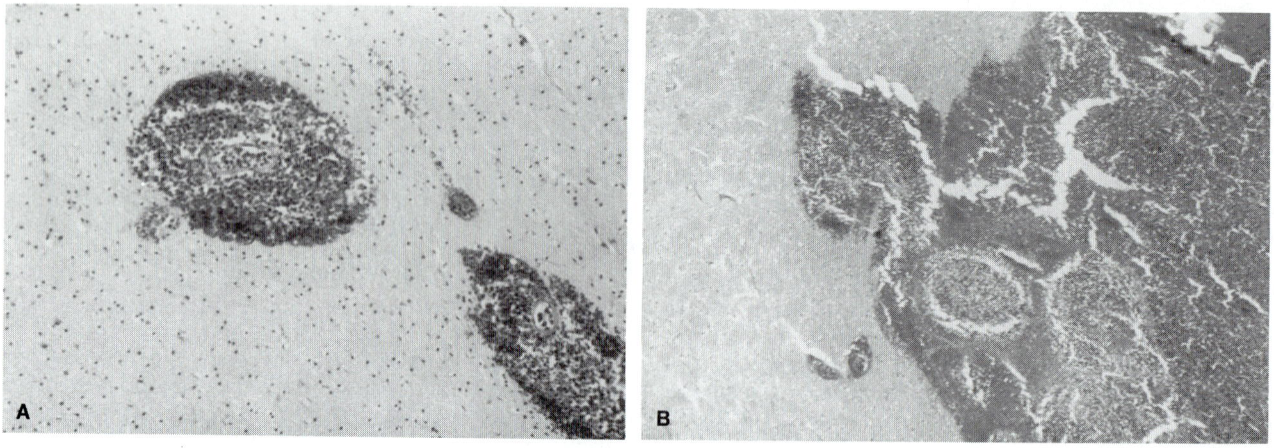

FIGURE 18-4. Central nervous system leukostasis in a patient with acute myelogenous leukemia. (**A**) Plugging of vessels by myeloblasts. (**B**) Hemorrhage and infarction.

About two thirds of patients who achieve complete remission do so after one cycle of induction, and the remainder of patients destined to respond do so after a second cycle.

Current induction protocols (Tables 18-8 and 18-9) for patients with AML usually involve drug regimens with two or more agents, including anthracycline and cytarabine. Cytarabine (ara-C) was introduced into clinical trial in the 1960s and remains the single most effective drug in the treatment of AML.[327] The original studies with ara-C were patterned after preclinical trials in mice bearing the L1210 leukemia, which illustrated significant schedule dependency.[388] This provided the basis for prolonged exposure (5 to 10 days) to ara-C at the commonly used dosages of 100 to 200 mg/m^2/d.[389] It was subsequently shown by CALGB that the combination of ara-C and thioguanine was superior to single-agent ara-C for inducing complete remission.[390]

After daunorubicin and doxorubicin were shown to be useful in the treatment of AML,[328,391] subsequent induction regimens added daunorubicin to ara-C and thioguanine (DAT) and showed that the three-drug regimen was superior to the two-drug regimen.[392] At about the same time, other investigators demonstrated the efficacy of 3 days of daunorubicin combined with a 7-day continuous infusion of ara-C (7-and-3 regimen).[393] The 7-and-3 combination has been compared with DAT in several randomized clinical trials and were found to be of equal efficacy.[394] Nevertheless, many AML induction regimens still use DAT. Subsequent studies have attempted to define the optimal dose and schedule of ara-C as well as the choice of anthracycline (daunorubicin or doxorubicin). Results of several randomized clinical trials have shown a slight advantage for continuous infusion versus twice-daily intravenous bolus ara-c and a statistically significant advantage for a 7-and-3 versus a 5-and-2 schedule.[395] CALGB could not demonstrate a further advantage for a more prolonged course of ara-C (10-and-3).[394]

Several cooperative group studies have shown that daunorubicin is preferable to doxorubicin when three daily equally myelosuppressive doses of either anthracycline are combined with a 7-day infusion of ara-C.[396] There has been less oral mucositis and gastrointestinal toxicity (necrotizing enterocolitis) with daunorubicin compared with doxorubicin, especially in patients over 60 years of age and in infants. The increased toxicity associated with doxorubicin led to more deaths during induction and a lower overall complete remission rate. Data from the Children's Cancer Study Group (CCSG) were similar to the adult experience but also showed greater toxicity of the 7-and-3 regimen in infants when doses were calculated by milligram per square meter rather than by milligram per kilogram.[397] It has been recommended that children under than 1 year of age or smaller than 0.6 m^2 should have doses of chemotherapy calculated on a milligram-per-kilogram basis.

Several newer chemotherapeutic agents, including mitoxantrone and idarubicin, have been combined with ara-C and compared with daunorubicin and ara-C for remission-induction efficacy as well as toxicity.[330,398,399] These new combinations have not resulted in higher complete remission rates but may have other advantages. For ex-

TABLE 18-8. AML Remission-Induction Regimens

Drug	Dosage (mg/m^2)	Route	Course 1 (d)	Course 2 (d)
Daunorubicin	45	IV	1, 2, 3	1, 2
Cytarabine (7-and-3)	100–200	Continuous IV infusion	1–7	1–5
Daunorubicin	60	IV	1, 2, 3	1, 2
Cytarabine	100	IV q 12 h	1–7	1–5
Thioguanine	100	PO q 12 h	1–7	1–5
Mitoxantrone	12	IV	1, 2, 3	1, 2
Cytarabine	100	Continuous IV infusion	1–7	1–5
Cytarabine	3000	IV q 12 h	1, 2	8, 9
L-Asparaginase	6000 U/m^2	IM	*	*

* L-Asparaginase is administered at hour 42.

TABLE 18-9. Remission-Induction Results in Untreated Patients With AML

Regimen	Percentage Achieving Complete Remission: Children	Age <60 Years	Age >60 Years	References
7-and-3 (cytarabine and daunorubicin)	79	70	31	399, 401, 403
7-and-3 (cytarabine and doxorubicin)	73	58	34	402
Daunorubicin, thioguanine, and cytarabine	82	70	51	398, 400
Cytarabine and mitoxantrone	—	80	46	405
High-dose cytarabine	—	67*		315

* Mean age, 54 ± 17.5 years. Data not shown for less than or more than 60 years of age.

ample, a significantly higher percentage of patients achieved complete remission after a single induction course of mitoxantrone and ara-C compared with daunorubicin and ara-C in one randomized trial.[399] This result may indicate a greater antileukemic efficacy of mitoxantrone compared with daunorubicin at doses that produced comparable toxicity. Since the median time to complete remission was shorter in patients treated with mitoxantrone compared with daunorubicin (35 versus 43 days), there was less supportive care required during induction.

The epipodophyllotoxins (VP 16 or VM 26) have been increasingly used in AML protocols.[400,401] They are particularly active single agents in patients with M4 and M5 AML. The addition of etoposide (VP 16) to daunorubicin and ara-C during induction, however, did not improve the induction response in an adult AML, randomized study.[401]

In an attempt to increase the complete remission rate or achieve greater leukemic cell kill early during induction, several groups have intensified therapy by using high-dose ara-C alone or in combination with either daunorubicin, amsacrine, or L-asparaginase.[402–405] There is sufficient clinical pharmacologic and biochemical data to suggest that intermittent infusions of high-dose ara-C, 1 to 3 g/m^2 given as a 1- to 3-hour infusion every 12 hours for 8 to 12 doses, may be more optimal than standard dosing.[406] Clinical responses to high-dose ara-C have been observed in patients with AML who were refractory to standard doses.[404,405] Early data from these high-dose ara-C studies show complete remission rates comparable to those achieved after standard-dose ara-C. Serious nonhematologic toxicity of high-dose ara-C has been limited to cerebellar dysfunction.[407] Most studies indicate that age over 50 years is the major risk factor for cerebellar toxicity. It is too early to assess the impact of these intensive regimens on remission duration.

Other novel approaches that have been used to increase leukemia cell kill during the induction phase have been based on leukemia cell kinetics and biochemistry. Researchers at Johns Hopkins Medical Center designed a study for adults with AML based on both a rodent model of AML[408] and principles developed in the laboratory.[409] In this model, initial reduction of leukemia with intensive chemotherapy results in predictable leukemic regrowth that is stimulated by host-derived humoral stimulatory activities. A second cycle of chemotherapy is timed to coincide with this increase in DNA synthesis in the blast population. This approach has been termed *timed sequential chemotherapy*. The original study that tested this concept achieved only a modest remission rate but long, unmaintained durations of remission in a small fraction of patients.[410] In a follow-up study, patients who entered complete remission received a second course of timed sequential chemotherapy. There was an impressive long-term leukemia-free survival for the patients who were able to receive the second cycle.[411] It is not known if this timed sequential therapy is more effective than conventionally timed high-dose intensive therapies for patients with AML.

Other experimental remission-induction approaches have included the use of colony-stimulating or hematopoietic growth factors (G-CSF or GM-CSF) to recruit leukemic cells into cycle to enhance their susceptibility to certain cell cycle–specific drugs.[133] Hematopoietic growth factors have also been used in combination with standard chemotherapy in an attempt to shorten the period of chemotherapy-induced pancytopenia, especially in the higher-risk elderly population.[412]

Postremission Management

Most patients with AML who enter complete remission still have occult residual leukemia. Regrowth of these leukemic cells leads to relapse in most patients. Consequently, several postremission strategies have emerged to prevent relapse. These include maintenance, consolidation, or intensification chemotherapy or marrow ablation followed by either allogeneic or autologous bone marrow transplantation. Consolidation generally refers to repetitive course of the induction regimen, and intensification refers to giving higher doses (with or without different drugs) than used during induction.[413] Consolidation and intensification courses both result in severe myelosuppression. Maintenance chemotherapy includes weekly or monthly cycles of therapy for several months or years and is less myelosuppressive.

Because the type of induction regimen (eg, single-agent versus intensive combination chemotherapy) impacts on the subsequent duration of remission, postremission therapies must be evaluated in the context of the induction therapy.[410,414] The more intensive induction programs have been associated with longer durations of unmaintained remission because of a presumed greater leukemia cell kill during the first several weeks of treatment.

By the early 1970s, it was clear that patients induced into remission with one or more courses of remission-induction therapy were almost certain to relapse within a few months if they received no further treatment. However, there were no successfully conducted randomized trials that objectively assessed the merits of maintenance therapy only after remission was achieved. Moreover, the results of one nonrandomized study suggested that no further therapy after initial remission provided a median duration of remission comparable to the results of maintenance therapy.[410] Therefore, the Eastern Cooperative Oncology Group (ECOG)[415] in 1984 began a randomized study comparing no postremission therapy to prolonged maintenance therapy (Table 18-10). Induction therapy consisted of one or two courses of daunorubicin, cytarabine, and thioguanine (5 days). The maintenance therapy consisted of thioguanine, 40 mg/m^2 orally every 12 hours for 4 days of the week, followed by ara-C, 60 mg/m^2 on the fifth day of the week subcutaneously (total duration of 2 years). Patients receiving no postremission therapy experienced significantly shorter remission durations compared with patients receiving maintenance. Each of the 26 patients in the group who were administered no postremission therapy relapsed (median remission duration of 4 months). In contrast, 16% of the patients who received maintenance therapy remained disease-free with, a median duration of remission of 8 months. In view of these results, there was early termination of this trial. CALGB[395,396] studied the optimal duration of maintenance treatment in patients with AML. Maintenance consisted of 8 to 36 months of rotating pairs of drug combinations. These studies did not show a benefit for prolonged maintenance therapy.

In the early 1980s, the contribution of maintenance therapy after one or more courses of consolidation was also prospectively evaluated. In a Swiss study,[416] patients were randomized to receive maintenance therapy or no therapy after one to three cycles of consolidation therapy. There was no improvement in duration of complete remission (median, 18 months) in the maintenance therapy group. Patients who relapsed before randomization were excluded from the analysis, leading to longer remission durations than those reported in other studies. In contrast, Buechner and colleagues[417,418] gave only one course of consolidation before randomizing patients to maintenance or no further therapy. In the patients receiving maintenance, the median duration of remission was 15 months and the probability of remission after 7 years was 22% versus, 7 months and 6%, respectively, for the observation arm. The monthly maintenance courses in this study were more myelosuppressive than several of the previously described maintenance regimens. This study has been criticized because the median duration of remission in the no maintenance arm was inferior to that reported for several uncontrolled trials of consolidation therapy alone.

The ECOG[419] and the British Medical Research Council (MRC)[420] both prospectively assessed the contribution of consolidation therapy in adults who were receiving maintenance chemotherapy (see Table 18-10). In these two large clinical trials, there was no statistically significant benefit for consolidation as defined by either two or six cycles of additional DAT induction courses. The median durations of remission ranged from 8 to 15 months, with less than 30% of complete responders still in remission after 2 years.

Data from these well-conducted randomized trials indicate that consolidation of remission (repetition of the induction regimen) for one or more courses offers a similar outcome compared with less intensive maintenance therapy continued for months or years. There was also increasing evidence that increasing the intensity of consolidation increased the median duration of remission, but most patients still relapsed.

In one of the earlier studies to employ the concept of intensification, both children and young adults (under 50 years of age) with AML were treated with 16 months of sequentially administered combinations of active, non–cross-resistant drugs.[421] Ara-C was given at two times the induction dose. In adults, the relapse-free survival was comparable to studies using short-course consolidation therapy, but the results in children were more impressive. Their 5-year probability of relapse-free survival was 45%, with an event-free survival of 31%. The German BFM Study Group[313] also completed several studies for childhood AML that included prolonged induction and consolidation over 8 weeks, followed by 2 years of maintenance treatment. This approach has been promising for children with AML. Results of selected chemotherapy protocols for AML in children are summarized in Table 18-11.

Subsequent clinical trials have intensified therapy with high-dose ara-C, 1 to 3 g/m^2, alone or combined with an anthracycline, amsacrine, or L-asparaginase[314,411,425–427] (Table 18-12). Ara-C has been the prototype drug for dose intensification. It is the single most active agent in AML, and laboratory and clinical studies have indicated that at least a log increase in its dose can overcome certain patterns of resistance and lead to complete remission in patients with AML who were previously refractory to conventional ara-C treatment. Intensification therapy has been given for one to three courses. Death secondary to drug toxicity or infection occurred in 5% to 17% of patients. The prolonged periods of pancytopenia have necessitated long hospitalizations. These studies have been uncontrolled and biased with a young patient population but nevertheless have produced encouraging early results (see Table 18-12). Several ongoing prospective randomized clinical trials (CALGB, ECOG) are comparing intensification with high-dose ara-

TABLE 18-10. Contribution of Maintenance or Consolidation Therapy to Remission Duration in Adult AML

Induction	CR (%)	Consolidation	Maintenance	Median Duration of CR (mo)	Actuarial DFS (y)	Reference
DAT	66	No	No treatment versus 6-TG, ara-C for 2 y	4 8	2 (0%) 2 (15%)	421
TAD 9	65	TAD 9—one cycle	No treatment versus ara-C alternated with daunorubicin, 6-TG, and cyclophosphamide for 3 y	7 15	7 (6%) 7 (22%)	423
7-and-3	72	7-and-3—two cycles	No treatment versus ara-C, 6-TG, vincristine, and prednisone for 2 y	18 18	2 (33%) 2 (42%)	422
DAT	67	DAT × 2 versus DAT × 6	Ara-C, 6-TG ± COAP (late intensification)	15 15	2 (21%) 2 (26%)	426

CR, complete remission; DFS, disease-free survival; DAT, daunorubicin, ara-C, and thioguanine; TAD, 6-thioguanine (6-TG), ara-C, and daunomycin; COAP, cyclophosphamide, Oncovin (vincristine), ara-C, and prednisone.

TABLE 18-11. Comparison of Treatment Results in Clinical Trials for Pediatric AML

Trial	No Patients	Complete Remission (%)	Actuarial DFS (%)	Actuarial EFS (%)
BFM-78[297]	151	80	47	38 (6 y)
BFM-83[297]	182	80	61	49 (4 y)
DFCI-VAPA[405]	125	72	45	31 (5 y)
POG-8498 (II)[408]	145	85	41	38 (2 y)
St. Jude (ANLL-83)[406]	68	85	—	33 (2 y)
LAM-8204[407]	133	80	41	33 (3 y)

DFS, disease-free survival (measured from the time of complete remission; failure is defined as relapse or death in remission from any cause; EFS, event-free survival (measured from the time of initial therapy; failure is defined as induction failure for any reason or termination of remission).

C to more conventional consolidation. The results of these studies should provide more definitive data on the contribution of intensification with high-dose ara-C to remission duration. Early results from a CALGB randomized trial show a dose response effect for cytarabine.. The projected probabilities for continuous remission after 3 years for patients under 60 years of age are 44%, 38%, and 24% for patients who received 3 g/m^2, 400 mg/m^2, and 100 mg/m^2, respectively (P = .004).[428] In the interim, a reasonable option is to treat patients under 50 years of age who have a good performance status with one to two cycles of post-complete remission high-dose ara-C and daunorubicin.[314,425]

TREATMENT OF THE ELDERLY

Treatment of elderly patients with AML requires special considerations because of both patient- and leukemia-related factors.[311] Elderly patients often have a poor performance status and therefore do not tolerate intensive chemotherapy. Therapy is frequently complicated by concomitant organ system (especially cardiovascular, pulmonary, and renal) disease. As mentioned earlier, AML in older patients is also associated with poor prognostic characteristics.

Because of these factors, elderly patients have a greater risk of early death from drug toxicity or infection. They also have more resistant leukemia than do younger patients. Therefore, the complete remission rates for patients over 60 years of age have ranged between 40% and 50%, well below that observed in younger patients.

Although a large proportion of patients with AML are over 65 years of age, few studies have specifically addressed optimal therapy for this age group. Some investigators have questioned whether older patients with AML should be treated at all. A recently reported study compared immediate standard induction chemotherapy versus supportive care with or without mild cytotoxic therapy (given only for relief of progressive symptoms related to an increased leukemic cell burden).[429] This study showed that a strategy based on supportive care only yielded extremely poor results. Complete remission was not achieved in the supportive care group, compared with a 58% complete remission rate in the chemotherapy-treated group. There was also a significantly longer survival for the latter group (median survival 21 versus 11 weeks).

Another approach used for elderly patients and others in poor-risk categories has been treatment with low-dose ara-C.[430,431] Low-dose ara-C has been used on the assumption that it is less toxic than conventional-dose ara-C. There is also in vitro but not in vivo evidence that low-dose ara-C induces differentiation of leukemic blasts.[432] In a recently reported randomized trial comparing low-dose ara-C (20 mg/m^2 for 21 days) with an intensive chemotherapy regimen (rubidazone, 100 mg/m^2 for 4 days, and ara-C, 200 mg/m^2 for 7 days) in patients over 65 years of age with de novo AML, there were a higher number of cases of complete remission with intensive chemotherapy; but with low-dose ara-C, there was a lower early death rate, thereby resulting in similar overall survivals.[430] Since the optimal therapy for elderly patients with AML remains controversial, a reasonable option is to treat patients who have a good perfor-

TABLE 18-12. Short-course Intensification or Consolidation Therapy for Adults With AML

Induction (CR%)	Median Age (y)	Postremission Treatment	Median Duration of CR	Actuarial DFS (%)	Reference
7-and-3 or 10-and-3*	38 (7–71)	One to three cycles: high-dose ara-C and daunorubicin	—	49 at 3.5 y	431
DAT (70)	46 (18-69)	One cycle: high-dose ara-C and amsacrine	1 y	30 at 3 y	432
Timed sequential daunorubicin and ara-C (55)	36	One cycle: ara-C and daunorubicin	2.5 y	41 at 8 y	417
Doxorubicin, ara-C, and 6-TG (63)	44	Zero to five cycles: doxorubicin, ara-C, and 6-TG	1 y	37 at 5 y	433
TAD (63)	47 (16–84)	Two cycles: high-dose ara-C and daunorubicin and standard-dose ara-C and daunorubicin	23 mo	32 at 5 y	320

CR, complete remission; DFS, disease-free survival; DAT, daunorubicin, ara-C, and thioguanine; TAD, 6-thioguanine (6-TG), ara-C, and daunomycin.

* Eligible patients were already in first remission before entering the study.

mance status with a modified 7-and-3 regimen[396] (reduced daunorubicin dose). Patients in poor clinical condition do poorly with any form of therapy, and there is no apparent advantage of low-dose chemotherapy over standard treatments.

Central Nervous System Prophylaxis

In contrast to studies in ALL,[433,434] early treatment or prophylaxis of the CNS with either intrathecal chemotherapy (methotrexate or ara-C) alone or combined with cranial irradiation has not been shown to prolong disease-free survival in either children or adults with AML. Most pediatric AML studies, however, include some form of CNS prophylaxis.[244,313,315,316] This practice evolved because childhood AML studies that did not include CNS prophylaxis reported as many as 20% of children having isolated CNS relapse during their first hematologic remission.[315] CNS prophylaxis included intrathecal chemotherapy (methotrexate or ara-C) alone or intrathecal methotrexate combined with cranial irradiation. These treatments have resulted in little additional acute toxicity and a low incidence of CNS relapse. Most adult therapy studies do not employ CNS prophylaxis but rely on systematically administered chemotherapy (ara-c) to eradicate occult meningeal leukemia. Ultimately, 5% to 10% of adults manifest meningeal involvement, usually in the setting of bone marrow relapse. Patients with high peripheral blast counts at diagnosis and M4 or M5 AML have the highest incidence of CNS leukemia.[264,435] The recommended therapy for CNS relapse includes four to six doses of intrathecal chemotherapy (methotrexate or ara-C) and an intensified regimen of systemic reinduction. This is sometimes followed by cranial spinal irradiation or bone marrow transplantation.

Myeloblastomas

Since most patients with isolated myeloblastomas eventually manifest bone marrow involvement, immediate systemic AML treatment has been recommended for these patients.[248,249] There is, however, little data to indicate that this approach has been successful. In most patients with AML and a myeloblastoma, it has not been necessary to administer local radiation therapy in addition to chemotherapy to achieve local control. In an emergency situation (ie, acute spinal cord compression secondary to an epidural myeloblastoma), however, several days of local irradiation, 175 to 250 cGy/d may be indicated.

Hypercalcemia secondary to ectopic production of parathyroid hormone or osteoclast-activating factor has been observed on rare occasion in patients with AML.[377]

Bone Marrow Transplantation in First Remission

Marrow ablative doses of chemotherapy with or without total-body irradiation followed by bone marrow transplantation from an HLA-matched sibling donor has been increasingly applied to young adults and children with AML in first remission.[436,437] Only a small proportion of patients with AML are considered for an allogeneic bone marrow transplantation because of age restrictions (under 50 years) and the lack of a histocompatible donor. The initial transplantation studies for AML involved patients with advanced refractory leukemia who had failed to respond or relapsed after multiple courses of chemotherapy.[438] Even in this desperate setting, 10% to 15% of patients with AML became long-term disease-free survivors. Beginning in the mid-1970s, allogeneic marrow transplantation for young patients with AML in first remission was investigated.[439–441] It was hoped that an allogeneic transplantation early in the course of the disease would be associated with less infectious morbidity and mortality and a lower leukemic relapse rate. Several conclusions became apparent from these early uncontrolled studies. The actuarial relapse rates (15% to 25%) were lower for patients who underwent transplantation in first remission compared with second or subsequent remissions, and the relapse rates were also lower than those achieved after consolidation or maintenance chemotherapy. Outcome was also related to recipient age in most studies, with 50% to 70% relapse-free survival in patients under age 30 years, and 30% to 50% relapse-free survival for patients between 30 and 50 years of age.

These studies were criticized because of the bias in timing and selection of patients referred for marrow transplantation. The median age of the patients who underwent transplantation was less than 35 years. The average time between documenting complete remission and referral to a transplantation center was several months (range, 1 month to 1 year), and therefore, patients who had more resistant or aggressive AML would most likely have relapsed before undergoing transplantation. Because of these controversies, several prospective studies in adults and children with AML were initiated to compare the outcomes of allogeneic bone marrow transplantation and chemotherapy.[442–444]

Several of these studies have reported a statistically significant leukemia-free survival advantage for the transplant recipients compared with those receiving chemotherapy. These studies have also been criticized for lack of intensity in the chemotherapy regimens, the unusually high percentage of patients with histocompatible donors, and the young patient population.

Based on the cumulative published experience, it appears that patients less than 30 years of age with AML in first remission are the most likely to benefit from allogeneic marrow transplantation.[436,445] Because of the higher mortality associated with bone marrow transplantation in the 30-to 50-year-old group, there is less of a survival advantage for those receiving transplants compared with chemotherapy. Not all studies, however, have reported an adverse effect of increasing age on outcome after allogeneic transplantation.[441] The preliminary data from intensive chemotherapy protocols are comparable to results achieved after allogeneic bone marrow transplantation, especially in the 30- to 50-year-old group.[411,425,428] Additional follow-up of these studies is needed before further recommendations can be made.

In an effort to reduce the mortality and morbidity of allogeneic bone marrow transplantation, attempts have been made to modify or prevent GVHD through the ex vivo depletion of T lymphocytes[446] from donor marrow or intensifying pharmacologic approaches.[447] Although these methods have been successful in reducing the incidence and severity of GVHD, fewer cases of this disease in some studies has resulted in an increased probability of post-transplantation leukemic relapse (ie, loss of graft-versus-leukemia effect). Because of the higher likelihood of relapse and an increased risk of graft failure, ex vivo T-cell depletion of donor marrow has not resulted in a survival advantage for patients with leukemia.[448]

Stimulated by the promising results of allogeneic marrow transplantation, an increasing number of patients with AML have been treated with cytoreductive therapy followed by autologous marrow rescue.[449–452] The advantages of autologous marrow transplantation or rescue include the elimination of problems associated with GVHD and the expansion of patient eligibility. Disadvantages include possible leukemic contamination of infused marrow and the loss of the graft-versus-leukemia effect. The early experience with autologous marrow transplantation included several uncontrolled clinical trials in adults with AML.[450,451] Transplantation preparation regimens included chemotherapy and total-body irradiation or high-dose chemotherapy alone. Purged (pharmacologic or monoclonal antibody–treated) and unpurged autologous marrow were used in these studies. The actuarial relapse rates were about 50%, with 30% to 65% of patients remaining in remission 2 to 4 years after transplantation, and the outcome appeared to be related to the timing of the transplantation. For patients who underwent transplantation within 3 months of achieving remission, there was only a 30% disease-free survival, compared with 50% to 60% for patients who underwent transplantation later in first remission (more than 9 months).[451] It was argued by many that the latter patients were already cured by the time they underwent transplantation. Whether marrow purging contributed to the success of these autologous transplants remains unknown, but a recent retrospective review suggests a benefit of purging for a subset of patients in first remission.[451] Several prospective studies have recently been initiated to compare autologous bone marrow transplantation to either allogeneic bone marrow transplantation or chemotherapy. In a Dutch AML study, allogeneic bone marrow transplantation resulted in more rapid hematopoietic reconstitution, was followed by fewer relapses, and provided better survival than autologous bone marrow transplantation.[452] A recently reported pediatric study showed comparable results (50% disease-free survival) after autologous and allogenic marrow transplantation.[453]

Refractory AML

Patients with refractory or resistant AML include those who survived the initial induction chemotherapy but failed to achieve complete remission and those who achieved a remission but eventually relapsed. Only a few studies[454,455] provide therapeutic guidelines for these patients. The initial management choices include reusing previously effective drugs, employing new classes of drugs, or proceeding directly to bone marrow transplantation. Bone marrow transplantation probably offers the greatest likelihood for a long-term second remission in this setting.[437,449]

Patients treated with chemotherapy alone for refractory (induction failure) or relapsed AML have little possibility of long-term disease-free survival.[456] In most of the reported studies, there have been few relapsed patients with second remissions lasting longer than the initial remission. The likelihood of achieving a second complete remission is lowest in patients with primary refractory AML and in patients who had short initial remission durations (less than 6 months). Patients in whom AML developed secondary to MDS or was therapy-induced were relatively resistant to primary therapy and particularly resistant to subsequent therapy. Results from the MRC[420] support these generalizations. In the eighth MRC trial, 155 of 531 relapsed patients (29%) achieved a second complete remission. Age above 60 years in addition to short initial complete remission duration adversely influenced second complete remission rates in that study. The M.D. Anderson Hospital[455] data are in accord with MRC results and also indicate longer second complete remission durations in the group of patients with longer first remissions.

A variety of different reinduction regimens were used in these patients. Is there a best second-line induction regimen, and in what circumstance should the initial induction regimen be used? Several factors, including duration of first complete remission and significant other medical problems, such as cardiac dysfunction or liver disease, influence subsequent choice of therapy. For patients who have had long initial remissions (more than 12 months) and who have not had high cumulative doses of an anthracycline nor cardiac toxicity, it is reasonable to reutilize the original effective remission-induction regimen. For the remainder of patients, newer treatment approaches should be considered. It could also be argued to test new drugs in a favorable group of relapsed patients because the goal is to identify active agents that might eventually be used as initial therapy.

High-dose cytosine arabinoside has been extensively studied in patients with refractory AML.[402,404,405] The mechanism of leukemia cell resistance to standard-dose ara-C (100 to 200 $mg/m^2/d$ for 5 to 7 days by intermittent or continuous parenteral administration) is not completely understood but may be overcome by using very high doses of ara-C (2 to 3 g/m^2 every 12 hours for 8 to 12 doses). Although complete remission can be achieved in this setting, it is not clear that the high-dose ara-C approach is of long-term value in such patients. Other active drugs include VP 16,[401] idarubicin,[457] diaziquone,[458] mitoxantrone, amsacrine,[403] and azacitidine.[459,460] Both the prednisone, vincristine, mercaptopurine, and methotrexate combination[461] and the regimen of methotrexate and L-asparaginase[462] have been effective in patients with either refractory or relapsed AML.

Allogeneic or autologous bone marrow transplantation appears to offer the possibility of long-term survival in 20% to 35% of patients with advanced AML.[437,449,463–465] The best timing of an allogeneic transplantation (at initial relapse or in second remission) and the potential benefit of in vitro treatment (purging) of marrow for an autologous transplantation remain unanswered questions. The Seattle and Johns Hopkins bone marrow transplantation groups have reported that the results of allogeneic transplantation in early relapse were equivalent to those achieved in second remission.[437,463] Because of these data, it may be prudent to follow the marrow status of patients closely to identify early relapse and to be able quickly to refer such patients for transplantation. This approach would especially apply to patients with an initial short remission because of their low likelihood of achieving a second remission.

Autologous bone marrow transplantation for patients who lack HLA-matched donors also appears promising.[449,455,464] Most of these transplantations, however, have been performed in second remission, thereby selecting a group of patients with less resistant leukemia. In addition, the second remissions have been durable enough to be able to refer the patients to a transplantation center. Not unlike the situation in first remission, the role of marrow purging with drugs or antimyeloid monoclonal antibodies is unknown. Purging of marrow appears to delay engraftment and therefore should be prospectively studied before it is more widely applied.[449]

Biologic Response Modifiers

During the past two decades, there have been extensive attempts to use immunologic agents to treat AML. The early studies used adjuvant and nonspecific agents such as *Corynbacterium parvum* and bacillus Calmette-Guérin alone or in combination with chemotherapy to enhance antileukemic immunity.[466,467] The administration of irradiated or chemically modified autologous or allogeneic leukemia cells was part of some of these protocols.[468] These forms of immunotherapy failed to improve the long-term disease-free survival of patients with AML. Interferon has also been used in the treatment of AML, but the data do not indicate that it is an active drug.[469] Recent investigational efforts have focused on enhancing the activity of lymphokine-activated killer cells or natural killer cells using IL-2 in patients with AML in remission.[470] Phase I and II studies using such approaches are underway.

Another experimental approach has been to use growth factors (ie, G-CSF or GM-CSF) either to recruit malignant myeloblasts into cell cycle or to shorten the duration of neutropenia associated with chemotherapy protocols.[133,412] As discussed earlier in the chapter, these growth factors may induce proliferation of myeloblasts and therefore have the potential to increase blast counts in these patients. Nevertheless, these innovative studies are proceeding with caution in relapsed or high-risk, newly diagnosed patients (over 60 years of age) with AML.

Differentiation Agents

Another potential approach to the treatment of AML is to induce maturation of leukemic blasts to terminal, nonproliferating cells.[163] Many agents can induce myeloid leukemic cells to differentiate in vitro, including vitamin D analogues, phorbol esters, retinoid agents, and low doses of chemotherapy drugs (eg, ara-C). Retinoic acid has been studied in patients with AML and MDS and with rare exceptions has not resulted in complete remission. Several recent reports, however, indicate that all-*trans*-retinoic acid rather than the commonly used *cis*-isomer is a very effective agent for inducing complete remission in patients with M3 AML.[471] Clinical response to this agent is associated with leukemic cell differentiation and is linked to the expression of an aberrant RAR nuclear receptor.[472–474] The proper role of all-*trans*-retinoic acid in the treatment of patients with M3 AML is being explored in a prospective clinical trial. Low-dose ara-C has also been extensively studied and is active in about 20% of patients with AML, but it probably acts through cytotoxicity rather than differentiation.[431]

TREATMENT OF PREGNANT PATIENTS

Although there have been no systematic studies of the effects of leukemia or its treatment on pregnancy, delivery, the fetus, or postnatal development, the data indicate that standard antileukemic chemotherapy can be administered safely during the second and third trimesters.[475] Cytarabine and the anthracyclines, the two most active drugs for patients with AML, have not been associated with birth defects. The risk for premature delivery, spontaneous abortion, a higher perinatal mortality, and lower birthweights for gestational age are increased in women treated for leukemia during pregnancy.[476] Growth and development of the newborn exposed to chemotherapy during the second and third trimesters appear to be normal. Issues such as elective delivery before term and vaginal delivery versus cesarean section should be individualized. Only one reasonably well-documented case of maternal–fetal transmission of AML has been reported.[477]

LONG-TERM SURVIVAL

During the past 20 years, the long-term prognosis for patients with AML has improved considerably. The CCSG reported an increase in 4-year survival probabilities from 19% to 36% for 1000 children with AML who were treated on CCSG protocols between 1972 and 1983.[478] The risk of death or relapse in each year of follow-up decreased progressively from a high of 43% in the first year to 8% by the fourth year and remained close to 5% for the next 5 years. The German BFM Study Group treated more than 300 children with AML between 1978 and 1986 with intensive induction and consolidation chemotherapy followed by 2 years of maintenance and demonstrated an improvement in event-free survival from 38% to 49%.[313]

The overall survival for adults with AML treated according to CALGB protocols between 1974 and 1985 increased from less than 10% to about 25% (Fig. 18-5). Age over 60 years was an adverse prognostic factor for relapse-free survival in the CALGB trials (see Fig. 18-3) as well as in other studies of elderly adults with AML. In the early CALGB studies (7421, 7521, 7721), the relapse curves did not plateau until the eighth year of remission.[479]

As previously discussed, survival following a relapse of AML is very poor. The M.D. Anderson Hospital reviewed their treatment experience for adults with AML in first relapse.[455,456] Thirty-three percent of patients obtained a second complete remission. The median survival after relapse was only 18 weeks. The overall survival at 5 years from relapse was 5%, and the 5-year survival probability for the complete remission patients was 16%.

LATE EFFECTS OF AML AND ITS TREATMENT

Relatively little is known about the late effects of therapy in long-term survivors of AML. This is not surprising since most patients with AML have not remained in remission

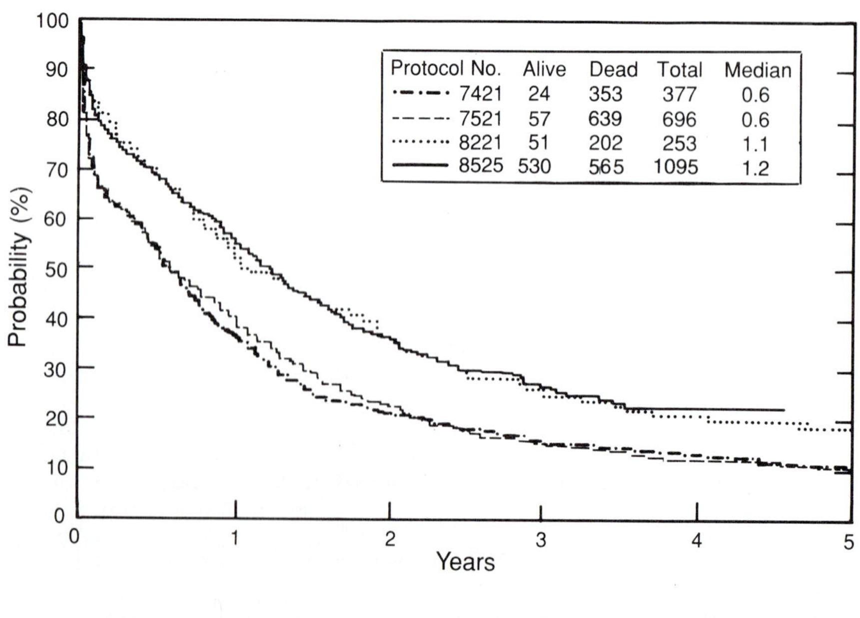

FIGURE 18-5. Kaplan-Meier analysis of survival for adults with acute myelogenous leukemia who were treated according to CALGB protocols between 1974 and 1985. (Data courtesy of Drs. Roger Davis and Charles Schiffer, Cancer and Leukemia Group B)

for 5 or more years. The biologic and psychologic late effects of surviving childhood ALL and its treatment have been well studied in the recent past (see Chap. 27). Somatic complications have included inhibition of linear growth, sterility, CNS and cardiac dysfunction, hepatic and renal toxicities, and second malignancies. The psychologic problems have included learning disabilities, academic failure, behavioral and other adjustment problems, and depression. There are no studies reporting late neuropsychological effects or brain abnormalities after treatment for AML. This probably reflects the minimal use of CNS therapy (cranial irradiation or intrathecal chemotherapy).

Infertility in leukemia survivors is a major concern. Results from a large retrospective cohort study of fertility in survivors of cancer during childhood and adolescence demonstrated that prior therapy with alkylating agents reduced fertility by about 60% in men, and there was no apparent effect among women.[480] Previous therapy with nonalkylating agents resulted in no apparent decrease in fertility in either sex. Further screening for gonadal toxicity caused by anthracyclines and cytarabine is necessary to assess reproductive function and pregnancy outcome in treated patients.

Second malignant tumors have rarely been reported in survivors of AML. This is not surprising since there have been few long-term survivors and since a limited number of patients have been treated with alkylating agents or irradiation (except in bone marrow transplantation studies).

Because the percentage of long-term survivors with AML is steadily increasing, studies should be initiated to examine the late sequelae of AML and its treatment as well as issues such as libido, sexual image, marital patterns, and overall psychological adjustment.

REFERENCES

1. Virchow R. Weisses Blut and Milztumoren. Med Z 1847;16:19.
2. Freidreich N. Ein neuer Fall von Leukamie. Arch Pathol Anat 1857;12:37.
3. Naegeli O. Ueber rotes Knochenmark und myeloblasten. Dtsch Med Wochenschr 1900;26:287.
4. Reschad H, Schilling-Torgau V. Ueber eine neue Leukamie durch echte uebergangsformen (Splenocytenleukamie) und ihre Bedeutung fur die Selbstandigkeit dieser Zellen. Munchen Med Wchnschr 1913;60:1981.
5. Watkins CH, Hall BE. Monocytic leukemia of the Naegeli and Schilling types. Am J Clin Pathol 1940;10:387.
6. DiGuglielmo G. Les maladies erythremisques. Rev Hematol 1946;1:355.
7. Hillstad LK. Acute promyelocytic leukemia. Acta Med Scand 1957;159:189.
8. Lewis SM, Szur L. Malignant myelosclerosis. Br Med J 1963;2:472.
9. Golomb HM, Rowley JD, Vardiman J, et al. "Microgranular" acute promyelocytic leukemia: a distinct clinical, ultrastructural, and cytogenetic entity. Blood 1980;55:253.
10. Bennett JM, Catovsky D, Daniel MT, et al. Proposals for the classification of the acute leukemias. Br J Haematol 1976;33:451.
11. Bennett JM, Catovsky D, Daniel MT, et al. Proposed revised criteria for the classification of acute myeloid leukemia. Ann Intern Med 1985;103:626.
12. Bennett JM, Catovsky D, Daniel MT, et al. Criteria for the diagnosis of acute leukemia of megakaryocytic lineage (M7). Ann Intern Med 1985;103:460.
13. San Miguel JF, Gonzalez M, Canizo MC, et al. Leukemias with megakaryoblastic involvement: clinical, hematologic, and immunologic characteristics. Blood 1988;74:402.
14. Stanley M, McKenna RW, Ellinger G, Brunning RD. Classification of 358 cases of acute myeloid leukemia by FAB criteria: analysis of clinical and morphologic features. In: Bloomfield CD, ed. Chronic and acute leukemias in adults. Boston, Martinus Niijhoff, 1985:147–174.
15. Cutler SJ, Young JL, eds. Third national cancer: incidence data. National Cancer Institute Monograph No. 41. Washington, DC, US Government Printing Office, 1975.
16. Young JL, Ries LG, Silverberg E, et al. Cancer incidence, survival, and mortality for children younger than age 15 years. Cancer 1986;58:598.
17. Linet MS. The leukemias: epidemiologic aspects. In: Lilienfeld AM, ed. Monographs in epidemiology and biostatistics. New York, Oxford University Press, 1985:1.
18. Cavdar AO, Arcasoy A, Babacan E, et al. Ocular granulocytic sarcoma (chloroma) with acute myelomonocytic leukemia in Turkish children. Cancer 1978;41:1606.
19. Committee on the Biological Effects of Ionizing Radiations, National Research Council. Health effects of exposure to low levels of ionizing radiation (BEIRV). Washington, DC, National Academy Press, 1990.
20. Matanoski GM, Seltser R, Sartwell PE. The current mortality rates of radiologists and other physician specialists: specific causes of death. Am J Epidemiol 1975;101:199.
21. Court-Brown WM, Doll R. Mortality from cancer and other causes after radiotherapy for ankylosing spondylitis. Br Med J 1965;2:1327.
22. Ichimaru M, Ishimaru T, Belsky JL. Incidence of leukemia in atomic bomb survivors belonging to a fixed cohort in Hiroshima and Nagasaki, 1950–1971: radiation dose, years after exposure, age at exposure, and type of leukemia. J Radiat Res 1978;19:262.
23. Shimizu Y, Schull WJ, Kato H. Cancer risk among atomic bomb survivors: the RERF Life Span Study. JAMA 1990;264:601.
24. Stewart A, Webb J, Hewitt D. A survey of children malignancies. Br Med J 1958;1:1495.
25. Graham S, Levin M, Lilienfeld A, et al. Preconception, intra-uterine, and postnatal irradiation as related to leukemia. Natl Cancer Inst Monogr 1966;19:347.
26. Gilbert ES, Marks S. An analysis of the mortality of workers in a nuclear facility. Radiat Res 1979;79:122.
27. Savitz DA, Calle E. Leukemia and occupational exposure to electromagnetic fields: review of epidemiologic surveys. J Occup Med 1987;29:47.
28. Severson, RK, Stevens RG, Kaune WT, et al. Acute non-lymphocytic leukemia and residential exposure to power frequency magnetic fields. Am J Epidemiol 1988;128:10.
29. Adamson RH, Seiber SM. Chemically induced leukemia in humans. Environ Health Perspect 1981;39:93.
30. Austin A, Delzell E, Cole P. Benzene and leukemia: a review of the literature and risk assessment. Am J Epidemiol 1988;127:419.
31. Cohen HJ, Huang ATF. A marker chromosome abnormality: occurence in chloramphenicol-associated acute leukemia. Arch Intern Med 1973;132:440.
32. Friedman GD. Phenylbutazone, musculoskeletal disease, and leukemia. J Chronic Dis 1982;35:233.
33. Tucker MA, Meadows AT, Boice JD , et al. Leukemia after therapy with alkylating agents for childhood cancer. J Natl Cancer Inst 1977;78:459.
34. Kaldor JM, Day NE, Clarke EA, et al. Leukemia following Hodgkin's disease. N Engl J Med 1990;322:7.
35. Kaldor JM, Day NE, Pettersson F, et al. Leukemia following chemotherapy for ovarian cancer. N Engl J Med 1990;322:1–6.
36. Pui CH, Behm FG, Raimondi SC, et al. Secondary acute myeloid leukemia in children treated for acute lymphoid leukemia. N Engl J Med 1989;321:136.
37. Ratain MJ, Kaminer LS, Bitran JD, et al. Acute nonlymphocytic leukemia following etoposide and cisplatin combination chemotherapy for advance non-small-cell carcinoma of the lung. Blood 1987;70:1412.
38. Gallo C, Wong-Staal F. Retroviruses and etiologic agents of some animal and human leukemias and lymphoma and as tools for elucidating the molecular mechanism of leukemogenesis. Blood 1982;60:545.
39. Deinhardt F, Wolfe LG, Theilen GH, Synder SP. ST-feline fibrosarcoma virus: induction of tumors in Marmoset monkeys. Science 1970;167:881.
40. Poiesz BJ, Ruscetti FW, Gazdar AF, et al. Detection and isolation of type C retrovirus particles from fresh and cultured lymphocytes of a patient with cutaneous T-cell lymphoma. Proc Natl Acad Sci USA 1980;77:7415.
41. Wong Staal F, Gallo RC. Human T-lymphotropic retroviruses. Nature 1985;317:395.
42. Bishop JM. Viral oncogenes. Cell 1985;42:23.
43. Varmus HE. The molecular genetics of cellular oncogenes. Annu Rev Genet 1984;18:553.
44. Weinberg RA. The action of oncogenes in the cytoplasm and nucleus. Science 1985;230:770.
45. Bishop JM. The molecular genetics of cancer. Science 1987;235:305.
46. Friend SH, Horowitz JM, Gerber MR, et al. Deletions of a DNA sequence in retinoblastomas and mesenchymal tumors: organization of the sequence and its encoded protein. Proc Natl Acad Sci USA 1987;84:9059.
47. Finlay CA, Hinds PW, Levine AJ. The p53 proto-oncogene can act as a suppressor of transformation. Cell 1989;57:1083.
48. Blasi E, Mathieson BJ, Varesio L, et al. Selective immortalization of murine macrophages from fresh bone marrow by a raf/myc recombinant murine retroviruses. Nature 1985;18:667.
49. Graf T, von Kirchbach A, Beug H. Characterization of the hematopoietic target cells of AEV, MC29, and AMV avian leukemia viruses. Exp Cell Res 1981;131:331.
50. Bartram CR, de Klein A, Hagemeijer A, et al. Translocation of the c-abl oncogene correlates with the presence of a Philadelphia chromosome myelocytic leukemia. Nature 1983;306:239.
51. Heisterkamp N, Stephenson JR, Groffen J, et al. Localization of the c-abl oncogene adjacent to a translocation break point in chronic myelocytic leukemia. Nature 1983;306:277.
52. Bos JL, Toksoz D, Marchall CJ, et al. Amino-acid substitutions at codon

13 of the N-ras oncogene in human acute myeloid leukemia. Nature 1985;315:726.
53. Needleman SW, Kraus MH, Srivastava SK, et al. High frequency of N-ras activation in acute myelogenous leukemia. Blood 1986;67:753.
54. Farr CJ, Saiki RK, Erlich HA, et al. Analysis of RAS gene mutations in acute myeloid leukemia by polymerase chain reaction and oligonucleotide probes. Proc Natl Acad Sci USA 1988;85:1629.
55. Barbicid M. Ras genes. Annu Rev Biochem 1987;56:779.
56. Varmus HE. The molecular genetics of cellular oncogenes. Annu Rev Genet 1984;18:553.
57. Satoh T, Nakafuku M, Miyajima A, Kaziro Y. Involvement of *ras* p21 protein in dsignal transduction pathways from interleukin 2, interleukin 3, and granulocyte/macrophage colony-stimulating factor, but not from interleukin 4. Proc Natl Acad Sci USA 1991;88:3314.
58. Lochrie MA, Simon MI. G. protein multiplicity in eukaryotic signal transduction systems. Biochemistry 1988;27:4957.
59. DeVos AM, Tong L, Milburn MV, et al. Three dimensional structure of an oncogene protein: catalytic domain of human c-H-vas p21. Science 1988;239:888.
60. Bos JL, Verlaan-de Vries M, van der Eb AJ, et al. Mutations in N-ras predominate in acute myeloid leukemia. Blood 1987;69:1237.
61. Senn HP, Jiricny J, Fopp M, et al. Relapse cell population differ from acute onset clone as shown by absence 6f the initially activated N-ras oncogene in a patient with acute myelomonocytic leukemia. Blood 1988;72:931.
62. Borrow J, Goddard AD, Sheer D, Solomon E. Molecular analysis of acute promyelocytic leukemia breakpoint cluster region on chromosome 17. Science 1990;240:1577.
63. Alcalay M, Zangrilli D, Pandolfi PP, et al. Translocation breakpoint of acute promyelocytic leukemia lies within the retinoic acid receptor alpha locus. proc Natl Acad Sci USA 1991;88: 1977.
64. de The H, Chomienne C, Lanotte M, Degos L, Dejean A. The t(15;17) translocation of acute promyelocytic leukaemia fuses the retinoic acid receptor gene to a novel transcribed locus. Nature 1990;347:558.
65. von Lindern M, Poutska AM, Lehrach H, Grosveld G. The (6;9) chromosome translocation, associated with a specific subtype of acute nonlymphocytic leukemia, leads to aberrant transcription of a target gene on 9q34. Mol Cell Biol 1990;10:4016.
66. Miyoshi H, Shimizu K, Kozu T, Maeski N, Kaneko Y, Ohki M. The t (8;21) breakpoints on chromosome 21 in acute myeloid leukemia clustered within a limited region of a novel gene AMLI. Proc Natl Acad Scie USA 1991;88:10431.
67. Gao J, Erickson P, Gardiner K, et al. Isolation of a yeast artificial chromosome spanning the 8;21 translocation breakpoint, t(8;21)(q22.3) in acute myelogenous leukemia. Proc Natl Acad Sci USA 1991;88:4882.
68. Erickson P, Gao J, Chang K-S, et al. Identification of breakpoints in t(8;21) AML and isolation of a fusion transcript with similarity to *Drosophila* segmentation gene runt. Blood 1992;80:1825.
69. Nucifora G, Larson RA, Rowley JD. Persistence of the 8;21 translocation in patients with acute myeloid leukemia type M2 in long-term remission. Blood 1993;82:712.
70. Kozu T, Miyoshi H, Shimizu K, et al. Junction sof the AML 1/MTG8(ETO) fusion are constant in t(8;21) acute myeloid leukemia detected by reverse transcription polymerase chain reaction. Blood 1993;82:1270.
71. Liu P, Tarle SA, Hajra A, et al. Fusion between transcription factor CBF beta/PEBA2 beta and a myosin heavy chain in acute myeloid leukemia. Science 1993;261:1041.
72. Domer PH, Fakharzadeh SS, Chen CSm et al. Acute mixed-lineage leukemia t(4;11)(q21;q23) generates an MLL-AF4 fusion product. Proc Natl Acad Sci USA 1993;90:7884.
73. Thirman MJ, Gill HJ, Burnett RC, et al. Rearrangement of the MLL gene in acute lymphoblastic and acute myeloid leukemias with 11q23 chromosomal translocations. N Engl J Med 1993;329:909.
74. Kobayashi H, Espinosa R III, Thirman MJ, et al. Heterogenity of breakpoints of 11q23 rearrangements in hematologic malignancies identified with fluoresence in situ hybridization. Blood 1993;82:547.
75. McCabe NR, Burnett RC, Gill HJ, et al. Cloning of cDNAs of the MLL gene that detect DNA rearrangements and altered RNA transcripts in human leukemic cells with 11q23 translocations. Proc Natl Acad Sci USA 1992;89:11794.
76. Zieman-van der Poel S, McCabe NR, Gill HJ, et al. Identification of a gene, MLL, that spans the breakpoint in 11q.23 translocations associated with human leukemias. Proc Natl Acad Sci USA 1991;88:10735.
77. Ahuja HG, Jat PS, Foti A, Bar-Eli M, Cline MJ. Abnormalities of the retinoblastoma gene in the pathogenesis of acute leukemia. Blood 1991;78:3259.
78. Ahuja HG, Bar-Eli M, Advani SH, Benchimol S, Cline MJ. Alterations in the p53 gene and the clonal evolution of the blast crisis of chronic myeloid leukemia. Proc Natl Acad Sci USA 1989;86:6783.
79. Willman CL, Sever CE, Pallavisini MG, et al. Deletion of IRF-1, mapping to chromosome 5q31.1, in human leukemia and preleukemia myelodysplasia. science 1993;259:968.
80. Harada H, Kitagawa M, Tanaka N, et al. Antioncogenic and oncogenic potentials of interferon regulatory factors 1 and 2. Science 1993;259: 971.
81. Linet MS. The leukemias: epidemiologic aspects. In: Lilienfeld AM, ed. Monographs in epidemiology and biostatistics. New York, Oxford University Press, 1985:1.
82. Mulvihill JJ. Congenital and genetic diseases. In: Fraumeni JF, ed. Persons at high risk of cancer. San Diego, Academic Press, 1975:3.
83. Garriga S, Crosby WH. The incidence of leukemia in families of patients with hypoplasia of the marrow. Blood 1959;14:1008.
84. Rosen RB, Kang S-JA. Congenital agranulocytosis terminating in acute myelomonocytic leukemia. J Pediatr 1979;94:406.
85. Rosner F, Lee SL. Down's syndrome and acute leukemia: myeloblastic or lymphoblastic? Am J Med 1972;53:203.
86. Weinstein HJ. Congential leukemia and the neonatal myeloproliferative disorders associated with Down's syndrome. Clin Hematol 1978;7:147.
87. Hayashi Y, Eguchi M, Sugita K, et al. Cytogenetic findings and clinical features in acute leukemia and transient myeloproliferative disorder in Down's syndrome. Blood 1988;72:15.
88. Eguchi M, Sakakibara H, Suda J , et al. Ultrastructual and ultracytochemical differences between transient myeloproliferative disorder and megakaryoblastic leukemia in Down's syndrome. Br J Haematol 1989;73:315.
89. Kurahashi H, Hara J, Yumura-Yagi K, et al. Monoclonal nature of transirent abnormal myelopoiesis in Down's syndrom. Blood 1991;77:1161.
90. Seibel NL, Sommer A, Miser J. Transient neonatal leukemoid reactions in mosaic trisomy 21. J Pediatr 1984;104:251.
91. Brodeur GM, Dahl GV, Williams DL, et al. Transient leukemoid reaction and trisomy 21 mosaicism in a phenotypically normal newborn. Blood 1980;55:691.
92. Zipursky A, Peeters M, Poon A. Megakaryoblastic leukemia and Down's syndrome: a review. Proc Clin Biol Res 1987;246:33.
93. Homans A, Verissimo AM, Vlacha V. Transient abnormal myelopoiesis of infancy associated with trisomy 21. Am J Pediatr Hematol Oncol 1993;15:392.
94. Till JE, McCulloch EA. A direct measurement of the radiation sensitivity of normal mouse bone marrow cells. Radiat Res 1961;14:213
95. Pluznik DH, Sachs L. The cloning of normal "mast" cells in tissue culture. J Cell Physiol 1965;66:319.
96. Pike BL, Robinson WA. Human bone marrow colony growth in agargel. J Cell Physiol 1970;76:77.
97. Becher AJ, McCulloch EA, Till JE. Cytological demonstration of the clonal nature of spleen colonies derived from transplanted mouse marrow cells. Nature 1963;197:452.
98. Bradley TR, Metcalf D. The growth of mouse bone marrow cells in vitro. Aust J Exp Biol Med Sci 1966;44:287.
99. Chervenick PA, Boggs DR. Bone marrow colonies: stimulation in vitro by supernatant from incubated human blood cells. Science 1970;69: 691.
100. Sheridan JW, Stanley ER. Tissue sources of bone marrow colony stimulating factor. J Cell Physiol 1971;78:451.
101. Golde DW, Clive MJ. Identification of the colony-stimulating cell in human peripheral blood. J Clin Invest 1972;51:2981.
102. Suda J, Suda T, Ogawa M. Analysis of differentiation of mouse hemopoietic stem cells in culture by sequential replating of paired progenitors. Blood 1984;64:393.
103. Spangrude GJ, Heimfeld S, Weissman IL. Purification and characterization of mouse hematopoietic stem cells. Science 1988;241:58.
104. Fauser AA, Messner HA. Identification of megakaryocytes, macrophages and eosinophils in colonies of human bone marrow containing neutrophilic granulocytes and erythroblasts. Blood 1979;53:1023.
105. Till JE, McCulloch EA. Hematopoietic stem cell differentiation. Biochem Biophys Acta 1980;605:431.
106. Ogawa M, Porter PN, Nakahata T. Renewal and commitment to differentiation of hemopoietic stem cells. (Review) Blood 1983;61:823.
107. Stephenson JR, Axelrod AA, McLeod DL, Shreeve MM. Induction of colonies of hemoglobin synthesizing cells by erythropoietin in vitro. Proc Natl Acad Sci USA 1971;68:1542.
108. Griffin JD, Lowenberg B. Clonogeneic cells in acute myeloblastic leukemia. Blood 1986;68:1185.
109. Metcalf D. The granulocyte-macrophage colony stimulating factors. Science 1985;229:16.
110. Dinarello CA, Mier JW. Lymphokines. N Engl J Med 1987;317:940.
111. Nienhuis AW. Hematopoietic growth factors. Biological complexity and clinical promise. N Engl J Med 1988;318:916.
112. Clark SC, Kamen R. The human hematopoietic colony-stimulating factors. Science 1987;236:1229.
113. Metcalf D. The molecular biology and functions of the granulocyte colony-stimulating factors. Blood 1986;67:257.
114. Sieff CA. Hematopoietic growth factors. J Clin Invest 1987;79:1549.
115. Bronchud MH, Scarffe JH, Thatcher N, et al. Phase I/II study of recombinant human granulocyte colony-stimulating factor in patients receiving intensive chemotherapy for small cell lung cancer. Br J Cancer 1987;56:809.
116. Gabrilove JL, Jakubowski A, Scher H, et al. Effect of granulocyte colony-stimulating factor on neutropenia and associated morbidity due to chemotherapy for transitional—cell carcinoma of the urothelium. N Engl J Med 1988;318:1414.
117. Antman KS, Griffin JD, Elias A, et al. Effect of recombinant human granulocyte-macrophage colony-stimulating factor on chemotherapy-induced myelosuppression. N Engl J Med 1988;319:593.

118. Ganser A, Volkers B, Ottmann OG, et al. Recombinant human granulocyte-macrophage colony-stimulating factor in patients with myelodysplastic syndromes: a phase I/II trial. Blood 1989;73:31.
119. Leischke GJ, Maher D, Cebon J, et al. Effects of bacterially synthesized recombinant human granulocyte-macrophage colony stimulating factor in patients with advanced malignancy. Ann Intern Med 1989;110:357.
120. Moore MAS, Williams N, Metcalf D. In vitro colony formation by normal and leukemic human hematopoietic cells: characterization of the colony forming cells. J Natl Cancer Inst 1973;50:603.
121. Minden MD, Till JE, McCulloch EA. Proliferative state of blast cells progenitors in acute myeloblastic leukemia (AML). Blood 1978;52:592.
122. Wouters R, Lowenberg B. On the maturation order of AML cells: a destruction on the basis of self renewal properties and immunologic phenotypes. Blood 1984;63:684.
123. Griffin JD, Larcom P, Schlossman SF. Use of surface markers to identify a subset of acute myelomonocytic leukemia cells with progenitor cells properties. Blood 1983;62:1300.
124. Koeffler HP, Golde DW. Human myeloid leukemia cell lines: a review. Blood 1980;56:344.
125. Greenberg PL. The smouldering myeloid leukemic states: clinical and biologic features. (Review) Blood 1983;61:1035.
126. Verma DS, Spitzer G, Dicke KA, McCredie KS. In vitro agar culture patterns in preleukemia and their clinical significance. Leuk Res 1979 3:41.
127. McCulloch EA, Curtis JE, Messner HA, Senn JS, Germanson TD. The contribution of blast cell properties to outcome variation in acute myeloblastic leukemia. Blood 1982;59:601.
128. Clarkson B, Fried J, Strife A, Sakai Y, Ota K, Ohkita T. Studies of cellular proliferation in human leukemia. III. Behavior of leukemic cell in three adults with acute leukemia given continuous infusions of 3H-thymidine for 8 or 10 days. Cancer 1970;25:1237.
129. Killmann SA. Proliferative activity of blast cells in leukemia and myelopoiesis: morphological differences between proliferating and non-proliferating blast cells. Acta Med Scand 1965;178:263.
130. Mauer AM, Saunders EF, Lampkine BC. Possible significance of non-proliferating leukemia cells. Natl Cancer Inst Monogr 1969;30:63.
131. Raza A, Maheshwari Y, Ucar K, Mayers G, Preisler, HD. Proliferative characteristics of acute nonlymphocytic leukemia in vivo. Acta Haematol (Basel) 1987;77:140.
132. Raza A, Maheshwari Y, Yasin Z, Madave N, Mayers GL, Preisler HD. A new method for studying cell cycle characteristics in ANLL using double-labeling with BrdU and 3 HHTdr. Leuk Res 1987;11:1079.
133. Cannistra SA, Groshek P, Griffin JD. Granulocyte-macrophage colony-stimulating factor enhances the cytotoxic effects of cytosine arabinoside in acute myeloblastic leukemia and in the myeloid blast crisis phase of chronic myeloid leukemia. Leukemia 1989;3:328.
134. Vellenga E, Young DC, Wagner K, Wiper D, Oslapovicz D, Griffin JD. The effects of GM-CSF and G-CSF in promoting growth of clonogenic cells in acute myeloblastic leukemia. Blood 1987;69:1771.
135. Vellenga E, Ostapovicz D, O'Rourke B, Griffin JD. Effects of recombinant IL-3, GM-CSF and G-CSF on proliferation of leukemic clonogenic cells in short-term and long-term cultures. Leukemia 1987;1:584.
136. Hoang T, Nara N, Wong G, et al. Effects of recombinant GM-CSF on the blast cells of acute myeloblastic leukemia. Blood 1986;68:313.
137. Hoang T, Haman A, Goncalves O, Leteudre F, Mathieu M, Wong GG, Clark SC. Interleukin 1 enhances growth factor-dependent proliferation of the clonogenic cells in acute myeloblastic leukemia and of normal human hemopoietic precursors. J Exp Med 1988;168:463.
138. Vadhan-Raj S, Keating M, LeMaistre A, et al. Effects of recombinant human granulocyte-macrophage colony-stimulating factor in patients with myelodysplastic syndromes. N Engl J Med 1987;317:1545.
139. Ganser A, Volkers B, Greher J, et al. Recombinant human granulocyte-macrophage colony-stimulating factor in patients with myelodysplastic syndromes: a phase I/II trial. Blood 1988;73:31.
140. Kobayashi Y, Okabe T, Ozawa K, et al. Treatment of myelodysplastic syndromes with recombinant human granulocyte colony-stimulating factor: a preliminary report. Am J Med 1989;86:178.
141. Negrin RS, Haeuber DH, Nagler AN, et al. Treatment of myelodysplastic syndromes with recombinant human granulocyte colony-stimulating factor: a phase I-II trial. Ann Intern Med 1989;110:976.
142. Herrmann F, Lindermann A, Klein H, et al. Effect of recombinant human granulocyte-macrophage colony-stimulating factor in patients with myelodysplastic syndrome with excess of blasts. Leukemia 1989;3:335.
143. Ganser A, Seipelt G, Lundermann A, et al. Effects of recombinant human interleukin 3 in patients with myelodysplastic syndromes. Blood 1990;76:455.
144. Cannistra SA, DiCarlo J, Groshek P, et al. Simultaneous administration of granulocyte-macrophage colony stimulating factor and cytosine arabinoside for the treatment of relapsed acute myeloid leukemia. Leukemia 1991;5:230.
145. Dexter TM, Garland J, Scott D, et al. Growth factor-dependent hemopoietic precursor cell lines. J Exp Med 1980;152:1036.
146. Lang RA, Metcalf D, Gough NM, Dunn AR, Gonda TJ. Expression of a hemopoietic growth factor cDNA in a factor-dependent cell line results in autonomous growth and tumorigenicity. Cell 1985;43:531.
147. Adkins B, Leutz A, Graf T. Autocrine growth factor induced by svc-related oncogenes in transformed chicken myeloid cells. Cell 1984;39: 439.
148. Baumbach WR, Stanley ER, Cole MD. Induction of clonal monocyte-macrophage tumors in vivo by mouse c-myc retrovirus: rearrangement of the CSF-1 gene as a secondary transforming event. Mol Cell Biol 1987;7:664.
149. Ymer S, Tucker WQJ, Sanderson CJ, Hapel AJ, Campbell HD, Young IG. Constitutive synthesis of interleukin 3 by leukemia cell line WEHI-3B is due to retroviral insertion near the gene. Nature 1985;317:255.
150. Young DC, Griffin JD. Autocrine secretion of GM-CSF in acute myeloblastic leukemia. Blood 1986;68:1178.
151. Young DC, Wagner K, Griffin JD. Constitutive expression of the granulocyte-macrophage colony-stimulating factor gene in acute myelocytic leukemia. J Clin Invest 1987;79:100.
152. Kaufman DC, Baer MR, Gao XZ, Wang Z, Preisler HD. Enhanced expression of the granulocyte-macrophage colony-stimulating factor gene in acute myelocytic leukemia cells following in vitro blast cell enrichment. Blood 1988;1329:1332.
153. Oster W, Lindemann A, Ganser A, Mertelsmann R, Herrmann FR. Constitutive expression of hematopoietic growth factors in acute myeloblastic leukemia cells. Behring Inst Mitt 1987;83:68.
154. Griffin JD, Rambaldi A, Vellenga E, Young DC, Ostapovicz D, Cannistra SA. Secretion of interleukin 1 by acute myeloblastic leukemia cells in vitro induces endothelial cells to secrete colony-stimulating factors. Blood 1987;70:1218.
155. Watari K, Asano S, Shirafuji N, et al. Serum granulocyte colony stimulating factor levels in healthy volunteers and patients with various disorders as estimated by enzyme immunoassay. Blood 1989;73:117.
156. Lowenberg B, van Putten WL, Touw IP, Delwel R, Santini V. Autonomous proliferation of leukemic cells in vitro as a determinant of prognosis of prognosis in adult acute myeloid leukemia. N Engl J Med 1993;328:614.
157. Collins SJ, Gallo RC, Gallagher RE. Continuous growth and differentiation of human myeloid leukemic cells in suspension culture. Nature 1977;270:347.
158. Koeffler HP, Golde DW. Acute myelogenous leukemia: a human cell line responsive to colony-stimulating activity. Science 1978;200:1153.
159. Lozzio CB, Lozzio BB. Human chronic myelogenous leukemia cell line with positive Philadelphia chromosome. Blood 1975;45:321.
160. Sundstrom C, Nilsson K. Establishment and characterization of a human histocytic lymphoma cell line (U-937). Int J Cancer 1976;17:565.
161. Tsuchiya S, Yamabe M, Yamaguchi Y, et al. Establishment and characterization of a human acute monocytic leukemic cell line (THP-1). Int J Cancer 1980;26:171.
162. Collins SJ. The HL-60 promyelocytic leukemia cell line: proliferation, differentiation, and cellular oncogene expression. Blood 1987;70:1233.
163. Hoffman SJ, Robinson WA. Use of differentiation-inducing agents in the myelodysplastic syndrome and acute non-lymphocytic leukemia. Am J Hematol 1988;28:124.
164. Huang ME, Ye YC, Chen SR, et al. Use of all-trans retinoic acid in the treatment of acute promyelocytic leukemia. Blood 1988;72:567.
165. Wang ZY, Sun GL, Lu JX, Gu LJ, Huang ME, Chen SR. Treatment of acute promyelocytic leukemia with all-trans retinoic acid in China. Nouv Rev Fr Hematol 1990;32:34.
166. Fialkow PJ, Singer JW, Adamson JW, et al. Acute nonlymphocytic leukemia: heterogeniety of stem cell origin. Blood 1981;57:1068.
167. Fialkow PJ, Singer JW, Raskind WH, et al. Clonal development, stem cell differentiation, and clinical remissions in a acute nonlymphocytic leukemia. N Engl J Med 1987;317:468.
168. Rowley JD. Recurring chromosome abnormalities in leukemia and lymphoma. Semin Hematol 1990;27:122.
169. Rowley JD, LeBeau MM. Cytogenetic and molecular analysis of therapy-related leukemia. Ann NY Acad Sci 1989;567:130.
170. Yunis JJ, Brunning RD. Prognostic significance of chromosomal abnormalities in acute leukaemias and myelodysplastic syndromes. Clin Haematol 1986;15:597.
171. Bloomfield CD, de la Chapelle A. Chromosome abnormalities in acute nonlymphocytic leukemia: clinical and biological significance. Semin Oncol 1987;14:372.
172. Fearon ER, Burke PJ, Schiffer CA, et al. Differentiation of leukemia cells to polymorphonuclear leukocytes in patients with acute nonlymphocytic leukemia. N Engl J Med 1986;315:15.
173. Jacobsen RJ, Temple MJ, Singer JW, et al. A clonal complete remission in a patient with acute nonlymphocytic leukemia originating in a multipotent stem cell. N Engl J Med 1984;310:1513.
174. LoCoco F, Pelicci PG, D Adamo F, et al. Polyclonal hematopoietic reconstitution in leukemia patients at remission after suppression of specific gene rearrangements. Blood 1993;82:606.
175. Busque L, Gilliland DG. Clonal evolution in acute myeloid leukemia. Blood 1993;82:337.
176. Fialkow PJ, Gartler SM, Yoshida A. Clonal origin of chronic myelocytic leukemia in man. Proc Natl Acad Sci USA 1967;58:1468.
177. Sabbath KD, Ball ED, Larcom P, Davis RB, Griffin JD. Heterogeniety of clonogenic cells in AML. J Clin Invest 1985;75:746.
178. Cheson BD, Cassiloth PA, Head Dr, et al. Report of the National Cancer Institute-sponsored workshop on definitions of diagnosis and response in acute myeloid leukemia. J Clin Oncol 1990;8:813.

179. Chan LC, Pegram SM, Greaves MF. Contribution of immunophenotype to the classification and differential diagnosis of acute leukemia. Lancet 1985;i:475.
180. Freedman AS, Nadler LM. Cell surface markers in hematologic malignancies. Semin Oncol 1987;14:193.
181. Drexter HG, Minowada J. The use of monoclonal antibodies for the identification and classification of acute myeloid leukemias. Leuk Res 1986;10:279.
182. Foon KA, Todd RF. Immunologic classification of leukemia and lymphoma. Blood 1986;68:1.
183. McMichael AJ, ed. Leucocyte typing. III. White cell differentiation antigens. Oxford, UK, Oxford University Press, 1987.
184. Griffin JD, Ritz J, Nadler LM, Schlossman SF. Expression of myeloid differentiation antigens on normal and malignant myeloid cells. J Clin Invest 1981;68:932.
185. Griffin JD, Davis R, Nelson DA, et al. Use of surface marker analysis to predict outcome of adult acute myeloblastic leukemia. Blood 1986;68:1232.
186. Drexter HG. Classification of acute myeloid leukemias: a comparison of FAB and immunophenotyping. Leukemia 1987;1:697.
187. Campos L, Guyotat D, Archimbaud E, et al. Surface marker expression in adult acute myeloid leukemia: correlations with initial characteristics, morphology and response to therapy. Br J Haematol 1989;72:161.
188. Schwarzinger I, Valent P, Koller U, et al. Prognostic significance of surface marker expression on blasts of patients with de novo acute myeloblastic leukemia. J Clin Oncol 1990;8:423.
189. Borowitz MJ, Gockerman JP, Moore JP, et al. Clinicopathologic and cytogenetic features of CD34 (My10)-positive acute nonlymphocytic leukemia. Am J Clin Pathol 1989;91:265.
190. Greaves MF, Chan LC, Furley AJW, Watt SM, Molgaard HV. Lineage promiscuity in hemopoietic differentiation and leukemia. Blood 1986;67:1.
191. Paietta F, Bettleheim P, Schwarzmeier JD, et al. Distinct lymphoblastic and myeloblastic populations in TdT positive acute myeloblastic leukemia: evidence by double fluorescence staining. Leuk Res 1983;7:301.
192. Cross AH, Goorha RM, Nuss R, et al. Acute myeloid leukemia with T-lymphoid features: A distinct biological and clinical entity. Blood 1988;72:579.
193. Hurwitz C, Raimondi S, Head D, et al. Distinctive immunophenotypic features of t(8;21) (q22;q22) acute myeloblastic leukemia in children. Blood 1992;80:3182.
194. Pui CH, Raimondi SC, Head D, et al. Characterization of childhood acute leukemia with multiple myeloid and lymphoid markers at diagnosis and relapse. Blood 1991;78:1327.
195. Smith FO, Lampkin BC, Versteeg C, et al. Expression of lymphoid-associated cell surface antigens by childhood acute myeloid leukemia cells lacks prognostic significance. Blood 1992;79:2415.
196. Jensen AW, Hokland M, Jorgensen H, et al. Solitary expression of CD7 among T-cell antigens in acute myeloid leukemia: Identification of a group of patients with similar T cell receptor beta and delta rearrangements and course of disease suggestive of poor prognosis. Blood 1991;78:1292.
197. Smith LJ, Curtis JE, Messner HA, Senn JS, et al. Lineage infidelity in acute leukemia. Blood 1983;61:1138.
198. Hershfield MS, Kurtzberg J, Harden E, et al. Conversion of a stem cell leukemia from a T-lymphoid to a myeloid phenotype induced by the adenosine deaminase inhibitor 2′-deoxycoformycin. Proc Natl Acad Sci USA 1984;81:253.
199. Pui CH, Frankel LS, Carroll AJ, et al. Clinical charactersitics and treatment outcome of childhood acute lymphoblastic leukemia with the t(4;11) (q21;q23): A collaborative study of 40 cases. Blood 1991;77:440.
200. Sobol RE, Mick R, Royston I, et al. Clinical importance of myeloid antigen expression in adult acute lymphoblastic leukemia. N Engl J Med 1987;316:1111.
201. Ball ED, Davis RB, Griffin JD, et al. Prognostic value of lymphocyte surface markers in acute myeloid leukemia. Blood 1991;77:2242.
202. Lee EJ, Pollak A, Leavitt RD, Testa JR, Schiffer CA. Minimally differentiated acute nonlymphocytic leukemia: a distinct entity. Blood 1987;70:1400.
203. Raghavachar A, Bartram CR, Ganser A, Heil G, Kleihauer E, Kubanek B. Acute undifferentiated leukemia: implications for cellular origin and clonality suggested by analysis of surface markers and immunoglobulin gene rearrangement. Blood 1986;68:658.
204. Pombo de Oliveira MS, Matutes E, Rani S, Morilla R, Catovsky D. Early expression of MCS2 (CD13) in the cytoplasm of blast cells from acute myeloid leukemia. Acta Haematol (Basel) 1988;80:61.
205. Parreira A, Pombo de Oliveira MS, Matutes E, Foroni L, Morilla R, Catovsky D. Terminal deoxynucleotidyl transferase positive acute myeloid leukemia: an association with immature myeloblastic leukaemia. Br J Haematol 1988;69:219.
206. Vainchenker W, Villeval JL, Tabilio A, et al. Immunophenotype of leukemic blasts with small peroxidase-positive granules detected by electron microscopy. Leukemia 1988;2:274.
207. Lo Coco F, De Rossi G, Pasqualetti D, et al. CD7 positive acute myeloid leukaemia: a subtype associated with cell immatirity. Br J Haematol 1989;73:480.
208. Matutes E, Pombo de Oliveira M, Foroni L, Morilla R, Catovsky D. The role of ultrastructural cytochemistry and monoclonal antibodies in clarifying the nature of undifferentiated cells in acute leukaemia. Br J Haematol 1988;69:205.
209. Larson RA, LeBeau MM, Vardiman JW, et al. The predictive value of initial cytogenetic studies in 148 adults with acute nonlymphocytic leukemia: A 12 year study (1970–1982). Cancer Genet Cytogenet 1983;10:219.
210. Berger R, Bernheim A, Flandrin G, et al. Valeur pronostique de anomalies chromosomiques dans les leucemies aigues non lymphoblastiques. Nouv Rev Fr Hematol 1983;25:87.
211. Keating MJ, Cork A, Broach Y, et al. Toward a clinically relevant cytogenetic classification of acute myelogenous leukemia. Leuk Res 1987;11:119.
212. The Fourth International Workshop on Chromosomes in Leukemia: a prospective study of acute nonlymphocytic leukemia. Cancer Genet Cytogenet 1984;11:249.
213. Yunis JJ, Brunning RD, Howe RB, Lobell M. High-resolution chromosomes as an independent prognostic indicator in adult acute nonlymphocytic leukemia. N Engl J Med 1984;311:812.
214. Arthur DC, Berger R, Golcomb HM, et al. The clinical significance of karyotype in acute myelogenous leukemia. Cancer Genet Cytogenet 1989;40:203.
215. Goddard AD, Borrow J, Freemont PS, Solomon E. Characterization of a zinc finger gene disrupted by the t(15;17) in acute promyelocytic leukemia. Science 1991;4:1371.
216. Kakizuka A, Miller WH, Umesono K, et al. Chromosomal translocation t(15;17) in human acute promyelocytic leukemia fuses RARa with a novel putative transcription factor, PML. Cell 1991;66:663.
217. de The H, Lavau C, Marchio A, Chomienne C, Degos L, Dejean A. The PML-RAR alpha fusion mRNA generated by the t(15;17) translocation in acute promyelocytic leukemia encodes a functionally altered RAR. Cell 66:675, 1991.
218. Huang M-E, Ye Y-C, Chen S-R, et al. Use of all-*trans* retinoic acid in the treatment of acute promyelocytic leukemia. Blood 1988;72:567.
219. Diaz MO, LeBeau MM, Pitha P, et al. Interferon and c-ets-1 genes in the translocation (9;11) (q22;q23) in human acute monocytic leukemia. Science 1986;265.
220. Arthur DC, Bloomfield CD. Partial deletion of the long arm of chromosome 16 and bone marrow eosinophilia in acute nonlymphocytic leukemia: a new association. Blood 1983;61:994.
221. LeBeau MM, Larson RA, Bitter MA, et al. Association of an inversion of chromosome 16 with abnormal marrow eosinophils in acute myelomonocytic leukemia. N Engl J Med 1983;309:630.
222. Holmes R, Keating MJ, Cork A, et al. A unique pattern of central nervous system leukemia in acute myelomonocytic leukemia associated with inv(16) (p13q22). Blood 1985;65:1071.
223. LeBeau MM, Diaz MO, Karin M, Rowley JD. Metallothionein gene cluster is split by chromosome 16 rearrangements in myelomonocytic leukaemia. Nature 1985;313:709.
224. Le Beau MM, Albain KS, Larson RA, et al. Clinical and cytogenetic correlation in 63 patients with therapy-related myelodysplastic syndromes and acute non-lymphocytic leukemia: further evidence for characteristic abnormalities of chromosomes no. 5 and 7. J Clin Oncol 1986;4:325.
225. Rowely JJ. Recurring chromosome abnormalities in leukemia and lymphoma. Semin Hematol 1990;27:122.
226. Levine EG, Bloomfield CD. Secondary myelodysplastic syndromes and leukemias. Clin Haematol 1986;15:1037.
227. Mitelman F, Nilsson PG, Brandt L, et al. Chromosome pattern, occupation and clinical features in patients with acute nonlymphocytic leukemia. Cancer Genet Cytogenet 1981;4:197.
228. Nimer SD, Golde DW. The 5q- abnormality. Blood 1987;70:1705.
229. Yang YC, Kovacic S, Kriz R, et al. The human genes for GM-CSF and IL-3 are closely linked in tandem on chromosome 5. Blood 1988;71:958.
230. Roberts WM, Look AT, Roussel MF, Sherr CJ. Tandem linkage of human CSF-1 receptor (c-fms) and PDGF receptor genes. Cell 1988;55:655.
231. Kurzrock R, Shtalrid M, Talpaz M, Kloetzer WS, Gutterman JU. Expression of c-abl in Philadelphia-positive acute myelogenous leukemia. Blood 1987;70:1584.
232. Kurzrock R, Gutterman JU, Talpaz M. The molecular genetics of Philadelphia-positive leukemias. N Engl J Med 1988;319:990.
233. Oshimura M, Freeman AI, Sandberg AA. Chromosomes and causation of human cancer and leukemia (ALL). Cancer 1977;40:1161.
234. Van den Berghe H, Broeckaert-Van Orsheven A, Louwagie A, et al. A new chromosome anomaly in acute lymphoblastic leukemia (ALL). Hum Genet 1979;46:173.
235. Arthur DC, Bloomfield CD, Lindquist LL, Nesbit ME. Translocation 4:11 in acute lymphoblastic leukemia: clinical characteristics and prognostic significance. Blood 1982;59:96.
236. Nagasaka M, Maeda S, Maeda H, et al. Four cases of t(4;11) acute leukemia and its myelomonocytic nature in infants. Blood 1983;61:1174.
237. Boggs DR, Wintrobe MM, Cartwright GE. The acute leukemias. Analysis of 322 cases and review of the literature. Medicine 1987;41:163.

238. Choi S-I, Simone JV. Acute non-lymphoblastic leukemia in 171 children. Med Pediatr Oncol 1976;2:119.
239. Bunin NJ, Pui CH. Differing complications in hyperleukocytosis in children with acute lymphoblastic leukemia or acute nonlymphoblastic leukemias. J Clin Onocl 1985;3:1590.
240. Ventura GJ, Hestar JP, Smith TL, Keating MJ. Acute myeloblastic leukemia with hyperleukocytosis: risk factors for early mortality in induction. Am J Hematol 1988;27:34.
241. Creutzig U, Ritter J, Budde M, et al. Early deaths due to hemorrhage and leukostasis in childhood acute myelogenous leukemia. Cancer 1987;60:3071.
242. Stanley M, McKenna RW, Ellinger G, et al. Classification of 358 cases of acute myeloid leukemia by FAB criteria: analysis of clinical and morphologic features. In: Bloomfield CD, ed. Chronic and acute leukemia in adults. Hingham, MA, Marinus Nijhoff, 1985:155.
243. Straus DJ, Mertelsmann R, Koziner B, et al. The acute monocytic leukemias: multidisciplinary studies in 45 patients. Medicine 1980;59: 409.
244. Pui CH, Dahl GV, Kalwinksy DK, et al. Central nervous system leukemia in children with nonlymphoblastic leukemia. Blood 1982;66:1062.
245. Pui CH, Kalwinsky D, Schell MJ, et al. Acute nonlymphoblastic leukemia in infants. J Clin Oncol 1988;6:1008.
246. Muss H, Moloney W. Chloroma and other myeloblastic tumors. Blood 1973;42:721.
247. Neiman RS, Barcos M, Berard C, et al. Granulocytic sarcoma: a clinicopathologic study of 61 biopsied cases. Cancer 1981;48:1426.
248. Eshghabadi M, Shojania AM, Carr I. Isolated granulocytic sarcoma: report of a case and review of the literature. J Clin Oncol 1986;4:912.
249. Meiss JM, Butler JJ, Osborne BM, et al. Granulocytic sarcoma in nonleukemic patients. Cancer 1986;56:2697.
250. Burns P, Armitage JU, Frey AL, et al. Analysis of presenting features of adult leukemia. Cancer 1981;47:2460.
251. Rowe JM. Clinical and laboratory feature of the myeloid and lymphoid leukemias. Am J Med Technol 1983;49:103.
252. Kaneko Y, Maseki N, Takasakin, et al. Clinical and hematologic characteristics in acute leukemia with 11q23 translocations. Blood 1986;67: 484.
253. McKenna RW, Parkin J, Bloomfield C, et al. Acute promyelocytic leukemia: a study of 39 cases with identification of a hyperbasophilic microgranular variant. Br J Haematol 1982;50:201.
254. Suda T, Onai T, Maekawa T. Studies on abnormal polymorphonuclear neutrophils in acute myelogenous leukemia. Am J Hematol 1983;15: 45.
255. Cowan DH. Thrombokinetics in acute non-lymphocytic leukemia. J Lab Clin Med 1973;82:911.
256. Woodcock BE, Cooper PC, Brown PR, et al. The platelet defect in acute myeloid leukemia. J Clin Pathol 1984;37:1339.
257. Gavosto F, Gabritti V, Masera P, Pileri A. The problem of anaemia in the acute leukemias. Eur J Cancer Clin Oncol 1970;6:33.
258. Bauer KA, Rosenberg RD. Thrombin generation in acute promyelocytic leukemia. Blood 1984;64:791.
259. Kantarjian HM, Keating MJ, Walters RS. Acute promyelocytic leukemia. Am J Med 1986;80:789.
260. McKenna RW, Bloomfield CD, Dick F, et al. Acute monoblastic leukemia: diagnosis and treatment of ten cases. Blood 1975;46:481.
261. Needleman SW, Burns CP, Dick FR, Armitage JO. Hypoplastic acute leukemia. Cancer 1981;48:1410.
262. Howe RB, Bloomfield CD, McKenna RW. Hypocellular acute leukemia. Am J Med 1982;72:391.
263. Carson JD, Trujillo JM, Estey EH, et al. Peripheral acute leukemia: high pest count. Blood 1989;74:1758.
264. Peterson BA, Levine EG. Uncommon subtypes of acute non-lymphocytic leukemia: clinical features and management of FAB M5, M6, and M7. Semin Oncol 187;14:425.
265. Babapulle FB, Catovsky D, Galton DAG. Clinical and laboratory features of de novo acute myeloid leukaemia with trilineage myelodysplasia. Br J Haematol 1987;66:445.
266. Fohlmeister F, Fischer R, Modder B, et al. Aplastic anemia and the hypocellular myelodysplastic syndrome. J Clin Pathol 1985;38:1218.
267. Swirsky DM, Li YS, Matthews JG, et al. 8;21 translocation in acute granulocytic leukemia: cytological, cytochemical, and clinical features. Br J Haematol 1984;56:199.
268. Lanham GR, Dahl GV, Billings FT, Stass SA. Pseudomonas aeruginosa infection with marrow suppression simulating acute promyelocytic leukemia. Am J Med 1983;14:147.
269. Sanal SM, Campbell EW, Bowdler AJ, Brat PJ. Pseudoleukemia. Postgrad Med 1983;65:143.
270. Peterson BA, Brunning RD, Bloomfield CD, et al. Central nervous system involvement in acute nonlymphocytic leukemia: a prospective study of adults in remission. Am J Med 1987;83:464.
271. Pui CA, Dahl GV, Kalwinnsky DK, et al. Central nervous system leukemia in children with acute nonlymphoblastic leukemia. Blood 1985;66:1062.
272. Meyer RJ, Ferreira P, Cuttner J, et al. Central nervous system involvement at presentation in acute granulocytic leukemia: a prospective cytocentrifuge study. Am J Med 1980;68:691.
273. Takave Y, Culbert S, Baram T, et al. Therapeutic modalities for central nervous system involvement by granulocytic sarcoma (chloroma) in children with acute nonlymphocytic leukemia. J Neurooncol 1987;4: 371.
274. Fritz RD, Forkner CD Jr, Freireich EJ. The association of fatal intracranial hemorrhage and "blastic crisis" in patients with acute leukemia. N Engl J Med 1959;261:59.
275. Price RA, Johnson WW. The central nervous system in childhood leukemia. I. The arachnoid. Cancer 1973;31:520.
276. Wiernik PH, Serpick AA. Clinical significance of serum and urinary muramidase activity in leukemia and other hematologic malignancies. Am J Med 1969;46:330.
277. Woodruff KH. Cerebrospinal fluid cytomorphology using cytocentrifugation. Am J Clin Pathol 1973;60:621.
278. Beuchner SA, Li C-Y, Su WPD. Leukemia cutis. Am J Dermatol 1985;7: 109.
279. Long JC, Mihm MC. Multiple granulocytic sarcomas of the skin: report of six cases of myelogenous leukemia with initial manifestation in the skin. Cancer 1977;39:2004.
280. Cooper PH, Innes DJ, Greer KE. Acute febrile neutorphilic dermatosis (Sweet's syndrome) and myeloproliferative disorders. Cancer 1983;51: 1518.
281. Roberts WC, Bodey GD, Wertlake PT. The heart in acute leukemia: a study of 420 autopsy cases. Am J Cardiol 1968;21:338.
282. Wiernik PH, Sutherland JC, Stechmiller BK, et al. Clinically significant cardiac infiltration in acute leukemia, lymphocytic lymphoma, and plasma cell myeloma. Med Pediatr Oncol 1976;2:75.
283. Ti M, Villafuerte R, Chase PH, Dosik H. Acute leukemia presenting as laryngeal obstruction. Cancer 1974;34:427.
284. Wukk, Burns CP. Leukemic pleural infiltrates during bone marrow remission of acute myelocytic leukemia. Cancer 1974;33:1179.
285. Armstrong P, Dyer R, Alford BA, O'Hara M. Leukemic pulmonary infiltrates: rapid development mimicking pulmonary edema. AJR 1980;135:373.
286. Nagler A, Brenner B, Zuckerman E, et al. Acute respiratory failure in hyperleukocytic acute myeloid leukemia. Am J Hematol 1988;27:65.
287. Lester TJ, Johnson JW, Cuttner J. Pulmonary leukostasis as the single worst prognostic factor in patients with acute myelocytic leukemia and hyperleukocytosis. Ann Intern Med 1985;79:43.
288. Duffy JH, Driscoll EJ. Oral manifestations of leukemia. Oral Surg 1958;11:484.
289. Hunter TB, Bjelland JC. Gastrointestinal complications of leukemia and its treatment. AJR 1984;142:513.
290. Norris NH, Weiner J. The renal lesions in leukemia. Am J Med Sci 1961;241:512.
291. Frame R, Head D, Lee R, et al. Granulocytic sarcoma of the prostate: two cases causing urinary obstruction. Cancer 1987;59:142.
292. Odom LF, Gordon EM. Acute monoblastic leukemia in infancy and early childhood: successful treatment with an epipodophyllotoxin. Blood 1984;64:875.
293. Spilberg I, Meyer GJ. The arthritis of leukemia. Arthritis Rheum 1972;15: 630.
294. Parker BR, Marglin S, Castellino RA, et al. Skeletal manifestations of leukemia, Hodgkin's disease, and non-Hodgkin lymphoma. Semin Roentgenol 1980;4:302.
295. Karesh JW, Goldman EJ, Reck K, et al. A prospective opthalmic evaluation of patients with acute myeloid leukemia: correlation of ocular and hematologic findings. J Clin Oncol 1989;7:1528.
296. Guyer DR, Schachat AP, Vitale S, et al. Leukemic retinopathy: relationship between fundus lesions and hematologic parameters at diagnosis. Opthalmology 1989;96:860.
297. Rowan PJ, Sloan JB. Iris and anterior chamber involvement in leukemia. Ann Opthalmol 1976;8:1081.
298. Estey E, Smith TL, Keating M, et al. Prediction of survival during induction therapy in patients with newly diagnosed acute myeloblastic leukemia. Leukemia 1989;3:257.
299. Keating MJ, Smith TL, Kantarjian H, et al. Cytogenetic pattern in acute myelogenous leukemia: a major reproducible determinant of outcome. Leukemia 1988;2:403.
300. Schiffer CA, Lee EJ, Tomiyasu T, et al. Prognostic impact of cytogenetic abnormalities in patients with de novo acute non-lymphocytic leukemia. Blood 1989;73:63.
301. Billstrom R, Nilsson PG, Mitelman F. Chromosomes, Auer rods, and prognosis in acute myeloid leukemia. Eur J Haematol 1988;40:273.
302. Swirsky DM, de Bastos M, Parish SE, et al. Features affecting outcome during remission induction of myeloid leukemia in 619 adult patients. Br J Hameatol 1986;64:435.
303. Cheson BD: The myelodysplastic syndomes: current approaches to therapy. Ann Intern Med 1990;112:932.
304. Hoyle CF, de Bastos M, Wheatley K, et al. AML associated with previous cytotoxic therapy, MDS, or myeloproliferative disorders: results from the MRC's 9th AML trial. Br J Haematol 1989;72:45.
305. Gajewski JL, Ho WG, Nimer SD, et al. Efficacy of intensive chemotherapy for acute myelogenous leukemia associated with a preleukemic syndrome. J Clin Oncol 1989;7:1637.
306. Mertelsmann R, Thaler HT, To L, et al. Morphological classification, response to therapy, and survival in 263 adult patients with acute nonlymphoblastic leukemia. Blood 1980;56:773.

307. Report of the Medical Research Council's Working Party on Leukemia in Adults: the relationship between morphology and other features of acute myeloid leukemia, and their prognostic significance. Br J Haematol 1975;31:165.
308. Preisler HD, Azarnia N, Raza A, et al. Relationship between the percent of marrow cells in S phase and the outcome of remission-induction therapy of acute myelogenous leukemia. Br J Haematol 1984;56:399.
309. Curtis JE, Messner HA, Mindin MD, et al. High-dose cytosine arabinoside in the treatment of acute myelogenous leukemia: contributions to the outcome of clinical and laboratory attributes. J Clin Oncol 1987;5:532.
310. Frei E, Yankee R, Krishan A. Cytokinetic evaluation of the effectiveness of remission induction treatment in patients with acute leukemia. Adv Biosci 1975;14:15.
311. Champlin RE, Gajewski JL, Golde DW. Treatment of acute myelogenous leukemia in the elderly. Semin Oncol 1989;16:51.
312. Keating MJ, Smith TL, Gehan EL, et al. A prognostic factor analysis for use in the development of predictive models for response in adult leukemia. Cancer 1982;50:457.
313. Creutzig U, Ritter J, Schellong G, for the AML-BFM Study Group. Identification of two risk groups in childhood acute myelogenous leukemia after therapy intensification in study AML-BFM-83 as compared with study AML-BFM-78. Blood 1990;75:1932.
314. Champlin R, Gajewski J, Nimer S, et al. Postremission chemotherapy for adults with acute myelogenous leukemia: improved survival with high-dose cytarabine and daunorubicin consolidation treatment. J Clin Oncol 1990;8:1199.
315. Grier HE, Gelber RD, Camitta BM, et al. Prognostic factors in childhood acute myelogenous leukemia. J Clin Oncol 1987;5:1026.
316. Dahl GV, Kalwinsky DK, Mirro J Jr, et al. Allogeneic bone marrow transplantation in a program of intensive sequential chemotherapy for children and young adults with acute non-lymphocytic leukemia in first remission. J Clin Oncol 1990;8:295.
317. Cunningham I, Gee TS, Reich LM, et al. Acute promyelocytic leukemia: treatment results during a decade at Memorial Hospital. Blood 1989;13:1116.
318. Kalwinsky DK, Raimondi SC, Schell MT, et al. Prognostic importance of cytogenetic subgroups in de novo pediatric acute non-lymphocytic leukemia. J Clin Oncol 990;8:75.
319. Barlogie B, Johnston DA, Keating M, et al. Evolution of oligoleukemia. Cancer 1984;53:2115.
320. Ifrah N, James J-M, Viguie J-PM, et al. Spontaneous remission in adult acute leukemia. Cancer 1985;56:1187.
321. Robert EE. Spontaneous complete remission in acute promyelocytic leukemia. NY State J Med 1985;86:622.
322. Wetherly-Mein G, Cottom DG. Fresh blood transfusion in leukemia. Br J Haematol 1956;2:25.
323. Ridings GR. Radiotherapy in the leukemias. Radiol Clin North Am 1968;6:83.
324. Thomas E, Epstein RB, Eschbach JW, et al. Treatment of leukemia by extracorporeal irradiation. N Engl J Med 1965;273:6.
325. Farber S, Diamond LK, Mercer RD, et al. Temporary remissions in acute leukemia in children produced by folic acid antagonist 4-aminopteroyl-glutamic acid (aminopterin). N Engl J Med 1948;238:787.
326. Marsoni S, Hoth D, Simon R, et al. Clinical drug development: an analysis of phase II trials, 1970–1985. Cancer Treat Rep 1987;71:71.
327. Ellison RR, Holland JF, Weil M, et al. Arabinoside cytosine, a useful agent in the treatment of acute leukemia in adults. Blood 1986;4:507.
328. Weil M, Glidewell OJ, Jacquillant CL, et al. Daunorubicin in the treatment of acute granulocytic leukemia. Cancer Res 1973;33:921.
329. Lewis JP. Clinical trials of adult acute non-lymphocytic leukemia: evidence of progress. Cancer Treat Rev 1985;12:133.
330. Clarkson BD, Gee T, Mertelsmann R, et al. Current status of treatment of acute leukemia in adults: an overview of the Memorial experience and review of the literature. Crit Rev Oncol Hematol 1986;4:221.
331. Peterson BA, Bloomfield CD. Long-term disease-free survival in acute non-lymphocytic leukemia. Blood 1981;6:1144.
332. Baehner RL, Kennedy MD, Sather H, et al. Characteristics of children with acute non-lymphocytic leukemia in long-term continuous remission: a report for the Children's Cancer Study Group. Med Pediatr Oncol 1981;9:393.
333. Wade JC, Newman KA, Schimpff SC, et al. Two methods for improved venous access in acute leukemia patients. JAMA 1981;246:140.
334. Mirro J, Bhaskar NR, Stokes DC, et al. A prospective study of Hickman/Broviac catheters and implantable ports in pediatric oncology patients. J Clin Oncol 1989;7:214.
335. Allegretta GJ, Weisman SJ, Altman AJ. Hematologic and infectious complications of cancer and cancer treatment. Pediatr Clin North Am 1985;32:613.
336. Neiburg PI, Stockman JA III. Rapid correction of anemia with partial exchange transfusion. Am J Dis Child 1977;131:60.
337. Hughes ASB, Brozovic B. Leucocyte depleted blood: an appraisal of available techniques. Br J Haematol 1982;50:381.
338. Chaplin H Jr. The proper use of previously frozen red blood cells for transfusion. Blood 1982;59:1118.
339. Schiffer CA, Wade JC. Supportive care: issues in the use of blood products and treatment of infection. Semin Oncol 1987;14:454.
340. Anderson K, Weinstein HJ. Transfusion associated graft-versus-host disease. N Engl J Med 1990;323:315.
341. Avvisati G, Wouter Ten Cate J, Buller HR, Mandelli F. Tranexamic acid for control of haemorrhage in acute promyelocytic leukemia. Lancet 1989;1:122.
342. Gaydos AL, Freireich EJ, Mantel N. The quantitative relation between platelet count and hemorrhage in patients with acute leukemia. N Engl J Med 1962;266:905.
343. Feusner J. The use of platelet transfusion. Am J Pediatr Hematol Oncol 1984;6:255.
344. Aderka D, Praff G, Santo M, et al. Bleeding due to thrombocytopenia in acute leukemias and reevaluation of the prophylactic platelet transfusion policy. Am J Med Sci 1986;291:147.
345. Ribeiro R, Pui CH. The clinical and biologic correlates of coagulopathy in children with acute leukemia. J Clin Oncol 1986;4:1212.
346. Fenaux P, Vanhaesbroucke C, Estienne MH, et al. Acute monocytic leukemia in adults: treatment and prognosis in 99 cases. Br J Haematol 1990;75:41.
347. Gralnick HR, Bagley J, Abrell E. Heparin treatment for the hemorrhagic diathesis of acute promyelocytic leukemia. Br J Haematol 1990;75:41.
348. Hayle CF, Swirsky DM, Freedman L, Hayhoe FGJ. Beneficial effects of heparin in the management of patients with APL. Br J Haematol 1988;68:283.
349. Goldberg MA, Ginsburg D, Mayer RJ, et al. Is heparin administration necessary during induction chemotherapy for patients with acute promyelocytic leukemia? Blood 1987;69:187.
350. Pizzo PA, Robichaud KJ, Wesley R, et al. Fever in the pediatric and young adult patient with cancer: a prospective study of 1001 episodes. Medicine 1982;61:153.
351. Schimpff SC. Overview of empiric antibiotic therapy for the febrile neutropenic patient. Rev Infect Dis 1985;7:5734.
352. Pizzo PA, Robichaud KJ, Gill FA, et al. Empiric antibiotic and antifungal therapy for cancer patients with prolonged fever and granulocytopenia. Am J Med 1982;72:101.
353. Sickles EA, Greene WH, Wiernik PH. Clinical presentation in granulocytopenic patients. Arch Intern Med 1975;135:715.
354. Hughes WT, Bodey G, Feld G, et al. Guidelines for the use of antimicrobial agents in neutropenic patients with unexplained fever. J Infect Dis 1990;161:381.
355. Hiemenz J, Skelton J, Pizzo PA. Perspective on the management of catheter related infections in cancer patients. Pediatr Infect Dis J 1986;5:6.
356. Kirby BD, Synder KM, Meyer RD, et al. Legionnaire's disease: report of sixty-five nosocomially acquired cases and review of the literature. Medicine 1980;59:188.
357. Kostiala I, Kostiala AAI, Kahanpaa A, et al. Acute fungal stomatitis in patients with hematologic malignancies: quantity and species of fungi. J Infect Dis 1982;146:101.
358. Lam MT, Pazin GJ, Armstrong JA, et al. Herpes simplex infection in acute myelogenous leukemia and other hematologic malignancies: A prospective study. Cancer 1981;48:2169.
359. Meyers JD, Wade JC, Mitchell CD, et al. Multicenter collaborative trial of intravenous acyclovir for treatment of mucocutaneous herpes simplex infection in the immunocompromised host. Am J Med 1982;73:229.
360. Buss DH, Scharyj M. Herpes virus infection of the esophagus and other visceral organs in adults: incidence and clinical significance. Am J Med 1979;66:457.
361. Skibber JM, Matler GJ, Lotze MT, et al. Right lower quandrant complications in young patients with leukemia: a surgical prospective. Ann Surg 1987;206:711.
362. Shamberger RC, Weinstein HJ, Delorey MJ, and Levey RH. The medical and surgical management of typhlitis in children with acute non-lymphocytic (myelogenous) leukemia. Cancer 1986;57:603.
363. Moir CR, Scudamore CH, Benny WB. Typhilitis: selective surgical management. Am J Surg 1986;151:563.
364. Alexander JE, Williamson SL, Seibert JJ, et al. The ultrasonographic diagnosis of typhlitis (neutropenic colitis). Pediatr Radiol 1988;18:200.
365. O'Regan S, Carson S, Chesney RW, Drummond KN. Electrolyte and acid base disturbances in the management of leukemia. Blood 1977;49:345.
366. Mir WA, Delamore IW. Metabolic disorders in acute myeloid leukemia. Br J Haematol 1978;40:79.
367. Zusman J, Brow DM, Nesbit ME. Hyperphosphatemia, hyperphosphaturia, and hypocalcemia in acute lymphoblastic leukemia. N Engl J Med 1973;289:1335.
368. Kjellstrand CM, Campbell DC, Von Hartitzsch B, Buselmeier TJ. Hyperuricemic acute renal failure. Arch Intern Med 1974;133:349.
369. Salomon J. Spurious hypoglycemia and hyperkalemia in myelomonocytic leukemia. Am J Med Sci 1974;267:359.
370. Bellvue R, Dosik H, Speigel G, Gussoff BD. Pseudohyperkalemia and extreme leukocytosis. J Lab Clin Med 1975;85:660.
371. Fox MJ, Brody JS, Weintraub LR, et al. Leukocyte larceny: a cause of spurious hypoxia. Am J Med 1979;67:742.
372. Palva IP, Salokannel SJ. Hypercalcemia in acute leukemia. Blut 1972;24:209.
373. Gewirtz AM, Stewart AF, Vignery A, et al. Hypercalcemia complicating

acute myelogenous leukemia: a syndrome of multiple aetiologies. Br J Haematol 1983;54:133.
374. Zidar BL, Shadduck RK, Winkelstein A, et al. Acute myeloblastic leukemia and hypercalcemia. N Engl J Med 1976;295:692.
375. Bergman GE, Balvarte HJ, Naiman JL. Diabetes insipidus as a presenting manifestation of acute myelogenous leukemia. J Pediatr 1976;88:355.
376. Dutcher J, Schiffer CA, Wiernik PH. Hyperleukocytosis in adult acute nonlymphocytic leukemia: impact on remission rate, duration and survival. J Clin Oncol 1987;5:1364.
377. Dearth J, Salter M, Wilson E, et al. Early death in acute leukemia in children. Med Pediatr Oncol 1983;11:225.
378. Wald BR, Heisel MA, Ortega JA. Frequency of early death in children with acute leukemia presenting with hyperleukocytosis. Cancer 1982;50:150.
379. Freireich EJ, Thomas LB, Frei E III, et al. A distinctive type of intracerebral hemorrhage associated with "blastic crisis" in patients with leukemia. Cancer 1960;13:146.
380. Mckee LC, Collins RD. Intravascular leukocyte thrombi and aggregates as a cause of morbidity and mortality in leukemia. Medicine 1974;53: 463.
381. Grund FM, Armitage JU, Burns CP. Hydroxyurea in the prevention of the effects of leukostasis in acute leukemia. Arch Intern Med 1977;137: 1246.
382. Cuttner J, Holland JF, Norton L, et al. Therapeutic leukapheresis for hyperleukocytosis in acute myelocytic leukemia. Med Pediatr Oncol 1983;11:76.
383. Frei E III, Freireich EJ. Progress and perspectives in the chemotherapy of acute leukemias. Adv Chemother 1965;2:269.
384. Champlin RE, Gale RP. Acute myelogenous leukemia. Blood 1987;69: 1551.
385. Mayer RJ. Current chemotherapeutic treatment approaches to the management of previously untreated adults with de novo acute myelogenous leukemia. Semin Oncol 1987;14:384.
386. Worsely A, Mufti GJ, Copplestone JA, et al. Very-low-dose cytarabine for myelodysplastic syndromes and acute myeloid leukemia in the elderly. Lancet 1986;1:966.
387. Stone RM, Maguire M, Goldberg MA, et al. Complete remission in acute promyelocytic leukemia despite persistence of abnormal marrow promyelocytes during induction therapy: experience in 34 patients. Blood 1988;71:690.
388. Skipper HE, Schabel FM, Wilcox WS. Experimental evaluation of potential anti-cancer agents. XXI. Scheduling of arabinosylcytosine to take advantage of its S phase specificity against leukemic cells. Cancer Chem Rep 1967;51:125.
389. South West Oncology Group. Cytarabine for acute leukemia in adults: effect of schedule on therapeutic response. Arch Intern Med 1974;133: 251.
390. Carey RW, Ribas-Mundo M, Ellison RR, et al. Comparative study of cytosine arabinoside therapy alone and combined with thioguanine, mercaptopurine, or daunorubicin in acute myelocytic leukemia. Cancer 1975;36:1560.
391. Wilson HE, Bodey GP, Moon TE, et al. Adriamycin therapy in previously treated adult acute leukemia. Cancer Treat Rep 1977;61:905.
392. Gale RP, Cline MS. High remission-induction rate in acute myeloid leukemia. Lancet 1977;1:497.
393. Yates JW, Wallace JH, Ellison RR, et al. Cytosine arabinoside (NSC-63878) and daunorubicin (NSC-83142) therapy in acute non-lymphocytic leukemia (part 1). Cancer Chemother Rep 1973;57:485.
394. Preisler H, Davis RB, Krishner J, et al. Comparison of three induction regimens and two postinduction strategies for the treatment of acute non-lymphocytic leukemia: a Cancer and Leukemia Group B study. Blood 1987;69:1441.
395. Rai KR, Holland JF, Glidewell OJ, et al. Treatment of acute myelocytic leukemia: a study by Cancer and Leukemia Group B. Blood 1981;58: 1203.
396. Yates J, Glidewell OJ, Wiernik P, et al. Cytosine arabinoside with daunorubincin or Adriamycin for therapy of acute myelocytic leukemia: a CALGB study. Blood 1982;60:454.
397. Buckley JD, Lampkin BC, Nesbit ME, et al. Remission induction in children with acute non-lymphocytic leukemia using cytosine arabinoside and doxorubicin or daunorubicin: a report from the Children's Cancer Study Group. Med Pediatr Oncol 1989;17:382.
398. Vogler WR, Velex-Garcia E, Omura G, et al. A phase III trial comparing daunorubicin and idarubicin in combination with cytosine arabinoside as induction therapy for acute myelogenous leukemia. Blood 1987;70: 240.
399. Arlin Z, Case DC, Moore J, et al. Randomized multi-center trial of cytosine arabinoside with mitoxantrone or daunorubicin in prevously untreated adult patients with acute nonlymphocytic leukemia (ANLL). Leukemia 1990;4:177.
400. Mathe G, Schwarzenberg L, Pouillart P, et al. Two epipodophyllotoxin derivatives, VM 26 and VP 16213, in the treatment of leukemias, hematosarcomas, and lymphomas. Cancer 1974;34:985.
401. Bishop JF, Lowenthal RM, Joshua D, et al. Etoposide in acute nonlymphocytic leukemia. Blood 1990;75:21.
402. Herzig RH, Lazarus HM, Wolff SM, et al. High-dose cytosine arabinoside therapy with and without anthracycline antibiotics for remission reinduction of acute non-lymphoblastic leukemia. J Clin Oncol 1985;3: 992.
403. Arlin ZA, Ahmed T, Mittelman A, et al. A new regimen of amsacrine with high dose cytarabine is safe and effective therapy for acute leukemia. J Clin Oncol 1987;5:371.
404. Capizzi RL, Davis R, Powell B, et al. Synergy between high-dose cytarabine and asparaginase in the treatment of adults with refractory and relapsed acute myelogenous leukemia: a Cancer and Leukemia Group B study. J Clin Oncol 1988;6:499.
405. Rudnick S, Cadman EC, Capizzi RL, et al. High dose cytosine arabinoside in refractory acute leukemia. Cancer 1979;44:1189.
406. Capizzi RL, Yang JL, Rathmell JP, et al. Dose-related pharmacologic effects of high dose ara-C and its self potentiation. Semin Oncol 1985;12: 65.
407. Herzig RH, Hines JD, Herzig GP, et al. Cerebellar toxicity with high dose cytosine arabinsoide. J Clin Oncol 1987;5:927.
408. Martens ACM, Van Bekkum DW, Hagenbeek A. The BN acute myelocytic leukemia (BNML): a rat model for studying human acute myelocytic leukemia. Leukemia 1990;4:244.
409. Karp JE, Donehower RC, Dole GB, et al. Correlation of drug perturbed marrow cell growth kinetics and intracellular 1-B-D-arabino furanosylcytosine metabolism with clinical response in adult acute myelogenous leukemia. Blood 1987;69:1134.
410. Vaughn WP, Karp JE, Burke PJ. Long chemotherapy-free remissions after single cycle timed sequential chemotherapy for acute myelocytic leukemia. Cancer 1980;45:859.
411. Burke PJ, Karp JE, Geller RB, Vaughn WP. Cures of leukemia with aggressive postremission treatment: an update of timed sequential therapy (Ac-D-Ac). Leukemia 1989;3:692.
412. Estey EH, Dixon D, Kantarjian HM, et al. Treatment of poor-prognosis, newly diagnosed acute myeloid leukemia with ara-C and recombinant human granulocyte-macrophage colony-stimulating factor. Blood 1990;75:1766.
413. Bloomfield CD. Postremission therapy in acute myeloid leukemia. J Clin Oncol 1985;3:1570.
414. Wiernik PH, Serpick AA. A randomized trial of daunorubicin and a combination of prednisone, vincristine, 6-mercaptopurine, and methotrexate in adult non-lymphocytic leukemia. Cancer Res 1972;32:2032.
415. Cassileth P, Harrighton DP, Hines JD, et al. Maintenance chemotherapy prolongs initial complete remission duration in adult acute non-lymphocytic leukemia. J Clin Oncol 1988;6:583.
416. Sauter C, Berchtold W, Foop M, et al. Acute myelogenous leukemia: maintenance chemotherapy after early consolidation does not prolong survival. Lancet 1984;1:379.
417. Buechner T, Urbanitz D, Hiddleman W, et al. Intensified induction and consolidation with or without maintenance chemotherapy for acute myeloid leukemia (AML): two multicenter studies of the German AML Cooperative Group. J Clin Oncol 1985;3:1583.
418. Buechner T, Hiddeman W, Nowrousian M, et al. Long-term effect on monthly myelosuppressive maintenance chemotherapy in acute myeloid leukemia (AML): a randomized study by the AMLCG. Proc Am Soc Clin Oncol 1990;9:202.
419. Cassileth PA, Begg CB, Bennett JM, et al. A randomized study of the efficacy of consolidation therapy in adult acute non-lymphocytic leukemia. Blood 1984;63:843.
420. Rees JKH, Gray RG, Swirsky D, et al. Principal results of the Medical Research Council's 8th acute myeloid leukaemia trial. Lancet 1986;2: 1236.
421. Weinstein HJ, Mayer RJ, Rosenthal DS, et al. Chemotherapy for acute myelogenous leukemia in children and adults: VAPA udpdate. Blood 1983;62:315.
422. Kalwinksy D, Mirro J, Schell M, et al. Early intensification of chemotherapy for childhood acute nonlymphoblastic leukemia: improved remission induction with a five drug regimen including etoposide. J Clin Oncol 1988;6:1134.
423. Amadori S, Ceci A, Correlli A, et al. Treatment of acute myelogenous leukemia in children: results of the Italian Cooperative study AISOP/ LAM8204. J Clin Oncol 1987;5:1356.
424. Steuber CP, Culbert SJ, Ravindranath Y, et al. Therapy of Childhood Acute Nonlymphocytic Leukemia: the Pediatric Oncology Group Experience (1977–1988). In: Buechner T, Schellong G, Hiddeman W, eds. Haematology and blood transfusion acute leukemias II. New York, Springer-Verlag, 1990;33:198.
425. Wolff SW, Herzig RN, Fay JW, et al. High-dose cytarabine and daunorubicin as consolidation therapy for acute myeloid leukemia in first remission: long-term follow-up and results. J Clin Oncol 1989;7:1260.
426. Cassileth PA, Begg CB, Silber R, et al. Prolonged unmaintained remission after intensive consolidation therapy in adult acute nonlymphocytic leukemia. Cancer Treat Rep 1987;71:137.
427. Rohatiner AZS, Gregory WM, Bassan R, et al. Short-term therapy for acute myelogenous leukemia. J Clin Oncol 1988;6:218.
428. Stone R, Mayer R. Treatment of the newly diagnosed adult with de novo acute myeloid leukemia. Hematol Oncol Clin North Am 1993; 7:47.
429. Lowenberg B, Zittoun R, Kerkhofs H, et al. On the value of intensive remission-induction chemotherapy in elderly patients of 65+ years with acute myeloid leukemia: a randomized phase III study of the

European organization for research and treatment of Cancer Leukemia Group. J Clin Oncol 1989;7:1268.
430. Tilly H, Castaigne S, Bordessoule D, et al. Low-dose cytarabine versus intensive chemotherapy in the treatment of acute nonlymphocytic leukemia in the elderly. J Clin Oncol 1990;8:272.
431. Cheson BD, Jasperse DM, Simon R, et al. A critical appraisal of low-dose cytosine arabinoside in patients with acute non-lymphoctyic leukemia and myelodysplastic syndromes. J Clin Oncol 1986;4:1857.
432. Sachs L. The differentiation of myeloid leukemia cells: new possibilities for therapy. Br J Haematol 1978;40:509.
433. Aur RJA, Simone JV, Husto HO, et al. Central nervous system therapy and combination chemotherapy of childhood lymphocytic leukemia. Blood 1971;37:272.
434. Nesbit ME, Sather HN, Robison LL, et al. Presymptomatic central nervous system therapy in previously untreated childhood acute lymphoblastic leukemia: comparison of 1800 rad and 2400 rad. A report for the Children's Cancer Study Group. Lancet 1981;1:461.
435. Cassileth PA, Sylvester LS, Bennett JM, Begg CB. High peripheral blast count in adult acute myelogenous leukemia is a primary risk factor for CNS leukemia. J Clin Oncol 1988;6:495.
436. Santos GW. Marrow transplantation in acute nonlymphocytic leukemia. Blood 1989;74:901.
437. Clift RA, Buckner CD, Thomas ED, et al. The treatment of acute non-lymphoblastic leukemia by allogeneic marrow transplantation. Bone Marrow Transplant 1987;2:243.
438. Thomas ED, Buckner CD, Banaji M, et al. One hundred patients with acute leukemia treated by chemotherapy, total body irradiation, and allogeneic marrow transplantation. Blood 1977;49:511.
439. Thomas ED, Buckner CD, Clift RA, et al. Marrow transplantation for acute non-lymphoblastic leukemia in first remission. N Engl J Med 1979;301:597.
440. Dinsmore R, Kirkpatrick D, Flomenberg N, et al. Allogeneic bone marrow transplantation for patients with acute nonlymphocytic leukemia. Blood 1984;63:649.
441. McGlave PB, Haake RJ, Bostrom BC, et al. Allogeneic bone marrow transplantation for acute nonlymphocytic leukemia in first remission. Blood 1988;72:1512.
442. Applebaum FR, Fisher LD, Thomas ED. Chemotherapy or marrow transplantation for adults with acute non-lymphocytic leukemia: a five year follow-up. Blood 1988;72:179.
443. Champlin RE, Ho WG, Gale RP, et al. Treatment of acute myelogenous leukemia: a prospective controlled trial of bone marrow transplantation versus consolidation chemotherapy. Ann Intern Med 1985;102:285.
444. Nesbit M, Buckley J, Feig S, et al. Chemotherapy for induction of remission of childhood acute myeloid leukemia followed by marrow transplantation or multiagent chemotherapy: a report from the Children's Cancer Group. J Clin Oncol 1994;12:127.
445. Hurd DD. Allogeneic and autologous bone marrow transplantation (BMT) for acute nonlymphocytic leukemia. Semin Oncol 1987;14:407.
446. Gale RP. T cells, bone marrow transplantation and immunotherapy. Ann Intern Med 1987;106:257.
447. Storb R, Deeg HJ, Whitehead J, et al. Methotrexate and cyclosporine compared with cyclosporine alone for prophylaxis of acute graft-versus-host disease after marrow transplantation for leukemia. N Engl J Med 1986;314:729.
448. Mitsuyasu R, Champlin RE, Gale RP, et al. Depletion of T lymphocytes from donor bone marrow for prevention of graft-versus-host disease following bone marrow transplantation. Ann Intern Med 1986;105:20.
449. Yeager AM, Kaizer H, Santos GW, et al. Autologous bone marrow transplantation in patients with acute nonlymphocytic leukemia: a phase II study of ex vivo marrow treatment with 4-hydroperoxycyclophosphamide. N Engl J Med 1986;315:141.
450. McMillan AK, Goldstone AH, Linch DC, et al. High-dose chemotherapy and autologous bone marrow transplantation in acute myeloid leukemia. Blood 1990;76:480.
451. Gorin NC, Aegerter P, Auvert B, et al. Autologous bone marrow transplantation for acute myelocytic leukemia in first remission: a European survey of the role of marrow purging. Blood 1990;75:1606.
452. Lowenberg B, Verdonck LG, Dekker AdW, et al. Autologous bone marrow transplantation in acute myeloid leukemia in first remission: results of a Dutch prospective study. J Clin Oncol 1990;8:287.
453. Woods W, Kobrinsky N, Neudorf S, et al. Intensively timed induction therapy followed by autologous or allogenic bone maroow transplantation for children with acute myeloid leukemia or myelodysplastic syndrome: a Children's Cancer Group pilot study. J Clin Oncol 1993;11:1448.
454. Giever MR. Treatment of patients with acute nonlymphocytic leukemia not in remission. Semin Oncol 1987;14:416.
455. Keating MJ, Kantarjian H, Smith TL, et al. Response to salvage therapy and survival after relapse in acute myelogenous leukemia. J Clin Oncol 1989;7:1071.
456. Kantarjian HM, Keating MJ, Walters RS, et al. The characteristics and outcome of patients with late relapse acute myelogenous leukemia. J Clin Oncol 1988;6:232.
457. Carella AM, Santini G, Martinengo M, et al. 4-Demethoxy daunorubicin (idarubicin) in refractory or relapsed acute leukemia: a pilot study. Cancer 1985;55:1452.
458. Lee EJ, Van Echo DA, Egorin MJ, et al. Diaziquone given as a continuous infusion is an active agent for relapsed adult acute nonlymphocytic leukemia. Blood 1986;67:182.
459. Glover AB, Leyland-Jones BR, Chun HG, et al. Azacytidine: 10 years later. Cancer Treat Rep 1987;71:737.
460. Kalwinsky DK, Dahl GV, Mirro J, et al. Induction failures in childhood acute nonlymphocytic leukemia: etoposide/5-azacytidine for cases refractory to daunorubicin/cytarabine. Med Pediatr Oncol 1986;14:245.
461. Leone G, Pagano L, Marra R, et al. Combination of 6-mercaptopurine, vincristine, methotrexate, and prednisone in resistant or relapsed acute nonlymphoid leukemia. Cancer Treat Rep 1987;71:751.
462. Amadori S, Tribalto M, Pastore S, et al. Sequential combination of methotrexate (mtx) and L-asparaginase (asp) in advanced acute nonlymphocytic leukemia (ANLL). (Abstract) Am Assoc Cancer Res 1980;21:131.
463. Geller RB, Saral R, Piantadosi S, et al. Allogeneic bone marrow transplantation after high-dose busulfan and cyclosphosphamide in patients with acute nonlymphocytic leukemia. Blood 1989;73:2209.
464. Korbling M, Hunstein W, Fliedner TM, et al. Disease-free survival after autologous bone marrow transplantation in patients with acute myelogenous leukemia. Blood 1989;74:1898.
465. Ball ED, Mills LE, Cornwell III GG, et al. Autologous bone marrow transplantation for acute myeloid leukemia using monoclonal antibody-purged bone marrow. Blood 1990;75:1199.
466. Baehner RL, Bernstein ID, Sather H, et al. Improved remission induction rate with D-ZAPO but unimproved remission duration with addition of immunotherapy to chemotherapy in previously untreated children with ANLL. Med Pediatr Oncol 1979;7:127.
467. Lister TA, Whitehouse JMA, Oliver RTD, et al. Chemotherapy and immunotherapy for acute myelogenous leukemia. Cancer 1980;46:2142.
468. Holland JF, Bekesi JG, Cuttner J, et al. Chemoimmunotherapy in acute myelocytic leukemia. Isr J Med Sci 1977;13:694.
469. Mirro J, Dow LW, Kalwinsky DK, et al. Phase I–II study of continuous-infusion high-dose human lymphoblastoid interferon and the in vitro sensitivity of leukemic progenitors in nonlymphocytic leukemia. Cancer Treat Rep 1986;70:363.
470. Adler A, Albo V, Blatt J, et al. Interleukin-2 induction of lymphokine-activated killer (CAk) activity in the peripheral blood and bone marrow of acute leukemia patients. II. Feasibility of LAK generation in children with active disease and in remission. Blood 1989;74:1690.
471. Meng-er H, Yu-chen Y, Shu-rong C, et al. Use of all-trans retinoic acid in the treatment of acute promyelocytic leukemia. Blood 1988;72:567.
472. Warrell R, Frankel S, Miller W, et al. Differentiation therapy of acute promyelocytic leukemia with tretinoin (all-*trans*-retinoic acid). N Engl J Med 1991;324:1385.
473. Fenaux P, Castaigne S, Dombret H, et al. All-transretinoic acid followed by intensive chemotherapy gives a high complete remission rate and may prolong remissions in newly diagnosed acute promyelocytic leukemia: A pilot study on 26 cases. Blood 1992;80:2176.
474. LoCoco F, Avvisati G, Diverio D, et al. Molecular evaluation of response to all-*trans*-retinoic acid therapy in patients with acute promyelocytic leukemia. Blood 1991;77:1657.
475. Doll DC, Ringenberg QS, Yarbro JW. Antineoplastic agents and pregnancy. Semin Oncol 1989;16:337.
476. Caligiuri MA, Mayer RJ. Pregnancy and leukemia. Semin Oncol 1989;16:388.
477. Osada S, Horibe K, Oiwak K, et al. A case of infantile acute monocytic leukemia caused by vertical transmission of the mother's leukemia cells. Cancer 1990;65:1146.
478. Buckley JD, Chard RL, Baehner RL, et al. Improvement in outcome for children with acute nonlymphocytic leukemia. Cancer 1989;63:1457.
479. Preisler HD, Anderson K, Rai K, et al. The frequency of long-term remission in patients with acute myelogenous leukemia treated with conventional maintenance chemotherapy: a study of 760 patients with a minimal follow-up time of 6 years. Br J Haematol 1989;71:189.
480. Byrne J, Mulvihill JJ, Myers MH, et al. Effects of treatment on fertility in long-term survivors of childhood or adolescent cancer. N Engl J Med 1987;317:135.

Blood: Principles and Practice of Hematology,
edited by Robert I. Handin, Thomas P. Stossel, and Samuel E. Lux.
J.B. Lippincott Company, Philadelphia © 1995.

19

Structure, Function, and Functional Disorders of the Phagocyte System

Thomas P. Stossel
Bernard M. Babior

The phagocyte system consists of bone marrow–derived cells with the common feature of efficient engulfment of particulate material. The development of these cells from the pluripotent and committed stem cells, covered in detail in Chapter 8, leads to the deployment of two major phagocyte classes: the neutrophilic polymorphonuclear leukocytes (PMNs) and the mononuclear phagocytes (MNPs). These consist of two morphologically distinct cell types: the blood monocytes and the tissue macrophages into which they develop. Eosinophilic polymorphonuclear leukocytes (eosinophils) qualify as phagocytes, but because they seem to have functions distinct from neutrophilic PMNs, they are usually separated conceptually from the phagocyte system (see Chap. 20). This chapter describes structural and functional properties of mature PMNs and MNPs. Other chapters discuss the life cycle of these cells and disorders affecting this cycle (Chap. 17), as well as neoplastic diseases of the phagocyte system (Chap. 18).

Although many have attributed the discovery of phagocytosis to the Russian comparative zoologist Elie Metchnikoff, it was a German clergyman and amateur naturalist named Johann Goeze[1] (1731 to 1793) who in 1777 published the first account of protists ingesting other protists (Fig. 19-1). In the following year, a German nobleman, Wilhelm F. von Gleichen-Russworm[2] (1717 to 1783) described his experiments feeding carmine particles to lower eukaryotes. The emigration of leukocytes from blood into tissues was observed by Waller and by Addison in the early part of the 19th century, and Schultze first described phagocytosis by human leukocytes in 1865.[3] Metchnikoff, however, deserves (and received) much credit for recognizing, beginning in 1888, the significance of this system of cells in physiology and pathology. Metchnikoff consolidated his theory that phagocytes mediate host defense and cause inflammation by a series of brilliant experiments using comparative pathology. By showing that animals without circulatory systems exhibited collections of phagocytes at sites of inflammation, Metchnikoff overcame the objection by his critics who espoused the earlier views of Virchow and Cohnheim that vascular permeability was the cause, not the effect, of phagocyte emigration.[4] The discovery of serum opsonins by Wright and Douglas and their identification as antibody and complement by Ward and Enders and others in the early 20th century provided an important step in ascertaining how phagocytes act specifically against pathogens and pointed to a source other than the phagocytes for that specificity.

The modern era of phagocytosis research began in the 1950s and 1960s with a number of important advances. One was recognition by Robert McKannes and his colleagues of macrophage activation in the containment of facultative intracellular parasites. Another was the cultivation and extensive characterization of mononuclear phagocytes by Zanvil Cohn and coworkers at Rockefeller University. Still another was the beginning use of phagocytes as subjects of biochemical research by Manfred Karnovsky at Harvard, who was interested in the metabolic basis of ingestion. These investigations and others by Filipo Rossi in Trieste led to new insights into the molecular mechanisms of microbicidal and inflammatory activities of phagocytes, especially the importance of oxygen metabolites. The elucidation of the antimicrobial myeloperoxidase (MPO) and hydrogen peroxide system by Seymour Klebanoff had a major influence in the development of this field. James Hirsch, Cohn, and later, Marco Baggiolini at Rockefeller, Dorothy Bainton and Marilyn Farquhar at the University of California, and John Spitznagel in Chapel Hill contributed landmark investigations on the composition and microbicidal function of phagocyte subcellular organelles. Peter Elsbach at New York University and, later, Bengt Samuelsson at the Karolinska Institute made phagocyte lipids important focuses of research. The introduction by Stephen Boyden in 1963 of a simple method for measuring leukocyte locomotion in vitro was the impetus for studies by Elmer Becker and Peter Ward at Walter Reed Army Institute for Medical Research and ultimately led to the discovery of a large number of humoral factors, chemoattractants, that controlled the direction of migration of leukocytes. Nobuyuki Senda in Osaka, Japan, pioneered studies on the role of contractile proteins in phagocyte motility. Also of great importance was the recognition that a qualitative disorder of phagocytes, chronic granulomatous disease, first described by Robert Good and colleagues at the University of Minnesota, led to susceptibility to infection. This group and others later documented that this disease resulted from a disorder of phagocyte bactericidal deficiency related to faulty oxygen metabolism.

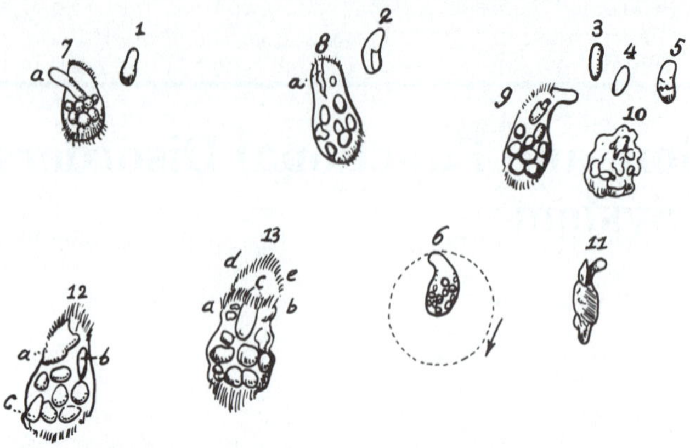

FIGURE 19-1. Original description of phagocytosis: reproduction by Joy Marlowe of drawings by Johann Goeze,[1] showing small protists, which Goeze called "small oval animals," ingested by larger ones, which he called "Haarwanzen" ("hairbugs").

GENERAL FUNCTIONS AND CLASSIFICATION OF PHAGOCYTES

The most clearly defined function of the phagocyte system is as a scavenger of senescent or damaged cells and macromolecules and as a powerful defense mechanism against infection by microorganisms. To the extent that these cells must use biochemical activities that are cytolytic or destructive of macromolecules in their degrading and defensive roles, they have the capacity to damage host tissue. When this destruction occurs, either as a by-product of the combat between phagocytes and invading microorganisms or as a direct attack on the host in autoimmune disorders, the phagocytes contribute importantly to inflammation and host cell destruction. The target range of phagocytes is relatively nonspecific, and the cells depend heavily on the lymphoid system (see Chap. 21) for directions.

Less well understood but increasingly apparent is the capacity of phagocytes to elaborate an enormous variety of compounds (Table 19-1), some of which participate in the local regulation of cell growth and development, in immune responses, in blood coagulation, and possibly even in atherogenesis and carcinogenesis.

Because PMNs and MNPs arise from a common committed stem cell, it is not surprising that they share many characteristics. Indeed, their functional similarities outweigh their differences sufficiently that it is reasonable to economize by summarizing much of their physiology together. Nevertheless, PMNs and MNPs have important differences. In addition to indicating these variations throughout the chapter, we highlight major differences here.

Mobility

Both PMNs and MNPs arise from the bone marrow and circulate. In their life cycles, both exhibit invasive properties when they enter the blood from the marrow sinuses and leave it to penetrate body tissues by active motility. In this motile activity, PMNs are more active than monocytes; indeed, PMNs are the most motile eukaryotic cells in the human body. As monocytes become macrophages, they lose most of their capacity to move translationally (mobility), although they remain actively *motile* in terms of surface ruffling, spreading, and phagocytosis.

Life Cycle

The growth and development of phagocytes are described in detail in Chapter 17. Although neither mature PMNs nor MNPs are able to self-replicate, they differ in the degree to which they are end cells. A relatively brief lifetime (days

TABLE 19-1. Substances Secreted by Mononuclear Phagocytes

CYTOKINES
Thymosin B_4
Interferon
IL-6
Tumor growth factor α, β
Fibroblast growth factor
Erythropoietin
IL-$1_{\alpha,\beta}$
Tumor necrosis factor
Platelet-derived growth factor
IL-8
IL-1 growth factor
Bombesin
Granulocyte-macrophage CSF
Granulocyte CSF
Macrophage CSF
IL-1 inhibitor
COMPLEMENT SYSTEM PROTEINS
C1, C4, C2, C3, C5
Factors B, D, H
Properdin
C3b inactivator
BINDING PROTEINS
Transcobalamin II
Haptoglobin
Transferrin
α_1-Antiprotease
α_2-Macroglobulin
α_1-Antichymotrypsin
Gelsolin
Apolipoprotein E
ENZYMES
Lysozyme
Arginase
Angiotensin-converting enzyme
Acid lipase
Acid phosphatase
Acid RNAase
Acid DNAase
α-Naphthylesterase
Leucine-2-naphthylaminidase
Acid deramidase
Sphingomyelinase
Phospholipase A_2
Elastase
Collagenase
Acid sulfatase
Aryl sulfatase A, B
ENZYMES (Continued)
Iduronate sulfatase
Heparan-N-sulfatase
N-acetylgalactosamine-6-sulfate sulfatase
N-acetylglucosamine sulfatase
β-Glucuronidase
Lipoprotein lipase
β-Glucosidase
β-Galactosidase
α-Mannosidase
α-L-Fucosidase
α-Iduronidase
α-Neuraminidase
Aspartylglycosaminidase
N-acetyl-β-glucosaminidase
N-acetyl-β-galactosaminidase
OXIDANTS
Superoxide
Hydroxyl radical
Hydrogen peroxide
Hypohalous acids
Nitrous oxide
COAGULATION SYSTEM PROTEINS
Factors V, VII, IX, X, XIII
Tissue factor
Plasminogen activator
Urokinase
Thrombospondin
LIPID METABOLITES
Prostaglandin E_2, $F_{2\alpha}$, I
Thromboxane A_2
Leukotriene B, C, D, E
Malonyldialdehyde
Mon-, di-HETE
Platelet-activating factor
OTHER METABOLITES, PEPTIDES, AND PROTEINS
Glutathione
Purines
Pyrimidines
Biopterin
Serum amyloid A, P
Fibronectin
Defensins
1,25-hydroxyvitamin D_3
Renin
Chondroitin sulfate proteoglycan

IL, interleukin; CSF, colony-stimulating factor; HETE, hydroxyeicosatetraenoic acid.

at most) is characteristic of PMNs, whereas MNPs persist for months as macrophages in the tissues. Nearly all the biosynthetic activity of PMNs takes place during their period of maturation in the bone marrow, whereas MNPs retain the ability to make an amazing variety of products throughout their lifetime. Both PMNs and MNPs are relegated to function in their final resting place in the tissue, in contrast to free-living phagocytic cells such as amebae, which they resemble in many other ways and which have the ability to crawl about and ingest particulate matter wherever they please. This apparent lack of economy in the failure to recycle phagocytic cells, which requires the human organism to generate billions of PMNs daily, seems wasteful at face value.

Functional Versatility

In keeping with their short life-span and limited biosynthetic capacity, PMNs have a narrower spectrum of functional roles than do MNPs. PMNs are of prime importance in the defense against many species of bacteria, and their rapid concentration in huge numbers at the site of attack by such organisms in the form of pus explains whey these microbes are called *pyogenic*. PMNs also collect in necrotic tissues, where they participate in the digestion of macromolecules. In these activities, PMNs depend on immunoproteins, immunoglobulin M (IgM), IgG, and complement protein fragments to recognize where to mobilize (see Chap. 16 and later discussion). MNPs also participate in the defense against pyogenic infection and in the digestion of denatured macromolecules, and they become increasingly prominent when such processes become chronic. Unlike PMNs, however, MNPs, in the form of tissue macrophages, have the major share of the task of clearance of senescent cells and macromolecules under normal circumstances. Moreover, MNPs play an important role in the containment and eradication of so-called facultative intracellular parasites and interact in the exercise of this function with T lymphocytes (see Chap. 21). In light of the numerous digestive enzymes, binding proteins, and cytokines produced by MNPs (see Table 19-1), these remarkable cells undoubtedly have many functions that are yet to be defined.

Why More Than One Kind of Phagocyte?

Relatively little comparative hematology has employed modern tools of cell biology, so we can only speculate about reasons for different characteristics of phagocytes in various species. Some of the mysteries include the absence of MPO in chicken phagocytes, the abundant neutral protease content of human PMNs but not of PMNs from other species, the lack of N-formyloligopeptide (FMLP) chemotactic factor receptors in bovine phagocytes, and the residence of MNPs in the lumen of pulmonary blood vessels of horse, sheep, pig, dogs, and cats, but not rabbits or humans.[5,6] Most curious of all is that only mammals have clearly defined populations of PMNs and MNPs. Lower organisms have phagocytes with characteristics resembling PMNs, but the phagocytes are more nearly akin to MNPs, and only mammals form true pus. It may be that the need for this particularly aggressive phagocyte evolved from the high risk of tissue infection associated with mammalian parturition.

PHAGOCYTIC FUNCTION: INTRACELLULAR SIGNALING

The many functional activities of phagocytes share certain common features. Most phagocyte functions are not constitutive but rather become manifest when soluble or particulate molecules in the environment of the cell perturb externally disposed plasma membrane receptors on the phagocyte[7] (Table 19-2). We allude to the acute initiation of such functions as phagocyte *excitation* to distinguish it from the phenomena to be defined below and known respectively as *stimulation* and *activation* of mononuclear phagocytes.

PMNs, monocytes, and macrophages can ingest a wide variety of pathogenic microorganisms, but many of these, known as facultative intracellular parasites, are not contained or killed after ingestion. Examples of such microorganisms include *Listeria monocytogenes*, *Salmonella* sp, mycobacteria causing tuberculosis and leprosy, certain fungi such as *Candida albicans*, and metazoan parasites like *Toxoplasma gondii* and *Leishmania donovanii*. Macrophages that have interacted with T lymphocytes from immunocompetent subjects previously exposed to these microorganisms acquire the ability to deal with them. This acquisition of defensive function is part of a cellular program known as MNP *activation* (Table 19-3). Activated MNPs also demonstrate enhanced cytotoxicity against mammalian cells, especially neoplastic cells, a phenomenon of great interest regarding immunity against malignant tumors. MNP activation is to be distinguished from the phenomenon known as MNP *stimulation*, the panel of alterations that takes place when MNPs ingest digestible material (see Table 19-3). A commonly applied experimental technique for preparing stimulated MNPs is to harvest them from the peritoneal cavities of mice 12 hours after intraperitoneal injection of thioglycolate broth.

T cells activate MNPs by secretion of interferon-γ (IFN-γ), which interacts with receptors on the MNP surface. One of the most important consequences of IFN-γ action on MNPs is stimulation of synthesis of components of the respiratory burst superoxide-producing NADPH oxidase, described in more detail later. Although monocytes respond acutely to stimuli with a respiratory burst, unactivated monocyte-derived macrophages do not, unless activated by IFN-γ. Another antimicrobial effector system of MNPs induced by activation is a biopterin-linked metabolic pathway that catalyzes the oxidation of arginine to citrulline concomitant with the elaboration of cytotoxic nitrogen dioxide. T cells elaborate other mediators, such as tumor necrosis factor (TNF), macrophage colony-stimulating factor (M-CSF), and interleukin-2 (IL-2), which may contribute to macrophage activation. Because activated MNPs have increased expression of TNF, this may explain in part enhanced MNP cytotoxicity against tumor cells. Other alterations in MNPs associated with activation are listed in Table 19-3. Presumably, the activation process is a mechanism for limiting autotoxicity of MNPs and eliciting the numerous cytotoxic products of MNPs only in the face of microbial challenge. The activation of MNPs can be inhibited by glucocorticosteroids. Interestingly, tumor cells release factors that deactivate MNPs. The cytokines, tumor growth factor-β (TGF-β), and IL-4 also deactivate MNPs.[8]

The number of agonists that affect phagocytes and the membrane receptors that these agents bind is large and growing (see Table 19-2). Receptor-ligand complexes initiate the various responses of phagocytes, which include adhesion, locomotion, phagocytosis, pinocytosis, and the secretion of many substances, either by exocytosis of preformed constituents or by the biosynthesis of molecules in the membrane, such as oxygen reduction products or metabolites of arachidonic acid. The numerous molecules that affect phagocytes appear to work through molecular events in the plasma membrane and subjacent cytoplasm, known collectively as *transmembrane signaling*, and phagocytes are a particularly active area of research in this realm. The diverse agonists affecting phagocytes appear to use common signals in eliciting varied responses.

TABLE 19-2. Receptors on Phagocyte Cell Surfaces*

Designations	Ligands and Special Functions
OPSONIN AND ADHESION RECEPTORS	
CR1 Receptor	
CR1, CD35	C3b, C4b, *Leishmania promastigotes* Cofactor for decay-accelerating factor (DAF)
C3b Receptor (β_2-integrin) Family	
CD11a/CD18, LFA-1, CR3	I-CAM, LPS, C3bi, *Escherichia coli, Leishmania* sp, *Histoplasma capsulatum, Staphylococcus aureus,* fibrinogen
CD11b/CD18, Mac-1, Mo-1, CR3	C3bi, LPS, *E coli, Leishmania, H capsulatum, S aureus,* fibrinogen, factor X
CD11c/CD18, p150,95	?C3bi, LPS, *E coli, Leishmania* sp, *H capsulatum, S aureus,* fibrinogen
C3d	C3bi, C4b, C3d
Fc Receptor Family	
CD64	IgG, high-affinity binding of monomeric IgG_1 and IgG_3
CDw32, FcγRII, NA2	IgG, opsonin receptor for immune complexes
CD16, FcγRII, NA1, NA2, (PI-linked and transmembrane protein)	IgG, opsonin receptor for immune complexes
Fcα	Monomeric or polymeric IgA_1 and IgA_2
FcϵRII, CD23	IgE. Receptor on lung macrophages from allergic but not normal subjects
Other Adhesins	
Mac-2	Galactose; IgE, laminin
CD49e, VLA-5 β_1-integrin	Fibronectin, up-regulates chemotaxis receptors and couples CR1 and CR3 for ingestion
Vitronectin B_3-Integrin	Vitronectin, senescent cells
CD49d/CD29, VLA-4	Extracellular matrix, VCAM-1 on endothelial cells
VLA-6, CD49f	Laminin
VLA-2	Collagen and/or laminin
MEL-14, LAM-1, TQ-1, Leu-8	Endothelial addressin
PADGEM ligand	Mediates phagocyte attachment to activated platelets through PADGEM (GMP140, CD62)
CD44, gp80-95, Pgp-1	Collagen
Hyaluronate, sulfated polysaccharide	Various extracellular matrix components
β-Glucan	β 1,3- and 1,6-Linked glucans, mediates zymosan binding
Polymannose	?Opsonin receptor for α-mannans and high-mannose-bearing particles, ?for particles coated with serum mannose–binding protein
C-reactive protein	CRP, ?opsonin receptor for CRP bound to bacteria
LPS-binding protein	Opsonin for LPS-binding protein (an acute phase reactant) bound to bacteria
C1q	Opsonin for C1q-coated parasites
CD36, gp90 (GP IV)	Thrombospondin; ?opsonin for malaria-infected erythrocytes
RECEPTORS MEDIATING ENDOCYTOSIS (PINOCYTOSIS)	
Mannose-6-phosphate	Lysosomal enzymes involved in receptor-mediated endocytosis and intracellular membrane traffic
CD74, class II, HLA-DR, DP, DQ, Ia	Antigens, receptors for antigen processing, and MNP-lymphocyte interactions
CD4, class II gp59	gp120 of HIV-I, mediates uptake of AIDS virus; class II accessory molecule
LDL	LDL, β-VLDL, triglyceride-rich VLDL, atypical dys-β-LDL
Scavenger	Acetyl-LDL, maleyl-LDL, dextran-LDL, maleyl-albumin
Protease and antiprotease	α_1-Antiprotease–elastase complexes
AGE receptor	Receptor on MNP for glucose-modified proteins
Galactose (equivalent to cell-associated CRP)	Receptor on MNP for galactose-bearing particles
Fucose	Receptor for L-fucosyl-glycoconjugates
CD71, transferrin	Transferrin-iron; up-regulated during MNP maturation
RECEPTORS MEDIATING† CHEMOTAXIS (1), STIMULATION (2), ACTIVATION (3), PRIMING (4), BLOOD COAGULATION (5), OR MOBILIZATION (6)	
FMLP	FMLP (1, 2, 4)
Leukotriene B_4	LTB_4 (1, 2, 4)
Leukotriene D_4	
Leukotriene E_4	

(continued)

TABLE 19-2. *(Continued)*

Designations	Ligands and Special Functions
RECEPTORS MEDIATING† CHEMOTAXIS (1), STIMULATION (2), ACTIVATION (3), PRIMING (4), BLOOD COAGULATION (5), OR MOBILIZATION (6) (Continued)	
C5a	C5a (1, 2, 4)
IL-8	IL-8: NAF, MDNCF, MONAP, NAP-1 (1, 2, 4)
IL-6	IL-6
Platelet-derived growth factor	PDGF (1, 2, ?4)
Platelet-activating factor	1-0-alkyl-2-acetyl-sn-glycero-3-phosphocholine (PAF) (1, 2, 4)
Protein kinase C	Phorbol esters (2, 4)
Granulocyte colony-stimulating factor	G-CSF (4, 6)
Granulocyte-macrophage colony-stimulating factor	GM-CSF (4, 6)
c-fms Tryosine kinase	M-CSF (1, 3, 4, 6)
Interferon-γ	IFN-γ (3)
IL-1	IL-1 (4, ?3)
Tumor necrosis factor (cachectin)	TNF (?1, 4, ?3)
Tumor growth factor-β	TGF-β (1)
CD25, gp^{55}	β Chain of IL-2, on activated monocytes
CD43, sialophorin	Missing in Wiskott-Aldrich syndrome, natural ligand unknown, anti-CD43 (3)
P2, purinergic	Adenosine, mediate metabolic effects of pyrimidine and purine nucleotides (3)
Factor Va–like molecule	Factor Xa (5)
Tissue factor	Factor VII (5)
Thrombin	Thrombin
C3d-K	C3-derived fragment (6)
CD55, DAF (PI-linked)	Accelerate decay of bound C3
RECEPTORS FOR WHICH FUNCTIONS ARE NOT KNOWN ON PHAGOCYTES	
CD9, P24	On monocytes
CDw17 (lactosylceramide)	
CDw12, p90-120	
CD45 (leukocyte common antigen, T200)	Has tyrosine phosphatase activity, up-regulated by secretagogues
CD10, CALLA	Has metalloendopeptidase activity
CD14, gp55 (PI-anchored)	
CD24, gp41/38	
gp140 (PMN)	Wheat germ agglutinin
β_2-Adrenergic	β_2-Adrenergic agonists
TSH-like	Target of anti-PMN autoantibodies
H_1, H_2	Histamine
Metabolic hormones	Insulin, glucagon
VIP, substance P	Neuropeptides
Serotonin, enkaphalins, endorphins, argipressin	Vasoactive amines
CD13, gp150	Has aminopeptidase activity; possibly related to degradation of peptide chemotactic factors
CD30	Detected on Reed-Sternberg cells of Hodgkin's disease
CD44, gp80-95	
CD63, gp53	
CDw65	Ceramide-dodecasaccharide 4c
CD66, gp180-200	
CD67, p100	PI-linked
CD68, gp100	

LPS, lipopolysaccharide; Ig, immunoglobulin; VLA, very late antigen; CRP, C-reactive protein; LDL, low-density lipoprotein; VLDL, very-low-density lipoprotein; FMLP, N-formyloligopeptides; IL, interleukin; CALLA, common acute lymphoblastic leukemia antigen; TSH, thyroid-stimulating hormone; VIP, vasoactive intestinal polypeptide.

* The table includes receptors identified by ligand-binding properties, reactivity with specific antibodies, isolation, molecular cloning, or a combination of these. For reference to specific receptors see text or reference 7.

† Sorting out what agonist-receptor complexes do is complicated by the fact that recombinant factors are often contaminated with endotoxin and by the fact that one agonist may cause PMN to generate one or more additional endogenously derived agonists.

TABLE 19-3. Characteristics of Activated and Stimulated Mononuclear Phagocytes

ACTIVATED
Increased killing of facultative parasites
Increased superoxide anion production
Increased plasminogen-activator secretion
Increased tissue transglutaminase activity
Increased neopterin secretion
Increased expression of IgA receptors, class II HLA antigens, FcRI receptors
Decreased endocytosis of mannose glycoconjugates
Synthesis of macrophage-inflammatory proteins
Increased metabolism of vitamin D_3
Increased TGF-β synthesis
Increased TNF and IL-1 secretion, PAF-related proteins
Increased α_1-proteinase–inhibitor secretion
Increased nitrate and nitrite secretion
Decreased transferrin receptor expression
Decreased CD4 expression
Increased C2 and factor B synthesis
Increased expression of Mo-3 antigen
STIMULATED
Increased CR1- and CR3-mediated phagocytosis
Increased acid hydrolase content
Increased elastase and collagenase secretion
Decreased icosanoid synthesis
Decreased PAF accumulation
Decreased 5′ nucleotide activity
Increased apoprotein E secretion
Increased synthesis of complement factor proteins
Increased glutathione release
Increased expression of heat-shock proteins

Ig, immunoglobulin; TGF, tumor growth factor; TNF, tumor necrosis factor; IL, interleukin; PAF, platelet-activating factor.

General Features

The concentration of agonist, the affinity of the receptor for the agonist, and the association and dissociation rates between receptor and ligand all influence subsequent events. These factors determine the extent to which the receptor exists in a state that leads to the generation of signals. Agonists, receptors, and signals interact in remarkably complex patterns. In some cases, a single agonist may act through a single receptor to elicit multiple responses, although the number of receptors occupied may determine which response predominates. For example, low concentrations (about 10 nmol) of the agonists C5a, FMLP, platelet-activating factor (PAF), and monocyte-derived chemotactic factors have chemotactic activities, whereas higher concentrations (100 to 1000 nmol/L) elicit secretion and the respiratory burst of phagocytes. In other instances, agonists elicit more limited effects.[9,10]

An additional element of complexity is the phenomenon known as *priming*.[11–16] Phagocytes may respond to agonists only if some predisposing event has occurred, presumably one that altered the intracellular set of signals or the responsiveness of intracellular signal targets. For example, PMNs carefully prepared using endotoxin-free solutions do not release superoxide in response to chemotactic peptides but will do so if first allowed to spread on protein-coated glass or if exposed to lipopolysaccharide (LPS) endotoxin. Other agents that prime phagocytes for these responses are tumor-promoting compounds derived from plants of the phorbacea family, such as tetradecanoyl phorbol myristate acetate (usually abbreviated TPA or PMA), purine and pyrimidine nucleotides, serine proteinases, granulocyte-macrophage colony-stimulating factor (GM-CSF), cytochalasins, and substance P. Spreading of cells on a surface can also have a priming effect. The responses induced by agonists with or without priming usually occur rapidly (within seconds) and are of short duration (minutes). As an exception, millimolar sodium fluoride concentrations slowly (over hours) elicit responses that persist for long periods.[17]

G Proteins

Increasing evidence points to an amplification step between receptor occupancy and signal transduction that is mediated by a large family of proteins known as *G proteins* because of their guanosine triphosphate (GTP) binding properties. G proteins amplify signal production since they cycle on and off activated receptors (Fig. 19-2).

The amplifying role of G proteins helps to explain why chemotactic oligopeptides can cause structural changes in PMNs when as few as 1% of the receptors for that peptide are ligated. The most completely understood class of G proteins consists of three polypeptide subunits of about 40 kd, designated α, β, and γ.[18,19] The α subunit is generally the module that interacts with targets such as the signal transducing enzyme adenylate cyclase or phospholipases A_2 or C. The way in which G proteins amplify signaling is that the trimeric complex binds to the cytoplasmic domain of transmembrane receptors activated by bound ligands. This binding causes the exchange of guanosine diphosphate (GDP) bound to the α subunit for GTP, and the α subunit complex dissociates from the β and γ subunits. The free α subunit activates or inhibits its target, dependent on the particular G protein; stimulatory G proteins are designated G_S, inhibitory G_i. Hydrolysis of the bound GTP to GDP and Pi restores the α subunit to a conformation in which it binds β and γ partners. Some evidence, therefore, for involvement of G proteins in phagocyte functions is documentation of GTP binding to and the GTPase activity of isolated membranes or partially purified receptor-ligand

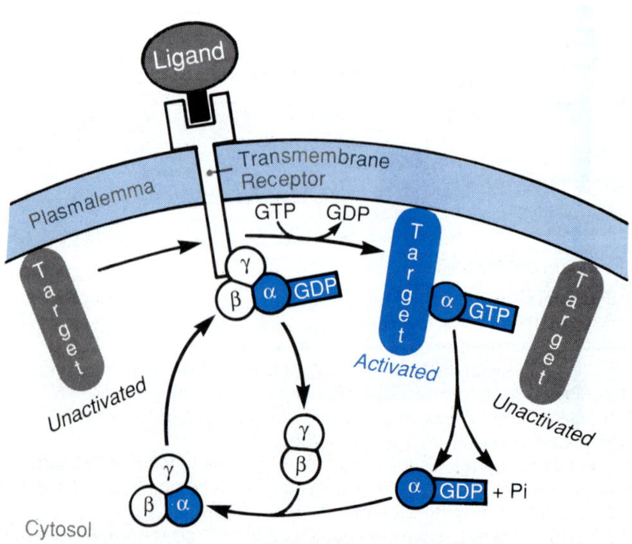

FIGURE 19-2. Role of heterotrimeric GTP-binding proteins (G proteins) in phagocyte signal–response coupling. Regulation of small monomeric GTP-binding proteins is similar. Not shown is that additional cofactors, GTPase activating proteins, stimulate GTP hydrolysis; others, GTP dissociation inhibitors, inhibit GTP/GDP exchange.

complexes from phagocytic cells.[20-23] The reformation of the trimeric complex terminates signal transduction and restores the G protein to a form ready for further messages from receptors. Thus, a single ligated receptor can excite multiple cycles of G-protein activation of target enzymes. Nonhydrolyzable GTP analogues lock G-protein α subunits in a conformation where they cannot reassociate, and signal generation is inhibited. Another group of G proteins are about 20 kd and are of interest since they are homologous to the oncogene product H_{ras}.

One experimentally useful property of some G proteins is that their α subunits are targets of an adenosine diphosphate (ADP) ribosylation reaction catalyzed by bacterial toxins. Depending on the toxin and the G protein, the consequence of ADP ribosylation varies. *Vibrio cholera* toxin, for example, causes the permanent activation of the G protein, which stimulates adenylate cyclase, causing the accumulation of large quantities of intracellular cyclic AMP (cAMP) in the poisoned target cell. Conversely, *Bordetella pertussis* toxin is proposed to inactivate G proteins that transduce activation signals for several phagocyte functions mediated by calcium transients and phosphoinositide turnover (discussed later). *Clostridium botulinum* exoenzyme 3 ADP ribosylates and inactivates the small G protein called *rho*.

Calcium Transients and Phosphoinositide Metabolism

One of the most frequent responses of phagocytes to binding of an agonist is a transient rise in cytosolic calcium (Fig. 19-3). Mammalian phagocytes live in an environment that contains millimolar ionized calcium concentrations. This calcium can slowly leak down a concentration gradient across lipid bilayers from the outside of the cell or from internalized membrane vesicles within. The resting cell, however, keeps its cytosolic calcium in the nanomolar range by several mechanisms. First, the cell contains many macromolecules with calcium-binding properties. These include negatively charged membrane phospholipids and abundant cytoplasmic proteins such as actin, which do not appear to be affected functionally by the presence or absence of calcium. Second, the cell actively extrudes calcium against a 1000-fold concentration gradient with an adenosine triphosphate (ATP) driven plasma membrane pump.[24] Should the calcium concentration rise into the micromolar range, four calcium atoms can bind to a high-affinity calcium-binding protein, calmodulin. The calcium–calmodulin complex is involved in triggering some responses, but it also promotes the removal of calcium by activating the membrane extrusion pump.[25-27] Third, the cell sequesters calcium in internal compartments. Mitochondria represent a low-affinity reservoir for calcium, but other vesicular structures analogous to the sarcoplasmic reticulum or striated muscle cells take up calcium with high avidity. In phagocytes, such vesicles have been shown to contain a protein immunoreactive with calsequestrin, the low-affinity, high-capacity, calcium-binding protein of striated muscle, and these vesicles have been named *calciosomes*.[28]

Stimulation of many cell receptors leads to activation of G proteins that increase the activity of cytoplasmic phospholipase C enzymes. These enzymes catalyze the hydrolysis of the phosphodiester bond between the glycerol backbone and the head group of membrane phospholipids, generating water-soluble base phosphates and diacylglycerols (DAG), the latter of which remain in the membrane bilayer.[29-31] Phospholipase C appears to be specific for particular phospholipids, but the most important for signal transduction hydrolyze phosphatidylinositol-4,5-bisphosphate (PIP_2) and phosphatidylcholine. Both phospholipases lead to DAG, which is important for one signal transduction

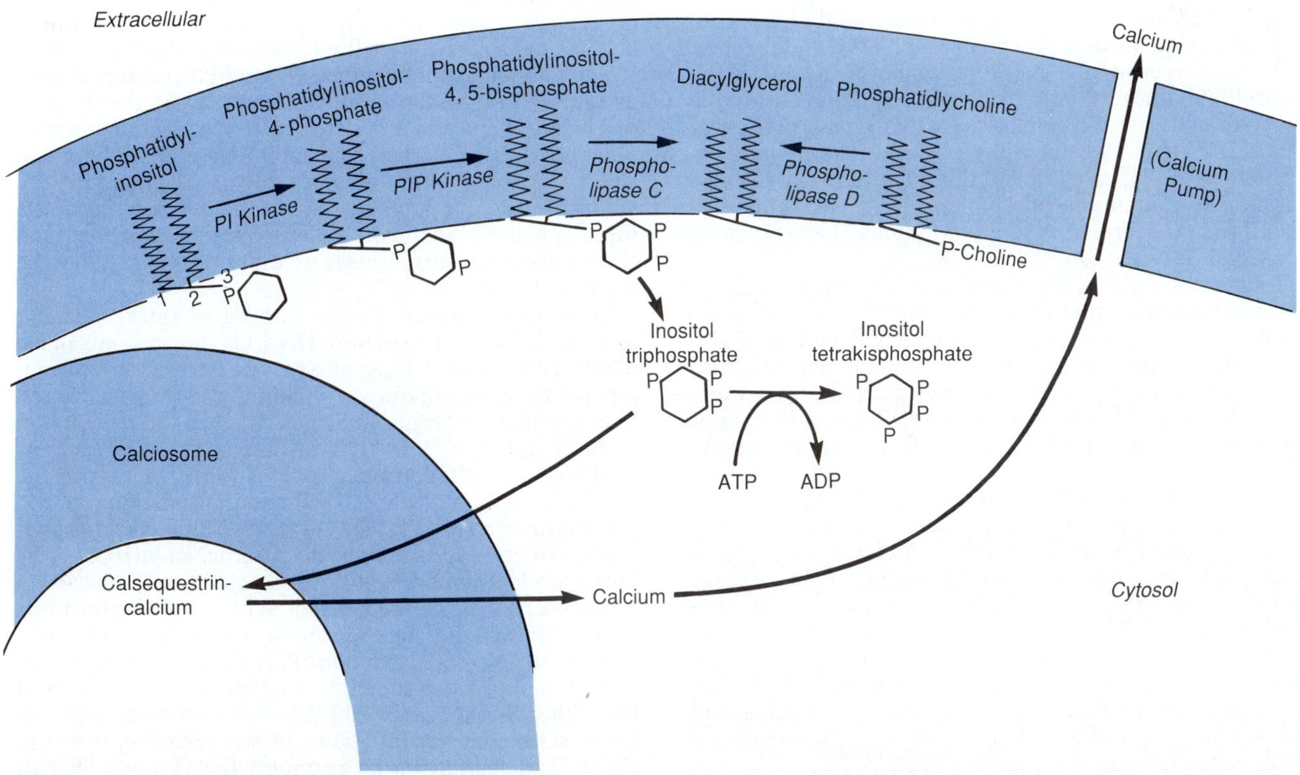

FIGURE 19-3. Signal transduction pathways in phagocytes showing the interrelation between membrane phospholipid metabolism and the regulation of cytosolic calcium concentrations.

pathway described later. PIP_2 breakdown, however, leads to the accumulation of inositol-4,5-triphosphate (IP_3), which has the important property of releasing calcium from the high-affinity intracellular vesicles. This mechanism is the basis for rises in cytosolic calcium accompanying cell stimulation, even when calcium is removed from the extracellular medium. When extracellular calcium is present, however, receptor perturbation also opens a channel in the membrane that permits calcium to pour down its concentration gradient. One effect of cytoplasmic calcium is that it increases the patency of this calcium leak.[32] The efficiency, therefore, of this pathway in increasing cytosolic calcium allows much lower agonist concentrations to elicit responses in the presence than in the absence of extracellular calcium.

As the free calcium rises in the cytosol, mechanisms come into play to remove the ion, such as the activation of the extrusion pump. In addition, a variety of reactions destroys the calcium-releasing isomer of IP_3 by dephosphorylation, isomerization to inositol-3,4-triphosphate, and even phosphorylation to inositol tetrakisphosphate (IP_4). Another source of IP_4 may be degradation of a recently discovered polyphosphoinositide, PIP_3, which appears in small amounts in stimulated neutrophils.[33] Some have proposed that IP_4, derived from the phosphorylation of IP_3, is a cofactor with cytosolic calcium in promoting calcium influx. The interplay of factors inciting accumulation versus removal of calcium determines the balance that cytoplasmic calcium attains. Even in the persisting presence of a calcium-increasing agonist, however, the cytosolic calcium concentration may fall to baseline, suggesting that the mechanism promoting calcium rises becomes refractory, that removal becomes more effective, or both. As discussed later, a sustained elevation of cytosolic calcium is not necessary for continuing cellular responses.[34–37]

Just as the cell performs ATP-consuming work to keep cytosolic calcium at low levels, so does it dispose of DAG and regenerate the phospholipids hydrolyzed during the first phase of the cellular response to agonist. Separate ATP-dependent kinases phosphorylate phosphatidylinositol to phosphatidylinositol-4-phosphate (PIP), PIP_2, and presumably PIP_3, respectively, and it is possible that some of the phosphotidylinositol and PIP kinases respond to unique receptor-activated G proteins.[38] A DAG kinase phosphorylates DAG to produce phosphatidic acid. The rise and decline in cytosolic calcium and the reciprocal fall and restoration of membrane phospholipids can sometimes be manifest in the form of *oscillations* that may have meaning for signal transduction.[39]

Calcium is a pleiotropic signal that can theoretically influence metabolic, motile, and membrane reactions. It activates enzymes of phospholipid metabolism and of glycogenolysis, and it regulates some proteins important for cell motility, as described later. Certain phagocyte functions, however, do not absolutely require a sustained or possibly even an acute rise in cytosolic calcium. Exposure of PMNs to chemotactic peptides induces an abrupt increase in cytosolic calcium, after which the calcium level falls to baseline, yet PMN locomotion continues. Lowering of the cytosolic calcium of PMNs and macrophages to nanomolar levels does not impair the extent of phagocytosis nor the initial response of PMNs to migrate toward chemoattractants.[34,35,40,41] As discussed later, PMNs express an exuberant respiratory burst without increasing intracellular calcium levels.[42] Secretion by exocytosis, however, appears to require that the cytosolic calcium increase, and raising the intracellular free calcium with ionophoric compounds induces exocytosis in PMNs.[43–45]

Diradylglycerols, where *radyl* refers to acyl, alkyl, or alk-1′-enyl groups, accumulate after the breakdown of PIP_2 during receptor-mediated cell stimulation. Recent evidence, however, points to hydrolysis of phosphatidylcholine as another source of DAG as well as of phosphatidic acid and phosphatidylethanol.[46] DAG activates a phosphatidylserine and calcium-activating protein kinase (protein kinase C). Ordinarily, this enzyme resides in the cytosol, but it moves to the plasma membrane to bind DAG as the latter accumulates during cell excitation.[47,48] The importance of DAG-activated protein kinase C for signal transduction is inferred from the ability of PMA to stimulate many functions of phagocytes and to substitute for DAG as a protein kinase C activator. Short-chain DAG, such as *O*-acetyl acylglycerol (OAG), are also experimentally useful probes for examining the role of DAG in cells.[47,48] DAG has also been reported to bind specifically to an intracellular actin-binding protein, α-actinin.[49] Sphingolipids, which are abundant in phagocytes and which interfere with phagocyte functions in vitro, reportedly inhibit the protein kinase C–inhibiting action of DAG.[50]

TPA or OAG in the absence of other agonists can stimulate phagocytes with respect to spreading, adhesion, exocytosis, and especially superoxide anion secretion. They also affect the function of certain receptors and promote marked vacuolization of the cells.[51,52] TPA does not stimulate phagocytosis, nor does it have chemotactic activity. In exerting its effects, TPA causes no detectable increase in cytosolic calcium; if anything, TPA stimulates the extrusion or sequestration of calcium by the cell, providing additional evidence that calcium transients are not always necessary for cell stimulation. It follows, moreover, that protein kinase C or some other ligand of DAG can initiate these cellular events directly. There is also evidence that DAG may be involved in inhibiting signal generation or promoting the destruction of signals, thereby acting as a terminator of transmembrane activation.[53] Protein kinase C phosphorylates many proteins in vitro, and certain polypeptides of phagocytes become heavily phosphorylated after treatment of the cells with TPA. The functional targets, however, of protein kinase C phosphorylation in phagocytes are presently unknown, although a number of polypeptides become phosphorylated after treatment of cells with TPA.

The polyphosphoinositides, PIP and PIP_2, interact with certain actin-binding proteins thought to be involved in phagocyte shape and motility. The activities of these phospholipids depend on their concentrations and their physical states. Although some agonists reportedly increase the concentration of polyphosphoinositides, many agonists initially cause breakdown of these phosphoinositides, and their subsequent resynthesis by different kinases may be important in signaling.[54]

In addition to phospholipases C and D, receptor activation activates another phospholipid hydrolyzing enzyme, phospholipase A_2 (PLA_2). PLA_2 cleaves the fatty acid in the sn-2 position of phospholipids, yielding free fatty acids and lysophosphatides; other enzymes catalyze the reacylation of the lysophosphatides.[55–57] PLA_2 is activated by receptor-mediated perturbation of phagocytes and by increasing the cytosolic calcium of the cell with appropriate ionophores.

It has been speculated for many years that lysophospholipids, which induce membrane disorder in vitro, may be important for membrane fusions associated with phagocyte responses, but there is no direct evidence to support this idea. Attention has focused more on the free fatty acid product of the PLA_2 reaction. Polyphosphoinositides are preferred substrates for PLA_2, and the sn-2 fatty acid of these phospholipids is arachidonate. Arachidonic acid can have two messenger functions. In one function, the fatty acid is the substrate of the enzyme 5′ lipoxygenase, which catalyzes the first of a series of reactions in phagocytes, leading to the biosynthesis of the bioactive metabolites, the *leukotrienes*. Leukotrienes, the synthetic pathways for which are described later, either directly or after subsequent metabolism by neighboring cells, act as potent mediators of inflammation. Because phagocytes have leukotriene receptors, this pathway can be seen as autostimulatory. In another function, arachidonic acid has been shown to participate as one cofactor in activation of the respiratory burst oxidase of phagocytes (described later).

Stimulated phagocytes also release free arachidonic acid, which can activate cellular responses, but lipid-binding proteins such as albumin can modulate this activity and its physiologic importance is unclear. When PLA_2 attacks the membrane phospholipid alkylacylphosphatidylcholine, the resulting reactions (described later) lead to the synthesis of acetyl glyceryl phosphatidylcholine, also known as PAF or PAF acether. PAF is a potent bioactive compound that, like the leukotrienes, can act on phagocyte receptors (see Table 19-2).

Other Signals

Prostaglandins of the E series, β-adrenergic agonists, cholera toxin, and some phagocytic stimuli result in the transient accumulation of intracellular cAMP in phagocytes, which leads to the phosphorylation of serines of selected cellular proteins and the concomitant activation of metabolic pathways such as glycogenolysis.[58] Because permeant forms of cAMP inhibit a variety of phagocytic functions,[59] the rise in this messenger may have a role in the termination or modulation of cellular responses.[60]

As is seen with mitogen-stimulated cultured cells, phagocytes respond to some agonists with proton extrusion, resulting in temporary rise in intracellular pH, presumably mediated by an Na^+-H^+ antiporter.[61–63] The importance of this alkalinization is unclear since its prevention by inhibitors does not impair the polymerization of actin associated with neutrophil stimulation.[64] In contrast to excitable cells such as nerve and muscle, phagocytes appear functionally impervious to broad variations in their intracellular monovalent ion composition and engage in acute responses to agonists, with either Na^+ or K^+ as the dominant extracellular cation. On the other hand, more delayed effects of agonists, such as the activation of mononuclear phagocytes by IFN-γ, may be influenced by monovalent cations since inhibition of Na^+ and H^+ exchange in macrophages prevented the induction of gene products associated with macrophage activation by this lymphokine.[65] In addition, changes in cytoplasmic pH were associated with marked alterations in membrane movement and the distribution of lysosomes in cultured macrophages.[66]

Reversible phosphorylation of tyrosine residues is thought to be important for transmembrane signaling by means of growth factor and insulin receptors, and such phosphorylation of phagocyte proteins has been documented.[67] The leukocyte glycoprotein CD45 (see Table 19-2) has been shown to express tyrosine dephosphorylation activity, and the activation of electropermeabilized PMNs by inhibitors of phosphotyrosine phosphatases is consistent with a role for tyrosine phosphorylation in signaling.[68]

Another interesting cell modification associated with phagocyte excitation is the acylation of certain intracellular polypeptides,[69] which causes a fatty acid to be added covalently to proteins, possibly enhancing their association with hydrophobic lipid membranes. In fact, one protein that becomes acylated in stimulated phagocytes acquires a membrane localization in association with myristoylation and is also a target for phosphorylation by protein kinase C.

Irreversible proteolysis of intracellular proteins has been proposed by one group as a mechanism for cellular excitation. It is claimed that cell excitation activates a calcium-dependent proteinase (calpain) that degrades a number of proteins, including protein kinase C, rendering it constitutively active rather than capable of being regulated by its usual cofactors.[70,71]

PHAGOCYTE MOBILITY

Little information exists about the movements other than cell division, if any, of phagocytes as they mature in the bone marrow. What is known is that translational movement as a prominent feature of what the cell *can* do becomes manifest at the band state of PMN development. Some fraction of PMNs and monocytes move out of the bone marrow. This form of motility involves active crawling. The cell extends one or more organelle-excluding pseudopodia in the direction of locomotion, and these attach to the surface (Fig. 19-4*A*). The cell body is drawn forward toward the pseudopodia, which extend outward again. In addition to actual movement, the phagocytes cause the lining cells of the bone marrow to separate and to be sufficiently pliable so they can negotiate the marrow–blood barrier and enter the peripheral circulation. Then, they actively migrate by crawling out of the bone marrow.

Once in the peripheral blood, the asymmetry of the extruded phagocytes dissipates, and the cells appear round as they roll along the walls of blood vessels in the so-called marginal blood pool. At some time during the cells' circulation time, some phagocytes attach to the endothelium with sufficient avidity to resist being moved by the flow of blood, and they leave the circulation by the process known as *diapedesis*. At this point, the cells again acquire the elongated configuration of motility and extend pseudopodia in the direction of movement. Insofar as phagocytes move several millimeters into the tissues, the daily net movement of billions of these cells in an adult amounts to a distance greater than the circumference of the earth.

Structural Aspects

The shape of phagocytes is determined by a cortical layer of cytoplasm that contains predominantly the protein actin in nearly millimolar concentrations. Actin, a slightly asymmetric 42.5-kd monomer, polymerizes reversibly into linear and three-dimensional polymers, and the balance between these states accounts for changes in cell-surface configuration associated with phagocyte movements. A number of actin-binding proteins control the interconversion between the states of actin, and these proteins are in turn regulated by the signal molecules, calcium, and polyphosphoinositides discussed previously (Table 19-4). Actin-binding alkaloids, such as the fungal metabolites known as *cytochalasins*, inhibit actin assembly and agonist-elicited phagocyte movements.[72]

Actin assembles by a nucleation condensation mechanism in which spontaneous nucleation in vitro is highly unfavorable. Elongation is more efficient than nucleation and is proportional to the monomer concentration, although the rate of growth is asymmetric on an actin polymer. Actin filaments to which myosin head fragments are bound look like strings adorned with arrowheads, and such decoration of actin filaments defines a "barbed" and "pointed" polarity. The growth of actin is 15 to 20 times faster at the barbed ends than at the pointed ends of actin filaments. Each actin monomer contains an ATP prosthetic group, which hydrolyzes to ADP and Pi during assembly. When ADP monomers dissociate from filaments, ambient ATP rapidly exchanges with the ADP to yield ATP-monomers. At steady state, therefore, actin exists in an ATP-consuming dynamic equilibrium, and a lower than micromolar concentration

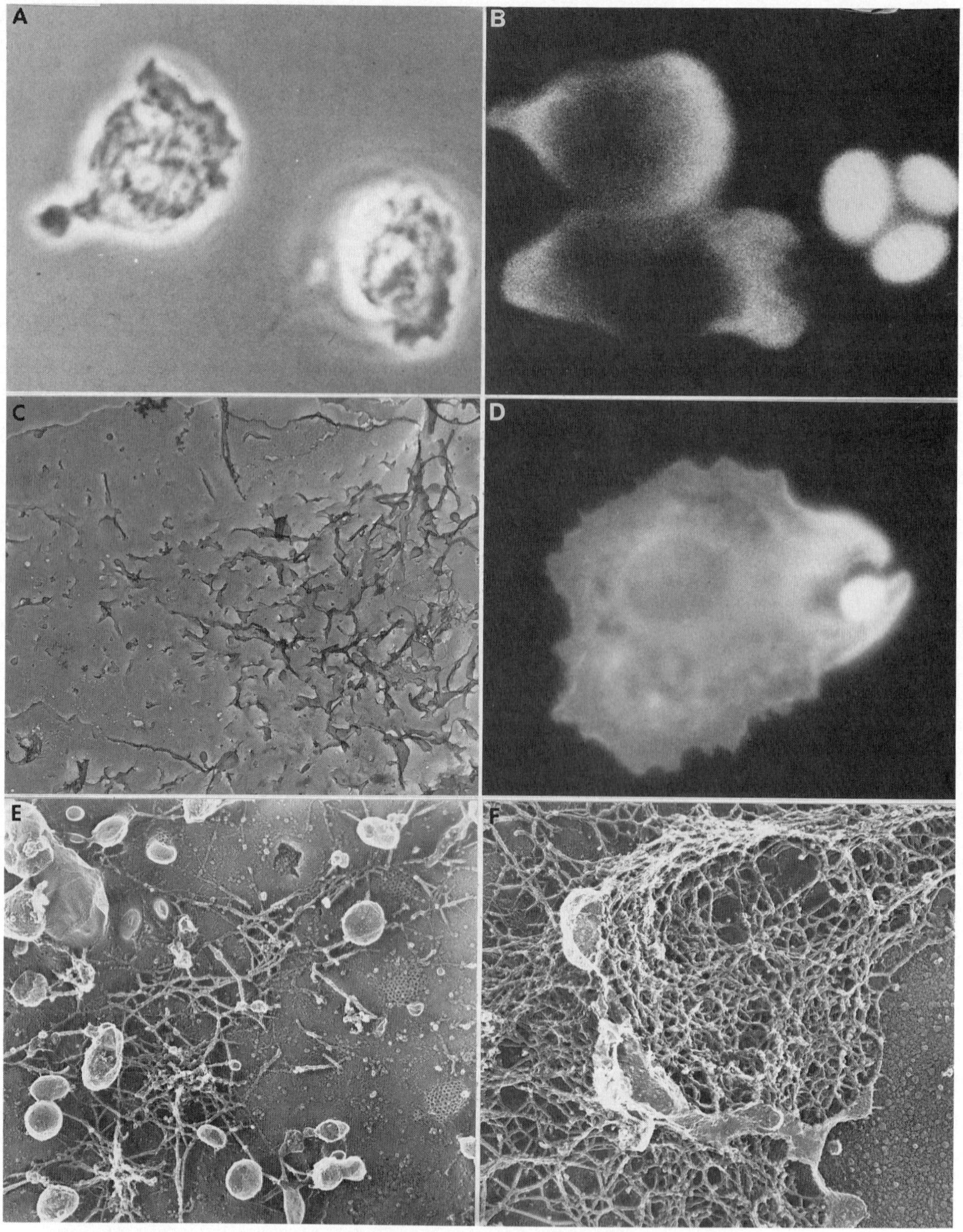

FIGURE 19-4. Morphology of neutrophils and mononuclear phagocytes. (**A**) Phase contrast photomicrograph of a neutrophil in the characteristic pose of locomotion. Note the asymmetric shape, anterior pseudopod, and posterior knob-like tail. (**B**) Immunofluorescence photomicrograph showing rhodamine staining of myosin in the pseudopodia of a neutrophil undergoing chemotaxis toward a fluorescein-stained yeast particle. (**C**) Scanning electron photomicrograph of the surface of a monocyte or macrophage revealing pleats and ruffles extended from the surface. (**D**) Immunofluorescence photomicrograph of a macrophage stained with rhodamine for actin-binding protein showing pseudopodia engulfing a fluorescein-stained yeast particle. (**E**) Cytoplasmic membrane surface of an adherent macrophage revealed by tearing of part of the membrane, rapid freezing, and metal casting. Actin filaments and basket-like clathrin-coating of endocytic vesicles are visible. (**F**) The cortical orthogonal actin network of a macrophage shown in a detergent-permeabilized cell that was then rapidly frozen and metal-shadowed. (Courtesy of John Hartwig, PhD, Division of Experimental Medicine, Brigham and Women's Hospital, Boston)

TABLE 19-4. **Actin-Binding Proteins Involved in Phagocyte Responses**

Protein	Function	Regulator
Profilin, cofilin, thymosin	Control polymerizability of monomeric actin	Polyphosphoinositides
Gelsolin, gcap39	Regulate actin filament length and number	Calcium and polyphosphoinositides
Tropomyosin	Stabilize actin filaments	
Actin-binding protein (filamin)	Cross-link actin filaments into orthogonal networks; link actin filaments to membrane glycoproteins	?Phosphorylation by calcium-calmodulin–dependent kinase
α-Actinin	Cross-link actin filaments into bundles	Calcium

of monomeric actin coexists with actin filaments in vitro. By contrast, nearly half the millimolar actin in resting phagocytes is unpolymerized, indicating that control of the competence of actin monomers to assemble in filaments is fundamental to the control of actin assembly in phagocytic cells.

One abundant actin-binding protein, profilin, has been the main candidate for the responsible agent for keeping cellular actin unpolymerized by stoichiometric formation of an equimolar complex in which the actin was kept sequestered, unable to nucleate or add on to filaments. The fact that PIP_2 dissociates actin–profilin complexes to yield profilin and actin monomers competent to polymerize provides a possible link between signal transduction and intracellular structural changes.[73] Information suggests that the unpolymerized actin concentration in platelets and neutrophils exceeds that of profilin by four-fold, suggesting that profilin keeps only some of the cellular actin unpolymerized; that it works catalytically to promote exchange of ATP for ADP active subunits; and that other factors, such as cofilin or β_4-thymosin, which also bind tightly to monomeric actin,[74] regulate actin monomer polymerizability.

Evidence indicates that the assembly of actin in the cell takes place when and where polyphosphoinositides accumulate in the membrane and interact with profilin and with another actin-modulating protein called *gelsolin*[75] (Fig. 19-5). In the presence of micromolar calcium, which appears in cytoplasm in response to cell activation, gelsolin noncovalently severs actin filaments and remains tightly bound to the barbed ends of the broken filaments. This action destroys the preexisting actin cortical network, maintaining the turgidity of the peripheral cytoplasm, and primes the cell for secretion by allowing granules to access the plasmalemma. Actin oligomers capped by gelsolin or by another protein called MCP or gCap39 diffuse to the plasma membrane, where the gelsolin or MCP binds polyphosphoinositides and concomitantly dissociates from the ends of the actin filaments, leaving many nucleation sites for rapid growth in the barbed direction. Profilin–actin complexes also migrate to the membrane, dissociate under the influence of polyphosphoinositides, and provide a monomer pool to grow on the filament ends provided by removal of gelsolin. This mechanism for actin assembly keeps actin polymerization at the plasma membrane and allows precise control over the rate of actin assembly and disassembly since the number of barbed ends, like the number of polymerization-competent monomers, is a modifiable variable in actin assembly and since a number of filament ends can be generated by activating nuclei in proportion to the signals evoked at the plasmalemma.

Once actin filaments assemble, they are cross-linked into various kinds of three-dimensional networks by actin–cross-linking proteins. In phagocytes, a high M_r protein called *actin-binding protein* causes actin filaments to form an elastic perpendicular branching network[76,77] (see Fig. 19-4). Another, α-actinin, promotes the formation of actin bundles.[78] An orthogonal network of actin cross-linked by

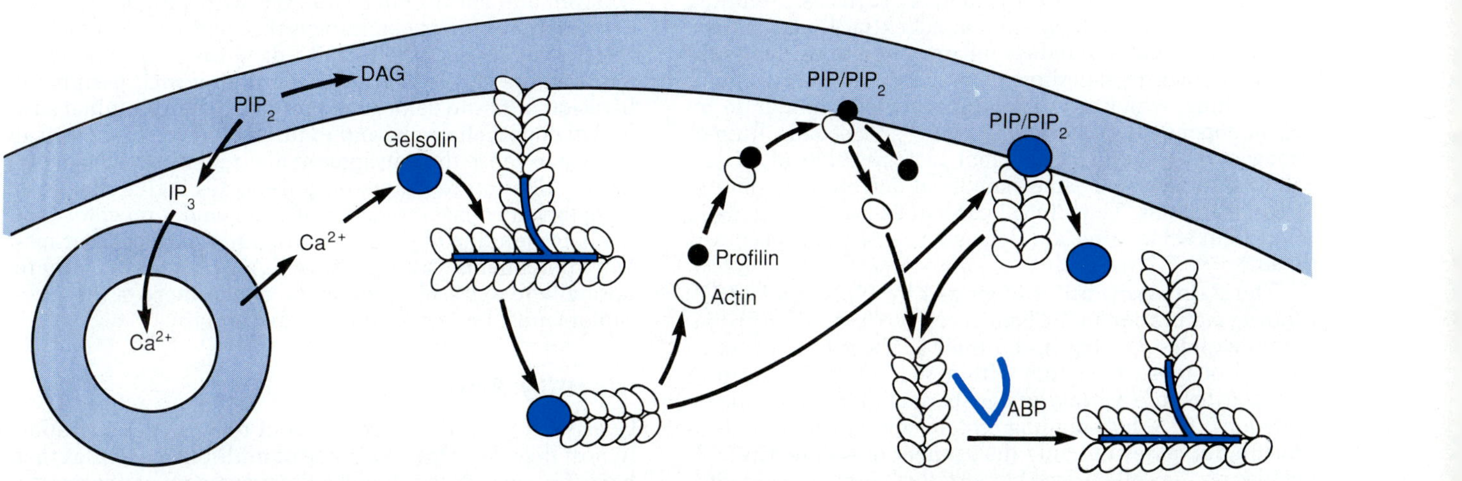

FIGURE 19-5. Postulated mechanism for regulation of actin assembly coordinated with signal–response coupling in phagocytes. The major actin subunit buffering protein is β-thymosin (not shown). IP_3, inositol triphosphate; ABP, actin-binding protein.

actin-binding protein is a strong yet porous structure that can immobilize and exclude organelles yet allow the permeation of water and small molecules. Actin bundles, on the other hand, can confer tensile strength on fine filopodia extended from the cell.

Adhesion of Phagocytes

Because phagocytes actively move by crawling rather than by swimming, the first step in diapedesis and indeed in locomotion and ingestion is adhesion. Sticking of phagocytes to substrates or to particulate objects can arise from changes in the phagocyte, in the adhesiveness of the surface, or in both.

Several of the receptors on phagocyte surfaces listed in Table 19-2 promote adhesion of the cells to complementary ligands attached to surfaces. Examples include the binding of the Fc domain of IgG molecules on glass to Fc receptors, or of iC3b- or C3b-coated erythrocytes to CR3 and CR1 receptors, respectively. The structure of phagocyte Fc and C receptors is described in detail in Chapter 16. The CR3 receptor has broad specificity, including, in addition to the iC3b fragment of C3, fibrinogen, protein-coated glass, certain microbial coat components, and a 90-kd glycoprotein I-CAM-1, which is found on the surface of a variety of human cells, including endothelial cells.[79,80] CR3 belongs to the *integrin* class of adhesion receptors, a superfamily of heterodimeric molecules that includes the fibronectin receptor, platelet glycoprotein IIb/IIIa, and receptors first identified on activated lymphocytes, called *very late antigens* (VLA).[81] Common to the integrin family is an amino acid sequence arg-gly-asp-ser in the externally disposed domain of the larger subunit. The receptor family that includes CR3 is designated β_2-integrin; its members include LFA-1, Mac-1, and gp150,95. The larger (α chain) of the two transmembrane polypeptide subunits that characterize Leu-CAM determines the specific identity of these receptors since they all express an identical β chain, designated CD18. The α chains of LFA-1 (CD11a), Mac-1 (CD11b), and gp150,95 (CD11c) have molecular masses of 180, 170, and 150 kd, respectively. The various members of this Leu-CAM family may interact cooperatively to mediate adhesion under different circumstances.[82]

Two lines of evidence show convincingly that the β_2-integrins, especially CD11b and CD18, are physiologically important for emigration of phagocytes out of blood vessels into all tissues, with the possible exception of the lung. First, antibodies against them inhibit phagocyte adhesion, locomotion, and phagocytosis to many surfaces, including vascular endothelium in vitro but not extracellular matrix. These antibodies also reduce inflammation in many tissues of live animals in experimental models, with the exception of the lung, which may allow phagocytes to emigrate by an independent adhesion system.[83–85] Second, human phagocytes genetically deficient in expression of CD11b and CD18 have the same functional defects as antibody-treated animals. The clinical consequences of this genetic trait (leukocyte adhesion deficiency, LAD) are discussed later.

The β_2-integrins are synthesized by PMNs and MNPs during maturation in the bone marrow. Circulating phagocytes express β_2-integrins on their surfaces but also have a pool of these receptors within the cell.[86] Exposure of phagocytes to a variety of agents, including chemotactic peptides, TPA, LPS-binding protein complexes, and fibronectin, increases not only the number of β_2-integrin molecules on the cell surface but also their functional avidity for ligands.[87] This up-regulation of phagocyte adhesion receptors on circulating phagocytes is demonstrable in humans after exposure of their circulation to foreign surfaces such as hemodialysis coils or extracorporeal cardiopulmonary assist devices. There is evidence that these maneuvers activate the alternative pathway of complement (see Chap. 16), which generates the chemotactic polypeptide C5a, which in turn up-regulates the β_2-integrins. The increased concentration of receptors correlates with a functional enhancement in cell adhesion to a variety of surfaces in vitro. Increased adhesiveness of interactions between the β_2-integrins and their ligands after excitation of phagocytes, however, is a result of an increase in their number and an increase in their binding affinity. The mechanism of this change in avidity is unknown. The β_2-integrin subunits are phosphorylated by exposure to agonists that excite phagocytes,[88] but β_2-integrin subunits made to lack phosphorylation sites by genetic mutation are able to change binding affinity as well as phosphorylatable receptors.[89,90]

The transmembrane polypeptides of the CR3 family are neither necessary nor sufficient to mediate phagocyte adhesion to endothelial cells, but they play an important role in that adherence. An additional factor involved in phagocyte–vessel interaction is the ability of agonists to distort phagocyte shape and stiffen them (responses related to intracellular actin assembly), and there is evidence that these mechanical changes in phagocytes can cause their retention in pulmonary capillaries independent of changes in cell-surface adhesiveness related to β_2-integrins.[91] In the absence of cell excitation, however, phagocytes roll along the walls of endothelial cells, and a nonintegrin class of surface receptors, known as *selectins*, appears to mediate this interaction.[92] One of these is MEL-14, which is homologous to the lymphocyte homing receptor for high endothelial cells in venules. Another, known as PADGEM, P-selectin, CD62, or GMP-140, mediates the binding of platelets to MNP.[93,93a] A third receptor of this class on endothelial cells, called ELAM-1 or E-selectin, appears slowly after exposure of the endothelium to the inflammatory cytokine IL-1.[94] The selectins bind fucosyl groups expressed on the surface of the partner cell that the selectin-bearing cell ligates, and these are part of O-linked mucin-like molecules that represent the blood group sialyl-Le^x.[95–97]

Most inflammatory or infectious insults are localized, however, and originate in the tissues, not in the circulation. If infection or injury damages the integrity of blood vessels, phagocytes can come into contact with the underlying matrix, where components such as fibronectin and laminin can bind complementary receptors on the phagocytes or where C3 fragments or other plasma proteins adherent to collagen and elastin might interact with CR3 or other receptors. It has long been known that phagocytes attach to intact capillary endothelium at a distance from an imposed tissue injury. Little is known about how such peripheral invasion or tissue damage is sensed by the abluminal surface of endothelial cells and in turn conveyed to the apical surface to cause the entrapment of circulating phagocytes. Other adhesion receptors on phagocytes include laminin receptors, a collagen receptor (CD44), and a receptor that mediates binding of phagocytes to other extracellular matrix components (VLA_4). Since LAD phagocytes adhere normally to extracellular matrix, one or more of these receptors must be responsible for this activity.

Motility Agonists

Consistent with the importance of phagocyte emigration in host defense is the existence of multiple molecules that have the capacity to influence the movement of phagocytes throughout their life cycle so as to guide them from bone marrow to appropriate tissue sites. Most of the agents listed in Table 19-1 are *chemotactic factors*, that is, molecules that, when originating from a source in a gradient, focus the direction of phagocytes up the concentration gradient. Most chemotactic factors attract both PMNs and MNPs, although some appear to be specific for MNPs or PMNs. A few other factors are *chemokinetic agents*, molecules that increase the speed at which phagocytes move; and yet others, fragments of C3, are *mobilizing compounds*, substances that cause phagocytes to leave the bone marrow to enter the circulation.[98,99] There are also *inhibitors of phagocyte mobility*. Interestingly, one of these, $(Ala\text{-}IL\text{-}8)_{77}$,[100] is a close relative of IL-8, a chemotactic and neutrophil-exciting factor.

Table 19-5 shows that chemoattractants arise from microorganisms and degraded and denatured tissue components as well as many sources that are likely to be involved in defense and inflammatory functions of the host. These include products of the complement system, the coagulation system, and the lipoxygenase pathway of arachidonic acid metabolism. Of special note is the central role of MNPs in generating chemotactic molecules, either by producing them in response to stimulation or by processing plasma protein. This involvement of MNPs is teleologically reasonable in view of the wide distribution of these cells in a sentry network poised for first exposure to pathogens.

Chemoattractant Receptors

Some of the agents described in Table 19-5 bind specific and distinct receptors on phagocytes. cDNAs encoding the receptors for C5a, FMLP, MCP-1, PAF, and IL-8 have been cloned, and the inferred amino acid sequences predict multiple-membrane spanning domains reminiscent of rhodopsin or β-adrenergic receptors.[101–103] In equilibrium binding studies, the K_d for agonist binding agrees reasonably with the ED_{50} for potency in assays of chemotaxis. The physiology of ligand–receptor interaction, however, is more complex than can be ascertained by equilibrium binding studies, since the on and off rates of the ligands appear to be important and because enzymatic hydrolysis of ligands, as well as internalization of receptor–ligand complexes by receptor-mediated endocytosis, occurs under physiologic conditions. Collectively, these effects have been grouped under the term *desensitization*.

The chemotactically active state of the N-formylpeptide chemotactic receptor is a rapidly dissociating one that becomes converted to a slowly dissociating form that is inactive in inducing cellular responses. In addition, two binding affinities can be identified, the higher of which mediates chemotaxis, the lower exocytosis. Whether these two states represent different receptors or different states of the same receptors is unresolved.[104] The chemotactic factor receptors induce signaling through G proteins, as evidenced by inhibition of responses by pertussis toxin and association of a variety of G proteins with partially purified receptors. The inactive form of the receptor is, in contrast to the active one, not associated with G protein and may be bound to actin filaments.[105]

Cellular Response to Chemotactic Factors

When chemotactic factors engage phagocytes that are in a rounded state, they first "cringe" by wrinkling their surface, and then they begin to spread uniformly on the substrate. PMNs and monocytes soon acquire the characteristic polarity of locomotion in which pseudopodia extend in a preferred direction, even when the chemotactic factor is not present in a gradient. If such a gradient exists, PMNs move toward it, not in a straight line, but with frequent deviations from the gradient source; as they approach higher concentrations of the factor, however, their turn angles decrease. If the chemoattractant is removed and replaced by a new supply, but from the opposite side, PMNs may round up and extend a pseudopod in the direction of the new gradient, but they prefer to retain their original polarity and make a U-turn. Macrophages tend to remain uniformly spread, but they have a limited capacity for slow locomotion.

Organelle-excluding pseudopodia can be dissociated from the cell by heat treatment, and these structures exhibit rudimentary locomotion,[106] suggesting that all the sensory and motor components reside in the cortical regions of the cell.[107] The mechanisms underlying the cell-surface shape changes involve focal increases in the turgor of the peripheral cytoplasm, and evidence indicates that the assembly of actin, by mechanisms discussed previously, is responsible for these increases.[108,109] It is unclear whether actin assembly mechanically pushes against the membrane to effect propulsion of pseudopodia or whether a transient dissociation of actin and profilin from each other and of profilin from the membrane generates osmotic particles that

TABLE 19-5. Molecules That Attract Phagocytes (Chemoattractants)

Source	Molecules
Complement system (plasma and MNP)	C5a, C5a-des-arg plus vitamin D–binding protein
Membrane phospholipids	Leukotriene B_4, lipoxin A and B, acetylglycerophosphatidylcholine (platelet-activating factor), diacylglycerol, lysophosphatidylcholine
Coagulation system (plasma and platelets)	Thrombin,* fibrinopeptides A and Bb1-42, platelet factor 4, platelet-derived growth factor, urokinase, heparin cofactor II–reaction products, interleukin-8–like peptide derived from platelet factor 4 by monocyte proteinases
Mononuclear phagocytes, tumor cells, endothelial cells, lymphocytes, epithelial cells	Interleukin-8 (monocyte-derived chemotactic factor),† tumor necrosis factor, ?macrophage colony-stimulating factor, oxidized low-density lipoprotein, ENA-78,† MCP-1,* RANTES,* 1-309,* KC/gro-related protein
Neutrophils	Defensins*
Denatured proteins	Maleyl albumin, casein, collagen fragments, elastase–α_1-proteinase inhibitor complex
Bacteria, mitochondria	N-formyloligopeptides
Metabolites, alkaloids	Adenosine, nicotine

* Reportedly chemotactic only for monocytes.
† Only for neutrophils.

lead to localized water influx and hydraulic propulsion.[110] According to this view, the adjacent actin gel, which has the capacity to retain water,[111] resists deformation and serves as a fulcrum such that propulsion is in the direction of the membrane bilayer.

The sequence of events in translational locomotion appears to be that pseudopodia extend in the direction of movement, they attach to the substrate, and then the cell body is pulled forward. If attachment fails, then the pseudopod may be retracted. These findings suggest that a contractile mechanism within the cytoplasm is operative, and myosin molecules that exert contractile forces on actin have been isolated from mammalian phagocytes. Unlike the situation in striated muscles, where myosin molecules are constitutively organized into bipolar filaments that interact with adjacent actin filaments, phagocyte myosin molecules are presumed, based on studies with myosins from smooth muscle and platelets, to be hexameric in the resting state with two 220-kd heavy and four 15- to 20-kd light subunits. The heavy chains have globular domains at their N terminals and helical tails extending to the C terminals. The tails fold over and bind to the two larger of the light chains, which cluster about the globular head of the myosin molecule, which is the domain that is capable of interacting with actin filaments to transduce ATP hydrolysis into mechanical force for movements. Cellular stimulation, by increasing cytosolic free Ca^{2+}, results in the phosphorylation of the 20-kd light chains, a reaction mediated by calmodulin and a specific myosin light-chain kinase. The phosphorylated light chains no longer bind the myosin heavy-chain tails, which now extend and are capable of self-associating with other phosphorylated myosins to form bipolar filaments. The phosphorylated light chains also render the myosin heads competent to hydrolyze ATP in the presence of actin filaments.[112] Non–filament-forming single- and double-headed myosins may also be involved in this contractile activity.

The translational movement of PMNs requires that they adhere to the substrate in vitro or to the fibers of connective tissue in vivo. The advancing pseudopod attaches to surfaces, and the cell body drags along behind. The adherent regions must then become unattached for the cell to move, and the mechanism of letting go is unknown. Proteases may digest adhesion proteins or else some more complex process may cause them to lose their avidity for their ligands. In some instances, parts of the cell fail to disengage, and long processes are drawn out; these may either break off or tether the cell, preventing its forward progress.

Measurement of Phagocyte Locomotion

Of many methods applicable to the study of leukocyte movement in vitro, the simplest is to observe cells directly under the phase-contrast microscope. One way to do this is to allow blood taken by finger prick to clot on a slide in a humidified Petri dish, wash off the clot with 10% autologous plasma in buffered salt solution over which is placed a cover slip, and then look for characteristic polarized shapes and movements of the PMNs and monocytes, preferably at 37°C. This method detects gross defects in leukocyte adhesion and motility in that cells appear rounded, fail to attach to the surface, and do not move translationally. For more sophisticated laboratory assessment of leukocyte locomotion, a system devised by Zigmond, in which a cell monolayer is separated by a slit from the source of a chemotactic factor, allows quantitation of the fraction of cells that polarize in the direction of the gradient. A two-compartment chamber first designed by Boyden, in which cells crawl through porous filters toward the source of a chemotactic gradient, has been employed extensively in chemotaxis studies. Another technique is to inject leukocytes under one part of an agarose sheet and chemotactic factor under another part and to stain the sheet after a suitable time and observe the extent to which the front of leukocytes has moved away from the site of injection.[113,114]

The techniques used for the assessment of phagocyte locomotion in vivo are semiquantitative at best. One time-honored method is to abrade the skin of a subject and apply a coverslip or sponge, sometimes impregnated with a chemotactic agent, and to assess by microscopy the number of cells in the inflammatory exudate. A more complex variation is to use a subcutaneous chamber and count the cells in the accumulated fluid. Some advocate the counting of leukocytes in isotonic salt solution mouthwashes as an index of phagocyte exudation. With all these approaches, it must be remembered that the supply of phagocytes in the circulation ultimately determines the number of cells available to the tissues, so that the measurement of locomotion in vivo in leukopenic patients yields abnormal results.[115]

PHAGOCYTOSIS

Despite many mechanistic similarities, it is increasingly clear that phagocytosis involves ligands, receptors, and signaling processes that are different from chemotaxis.

Opsonins

Opsonins are molecules that promote phagocytosis. Opsonins and their homologous receptors may be *incomplete*, mediating primarily cell-particle attachment, or *complete*, promoting attachment and ingestion. The Fcγ receptors of phagocytes (see Table 19-2), the structures of which were detailed in Chapter 16, are complete. Not only do they induce phagocytosis by interaction with the Fc domains of IgG molecules attached to particles, but FcγRIII induces phagocytosis when high mannose sugars in its externally disposed domain bind to lectins such as concanavalin A.[116] What is especially interesting about this receptor is that it is not necessarily a transmembrane protein but can be a phospholipid-linked protein, implying that it signals ingestion by binding to some other membrane component. A polypeptide component of the tetrameric mast cell IgE receptor (FcϵRI,), the γ-chain, was identified as a part of the macrophage Fc RIII receptor.[117] The mannose receptor that binds to mannose residues on the surface of microorganisms such as yeasts is also a complete opsonin.[118,119]

Receptors for fibronectin, LPS-binding protein, and mannose-binding protein are incomplete and mediate only attachment of phagocytes to their homologous ligand-coated surfaces or particles. The C3-derived fragments, C3b and C3bi, which affix to objects such as blood cells or microorganisms by activation of the classic or alternative complement pathways, are also opsonins (see Chap. 16). The C3-fragment receptors, CR1 and CR3 (see Chap. 16), may be complete or incomplete depending on the state of the phagocyte. CR1 (C3b) receptors primarily mediate attachment, but they may signal ingestion in PMNs if the cells are previously exposed to TPA or to fibronectin. Resting mouse macrophages attach only to C3b-coated erythrocytes, but they ingest them if previously stimulated by exposure to denatured proteins. The reason for these effects is unknown. Some of the treatments that render CR1 and CR3 molecules competent to signal ingestion switch them from being dispersed in the plasma membrane to being aggregated in concert with phosphorylation of their cytoplasmic domains.[120,121] Incomplete opsonin–receptor complexes may act cooperatively to permit small numbers of complete complexes to trigger ingestion.

The phagocytic response is localized to the region of receptor–ligand interaction such that particles are engulfed by the progressive extension of pseudopodia around recognition molecules on the particle surface, a phenomenon known as *zippering*.[122] The mechanism of pseudopod extension that leads to the enclosure of objects within phagocytic vacuoles is similar to that encountered in locomotion, in that actin assembly occurs in the submembrane zone of particle contact, although, as summarized previously, the signals used to elicit this actin assembly may be different in phagocytosis.

Exocytosis and Endocytosis

At the pit of forming phagocytic vacuoles in PMNs, cytoplasmic granules fuse with the plasma membrane and secrete their contents onto the engulfed particle, and the phagocytic vesicle becomes a phagolysosome, the inside of which contains the secretory products of the granules and the membrane of which acquires proteins previously embedded in the granule membrane. The secretion of large granules, which can be seen with the light microscope, is known as *degranulation*. The vesicle contents are discharged into phagocytic vacuoles. Some of this material leaks out of incompletely closed vacuoles into the extracellular medium. Direct fusion of granules with the plasma membrane can also occur, resulting in exocytosis. This phenomenon, part of the digestive and microbicidal action of phagocytes (discussed later), is representative of a more general class of membrane fusion events in phagocytes and other cells. As mentioned previously, for example, chemotactic factor–receptor complexes are internalized in less than 0.1-μm diameter structures known as *coated pits*. The "coats" of these vesicles were first recognized as electron-dense particles lining their cytoplasmic surfaces and are basket-like networks composed mainly of a complex of proteins collectively called *clathrin*. MNPs also endocytose IgG-containing immune complexes in coated pits, and a specific determinant in the cytoplasmic domain of the transmembrane tail of Fc RII mediates this process. Macrophages internalize and return to the surface their entire plasma membrane every 20 minutes in the form of such vesicles, called *endosomes*, some coated and some not. The membrane cycling process in which membrane is shuttled among intracellular compartments, especially the Golgi cisternae, is somewhat vectorial, in that it concentrates near areas of cell interaction with surfaces or with phagocytic particles.[123]

The form of endocytosis just described, known as *receptor-mediated endocytosis*, is constitutive and is not inhibited by cytochalasins and therefore presumably does not involve the reversible assembly of cortical actin. Another form of endocytosis, probably equivalent to what classically was known as *pinocytosis* (cell drinking), is induced by various agents, including M-CSF and phorbol esters, and is inhibited by cytochalasins. This endocytic process may therefore be mediated by small protrusions of actin-rich cytoplasm and is functionally equivalent to the phagocytosis of small particles.[124]

The distribution of intracellular organelles involved in endocytosis and exocytosis involves in part the function of *microtubules*.[125] Microtubules are hollow fibers composed of helical assemblies of *tubulin* heterodimers, and their outer surfaces are coated with a large number of proteins known as *microtubule-associated proteins*. In interphase cells, like phagocytes, microtubules originate in a perinuclear structure, the *centriole*, and radiate outward to enter the actin-rich cell periphery. One species of microtubule-associated proteins, known as *dyneins* and *kinesins*, may attach large intracellular secretory granules (described later) and, using ATP as an energy source, motor the granules outward (kinesin) and inward (dynein). Localized disaggregation of the submembrane actin networks permits the granules to approach the plasmalemma for fusion. Gelsolin activated by calcium can destroy the actin network by severing actin filaments, which may explain why there is a calcium requirement for this kind of exocytosis.[43] Smaller vesicles presumably can percolate through the network. The intracellular pH affects the distribution of intracellular granules.[66]

Although the molecular mechanism for membrane fusion involved in endocytosis and exocytosis is unclear, recent evidence indicates that it involves GTP-binding proteins.[126] The fusion of coated vesicles involves ATP-dependent removal of clathrin from the endosome surface, and the pH of the vesicle regulates the uncoating process. A protein that mediates intracellular membrane fusions of macrophages has been identified. This protein is a tetramer composed of 70-kd subunits, uses acetyl coenzyme A in its action, and is inhibited by the sulfhydryl-alkylating compound, N-ethylmaleimide.[127,128] Approximation of granules to the membrane before fusion may also be facilitated by a family of calcium- and phospholipid-binding proteins. Phagocytes have at least two of these, lipocortin (annexin III) and synexin,[129] and lipocortin accumulates at regions where granules fuse with phagosomes during phagocytosis.[130]

A variety of pharmacologic agents inhibit endosome–lysosome fusion, but the mechanism by which they do so is unclear.[128] Some of these effects may be clinically important because certain microorganisms have the capacity to prevent fusion in some cases and acidification of the endosome in others. The molecular basis of these actions is not known.[131–135]

Measurement of Phagocytosis and Secretion

Few situations arise in which evaluation of patients requires measurement of these parameters because all clinical disorders associated with cell-based abnormalities of phagocytosis or exocytosis have even more profound impairments of adhesion and locomotion. For laboratory assessment of phagocytosis and exocytosis, a variety of methods are available. The simplest involve morphologic observation of ingestion by phagocytes by light microscopy. More-sophisticated assays measure the uptake of radioactively or otherwise labeled particles by the cells. Detection of granule contents, usually hydrolytic enzymes, in the extracellular medium is a simple method of measuring phagocyte exocytosis.[136]

DISORDERS OF PHAGOCYTE MOTILITY AND INGESTION

Chapter 24 describes diseases in which deficient synthesis of the immunoproteins IgM, IgG, or C3 leads to the impairment of opsonic function. Microorganisms are not rendered recognizable to phagocytic cells, and affected patients suffer from recurrent or severe infections, usually caused by encapsulated bacteria. From the pattern of infections, one can infer that the role of these immunoproteins in phagocytosis is primarily to promote clearance of certain pathogenic bacteria by mononuclear phagocytes and is less directed toward defending the tissue–environmental interfaces. This latter task appears to be the responsibility of the moving phagocytes, the neutrophils, and the monocytes since, as described in Chapter 17, neutropenia and monocytopenia predispose to bacterial infections affecting the skin, lungs, and gastrointestinal tract.

Leukocyte Adhesion Deficiency

In 1978, a boy was encountered who suffered from recurrent tissue bacterial infections. The patient had a neutrophilic leukocytosis, but the blood neutrophils did not enter infected sites and were deficient in migration assays in vitro. The locomotion defect was localized to an inability of the cells to adhere to surfaces. A surface glycoprotein of normal PMNs was missing from the PMNs of this patient, and the PMNs of the boy's parents had this glycoprotein in reduced amounts compared with normal, indicating autosomal recessive inheritance.[137] This was the first example of what has become established as a rare but conceptually important genetic disease affecting phagocytes. Subsequent work has shown that this disorder is actually a family of related diseases affecting the CR3 receptor molecule.[138]

As described previously and in more detail in Chapter 16, CR3 is a heterodimer composed of an invariant β chain and an α chain, the latter of which determines which member of the family comprising LFA-1, Mac-1, or gp150,95 the particular molecule represents. All cases of the disease under discussion arise from defects affecting β-chain synthesis or its primary amino acid sequence, but the dimeric complex is either totally or partially missing, suggesting that both components must be present for normal deployment to the cell surface.[139–141] For this reason, affected patients underexpress all members of the adhesion molecule family, although the degree of reduced expression varies depending on the underlying biosynthetic defect.[142]

The clinical manifestations of LAD (Table 19-6) are similar to those seen in neutropenic patients, but LAD patients have normal to elevated peripheral blood phagocyte counts. The findings underscore that CR3 has a more generalized role in adhesion than as an opsonin for iC3b-coated bacteria. The major functional defect appears to be that mobile phagocytes simply do not enter the tissues to control microorganisms, and the bone marrow attempts to compensate by increasing phagocyte production. These facts tend to minimize the importance of some of the other phagocyte adhesion molecules that have been identified by their activities in vitro. Recent fascinating evidence suggests, however, that the lung is an exception to this rule, implying that a different adhesion and recognition system mediates transit of phagocytes into that organ, but their phagocytic function may be impaired even if they access the lung. LAD phagocytes are also variably defective in phagocytosis of a variety of particles, not just iC3b-opsonized ones, indicating that adhesion required for phagocytosis is a cooperative phenomenon. The clinical severity of LAD correlates well with the extent of expression of β_2-integrin on the phagocyte surface. Patients with mildly reduced β_2-integrin expression may only have neutrophilia, gingivitis, and moderate infections, whereas patients with severely deficient phagocytes have life-threatening infections, especially necrotizing enterocolitis, and have died from such infections.

Leukocyte Actin Dysfunction

A male infant was described in 1974 who suffered from severe tissue infections and did not mobilize PMNs to make pus. Like LAD patients, this patient had a peripheral blood neutrophilia. The infant's PMNs were quantitatively defective in adhesion and locomotion and less so in phagocytosis. A severe deficiency in the extent of actin assembly was detected in PMN extracts of the patient, and a partial deficiency was identified in both intact and extracts of the PMNs of the patient's parents and siblings. The patient's father's PMNs expressed CD11c and CD18 receptors at about half normal levels. The basis of the actin polymerization deficiency is not known, and since most LAD patients polymerize actin normally in response to various stimuli, the relation of this disorder to LAD is unclear.[143–145] Two additional families with patients and relatives demonstrating this constellation of findings have been identified, and their PMNs have been shown to contain supranormal quantities of LSP-1, an actin-binding protein.[145a]

Other Disorders

The complexity of phagocyte locomotion causes considerable variation in the results of assays measuring it, and as a result, the literature contains numerous reports correlating phagocyte (especially PMN) chemotaxis deficiency with various diseases for which a clearcut linkage is unclear. Examples include reduced in vitro PMN motility associated with neutropenia (lazy leukocyte syndrome), with periodontal disease, with the hyper IgE syndrome (see Chap. 24), and with a variety of systemic disorders, including bacterial sepsis, burns, malnutrition, rheumatoid arthritis, systemic lupus erythematosus, multiple myeloma, and hepatic cirrhosis.[146] The neutrophils of newborns also have functional abnormalities detectable in in vitro assays. It is possible that these findings reflect the stress of childbirth and infusion of substances released from the destruction of the placenta and umbilical cord.

PHAGOCYTE GRANULES

Neutrophil Granules

Neutrophil granules fall into two general categories: secretory granules, whose contents are mostly secreted into the external medium, and lysosome-like granules, whose contents are mostly used within the neutrophil. The secretory granules include the *specific granules* (also called secondary granules) and the recently described tertiary granules, which may actually be a subset of the specific granules. There is only one type of lysosome-like granule—the primary or *azurophil granule.*

TABLE 19-6. Phagocyte Adhesion Molecule (Leu-CAM) Deficiency

Clinical Features	Laboratory Features
Autosomal recessive inheritance	Neutrophilic and monocytic leukocytosis
Delayed separation of umbilical stump	Variably impaired adhesion, locomotion, spreading, phagocytosis by neutrophils and monocytes
Variable incidence of pyogenic infections	
Periodontal disease	Variably decreased expression of Leu-CAM (CR3) subunits

Azurophil Granules

The azurophil granules are the blue-staining granules seen in neutrophils as they appear in blood films treated with Wright's stain. These granules, generally about 0.5 μm in diameter,[147] are first detected in the promyelocyte, where, on staining with Wright-Giemsa, they are recognized as purple granules that are dark in hue compared with their appearance in more mature stages of the neutrophil. Their biosynthesis ceases at the myelocyte stage,[147] by which time they have taken on their final staining characteristics.

The contents of the azurophil granules are used almost exclusively for the disposal of ingested microorganisms. Accordingly, these granules almost invariably deliver their contents into phagocytic vesicles, with little discharge outside the cell except for release from disintegrating neutrophils or leakage as the granules expel their contents prematurely into developing vesicles still in communication with the exterior. Some of the azurophil granule components, however, are highly corrosive, and the portions of these that manage to escape from the neutrophils are responsible for much of the damage sustained by tissues in the neighborhood of an inflammatory reaction.[148–150] In functional terms, the azurophil granules contain two groups of constituents: microbicidal agents, which kill ingested microorganisms, and hydrolytic enzymes, which dispose of the remains. They also contain proteoglycans, which curb the activity of the hydrolases before their release from the granules.

Microbicidal Agents

Four kinds of microbicidal agents are known to occur in the azurophil granules. All are cationic at physiologic pH, so they all adhere firmly to the negatively charged surfaces of their targets. One of these microbicidal agents, MPO, is involved in the oxygen-dependent microbicidal mechanisms that account for much of the killing power of neutrophils. These are discussed in detail in a subsequent section. The rest are able to destroy bacteria under anaerobic conditions.

Oxygen-Independent Microbicidal Agents

DEFENSINS. The defensins are a group of three small peptides with potent lethal activity against a wide variety of microorganisms, including bacteria, viruses, and fungi.[151] Identical except for their N-terminal amino acids, the three peptides are all rigid bicyclic structures with positively charged amino acids at one end and hydrophobic amino acids at the other (Fig. 19-6), a distribution that gives them the properties of cationic detergents. In the neutrophil, the defensins occur at high concentrations, constituting over 5% of the total protein of the cell. They are not uniformly distributed among the azurophil granules, however, but are found only in a morphologically distinct subset (Fig. 19-7).

The defensins appear to kill bacteria by destroying the barrier function of their membranes. Defensins only affect bacteria that are engaged in energy production; bacteria maintained in a nutrient-free environment are resistant to their action.[152] One of the principal uses of metabolic energy in a microorganism is for the maintenance of the transmembrane potential. It may be that, as with mellitin, one of the active principals of bee venom, the membrane-permeabilizing activity of the defensins is only expressed in the presence of a transmembrane potential of a certain magnitude. Some microorganisms manage to synthesize specific gene products under direction of a transcriptional regulatory protein known as PhoP, which renders them resistant to the microbicidal action of defensins.

BACTERICIDAL PERMEABILITY-INCREASING PROTEIN. Bactericidal permeability-increasing protein (BPI) is a 60-kd cationic protein of known sequence.[153] Like the defensins, BPI kills by causing the membranes of its targets to become leaky.[154] Whereas the target range of the defensins is broad, BPI is only active against gram-negative bacteria. In a process antagonized by Ca^{2+} and Mg^{2+}, it binds to the outer walls of these bacteria (ie, their LPS),[155] then works its way through these walls to disorganize their cell membranes. Within minutes of exposure to BPI, the membrane barrier becomes sufficiently dysfunctional to allow actinomycin C to leak in, but macromolecule synthesis remains intact for some hours.[156] The membrane leak, however, destroys the microorganism as a colony-forming unit.

LYSOZYME. The interior of a bacterium is hypertonic with respect to its environment, and as a result, the microorganism tends to take in water from surrounding fluids. Rupture of the organism through the unopposed influx of water is prevented, however, by peptidoglycan, a vast polymer of N-acetylglucosamine and muramic acid exten-

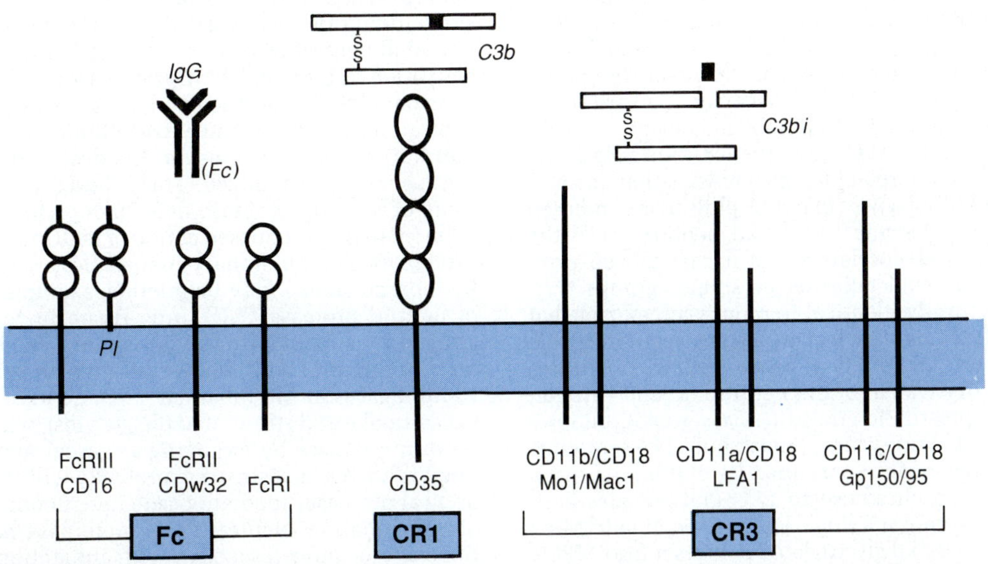

FIGURE 19-6. Schematic summary of the major opsonins and their receptors on phagocytic cells.

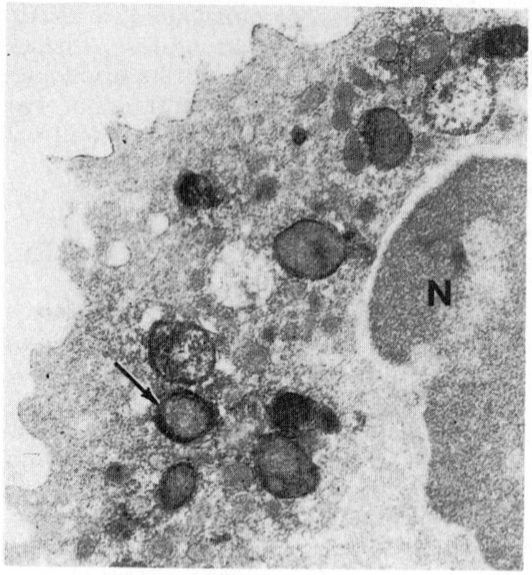

FIGURE 19-7. Morphologic characteristics of defensin-containing azurophil granules. In this section of a neutrophil stained for peroxidase and viewed by electron microscopy, azurophil granules appear black because of their myeloperoxidase content. Defensin-containing granules are stained only at the periphery because myeloperoxidase is excluded from their centers, possibly by crystals of defensin (*arrow*). N, nucleus.

sively cross-linked by short peptides that lies between the cell wall and the plasma membrane. The densely woven peptidoglycan forms a strong nonexpandable net that envelops the microorganism and protects it from the hypotonic medium in which it lives.

Lysozyme, a 14-kd enzyme found in both the azurophil and specific granules,[157] destroys peptidoglycan by hydrolyzing the glycosidic bonds in the glucosamine–muramic acid polymers. It operates most effectively at pH 4 to 5, the typical pH in the interior of the phagosome.[158] With the lysis of the peptidoglycan, the force opposing the osmotic gradient between the microorganism and its environment is lost. Water then moves freely into the bacterium, causing it to swell and burst.

The peptidoglycans of most bacteria contain substituents that render them resistant to the action of lysozyme.[159,160] Their resistance to lysozyme is broken down, however, by exposure to oxidants of the kind generated by stimulated neutrophils. In these cases, lysozyme appears to serve an auxiliary role, acting in concert with the oxidants to destroy the targets. In a few microorganisms, however, the peptidoglycan is readily hydrolyzed by lysozyme. Toward these, the enzyme alone is a potent microbicidal agent.

Myeloperoxidase. MPO plays an important role in the oxygen-dependent microbicidal mechanisms that account for much of the killing power of neutrophils. It is composed of two 60-kd peptides and two 12-kd peptides,[161,162] the larger of which is glycosylated, and it carries two iron-containing chlorin molecules as prosthetic groups.[163,164] Chlorin is structurally identical to prophyrin, except that the outer double bonds of each of an opposing pair of pyrrole rings are reduced. An abundant protein, MPO constitutes over 5% of the dry weight of the neutrophil, and through the color of its prosthetic groups (ξλωροσ,green), endows the cell with its characteristic greenish hue. The sequence of the enzyme has been determined by cloning its gene, which is located on chromosome 17[162] and encodes both subunits of the enzyme as a single long polypeptide.[165] MPO is synthesized as a 92-kd glycosylated precursor (pro-MPO), then undergoes limited deglycosylation followed by proteolysis to release a short glycopeptide and cut the remaining fragment into the 60-kd and 12-kd peptides.[166,167] Dimerization and delivery to the azurophil granule complete the formation of the enzyme.

MPO catalyzes the oxidation of Cl^- by the H_2O_2 generated by neutrophils when they are exposed to a target microorganism. This oxidation produces hypochlorous acid, a powerful microbicidal oxidant:

$$Cl^- + H_2O_2 \xrightarrow{MPO} HOCl + OH^-$$

The microbicidal role of MPO is aided by a high isoelectric point that confers a positive charge on the enzyme at physiologic pH, allowing it to bind directly to the negatively charged surface of an ingested microorganism. From this location, it can deliver its lethal products to the target with maximal efficiency. MPO can also catalyze the oxidation of Br^- and I^- to the corresponding hypohalous acids,[168] but Cl^- is its physiologic substrate. Like many lysosomal enzymes, it operates best at pH 4 to 5.

Hydrolytic Enzymes. The azurophil granules contain a battery of hydrolytic enzymes that act on a wide variety of substrates, including proteins, polysaccharides, lipids, and nucleic acids. These enzymes play a major role in the disposal of phagocytized bacteria and other ingested particles. Some (eg, lysozymes) may also participate in killing, particularly of organisms whose defenses have been weakened by microbicidal oxidants.

Neutral Proteases. The term *neutral proteases* refers to a group of proteolytic enzymes whose activities are maximum at pH values around neutrality, a pH optimum that distinguishes them from the other azurophil granule hydrolases, most of which show optimal activity at pH near 4 or 5. Three neutral proteases are found in the azurophil granules[169]—*elastase*,[170] *cathepsin G*,[171] and *proteinase 3*.[172] The exact physiologic function of these proteases has not yet been established, but their pH optimum suggests that they act during the earliest stages of phagocytosis, before the phagosomes have become acidified. Why proteolysis should be necessary at this stage of phagocytosis is not clear, although it can be speculated that the neutral proteases might inactivate microbial toxins that could otherwise destroy a neutrophil before it could kill the ingested target.[173,174] Cathepsin G also displays microbicidal properties that are independent of its catalytic activity.[156]

Although their physiologic role is unclear, it is evident that these proteases, as enzymes of broad specificity active at physiologic pH, have the potential to inflict considerable damage when they are released from the neutrophil into surrounding tissues. Normally, tissue destruction by the liberated neutral proteases is controlled through rapid inactivation by a group of antiproteinases (α_1-antiproteinase, α_2-macroglobulin, and so forth) that are found at high concentrations in plasma and extracellular fluids.[175] When the antiproteinases fail, however, the destructive potential of these enzymes is realized. This is best seen in the emphysema of α_1-antiproteinase deficiency, which has been attributed to the unopposed action of neutrophil elastase and proteinase 3 on pulmonary tissues. Destruction of the lung by tobacco smoke may be another example of the effects of neutral proteases[176,177]; lung tissue in this case is destroyed by a smoldering inflammatory reaction featuring an abundance of both neutrophils, which bring their neutral proteases to the inflamed site, and oxidants (from tobacco smoke and stimulated phagocytes), which inactivate α_1-antiproteinase by oxidizing a critical methionine residue.[178] Further investigation probably will show that these neutral proteases mediate tissue destruction at other sites of inflammation. Neutral PMN proteinase has been identified as one antigen reactive with autoantibodies found in the plasma of patients with Wegener's granulomatosis.[179,180]

Acid Hydrolases. The azurophil granules are the lysosomes of the neutrophils and as such contain a wide variety of hydrolytic enzymes that are maximally active at the relatively low pH of a fully acidified phagocytic vesicle.[157,181,182] These enzymes are responsible for breaking down the macromolecules of the ingested targets to their low-molecular-weight constituents. Included among the acid hydrolases of the azurophil granules are proteases (eg, cathepsin D, an aspartate protease active at pH 4.0 to 5.0),[183,184] glycosidases (eg, lysosome, lipid-hydrolyzing enzymes,[185,186] and RNAse).[187] Neutrophils have surprisingly little ability to degrade DNA.[188,189] A partial listing of acid hydrolases is given in Table 19-7.

Proteoglycans. Proteoglycans, or mucopolysaccharides, are molecules composed of a serine- and glycine-rich polypeptide[190] extensively substituted with highly anionic polysaccharide chains rich in uronic acids and sulfate groups. In neutrophils and their precursors, the azurophil granules (but not the specific granules) contain substantial concentrations of proteoglycans, principally chondroitin sulfate. The rich purple color of the azurophil granules in the promyelocytes is due to their proteoglycan content, and the loss of color as the cells mature is thought to result from the masking of the proteoglycan sulfate groups as the granules mature.[191]

TABLE 19-7. Contents of Human Neutrophil Secretory Granules

PRIMARY (AZUROPHILIC) GRANULES
Acid phosphatase
N-acetyl-β-glucosaminidase
α-Mannosidase
β-Glucuronidase
Cathepsins B, D, and G
Elastase
Proteinase 3
Azurocidin
Azurophil granule protein 7
Bacterial permeability inducer
Lysozyme
Defensins
(Myelo)peroxidase
SECONDARY (SPECIFIC) GRANULES
Vitamin B_{12}–binding protein
N-formyloligopeptide receptors
Laminin receptors
Lactoferrin
Collagenase
Lysozyme
NADPH oxidase (cytochrome *b*)
β_2-Microglobulin
Gelatinase
CD11b/CD18 (CR3 receptors)
Vitronectin receptors
TERTIARY (MICROVESICULAR) GRANULES
Class 1
Gelatinase
CD11b/CD18
Plasminogen activator
Class 2
Alkaline phosphatase
Tetranectin

In proteoglycan-containing granules, not only in phagocytes but also in mast cells and natural killer (NK) cells, hydrolases and other positively charged proteins are held as complexes in a dense network of anionic polysaccharide chains.[192,193] Although the hydrolases are active when complexed to proteoglycan, their access to substrates is greatly restricted; the attachment of the enzymes to the proteoglycan matrix prevents them from diffusing to potential substrates, whereas substrate molecules more than a few kilodaltons are screened away from the active sites of the complexed enzymes by the close mesh of the polysaccharide network.[193] Autolysis of the granules is therefore prevented by the proteoglycan, which appears to be largely responsible for maintaining the structural integrity of granules despite their content of potentially destructive hydrolytic enzymes.

Specific Granules

The specific granules are smaller than the azurophil granules (average size about 0.2 μm) and appear pink on Wright-stained blood films. They are first seen in the myelocytes, but unlike the azurophil granules, whose production ceases at the myelocyte stage, their numbers continue to increase throughout most of the later stages of neutrophil maturation.[147] By the time the cell is mature, it contains about two specific granules for every azurophil granule.

The specific granules resemble the azurophil granules in delivering their contents into phagocytic vesicles. Unlike the azurophil granules, however, the specific granules also secrete their contents deliberately into the extracellular medium.[194,195] Secretion occurs in response to many agents, including such physiologic stimuli as the anaphylotoxin C5a, liberated during complement activation[196,197]; FMLP, released from bacteria and from the mitochondria of damaged cells; and lipid mediators,[86,198,199] such as leukotriene B_4 and PAF.[198,200] Secretion takes place by the fusion of the specific granule with the plasma membrane, a process that transfers the granule membrane, with its complement of proteins, to the plasma membrane. Accordingly, secretion releases proteins into the extracellular medium and transfers other proteins to the outer layer of the neutrophil.[201] Among the specific granule membrane components relocated in this way are the C5a receptor,[202] the CD11/CD18 family of adhesion glycoproteins (discussed previously) and cytochrome b_{558}, a heme protein that participates in microbicidal oxidant production, as explained later.[203,204]

The contents of the specific granule include lysozyme, also found in the azurophil granules; certain ligand-binding proteins; and a few proteases with highly restricted substrate specificities. Lysosomal hydrolases and microbicidal cationic proteins are absent from this granule.

Ligand-Binding Proteins. The specific granules contain two ligand-binding proteins: apolactoferrin and cobalamin-binding protein. One binds iron tightly, and the other takes up cobalamin and related corrinoids.

Apolactoferrin. Apolactoferrin is the iron-binding protein of the specific granules.[205,206] Each molecule of apolactoferrin contains two sites that bind ferric (Fe^{3+}) iron with very high affinity (K_a 10^{22} mol^{-1}).[206,207] When one or both of these sites is occupied, the protein is called *lactoferrin*.

Some have proposed that the iron bound to the protein in its lactoferrin form catalyzes the production of the very reactive hydroxyl radical (OH·) from the oxidants generated by stimulated neutrophils (the so-called Haber-Weiss reaction, discussed later).[208,209] It is more likely, however, that lactoferrin-bound iron is unable to participate in the Haber-Weiss reaction. Apolactoferrin may therefore play a protective role at sites of inflammation, controlling nonspecific oxidant damage by sequestering loose iron and suppressing its reactivity.[210] The protein may also potentiate microbial killing by preventing the ingested bacteria from obtaining the iron they required metabolically.[211] Finally, lactoferrin appears to exert some control over granulopoiesis by inhibiting GM-CSF secretion by mononuclear phagocytes.

Cobalamin-Binding Protein. The corrinoids are a family of compounds that all contain a *corrin ring*, a partly reduced tetrapyrrole with a cobalt at its center. Biologic systems contain many kinds of corrinoids, some direct products of biosynthesis and others arising through chemical modification of the biosynthetically produced compounds.[212] Only one group of corrinoids, however, is active in humans; these are the *cobalamins*. Humans assimilate other classes of corrinoids,[208,213] acquiring them in part from bacteria.[214,215] These nonphysiologic corrinoids must be disposed of to prevent them from interfering with the function of the cobalamins in the tissues.

The specific granules contain a cobalamin-binding glycoprotein, sometimes called *transcobalamin III*, that is closely related to transcobalamin I, the principal cobalamin-binding protein of plasma.[216,217] The specific granule cobalamin binder takes up a wide variety of corrinoids with high affinity.[218,219] It is thought that this protein aids in the elimination of nonphysiologic corrinoids by binding them where they are released and transporting them to the liver, which excretes them in bile.[220,221]

Proteases

Collagenase and Gelatinase. As their names imply, these two enzymes catalyze the hydrolysis of native (collagenase) and denatured (gelatinase) collagens.[222,223] Like other collagenases, the specific granule collagenase splits the collagen molecule asymmetrically into two fragments by hydrolyzing a specific peptide bond; further degradation of the incised collagen molecule is accomplished by other proteases.[224,225] Whether gelatinase is similarly restricted in its specificity is not known. It is likely that these enzymes serve as demolition units, helping to clear away debris at damaged and inflamed sites preparatory to reconstruction. By digesting basement membrane beneath the endothelial cell layer, gelatinase may also participate in the egress of neutrophils from the vascular tree.[226]

Both collagenase and gelatinase are metalloproteases, bearing a Ca^{2+} ion at their active sites.[227,228] They exist in the specific granules as proenzymes but are converted to the active enzymes by exposure to the microbicidal oxidants manufactured by stimulated neutrophils. Both enzymes are secreted when the neutrophils are exposed to activators of degranulation, gelatinase in particular being liberated in response to stimuli too weak to cause generalized release of the specific granule contents.[229,230] The latter finding has suggested that gelatinase resides in a special granule population known as the *tertiary granules*.[230] It is not yet known, however, whether these highly secretory gelatinase-containing granules actually represent a distinct granule population or are only a subset of the specific granules.[231]

C5-Activating Protease. Contained within the specific granules and released into the extracellular medium when neutrophils are stimulated is a protease that splits the circulating complement component C5 into C5a and C5b.[232] The C5a liberated through the action of this enzyme is both a chemotactic factor that calls more neutrophils to its site of production and (at higher concentrations) a stimulating agent that induces the newly arrived neutrophils to release their specific granule contents, including the C5-activating protease. The release of the C5a-activating enzyme therefore introduces a positive feedback loop that amplifies the inflammatory reaction, drawing progressively increasing numbers of neutrophils into the inflamed site.

Granules of Mononuclear Phagocytes

Unlike neutrophils, mononuclear phagocytes contain only one type of granule.[2] Sometimes, a distinction is made between an early MPO-containing granule that occurs in monocytes and the later MPO-free granule that is found in macrophages. Apart from their differences in peroxidase content, however, the two kinds of granules are similar in composition and function and therefore are considered to represent a single granule type. Although this granule has not been as well characterized as those of the neutrophil, studies have shown that it closely resembles the neutrophil azurophil granule. Like the latter, the granule of the mononuclear phagocyte contains a large number of acid hydrolases, giving it the character of a lysosome.[233,234] In addition, it contains several other constituents found in azurophil granules, including several microbicidal proteins: the defensins,[235] lysozyme,[233] and (at certain stages) MPO.[236] Because of their content of microbicidal proteins, these granules, like the azurophil granules of the neutrophil, are able to participate in the killing of ingested microorganisms. In addition, the acid hydrolases in these granules are responsible for the degradation of materials ingested by the cell, which in the case of mononuclear phagocytes include invading microorganisms and superannuated cells (eg, red blood cells [RBCs] at the end of their life-spans and assorted debris that accumulate at sites of injury). The various lipid storage diseases (eg, Gaucher's disease, Neimann-Pick disease) are caused by deficiencies of one or another of these lysosomal acid hydrolases (see Chap. 32).

During their lifetimes, which may last months, mononuclear phagocytes can undergo many changes in morphology and function in response to exogenous influences (eg, LPS, IFN-γ) as they transform from circulating monocytes to tissue macrophages[237,238] (see Table 19-2). Included among these changes are major alterations affecting their granules. Granule numbers increase continuously[239,240] as the monocyte, maturing under the influence of cytokines and tissue location, enlarges to a macrophage (first resting, then activated), then with continued stimulation to an epithelioid cell, and finally to a giant cell, the latter arising through the fusion of epithelioid cells that have been subjected to prolonged stimulation by cytokines[241] (Fig. 19-8). The composition of the granules also changes; for example, levels of defensins and acid hydrolases increase,[239,242] whereas MPO, abundant in monocyte granules, declines greatly as the cell transforms into a macrophage.[236] These changes and others that occur as mononuclear phagocytes come under the influence of their local environment may enable them to accomplish their tasks of demolition and destruction in an optimal fashion regardless of the circumstances or the targets.

Macrophages are highly secretory cells, releasing a large number of substances into their environment when appropriately stimulated[243] (see Table 19-1). Among these substances are the acid hydrolases, which, unlike most of these secreted materials (discussed later), are not synthesized de novo in response to the stimulus but exist as preformed proteins in the macrophage granules.[244,245] Release of these lysosomal hydrolases takes place in part through leakage due to premature fusion of the granules with partly formed phagocytic vesicles and in part through deliberate exocytosis of the granule contents.[234,244,246,247] The liberated hydrolases, which include cathepsins, glycosidases, aryl sulfatases, and other catabolic enzymes, participate in the

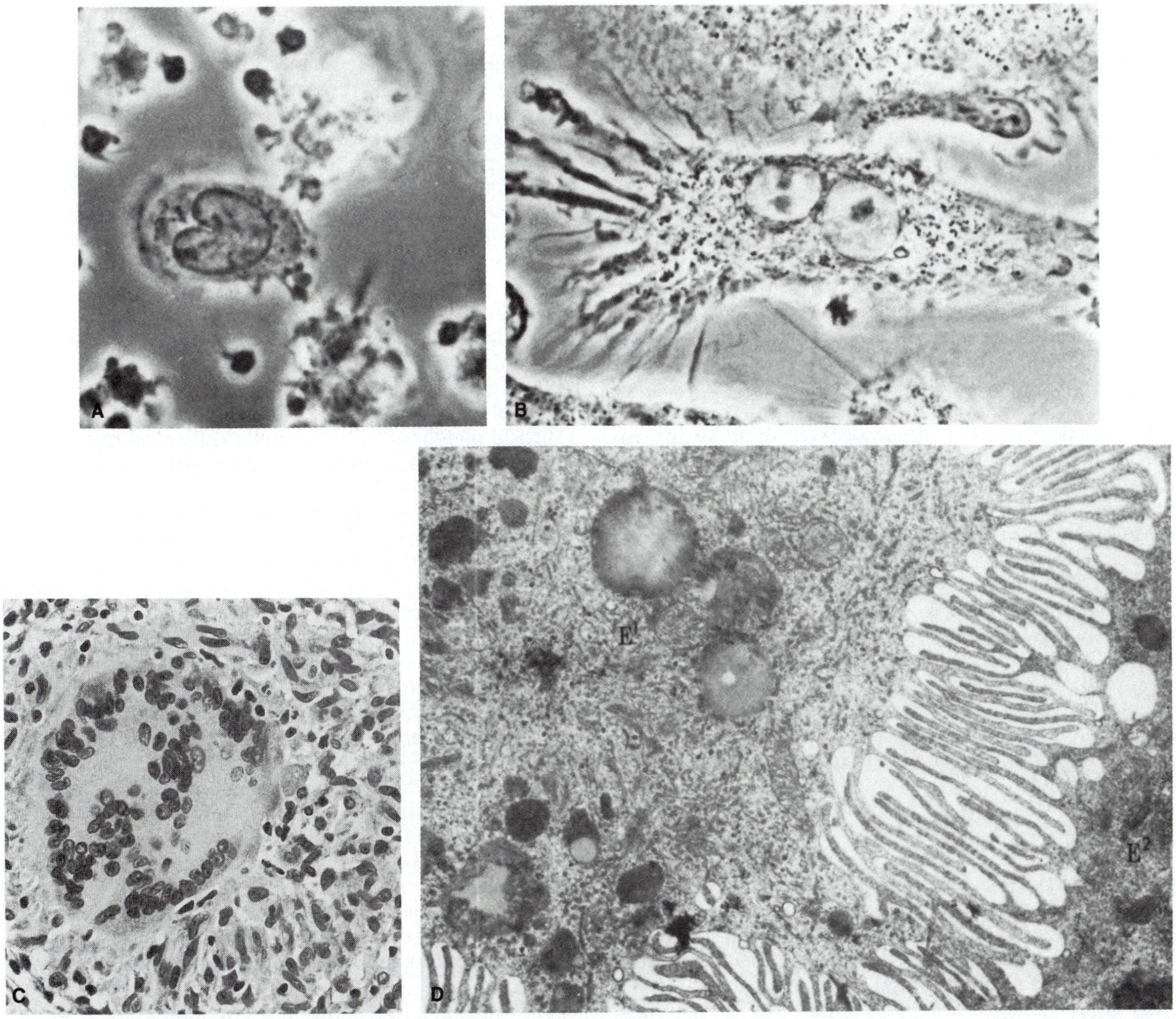

FIGURE 19-8. Stages in the transformation of a monocyte to a giant cell at an inflammatory site. (**A**) Monocyte. (**B**) Macrophage. This cell is much larger and more granular than the monocyte. Its membrane is thrown into irregular folds and projections, through which it adheres to nearby cells and substratum. (**C**) Granuloma, showing a large giant cell surrounded by tightly packed epithelioid cells. (**D**) The junction between two epithelioid cells, showing that they are tightly joined through a complex system of interdigitating membrane folds. E^1, first epithelioid cell; C^2, second epithelioid cell.

tissue repair process at inflammatory sites and also alter the nature of the inflammatory reaction by destroying protein mediators such as C5a and immunoglobulins.

DISEASES AFFECTING PHAGOCYTE GRANULES

Chédiak-Higashi disease is an inherited disorder of granule morphogenesis affecting tissues throughout the body. Its most prominent and dangerous clinical manifestations are a greatly increased susceptibility to bacterial infections resulting from serious abnormalities in the function of affected phagocytes and a lymphoma-like illness that eventually kills most patients who survive the bacterial infections.[248,249]

Pathogenesis

The pathogenetic basis for Chédiak-Higashi disease is readily apparent on inspecting affected cells under the microscope. Phagocytes, instead of containing granules that are relatively regular in size and shape, contain a highly inhomogeneous population of granules, some normal but many huge and misshapen. These grossly distorted granules are also seen in other cells, including melanocytes, platelets, lymphocytes, and cells of the nervous system, all of which contribute to the clinical manifestations of the disease. In neutrophils, the defective organelles contain constituents from both the azurophil and specific granules,[250] some in decreased amounts,[251] whereas some components (eg, cathepsin G and elastase)[252,253] are absent altogether. The abnormal granules are seen in mature cells, in myeloid precursors,[254] and in colonies derived from affected marrow stem cells.[255]

These abnormal granules cause disturbances in the function of various types of blood cells in Chédiak-Higashi patients. In *neutrophils*, both phagocytosis and O_2^- production are normal,[256] but bacterial killing is impaired, degranulation is delayed and incomplete, and chemotaxis is defective,[257] perhaps because the enlarged granules pass only with difficulty through the narrow spaces of the tissues. Defects in degranulation and chemotaxis may be partly attributable to disruption in the function of the microtubules, which show abnormalities in polymerization and in interaction with the granule membranes.[258,259] A high proportion of the cells are destroyed in the marrow (ineffective granulopoiesis), leading to a mild to moderate neutropenia and the excretion of abnormally large amounts of lysozyme (muramidase) in the urine. In the *platelets*, storage pools of ADP and serotonin are decreased[260,261] possibly because of a deficiency in dense granule precursors in the megakaryocytes.[262] Lymphocytes show an impairment of both antibody-dependent (ADCC) and NK cell–mediated cytotoxicity,[263,264] demonstrating in particular a problem in handling Epstein-Barr virus infections that can lead to serious clinical consequences late in the course of the disease.[265]

Studies with myeloid precursors have suggested that the giant granules of Chédiak-Higashi disease arise through the progressive coalescence of smaller granules as the defective cells mature.[254] The molecular lesion underlying this abnormality in granule morphogenesis is not known. It seems reasonable to speculate, however, that the affected component is a protein in the membranes of the abnormal granules, possibly involved in the regulation of degranulation.

Clinical Features

Chédiak-Higashi is a rare disorder inherited as an autosomal recessive trait. In the past, patients with Chédiak-Higashi disease have typically died of bacterial infections in their first or second decade. The prevention of infections by prophylactic antibiotics and other measures have recently altered this pattern, and patients are living longer. Of those who survive the infections, however, most succumb to the *accelerated phase*, a progressive lymphoproliferative syndrome that leads inevitably to death through pancytopenia.[266]

Infections begin in early infancy. They are serious and recurrent, typically involving the skin and subcutaneous tissues (abscess and pyoderma) and the upper and lower respiratory tracts (sinusitis, otitis media, pneumonia).[208] Severe gum disease with bone atrophy and loss of teeth is also seen in Chédiak-Higashi disease, as it is in several other disorders of neutrophil function. *Staphylococcus aureus* is the most frequent pathogen, but infections by other bacteria (eg, *Streptococcus pneumoniae, Streptococcus pyogenes*) are also seen, as well as infections by *Aspergillus* and *Candida* sp. The infections tend to be protracted, responding only slowly to antibiotic treatment.

Other signs of the disease also appear in infancy. Diffuse hypopigmentation (partial albinism) is evident at birth, with pale skin and eyegrounds and a silvery sheen to the hair. These pigmentary abnormalities are manifestations of the granular abnormalities that occur in Chédiak-Higashi melanocytes. Neurologic signs, which are manifestations of abnormalities affecting the neurons, glia, and Schwann's cells, may include peripheral neuropathy, ataxia, weakness, and seizures.[266,267]

Total leukocyte counts of Chédiak-Higashi patients are low (1000 to 3000/μL), and urine muramidase is high, both reflecting intramedullary destruction of granulocytes. The bleeding time is prolonged, and platelet aggregation is abnormal as a result of the storage pool defect in Chédiak-Higashi platelets,[260] although clinically significant bleeding is usually not a problem. The diagnosis is made by examination of the blood film, which shows the pathognomonic giant granules in most members of the leukocyte series, including neutrophils, eosinophils, monocytes, and occasional granular lymphocytes (Fig. 19-9). The giant granules are also seen in hematopoietic precursors in the marrow.

In most Chédiak-Higashi patients who survive for a sufficiently long time, the disease enters an accelerated phase.[266] This is a lymphoma-like illness characterized by an uncontrolled and ultimately fatal proliferation of normal-appearing lymphocytes and histiocytes (Fig. 19-10), possibly in response to an Epstein-Barr virus infection that the defective lymphocytes are unable to control.[265,268] Affected patients begin to develop recurrent fevers, rash, and prostration, perhaps due to the release of lymphokines from the proliferating cells, and infections increase in frequency. The neutrophil counts begin to decline from their already diminished levels, and anemia and (less often) thrombocytopenia appear. The liver, spleen, and lymph nodes enlarge as they become infiltrated with the proliferating cells, which also fill the marrow, accounting for the progressively worsening pancytopenia. Death from the complications of pancytopenia is inevitable after a relentless downhill course of a few months to 2 years.

Treatment

The treatment of Chédiak-Higashi disease amounts to the prevention and treatment of the infectious complications. Patients should be placed on prophylactic antibiotic therapy: trimethoprim, 160 mg/d, plus sulfamethoxazole, 800 mg/d (the combination is available as Septra, Bactrim, or generic equivalents, and all are sold as elixirs for children, in whom the dose is 5 mL per 10 kg); or for patients with allergy to sulfonamides, dicloxacillin, 500 mg (250 mg in children) twice daily. Infections that develop should be

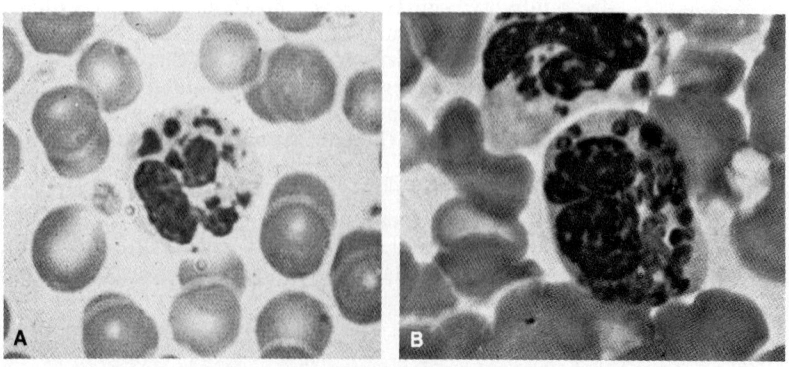

FIGURE 19-9. Neutrophils in Chédiak-Higashi disease. (**A**) Peripheral blood. (**B**) Bone marrow. The large, malformed granules that are pathognomonic of Chédiak-Higashi disease are readily identified. In the bone marrow, precursors as well as mature cells contain the defective granules, which are found in all leukocyte lines.

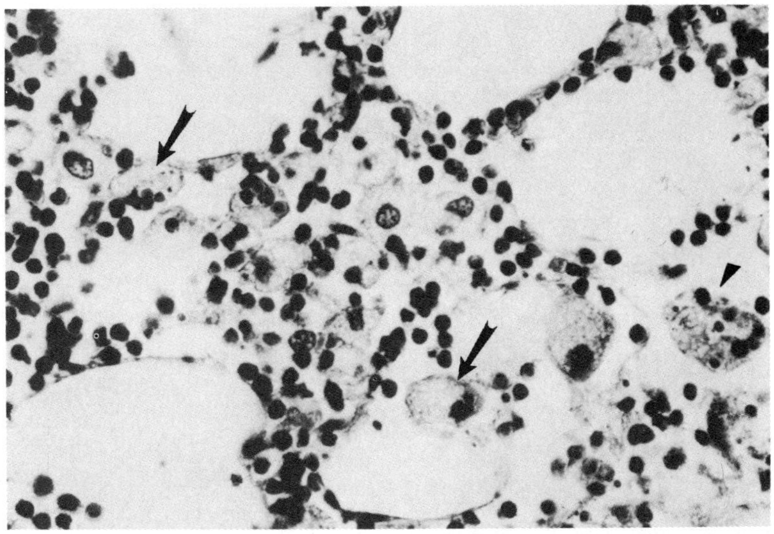

FIGURE 19-10. The accelerated phase of Chédiak-Higashi disease. The involved bone marrow infiltrated with large, benign-appearing mononuclear cells (*arrows*). This marrow also shows hematophagocytosis (*arrowheads*), another typical feature of the accelerated phase of Chédiak-Higashi disease.

treated vigorously with high doses of appropriate antibiotics and surgical drainage as necessary. High-dose ascorbic acid, 200 mg/d, improves neutrophil function and ameliorates the clinical manifestations in some patients.[269,270] As to the accelerated phase, steroids, vincristine, and antithymocyte globulin have been used for treatment but with only modest success. Some patients entering the accelerated phase have been successfully treated by marrow transplantation from HLA-compatible donors.

Specific Granule Deficiency

Inherited

Inherited specific granule deficiency is a condition whose most characteristic feature is the absence of specific granules from affected neutrophils.[271] In these cells, specific granules cannot be detected by either light or electron microscopy (Fig. 19-11). Cells from one patient contained small flat vesicles that were tentatively identified as empty specific granules. Moreover, many individual specific granule components are missing from these cells. Cobalamin-binding protein and lactoferrin are absent, as is gelatinase, ordinarily found in a readily discharged subset of specific granules (perhaps tertiary granules). Lactoferrin mRNA is greatly diminished in marrow cells from patients deficient in specific granules. In addition, unlike normal neutrophils, specific granule-deficient cells fail to deliver additional CD11/CD18, FMLP receptors, and cytochrome b_{558} (part of the O_2^--forming apparatus, discussed later) to the plasma membrane in response to stimuli, suggesting that pools of these components normally found in the specific granule membranes are also missing from these cells.

The term *specific granule deficiency* is somewhat of a misnomer because several other structures are also involved. In the *azurophil granules*, complex carbohydrates stain abnormally, and the defensins, a group of potent antimicrobial peptides restricted to the azurophil granules, are completely absent,[253] although MPO appears to be normal. *Nuclei* are abnormal in shape, frequently bilobed (pseudo–Pelger-Huët), with redundant membranes (Fig. 19-12). Finally, leukocyte alkaline phosphatase activity is absent from the *plasma membrane*.[272] These findings suggest that inherited specific granule deficiency actually represents a general defect in membrane biosynthesis that affects all the membranes of the neutrophil.

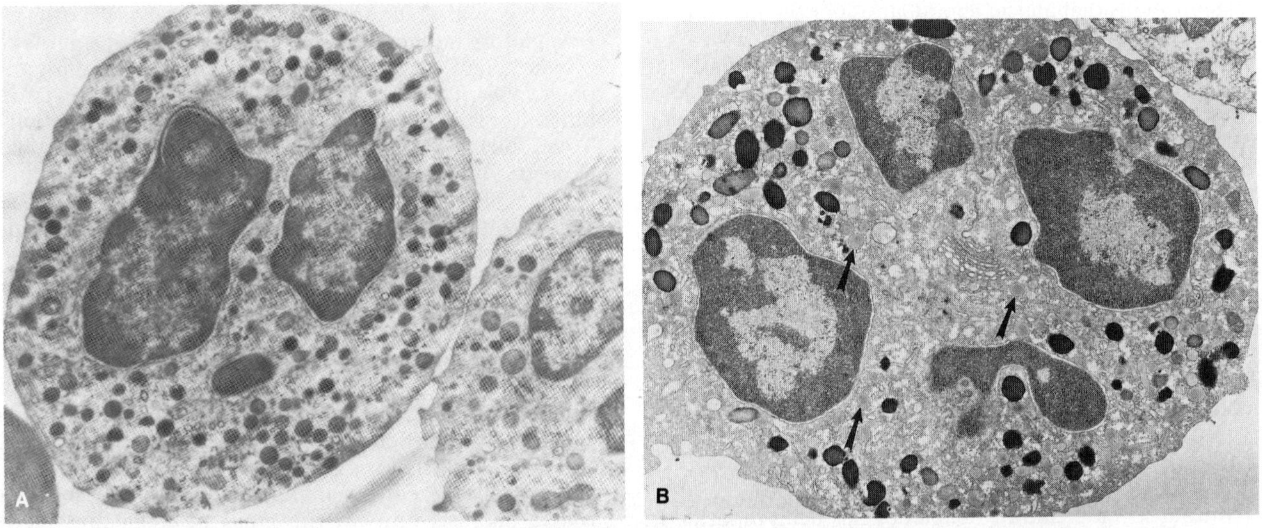

FIGURE 19-11. Electron micrographs of neutrophils from a patient with specific granule deficiency (**A**) and a normal patient (**B**). Darkly stained azurophil granules are present in both neutrophil profiles, but smaller, lighter-staining specific granules (*arrow*) are seen only in the normal cell.

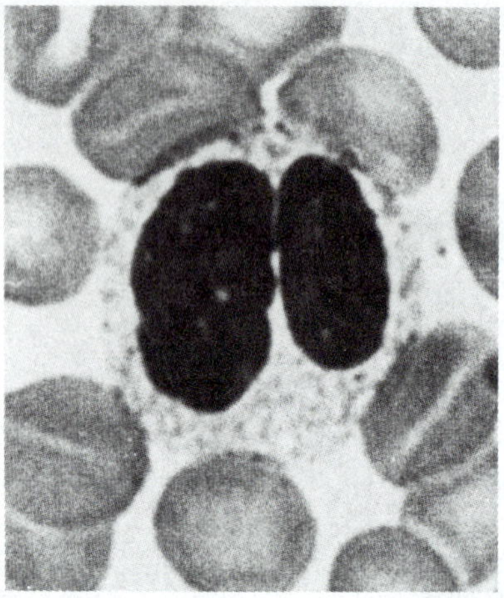

FIGURE 19-12. A specific granule-deficient neutrophil, showing its abnormal nucleus. The nucleus is much larger than normal, bilobed, and highly atypical in appearance.

The biochemical deficiencies in inherited specific granule deficiency result in characteristic abnormalities in neutrophil function. Chemotaxis is abnormal[273] possibly because of defects in neutrophil adherence and chemotactic sensing due to the failure of the defective neutrophils to up-regulate CD11/CD18 adherence proteins and chemotactic receptors on activation. In contrast, no consistent abnormality in O_2^- production has been demonstrated,[274,275] and MPO levels are normal.[248] Bacterial killing (*S aureus, Escherichia coli*), however, is depressed in specific granule-deficient neutrophils despite the presence of normal oxidative killing mechanisms probably because of the lack of defensins in these cells.

Inherited specific granule deficiency is rare, having been reported in only five patients to date.[271,273,274,276–278] Genetic transmission appears to occur by an autosomal recessive mechanism. As with other inherited disorders of neutrophils, patients with specific granule deficiency show a marked susceptibility to recurrent bacterial infections involving the skin, subcutaneous tissues, and upper and lower respiratory tracts. *S aureus* is the most common infecting organism, but enterobacterial and candidal infections have also been seen. In the appropriate clinical setting, the diagnosis of inherited specific granule deficiency is suggested by neutrophils that appear agranular under the microscope (Wright's stain normally reveals specific but not azurophil granules), with bilobed nuclei. The cells stain normally for MPO, but leukocyte alkaline phosphatase is usually low. If necessary, the diagnosis of specific granule deficiency can be established definitively either by demonstrating that the neutrophils are deficient in a specific granule component (lactoferrin or cobalamin-binding protein) or by showing through electron microscopy that the specific granules are missing from the neutrophils. Management involves vigorous antibiotic treatment of infections, with drainage of abscesses as necessary. Prophylactic antibiotics may be useful in this condition as they are in other abnormalities of neutrophil function. With proper treatment, the prognosis of inherited specific granule deficiency is good.

Acquired

Acquired specific granule deficiency has been reported in neonates[273] and in burned patients.[279,280] In the latter group, the deficiency may reflect the presence in the circulation of neutrophils that have undergone partial degranulation in response to the thermal injury. Neutrophils from both groups show decreased chemotaxis. Acquired specific granule deficiency is also seen in patients with certain stem cell disorders. This is discussed later.

GRANULE-INDEPENDENT SECRETION

In addition to secreting substances produced at an earlier time and stored in secretory granules until needed, phagocytes are also able to secrete freshly synthesized materials. These materials include a large number of proteins, an array of lipid mediators, and a group of low-molecular-weight oxygen- and nitrogen-containing compounds, some of which are used as microbicidal agents. Some of these materials exert their effects only in the immediate vicinity of the secreting cell, whereas others are distributed throughout the tissues by the circulation and operate far from their site of production.

Proteins

Newly synthesized proteins are secreted by both neutrophils and mononuclear phagocytes, usually in response to stimulation by an external agent. Mononuclear phagocytes secrete a remarkable number of peptides with diverse functions, most related to aspects of host defense and inflammation (see Table 19-1). Neutrophils are generally thought to have little capacity for protein synthesis, but recent work has shown that these cells too are able to manufacture and secrete certain proteins when the need arises.

Mononuclear Phagocytes

Cytokines. Cytokines are intercellular messengers that coordinate the host response to infection or injury. They are released in small amounts by cells that participate in this response (eg, inflammatory cells, endothelial cells, fibroblasts), then bind to specific receptors on target cells (often including the secreting cells themselves) and instruct these cells to alter their growth and function. At last count, the cytokines numbered over two dozen, each produced by many types of cells and each binding to many kinds of targets. Moreover, many different cytokines are generated by each type of producer cell, whereas each target cell responds to many different cytokines, each of which affects the target's response to all the others.[281] It is clear that the cytokines with their array of producer and target cells form a regulatory network of fantastic intricacy and complexity.

Nearly half the cytokines are produced by mononuclear phagocytes. As a rule, these cells generate the cytokines only after stimulation, either by direct interaction with a T cell during antigen presentation (discussed later) or by exposure to cytokines secreted by other cells (eg, the T-lymphocyte product IFN-γ, usually in the presence of LPS). The cytokines known to be produced by mononuclear phagocytes are listed in Table 19-1. A few deserve special mention.

Interleukin-1 and Tumor Necrosis Factor (Cachectin). These peptides, both 17-kd, are regarded as the major proinflammatory peptides released by mononuclear phagocytes. IL-1, originally known as leukocyte pyrogen, consists of two 17-kd peptides, designated IL-1α and IL-1β, with considerable sequence homology and similar actions.[282] TNF was initially recognized for two of its activities: its ability to cause certain malignancies to undergo hemorrhagic necrosis and (in the guise of cachectin) its role in the pathogenesis of wasting in trypanosome-infected mice.[281,283,284]

Both IL-1 and TNF are produced by mononuclear phagocytes in response to stimulation by endotoxin or IFN-γ[281,282,285]; in combination, endotoxin and IFN-γ act synergistically to amplify cytokine production.[286] Corticosteroids antagonize the effects of endotoxin and IFN-γ on mononuclear phagocytes, suppressing the production of both cytokines.[282,286] IL-1 production is also stimulated by phagocytosis,[283] leukotrienes,[287] C5a,[285] and GM-CSF,[288] whereas TNF production is stimulated by the combination of GM-CSF and IL-3 (multi-CSF) but not by either agent acting individually.[289] Finally, IL-1 and TNF each stimulate the production of the other.[288,290,291]

Extensive studies of both IL-1 and TNF have shown them to have similar effects on a wide variety of cells and tissues.[281,283,292] A partial list of these effects is given in Table 19-8. It is evident from this list that the actions of these two cytokines are responsible for many of the systemic manifestations of inflammation. In particular, TNF appears to be largely responsible for septic shock, the systemic catastrophe that accompanies massive endotoxemia.

Colony-Stimulating Factors. The colony-stimulating factors are a group of peptide hormones that are necessary for the production of neutrophils and mononuclear phagocytes. These factors include IL-3 and GM-CSF, which stimulate the growth and differentiation of early hematopoietic precursors, and G-CSF and M-CSF, which act on hematopoietic precursors that are already committed to the phagocyte lineage, directing them to differentiate into neutrophils and monocytes, respectively. Of these four colony-stimulating factors, all but IL-3 are made by mononuclear phagocytes.[293,294] For the production of G-CSF and GM-CSF, the mononuclear phagocytes must be stimulated by other cytokines (IL-3, IFN-γ) or by LPS[295,296]; M-CSF, however, is made by unstimulated mononuclear phagocytes,[293,295] although its production is increased when the cells are exposed to cytokines (eg, IL-3).[296]

In addition to influencing cell proliferation and differentiation, the colony-stimulating factors exert many effects on the function and behavior of mature phagocytes. These effects are discussed elsewhere in the chapter.

Tissue Factor. Mononuclear phagocytes make a number of procoagulant proteins. Of these, the most important is tissue factor.[297] Unlike the other proteins discussed in this section, tissue factor is not a secreted protein but rather is associated with the cell surface, where its active site faces the exterior. Here, tissue factor accelerates clotting by binding factor VII to its active site to form a tissue factor–factor VII complex that is much more effective than free factor VII as an activator of factor X.[298]

Tissue factor is found in both monocytes and macrophages. On the surface of unstimulated mononuclear phagocytes, it is detectable in only small amounts, but its surface expression increases sharply over a few hours when the phagocytes are activated by exposure to IFN-γ plus LPS,[299] to TNF,[300] or to 12-hydroxyeicosatetraenoic acid (12-HETE), which is released by activated platelets.[301] Much of the coagulation that occurs in regions of inflammation may be due to the increased surface tissue factor activity

TABLE 19-8. Some Actions of Interleukin-1 and Tumor Necrosis Factor

INTERLEUKIN-1 (IL-1)
Central nervous system
Pyrogenic
Induces slow-wave sleep
Suppresses appetite
Liver: acute-phase response
Fat and muscle: induces catabolic state
Endothelial cells: induces procoagulant state (tissue factor, plasminogen-activator inhibitor)
Lymphocytes: activates IL-2 production and expression of IL-2 receptors
Endocrine system: stresses hormone response (secretion of endorphins, corticotropin-releasing factor, ACTH, somatostatin)
TUMOR NECROSIS FACTOR
Central nervous system
Pyrogenic
Suppresses appetite
Liver: actue-phase response
Fat: induces catabolic state*
Bone and cartilage: promotes resorption*
Endothelial cells
Stimulates IL-1 production
Induces procoagulant state*
Increases surface adhesion proteins (integrins)*
Phagocytes: causes general increase in PMN and monocyte and macrophage activity (adhesion, phagocytosis, respiratory burst)
Bone marrow: a cause of the anemia of chronic disease (suppresses erythropoiesis, shortens red blood cell life-span)
Miscellaneous
Kills tumor cells with fragmentation of DNA (apoptosis)
Causes hypotension and capillary leak (responsible for many of the manifestations of endotoxin shock)*
No effect on lymphocytes

* Potentiated by IL-1.

of mononuclear phagocytes activated by cytokines released into the inflamed tissues. The hypercoagulable state seen in patients with inflammatory diseases may be attributable in part to the same cause.

Complement Components. Mononuclear phagocytes are important sources of early complement components. Components C2 through C5 are manufactured by mononuclear phagocytes (see Chap. 16), as are the specific alternative pathway components: factor B, factor D, and properdin. Factors H and I, which together greatly accelerate the destruction of component C3b, are also produced by mononuclear phagocytes. The production of some of these factors is augmented by exposure of the cells to LPS.[302] IFN-γ also augments the secretion of complement components by mononuclear phagocytes.[303,304]

Proteases and Protease Antagonists. Mononuclear phagocytes synthesize a variety of proteases and antiproteases that participate in the demolition necessary for tissue repair at inflammatory sites. These include elastase[305] and collagenase,[306,307] which degrade connective tissue, and tissue plasminogen activator,[308] which binds to the fibrin in a thrombus and there initiates lysis of the thrombus by activating the fibrin-splitting enzyme plasmin. Antagonists of these proteases are also manufactured by mononuclear phagocytes. Among these antagonists are α_1-antiproteinase[309] and α_2-macroglobulin,[310] which inactivate serine proteases such as phagocyte elastase; a collagenase inhibitor; and inhibitors of fibrinolysis, including plasminogen activator inhibitor[308,311] and α_2-antiplasmin.[312] α_2-Antiplasmin is a powerful, specific, and rapidly acting inactivator of circulating plasmin that has relatively little effect on fibrin-bound plasmin.[313,314] Deficiency of plasminogen-activator inhibitor leads to a hypercoagulable state,[315] whereas α_2-antiplasmin deficiency results in a severe bleeding disorder in which all the usual coagulation screening tests are normal.[313]

Lysozyme. Lysozyme, whose properties were discussed previously, is secreted continuously by mononuclear phagocytes. Its rate of secretion remains invariant regardless of whether the phagocytes have been exposed to cytokines, LPS, or other modifying influences.[245,316] Lysozyme is able to destroy bacteria, sometimes as a single agent but more often in concert with antimicrobial oxidants of phagocytic origin. The steady release of lysozyme into the tissues thus provides extracellular fluids with a certain degree of intrinsic antimicrobial activity.

Neutrophils

Neutrophils also secrete newly synthesized proteins into the surrounding medium but to a much smaller extent than mononuclear phagocytes. In response to stimuli present at an inflamed site, neutrophils manufacture and secrete cytokines that further influence the nature of the inflammatory and repair processes occurring at that site.[288] Activated neutrophils also secrete fibronectin.[317] Further investigations likely will reveal other proteins that are secreted by neutrophils under appropriate circumstances.

Lipid Agonists

Phagocytes secrete lipid agonists that can exert powerful effects on surrounding cells. These lipid agonists include leukotrienes, prostaglandins, thromboxanes, and PAF. All are derived from arachidonic acid except PAF, which is generated from a phospholipid.

Leukotrienes

Leukotrienes are the principal arachidonate-derived inflammatory mediators manufactured by phagocytes.[318] Their production begins with the phospholipase A_2–catalyzed release of arachidonic acid from a phospholipid (a phosphatidylcholine or phosphatidylinositol)[319] in response to a stimulus that raises the intracellular concentration of Ca^{2+}, a cofactor for the phospholipase. Commitment to the leukotriene pathway occurs with the 5-lipoxygenase catalyzed conversion of the arachidonate to leukotriene A_4 (LTA_4), an oxidation in which the double bonds of the arachidonate are shifted and a 5,6-epoxide group is introduced into the molecule[320,321] (Fig. 19-13). Activation of the 5-lipoxygenase is associated with its translocation from the cytosol to the plasma membrane and requires a cofactor protein of 18 kd.[322] The unstable LTA_4 is then rapidly converted into the inflammatory mediators: leukotriene B_4 (LTB_4), an agent with powerful pleiotropic effects on the phagocytes; and the cysteine-containing leukotrienes LTC_4, LTD_4, and LTE_4, which permeate small blood vessels and cause protracted spasms of the bronchi, arterioles, and intestine through their agonist effect on smooth muscle, but do little to phagocytes. LTB_4 is produced through the action of an epoxide hydrolase,[323] which opens the epoxide ring and places a hydroxyl group at the 12 position of the molecule, whereas LTC_4 is generated by a glutathione S-transferase cytochrome P-450_{LTB} of neutrophils to 12,20-diHETE and then further to the inactive 12-HETE-1,20-dioic acid.[341] Conversely, the phagocyte product 5-HETE is converted by platelets to 5,12-diHETE. Pulmonary epithelial cells release arachidonic acid, which is converted by alveolar macrophages to LTB_4,[342] whereas neutrophils feed LTA_4 to pulmonary tissues, which converts it to LTB_4, 20-OH LTB_4, and the cysteine leukotrienes LTC_4, LTD_4, and LTE_4.[326] It is likely that increasing numbers of these transcellular interactions will be recognized as more is learned about these lipid mediators.

Other Arachidonate-Derived Agonists

Other arachidonate-derived agonists manufactured by phagocytes include *prostaglandins*, which increase intracellular cAMP levels in many tissues by activating membrane adenylate cyclase, and *thromboxanes*, which act on platelets to promote thromboxane A_2 (TxA_2) or inhibit prostacyclin aggregation.[343] Prostaglandin E_2 (PGE_2) is released in large amounts by macrophages in response to many kinds of stimuli:

- Opsonized zymosan
- Unopsonized zymosan (through the α-glucan receptor)
- Endotoxin
- IL-1
- C3b
- Late complement components
- PAF
- Immune complexes

The production of PGE_2 is suppressed, however, by exposure of the macrophage to IFN-γ,[344] perhaps a result of the maturation of the macrophage into an epithelioid-like cell under the influence of the cytokine.[345,346] Most of the agents that elicit PGE_2 formation also stimulate macrophages to produce TxA_2 (detected as its footprint, TxB_2).[344,347,348] TxA_2 is also manufactured by neutrophils; its production in these cells does not require the activity of the O_2^--forming respiratory burst oxidase.[349] Prostacyclin (detected as 6-keto$PGF_{1\alpha}$) is also formed by macrophages under certain circumstances.[350,351]

Platelet-Activating Factor

Another lipid mediator of inflammation is PAF. An exceedingly powerful inflammatory agonist, PAF exerts major

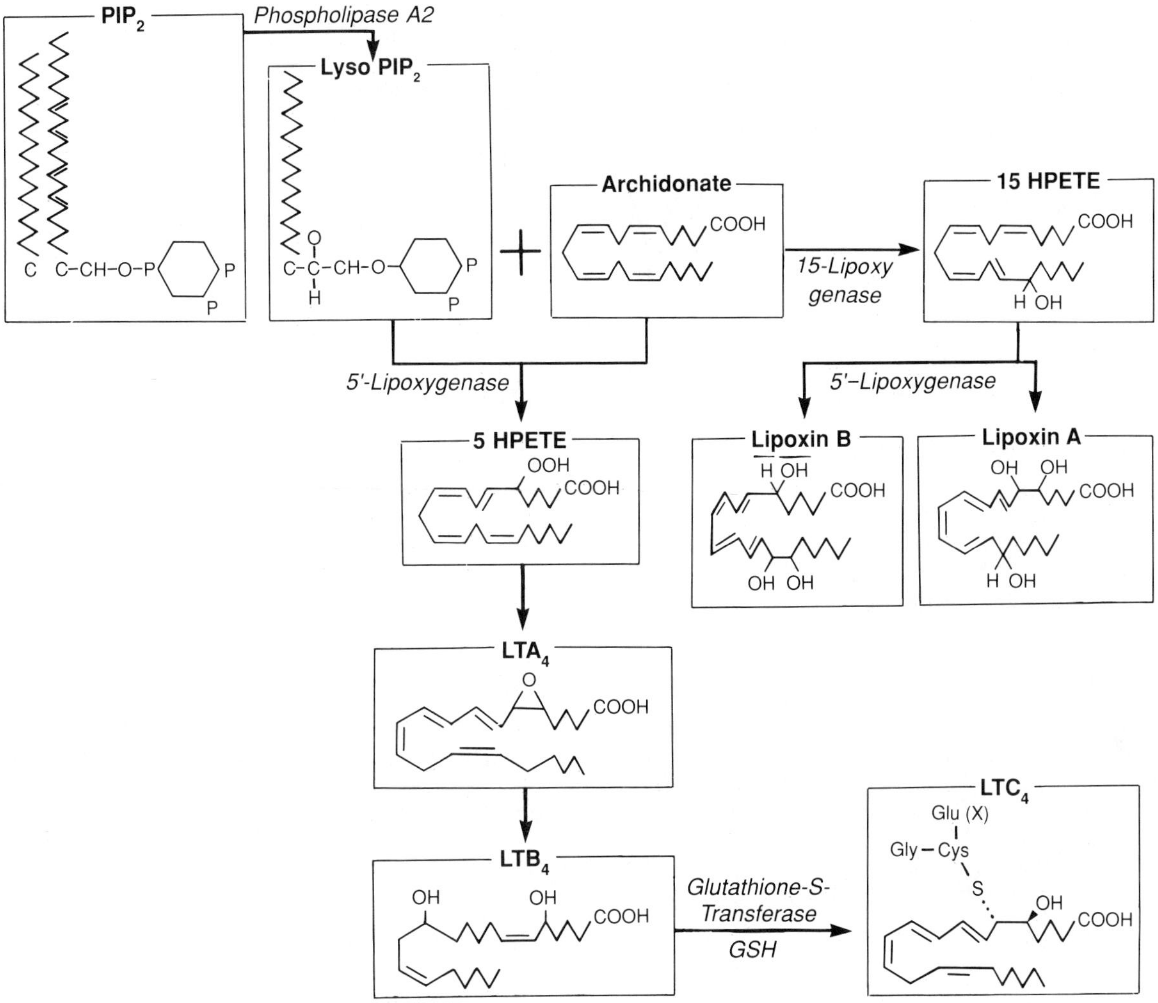

FIGURE 19-13. Biosynthesis of the leukotrienes.

effects on a variety of cells and tissues.[352] Its potency is such that when given intravenously to baboons in submilligram quantities, it is able to cause an immediate and highly lethal anaphylactic reaction.[353]

PAF is 1-O-alkyl-2-acetylglycero-3-phosphocholine, a phospholipid that bears a structural resemblance to the common phospholipid phosphatidylcholine. It is manufactured by both neutrophils and mononuclear phagocytes. In the principal route of PAF synthesis, lyso-PAF is formed by the release of arachidonate from 1-O-alkyl-2-arachidonylphosphatidylcholine, an abundant membrane lipid.[354,355] The lyso-PAF is then acylated with acetyl coenzyme A to yield the final product (Fig. 19-14). The release of arachidonic acid from the alkylacylphospholipid is accomplished by means of a Ca^{2+}-activated cytosolic phospholipase A_2,[356] whereas the subsequent acetylation is catalyzed by a highly specific membrane-associated acetyltransferase.[357]

The newly synthesized PAF is initially found in the membrane of the cell that produced it.[357,358] There, it is rapidly inactivated by removal of the acetate group and reacylation with long-chain fatty acids to regenerate alkylacylphosphatidylcholine, the starting material from which PAF was originally formed.[359,360] The fraction of PAF that is not inactivated is released over minutes into the extracellular medium, where it can act on other cells.

PAF is not manufactured by resting phagocytes[358,361] but only by phagocytes that have been suitably stimulated. A variety of agents induce PAF production by neutrophils, including opsonized zymosan, 5-HETE, LTB_4, FMLP, C5a, TNF, and PAF.[358,362–364] PAF production elicited by FMLP and C5a is greatly increased by prior exposure of the cells to GM-CSF.[365] Agents that stimulate PAF production by mononuclear phagocytes include opsonized zymosan and TNF.[361,362] PAF production in stimulated phagocytes appears to result from a rapid increase in acetyltransferase activity[361,363,366] combined with a decrease in the activity of acetylhydrolase, the enzyme that converts PAF to lyso-PAF.[363] Synthesis of PAF declines greatly as monocytes mature into macrophages, a feature ascribed to an increase in acetylhydrolase that occurs during the monocyte-to-macrophage transition.[367] As with leukotrienes, the biosynthesis of PAF is suppressed in subjects on diets containing large amounts of eicosapentaenoic acid.[368]

PAF has significant effects on phagocytes, binding to specific receptors to stimulate many functions directly[369,370] and priming the cells for augmented responses to other stimuli.[371,372] The ability of PAF to stimulate its own synthesis lends a self-reinforcing character to inflammatory processes in which this mediator is released.

Oxidases of Nitrogen

Certain cells are able to manufacture a number of oxides of nitrogen, including nitrite (NO_2^-), nitrate (NO_3^-), and the toxic radical nitric oxide (NO·). The production of NO was

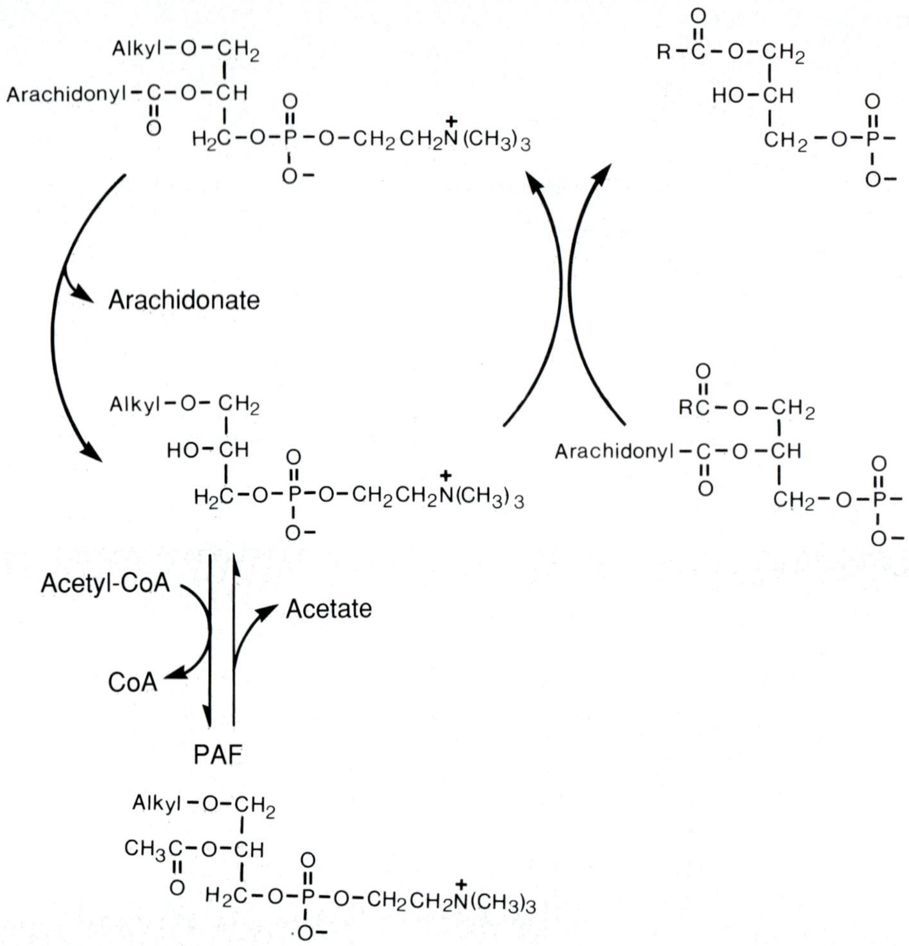

FIGURE 19-14. Biosynthesis of platelet-activating factor.

first demonstrated in endothelial cells, in which it was found to be identical to endothelium-derived relaxation factor, the short-lived vasodilator released by these cells on stimulation with cholinergic agents.[373,374] More recently, NO has been found to be generated by activated (ie, IFN-γ–treated) mononuclear phagocytes,[375] and in much smaller quantities, by neutrophils.[376,377] The production of NO by neutrophils is stimulated by several inflammatory mediators, including LTB_4, FMLP, and PAF.[377]

The biochemical source of NO is arginine; one of the guanidine nitrogens of arginine is oxidized, and the remainder of the molecule is converted to citrulline.[378,379] The oxidation of arginine to NO and citrulline is blocked by methotrexate, perhaps an explanation for the unexpected antiinflammatory effect of this drug. Once formed, the NO can exert its direct biologic effects.[380] Alternatively, it can be oxidized further to NO_2^- and NO_3^-[381,382] or destroyed by O_2^-.[383]

The principal known biologic effect of NO is its well-established ability to activate guanylate cyclase.[384,385] Its action on blood vessels appears to be mediated through this effect. As a highly reactive compound, NO is also a toxin, but only at much higher concentrations than occur normally in tissues. NO_2^- is also potentially dangerous because at low pH it can add to amino nitrogens to form carcinogenic nitrosamines[381,382]; the extent to which nitrosamines formed in this way are responsible for endogenous carcinogenesis is not known. NO_3^- is excreted in the urine, and its excretion increases greatly in infection,[386] perhaps a result of an increase in the rate of production of NO and its derivatives by macrophages activated by the cytokines (especially IFN-γ) released during infection.[387] Other biologic effects of these oxides of nitrogen likely will be discovered as this interesting group of compounds is further explored.

MICROBICIDAL OXIDANT PRODUCTION AND THE RESPIRATORY BURST

When exposed to appropriate stimuli, most phagocytes change their pattern of oxygen metabolism, increasing their oxygen uptake sharply and at the same time releasing large amounts of superoxide (O_2^-) and hydrogen peroxide (H_2O_2) into their environment. This change in oxygen metabolism, which usually lasts from a few seconds to 10 to 15 minutes, is known as the *respiratory burst*. Its purpose is the production of microbicidal oxidants by the partial reduction of oxygen. Mature PMNs and blood monocytes constitutively express the components required to engage in the respiratory burst in response to excitation of appropriate receptors. As monocytes mature into macrophages in vitro, they lose the capacity to have a respiratory burst unless exposed to the cytokine IFN-γ, although Kupffer cells do not develop a respiratory burst ability even after cultivation with IFN-γ. Considerable evidence indicates that the phenomenon of macrophage activation, in which these cells acquire the ability to contain or kill a variety of facultative intracellular parasites, depends on this development of a respiratory burst in response to IFN-γ.[243]

Respiratory Burst Oxidase

The key reaction of the respiratory burst is the one-electron reduction of oxygen to O_2^- at the expense of NADPH[388,389]:

$$2O_2 + NADPH \rightarrow 2O_2^- + NADP^+ + H^+$$

The O_2^- produced in this reaction serves as the precursor of a group of powerful microbicidal oxidants that are deployed by the phagocyte as microbicidal agents, whereas the $NADP^+$ is reconverted to NADPH by glucose-6-phosphate dehydrogenase and 6-phosphogluconate dehydrogenase, the first two enzymes of the hexosemonophosphate shunt. The increase in hexosemonophosphate shunt activity that occurs during the respiratory burst is detectable as an increase in CO_2 production from the six-carbon of glucose, a feature that has been used as a way of measuring the respiratory burst.[390]

The reduction of oxygen to O_2^- is catalyzed by a membrane-bound enzyme known as the respiratory burst oxidase.[391] This enzyme is dormant in resting cells but acquires catalytic activity when the cells are exposed to certain activating agents. A wide variety of agents are able to activate the oxidase, including particulate (eg, opsonized bacteria)[392] and soluble stimuli (eg, C5a)[393] or the FMLP intermediates of bacterial protein synthesis.[393,394] With agents whose association with the phagocyte can be reversed (eg, F^-, or N-formylpeptides), oxidase activation may also be reversed, the enzyme returning to the dormant state on removal of the activating agent.[395] With other activators, especially particulate agents, activation is irreversible; oxidase activated by these agents continues to manufacture O_2^- until the enzyme is eventually destroyed by its own products.[396]

The activation of the oxidase involves an assembly of components. The electron transporting oxidase is cytochrome b558, a membrane-associated complex of 90- and 20-kd polypeptides that binds heme and FAD. Its activity requires its binding to a number of initially cytosolic molecules that become membrane attached following activation. These molecules include two phosphoproteins, p47-*phox* and p67-*phox*, and two small GTP-binding proteins, Rac 2 and Rap 1A. During activation Rap 1A exchanges a bound GDP for GTP and Rac 2 dissociates from an inhibitor GDI and also exchanges bound GDP for GTP. Posttranslationally added isoprenyl groups are involved in the membrane binding of the two GTP-binding proteins.[396a–398]

Oxidase activity begins to decline, even with continued exposure to the activating agent, until by 1 week the cells are no longer able to express a respiratory burst. In other respects, however, the macrophages are at this point highly activated and well on their way to the epithelioid state. Macrophages are thus only transiently capable of expressing a respiratory burst, with oxidase activity appearing and disappearing during the first week of activation.

In cells containing a competent oxidase, O_2^- production is stimulated by a broad range of agents. Those that evoke the largest O_2^- responses are particulate stimuli such as opsonized bacteria and yeast cell walls.[196,392] Soluble stimuli such as immune complexes, C5a, FMLP, and leukotriene B_4 also elicit O_2^- production, but generally for a much shorter period of time than the particulate stimuli.[411] Neutrophils incubated with a substimulatory concentration of a soluble stimulus, however, produce much more O_2^- than usual when previously primed (discussed earlier).

Reactive Oxidants

The O_2^- produced in the respiratory burst has little antimicrobial activity of its own. Rather, it is the precursor of a complex battery of reactive oxidants that together represent the real microbicidal oxidizing power of the phagocyte. These reactive oxidants fall into two groups: the oxidized halogens and the oxidizing radicals.

The production of both groups of microbicidal oxidants begins with the dismutation of O_2^- to oxygen and H_2O_2:

$$2O_2^- \rightarrow O_2 + H_2O_2$$

Oxidized halogen production is then initiated by the H_2O_2-mediated oxidation of Cl^- to hypochlorite (OCl^-), a reaction catalyzed by MPO (described previously)[412,413]:

$$H_2O_2 + Cl^- \xrightarrow{MPO} OCl^- + H_2O$$

OCl^- itself is a powerful microbicidal agent. It also reacts with the many amines that occur in biologic systems, producing a vast number of chloramines[414,415]:

$$OCL^- + R\text{-}NH_2 \rightarrow R\text{-}NHCl + OH^-$$

$$OCl^- + R\text{-}NHCl \rightarrow R\text{-}NCl_2 + OH^-$$

Some of these chloramines, especially those that are lipid-soluble (eg, NH_2Cl), are even more toxic than OCl^-; others such as taurine chloramine are stable and may furnish protection for the phagocyte against the potentially lethal products of its own metabolism.[416] The reactive oxidized halogens then kill by inactivating proteins and other susceptible molecules in the target through oxidation and halogenation. Iron-sulfur proteins are particularly liable to inactivation by oxidized halogens.[417]

The production of oxidizing radicals is generally ascribed to the Haber-Weiss reaction, in which a metal ion (iron or copper) catalyzes the oxidation of O_2^- by H_2O_2, yielding oxygen and hydroxyl radical ($OH\cdot$).[418,419] For example:

$$O_2^- + Fe^{3+} \rightarrow O_2 + Fe^{2+}$$

$$H_2O_2 + Fe^{2+} \rightarrow OH\cdot + Fe^{3+} + OH^-$$

$$O_2^- + H_2O_2 \rightarrow OH\cdot + O_2 + OH^-$$

Other oxidizing radicals are manufactured by phagocytes, but radicals other than $OH\cdot$ have not been specifically identified as yet, nor have their routes of production been elucidated. The oxidizing radicals provide a backup system to the oxidized halogens, killing less rapidly but just as efficiently as the oxidized halogens. One particularly important target of hydroxyl radicals is the bases comprising DNA.[420] Phagocyte-induced DNA damage may account in part for the association between chronic inflammation and malignancy.[421]

Antioxidant Defenses

Like other cells, phagocytes are equipped with systems that destroy the highly reactive oxidants that arise in the course of the cells' activity. These include enzymes and low-molecular-weight antioxidants.

Antioxidant Enzymes

Phagocytes contain antioxidant enzymes that can destroy O_2^- and H_2O_2, the two compounds that together represent the ultimate source of all the microbicidal oxidants deployed in the respiratory burst.

Superoxide Dismutase. Superoxide dismutase catalyzes a reaction in which one molecule of O_2^- is reduced by another, converting the two O_2^- molecules into H_2O_2 and oxygen, respectively:[422]

$$2O_2^- + 2H^+ \rightarrow O_2 + H_2O_2$$

This enzyme is present in virtually all prokaryotic and eukaryotic cells,[423] where it protects them from the deleterious effects of O_2^-. Its importance in antioxidant defense has been best shown in *E coli* dismutase-less mutants, which grow poorly in the presence of oxygen and are highly susceptible to further mutation.[424] Phagocytes, like most mammalian cells, contain two forms of the dismutase: a copper- and zinc-containing enzyme that is found in the cytosol and a manganese-containing enzyme located in the mitochondria.[425] These enzymes protect the cells from the O_2^- routinely generated in the course of mitochondrial oxygen metabolism and from the O_2^- that leaks back into the cytoplasm during the respiratory burst. Not surprisingly, the phagosomes containing the target organisms are free of phagocyte superoxide dismutase.

Glutathione Peroxidase–Glutathione Reductase System. In this system, glutathione and the enzymes glutathione peroxidase and glutathione reductase catalyze the reduction of H_2O_2 to H_2O using NADPH as electron donor.[426,427] The first step in this system is the reduction of H_2O_2 to H_2O by glutathione, a reaction catalyzed by glutathione peroxidase, a selenium-containing enzyme. Glutathione peroxidase is the only selenium-containing enzyme known to occur in mammalian cells[428] and appears to explain the requirement for selenium in the human diet:

$$2GSH + H_2O_2 \xrightarrow{\text{GSH peroxidase}} GSSG + H_2O$$

where:
GSH = reduced glutathione and
GSSG = oxidized glutathione

In the second step, the oxidized glutathione is converted back to the reduced form by NADPH in a reaction catalyzed by glutathione peroxidase:

$$GSSG + NADPH + H^+ \xrightarrow{\text{GSH reductase}} 2GSH + NADP^+$$

Because glutathione peroxidase has a high turnover number, the glutathione peroxidase–glutathione reductase system is an efficient scavenger of H_2O_2, eliminating it even when it is present at low concentrations.[429] Lipid hydroperoxides, readily formed in biologic systems by the autoxidation of polyunsaturated fatty acids, are also detoxified by this system through the ability of glutathione peroxidase to use organic hydroperoxides as substrates[430]:

$$2GSH + ROOH \xrightarrow{\text{GSH peroxidase}} GSSG + ROH + H_2O$$

Catalase. Catalase is a large heme-containing protein that catalyzes the conversion of H_2O_2 to oxygen and water[431]:

$$2H_2O_2 \rightarrow O_2 + 2H_2O$$

The enzyme is found in the cytoplasm of phagocytes and other cells. It has a high turnover number, but under the usual assay conditions, it also shows a high K_m (ie, a low affinity) for its substrate[432] and therefore has been thought to be specialized for handling large peroxide fluxes that result in high steady-state concentrations of H_2O_2.[433] Catalase, however, possesses a tightly bound NADPH that prevents inactivation of the enzyme by H_2O_2.[434] It is therefore likely that under physiologic conditions, catalase is able to deal effectively with H_2O_2 even at the relatively low concentrations that are likely to prevail in tissues.

A few families have been reported whose tissues contain very low levels of catalase. Members of these families show little pathology except for oral ulcerations.[435] The lack of unusual susceptibility to bacterial infections in patients with acatalasemia indicates that the glutathione peroxidase–glutathione reductase system alone is sufficient to protect the phagocytes from the peroxide stress to which they are normally exposed.

Low-Molecular-Weight Antioxidants

The major low-molecular-weight oxidants found in the neutrophil are ascorbic acid, taurine, and α-tocopherol. In the form of dehydroascorbate, ascorbic acid is actively transported into the cytosol of the phagocyte, where it is found in high concentrations. It is highly effective as an antioxidant[436] and is probably the principal scavenger of reactive radicals in the phagocyte cytosol. Taurine, also present in phagocytes in high concentrations, reacts readily with OCl^- to form the relatively stable taurine chloramine ($=O_3S-CH_2CH_2-NHCl$), protecting the phagocyte from the harmful effects of OCl^- and at the same time providing a relatively long-lived source of oxidized halogen.[414]

α-Tocopherol (vitamin E) is a lipid-soluble antioxidant that is found in the organelles and plasma membranes of the phagocytes.[437] It reacts rapidly with oxidizing radicals[438] and, like ascorbate, serves as a primary radical scavenger, but in lipid rather than aqueous environments.[436,439,440] In neonates and infants, α-tocopherol deficiency causes a hemolytic anemia that appears to arise because of oxidant damage to the red-cell membrane (see Chap. 58).

Methods for Measuring Components of Phagocytic Oxygen Metabolism

Myeloperoxidase activity of phagocytes is easily determined histochemically on air-dried blood smears. The respiratory burst requires isolation and appropriate stimulation of phagocytic cells and is quantifiable by detection of oxygen consumption; reduction of nitroblue tetrazolium (NBT) or cytochrome *c* by superoxide released from the cells; scopoletin oxidation by released hydrogen peroxide; or oxidation of ^{14}C-1-glucose through the hexose monophosphate shunt, which is activated by the detoxification of hydrogen peroxide, as described previously. In the clinical laboratory, a histochemical application of NBT reduction is easy to perform and is described later as the diagnostic test for chronic granulomatous disease (CGD).

DISORDERS OF THE OXYGEN-DEPENDENT MICROBICIDAL SYSTEM

Myeloperoxidase Deficiency

Myeloperoxidase deficiency is the most common inherited disorder of phagocytes. Its estimated prevalence is about 1 in 2000,[441–443] but only a small number of MPO-deficient patients are clinically ill from the disease.

Pathogenesis

Inherited MPO deficiency has been shown to be caused by any of several mutations affecting the MPO gene. In five unrelated patients, the genetic defects resulted in a post-translational processing abnormality because pro-MPO was detected in their phagocytes but MPO was not. Restriction maps of the MPO genes from these patients gave three different fragment patterns.[444] Cells from a sixth patient contained neither MPO, pro-MPO, nor processed MPO mRNA, although unprocessed message was detected.[445] These findings suggest the existence of at least four different kinds of genetic lesions in patients with MPO deficiency.

The deficiency of the enzyme can be partial or complete; the aggregate ratio of partial to complete deficiency in two recent series was about 3:1.[442,443] In terms of neutrophil function, MPO-deficient cells show normal phagocytosis,[443,446] but the respiratory burst is significantly altered. O_2^- and H_2O_2 production are increased in amount and duration[447,448] probably because the usual MPO-mediated inactivation of the respiratory burst oxidase is retarded,[396] but OCl^- production is low to nil depending on the level of residual MPO. Killing of bacteria (*S aureus, E coli*) by MPO-deficient phagocytes, although significantly retarded at early times, reaches normal values by 1 hour.[449–451] On the other hand, certain fungi that are readily killed by normal neutrophils, such as the hyphal stages of *C albicans* and *Aspergillus fumigatus*, are highly resistant to killing by MPO-deficient cells.[443,450,452,453]

MPO deficiency can also be an acquired condition. It is a frequent accompaniment of myeloproliferative disorders (discussed later). In newborns, neutrophil MPO levels are normal at birth, fall by 75% after 1 to 2 days, then return to normal levels at 1 week.[454]

Clinical Features

Most patients with MPO deficiency suffer no ill effects from their condition. This fact attests to the redundancy of the microbicidal mechanisms of phagocytes, which include oxidizing radicals and several microbicidal proteins in addition to the MPO-dependent microbicidal agents. In those rare patients in whom MPO deficiency results in clinical disease, the most frequent manifestation has been disseminated candidiasis, usually in patients who also have diabetes mellitus.[443,450,455] A few other patients have been described in whom MPO deficiency has been associated with recurrent bacterial infections, most frequently skin infections, sometimes combined with *Candida* infections of the perianal region.[167,456–458] It is not known why this small minority of MPO-deficient patients is so susceptible to infections, although mixed defects in phagocyte function have been postulated.[167,456]

Diagnosis

The diagnosis is made by demonstrating that peroxidase in the neutrophils and monocytes is deficient or absent. This can be accomplished by a spectrophotometric assay or by staining a blood film for MPO; the latter is probably better because eosinophil peroxidase, a distinct enzyme that is unaltered in MPO deficiency,[459] can be a source of confusion in a spectrophotometric assay but does not affect an assay in which the peroxidase-positive cells are individually identified. MPO deficiency can also be diagnosed using the Hemalog D automated blood counter, which employs an MPO stain as a means of identifying neutrophils. With this instrument, MPO-deficient neutrophils are recorded as large, unidentified cells. Through screening with the Hemalog D, the surprisingly high prevalence of asymptomatic MPO deficiency was established.[441,443]

Treatment

Because MPO deficiency is a silent abnormality in most patients, treatment is usually not necessary. In those few patients with recurrent infections, management is based on the usual measures of vigorous antibiotic therapy and drainage of abscesses as indicated. If recurrent bacterial infections are a problem, prophylactic antibiotics may be tried, but these are of no value for the prevention of fungal infections. In patients with diabetes mellitus, control of blood glucose levels should be optimized.

Chronic Granulomatous Disease

Chronic granulomatous disease is an inherited disorder in which phagocytes are unable to express a respiratory burst. As a result, all oxygen-dependent microbial killing is ablated, and patients suffer recurrent infections that eventually lead to chronic organ pathology and an early death.[460–462]

Pathogenesis

Chronic granulomatous disease results when the respiratory burst oxidase or its activating apparatus is defective. Four types of CGD have been described, each caused by an abnormality affecting one of the four oxidase polypeptides identified to date. The most common type of CGD, accounting for about two thirds of reported cases,[401,459] is due to an abnormality involving the 91-kd subunit of the cytochrome. Phagocytes from most patients with this type lack cytochrome b_{558}.[404,463] The gene encoding the 91-kd subunit is on the X chromosome,[464] so transmission of this type of the disease is X-linked. Most of the remaining patients lack the 47-kd phosphoprotein.[401] In these patients, the disease is inherited as an autosomal recessive trait, and cytochrome b_{558} is present. A few patients have been described in whom the primary lesion affects the 67-kd cytosolic polypeptide or the 22-kd subunit of the cytochrome.[400,465–467] These rare types of CGD are transmitted according to an autosomal recessive pattern. Cytochrome b_{558} is present in neutrophils deficient in the 67-kd polypeptide and absent from neutrophils lacking the 22-kd subunit. In each of the cytochrome b_{558}–deficient types of CGD, both cytochrome subunits are missing[466,467] possibly because in the absence of one subunit the other is unstable and is destroyed by intracellular proteases. The various types of CGD are summarized in Table 19-9.

In the X chromosome, the gene encoding the 91-kd subunit is located on the short arm at Xp21.1. Nearby are other genes that, when defective, result in clinical abnormalities, and several patients have been reported with multiple diseases caused by an abnormality that simultaneously affects two or more of these genes. The most common inherited disorder associated with CGD is the McLeod phenotype, a condition that results from a deficiency of the K_x antigen, a precursor of the Kell blood group antigen family.[468,469] K_x, encoded by a gene that is closely linked to the 91-kd gene on the X-chromosome, is normally found on the surfaces of RBCs and phagocytes but is missing from one or both in most patients with X-linked CGD.[470,471] Its absence from

TABLE 19-9. Types of Chronic Granulomatous Disease

Mode of Inheritance	Status of Cytochrome b-558	Deficient Components*	Abnormal Gene
X-linked	Absent	p22 and gp91	*gp91*
X-linked	Present	gp91 (his → pro)	*gp91* (missense)
Autosomal recessive	Absent	p22 and gp91	*p22*
Autosomal recessive	Present	p47	*p47*
Autosomal recessive	Present	p67	*p67*

* Cytochrome b-558 is a membrane-associated component made up of gp91 and p22, whereas p47 and p67 are found in the cytosol; p47 is phosphorylated during oxidase activation.

the RBCs results in a mild hemolytic anemia. Inherited disorders less frequently combined with CGD include retinitis pigmentosa and Duchenne's muscular dystrophy. Combinations of X-linked CGD, the McLeod phenotype, and retinitis pigmentosa, with or without Duchenne's muscular dystrophy, have been reported in unfortunate patients with small deletions involving the Xp21 locus.[472–473]

The motor functions of CGD neutrophils (chemotaxis, phagocytosis, and degranulation) are normal. Respiratory burst activity, however, is grossly deficient, whether determined as O_2^- production, H_2O_2 production, or oxygen uptake, and whether measured in neutrophils, monocytes, or eosinophils. Because they are unable to produce microbicidal oxidants, neutrophils from patients with CGD have great difficulty killing most species of bacteria, including *S aureus* and *Enterobacteriaceae* sp. Fungal killing is also defective. CGD neutrophils, however, have no problem with catalaseless organisms such as *S pneumoniae* and *S pyogenes*, in part perhaps because these bacteria excrete H_2O_2 into the surrounding medium, thereby providing the defective neutrophils with the OCl^- precursor they cannot produce.

Clinical Features

Recurrent infection beginning in infancy is the major clinical manifestation of CGD,[474–476] although in mild cases, the presentation may be delayed until adolescence or even adulthood.[477,478] Infections usually take the form of abscesses involving deep subcutaneous tissues, lymph nodes, or liver or serious respiratory tract infections involving the sinuses or lungs. They are long-lasting and respond only sluggishly to antibiotic therapy. Because these repeated infections lead to chronic activation of the immune system, most patients with CGD also manifest generalized lymphadenopathy, sometimes prominent, as well as enlarged livers and spleens.[474]

The organism found most frequently in these infections is *S aureus*, but infections due to enterobacteria[476,479] and certain fungi (*Aspergillus* sp in particular)[480–482] are also common. Infections with unusual microorganisms, however, are also to be expected.[483–485] In particular, *Pseudomonas cepacia* infections, rare under other circumstances, are characteristic of CGD perhaps because this species may be unusually resistant to the anaerobic mechanisms that represent the residual microbicidal capacity of CGD phagocytes. Mycobacterial infections also occur at a greater-than-normal frequency, and death at an early age from miliary tuberculosis has been described. On the other hand, infections with streptococci (including pneumococci) are not a problem, a clinical reflection of the ability of CGD cells to kill bacteria of this genus.

In addition to abscesses and other acute infections, patients with CGD also develop chronic inflammatory processes, probably the result of granulomatous reactions and fibrosis in the neighborhood of imperfectly suppressed infections.[476,486] These inflammatory processes may lead to masses and strictures affecting a variety of hollow organs, including the stomach,[487] intestine, ureter, and bladder (Fig. 19-15). Recurrent vomiting may suggest gastric obstruction, whereas a patient with obstruction of the urogenital tract

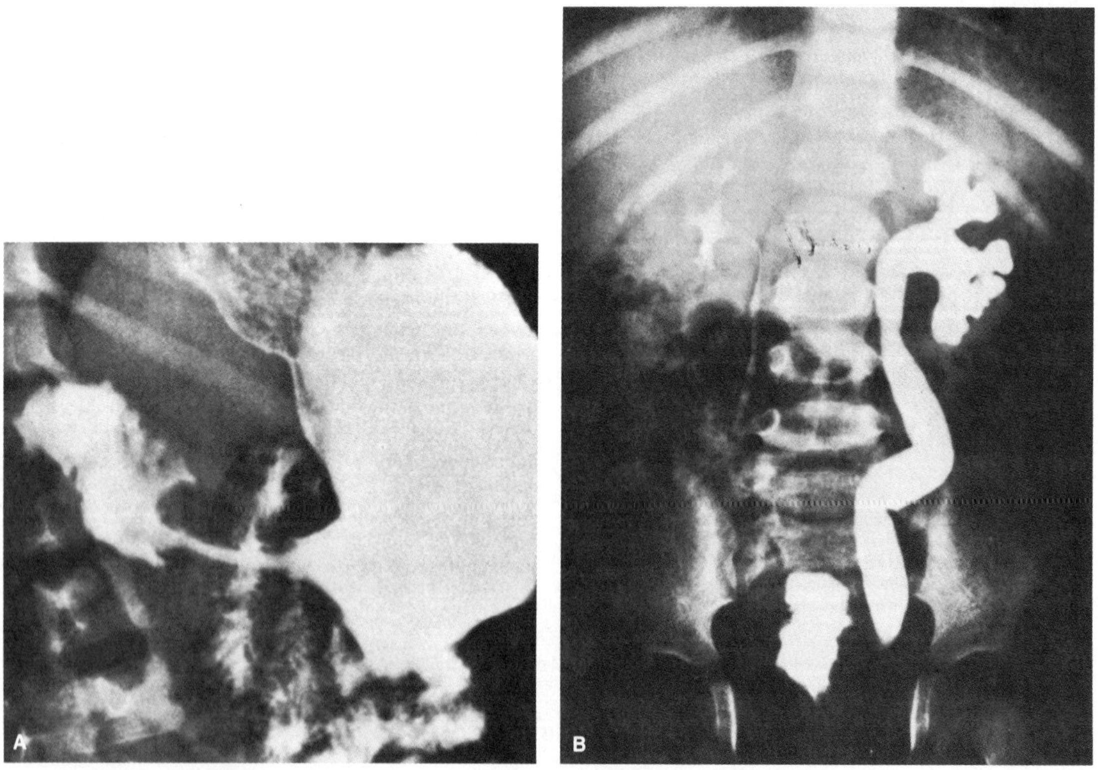

FIGURE 19-15. Some complications of chronic granulomatous disease (CGD). **(A)** Gastric antral lesion. Characteristic roentgenographic appearance of the gastric antral lesion in a 4-year-old boy with X-linked CGD who presented with persistent vomiting. A concentric prepyloric narrowing was associated with delayed gastric emptying. Biopsy of the lesion revealed granulomatous inflammation. Cultures for bacteria and fungi were negative. The patient was managed conservatively with small frequent feedings. The lesion spontaneously improved over 1 year. **(B)** Obstructive uropathy. Intravenous pyelogram of a boy with X-linked CGD demonstrating hydronephrosis and hydroureter on the left side. The obstruction was due to compression by a large inflammatory mass in the pelvis between the rectum and the bladder.

may present with symptoms of chronic cystitis or pyelonephritis. Intractable chronic pulmonary inflammation leads through bronchiectasis and emphysema to the eventual destruction of the lung. With the recent practice of treating these patients with prophylactic antibiotics, these chronic processes have become more common. In addition, *Aspergillus* sp pneumonia has become a frequent cause of death in these patients as their incidence of acute bacterial infections has declined.

Diagnosis

The diagnosis of CGD is usually made by means of the NBT test.[488] In this test, neutrophils are incubated with an activating agent in the presence of NBT, a yellow dye that is readily soluble in water. The O_2^- liberated from the activated neutrophils reduces the dye to an insoluble dark blue formazan that is deposited on the activated cells as a granular precipitate, easily seen under the microscope (Fig. 19-16*A*). Because they are unable to manufacture O_2^-, neutrophils from patients with CGD form no formazan precipitate when activated in the presence of NBT (see Fig. 19-16*B*). Appropriate radiologic examinations are employed to identify the abscesses and obstructive complications that occur frequently in patients with CGD.

Female carriers of the X-linked type of CGD can be identified by the NBT test. Because of random X-chromosome inactivation, the gene encoding the *normal* 91-kd subunit is expressed in about half the neutrophils of such a carrier, whereas the gene encoding the *defective* subunit is expressed in the remainder of the cells. Therefore, the NBT test shows two populations of neutrophils in a carrier of X-linked CGD: a normal population that reduces NBT and an abnormal population that does not (see Fig. 19-16C). Although the diagnosis of CGD can also be made by measuring O_2^- production, H_2O_2 production, oxygen uptake, or hexosemonophosphate shunt activity (assayed as the release of $^{14}CO_2$ from glucose-1-^{14}C) in activated neutrophils, the NBT test is generally used because of its simplicity and its ability to detect the carrier state.

Prenatal diagnosis can be made by performing an NBT test on blood obtained at fetoscopy.[489] It is necessary to wait until the 18th week of pregnancy to obtain fetal blood by this procedure, which carries a small but distinct risk of fetal loss. The recent report of a restriction fragment length polymorphism involving the gene encoding the 91-kd subunit of cytochrome b_{558} offers the promise that, in at least some instances, prenatal diagnosis of the X-linked form of CGD can be made by restriction mapping of fetal DNA obtained by the much less hazardous procedure of amniocentesis.

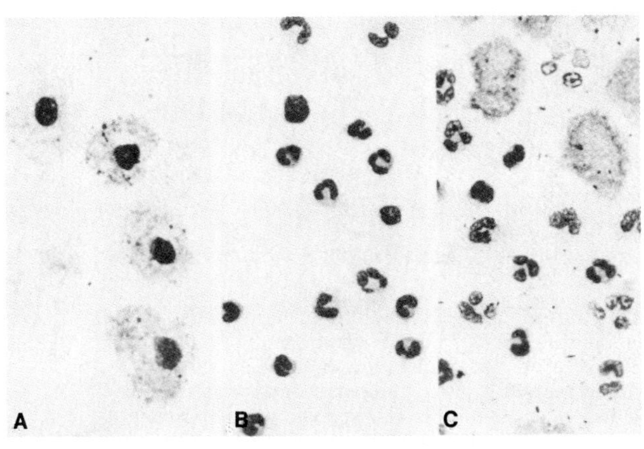

FIGURE 19-16. Nitroblue tetrazolium (NBT) test for the diagnosis of chronic granulomatous disease (CGD). A drop of blood is placed on an endotoxin-coated coverslip and incubated to allow the granulocytes and monocytes to adhere to the glass surface. The coverslip is then incubated with a solution of serum and NBT dye, then washed, fixed, counterstained, and mounted. (**A**) Normal control. All the neutrophils are NBT-positive, appearing as large, exploded cells with cytoplasm stained blue by reduced NBT. (**B**) Patient with CGD. All the neutrophils are NBT-negative. They retain their typical morphologic appearance and show no blue (reduced) dye. (**C**) Carrier of CGD. Two populations of cells coexist, one NBT-positive and the other NBT-negative.

The only other condition in which the respiratory burst may be impaired enough to affect microbial killing is severe glucose-6-phosphate dehydrogenase (G6PD) deficiency. A few patients with G6PD deficiency have displayed a CGD-like picture, presenting with recurrent bacterial infections and a greatly diminished respiratory burst.[490–495] It is likely that in the neutrophils of these patients, G6PD levels were so low that NADPH production was severely curtailed, leading to a failure of O_2^- generation because of a deficiency of reducing agent. The clue that the disease responsible for the recurrent infections in this group of patients was something other than CGD was the simultaneous existence in each of the patients of a hemolytic anemia, a feature that is typical of G6PD deficiency but not of CGD. The diagnosis is easily made by measuring red-cell G6PD levels.

Treatment

As with other disorders of phagocyte function, the treatment of CGD mainly involves the prevention and treatment of the infections that complicate the disorder. Prophylactic antibiotics have been shown to reduce inpatient days and prolong life expectancy in patients with CGD[476,496,497] and are employed routinely in this and other disorders of phagocyte function. The usual program is similar to that used for Chédiak-Higashi disease: trimethoprim, 160 mg/d, plus sulfamethoxazole, 800 mg/d, with a reduced dose for children; or, for patients allergic to sulfonamides or trimethoprim, dicloxacillin, 500 mg (250 mg for children) twice daily. When infections occur, vigorous therapy must be applied using large doses of appropriate antibiotics. Surgery may be required to drain collections.[498,499] Although relief of obstructions may require surgery,[499] such obstructions may gradually resolve under long-term antibiotic therapy to treat the underlying infection, plus or minus steroids; the choice between medical and surgical therapy for such a complication can be difficult. Granulocyte transfusions have been employed as adjunct therapy, but with equivocal results.[499,500] Bone marrow transplantation has cured some patients with CGD, but some patients have died as a result of the procedure.

Reports that O_2^- production, cytochrome b_{558} content, and bacterial killing by both normal and CGD neutrophils could be increased by treating the cells with recombinant IFN-γ[501,502] led to considerable interest in the possible use of IFN-γ in the treatment of CGD. A multicenter placebo-controlled clinical trial of 128 patients with X-linked or autosomal CGD led to the conclusion that recombinant IFN-γ, 50 $\mu g/m^2$ subcutaneously three times per week, was well tolerated and reduced the number of serious infections by about half. Despite the clinical benefits, none of the IFN-treated patients' phagocytes showed any improvement in respiratory activity.[503]

Miscellaneous Granulocyte Abnormalities

Morphologic Variants

Inherited. There are a few inherited conditions in which normally functioning neutrophils show well-defined morphologic abnormalities.

Pelger-Huët Anomaly. The Pelger-Huët anomaly is an inherited trait in which the nuclei in most neutrophils of heterozygotes are hyposegmented, having only one or two lobes instead of the usual three to five.[504,505] In Pelger-Huët homozygotes, neutrophil nuclei are uniformly unsegmented[504] (Fig. 19-17*A*). The incidence of this trait has been estimated at 1 in 5000.[504,505] Pelger-Huët neutrophils are normal in size and show fully condensed chromatin, features that serve to distinguish them from normal neutrophil precursors such as myelocytes and metamyelocytes. The function of Pelger-Huët neutrophils is entirely normal, and the trait is of no clinical significance.[504,506]

An acquired Pelger-Huët anomaly, usually termed *pseudo–Pelger-Huët,* has been reported in a remarkably large number of conditions.[507] Most frequently seen in disorders of myeloid stem cells,[508] it has also been described inter alia in infections such as tuberculosis,[509] mycoplasma pneumonia,[510] allergic reactions,[511] and lymphoid malignancies.[512,513]

May-Hegglin Anomaly. The May-Hegglin anomaly is a rare but dominantly inherited trait affecting neutrophils and platelets. On a Wright-stained blood film, most of the neutrophils are seen to contain small homogeneous blue inclusions (Döhle bodies) that actually represent aggregates of RNA (see Fig. 19-17*B*). The platelets are abnormally large (as large as in Bernard-Soulier disease) and hypogranular, the platelet counts are low, and platelet survival is shortened by about half.[514] In about half of cases, the May-Hegglin anomaly is associated with a bleeding disorder,[515] usually mild (epistaxis, bruising)[516–518] but sometimes more serious. The bleeding time is prolonged to a value consistent with the reduced platelet count, but platelet function studies have been variable.[517–519] The May-Hegglin anomaly has also been reported in a few patients with hereditary nephritis (Alport's syndrome)[519,520]; the term *Fechtner's syndrome* has been used to refer to this combination of Alport's nephritis and May-Hegglin anomaly.

Alder-Reilly Anomaly. Alder-Reilly bodies are deeply basophilic granules that are sometimes seen in neutrophils from patients with disorders of mucopolysaccharide degradation (eg, Hunter's, Hurler's, and Maroteaux-Lamy syndromes; see Fig. 19-17*C*). These granules may also be present in lymphocytes and monocytes. Although often absent from circulating leukocytes, Alder-Reilly bodies can usually be found in the marrow, where they appear as darkly staining granules in mononuclear cells (Buhot cells). Alder-Reilly bodies appear to be lysosomes that stain abnormally due to their content of incompletely degraded mucopolysaccharides.

Toxic Phagocytes. Circulating neutrophils from patients with a variety of inflammatory conditions can show characteristic morphologic changes (see Fig. 19-17*D*). These include cytoplasmic vacuoles, Döhle bodies, and toxic granules. Döhle bodies appear as greenish inclusions on Wright-stained smears, and electron micrographs reveal them to be aggregates of rough endoplasmic reticulum.[521] Toxic granules are azurophilic granules that do not appear stained in normal neutrophils. Because of a degree of immaturity of neutrophils produced in response to inflammatory demands, however, the mucopolysaccharide content of the toxic neutrophils is increased, causing them to appear as dark dots in the cytoplasm.[522] They do not take on the deep violet hue of azurophilic granules seen in the normal promyelocyte.

The toxic changes seen in neutrophils are nonspecific in that they are often associated with, but do not necessarily reflect, the presence of bacterial infections.[523] From a functional standpoint, toxic neutrophils appear "primed" and excited. They have abnormally high resting rates of oxygen consumption, reactive oxygen metabolite release, and sur-

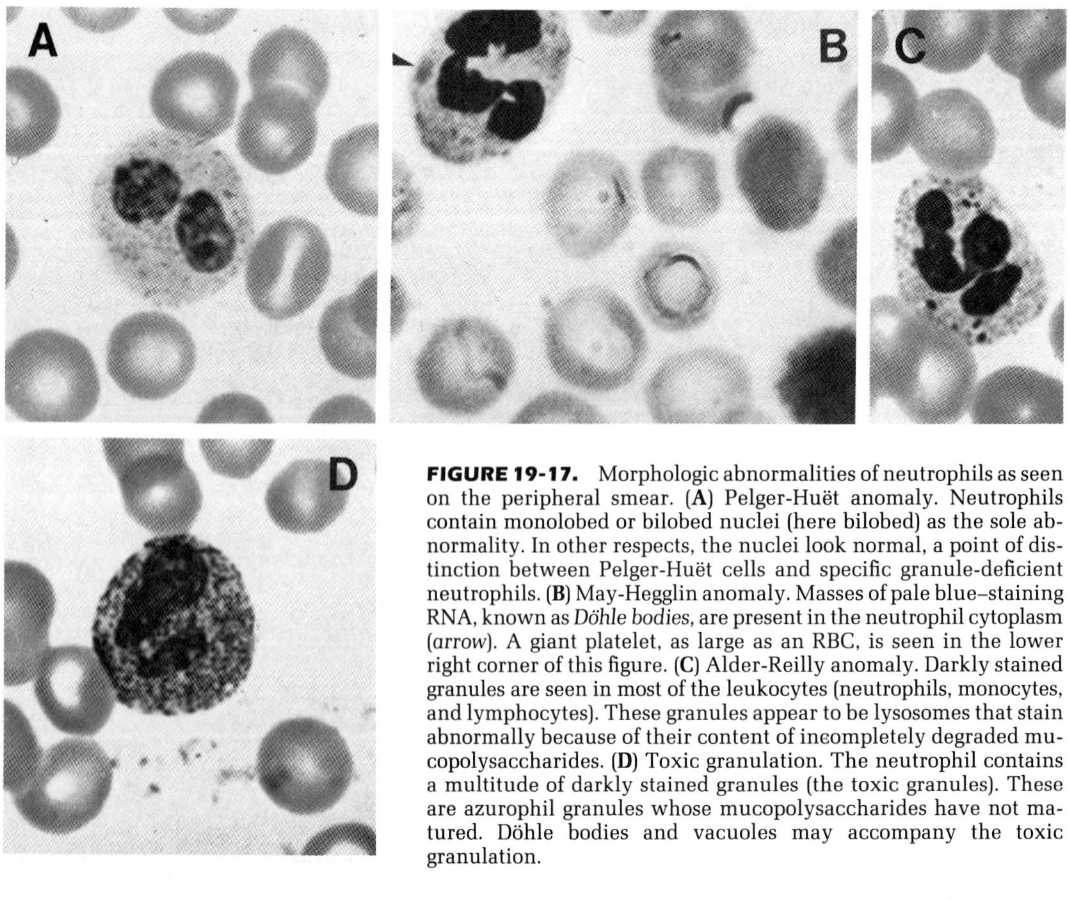

FIGURE 19-17. Morphologic abnormalities of neutrophils as seen on the peripheral smear. (**A**) Pelger-Huët anomaly. Neutrophils contain monolobed or bilobed nuclei (here bilobed) as the sole abnormality. In other respects, the nuclei look normal, a point of distinction between Pelger-Huët cells and specific granule-deficient neutrophils. (**B**) May-Hegglin anomaly. Masses of pale blue–staining RNA, known as *Döhle bodies,* are present in the neutrophil cytoplasm (*arrow*). A giant platelet, as large as an RBC, is seen in the lower right corner of this figure. (**C**) Alder-Reilly anomaly. Darkly stained granules are seen in most of the leukocytes (neutrophils, monocytes, and lymphocytes). These granules appear to be lysosomes that stain abnormally because of their content of incompletely degraded mucopolysaccharides. (**D**) Toxic granulation. The neutrophil contains a multitude of darkly stained granules (the toxic granules). These are azurophil granules whose mucopolysaccharides have not matured. Döhle bodies and vacuoles may accompany the toxic granulation.

face expression of Fc and complement receptors. They also may have reduced contents of granule enzymes. These changes presumably represent exposure of the neutrophils to bacteria or to microbial products such as LPS endotoxin. Toxic neutrophils appear to characterize neutrophils that are in a state of heightened responsiveness to an infection, but whether neutrophils in such a condition in the circulation can get to the source of infection is unclear.

In patients with rheumatoid arthritis, neutrophils may contain amorphous eosinophilic material, presumably representing ingested rheumatoid factor immune complexes. Such neutrophils, as well as those from patients with systemic lupus erythematosus, another immune complex disorder, reportedly have reduced antimicrobial functional activity. Whether these abnormalities are of clinical importance is not clear.

Monocytes from patients with infections or with other inflammatory conditions may also appear abnormal. They tend to resemble macrophages on Wright-stained smears in that they are larger than monocytes; they have a rounder, more eccentric nucleus with more condensed chromatin than monocyte nuclei; and, rather than the characteristic gray hue of the monocyte cytoplasm, they have a bluish tinge with prominent azurophilic cytoplasmic granules.

Myelodysplasia and Myeloproliferative Disorders. Neutrophils and neutrophil precursors derived from abnormal stem cells frequently show morphologic abnormalities. These may include pseudo Pelger-Huët changes in the nucleus,[508,524–526] an agranular appearance due to loss of the specific granules,[526] and loss of stainable MPO on the blood film.[527,528] These abnormalities may be seen in any stem cell disorder: aplastic anemia, myeloid metaplasia, and acute and chronic myelogenous leukemia. They are perhaps most characteristic of myelodysplasia, where their presence indicates clinically significant involvement of the myeloid series, a finding that places the disorder into the *excess blasts* or the *chronic myelomonocytic leukemia* category. PMNs from patients with chronic myelogenous leukemia have, in addition to low or absent alkaline phosphatase activity (see Chap. 15), moderately reduced locomotion, phagocytosis, and oxidant release in response to excitation.[529–531] These functional abnormalities detectable in vitro do not appear to predispose patients with this disease to pyogenic infection so long as they have normal or high peripheral blood neutrophil counts.

Phagocytes in Atherosclerosis

It is believed that MNPs play an important role in atherogenesis[532] (Fig. 19-18). The first event is invasion of the arterial endothelial lining by monocytes. The monocytes enter the arterial wall, where they mature into macrophages.[533,534] Cholesterol-rich low-density lipoprotein (LDL) and β very-low-density lipoprotein (VLDL) filtered from the lumen into the artery can be modified in at least two ways by resident MNPs: the respiratory burst oxidase may oxidize the lipids; and malonyldialdehyde, a product of MNP arachidonate peroxidation, can alkylate them. Such altered lipids have been shown to be chemotactic for monocytes, thereby accelerating influx of offending MNPs.[535] Modified lipids are also taken up by the scavenger receptor of MNPs. MNPs also endocytose hypertriglyceridemic VLDL and atypical dys-β LDL through the LDL receptor.[508,536] Lipoprotein-derived cholesterol is esterified in MNPs by arylcoenzyme A; cholesterol acyltransferase[537] and cholesterol esters accumulate in vacuoles, producing characteristic foam cells of the atherosclerotic fatty streak. Foam cell formation is reversible in that MNP-derived apolipoprotein E can abstract free cholesterol from MNPs when it becomes incorporated into high-density lipoprotein, which transports it to the liver. Stimulated by the ingestion of fatty particles and fatty conjugates with extracellular matrix, MNPs secrete their effector products, which damage the arterial cells. MNPs also release growth factors in this setting, which causes migration and proliferation of fibroblasts and smooth muscle cells. The result is the mature proliferating and ulcerated atherosclerotic lesion, which promotes thrombosis and ischemic disease.[538–540]

Phagocytes and the Immune Response

Mononuclear phagocytes play a central role as antigen-presenting cells in the immune response. MNPs internalize and degrade antigens into fragments that recycle by vesicular transport to the plasma membrane. This recycling of antigens may occur within a novel endosome pathway in which cathepsin D (aspartyl protease) partially degrades intravesicular proteins but does not fuse with lysosomes, thereby escaping total annihilation.[541] Once returned to the external cell surface, partially hydrolyzed antigens bind class II HLA, and the HLA complex interacts with the an-

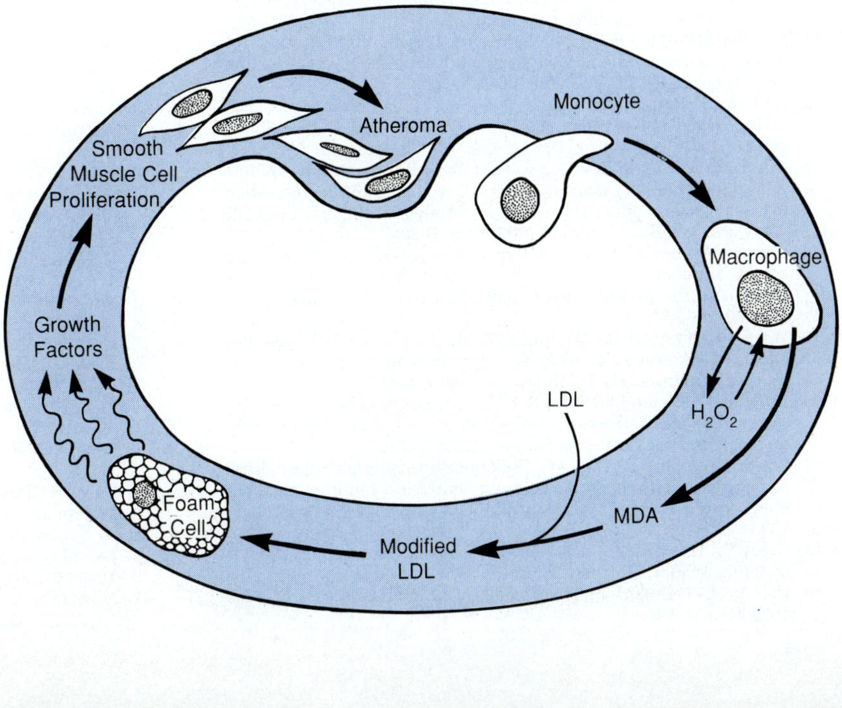

FIGURE 19-18. Role of mononuclear phagocytes in the pathogenesis of atherosclerosis.

tigen receptor complexes of T and B cells to elicit immunoglobulin-producing or specifically cytotoxic cells.[542,543] Other receptors on the surface of MNPs influence the efficiency of antigen presentation. Some receptors shown to be important are the β_2-integrin LFA-1 (CD11a/CD18) expressed on both MNPs and lymphocytes, which interacts either with ICAM-1 on MNPs or with the T-cell surface proteins CD3 and CD4 on the MNP surface, which bind to the T-cell receptor complex.[79] Antigen processing is subject to modulation by molecules in the environment. TNF and GM-CSF, for example, enhance MNP major histocompatibility complex expression and antigen presentation.[544,545] LTB_4 released by MNPs induces T cells to produce IFN-γ, which in turn also enhances MNP antigen presentation function by up-regulation of class II antigens.[546] On the other hand, PGE_2, which is synthesized by MNPs, inhibits the activity of T lymphocytes. Phagocytes can also inhibit immune responses in vitro, as evidenced by PMN cytotoxicity against T cells. This phenomenon may underlie the observation of anergy in patients with various chronic inflammatory states associated with neutrophilia and the enhancement of an immune response by macrophage ablation in mice.[547]

REFERENCES

1. Goeze JAE. Infusionsthierchen die Andre fressen. Beschaftigungen der Berlinishen Gesellschaft naturforschender Freunde. 1777;3:373–384.
2. von Gleichen FF. Abhandlung uber die Saamen und Beobachtungen des Saamens der Thiere, und verschiedener Infusionen. Winterschmidt, AW Nuremberg, 1778.
3. Rather LJ. Addison and the white corpuscles: an aspect of nineteenth-century biology. Berkeley, University of California Press, 1972.
4. Tauber AI, Chernyak L. The birth of immunology. II. Metchnikoff and his critics. Cell Immunol 1989;121:447–473.
5. Warner AE, Brain JD. Intravascular pulmonary macrophages: novel cell removes particles from blood. Am J Physiol 1986;19:R728–R732.
6. Miyamoto K, Schultz E, Heath T, Mitchell MD, Albertine KJ, Staub NC. Pulmonary intravascular macrophages and hemodynamic effects of liposomes in sheep. J Appl Physiol 1988;64:1143–1152.
7. Horejsi V. Surface antigens of human leukocytes. Adv Immunol 1991;49:75–147.
8. Lehn M, Weisner WY, Engelhorn S, Gillis S, Remold HG. IL-4 inhibits H_2O_2 production and antileishmanial capacity of human cultured monocytes mediated by IFN-γ. J Immunol 1989:143:3020–3024.
9. Dewald B, Thelen M, Baggiolini M. Two transduction sequences are necessary for neutrophil activation by receptor agonists. J Biol Chem 1988;263:16179–16184.
10. Omann GM, Sklar LA. Response of neutrophils to stimulus infusion: differential sensitivity of cytoskeletal activation and oxidant production. J Cell Biol 1988;10:7951–7958.
11. Doerfler ME, Danner RL, Shelhamer JH, Parrillo JE. Bacterial lipopolysaccharides prime human neutrophils for enhanced production of leukotriene B4. J Clin Invest 1989;83:970–977.
12. Nathan CF. Respiratory burst in adherent human neutrophils: triggering by colony-stimulating factors CSF-GM and CSF-G. Blood 1989;73:301–306.
13. Seifert R, Wenzel K, Eckstein F, Schultz G. Purine and pyrimidine nucleotides potentiate activation of NADPH oxidase and degranulation by chemotactic peptides and induce aggregation of human neutrophils via G proteins. Eur J Biochem 1989;181:277–285.
14. Khawaja A, Carver J, Linch D. Interactions of granulocyte-macrophage colony-stimulating factor (CSF), granulocyte CSF, and tumor necrosis factor α in the priming of the neutrophil respiratory burst. Blood 1992;79:745–753.
15. Ward PA, Cunningham TW, McCullough KK, Johnson KJ. Regulatory effects of adenosine and adenine nucleotides on oxygen radical responses of neutrophils. Lab Invest 1988;58:438–447.
16. Aderem AA, Keum MM, Pure E, Cohn ZA. Bacterial lipopolysaccharides prime macrophages for enhanced release of arachidonic acid metabolites. Proc Natl Acad Sci 1986;83:5817–5821.
17. English D, Debono DJ, Gabig TG. Relationship of phosphatidylinositol bisphosphate hydrolysis to calcium mobilization and functional activation in fluoride-treated neutrophils. J Clin Invest 1987;80:145–153.
18. Casey PJ, Gilman AG. G protein involvement in receptor–effector coupling. J Biol Chem 1988;263:2577–2580.
19. Hall A. The cellular function of small GTP-binding proteins. Science 1990;249:635–640.
20. Bokoch GM. The presence of free G protein β/γ subunits in human neutrophils results in suppression of adenylate cyclase activity. J Biol Chem 1987;262:589–594.
21. Imamura K, Sherman JL, Spriggs D, Kufe DW. Effect of tumor necrosis factor on GTP binding and GTPase activity in HL-60 and L929 cells. J Biol Chem 1988;263:10247–10253.
22. Rotrosen D, Gallin JI, Spiegel AM, Malech HL. Subcellular localization of Giα in human neutrophils. J Biol Chem 1988;263:10958–10964.
23. Volpp BD, Nauseef WM, Clark RA. Subcellular distribution and membrane association of human neutrophil substrates for ADP-ribosylation by pertussis toxin and cholera toxin. J Immunol 1989;142:3206–3212.
24. Krause K-H, Lew PD. Subcellular distribution of Ca2+ pumping sites in human neutrophils. J Clin Invest 1987;80:107–116.
25. Lagast H, Lew PD, Waldvogel FA. Adenosine triphosphate–dependent calcium pump in the plasma membrane of guinea pig and human neutrophils. J Clin Invest 1984;73:107–115.
26. Lew PD, Stossel TP. Calcium transport by macrophage plasma membranes. J Biol Chem 1980;255:5841–5846.
27. Hirata M, Hamachi T, Hashimoto T, Suematsu E, Koga T. Ca2+ release in the endoplasmic reticulum of guinea pig peritoneal macrophages. J Biochem 1983;94:1155–1163.
28. Volpe P, Krause K-H, Hashimoto S, et al. Calciosome, a cytoplasmic organelle: the inositol 1,4,5-triphosphate-sensitive Ca2+ store of non-muscle cells. Proc Natl Acad Sci USA 1988;85:1091–1095.
29. Berridge M. Inositol trisphosphate and calcium signalling. Nature 1993;361:315–325.
30. Abdel-Latif AA. Calcium-mobilizing receptors, polyphosphoinositides, and the generation of second messengers. Pharmacol Rev 1986;38:228–272.
31. Exton JH. Mechanisms of action of calcium-mobilizing agonists: some variations on a young theme. FASEB J 1988;2:2670–2676.
32. von Tscharner V, Prod'hom B, Baggiolini M, Reuter H. Ion channels in human neutrophils activated by a rise in free cytosolic calcium concentration. Nature 1986;324:369–372.
33. Traynor-Kaplan AE, Harris AL, Thompson BL, Taylor P, Sklar LA. An inositol tetrakisphosphate-containing phospholipid in activated neutrophils. Nature 1988;334:353–356.
34. Bengtsson T, Rundquist I, Stendahl O, Wymann MP, Andersson T. Increased breakdown of phosphatidylinositol 4,5-bisphosphate is not an initiating factor for actin assembly in human neutrophils. J Biol Chem 1988;263:17385–17389.
35. Perez HD, Elfman F, Marder S, Lobo E, Ives HE. Formyl peptide-induced chemotaxis of human polymorphonuclear leukocytes does not require either marked changes in cytosolic calcium or specific granule discharge: role of formyl peptide receptor expression (or recycling). J Clin Invest 1989;83:1963–1970.
36. Sha'afi RI, Shefcyk J, Yassin R, et al. Is a rise in intracellular concentration of free calcium necessary or sufficient for stimulated cytoskeletal-associated actin. J Cell Biol 1986;102:1459–1463.
37. Sklar LA, Omman GM, Painter RG. Relationship of actin polymerization and depolymerization to light scattering in human neutrophils: dependence on receptor occupancy and intracellular Ca2+. J Cell Biol 1985:101:1161–1166.
38. Pike MC, Arndt C. Characterization of phosphatidylinositol and phosphatidylinositol-4-phosphate kinases inhuman neutrophils. J Immunol 1988;140:1967–1973.
39. Schlegel W, Winiger BP, Mollard P, et al. Oscillations of cytosolic Ca2+ in pituitary cells due to action potentials. Nature 1987:329:719–721.
40. Marks P, Maxfield F. Transient increases in cytosolic free calcium appear to be required for the migration of adherent human neutrophils. J Cell Biol 1990;110:43–52.
41. Marks P, Hendley B, Maxfield F. Attachment to fibronectin or vitronectin makes human neutrophil migration sensitive to alterations in cytosolic free calcium concentration. J Cell Biol 1991;112:149–158.
42. Pozzan T, Lew PD, Wollheim CB, Tsien RY. Is cytosolic ionized calcium regulating neutrophil activation? Science 1983;221:1413–1415.
43. Lew PD, Monod A, Waldvogel FA, Dewald B, Baggiolini M, Pozzan T. Quantitative analysis of the cytosolic free calcium dependency of exocytosis from three subcellular compartments in intact human neutrophils. J Cell Biol 1986;102:2197–2204.
44. Jaconi MEE, Lew DP, Carpentier J, Magnusson KE, Sjogren M, Stendahl O. Cytosolic free calcium elevation mediates the phagosome–lysosome fusion during phagocytosis in human neutrophils. J Cell Biol 1990;110:1555–1564.
45. Jaconi M, Theler J, Schlegel W, Appel R, Wright S, Lew P. Multiple elevations of cytosolic-free Ca2+ in human neutrophils: initiation by adherence receptors of the integrin family. J Cell Biol 1991;112:1249–1257.
46. Korchak HM, Vosshal LB, Haines KA, Wilkenfeld C, Lundquist KF, Weissmann G. Activation of the human neutrophil by calcium-mobilizing ligands. II. Correlation of calcium, diacyl glycerol and phosphatidic acid generation with superoxide generation. J Biol Chem 1988;263:11098–11105.
47. Nishizuka Y. Studies and perspectives of protein kinase C. Science 1986;233:305–312.

48. Nishizuka Y. Intracellular signalling by hydrolysis of phospholipids and activation of protein kinase C. Science 1992;258:607–614.
49. Burn P. Phosphatidylinositol cycle and its possible involvement in the regulation of cytoskeletal-membrane interactions. J Cell Biochem 1988;36:15–24.
50. Lambeth JD, Burnham DN, Tyagi SR. Sphinganine effects on chemoattractant-induced diacylglycerol generation, calcium fluxes, superoxide production, and on cell viability in the human neutrophil: delivery of sphinganine with bovine serum albumin minimizes cytotoxicity. J Biol Chem 1988;263:3818–3822.
51. Phaire-Washington L, Wang E, Silverstein SC. Phorbol myristate acetate stimulates pinocytosis and membrane spreading in mouse peritoneal macrophages. J Cell Biol 1980;86:634–640.
52. Repine JE, White JG, Clawson CC, Holmes BM. Effects of phorbol myristate acetate on the metabolism and ultrastructure of neutrophils in chronic granulomatous disease. J Clin Invest 1974;54:83–90.
53. Yamazaki M, Gomez-Cambronero J, Durstin M, Molski TFP, Becker EL, Sha'afi RI. Phorbol 12-myristate 13-acetate inhibits binding of leukotriene B4 and platelet-activating factor and the responses they induce in neutrophils: site of action. Proc Natl Acad Sci USA 1989;86: 5791–5794.
54. Varticovski L, Druker B, Morrison D, Cantley L, Roberts T. The colony-stimulating factor-1 receptor associates with and activates phosphatidylinositol-3 kinase. Nature 1989;342:699–702.
55. Billah MM, Pai J-K, Mullmann TJ, Egan RW, Siegel MI. Regulation of phospholipase D in HL-60 granulocytes: activation by phorbol esters, diglyceride, and calcium ionophore via protein kinase C-independent mechanisms. J Biol Chem 1989;264:9069–9076.
56. Dougherty RW, Dubay GR, Niedel JE. Dynamics of the diradylglycerol responses of stimulated phagocytes. J Biol Chem 1989;264:11263–11269.
57. Balsinde J, Diez E, Schuller A, Mollinedo F. Phospholipase A2 activity in resting and activated human neutrophils: substrate specificity, pH dependence and subcellular localization J Biol Chem 1988;263:1929–1936.
58. Stossel TP. The molecular biology of phagocytes and molecular basis of nonneoplastic phagocyte disorders. In: Stamatoyannopoulos G, Nienhuis AW, Leder P, Majerus PW, eds. The molecular basis of blood diseases. Philadelphia, WB Saunders, 1987.
59. Andersson T, Schlegel W, Monod A, Krause K-H, Stendahl O, Lew PD. Leukotriene B4 stimulation of phagocytes results in the formation of inositol 1,4,5-triphosphate: a second messenger for Ca2+ mobilization. Biochem J 1986;240:333–340.
60. Confer DL, Eaton JW. Phagocyte impotence caused by an invasive bacterial adenylate cyclase. Science 1982;217:948–951.
61. Bidani A, Brown SES, Heming TA, Gurich R, DuBose TD J. Cytoplasmic pH in pulmonary macrophages: recovery from acid load is N2+ independent and NEM sensitive. Am J Physiol 1989;257:C56–C76.
62. Gallin E. Ion channels in leukocytes. Physiol Rev 1991;71:775–811.
63. Swallow CJ, Grinstein S, Rotstein OD. Cytoplasmic pH regulation in macrophages by an ATP-dependent and N,N'-dicyclohexylcarbodiimide-sensitive mechanism: possible involvement of a plasma membrane proton pump. J Biol Chem 1988;263:19558–19563.
64. Downey GP, Grinstein S. Receptor-mediated actin assembly in electropermeabilized neutrophils: role of intracellular pH. Biochem Biophys Res Commun 1989;160:18–24.
65. Prpic V, Yu S-F, Figueiredo F, et al. Role of Na+/H+ exchange by interferon-γ in enhanced expression of JE and I-Ab genes. Science 1989;244:469–471.
66. Heuser J. Changes in lysosome shape and distribution correlated with changes in cytoplasmic pH. J Cell Biol 1989;108:855–864.
67. Kraft AS, Berkow RL. Tyrosine kinase and phosphotyrosine phosphatase activity in human promyelocytic leukemia cells and human polymorphonuclear leukocytes. Blood 1987;70:356–362.
68. Grinstein S, Hill H, Furuya W. Activation of electropermeabilized neutrophils by adenosine 5'-[γ-thio]triphosphate (ATP[S]): role of phosphatases in stimulus-response coupling. Biochem J 1989;261:755–759.
69. Aderem A. The MARCKS brothers: a family of protein kinase C substrates. Cell 1992;71:713–716.
70. Pontremoli S, Melloni E, Damiani G, et al. Effects of a monoclonal anti-calpain antibody on responses of stimulated human neutrophils: evidence for a role for proteolytically modified protein kinase C. J Biol Chem 1988;263:1915–1919.
71. Pontremoli S, Melloni E, Michetti M, Salamino F, Sparatore B, Horecker BL. An endogenous activator of the Ca2+-dependent proteinase of human neutrophils that increases its affinity for Ca2+. Proc Natl Acad Sci USA 1988;85:1740–1743.
72. Stossel TP. From signal to pseudopod: how cells control cytoplasmic actin assembly. J Biol Chem 1989;264:18261–18264.
73. Lassing I, Lindberg U. Specificity of the interaction between phosphatidylinositol 4,5-bisphosphate and the profilin:actin complex. J Cell Biochem 1988;37:255–267.
74. Safer D, Elzinga M, Nachmias V. Thymosin β4 and Fx, an actin-sequestering peptide, are indistinguishable. J Biol Chem 1991;266: 4029–4032.
75. Matsudaira P, Janmey PA. Pieces in the actin severing puzzle. Cell 1989;54:139–140.
76. Hartwig JH, Shevlin P. The architecture of actin filaments and the ultrastructural location of actin-binding protein in the periphery of lung macrophages. J Cell Biol 1986;103:1007–1020.
77. Gorlin J, Yamin R, Egan S, et al. Human endothelial actin-binding protein (ABP, nonmuscle filamin): a molecular leaf spring. J Cell Biol 1990;111:1089–1105.
78. Bennett JP, Zaner KS, Stossel TP. Isolation and some properties of macrophage α-actinin: evidence that it is not an actin gelling protein. Biochem 1984;23:5081–5086.
79. Springer T. Traffic signals for lymphocyte recirculation and leukocyte emigration: the multistep paradigm. Cell 1997;76:301–314.
80. Makgoba MW, Sanders ME, Ginther Luce GE, et al. ICAM-1, a ligand for LFA-1-dependent adhesion of B, T and myeloid cells. Nature 1988;331:86–88.
81. Hemler ME. VLA proteins in the integrin family: structures, functions and their role on leukocytes. Annu Rev Immunol 1990;8:365–400.
82. Smith CW, Martin SD, Rothlein R, Toman C, Anderson DC. Cooperative interactions of LFA-1 and Mac-1 with intercellular adhesion molecule-1 in facilitating adherence and transendothelial migration of human neutrophils in vitro. J Clin Invest 1989;83:2008–2017.
83. Ismail G, Morganroth ML, Todd RF I, Boxer LA. Prevention of pulmonary injury in isolated perfused rat lungs by activated human neutrophils preincubated with anti-Mo 1 antibody. Blood 1987;69: 1167–1174.
84. Simpson PJ, Todd RF I, Fantone JC, et al. Reduction of experimental canine myocardial reperfusion injury by a monoclonal antibody (anti-Mo 1, anti-CD11b) that inhibits leukocyte adhesion. J Clin Invest 1989;81:624–629.
85. Vedder NB, Winn RK, Rice CL, Chi Y, Arfors K-E, Harlan JM. A monoclonal antibody to the adherence-promoting leukocyte glycoprotein CD 18, reduces organ injury and improves survival from hemorrhagic shock and resuscitation in rabbits. J Clin Invest 1988;81: 939–944.
86. Borregaard N, Kjeldsen L, Rygaard K, et al. Stimulus-dependent secretion of plasma proteins from human neutrophils. J Clin Invest 1992;90:86–96.
87. Hermanowski-Vosatka A, Van Strijp J, Swiggard W, Wright S. Integrin modulating factor-1: a lipid that alters the function of leukocyte integrins. Cell 1992;68:341–352.
88. Buyon JP, Slade SG, Reibman J, et al. Constitutive and induced phosphorylation of the α- an β-chains of the CD11/CD18 leukocyte integrin family: relationship to adhesion-dependent functions. J Immunol 1990;144:191–197.
89. Hibbs M, Xu H, Stackler S, Springer T. Regulation of adhesion to ICAM-1 by the cytoplasmic domain of LFA-1 integrin β subunit. Science 1991;251:1611–1613.
90. Diamond M, Staunton D, Marlin S, Springer T. Binding of the integrin Mac-1 (CD11b/CD18) to the third immunoglobulin-like domain of ICAM-1 (CD54) and its regulation by glycosylation. Cell 1991;65:961–971.
91. Worthen GS, Schwab BI, Elson EL, Downey GP. Mechanics of stimulated neutrophils: cell stiffening induces retention in capillaries. Science 1989;245:183–186.
92. Lawrence M, Springer T. Leukocytes roll on a selectin at physiologic flow rates: distinction from and prerequisite for adhesion through integrins. Cell 1991;65:859–873.
93. Ley K, Gaehtgens P, Fennie C, Singer M, Lasky L, Rosen S. Lectin-like cell adhesion molecule 1 mediates leukocyte rolling in mesenteric venules in vivo. Blood 1991;77:2553–2555.
93a. Larsen E, Palabrica T, Sajer S, et al. PADGEM-dependent adhesion of platelets to monocytes and neutrophils is mediated by a lineage-specific carbohydrate, LNF III (CD15). Cell 1990;63:467–474.
94. Bevilacqua MP, Stengelin S, Gimbrone MA J, Seed B. Endothelial leukocyte adhesion molecule 1: an inducible receptor for neutrophils related to complement regulatory proteins and lectins. Science 1989;243:1160–1165.
95. Brandley BK, Swiedler SJ, Robbins PW. Carbohydrate ligands of the LEC cell adhesion molecules. Cell 1990;63:861–863.
96. Goelz SE, Hession C, Goff D, et al. ELFT: a gene that directs the expression of an ELAM-1 ligand. Cell 1990;63:1349–1356.
97. Polley M, Philips M, Wayner E, et al. CD62 and endothelial cell-leukocyte adhesion molecule 1 (ELAM-1) recognize the same carbohydrate ligand, sialyl-Lewis x. Proc Nat Acad Sci USA 1991;88: 6224–6228.
98. Hoeprich PD, Dahinden CA, Lachmann PJ, Davis AE I, Hugli TE. A synthetic nonapeptide corresponding to the NH2-terminal sequence of C3d-K causes leukocytosis in rabbits. J Biol Chem 1985;260:2597–2600.
99. Shigeoka AO, Gobel J, Janatova J, Hill HR. Neutrophil mobilization induced by complement fragments during experimental group B streptococcal (GBS) infection. Am J Pathol 1988;133:623–629.
100. Hechtman D, Cybulsky M, Fuchs H, Baker J, Gimbrone M Jr. Intravascular IL-8: inhibitor of polymorphonuclear leukocyte accumulation at sites of acute inflammation. J Immunol 1991;147:883–892.
101. Thomas K, Pyun H, Navarro J. Molecular cloning of the f-met-leu-phe receptor from neutrophils. J Biol Chem 1990;265:20061–20064.
102. Gerard N, Gerard C. The chemotactic receptor for human C5a anaphylatoxin. Nature 1991;349:614–617.

103. LaRosa G, Thomas K, Kaufmann M, et al. Amino terminus of the interleukin-8 receptor is a major determinant of receptor subtype specificity. J Biol Chem 1992;267:25402–25406.
104. Snyderman R, and Uhing R. Chemoattractant stimulus-response coupling. In: Inflammation: basic principles and clinical correlates. New York, Raven Press, 1992:421–440.
105. Jesaitis AJ, Tolley JO, Bokoch GM, Allen RA. Regulation of chemoattractant receptor interaction with transducing proteins by organizational control in the plasma membrane of human neutrophils. J Cell Biol 1989;109:2783–2790.
106. Malawista SE, van Blarikom G. Cytoplasts made from human blood polymorphonuclear leukocytes with or without heat: preservation of both mile function and respiratory burst oxidase activity. Proc Natl Acad Sci USA 1987;84:454–458.
107. Stossel T. On the crawling of animal cells. Science 1993;260:1086–1094.
108. Howard TH, Wang D. Calcium ionophore, phorbol ester, and chemotactic peptide-induced cytoskeleton reorganization in human neutrophils. J Clin Invest 1987;79:1359–1364.
109. Stossel TP. The mechanical responses of white blood cells. In: Gallin JI, Goldstein IM, Snyderman R, eds. Inflammation: basic principles and clinical correlates. New York, Raven Press, 1992:459–476.
110. Oster GF, Perelson AS. The physics of cell mility. J Cell Sci 1987;8:35–54.
111. Ito T, Zaner KS, Stossel TO. Non-ideality of volume flows and phase transitions of F-actin solutions in response to osmotic stress. Biophys J 1987;51:745–753.
112. Trybus K. Assembly of cytoplasmic and smooth muscle myosins. 1991;3:105–111.
113. Devreotes PN, Zigmond SH. Chemotaxis in eukaryotic cells: a focus on leukocytes and Dictyostelium. Annu Rev Cell Biol 1988;4:649–686.
114. Lauffenburger D, Rothman C, Zigmond SH. Measurement of leukocyte motility and chemotaxis parameters with a linear under-agarose migration assay. J Immunol 1983;131:940–947.
115. Rebuck JW, Crowley JH. A method of studying leukocyte functions in vivo. Ann NY Acad Sci 1955;59:757–793.
116. Edberg JC, Redecha PB, Salmon JE, Kimberley RP. Human FcγRIII[CD16]: isoforms with distinct allelic expression, extracellular domains, and membrane linkages on polymorphonuclear and natural killer cells. J Immunol 1989;143:1642–1649.
117. Ra C, Jouvin M-H E, Blank U, Kinet J-P. A macrophage Fcγ receptor and the mast cell receptor for IgE share an identical subunit. Nature 1989;341:752–754.
118. Ezekowitz RAB, Sastry K, Bailly P, Warner A. Molecular characterization of the human macrophage mannose receptor: demonstration of multiple carbohydrate recognition-like domains and phagocytosis of yeasts in Cos-1 cells. J Exp Med 1990;172:1785–1794.
119. Ezekowitz R, Williams D, Koziel H, Armstrong M, Warner A, Richards F, Rose R. Uptake of *Pneumocystis carinii* mediated by macrophage mannose receptor. Nature 1991;351:155–158.
120. Wright SD, Detmers PA. Adhesion-promoting receptors on phagocytes. J Cell Sci 1988;9:99–120.
121. Bussolino F, Fischer E, Turrin F, Kazatchkine ME, Arese P. Platelet activating factor enhances complement-dependent phagocytosis J Biol Chem 1989;264:21711–21719.
122. Silverstein SC, Steinman RM, Cohn ZA. Endocytosis. Annu Rev Biochem 1977;46:669–691.
123. Werb Z, Takemura R, Sternberg PE, Bainton DF. Directed exocytosis of secretory granules containing apolipoprotein E to the adherent surface and basal vacuoles of macrophages spreading on immobile immune complexes. Am J Pathol 1989;134:661–670.
124. Racoosin E, Swanson JA. Macrophage colony-stimulating (rM-CSF) stimulates pinocytosis in bone marrow–derived macrophages. J Exp Med 1989;170:1635.
125. Rothwell SW, Nath J, Wright DG. Interactions of cytoplasmic granules with microtubules in human neutrophils. J Cell Biol 1989;108:2313–2326.
126. Diaz R, Mayorga LS, Weidman PJ, Rothman JE, Stahl PD. Vesicle fusion following receptor-mediated endocytosis requires a protein active in Golgi transport. Nature 1989;339:398–400.
127. Mayorga LS, Diaz R, Stahl PD. Plasma membrane-derived vesicles containing receptor-ligand complexes are fusogenic with early endosomes in a cell-free system. J Biol Chem 1988;263:17213–17216.
128. Hart PD, Young MR, Jordan MM, Perkins WJ, Geisow MJ. Chemical inhibitors of phagosome-lysosome fusion in cultured macrophages also inhibit saltatory lysosomal movements. J Exp Med 1983;158:477–492.
129. Meers P, Ernst JD, Duzgunes N, Hong K, Fedor J, Goldstein IM, Papahadjopoulos D. Synexin-like proteins from human polymorphonuclear leukocytes: identification and characterization of granule-aggregating and membrane-fusing activities. J Biol Chem 1987;262:7850–7858.
130. Ernst J. Annexin III translocates to the periphagosomal region when neutrophils ingest opsonized yeast. J Immunol 1991;146:3110–3114.
131. Black CM, Paliescheskey M, Beaman BL, Donovan RM, Goldstein E. Acidification of phagosomes in murine macrophages: blockage by Nocardia asteroides. J Infect Dis 1986;154:952–958.
132. Hart PD, Young MR, Gordon AH, Sullivan KH. Inhibition of phagosome-lysosome fusion in macrophages by certain mycobacteria can be explained by inhibition of lysosomal movements observed after phagocytosis. J Exp Med 1987;166:933–946.
133. Horwitz MA, Maxfield FR. *Legionella pneumophilia* inhibits acidification of its phagosome in human monocytes. J Cell Biol 1984;99:1936–1943.
134. Joiner KA, Ganz T, Albert J, Rotrosen D. The opsonizing ligand on *Salmonella typhimurium* influences incorporation of specific, but not azurophil, granule constituents into neutrophil phagosomes. J Cell Biol 1989;109:2771–2782.
135. Sibley DL, Weidner E, Krahenbuhl JL. Phagosome acidification blocked by intracellular *Toxoplasma gondii*. Nature 1985;315:416–419.
136. Kravet RI, Brain JD. Methods to quantify endocytosis: a review. J Reticuloendothelial Soc 1980;27:201–221.
137. Anderson DC, Springer TA. Leukocyte adhesion deficiency: an inherited defect in the Mac-1, LFA-1, and p150,195 glycoproteins. Annu Rev Med 1987;38:175–194.
138. Crowley CA, Curnutte JT, Rosin RE, et al. An inherited abnormality of neutrophil adhesion: its genetic transmission and association with a missing protein. N Engl J Med 1980;291:1163–1169.
139. Sligh JJ, Hurwitz M, Zhu C, Anderson D, Beaudet A. An initiation codon mutation in CD18 in association with the modeate phenotype of leukocyte adhesion deficiency. J Biol Chem 1992;267:714–718.
140. Kishimoto TK, O'Connor K, Springer TA. Leukocyte adhesion deficiency: aberrant splicing of a conserved integrin sequence causes a moderate deficiency phenotype. J Biol Chem 1989;264:3588–3595.
141. Arnaout MA, Dana N, Gupta SK, Tenen DG, Fathallah DM. Point mutations impairing cell surface expression of the common b subunit (CD18) in a patient with leukocyte adhesion molecule (Leu-CAM) deficiency. J Clin Invest 1990;85:977–981.
142. Arnaout MA. Structure and function of the leukocyte adhesion molecules CD11/CD18. Blood 1990;75:1037–1050.
143. Boxer LA, Hedley-White TE, Stossel TP. Neutrophil actin dysfunction and abnormal neutrophil behavior. N Engl J Med 1974;291:1093–1098.
144. Southwick FS, Dabiri GA, Stossel TP. Neutrophil actin dysfunction (NAD) is a genetic disorder associated with partial impairment of actin assembly in three family members. J Clin Invest 1988;82:15225–15229.
145. Southwick FS, Howard TH, Holbrook T, Anderson DC, Stossel TP, Arnaout MA. The relationship between CR3 deficiency and neutrophil actin assembly. Blood 1989;73:1973–1979.
145a. Howard T, Li Y, Torres M, Guerrero A, Coates T. The 47-kD protein increased in neutrophil actin dysfunction with 47- and 89-kD protein abnormalities is lymphocyte-specific protein. Blood. 1994;83:231–241.
146. Rotrosen D, Gallin JI. Disorders of phagocytic function. Adv Immunol 1987;5:1276–2105.
147. Bainton DF, Ullyot JL, Farquhar MG. The development of neutrophilic polymorphonuclear leukocytes in human bone marrow. J Exp Med 1971;2673:907.
148. Henson PM. The immunological release of constituents from neutrophil leukocytes. J Immunol 1971;107:1535.
149. Schraufstatter IU, Revak SD, Cochrane CG. Proteases and oxidants in experimental pulmonary inflammatory injury. J Clin Invest 1984;73:1175.
150. Henson PM, Johnston RB J. Tissue injury in inflammation: oxidants, proteinases, and cationic proteins. J Clin Invest 1987;79:669–674.
151. Lehrer R, Ganz T, Selsted M. Defensins: endogenous antibiotic peptides of animal cells. Cell 1991:64:229–230.
152. Lichtenstein AK, Ganz T, Nguyen TM, Selsted ME, Lehrer RI. Mechanism of target cytolysis by peptide defensins: target cell metabolic activities, possibly involving endocytosis, are crucial for expression of cytotoxicity. J Immunol 1988;140:2686–2694.
153. Gray PW, Flaggs G, Leong SR, et al. Cloning of the cDNA of a human neutrophil bactericidal protein. J Biol Chem 1989;264:9505–9509.
154. Zeya HI, Spitznagel JK. Cationic proteins of polymorphonuclear leukocyte lysosomes. I. Resolution of antibacterial and enzymatic activities. J Bacteriol 1966;91:750–754.
155. Weiss J, Hutzler M, Kao L. Environmental modulation of lipopolysaccharide chain length alters the sensitivity of *Escherichia coli* to the neutrophil bactericidal/permeability-increasing protein. Infect Immun 1986;51:594–599.
156. Weiss J, Franson RC, Beckerdite S, et al. Partial characterization and purification of a rabbit granulocyte factor that increases permeability of *Escherichia coli*. J Clin Invest 1975;55:33–42.
157. Wile CG, Snable JL, Scott RW. Characterization of two azurophil granule proteases with active-site homology to neutrophil elastase. J Biol Chem 1990;265:2038.
158. Jensen MS, Bainton DF. Temporal changes in pH within the phagocytic vacuole of the polymorphonuclear neutrophilic leukocyte. J Cell Biol 1973;56:379–388.
159. Strominger JL, Ghuysen J-M. Mechanisms of enzymatic bacteriolysis: cell walls of bacteria are solubilized by action of either specific carbohydrases or specific peptidases. Science 1967;156:213.
160. Salton MRJ. The properties of lysozyme and its action of microorganisms. Bact Rev 1957;21:82–99.
161. Apfeldorf WJ, Melnick DA, Meschulam T, Rasmussen H, Malech HL. A transient rise in intracellular free calcium is not a sufficient stimulus

for respiratory burst activation in human polymorphonuclear leukocytes. Biochem Biophys Res Commun 1985;132:674–680.
162. Ohlsson K. Granulocyte collagenase and elastase and their interactions with alantitrypsin and α2-macroglobulin. In: Reich E, Rifkin D, Shaw G, eds. Proteases and biological control. Cold Spring Harbor, NY, Cold Spring Harbor Press, 1975.
163. Sibbett SS, Hurst JK. Structural analysis of myeloperoxidase by resonance Raman spectroscopy. Biochemistry 1984;23:3007–3013.
164. Babcock GT, Ingle RT, Oertling WA, et al. Raman characterization of human leukocyte myeloperoxidase and bovine spleen greem haemoprotein: insight into chromophore structure and evidence that the chromophores of myeloperoxidase are equivalent. Biochim Biophys Acta 1985;828:58–66.
165. Nauseef WM, Olsson I, Arnljots K. Biosynthesis and processing of myeloperoxidase: a marker for myeloid cell differentiation. Eur J Haematol 1988;40:97–110.
166. Nauseef WM. Posttranslational processing of a human myeloid lysosomal protein, myeloperoxidase. Blood 1987;70:1143–1150.
167. Nauseef WM. Myeloperoxidase deficiency. Hematol Oncol Clin North Am 1988.
168. Klebanoff SJ, Hamon CB. Role of myeloperoxidase-mediated antimicrobial systems in intact leukocytes. J Reticuloendo Soc 1972;12:170.
169. Dewald B, Linkler-Ludwig R, Bretz U, Baggiolini M. Subcellular localization and heterogeneity of neutral proteases in neutrophilic polymorphonuclear leukocytes. J Exp Med 1975;141:709–723.
170. Sinha S, Watorek W, Karr S, Giles J, Bode W, Travis J. Primary structure of human neutrophil elastase. Proc Natl Acad Sci 1987;84:2228–2232.
171. Noble EP, Stjernholm RL, Weisberger AS. Carbohydrate metabolism in leukocytes. I. The pathway of two- and three-carbon compounds in the rabbit polymorphonuclear leukocyte. J Biol Chem 1960;235:1261.
172. Rao N, Wehner N, Marshall B, Gray W, Gray B, Hoidal J. Characterization of proteinase-3 (PR-3), a neutrophil serine proteinase: structural and functional properties. J Biol Chem 1991;266:9540–9548.
173. Bjornson HS. Enzymes associated with the survival and virulence of gram-negative anaerobes. Rev Infect Dis 1984;1:S21–24.
174. Brubaker RR. Mechanisms of bacterial virulence. Annu Rev Microbiol 1985;39:21–50.
175. Travis J, Salvesen GS. Human plasma proteinase inhibitors. Annu Rev Biochem 1983;52:655–709.
176. Janoff A, Carp H, Laurent P, Raju L. The role of oxidative processes in emphysema. Am Rev Respir Dis 1983;127:S31–S38.
177. Swain MW, Pizzo SV. Methionine sulfoxide and the oxidative regulation of plasma proteinase inhibitors. J Leukocyte Biol 1988;43:365–379.
178. Gabig TG, Schervish EW, Santinga JT. Functional relationship of the cytochrome b to the superoxide-generating oxidase of human neutrophils. J Biol Chem 1982;257:4114–4119.
179. Bini P, Gabay J, Teitel A, Melchior M, Zhou JL, Elkon K. Antineutrophil cytoplasmic autoantibodies in Wegener's granulomatosis recognize conformational epitope(s) on proteinase 3. J Immunol 1992;149:1409–1415.
180. Goldschmeding R, van der Schoot CE, ten Bokkel Huinink D, et al. Wegener's granulomatosis autoantibodies identify a novel diisopropylfluorophosphate-binding protein in the lysosomes of normal human neutrophils. J Clin Invest 1989;84:1577–1587.
181. Borregaard N, Christensen L, Bjerrum OW, Birgens HS, Clemmensen I. Identification of a highly mobilizable subset of human neutrophil intracellular vesicles that contain tetranectin and latent alkaline phosphatase. J Clin Invest 1990;85:408.
182. Geisow MJ, Hart PD, Young MR. Temporal changes in lysosome and phagosome pH during phagolysosome formation in macrophages: studies by fluorescence spectroscopy. J Cell Biol 1981;89:645–652.
183. Ishikawa I, Cimasoni G. Isolation of cathepsin D from human leukocytes. Biochim Biophys Acta 1977;480:228–240.
184. Levy J, Kolski GB, Douglas SD. Cathepsin D-like activity in neutrophils and monocytes. Infect Immun 1989;57:1632–1634.
185. Hack NJ, Smith GP, Peters TJ. Subcellular localization and properties of lipase activities in human polymorphonuclear leukocytes. Biochim Biophys Acta 1985;833:406–411.
186. Patsch W, Rindler-Ludwig R, Sailer S, Braunsteiner H. Avid cholesterol ester and glycerol ester hydrolase activities: evidence for the individuality of these enzymes in human mononuclear leukocytes. Biochim Biophys Acta 1980;618:337–346.
187. Sznajd J, Naskalski JW. Ribonuclease from human granulocytes. Biochim Biophys Acta 1973;302:282–292.
188. Fox HB, DeTogni P, McMahon G, et al. Fate of the DNA in plasmid-containing *E coli* minicels ingested by human neutrophils. Blood 1987;69:1394–1400.
189. Lamers MC, DeGroot ER, Roos D. Phagocytosis and degradation of DNA-anti-DNA complexes by human phagocytes. I. Assay conditions, quantitative aspects and differences between human blood monocytes and neutrophils. Eur J Immunol 1981;11:757–764.
190. Stevens RL, Avraham S, Gartner MC, Bruns GA, Austen KF, Weis JH. Isolation and characterization of a cDNA that encodes the peptide core of the secretory granule proteoglycan of human promyelocytic leukemia HL-60 cells. J Biol Chem 1988;263:7287–7291.
191. Parmley RT, Hurst RE, Takagi M, Spicer SS, Austin RL. Glycosaminoglycans in human neutrophils and leukemic myeloblasts: ultrastructural, cytochemical, immunologic, and biochemical characterization. Blood 1983:61:257.
192. Kamada MM, Michon J, Ritz J, et al. Identification of carboxypeptidase and tryptic esterase activities that are complexed to proteoglycans in the secretory granules of human cloned natural killer cells. J Immunol 1989;142:609–615.
193. Deshpande KL, Fried VA, Ando M, Webster RG. Glycosylation affects cleavage of an H5N5 influenza virus hemagglutinin and regulates virulence. Proc Natl Acad Sci 1987;84:36–40.
194. Bainton DF. Sequential degranulation of the two types of polymorphonuclear leukocyte granules during phagocytosis of microorganisms. J Cell Biol 1973;58:259–264.
195. Wright DG, Gallin JI. Secretory responses of human neutrophils: exocytosis of specific (secondary) granules by human neutrophils during adherence in vivo and during exudation in vivo. J Immunol 1979;123:285.
196. Whitin JC, Ryan DH, Cohen HJ. Graded responses of human neutrophils induced by serum-treated zymosan. Blood 1985;66:1182–1188.
197. Goldstein IM, Hoffstein ST, Weissmann G. Influence of divalent cations upon complement-mediated enzyme release from human polymorphonuclear leukocytes. J Immunol 1975;115:665–670.
198. Naccache PH, Molski TFP, Borgeat P, White JR, Sha'afi RI. Phorbol esters inhibit the fMet-Leu-Phe- and leukotriene Br-stimulated calcium mobilization and enzyme secretion in rabbit neutrophils. J Biol Chem 1985;260:2125–2131.
199. Omann GM, Traynoro AE, Harris AL, Sklar LA. LTB4-induced activation signals and responses in neutrophils are short-lived compared to formylpeptide. J Immunol 1987;138:2626–2632.
200. O'Flaherty JT, Nishihira J. Arachidonate metabolites, platelet-activating factor, and the mobilization of protein kinase C in human polymorphonuclear neutrophils. J Immunol 1987;138:1889–1895.
201. Hughes B, Hollers J, Crockett-Torabi E, Smith C. Recruitment of CD11b/CD18 to the neutrophil surface and adherence-dependent cell locomotion. J Clin Invest 1992;90:1687–1696.
202. Berger M, Birx DL, Wetzler EM, O'Shea JJ, Brown EJ, Cross AS. Calcium requirements for increased complement receptor expression during neutrophil activation. J Immunol 1985;135:1342–1348.
203. Higson FK, Durbin L, Pavlotsky N, Tauber AI. Studies of cytochrome b-245 translocation in the PMA stimulation of the human neutrophil NADPH-oxidase. J Immunol 1985;135:519–524.
204. Borregaard N, Heiple JM, Simons ER, Clark RA. Subcellular localization of the b-cytochrome component of the human neutrophil microbicidal oxidase: translocation during activation. J Cell Biol 1983;97:52–61.
205. Cramer E, Pryzwansky KB, Villeval J-L, Testa U, Breton-Gorius J. Ultrastructural localization of lactoferrin and myeloperoxidase in human neutrophils by immunogold. Blood 1985;65:423–432.
206. Anderson BF, Baker HM, Dodson EJ, et al. Structure of human lactoferrin at 32-A resolution. Proc Natl Acad Sci 1987;84:1969–1773.
207. Parry J, Brown RM, Brown EM. Lactoferrin conformation and metal binding properties. Adv Exp Med Biol 1974;48:141–160.
208. Ambruso DR, Johnston RB J. Lactoferrin enhances hydroxyl radical production by human neutrophils, neutrophil particulate fractions, and an enzymatic generating system. J Clin Invest 1981;67:352–360.
209. Vercellotti GM, Van Asbeck BS, Jacob HS. Oxygen radical-induced erythrocyte hemolysis by neutrophils: critical role of iron and lactoferrin. J Clin Invest 1985;76:956–962.
210. Weinberg ED. Iron withholding: a defense against infection and neoplasia. Physiol Rev 1984;64:65–102.
211. Letendre ED. The importance of iron in the pathogenesis of infection and neoplasia. Trends Biochem Sci 1985;10:166–168.
212. Babior BM. Cobamides as cofactors: adenosylcobamide-dependent rearrangements. In: Cobalamin: biochemistry and pathophysiology. New York, John Wiley, 1975.
213. Kolhouse JF, Kondo H, Allen NC, Podell E, Allen RH. Cobalamin analogues are present in human plasma and can mask cobalamin deficiency because current radioisotope dilution assays are not specific for true cobalamin. N Engl J Med 1978;299:785–792.
214. Murphy MF, Sourial NA, Burman JF, et al. Megaloblastic anaemia due to vitamin B12 deficiency caused by small intestinal bacterial overgrowth: possible role of vitamin B12 analogues. Br J Haematol 1986;62:7–12.
215. Herbert V, Drivas G, Manusselis C, Mackler B, Eng J, Schwartz E. Are colon bacteria a major source of cobalamin analogues in human tissues? 24-hr human stool contains only about 5 micrograms of cobalamin but about 100 micrograms of apparent analogue (and 200 micrograms of folate). Trans Assoc Am Physicians 1984;97:161–171.
216. Kane SP, Peters TJ. Analytical subcellular fractionation of human granulocytes with reference to the localization of vitamin B12-binding proteins. Clin Sci Mol Med 1975;49:171–182.
217. Allen RH, Majerus PW. Isolation of vitamin B12-binding proteins using affinity chromatography. II. Purification and properties of a human granulocyte vitamin B12–binding protein. J Biol Chem 1972;247:7702–7708.
218. Allen RH. Human vitamin B12 transport proteins. Prog Hematol 1975;9:57–84.

219. Burger RL, Mehlman CS, Allen RH. Human plasma R-type vitamin B12-binding proteins. I. Isolation and characterization of transcobalamin I: transcobalamin III and the normal granulocyte vitamin B12-binding protein. J Biol Chem 1975;250:7700–7706.
220. Gueant JL, Monin P, Boissel P, Gaucher P, Nicolas JP. Biliary excretion of cobalamin and cobalamin analogues in man. Digestion 1984;30: 151–157.
221. Kanazawa S, Herbert V, Herzlich B, Drivas G, Manusselis C. Removal of cobalamin analogue in bile by enterohepatic circulation of vitamin B12. (Letter) Lancet 1983;1:707–708.
222. Murphy G, Reynolds JJ, Bretz U, Baggiolini M. Partial purification of collagenase and gelatinase from human polymorphonuclear leukocytes: analysis of their actions on soluble and insoluble collagens. Biochem J 1982;203:209–221.
223. Devarajan P, Mookhtiar K, Van Wart H, Berliner N. Structure and expression of the cDNA encoding human neutrophil collagenase. Blood 1991;77:2731–2738.
224. Weiss SJ, Peppin GJ. Collagenolytic metalloenzymes of the human neutrophil: characteristics, regulation and potential function in vivo. Biochem Pharmacol 1986;35:3189–3197.
225. Sellers A, Murphy G. Collagenolytic enzymes and their naturally occurring inhibitors. Int Rev Connect Tissue Res 1981;9:151–190.
226. Baggiolini M, Schnyder J, Bretz U, Dewald B, Ruch W. Cellular mechanisms of proteinase release from inflammatory cells and the degradation of extracellular proteins. Ciba Found Symp 1979:105–121.
227. Shah SV, Baricos WH, Basci A. Degradation of human glomerular basement membrane by stimulated neutrophils: activation of a metalloproteinase(s) by reactive oxygen metabolites. J Clin Invest 1987;79: 25–31.
228. Peppin GJ, Weiss SJ. Activation of the endogenous metalloproteinase, gelatinase, by triffered human neutrophils. Proc Natl Acad Sci 1986;83: 4322–4326.
229. Petrequin PE, Todd RF I, Devall LJ, Boxer LA, Curnutte JT I. Association between gelatinase release and increased plasma membrane expression of the Mo1 glycoprotein. Blood 1987;69:605–610.
230. Dewald B, Bretz U, Baggiolini M. Release of gelatinase from a novel secretory compartment of human neutrophils. J Clin Invest 1982;70: 518–525.
231. Hibbs MS, Bainton DF. Human neutrophil gelatinase is a component of specific granules. J Clin Invest 1989;84:1395.
232. Wright DG, Gallin JI. A functional differentiation of human neutrophil granules: generation of C5a by a specific (secondary) granule product and inactivation of C5a by azurophil (primary) granule products. J Immunol 1977;119:1068–1076.
233. Cohn ZA, Wiener E. The particulate hydrolases of macrophages. I. Comparative enzymology, isolation, and properties. J Exp Med 1963;118:991–1004.
234. Weissman G, Dukor P, Zurier RB. Effect of cyclic AMP on release of lysosomal enzymes from phagocytes. Nature 1971;231:131–133.
235. Selsted ME, Brown DM, DeLange RJ, Lehrer RI. Primary structures of MCP-1 and MCP-2, natural peptide antibiotics of rabbit lung macrophages. J Biol Chem 1983;258:14485–14489.
236. Johnson J, Mei B, Cohn ZA. The separation, long-term cultivation and maturation of the human monocyte. J Exp Med 1977;146:1613–1630.
237. Lasser A. The mononuclear phagocytic system: a review. Philadelphia, WB Saunders, 1982.
238. Johnston RB. Monocytes and macrophages. N Engl J Med 1988;318: 747–752.
239. Karnovsky ML, Lazdins JK. Biochemical criteria for activated macrophages. J Immunol 1978;121:809–813.
240. Adams DO, Hamilton TA. The cell biology of macrophage activation. Annu Rev Immunol 1984;2:283–318.
241. MacDonald BR, Mundy GR, Clark S, et al. Effects of human recombinant CSF-GM and highly purified CSF-1 on the formation of multinucleated cells with osteoclast characteristics in long-term bone marrow cultures. J Bone Mineral Res 1986;1:227–233.
242. Lehrer RI, Szklarek D, Selsted ME, Fleischmann J. Increased content of microbicidal cationic peptides in rabbit alveolar macrophages elicited by complete Freund adjuvant. Infect Immun 1981;33:775–778.
243. Nathan CF. Secretory products of macrophages. J Clin Invest 1987;79: 319–326.
244. Cohn ZA, Wiener E. The particulate hydrolases of macrophages. II. Biologic and morphological responses to particulate ingestion. J Exp Med 1963;118:1009.
245. Schnyder J, Baggiolini M. Secretion of lysosomal hydrolases by stimulated and nonstimulated macrophages. J Exp Med 1978;148:435.
246. Candella CJ, Davies P, Allison AC. Immune complexes induce selective release of lysosomal hydrolases from macrophages. Nature 1974;247:46.
247. Takemura R, Werb Z. Secretory products of macrophages and their physiological functions. Am J Physiol 1984;246:C1–C9.
248. Weiss J. Leukocyte-derived antimicrobial proteins. Curr Opin Hematol 1994;1:78.
249. Henson P, Henson J, Fittschen C, Bratton D, Riches D. Degranulation and secretion by phagocytic cells. In: Inflammation: basic principles and clinical correlates. New York, Raven Press, 1992:511–540.
250. Rausch PG, Pryzwansky KB, Spitznagel JK. Immunocytochemical identification of azurophilic and specific granule markers in the giant granules of Chediak-Higashi neutrophils. N Engl J Med 1978;298:693–698.
251. Kimball HR, Ford GH, Wolff SM. Lysosomal enzymes in normal and Chediak-Higashi blood leukocytes. J Lab Clin Med 1975;86:616–630.
252. Ganz T, Metcalf JA, Gallin JI, et al. Two genetic disorders that affect human neutrophils (PMN) are associated with deficiencies of microbicidal and cytotoxic granule proteins. Clin Res 1987;35:424A.
253. Ganz T, Metcalf JA, Gallin JI, Boxer LA, Lehrer RI. Microbicidal/cytotoxic proteins of neutrophils are deficient in two disorders: Chediak-Higashi syndrome and specific granule deficiency. J Clin Invest 1988;82:552–556.
254. Oliver C, Essner E. Formation of anomalous lysosomes in monocytes, neutrophils, and eosinophils from bone marrow of mice with Chediak-Higashi syndrome. Lab Invest 1985;32:17–30.
255. Barak Y, Karov Y, Nir E. Chediak-Higashi syndrome: expression of the cytoplasmic defect by in vitro cultures of bone marrow progenitors. Am J Pediatr Hematol Oncol 1986;8:128–133.
256. Rott RK, Rosenthal AS, Balestra DJ. Abnormal bactericidal, metabolic and lysosomal function of Chediak-Higashi syndrome leukocytes. J Clin Invest 1972;51:649–655.
257. Clark RA, Kimball HR. Defective granulocyte chemotaxis in the Chediak-Higashi syndrome. J Clin Invest 1971;50:2645.
258. Ostland ER, Tucker RW, Leong JT, et al. The cytoskeleton in Chediak-Higashi syndrome fibroblasts. Blood 1980;56:806–817.
259. Pryzwansky KB, Schliwa M, Boxer LA. Microtubule organization of unstimulated and stimulated adherent human neutrophils in Chediak-Higashi syndrome. Blood 1985;66:1398–1403.
260. Boxer GJ, Holmsen H, Robkin K, et al. Abnormal platelet function in Chediak-Higashi syndrome. Br J Haematol 1977;35:521.
261. Buchanan GB, Handin RI. Platelet function in the Chediak-Higashi syndrome. Blood 1976;47:941–951.
262. Menard M, Meyers KM. Storage pool deficiency in cattle with the Chediak-Higashi syndrome results from an absence of dense granule precursors in their megakaryocytes. Blood 1988;72:1726–1734.
263. Klein M, Roder J, Haliotis T, et al. Chediak-Higashi gene in humans. II. The selectivity of the defect in natural-killer and antibody-dependent cell-mediated cytoxicity function. J Exp Med 1980;151:1049–1062.
264. Nair MPN, Gray RH, Boxer LA, et al. Deficiency of inducible suppressor cell activity in Chediak-Higashi syndrome. Am J Hematol 1987;26:55–60.
265. Rubin CM, Burke BA, McKenna RW, et al. The accelerated phase of Chediak-Higashi syndrome: an expression of the virus-associated hemophagocytic syndrome. Cancer 1985;56:524–530.
266. Blume RS, Wolff S. The Chediak-Higashi syndrome: studies in four patients and a review of the literature. Medicine 1972;512:47–280.
267. Pettit RE, Berdal KG. Chediak-Higashi syndrome: neurologic appearance. Arch Neurol 1984;41:1001–1005.
268. Merino F, Henle W, Ramirez Duque P. Chronic active Epstein-Barr virus infection in patients with Chediak-Higashi syndrome. J Clin Immunol 1986;6:299.
269. Boxer LA, Watanabe AM, Rister M. Correction of leukocyte function in Chediak-Higashi syndrome by ascorbate. N Engl J Med 1976;39: 1041–1046.
270. Weening RS, Schoorel ER, Roos D, et al. Effect of ascorbate on abnormal neutrophil, platelet, and lymphocyte function in a patient with the Chediak-Higashi syndrome. Blood 1981;57:856–866.
271. Gallin JI. Neutrophil specific granule deficiency. Annu Rev Med 1985;36:263–274.
272. Parmley RT, Tzeng DY, Baehner RL, Boxer LA. Abnormal distribution of complex carbohydrates in neutrophils of a patient with lactoferrin deficiency. Blood 1983;62:538–548.
273. Gallin JI, Fletcher MP, Seligmann BE, Hoffstein S, Cehrs K, Mounessa N. Human neutrophil-specific granule deficiency: a model to assess the role of neutrophil-specific granules in the evolution of the inflammatory response. Blood 1982;59:1317–1329.
274. Boxer LA, Coates TD, Haak RA, et al. Lactoferrin deficiency associated with altered granulocyte function. N Engl J Med 1982;307:404.
275. Gallin JI, Elin RJ, Rubert RT, et al. Efficacy of ascorbic acid in Chediak-Higashi syndrome (CHS): studies in humans and mice. Blood 1979;53: 226.
276. Ambruso DR, Sasada M, Nishiyama H, et al. Defective bacterial activity and absence of specific granules in neutrophils from a patient with recurrent bacterial infections. J Clin Immunol 1984;4:23.
277. Spitznagel JK. Nonoxidative antimicrobial reactions of leukocytes. Contemp Top Immunobiol 1984;14:283.
278. Stewart DIH, Crawford N. Redistribution of membrane-bound and cytosolic actin in rabbit polymorphonuclear leukocytes during phagocytosis. Biochem J 1985;225:807.
279. Davis JM, Dineen J, Gallin JI. Neutrophil degranulation and abnormal chemotaxis after thermal injury. J Immunol 1980;124:1467–1471.
280. Wolach B, Coates TD, Hugli TE, Baehner RL, Boxer LA. Plasma lactoferrin reflects granulocyte activation via complement in burn patients. J Lab Clin Med 1984;103:284–293.

281. Beutler B, Cerami A. The history, properties, and biological effects of cachectin. Biochemistry 1988;27:7575–7582.
282. Dinarello CA. Biology of interleukin I. FASEB J 1988;2:198–215.
283. Sherry B, Cerami A. Cachectin/tumor necrosis factor exerts endocrine, paracine, and autocrine control of inflammatory responses. J Cell Biol 1988;107:1269–1277.
284. Vilcek J, Lee T. Tumor necrosis factor: new insights into the molecular mechanisms of its multiple actions. J Biol Chem 1991;266:7313–7316.
285. Hart PH, Whitty GA, Piccoli DS, Hamilton JA. Synergistic activation of human monocytes by granulocyte-macrophage colony-stimulating factor and IFN-gamma: increased TNF-alpha but not IL-1 activity. J Immunol 1988;141:1516–1521.
286. Beutler B, Cerami A. Tumor necrosis, cachexia, shock, and inflammation: a common mediator. Annu Rev Biochem 1988;57:505–518.
287. Goodman MG, Chenoweth DE, Weigle WO. Induction of interleukin 1 secretion and enhancement of humoral immunity by binding of human C5a to macrophage surface C5a receptors. J Exp Med 1982;156: 912–917.
288. Lindemann A, Riedel D, Oster W, et al. Granulocyte/macrophage colony-stimulating factor induces interleukin 1 production by human polymorphonuclear neutrophils. J Immunol 1988;140:837–839.
289. Grau GE, Kindler V, Piguet PF, Lambert PH, Vassalli P. Prevention of experimental cerebral malaria by anticytokine antibodies: interleukin 3 and granulocyte macrophage colony-stimulating factor are intermediates in increased tumor necrosis factor production and macrophage accumulation. J Exp Med 1988;168:1499–1504.
290. Dinarello CA, Cannon JG, Wolff SM, et al. Tumor necrosis factor (cachectin) is an endogenous pyrogen and induces production of interleukin 1. J Exp Med 1986;163:1433–1450.
291. Le J, Vilcek J. Accessory function of human fibroblasts in mitogen-stimulated interferon-gamma production by T lymphocytes: inhibition by interleukin 1 and tumor necrosis factor. J Immunol 1987;139:3330–3337.
292. Dinarello CA, Mier JW. Lymphokines. N Engl J Med 1987;317:940–945.
293. Clark SC, Kamen R. The human hematopoietic colony-stimulating factors. Science 1987;236:1229–1237.
294. Sugimoto M, Wakabayashi Y, Hirose S, Murphy MJ J. Mouse peritoneal macrophages produce CFU-gm and CFU-meg growth-promoting factors. Exp Cell Biol 1988;56:29–38.
295. Sieff CA, Niemeyer CM, Mentzer SJ, Faller DV. Interleukin-1, tumor necrosis factor, and the production of colony-stimulating factors by cultured mesenchymal cells. Blood 1988;72:1316–1323.
296. Vellenga E, Rambaldi A, Ernst TJ, Ostapovicz D, Griffin D. Independent regulation of M-CSF and G-CSF gene expression in human monocytes. Blood 1988;71:1529–1532.
297. Schwartz BS, Levy A, Fair DS, Edgington TS. Murine lymphoid procoagulant activity induced by bacterial lipopolysaccharide and immune complexes in a monocyte prothrombinase. J Exp Med 1982;155: 1464–1479.
298. Rao LV, Rapaport SI. Activation of factor VII bound to tissue factor: a key early step in the tissue factor pathway of blood coagulation. Proc Natl Acad Sci 1988;85:6687–6691.
299. Moon DK, Geczy CL. Recombinant IFN-gamma synergizes with lipopolysaccharide to induce macrophage membrane procoagulants. J Immunol 1988;141:1536–1542.
300. Conkling PR, Chua CC, Nadler P, et al. Clinical trials with human tumor necrosis factor: in vivo and in vitro effects on human mononuclear phagocyte function. Cancer Res 1988;48:5604–5609.
301. Lorenzet R, Niemetz J, Marcus AJ, Broekman MJ. Enhancement of mononuclear procoagulant activity by platelet 12-hydroxyeicosatetraenoic acid. J Clin Invest 1986;78:418–423.
302. Strunk RC, Whitehead AS, Cole FS. Pretranslational regulation of the synthesis of the third component of complement in human mononuclear phagocytes by the lipid A portion of lipopolysaccharide. J Clin Invest 1985;76:985–990.
303. Colten HR, Strunk RC, Perlmutter DH, Cole FS. Regulation of complement protein biosynthesis in mononuclear phagocytes. Ciba Found Symp 1986;118:141–154.
304. Hamilton AO, Jones L, Morrison L, Whaley K. Modulation of monocyte complement synthesis by interferons. Biochem J 1987;242:809–815.
305. Werb Z, Gordon S. Elastase secretion by stimulated macrophages: characterization and regulation. J Exp Med 1975;142:361–377.
306. Wahl LM, Wahl S, Mergenhagen SE, Martin GE. Collagenase production by endotoxin-activated macrophages. Proc Natl Acad Sci 1974;71:3598–3601.
307. Welgus HG, Campbell EJ, Bar-Shavit Z, Senior RM, Teitelbaum SL. Human alveolar macrophages produce a fibroblast-like collagenase and collagenase inhibitor. J Clin Invest 1985;76:219–224.
308. Vassalli J, Dayer J, Wohlwend A, Belin D. Concomitant secretion of prourokinase and of plasminogen activator-specific inhibitor by cultured human monocytes-macrophages. J Exp Med 1985;159:1653–1668.
309. Mornex J-F, Chytil-Weir A, Martinet Y, Courtney M, LeCocq J-P, Crystal RG. Expression of the alpha-1-antitrypsin gene in mononuclear phagocytes of normal and alpha-1-antitrypsin-deficient individuals. J Clin Invest 1986;77:1952–1961.
310. Hovi T, Mosher D, Vaheri A. Cultured human monocytes synthesize and secrete alpha-2-macroglobulin. J Exp Med 1977;145:1580–1589.
311. Chapman HA, Stone OL. Characterization of a macrophage-derived plasminogen-activator inhibitor: similarities with placental urokinase inhibitor. Biochem J 1985;230:109–116.
312. Klimetzek V, Sorg C. The production of fibrinolysis inhibitors as a parameter of the activation state in murine macrophages. Eur J Immunol 1979;9:613–619.
313. Saito H. Alpha 2-plasmin inhibitor and its deficiency states. J Lab Clin Med 1988;112:671–678.
314. Aoki N, Harpel PC. Inhibitors of the fibrinolytic enzyme system. Semin Thromb Hemost 1984;10:24–41.
315. Kitchens CS. Concept of hypercoagulability: a review of its development, clinical application, and recent progress. Semin Thromb Hemost 1985;11:293–315.
316. Cohn ZA. Macrophage physiology. Fed Proc 1975;34:1725–1729.
317. LaFleur M, Beaulieu AD, Kreis C, Poubelle P. Fibronectin gene expression in polymorphonuclear leukocytes: accumulation of mRNA in inflammatory cells. J Biol Chem 1987;262:2111–2115.
318. Samuelsson B, Dahlen S-E, Lindgren J-A, Rouzer CA, Serhan CN. Leukotrienes and lipoxins: structures, biosynthesis and biological effects. Science 1987;237:1171–1176.
319. Scott WA, Rouzer CA, Cohn ZA. Leukotriene C release by macrophages. Fed Proc 1983;42:129–133.
320. Rouzer CA, Matsumoto T, Samuelsson B. Single protein from human leukocytes possesses 5-lipoxygenase and leukotriene A4 synthase activities. Proc Natl Acad Sci 1986;83:857–861.
321. Soberman RJ, Harper TW, Betteridge D, Lewis RA, Austen KF. Characterization and separation of the arachidonic acid 5-lipoxygenase and linoleic acid omega-6 liposygenase (arachidonic acid 15-lipoxygenase) of human polymorphonuclear leukocytes. J Biol Chem 1985;260:4508–4515.
322. Miller DK, Gillard JW, Vickers PJ, et al. Identification and isolation of a membrane protein necessary for leukotriene production. Nature 1990;343:278.
323. Rådmark O, Shimizu T, Jornvall H, Samuelsson B. Leukotriene A4 hydrolase in human leukocytes: purification and properties. J Biol Chem 1984;259:12339–12345.
324. Jakschik BA, Harper T, Murphy RC. Leukotriene C4 and D4 formation by particulate enzymes. J Biol Chem 1982;257:5346–5349.
325. Lewis RA, Austen KF. The biologically active leukotrienes: biosynthesis, metabolism, receptors, functions, and pharmacology. J Clin Invest 1984;73:889–897.
326. Grimminger F, Menger M, Becker G, Seeger W. Potentiation of leukotriene production following sequestration of neutrophils in isolated lungs: indirect evidence for intercellular leukotriene A4 transfer. Blood 1988;72:1687–1692.
327. Samuelsson B, Funk CD. Enzymes involved in the biosynthesis of leukotriene B4. J Biol Chem 1989;264:19469–19472.
328. Peveri P, Walz A, Dewald B, Baggiolini M. A novel neutrophil-activating factor produced by human mononuclear phagocytes. J Exp Med 1988;167:1547–1559.
329. Dessein AJ, Lee TH, Elsas P, et al. Enhancement by monokines of leukotriene generation by human eosinophils and neutrophils stimulated with calcium ionophore A23187. 1986;136:3829–3838.
330. Haurand M, Flohe L. Leukotriene formation by human polymorphonuclear leukocytes from endogenous arachidonate: physiological triggers and modulation. Biochem Pharmacol 1989;38:2129–2137.
331. Dahinden CA, Zingg J, Maly FE, deWeck AL. Leukotriene production in human neutrophils primed by recombinant human granulocyte/macrophage colony-stimulating factor and stimulated with the complement component C5A and FMLP as second signals. J Exp Med 1988;167:1281–1295.
332. Rouzer CA, Scott WA, Hamill AL, et al. Secretion of leukotriene C and other arachidonic acid metabolities by macrophages challenged with immunoglobulin E immune complexes. J Exp Med 1982;56:1077–1086.
333. Ouwendijk RJ, Zijlstra FJ, van den Broek AM, et al. Comparison of the production of eicosanoids by human and rat peritoneal macrophages and rat Kupffer cells: prostaglandins 1988;35:437–446.
334. Fuller RW, Kelsey CR, Cole PJ, Dollery CT, MacDermott J. Dexamethasone inhibits the production of thromboxane B2 and leukotriene B4 by human alveolar and peritoneal macrophages in culture. Clin Sci 1984;67:653–656.
335. Bertram TA, Overby LH, Danilowicz R, Eling TE, Brody AR. Pulmonary intravascular macrophages metabolize arachidonic acid in vitro: comparison with alveolar macrophages. Am Rev Respir Dis 1988;138:936–944.
336. Lee TH, Hoover RL, Williams JD, et al. Effect of dietary enrichment with eicosapentaenoic and docosahexaenoic acids on in vitro neutrophil and monocyte leukotriene generation and neutrophil function. N Engl J Med 1985;312:1217–1224.
337. Soberman RJ, Sutyak RT, Okite I, Wendelborn DF, Roberts LJ, Austen KF. The identification and formation of 20-aldehyde leukotriene B4. J Biol Chem 1988;263:7996–8002.
338. Sumimoto JK, Takeshige K, Minakami S. Characterization of human neutrophil leukotriene B4 omega-hydroxylase as a system invovling

a unique cytochrome P-450 and NADPH–cytochrome P-450 reductase. Eur J Biochem 1988;172:315–324.
339. Lee CW, Lewis RA, Tauber AI, et al. The myeloperoxidase-dependent metabolism of leukotrienes C4, D4, and E4 to 6-trans-leukotriene B4 diastereoisomers and the subclass-specific S-diastereoisomeric sulfoxides. J Biol Chem 1983;258:15004–15010.
340. Marcus AJ. Transcellular metabolism of eicosanoids. Prog Hemost Thromb 1986;262:127–142.
341. Marcus AJ. Eicosanoids as bioregulators in clinical medicine. Am J Med 1985;78:805–810.
342. Chauncey JB, Simon RH, Peters-Golden M. Rat alveolar macrophages synthesize leukotriene B4 and 12-hydroxyeicosatetraenoic acid from alveolar epithelial cell–derived arachidonic acid. Am Rev Resp Dis 1988;138:928–935.
343. Samuelsson B, Goldyne M, Granstrom E, Hamberg M, Sammarstrom S, Malmsten C. Prostaglandins and thromboxanes. Annu Rev Biochem 1978;47:997–1029.
344. Browning JL, Ribolini A. Interferon blocks interleukin 1-inducted prostaglandin release from human peripheral monocytes. J Immunol 1987;138:2857–2863.
345. Scott WA, Pawlowski NA, Murray HW, Andreach M, Zrike J, Cohen ZA. Regulation of arachidonic acid metabolism by macrophage activation. J Exp Med 1982;155:1148–1160.
346. Chensue SW, Kunkel SL, Higashi GI, Ward PA, Boros DL. Production of superoxide anion, prostaglandins, and hydroxy eicosatetraenoic acids by macrophages from hypersensitivity-type (Schistosoma mansoni egg) and foreign body-type granulomas. Infect Immun 1983;42: 1116–1125.
347. Hansch BM, Seitz M, Martinotti G, et al. Macrophages release arachidonic acid, prostaglandin E2, and thromboxane in response to late complement components. J Immunol 1984;133:2145–2150.
348. Wood JN, Coote PR, Rhodes J. Hydrocortisone inhibits prostaglandin production but not arachidonic acid release from cultured macrophages. FEBS Lett 1984;174:143–146.
349. Segal ML, Fertel RH, Kraut EH, Sagone AL. The role of reactive oxygen species in thromboxane b2 generation by polymorphonuclear leukocytes. J Lab Clin Med 1983;102:788–794.
350. Schade UF. Involvement of lipoxygenases in the activation of mouse macrophages by endotoxin. Biochem Biophys Res Commun 1986;138: 842–849.
351. Lim LK, Hunt NH, Eichner RD, Weidemann MJ. Cyclic AMP and the regulation of prostaglandin production by macrophages. Biochem Biophys Res Commun 1983;114:248–254.
352. Hanahan DJ. Platelet-activating factor: a biologically active phosphoglyceride. Annu Rev Biochem 1986;55:483–509.
353. McManus LM, Pinckard N, Fitzpatrick FA, O'Rourke RA, Crawford MH, Hanahan DJ. Acetyl glyceryl ether phosphorylcholine: intravascular alterations following intravenous infusion into the baboon. Lab Invest 1981;45:303–307.
354. Nakagawa Y, Sugiura T, Waku K. The molecular species composition of diacyl-, alkylacyl- and alkenylacylglycerophospholipids in rabbit alveolar macrophages: high amounts of 1-O-hexadecyl-2-arachidonyl molecular species in alkylacylglycerophosphocholine. Biochim Biophys Acta 1985;833:323–329.
355. Leslie CC, Detty DM. Arachidonic acid turnover in response to lipopolysaccharide and opsonized zymosan in human monocyte-derived macrophages. Biochem J 1986;236:251–259.
356. Alonso F, Henson PM, Leslie CC. A cytosolic phospholipase in human neutrophils that hydrolyzes arachidonoyl-containing phosphatidylcholine. Biochim Biophys Acta 1986;878:273–280.
357. Mollinedo F, Gomez-Cambronero J, Cano E, Sanchez-Crespo M. Intracellular localization of platelet-activating factor synthesis in human neutrophils. Biochem Biophys Res Commun 1988;154:1232–1239.
358. Lynch JM, Henson PM. The intracellular retention of newly synthesized platelet-activating factor. J Immunol 1986;37:2653–2661.
359. Ramesha CS, Pickett WC. Metabolism of platelet-activating factor by arachidonic acid–depleted rat polymorphonuclear leukocytes. J Biol Chem 1986;261:15519–15523.
360. Sugiura T, Masuzawa Y, Nakagawa Y, Waku K. Transacylation of lyso platelet-activating factor and other lysophospholipids by macrophage microsomes: distinct donor and acceptor selectivities. J Biol Chem 1987;262:1199–1205.
361. Roubin R, Dulioust A, Haye-Legrand I, NMinio E, Benveniste J. Biosynthesis of pafacether. VIII. Impairment of paf-acether production in activated macrophages does not depend upon acetyltransferase activity. J Immunol 1986;136:1796–1802.
362. Camussi G, Bussolini F, Salvidio G, Baglioni C. Tumor necrosis factor/cachectin stimulates peritoneal macrophages, polymorphonuclear neutrophils, and vascular endothelial cells to synthesize and release platelet-activating factor. J Exp Med 1987;166:1390–1404.
363. Tessner TG, O'Flaherty JT, Wykle RL. Stimulation of platelet-activating factor synthesis by a nonmetabolizable bioactive analog of platelet-activating factor and influence of arachidonic acid metabolites. J Biol Chem 1989;264:4794–4799.
364. Doebber TW, Wu MS. Platelet-activating factor (PAF) stimulates the PAF-synthesizing enzyme acetyl-CaA:1-alkyl-sn-glycero-3-phosphocholine O2-acetyltransferase and PAF synthesis in neutrophils. Proc Natl Acad Sci 1987;84:7557–7561.
365. Wirthmueller U, deWeck AL, Dahinden CA. Platelet-activating factor production in human neutrophils by sequential stimulation with granulocyte-macrophage colony-stimulating factor and the chemotactic factors C5A or formyl-methionyl-leucyl-phenylalanine. J Immunol 1989;142:3213–3218.
366. Sisson JH, Prescott SM, McIntyre TM, Zimmerman GA. Production of platelet-activating factor by stimulated human polymorphonuclear leukocytes: correlation of synthesis with release, functional events, and leukotriene B4 metabolism. J Immunol 1987;138:3918–3926.
367. Elstad MR, Stafforini DM, McIntyre TM, Prescott SM, Zimmerman GA. Platelet-activating factor acetylhydrolase increases during macrophage differentiation: a novel mechanism that regulates accumulation of platelet-activating factor. J Biol Chem 1989;264:8467–8470.
368. Sperling RI, Robin JL, Kylander KA, et al. The effects of N-3 polyunsaturated fatty acids on the generation of platelet-activating factor acether by human monocytes. J Immunol 1987;139:4186–4191.
369. Dewald B, Baggiolini M. Platelet-actiating factor as a stimulus of exocytosis in human neutrophils. Biochim Biophys Acta 1986;888:42–48.
370. Conrad GW, Rink TJ. Platelet activating factor raises intracellular calcium ion concentration in macrophages. J Cell Biol 1986;103:439–450.
371. Gay JC, Beckman JK, Zaboy KA, Lukens JN. Modulation of neutrophil oxidative responses to soluble stimuli by platelet-activating factor. Blood 1986;67:931–936.
372. Ingraham LM, LaFuze JE, Boxer LA, Baehner RL. In vitro and in vivo effects of treatment by platelet-activating factor on N-formyl-metleuphe-mediated responses of polymorphonuclear leukocytes. Br J Haematol 1987;66:219–225.
373. Palmer RMJ, Ferrige AG, Moncada S. Nitric oxide release accounts for the biological activity of endothelium-derived relaxing factor. Nature 1987;327:524–526.
374. Ignarro LJ. Endothelium-derived nitric oxide: actions and properties. FASEB J 1989;3:31–36.
375. Stuehr DJ, Gross SS, Sakuma I, Levi R, Nathan CF. Activated murine macrophages secrete a metabolite of arginine with the bioactivity of endothelium-derived relaxing factor and the chemical reactivity of nitric oxide. J Exp Med 1989;169:1011–1120.
376. Wright CD, Mulsch A, Busse R, Osswald H. Generation of nitric oxide by human neutrophils. Biochem Biophys Res Commun 1989;160:813–819.
377. Schmidt HH, Seifert R, Bohme E. Formation and release of nitric oxide from human neutrophils and HL-60 cells induced by a chemotactic peptide, platelet activating factor and leukotriene B4. FEBS Lett 1989;44:357–360.
378. Sakuma I, Stuehr DJ, Gross SS, Nathan C, Levi R. Identification of arginine as a precursor of endothelium-derived relaxing factor. Proc Natl Acad Sci 1988;85:8664–8667.
379. Moncada S, Palmer RM, Higgs EA. Biosynthesis of nitric oxide from L-arginine: a pathway for the regulation of cell function and communication. Biochem Pharmacol 1989;38:1709–1715.
380. Stuehr DJ, Nathan CF. Nitric oxide: a macrophage product responsible for cytostasis and respiratory inhibition in tumor target cells. J Exp Med 1989;169:1543–1555.
381. Iyengar R, Stuehr DJ, Marletta MA. Macrophage synthesis of nitrite, nitrate, and N-nitrosamines: precursors and role of the respiratory burst. Proc Natl Acad Sci 1987;84:6369–6373.
382. Miwa M, Stuehr DJ, Marletta MA, Wishnok JS, Tannenbaum SR. Nitrosation of amines by stimulated macrophages: carcinogenesis 1987;8: 955–958.
383. Ignarro LJ, Gold ME, Buga GM, et al. Basic polyamino acids rich in arginine, lysine or ornithine cause both enhancement of and refractoriness to formation of endothelium-derived nitric oxide in pulmonary artery and vein. Circ Res 1989;64:315–329.
384. Vanhoute PM. The end of the quest? Nature 1987;327:459–460.
385. Arnold WP, Mittal CK, Katsuki S, Murad F. Nitric oxide activates guanylate cyclase and increases guanosine 3′:5′-cyclic monophosphate levels in various tissue preparations. Proc Natl Acad Sci 1977;74:3203–3207.
386. Stuehr DJ, Marletta MA. Mammalian nitrate biosynthesis: mouse macrophages produce nitrite and nitrate in response to *Escherichia coli* lipopolysaccharide. Proc Natl Acad Sci 1985;82:7738–7742.
387. Stuehr DJ, Marletta MA. Induction of nitrite/nitrate synthesis in murine macrophages by BCG infection, lymphokines, or interferon-gamma. J Immunol 1987;139:518–525.
388. Babior BM. The respiratory burst oxidase. Trends Biochem Sci 1987;12: 241–243.
389. Segal AW. The electron transport chain of the microbicidal oxidase of phagocytic cells and its involvement in the molecular pathology of chronic granulomatous disease. J Clin Invest 1989;83:1785–1793.
390. Babior BM. Oxygen-dependent microbial killing by phagocytes. N Engl J Med 1978;298:659–668.
391. Dewald B, Baggiolini M, Curnutte JT, Babior BM. Subcellular localization of the superoxide-forming enzyme inhuman neutrophils. J Clin Invest 1979;63:21–29.
392. Curnutte JT, Babior BM. Biological defense mechanisms: the effect of bacteria and serum on superoxide production by granulocytes. J Clin Invest 1974;53:1662–1672.

393. Wymann MP, von Tscharner V, Deranleau DA, Baggiolini M. The onset of the respiratory burst in human neutrophils: real-time studies of H2O2 formation reveal a rapid agonist-induced transduction process. J Biol Chem 1987;262:12048–12053.
394. Sklar LA, Hyslop PA, Oades ZG, Omann GM, Jesaitis AJ, Painter RG, Cochrane CG. Signal transduction and ligand-receptor dynamics in the human neutrophil: transient responses and occupancy-response relations at the formyl peptide receptor. J Biol Chem 1985;260:11461–11468.
395. Curnutte JT, Babior BM, Karnovsky LM. Fluoride-mediated activation of the respiratory burst in human neutrophils. J Clin Invest 1979;63: 637–647.
396. Jandl RC, Andre-Schwartz J, Borges-Dubois L, Kipnes L, McMurrich BJ, Babior BM. Termination of the respiratory burst in human neutrophils. J Clin Invest 1978;61:1176–1185.
396a. Bokoch G, Knaus U. Ras-related GTP-binding proteins and leukocyte signal transduction. Curr Opin Hematol 1994;1:53.
397. Royer-Pokora B, Kunkel LM, Monaco AP, et al. Cloning the gene for an inherited human disorder—chronic granulomatous disease—on the basis of its chromosomal location. Nature 1986;322:32–38.
398. Parkos CA, Allen RA, Cochrane CG, Jesaitis AJ. Purified cytochrome b from human granulocyte plasma membrane is comprised of two polypeptides with relative molecular weights of 91,000 and 22,000. J Clin Invest 1987;80:732–742.
399. Hayakawa T, Suzuki K, Suzuki S, Andrews PC, Babior BM. A possible role for protein phosphorylation in the activation of the respiratory burst in human neutrophils. J Biol Chem 1986;261:9109–9115.
400. Nunoi H, Rotrosen D, Gallin JI, Malech HL. Two forms of autosomal chronic granulomatous disease lack distinct neutrophil cytosol factors. Science 1988;242:1298–1301.
401. Clark RA, Malech HL, Gallin JI, et al. Genetic variants of chronic granulomatous disease: prevalence of deficiencies of two discrete cytosolic components of the NADPH oxidase system. N Engl J Med 1989;321:647.
402. Abo A, Boyhan A, West I, Thrasher A, Segal A. Reconstitution of neutrophil NADPH oxidase activity in the cell-free system by four components: p67-*phox*, p47-*phox*, p21*rac*1, and cytochrome b-245. J Biol Chem 1992;267:16767–16770.
403. Leto TL, Lomax KJ, Volpp BD, et al. Cloning of a 67-kD neutrophil oxidase factor with similarity to a noncatalytic region of p60c-src. Science 1990;248:727.
404. Okamura N, Malawista SE, Roberts RL, et al. Phosphorylation of the oxidase-related 48K phosphoprotein family in the unusual autosomal cytochrome-negative and X-linked cytochrome-positive types of chronic granulomatous disease. Blood 1988;72:811–816.
405. Smith RM, Curnutte JT, Babior BM. Affinity labeling of the cytosolic and membrane components of respiratory burst oxidase by the 2′,3′-dialdehyde derivative of NADPH: evidence for a cytosolic location of the nucleotide-binding site in the resting cell. J Biol Chem 1989;264: 1958–1962.
406. Suzuki H, Pabst MJ, Johnston RB. Enhancement by Ca2+ or Mg2+ of catalytic activity of the superoxide-producing NADPH oxidase in membrane fractions of human neutrophils and monocytes. J Biol Chem 1985;260:3635–3639.
407. Zakhireh B, Root RK. Development of oxidase activity by human bone marrow. Blood 1979;54:429–439.
408. Johnston J, Oxygen RB. metabolism and the microbicidal activity of macrophages. Fed Proc 1978;37:2759–2764.
409. Kitagawa S, Johnston RB. Relationship between membrane potential changes and superoxide-releasing capacity in resident and activated mouse pepritoneal macrophages. J Immunol 1985;135:3417–3423.
410. Murray HW, Scavuzzo D, Jacobs JL, et al. In vitro and in vivo activation of human mononuclear phagocytes by interferon-gamma: studies with normal and AIDS monocytes. J Immunol 1987;138:2457–2462.
411. Jesaitis AJ, Tolley JO, Allen RA. Receptor-cytoskeleton interactions and membrane traffic may regulate chemoattractant-induced superoxide production in human granulocytes. J Biol Chem 1986;261:13662–13669.
412. Thomas EL, Fishman M. Oxidation of chloride and thiocyanate by isolated leukocytes. J Biol Chem 1986;261:9694–9702.
413. Klebanoff SJ. Oxygen-dependent cytotoxic mechanisms of phagocytes. Adv Host Defense Mech 1982:1:111.
414. Weiss SJ, Peppin G, Ortiz X, Ragsdale C, Test ST. Oxidative autoactivation of latent collagenase by human neutrophils. Science 1985;227: 747–749.
415. Thomas EL, Jefferson MM, Grisham M. Myeloperoxidase-catalyzed incorporation of amino acids into proteins: role of hypochlorous acid and chloramines. Biochemistry 1982;21:6299–6308.
416. Weiss SJ, Klein R, Slivka A. Chlorination of taurine by human neutrophils. J Clin Invest 1982;70:598.
417. Rosen H, Rakita RM, Waltersdorph AM, Klebanoff SJ. Myeloperoxidase-mediated damage to the succinate oxidase system of *Escherichia coli*: evidence for selective inactivation of the dehydrogenase component. J Biol Chem 1987;242:15004–15010.
418. Green MR, Hill HAO, Okolow-Zublowska MJ, Segal AW. The production of hydroxyl and superoxide radicals by stimulated human neutrophils: measurement by EPR spectroscopy. FEBS Lett 1979;100: 23–26.
419. Samuni A, Black CDV, Krishna CM, Malech HL, Bernstein EF, Russo A. Hydroxyl radical production by stimulated neutrophils reappraised. J Biol Chem 1988;263:13797–13801.
420. Jackson JH, Gajewski E, Schraufstatter IV, et al. Damage to the bases in DNA induced by stimulated human neutrophils. J Clin Invest 1989;84:1644–1649.
421. Weitzman SA, Weitberg AB, Clark EP, Stossel TP. Phagocytes as carcinogens: malignant transformation produced by human neutrophils. Science 1985;227:1231–1233.
422. McCord JM, Fridovich I. Superoxide dismutase: an enzymic function for erythrocuprein. J Biol Chem 1969;244:6049–6055.
423. McCord JM, Keele BB J, Fridovich I. An enzyme-based theory of obligate anaerobiosis: the physiological function of superoxide dismutase. Proc Natl Acad Sci 1971;68:1024–1027.
424. Farr SB, D'Ari R, Touati D. Oxygen-dependent mutagenesis in Escherichia coli lacking superoxide dismutase. Proc Natl Acad Sci 1986;83: 8268–8272.
425. Fridovich I. Superoxide dismutases: an adaptation to a paramagnetic gas. J Biol Chem 1989;264:7761–7764.
426. Bass DA, DeChatelet LR, Burk RF, Shirley P, Szejda P. Polymorphonuclear leukocyte bactericidal activity and oxidative metabolism during glutathione peroxidase deficiency. Infect Immun 1989;18:78–84.
427. Takahashi K, Cohen HJ. Selenium-dependent glutathione peroxidase protein and activity: immunological investigations on cellular and plasma enzymes. Blood 1986;68:640–645.
428. Tappel AL. Selenium—glutathione peroxidase: properties and synthesis. Curr Top Cell Regul 1984;24:87–97.
429. Awasthi YC, Beutler E, Srivastava SK. Purification and properties of human erythrocyte glutathione peroxidase. J Biol Chem 1975;250: 5144–5149.
430. Forstrom JW, Stults FH, Tapel AL. Rat liver cytosolic glutathione peroxidase: reactivity with linoleic acid hydroperoxide and cumene hydroperoxide. Arch Biochem Biophys 1979;193:51–55.
431. Deisseroth A, Dounce AL. Catalase: physical and chemical properties, mechanism of catalysis, and physiological role. Physiol Rev 1970;50: 319–375.
432. Nicholls P, Schonbaum GR. Catalases. In: Boyer L, Lardy H, Myrback E, eds. The enzymes. New York, Academic Press, 1963.
433. Voetman AA, Roos D. Endogenous catalase protects human blood phagocytes against oxidative damage by extracellularly generated hydrogen peroxide. Blood 1980;56:846–852.
434. Gaetani GF, Galiano S, Canepa L, Ferraris AM, Kirkman HN. Catalase and glutathione peroxidase are equally active in detoxification of hydrogen peroxide in human erythrocytes. Blood 1989;73:334–339.
435. Aebi H, Suter H. Acatlasemia. Adv Hum Genet 1971;2:143–199.
436. Frei B, Stocker R, Ames BN. Antioxidant defenses and lipid peroxidation in human blood plasma. Proc Natl Acad Sci 1988;85:9748–9752.
437. Baehner RL, Boxer LA. Role of membrane vitamin E and cytoplasmic glutathione in the regulation of phagocytic functions of neutrophils and monocytes. Am J Pediatr Hematol Oncol 1979;1:71–76.
438. Mukai K, Nishimura M, Ishizu K, Kitamura Y. Kinetic study of the reaction of vitamin C with vitamin E radicals (tocopheroxyls) in solution. Biochim Biophys Acta 1989;991:276–279.
439. Liebler DC, Kling DS, Reed DJ. Antioxidant protection of phospholipid bilayers by alpha-tocopherol: control of alpha-tocopherol status and lipid peroxidation by ascorbic acid and glutathione. J Biol Chem 1986;261:12114–12119.
440. Barclay LR. The cooperative antioxidant role of glutathione with a lipid-soluble and a water-soluble antioxidant peroxidation of liposomes initiated in the aqueous phase and in the lipid phase. J Biol Chem 1988;263:16138–16142.
441. Cramer R, Soranzo MR, Dri P, et al. Incidence of myeloperoxidase deficiency in an area of northern Italy: histochemical, biochemical and functional studies. Br J Haematol 1982;51:81.
442. Kitahara M, Eyre HJ, Simonian Y, et al. Hereditary myeloperoxidase deficiency. Blood 1981;57:888.
443. Parry MF, Root RK, Metcalf JA, et al. Myeloperoxidase deficiency: prevalence and clinical significance. Ann Intern Med 1981;95:283.
444. Nauseef WM. Aberrant restriction endonuclease digests of DNA from subjects with hereditary myeloperoxidase deficiency. Blood 1989;73: 290–295.
445. Tobler A, Selsted ME, Miller CW, et al. Evidence for a pretranslational defect in hereditary and acquired myeloperoxidase deficiency. Blood 1989;73:1980–1986.
446. Cech P, Papathanassiou A, Boreaux G, et al. Hereditary myeloperoxidase deficiency. Blood 1979;53:403.
447. Rosen H, Klebanoff SJ. Chemiluminescence and superoxide production by myeloperoxidase-deficient leukocytes. J Clin Invest 1976:58:50.
448. Stendahl O, Coble B-I, Dahlgren C, et al. Myeloperoxidase modulates the phagocytic activity of polymorphonuclear leukocytes: studies with cells from a myeloperoxidase-deficient patient. J Clin Invest 1984;73: 366.
449. Klebanoff SJ. Myeloperoxidase: contribution to the microbicidal activity of intact leukocytes. Science 1970;169:1095.
450. Lehrer RI, Cline MJ. Leukocyte myeloperoxidase deficiency and dis-

seminated candidasis: the role of myeloperoxidase in resistance to Candida infection. J Clin Invest 1969;48:1478.
451. Lehrer RI, Hanifin J, Cline MJ. Defective bactericidal activity in myeloperoxidase-deficient human neutrophils. Nature 1969;223:78.
452. Lehrer RI, Landra KM, Hake RB. Nonoxidative fungicidal mechanisms of mammalian granulocytes: demonstration of components with candidacidal activity in human, rabbit, and guinea pig leukocytes. Infect Immun 1975;11:226.
453. Diamond RD, Clark RA, Haudenschild CC. Damage to *Candida albicans* hyphae and pseudohyphae by the myeloperoxidase system and oxidative products of neutrophil metabolism in vitro. J Clin Invest 1980;66:908.
454. Rider ED, Christensen RD, Hall DC, Rothstein G. Myeloperoxidase deficiency in neutrophils of neonates. J Pediatr 1988;112:648–651.
455. Cech P, Stalder H, Widmann JJ, et al. Leukocyte myeloperoxidase deficiency and diabetes mellitus associated with Candida albicans liver abcess. Am J Med 1979;66:149.
456. Robertson, CF, Thong YH, Hodge GL, et al. Primary myeloperoxidase deficiency associated with impaired neutrophil margination and chemotaxis. Acta Pediatr Scand 1979;68:915.
457. Kussenbach G, Rister M. Der Myeloperoxidase-Mangel als Ursache rezidivierende Infektionen. Klin Paediatr 1985;197:443.
458. Stendahl O, Lindgren S. Function of granulocytes with deficiency of myeloperoxidase-mediated iodination in a patient with generalized pustular psoriasis. Scand J Haematol 1976;16:144.
459. Salmon SE, Cline MJ, Schultz J, Lehrer RI. Myeloperoxidase deficiency: immunological study of a genetic leukocyte defect. N Engl J Med 1970;282:250.
460. Malech HL, Gallin JI. Current concepts: immunology. Neutrophils in human disease. N Engl J Med 1987;317:687–694.
461. Boxer LA, Morganroth ML. Neutrophil function disorders. Dis Mon 1987;33:681–780.
462. Smith R, Curnutte J. Molecular basis of chronic granulomatous disease. Blood 1991;77:673–686.
463. Segal AW, Cross AR, Garcia RC, et al. Absence of cytochrome b-245 in chronic granulomatous disease: a multicenter European evaluation of its incidence and relevance. N Engl J Med 1978;308:245–251.
464. Dinauer MC, Orkin SH, Brown R, Jesaitis AJ, Parkos CA. The glycoprotein encoded by the X-linked chronic granulomatous disease locus is a component of the neutrophil cytochrome b complex. Nature 1987;327:717–720.
465. Volpp BD, Nauseef WM, Clark RA. Two cytosolic neutrophil oxidase components absent in autosomal chronic granulomatous disease. Science 1988;242:1295–1297.
466. Parkos CA, Dinauer MC, Jesaitis AJ, Orkin SH, Curnutte JT. Absence of both the 91kD and 22kD subunits of human neutrophil cytochrome b in two genetic forms of chronic granulomatous disease. Blood 1989;73:1416–1420.
467. Segal AW. Absence of both cytochrome b-245 subunits from neutrophils in X-linked chronic granulomatous disease. Nature 1987;326: 88–92.
468. Marsh WL. Chronic granulomatous disease, the McLeod syndrome, and the Kell blood groups. Birth Defects 1978;14:9–25.
469. Marsh WL, Oyen R, Nichols ME, Allen FH. Chronic granulomatous disease and the Kell blood groups. Br J Haematol 1975;29:247–262.
470. Densen P, Wilkinson-Kroovand S, Mandell GL, Sullivan G, Oyen R, Marsh WL. Kx: its relationship to chronic granulomatous disease and genetic linkage with Xg. Blood 1981;58:34–37.
471. Woodruff RK, Wiley JS, Bell WR, McPherson AJ, Ford DS. Acanthocytosis and haemolytic anaemia due to the McLeod blood groups. Aust N Z J Med 1981;11:184–187.
472. deSaint-Basile G, Bohler MC, Fischer A, et al. Xp21 DNA microdeletion in a patient with chronic granulomatous disease, retinitis pigmentosa, and McLeod phenotype. Hum Genet 1988;80:85–90.
473. Baehner RL, Kunkel LM, Monaco AP, et al. DNA linkage analysis of X chromosome-linked chronic granulomatous disease. Proc Natl Acad Sci 1986;83:3398–3401.
474. Johnston RB, Newman SL. Chronic granulomatous disease. Pediatr Clin North Am 1977;24:365–376.
475. Baehner RL. Neutrophil dysfunction associated with states of chronic and current infection. Pediatr Clin North Am 1980;27:377–401.
476. Forrest CB, Forehand JR, Axtell RA, Roberts RL, Johnston RB. Clinical features and current management of chronic granulomatous disease. Hematol Oncol Clin North Am 1988:2;253–266.
477. Dilworth JA, Mandell GL. Adults with chronic granulomatous disease of childhood. Am J Med 1977;63:233–266.
478. Perry HB, Boulanger M, Pennoyer D. Chronic granulomatous disease in an adult with recurrent abcesses. Arch Surg 1980;115:200–202.
479. Burniat W, Toppet M, DeMol P. Acute and recurrent salmonella infections in three children with chronic granulomatous disease. J Infect 1980;2:263–268.
480. Cohen MS, Isturiz RE, Malech HL, et al. Fungal infection in chronic granulomatous disease: the importance of the phagocyte in defense against fungi. Am J Med 1981;71:59–66.
481. Elgefors B, Haugstvedt S, Brorsson JE, Esbjorner E. Disseminated aspergillosis treated with amphotericin B and surgery in a boy with chronic granulomatous disease. Infection 1980;8:174–176.
482. Corrado ML, Cleri D, Fikrig SM, Phillips JC, Ahonkhai VI. Aspergillosis in chronic granulomatous disease: therapeutic considerations. Am J Dis Child 1980;134:1092–1094.
483. Peerless AG, Liebhaber M, Anderson S, Lehrer RI, Stiehm ER. Legionella pneumonia in chronic granulomatous disease. J Pediatr 1985;106:783–785.
484. White CJ, Kwon-Chung KJ, Gallin JI. Chronic granulomatous disease of childhood: an unusual case of infection in a child with chronic granulomatous disease. Am J Clin Pathol 1988;90:312–316.
485. McGinnis MR, Walker DH, Folds JD. Hansenula polymorpha infection in a child with chronic granulomatous disease. Arch Pathol Lab Med 1980;104:290–292.
486. Schmidt I, Poncz M, Russell MO, Schwartz E. Unusual manifestations of chronic granulomatous disease. Am J Dis Child 1981;135:376–377.
487. Bowen I, Gibson A. Chronic granulomatous disease with gastric antral narrowing. Pediatr Radiol 1980;10:119–120.
488. MacPherson BR. The clinical laboratory diagnosis of chronic granulomatous disease in childhood. CRC Crit Rev Clin Lab Sci 1977;8:81–103.
489. Alter BP. Advances in the prenatal diagnosis of hematologic diseases. Blood 1984;64:329–340.
490. Gray GR, Stamatoyannopoulos G, Naiman SC, et al. Neutrophil dysfunction, chronic granulomatous disease, and nonspherocytic hemolytic anemia caused by complete deficiency in glucose-6-phosphate dehydrogenase. Lancet 1972;2:530.
491. Baehner RL, Johnston RB, Nathan DG. Reduced pyridine nucleotide (RPN) content in G6PD-deficient granulocytes (PMN): an explanation for their defective bactericidal function. J Clin Invest 1971;50:4A.
492. Baehner RL, Johnston RB, Nathan DG. Comparative study of the metabolic and bactericidal characteristics of severely glucose-6-phosphate dehydrogenase-deficient polymorphonuclear leukocytes and leukocytes from children with chronic granulomatous disease. J Reticuloendothelial Soc 1972;12:150.
493. Cooper MR, DeChatelet LR, McCall CE, LaVia MF, Spurr CL, Baehner RL. Complete deficiency of leukocyte glucose-6-phosphate dehydrogenase with defective bactericidal activity. J Clin Invest 1972;51:769.
494. Cooper MR, DeChatelet LR, McCall CE, LaVia M, Spurr CL, Baehner RL. Leukocyte G-6-PD deficiency. Lancet 1970;2:110.
495. Cooper MR, DeChatelet LR, LaVia MF, McCall CE, Spurr CL, Baehner RL. Complete deficiency of leukocyte glucose-6-phosphate dehydrogenase with defective bactericidal activity. J Clin Invest 1970;49: 21A.
496. Gonzalez LA, Hill HR. Advantages and disadvantages of antimicrobial prophylaxis in chronic granulomatous disease in childhood. Pediatr Infect Dis J 1988;7:83–85.
497. Quie PG. Phagocytic cell dysfunction. J Allergy Clin Immunol 1988;77: 387–398.
498. Leonard AS, Mulholland MW, Filipovich AH. Surgery of the immunodeficient child. Surg Clin North Am 1985;65:1505–1525.
499. Fanconi S, Seger J, Gmur J, et al. Surgery and granulocyte transfusions for life-threatening infections in chronic granulomatous disease. Helv Paediatr Acta 1985;40:277–284.
500. dePlanque MM, Brand A, Kluin-Nelemans HC, et al. Haematopoietic and immunologic abnormalities in severe aplastic anaemia patients treated with anti-thymocyte globulin. Br J Haematol 1989;71:421–430.
501. Ezekowitz RA, Newburger PE. New perspectives in chronic granulomatous disease. J Clin Immunol 1988;8:419–425.
502. Sechler JM, Malech HL, White CJ, Gallin JI. Recombinant human interferon-gamma reconstitutes defective phagocyte function in patients with chronic granulomatous disease of childhood. Proc Natl Acad Sci 1988;85:4874–4878.
503. Group TICGDS. A controlled trial of interferon gamma to prevent infection in chronic granulomatous disease. N Engl J Med 1991;324: 509–516.
504. Aznar J, Vaya A. Homozygous form of the Pelger-Huet leukocyte anomaly in man. Acta Haematol 1981;66:59–62.
505. Matsumoto T, Harada Y, Yamaguchi K, et al. Cytogenetic and functional studies of leukocytes with Pelger-Huet anomaly. Acta Haematol 1984;72:264–273.
506. Johnson CA, Bass DA, Trillo AA, Snyder MS, DeChatelet LR. Functional and metabolic studies of polymorphonuclear leukocytes in the congenital Pelger-Huet anomaly. Blood 1980;55:466–469.
507. Liesveld J, Smith BD. Acquired Pelger-Huet anomaly in a case of non-Hodgkin's lymphoma. Acta Haematol 1988;79:46–49.
508. Dorr AD, Moloney WC. Acquired pseudo-Pelger anomaly of granolocytic leukocytes. N Engl J Med 1959;261:742–748.
509. Shenkenberg TD, Rice L, Waddell CC. Acquired Pelger-Huet nuclear anomaly with tuberculosis. Arch Intern Med 1982;142:153–154.
510. vanHook L, Spivack C, Duncanson FP. Acquired Pelger-Huet anomaly associated with *Mycoplasma pneumoniae* pneumonia. Am J Clin Pathol 1985;84:248–251.
511. Deutsch PH, Mandell GL. Reversible Pelger-Huet anomaly associated with ibuprofen therapy. Arch Intern Med 1985;145:166.
512. Oneson R, Sabio H, Innes J, DJ. Acute lymphoblastic leukaemia in a child with familial Pelger-Huet anomaly. Br J Haematol 1987;66:193–197.

513. Kornberg A, Goldfarb A, Shalev O. Pseudo-Pelger-Huet anomaly in chronic lymphocytic leukemia. Acta Haematol 1981;66:127–128.
514. Heyns ADP, Badenhorst PN, Wessels P, Pieters H, Lotter MG. Kinetics, in vitro redistribution and sites of sequestration of indium-111–labeled platelets in giant platelet syndromes. Br J Haematol 1985;60: 323–330.
515. Cabrera JR, Fontan G, Lorente F, Regidor C, Fernandez MN. Defective neutrophil mobility in the May-Hegglin anomaly. Br J Haematol 1981;47:337–343.
516. Coller BS, Zarrabi MH. Platelet membrane studies in the May-Hegglin anomaly. Blood 1981;58:279–284.
517. Djaldletti M, Creter D, Bujanover Y, Elian E. Ultrastructural and functional studies of the platelets in patients with May-Hegglin anomaly. Haematologica 1982;67:530–538.
518. Milton JG, Hutton RA, Tuddenham EG, Frojmovic MM. Platelet size and shape in hereditary giant plate syndromes on blood smear and in suspension: evidence for two types of abnormalities. J Lab Clin Med 1985;106:326–335.
519. Brivet F, Girot R, Barbanel C, et al. Hereditary nephritis associated with May-Hegglin anomaly. Nephron 1981;29:59–62.
520. Peterson LC, Rao KV, Crosson JT, White JG. Fechtner syndrome: a variant of Alport's syndrome with leukocyte inclusions and macrothrombocytopenia. Blood 1985;65:397–406.
521. McCall CE, Katayama I, Cotran S, Finland M. Lysosomal and ultrastructural changes in human "toxic" neutrophils during bacterial infection. J Exp Med 1969;129:267–293.
522. Schofield KP, Stone PCW, Beddall AC, Stuart J. Quantitative cytochemistry of the toxic granulation blood neutrophil. Br J Haematol 1983;53:15–22.
523. Simms HH, Frank MM, Quinn TC, Hollan S, Gaither T. Studies on phagocytosis in patients with acute bacterial infections. J Clin Invest 1989;83:252–260.
524. Vandermolen L, Rice L, Rose MA, Lynch EC. Ringed sideroblasts in primary myelodysplasia: leukemic propensity and prognostic factors. Arch Intern Med 1988;148:653–656.
525. O'Donnell JR, Farrell MA, Fitzgerald MX, O'Connell LG. Agnogenic myeloid metaplasia preceded by repeated leukemoid reactions and persistent acquired Pelger-Hüet anomaly of granulocytes: case report with review of acquired Pelger-Hüet anomaly. Cancer 1982;50:1498–1505.
526. Kuriyama K, Tomonaga M, Matsuo T, Ginnai I, Ichimaru M. Diagnostic significance of detecting pseudo-Pelger-Huet anomalies and micromegakaryocytes in myelodysplastic syndrome. Br J Haematol 1986;63: 665–669.
527. Davey FR, Erber WN, Gatter KC, Mason DY. Abnormal neutrophils in acute myeloid leukemia and myelodysplastic syndrome. Hum Pathol 1988;19:454–459.
528. Bizzaro N, Briani G, Boccato P. Acquired myeloperoxidase deficiency of neutrophils in a patient with aplastic anemia (idiopathic marrow aplasia). Acta Haematol 1988;80:71–73.
529. Naik N, Bhisey A, Advani S. Flow cytometric studies on actin polymerization in PMN cells from chronic myeloid leukemia (CML) patients. Leuk Res 1990;14:921–930.
530. Naik N, Advani S, Bhisey A. PMN cells from chronic myeloid leukemia (CML) patients show defective chemotaxis in remission. Leuk Res 1989;13:959–965.
531. Olofsson T, Odeberg H, Olsson I. Granulocyte function in chronic granulocytic leukemia. II. Bactericidal capacity, phagocytic rate, oxygen consumption and granule protein composition in isolated granulocytes. Blood 1976;48:581–593.
532. Brown MS, Goldstein JL. Lipoprotein metabolism in the macrophage: implications for cholesterol deposition in atherosclerosis. Annu Rev Biochem 1983;52:223–261.
533. Ellsworth JL, Karemer FB, Cooper AD. Transport of β very low density lipoproteins and chylomicron remnants is mediated by the low density lipoprotein receptor pathway. J Biol Chem 1987;262:2316–2325.
534. Gerrity RG. The role of the monocyte in atherogenesis. I. Transition of blood-borne monocytes into foam cells in fatty lesions. Am J Pathol 1981;103:181–190.
535. Gerrity RG, Goss JA, Soby L. Control of monocyte recruitment by chemotactic factor(s) in lesion-prone areas of swine aorta. Arteriosclerosis 1985;5:55–66.
536. Montgomery RR, Cohn ZA. Endocytic and secretory repertoire of the lipid-loaded macrophage. J Leuk Biol 1989;45:129–138.
537. Ross R. The pathogenesis of atherosclerosis. N Engl J Med 1986;314: 488–500.
538. Steinberg D, Parthasarathy S, Carew TE, Khoo JC, Witzum JL. Beyond cholesterol: modifications of low-density lipoprotein that increase its atherogenicity. N Engl J Med 1989;320:915–924.
539. Suits AG, Chait A, Aviram M, Heinecke JW. Phagocytosis of aggregated lipoprotein by macrophages: low density lipoprotein receptor-dependent foam-cell formation. Proc Natl Acad Sci 1989;86:2713–2717.
540. Tabas I, Boykow GC. Protein synthesis inhibition in mouse peritoneal macrophages results in increased acyl coenzyme A: cholesterol acyl transferase activity and cholesteryl ester accumulation in the presence of native low density lipoprotein. J Biol Chem 1987;262:12175–12187.
541. Mayorga L, Bertini F, Stahl P. Fusion of newly formed phagosomes with endosomes in intact cells. J Biol Chem 1991;266:6511–6517.
542. Unanue ER, Allen PM. The basis for the immunoregulatory role of macrophages and other accessory cells. Science 1987;236:551–557.
543. Unanue ER, Cerottini JC. Antigen presentation. FASEB J 1989;3:2496–2502.
544. Arenzan-Seisedos F, Mogensen SC, Vuillier F, Fiers W, Virelizier J-L. Autocrine secretion of tumor necrosis factor under the influence of interferon-γ amplifies HLA-DR gene induction in human monocytes. Proc Natl Acad Sci USA 1988;85:6087–6091.
545. Fischer H-G, Frosch S, Reske K, Reske-Kunz AB. Granulocyte-macrophage colony-stimulating factor activates macrophages derived from bone marrow cultures to synthesis of MHC class II molecules and to augmented antigen presentation function. J Immunol 1988;141: 3882–3888.
546. Rola-Plesczynski M, Bouvrette L, Gingras D, Girard M. Identification of interferon-γ as the lymphokine that mediates leukotriene B4–induced immunoregulation. J Immunol 1987;139:513–517.
547. Thepen T, vanRooijen N, Kraal G. Alveolar macrophage elimination in vivo is associated with an increase in pulmonary immune response in mice. J Exp Med 1989;170:499–509.

Blood: Principles and Practice of Hematology,
edited by Robert I. Handin, Thomas P. Stossel, and Samuel E. Lux.
J.B. Lippincott Company, Philadelphia © 1995.

20

Eosinophils, Basophils, and Mast Cells

Stephen J. Galli
Edward J. Goetzl

EOSINOPHILS

The eosinophil is a normal constituent of blood and some tissues, with a predominant distribution in the skin, lungs, intestines, and genitourinary tract. The clinical laboratory evaluation of eosinophils usually is confined to quantification of the blood concentration, an increase in which suggests the possibility of allergic or other hypersensitivity states, parasitic infections, or one of the tissue hypereosinophilic syndromes. The recent application of techniques of modern cellular and molecular biology has increased immensely our understanding of the properties and functions of eosinophils and has suggested new approaches to the assessment and treatment of human diseases characterized by deficient or excessive responses of eosinophils.

Production, Cellular Cycle and Kinetics, and Tissue Distribution

Eosinophils are produced in the bone marrow of normal adult mammals in a series of stages, which resemble those of other granulocytes and progress from multipotent stem cells to committed stem cells to recognizable eosinophil precursors to mature bone marrow eosinophils to peripheral blood eosinophils—both in marginated pools and in the circulation—to tissue eosinophils.[1–3] The results of in vitro studies and observations of abnormalities of human eosinophilopoiesis suggested initially that bone marrow progenitors of eosinophils are different from those of other leukocytes and are controlled independently by one or more distinct eosinophilopoietic factors.[4–7] Bone marrow–derived eosinophil colony-forming cells or units of some species may be resolved by physical techniques from stem cells committed to developing into neutrophil and macrophage colonies. The circulating level of eosinophils is not diminished in patients with congenital or acquired agranulocytosis or neutropenia.[8–10] Eosinophil granule enzymes are present in normal amounts in states of genetically determined absence of the same constituents from other granulocytes.[3,11]

Evidence from experimental systems strongly supports the existence of two separate pathways for the generation of factors that stimulate bone marrow eosinophilopoiesis (Fig. 20-1). The first pathway is composed of T-lymphocyte–dependent immunologic mechanisms. Intravascular injection of immunogenic particles and incubation of soluble antigens with mixtures of marrow cells and lymphocytes of sensitized animals in vitro both induce eosinophilia with a time course and dependence on antigen and T lymphocytes similar to that seen in other immune responses.[11–13] In rodents genetically deficient in specific components of the immune system or irradiated to induce immunodeficiency, the eosinophilic responses are diminished and can be reconstituted by T lymphocytes. Immunologically evoked eosinophilia is largely independent of B lymphocytes and antibody formation. B-lymphocyte deficiency early in the development of some species is associated with eosinophilia, which increases after introduction of soluble antigens, suggesting that B lymphocytes may regulate eosinophil production or turnover in some circumstances.[14] The second pathway consists of a series of T-lymphocyte–independent mechanisms, invoked either by eosinopenia, as in mice after the administration of specific antieosinophil serum[15] or by helminthic parasite infections in patients and mice.[16,17]

Low-molecular-weight peptides appear to be the critical mediators of eosinophilopoiesis elicited by the non–T-lymphocyte pathway.[16,17] IgE antibodies to the parasites have no role in the second pathway, as evidenced by the identical levels and kinetics of eosinophilia in selectively IgE-deficient SJA/9 and normal IgE congenic SJL/J mice resulting from infections with either *Trichinella spiralis* or *Nippostrongylus brasiliensis*.[18]

Diverse cytokines from T lymphocytes mediate eosinophilopoiesis with differing potencies and target cellular specificities (see Fig. 20-1). Interleukin-5 (IL-5) is a homodimeric 45-kd glycosylated protein, encoded by a gene on human chromosome 5, which stimulates mouse and human bone marrow to produce eosinophils.[7] IL-5 has no effect on neutrophil or monocyte production, and in humans it also lacks prominent B-lymphocyte activity or T-lymphocyte replacing factor activity. IL-5 augments several functions of mature eosinophils, and also stimulates proliferation.[7] Other T-lymphocyte–derived cytokines capable of initiating production of eosinophils are interleukin-3 (IL-3), interleukin-4 (IL-4), and granulocyte-macrophage colony-stimulating factor (GM-CSF), but all these are less potent and selective than IL-5 or require the presence of accessory cells for maximal activity.[19–22] IL-3 is more effective than IL-5 at promoting the development of IL-5–responsive, eosinophil-committed progenitors from multipotent stem cells, so that these cytokines may act synergistically in the overall production of eosinophils by bone marrow.[22]

The few studies of eosinophil kinetics conducted in hu-

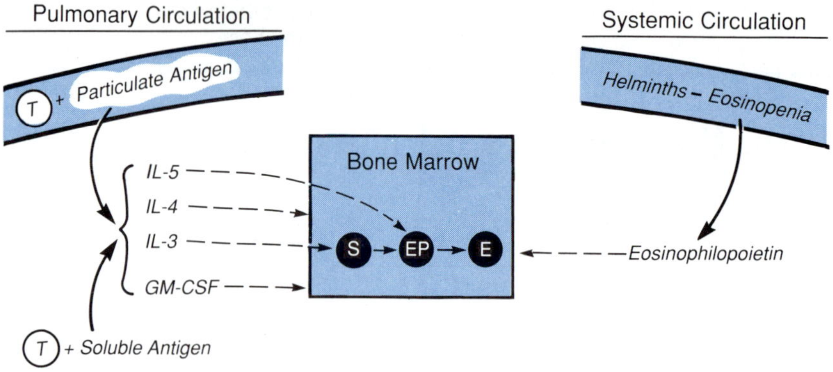

FIGURE 20-1. Regulation of eosinophilopoiesis by T-lymphocyte–dependent and T-lymphocyte–independent pathways. T, T lymphocyte; S, stem cell; E, eosinophil; EP, eosinophil precursor; long arrows, release of a factor; short arrows, cellular maturation; dashed arrows, stimulation.

mans and those in other adult mammals have shown an emergence time for release into blood of 48 to 80 hours, a half-life in circulation of 6 to 12 hours, and a tissue half-life of about 1 to 5 days.[3,23–26] In one study, a small subset of eosinophils emerged in 10 hours. These emergence times depend on species, levels of activity of different eosinophilopoietic factors, and contributions of margination and recirculation. The tissue compartment is the most difficult to assess, especially in humans, and represents a much larger population than that of other granulocytes. The eosinophil is principally a tissue cell, since the nonmarrow pool is nearly equal to that in bone marrow, which exceeds 100 to 400 times the number of eosinophils in blood.[27,28]

Only one patient with an intrinsic cellular deficiency of eosinophils alone has been described,[29] but patients with two different types of immune disorders may develop complete absence of eosinophils in tissues, blood, and bone marrow. Persons with diverse allergic diseases may acquire an IgG antieosinophil antibody that is selectively cytotoxic for mature eosinophils and eosinophil precursors by a complement-dependent mechanism.[30] One patient with hypogammaglobulinemia and a thymoma became deficient in eosinophils and basophils in association with the development of excessive suppressor T-lymphocyte activity.[31] The relation of the cellular immune abnormality to the absence of eosinophils was not established. Similarly, the noncytolytic and selective eosinopenia evoked by corticosteroids, β-adrenergic agents, and some prostaglandins are not understood in terms of the two classes of eosinophilopoietins or other determinants of eosinophil homeostasis. Corticosteroids appear to act directly on eosinophil progenitors and not by an effect on T-lymphocyte function.[32]

Cellular Constituents and Biochemical Properties

The eosinophil has a polymorphic cellular shape typical of all granulocytes, but the nucleus is bilobed and lacks a nucleolus[33,34] (Fig. 20-2). The most distinctive microscopic

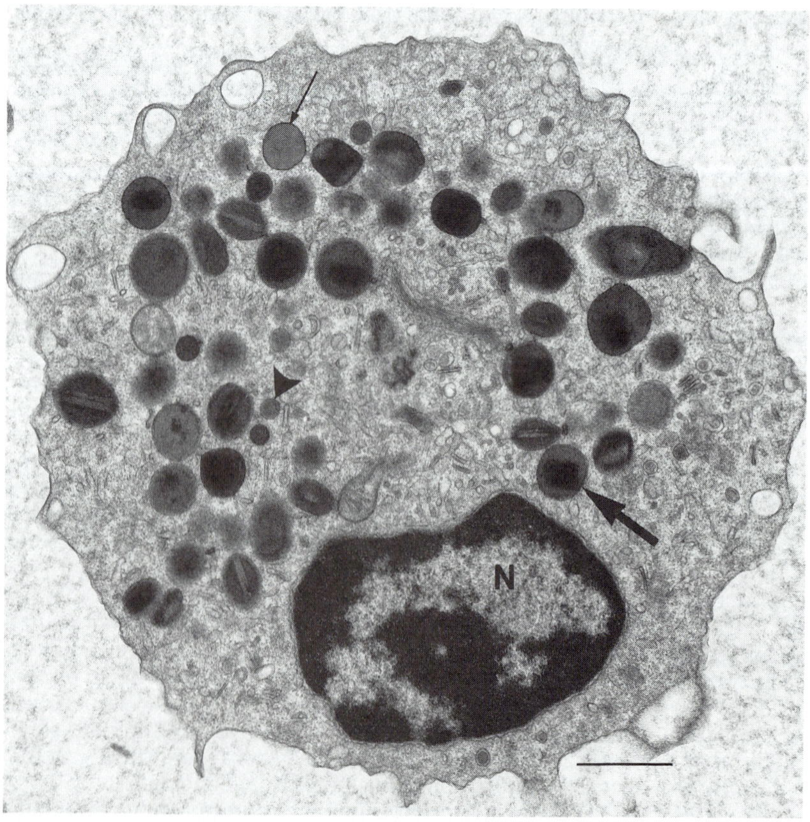

FIGURE 20-2. Transmission electron micrograph of a peripheral blood eosinophil from a patient with the hypereosinophilic syndrome. Cytoplasmic granules include many containing a central crystalloid core (*large arrow*), other large granules lacking a crystalloid core (*small arrow*), and occasional small granules (*arrowhead*). N, nucleus; bar = 1 μm. (Dvorak AM, Letourneau L, Login GR, Weller PF, Ackerman SJ. Ultrastructural localization of the Charcot-Leyden crystal protein [lysophosphatase] to a distinct crystalloid-free granule population in mature human eosinophils. Blood 1988;72:150)

feature of the eosinophil is a class of large ellipsoid cytoplasmic granules, termed *secondary* or *specific granules*, which contain an electron-dense crystalloid core enclosed in a less dense matrix.[2,3,33,35] Large spherical primary lysosomal granules proliferate during the early development of eosinophils, and many mature into crystalloid granules after the myelocyte stage. A separate class of small and homogeneously dense cytoplasmic granules develops during the metamyelocyte stage and increases in number progressively with eosinophil maturation in marrow and later in other tissues. The need for continued synthesis of protein constituents of such granules may explain the greater density of endoplasmic reticulum and Golgi's lamellae in mature eosinophils of blood and tissues than in neutrophils.[3,34]

Eosinophil granules contain an array of enzymes comparable to those in neutrophil lysosomes, but the eosinophil lacks lysozyme, and the content of peroxidase, β-glucuronidase, and acid phosphatase exceeds that of neutrophils two- to three-fold[11,34,35] (Table 20-1). Eosinophils from human pulmonary airways also contain a collagenase that cleaves human collagen types I and III preferentially, but eosinophils do not express an elastase or an unspecific neutral proteinase.[36] Some eosinophil granule enzymes and several cationic polypeptides, present predominantly in eosinophils, are of special importance in tissue eosinophilias and hypersensitivity reactions. Eosinophil peroxidase is a protein composed of a single chain of 75 kd[35] that is localized in the matrix of secondary granules. Eosinophil peroxidase exhibits microbicidal and cytotoxic activities in the presence of a halide and H_2O_2, of which eosinophils generate a large quantity, but it differs in several structural and catalytic respects from neutrophil myeloperoxidase.[11,35] Of the several uniquely expressed eosinophil enzymes capable of degrading phospholipids, the most active are the 13- to 17-kd lysophospholipase found in the plasma membrane and a 60-kd phospholipase D present in one or more populations of granules.[34] The lysophospholipase is identical with the protein of Charcot-Leyden crystals found in basophils in amounts similar to those in eosinophils.[37] A granule-derived histaminase of 160 to 200 kd has not been studied in sufficient detail for comparison with that of neutrophils.

At least three different cationic polypeptides are major constituents of eosinophil granules and are found in far smaller quantities in other granulocytes (see Table 20-1). Major basic protein (MBP) is an arginine-rich polypeptide of about 14 kd that makes up 95% of the protein content of the core of secondary granules.[35] As for the lysophospholipase, MBP is also present in basophils, but the amount per cell is 3% to 4% of that found in eosinophils. The nucleotide sequence of a cDNA for MBP has revealed a 25-kd preprotein from which MBP is released proteolytically.[38,39] MBP is toxic to a wide variety of cells from parasites to mammalian epithelial cells, and it evokes mediator release from basophils and mast cells noncytotoxically.[40,41] Two eosinophil cationic proteins of 21 to 29 kd are contained in the matrix of eosinophil secondary granules. Eosinophil cationic proteins and MBP share a range of cell-directed activities, but the cationic proteins alone alter Hageman's factor function in blood clotting, kinin generation, and possibly fibrinolysis, and they exhibit neurotoxic activity.[42,43] Eosinophil-derived neurotoxin (EDN) and a probably identical protein X are 18- to 19-kd components of the matrix of eosinophil secondary granules with distinctive toxicity for the central nervous system.[35] Both the cationic proteins and EDN possess RNase activity, and EDN is structurally identical to an RNase.[44,45]

General Functions, Synthetic Pathways, and Mechanisms of Activation

Optimal expression of the unique functional capabilities of eosinophils requires directed influx, accumulation, and activation at sites of specific tissue reactions. Structurally

TABLE 20-1. Principal Proteins of Human Eosinophils

Constituent	Cellular Localization	Structure	Functions
ENZYME			
Peroxidase	Secondary granules, matrix	75 kd pI >11	Microbicidal and cytotoxic with H_2O_2 and halide
Lysophospholipase (Charcot-Leyden crystal protein)	Plasma membrane	13–17 kd pI 5.1–5.7	Inactivates lysophospholipids
Phospholipase D	Granules	~60 kd pI 5.8–6.2	Inactivates platelet-activating factor
Histaminase	Granules	~160 kd	Inactivates histamine
CATIONIC POLYPEPTIDES			
Major basic protein	Secondary granules, >95% of core protein	14 kd pI 11.6, arginine rich	Mediates eosinophil adherence and toxicity for helminths and other cells
Eosinophil cationic proteins	Secondary granules, matrix	21–29 kd	Affects Hageman factor and plasmin activity, helminthicidal, neurotoxic, activates mast cells
Eosinophil-derived neurotoxin	Secondary granules, matrix	19 kd	Centrally neurotoxic
Eosinophil protein X	—	—	—
RECEPTORS			
Cb3R (CR1)	Plasma membrane	~250 kd	Enhances phagocytosis
C3biR (CR3)	Plasma membrane	2 chains of 165 and 95 kd	Enhances phagocytosis and leukocyte adhesion to surfaces
$Fc_{\gamma}RII$	Plasma membrane	42 kd	Low-affinity binding of IgG
$Fc_{\gamma}RIII$	Plasma membrane	50–70 kd	Low-affinity binding of IgG, associates with C3b receptors
$Fc_{\epsilon}RII$	Plasma membrane	45–50 kd	Low-affinity binding of IgE

distinct factors from several different sources are selectively chemotactic for eosinophils[34,46] (Table 20-2). Of these, the C5a fragment of the fifth component of complement, the peptides of the eosinophil chemotactic factor of anaphylaxis (ECF-A) and larger peptides from mast cells, leukotriene B_4 (LTB_4) and the phospholipid platelet-activating factor (PAF) from mast cells and mononuclear phagocytes, and proteins from stimulated lymphocytes are potent and necessary participants of many tissue eosinophilias. As for other leukocytes, eosinophils respond to a variety of fluid-phase and particulate stimuli with increased adherence, modified expression of membrane receptors, phagocytosis, enhancement of synthetic activities, lysosomal degranulation, and oxidative metabolism (see Table 20-2). PAF is a selective and potent stimulus for eosinophil chemotaxis,[47,48] degranulation,[49] and adherence to vascular endothelial cells.[50] Several cytokines have eosinophil chemotactic activity similar in magnitude and leukocytic specificity to that of PAF. The most potent of these are IL-5[51] and RANTES.[52] Neither attracts neutrophils in vitro, but RANTES is a chemoattractant for memory-type T lymphoctyes. IL-5 also induces eosinophil proliferation and differentiation, and enhances the cytotoxicity and degranulation of human eosinophils mediated by antibody,[53] whereas RANTES has not been examined for these activities. The eosinophil functional specificity of cytokines is further emphasized by the distinctive capacities of TNF and IFN-γ to augment the expression of surface proteins on human eosinophils.[54] Eosinophil surface levels of ICAM-1 were increased by TNF and IFN-γ separately, but only the effects of TNF were enhanced synergistically by concentration of IL-3, IL-5, or GM-CSF that lacked activity alone. In contrast, IL-3, but not IL-5 or GM-CSF, augmented synergistically the increases in eosinophil surface levels of HLA-DR elicited by IFN-γ, without altering those similarly elicited by TNF. Eosinophils adhere to and phagocytose particles opsonized with IgG and C3b at far greater rates than unopsonized particles. The facilitative effect of opsonization is attributable to the presence on eosinophils of receptors for the Fc portion of IgG, C3bi, and C3b/C4 (see Table 20-1).

The human eosinophil Fc receptors for IgG consist of low- and high-affinity subsets that may also exhibit IgG subclass specificity.[55] Immune complexes containing IgE activate eosinophils preferentially and antibodies to the type 2 receptor for IgE-Fc block eosinophil, but not mast cell, recognition of IgE.[56] Human eosinophils recently have been found to express CD4 proteins and to bind the gp 120 of human immunodeficiency virus 1 in a manner that permits cellular infection.[57]

Patients with hypereosinophilic states have two populations of peripheral blood eosinophils, consisting of low-density or hypodense and normodense eosinophils, as assessed by centrifugation on metrizamide or Percoll gradients.[58–61] The number of hypodense eosinophils varies directly according to the level of eosinophilia and the severity of the disease. Although the source of hypodense eosinophils is not yet established, these eosinophils appear to be activated functionally with greater levels of oxidative and other types of metabolism, increased rates of synthesis of mediators, and greater cytotoxicity relative to normodense eosinophils.[62,63] The normodense eosinophils have more active chemotactic responses to PAF and some other stimuli,[47] but little or no expression of $Fc\epsilon_2$ and $Fc\gamma$ receptors, suggesting that hypodense eosinophils are derived from normodense eosinophils by exposure to chemotactic and other stimuli to which they become less responsive.

Eosinophils generate superoxide and hydroxyl radicals at rates equal to or higher than those observed for neutrophils. More important, the production of superoxide by eosinophils remains at a maximum level for over 3 hours, whereas superoxide production by similarly stimulated neutrophils falls dramatically within 1 hour. The difference in time course of oxidative metabolism appears to be partly attributable to the greater resistance of eosinophils to superoxide and other products, which are cytotoxic for neutrophils and many other types of cells. A broad spectrum of other enzymatic activities of eosinophils is devoted to the oxygenation of arachidonic acid in plasma membranes and cytoplasmic lipid bodies,[64] which is the source of numerous potent mediators (see Table 20-2).

The eosinophil cyclooxygenase pathway produces

TABLE 20-2. Synthetic and Functional Activities of Human Eosinophils

CELLULAR AND METABOLIC FUNCTIONS	STIMULI OR TARGETS
Chemotaxis	PAF, C5a, LTB_4, ECF-A, lymphokines
Adherence	IgG, IgE, C3b
Phagocytosis	Opsonized particles
Degranulation, oxidative metabolism	Opsonized particles, immune complexes, chemotactic factors
SYNTHETIC PATHWAYS	**PRODUCTS OF ARACHIDONIC ACID AND PHOSPHOLIPIDS**
5-Lipoxygenase	LTC_4, LTB_4, 5-HETE
15-Lipoxygenase	15-HETE, 8,15-diHETEs, 14,15-diHETEs
Cyclooxygenase	PGE_2
Phospholipase, acetyltransferase	PAF
SPECIAL ACTIVITIES	**FUNCTIONS AND MECHANISMS**
Defense against helminths and ticks	Chemotaxis, adherence, release of MBP, ECP, EPO, oxygen radicals, cytokines (eg, TNF-α)
Suppression of hypersensitivity reactions	Destruction of histamine, LTs, PAF, lysophospholipids, cytokines (eg, TGF-β)
Enhancement of hypersensitivity reactions	Production of LTC_4, activation of mast cells by MBP, ECPs, EPO, cytokines (eg, TNF-α, MIP-1α, IL-3, GM-ESF)

PAF, platelet-activating factor; LTB_4, leukotriene B_4; ECF, eosinophil chemotactic factor of anaphylaxis; MBP, major basic protein.

predominantly prostaglandin E_2 (PGE_2). The ratio of 15-lipoxygenase to 5-lipoxygenase activity is a function of the stage of differentiation and the nature of stimulation of the eosinophils. In most instances, 15-lipoxygenation predominates and results in generation of the metabolites 15-hydroxyeicosatetraenoic acid (15-HETE), 8,15-di-HETEs, and 14,15-di-HETEs.[65,66] One of the 14,15-di-HETEs suppresses natural killer cell activity, whereas 15-HETE exerts selective effects on the expression of 5-lipoxygenase activity. 15-HETE suppresses 5-lipoxygenase activity in polymorphonuclear leukocytes and mononuclear phagocytes, but it enhances the activity in some types of mast cells. The 5-lipoxygenase pathway of eosinophils generates principally the LTC_4 smooth muscle contractile and vasoactive factor, with lesser amounts of LTD_4, LTE_4, and the LTB_4 leukocyte-activating factor.[66] Diverse chemotactic factors, IgG-containing immune complexes, and GM-CSF enhance the rates of lipoxygenation of arachidonic acid by eosinophils.[67,68] The level of production of LTC_4 again is greater for hypodense than for normodense eosinophils.[69]

The specificity and intensity of microbicidal activities of eosinophils differ substantially from those of other leukocytes. The bactericidal capabilities of eosinophils, with rare exceptions, are less efficient than those of neutrophils.[70] This difference is at a cellular level and is not a function of any specific enzymatic deficiencies of eosinophils. In fact, eosinophil peroxidase is more actively bactericidal than myeloperoxidase, since it adheres to *Staphylococcus aureus* and some other bacteria and exhibits both direct oxidative cytotoxicity and the capacity to potentiate the bactericidal functions of mononuclear phagocytes.[71] The weight of recent evidence suggests that the major protective role of eosinophils in host defense is the containment and destruction of metazoan parasites.

Specialized Effector Functions

The most common causes of blood and tissue eosinophilia in humans are hypersensitivity reactions and metazoan parasite infections.[72–75] The two types of conditions share many mechanisms of induction and function. For example, the bulk of the eosinophil chemotactic activity generated by helminth infections is dependent on the responses of mast cells, macrophages, and lymphocytes of sensitized hosts to parasite antigens. Eosinophil interactions with the surface of helminths also is a function of surface IgG and C3b. Mast cell activation by eosinophils is mediated partly by granule proteins, which also induce the formation of functional channels in membranes of helminths in the process of antibody-dependent cytotoxicity.[41,76]

The eosinophil is a central component of the inflammation typical of late-phase cutaneous allergic reactions to environmental antigens. When allergic patients were challenged with pollen or mite antigen, a population of predominantly CD4+ T lymphocytes and eosinophils constituted the infiltrate at 6 hours after antigen.[77] The number of eosinophils in such lesions correlated with the diameter of the late-phase reaction. The concentration of eosinophil cationic protein in nasal secretions also relates significantly to the intensity of the nasal response to antigen and the late-phase inflammatory reaction.[78]

The modulation of mast cell–dependent hypersensitivity reactions by eosinophils is complex and includes both stimulatory and inhibitory aspects (see Table 20-2). As for reactions to helminth infections, the eosinophils are attracted to and activated at the sites of immediate-type hypersensitivity responses predominantly by mast cell–derived mediators, such as PAF, ECF-A, and LTB_4. The down-regulatory components of eosinophil activities are attributable to both cellular activities and specific factors. PGE_2 from eosinophils suppresses the release of mediators by mast cells. Intact eosinophils ingest mast cell granules. MBP binds and thus inactivates heparin. A set of highly specific eosinophil enzymes is capable of degrading mediators. Eosinophil-derived histaminase inactivates histamine, and phospholipase D cleaves PAF. Eosinophil peroxidase, in the presence of H_2O_2 and a halide, oxidizes the C6-peptide leukotrienes to less potent or inactive sulfones. Eosinophil granule cationic proteins also may limit indirectly the activation of basophils by complement-derived C3a and C5a as a result of inhibition of formation of the cell-bound alternative pathway C3 convertase that generates C3a and C5a.[79]

The capability of eosinophils to initiate or enhance hypersensitivity reactions is a function both of mast cell and basophil stimulation by eosinophil-derived factors and of the primary effects on target organs of eosinophil-derived mediators (see Table 20-2). Eosinophil cationic proteins, MBP, eosinophil peroxidase, with H_2O_2 and a halide and substance P (SP) from eosinophils, all are able to stimulate mast cells to release mediators. The LTC_4 and SP from eosinophils are potent direct bronchoconstrictors and active secretagogues for bronchial epithelial cells and glands independent of mast cells. At concentrations attained in the airways in some hypersensitivity diseases, MBP injures the bronchial epithelial cells and increases airway permeability to luminal factors.[35] Eosinophil degranulation commonly occurs in the airways in asthma.[80] Another mechanism for eosinophil–mast cell interaction is the transformation of mast cell–derived PGD_2 into isomeric PGF_2 compounds, such as $9\alpha,11\beta$-PGF_2, by human eosinophils.[81] Both PGD_2 and $9\alpha,11\beta$-PGF_2 contract human bronchioles with equal potency, but PGD_2 dilates and $9\alpha,11\beta$-PGF_2 constricts systemic blood vessels. Human eosinophils recently have been shown to produce many cytokines, including TGF-α,[82] TGF-β,[83,84] GM-CSF,[85,86] IL-1α,[87] IL-3,[85] IL-5,[88] IL-6,[89] TNF-α,[90] and MIP-1α[90] The generation of IL-5 and GM-CSF by eosinophils at sites of allergic inflammation, evoked by endobronchial antigen challenge of asthmatics, represents a source of cytokines capable of autocrine recruitment of eosinophils and the activation of their effector functions.[91] The local concentrations of IL-5 and GM-CSF, as well as IL-3 and IL-4, at sites of allergic inflammation in human airways correlate well with the number of activated eosinophils.[92] Other contributions of eosinophil-derived cytokines may include the augmentation of bronchial reactivity by TNF-α,[90] and changes in epithelial cells and extracellular matrix by TGF-α[84] and TGF-β[85,86] in asthma and other disorders characterized by eosinophil infiltration. Eosinophil-derived IL-1α,[87] TNF-α,[90] MIP-1α,[90] and IL-6[89] also may promote and prolong the inflammation at sites of eosinophil infiltration. The factors that regulate eosinophil cytokine production in vivo remain to be defined, but several lines of evidence indicate that eosinophils that have infiltrated into tissues, or the circulating eosinophils of patients with the idopathic hypereosinophilic syndrome, exhibit higher levels of cytokine production than do the blood eosinophils of normal donors.[82,83,90]

Eosinophils are clearly tissue cells, which have the capacity to augment and prolong or inhibit and terminate immediate and later reactions evoked by mast cells and basophils. The net outcome of eosinophil–mast cell interactions at any time during a hypersensitivity response is a function of the relative number of each type of cell, their respective degrees of activation, and the contributions of other factors and cells to the overall reaction. Eosinophils alone and in concert with mast cells and macrophages thus have the potential to participate in host defense or to promote processes that injure host tissues. The possibilities that eosinophils may also be involved in tissue fibrosis, coagulation and fibrinolytic abnormalities, and regulation of cellular immunity are suggested by results of some preliminary studies that require verification and extension. The finding of elevated concentrations of specific eosinophil constituents in lesional tissues and fluids of allergic cutaneous diseases, as well as in sputum and lung tissue of patients with asthma and other inflammatory lung diseases of suspected allergic origin, emphasizes the importance of further analyses of the eosinophil in normal organ function and diseases.

Eosinophil infiltrates around invading helminths and ticks were documented many years ago, but a possible protective role for eosinophils in damaging the parasites was suggested only recently. The capacity of antieosinophil sera to deplete eosinophils selectively and to concurrently diminish the resistance of animals to infections with *Schistosoma mansoni*, *T spiralis*, and *Amblyomma americanum* supported a protective role for the eosinophil.[3] That eosinophils selectively injure helminths in vitro confirmed the possibility of their central involvement in host defense against parasites. Eosinophils adhere to helminths by C3b- and IgG-dependent mechanisms, degranulate, and deposit granule proteins on the surface of the helminth, leading to the appearance of microscopic defects in the cuticle.[35,76] Eosinophil cationic proteins are 10 times more active than MBP in killing schistosomes and other helminths. Concentrations of eosinophil cationic proteins as low as 10^{-7} mol/L are optimally cytotoxic by creating transmembrane functional pores, which serve as voltage-insensitive and non–ion-selective channels.[93]

In contrast, eosinophil peroxidase exhibits toxicity for helminths that is both direct and mediated by an H_2O_2–halide mechanism. Eosinophil peroxidase adheres to many types of mammalian cells but exerts cytotoxic effects on only a few in the absence of exogenous H_2O_2.[94] The efficiency of the helminthicidal activity of eosinophils is enhanced markedly by ECF-A and LTB_4, which augment the expression of C3b receptors,[95] and by colony-stimulating factors of the α type, which also increase eosinophil adherence to helminths.[96] Eosinophil helminthicidal activity is also enhanced by several distinct monokines and T lymphokines such as the eosinophil stimulation promoter[97] and tumor necrosis factor (TNF).[98]

Spectrum of Eosinophilic Syndromes

Blood and tissue eosinophilia are characteristic of a wide range of different parasitic, neoplastic, collagen–vascular, allergic, and other systemic diseases, in which excessive, deficient, or otherwise abnormal immunologic responses stimulate increased production and tissue localization of eosinophils.[3,34,99–102] The expression of some surface proteins, such as CD69, on eosinophils recovered from lungs and other organs involved in allergic reactions with eosinophilia—but not on those eosinophils recovered from blood—suggests that readily quantifiable markers may reflect different aspects of the functional activation of eosinophils.[103] Many of these secondary or reactive eosinophilias are transient manifestations that apparently do not injure the host, whereas others are associated with functionally deleterious inflammation and fibrosis. An exhaustive list of all reported causes of eosinophilia is available, but is unrevealing mechanistically and may discourage appropriate investigations of the more serious infections and neoplastic causes.[3] The primary or idiopathic eosinophilias, such as the hypereosinophilic syndromes, most often result in tissue injury and altered organ function. Although many different systems can be the principal focus of eosinophilic infiltration, the most frequently affected are lungs, skin, intestines, brain or peripheral nerves, and kidneys.

Pulmonary Eosinophilias

The present classification of pulmonary diseases with parenchymal infiltration of eosinophils and peripheral blood eosinophilia is based principally on clinical features such as time course, the histopathology, and the perceived primary etiologic agent (see Table 20-3). Particularly interesting is the fact that many of the patients with different types of reactive pulmonary eosinophilia exhibit similar immunologic abnormalities such as early- and late-phase IgE-mediated tissue responses, and elevated serum concentration of IgE. The likely involvement of cytokines capable of stimulating both eosinophil and IgE responses, such as IL-4, implies a fundamental role for T lymphocytes that remains to be elucidated. Acute pulmonary eosinophilia (Löffler's syndrome) involves diverse possible causes, rang-

TABLE 20-3. Pulmonary Hypereosinophilic Syndromes

Disease	Pathogenesis and Usual Causes	Clinical Characteristics	Laboratory Findings
Acute pulmonary eosinophilic infiltrates with blood eosinophilia	Immune reaction to antigens localized in the lung; drugs, parasites, heavy metals, blood transfusion, radiocontrast media	Fever, malaise, dry cough	Lung tissue eosinophilia and vascular inflammation; increased serum IgE
Allergic bronchopulmonary aspergillosis	Early- and late-phase IgE-mediated reactions; immune complexes; T-lymphocyte responses	Worsening of asthma with early and late bronchospasm after *Aspergillus* inhalation	Lung tissue eosinophilia and central bronchiectasis; IgG and IgE antibodies to *Aspergillus;* increased serum IgE
Tropical filarial eosinophilia	Early- and late-phase IgE-mediated reactions	Fever, weight loss, fatigue; episodes of dyspnea and cough, adenopathy; bibasilar infiltrates	Lung tissue eosinophilia and granuloma; increased serum IgE and IgE antifilaria
Chronic eosinophilic pneumonia	Fixed IgE- and occasionally IgG-mediated reactions, antigens unknown, background of asthma	Subacute to chronic high fevers, weight loss, night sweats, peripheral field infiltrates	Lung tissue eosinophilia with giant cells, vasculitis, bronchiolitis obliterans
Allergic granulomatosis (Churg-Strauss syndrome)	IgE-mediated reactions and immune complexes	Fever, weight loss, anemia, asthma	Lung tissue eosinophilia; granulomatous vasculitis; infarction; increased serum IgE
Disseminated hypereosinophilic syndrome	Eosinophil disorder	Multisystem disease; cutaneous urticaria and angioedema	Lung tissue eosinophilia; necrosis; endomyocardia fibrosis; increased serum IgE

ing from drugs and parasite infections to foreign proteins and heavy metals.[104] All other pulmonary eosinophilias are characterized by chronic or recurrent courses, and the possibility of parenchymal and vascular injury and fibrosis (see Table 20-3). Although sometimes included in this set of diseases, eosinophilic granuloma of the lung is distinct in many ways, including mixed cellular infiltrates in tissues, the absence of peripheral blood eosinophilia, and the frequent involvement of bone and the occasional involvement of other organs.[34,105,106]

Eosinophilia–Myalgia Syndrome

In late 1989, physicians began to see patients with the common features of fatigue, severe myalgia and peripheral blood eosinophilia, and a history of having consumed large quantities of products containing L-tryptophan, which was being used as a sedative.[107,108] The signs and symptoms of this disorder developed over a period of weeks and sometimes included arthralgias, dyspnea, cough, swelling of the extremities, and maculopapular, urticarial, or vesicular rash. Some patients had hepatomegaly, cardiac failure, and arrhythmias. The eosinophil count was usually more than 2000/μL but sometimes much higher (10,000 to 30,000/μL). Histologic specimens of muscle revealed perivascular infiltrates of eosinophils. The documentation of elevated levels of some metabolites and contaminants in preparations of L-tryptophan associated with this syndrome has implicated traces of toxins, as well as host factors, in the etiology. Discontinuation of L-tryptophan led to rapid complete remission of the disease in a minority of patients, but many patients had slow regression or even progression of the disorder and some had cutaneous sclerosis or ascending polyneuropathy. Experience with this newly recognized syndrome is too limited for specific therapeutic guidelines other than elimination of the L-tryptophan. Some patients seem to have benefited from treatment with corticosteroids.[109]

Hypereosinophilic Syndrome

Hypereosinophilic syndrome is characterized predominantly by eosinophilic pulmonary infiltrates and peripheral blood eosinophilia but usually involves other organs as well.[101,102] The most benign variant is eosinophilic infiltrates in the bases and periphery of the lungs, with recurrent angioedema. Other forms may begin with the same manifestations but develop into severe cardiac or central nervous system disease. Frequent thrombotic episodes and splenomegaly early in the course distinguish this condition from the spectrum of reactive pulmonary eosinophilias (see Table 20-3). Over half of the more than 100 patients evaluated have experienced anorexia, weight loss, fever, sweating, splinter hemorrhages, thromboembolic episodes, lesions of the skin and retina, splenic and lymphatic involvement, and central nervous system disease. The peripheral blood eosinophils are predominantly the hypodense type and have a variety of cellular abnormalities but the chromosomes are apparently normal. T lymphocytes are a source of the eosinophilopoietic factors in some patients with hypereosinophilic syndrome.[110]

Management of the idiopathic hypereosinophilic syndrome is based on its general features of chronicity, frequent remissions and relapses, and diverse complications that damage tissues in multiple organ systems. Accordingly, a program of medications is designed and revised as frequently as necessary to contain the process with the fewest harmful side effects of treatment. Only general guidelines may be offered without knowledge of a specific patient. Low doses of corticosteroids equivalent to 20 mg/d of prednisone are used to control symptoms and mild tissue infiltration; moderate doses equivalent to 40 to 60 mg/d of prednisone are needed for persistent tissue involvement; 60 to 100 mg/d of prednisone is needed for progressive tissue damage; prednisone, 60 to 100 mg/d, is the initial drug of choice in severe disease of critical organs. Intermittent courses of hydroxyurea, 1 to 2 g/d, can be added to reduce corticosteroid doses. Continuous hydroxyurea is the drug of choice for corticosteroid failures. Limited responses of eosinophilia to hydroxyurea, incompletely controlled severe organ complications, or thrombocytopenia should prompt consideration of the addition of 1.5 mg vincristine every 2 weeks.

All patients with hypereosinophilic syndrome are at risk for thrombotic and embolic complications and should receive warfarin continuously with the addition of low-dose aspirin or dipyridamole at times of highest eosinophilia. The roles of plasmapheresis and leukopheresis are still undefined.

Cutaneous Eosinophilias

A complex array of cutaneous disorders with blood and tissue eosinophilia ranges from disorders with persistent but benign lesions to those with tissue damage and chronic fibrosis (Table 20-4). Some patients with cutaneous eosinophilia have constitutional manifestations of disease or involvement of other organs. Eosinophilic lymphofolliculosis is a disease of males consisting of facial, axillary, and inguinal eosinophilic furunculosis with granulomatous hyperplasia of the draining lymph nodes.[111] Subcutaneous eosinophilic angiolymphoid hyperplasia is a similar condition with eosinophilic lymphoid nodules on the head and neck, which contain foci of capillary hyperplasia.[112] Patients with bullous pemphigoid develop IgG antibodies to constituents of the dermal–epidermal junction, detected at the bases of bullous lesions and in the circulation.[113,114] This disorder resembles immunohistochemically some of the reactive pulmonary eosinophilias, since some patients have elevated serum levels of IgE, as well as the presence of IgE, degranulated mast cells, and eosinophil chemotactic activity in the lesions.[115]

Substantial fever, chills, myalgias, and arthralgias are typical of both recurrent granulomatous dermatitis (Well's disease[116]), and eosinophilic fasciitis or Shulman's syndrome.[117] These diseases present acutely, follow a subacute or relapsing course, and show serum polyclonal hypergammaglobulinemia and lesional IgG and C3.[118] Patients with eosinophilic fasciitis present with thickening of the skin due to edema, which can evolve to sclerosis and hyperpigmentation. Unlike scleroderma, cutaneous fibrosis

TABLE 20-4. Cutaneous Hypereosinophilic Syndromes

SKIN INVOLVEMENT ALONE
Eosinophilic lymphofolliculosis (Kimura's disease)
Subcutaneous eosinophilic angiolymphoid hyperplasia
Bullous pemphigoid
SKIN INVOLVEMENT AND CONSTITUTIONAL SYMPTOMS
Granulomatous dermatitis with eosinophilia (Well's disease)
Eosinophilic fasciitis (Shulman's syndrome)
SYSTEMIC HYPEREOSINOPHILIC SYNDROME WITH ENDOMYOCARDIAL FIBROSIS
Papulonodular lesions
Urticaria and angioedema

spares the perivenous tissue, and raising an affected extremity causes grooves to form where the veins collapse. Carpal tunnel syndrome affects 30% of patients, and 10% of reported cases have had associated hematologic disorders, including aplastic anemia and thrombocytopenia.[119] About 30% of patients with primary hypereosinophilic syndrome and cutaneous involvement have high serum concentrations of IgE, but the incidence of elevated serum IgE is no different for patients with predominantly urticarial lesions than for those with papulonodular lesions.[120]

BASOPHILS AND MAST CELLS

Basophils are circulating granulocytes that can infiltrate tissues or appear in exudates during a variety of inflammatory or immunologic processes. By contrast, morphologically identifiable mast cells do not normally circulate but reside in virtually all normal vascularized tissues. Despite significant differences in their natural history and distribution, both basophils and mast cells have prominent cytoplasmic granules with affinity for certain basic dyes. They store or release, on appropriate stimulation, a similar (not identical) pattern of biochemical mediators, and they express cell surface receptors ($Fc_{\epsilon}RI$) that bind the Fc portion of IgE class antibodies with high affinity. Most important, they participate both in mechanisms of host defense and in allergic disorders with components of immediate hypersensitivity. To highlight their many similarities, and also to emphasize their differences, the features of basophils and mast cells are presented together.

Production, Cellular Cycle and Kinetics, and Tissue Distribution

The derivation of basophils from precursors shared by other granulocytes and monocytes is suggested by cytogenetic evidence,[121,122] analyses of cell surface phenotype,[123] and observations made in vitro in which colonies of bone marrow–derived cells that include basophils also usually contain eosinophils and other granulocytes.[124,125] Studies of the production and circulation of human basophils have been limited but suggest that the kinetics of basophil production and peripheral circulation are similar to those of eosinophils.[24,126] Basophils and eosinophils share certain biochemical constituents, exhibit some similarities in the regulation of their numbers in the circulation (see section about basophilopenia and basophilia), and often represent the two most prevalent lineages when human hematopoietic cells are cultured in suspension in the presence of T-cell–associated products, including IL-3 and IL-4.[123,127,128] In addition, a single family has been reported with a hereditary syndrome in which crystalline inclusions appear in the cytoplasmic granules of eosinophils and basophils but not in neutrophils or mast cells.[129] Taken together, these findings suggest that basophils and eosinophils may be more closely related to each other than to neutrophils or other differentiated products of the hematopoietic system.

The basophil is the least common of human blood granulocytes, with a normal mean incidence of less than 0.5% of total circulating leukocytes and about 0.3% of total nucleated bone marrow cells.[130] The basophil's prominent, metachromatic cytoplasmic granules permit it to be identified easily in Wright-Giemsa–stained preparations of peripheral blood or bone marrow cells, but because of the cell's rarity, accurate estimates of basophil numbers require absolute counting methods.[130,131] The absolute numbers of circulating basophils exhibit wide individual variation, with normal ranges in two studies of 20 to 45/μL and 10 to 80/μL.[121,131] Unlike the eosinophil, the basophil ordinarily does not occur in peripheral tissues in significant numbers. Basophils can infiltrate sites of many immunologic or inflammatory processes (often in association with eosinophils) and are represented in the reactions to some tumors.[132,133] In such cases, the basophils are readily distinguishable from mast cells residing in the same tissues.[134]

In contrast to the basophil, mast cells do not normally circulate in mature form. Although the circulating precursor of the mast cell has not been identified in any species, studies in mice indicate that the mast cell precursor is a bone marrow–derived cell lacking morphologically identifiable cytoplasmic granules.[135,136] The hypothesis that basophils represent the circulating precursors of mast cells has not been formally excluded, but it seems unlikely for several reasons:

1. No evidence has been presented indicating that mature circulating basophils are capable either of division or of differentiation into mast cells.
2. The rare reports of patients with hereditary or acquired abnormalities affecting basophil numbers or morphology indicate that eosinophils but not mast cells may also be affected in these disorders.[31,129,137]
3. Morphologically identifiable human tissue mast cells can exhibit mitotic activity, indicating that this lineage can replicate independently of a stage resembling the circulating basophil.[138]

Mast cells occur throughout virtually all vascularized tissues, although their numbers in individual anatomic sites exhibit considerable variation.[132,139–142] In humans and many other mammalian species, mast cells are particularly abundant near surfaces exposed to environmental antigens or parasites, such as the skin, gastrointestinal tract, and respiratory system. Mast cells also represent a numerically minor component of human bone marrow (0.02% or less of nucleated cells in sternal aspirates[130]). The anatomic distribution of mast cells within individual organs or tissues varies, although in most sites mast cells occur in close association with blood vessels or nerves.[95,139,140,143]

Under some circumstances, such as in association with certain inflammatory or immunologic reactions, mast cells can appear within the respiratory or gastrointestinal epithelium and in secretions at these sites.[144] The numbers of mast cells at sites of chronic inflammation due to a variety of different causes can often be many times higher than in the corresponding normal tissues.[95,139,140,143,144] The extent to which such changes in mast cell number reflect proliferation of resident mast cell populations, compared with recruitment and differentiation of mast cell precursors, remains to be determined.

Variation in multiple morphologic, biochemical, or functional characteristics, including sensitivity to pharmacologic agents, has been identified in mast cells derived from different anatomic locations (and even among mast cells in the same tissue or organ) in humans and several other mammalian species.[95,140–142,144–148] This phenomenon, called *mast cell heterogeneity*, suggests that mast cells of different phenotype may express different functions in health and disease. Mast cell phenotype may be regulated by multiple mechanisms influencing the maturation/differentiation or function of the cells.[141,142,149–153]

In mice, T-cell–associated products (eg, IL-3 and IL-4) and stem cell factor (SCF; also named mast cell growth factor [MGF], *kit* ligand [KL], and steel factor [SLF]), the ligand for the c-*kit* tyrosine kinase growth factor receptor[136,141,151–154] importantly regulate the development of various mast cell populations. SCF also promotes mast cell development in rats[155] and nonhuman primates.[156] In humans, IL-3 promotes basophil production and survival in vitro[123,128] and can induce basophilia in vivo.[157] These findings suggest that IL-3 may contribute to the regulation of normal levels of blood basophils and raise the possibility that increased production of IL-3 by T cells may promote the basophilia associated with certain immunologic responses. Basophils also express receptors for several other cytokines, including IL-2 (CD25), IL4, IL5, and IL8,[123,142] and some basophils express small numbers of receptors for SCF.[158] IL-3 and some of these other cytokines can modulate basophil function, for example, by inducing mediator release directly or by augmenting the cell's ability to release mediators in response to challenge with IgE and specific antigen.[123,157,159,160]

Recent in vitro and in vivo studies in murine rodents, nonhuman primates, and humans indicate that many individual aspects of mast cell development are critically regulated by SCF.[151–153] SCF is produced in both membrane-associated and soluble forms, both of which are biologically active.[151–153] Notably, SCF is the first defined growth factor that has been shown to induce human mast cell development in vitro[161–164] and in vivo.[165] In addition to promoting the migration, survival, proliferation, and maturation of cells in the mast cell lineage, SCF also can directly promote mast cell mediator release[158,166,167] and, at even lower concentrations, can augment mast cell mediator release in response to stimulation by IgE and antigen.[158,167,168] Thus, SCF not only regulates the normal development of mast cells but also influences the functional repertoire of these cells. It appears likely that alteration in the production of SCF by fibroblasts and other cells contributes to the changes in mast cell numbers that occur during many chronic inflammatory conditions and other pathologic responses. Similarly, variation in the normal levels of SCF pródu̇ction in different tissues may contribute to the wide variation in the normal densities of mast cells obseved in different anatomic sites.[151–153,156] Factors in addition to SCF may also contribute to mast cell development of survival in humans. For example, the numbers of one mast cell subpopulation, containing cytoplasmic granules with little or no chymase, is markedly reduced in the intestinal mucosa and submucosa of patients with either congenital combined immunodeficiency disease or the acquired immunodeficiency syndrome.[169] The molecular basis for this observation has not been determined.

Morphology, Cellular Constituents, and Biochemical Properties

Morphologic distinctions between mature basophils and mast cells have been appreciated in all mammalian species that have been carefully studied.[132,134,170–175] Typical human basophils and mast cells can be distinguished from each other in appropriately fixed and processed light microscopic sections,[132] but the differences between the two cell types are particularly evident by transmission electron microscopy.[132,134,175] Mature human basophils contain round cytoplasmic granules with electron-dense particles and, rarely, large crystals[134,170–172] (Fig. 20-3). As in other mature granulocytes, the nucleus is segmented and the chromatin is heavily condensed, the cytoplasm contains glycogen particles and aggregates, and the rough endoplasmic reticulum and Golgi apparatus are inconspicuous.

Human mast cells generally appear larger than basophils and contain a round-to-oval nucleus that is not segmented and generally occupies an eccentric location within the cell[132,134,174,175] (Fig. 20-4). Mature human mast cells have granules that are more numerous, smaller, and more variable in shape than those of basophils. The granule content also is much more heterogeneous and can appear as scrolls, particles, or crystals, either alone or in combination.[132,134,173–175] Human basophil granules can also contain occasional multilamellar arrays and scroll-like structures.[173,175–177] In contrast to the blunt surface projections of basophils, quiescent mast cells (those not participating in a degranulation event) are covered by uniformly distributed, thin surface processes. Mast cells also differ from basophils in having many more cytoplasmic filaments and in lacking cytoplasmic glycogen deposits.[132,134,174,175] Human mast cells can also contain numerous cytoplasmic lipid bodies, structures uncommonly observed in basophils.[176,178,179]

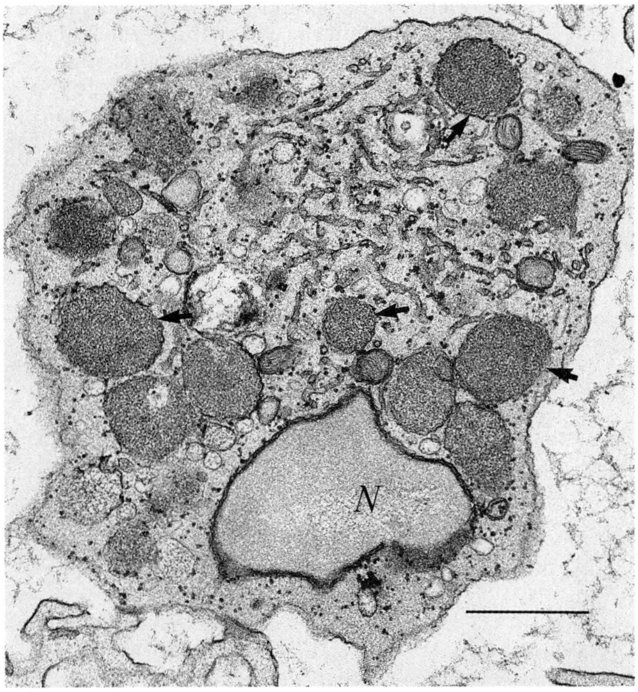

FIGURE 20-3. Transmission electron micrograph of a human basophil in a preparation of peripheral blood leukocytes obtained by separation over Ficoll-Hypaque. All cytoplasmic granules (some indicated by *solid arrows*) contain particulate electron-dense material. N, nucleus; bar = 1 μm. (Dvorak AM, Newball HH, Dvorak HF, Lichtenstein LM. Antigen-induced IgE-mediated degranulation of human basophils. Lab Invest 1980;43:126)

Basophils and mast cells contain or elaborate on appropriate stimulation, a diverse array of potent, biologically active mediators[140,150,180,181] (Table 20-5). Some of these are stored preformed in the cells' cytoplasmic granules (proteoglycans, proteases, histamine); others are synthesized on activation of the cell by IgE and antigen or other stimuli (products of arachidonic acid oxidation through the cyclooxygenase or lipoxygenase pathways, and, in some cells, PAF). Individually, these agents can have diverse effects in inflammation, immunity, and tissue remodeling, and can influence the clotting, fibrinolytic, complement, and kinin systems.[140,150,180,181]

Human mast cell populations contain variable mixtures of heparin and chondroitin sulfate proteoglycans.[182,183] Although the sulfated glycosaminoglycans of normal human blood basophils have not been characterized, heparin has not been detected consistently in basophils of patients with myelogenous leukemia.[184,185]

Both human basophils and mast cells synthesize histamine and store histamine in their cytoplasmic granules in ionic association with the granule proteoglycans.[140,180,181] Basophils are the source of most, if not all, of the histamine present in normal human blood.[186] Studies in genetically mast cell–deficient and congenic normal mice indicate that mast cells represent the source of virtually all of the his-

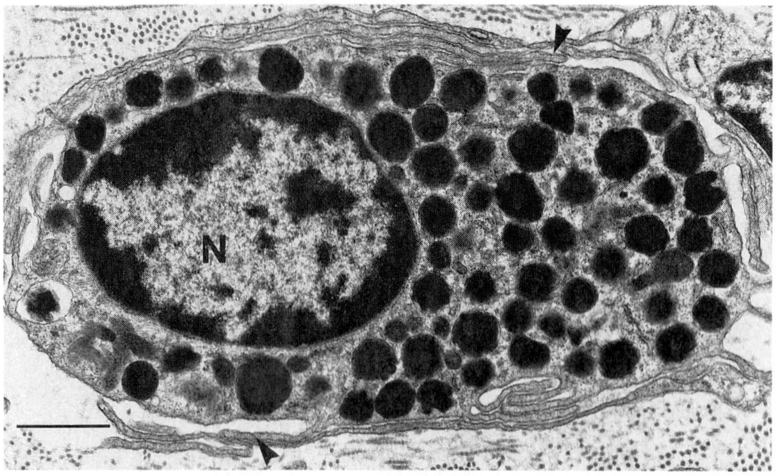

FIGURE 20-4. Transmission electron micrograph of a human mast cell from a breast fibroadenoma specimen. The nucleus (N) is monolobed, narrow surface folds (*arrowheads*) and numerous cytoplasmic granules are seen. Bar = 1 μm. (Dvorak AM. Human mast cells. In: Beck F, Hild W, Kriz W, Ortmann R, Pauly JE, Schiebler TH, eds. Advances in anatomy embryology and cell biology, vol. 114. Berlin, Springer-Verlag, 1989:1)

tamine stored in normal tissues, with the notable exceptions of the stomach and the central nervous system.[187] Mouse and rat mast cells contain significant quantities of serotonin, but this amine has not been detected in populations of human mast cells or basophils.[140,180,181]

Neutral proteases represent the major protein component of mast cell secretory granules. Human mast cell tryptase is a serine endopeptidase that exists in the granule in active form as a tetramer of 134 kd containing subunits of 31 to 35 kd, each of which contains an active site.[148] Negligible amounts of tryptase have been identified in normal human basophils by immunoassay, but it is not clear whether this activity represents an enzyme identical with that present in the mast cell.[148] Because the enzyme is at least highly concentrated in, and may be unique to, the human mast cell, the levels of mast cell tryptase in biologic fluids such as plasma, serum, or inflammatory exudates have been used as a specific indicator of mast cell activation.[188] The active tetrameric form of tryptase is stabilized by its association with heparin and perhaps other proteoglycans within the mast cell granule.[189]

Mast cell chymase is also a serine protease that is stored in active form in the mast cell granule but as a monomer with a molecular weight of 30 kd.[190,191] Chymase is present

TABLE 20-5. Principal Mediators of Human Basophils and Mast Cells

Mediator	Subcellular Localization or Origin	Basophils	Mast Cells
Histamine	Cytoplasmic granules	+	+
Heparin	Cytoplasmic granules	?	+
Chondroitin sulfates	Cytoplasmic granules	+	+
Chymase	Cytoplasmic granules	±	+
Tryptase	Cytoplasmic granules	ND	+
Carboxypeptidase	Cytoplasmic granules	NE	+
Lysophospholipase	Cytoplasmic granules	+	ND
PGD_2	Membrane lipids	ND	+
LTC_4	Membrane lipids	+	+
PAF-acether		ND	±*
TNF-α	Cytoplasmic granules	NE	+
IL-4	Unknown	+	+

ND, not detected; NE, not examined.
* Purified human lung mast cells may be able to synthesize PAF-acether that remains cell associated.

in relatively high levels of some mast cell populations, including those of the skin and gastrointestinal submucosal tissue, but is present in low or undetectable levels in many of the mast cells in other anatomic sites such as the lung and gastrointestinal mucosa.[148,192,193]

Human mast cells contain a cytoplasmic granule-associated carboxypeptidase that can convert angiotensin I to des-leu$_{10}$ angiotensin I.[194] Human basophils, like eosinophils, can form Charcot-Leyden crystals[37,195,196] and contain Charcot-Leyden crystal protein (lysophospholipase) in quantities similar to that of eosinophils.[37] Although Charcot-Leyden crystal protein has been localized ultrastructurally to the major cytoplasmic granule population of basophils, it is not clear whether basophils synthesize Charcot-Leyden crystal protein or internalize product derived from eosinophils.[197]

In addition to the preformed, cytoplasmic granule-associated mediators, basophils and mast cells can release products of arachidonic acid oxidation after appropriate stimulation (eg, with IgE and specific antigen).[150,180,181] The specific products released by different populations of mast cells or by blood basophils vary considerably.[150] For example, mast cells isolated from a variety of different human tissues release both LTC_4 and PGD_2, whereas peripheral blood basophils release LTC_4 but no detectable PGD_2.

Platelet-activating factor (originally PAF, more recently designated PAF-acether or alkylglycerylhetherphosphorylcholine [AGEPC]) and its inactive derivative, lyso-PAF, appear in biologic fluids after antigen challenge in humans,[198] but it is unclear whether human basophils or mast cells represent important potential sources of this mediator. Production of AGEPC by human basophils has not been demonstrated.[199] Purified human lung mast cells can generate AGEPC on immunologic activation, but the compound apparently remains cell associated.[200]

Recent work, much of it conducted with mouse mast cells, indicates that mast cells represent a source of multifunctional cytokines.[201,202] For example, appropriately stimulated mouse or human mast cells can release the cytokine tumor necrosis factor-α (TNF-α),[40–42,142,201–204] and both mouse and human mast cells and basophils can produce interleukin-4 (IL-4).[142,205–208] Work with mouse mast cells indicates that mast cells may also represent a potential source of several additional cytokines with effects in inflammation, immunity, hematopoiesis, tissue remodeling, and many other biologic processes.[142,201,202,209–211] At least one of the mast cell–associated cytokines, TNF-α, can be released by mast cells from both preformed, cytoplasmic, granule-associated stores and, in even larger amounts, from a newly synthesized pool.[203,204,212,213] Thus, TNF-α represents a mast cell–associated mediator that is both preformed and newly synthesized.

General Functions, Synthetic Pathways, and Mechanisms of Activation

The actual roles of basophils and mast cells in health and host defense have been remarkably difficult to ascertain. In part, this reflects the rarity of "experiments of nature" affecting these populations. Few patients lacking basophils have been reported, and these persons usually also have other abnormalities that potentially affect immune or inflammatory responses.[31,137] Thus, the role of the basophil defect in any clinical problems expressed by those patients is uncertain. We are not aware of reports of humans with a profound mast cell deficiency.

In the absence of information derived from patients with isolated abnormalities of basophil or mast cell numbers or function, concepts of the roles of these cells in human health and disease have been developed based on more indirect lines of evidence, including animal experiments. This work indicates that the major roles of basophils and mast cells in host defense are in the orchestration of local immunologic and inflammatory reactions, especially those associated with parasitic infections, and that their major role in disease is to represent an important source of the mediators responsible for many reactions of immediate hypersensitivity and related disorders.[9,140–142,150,180,214] In both of these contexts—host defense against parasites and immediate hypersensitivity—the roles of basophils and mast cells are expressed primarily by the release to the exterior of preformed, granule-associated mediators, cytokines, or newly generated (lipid) mediators. Although the limited ability of basophils or mast cells to phagocytose bacteria and other particles has been reported, little evidence suggests that this represents an important aspect of their contribution to host defense or pathology.[215,216]

Experimental studies also indicate that basophils and mast cells can internalize and store in their granules certain products of other cell types, including eosinophil peroxidase.[217,218] This mechanism may contribute to the limitation of the toxicity or other biologic activities of the internalized compounds, or alternatively may place the expression of the compounds' biologic activity under the regulation of signals that elicit basophil or mast cell degranulation.

The dominant cellular event that underlies expression of basophil or mast cell function is the process of *degranulation*, a stereotyped constellation of stimulus-activated biochemical[219] and morphologic[132,175,221] events that result in the fusion of the cytoplasmic granule membranes with the plasma membrane (with external release of granule-associated mediators), associated with the generation and release of products of arachidonic acid oxidation (Fig. 20-5). Although a variety of stimuli can initiate basophil or mast cell degranulation (Table 20-6), the best-studied pathway of stimulation is that transduced through $Fc_{\epsilon}RI$ expressed on the basophil or mast cell surface.[219,220] Human basophils generated in vitro express about 2.7×10^5 $Fc_{\epsilon}RI$ per cell, which bind monovalent IgE immunoglobulin with a K_A of about 2.8×10^9 mol/L.[222] Similar values have been obtained for the $Fc_{\epsilon}RI$ of rat and mouse mast cells.[219] The $Fc_{\epsilon}RI$ consists of one α, one β, and two identical disulfide-linked γ chains, all components of which recently have been cloned and sequenced.[220,223–225] When adjacent $Fc_{\epsilon}RIs$ are bridged, either by bivalent or multivalent antigen interacting with receptor-bound IgE, or by antibodies directed against receptor-bound IgE or the receptor itself, activation of the cells for release of stored and newly generated mediators is rapidly triggered.[219] This process is physiologic and temperature-dependent, occurring without evidence of toxicity to the responding cell, and requires energy and the uptake of extracellular calcium.[219]

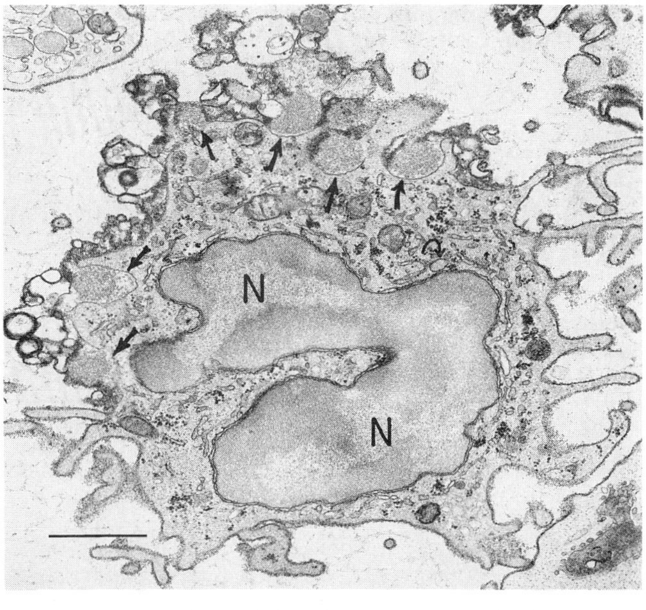

FIGURE 20-5. Transmission electron micrograph of a human basophil 2 minutes after exposure to antigen in vitro. Cell exhibits extrusion of granules from six separate sites on plasma membrane (*arrows*). At this time after cell stimulation, particle-filled granules retain shape and characteristic structure even after exposure to extracellular milieu. Electron-dense deposits of cationized ferritin coats cell surface and enters cul-de-sacs that contain exteriorized granules. Cell exhibits no fully intracytoplasmic, typical basophilic granules, but one of the smaller kind of granules (*curved arrow*) can be observed in perinuclear region. N, nucleus; bar = 1 μm. (Dvorak AM, Newball HH, Dvorak HF, Lichtenstein LM. Antigen-induced IgE-mediated degranulation of human basophils. Lab Invest 1980;43:126)

Degranulation by the $Fc_{\epsilon}RI$ is also associated with activation of membrane-associated serine proteases, phospholipase C, methyltransferase and adenylate cyclase, the stimulation of phosphatidylinositol turnover and generation of diacylglycerol, and activation of protein kinase C and phospholipase A_2.[219,220] The precise manner in which the biochemical events associated with $Fc_{\epsilon}RI$-mediated basophil and mast cell activation are coordinated to orchestrate the cellular response, although not elucidated in every detail, is the subject of intense investigation.

In addition to IgE and specific antigen, a variety of biologic substances, chemical agents, and physical stimuli can elicit release of basophil or mast cell mediators (see Table 20-6). The responsiveness of basophils and mast cells to individual examples of these stimuli varies, and significant differences have been reported in the responses of mast cells derived from different anatomic sites.[141,142,144–148] Some of these agents, when administered systemically, can induce a clinical picture indistinguishable from IgE-dependent anaphylaxis.[226] Others may release proportionately more histamine than products of arachidonic acid oxidation.[150,227]

A variety of cell types, including peripheral blood mononuclear cells, bronchoalveolar lavage cells, neutrophils, vascular endothelial cells, and platelets have been shown to produce several specific cytokines and perhaps additional histamine-releasing factors (HRFs) which have not yet been specifically identified, all of which are capable of inducing noncytolytic release of histamine from human

TABLE 20-6. Stimuli of Human Basophil or Mast Cell Mediator Release

Stimulus	Basophils	Mast Cells
IgE and specific divalent or multivalent antigen, or anti-IgE	+	+
C5a	+	+*
f-Met Leu Phe	+	+*
Mannitol (hyperosmolar)	+	+
Substance P	0	+*
Morphine	0	+*
Histamine-releasing factors (see text)†	+	±
Stem cell factor	±	+

* Purified skin mast cells are much more responsive than lung or gut mast cells.[126]

† Some histamine-releasing factors may stimulate mediator release by interacting with a subclass of IgE bound to the basophil surface (see text).

basophils.[160,228–230] Some of these agents can stimulate histamine release from all basophils tested[228,231–233]; others release histamine from the basophils of allergic patients preferentially.[229,230,234] It has been proposed that the latter agents may stimulate basophil histamine release by binding to a subclass of IgE antibodies on the surface of basophils of some allergic patients.[229,230] HRFs may be important in the regulation of basophil function at sites of allergic disease, for example, during asthma.

Specialized Effector Functions

The rapid release of mediators from IgE-primed basophils and mast cells activated by exposure to parasite-associated antigens is thought to contribute significantly to the local inflammation associated with IgE-dependent immune responses to parasites.[142,235,236] When the same events are triggered by antigens that are intrinsically innocuous or of limited toxicity, such as pollen, food components, pharmacologic agents, or insect venom, the result is a disorder of immediate hypersensitivity. The latter can range in severity from the simply annoying (allergic rhinitis) to the catastrophic and life-threatening (systemic anaphylaxis).[226] In addition to such acute manifestations of IgE-dependent disorders, basophils and mast cells also contribute significantly to late-phase reactions (LPRs), inflammatory reactions involving the skin, respiratory tract, or gastrointestinal tract, which follow by hours the exposure of sensitive subjects to specific antigen.[142,150,237]

It is widely believed that much of the morbidity associated with chronic allergic conditions, such as allergic asthma, reflects the actions of leukocytes recruited to sites of LPRs.[142,150,237] Studies in genetically mast cell–deficient mice that are mast cell reconstituted ("mast cell knock-in mice") indicate that mast cells are responsible for virtually all of the vascular permeability changes and leukocyte infiltration associated with experimental cutaneous LPRs and that TNF-α contributes to these responses.[238,239] It is likely that mast cell TNF-α production also helps to initiate LPRs in humans[142,202,204] and that basophils, eosinophils, and other leukocytes that are recruited to these reactions produce cytokines and other mediators that regulate the further development and, ultimately, the resolution of these reactions.[142,202] This sequence of events in the pathogenesis of LPRs is termed the mast cell–leukocyte–cytokine cascade.[142,202]

Mast cell activation and infiltration of circulating basophils also can occur during a variety of T-cell–dependent immunologic responses in both humans and experimental animals.[132,133] However, genetically mast cell–deficient mice express apparently unimpaired T-cell–dependent responses.[142,236,240] Accordingly, the specific roles of mast cells and basophils in such responses remain to be determined.

Theories about the specific functions and potential importance of basophils and mast cells in parasite infections have far outdistanced hard evidence documenting the cells' actual contributions. This reflects, in large part, the difficulties of effectively manipulating these populations in vivo.[141,142,151,236,241,242] The most compelling evidence for a role for basophils and mast cells in defense against parasites is in immune responses to ectoparasites such as ticks. The relative importance of basophils or mast cells in orchestrating the effector limb of the immune response to ticks may vary, according to species of host and species of tick.[142,151,236,243–245]

In addition to their participation in immune responses, basophils or mast cells have been implicated in a wide variety of biologic responses including acute inflammatory responses elicited independently of the immune response, angiogenesis and wound healing, and inflammatory bowel disease, scleroderma, and in the reactions to certain neoplasms.[132,133,139,141,142,144,145,151,236,241,246,247] Although the roles for basophils or mast cells in most of the responses mentioned are uncertain, studies in mast cell knock-in mice indicate that mast cells can augment the intensity or rate of development of immunologically nonspecific acute inflammatory reactions and also may accelerate the development of blood vessels in association with certain experimental tumors.[246,248–250]

Basophilopenia and Basophilia

Except when numbers of basophils are extraordinarily elevated, such as in chronic myelogenous leukemia (CML) and other myeloproliferative disorders, accurate determination of blood basophil levels requires absolute methods of quantification.[130,131] Since most laboratories do not routinely perform such determinations, information about conditions associated with elevation or diminution of numbers of basophils is more limited than it is in other granulocytes (Table 20-7). Basophilopenia has been recorded immediately after anaphylaxis and in urticaria, especially when angioedema is present.[251,252] These findings probably reflect, at least partly, a loss of metachromatic staining of degranulated basophils, rather than an actual drop in basophil numbers.[251] Diurnal variations in basophil levels, with lowest levels in the morning, have been reported in some persons[251,253] but not in others.[251] Some authors have detected slight variations in adult basophil counts with age or sex, whereas this was not observed in other studies.[251,254,255] Basophils have been reported to almost double within 24 hours of birth, to drop to values less than half of the adult levels by 1 week, then to increase nearly to adult levels by 6 weeks after birth.[254] Most authors found blood basophil levels in children to be similar to those of adults.[251,254]

Perhaps the most common clinical settings in which basophilopenia can be documented, often in association with a parallel eosinophilopenia, are during the reactive leukocytoses associated with disorders such as acute myocardial infarction, lobar pneumonia, and bleeding peptic ulcer.[256,257] These findings may reflect effects of release of increased levels of corticosteroids during these conditions, since administration of ACTH or corticosteroids results in marked reductions in basophil and eosinophil

TABLE 20-7. **Conditions Associated With Basophilopenia or Basophilia**

Condition	Effect on Blood Basophil Levels
Anaphylaxis, urticaria (certain cases)	Decreased
Severe acute illnesses (myocardial infarction, pneumonia, bleeding peptic ulcer)	Decreased during acute phases Increased during recovery
Administration of ACTH or corticosteroids	Decreased
Administration of thyroid hormone, thyrotoxicosis	Decreased
Ovulation	Decreased
Lipemia	Decreased
Chronic myeloid leukemia (and basophilic leukemia)	Markedly increased, especially terminally
Other myeloproliferative disorders (myeloid metaplasia, polycythemia vera)	Moderately increased
Systemic mast cell disease	Increased in a minority of patients
Drug allergies	Slightly increased during chronic phase
Ulcerative colitis	Slightly increased
Juvenile rheumatoid arthritis	Slightly increased
Myxedema	Slightly increased

counts.[258-260] Basophils can be greatly diminished in thyrotoxicosis or after treatment with thyroid hormones and may be increased after ablation of thyroid function or in myxedema.[256,257,261] Ovulation has been associated with a rapid and significant (up to 50%) drop in basophil levels; the mechanisms and significance of this phenomenon are not clear.[262] Basophil degranulation can also be observed during lipemia.[121,263] One study has reported that patients with solid malignant tumors exhibited a modest (around 30% to 40%) diminution of levels of blood histamine, basophils, and eosinophils compared with those of control groups.[264]

Basophil levels are variably increased in patients with chronic myeloproliferative disorders, a finding that can be useful in distinguishing these conditions from leukemoid reactions in which absolute basophil levels generally are low.[265] Basophils may be moderately elevated to 1000/μL or more in myeloid metaplasia and polycythemia vera,[265] and can be strikingly elevated in CML, in which basophils often account for 2% to 20% of circulating leukocytes.[121,265] Basophil counts exceeding 30% can occur intermittently during the course of CML, particularly late in the disease, often in association with its terminal phase.[266] The basophils found in CML patients are best considered neoplastic cells, which in some patients have been reported to possess the Ph chromosome[121,131] and which can exhibit a variety of morphologic and histochemical alterations.[121,267] At least some basophils from patients with CML can be triggered to degranulate in vitro.[268-270] Immature forms may circulate, particularly during the terminal basophil crisis,[121] and some cases of apparently acute myelogenous leukemia with high levels of immature basophils have been reported.[121,267,271]

Cells resembling normal basophils may rarely account for over 80% of circulating leukocytes even early in CML.[121,272] Such cases sometimes have been designated *basophil leukemia*. Occasional patients with CML with extremely high levels of circulating basophils may exhibit clinical effects attributable to the liberation of histamine and perhaps other basophil mediators.[273,274] The treatment of patients with extremely high levels of circulating basophils is particularly problematic, since the cytolysis of these basophils during chemotherapy can result in shock as a result of the massive release of histamine and perhaps other basophil-associated mediators.[273]

Basophilia has been reported in patients in the chronic phases of drug allergies,[274-276] in those with ulcerative colitis[256] and myxedema,[256,257,261] in those recovering from acute illnesses,[257] and in those with juvenile rheumatoid arthritis.[277] Generally, the recorded elevations in basophil counts were modest and overlapped the normal range. A single report has been made of a patient with a leukemoid reaction in association with disseminated tuberculosis, whose basophil count was markedly elevated (11% to 56%).[278]

Reactive Mastocytosis and the Spectrum of Mast Cell Neoplasia

The factors regulating the numbers and phenotype of the mast cells that occur normally in various human tissues and the factors that influence changes in mast cell numbers or phenotypes during immunologic or pathologic processes have not been defined. It has been extraordinarily difficult to generate normal human mast cells in vitro using techniques that readily result in the successful growth of mouse or rat mast cells.[128] The generation of a mast cell line from a patient with mastocytosis has been reported,[279] as has the establishment of a long-term cell line from a patient with mast cell leukemia.[280] Initial attempts to grow mast cells in suspension culture from normal human bone marrow or umbilical cord blood cells have generated basophils and eosinophils but not mast cells.[125,127,128] A recent report described the development of colonies of cells with morphologic and histochemical characteristics of mast cells in semisolid agar cultures of human bone marrow or cord blood cells.[281] These candidate mast cells exhibited reactivity with a monoclonal antibody reported to be specific for human mast cells,[282] but did not react with a monoclonal antibody reactive with human basophils.[283]

As noted earlier, several groups recently showed that human mast cells can be generated from various sources of hematopoietic cells in vitro in the presence of the c-*kit* ligand, SCF.[161-164] Moreover, the subcutaneous administration of recombinant human SCF to humans results in a significant increase in the number of cutaneous mast cells.[165] These findings indicate that SCF can regulate mast cell development in humans and suggest that excessive or dysregulated production of SCF, or mutations involving the c-*kit* receptor that promote its constitutive activation or augment its sensitivity to SCF, might accout for some cases of disordered mast cell proliferation. Constitutive activation of c-*kit* has been reported in one mouse mastocytoma cell line,[284] and a single human mast cell leukemia cell line[280] has been found to exhibit mutations in the coding sequence of c-*kit* that are associated with the ligand-independent activation of the c-*kit* receptor.[285]

It will be of interest to evaluate to what extent abnormalities in SCF production or c-*kit* function are involved in the spontaneous development of abnormal proliferations of mast cells. However, until the factors regulating the proliferation of neoplastic human mast cells have been better defined, analysis of changes in the numbers of mast cells, and identification of neoplasms involving the cell type, will continue to depend on careful morphometric analysis of mast cell numbers and, in the case of neoplasms, appreciation of the clinical features of the diseases. Increased numbers of mast cells have been reported in association with a variety of diseases with components of immediate hypersensitivity, including allergic rhinitis[139,286–288] and certain forms of asthma and urticaria, in the lymph nodes of patients with filariasis and other parasitic diseases,[139,289] in association with Hodgkin's disease and lymphoproliferative disorders[290] and in lymph nodes draining breast carcinoma,[290] in the connective tissue associated with some benign and malignant neoplasms,[289,290] in neurofibromas,[291] in scleroderma,[247] in inflammatory bowel disease and peptic ulcers,[292,293] in the synovium of joints with rheumatoid arthritis,[294,295] and in association with osteoporosis[296] and the osteitis fibrosa associated with renal failure.[297] Based on observations in animals, it would not be unreasonable to consider that modest elevations in mast cell numbers may occur in association with most conditions associated with chronic inflammation or tissue remodeling.[132,139,140] It is likely that the elevations in mast cell numbers observed in at least some of these conditions reflect the increased production of SCF by fibroblasts and other cells at the involved sites.[152,153]

Relatively few conditions that are associated with diminished numbers of mast cells have been reported. Mast cells become difficult to identify histologically after extensive degranulation in response to IgE and specific antigen or other signals.[239,298] The chronic administration of corticosteroids to the skin using occlusive dressings also results in a marked local diminution in the number of identifiable dermal mast cells.[299]

The spectrum of neoplastic disorders involving mast cell proliferation is broad, ranging from isolated benign cutaneous mastocytomas that resolve spontaneously to rapidly fatal mast cell leukemia.[289,300–303] Between these extremes of clinical presentation are a variety of clinical conditions that vary in the number and anatomic distribution of lesions, clinical course, and prognosis. Although some of these conditions are clearly neoplastic based on the biologic behavior of the mast cell populations, no direct evidence exists that the mast cell populations constituting the more benign lesions are actually clonal. Nevertheless, these lesions are conventionally considered to represent neoplasms.

Solitary benign cutaneous mastocytomas can be present at birth or develop later in life.[290,302] Generally, the lesions are small and regress spontaneously. The most common disorder associated with multiple mast cell lesions is cutaneous mastocytosis or *urticaria pigmentosa*.[289,302,303] The lesions of urticaria pigmentosa are most typically small red to brown macules or papules that, when subjected to mild trauma such as rubbing, develop edema and erythema at their periphery (Darier's sign). The lesions may be pruritic, a symptom that can be exacerbated by trauma, changes in temperature, and ingestion of certain foods or drugs. Typically, patients have multiple individual lesions widely distributed over the trunk and extremities. Diffuse cutaneous involvement also can occur,[289,302,303] and a few cases of familial urticaria pigmentosa have been reported.[302] Diagnosis of urticaria pigmentosa is made by skin biopsy demonstrating increased numbers of dermal mast cells, particularly in the papillary dermis.[289,302,303] Some patients with clinical evidence of urticaria pigmentosa may not demonstrate increased numbers of mast cells on skin biopsy.[302]

More than half of all children presenting with cutaneous mastocytosis experience resolution of their cutaneous lesions by adulthood; a subset of children progress to systemic disease. In adults, skin disease virtually always persists and may be followed years later by systemic mastocytosis, with gastrointestinal and skeletal involvement.[289,302,303] Affected persons can develop gastric hypersecretion as a result of elevated plasma histamine, peptic ulcer disease, malabsorption, and abdominal cramps.[303,304] Up to 70% of patients with bone marrow involvement during systemic mastocytosis have changes detectable radiographically, particularly in the long bones, pelvis, ribs, and skull.[303] Bone pain is the most common symptom. The bone marrow lesions consist of aggregates of spindle-shaped mast cells, often mixed with lymphocytes, eosinophils, and fibroblasts.[289,302,303] Hepatic fibrosis associated with mast cell involvement of the liver can lead to portal hypertension and ascites.[289,302,303,305] Patients with systemic mastocytosis also may experience flushing or overt anaphylaxis, which occasionally may be provoked by identifiable stimuli such as aspirin, infection, exercise, or alcohol.[303]

Although some patients who present with urticaria pigmentosa progress to systemic mast cell disease, up to half of patients with systemic mast cell disease lack clinically evident cutaneous involvement.[302] The clinical presentation of such patients varies considerably, including anaphylaxis, findings related to bone or gastrointestinal involvement, or a hematologic or solid malignancy.[302]

Twenty-two of a series of 66 patients with systemic mast cell disease had associated hematologic disorders, including dysmyelopoietic syndromes,[10] myeloproliferative disorders,[5] acute leukemias,[3] lymphomas,[3] and chronic neutropenia.[1,305] Roughly one third of these patients exhibited lesions of urticaria pigmentosa, but most diagnoses of mastocytosis in this group were made as a result of bone marrow aspiration and biopsy performed for the primary hematologic disorder.[305]

Given the likelihood that cytokines with actions on the hematopoietic system may influence human mast cell proliferation and differentiation, it is possible that some of the mastocytosis that develops in association with other hematologic disorders represents a proliferation of nonneoplastic cells. In patients with mastocytosis associated with other hematologic disorders, the prognosis is that of the primary disease process.

In recent studies, basophilia has been seen in up to 7% of patients with systemic mast cell disease; circulating mast cells have been found in less than 4%.[302] Poor prognostic factors in systemic mast cell disease include constitutional symptoms, anemia, thrombocytopenia, abnormal liver function tests, lobulated nuclei in mast cells, low percentage of bone marrow fat cells, and associated hematologic disorders.[302] Although a previous classification of systemic mastocytoses divided the patients into those with benign and those with malignant disorders,[289] Travis and colleagues[302] have suggested that the former would be better classified as *indolent*. This designation indicates that a subset of patients with systemic mast cell disease can be expected to have a favorable long-term survival but that even those patients with the most favorable prognostic features may develop a more aggressive form of their disease or an associated hematologic malignancy.[302]

The rarest general category of mast cell disease is mast

cell leukemia.[301] Mast cells of abnormal morphology are present in the peripheral blood (10% to 96% of nucleated cells), a finding that virtually never occurs in the other categories of mastocytosis. Moreover, when mast cells appear in the blood of patients with systemic mast cell disease, they generally represent less than 10% of nucleated cells.[301,302] Patients with mast cell leukemia generally do not exhibit urticaria pigmentosa. Peptic ulcer disease, constitutional symptoms, anemia, and hepatosplenomegaly are common. Duration of survival is generally less than 6 months. By morphology, the circulating mast cells can resemble normal mast cells or can represent aberrant forms with only a few metachromatic cytoplasmic granules. Erythrophagocytosis has been reported.[289] Mast cell leukemia should be distinguished from the acute nonlymphocytic leukemia that can develop in association with systemic mast cell disease,[289,296] and from the reactive proliferation of normal-appearing mast cells that can be seen in the bone marrow of patients with leukemic or preleukemic disorders.[306–308] One case of mast cell sarcoma has been reported[289]; an elderly woman presented with a subglottal tumor, then with two skin lesions, and finally with involvement of multiple organ systems. Terminally, the blood contained 95% immature mast cells.

A final category of patients with systemic mast cell disease exhibits an aggressive clinical course in the absence of mast cell leukemia or an associated hematologic disease. Patients with this disorder, designated lymphadenopathic mastocytosis with eosinophilia,[303,309] rarely exhibit urticaria pigmentosa but have peripheral eosinophilia, anemia, hepatosplenomegaly and lymphadenopathy, and bone marrow lesions of mastocytosis. Gastrointestinal disease has been reported, and patients often also develop hepatic and splenic fibrosis and portal hypertension.

Treatment of patients with various forms of systemic mastocytosis consists of control of mast cell mediator–associated signs and symptoms, management of mastocytosis-associated gastrointestinal problems, and specific therapy of any associated hematologic disorder.[301–305] H_1 receptor antagonists can be helpful in reducing pruritus, tachycardia, and flushing, whereas gastric acid hypersecretion and associated gastric ulceration can be controlled with H_2 antagonists. Systemic steroids may be useful in severe malabsorption. The diarrhea associated with mastocytosis can be particularly difficult to manage. Chemotherapy has not proved to be of benefit in patients with mast cell leukemia, nor is it indicated in treatment of indolent systemic mastocytosis. Preliminary data suggest that patients with aggressive mastocytosis who had splenectomy for hypersplenism or other purposes exhibited prolonged survival and better tolerance of chemotherapy compared with those who did not receive splenectomy.[303]

Acknowledgments

We thank the many colleagues who critically read the chapter, and Ann M. Dvorak for the electron micrographs.

REFERENCES

1. Hudson G. Quantitative study of the eosinophil granulocytes. Semin Hematol 1968;5:166.
2. Bainton DF, Farqhuar MG. Segregation and packaging of granule enzymes in eosinophilic leukocytes. J Cell Biol 1970;45:54.
3. Spry JFS. Eosinophils: a comprehensive review, and guide to scientific and medical literature. Oxford, Oxford University Press, 1988.
4. Dresch C, Johnson GR, Metcalf D. Eosinophil colony formation in semisolid cultures of human bone marrow cells. Blood 1977;49:835.
5. Dao C, Metcalf D, Bilski-Pasquier G. Eosinophil and neutrophil colony-forming cells in culture. Blood 1977;50:833.
6. Metcalf D, Cutler RL, Nicola NA. Selective stimulation by mouse spleen cell conditioned medium of human eosinophil colony formation. Blood 1983;61:999.
7. Lopez AF, Begley CG, Williamson DJ, et al. Murine eosinophil differentiation factor: an eosinophil-specific colony-stimulating factor with activity for human cells. J Exp Med 1986;163:1085.
8. L'Esperance P, Brunning R, Good RA. Congenital neutropenia: in vitro growth of colonies mimicking the disease. Proc Natl Acad Sci USA 1973;70:669.
9. Zucker-Franklin D, L'Esperance P, Good RA. Congenital neutropenia: an intrinsic cell defect demonstrated by electron microscopy of soft agar colonies. Blood 1977;49:425.
10. Parmley RT, Crist WM, Ragab AH, et al. Congenital dysgranulopoietic neutropenia: clinical, serologic, ultrastructural, and in vitro proliferative characteristics. Blood 1980;56:465.
11. Slifman NR, Adolphson CR, Gleich GJ. Eosinophils: biochemical and cellular aspects. In: Middleton E, Reed CE, Ellis EF, Adkinson NF Jr, Yunginger JW, eds. Allergy principles and practice, ed 3. St Louis, CV Mosby, 1988:179–205.
12. Basten A, Beeson PB. Mechanisms of eosinophilia. II. Role of the lymphocyte. J Exp Med 1970;131:1288.
13. Ruscetti FW, Cypress RH, Chervenick PA. Specific release of neutrophilic- and eosinophilic-stimulating factors from sensitized lymphocytes. Blood 1976;47:757.
14. Korpela R, Jalkanen S, Paljärvi L, et al. Early embryonic bursectomy induces eosinophilia. J Immunol 139:3915.
15. Mahmoud AAF, Stone MK, Kellermeyer RW. Eosinophilopoietin: a circulating low molecular weight peptide-like substance which stimulates the production of eosinophils in mice. J Clin Invest 1977;60:675.
16. Mahmoud AAF, Stone MK, Tracy JW. Eosinophilopoietin production: relationship to eosinophilia of infection and thymus function. Trans Assoc Am Phys 1979;92:355.
17. Bartelmez SH, Dodge WH, Mahmoud AAF, et al. Stimulation of eosinophil production in vitro by eosinophilopoietin and spleen cell-derived eosinophil growth-stimulating factor. Blood 1980;56:706.
18. Watanabe N, Katakura K, Kobayashi A, et al. Protective immunity and eosinophilia in IgE-deficient SJA/9 mice infected with *Nippostrongylus brasiliensis* and *Trichinella spiralis*. Proc Natl Acad Sci USA 1988;85:4460.
19. Ihle JN, Weinstein Y. Immunological regulation of hematopoietic/lymphoid stem cell differentiation by interleukin 3. Adv Immunol 1986;39:1.
20. Sanderson CJ, O'Garra A, Warren DJ, et al. Eosinophil differentiation factor also has B-cell growth factor activity: proposed name interleukin 4. Proc Natl Acad Sci USA 1986;83:437.
21. Owen WF, Rothenberg ME, Silberstein DS, et al. Regulation of human eosinophil viability, density, and function by granulocyte/macrophage colony-stimulating factor in the presence of 3T3 fibroblasts. J Exp Med 1987;166:129.
22. Warren DJ, Moore MAS. Synergism among interleukin 1, interleukin 3, and interleukin 5 in the production of eosinophils from primitive hemopoietic stem cells. J Immunol 1988;140:94.
23. Parwaresch MR, Walle AJ, Arndt D. The peripheral kinetics of human radiolabelled eosinophils. Virchows Arch (B) 1957;21:57.
24. Steinbach KH, Schick P, Trepel F, et al. Estimation of kinetic parameters of neutrophilic, eosinophilic, and basophilic granulocytes in human blood. Blut 1979;39:27.
25. Herion JC, Glasser RM, Walker RI, et al. Eosinophil kinetics in two patients with eosinophilia. Blood 1970;36:361.
26. Dale DC, Hubert RT, Fauci A. Eosinophil kinetics in the hypereosinophilic syndrome. J Lab Clin Med 1976;87:487.
27. Osgood EE. Number and distribution of human hemic cells. Blood 1954;9:1141.
28. Rytömaa T. Organ distribution and histochemical properties of eosinophil granulocytes in rat. Acta Pathol Microbiol Scand 1960;50(Suppl 140):1.
29. Telerman A, Amson RB, Delforge A, et al. A case of chronic aneosinocytosis. Am J Hematol 1982;12:187.
30. Nakahata T, Spicer SS, Leary AG, et al. Circulating eosinophil colony-forming cells in pure eosinophil aplasia. Ann Intern Med 1984;101:321.
31. Mitchell EB, Platts-Mills TAE, Pereira RS, et al. Acquired basophil and eosinophil deficiency in a patient with hypogammaglobulinaemia associated with thymoma. Clin Lab Haematol 1983;5:253.
32. Bjornson BH, Harvey JM, Rose L. Differential effect of hydrocortisone on eosinophil and neutrophil proliferation. J Clin Invest 1985;76:924.
33. Beeson PB, Bass DA. The eosinophil. Philadelphia, WB Saunders, 1977.
34. Weller PF, Goetzl EJ. The human eosinophil. Roles in host defense and tissue injury. Am J Pathol 1980;100:793.
35. Gleich GJ, Loegering, DA. Immunobiology of eosinophils. Ann Rev Immunol 1984;2:429.
36. Davis WB, Fells GA, Sun X-H, et al. Eosinophil-mediated injury to lung parenchymal cells and interstitial matrix. A possible role for eosinophils in chronic inflammatory disorders of the lower respiratory tract. J Clin Invest 1984;74:269.
37. Ackerman SJ, Weil GJ, Gleich GJ. Formation of Charcot-Leyden crystals by human basophils. J Exp Med 1982;155:1597.
38. Barker RL, Gleich GJ, Pease, LR. Acidic precursor revealed in human eosinophil granule major basic protein cDNA. J Exp Med 1988;168:1493.

39. McGrogan M, Simonsen C, Scott R, et al. Isolation of a complementary DNA clone encoding a precursor to human eosinophil major basic protein. J Exp Med 1988;168:2295.
40. O'Donnell MC, Ackerman SJ, Gleich GJ, et al. Activation of basophil and mast cell histamine release by eosinophil granule major basic protein. J Exp Med 1983:157:1981.
41. Zheutlin LM, Ackerman SJ, Gleich GJ, et al. Stimulation of basophil and rat mast cell histamine release by eosinophil granule-derived cationic proteins. J Immunol 1984;133:2180.
42. Venge P, Dahl R, Hallgren R. Enhancement of factor XII-dependent reactions by eosinophil cationic protein. Thromb Res 1979;14:641.
43. Fredens K, Dahl R, Venge P. The Gordon phenomenon induced by the eosinophil cationic protein and eosinophil protein X. J Allergy Clin Immunol 1982;70:361.
44. Slifman NR, Loegering DA, McKean DJ, et al. Ribonuclease activity associated with human eosinophil-derived neurotoxin and eosinophil cationic protein. J Immunol 1986;137:2913.
45. Sorrentino S, Glitz DG, Hamann KJ, Loegering DA, Checkel JL, Gleich GJ. Eosinophil-derived neurotoxin and human liver ribonuclease: identity of structure and linkage of neurotoxicity to nuclease activity. J Biol Chem 1992;267:14859.
46. Weller PF, Goetzl EJ. The regulatory and effector roles of eosinophils. Adv Immunol 1979;27:339.
47. Sigal CE, Valone FH, Holtzman MJ, Goetzl, EJ. Preferential human eosinophil chemotactic activity of the platelet-activating factor (PAF) 1-*0*-hexadecyl-2-acetyl-*sn*-glyceryl-3-phosphocholine (AGEPC). J Clin Immunol 1987;7:179.
48. Wardlaw AJ, Moqbel R, Cromwell O, et al. Platelet-activating factor: a potent chemotactic and chemokinetic factor for human eosinophils. J Clin Invest 1986;78:1701.
49. Kroegel C, Yukawa T, Dent G, et al. Platelet-activating factor induces eosinophil peroxidase release from purified human eosinophils. Immunology 1988;64:559.
50. Kimani G, Tonnesen MG, Henson PM. Stimulation of eosinophil adherence to human vascular endothelial cells in vitro by platelet-activating factor. J Immunol 1988;140:3161.
51. Wang JM, Rambaldi A, Biondi J, Chen ZG, Sanderson CJ, Mantovani A. Recombinant human interleukin 5 is a selective eosinophil chemoattractant. Eur J Immunol 1989;19:701.
52. Kameyoshi Y, Dorschner A, Mallet AI, Christophers E, Schroder JM. Cytokine RANTES released by thrombin-stimulated platelets is a potent attractant for human eosinophils. J Exp Med 1992;176:587.
53. Kita H, Weiler DA, Abu-Ghazaleh R, Sanderson CJ, Gleich GJ. Release of granule proteins from eosinophils cultured with IL-5. J Immunol 1992;149:625.
54. Hansel TT, DeVries JM, Carballido JM, et al. Induction and function of eosinophil intercellular adhesion molecule-1 and HLA-DR. J Immunol 1992;149:2130.
55. Khalife J, Capron M, Grzych J-M, et al. Fcγ receptors on rat eosinophils: isotype-dependent cell activation. J Immunol 1985;135:2780.
56. Metzger H. Molecular aspects of receptors and binding factors for IgE. Adv Immunol 1988;43:277.
57. Lucey DR, Dorsky DI, Nicholson-Weller A, et al. Human eosinophils express CD4 protein and bind human immunodeficiency virus 1 gp120. J Exp Med 1989;169:327.
58. Bass DA, Grover WH, Lewis JC, et al. Comparison of human eosinophils from normals and patients with eosinophilia. J Clin Invest 1980;66:1265.
59. Winqvist I, Olofsson T, Olsson I, et al. Altered density, metabolism and surface receptors of eosinophils in eosinophilia. Immunology 1982;47:531.
60. Prin L, Capron M, Tonnel A-B, et al. Heterogeneity of human peripheral blood eosinophils: variability in cell density and cytotoxic ability in relation to the level and the origin of hypereosinophilia. Int Arch Allergy Appl Immunol 1983;72:336.
61. Fukuda T, Dunnette SL, Reed CE, et al. Increased numbers of hypodense eosinophils in the blood of patients with bronchial asthma. Am Rev Respir Dis 1985;132:981.
62. Pincus SH, Schooley WR, DiNapoli AM, et al. Metabolic heterogeneity of eosinophils from normal and hypereosinophilic patients. Blood 1981;8:1175.
63. Kajita T, Yui Y, Mita H, et al. Release of leukotriene C_4 from human eosinophils and its relation to the cell density. Int Arch Allergy Appl Immunol 1985;78:406.
64. Weller PF, Dvorak AM. Arachidonic acid incorporation by cytoplasmic lipid bodies of human eosinophils. Blood 1985;65:1269.
65. Turk J, Maas RL, Brash AR, et al. Arachidonic acid 15-lipoxygenase products from human eosinophils J Biol Chem 1982;257:7068.
66. Henderson WR, Harley JB, Fauci AS. Arachidonic acid metabolism in normal and hypereosinophilic syndrome human eosinophils: generation of leukotrienes B_4, C_4, D_4, and 15-lipoxygenase products. Immunology 1984;51:679.
67. Silberstein DS, Owen WF, Gasson JC, et al. Enhancement of human eosinophil cytotoxicity and leukotriene synthesis by biosynthetic (recombinant) granulocyte-macrophage colony-stimulating factor. J Immunol 1986;37:3290.
68. Cromwell O, Moqbel R, Fitzharris P, et al. Leukotriene C_4 generation from human eosinophils stimulated with IgG–*Aspergillus fumigatus* antigen immune complexes. J Allergy Clin Immunol 1988;82:535.
69. Kauffman HF, van der Belt B, de Monchy JGR, et al. Leukotriene C_4 production by normal-density and low-density eosinophils of atopic individuals and other patients with eosinophilia. J Allergy Clin Immunol 1987;79:611.
70. Yazdanbakhsh M, Eckmann CM, Bot AAM, et al. Bactericidal action of eosinophils from normal human blood. Infect Immun 1986;53:192.
71. Ramsey PG, Martin T, Chi E, et al. Arming of mononuclear phagocytes by eosinophil peroxidase bound to *Staphylococcus aureus*. J Immunol 1982;128:415.
72. Crofton JW, Livingston JL, Oswald NC, et al. Pulmonary eosinophilia. Thorax 1952;7:1.
73. Sovijarvi ARA, Lemola M, Stenius B, et al. Nitrofurantoin-induced acute, subacute, and chronic pulmonary reactions. Scand J Respir Dis 1977;58:41.
74. Neva FA, Ottesen EA. Tropical (filarial) eosinophilia. N Engl J Med 1978;298:1129.
75. Hendrick DJ, Ellithorpe DB, Lyon F, et al. Allergic bronchopulmonary helminthosporiosis. Am Rev Respir Dis 1982;126:935.
76. Butterworth AE, Wassom DL, Gleich GJ, et al. Damage to schistosomula of *Schistosoma mansoni* induced directly by eosinophil major basic protein. J Immunol 1979;122:221.
77. Frew AJ, Kay AB. The relationship between infiltrating $CD4^+$ lymphocytes, activated eosinophils, and the magnitude of the allergen-induced late phase cutaneous reaction in man. J Immunol 1988;141:4158.
78. Linder A, Venge P, Deuschl H. Eosinophil cationic protein and myeloperoxidase in nasal secretion as markers of inflammation in allergic rhinitis. Allergy 1987;42:583.
79. Weiler JM, Edens RE, Gleich GJ. Eosinophil granule cationic proteins regulate complement. I. Activity on the alternative pathway. J Immunol 1992;149:643.
80. Gleich GJ, Motojima S, Frigas E, et al. The eosinophilic leukocyte and the pathology of fatal bronchial asthma: evidence for pathologic heterogeneity. J Allergy Clin Immunol 1987;80:412.
81. Parsons WG III, Roberts LJ II. Transformation of prostaglandin D_2 to isomeric prostaglandin F_2 compounds by human eosinophils. J Immunol 1988;141:2413.
82. Wong DTW, Weller PF, Galli SJ, et al. Human eosinophils express transforming growth factor-alpha. J Exp Med 1990;172:673.
83. Wong DTW, Elovic A, Matossian K, et al. Eosinophils from patients with blood eosinophilia express transforming growth factor β1. Blood 1991;8:2702.
84. Ohno I, Lea RG, Flanders KC, et al. Eosinophils in chronically inflamed human upper airway tissue express transforming growth factor β1 gene (TGFβ1). J Clin Invest 1992;89:1662.
85. Kita H, Ohnishi T, Okubo Y, Weiler D, Abrams JS, Gleich GJ. Granulocyte/macrophage colony-stimulating factor and interleukin 3 release from human peripheral blood eosinophils and neutrophils. J Exp Med 1991;174:745.
86. Moqbel R, Hamid Q, Ying S, et al. Expression of mRNA and immunoreactivity for the granulocyte/macrophage colony-stimulating factor in activated human eosinophils. J Exp Med 1991;174:749.
87. Weller PF, Rand TH, Barrett T, Elovic A, Wong DTW, Finberg RW. Accessory cell funtion of human eosinophils: HLA-DR-dependent, MHC-restricted antigen presentation and interleukin-α expression. J Immunol 1993;150:2554.
88. Desreumaux P, Janin A, Colombel JF, et al. Interleukin 5 messenger RNA expression by eosinophils in the intestinal mucosa of patients with coeliac disease. J Exp Med 1992;75:293.
89. Hamid Q, Barkans J, Meng Q, et al. Human eosinophils synthesize and secrete interleukin-6, *in vitro*. Blood 1992;80:1496.
90. Costa JJ, Matossian K, Resnick MB, et al. Human eosinophils can express the cytokines tumor necrosis factor-α and macrophage inflammatory protein-1α. J Clin Invest 1993;91:2673.
91. Broide DH, Paine MM, Firestein GS. Eosinophils express interleukin 5 granulocyte-macrophage-colony-stimulating factor mRNA at sites of allergic inflammation in asthmatics. J Clin Invest 1992;90:1414.
92. Durham SR, Ying S, Varney VA, et al. Cytokine messenger RNA expressing for IL-3, IL-4, IL-5 and granulocyte/macrophage colony-stimulating factor in the nasal mucosa after local allergen provocation: relationship to tissue eosinophilia. J Immunol 1992;148:2390.
93. Young JD-E, Peterson CGB, Venge P, et al. Mechanisms of membrane damage mediated by human eosinophil cationic protein. Nature 1986;321:613.
94. Samoszuk MK, Petersen A, Gidanian F, et al. Cytophilic and cytotoxic properties of human eosinophil peroxidase plus major basic protein. Am J Pathol 1988;132:455.
95. Moqbel R, Sass-Kuhn SP, Goetzl EJ, et al. Enhancement of neutrophil- and eosinophil-mediated complement-dependent killing of schistosomula of *Schistosoma mansoni in vitro* by leukotriene B_4. Clin Exp Immunol 1983;52:519.
96. Dessein AJ, Vadas MA, Nicola NA, et al. Enhancement of human blood eosinophil cytotoxicity by semi-purified eosinophil colony-stimulating factor(s). J Exp Med 1982;156:90.
97. Colley DG. Eosinophils and immune mechanisms. I. Eosinophil stim-

ulation promoter (ESP): a lymphokine induced by specific antigen or phytohemagglutinin. J Immunol 1973;110:1419.
98. Silberstein DS, David JR. Tumor necrosis factor enhances eosinophil toxicity to *Schistosoma mansoni* larvae. Proc Natl Acad Sci 1986 83: 1055.
99. Ford RM. Transient pulmonary eosinophilia and asthma: a review of 20 cases occurring in 5,702 asthma sufferers. Am Rev Respir Dis 1966;93: 797.
100. Hardy WR, Anderson RE. The hypereosinophilic syndromes. Ann Intern Med 1968;68:1220.
101. Chusid MJ, Dale DC, West BC, et al. The hypereosinophilic syndrome: analysis of fourteen cases with review of the literature. Medicine 1975;54:1.
102. Spry CJF. The hypereosinophilic syndrome: clinical features, laboratory findings and treatment. Allergy 1982;37:539.
103. Nishikawa K, Morii T, Ako H, Hamada K, Saito S, Narita N. In vivo expressing of CD69 on lung eosinophils in eosinophilic pneumonia: CD69 as a possible activation marker for eosinophils. J Allergy Clin Immunol 1992;90:169.
104. Schatz M, Wasserman S, Patterson R. Eosinophils and immunologic lung disease. Med Clin North Am 1981;65:1055.
105. Lewis JG. Eosinophilic granuloma and its variants with special reference to lung involvement: a report of 12 patients. Q J Med 1964;131:337.
106. Hoffman L, Cohn JE, Gaensler EA. Respiratory abnormalities in eosinophilic granuloma of the lung: long-term study of five cases. N Engl J Med 1962;267:577.
107. Hertzman PA, Blevins WL, Mayer J, Greenfield B, Ting M, Gleich GL. Association of the eosinophilia-myalgia syndrome with the ingestion of tryptophan. N Engl J Med 1990;322:869.
108. Silver RM, Heyes MP, Maize MC, Quearry B, Vionnet-Fuasset M, Sternberg EM. Scleroderma, fasciitis, and eosinophilia associated with the ingestion of tryptophan. N Engl J Med 1990;322:874.
109. Kilbourne EM, Swygert LA, Philen RM, et al. Interim guidance on the eosinophilia-myalgia syndrome. Ann Intern Med 1990;112:85.
110. Raghavachar A, Fleischer S, Frickhofen N, et al. T lymphocyte control of human eosinophilic granulopoiesis: clonal analysis in an idiopathic hypereosinophilic syndrome. J Immunol 1987;139:3753.
111. Kimura T, Yoshimura S, Ishikawa E. Unusual granulation combined with hyperplastic changes of lymphatic tissue. Trans Soc Pathol Japan 1948;37:179.
112. Wells GC, Whimster IW. Subcutaneous angiolymphoid hyperplasia with eosinophilia. Br J Dermatol 1969;81:1.
113. Beutner EH, Jordon RE, Chorzelski TP. The immunopathology of pemphigus and bullous pemphigoid. J Invest Dermatol 1968;51:63.
114. Provost TT, Tomasi TB Jr. Immunopathology of bullous pemphigoid: basement membrane deposition of IgE, alternate pathway components and fibrin. Clin Exp Immunol 1974;18:193.
115. Wintroub BU, Mihm MC Jr, Goetzl EJ, et al. Morphologic and functional evidence for release of mast-cell products in bullous pemphigoid. N Engl J Med 1978;298:417.
116. Wells GC. Recurrent granulomatous dermatitis with eosinophilia. Trans St John's Hosp Dermatol Soc 1971;57:46.
117. Shulman LE. Diffuse fasciitis with eosinophilia: a new syndrome? Trans Assoc Am Phys 1975;88:70.
118. Shewmake SW, Lopez DA, McGlamory JC. The Shulman syndrome. Arch Dermatol 1978;114:556.
119. Lakhanpal S, Ginsburg WW, Michet CJ, Doyle JA, Moore SB. Eosinophilic fascitis: clinical spectrum and therapeutic response. Semin Arthritis Rheum 1988;17:221.
120. Kazmierowski JA, Chusid MJ, Parrillo JE, Fauci AS, Wolff SM. Dermatologic manifestations of the hypereosinophilic syndrome. Arch Dermatol 1978;114:531.
121. Parwaresch MR. The human blood basophil. New York, Springer-Verlag, 1976.
122. Denegri JF, Naiman SC, Gillen J, Thomas JW. *In vitro* growth of basophils containing the Philadelphia chromosome in the acute phase of chronic myelogenous leukemia. Br J Haematol 1978;40:351.
123. Valent P, Bettelheim P. The human basophil. Crit Rev Oncol Hematol 1990;10:327.
124. Denburg JA, Tanno Y, Bienenstock J. Growth and differentiation of human basophils, eosinophils, and mast cells. In: Befus AD, Bienenstock J, Denburg JA, eds. Mast cell differentiation and heterogeneity. New York, Raven Press, 1986:71.
125. Ishizaka T, Dvorak AM, Conrad DH, Niebyl JR, Marquette JP, Ishizaka K. Morphological and immunological characterization of human basophils developed in cultures of cord blood mononuclear cells. J Immunol 1985;134:532.
126. Murakami I, Ogawa M, Amo H, Ota K. Studies on kinetics of human leukocytes *in vivo* with ^{3}H-thymidine autoradiography. II. Eosinophils and basophils. Acta Haematol 1969;32:384.
127. Saito H, Hatake K, Dvorak AM, et al. Selective differentiation and proliferation of hematopoietic cells induced by recombinant human interleukins. Proc Natl Acad Sci 1988;85:2288.
128. Ishizaka T, Saito H, Furitsu T, Dvorak AM. Growth of human basophils and mast cells *in vitro*. In: Galli SJ, Austen KF, eds. Mast cell and basophil differentiation and function in health and disease. New York, Raven Press, 1989:39.
129. Tracey R, Smith H. An inherited anomaly of human eosinophils and basophils. Blood Cells 1978;4:291.
130. Juhlin L. Basophil leukocyte differential in blood and bone marrow. Acta Haematol 1963;29:89.
131. Gilbert HS, Ornstein L. Basophil counting with a new staining method using alcian blue. Blood 1975;46:279.
132. Galli SJ, Dvorak AM, Dvorak HF. Basophils and mast cells: morphologic insights into their biology, secretory patterns and function. Prog Allergy 1984;34:1.
133. Galli SJ, Askenase PW. Cutaneous basophil hypersensitivity. In: Abramoff P, Phillips SM, Escobar MR, eds. The reticuloendothelial system: a comprehensive treatise, vol 9. New York, Plenum Press, 1986:321.
134. Dvorak AM, Dvorak HF, Galli SJ. Ultrastructural criteria for identification of mast cells and basophils in humans, guinea pigs, and mice. Am Rev Respir Dis 1983;128:S49.
135. Nakano T, Kanakura Y, Nakahata T, Matsuda H, Kitamura Y. Genetically mast cell–deficient W/W^v mice as a tool for studies of differentiation and function of mast cells. Fed Proc 1987;46:1920.
136. Kitamura Y, Nakayama H, Fujita J. Mechanism of mast cell deficiency in mutant mice of W/W^v and Sl/Sl^d genotype. In: Galli SJ, Austen KF, eds. Mast cell and basophil differentiation and function in health and disease. New York, Raven Press, 1989:15.
137. Juhlin L, Michaëlsson G. A new syndrome characterized by absence of eosinophils and basophils. Lancet 1977;1:1233.
138. Dvorak AM, Mihm MC Jr, Dvorak HF. Morphology of delayed-type hypersensitivity reactions in man. II. Ultrastructural alterations affecting the microvasculature and the tissue mast cells. Lab Invest 1976;34:179.
139. Selye H. The mast cells. Washington, DC, Butterworths, 1965.
140. Metcalfe DD, Kaliner M, Donlon MA. The mast cell. CRC Crit Rev Immunol 1981;2:23.
141. Galli SJ. New insights into "the riddle of the mast cells": microenvironmental regulation of mast cell development and phenotypic heterogeneity. Lab Invest 1990;62:5.
142. Galli SJ. New concepts about the mast cell. N Engl J Med 1993;328: 257.
143. Bienenstock J, Blennerhassett M, Kakuta Y, et al. Evidence for central and peripheral nervous system interaction with mast cells. In Galli SJ, Austen KF, eds. Mast cell and basophil differentiation and function in health and disease. New York, Raven Press, 1989:275.
144. Enerbäck L, Pipkom U, Aldenborg F, Wingren U. Mast cell heterogeneity in man: properties and function of human mucosal mast cells. In: Galli SJ, Austen KF, eds. Mast cell and basophil differentiation and function in health and disease. New York, Raven Press, 1989:27.
145. Bienenstock J, Befus AD, Denburg JA. Mast cell heterogeneity: basic questions and clinical implications. In: Befus AD, Bienenstock J, Denburg JA, eds. Mast cell differentiation and heterogeneity. New York, Raven Press, 1986:391.
146. Church MK, Benyon RC, Rees PH, et al. Functional heterogeneity of human mast cells. In: Galli SJ, Austen KF, eds. Mast cell and basophil differentiation and function in health and disease. New York, Raven Press, 1989:161.
147. Cohan VL, Massey WA, Gittlen SD, et al. The heterogeneity of human histamine containing cells. In: Galli SJ, Austen KF, eds. Mast cell and basophil differentiation and function in health and disease. New York, Raven Press, 1989:149.
148. Schwartz LB. Heterogeneity of mast cells in humans. In: Galli SJ, Austen KF, eds. Mast cell and basophil differentiation and function in health and disease. New York, Raven Press, 1989:93.
149. Galli SJ. Mast cell heterogeneity: can variation in mast cell phenotype be explained without postulating the existence of distinct mast cell lineages? In: Befus AD, Bienenstock J, Denburg JA, eds. Mast cell differentiation and heterogeneity. New York, Raven Press, 1986:167.
150. Galli SJ, Lichtenstein LM. Biology of mast cells and basophils. In: Middleton E Jr, Reed CE, Ellis EF, Adkinson NF Jr, Yunginger JW, eds. Allergy: principles and practice, ed 3. St Louis, CV Mosby, 1988:71.
151. Galli SJ, Geissler EN, Wershil BK, Gordon JR, Tsai M, Hammel I. Insights into mast cell development and function derived from analyses of mice carrying mutation at beige, *W/c-kit* or *Sl/SCF* (*c-kit* ligand) loci. In: Kaliner MA, Metcalfe DD, eds. The role of the mast cell in health and disease. New York, Marcel Dekker, 1992:129.
152. Galli SJ, Tsai M, Wershil BK. The c-*kit* receptor, stem cell factor, and mast cells: what each is teaching us about the others. Am J Pathol 1993;142:965.
153. Galli SJ, Zsebo KM, Geissler EN. The kit ligand, stem cell factor. Adv Immunol 1994;55:1.
154. Stevens RL, Serafin WE, Reynolds DS, Dayton ET, Gravallese PM, Austen KF. Development and characterization of *in vitro*–differentiated transformed and non-transformed mouse connective tissue-like mast cells, and the regulation of fibroblasts by these mast cells. In: Galli SJ, Austen KF, eds. Mast cell and basophil differentiation and function in health and disease. New York, Raven Press, 1989:1.
155. Tsai M, Shih LS, Newlands GFJ, et al. The rat *c-kit* ligand, stem cell factor, induces the development of connective tissue–type and mucosal mast cells *in vivo*: analysis by anatomical distribution, histochemistry, and protease phenotype. J Exp Med 1991;174:125.
156. Galli SJ, Iemura A, Garlick DS, Gamba-Vitalo C, Zsebo KM, Andrews

RG. Reversible expansion of primate mast cell populations *in vivo* by stem cell factor. J Clin Invest 1993;91:148.
157. Ganser A, Lindemann A, Seipelt G, et al. Effects of recombinant human interleukin-3 in patients with normal hemopoiesis and in patients with bone marrow failure. Blood 1990;76:666.
158. Columbo M, Horowitz EM, Botana LM, et al. The human recombinant *c-kit* receptor ligand, rhSCF, induces mediator release from human cutaneous mast cells and enhances IgE-dependent mediator release from both skin mast cells and peripheral blood basophils. J Immunol 1992;149:599.
159. Kurimoto Y, de Weck AL, Dahinden CA. The effect of interleukin 3 upon IgE-dependent and IgE-independent basophil degranulation and leukotriene generation. Eur J Immunol 1991;21:361.
160. Alam R, Welter JB, Forsythe PA, Lett-Brown MA, Grant JA. Comparative effects of recombinant IL-1, -2, -3, -4, and -6, INF-γ, granulocyte-macrophage-colony-stimulating factor, tumor necrosis factor-α, and histamine-releasing factors on the secretion of histamine from basophils. J Immunol 1989;142:3431.
161. Kirshenbaum AS, Goff JP, Kessler SW, Mican JM, Zsebo KM, Metcalfe DD. Effect of IL-3 and stem cell factor on the appearance of human basophils and mast cells from CD34+ pluripotent progenitor cells. J Immunol 1992;148:772.
162. Ishizaka T, Furitsu T, Mitsui H, et al. Development of human mast cells from umbilical cord cells by human and murine c-*kit* ligand. (Abstract) FASEB J 1992;6:A1403.
163. Nilsson G, Irani AA, Ishizaki T, Schwartz LB. Human recombinant stem cell factor (SCF), the ligand for c-*kit*, induces development of human mast cells whereas IL-3 induces basophil-like cells from fetal liver cells (FLC). (Abstract) FASEB J 1992;6:A1722.
164. Valent P, Spanblöchl E, Sperr WR, et al. Induction of differentiation of human mast cells from bone marrow and peripheral blood mononuclear cells by recombinant human stem cell factor/*kit*-ligand in long-term culture. Blood 1992;80:2237.
165. Costa JJ, Demetri GD, Hayes DF, Merica EA, Menchaca DM, Galli SJ. Increased skin mast cells and urine methyl histamine in patients receiving recombinant methionyl human stem cell factor. Cancer Res (in press).
166. Wershil BK, Tsai M, Geissler EN, Zsebo KM, Galli SJ. The rat *c-kit* ligand, stem cell factor, induces *c-kit receptor*–dependent mouse mast cell activation *in vivo*: evidence that signalling through the *c-kit* receptor can induce expression of cellular function. Exp Med 1992;175: 245.
167. Coleman JW, Holliday MR, Kimber I, Zsebo KM, Galli SJ. Regulation of mouse peritoneal mast cell secretory function by stem cell factor, IL-3 or IL-4. J Immunol 1993;150:556.
168. Bischoff SC, Dahinden CA. *c-kit* Ligand: a unique potentiator of mediator release by human lung mast cells. J Exp Med 1992;175:237.
169. Irani AA, Craig SS, DeBlois G, Elson CO, Schechter NM, Schwartz LB. Deficiency of the tryptase-positive, chymase-negative mast cell type in gastrointestinal mucosa of patients with defective T lymphocyte function. J Immunol 1987;138:4381.
170. Zucker-Franklin D. Electron microscopic study of human basophils. Blood 1967;29:878.
171. Hastie R. A study of the ultrastructure of human basophil leukocytes. Lab Invest 1974;31:223.
172. Dvorak AM, Monahan RA. Crohn's disease: ultrastructural studies showing basophil leukocyte granule changes and lymphocyte parallel tubular arrays in peripheral blood. Arch Pathol Lab Med 1982;106: 145.
173. Kawanami O, Ferrans VJ, Fulmer JD, Crystal RG. Ultrastructure of pulmonary mast cells in patients with fibrotic lung disorders. Lab Invest 1979;40:717.
174. Dvorak AM. Human mast cells. In: Beck F, Hild W, Kriz W, Ortmann R, Pauly JE, Schiebler TH, eds. Advances in anatomy, embryology and cell biology, vol 114. Berlin, Springer-Verlag, 1989:1.
175. Dvorak AM. Blood cell biochemistry: basophil and mast cell degranulation and recovery, vol 4. New York, Plenum Press, 1991.
176. Dvorak AM, Monahan RA, Osage JE, Dickersin GR. Crohn's disease: transmission electron microscopic studies. II. Immunologic inflammatory response: alterations of mast cells, basophils, eosinophils, and the microvasculature. Hum Pathol 1980;11:606.
177. Dvorak AM, Mihm MC Jr, Osage JE, Kwan TH, Austen KF, Wintroub BU. Bullous pemphigoid, an ultrastructural study of the inflammatory response: eosinophil, basophil, and mast cell granule changes in multiple biopsies from one patient. J Invest Dermatol 1982;78:91.
178. Dvorak AM, Hammel I, Schulman ES, et al. Differences in the behavior of cytoplasmic granules and lipid bodies during human lung mast cell degranulation. J Cell Biol 1984;99:1678.
179. Hammel I, Dvorak AM, Peters SP, et al. Differences in the volume distributions of human lung mast cell granules and lipid bodies: evidence that the size of these organelles is regulated by distinct mechanisms. J Cell Biol 1985;100:1488.
180. Schwartz LB, Austen KF. Structure and function of the chemical mediators of mast cells. Prog Allergy 1984;34:271.
181. Holgate ST, Robinson C, Church MK. Mediators of immediate hypersensitivity. In: Middleton E Jr, Reed CE, Ellis EF, Adkinson NF Jr, Yunginger JW, eds. Allergy: principles and practice, ed 3. St Louis, CV Mosby, 1988:135.
182. Stevens RL, Fox CC, Lichtenstein LM, Austen KF. Identification of chondroitin sulfate E proteoglycans and heparin proteoglycans in the secretory granules of human lung mast cells. Proc Natl Acad Sci USA 1988;85:2284.
183. Thompson HL, Schulman ES, Metcalfe DD. Identification of chondroitin sulfate E in human lung mast cells. J Immunol 1988;140:2708.
184. Metcalfe DD, Bland CE, Wasserman SI. Biochemical and functional characterization of proteoglycans isolated from basophils of patients with chronic myelogenous leukemia. J Immunol 1984;132:1943.
185. Rothenberg ME, Caulfield JP, Austen KF, Hein A, Edmiston K, Newburger PE, Stevens RL. Biochemical and morphological characterization of basophilic leukocytes from two patients with myelogenous leukemia. J Immunol 1987;138:2616.
186. Porter JF, Mitchell RGL. Distribution of histamine in human blood. Physiol Rev 1972;52:361.
187. Yamatodani A, Maeyama K, Watanabe T, Wada H, Kitamura Y. Tissue distribution of histamine in a mutant mouse deficient in mast cells: clear evidence for the presence of non-mast cell histamine. Biochem Pharmacol 1982;31:305.
188. Schwartz LB, Metcalfe DD, Miller JS, Earl H, Sullivan T. Tryptase levels as an indicator of mast cell activation in systemic anaphylaxis and mastocytosis. N Engl J Med 1987;316:1622.
189. Schwartz LB, Bradford TM. Regulation of tryptase from human lung mast cells by heparin: stabilization of the active tetramer. J Biol Chem 1986;261:7372.
190. Schechter NM, Franki JE, Geesin JC, Lazarus GS. Human skin chymotryptic proteinase. I. Isolation and relation to cathepsin G and rat mast cell protease. J Biol Chem 1983;31:276.
191. Johnson LA, Moon KE, Eisenberg M. Purification to homogeneity of the human skin chymotryptic proteinase "chymase." Anal Biochem 1986;155:358.
192. Craig SS, Schechter NM, Schwartz LB. Ultrastructural analysis of human T and TC mast cells identified by immunoelectron microscopy. Lab Invest 1988;58:682.
193. Craig SS, Schechter NM, Schwartz LB. Ultrastructural analysis of maturing human T and TC mast cells in situ. Lab Invest 1989;60:147.
194. Goldstein SM, Kaempfer CE, Proud D, Schwartz LB, Irani AA, Wintroub BU. Detection and partial characterization of a human mast cell carboxypeptidase. J Immunol 1987;139:2724.
195. Bessis M, Tabuis J. Formation des crysteaux à partir des leucocyte basophils. CR Soc Biol 1955;149:873.
196. Archer GT, Blackwood A. Formation of Charcot-Leyden crystals in human eosinophils and basophils and study of the composition of isolated crystals. J Exp Med 1965;122:173.
197. Dvorak AM, Ackerman SJ. Ultrastructural localization of the Charcot-Leyden crystal protein (lysophospholipase) to granules and intragranular crystals in mature human basophils. Lab Invest 1989;60:557.
198. Hammarström S, Lindgren JA, Marcelo C, Duell EA, Anderson TF, Voorhees JJ. Arachidonic acid transformations in normal and psoriatic skin. J Invest Dermatol 1979;73:180.
199. Betz SJ, Lotner GZ, Henson PM. Generation and release of platelet-activating factor (PAF) from enriched preparations of rabbit basophils; failure of human basophils to release PAF. J Immunol 1980;125:2749.
200. Schleimer RP, MacGlashan DW, Peters SP, Pinckard RN, Adkinson NF Jr, Lichtenstein LM. Characterization of inflammatory mediator release from purified human lung mast cells. Am Rev Respir Dis 1986;133:614.
201. Gordon JR, Burd PR, Galli SJ. Mast cells as a source of multifunctional cytokines. Immunol Today 1990:11;458.
202. Galli SJ, Gordon JR, Wershil BK. Cytokine production by mast cells and basophils. Curr Opin Immunol 1991;3:865.
203. Gordon JR, Galli SJ. Mast cells as a source of both preformed and immunologically inducible TNF-α/cachectin. Nature 1990;346:274.
204. Walsh LJ, Trincheri G, Waldorf HA, Whitaker D, Murphy GF. Human dermal mast cells contain and release tumor necrosis factor α, which induces endothelial leukocyte adhesion molecule 1. Proc Natl Acad Sci USA 1991;88:4220.
205. Seder RA, Paul WE, Dvorak AM, et al. Mouse splenic and bone marrow cell populations that express high-infinity Fc_{ϵ} receptors and produce interleukin 4 are highly enriched in basophils. Proc Natl Acad Sci USA 1991;88:2835.
206. Dvorak AM, Seder RA, Paul WE, Kissell-Rainville S, Plaut M, Galli SJ. Ultrastructural characteristics of Fc_{ϵ}R-positive basophils in the spleen and bone marrow of mice immunized with goat anti-mouse IgD antibody. Lab Invest (in press).
207. Bradding P, Feather IH, Howarth PH, et al. Interleukin 4 is localized to and released by human mast cells. J Exp Med 1992;176:1381.
208. Brunner T, Heusser CH, Dahinden CA. Human peripheral blood basophils primed by interleukin 3 (IL-3) produce IL-4 in response to immunoglobulin E receptor stimulation. J Exp Med 1993;177:605.
209. Burd PR, Rogers HW, Gordon JR, et al. IL-3–dependent and –independent mast cells stimulated with IgE and antigen express multiple cytokines. J Exp Med 1989;170:245.
210. Plaut M, Pierce JH, Watson CJ, Hanley-Hyde J, Nordan RP, Paul WE.

Mast cell lines produce lymphokines in response to cross-linkage of Fc$_\epsilon$RI or to calcium ionophores. Nature 1989;339:64.
211. Wodnar-Filipowicz A, Heusser CH, Moroni C. Production of the haemopoietic growth factors GM-CSF and interleukin-3 by mast cells in response to IgE receptor–mediated activation. Nature 1989;339:150.
212. Young JD-E, Liu CC, Butler G, Cohn ZA, Galli SJ. Identification, purification, and characterization of a mast cell–associated cytolytic factor related to tumor necrosis factor. Proc Natl Acad Sci USA 1987;84:9175.
213. Gordon JR, Galli SJ. Release of both preformed and newly synthesized tumor necrosis factor α (TNF-α)/cachetin by mouse mast cells stimulated by the Fc$_\epsilon$RI: a mechanism for the sustained action of mast cell–derived TNF-α during IgE-independent biological responses. J Exp Med 1991;174:103.
214. Woodbury RG, Le Trong H, Cole K, Neurath H, Miler HRP. Rat mast cell proteases. In: Galli SJ, Austen KF, eds. Mast cell and basophil differentiation and function in health and disease. New York, Raven Press, 1989:71.
215. Sampson D, Archer GT. Release of histamine from human basophils. Blood 1967;29:722.
216. Padawer J. The mast cell and immediate hypersensitivity. In: Bach MK, ed. Immediate hypersensitivity: modern concepts and developments. New York, Marcel Dekker, 1978:301.
217. Dvorak AM, Klebanoff SJ, Henderson WR, Monahan RA, Pyne K, Galli SJ. Vesicular uptake of eosinophil peroxidase by guinea pig basophils and by cloned mouse mast cells and granule-containing lymphoid cells. Am J Pathol 1985;118:425.
218. Dvorak AM, Ishizaka T, Galli SJ. Ultrastructure of human basophils developing in vitro. Evidence for the acquisition of peroxidase by basophils, and for different effects of human and murine growth factors on human basophil and eosinophil maturation. Lab Invest 1985;53:57.
219. Ishizaka T. Mechanisms of IgE-mediated hypersensitivity. In: Middleton E Jr, Reed CE, Ellis EF, Adkinson NF Jr, Yunginger JW, eds. Allergy: principles and practice, ed 3. St Louis, CV Mosby, 1988:71.
220. Kinet J-P. The high-affinity receptor for IgE. Curr Opin immunol 1989;2: 499.
221. Röhlich R, Anderson P, Uvnäs B. Electron microscopic observations on compound 48/80-induced degranulation in rat mast cells: evidence for sequential exocytosis of storage granules. J Cell Biol 1971;51:465.
222. Ogawa M, Nakahata T, Leary AG, Sterk AR, Ishizaka K, Ishizaka T. Suspension culture of human mast cells/basophils from umbilical cord blood mononuclear cells. Proc Natl Acad Sci USA 1983;80:4494.
223. Shimizu A, Tepler I, Benfey PN, Berenstein EH, Siraganian RP, Leder P. Human and rat mast cell high-affinity immunoglobulin E receptors: characterization of putative α-chain gene products. Proc Natl Acad Sci USA 1988;85:1907.
224. Blank U, Ra C, Miller L, White K, Metzger H, Kinet J-P. Complete structure and expression in transfected cells of high affinity IgE receptor. Nature 1989;337:187.
225. Miller L, Blank U, Metzger H, Kinet J-P. Expression of high-affinity binding of human immunoglobulin E by transfected cells. Science 1989;244:334.
226. Wasserman SI, Marquardt DL. Anaphylaxis. In: Middleton E Jr, Reed CE, Ellis EF, Adkinson NF Jr, Yunginger JW, eds. Allergy: principles and practice, ed 3. St Louis, CV Mosby, 1988:1365.
227. Benyon RC, Robinson C, Church MK. Differential release of histamine and eicosanoids from human skin mast cells activated by IgE-dependent and non-immunological stimuli. Br J Pharmacol 1989;97:898.
228. Thueson DO, Speck LS, Lett-Brown MA, Grant JA. Histamine releasing activity (HRA). I. Production by mitogen- or antigen-stimulated human mononuclear cells. J Immunol 1979;123:626.
229. MacDonald SM, Lichtenstein LM, Proud D, et al. Studies of IgE-dependent histamine releasing factors: heterogeneity of IgE. J Immunol 1987;139:506.
230. Lichtenstein LM. Histamine releasing factors and IgE heterogeneity. J Allergy Clin Immunol 1988;81:814.
231. Alam R, Lett-Brown MA, Forsythe PA, et al. Monocyte chemotactic and activating factor is a potent histamine-releasing factor for basophil. J Clin Invest 1992;89:723.
232. Bischoff SC, Krieger M, Brunner T, Dahinden CA. Monocyte chemotactic protein 1 is a potent activator of human basophils. J Exp Med 1992;175:1271.
233. Reddigari SR, Kuna P, Miragliotta GF, et al. Connective tissue–activating peptide III and its derivative, neutrophil-activating peptide-2, release histamine from human basophils. J Allergy Clin Immunol 1992;89:666.
234. Alam R, Forsythe PA, Stafford S, Lett-Brown MA, Grant JA. Macrophage inflammatory protein-1α activates basophils and mast cells. J Exp Med 1992;176:781.
235. Askenase PW. Immunopathology of parasitic diseases: involvement of basophils and mast cells. Semin Immunopathol 1980;2:417.
236. Wershil BK, Mekori YA, Galli SJ. The contribution of mast cells to immunological responses with IgE- and/or T cell–mediated components. In: Galli SJ, Austen KF, eds. Mast cell and basophil differentiation and function in health and disease. New York, Raven Press, 1989:229.
237. Lemanske RF Jr, Kaliner MA. Late-phase allergic reactions. In: Middleton E Jr, Reed CE, Ellis EF, Adkinson NF Jr, Yunginger JW, eds. Allergy: principles and practice, ed 3. St Louis, CV Mosby, 1988:224.
238. Wershil BK, Mekori YA, Murakami T, Galli SJ. ^{125}I-fibrin deposition in IgE-dependent immediate hypersensitivity reactions in mouse skin: demonstration of the role of mast cells using genetically mast cell–deficient mice locally reconstituted with cultured mast cells. J Immunol 1987;139:2605.
239. Wershil BK, Wang Z-S, Gordon JR, Galli SJ. Recruitment of neutrophils during IgE-dependent cutaneous late phase responses in the mouse is mast cell dependent: partial inhibition of the reaction with antiserum against tumor necrosis factor-alpha. J Clin Invest 1991;87:446.
240. Galli SJ, Hammel I. Uniequivocal delayed hypersensitivity in mast cell–deficient and beige mice. Science 1984;226:710.
241. Galli SJ, Wershil BK, Yano H, Arizono N, Gordon JR, Murakami T. Analysis of the roles of phenotypically distinct mast cell populations in non-immunological responses. In: Galli SJ, Austen KF, eds. Mast cell and basophil differentiation and function in health and disease. New York, Raven Press, 1989:255.
242. Reed ND. Function and regulation of mast cells in parasite infections. In: Galli SJ, Austen KF, eds. Mast cell and basophil differentiation and function in health and disease. New York, Raven Press, 1989:205.
243. Brown SJ, Galli SJ, Gleich GJ, Askenase PW. Ablation of immunity to *Amblyomma americanum* by anti-basophil serum: cooperation between basophils and eosinophils in expression of immunity to ectoparasites (ticks) in guinea pigs. J Immunol 1982;129:790.
244. Matsuda H, Nakano T, Kiso Y, Kitamura Y. Normalization of anti-tick response of mast cell–deficient W/W^v mice by intracutaneous injection of cultured mast cells. J Parasitol 1987;73:155.
245. Matsuda H, Watanabe N, Kiso Y, et al. Necessity of IgE antibodies and mast cells for manifestation of resistance against larval *Haemaphysalis longicornis* ticks in mice. J Immunol 1990;144:259.
246. Crowle PK, Starkey JR. Mast cells and tumor-associated angiogenesis. In: Galli SJ, Austen KF, eds. Mast cell and basophil differentiation and function in health and disease. New York, Raven Press, 1989:307.
247. Hawkins RA, Claman HN, Clark RAF, Steigerwald JC. Increased dermal mast cell populations in progressive systemic sclerosis: a link in chronic fibrosis. Ann Intern Med 1985;102:182.
248. Wershil BK, Murakami T, Galli SJ. Mast cell–dependent amplification of an immunologically nonspecific inflammatory response: mast cells are required for the full expression of cutaneous acute inflammation induced by phorbol 12-myristate 13-acetate. J Immunol 1988;140:2356.
249. Yano H, Wershil BK, Arizono N, Galli SJ. Substance P-induced augmentation of cutaneous vascular permeability and granulocyte infiltration in mice is mast cell–dependent. J Clin Invest 1989;84:1276.
250. Qureshi R, Jakschik BA. The role of mast cells in thioglycollate-induced inflammation. J Immunol 1988;141:2090.
251. Rorsman H. Studies on basophil leukocytes with special reference to urticaria and anaphylaxis. Acta Derm Venereol 1962;42(Suppl 48):1.
252. Shelley WB, Juhlin L. New test for detecting anaphylactic sensitivity: basophil reaction. Nature 1961;191:1056.
253. Osada Y. Diurnal rhythms of the numbers in circulating basophils and eosinophils in healthy adults. Bull Inst Public Health 1956;5(4):5.
254. Mitchell RG. Circulating basophilic leukocyte counts in the newborn. Arch Dis Child 1955;30:130.
255. Thonnard-Neumann E. Studies of basophils: variations with age and sex. Acta Haematol 1963;30:221.
256. Juhlin L. Basophil and eosinophil leukocytes in various internal disorders. Acta Med Scand 1963;174:249.
257. Mitchell RG. Basophilic leukocytes in children in health and disease. Arch Dis Child 1958;33:193.
258. Kelemen E, Bikich G. Insufficiency of acute response of basophil and eosinophil leukocytes and of blood histamine after the administration of ACTH and cortisone in untreated myelocytic leukemia. Acta Haematol 1956;15:202.
259. Boseila A-WA, Uhrbrand H. Basophil-eosinophil relationship in human blood. Studies on the effect of corticotrophin (ACTH). Acta Endocrinol 1958;28:49.
260. Juhlin L. The effect of corticotropin and corticosteroids on the basophil and eosinophil granulocytes. Acta Haematol 1963;29:157.
261. Inagaki S. The relationship between the level of circulating basophil leucocytes and thyroid function. Acta Endocrinol 1957;26:477.
262. Mettler L, Shirwani D. Direct basophil count for timing ovulation. Fertil Steril 1974;25:718.
263. Shelley WB, Juhlin L. Degranulation of the basophil of man induced by lipemia. Am J Med Sci 1961;242:211.
264. Galoppin L, Noirot C, Wastiaux JP, Scheinmann P, Paupe J, Burtin C. Comparison between number of basophils, blood histamine, and histamine release in cancer and non cancer patients. J Allergy Clin Immunol 1989;84:501.
265. Fredericks RE, Moloney WC. The basophilic granulocyte. Blood 1959;14: 571.
266. Doan CA, Reinhart HL. The basophil granulocyte, basophilicytosis and myeloid leukemia basophil and mixed granule types: an experimental, clinical and pathological study, with the report of a new syndrome. Am J Clin Pathol 1941;11:1.
267. Dvorak AM, Monahan RA, Dickersin GR. Diagnostic electron microscopy. I. Hematology: differential diagnosis of acute lymphoblastic and acute myeloblastic leukemia—use of ultrastructural peroxidase cy-

tochemistry and routine electron microscopic technology. In: Sommers SC, Rosen PP, eds. Pathology annual, part I. New York, Appleton-Century-Crofts, 1981;16:101.
268. Dvorak AM, Dickersin GR, Connell AB, Carey RW, Dvorak HF. Degranulation mechanisms in human leukemic basophils. Clin Immunol Immunopathol 1976;5:235.
269. Lichtenstein LM, Sobotka AK, Malveaux FJ, Gillespie E. IgE-induced changes in human basophil cyclic AMP levels. Int Arch Allergy Appl Immunol 1978;56:473.
270. Lewis RA, Goetzl EJ, Wasserman SI, Valone FH, Rubin RH, Austen KF. The release of four mediators of immediate hypersensitivity from human leukemic basophils. J Immunol 1975;114:87.
271. Mitrakul C, Othaganonda BO, Manothal P, Bhanichaya-Bhongsa S. Basophilic leukemia: report of a case. Clin Pediatr 1969;8:178.
272. Lennert K, Koster E, Martin H. Über die Mastzellen-leukaemie. Acta Haematol 1956;16:255.
273. Youman JD, Taddeini L, Cooper T. Histamine excess, symptoms in basophilic chronic granulocytic leukemia. Arch Intern Med 1973;131:560.
274. Rosenthal S, Schwartz JH, Canellos GP. Basophilic chronic granulocytic leukaemia with hyperhistaminaemia. Br J Haematol 1977;36:367.
275. Shelley WB. The circulating basophil as an indicator of hypersensitivity in man. Arch Dermatol 1963;88:759.
276. Shelley WB, Parnes HM. The absolute basophil count. JAMA 1965;192:368.
277. Athreya BH, Moser G, Raghavan TES. Increased circulating basophils in juvenile rheumatoid arthritis: a preliminary report. Am J Dis Child 1975;129:935.
278. Paar JA, Scheinman MM, Weaver RA. Disseminated nonreactive tuberculosis with basophilia, leukemoid reaction and terminal pancytopenia. N Engl J Med 1966;274:335.
279. Horton MA, O'Brien HAW. Characterization of human mast cells in long-term culture. Blood 1983;62:1251.
280. Butterfield JH, Weiler D, Dewald G, Gleich GJ. Establishment of an immature mast cell line from a patient with mast cell leukemia. Leuk Res 1988;12:345.
281. Yuen E, Brown RD, van der Lubbe L, Rickard KA, Kronenberg H. Identification and characterization of human hemopoietic mast cell colonies. Exp Hematol 1988;16:896.
282. Mayrhofer G, Gadd SJ, Spargo LDJ, Ashman LK. Specificity of a mouse monoclonal antibody raised against acute myeloid leukaemia cells for mast cells in human mucosal and connective tissues. Immunol Cell Biol 1987;65:241.
283. Bodger MP, Mounsey GL, Nelson J, Fitzgerald PH. A monoclonal antibody reacting with human basophils. Blood 1987;69:1414.
284. Rottapel R, Reedijk M, Williams DE et al. The *Steel/W* transduction pathway: kit autophosphorylation and its association with a unique subset of cytoplasmic signaling proteins is induced by the Steel factor. Mol Cell Biol 1991;11:3043.
285. Furitsu T, Tsujimura T, Tono T, et al. Identification of mutations in the coding sequence of the protooncogene c-*kit* in a human mast cell leukemia cell line causing ligand-independent activation of c-*kit* product. Blood 1992;80:302a.
286. Tomioka M, Ida S, Yuriko S, Ishihara T, Takashima T. Mast cells in bronchoalveolar lumen of patients with bronchial asthma. Ann Rev Respir Dis 1984;129:1000.
287. Natbony SF, Phillips M, Elias JM, Godfrey HP, Kaplan AP. Histologic studies of chronic idiopathic urticaria. J Allergy Clin Immunol 1983;71:177.
288. Connell JT. Nasal disease: mechanisms and classification. Ann Allergy 1983;50:227.
289. Lennert K, Parwaresch MR. Mast cells and mast cell neoplasia: a review. Histopathology 1979;3:349.
290. Parwaresch MR, Horny H-P, Lennert K. Tissue mast cells in health and disease. Pathol Res Pract 1985;179:439.
291. Olsson Y. Mast cells in human peripheral nerve. Acta Neurol Scand 1971;47:357.
292. Hiatt RB, Katz L. Mast cells in inflammatory conditions of the gastrointestinal tract. Am J Gastroenterol 1962;37:541.
293. Dvorak AM, Monahan RA. Crohn's disease: mast cell quantitation using one micron plastic sections for light microscopic study. Pathol Annu 1983;18:181.
294. Crisp AJ, Chapman CM, Kirkham SE, Schiller AL, Krane SE. Articular mastocytosis in rheumatoid arthritis. Arthritis Rheum 1984;27:845.
295. Godfrey HP, Ilardi C, Engber W, Graziano FM. Quantitation of human synovial mast cells in rheumatoid arthritis and other rheumatic diseases. Arthritis Rheum 1984;27:852.
296. Frame B, Nixon RK. Bone marrow mast cells in osteoporosis of aging. N Engl J Med 1968;279:626.
297. Peart KM, Ellis HA. Quantitative observations on the iliac bone marrow mast cells in chronic renal failure. J Clin Pathol 1975;28:947.
298. Mota I, Vugman I. Effects of anaphylactic shock and compound 48/80 on the mast cells of the guinea pig lung. Nature 1956;177:427.
299. Lavker RM, Schechter NM. Cutaneous mast cell depletion results from topical steroid usage. J Immunol 1985;135:2368.
300. Travis WD, Li C-Y, Su WPD. Adult-onset urticaria pigmentosa and systemic mast cell disease. Am J Clin Pathol 1985;84:710.
301. Travis WD, Li C-Y, Hoagland HC, Travis LB, Banks PM. Mast cell leukemia: report of a case and review of the literature. Mayo Clin Proc 1986;61:957.
302. Travis WD, Li C-Y, Bergstralh EJ, Yam LT, Swee RG. Systemic mast cell disease: analysis of 58 cases and literature review. Medicine 1988;67:345.
303. Kirshenbaum AS, Metcalfe DD. The biology and therapy of mastocytosis. In: Galli SJ, Austen KF, eds. Mast cell and basophil differentiation and function in health and disease. New York, Raven Press, 1989:317.
304. Cherner JA, Jensen RT, Dubois A, O'Dorisio TM, Gardner JD, Metcalfe DD. Gastrointestinal dysfunction in systemic mastocytosis: a prospective study. Gastroenterology 1988;95:657.
305. Travis WD, Li C-Y, Yam LT, Bergstralh EJ, Swee RG. Significance of systemic mast cell disease with associated hematologic disorders. Cancer 1988;62:965.
306. Prokocimer M, Polliack A. Increased bone marrow mast cells in preleukemic syndromes, acute leukemia, and lymphoproliferative disorders. Am J Clin Pathol 1981;75:34.
307. Yoo D, Lessin LS. Bone marrow mast cell content in preleukemic syndrome. Am J Med 1982;73:539.
308. Fohlmeister I, Reber T, Fischer R. Bone marrow mast cell reaction in preleukaemic myelodysplasia and in aplastic anaemia. Virchows Arch (A) 1985;405:503.
309. Meggs WJ, Macher AM, Friedman MM, Kramer N, Metcalfe DD. Lymphadenopathic mastocytosis with eosinophilia. Clin Res 1985;33:162A.

Blood: Principles and Practice of Hematology,
edited by Robert I. Handin, Samuel E. Lux, and Thomas P. Stossel.
J.B. Lippincott Company, Philadelphia © 1995.

21

Cellular and Molecular Biology of Lymphoid Cells

Manlio Ferrarini
Carlo E. Grossi
Max D. Cooper

All vertebrates have a sophisticated immune system that is capable of defense against invading microorganisms and potentially capable against malignant cells. The distinctive property of the immune system is its capacity to discriminate between self and foreign molecules (collectively termed *antigens*) and to recall previous antigen encounters by heightened immune responses (*immunologic memory*).[1] The central recognition and responsive elements of the immune system are the T and B lymphocytes. They are aided by a population of lymphoid cells called *natural killer* (NK) cells, which represent a more primitive recognition and effector system. All these cells derive from a common progenitor cell that may enter separate developmental pathways in different microenvironments.

T and B cells derive their name from the central lymphoid organs in which they are generated, namely, the thymus and the bone marrow in mammals.[2–4] For a limited time during early development, B cells are produced in the fetal liver.[5] NK cells are also produced in the bone marrow and perhaps earlier in the fetal liver. Mature T, B, and NK cells circulate throughout the body with homing preference for the various peripheral lymphoid tissues such as the spleen, lymph nodes, and intestinal Peyer's patches[6] (Fig. 21-1).

T and B lymphocytes are capable of binding antigens by means of their specialized antigen receptors, and they collaborate in the immune response. The antigen receptor of B cells is an immunoglobulin (Ig) molecule; that of T cells is a related molecule of different structure called the T-cell receptor (TcR). B cells can use their Ig receptors to recognize native antigenic molecules, whereas T cells can recognize only peptide fragments of antigens that have been partially degraded by antigen-presenting cells, which include cells of macrophage–monocyte lineages and the B cells themselves.[7]

Certain common features characterize the mode of antigen recognition. First, all the thousands of cell surface receptors expressed by an individual T or B cell are identical, thus conferring specificity for the cell to respond to a single antigen or to limited numbers of cross-reactive antigens. The great diversity required for body defense is based on the development of highly diversified populations of T and B cells, each of which may express receptor molecules of different antigen specificity. Second, the antigen receptors are synthesized and expressed prior to actual encounter with antigens. The immune system thus prearms itself with a vast array of antigen receptor specificities. Third, on encounter with an appropriate antigen, a T or a B lymphocyte is stimulated to proliferate and differentiate into mature effector cells. This leads to the expansion of clones of cells with specificity for the stimulating antigen and to an effective immune response. Alternatively, the antigen encounter can lead to cell inactivation or cell death, thus resulting in specific immune tolerance to the challenging antigen. This is likely to occur when T or B cells encounter self-antigens as immature, newly formed cells. These basic concepts, originally formulated on theoretical grounds as the *clonal selection theory*, are now supported by extensive experimental evidence.[8] These concepts provide the basic framework for understanding the fine recognition capacities of the immune system.[8–10]

T and B lymphocytes regulate most of the effector mechanisms that neutralize and eventually dispose of invading microorganisms. B cells exert this control primarily by secreting antibody molecules that bind to the foreign particles or microorganisms and facilitate their elimination by complement-mediated lysis and by phagocytic cells. Reactions initiated by antibodies are collectively termed *humoral immunity*.

An efficient humoral response does not occur in the absence of T cells because they provide the help needed to promote B-cell proliferation and differentiation into plasma cells.[11] T cells thus play a central role in the immune response. To achieve their diverse functions, T cells develop along specialized sublineages to become helper (T_H) or cytotoxic (T_C) T cells.[12–14] T cells exert their regulatory function by producing biologically active peptides called *lymphokines*.[15] These soluble factors bind to receptors on the surface of effector cells such as macrophages, and deliver activation signals to facilitate killing of pathogens after endocytosis. T_C cells themselves may kill virus-infected or malignant cells. The immune responses mediated by T cells and their macrophage collaborators are called *cellular immunity*.

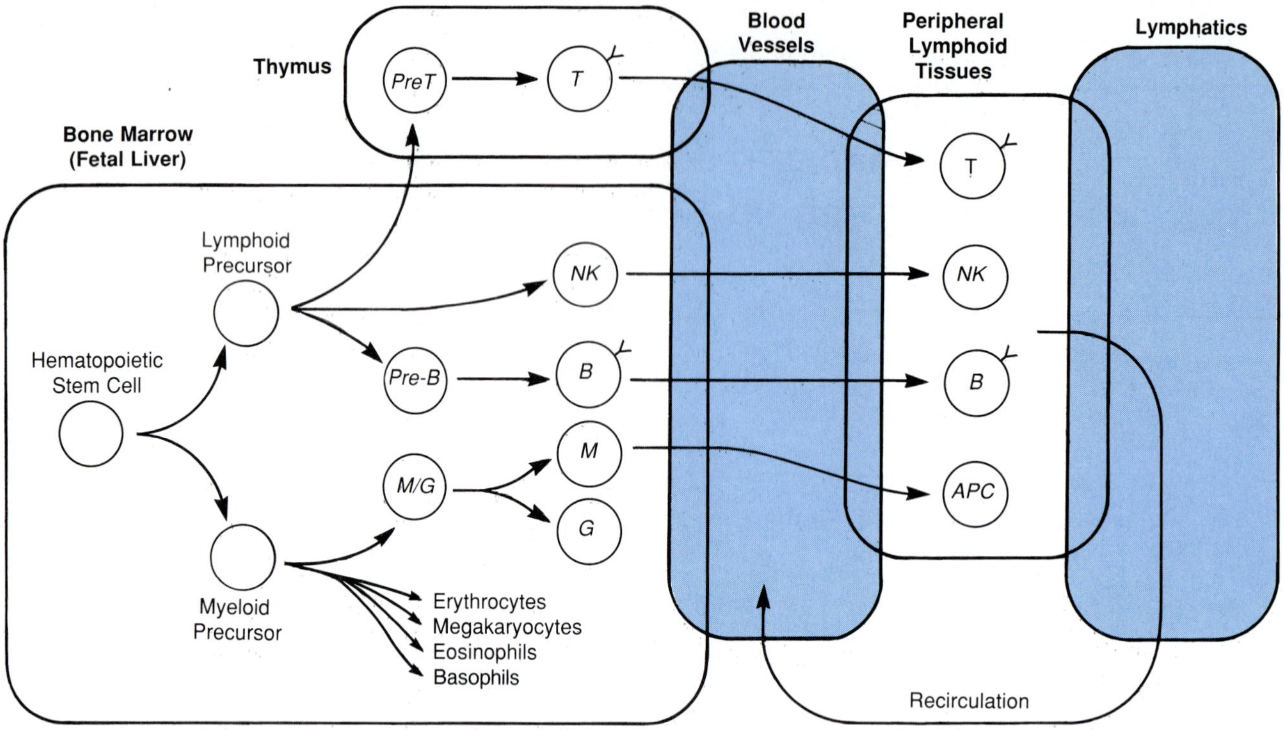

FIGURE 21-1. Immune system development and distribution. T, T lymphocytes; B, B lymphocytes; NK, natural killer cells; M/G, monocytes/granulocytes; APC, antigen-presenting cells.

The most recently recognized component of the immune system is the NK cell. Lymphoid cells of this lineage lack the specific antigen receptors of their T- and B-cell relatives, but they have a more general recognition capability, which may allow them to kill virus-infected or neoplastic cells.[16]

The progenitors of T, B, and NK lymphocytes derive from self-replicating hematopoietic stem cells that also give rise to myeloid and erythroid progenitors (see Chap. 7). Hematopoietic stem cells originate in the mesenchyme near the embryonic aorta, then migrate into the yolk sac, where hematopoietic islands are formed. In these blood islands, the stem cells enter the erythroid and myeloid differentiation compartments. Later in embryonic life, the pluripotent stem cells migrate to the liver, then to the bone marrow when this becomes the primary site of hematopoiesis. Although an early developmental dichotomy appears to exist between lymphoid and myeloid progenitor cells (see Fig. 21-1), immature cells of T-, B-, and NK-cell lineages may share a number of cell surface molecules in common with myelomonocytic cells.

B LYMPHOCYTES

Stem cells begin to generate B-cell precursors when they migrate into the fetal liver and continue to do so when they seed the bone marrow. In the bone marrow, stem cell progeny continuously enter the B-cell pathway of differentiation throughout life (Fig. 21-2). The life history of B-lineage cells can be conveniently divided into antigen-dependent and antigen-independent phases of development.[17] The antigen-independent phase includes the pre–B cells and immature B cells characterized by their surface expression of IgM antibody receptors. The second phase involves those B cells that are stimulated by antigen and T cells to undergo proliferation and differentiation. The end-stage cell is the mature plasma cell, which produces and secretes thousands of antibody molecules per second during its relatively short life-span that usually lasts for only a few days.[18]

Although all the stages in B-cell differentiation are ultimately represented in the bone marrow, this hematopoietic tissue is concerned with the generation of pre–B and B cells. The earliest stages in development of B-lineage cells are thus confined to the bone marrow in postnatal life. The precursor B-cells (referred to as pre–B cells) are characterized by polyclonal cell growth during which the genes encoding for the Ig heavy and light chains are rearranged for diversification and expression. An estimated 10 billion B cells are produced daily in the bone marrow of a normal person. In this way, a vast array of B-cell clones are being continuously generated, each of which expresses surface IgM antibodies of unique specificity.[19–22]

Intimate interaction with bone marrow stromal cells is crucial to the polyclonal pre–B cell growth and differentiation. The relation between these two cell types depends in part on cell adhesion molecules present on the precursor B cells and their interaction with complementary molecules on the surface of the stromal cells.[23,24] In addition, the stromal cells produce soluble growth and differentiation factors for pre–B cells. The best defined of these is interleukin-7, a molecule of 25 kd, which binds to a specific receptor that is present on pre–B cells (T cells may also express this receptor).[25]

The differentiation of pre–B cells into IgM-bearing B cells follows an orderly program of linked external and internal signals. The rearrangement and expression of genes encoding the μ heavy chain usually occur first, and this is reflected by the cytoplasmic expression of μ chains.[17,19–22] Few of the cytoplasmic μ chains reach the surface of the pre–B cell before the rearrangement and expression of a light chain (κ or λ). Both heavy- and light-chain genes must be productively rearranged before cells acquire the potential to respond to antigens via expression of cell surface antibody receptors.

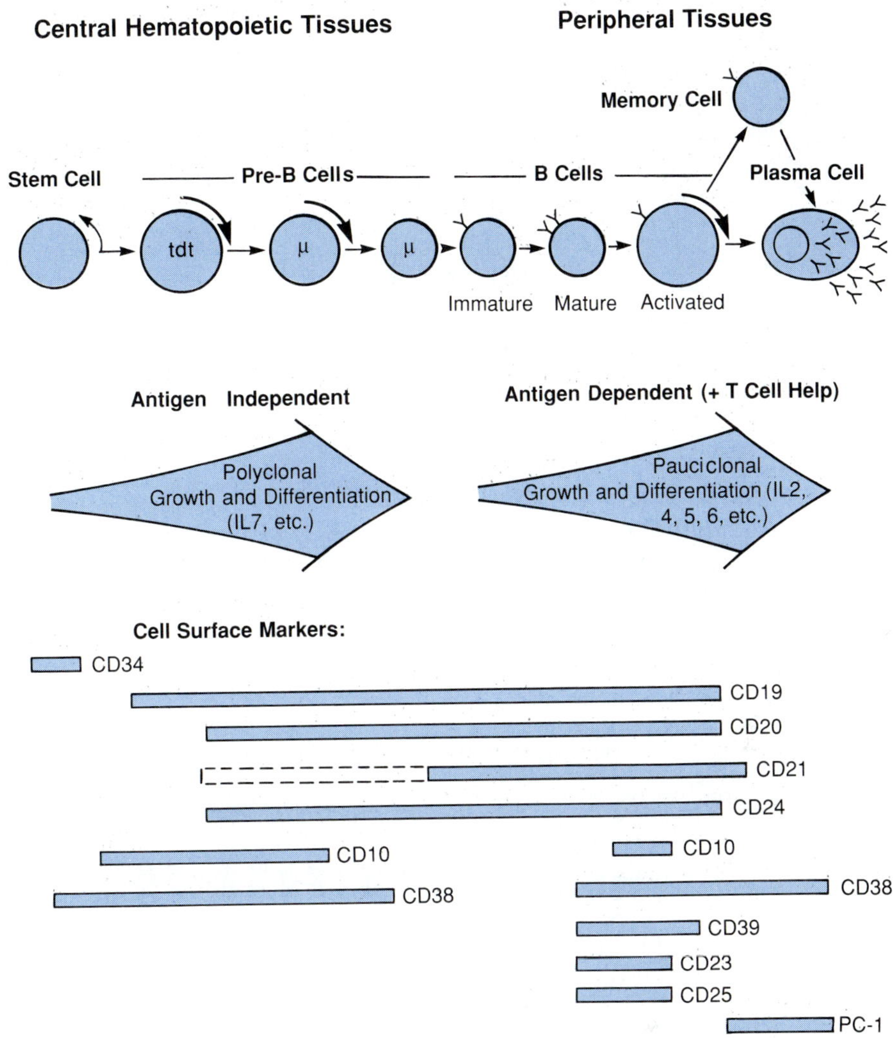

FIGURE 21-2. Stages of B-cell development and differentiation.

Immunoglobulin Gene Rearrangement in Preparation for Antibody Production

Antibodies are glycoproteins that are formed by pairs of heavy and light chains (Fig. 21-3). The antigen binding sites of an antibody molecule are formed by the three hypervariable amino acid sequences of the heavy chain and the three analogous hypervariable sequences located near the N terminal of the light chain. These hypervariable regions are separated by relatively conserved sequences. In the fully assembled Ig molecule, the hypervariable regions, also called *complementarity-determining regions* (CDRs), form a cleft into which a particular antigen can fit.

The first two CDRs of the heavy chain are encoded by one of about 50 V_H (variable) region genes located upstream (5′) from the heavy-chain constant region (C) genes on chromosome 14.[19–22] The V_H genes are grouped into seven families, composed of 1 to more than 12 related V_H genes. Downstream from the V_H gene families is a family of diversity (D) gene segments followed by a family of J_H (joining) gene segments, all of which are separated by intervening DNA sequences. The distance between the last V_H gene and the first J_H gene segment is about 100 kb. The third CDR of the antibody heavy chain is formed by sequences derived by the joining of the V_H, D, and J_H gene segments.

The genes encoding the κ and λ light chains are located on chromosomes 2 and 22, respectively, and their basic organization is similar to that of the heavy-chain genes. The first two CDRs are encoded by one of many variable region (V_L) gene segments, whereas the joining of a V_L gene with one of several joining (J_L) gene segments generates the coding sequence for the third CDR. Before antibodies can be produced, the genes encoding different parts of the heavy and light chains must be rearranged, and the V region genes selected for rearrangement and expression in a particular cell determine its antibody specificity.[19–22]

The Ig gene rearrangement usually begins with the joining of one of the D segments of the heavy-chain locus to one of the J segments and the deletion of the DNA between the translocated gene segments, which may include intervening D and J segments (Fig. 21-4). The rearrangement process continues with the joining of a V_H gene to the DJ_H complex. These rearrangements involve a set of recombinase proteins not yet defined precisely but which appear to operate for both Ig and TcR gene rearrangements.[26,27]

Two proteins of 119 and 59 kd encoded by the recombination-activating genes RAG-1 and the RAG-2, respectively, activate the expression of the recombinase activity exclusively in the maturing lymphoid cells. These two proteins may also participate in the recombinase reaction.[28]

The V, D, and J gene segments are flanked by palindromic recombination signal sequences separated by spacers of 12 or 23 base pairs (see Fig. 21-4). These elements serve as the recognition sites for the recombinase proteins. The rule for V(D)J joinings requires that splicing is accomplished only when the recombination signal sequences are separated by unequal spacers, that is, 12 to 23 or 23 to 12 (see Fig. 21-

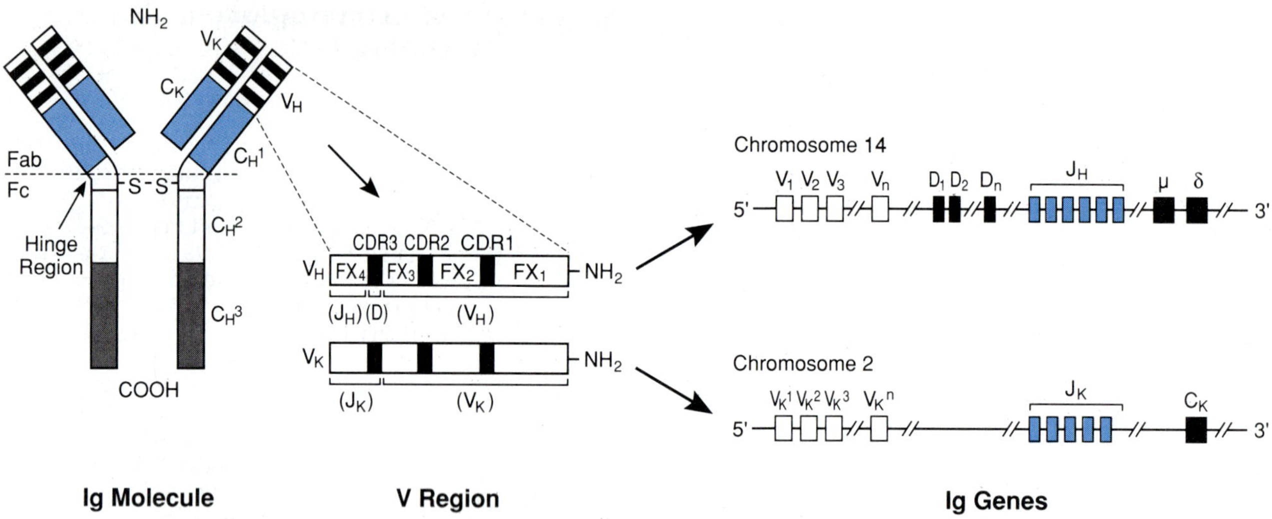

FIGURE 21-3. Molecular basis for antibody specificity. The complementarity-determining regions (CDR) are indicated in the immunoglobulin molecule, and details are provided in the V region map. The chromosomal arrangement of Ig genes encoding for heavy and one light chain (κ) is indicated.

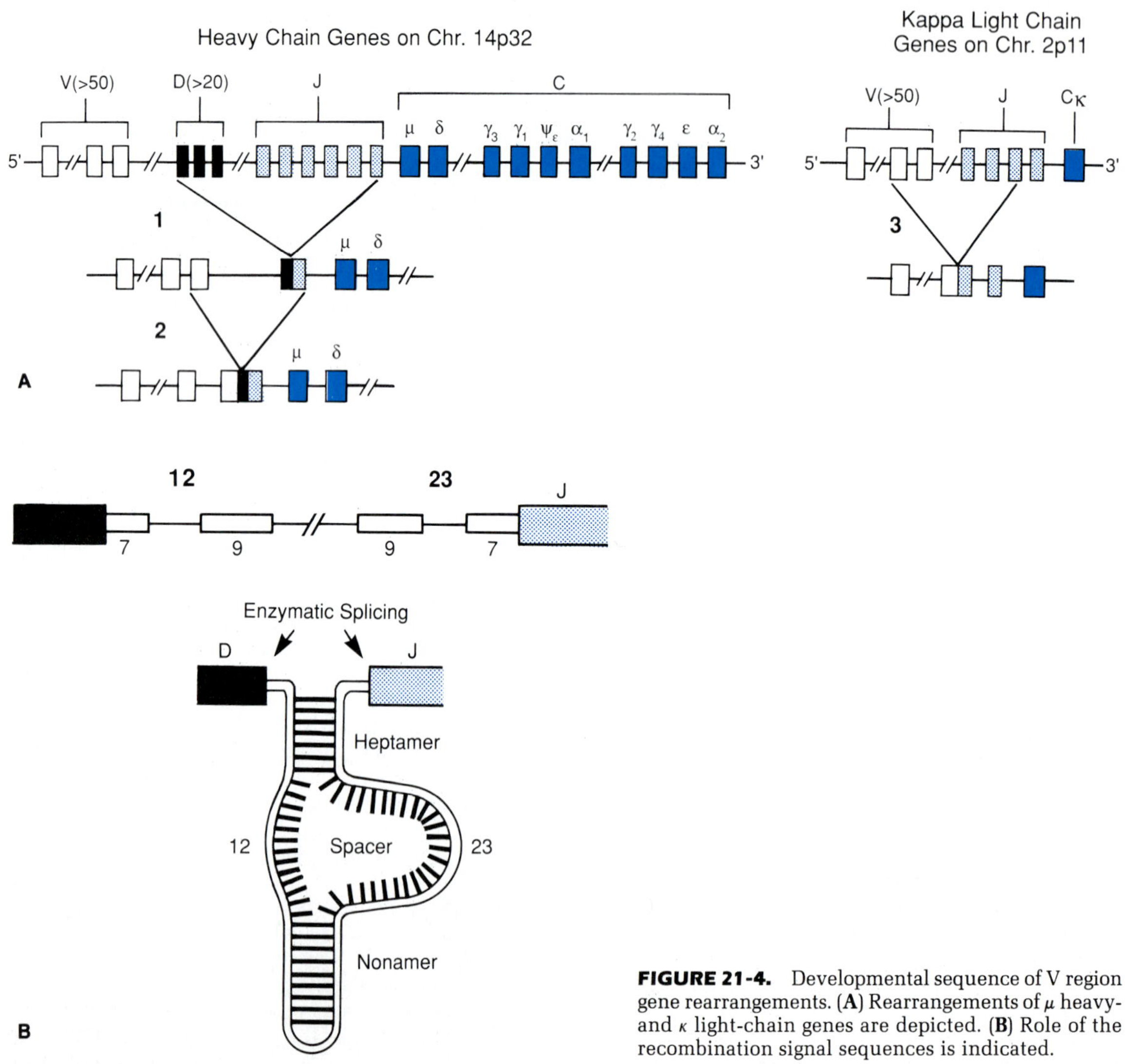

FIGURE 21-4. Developmental sequence of V region gene rearrangements. (**A**) Rearrangements of μ heavy- and κ light-chain genes are depicted. (**B**) Role of the recombination signal sequences is indicated.

4). This rule dictates the joining of V to D and of D to J gene segments.

The random combination of one of approximately 50 V_H genes with an equally random D–J combination in each cell leads to the generation of a large array of cells expressing different antibody specificities. The D–J rearrangements take place in a proliferating pre–B cell that gives rise to progeny with the same DJ rearrangement. Each of these daughter cells can then select a different V_H gene segment for rearrangement; thus, a single progenitor cell can generate cells with different antibody specificities. Additional mechanisms contribute to the generation of antibody diversity and greatly amplify the antibody repertoire. First, the VDJ joinings are often imprecise, resulting in loss of nucleotides from the coding partners and creating additional diversity. During repair of the DNA splice site, the terminal deoxynucleotidyl transferase (TdT) enzyme that operates without a preformed DNA template may add new nucleotides (N segments) to contribute further to sequence diversification in the CDR3.[29,30]

After successful V(D)J joining in a productive reading frame, rearrangement begins in one of the light-chain gene loci, usually κ before λ.[31,32] Rearrangement of light-chain V_L and J_L segments is accomplished by the recombination signal sequences that are used by recombinase enzymes to join them. Light-chain diversity is generated by random pairing of different V_L and J_L genes, by imprecision in their splicing, and by the insertion of N sequences in the join.[19–22] Because TdT activity is usually diminished by the time the pre–B cell rearranges its light-chain genes, the insertion of new nucleotides contributes much less to the light-chain diversification process. The order of Ig gene rearrangements is usually, but not always, as outlined already: D to J_H, V_H to DJ_H, V_κ to J_κ and, if necessary, V_λ to J_λ.

If the VDJ_H rearrangement is productive (in a correct DNA reading frame) on one chromosome, the V_H gene rearrangement process does not continue on the other allele. Similarly, a productive V_L to J_L rearrangement inhibits the light-chain gene rearrangement process. This phenomenon, the mechanism for which is incompletely understood, is called *allelic exclusion*.[33–35] In this way, each B cell expresses only one heavy-chain VDJ-C_μ and one light-chain VJ-C_κ or C_λ product, which combine to form an IgM antibody of one specificity. At this point in the differentiation process, the pre–B cell begins to express the complete IgM molecule on the cell surface to become a B cell.

Regulation of Immunoglobulin Gene Expression During B-Cell Differentiation

After successful VDJ rearrangement in a pre–B cell, transcription is initiated upstream of the leader sequence that precedes each V_H gene segment. Regulatory sequences located 5′ to each leader sequence and enhancer sequences located in the intron between the J_H genes and the C_μ region gene segments influence the transcriptional process. The transcription is initiated by the collective binding of a family of nuclear proteins to these regulatory sequences to expose an upstream promoter to RNA polymerase II.[36,37] Since transcription of μ chains usually precedes light-chain gene rearrangement, a pre–B cell can be recognized through the presence of intracytoplasmic μ chains (see Fig. 21-2).

In the case of μ chains, as well as for heavy chains of other Ig classes, amino acid sequences at the C terminal determine whether the complete Ig molecule is membrane-bound or secreted (Fig. 21-5). The synthesis of heavy chains with different C-terminal sequences is made possible by selective posttranscriptional processing of mRNA potentially capable of coding for either membrane or secretory chains. The membrane form of the heavy chain includes a hydrophobic transmembrane segment followed by a short cytoplasmic tail of only a few amino acids. The secretory form of the heavy chain lacks the transmembrane region, instead having an abbreviated, relatively hydrophobic tail.[38]

Pre–B cells synthesize predominantly the membrane form of the μ chain. In the absence of light-chain synthesis, the μ chains are largely retained in the endoplasmic reticulum and subsequently degraded. Retention is caused by μ-chain binding to a 78-kd glycoprotein, which belongs to the family of heat shock proteins and is called BiP for binding protein.[39,40] Neoplastic pre–B cells that have not undergone light-chain gene rearrangement may express small amounts of μ chains on their surface. In this case, the μ chain bond with BiP is displaced by a surrogate light-chain complex that is encoded by V pre–B and λ-like genes that do not require rearrangement to be expressed.[41,42] This step also occurs during normal pre–B-cell differentiation; it is postulated that the μ chain/surrogate–light-chain complex serves as the receptor for signals that promote survival during the light-chain gene rearrangements. The subsequent onset of light-chain synthesis results in efficient displacement of BiP and the formation of fully assembled IgM

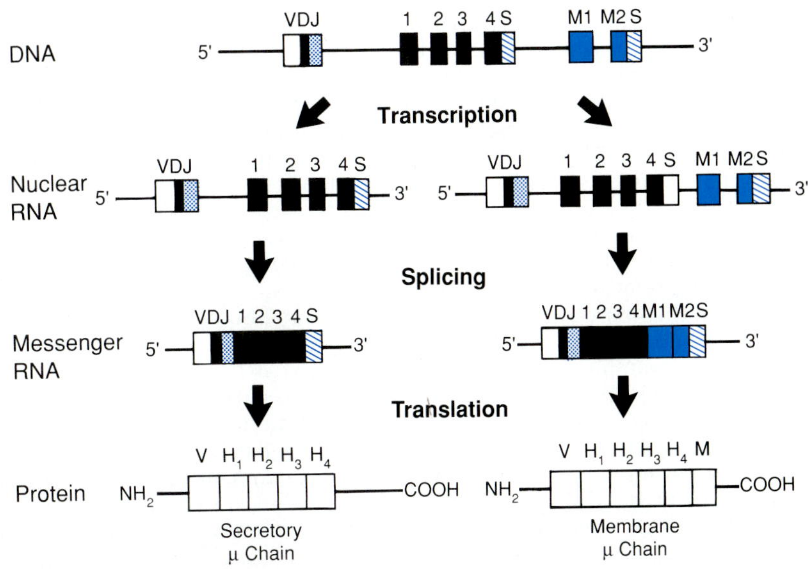

FIGURE 21-5. Synthesis of membrane and secretory forms of an IgM antibody requires differential transcription and RNA splicing.

molecules of the membrane bound form that characterize the newly formed B cell.[39,40]

Immunoglobulin Isotype Switching

Immunoglobulin isotype switching is a process by which B cells within each clone can switch from the production of IgM to that of molecules of different isotypes while retaining their antibody specificity.[21,43,44]

Two types of isotype switching occur. The first takes place in immature IgM+ B cells when they begin to express membrane IgD. These cells produce long nuclear transcripts that include the VDJ together with C_μ and C_δ RNA. The long transcript is subsequently spliced into shorter messengers for either μ or δ chains, each sharing the same VDJ mRNA (Fig. 21-6A). The messengers are subsequently translated in the endoplasmic reticulum to yield μ and δ chains in variable proportions.

The other type of switching involves a DNA rearrangement and deletional process. In this case, a region of repetitive DNA sequences (switch [S] regions) located upstream of the C_μ gene is joined with an S region located upstream of another C_H gene, and the intervening DNA is deleted. Figure 21-6B depicts an example of switching from IgM to IgG1, which involves deletion of the intervening C_μ, C_δ, and $C_\gamma 3$ genes. This type of switch may take place any time after successful VDJ rearrangement, but is far more frequent in maturing B cells within germinal centers. It is facilitated by antigenic stimulation, T-cell help, and lymphokines. Interleukin-4 (IL-4), for example, may selectively enhance the IgE component of the antibody response.[15]

Because no well-formed switch sequence is located between the C_μ and C_δ genes, few B cells switch by the DNA deletion mechanism to give rise to IgD-producing cells.

Positive and Negative Selection of B-Cell Clones

Although millions of cells with differing antibody specificities are generated daily in an apparently random fashion, the process of selection of B-cell clones is highly regulated from its onset, early in embryonic life. Orderly regulation of the development of the B-cell compartment is obtained by both negative and positive selection.

Failure to achieve productive rearrangement of both heavy- and light-chain genes, which may occur frequently, apparently dooms the pre–B cells to an early death.[21] Negative selection continues to take place on newly formed immature B cells to eliminate self-reactive clones.[45–47] As a consequence of the mechanisms governing the acquisition of the antibody repertoire, any B cell can become equipped with surface receptors directed against exogenous as well as self-antigens. When the antibody receptors on the surface of an immature B cell are cross-linked by the self-antigens constantly present (or experimentally by an anti-Ig antibody), the cell is killed. This type of clonal abortion may involve the activation of endonucleases, causing programmed cell death (apoptosis). Alternatively, such contact may render the cell unresponsive to subsequent stimuli, a phenomenon referred to as *clonal anergy*.[45–47]

A bias in the expression of V_H region genes may also be part of the orderly process of maturation of the immune system. For example, during ontogeny, the first B cells preferentially use those V_H region families located closest to the D–J region segments.[48,49] This biased V_H gene utilization is not apparent in the normal pool of mature B cells, where the expressed V_H gene repertoire reflects the number of V_H genes in the different V_H gene families. This normalization of the gene repertoire may in part involve selective pressure by antigen and in part be related to the overrepresentation in the early stages of ontogeny of B cells characterized by the surface expression of the CD5 surface marker.[50] These CD5+ cells, which represent a discrete B-cell subset population, are characterized by the capacity to produce antibodies, mainly of the IgM isotype, which bind to a variety of self-antigens with a low intrinsic affinity. In addition, CD5+ cells predominate in the malignant cell clones of the chronic lymphocytic leukemia and may participate in the pathogenesis of autoimmune rheumatic disorders.[50]

The expression of CD5 may distinguish a subset of B cells with homing properties, self-renewal features, and functional features different from those of other (conventional) B cells. Their predominance in neonatal tissues also suggests a special role for CD5+ cells, perhaps related to the production of natural antibodies. However, CD5 expression can be induced by B-cell activation, and the precise physiologic role of CD5+ B cells remains uncertain.

Phenotypic Markers of B-Lineage Cells

The most reliable marker of early B-lineage commitment is a productive VDJ gene rearrangement that is reflected by the synthesis of μ chains. In addition, a variety of cell surface and cytoplasmic molecules mark the orderly sequence of differentiation events, the definition of which allows diagnosis and classification of leukemic cell counterparts.[53] The CD34 cell surface glycoprotein is expressed on early precursor cells of B lineage, and of other hematopoietic lineages, before expression of surface IgM.

Several stages of pre–B-cell maturation can be identified by other cell surface (or nuclear) markers (see Fig. 21-2). Even before the CD10+ stage, B-cell precursors undergoing rearrangement of their Ig genes, currently termed pro–B cells, may express high levels of nuclear TdT and HLA-DR. The CD19 and CD24 surface markers are then acquired.* Together, these markers allow the distinction of early B lineage cells from early hematopoietic cells of other lineages.

The CD10 antigen, a cell surface ectoenzyme (neutral endopeptidase) originally identified as an acute lymphoblastic leukemia antigen, is acquired before the appearance of Ig heavy chains in the cytoplasm.[54,55] In the absence of conventional light chains, pre–B cells express little or no surface Ig, are rarely positive for TdT, and can be divided into large, lymphoid precursors of the small, postmitotic pre–B cells. Large pre–B cells exhibit a characteristic cerebriform nucleus with deep clefts and indentations. CD38, a nonlineage-specific marker expressed during early stages of B-cell differentiation, disappears with B-cell maturation, only to be reexpressed at high level on the surface of mature plasma cells.[56] Other surface markers expressed during and beyond the pre–B-cell stage are CD20 and CD21 (CR2/EBV receptor).[57] CD21 is usually not present in amounts sufficient for immunofluorescence detection until the B cells express both surface IgM and IgD.

Antigen-Driven B-Cell Differentiation

The interaction of antigens with surface Igs begins the chain of events leading to B-cell activation. These events have been elucidated by in vitro studies with polyclonal B-cell activators, such as insolubilized anti-IgM antibodies or

* The CD22 antigen, expressed in the cytoplasm of pre–B cells is first expressed on the surface immediately after the acquisition of surface IgD and disappears after B-cell activation.

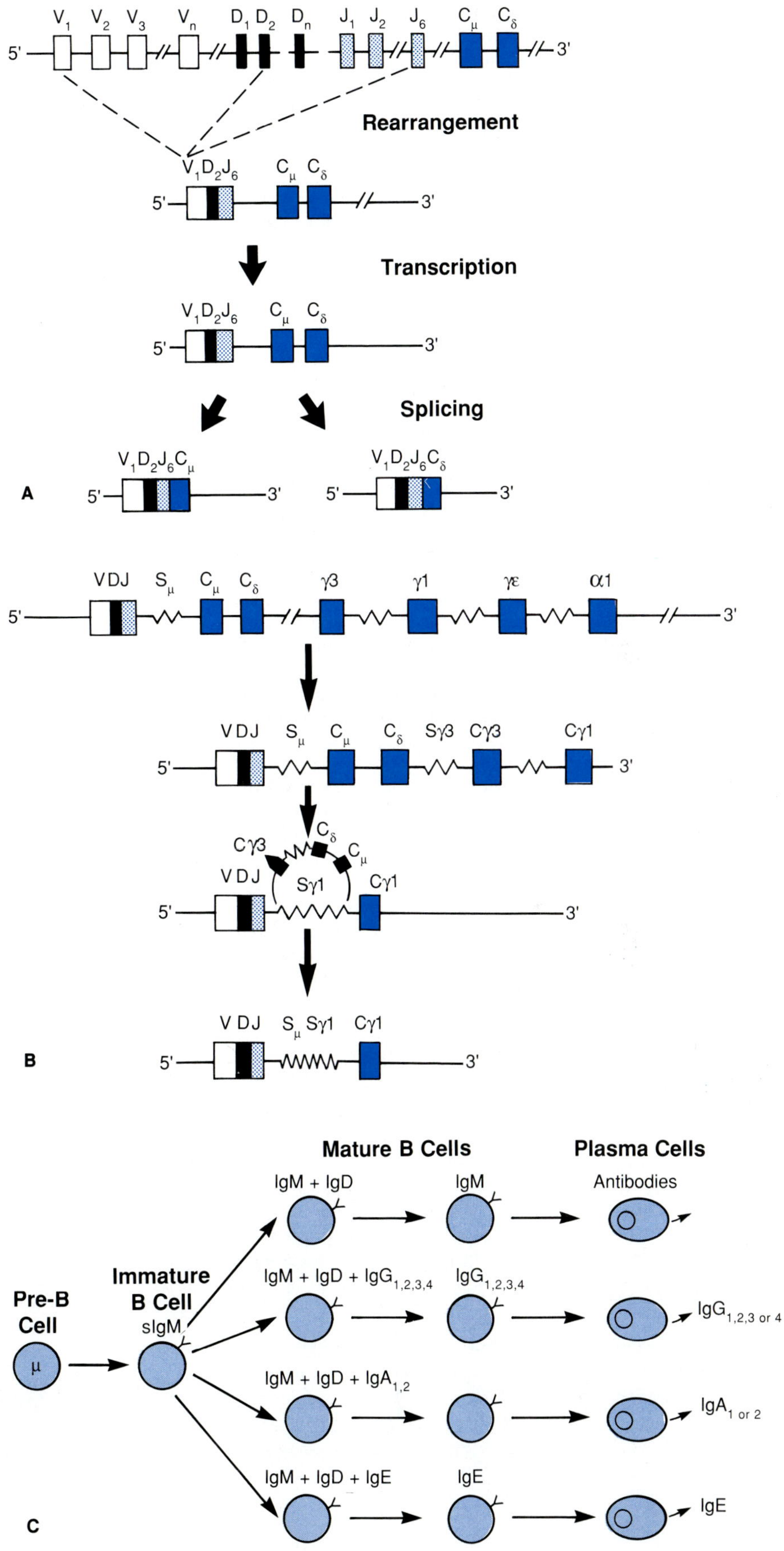

FIGURE 21-6. Two types of immunoglobulin isotype switching. (**A**) Switch from B-cell expression of IgM to expression of both IgM and IgD is shown by the formation of two different cytoplasmic mRNAs for μ and δ chains. (**B**) Permanent switch from IgM to other immunoglobulin isotypes occurs by a mechanism that results in deletion of C_H gene DNA. (**C**) In this example, the switching events allow the expression of all of the different isotypes by members of a single B-cell clone.

Staphylococcus aureus Cowan, which mimic the antigenic signal by cross-linking membrane Ig and offer the advantage of binding to a large number of cells.[11,58–61]

Membrane-bound immunoglobulins have long been thought to represent the complete B-cell antigen receptor. It has now been shown that they are part of a more complex receptor structure that includes the Igα and Igβ chains encoded by the mb-1 and b29 genes, respectively.[58–61] In murine B cells, Igα has a molecular weight of 34 kd and Igβ of 38 kd[58–60]; in human B cells, these molecules display a higher molecular weight and greater heterogeneity, related in part to a higher level of glycosylation.[61] Igα (CD79a) and Igβ (CD79b) are transmembrane molecules, noncovalently linked to membrane-bound Ig, that subserve the function of transducing activation signals delivered by encounter with antigen. Igα and Igβ expression is lost during terminal plasma cell differentiation, a finding that accounts for the inability of these cells to express surface Ig.[61,62] Each of the Ig isotypes is capable of forming a complex with Igα and Igβ.

Ligation of the B-cell antigen receptor complex leads to activation of several tyrosine kinases. Three tyrosine kinases of the src family (lyn, blk, and lck) are associated with the antigen receptor complex, and additional tyrosine kinases are also involved. Moreover, protein phosphorylation is finely tuned by the activity of tyrosine phosphatase enzymes: cells lacking the CD45 transmembrane protein with phospahatase activity have impaired signal-transducing capacities.[58–60]

Tyrosine phosphorylation causes the activation of phospholipase C, which hydrolyzes polyphosphoinositides into inositol-3-phosphate and diacylglycerol (DAG).[59,60] Formation of these products induces the release of Ca^{2+} stores from the endoplasmic reticulum as well as influx of extracellular Ca^{2+}. Ca^{2+} and DAG act in concert to activate phosphokinase C. Some of the subsequent phosphorylation reaction products reach the nucleus and induce the transcription of selected genes to cause cell activation.

An activated B cell can be recognized by the expression of surface markers detectable by antibodies such as CD23 (low-affinity receptor for IgE), CD25 (low-affinity receptor for interleukin-2 [IL-2]; see text that follows), CD38, CD39, CD69, and CD71 (transferrin receptor). Many are lost during terminal differentiation (CD25 and CD23) and are substituted by markers specific for this maturational stage (eg, PC-1).

Activated B cells become responsive to factors that can be operationally divided into three broad categories: (1) conditioning factors that participate in B-cell activation; (2) factors that induce proliferation (termed collectively *B-cell growth factors* [BCGFs]); and (3) factors that induce terminal B-cell differentiation (BCDFs).[11] Although this subdivision is convenient, it cannot be considered absolute. IL-4 and interferon-γ are examples of the first category, but they may also exert BCGF or BCDF activities, depending on prior signals received by the responding B cell. IL-2 promotes B-cell proliferation and has a BCDF activity on cells at late activation stages. Interleukin-6 (IL-6), although a typical BCDF, may also exert a BCGF effect. In reality, the activation of B cells usually involves a complex cascade of signals generated by several ligand stimuli.

Some of the key events in B-cell activation, proliferation, and differentiation are depicted in Figure 21-7. Interleukin-5 (IL-5), although a major growth factor for murine B cells, has not been shown to have the same effects on human B cells. Other accessory factors that have not been fully characterized are low-molecular-weight and high-molecular-weight BCGFs. Accessory factors like interleukin-1 (IL-1), tumor necrosis factor (TNF), interferon-α (IFN-α), and split products of C3 (C3d) that are present at inflammatory sites may amplify an ongoing B-cell response. The receptors for some of these factors are expressed continuously by B cells, as in the case of IL-4 receptors, whereas the expression of receptors for other factors is induced during activation.

The response to the various factors differs according to the conditioning signals that the B cell has received earlier. In the natural scheme of an antibody response, the antigen serves as an initial activating signal for B cells. Although a proportion of activated B cells responds to BCDFs and BCGFs with differentiation into end-stage plasma cells, some of the members of an activated clone of B cells undergo proliferation only, then return to the resting state to constitute a memory B-cell pool. Activation of a B cell that bears IgM and IgD may result in proliferation and loss of IgD expression in preparation for the final differentiation response. Memory cells that have switched to the production of another Ig class express a single membrane isotype.

The binding of antigen to membrane Ig followed by stimulation with soluble factors is sufficient to induce B-cell proliferation. A successful antibody response usually requires the physical presence of T cells as well as their sol-

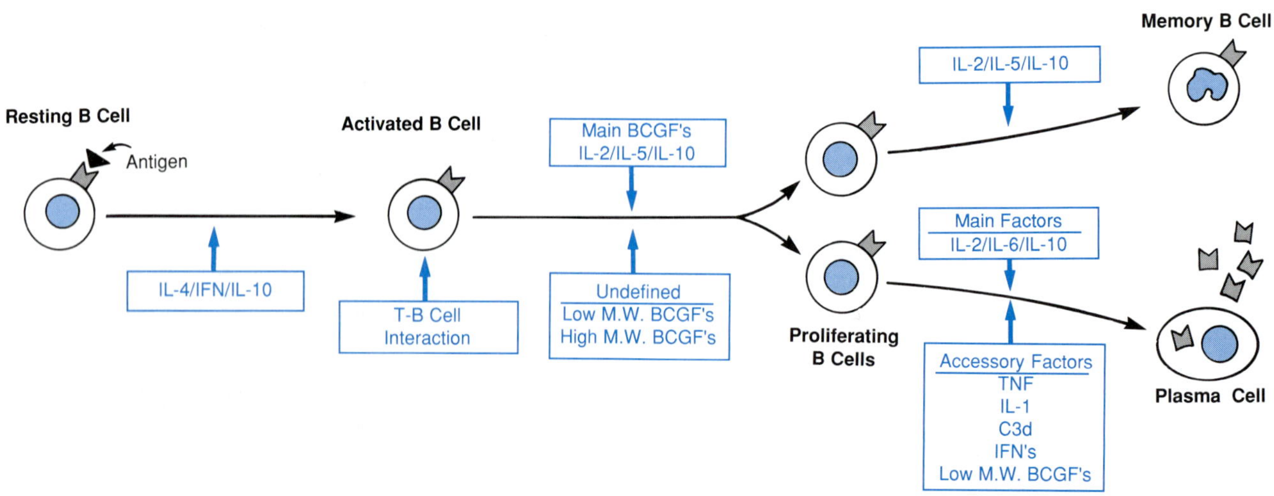

FIGURE 21-7. A model indicating the differential roles of cytokines in the process of antigen-driven B-cell differentiation. IFN, interferon; IL, interleukin; BCGF, B-cell growth factor.

uble BCGF and BCDF products.[62] T cells may deliver additional signals while recognizing the antigenic peptide presented by the class II molecules on the B-cell surface (see section on antigen recognition of T cells).

These signals may be delivered by the interaction of certain molecules on B cells with complementary surface structures expressed by T cells. For example, the CD40 molecule expressed on B cells interacts with a 39-kd glycoprotein ligand (CD40L) on T cells, T cell CD28 interacts with a membrane structure on B cells recognized by monoclonal antibodies. Another example of B7 (CD80) B-cell–T-cell interaction is represented by the mutual recognition of CD5 on T cells and CD72 on B cells. The precise function of some of these interactions is not fully understood, although recent observations in patients with Ig deficiency and increased IgM indicate that interaction between CD40 and its natural ligand on T cells is essential for promoting a switch from the production of IgM to that of other Ig isotypes.[63–65]

In the course of humoral responses, a progressive replacement of IgM antibodies with antibodies of other Ig classes (particularly IgG) occurs. This is accompanied by an increase in the affinity of the antibodies for the stimulating antigen. The first event is a consequence of the Ig heavy-chain switch, which may occur stochastically in the responsive clone or clones of proliferating cells and may be directed by lymphokines that act as preferential switch factors.

Changes in antibody affinity are related to a somatic mutation in the V region gene together with selection operated by the antigen.[22] This occurs in the germinal centers of secondary follicles in the peripheral lymphoid organs. It has been suggested that this process may occur according to the following scheme.[66] After stimulation with antigen, centroblasts, which represent a particular stage of activated B cells, accumulate in the dark zone of the germinal center and their V_H and V_L gene segments undergo somatic hypermutation. This results in the production of membrane Ig with different affinity for the stimulating antigen. Soon thereafter, centroblasts revert to the relative quiescent state of centrocytes in the light zone of germinal centers and undergo apoptosis (a programmed cell death that is characterized by internucleosomal DNA fragmentation), unless they are stimulated by the encounter with the specific antigen presented by dendritic cells in the presence of lymphokines (IL2, IL4, or IL1α). These events result in increased expression of the bcl2 oncogene product and inhibition of apoptosis.[66] Therefore, only those cells that express a receptor with higher affinity for the stimulating antigen are rescued from apoptosis.

With progression of an immune response, the antigen is eliminated by effector mechanisms, and its concentration

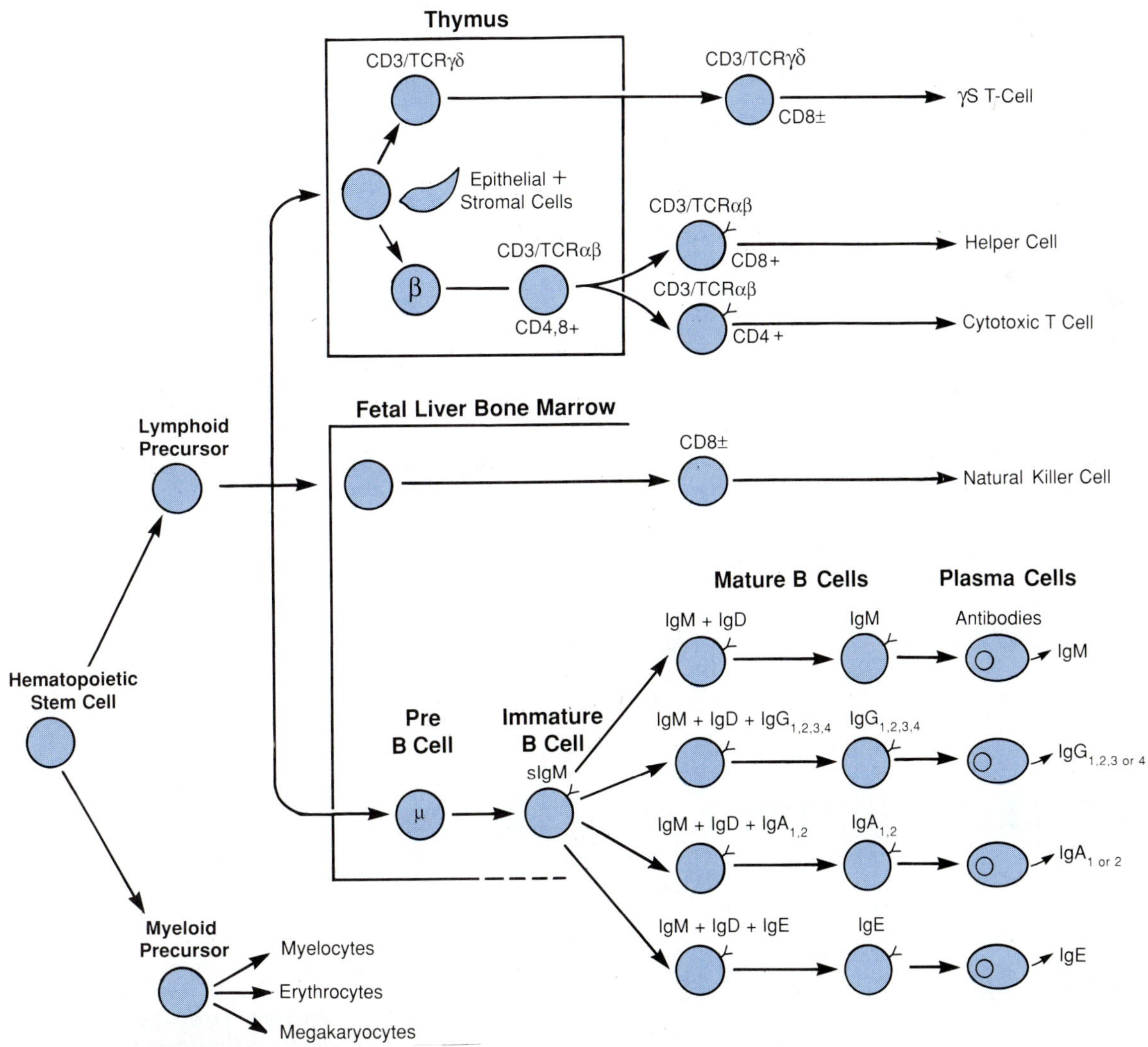

FIGURE 21-8. A scheme summarizing the maturational pathways of T cells, B cells, and natural killer cells.

in the lymphoid organs decreases progressively. This causes further competition for antigen among the specific B cells and results in the selective stimulation of cells equipped with higher-affinity receptors.

Termination of the antibody response is mediated by antigen elimination and in part by a feedback mechanism initiated by IgG antibodies. In this case, IgG antibodies linked to the antigen bind to the Fc γ receptors on B cells to form an antigen bridge with membrane-bound antibody and thus generate an inhibitory signal.

T LYMPHOCYTES

Development of the Thymus

The embryonic thymus, which provides the microenvironment in which bone marrow-derived precursors are induced to begin their differentiation into immunocompetent T cells, originates from the epithelial lining of the third and fourth pharyngeal pouches.[67] During the sixth week of gestation, these specialized epithelial cells begin their migration into the thoracic cavity. During the eighth week of gestation, the epithelial anlage is invaded by bone marrow-derived precursor cells, macrophages, and local mesenchymal cells, which give rise to the blood vessels and connective tissue of the thymus. Lymphoid progenitors are attracted by soluble chemoattractants produced by the epithelial cell. Within the thymus, these lymphoid precursors are induced to divide and to differentiate along one of two basic pathways of T-cell differentiation (Fig. 21-8). The expanding population of thymocytes contributes to the development of distinct cortical and medullary zones in the thymic lobules. This structure is maintained throughout basic life, although gradual involution of the thymus begins early in life.

In fully differentiated thymic lobules, the outer cortex is occupied by immature thymocytes. These give rise to the dividing cells of intermediate maturity in the midcortical areas, whereas the deeper cortex contains small postmitotic thymocytes with dense nuclear heterochromatin and a thin layer of relatively undifferentiated cytoplasm. The cortical epithelial network is made up by cells linked together by desmosomes. The thymic epithelial cells, which contain secretory granules, define the tridimensional spaces occupied by the developing thymocytes. In this manner, a large epithelial surface is available for direct contact through complementary molecules expressed on the surface of developing thymocytes.

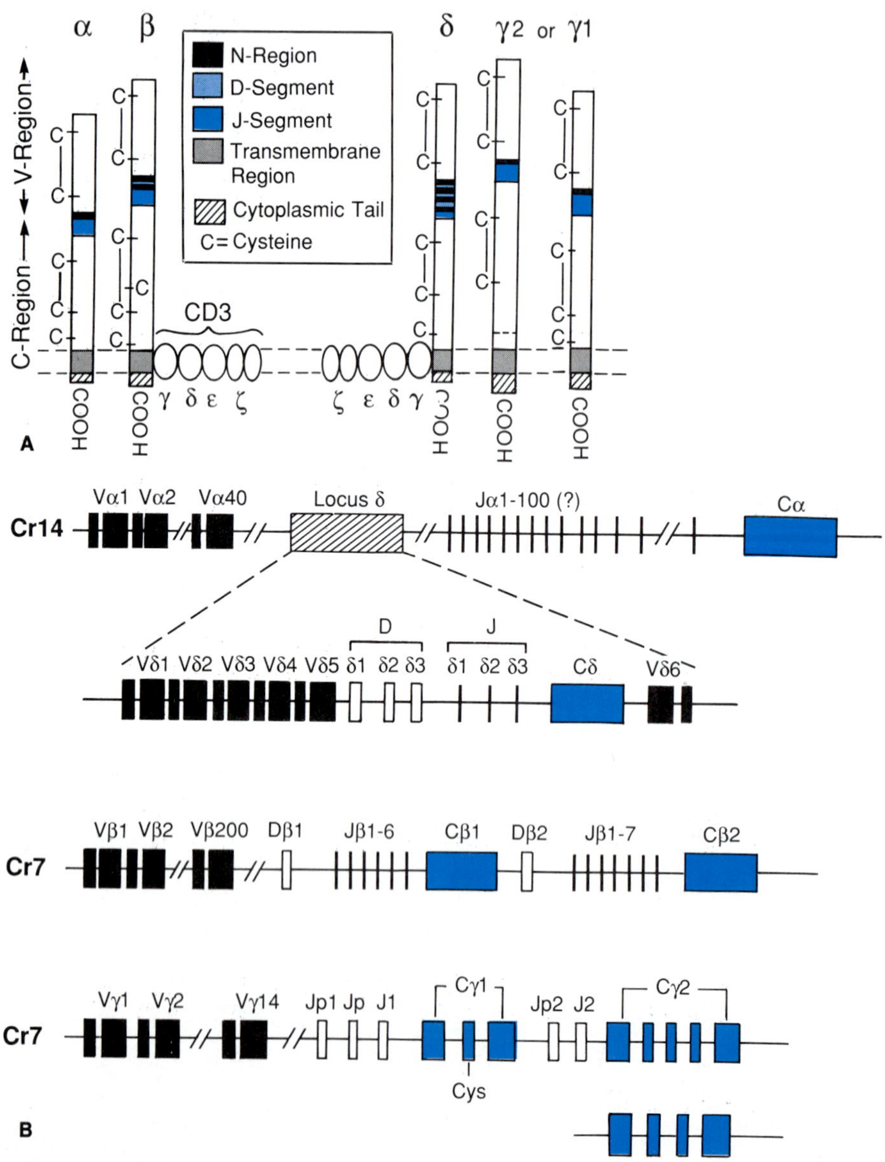

FIGURE 21-9. (A) Molecular organization of the $\alpha\beta$ and $\gamma\delta$ TcR and the associated CD3 molecular complex. (B) Organization of the TcR genes.

The medulla is occupied by relatively mature thymocytes that are derived from cortical thymocytes. The medullary epithelial cells, pleomorphic in shape and structure, are sometimes wrapped around one another to form structures known as Hassall's corpuscles. These consist of a concentric array of squamous cells that contain bundles of heavy keratin filaments and keratohyalin granules. Macrophages are located predominantly at the corticomedullary junction, around the postcapillary venules, which are the major site of exit for mature thymocytes. Interdigitating dendritic cells in the medulla may be responsible for the presentation of self-peptides to mature thymocytes.

T-Cell Receptor

The TcR is formed by two disulfide-linked chains, which are noncovalently associated with the CD3 complex of proteins that subserve a signal-transducing function.[68–71] The CD3 complex is composed of five different proteins of 20 to 30 kd named γ, δ, ϵ, and two subunits forming the ζ complex (Fig. 21-9*A*).

The two types of TcR are termed $\alpha\beta$ and $\gamma\delta$ TcR, respectively.[69–71] Most T cells bear the $\alpha\beta$ heterodimer. A smaller subpopulation of T cells expresses $\gamma\delta$ TcR. Figure 21-9*A* illustrates the basic polypeptide structure of the $\alpha\beta$ and the $\gamma\delta$ TcR, which share many similarities with Ig molecules. The TcR polypeptide chains have a variable (V) region located at the N terminal and a constant (C) portion at the C terminal. In the proximity of the membrane, a hinge or connecting peptide of the C portion has a cysteine residue for the interchain disulfide bond. All chains have a transmembrane portion, whereas only the $\alpha\beta$ and $\gamma\delta$ chains of TcR possess short intracycloplasmic tails. In the outermost V regions, hypervariable segments are interspaced between conserved sequences. The TcR chains are folded so that the hypervariable complementarity-determining regions (CDR), form the combining site for antigens. Three CDR are present in each chain.

Molecular Basis for Generation of the TcR Repertoire

The maturation of T cells involves polyclonal cell proliferation and the concomitant rearrangement of gene segments encoding for the TcR molecules. The organization of the TcR gene loci is similar to that of the Ig heavy- and light-chain gene loci in that the β and δ genes consist of minigene families encoding the V, D, and J regions and nearby C region genes, whereas the α and γ gene loci contain only V and J minigene families together with their respective C region genes[69,71,72] (see Fig. 21-9*B*). The initial TcR diversity is generated by the joining of one of the V region genes (which encodes for the first two CDR) with a J or with rearranged DJ gene segments that contribute to the formation of the third CDR. The rearrangements are catalyzed by the same recombinases that are involved in Ig gene rearrangements. This is because the TcR genes are flanked by the same recombination signal sequences, namely conserved heptamer and nonamer sequences spaced by 12 or 23 nucleotides[26–28] (see Fig. 21-4).

The random pairing of V, D, and J gene segments may yield only about 2500 and 70 specificities for $\alpha\beta$ TcR and $\gamma\delta$ TcR, respectively. The generation of a much larger repertoire is ensured by varying the V(D)J splicing sites and by insertion of new nucleotides during the splicing process. The synthesis of these N regions is catalyzed by the enzyme TdT, as in the case of B cells. Both processes contribute greatly to the diversity of CDR3 of the TcR, bringing the number of possible specificities to as many as 10^{15} and 10^{18} for the $\alpha\beta$ TcR and $\gamma\delta$ TcR, respectively.

The α-chain locus on chromosome 14 contains the δ-chain loci in its midst, between the V_α and J_α genes (see Fig. 21-9*B*). The rearrangement of the V_α and J_α genes thus results in the deletion of δ-chain genes, preventing the possibility of δ-chain expression by the $\alpha\beta$ T cells. A successful δ-chain gene rearrangement must precede that of the α-chain genes. A definite order of TcR gene rearrangements is observed during ontogeny. The productive rearrangement of γ- and δ-gene loci occurs first to result in the generation of an initial wave of $\gamma\delta$ T cells.[71,73] Other T cells undergo productive rearrangement of V, D, and J to express TcR β chains in their cytoplasm. Later, these cells achieve a productive VJ rearrangement in their α locus to express both α and β chains together with the CD3 protein complex on their surface. Because of this developmental sequence of rearrangements, the $\gamma\delta$ TcR is sometimes referred to as TcR-1 and the $\alpha\beta$ TcR as TcR-2.[73] Although the TcR-1 and TcR-2 cells are known to represent separate sublineages, the deciding mechanism for choosing the TcR gene rearrangements is presently unclear. Silencer regions located 3′ to the α and γ gene loci may be involved in the decision making by these cells after a successful α or γ VJ rearrangement event.

Nonproductive rearrangements of the γ loci are frequently observed in cells bearing $\alpha\beta$ TcR. These data, together with observations in TcR transgenic mice, suggest that the process of T-cell maturation begins with rearrangement of γ-chain loci followed by that of δ-chain loci.[74] In nonproductive VJγ rearrangements, thymocytes may begin to rearrange their β-chain genes and then their α-chain genes.

TcR genes usually follow the rule of allelic exclusion in that one of the two alleles encoding for a given TcR chain is productively rearranged, whereas the other remains unrearranged or is rearranged nonproductively. This is best demonstrated for TcR β chains. In the TcR-2 clones, one of the β-chain alleles is productively rearranged, whereas the other allele may be unrearranged, may show an incomplete DJ joining, or may have a nonproductive VDJ rearrangement.[69,71] T cells in transgenic mice that express an exogenous, rearranged copy of a β-chain gene rarely undergo productive rearrangements of the endogenous VDJ_β genes.[72] These data imply that successful rearrangement of one V_β allele makes the rearrangement of the other allele unlikely, so that most T cells express the product of a simple rearranged allelic locus.

Markers of Maturing Thymocytes

T-cell precursors acquire the CD7 antigen prior to entering the thymus and continue to express this cell surface molecule as their progeny begin T-cell development in the

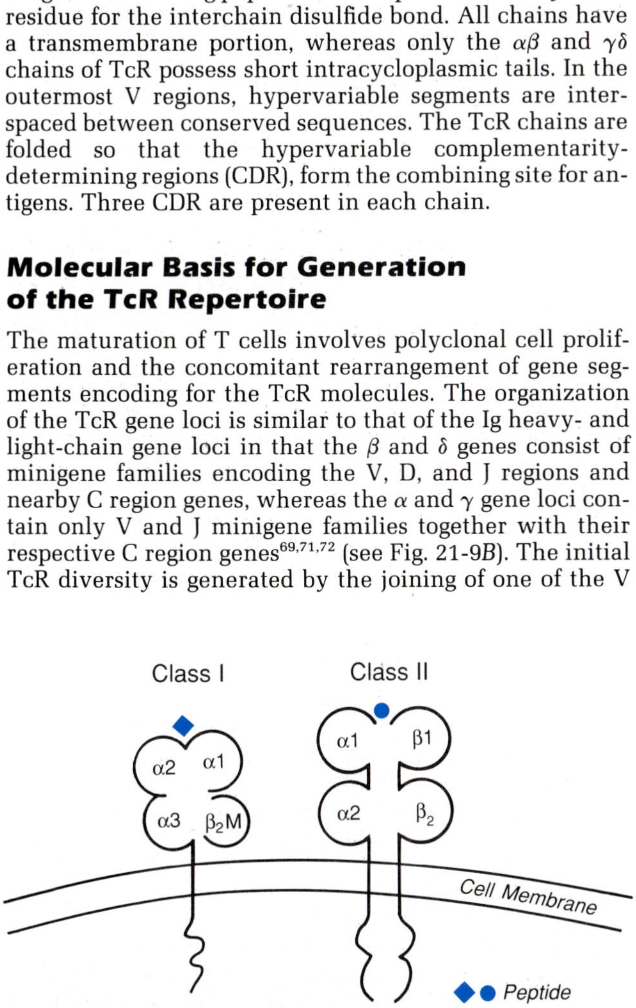

FIGURE 21-10. Class I and II MHC molecules. The groove containing the antigen peptide is indicated.

thymus and complete their life history in the periphery.[67] On entering the thymus, pre–T cells begin the orderly process of maturation characterized by the sequential rearrangement and expression of TcR genes and expression of other genes encoding a diverse spectrum of cell surface glycoproteins. These cell surface molecules can be identified by monoclonal antibodies, which can serve as practical differentiation markers.

Thymocyte maturation is traditionally divided into three distinct stages, each of which is characterized by the expression of a particular combination of markers.[14,67,71] The classic thymocyte maturational stages are those defined for the predominant subpopulation of cells destined to express $\alpha\beta$ TcR/CD3 receptors. (The developmental pattern of $\gamma\delta$ T cells is different and is discussed later in this chapter).

Thymocyte Stage I

Stage I cells express membrane-bound CD7, CD2, and CD5 molecules, and are negative for cell surface TcR/CD3 receptor complexes. Except perhaps early in embryonic life, these cells are also TdT-positive.

Thymocyte Stage II

Most cortical thymocytes, numerically the largest thymocyte subpopulation, represent the stage II maturational stage. This proliferating subpopulation of cells expresses the CD1 thymocyte-specific surface molecule and is TdT-positive. Most cells express both the CD8 and the CD4 markers, CD8 expression being evident before CD4 expression. CD4 is a 55-kd membrane glycoprotein, whereas CD8 is a heterodimer that consists of two distinct polypeptide chains of 30 and 35 kd. Many thymocytes at this stage have already accomplished VDJ_β rearrangements and express the TcR β chain in their cytoplasm. Productive VJ_α rearrangements occur next in a subpopulation of the innermost cortical thymocytes, which then begin to express the TcR-2/CD3 complex of proteins in low levels. Clonal selection begins during this stage in development and involves interactions between both the $\alpha\beta$ TcR and the CD4 and CD8 coreceptors with major histocompatibility complex (MHC) class II or class I molecules, respectively.

Thymocyte Stage III

Higher surface levels of the TcR-2/CD3 expression mark stage III, the final stage of thymocyte maturation by cells that express exclusively either the CD4 or the CD8 accessory molecules.

The cortical development of the TcR-1 cells precedes TcR-2 development as they rearrange and immediately express both γ- and δ-chain genes. Thus, the $\gamma\delta$/CD3 receptor complex is expressed in relatively high levels even on TcR-1 cells in the outer cortex of the thymus. The TcR-1 cells lack both the CD4 and CD8 accessory molecules during their relatively rapid transit through the cortex to enter the medulla and exit via corticomedullary vessels to reach the periphery.[75]

Less than 1% of the TcR-2 cells estimated to be generated in the thymus actually survive to migrate to the periphery. Most of the TcR-2 cells are killed by apoptosis. Programmed cell death may be triggered by encounter with self-antigens and is characterized by an increase in intracellular calcium and DNase activity that fragments the nuclear DNA.[76,77]

Both TcR-1+ and TcR-2+ cells are probably generated throughout life; although the peak of thymopoietic activity is reached during infancy. Because the life-span of peripheral T lymphocytes can be counted in decades, the need for continued thymocyte production normally is not great in adulthood. Information on the precise duration of thymic regenerative capacity is limited, but the atrophic nature of the adult thymus suggests that thymopoietic function is greatly diminished with advancing age.

Antigen Recognition by T Cells

T cells do not recognize intact proteins as antigens. Instead, they recognize short peptide fragments of the partially degraded antigen that are presented on the surface of specialized antigen-presenting cells. Through their TcR, T cells recognize the foreign peptides in the groove of cell surface molecules encoded by genes of the MHC.[70,78,79] The two types of MHC-encoded molecules are called class I and class II molecules (Fig. 21-10). Class I molecules, expressed by virtually all cell types, are formed by two noncovalently linked polypeptide chains of 45 and 11 kd, respectively. The heavier chain is encoded by MHC class I genes on chromosome 6, whereas the smaller chain, B_2 microglobulin, is encoded by a gene located on chromosome 15. Three different and closely linked loci on the short arm of chromosome 6 encode the class I molecule heavy chain. These loci, defined as HLA-A, HLA-B, and HLA-C, encode the corresponding HLA (human leukocyte antigen) membrane antigens. The HLA-A, HLA-B, and HLA-C loci are highly polymorphic in that multiple alleles at each locus account for a large number of serologically identifiable molecules in humans.[80]

Class II molecules are constitutively expressed on a limited number of cell types. They are composed of two noncovalently linked peptide chains of 33 kd (α chains) and 28 kd (β chains). Human class II molecules are encoded by genes located at three closely linked regions (DP, DR, DQ) near the HLA-A, HLA-B, and HLA-C loci. Each of these loci contains genes that encode one or more α or β chains. The general rule is that α and β chains encoded by neighboring genes are coordinately transcribed to yield a complete class II molecule termed HLA-DP, HLA-DR, or HLA-DQ.[80] Because of the large number of alleles at each locus, class II molecules are highly polymorphic. Since heterozygosity at these loci is typical in man, additional phenotypic polymorphism is generated by the random combination of the α chains encoded in a given locus with the β chains encoded by a gene on the homologous or allelic chromosome.

Peptide fragments of the antigens are bound within a groove on the exposed surface of the MHC molecule, thereby allowing the TcR to bind both the antigen peptide and the self MHC molecule. An important rule of this T-cell recognition is that T cells can recognize antigens that are presented by autologous antigen-presenting cells, but not by allogeneic antigen-presenting cells.[4,12,69–71] Partial MHC homology between T cells and antigen-presenting cells can be sufficient for successful antigen presentation. This associative recognition is often referred to as *cognate recognition* or *MHC restriction*.

Some T cells can recognize antigens only in association with class II molecules, whereas others preferentially recognize antigens in combination with class I molecules.[69,71] T cells restricted for class II molecules express the CD4 marker, together with the $\alpha\beta$ TcR. Cells that are restricted for class I molecules express the CD8 surface marker. In mature T cells, expression of the CD4 or CD8 accessory molecules is mutually exclusive. These two molecules are closely involved in the process of class I (CD8)- or class II (CD4)- restricted antigen recognition by $\alpha\beta$ TcR+ cells. The CD4 molecule functions as a coreceptor by binding to the MHC class II molecule on the antigen-presenting cell, whereas the CD8 molecule has an affinity for class I molecules. Although these rules have been defined for the TcR-2+ cells, the expression of CD8 by TcR-1+ cells in the peripheral lymphoid tissues suggests that these may preferentially recognize peptide fragments in association with class I or class I–like cell surface molecules.

The cells that present antigen to class II–restricted, CD4+ cells possess high concentrations of membrane class II molecules, have a well-developed lysosomal apparatus, and are capable of causing phagocytosis or pinocytosis of soluble antigens. These are typical properties of macrophage–monocytes and of other antigen-presenting cells, including Langerhans cells, interdigitating cells, and dendritic cells. B cells also serve as antigen-presenting cells. They constitutively express class II molecules and bind antigens by means of their membrane-bound antibody receptors. Other cells may occasionally serve as antigen-presenting cells. An example is intestinal epithelial cells that can be induced by interferon-γ (IFN-γ) to express membrane class II molecules. Thus, for the epithelial cell, an inflammatory stimulus is required to initiate IFN-γ production.[78,79]

In antigen-presenting cells, the α and β chains of the class II molecules are assembled in the endoplasmic reticulum where a third chain, the γ (invariant) chain, is added to the molecular complex. The γ chain prevents the binding of peptides to the $\alpha\beta$-chain dimers and facilitates their transport to the endocytic pathway. From the endoplasmic reticulum, the $\alpha\beta\gamma$-chain complex is transported to the endosome compartment through the Golgi and the trans-Golgi reticulum. In the endosomes, the γ chain is degraded, thus allowing the $\alpha\beta$ class II dimers to bind the endocytosed antigenic peptides.[81]

The predigested peptides and class II molecules have a slow association rate, but after these complexes are formed they are highly stable, allowing transport to the outer cell membrane. Endogenous as well as exogenous peptides can be similarly processed and presented on MHC class II molecules to the CD4+ T cells. This is true for virally coded proteins synthesized within an infected cell, antigens of parasites harbored within the cell cytoplasm, or even self-antigens.[81,82]

There are several differences in the mode of antigen presentation to class I–restricted, CD8+ T cells:

1. Class I molecules are expressed by virtually all types of cells (therefore, any nucleated cell is a potential antigen-presenting cell).
2. Class I–restricted CD8+ T cells exert primarily a cytotoxic function against virally infected or neoplastic cells.
3. The antigenic peptide to be associated with the class I molecule is almost always produced by the antigen-presenting cell itself.
4. In the cell that serves the function of antigen-presenting cell, cytoplasmic proteins are degraded into peptides by proteasomes, multimolecular structures with proteolytic activity, some components of which are encoded by genes located in the MHC (LMP genes). The resulting peptides bind to transporter molecules encoded by MHC genes (Tap 1 and Tap 2 genes), which serve to transport the peptides into the lumen of the endoplasmic reticulum where they bind to class I molecules. Class I molecules loaded with peptides are subsequently exported to the cell surface.[82,83]

Besides the CD4, CD8, and MHC molecules, other cell surface structures have been shown to be involved in the interaction between the T cell and the antigen-presenting cell. These include molecules such as LFA-3 or CD2 that enhance cell-to-cell adhesion, as well as the LFA-1 and ICAM-1 molecular interaction. In the collaborative interaction between CD4+ T cells and antigen-presenting B cells, the responding T cell expresses the CD40 ligand, which binds to the CD40 molecule on the B cell to deliver essential activation signals. In turn, the activated B cell expresses the CD80 antigen that interacts with the CD28 molecule on the T cell. This elicits an essential second signal that allows the T cell to escape the anergic state and to respond positively to the antigen.

Negative and Positive Selection of T Cells in the Thymus

The negative and positive selection processes that take place within the thymus during thymocyte development are well documented for TcR-2+ cells, but not for TcR-1+ cells.[45,46,74,84]

Elimination of self-reactive clones by an apoptotic mechanism is shown most clearly by experiments in transgenic mice.[74] Mice have been made transgenic by the insertion of genes encoding TcR α and β chains that have specificity for the Y antigen selectively expressed by male cells. In such female transgenic mice, a large proportion of thymocytes at various stages of maturation, as well as the peripheral T cells express the anti–Y antigen TcR. By contrast, in male transgenic mice, the same TcR is detected on many thymocytes, but not on peripheral T cells. These findings indicate that autoreactive (anti–Y antigen) T cells have been selectively eliminated when encountered with the Y antigen during intrathymic maturation.

Positive selection favors the survival of T cells capable of cognate recognition and contributes to the elimination of cells that lack this property. The process of positive selection is dependent on two variables: the binding capacity of the TcR expressed by T cells and the peptide-loaded MHC molecules encountered by T cells during maturation. Because of the polymorphism within MHC molecules, each individual has its own set of MHC molecules, and the T cells that mature in the thymus of that particular individual learn to recognize antigenic peptides only in conjunction with self MHC molecules.

A second aspect of positive T-cell selection involves expression of the CD4 or CD8 molecules that enhance the bonding between the TcR and the MHC molecule–antigenic determinant complex. The expression of CD4 or CD8 molecules by a given cell is dictated by the type of restriction of its TcR. This principle can be demonstrated in transgenic mice.[74] In mice made transgenic by transferring the α and β chain coding genes from a murine T-cell clone that is CD8-positive and class I–restricted, all of the T cells that express the transgenic TcR, besides having the same antigenic specificity and MHC restriction of the clone that served as gene donor, also express CD8 molecules. This selection process begins in the population of intermediate thymocytes that express TcR plus both the CD4 and CD8 coreceptors, and it results in the development of restricted subpopulations of mature CD4+ and CD8+ cells.

T-Cell Proliferation

In the peripheral lymphoid organs, the activation and proliferation of appropriate T-cell clones are initiated by encounter with the antigen-presenting cell bearing the appropriate peptide fragment. The interaction between the TcR and the MHC-antigenic peptide triggers the T-cell activation process.[60,85]

Antigen binding to the TcR/CD3 receptor complex leads to activation of several tyrosine kinases, including those of the Src family, such as lck and fyn.[60,86–88] Tyrosine kinase activation initiated through the TcR is followed by phosphatidylinositol turnover and Ca^{2+} mobilization. The activation of tyrosine kinases leads to the phosphorylation of many intracellular substrates, including the CD3 ζ chain, CD4, CD8, CD5, and phospholipase C, to initiate a cascade of events leading to T-cell activation. These events can be mimicked in vitro by treatment of T cells with anti-TcR antibodies that cross-link the TcR molecules. Insolubilized anti-CD3 monoclonal antibodies and plant lectins, such as phytohemagglutinin and concanavalin A, which bind to membrane glycoproteins, also deliver activation signals and cause cell proliferation. Certain bacterial toxins and viral components can form bridges between T cells and antigen-presenting cells. These substances, called "superantigens," do not require processing, as they bind directly to class II molecules outside the cleft used for peptide presentation. Superantigens bind to the TcR outside the antigen combining site but have specificity for certain V_β gene products. Thus, the superantigens can induce the proliferation of selected families of T cells.[89]

IL-1 that is produced by the antigen-presenting cell (APC) and other T-cell–APC interaction molecules are involved in the transmission of signals to the cell. Both resting and activated T cells have surface receptors for IL-1. Interaction between the surface receptor and IL-1 may be essential for the T cells to enter the cell cycle.[90] The signal delivered by IL-1 contributes to phosphokinase C activation, which is instrumental in inducing both the synthesis of IL-2 and of IL-2 receptors. IL-1 plays a major role in initiating inflammatory reactions and acute phase responses, and its participation in T-cell stimulation ensures that immune responses are initiated together with a more generalized reaction of the organism to the insulting agent. IL-6 and TNF-α, which share some of the inflammatory properties of IL-1, may also promote T-cell responses.

In addition to the high-affinity IL-2 receptor, activated T cells express other markers such as class II molecules, the transferrin receptor (CD71), and the CD26, CD30, CD38, and CD69 antigens.[85] The activated T cell does not enter the DNA synthesis phase of the cell cycle unless it receives the signal delivered by IL-2. IL-2 is produced by a subpopulation of appropriately stimulated CD4+ T cells, which may govern the growth of a neighboring T cell, such as a CD8+ T_C cell, or a B cell. The ordered expression of the IL-2 receptors (IL-2R) and the release of IL-2 thus regulate to a large extent the final step leading to T-cell proliferation and differentiation.[88]

The IL-2R is made up by several subunits, termed α, β, and γ. IL-2Rα, a polypeptide chain of 55 kd that is recognized by CD25 monoclonal antibody, is also known as the *low-affinity IL-2R*. IL-2Rβ, known as the *intermediate affinity IL-2R*, is a polypeptide chain of about 75 kd, which is constitutively expressed by a number of T cells. IL-2Rγ, the most recently recognized member of this complex, is a polypeptide chain of 54 kd that forms another essential part of the IL-2 binding cell surface complex.[88]

IL-2Rα is not expressed by most resting T cells, and its absence precludes expression of high-affinity IL-2R. Because the IL-2Rα gene is highly inducible, it plays a major role in the dynamic expression of high-affinity IL-2R. The regulator nucleotide sequences upstream of the IL-2Rα gene include binding sites for NF-κB (nuclear factor-κ B), NF-AT (nuclear factor–activating T), and other nuclear proteins that can influence transcription of the appropriate T-cell genes.

The initial polyclonal proliferation of immature thymocytes is dependent on non–TcR/CD3 initiated signals. One of the important receptors for immature thymocytes is the 50-kd CD2 molecule by which they interact with the 60-kd LFA-3 glycoprotein on thymic epithelial cells. This surface structure is traditionally known as the *sheep erythrocyte receptor*. Cross-linkage of the thymocyte CD2 receptor induces the activation process characterized by increased phosphatidylinositol turnover, Ca^{2+} mobilization, and phosphokinase C activation.[91] Unlike thymocytes, mature T cells cannot be induced to proliferate by ligands that bind to CD2. However, signals delivered via surface CD2 can amplify the responses of mature T cells stimulated through different pathways. Activated thymocytes may also receive signals delivered by IL-1, IL-2, IL-4, IL-7, TNF-α, and other cytokines that may be involved in regulating thymocyte growth and maturation.[67] Thymic epithelial cells may release several thymic hormones, the precise function of which is still unknown.

Markers of Virgin and Memory T Cells

Antigen priming causes changes in the expression of certain surface molecules of T cells.[92] On leaving the thymus, virgin T cells express high levels of a 200- to 220-kd surface glycoprotein, an isoform of a molecular structure known as the common leukocyte antigen that is recognized by CD45RA antibodies. Memory T cells express little CD45RA but express a different isoform (180 kd) of the same antigen that is recognized by the CD45RO antibody. This switch in gene products is the consequence of a change in RNA splicing of transcripts from the same gene. The availability of such surface markers has led to the definition of other properties of both virgin and memory T cells. For example, memory T cells can be more easily stimulated through their TcR/CD3 and CD2 receptors without the requirement of exogenous IL-2 for cell proliferation.[93]

Notably, most immature thymocytes have a memory T-cell phenotype (CD45RA low; CD45RO high), and these either die or revert to the virgin phenotype as they mature to leave the thymus.

T-Cell Kinetics

The thymus is colonized by waves of hematopoietic precursors derived first from the fetal liver, beginning around the seventh to eighth week of gestation, and later from the bone marrow. These CD7+ cells migrate through the perithymic mesenchyme to enter the epithelial thymus anlage and to begin their proliferation and differentiation as T cells.[67] Successive waves of precursor cells are attracted by chemotactic peptides produced by the thymic epithelium. In lower vertebrates, and presumably in humans, each wave of progeny T cells requires approximately 3 weeks to progress through the thymus selection and maturation process before seeding to the peripheral lymphoid tissues. As long as the thymus retains its lymphoid nature, it is assumed to continue to receive precursor cells and produce their T-cell progeny.

Mature T cells leave the thymus by means of the circulation to seed the peripheral lymphoid organs.[94,95] The initial postthymic T-cell pool thus consists of cells produced in the thymus; in subsequent periods, both thymic output and self-renewal of peripheral T cells are responsible for the maintenance of peripheral T cells. The contribution of memory T cells is indicated by the progressive accumulation of CD45RO T cells in the circulation and peripheral lymphoid tissues as a function of age. The peripheral T-cell pool in adult humans is estimated to contain more than 10^{11} cells, most of which are long-lived. The thymus appears to show little lymphopoietic activity in adults, and its removal does not result in significant alteration of the peripheral T-cell pool, consistent with the idea that, after it is filled, the peripheral T-cell pool is self-maintained for several decades.

T-Cell Subpopulations

The two major subpopulations of TcR-2 cells are the T_H and T_C cells. T_H cells recognize antigens in conjunction with class II molecules, express membrane CD4, and release lymphokines that help to induce B-cell responses, other T-cell responses, the inflammatory response of nonlymphoid cells, and the process of hematopoiesis.

Whereas virgin T cells can produce a variety of cytokines on stimulation with antigen (or mitogen), memory T cells tend to become specialized in producing either inflammatory lymphokines (ie, IL-2 and IFN-γ) or lymphokines that act primarily on B-cell growth or differentiation (IL-4, IL-5, IL-6, and IL-10). According to the current nomenclature, T cells that produce IFN-γ and IL-2 are called T_H1 cells, whereas those producing IL-4 and IL-5 are called T_H2 cells. T cells that are not specialized to produce a particular lymphokine group are termed T_H0 cells.[96,97]

T_C cells express CD8 and are restricted for the recognition of peptides presented within the groove of class I molecules. After appropriate antigenic stimulation, T_C cells acquire a cytoplasmic granular apparatus containing acid hydrolases and other substances that can result in lysis of their target cells. This cytotoxic apparatus is similar to that of NK cells. The target cells of T_C lymphocytes can be virus-infected or malignant cells. Cells infected with parasites or altered by contact with certain chemicals may also represent suitable targets. T_C cells are generally poor producers of lymphokines and may require T_H cells for their activation and proliferation.[12,13,98]

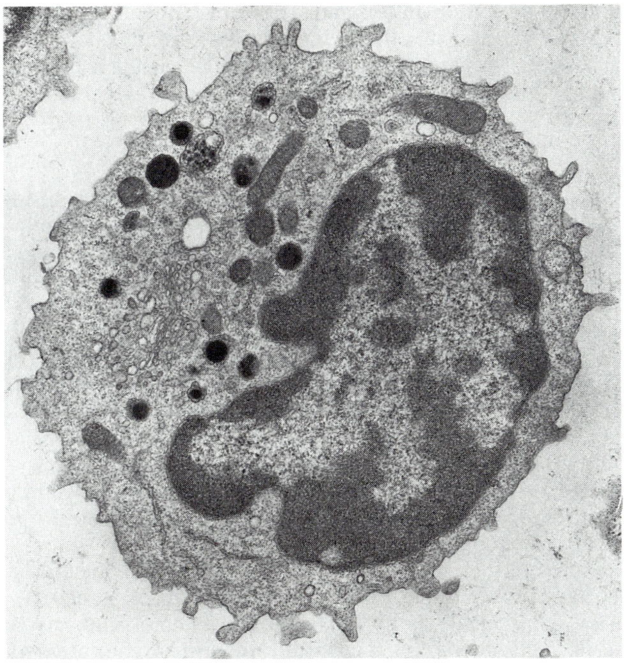

FIGURE 21-11. Ultrastructural features of a large granular lymphocyte.

NATURAL KILLER CELLS

Natural killer cells were first identified by their spontaneous capacity to kill virus-infected cells or neoplastic cells in the absence of a previous priming exposure.[16,99] Other functional characteristics are the absence of obvious clonal distribution, an ability to bind to cell targets by means of structures other than Ig molecules or TcR, and a lack of MHC–antigen restriction for target specificity. NK cells are now defined as a special cell type with distinctive morphology and cell surface antigen profile. NK cells lack the T-cell and B-cell antigens such as CD3, CD19, and CD20, and they do not react with monoclonal antibodies specific for most antigens on macrophage–monocytes. NK cells express the CD56 and CD16 antigens. CD56 defines an isoform of the neural adhesion molecule N-CAM.[100] CD16 recognizes the IgG Fc receptor (FcRγIII), which is present on most NK cells.[16] CD16 is also expressed by most granulocytes and by resident macrophages.

A subset of circulating CD8+ T_c cells expresses both CD16 and CD56, and the IL-2Rβ.[101] These cells may represent the normal counterpart of the aberrant population of cells in patients with the so-called large granular lymphocyte lymphocytosis.

The NK cells contain azurophilic, electron-dense intracytoplasmic granules that confer their typical granular lymphocyte morphology[102] (Fig. 21-11). These granules contain acid hydrolases but are negative for peroxidase, another feature that distinguishes them from monocytes. NK cells have also been called *large granular lymphocytes* (LGL), and the terms LGL and NK cells are used interchangeably. Since a proportion of both CD4+ and CD8+ cells and most T_cR1+ cells have an LGL morphology (without NK cell activity), the unqualified definition of NK cells as LGL may be misleading.

NK cells are also derived from hematopoietic stem cells (see Figs. 21-1 and 21-7) and represent a distinctive lineage of bone marrow–derived cells. NK cells constitute about 5% to 15% of the circulating lymphocytes. Marginally higher proportions of these cells may be found in the spleen, whereas mature NK cells are virtually absent from the lymph nodes, bone marrow, and thymus.

The relevance of the cytotoxic function of NK cells for survival is indicated by several observations.[99] In experimental animals, the survival of tumor transplants and their metastatic spread are enhanced by treatments that suppress NK-cell function. Treatment of animals with antibodies to NK cells also increases susceptibility to viral infections. In humans with the Chédiak-Higashi syndrome and in beige mice, where the cytotoxic functions of NK cells are impaired because of an abnormality of granule formation,[103] a higher incidence of lymphoproliferative disorders is found. NK cells seem to confer special protection against hematopoietic malignancies, in keeping with the fact that NK cells manifest relatively efficient cytotoxicity against cells of hematopoietic lineages.[104]

NK cells may also regulate the growth of hematopoietic cell lineages by the production of soluble factors that promote the growth of erythroid and myeloid cells. An example is their production of granulocyte-macrophage colony-stimulating factor.[104,105] After stimulation with NK-sensitive target cells, NK cells may also release factors that inhibit hematopoiesis. One such factor has been identified as the TNF.[104,105] Therefore, in addition to their primary role in host defense, NK cells may function to regulate the growth of hematopoietic cells and to eliminate aberrant cells that may arise in the course of hematopoietic differentiation.

LYMPHOCYTES AS CYTOTOXIC EFFECTOR CELLS

Mechanisms of Lymphocyte Cytotoxicity

The selective destruction of nucleated cells is primarily accomplished by T_C and NK cells, two cell types that share the same cytotoxic machinery.[106] The lysis of target cells is the end result of an ordered sequence of events: (1) target cell recognition, (2) effector cell–target cell adhesion, and (3) lysis of the target cell. The effector cell itself is not destroyed and can move on in search of a new target cell.

Target Cell Recognition

Target cell recognition is accomplished by the interaction between exterior membrane structures of the cytotoxic lymphocytes that are complementary to surface molecules on the target cell. T_C cells recognize molecules on the surface of the target by means of specific $\alpha\beta$ or $\gamma\delta$ TcR. Antibody molecules, primarily those of IgG classes, may also serve as recognition elements. The antibody molecules do this by binding first to antigens on the target cell surface, then, by means of their Fc portion, to the NK cell or a T_C cell bearing Fc receptors.[107] This mode of cytotoxicity is defined as antibody-dependent cell-mediated cytotoxicity, or ADCC. NK cells may also recognize their targets in the absence of such opsonizing antibodies. This recognition process is mediated by NK-cell surface structures that are complementary to surface molecules of virus-infected or malignant cells. The nature of these recognition structures is still imprecisely defined. The membrane molecules used by NK cells for target recognition may also be expressed by activated T cells, since certain T-cell lines can bind to and kill a variety of NK-sensitive targets.[108–110]

Notably, target cell recognition by NK cells is also regulated in a "negative" manner (i.e., NK cells fail to kill target cells that express particular surface molecules). For example, the expression of HLA-molecules, particularly of those encoded by the HLA-C locus, inhibits the killing of a given target by autologous NK cells. This mechanism ensures that normal target cells are not damaged by NK cells, while malignant cells that often fail to express HLA-molecules can be eliminated.[111]

Adhesion of Cytotoxic Cells to Target Cells

The effector cells adhere to their targets to form stable conjugates and to activate the lytic process. Adhesion structures on the effector cells include molecules of the β_2 integrin family: LFA-1, the CR2 receptor for the C3b fragment of complement, and the p150,95 complex.[112] These structures are heterodimers that share a β_2 chain of 95 kd in common, but each contains a distinctive α chain. The common β_2 chain is recognized by CD18 antibodies. The LFA-1 α chain, a 180-kd glycoprotein, is recognized by CD11a antibodies. The α chain of CR2 has a mass of 170 kd and reacts with CD11b antibodies. p150,90 has an α chain of 150 kd, which is recognized by CD11c antibodies. All of these α chains are encoded by closely linked genes located on the short arm of chromosome 16. LFA-1 has complementarity for the intercellular adhesion molecule-1 or ICAM-1 (CD54), a glycosylated structure usually found on the targets of cytotoxic lymphocytes. p150,90 and CR2 appear to be less important in the cytotoxic reactions.

The CD2 molecule on T_C and NK cells is also an important adhesion molecule that can bind to LFA-3 molecules on the target cells. Antibodies to these complementary adhesion structures inhibit cell cytotoxicity, and the absence of these adhesion structures on neoplastic cells may correlate with their enhanced growth and metastasis.[112] On binding to their ligands, the adhesion molecules may also transmit activation signals to the cytotoxic cells. For example, antibodies to CD2 may induce the release of cytotoxic elements and cell proliferation.[113]

These cell adhesion structures may also play a role in the process of lymphocyte activation by antigens, by facilitating the binding of T cells to the antigen-presenting cell.[114] This role is best demonstrated by observations in patients with lymphocyte adhesion deficiency, which is featured by the absence of the LFA-1 family of membrane molecules due to the failure to express the shared β_2 chain. This genetic defect results in impaired immune responsiveness, phagocytic inefficiency, and cytotoxic lymphocyte impairment.[115]

Target Cell Killing

After the formation of effector–target cell conjugates, exocytosis of the granule content of the cytotoxic cell occurs at those sites of close contact between targets and effectors. This allows elements in the granules to bind to the target cell membrane to form pores that cause cell death through osmotic lysis. The term *perforins* refers to the molecules in the granules that are responsible for pore formation.[106] In the granules, perforins are found in monomeric form, but after secretion they are polymerized in the presence of Ca^{2+}. These polymers form transmembrane pores in the target cell membrane similar to those formed by the ninth component of activated complement with which they share antigenic and structural similarities. The granules of cytotoxic lymphocytes also contain at least two serine esterases that may participate in the cytotoxic process.[116]

Potentiation of Cytotoxic Activities

IFN-γ and IL-1α (NKSF)[117] are two of the cytokines that can potentiate NK-cell function. Because NK cells are responsive to IL-2, it is possible to expand NK cells from a cancer patient in culture and to reinfuse them into the same patient. Regression of tumor masses has been obtained in some patients on infusion of these cells together with IL-2.[118] NK cells activated by IL-2 are called *lymphokine-activated killer (LAK) cells.* Besides their powerful cytotoxic potential, LAK cells may display a broader range of target cell specificity than do ordinary NK cells.[119] Certain subpopulations of T_C cells may also respond to IL-2 to become LAK cells. These T cells may include subsets of $\gamma\delta$ TcR+ cells and CD8+ $\alpha\beta$ TcR+ cells, which express the CD11b antigen and other cell surface molecules shared by NK cells.[120,121]

IMMUNE RESPONSE

The immune response takes place primarily in the peripheral lymphoid organs where antigen is taken up by the antigen-presenting cells. Recognition of the processed antigen by T cells leads to a clonal expansion of activated T cells, which release lymphokines that subserve several functions. First, the T cells and their lymphokine products contribute to the induction of a local reaction, which is instrumental in recruiting more immunocompetent cells in the site. Second, they activate neighboring macrophages to begin disposition of the antigen and to release their cytokines with inflammatory functions. Third, the activated T cells provide help for antigen-reactive B cells, inducing them to proliferate and differentiate into antibody-producing plasma cells.

After contact with antigen, some activated cells may leave the lymphoid tissues where the response originated and seed to other lymphoid sites, ensuring generalized protection. B cells thus differentiate into plasma cells in the red pulp of the spleen, in the medullary cords of the lymph nodes, in the bone marrow, in the mucosal lamina propria, and in the connective interstitium of other organs.

During B-cell proliferation and differentiation in germinal centers, somatic mutations and selection by antigen lead to an increased antibody affinity, and isotype switches also take place. Not all the cells undergo terminal differentiation outside of the germinal centers, and an expansion of these memory B cells during a primary response ensures a more rapid response and prompt activation of effector mechanisms on a second challenge with the same antigen.

A timely inhibition of the immune response is required if excessive antibody and lymphokine production or unwanted side effects, such as autoimmunity, deposition of immune complexes, and amyloid formation, are to be avoided. Several mechanisms participate in the regulation and eventual termination of a successful immune response. The production of high-affinity antibodies causes feedback inhibition by competing with the immunocompetent cells for antigens and by binding to their Fc receptor to elicit a negative signal.[66] As a consequence, competent cells may receive progressively fewer stimulatory signals. Antigen opsonization by antibodies also contributes to its removal by Fc receptor–bearing cells of the phagocyte system. T_C lymphocytes may contribute to the inhibition of an ongoing response by attacking other cells involved in the response. The lymphokines produced during the immune response are rapidly degraded, preventing them from reaching physiologically significant levels at distant sites. Moreover, certain lymphokines released by activated T_H cells such as IL-10 have the capacity to inhibit lymphokine production by other T cells, thus contributing to the inhibition of an ongoing response.[122]

Several sophisticated models have been proposed to explain the fine tuning and termination of the immune response. One such model postulates that antibodies produced in the course of the response become antigenic for the immune system.[123–125] This is possible since the antibody combining site is unique for each antibody produced, and the immune system does not become tolerant to it. The antigenic determinants of the antibody-combining site are called *idiotypes*.[123] In the course of a response to antigen, the increasing concentration of a given antibody induces an antiidiotypic response, the function of which would be that of modulating the first response. The same theoretical approach might be used for the TcR expressed by T-cell clones arising during the immune response, by postulating the production of anti-TcR antiidiotypic antibodies or the existence of anti-TcR cell–mediated responses.

Regulation by means of idiotypic recognition could exert either a positive or a negative influence. For example, antiidiotypic antibodies could bind to the B-cell surface Ig to deliver an activation signal or, by additionally binding to an Fc γ receptor on the B cell, a negative signal. T_c cells with specificity for degradation fragments of TcR or surface Ig could eliminate the relevant T or B cells. Extension of this model suggests that the antiidiotypic responses are in turn regulated by anti-antiidiotypic responses. This network hypothesis postulates the existence of a complex network of both humoral and cell-mediated reactions, with the aim of fine tuning the immune system.

The idea that T cells with suppressor functions play a major role in terminating the immune response is no longer fashionable because it has not been possible to identify specific suppressor factors or to distinguish cells with putative suppressor function among the T cells.[126] Immune suppression could be a function of T_c cells, which can eliminate any type of cell that goes through endocytosis and presents the relevant antigenic peptide.

REFERENCES

1. Nossal GJV. The basic components of the immune system. N Engl J Med 1987;316:1320.
2. Mitchell GF, Miller JFAP. Cell-to cell interaction in the immune response. II. The source of hemolysin-forming cells in irradiated mice given bone marrow and thymus or thoracic duct lymphocytes. J Exp Med 1968;128, 821.
3. Peterson RD, Cooper MD, Good RA. The pathogenesis of immunologic deficiency diseases. Am J Med 1965;38:579.
4. Paul WE, Benacerraf B. Functional specificity of thymus-dependent lymphocytes. Science 1977;195:1293.
5. Cooper MD. Pre-B cells: normal and abnormal development. J Clin Immunol 1981;1:81.
6. Howard JC, Hunt SV, Gowans JL. Identification of marrow-derived and thymus-derived small lymphocytes in the lymphoid tissue and thoracic duct lymph of normal rats. J Exp Med 1972;135:200.
7. Chestnut RW, Grey HN. Antigen presenting cells and mechanisms of antigen presentation. CRC Crit Rev Immunol 1985;5:263.
8. Burnet FM. The clonal selection theory of acquired immunity. Nashville, Vanderbilt University Press, 1959.
9. Billingham RE, Brent L, Medawar PB. Actively acquired tolerance of foreign cells. Nature 1953;172:603.
10. Jerne NK. The generative grammar of the immune system. Science 1985;229:1057.
11. Kishimoto T, Hirano T. Molecular regulation of B lymphocyte response. Annu Rev Immunol 1988;6:513.
12. Zinkernagel RM, Doherty PC. MHC-restricted cytotoxic cells: studies on the biological role of polymorphic major transplantation antigens determining T-cell restriction-specificity, function and responsiveness. Adv Immunol 1979;25:51.
13. Cerottini JC, Brunner KT. Cell-mediated cytotoxicity, allograft rejection, and tumor immunity. Adv Immunol 1974;18:67.
14. Reinherz E, Shlossman S. The differentiation and function of human T lymphocytes. Cell 1980;3:113.
15. Paul WE. Pleiotropy and redundancy: T cell–derived lymphokines in the immune response. Cell 1989;57:521.
16. Trinchieri G. Biology of natural killer cells. Adv Immunol 1989;47: 187.
17. Cooper MD. The B lymphocyte: normal development and function. N Engl J Med 1987;317:1452.
18. Osmond DG. Population dynamics of bone marrow B lymphocytes. Immunol Rev 1986;93:102.
19. Tonegawa S. Somatic generation of antibody diversity. Nature 1983;302: 575.
20. Leder P. The genetic of antibody diversity. Sci Am 1982;246:72.
21. Alt FW, Blackwell TK, Jancopoulos GD. Development of the primary antibody repertoire. Science 1987;238:1079.
22. Moller G, ed. Role of somatic mutation in the generation of lymphocyte diversity. Immunol Rev 1987;96:1.
23. Kincade PW. Experimental models for understaining B lymphocyte formation. Adv Immunol 1987;41;181.
24. Edelman GM. CAMs and Igs: cell adhesion and the evolutionary origins of immunity. Immunol Rev 1987;100:11.
25. Namen AE, Schmeirer AE, March CJ, et al. B cell precursor growth promoting activity. J Exp Med 1988;167:988.
26. Schatz DG, Oettinger MA, Baltimore D. The V(D)J recombination activating gene, RAG1. Cell 1989;59:1035.
27. Schuler W, Weiler IJ, Schuler A, et al. Rearrangement of antigen receptor genes is defective in mice with severe combined immunodeficiency. Cell 1986;46:963.
28. Oettinger MA, Schatz DG, Gorka C, Baltimore D. RAG-1 and RAG-2, adjacent genes that synergistically activate VDJ recombination. Science 1990;248:1517.
29. McCaffrey R, Harrison TA, Parkman R, Baltimore D. Terminal deoxynucleotidyl transferase activity in human leukemic cells and in normal human thymocytes. N Engl J Med 1975;292:775.
30. Greenwood MF, Coleman MS, Hutton JJ, et al. Terminal deoxynucleotidyl transferase distribution in neoplastic and hematopoietic cells. J Clin Invest 1977;59:889.
31. Hieter PA, Korsmeyer SJ, Waldmann TA, Leder P. Human Ig K light chain genes are detected or rearranged in λ producing B cells. Nature 1981;290:368.
32. Korsmeyer SJ, Hieter PA, Ravech JV, Poplack DG, Waldmann TA, Leder P. Developmental hierarchy of immunoglobulin gene rearrangements in human leukemic pre-B cells. Proc Natl Acad Sci USA 1981;78:7096.
33. Pernis B, Chiappino G, Kelus AS, Gell PGH. Cellular localization of immunoglobulins with different allotypic specificities in rabbit lymphoid tissues. J Exp Med 1965;122:853.
34. Natvig JB, Kunkel HG. Immunoglobulins: classes, subclasses, genetic variants and idiotypes. Adv Immunol 1973;16:1.
35. Early E, Hood L. Allelic exclusion and non productive immunoglobulin gene rearrangements. Cell 1981;24:1.
36. Calame K. Mechanisms that regulate Ig gene expression. Annu Rev Immunol 1985;3:159.
37. Cook GP, Mason JO, Neuberger MS. Immunoglobulin gene expression. In: Calabi F, Neuberger MS, eds. Molecular genetics of immunoglobulins. New Comprehensive Biochemistry 17. Amsterdam, Elsevier, 1988.
38. Early P, Rogers J, Davis M, et al. Two mRNAs can be produced from a single immunoglobulin μ gene by alternative RNA processing pathways. Cell 1980;20;313.
39. Hendershot LM, Bole D, Kearney JF. The role of immunoglobulin heavy

chain binding protein in immunoglobulin transport. Immunol Today 1987;8:111.
40. Gething M-J, Sambrook J. Transport and assembly processes in the endoplasmic reticulum. Semin Cell Biol 1990;1:65.
41. Pillai S, Baltimore D. Formation of disulphide-linked μ_2-ω_2 tetramers in pre-B cells by the 18 Kd ω Ig light chains. Nature 1987;329:172.
42. Sakaguchi N, Melchers F. λ_5, a new light chain–related locus selectively expressed in pre-B lymphocytes. Nature 1986;324:579.
43. Cooper MD, Kearney JF, Gathings WE, Lawton AR. Effects of anti Ig antibodies on the development and differentiation of B cells. Immunol Rev 1980;52:29.
44. Shimizu A, Honjo T. Immunoglobulin class switching. Cell 1984;36: 801.
45. Nossal GJV. Immunologic tolerance: collaboration between antigen and lymphokines. Science 1989;245:147.
46. Schwartz RH. Acquisition of immunologic self-tolerance. Cell 1989;57: 1073.
47. Goodnow CC, Crosbie J, Jorgensen H, Brink RA, Basten A. Induction of self tolerance in mature peripheral B lymphocytes. Nature 1989;342;84.
48. Perlmutter RH, Kearney JF, Chang SP, Hood LE. Developmentally controlled expression of Ig V_H genes. Science 1985;227:1597.
49. Bona CA. V genes encoding autoantibodies: molecular and phenotypic characteristics. Annu Rev Immunol 1988;6:327.
50. Casali P, Notkins AL. CD5+ B lymphocytes, polyreactive antibodies and the human B cell repertoire. Immunol Today 1989;10:364.
51. Kipps TJ. The CD5 B cell. Adv Immunol 1989;47:117.
52. Kantor AB. The development and repertoire of B-1 cells (CD5 B cells). Immunol Today 1991;12:389.
53. Greaves MF, Grossi CE, Ferrarini M, Jaffe ES, Zucker-Franklin D. The lymphocytes. In: Zucker-Franklin D, Greaves MF, Grossi CE, Marmont AM, eds. Atlas of blood cells: function and pathology. Philadelphia, Lea & Febiger, 1988.
54. Greaves MF, Hariri G, Newman RA, Sutherland DR, Ritter MA, Ritz J. Selective expression of the common acute lymphoblastic leukemia (gp100) antigen on immature lymphoid cells and their malignant counterparts. Blood 1983;61:628.
55. Letarte M, Vera S, Tran R, et al. Common acute lymphocytic leukemia antigen is identical to neutral endopeptidase. J Exp Med 1988;168: 1247.
56. Tedder TF, Clement LT, Cooper MD. Human lymphocyte differentiation antigens HB-10 and HB-11. I. Ontogeny of antigen expression. J Immunol 1985;134:2983.
57. Fingeroth JD, Weiss JJ, Tedder TF, Strominger JL, Biro PA, Fearon DT. Epstein-Barr virus receptor of human lymphocytes is the C3d receptor CR2. Proc Natl Acad Sci USA 1984;81:4510.
58. De Franco AL. Thyrosine phosphorylation and the mechanism of signal transduction by the B-lymphocyte antigen receptor. Eur J Biochem 1992;210:381.
59. Reth M. Antigen receptors on B lymphocytes. Ann Rev Immunol 1992;10:97.
60. Varmus HE, Lowell CD. Cancer genes and hematopoiesis. Blood 1994;83: 65.
61. Nakamura T, Kubagawa H, Cooper MD. Heterogeneity of Ig-associated molecules on human B cells identified by monoclonal antibodies. Proc Natl Acad Sci USA 1992;89:8522.
62. Mason DY, Van Noesel CJM, Cordell JL, et al. The B29 and mb-1 polypeptides are differentially expressed during human B cell differentiation. Eur J Immunol 1992;22:2753.
63. Clark EA, Lane PJL. Regulation of human B cell activation and adhesion. Ann Rev Immunol 1991;9:97.
64. Korthaner U, Graf D, Mages HW, et al. Defective expression of T cell CD40 ligand causes X-linked immunodeficiency with hyper IgM. Nature 1993;361:539.
65. Di Santo JP, Bonnefoy JY, Ganehat JF, Fisher A, de Saint Basile G. CD40 ligand mutations in X-linked immunodeficiency with hyper IgM. Nature 1993;361:541.
66. Liu YG, Johnson GD, Gordon J, MacLennan ICM. Germinal centers in T-cell–dependent antibody responses. Immunol Today 1992;13:17.
67. Lobach DF, Haynes BF. Ontogeny of the human thymus during fetal development. J Clin Immunol 1987;7:81.
68. Reinherz EL, Acuto O, Fabbi M, et al. Clonotypic surface structure on human T lymphocytes: functional and biochemical analysis of the antigen receptor complex. Immunol Rev 1984;81:95.
69. Davis MM, Bjorkman PJ. T-cell antigen receptor genes and T-cell recognition. Nature 1988;334:395.
70. Marrack P, Kappler J. The T cell repertoire for antigen and MHC. Immunol Today 1988;9:308.
71. Strominger JL. Developmental biology of T cell receptor. Science 1989;244:944.
72. Moller G, ed. The T cell repertoire. Immunol Rev 1988;101:1.
73. Sowder JT, Chen CL, Ager LL, Chan MM, Cooper MD. A large subpopulation of avian T cells express a homologous of the mammalian $T\gamma\delta$ receptor. J Exp Med 1988;167:315.
74. Von Boehmer H, Teh HS, Kisielow P. The thymus selects the useful, neglects the useless and destroys the harmful. Immunol Today 1989;10: 52.
75. Lafaille JJ, Haas W, Coutinho A, Tonegawa S. Positive selection of $\gamma\delta$ T cell. Immunol Today 1990;11:75.
76. Smith CA, Williams GT, Kingston EJ, Owen JJT. Antibodies to CD3/T cell receptor complex induce death by apoptosis in immature T cells in thymic cultures. Nature 1989;337:181.
77. Scollay R, Wilson A, D' Amico, et al. Developmental status and reconstitution potential of subpopulations of murine thymocytes. Immunol Rev 1988;104:81.
78. Moller G, ed. Antigenic requirements for activation of MHC restricted responses. Immunol Rev 1987;98:1.
79. Schwartz RH. T lymphocyte recognition of antigen in association with gene products of the major histocompatibility complex. Annu Rev Immunol 1985;3:237.
80. Trowsdale J, Campbell RD. Physical map of a human HLA region. Immunol Today 1988;9;34.
81. Neefjes JJ, Ploegh HL. Intracellular transport of MHC class II molecules. Immunol Today 1992;13:179.
82. Long EO, Jacobson S. Pathways of viral antigen processing and presentation to CTL. Immunol Today 1989;10:45.
83. Monaco JJ. A molecular model of MHC class-I–restricted antigen processing. Immunol Today 1992;13:173.
84. Kumar V, Kono DH, Urban JL, Hood L. The T-cell receptor repertoire and autoimmune diseases. Annu Rev Immunol 1989;9:657.
85. Crabtree GR. Contingent genetic regulatory events in T cell activation. Science 1989;243:355.
86. Beyers AD, Spruyt LL, Williams AF. Molecular association between the T lymphocyte antigen receptor complex and the surface antigens CD2, CD4 or CD8 and CD5. Proc Natl Acad Sci USA 1992;89:2945.
87. Osman N, Ley SC, Crumpton MJ. Evidence for an association between the T cell receptor/CD3 antigen complex and the CD5 antigen in human T lymphocytes. Eur J Immunol 1992;22:2995.
88. Greene WC, Bohnlein E, Ballard DW. HIV, HTLV I and normal T cell growth: transcriptional strategies and surprises. Immunol Today 1989;10:272.
89. Marrack P, Kappler J. The staphylococcal enterotoxins and their relatives. Science 1990;248:705.
90. Weaver CT, Unanue ER. The co-stimulatory function of antigen presenting cells. Immunol Today 1990;11:49.
91. Meuer SC, Hussey RE, Fabbi M, et al. An alternative pathway of T cell activation: a functional role for the 50 KD T11 sheep erythrocyte receptor protein. Cell 1984;36:891.
92. Saunders ME, Makgoba MW, Shaw J. Human naive and memory cells: reinterpretation of helper-inducer subsets. Immunol Today 1988;9:195.
93. Byrne JA, Butler JL, Cooper MD. Differential activation requirements for virgin and memory T cells. J Immunol 1988;141:3249.
94. Scollay R, Butcher E, Weissman I. Thymus migration: quantitative studies on the rate of migration of cells from the thymus to the periphery in mice. Eur J Immunol 1980;10:210.
95. Sprent J, Webb SR Function and specificity of T cell subsets in the mouse. Adv Immunol 1987;41:39.
96. Mossmann TR, Coffman RL. Heterogeneity of cytokine secretion patterns and functions of helper T cells. Adv Immunol 1989;46:111.
97. Romagnani S. Induction of T_H1 and T_H2 responses: a key role for the "natural" immune reponse? Immunol Today 1992;131:379.
98. Doherty PC, Allan JE, Lynch F, Ceredig R. Dissection of inflammatory processes induced by CD8+ T cells. Immunol Today 1990;11:55.
99. Herberman RB, Ortaldo JR. Natural killer cells: their role in defense against disease. Science 1981;214:24.
100. Lanier LL, Testi R, Binal J, Phillips JH. Identity of Leu 19 (CD56) leukocyte differentiation antigen and neural cell adhesion molecule. J Exp Med 1989;169:2233.
101. Zupo-Rocchi S, Azzoni L, Massara R, et al. Co-expression of Fcγ receptor IIIA and IL-2 receptor β chain by a subset of human CD3+/CD8+/CD11b+ lymphocytes. J Clin Immunol 1993 (in press).
102. Grossi CE, Cadoni A, Zicca A, Leprini A, Ferrarini M. Large granular lymphocytes in human peripheral blood: ultrastructural and cytochemical characterization of the granules. Blood 1982;59:277.
103. Grossi CE, Crist WM, Abo T, Velardi A, Cooper MD. Expression of the Chediak-Higashi lysosomal abnormality in human peripheral blood lymphocyte populations. Blood 1985;65:837.
104. Trincheri G, Murphy M, Perussia B. Regulation of hematopoiesis by T lymphocytes and Natural Killer cells. CRC Crit Rev Oncol Haematol 1987;7:219.
105. Pistoia V, Zupo S, Corcione A, et al. Production of colony stimulating activity by human NK cells. Analysis of the conditions that influence the release and detection of CSA. Blood 1989;74:156.
106. Podack ER. Killer lymphocytes and how they kill. Curr Opin Cell Biol 1989;1:929.
107. Perussia B, Starr S, Abraham S, Trincheri G. Human natural killer cells analyzed by B73.1, a monoclonal antibody blocking Fc receptor function. I. Characterization of the lymphocyte subset reactive with B73.1. J Immunol 1983;30:2133.
108. Moretta A, Pantaleo G, Moretta L, Mingari MC, Cerottini JC. Quantitative assessment of the pool size and subset distribution of cytolytic T lymphocytes within human resting and alloactivated peripheral blood T cell populations. J Exp Med 1983;158:571.

109. Faure F, Triebel F, Hercend J. MHC-unrestricted cytotoxicity. Immunol Today 1990;11:108.
110. Hersey P, Bolhuis RLH. MHC-unrestricted killing by T cells: multireceptor hypothesis. 1980;11:110.
111. Moretta L, Ciccone E, Moretta A, et al. Allorecognition by NK cells: nonself or noself? Immunol Today 1992;13:300.
112. Springer TA, Dustin ML, Kishimoto TK, Marlin JD. The lymphocyte function-associated LFA-1, CD2 and LFA-3 molecules: cell adhesion receptors of the immune system. Annu Rev Immunol 1987;5:223.
113. Schmidt RE, Michon JM, Woronicz J, Schlossman SF, Reinherz EL. Enhancement of natural killer function through activation of the T11 E rosette receptor. J Clin Invest 1987;79:305.
114. Bierer BE, Burakoff SJ, T cell adhesion molecules. FASEB J 1988;2:2584.
115. Fisher A, Lisowska-Grospierre B, Anderson DC, Springer IA. Leukocyte adhesion deficiency: molecular basis and functional consequences. Immunodef Rev 1988;1:39.
116. Krahenbuhl O, Rey C, Jenne D, et al. Characterization of granzymes A and B isolated from granules of cloned human cytotoxic T lymphocytes. J Immunol 1988;141:347.
117. Kobayashi M, Fitz L, Ryan M, et al. Identification and purification of natural killer cell stimulatory factor (NKSF), a cytokine with multiple biologic effects of human lymphocytes. J Exp Med 1989;170:827.
118. Rosenberg SA. The development of new immunotherapies for the treatment of cancer using interleukin 2. Ann Surg 1988;208:121.
119. Grimm EA, Mazumder A, Zhang HZ, Rosenberg SA. Lymphokine-activated killer cell phenomenon: lysis of natural killer-resistant fresh solid tumor cells by interleukin 2-activated autologous human peripheral blood lymphocytes. J Exp Med 1982;155:1823.
120. Dianzani U, Zarcone D, Pistoia V, et al. CD8+/CD16b+ peripheral blood T cells contain lymphokine-activated killer (LAK) cell precursors. Eur J Immunol 1989;19:1037.
121. Ferrini S, Zarcone D, Viale M, et al. Morphologic and functional characterization of human peripheral blood cells expressing the $\gamma\delta$ T cell receptor. Eur J Immunol 1989;19:1183.
122. Howard M, O'Garra A. Biological properties of interleukin 10. Immunol Today 1992;13:198.
123. Jerne NK. Towards a network theory of the immune system. Ann Immunol (Paris) 1974;125:373.
124. Paul WE, Bona CA. Regulatory idiotopes and immune networks: a hypothesis. Immunol Today 1982;3:230.
125. Dorf ME, Bonacerraf B. Suppressor cells and immunoregulation. Annu Rev Immunol 1984;2:127.
126. Green DR, Flood PM, Gershon RK. Immunoregulatory T cell pathways. Annu Rev Immunol 1983;1:439.

Blood: Principles and Practice of Hematology,
edited by Robert I. Handin, Thomas P. Stossel, and Samuel E. Lux.
J.B. Lippincott Company, Philadelphia © 1995.

22

Reactive Lymphocyte Disorders and Lymphadenopathy

Kenneth B. Miller

Lymphadenopathy and splenomegaly are two common hematologic disorders. This chapter reviews the history of the discovery of the lymphatic system and its function, the anatomy of lymphatic organs, and the causes and evaluation of lymphadenopathy and splenomegaly.

HISTORY

Long before the lymphatic system was recognized, the function of the mysterious spleen had been a subject of speculation. Throughout the centuries, the spleen was given many roles and names, reflecting its pivotal anatomic position but unknown functional importance.

The ancients considered the spleen to be part of the digestive system.[1] Galen, a father of modern science, believed the spleen functioned to extract liquid from the stomach. He was perplexed by this role, referring to the spleen as a "plenum mysterii organon," an organ filled with mystery.[2] Erasistratus, one of the first anatomists, saw the spleen as a counterbalance to the mighty liver, preserving the symmetry of the abdomen. Plato was also intrigued by the spleen and its proximity to the liver. He suggested that it served to keep the liver clean and healthy. Hippocrates believed that the spleen balanced the four essential humors of man: blood, phlegm, golden bile, and black bile. The liver was thought to be the source of the all-important golden bile, and the spleen the source of black bile. The Greeks and Romans believed that the spleen affected athletic ability, and they consumed certain beverages before athletic competition, purportedly to shrink the spleen and enhance their performance.

The spleen, as a ductless gland occupying so much of the anterior abdomen, has fascinated physician and philosopher alike. The spleen was considered as both the center of violent ill tempers, as in "venting one's spleen," and as the origin of amusement and laughter. The Talmud describes the spleen as the source of both laughter and joy.[3] *Melt* was an another word for the spleen, reflecting its key anatomic position. This term was derived from the verb *to melt*, meaning to knock down by a blow to the side.[4] In battle, a blow to the melt, or spleen, could be fatal. This anatomic weakness was well known in Southeast Asia, where massively swollen spleens were commonplace, presumably caused by malaria. A sharp blow to the left upper quadrant, rupturing the spleen, was a quick and effective tactic for assassins.[5]

The lymphatic system, from the Latin, *lympha*, meaning clear spring water, was recognized in the 17th century as distinct from the arterial and venous systems. Jean Pecquet[6] noted in 1651 that the lymphatics, like the venous system, are composed of numerous small vessels that gradually combine to form larger and larger trunks, eventually emptying into the subclavian vein through the thoracic duct. William Hewson,[7] one of the fathers of hematology, studied extensively the anatomy and function of the lymphatic system. In his treatise on the lymphatic system, Hewson described its anatomy in detail, including the basic architecture of the lymph nodes and the dual circulation within them.[7] He included the lymphatic vessels, lymphatic glands, thymus, and spleen in the lymphatic system.

Hewson[8] noted prominent lymphadenopathy in some patients with syphilis, cancer, and abscesses. He concluded that the primary function of the lymph nodes was to act as "absorbants," to drain adjacent areas of noxious agents. He observed that lymph nodes were common sites for residual cancer separate from the primary lesions, noting that

> *. . . the axillary glands are . . . frequently observed to swell in consequence of cancers in the breast, and it is found to be of no use to extirpate the breast itself, unless the infected glands can likewise be removed; for otherwise the cancerous humor left in the glands may renew the disease.*

He also noticed that the lymph fluid contains colorless nucleated cells, which he speculated were formed in the lymph nodes and thymus. He postulated that the entire hematopoietic system is derived from these colorless lymphocytes, calling the lymph corpuscles "central particles." The lymphocytes, according to Hewson, form the central colorless area of the red blood cells (RBCs), thus the term *central*. Noting the enlarged thymus in children, he speculated on its biologic importance in the normal development of the lymphoid system. Hewson's career was cut short when he died at the age of 35 from an infection sustained during a dissection. Unfortunately, many of his observations and theories were not accepted by the physicians of his day.

By the late 19th century, the spleen and lymph nodes were known to be involved in different disorders such as tuberculosis, leukemia, and cancer. Virchow,[9] a leading pathologist of the day, attempted to address the morphologic and biologic differences between lymphoid hyperplasia and neoplasia. Virchow studied the spleen in patients with leukemia. He commented on change in the normal architecture, using the word *neoplasia* to describe new growth and to distinguish these findings from hyperplasia. In 1875, Louis Antoine Ranvier,[10] a prominent and highly respected physician, published the then-definitive text on the lymphatic system. His 1100-page volume, *Traité technique d'histologie*, described the structure and function of the lymph nodes and lymphatic vessels. Ranvier speculated that the lymphocytes were involved in healing and tissue repair, presumably because of their ability to migrate through blood vessel walls. He asserted that the lymphocyte is a carrier cell that supplies nutrients and essential metabolites to tissues with sudden or unusual metabolic requirements. Fleming,[11] using new staining techniques developed by Ehrlich and newly improved microscopes, described the follicles in the spleen, lymph nodes, and tonsils. He called the central pale areas "germinal centers" because of their many dividing cells.

Ehrlich's method of staining thin dried films of blood had a profound influence on all areas of hematology, including studies of the lymphatics. He was able to clearly distinguish the lymphocyte from the leukocyte. Moreover, Ehrlich proposed that the lymphocyte represents a separate cell lineage, originating in the lymph nodes and spleen and separate from the cellular elements formed in the bone marrow. The lymphocyte had been considered the equivalent of the pluripotential stem cell, a precursor cell for the erythrocytes, leukocytes, and macrophages. The lymphocyte was also believed to have a role in controlling the size and growth of various organs.

In the 17th century, Marcello Malphigi[12] described the glandular appearance of the spleen and the densely packed cells now known as the *malphigian corpuscles*. In 1854, Theodor Billroth[13] identified the unique vascular structures of the spleen. He described the splenic red pulp, now called the *cords of Billroth*, and the splenic sinuses, referred to as the *sinuses of Billroth*.

The observations and analyses of the lymphatic system by these men of science have, over the centuries, laid the foundation for the study of immunology.

LYMPHOID CELLS AND THE LYMPHATIC SYSTEM

Lymph Nodes

The lymphatic system consists of the peripheral lymph nodes, the spleen, Waldeyer's ring (including the oropharyngeal lymphoid tissues), and lymphoid aggregates in the lamina propria and submucosa of the respiratory and gastrointestinal tract, including Peyer's patches. Afferent and efferent vessels carry lymph into and out of the nodes. Normal lymph nodes vary in size from 2 to 20 mm, averaging 15 mm in longitudinal diameter. Size and structure vary according to the node's location and the person's age. Lymph nodes draining areas of active antigenic stimulation, such as the neck, inguinal area, and abdomen, have proportionally larger and more numerous germinal centers, whereas mesenteric nodes have wider medullary sinuses and fewer germinal centers. Peripheral nodes are more common in younger persons and are absent in newborns.[14]

Evaluation of a lymph node traditionally addresses the changes that occur in the different anatomic and functional compartments (Fig. 22-1). The nodal architecture is important in the classification and evaluation of different lymphomas, and changes in the different nodal compartments are helpful in differentiating a reactive node from one involved with a lymphoproliferative disorder.[15] The lymph node has a limited repertoire of morphologic responses to the wide variety of specific and nonspecific stimuli that it receives.[16] Histochemistry, immunochemistry, and enzyme and molecular studies are therefore helpful in evaluating the pathologic changes in an enlarged lymph node.

Immunohistochemical markers, using monoclonal antibodies capable of recognizing differentiation antigens and surface markers on distinct populations of B, T, and natural killer cells and monocytes, have defined the distribution and compartmentalization of lymphocytes in normal lymph nodes. In peripheral lymph nodes, T cells are usually restricted to the paracortical or interfollicular areas, whereas B cells are concentrated in the lymphoid follicles and med-

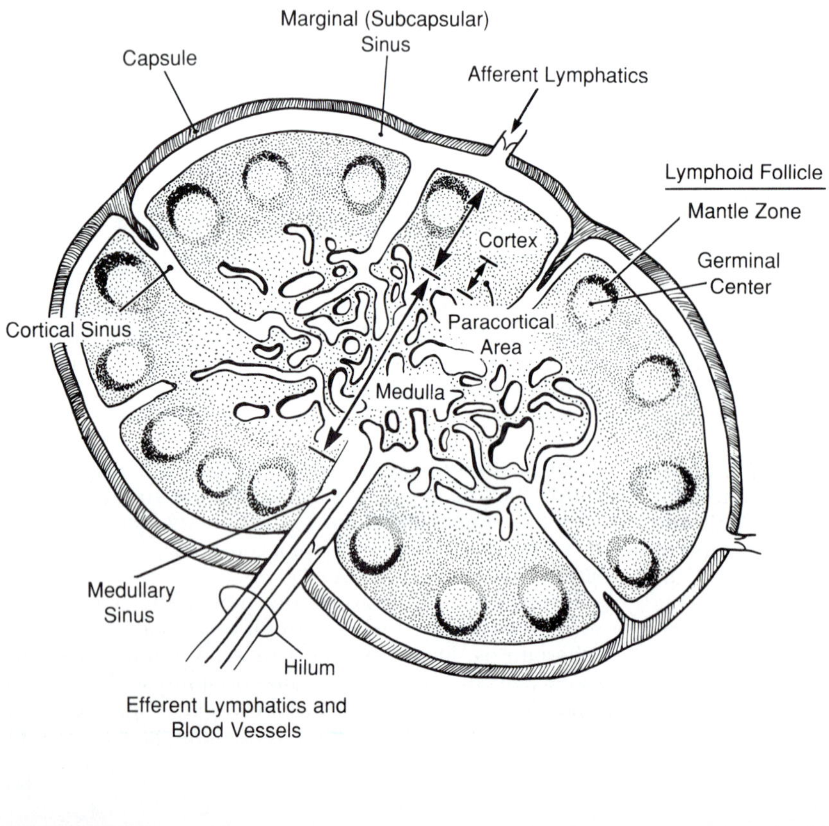

FIGURE 22-1. Schematic view of the organization of the human lymph node.

ullary zones. Most cells in the follicle area, which includes the mantle zone and the germinal centers, are B lymphocytes, positive for the pan–B-cell marker, B1 (CD20). The expression of surface immunoglobulins (Igs) is highly variable within these regions. The B cells in the mantle zone are positive for μ and δ heavy chains. The B-cell population of a normal lymph node is polyclonal and therefore contains roughly equal populations of cells that express either κ or λ light chains on their surfaces. The germinal centers reflect the events of antigenic stimulation and the normal differentiation steps of B lymphocytes.

Most of the B cells that express surface Ig are positive for IgD and IgM, with IgG-positive cells constituting less than 10% of the B cells. This distribution is consistent with the observation that the first class of IG to be expressed on the B-cell surface is IgM, followed by IgD.[17] Most B cells apparently acquire surface IgM followed by surface IgD and then switch to the expression of surface IgG or surface IgA. This sequence IgD expression is not a prerequisite for switching of B cells to the IgG or IgA isotypes.[18] Normally, B cells bearing IgG or surface IgA have lost the expression of surface IgM and surface IgD and express a single isotype. B lymphocytes bearing the surface IgM and surface IgD are found throughout the normal node but are concentrated primarily in the mantle zone. More mature lymphocytes bearing surface IgG or surface IgA are rarely found in the normal lymph node.

T cells present in the normal lymph node stain with a number of monoclonal antibodies.[19] T cells that mark with the pan–T-cell marker, CD2, are found diffusely throughout the paracortical and intrafollicular area of the normal lymph node. In the paracortical areas, CD4+ (helper and inducer T cells) and CD8+ (suppressor–cytotoxic cells), are normally present in a ratio of 2 to 3:1, respectively, a ratio similar to that found normally in the peripheral blood. The T cells in the germinal centers, although occurring infrequently, are usually of the helper–inducer phenotype (CD4); the suppressor–cytotoxic T cell (CD8+) is virtually absent.

In response to an antigenic stimulus, the lymph node rapidly increases the proportion of CD4+ cells two- to threefold. Rarely does an increase of the CD8+ population in hyperplastic nodes occur.[20] In the germinal centers and mantle zones, T cells make up between 5% and 20% of the total cells.[20] CD57 (Leu-7), which includes cells of the natural killer phenotype, can also be found in the germinal centers. Moreover, many of these CD57+ cells are localized to the upper poles of the germinal centers and double-stain with CD4.[20,21]

The interdigitating reticulum cells are usually strongly positive for HLA-DR and are most numerous in the paracortical area and germinal centers.[22] In many instances, the HLA-DR–positive reticulum cells are juxtaposed with the CD4+ T cells in the paracortical area, suggesting a functional relation.[23]

Spleen

The distribution of lymphocytes in the spleen closely resembles that in the normal lymph node. The splenic follicles, like the lymph node follicles, contain mostly B cells that stain with the pan–B-cell marker, B1 (CD20). The B lymphocytes in the mantle zone also express surface Ig of the μ and δ heavy chains. Most of the lymphocytes in the periarteriolar sheaths are CD4+ T cells and the ratio of CD4+ to CD8+ cells is about 3:1.[24] In the marginal zone, the T and B cells are mixed with occasional OM1+ and HLA-DR+ monocytes, reflecting the extensive blood supply to this area and the branching trabeculae. Within the splenic sinusoids and cords, T and B cells are randomly distributed. The red pulp contains few resident lymphocytes, most of which are cells that are CD8+, suppressor–cytotoxic T cells.

In the peripheral blood, lymphocytes make up 20% to 40% of total blood leukocytes. Most of the circulating lymphocytes are small (10 μm or less) and are referred to by their morphologic appearance (small, medium, large, clefted), their functional characteristics (helper, suppressor, or natural killer cells), or surface phenotype markers (eg, CD4, CD8). These characteristics have demonstrated that lymphocytes are a heterogeneous collection of cells with different origins, functions, and life-spans.

The small resting lymphocyte in the peripheral blood appears on the Wright-stained smear as a cell with a deep purplish-blue nucleus composed of dense aggregates of chromatin. The margin of the nucleus is usually sharply defined and is surrounded by a slightly indented and eccentrically placed sky blue cytoplasm. The nuclear/cytoplasmic ratio varies greatly in the normal lymphocyte population. The cytoplasm may form a fine rim around the nucleus, or it may occupy more than half of the cell. Granules are usually absent from the cytoplasm, but several bright, reddish violet, peroxidase-negative granules are seen in some cells.

Most circulating lymphocytes are long-lived, with an average life of 4.4 years.[25] Viral infections are the most common cause of transient lymphocytosis (Table 22-1). Varicella, mumps, cytomegalovirus, and Epstein-Barr virus are associated with a prominent lymphocytosis. Viral infections are characterized by the increased numbers of large, reactive, atypical-appearing lymphocytes. Lymphocytosis rarely occurs during most bacterial infections, with the exception of pertussis, in which the total white blood count may range between 20,000 and 50,000/μL, with 60% or more lymphocytes. Patients with hyposplenism have a persistently high lymphocyte count.[26] In these reactive settings, a polyclonal increase in lymphocytes is found, in contrast to that found in patients with early chronic lymphocytic leukemia and other lymphoproliferative disorders in which an increase in clonal populations of cells occurs. Monoclonal antibodies, immunohistochemical staining, and molecular studies demonstrating Ig or T-cell receptor (TCR) gene rearrangements have made it possible to distinguish a clonal lymphoproliferative disorder from a reactive lymphocytosis.[27] In most patients, a persistent chronic lymphocytosis is associated with an underlying monoclonal malignant lymphoproliferative disorder.[27]

TABLE 22-1. Causes of Lymphocytosis

INFECTIONS
Pertussis
Infectious mononucleosis
Mumps
Varicella
Hepatitis
Brucellosis
Congenital syphilis
HEMATOPOIETIC DISORDERS
Chronic lymphocytic leukemia
T-cell lymphocytosis
Sézary's syndrome
Hairy-cell leukemia
MISCELLANEOUS
Thyrotoxicosis

The percentage of circulating lymphocytes in the peripheral blood varies according to the person's age.[28] The lymphocyte concentration is high at birth and may rise to 22,000/μL in apparently healthy infants during the first year of life. Then, a gradual decline throughout childhood occurs, which stabilizes after age 7 years at about 4000/μL. The increased total lymphocyte count in infants reflects the high relative proportion of surface Ig–positive B cells with a relative decrease in circulating T cells. The percentage of T cells slowly increases after the second year of life to reach adult levels by the age of 7 years.[29] In adults, the total number of T or B lymphocytes does not appear to change with age.[30] The relative distribution of T lymphocytes in the peripheral blood does change with age; an increase in the number of CD4+ T cells and a decrease in the CD8+ cells occur.[31] The latter cells exhibit the phenotype of natural killer cells.[32] The lymphoid organs gradually decrease in size with advancing age with a decrease in the number and size of germinal centers in lymph nodes and an increase in plasma cells and both B and T lymphocytes in the bone marrow.

CLINICAL EVALUATION OF LYMPHOID TISSUES

Lymphadenopathy is frequently noted in patients with no evidence of active malignant, infectious, or autoimmune diseases. Palpable cervical nodes are not uncommon in young children and adults, for example. Soft movable lymph nodes between 0.5 and 1 cm are frequently felt in the submandibular and posterior cervical regions. The evaluation of these and other lymphoid tissues depends on a careful examination of the patient, a detailed medical history, and consideration of the different functions of the lymphatic system. A range of variables, including the patient's age and medical history, and the location, size, shape, and texture of enlarged nodes provide important clues to the cause of lymphadenopathy. The differential diagnosis must also consider the dual function of lymphatic organs, as both immunologic agents and as mechanical filters that trap foreign antigens and malignant cells.

Children and adolescents commonly have palpable lymph nodes that reflect exposure to new antigens or recurrent viral infections.[33] In adolescence, mononucleosis is a common cause of cervical lymphadenopathy, and although usually associated with an acute pharyngitis, it may occur without apparent pharyngeal symptoms. Toxoplasmosis or CMV infections may mimic mononucleosis. The likelihood of finding a malignant process in a palpable peripheral lymph node increases with age. In patients under the age of 20 years, 75% to 85% of all biopsy specimens of nodes are benign, whereas less than 30% of the specimens in patients over the age of 60 are benign.[34]

The location of the lymphadenopathy is extremely important. For example, large bilateral hilar nodes without other detectable lymphadenopathy in a young asymptomatic black patient is suggestive of sarcoidosis.[35] Mediastinal lymphadenopathy, even in the absence of other detectable adenopathy, suggests Hodgkin's disease or non-Hodgkin's lymphoma. Generalized tender lymphadenopathy is consistent with a bacterial or viral infection. Supraclavicular and scalene lymphadenopathy is more suggestive of carcinoma, whereas a solitary axillary node more frequently suggests Hodgkin's disease or non-Hodgkin's lymphoma. Inguinal nodes are more often involved with a reactive process (Table 22-2).

Superficial lymphadenopathy in the head and neck most often results from intercurrent or recovering acute bacterial or viral illness. Neoplasms or infectious processes originating in the lung or retroperitoneal area produce supraclavicular and scalene lymphadenopathy. Axillary lymphadenopathy occurs from changes in the upper extremities, including infections, trauma, or even insect bites to the extremities. Inguinal adenopathy is frequently noted in the form of 0.5- to 1-cm nontender nodes in the region of the inguinal ligament and femoral triangle and usually reflects ongoing inflammation in the perirectal and vaginal areas and the lower extremities. Small abrasions of the toes or infections in the nail beds can cause prominent reactive lymphadenopathy in the extremity involved.

The texture of the node may provide clues to its cause. Bacterial infections usually cause firm, tender enlargement from the draining area, whereas malignant diseases tend to present with firm, painless lymphadenopathy. Discrete, hard, fixed, or matted lymph nodes are highly suggestive of metastatic involvement of the lymph node.

Patients should be questioned about recent travel, immunizations, trauma, and exposure to infections. A history of exposure to different chemicals or multiple episodes of trauma to the hands or legs may affect the evaluation. A detailed drug history is important to rule out drug-associated lymphadenopathy. Reactive, hyperplastic lymphadenopathy has been associated with a number of drugs, including phenylbutazone, methyldopa, meprobamate, hydralazine, and the phenytoin derivatives.[36,37] Dilantin can produce a clinical syndrome that is similar to Hodgkin's disease, with the development of fever, eosinophilia, and lymphadenopathy occurring within weeks to months after starting the drug.[38,39]

Endocrine or autoimmune disorders can present with lymphadenopathy or splenomegaly. Patients with hyperthyroidism can present with findings suggestive of a lymphoproliferative disorder, including a history of weight loss, diffuse sweating, and generalized lymphadenopathy and splenomegaly. Autoimmune disorders such as systemic lupus erythematosus and Sjögren's syndrome may present with diffuse or localized lymphadenopathy.[40,41]

A partial list of conditions that lead to lymphadenopathy is noted in Table 22-2. The causes include infections, immune responses, malignant disease, drugs, and inflammation. The most common cause of lymphoid enlargement is the result of cellular proliferation in the lymph node in response to antigenic stimulation.

When and whether to perform a biopsy on an enlarged lymph node may present a difficult clinical decision. A patient with symptoms of weight loss, night sweats, or gradually enlarging nontender asymmetric lymphadenopathy without an obvious source of infection usually requires a lymph node biopsy. More difficult is the patient with a recent bacterial or viral infection with a residually enlarged isolated lymph node. An enlarged lymph node that does not decrease in size and is thought to be due to an infectious process should undergo biopsy if it does not diminish within 2 months after resolution of the infection.

The evaluation of a patient with lymphadenopathy usually begins well in advance of the decision to perform a biopsy on a lymph node. The patient who presents with a history of weight loss, fevers, and night sweats takes a different direction from the patient with asymptomatic lymphadenopathy noticed incidentally on a screening or routine physical examination.

As noted, a detailed medical history should be obtained for all patients. Patients should be specifically questioned regarding medication, smoking, alcohol use, family history of autoimmune or neoplastic diseases, and recent travel. Jet travel has changed the pattern and incidence of a number of infectious and parasitic diseases. A detailed sexual history is also needed on all patients with unexplained lymphadenopathy. Sexually transmitted disease such as syphilis, chancroid, and herpes simplex (type 2) can present

TABLE 22-2. Common Causes of Lymphadenopathy

Region	Etiology
Occipital lymph nodes	Scalp infections, insect bites (children), ringworm, very rarely lymphoma or metastatic tumors; cat-scratch fever
Posterior auricular	Rubella, oculoglandular syndromes
Anterior auricular	Infections of eyelids and conjunctiva, epidemic keratoconjunctivitis
Posterior and anterior cervical	Toxoplasmosis, adenovirus syndromes, infections of oral cavity and pharynx
Posterior cervical and submental	Scalp infections, dental infections, tuberculosis
Cervical (suppurative)	Tuberculosis
Supraclavicular (hard and fixed)	Metastases from intrathoracic or intraabdominal carcinoma, Hodgkin's disease
Axillary	Infection of upper extremities, cat-scratch disease, brucellosis, sporotrichosis, non-Hodgkin's lymphomas
Epitrochlear	
Unilateral	Infections of hands, Hodgkin's disease
Bilateral	Viral disease in children, sarcoidosis, tularemia
Inguinal	
Unilateral	Lymphogranuloma venereum, syphilis, chancroid; gonococcal, herpetic venereal infections; mycoplasma; urethritis, tularemia, plague, loiasis, onchocerciasis, lymphoma, metastatic pelvic carcinoma, gynecologic malignancies
Bilateral	
Pulmonary hilar	
Unilateral	Metastatic lung carcinoma
Bilateral	Sarcoidosis, tuberculosis, histoplasmosis, coccidioidomycosis
Mediastinal, symmetric	Hodgkin's disease and lymphoma
Intraabdominal and retroperitoneal	Lymphoma, metastatic carcinoma, tuberculosis in mesenteric lymph nodes
Regional involvement in systemic infections	Infectious mononucleosis, viral hepatitis, cytomegalovirus disease, rubella, influenza, leprosy, toxoplasmosis, acquired immunodeficiency syndrome
Generalized lymphadenopathy	Sarcoidosis, hyperthyroidism, systemic lupus erythematosus, lymphoma, syphilis

with lymphadenopathy.[42–44] Diffuse lymphadenopathy may be one of the early signs of an HIV-associated infection.[45,46]

The initial evaluation of a patient with lymphadenopathy should include a complete physical examination. The physician should carefully note the location, size, shape, and consistency of the enlarged lymph nodes. Whenever possible, the nodes should be measured in two dimensions. Close attention should be paid to the area draining the involved nodes. Isolated cervical lymphadenopathy requires a detailed head and neck examination, paying close attention to the tongue, gums, and hard and soft palates. For patients with a solitary submandibular or submental node, a thorough head and neck examination including indirect laryngoscopy is necessary before proceeding with a biopsy. Those patients with a history of tobacco use require a careful oral examination. In addition to cigarettes, chewing tobacco and use of snuff have been associated with an increased incidence of head and neck cancers.

Occipital lymphadenopathy requires a thorough examination of the head and scalp, since small areas of eczema on the hairline can produce localized cervical adenopathy. Supraclavicular nodes are more worrisome and suggest disease in the chest or retroperitoneum. Virchow's node, a supraclavicular node once considered diagnostic of a gastric malignancy, is found with many intraabdominal malignancies. As noted, reactive inguinal adenopathy is common in both children and adults. Nevertheless, these nodes may reflect infections in the inguinal, pelvic, and retroperitoneal areas.

Multiple studies have attempted to define algorithms for the evaluation of lymphadenopathy.[47–49] A patient with a node larger than 2 cm, an abnormal chest radiograph, and no high fevers or chills is likely to require a biopsy for diagnosis. An enlarged scalene, supraclavicular, or solitary axillary node is highly suggestive of a malignant or granulomatous disorder.

The initial investigation should focus on likely causes of infectious or reactive lymphadenopathy. The location of the lymphadenopathy should direct the evaluation. Supraclavicular adenopathy of more than 1 cm is highly suggestive of intrathoracic disease, and a chest radiograph or computed tomographic (CT) scan should be obtained. Patients with asymptomatic generalized symmetric cervical lymphadenopathy and a negative chest radiograph can usually be followed for 1 to 2 months before proceeding with a biopsy. If all evaluations are negative or nondiagnostic and the lymphadenopathy persists or increases, a biopsy should be obtained.

Lymph node biopsies provide information for diagnosis, treatment planning, and, if necessary, staging. A needle biopsy may be helpful in confirming a diagnosis of metastatic disease but is rarely sufficient to diagnose lymphoma or Hodgkin's disease. A needle biopsy also does not usually obtain sufficient cells for immunophenotyping or studies of nodal architecture or mitotic activity. In addition, a needle sample may not obtain enough representative material from certain pleomorphic malignancies, such as Hodgkin's disease, which may result in a misdiagnosis. If a high suspicion of an underlying malignant disease exists and no primary site is noted, it is best to proceed with a definitive biopsy rather than a needle biopsy. In certain diseases, such as head and neck cancers, needle biopsy actually increases the likelihood of spreading the disease because of the development of a nonhealing sinus tract.[49]

The diagnostic yield from the first node biopsy ranges from 37% to 63%,[34,50] depending on the location of the node. Inguinal nodes have the lowest yield, and supraclavicular and axillary nodes have the highest yield. In patients with a nondiagnostic or reactive node on the initial biopsy, about 20% have a specific diagnosis confirmed on a later biopsy.[64] Therefore, in patients with persistent lymphadenopathy, a second biopsy from a different nodal chain may be diagnostic.

LYMPHADENOPATHY DUE TO INFECTIONS

Lymphadenopathy due to an infection may be either localized, from draining an infected area, or generalized, from a systemic infection. It may result from a lymph node reaction or from direct involvement of a node resulting in lymphadenitis. The gross and microscopic changes in a node depend on the nature of the infectious organism, the host's defense, and the antimicrobial therapy that the patient receives.[50]

Certain infections produce distinctive pathologic findings. Caseous necrosis results from infections with *Mycobacterium tuberculosis, Histoplasma capsulatum, Coccidioides immitis,* and the various atypical mycobacteria.[51,52] Cat-scratch disease, tularemia, and lymphogranuloma venereum produce stellate abscesses surrounded by palisading epithelioid cells.[53–55] Toxoplasmosis produces follicular hyperplasia with reactive germinal centers and clusters of epithelial cells in the paracortex and germinal centers. Acute lymphadenitis due to pyogenic bacteria produces tender, enlarged nodes, firm or fluctuant to palpation, usually at least 3 cm in diameter. Acute lymphadenitis, more common in children than adults, is usually due to *Staphylococcus aureus* or group A streptococci.[56] The most common nodes of involvement, in descending order of rate of occurrence, are submandibular, anterior and posterior cervical, inguinal, and axillary. Cervical lymphadenopathy from these infections is usually unilateral and tender, and is often associated with swelling of the face or neck, sometimes pronounced enough to interfere with the opening of the mouth.

Lymphadenopathy is caused by lymphatic drainage of the involved area. The iliac nodes, located along the external and common iliac arteries, receive lymphatic drainage from the lower abdominal wall and superficial and deep inguinal structures. Iliac and inguinal lymphadenopathy reflect infections of the lower extremities, lower abdominal wall, perineum, and pelvis. Patients may develop limping, back pain, or hip pain because the lymphadenopathy causes pain on extension of the thigh.

A variety of organisms other than the common bacterial pathogens can produce localized lymphadenitis. These disorders may be characterized by a prolonged and indolent course, with intermittent fevers and involvement of atypical anatomic areas. Scrofula, or tuberculous cervical lymphadenopathy, was formerly common. It was frequently acquired from infected milk or bovine tuberculosis, or was lymphohematogenically spread from an initial pulmonary focus. Most mycobacterial cervical lymphadenitis is now caused by atypical mycobacteria, such as *Mycobacterium scrofulaceum* or *Mycobacterium avium-intracellulare,* rather than *M tuberculosis*.[57,58] Fevers and other systemic symptoms are usually absent early in the course of scrofula. An enlarging nontender cervical mass usually brings the patient to seek medical attention, and most patients have no additional clinical evidence of tuberculosis. Defining the species of mycobacteria is important. The atypical mycobacteria are frequently resistant to standard antituberculosis therapy.

The paratracheal and mediastinal nodes may be sites of tuberculosis adenitis. A large mediastinal mass may signal tuberculous involvement of mediastinal nodes.[58] On biopsy, the caseous necrosis characteristic of tuberculosis is coagulative, with total necrosis that leaves no cellular traces or nuclear debris. The diagnosis is confirmed by demonstrating the typical acid-fast bacilli on smears or sections of the node or by culturing the organism, which is more sensitive, since the smear may be positive in less than one third of patients with a positive culture.[59]

Cat-scratch fever is an indolent, self-limited disease, characterized by tender, regional lymphadenopathy. The presumed etiologic agent is a pleomorphic gram-negative bacillus, *Rochalimaea henselae*, identified by the Warthin-Starry silver stain.[60,61] Cultures of material aspirated from the node are usually nonrevealing, and the diagnosis is made on the basis of appropriated exposure and the clinical picture.[53] Patients are usually not ill, in spite of impressive regional lymphadenopathy. Some patients may complain of a recent influenza-like illness with diffuse myalgia and low-grade fever.[53] Over 90% of patients give a history of contact with a cat, and the mode of transmission is presumably from a scratch, bite, or lick of a cat. A primary lesion consisting of a small papule or vesicle that resembles an insect bite usually develops at the site of the scratch 7 to 14 days after contact with the cat. The primary lesion may persist for 1 to 3 weeks, and it heals without scar formation. Regional lymphadenopathy develops within 2 weeks of the appearance of the skin papule. Any peripheral lymph node may be involved, but axillary, cervical, and occipital nodes, respectively, are most frequently involved and are rarely tender.[53]

Epitrochlear adenopathy is rare, in spite of the frequent inoculation of the hands and forearms. The node biopsy reveals follicular hyperplasia, with little distortion of the general nodal architecture. The germinal centers are enlarged, with a diffuse proliferation of immunoblasts, macrophages, and scattered plasma cells. Later in the disease, granuloma forms with central microabscesses. The use of serologic and skin tests to diagnose this disease is still controversial.[53]

Bilateral inguinal adenopathy in a young, sexually active, otherwise healthy patient is frequently caused by one of several venereal diseases.[43] The primary lesion of syphilis, the *chancre*, is usually accompanied by discrete, firm, painless enlarged inguinal nodes.[62] Lymphogranuloma venereum results in large, tender, discrete, and movable bilateral inguinal nodes. Chancroid usually presents with painful, tender inguinal adenopathy. Primary herpetic infections are often associated with tender inguinal adenopathy. In many of these diseases, the primary lesion may have partially or completely resolved and therefore may not be readily apparent on physical examination. In patients with unexplained inguinal adenopathy, a careful examination of the genital and perirectal areas and a detailed history of recent infections are important.

Inguinal adenopathy can also be a manifestation of nonvenereal systemic infections. In bubonic plague, caused by *Yersinia pestis*, the inguinal nodes are frequently involved because the flea bite introducing the infection commonly occurs on the lower extremity.[55,63] The buboes of the plague produce rapidly enlarging tender lymphadenopathy that quickly becomes suppurative and frequently drains spontaneously. Tularemia may mimic some of the features of the plague and produce regional suppurative adenopathy. In these infections, blood cultures are usually positive early in the disease. Helminthic infections such as loiasis and onchocerciasis can produce impressive local lymphadenopathy.

A variety of bacterial, rickettsial, chlamydial, spirochetal, protozoal, and helminthic agents can cause localized and generalized lymphadenopathy (see Table 22-2). In many instances, the lymphadenopathy is a manifestation of widespread disease, as a result of dissemination either by the blood or by the lymphatic stream. Many common viral syndromes typically present with generalized prominent lymphadenopathy, including rubella, measles, HIV, infectious mononucleosis, and CMV infections.

EPSTEIN-BARR VIRUS: INFECTIOUS MONONUCLEOSIS

Pathogenesis

Infectious mononucleosis is caused by the Epstein-Barr virus (EBV), a member of the human herpesvirus group. EBV infections occur worldwide and usually result in subclinical early childhood infections. Over 90% of American adults have demonstrable antibodies to EBV.[64] The illness generally develops before age 30 years; in underdeveloped countries, it usually occurs by age 10 years (only 30% to 40% of American children are infected with EBV by age 10). In adolescence and early adulthood, a conversion rate to EBV occurs in about 12%.[64]

EBV is a DNA virus. EBV receptors have been detected on human B lymphocytes, complement receptor–positive non-B, non-T lymphocytes, and nasopharyngeal epithelial cells.[64,65] The EBV receptor is the receptor for the third complement component, the C3d receptor (also known as CR2 or CD21).[65–67] The virus interacts with the B cell in a number of defined steps. First, it attaches to the receptor; then, it gains entry into the susceptible B lymphocyte. Epstein-Barr nuclear antigens (EBNA) appear within cell nuclei within 6 hours of infection and before virus-directed protein synthesis is detectable.[68] At least five different EBNA proteins are coded for by EBV, each playing a different role in cellular transformation.[69–71] During the initial phase of primary EBV infection, up to 18% of peripheral B lymphocytes express one or more EBNA proteins.[72]

In the normal host, EBV infection results in the proliferation of transformed B cells, which are contained by a vigorous immune response involving both the T- and B-cell network. EBV in effect activates B cells, resulting in their polyclonal stimulation[71] (Fig. 22-2). This response elicits a corresponding polyclonal T-cell response.[71,72] T cells form most of the circulating atypical lymphocytes in patients with infectious mononucleosis. In the early phase of the illness, many T cells are cytotoxic toward EBV-containing B cells, or they inhibit B-cell activation.[72–75] The latter suppressor T cell most likely accounts for the depressed number of circulating Ig-secreting B cells found during the second week, and the subsequent decrease in polyclonal hypergammaglobulinemia. An abnormal suppressor T-cell response may also result in the rare cases of agammaglobulinemia.[76]

The serologic response includes production of neutralizing antibodies to glycoproteins on the cell membranes of EBV-infected cells. EBV infection also produces antibodies to a number of unrelated antigens found in sheep, horse, and beef RBCs.[77] These heterophile antibodies, which are detected as sheep and horse RBC agglutinins and beef cell hemolysins, do not cross-react with specific antibodies against EBV antigens. They are IgM antibodies with no clear role in the pathogenesis of the infection or in recovery.

Clinical Features

Infection with EBV causes a broad spectrum of illness in humans (Fig. 22-3). EBV is also associated with the development of African Burkitt's lymphoma and nasopharyngeal carcinoma.[78] The EBV genome has been demonstrated by DNA hybridization studies in biopsy specimens of African patients with Burkitt's lymphoma and nasopharyngeal carcinoma.[79,80] In addition, the virus can be recovered from biopsy specimens, and the EBNA is demonstrable in the nuclei of cells obtained from the involved nodes.[80] The geographic restriction of Burkitt's lymphoma in Africa suggests the role of associated genetic, environmental, and possibly other viral infections in the development of the

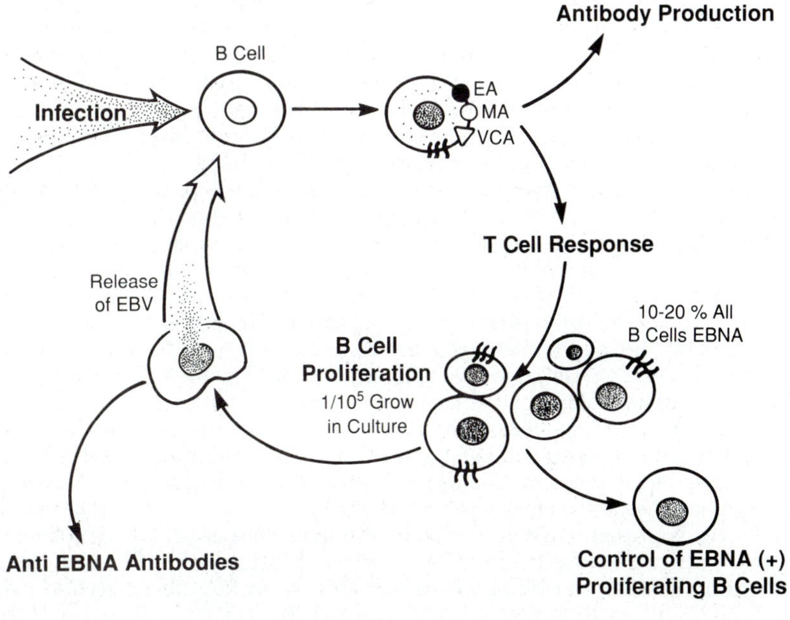

FIGURE 22-2. The cellular and humoral immune response in infectious mononucleosis. The immune response to Epstein-Barr virus (EBV) infects B cell and results in the synthesis of circulating antibodies directed against viral antigens as well as unrelated antigens. These later antigens are the heterophile antibodies. The responding T lymphocytes are cytotoxic to EBV-infected B cells and appear as atypical lymphocytes found in the peripheral blood. The T-cell response is important in the control of the EBV-infected B lymphocytes. EA, early antigen; EBNA, Epstein-Barr nuclear antigens; MA, latent membrane proteins; VCA, viral capsid antigen.

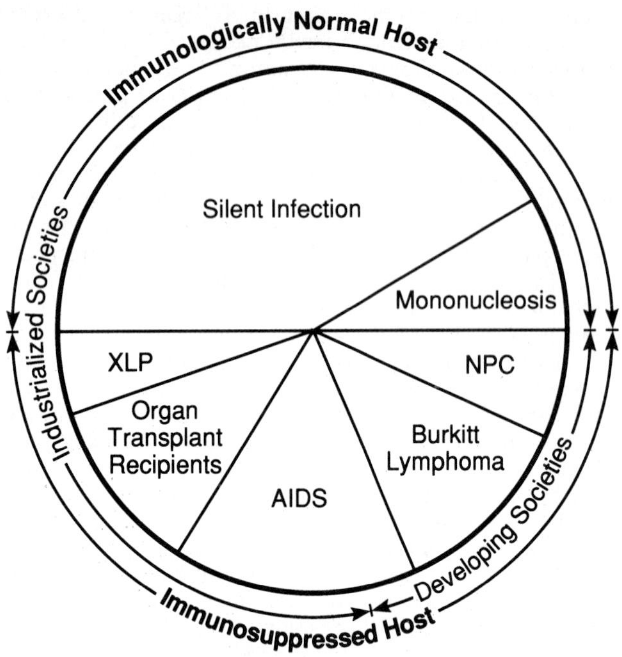

FIGURE 22-3. The spectrum of infections with Epstein-Barr virus (EBV). The immune status of the host determines the outcome of an EBV infection. NPC, nasopharyngeal carcinoma; XLP, X-linked lymphoproliferative disorder.

TABLE 22-3. Clinical Manifestation of Infectious Mononucleosis

Finding	Occurrence (%)
Lymphadenopathy	100
Malaise or fatigue	90–100
Fever	85–95
Sore throat or dysphagia	80–85
Pharyngitis	70–80
Splenomegaly	50–75
Anorexia or nausea	50–80
Chills	40–60
Periorbital edema	25–40
Hepatomegaly	10–25
Myalgia	10–25
Jaundice	06–12
Rash	03–06
Arthralgias	<5
Photophibia, diarrhea	<5

disease.[81] EBV does not appear to be associated with Burkitt's lymphoma in Americans.[82] In patients with Duncan's syndrome, a rare familial X-linked recessive lymphoproliferative disorder, EBV infection is overwhelming and may result in agammaglobulinemia, B-cell lymphomas, or death during the acute phase.[83,84] Primary EBV infections may also evolve into a fatal immunoblastic lymphoma.[85,86] Immunodeficient or immunosuppressed persons have been noted to develop EBV-related lymphomas and lymphoproliferative syndromes.[87–92] EBV-related lymphomas have been observed in patients after renal, cardiac, and bone marrow transplantation. Patients on prolonged immunosuppression, particularly with cyclosporine (Cyclosporin-A), are at risk for EBV-associated lymphoma,[91] which sometimes resolve when immunosuppressive therapy is stopped.[93]

The patient's age affects the clinical course of EBV infection. In children under 5 years of age, the primary EBV infection is usually asymptomatic or associated with mild, nonspecific symptoms such as a rash or mild pharyngitis.[94] In most children, the disease is self-limited and lasts 2 or 3 weeks. Adolescents and adults usually develop acute infectious mononucleosis. The incubation period is about 30 to 50 days. Clinical manifestations of mononucleosis are summarized in Table 22-3. Patients develop abrupt onset of sore throat, malaise, fatigue, and fever. Headache, diffuse myalgias, a feeling of abdominal fullness, and anorexia are common nonspecific symptoms.[95] The most common complaint is a severe sore throat with accompanying dysphagia, developing during the first week and lasting about 7 to 10 days. The pharynx is typically erythematous with a thick white exudate. Palatal petechiae are also common but are not diagnostic of infectious mononucleosis and can be seen in other viral illnesses. Tonsillar enlargement is prominent and may become severe enough to interfere with deglutition or cause respiratory obstruction.[96]

Fever is present early in the course in over 90% of patients with infectious mononucleosis. Cervical lymphadenopathy, present in 80% to 90% of patients, is symmetric and most frequently involves the posterior and anterior cervical chain. Axillary and inguinal adenopathy is usually present. Hilar adenopathy is rare, occurring in less than 1% of patients.[97,98] Splenomegaly is present in most cases and is usually maximal after 10 to 14 days. Generally, the spleen is only moderately enlarged, extending 2 to 3 cm below the left costal margin. Hepatomegaly is noted in 10% to 20% of cases and jaundice in 5% to 10%, which usually peaks in the second week of the illness. Mild to moderate hepatic dysfunction is common, and occasionally patients develop marked hyperbilirubinemia.[99] Liver biopsies have revealed infiltration of the sinusoids with atypical lymphocytes.[99,100] A macular papular rash is noted in about 5% of patients. A pruritic macular papular rash develops in 90% to 100% of patients who have been given ampicillin, presumably for misdiagnosis of a bacterial pharyngitis.[101]

Complications of infectious mononucleosis are outlined in Table 22-4. Hematologic complications occur in 0.5% to 5% of patients, the most common being the development of hemolytic anemia and thrombocytopenia.[97] Hemolytic anemia is usually mild and occurs in about 3% of all cases.[102,103] Rarely, severe hemolytic anemia has been noted in patients with mononucleosis.[104] In 70% of patients, the Coombs' test is positive. Seventy to 90% of patients develop a cold agglutinin, usually IgM and rarely of the IgG class, and specific for the RBC antigen i.[103] The anti-i antibodies are common in patients with infectious mononucleosis, but, as noted, hemolytic anemia is rare.[105] In only a few cases has the hemolytic anemia clearly been shown to be caused by the anti-i antibody.[106] The development of hemolysis may be related to the thermal amplitude of the antibody or other associated antibodies.[107,108] Thrombocytopenia is a frequent complication, more common in children than adults, but it is rarely sufficient to produce petechiae.[97,109] Usually occurring during the first 2 weeks of the illness, thrombocytopenia may be related to the development of antiplatelet–antibodies directed to antigenic determinants on the platelet membrane.[110] Mild neutropenia is frequently found in the first weeks of infection.[97] Antineutrophil antibodies are a common manifestation of the polyclonal B-cell activation induced by EBV.[111]

Aplastic anemia has been reported in association with EBV infections, possibly caused by direct viral infection of bone marrow progenitor cells or a suppressive effect of circulating reactive suppressor T cells.[111,112] Moreover, DNA hybridization studies have revealed EBV and protein in

TABLE 22-4. Complications of Infectious Mononucleosis

HEMATOLOGIC (0.5%–5%)	
Autoimmune hemolytic anemia	
Thrombocytopenia	
Neutropenia	
Aplastic anemia	
Splenic rupture (<1%)	
CARDIAC (1%–6%)	
Pericarditis	
Myocarditis	
Bradycardia	
ECG abnormalities	
NERVOUS SYSTEM (0.5%–2%)	
Encephalitis	
Meningitis	
Gullain-Barré syndrome	
Optic neuritis	
Cranial nerve palsies	
Myelitis—psychiatric disorders	
PULMONARY (1%–5%)	
Cough	
Interstitial infiltrate	
Adult respiratory distress syndrome	
Pleural effusions	

the bone marrow of patients with aplastic anemia who have no recent history of infectious mononucleosis.[111]

Rapid enlargement of the spleen during the course of infectious mononucleosis leaves it vulnerable to rupture. This is a rare but potentially fatal complication. The highest incidence of splenic rupture occurs during the second and third weeks of the illness. It may happen spontaneously or with minimal trauma to the left upper quadrant.[113] Abdominal pain is infrequent in patients with infectious mononucleosis. Therefore, the presence of pain may signal a potential splenic rupture, especially when accompanied by left shoulder pain. The onset of such pain may be insidious or abrupt. Signs of peritoneal irritation, such as rebound tenderness and shifting dullness from intraabdominal bleeding, may dominate the clinical picture. Laboratory findings include a falling hematocrit, frequently with neutrophilia.[113]

Neutrophilia is infrequent in uncomplicated mononucleosis; its presence may signal an abdominal catastrophe. The abdominal CT scan is the study of choice to confirm a ruptured spleen.[112] A liver and spleen scan or RUQ ultrasound may be helpful when CT is not available. On the other hand, interpretation of radionuclide spleen imaging in patients with infectious mononucleosis can be difficult. Splenic tears may be poorly defined, and the resulting splenic uptake may be nonhomogeneous.[114] Splenic rupture usually requires an emergency splenectomy. Patients should be warned of the potential for splenic rupture and told to avoid strenuous exercise for at least 1 month and contact sports for at least 3 months after onset of symptoms.[115]

Neurologic complications of infectious mononucleosis occur in less than 1% of all patients and may be the first or only manifestation of the illness.[116] The clinical picture may be atypical with minimal lymphadenopathy, a negative monospot test, and rare circulating atypical lymphocytes. The diagnosis, therefore, in many cases rests on changes in EBV-specific serologies.[117,118] Encephalitis is the most common neurologic complication.[117] It can be acute in onset and rapidly progressive, and may resemble aseptic meningitis. Spinal fluid analysis reveals a mononuclear pleocytosis with a normal to mildly elevated protein and normal glucose. The cerebrospinal fluid may have low titers of EBV viral capsid antigen (VCA).[118] Other neurologic complications are meningitis,[117] Guillain-Barré syndrome,[116] optic neuritis,[118] cranial nerve palsies,[119] and transverse myelitis.[120] Although neurologic complications account for most deaths from infectious mononucleosis, most patients with neurologic complications recover completely after variable periods of time.[116]

Hepatic involvement usually consists of self-limited elevations of hepatocellular enzymes. Most patients with uncomplicated infectious mononucleosis have mild elevations of liver enzymes (50% to 80%). The pattern is mainly cholestatic in type, but jaundice is infrequent.[121] Rare cases of severe hepatitis have occurred during the course of infectious mononucleosis.[122] Cardiac involvement is also rare and may represent with nonspecific chest pain, arrhythmias, EKG abnormalities, pericarditis, and myocarditis.[123,124] Pulmonary involvement may present as a diffuse interstitial infiltrate. Rare instances of fatal pneumonia and adult respiratory distress syndrome have been noted after infectious mononucleosis.[125]

Laboratory Features

The most common laboratory abnormalities associated with infectious mononucleosis occur in response to virally infected B cells, polyclonal B-cell proliferation, and specific antibodies to EBV. The infection usually produces a prominent lymphocytosis with circulating atypical lymphocytes. Total white blood cell count usually ranges from 12,000 to 25,000/μL, although counts as high as 80,000/μL have been noted.[126] Leukocytosis is usually due to a lymphocytosis, which represents 60% to 90% of the cells with a variety of circulating atypical lymphocytes. These lymphocytes have round or irregular nuclei with prominent clumped chromatin. The cytoplasm is intensely basophilic with numerous vacuoles. The many atypical cells may be confused with lymphoblasts. Some may appear as immature lymphocytes with coarsely reticular nuclei and abundant cytoplasm. These atypical lymphocytes are referred to as *nonleukemic lymphoblasts, Downey cells* (type I, II, or III) and *leukocytoid lymphocytes.* They are mostly activated T lymphocytes that are responding to the infected B lymphocytes. Monocyte counts may rise transiently, but the term *mononucleosis* refers to the rise of lymphocytes, not monocytes. These cytologic alterations are not pathognomonic of infectious mononucleosis and are noted in a number of viral illnesses, including CMV infections, hepatitis, varicella, and the occasional viral exanthema in children.

The neutrophil count is relatively and absolutely decreased in the first weeks of infectious mononucleosis. A shift to the left may occur with toxic granules and Döhle's bodies in circulating neutrophils. The platelet count is modestly depressed in over 90% of patients. A Coombs' test is frequently positive, but hemolysis is rare. Antinuclear antibodies may be present as well as cold agglutinins and cryoglobulins.

The heterophile antibody, first described by Paul and Bunnel[77] as sheep erythrocyte agglutinins, is present in the sera at some time during the course of infectious mononucleosis in 90% of patients. The presence of this antibody is not specific for infectious mononucleosis. In patients with infectious mononucleosis, the heterophile antibodies are absorbed by beef RBCs and not by other antigens such as those found in guinea pig kidneys (Table 22-5). This provides the basis for the sensitive monospot test. Test serum is mixed with a suspension of finely ground guinea pig kidney on one part of the slide and a suspension of beef erythrocyte stroma on the other. Horse erythrocytes, more sensitive than the originally described sheep RBCs, are added to each spot and mixed. The sera from a patient with infectious mononucleosis agglutinates with the horse erythrocytes in the serum absorbed with guinea pig kidney but not in the serum absorbed with beef erythrocyte stroma. This provides a highly specific and sensitive test.

False-negative tests occur mainly in young children who produce limited amounts of the IgM heterophile antibody. In these patients, the diagnosis requires the assay of specific antibodies to EBV. False-positive monospot tests have been noted rarely in patients with lymphomas and hepatitis.[127]

Several virus-specific antibodies produced by the host in response to EBV infection appear and disappear at different times during the course of the illness (Fig. 22-4). Determination of these antibodies is rarely necessary for diagnosis, since over 90% of cases are heterophile-positive and have a positive monospot test. In the atypical or heterophile-negative case, determination of EBV-specific antibodies may be helpful.[127] Antibodies to VCA occur early in the course of infectious mononucleosis in all patients. Those who are acutely ill already have IgG antibodies to VCA when they present for evaluation. The IgG anti-VCA persists for life and therefore is not helpful in establishing a diagnosis of an acute or ongoing infection. The IgM anti-VCA antibody is highly sensitive and specific for recent EBV infection. An antibody titer of more than 5, as measured by indirect immunofluorescence, is virtually diagnostic of an acute infection. The IgM anti-VCA falls rapidly after the first 4 to 8 weeks, and only 10% of patients have titers after 4 months.[127]

Serum antibodies to specific early antigens are demonstrable in the first month of infection. The presence of early antigens is variable and may correlate with severe disease or a protracted course.[128] The early antigen antibodies persist for only a few years. Specific antibodies to EBNA develop after the acute phase of the illness, usually after 4 weeks, and persist for life. The appearance of EBNA antibodies in an EBNA-negative, VCA-positive patient is diagnostic of recent EBV infection. Complement-fixing antigens (anti-S) and neutralizing antibodies also occur late in the course and reach maximal levels 6 to 8 weeks after onset of the illness. A rising titer of anti-S antibody is suggestive of a recent EBV infection. The EBV-specific antibodies occur independently of the heterophile antibody. These specific antibodies are useful in the evaluation of atypical, heterophile negative cases.

EBV may be cultured from oropharyngeal washings or cultured peripheral blood B lymphocytes from most patients with infectious mononucleosis.[129] On the other hand, many normal persons without an acute infection may shed the virus. Therefore, culturing the virus is of questionable clinical use.

TABLE 22-5. Heterophile Antibodies

		After Absorption*	
Source of Serum	**Unabsorbed***	**Beef RBCs**	**Guinea Pig Kidney**
Infectious mononucleosis†	++++	0	+++
Serum sickness	+++	0	0
Normal serum (Forssman)	+	+	0

* Sheep RBC agglutination.
† Sixty percent positive during first 2 weeks of Epstein-Barr virus infection; 80% to 90% positive by 1 month; usually negative after 3 to 6 months.

In most cases, the diagnosis of infectious mononucleosis is clear from the clinical manifestations, appropriate setting, circulating atypical lymphocytes, and positive heterophile monospot test. Diagnosis becomes difficult when clinical manifestations are atypical, blunted, or severe, and when they occur in heterophile-negative infections. CMV infection is the most common cause of heterophile-negative infectious mononucleosis. CMV can produce an illness that is similar clinically to EBV infection. CMV infection presents with less pharyngitis and lymphadenopathy and rarely induces anti-i-specific cryoglobulins.[130] Toxoplasmosis may mimic many of the features of infectious mononucleosis. In addition, many other viral illnesses may present with features of infectious mononucleosis, including hepatitis A and B, coxsackieviruses, and HIV infections. Bacterial pharyngitis and adenovirus pharyngitis can also mimic the early phases of infectious mononucleosis. In most cases, these disorders are confirmed by bacterial cultures or specific serologies.

Treatment

Infection with EBV causes a variety of clinical manifestations that are partly dependent on the immune response elicited in the infected host.[64] Most patients who develop infectious mononucleosis require no specific therapy. Most cases resolve spontaneously over a 2- to 3-week period. The sore throat is usually maximal for 3 to 5 days early in the course, then gradually resolves within 1 week to 10 days and responds to supportive therapy and mild analgesics. Bed rest is advisable during this course, and the patient should avoid all sports or strenuous activity because of the risk of splenic rupture. Some patients may experience severe tonsillar enlargement, which can result (rarely) in airway obstruction.[96,131]

Corticosteroids are effective for the treatment of impending airway obstruction in patients with infectious mononucleosis.[132] Prednisone or an equivalent steroid preparation, 40 to 80 mg/d in divided doses tapering over 7 to 10 days, can have a dramatic effect on tonsillar enlargement and pharyngitis. Corticosteroids do not appear to change the pattern of lymphocyte response during the early phase of the illness or to alter the serologic response to EBV. Corticosteroids are also generally administered for many of the complications associated with an acute EBV infection such as severe thrombocytopenia, hemolytic anemia, neurologic sequelae, myocarditis, and pericarditis.[133] Steroid therapy should generally be reserved for complicated or severe cases and should not be used in patients without complications and with acute infectious mononucleosis.

Treatment with acyclovir does not affect the clinical symptoms or laboratory parameters but may decrease oropharyngeal viral shedding early in the course in patients with infectious mononucleosis.[134] Antibiotics have no effect on the course of EBV infection. About 20% of patients during an acute infection have a concurrent β-hemolytic streptococcal pharyngitis and should therefore receive appropriate antibiotics. Almost all patients demonstrate a rash from ampicillin, but penicillin or erythromycin can be safely administered.

The other EBV-associated disorders are more difficult to treat. The aggressive and potentially fatal infectious mononucleosis that occurs in patients with the X-linked lymphoproliferative syndrome generally do not respond to acyclovir.[133] γ-interferon, interleukin-2, and intravenous

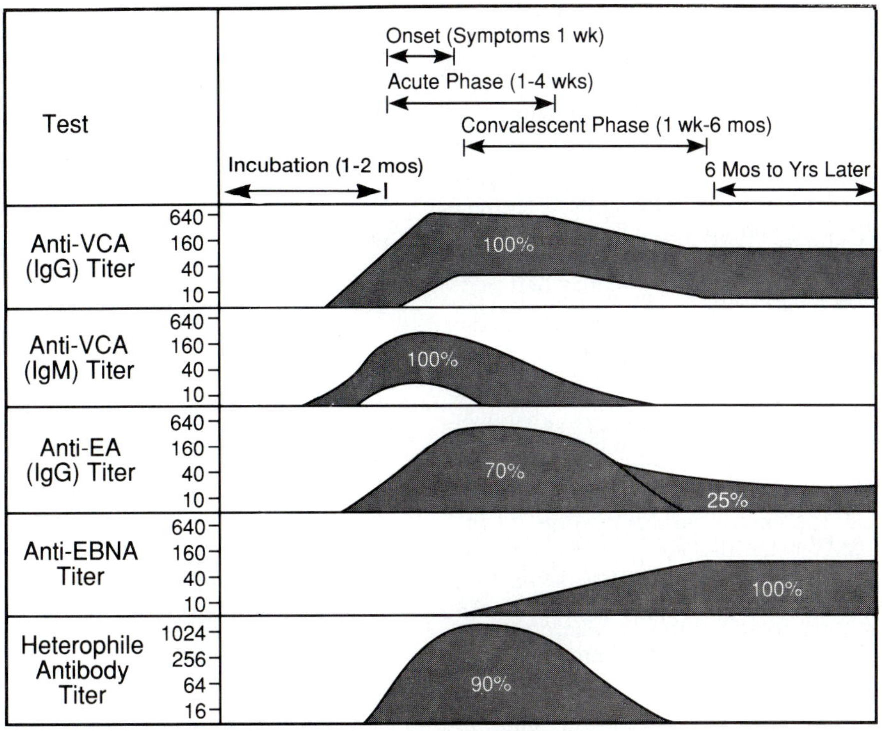

FIGURE 22-4. Antibody response to Epstein-Barr virus (EBV) infection. Antibodies to the viral capsid antigen (VCA) are measured by immunofluorescence and rise early in the course of the illness. IgG antibodies to the VCA are present in 100% of patients. The highest titers are found at the onset of clinical illness. The IgG VCA antibody is present for life after an EBV infection. The IgM anti-VCA antibodies are sensitive and specific. They are found in 100% of individuals and occur at the onset of infection. Titers usually fall within 4 weeks after the onset of infection, and most individuals have negative titers at 4 months. The presence of anti-VCA IgM titer is virtually diagnostic in an acute EBV infection. Anti–early antigen (anti-EA) antibodies persist for 3 to 6 months and correlate in part with the severity of the disease. Anti–Epstein-Barr nuclear antigen (anti-EBNA) is found in all patients, appearing late in the course of clinical infection. The peak titer occurs 2 to 4 weeks after the onset of clinical symptoms. EBNA persists for years and may be helpful in the diagnosis of heterophile-negative cases. The appearance of EBNA antibodies in a patient who was previously VCA-positive and EBNA-negative is strong evidence of recent EBV infection. (After Henle W, Henle GE, Horwitz CA. Epstein-Barr virus–specific diagnostic tests in infectious mononucleosis. Hum Pathol 1974;5:551)

immunoglobulin have been tried in selected cases of aggressive EBV infections with some limited success.[135–137] The EBV-associated lymphoproliferative disease in immunocompromised hosts may transiently respond to intravenous acyclovir given at 5 to 10 mg/kg every 8 hours.[138,139]

CHRONIC MONONUCLEOSIS SYNDROME

Chronic mononucleosis syndrome is a poorly defined clinical entity, linked to EBV because its symptoms are similar to the prodrome of infectious mononucleosis. It is marked by prolonged fever and malaise in young and middle-aged adults.[140] Other prominent symptoms are difficulty in concentrating, arthralgias, myalgias, recurrent sore throat, and fluctuating lymphadenopathy. Patients rarely experience weight loss or intermittent night sweats. Despite the similarities to infectious mononucleosis, a number of studies have suggested that EBV is not the etiologic agent. Although many patients exhibit antibody titers to EBV, the association of these antibodies to this disorder, if any, is not clear.[141]

At this point, no one etiologic agent has been identified for chronic mononucleosis syndrome. Possible infectious agents are CMV, HIV, influenza A, coxsackievirus, and *Borrelia burgdorferi*. Many studies of chronic mononucleosis and chronic fatigue syndrome are frustrated by a lack of objective findings. At this time, it is unlikely that EBV infection is the source of this disorder.[142]

CYTOMEGALOVIRUS

Pathogenesis and Clinical Features

Cytomegalovirus (CMV) is a member of the herpes group and produces a clinical syndrome similar to EBV. CMV presents many unique problems for the immunocompromised host, including bone marrow and organ transplant patients, immature neonates, and persons with acquired immunodeficiency syndrome.

The epidemiology of CMV infections is like that of other herpesviruses. The infection is widespread and usually unapparent. The percentage of antibodies in adults ranges from 40% to 100% and is significantly higher in third world countries than in the United States and Europe.[143] In Third World countries, between 30% to 50% of patients acquire the infection in the perinatal period. The infection rate increases slowly during the first year.

CMV can be transmitted through the contaminated uterine cervix during birth as well as through human milk.[144] Transmission is also common from exposure in nurseries and day care centers.[145] Infected children generally carry the virus for long periods in the respiratory tract and urine. Adults rarely shed the virus in urine or respiratory secretions.[146]

Another significant source of CMV transmission is through blood products. The risk of infection is proportional to the number of units received, with estimates varying from 3% to 12% per unit.[147] The overall risk of acquiring a CMV infection is 2 seroconversions per 100 units of red cells transfused.[148] Infection is usually asymptomatic. The risk of CMV transmission is decreased by using cryopreserved blood, leukocyte-poor blood, or blood from seronegative donors.[149] Many blood products are now being tested for CMV, and CMV-negative blood products are available for selected patients. Special care must be taken when blood products are used with seronegative neonates, because they are at high risk for primary fatal CMV infection.

CMV is also transmitted sexually. The incidence of asymptomatic CMV virus in the cervix ranges from 1% to 35% among different populations.[150] CMV has also been found in high titers in the semen of both heterosexual and homosexual males.[151] Liver, heart, and bone marrow transplant patients are at high risk for severe CMV infection.[152] Clinical manifestations of the reactivation of CMV infections include CMV hepatitis, pneumonitis, and colitis.[130] Most CMV infections are asymptomatic. Congenital CMV infections can produce jaundice, hepatosplenomegaly, and multiple system organ failures.[153] Macrocephaly, chorioretinitis, and cerebral calcification are also common.[153]

CMV infections are similar to EBV infections, with most adults presenting with fever, malaise, and splenomegaly. Pharyngitis and lymphadenopathy are less commonly seen with CMV infections. CMV infection may also be more prolonged than an EBV infection, with fevers persisting for 1 to 2 months. Like EBV, a number of complications have been reported in the normal host, including hepatitis, neurologic complications, pneumonitis, and gastroenteritis. Most normal, nonimmunosuppressed patients recover from CMV infection without difficulty.

CMV also has many of the laboratory features of EBV infections. Lymphocytosis is prominent, with an elevated total lymphocyte count and many circulating atypical lymphocytes. Immunologic features, including Coombs' test, cold agglutinins, and cryoglobulins, are less common in CMV-associated infections. Hepatitis is more common in patients with CMV. As with other herpesviruses, CMV can be cultured from urine, semen, white blood cells, and other infected tissues, but this does not necessarily reflect an acute infection. A four-fold rise in complement-fixing antibodies to CMV is considered diagnostic of a recent infection. The antibodies to the different CMV antigens are less well defined than are those to EBV.

Splenomegaly may be a prominent feature of CMV infections. The differential diagnosis includes hepatitis A and B virus, toxoplasmosis, HIV, and coxsackievirus infections, and, of course, EBV.

Therapy

Most patients with CMV infection recover without therapy. Treating immunocompromised patients with CMV infections presents a number of special problems. Gancyclovir may be effective in limited CMV disease (5 mg/kg/12 h for the first 2 weeks, followed by 5 mg/kg/d). Results in patients with CMV retinitis are encouraging, although responses with other serious CMV infections have been variable.[154,155] Gancyclovir, either alone or in combination with high-dose intravenous immunoglobulin (500 mg/kg/d), has been effective in selected immunosuppressed bone marrow transplant patients with CMV pneumonitis.[154–156] The dose of gancyclovir must be adjusted for renal function and the white blood count and platelets must be closely followed. The potential for treatment with immunoglobulin and gancyclovir in other immunosuppressed patients requires further study.

REFERENCES

1. Gray H. On the structure and use of the spleen. London, John W Parker, 1854:380.
2. May MT. Galen: on the usefulness of the parts of the body. Ithaca, NY, Cornell University Press, 1968:232.
3. Rosner F. The spleen in the Talmud and other early Jewish writing. Bull Hist Med 1972;40:82.
4. Crosby WH. The spleen. In: Wintrube MM, ed. Blood pure and eloquent. New York, McGraw-Hill, 1980.
5. Muller J. Uber die Strucktur der eigenthumlichen Korperchen in der Milz einiger planzefresser: Saugetiere. Arch Anat Physiol 1834;1:80.
6. Joffey JM, Courtice FC. Lymphocytes, lymph and the lymphomyeloid complex. London, Academic Press, 1970:942.
7. Hewson W. In: Falconar M, ed. Experimental inquiries. Part the Third, containing a description of the red particles of the blood in the human subject and other animals, with an account of the structure and offices of the lymphatic gland, of the thymus gland, and of the spleen. London, T Longman 1777:133.
8. Gulliver G, ed. The works of William Hewson FRS. London, Sydenham Society, 1848:360.
9. Virchow R. Die Leukämie, in Gesammelte Abhandlungen zur wissenschaftlichen Medizin. Frankfurt, Meidinger, 1956:190.
10. Ranvier LA. Triate technique d'histologie. Paris, Librairie F Savy, 1875.
11. Fleming W. Studien über Regeneration der Gewebe. I. Die Zellvermebrung in den lymphdrusen and verwandten Organen, und ihr Einflus auf Deren Bau. Bonn, Max Cohen & Sohn, 1885:66.
12. Malphighi M. De Viscerum structura exercitatio anatomica, Chapter IV, Bonn, De Liene, 1666:101.
13. Billroth T. Neue Beitragezur vergleichenden Histologie der Milz. Arch Anat Physiol 1857;24:88.
14. MacDonald RH, Moretta L. The definition of lymphocyte subpopulations: new approaches to an old problem. Semin Oncol 1984;21:223.
15. Lennert K, Stein HH. The germinal center: morphology, histochemistry, and immunohistology. In: Goos M, Christophe E, eds. Lymphoproliferative diseases of the skin. Berlin, Springer-Verlag, 1982:3.
16. Mann RB, Jaffe Es, Berard CW. Malignant lymphomas: a conceptual understanding of morphological diversity. Am J Pathol 1979;94:105.
17. Hsu S, Cossman J, Jaffe ES. Lymphocyte subpopulation in normal human lymphoid tissues. Am J Clin Pathol 1983;80:21.
18. Gathings WE, Kubagawa H, Cooper MD. A distinctive pattern of B cell immaturity in perinatal humans. Immunol Rev 1981;57:107.
19. Aisenber AC. Current concepts in immunology: cell-surfaced markers in lymphoproliferative disease. N Engl J Med 1981;304:331.
20. Hsu S, Cossman J, Jaffe ES. Lymphocyte subsets in normal lymphoid tissues. Am J Clin Pathol 1983;80:21.
21. Janossy G, Tidman N, Selby W, et al. Human T lymphocytes of inducer and suppressor type occupy different microenvironments. Nature 1980;287:81.
22. Klaus GGR, Humphrey JH, Kunkl A, Dongwor DW Jr. The follicular dendritic cell: its role in antigen presentation in the generation of immunological memory. Immunol Rev 1980;53:3.
23. Pizzolo G, Chilosi M. Double immunostaining of lymph node sections by monoclonal antibodies using phycoerythrin labeling and haptenated reagents. Am J Clin Pathol 1984;82:44.
24. Stein H, Gerdes J, Mason DY. The normal and malignant germinal centre. Clin Haematol 1982;11:531.
25. Craddock CG. Kinetics of lymphoreticular tissue. Semin Hematol 1967;4:387.
26. Wilkinson L, Tang A, Gjedrteda A. Marked lymphocytosis suggesting chronic lymphocytic leukemia in three patients with hyposplenism. Am J Med 1983;75:1053.
27. Tefferi A, Phyliky R. Role of immunotyping in chronic lymphocytosis: review of the natural history of the condition in 145 adult patients. Mayo Clin Proc 1988;63:801.
28. Katu K. Leucocytes in infancy and childhood. J Pediatr 1935;7:7.
29. Falcao RP. Human blood lymphocytes subpopulations from birth to eight years. Clin Exp Immunol 1980;39:203.
30. Weksler ME. Senescence of the immune system. Med Clin North Am 1983;67:263.
31. Moody CE, Innes JB, Staiano-Coico L, et al. Lymphocyte transformation induced by autologous cells. XI. The effect of age on the autologous mixed lymphocyte reaction. Immunology 1981;44:431.
32. Ales MJE, Alvarez MM, Merino F, et al. Decreased TcR-CD3+ T cell numbers in healthy aged humans: evidence that T cell defects are masked by a reciprocal increase of TcR-CD3-CD2+ natural killer cells. Eur J Immunol 1988;18:1827.
33. Dajani AS, Garcia RE, Wolinski E. Etiology of cervical lymphadenitis in children. N Engl J Med 1963;268:1329.
34. Lee YN, Terry R, Lukes RJ. Lymph node biopsy for diagnosis: a statistical study. J Surg Oncol 1980;14:53.
35. Sap GB, Brooks JSJ, Schwartz J. When to perform biopsies of enlarged peripheral lymph nodes in young patients. JAMA 1984;252:1321.

36. Schen RJ. Lymphadenopathy due to drug: a survey of the literature. Isr J Med Sci 1904;23:129.
37. Weisenburger DD. Immunoblastic lymphadenopathy associated with methyldopatherapy. Cancer 1978;42:2322.
38. Gams RA, Neal JA, Conrad FG. Hydantoin-induced pseudolymphoma. Ann Intern Med 1968;69:557.
39. Saltzstein SL, Ackerman LV. Lymphadenopathy induced by anticonvulsant drugs and mimicking clinically and pathologically malignant lymphomas. Cancer 1959;12:104.
40. Estes D, Christian CL. The natural history of systemic lupus erythematosis. Medicine 1971;50:85.
41. Moutsopoulos HM, Chiesed TM, Mann DL, et al. Sjögren syndrome: current issues. Ann Intern Med 1980;92:212.
42. Drusin LM, Singer C, Valtni AJ, et al. Infectious syphillis mimicking neoplastic disease. Arch Intern Med 1977;137:156.
43. Holmes KK, Mardh PA, Sparling PF, et al. Sexually transmitted diseases. New York, McGraw-Hill, 1984.
44. Epstein JI, Ambinder RF, Kuhajda, et al. Localized herpes simplex lymphadenitis. Am J Clin Pathol 1986;86:444.
45. Metroka CE, Cunningham-Rundles S, Pollack MS, et al. Generalized lymphadenopathy in homosexual men. Ann Intern Med 1983;99:585.
46. Tindall B, Barker S, Donovan B, et al. Characterization of the acute clinical illness associated with human immunodeficiency virus infection. Arch Intern Med 1988;148:945.
47. Sinclair S, Beckman E, Ellman L. Biopsy of enlarged, superficial lymph nodes. JAMA 1974;228:602.
48. Greenfield S, Jordan C. The clinical investigation of lymphadenopathy in primary care practice. JAMA 1978;240:1388.
49. Knight PJ, Mulne AF, Vassy LE. When is lymph node biopsy indicated in children with enlarged peripheral nodes? Pediatrics 1982;69:391.
50. Zaelzer WW, Kaplan J. The child with lymphadenopathy. Semin Hematol 1975;112:323.
51. Swartz M. Lymphadenitis and lymphangitis. V. New York, McGraw-Hill, 1990:818.
52. Iles PB, Emerson PA. Tuberculous lymphadenitis. Br Med J 1974;1: 143.
53. Carithers HA. Cat-scratch disease: an overview based on a study of 1,200 patients. Am J Dis Child 1985;139:1124.
54. Becker LE. Lymphogranuloma venereum. Int J Dermatol 1976;15:26.
55. Young LS, Bicknell DS, Archer BG, et al. Tularemia epidemic: Vermont 1968: forty-seven cases linked to contact with muskrats. N Engl J Med 1969;280:1253.
56. Scobie WG. Acute suppurative adenitis in children. Scott Med J 1969;14: 352.
57. Lincoln EM, Gilbert LA. Disease in children due to mycobacteria other than Mycobacterium tuberculosis. Am Rev Respir Dis 1972;683:105.
58. Spark RP, Fried ML, Bean CK, et al. Nontuberculous mycobacterial adenitis of childhood: the ten-year experience at a community hospital. Am J Dis Child 1988;142:106.
59. Boyd JC, Marr JJ. Decreasing reliability of acid fast smear techniques for detection of tuberculous. Ann Intern Med 1975;82:481.
60. Tappero JN, Mohle-Boetani J, Koehler JE, et al. The epidemiology of bacillary angiomatosis and bacillary peliosis. JAMA 1993;269:770.
61. Dolan MJ, Wong MT, Regnery RL, et al. Syndrome of *Rochalimaea henselae* adenitis suggesting cat scratch disease. Ann Intern Med 1993;118:331.
62. Dorfman RF, Warnke R. Lymphadenopathy simulating the malignant lymphomas. Hum Pathol 1974;5:519.
63. Reed WBC, Palmer DL, Williams RC, et al. Bubonic plague in southwestern Unites States. Medicine 1970;49:465.
64. Straus S, Cohen JI, Tosato G, Meier J. Epstein-Barr virus infections: biology, pathogenesis and management. Ann Intern Med 1993;118:45.
65. Sixbey JW, Davis DS, Young LS, et al. Human epithelial cell expression of an Epstein Barr virus receptor. J Gen Virol 1987;68:805.
66. Jondal M, Klein G. Surface markers on human B and T lymphocytes. II. Presence of Epstein Barr virus receptors on B lymphocytes. J Exp Med 1973;138:1365.
67. Fingeroth JD, Weiss JJ, Tedder TF, et al. Epstein-Barr virus receptor of human B lymphocytes is the C3d receptor CR2. Proc Natl Acad Sci USA 1984;81:4510.
68. Hennesy K, Kieff E. One of two Epstein-Barr virus nuclear antigens contains a glycine-alanine copolymer domain. Proc Natl Acad Sci USA 1983;80:5665.
69. Hennessy K, Wang F, Bushman EW, et al. Definitive identification of a member of the Epstein-Barr virus nuclear protein 3 family. Proc Natl Acad Sci USA 1986;83:5693.
70. Killner J, Kallin B, Alexander H, et al. An Epstein-Barr virus (EBV)-determined nuclear antigen (EBNA5) partly encoded by the transformation-associated Bam WYH region of EBV DNA: preferential expression in lymphoblastoid cell lines. Proc Natl Acad Sci USA 1986;83: 6641.
71. Thorley-Lawson DA, Mann KP. Early events in Epstein-Barr virus infection provide a model for B cell activation. J Exp Med 1985;162:45.
72. Robinson J, Smith RW, Niederman JC. Mitotic EBNA-positive lymphocytes in peripheral blood during infectious mononucleosis. Nature 1980;287:334.
73. De Waele M, Theilemans C, VanCamp BKG. Characterization of immunoregulatory T cells in EBV-induced infectious mononucleosis by monoclonal antibodies. N Engl J Med 1981;304:460.
74. Svedmyr E, Jondal M. Cytotoxic effector cells specific for B cell lines transfored by Epstein-Barr virus are present in patients with infectious mononucleosis. Proc Natl Acad Sci USA 1975;72:1622.
75. Tosato G, Magrath I, Kiski I, et al. Activation of suppressor T cells during Epstein-Barr virus–induced infectious mononucleosis. N Engl J Med 1979;301:1133.
76. Provisor AJ, Iacuone JJ, Chilcote RR, et al. Acquired gammaglobulinemia after a life-threatening illness with clinical and laboratory features of infectious mononucleosis in three related male children. N Engl J Med 1975;293:62.
77. Paul JR, Bunnel WW. The presence of heterophile antibodies in infectious mononucleosis. Am J Med Sci 1932;183:90.
78. Strauss SE, Cohen JI, Tosato G, Meier J. Epstein-Barr virus infections: biology, pathogenesis, and management. Ann Intern Med 1993;118:45.
79. Zur Hausen H, Schulte-Holthausen H, Klein G, et al. EBV DNA in biopsies of Burkitt's tumors and anaplastic carcinomas of the nasopharynx. Nature 1970;228:1056.
80. Lindahl T, Klein G, Reedman BM, et al. Relationship between Epstein-Barr virus (EBV) DNA and the EBV determined nuclear antigen (EBNA) in Burkitt's lymphoma biopsies and other lymphoproliferative malignancies. Int J Cancer 1974;13:764.
81. deThe G, Geser A, Day NE, et al. Epidemiological evidence for causal relationship between Epstein-Barr virus and Burkitt's lymphoma from a Ugandan prospective study. Nature 1978;274:756.
82. Pagano JS, Huang CH, Levine P. Absence of Epstein-Barr viral DNA in American Burkitt's lymphoma. N Engl J Med 1973;289:1395.
83. Sullivan JL, Byron KS, Brewster FE, et al. X-linked lymphoproliferative syndromes: natural history of the immunodeficiency. J Clin Invest 1983;71:1765.
84. Grierson H, Purtilo DT. Epstein-Barr virus infection in males with the X-linked lymphoproliferative syndrome. Ann Intern Med 1987;106: 538.
85. Snydman DR, Rudders RA, Daoust P, et al. Infectious mononucleosis in an adult progressing to fatal immunoblastic lymphoma. Ann Intern Med 1982;96:737,.
86. Robinson JE, Brown N, Andimauw et al. Diffuse polyclonal B-cell lymphoma during primary infection with Epstein-Barr virus. N Engl J Med 1980;302:1293.
87. Andiman W, Gradonville L, Heston L, et al. Use of clonedprobes to detect Epstein-Barr viral DNA in tissues of patients with neoplastic and lymphoproliferative disease. J Infect Dis 1983;148:967.
88. Hanto DW, Frizzera G, Gajl-Peczalska KJ, et al. Epstein-Barr virus induced B-cell lymphoma after renal transplantation: acyclovir therapy and transition from polyclonal to monoclonal B-cell proliferation. N Engl J Med 1982;306:913.
89. Frizzera G, Hanto DW, Gajl-Peczalska J, et al. Polymorphic diffuse B-cell hyperplasias and lymphomas in renal transplant recipients. Cancer Res 1981;41:4262.
90. Hanto DW, Frizzera G, Gajl-Peczalska J, et al. The Epstein-Barr virus in the pathogenesis of post-transplant lymphoma. Transplant Proc 1981;13:756.
91. Crawford DH, Thomas JA, Janossy G, et al. Epstein-Barr virus nuclear antigen positive lymphoma after cyclosporin: a treatment in a patient with a renal allograft. Lancet 1980;1:1355.
92. Zeigler JL, Miner RC, Rosenbaum E, et al. Outbreaks of Burkitt's-like lymphoma in homosexual men. Lancet 1982;2:631.
93. Ho M, Jaffe R, Miller G, et al. The frequency of Epstein-Barr virus infection and associated lymphoproliferative syndrome after transplantation and its manifestations in children. Transplantation 1988;45: 719.
94. Fleisher GR, Pasquariello PS, Warren WS, et al. Intrafamilial transmission of Epstein-Barr virus infections. J Pediatr 1981;98:16.
95. Sumaya CV, Ench Y. Epstein-Barr virus infectious mononucleosis in children. I. Clinical and general laboratory findings. Pediatrics 1985;75: 1003.
96. Catling SJ, Astbury AJ, Latif M. Airway obstruction in infectious mononuclosis. Anaesthesia 1984;39:699,.
97. Hoagland RJ. Infectiouis mononucleosis. New York, Grune & Stratton, 1967:52.
98. Rosenthal T, Hertz M. Mediastinal lymphadenopathy in infectious mononucleosis. JAMA 1975;233:1300.
99. Kilpatrick ZM. Structural and functional abnormalities of the liver in infectious mononucleosis. Arch Intern Med 1966;117:47.
100. Fuhrman SA, Gill R, Horowitz CA, et al. Marked hyperbilirubinemia in infectious mononucleosis: analysis of laboratory data in seven patients. Arch Intern Med 1987;147:850.
101. Pullen H, Wright N, Murdock J McC. Hypersensitivity reactions to antibacterial drugs in infectious mononucleosis. Lancet 1967;2:1176.
102. Troxel DB, Innella F, Cohen RJ. Infectious mononucleosis complicated by hemolytic anemia due to anti-i. Am J Clin Pathol 1966;46:625.
103. Horwitz CA, Moulds J, Henle W, et al. Cold agglutinins in infectious mononucleosis and heterophile antibody negative mononucleosis-like syndromes. Blood 1977;50:195.
104. Silber M, Richards JD, Jacobs P. Life threatening haemolytic anemia and infectious mononucleosis: a case report. S Afr Med J 1985;07:183.

105. Wilkinson LS Petz, LD Garraty, G. Reappraisal of the role of anti-i in haemolytic anemia in infectious mononucleosis. Br J Haematol 1973;25: 715.
106. Sutton RNP. The occurrence of autoantibodies in infectious mononucleosis. Clin Exp Immunol 1974;17:427.
107. Woodruff RK, McPherson AJ. Severe hemolytic anemia complicating infectious mononucleosis. Aust NZ J Med 1976;6:509.
108. Horowitz CA, Moulds J, Henle W, et al. Cold agglutinins in infectious mononucleosis and heterophil-antibody–negative mononucleosis-like syndromes. Blood 1977;50:195.
109. Clark BF, Davies SH. Severe thrombocytopenia in infectious mononucleosis. Am J Med Sci 1964;248:703.
110. Winiarski J. Antibodies to platelet membrane glycoprotein antigens in three cases of infectious mononucleosis–induced thrombocytopenic purpura. Eur J Haematol 1989;43:29.
111. Schooley RT, Densen P, Harmon D, et al. Antineutrophil antibodies in infectious mononucleosis. Am J Med 1984;76:85.
112. Baranski B, Armstrong G, Truman JT, et al. Epstein-Barr virus in the bone marrow of patients with aplastic anemia. Ann Intern Med 1988;109:695.
113. Frecentese DF, Cogbill TH. Spontaneous splenic rupture in infectious mononucleosis. Am Surg 1987;53:521.
114. Vezina WC, Nicholson RL, Cohen P, et al. Radionuclide diagnosis of splenic rupture in infectious mononucleosis. Clin Nucl Med 1984;9: 341.
115. Haines JD Jr. When to resume sports after infectious mononucleosis: how soon is safe? Postgrad Med 1987;81:331.
116. Silverstein A, Steinberg S, Nathanson M. Nervous system involvement in infectious mononucleosis: the heralding and/or major manifestation. Arch Neurol 1972;26:353.
117. Grose C, Henle W, Henle G, et al. Primary Epstein-Barr virus infections in acute neurologic diseases. N Engl J Med 1975;292:392.
118. Joncas JH, Chicoine L, Thivierge R, et al. Epstein-Barr virus antibodies in the cerebrospinal fluid. Am J Dis Child 1974;127:282.
119. Tanner OR. Ocular manifestations of infectious mononucleosis. Arch Ophthalmol 1954;51:229.
120. Silber MH. Acute transverse myelopathy in Epstein-Barr virus infection: case reports. S Afr Med J 1983;64:753.
121. Finkel M, Parker GW, Fanselau HA. The hepatitis of infectious mononucleosis: experience with 235 cases. Milit Med 1964;129:533.
122. Markin RS, Linder J, Zuerlein K, et al. Hepatitis in fatal infectious mononucleosis. Gastroenterology 1987;93:1210.
123. Cheng TC. Severe chest pain due to infectious mononucleosis. Postgrad Med 1983;73:149.
124. Butler T, Pastore J, Simon G, et al. Infectious mononucleosis myocarditis. J Infect 1981;3:172.
125. Pether JV, Caul EO, Betteridge TJ, et al. Fatal pneumonia after glandular fever and rubella. (Letter) Lancet 1989;1:1210.
126. Henry JB. Clinical diagnosis and management by laboratory methods. Philadelphia, WB Saunders, 1984:715.
127. Halpring J, Scott AL, Jacobson L, et al. Enzyme-linked immunosorbent assay of antibodies to Epstein-Barr virus nuclear and early antigens in patients with infectious mononucleosis and nasopharyngeal carcinoma. Ann Intern Med 1986;104:331.
128. Horowitz CA, Henle W, Henle G, et al. Clinical and laboratory evaluation of elderly patients with heterophil-antibody positive infectious mononucleosis. Am J Med 1976;61:333.
129. Niederman JC, Miller G, Pearson HA, et al. Infectious mononucleosis: Epstein-Barr virus shedding in saliva and the oropharynx. N Engl J Med 1976;294:1355.
130. Betts RF. Syndrome of cytomegalovirus infection. Adv Intern Med 1980;26:447.
131. Synderman NL, Stool SE. Management of airway obstruction in children with infectious mononucleosis. Otolaryngol Head Neck Surg 1982;90: 168.
132. Brandfonbrener A, Epstein A, Wu S, Phair J. Corticosteroid therapy in Epstein-Barr virus infection: effect on lymphocyte class, subset, and response to early antigen. Arch Intern Med 1986;146:337.
133. Andersson J, Ernberg I. Management of Epstein-Barr virus infections. Am J Med 1988;85:107.
134. Andersson J, Britton S, Ernberg I, et al. Effect of acyclovir on infectious mononucleosis: a double-blind, placebo-controlled study. J Infect Dis 1986;153:283.
135. Okano M, Thiele GM, Kobayashi RH, et al. Interferon-gamma in a family with X-linked lymphoproliferative syndrome with acute Epstein-Barr virus infection. J Clin Immunol 1989;9:48.
136. Aronson FR, Dempsey RA, Allegretta M, et al. Malignant granular lymphoproliferation after Epstein-Barr virus infection: partial immunologic reconstitution with interleukin-2. Am J Hematol 1987;25:427.
137. Duncombe AS, Amos RJ, Metcalfe P, et al. Intravenous immunoglobulin therapy in thrombocytopenic infectious mononucleosis. Clin Lab Haematol 1989;11:11.
138. Purtilo DT. Epstein-Barr virus: the spectrum of its manifestations in human beings. South Med J 1987;80:943.
139. Hanto DW, Najarian JS. Advances in the diagnosis and treatment of EBV-associated lymphoproliferative diseases in immunocompromised hosts. J Surg Oncol 1985;30:215.
140. Straus SE. The chronic mononucleosis syndrome. J Infect Dis 1988;157: 405.
141. Merlin TL. Chronic mononucleosis: pitfalls in the laboratory diagnosis. Hum Pathol 1986;17:2.
142. Schooley RT. Chronic fatigue syndrome: a manifestation of Epstein-Barr virus infection? Curr Clin Top Infect Dis 1988;9:126.
143. Krech U. Complement-fixing antibodies against cytomegalovirus in different parts of the world. Bull WHO 1973;49:103.
144. Stagno S, Reynolds DW, Pass RF, et al. Breast milk and the risk of cytomegalovirus infection. N Engl J Med 1980;312:1073.
145. Pass RF, August AM, Dworsky M, et al. Cytomegalovirus infection in a day care center. N Engl J Med 1982;307:477.
146. Dworsky ME, Welder K, Cassaday G, et al. Occupational risk for primary cytomegalovirus infection among pediatric health care workers. N Engl J Med 1983;309:950.
147. Prince AM, Szmuness W, Millian SJ, et al. A serologic study of cytomegalovirus infections associated with blood transfusions. N Engl J Med 1971;284:1125.
148. Chou S, Kim DY, Normal DJ. Transmission of cytomegalovirus by pretransplant leukocyte transfusions in renal transplant candidates. J Infect Dis 1987;155:565.
149. Bowden Ra, Slichter SJ, Sayers MH, Mori M, Cays MJ, Meyers JD. Use of leukocyte-depleted platelets and cytomegalovirus-seronegative red blood cells for prevention of primary cytomegalovirus infection after marrow transplant. Blood 1991;79:246.
150. Stagno S, Reynolds D, Tsiantos A, et al. Cervical cytomegalovirus excretion in pregnant and non-pregnant women: suppression in early gestation. J Infect Dis 1975;131:522.
151. Lang DJ, Kummer JF. Demonstration of cytomegalovirus in semen. N Engl J Med 1972;287:756.
152. Neiman P, Wasserman PB, Wentworth BB, et al. Interstitial pneumonia and cytomegalovirus infection as complications of human marrow transplantation. Transplantation 1973;15:478.
153. Drew WL, Buhles W, Erlich KS. Herpes virus invections (cytomegalovirus, herpes simplex virus, varicella-zoster virus): how to use ganciclovir (DHPG) and acyclovir. Infect Dis Clin North Am 1988;2:495.
154. Mai M, Nery J, Sutker W, et al. DHPG (gancyclovir) improves survival in CMV pneumonia. Transplant Proc 1989;21:2263.
155. Winston DJ, Ho WG, Bartoni K, et al. Ganciclovir prophylaxis of cytomegalovirus infection and disease in allogeneic bone marrow transplant recipients: results of a placebo-controlled, double-blind trial. Ann Intern Med 1993;118:179.
156. Zaid JA. Prevention and treatment of cytomegalovirus pneumonia in transplant recipients. Clin Infect Dis 1993;17(Suppl 2):392.

Blood: Principles and Practice of Hematology,
edited by Robert I. Handin, Thomas P. Stossel, and Samuel E. Lux.
J.B. Lippincott Company, Philadelphia © 1995.

23

Autoimmunization

Robert S. Schwartz

Immunologic mechanisms participate in causing or aggravating a wide range of blood diseases. Among these mechanisms, autoimmunization is of particular clinical importance. Autoimmune diseases of the blood are encountered infrequently in general medical clinics, but they constitute an important aspect of any hematology consultation service (Table 23-1). Autoimmune thrombocytopenia, autoimmune hemolytic anemia, and the immunologic complications of chronic lymphocytic leukemia (CLL) are at the core of clinical hematology. This chapter aims to summarize the bases of contemporary thinking about the origins of these diseases.

DEVELOPMENT OF IDEAS ABOUT AUTOIMMUNITY

Nourished for almost 100 years by the same root, the intertwined branches of hematology and immunology have borne many fruits of discovery: human blood groups (1900), the first recognized autoimmune disease (paroxysmal cold hemoglobinuria [PCH]; 1904), the identification of antibodies as γ-globulins (1939), immunologic tolerance (erythrocyte chimerism; 1945), diagnostic testing for autoimmune diseases (the antiglobulin test; 1946), the pathogenic properties of autoantibodies (autoimmune thrombocytopenic purpura; 1951), the human major histocompatibility system (1954), animal models of genetically determined spontaneous autoimmune diseases (New Zealand black [NZB] mice, 1959), the complete structure of an immunoglobulin molecule (1962), and immunoglobulin idiotypes (1963).

Paul Ehrlich, one of the founders of contemporary immunology, began his career as a hematologist. His method of staining cells and tissues with organic dyes quickly led him to the discovery of the reticulocyte, the eosinophil, the neutrophil, the basophil, and the mast cell.[1] Ehrlich's studies of the immune response to red blood cells (RBCs) defined the difference between isoantibodies and autoantibodies[2] and culminated in his dictum of "horror autotoxicus," the earliest attempt to formulate a theoretical solution to the problem of autoimmunization.[3] Equally notable but not as widely known in these classical papers is that of the first recorded examples of antiidiotypes—the demonstration that anti-antibodies blocked the lytic action of antierythrocyte antibodies in vitro.[4]

Ehrlich arrived at his ideas about autoimmunization by a powerful combination of experimentation and intuition. He knew, from his work on isoantibodies with Morgenroth, that goats that were immunized with the RBCs of other goats never made antibodies against their own erythrocytes; that is, they never produced autoantibodies. To explain this remarkable phenomenon, Ehrlich used a metaphor—horror autotoxicus—for the mechanisms that prevent autoimmunization, two of which were of great significance: the absence of cell surface receptors for autoantigens and regulatory antiidiotypes. Later in this chapter, these two ideas, formulated almost 90 years ago, are shown to be the major currents of present-day research on autoimmunity.

Ehrlich's clinical investigations included studies of PCH, the rapid development of intravascular hemolysis after exposure to cold. A finger of a patient with PCH was ligated with an elastic band and immersed in ice water; Ehrlich observed that blood from the finger was hemolyzed and, on microscopic examination, he found erythrophagocytosis.[5,6] The disease was also studied by Karl Landsteiner, discoverer of the ABO blood group system and a pioneer in the science of immunochemistry. Soon after Ehrlich had written that "it would be difficult to believe" that autoantibodies could be formed against one's own RBCs,[3] Donath and Landsteiner[7] discovered the immunologic basis of PCH: a complement-fixing autoantibody. Ehrlich had ignored the possibility that an autoantibody could mediate the disease, which he attributed to toxins produced by blood vessels as a result of cold.[8] The connection between PCH and syphilis, recognized in 1884 by Götze,[9] is notable as the first example of a link between an autoimmune disease and an infectious agent.

These exciting observations on PCH—which had established a new principle of disease (autoimmunization), demonstrated two important mechanisms of immune destruction of blood cells (lysis and opsonization), and made an unequivocal connection between an autoimmune disorder and an infectious disease (syphilis)—might have opened a new era in immunohematology, if not immunology itself. On the contrary, the idea that autoimmunization could account for the mechanism of a variety of diseases, then of unknown cause, was authoritatively renounced. As a result, the field stagnated for the next 50 years. If this repudiation was due to Ehrlich's influence (horror autotoxicus), as many believe, it is ironic that Ehrlich's own side-chain theory,[10] an unmistakable forerunner of the foundation of modern cellular immunology (clonal selection theory), was equally rejected, and by no less a figure than Landsteiner himself.[11] In the years just preceding World War I, the groundwork was prepared for a major advance in immunology, but it languished unnoticed.

TABLE 23-1. Autoimmune Diseases in Hematology

AUTOIMMUNE HEMATOLOGIC DISEASES

Autoimmune hemolytic anemia
- IgG (warm) autoantibodies
- IgM (cold) autoantibodies
- IgG Donath-Landsteiner autoantibodies
- Drug induced (α-methyldopa)

Autoimmune thrombocytopenia

Autoimmune neutropenia

Pure red cell anemia

? Aplastic anemia

Monoclonal gammopathies with autoantibody activity
- Cold agglutinins
- Anti–peripheral nerve autoantibodies
- Other rare monoclonal autoantibodies

Antiphospholipid antibody syndrome (lupus anticoagulant)

Acquired anticoagulant autoantibodies
- Anti–factor VIII
- Anti–factor XIII

DISEASES ASSOCIATED WITH AUTOIMMUNE HEMATOLOGIC DISORDERS

Chronic lymphocytic leukemia

B-cell lymphomas

Acquired immunodeficiency syndrome

Systemic lupus erythematosus

Granulated T-cell lymphocytosis

Thymoma

Research on autoimmunity in the years between the two world wars yielded two important advances: the development of experimentally induced animal models of autoimmune diseases, most notably experimental allergic encephalomyelitis,[12] which is an organ-specific autoimmune disease, and the demonstration in 1938 by Dameshek and Schwartz[13] that all hematologic features of autoimmune hemolytic anemia, including the spherocytosis and increased red-cell fragility of the disorder, could be reproduced in guinea pigs by injection of an antierythrocyte heteroantibody. Even so, identification of cases of antibody-mediated hemolytic anemia was difficult because only cold agglutinins or rare forms of other hemagglutinating antibodies were detectable in the laboratory.

The antiglobulin test devised by Coombs, Mourant, and Race,[14] a landmark in immunohematology, solved the problem of detecting nonagglutinating antibodies in 1945. Within 1 year, Boorman, Dodd, and Loutit[15] reported its application in the differential diagnosis of hemolytic anemia. With the antiglobulin test they were able to distinguish for the first time congenital hemolytic anemia (eg, hereditary spherocytosis) from autoimmune hemolytic anemia due to incomplete (nonagglutinating) autoantibodies. Before the invention of the antiglobulin test, the two types of anemia were often indistinguishable; in almost every instance, the clinician had the difficult task of sorting out such nonspecific findings as jaundice, splenomegaly, anemia, spherocytosis, and reticulocytosis. With the antiglobulin technique, which was the first diagnostic test for an autoimmune disease, a logical framework for diagnosing these disorders was quickly evident.

In *Who Goes First?*, Lawrence Altman recounts in detail William Harrington's dramatic demonstration of the presence of antiplatelet autoantibodies in autoimmune thrombocytopenia.[16] Harrington volunteered to receive an infusion of plasma (administered by James Hollingsworth, another Hematology Fellow [with Harrington] at the Barnes Hospital) from a patient with a severe manifestation of the disease. Within hours of receiving the plasma, Harrington's platelet count fell precipitously; a bone marrow aspirate obtained by Hollingsworth while Harrington was still thrombocytopenic showed no effect on megakaryocytes. The results substantiated Harrington's idea that a factor in the plasma of patients with idiopathic thrombocytopenia, which he and Hollingsworth thought was an antibody, destroys circulating platelets. These experiments, reported in 1951 and no longer permitted by human experimentation committees, established both the mechanism of platelet destruction in autoimmune thrombocytopenia and the principle that an autoantibody can be pathogenic.[17]

Soon thereafter, Noel Rose and Ernest Witebsky,[18] at the University of Buffalo, developed their model of experimental autoimmune thyroiditis. They found that injection of rabbits with rabbit thyroglobulin caused lesions almost identical with those of Hashimoto's thyroiditis in humans. Equally important was their finding of a regular association between development of thyroid lesions and production of antithyroglobulin autoantibodies. Here began a chain of events: autoimmunization → autoantibody → disease. The impact of the thyroiditis model was reinforced in the same year (1956) by Roitt and colleagues,[19] who were able to demonstrate antithyroglobulin antibodies in the serum of patients with Hashimoto's disease. In the following year, anti-DNA antibodies were discovered in the serum of patients with systemic lupus erythematosus (SLE), thus opening the way for exacting analysis of the prototypic systemic autoimmune disease.[20–23]

A spontaneous animal model of autoimmune disease was the one decisive element required for further progress in studies of autoimmunization. This was finally provided in 1959 from the University of Otago in NZB mice.[24] This strain, originally bred for the color of its coat, was found to develop autoimmune hemolytic anemia spontaneously without any experimental manipulation. Moreover, when NZB mice were mated with New Zealand white (NZW) mice, the B/W F_1 progeny had a different disease: severe, usually lethal lupus nephritis.[25] This observation made it evident that genetic factors can dictate both the susceptibility and the phenotypic expression of spontaneous autoimmune diseases.

By the end of the 1950s, a half-century after Ehrlich's work, the main features of autoimmunity had become evident and widely accepted. For clinicians, the laboratory diagnosis of autoimmune diseases was now possible with tests for LE cells, antinuclear antibodies, rheumatoid factor, antithyroglobulin antibodies, anti-RBC antibodies and other autoantibodies. The clinical importance of these diagnostic tests was further emphasized by the favorable results of corticosteroid treatment of patients with autoimmune diseases. For immunologists, the basic mechanisms of immune injury—anaphylaxis, lysis, opsonization, immune complexes, and delayed hypersensitivity—had been established. With an easily bred animal model, it was possible to design experiments that would define the genetic and, ultimately, the molecular basis of autoimmunization. Yet, more than 30 years later, those expectations have not been fully realized. For clinicians, the diagnostic tests for autoimmune diseases are not as telling as they first seemed, and effective treatment remains a common problem.

For immunologists, the problems of autoimmunity and immunologic tolerance are inextricable: one cannot be solved without the other, and neither has been settled.

IMMUNOLOGIC TOLERANCE

In 1945, R.D. Owen discovered that the blood of genetically dissimilar dizygotic cattle twins contained a mixture of erythrocytes with distinctly different blood groups. This unusual condition, he concluded, must have arisen as a result of the passage of "embryonal cells ancestral to the erythrocytes of the adult animal" through the vascular anastomoses of the single placenta that joined the twins in utero.[26] The immunologic consequences of erythrocyte chimerism did not escape Owen, who found no isohemagglutinins in such cattle twins despite the presence of foreign RBCs in their circulation. His observation played a key role in the theory of immunologic tolerance formulated by Burnet and Fenner.[27] They postulated that the immunologic distinction between self and nonself is established through contacts of the embryonic immune system with the antigens in its environment. The outlines of this theory, first advanced in 1949, have been validated by a large body of experimental evidence, most recently through immunologic studies of transgenic mice in which a gene foreign to the animal is implanted at the blastocyst stage of ontogeny.[28] If the protein encoded by such a gene, even a viral gene, is expressed early in embryogenesis, it elicits no detectable immune response in the transgenic animal.[28]

Tolerance of Blood Group Antigens

A naturally occurring counterpart of the genetically engineered immunologic tolerance in transgenic mice can be found in the immunology of the ABO blood group system. The serologic specificity of the ABO blood group substances is determined by their oligosaccharide components. The immunodominant sugar of the A antigen is N-acetylglucosamine and the B determinant is galactose. The embryo synthesizes A or B antigens before the first lymphocyte appears, as early as 5 weeks after implantation.[29] Expression of blood group antigens so early in ontogeny is a plausible explanation for the infallible ability of the immune system to discriminate between the A and B substances, which differ by only a single acetyl group. The rarity of autoimmune hemolytic anemia due to anti-A or anti-B autoantibodies implies that B cells capable of producing such autoantibodies are eliminated from the immune repertoire during fetal development, that is, by *clonal deletion*, which was originally postulated by Burnet and Fenner.[27]

The presence in all human serum of IgG antibodies with anti-α-galactosyl specificity is another illustration of the fidelity of immunologic tolerance to ABO antigens.[30] These antibodies presumably arise as a result of immune stimulation by lipopolysaccharides of endogenous bacterial flora. Various animal species have the capacity to produce such antibodies but only if their own tissues lack galactose $\alpha1 \rightarrow 3$ galactose. In contrast to group A subjects, group B subjects produce anti-α-galactosyl antibodies that do not cross-react with galactose $\alpha1 \rightarrow 3$(fucose $\alpha1 \rightarrow 2$) galactose, the blood group B substance.[31] Tolerance of particular sugar epitopes in tissues or on erythrocytes thus creates a "hole" in the immune repertoire, which restricts the immune response against certain bacterial $\alpha1 \rightarrow 3$ terminal residues.

The I/i blood group system is another instructive example of *natural tolerance*. Wiener and associates[32] tested more than 22,000 people before finding 5 whose erythrocytes were not agglutinated by a cold agglutinin from a patient with autoimmune hemolytic anemia. The five negative samples were called *i*, and the antigen found on the other 99.9% of the panel was termed *I*. Fetal erythrocytes lack the enzyme responsible for converting the unbranched i ganglioside antigen to the antigenically different branched ganglioside structure of I; they are I−/i+, whereas adult RBCs are the reverse.[33] Because of its inability to synthesize the I antigen, the fetus acquires no tolerance of that erythrocyte ganglioside and, unlike their anti-A or anti-B counterparts, clones of B cells capable of producing anti–I antibodies are not deleted from the repertoire. This explains why anti–I cold agglutinins are usually found in normal serum and why autoimmune hemolytic anemia due to anti–I autoantibodies (cold agglutinin disease) is not unusual (anti–i autoantibodies, by contrast, are rare). The fact that about 10% of the monoclonal IgM immunoglobulins in Waldenström's macroglobulinemia are anti–I cold agglutinins[34] is probably a manifestation of the high frequency with which anti–I B-cell clones occur in the immune repertoire. By contrast, no recorded example exists of a monoclonal macroglobulin (or myeloma protein) with ABO specificity.

T Cells and Immunologic Tolerance

Intrathymic Acquisition of Immunologic Tolerance

The role of the thymus in the acquisition of immunologic tolerance by the T-cell compartment has been definitively established by experiments carried out in mice, but the similarities between murine and human T cells are persuasive enough to permit extrapolation of the murine data to humans. Before proceeding with this topic, review of some pertinent aspects of T-cell differentiation and function is helpful.

T cells arise from immature lymphocytes that migrate from the bone marrow to the thymus. Within the thymic cortex, these precursors begin to acquire two of the major properties of mature T cells: receptors for antigens (*T-cell receptor* [TCR]) and expression of the CD4 and CD8 antigens—membrane glycoproteins that determine either helper or cytotoxic/suppressor activity. The antigen receptors of most T cells consist of two polypeptide chains, α and β; a small subset of T cells uses a different kind of receptor, consisting of γ and δ chains. These highly variable structures associate on the T-cell membrane with the *CD3 complex*, a group of polypeptides that inform the interior of the cell that its surface receptors are occupied.

Theoretically, at least 2500 mature α genes can arise from rearrangements among 50 different α chain V (variable) region genes and a similar number of α chain J (joining) region genes in the human germline. At least 4000 different human β-chain genes can arise from combinations selected from 50 V region genes, two D (diversity) genes, and 13 J region genes. In principle, a census of the human T-cell repertoire would reveal more than 10^7 $\alpha\beta$ receptors—a population comparable to the number of different immunoglobulin V regions.[35]

The T cell depends on interactions at cell surfaces. Its receptor cannot bind to native antigen in solution, unlike the immunoglobulin V region. Binding occurs only when a cell membrane glycoprotein that is encoded by a gene of the major histocompatibility complex (MHC) presents the antigen to the T cell (Fig. 23-1). The response of the T cell is thus restricted by the molecular composition of the MHC glycoprotein on the antigen-presenting cell (*MHC restriction*). The actual structure recognized by the TCR is compounded of a peptide derivative of the intact immunogen and a portion of an MHC molecule (Fig. 23-2). The peptide/MHC conjugate is brought to the surface of an antigen-presenting cell by the MHC glycoprotein after the immunogen has undergone endocytosis (or phagocytosis) and partial proteolytic digestion[36] (Fig. 23-3).

The ability of MHC glycoproteins to bind immunogenic peptides is broad but specific. Not all MHC molecules bind all peptides. This fact accounts for the genetic basis of immunologic responsiveness.[37] Of two persons, *A* and *B*, with different MHC phenotypes (*haplotypes*), *A* may respond to a particular peptide antigen, whereas *B* may not. *A* possesses an MHC structure that can present the peptide in an immunogenic configuration to T cells with appropriate receptors, whereas *B* lacks such an MHC. The controlling role of MHC glycoproteins in immunologic responsiveness accounts for one of the major genetic factors determining

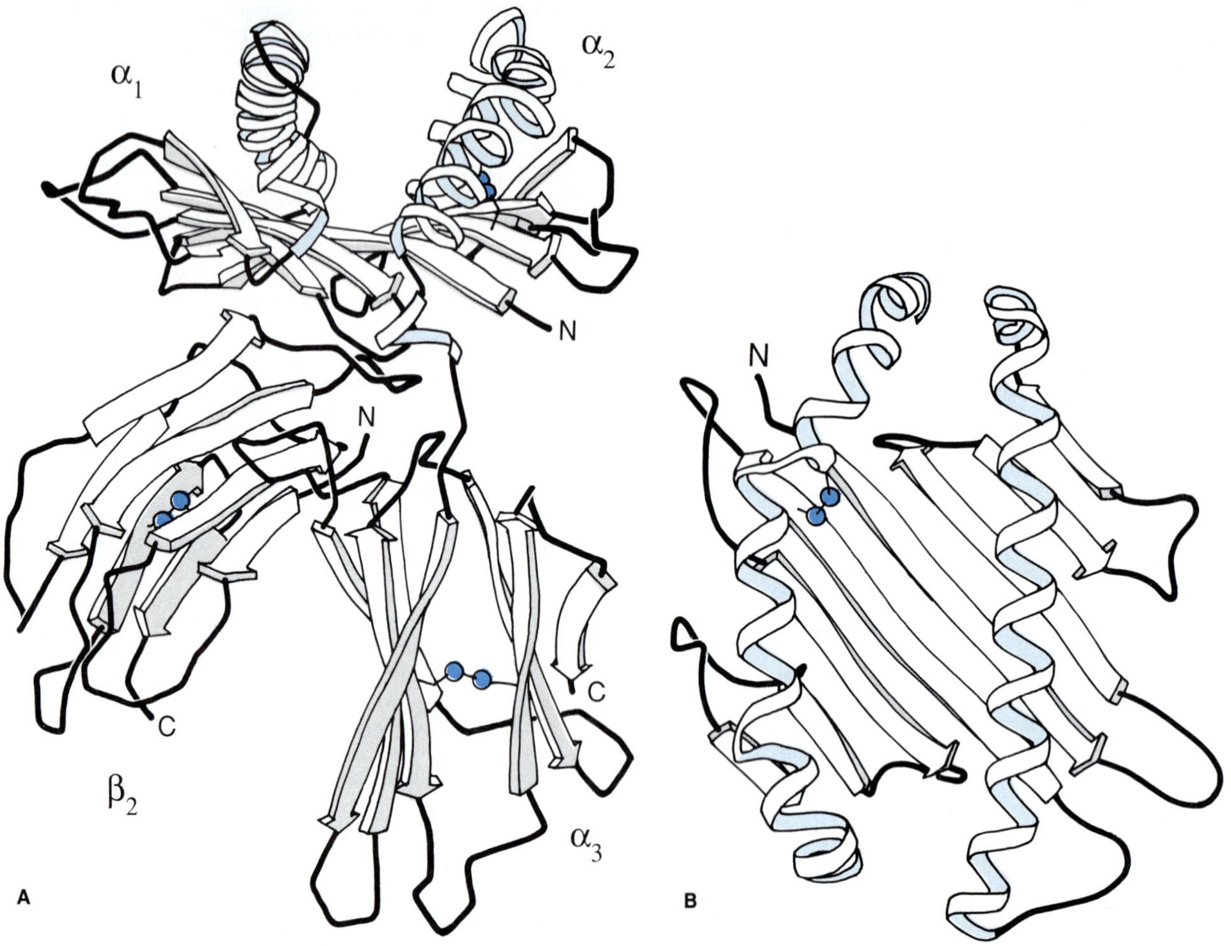

FIGURE 23-1. Side (**A**) and top (**B**) views of the structure of a class I MHC molecule, showing the antigen-binding pocket. A molecule of β_2 microglobulin anchors the α_3 chain to the cell membrane. The α_1 and α_2 domains form a deeply grooved β sheet (**B**), which can accommodate a processed peptide. The general features of a class II MHC molecule are similar. N, (Adapted from Bjorkman PJ, et al. Structure of the human class I histocompatibility antigen, HLA-A2. Nature 1987;329:506)

susceptibility to several different kinds of autoimmune diseases.[37]

The two major classes of MHC glycoproteins, class I and class II, differ in their antigen-presenting functions. The former makes contacts with CD8 T cells, whereas the latter engages CD4 T cells. Thus, the precision built into the antigen-presenting system is related to the T-cell adhesion molecules, CD8 and CD4, which bind to either class I (CD8) or class II glycoproteins (CD4) on antigen- presenting cells.[38] Except in the thymus, only B cells, dendritic cells, and macrophages express class II MHC molecules; therefore, these cells present antigen to helper (CD4+) T cells. All other nucleated cells, by contrast, normally express only class I molecules. A virus-infected epithelial cell can be the target of a specifically sensitized CD8+ cell, but a normal epithelial cell cannot present antigen to a CD4+ cell.

Let us consider how the thymus shapes the T-cell repertoire. Epithelial cells, macrophages, and dendritic cells embedded throughout the cortex and medulla of the gland display class II MHC membrane glycoproteins.[39] These cells can endocytose, digest, and position self-peptides in the clefts of their class II MHC molecules (see Fig. 23-1). For example, epithelial cells, macrophages, and dendritic cells within the fetal thymus digest hemoglobin and present the resulting self-peptides in their class II MHC molecules.[40] Percolating through these same regions of the thymus are T cells, which, in the aggregate, have generated 10^7 different $\alpha\beta$ receptors, a number sufficiently high to include, by chance, receptors capable of recognizing either a self-peptide/class II MHC amalgam or a portion of the MHC molecule itself.

How is it that inadvertently generated antiself T cells do not enter the periphery, where they could instigate an autoimmune response? Such cells are clearly deleted within the thymus at a relatively immature stage of development[41] (Fig. 23-4). The molecular mechanism of intrathymic clonal deletion may depend on the affinity of the receptor for a self-peptide/MHC complex or for the MHC glycoprotein itself. The affinity of the randomly generated receptors for their ligands range from very high to very low, and some $\alpha\beta$ combinations may not bind at all to an MHC-related configuration within the thymus. T cells with high-affinity receptors would be destroyed (*negative selection*), whereas those with receptors of moderate or low affinity would be allowed to differentiate[42] (*positive selection*; Fig. 23-5). The numerous immature cortical thymocytes that express very low levels of the $\alpha\beta$ receptor polypeptides are highly susceptible to phagocytosis and destruction by thymic macrophages.[43] This plausibly accounts for the extraordinary turnover of thymocytes. Over 95% of the proliferating cells in the murine thymus never leave the gland.[44] Thus, by measures that may seem draconian, these three mechanisms of intrathymic selection result in a population of mature T cells whose receptors recognize class II MHC

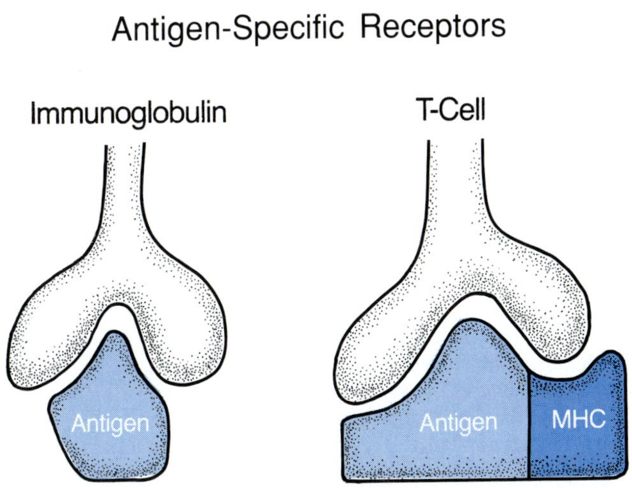

FIGURE 23-2. Immunoglobulin and T-cell V regions. The antibody molecule can bind to antigen in solution, whereas the T-cell receptor recognizes a compound structure consisting of a peptide derivative of the antigen plus a portion of the MHC glycoprotein.

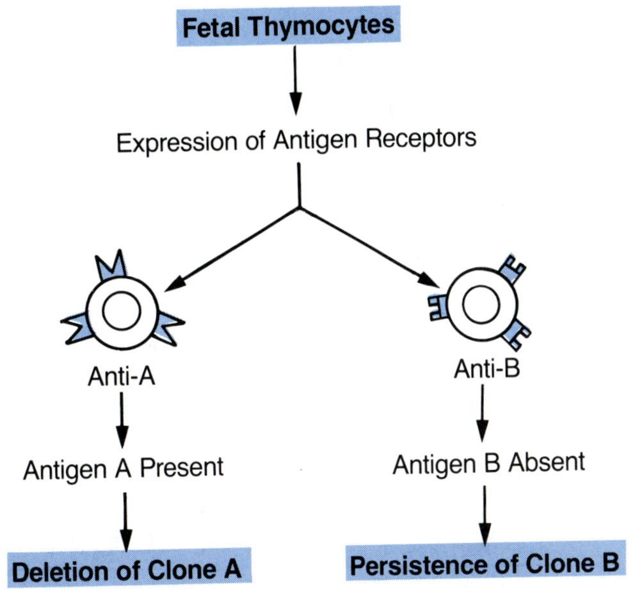

FIGURE 23-4. Acquisition of immunologic tolerance within the fetal thymus. T cells with receptors capable of binding antigens that are presented in potentially immunogenic form by intrathymic macrophages, dendritic cells, and epithelial cells are deleted. In the absence of contact with such antigens, T cells escape into the periphery.

structures with just the right affinity to allow immune responses only to foreign peptide/class II MHC complexes.

Escape From Tolerance

The intrathymic purging of T cells offers substantial protection against autoimmunization, but does it delete all self-reactive T cells from the immune system? This clearly cannot be the case. The human body produces more than 10^5 different proteins, each of which can generate at least three MHC-binding peptides.[45] The thymus cannot possibly express (or extract from the blood) all 300,000 self-determinants. Many of these self-reactive T cells, which are within organs like the brain or the eye or are hidden inside cells, sequestered from the circulation; others may enter the blood, only to be degraded by proteolytic enzymes or nucleases. Still others, like the I blood group antigen, appear exclusively after the fetus has completed its survey of self. We can surmise that the peripheral pool of mature T cells contains at least some that are self-reactive.

What prevents the self-reactive cells from initiating an autoimmune response? The rule that CD4+ T cells can recognize antigens only when they are bound to a class II MHC molecule is thought to be a powerful safeguard. Since class II MHC molecules occur only on macrophages, dendritic cells, and B cells, autoantigens exposed on the surface of other cells are ignored by potentially self-reactive CD4+

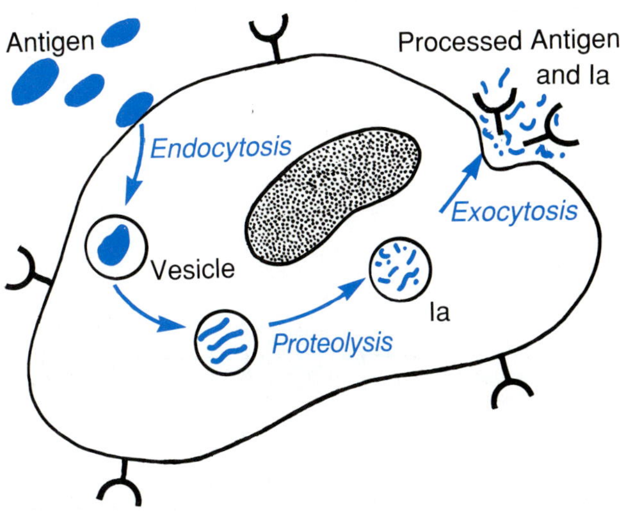

FIGURE 23-3. Antigen processing. After pinocytosis (or phagocytosis), the antigen is taken up in endosomes (vesicle), where it undergoes limited proteolysis. Within the cytoplasm, the resulting peptides bind to class II MHC molecules (also called Ia molecules). The Ia–peptide complex is transported to the cell membrane for presentation to T cells.

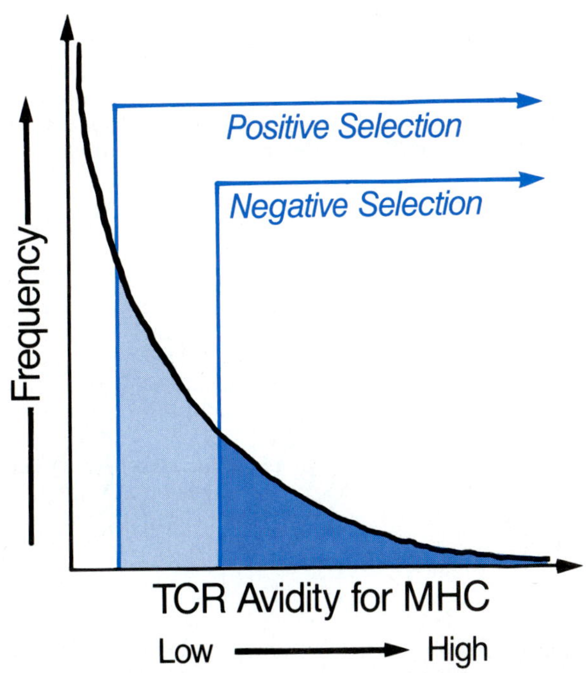

FIGURE 23-5. Molecular mechanism for positive and negative selection of thymocytes. T cells with highly avid MHC-binding receptors are deleted, whereas those with receptors of low avidity are positively selected.

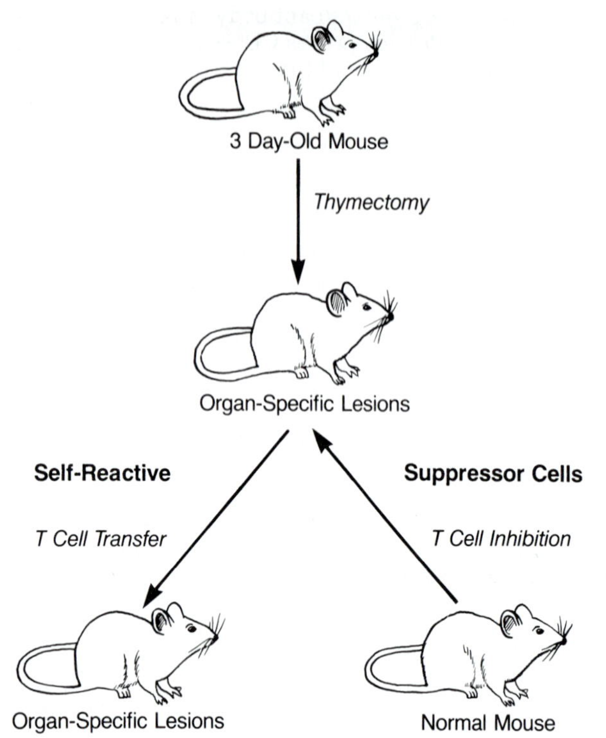

FIGURE 23-6. Development of organ-specific autoimmune lesions following thymectomy. The lesions can be prevented by suppressor cells from normal mice (*right*) or transferred to normal mice from T cells from diseased animals (*left*).

T cells. If such T cells enter the thyroid, for example, they would be "blind" to antigens of the gland because of the absence of class II MHC glycoproteins.

The aberrant expression of class II MHC molecules could instigate autoimmunization against thyroid antigens. A local viral infection would, it has been proposed, induce the production of γ-interferon which in turn initiates expression of class II MHC antigens by thyroid epithelial cells. The epithelial cells thus acquire the property of antigen-presenting cells and the potential to trigger antithyroglobulin CD4+ T cells.[46] This is an appealing hypothesis about the origins of organ-specific autoimmune diseases, but much of the supporting evidence remains circumstantial.

Suppressor Cells

Intensively investigated since Gershon and Kondo[47] discovered them in 1971 by transferring immunologic tolerance with lymphocytes from tolerant to naive mice (infectious immunologic tolerance), suppressor cells represent another system of protection against autoimmunization. Although the very existence of antigen-specific suppressor cells has been called into question, recent evidence implicates them directly in the defense against autoimmunization.[48]

Removal of the thymus from mice 2 to 4 days after birth results in the development of organ-specific autoimmune diseases of the ovary, stomach, thyroid, epididymis, testis, or prostate.[49,50] The lesions can be induced in normal animals by T cells from diseased thymectomized mice, and they can be prevented in neonatally thymectomized animals by inoculation of T cells from normal mice.[51] The implications of these results are that (1) the thymus *does* export T cells with the potential for self-reactivity and (2) those T cells are held in abeyance by other T cells—suppressor cells—which, in mice, emigrate from the thymus soon after birth. Removal of the thymus before the suppressor cell population has entered the periphery (2 to 4 days after birth) gives the self-reactive helper population unrestricted access to respond to extrathymic autoantigens that are sequestered in such organs as the testis or ovary (Fig. 23-6).

An unusually interesting counterpart to the thymectomy experiments has been found in animals treated with cyclosporine. Treatment of mice, rats, and humans with this potent immunosuppressive agent can result in a paradoxical outcome: the development of a graft-versus-host–like disorder.[52–54] T cells from cyclosporine-treated donors can transfer the syndrome to normal animals, and normal thymocytes can prevent it in cyclosporine-treated mice.[55] The drug has been shown to inhibit selectively the development of mature CD4 and CD8 thymocytes and to interfere with the elimination of self-reactive T cells.[56]

Convincing evidence of the identity and function of human suppressor cells has also been developed recently (Fig. 23-7). Human CD4+ T cells can be divided into two subsets by means of monoclonal antibodies. Anti-2H4 identifies a 200- to 220-kd membrane glycoprotein (T200; also called CD45R), and anti-4B4 defines a 135-kd protein, widely distributed on hematopoietic cells. The CD4+/2H4−/4B4+ T cells provide helper functions to B cells (helper–inducer

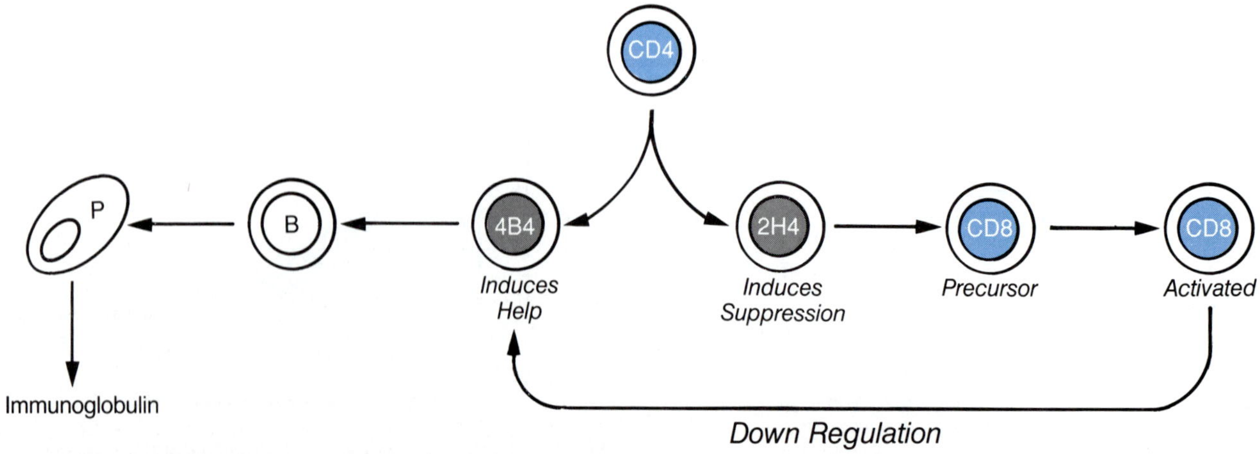

FIGURE 23-7. Functional subdivisions of CD4 cells. The CD4+/4B4+/2H4− cell provides help to antibody-producing B cells (B); the CD4+/4B4−/2H4− T cell induces suppressor activity in a CD8+ precursor. P, plasma cell.

T cells), whereas the CD4+/2H4+/4B4− T cells have the ability to activate CD8+ suppressor cells (suppressor-inducer cells).[57–59] The targets of the latter, CD8+ T cells, vigorously suppress antibody synthesis in vitro. A cloned human suppressor cell has been shown to express an $\alpha\beta$ TCR, to specifically inhibit synthesis of antihemocyanin antibodies by cultured B cells, and to cancel the helper effects of CD4+/4B4+ T cells.[60] The demonstration of reduced numbers of CD4+/2H4+ T cells in the blood of patients with multiple sclerosis[61] and SLE[62] supports the clinical relevance of these in vitro effects. How such an imbalance in T-cell populations develops in the first place remains an enigma.

B Cells and Immunologic Tolerance

B-Cell Tolerance

The molecular mechanisms responsible for generating the diversity of immunoglobulin V regions inevitably by chance result in heavy- and light-chain combinations with the properties of autoantibodies. By contrast with what occurs with T cells, B cells with self-reactive antigen receptors (surface immunoglobulins) are not usually targets of a clonal deletion mechanism. The apparent elimination from the immune repertoire of B-cell clones with antiself ABO blood group activity, already discussed, is not the rule. On the contrary, numerous kinds of natural autoantibodies, usually of the IgM isotype, are present in low levels in virtually all sera from normal humans and animals.[63] Furthermore, polyclonal activation of normal B cells in vitro, with mitogenic stimuli or the Epstein-Barr virus, regularly provokes the production of rheumatoid factor, anti-DNA antibodies, and other autoantibodies.[64–66] These autoantibodies are unlikely to result from stimulation by microbial antigens because B cells from newborn[67] and even germ-free mice[68] can produce them.

Monoclonal gammopathies with autoantibody activity are common in Waldenström's macroglobulinemia; rheumatoid factor and autoantibodies against the I RBC antigen, DNA, a glycoprotein of peripheral nerve, and the Ro ribonucleoprotein autoantigen are examples.[69–73] The monoclonal autoantibodies presumably arise from the B cells in the preimmune repertoire, which normally produce natural autoantibodies. Such autoantibodies are so prevalent that they may have some physiologic role, perhaps in the elimination of degraded autoantigens and senescent cells.[74–76]

A peculiar subset of B cells, marked by the CD5 membrane protein (also called Ly-1), is relevant to the production of natural autoantibodies. These cells make up only a minority of the B cells in adults, whereas most fetal B cells are CD5+.[77] CD5+ B cells typically, but not exclusively, produce rheumatoid factor, anti-DNA, antiinsulin, and antithyroglobulin autoantibodies.[78] In rheumatoid arthritis patients, the CD5+ population is increased, is activated, and secretes rheumatoid factor.[79] A substantial proportion of the CD5+ population of B cells in normal mice produces antiphosphatidylcholine antibodies that bind to protease-treated autologous erythrocytes,[80] and clonal populations of CD5+ B cells in the autoimmune NZB strain are greatly increased.[81]

Taken together, these observations point to the participation of the CD5+ B cell in autoimmune diseases. They can plausibly explain the previously discussed high incidence of autoantibodies in certain B-cell neoplasms: the malignant B cells of almost all cases of CLL and of about 25% of other B-cell malignancies are CD5+.[82] The role of this subset in other autoimmune diseases is problematic. CD5+ B cells usually produce only IgM antibodies, whereas the typical pathogenic autoantibody is IgG in type. Furthermore, no evidence proves CD5+ B cells can undergo the maturation required for the production of high-affinity antibodies—the kind of antibodies most likely to cause an immune lesion (see section on affinity maturation of the immune response).

Autoantibody Genes

Susceptibility to an autoimmune disease can have an inherited basis, as we have seen in the case of MHC genes, but no evidence exists for unique autoantibody or TCR genes in either humans or lupus-prone mice. Analysis of the amino acid or nucleic acid sequences of the heavy and light chains of several human rheumatoid factors and anti-DNA autoantibodies have shown that they are encoded by germline V genes.[83] Cold agglutinins are probably also encoded by germline genes, and their association with B-cell lymphomas most likely reflects the expansion of a germline clone of B cells.[84] V genes related to autoantibodies are represented not only in genomic DNA. They are rearranged in expressible form by mature B cells. For example, a germline gene, V_κRF, which encodes a rheumatoid factor light chain, is expressed by a large proportion of κ light-chain–producing CLL cells[85]; another unmutated germline V_κ gene was cloned from the rearranged light-chain gene of CLL cells, which produced a monoclonal rheumatoid factor.[86]

Polyclonal B-Cell Activation

The evidence that the germline has preserved autoantibody V genes is convincing, but the reasons for the conservation of such genes in the genome are unclear. Their survival through darwinian selection seems paradoxical. Whatever the explanation for these events, the fact is that about 1 in 1000 B cells in normal mice have the potential to produce anti-DNA antibodies[87]; a similar number may be expected in humans.[88]

From what has been recounted thus far, we can assume that these antiself B cells are normally held in tether by immunoregulatory T cells. What mechanism allows their activation in a person with an autoimmune disease? B cells can be triggered either by the classic antigen-dependent mechanisms, which the immune system uses in its response to exogenous antigens, or by one or more antigen-independent mechanisms, collectively referred to as polyclonal B-cell activation. B-cell activation can be initiated by T-cell lymphokines or mitogenic bacterial products such as lipopolysaccharides, or it may result from an inherently abnormal hyperactivity of B cells, as has been noted in SLE.[89]

As mentioned, polyclonal B-cell activation stimulates the production of certain types of autoantibodies in vitro; an in vivo counterpart of this phenomenon is the production of autoantibodies in malaria and other parasitic diseases associated with marked hypergammaglobulinemia.[90] The presence in human immunodeficiency virus infection of hypergammaglobulinemia[91] and of autoantibodies, including antinuclear[92] and antiphospholipid[93] antibodies, as well as antierythrocyte[94] and antiplatelet[95] antibodies may have a similar basis. In some patients, the clinical and laboratory pictures can be confused with that of SLE.[92] The dysfunction of T cells in human immunodeficiency virus infection could destabilize the B-cell population, leading to polyclonal B-cell activation; nevertheless, a direct effect of the virus on B cells cannot be excluded. An extraordinary case in which a patient with an interleukin-6 (IL-6)–secreting atrial myxoma produced multiple autoantibodies has been reported.[96] The development of thyroiditis in cancer patients treated with high doses of interleukin-2, a potent T-cell activator, suggests that polyclonal activation of helper T cells by lymphokines might be a factor leading toward some instances of autoimmunization.[97]

An inherent abnormality of CD5+ B cells could explain the remarkable increase of that population in the NZB strain, which may have a condition analogous to the lymphoproliferative disorder CLL.[81] The autoimmune hemolytic anemia in these animals has been attributed to autoantibodies produced by the greatly expanded set of CD5+ B cells. However, the pathogenic autoantibodies in NZB mice are IgG antibodies with specificity for an erythrocyte glycoprotein, whereas the CD5+ B cells produce IgM antibodies against a cryptic phospholipid exposed on the RBC membrane after in vitro treatment with a proteolytic enzyme.[98] The parallel with CLL in humans is striking: the autoimmune hemolytic anemia in CLL is usually mediated by IgG antibodies, whereas the neoplastic CD5+ B cells produce only IgM antibodies. The latter are often autoantibodies against DNA or rheumatoid factors, yet their pathogenic consequences are rarely noticed.[99] Thus, if polyclonal, oligoclonal, or even monoclonal B-cell activation is involved in the autoimmune disease of NZB mice (or CLL patients), it must exert its effects only indirectly.

Polyclonal B-cell activation is also prominent in MRL-*lpr*/*lpr* mice, a strain that uniformly and rapidly develops a lethal form of SLE. Even more prominent is the proliferation of T cells, which accounts for the development of huge lymph nodes and massive splenomegaly in these animals. The lymphoproliferative disorder has been traced to homozygosity for the recessive *lpr* gene.[100] Many of the proliferating MRL-*lpr*/*lpr* T cells are released from the thymus prematurely, and they secrete the potent B-cell differentiating factor, IL-6.[101] When cultured with resting MRL-*lpr*/*lpr* B cells, these immature T cells, as well as mature CD4+ T cells, have been shown to induce the production of IgG anti-DNA antibodies of the type that has been implicated in the development of lupus nephritis.[102] In this animal model, therefore, polyclonal T-cell activation due to an abnormal gene (*lpr*) may be the underlying cause of polyclonal B-cell activation.

Chronic Graft-Versus-Host Disease

If lymphocytes are injected into histocompatible hosts that cannot reject the grafted cells, a graft-versus-host reaction occurs. The ensuing disorder is caused by T cells in the grafted inoculum, which respond to histocompatibility antigens of the recipient. A severe form of the disease occurs when class II MHC differences are present between donor and host. Chronic graft-versus-host disease (GVHD) can be induced in F_1 hybrid mice by injection of lymphocytes from one of the parental strains: $A \rightarrow (A \times B)F_1$, where the A graft is not rejected because the hybrid already has A antigens. This form of graft-versus-host reaction induces an autoimmune disease whose manifestations depend on genes present in both the donor and the recipient. The major manifestations of chronic GVHD are either autoimmune hemolytic anemia[103] or immune-complex nephritis,[104] with either anti-RBC[105] or anti-DNA antibodies, or both.[106] Some animals with chronic GVHD develop a persistent lymphoproliferative disorder of B cells, which culminates as a malignant lymphoma.[107]

The numerous donor T cells engaged in a response to the recipient's class II MHC antigens produce large amounts of IL-6,[108] which in turn causes polyclonal activation of the host's B cells and hence production of autoantibodies. Autoimmunization does not occur in this experimental model if the recipient is genetically deficient in B cells.[109] No exogenous antigen is required for the disease to occur, nor is release of autoantigens due to tissue destruction by the grafted cells necessary.[110] This model is the most convincing example of the experimental induction of an autoimmune disease by polyclonal B-cell activation. The development of autoimmune thrombocytopenia after allogeneic bone marrow transplantation in humans is a human counterpart of the murine model[111]; scleroderma, sicca syndrome, and other chronic complications of human GVHD may have a similar basis.[112]

T-CELL AND B-CELL COLLABORATION IN AUTOIMMUNIZATION

Affinity Maturation of the Immune Response

The production of high-affinity IgG antibodies, the usual mediators of autoimmune lesions, requires a collaboration between helper T cells and B cells. The two cells interact with different structures on the immunogen. For the helper T cell, the relevant portion of the immunogen is the *carrier*, whose amino acid sequence is crucial for T-cell recognition.[113] The surface immunoglobulin of the B cell (or antibody), by contrast, is often specific for a three-dimensional configuration on the immunogen. In addition to T-cell help, two other mechanisms are required: somatic mutation of immunoglobulin V genes and the selection of B-cell clones whose mutated V genes specify surface immunoglobulins with high affinity for the immunizing antigen. Note that selection of B-cell clones is antigen-dependent[114] (Fig. 23-8).

Molecular analysis of autoantibodies produced by MRL-*lpr*/*lpr* mice indicates that they arise as a result of the preceding mechanism: the V genes encoding MRL-*lpr*/*lpr* anti-DNA antibodies and rheumatoid factors have mutations of the type expected in an antigen-driven process.[115] The epitope (antigenic determinant) responsible for initiating that process is enigmatic. One of the major challenges in the field of autoimmunization is to identify the immunogens that provoke and drive the affinity maturation of autoantibodies. What stimulates the T cells? The immunogens in

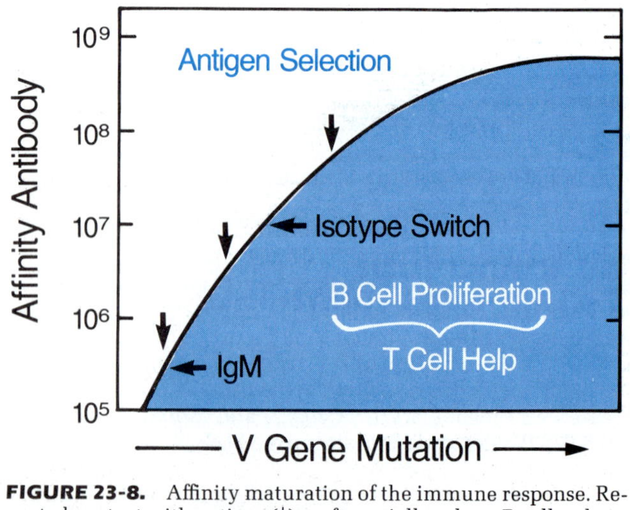

FIGURE 23-8. Affinity maturation of the immune response. Repeated contact with antigen (↓) preferentially selects B cells whose receptors best fit the immunogen, thus causing a progressive increase in the affinity of antibodies against the immunizing stimulus. Within germinal centers, B cells mutate their V genes; mutants with low (or no) affinity for the immunogen are not selected, whereas those with high affinity are stimulated to proliferate. Lymphokines produced by T cells trigger B-cell differentiation, proliferation, and isotype switching (eg, IgM → IgG).

autoimmune hemolytic anemia, autoimmune thrombocytopenia, SLE, type I diabetes, rheumatoid arthritis, and multiple sclerosis, for example, are unknown.

The antigens that bind to the autoantibodies of some of these diseases have been studied in great detail, but no evidence proves that they are the instigating immunogens. Native, double-stranded DNA is the emblematic autoantigen of SLE, but it is barely immunogenic, even in lupus-prone MRL-*lpr/lpr* mice.[116]

Antigenic Mimicry

The microbial world is an interesting source of potential autoimmunogens. Proteins of a number of bacteria and viruses have structural homologies with mammalian proteins[117]; such amino acid sequences could subvert immunologic tolerance if adjacent foreign peptides in the microbial protein were recognized by T cells. The latter would serve as carriers, whereas B cells with self-reactive surface immunoglobulins would bind the autoantigen-mimicking sequences (see Fig. 23-7). This kind of mechanism may explain (1) the induction of autoimmune hemolytic anemia in mice by repeated injections of haptenated (trinitrophenol) mouse erythrocytes,[118] (2) the relation between infection by group A streptococci and rheumatic carditis,[119] and (3) the autoimmune complications of infection by bacilli of *Yersinia*.[120]

Immunologic Reconstruction of Paroxysmal Cold Hemoglobinuria

We are now able to attempt an explanation of the first autoimmune disease to be recognized, PCH. The association of PCH with syphilis is classic. However, only a rare victim of that infection has the bad luck to develop PCH. Therefore, factors other than the spirochete must be considered. From what we have reviewed here, we can replace the idea of bad luck with the concept of "gene." The latter involves, as a minimum, the class II MHC genes that govern the immune response. If the antigenic constituents of *Treponema pallidum* contain a foreign carrier (the T-cell epitope) together with a structure that can mimic an autoantigen (the B-cell epitope), T–B collaboration (foreign epitope/self-mimicking epitope) can proceed.

An autoimmune response can occur only in a patient with a class II MHC structure that binds to the appropriate T-cell epitope of the spirochete. *T pallidum* appears to contain at least two T-cell epitopes that promote autoimmunization. One of these epitopes, which might be thought of as a universal epitope, leads to the production of antiphospholipid autoantibodies in essentially all patients with syphilis. These autoantibodies are the basis for the serologic diagnosis of the disease. There should also be a private T-cell epitope, responsible for driving production of the IgG Donath-Landsteiner autoantibodies of PCH. The universal epitope must bind to all class II MHC molecules, whereas only a rare class II MHC haplotype binds the private epitope. That rare haplotype is the patient's bad luck.[121]

AUTOANTIBODY IDIOTYPES

Definition

An idiotype is a serologically defined marker of the immunoglobulin V region. It is recognized by an antiidiotype, usually prepared by immunization of one species (eg, rabbit) with a monoclonal antibody from another species (eg, human). The antiidiotype can recognize a determinant (eg, an amino acid sequence) on either the heavy- or the light-chain portion of the V region or a three-dimensional configuration composed of both chains. The idiotype may be present in the antigen-binding site (hypervariable region) of the molecule or in the framework structures of the V region. In any case, its determinant must reside on the surface of the immunoglobulin to allow binding to the antiidiotype. Discrete antigenic determinants of the idiotype are termed *idiotopes*. The term *idiotype* has traditionally referred to the immunoglobulin V region, but it has recently been extended to include serologically defined regions of the TCR.

The word idiotype is derived from the Greek, διο, meaning personal and distinct, and it implies a unique structure. *Private idiotypes* are found only on one or extremely few immunoglobulins. *Public idiotypes* are the most useful markers for analytic work. If two different antibodies share the same heavy (or light) chain, they may also share the same idiotype.[122] An idiotype, therefore, does not necessarily define the antigen-binding property of the antibody, nor is it a gene probe. The idiotypes of rheumatoid factors in the serum of patients with rheumatoid arthritis are largely private, indicating extensive structural diversity in those autoantibodies.[123] By contrast, the idiotypes of the monoclonal rheumatoid factors of Waldenström's macroglobulinemia are public; that is, macroglobulins from different patients have been shown to cross-react extensively with certain antiidiotypes.[124] Many of the anti-DNA antibodies in SLE serum also share public idiotypes, an indication of their origins from a common precursor.[125] The presence of these shared idiotypes in genetically unrelated patients is consistent with the idea that the autoantibodies arise from germline genes (see section on autoantibody genes).

Idiotype Networks

Niels Jerne's idea that the immune system is organized into networks of V regions with complementary idiotypes has had a powerful influence on experimental and theoretical immunology.[126] The basic components of an idiotypic network are antibody-1 and antibody-2. Antibody-1 produces its effects (stimulation or suppression) on the production of antibody-2 by interacting with the idiotype of antibody-2 on the surface of a B cell. The idiotype of antibody-1 can also influence antibody-2 by interacting with a complementary idiotype in the V region of a TCR. Antibody-2 can in turn stimulate antibody-3, but there the circuit usually ends because, in principle, antibody-3 (also termed *antibody-1′*) is idiotypically similar to antibody-1: antibody-1 → antibody-2 → antibody-3. The designations, antibody-1 and antibody-2, are arbitrary; any idiotype is a potential antiidiotype and vice versa.[127] Antibody-2 is called an *auto-antiidiotype* when it is thought to participate in the physiologic regulation of immune responses by antibody-1 → antibody-2 circuits.[128] Putative immunoregulatory auto-antiidiotypes have been found in patients with SLE,[129] myasthenia gravis,[130] and autoimmune thyroid diseases.[131] The suppression of autoantibodies to factor VIII by treatment with large amounts of intravenous γ-globulin, which was observed in two patients with acquired hemophilia, may have been due to naturally occurring antiidiotypes (antibody-2) against idiotypes expressed by anti-VIIIc autoantibodies (antibody-1) in the pooled normal γ-globulin preparation.[132] The spontaneous reversal of autoimmune dysfibrinogenemia, which was associated with a severe hemorrhagic disorder, coincided with the appearance in the patient's serum of auto-antiidiotypes to the antifibrinogen autoantibodies.[133]

A topic of substantial interest is the induction of autoantibodies by an antibody-2 whose V region imitates the structure of an autoantigen (the *internal image effect*[134];

Fig. 23-9). An example of this phenomenon is the development of myasthenia gravis in rabbits immunized with BisQ, a synthetic compound that binds to the acetylcholine receptor. A population of antibody-2 against anti-BisQ antibodies (antibody-1) in the serum of the affected rabbits had properties of antiacetylcholine receptor antibodies.[135] Mice immunized with insulin can produce not only antiinsulin antibodies but also anti-(antiinsulin) antibodies, which bind the insulin receptor.[136] A similar network occurs spontaneously in BB/E rats that develop autoimmune diabetes; its mechanism depends on the recognition by autoantibody-1 (antiinsulin) of an epitope on insulin that binds to the insulin receptor.[137] Another example of the induction of autoimmunity by means of idiotypes was found in mice immunized with the human monoclonal anti-DNA antibody bearing the 16/6 idiotype. The animals produced high levels of anti-16/6 idiotype antibodies and also anti–(anti-16/6 idiotype) antibodies that had anti-DNA activity. Other autoantibodies, including anti-Sm/RNP, anti-Ro, anti-La, and anticardiolipin autoantibodies were also found.[138]

Of even greater significance is the development of immune complex nephritis in these animals, with mouse 16/6 idiotype in the renal lesion.[132] In this model, the human 16/6 idiotype (antibody-1) probably evoked an antibody-2 population that mimicked the V region of the human autoantibody; these in turn elicited a population of pathogenic Ab-3 with the 16/6 idiotype.

GENETIC COMPLEXITY OF AUTOIMMUNE DISEASES

The issues we have dealt with thus far are relatively straightforward when compared with actual clinical events. When we turn from molecular aspects of the immune system or from the immune responses of inbred laboratory mice to patients with autoimmune diseases, we see phenomena that have thus far defied adequate explanations. An example is the preponderance of women in most autoimmune diseases, with the classic example being SLE in which the female/male ratio is 9:1. Despite numerous investigations, the mechanism accounting for the influence of sex hormones on susceptibility to autoimmunization remains unknown.[139]

Another example is the discordance of type I diabetes in identical twins, even in twins raised in the same environment. Susceptibility to that autoimmune disease is strongly influenced by genetic factors, especially the HLA genotype.[37] Even so, apparently random events seem to impose themselves on the phenotypic expression of the disease. If polyclonal B-cell activation is the underlying disturbance in SLE, why is the clinical picture dominated by immune thrombocytopenia in one patient and glomerulonephritis in another?

An examination of the variety of autoimmune diseases in NZB mice and their F_1 hybrid progeny can be instructive.[140] The autoimmune disease in the NZB strain is autoimmune hemolytic anemia; by contrast, progeny of the crossbreed (NZB × BXSB) develop autoimmune thrombocytopenia.[141] The (NZB × NZW)F_1 animal develops chronic, usually fatal lupus nephritis relatively late in life, whereas nephritis is rare in both parental strains. No autoimmune disease develops in (NZB × C57B1)F_1 mice. The (NZW × BXSB)F_1 hybrid develops an acute form of lupus nephritis with vasculitis of the coronary vessels early in life.[142]

From these examples, we can see that genetic information from both parents influences the outcome. The (NZB × SWR)F_1 is particularly revealing in this regard. The SWR strain, unlike NZW and BXSB, has no tendency whatsoever to develop autoimmune diseases or autoantibodies, yet when crossed with the NZB strain the progeny develop severe lupus nephritis.[143] Furthermore, the pathogenic anti-DNA antibodies in these F_1 mice bear genetic (allotypic) markers of both the NZB and the SWR parent.[144] In this model, the dormant potential to produce nephritogenic autoantibodies, present in the genomes of both parental lines, is activated in the F_1. The inherent tendency toward autoimmunization of the NZB parent, which rarely develops nephritis, not only takes on a form not found in the NZB animal but also evokes the expression of latent genes inherited from normal SWR mice. Under the influence of NZB genes, these normal genes can give rise to pathogenic autoantibodies.

The nature and number of the genes that enhance, modify, or suppress autoimmunization in animal models (and in humans) is unknown. In NOD mice, which spontaneously develop type I diabetes, at least three recessive genetic loci (gene clusters) contribute to the disease, one of which is the MHC; the others are known only by their linkage to other loci.[145]

FUTURE DIRECTIONS

In this chapter, we have seen that the immune system undergoes a radical change during ontogeny. A complete about-face occurs from the acquisition of immunologic tolerance—the major task of fetal lymphocytes—to the development of immunity against the hostile environment in store for the infant. Despite its elaborate mechanism for the deletion of autoreactive lymphocytes, the immune system retains the capacity to form numerous kinds of autoantibodies as well as all the elements required for an immune attack against self (Fig. 23-10). Autoimmunity is thus a normal condition, but when the forces that regulate it are weakened, it can become pathologic.

Elucidation of these forces is the major task in autoimmunity research. Identification of the contribution of the HLA locus to susceptibility to autoimmune diseases has

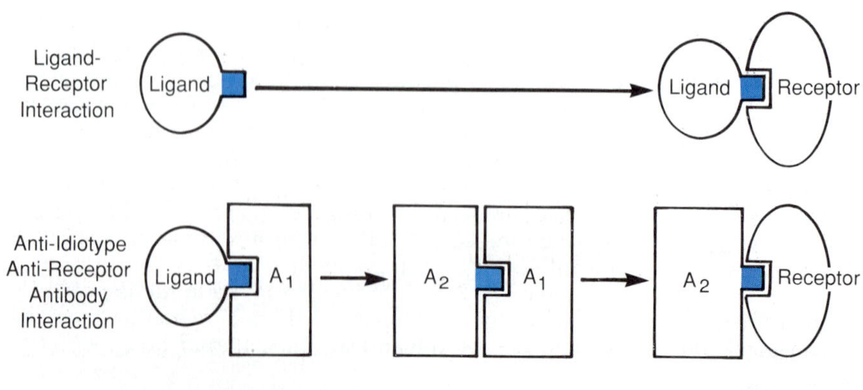

FIGURE 23-9. Idiotypes as surrogate antigens. A configuration (or sequence) in the V region of antibody-2 (A_2) resembles an antigenic determinant (epitope) of the immunogenic ligand—the internal image effect. A_2 can thus bind to the natural receptor for the ligand.

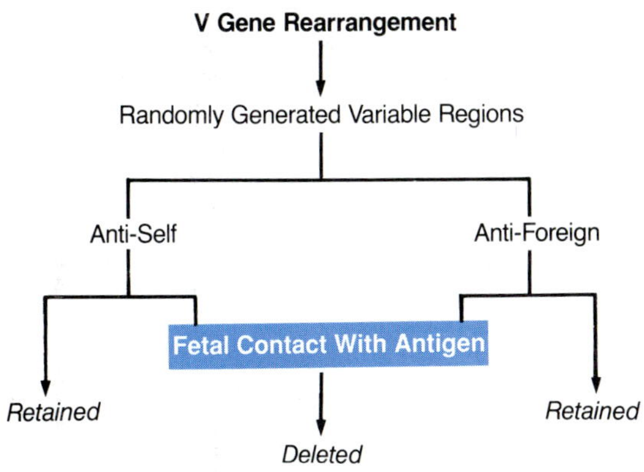

FIGURE 23-10. A summary of natural tolerance. Randomly generated V regions produce both antiforeign and antiself T cells and B cells. Those cells are deleted in the fetus if they contact the corresponding antigens. If such contacts are not made, the postnatal population of lymphocytes in the periphery harbors antiself and antiforeign T cells and B cells.

been a major achievement, but clearly many other genetic determinants are involved, some of which may not be directly or primarily engaged in immunity. The instigating immunogens of autoimmune diseases represent another major challenge: Are they environmental microbes or chemicals that mimic autoantigens? Are they derived from endogenous self-antigens? What accounts for the apparent randomness of autoimmunization? Could the stochastic generation of V region networks provide the explanation? Can we logically explain the development of autoimmune thrombocytopenia in a previously healthy woman, or is it merely bad luck?

REFERENCES

1. Ehrlich P, Lazarus A. Histology of the blood: normal and pathological. Cambridge, Cambridge University Press, 1900.
2. Ehrlich P, Morgenroth J. On hemolysins: third communication. In: The collected papers of Paul Ehrlich, vol 2. London, Pergamon Press, 1957:205.
3. Ehrlich P, Morgenroth J. On hemolysins: fifth communication. In: The collected papers of Paul Ehrlich, vol 2. London, Pergamon Press, 1957: 253.
4. Ehrlich P, Morgenroth J. On hemolysins: Sixth communication. In: The collected papers of Paul Ehrlich, vol 2. London, Pergamon Press, 1957:256.
5. Ehrlich P. Über paroxysmale Hämoglobinurie. Z Klin Med 3:383, 1881.
6. Ehrlich P. Über paroxysmale Hämoglobinurie. In: Farbeanalaytische Untersuchungen zur Histologie und Klinik des Blutes. Berlin, August Hirschwald, 1891:110.
7. Donath J, Landsteiner K. Über paroxysmale Hämoglobinurie. Muench Med Wochenschr 1904;51:1590.
8. Ehrlich P, Morgenroth J. Über Hämolysine: zweite Mittheilung. Berl Klin Wochenschr 1899;36:481.
9. Götze L. Beitrag zur Lehre von der paroxysmalen Haemoglobinurie. Berl Klin Wochenschr 1884;21:716.
10. Ehrlich P. On immunity with special reference to cell life: Croonian lecture. In: The collected papers of Paul Ehrlich, vol 2. London, Pergamon Press, 1957:178.
11. Landsteiner K. The specificity of serological reactions. New York, Dover Publications, 1936:148.
12. Rivers TM, Sprunt DH, Berry GP. Observations on attempts to produce acute disseminated encephalomyelitis in monkeys. J Exp Med 1933;58: 39.
13. Dameshek W, Schwartz SO. Hemolysins as the cause of clinical and experimental hemolytic anemias, with particular reference to the nature of spherocytosis and increased fragility. Am J Med Sci 1938;196: 769.
14. Coombs RRA, Mourant AE, Race RR. A new test for the detection of weak and incomplete Rh agglutinins. Br J Exp Pathol 1945;26:255.
15. Boorman KE, Dodd BE, Loutit JF. Hemolytic icterus (acholuric jaundice) congenital and acquired. Lancet 1946;1:812.
16. Altman LK. Who goes first? The story of self-experimentation in medicine. New York, Random House, 1987.
17. Harrington WJ, Minnich V, Hollingsworth JW, et al. Demonstration of a thrombocytopenic factor in the blood of patients with thrombocytopenic purpura. J Lab Clin Med 1951;38:1.
18. Rose NR, Witebsky E. Studies on organ specificity. V. Changes in the thyroid glands of rabbits following acute immunization with rabbit thyroid extracts. J Immunol 1956;76:417.
19. Roitt IM, Doniach D, Campbell B, et al. Autoantibodies in Hashimoto's disease (lymphadenoid goitre). Lancet 1956;2:820.
20. Miescher P, Strassle R. New serological methods for the detection of the L.E. factor. Vox Sang 1957;2:283.
21. Robbins WC, Holman HR, Deicher H, et al. Complement fixation with cell nuclei and DNA in lupus erythematosus. Proc Soc Exp Biol Med 1957;96:575.
22. Cepellini R, Polli E, Celada FA. DNA-reacting factor in serum of a patient with lupus erythematosus diffusus. Proc Soc Exp Biol Med 1957;96:572.
23. Seligmann M. Mise en évidence dans le sérum de malades atteints de lupus érythemateux dissémine d'une substance déterminant une réaction de précipitation avec l'acide desoxyribonucléique. CR Acad Sci 1957;245:243.
24. Bielschowsky M, Helyer BJ, Howie JB. Spontaneous hemolytic anemia in mice of the NZB/B1 strain. Proc Univ Otago Med Sch 1959;37:9.
25. Helyer BJ, Howie JB. Renal disease associated with positive lupus erythematosus tests in a cross-bred strain of mice. Nature 1963;197: 197.
26. Owen RD. Immunogenetic consequences of vascular anastomoses between bovine cattle twins. Science 1945;102:400.
27. Burnet FM, Fenner F. The production of antibodies. London, Macmillan, 1949.
28. Cuthbertson A, Klintworth GK. Transgenic mice: a gold mine for furthering knowledge in pathobiology. Lab Invest 1988;58:484.
29. Szulman AE. The histologic distribution of blood group substances in man as disclosed by immunofluorescence. IV. The ABH antigens in embryos as the fifth week postfertilization. J Exp Med 1964;119:503.
30. Galili U, Rachmilewitz EA, Peleg A, et al. A unique natural human IgG antibody with anti-α-galactosyl specificity. J Exp Med 1984;160: 1519.
31. Galili U, Macher BA, Buehler J, at al. Human natural anti-α galactosyl IgG. III. The subtlety of immune tolerance in man as demonstrated by cross-reactivity between natural anti-Gal and anti-B antibodies. J Exp Med 1987;165:693.
32. Wiener AS, Unger LJ, Cohen L, et al. Type-specific cold-autoantibodies as a cause of acquired hemolytic anemia and hemolytic transfusion reactions: biologic test with bovine red cells. Ann Intern Med 1956;44: 221.
33. Hakamori S. Blood group ABH and Ii antigens of human erythrocytes: chemistry, polymorphism, and their developmental changes. Semin Hematol 1981;18:39.
34. Merlini G, Farhangi M, Osserman EF. Monoclonal immunoglobulins with antibody activity in myeloma, macroglobulinemia and related plasma cell dyscrasias. Semin Oncol 1986;13:350.
35. Marrack P, Kappler J. The T cell receptor. Science 1987;238:1073.
36. Unanue ER, Allen P. The basis for the immunoregulatory role of macrophages and other accessory cells. Science 1987;236:551.
37. Todd JA, Acha-Orbea H, Bell JI, et al. A molecular basis for MHC class II-associated autoimmunity. Science 1988;240:1003.
38. Bierer BA, Burakoff SJ. T cell adhesion molecules. FASEB J 1988;2: 2584.
39. Lo D, Sprent J. Identity of cells that imprint H-2 restricted T cell specificity in the thymus. Nature 1986;319:672.
40. Lorenz RG, Allen PM. Thymic cortical epithelial cells can present self antigens in vivo. Nature 1989;337:560.
41. Von Boehmer H, Teh HS, Kisielow P. The thymus selects the useful, neglects the useless and destroys the harmful. Immunol Rev 1989;10: 57.
42. Fink P. Stop and go in the thymus. Immunol Today 1988;9:377.
43. Inaba K, Inaba M, Kinashi T, et al. Macrophages phagocytose thymic lymphocytes with productively rearranged T cell receptor α and B genes. J Exp Med 1988;168:2279.
44. McPhee D, Pye J, Shortman K. The differentiation of thymocytes. V. Evidence for intrathymic death of most thymocytes. Thymus 1979;1: 151.
45. Marrack P, Kappler J. The T cell repertoire for antigen and MHC. Immunol Today 1988;9:308.
46. Bottazzo GF, Pujol-Borrell R, Hanafusa T, et al. Role of aberrant HLA-DR expression and antigen presentation in induction of endocrine autoimmunity. Lancet 1983;2:1115.
47. Gershon RK, Kondo K. Infectious immunological tolerance. Immunology 1971;21:903.
48. Moller G. Do suppressor T cells exist? Scand J Immunol 1988;27:247.
49. Sakaguchi S, Fukuma K, Kuribayashi K. Organ-specific autoimmune diseases induced in mice by elimination of T cell subsets. I. Evidence for the active participation of T cells in natural self tolerance. J Exp Med 1985;161:72.
50. Tung KSK, Smith S, Teuscher C, et al. Murine oophoritis, epididymoorchitis and gastritis induced by day 3 thymectomy. Am J Pathol 1987;126:293.
51. Taguchi O, Nishizuka Y. Self tolerance and localized autoimmunity:

mouse models of autoimmune disease that suggest tissue-specific suppressor T cells are involved in self tolerance. J Exp Med 1987;165:146.
52. Glazier A, Tutschka PJ, Farmer ER, et al. Graft-versus-host disease in cyclosporin A–treated rats after syngeneic and autologous bone marrow reconstitution. J Exp Med 1983;158:1.
53. Sorokin R, Kimura H, Schroder K, et al.Cyclosporine-induced autoimmunity: conditions for expressing disease, requirement for intact thymus, and potency estimates of autoimmune lymphocytes in drug-treated rats. J Exp Med 1986;164:1615.
54. Hood AF, Vogelsgang GB, Black LP, et al. Acute graft-versus-host disease: development following autologous and syngeneic bone marrow transplantation. Arch Dermatol 1987;123:745.
55. Sakaguchi S, Sakaguchi N. Transplantation of the thymus from cyclosporine A-treated mice causes organ-specific autoimmune disease in athymic nude mice. J Exp Med 1988;167:1479.
56. Jenkins MK, Schwartz RH, Pardoll DM. Effects of cyclosporin A on T cell development and clonal deletion. Science 1988;241:1655.
57. Morimoto C, Letvin NL, Distaso JA, et al. The isolation and characterization of the human suppressor inducer T cell subset. J Immunol 134:1515, 1985.
58. Takeuchi T, Rudd CE, Tedder TF, et al. Amplification of suppressor inducer pathway with monoclonal antibody, anti-2H4, identifying a novel epitope of the common leukocyte antigen/T200 antigen. Cell Immunol 1989;118:68.
59. Morimoto C, Letvin NL, Boyd AW, et al. The isolation and characterization of the human helper inducer T cell subset. J Immunol 1985;134: 3762.
60. Takeuchi T, Schlossman SF, Morimoto C. Development of an antigen-specific CD8 suppressor effector clone in man. J Immunol 1988;141: 3010.
61. Chofflon M, Weiner HL, Morimoto C, Hafler DA. TI Loss of functional suppression is linked to decreases in circulating suppressor inducer (CD4+ 2H4+) T cells in multiple sclerosis. Ann Neurol 1988;24:185.
62. Morimoto C, Steinberg AD, Letvin NL, et al. A defect of immunoregulatory T cell subsets in systemic lupus erythematosus demonstrated with anti-2H4 antibody. J Clin Invest 1987;79:762.
63. Gilbert B, Dighiero G, Avrameas S. Naturally occurring antibodies against nine common antigens in human sera. J Immunol 1982;128: 2779.
64. Levinson AI, Dalal N, Hardar M, et al. Prominent IgM rheumatoid factor production by human cord blood lymphocytes stimulated in vitro with *Staphylococcus aureus*: Cowan I. J Immunol 1987;139:2237.
65. Cairns E, St Germain J, Bell DA. The in vitro production of anti-DNA antibody by cultured peripheral blood or tonsillar lymphoid cells from normal donors and SLE patients. J Immunol 1985;135:3839.
66. Garzelli C, Taub FE, Scharff JE, et al. Epstein-Barr virus transformed lymphocytes produce monoclonal autoantibodies that react with antigens in multiple organs. J Virol 1984;52:722.
67. Dighiero G, Lymberi P, Holmberg D, et al. High frequency of natural autoantibodies in normal newborn mice. J Immunol 1985;134:765.
68. Underwood JR, Pedersen PJ, Chalmers PJ, et al. Hybrids from normal, germ-free, nude and neonatal mice produce monoclonal autoantibodies to eight different intracellular structures. Clin Exp Immunol 1985;68: 417.
69. Seligmann M, Brouet JC. Antibody activity of human myeloma globulins. Semin Hematol 1973;10:163.
70. Rauch J, Schwartz RS, Stollar BD. Applications of hybridoma technology to autoimmunity. In: Katz DH, ed. Monoclonal antibodies and T cell products. Boca Raton, CRC Press, 1982:91.
71. Dighiero G, Guilbert B, Fermand JP, et al. Thirty-six human monoclonal immunoglobulins with antibody activity against cytoskeletal proteins, thyroglobulin, and native DNA. Blood 1983;264:62.
72. Freddo L, Ariga T, Saito M, et al. The neuropathy of plasma cell dyscrasias: binding of IgM M-proteins to peripheral nerve glycolipids. Neurology 1985;35:1420.
73. Sestak AL, Harley JB, Yoshida S, et al. Lupus/Sjogren's autoantibody specificities in sera with paraproteins. J Clin Invest 1987;80:138.
74. Grabar P. Autoantibodies and the physiological role of immunoglobulins. Immunol Today 1983;4:337.
75. Naparstek Y, André-Schwartz J, Manser T, et al. A single germline VH gene segment of normal A/J mice encodes autoantibodies characteristic of systemic lupus erythematosus. J Exp Med 1986;164:614.
76. Cohen IR, Cooke A. Natural autoantibodies might prevent autoimmune disease. Immunol Today 1987;7:363.
77. Antin JH, Emerson SG, Martin P, et al. Leu-1+ (CD5+) B cells: a major lymphoid subpopulation in human fetal spleen: phenotypic and functional studies. J Immunol 1986;136:505.
78. Casali P, Prabhakar BS, Notkins AL. Characterization of multireactive autoantibodies and identification of Leu 1+ B lymphocytes as cells making autoantibodies binding multiple self and exogenous molecules. Int Rev Immunol 1988;3:17.
79. Burastero SE, Casali P, Wilder RL, et al. Monoreactive high affinity and polyreactive low affinity rheumatoid factors are produced by CD5+ B cells from patients with rheumatoid arthritis. J Exp Med 1988;168: 1979.
80. Mercolino TJ, Arnold LW, Hawkins LA, et al. Normal mouse peritoneum contains a large population of Ly-1+ (CD5) B cells that recognize phosphatidyl choline. J Exp Med 1988;168:687.
81. Stall AM, Fariñas MC, Tarlinton DM, et al. Ly-1 B cell clones similar to human chronic lymphocytic leukemias routinely develop in older normal mice and young autoimmune (New Zealand black–related) animals. Proc Natl Acad Sci USA 1988;85:7312.
82. Caligaris-Cappio F, Janossy G. Surface markers in chronic lymphocytic leukemia of B cell type. Semin Hematol 1985;22:1.
83. Stewart AK, Huang C, Long AA, Stollar BD, Schwartz RS. VH gene representation in autoantibodies reflects the normal B cell repertoire. Immunol Rev 1992;128:101.
84. Silverman GJ, Goni F, Fernandez J, et al. Distinct patterns of heavy chain variable region subgroup use by human monoclonal autoantibodies of different specificity. J Exp Med 168:2361, 1988.
85. Kipps TJ, Fong S, Tomhave E, et al. High-frequency expression of a conserved light-chain variable-region gene in chronic lymphocytic leukemia. Proc Natl Acad Sci USA 1987;84:2916.
86. Jirik FR, Sorge J, Fong S, et al. Cloning and sequence determination of a human rheumatoid factor light-chain gene. Proc Natl Acad Sci USA 1986;83:2195.
87. Souroujon M, White-Scharff ME, André-Schwartz J, Gefter ML, Schwartz RS. Preferential autoantibody reactivity of the preimmune B cell repertoire in normal mice. J Immunol 1988;140:4173.
88. Cairns E, St Germain J, Bell DA. The in vitro production of anti-DNA antibody by cultured peripheral blood or tonsillar lymphoid cells from normal donors and SLE patients. J Immunol 1985;135:3839.
89. Suzuki N, Sakane T. Induction of excessive B cell proliferation and differentiation by an in vitro stimulus in culture in human systemic lupus erythematosus. J Clin Invest 1989;83:937.
90. McGregor IA. The significance of parasitic infections in terms of clinical disease. Parasitology 1987;94:5159.
91. Ammann AJ, Abrams D, Conant M, et al. Acquired immune dysfunction in homosexual men: immunologic profiles. Clin Immunol Immunopathol 1983;27:315.
92. Kopelman R, Zolla-Pazner S. Association of human immunodeficiency virus infection and autoimmune phenomena. Am J Med 1988;84:82.
93. Bloom EJ, Abrams DI, Rogers G. Lupus anticoagulant in the acquired immunodeficiency syndrome. JAMA 1986;256:491.
94. Toy TCY, Reid ME, Burns M. Positive direct antiglobulin test associated with hyperglobulinemia in acquired immunodeficiency syndrome (AIDS). Am J Hematol 1985;19:145.
95. Stricker RB, Abrams DI, Corash L, et al. Target platelet antigen in homosexual men with immune thrombocytopenia. N Engl J Med 1985;313:1375.
96. Hirano T, Taga T, Yasukawa K, et al. Human B cell differentiation factor defined by an anti-peptide antibody and its possible role in autoantibody production. Proc Natl Acad Sci USA 1987;31:228.
97. Atkins MB, Mier JW, Parkinson DR, et al. Hypothyroidism after treatment with interleukin-2 and lymphokine-activated killer cells. N Engl J Med 1988;318:1557.
98. Moore JS, Calkins CE. In vitro regulation of the pathogenic anti-erythrocyte autoantibody response of New Zealand black mice. J Immunol 1985;134:3838.
99. Sthoeger ZM, Wakai M, Tse DB, et al. Production of autoantibodies by CD5-expressing B lymphocytes from patients with chronic lymphocytic leukemia. J Exp Med 1989;169:255.
100. Murphy ED, Roths JB. Autoimmunity and lymphoproliferation-Induction by mutant gene lpr and acceleration by a male-associated factor in strain BXSB mice. In: Rose NR, Bigazzi PE, Warner NL, eds. Genetic control of autoimmune disease. Amsterdam, Elsevier, 1979: 207.
101. Dobashi K, Ono S, Mirakami S, et al. Polyclonal B cell activation by a B cell differentiation factor, B151-TRF2 IV. B151-TRF2 as a B cell differentiation factor closely associated with autoimmune disease. J Immunol 1987;138:780.
102. Datta SK, Patel H, Berry D. Induction of a cationic shift in IgG anti-DNA autoantibodies: role of T helper cells with classical and novel phenotypes in three murine models of lupus nephritis. J Exp Med 1987;165:1252.
103. Oliner H, Schwartz R, Dameshek W. Studies in experimental autoimmune disorders. I. Clinical and laboratory features of autoimmunization (runt disease) in the mouse. Blood 1961;17:20.
104. Gleichmann H, Gleichmann E, André-Schwartz J, et al. Chronic allogeneic disease. III. Genetic requirements for the induction of glomerulonephritis. J Exp Med 1972;135:516.
105. Streilein JW, Stone MJ, Duncan WR. Studies on the specificity of autoantibodies produced in systemic graft-versus-host disease. J Immunol 1975;114:255.
106. Van-der-Veen F, Rolink AG, Gleichmann E. Diseases caused by reactions of T lymphocytes to incompatible structures of the major histocompatibility complex. IV. Autoantibodies to nuclear antigens. Clin Exp Immunol 1981;46:589.
107. Schwartz RS, Beldotti L. Malignant lymphomas following allogeneic disease: transition from an immunological to a neoplastic disorder. Science 1965;149:1511.
108. Dobashi K, Ono S, Mirakami S, et al. Polyclonal B cell activation by a

B cell differentiation factor, B151-TRF2. IV. B151-TRF2 as a B cell differentiation factor closely associated with autoimmune disease. J Immunol 1987;138:780.
109. Reeves JP, Steinberg AD. Effect of the xid gene on graft-versus-host–induced autoantibody production in nonautoimmune mice. Clin Immunol Immunopathol 1985;36:320.
110. Rolnik AG, Pals S, Gleichmann, E. Allosuppressor and allohelper T cells in acute and chronic graft-versus-host disease. II. F_1 recipients carrying mutations at H-2K and/or I-A. J Exp Med 1983;157:755.
111. Anasetti C, Rybka W, Sullivan KM, et al. Graft-v-host disease is associated with autoimmune-like thrombocytopenia. Blood 1989;73:1054.
112. Sullivan KM, Shulman HM, Storb R, et al. Chronic graft versus host disease in 52 patients: adverse natural course and successful treatment with combination immunosuppression. Blood 1985;66:921.
113. Berzofsky JA. Structural basis of antigen recognition by T lymphocytes. J Clin Invest 1988;82:1811.
114. Rajewsky K, Förster I, Cumano A. Evolutionary and somatic selection of the antibody repertoire in the mouse. Science 1987;238:1088.
115. Shlomchik MJ, Marshak-Rothstein A, Wolfowicz CB, et al. The role of clonal selection and somatic mutation in autoimmunity. Nature 1987;328:805.
116. Madaio MP, Hoder S, Stollar BD, Schwartz RS. Responsiveness of autoimmune and normal mice to nucleic acid antigens. J Immunol 1984;132:872.
117. Oldstone MBA. Molecular mimicry and autoimmune disease. Cell 1987;50:819.
118. Sharon R, Giloh H, Naor D. Experimental autoimmune hemolytic anemia induced with haptenated syngeneic mouse red blood cells and low dose X-radiation. Clin Immunol Immunopathol 1988;47:310.
119. Zabriskie JB. Rheumatic fever: a model for the pathological consequences of microbial-host mimicry. Clin Exp Rheumatol 1986;4:65.
120. Editorial. Yersiniosis today. Lancet 1984;1:84.
121. Fathman CG, Goronzt J, Weyand C. Gene conversion: a mechanism to explain HLA-D region and disease association. Ann NY Acad Sci 1986;475:24.
122. Oudin J, Cazenave PA. Similar idiotypic specificities in immunoglobulin fractions with different antibody functions or even without detectable antibody function. Proc Natl Acad Sci USA 1971;68:2616.
123. Nelson JL, Nardella FA, Oppliger IR, et al. Rheumatoid factors from patients with rheumatoid arthritis possess private repertoires of idiotypes. J Immunol 1987;138:1391.
124. Chen PP, Goni F, Fong S, et al. The majority of human monoclonal IgM rheumatoid factors express a "primary structure–dependent" cross-reactive idiotype. J Immunol 1985;134:3281.
125. Isenberg DA, Shoenfeld Y, Madaio M, et al. Anti-DNA antibody idiotypes in systemic lupus erythematosus. Lancet 1984;2:417.
126. Jerne NK. Towards a network theory of the immune system. Ann Immunol Inst Pasteur 1974;125c:373.
127. Burdette S, Schwartz RS. Idiotypes and idiotypic networks. N Engl J Med 1987;317:219.
128. Geha RS. Presence of auto-anti-idiotypic antibody during the normal human immune response to tetanus toxoid antigen. J Immunol 1982;129:139.
129. Silvestres F, Bankhurst RD, Searles RP, et al. Studies of anti-F $(ab')_2$ antibodies and possible immunologic control mechanisms in systemic lupus erythematosus. Arthritis Rheum 1984;27:1387.
130. Dwyer DS, Bradley RJ, Urquhart CK, et al. Naturally occurring anti-idiotypic antibodies in myasthenia gravis patients. Nature 1983;301:611.
131. Sikorska HM. Anti-thyroglobulin anti-idiotypic antibodies in sera of patients with Hashimoto's thyroiditis and Graves' disease. J Immunol 1986;137:3786.
132. Sultan Y, Kazatchkine MD, Maisonneuve P, et al. Anti-idiotypic suppression of autoantibodies to factor VIII (antihaemophilic factor) by high-dose intravenous gammaglobulin. Lancet 1984;2:765.
133. Ruiz-Arguelles A. Spontaneous reversal of acquired autoimmune dysfibrinogenemia probably due to an antiidiotypic antibody directed to an interspecies cross reactive idiotype expressed on antifibrinogen antibodies. J Clin Invest 1988;82:958.
134. Cooke A, Lydyard PM, Roitt IM. Autoimmunity and idiotypes. Lancet 1984;2:723.
135. Wasserman NH, Penn AS, Freimuth PI, et al. Anti-idiotypic route to anti-acetylcholine receptor antibodies and experimental myasthenia gravis. Proc Natl Acad Sci USA 1982;79:4810.
136. Shechter Y, Maron R, Elias D, et al. Autoantibodies to insulin receptor spontaneously develop as anti-idiotypes in mice immunized with insulin. Science 1982;216:542.
137. Elias D, Bone AJ, Baird JD, et al. Insulin-mimicking anti-idiotypic antibodies accompany the development of spontaneous autoimmune diabetes in BB/E rats. Diabetes 1990;39:1467.
138. Mendlovic S, Brocke S, Shoenfeld Y, et al. Induction of a systemic lupus erythematosus-like disease in mice by a human common anti-DNA idiotype. Proc Natl Acad Sci USA 1988;85:2260.
139. Ahmed SA, Penhale WJ, Talal N. Sex hormones, immune responses, and autoimmune diseases. Am J Pathol 1985;121:531.
140. Theofilopoulos AN, Dixon FJ. Murine models of systemic lupus erythematosus. Adv Immunol 1985;37:269.
141. Oyaizu N, Yasumizu R, Miyama-Inaba M, et al. (NZB $\times$ BXSB)F_1 mouse: a new model of idiopathic thrombocytopenic purpura. J Exp Med 1988;167:2017.
142. Hang LM, Izui S, Dixon FJ. (NZW $\times$ BXSB)F_1 hybrid: a model of acute lupus and coronary vascular disease with myocardial infarction. J Exp Med 1981;154:216.
143. Datta SK, Schwartz RS. Genetics of expression of xenotropic virus and autoimmunity in NZB mice. Nature 1976;263:412.
144. Gavalchin J, Nicklas JA, Eastcott JW, et al. Lupus prone (SWR $\times$ NZB)F_1 mice produce potentially nephritogenic autoantibodies inherited from the normal SWR patient. J Immunol 1985;134:885.
145. Prochazka M, Leiter EH, Serreze DV, et al. Three recessive loci required for insulin dependent diabetes in non-obese diabetic mice. Science 1987;237:286.

Blood: Principles and Practice of Hematology,
edited by Robert I. Handin, Thomas P. Stossel, and Samuel E. Lux.
J.B. Lippincott Company, Philadelphia © 1995.

24

Primary Immunodeficiency Diseases

Fred S. Rosen

The immune system is a complex of interacting factors that provide protection against infections. The system is composed of elements that are specific in their interactions with microbes and other elements that become nonspecifically engaged during immune reactions. The specificity of immunity resides in antibodies and the T-cell antigen receptor. Thus, defects in T lymphocytes or B lymphocytes, which make antibodies, result in deficiencies of specific immune responses.[1] Repeated bacterial, fungal, and viral infections of varying severity are the consequences of these deficiencies.

SEVERE COMBINED IMMUNODEFICIENCY

The term *severe combined immunodeficiency* (SCID) describes a clinical phenotype that is genetically determined but has many different genetic bases. The X-linked form of the disease is distinctive from the autosomal recessive form, and the latter form may result from a deficiency in the purine degradation enzymes, adenosine deaminase (ADA) or purine nucleoside phosphorylase (PNP), or from other rare, specific defects. SCID is characterized by a profound absence of T lymphocytes and an absence of cell-mediated immunity; it is invariably fatal to affected infants.[2]

Clinical Course and Laboratory Findings

Infants with SCID develop persistent infection, usually by 3 months of age. The most common infections are moniliasis of the mouth and skin, protracted diarrhea, and severe, pertussis-like cough due to interstitial pneumonia. The interstitial pneumonia is most frequently caused by *Pneumocystis carinii* and, left untreated, is the most frequent cause of death. In European countries where universal bacille Calmette-Guérin (BCG) vaccination is practiced, progressive infection with BCG is fatal to infants with SCID. In earlier times, when smallpox vaccination was universally applied, infants with SCID died of progressive vaccinia. Infection with varicella, herpes, and adenoviruses also is a frequent cause of death. In contrast to males with X-linked agammaglobulinemia who are extremely susceptible to pyogenic infections, infants with SCID almost invariably succumb to opportunistic infections.

Since these infants are immunologically incompetent, they are also extremely susceptible to the development of graft-versus-host (GVH) disease when they are transfused with immunologically competent cells. Blood transfusions are the most frequent sources of immunologically competent cells (ie, lymphocytes), and therefore, blood must be oxygenated and irradiated to inactivate lymphocytes before administration to infants with SCID to avoid GVH disease.

Infants with SCID have no cell-mediated immunity. They are therefore unable to reject tissue grafts (eg, of skin). The blood mononuclear cells are unresponsive to nonspecific mitogens, such as phytohemagglutinin, and to specific antigens, such as tetanus or diphtheria toxoids. Although their mononuclear cells are capable of stimulating allogeneic cells in vitro, their own cells do not respond to such a stimulus. Infants with SCID are profoundly lymphopenic (fewer than 3000 lymphocytes/μL), and when CD3+ T cells are encountered in the circulation, they usually are of maternal origin. When a weak response is found in vitro to any stimulus, one must be certain that the cells responding are not of maternal origin. The pathognomonic finding in infants with SCID is the histopathology of the thymus gland. Remnants of thymus are usually found in the neck; the organ fails to become lymphoid and to descend into the anterior mediastinum. The stroma of the thymus gland is formed from endodermal elements of the third and fourth pharyngeal pouches. By 6 to 8 weeks of human gestation, the organ becomes lymphoid as stem cells from the yolk sac and subsequently from fetal liver immigrate into the thymus gland. These normal events in thymus ontogeny fail to occur in infants with SCID, leaving the thymus gland bereft of lymphoid elements and Hassall's corpuscles. Sometimes, when it is difficult to establish the diagnosis of SCID, a skilled surgeon can obtain a thymus biopsy specimen by the aid of fiber optics. The thymus cannot be seen in a chest radiograph of an SCID patient, and this helps in the diagnosis. Although the lymph nodes are also devoid of lymphoid elements, it is difficult to find them because they are so small, and the biopsy of lymph nodes is not recommended since it frequently provides a portal for the entry of infection.

Genetics

The X-linked form of SCID has been mapped to chromosome Xq13, close to the locus for phosphoglucokinase. A defect in the γ chain of the IL-2 receptor, whose gene maps to Xq13, has been found in X-linked SCID. This γ chain is also found in the IL-4 and IL-7 receptors.[2a] The prenatal diagnosis has been established with restriction fragment length polymorphism (RFLP). The obligate maternal heterozygotes can also be detected by failure of random X inactivation in T-lymphocyte lines. The X-linked form of SCID is characterized by the normal number of B lymphocytes in the blood, in contrast to the autosomal recessive forms, in which both T and B lymphocytes are profoundly deficient.[3] In some cases of X-linked SCID, oligoclonal or polyclonal immunoglobulins are found in the blood, and this has been called *Nezelof's syndrome*, but there is no reason to think that this is a distinct entity.

As mentioned, the autosomal recessive form of SCID can be due to an absence of the purine degradation enzymes, ADA or PNP.[4,5] These enzyme deficiencies account for about half of the autosomal recessive cases of SCID. ADA is composed of a single polypeptide chain of 363 amino acid residues whose gene maps to chromosome 20q13-ter. Several mutations have been observed in this gene that do not have clinical consequences but result in an absence of ADA from red blood cells; apparently, there is enough residual ADA activity in the lymphocytes to prevent the untoward biochemical consequences that result in SCID.[6] Several successful attempts have been made to insert the ADA gene into a retroviral vector with the aim of transfecting deficient lymphoid cells for therapeutic purposes.[7] Indeed, successfult results have been seen with this therapy in children with adenosine deaminase deficiency.[8]

PNP is a trimer of polypeptide chains, each of which is composed of 289 amino acid residues. The gene encoding this polypeptide chain maps to chromosome 14q13.1. PNP deficiency is relatively rare compared with the incidence of ADA deficiency, but the frequency of these defects in the population is not known. The biochemical consequences of ADA and PNP deficiencies are of some interest because it was not anticipated a priori that such deficiencies would result in profound defects of lymphocyte function, and at first, this appeared so mysterious as to be a mere coincidence. This proved not to be the case.

Biochemical Considerations

Adenosine deaminase is ubiquitously distributed in mammalian cells, but there is about 13 times more ADA in thymocytes than in other cells. ADA catalyzes the deamination of adenosine and deoxyadenosine to inosine and deoxyinosine. In the absence of this enzyme, adenosine and deoxyadenosine accumulate within cells and are converted to adenosine triphosphate and deoxyadenosine triphosphate (dATP). The latter is particularly toxic to ribonucleotide reductase, the enzyme required for DNA synthesis. In addition, high amounts of adenosine inside cells inhibit the enzyme S-adenosyl homocysteine hydrolase, which is required for the methylation of DNA. These biochemical consequences of ADA deficiency are especially noxious to lymphoid cells because they are relatively lacking in ribonucleotidase activity, which would prevent accumulation of deoxyadenosine monophosphate, and thus dATP.[6]

PNP catalyzes the phosphorolysis of guanosine and inosine as well as of deoxyguanosine and deoxyinosine. Analogous to the consequences of ADA deficiency, PNP deficiency results in an accumulation of guanosine triphosphate and deoxyguanosine triphosphate. The latter has the same effects as dATP in inhibiting ribonucleotide reductase.

Therapy

The most successful therapy of SCID results from the transplantation of histoidentical bone marrow, usually from a matched sibling.[9] It is relatively easy to render a SCID patient with a histoidentical bone marrow donor into a lymphoid chimera, but only 40% of affected children have a matched donor. In light of this, successful attempts have been made to use haploidentical bone marrow donors. In practice, this usually involves one of the parents. The donated bone marrow must be rendered free of T lymphocytes so as to avoid GVH disease. This has been accomplished by two means: treatment of the bone marrow from the donor with a monoclonal antibody to mature T lymphocytes or depletion of T lymphocytes by passing the donor marrow over lectin columns that bind T lymphocytes. With both approaches, numerous infants with SCID have been rendered into bone marrow chimeras with outstanding results. In most cases, B lymphocyte engraftment does not occur, and intravenous γ-globulin substitution must be maintained.[10]

It is apparent that SCID associated with ADA or PNP deficiency results from the accumulation of toxic metabolites. Transfusions of red blood cells first acted beneficially as a source of these enzymes and depleted affected infants of the burdensome metabolites. More recently, ADA bound to polyethylene glycol has proved to be effective therapy for ADA deficiency.[11]

Rare cases of SCID have been observed to result from failure of interleukin-2 (IL-2) synthesis,[12] absence of the CD3 γ chain,[13] and failure of the transduction mechanism in T-cell activation,[14] which mobilizes intracellular calcium. In these rare instances, other therapies, such as administration of recombinant IL-2, may prove effective.

A rapidly fatal form of SCID in which not only T and B lymphocytes but also myeloid cells are absent is called *reticular dysgenesis*.[15] It was thought to be inherited as an autosomal recessive phenomenon, but it has recently been suggested that the myeloid aplasia results from destruction of myeloid elements in utero by maternal lymphocytes that have crossed the placenta.

MAJOR HISTOCOMPATIBILITY COMPLEX CLASS II DEFICIENCY

Recently, a number of children have been described with a genetically determined deficiency of major histocompatibility complex (MHC) class II molecules. The deficiency is inherited as an autosomal recessive trait, but the gene defect is not linked to the MHC, whose genes map to the short arm of chromosome 6. Most of the affected kindred have been from North Africa, and the affected offspring have been the result of consanguineous mating. A few cases have been observed in western Europeans and North Americans.

Affected cases sustain severe viral and bacterial infections. Diarrhea has been a prominent finding in most cases due to intestinal candidiasis and cryptosporidiosis. Flattening of the intestinal villi has been observed in biopsy specimens. None of the cases has developed progressive BCG infection after neonatal vaccination with BCG, nor has any developed GVH disease after blood transfusion. In both these regards, MHC class II deficiency is different from SCID.

Normal numbers of T and B lymphocytes are found in the blood of these patients, but there are decreased numbers of CD4+ cells and increased numbers of CD8+ cells. Similar findings have been established in mice given antibody to class II MHC molecules; there is a resultant diminution of CD4+ cells. Expression of class I MHC molecules is normal or slightly decreased. Affected infants have no cell-mediated immune responses to skin test antigens, and they are hypogammaglobulinemic. The responses in mixed lymphocyte cultures in vitro are normal, however, as are cytotoxicity responses of T lymphocytes. Epstein-Barr virus (EBV) transformed B lymphocytes have been found to contain no mRNA transcripts of class II molecules; neither the α nor the β chains of DR, DP, or DQ are present. Furthermore, expression of these molecules cannot be elicited by treatment of cells with interferon-γ (IFN-γ), as occurs in normal cells. Since the defect is not linked to the MHC, some other molecular basis for the defect must pertain. It appears certain that a promoter-binding protein is deficient since there is no band shift in the DNA promoter region on mixing the relevant DNA with extracts of patients' cells. This disease is the first genetic defect in which a promoter-binding protein is deficient.[16]

X-LINKED AGAMMAGLOBULINEMIA

Clinical Course and Laboratory Findings

X-linked agammaglobulinemia (XLA) was described in 1952 and was the first well-defined immunodeficiency disease. It was immediately apparent that only males were affected, and family studies revealed that XLA is inherited as an X-linked recessive phenomenon. Affected males are well during the first 9 to 12 months of life presumably because of passive protection provided by transplacentally passed immunoglobulin G (IgG). Subsequently, these boys develop recurrent pyogenic infections of the upper and lower respiratory tracts, the skin, and the middle ear. They are strikingly free of urinary tract infections and diarrhea and recover from the ordinary viral infections of childhood in the usual manner, although they may be prone in such situations to secondary pyogenic infections. The most common pyogen found in affected males is *Haemophilus influenzae*, but they are also susceptible to repeated infections with pneumococci, streptococci, and staphylococci, and to a lesser extent with *Pseudomonas* sp. Although these infections can be controlled with antibiotics, they are anatomically destructive, and most commonly result in chronic obstructive pulmonary disease. This can be readily prevented with γ-globulin rendered suitable for intravenous administration at a dose of at least 300 mg/kg every month. The optimal dose of γ-globulin for each patient with XLA must be determined empirically by achieving freedom from pyogenic infections; the optimal dose usually exceeds the minimal dose cited previously.[17]

In addition to the aforementioned pyogenic infections, other interesting clinical observations have been made in males with XLA. Before treatment, they tend to develop joint swelling, particularly of the large joints; the cause of this has never been clarified, and the symptoms and signs of arthritis promptly vanish after the institution of γ-globulin therapy. A syndrome, much resembling dermatomyositis, was noted in affected males 30 years ago. It subsequently turned out to be due to infection of the central nervous system with echoviruses, which can be readily recovered from cerebrospinal fluid.[18] These infections were invariably fatal but are now readily controlled with high doses of intravenous γ-globulin; it is important to test the various products for the best titer against the relevant echovirus in each patient. Another rare finding in XLA (as well as in common variable immunodeficiency [CVID]) is the occurrence of sarcoid-like granulomas in the skin and viscera; the cause of this is unknown. Patients with all forms of agammaglobulinemia are extremely susceptible to infection with *Giardia lamblia*, which causes diarrhea, steatorrhea, and weight loss. It is unusual, however, to find this in young males with XLA.

The only striking and consistent finding on physical examination of boys with XLA is the virtual absence of tonsillar tissue, which is composed mostly of B lymphocytes. Their blood contains no B lymphocytes, nor do their lymph nodes, as a consequence of which there is little architectural organization and an absence of follicular structures. Plasma cells cannot be found in the lymphoid tissue and in the bone marrow. The bone marrow contains normal numbers of pre–B cells, but there is a failure of maturation of these cells, and this remains the central mystery of XLA.[19] The serum contains little IgG (about 10% of normal) and no IgA, IgM, IgD, and IgE (Fig. 24-1).

T-cell number and function is normal in XLA. Normal delayed-type hypersensitivity can be elicited with the usual skin test antigens. Skin grafts are rejected in the usual manner. Observation of affected males over many years leads to the impression that their cell-mediated immunity is supernormal. They tend to have more poison ivy and drug reactions than age-matched cohorts; about 70% have severe reactions to trimethoprim and sulfa.

Genetics

X-linked agammaglobulinemia is the only disease model in which there is a complete absence of B lymphocytes. As already mentioned, it is transmitted as an X-linked phenomenon. Obligate heterozygous carriers of the defect are immunologically normal. The question arises as to whether the defect is intrinsic to the B-lymphocyte lineage; three lines of evidence indicate that this is so. There is nonrandom inactivation of the X chromosome in female obligate heterozygotes. That is, in normal females, one would anticipate that B-cell lines obtained by EBV transformation would be composed of half with one X chromosome and half with the other. In obligate heterozygous carriers of XLA, all the B-cell lines established have only the normal X chromosome, not the X chromosome bearing the XLA defect, as determined by DNA methylation patterns or by RFLP or linkage to a known marker on the X chromosome, such as glucose-6-phosphate dehydrogenase.[20,21] Furthermore, abnormal pre- or early B cells have been found in obligate heterozygotes; these abnormal cells do not mature to function, that is, synthesize and secrete antibody.[22] Thus, the defect appears to be intrinsic to cells of B-lymphocyte lineage. All other lineages tested reveal nonrandom X inactivation.

The gene for XLA has been mapped to chromosome Xq21.3-22 by RFLP. The original markers that were used to localize XLA, DXS3 and DXS17, now appear clearly to flank the gene defect. Another probe, DXS178, appears close

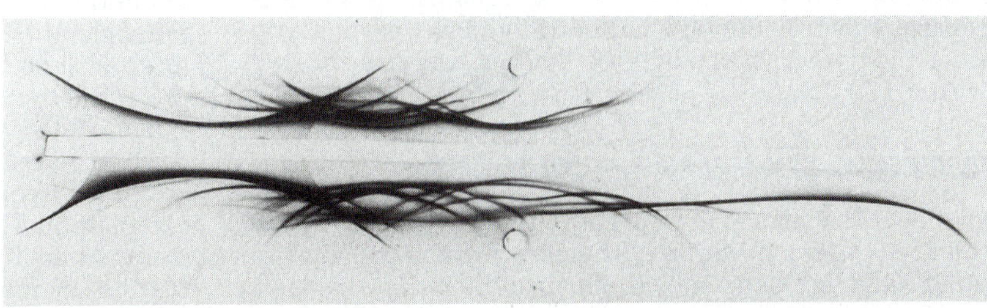

FIGURE 24-1. Immunoelectrophoresis of the serum of an agammaglobulinemic person (*top*) and a normal subject (*bottom*). The anode is to the left. The pattern was developed with horse antihuman serum. The precipitin bands for IgG, IgA, and IgM are missing from the agammaglobulinemic serum.

to XLA, so that a lod score of 10.24 has been obtained; this makes the odds in favor of linkage 1.7×10^{10}.[23] From a yeast artificial chromosome (YAC) containing the DXS178 marker, a gene has been identified that is defective in X-linked agammaglobulinemia.[24] It is a unique tyrosine kinase. Its precise role in the maturation of B lymphocytes is not yet clear. This is the first example of a genetic defect of a member of the tyrosine kinase family.[25]

IMMUNOGLOBULIN G DEFICIENCY WITH INCREASED IMMUNOGLOBULIN M (HYPER-IgM SYNDROME)

Several males have been described in whom there is a deficiency of IgG and IgA and a marked increase in IgM (more than 300 mg/dL) and sometimes of IgD. Although it was first thought that this disease was also transmitted as an X-linked recessive trait, several females with the disease have been described; it appears to be transmitted in some families as an autosomal recessive. There are also many sporadic cases. In addition to susceptibility to pyogenic infection, as is observed in males with XLA, patients with this syndrome almost always develop autoimmune neutropenia, thrombocytopenia, and hemolytic anemia with IgM antibodies to various cell membrane components. Treatment for this syndrome is as outlined for treatment of XLA. Large doses of intravenously administered γ-globulin may result in a decrease in serum IgM.

It had been assumed that these patients have an intrinsic B-cell defect that prevents class switching from IgM and IgD to the other heavy-chain genes. A T-cell lymphoma, however, was found to induce the switching in these patients in vitro, and these findings suggest that the syndrome is due to a failure of some T-lymphocyte subpopulation that induces class switching.[26]

The defective T-cell protein has been identified as the CD40 ligand. A cell surface molecule of B lymphocytes, CD40, must be engaged by a ligand expressed on activated T lymphocytes for successful isotype switching.[27] The CD40 ligand, encoded by a gene that maps Xq26, is defective in the hyper-IgM syndrome.[28] Successful isotype switching from IgM and IgD synthesis to IgG, IgA, and IgE synthesis requires not only the engagement of CD40 and its ligand but also cytokines such as IL-2, IL-4, and, possibly, IL-10.

IMMUNOGLOBULIN G HEAVY-CHAIN AND κ LIGHT-CHAIN DELETIONS

It is curious that few immunodeficiency diseases result from gene deletions in the immunoglobulin heavy-chain locus or at the various loci that encode the T-cell antigen receptor. About 10% of the population bears such deletions on one of their two chromosome, and this is without clinical consequences. A few homozygotes have been identified, however, who are deficient in IgG1 or IgG2, and in cases with extensive deletions, additional deficiencies of IgE and IgA2 have also been observed.

A few families have been found to have point mutations at chromosome 2p11, to which the κ gene maps, and they cannot make antibodies bearing κ light chains. The clinical consequences of this are not entirely clear, particularly since the patient in one of these kindred was also affected with cystic fibrosis.

IMMUNOGLOBULIN A DEFICIENCY

One in 700 whites is IgA deficient; thus, IgA deficiency is the most common immunodeficiency in humans. On the other hand, IgA deficiency is not encountered in Africans. There are no apparent clinical consequences of note in patients with IgA deficiency unless they have a concomitant deficiency of IgG2 or IgG4, as is found in patients with ataxia telangiectasia and others with IgG-subclass deficiencies. In a survey of patients with rheumatoid arthritis, it was found that IgA deficiency was more frequent than in the normal control population. This is true of most autoimmune diseases, which occur with greater frequency in IgA-deficient persons. Furthermore, the extended haplotype HLA-B8, DR3, complotype SC01 is found frequently in IgA-deficient patients, and this haplotype is associated with several autoimmune diseases, such as gluten-sensitive enteropathy, dermatitis herpetiformis, and insulin-dependent diabetes mellitus.

Patients with IgA deficiency tend to form antibodies to IgA and may sustain severe anaphylactic reactions when given transfusions of whole blood or plasma. These reactions are apparently due to IgE antibodies to IgA.

The inheritance of IgA deficiency is variable and defies simple mendelian analysis. IgA-deficient patients have normal numbers of circulation B cells bearing surface α chains. Why they fail to differentiate terminally into IgA-secreting plasma cells is not known.[29]

SELECTIVE DEFICIENCY OF IMMUNOGLOBULIN G SUBCLASSES

Selective deficiency of IgG2 or IgG3 renders patients susceptible to recurrent pyogenic infections. Selective deficiency of IgG4 appears to be without clinical consequences, and selective deficiency of IgG1 would be indistinguishable from CVID or acquired agammaglobulinemia because IgG1 constitutes about 75% of the total IgG in the blood. Patients with selective deficiency of IgG2 or IgG3 respond well clinically to intravenous administration of γ-globulin.[30]

COMMON VARIABLE IMMUNODEFICIENCY

Common variable immunodeficiency may be acquired at any time in life and affects males and females equally. There is no clear inheritance pattern for the acquisition of CVID, and the cause of the disease is unknown, although it may follow an infection with EBV or hepatitis virus in rare instances. Patients with CVID are susceptible to recurrent pyogenic infections, as are males with XLA, and any survey of a population with chronic obstructive pulmonary disease reveals some patients with undiagnosed CVID. These patients are prone to developing pernicious anemia and becoming vitamin B_{12} dependent. This complication should always be suspected when a serious infection does not respond to antibiotic therapy in a patient with CVID who is receiving adequate γ-globulin replacement. Rarely, patients with CVID develop warm hemolytic anemia as a result of an antibody to the Landsteiner-Weiner antigen, the public antigen of the Rh blood groups.

In contrast to males with XLA who lack B lymphocytes, patients with CVID usually have B lymphocytes that do not function properly in responding to growth and differentiation cytokines or synthesize but fail to secrete immunoglobulin. In rare instances, the disease may be due to an absence of helper T cells or excessive T-cell suppressor activity or to the presence of autoantibodies to B lymphocytes.[31] Sometimes, their lymphoid tissue is abundant, and patients may develop splenomegaly and giant lymphoid hyperplasia of the intestine, which gives a characteristic moth-eaten appearance to the gut in a barium study. As mentioned, a noncaseating granulomatous disease may be encountered in the skin or viscera; it responds well to steroid therapy. There appears to be an increased incidence of gastrointestinal malignancy in patients with CVID. Diarrhea and steatorrhea are common and usually are due to infestation with G *lamblia*.

CVID should be treated with regular intravenous administration of γ-globulin. Because most patients with CVID are adults, it is preferable to give the γ-globulin at biweekly intervals to sustain an adequate blood level of IgG. As stated for XLA, the minimal dose is 300 mg/kg/mo. The optimal dose has to be determined for individual patients since some may require twice the recommended minimal dose.

TRANSIENT HYPOGAMMAGLOBULINEMIA OF INFANCY

During the last trimester of pregnancy, IgG, but no other immunoglobulin, crosses the placenta in great quantity by an active transport mechanism, so that the concentration of IgG in the maternal blood becomes equilibrated with that in the fetal blood. This dowry of IgG is catabolized by the newborn, but substantial passive protection can be achieved for months. Nonetheless, by the third month of life, infants begin to synthesize their own immunoglobulin, and by the end of the first year, IgG concentrations are near normal. When the onset on IgG synthesis is delayed in certain infants, they become vulnerable to pyogenic infection. Whether to administer γ-globulin to affected infants is always a difficult decision because the disease is self-limited and infants recover from this by 36 months of age at the latest. The delay in the onset of IgG synthesis has been attributed to a failure of T-cell help because affected infants have normal numbers of B lymphocytes that synthesize IgG normally in the presence of normal mature CD4 T cells.[32]

WISKOTT-ALDRICH SYNDROME

The Wiskott-Aldrich syndrome is a rare, X-linked immunodeficiency. Affected males have thrombocytopenia, eczema, and recurrent bacterial infections. The gene for Wiskott-Aldrich syndrome maps to chromosome Xp11.22 by the use of RFLP.[33] The number of platelets in the blood of these children is markedly decreased, and the platelets are abnormally small (effective average diameter 1.82 + 0.1 μm compared with the normal diameter of 2.23 + 0.1 μm). The platelets are also coated with IgG. The size of the platelets has been noted to increase after splenectomy, and the amount of surface IgG decreases to normal.[34] Cell-mediated immunity progressively declines with age, but the number and phenotype of the blood lymphocytes are generally normal. Like the platelets, the blood lymphocytes are also small, and their size increases after splenectomy. By scanning electron microscopy, these blood elements have a characteristically abnormal appearance, and this has proved useful in the perinatal and prenatal diagnosis of Wiskott-Aldrich syndrome[35] (Fig. 24-2). The serum immunoglobulins are abnormal in that the concentrations of IgA and IgE are elevated and the concentration of IgM is decreased; IgG is normal. Affected males do not respond to polysaccharide antigens, whereas the response to protein antigens is normal or nearly so. Several affected males have received successful bone marrow transplantations from histoidentical siblings after lethal doses of irradiation or busulfan. Their immunologic function and platelet number and function is subsequently normal.[36] For reasons that are unclear, it has been difficult to perform transplantations in patients with Wiskott-Aldrich syndrome with haploidentical marrow; this procedure has succeeded in only a few instances.[37] In some cases, recipients have been rendered partial T-cell chimeras, without correction of the hematologic abnormalities; but the eczema disappeared,

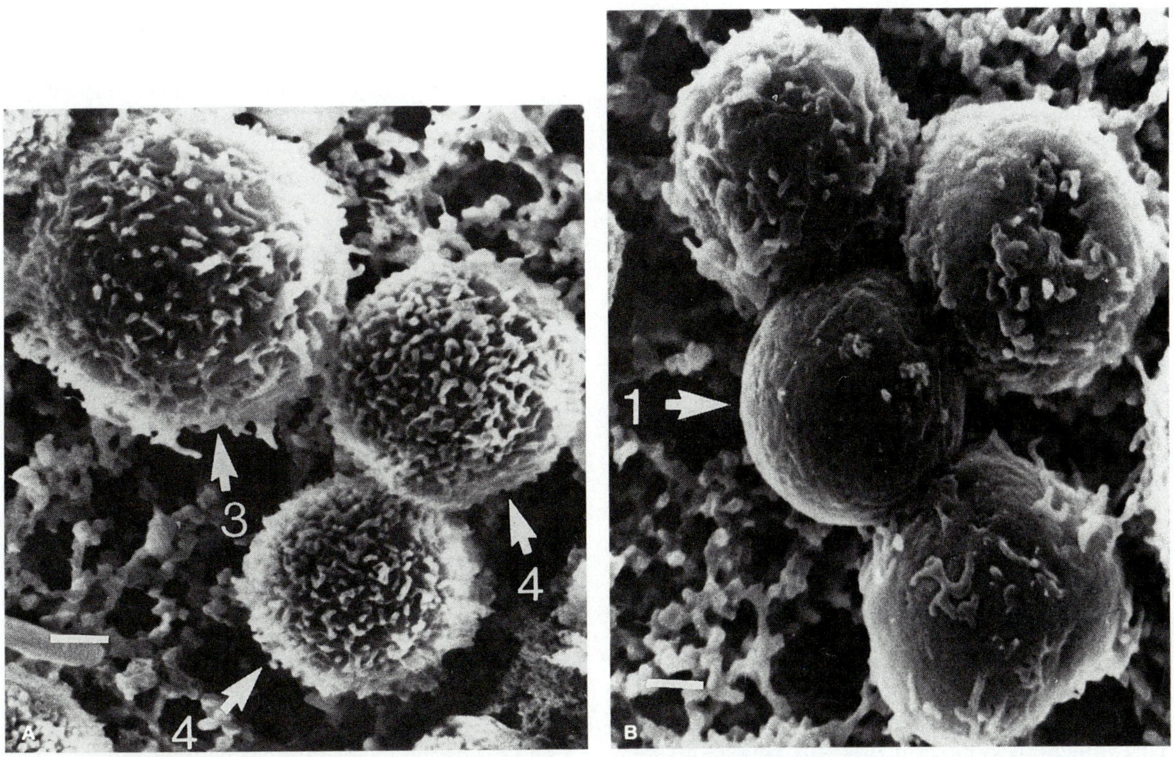

FIGURE 24-2. Scanning electron micrograph of lymphocytes from a normal subject (**A**) and from a patient with Wiskott-Aldrich syndrome (**B**). Note the baldness of the affected cells. (Kenney D, Cairns L, Remold-O'Donnell E, Peterson J, Rosen FS. Morphological abnormalities in the lymphocytes of patients with Wiskott-Aldrich syndrome. Blood 1986;68:1329)

serum immunoglobulin concentrations became normal, and a normal response to polysaccharide antigens was noted.

Abnormality in CD43

The abnormality in the size of the lymphocytes prompted an examination of the cell membranes from lysates of radioiodinated cells. A band of 115 kd was identified under both reducing and nonreducing conditions in normal lymphocyte membranes but not in preparations from lymphocytes of a boy with Wiskott-Aldrich syndrome. The protein thus first identified was called gpL115. By virtue of its adherence to wheat germ lectin and peanut lectin, gpL115 was purified; it was found to have a high content of sialic acid and was therefore named *sialophorin.* Several monoclonal antibodies to sialophorin were generated; it subsequently became apparent that several investigators had monoclonal antibodies to this same glycoprotein; it was assigned the designation CD43 at the Oxford workshop.

CD43 is present not only in the membranes of both CD4 and CD8 subsets of T lymphocytes but also in the membranes of mononuclear phagocytes, a portion of B lymphocytes, neutrophils, natural killer cells, and platelets. CD43 is not present on erythrocytes nor on any other cell type thus far tested (eg, fibroblasts, glioblasts, or rhabdomyoblasts).

A monoclonal antibody (L10) to CD43 activates and induces proliferation of blood mononuclear cells. The stimulation appears to be independent of the CD3-Ti complex. L10 induces increased secretion of IL-2 and an increase in intracellular calcium and phosphorylation of CD43. L10 also increases the adhesiveness of blood monocytes and causes homotypic adhesion of these cells. This requires magnesium ions and LFA-1. Moreover, L10 increases hydrogen peroxide production in mononuclear phagocytes challenged with PMA. This action of L10 thus resembles that of IFN-γ.

Clones of cDNA reveal that CD43 is composed of 400 amino acid residues. The amino-terminal 235 residues form a mucin-like extracellular domain followed by a putative 23-residue transmembrane region and a 123-residue carboxy-terminal intracellular domain; the signal sequence is presumed to contain 19 residues. The extracellular domain of 235 residues contains 46 serines and 47 threonines; it appears that 84 of these 93 residues are O-glycosylated with sialylated Gal–GalNAc side chains. More complex O-linked saccharides are present on activated T lymphocytes. Residues 135 to 224 form a 90–amino acid stretch containing five repeats of 19 residues. The function of the stretch containing these repeating elements is not known. Because the gene encoding CD43 maps to chromosome 16 at band p11.2, the defect in CD43 observed in the Wiskott-Aldrich syndrome cannot be the primary defect. The basic defect in Wiskott-Aldrich syndrome that causes the instability of surface CD43 remains an enigma.[38]

HEREDITARY ATAXIA TELANGIECTASIA

Hereditary ataxia telangiectasia is inherited as an autosomal recessive characteristic. Affected children first develop ataxia after 18 months of age, that is, after they have started walking. In the sixth year, fine telangiectases develop in the conjunctivae, on the ear lobes, and on other exposed parts of the body. Most patients develop persistent sinopulmonary infections. The diagnosis can be established early by the elevation of serum α-fetoprotein. About 80% of patients are deficient in IgA. Some of these patients have a concomitant deficiency of IgG4 and IgG2, and these susceptibility to infection is most frequently encountered in these patients. Patients with ataxia telangiectasia develop malignancies, principally of the lymphoreticular organs, usually by the end of the second decade of life.

Patients with ataxia telangiectasia are susceptible to the effects of ionizing radiation. Cultured cells, such as fibroblasts, exhibit many chromosomal breaks after exposure to ionizing irradiation. Lymphocytes frequently exhibit breaks at the chromosome map location of the T-cell–antigen receptor genes, that is, 14q11-12, 7q32-35, and 7p15, as well as at the immunoglobulin gene loci, that is, 2p11, 14q32.3, and 22p11.

There are six known complementation groups among ataxia telangiectasia patients, and the most common has been mapped to chromosome 11q22.3, where it is linked to the locus for *thy-1*.[39] The molecular basis for the failure of repair of chromosomal breaks in ataxia telangiectasia is unknown.

DiGEORGE'S SYNDROME

The thymus gland is derived early in embryogenesis from the third and fourth pharyngeal arches. From these same embryonic structures are derived the parathyroid glands, the cardiac outflow vessels, and the hyomandibular elements of the face. By the sixth week of human gestation, the thymus becomes lymphoid due to an immigration of lymphoid stem cells from the yolk sac and subsequently from the fetal liver. By 20 weeks of gestation, fully competent T lymphocytes begin to emigrate from the thymus to populate the secondary lymphoid organs. Because of an unclear in utero event, there may be faulty development of the organs derived from the third and fourth pharyngeal arches. This results in neonatal tetany, as a result of hypoplasia of the parathyroids, and an absence of severe hypoplasia of the thymus. Affected infants may have poor cell-mediated immunity and a decrease in the number of circulating T cells. They also have anomalies of the great vessels and tetralogy of Fallot as well as peculiar facies characterized by low-set ears, shortened filtrum of the upper lip, and an increased interocular space. Midline clefts in the nose are sometimes present, and absence of the corpus callosum has been observed. The major cause of death in affected infants is due their cardiac abnormalities. In some, opportunistic infections, characteristic of T-cell deficiency, are encountered. In these infants, cell-mediated immunity has been improved by transplantations of fetal thymus gland. Blood transfusions in newborns with DiGeorge's syndrome have caused fatal GVH disease.

HYPER-IgE SYNDROME

The hyper-IgE syndrome is characterized by severe infections, skin lesions, and extremely high serum concentrations of IgE. The cause of this concatenation of findings is not known. Furthermore, there is no apparent mendelian inheritance of the syndrome. The skin abscesses, which are commonly found in these patients, are unaccompanied by erythema and heat and have been called *cold abscesses.* The patients also have chronic eczematoid dermatitis. Infection of the viscera is also common. The age of onset of the syndrome is usually in early infancy. The major bacterial pathogen recovered from sites of infection is *Staphylococcus aureus*, but other pyogens may also be found. Chronic candidal infections of the skin, nails, and mouth are present in almost all patients.

The serum IgE levels in these patients mount rapidly in infancy to greater than 2500 IU/mL. Normal infants have IgE levels of less than 4 IU/mL. Eosinophilia is commonly found, particularly during infections. T lymphocytes respond poorly to specific antigens but respond normally to

TABLE 24-1. Other Syndromes Associated With Immunodeficiency

CHROMOSOMAL ABNORMALITIES
Bloom's syndrome
Fanconi's anemia
Down's syndrome
MULTIPLE ORGAN SYSTEM ABNORMALITIES
Partial albinism
Short-limbed dwarfism
Cartilage hair hypoplasia
Agenesis of the corpus callosum
HEREDITARY METABOLIC DEFECTS
Transcobalamin-2 deficiency
Acrodermatitis enteropathica
Type I orotic aciduria
Biotin-dependent carboxylase deficiency
HYPERCATABOLISM OF IMMUNOGLOBULIN
Familial hypercatabolism of immunoglobulin
Myotonic dystrophy
Intestinal lymphagiectasia
OTHER
Hyper-IgE syndrome
Chronic mucocutaneous candidiasis
Thymoma
Immunodeficiency following hereditarily determined susceptibility to Epstein-Barr virus

nonspecific mitogens and other nonspecific agonists. It has been postulated that the syndrome results from a deficiency of those T lymphocytes that suppress IgE synthesis. It is also presumed that inflammation in these patients is poor because IgE antibodies to *S aureus* and other bacteria do not fix complement.

There is no specific therapy for the hyper-IgE syndrome.

Several other disease entities associates with immunodeficiency are listed in Table 24-1.

REFERENCES

1. Eibl M, Griscelli C, Seligmann M. Primary immunodeficiency diseases: report of a WHO Scientific Group. Immunodefic Rev 1989;1:173.
2. Rosen FS, Cooper MD, Wedgwood JR. The primary immunodeficiencies, part 2. N Engl J Med 1984;311:300.
2a. Kondo M, Takeshita T, Higuchi M, et al. Functional participation of the IL-2 receptor γ chain in IL-7 receptor complexes. Science 1994;263:1453.
3. Puck JM, Nussbaum RL, Conley ME. Carrier detection in X-linked severe combined immunodeficiency based on patterns of X chromosome inactivation. J Clin Invest 1987;79:1395.
4. Giblett ER, Anderson JE, Cohen F, et al. Adenosine-deaminase deficiency in two patients with severely impaired cellular immunity. Lancet 1972;2:1067.
5. Giblett ER, Ammann AJ, Wara DW, et al. Nucleoside-phosphorylase deficiency in a child with severely defective T-cell immunity and normal B-cell immunity. Lancet 1975;1:1010.
6. Hirschhorn R. Adenosine deaminase deficiency. Immunodefic Rev 1990;2:175.
7. Williams DA, Orkin SH, Mulligan RC. Retrovirus-mediated transfer of human adenosine deaminase gene sequences into cells in culture and into murine hematopoietic cells *in vivo*. Proc Natl Acad Sci USA 1986;83:2566.
8. Blaese RM, Culver KW. Gene therapy for primary immunodeficiency disease. Immunodefic Rev 1992;3:329.
9. Parkman R, Gelfand EW, Rosen FS, et al. Severe combined immunodeficiency and adenosine deaminase deficiency. N Engl J Med 1975;292:714.
10. O'Reilly, RJ, Keever CA, Small TN, Brochstein J. The use of HLA-nonidentical T-cell–depleted marrow transplants for correction of severe combined immunodeficiency disease. Immunodefic Rev 1989;1:273.
11. Hershfield MS, Buckley RH, Greenberg ML, et al. Treatment of adenosine deaminase deficiency with polyethylene glycol-modified adenosine deaminase. N Engl J Med 1987;316:589.
12. Pahwa R, Chatila T, Pahwa S, et al. Recombinant interleukin 2 therapy in severe combined immunodeficiency disease. Proc Natl Acad Sci USA 1989;86:5069.
13. Alarcon B, Terhorst C, Arnaiz-Villena A, et al. Congenital T-cell receptor immunodeficiencies in man. Immunodefic Rev 1990;2:1.
14. Chatila T, Wong R, Young M, et al. An immunodeficiency characterized by defective signal transduction in T lymphocytes. N Engl J Med 1989;320:696.
15. Levinsky RJ, Tiedemann K. Successful bone-marrow transplantation for reticular dysgenesis. Lancet 1983;1:671.
16. Griscelli C, Lisowska-Grospierre B, Mach B. Combined immunodeficiency with defective expression in MHC class II genes. Immunodefic Rev 1989;1:135.
17. Rosen FS, Cooper MD, Wedgwood RJP. The primary immunodeficiencies, part 1. N Engl J Med 1984;311:235.
18. Wilfert CM, Buckley RH, Monanakumar T, et al. Persistent and fatal central-nervous-system echovirus infections in patients with agammaglobulinemia. N Engl J Med 1977;296:1485.
19. Pearl E, Vogler L, Okos A, et al. B lymphocytes precursors in human bone marrow. J Immunol 1976;120:1169.
20. Conley M, Brown P, Pickard A, et al. Expression of the gene defect in X-linked agammaglobulinemic lymphocytes. J Clin Invest 1968;47:836.
21. Fearon E, Winkelstein J, Civin C, et al. Carrier detection in X-linked agammaglobulinemia by analysis of X-chromosome inactivation. N Engl J Med 1987;316:427.
22. Schwaber J, Payne J, Chen R. B lymphocytes from X-linked agammaglobulinemia: delayed expression of light chain and demonstration of lyonization in carriers. J Clin Invest 1988;81:514.
23. Kwan S-P, Terwilliger J, Parmley R, et al. Identification of a closely linked DNA marker, DXS178, to further refine the X-linked agammaglobulinemia locus. Genomics 1990;6:238.
24. Vetrie D, Vorechovsky I, Sideras P, et al. The gene involved in X-linked agammaglobulinaemia is a member of the src family of protein-tyrosine kinases. Nature 1993;361:226.
25. Tsukuda S, Saffran DC, Rawlings DJ, et al. Deficient expression of a B cell cytoplasmic tyrosine kinase in human X-linked agammaglobulinemia. Cell 1993;72:279.
26. Mayer L, Kwan S-P, Thompson C, et al. Evidence for a defect in "switch" T cells in patients with immunodeficiency and hyperimmunoglobulinemia M. N Engl J Med 1986;314:409.
27. Fuleihan R, Ramesh N, Low R, et al. Defective expression of the CD40 ligand in X chromosome–linked immunoglobulin deficiency with normal or elevated IgM. Proc Natl Acad Sci USA 1993;90:2170.
28. Ramesh N, Fuleihan R, Ramesh V, et al. Deletions in the ligand for CD40 in X-linked immunoglobulin deficiency with normal or elevated IgM (HIGMX-1) Immunol Int (in press).
29. Conley ME, Cooper MD. Immature IgA B cells in IgA-deficient patients. N Engl J Med 1981;305:495.
30. Preud'Homme JL, Hanson LA. IgG subclass deficiency. Immunodefic Rev 1990;2:129.
31. Geha RS, Schneeberger E, Merler E, Rosen FS. Heterogeneity of "acquired" or common variable agammaglobulinemia. N Engl J Med 1974;291:1.
32. Siegel RL, Issekutz T, Schwaber J, et al. Deficiency of T helper cells in transient hypogammaglobulinemia of infancy. N Engl J Med 1981;305:1307.
33. Kwan S-P, Sandkuyl LA, Blaese M. Genetic mapping of the Wiskott-Aldrich syndrome with two highly-linked polymorphic DNA markers. Genomics 1988;3:39.
34. Lum LG, Tubergen DG, Corash L, et al. Splenectomy in the management of the thrombocytopenia of the Wiskott-Aldrich syndrome. N Engl J Med 1980;302:892.
35. Kenney D, Cairns L, Remold-O'Donnell E, et al. Morphological abnormalities in the lymphocytes of patients with Wiskott-Aldrich syndrome. Blood 1986;68:1329.
36. Parkman R, Rappeport J, Geha RS, et al. Complete correction of the Wiskott-Aldrich syndrome by allogenic bone marrow transplantation. N Engl J Med 1978;298:921.
37. Rumelhart SL, Trigg ME, Horowitz SD, Hong R. Monoclonal antibody T-cell-depleted HLA-haploidentical bone marrow transplantation for Wiskott-Aldrich syndrome. Blood 1990;75:1031.
38. Remold-O'Donnell E, Rosen FS. Sialophorin (CD43) and the Wiskott-Aldrich syndrome. Immunodefic Rev 1990;2:151.
39. Gatti RA, Berkel E, Braedt G, et al. Localization of an ataxia-telangiectasia gene to chromosome 11q22-23. Nature 1988;336:577.
40. Geha RS, Leung DYM. Hyper immunoglobulin E syndrome. Immunodefic Rev 1989;1:155.

Blood: Principles and Practice of Hematology,
edited by Robert I. Handin, Thomas P. Stossel, and Samuel E. Lux.
J.B. Lippincott Company, Philadelphia © 1995.

25

Acquired Immunodeficiency Syndrome

David T. Scadden
Jerome E. Groopman

HISTORY OF THE ACQUIRED IMMUNODEFICIENCY SYNDROME EPIDEMIC

The acquired immunodeficiency syndrome (AIDS) was initially recognized as a small cluster of unusual infections occurring among homosexual men in Los Angeles and New York. It has clearly emerged as a major and complex disease of global proportions[1-6] (Fig. 25-1). The history of the AIDS epidemic is still being written and, as with all history, it is viewed from many different perspectives and is prone to revision. Nonetheless, certain common lessons have been learned during the evolution of a communicable disease that rapidly spread among certain populations in the late 1970s in the United States, the Caribbean, and Europe. These generally young and otherwise previously healthy persons with AIDS manifested infectious or neoplastic maladies such as oral candidiasis, *Pneumocystis carinii* pneumonia, severe perianal herpes simplex, and Kaposi's sarcoma, disorders that had been associated with significant cellular immunodeficiency conditions[7-9] (Table 25-1).

Early efforts to understand the basis of these unusual cases included lymphocyte phenotyping, a frequently applied laboratory tool of the clinical immunologist in 1981. It revealed an inversion of the ratio of helper–inducer CD4+ to suppressor–cytotoxic CD8+ peripheral T cells, with an absolute decrease in the number of helper T cells in the blood of those afflicted.[10] This correlated with anergy to skin testing with recall antigens and reduced lymphocyte proliferative responses to mitogens and antigens.

Many causes were invoked to explain this new syndrome, some of them derived from delving into the subculture of a largely previously covert male homosexual life-style in the United States. Loss of immune function was postulated to represent a breakdown in defense consequent to the assault by certain behaviors common in this group. It was hypothesized that antigenic overload due to exposure to allogeneic semen or that toxicity due to recreational drugs, such as inhaled nitrites, resulted in severe cellular immunodeficiency. Critical to the ultimate discovery of the cause of AIDS were two factors: the apparent transmission of the syndrome by transfused blood products and its traceability among direct sexual partners of index cases. These epidemiologic clues firmly established AIDS as a communicable disease.

A virus as the communicable agent became the leading suspect in this medical mystery. Because certain DNA viruses of the herpes family, such as cytomegalovirus (CMV), were known to cause transient immunosuppression, consideration was given to new strains of CMV or other DNA viruses as etiologic agents in AIDS. Other researchers, looking at the reactivity of sera from AIDS patients with T-cell lines infected with the retrovirus human T-cell leukemia/lymphoma virus type I (HTLV-I), reported weak reactivity to retroviral proteins and postulated that an aberrant or related form of HTLV had emerged.

Methods that were developed in the 1970s for the isolation and propagation of human T cells in vitro proved important in unraveling the AIDS story. Such methods used growth factors, particularly the T-cell growth factor, interleukin-2 (IL-2), which supported the continuous replication of lymphocytes that had been stimulated with mitogens or antigens. Furthermore, permanent T-cell lines of different phenotypes had been derived from various T-cell malignancies, and several of these lines were recognized to support the growth of HTLV-I.

The story of the discovery of the viral cause of AIDS is now well known. Two independent groups, one working under Dr. Luc Montagnier at the Institut Pasteur in Paris[11] and the other under Dr. Robert Gallo at the National Cancer Institute in Bethesda[12] reported a new retrovirus that could be propagated in fresh peripheral blood T cells as well as in permanent T-cell lines. The identification of permanent T-cell lines capable of supporting continuous replication of the AIDS virus proved to be key to its ultimate identification and characterization. The initial difficulties in maintaining cultures of the virus were related to its relatively rapid destruction of fresh peripheral blood T cells grown in vitro in the presence of IL-2 and mitogens. The fortuitous concurrence of several relatively recent advances in cell biology, as well as the excitement in 1980 of the discovery of the first human retrovirus, HTLV-I, had clearly positioned the scientific community to identify in a relatively rapid time frame the etiologic agent of this disease.

Certain sexual practices and intravenous drug abuse were ultimately determined to be major vectors for the transmission of the AIDS virus. The cultural revolution of the 1960s and 1970s, together with an increasingly mobile society, allowed for rapid penetration and dissemination of the AIDS virus. What began as an unusual cluster of unexplained and previously rare infectious and malignant disorders in young homosexual men on both coasts of the United States is now a public health threat of huge proportions and a clinical disorder that virtually every prac-

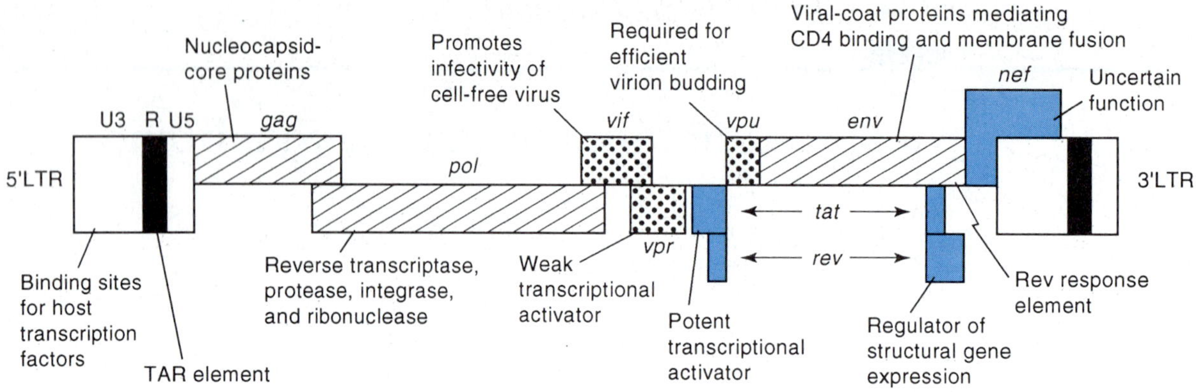

FIGURE 25-1. Organization of the proviral genome.

ticing physician will encounter. Its importance for the hematologist is clear, given its potential transmission by blood products as well as its association with cytopenias and lymphatic neoplasms.

GENETICS OF THE HUMAN IMMUNODEFICIENCY VIRUS

Now recognized are two pathogenic human retroviruses, termed *human immunodeficiency virus type I* (HIV-1) and *type II* (HIV-2), which result in the clinical syndrome of AIDS. These two viruses are similar in their molecular organization, although they differ in at least one open reading frame, which encodes a protein recognized by sera from

TABLE 25-1. Conditions Included in the 1993 AIDS Surveillance Case Definition

Candidiasis of bronchi, trachea, or lungs
Candidiasis, esophageal
Cervical cancer, invasive
Coccidioidomycosis, disseminated or extrapulmonary
Cryptococcosis, extrapulmonary
Cryptosporidiosis chronic intestinal (>1 month's duration)
Cytomegalovirus disease (other than liver, spleen, or nodes)
Cytomegalovirus retinitis (with loss of vision)
Encephalopathy, HIV related
Herpes simplex: chronic ulcers (>1 month's duration) or bronchitis, pneumonitis, or esophagitis
Histoplasmosis, disseminated or extrapulmonary
Isosporiasis, chronic intestinal (>1 month's duration)
Kaposi's sarcoma
Lymphoma, Burkitt's (or equivalent term)
Lymphoma, immunoblastic (or equivalent term)
Lymphoma, primary, of brain
Mycobacterium avium complex or *Mycobacterium kansasii* infection, disseminated or extrapulmonary
Mycobacterium tuberculosis infection, any site (pulmonary* or extrapulmonary)
Mycobacterium infection, other species or unidentified species, disseminated or extrapulmonary
Pneumocystis carinii pneumonia
Pneumonia, recurrent
Progressive multifocal leukoencephalopathy
Salmonella septicemia, recurrent
Toxoplasmosis of the brain
Wasting syndrome due to HIV

* Added in 1993 expansion of the AIDS surveillance case definition. (Statistics from the Center for Disease Control. AIDS 1992;6:145)

infected persons. A schematic depiction of the HIV genome is shown in Figure 25-1.[12a]

Human immunodeficiency virus is 9.2 kb long and contains certain genes common to retroviruses but also has distinct functional genes. Although HIV has been cloned and sequenced, functional genetic elements may be within the virus that have not been recognized. Like all retroviruses, HIV is composed of RNA. A genetic element within the RNA termed *pol* codes for the enzyme reverse transcriptase. The reverse transcriptase forms the DNA copy from the viral RNA template after the virus enters the cytoplasm of the target cell. Both circularized and linear DNA copies of the virus are generated, and some are transported to the nucleus and subsequently integrated into the host cell genome. The term *provirus* is used to identify the viral DNA that is integrated within the host nuclear DNA. In an acutely infected host cell, forms of viral DNA not only are integrated as provirus but also are present within the cytoplasm, along with viral RNA within cytoplasm. The integration of the viral DNA as a provirus does not occur at a unique site within the host cellular DNA but appears to be a random or semirandom process mediated by a viral encoded integrase.[13] This provirus is able to harness the cellular machinery to make viral RNA and subsequently viral protein. The viral protein assembles around the newly formed viral RNA and yields infectious particles through a process of budding from the cell surface membrane.

The viral genome can best be divided into two major categories. The first category includes viral genes that code for structural elements of the virus; the second includes genes that encode regulatory elements. Like all other retroviruses, HIV has a core structure that is encoded by the *gag* gene and has an envelope encoded by the *env* gene. The *gag* gene product is initially made as a fusion protein that includes the structural core proteins as well as the reverse transcriptase and a protease that is capable of cleaving this fusion molecule into the appropriate subunits.[14] The major core protein is 24 kd and represents one of the major viral gene products. The *env* gene encodes a large and heavily glycosylated exterior envelope protein that is termed *gp120* because it is 120 kd. This large exterior glycoprotein is anchored by a transmembrane protein of 41 kd termed *gp41*. The gp41 is hydrophobic in composition, allowing for its stable placement within the lipid membrane.

As can be seen in Figure 25-1, open reading frames are present within the viral genome that overlap other genetic elements. Long precursor forms of RNA appear to be made, and these are then differentially spliced to yield messenger RNAs that encode distinct proteins. This differential splicing of RNA, as well as shifts in the reading frame of the transcript, led to the identification of previously unrecognized protein products of the virus that may have important functions. Thus, the full description and understanding of the structure and function of the HIV genome may not yet have been completed.

HIV gene products are capable of modulating transcription and possibly translation, providing the machinery whereby the virus may regulate its own expression and possibly sustain a state of relative latency.[15,16] The flanking sequences of the HIV genome are termed *long terminal repeats* (LTR). The structure of the HIV-LTR is similar to that seen with other retroviruses and contains genetic elements that are responsive to positive and negative signals that regulate transcription. The *tat* gene derived its name from its function as a transcriptional activator.[17,18] In a variety of in vitro model systems, *tat* appears to increase the steady-state level of messenger RNA and increase translational use of HIV-LTR–directed transcription.[19] The *tat* RNA and *tat* protein are among the first products to appear after viral infection of host T lymphocytes.

Certain cofactors may increase HIV replication within infected cells, such as T-cell mitogens, cytokines such as tumor necrosis factor (TNF), and the gene products of certain DNA viruses.[20–22] These may activate latent HIV provirus. Up-regulation of HIV by *tat* is believed to occur by means of an element within the LTR termed *tar*.[23] The *tar* element is 3′ to the transcriptional start site, is dependent with respect to position and orientation, and has a characteristic "stem loop" structure that must be maintained for its activity. That *tat* directly binds to the *tar* element is clear, but whether *tat* mediates its effects alone or in conjunction with other cellular proteins remains open to question.[24]

Another important regulatory viral gene is termed *rev*. This gene product is absolutely required by the virus for production of the *gag* and *env* proteins as well as the reverse transcriptase encoded by *pol*.[25] The apparent function of *rev* is complex and appears to involve reduction in synthesis of HIV proteins translated from multiply spliced messenger RNAs. The HIV proteins that are translated from multiply spliced mRNAs are predominantly *tat*, *rev*, and the open reading frame in the 3′ position termed *nef*. The region of the viral genome that interacts with *rev* is termed the *rev-response element* and includes a 240–base pair segment within the *env* gene.[26] The *rev* protein appears to oligomerize and bind to the *rev*-response element. In doing so, *rev* appears both to inhibit the splicing of the RNA and to reduce its transport from nucleus to cytoplasm.[27–29]

Considerable controversy exists regarding the open reading frame at the 3′ position of HIV. Originally termed *nef* for a negative regulatory gene, this gene product was believed to appear early after viral infection and reduce viral transcription, thereby sustaining viral latency.[30] It is not clear whether the protein has this function,[31,32] and recent animal studies of viruses in which *nef* has been deleted suggest an opposite effect—that *nef* may enhance the replicative activity of the closely related virus, simian immunodeficiency virus (SIV).[33]

Other recently recognized viral genes are *vif*, *vpu*, and *vpr*. The *vif* gene product appears to be important in the infectivity of virion particles. The *vpr* gene may function in some way to increase the cytopathic effect of the virus on host T lymphocytes.[34] The *vpu* gene is present within the HIV-1 genome but not within the HIV-2 genome. The function of the *vpu* gene is not understood but may involve integration of its protein product into the membrane of the infected cell.[35,36] The *vpu* protein is found in significant quantities in virus-producing cells, but the protein has not been detected in cell-free culture fluid so it is probably not associated with the virion. *Vpu* may function in the release of the virus particles from infected cells.

The genomes of HIV-1 and HIV-2 differ with respect to the above-mentioned *vpu* gene product. In addition, the HIV-2 genome (as well as SIV) contains a gene product termed *vpx* not found in HIV-1.[37,38] HIV-2 may be less pathogenic than HIV-1, and differences in pathogenicity may in some way relate to these differences in the viral genomes. With regard to the relation of HIV-1 and HIV-2 to the leukemogenic human retrovirus HTLV-I, HIV was originally postulated to be a member of the HTLV family. Based on both genome structure and protein products, the relation between HIV and HTLV is now considered distant. Nonetheless, some broad similarities exist in patterns of gene expression between HIV and HTLV. HTLV-I encodes a transcriptional transactivator termed *tax*, which is similar to the HIV *tat* protein because it can function to augment viral gene expression. HTLV-I also encodes a transactivator termed *rex*, which is needed for expression of the unspliced messenger RNAs that encode the *gag*, *pol*, and *env* products of HTLV-I. Functional parallels exist between HTLV-I *rex* and HIV *rev* genes, although they do not manifest sequence homology.[39]

Structural Molecules of Human Immunodeficiency Virus and Tests for Infection

The two major components of the virus structure are the exterior envelope encoded by the *env* gene and the core encoded by the *gag* gene. The diagnosis of HIV infection by serologic assays depends on a detectable antibody response to these two viral structures. In some persons, before the detection of antibody, free viral core (p24) antigen can be detected in the plasma using an antigen capture assay. Several weeks after primary infection, usually antibody to the p24 structure appears, with concurrent loss of detectable antigen. The antigen is believed to be now complexed by the antibody and no longer available for capture in the assay. Antibody to HIV envelope proteins of 120 and 41 kd appears as another early event after primary infection. This antibody generally persists throughout the course of the illness, as the patient progresses from an asymptomatic infected state to symptomatic disease defined as AIDS. In many persons, a decline in titer of antibody occurs to the core p24 antigen with subsequent reappearance of p24 antigenemia. This is often a negative prognostic event, which may predate by months to years accelerated clinical deterioration. This particular pattern is certainly not a uniform finding. Many patients do not have detectable p24 antigen prior to antibody seroconversion with primary infection, and also a significant number of persons, estimated at about 40% to 50%, do not manifest the reappearance of p24 antigen in the later stages of HIV infection. Newer laboratory methods that dissociate antigen–antibody complexes by acid treatment[40] have increased the frequency of detectable p24 antigen levels to 60% to 80% of patients.

The serologic test used for initial screening for antibody to HIV is an enzyme-linked immunosorbent assay (ELISA). Guidelines for the use of this test and the confirmatory Western blot have been published by the Centers for Disease Control and Prevention (CDC).[41] The ELISA assay uses antigen prepared from whole virus harvested from tissue culture. More recent assays use envelope and core antigens prepared by recombinant DNA technology. A positive ELISA test is scored as such according to increased reactivity above background. Each ELISA has its own set of criteria with regard to the degree of increased reactivity that represents a positive reaction. Generally, a serum sample is tested in duplicate, and if a positive reaction results in both tests, the person is said to be HIV ELISA reactive. All repeatedly reactive ELISA tests must be confirmed using a second method to validate that a person has antibody to HIV. The profound personal, social, and medical implications of this serologic finding underscore the need for accurate testing using more than one method and correct interpretation of the results.

The Western, or immunoblot, assay is the most frequently used secondary test for antibody to HIV. This method involves native or recombinant antigens that are separated by electrophoretic mobility and apparent size on a gel and then transferred to nitrocellulose paper. The serum sample is layered over this paper and the reaction developed. The interpretation of the Western blot is therefore subjective, since the viewer must determine whether reactivity is present. The criteria for scoring a positive Western blot involve determination of reactivity at molecular weights, which represents core (24 kd) and envelope (41 and 120 kd) proteins. In addition, frequently reactions are seen with the HIV polymerase and gag precursor (53 to 55 kd and 65 kd). Detailed recommendations for interpretation of Western blot assays and management of those patients with an indeterminate Western blot have been prepared by the CDC.[42–47]

The core antigen (p24) capture assay has not been verified to be useful for diagnosis of HIV infection in the absence of detectable antibody. This assay is not likely to be broadly useful for screening blood donors or high-risk persons, since the period of antigenemia after primary infection is relatively short, and the rate of antigen detection is relatively low even among persons who later undergo antibody seroconversion. Recently, several studies have used other methods to detect HIV. These include culturing cell-free plasma for HIV and the polymerase chain reaction (PCR).[48–50] The former is a relatively simple technique in which plasma is serially diluted and then inoculated into cultures of stimulated peripheral blood mononuclear cells from healthy HIV-negative donors. The highest dilution that yields detectable virus in these cultures is taken as the titer of plasma viremia. Most HIV-infected persons have detectable plasma virus using this assay, and the titer of plasma virus increases as the clinical stage of HIV disease progresses.[48,49] This method is not practical for general screening but may prove useful in clinical studies of antiviral drugs, since preliminary data indicate that the titer of plasma viremia declines with effective anti-HIV therapy.

The PCR technique involves amplification of DNA or RNA sequences and detection using specific oligonucleotide primers derived from conserved sequences of the HIV genes. The PCR technique is particularly powerful, since it is capable of detecting sequences of DNA or RNA present at very low levels. Methods using PCR to quantitate the amount of circulating viral RNA have recently been developed and are being used to assess the effect of antiviral therapies.[51,52] The use of this technique in HIV diagnosis is still experimental. The major concern with the PCR method is false-positive results. Even minor contamination can lead to significant amplification and an apparent positive reaction. Nonetheless, application of PCR analysis to high-risk persons who were serologically negative for HIV antibody has revealed some to have detectable viral DNA months to years before results for Western blot or ELISA are positive.[53–55] The incidence of this phenomenon is not known, nor is it clear what potential for transmitting virus these persons represent.

A false-negative antibody screen may also occur during the "window period" after HIV infection before an antibody response is detectable. Among the general population recruited as blood donors who were initially self-screened about risk behavior for HIV on a questionnaire, a low incidence of HIV infection was found.[56,57] With improved blood donor education and antibody screening, the occurrence of HIV transmission by blood transfusion declined 30% per year between 1985 and 1987 and is currently estimated to occur in no more than 1 in 36,000 to 153,000 units transfused.[57–60] The sensitivity of PCR analysis could be used to reduce this risk even lower; nevertheless, many logistic hurdles, particularly the issue of false-positives, need to be overcome before this method can be practically applied. The false-positive rate using sequential ELISA and Western blot testing among self-screened blood donors is extremely low, estimated to be 0% to 0.0006%.[61] The recommended screening protocols for blood donors have been detailed by the CDC.[62] One caveat in screening procedures is that HIV-2 is poorly detected by the current ELISA and Western blot methods of testing blood products. This virus has been extremely rare in the United States, but given the potential for spread by transfusion, tests specifically designed to detect anti–HIV-2 antibody are likely to be added to the panel of screening procedures.

PATHOGENESIS

The in vivo targets of HIV infection include the CD4 bearing lymphocyte and the macrophage–monocyte. Although other cells appear susceptible to infection with HIV in vitro, including neuronal cells, fibroblasts, and astrocytes, no direct evidence of in vivo infection of these cell types exists. The CD4 structure on the surface of lymphocytes and monocytes acts as the major viral receptor for both HIV-1 and HIV-2. Recent work has helped to map the specific domains of surface CD4 that interact with the HIV envelope.[63–65] This has been accomplished both by monoclonal antibody analysis of inhibition of gp120 binding to CD4[66] and by deletion and point mutagenesis of the CD4 and gp120 molecules. The affinity of HIV-1 gp120 and CD4 is high, with an affinity constant on the order of 10^{-9} mol.[67]

In vitro, cells that do not bear the CD4 structure may be susceptible to infection.[68–70] Productive infection is not blocked by monoclonal antibodies to the CD4 protein or by soluble recombinant CD4 that binds to the HIV envelope and blocks interaction with the natural receptor. The process of entry of virus into CD4− cells is not known. A second surface structure is probably important in viral entry.

Different isolates of HIV have a differential capacity to infect target lymphocytes versus monocytes. Such strains are termed *tropic* for T lymphocytes or for macrophage–monocytes. Despite the marked differences in ability to infect these cells, the HIV isolates apparently bind with equal efficiency to the surface CD4 structure of both cell types. The major determinant of tropism appears to reside early in the virus life cycle after CD4 binding. Single mutations in the HIV envelope can alter the tropism of the particular isolate, rendering it incapable of productive infection, despite binding to CD4.[71,72] Tropism appears to be important with respect to the pathophysiology of certain HIV-related conditions.[73] Viral isolates that preferentially infect target macrophage–monocytes are often derived from patients with central nervous system (CNS) manifestations of HIV.[74,75] These observations are preliminary and require more detailed investigation. Nonetheless, differences in viral tropism and differences with respect to infection of cell populations may prove to be important in the pathophysiology of certain HIV-related disorders.

The major manifestations of immunodeficiency associated with HIV infection are related to impaired T-cell function. The CD4+ lymphocyte population is clearly susceptible to HIV infection, but controversy exists about the pathophysiology of T-cell dysfunction after HIV infection.[76–78] The crux of the controversy involves direct versus indirect effects of the retrovirus. If only a small proportion of circulating helper–inducer CD4+ lymphocytes carries HIV, what causes the dramatic loss of T-cell number as well as T-cell dysfunction? If a significant proportion of circulating T cells is infected or if substantial quantities of free virus are able to infect uninfected cells, the progressive loss of the helper–inducer T-lymphocyte population and the subsequent dysfunction of cells may be explicable by direct infection. Recent studies indicate that a higher proportion of circulating cells is infected than previously thought,[49,79–80b] that virus is circulating free in plasma,[81] and that active viral production is ongoing in lymphoid organs throughout the stages of HIV disease.[78,82,82a]

Direct HIV-1–mediated effects hypothesized to lead to immunologic deterioration include CD4-gp120–mediated fusion events resulting in single-cell lysis or syncytia formation.[83] The role of this form of cytopathology has recently been supported by documentation of clinical decline associated with an in vitro syncytia-forming phenotype of HIV-1.[84]

Many models of the indirect effects of HIV-1 on immune function have been proposed. For example, free envelope protein gp120 may interact with the CD4 structure on uninfected cells, leading to impaired lymphocyte function resulting from blockade of this surface molecule.[85–87] The blockade of CD4 may disable even uninfected cells, causing a type of anergy.[88] Alternatively, interactions of HIV-1 with T cells may induce a hyperstimulatory effect[89] through binding to a shared portion of the T-cell receptor β chain inducing a superantigen-like overdrive and subsequent depletion of cells. Recent data on selected depletion of β-chain subsets of T cells in AIDS support this possibility.[90] Either type of cell surface interaction may trigger a series of events within T cells resulting in cell death. This normal mechanism of eliminating cells, called *apoptosis* or *programmed cell death*, may be unusually active in the setting of HIV infection, resulting in the depletion of even uninfected T cells.[91,92]

Other indirect mechanisms of cell destruction may be through the binding of gp120 on cell surface acting as a target for immune attack.[93] T cells may thereby become "innocent bystanders" and may be destroyed either by cytotoxic T cells that recognize the HIV gp120 on the cell surface or by antibodies to HIV that complex with the envelope protein, leading to phagocytosis or lysis of the coated uninfected cell.[93,94]

The clinical outcome of cellular immune deficiency with helper–inducer T-cell depletion are opportunistic infections and neoplasms. The infectious agents include protozoa, mycobacteria, herpesviruses, and fungi. The neoplasms that arise as a result of the cellular immune deficiency include Kaposi's sarcoma, aggressive B-cell lymphoma, and squamous cell neoplasia. The interval between HIV infection and the development of these complications is variable; the median time between seroconversion and AIDS has been estimated to be between 5 and 10 years.[97,98] The pathophysiologic basis for development of certain opportunistic infections and neoplasms, and not others, in the context of HIV infection is not understood. For example, fungal infections such as oral and esophageal candidiasis are common in immunodeficient patients with HIV, whereas disseminated candidiasis or other fungal disorders such as aspergillosis are rare. What prevents *Candida albicans* from disseminating from mucosal surfaces into the blood stream in patients with AIDS is not known. (The major clinical manifestations of AIDS and AIDS-related complex [ARC] are summarized in the following section.)

In addition to T-cell depletion, another manifestation of AIDS is T-cell dysfunction. This dysfunction is generally manifested as impaired ability to respond to soluble antigen.[85,86,99] Interference with the CD4 structure due to anti-gp120 antibody complexed with antigen may impair cell-signaling processes that are required for an appropriate antigen response. The failure of T lymphocytes to respond to antigen by proliferation and production of regulatory cytokines may be important in the impairment of host defense. In addition to defects in T-cell function, abnormalities have been described in macrophage–monocytes. The basis of these monocyte defects is less clear but may result from direct HIV infection of these cells.[100–102] The defects mainly involve macrophage–monocyte chemotaxis or killing of obligate intracellular parasites.[103,104]

Following HIV infection, a derangement of the humoral immune system occurs. Many patients manifest clonal hypergammaglobulinemia. This could result from reactivation of latent Epstein-Barr virus (EBV), a common infection in HIV risk groups, or direct mitogenic effects of HIV on B cells. Note that patients with HIV infection often fail to mount an appropriate antibody response to neoantigens, such as pneumococcal polysaccharide. Vaccination is thus only variably effective in eliciting a protective humoral response.[105] Moreover, a subset of persons with HIV infection develop recurrent infections with encapsulated bacteria such as *Haemophilus influenzae* and *Staphylococcus pneumoniae*. These persons appear to have major problems in mobilizing a sufficient humoral response to protect against these pathogens.

Some signs and symptoms of HIV infection cannot be directly ascribed to an opportunistic infection or neoplasm. Foremost among these are dementia, persistent fever, weight loss, and a wasting syndrome. Although the pathophysiology of the dementia appears to be related to HIV infection of the brain, the molecular consequences of that infection with respect to neurotransmitters or production of toxic factors that may cause demyelination or neuronal cell dysfunction have not been elucidated.[106,107] The wasting syndrome, fever, and anorexia associated with HIV may be due to production of certain cytokines such as TNF by HIV-infected macrophage–monocytes. Although some investigators have found that HIV infection or HIV envelope interaction with CD4 resulted in augmented production of TNF and other inflammatory cytokines such as interleukin-1 (IL-1) and interleukin-6 (IL-6), others have not confirmed these findings.[108–110] TNF is identical with cachectin and induces anorexia, fever, and wasting in experimental animals. Further work is required to better define the importance of cytokines in the manifestations of HIV disease.

CLINICAL FEATURES

Acquired immunodeficiency syndrome is defined on the basis of its clinical manifestations. AIDS represents a clinical state of severe immunodeficiency manifested as life-threatening opportunistic infections or neoplasms. The CDC definition for AIDS is provided in Table 25-2. Other clinical conditions may result from HIV immune deficiency but do not qualify as AIDS according to the current definition. These include lymphadenopathy, neurologic dysfunction, and opportunistic infections that are not life-threatening such as oral candidiasis, and herpes zoster. Although several staging systems are used by different groups to classify HIV disease, most investigators use the CDC classification (Table 25-3). Symptomatic HIV-infected persons who have suffered weight loss, significant fatigue, unexplained fever, or low-grade opportunistic infections such as oral candidiasis or herpes zoster are grouped under the rubric of ARC. ARC generally precedes AIDS, although some persons may present with Kaposi's sarcoma or B-cell lymphoma without a prodrome or ARC. The earlier stages of HIV disease include asymptomatic persons who may or may not have generalized lymphadenopathy. Some inves-

TABLE 25-2. The Full Definition of AIDS

A case of AIDS is defined as an illness characterized by one or more of the following "indicator" diseases, depending on the status of laboratory evidence for HIV infection:

1. WITHOUT LABORATORY EVIDENCE OF HIV INFECTION

If laboratory tests for HIV were not performed or gave indeterminate results, any of the conditions in the following list indicates AIDS if diagnosed by a *definitive* method and if the patient had none of the other causes of immunodeficiency listed below that could explain the occurrence of the indicator disease.

- *Pneumocystis carinii* pneumonia
- Toxoplasmosis of the brain in a patient more than 1 year of age
- Cryptosporidiosis with diarrhea present from more than 1 month
- Candidiasis of the esophagus, trachea, bronchi, or lungs
- Extrapulmonary cryptococcosis
- *Mycobacterium avium* complex or *Mycobacterium kansasii* disease at a site other than the lungs or lymph nodes
- Cytomegalovirus infection of an internal organ other than the liver in a patient more than 1 month old
- Herpes simplex infection causing a mucocutaneous ulcer that persists for more than 1 month, or bronchitis, pneumonitis, or esophagitis for any duration in a patient more than 1 month old
- Progressive multifocal leukoencephalopathy
- Primary lymphoma of the brain in a patient less than 60 years old
- Kaposi's sarcoma in a patient less than 60 years old
- Pulmonary lymphoid hyperplasia or lymphoid interstitial pneumonia (PLH/LIP complex) in a child less than 13 years old

Causes of Immunodeficiency That Disqualify Diseases as Indicators of AIDS in the Absence of Antibody Evidence for HIV Infection

- High-dose or long-term systemic corticosteroid therapy or other immunosuppressive/cytotoxic therapy within 3 months before onset of the indicator disease
- Hodgkin's disease, non-Hodgkin's lymphoma (other than primary brain lymphoma), lymphocytic leukemia, multiple myeloma, or another cancer of lymphoreticular or histiocytic tissue, or angioimmunoblastic lymphadenopathy, diagnosed before or within 3 months after diagnosis of the indicator disease
- A genetic (congenital) immunodeficiency syndrome or an acquired immunodeficiency syndrome atypical of HIV infection, such as one involving hypogammaglobulinemia

2. WITH LABORATORY EVIDENCE OF HIV INFECTION

In the presence of antibody evidence for HIV infection, any of the conditions listed above or below indicates AIDS regardless of the presence of other causes of immunodeficiency.

Diseases Diagnosed Definitively

- Isosporiasis with diarrhea persisting for more than 1 month
- Extrapulmonary or disseminated histoplasmosis
- Extrapulmonary or disseminated coccidioidomycosis
- Extrapulmonary or disseminated tuberculosis
- Any noncutaneous extrapulmonary or disseminated mycobacterial infection other than tuberculosis or leprosy
- Recurrent nontyphoid *Salmonella* septicemia
- Multiple or recurrent bacterial infections (any combination of more than 2 within a 2-year period) of the following types in a child less than 13 years old:
  - Septicemia, pneumonia, meningitis, bone or joint infection, or abscess of an internal organ or body cavity (excluding otitis media or superficial skin or mucosal abscesses), caused by *Haemophilus, Streptococcus* (including pneumococcus), or other pyogenic bacteria
- Kaposi's sarcoma at any age
- Primary lymphoma of the brain at any age
- Other non-Hodgkin's lymphoma of B-cell immunologic phenotype*:
  - Small noncleaved lymphoma (Burkitt's tumor or Burkitt-like lymphoma)
  - Immunoblastic sarcoma (large-cell lymphoma, diffuse histiocytic lymphoma, diffuse undifferentiated lymphoma, reticulum cell sarcoma, or high-grade lymphoma)
- HIV encephalopathy (AIDS demential complex)†
- HIV wasting syndrome‡

Diseases Diagnosed Presumptively

- *Pneumocystis carinii* pneumonia
- Toxoplasmosis of the brain in a patient more than 1 month old
- Esophageal candidiasis
- Extrapulmonary or disseminated mycobacterial infection (acid-fast bacilli of undetermined species)
- Kaposi's sarcoma
- PLH/LIP complex in a child less than 13 years old

3. WITH EVIDENCE AGAINST HIV INFECTION

With laboratory test results negative for HIV infection, AIDS is ruled out for surveillance purposes unless the patient has had either of the following:

- *Pneumocystis carinii* pneumonia diagnosed by a definitive method
- Any of the other diseases indicative of AIDS listed in section 1 diagnosed by a definitive method and a helper T (T4) lymphocyte count below 400/μL

In addition, the patient must not have any of the other causes of immunodeficiency listed in section 1.

* Lymphomas are not included if they are of T-cell immunologic phenotype or are described as lymphocytic, lymphoblastic, small cleaved, or plasmacytoid lymphocytic.

† Clinical findings of disabling cognitive or motor dysfunction that interferes with occupation or the activities of daily living, or loss of behavioral developmental milestones in a child, progressing over weeks to months, in the absence of a concurrent illness or condition other than HIV infection that could explain the findings. Methods to rule out such concurrent illnesses and conditions must include cerebrospinal fluid examination and other brain imaging (computed tomography or magnetic resonance) or autopsy.

‡ Findings of profound involuntary weight loss (more than 10% of baseline body weight) plus other chronic diarrhea (lasting more than 1 month) or documented chronic fever and weakness (lasting more than 1 month) in the absence of a concurrent illness or condition other than HIV infection that could explain the findings (eg, cancer, tuberculosis, cryptosporidiosis, or other specific enteritis).

(MMWR 1987;36[Suppl 15]:100–101)

TABLE 25-3. 1993 Revised Classification System for HIV Infection and Expanded AIDS Surveillance Case Definition for Adolescents and Adults

	Clinical Categories*		
CD4+ T-Cell Count	**A: Asymptomatic, Acute (Primary) HIV or PGL†**	**B: Symptomatic, Not Category A or C Conditions‡**	**C: AIDS-Indicator Conditions§**
≥500 μL	A1	B1	C1
200–499/μL	A2	B2	C2
<200/μL AIDS indicator T-cell count	A3	B3	C3

PGL, persistent generalized lymphadenopathy.
* The shaded cells illustrate the expanded AIDS surveillance case definition. Persons with AIDS-indicator conditions (category C) as well as those with CD4+ T-lymphocyte counts below 200 μ/L (categories A3 or B3) are reportable as AIDS cases in the United States and Territories, effective January 1, 1993.
† Clinical category A includes acute (primary) HIV infection.
‡ See text for discussion.
§ See Table 25-1.

tigators designate a subgroup that is asymptomatic with generalized lymphadenopathy and apply the term *persistent generalized lymphadenopathy*. Others have not found particular prognostic significance to the lymphadenopathy and therefore group patients into those with and those without enlarged lymph nodes.

A general correlation exists between the decrease in CD4 lymphocyte number and the clinical manifestations of HIV disease.[111-113] Most patients with symptoms have less than 200 to 300 helper–inducer CD4+ lymphocytes per microliter, whereas those who are asymptomatic or have persistent generalized lymphadenopathy generally have more than 400 CD4+ lymphocytes per microliter. The general relation of CD4 counts, plasma virus titers, and disease manifestations to time after infection are shown in Figure 25-2.

EPIDEMIOLOGY OF HUMAN IMMUNODEFICIENCY VIRUS INFECTION

Human immunodeficiency virus is transmitted by sexual contact, by contaminated blood during transfusion or sharing of intravenous drug apparatus, and by mother to fetus during the birth process. It is not transmitted by aerosol or casual contact such as shaking hands. The virus has been identified in blood, semen, cervical secretions, saliva, and feces. It is not clear whether certain strains of the virus may be particularly transmissible through specific routes, particularly sexual. It is clear that transmission of HIV by blood product transfusion is extremely efficient and that nearly 100% of recipients of HIV-contaminated blood become infected.[114] Sexual contact, specifically vaginal and anal intercourse, are also relatively efficient at transmitting the virus, with estimates of 25% to 75% infection of regular sexual partners who have repeated exposure with intercourse. Orogenital sexual contact can transmit the virus but apparently less efficiently. No cases are documented of transmission by kissing, probably because of the extremely low titer of virus in saliva and the presence of putative blocking factors or proteases that can inactivate virus.

The major populations infected with HIV in the United States and western Europe are homosexual and bisexual men,[1] intravenous drug abusers,[115] recipients of blood products,[114] particularly hemophiliacs,[116] female prostitutes (many of whom also use intravenous drugs), and infants born to HIV-infected mothers.[117,118] The rate of transmission from mother to child is 7% to 39%.[119-123] Spread of HIV among the general population by heterosexual intercourse has been limited, but the exact dimensions of this spread are not well defined because of the absence of widespread testing for HIV.[124] In certain communities, particularly

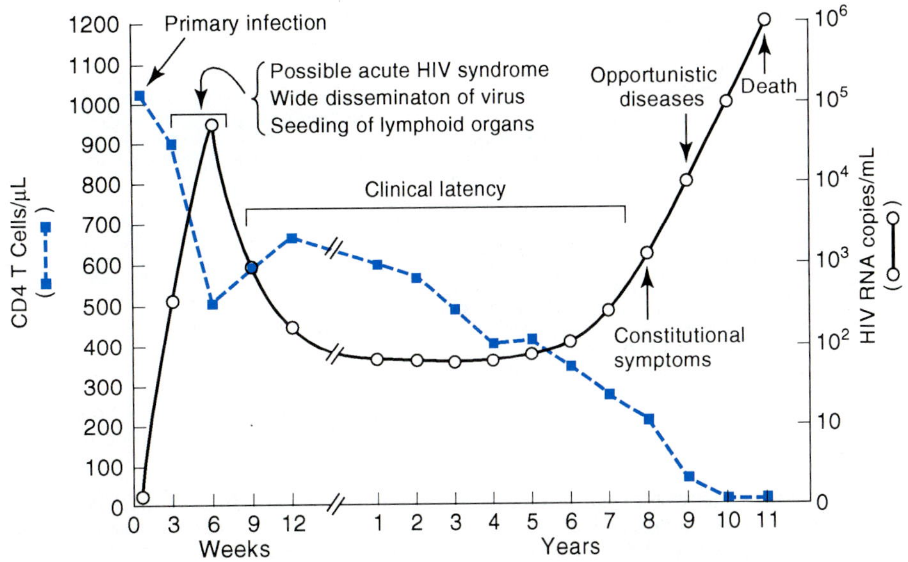

FIGURE 25-2. After primary infection, there is widespread dissemination of virus and a sharp decrease in the number of CD4 T cells in peripheral blood. An immune response to HIV ensues, with a decrease in detectable viremia followed by a prolonged period of clinical latency. The CD4 T-cell count continues to decrease during the following years, until it reaches a critical level below which there is a substantial risk of opportunistic diseases. (Pantaleo G, Graziosi C, Fauci AS. Mechanisms of disease: the immunopathogenesis of human immunodeficiency virus infection. N Engl J Med 1993;328:329).

lower socioeconomic groups in cities on the east coast of the United States, a relatively high incidence of infection is found among young women who do not use intravenous drugs; this is caused by sexual intercourse with men who have used or currently use drugs.

Central Africa is suffering an AIDS epidemic of major proportions among the general heterosexual population. Estimates of HIV infection of 3% to 5% of the adult male and female population in countries like Zaire, Uganda, and Rawanda are relatively conservative.[3,5,125] The World Health Organization estimates that 6 million people are infected in Sub-Saharan Africa (Fig. 25-3). The major route of transmission in Africa appears to be heterosexual intercourse, although contaminated blood products and contaminated needles used in hospitals and clinics may also transmit the virus. The transmission from woman to man also appears to be much higher in Central Africa than in Europe and the United States. This may be related to the high incidence of genital ulceration among men and women in developing countries of Africa.[126] Such ulcers may impair the mucosal barrier and allow for more ready transmission of HIV from vaginal fluids to the male urethra during intercourse.

Detailed studies have been conducted among health care personnel with respect to occupational risks for HIV.[127,128] The health care workers who have become infected with the retrovirus have generally contracted the infection after traumatic puncture wounds. Current estimates of the risk of transmission through a needlestick injury from an HIV-1 infected person are about 1 in 300.

The precautions recommended by the CDC for health care workers include wearing latex gloves for performing a procedure that might lead to exposure of body fluids, wearing masks and goggles when exposed to effluent such as during a colonoscopy, and inactivation of potentially contaminated instruments by sterilization. The virus is inactivated by detergents, bleach, and alcohols such as isopropyl. Surfaces that may be exposed to contaminated fluids can be effectively sterilized using these materials. A detailed discussion of the rationale for specific precautions and recommendations for counseling exposed health care workers is provided by the CDC.[129,130] The use of postexposure zidovudine (azidothymidine [AZT]) is controversial and requires an assessment of the infectious potential of the material (fresh blood versus other body fluids) and the severity of the exposure (exposed skin versus injection by needle stick). Particular caution must be used when considering treatment of women of childbearing age for whom AZT may pose a greater risk.[131]

TREATMENT

Vaccine Development

The immunologic basis of protection against challenge with the HIV pathogen is not fully understood. Both cellular and humoral immune responses are believed to be important, with development of cytotoxic T cells and neutralizing antibodies, respectively.[132] Studies of HIV-infected persons show significant levels of cytotoxic T cells in the circulation but a modest humoral response in terms of neutralizing antibody titer.[133,134] Furthermore, in vitro and in vivo studies have demonstrated the capacity of HIV to mutate to escape neutralization by antibodies. This is not surprising,

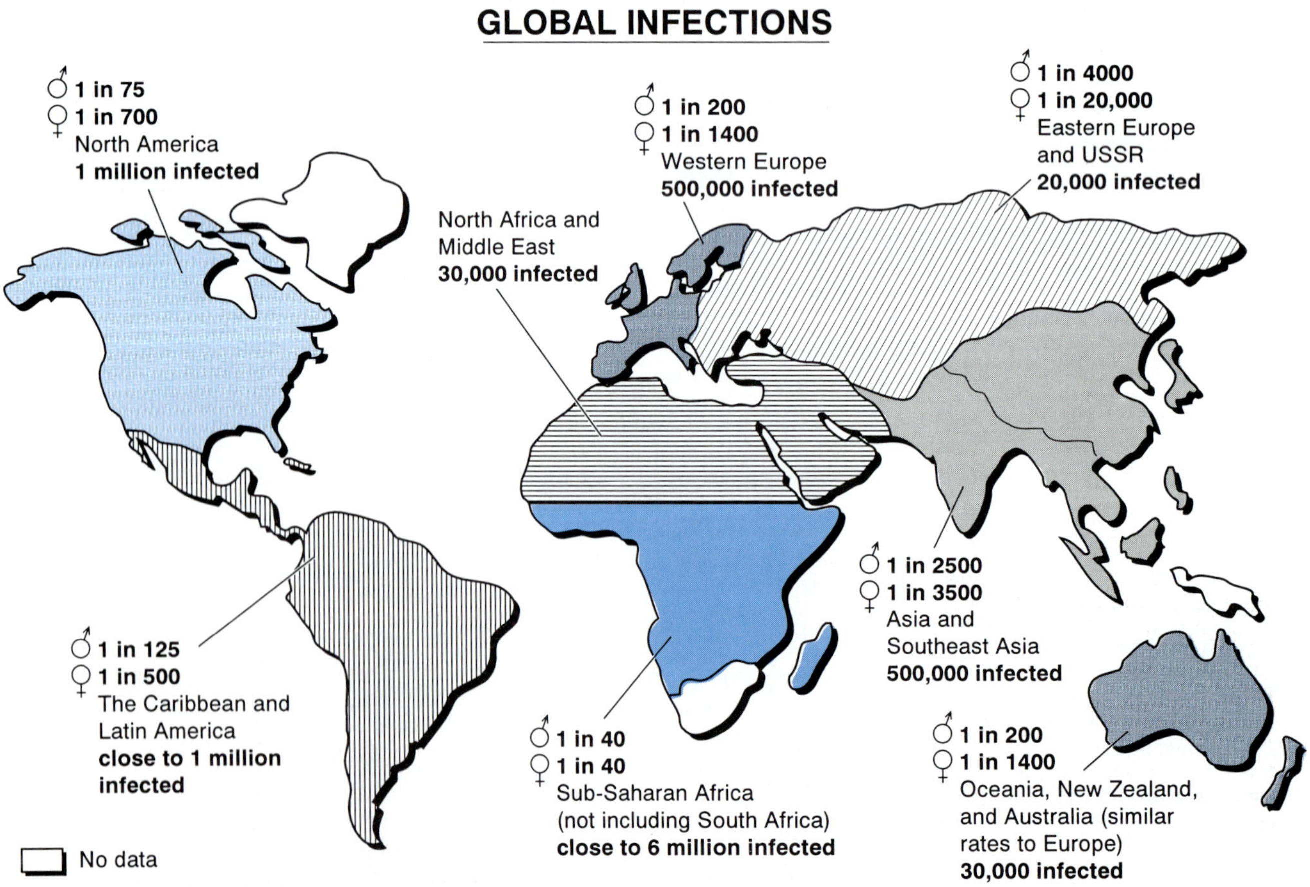

FIGURE 25-3. Although sub-Saharan Africa still has the most infections, other regions appear to be catching up. Incidence is by sex for adults aged 15 to 49. (Palca J. The sobering geography of AIDS. Science 1993;252:372)

since the primary neutralization response is directed against the exterior envelope glycoprotein, which has a considerable degree of variability.[135] Although the predominant epitope recognized by neutralizing antibodies appears to be a loop structure in the viral envelope, studies with neutralizing monoclonal antibodies directed against this relatively conserved immunodominant loop have revealed that mutations in epitopes outside the loop can readily lead to escape from neutralization, presumably because of secondary changes in the loop structure after adjacent mutations.[72,136] Thus, considerable pessimism persists over whether an effective vaccine can be developed that will protect against the potentially infinite number of HIV strains that might arise.

Despite the pessimism, recent studies using SIV in rhesus macaques may provide models for ultimate development of HIV vaccines. In these SIV models, it has been demonstrated that whole inactivated virus or fixed inactivated cells were capable of protecting some monkeys against challenge with the strain of SIV that was used to prepare the vaccine.[137,138] In addition, live, attenuated SIV has protected Rhesus monkeys against intravenous inoculation with live, pathogenic SIV.[139] Importantly, mucosal and systemic immunity has also been reported in vaccinated macaques.[140] Vaccination of chimpanzees, the only primate species other than humans that is susceptible to HIV-1, with recombinant HIV-1 envelope gp120 was capable of protecting the animals from infection after challenge.[141] In another study, chimpanzees that received a mixture of HIV-1 antigens appeared to be protected for as long as 1 year after vaccination.[142] A number of phase I and II vaccination studies of human HIV-seronegative volunteers using HIV envelope glycoproteins are underway, but preliminary results indicate that the prototype vaccine antigens are weak in eliciting a high titer neutralizing antibody response in humans.[143] Whether vaccine preparations may be useful in boosting beneficial immune responses in already infected persons is not clear. It does appear that cytotoxic T-cell responses to HIV can be generated by vaccination, but concern remains about virus escape from the specific targets recognized by the T cell.[144]

Antiviral Therapy

The established drug treatments of HIV infection are the nucleoside derivatives AZT, didioxyinosine (ddI), and dideoxycytidine (ddC). The AZT nucleoside has an azide moiety that leads to chain termination when AZT is incorporated into DNA during the process of viral reverse transcription.[145] This phenomenon is clearly seen in vitro, and inhibition of the viral reverse transcriptase by AZT is believed to be the major mechanism of action of the drug. AZT has been shown to be effective in symptomatic persons with either AIDS or ARC.[146–150] The major effects of drug treatment are reduction in the rate of decline of immunologic function measured by CD4 cell numbers, reduction in the incidence of opportunistic infections, improvement in CNS function in patients who have HIV-related dementia, and improvement in survival. Whether asymptomatic persons with less than 500 circulating CD4+ lymphocytes benefit from AZT therapy is controversial.[151–163b]

AZT inhibits not only the formation of viral DNA from the RNA template during reverse transcription but also the mammalian DNA polymerase during the process of cell division. The major toxicity of the drug is thus seen in the hematopoietic system that has a relatively rapid turnover of cells. Significant anemia and leukopenia are the major dose-limiting toxicities of AZT for a large number of patients.[164,165] Another toxicity that is not understood is that of AZT-induced myopathy.[166,167] Although the hematologic toxicity is usually seen within the first 6 months of treatment with the agent, the myopathy generally occurs after prolonged treatment for 12 months or more.

The recommendations for use of AZT in HIV-infected adults are limited to those with symptoms or those asymptomatic adults in whom the CD4 cell count has fallen to below 500/μL. The dose recommended for symptomatic adults is AZT, 200 mg orally every 4 hours for 1 month, then 100 mg every 4 hours. For asymptomatic persons, the dose is 100 mg every 4 hours during waking hours. The recommendations as to whom should be treated with AZT and at what dose have only recently evolved and will undergo revision as more information becomes available. In particular, the use of AZT in asymptomatic patients is highly controversial because of a European study, the Concorde trial, that showed no sustained benefit of AZT therapy.[153]

The nucleoside derivative ddI has been approved for the treatment of patients with HIV infection who either are intolerant of AZT or have experienced significant immunologic deterioration while receiving AZT.[168,169] Zalcitabine, or ddC, is approved both in combination with AZT for patients who experience immunologic decline while on AZT therapy alone[170,171] and as a single agent for indications similar to those for ddI.[171a] Multiple ongoing studies of monotherapy and 2- and 3-day combinations are in progress and will probably result in revised recommendations for the use of these agents. ddI and ddC work in the same way as AZT with respect to inhibition of the reverse transcriptase.[145] The toxicities of ddI and ddC are different from those of AZT. Hematologic toxicity appears not to occur with ddI or ddC, but pancreatitis (particularly with ddI) and neuropathy are more prominent complications. ddI also often induces gastrointestinal (GI) distress, and ddC may cause mucosal ulcerations. Effective therapy of HIV infection is likely to require several different nucleoside derivatives, since virus becomes resistant after 6 to 12 months of antiviral nucleoside therapy in many patients.[172–174] Isolates of HIV that appear resistant to AZT have remained sensitive to inhibition by ddI. As in other situations with antiinfective therapy, use of combinations of different antiviral nucleosides are possible to present significant obstacles to the virus with regard to mutation in the polymerase gene and subsequent emergence of resistance.

Based on the life cycle of the virus, numerous points of intervention could lead to the development of effective drugs (Fig. 25-4). These include inhibition of *tat* function with specific antagonists, disruption of HIV RNA transport and processing through interference with *rev* function,[175] the use of mutant *gag* molecules that impair proper virus assembly,[176] and inhibition of the protease, which would prevent the *gag* precursor from being appropriately processed and lead to aborted infection.[177–179] Recent crystallization of the protease has launched a major effort to identify drugs capable of specifically inhibiting this enzyme.[180,181]

Another strategy is that of blocking binding of HIV to the surface CD4 structure. Several groups have developed soluble recombinant forms of CD4 that are capable of protecting T cells and macrophage–monocytes from in vitro infection with HIV.[63,182] Clinical studies were disappointing, however.[183,184]

A chimeric molecule consisting of the heavy chain of immunoglobulin G (IgG) subclass 1 fused to CD4, termed an *immunoadhesin*, has also undergone clinical study.[185] The appeal of this hybrid molecule is its pharmacokinetics, which resemble those of antibody, so that significant plasma levels can be achieved with intermittent administration. The immunoadhesin also is capable of crossing the placenta

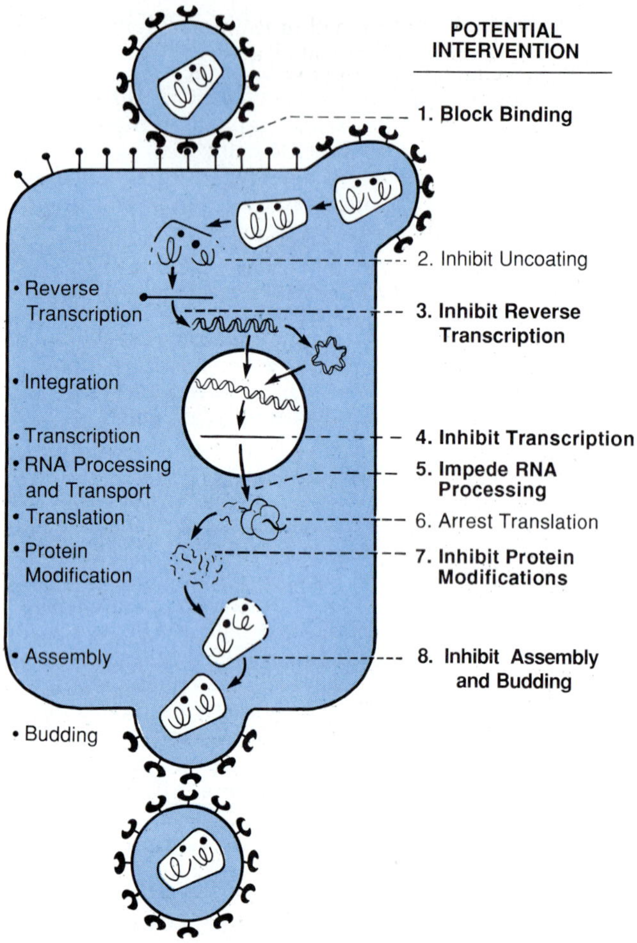

FIGURE 25-4. HIV life cycle and potential sites of intervention. (*Left*) The major steps in the virus life cycle. (*Right*) Sites of possible therapeutic intervention. Interventions tested or currently in clinical trial are in bold: soluble CD4 for blocking of virus binding to receptor, nucleoside analogues (ZDV, ddI, ddC), nonnucleoside inhibitors of reverse transcription, *tat* inhibitors, anti-*rev* oligonucleotides, proteinase inhibitors, interferon-α inhibiting virus assembly and budding.

and might afford some degree of protection to a developing fetus from HIV infection transmitted from the mother. These hybrid molecules also are capable of mediating antibody-dependent cellular cytotoxicity, with in vitro lysis of HIV-infected target cells.[186] The in vivo significance of antibody-dependent cellular cytotoxicity is not known but is believed by some to be an important link between humoral and cellular immune defense. Hybrid molecules that combine the HIV binding site of CD4 and a cytotoxic element such as the ricin A chain or *Pseudomonas* exotoxin have also been designed.[187,188] These molecules are capable of selectively killing HIV-infected cells and can theoretically act to eliminate the cellular sources of the virus.

Other sites of potential interference with the virus life cycle are altered posttranslational modification and therefore function of viral proteins,[189] interference through a new class of TIBO compounds, and nonnucleoside reverse transcriptase inhibitor action.[190] Compound Q has been reported to preferentially inhibit virus production in macrophage–monocytes and is in the process of clinical evaluation.[191] The interferons are capable of inhibiting HIV infection of target T cells and macrophage–monocytes, possibly interfering with the process of viral assembly.[192] Recombinant interferon-α has been developed for the therapy of Kaposi's sarcoma (see section about Kaposi's sarcoma) but also may have direct anti-HIV effects.[193] Recent experimental clinical trials have used low doses of AZT with recombinant interferon-α, since there is synergy in vitro with this particular combination. An antiviral effect in vivo appears promising from results of this study.[194]

Effective therapy of HIV disease is likely to require multiple drugs used in combination, particularly those that interfere with different steps in the life cycle of virus and make viral resistance more difficult to achieve. Similar to combination chemotherapy regimens that have been successfully developed for diseases like Hodgkin's disease or testicular cancer, anti-HIV therapy will probably include drugs not only with different mechanisms of action but also with different levels of toxicity. Furthermore, the complex opportunistic infections and neoplasms that AIDS patients suffer require therapy as well. Drug regimens for HIV must be integrated into the general treatment program. Prophylaxis against *P carinii* pneumonia with aerosolized pentamidine or oral trimethoprim–sulfamethoxazole (the more effective prophylactic therapy) has shown benefit for many patients with CD4 counts below 200 cells/μL. Rifabutin decreases the incidence of *Mycobacterium avium-intracellulare* infection, and trimethoprim–sulfamethoxazole decreases the incidence of toxoplasmosis. The optimal integration of such prophylactic or active treatment regimens into the broad context of anti-HIV therapy is still being evaluated. Many of these treatments are likely to be significantly toxic to the bone marrow, resulting in dose-limiting cytopenias. For that reason, interest has been directed toward the use of hematopoietic growth factors in conjunction with antiviral, antiinfective, and antineoplastic therapy in AIDS and ARC. This is discussed in greater detail later in this chapter.

HEMATOLOGIC ASPECTS

General Features

One of the hallmarks of HIV infection is a gradual progressive decline in the number of CD4 lymphocytes. Decreases in other circulating cells also occur, with anemia reported in 60%, thrombocytopenia in 40%, and neutropenia in 50% of patients with AIDS.[195–198] Cytopenia tends to develop coincident with progressive deterioration of the immune system of these patients, occurring less frequently in earlier stages of HIV-related illness. Thrombocytopenia is the exception to this generalization, since it may be the presenting manifestation of HIV infection. Potential mechanisms for thrombocytopenia in this setting and its management are discussed in the next section.

The cytopenias seen in advanced HIV infection may be the result of multiple interacting factors.[199] In addition to possible direct and indirect roles for the virus, complicating opportunistic infections, neoplasms, and myelotoxic antiretroviral, antimicrobial, and antitumor therapies are frequently important. The differential diagnosis of low blood counts in HIV-infected patients is broad. The diagnostic approach to a patient with low blood counts who is known to be HIV-infected differs from that in uninfected persons primarily in its emphasis on a careful evaluation for infectious causes and attention to the possible myelotoxic effect of intercurrent therapy.

Standard laboratory approaches to cytopenias should be undertaken; blood cultures for fungi and mycobacteria and buffy coat cultures for CMV should be added to these. When proceeding with bone marrow sampling, cultures for fungi and mycobacteria and stains for their presence histologically are essential. *M avium-intracellulare, Mycobacterium tuberculosis, Cryptococcus neoformans, Histoplasma capsulatum, P carinii,* and *Ehrlichia* sp are associated with hematologic abnormalities and may be found on examination of the bone marrow.[200–204] Parvovirus infection is associated with giant pronormoblasts on histologic study and may cause profound anemia in patients with AIDS. CMV does not induce specific morphologic changes of the bone marrow but does alter hematopoiesis and may be cultured from the buffy coat. In addition, bone marrow involvement by non-Hodgkin's lymphoma (NHL) may be the presenting site for that diagnosis since marrow infiltration is common in HIV-infected patients with this neoplasm. Kaposi's sarcoma, the other major neoplastic complication of HIV infection, has only rarely been reported in the bone marrow.[205]

Guidelines for proceeding with bone marrow aspirate and biopsy in an HIV-infected patient with low blood counts have not been well defined but may include the following: (1) cytopenia out of proportion to the stage of HIV-related illness; (2) rapidly developing cytopenia (other than anemia due to blood loss); (3) severe systemic symptoms such as fever with an otherwise negative evaluation; and (4) use of aspirate and biopsy as a staging modality in patients with a known malignancy. Although the use of bone marrow evaluation appears to be only equally sensitive to routine blood culture for the diagnosis of mycobacterial or fungal disease, the rapidity with which a histologic diagnosis can be made is often advantageous in AIDS patients with systemic symptoms.[206]

Even in the absence of the identifiable pathogenetic processes already described, morphologic abnormalities are present in the bone marrow in most patients. However, there is no pathognomonic appearance to an HIV-positive bone marrow sample; the abnormalities are nonspecific. Cellularity tends to be increased or normal, with only 1 in 20 marrow specimens appearing hypocellular.[197,207–209] The myeoloid/erythroid ratio ranges from 2:1 to 5:1.[197,210] Abnormalities in cell maturation are common, with megaloblastic changes, ringed sideroblasts, and other dysplastic features identified.[211–214] All cell types may be affected and typically show high nuclear/cytoplasmic ratios and aberrant nuclear contours. Morphologic abnormalities tend to increase with advanced immunosuppression as patients with isolated thrombocytopenia occurring relatively early in HIV-1 disease often have increased megakaryocytes but otherwise unremarkable bone marrow histology. Increased plasma cells, lymphoid aggregates, increased eosinophils, and a focal or diffuse increase in reticulin are also frequently seen. There may be granuloma-like collections of cells and a general increase in marrow histiocytes. Large foamy histiocytes (pseudo-Gaucher cells) have been associated with infiltration of the marrow with *M avium-intracellulare*.[215] The presence of lymphoid aggregates is common (reported in up to 50% of patients) and is nonspecific.[197,207–210] The presence of paratrabecular lymphoid aggregates has been associated with lymphoma. Because the non-Hodgkin's lymphoma that occurs in AIDS is often extranodal and involves the bone marrow in about 25% of patients, this finding should raise the suspicion of a lymphomatous process.

The mechanisms for the morphologic abnormalities and the clinically apparent dysregulation of blood cell production are poorly understood. Laboratory investigations into the cause of abnormal hematopoiesis in these patients have yielded only suggestive, at times contradictory, results. Laboratory studies have focused on three main areas of potential abnormality: the blood cell progenitor, the stromal environment, and the immunologic background.

A number of studies have evaluated whether HIV-exposed bone marrow or blood cells form normal numbers of blood cell colonies when cultured under the appropriate laboratory conditions. The results have been variable, but most of the data suggest a modest decrease in the colony-forming capacity of blood cell progenitors of multiple lineages.[216–226] One study indicated a specific defect in the megakaryocytic colony (CFU-MEG)–forming cells among patients with thrombocytopenia.[227] In addition, data suggest that the CD34+ population of bone marrow progenitors may have an altered ability to survive in liquid culture after exposure to HIV.[221] The basis for disordered growth characteristics of progenitor cells has not been well defined and remains controversial. Several lines of evidence point away from direct infection of HIV as a major contributing factor.[220,224–226,228] If HIV infection of early progenitor cells occurs, it does so infrequently. This is in contrast to the ready infection of later, more differentiated cells of monocytic or megakaryocytic lineage.[229–232] Although infection of early progenitors by HIV is uncommon, it may be that other direct interactions of the virus with these cells induce alterations in their physiology. The possibility that virus perturbs the cellular differentiation program through interactions at the cell surface is an area of active research.[233]

The microenvironment of the bone marrow has several cellular constituents that are ready targets of HIV (lymphocytes and monocytes) and some that have been reported to be infectible under in vitro conditions (fibroblasts and endothelial cells).[233,234] Infection of these accessary cells of the bone marrow stroma may result in an altered mileau in which hematopoietic cells mature. Testing such a hypothesis has been done in two ways—long-term bone marrow culture techniques and measurement of cytokines released by individual accessory cell types. Some data suggest that infection of bone marrow stroma may alter the in vitro support of erythroid progenitors in long-term bone marrow culture.[235] Evidence for an altered production of cytokines in the presence of HIV or HIV products is more controversial. Ambiguity remains as to whether HIV directly induces cytokine alterations or whether they may be induced secondarily as the result of coincident effects on other aspects of immune function or intercurrent infections.[108–110,236,237] However, patients with HIV disease have abnormally elevated levels of certain cytokines, such as tumor necrosis factor-α, IL-6, transforming growth factor-β, and interferon-α.[238–241] It has also been observed that serum erythropoietin levels are abnormally depressed in patients with AIDS.[242,243] The clinical relevance of these changes in unknown, but dysregulation of cytokine production probably contributes to the altered hematopoiesis of HIV disease.

More difficult to evaluate is the role of immune phenomena on the bone marrow or mature blood cells in AIDS. It has been reported that the immunoglobulin fraction of the sera of AIDS patients or of an 84-kd glycoprotein derived from mononuclear cells of patients with AIDS are capable of inhibiting in vitro colony formation.[216,217] Also, T-cell depletion has been reported to enhance colony growth of AIDS patients' bone marrow.[219] Others have found that the changes in subsets of T cells are more closely linked to effects on colony formation and have proposed a causative role.[226] The complex interactions of T cells with other bone marrow elements are difficult to dissect experimentally. Until better methods of analysis are developed, understanding of the interplay between HIV, T cells, and hematopoiesis will remain frustratingly limited.

Thrombocytopenia

Thrombocytopenia may occur as either an isolated hematologic abnormality at any stage of HIV disease or with other cytopenias in patients with advanced immunodeficiency. In one study evaluating the epidemiology of thrombocytopenia in HIV-seropositive patients, the incidence of a platelet count below 150,000/μL was 11%, below 100,000/μL was 4.2%, and below 50,000/μL was 1.5%.[214]

All risk groups for HIV disease may develop thrombocytopenia, but the incidence may be slightly higher among whites and lower in patients whose risk factor for HIV infection was heterosexual contact.[214]

Because thrombocytopenia may be the clinical finding that first brings an HIV-infected person to medical attention, HIV infection should be considered in patients presenting with low platelet counts. Participation in high-risk behaviors should be specifically addressed when obtaining a history from a patient with unexplained thrombocytopenia. Those patients with isolated thrombocytopenia who are found to be HIV-seropositive and have no other HIV-related diseases apparently have the same risk over time for the development of AIDS as asymptomatic HIV-seropositive persons.[245] The presence of thrombocytopenia does not define advanced HIV disease by CDC criteria.

Thrombocytopenia in HIV infection may have multiple causes, including immune-mediated destruction, impaired hematopoiesis, or, rarely, syndromes resembling hemolytic uremic syndrome or thrombotic thrombocytopenic purpura.[246,247] Isolated thrombocytopenia is generally associated with a clinical picture resembling that of classic autoimmune thrombocytopenic purpura (AITP). Affected patients have a normal to increased number of megakaryocytes in the bone marrow and elevated levels of platelet-bound immunoglobulin. The platelet-bound protein has been identified in homosexual men as immune complexes.[248] The platelet adherent immune complexes have been shown to include anti-HIV antibodies and antibodies directed against them.[250–251b] Some cross-reactivity between anti-HIV antibodies and platelet antigen has been demonstrated.[251b,252] There appear to be shared epitopes between HIV gp120 and platelet GP and HIV p25 and platelets that may account for the specific antiplatelet antibodies documented in some patients.[251b,252] The presence of immune complexes bound to platelet surfaces is inconsistently associated with low platelet numbers in HIV-infected persons. One potential mechanism for patients with platelet-bound proteins being protected from thrombocytopenia is the abnormal reticuloendothelial cell function documented in HIV infection.[253–255] Some patients with cell-associated antibodies may maintain higher cell counts because of impairment of the Fc receptor–mediated clearance of these cells.

Thrombocytopenic, HIV-positive patients have been shown to have abnormalities in platelet production as well as decreased platelet survival times.[231] Megakaryocytes appear to be susceptible to HIV-1 infection, possibly resulting in diminished platelet formation.[232]

The complications from thrombocytopenia in HIV-infected patients are similar to those in uninfected persons with AITP. Fortunately, severe thrombocytopenia is uncommon in these patients. More problems may occur with HIV-infected hemophiliacs who develop complicating thrombocytopenia. The mechanism for thrombocytopenia in these patients appears to be similar to that seen in other subgroups of HIV-positive patients.[256] Complications from thrombocytopenia may be severe in this population; therefore, maintenance of a more conservative threshold for initiation of therapy is recommended.[257]

Therapeutically, an important distinction in approaching HIV thrombocytopenic patients as opposed to seronegative patients with AITP is the improvement in platelet numbers documented with AZT therapy.[150,164,258–261] About half of HIV-positive patients have been reported to increase their platelet counts (a three-fold mean increase) within 12 weeks of initiating AZT therapy.[261–262b] For HIV-positive patients who do not respond to AZT and who have symptomatic thrombocytopenia, the range of therapeutic modalities used in AITP such as corticosteroids,[263–265] splenectomy,[266–269] γ-globulin,[270–272] anti-RhD,[273,274] danazol,[275] and vincristine[276] have been shown to be of some usefulness. Recently, interferon-α[277,278] and dapsone[279] have been reported to increase platelet numbers in some patients. One caveat when treating this already immunocompromised population is the theoretical risk of long-term use of immunosuppressive therapies such as corticosteroids. Other than possible exacerbation of Kaposi's sarcoma,[280] adverse effects have not been seen with short-term use of immunomodulatory agents, but long-term consequences have not been defined. Further, when the use of an immunosuppressive agent or splenectomy is contemplated, excluding an infectious cause for the thrombocytopenia, such as mycobacteria, takes on even greater importance. Appropriate treatment of the infection may correct the thrombocytopenia, and immunosuppressive therapy and splenectomy are clearly undesirable in the setting of disseminated mycobacterial disease.

A number of cases of thrombotic thrombocytopenic purpura (TTP) and hemolytic uremic syndrome have been reported in patients with AIDS.[246,247] Whether there is an increased incidence of these events in AIDS patients has not been defined. When TTP occurs, it generally does so late in the course of HIV disease. Therapies used in TTP outside the setting of HIV infection have met with some clinical improvement in patients with AIDS, but the successes are generally short-lived and the overall outlook is poor.

Anemia

Anemia is the most common hematologic abnormality seen in HIV-infected patients. It occurs coincidently with the development of advanced stages of immunosuppression. Typically, the anemia is normochromic and normocytic anemia, with a depressed reticulocyte index and iron studies that are either normal or consistent with that of chronic disease. Antiglobulin tests have been reported to be positive in up to 85% of AIDS patients and 44% of asymptomatic homosexual men.[281,282] The antibodies are occasionally of anti-i or other specificity, but nonspecific binding of antiphospholipid antibodies or immune complexes to erythrocytes is more common. As with platelets, the presence of red blood cell (RBC)–associated antibody does not correlate well with anemia and hemolysis is rare.[283]

The predominant mechanism resulting in anemia in HIV disease is inadequate erythropoiesis. A range of potential factors contribute to this problem and should be considered in the differential diagnosis. In addition to the complex changes in the bone marrow discussed earlier, toxic, infectious, endocrine, or nutritional abnormalities may play contributing roles.

Many patients with HIV disease experience GI disorders that may affect the hematopoietic system. Chronic blood loss from Kaposi's sarcoma, lymphoma, or infections of the gut may result in depletion of iron stores. A range of infectious intestinal insults or HIV itself may alter nutrient absorption and result in other deficiencies, particularly in the context of poor food intake that often occurs in persons with AIDS. Measurements of iron, folate, and B_{12} are important to exclude these treatable causes of anemia.

A caveat to the interpretation of an abnormal serum B_{12} level in patients with AIDS has been raised by one report.[284] Rather than a physiologic deficiency of B_{12}, transcobalamin transport was shown to be affected and supplemental B_{12} did not improve the patients' anemia. Nevertheless, appropriate diagnostic measures should be undertaken to exclude a physiologically significant B_{12} deficiency.

Serum erythropoietin levels have been reported to be disproportionately low for the degree of anemia in AIDS patients compared with a control group.[285] These alterations have been noted despite the absence of evidence for renal dysfunction, and the cause is not clear. One in vitro model system for this phenomenon suggested that it may be due to a direct action of HIV on the posttranslational events important in erythropoietin production.[286] In addition, parvovirus infection has been documented as a cause of RBC aplasia in patients with AIDS and may be diagnosed by bone marrow examination or appropriate serologic tests. γ-Globulin has been reported to reverse this unusual cause of severe anemia.[287]

Drug-induced anemia is particularly common in HIV-infected patients. AZT, which remains the antiretroviral therapy in widest use, frequently causes anemia.[164,165] The degree to which AZT affects the bone marrow is clearly dose related and varies widely, with the most severely immunocompromised tolerating the drug least well. At currently recommended doses, AZT is associated with the development of anemia (hemoglobin levels below 8 g/dL) in 29% of AIDS patients (compared with 34% to 39% using the previously recommended AZT dose of 1200 to 1500 mg/d). The anemia associated with AZT is usually macrocytic, although some patients have normal mean corpuscular volumes. The normocytic anemia of AZT is often more severe and refractory to erythropoietin therapy. Rarely, AZT may induce a profound depression of erythropoietin resembling pure red cell aplasia.[288] Whereas anemia associated with AZT generally responds to the withdrawal of AZT, this latter group may have a persistent defect in RBC production.

The changes AZT induces in blood cell formation are probably due to its effects on DNA synthesis. AZT is a thymidine anologue that functions both to competitively inhibit thymidine kinase and to induce DNA chain termination when incorporated into nascent DNA. The kinetics of its incorporation into DNA by the viral reverse transcriptase are one or two orders of magnitude above its incorporation by cellular DNA polymerases.[289] However, inhibition of cellular proliferation occurs, and occurs preferentially in erythroid cells compared with granulocytic cells.[290,291] Anemia or other cytopenias do not appear to be toxicities common to all nucleoside analogues since ddC and ddI do not induce bone marrow depression.

Recombinant erythropoietin has been shown to decrease the transfusion requirement and increase hemoglobin and hematocrit in anemic AIDS patients even if their anemia was precipitated by AZT.[292,293] Thus, erythropoietin may be an alternative to AZT dose reduction in some patients and an important adjunctive measure in the case of HIV-infected patients requiring frequent RBC transfusion. The benefits of exogenous erythropoietin are apparently limited to those in whom the pretreatment serum erythropoietin level is below 500 mU/mL.[293]

Neutropenia

Neutropenia in association with decreases in other cell counts is seen with progressive deterioration of the immune system in HIV-infected patients. As with other cytopenias, neutropenia may be caused by a combination of decreased production and increased clearance of these cells. Antibody bound to granulocyte cell surfaces has been detected in about one third of HIV-infected persons.[282,294] The presence of neutrophil-associated antibodies in these studies again did not directly correlate with the presence of decreased neutrophil cell counts. The abnormalities in bone marrow function described earlier are likely to be major contributors to the neutropenia observed in HIV disease.

It is perhaps these underlying abnormalities in hematopoiesis that account for the particular sensitivity to the myelotoxic effects of drug therapies observed in patients with AIDS. Neutropenia accompanies the use of many common therapies in AIDS and often limits their use. Although ddI and ddC are not implicated in myelosuppresssion, AZT is at times dose limited by neutropenia or anemia.[164,165] In addition, therapy with trimethoprim-sulfamethoxazole for *P carinii* pneumonia, pyrimethamine-sulfadiazine for CNS toxoplasmosis, ganciclovir (DHPG) for CMV retinitis, and acyclovir for disseminated herpes simplex or herpes zoster may be complicated by dose-limiting neutropenia. Ganciclovir is particularly toxic for neutrophils, and isolated severe neutropenia is common when using this medication. Antitumor therapy is also often frustrated by neutropenia. Myelosuppression is therefore a fundamental problem in the treatment of both the underlying HIV infection and its complicating infectious or neoplastic diseases. Attempts to overcome this problem are the development of less myelotoxic antiretroviral therapies and the use of hematopoietic growth factors.

In addition to low cell numbers, abnormalities in neutrophil function have been documented.[295] Phagocytic and intracellular killing of microbes may be impaired in HIV disease. The extent to which these abnormalities contribute to the susceptibility of the patients to infection is not clear. A subset of AIDS patients seems particularly susceptible to recurrent infections with encapsulated bacteria, but no correlation with neutrophil dysfunction has been documented.

Hematopoietic Growth Factors

Because of the sensitivity of the bone marrow in HIV-infected persons to the toxic effects of therapy or coincident illness, hematopoietic growth factors have been used in the care of these patients. Erythropoietin,[292–293a] granulocyte-macrophage colony-stimulating factor (GM-CSF)[296–297f] granulocyte colony-stimulating factor (G-CSF),[293a] and IL-3[298] have been tested in patients with AIDS. Erythropoietin has been evaluated in four randomized, placebo-controlled trials and one expanded-access trial of patients experiencing anemia while receiving AZT.[292] Analysis of the experience in the randomized trials indicated that benefit was significant only if the pretreatment serum erythropoietin level was below 500 mU/mL. (The previously stated depression of serum erythropoietin levels in AIDS patients who were anemic before AZT therapy does not hold when AZT therapy is introduced; in that setting, serum erythropoietin levels rise markedly.) Before considering erythropoietin therapy, a serum erythropoietin level should be obtained since little benefit can be expected if the level is above 500 mU/mL. About two thirds of anemic AIDS patients receiving AZT fall into the group with erythropoietin levels below 500 mU/mL. In the subset of patients with hematocrits below 30% and erythropoietin levels below 500 mU/mL, recombinant human erythropoietin at a dose of 4000 U/d 6 days a week has been shown to improve the hematocrit and reduce transfusion requirements.

GM-CSF and G-CSF have been evaluated in neutropenic AIDS patients and are capable of improving neutrophil counts at relatively low doses. This ability to mitigate myelosuppression is apparent even in the presence of myelotoxic agents such as AZT, interferon-α, or ganciclovir.[297–297f] The hematologic effects have been sustained despite chronic usage of the growth factors without evidence for tachyphylaxis or antibody formation.[299] One note of concern was the development of thrombocytopenia in 5 of 17 patients treated with GM-CSF while receiving AZT.[297] Although effects on hematologic parameters have been well documented, other clinical outcomes have been less well studied. Randomized trials have been completed in AIDS patients with cytomegalovirus retinitis who were receiving ganciclovir[297c] and in AIDS patients with lymphoma who were receiving CHOP.[297d] The subjects were randomly assigned to receive GM-CSF or to a control group. The data in the cytomegalovirus trial indicated reduced days with ANC below 750 cells/μL, but did not demonstrate a statistically significant benefit in either drug delivery or preservation of vision with GM-CSF. In the lymphoma trial, GM-CSF did result in improvements in days of fever and neutropenia, in days of hospitalization, and in drug delivery. Further randomized trials using GM-CSF in the setting of lymphoma and G-CSF in the setting of Kaposi's sarcoma or moderate neutropenia are in progress.

The side effect profile of recombinant growth factors in this patient population is similar to that of other patient groups. Several issues about growth factor use in HIV disease distinguish it from other clinical situations, however. Specifically, the growth factors may interact with the virus or with the other drugs that are frequently in concurrent use. In vitro data conflict but suggest that certain growth factors—most notably GM-CSF, IL-3, and M-CSF—are capable of enhancing HIV replication.[301–305] The clinical data regarding this issue also conflict, with some studies suggesting that GM-CSF increases virologic parameters and others reporting no such changes.[297b–297d] In the absence of more definitive data, caution suggests that GM-CSF should be used in conjunction with antiretroviral therapy. Neither G-CSF nor erythropoietin is associated with effects on HIV-1 replication.

Because growth factors are often used coincidently with myelosuppressive medications in AIDS patients, the interactions of these agents may have clinical significance. In vitro data suggest that some of these interactions may be substantial. For example, the metabolism of AZT appears to be altered in monocytic cells in the presence of GM-CSF, with increased cellular levels of AZT and its active triphosphylated form resulting in a marked enhancement of anti-HIV activity.[304–307] Although this issue has been explored only in in vitro studies, the possibility that these phenomena may be exploited in vivo are intriguing and are the basis for ongoing clinical trials.

Future uses of growth factors in HIV disease depend on the ability of randomized studies to demonstrate a clinical benefit beyond that of the hematologic parameters. No data have been compiled reporting an impact on survival with the use of these proteins in AIDS patients, but other clinical benefits have been demonstrated as noted earlier. Drug interactions need to be further explored, research that may lead to novel applications of growth factors. Furthermore, the augmentation of mature cell function, such as intracellular killing by macrophages or neutrophils, may be an area in which growth factors prove clinically useful in AIDS, particularly in patients with drug-resistant tuberculosis or other intracellular pathogens for which drug therapies alone are inadequate. Finally, as more early acting growth factors are developed, it is conceivable that stimulation of lymphopoiesis will be attempted—that growth factors may be ultimately used to affect the inexorable decline of certain lymphocytes central to the pathophysiology of AIDS.

GAMMOPATHY AND COAGULOPATHY

The spectrum of immunohematologic abnormalities induced by HIV-1 is extremely broad and includes a variety of abnormalities in B-cell function such as antibody production and proliferation. Elevation of immunoglobulin levels is a virtually uniform laboratory abnormality seen in HIV-1–seropositive people regardless of the stage of HIV disease. Generally, the immunoglobulins are polyclonal, but the incidence of oligoclonal or monoclonal increases has been reported to be as high as 9%,[308–314] and some of the clones appear to be specifically reactive to HIV-1.[315] These elevations are generally not accompanied by a decrease in other immunoglobulins and only rarely result in hyperviscosity.[316] The abnormalities associated with the dysregulated immunoglobulins are the increased cell-associated immunoglobulin noted earlier and the formation of antibodies affecting coagulation.

Antiphospholipid antibodies have been reported in 20% to 70% of HIV-seropositive individuals.[317–321] They generally are associated with laboratory findings of a lupus anticoagulant—namely, a prolonged activated partial thromboplastin time not corrected by normal plasma, often an increased prothrombin time, and an abnormal Russell's viper venom time. The antibodies mediating these abnormalities are often IgM[317] and are common in symptomatic and asymptomatic patients alike, with a reported incidence in asymptomatic patients as high as 43%.[322,323]

A subset of patients with antiphospholipid antibodies have anticardiolipin antibodies, which may or may not be associated with lupus anticoagulant characteristics. These appear to be unrelated in frequency to the clinical status of the patient and do not correlate with the risk of progression to AIDS or with thrombocytopenia.[321,322] Indeed, some studies have documented a high incidence of ACAs in patients at risk of, but negative for, HIV.[322] There does not appear to be an associated increase in the false-positive rate of the Venereal Disease Research Laboratory (VDRL) test.[317] Slight elevations (1:20 and, rarely, 1:160) of antinuclear antibodies have been reported in 13% of symptomatic HIV-positive patients. The correlation of these with anticardiolipin antibodies has not been defined in HIV disease.

Strong clinical associations with these laboratory abnormalities are not apparent. Thrombosis and embolism have been reported,[318] but there does not appear to be an unusual predisposition to these events. Similarly, abnormal bleeding is uncommon, although one case in a patient with a decreased factor VII level has been reported[325] and qualitative platelet function abnormalities were documented.[317] The most problem-filled scenario is that of patients with inherited coagulation disorders in whom the antibodies may distort the laboratory parameters used to measure replacement therapy.

The mechanisms underlying the abnormal development of antibodies in HIV disease remains obscure. Associations with opportunistic infections have been noted, but the incidence of the antibodies in asymptomatic individuals suggests otherwise.[326] Rather, there appears to be a poorly understood dysregulation of the interactions between T cells and B cells that normally govern the modulation of B-cell proliferation and the antibodies their progeny produce.

LYMPHADENOPATHY

Depletion of the CD4 T lymphocyte, the primary target of HIV, is accompanied by altered function of other elements of the immune system. B-cell growth and immunoglobulin production are markedly abnormal, which may result in the hypergammaglobulinemia and lymphadenopathy that are common features of HIV infection.

Lymphadenopathy occurs in most patients infected with HIV at some time during the course of their illness. The possible causes of this abnormality are multiple, including HIV infection and a host of secondary infections such as EBV, CMV, *M avium-intracellulare, M tuberculosis, C neoformans, H capsulatum*, and syphilis. In addition, lymphoma and Kaposi's sarcoma occur dramatically more frequently in HIV-infected persons and may result in marked lymph node enlargement.

The mechanism by which HIV affects B-cell function has not been well defined, but dysregulation of activation is apparent.[327,328] Early in HIV infection, IgG and IgA antibody production is nonspecifically elevated (IgM synthesis may be decreased) and antigen-specific B-cell clonal proliferation occurs.[134] Lymphadenopathy is clinically apparent during this phase of HIV infection and may persist for months to years. The presence of lymphadenopathy in two or more noninguinal lymph node sites of at least 3 months' duration without other secondary causes of adenopathy has been defined by the CDC as persistent generalized lymphadenopathy. This phase of HIV infection has not been associated with a high incidence of opportunistic infection and is apparently not a harbinger of the imminent onset of an AIDS-defining illness.[329–331]

Differentiating between HIV-related and secondary causes of lymph node enlargement is complex and may require lymph node biopsy. Reports have indicated that otherwise clinically indistinguishable patients undergoing lymph node biopsy may reveal a secondary cause of lymphadenopathy in about 15% of patients.[332] The incidence of secondary conditions that result in a different treatment plan based on this diagnostic procedure is considerably lower. The site of lymph node enlargement is of little help in selecting patients for biopsy, since virtually any site (including the spleen) may be abnormal without a specific secondary cause. Cervical, axillary, and inguinal lymph nodes enlarge at some time in almost all persistent generalized lymphadenopathy and most HIV-infected patients. Guidelines for deciding which patients should undergo lymph node biopsy, modified from those proposed by Abrams,[333] are the following:

- Disproportionate localized lymph node enlargement
- Rapidly evolving lymphadenopathy
- Marked constitutional symptoms with negative cultures including bone marrow
- Bulky mediastinal or abdominal adenopathy or a splenic mass

Patients with persistent generalized lymphadenopathy have nonspecific histologic features on lymph node biopsy. These hyperplastic nodes have several atypical features.[334–338] Prominent follicular hyperplasia with disruption of the follicular structure or dendritic network, attenuation of mantle zones, multinucleated cells and monocytoid cells are commonly noted. In addition, alterations in CD4 and CD8 lymphocyte populations within nodal zones are documented and reflect the decline in CD4 and increase in CD8-bearing lymphocytes seen in the circulation.[339] With progression of the stage of HIV infection, lymphadenopathy tends to resolve, with involution of follicles, hyperplasia of paracortical histiocytes and blood vessels, and depletion of lymphocytes.[340] Lymph nodes in AIDS frequently reveal absent or markedly atrophic follicles, a fibrotic capsule, and prominent sinus histiocytosis.[341] Clinically, lymphadenopathy becomes less prominent with progression to AIDS unless involved with a previously noted secondary cause of lymph node enlargement.

Abundant HIV is found within the lymph nodes throughout the course of HIV disease.[95,96] Early in infection, follicular dendritic cells are coated with viral particles and probably serve as a reservoir for infecting T cells that traffic through the lymph node follicle. As the disease progresses, dendritic cells are lost and plasma virus levels increase while HIV in lymph node T cells can still be detected. The lymphoid organs appear to play a critical role in the pathophysiology of HIV disease, though the specific mechanisms that result in depletion of certain cell types remain to be elucidated.

NON-HODGKIN'S LYMPHOMA

Lymphoproliferation may occur when select subcomponents of the immune system are dysfunctional, whether from HIV infection, from immunosuppressive drugs as used after organ transplant, or from the genetic immunodeficiency states such as Wiskott-Aldrich syndrome and ataxic telangiectasia[342] (Table 25-4). Against these backgrounds, B-cell proliferation and malignant transformation to NHL occur with increased frequency. Levine and colleagues[341] have estimated that the rate of conversion from persistent generalized lymphadenopathy to lymphoma is about 3% per person per year, placing the relative risk of lymphoma in patients with persistent generalized lymphadenopathy at 850 times the expected rate for non–HIV-infected persons of comparable age. Other studies have estimated the risk of lymphoma in advanced HIV disease as 3% to 12% at 24 months.[343,344] The contribution of AIDS-related lymphoma NHL in the United States has been estimated at 8% to 27%.[345]

The one clear feature of the pathophysiology of AIDS lymphoma is that HIV is not directly involved. There is no HIV in B-cell lymphoma cells; rather, the virus plays an indirect role, providing the immunodeficiency in which B-cell malignancy may occur. These tumors appear to be opportunistic neoplasms in a fashion similar to the multiple infectious agents these patients acquire. NHL in an HIV-positive person is now considered an AIDS-defining illness.

The role of EBV in the pathogenesis of NHL in HIV-positive persons is not clear.[346–349] EBV-induced B-cell pro-

TABLE 25-4. Relative Risk (RR) of Lymphoma Associated With Selected Conditions That Entail Altered Immunity*

Magnitude of Relative Risk of Lymphoma		
High (RR > 15)	**Intermediate (RR > 2)**	**Low (RR ≤ 2)**
Multiple transplants	Sibling transplant	Splenectomy
Cadaver transplant	Mild sicca syndrome	Sarcoidosis
Severe sicca syndrome	Nontropical sprue	Hyperimmunization
Wiskott-Aldrich syndrome	Crohn's disease	Asthma
Ataxia-telangiectasia	Short-term HIV infection	Hansen's disease
Long-term HIV infection	Rheumatoid arthritis	Cytotoxic drug therapy
		Systemic lupus

* Risk of lymphoma in patients with the condition relative to a risk of 1.0 to comparable individuals without the condition.

(Hoover RN. Lymphoma risks in populations with altered immunity: a search for mechanism. Cancer Res 1992;52:5477S) liferation has been suggested to be florid in an HIV setting, unchecked because of alterations in T-cell function, resulting in a mitotically active polyclonal B-cell population.[346] This pool may serve as an expanded target for the genetic abnormalities leading to malignant conversion. The multiple (rather than single) clonal populations of B cells seen in some HIV patients with NHL lends support to this model.[350,351] EBV does not appear to be necessary for AIDS lymphoma, however, since only 39% to 68% of tumors contain the EBV genome.[348,350–354] Cytogenetic abnormalities typically found in these clonal outgrowths involve chromosome 8 (8:14;8:22,8:2 translocations), the site of the c-*myc* oncogene, rearranging with loci encoding immunoglobulin genes.[355–359] The nature of the *myc* rearrangement more closely resembles that seen in sporadic rather than endemic Burkitt's lymphoma and suggests a more mature B cell as the cell of origin.[358]

In addition, other coincident viral infections such as HTLV-I[360] or the DNA human herpesvirus-6,[361] have been hypothesized to also play a role in the pathophysiology of HIV-associated NHL. Whether infectious cofactors are important in AIDS lymphoma is still conjectural. Unlike Kaposi's sarcoma, no particular subgroup of HIV-infected persons seems to have a higher predilection for developing NHL, and the clinical and pathologic features of AIDS lymphoma are similar across risk groups.

Parallels between the lymphoma seen in HIV-infected patients and other immunocompromised persons extend to the high-grade histologic pattern of the lymphoma and the associated aggressive clinical course. Estimates of the incidence of specific histologies in NHL in this population have varied. Most patients clearly have high-grade malignancies[362–368] (Table 25-5). Small, noncleaved or immunoblastic–plasmacytoid histologies (both high grade according to the Working Formulation of Non-Hodgkin's Lymphomas for Clinical Use) account for 60% to 70% of all NHL in this setting. The remaining histologies are almost entirely diffuse and large cell (intermediate grade) although lower-grade lymphomas have been reported, as have Ki-1–positive and T-cell lymphomas. Rarely, B-cell acute lymphocytic leukemia has been described.[369,370] T-cell lymphomas may be associated with an oncogenic transformation induced by HIV integration into the host cell genome.[370a]

Apart from the unusual case of low-grade lymphoma that may be associated with a less aggressive clinical cause and perhaps a different pathogenesis, the histologic classification of HIV-associated NHL has not been consistently correlated with prognosis. Conflicting data have been presented and require further compilation of patient information to be clarified.[364,366,371,372] In general, NHL in this setting is highly aggressive regardless of histologic grade.

Sites of involvement in HIV, as in other settings of immunocompromised associated NHL, are often outside the confines of the lymphatic system. Extranodal disease is present in most patients, often involving the GI tract, bone marrow, CNS, liver, and soft tissues (Table 25-6). Two thirds of all patients in one large series were diagnosed with NHL based on biopsies of nonnodal anatomic sites.[365] The site of extranodal disease may correlate with histologic type as in one series in which about 40% of patients with small, noncleaved cells had bone marrow involvement. This is a less common event in patients with an immunoblastic histology and rare in patients with a diffuse large-cell histology.[365] In contrast, GI involvement is noted more frequently with immunoblastic (48%) and diffuse large, noncleaved cells (36%) than with small, noncleaved cells (8%). GI involvement may occur anywhere from esophagus to anus with an unusual predilection for anal or rectal involvement in homosexual males.[373]

The site of CNS involvement may vary according to the status of the patient's lymphoma. That is, patients presenting with primary CNS lymphoma (almost uniformly an immunoblastic histology and associated with EBV[374]) tend to have mass lesions in the parenchyma of the brain, whereas CNS involvement in conjunction with systemic lymphoma favors meningeal sites. The incidence of CNS involvement in patients with systemic lymphoma has been estimated at 20%[375]: thus, all HIV-positive patients presenting with systemic NHL should undergo careful assessment of the CNS.

At presentation, most HIV-infected patients with NHL have advanced-stage lymphoma. Systemic "B" symptoms (fever, weight loss, anorexia, malaise) are particularly common, although secondary infectious causes must be vigorously excluded. Staging the extent of tumor involvement should follow guidelines that are followed for NHL in other settings, with particular attention to the CNS, GI tract, and bone marrow. As with histologic classification, whether tumor stage affects the prognosis is not clear.[362,367,371] Study has found that prior AIDS, a low CD4 count, and performance status predicted a shorter survival time, whereas B symptoms, mass size, LDH levels, histologic

TABLE 25-5. Histologic Grade of Non-Hodgkin's Lymphoma in AIDS Patients

Study	Patients	SNCC	Histology IBS/ALC	LC
Levine et al	27	10	13	—
Kalter et al	14	7	1	5
Gill et al	22	16	6	—
Knowles et al	89	36	25	25
Ziegler et al	90	32	24	17
Bermudez et al	31	8	6	10
Lowenthal et al	43	16	8	16
Kaplan et al	84	29	36	17
Kaplan et al	30	7	16	3
Levine et al	42	17	14	4
Remick et al	18	0	7	10
Raphael et al	113	41	33	35
TOTAL	603	219 (36%)	189 (31%)	142 (24%)

SNCC, small noncleaved cell; IBS, immunoblastic; ALC, anaplastic large cell; LC, large cell.

TABLE 25-6. Location and Stage of Non-Hodgkin's Lymphoma in AIDS Patients

Study	Patients	Extranodal Sites				Stage	
		GI	Liver	CNS	Marrow	I or II	III or IV
Levine et al	27	6	1	8	5	7	20
Kalter et al	14	2	2	8	4	1	13
Gill et al	22	5	5	3	7	1	21
Knowles et al	89	14	14	19	19	27	57
Ziegler et al	90	8	8	38	30	38	52
Bermudez et al	31	6	6	8	10	1	30
Lowenthal et al	43	11	6	11	13	9	26
Kaplan et al	84	7	22	10	26	14	69
Kaplan et al	30	?	?	?	7	12	14
Levine et al	42	5	11	6	6	11	24
Remick et al	18	5	?	?	?	5	13
Raphael et al	113	18	3	22	17	—	—
TOTAL	603	124 (21%)	78 (13%)	133 (23%)	138 (23%)	126 (27%)	339 (73%)

type, and even the presence of leptomeningeal disease had no prognostic significance.[371]

The unusual sites of involvement by NHL can pose difficult diagnostic problems. Particularly, primary CNS disease may be difficult to differentiate from progressive multifocal leukoencephalopathy or infection with *Toxoplasma gondii* or *M tuberculosis*. Radiographically, progressive multifocal leukoencephalopathy may be distinguished by its lack of enhancement with gadolinium on nuclear magnetic resonance imaging. Lymphomatous lesions may be isodense or hypodense and contrast enhancing on computed tomographic scans and enhancing on magnetic resonance imaging scans, but so may toxoplasmal abscess.[376] Other features may help discriminate among these diagnoses such as the number of lesions (usually single in lymphoma, multiple in toxoplasmosis) and their location (lymphoma tends to be paraventricular), but there is no definitive radiographic appearance. Frequently, biopsy is necessary, particularly in the setting of continued progression despite empiric antiinfective therapy.

Treatment of patients with HIV-associated NHL is complicated by the limited tolerance for chemotherapy in this patient population as well as the aggressive biology of the malignancy. Bone marrow suppression and opportunistic infection commonly limit treatment, impeding optimal delivery of antitumor therapy. These complications occur more commonly with more advanced HIV disease. Thus, selecting a treatment for patients with NHL should include consideration of the status of the HIV disease. Patients with prior AIDS-defining illnesses (opportunistic infection or Kaposi's sarcoma) or CD4 counts below 200/μL have a worse prognosis.[371] Patients in whom lymphoma is the AIDS-defining illness generally tolerate chemotherapy well, without severe myeolosuppression of mucositis. Overall, tumor response rates to chemotherapy in AIDS lymphoma are comparable to that seen in NHL patients without HIV infection but with similar-grade malignancies.[367] Responders may have prolonged disease-free survival.[367,375]

Although there may be differing molecular characteristic to the tumors,[377] clinical experience suggests that it may be reasonable to approach the subset of patients with a good performance status despite HIV disease in a manner similar to that of NHL patients without HIV. Two important caveats have generally been adopted though not well studied: prophylaxis for *P carinii* should probably be administered to all patients, and some form of intrathecal prophylaxis for CNS disease is generally given.[375]

The optimal chemotherapy for AIDS lymphoma remains ill defined, and patients should be encouraged to participate in clinical trials whenever feasible. Two general approaches have emerged. In Europe, an intensive combination chemotherapy regimen has been tested with a complete remisssion rate of 63% and median disease-free survival of 16 months.[378] Overall survival was only 9 months, however, often because of opportunistic infection. In the United States, adverse experience with aggressive protocols early in the epidemic[365,379–381] led efforts to use minimally toxic regiments to avoid the high rates of chemotherapy-associated morbidity and mortality. A pilot study of low-dose m-BACOD resulted in a complete remission rate of 50%, with a median survival of 15 months for responders and 6.5 months overall.[375] A randomized, controlled trial is in progress to compare this modified m-BACOD regimen with full-dose m-BACOD plus growth factor support by the multicenter AIDS Clinical Trials Group (ACTG) of the National Institute of Allergy and Infectious Disease (NIAID).

In addition to the issue of chemotherapy dosing, other issues, such as the role of antiretroviral therapy and salvage treatments, require further definition. With relapse occurring in about half of patients achieving remission as well as a considerable fraction of nonresponding patients, better treatment approaches are clearly needed. In this setting, where failed immune surveillance may be playing a key role, immune-based strategies can be expected to be tested.

The challenge for new therapies is particularly keen in the area of primary CNS AIDS lymphoma. Patients with this diagnosis are generally far advanced in their immunosuppression, with an approximate median survival of 1 month without therapy and 2 to 4 months with treatment. Although some durable remissions with radiation therapy have been documented, mortality from opportunistic infections has been daunting.[383,384] Current treatment consists of choosing between observation, corticosteroids, or radiation plus corticosteroids; selection should be made with consideration of the patient's overall outlook. Investigational approaches evaluating systemic therapy plus chemotherapy or intraarterial chemotherapy infusions are in development.

HODGKIN'S DISEASE

The incidence of Hodgkin's disease appears to be slighlty increased in the setting of HIV infection.[385,386] The clinical course of the disease in HIV-positive persons is substantially different from uninfected counterparts with a higher incidence of advanced-stage disease, extranodal disease, and mixed-cellularity histology.[387–389] AIDS patients with Hodgkin's disease appear to have a decreased tolerance for chemotherapy and a high incidence of tumor relapse. A treatment plan for HIV-positive patients with Hodgkin's disease should follow the same principle of treatment as appropriate for stage applied to non–HIV-infected patients. However, aggressive chemotherapeutic regimens may need to be modified according to the patient's stage of HIV infection and PCP prophylaxis should be included. Hodgkin's patients with advanced AIDS may be more likely to experience opportunistic infections and severe bone marrow depression from standard chemotherapeutic regimens. Treatment programs must balance the risk of relapse from compromised dose intensity and the risk of opportunistic infection from an aggressive drug regimen.

OTHER MALIGNANCIES

In addition to lymphomas, patients with HIV may have an increased incidence of premalignant squamous cell neoplasia, probably because of the high occurrence of papillomavirus infection. This problem is particularly acute among HIV-infected women who have a high incidence of cervical dysplasia and intraepithelial neoplasia.[390] It is often multifocal and usually human papillomavirus related—often oncogenic strains 16 and 18. Although an increase in frank carcinoma has not yet been documented, concern and surveillance for such is indicated. The presence of cervical cancer is an AIDS-defining diagnosis. Similar concerns may be appropriate for homosexual men, in whom anal dysplasia has been documented in up to 40%.[391–396] Indeed, it has recently been reported that the incidence of anal cancer is markedly increased in AIDS.[296a] The frequency and manifestations of both these problems appear to be related to severity of immunosuppression. Scattered reports of other tumors in HIV-positive patients have been published[385,397–400]; whether their incidence is statistically above that of the general population is unclear. In general, treatment of patients with any malignant condition who have coincident AIDS may be complicated by a higher rate of complications from chemotherapy. The aggressiveness with which to address the malignant diagnosis must be determined in light of the severity of the HIV disease.

KAPOSI'S SARCOMA

General Features

Kaposi's sarcoma is the most common neoplastic complication of HIV infection. When present, it defines an HIV-infected patient as having AIDS according to CDC criteria. Kaposi's sarcoma appears in multiple other settings, and its epidemiology highlights some of the important biologic features of this tumor.

Moricz Kaposi,[401] a Hungarian dermatologist, first described an abnormality in 1872 as an "idiopathic, multiple pigmented sarcoma" (p. 265) occurring predominantly in the lower extremities of elderly men of Mediterranean and Jewish extraction. This classic form of Kaposi's sarcoma has a high male/female ratio, is associated with the HLA-DR5 locus, and is associated with other malignant neoplasms, particularly of the lymphoid type, in 30% of cases. The latter features suggest a strong influence of genetic background and underlying immune dysregulation in the etiology of this process.

An endemic form of Kaposi's sarcoma has also been documented to occur in restricted geographic locations in Central Africa. Documentation of this problem in Africa antedated the recent epidemic of HIV-related disease in the same region. A high male/female ratio was found among these persons, but the ratio was diminished in the rare cases involving children. The association of male gender and adulthood with the disease suggests a role for hormonal as well as genetic influences in the biology of the tumor. In addition, the lack of this tumor in Asians or Europeans living within the endemic area and the lack of the development of this process in persons from this area who move elsewhere, suggests that the cause may be an infectious agent (perhaps transmitted in a manner similar to HIV) or some other culturally restricted environmental agents.

The other most relevant setting in which Kaposi's sarcoma has been documented may be that of patients who are receiving immunosuppressive agents for organ transplantation. Renal transplant patients develop Kaposi's sarcoma when on high-dose single- or multiple-agent immunosuppressive drugs. Their lesions tend to resolve with modulation or discontinuation of immunosuppressive drugs.[402,403] The role of immunosuppression is clearly predominant in developing Kaposi's sarcoma in this setting. Nevertheless, other genetic or environmental factors play a role, since the incidence of Kaposi's sarcoma is increased about 50-fold in renal transplantation patients in Saudi Arabia compared with those in the United States.[404] Kaposi's sarcoma may also rarely complicate other diseases of immune dysregulation including Hodgkin's disease, NHL, systemic lupus erythematosus, pemphigus vulgaris, and mycobacterium tuberculosis infection. Although rare, these associations should be kept in mind when first evaluating a patient with Kaposi's sarcoma who denies involvement in a group that is high risk for HIV.

The incidence of Kaposi's sarcoma is clearly highest in the setting of HIV infection (estimated to be 20,000 times greater than in the general population). Kaposi's sarcoma was originally noted in 40% of AIDS patients when first reported in 1981. The incidence has been on a steady decline and now involves about 15% of all US AIDS patients.[405] This change in the epidemiology of AIDS-related Kaposi's sarcoma is apparently not due to altered reporting patterns of the disease.[406] When it does occur, AIDS-associated Kaposi's sarcoma is highly associated with homosexual or bisexual men rather than other HIV risk groups, suggesting that immunosuppression alone is insufficient to account for this disease. As in the non–HIV-associated Kaposi's sarcoma, other coincident factors need to be present. Early investigations into the nature of these cofactors suggested an association with either CMV infection or the use of volatile alkyl nitrates. A parallel decline has occurred in the incidence of the possible linked cofactors and a decline in the incidence of Kaposi's sarcoma. The decline in these cofactors also parallels the decrease in incidence of new cases of HIV infection and suggests altered patterns of sexual behavior within this high-risk group. Reports of HIV-seronegative homosexual men with Kaposi's sarcoma and an increased incidence in gay men practicing oral–anal sex has lent support to the hypothesis of an independent sexually transmitted infectious agent as an essential cofactor.[407,408] A direct role for infection by known viruses in the development of this process has not been supported by evaluation of involved tissue. Neither HIV nor CMV has been consistently found in those with Kaposi's sarcoma lesions.

The epidemiologic features of Kaposi's sarcoma suggest an important interplay of infectious, genetic, hormonal, and environmental factors with a common underlying theme of immune dysregulation.[408a] The complex interaction of multiple factors is mirrored by the histologic appearance of these lesions. Unlike most sarcomas, these lesions appear as a conglomerate of different cell types. Prominent within these lesions are cells of endothelial origin forming nests of microvascular structures. These structures are surrounded by a prominent spindle cell component admixed with extravasated RBCs and cells of macrophage–monocyte origin.[409,410] The endothelial cells lack Weibel-Palade bodies that are characteristic of normal vascular endothelial cells, suggesting an origin from lymphatic endothelium. This composite of cells of different lineages suggests the outgrowth of otherwise normal tissue. No evidence is found for this process representing the clonal expansion of a single transformed cell,[411] and it is not clear whether it is a true malignancy. Characterization of this tumor as a sarcoma may be misleading, and the process is perhaps more accurately characterized as Kaposi's disease rather than Kaposi's sarcoma.

Several lines of investigation have recently provided further insight into the nature of this process of formation of Kaposi's sarcoma. Mice transgenic for the HIV *tat* gene were found to express this gene primarily in cutaneous sites.[412] Founder mice of exclusively male gender were found to develop cutaneous lesions histologically resembling those of Kaposi's sarcoma. This is the first evidence of an HIV-specific effect, although the relation of this mouse model to human Kaposi's sarcoma and whether *tat* acted directly or by influencing the expression of other host genes remain ill defined. Efforts to evaluate Kaposi's sarcoma tumor tissue in vitro have only recently been successful by cultivating biopsy-derived cells with supernatants from retrovirally infected T lymphocytes.[413] Cells cultivated under these conditions resemble the spindle cells seen histologically in Kaposi's sarcoma lesions. These cells have been shown to express high levels of basic fibroblast growth factor and IL-1 RNA—factors known to induce vascular proliferation.[414,415] In addition, these cells secrete and respond to IL-6 and are responsive to Oncostatin M.[416,417] Therefore, one model for the pathophysiology of these lesions is that retroviral infection induces the immune perturbation necessary for the abnormal expression of growth stimulatory cytokines. Dysregulation of these controlling factors may lead to outgrowth of multiple cell types in a paracrine or even autocrine fashion. Complex factors appear to interact in the development of these lesions, and a satisfactory model that can be tested in vitro will be difficult to develop.[408a]

Clinical Features

Clinically, cutaneous Kaposi's sarcoma appears as a cutaneous nonblanching erythematous macule or occasionally as a subcutaneous nodule with only faint overlying pigmentation. As these lesions evolve, they become maculopapular, increase in diameter and nodularity, and usually develop a more violaceous pigmentation. Rapidly expanding lesions often have a surrounding ecchymotic halo. Some lesions evolve to become heaped up or even pedunculated nodules and occasionally become necrotic. Clusters of lesions may become confluent, and large plaque-like lesions may develop, particularly on the lower extremities. In general, this tumor tends to appear at multiple sites independently with no orderly tumor progression. Removal of the initial site or sites of involvement appears to be irrelevant to the development of future lesions. Lesions occur sporadically, may remain stable for long periods of time, rarely resolve spontaneously, or may rapidly proliferate and conglomerate. Factors that may influence the pattern of disease are poorly understood. The recent description of cutaneous pigmented lesions in AIDS patients caused by *Rochalimaea* sp or by cutaneous *P carinii* has affirmed the need for biopsy on first clinical presentation.[418,419] Bacillary angiomatosis due to *Rochalimaea* requires antibiotics and clearly has different clinical implications than the AIDS-defining diagnosis of Kaposi's sarcoma.

Kaposi's sarcoma lesions can occur on any cutaneous site. They frequently occur on the face, and they have a predilection for the pinnae of the ears and the distal portion of the nose. Mucous membrane involvement is common, with lesions occurring on the oropharynx, conjunctiva and, less commonly, urethral meatus surfaces. Involvement of these areas can obviously lead to local complications, whereas cutaneous lesions are mostly of cosmetic concern. Given the diagnosis underlying these lesions, the psychological weight of these cosmetic concerns cannot be overstated. Effectively treating these cutaneous lesions can overcome a major cause of distress for these patients.

In addition to cutaneous involvement, Kaposi's sarcoma occurs in viscera, particularly those richly endowed with lymphatics. Common sites are the tracheobronchial tree, the lungs, and the GI tract. Involvement of virtually every organ has been reported. Pulmonary involvement may involve airways, air space, and pleural surfaces; clinical manifestations may range from hemoptysis to reactive airways disease to parenchymal infiltration with poor gas exchange to symptomatic pleural effusions. Discriminating between Kaposi's sarcoma and infectious causes of these abnormalities is frequently difficult, and Kaposi's sarcoma is often a diagnosis of exclusion. One potentially useful criterion is that Kaposi's sarcoma lesions are not gallium-avid,[420] but biopsy is necessary to confirm the diagnosis. Symptomatic pulmonary involvement is generally a poor prognostic sign and is indicative of the requirement for the institution of chemotherapy.[421]

GI involvement is generally asymptomatic but can lead to multiple nonspecific symptoms, occasionally to volvulus and to chronic low-grade GI blood loss. Rarely, fatal uncontrolled GI blood loss has occurred. The presence of GI involvement with Kaposi's sarcoma is correlated with extensive oropharyngeal Kaposi's sarcoma. Kaposi's sarcoma as a cause for GI symptoms, anatomic evaluation, and exclusion of other possible contributing infectious agents is required.

Lymph node involvement is the most common cause of morbidity from Kaposi's sarcoma. Lymph node enlargement is particularly common in the groin and on the head and neck, frequently inducing marked local edema or debilitating lower extremity or periorbital edema. In addition to superficial nodal involvement, visceral nodes in the chest and abdomen can be seen radiographically; in the abdomen, these nodes are often associated with hepatic and splenic enlargement.

Differentiating lymphadenopathy induced by Kaposi's sarcoma from that of lymphoma or other infectious processes is difficult. The progression of Kaposi's sarcoma–related lymphadenopathy is generally slower, and constitutional symptoms are less common than that which occurs from lymphoma or infectious causes. Distinguishing between these entities frequently requires lymph node biopsy.

Management

In evaluating and treating a patient with AIDS-associated Kaposi's sarcoma, several important distinctions are made in managing this as opposed to other neoplasms that a hematologist may confront. First, patients generally do *not* die of Kaposi's sarcoma but from infectious complications of their immune deficiency.[422] Prognosis has been shown to be more closely correlated with the stage of HIV infection than that of the tumor.[423] Staging systems must therefore emphasize immunologic parameters and systemic symp-

TABLE 25-7. Kaposi's Sarcoma: Recommended Staging Classification

	Good Risk (0) (All of the Following)	Poor Risk (1) (Any of the Following)
Tumor (T)	Confined to skin or lymph nodes or minimal oral disease*	Tumor-associated edema or ulceration Extensive oral KS Gastrointestinal KS KS in other nonnodal viscera
Immune system (I)	CD4 cells ≥200/μL	CD4 cells <200/μL
Systemic illness (S)	No history of OI or thrush No B symptoms† Performance status ≥70 (Karnofsky)	History of OI or thrush B symptoms present Performance status <70 Other HIV-related illness (eg, neurologic disease, lymphoma)

KS, Kaposi's sarcoma; OI, opportunistic infection.
* Minimal oral disease is nonnodular KS confined to the palate.
† B symptoms are unexplained fever, night sweats, more than 10% involuntary weight loss, or diarrhea persisting more than 2 weeks.
(Krown SE, Metroka C, Wernz J. Kaposi's sarcoma in the acquired immune deficiency syndrome: a proposal for uniform evaluation, response, and staging criteria. J Clin Oncol 1989;7:1201)

toms in addition to the extent of the Kaposi's sarcoma. A recently proposed tumor (T), immunologic status (I), and systemic symptoms (S) classification (TIS) may be useful in evaluating these patients[424] (Table 25-7). It follows from such a staging system that treatment for patients with Kaposi's sarcoma should include antiretroviral as well as antineoplastic components. Use of antiretroviral agents should be considered a priority in these patients, despite the lack of evidence for a direct antitumor effect of these drugs.

The range of therapeutic options in Kaposi's sarcoma is broad, ranging from observation to systemic chemotherapy.[424a,426] In deciding the appropriate approach, the severity of the patient's immunodeficiency and the severity of the symptoms from Kaposi's sarcoma are to be considered (Fig. 25-5). Patients with symptomatic visceral disease or rapidly evolving Kaposi's sarcoma–associated edema generally require chemotherapy. Several different chemotherapeutic agents have been effective, including single-agent doxorubicin, VP-16, vinblastine, and vinblastine alternating with vincristine, or the combination of doxorubicin, bleomycin, and vincristine[425–429d] (Table 25-8). The combination of bleomycin and vincristine generally provides a fairly prompt therapeutic benefit in most patients and is minimally myelotoxic, a feature that is particularly appealing because it permits coincident treatment with AZT. Liposomal formulations of anthracyclines are in clinical trial and may also be well-tolerated, effective drugs.[429e] Use of chemotherapy generally results in a fairly rapid im-

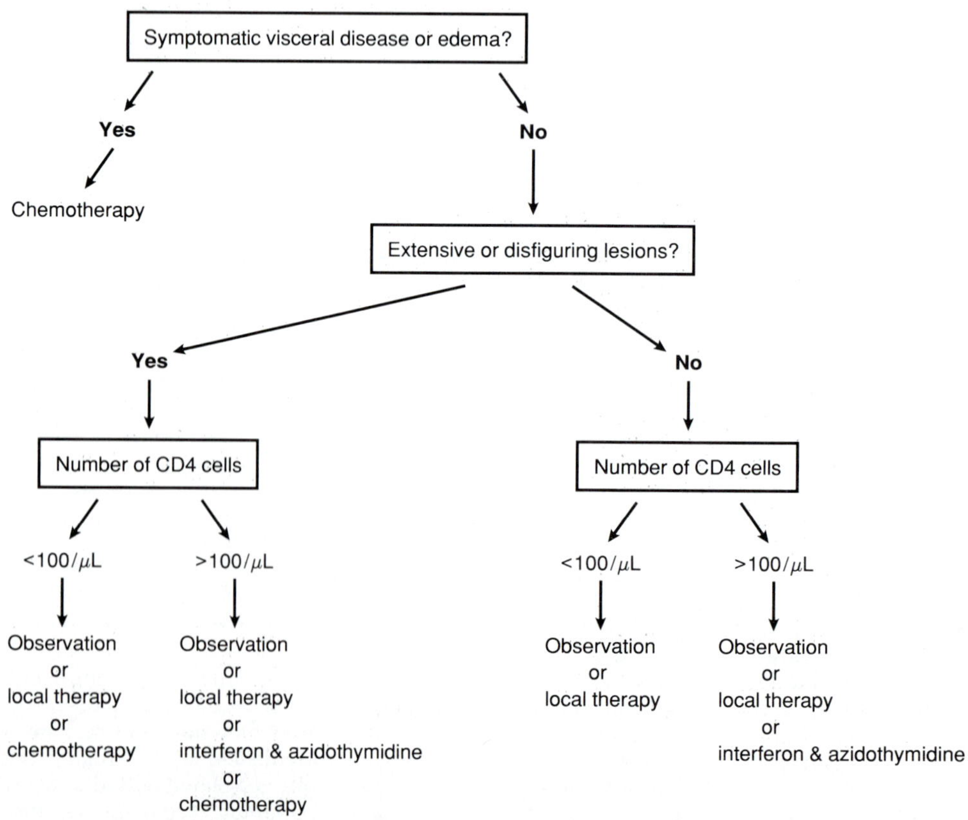

FIGURE 25-5. Treatment recommendations for Kaposi's sarcoma.

TABLE 25-8. Treatment for Kaposi's Sarcoma: Dosage Recommendations

INTERFERON-α	
Single agent	
Alpha-2a (Roche)	18–36 million U SC/d for 8 wk, then 3 times weekly
Alpha-2b (Schering)	30 million U SC 3 times weekly
Combined therapy	
Zidovudine	Zidovudine, 100 mg PO every 4 hours while awake; interferon-α, 5–10 mIU SC 3 times weekly
CHEMOTHERAPY	
Single agent	
Adriamycin	10–40 mg/m² IV every 2–3 wk
VP-16	100 mg/m² IV every 2–3 wk or 50 mg PO daily as tolerated
Vinblastine	2–8 mg IV weekly
Combined therapy	
Vincristine/vinblastine	Vincristine, 2 mg IV every 2 wk
	Vinblastine, 2–8 mg IV on alternate weeks
Adriamycin/bleomycin/vincristine	Adriamycin, 20 mg/m² IV every 3 wk
	Bleomycin, 15 U/m² IV every 3 wk
	Vincristine, 2 mg IV every 3 wk
Bleomycin/vincristine	Bleomycin, 15 U IV every 2–3 wk
	Vincristine, 2 mg IV every 2–3 wk

SC, subcutaneously; PO, by mouth.

provement of Kaposi's sarcoma lesions, which is marked by a loss of the surrounding ecchymotic halo, a decrease in the thickness of the lesions, and a change of the pigment to a gray-brown color. Recently acquired lesions may entirely resolve, but complete disappearance of lesions is uncommon. Patients should be counseled that lesions often thin out and leave a residual pigment stain. Biopsy of such lesions may show remaining hemosiderin and some vascular proliferation but may lack the spindle cell component. These histologic complete remissions may leave improved but still disfiguring cosmetic effects. With rare exceptions, lesions regrow when chemotherapy is interrupted.

Because chemotherapy is palliative, because death due to the tumor is uncommon, and because it may be a nonmalignant condition, the principles of chemotherapy use in this setting are often different than with other tumors. Experience with chemotherapy interrupted because of intercurrent illness then reinstituted with equivalent effectiveness in tumor regression suggests that the concern may be less with selection of a drug-resistant cell clone than with the toxic effects of therapy. Sparing use of low doses of chemotherapy titrated to the patient's response and tolerance has been a reasonable approach in our experience.

Patients who do not require immediate intervention because of the extent of their tumor have several other therapeutic options: observation, interferon-α, or local therapies such as radiation, intralesional chemotherapy, cryotherapy, and surgery.

Patients who fall into the good-risk category by TIS staging are also good candidates for a response to interferon-α.[194,430–432] This agent has been shown at higher doses to have both antiviral and antitumor effects.[433,434] Interferon-α may be similarly beneficial at lower doses when used in combination with AZT,[194,297a,297f] although with substantial hematologic toxicity. Interferon-α inhibits viral assembly, and in vitro it has a synergistic antiviral effect when used with the reverse transcriptase inhibitor, AZT.[435] GM-CSF is able to overcome the neutropenia that frequently accompanies the clinical use of these combined agents.[297a,297e,297f] Although appealing for its antiviral and antitumor effects, interferon-α is associated with a high incidence of flu-like symptoms, is costly, has a median time to response of 10 weeks, and is unlikely to benefit patients with CD4 counts below 100 cells/μL. Whether it offers survival benefit must be answered in comparative trials.

For Kaposi's sarcoma patients who are considered poor risk by TIS staging, antiretroviral therapy is of high priority. Local treatment of cosmetically troublesome lesions or judicious use of chemotherapy may be used as necessary. Local treatment options include intralesional injection of vinblastine,[436] radiation therapy,[437] cryotherapy,[438] and surgery (less satisfactory). Radiation therapy must be used cautiously, particularly on mucous membranes because of an observed unusual radiosensitivity in AIDS patients. Other agents with antiangiogenic potential or cytokines or *tat* antagonists may also ultimately prove to be useful and are in clinical trial. Improved understanding of the biology of Kaposi's sarcoma and emerging treatment options make the management of Kaposi's sarcoma an area likely to undergo rapid evolution.

REFERENCES

1. Statistics from the Centers for Disease Control. AIDS 1994;8:399.
2. Centers for Disease Control and Prevention. 1993 revised classification system for HIV infection and expanded surveillance case definition for AIDS among adolescents and adults. MMWR 1992;41:1.
3. Rwandan HIV Seroprevalence Study Group. Nationwide community-based serological survey of HIV-1 and other human retrovirus infections in a central African country. Lancet 1989;2:941.
4. McNeil JG, Brundage JF, Wann ZF, Burke DS, Miller RN, Walter Reed Retrovirus Research Group. Direct measurement of human immunodeficiency virus seroconversions in a serially tested population of young adults in the United States Army, Oct 1985 to Oct 1987. N Engl J Med 1989;320:1581.
5. DeCock KM, Odehouri K, Moreau J, et al. Rapid emergence of AIDS in Abidjan Ivory Coast. Lancet 1989;2:408.
6. Cortes E, Detels R, Aboulafia D, et al. HIV-1, HIV-2 and HTLV-I infection in high-risk groups in Brazil. N Engl J Med 1989;320:953.
7. Masur H, Michelis MA, Greene JB, et al. An outbreak of community-acquired *Pneumocystis carinii* pneumonia. N Engl J Med 1981;305:1431.
8. Siegal FP, Lopez C, Hammer GS, et al. Severe acquired immunodeficiency in male homosexuals, manifested by chronic perianal ulcerative herpes simplex lesions. N Engl J Med 1981;305:1439.
9. Gottlieb MS, Schroff R, Schanker HM, et al. *Pneumocystis carinii* pneumonia and mucosal candidiasis in previously healthy homosexual men. N Engl J Med 1981;305:1425.

10. Ammann AJ, Abrams D, Conant M, et al. Acquired immune dysfunction in homosexual men: immunologic profiles. Clin Immunol Immunopathol 1983;27:315.
11. Barré-Sinoussi F, Chermann JC, Rey F, et al. Isolation of a T-lymphotropic retrovirus from a patient at risk for acquired immunodeficiency syndrome (AIDS). Science 1983;220:868.
12. Gallo RC, Salahuddin SZ, Popovic M, et al. Frequent detection and isolation of cytopathic retroviruses (HTLV-III) from patients with AIDS and at risk for AIDS. Science 1984;224:500.
12a. Green WC. The molecular biology of human immunodeficiency virus type 1 infection. N Engl J Med 1993;324:308.
13. Chow SA, Vincent KA, Ellison V, Brown PO. Reversal of integration and DNA splicing mediated by integrase of human immunodeficiency virus. Science 1992;255:723.
14. Skalka AM. Retroviral proteases: first glimpses at the anatomy of a processing machine. Cell 1989;56:911.
15. Cullen BR, Greene WC, Hughes H. Regulatory pathways governing HIV-1 replication. Cell 1989;58:423.
16. Varmus B. Regulation of HIV and HTLV gene expression. Genes Dev 1988;2:1055.
17. Ayra SK, Guo C, Josephs SJ, Wong-Staal F. Transactivator gene of human T-lymphotropic virus type III (HTLV-III). Science 1985;229:69.
18. Sodroski J, Rosen C, Wong-Staal F, et al. Trans-acting transcriptional regulation of human T-cell leukemia virus type III long terminal repeat. Science 1985;227:171.
19. Cullen BR. Trans-activation of human immunodeficiency virus occurs via a bimodel mechanism. Cell 1986;46:973.
20. Folks TM, Justement J, Kinter A, Dinarello CA, Fauci AS. Cytokine-induced expression of HIV-1 in a chronically-infected promonocyte cell line. Science 1987;238:800.
21. Albrecht MA, DeLuca NA, Byrn RA, Schaffer PA, Hammer SM. The herpes simplex virus immediate-early protein, ICP4, is required to potentiate replication of human immunodeficiency virus in CD4+ lymphocytes. J Virol 1989;63:1861.
22. Nabel G, Baltimore D. An inducible transcription factor activates expression of human immunodeficiency virus in T cells. Nature 1987;326:711.
23. Muesing MA, Smith DH, Cabradill CD, Benton CV, Lasky LA, Capon DJ. Nucleic acid structure and expression of the human AIDS/lymphadenopathy retrovirus. Nature 1985;313:450.
24. Nelbock P, Dillon PJ, Perkins A, Rosen CA. A cDNA for a protein that interacts with the human immunodeficiency virus tat transactivator. Science 1990;248:1650.
25. Feinberg MB, Jarrett RF, Aldovini A, et al. HTLV-III expression and production involve complex regulation at the levels of splicing and translation of viral RNA. Cell 1986;46:807.
26. Dayton ET, Powell DM, Dayton AI. Functional analysis of rar, the target sequence for the rev protein of HIV-1. Science 1989;246:1625.
27. Malim MH, Hauber J, Le SY, Maizel JV, Cullen BR. The HIV-1 rev trans-activator acts through a structured target sequence to activate nuclear export of unspliced viral mRNA. Nature 1989;338:254.
28. Chang DD, Sharp PA. Regulation by HIV rev depends upon recognition of splice sites. Cell 1989;59:789.
29. Chang DD, Sharp PA. Messenger RNA transport and HIV rev regulation. Science 1990;249:614.
30. Ahmad N, Maitra RK, Venkatesan S. Rev-induced modulation of nef protein underlies temporal regulation of human immunodeficiency virus replication. Proc Natl Acad Sci USA 1989;86:6111.
31. Cheng-Mayer C, Iannello P, Shaw K, Luciw PA, Levy JA. Differential effects of nef on HIV replication: implications for viral pathogenesis in the host. Science 1989;246:1629.
32. Kim S, Ikeuchi K, Byrn R, Groopman JE, Baltimore A. Lack of a negative influence on viral growth by the nef gene of human immunodeficiency virus type 1. Proc Natl Acad Sci USA 1989;86:9544.
33. Kestler HW III, Ringler DJ, Mori K, et al. Importance of the nef gene for maintenance of high virus loads and for development of AIDS. Cell 1991;65:651.
34. Ogawa K, Shibata R, Kiyomasu T, et al. Mutational analysis of the human immunodeficiency virus vpr open reading frame. J Virol 1989;63:4110.
35. Strebel K, Klimkait T, Maldarelli F, Martin MA. Molecular and biochemical analyses of human immunodeficiency virus type 1 vpu protein. J Virol 1989;63:3784.
36. Terwilliger EF, Cohen EA, Lu Y, Sodroski JG, Haseltine WA. Functional role of human immunodeficiency virus type 1 vpu. Proc Natl Acad Sci USA 1989;86:5163.
37. Guyader M, Emerman M, Sonigo P, Clavel F, Montagnier L, Alizon M. Genome organization and transactivation of the human immunodeficiency virus type 2. Nature 1987;326:662.
38. Hirsch VM, Olmsted RA, Corb MM, Purcell RH, Johnson PR. An African primate lentivirus (SIV_{sm}) closely related to HIV-2. Nature 1989;339:389.
39. Rimsky L, Hauber J, Dukovich M, et al. Functional replacement of the HIV-1 rev protein by the HTLV-1 rex protein. Nature 1988;335:738.
40. Miles SA, Balden E, Magpantay L, et al. Rapid serologic testing with immune-complex–dissociated HIV p24 antigen for early detection of HIV-infection in neonates. N Engl J Med 1993;328:297.
41. Centers for Disease Control. Update: serologic testing for antibody to human immunodeficiency virus. MMWR 1988;36:833.
42. Centers for Disease Control. Interpretation and use of the Western blot assay for serodiagnosis of human immunodeficiency virus Type 1 infections. MMWR 1989;38:5.
43. Leitman SF, Klein HG, Melpolder JJ, et al. Clinical implications of positive tests for antibodies to human immunodeficiency virus type 1 in asymptomatic blood donors. N Engl J Med 1989;321:917.
44. Genesca J, Shih JWK, Jett BW, Hewlett IK, Epstein JS, Alter HJ. What do Western blot indeterminate patterns for human immunodeficiency virus mean in EIA-negative blood donors? Lancet 1989;2:1023.
45. Jackson JB, MacDonald KL, Cadwell J, et al. Absence of HIV infection in blood donors with indeterminate Western blot tests for antibody to HIV-1. N Engl J Med 1990;322:217.
46. Celum CL, Coombs RW, Lafferty W, et al. Indeterminate human immunodeficiency virus type 1 Western blots: seroconversion risk, specificity of supplemental tests, and an algorithm for evaluation. J Infect Dis 1991;164:656.
47. Laurence J. Search for HIV in HIV-seronegative individuals. AIDS Reader 1992;May/June:104.
48. Ho DD, Moudgil T, Alam MS, Alam M. Quantitation of human immunodeficiency virus type 1 in the blood of infected persons. N Engl J Med 1989;321:1621.
49. Coombs RW, Collier AC, Allain JP, et al. Plasma viremia in human immunodeficiency virus infection. N Engl J Med 1989;321:1626.
50. Ou C-Y, Swok S, Mitchell SW, et al. DNA amplification for direct detection of HIV-1 in DNA of peripheral blood mononuclear cells. Science 1988;239:295.
51. Holodniy M, Katzenstein DA, Sengupta S, et al. Detection and quantification of human immunodeficiency virus RNA in patient serum by use of the polymerase chain reaction. J Infect Dis 1991;163:862.
52. Scadden DT, Wang Z, Groopman JE. Quantitation of plasma human immunodeficiency virus type 1 RNA by competitive polymerase chain reaction. J Infect Dis 1992;165:1119.
53. Loche M, Mach B. Identification of HIV-infected seronegative individuals by a direct diagnostic test based on hybridisation to amplified viral DNA. Lancet 1988;2:418.
54. Imagawa DT, Lee MH, Wolinsky SM, et al. Human immunodeficiency virus type 1 infection in homosexual men who remain seronegative for prolonged periods. N Engl J Med 1989;320:1458.
55. Wolinsky SM, Rinaldo CR, Kwok S, et al. Human immunodeficiency virus type 1 (HIV-1) infection a median of 18 months before a diagnostic Western blot. Ann Intern Med 1989;111:961.
56. Menitove JE. The decreasing risk of transfusion-associated AIDS. N Engl J Med 1989;321:966.
57. Cumming PD, Wallace EL, Schorr JB, Dodd RY. Exposure of patients to human immunodeficiency virus through the transfusion of blood components that test antibody-negative. N Engl J Med 1989;321:941.
58. Cohen ND, Munoz A, Reitz BA, et al. Transmission of retroviruses by transfusion of screened blood in patients undergoing cardiac surgery. N Engl J Med 1989;320:1172.
59. Donahue JG, Nelson KE, Munoz A, et al. Transmission of HIV by transfusion of screened blood. N Engl J Med 1990;323:1709.
60. Busch MP, Eble BE, Khayam-Bashi H, et al. Evaluation of screened blood donations for human immunodeficiency virus type 1 infection by culture and DNA amplification of pooled cells. N Engl J Med 1990;323:1709.
61. MacDonald KL, Jackson B, Bowman RJ, et al. Performance characteristics of serologic tests for human immunodeficiency virus type 1 (HIV-1) antibody among Minnesota blood donors. Ann Intern Med 1989;110:617.
62. Centers for Disease Control. Provision Public Health Service interagency recommendations for screening donated blood and plasma for antibody to the virus causing acquired immunodeficiency syndrome. MMWR 1985;34:1.
63. Arthos J, Deen KC, Chaikin MA, et al. Identification of the residues in human CD4 critical for the binding of HIV. Cell 1989;57:469.
64. Peterson A, Seed B. Genetic analysis of monoclonal antibody and HIV binding sites on the human lymphocyte antigen CD4. Cell 1988;54:65.
65. Clayton LK, Sieh M, Pious DA, Reinherz EL. Identification of human CD4 residues affecting class II MHC versus HIV-1 gp120 binding. Nature 1989;339:548.
66. Sattentau Q, Dalgleish AG, Weiss RA, Beverley PCL. Epitopes of the CD4 antigen and HIV infection. Science 1986;234:1120.
67. Smith DH, Byrn RA, Marsters SA, Gregory T, Groopman J, Capon DJ. Blocking of HIV-1 infectivity by a soluble, secreted form of the CD4 antigen. Science 1987;238:1704.
68. Kunsch C, Hartle HT, Wigdahl B. Infection of human fetal dorsal root ganglion glial cells with human immunodeficiency virus type 1 involves an entry mechanism independent of the CD4 T4A epitope. J Virol 1989;63:5054.
69. Tateno M, Scarano FG, Levy JA. Human immunodeficiency virus can infect CD4-negative human fibroblastoid cells. Proc Natl Acad Sci USA 1989;86:4287.

70. Harouse JM, Kunsch C, Hartle HT, et al. CD4-Independent infection of human neural cells by human immunodeficiency virus type 1. J Virol 1989;63:2527.
71. Cordonnier A, Montagnier L, Emerman M. Single amino-acid changes in HIV envelope affect viral tropism and receptor binding. Nature 1989;340:571.
72. Cordonnier A, Riviere Y, Montagnier L, Emerman M. Effects of mutations in hyperconserved regions of the extracellular glycoprotein of human immunodeficiency virus type 1 on receptor binding. J Virol 1989;63:4464.
73. Ho DD, Pomerantz RJ, Kaplan JC. Pathogenesis of infection with human immunodeficiency virus. N Engl J Med 1987;317:278.
74. Ho DD, Rota TR, Schooley RT, et al. Isolation of HTLV-III from cerebrospinal fluid and neural tissues of patients with neurologic syndromes related to the acquired immunodeficiency syndrome. N Engl J Med 1985;313:1493.
75. Koenig S, Gendelman HE, Orenstein JM, et al. Detection of AIDS virus in macrophages in brain tissue from AIDS patients with encephalopathy. Science 1986;233:1089.
76. Baltimore D, Feinberg MB. HIV revealed. N Engl J Med 1989;321: 1673.
77. Fauci AS. The human immunodeficiency virus: infectivity and mechanisms of pathogenesis. Science 1988;239:617.
78. Pantaleo G, Graziosi C, Fauci AS. The immunopathogenesis of human immunodeficiency virus infection. In: Epstein FH, eds. Mechanisms of Disease 328:327,1993.
79. Pantaleo G, Graziosi C, Butini L, et al. Lymphoid organs function as major reservoirs for human immunodeficiency virus. Proc Natl Acad Sci USA 1991;88:9838.
80. Embretson J, Zupancic M, Ribas JL, et al. Massive covert infection of helper T lymphocytes and macrophages by HIV during the incubation period of AIDS. Nature 1993;362:359.
80a. Wood R, Dong H, Katzenstein D, Merigan T. Quantification and comparison of HIV-1 proviral load in peripheral blood mononuclear cells and isolated CD4+ T cells. J Acquir Immune Defic Syndr 1993;6:237.
80b. Patterson B, Till M, Otto P, et al. Detection of HIV-1 DNA and messenger RNA in individual cells by PCR-driven in situ hybridization and flow cytometry. Science 1993;260:9776.
81. Piatak Jr. M, Saag MS, Yang LC, et al. High levels of HIV-1 in plasma during all stages of infection determined by competitive PCR. Science 1993;259:1749.
82. Donaldson YK, Bell JE, Ironside JW, et al. Redistribution of HIV outside the lymphoid system with onset of AIDS. Lancet 1994;343:382.
82a. Freedman AR, Scadden DT. Viral activity in early HIV disease. Curr Opin Hematol 1994;1:19.
83. Lifson JD, Reyes GR, McGrath MS, et al. AIDS retrovirus–induced cytopathology: giant cell formation and involvement of CD4 antigen. Science 1986;232:1123.
84. Tersmette M, Gruters RA, deWolf F, et al. Evidence for a role of virulent human immunodeficiency virus (HIV) variants in the pathogenesis of acquired immunodeficiency syndrome: studies on sequential HIV isolates. J Virol 1989;63:2118.
85. Chirmule N, Kalyanaraman VS, Oyaizu N, Slade HB, Pahwa S. Inhibition of functional properties of tetanus antigen-specific T-cell clones by envelope glycoprotein GP120 of human immunodeficiency virus. Blood 1990;75:152.
86. Gurley RJ, Ikeuchi K, Byrn RA, Anderson K, Groopman JE. CD4+ lymphocyte function with early human immunodeficiency virus infection. Proc Natl Acad Sci USA 1989;86:1993.
87. Mittler RS, Hoffman MK. Synergism between HIV gp120 and gp120-specific antibody in blocking human T cell activation. Science 1989;245:1380.
88. Amadori A, deSilvestro G, Zamarchi R, et al. CD4 epitope masking by gp120/anti-gp120 antibody complexes: a potential mechanism for CD4+ cell function down-regulation in AIDS patients. J Immunol 1992;148:2709.
89. Kornfeld H, Cruikshank WW, Pyle SW, Berman JS, Center DM. Lymphocyte activation by HIV-1 envelope glycoprotein. Nature 1988;335: 445.
90. Imbert L, Scottini A, Bettinard A, et al. Selective depletion in HIV infection of T cells that bear specific T cell receptor Vβ sequences. Science 1992;254:860.
91. Groux H, Torpier G, Monte D, et al. Activation-induced death by apoptosis in CD4+ T cells from human immunodeficiency virus–infected asymptomatic individuals. J Exp Med 1992;175:331.
92. Meyaard L, Otto SA, Jonker RR, et al. Programmed death of T cells in HIV-1 infection. Science 1992;257:217.
93. Lyerly HK, Matthews TJ, Langlois AJ, Bolognesi DP, Weinhold KJ. Human T-cell lymphotropic virus III_B glycoprotein (gp120) bound to CD4 determinants on normal lymphocytes and expressed by infected cells serves as target for immune attack. Proc Natl Acad Sci USA 1987;84:4601.
94. Siliciano RF, Lawton T, Kanll C, et al. Analysis of host-virus interactions in AIDS with anti-gp120 T cell clones: effect of HIV sequence variation and a mechanism for CD4+ cell depletion. Cell 1988;54: 561.
95. Schnittman SM, Psallidopoulos MC, Lane HC, et al. The reservoir for HIV-1 in human peripheral blood is a T cell that maintains expression of CD4. Science 1989;245:305.
96. Psallidopoulos MC, Schnittman SM, Thompson LM, et al. Integrated proviral human immunodeficiency virus type 1 is present in CD4+ peripheral blood lymphocytes in healthy seropositive individuals. J Virol 1989;63:4626.
97. Bacchetti P, Moss AR. Incubation period of AIDS in San Francisco. Nature 1989;338:251.
98. Costagliola D, Mary JY, Brouard N, Laporte A, Valleron AJ. Incubation time for AIDS from French transfusion-associated cases. Nature 1989;338:768.
99. Shalaby MR, Krowka JF, Gregory TJ, et al. The effects of human immunodeficiency virus recombinant envelope glycoprotein on immune cell functions in vitro. Cell Immunol 1987;110:140.
100. Gartner S, Markovits P, Markovitz DM, Kaplan MH, Gallo RC, Popovic M. The role of mononuclear phagocytes in HTLV-III/LAV infection. Science 1986;233:215.
101. Ho DD, Rota TR, Hirsch MS. Infection of monocyte/macrophages by human T-lymphotropic virus type III. J Clin Invest 1986;77:1712.
102. Popovic M, Gartner S. Isolation of HIV-1 from monocytes but not T lymphocytes. Lancet 1987;2:916.
103. Poli G, Bottazzi B, Acero R, et al. Monocyte function in intravenous drug abusers with lymphadenopathy syndrome and in patients with acquired immunodeficiency syndrome: selective impairment of chemotaxis. Clin Exp Immunol 1985;62:136.
104. Gendelman HE, Orenstein JM, Baca LM, et al. The macrophage in the persistence and pathogenesis of HIV infection. AIDS 1989;3: 475.
105. Miotti, PG, Nelson KE, Dallabetta GA, Farzadegan H, Margolick J, Clements ML. The influence of HIV infection on antibody responses to a two-dose regimen of influenza vaccine. JAMA 1989;262:779.
106. Ho DD, Bredesen DE, Vinters HV, Daar ES. The acquired immunodeficiency syndrome (AIDS) dementia complex. Ann Intern Med 1989;111:400.
107. Pang S, Koyanagi Y, Miles S, Wiley C, Vinters HV, Chen ISY. High levels of unintegrated HIV-1 DNA in brain tissue of AIDS dementia patients. Nature 1990;343:85.
108. Wahl LM, Corcoran ML, Pyle ST, Arthur LO, Bellan AH, Farrar WL. Human immunodeficiency virus glycoprotein (gp120) induction of monocyte arachidonic acid metabolites and interleukin 1. Proc Natl Acad Sci USA 1989;86:621.
109. Merrill JE, Koyanagi Y, Chen ISY. Interleukin-1 and tumor necrosis factor alpha can be induced from mononuclear phagocytes by human immunodeficiency virus type 1 binding to the CD4 receptor. J Virol 1989;63:4404.
110. Molina JM, Scadden DT, Amirault C, et al. Human immunodeficiency virus does not induce interleukin-1, interleukin-6, or tumor necrosis factor in mononuclear cells. J Virol 1990;64:2901.
111. Fahey JL, Taylor JMG, Detels R, et al. The prognostic value of cellular and serologic markers in infection with human immunodeficiency virus type 1. N Engl J Med 1990;322:166.
112. Phair J, Munoz A, Detels R, Kaslow R, Rinaldo C, Saar A, Multicenter AIDS Cohort Study Group: the risk of *Pneumocystis carinii* pneumonia among men infected with human immunodeficiency virus type 1. N Engl J Med 1990;322:161.
113. Eyster ME, Ballard JO, Gail MH, Drummond JE, Goedert JJ. Predictive markers for the acquired immunodeficiency syndrome (AIDS) in hemophiliacs: persistence of p24 antigen and low T4 cell count. Ann Intern Med 1989;110:963.
114. Ward JW, Bush TJ, Perkins HA, et al. The natural history of transfusion-associated infection with human immunodeficiency virus. N Engl J Med 1989;321:947.
115. Schoenbaum EE, Hartel D, Selwyn PA, et al. Risk factors for human immunodeficiency virus infection in intravenous drug users. N Engl J Med 1989;321:874.
116. Goedert JJ, Kessler CM, Aledort LM, et al. A prospective study of human immunodeficiency virus type 1 infection and the development of AIDS in subjects with hemophilia. N Engl J Med 1989;321:1141.
117. Selwyn PA, Schoenbaum EE, Davenny K, et al. Prospective study of human immunodeficiency virus infection and pregnancy outcomes in intravenous drug users. JAMA 1989;261:1289.
118. Koonin LM, Ellerbrock TV, Atrash HK, et al. Pregnancy-associated deaths due to AIDS in the United States. JAMA 1989;261:1306.
119. Goedert JJ, Mendez H, Drummond JE, et al. Mother-to-infant transmission of human immunodeficiency virus type 1: association with prematurity or low anti-gp120. Lancet 1989;2:1351.
120. Rogers MF, Ou CY, Rayfield M, et al. New York City Collaborative Study of Maternal HIV Transmission and Montefiore Medical Center HIV Perinatal Transmission Study Group: use of the polymerase chain reaction for early detection of the proviral sequences of human immunodeficiency virus in infants born to seropositive mothers. N Engl J Med 1989;320:1649.
121. Blanche S, Rouzioux C, Moscato MLG, et al. HIV Infection in Newborns French Collaborative Study Group: a prospective study of infants born to women seropositive for human immunodeficiency virus type 1. N Engl J Med 1989;320:1643.
122. Ryder RW, Nsa W, Hassig SE, et al. Perinatal transmission of the

human immunodeficiency virus type 1 to infants of seropositive women in Zaire. N Engl J Med 1989;320:1637.
123. Newell ML, Dunn D, Peckham CS, et al. Risk factors for mother-to-child transmission of HIV-1. Lancet 1992;339:1007.
124. Rhame FS, Maki DG. The case for wider use of testing for HIV infection. N Engl J Med 1989;320:1248.
125. Mann JM, Francis H, Quinn T, et al. Surveillance for AIDS in a central African city: Kinshasa, Zaire. JAMA 1986;255:3255.
126. Cameron DW, D'Costa LJ, Maitha GM, et al. Female to male transmission of human immunodeficiency virus type 1: risk factors for seroconversion in men. Lancet 1989;2:403.
127. Becker CE, Cone JE, Gerberding J. Occupational infection with human immunodeficiency virus (HIV): risks and risk reduction. Ann Intern Med 1989;110:653.
128. Scannell KA. Surgery and human immunodeficiency virus disease. J AIDS 1989;2:43.
129. Centers for Disease Control. Guidelines for prevention of transmission of human immunodeficiency virus and hepatitis B virus to health-care and public-safety workers. MMWR 1989;38:June 23.
130. Centers for Disease Control. Public health service statement on management of occupational exposure to human immunodeficiency virus, including considerations regarding zidovudine postexposure use. MMWR 1990;39:January 26.
131. Sperling RS, Stratton P, O'Sullivan MJ, et al. A survey of zidovudine use in pregnant women with human immunodeficiency virus infection. N Engl J Med 1992;326:857.
132. Fauci AS, Gallo RC, Koenig S, Salk J, Purcell RH. Development and evaluation of a vaccine for human immunodeficiency virus (HIV) infection. Ann Intern Med 1989;110:373.
133. Walker BD, Chakrabarti S, Moss B, et al. HIV-specific cytotoxic T lymphocytes in seropositive individuals. Nature 1987;328:345.
134. Wigzell H. Immunopathogenesis of HIV infection. J AIDS 1988;1:559.
135. Berman PW, Riddle L, Nakamura G, et al. Expression and immunogenicity of the extracellular domain of the human immunodeficiency virus type 1 envelope glycoprotein, gp160. J Virol 1989;63: 3489.
136. Javaherian K, Langlois AJ, McDanal C, et al. Principal neutralizing domain of the human immunodeficiency virus type 1 envelope protein. Proc Natl Acad Sci USA 1989;86:6768.
137. Desrosiers RC, Wyand MS, Kodama T, et al. Vaccine protection against simian immunodeficiency virus infection. Proc Natl Acad Sci USA 1989;86:6353.
138. Stott EJ, Chan WL, Mills KHG, et al. Preliminary report: protection of cynomolgus macaques against simian immunodeficiency virus by fixed infected-cell vaccine. Lancet 1990;336:1538.
139. Daniel MD, Kirchhoff F, Czajak SC, et al. Protective effects of a live attenuated HIV vaccine with a deletion in the *nef* gene. Science 1992;258:1938.
140. Lehner T, Bergmeier LA, Panagiotidi C, et al. Induction of mucosal and systemic immunity to a recombinant simian immunodeficiency viral protein. Science 1992;258:1365.
141. Berman PW, Gregory TJ, Riddle L, et al. Protection of chimpanzees from infection by HIV-1 after vaccination with recombinant glycoprotein gp120 but not gp160. Nature 1990;345:622.
142. Fultz PN, Nara P, Barre-Sinoussi F, et al. Vaccine protection of chimpanzees against challenge with HIV-1–infected peripheral blood mononuclear cells. Science 1992;25:1687.
143. Dolin R, Graham BS, Greenberg SB, et al. The safety and immunogenicity of a human immunodeficiency virus type 1 (HIV-1) recombinant gp160 candidate vaccine in humans. Ann Intern Med 1991;114: 119.
144. Phillips RE, Rowland-Jones S, Nixon DF, et al. Human immunodeficiency virus genetic variation that can escape cytotoxic T cell recognition. Nature 1991;354:453.
145. Yarchoan R, Mitsuya H, Myers CE, Broder S. Clinical pharmacology of 3′-azido-2′, 3′-dideoxythymidine (zidovudine) and related dideoxynucleosides. N Engl J Med 1989;321:726.
146. Volberding PA, Lagakos ST, Koch MA, et al. Zidovudine in asymptomatic human immunodeficiency virus infection: a controlled trial in persons with fewer than 500 CD4-positive cells per cubic millimeter. N Engl J Med 1990;322:941.
147. Fischl MA, Richman DD, Grieco MH, et al. The efficacy of azidothymidine (AZT) in the treatment of patients with AIDS and AIDS-related complex: a double-blind, placebo-controlled trial. N Engl J Med 1987;317:185.
148. Dournon E, Rozenbaum W, Michon C, et al. Effects of zidovudine in 365 consecutive patients with AIDS and AIDS-related complex. Lancet 1988;2:1297.
149. Creagh-Kirk T, Doi P, Andrews E, et al. Survival experience among patients with AIDS receiving zidovudine: follow-up of patients in a compassionate plea program. JAMA 1988;260:3009.
150. Schmidt FA, Bigley JW, McKinnis R, et al. Neuropsychological outcome of zidovudine (AZT) treatment of patients with AIDS and AIDS-related complex. N Engl J Med 1988;319:1573.
151. Volberding PA, Lagakos SW, Koch MA, et al. Zidovudine in asymptomatic human immunodeficiency virus infection: a controlled trial in persons with fewer than 500 CD4-positive cells per cubic millimeter. N Engl J Med 1990;332:941.
152. Merigan TC, Amato DA, Balsley J. Placebo-controlled trial to evaluate zidovudine in treatment of human immunodeficiency virus infection in asymptomatic patients with hemophilia. Blood 1991;78:900.
153. Aboulker JP, Swart AM. Preliminary analysis of the Concorde trial. Lancet 1993;341:889.
154. Lagakos S. Fischl MA, Stein DS, et al. Effects of zidovudine therapy in minority and other subpopulations with early HIV infection. JAMA 1991;266:2709.
155. Easterbrook PJ, Keruly JC, Creagh-Kirk T, et al. Racial and ethnic differences in outcome in zidovudine-treated patients with advanced HIV disease. JAMA 1991;266:2713.
156. Volberding PA, Lagakos SW, Koch MA, et al. Zidovudine in asymptomatic human immunodeficiency virus infection. N Engl J Med 1990;322:941.
157. Moore RD, Hidalgo J, Sugland BW, et al. Zidovudine and the natural history of the acquired immunodeficiency syndrome. N Engl J Med 1991;324:1412.
158. Fischl MA, Richmand DD, Hansen N, et al. The safety and efficacy of zidovudine (AZT) in the treatment of subjects with mildly symptomatic human immunodeficiency virus type 1 (HIV) infection. Ann Intern Med 1991;112:727.
159. Hamilton JD, Hartigan PM, Simberkoff MS, et al. A controlled trial of early versus late treatment with zidovudine in symptomatic human immunodeficiency virus infection. N Engl J Med 1992;326:437.
160. Vella S, Giuliano M, Pezzotti P, et al. Survival of zidovudine-treated patients with AIDS compared with that of contemporary untreated patients. JAMA 1992;267:1232.
161. Merigan TC, Amato DA, Balsley J, et al. Placebo-controlled trial to evaluate zidovudine in treatment of human immunodeficiency virus infection in asymptomatic patients with hemophilia. Blood 1991;78: 900.
162. Cooper DA, Pehrson PO, Pedersen C, et al. The efficacy and safety of zidovudine alone or as cotherapy with acyclovir for the treatment of patients with AIDS and AIDS-related complex: a double-blind, randomized trial. AIDS 1993;7:197.
163. McLeod GX, Hammer SM. Zidovudine: five years later. Ann Intern Med 1992;117:487.
163a. Sande MA, Carpenter CCJ, Cobbs CG, Holmes KK, Sanford JP. Antiretroviral therapy for adult HIV-infected patients: recommendations from a state-of-the-art conference. JAMA 1993;270:2583–2589.
163b. Lenderking WR, Gelber RD, Cotton DJ, Cole BF, Goldhirsch A, Volberding PA, Testa MA. Evaluation of the quality of life associated with zidovudine treatment in asymptomatic human immunodeficiency virus infection. N Engl J Med 1993;738.
164. Richman DD, Fischl MA, Grieco MH, et al. The toxicity of azidothymidine (AZT) in the treatment of patients with AIDS and AIDS-related complex: a double-blind, placebo-controlled trial. N Engl J Med 1987;317:192.
165. Walker RE, Parker RI, Kovacs JA, et al. Anemia and erythropoiesis in patients with the acquired immunodeficiency syndrome (AIDS) and Kaposi sarcoma, treated with zidovudine. Ann Intern Med 1988;108:372.
166. Bessen LJ, Greene JB, Louie E, Seitzman P, Weinberg H. Severe polymyositislike syndrome associated with zidovudine therapy of AIDS and ARC. (Letter) N Engl J Med 1988;318:708.
167. Dalakos MC, Illa I, Pezeshkpour GH, Laukaitis JP, Cohen B, Griffin JL. Mitochondrial myopathy caused by long-term zidovudine therapy. N Engl J Med 1990;322:1098.
168. Kahn JO, Lagakos SW, Richman DD, et al. A controlled trial comparing zidovudine with didanosine in human immunodeficiency virus infection. N Engl J Med 1992;327:581.
169. Groopman JE, Molina J-M. Nucleoside therapy for HIV infection: some answers, many questions. N Engl J Med 1992;327:639.
170. Fischl MA, Olson RM, Follansbee SE, et al. Zalcitabine compared with zidovudine in patients with advanced HIV-1 infection who received previous zidovudine therapy. Ann Intern Med 1993;118:762.
171. Meng T-C, Fischl MA, Boota AM. Combination therapy with zidovudine and dideoxycytidine in patients with advanced human immunodeficiency virus infection. Ann Intern Med 1992;116:13.
171a. Abrams DI, Goldman AI, Launder C, et al. A comparative trial of didanosine or zalcitabine after treatment with zidovudine in patients with human immunodeficiency virus infection. N Engl J Med 1994;330:657.
172. Larder BA, Darby G, Richman DD. HIV with reduced sensitivity to zidovudine (AZT) isolated during prolonged therapy. Science 1989;243:1731.
173. Larder BA, Kemp SD, Purifoy DJM. Infectious potential of human immunodeficiency virus type 1 reverse transcriptase mutants with altered inhibitor sensitivity. Proc Natl Acad Sci USA 1989;86:4803.
174. Rooke R, Tremblay M, Soudeyns H, et al. Canadian Zidovudine Multi-Centre Study Group: isolation of drug-resistant variants of HIV-1 from patients on long-term zidovudine therapy. AIDS 1989;3:411.
175. Matsukura M, Zon G, Shinozuka K, et al. Regulation of viral expression of human immunodeficiency virus in vitro by an antisense phospho-

rothioate oligodeoxynucleoside against rev (art/trs) in chronically infected cells. Proc Natl Acad Sci USA 1989;86:4244.
176. Trono D, Feinberg MB, Baltimore D. HIV-1 gag mutants can dominantly interfere with the replication of the wild-type virus. Cell 1989;113.
177. Dreyer GB, Metcalf BW, Tomaszek TA Jr, et al. Inhibition of human immunodeficiency virus 1 protease in vitro: rational design of substrate analogue inhibitors. Proc Natl Acad Sci USA 1989;86:9752.
178. Meek TD, Lambert DM, Dreyer GB, et al. Inhibition of HIV-1 protease in infected T-lymphocytes by synthetic peptide analogues. Nature 1990;343:90.
179. Weber IT, Miller M, Jaskolski M, Leis J, Skalka AM, Wlodawer A. Molecular modeling of the HIV-1 protease and its substrate binding site. Science 1989;243:928.
180. Wlodawer A, Miller M, Jaskolski M, et al. Conserved folding in retroviral proteases: crystal structure of a synthetic HIV-1 protease. Science 1989;245:616.
181. Navia MA, Fitzgerald P, McKeever BM, et al. Three-dimensional structure of aspartyl protease from human immunodeficiency virus (HIV-1). Nature 1989;337:615.
182. Byrn RA, Sekigawa I, Chamow SM, et al. Characterization of in vitro inhibition of human immunodeficiency virus by purified recombinant CD4. J Virol 1989;63:4370.
183. Schooley RT, Merigan TC, Gaut P, et al. Recombinant soluble CD4 therapy in patients with the acquired immunodeficiency syndrome (AIDS) and AIDS-related complex: a phase I-II escalating dosage trial. Ann Intern Med 1990;112:247.
184. Kahn JO, Allan D, Hodges TL, et al. The safety and pharmacokinetics of recombinant soluble CD4 (rCD4) in subjects with the acquired immunodeficiency syndrome (AIDS) and AIDS-related complex: a phase I study. Ann Intern Med 1990;112:254.
185. Capon DJ, Chamow SM, Mordenti J, et al. Designing CD4 immunoadhesins for AIDS therapy. Nature 1989;337:525.
186. Byrn RA, Mordenti J, Lucas C, et al. Biological properties of a CD4 immunoadhesin. Nature 1990;344:667.
187. Till MA, Ghetie V, Gregory T, et al. HIV-infected cells are killed by rCD4-ricin A chain. Science 1988;242:1166.
188. Chaudhary VK, Mizukami T, Fuerst TR, et al. Selective killing of HIV-infected cells by recombinant CD4–*Pseudomonas* exotoxin hybrid protein. Nature 1988;335:369.
189. Walker BD, Kowalski MM, Goh WC, et al. Inhibition of human immunodeficiency virus syncytium formation and virus replication by castanospermine. Proc Natl Acad Sci USA 1987;84:8120.
190. Pauwels R, Andries K, Desmyter J, et al. Potent and selective inhibition of HIV-1 replication in vitro by a novel series of TIBO derivatives. Nature 1990;343:470.
191. McGrath MS, Hwang KM, Caldwell SE, et al. GLQ223: an inhibitor of human immunodeficiency virus replication in acutely and chronically infected cells of lymphocyte and mononuclear phagocyte lineage. Proc Natl Acad Sci USA 1989;86:2844.
192. Kornbluth RS, Oh PS, Munis JR, Cleveland PH, Richman DD. Interferons and bacterial lipopolysaccharide protect macrophages from productive infection by human immunodeficiency virus in vitro. J Exp Med 1989;169:1137.
193. Poll G, Orenstein JM, Kinter A, Folks TM, Fauci AS. Interferon-alpha but not AZT suppresses HIV expression in chronically infected cell lines. Science 1989;224:575.
194. Kovacs JA, Deyton L, Falloon DR, et al. Combined zidovudine and interferon-alpha therapy in patients with Kaposi sarcoma and the acquired immunodeficiency syndrome (AIDS). Ann Intern Med 1989;111:280.
195. Spivak JL, Sclonick SE, Quinn TC. Acquired immune deficiency syndrome and pancytopenia. JAMA 1983;250:3084.
196. Spivak JL, Bender BS, Quinn TC. Hematologic abnormalities in the acquired immune deficiency syndrome. Am J Med 1984;77:224.
197. Zon LI, Arkin C, Groopman JE. Haematologic manifestations of the human immune deficiency virus (HIV). Br J Haematol 1987;66:251.
198. Treacy M, Lai L, Costello C, Clark A. Peripheral blood and bone marrow abnormalities in patients with HIV-related disease. Br J Haematol 1987;65:289.
199. Scadden, DT, Zon LI, Groopman JE. Pathophysiology and management of HIV-associated hematologic disorders. Blood 1989;74:1455.
200. Solis OC, Belmonte AH, Ramaswamy G. Pseudogaucher cells in *Mycobacterium avium-intracellulare* infections in acquired immune deficiency syndrome (AIDS). Am J Clin Pathol 1986;85:233.
201. Kovacs JA, Kovacs AA, Polis M, et al. Cryptococcosis in the acquired immunodeficiency syndrome. Ann Intern Med 1985;103:533.
202. Mandell W, Goldberg DM, Neu HC. Histoplasmosis in patients with the acquired immunodeficiency syndrome. Am J Med 1986;81:974.
203. Rossi JF, Dubois A, Bengler C, et al. *Pneumocystis carinii* in bone marrow. Ann Intern Med 1985;102:868.
204. Raviglione MC, Garner GR, Mullen MP. *Pneumocystis carinii* in bone marrow. Ann Intern Med 1988;109:253.
205. Little BJ, Spivak JL, Quinn TC, et al. Kaposi's sarcoma with bone marrow involvement: occurrence in a patient with the acquired immunodeficiency syndrome. Am J Med Sci 1986;292:44.
206. Northfelt DW, Mayer A, Kaplan LD, et al. The usefulness of diagnostic bone marrow examination in patients with human immunodeficiency virus (HIV) infection. J AIDS 1991;4:659.
207. Mir N, Costello C, Luckit J, Lindley R. HIV-disease and bone marrow changes: a study of 60 cases. Eur J Haematol 1989;42:339.
208. Osborne BM, Guarda LA, Butler JJ. Bone marrow biopsies in patients with the acquired immunodeficiency syndrome. Hum Pathol 1984;15:1048.
209. Costella A, Croxson TS, Mildvan D, et al. The bone marrow in AIDS: a histologic, hematologic and microbiologic study. Am J Clin Pathol 1985;84:425.
210. Perkocha LA, Rodgers GM. Hematologic aspects of human immunodeficiency virus infection: laboratory and clinical considerations. Am J Hematol 1988;29:94.
211. Franco CM, Hendrix LE, Lokey JL. Bone marrow abnormalities in the acquired immunodeficiency syndrome. (Letter) Ann Intern Med 1984;101:275.
212. Geller SA, Muller R, Greenberg ML, Siegal FP. Acquired immunodeficiency syndrome: distinctive features of bone marrow biopsies. Arch Pathol Lab Med 1985;109:138.
213. Hromas RA, Murray JL. Bone marrow in the acquired immunodeficiency syndrome. (Letter) Ann Intern Med 1984;101:877.
214. Schneider DR, Picker LJ. Myelodysplasia in the acquired immune deficiency syndrome. Am J Clin Pathol 1985;84:144.
215. Solis OG, Belmonte AH, Ramaswamy G, Tchertkoff V. Pseudogaucher cells in *Mycobacterium avium-intracellulare* infections in acquired immune deficiency syndrome (AIDS). Am J Clin Pathol 1986;85:233.
216. Donahue RE, Johnson MM, Zon LI, Groopman JE. In vitro suppression of hematopoiesis after human immunodeficiency virus infection. Nature 1987;326:200.
217. Leiderman IZ, Greenberg ML, Adelsberg BR, Siegal FP. A glycoprotein inhibitor of in vitro granulopoiesis associated with AIDS. Blood 1987;70:1267.
218. Sloand EM. Epidemiology of thrombocytopenia in HIV infection. Eur J Haematol 1992;48:168.
219. Stella CC, Ganser A, Hoelzer D. Defective in vitro growth of the hemopoietic progenitor cells in the acquired immunodeficiency syndrome. J Clin Invest 1987;80:286.
220. Molina JM, Scadden DT, Sakaguchi M, Fuller B, Woon A, Groopman JE. Growth of hematopoietic progenitor cells after in vivo or in vitro exposure to human immunodeficiency virus. Blood 1990;76:2776.
221. Von Laer D, Hufert FT, Fenner TE, et al. CD34+ hematopoietic progenitor cells are not a major reservoir of the human immunodeficiency virus. Blood 1990;76:1281.
222. Davis BR, Marx JC, Johnson CE, et al. Absent or rare HIV infection of bone marrow stem/progenitor cells in vivo. J Virol 1991;65:1985.
223. Steinberg HN, Crumacker CS, Chatis PA. In vitro suppression of normal human bone marrow progenitor cells by human immunodeficiency virus. J Virol 1991;65:1765.
224. Zauli G, Re MC, Visani G, et al. Evidence for an human immunodeficiency virus-type 1 mediated suppression of uninfected hematopoietic (CD34+) progenitor cells in AIDS patients. J Infect Dis 1992;166:710.
225. Zauli G, Vitale M, Re MC, et al. In vitro exposure to human immunodeficiency virus type 1 induces apoptotic cell death of the factor-dependent TF-1 hematopoietic cell line. Blood 1994;83:167.
226. Ganser A, Ottman OG, Briesen HV, et al. Changes in the hematopoietic progenitor cell compartment in the acquired immunodeficiency syndrome. Res Virol 1990;141:185.
227. Please provide.
228. Folks TM, Kessler SW, Orenstein JM, Justement JS, Jaffe ES, Fauci AS. Infection and replication of HIV-1 in purified progenitor cells of normal human bone marrow. Science 1988;242:919.
229. Kitano K, Abboud CN, Ryan DH, Quan SG, Baldwin GC, Golde DW. Macrophage-active colony-stimulating factors enhance human immunodeficiency virus type 1 infection in bone marrow stem cells. Blood 1991;77:1699.
230. Schuitemaker H, Kootstra NA, Koppelman MHGM, et al. Proliferation-dependent HIV-1 infection of monocytes occurs during differentiation into macrophages. J Clin Invest 1992;89:1154.
231. Louache F, et al. Infection of megakaryocytes by human immunodeficiency virus in seropositive patients with immune thrombocytopenic purpura. Blood 1991;78:1697.
232. Zauli G, et al. Lack of compensatory megakaryocytopoiesis in HIV-1–seropositive thrombocytopositive thrombocytopenic purpura patients. AIDS 1991;5:1345.
233. Scadden DT, Zeira M, Woon A, et al. Human immunodeficiency virus infection of human bone marrow stromal fibroblasts. Blood 1990;76:317.
234. Steffan AM, Lafon ME, Gendrault JL, et al. Primary cultures of endothelial cells from the human liver sinusoid are permissive for human immunodeficiency virus type 1. Proc Natl Acad Sci 1992;89:1582.
235. Calenda V, Sebahoun G, Chermann JC. Modulation of normal human erythropoietic progenitor cells in long-term liquid cultures after HIV-1 infection. AIDS 1992;8:61.
236. Zauli G, Davis BR, Carla Re M, et al. *tat* Protein stimulates production of transforming growth factor-$\beta 1$ by marrow macrophages: a potential

mechanism for human immunodeficiency virus-1–induced hematopoietic suppression. Blood 1992;80:3036.
237. Molina JM, Scadden DT, Byrn RA, Dinarello CA, Groopman JE. Production of tumor necrosis factor and interleukin-1 by monocytic cells infected with human immunodeficiency virus. J Clin Invest 1989;84:733.
238. Ladevirta J, Maury CPJ, Teppo A-M, Repo H. Elevated levels of circulating cachectin/tumor necrosis factor in patients with acquired immunodeficiency syndrome. Am J Med 1988;85:289.
239. Reddy MM, Sorrell SJ, Lange M, Grieco MH. Tumor necrosis factor and HIV P24 antigen levels in serum of HIV-infected populations. J AIDS 1988;1:436.
240. Breen EC, Rezai AR, Nakajima K, et al. Infection with HIV is associated with elevated IL-6 during human immunodeficiency virus infection. J Immunol 1990;144:480.
241. Kekow J, Wachsman W, McCutchan JA, et al. Transforming growth factor beta and noncytopathic mechanisms of immunodeficiency virus infection. Proc Natl Acad Sci 1991;87:8321.
242. Spivak JL, Barnes D, Fuchs E, Quinn TC. Serum immunoreactive erythropoietin in HIV-infected patients. JAMA 1989;261:3104.
243. Rarick MU, Loureiro C, Groshen S, et al. Serum erythropoietin titers in patients with human immunodeficiency virus (HIV) infection and anemia. J AIDS 1991;4:593.
245. Holzman RS, Walsh CM, Karpatkin S. Risk for the acquired immunodeficiency syndrome among thrombocytopenic and nonthrombocytopenic homosexual men seropositive for the human immunodeficiency virus. Ann Intern Med 1987;106:383.
246. Boccia RV, Gelmann EP, Baker CC, Marti G, Longo DL. A hemolytic uremic syndrome with the acquired immunodeficiency syndrome. Ann Intern Med 1984;101:716.
247. Jokela J, Flynn T, Henry K. Thrombotic thrombocytopenic purpura in a patient who subsequently developed the acquired immunodeficiency syndrome (AIDS). Ann Intern Med 1988;109:242.
248. Walsh CM, Nardi MA, Karpatkin S. On the mechanism of thrombocytopenic purpura in sexually active homosexual men. N Engl J Med 1984;311:635.
249. Stricker RB, Abrams DI, Corash L, Shuman MA. Target platelet antigen in homosexual men with immune thrombocytopenia. N Engl J Med 1985;313:1375.
250. Yu JR, Lennette ET, Karpatkin S. Anti-F(ab')2 antibodies in thrombocytopenic patients at risk for acquired immunodeficiency syndrome. J Clin Invest 1986;77:1756.
251. Karpatkin S, Nardi M, Lennette ET, Byrne B, Poiesz B. Anti-human immunodeficiency virus type 1 antibody complexes on platelets of seropositive thrombocytopenic homosexuals and narcotic addicts. Proc Natl Acad Sci USA 1988;85:9763.
251a. Bettaieb A, Fromont P, Louache F, et al. Presence of cross-reactive antibody between human immunodeficiency virus (HIV) and platelet glycoproteins in HIV-related immune thrombocytopenic purpura. Blood 1992;80:162.
251b. Hohmann AW, Booth K, Peters V, Gordon DL, Comacchio RM. Common epitope on HIV p24 and human platelets. Lancet 1993;342:1274.
252. Bettaieb A, et al. Presence of cross-reactive antibody between human immunodeficiency virus (HIV) and platelet glycoproteins in HIV-related immune thrombocytopenic purpura. Blood 1992;80:162.
253. Bender BS, Frank MM, Lawley TJ, Smith WJ, Brickman CM, Quinn TC. Defective reticuloendothelial system Fc-receptor function in patients with acquired immunodeficiency syndrome. J Infect Dis 1985;152:409.
254. Bender BS, Quinn TC, Spivak JL. Homosexual men with thrombocytopenia have impaired reticuloendothelial system Fc receptor–specific clearance. Blood 1987;70:392.
255. Kelton JG, Carter CJ, Rodger C, et al. The relationship among platelet-associated IgG, platelet lifespan, and reticuloendothelial cell function. Blood 1984;63:1434.
256. Karpatkin S, Nardi M. Immunologic thrombocytopenic purpura in human immunodeficiency virus–seropositive patients with hemophilia: comparison with patients with classic autoimmune thrombocytopenic purpura, homosexuals with thrombocytopenia, and narcotic addicts with thrombocytopenia. J Lab Clin Med 1988;111:441.
257. Ragni M, Pontempo F, Myers D, Kiss J, Oral A. Hemorrhagic sequelae of immune thrombocytopenic purpura (ITP) in HIV infected hemophiliacs. Blood 1989;90(Suppl 1):127a.
258. Pottage JC, Benson CA, Spear JB, Landay AL, Kessler HA. Treatment of human immunodeficiency virus–related thrombocytopenia with zidovudine. JAMA 1988;260:3045.
259. Gottlieb MS, Wolfe PR, Chafey S. Response of AIDS-related thrombocytopenia to intravenous and oral azidothymidine (3'-azido-3'deoxythymidine). AIDS Res Hum Retroviruses 1987;3:109.
260. Fischl MA, Parker CB, Pettinelli C, et al. A randomized controlled trial of a reduced daily dose of zidovudine in patients with the acquired immunodeficiency syndrome. N Engl J Med 1990;323:1009.
261. Oksenhendler E, Bierling P, Ferchal F, Chauvel J, Seligmann. Zidovudine for thrombocytopenia related to human immunodeficiency virus infection. Ann Intern Med 1989;110:366.
262. Hymes KB, Greene JB, Karpatkin S. The effect of azidothymidine on HIV-related thrombocytopenia. N Engl J Med 1988;318:516.
262a. Pottage JC, Benson CA, Spear JB, Landay AL, Kessler HA. Treatment of human immunodeficiency virus–related thrombocytopenia with zidovudine. JAMA 1988;260:3045.
262b. Swiss Group for Clinical Studies on the Acquired Immunodeficiency Syndrome (AIDS). Zidovudine for the treatment of thrombocytopenia associated with human immunodeficiency virus (HIV). Ann Intern Med 1988;109:718.
263. Rosenfelt FP, Rosenbloom BE, Weinstein IM. Immune thrombocytopenia in homosexual men. Ann Intern Med 1984;104:583.
264. Ratner L. Human immunodeficiency virus-associated autoimmune thrombocytopenic purpura: a review. Am J Med 1989;86:194.
265. Walsh C, Krigel R, Lennette E, Karpatkin S. Thrombocytopenia in homosexual patients: prognosis, response to therapy, and prevalence of antibody to the retrovirus associated with the acquired immunodeficiency syndrome. Ann Intern Med 1985;103:542.
266. Goldsweig HG, Grossman R, William D. Thrombocytopenia in homosexual men. Am J Hematol 1986;21:243.
267. Costello C, Treacy M, Lai L. Treatment of immune thrombocytopenia in homosexual men. Scand J Haematol 1986;36:507.
268. Schneider PA, Abrams DI, Rayner AA, Hohn DC. Immunodeficiency-associated thrombocytopenic purpura (IDTP): response to splenectomy. Arch Surg 1987;122:1175.
269. Barbui T, Cortelazzo S, Minetti B, Galli M, Buelli M. Does splenectomy enhance risk of AIDS in HIV-positive patients with chronic thrombocytopenia? (Letter) Lancet 1987;2:342.
270. Tertian G, Boue F, Lebras P, et al. Thrombocytopenia in ARC: management with high dose IV IgG. Vox Sang 1987;52:170.
271. Beard J, Savidge GF. High-dose intravenous immunoglobulin and splenectomy for the treatment of HIV-related immune thrombocytopenia in patients with severe haemophilia. Br J Haematol 1988;68:303.
272. Pollak AN, Janinis J, Green D. Successful intravenous immune globulin therapy for human immunodeficiency virus–associated thrombocytopenia. Arch Intern Med 1988;148:695.
273. Oskenhendler E, Bierling P, Brossard Y, et al. Anti-Rh immunoglobulin therapy for human immunodeficiency virus–related immune thrombocytopenia. Blood 1988;71:1499.
274. Biniek R, Malessa R, Brockmeyer NH, Luboldt W. Anti-Rh(D) immunoglobulin for AIDS-related thrombocytopenia. Lancet 1986;2:627.
275. Fischl MA, Ahn YS, Klimas N, Harrington WJ, Fletcher MA. Use of Danazol in autoimmune thrombocytopenic purpura associated with the acquired immunodeficiency syndrome. (Abstract) Blood 1984;64:236a.
276. Mintzer DM, Real FX, Jovino L, Krown SE. Treatment of Kaposi's sarcoma and thrombocytopenia with vincristine in patients with the acquired immunodeficiency syndrome. Ann Intern Med 1985;102:200.
277. Ellis ME, Neal KR, Leen CLS, Newland AC. Alfa-2a recombinant interferon in HIV-associated thrombocytopenia. Br Med J 1987;295:1519.
278. Lever AML, Brook MG, Yap I, Thomas HC. Treatment of thrombocytopenia with alpha interferon. Br Med J 1987;295:1519.
279. Durand JM, Lefevre P, Hovette P, et al. Dapsone for thrombocytopenic purpura related to human immunodeficiency virus infection. Am J Med 1991;90:675.
280. Gill PS, Loureiro C, Bernstein-Singer M, Rarick MU, Satter F, Levine AM. Clinical effect of glucocorticoids on kaposi sarcoma related to the acquired immunodeficiency syndrome (AIDS). Ann Intern Med 1989;110:937.
281. Toy PT, Reid ME, Burns M. Positive direct antiglobulin test associated with hyperglobulinemia in acquired immunodeficiency syndrome (AIDS). Am J Hematol 1985;19:145.
282. McGuinniss MH, Macher AM, Rook AH, Alter HJ. Red cell autoantibodies in patients with acquired immune deficiency syndrome. Transfusion 1986;26:405.
283. Simpson MB, Delong N. Autoimmune hemolytic anemia in a patient with acquired immunodeficiency syndrome. Blood 1987;705:127.
284. Burkes RL, Cohen H, Krailo M, Sinow RM, Carmel R. Low serum cobalamin levels occur frequently in the acquired immune deficiency syndrome and related disorders. Eur J Haematol 1987;38:141.
285. Spivak JL, Barnes DC, Fuchs E, Thomas C, Quinn C. Serum immunoreactive erythropoietin in HIV-infected patients. JAMA 1989;261:21.
286. Wang Z, Goldberg MA, Scadden DT. HIV-1 suppresses erythropoietin production in vitro. Exp Hematol 1993;21:683.
287. Frickhofen N, Abkowitz J, King L, Astrow A, Halperin I, Young N. Red cell aplasia due to persistent B19 parvovirus infection in HIV-infected patients and its treatment with immunoglobulin. (Abstract) Blood 1989;74(Suppl 1):44a.
288. Forester G. Profound cytopenia secondary to azidothymidine. (Letter) N Engl J Med 1987;317:772.
289. Palefsky JM. Anal human papillomavirus infection and anal cancer in HIV-positive individuals: an emerging problem. AIDS 1994;8:283.
290. Scadden DT, Wang A, Zsebo K, et al. In vitro effects of stem cell factor

or interleukin-3 on myelosuppression associated with AIDS. AIDS (in press).

291. Dainiak N, Worthington M, Riordan MA, et al. 3′-azido-3′-deoxythymidine (AZT) inhibits proliferation in vitro of human hematopoietic progenitor cells. Br J Haematol 1988;69:299.

292. Henry DH, Beall GN, Benson CA, et al. Recombinant human erythropoietin in the treatment of anemia associated with human immunodeficiency virus (HIV) infection and zidovudine therapy. Ann Intern Med 1992;117:739.

293. Phair JP, Abels RI, McNeill MV, Sullivan DJ. Recombinant human erythropoietin treatment: investigational new drug protocol for the anemia of the acquired immunodeficiency syndrome. Arch Intern Med 1993;153:2669.

293a. Miles SA, Mitsuyasu RT, Moreno J, et al. Combined therapy with recombinant G-CSF and EPO decreases hematologic toxicity from zidovudine. Blood 1991;77:2109.

294. Murphy MF, Metcalfe P, Walters AH, et al. Incidence and mechanism of neutropenia and thrombocytopenia in patients with human immunodeficiency virus infection. Br J Haematol 1987;66:337.

295. Baldwin GC, Gasson JC, Quan SG, et al. Granulocyte-macrophage colony-stimulating factor enhances neutrophil function in acquired immunodeficiency syndrome patients. Proc Natl Acad Sci USA 1988;85:2763.

296. Groopman JE, Mitsuyasu RT, DeLeo MJ, Oette DH, Golde DW. Effect of recombinant human granulocyte-macrophage colony-stimulating factor on myelopoiesis in the acquired immunodeficiency syndrome. N Engl J Med 1987;317:593.

296a. Melbye M, Cote TR, Kessler L, et al. High incidence of anal cancer among AIDS patients. Lancet 1994;343:636.

297. Levine JD, Allan JD, Tessitore JH, et al. Recombinant human granulocyte-macrophage colony-stimulating factor ameliorates zidovudine-induced neutropenia in patients with acquired immunodeficiency syndrome (AIDS)/AIDS-related complex. Blood 1991;78: 3148.

297a. Scadden DT, Bering HA, Levine JD, et al. Granulocyte-macrophage colony-stimulation factor mitigates the neutropenia of combined interferon alfa and zidovudine treatment of acquired immune deficiency syndrome–associated Kaposi's sarcoma. J Clin Oncol 1993;9:802.

297b. Pluda JM, Yarchoan Y, Smith PD. Subcutaneous recombinant granulocyte-macrophage colony-stimulating factor used as a single agent and in an alternative regimen with azidothymidine in leukopenia patients with severe human immunodeficiency virus infection. Blood 1990;76:2303.

297c. Hardy WD. Combined ganciclovir and recombinant granulocyte-macrophage colony-stimulating factor in the treatment of cytomegalovirus retinitis in AIDS patients. J Acquir Immune Defic Syndr 1991;4:S22.

297d. Kaplan LD, Kahn JO, Crose S, et al. Clinical and virologic effects of recombinant human granulocyte-macrophage colony-stimulating factor in patients receiving chemotherapy for human immunodeficiency virus–associated non-Hodgkin's lymphoma: results of a randomized trial. J Clin Oncol 1991;9:929.

297e. Davey RT, Davey VJ, Metcalf JA, et al. A phase I/II trial of zidovudine, interferon-α, and granulocyte-macrophage colony-stimulating factor in the treatment of human immunodeficiency virus type 1 infection. J Infect Dis 1991;164:43.

297f. Krown SE, Paredes J, Bundow D, et al. Interferon-α, zidovudine, and granulocyte-macrophage colony-stimulating factor: a phase I AIDS Clinical Trials Group study in patients with Kaposi's sarcoma associated with AIDS. J Clin Invest 1992;10:1344.

298. Scadden DT, Levine JD, Hammer S, McGrath J, Bresnahan J, Young DC. Recombinant human interleukin-3 for cytopenia in AIDS. Blood 1992;80(suppl 1):515a.

299. Scadden DT, Agosti J. No antibodies to granulocyte-macrophage colony-stimulating factor with prolonged use in AIDS. (Letter) AIDS 1993;7:438.

301. Hammer SM, Gillis JM, Groopman JE, Rose RM. In vitro modification of human immunodeficiency virus infection by granulocyte-macrophage colony-stimulating and gamma interferon. Proc Natl Acad Sci USA 1986;83:8734.

302. Koyanagi Y, O'Brien WA, Zhao JQ, Golde DW, Gasson JC, Chen IS. Cytokines alter production of HIV-1 from primary mononuclear phagocytes. Science 1988;241:1673.

303. Perno CF, Cooney DA, Gao WY, et al. Effects of bone marrow stimulatory cytokines on human immunodeficiency virus replication and the antiviral activity of dideoxynucleosides in cultures of monocyte/macrophages. Blood 1992;80:995.

304. Perno CF, Yarchoan R, Cooney DA, et al. Replication of human immunodeficiency in monocytes. J Exp Med 1989;169:933.

305. Schuitemaker H, Kootstra NA, van Oers MHJ, et al. Induction of monocyte proliferation and HIV expression by IL-3 does not interfere with anti-viral activity of zidovudine. Blood 1990;76:1490.

306. Hammer SM, Gillis JM. Synergistic activity of granulocyte-macrophage colony-stimulating factor and 3′-azido-3′ deoxythymidine against human immunodeficiency virus in vitro. Antimicrob Agents Chemother 1987;31:1046.

307. Dhawan RK, Kharbanda S, Makamura M, et al. Effects of granulocyte-macrophage colony-stimulating factor on 3′-azido-3′-deoxythymidine uptake, phosphorylation and nucleotide retention in human U-397 cells. Bio Pharm 1990;40:2695.

308. Turbat-Herrera EA, Hancock C, Cabello-Inchausti B, Herrera GA. Plasma cell hyperplasia and monoclonal paraproteinemia in human immunodeficiency virus–infected patients. Arch Pathol Lab Med 1993;117:497.

309. Sala PG, Mazzolini S, Tonutti E, Bramezza M. Monoclonal immunoglobulins in HTLV-III-positive sera. Clin Chem 1986;32:574.

310. Papadopoulos NM, Lane HC, Costello HC, et al. Oligoclonal immunoglobulins in patients with the acquired immunodeficiency syndrome. Clin Immunol Immunopathol 1985;35:43.

311. Crapper RM, Deam DR, Mackay IR. Paraproteins in homosexual men with HIV infection: lack of association with abnormal clinical or immunologic findings. Am J Clin Pathol 1987;88:348.

312. LeFrere J-J, Fine J-M, Lambin P, et al. Monoclonal gammopathies in asymptomatic HIV-seropositive patients. Clin Chem 1987;33:1697.

313. Kouns DM, Marty AM, Sharpe RW. Oligoclonal bands in serum protein electrophoretograms of individuals with human immunodeficiency virus antibodies. JAMA 1986;256:2343.

314. Heriot K, Harrquist AE, Tomar RH. Paraproteinemia in patients with acquired immunodeficiency syndrome (AIDS) or lymphadenopathy syndrome (LAS). Clin Chem 1985;31:1224.

315. Ng VL, Hwang KM, Reyes GR, et al. High-titer anti-HIV antibody reactivity associated with a paraprotein spike in a homosexual male with AIDS-related complex. Blood 1988;71:1397.

316. Martin CM, Matlow AG, Chew E, et al. Hyperviscosity syndrome in a patient with acquired immunodeficiency syndrome. Arch Intern Med 1989;149:1435.

317. Cohen AJ, Philips TM, Kessler CM. Circulating coagulation inhibitors in the acquired immunodeficiency syndrome. Ann Intern Med 1986;104:175.

318. Bloom EJ, Abrams DI, Rodgers G. Lupus anticoagulant in the acquired immunodeficiency syndrome. JAMA 1986;256:491.

319. Canoso RT, Zon LI, Groopman JE. Anticardiolipin antibodies associated with human T-lymphotropic virus type III infection. Br J Haematol 1987;65:495.

320. Canoso RT, Zon LI, Groopman JE. Anticardiolipin antibodies associated with HTLV-III infection. Br J Haematol 1988;68:270.

321. Intrator L, Oksenhendler E, Desforges L, et al. Anticardiolipin antibodies in HIV-infected patients with or without immune thrombocytopenic purpura. Br J Haematol 1988;68:269.

322. Panzer S, Stain C, Harly H, et al. Anticardiolipin antibodies are elevated in HIV-1–infected hemophiliacs but do not predict for disease progression. Thomb Hamost 1989;61:81.

323. LeFrere J-J, Gozin D, Modai J, Vittecoq D. Circulating anticoagulant in the acquired immunodeficiency syndrome. Ann Intern Med 1987;107:429.

324. Kopelman RG, Zolla-Pazner S. Association of human immunodeficiency virus infection and autoimmune phenomena. Am J Med 1988;84:82.

325. Ndimbie OK, Raman BKS, Saseed SM. Lupus anticoagulant–associated with specific inhibition of factor VII in a patient with AIDS. Am J Clin Pathol 1989;91:491.

326. DiPrima MA, Sorice M, Vullo V, et al. Anticardiolipin antibody in the acquired immunodeficiency syndrome: a marker of *Pneumocystis carinii* infection? J Infect 1989;18:100.

327. Lane HC, Masur H, Edgar LC, et al. Abnormalities of B-cell activation and immunoregulation in patients with the acquired immunodeficiency syndrome. N Engl J Med 1983;309:453.

328. Yarchoan R, Redfield RR, Brodr S. Mechanisms of B cell activation in patients with acquired immunodeficiency syndrome and related disorders. J Clin Invest 1986;78:439.

329. Mathur-Wagh U, Enlow RW, Spigland I, et al. Longitudinal study of persistent generalized lymphadenopathy in homosexual men: relation to the acquired immunodeficiency syndrome. Lancet 1984;1: 1033.

330. Fishbein DB, Kaplan JE, Spira TJ, et al. Unexplained lymphadenopathy in homosexual men: a longitudinal study. JAMA 1985;254:930.

331. Abrams DI, Lewis BJ, Beckstead JF, et al. Persistent diffuse lymphadenopathy in homosexual men: endpoint or prodrome? Ann Intern Med 1984;100:801.

332. Levine AM, Meyer PR, Gill PS, et al. Results of initial lymph node biopsy in homosexual men with generalized lymphadenopathy. J Clin Oncol 1986;4:165.

333. Abrams DI. AIDS-related lymphadenopathy: the role of biopsy, J Clin Oncol 1986;4:126.

334. Brynes RK, Chan WC, Spira TJ, et al. Value of lymph node biopsy in unexplained lymphadenopathy in homosexual men. JAMA 1983;250: 1313.

335. Burns BF, Wood GS, Dorfman RF. The varied histopathology of lymphadenopathy in the homosexual male. Am J Surg Pathol 1985;9: 287.

336. Fernandez R, Mouradian J, Metroka C, et al. The prognostic values of histopathology in persistent generalized lymphadenopathy in homosexual men. (Letter) N Engl J Med 1983;309:185.

337. Ewing EP, Chandler FW, Spira TJ, et al. Primary lymph node pathology

in AIDS-related lymphadenopathy. Arch Pathol Lab Med 1985;109:977.
338. Ioachim HL, Lerner CW, Tapper ML. The lymphoid lesions associated with AIDS. Am J Surg Pathol 1983;7:543.
339. Wood GS, Garcia CF, Dorfman RF, et al. The immunohistology of follicle lysis in lymph node biopsies from homosexual men. Blood 1985;66:1092.
340. O'Hara CT. The lymphoid and hematopoietic systems. In: Harawi SJ, O'Hara CJ, eds. Pathology and pathophysiology of AIDS and HIV-related diseases. London, Chapman & Hall, 1989:135.
341. Levine AM, Gill PS, Krailo M, et al. Natural history of persistent, generalized lymphadenopathy (PGL) in gay men: risk of lymphoma and factors associated with development of lymphoma. (Abstract) Blood 1986;68:130a.
342. Hoover RN. Lymphoma risks in populations with altered immunity: a search for mechanism. Cancer Res 1992;52:5477.
343. Pluda JM, Yarchoan R, Jaffe ES, et al. Development of non-Hodgkin's lymphoma in a cohort of patients with several human immunodeficiency virus (HIV) infections on long-term antiretroviral therapy. Ann Intern Med 1990;113:246.
344. Moore RD, Kessler H, Richman DD, et al. Non-Hodgkin's lymphoma in patients with advanced HIV infection treated with zidovudine. JAMA 1991;265:2208.
345. Gail MH, Pluda JM, Rabkin CS, et al. Projections of the incidence of non-Hodgkin's lymphoma related to acquired immunodeficiency syndrome. J Natl Cancer Inst 1991;83:695.
346. Birx DL, Redfield RR, Tosato G. Defective regulation of Epstein-Barr infection in patients with acquired immunodeficiency syndrome (AIDS) or AIDS-related disorders. N Engl J Med 1986;314:874.
347. Peterson JM, Tubbs RR, Savage RA, et al. Small noncleaved B-cell Burkitt-like lymphoma with chromosome t(8;14) translocation and Epstein Barr virus nuclear-associated antigen in a homosexual man with acquired immune deficiency syndrome. Am J Med 1985;78:141.
348. Subar M, Neri A, Inshirami G, Knowles DM, Dalla-Favera R. Frequent c-*myc* oncogene activation and infrequent presence of Epstein-Barr virus genome in AIDS-associated lymphoma. Blood 1988;72:667.
349. Shibata D, Weiss LM, Nathwani BN, et al. Epstein-Barr virus in benign lymph node biosis from individuals infected with the human immunodeficiency virus is associated with concurrent or subsequent development of non-Hodgkin's lymphoma. Blood 1991;77:1526.
350. Pelicci P, Knowles DM, Arlin ZA, et al. Multiple monoclonal B cell expansions and c-*myc* oncogene rearrangements in acquired immune deficiency syndrome–related lymphoproliferative disorders: implications for lymphomagenesis. J Exp Med 1986;164:2049.
351. Shiramizu B, Herndier B, Meeker T, et al. Molecular and immunophenotypic characterization of AIDS-associated, Epstein-Barr virus–negative, polyclonal lymphoma. J Clin Oncol 1992;10:383.
352. Meeker TC, Shiramizu B, Kaplan L, et al. Evidence for molecular subtypes of HIV-associated lymphoma: division into peripheral monoclonal, polyclonal and central nervous system lymphoma. AIDS 1991;5:669.
353. Levine AM, Shibata D, Sullivan-Halley J, et al. Case control study of HIV-positive and HIV-negative lymphoma in Los Angeles County. Proc ASCO 1992;11:333.
354. Raab-Traub N, Flynn K. The structure of the terminal of the Epstein-Barr virus as a marker of clonal cellular proliferation. Cell 1986;47:883.
355. Wang PG, Lee EC, Sieverts H, et al. Burkitt's lymphoma in AIDS: cytogenetic study. Blood 1984;63:190.
356. Chaganti RSK, Jhanwar SC, Koziner B, et al. Specific translocations characterize Burkitt's-like lymphoma of homosexual men with the acquired immunodeficiency syndrome. Blood 1983;61:1265.
357. Bernheim A, Berger R. Cytogenetic studies of Burkitt lymphoma/leukemia in patients with acquired immunodeficiency syndrome. Cancer Genet Cytogenet 1988;32:67.
358. Neri A, Barriga F, Knowles DM, et al. Different regions of the immunoglobulin heavy-chain locus are involved in chromosomal translocations in distinct pathogenetic forms of Burkitt lymphoma. Proc Natl Acad Sci 1988;85:2748.
359. Ballerini P, Gaidano G, Gong JZ, et al. Multiple genetic lesions in acquired immunodeficiency syndrome-related non-Hodgkin's lymphoma. Blood 1993;81:166.
360. Mann DL, DeSantis P, Mark G, et al. HTLV-1 associated B-cell CLL: Indirect role for retrovirus in leukemogenesis. Science 1987;236:1103.
361. Salahuddin SZ, Ablashi DV, Markham PD, et al. Isolation of a new virus, HBLV, in patients with lymphoproliferative disorders. Science 1986;234:596.
362. Ziegler JL, Beckstead JA, Volberding PA, et al. Non-Hodgkin's lymphoma in 90 homosexual men: relationship to generalized lymphadenopathy and acquired immunodeficiency syndrome (AIDS). N Engl J Med 1984;311:565.
363. Levine, AM, Gill PS, Meyer PR, et al. Retrovirus and malignant lymphoma in homosexual men. JAMA 1985;254:1921.
364. Kalter SP, Riggs SA, Cabanillas F, et al. Aggressive non Hodgkin's lymphomas in immunocompromised homosexual males. Blood 1985;66:655.
365. Gill PS, Levine AM, Krailo M, et al. AIDS-related malignant lymphoma: results of prospective treatment trials. J Clin Oncol 1987;5:1322.
366. Knowles DM, Chamulak GA, Subar M, et al. Lymphoid neoplasia associated with the acquired immunodeficiency syndrome (AIDS). Ann Intern Med 1988;108:744.
367. Lowenthal DA, Straus DJ, Campbell SW, et al. AIDS-related lymphoid neoplasia: the Memorial Hospital experience. Cancer 1988;61:2325.
368. Bermudez MA, Grant KM, Rodvien R, et al. Non-Hodgkin's lymphoma in a population with or at risk for acquired immunodeficiency syndrome. Am J Med 1989;86:71.
369. Rossi G, Gorla R, Cadeo GP, Stellini R, Marinone G. Acute lymphoblastic leukaemia of B cell origin in an anti-HIV positive intravenous drug abuser. Br J Haematol 1988;68:140.
370. Gill PS, Meyer PR, Pavlova Z, et al. B-cell acute lymphocytic leukemia in adults: clinical, morphologic and immunologic findings. J Clin Oncol 1986;4:737.
370a. Herndier BG, Shiramizu BT, Jewett NE, Aldape KD, Reyes GR, McGrath MS. Acquired immunodeficiency syndrome–associated T-cell lymphoma: evidence for human immunodeficiency virus type 1–associated T-cell transformation. Blood 1992;79:1768.
371. Levine AM, Sullivan-Halley J, Pike MC, et al. HIV-related lymphoma: prognostic factors predictive of survival. Cancer 1991;68:2466.
372. Levine AM. Acquired immunodeficiency syndrome–related lymphoma. Blood 1992;80:8.
373. Burkes RL, Meyer PR, Gill PS, et al. Primary rectal lymphoma in homosexual men. Arch Intern Med 1986;146:913.
374. MacMahon EME, Glass JD, Hayward SD, et al. Epstein-Barr virus in AIDS-related primary central nervous system lymphoma. Lancet 1991;338:969.
375. Levine AM, Wernz JC, Kaplan L, et al. Low dose chemotherapy with central nervous system prophylaxis and azidothymidine maintenance in AIDS-related lymphoma: a prospective multi-institutional trial. JAMA 1991;266:84.
376. Gill PS, Levine AM, Meyer PR, et al. Primary central nervous system lymphoma in homosexual men: clinical, immunologic, and pathologic features. Am J Med 1985;78:742.
377. Levine AM, Shibata D, Weiss LM, et al. Molecular characteristics of intermediate/high (I/H) grade lymphomas (NHL) arising in HIV-positive vs. HIV-negative PTS: preliminary data from a population (POP) based study in the county of Los Angeles. Blood 1992;80:1028.
378. Gisselbrecht C, Lepage E, Tirelli U, et al. Human immunodeficiency virus–related lymphoma treatment with intensive combination chemotherapy. ASCO 1993;12:1227.
379. Dugan M, Subar M, Odajnyk C, et al. Intensive multiagent chemotherapy for AIDS related diffuse large cell lymphoma. (Abstract) Blood 1986;68:124.
380. Odajnyk C, Subar M, Dugan M, et al. Clinical features and correlates with immunopathology and molecular biology of a large group of patients with AIDS associated small non-cleaved lymphoma (SNCL). (Abstract) Blood 1986;68:131.
381. Kaplan LD, Abrams DI, Feigal E, et al. AIDS-associated non-Hodgkin's lymphoma in San Francisco. JAMA 1989;261:719.
382. Gill PS, Levine AM, Krailo M, et al. AIDS-related malignant lymphoma: results of prospective treatment trials. J Clin Oncol 1987;5:1322.
383. Formenti SC, Gill PS, Lean E, et al. Primary central nervous system lymphoma in AIDS: results of radiation therapy. Cancer 1989;63:1101.
384. Baumgartner JE, Rachlin JR, Beckstead JH, et al. Primary central nervous system lymphomas: natural history and response to radiation therapy in 55 patients with acquired immunodeficiency syndrome. J Neurosurg 1990;73:206.
385. Kaplan MH, Susin M, Pahwa SG, et al. Neoplastic complications of HTLV-III infection: lymphomas and solid tumors. Am J Med 1987;82:389.
386. Tirelli A, Serraino D, Carbone A. Hodgkin disease and AIDS. Ann Intern Med 1993;118:313.
387. Scheib RG, Siegel RS. A typical Hodgkin's disease and the acquired immunodeficiency syndrome. (Letter) Ann Intern Med 1985;102:554.
388. Schoeppel SL, Hoppe RT, Dorfman FT, et al. Hodgkin's disease in homosexual men with generalized lymphadenopathy. Ann Intern Med 1985;102:68.
389. Robert NJ, Schneiderman H. Hodgkin's disease and the acquired immunodeficiency syndrome. (Letter) Ann Intern Med 1984;101:142.
390. Maiman M, Fruchter RG, Serur E, et al. Human immunodeficiency virus infection and cervical neoplasia. Gynecol Oncol 1990;38:377.
391. Li FP, Osborn D, Cronin CM. Anorectal squamous carcinoma in two homosexual men. Lancet 1982;2:391.
392. Gal AA, Meyer PR, Taylor CR. Papillomavirus antigens in anorectal condyloma and carcinoma in homosexual men. JAMA 1987;257:337.
393. Daling JR, Weiss NS, Klopfenstein LL et al. Correlates of homosexual behavior and the incidence of anal cancer. JAMA 1982;247:1988.
394. Kiviat N, Rompalo A, Bowden R, et al. Anal human papilloma-virus infection among human immunodeficiency virus–seropositive and –seronegative men. J Infect Dis 1990;162:358.
395. Conant MC, Volberding P, Fletcher V, et al. Squamous cell carcinoma in sexual partner of Kaposi's sarcoma patient. Lancet 1982;1:286.
396. Palefsy JM, Gonzales J, Greenblatt RM, et al. Anal intraepithelial neoplasia and anal papillomavirus infection among homosexual males with group IV HIV disease. JAMA 1990;263:2911.
397. Irwin LE, Bergandy MK, Moore TML. Adenosquamous carcinoma of

the lung and the acquired immunodeficiency syndrome. Ann Intern Med 1984;100:158.
398. Logothetis CJ, Newell GY, Samuels ML. Testicular cancer in homosexual men with cellular immune deficiency: report of two cases. J Urol 1985;133:484.
399. Ravalli S, Chabon AB, Khan AA. Gastrointestinal neoplasia in young HIV antibody-positive patients. Am J Clin Pathol 1989;91:458.
400. Vandermolen LA, Fehir KM, Rice L. Multiple myeloma in a homosexual man with chronic lymphadenopathy. Arch Intern Med 1986;145:745.
401. Kaposi M. Idiopathisches multiples pigmentsarkom der haut. Arch Dermatol Syph 1872;4:265.
402. Harwood AR, Osoba D, Hofstader SL, et al. Kaposi's sarcoma in recipients of renal transplants. Am J Med 1979;67:759.
403. Penn I. Kaposi's sarcoma in organ transplant recipients. Transplantation 1979;27:8.
404. Qunibi W, Akhtar M, Sheth K, et al. Kaposi's sarcoma: the most common tumor after renal transplantation in Saudi Arabia. Am J Med 1988;84:225.
405. Chow WH, Liff JM, Greenberg RS, Williams BO. A comparison of acquired immunodeficiency syndrome and Kaposi's sarcoma incidence rates, Atlanta, 1983. Am J Public Health 1989;79:503.
406. Rutherford GW, Schwarcz SK, Lemp GF, et al. The epidemiology of AIDS-related Kaposi's sarcoma in San Francisco. J Infect Dis 1989;159:569.
407. Friedman-Kien AE, Salzman BR, Cao Y, Mirabile M, Li JJ, Peterman TA. Kaposi's sarcoma in HIV-negative homosexual men. Lancet 1990;1:168.
408. Beral V, Peterman TA, Berkelman RL, Jaffe HW. Kaposi's sarcoma among persons with AIDS: a sexually transmitted infection. Lancet 1990;335:123.
408a. Roth WK, Brandstetter H, Sturzl M. Cellular and molecular features of HIV-associated Kaposi's sarcoma. AIDS 1992;6:895.
409. Harawi SJ. Kaposi's sarcoma. In: Harawi SJ, O'Hara CJ, eds. Pathology and pathophysiology of AIDS and HIV-related diseases. London, Chapman & Hall, 1989:83.
410. Nickoloff BJ, Griffiths CE. Factor XIIIa–expressing dermal dendrocytes in AIDS-associated cutaneous Kaposi's sarcomas. Science 1989;31:243.
411. Delli Bovi P, Donti E, Knowles DM, et al. Presence of chromosomal abnormalities and lack of AIDS retrovirus DNA sequences in AIDS-associated Kaposi's sarcoma. Cancer 1986;46:6333.
412. Vogel J, Hinrichs SH, Reynolds RK, Luciw PA, Jay G. The HIV tat gene induces dermal lesions resembling Kaposi's sarcoma in transgenic mice. Nature 1988;13:335:606.
413. Nakamura S, Salahuddin SZ, Biberfeld P, et al. Kaposi's sarcoma cells: long-term culture with growth factor from retrovirus-infected CD4+ T cells. Science 1988;21:242:426.
414. Salahuddin SZ, Nakamura S, Biberfeld P, et al. Angiogenic properties of Kaposi's sarcoma-derived cells after long-term culture in vitro. Science 1988;21:242.
415. Ensoli B, Nakamura S, Salahuddin SZ, et al. AIDS-Kaposi's sarcoma-derived cells express cytokines with autocrine and paracrine growth effects. Science 1989;13:243.
416. Miles SA, Rezai AR, Salazar-Gonzalex JF, et al: AIDS Kaposi's sarcoma–derived cells produce and respond to interleukin 6. Proc Natl Acad Sci USA 1990;87:4068.
417. Miles SA, Martinex-Maza O, Rezai A, et al. Oncostatin M as a potent mitogen for AIDS Kaposi's sarcoma–derived cells. Science 1992;255:1432.
418. Koehler JE, Quinn FD, Berger TG, et al. Isolation of *Rochalimaea* species from cutaneous and osseous lesions of bacillary angiomatosis. N Engl J Med 1992;327:1625.
419. Litwin MA, Williams CM. Cutaneous *Pneumocystis carinii* infection mimicking Kaposi's sarcoma. Ann Intern Med 1992;117:48.
420. Woolfenden JM, Carrasquillo JA, Larson SM, et al. Acquired immunodeficiency syndrome: [^{67}Ga] citrate imaging. Radiology 1987;162:383.
421. Gill PS, Akil B, Colletti P, et al. Pulmonary Kaposi's sarcoma: Clinical findings and results of therapy. Am J Med 1989;87:57.
422. Krown SE. AIDS-associated Kaposi's sarcoma: pathogenesis, clinical course and treatment. AIDS 1988;2:71.
423. Chachoua A, Krisel R, Lafleur F, et al. Prognostic factors and staging classification of patients with epidemic Kaposi's sarcoma. J Clin Oncol 1989;7:774.
424. Krown SE, Metroka C, Wernz J. Kaposi's sarcoma in the acquired immune deficiency syndrome: a proposal for uniform evaluation, response, and staging criteria. J Clin Oncol 1989;7:1201.
424a. Lilenbaum RC, Ratner L. Systemic treatment of Kaposi's sarcoma: current status and future directions. AIDS 1994;8:141.
425. Volberding PA, Abrams DI, Conant M, et al. Vinblastine therapy for Kaposi's sarcoma in acquired immunodeficiency syndrome. Ann Intern Med 1985;103:335.
426. Groopman JE. Therapy of epidemic Kaposi's sarcoma. Semin Hematol 1986;23(Suppl 1):14.
427. Schwarstmann G, Springz E, et al. Phase II study of tenopiside in patients with AIDS-related Kaposi's sarcoma. Eur J Cancer 1991;27:1637.
428. Lassoued K, Clauvel J-P, Katlama C, et al. Treatment of the acquired immune deficiency syndrome-related Kaposi's sarcoma with bleomycin as a single agent. Cancer 1990;66:1869.
429. Fischl MA, Krown SE, O'Boyle KP, et al. Weekly doxorubicin in the treatment of patients with AIDS-related Kaposi's sarcoma. J Acquir Immune Defic Syndr 1993;6:249.
429a. Gelmann EP, Longo D, Lane HC, et al. Combination chemotherapy of disseminated Kaposi's sarcoma patients with the acquired immune deficiency syndrome. Am J Med 1987;82:456.
429b. Gill PS, Rarick M, McGutchan JA, et al. Systemic treatment of AIDS-related Kaposi's sarcoma: results of a randomized trial. Am J Med 1991;90:427.
429c. Kaplan L, Abrams D, Volberding P. Treatment of Kaposi's sarcoma in acquired immunodeficiency syndrome with an alternating vincristine-vinblastine regimen. Cancer Treat Rep 1986;70:1121.
429d. Gill PS, et al. Treatment of advanced Kaposi's sarcoma using a combination of bleomycin and vincristine. Am J Clin Oncol 1990;13:315.
429e. Presant CA, Scolaro M, Kennedy P, et al. Liposomal daunorubicin treatment of HIV-associated Kaposi's sarcoma. Lancet 1993;341:1242.
430. Krown SE, Real FX, Cunningham-Rundles S, et al. Preliminary observations on the effect of recombinant leukocyte A interferon in homosexual men with Kaposi's sarcoma. N Engl J Med 1983;308:1071.
432. Groopman JE, Scadden DT. Interferon therapy for Kaposi sarcoma associated with the acquired immunodeficiency syndrome (AIDS). Ann Intern Med 1989;110:335.
433. Lane HC, Kovacs JA, Feinberg J, et al. Anti-retroviral effects of interferon-alpha in AIDS-associated Kaposi's sarcoma. Lancet 1988;2:1218.
434. de Wit R, Schattenkerk JK, Boucher CA, Bakker PJ, Veenhof KH, Danner SA. Clinical and virological effects of high-dose recombinant interferon-alpha in disseminated AIDS-related Kaposi's sarcoma. Lancet 1988;2:1214.
435. Hartshorn KL, Vogt MW, Chou TC, et al. Synergistic inhibition of human immunodeficiency virus in vitro by azidothymidine and recombinant alpha A interferon. Antimicrob Agents Chemother 1987;31:168.
436. Galzagorry MA, Illeman M. Intralesional vinblastine (Velban) treatment of lesion of Kaposi's sarcoma. Fifth International Conference on AIDS. Montreal, 1989:550.
437. Chak LY, Gill PS, Levine AM, Meyer PR, Anselmo JA, Petrovich Z. Radiation therapy for acquired immunodeficiency syndrome–related Kaposi's sarcoma. J Clin Oncol 1988;6:863.
438. Tappero JW, Berger TG, Kaplan LD, et al. Cryotherapy for cutaneous Kaposi's sarcoma (KS) associated with acquired immune deficiency syndrome (AIDS): a phase II trial. J AIDS 1991;4:9.

Blood: Principles and Practice of Hematology,
edited by Robert I. Handin, Thomas P. Stossel, and Samuel E. Lux.
J.B. Lippincott Company, Philadelphia © 1995.

26

Biology and Classification of Lymphoid Neoplasia

Stanley J. Korsmeyer

The last two decades have provided enormous advances in understanding of the immunology and molecular biology of human lymphoid neoplasms. The realization that lymphomas and leukemias represented distinct stages of normal lymphocyte development profoundly affected concepts of their cellular origin. The generation of monoclonal antibodies to lymphoid cell surface antigens made it plausible to equate many of these neoplasms with distinct stages of either B- or T-lymphocyte maturation. Some of these lineage-restricted antigens even provide potential targets for tumor-directed immunotherapy.

DNA rearrangements that assemble the antigen-specific genes in B and T cells have proved to be particularly useful as molecular markers unique to individual neoplasms. These immunoglobulin and T-cell receptor (TCR) genes are composed of separated gene subsegments in their germline or embryonic form. A rearrangement at the level of DNA assembles these subcomponents of immunoglobulin (Ig) genes in B cells and TCR genes in T cells. Much knowledge concerning the basic mechanisms of Ig or TCR gene recombination and expression was gleaned from an examination of the clonally expanded cells provided by lymphoid tumors. In return, these gene recombination events provide sensitive and specific markers for the clonality, lineage, and stage of development of lymphocyte malignancies. Some neoplasms of uncertain cellular origin can now be classified by the determination of their gene rearrangement pattern.

Gene rearrangement enabled T-lineage as well as B-lineage expansions of lymphocytes to be assessed for their polyclonal and monoclonal compositions. Both Ig and TCR genes rearrange in an ordered cascade. An examination of acute lymphoblastic leukemia indicated that the leukemia cells represent a developmental hierarchy of Ig and TCR rearrangements. Moreover, errors in Ig gene recombination and expression have been defined, which account for the truncated proteins of human heavy-chain diseases. Finally, because gene rearrangement patterns are unique to each tumor, they serve as markers to follow the natural history of tumors and to search for minimal residual disease.

The study of Ig and TCR genes in lymphoid tumors has paid an even greater dividend. These genes proved to be the sites of illegitimate interchromosomal translocations. This rearrangement occurs between nonhomologous chromosomes in malignant cells, but not in their normal cellular counterparts. In addition, specific translocations are found recurrently with distinct types of neoplasms, suggesting that they participate in the malignant process. These unanticipated rearrangements of Ig and TCR genes often juxtapose these loci with new protooncogenes that have been shown in some instances to contribute directly to the malignant phenotype.

Classification schemes for leukemias and lymphomas are still predominantly based on morphology and histology. This chapter reviews these schemes, which can be used to dictate how individual cases are grouped. An understanding and continued reexamination of these categorization systems are crucial. These systems compromise the framework for defining the biologic behavior and responsiveness of neoplastic subgroups; they have already undergone several revisions. More refinements in classification can be anticipated because immunologic and molecular dissection provides further insights into pathogenesis and prognosis.

HISTORICAL CLASSIFICATION SCHEMES

Non-Hodgkin's Lymphomas

The non-Hodgkin's lymphomas (NHLs) are a heterogeneous set of tumors that are diverse in their cellular origin, morphology, response to treatment, and prognosis. This diversity has prompted multiple different classification schemes and subsequent revisions over the years. Thomas Hodgkin[1] is often credited with the first report in 1832 of malignancies of the lymphoreticular system. Attempts to subdivide malignant lymphoma followed, which were based predominantly on histology and patterns of spread. Sternberg and Reed subsequently described a giant cell, which bears their names and separates Hodgkin's disease as a distinct entity. Out of this initial era evolved four cytologic categories of malignant lymphoma: Hodgkin's disease, nodular lymphoma, lymphosarcoma, and reticulum cell sarcoma.[1] The NHLs are still subdivided mostly by morphologic criteria. The major determinants are follicular versus diffuse architecture, cell size, cell shape, nuclear and nucleolar appearance, chromatin distribution, and cytoplasmic characteristics. After the definition of T and B lymphocytes and their geographic distribution, immunologic parameters have been incorporated into some schemes. These classifications include the Rappaport,[2] Lukes and Collins,[3] Kiel,[4] British National Lymphoma Investigation, Dorfman,[5] and the WHO classification. Several attempts have been made to develop uniform terminologies for these classification systems and to allow translation among the systems. In 1982, a large multiinstitutional study sponsored by the National Cancer Institute (NCI), developed the Working Formulation for Clinical Usage as a classification scheme to help standardize patients in clinical trials.[6]

Rappaport Classification

Although a number of classification proposals had been offered for NHLs, the one proposed by Rappaport[2] in 1956 was the first to gain wide acceptance and use. It provided a framework of terms to subdivide the disease into clinically meaningful subgroups. The original Rappaport system as well as subsequent revisions divided the NHLs into two major groups, nodular and diffuse, based on the architecture of their growth patterns. Further subgroups were generated based on concepts of the day concerning their cellular origin and degree of differentiation. As the knowledge of the immune system advanced, the Rappaport classification has undergone numerous modifications by Berard, Dorfman,[5] and Rappaport himself.[7,8] A considerable amount of descriptive terminology has been retained even though more biologically important immunologic subsets can be defined.

The *modified Rappaport system* divides NHLs into 12 morphologic subtypes (Table 26-1). The five nodular or diffuse subtypes of NHL are the following:

- Nodular poorly differentiated lymphocytic
- Mixed
- Histiocytic
- Burkitt's
- Undifferentiated non-Burkitt's

The following seven NHL morphologic subtypes are characterized by diffuse involvement of the lymph node:

- Well-differentiated lymphocytic
- Intermediate lymphocytic
- Lymphoblastic
- Immunoblastic
- Diffuse epithelioid histiocytic (Lennert type)
- Mycosis fungoides
- Unclassifiable

The diffuse lymphomas have proved to be more heterogeneous with respect to their cellular origin and clinical characteristics than those of nodular pattern.

Lukes and Collins Classification

The Lukes and Collins classification system focused more on the evolving concepts concerning immunologic subsets of cells[3] (Table 26-2). Observations concerning separate B- and T-cell lineages, their distinct distribution within lymphoid tissue, and the transformation of normal lymphocytes with mitogens prompted this scheme. This system more accurately reflects the cellular origin of the various neoplasms. It subsequently relies on morphologic descriptions of cell size and on whether the nuclei are cleaved or noncleaved to further subdivide these disorders. Investigators also incorporated knowledge of the normal follicular center or germinal center cells of lymph nodes.[3] They refined the terminology of nodular neoplasms to indicate that these NHLs represent tumors of follicular center cells, which proved to be early B cells. The T-cell neoplasms were separated to acknowledge their different cellular origin, but their subclassification remained less defined awaiting further dissection of the T-cell subsets.

Kiel Classification

The Kiel classification system developed by Lennert has enjoyed considerable use in Europe[4] (Table 26-3). This scheme is also founded on the biology and immunologic markers of normal lymphocytes. It relies heavily on the distinction between centroblasts and centrocytes to subdivide the follicular center cell lymphomas. Moreover, this

TABLE 26-1. The Rappaport Classification of Non-Hodgkin's Lymphomas

Type/Subtype of Lymphoma	Cell of Origin	Growth Pattern/Morphology
Nodular or diffuse poorly differentiated lymphocytic (NPDL)	Follicular center (B cell)	Small cleaved lymphoid cells
Mixed		Small and large lymphoid cells in a nodular or nodular and diffuse growth pattern
Histiocytic		Large cleaved or noncleaved cells, frequent mitoses; rarely purely nodular pattern
Burkitt's	Early B cell	Undifferentiated, rarely nodular; small noncleaved cells, prominent nucleoli, starry-sky appearance
Undifferentiated, non-Burkitt's		Pleomorphic, noncleaved nuclei, starry-sky appearance; diffuse growth pattern
Diffuse, well-differentiated lymphocytic (DWDL)1	Small B-cell medullary cords of lymph nodes	Small round lymphoid cells, pseudofollicular growth centers
Intermediate lymphocytic	B cells of primary follicles and mantle zones of lymph nodes	Intermediate differentiation between DWDL and PDL; small cleaved and noncleaved cells
Lymphoblastic	T cell/thymocyte, rarely pre–B cell	Lymphoblastic; convoluted and nonconvoluted nuclei with fine chromatin; no nucleoli, starry-sky appearance
Immunoblastic	B cell Peripheral T cell or T-dependent areas of lymph nodes and spleen	Plasmacytoid Polymorphous or clear cell or epithelioid.
NHL with diffuse epithelioid histiocytic reaction (Lennert's type)	Peripheral T cell	Mixed cells and transitional forms
Mycosis fungoides	Mature peripheral helper T cell	Cerebriform nuclei; aggregates in the epidermis (Pautrier's microabscesses)
Unclassifiable		

TABLE 26-2. Lukes and Collins Classification

B CELL	
Small lymphocytic	
Plasmacytoid lymphocytic	
Follicular center cell, small cleaved	
Follicular center cell, large cleaved	
Follicular center cell, small noncleaved	
Follicular center cell, large noncleaved	
Subtypes of follicular center cell lymphomas:	
	Follicular
	Follicular, diffuse
	Diffuse
	Sclerotic with follicles
	Sclerotic without follicles
Immunoblastic sarcoma (B cell)	
T CELL	
Small lymphocytic	
Sézary–mycosis fungoides (cerebriform)	
Convoluted lymphocytic	
Immunoblastic sarcoma (T cell)	
OTHER	
Histiocytic	
Malignant lymphoma, unclassified	

system places each morphologic subset into either a low-grade or high-grade category in an attempt to convey prognostic information.

The existence of multiple classification schemes and the impossibility of clearly translating one type of classification to another have generated some confusion over the years. This diversity has been most frustrating when the results of clinical trials in NHL are compared. No consensus emerged as to whether the Rappaport, Lukes and Collins, or Kiel classification system was the most accurate. Subsequently, the NCI sponsored a multiinstitutional study to establish a unified system that generated the Working Formulation of Non-Hodgkin's Lymphoma for Clinical Usage[6] (Table 26-4). This common language has been important in enabling the results of clinical studies from different groups and institutions to be compared. Classic examples of two major categories of lymphoma—follicular, small cleaved cell and diffuse large cell—are shown in Figure 26-1. A sobering aspect of the multiinstitutional NCI study was the lack of reproducibility among highly trained hematopathologists in the further subclassification of individual cases.

TABLE 26-3. Kiel Classification

LOW-GRADE MALIGNANCY
Lymphocytic, chronic lymphocytic leukemia
Lymphocytic, other
Lymphoplasmacytoid
Centrocytic
Centroblastic–centrocytic, follicular, without sclerosis
Centroblastic–centrocytic, follicular, with sclerosis
Centroblastic–centrocytic, follicular and diffuse, without sclerosis
Centroblastic–centrocytic, follicular and diffuse, with sclerosis
Centroblastic–centrocytic, diffuse
Low-grade malignant lymphoma, unclassified
HIGH-GRADE MALIGNANCY
Centroblastic
Lymphoblastic, Burkitt's type
Lymphoblastic, convoluted cell type
Lymphoblastic, other (unclassified)
Immunoblastic
High-grade malignant lymphoma, unclassified
MALIGNANT LYMPHOMA, UNCLASSIFIED
Unable to specify high grade or low grade
COMPOSITE LYMPHOMA

IMMUNOLOGIC CLASSIFICATION OF NEOPLASIA

Advances in cellular immunology have provided insights into the normal pathways of lymphocyte development and the cellular origin of lymphoid neoplasms. Monoclonal an-

TABLE 26-4. Working Formulation of Non-Hodgkin's Lymphomas for Clinical Usage

LOW GRADE	
Small lymphocytic	
	Consistent with chronic lymphocytic leukemia
	Plasmacytoid
Follicular small cleaved cell	
	Diffuse areas
	Sclerosis
Follicular mixed small cleaved and large cell	
	Diffuse area
	Sclerosis
INTERMEDIATE GRADE	
Follicular predominantly large cell	
	Diffuse areas
	Sclerosis
Diffuse small cleaved cell	
	Sclerosis
Diffuse mixed, small and large cell	
	Sclerosis
	Epithelial cell component
Diffuse large cell	
	Cleaved cell
	Noncleaved cell
	Sclerosis
HIGH GRADE	
Large cell, immunoblastic	
	Plasmacytoid
	Clear cell
	Polymorphous
	Epithelial cell component
Lymphoblastic	
	Convoluted cell
	Nonconvoluted cell
Small noncleaved cell	
	Burkitt's
	Follicular areas
MISCELLANEOUS	
Composite	
Mycosis fungoides	
Histiocytic	
Extramedullary plasmacytoma	
Unclassifiable	

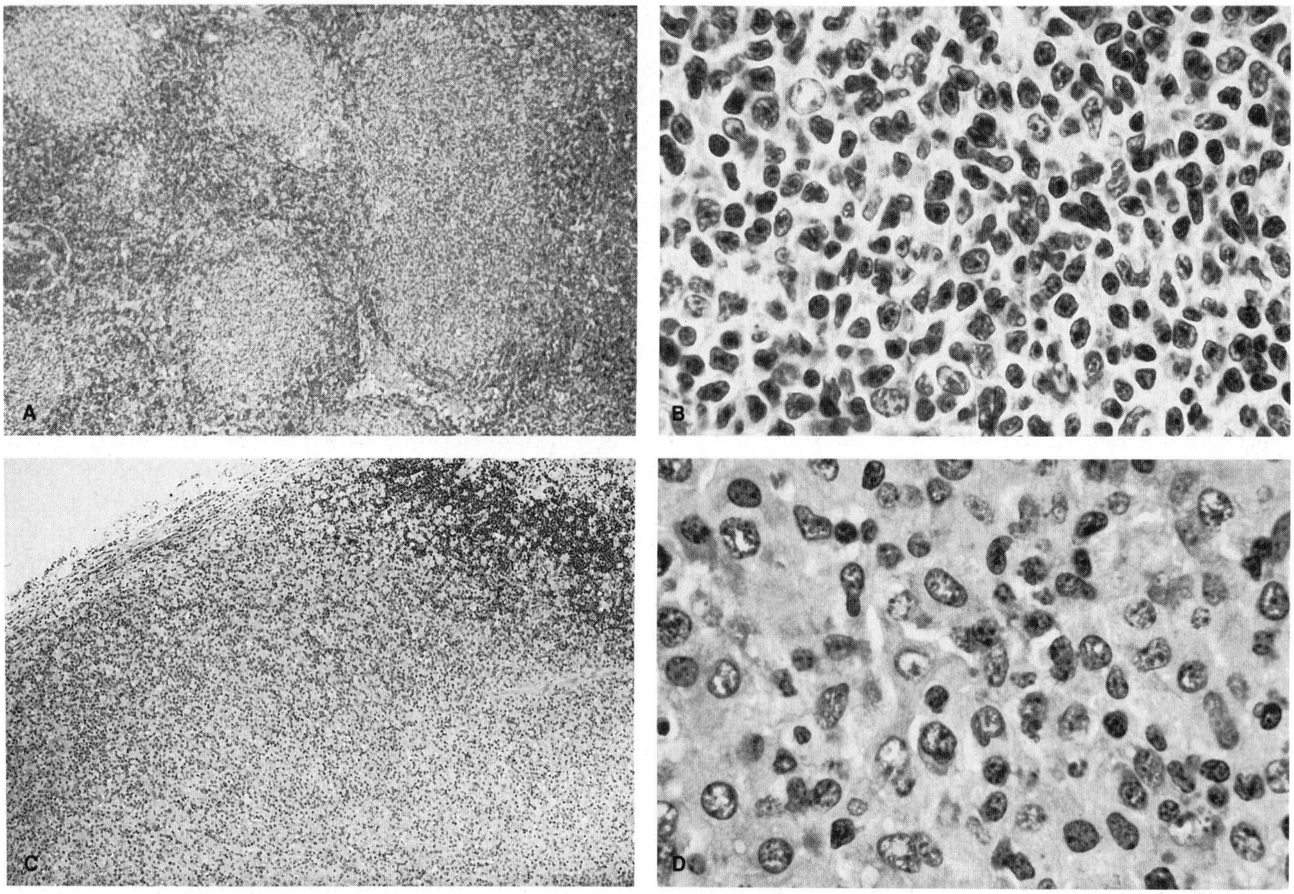

FIGURE 26-1. Histology of non-Hodgkin's lymphoma. Hematoxylin and eosin-stained section of lymph node biopsy reveals a follicular pattern of lymphoma (**A**), which is composed of small cleaved cells demonstrated by higher magnification (**B**). Lymph node biopsy reveals diffuse pattern of lymphoma (**C**) composed of large cells demonstrated by higher magnification (**D**). (See Color Fig. 26-1.)

tibodies directed against cell surface antigens have defined the differentiation stages of lymphocytes. Accompanying chapters detail the normal developmental biology of the immune system and any known functional roles of the cell surface antigens. Lymphoid neoplasms represent monoclonal expansions of cells relatively arrested at a certain stage of maturation. Consequently, numerous attempts have been made to assign leukemias and lymphomas an immunologic classification.[9–11] The following section summarizes this information.

Acute Lymphoblastic Leukemia

Acute lymphoblastic leukemias (ALL) are distributed over a wide range of B- and T-cell development. About 80% of ALLs lack definitive T-cell markers and have been termed *non–T-cell* or *non–T-, non–B-cell* (*null cell*) ALL. The advent of monoclonal antibodies recognizing B-cell surface antigens and Ig gene rearrangement studies have provided evidence for their B-lineage commitment. (See later sections for detailed discussion of the current uncertainty as to whether these ALLs fully represent normal B precursor cells.) The most mature cells classified as ALL possess HLA-DR surface determinants and the intracellular enzyme terminal deoxynucleotidyl transferase (TdT) postulated to have a role in N segment addition at Ig gene joints.[12] Subsequent steps in B-cell lineage maturation are characterized by the acquisition of CD19 (B4 antigen), followed by CD10 (common ALL antigen [CALLA]) and subsequently CD20 (B1 antigen).[13] Antigenic addition occurs in a cascade of events that is roughly coordinated with evolving Ig gene rearrangements. Most (70%) of non–T-cell ALLs bear CD10 reactivity,[14] but CD10 is missing from the least mature subsets of ALL.[13] In addition, about 15% to 20% of non–T-cell ALLs demonstrate cytoplasmic μ chain, which indicates that they are pre–B cells.[15] HLA-DR and CALLA antigens are predominantly found on pre–B-cell ALLs, but are occasionally noted on cases otherwise bearing markers associated with T-cell ALLs. Overall, the B4 antigen is the more B-cell–restricted marker.

Other early ALLs possess TdT and bear only CD7, suggesting they belong to the T-cell lineage.[16] Such cells subsequently add CD2 (sheep erythrocyte receptor) and CD5 (T1 antigen). With the completion of an $\alpha\beta$ or $\gamma\delta$ heterodimeric antigen receptor, cell surface CD3 is displayed. ALLs with double positive (CD4+, CD8+) or double negative (CD4−, CD8−) phenotype are noted (see Fig. 26-1).[17] Subsequently, thymocytes make a commitment to the single positive CD8+ lineage or CD4+ lineage. Most lymphoblastic lymphomas also express TdT and occupy positions similar to those of T-cell acute lymphoblastic leukemias (T-ALL) along this developmental scheme.[9–11]

Mature T-Cell Leukemia and Lymphoma

About 5% of chronic lymphocytic leukemias (CLLs) may be of T-cell origin.[18] Both CD4 and CD8 types have been noted. The CD8 lymphocytosis syndromes often associated with hematocytopenias, especially neutropenia, were previously referred to as Tγ lymphoproliferative diseases because of the frequent presence of Fcγ receptors. The lymphoid cells in this disorder are often large granular lymphocytes and can bear Leu-7, a natural killer cell–associated antigen.[19]

The cutaneous T-cell lymphomas contain cases classified as mycosis fungoides and Sézary cell leukemia.[20] A spectrum of skin lesions—from limited plaques to cutaneous nodules—are evident. T cells with cerebriform nuclei almost always belong to the CD4 lineage. Note that CD7 antigen is usually absent from Sézary cells.[21]

The high-grade peripheral T-cell lymphomas are thought to originate from peripheral rather than thymic T cells.[22] They often mark for CD4, but the lesions are noteworthy for an admixture of epithelioid histiocytes.

Adult T-cell leukemia is the result of HTLV-1 (human retroviral infection).[23] The malignant T cells usually demonstrate CD4 as well as CD25 (the α chain of the IL-2 receptor).[24]

Most CLLs are proliferations of mature B cells with low levels of surface Ig that is classically IgM, although IgM/IgD and occasionally IgG/IgA can be noted.[25] B-cell CLLs represent the subpopulation of B cells displaying CD5.[26] CLLs are generally nonsecretory, but can be driven in differentiation with phorbol ester. Patients classified as having prolymphocytic leukemia often have higher blast cell counts and splenomegaly, but no lymphadenopathy.[27] These cells often demonstrate more surface Ig than CLL, lack CD5, and display FMC-7 reactivity as a distinguishing feature.

Immunophenotypic and gene rearrangement studies indicate that the bizarre cells of hairy-cell leukemia (HCL) are clonal B cells.[28–30] Nearly all of these cells demonstrate the tartrate-resistant isoenzyme of acid phosphatase. Most HCL also demonstrate CD25 or Tac, the α chain of the IL-2 receptor. IL-2 receptors are found on activated normal B cells, suggesting that HCL corresponds to an activated stage of B cells. Several antibodies reactive with HCL (HCL-2, αS-HCL) have also been developed.[28]

Follicular and Diffuse Lymphomas

Follicular lymphomas are believed to be a proliferation of follicular center B cells. These cells usually express surface IgM and a small quantity of IgD, although surface Ig negative cases occur. They usually display HLA-DR, CD19, and CD20. Moreover, about 50% demonstrate CD10.[31] Diffuse lymphomas also usually display surface Ig, although examples of acquired Ig defects are noted. These lymphomas possess HLA-DR, CD19, CD20, and CD21 but lack CD10.

Waldenström's macroglobulinemia is characterized by plasmacytoid B cells secreting large amounts of IgM. These cells still display surface IgM, HLA-DR, CD19, and CD20 but also possess the PCA-1 antigen.[32] In contrast, multiple myeloma reflects a malignancy of true plasma cells. They lack surface Ig, HLA-DR, CD19, CD20, and CD21.[33]

MOLECULAR CLASSIFICATION OF NEOPLASIA

Immunoglobulin Gene Subsegments Rearrange to Generate Antibody Diversity

The molecular dissection of the immune response has revealed the mechanisms that enable humans to generate a seemingly unlimited number of different antibody specificities (10^6 to 10^9).[34,35] The final antibody molecule is composed of two identical heavy chains of disulfide linked to two identical light chains. The N-terminal variable (V) portion of each chain possesses the antigen recognition site, whereas the C-terminal constant (C) portion is invariant in sequence and performs effector functions. In 1965, Dreyer and Bennett[36] examined limited peptide map information and correctly surmised that this unusual immunoglobulin molecule would be encoded by at least two separate gene segments. Studies by Leder[34] and Tonegawa[35] and their colleagues using recombinant DNA technology discovered that Ig genes were organized as discontinuous DNA segments in their embryonic or germline form that were assembled during B-cell development.

The V portion of the human heavy-chain gene is generated from families of variable (V_H) regions, a set of internal diversity (D_H) regions, and a strip of six alternative joining (J_H) gene segments located on chromosomal segment 14q32 (Fig. 26-2). The first step of Ig gene assemblage is usually to rearrange a D_H region together with a J_H region to produce a D_H/J_H intermediate rearrangement.[37] Subsequently, a V_H region fuses with the D_H/J_H combination to create the functional $V_H/D_H/J_H$ responsible for the cells heavy-chain protein. Inserted extranucleotides are frequently found at the site of each juncture and have been referred to as N segments.[12] These bases contribute to antibody diversity in that they are located at a site within the antibody molecule that has contact with an antigen. In addition, a somatic hypermutation mechanism is activated at a later stage of B-cell development, which alters the VDJ sequence and can improve the antigen-binding affinity.[38,39] Most human B cells have needed to rearrange both of their Ig heavy-chain alleles to create a workable $V_H/D_H/J_H$ recombination. The other allele often possesses an intermediate D_H/J_H or invalid rearrangement.

The earliest recognizable B cells display only surface IgM and thus use the most proximal constant region (C_H), which is C_μ (see Fig. 26-2). Subsequently, these cells exploit an alternative splicing mechanism to place either C_μ or C_δ with the same V/D/J specificity and display simultaneous surface IgM and IgD.[40,41] Finally, a heavy-chain class switch

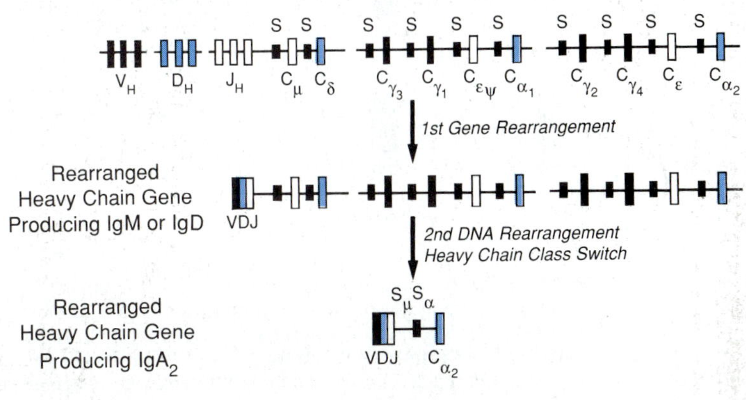

FIGURE 26-2. Schematic representation of human embryonic or germline heavy-chain gene locus on chromosome segment 14q32. The first DNA rearrangement assembles the variable (V), diversity (D), and joining (J) segments to complete the variable portion of the molecule. Later in development, a second DNA rearrangement may occur between the homologous switch sites flanking each construct (C) region. The heavy-chain class switch moves a distal C region next to the assembled VDJ.

may occur, which moves a more distal region of C_γ, $C_\epsilon 8$, or C_α next to that same V/D/J.[42–44] The heavy-chain class switch enables the same antigen specificity to be linked with a new C_H, providing the different physiologic function of an IgG, IgE, or IgA molecule.

Mature B cells produce but one of the two available light-chain classes, κ or λ, referred to as *isotypic exclusion*. From that selected light-chain class, the cell expresses only the maternal or paternal allele, referred to as *allelic exclusion*. Human B cells display κ in 60% of cases and λ in 40%. If a B cell is to ultimately produce κ light chain, it rearranges its κ gene locus immediately after heavy-chain rearrangement. The human κ gene locus is located on the short arm of chromosome 2 at band 2p11[45] (Fig. 26-3). Multiple different V_k segments exist in humans, but each is foreshortened, contributing only the N-terminal 95 amino acids of the 108 amino acids that constituted the V portion of the protein. The remaining 13 amino acids are contributed by one of five alternative joining (J_k) gene segments. Only one constant (C_k) gene region is present on each allele. Again, a process of V/J rearrangement completes the coding sequence for the V portion and activates this gene. The alternative λ light-chain gene is located on chromosome segment 22q11.[46] Similarly, it assembles V_λ/J_λ segments to activate this gene. It is slightly more complex because it is composed of multiple J_λ–C_λ clusters (six to nine in humans), which have a common pool of V_λ regions. An analysis of clonal pre–B-cell and B-cell malignancies revealed an ordered sequence of light-chain rearrangement in which κ preceded λ.

Immunoglobulin Gene Rearrangements

The molecular event that moves and combines a V and J segment results in the relocation of restriction endonuclease sites at the DNA level. Consequently, the DNA restriction fragment that bears an Ig gene in its rearranged form is of altered size compared with the germline form of the gene (see Fig. 26-3). Classic B-cell malignancies represent clonal expansions of a single progenitor cell. Each tumor possesses multiple copies of an identical V/J rearrangement. This expanded copy number makes it possible to detect such rearrangements by routine Southern blots. Because each B cell uses one V and one J of the many possibilities, the pattern of its gene rearrangement is unique to that cell. Thus, these rearrangements serve as tumor-associated molecular markers useful in determining clonality and lineage commitment.[47–49]

An Ig or a TCR rearrangement is a moderately sensitive and specific marker, and detection of such may enable identification of minority populations (1% to 5%) of clonal cells in tissues of mixed cellularity. Clonality is not necessarily tantamount to a verdict of malignancy. Lymphoproliferation, particularly in the setting of immunodeficiency, can result in the emergence of transient clones, which need not result in malignancy.[48,50] The molecular rearrangement markers are unique to these cells and provide the capacity to follow the natural history of such clones.

Because DNA rearrangement markers do not require the production of the final protein, they are applicable to the entire spectrum of neoplasia including pre–B-cell and pre–T-cell neoplasms. Gene rearrangements have proved to be instructive for examining the cellular origin of lymphoid neoplasms lacking lineage restricted surface antigens. Moreover, a developmental hierarchy for both the Ig and TCR gene rearrangements is manifest during early B- and T-cell maturation and provides a means of categorizing the developmental stage of each neoplasm. Finally, a number of the unexpected rearrangements of Ig and TCR genes noted in lymphoid tumors have proved to be the sites of interchromosomal translocation.

Non–T-, Non–B-Cell Acute Lymphoblastic Leukemia: A Developmental Series of Lymphoid Precursors

Before the era of gene rearrangement analysis, little was known of the cellular origin of most (80%) ALL that lacked surface Ig and T-cell antigens. Consequently, ALLs had been referred to as non–T-, non–B-cell ALL, or even null cell ALL. Analysis of their Ig genes revealed that these ALLs appeared to represent a developmental cascade of B-cell precursors[47,51] (Fig. 26-4). Rarely found are leukemias of immature cells that represent uncommitted progenitors retaining all Ig and TCR genes in the germline form. These leukemias are often in children under 2 years of age.[52] Regardless of the age of the patient, this germline genotype for all receptors is a subgroup of ALL based on gene rearrangement and has the worst prognosis. The remainder of the non–T-, non–B-cell ALLs all possess rearranged Ig heavy-chain genes. Sixty percent of these retain germline κ and λ light-chain genes, providing the first evidence in humans that heavy-chain rearrangement precedes light-chain rearrangement.[47,51] Moreover, the patterns of light-chain rearrangement in the remaining 40% can be

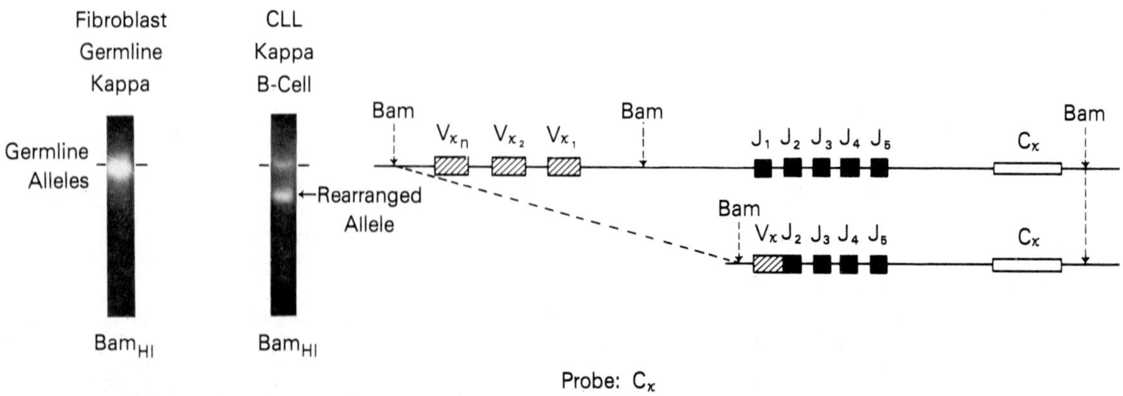

FIGURE 26-3. Southern blot detection of a rearranged human κ gene. The upper schematic denotes a germline configuration of the κ gene in which a C_κ probe recognizes a 12-kb sized BamHI fragment. Activation of a kappa allele juxtaposes one of many V_κ regions with one of five alternative J_κ segments. This V_κ/J_κ rearrangement introduces a new 5′ BamHI restriction site. Consequently, a rearranged kappa allele is altered in size compared with a germline allele.

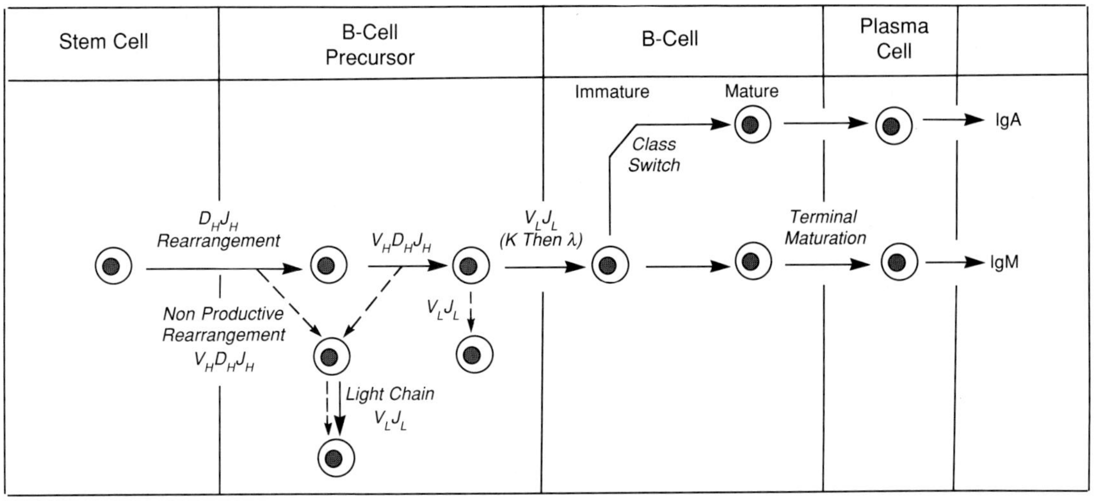

FIGURE 26-4. Solid lines reflect the pathway of correct Ig gene rearrangements during development in which heavy-chain diversity (D) segments rearrange to joining (J_H) segments followed by the addition of variable (V_H) segments. Subsequently, light chains rearrange generally in a kappa before lambda order. B-cell precursor leukemia may possess correct or nonproductive, aberrantly rearranged genes (*dashed lines*). Mature B-cell malignancies possess effective heavy- and light-chain rearrangements and surface IgM or other isotypes (eg, IgA) if they have undergone a heavy-chain class switch. Multiple myeloma corresponds to the terminally differentiated plasma cell stage.

construed as representing B-cell precursors arrested at sequential stages in a κ before λ sequence. The immunoglobulin gene pattern within these pre–B-cell ALLs has revealed a hierarchy of rearrangements in which heavy-chain genes preceded λ and κ rearrangements preceded λ.

A coordinate sequence of cell surface antigen expression accompanies this cascade of gene rearrangements during B-cell differentiation.[13] The earliest identifiable B-cell precursors possess the histocompatibility antigen, HLA-DR, and a B-cell–associated antigen, B4. Subsequently, a cell surface neutral endopeptidase, the CALLA, is expressed and the B1 B-cell–associated antigen is added later. The gene for J chain, a small glycoprotein that ultimately connects pentameric IgM and dimeric IgA, may also be expressed in human pre–B-cell ALLs.[53] Despite the presence of heavy-chain rearrangements in pre–B-cell ALLs, only about 25% actually produce cytoplasmic immunoglobulin μ chain protein.[15] This subset appears to have a worse prognosis that is intermediate between pre–B-cell ALLs without μ chain and mature B-cell ALL with L3 morphology.[54,55] Genetic explanations such as the presence of only intermediate D_H/J_H or aberrant $V_H/D_H/J_H$ rearrangements would account for the inability to produce μ chain in some ALLs. Others appear to possess effective $V_H/D_H/J_H$ rearrangements but fail to make μ chain at their arrested maturational stage of development.[56] Overall, the B-cell precursor ALLs have provided important details concerning normal and mistaken events of early B-cell differentiation.

Although TCR gene rearrangements are mandatory in T-cell development and Ig gene rearrangements are required in B-cell development, some spillover of Ig and TCR rearrangements also occurs into the opposite lineage.[57–59] About 10% of true T cells and occasional myeloid cells possess an Ig heavy-chain rearrangement. These are frequently incomplete D/J type rearrangements. Fortunately, the later B-cell developmental event of Ig light-chain rearrangement is usually restricted to the B-cell series. The lineage crossover of antigen receptor rearrangements can be seen within normal as well as malignant cells. This may reflect the presence of a single recombinase that mediates rearrangement of both Ig and TCR loci.[60] Such rearrangements occur early in development and perhaps at times before full lineage commitment has occurred. Because of the lineage spillover of TCR and Ig gene rearrangement, caution must be used when applying such markers to determine cellular type.

The presence of Ig κ or λ light-chain rearrangement is strong evidence of B-cell commitment. Similarly, the presence of TCR utilization in the absence of Ig gene rearrangement is almost conclusive for a T-cell origin. A most dramatic finding has been the occurrence of some TCR rearrangements within what had been genetically classified as pre–B-cell ALL. After the molecular cloning of the γ and δ TCR gene, the first to rearrange in development, it has become apparent that the so-called pre–B-cell ALLs have an inordinately high incidence of γ TCR (about 45%) and δ TCR (up to 90%) rearrangements.[52,59] Once again, the δ TCR rearrangements are predominantly incomplete, intermediate rearrangements. These cells possess other evidence of being more B- than T-lineage–committed. These cells bear HLA-DR, B4, and often B1, which are rarely seen on T cells, and they have uniform heavy-chain and at times light-chain rearrangements.

The high incidence of δ TCR rearrangements was not witnessed in mature B-cell neoplasms or cell lines. This indicates that this group of pre–B-cell ALLs does not represent the progenitor cells that give rise to more mature B cells. Moreover, further studies of cell surface antigens in pre–B-cell ALL and normal bone marrow suggest an asynchrony in the appearance of surface markers in this leukemia. Thus, pre–B-cell ALL may prove to be a rare subpopulation of cells made evident only by malignant transformation. On the other hand, ongoing gene rearrangement and inappropriate antigen expression may be consequences of transformation and immortalization at this immature stage.

The lack of tumor-restricted surface markers in ALL has prompted the use of gene rearrangement patterns to follow the natural history of this disease. A comparison of specific Ig heavy-chain and light-chain patterns at diagnosis and relapse indicated that most leukemic episodes of ALL represented the same clone. Occasionally, variation in Ig gene rearrangements may be seen over time, but even these shared at least one identical Ig gene rearrangement. Therefore, all episodes of clinical leukemia in an ALL patient appears to arise from a common clonal progenitor cell. This suggests that these leukemias are not truly biclonal because they do not arise from entirely independent transformation events.[61–63] The variation in Ig gene pattern may reflect accompanied alterations of other genes that confer a growth advantage and account for the emergency of these clonal subpopulations.

Multivariate analyses of children and adults with ALL have identified important, independent prognostic factors beyond the configuration of Ig genes. A markedly elevated white blood cell count (more than 50×10^9/L) at presentation has been known to inversely correlate with prognosis for some time. Age is also an important parameter, with patients 11 years of age or over and infants less than 1 year who demonstrate lower remission rates and shorter remission duration.[55] Males have a shorter duration of remission. An additional immunophenotypic parameter that is associated with a worse prognosis in adult ALL is the presence of myeloid antigens on the lymphoblasts.[64]

Cytogenetic abnormalities have been extensively studied in ALL, and recurrent translocations are common.[65,66] The most common translocations in pre–B type ALL are the t(1;19), t(9;22), and abnormalities of 11q23 including the t(4;11). About 5% of children and 25% of adults with ALL have the t(9;22)(q34;q11) Ph chromosome. The adult ALLs with the t(9;22) can be subdivided into two major molecular subtypes, depending on where they break within the breakpoint cluster region (*bcr*) gene. In about half of cases, the breakpoint is similar to chronic myelogenous leukemia and results in a 210-kd chimeric *bcr/abl* peptide, whereas the other portion resemble childhood ALL in which the breakpoint is further 5′ and manifests as a 190-kd *bcr/abl* protein. Prospective studies are underway to determine whether a substantial prognostic difference exists between these two translocation breakpoints. Mature B-cell ALL or Burkitt's leukemia typically possesses a c-*myc* to Ig locus translocation of the t(8;14), t(2;8), or t(8;22) variety. Beyond those specific interchromosomal aberrations, large studies have also indicated that pseudodiploidy has an unfavorable prognosis, whereas hyperdiploidy has a marginally better outcome.[65] Determining the molecular basis of these translocations holds the promise of providing better insights into the pathogenic subsets of ALL.

Lymphoid Blast Crisis in Chronic Myelogenous Leukemia

Chronic myelogenous leukemia (CML) is a clonal proliferation of cells arising from a remarkably pluripotent stem cell. Examination of G6PD alleles and the t(9;22) Ph chromosomal marker has revealed that numerous hematopoietic lineages could be clonally involved.[67] Because of the multipotential involvement in this disease, the exact lineage and stage of development of the blast crisis phases were often uncertain. A small percentage of lymphoid blast crises demonstrate cytoplasmic μ chain, indicating that this subset can be categorized as pre–B cells. The demonstration of rearranged heavy-chain and often light-chain immunoglobulin genes in most lymphoid crises argued that these cells are genetically committed B-cell precursors.[68,69] A soundly documented T-cell blast crisis has also been described.[70] In addition, the clonal cells in CML have proved capable of differentiation.

Similar to that seen in the clonal evolution in pre–B-cell ALL patients, CML patients may demonstrate several lymphoid blast crisis episodes over time. Serial examination of such CML crises revealed that separate lymphoid crises arise from a common B-lymphocyte progenitor with identical heavy-chain rearrangements; intact differentiation capacity manifested as a progression to light-chain rearrangement in some crises.[69] As the accompanying chapters detail the characteristic t(9;22)(q34;q11) results in a p210 *bcr/abl* fusion peptide with exaggerated tyrosine kinase activity. The predilection of CML for B-cell as opposed to T-cell lineage crises and the proclivity of Abelson murine leukemia virus to produce pre–B-cell lines furnish good arguments that this deregulated kinase may favor the B-cell pathway.

Chronic Lymphocytic Leukemia

Mature B cells must possess the obligate rearrangement of heavy-chain and light-chain immunoglobulin genes corresponding to their cell surface antibody (see Figs. 26-2 and 26-3). In addition to the first DNA rearrangement that assembles the V/D/J, such cells may demonstrate a second rearrangement known as the heavy-chain class switch (see Fig. 26-2). This enables the efficient production of the more 3′ C_H regions responsible for IgG, IgA, or IgE. Mature B cells often display archaeologic evidence of the ordered rearrangement of light-chain genes. In general, κ-producing cells often retain germline λ genes, whereas λ-producing cells have usually deleted their κ genes.

The mature B-cell leukemia, CLL, represents a clonal expansion of a novel subset of B cells. Most CLLs (more than 95%) bear CD5 (Leu-1, OKT-1) a 67-kd surface protein. CLLs are felt to represent a malignant expansion of the CD5 subset of B cells that account for less than 15% of B cells in normal persons. CD5 B cells are associated with the production of autoantibodies such as rheumatoid factor (RF) and anti-DNA Abs frequently of the spontaneously secreted IgM type. κ-producing CLL cells have been shown to express a single V_κIIIb region in about 25% of cases.[71] This HumKu 325 subgroup encodes the idiotype found in most monoclonal RFs. Recently, other cross-reactive idiotypes found on human IgM RF paraproteins have also been found to be overrepresented in CLL.[72] Moreover, CLLs do not appear to possess hypermutational activity for Ig genes and retain the germline sequence for these immunoglobulins. These findings indicate that CLL arises from a distinct subpopulation of B cells possessing a restricted Ig gene repertoire.

Follicular Lymphoma as a Hypermutational B-Cell Stage

Follicular lymphomas are monoclonal expansions of B cells thought to represent follicular center cells. This proliferation results in a nodular pattern caused by the expansion of the B-cell zone of a lymphoid follicle. These cells commonly display surface IgM often with low levels of IgD or occasionally IgG. In addition to other B-cell lineage markers, follicular lyphomas are the only mature B-cell malignancy frequently positive for CD10. Although the initial clinical course of follicular lymphoma is often indolent, the neoplastic cells are usually widely distributed, including into bone marrow and blood. During a normal primary immune response, a population of memory B cells is generated that is relatively long-lived and enables a higher-affinity secondary response on reexposure to antigen. Part of this maturation of the Ig response is related to the presence of extensive somatic mutation within V regions. Follicular lymphomas have been shown to display clonal variation with respect to their Ig idiotype (id; a measurement of the uniqueness of an antibody molecule). This has been shown to result in a high rate of V region somatic mutation that is ongoing within the tumors.[73] Unfortunately, this mutation often enables these tumors to escape from anti-id antibody therapy.[74] In contrast, the rate of somatic mutation in other B-cell tumors including CLL, pre–B ALL, and Burkitt's leukemia-lymphoma have been shown to be low.[75–77] This suggests that follicular B-cell lymphoma represents a neoplasm of a developmental stage characterized by selective hypermutation of Ig genes.

Heavy-Chain Disease: Defects in Immunoglobulin RNA Splicing

A subset of B-cell lymphoproliferative disorders demonstrate only surface Ig heavy chain, but no associated light chain.[78] Such heavy-chain diseases (HCD) have been described for all three major Ig classes (IgM, IgG, IgA). Studies of these heavy-chain proteins revealed them to be truncated and lacking all or most of the V region. They often began at sites of interdomain, exon boundaries, within the C region.[78] Three generalized mechanisms could be envisioned as the cause of these shortened heavy chains: postsynthetic degradation, DNA deletion, and an RNA splicing abnormality. The precise molecular basis for this event has been detailed in both a μ and a γ HCD.[79–82]

The initially synthesized heavy-chain protein in all cases of HCD examined has been small, indicating no role for extensive postsynthetic degradation. Any number of defects within the complex process of correctly expressing a heavy chain could prove responsible for HCD. Mistaken VDJ rearrangement or heavy-chain class switching might delete important regions and result in an incorrectly initiated RNA or an RNA splicing abnormality. Alternatively, simple somatic mutation could also eliminate donor or acceptor splice sites and consequently remove the corresponding V or C subsegments. A molecular dissection of HCDs has revealed multiple different defects.

A μ HCD protein was shown to arise from an aberrant RNA splice between the leader sequence and the constant μ (C_μ) region[79] (Fig. 26-5). This proved to be secondary to a small DNA insertion–deletion event that removed the J region's donor splice site and necessitated an aberrant RNA splice between the leader region and the first exon (CH1) of C_μ. This direct fusion of leader and C region sequence created a recognition sequence for signal peptidase cleavage

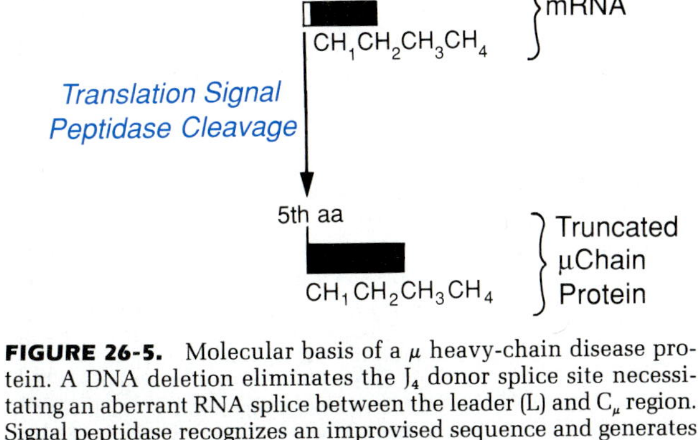

FIGURE 26-5. Molecular basis of a μ heavy-chain disease protein. A DNA deletion eliminates the J_4 donor splice site necessitating an aberrant RNA splice between the leader (L) and C_μ region. Signal peptidase recognizes an improvised sequence and generates a truncated μ chain that begins at the fifth amino acid (5th aa) of the CH1 domain.

at the fifth amino acid of the first exon (CH1) of the region C_μ. The product is a truncated μ chain that possesses only C region, lacks V region, and consequently fails to assemble with light chain.

Several γ HCD lymphomas have also been examined that demonstrate abnormal DNA deletions of portions of their utilized V region.[80,81] In one example, sequences apparently of nongenomic origin have been inserted into an assembled V region. This was compounded by an abnormal heavy-chain class switch event that eliminated the CH1 acceptor splice site. The molecular consequence is redirected RNA splicing between the leader and hinge exon of C_γ. This accounts for the $\gamma 1$ HCD protein that begins within the hinge. These well-studied examples suggest a common mechanism for the generation of HCD proteins that initiate at the boundaries of Ig domains. Step 1 would be the elimination of effective donor or acceptor splice sites at the DNA level by an inappropriate Ig rearrangement, by an insertion/deletion, or perhaps by somatic mutation. This forces step 2, an alternative RNA processing in which the leader exon is spliced to the next available Ig exon, accounting for the common features of HCD protein: truncated Ig heavy chains that fail to assemble light chains and are present both on the surface of the B cells and in the serum.

An important molecular difference exists between μ HCD and γ and α HCDs. Most μ HCD cells secrete a normal-sized free light chain, which is filtered into the urine as a Bence Jones protein. In contrast, most γ and α HCD cells synthesize no complete light chain.[78] Examination of a γ HCD revealed a defective κ light chain with extensive somatic mutation that eliminated acceptor and donor splice sites.[82] This γ HCD has defects in both heavy-chain and light-chain genes, raising important questions as to which gene defect occurs first. Evidence exists that free intact heavy chains can be toxic to cells, whereas free light chain is easily tolerated. This argues for a model in which light-chain abnormalities might arise first. This event would rapidly select subclones with an acquired γ gene defect that permitted the transport and secretion of a truncated heavy chain. Thus, α and γ HCD might also be thought of as a light-chain absence disease. The simultaneous heavy-chain and light-chain defects may prove to reflect a hypermutational process operative in the γ and α HCD B cells, but not in the μ HCD B cells that often resemble CLL.

Sjögren's Syndrome as a Preneoplastic Model

Sjögren's syndrome, long regarded as an autoimmune disorder, is also characterized by lymphoid cell overgrowth and infiltration of tissues. The salivary and lacrimal glands are the initial sites of an infiltrate of B and T cells, which result in a glandular destruction called the *benign lymphoepithelial lesion*. Some patients develop extraglandular lymphoid aggregates termed *pseudolymphoma*, which usually follow a benign course. Over time, Sjögren's syndrome patients also demonstrate an increased incidence of NHLs. Application of molecular technology has indicated that Ig gene rearrangements, and thus clonal B cells, are already present at the stage of the benign lymphoepithelial lesion.[83] The light-chain rearrangements were disproportionately κ and not λ in type. Moreover, the lymphomas from Sjögren's patients usually display κ rather than λ light chain.[84] Evidence is emerging that sera of Sjögren's patients often possess a V_κ-encoded rheumatoid factor and that their B-cell lymphomas often used the same RF encoding V_κIIIb region associated with CLL.[85] Therefore, molecular genetic data suggest that Sjögren's syndrome may provide a model of multistep malignancy. The early benign lymphoepithe-

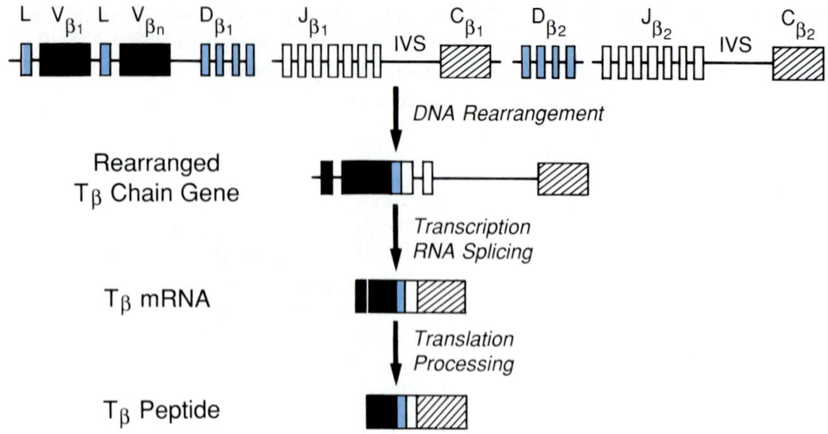

FIGURE 26-6. Schematic representation of the human β-chain gene of the T-cell receptor. Two constant regions ($C_{\beta 1}$ and $C_{\beta 2}$) possess their own set of joining ($J_{\beta 1}$ and $J_{\beta 2}$) as well as diversity ($D_{\beta 1}$ and $D_{\beta 2}$) segments. A common pool of variable (V_β) segments is assembled by a rearrangement process, followed by transcription RNA splicing, translation, and processing to generate the final β chain.

lial lesion already possesses a clonal outgrowth of a distinct B-cell subset. These clones may be subject to continued proliferation, providing the opportunity for genetic alterations that account for the high incidence of lymphoma in Sjögren's syndrome.

A DEVELOPMENTAL SEQUENCE OF T-CELL RECEPTOR GENE ACTIVATION

T cells also demonstrate antigen-specific recognition through a cell surface T_3–Ti (idiotype) complex. The Ti portion is the antigen receptor and is composed of either α plus β TCR chains or alternative γ plus δ heterodimeric TCR chains. The genes for α, β, γ, and δ TCR chains have been cloned and characterized. These genes are evolutionarily related but distinct from Ig genes, and they also rearrange to assemble gene subsegments. The β TCR gene located on chromosome segment 7q35 is diagrammed in Figure 26-6.[86,87] It has two available constant regions, $C_\beta 1$ and $C_\beta 2$, sets of diversity (D_β) and joining (J_β) segments as well. The γ TCR complex is located on chromosome segment 7p15 and is rearranged and expressed early in T-cell development.[88–90] The α and δ TCR loci have the most novel organization. The δ TCR is a gene within a gene located within the heart of the α TCR complex on chromosome segment 14q11.[91,92] An important advantage must exist for embracing this complexity. The rationale is not immediately obvious, since the δ and α loci most often use unique rather than shared sets of Vs, Ds, and Js. One possible explanation is that the δ within α TCR design is intentional to ensure that an early T cell can make only α or δ (Fig. 26-7).

Some evidence is emerging that suggests that the $\gamma\delta$ and $\alpha\beta$ TCR pathways are distinct rather than sequential lineages.[93] Since the δ TCR locus is located between V_α and J_α region, any V_α/J_α rearrangement would loop out and delete the δ TCR locus. Moreover, specialized sequences known as δ deleting elements flank the δ TCR locus and rearrange in thymus to eliminate the possibility of making δ but not α. One intriguing possibility is that an early decision to rearrange rather than eliminate the δ TCR locus may provide a pivotal event in choosing between the $\gamma\delta$ and the $\alpha\beta$ lineages.

T-Cell Receptor Rearrangements

The TCR genes provided the first uniformly applicable clonal markers for T cells and proved that most T-cell neoplasms were of clonal origin.[57,58,94–99] The TCR genes enable issues of lineage commitment, clonality, stage of develop-

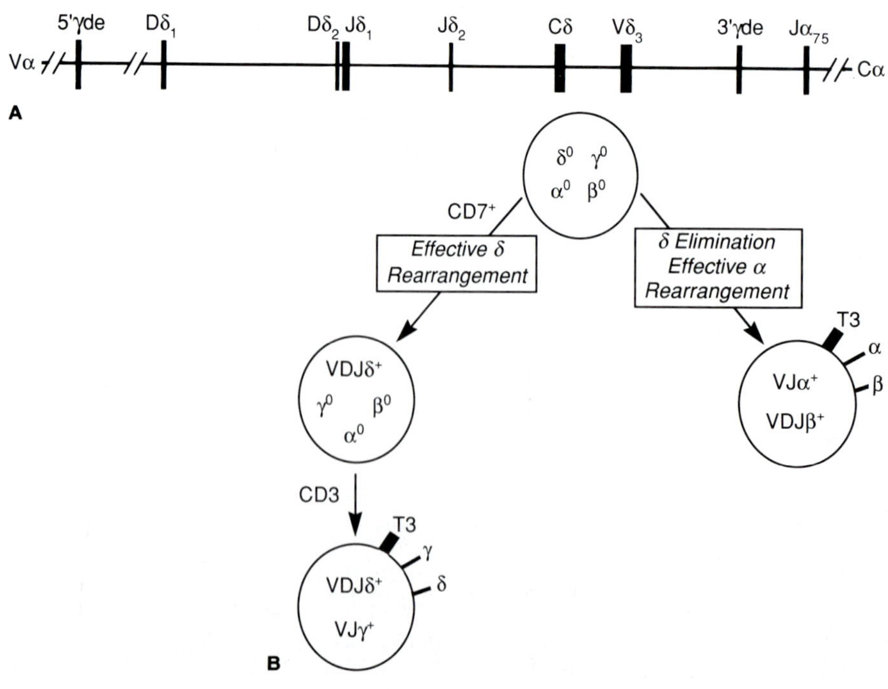

FIGURE 26-7. (**A**) Schematic organization of the germline human α/δ T-cell receptor locus at 14q11. (**B**) Proposed scheme of lineage determination starting with pluripotent T stem cell with germline $\delta^0\gamma^0\alpha^0$ and β^0 TcR genes. The effective rearrangement of VDJδ+ or δ elimination and α rearrangement may help select the $\gamma\delta$ versus $\alpha\beta$ cell pathways.

ment, and site of translocation to be addressed in T-cell neoplasms parallel with the use of Ig genes in B cells. The assessment of TCR genes has been useful in addressing whether T-cell lymphoproliferations are polyclonal expansions of regulatory T cells or monoclonal proliferations. TCR genes were instructive in the CD8 (Tγ) lymphocytosis often associated with hematocytopenias, especially granulocytopenia. The regulatory capacities of these large granular lymphocytes and the often indolent course raised questions as to whether the leukemia was a chronic or a reactive process. Most of these patients (about 80%) have revealed clonal β or γ (or both) TCR rearrangements, indicating a clonal neoplasia.[94,97,99]

T-cell acute lymphoblastic leukemia (T-ALL) represents clonal expansion of maturationally arrested cells at specific stages of thymic ontogeny as schematized in Figure 26-7. T-ALLs are seen that have only rearranged the δ TCR and express CD7.[92] $\gamma\delta$ T-ALLs possessing the subsequent CD2 and CD3 molecules also exist. Moreover, the T-ALLs revealed monoclonal CD3-T cells that had deleted the δ TCR and other more mature T cells with CD3 together with CD4 or CD8 that demonstrated $\alpha\beta$ heterodimers.[92] The adoption of intensive treatment regimens has markedly improved the response and duration of remission for T-ALLs. Preliminary studies indicate that the most immature T-ALLs with only the CD7 marker are a subgroup with a poorer response to chemotherapeutic regimens.[16,100]

CHROMOSOMAL TRANSLOCATIONS

Immunoglobulin Gene Loci

Specific interchromosomal translocations are uniquely or highly associated within distinct types of neoplasms.[101,102] Within mature B-cell malignancies, the most common sites of translocation involve the cytogenetic bands that possess the Ig gene loci (Table 26-5). The most common translocation in Burkitt's lymphoma, a t(8;14) reciprocal translocation, involves 14q32, the home of the Ig heavy-chain gene. The variant translocations present in about 15% of Burkitt's lymphomas were shown to involve the site of the κ gene at 2p11 or λ light-chain gene at 22q11.[103] The t(8;14) of Burkitt's lymphoma was the first interchromosomal translocation to be characterized at a molecular level (Fig. 26-8). This translocation juxtaposed the Ig heavy-chain, κ, or λ loci with the c-*myc* cellular protooncogene from chromosome segment 8q24.[104–106] Thus, Burkitt's lymphoma represents the first technical generation of translocation breakpoints in which two known genes were relocated onto a common DNA fragment.

Further dissection of the Burkitt's chromosomal translocation has revealed important insights concerning the role of the Ig-*myc* translocation in the genesis of neoplasia. Analysis of multiple t(8;14) breakpoints revealed that they break 5′ to *myc* protein encoding exons II and III, whereas the t(8;22) and t(2;8) breakpoints lie 3′ to c-*myc*. These experiments of nature revealed that the *myc* protein-encoding region itself was never interrupted, indicating that it was the critically important gene on chromosome segment 8q24.

The target site for rearrangement within the Ig locus at 14q32 can vary. The endemic Burkitt's lymphomas of Central Africa, which are epidemiologically associated with Epstein-Barr virus and malaria, are frequently more immature in phenotype and juxtapose a heavy-chain joining region with 8q24. Conversely, the sporadic cases of Burkitt's lymphoma in the United States frequently involve the μ switch region of the heavy-chain locus. In the latter cases, the Ig enhancer region capable of increasing the transcription of unrelated promoters would not be on the same chromosome as the *myc* gene. This was some of the first evidence to indicate that the deregulation of c-*myc* would involve mechanisms other than overexpression secondary to the Ig enhancer sequence.

Detailed analysis of the 5′ end of translocated *myc* genes has revealed a high incidence of somatic mutation flanking a Pvu II site at the end of exon I and the beginning of intron I.[107] Normally, mature B cells attenuate the elongation of their c-*myc* RNAs within this region. In contrast, Burkitt's lymphoma cells that possess altered nucleotides at these regulatory sites are capable of elongating their c-*myc* RNA transcripts. Therefore, the acquisition of somatic mutations may also play a role in deregulating c-*myc* in Burkitt's lymphoma.

The prospective importance of the c-*myc* translocation in lymphoid neoplasia was established by placing a deregulated *myc* gene construct into the germline of mice.[108,109] Transgenic mice possessing a *myc* gene fused to an Ig enhancer (Eμ-*myc*) developed an initial polyclonal pre–B-cell hyperplasia that progressed over a short period of time to monoclonal life-threatening malignancies. The time course of tumor development suggested that other genetic abnormalities were required for full tumorigenesis. This experimental system is being exploited to define the specific genes capable of complementing *myc* in tumorigenesis. Moreover, tumorigenesis studies using human lymphoblastoid cell lines revealed that the addition of deregulated *myc* could complement Epstein-Barr virus, providing experimental evidence for two of the major etiologic events in Burkitt's lymphoma.[110]

TABLE 26-5. Chromosomal Translocations in B-Lymphoid Neoplasms

Translocation	Type of Neoplasm
t(8;14)(q24;q32) t(8;22)(q24;q11) t(2;8)(p11;q24)	Burkitt's lymphoma
t(11;14)(q13;q32)	Multiple myeloma
	B-cell chronic lymphocytic leukemia
	Small-cell lymphocytic lymphoma
	Diffuse large-cell lymphoma
t(14;18)(q32;q21)	Follicular small cleaved-cell lymphoma
	Follicular mixed-cell lymphoma
	Follicular large-cell lymphoma
	Diffuse large-cell lymphoma

bcl-2 Protooncogene in Follicular Lymphoma

A second technologic generation of translocations juxtaposes a known gene on one side of the chromosomal breakpoint with a new putative protooncogene on the other. The quintessential example of this is the t(14;18) (q32;q21) of follicular lymphoma, a neoplasm of early follicular center B cells. The typical lymphoma has a normal chromosome 14, a normal chromosome 18, and two reciprocal products including the derivative (der) 14 that introduces the *bcl*-2 gene into the Ig heavy-chain locus[111–113] (Fig. 26-9). Despite the mature B-cell phenotype of t(14;18)-bearing lymphomas, the translocation appears to occur earlier in development at pre–B-cell stage.[114] Ig recombinase initiates the first attempted rearrangement in pre–B development by cleaving at a D and J segment. Instead of completing that recombination, progenitor cells of follicular lymphoma introduce a broken *bcl*-2 gene from 18q21 into these Ig sites. Less than 70% of breakpoints on chromosome 18 occur within a major breakpoint region in the 3′ untranslated region of the *bcl*-2 gene. The molecular consequence is to

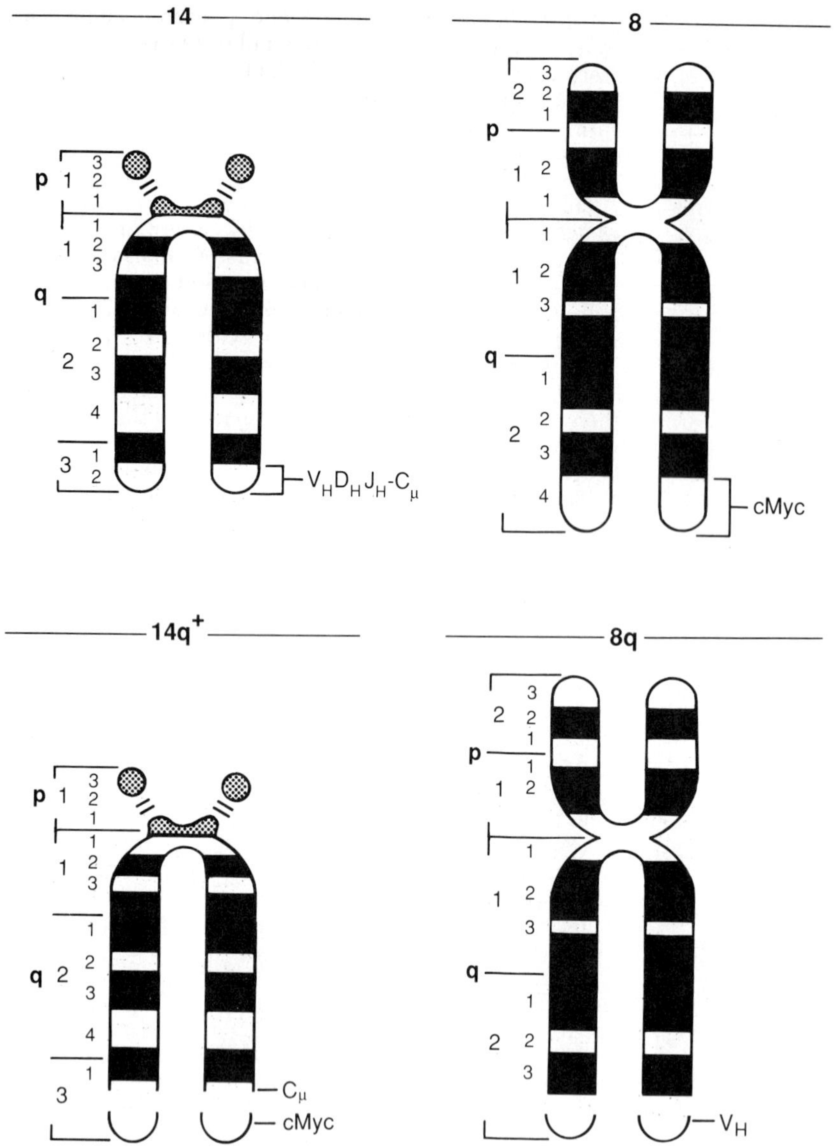

FIGURE 26-8. Schematic molecular karyotype of Burkitt's lymphoma t(8;14). The normal chromosome 14 possesses an effectively rearranged $V_H/D_H/J_H$ responsible for IgM production. The normal chromosome 8 retains a germline copy of the c-*myc* oncogene. The 14q+ chromosome at band 14q32 introduces the c-*myc* gene from chromosome 8. The 8q− chromosome reciprocally receives a portion of chromosome 14 usually including V_H segments.

move *bcl*-2 from its native home on chromosome 18 to the J_H region on chromosome 14 and to generate a *bcl*-2–Ig fusion gene.[115,116] Placing *bcl*-2 into the geographic locale of the Ig locus markedly deregulates the gene by altering both its transcription and its RNA processing. The result is an inappropriately increased amount of *bcl*-2–Ig chimeric RNA as well as the 25-kd *bcl*-2 protein.

The cloning of this second generation breakpoint provided a new gene, *bcl*-2, for assessment. The *bcl*-2 gene encodes a unique 25-kd membrane associated intracellular protein with no significant homology to other protooncogenes. The expression of the normal *bcl*-2 gene is associated with B-cell activation. The *bcl*-2 gene is quiescent in resting B cells, but is expressed after activation with antigen and B-cell growth factors. It is subsequently down-regulated as the B-cell differentiates.

A major question still remained as to whether any of the newly discovered genes, including *bcl*-2, found at the sites of chromosomal translocation would prove to be transforming in a prospective fashion. When *bcl*-2 was placed into human B lymphoblastoid lines, it consistently improved their growth in soft agar.[117,118] Although it was insufficient as a single agent to fully transform such cells, *bcl*-2 was able to complement the c-*myc* gene in inducing tumors.[117] A further dissection of *bcl*-2's mechanism of action reveals that it provides a survival advantage to certain growth factor–starved cells.[119] Cells that would normally die in the absence of an interleukin are spared from death but remain in a G0 resting state.

A transgenic mouse model has convincingly been generated with a *bcl*-2–Ig minigene within its germline, which recreates the molecular consequence of the t(14;18) translocation.[120] These mice uniformly develop a follicular lymphoproliferation, which selectively expands a small resting IgM/IgD B cell. Again, these cells demonstrate no proliferative advantage but show extended survival. The result is the accumulation of excess B cells in the spleen, lymph nodes, and bone marrow. Over time, these B cells acquire secondary genetic events and progress to monoclonal, often high-grade lymphoma. This provides an animal model that is highly reminiscent of human follicular lymphoma, which is often indolent for years before progressing to a threatening diffuse large-cell lymphoma.

T-Cell Translocations

The most common interchromosomal translocation within T-lymphoid neoplasms also involves their antigen receptor genes. Chromosome segment 14q11, the home of the $\alpha\delta$ TCR, is most frequently involved. In fact, the fact that many

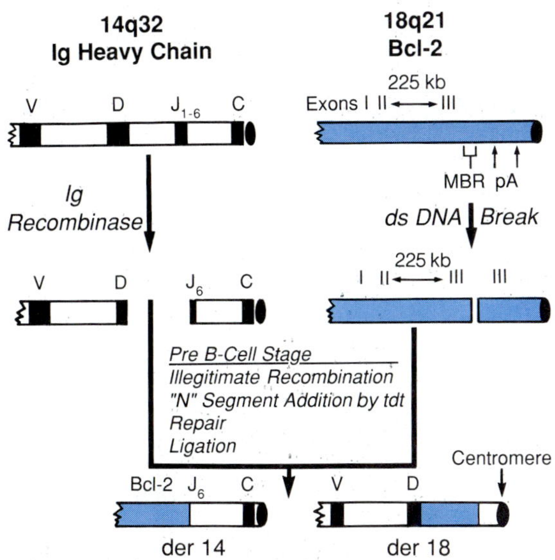

FIGURE 26-9. Mechanism of the t(14;18) recombination. Der 14 chromosomes demonstrate breakpoints at J segments, whereas der 18 breakpoints are at D segments. This suggests that the translocation occurs at a pre–B-cell stage when Ig recombinase has cleaved at a D and J segment and these ends recombine with a break at 18q21 within the major breakpoint region (MBR) of *bcl*-2 exon III.

of the T-cell leukemias with 14q11 breakpoints lacked $\alpha\beta$ TCRs and often CD3 suggested that they might be arrested during their attempts to assemble the δ TCR. The small size of the δ TCR locus has enabled a number of interchromosomal translocations to be cloned.[121–125] Analysis of transcripts from the far side of these chromosomal breakpoints has proved to be rewarding. Many of these protooncogene candidates are normally expressed in cell types other than T cells. Their introduction into the TCR locus markedly deregulates them and transfers their function to the T-cell lineage.

The t(11;14) (p15;q11) translocation in a T-ALL provided a new gene, Ttg-1, a 17-kd nuclear protein that demonstrates a zinc finger-like motif.[123] Another breakpoint in T-ALL, the t(7;19), identified the Lyl-1 gene with a helix–loop–helix DNA binding motif.[126] Moreover, the t(7;9) (q34;q34.3) has revealed a unique gene-bearing homology to the *Drosophila* notch locus.[127] In addition, molecular cloning of the t(10;14) has provided a new locus, HOX11, at 10q24.[124,125] Therefore, the incidence in which any single chromosomal segment is involved in T-cell neoplasia is lower than that seen in B-cell tumors. The greater number of recurrent translocations in these neoplasms is providing the opportunity to assess the contribution of a variety of new genes to T-cell neoplasia.

Diagnostic Applications of Interchromosomal Translocations

The detection of Ig and TCR gene rearrangements has led to increasing use in the molecular definition of lymphoid neoplasms, providing a great deal of insightful information. TCR and Ig genes also rearrange within normal lymphocytes and have a wide repertoire of potential recombinations. Although the Ig or TCR pattern is distinct for an individual tumor cell, the detection of these rearrangements by Southern blot techniques is only relatively sensitive, requiring 1% to 5% of all cells examined to be clonal. This limited sensitivity has hampered the capacity of these markers to detect minimal numbers of tumor cells.[62] Moreover, amplification of the TCR and Ig rearrangements also includes the possibility that similar rearrangements in normal cells may also be amplified.

In contrast, interchromosomal translocations appear to be limited to a malignant clone of cells and are not present (at least in detectable numbers) in normal cells. Many of these breakpoints are also restricted in their sites of cleavage. This makes it possible to design universal diagnostic tests that can be applied to a variety of cases. As illustrated in Figure 26-10, at t(14;18), the clustering of breakpoints within the *bcl*-2 major breakpoint region on chromosome 18 and at the Ig J_H sequence on chromosome 14 generates a rearranged restriction fragment with the *bcl*-2–Ig junction.[128] This rearrangement is specific to the malignant clone. Such molecular markers for *bcl*-2, *myc*, and *bcr-abl* translocations have been useful in resolving complex translocations in which routine cytogenetics was indeterminate. Improvements in the capacity to place fluorescent tags on such DNA probes and advances in confocal microscope technology may ultimately enable interchromosomal translocations to be directly diagnosed in interphase cells.

POLYMERASE CHAIN REACTION AND THE DETECTION OF MINIMAL RESIDUAL DISEASE

The capacity to detect minimal numbers of neoplastic cells is of major diagnostic importance for cancer patients. The ability to identify and distinguish patients after therapy who are truly cured from those with minimal residual disease is a major goal. Such information might spare patients without disease from needless maintenance therapy and allow patients with residual disease to be stratified into more innovative treatment regimens.

The focused nature of many chromosomal translocations provides an amplifiable site of interchromosomal juncture (see Fig. 26-10). This is accomplished by a DNA polymerase chain reaction (PCR).[129,130] As illustrated for the t(14;18) breakpoint in Figure 26-11, short oligonucleotide primers are synthesized that anneal to *BCL*-2 sequences or Ig J_H sequences flanking the breakpoint. To initiate the reaction, a source of lymphoma DNA possessing the t(14;18) juncture

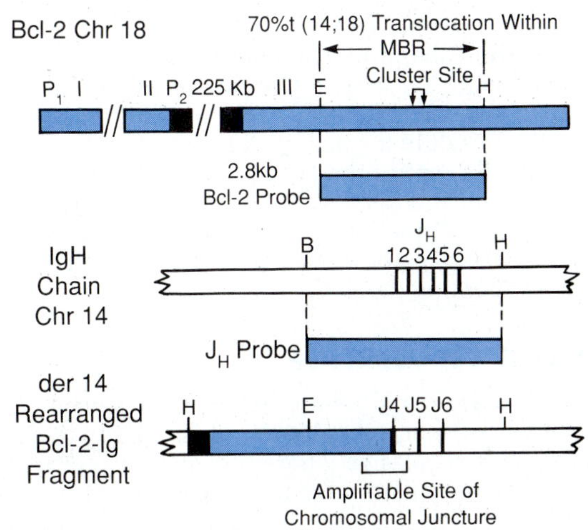

FIGURE 26-10. Schematic representation of a molecular marker for the t(14;18) interchromosomal breakpoint. The der (14) chromosome possesses an altered size HindIII (H) DNA fragment that will hybridize to both a chromosome 18 *bcl*-2 probe or a chromosome 14 J_H probe. The focusing of the breakpoints on chromosome 14 and chromosome 18 results in an amplifiable site of chromosomal juncture.

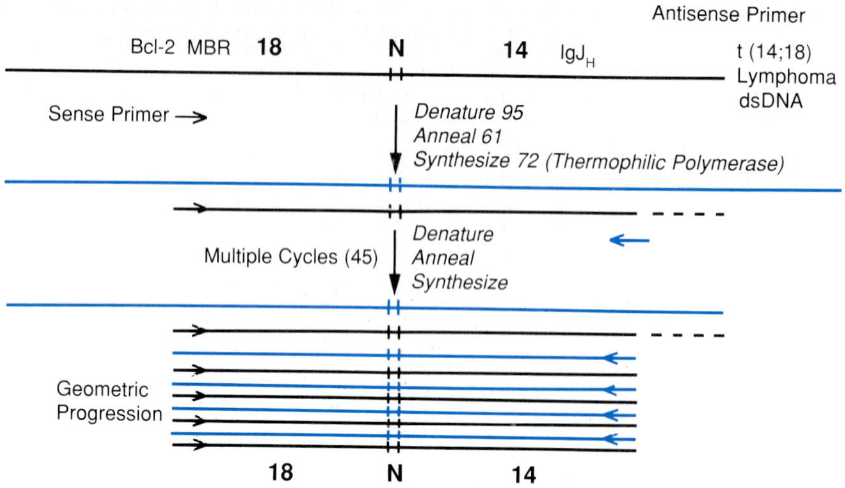

FIGURE 26-11. Schematic representation of polymerase chain reaction amplification of the t(14;18) breakpoint. A sense oligonucleotide primer 5′ to the *bcl*-2 major breakpoint region (MBR) is used together with an antisense primer complementary to the J_H region on chromosome 14. Successive cycles of denaturation, primer annealing, and synthesis with polymerase results in the specific amplification of a fragment possessing chromosome 18, N segment, and chromosome 14 information.

is denatured into single strands and the specific primers are annealed. The use of a thermostable form of DNA polymerase allows annealing and synthetic steps at high temperatures ensuring that this breakpoint is the only region amplified of the 3-by-10^9 base pairs of the human genome. Multiple cycles of the PCR result in the geometric amplification of a fragment containing the chromosomal breakpoint. This provides a sensitive and specific assay capable of amplifying one template copy of the breakpoint. In practical terms, PCR can detect 1 lymphoma cell in 1 million normal cells.[130] Similarly, PCR amplification can be applied to other translocations, provided that their DNA breakpoints are focused so that a few primers can be universally applied. In addition, it has been possible to amplify the hybrid RNA transcripts of the *bcr-abl* fusion in CML and ALL by first converting mRNA to cDNA with reverse transcriptase and then proceeding with the PCR.[131]

PCR reaction assays that amplify DNA breakpoints can also be performed on DNA extracted from fixed tissue blocks, enabling diagnostic studies on such samples. PCR assays of chromosomal breakpoints have identified subclinical leukemic cells and also provide the capability of quickly assessing protocols designed to purge malignant cells from bone marrow. Several caveats exist concerning the PCR technique. Although its usefulness is its exquisite sensitivity, its sensitivity makes it very vulnerable to false-positives from laboratory contamination.

It is theoretically possible that rare progenitor cells may possess the translocation but lack the additional genetic defects that result in the final malignancy. Unquestionably, PCR markedly refines the capacity to detect minimal residual disease. Prospective clinical trials will determine whether this information is important in clinical decisions related to the stage of disease, the stratifying treatment, and the evaluating therapy.

FUTURE CHALLENGE

Various histologic and immunophenotypic schemes have contributed an enormous amount to our ability to classify the lymphoid neoplasms. These schemes have provided a framework to compare the natural history and treatment responses of these diseases. The current challenge is to move beyond descriptive phenotypic stages and to identify the genetic basis for each tumor. A variety of approaches are helping to define the series of molecular transforming events within malignancies. This knowledge may provide the key to better predictions of biologic behavior, responsiveness to therapies, and prognosis. Molecular facts that can be translated into clinically relevant information will provide the basis for tomorrow's classification schemes.

REFERENCES

1. Mann RB, Jaffe ES, Berard CW. Malignant lymphoma: a conceptual understanding of morphologic diversity. Am J Pathol 1979;94:105.
2. Rappaport H. Tumors of the hematopoietic system. In: Atlas of tumor pathology, section III, fasc 8. Washington, DC, Armed Forces Institute of Pathology, 1966.
3. Lukes RJ, Collins RD. Immunologic characterization of human malignant lymphomas. Cancer 1974;34:1488.
4. Lennert K, Stein H, Kaiserling E. Cytological and functional criteria for the classification of malignant lymphomata. Br J Cancer 1975;31:29.
5. Dorfman RF. Classification of non-Hodgkin's lymphomas. Lancet 1974;1:1295.
6. The non-Hodgkin's lymphoma pathologic classification project: National Cancer Institute sponsored study of classifications of non-Hodgkin's lymphomas: summary and description of a working formulation for clinical usage. Cancer 1982;49:2112.
7. Nathwani B. The Rappaport classification of the non-Hodgkin's lymphomas: is it pertinent for the 1980's? In: Bennet JM, ed. Controversies in the management of lymphomas. Boston, Martinus Nijhoff, 1983.
8. Mann RB, Jaffe ES, Berard CW. Malignant lymphomas: a conceptual understanding of morphologic diversity—a review. Am J Pathol 1979;94:105.
9. Aisenberg AC. Cell surface markers in lymphoproliferative disease. N Engl J Med 1978;304:331.
10. Foon KA, Todd RF. Immunologic classification of leukemia and lymphoma. Blood 1986;68:1.
11. Foucar K, Chen I-Ming, Crago S. Organization and operation of a flow cytometric immunophenotyping laboratory. Semin Diagn Pathol 1989;6:13.
12. Desiderio S, Yancopoulos GD, Paskind M, et al. Insertion of N regions into heavy-chain genes is correlated with expression of terminal deoxytransferase in B cells. Nature 1984;311:752.
13. Nadler LM, Korsmeyer SJ, Anderson KC, et al. The B cell origin of non-T acute lymphoblastic leukemia: a model for discrete stages of neoplastic and normal pre-B cell differentiation. J Clin Invest 1984;74:332.
14. Greaves MF, Brown G, Rapson NT, et al. Antisera to ALL cells. Clin Immunol Immunopathol 1975;4:67.
15. Vogler LB, Crist WB, Bockman DE, et al. Pre-B cell leukemia: a new phenotype of childhood lymphoblastic leukemia. N Engl J Med 1978;298:872.
16. Kurtzberg J, Waldmann TA, Davey MP, et al. CD7+, CD_4−, CD8− acute leukemia: a syndrome of malignant, pluripotent lymphohematopoietic cells. Blood 1989;73:381.
17. Reinherz EL, Kung PC, Goldstein G, et al. Discrete stages of human intrathymic differentiation: analysis of normal thymocytes and leukemic lymphoblasts of T-cell lineage. Proc Natl Acad Sci USA 1980;77:1588.
18. Brouet JC, Flandrin G, Sasportes M, et al. Chronic lymphocytic leukemia of T-cell origin: immunologic and clinical evaluation in eleven patients. Lancet 1975;2:890.
19. Reynolds CW, Foon KA. Tγ-lymphoproliferative disease and related disorders in man and experimental animals: a review of the clinical, cellular and functional characteristics. Blood 1984;64:1146.

20. Bunn PA, Huberman MS, Wang-Peng J, et al. Prospective staging evaluation of patients with cutaneous T-cell lymphoma: demonstration of a high frequency of extracutaneous dissemination. Ann Intern Med 1980;93:223.
21. Haynes BF, Bunn P, Mann D, et al. Cell surface differentiation antigens of the malignant T cell in Sezary syndrome and mycosis fungoides. J Clin Invest 1981;67:523.
22. Green JP, York JC, Consar JB, et al. Peripheral T cell lymphoma: a clinicopathologic study of 42 cases. J Clin Oncol 1984;2:788.
23. Poiesz BJ, Ruscetti FW, Gazdar AF, et al. Detection and isolation of type C retrovirus particles from fresh and cultured lymphocytes of a patient with cutaneous T cell lymphoma. Proc Natl Acad Sci USA 1980;77:7415.
24. Tsudo M, Uchiyama T, Uchino H, Yodoi, J. Failure of regulation of Tac antigen-TCGF receptor in adult T-cell leukemia cells by the anti-Tac monoclonal antibody. Blood 1983;62:1014.
25. Ligler FS, Kettman JR, Smith G, Frenkel EP. Immunoglobulin phenotype on B cells correlates with clinical stage of chronic lymphocytic leukemia. Blood 1983;62:256.
26. Royston I, Majda JA, Baird SM, et al. Human T cell antigens defined by monoclonal antibodies: the 65,000-dalton antigen of T cells (T65) is also found on chronic lymphocytic leukemia cells bearing surface immunoglobulin. J Immunol 1980;125:725.
27. Melo JV, Foroni L, Babapulle B, et al. Prolymphocytic leukemia of B cell type: rearranged immunoglobulin (Ig) genes with defective Ig production. Blood 1985;66:391.
28. Posnett DN, Chiorazzi N, Kunkel HG. Monoclonal antibodies with specificity for hairy cell leukemia cells. J Clin Invest 1982;70:254.
29. Korsmeyer SJ, Greene WC, Cossman J, et al. Rearrangement and expression of immunoglobulin genes and expression of Tac antigen in hairy cell leukemia. Proc Natl Acad Sci USA 1983;80:4522.
30. Cleary ML, Wood GS, Warnke R, et al. Immunoglobulin gene rearrangements in hairy cell leukemia. Blood 1984;64:99.
31. Anderson KC, Bates MP, Slaughenhoupt BL, et al. Expression of human B cell–associated antigens on leukemias and lymphomas: a model of human B cell differentiation. Blood 1984;63:1424.
32. Koziner B, Kempin S, Passe S, et al. Characterization of B-cell leukemias: a tentative immunomorphological scheme. Blood 1980;56:815.
33. Foon KA, Schroff RW, Fligiel S. Monoclonal antibody characterization of plasmacytoma cells associated with T lymphocytes with a suppressor phenotype. Clin Immunol Immunopathol 1982;25:59.
34. Leder P. The genetics of antibody diversity. Sci Am 1982;246:102.
35. Tonegawa S. Somatic generation of antibody diversity. Nature 1983;302: 575.
36. Dreyer WJ, Bennet JC. The molecular basis of antibody formation: a paradox. Proc Natl Acad Sci USA 1965;54:864.
37. Ravetch JV, Siebenlist U, Korsmeyer SJ, et al. The structure of the human immunoglobulin μ locus: characterization of embryonic and rearranged J and D genes. Cell 1981;27:583.
38. Cook WD, Scharff MD. Antigen-binding mutants of mouse myeloma cells. Proc Natl Acad Sci USA 1977;74:5687.
39. Kim S, David M, Sinn E, et al. Antibody diversity: somatic hypermutation of rearranged VH genes. Cell 1981;27:573.
40. Knap MR, Liu C-P, Newell N, et al. Simultaneous expression of immunoglobulin μ and heavy chains by a cloned B cell lymphoma: a single copy of the V_H gene is shared by two adjacent C_H genes. Proc Natl Acad Sci USA 1982;79:2996.
41. Moore KW, Rogers J, Hunkapiller T, et al. Expression of IgD may use both DNA rearrangement and RNA splicing mechanisms. Proc Natl Acad Sci USA 1981;78:1800.
42. Davis MM, Kim SK, Hood LE. DNA sequences mediating class switching in α-immunoglobulins. Science 1980;209:1360.
43. Kataoka T, Miyata T, Honjo T. Repetitive sequences in class switch recombination regions of immunoglobulin heavy chain genes. Cell 1981;23:357.
44. Ravetch JV, Kirsch IR, Leder P. Evolutionary approach to the question of immunoglobulin heavy chain switching: evidence from cloned human and mouse genes. Proc Natl Acad Sci USA 1980;77:6734.
45. Malcolm S, Barton P, Murphy C, et al. Localization of human immunoglobulin κ light chain variable region genes to the short arm of chromosome 2 by in situ hybridization. Proc Natl Acad Sci USA 1982;79: 4957.
46. Hieter PA, Hollis GF, Korsmeyer SJ, et al. Clustered arrangement of immunoglobulin λ constant region genes in man. Nature 1981;294: 536.
47. Korsmeyer SJ, Hieter PA, Ravetch JV, et al. Developmental hierarchy of immunoglobulin gene rearrangements in human leukemic pre-B cells. Proc Natl Acad Sci USA 1981;78:7096.
48. Arnold A, Cossman J, Bakhshi A, et al. Immunoglobulin gene rearrangements as unique clonal markers in human lymphoid neoplasms. N Engl J Med 1983;309:1593.
49. Cleary ML, Chao J, Warnke R, Sklar J. Immunoglobulin gene rearrangement as a diagnostic criterion of B cell lymphoma. Proc Natl Acad Sci USA 1984;81:593.
50. Cleary ML, Warnke R, Sklar J. Monoclonality of lymphoproliferative lesions in cardiac-transplant recipients on immunoglobulin gene rearrangements. N Engl J Med 1984;310:477.
51. Korsmeyer SJ, Arnold A, Bakhshi A, et al. Immunoglobulin gene rearrangement and cell surface antigen expression in acute lymphocytic leukemias of T-cell and B-cell precursor origins. J Clin Invest 1983;71: 301.
52. Felix CA, Poplack DG, Kirsch IR. Characterization of immunoglobulin and T cell receptor gene patterns in B cell precursor acute lymphoblastic leukemia of childhood. J Clin Oncol 1989.
53. Max EE, Korsmeyer SJ. The human J chain gene: structure and expression in B lymphoid cells. J Exp Med 1985;161;832.
54. Crist W, Boyett J, Jackson J, et al. Prognostic importance of the pre B cell immunophenotype and other presenting features in B-lineage childhood acute lymphoblastic leukemia: a Pediatric Oncology Group study. Blood 1989;74:1252.
55. Jackson J, Dowell B, Frankel L, et al. Clinical and biologic features predict a poor prognosis in acute lymphoid leukemias in infants: a Pediatric Oncology Group review. Blood 1986;67:135.
56. Cossman J, Neckers LM, Arnold A, et al. Induction of differentiation in the primitive B-cell of common acute lymphoblastic leukemia. N Engl J Med 1982;307:1251.
57. Griesser H, Tkachuk D, Reis MD, et al. Gene rearrangements and translocations in lymphoproliferative diseases. Blood 1989;73:1402.
58. Waldman TA. The arrangement of immunoglobulin and T cell receptor genes in human lymphoproliferative disorders. Adv Immunol 1987;40: 247.
59. Felix CA, Wright JJ, Poplack DG, et al. T cell receptor α-, β-, and γ-genes in T cell and pre-B cell acute lymphoblastic leukemia. J Clin Invest 1987;80:545.
60. Yoncopoulos G, Blackwell TK, Suh H, et al. Introduced T cell receptor variable region gene segments in pre-B cells: evidence that B and T cells use a common recombinase. Cell 1986;44:251.
61. Sklar J, Cleary ML, Thielemans K, et al. Biclonal B cell lymphoma. N Engl J Med 1984;311:20.
62. Wright JJ, Poplack DG, Bakhshi A, et al. Gene rearrangements as markers of clonal variation and minimal residual disease in acute lymphoblastic leukemia. J Clin Oncol 1987;5:735.
63. Raffeld M, Wright JJ, Lipford E, et al. Clonal evolution of t(14;18) follicular lymphomas demonstrated by immunoglobulin genes and an 18q21 breakpoint region. Cancer Res 1987;47:2537.
64. Sobol RE, Mick R, Royston I, et al. Clinical importance of myeloid antigens expression in adults acute lymphoblastic leukemia. N Engl J Med 1987;316:1111.
65. Look AT. The cytogenetics of childhood leukemia: clinical and biologic implications. Pediatr Clin North Am 1988;35:723.
66. Champlin R, Gale RP. Acute lymphoblastic leukemia: recent advances in biology and therapy. Blood 1989;73:2051.
67. Barr RD, Fialkow PF. Clonal origin of chronic myelocytic leukemia. N Engl J Med 1973;289:307.
68. Ford AM, Molgaard HV, Greaves MF, et al. Immunoglobulin gene organization and expression in hematopoietic stem cell leukemia. EMBO J 1983;2:997.
69. Bakhshi A, Minowada J, Arnold A, et al. Lymphoid blast crises of chronic myelogenous leukemia represent stages in the development of B-cell precursors. N Engl J Med 1983;309:826.
70. Chan LC, Furley AJ, Ford AM, et al. Clonal rearrangement and expression of T cell receptor β gene and involvement of the breakpoint cluster region in blast crises of CGL. Blood 1986;67:533.
71. Kipps TJ, Fong S, Tomhove E, et al. High frequency expression of a conserved κ light chain variable-region gene in chronic lymphocytic leukemia. Proc Natl Acad Sci USA 1987;84:2916.
72. Kipps TJ, Robbins BA, Kuster P, Corsan DA. Auto-antibody associated cross-reactive idiotypes expressed at high frequency in chronic lymphocyte leukemia relative to B cell lymphomas of follicular center cell origin. Blood 1988;72:422.
73. Cleary ML, Meeker TC, Levy S, et al. Clustering of extensive somatic mutations in the variable region of an immunoglobulin heavy chain gene from a human B cell lymphoma. Cell 1986;44:97.
74. Meeker T, Lowder J, Cleary ML, et al. Emergence of idiotype variants during treatment of B cell lymphoma with anti-idiotype antibodies. N Engl J Med 1985;312:1658.
75. Meeker TC, Grimaldi JC, O'Rourke R, et al. Lack of detectable somatic hypermutation in the V region of the Ig H chain gene of a human chronic B lymphocytic leukemia. J Immunol 1988;141:3994.
76. Bird J, Galili N, Link M, et al. Continuing rearrangement but absence of somatic hypermutation in immunoglobulin genes of human B cell precursor leukemia. J Exp Med 1989;168:229.
77. Carroll WL, Yu M, Link MP, Korsmeyer SJ. Absence of Ig V region gene somatic hypermutation in advanced Burkitt's lymphoma. J Immunol 1989;143:692.
78. Seligman M, Mihaesco E, Preud'homme JL, et al. Heavy chain disease: current findings and concepts. Immunol Rev 1979;48:145.
79. Bakhshi A, Guglielmi P, Siebenlist U. A DNA insertion/deletion necessitates an aberrant splice accounting for a human mu heavy chain disease protein. Proc Natl Acad Sci USA 1986;83:2689.
80. Alexander A, Steinmetz A, Barritault D, et al. γ Heavy chain disease in man: cDNA sequence supports partial gene deletion model. Proc Natl Acad Sci USA 1982;79:3260.
81. Guglielmi P, Bakhshi A, Cogne M, et al. Multiple genomic defects

result in an alternative RNA splice creating a human gamma heavy chain disease protein. J Immunol 1988;141:1762.
82. Cogne M, Bakhshi A, Korsmeyer SJ, Guglielmi P. Gene mutations and alternate RNA splicing result in truncated Igl chains in human γ H chain disease. J Immunol 1988;141:1738.
83. Fishleder A, Tubbs R, Hesse B, Levin H. Uniform detection of immunoglobulin gene rearrangement in benign lymphoepithelial lesions. N Engl J Med 1987;316:1118.
84. Zulman J, Jaffe R, Talal N. Evidence that the malignant lymphoma of Sjogren's syndrome is a monoclonal B cell neoplasm. N Engl J Med 1978;299:1215.
85. Fong S, Chen PP, Gilbertson TA, et al. Expression of three cross reactive idiotypes on rheumatoid factor autoantibodies from patients with autoimmune diseases and sero-positive adults. J Immunol 1986;137:122.
86. Yanagi Y, Yoshikai Y, Leggett K, et al. A human T-cell specific cDNA clone encodes a protein having extensive homology to immunoglobulin chains. Nature 1984;308:145.
87. Hedrick SM, Cohen DI, Nielson EA, et al. Isolation of cDNA clones encoding T-cell specific membrane-associated proteins. Nature 1984;308:149.
88. Hayday AC, Saito H, Gillies SD, et al. Structure, organization and somatic rearrangement of T-cell γ genes. Cell 1985;40:259.
89. Lefranc MP, Rabbitts TH. Two tandemly organized human genes encoding the T-cell γ constant region sequences show multiple rearrangement in different T-cell lines. Nature 1985;316:464.
90. Quertermous T, Murre C, Dialynas D, et al. Human T-cell gamma genes: organization, diversity and rearrangement. Science 1986;231:252.
91. Chien Y, Iwashima M, Kaplan KB, et al. A new T-cell receptor gene located within the alpha locus and expressed early in T-cell differentiation. Nature 1987;327:677.
92. Hockett RD, deVillartay JP, Pollock K, et al. Human T-cell antigen receptor (TCR) delta-chain locus and elements responsible for its deletion are within the TCR alpha-chain locus. Proc Natl Acad Sci USA 1988;85:9694.
93. Brenner MB, McLean J, Dialynas DP, et al. Identification of a putative second T-cell receptor. Nature 1986;322:145.
94. Waldmann TA, Davis MM, Bongiovanni KF, et al. Rearrangements of genes for the antigen receptor on T cells as markers of lineage and clonality in human lymphoid neoplasms. N Engl J Med 1985;313:776.
95. Minden MD, Toyonaga B, Ha K, et al. Somatic rearrangement of T-cell antigen receptor gene in human T-cell malignancies. Proc Natl Acad Sci USA 1985;82:1224.
96. Rabbitts TH, Stinson A, Forster A, et al. Heterogeneity of T-cell β chain gene rearrangements in human leukemias and lymphomas. EMBO J 1985;4:2217.
97. Aisenberg AC, Krontiris TG, Mak T, et al. Rearrangement of the gene for the beta chain of the T-cell receptor in T-cell chronic lymphocytic leukemia and related disorders. N Engl J Med 1985;313:529.
98. Bertness V, Kirsch I, Hollis G, et al. T-cell receptor gene rearrangements as clinical markers of human T-cell lymphomas. N Engl J Med 1985;313:534.
99. Flug F, Pelicci P-G, Bonetti F, et al. T-cell receptor gene rearrangements as markers of lineage and clonality in T-cell neoplasms. Proc Natl Acad Sci USA 1985;82:3460.
100. Crist WM, Shuster JJ, Falletta J, et al. Clinical features and outcome in childhood T cell leukemia-lymphoma according to stage of thymocyte differentiation in a pediatric oncology group study. Blood 1988;72:1891.
101. Rowley JD, Testa JR. Chromosome abnormalities in malignant hematologic diseases. Adv Cancer Res 1982;36:103.
102. Yunis JJ. Chromosomal basis of human neoplasia. Science 1983;221:227.
103. Lenoir GM, Preud'homme JL, Bernheim A, et al. Correlations between immunoglobulin light chain expression and variant translocation in Burkitt's lymphoma. Nature 1982;298:474.
104. Taub R, Kirsch I, Morton C, et al. Translocation of the *c-myc* gene into the immunoglobulin heavy chain locus in human Burkitt lymphoma and murine plasmacytoma cells. Proc Natl Acad Sci USA 1982;79:7837.
105. Dalla-Favera R, Bregni M, Erikson J, et al. Human *c-myc* oncogene is located on the region of chromosome 8 that is translocated in Burkitt lymphoma cells. Proc Natl Acad Sci USA 1982;79:7824.
106. Adams JM, Gerondakis S, Webb E et al. Cellular *myc* oncogene is altered by chromosome translocation to an immunoglobulin locus in murine plasmacytomas and is rearranged similarly in human Burkitt lymphomas. Proc Natl Acad Sci USA 1983;80:1982.
107. Cesarman E, Dalla-Favera R, Bently D, Groudine M. Mutations in the first exon are associated with altered transcription of *c-myc* in Burkitt lymphoma. Science 1987;238:1272.
108. Adams JM, Harris AW, Pinkert CA, et al. The *c-myc* oncogene driven by immunoglobulin enhancers induces lymphoid malignancy in transgenic mice. Nature 1985;318:533.
109. Leder A, Pattengale PK, Kuo A, et al. Consequences of widespread deregulation of the *c-myc* gene in transgenic mice: multiple neoplasms and normal development. Cell 1986;45:485.
110. Lombardi L, Newcomb EW, Dalla-Favera R. Pathogenesis of Burkitt lymphoma: expression of an activated *c-myc* oncogene causes the tumorigenic conversion of EBV-infected human B lymphoblasts. Cell 1987;49:161.
111. Tsujimoto Y, Gorham J, Cossman J, et al. The t(14;18) chromosome translocations involved in B-cell neoplasms result from mistakes in VDJ joining. Science 1985;229:1390.
112. Cleary ML, Sklar J. Nucleotide sequence of a t(14;18) chromosomal breakpoint in follicular lymphoma and demonstration of a breakpoint cluster region near a transcriptionally active locus on chromosome 18. Proc Natl Acad Sci USA 1985;82:7439.
113. Bakhshi A, Jensen JP, Goldman P, et al. Cloning the chromosomal breakpoint of t(14;18) human lymphomas: clustering around J_H on chromosome 14 and near a transcriptional unit on 18. Cell 1985;41:889.
114. Bakhshi A, Wright JJ, Graninger W, et al. Mechanism of the t(14;18) chromosomal translocation: structural analysis of both derivative 14 and 18 reciprocal partners. Proc Natl Acad Sci USA 1987;84:2396.
115. Cleary ML, Smith SD, Sklar J. Cloning and structural analysis of cDNAs for *bcl*-2 and a hybrid *bcl*-2/immunoglobulin transcript resulting from the t(14;18) translocation. Cell 1986;47:19.
116. Seo M, Jaeger U, Hockett RD, et al. Alternative promoters and exons, somatic mutation and transcriptional deregulation of the *bcl*-2-Ig fusion gene in lymphoma. EMBO J 1988;7:123.
117. Nunez G, Seto M, Seremetis S, et al. Growth and tumor-promoting effects of deregulated *bcl*-2 in human B lymphoblastoid cells. Proc Natl Acad Sci USA 1989;86:4589.
118. Tsujimoto Y. Overexpression of the human *bcl*-2 gene product results in growth enhancement of Epstein-Barr virus–immortalized B cells. Proc Natl Acad Sci USA 1989;86:1958.
119. Vaux DL, Cory S, Adams JM. Bcl-2 gene promotes haematopoietic cell survival and cooperates with *c-myc* to immortalize pre-B cells. Nature 1988;335:440.
120. McDonnell TJ, Deane N, Platt FM, et al. *bcl*-2-Immunoglobulin transgenic mice demonstrate extended B cell survival and follicular lymphoproliferation. Cell 1989;57:79.
121. Boehm T, Baer R, Lavenier I. The mechanism of chromosomal translocation t(11;14) involving the T-cell receptor C_δ locus on human chromosome 14q11 and a transcribed region of chromosome 11p15. EMBO J 1988;7:385.
122. Boehm T, Buluwela L, Williams D, et al. A luster of chromosome 11p13 translocations found via distinct D–D and D–D–J rearrangements of the human T cell receptor delta chain gene. EMBO J 1988;7:2011.
123. McGuire EA, Hockett RD, Pollock KM, et al. The t(11;14)(p15;q11) in a T-cell acute lymphoblastic leukemia cell line activates multiple transcripts, including Ttg-1, a gene encoding a potential zinc finger protein. Mol Cell Biol 1989;9:2124.
124. Kagan J, Finger LR, Letofsky J, et al. Clustering of breakpoints on chromosome 10 in acute T-cell leukemias with the t(10q14) chromosome translocation. Proc Natl Acad Sci USA 1989;86:4161.
125. Zutter M, Hockett RD, Roberts CWM. The t(10;14)(q24(q24;q11) of T cell acute lymphoblastic leukemia juxtaposes the δ T cell receptor with a conserved and activated locus, TCL-3 at 10q24. Proc Natl Acad Sci USA 1989;87:3161.
126. Mellentin JD, Smith SD, Cleary ML. lyl-1, a novel gene altered by chromosomal translocation in T cell leukemia: codes for a protein with a helix–loop–helix DNA binding motif. Cell 1989;58:77.
127. Reynolds TC, Smith SD, Sklar J. Analysis of DNA surrounding the breakpoints of chromosomal translocations involving the beta T cell receptor gene in human lymphoblastic neoplasms. Cell 1987;50:107.
128. Lipford E, Wright JJ, Urba W, et al. Refinement of lymphoma cytogenetics by the 18q21 major breakpoint region. Blood 1987;70:1816.
129. Lee MS, Chang KS, Cabanillas F. Detection of minimal residual cells carrying the t(14;18) by DNA sequence amplification. Science 1987;237:175.
130. Crescenzi M, Seto M, Herzig GP, et al. Thermostable DNA polymerase chain amplification of t(14;18) chromosome breakpoints and detection of minimal residual disease. Proc Natl Acad Sci USA 1988;85:4869.
131. Hooberman AL, Carrino JJ, Leibowitz D. Unexpected heterogeneity of BCR-ABL fusion mRNA detected by polymerase chain reaction in Philadelphia chromosome–positive acute lymphoblastic leukemia. Proc Natl Acad Sci USA 1989;86:4259.

Blood: Principles and Practice of Hematology,
edited by Robert I. Handin, Thomas P. Stossel, and Samuel E. Lux.
J.B. Lippincott Company, Philadelphia © 1995.

27

Acute Lymphoblastic Leukemia

Gaston K. Rivera
William M. Crist

The development of effective therapy for patients with acute lymphoblastic leukemia (ALL) is one of the undisputed successes of modern clinical hematology. Three decades ago, this disease was uniformly fatal. Now, virtually all patients are treatable, and about one third of adults and two thirds of children are curable. This extraordinary achievement resulted from a series of studies that helped to clarify the pathophysiology of ALL and demonstrated how combinations of antileukemic drugs, radiation, and supportive measures could be applied with curative intent. More recently, advances in the understanding of leukemia cell biology and clinical risk factors have made it possible to recognize a spectrum of ALL subtypes and to predict treatment outcome with greater precision. This has led in turn to the development of therapy more appropriate to the patient's risk of failure. In poor-prognosis ALL, the goal has been to sufficiently intensify treatment to overcome drug resistance, which continues to account for most relapses. This strategy has contributed importantly to treatment success, increasing the cure rate among children with high-risk ALL from about 30% to almost 70% in some recent trials. Conversely, use of less intensive therapy for patients with a relatively low risk of failure has resulted in decreased acute and late toxic effects and in an improved quality of life achievements that assume special significance in children. Bone marrow transplantation and other treatment approaches, including the use of biologic-response modifiers, are continuing to evolve as promising therapeutic innovations and within the next decade can be expected to boost cure rates still further. This chapter reviews the epidemiology, classification, and clinical management of ALL, concentrating on the principles and strategies of therapy, with particular attention given to unresolved controversies.

DEFINITION

Acute leukemia refers to clonal malignant disorders of lymphoid or myeloid progenitor cells, which in most cases have definable genetic and immunologic characteristics. In ALL, abnormalities of lymphoid cell differentiation, proliferation, or both lead to excessive infiltration and accumulation of leukemic lymphoblasts in multiple organs, with resultant organomegaly and bone marrow failure. If untreated, the disease has a rapidly fatal course, with death caused by infection or bleeding. About 80% of the childhood leukemias in the United States are classified as ALL; the remaining 20% originate in cells of the myeloid lineage and collectively are called *acute myelogenous leukemia* (AML).[1] This ratio is reversed in adults.[2]

The available evidence indicates that the transforming event in ALL could occur in any cell in the lymphoid pathway of hematopoietic stem cell differentiation (Fig. 27-1). Over 80% of pediatric cases involve B-lineage progenitor cells; about 15% involve thymocytes; 1% involve B cells; and less than 5% have an uncertain cellular origin.[3] A small proportion of pediatric cases (fewer than 10%) and perhaps more adult cases are characterized by expression of both myeloid- and lymphoid-associated cell-surface markers, either on the same cells (mixed lineage or biphenotypic leukemia), suggesting dysregulation of differentiation-specific genes, or on different but coexisting subpopulations of cells (bilineal or biclonal leukemia), suggesting two independent clones.[4] Adult cases appear to have a similar distribution of immunophenotypes (ie, subtypes of ALL defined by immunologic marker expression), except that the proportion of non–B-cell, non–T-cell cases that fail to express the common ALL antigen (CALLA; CD10) is much higher, and the proportion of T-cell cases is slightly higher.[2] Progenitor B-cell ALL is thought to arise primarily in the bone marrow, in contrast to B-cell ALL, which may arise in lymphoid tissue within the gut. T-cell ALL probably arises in thymic or peripheral lymphoid tissue, often spreading to bone marrow early in the clinical course.

B- and T-cell ALL are virtually indistinguishable, both cytologically and cytogenetically, from disseminated Burkitt's and lymphoblastic non-Hodgkin's lymphoma, respectively.[3,5] The diagnosis of leukemia is usually based on more than 25% blast cells in bone marrow; lesser involvement indicates marrow infiltration by non-Hodgkin's lymphoma. Although arbitrary, this distinction can be important for stratification of patients in clinical trials and for treatment planning.

EPIDEMIOLOGY

About 2000 cases of childhood ALL are diagnosed in the United States each year, making this the most common form of cancer in children. Over the past 50 years, the incidence of childhood ALL appears to have increased,

This work was supported in part by grants CA-20180, CA-15989, CA-31566, and CA-21765 from the National Cancer Institute and by the American Lebanese Syrian Associated Charities.

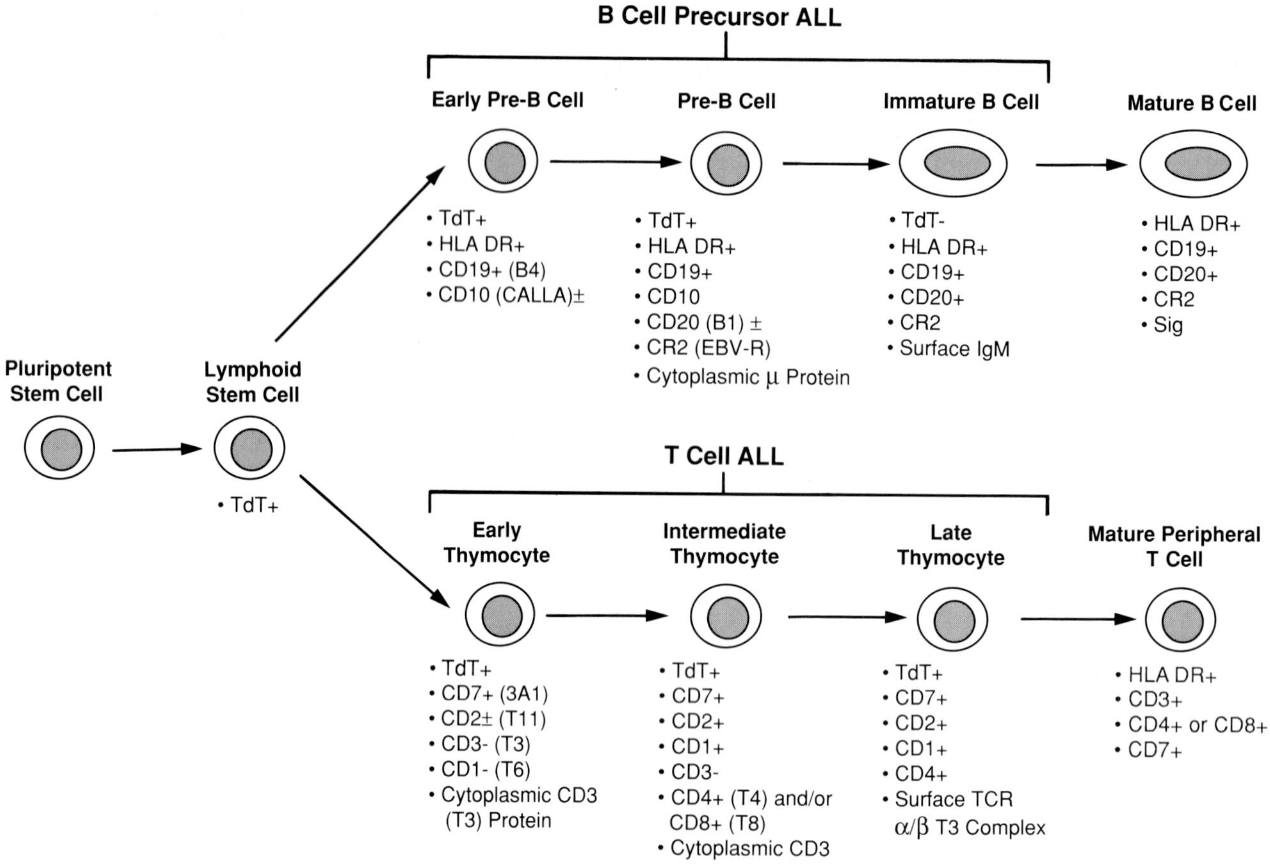

FIGURE 27-1. Model of lymphoid cell differentiation showing stages of cellular development based on terminal deoxynucleotidyl transferase (TdT) activity, binding to commonly used monoclonal antibodies, T-cell receptor gene rearrangement, and the presence of immunoglobulin molecules. CD, cluster of differentiation group.

probably as a result of better diagnostic techniques and case reporting. The annual incidence of ALL among children 15 years of age or younger is 29.4 cases per 1 million population in whites and 13.7 cases per 1 million population in blacks.[1] In contrast to epidemiologic findings in the United States, childhood ALL is less frequent than AML in Turkey and in parts of China, and cases of B- and T-cell ALL are more frequent than the progenitor B-cell subtype among African blacks and Arabs in the Gaza Strip.[6,7] Reasons for this geographic variation are unclear; more exact comparisons await better methods of studying large groups of patients worldwide. The age-adjusted incidence of ALL in adults (over 15 years of age) is 7 cases per 1 million population.[8]

The peak incidence of childhood ALL in the United States occurs in children between the ages of 3 and 5 years; a similar age distribution has been noted in England and Wales.[9] The age distribution at diagnosis of ALL in children with different immunologic subtypes is shown in Table 27-1. T-cell ALL occurs more often in older children, whereas early pre–B-cell or pre–B-cell ALL usually develops in children younger than 7 years. No obvious peak incidence of ALL is observed during adulthood, although incidence decreases with increasing age.[8]

ALL affects males more often than females in all age groups except infants. About 20% to 30% more males than females develop this leukemia. Male predominance has been observed in virtually all series of patients, including adults; it extends to all immunophenotypic categories of childhood ALL and is exaggerated in B-cell and T-cell ALL (see Table 27-1). In the United States, white children have a higher incidence of ALL than do black children, an observation that lacks a clear explanation.

The striking associations of ALL with certain risk groups has provided valuable clues to its cause. Siblings of leukemia patients are four times more likely to develop the disease than are people in the general population. About 20% of monozygotic twins of children with ALL develop leukemia within the first 6 years of life; their symptoms usually appear within several months after the diagnosis of leukemia in the other sibling.[10] Concordant leukemia in monozygotic twins may reflect a common prezygotic determinant, shared intrauterine leukemogenic event, or spread of the disease from one twin to the other.

Children with certain genetic disorders[11–13] (Table 27-2) have an increased risk of developing ALL,[10] as do people exposed to irradiation. Among Japanese within 1000 meters of the hypocenters of atomic bomb blasts in Nagasaki and Hiroshima, the risk of ALL was 1 in 60 over 12 years.[10] Environmental carcinogens, such as hydrocarbons, have also been implicated in leukemogenesis.[14]

Parasitic and viral infections have been linked to the pathogenesis of certain types of lymphoid cancer. Specifically, malarial infestation and Epstein-Barr virus (EBV) infection early in life are thought to increase the risk of B-cell lymphoid tumors.[15] EBV-infected B lymphocytes have an increased proliferative rate, increasing the risk of genetic error during DNA replication. Moreover, depression of cellular immunity due to malaria may increase the likelihood that altered lymphoid cells with specific chromosomal translocations, such as t(8;14), t(2;8), or t(8;22), will escape from cellular immune surveillance and give rise to leu-

TABLE 27-1. Initial Clinical and Laboratory Findings in Children With Acute Lymphoblastic Leukemia According to Immunophenotype

Characteristic	Immunophenotype				P Value for Statistical Comparison*	
	Early Pre-B	Pre-B	T	B	Early Pre-B Versus Pre-B	Non-T, Non-B Versus T
Sex						
Male	521 (54%)	144 (52%)	131 (68%)	6 (67%)	.66	.0001
Female	450 (46%)	132 (48%)	62 (32%)	3 (33%)		
Race						
White	781 (80%)	202 (73%)	136 (70%)	7 (78%)	.02	.0001
Black	89 (9%)	36 (13%)	36 (19%)	1 (11%)		
Hispanic	69 (7%)	30 (11%)	9 (5%)	1 (11%)		
Other	33 (4%)	9 (3%)	12 (6%)	0 (0%)		
Age (y)						
<1.5	60 (6%)	25 (9%)	5 (2%)	3 (18%)	.28	.0001
1.5–7	654 (66%)	175 (61%)	98 (45%)	8 (47%)		
7–10	130 (13%)	43 (15%)	56 (26%)	2 (12%)		
≥10	149 (15%)	42 (15%)	57 (26%)	4 (24%)		
Leukocyte count (×10⁸/L)						
<10	493 (50%)	122 (43%)	43 (20%)	5 (31%)	.003	.0001
10–50	348 (35%)	93 (33%)	63 (29%)	6 (38%)		
50–100	82 (8%)	33 (12%)	27 (13%)	3 (19%)		
>100	71 (7%)	37 (13%)	83 (38%)	2 (13%)		
Platelet count ($\times 10^9$/L)						
<20	201 (21%)	64 (23%)	25 (13%)	3 (38%)	.25	.0001
20–100	514 (53%)	130 (47%)	85 (44%)	5 (62%)		
<100	252 (26%)	80 (29%)	84 (43%)	0 (0%)		
Hemoglobin (g/dL)						
<7.5	482 (50%)	120 (44%)	50 (27%)	4 (50%)	.001	.0001
7.5–10	311 (32%)	76 (28%)	42 (22%)	1 (12%)		
>10	167 (17%)	75 (28%)	95 (51%)	3 (38%)		
Hepatomegaly						
No	923 (93%)	263 (92%)	187 (87%)	13 (81%)	.74	.001
Yes†	71 (7%)	22 (8%)	27 (13%)	3 (19%)		
Splenomegaly						
No	905 (91%)	254 (89%)	170 (79%)	14 (87%)	.46	.0001
Yes*	86 (9%)	31 (11%)	44 (21%)	2 (13%)		
Lymphadenopathy						
None	385 (39%)	101 (35%)	48 (22%)	2 (12%)	.72	.0001
Minimal	392 (39%)	114 (40%)	59 (27%)	10 (59%)		
Moderate	190 (19%)	61 (21%)	64 (30%)	1 (6%)		
Marked	28 (3%)	9 (3%)	44 (20%)	4 (24%)		
Mediastinal mass						
No	990 (95%)	284 (99%)	104 (48%)	17 (100%)	.69	.0001
Yes	5 (5%)	2 (1%)	112 (52%)	0 (0%)		
CNS disease						
No	954 (96%)	272 (95%)	205 (95%)	14 (72%)	—	—
Yes	41 (4%)	13 (5%)	11 (5%)	3 (18%)		
PAS stain						
Positive (>50)	641 (65%)	170 (60%)	74 (35%)	3 (19%)	.12	.0001
Negative	347 (35%)	114 (40%)	140 (65%)	13 (81%)		
Glucocorticoid (receptors/cell)						
<2500	18 (5%)	7 (7%)	27 (25%)	4 (31%)	.57	.0001
2500–6000	80 (20%)	26 (25%)	54 (49%)	3 (23%)		
6000–10,000	102 (26%)	27 (25%)	16 (15%)	2 (15%)		
10,000–20,000	159 (41%)	35 (33%)	11 (10%)	4 (31%)		
>20,000	33 (8%)	11 (10%)	2 (2%)	0 (0%)		
CALLA						
Positive	895 (90%)	260 (91%)	65 (30%)	8 (50%)	.58	.0001
Negative	98 (10%)	25 (9%)	150 (70%)	8 (50%)		
HLA-DR						
Positive	974 (98%)	277 (97%)	36 (17%)	15 (94%)	.36	.0001
Negative	19 (2%)	8 (3%)	180 (83%)	1 (6%)		

PAS, periodic acid–Schiff; CALLA, common acute lymphoblastic leukemia antigen.
* There were too few patients with B-cell ALL for statistical comparisons.
† Palpable to below umbilicus.
(Pullen DJ, Boyett JM, Crist WM, et al. Pediatric Oncology Group utilization of immunologic markers in the designation of acute lymphocytic leukemia subgroups: influence on treatment response. Ann NY Acad Sci 1984;428:26)

TABLE 27-2. Congenital Disorders Associated With an Increased Risk of Leukemia or Lymphoma

Disorder	Estimated Risk	Reference
Down's syndrome	1 in 74 before age 10 y	11
Fanconi's syndrome	1 in 12 before age 21 y	11
Bloom's syndrome	1 in 8 before age 26 y	11
Ataxia telangiectasia	12 in 100	12
Immunoglobulin A deficiency	Unknown	
Wiskott-Aldrich syndrome	12 in 100	13

kemic clones. These translocations rearrange elements of immunoglobulin (Ig) genes to the vicinity of the c-*myc* oncogene, leading to its constitutive expression. In this indirect way, EBV probably contributes to the pathogenesis of African Burkitt's lymphoma and B-cell ALL in children and adults.[15,16] Retroviruses, such as human T-cell leukemia/lymphoma virus type 1, have a direct causative role in leukemogenesis in some adults, but they have not been convincingly linked to the childhood leukemias.[17]

Attempts to identify common exposures, either infections or environmental, for clusters of leukemia cases developing over a short time have not yielded consistent results. The difficulties inherent in identifying time and space clusters of leukemia cases, including the definition of the population at risk, are well illustrated by experience with nonionizing radiation. Wertheimer and Leeper[18] reported an association between proximity to high-current electrical wiring and childhood cancer incidence in Colorado, whereas Fulton and colleagues,[19] using the Wertheimer-Leeper method, failed to show a similar relation in Rhode Island.

Random mutations may account for most cases of ALL. As argued by Greaves,[6] the immune system of children affords an ideal stage for genetic error, owing to the high proliferative rate of lymphoid cells with their rearranging Ig or T-cell receptor gene segments, which are necessary for the production of Ig and the development of T-cell function, respectively. Others have hypothesized that two mutations in or near key regulatory genes are required for the induction of leukemia.[20] This theory allows for exceptional cases in which genetic predisposition and environmental exposure play important roles in malignant transformation. The lower incidence of ALL in adults as compared with children[21] might also be predicted from this hypothesis since the adult immune system is more fully developed and its cells less rapidly proliferating.

The risk of vertical transmission of ALL appears low. Among 119 pregnant women with leukemia, including ALL, none had offspring with this disease[22]; however, there have been isolated reports of leukemia in infants whose mothers had the disease.[23–25]

CLASSIFICATION

As detailed later, ALL is a diverse group of hematologic diseases composed of many recognizable subtypes. Continued study of these subtypes may further improve classification systems, provide information of prognostic importance, and lead to an understanding of the mechanisms of leukemic transformation.

Recent applications of monoclonal antibodies and other biologic probes in the analysis of leukemic lymphoblasts and their normal counterparts have greatly improved the precision with which particular cell types can be identified, isolated, and characterized.[26] Initially, the detection of B-lineage–associated determinants, including the human leukocyte antigen (HLA) DR-related, Ia-like antigens[27] and CALLA (CD10; neutral endopeptidase)[28] on the surface of non–T lymphoblasts from patients with ALL suggested that these cases might be of B-cell origin. It was also found that about one fourth of these leukemias were characterized by cytoplasmic μ heavy chains of the Ig molecule, and over 90% expressed B-cell–*associated* surface antigens, including CD19.[29,30] Both sets of observations supported the idea that most cases of non–T-cell ALL arise in B-cell precursors, preceding the pre–B-cell stage of development in which the cells are positive for cytoplasmic Ig. Subsequently, analysis of Ig gene rearrangements has demonstrated that most of these cases have rearranged heavy-chain genes with or without rearranged light-chain genes consistent with their origin in a progenitor B cell.[31] Figure 27-1 shows the combinations of biologic probes used to distinguish among leukemic subgroups that correspond to relatively distinct stages of normal progenitor B-cell differentiation.

Morphology

Because leukemic lymphoblasts are morphologically indistinguishable from immature normal lymphoid cells, attempts to subclassify these cells on the basis of size, nuclear/cytoplasmic ratio, presence of cytoplasmic granules, or other features have been largely unsuccessful. A morphologic classification system devised by the French-American-British (FAB) Cooperative Working Group (Fig. 27-2) has gained wide acceptance.[32] About 90% of cases of childhood ALL are of the FAB L1 subtype, characterized by relatively small lymphoblasts with scanty cytoplasm and inconspicuous nucleoli. Cells in the L2 category, found in 5% to 15% of cases, are larger than those classified as L1, show marked variability in size, and have prominent nucleoli and more abundant cytoplasm. Only 1% or less of ALL cases in children have L3 lymphoblasts, which appear identical to Burkitt's lymphoma cells. The distribution of FAB subtypes in adult ALL differs strikingly from that in children in that a much higher percentage of cases are classified as L2.[2] Other morphologic variants of ALL, including ALL with "hand-mirror" cells or granules, have been described but are of uncertain significance.[33,34]

Cytochemistry

A variety of cytochemical stains have been studied for their ability to delineate lineage-specific or lineage-related components of leukemic blast cells. Although some strong correlations between blast cell–staining characteristics and subtype of ALL have been noted, the practical value of this type of information is limited. The acid phosphatase reaction, for example, can be used to distinguish cases of T-cell ALL from other immunologic subtypes; but it is not specific for the lymphoid lineage, nor does it identify all cases that express T-cell–specific antigens.[35,36] Terminal deoxynucleotidyl transferase, an unusual enzyme that catalyzes the polymerization of deoxynucleoside monophosphates into a single-strand DNA primer, can be demonstrated in the nuclei of both T- and B-cell leukemic precursors and is rarely present in cases of myeloid leukemia.[37–40] This activity appears more relevant to identifying a cell's maturational stage than to specifying its lineage. Myeloperoxidase is often helpful in ruling out lymphoblastic leukemia because it is specific for myeloid cells and does not stain lymphoblasts; Sudan black B, a lipid stain, often reacts with leukemic myeloid cells but must be interpreted with caution because of its occasional reactivity with leukemic lymphoblasts.

Immunophenotype

Differences in surface membrane or cytoplasmic components of T and B lymphocytes (immunophenotype) can be used to identify and classify lymphoproliferative diseases

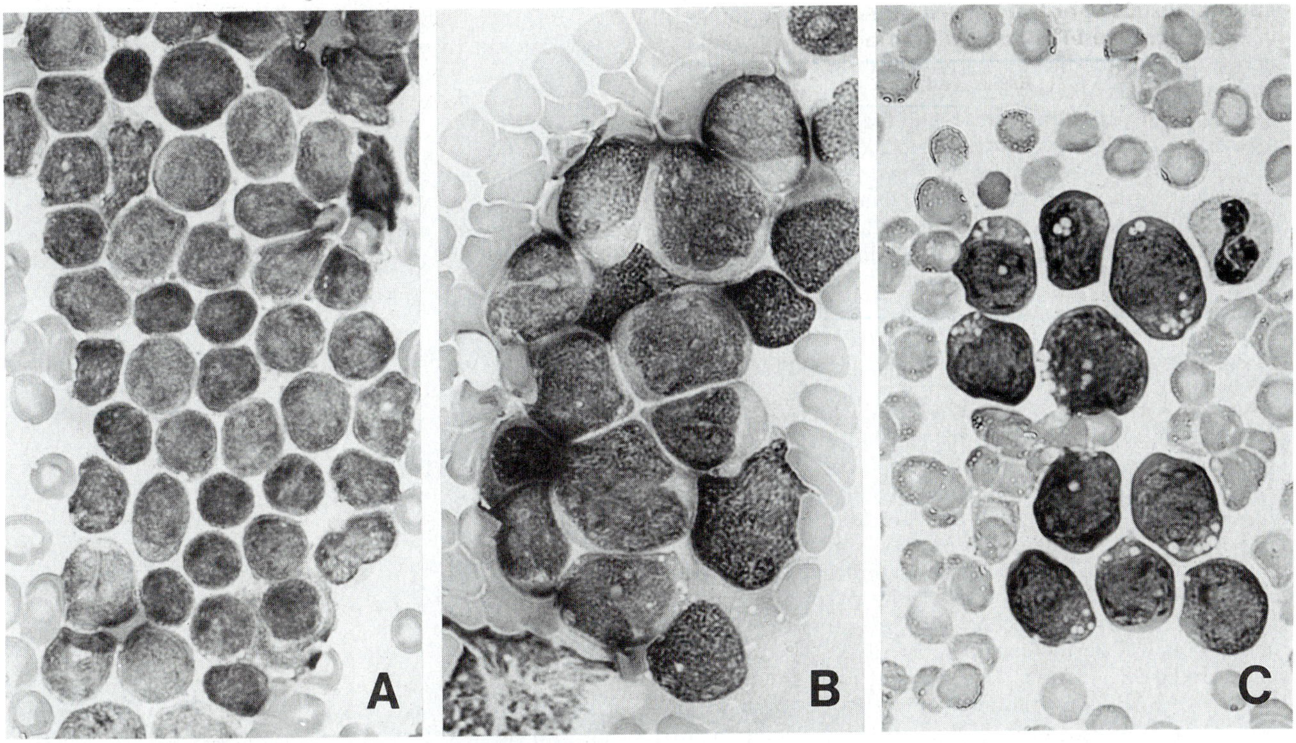

FIGURE 27-2. Morphologic appearance of leukemic lymphoblasts according to the French-American-British (FAB) classification system. (**A**) L1 blasts are small with scanty cytoplasm. (**B**) L2 blasts are larger with increased amounts of cytoplasm, irregular nuclear membranes, and prominent nucleoli. (**C**) L3 blasts have basophilic cytoplasm with vacuolization. (Rivera G, Pui C-H. Acute lymphoblastic leukemia. In: Rudolph AM, ed. Pediatrics. Norwalk, CT, Appleton-Century-Crofts, 1987:1098)

as to cell of origin and stage of maturation (see Fig. 27-1). Markers that are specific for or closely related to cell lineage or stage of differentiation have proved especially useful in this regard.[3,41] The proportions of children and adults with specific immunophenotypes of newly diagnosed ALL are shown in Table 27-3, according to age group.[3,41,42]

B-Cell ALL

The B-cell phenotype characterizes less than 1% of newly diagnosed cases of childhood ALL and 4% of adult cases in the United States.[3,43] Many of these patients probably had Burkitt's lymphoma that spread to the bone marrow, blood, or both before presentation.[44] Morphologically, the blast cells tend to have FAB L3 features, with intensely staining cytoplasmic basophilia similar to that of erythroblasts (see Fig. 27-2). In a significant minority of cases, one finds L1 or L2 blasts, making it difficult to diagnose B-cell ALL on morphologic grounds alone. Rather, immunologic marker analysis is needed to demonstrate cell surface Ig, which in most cases consists of μ heavy chains and κ or λ light chains.[44] Many of these cases have a characteristic 8;14 translocation, which also is observed in the blasts of most patients with Burkitt's lymphoma.

Pre–B-Cell and Early Pre–B-cell Acute Lymphoblastic Leukemia

Vogler and colleagues[45] were the first to recognize pre–B-cell ALL. In 1978, they reported on a small cohort of childhood leukemia patients whose bone marrow lymphoblasts (over 10%) expressed cytoplasmic Ig heavy chains (cμ+)

TABLE 27-3. Percentage Distribution of Immunophenotypes of Acute Lymphoblastic Leukemia Among Different Age Groups

Immunophenotype	Infants (<1.5 y; n = 70)	Children (1.5 to 10 y; n = 1006)	Adolescents (>10 y; n = 225)	Adults* (>15 y; n = 1145)
Early pre-B	64	68	58	51†
CD10+	49	94	87	
CD10−	51	6	13	
Pre-B	26	18	18	Unknown
T	6	13	23	22
B	4	1	1	4

* Numbers shown are weighted means from eight different studies.

† About half of adult cases are common ALL (CALLA+) and one fourth are null-cell ALL (CALLA−; non-T, non-B phenotypes).

(Modified from Crist W, Rivera G, Pullen J, Weinstein H. The leukemias of childhood. In: Rosenthal DS, Feinstein DI, Goodnight S, et al, eds. Hematology: 1985. Education Program, American Society of Hematology, 1985:48) but lacked surface Ig (cμ+, sIg−), a characteristic feature of pre–B cells. Use of heterologous antisera and, later, monoclonal antibodies disclosed CD10 on the surface of leukemic lymphoblasts in about 90% of children with ALL, including the group with pre–B-cell features (18% to 25% of cases).[42] This subset was designated *common ALL* to distinguish it from cases defined by T-cell features or the apparent lack of either T-cell or B-cell characteristics. Thus, in 80% to 85% of children with ALL, the leukemia represents monoclonal proliferation of B-cell precursors in different stages of differentiation. Cells expressing cIg are more mature than those with CD10 expression only but are not as mature as those expressing sIg. No comprehensive studies have been done on the pre–B-cell immunophenotype in adults.

Studies performed by the Pediatric Oncology Group (POG) during the past decade have demonstrated that the clinical features of children with pre–B-cell or early pre–B-cell ALL do not differ significantly, except for higher leukocyte levels at presentation, a higher frequency of black patients, and higher hemoglobin levels in the pre–B-cell group[3,41,45–50] (see Table 27-1). No significant differences have been found between these two phenotypically defined groups in number of glucocorticoid receptors in blasts or the incidence of periodic acid–Schiff reactivity or expression of HLA-DR antigens. Over 90% of both groups have blasts with FAB L1 morphology, and about one fourth of children with pre–B-cell ALL have a t(1;19).[51,52] A recent report indicates that all the adverse features previously associated with the pre–B-cell phenotype are entirely due to the subset with the t(1;19) and that the adverse prognosis ascribed to this phenotype of ALL is also due to the subgroup with this translocation.[30] Cases of early pre–B-cell ALL with the same cytogenetic abnormality (about 1% of the total cases) lack these molecular findings, and the early pre–B-cell cases do not appear to share the worse prognosis of pre–B-cell cases with this translocation.[53] Molecular studies demonstrate that a homeobox gene on chromosome 1 band q23 (*prl*, pre–B-cell leukemia) fuses with the transcription factor encoding gene *E2A*, located at 19p13, to form a novel fusion gene in all cases of pre–B-cell ALL with the t(1;19)(q23:p13); a novel fusion protein is always expressed,[54–56] implying that this translocation is involved in the pathogenesis of this form of ALL.

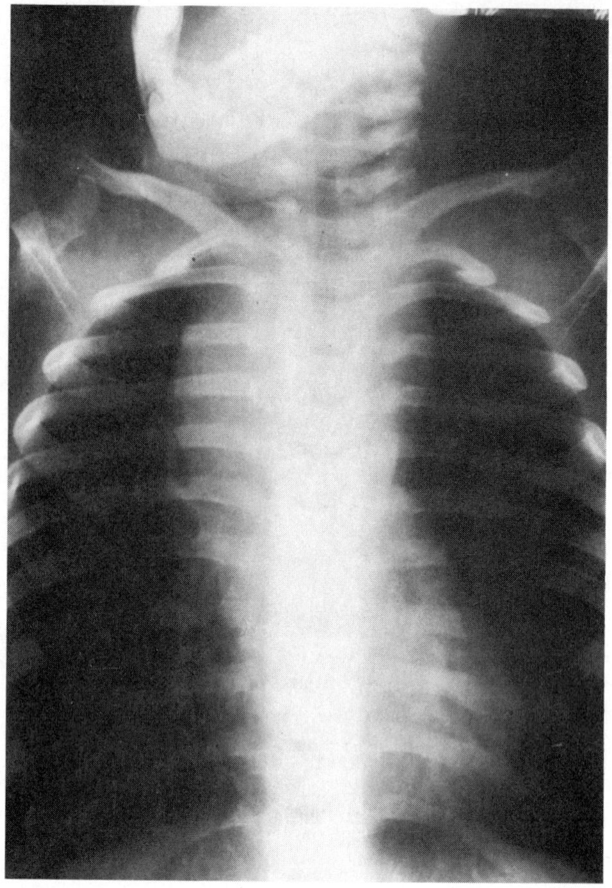

FIGURE 27-3. Chest roentgenogram showing an anterior mediastinal mass in a child with newly diagnosed acute lymphoblastic leukemia.

T-Cell ALL

Recognition of T-cell leukemia can be credited to Borella and Sen,[57] who in 1973 reported on a boy with a very high initial leukocyte count and lymphoblasts that formed rosettes with sheep erythrocytes (SER+), a characteristic of T cells but not of B cells. Subsequently, Kersey, Dow, and others[58–62] emphasized the clinical importance of T-cell markers in childhood ALL, noting a male sex predominance, high leukocyte count, high incidence of mediastinal mass (Fig. 27-3), and generally poor responses to therapy. The frequency of T-cell ALL in large pediatric series ranges from 12% to 18% and in adults from 20% to 25%[2] (see Table 27-1).

Use of anti–T-cell heteroantisera with pan-T specificity and, more recently, monoclonal antibodies directed against epitopes of T-cell–associated antigens[63,64] has improved the detection of leukemic T lymphoblasts; hence, cases formerly overlooked because of their SER$^-$ phenotype are now known to have T-cell markers. T-cell ALL can be subclassified by using monoclonal antibodies that recognize surface antigens expressed during discrete stages of normal T-cell development.[65] Most investigators regard T-cell ALL as deriving from thymocytes in one of three maturational stages (see Fig. 27-1): early (stage I), intermediate (stage II), or late (stage III). Stage II cases occur more often than stage I cases, and stage III cases are the least frequent. The ultimate clinical relevance of this subclassification scheme remains to be established[5,65]; however, recent information indicates that patients whose T-cell disease involves early thymocytes enter remission less often than those with other subtypes.[5]

In comparison with patients having early pre–B-cell or pre–B-cell ALL, children with T-cell leukemia are more often older boys with high leukocyte counts and extensive bulky disease, including lymphadenopathy, hepatosplenomegaly, and a thymic mass (more than half of patients). This pattern of distinctive clinical features is shared by adults with T-cell disease.

Null-Cell ALL

The proportion of patients whose lymphoblasts fail to display any recognizable T-cell or B-cell features continues to decrease as more lineage-specific cell markers are identified. Nevertheless, if one employs a limited battery of immunologic markers, including anti-CD10, pan-T antibodies, and anti-sIg, about 5% of children and 23% of adults will have blasts lacking the molecules recognized by these reagents. Their leukemia has been designated *null-cell ALL* in many reports.[3,43] Some CD10 cells express cytoplasmic μ heavy chains, indicating a pre–B-cell classification, or have other characteristics of early pre–B-cell leukemia.[3] Clinical and nonimmunologic criteria do not distinguish patients with null-cell ALL from those with cμ− (early pre–B-cell) or cμ+ (pre–B-cell) ALL. Recent evidence suggests that the increased frequency of null-cell ALL in adults may be due to masked forms of myeloid or hybrid leukemias, as described later.[66]

Mixed Lineage and Bilineal Leukemias

Mixed lineage (biphenotypic) *leukemia* refers to cases in which both lymphoid- and myeloid-associated surface antigens are expressed on the same cells. The incidence of mixed lineage leukemia has been estimated to be as high as 15% to 20% in some studies but generally ranges from 5% to 10% of pediatric and adult cases of ALL, although the percentage may be higher in adults.[2,4,67] This variability appears to reflect differences in specific diagnostic criteria. Occasionally, one subpopulation of blasts may express lymphoid-associated markers and another myeloid-associated markers; such cases have been called *bilineal* (biclonal) *leukemia* and are thought to arise from separate transformation events.[67]

Studies with dual labeling techniques, using fluorochrome–monoclonal antibody conjugates, have made it possible to determine if differentiation antigens reside on the same or different blasts. The clinical features of patients with mixed lineage leukemia do not distinguish them from others with ALL; however, such cases have a high frequency of 11q23 karyotypic abnormalities, such as the t(4;11) or t(9;11).[67] Mixed lineage leukemia could arise from a transformed pluripotent stem cell capable of differentiation in either the lymphoid (see Fig. 27-1) or myeloid pathway, from aberrant gene expression in a committed precursor cell, or from transformation of a normal biphenotypic cell.[68]

Cytogenetics and Molecular Genetics

Recently improved techniques for determining chromosome number (ploidy) and identifying structural changes in chromosomes (eg, translocations, inversions, and deletions) have been applied to the study of leukemic cells from large numbers of patients with ALL. These studies have revealed abnormalities in leukemic cells from more than 90% of children and at least 65% of adults with ALL.[43,69–72] Because most children and adults with leukemia have normal constitutional karyotypes, the presence of clonal karyotypic abnormalities in bone marrow cells often provides definitive evidence of malignancy, especially in situations in which leukemic cells have only partially infiltrated the bone marrow.[72]

Table 27-4 documents the close relation between ploidy and immunophenotype in pediatric ALL.[69] Hyperdiploidy (more than 50 chromosomes) occurs less often in B-cell, T-cell, CD10– early pre–B-cell, and pre–B-cell cases than in CD10+ early pre–B-cell cases.[69,73] Both adults and children with B-cell ALL typically have a pseudodiploid karyotype with a t(8;14)(q24;q23), t(2;8)(p11–13;q24) or t(8;22)(q24;q11).[72] Table 27-5 shows the distribution of chromosomal translocations, genes affected, and incidence of each genetic abnormality in childhood ALL and the association of these changes with immunophenotype.[69,72,74–84] Children with CD10+ early pre–B-cell ALL have clinically unfavorable chromosomal translocations significantly less often than children with pre–B-cell ALL or CD10– early pre–B-cell ALL.[69] Recurring chromosomal abnormalities have made it possible to pinpoint genetic lesions that appear to be involved in the molecular origin or progression of leukemia. For example, immunophenotype-specific translocations often have breakpoints that involve genes encoding Ig or T-cell receptor genes (see Table 27-5). Also, several protooncogenes, including c-*myc* in Burkitt's lymphoma and c-*abl* in ALL with the Philadelphia (Ph) chromosome [t(9;22)], have been linked to malignant transformation.[16,72,75,76,78,80,82,85,86]

Further identification and molecular characterization of such genes promise major advances in the understanding and treatment of ALL. Most of the nonrandom structural chromosomal abnormalities found in children with ALL are also found in adults with this disease, although the frequency of specific abnormalities may differ considerably.[2,71,72] For example, the proportion of adults with ALL who have the Ph chromosome has been estimated at 12% or more, as compared with a frequency of about 2% to 5% in children.[43,87] The Third International Workshop on Chromosomes in Leukemia has recorded in considerable detail the karyotypic features of 330 cases of children and adults with ALL and has related these characteristics to other features of the patients, including treatment outcome.[71] These data provide a reliable estimate of the frequency of recurring structural chromosomal abnormalities in both age groups of patients and indicate the independent adverse prognostic influence of certain karyotypic features, particularly the t(9;22)(q34;q11), 8q24, and t(4;11)(q21;q23), in both adults and children.

The issue raised by ALL with the Ph chromosome, that is, whether such cases denote the lymphoid acute phase of chronic myelogenous leukemia (CML) or a distinct disorder, deserves special mention. The t(9;22)(q34;q11) translocation in CML results in a chromosomal break that is usually within the breakpoint cluster region (*bcr*) gene on chromosome 22 and transfer of some or all of the c-*abl* protooncogene from chromosome 9 to a position adjacent to the truncated *bcr* gene, forming a chimeric *bcr/abl* gene. The translocation is similar in most cases of ALL except that typically the breakpoint on chromosome 22 occurs outside the *bcr* gene, resulting in a smaller mRNA tran-

TABLE 27-4. Distribution of Ploidy Groups According to Immunophenotype in Children With Acute Lymphoblastic Leukemia

		Early Pre-B				
Ploidy Group	**Total Cases (n = 364)**	**CALLA⁺ (n = 188)**	**CALLA⁻ (n = 21)**	**Pre-B (n = 79)**	**B (n = 12)**	**T (n = 64)**
Hyperdiploid (>50 chromosomes)	79	62	0	14	0	3
Hyperdiploid (47–50 chromosomes)	57	36	5	13	0	3
Pseudodiploid	162	61	14	39	12	36
Normal	38	12	2	5	0	19
Hypodiploid	28	17	0	8	0	3

CALLA, common acute lymphoblastic leukemia antigen.
(Pui C-H, Williams DL, Roberson PK, et al. Correlation of karyotype and immunophenotype in childhood acute lymhoblastic leukemia. J Clin Oncol 1988;6:56)

TABLE 27-5. Nonrandom Chromosomal Translocations in Childhood Acute Lymphoblastic Leukemia

Nonrandom Translocation	Involved Genes*		Predicted Protein Product	Frequency (%)
PRE-B AND EARLY PRE-B CELLS				
t(9;22)(q34;q11)	*abl*	*bcr*	P185[bcr/abl]	3–5
t(1;19)(q23;p13)	*prl*	*E2A*	E2A-PRL fusion protein	5–6
t(11;V)(q23;V)	Unknown	Unknown		3
t(4;11)(q21;q23)	Unknown	Unknown		2
t(1;11)(p32;q23)	Unknown	Unknown		<1
t(10;11)(p14-p15;q22)	Unknown	Unknown		<1
t(11;19)(q23;p13)	Unknown	Unknown		<1
t(9;11)(p21-p22;q23)	Unknown	Unknown		<1
t(12;V)(p12-p13;V)	Unknown	—		5
dic(9;12)(p11-p12;p12)	Unknown	Unknown		1–2
dic(7;9)(p13;p11)	Unknown	Unknown		<1
T CELLS				
t(11;14)(p13;q11)	Unknown	*tcra/tcrd*		1
t(11;14)(p15;q11)	*ttg-1*	*tcra/tcrd*	Zinc finger protein (rhombotin)	Rare
t(10;14)(q24;q11)	Unknown	*tcra/tcrd*		<1
inv(14)(q11;q32.3)	*tcra/tcrd*	Unknown		<1
t(1;14)(p32-p34;q11)	*tal-1*	*tcra/tcrd*	Helix-loop-helix protein	Rare
t(8;14)(q24;q11)	*myc*	*tcra/tcrd*	Helix-loop-helix protein	Rare
t(7;V)(q35;V)	*tcrb*	—		2
t(7;9)(q34-q36;q34)	*tcrb*	Unknown		Rare
t(7;9)(q34-q36;q32)	*tcrb*	—		Rare
t(7;19)(q35;p13)	*tcrb*	*lyl-1*	Helix-loop-helix protein	Rare
B CELLS				
t(8;14)(q24;q32.3)	*myc*	*igh*	Helix-loop-helix protein	2
t(8;22)(q24;q11)	*myc*	*igl*	Helix-loop-helix protein	0.3
t(2;8)(p11-p12;q24)	*igk*	*myc*	Helix-loop-helix protein	Rare

abl, cellular homologue of the Abelson murine leukemia virus oncogene; *bcr*, gene containing the breakpoint cluster region involved in Ph translocation; *prl*, pre–B-cell leukemia gene; *E2A*, gene for immunoglobulin enhancer binding proteins E12/E47; *tcr*, T-cell receptor gene; *ttg*, T-cell translocation gene; *igh*, immunogloublin heavy-chain gene; *tal*, T-cell acute leukemia gene; *myc*, cellular homologue of the transforming sequence of the avian myelocytomatosis virus; *igk*, immunogloublin κ light-chain gene; *igl*, immunoglobulin λ light-chain gene; *lyl*, lymphoid leukemia gene.

* The order of genes listed in the two columns corresponds to the order of breakpoints shown in the set of parentheses describing the chromosomal rearrangement.

(Crist WM, Pui C-H. Clinical implications of cytogenetic and molecular analyses of pediatric acute lymphoblastic leukemia. Stem Cells 1993;11:81)

script.[75] In cases of CML, the rearrangement results in the expression of a 210-kd chimeric protein, whereas in ALL, it usually leads to expression of a 185-kd *bcr/abl* protein in pediatric cases (the frequency of expression of the two forms of the protein is about equal in adult cases). Both proteins are constitutively expressed and are tyrosine kinases, leading to speculation that they may be involved in intracellular signaling.[75] Also, because the kinases differ, one could speculate that the different clinical manifestations associated with the Ph chromosome stem from these molecular differences. Patients with the variant Ph chromosomes without obvious involvement of chromosome 9 generally lack the molecular abnormalities cited previously and do not appear to share the poor prognosis of Ph ALL.[88] This finding underscores the importance of molecular genetic studies in ALL and the possibility of explaining the various presentations of this disease through detection of specific genetic changes.

DIAGNOSIS

The diagnosis of ALL can be made in most patients by physical examination and assessment of the complete blood count and bone marrow specimen. Although lymphoblasts are usually evident in a stained peripheral blood smear, they may be absent in certain unusual cases termed *aleukemic leukemia*. Children often have activated blood lymphocytes due to viral infections, a finding that may confuse even experienced hematologists. Regardless of the involvement of peripheral blood, it is important to study an adequate sample of well-stained bone marrow. In most cases, marrow is hypercellular with 60% to 100% blast cells, scattered normal myeloid or erythroid precursors, and few or no detectable megakaryocytes. By convention, at least one fourth of the nucleated marrow cells must be blasts to establish the diagnosis of acute leukemia; if the FAB morphologic subtype is lymphoid and the myeloperoxidase stain is negative (ie, less than 3% of blasts are positive), a diagnosis of ALL can be made. Blood transfusion rarely alters bone marrow morphologic findings; hence, this supportive therapy can be given before marrow aspiration.

About 5% to 10% of cases are more diagnostically challenging. In some patients, bone marrow aspiration may be difficult, resulting in a poor sample for examination. In others, the leukemic blasts may be large, with abundant cytoplasm and prominent nucleoli resembling poorly differentiated myeloblasts. In such cases, a myeloperoxidase stain can be useful since the enzyme is expressed only in myeloid cells. Anemia, generally normochromic and normocytic, is present. Teardrop and nucleated red blood cell precursors may betray the presence of disturbed marrow architecture caused by proliferating leukemic cells.

The frequencies of clinical and laboratory abnormalities commonly observed in children with ALL are shown in Table 27-1, according to immunophenotype.[89] No indication has been found that these features differ substantially in adults. The differences noted among the immunophenotypic groups probably reflect basic biologic differences in these ALL subtypes. Peripheral blood counts and physical findings are almost universally abnormal at the time of presentation, although the degree of abnormality varies widely.[90] Among 584 consecutive children with ALL treated at St Jude Children's Research Hospital in the 1980s, the most common presenting signs and symptoms were fever and malaise, followed by bleeding, usually into skin or mucous membranes[90] (Table 27-6). Bone and joint pain were also frequent. Pallor, which is seen in most patients, is caused by low hemoglobin levels due to bone marrow infiltration by leukemic cells, leading to inadequate erythrocyte production.

Fever at presentation may be due to infection (usually viral or bacterial) or to undetermined causes. Rarely, such fever reflects fungal or protozoan infections. Establishing a precise cause of fever is often difficult, but it should be attempted.

Malaise may be due to anemia, infection, or unknown causes. Bleeding is usually secondary to thrombocytopenia resulting from marrow failure, but it is occasionally caused by consumptive coagulopathy, with or without thrombocytopenia, especially in patients with T-cell ALL.[91] Bone and joint pain are thought to reflect leukemic infiltration with secondary stretching of the periosteum or joint capsule, which contains sensory nerve endings. Lymphadenopathy and hepatosplenomegaly, two frequently observed signs of ALL, often result from infiltration by leukemic cells. In rare cases, peripheral blood findings or physical examination may be normal.[92]

Children with ALL usually have normal cardiovascular systems and tolerate anemia surprisingly well; adults with cardiovascular or pulmonary disease tend to tolerate this complication less well. It is therefore necessary to use clinical judgment, in addition to measurements of hemoglobin level, when making decisions about the need for blood product transfusion. Because anemia is due to gradual interference with erythropoiesis as leukemic cells infiltrate the marrow and replace normal marrow elements, patients often have sufficient time to develop compensatory mechanisms to offset, in part, decreases in oxygen-carrying capacity. Restlessness due to hypoxia may occur in any patient but is often overlooked in small children, who are especially anxious in a hospital setting.

TABLE 27-6. Most Common Presenting Signs and Symptoms in Childhood Acute Lymphoblastic Leukemia

Feature	Frequency (%)
Fever	55
Malaise	50
Bleeding	42
Bone or joint pain	27
Anorexia	20
Abdominal pain	10

(Rivera G, Pui C-H. Acute lymphoblastic anemia. In: Rudolph AM, ed. Pediatrics. Norwalk, CT, Appleton-Century-Crofts, 1987:1098)

Some patients may swallow a substantial amount of blood as a result of epistaxis, leading to gastric irritation with nausea and vomiting and to elevation of the blood urea nitrogen level. The psychological as well as physical effects of hematemesis may be appreciable; therefore, every effort should be made to control bleeding quickly. Bleeding may also result in melena, grossly bloody stools, or diarrhea, depending on the bleeding rate. Digested blood may cause considerable flatus and distention. Because bleeding can usually be controlled by platelet transfusion, it is an infrequent cause of death in newly diagnosed patients. An exception is the severe hemorrhagic disorder called *disseminated intravascular coagulation*, which may develop in T-cell ALL patients as a result of thromboplastic substances released from T lymphoblasts.[91]

Some patients complain of nonspecific abdominal pain, presumably resulting from areas of inflammation or nodal involvement within the intestinal tract. Others complain of rectal pain due to proctitis. These lesions are not easily seen unless the perianal area is examined carefully, averting the anorectal skin to observe the mucocutaneous junction.

Any break in skin is a potential opening for bacterial invasion; it is not unusual to see paronychia, infected insect bites, or cellulitis secondary to minor abrasions. Deep infection may be seen at the sites of intramuscular injections of medications. Figure 27-4 illustrates the important steps in the initial evaluation of a patient with suspected ALL.

DIFFERENTIAL DIAGNOSIS

Most cases of ALL can be readily identified and the cell lineage definitively established by a series of laboratory studies considered with the patient's clinical features.[3] A relatively small number of pediatric cases and a somewhat larger number of adult cases have ambiguous morphologic findings, negative myeloperoxidase staining, and markers associated with two different cell lineages, which may be present on the surface of individual blast cells or on subpopulations of blasts coexisting in the same patient.[3,43] Such cases represent newly identified subgroups of acute leukemia in both age groups.[67] The cytogenetic features of many cases of ALL have been shown to be closely associated with specific immunophenotypes[59] (see Tables 27-4 and 27-5) and therefore may be helpful in providing corroborative information regarding the biologic nature of a particular case.

Differential diagnoses include other forms of leukemia, non-Hodgkin's lymphoma, idiopathic thrombocytopenic purpura (ITP), metastatic solid tumors with marrow involvement, juvenile rheumatoid arthritis (JRA), aplastic anemia, acute infectious mononucleosis, neutropenic conditions, and certain infectious disorders associated with lymphocytosis.

The morphology of lymphoblasts in ALL is generally sufficiently different from that of Sézary cells, plasma cells, or hairy cells to avoid confusion with these disorders. Oc-

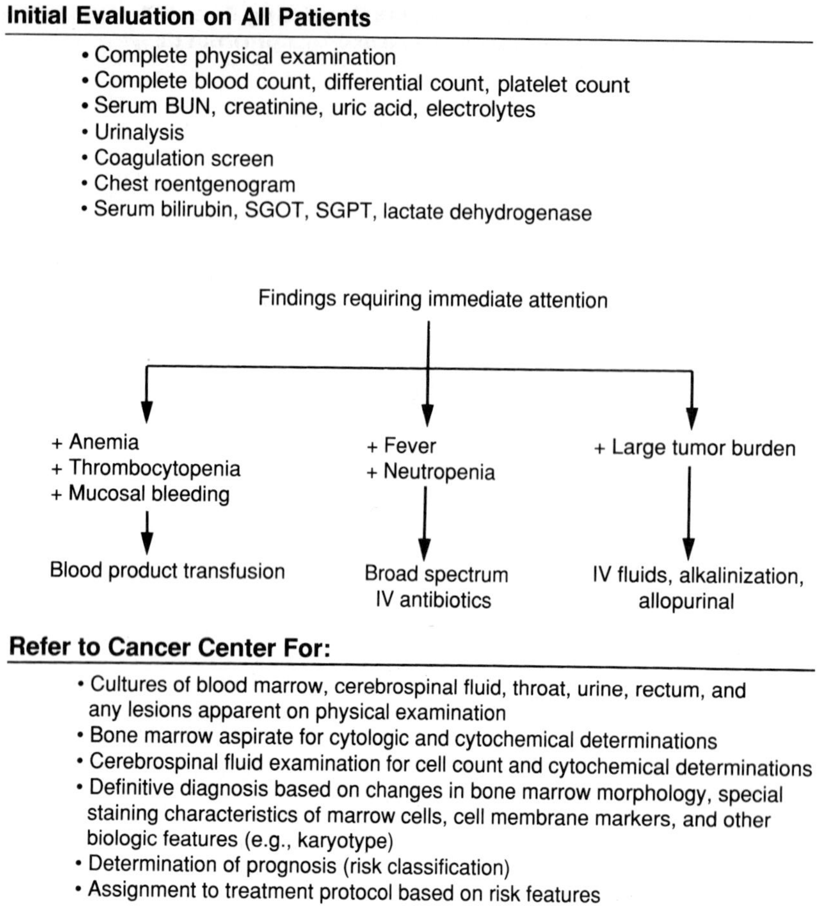

FIGURE 27-4. Flow diagram of the important steps in the initial evaluation and management of patients with newly diagnosed acute lymphoblastic leukemia.

casionally, a case of ALL has relatively mature-appearing lymphoid cells, leading to some difficulty, on morphologic grounds alone, in distinguishing between this disease and chronic lymphocytic leukemia (CLL), which is characterized by relatively mature cells. The vastly different age ranges (0 to 30 years for ALL and 30 or more years for CLL), presenting features, clinical courses, and complications of these two diseases make a distinction relatively easy.

The most difficult differential diagnosis is non-Hodgkin's lymphoma in an advanced stage with bone marrow and blood involvement. Such cases are impossible to distinguish from their immunophenotypically identical ALL counterparts (ie, T- and B-cell ALL). This lack of distinctive features does not appear to be clinically important because methods of classification (morphologic, immunophenotypic, and karyotypic) suggest that the essential difference in these diseases lies in their extent at presentation. Thus, decisions regarding appropriate management can be based on biologic features and extent of disease progression.

ITP can be distinguished from ALL with relative ease because isolated thrombocytopenia, often with large platelets seen on a blood smear, contrast sharply with the more generalized blood cell abnormalities and small platelets typically observed in patients with ALL. Physical findings in ITP are usually limited to bruising or bleeding associated with thrombocytopenia. An occasional patient develops modest splenomegaly, probably caused by a recent viral infection. In most cases, the leukocyte level and differential count is unremarkable, and there is no anemia unless bleeding has been substantial or an unrelated anemia is present. If doubt exists, a bone marrow aspirate is diagnostic because the marrow elements appear normal or show increased megakaryocytes. Adults with ITP are more likely to have associated serious diseases, such as malignancy or collagen vascular disease, than are children.

Children with neuroblastoma frequently have malignant involvement of liver, lymph nodes, bone, or bone marrow; the marrow involvement may be extensive. Occasionally, neuroblasts are found on a peripheral blood smear, and their appearance may resemble that of lymphoblasts.[93] A palpable or radiographically demonstrable abdominal nonhepatic mass is usually discernible, suggesting the true diagnosis. Neuroblasts tend to cluster and form pseudorosettes, in contrast to the diffuse involvement generally observed in ALL. The diagnosis can be confirmed by measurement of urinary catecholamines, radiologic examination, and biopsy of the mass. Other tumors (rhabdomyosarcoma, Ewing's sarcoma, or carcinomas in adults) with extensive marrow involvement may also enter the differential diagnosis. If questions remain after bone marrow examination, including cytochemical, immunophenotypic, and cytogenetic evaluations, electron microscopy may disclose neurosecretory granules or other features helpful in specific diagnosis; use of monoclonal antibodies (conjugated to fluorochromes) to lineage-specific or lineage-associated cell-surface antigens may also be useful.

Patients with aplastic anemia usually present with pancytopenia without blast cells in blood or bone marrow; blood cell precursors are either decreased or absent in a bone marrow biopsy specimen. Organs are not usually enlarged. Rarely, patients with ALL present with pancytopenia and have areas of bone marrow that are fibrotic and empty, impeding diagnosis. Repeated bone marrow aspirates or biopsies establish the correct diagnosis by demonstrating areas of marrow that are infiltrated with blast forms.

JRA may mimic ALL in children because of lymphadenopathy, splenomegaly, pallor, fever of unknown origin, neutrophilia, and joint pain. Because no conclusive test for the presence of JRA is available, bone marrow aspiration is recommended to establish the diagnosis. Some patients with positive antinuclear antibody tests have been later shown to have ALL.[94]

Patients with acute infectious mononucleosis syndrome due to EBV, cytomegalovirus, or *Toxoplasma* infection may have symptoms and signs similar to those seen in patients with ALL. Usually, the neutrophil and platelet counts remain normal in infectious mononucleosis, even if there is marked leukocytosis with bizarre mononuclear cells.[15] The diagnosis of infectious mononucleosis can be serologically confirmed; if doubt remains, normal findings on bone marrow examination rule out ALL. Patients with ALL may also have coexisting infectious mononucleosis.

Patients with congenital or acquired neutropenia or sepsis may present with neutropenia. No proliferation of lymphoid cells occurs, so that confusion with ALL is unlikely in most cases. For the few patients with ALL who present with neutropenia as the primary abnormality, a bone marrow examination usually provides a definitive diagnosis because septic patients without leukemia lack substantial numbers of lymphoblasts.

Patients with pertussis, parapertussis, or a similar syndrome or with infectious lymphocytosis may present with marked lymphocytosis; however, unlike lymphoblasts, the lymphocytes appear small and mature with tightly packed chromatin, and the patients lack symptoms of marrow failure (pancytopenia). Characteristic paroxysmal cough suggests the presence of the pertussis-like syndromes. Patients with infectious lymphocytosis are either asymptomatic or have mild respiratory or gastrointestinal symptoms; other family members are often affected as well.

TABLE 27-7. Factors Predicting Event-Free Survival in Children With Acute Lymphoblastic Leukemia*

Feature	Relative Risk†
Leukocyte count ($\times 10^9$/L)	>20/<20 = 2.2
Mediastinal mass	Yes/no = 2.8
Sex	M/F = 1.8
Splenomegaly	Mark/norm + mod = 1.9
Age (years)	<1/1–9 = 4.1
	≥10/1–9 = 2
Day-14 marrow	M3/M1 = 2.7
	M2/M1 = 1.7
Hepatosplenomegaly	Mark/norm + mod = 1.6
Platelet count ($\times 10^9$/L)	<50/>50 = 1.4
Node enlargement	Mark/norm + mod = 1.8
Blast morphology (FAB)	L2/L1 = 1.9
	L1 + L2/L1 = 1.5
IgM level	Depr/norm = 1.4
E-rosette reactivity	Pos/neg = 1.5
Race	Nonwhite/White = 1.3
Hemoglobin level (g/dL)	>8/<8 = 1.2
CNS leukemia at diagnosis	Yes/no = 1.5
IgA level	Depr/norm = 1
IgG level	Depr/norm = 1

FAB, French-American-British classification system; Ig, immunogloublin; mod, moderate; M/F, male/female ratio; Mark, marked; norm, normal; Depr, depressed.

* Univariate log-rank analysis of Kaplan-Meier life-table data for 1490 patients treated in consecutive clinical trials of the Children's Cancer Study Group from 1978 to 1983.

† Relative risk of relapse (at any site) of death, comparing treatment results for patients with different values of the same features.

(Hammond D, Sather H, Nesbit M, et al. Analysis of prognostic factors in acute lymphoblastic leukemia. Med Pediatr Oncol 1986;14:124)

PROGNOSTIC FACTORS

Despite remarkable improvement in the prognosis for patients with ALL, about one third of children and more than one half of adults continue to die from the complications of relapse or, less commonly, from the side effects of treatment.[2,89] Most patients can be assigned, at diagnosis, to favorable or unfavorable risk groups by analysis of presenting clinical and laboratory features. The ability to identify reliable prognostic factors has contributed importantly to explanations of disease outcome and to the design and evaluation of treatment protocols. An array of clinical and lymphoblast biologic features has been related to the results of therapy (Table 27-7); however, the interdependence of these factors suggests that only a small number are of genuine value in treatment planning. It is important to recognize that the impact of any prognostic factor depends on the efficacy of therapy—the single most influential predictor of clinical outcome. In the following sections, we discuss only those factors that have shown statistically significant prognostic value in large numbers of clinical trials.

Age

The age of patients with ALL exerts a striking effect on clinical outcome (Fig. 27-5). Children younger than 2 years and those older than 10 have a relatively poor prognosis in comparison with patients in the intermediate age group.[49] The worst prognosis is for infants younger than 1 year of age at diagnosis, whose leukemia appears to be biologically unique. ALL in infants is clinically aggressive, frequently presenting with central nervous system (CNS) leukemia, massive hepatosplenomegaly, and high leukocyte levels. In two large series of infants recently studied by investigators of the Children's Cancer Group and the POG, the event-free survival rate at 4 years from diagnosis did not exceed 34%, a poor result in view of the generally favorable outlook for children with ages between 2 and 10 years.[95–99] Recent observations in a clinical trial of aggressive multiagent chemotherapy suggest a modest improvement in the long-term outcome for this poor-risk group.[100]

Of all patients less than 21 years of age with newly diagnosed ALL, about 15% are adolescents (over 10 years of age), whose prognosis is poorer than in the 2- to 10-year-old group. Because of their unique stage of psychologic and physical development, adolescents often experience serious adjustment problems related to the diagnosis and treatment of ALL, leading in some cases to inadequate compliance with protocol-specified therapy. The influence of this factor on prognosis has not been carefully assessed. Adolescents also have an increased incidence of T-cell and CD10− early pre–B-cell ALL, both of which respond less readily to chemotherapy than does the more common CD10+ early pre–B-cell form of ALL. Regardless of immunophenotype, the leukemia in adolescents tends to be associated with features that predict an unfavorable prognosis: higher leukocyte levels, male predominance, and a higher incidence of hypodiploid and pseudodiploid karyotypes.[101] In nonrandomized clinical trials of intensified chemotherapy, an adolescent age lacked any demonstrable influence on prognosis.[102]

The comparatively poor prognosis of ALL in adults is well known. Recently, Hoelzer and colleagues[2] analyzed a number of factors that may explain this finding. Briefly, adults have a lower incidence of CD10+ ALL and a higher

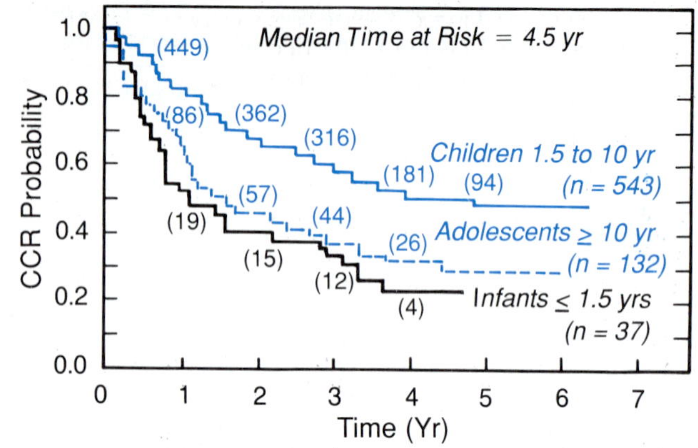

FIGURE 27-5. Probability of continuous complete remission (CCR) in children with acute lymphoblastic leukemia stratified into three age groups. The curves were constructed by the Kaplan-Meier procedure; numbers in parentheses indicate patients still at risk. Statistical comparisons: infants versus children, P = .0001; adolescents versus children, P = .0001. (Courtesy of D. J. Pullen, MD, the Pediatric Oncology Group)

incidence of Ph chromosome–positive ALL. In addition, a worse tolerance of chemotherapy and a longer time to achieve complete remission in adults may adversely affect clinical outcome.

Leukocyte Count

The initial leukocyte count remains among the most consistently reliable predictors of treatment outcome identified to date[49,103] (see Tables 27-7 and 27-8). Its relation to prognosis is linear; that is, outcome worsens as the leukocyte count increases. For each rise of 10×10^9/L in the initial leukocyte count, there is a stepwise worsening of prognosis.[104] Although, in the context of modern chemotherapy, investigators disagree over the prognostic significance of small increments in leukocyte count, there is general consensus on 50×10^9/L as the level separating patients with an unfavorable outlook from those more likely to have a durable response.

Immunophenotype

Stage of blast cell maturation has been shown to be an important determinant of treatment outcome in ALL, which is not surprising when one considers the marked differences in biologic features that characterize each of

TABLE 27-8. Criteria for Risk Assignment in a Clinical Trial for Children With Acute Lymphoblastic Leukemia*

Feature	"Worse" Category	Estimated Relative Risk
DNA index	≤1.15	4.7
Race	Black	2.5
Chromosomal translocation	Present	2.2
Leukocyte count	$>25 \times 10^9$/L	1.9
Age (years)	<2 or >10	1.8

* Probability of relapse, at any time, in a patient with a "worse" feature compared with that in a patient lacking that feature.
(Rivera GK, George SL, Williams D, et al. Early results of intensified remission induction chemotherapy for childhood acute lymphocytic leukemia. Med Pediatr Oncol 1986;14:177)

these immunologic subtypes. Virtually all cases of B-cell ALL have specific chromosomal translocations: t(8;14), t(8;22), or t(2;8).[72]

A rapid growth rate of malignant blast cells is seen in B-cell leukemia, which possibly adversely influences the clinical course by producing more extensive disease at diagnosis. Also, acute renal insufficiency and other intraabdominal complications often occur. Another characteristic of B-cell non-Hodgkin's lymphoma and leukemia is that patients who respond to therapy and do not relapse within a year after diagnosis are generally cured.[44] Until recently, these patients had a dismal prognosis, especially when they presented with CNS leukemia at diagnosis.

About one fourth of pre–B-cell cases, also considered to respond relatively poorly, possess a t(1:19).[105] Results of two recent studies show that the increased incidence of high-risk features, including high leukocyte count and black patients, and the worse treatment outcome of children with pre–B-cell ALL is strongly associated with the subset of patients with the t(1;19).[30,106] In early pre–B-cell cases, by contrast, the t(1;19) is generally lacking, and patients tend to have a favorable outcome.

The historically poor outcome for patients with T-cell ALL can be attributed to the large tumor burden that is usually associated with this subtype. Most patients present with leukocyte counts of more than 20×10^9/L, marked organomegaly, and mediastinal masses.[5] More recently, acute leukemia with the T-cell immunophenotype has proved susceptible to intensive treatment protocols, so that its previous dire outlook may be changing.[102,107] Interestingly, the T-cell phenotype in adults does not always connote a poor prognosis.[2]

Preliminary findings suggested that children and adults with mixed lineage or bilineal leukemia fare less well than other patients with ALL; however, a current study[108] shows no difference in outcome between children with or without mixed lineage leukemia treated with modern ALL-directed therapy. Children with AML characterized by low levels of myeloperoxidase activity and expression of the T-cell–associated antigen (T11; CD2) have been reported to respond to prednisone, vincristine, and L-asparaginase—drugs usually effective in ALL—but not to agents generally used to treat the myeloid leukemias.[109]

Genetics

Chromosome number has been shown to affect prognosis in ALL, with modal findings of 51 chromosomes or more conferring the most favorable outlook and the presence of structural abnormalities the worst[110] (Fig. 27-6). Hypodiploidy and near haploidy are unfavorable karyotypic features in patients with ALL.[111,112] Two translocations—the 4;11, and 9;22—are consistently linked to short remissions, whereas others have been related to variable outcomes.[113] This raises the important question of whether translocations should be uniformly considered to indicate a poor prognosis, as was suggested by Williams and colleagues.[114] At the Third International Workshop on Chromosomes in Leukemia, Bloomfield and coworkers[113] evaluated the significance of banded chromosomal analysis in patients with newly diagnosed ALL. By multivariant analysis, they found that karyotype was an independent prognostic factor influencing the duration of complete remission and survival. This result prompted the recommendation that chromosomal studies be performed at the time of diagnosis in all patients, since karyotypic findings may identify patients who, despite having better-risk clinical features, are in fact at high risk of relapse. In the experience of these investigators, treatment outcome was more accurately predicted when blast cell classification was based on the specific

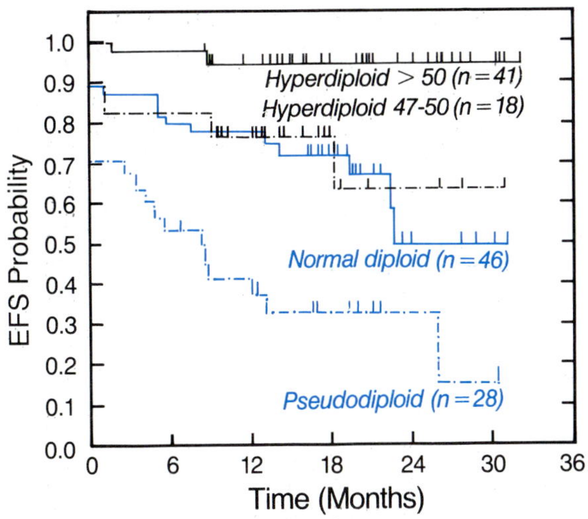

FIGURE 27-6. Event-free survival (EFS) for patients subdivided by ploidy group. Tick marks represent patients still at risk; curves constructed by the Kaplan-Meier method ($P < .001$). (After Williams DL, Tsiatis A, Brodeur GM, et al. Prognostic importance of chromosome number in 136 untreated children with acute lymphoblastic leukemia. Blood 1982;60:864)

chromosomal abnormality and not limited to modal number. For example, patients with the Ph chromosome fared poorly even when their modal chromosomal number was greater than 50.

The generally dismal prognosis of cases with the Ph chromosome [t(9;22)] has changed little with recent improvements in therapy.[87] In the Dana-Farber 81-01 study,[102] for example, five of six patients with this abnormality relapsed, despite good results for other risk groups. The prognostic influence of chromosomal deletions and inversions remains unclear.

Molecular genetic changes in ALL are only beginning to be catalogued, and considerably more time is needed to determine their relation to prognosis. One might predict that discovery of additional critical genes, such as c-*abl* in Ph chromosome–positive ALL, will correlate with the aggressiveness of particular cases.

Other Prognostic Factors

Race, gender, blast cell morphology, serum lactic dehydrogenase, and lymphomatous presentations (marked nodal and visceral enlargement) are prognostic variables that may independently influence treatment outcome.[102,107,115–118] The best example of racial variation in childhood ALL can be seen in a comparison of white and black children with ALL. Blacks present more often with hyperleukocytosis (leukocyte level 100×10^9/L or higher), a mediastinal mass, and FAB L2 blast cells, and they tend to have fewer favorable-risk cytogenetic features, such as hyperdiploid ALL. Results of multivariant analysis, however, indicate that no single feature accounts entirely for the worse outcome in blacks. Decreased drug absorption or metabolism may also contribute to the poor prognosis in black children.[119] In some pediatric clinical trials testing similar treatment regimens, it has not been possible to identify differences in outcome between male and female patients.[120] With use of modern intensive therapy, gender has not shown prognostic value in adults with ALL.[121]

Early evaluation of bone marrow response (eg, on day 14 or 15 of initial induction therapy) may provide important prognostic information. Patients with drug-sensitive disease at this interval are more likely to enter complete remission and to achieve prolonged disease-free survival. The outlook for slow responders is more guarded.[115]

The clinical utility of some prognostic factors in adult patients differs significantly from that in children.[2,71,103,121–127] Reasons for these discrepancies are not clear but may relate to the generally decreased efficacy of antileukemic therapy in adults, the smaller numbers of adults enrolled in clinical trials, and failure to study certain risk factors. The authors of a recent review of adult ALL concluded that higher leukocyte level, longer time to achieve complete remission, older age, and a CD10− or mixed lineage phenotype exert the most consistently negative prognostic influence in patients who have been intensively treated in contemporary clinical trials.[2] They stated further that prognostic factor analysis is appropriate and indicated in adult ALL to identify patients who might benefit from alternative therapy, such as bone marrow transplantation in first complete remission for those with the highest risk of early failure.

Prognostic Factor Analysis

It is common practice in therapeutic trials in ALL to analyze the impact of prognostic factors on clinical outcome. This serves at least four purposes. It allows investigators to identify variables that might explain the heterogeneity of responses to a given therapy; it permits an understanding of the interrelations of such factors, not just their individual or univariate effects; it provides a means of ensuring the comparability of patient groups resulting from randomization; and it may identify subsets of patients that would be best treated by different approaches. Unfortunately, no single factor possesses adequate predictive strength to be used as the sole criterion for risk assignment. This problem has led to the development of elaborate systems for defining favorable and unfavorable risks of treatment failure.

To illustrate this point, investigators at St Jude Children's Research Hospital, realizing the inadequacy of risk definitions used in their Total Therapy X study, sought to develop a model that would more reliably predict outcome in programs of intensive chemotherapy. From multivariate analysis of 15 clinical and biologic factors with potential prognostic value in 384 consecutive patients enrolled in study X, it was apparent that five variables needed to be considered for optimal assignment of patients to risk groups[128] (see Table 27-8). Three of the characteristics were standard factors in studies of childhood ALL (leukocyte count, age, and race), whereas two were cytogenetic features (DNA index and chromosomal translocations) that had not been identified in previous analyses. Patients with none or only one of the features shown in Table 27-8 were classified as better risk and those with two or more features were considered worse risk.

Similar analyses have given rise to diverse classification systems, making it difficult to compare results obtained by different cooperative study groups or at different treatment centers. Uniform patient eligibility criteria and uniform methods of clinical trial reporting are needed if this situation is to be corrected. A recent international workshop was convened in Rome to address these issues.[129] The participants agreed on methods for uniform recording of prognostic factors and on statistical methods for reporting clinical trial results. Specifically, they recommended that patients younger than 1 year at diagnosis and those with initial leukocyte counts of 50×10^9/L or higher be identified clearly in published reports because of their consistently higher risk of relapse.

Continued study of prognostic factors is important if leukemia specialists expect to improve the therapeutic index (toxicity versus efficacy) of intensive treatment regimens. The ultimate goal is to provide less toxic but highly effective therapy to patients with a relatively low risk of relapse and more aggressive (hence more toxic) treatment to those judged to have a poor prognosis.

BACKGROUND FOR TREATMENT

Chemotherapy for ALL has become increasingly complex since the initial observation of temporary remissions in patients treated with aminopterin, a folic acid antagonist. Five ideas have been pivotal in guiding the evolution of antileukemic treatment. First, combination chemotherapy is superior to single-agent treatment for inducing complete remissions,[130] and certain drugs may be more useful for maintaining remissions than for inducing them. Second, leukemic cells in the arachnoid tissue continue to proliferate and eventually cause relapse if treatment does not include a component specifically directed to clinically inapparent leukemia in the CNS.[131] Third, leukemia is a curable disease when combinations of effective agents are used to reduce the initial blast cell burden to a low level early in the clinical course and to suppress or eradicate residual leukemic cells during the period of continuation therapy.[132] Fourth, the various components of therapy are tightly interrelated,[133] so that weakness in any component is likely to decrease the odds for treatment success. Fifth is the recognition of ALL as a heterogeneous disease with different subtypes that respond differently to treatment.[57] The tendency of some cases of ALL to develop drug resistance more rapidly than others has led to the idea that intensive chemotherapy is needed to eradicate leukemic cells before they are able to mutate to a resistant state. Awareness that ALL is not one but several diseases has given rise to sophisticated techniques for classifying cases by cytogenetic, immunologic, and biochemical criteria. This development, together with the increased intensity of chemotherapy, has led to the practice of treating ALL in centers where specialists and modern technology are available.

A proper clinical trial of antileukemic therapy requires an enormous expenditure of time, energy, and resources. Furthermore, conclusions drawn from a trial may have a substantial ripple effect on other trials for years to come. Consequently, it is appropriate to underscore the difficulty of designing and executing a proper clinical trial from which justifiable and long-lasting generalizations can be made.[134] Clinical trials are relatively crude methods of investigation, particularly when multiple institutions are involved. Because they are the only method we have for reliably testing new modalities of treatment, however, it is imperative that the resources be expended appropriately to see that the results are reliable and reproducible. Trials with a poor design or incomplete analysis of data confound and mislead. Well-designed and well-analyzed trials, however, continue to pay dividends for many years because the information obtained provides a sound basis for future developments. The trend in clinical trial reporting is to express treatment outcome in terms of event-free survival, defined as survival without remission failure, relapse of any kind, development of a life-threatening secondary malignancy, or death due to any cause.

The following sections deal with the essential elements of contemporary treatment programs for patients with ALL, with emphasis on the practical aspects of selecting an appropriate plan of therapy. No single protocol can be recommended as superior to all others. Instead, clinical hematologists must weigh the advantages of several effective regimens and choose the one that appears best suited to their patients and to their available medical resources. Until therapy is greatly improved, however, patients will likely benefit more from enrollment in clinical trials than from non–protocol-controlled management.

REMISSION INDUCTION AND INTENSIFICATION (EARLY THERAPY)

The first aim of treatment for ALL is to induce a complete remission, defined as the absence of physical signs of leukemia, no leukemic cells in the peripheral blood, less than 5% blast forms in the bone marrow with evidence of hematopoietic recovery, and fewer than five mononuclear cells in 1 μL of cerebrospinal fluid (CSF). The peripheral leukocyte count should be near or within the range of normal values. Such therapy is designed to eradicate a large proportion of the initial leukemic cell burden (remission induction) and then secure that gain with a brief period of intensification (consolidation) treatment.

Prompt induction of complete remission is essential for successful long-term control of ALL; partial remissions are not clinically valuable. Thus, one should attempt to administer chemotherapy that will produce a 99% or greater reduction in the number of leukemic cells without unduly jeopardizing the return of bone marrow function.[135] The best results of initial treatment of ALL are being obtained in clinical trials that emphasize rapid early cytoreduction through addition of two or more drugs to a proven regimen of chemotherapy, followed by treatment that decreases the likelihood of drug cross-resistance. In adult patients, the evidence that early intensification of chemotherapy will significantly influence remission duration is less clear.

Basic Regimens for Remission Induction

In most patients with ALL, especially children, the leukemic blast cells are initially sensitive to chemotherapy. Among the drugs commonly used for remission induction (Table 27-9), prednisone,[23,136] a synthetic analogue of cortisone, and vincristine,[137–139] an alkaloid extracted from the plant *Vinca rosea* Linn, are highly effective.[23,136–139] In combination, these agents induce complete remissions in 85% to 90% of children within 4 to 6 weeks.[140] By binding to microtubules, vincristine inhibits the passage of dividing cells through mitosis, with arrest occurring mainly in metaphase.[141] The precise mechanism of action of the corticosteroids is poorly understood, although their lymphocytolytic action is well recognized.[142] Prednisone and vincristine act rapidly but do not greatly suppress bone marrow regeneration; their oncolytic effects, but not their toxicity, are additive. Prednisone is usually administered at dosages of 40 to 60 mg/m^2/d orally, and vincristine at about 1.5 mg/m^2/wk intravenously (maximum single dose, 2 mg).

Two active compounds, daunorubicin and L-asparaginase, were introduced in the 1960s as therapy for patients with lymphoid malignancies. The mechanisms of action and toxic effects of these agents differ from those of steroids, vincristine, cyclophosphamide, and antimetabolites. The antineoplastic activity of daunorubicin, an anthracycline antibiotic isolated from *Streptomyces*, was first demonstrated in experimental tumors[143] and then in patients with acute leukemia.[144] It is still considered one of the most effective agents for the treatment of acute lymphoblastic and myeloblastic leukemias. A second anthracycline compound, doxorubicin, is as effective as daunorubicin in treatment of the acute leukemias[145,146] but has a wider spectrum of activity, extending to solid tumors. The cytotoxicity of these drugs results from their tight binding to DNA; they also alter cell membrane function.

L-Asparaginase, an enzyme derived from *Escherichia coli* or *Erwinia carotovora*, has a unique mode of action. Its antitumor activity results from rapid depletion of extracellular pools of L-asparagine, a nonessential amino acid in normal cellular metabolism but a necessary nutrient for leukemic blasts.[147,148] Because of the highly selective cy-

TABLE 27-9. **Drugs Commonly Used in the Treatment of Acute Lymphoblastic Leukemia**

Decade Introduced	Mechanism of Action	Route	Dose per m²
1940s AND 1950s			
Methotrexate	Inhibits dihydrofolate reductase, thus limiting the one-carbon pathways required for pyrimidine and purine synthesis	PO, IM, IV, IT	7.5–33,000 mg
Prednisone	Unknown but may involve induction of aberrant protein synthesis	PO	40–60 mg
Mercaptopurine	Inhibits purine synthesis; also incorporated into DNA	PO, IV	50–90 mg
Cyclophosphamide	Reacts covalently with DNA, often cross-linking the strands	PO, IV	250–1800 mg
1960s			
Vincristine	Disrupts microtubules, producing metaphase arrest	IV	1–1.5 mg
Daunorubicin	Intercalates between base pairs in DNA; inhibits nucleic acid synthesis	IV	30–45 mg
Cytarabine	Competitively inhibits replicative DNA polymerase; also incorporated into DNA	IV, IT	100–3000 mg
L-asparaginase	Depletes extracellular fluids of L-asparagine, starving tumor cells for this amino acid	IM, IV	6000–25,000 IU
1970s			
Epipodophyllotoxins (teniposide and etoposide)	Interact with topoisomerase II to produce protein-associated cross-links and strand breaks in DNA	IV	150–200 mg

PO, orally; IM, intramuscularly; IV, intravenously; IT, intrathecally.

totoxicity of L-asparaginase, its introduction into clinical trials generated much enthusiasm among oncologists.

Addition of L-asparaginase or an anthracycline, or both, to a basic regimen of prednisone and vincristine, improves the remission-induction rate in childhood ALL from 85% to 90% to as high as 96% or 100%[149] (Table 27-10). To demonstrate that more than two drugs are needed for remission induction, investigators in the Children's Cancer Group (CCG) compared results of prednisone plus vincristine treatment in 499 children with those for 815 children who received these two agents plus L-asparaginase.[150] The dose of L-asparaginase was 6000 IU/m² given intramuscularly three times a week for a total of nine doses, starting on day 3. Regardless of their presenting features, patients enrolled in the three-drug trial entered complete remission significantly more often than did patients treated with two agents. Although toxicity was more pronounced in children given L-asparaginase, it was not dose-limiting. The CCG experience was confirmed in later cooperative clinical trials,[151,152] and L-asparaginase is now considered virtually indispensable in therapy for ALL.

The value of adding an anthracycline compound to the combination of prednisone and vincristine is more controversial.[145,153] European investigators were among the first to incorporate daunorubicin into antileukemic therapy. In a trial conducted at Hôpital St Louis in Paris, an apparent benefit of the three-agent regimen was reported, but patients were neither stratified nor randomized, making definitive interpretation of this trial difficult.[154] Because most leukemia therapists designing clinical trials in the 1990s—for children as well as adults—used at least three drugs during the first weeks of treatment, the issue is not whether to administer additional agents but how and when to add them.

Investigators of Acute Leukemia Group B (CALGB) opened a clinical trial for adult patients (over 20 years of age) with untreated ALL, in which they tested the efficacy of adding 3 consecutive days of daunorubicin, 45 mg/m² intravenously on days 1 through 3, to an otherwise standard regimen of vincristine, prednisone, and L-asparaginase.[155] One hundred seventy-seven patients were randomized to receive induction therapy with the three-drug combination, with or without daunorubicin. Only 47% of the group treated with vincristine, prednisone, and L-asparaginase achieved complete remission, compared with 83% of patients who received the three agents plus daunorubicin. The frequency of severe myelosuppression was significantly higher in patients receiving four agents, but this toxicity was not associated with a substantial increase in fatalities. The CALGB study demonstrated conclusively the efficacy of anthracycline therapy for remission induction in adult ALL in a randomized setting. Use of a four-drug induction regimen, including L-asparaginase and doxorubicin, yielded complete remissions in 75% of adult patients in a more recent trial.[118,156]

These results emphasize the marked difference in remission-induction rates obtained in children and adults with use of essentially identical chemotherapy. Whereas prednisone, vincristine, and L-asparaginase can be expected to induce complete remissions in about 93% of children with ALL, this combination was ineffective in more than half the adults treated in the CALGB study. Moreover, in contrast to the low fatality rate among children receiving three- or four-agent induction therapy, there were 20 early

TABLE 27-10. Results of Induction Therapy for Children With Newly Diagnosed Acute Lymphoblastic Leukemia

Drug Combination	Patients	Complete Remission Rate (%)	Study	Reference
Pred + VCR + Asp	815	93	CCG 101-143	150
Pred + VCR + DNR	162	93	Paris 06-LA-66	154
Pred + VCR + DNR + IT MTX	133	95	L2-L10	124, 161
Pred + VCR + DNR + Asp	277	96	BFM 70-76/76-79	107, 167
Pred + VCR + DNR + Cyclo	155	91	CCG 141	115
	53*	88	POG 7615	149
Pred + VCR + ADR + MTX + IT ara-C	289	96	DFCC 81-01	102
Pred + VCR + Asp + IT MTX + VM-26 + ara C	101	88	SJCRH XH	175
Pred + VCR + DNR + Cyclo + Asp + ara-C + IT MTX + IT ara-C	100†	96	CCG 192P	116
Pred + VCR + DNR + Asp + VM-26 + ara-C + IT MTX + IT HC + IT ara-C	358	96	SJCRH XI	179

Pred, prednisone; VCR, vincristine; Asp, L-asparaginase; DNR, daunorubicin; MTX, methotrexate; HD, hydrocortisone; Cyclo, cyclophosphamide; ara-C, cytarabine; VM-26, teniposide; ADR, doxorubicin (Adriamycin); IT, intrathecal.
* T-cell patients only.
† High-risk patients only.

deaths, mainly due to septicemia, in adults treated in this trial.

Intensive Multiagent Regimens

Although complete remissions can be readily induced with vincristine, prednisone, and one or two other drugs, the need for maximum initial cell kill has become obvious as a result of findings in experimental systems and in more recent clinical trials. Skipper and colleagues,[157] using mice with L1210 leukemia, demonstrated a direct relation between the dosage of an effective drug (1 mg/kg) and the percentage kill of leukemic cells by a single injection of that agent. In the 1970s, several groups of investigators published reports indicating that the resistance of mammalian cell lines to antineoplastic drugs arose in a spontaneous, random fashion similar to resistance in bacterial cells. Goldie and coworkers[158] exploited these observations to devise a mathematic model that predicted an increase in drug-resistant cells as the mutation rate increased; the fraction of resistant cells was postulated to depend on whether the drug-resistant mutant emerged early or late in the treatment course. These studies suggested that early *intensified* therapy may decrease the likelihood of the development of drug resistance.

Historical Precedents

Most intensive regimens of chemotherapy are indebted to studies conducted at St Jude Children's Research Hospital and at Memorial Sloan-Kettering Cancer Center (MSKCC) in the late 1960s. In St Jude Total Therapy Study V, all patients received an intensive phase of chemotherapy early in remission that consisted of 1 week of high-dose mercaptopurine, methotrexate, and cyclophosphamide; this was followed by CNS prophylaxis, 2400 cGy of cranial irradiation, combined with intrathecal methotrexate and multiagent continuation therapy.[159] Of 35 children, 31 achieved complete remission; 19 of these responders remained alive and free of leukemia for more than 25 years. This result suggested that the cure rate for childhood ALL could be significantly boosted by intensification of chemotherapy early in remission.

Aur and coworkers,[160] in 1968, devised the first clinical protocol featuring risk-oriented therapy with a four-drug induction regimen. Based on an astute clinical observation by this group, 11 children with florid leukemia were prospectively identified as being at high risk for early relapse; hence, they were treated more intensively than other patients, beginning early in the clinical course. Each child entered complete remission with administration of standard doses of vincristine and prednisone, four to six intravenous doses of daunorubicin, 25 mg/m²/wk, and two intravenous doses of L-asparaginase, 10,000 to 20,000 IU/m²/wk intravenously. Drug-induced toxic effects were reversible, and all patients were able to begin to receive postinduction therapy without delay. Three of these children are long-term survivors, 20 years after diagnosis.

In an effort to induce maximal cell kill during the first 12 to 13 weeks of therapy, MSKCC investigators used a cell kinetic rationale to devise a novel eight-drug induction–consolidation regimen that combined cell-cycle–specific and nonspecific agents. Termed L-2, this protocol relied exclusively on chemotherapy for CNS prophylaxis; no irradiation was employed.[161] All patients received prednisone, vincristine, daunorubicin, and intrathecal methotrexate during weeks 1 to 4 of therapy, and cytarabine, thioguanine, L-asparaginase, and bischloroethylnitrosourea from weeks 4 to 13. This nonrandomized clinical trial was the first to include intrathecal therapy as early as the fourth day of induction treatment and to use intravenous doses of L-asparaginase as high as 60,000 IU/m² three times a week for 4 weeks. Initially, 23 adults (15 years of age or older) and 75 children received the L-2 treatment, which yielded a remission-induction rate of 78% in adults and 98% in children. Similarly, the proportion of children who attained long-term leukemia-free survival was substantially higher than the results for adults: 55% versus 26%. Although the L-2 regimen was clearly effective therapy for ALL, the end results were no better than those being reported for less intensive and less complex treatments.[162]

Refinements of the MSKCC treatment strategy from 1973 to 1979 emphasized greater intensification with an extra dose of anthracycline and earlier administration of cyclophosphamide during the induction phase, six instead of three cycles of consolidation therapy administered to all patients, and more prolonged intrathecal prophylaxis given throughout the continuation phase. Irradiation to areas of bulky disease was also used. Early results for 72 adult patients treated in two studies (L-10 and L-10M) included an 85% complete remission rate, a median remission duration of 51 months, and disease-free intervals of 2 to 4 years for 60% of the patients, excluding those with the Ph chromosome.[124]

Although considered among the best treatment experiences in adult ALL, these trials were still marked by a high rate of marrow relapse, mainly during the consolidation phase and the first months of maintenance therapy. Major treatment complications were acute infections secondary to chemotherapy-induced myelosuppression. Sixty-five percent of the patients had sepsis during induction treatment (median hospitalization time, 1 month); hepatitis, *Pneumocystis carinii* pneumonia, and herpes zoster were noted during periods of complete remission. This toxicity was considered manageable and justifiable based on the marked improvement in therapeutic outcome. Use of prolonged CNS prophylaxis with chemotherapy only was judged to be both safe and efficacious. This MSKCC experience demonstrated the superiority of intensified chemotherapy in securing higher rates of leukemia-free survival and suggested, at the time, that childhood and adult ALL might be treated with comparable success.

The L series of MSKCC clinical trials was recently reviewed and updated by Clarkson and colleagues,[163,164] who concluded that improvements in outcome had indeed been produced by intensification of therapy but that no gains were apparent after the development of the L-10 regimen in the mid-1970s. To confirm the MSKCC reports, investigators of the Southwest Oncology Group (SWOG) conducted a large cooperative trial that included consecutive patients with ALL irrespective of age and cytogenetic characteristics. The treatment regimen they used was identical to the L-10 protocol. Of 168 patients treated between 1980 and 1985, 115 (68%) achieved complete remission, and 29 (17%) died early in the induction phase; the median disease-free survival time was only 23 months, less than half the interval achieved in the original L-10 study.[165] Possible explanations for this discrepancy include differences in the composition of the study groups; for example, the SWOG trial had a higher proportion of patients over 50 years of age and included patients with Ph chromosome–positive ALL. For patients between 20 and 50 years of age who presented with leukocyte counts less than $15 \times 10^9/L$, however, the 4-year disease-free survival rate was 58%, an exceptionally good result.

Despite wide agreement on the need to intensify early chemotherapy for ALL, there is no consensus on the best way to achieve this objective. The evolution of contemporary regimens began as early as 1970, a turning point at which antileukemic treatment began to be curative for increasing numbers of patients.

Multiple Agents Given at Maximally Tolerated Dosages

Stimulated by results of the St Jude and MSKCC trials, Riehm and coworkers[166] in the Berlin–Frankfurt–Münster (BFM) study group began a series of investigations in which children with ALL received intensive multidrug therapy during the first 2 to 4 months of treatment, regardless of their risk status. As in the MSKCC trials, this approach represented a departure from conventional protocols, if not in the actual schema of chemotherapy, in the idea to treat all patients intensively and early. Induction chemotherapy featured four drugs—a steroid, vincristine, daunorubicin, and L-asparaginase. The consolidation phase was identical to that in the MSKCC protocols, and continuation treatment was conventional. CNS prophylaxis consisted of a combination of irradiation and intrathecal chemotherapy and did not rely exclusively on chemotherapy as in the MSKCC trials.

Results of the first BFM trial, conducted from 1970 to 1976, were not significantly better than those reported earlier.[166] Since 1976, however, this study group has convincingly demonstrated the efficacy of intensive early therapy for childhood ALL.[107,167] Their unique contribution was the concept of reinduction therapy, or virtually repeating the initial induction–consolidation phase at a strategic point in the treatment course. The BFM group has consistently reported 5-year event-free survival rates of about 65%. Importantly, patients with high-risk ALL benefited most from this therapy, achieving essentially the same outcome as patients with less resistant leukemia. In other words, the treatment had converted high-risk ALL to standard-risk ALL. The advantage of the BFM regimens for children with an average or lower risk of relapse was less obvious. These results should be interpreted with the realization that black patients, a group known to have a poor prognosis,[168,169] were absent from the BFM trials, and that these were nonrandomized studies. Recent reports from the CCG confirm the BFM results for high-risk patients and indicate that another intensive multiagent regimen, termed the *New York regimen*, is equally effective.[170]

The relevance of the BFM series of clinical trials for adults with ALL was demonstrated by Hoelzer and colleagues, also in Germany.[2,121] From 1978 to 1983, they conducted a large, prospective, multicenter trial that included 384 patients between 15 and 65 years of age. Marked differences in outcome as compared with experience in children were noted from the outset of treatment. For example, the death rate during induction treatment was three-fold higher in adults: 8% to 10% versus less than 3%. Both the remission-induction rate (74%) and event-free survival at 5 years (37% ± 7% SE) were inferior to results reported for childhood ALL. By segregating patients into standard- and high-risk groups, however, it was possible to distinguish a subgroup with a 5-year event-free survival rate of 60%. By improving the risk classification of adults with ALL, these investigators were able to identify patients who might require alternative therapy, such as bone marrow transplantation. Nonrandomized trials such as the MSKCC and German studies suggest that intensified consolidation therapies may be useful in adults, but neither the optimal combination of drugs nor the schedule of administration is known.

For the past 10 years, CCG investigators have conducted large pediatric clinical trials based in part on the MSKCC and BFM treatment strategies. The New York regimen, for example, features multimodal therapy derived from earlier MSKCC trials, namely the LSA_2L_2 studies.[116] High-dose cyclophosphamide and irradiation (1500 cGy) are administered to sites of bulky disease early in treatment. Seven drugs are given during the first 4 weeks of therapy, and intrathecal chemotherapy is started on the first day of treatment. The second phase of the New York regimen is analogous to both the BFM and MSKCC L-10 studies in that AML-like therapy with thioguanine and cytarabine infusions is given with methotrexate and additional L-asparaginase. As in most of the BFM studies, but in contrast to the MSKCC trials, CNS irradiation with intrathecal methotrexate is administered to all patients. Remission continuation therapy is given in 2-month cycles for 36 months. From 1979 to 1983, 100 previously untreated patients at high risk for early relapse, excluding infants, were treated; 96% of the patients entered complete remission with an estimated 4-year event-free survival of 69% ± 5% SE. Despite the intensity of therapy, tolerance was judged as adequate.

Few studies have prospectively compared regimens of intensive chemotherapy or, for that matter, regimens of intensive and standard therapy. Hence, the recent availability of findings in a CCG clinical trial (CCG-106 protocol) assessing the New York and BFM 76/79 regimens against each other, as well as against a control group treated in a standard fashion, has generated much interest.[170] Control patients were almost three times more likely to fail induction therapy or to relapse than were patients treated intensively. remission-induction rates were: BFM, 99%; New York, 97%; and control, 84%. Three-year event-free survival rates were 77% for BFM, 79% for New York, and 49% for the control regimen. Comparisons with other pediatric trials are difficult mainly because of differences in risk-group definitions; however, these results undoubtedly represent a therapeutic gain for children and adolescents with high-risk ALL (38% of the patients were between 10 and 22 years of age). This study included randomized controls, avoiding the usual difficulty of using historical controls in comparisons of treatment outcome.

Intensification With Two Drugs

Alternatives to the multiagent MSKCC, BFM, and CCG protocols were developed by investigators at the Dana-Farber Cancer Center and St Jude Children's Research Hospital. The Dana-Farber 81-01 protocol differs from the BFM and New York regimens in that the initial 4 weeks of therapy include one dose of methotrexate, 40 mg/m^2 to 33 g/m^2, followed 4 days later by a single dose of doxorubicin, 45 mg/m^2, and intrathecal cytarabine; the remaining 28 days of prednisone with four weekly doses of vincristine can be characterized as conventional. Intensification, which begins after patients achieve hematologic remission, consists of weekly high-dose L-asparaginase, 25,000 IU/m^2/dose, administered for about 20 weeks with vincristine, prednisone, methotrexate, and doxorubicin. Thus, to improve results, the Dana-Farber group relied mainly on an anthracycline and high-dose L-asparaginase added to an otherwise conventional treatment.[102]

From 1981 to 1985, 289 newly diagnosed pediatric patients were enrolled on the study; high-risk and standard-risk patients were treated similarly with small dosage variations. Encouraging results were obtained: 4-year event-free survival of 77% ± SE 3% for all patients; 71% ± 4% SE for high-risk patients; and 86% ± 4% SE for standard-risk patients. Less than 1% of patients enrolled on this trial were black, and the study was not randomized.

About one third of the patients developed mild to severe L-asparaginase–induced toxicity (one death). During remission, 10 patients had treatment-related fatal complications, usually infections. The authors contend that the risk/benefit ratio in this study favors continued use of weekly high-dose L-asparaginase. Randomized trials evaluating the efficacy of L-asparaginase therapy in a large number of patients are being conducted by a pediatric cooperative group.

St Jude investigators introduced the concept of adding an investigational drug combination, at the outset of treatment, to an otherwise basic plan of chemotherapy. Cytarabine was used with VM-26, one of a newer class of agents, the epipodophyllotoxins, which interact with topoisomerase II to produce cross-links and strand breaks in DNA.[171] The rationale for combining these two agents was the marked synergistic activity they had shown in animal models[172] and in treatment of patients with refractory ALL.[173,174] When administered to 57 consecutive patients with very-high-risk ALL (median leukocyte count, 199 × 10^9/L; range 100 to 1000 × 10^9/L), both before and after induction treatment, cytarabine and VM-26 were associated with striking antileukemic effects.[175] At a median follow-up time of 6 years, 44% of the 57 patients with high-risk ALL were event-free survivors, compared with only 10% in the historical control group.

Based on the St Jude series of studies with VM-26 and cytarabine, several groups of hematologists in the United States and elsewhere have included this combination in their protocols for adults with ALL. Linker and coworkers,[176] for example, reported the results of a study incorporating VM-26 and cytarabine into intensified regimens, including a four-drug induction treatment with steroids, vincristine, daunorubicin, and L-asparaginase (4 to 6 weeks) and a prolonged 10-month consolidation therapy featuring VM-26 and cytarabine as one of three different drug combinations. Patients over 50 years of age and those presenting with Ph chromosome–positive leukemia were excluded. Of 81 patients, 94% entered complete remission; these authors project a 3-year disease-free survival of 50% ± 9% SE. These preliminary yet encouraging results suggest that intensified treatment including VM-26 and cytarabine may also influence clinical outcome in adults with ALL.

Rapid Rotation of Effective Drug Combinations

Theoretically, the alternating use of non–cross-resistant pairs of drugs should provide a distinct advantage in leukemia therapy. Identification of the epipodophyllotoxins as active new agents in childhood ALL permitted the St Jude group to design a multiagent clinical trial testing the efficacy of rotational combination chemotherapy.[177,178] This trial was open to all patients, including infants, blacks, and those with Ph chromosome–positive ALL. In contrast to other trials in ALL, the St Jude Total XI study features a seven-drug induction regimen and eight-drug postremission therapy. Intensified chemotherapy is administered to all patients, regardless of risk status, for the entire 128 weeks of treatment. Short exposure to effective drugs is emphasized.

Opened in 1984, this study has accrued 358 consecutive children and adolescents with newly diagnosed ALL; the overall rate of complete remission induction is 96%. At a median follow-up time of 50 months, the estimated 4-year event-free survival is 72 ± 4% SE.[178,179] They indicate the efficacy of continuous administration of intensive chemotherapy throughout all treatment phases, a finding recently confirmed by other investigators.[179]

Single Agents at Increased Dosage

A less complex method of treatment intensification has been to increase, by about 10- to 40-fold, the dosage of a limited number of antileukemic agents in an otherwise standard and easily administered regimen. The best example of this strategy is the use of periodic infusions of high-dose intravenous methotrexate, pioneered by investigators at Roswell Park Memorial Institute.[180] First devised as alternative CNS prophylaxis to replace irradiation to the brain, this approach has been possible because of the availability of chemical rescue with leucovorin to avoid serious side effects. Such therapy should be attempted only in settings where adequate pharmacokinetic support is available. If carefully monitored, methotrexate-induced toxicity is predictable and reversible. The initial purpose of high-dose methotrexate therapy was to achieve and maintain high serum concentrations of the drug, sufficient for adequate penetration of the CNS and other organs, such as the testes. This method of intensification has been recognized to have significant systemic antileukemic effects and is used largely for that reason. A detailed discussion of the efficacy of high-dose methotrexate as CNS prophylaxis in leukemia patients is presented in a later section.

Investigators at the Baltimore Cancer Research Center assessed the value of methotrexate therapy administered during different treatment phases at different dosages to adults with ALL. This protocol, termed *MOAD*, featured a combination of methotrexate, Oncovin (vincristine), L-asparaginase, and dexamethasone as remission-induction therapy.[181] Methotrexate dosages were increased according to patient tolerance, from 100 to 225 mg/m² by intravenous push; this was followed by L-asparaginase therapy as initially described by Capizzi and coworkers.[182] Postremission treatment included a consolidation phase and cytoreductive therapy with methotrexate administered intravenously at 100 mg/kg over 6 hours followed by leucovorin rescue. During the continuation period, methotrexate was used at a low dosage, 15 mg/m², given orally once a week. Eighteen of 24 previously untreated patients (75%) achieved a complete remission, but overall disease control thereafter was unremarkable.

After inducing initial remissions with prednisone, vincristine, and doxorubicin, the EORTC Leukemia Lymphoma Study Group compared two forms of treatment intensification in adults.[183] The patients were randomized to receive or not receive (1) a dose of high-dose cytarabine at 2.5 g/m² by intravenous bolus on day 1, and (2) brief intensification treatment with L-asparaginase and cyclophosphamide or more prolonged five-agent intensification chemotherapy treatment with L-asparaginase, cyclophosphamide, thioguanine, methotrexate, and cytarabine. The complete remission rate was 71% and the median length of complete remission 22 months; neither the high-dose cytarabine nor the prolonged consolidation significantly influenced treatment outcome.

Summary of Early Therapy

A single optimal approach to treatment intensification cannot be recommended. The theoretic basis for this strategy appears sound, and the emerging data warrant continued testing in clinical trials.[184] Ideally, intensive chemotherapy should be reserved for the subset of patients who cannot be cured by conventional means, yet methods for prospectively identifying these children, although much improved, remain imprecise. Any program of intensified chemotherapy may produce excessive morbidity and mortality.[185] Prohibitive gastrointestinal toxicity, for example, led to extensive modification of a St Jude clinical trial shortly after it had opened.[186] Methods for controlling the complications most often associated with intensive chemotherapy are described in the section on supportive care.

THERAPY FOR INDUCTION FAILURES AND OVERT CENTRAL NERVOUS SYSTEM LEUKEMIA AT DIAGNOSIS

Failure to respond promptly to early therapy may be caused by death, treatment complications, or resistant leukemia. Patients who do not achieve a complete remission develop progressive disease, followed rapidly by the usually fatal complications of bone marrow failure. Few reports are available on the results of secondary treatment for this group of patients, often termed *induction failures*. In an Australian trial, cytarabine and a combination of cyclophosphamide and L-asparaginase was effective therapy for a group of six children who had not attained complete remission with prednisone, vincristine, and daunorubicin.[187] Of 14 patients with initially refractory disease who did not attain remission after 6 to 12 weeks of treatment with prednisone, vincristine, daunorubicin, and L-asparaginase, with or without cytarabine, nine responded to VM-26 plus cytarabine. Treatment consisted of 4 weeks of combination chemotherapy, given together twice weekly at dosages of 165 and 300 mg/m², respectively. Previous failure to respond to cytarabine did not preclude responses when cytarabine was combined with teniposide.[174]

Because the treatment of overt CNS leukemia remains difficult and complex, the methods employed for CNS prophylaxis are particularly important in determining eventual outcome. The proportion of patients presenting with leukemic blasts in the CSF is low, about 3% to 4%. Certain subsets of patients (eg, infants and patients with high leukocyte counts or T-cell ALL) have an increased likelihood of developing this complication. After inducing a complete remission, both hematologic and CNS, with use of intravenous and intrathecal chemotherapy, most investigators treating patients with CNS leukemia at diagnosis administer CNS irradiation at some point in the clinical course, usually during the first year. Hoelzer and colleagues,[121] for example, reported satisfactory results in adult patients with initial CNS leukemia, using intrathecal methotrexate until the spinal fluid was free of blast cells and then administering skull and spinal irradiation (3000 cGy).

THERAPY FOR SUBCLINICAL CENTRAL NERVOUS SYSTEM LEUKEMIA

Meningeal involvement by leukemic cells first became apparent when CSF began to be routinely examined at diagnosis and when bone marrow remissions were becoming more durable.[188] George and Pinkel[189] hypothesized that leukemic blasts invaded the CNS before any treatment was given and that agents used for systemic therapy did not penetrate the meninges in therapeutic concentrations. Because of its morbidity and implications for systemic relapse, leukemic involvement of the CNS represents a major clinical problem. Any proposed treatment of ALL must include specific CNS therapy because leukemic cells, often undetected at diagnosis, may be protected in a pharmacologic "sanctuary site." The introduction of effective therapy for subclinical CNS leukemia was a pivotal step in boosting long-term disease-free survival rates to 50% in childhood ALL.

Studies performed at St Jude Children's Research Hospital demonstrated that overt leukemic infiltration of the meninges could be prevented by early use of 2400 cGy of craniospinal irradiation or 2400 cGy of cranial irradiation plus intrathecal methotrexate.[132,159] Subsequently, most regimens included some form of local treatment for prevention of overt CNS leukemia, usually intrathecal injections of antileukemic drugs or gamma radiation, or both.

The need for early treatment of subclinical CNS leukemia is undisputed; however, the search for more effective and less toxic regimens continues. The incidence of overt CNS leukemia at diagnosis and of isolated CNS relapse varies with the clinical risk status and blast cell immunophenotype of patients. Those with unusually high leukocyte counts (over 100×10^9/L), those with T-cell ALL and a leukocyte count of more than 50×10^9/L, those with Ph chromosome–positive ALL, and infants (over 1 year of age) are at especially high risk for meningeal involvement.[95,98,190] The incidence of CNS leukemia varies among study groups and may depend in part on the diagnostic criteria employed. Methods of detecting leukemic cells in the CSF have improved since the 1960s, yet the definition of CNS leukemia has remained inconsistent and controversial. Patients with this complication are usually asymptomatic; only rarely do they present with cranial nerve palsies without leukemic blasts in the CSF. Thus, criteria for the diagnosis of meningeal leukemia are based on microscopic findings, that is, the unequivocal presence of blast cells and more than five mononuclear cells per milliliter in a cytospin preparation of CSF.

Three general approaches to CNS prophylaxis—irradiation, intrathecal chemotherapy, and high-dose intravenous chemotherapy—are commonly used. Systemic treatment with agents that penetrate the CNS, such as high-dose cytarabine, may contribute to the overall effectiveness of preventive CNS treatment. The intent of any form of prophylactic CNS therapy should be to limit the CNS relapse rate to less than 10%, without producing long-term toxic effects. Specific methods for achieving this goal are summarized in Table 27-11.[161,191]

The acute side effects of prophylactic irradiation and intrathecal chemotherapy may be local (alopecia and hyperpigmentation of the scalp), systemic (anorexia, nausea, vomiting, and fever), or neurologic (somnolence syndrome[192,193] and seizure disorders[194]).

Irradiation

Radiation therapy was tested as CNS prophylaxis in early clinical trials because of experiments demonstrating that L1210 murine leukemia could be cured by addition of cranial irradiation to systemic treatment with cyclophosphamide.[195] Although intrathecal chemotherapy was believed to be sufficient for disease that was limited to the subarachnoid space, it was not considered adequate for perivascular arachnoid leukemia, deep in the cerebral hemispheres. In such patients, the flow of spinal fluid could be altered because of leukemic infiltration and swelling of the tissues. By contrast, external megavoltage irradiation would have the advantage of providing uniform antileukemic effects to the entire cranial or craniospinal contents, including both superficial and deep arachnoid membranes.[196]

Investigators at St Jude Children's Research Hospital were the first to document the effectiveness of CNS preventive therapy,[197] relying on a series of comparative studies that began 30 years ago. In Study V,[159] they administered 2400 cGy to the cranium with five doses of intrathecal methotrexate (12 mg/m^2; maximum single dose, 15 mg) over 18 days. This treatment, given early in remission, was associated with cure rates of 50% and a decrease in the incidence of meningeal relapse from 60% to 8%. The impact of this CNS therapy on clinical outcome was investigated further in Study VI.[198] Patients were randomized to receive or not to receive 2400 cGy of preventive craniospinal irradiation, with the thought that craniospinal irradiation would avoid any confounding effects of intrathecal methotrexate. Patients in the nonirradiated group received therapeutic irradiation only if they developed an overt meningeal relapse. The difference in CNS relapse rates was striking: only 2 (4%) of 45 irradiated patients had their initial complete remissions ended by meningeal relapse, compared with 33 (67%) of 49 nonirradiated patients. The median time to CNS relapse was 8 months (range, 2 to 29 months). Moreover, 31 of the patients who received prophylactic irradiation continue to survive after 18 to 20 years; only 10 patients in the comparison group are alive.

This study established the importance of administering CNS therapy before the development of overt CNS leukemia, and it demonstrated the relation of effective CNS prophylaxis to clinical outcome in general. It did not show, however, that craniospinal irradiation was the only effective method of CNS prophylaxis. To assess the contribution of intrathecal methotrexate to the prevention of CNS leukemia, the same group of investigators randomized patients to receive 2400 cGy of cranial irradiation with intrathecal methotrexate or 2400 cGy of craniospinal irradiation with-

TABLE 27-11. Outline of Presymptomatic CNS Therapy for Children With Acute Lymphoblastic Leukemia

	Postinduction Therapy			
During Induction	**Early Only**	**Throughout**	**Study**	**Reference**
INTRATHECAL THERAPY				
None	IT MTX × 6	None	CCG-101	191
None	None	Monthly IT MTX × 4 y	06-LA-66	154
IT MTX	IT MTX	± IT MTX ± ara-C every 8 wk × 3 y	L2-10	124, 161
± IT MTX + HC + ara-C	IT MTX + HC + ara-C × 6	IT MTX + HC + ara-C every 8 wk × 1–3 y	ALinC series (POG)	204
INTRATHECAL PLUS HIGH-DOSE SYSTEMIC CHEMOTHERAPY				
IT MTX	↑ Dose IV MTX + IT MTX every 3 wk × 3	None	ALGB 7611	180
IT MTX	↑ Dose IV MTX + IT MTX weekly × 3	↑ Dose IV MTX + IT MTX every 6 wk × 12	SJCRH XS	128
None	IT MTX + HC + ara-C × 6	± ↑ Dose IV MTX + IT MTX + HC + ara-C every 8 wk × 1 y	ALinC 13	50
RADIATION WITH OR WITHOUT CHEMOTHERAPY				
None	Radiation alone, 24 Gy	None	SJCRH VI	198
None	Radiation 24 Gy + IT MTX	None	SJCRH V, VIII (BFM studies)	159, 215 107, 167
None	Radiation 18 Gy + IT MTX	None	CCG 143	200
IT ara-C	Radiation 18 to 28 Gy + IT MTX	IT MTX every 18 wk × 30 mo	SFCC 81-01	102
IT MTX	IT MTX every 10 wk × 7	Radiation 24 Gy + IT MTX	SJCRH XH	175

IT MTX, intrathecal methotrexate; HC, hydrocortisone; ara-C, cytarabine; POG, Pediatric Oncology Group; BFM, Berlin–Frankfurt–Münster study group.

out intrathecal chemotherapy.[199] Neither treatment proved superior to the other. Cranial irradiation combined with intrathecal chemotherapy is favored over craniospinal irradiation because of the increased toxicity—excessive myelosuppression and spinal growth retardation—associated with the latter modality. The St Jude findings have been confirmed by oncologists worldwide, to the extent that cranial irradiation plus intrathecal methotrexate was considered standard CNS prophylaxis in most protocols for patients with ALL until recently.

In an effort to decrease the incidence of long-term toxicity associated with irradiation of the brain, especially in young children, leukemia therapists have tested lower doses of radiation as alternatives to 2400 cGy. The CCG was able to show that cranial irradiation can be safely decreased to 1800 cGy[200]; the BFM group in Germany is evaluating dose reductions to 1200 cGy. Although ineffective in clinical trials of the early 1960s,[201] lower radiation doses might be useful now that intensive systemic chemotherapy has improved control of hematologic relapse.

Intrathecal Chemoprophylaxis

Recent studies of intensive systemic therapy have indicated that intrathecal chemotherapy is adequate CNS prophylaxis for most patients with ALL.[152,202,203] Selected patient subgroups, however, as mentioned previously, continue to require CNS irradiation in addition to intrathecal therapy. Four consecutive studies conducted by the POG from 1974 to 1990 have provided important information on the efficacy of chemoprophylaxis for CNS leukemia.[152,202–205] These investigators evaluated periodic use of triple intrathecal combination chemotherapy, consisting of methotrexate 15 mg/m^2 (maximum single dose, 15 mg), hydrocortisone 15 mg/m^2 (maximum single dose, 15 mg), and cytarabine 30 mg/m^2 (maximum single dose, 30 mg) given intrathecally on a weekly basis over 4 to 6 weeks during early therapy, followed by injections every 8 weeks for 1 to 3 years during continuation therapy. Toxicity appeared to be increased when chemoprophylaxis was begun during induction treatment; however, a 3- to 4-month delay increased the risk of CNS relapse. Thus, simultaneous administration of chemoprophylaxis early in therapy is recommended. The POG investigators originally concluded that 1 year of triple intrathecal chemotherapy is as effective as 3 years; however, subsequent studies and reanalysis led them to recommend at least 2 years. They also recommend combining intrathecal chemoprophylaxis with CNS irradiation for patients with T-cell ALL who present with leukocyte counts of 50 × 10^9/L or higher. In POG study ALinC 13, six doses of triple intrathecal chemotherapy during remission induction and consolidation treatment, followed by periodic low-dose intrathecal methotrexate combined with high-dose intravenous methotrexate, was less effective than continued triple intrathecal chemoprophylaxis alone.[205] From these findings, it appears that triple intrathecal chemotherapy, administered periodically for about 2 years, offers effective CNS prophylaxis for patients with early pre-B-cell or pre–B-cell ALL. More specific conclusions will be possible when information on long-term effects becomes available.

High-Dose Systemic Plus Intrathecal Chemotherapy

In 1972, investigators at Roswell Park Memorial Institute began a series of clinical and pharmacologic studies that introduced a new concept of CNS prophylaxis.[206] They revived the use of high-dose systemic methotrexate to achieve and maintain high plasma levels of the drug for adequate penetration into the CSF. The rationale was that chemoprophylaxis would not only be as effective in preventing meningeal relapse but also would lower the risk of neurotoxicity produced by cranial irradiation, a complication that was being recognized and reported in long-term survivors. After remission induction with prednisone, vincristine, and L-asparaginase (also three doses of intrathecal methotrexate), patients received intravenous methotrexate, 500 mg/m^2, over 24 hours with simultaneous intrathecal methotrexate and leucovorin rescue every 3 weeks early in remission; no other CNS therapy was given during the continuation phase. Termed *intermediate-dose methotrexate*, this treatment resulted in cytotoxic levels of the drug in CSF and was adequately tolerated by most patients; the effect on the CNS relapse rate was initially favorable.

A critical comparison of intermediate-dose methotrexate and the standard form of CNS irradiation was made by investigators of Cancer and Leukemia Group B. Five hundred forty-one children in complete remission, who had been stratified by age and leukocyte count, were randomized to receive either method of CNS prophylaxis.[180] Initially, the combination of intrathecal and intravenous methotrexate appeared effective as prophylactic CNS therapy in standard-risk but not in high-risk patients. To improve results in the latter group, the dosage of methotrexate, the number of cycles of therapy, and the number of intrathecally administered agents were increased, but none of these changes convincingly improved clinical outcome. An update of the study,[207] published in 1985, showed conclusively that six doses of intrathecal methotrexate with three courses of intermediate-dose methotrexate was inferior to prophylactic CNS irradiation, regardless of the risk status of patients (CNS relapse rates, about 30% versus less than 10%). Intermediate-dose methotrexate therapy, however, was significantly related to longer periods of remission in standard-risk patients and provided effective protection against testicular relapse. The end results of this study failed to show a significant therapeutic gain over other contemporary trials, casting doubt on the long-term benefits of intermediate-dose methotrexate administered as CNS prophylaxis.

Intensified regimens of intravenous methotrexate have been tested by investigators at St Jude Hospital and POG. In the former studies, methotrexate, 1 g/m^2, given intravenously over 24 hours, followed by leucovorin rescue, was administered with intrathecal methotrexate in 12 postinduction courses to 154 patients.[128] This study demonstrated adequate CNS protection for a selected group of good-risk patients, as defined by a leukocyte count lower than 25 × 10^9, age between 2 and 10 years, white race, and hyperdiploid leukemic blasts without chromosomal translocations. Additional analysis indicated that cranial irradiation affords better protection against CNS relapse in a small subset of higher-risk patients than does the high-dose methotrexate regimen, which was most beneficial for patients with leukocyte counts lower than 25 × 10^9/L and prognostically favorable ages and cytogenetic features. Administering methotrexate in increased dosages (eg, 4 to 8 to 33 g/m^2) has not improved results over those in more conventional trials.[208] The POG has concluded that triple intrathecal chemoprophylaxis is superior to intravenous high-dose methotrexate with low-dose intrathecal methotrexate.

With long-term follow-up, studies thought to demonstrate an advantage of intrathecal or high-dose systemic chemotherapy for prevention of CNS leukemia have not proved as conclusive as initially reported.[209] Moreover, the argument that most isolated CNS relapses can be treated successfully and therefore do not affect cure rates has been discounted.[210] Among 107 children with an isolated CNS relapse as their first adverse event in St Jude Total Therapy Studies I to IX, 83% had a subsequent relapse.[211] These data, which have been confirmed in more recent CCG trials, underscore the advantages of preventing meningeal relapses rather than attempting to treat them later in the clinical course.[212] Because cranial irradiation was used in most treatment programs with the highest rates of event-free survival, we believe that any decision to eliminate this method from protocols for very-high-risk patients would be unwise without further investigation.

Fewer studies in adults have addressed questions related to CNS prophylaxis. In adults not receiving CNS prophylaxis, the incidence of CNS leukemia ranges from 20% to 60%, with a trend toward increased CNS involvement as systemic chemotherapy has become more effective. It has been assumed that the benefits of CNS prophylaxis for children with ALL would apply equally to adults. When patients aged 15 years or greater were randomized to receive or not to receive intrathecal methotrexate and 2400 cGy of cranial irradiation, imposed on identical regimens of intensive multiagent systemic therapy, the former group attained significantly longer periods of CNS remission. Gains in length of marrow remission and survival were not apparent. This study, conducted by the Southwest Cancer Study Group, established the value of CNS prophylaxis in decreasing the rate of meningeal relapse in adults, but the full impact of CNS prophylaxis could not be appreciated because of the lack of control of marrow involvement.[213]

More recently, investigators from the MD Anderson Hospital and Tumor Institute reported that despite use of an intensive regimen of systemic chemotherapy, the incidence of CNS relapse was high in patients not receiving CNS prophylaxis (20% at a median follow-up of 6 months).[214] Although this experience is limited, it indicates the need for effective CNS prophylaxis in adults. The efficacy of particular methods, however, may differ somewhat among age groups.

THERAPY DURING REMISSION

Components and Rationale

Even when treated with intensive and effective early therapy, all patients with ALL relapse within a median of 4 to 6 months if treatment is not continued. The need for systemic treatment after induction of complete remission in patients with ALL was established as early as the 1950s, and attempts to refine this phase of therapy are still under way. In contrast to treatment for AML, there is little controversy over the value of continuation therapy for ALL. It is ironic, however, that among the recognized phases of ALL therapy, continuation treatment has received the least attention, even though most failures occur during the post-induction period.

Given the need for prolonged chemotherapy, the selection of suitable agents, dosages, scheduling, and treatment duration becomes pivotal. These choices are difficult because it is not possible to assess accurately the contribution of each compound in multidrug combinations to the observed oncolytic and toxic effects. The possibilities of drug interaction, whether favorable or not, expand rapidly as drugs are added to a therapeutic regimen, increasing the complexity of analysis and interpretation of results.

Antileukemic drugs are not equally effective for prolonging remissions. For example, the combination of vincristine and prednisone, although highly effective against newly diagnosed ALL, cannot be administered as continuation therapy. For most agents, myelosuppression is the dose-limiting factor. When used in combination chemotherapy, however, a nonmyelosuppressive agent may become cytotoxic to the marrow.

The selection of drugs for continuation therapy has been basically empiric. Thirty months of continuous combination chemotherapy with the purine antagonist 6-mercaptopurine, 50 to 90 mg/m^2/d, and the antifolate methotrexate, 20 to 40 mg/m^2/wk, constitutes standard continuation therapy in many centers. Evidence favoring this two-drug regimen over more complex combinations was convincing, and its administration is convenient and relatively uncomplicated. St Jude Study VIII (1972 to 1975),[215] for example, addressed the question of whether the advantages of multiagent chemotherapy outweighed the disadvantages of reducing the dosages of more effective agents. After receiving identical three-drug induction therapy and CNS prophylaxis, 228 patients were randomized to receive one, two, three, or four drugs during continuation treatment. The best outcome—a 10-year complete remission rate of 53% ± 6%—was achieved in patients receiving 6-mercaptopurine and methotrexate. Methotrexate alone was insufficient therapy, and addition of cyclophosphamide and cytarabine as third and fourth agents increased toxicity but did not favorably influence event-free survival.

More recent evaluation of patients treated in the 1970s with 6-mercaptopurine and methotrexate has disclosed disturbing information. In a group of 261 patients followed for a median of 10 years, more than half have relapsed despite 2 to 3 years of continuation therapy with this two-drug combination. Predictably, the best results were obtained in patients with leukocyte counts lower than 25 × 10^9/L at the time of diagnosis: 42% event-free survival versus 16% for all others. In patients with higher leukocyte counts at diagnosis, induction therapy evidently failed to reduce the initial leukemic cell burden to a level that could be eradicated by 6-mercaptopurine and methotrexate. Thus, to boost cure rates, it may be necessary to intensify continuation treatment as intensively as early therapy. Similarly, the inadequacy of a 6-mercaptopurine and methotrexate–based continuation regimen with periodic reinforcement courses of prednisone and vincristine is well illustrated by the experience of CALGB investigators. Despite a high remission-induction rate of 83%, the 4-year event-free survival in their patients was only 25%.[155] The risk of relapse has proved excessive when standard continuation chemotherapy regimens are used. Results of selected treatment programs for ALL in adults are summarized in Table 27-12.[216–218]

Attempts to improve continuation treatment have generally consisted of intensification of therapy using agents and schedules designed to minimize the development of drug resistance. Whether such strategies have contributed to recently reported gains in event-free survival in international studies[219] (Table 27-13) is not clear because of the scarcity of randomized trials evaluating alternative approaches to postinduction intensification of therapy. Nonetheless, regimens in which periodic phases of reinduction or reconsolidation therapy are added to a backbone of methotrexate and 6-mercaptopurine have become more common in leukemia therapy. Agents selected for cyclic intensification of continuation treatment include teniposide,[175] cytarabine,[215] high-dose methotrexate,[128,180] cyclophosphamide,[161] anthracycline compounds,[102] and L-asparaginase.[102] Of all the variables that influence treatment outcome, drug dosage is perhaps the most critical. Steep dose–response curves have been demonstrated for most therapeutic and toxic effects.[220–222] In animal models, moreover, it has been shown that small variations in dosage can significantly alter response to chemotherapy.[223] In clinical trials, dose–response correlations can best be shown in drug-sensitive malignancies, such as lymphomas and

TABLE 27-12. Results of Selected Treatment Programs for Acute Lymphoblastic Leukemia in Adults (1980–1989)

Study	Patients	Median Age (y)	Remission Induction Rate (%)	Clinical Outcome
Omura et al[213]	99	23	80	17% 5-y DFS
Blacklock et al[216]	73	24	89	61% 5-y survival
Gottlieb et al[155]	46	30	83	25% 3-y DFS
Baccarani et al[122]	293	35	79	25% 5-y survival
Carella et al[217]	125	22	87	19-mo median survival
Shauer et al[218]	73	26	85	45% 5-y DFS
Hoelzer et al[2]	368	25	74	35% 5-y DFS
Linker et al*[176]	81	24	94	50% 3-y DFS
Radford et al[118]	59	37	75	35% 5-y DFS

DFS, disease-free survival.
* Excludes patients with Philadelphia chromosome–positive acute lymphoblastic leukemia.

leukemias, testicular cancer, and small cell lung cancer.[222] Recently, findings in randomized trials comparing different treatments for breast cancer have shown that higher doses of chemotherapy are superior.[224]

The first study to show how drug dosage is related to length of complete remission was designed by Pinkel and coworkers in 1965.[225] At the time they achieved complete remission, 42 patients were randomized to receive maximally tolerated (full-dosage) combination chemotherapy or the same drugs at half dosage. The median duration of complete remission was 15 months in the group receiving full dosages compared with only 6 months in the half-dosage group. These data represent the first evidence supporting the value of dose intensity in the treatment of human leukemia.

The observation that blood levels of antileukemic drugs may vary as much as four- to six-fold among patients receiving the same planned dosage has far-reaching implications for the development of future protocols. In two studies conducted at St Jude Children's Research Hospital, it was shown that blood concentrations of methotrexate or teniposide influence the clinical outcome of therapy.[226–228] These results are provocative and suggest that individualization of drug dosages to attain a predetermined systemic dose intensity might strengthen current regimens of continuation treatment. This hypothesis is under investigation.

The scheduling of combination chemotherapy is another factor that can influence the length of remission. British investigators have been particularly interested in testing the impact of scheduling of chemotherapy in patients with leukemia.[229] From well-designed and well-analyzed trials, two important conclusions were reached. First, intermittent administration of continuation chemotherapy—as 5-day "pulsed" treatment every 3 weeks—is less immunosuppressive than continuous chemotherapy. The degree of lymphopenia and the incidence of severe, life-threatening infections were lower in patients treated intermittently; however, these benefits were outweighed by a significantly higher leukemia relapse rate. With a minimal follow-up of 7 years, for example, the results of the UKALL Study V, which included 496 patients, demonstrated that intermittent chemotherapy is less immunosuppressive, but also less effective, than conventional continuous therapy in the treatment of ALL.

Delayed intensification for patients who initially received inadequate early therapy appears to be a futile exercise. In St Jude Study IX, conducted in the mid-1970s, an unsatisfactory interim result led to the decision to begin late intensification of chemotherapy. This attempt failed to improve outcome over that in a matched control group.[230] Thus, it would seem that once drug resistance has developed, late therapeutic manipulations do not significantly

TABLE 27-13. Current Results of International Studies of Childhood Acute Lymphoblastic Leukemia*

Study	Children	Event-Free Survival (%)	Reference
Dana-Farber 81-01 (1981–1985)†	289	70 at 6 y	388
BFM (1983–1986)†	653	64 at 5 y	167, 389
CCG 100 series (1983–1989)‡	3544	66 at 5 y	—
FRALLE 83-87 (1983–1987)	559	57 at 5 y	390
St Jude XI (1984–1988)	358	71 at 5 y	179
POG ALinC 14 + T-cell + Infant Protocol (1986–1991)§	2062	67 at 4 y	—
MRC ALL X (1985–1990)	1614	66 at 4 y	391

CCG, Children's Cancer Study Group; POG, Pediatric Oncology Group, St Jude, St Jude Children's Research Hospital.
* Results shown are latest data available to us; the length of follow-up among these trials varies considerably.
† Few or no black patients.
‡ Unpublished data from A. Bleyer for Childrens Cancer Group (1993).
§ Unpublished data from POG studies 8602, 8691, 8704, 8493, and 8398, P. Steuber.

alter the disease course but may add toxicity. Furthermore, in a subsequent trial, St Jude study X, continuation therapy with 6-mercaptopurine and methotrexate was interrupted at 9 and 13 months by adding two additional drug pairs. The timing of the drug switch was too late and did not prove particularly effective.[231] In St Jude study XI, however, which used four drug pairs given in rotation early in the course of therapy, treatment outcome was significantly better.[179] Finally, the route of administration of antileukemic drugs and protocol compliance should also be considered. Methotrexate, for example, may be more effective when used parenterally rather than orally.[232,233]

Duration of Treatment

Continuation chemotherapy should not be administered indefinitely because all antileukemic drugs produce toxic effects and their long-term sequelae may be life-threatening.[234] Theoretically, antileukemic agents should be administered long enough to destroy the leukemic cell populations, but no longer. Unfortunately, there is no reliable way to detect minimal residual disease, although new methods appear promising.[235,236] Evidence from randomized clinical trials indicates that therapy can be stopped at some point between 2 and 5 years without undue risk of relapse.[237,238] Most therapists use a guideline of 2 to 3 years for all patients. Others treat boys longer than girls (5 versus 3 years).[239] An exception is the treatment of children with B-cell ALL, who require intensive therapy of brief duration (4 to 12 months).[240,241] At St Jude Children's Research Hospital, all therapy is electively stopped in non–B-cell ALL patients who have been in continuous complete remission for 30 months and in extramedullary remission for at least 1 year after an isolated CNS or testicular relapse.

Of 518 patients treated in 10 consecutive total therapy studies for ALL at St Jude Hospital, 83 have been off therapy for 15 to 22 years, 230 for 7 to 15 years, and 201 for 2 to 7 years. None of the presenting features of this group, other than gender (33% males versus 15% females) have been associated with a higher frequency of relapse after cessation of therapy. This difference remains significant when patients with isolated testicular relapses are excluded from comparison. The relapse rate after cessation of therapy is highest during the first year, decreasing to 3% during the second year and 2% during the third year.[237,238] Although late relapses are being reported,[242] patients rarely relapse after they have been off therapy for as long as 5 to 6 years.

Reports of relapse frequencies after cessation of therapy are remarkably similar. Mandelli and coworkers[243] from the Italian Cooperative Group discontinued therapy in 122 of 247 pediatric patients; 27 children (22%) relapsed at 1 to 32 months after cessation of therapy (median time, 10 months). Neither the patients presenting features nor the treatment administered predicted relapse after therapy was stopped. Moe[156] reported on a series of 277 patients, also children, from five Scandinavian countries who had been taken off therapy after 3 years of remission. Of these, 64 (23%) relapsed, mainly in the first year. In a British trial,[229] 292 children in remission at 2 years were randomized to receive no further treatment or an additional year of therapy; an overall benefit was apparent in the group treated for 3 years. Finally, the CCG[244] and the POG[245] conducted randomized studies for cessation of therapy after 3, 5, or 6 years; a recent assessment indicates no difference between 3 and 5 years.[120]

Given the worse treatment outcome in older patients, there are few data on the outcome of stopping antileukemic therapy after prolonged initial remission. Italian and Dutch investigators,[246] however, reported the results of stopping therapy in 45 adolescents and adult patients (more than 11 years of age) who had treatments discontinued after 2 to 5 years of therapy. After 4 to 32 months, seven patients relapsed during unmaintained remission, primarily in the marrow, and during the first year off drugs. The pattern of relapses off therapy was remarkably similar to those reported for children with ALL. These data refer to treatment programs designed and conducted during the 1970s. It is too early to determine if relapse rates after cessation of intensified therapy as given in the 1980s will differ significantly from past experience. Nonetheless, as illustrated in Figure 27-7, the trend toward more intensified chemotherapy has yielded progressively larger proportions of event-free survivors.

THERAPY AFTER RELAPSE

Bone Marrow

The clinical management of patients with ALL in hematologic relapse is an excellent example of how treatment history and prior outcome can dictate the selection of sec-

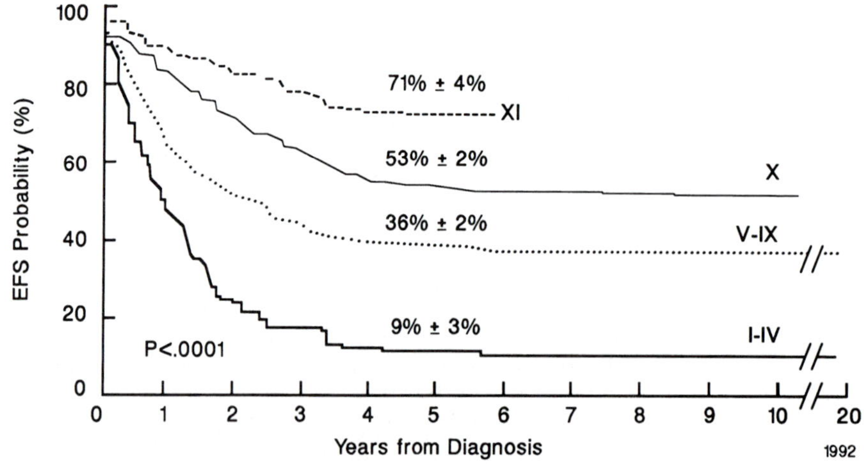

XI	358	315	296	243	159	93	25	-	-	-	-	-
X	428	353	299	262	233	225	217	190	136	85	43	-
V-IX	825	533	414	347	305	294	284	280	273	270	265	47
I-IV	91	42	20	15	10	9	8	8	8	8	8	6

FIGURE 27-7. Cumulative experience in the treatment of childhood acute lymphoblastic leukemia at St Jude Children's Research Hospital. The Kaplan-Meier curves show progressive improvement ($P < .0001$) in event-free survival (EFS) in successive clinical trials spanning 30 years. Numbers in parentheses indicate patients still at risk; bars denote 1 SEM.

ondary therapy. In choosing effective chemotherapy for relapsed ALL, it is important to consider the length of the initial bone marrow remission. Relapses during therapy are much more drug resistant than those occurring 6 months or more after the cessation of treatment.[247,248] New and relatively long remissions were reinduced with intensive chemotherapy in patients who received primary therapy in the 1970s and early 1980s, but the prospects for cure were markedly diminished (Fig. 27-8). In contrast to lymphoblasts present at diagnosis, those seen at relapse appear to represent a selected subpopulation that has become resistant to primary chemotherapy. Comparison of the biologic characteristics of leukemic cells at diagnosis and relapse has revealed an unexpectedly high proportion of patients with secondary AML in two sequential St Jude studies.[249] Treatment regimens associated with weekly or biweekly administration of epipodophyllotoxins were associated with an especially high frequency of this complication.[250] Secondary AML has proved difficult to treat.[249] Similar findings have not been reported in most other large trials for children with ALL, but this report suggests that close examination of the biologic features of ALL in relapse is indicated, especially in children receiving therapy as described previously.

For patients initially treated in the 1970s and early 1980s, the results of conventional secondary chemotherapy were unsatisfactory. The first objective of secondary treatment is to induce a new remission. The POG completed a study in which a four-drug reinduction regimen consisting of prednisone and vincristine, combined with daunorubicin, 25 mg/m²/wk for 4 weeks, and L-asparaginase, 10,000 IU/m² intramuscular three times a week for 4 weeks, induced second remissions in 245 (82%) of 297 patients.[251] Remission reinduction rates in adults with relapsed ALL rarely exceeded 50%.

The end results of secondary chemotherapy were uniformly poor. Kimball and coworkers[252] reported a median length of second remission of 35 weeks in children treated with monthly cycles of methotrexate, 150 mg/m², followed by a combination of prednisone, vincristine, 6-mercaptopurine, and daunorubicin. Based on the work of Capizzi and colleagues,[182] investigators from the CCG have recommended the use of methotrexate, vincristine, and L-asparaginase for continuation therapy during sec-

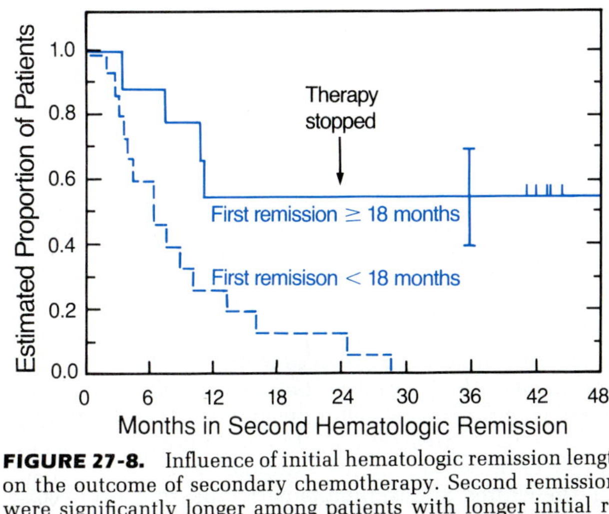

FIGURE 27-8. Influence of initial hematologic remission length on the outcome of secondary chemotherapy. Second remissions were significantly longer among patients with longer initial remissions ($P = .004$ by Cox life-table regression analysis). Tick marks represent patients still at risk; the bar at 36 months denotes the 95% confidence limit. (After Rivera GK, Buchanan G, Boyett JM, et al. Intensive retreatment of childhood acute lymphoblastic leukemia in first bone marrow relapse. N Engl J Med 1986;315:273)

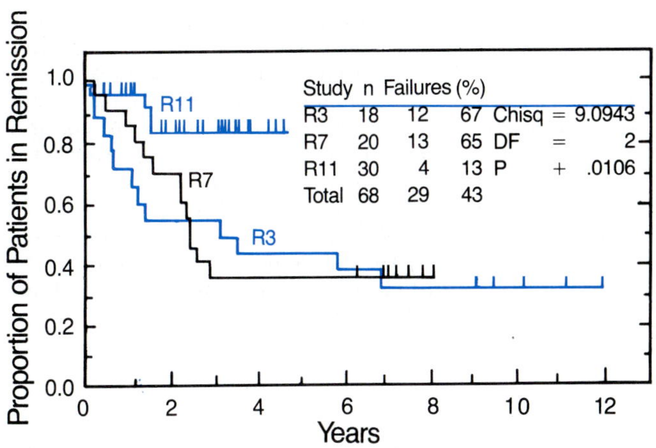

FIGURE 27-9. Kaplan-Meier analysis of disease-free survival (DF) among 30 children with late-relapsing acute lymphoblastic leukemia treated with intensive chemotherapy. The initial relapses in this group of patients occurred in the bone marrow from 34 to 102 months (median, 44 months) after the date of remission induction. None of the patients had an adverse event other than leukemic relapse. Tick marks represent disease-free survivors. Chisq, chi-square. (After Rivera GK. Cyclophosphamide and bone marrow transplantation. [Letter] N Engl J Med 1988;318:1541).

ond remissions[253]; however, Amadori and coworkers[254] using a similar regimen in adults—methotrexate and L-asparaginase without vincristine—obtained a median remission length of only 10 weeks. High-dose methotrexate, 2 to 8 g/m², for refractory adult ALL, has had only marginal effectiveness.[255]

Use of investigational agents may contribute significantly to improved results in patients with relapsed ALL. The combination of VM-26 and cytarabine is a case in point. This therapy induces complete remissions in some patients with initially refractory leukemia, and it appears to prolong second remissions when added to more conventional continuation regimens.[173,174,256] The value of this drug pair lies in the unique mechanism of action of VM-26 and its ability to potentiate the cytotoxicity of cytarabine. Clinical application of VM-26 plus cytarabine has been extended to adults with ALL, with some reports indicating improved results. Other agents (eg, VP-16,[257] high-dose cytarabine,[258] and the acridine derivative amsacrine[259]) have also been incorporated into protocols for relapsed ALL, but end results were not significantly better than those obtainable with more conventional therapy or with VM-26 plus cytarabine. Most investigators agree that patients who experience an early marrow relapse after intensive, contemporary treatment have a poor prognosis, justifying an allogenic bone marrow transplant.

Patients who develop late bone marrow relapses (more than 36 months from diagnosis) represent a distinct subgroup with an improved prognosis. Among 30 children in this category who were retreated with intensified chemotherapy, the probability of remaining in second remission for 4 years was 76% ± 18% SE (Fig. 27-9), a result that compares favorably with the eventual outcome in newly diagnosed patients. A recent report from the POG, which included 102 children treated with moderately intensive chemotherapy, produced a 4-year event-free survival of 37% ± 6%.[260] The option of bone marrow transplantation for children with relapsed ALL may appear attractive, but evidence that it is superior to chemotherapy only is conflicting.[261] From a review of the International Bone Marrow Transplant Registry for pediatric patients, it was concluded that transplantation was superior in patients with short initial remissions but not for those who experienced relapse at 18 months or more after initial remission induction. Henze and colleagues[262] demonstrated that patients with late relapse fare as well when treated with intensive chemotherapy or allogeneic bone marrow transplantation. Therefore, the choice of therapy for relapsed ALL must be made on an individual basis until we are able to identify at diagnosis those patients who are apt to benefit most from transplantation or chemotherapy.[263] We favor intensive chemotherapy over transplantation for cases of late bone marrow relapses[264] (more than 36 months of initial remission) because of the persistently high rates of peritransplantation morbidity and mortality. Whether either modality is adequate for patients relapsing on current programs of intensive chemotherapy remains to be determined. The results of transplantation for children in second or third remission are not significantly different.[265] Thus, some investigators use chemotherapy to treat patients in second remission, reserving transplantation for those in third remission, provided the reinduction therapy is effective.

Central Nervous System

The clinical outcome of therapy for patients who develop an isolated CNS relapse as a first event during initial hematologic remission depends mainly on the first method of CNS prophylaxis employed. In the past, some patients who experienced relapse after suboptimal prophylaxis were salvaged with intensified secondary treatments. Secondary treatment of children who experienced CNS relapse after initially receiving only six doses of intrathecal methotrexate therapy was thought to be satisfactory, even curative in some cases[266]; however, longer follow-up observation has shown that CNS relapse adversely influences cure rates.[212]

In view of the good penetration of systemic high-dose cytarabine into the CNS, Morra and coworkers[258] administered this agent to 15 adult patients with overt meningeal leukemia, using 3 g/m^2 intravenous every 12 hours (3-hour infusion for eight doses followed in 3 weeks by a second course of four doses). Thirteen patients attained second CNS remission, but 11 experienced relapse again in a median time of 5 months (range, 2 to 8 months).

Most available information indicates that to cure a patient with a CNS relapse, it is necessary to use CNS irradiation. Both craniospinal irradiation and cranial irradiation, combined with intrathecal methotrexate, have been used for this purpose, yielding cure rates of about 30%.[267] Investigators in the POG and in the United Kingdom have reported on these therapies.[268,269] Improved outcomes have been noted, even in patients with isolated meningeal relapses who require a second course of CNS irradiation; however, end results for this group are still unavailable. A recent POG study of 120 patients yielded a 3-year event-free survival of 48% ± 6%.[270] At St Jude Children's Research Hospital, the recommended therapy for CNS relapse includes an intensified regimen of chemotherapy for systemic reinduction, administered with four to six doses of weekly triple chemotherapy (methotrexate, hydrocortisone, and cytarabine). Patients who attain a second CNS remission are treated with craniospinal irradiation at doses of 2400 and 1500 cGy, respectively. Continuation therapy based on rotation of combination treatments has been both effective and safe.[271] Information on the treatment of CNS relapses in adult patients is unavailable.

Testes

Boys rarely had overt testicular leukemia at the time of diagnosis, but as systemic control of bone marrow relapse became more effective, testicular infiltration began to emerge as an important cause of extramedullary disease. The diagnosis should be confirmed by bilateral wedge biopsy because of the strong probability of occult disease in the uninvolved testis. Detailed reviews,[196,272] summarizing two large series of patients, have been published on this subject, including the factors that predispose patients to relapse in this organ. Prompt induction of a new systemic remission is recommended because testicular relapse tends to be followed by bone marrow relapse within 3 to 4 months. In asymptomatic patients treated with intensive chemotherapy, elective testicular biopsies at the completion of therapy have not been clinically useful.[273] A recently reported POG study from Wofford and coworkers[274] showed a 3-year event-free survival of 63% ± 7% among boys with occult testicular leukemia.

With current regimens of intensified chemotherapy, one rarely encounters testicular relapse as a first event ending hematologic remission.[184] Patients who develop testicular leukemia while receiving chemotherapy have a worse prognosis than those with an isolated testicular relapse during unmaintained remission.[275] Among this latter group of patients, the POG study by Wofford and coworkers[274] produced a 3-year event-free survival of 88% ± 9%. Optimal therapy for testicular relapse includes both local radiation therapy and systemic chemotherapy. Radiation doses of 2400 cGy to both testes have been considered adequate.[272] Hormonal dysfunction usually follows gonadal irradiation.[276]

Unusual Sites of Extramedullary Relapse

Infiltration of different organs and tissues by leukemic blasts is well documented clinically.[277,278] Involvement of the kidneys, ovaries, eyes, and bones may become apparent as the initial relapse or as a late event after multiple recurrences.[279-282] One might predict a higher incidence of unusual extramedullary relapses as the proportion of long-term event-free survivors grows larger. Isolated ocular relapses are usually followed by an overt CNS relapse. As with other extramedullary relapses, a course of systemic reinduction therapy and local irradiation therapy, about 1000 cGy, are recommended.

SPECIAL PROTOCOLS

B-cell ALL presents a difficult challenge to leukemia therapists, justifying the development of separate clinical trials. The recommended approach to therapy is a relatively brief (4- to 12-month) course of high-dose chemotherapy with rest periods of 2 to 3 weeks to prevent life-threatening myelosuppression.[240] The most active known agents against B-cell ALL are cyclophosphamide, methotrexate, and cytarabine; combinations of intravenous and intrathecal chemotherapy appear to provide the most effective CNS prophylaxis.[44,240] French investigators developed an intensive multidrug regimen, termed *LMB 89*, that yielded an event-free survival of about 80% among 31 children with B-cell ALL[283]; the event-free survival was 57% for adults treated with a similar approach based on their earlier pediatric studies (LMB 81 and 84).[284] Comparable results were reported by Reiter and coworkers for 39 children[285]; however, none of these children had initial CNS leukemia, a known poor prognostic factor. In addition, these acutely ill patients must be treated in modern centers by investigators capable of providing intensive supportive care.

In the United States, infants with leukemia are usually treated in separate, specially designed clinical trials.[95,100] Intensive chemotherapy modeled on the New York regimen has proved superior to more conventional regimens, although end results remain unsatisfactory. A major problem in treating infants is to control CNS leukemia without inducing serious neurotoxicity.[100]

It is possible that in the future, patients with Ph chromosome–positive ALL or hybrid leukemia may also require special protocols. Some investigators treat hybrid cases with combinations of drugs that are active against both lymphoid and myeloid leukemias; however, little information on the optimal therapy for this unusual disease is available.

BONE MARROW TRANSPLANTATION

Allogeneic

Although used increasingly as alternative therapy for patients who are not likely to have durable responses to chemotherapy, allogeneic bone marrow transplantation is still regarded as investigational treatment for patients with ALL in first remission.[286] This approach, which entails administration of intensive (ablative) chemotherapy followed by hematopoietic rescue with intravenously infused bone marrow from an appropriately matched donor, imposes the risk of excessive morbidity and mortality.[287–290] Recent progress in the biology of marrow transplantation has begun to reduce the risk of lethal toxicity, raising the possibility of transplantation for larger numbers of patients with either completely or incompletely HLA-matched donors (see Chap. 2).

Herzig and coworkers[291] summarized the results of allogeneic bone marrow transplantation in patients with ALL who had been treated at 101 transplantation centers worldwide. The justification for this procedure was the attending physician's impression of high-risk leukemia, based on one or more of the following criteria: age less than 2 or more than 16 years; leukocyte count higher than 50 $\times 10^9$/L; CNS involvement; B-cell immunophenotype or FAB L3 morphologic subtype; and the presence of the t(4;11), t(9;22), or t(8;14) chromosomal translocation. Of the 444 patients judged to be at high risk for early failure on chemotherapy, 236 were in first marrow remission, and 208 were in second remission. The 4-year probability of event-free survival was significantly higher in the group in first remission (45% ± 9% SE versus 22% ± 7% SE), demonstrating the greater efficacy of transplantation in patients who have not relapsed.

Zander and coworkers[292] from the MD Anderson Hospital and Tumor Institute developed a predictive model to aid in the selection of adults with either myeloid or lymphoid leukemia, for allogeneic marrow transplantation in first remission. The conditioning regimen included piperazinedione and fractionated total-body irradiation. Encouraged by the early results of a controlled pilot study, they expanded patient eligibility from very-poor-risk patients to include intermediate- and good-prognosis groups. In all subgroups, the leukemia relapse rate was low, but advantages in terms of overall survival were less clear. A particularly interesting group was the cohort of good-prognosis patients in first remission, whose survival was not improved by transplantation. This relatively poor result was attributed to an increase in morbidity and mortality, apparently secondary to the effects of in vitro depletion of T cells.[293–295]

Interpretation of this trial is complicated by the inclusion of multiple regimens of chemotherapy in the control group, contrasted with uniform management of allografted patients, and the lack of separate analyses for patients with AML and ALL. A more valid comparative analysis would have been possible had optimal chemotherapy and transplantation procedures been available. Predictive models that identify patients at high risk for transplant-induced morbidity and mortality would be desirable, so that transplantation could be reserved for treatment after relapse.

No best choice of therapy has been determined for ALL in adults in first remission, with chemotherapy and transplantation producing about equivalent end results[296,297] (Table 27-14). Gale and Butturini[298] reviewed the international experience in allogeneic marrow transplantation and chemotherapy. For adults with ALL in first remission, the 3- to 5-year disease-free survival rate in the chemotherapy-only group was 35%, even with intensive therapy, and 45% in studies with HLA-identical donors. Although chemotherapy was associated with a higher incidence of leukemic relapse, transplantation produced more severe (sometimes fatal) toxicity, primarily interstitial pneumonias and graft-versus-host disease. As a result, survival rates in the two groups were about equal. In this series, most marrow transplantations were performed after standard preparatory treatment with cyclophosphamide and total-body irradiation. Similar transplantation for adults in second remission yielded a 3-year disease-free survival of about 20%. The authors recommended transplantation only for children in second remission who relapse early during initial administration of chemotherapy. Children relapsing off therapy should receive intensified chemotherapy, with transplantation reserved for those who relapse and achieve a third remission.

In a recently published study by French investigators,[299] 27 patients between the ages of 15 and 40 years received marrow transplants from HLA-A, B, and D genotypically identical siblings during first complete remission of ALL. Although pretransplantation therapy differed markedly, all patients were treated with the same cytoreductive regimen: cyclophosphamide followed by total-body irradiation. Methotrexate was added to avoid severe graft-versus-host disease. With a median follow-up of 56 months, the 3-year disease-free survival rate among the 27 subjects was 59% ± 18% SE. This study was not controlled, and eight patients received their transplants after being in remission for more than 6 months (range, 2 to 19 months). Patients relapsing soon after complete remission were not given transplants.

TABLE 27-14. Results of Alternative Approaches to the Management of Adults With Acute Lymphoblastic Leukemia in First Remission

Source	Patients	Median Follow-Up (mo)	Median Age (y)	Relapsed Patients	Probability of 3-Year Disease-Free Survival (%)
Allogeneic bone marrow transplantation					
Seattle	34	47	22	8 (24%)	38
Westminster Hospital (London)	23	43	26	7 (30%)	44
City of Hope	39	28	23	4 (10%)	63
Intensive chemotherapy					
German studies	272	>60	25	156 (57%)	42
Memorial Hospital	163	>60	~27	92 (57%)	40

(Courtesy of R. Mayer, MD, Dana Farber Cancer Center, Boston)

A new controlled study designed to transplant patients earlier in remission is underway. A regimen of fractionated total-body irradiation and high-dose VP-16, 60 to 70 mg/kg, followed by allogeneic transplantation, has been reported to be highly effective.[300]

Results of allogeneic marrow transplantation with a conditioning regimen of ablative combination chemotherapy (cytarabine and cyclophosphamide) have also been reported by Blume and coworkers.[301] Among 13 adults with high-risk ALL in first remission (median age, 24 years) in whom transplantation was attempted at a median of 2 months after the date of remission induction, the actuarial survival at a median follow-up time of about 2 years was 57% ± 13% SE, in contrast to only 34% ± 12% SE for a comparison group of 20 additional patients who received similar treatment but underwent marrow transplantation when in second or subsequent remission. In a contemporary British clinical trial,[302] 20 high-risk patients, including children, adolescents, and young adults, were treated with a five-drug preparatory regimen, intrathecal methotrexate, and total-body irradiation. The efficacy of marrow transplantation for patients in first remission was superior to that for those in second or third remission.

Better results of allogeneic bone marrow transplantation for children with ALL in second marrow remission have been obtained in patients who received conditioning regimens modified somewhat from those originally described by Thomas and coworkers in Seattle.[287] Employing hyperfractionated total-body irradiation, booster doses of radiation to the testes, high doses of cyclophosphamide, and non–T-cell–depleted marrows, the group from MSKCC obtained a 5-year disease-free survival rate of 64% ± 9% SE for a group of 31 children in second remission.[265] Coccia and coworkers[303] devised a regimen based on 12 doses of cytarabine therapy as high as 3000 mg/m²/dose, followed by 1200 cGy total body irradiation and allogeneic marrow transplantation. In 18 children in second remission, they achieved a 5-year disease-free survival rate of 58%, with surprisingly good treatment tolerance. Twelve of these 18 patients had not received previous therapy with cytarabine.

Aware of the trend toward smaller families in the United Kingdom, British investigators evaluated the scope of allogeneic marrow transplantation, using an unselected group of 56 children with ALL in first marrow relapse, who presented to a single cancer center from 1980 to 1984.[304] After failing on conventional chemotherapy during first remission, the patients received similar reinduction and consolidation treatments. Comparison of outcome in children with and without an HLA-compatible sibling donor disclosed a high overall rate of second remission induction (95%). After 1 to 5 years of follow-up, 5 of 13 patients eligible for transplantation, as compared with 16 of 40 who received only chemotherapy, were long-term survivors. From these results, the authors concluded that marrow transplantation has a limited role in prolonging second remissions. The pool of potential bone marrow recipients, however, may expand in the future if investigations with allografts using partially matched family members or matched unrelated donors prove as effective as those with histocompatible donors.[305]

The available data indicate that allogeneic bone marrow transplantation is a reasonable option for adults who have an HLA-identical donor. Whether this generalization holds for adolescents and young adults is still unclear and cannot be resolved until better methods of prospectively identifying high-risk groups become available. Most children with ALL in first remission can be expected to respond well to chemotherapy and do not require transplantation.[306] Perhaps in an experimental setting, judiciously selected subjects, such as children with hyperleukocytosis (more than 200 × 10⁹/L) or Ph chromosome–positive blast cells, might benefit from allogeneic transplantation.[190,306a] Several reports have documented the dire prognosis for children with Ph chromosome–positive ALL, even in treatment programs relying on intensive chemotherapy.[102,190] In a small group of 10 patients with Ph chromosome–positive ALL, Forman and coworkers[307] recently reported the treatment outcome of allogeneic marrow transplantation. Four patients died with transplant-related complications,and six remained alive and well for 6 to 30 months (median, 19 months). This encouraging observation is being closely followed. As discussed earlier, marrow transplantation may also be advantageous in children in second marrow remission whose initial remission did not exceed 18 months.

Autologous

The role of autologous transplantation in ALL in first remission is difficult to evaluated because of the scarcity of available information.[308] Few adult patients with ALL in first or second remission have received autografts.[309] In this procedure, pretransplantation preparatory high-dose chemotherapy is followed by infusion of cryopreserved remission marrow, usually treated with either antileukemic drugs or leukemia-associated monoclonal antibodies to remove potentially contaminating leukemic cells. Recombinant hematopoietic growth factors have been shown to be clinically useful for marrow rescue and therefore may decrease the morbidity associated with autologous marrow transplantation in ALL. Moreover, peripheral blood stem cells are being investigated as an alternative of hematopoietic rescue, especially in patients not able to receive an autologous bone marrow transplant.[310]

Overall, the results obtained with autologous marrow transplantation in patients with ALL in second remission are less promising. Within the past 5 years, however, Kersey and other investigators[311] at the University of Minnesota have made progress, reporting a decrease in both time to engraftment and early death rates. Important differences among patients receiving autografts versus allogeneic bone marrow transplants were recently reported by investigators at Fred Hutchison Cancer Research Center.[290] Two studies provided evidence that with reinstitution of standard chemotherapy, one third to one half of patients with ALL who relapse after bone marrow transplantation may attain a new remission.[312,313]

COMPLICATIONS

The most frequent complications in patients with newly diagnosed ALL are infection and bleeding, which stem from the almost total replacement of normal marrow elements by leukemic blasts. This overgrowth compromises normal hematopoiesis, leading to thrombocytopenia, neutropenia, and anemia. Most bleeding disorders are related to thrombocytopenia, with increased capillary fragility and systemic infection contributing in some cases. Disseminated intravascular coagulation occurs in a small proportion of patients with ALL, mainly those with T-cell disease.[91] To identify this complication with certainty, one should evaluate prothrombin and partial thromboplastin times, fibrinogen, and fibrin split product levels and platelet counts in patients with T-cell ALL. If hypoprothrombinemia and bleeding develop after prolonged antibiotic therapy, malabsorption, or hepatic damage from chemotherapy, treatment with vitamin K is usually adequate. Anemia is rarely life-threatening in patients with ALL because its onset tends to be gradual, and compensatory mechanisms can be activated to diminish the adverse effects of a decreased red-cell mass. Pseudohypoglycemia, resulting from glucose use by leukemic cells in vitro, may be observed in patients with extreme leukocytosis.[314]

Viral and bacterial infections are the most serious complications in patients with ALL. Increased susceptibility to infection in leukemia patients probably involves several different factors: malnutrition, loss of neutrophil reserves in bone marrow due to leukemic infiltration and myelosuppressive treatment, and immunosuppression due to the effects of therapy. Any episode of fever and neutropenia (fewer than 500 neutrophils/μL) should be regarded as a sign of infection, regardless of other clinical findings. Bacterial infections most often involve staphylococci or enteric gram-negative organisms and should be treated empirically with effective broad-spectrum antibiotic therapy as soon as they are suspected. The specific source of infection should be diligently sought by chest roentgenography and cultures of blood, throat, urine, and other sites. Meningitis is rare and can be easily ruled out by examining spinal fluid for pathogens after routine lumbar punctures to detect leukemia cells. The causes and appropriate treatment of specific infections are reviewed elsewhere in this textbook.

Central Nervous System

In the 1940s, Evans and colleagues[188] reported a 10% incidence of meningeal infiltration in children with leukemia. Leukemic involvement of the CNS was demonstrated in that same decade in 83% of children who were examined at the time of autopsy; only 35% had been symptomatic.[315] The overall incidence of meningeal leukemia in children with ALL was 56% in a study conducted by the Children's Cancer Study Group in 1970.[188] Recognition of the CNS as a "sanctuary" for leukemic cells led to specific therapy for this complication (see previous section on therapy for subclinical CNS leukemia).

Although the definition of CNS leukemia has been controversial[149,191,219] (Table 27-15), most investigators use the criterion of unequivocal blast cells observed in a stained cytospin preparation of spinal fluid and greater than five mononuclear cells per microliter in a spinal fluid cell count. If CNS infection is suspected, specimens should be cultured and appropriately stained for bacteria, fungi, and acid-fast organisms and assessed for protein and glucose levels. Some cases of tumor meningitis mimic bacterial meningitis in that the glucose level in CSF is low and the protein level frequently elevated.[316]

The most common symptoms of meningeal leukemia—early-morning headache, nausea, vomiting, irritability, lethargy, nuchal rigidity, strabismus, and facial nerve palsy—result from increased intracranial pressure. The onset of symptoms and signs may be indolent.[316] As intracranial pressure increases in infants, sutures may separate, and the head circumference may increase in size; this complication can lead to papilledema or cranial nerve palsy in a child of any age. An abnormal appetite and unusual weight gain may be the primary features of meningeal leukemia in obese patients with leukemic infiltration of the hypothalamus.[317] Diabetes insipidus has also been reported.[318]

Few patients develop CNS hemorrhage.[319] Those with low platelet counts (less than 20×10^9/L) or high leukocyte counts (100×10^9/L or higher) are most susceptible, and the risk is further increased by disseminated intravascular coagulation. Recognizing the rarity of CNS hemorrhage, regardless of platelet count, many investigators reserve the use of platelet concentrates for active bleeding or coagulopathy. It is advisable to avoid intramuscular injections and drugs with antiplatelet effects, such as aspirin, especially in patients with low platelet counts. Therapeutic pheresis followed by cytoreductive chemotherapy has been useful in reducing high leukocyte levels (more than 200×10^9/L).[319]

Genitourinary Tract

With longer durations of CNS and bone marrow remissions, testicular infiltration by leukemic cells has become more common,[320] occurring in 5% to 30% of pediatric patients.[245] Although not clinically obvious in all cases, this complication typically presents as a firm, painless, unilateral or bilateral testicular swelling. The extent of infiltration tends to be bilateral. Among 24 boys with ALL who lacked any symptoms of testicular involvement, four had evidence of this complication in pretreatment biopsy specimens.[320] About 7% of boys completing therapy in another study had positive biopsies without clinical evidence of disease; some investigators reported a much lower prevalence in their posttreatment samples.[321,322] Less information on leukemic infiltration of the testes is available for adults; however, this complication can occur in older age groups, and the approaches to prevention and treatment should probably follow those recommended for children (see previous sec-

TABLE 27-15. Definition and Incidence of Central Nervous System Leukemia at Diagnosis in Children

Study Group and Clinical Trials	Patients	Criteria	Incidence (%)	Reference
CCG				
101	724	>10 mononuclear cells and any number of blasts	1.5	191
161–163	2210	>5 mononuclear cells and any number of blasts	3.8	219
POG				
ALinC 11	408	Any number of blasts	1	204
7615*	53	Not defined	15	149
St Jude				
I–VI	250	>10 mononuclear cells and any number of blasts	3	131
VII–IX	671	Any number of blasts	2.3	230

CCG, Children's Cancer Study Group; POG, Pediatric Oncology Group; St Jude, St Jude Children's Research Hospital.
* T-cell only.

tion on therapy after relapse). Priapism is rare in patients with ALL, occurring mainly in patients with a leukocyte level higher than 100 × 10^9/L, and its pathogenesis is unclear.[323]

The prevalence of leukemic involvement of the ovary in one autopsy study was 35%, as compared with testicular involvement in 57% of male cases.[324] The actual incidence of ovarian involvement has been estimated to be 17%,[282] but this figure may not apply to patients receiving modern therapy. More reliable information would be useful because leukemic cells sequestered in this site could become drug resistant and eventually reseed the bone marrow, leading to systemic relapse. Noninvasive methods of detection are too insensitive for accurate assessment, and invasive study of the ovaries in girls is not likely to be attempted because of the generally excellent end results of therapy for childhood ALL. Too little is known about this complication in adult women to establish clinical significance.

Many patients with ALL show marked enlargement of the kidneys during the course of their disease.[282] Usually, no associated symptoms occur, although acute renal failure may occur in some cases. This complication is thought to arise from high levels of uric acid or other metabolic products of purine metabolism that obstruct the renal tubules, leading to renal vasospasm. Patients with a high leukemic cell burden (eg, high leukocyte level and organomegaly) are most likely to be affected.

Heart

Pericardial tamponade and myocardial infiltration have been observed in patients with newly diagnosed ALL but rarely in those who have attained complete remission.[325] The latter complication is seen at autopsy in one half to two thirds of patients, although symptomatic heart disease occurs in less than 5%.[326] Pathologic cardiac involvement is thought to result from obstruction of normal lymphatic flow between the endocardium and epicardium. Cardiomyopathy in patients with ALL most often follows treatment with an anthracycline compound but occasionally reflects an underlying infection.[326]

Lungs

Leukemic involvement of the lungs rarely produces clinical symptoms in patients with ALL. When present, even during remission, such symptoms may be confused with interstitial pneumonia due to infection or may be secondary effects of chemotherapy with methotrexate or other antineoplastic drugs.[327–329] Some patients may have pulmonary hemorrhage during periods of thrombocytopenia, and this complication is found in about half of patients at autopsy.[327] Because the lungs are a frequent site of infection, it may be impossible to distinguish among leukemic infiltration, hemorrhage, and infection in this organ.

Thymus

Leukemic infiltration of the thymus appears to be a relatively common consequence of ALL. Gilmartin[330] reported abnormally large thymic shadows in 15% of children with newly diagnosed ALL (see Fig. 27-3). In 5 of 12 patients, the shadows were present before abnormal blood counts were observed, suggesting the thymus as a primary site of involvement. All these patients were found to have T-cell ALL; in fact, there is an almost perfect correlation between a thymic mass and the T-cell phenotype (see Table 27-1).

Eye

Retinal hemorrhage secondary to thrombocytopenia, vessel infiltration, coagulopathy, and papilledema due to CNS leukemia are the most common ocular findings in patients with ALL. Marked scleral erythema with leukemic cell infiltration is rarely seen. An occasional patient may have clouding of the anterior chamber (hypopyon; Fig. 27-10) or retinal infiltration, both of which can lead to CNS relapse even when the spinal fluid is free of lymphoblasts.[331] If ocular involvement is suspected, the diagnosis can be made by examining aspirates from the anterior chamber. Leukemic iritis may be associated with glaucoma.[332]

Bones and Joints

Bone or joint pain is a major complaint of many children and adults presenting with ALL; other patients have characteristic radiologic changes with or without complaints or pain.[333,334] These changes are easily seen in the long bones, especially near the knees, ankles, or wrists. Bone necrosis may produce bone pain, often during a period of leukopenia.[335] Unlike leukemic infiltration, it does not respond to irradiation. Pathologic bone fractures have been observed in some patients, especially those receiving long-term methotrexate or corticosteroid therapy.[234] Point ten-

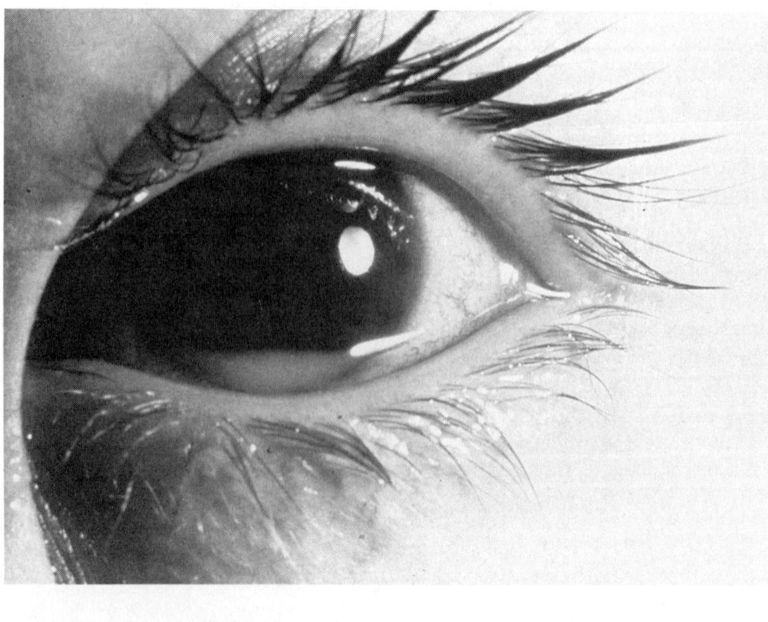

FIGURE 27-10. Hypopyon in the left eye of a child with acute lymphoblastic leukemia. Milky material can be seen at the base of the iris within the anterior chamber.

derness, possibly due to periosteal elevation caused by infiltrates of leukemic cells or by hemorrhage, is common. Pain or swelling of a joint due to leukemic infiltration can be confused with other diseases related to arthritis, such as rheumatic fever or rheumatoid arthritis. The pain is sometimes migratory and is probably caused by periosteal elevation accompanying leukemic cell infiltration, bone infarction, or expansion of the marrow space with leukemic cells.[336]

Gastrointestinal Tract

Children with ALL commonly have abdominal pain; gastrointestinal bleeding can occur in either children or adults and typically reflects thrombocytopenia, coagulopathy, or toxic effects of chemotherapy on the gastrointestinal mucosa. *Typhlitis*, or *necrotizing enterocolitis*, refers to a specific syndrome of right lower quadrant pain with rebound tenderness, abdominal distention, vomiting, and sepsis.[337–339] Abdominal radiographs sometimes show decreased amounts of air in the right lower quadrant, a condition probably related to mucosal and bowel wall damage secondary to chemotherapy. It is seen most often during periods of prolonged neutropenia. Bowel rest, intravenous fluids, and broad-spectrum antibiotic therapy are recommended for this complication; surgery is reserved for patients with evidence of bowel perforation, uncontrolled bleeding, or abdominal wall cellulitis. Other common complications of the gastrointestinal tract that may require surgery are appendicitis and intussusception; however, unusual side effects of leukemia treatment, such as pancreatitis or acute cholangitis, must be considered and ruled out.

Other gastrointestinal lesions encountered in patients with ALL include mucositis or esophagitis secondary to infection or chemotherapy, often occurring during periods of severe neutropenia.[340,341] Oral moniliasis, a complication of prolonged corticosteroid or antibiotic administration, is also seen. Some patients with leukemia develop lactose malabsorption with cramps and diarrhea.[342] Mikulicz's syndrome, or bilateral enlargement of the salivary and lacrimal glands generally due to leukemic infiltration,[343] has been reported, but only rarely.

Other Sites

Hepatic fibrosis may be associated with 6-mercaptopurine or methotrexate therapy or may be observed at autopsy, but usually it is of no clinical significance.[344,345] Skin infiltration is uncommon in ALL, occurring mainly in infants and children with T-cell or pre–B-cell ALL[346] (Fig. 27-11). Pleural effusions may be associated with an anterior mediastinal mass. Involvement of the inner ear causes vertigo or hearing loss in rare cases.[347] Leukemic infiltration of the breasts has also been reported.[348]

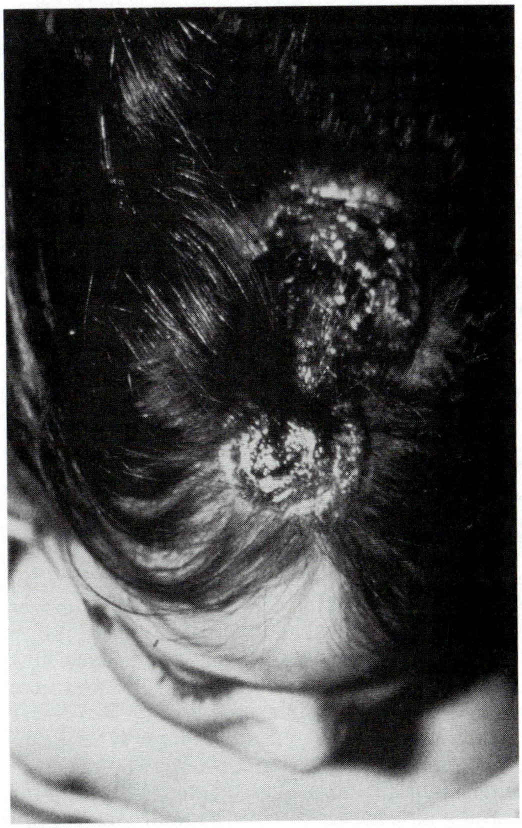

FIGURE 27-11. Infiltrative cutaneous mass in the scalp in a patient with pre–B-cell acute lymphoblastic leukemia.

SUPPORTIVE CARE

During remission induction, hyperkalemia, hyperphosphatemia, and hyperuricemia develop in some intensively treated patients due to rapid destruction of leukemic blast cells. Often termed *acute tumor cell lysis syndrome*, this complication may be treated by vigorous hydration (about 3 L/m^2), maintenance of an alkaline urine, and administration of allopurinol, a purine isomer that inhibits xanthine oxidase and prevents the conversion of hypoxanthine and xanthine to uric acid. Some patients may require renal dialysis in addition to medical treatment. Hyperleukocytosis (leukocyte level 100 $\times$ 10^9/L or higher) may lead to early morbidity and mortality as a result of metabolic complications due to rapid blast cell lysis or leukostasis in the cerebral and pulmonary vasculature. Cytoreductive procedures have been employed to prevent the serious consequences of hyperleukocytosis.[349] In a study of 35 pediatric patients with acute leukemia and leukocyte counts 100 $\times$ 10^9/L or higher at diagnosis, it was concluded that cytoreduction could be performed safely and efficiently.[319] Another recent study demonstrated that patients presenting with severe hyperuricemia and renal dysfunction may benefit from leukapheresis. Small initial doses of prednisone or emergency cranial irradiation do not appear to be effective.[350] An occasional patient develops hypercalcemia, presumably due to circulating tumor products that increase bone resorption and renal tubular calcium reabsorption and lead to increased levels of calcium in extracellular fluids. Treatment consists of rapid infusion of normal saline, hydrocortisone, and sometimes calcitonin.

Intravenous antibiotic therapy should be administered immediately to patients with suspected or proven infections.[351] The addition of vancomycin to ticarcillin and amikacin has proved advantageous in reducing the incidence of breakthrough bacteremia in febrile neutropenic patients.[352] Intermittent chemoprophylaxis with trimethoprim-sulfamethoxazole successfully prevents *P carinii* pneumonia; a treatment schedule of 3 days a week is particularly effective.[353]

Platelet and erythrocyte infusions are required for adequate hematologic support in patients with ALL. For long-term vascular access, the use of indwelling lines (ie, Hickman and Broviac right atrial catheters or subcutaneously placed Port-A-Caths) has become more common in patients with leukemia. Although by comparison with historical controls, the overall incidence of bacteremia in neutropenic patients has not changed significantly with the introduction of Hickman catheters, it is essential that patients be monitored closely for infection and be taught to care for their catheters. No obvious correlation has been found between the incidence of catheter-related infections and the length of time the device is in place. The daily risk of catheter-induced infection remains relatively constant regardless of the duration of catheter placement. Thrombotic occlusion of indwelling lines has been associated with increased susceptibility to bacterial colonization. Catheters may be replaced shortly after their removal if a second catheter is considered necessary.[354]

With increased experience in the administration of intensive chemotherapy, many of the previously unexpected side effects can be avoided. Nevertheless, the well-documented toxicity that has been associated with aggressive treatment of ALL serves as a reminder that such therapy is highly toxic and that the therapeutic index is often narrow.

LATE SEQUELAE OF ACUTE LYMPHOBLASTIC LEUKEMIA AND ITS TREATMENT

Disabilities with significant effects on quality of life can be anticipated in a variable proportion of ALL survivors. Antimetabolites such as methotrexate, cytarabine, and 6-mercaptopurine have been reported to induce functional and fibrotic changes in the liver.[234,355] By and large, this hepatotoxicity is reversible, especially after cessation of treatment. It is advisable to assess liver function periodically during prolonged chemotherapy.

Urinary bladder fibrosis associated with long-term cyclophosphamide therapy has been reported.[356] The resulting complications may also include chronic cystitis and ureteric reflux. 6-Mercaptopurine may also cause long-term genitourinary sequelae such as renal tubular defects, chronic glomerulonephritis, and nephrosis.[357] Infertility in leukemia survivors is a serious concern. Two commonly used drugs, cyclophosphamide and cytarabine, are known to impair reproductive function, primarily in males.[358] Apparently, ova are more resistant to chemotherapy-induced damage than are spermatogonia. Most women who receive chemotherapy before gestation or after the first trimester of pregnancy have uncomplicated pregnancies.

The anthracycline antibiotics are the antileukemic drugs most often associated with cardiotoxicity,[359] although cyclophosphamide has been implicated in some patients.[360] As in cases of cystitis, cardiotoxicity is more likely to occur when patients have received simultaneous irradiation. Histologic examination may disclose degenerating cardiac fibers, mitochondrial swelling, and alterations in nuclear chromatin. Cardiotoxicity, which may be reversible, can present as pericarditis, congestive heart failure, or both. Long-term follow-up of patients receiving chemotherapy and irradiation is mandatory because of the unpredictable nature of late cardiac complications.[361,362] Lipshultz and colleagues[361] assessed the cardiac status of 97 children who had been treated for ALL with doxorubicin (median total dose, 360 mg/m^2) at a median interval of 6.4 years. They found that 65% of patients had evidence of left ventricular insufficiency and concluded that this agent impaired myocardial growth. Also, Steinherz and colleagues[362] studied 201 children with cancer who had received a median of 450 mg/m^2 of anthracycline and found a 23% incidence of late cardiac abnormalities. Therefore, serial assessment of cardiac function is recommended for patients receiving anthracyclines.

Prolonged use of corticosteroids and methotrexate may induce osteoporosis and pathologic fractures.[363] Avascular necrosis of long bones, secondary to steroid treatment, may also occur. Spinal deformities and shortening may be secondary to spinal irradiation, especially in young children. Thyroid and pituitary endocrinopathies may develop as a direct damage induced by irradiation. Growth retardation has been reported in a significant proportion of long-term survivors, as high as about one third.[364] Both irradiation and chemotherapy may be causative agents; the benefits of growth hormone therapy are still under investigation.

Delayed toxicities affecting the CNS in long-term survivors of ALL have received much attention. Initial assessments suggested that CNS prophylaxis with cranial irradiation and intrathecal chemotherapy was not followed by clinically significant long-term side effects.[365] With a larger number of subjects and longer follow-up periods, however, distinct forms of late CNS toxicity have been identified.[366]

Price and coworkers[367,368] studied necropsy specimens from children with leukemia who died and identified two main types of delayed neuropathologic changes, presumably induced by large cumulative doses of CNS irradiation and methotrexate.[369] The first, termed *subacute leukoencephalopathy*,[368] which begins about 6 to 12 months after CNS irradiation, is characterized pathologically by multifocal demyelination. Clinical manifestations vary greatly, from poor school performance to lethargy, ataxia, spasticity, and progressive dementia. Some patients may be completely asymptomatic. Intravenous methotrexate alone may also cause leukoencephalopathy in children with leukemia.[370] The process may be fatal, but apparently there are patients who have recovered and survived with no signs of permanent neurologic damage. The risk of leukoencephalopathy is virtually nil in patients treated with 1800 cGy or less of CNS irradiation.

The second neuropathologic lesion is a degenerative disorder of small vessels, so-called mineralizing microangiopathy,[367] which is usually accompanied by dystrophic calcifications of the brain, apparent on computed tomographic (CT) scan examinations. Unlike leukoencephalopathy, mineralizing microangiopathy predominantly affects CNS gray matter. Although this complication may produce permanent destructive changes, its clinical manifestations are minimal. Additional neurologic sequelae have been described by others.[371]

Abnormal CT brain scans in asymptomatic patients with ALL have been reported for over a decade.[209] Findings include ventricular dilation and widening of the subarachnoid spaces, hypodensities of white matter, and intracerebral calcifications.[372] Abnormalities in CT scans of the brain were also seen predominantly in patients who received 2400 cGy of cranial irradiation plus intrathecal chemotherapy, the standard therapy in the 1970s. As discussed earlier, most therapists currently treat with reduced dosages of CNS irradiation, about 1800 cGy, which appears safe.[200] Alternative methods of CNS prophylaxis employing high doses of intravenous chemotherapy or repeated intrathecal treatment may also result in neurotoxicity.[373]

Several reports have shown an association between brain abnormalities and neuropsychological dysfunction.[372] The neuropsychological consequences of CNS therapy for patients with ALL have become a major concern as the long-term survivor population grows.[374] Although the late neuropsychological effects of treatment for ALL have been evaluated by many investigators, the results are difficult to analyze because of different methodologies employed. Also, results have been inconsistent and several findings never replicated. For example, some investigators found intellectual deficits, but others did not. Williams and Davis[375] reviewed 28 studies of the effects of cranial irradiation, chemotherapy, or both on the CNS in children with ALL. Their findings indicate a lack of significant cognitive abnormalities and do not unequivocally show that cranial irradiation produces greater impairment than chemotherapy. Firm conclusions in this field are difficult to make because of the inability to separate treatment effects from those produced by the leukemia itself. One generality appears to hold regardless of the circumstances of treatment or the features of a given study population: children younger than 8 years have a worse neuropsychological outcome than do older patients, although both groups perform in the average range. In fact, younger children, especially those under 5 years of age treated with 2400 cGy of cranial irradiation, are thought to be more seriously damaged. To understand better the consequences of leukemia treatment on cognitive tests, new studies should be designed to include assessment of socioeconomic status, school attendance, ratings of behavior, and school grades.

In a recent study, 40 children with ALL in continuous complete remission were assessed for memory functioning 5 years after random assignment to receive CNS prophylaxis with either 1800 cGy cranial irradiation plus intrathecal methotrexate or intrathecal methotrexate plus high-dose intravenous methotrexate.[376] No differences between the two treatment groups were seen on 16 standardized memory measures or IQ tests. Only by measuring factors such as memory loss can the effects of CNS treatment on intellectual functioning be separated from the general effects of experiencing leukemia. It is helpful to understand that, overall, most leukemic children who receive CNS prophylaxis do not experience severe intellectual deficits. On the other hand, it is clear that the neurospsychosocial consequences of treatment in patients with CNS relapse are more severe than in patients who remain in remission. In a comparative study, children who were treated for CNS relapse scored significantly lower than a group of patients in remission. A second course of irradiation and young age at relapse predicted lower neuropsychological performance.[374]

Behavioral problems, impaired attainment of social skills, and poorer school performance have been reported among survivors of ALL who have been compared with matched groups of controls or with siblings.[377] Psychological evaluations and assistance is essential for patients with leukemia—not only during the difficult years of treatment administration but also after therapy is successfully completed—to assist the patient in becoming a productive member of society. An interesting report by Tebbi and coworkers[378] on long-term vocational adjustment of cancer survivors diagnosed during adolescence was recently published. Despite the disabilities related to their disease and a generally negative public attitude (discrimination in hiring and difficulties in obtaining health, life, and disability insurance), long-term survivors had a good outlook on life and were competitive members of the workplace and society.

The development of second malignant tumors is also of special concern.[379] The risk 20 years after the first malignancy is estimated to range from 3% to 12%.[380,381] Genetic and treatment factors have been implicated in the cause of second malignancies. Among the most common therapy-related agents are cyclophosphamide and ionizing irradiation.[382,383] In a recent review of second malignancies in childhood ALL, Ochs and Mulhern[384] identified a total of 111 cases. Malignancies involving hematopoietic or lymphatic tissues developed in a shorter median time after diagnosis (60 malignancies in 22 months) than did solid tumors (51 tumors in 77 months). More than one third of secondary solid tumors developed in the brain, especially in patients who received 2400 cGy cranial irradiation and intrathecal methotrexate as part of preventive CNS therapy. A case in point is a CCG study in which 9 biopsy-proven brain tumors were found among 468 long-term survivors.[385] It was estimated that this incidence represented a more than 200-fold increase over the expected number in a similar age-distributed normal population. No patient was older than 6 years at the time of irradiation. Secondary CNS tumors have also been reported in patients who have never received CNS irradiation—an indication that regardless of the therapy received, long-term survivors of leukemia may be at higher risk for developing a second tumor compared with nonleukemic children. The cumulative risk for developing a second tumor among 1866 patients with ALL, treated over 30 years, was 2% at 5 years postdiagnosis, increasing to 4% at 10 years and 6.3% at 15 years.[386]

FUTURE DIRECTIONS

Despite increasingly effective treatment, certain subsets of patients continue to relapse, requiring new emphasis on the development of protocols for high-risk ALL. Two research avenues are likely to yield clinically useful strategies. Recent studies indicate that variations in blood concentrations of antileukemic drugs may affect treatment outcome; thus, efforts to exploit pharmacokinetic and pharmacodynamic principles to improve the therapeutic index of effective agents have been given high priority. By targeting drug doses to achieve a predetermined serum concentration in individual patients, it may be possible to effectively increase dose intensity without the hazard of lethal toxicity and to control interpatient and intrapatient variability in drug disposition. Further intensification of chemotherapy in high-risk patients may be possible with use of molecularly cloned hematopoietic growth factors, such as granulocyte-macrophage colony-stimulating factor and granulocyte colony-stimulating factor, which hold the promise of decreasing both the duration and severity of drug-induced myelosuppression.

Moreover, the dismal long-term outlook for adults with ALL and for children who relapse early during initial chemotherapy may improve with refinements in both allogeneic and autologous marrow transplantation. New laboratory methods for purging potentially contaminating malignant cells from the bone marrow, combined with the ability to eradicate residual leukemia with intensive conditioning regimens, has made this approach an attractive option for the future. Patients will undoubtedly benefit from additional improvements in allogeneic marrow transplantation, namely, methods to avoid graft rejection and graft-versus-host disease as well as expansion of donor pools through use of marrow from similarly but not identically matched donors.

More sensitive techniques for early detection of minimal residual disease are urgently needed. Periodic bone marrow aspirations, at times combined with cytogenetic evaluations, are the only reliable way to monitor the pathophysiologic course of ALL, but even with these procedures, one often overlooks small numbers of leukemic cells. Molecular biologic assessment of genetic alterations, perhaps using polymerase chain-reaction technology, may be required.

Observations of transient decreases in circulating leukemic blasts in patients treated with monoclonal antibodies and certain lymphokines suggest that biologic response modifiers may have a role in future leukemia therapy. The most likely use of agents with immunomodulatory effects would be to augment rather than completely replace chemotherapy.

Finally, although scientific communications have improved remarkably over the past decade, there remains a need for a more universal language among leukemia therapists. Few investigators agree on the criteria for assigning patients to risk groups, resulting in confusion when clinical outcome data are compared. Consistent reporting of event-free survival for all patients enrolled in clinical trails, together with clear definitions of their clinical and biologic risk factors, would do much to facilitate better comparisons of end results of treatment and hence could speed the development of optimal therapy.

REFERENCES

1. Young JL Jr, Ries LG, Silverberg E, Horm JW, Miller RW. Cancer incidence, survival and mortality for children younger than age 15 years. Cancer 1986;58:598.
2. Hoelzer D, Gale RP. Acute lymphoblastic leukemia in adults: recent progress, future directions. Semin Hematol 1987;24:27.
3. Crist WM, Grossi CE, Pullen DJ, Cooper MD. Immunologic markers in childhood acute lymphocytic leukemia. Semin Oncol 1985;12:105.
4. Mirro J, Zipf TF, Pui C-H, et al. Acute mixed lineage leukemia: clinicopathologic correlations and prognostic significance. Blood 1985;66:1115.
5. Crist WM, Shuster JJ, Falletta J, et al. Clinical features and outcome in childhood T-cell leukemia-lymphoma according to stage of thymocyte differentiation: a Pediatric Oncology Group study. Blood 1988;72:1891.
6. Greaves MF. Speculations on the cause of childhood acute lymphoblastic leukemia. Leukemia 1988;2:120.
7. Miller RW. Ethnic differences in cancer occurrence: genetic and environmental influences with particular reference to neuroblastoma. In: Mulvihill JJ, Miller RW, Fraumeni JF Jr, eds. Genetics of human cancer. New York, Raven Press, 1977.
8. Division of Cancer Prevention and Control, Division of Cancer Treatment. 1987 annual cancer statistics review including cancer trends: 1950–1985. Bethesda, NIH Publication No. 88-2789, 1987.
9. Cooke JV. Incidence of acute leukemia in children. JAMA 1942;119:547.
10. Miller RW. Persons with exceptionally high risk of leukemia. Cancer Res 1967;27:2420.
11. Pendergrass TW. Epidemiology of acute lymphoblastic leukemia. Semin Oncol 1985;12:80.
12. Spector BD, Filipovich AH, Perry GS, et al. Epidemiology of cancer in ataxia-telangiectasia. In: Bridges BA, Harnden DG, eds. Ataxia-telangiectasia: a cellular and molecular link between cancer, neuropathology, and immune deficiency. New York, John Wiley & Sons, 1982.
13. Fahey JL, Zighelboim J. Tumor immunology. In: Parker CW, ed. Clinical Immunology, vol 1. Philadelphia, WB Saunders, 1980:445.
14. International Agency for Research on Cancer. IARC monographs on the evaluation of the carcinogenic risk of chemicals to humans: chemicals, industrial processes and industries associated with cancer in humans. Lyon, France, International Agency for Research on Cancer, 1982:1.
15. Sullivan JL. Epstein-Barr virus and lymphoproliferative disorders. Semin Hematol 1988;25:269.
16. Croce CM. Chromosome translocations and human cancer. Cancer Res 1986;46:6019.
17. Gallo RC. Human T-lymphotropic retroviruses. In: Gallo RC, Essex ME, Gross L, eds. Human t-cell leukemia/lymphoma virus. Cold Spring Harbor, New York, Cold Spring Harbor Laboratory, 1984:1.
18. Wertheimer N, Leeper E. Electrical wiring configurations and childhood cancer. Am J Epidemiol 1979;109:109.
19. Fulton JP, Cobb S, Preble L, et al. Electrical wiring configurations and childhood leukemia in Rhode Island. Am J Epidemiol 1980;111:292.
20. Knudson AG Jr. Mutation and cancer: a statistical study of retinoblastoma. Proc Natl Acad Sci 1971;68:820.
21. Boggs DR. The acute leukemias. Medicine 1962;41:163.
22. Harris LJ. Leukaemia and pregnancy. Cancer Med Assoc J 1953;68:234.
23. Bernard J, Boiron M, Weil M. Etude de la remission complete des leucemies aigues. Nouv Rev Fr Hematol 1962;2:195.
24. Bernard J, Jacquillat C, Chavelet F. Leucemie aigue d'une enfante de 5 mois nee d'une mere atteinte de leucemie aigue au moment de accouchement. Nouv Rev Fr Hematol 1964;4:130.
25. Cramblett HG, Friedman JL, Najjar S. Leukemia in an infant born of a mother with acute leukemia. N Engl J Med 1958;259:727.
26. Greaves MF. Differentiation-linked leukemogenesis in lymphocytes. Science 1986;234:696.
27. Schlossman SF, Chess L, Humphrey RE, Strominger JL. Distribution of Ia-like molecules on the surface of normal and leukemic human cells. Proc Natl Acad Sci 1976;73:1288.
28. Greaves MF, Harini G, Newman RA, et al. Selective expression of the common acute lymphoblast leukemia (gp100) antigens on immature lymphoid cells and their malignant counterparts. Blood 1983;61:628.
29. Crist W, Shuster J, Look AT, et al. Current results of studies of immunophenotype-, age- and leukocyte based therapy for children with acute lymphoblastic leukemia. Leukemia 1992;6:162.
30. Crist W, Carroll A, Shuster J, et al. Poor prognosis of children with pre-B acute lymphoblastic leukemia is associated with the t(1;19)(q23'3): a Pediatric Oncology Group study. Blood 1990;76:117.
31. Korsmeyer SJ, Hieter PA, Ravetch JV, et al. Immunoglobulin gene rearrangement and cell surface antigen expression in acute lymphoblastic leukemias of T cell and B cell precursor origins. J Clin Invest 1983;71:301.
32. Bennett JM, Catovsky D, Daniel MT, et al. Proposals for the classification of the acute leukaemias: French-American-British (FAB) Co-Operative Group. Br J Haematol 1976;33:451.
33. Miller DR, Steinherz PG, Feuer D, Sather H, Hammond D. Unfavorable prognostic significance of hand mirror cells in childhood acute lymphoblastic leukemia: a report from the Children's Cancer Study Group. Am J Dis Child 1983;137:346.
34. Rosen NR, DiFino S, Nelson DA. Acute leukemia with unusual cytoplasmic inclusions: a cytochemical and ultrastructural study. Cancer 1979;43:2405.
35. Head DR, Borowitz M, Cerezo L, et al. Acid phosphatase positivity in childhood acute lymphocytic leukemia. Am J Clin Pathol 1986;86:650.
36. Shaw MT. The cytochemistry of acute leukemia: a diagnostic and prognostic evaluation. Semin Oncol 1976;3:219.
37. Coleman MS, Greenwood MF, Hutton JJ, et al. Adenosine deaminase, terminal deoxynucleotidyl transferase (TdT), and cell surface markers in childhood acute leukemia. Blood 1978;52:1125.
38. Jani P, Verbi W, Greaves MF, Bevan D, Bollum F. Terminal deoxynucleotidyl transferase in acute myeloid leukaemia. Leuk Res 1983;7:17.
39. Kaplan SS, Penchansky L, Krause JR, Basford RE, Zdziarski U. Simultaneous evaluation of terminal deoxynucleotidyl transferase and myeloperoxidase in acute leukemias using an immunocytochemical method. Am J Clin Pathol 1987;87:732.
40. Seremetis SV, Pelicci PG, Tabilio A, et al. High frequency of clonal immunoglobulin or T cell receptor gene rearrangements in acute myelogenous leukemia expressing terminal deoxyribonucleotidyl transferase. J Exp Med 1987;165:1703.
41. Pullen DJ, Boyett JM, Crist WM, et al. Pediatric Oncology Group utilization of immunologic markers in the designation of acute lymphocytic leukemia subgroups: influence on treatment response. Ann NY Acad Sci 1984;428:26.
42. Crist W, Rivera G, Pullen J, Weinstein H. The leukemias of childhood. In: Rosenthal DS, Feinstein DI, Goodnight S, McArthus JR, eds. Hematology 1985. Education Program, American Society of Hematology, New Orleans, 1985:48.
43. Jacobs AD, Gale RP. Recent advances in the biology and treatment of acute lymphoblastic leukemia in adults. N Engl J Med 1984;311:1219.
44. Sullivan MP, Pullen J, Crist W, et al. Clinical and biological heterogeneity of childhood B-cell acute lymphocytic leukemia: implications for clinical trials. Leukemia 1990;4:6.
45. Vogler LB, Crist WM, Bockman DE, Pearl ER, Lawton AR, Cooper MD. Pre-B-cell leukemia: a new phenotype of childhood lymphoblastic leukemia. N Engl J Med 1978;298:872.
46. Crist W, Boyett J, Roper M, et al. Pre-B cell leukemia responds poorly to treatment: a Pediatric Oncology Group study. Blood 1984;63:407.
47. Pullen DJ, Falletta JM, Crist WM, et al. Southwest Oncology Group experience with immunological phenotyping in acute lymphocytic leukemia of childhood. Cancer Res 1981;41:4802.
48. Vogler LB, Crist WM, Sarrif AM, et al. An analysis of clinical and laboratory features of acute lymphocytic leukemias with emphasis on 35 children with pre-B leukemia. Blood 1981;58:135.
49. Crist W, Boyett J, Jackson J, et al. Prognostic importance of the pre-B-cell immunophenotype and other presenting features in B-lineage childhood acute lymphoblastic leukemia: a Pediatric Oncology Group study. Blood 1989;74:1252.
50. Pullen DJ. A Pediatric Oncology Group classification protocol for acute lymphocytic leukemia (ALinC 13): immunologic phenotypes and correlation with treatment results. In: Murphy SB, Gilbert JR, eds. Leukemia research: advances in cell biology and treatment. New York, Elsevier Biomedical, 1983:221.
51. Carroll AJ, Crist WM, Parmley RT, Roper M, Cooper MD, Finley WH. Pre-B cell leukemia associated with chromosome translocation 1;19. Blood 1984;63:721.
52. Williams DL, Look AT, Melvin SL, et al. New chromosomal translocations correlate with specific immunophenotypes of childhood acute lymphoblastic leukemia. Cell 1984;36:101.
53. Privitera E, Kamps MP, Hayashi Y, et al. Different molecular consequences of the 1;19 chromosomal translocation in childhood B-cell precursor acute lymphoblastic leukemia. Blood 1992;79:1781.
54. Mellentin JD, Murre C, Donlon TA, et al. The gene for enhancer binding proteins E12/E47 lies at the t(1;19) breakpoint in acute leukemias. Science 1989;246:379.
55. Kamps MP, Murre C, Sun X, Baltimore D. A new homeobox gene contributes the DNA binding domain of the t(1;19) translocation protein in pre-B ALL. Cell 1990;60:547.
56. Nourse J, Mellentin JD, Galili N, et al. Chromosomal translocation t(1;19) results in synthesis of a homeobox fusion mRNA that codes for a potential chimeric transcription factor. Cell 1990;60:535.

57. Borella L, Sen L. T cell surface markers on lymphoblasts from acute lymphocytic leukemia. J Immunol 1973;111:1257.
58. Brouet JC, Flandrin G. Clinical and hematological heterogeneity of T-cell derived lymphoproliferative diseases. Bull Cancer (Paris) 1977;64:267.
59. Dow LW, Borella L, Sen L, et al. Initial prognostic factors and lymphoblast-erythrocyte rosette formation in 109 children with acute lymphoblastic leukemia. Blood 1977;50:671.
60. Kersey J, Nesbit M, Hallgren H, Sabad A, Yunis E, Gajl-Peczalska K. Evidence for origin of certain childhood acute lymphoblastic leukemias and lymphomas in thymus-derived lymphocytes. Cancer 1975;36:1348.
61. Tsukimoto I, Wong KY, Lampkin BC. Surface markers and prognostic factors in acute lymphoblastic leukemia. N Engl J Med 1976;294:245.
62. Kersey JH, Nesbit ME, Luckasen JR. Acute lymphoblastic leukemia and lymphoma cells with thymus-derived T-markers. Mayo Clin Proc 1974;49:584.
63. Borowitz MJ, Dowell BL, Boyett JM, et al. Monoclonal antibody definition of T cell acute leukemia: a Pediatric Oncology Group study. Blood 1985;65:785.
64. Pincus JK, Falletta FM, Metzgar R. The accuracy of identifying T cell leukemia using E rosetting of bone marrow lymphoblasts. (Abstract) Pediatr Res 1981;15:4.
65. Roper M, Crist WM, Metzgar R, et al. Monoclonal antibody characterization of surface antigens in childhood T-cell lymphoid malignancies. Blood 1983;61:830.
66. Sobol RE, Royston I, LeBien TW, et al. Adult acute lymphoblastic leukemia phenotypes defined by monoclonal antibodies. Blood 1985;65:730.
67. Mirro J, Kitchingman GR. The morphology, cytochemistry, molecular characteristics and clinical significance of acute mixed lineage leukemia. In: Scott S, ed. Leukaemia cytochemistry. Chichester, UK, Ellis Horwood, 1989:155.
68. Uckun FM, Muraguchi A, Ledbetter JA, et al. Biphenotypic leukemic lymphocytic precursors in CD2+, CD19+ acute lymphoblastic leukemia and their putative normal counterparts in human fetal hematopoietic tissues. Blood 1989;73:1000.
69. Pui C-H, Williams DL, Roberson PK, et al. Correlation of karyotype and immunophenotype in childhood acute lymphoblastic leukemia. J Clin Oncol 1988;6:56.
70. Williams DL, Raimondi S, Rivera G, George S, Berard CW, Murphy SB. Presence of clonal chromosome abnormalities in virtually all cases of acute lymphoblastic leukemia. N Engl J Med 1985;313:640.
71. Bloomfield CD, Goldman AI, Alimena G, et al. Chromosomal abnormalities identify high-risk and low-risk patients with acute lymphoblastic leukemia. Blood 1986;67:415.
72. Look AT. The cytogenetics of childhood leukemia: clinical and biologic implications. Pediatr Clin North Am 1988;35:723.
73. Jackson JF, Pullen J, Patterson R, Land V, Borowitz M, Crist W. Favorable prognosis associated with hyperdiploidy in children with acute lymphocytic leukemia correlates with extra chromosome 6: a Pediatric Oncology Group study. Cancer 1990;66:1183.
74. Barletta C, Pelicci PG, Kenyon LC, Smith SD, Dalla-Favera R. Relationship between the c-*myb* locus and the 6q-chromosomal aberration in leukemias and lymphomas. Science 1987;235:1064.
75. Clark SS, McLaughlin J, Crist WM, Champlin R, Witte ON. Unique forms of the abl tyrosine kinase distinguish Ph1-positive CML from Ph1-positive ALL. Science 1987;235:85.
76. Dalla-Favera R, Bregni M, Erikson J, Patterson D, Gallo RC, Croce CM. Human c-*myc* oncogene is located on the region of chromosome 8 that is translocated in Burkitt lymphoma cells. Proc Natl Acad Sci 1982;79:7824.
77. Diaz MO, Le Beau MM, Pitha P, Rowley JD. Interferon and c-*ets*-1 genes in the translocation (9;11)(p22;q23) in human acute monocytic leukemia. Science 1986;231:265.
78. Emanuel BS, Selden JR, Chaganti RS, Jhanwar S, Nowell PC, Croce CM. The 2p breakpoint of a 2;8 translocation in Burkitt lymphoma interrupts the V kappa locus. Proc Natl Acad Sci 1984;81:2444.
79. Erikson J, Williams DL, Finan J, Nowell PC, Croce CM. Locus of the alpha-chain of the T-cell receptor is split by chromosome translocation in T-cell leukemias. Science 1985;229:784.
80. Hollis GF, Mitchell KF, Battey J, et al. A variant translocation places the lambda immunoglobulin genes 3′ to the c-*myc* oncogene in Burkitt's lymphoma. Nature 1984;307:752.
81. Jhanwar SC, Neel BG, Hayward WS, Chaganti RS. Localization of c-*ras* oncogene family on human germ-line chromosomes. Proc Natl Acad Sci 1983;80:4794.
82. Kurzrock R, Shtalrid M, Romero P, et al. A novel c-*abl* protein product in Philadelphia-positive acute lymphoblastic leukaemia. Nature 1987;325:631.
83. Reynolds TC, Smith SD, Sklar J. Analysis of DNA surrounding the breakpoints of chromosomal translocations involving the beta T cell receptor gene in human lymphoblastic neoplasms. Cell 1987;50:107.
84. Yang-Feng TL, Francke U, Ullrich A. Gene for human insulin receptor: localization to site on chromosome 19 involved in pre-B-cell leukemia. Science 1985;228:728.
85. Lombardi L, Newcomb EW, Dalla-Favera R. Pathogenesis of Burkitt lymphoma: expression of an activated c-*myc* oncogene causes the tumorigenic conversion of EBV-infected human B lymphoblasts. Cell 1987;49:161.
86. Look AT. Genetic abnormalities in human leukemia. In: Mauer AM, ed. Biology of human leukemia. Baltimore, Johns Hopkins University Press, 1988:200.
87. Riberio RC, Abromowitch M, Raimondi SC, Murphy SB, Behm FG, Williams DL. Clinical and biologic hallmarks of the Philadelphia chromosome in childhood acute lymphoblastic leukemia. Blood 1987;70:948.
88. Crist W, Carroll A, Shuster J, et al. Philadelphia chromosome positive childhood acute lymphoblastic leukemia: clinical and cytogenic characteristics and treatment outcome—a Pediatric Oncology Group study. Blood 1990;76:489.
89. Crist WM, Pullen DJ, Rivera GK. Acute lymphocytic leukemias. In: Fernbach DJ, Vietti T, eds. Clinical pediatric oncology. St Louis, CV Mosby, 1988.
90. Rivera G, Pui C-H. Acute lymphoblastic leukemia. In: Rudolph AM, ed. Pediatrics. Norwalk, CT, Appleton-Century-Crofts, 1987:1098.
91. Ribeiro RC, Pui C-H. The clinical and biological correlates of coagulopathy in children with acute leukemia. J Clin Oncol 1986;4:1212.
92. Sallan SE, Weinstein HJ. Childhood acute leukemia. In: Nathan D, Oski F, eds. Hematology of infancy and childhood. Philadelphia, WB Saunders, 1987:1028.
93. Pereira F, Crist W, McKaig S. Neuroblastoma "leukemia": a rarity? Report of a case. Clin Pediatr 1978;17:701.
94. Saulsbury FT, Sabio H, Conrad D, Kesler RW, Levien MG. Acute leukemia with features of systemic lupus erythematosus. J Pediatr 1984;105:57.
95. Crist W, Pullen J, Boyett J, et al. Clinical and biologic features predict a poor prognosis in acute lymphoid leukemias in infants: a Pediatric Oncology Group study. Blood 1986;67:135.
96. Katz F, Malcolm S, Gibbons B, et al. Cellular and molecular studies on infant null acute lymphoblastic leukemia. Blood 1988;71:1438.
97. Pui C-H, Raimondi SC, Murphy SB, et al. An analysis of leukemic cell chromosomal features in infants. Blood 1987;69:1289.
98. Reaman G, Zeltzer P, Bleyer WA, et al. Acute lymphoblastic leukemia in infants less than one year of age: a cumulative experience of the Children's Cancer Study Group. J Clin Oncol 1985;3:1513.
99. Stark B, Vogel R, Cohen IJ, et al. Biologic and cytogenetic characteristics of leukemia in infants. Cancer 1989;63:117.
100. Reaman GH, Steinherz PG, Gaynon PS, et al. Improved survival of infants less than 1 year of age with acute lymphoblastic leukemia treated with intensive multiagent chemotherapy. Cancer Treat Rep 1987;71:1033.
101. Crist W, Pullen J, Boyett J, et al. Acute lymphoid leukemia in adolescents: clinical and biologic features predict a poor prognosis—a Pediatric Oncology Group study. J Clin Oncol 1988;6:34.
102. Clavell LA, Gelber RD, Cohen HJ, et al. Four-agent induction and intensive asparaginase therapy for treatment of childhood acute lymphoblastic leukemia. N Engl J Med 1986;315:657.
103. Gaynor J, Chapman D, Little C, et al. A cause-specific hazard rate analysis of prognostic factors among 199 adults with acute lymphoblastic leukemia: the Memorial Hospital experience since 1969. J Clin Oncol 1988;6:1014.
104. Hammond D, Sather H, Nesbit M, et al. Analysis of prognostic factors in acute lymphoblastic leukemia. Med Pediatr Oncol 1986;14:124.
105. Pui C-H, Williams DL, Kalwinsky DK, et al. Cytogenetic features and serum lactic dehydrogenase level predict a poor treatment outcome for children with pre-B-cell leukemia. Blood 1986;67:1688.
106. Raimondi SC, Behm FG, Roberson PK, et al. Cytogenetics of pre-B-cell acute lymphoblastic leukemia with emphasis on prognostic implications of the t(1;19). J Clin Oncol 1990;8:1380.
107. Riehm H, Gadner H, Henze G, et al. Acute lymphoblastic leukemia: treatment results in three BFM studies (1970–1981). In: Murphy SB, Gilbert JR, eds. Leukemia research: advances in cell biology and treatment. New York, Elsevier Biomedical, 1983:251.
108. Pui C-H, Behm FG, Singh B, et al. Myeloid-associated antigen expression lacks prognostic value in childhood acute lymphoblastic leukemia treated with intensive multiagent chemotherapy. Blood 1990;75:198.
109. Pui C-H, Behm FG, Kalwinsky DK, et al. Clinical significance of low levels of myeloperoxidase positivity in childhood acute nonlymphoblastic leukemia. Blood 1987;70:51.
110. Williams DL, Tsiatis A, Brodeur GM, et al. Prognostic importance of chromosome number in 136 untreated children with acute lymphoblastic leukemia. Blood 1982;60:864.
111. Pui C-H, Williams DL, Raimondi S, et al. Hypodiploidy is associated with a poor prognosis in childhood acute lymphoblastic leukemia. Blood 1987;70:247.
112. Nordenson I, Adrian BA, Holmgren G, Roos G, Rudolphi O, Wahlqvist Y. Near-haploidy in childhood leukemia: a high-risk component. In: Forestier E, ed. Pediatric hematology and oncology. Washington, DC, Hemisphere Publishing, 1988:309.
113. Bloomfield CD, Rowley JD, Goldmann AI. Third international workshop on chromosomes in leukemia: chromosomal abnormalities and their clinical significance in acute lymphoblastic leukemia. Cancer Res 1983;43:868.

114. Williams DL, Harber J, Murphy SB, et al. Chromosomal translocations play a unique role in influencing prognosis in childhood acute lymphoblastic leukemia. Blood 1986;68:205.
115. Miller DR, Leikin S, Albo V, Sather H, Karon M, Hammond D. Prognostic factors and therapy in acute lymphoblastic leukemia of childhood: CCG-141—a report from Children's Cancer Study Group. Cancer 1983;51:1041.
116. Steinherz PG, Gaynon P, Miller DR, et al. Improved disease-free survival of children with acute lymphoblastic leukemia at high risk for early relapse with the New York regimen: a new intensive therapy protocol—a report from the Children's Cancer Study Group. J Clin Oncol 1986;4:744.
117. Pui C-H, Dodge RK, Dahl GV, et al. Serum lactic dehydrogenase level has prognostic value in childhood acute lymphoblastic leukemia. Blood 1985;66:778.
118. Radford JE, Burns CP, Jones MP, et al. Adult acute lymphoblastic leukemia: results of the Iowa HOP-L protocol. J Clin Oncol 1989;7:58.
119. Kalwinsky DK, Rivera G, Dahl GV, et al. Variation by race in presenting clinical and biologic features of childhood acute lymphoblastic leukaemia: implications for treatment outcome. Leukemia Res 1985;9:817.
120. Miller DR, Leikin SL, Albo VC, Sather H, Hammond GD. Three versus five years of maintenance therapy are equivalent in childhood acute lymphoblastic leukemia: a report from the Children's Cancer Study Group. J Clin Oncol 1989;7:316.
121. Hoelzer D, Thiel E, Loffler H, et al. Prognostic factors in a multicenter study for treatment of acute lymphoblastic leukemia in adults. Blood 1988;71:123.
122. Baccarani M, Corbelli G, Amadori S, et al. Adolescent and adult acute lymphoblastic leukemia: prognostic features and outcome of therapy. A study of 293 patients. Blood 1982;60:677.
123. Bitran JD. Prognostic value of immunologic markers in adults with acute lymphoblastic leukemia. (Letter) N Engl J Med 1978;299:1317.
124. Schauer P, Arlin ZA, Mertelsmann R, et al. Treatment of acute lymphoblastic leukemia in adults: results of the L-10 and L-10M protocols. J Clin Oncol 1983;1:462.
125. Lister TA, Roberts MM, Brearley RL, Woodruff RK, Greaves MF. Prognostic significance of cell surface phenotype in adult acute lymphoblastic leukaemia. Cancer Immunol Immunother 1979;6:227.
126. Fasola G, Fanin R, Baccarani M, et al. Relationship of serum lactate dehydrogenase level with first remission length in adult acute lymphocytic leukaemia. Br J Haematol 1987;66:49.
127. Champlin R, Gale RP. Acute lymphoblastic leukemia: recent advances in biology and therapy. Blood 1989;73:2051.
128. Abromowitch M, Ochs J, Pui C-H, Fairclough D, Murphy SB, Rivera GK. Efficacy of high-dose methotrexate in childhood acute lymphocytic leukemia: analysis by contemporary risk classifications. Blood 1988;71:866.
129. Mastrangelo R, Poplack D, Bleyer A, Riccardi R, Sather H, D'Angio G. Report and recommendations of the Rome workshop concerning poor-prognosis acute lymphoblastic leukemia in children: biologic bases for staging, stratification, and treatment. Med Pediatr Oncol 1986;14:191.
130. DeVita VT, Schein PS. The use of drugs in combination for the treatment of cancer: rationale and results. N Engl J Med 1973;288:998.
131. Pinkel D. Five year follow-up of "total therapy" of childhood lymphocytic leukemia. JAMA 1971;216:648.
132. Pinkel D. Curing children of leukemia. Cancer 1987;59:1683.
133. Simone JV. Factors that influence haematological remission duration in acute lymphocytic leukaemia. Br J Haematol 1976;32:465.
134. George SL. Design and evaluation of leukaemia trials. Clin Haematol 1978;7:227.
135. Skipper HE, Schabel FM Jr, Wilcox WS. Experimental evaluation of potential anticancer agents. XIV. Further study of certain basic concepts underlying chemotherapy of leukemia. Cancer Chemother Rep 1965;45:5.
136. Vietti TJ, Starling K, Wilbur JR. Vincristine, prednisone and daunomycin in acute leukemia of childhood. Cancer 1971;27:602.
137. Haggard ME, Fernbach DJ, Holcomb TM, Sutow WW, Vietti TJ, Windmiller J. Vincristine in acute leukemia of childhood. Cancer 1968;22:438.
138. Evans AE, Farber S, Brunet S, Mariano PJ. Vincristine and the treatment of acute leukemia in children. Cancer 1963;16:1302.
139. Karon MR, Freirich EJ, Frei E III. A preliminary report on vincristine sulfate: a new active agent for the treatment of acute leukemia. Pediatrics 1962;30:79.
140. Selawry OS, Frei E III. Prolongation of remission in acute lymphocytic leukemia by alteration in dose schedule and route of administration of methotrexate. Clin Res 1964;12:231.
141. Wilson L, Anderson KA, Chin D. Nonstoichiometric poisoning of microtubule polymerization: a model for the mechanism of action of the vinca alkaloids, podophyllotoxin and colchicine. In: Goldman R, Pollard T, Rosenbaum J, eds. Cell proliferation. III. Cell motility. Cold Spring Harbor, New York, Cold Spring Harbor Laboratory, 1976:1051.
142. Sibley GH, Tomkins GM. Mechanism of steroid resistance. Cell 1974;2:221.
143. Di Marco A, Soldati M, Fioretti A, Dasdia T. Activity of daunomycin, a new antibiotic on normal and neoplastic cells grown in vitro. Cancer Chemother Rep 1964;38:39.
144. Tan C, Tasaka H, Yu KP, et al. Daunomycin and antitumor antibiotic in the treatment of neoplastic disease. Cancer 1967;20:333.
145. Shaw MT, Raab SO. Adriamycin in combination chemotherapy of adult acute lymphoblastic leukemia: a Southwest Oncology Group study. Med Pediatr Oncol 1977;3:261.
146. Sackman MF, Pavlosky S, Penalver JA, et al. Evaluation of induction of remissions, intensifications, and central nervous system prophylactic treatment in acute lymphoblastic leukemia. Cancer 1974;34:418.
147. Broome JD. Evidence that the L-asparaginase of guinea pig serum is responsible for its antilymphoma effects. I. Properties of the L-asparaginase of guinea pig serum in relation to those of the antilymphoma substance. J Exp Med 1963;118:99.
148. Oettgen HF, et al. Inhibition of leukemias in man by L-asparaginase. Cancer Res 1967;27:2619.
149. Pullen DJ, Sullivan MP, Falletta JM, et al. Modified LSA2-L2 treatment in 53 children with E-rosette-positive T-cell leukemia: results and prognostic factors—a Pediatric Oncology Group study. Blood 1982;60:1159.
150. Ortega JA, Nesbit ME Jr, Donaldson MH, et al. L-asparaginase, vincristine, and prednisone for induction of first remission in acute lymphocytic leukemia. Cancer Res 1977;37:535.
151. Jones B, Holland JF, Glidewell O, et al. Optimal use of L-asparaginase (NSC-109229) in acute lymphocytic leukemia. Med Pediatr Oncol 1977;3:387.
152. van Eys J, Berry D, Crist W, et al. A comparison of two regimens for high-risk acute lymphocytic leukemia in childhood: a Pediatric Oncology Group study. Cancer 1989;63:23.
153. Hitchcock-Bryan S, Gelber R, Cassady JR, Sallan SE. The impact of induction anthracycline on long-term failure-free survival in childhood acute lymphoblastic leukemia. Med Pediatr Oncol 1986;14:211.
154. Jacquillat C, Weil M, Gemon MF, et al. Combination therapy in 130 patients with acute lymphoblastic leukemia (protocol 06 LA 66-Paris). Cancer Res 1973;33:3278.
155. Gottlieb AJ, Weinberg V, Ellison RR, et al. Efficacy of daunorubicin in the therapy of adult acute lymphocytic leukemia: a prospective randomized trial by cancer and leukemia group B. Blood 1984;64:267.
156. Shinn LC, Cruz JM, Powell BL, et al. A dose-intense cyclic treatment (RX) program for adult acute lymphoblastic leukemia (ALL). (Abstract) Proc Am Soc Clin Oncol 1991;10:224.
157. Skipper HE, Schabel FM Jr, Wilcox WS. Experimental evaluation of potential anticancer agents. XII. On the criteria and kinetics associated with "curability" of experimental leukemia. Cancer Chemother Rep 1964;35:1.
158. Goldie JH, Coldman AJ, Gudauskas GA. Rationale for the use of alternating non-cross-resistant chemotherapy. Cancer Treat Rep 1982;66:439.
159. Aur RJ, Simone J, Hustu HO, et al. Central nervous system therapy and combination chemotherapy of childhood lymphocytic leukemia. Blood 1971;37:272.
160. Aur RJA, Simone JV, Pratt CB. Successful remission induction in children with acute lymphocytic leukemia at high risk for treatment failure. Cancer 1971;27:1332.
161. Haghbin M, Tan CC, Clarkson BD, Mike V, Burchenal JH, Murphy ML. Intensive chemotherapy in children with acute lymphoblastic leukemia (L-2 protocol). Cancer 1974;33:1491.
162. Haghbin M, Murphy ML, Tan CC, et al. A long-term clinical follow-up of children with acute lymphoblastic leukemia treated with intensive chemotherapy regimens. Cancer 1980;46:241.
163. Clarkson B, Ellis S, Little C, et al. Acute lymphoblastic leukemia in adults. Semin Oncol 1985;12:160.
164. Gulati SC, Gaynor J, Esseesse, et al. Use of prognostic factors in deciding therapy for adult acute lymphoblastic leukemia: new approaches at Memorial Sloan-Kettering Cancer Center (MSKCC). Bone Marrow Transplant 1989;4(suppl 1):86.
165. Hussein KK, Dahlberg S, Head D, et al. Treatment of acute lymphoblastic leukemia in adults with intensive induction, consolidation, and maintenance chemotherapy. Blood 1989;73:57.
166. Riehm H, Gadner H, Henze G. The Berlin childhood acute lymphoblastic leukemia study, 1970–1976. Am J Pediatr Hematol Oncol 1980;2:299.
167. Riehm H, Feickert H-J, Lampert F. Acute lymphoblastic leukemia. In: Voute PA, Barrett A, Bloom J, eds. UICC cancer in children: clinical management. Berlin, Springer-Verlag, 1986:101.
168. Kalwinsky DK, Roberson P, Dahl G, et al. Clinical relevance of lymphoblast biological features in children with acute lymphoblastic leukemia. J Clin Oncol 1985;3:477.
169. Walters TR, Bushmore M, Simone J. Poor prognosis in Negro children with acute lymphoblastic leukemia. Cancer 1972;29:210.
170. Gaynon PS, Steinherz PG, Bleyer WA, et al. Intensive therapy for children with acute lymphoblastic leukaemia and unfavorable presenting features early conclusions of study CCG-106 by the Children's Cancer Study Group. Lancet 1988;1:921.

171. Krishan A, Paika D, Frei EIII. Cytofluorometric studies on the action of podophyllotoxin and epipodophyllotoxins (VM-26, VP-16-213) on the cell cycle traverse of human lymphoblasts. J Cell Biol 1975;66: 521.
172. Rivera G, Avery T, Roberts DW. Response of L1210 to combinations of cytosine arabinoside and VM-26 or VP16-213. Eur J Cancer 1975;11: 639.
173. Rivera G, Aur RJ, Dahl GV, Pratt CB, Wood A, Avery TL. Combined VM-26 and cytosine arabinoside in treatment of refractory childhood lymphocytic leukemia. Cancer 1980;45:1284.
174. Rivera G, Dahl GV, Bowman WP, Avery TL, Wood A, Aur RJ. VM-26 and cytosine arabinoside combination chemotherapy for initial induction failures in childhood lymphocytic leukemia. Cancer 1980;46:1727.
175. Dahl GV, Rivera GK, Look AT, et al. Teniposide plus cytarabine improves outcome in childhood acute lymphoblastic leukemia presenting with a leukocyte count ≥ 100 × 10⁹/L. J Clin Oncol 1987;5:1015.
176. Linker CA, Levitt LJ, O'Donnell M, et al. Improved results of treatment of adult acute lymphoblastic leukemia. Blood 1987;69:1242.
177. Rivera GK, George SL, Williams D, et al. Early results of intensified remission induction chemotherapy for childhood acute lymphocytic leukemia. Med Pediatr Oncol 1986;14:177.
178. Rivera GK, Kovnar E, Pui C-H, et al. Limiting toxicities during intensified remission induction chemotherapy for childhood acute lymphocytic leukemia. Hamatol Bluttransfus 1987;30:156.
179. Rivera GK, Raimondi SC, Hancock ML, et al. Improved outcome in childhood acute lymphoblastic leukaemia with reinforced early treatment and rotational combination chemotherapy. Lancet 1991;337: 61.
180. Freeman AI, Weinberg V, Brecher ML, et al. Comparison of intermediate-dose methotrexate with cranial irradiation for the post-induction treatment of acute lymphocytic leukemia in children. N Engl J Med 1983;308:477.
181. Esterhay RJ Jr, Wiernik PH, Grove WR, Markus SD, Wesley MN. Moderate dose methotrexate, vincristine, asparaginase, and dexamethasone for treatment of adult acute lymphocytic leukemia. Blood 1982;59:334.
182. Capizzi RL. Schedule-dependent potentiation of the activity of methotrexate and high-dose ara-C by asparaginase in treatment of the acute leukemias. In: Murphy SB, Gilbert JR, eds. Leukemia research: advances in cell biology and treatment. New York, Elsevier Science Publishing, 1983:145.
183. Stryckmans P, Marie JP, Debusscher L, et al. Chemotherapy of adult acute lymphoblastic leukemia (ALL). (Abstract) Blood 1985;66:209a.
184. Rivera GK, Mauer AM. Controversies in the management of childhood acute lymphoblastic leukemia: treatment intensification, CNS leukemia, and prognostic factors. Semin Hematol 1987;24:12.
185. Sallan SE, Clavell LA, Gelber R. Intensive chemotherapy in childhood acute lymphoblastic leukemia. In: Wehinger H, ed. Leukamiebehandlung im kindesalter stand zu begin der 80 er Jugre (Wissenchafliche Information Juhrgang 10, Heft 2). Milupa AG, 6382 Friedrichsdorf/Taunus, 1984:35.
186. Rivera GK, Evans WE, Kalwinsky DK, et al. Unexpectedly severe toxicity from intensive early treatment of childhood lymphoblastic leukemia. J Clin Oncol 1985;3:201.
187. Lay HN, Ekert H, Colebatch JH. Combination chemotherapy for children with acute lymphocytic leukemia who fail to respond to standard remission-induction therapy. Cancer 1975;36:1220.
188. Evans AE, Gilbert ES, Zandstra R. The increasing incidence of central nervous system leukemia in children. (Children's Cancer Study Group A). Cancer 1970;26:404.
189. George P, Pinkel D. CNS radiation in children with acute lymphocytic leukemia in remission. Proc Am Assoc Cancer Res 1965;6:22.
190. Ribeiro RC, Abromowitch M, Raimondi SC, Murphy SB, Behm F, Williams DL. Clinical and biologic hallmarks of the Philadelphia chromosome in childhood acute lymphoblastic leukemia. Blood 1992;70:948.
191. Nesbit ME, Sather H, Robison LL, et al. Sanctuary therapy: a randomized trial of 724 children with previously untreated acute lymphoblastic leukemia. Cancer Res 1982;42:674.
192. Freeman JE, Johnston PG, Voke JM. Somnolence after prophylactic cranial irradiation in children with acute lymphoblastic leukaemia. Br Med J 1973;4:523.
193. Berg RA, Chi'en L, Lancaster W, et al. Neuropsychologic sequelae of postradiation somnolence syndrome. J Dev Behav Pediatr 1989;4: 103.
194. Ochs JJ, Pui C-H, Mason C, et al. Seizure in childhood lymphoblastic leukemia patients. Lancet 1984_{∞}:1422.
195. Johnson R. An experimental therapeutic approach to L1210 leukemia in mice: combination chemotherapy and central nervous system irradiation. J Natl Cancer Inst 1964;32:133.
196. Hustu HO, Aur RJ. Extramedullary leukaemia. Clin Haematol 1978;7: 313.
197. Hustu HO, Aur RJ, Verzosa MS, Simone JV, Pinkel D. Prevention of central nervous system leukemia by irradiation. Cancer 1973;32:585.
198. Aur RJA, Simone JV, Hustu HO, Verzosa MS. A comparative study of central nervous system irradiation and intensive chemotherapy early in remission of childhood acute lymphocytic leukemia. Cancer 1972;29:381.
199. Aur RJA, Hustu HO, Verzosa MS, Wood A, Simone JV. Comparison of two methods of preventing central nervous system leukemia. Blood 1973;42:349.
200. Nesbit ME Jr, Sather HN, Robison LL, et al. Presymptomatic central nervous system therapy in previously untreated childhood acute lymphoblastic leukaemia: comparison of 1800 rad and 2400 rad—a report for Children's Cancer Study Group. Lancet 1981;1:461.
201. Simone J. Acute lymphocytic leukemia in childhood. Semin Hematol 1974;11:25.
202. van Eys J, Berry D, Crist WM, et al. Treatment intensity and outcome for children with acute lymphocytic leukemia of standard risk: a Pediatric Oncology Group study. Cancer 1989;63:1466.
203. Trueworthy R, Shuster J, Look T, et al. Ploidy of lymphoblasts is the strongest predictor of treatment outcome in B-progenitor cell acute lymphoblastic leukemia of childhood: a Pediatric Oncology Group study. J Clin Oncol 1992;10:606.
204. Sullivan MP, Chen T, Dyment PG, et al. Equivalence of intrathecal chemotherapy and radiotherapy as central nervous system prophylaxis in children with acute lymphoblastic leukemia: a Pediatric Oncology Group study. Blood 1982;60:948.
205. Pullen J, Frankel L, Iyer R. Extended triple intrathecal (T.I.T.) chemotherapy provides effective central nervous system (CNS) prophylaxis for both good and poor prognosis patients with non-T, non-B acute lymphocytic leukemia (ALL): substitution of intermediate dose methotrexate (IDM) for T.I.T. after consolidation provides less effective protection for the CNS. (Abstract) Proc Am Soc Clin Oncol 1988;7: 681.
206. Wang JJ, Freeman AI, Sinks LF. Treatment of acute lymphocytic leukemia by high dose intravenous methotrexate. Cancer Res 1976;36: 1441.
207. Freeman AI. Intermediate dose methotrexate (IDM) in children with acute lymphocytic leukemia (ALL). Sangre 1985;30:1007.
208. Poplack DG, Reaman GH, Bleyer WA, et al. Central nervous system preventive therapy with high-dose methotrexate in acute lymphoblastic leukemia: a preliminary report. (Abstract) Proc Am Soc Clin Oncol 1984;3:204.
209. Green DM. Comparison of three methods of central nervous system prophylaxis in childhood acute lymphoblastic leukemia. Lancet 1980;1398.
210. Simone JV. Leukaemia remission and survival. (Letter) Lancet 1981;531.
211. George SL, Ochs JJ, Mauer AM, Simone JV. The importance of an isolated central nervous system relapse in children with acute lymphoblastic leukemia. J Clin Oncol 1985;3:776.
212. Ortega JA, Nesbit ME, Sather HN, Robison LL, D'Angio GJ, Hammond GD. Long-term evaluation of a CNS prophylaxis trial: treatment comparisons and outcome after CNS relapse in childhood ALL—a report from the Children's Cancer Study Group. J Clin Oncol 1987;5:1646.
213. Omura GA, Moffitt S, Vogler WR, Salter MM. Combination chemotherapy of adult acute lymphoblastic leukemia with randomized central nervous system prophylaxis. Blood 1980;55:199.
214. Kantarjian HM, Walters RS, Smith TL, et al. Identification of risk groups for development of central nervous system leukemia in adults with acute lymphocytic leukemia. Blood 1988;72:1784.
215. Aur RJ, Simone JV, Verzosa MS, et al. Childhood acute lymphocytic leukemia: study VIII. Cancer 1978;42:2123.
216. Blacklock HA, Matthews JRD, Buchanan JG, Ockelford PA, Hill RS. Improved survival from acute lymphoblastic leukemia in adolescents and adults. Cancer 1981;48:1931.
217. Carella AM, Nicolino M, Santini G, et al. Induction and consolidation combination chemotherapy with 8 drugs (L-10 protocol) for acute lymphoblastic leukemia. Haematologica 1981;66:311.
218. Schauer P, Arlin ZA, Mertelsman R, et al. Treatment of acute lymphoblastic leukemia in adults: results of the L-10 and L-10M protocols. J Clin Oncol 1983;1:462.
219. Coccia PF. Development and preliminary findings of Children's Cancer Study Group protocols (161, 162, and 163) for low-, average-, and high-risk acute lymphoblastic leukemia in children. In: Murphy SB, Gilbert JR, eds. Leukemia research: advances in cell biology and treatment. New York, Elsevier Science Publishing, 1983:241.
220. Hryniuk W. The importance of dose intensity in outcome of chemotherapy. In: Hellman S, DeVita V, Rosenberg S, eds. Advances in oncology. Philadelphia, JB Lippincott, 1988:121.
221. Hryniuk WM. More is better. (Editorial) J Clin Oncol 1988;6:1365.
222. DeVita VT. Dose response is alive and well. J Clin Oncol 1986;4:1157.
223. Schabel FM Jr, Simpson-Herren L. Some variables in experimental tumor systems which complicate interpretations of data from in vivo kinetic and pharmacologic studies with anticancer drugs. Antibiot Chemother 1978;23:113.
224. Tannock IF, Boyd NF, DeBoer G, et al. A randomized trial of two levels of CMF chemotherapy for patients with metastatic breast cancer. J Clin Oncol 1988;6:1377.
225. Pinkel D, Hernandez K, Borella L, et al. Drug dosage and remission duration in childhood lymphocytic leukemia. Cancer 1971;27: 247.

226. Evans WE. Clinical pharmacodynamics of anticancer drugs: a basis for extending the concept of dose-intensity. Blut 1988;56:241.
227. Rodman JH, Abromowitch M, Sinkule JA, Hayes FA, Rivera GK, Evans WE. Clinical pharmacodynamics of continuous infusion teniposide: systemic exposure as a determinant of response in a phase I trial. J Clin Oncol 1987;5:1007.
228. Evans WE, Crom WR, Abromowitch M, et al. Clinical pharmacodynamics of high-dose methotrexate in acute lymphocytic leukemia: identification of a relation between concentration and effect. N Engl J Med 1986;314:471.
229. Medical Research Council Leukaemia Trial. UKALL V: an attempt to reduce the immunosuppressive effects of therapy in childhood lymphoblastic leukemia. J Clin Oncol 1986;4:1758.
230. Pui C-H, Aur RJ, Bowman WP, et al. Failure of late intensification therapy to improve a poor result in childhood lymphoblastic leukemia. Cancer Res 1984;44:3593.
231. Abromowitch M, Ochs J, Pui C-H, et al. High-dose methotrexate improves clinical outcome in children with acute lymphoblastic leukemia: St Jude Total Therapy Study X. Med Pediatr Oncol 1988;16: 297.
232. The Medical Research Council's Working Party on Leukaemia in Childhood. Medical Research Council leukaemia trial, UKALL VII. Arch Dis Child 1985;6:1050.
233. Balis FM, Mirro J, Reaman G, et al. Pharmacokinetics of subcutaneous methotrexate. J Clin Oncol 1988;6:1882.
234. Nesbit M, Krivit W, Heyn R, Sharp H. Acute and chronic effects of methotrexate on hepatic, pulmonary, and skeletal systems. Cancer 1976;37:1048.
235. Lee MS, Chang KS, Freireich EJ, et al. Detection of minimal residual bcr/abl transcripts by a modified polymerase chain reaction. Blood 1988;72:893.
236. Hale G, Cobbold SP, Clark MR, et al. Monoclonal antibodies for conditioning prior to marrow transplantation. Bone Marrow Transplant 1989;Suppl 4:240.
237. George SL, Aur RJ, Mauer AM, Simone JV. A reappraisal of the results of stopping therapy in childhood leukemia. N Engl J Med 1979;300: 269.
238. Aur RJA, Simone JV, Hustu HO, Verzosa MS, Pinkel D. Cessation of therapy during complete remission of childhood acute lymphocytic leukemia. N Engl J Med 1974;291:1230.
239. Ortega JJ, Javier G, Olive T, Pethema Y. Treatment of high-risk acute lymphoblastic leukemia with protocols PETHEMA LAL 7/78 and LAL 17/84. Anal Espanol Pediatr 1988;29:72.
240. Murphy SB, Bowman WP, Abromowitch M, et al. Results of treatment of advanced-stage Burkitt's lymphoma and B cell (SIg+) acute lymphoblastic leukemia with high-dose fractionated cyclophosphamide and coordinated high-dose methotrexate and cytarabine. J Clin Oncol 1986;4:1732.
241. Patte C, Philip T, Rodary C, et al. Improved survival rate in children with stage III and IV B cell non-Hodgkin's lymphoma and leukemia using multi-agent chemotherapy: results of a study of 114 children from the French Pediatric Oncology Society. J Clin Oncol 1986;4: 1219.
242. Nygaard R, Moe PJ, Brincker H, et al. Late relapses after treatment for acute lymphoblastic leukemia in childhood: a population based study from the Nordic countries. Med Pediatr Oncol 1989;17:45.
243. Mandelli F, Amadori S, Rajnoldi AC, et al. Discontinuing therapy in childhood acute lymphocytic leukemia: a multicentric survey in Italy. Cancer 1980;46:1319.
244. Baum E, Sather H, Nachman J, et al. Relapse rates following cessation of chemotherapy during complete remission of acute lymphocytic leukemia. Med Pediatr Oncol 1979;7:25.
245. Land VJ, Berry DH, Herson J, et al. Long-term survival in childhood acute leukemia: "late" relapses. Med Pediatr Oncol 1979;7:19.
246. Amadori S, Meloni G, Baccarani M, et al. Long-term survival in adolescent and adult acute lymphoblastic leukemia. Cancer 1983;52: 30.
247. Rivera G, Aur RJ, Dahl GV, et al. Second cessation of therapy in childhood lymphocytic leukemia. Blood 1979;53:1114.
248. Rivera G, Pratt CB, Aur RJA. Recurrent childhood lymphocytic leukemia following cessation of therapy: treatment and response. Cancer 1976;37:1679.
249. Pui C-H, Behm FG, Raimondi SC, et al. Secondary acute myeloid leukemia in children treated for acute lymphoid leukemia. N Engl J Med 1989;321:136.
250. Pui C-H, Ribeiro RC, Hancock ML, et al. Acute myeloid leukemia in children treated with epipodophyllotoxins for acute lymphoblastic leukemia. N Engl J Med 1991;325:1682.
251. Buchanan GR, Rivera GK, Boyett JM, Chauvenet AR, Crist WM, Vietti TJ. Reinduction therapy in 297 children with acute lymphoblastic leukemia in first bone marrow relapse: a Pediatric Oncology Group study. Blood 1988;72:1286.
252. Kimball JC, Herson J, Sullivan MP. Favorable response to maintenance therapy of second or subsequent remissions in childhood acute lymphocytic leukemia. Cancer 1980;46:1093.
253. Baum E, Nachman J, Ramsay N, et al. Prolonged second remissions in childhood acute lymphocytic leukemia: a report from the Children's Cancer Study Group. Med Pediatr Oncol 1983;11:1.
254. Amadori S, Tribalto M, Pacilli L, De Laurentis C, Papa G, Mandelli F. Sequential combination of methotrexate and L-asparaginase in the treatment of refractory acute leukemia. Cancer Treat Rep 1980;64: 939.
255. Peterson BA, Bloomfield CD. High-dose methotrexate for the remission induction of refractory adult acute lymphocytic leukemia. Med Pediatr Oncol 1978;5:79.
256. Rivera GK. The epipodophyllotoxin teniposide in therapy for childhood acute lymphocytic leukemia. (Editorial) J Clin Oncol 1988;6: 191.
257. Morra E, Lazzarino M, Alessandrino EP, Inverardi D, Canevari A, Bernasconi C. VP 16-213 and cytosine-arabinoside combination chemotherapy for refractory acute lymphoblastic leukemia in adults. Eur J Cancer Clin Oncol 1984;20:1471.
258. Morra E, Lazzarino M, Brusamolino E, et al. Systemic high-dose cytosine arabinoside (HDARA-C) for treatment of central nervous system disease (CNS+) in adult acute lymphoblastic leukemia (ALL) and non-Hodgkin's lymphoma (NHL). Proc Am Soc Clin Oncol 1986;5:161.
259. Arlin ZA, Feldman E, Kempin S, et al. Amsacrine with high-dose cytarabine is highly effective therapy for refractory and relapsed acute lymphoblastic leukemia in adults. Blood 1988;72:433.
260. Sadowitz D, Smith SD, Shuster J, et al. Treatment of late bone marrow relapse in children with acute lymphoblastic leukemia: a Pediatric Oncology Group study. Blood 1993;81:602.
261. Pinkel D. Allogeneic bone marrow transplantation in children with acute leukemia: a practice whose time has gone. Leukemia 1989;3: 242.
262. Henze G, Fengler R, Hartmann R, et al. Six-year experience with a comprehensive approach to the treatment of recurrent childhood acute lymphoblastic leukemia (ALL-REZ BFM 85): a relapse study of the BFM Group. Blood 1991;78:1166.
263. Butturini A, Rivera GK, Bortin MM, Gale RP. Which treatment for childhood acute lymphoblastic leukaemia in second remission. Lancet 1987;1:429.
264. Rivera GK. Cyclophosphamide and bone marrow transplantation. (Letter) N Engl J Med 1988;318:1541.
265. Brochstein JA, Kernan NA, Groshen S, et al. Allogeneic bone marrow transplantation after hyperfractionated total-body irradiation and cyclophosphamide in children with acute leukemia. N Engl J Med 1987;317:1618.
266. Nesbit ME, D'Angio GJ, Sather HN, et al. Effect of isolated central nervous system leukaemia on bone marrow remission and survival in childhood acute lymphoblastic leukemia: a report from Children's Cancer Study Group. Lancet 1981;1:1386.
267. Kun LE, Camitta BM, Mulhern RK, et al. Treatment of meningeal relapse in childhood acute lymphoblastic leukemia. I. Results of craniospinal irradiation. J Clin Oncol 1984;2:359.
268. Land VJ, Thomas PR, Boyett JM, et al. Comparison of maintenance treatment regimens for first central nervous system relapse in children with acute lymphocytic leukemia: a Pediatric Oncology Group study. Cancer 1985;56:81.
269. Willoughby MLN. Treatment of overt meningeal leukemia in children: results of second MRC meningeal trial. Br Med J 1976;1:864.
270. Winick N, Smith SD, Shuster J, Wharam MD, Buchanan GR, Rivera GK. Treatment of central nervous system relapse in children with acute lymphoblastic leukemia: a Pediatric Oncology Group study. J Clin Oncol 1993;11:271.
271. Rivera GK, Ochs J, Roberson PK, et al. Intensive salvage therapy for isolated initial CNS relapses in childhood ALL. Blood 1986;68:802.
272. Nesbit ME, Robison LL, Ortega JA. Testicular relapse in childhood acute lymphoblastic leukemia: association with pretreatment patient characteristics and treatment. A report for Children's Cancer Study Group. Cancer 1980;45:2009.
273. Pui C-H, Dahl GV, Bowman WP, et al. Elective testicular biopsy during chemotherapy for childhood leukaemia is of no clinical value. Lancet 1985;2:410.
274. Wofford MM, Smith SD, Shuster JJ, et al. Treatment of occult or late overt testicular relapse in children with acute lymphoblastic leukemia: a Pediatric Oncology Group study. J Clin Oncol 1992;10:624.
275. Bowman WP, Aur RJ, Hustu HO, Rivera G. Isolated testicular relapse in acute lymphocytic leukemia of childhood: categories and influence on survival. J Clin Oncol 1984;2:924.
276. Shapiro E, Kinsella TJ, Makuch RW, et al. Effects of fractionated irradiation on endocrine aspects of testicular function. J Clin Oncol 1985;3:1232.
277. Mathe G, Schwarzenberg L, Mery AM, et al. Extensive histological and cytological survey of patients with acute leukaemia in complete remission. Br Med J 1966;5488:640.
278. Nies BA, Bodey GP. The persistence of extramedullary leukemic infiltrates during bone marrow remission of acute leukemia. Blood 1965;26:133.
279. Bunin NJ, Pui C-H, Hustu HO, Rivera GK. Unusual extramedullary relapses in children with acute lymphoblastic leukemia. J Pediatr 1986;109:665.
280. Chu J-Y, Cradock TV, Davis RK, Tennant NE. Ovarian tumor as a manifestation of relapse in acute lymphoblastic leukemia. Cancer 1981;48:377.
281. Cecalupo AJ, Frankel LS, Sullivan MP. Pelvic and ovarian extra-

medullary leukemia relapse in young girls: a report of four cases and review of the literature. Cancer 1982;50:587.
282. Zarrouk SO, Kim TH, Hargreaves HK, Ragab AH. Leukemic involvement of the ovaries of childhood acute lymphocytic leukemia. J Pediatr 1982;3:422.
283. Patte C, Michon J, Bouffet E, et al. High survival rate of childhood B-cell lymphoma and leukemia (ALL) as result of the LMB 89 Protocol of the SFOP (French Pediatric Oncology Society). Proc Am Soc Clin Oncol (Abstract) 1992;11:340.
284. Philip T, Meckenstock R, Deconnick E, et al. Treatment of poor prognosis Burkitt's lymphoma in adults with the Societe Francaise d'Oncologie Pediatrique LMB: a study of the Federation Nationale des Centres de Lutte Contre le Cancer (FNLCC). Eur J Cancer 1992;28A: 1954.
285. Reiter A, Schrappe M, Henze G, et al. B-cell acute lymphoblastic leukemia of childhood treatment strategy and results in three BFM trials. (Abstract) Haematologica 1992;76:105.
286. Scott EP, Forman SJ, Spruce WE, et al. Bone marrow ablation followed by allogeneic bone marrow transplantation for patients with high-risk acute lymphoblastic leukemia during complete remission. Transplant Proc 1983;15:1395.
287. Thomas ED, Sanders JE, Flournoy N, et al. Marrow transplantation for patients with acute lymphoblastic leukemia in remission. Blood 1979;54:468.
288. Gale RP, Kersey JH, Bortin MM, et al. Bone-marrow transplantation for acute lymphoblastic leukaemia. Lancet 1983;2:663.
289. O'Reilly RJ. Allogeneic bone marrow transplantation. Blood 1983;62: 941.
290. Bearman SI, Appelbaum FR, Buckner CD, et al. Regimen-related toxicity in patients undergoing bone marrow transplantation. J Clin Oncol 1988;6:1562.
291. Herzig R, Brotin MM, Gluckman E, et al. Optimal timing of bone marrow transplantation in patients with high risk acute lymphoblastic leukemia. Lancet 1987;1:786.
292. Zander AR, Keating M, Dicke K, et al. A comparison of marrow transplantation with chemotherapy for adults with acute leukemia of poor prognosis in first complete remission. J Clin Oncol 1988;6:1548.
293. Gale RP. Immune intervention in disease. Ann Intern Med 1987;106: 257.
294. Martin PJ, Hanson JA, Buckner CD, et al. Effects of in vitro depletion of T cells in HLA-identical allogeneic marrow grafts. Blood 1985;66: 664.
295. Marmont AM. T cell depletion in allogeneic bone marrow transplantation: progress and problems. Bone Marrow Transplant 1989;Suppl 4:229.
296. Buckner CD, Clift RA. Marrow transplantation for acute lymphoblastic leukemia. Semin Hematol 1984;21:43.
297. Mayer R. Allogeneic transplantation versus intensive chemotherapy in first-remission acute leukemia: is there a "best choice?" J Clin Oncol 1988;6:1532.
298. Gale RP, Butturini A. Acute lymphoblastic leukemia: chemotherapy versus transplantation. In: Gale RP, Champlin RE, eds. Bone marrow transplantation: current controversies, New York: Alan R Liss, 1989: 67.
299. Vernant JP, Marit G, Maraninchi D, et al. Allogeneic bone marrow transplantation in adults with acute lymphoblastic leukemia in first complete remission. J Clin Oncol 1988;6:227.
300. Schmitz N, Gassman W, Rister M, et al. Fractionated total body irradiation and high dose VP16-213 followed by allogeneic bone marrow transplantation in advanced leukemias. Blood 1988;72:1567.
301. Blume KG, Forman SJ, Snyder DS, et al. Allogeneic bone marrow transplantation for acute lymphoblastic leukemia during first complete remission. Transplantation 1987;43:389.
302. Barrett AJ, Kendra JR, Lucas CF, et al. Bone marrow transplantation for acute lymphoblastic leukaemia. Br J Haematol 1982;52:181.
303. Coccia PF, Strandjord SE, Warkentin PI, et al. High-dose cytosine arabinoside and fractionated total-body irradiation: an improved preparative regimen for bone marrow transplantation of children with acute lymphoblastic leukemia in remission. Blood 1988;71:888.
304. Chessells JM, Rogers DW, Leiper AD, et al. Bone-marrow transplantation has a limited role in prolonging second marrow remission in childhood lymphoblastic leukaemia. Lancet 1986;1:1239.
305. Beatty PG, Clift RA, Mickelson EM, et al. Marrow transplantation from related donors other than HLA-identical siblings. N Engl J Med 1985;313:765.
306. Rivera GK. Therapeutic options for children with acute lymphocytic leukemia who fail on contemporary protocols. In: Bone marrow transplantation: current controversies. Alan R Liss, 1989:31.
306a. Pui C-H, Carroll AJ, Raimondi SC, et al. Clinical presentation, karyotypic characterization, and treatment outcome of childhood acute lymphoblastic leukemia with a near-haploid or hypodiploid <45 line. Blood 1990;75:1170.
307. Forman SJ, O'Donnell MR, Nademanee AP, et al. Bone marrow transplantation for patients with Philadelphia chromosome-positive acute lymphoblastic leukemia. Blood 1987;70:587.
308. Cheson BD, Lacerna L, Leyland-Jones B, et al. Autologous bone marrow transplantation: current status and future directions. Ann Intern Med 1989;110:51.
309. Kaizer H, Stuart RK, Brookmeyer R, et al. Autologous bone marrow transplantation in acute leukemia: a phase II study of 4-hydroperoxycyclophosphamide to purge tumor cells. Blood 1985;65:1504.
310. Reiffers J, Marit G, Boiron JM, et al. The role of peripheral blood stem cells as rescue after myeloablative therapy. Bone Marrow Transplant 1989;Suppl 4:212
311. Kersey JH, Weisdorf D, Nesbit ME, et al. Comparison of autologous and allogeneic bone marrow transplantation for treatment of high-risk refractory acute lymphoblastic leukemia. N Engl J Med 1987;317: 461.
312. Mortimer J, Blinder MA, Schulman S, et al. Relapse of acute leukemia after marrow transplantation: natural history and results of subsequent therapy. J Clin Oncol 1989;7:50.
313. Bostrom B, Woods WG, Nesbit ME, et al. Successful reinduction of patients with acute lymphoblastic leukemia who relapse following bone marrow transplantation. J Clin Oncol 1987;5:376.
314. Miller AP, Stool JA, Brown WG. Pseudohypoglycemia in a child with chronic myelogenous leukemia. Med Rec Am 1966;59:402.
315. Leidler F, Fussell WO. The brain in leukemia. Arch Pathol 1945; 40:1.
316. Fernbach DJ. Natural history of acute leukemia. In: Sutow WW, Fernbach DJ, Vietti TJ, eds. Clinical pediatric oncology. St Louis, CV Mosby, 1984:332.
317. Greydanus DE, Burgert OE, Gilchrist GS. Hypothalamic syndrome in children with acute lymphoblastic leukemia. Mayo Clin Proc 1978;53: 217.
318. Miller VI, Campbell WG Jr. Diabetes insipidus as a complication of leukemia: a case report with a literature reviews. Cancer 1971;28: 666.
319. Bunin NJ, Pui C-H. Differing complications of hyperleukocytosis in children with acute lymphoblastic or acute nonlymphoblastic leukemia. J Clin Oncol 1985;3:1590.
320. Kim TH, Lui VK, Woodruff RD, Ragab AH. Testicular biopsy prior to termination of leukemic therapy. J Pediatr 1979;94:95.
321. Askin FB, Land VJ, Sullivan MP, et al. Occult testicular leukemia: testicular biopsy at three years continuous complete remission of childhood leukemia—a Southwest Oncology Group Study. Cancer 1981;47:470.
322. Mahoney DH Jr, Gonzales ET, Ferry GD, Sanjad SA, von Noorden GK, Fernbach DJ. Childhood acute leukemia: a search for occult extramedullary disease prior to discontinuation of chemotherapy. Cancer 1981;48:1964.
323. Vadakan VV, Ortega J. Priapism in acute lymphoblastic leukemia. Cancer 1972;30:373.
324. Chu JY, Craddock TV, Danis RK, Tennant NE. Ovarian tumor as manifestation of relapse in acute lymphoblastic leukemia. Cancer 1981;48:377.
325. Jaffe N, Traggis DG, Tefft M. Acute leukemia presenting with pericardial tamponade. Pediatrics 1970;45:461.
326. Roberts WC, Bodey GP, Wertlake PT. The heart in acute leukemia: a study of 420 autopsy cases. Am J Cardiol 1968;21:388.
327. Bodey GP, Powell RD Jr, Hersh EM, Yeterian A, Freireich EJ. Pulmonary complications of acute leukemia. Cancer 1966;19:781.
328. Klatte EC, Yardley J. The pulmonary manifestations and complications of leukemia. Am J Roentgenol 1963;89:598.
329. Wells RJ, Weetman RM, Ballantine TV, Grosfeld JL, Baehner RL. Pulmonary leukemia in children presenting as diffuse interstitial pneumonia. J Pediatr 1980;96:262.
330. Gilmartin D. Leukemic involvement of the thymus in children. Br J Radiol 1963;36:211.
331. Holbrook CT, Elsas FJ, Crist WM, Castleberry RP. Acute leukemia and hypopyon. J Pediatr 1978;93:626.
332. Fonken HA, Ellis PP. Leukemic infiltrates in the iris: successful treatment of secondary glaucoma with x-irradiation. Arch Ophthalmol 1966;76:32.
333. Simmons CR, Harle TS, Singleton EB. The osseous manifestations of leukemia in children. Radiol Clin North Am 1968;6:115.
334. Wilson JVK. The bone lesions of childhood leukemia: a survey of 140 cases. Radiology 1959;72:672.
335. Masera G, Carnelli V, Ferrari M, Recchia M, Bellini F. Prognostic significance of radiological bone involvement in childhood acute lymphoblastic leukaemia. Arch Dis Child 1977;52:530.
336. Schaller J. Arthritis as a presenting manifestation of malignancy in children. J Pediatr 1972;81:793.
337. Abramson SJ, Berdon WE, Baker DH. Childhood typhlitis: its increasing association with acute myelogenous leukemia—report of five cases. Radiology 1983;146:61.
338. Moir CR, Scudamore CH, Benny WB. Typhlitis: selective surgical management. J Surg 1986;151:563.
339. Shamberger RC, Weinstein HJ, Delorey MJ, Levey RH. The medical and surgical management of typhlitis in children with acute nonlymphocytic (myelogenous) leukemia. Cancer 1986;57:603.
340. al-Rashid RA, Harned RK. Dysphagia due to leukemic involvement of the esophagus. Am J Dis Child 1971;121:75.
341. Newburger PE, Cassady JR, Jaffe N. Esophagitis due to Adriamycin and radiation therapy for childhood malignancy. Cancer 1978;42:417.

342. Hyams JS, Batrus CL, Grand RJ, Sallan SE. Cancer chemotherapy-induced lactose malabsorption in children. Cancer 1982;49:646.
343. Cocchi R, Borgheresi S. The Mikulicz syndrome in the course of leukemia. Minerva Pediatr 1966;18:997.
344. Einhour M, Diards I. Hepatotoxicity of mercaptopurine. JAMA 1964;188:802.
345. Wetherley-Mein G, Cottom DG. Portal fibrosis in acute leukemia. Br J Haematol 1956;2:345.
346. Link MP, Roper M, Dorfman RF, Crist WM, Cooper MD, Levy R. Cutaneous lymphoblastic lymphoma with pre-B markers. Blood 1983;61:838.
347. LaVenuta F, Moore JA. Involvement of the inner ear in acute stem cell leukemia: report of two cases. Ann Otol Rhinol Laryngol 1972;81:132.
348. Kennedy BJ, Bornstein R, Brunning RD, Oines D. Breast involvement in acute lymphatic leukemia: daunorubicin-induced remission—*Pneumocystis carinii* pneumonia. Cancer 1970;25:693.
349. Eguiguren JM, Schell MJ, Crist WM, Kunkel K, Rivera GK. Complications and outcome in childhood acute lymphoblastic leukemia with hyperleukocytosis. Blood 1992;79:871.
350. Maurer HS, Steinherz PG, Gaynon PS, et al. The effect of initial management of hyperleukocytosis on early complications and outcome of children with acute lymphoblastic leukemia. J Clin Oncol 1988;6:1425.
351. Pizzo PA. Infectious complications in the child with cancer. II. Management of specific infectious organisms. J Pediatr 1981;98:513.
352. Shenep JL, Hughes WT, Roberson PK, et al. Vancomycin, ticarcillin, and amikacin compared with ticarcillin-clavulanate and amikacin in the empirical treatment of febrile, neutropenic children with cancer. N Engl J Med 1988;319:1053.
353. Hughes WT, Rivera GK, Schell MJ, Thornton D, Lott L. Successful intermittent chemoprophylaxis for *Pneumocystis carinii* pneumonitis. N Engl J Med 1987;316:1627.
354. Hughes WT, Feldman S, Gigliotti F, et al. Prevention of infectious complications in acute lymphoblastic leukemia. Semin Oncol 1985;12:180.
355. Hersh EM, Wong VG, Henderson ES, et al. Hepatotoxic effects of methotrexate. Cancer 1966;19:600.
356. Coggins PR, Ravdin RG, Eisman SM. Clinical pharmacology and preliminary evaluation of cytoxin (cyclophosphamide). Cancer Chemother Rep 1959;3:9.
357. Butler HE, Morgan JM, Smythe CM. Mercaptopurine and acquired tubular dysfunction in adult nephrons. Arch Intern Med 1965;116:853.
358. Warne GL, Fairley GF, Hobbs JB, et al. Cyclophosphamide-induced ovarian failure. N Engl J Med 1973;289:1159.
359. Blum RH, Carter SK. Review of Adriamycin, a new anticancer drug with significant clinical activity. Ann Intern Med 1974;80:249.
360. Mills BA, Roberts RW. Cyclophosphamide-induced cardiomyopathy: a report of two cases and review of the English literature. Cancer 1979;43:2223.
361. Lipshultz SE, Colan SD, Gelber RD, Perez-Atayde AR, Sallan SE, Sanders SP. Late cardiac effects of doxorubicin therapy for acute lymphoblastic leukemia in childhood. N Engl J Med 1991;324:808.
362. Steinherz LJ, Steinherz PG, Tan CTC, Heller G, Murphy L. Cardiac toxicity 4 to 20 years after completing anthracycline therapy. JAMA 1991;266:1672.
363. Ragab AH, Freich RS, Vietti TJ. Osteoporotic fractures secondary to methotrexate therapy of acute leukemia in remission. Cancer 1970;25:580.
364. Schriock EA, Schell MJ, Carter M, Hustu O, Ochs JJ. Abnormal growth patterns and adult short stature in 115 long-term survivors of childhood leukemia. J Clin Oncol 1991;9:400.
365. Soni SS, Martin GW, Pitner SE, et al. Effects of CNS irradiation on neuropsychologic functioning of children with acute lymphoblastic leukemia. N Engl J Med 1975;293:113.
366. Poplack DG, Brouwers P. Adverse sequelae of central nervous system therapy. Clin Oncol 1985;4:263.
367. Price RA, Birdwell DA. The central nervous system in childhood leukemia. III. Mineralizing microangiopathy and dystrophic calcification. Cancer 1978;42:717.
368. Price RA, Jamieson PA. The central nervous system in childhood leukemia. II. Subacute leukoencephalopathy. Cancer 1975;35:306.
369. Bleyer WA, Drake JCR, Chabner BA. Neurotoxicity and elevated cerebrospinal fluid methotrexate concentration in meningeal leukemia. N Engl J Med 1973;289:770.
370. Ch'ien LT, Aur RJA, Verzosa MS, et al. Progression of methotrexate-induced leukoencephalopathy in children with leukemia. Med Pediatr Oncol 1981;9:133.
371. Poplack DG. Acute lymphoblastic leukemia. In: Pizzo PA, Poplack DG, eds. Principles and practice of pediatric oncology. Philadelphia, JB Lippincott, 1989:323.
372. Brouwers P, Riccardi R, Fedio R, Poplack DG. Long-term neuropsychological sequelae of childhood leukemia: correlations with CT brain scan abnormalities. J Pediatr 1985;106:723.
373. Kay HEM, Knapton PJ, O'Sullivan JP, et al. Encephalopathy in acute leukemia associated with methotrexate therapy. Arch Dis Child 1972;47:344.
374. Rowland JH, Glidewell OJ, Sibley RF. Effects of different forms of central nervous system prophylaxis on neuropsychologic function in childhood leukemia. J Clin Oncol 1984;2:1327.
375. Williams JM, Davis KS. Central nervous system prophylactic treatment for childhood leukemia: neuropsychologic outcome studies. Cancer Treat Rev 1986;13:113.
376. Mulhern RK, Wasserman AL, Fairclough D, Ochs J. Memory function in disease-free survivors of childhood acute lymphocytic leukemia given CNS prophylaxis with or without 1,800 cGy cranial irradiation. J Clin Oncol 1988;6:315.
377. Kelaghan J, Myers MH, Mulvihill JJ, et al. Educational achievement of long-term survivors of childhood and adolescent cancer. Med Pediatr Oncol 1988;16:320.
378. Tebbi CK, Bromberg C, Peidmonte M. Long-term vocational adjustment of cancer patients diagnosed during adolescence. Cancer 1989;63:213.
379. Harris JR, Coleman CN. Estimating the risk of second primary tumors following cancer treatment. J Clin Oncol 1989;7:5.
380. Li FP, Cassady JR, Jaffe N. Risk of second tumors in survivors of childhood cancer. Cancer 1975;35:1230.
381. Mike V, Meadows AT, D'Angio GD. Incidence of second malignant neoplasms in children: results of an international study. Lancet 1982;ii:1326.
382. Refetoff S, Harrison J, Karanfilski BT, et al. Continuing occurrence of thyroid carcinoma after irradiation to the neck in infancy and childhood. N Engl J Med 1975;292:171.
383. Sieber SM, Adamson RH. Toxicity of antineoplastic agents in man: chromosomal aberrations, antifertility effects, congenital malformations and carcinogenic potential. Adv Cancer Res 1975;22:155.
384. Ochs J, Mulhern RK. Late effects of antileukemic treatment. Pediatr Clin North Am 1988;35:815.
385. Albo V, Muller P, Leiken S, et al. Nine brain tumors as a late effect in children "cured" of acute lymphoblastic leukemia from a single protocol. Proc Am Soc Clin Oncol (Abstract) 1985;4:172.
386. Pratt CB, George SL, Hancock ML. Second malignant neoplasms (SMNs) in survivors of childhood acute lymphoblastic leukemia (ALL). (Abstract) Pediatr Res 1988;23:345A.
387. Pui C-H, Crist WM, Look AT. Biology and clinical significance of cytogenetic abnormalities in childhood acute lymphoblastic leukemia. Blood 1990;76:1449.
388. Niemeyer CM, Reiter A, Riehm H, Donnelly M, Gelber RD, Sallan SE. Comparative results of two intensive treatment programs for childhood acute lymphoblastic leukemia. Ann Oncol 1991;2:745.
389. Ritter J, Creutzig U, Reiter A, Riehm H, Schelling G. Childhood leukemia: cooperative Berlin-Frankfurt-Münster trials in the Federal Republic of Germany. J Cancer Res Clin Oncol 1990;116:100.
390. Schaison G, Sommelet D, Bancillon A, et al. Treatment of acute lymphoblastic leukemia French protocol Fralle 83-87. Leukemia 1991;6:148.
391. Rivera GK, Buchanan GB, Boyett J, et al. Intensive retreatment of childhood acute lymphoblastic leukemia in first bone marrow relapse. A Pediatric Oncology Group study. N Engl J Med 1986;315:273.
392. Chessells JM, Bailey CC, Richards S. MRC UKALL X: the UK protocol for childhood ALL—1985–1990. Leukemia 1991;6:157.

Blood: Principles and Practice of Hematology,
edited by Robert I. Handin, Thomas P. Stossel, and Samuel E. Lux.
J.B. Lippincott Company, Philadelphia © 1995.

28

Chronic Lymphoid Leukemias

Kenneth A. Foon
Robert Peter Gale

Leukemia was first described clinically by Velpeau in 1827[1]; in 1844, Donne showed that increased leukocytes were responsible for the clinical features of leukemia.[2] The chronic leukemias were first described by Bennett and Virchow in 1847.[4,5] Both splenic and lymphoid types were identified, roughly corresponding to chronic myelogenous leukemia (CML) and chronic lymphoid leukemia (CLL), respectively. At that time, leukemia was thought to originate in the spleen or lymph node. In 1870, however, Neuman showed that blood cells arise from the bone marrow and suggested this as the site of transformation of leukemia. The distinction between CML and CLL became clearer in the latter part of the last century when histochemical stains became available.[8] By 1909, current notions of CML and CLL were described in popular medical texts.[9] The initial treatment of chronic leukemias involved arsenicals. This was followed by the introduction of radiation therapy in 1902.[10–12] The modern era of chronic leukemia treatment began with the use of nitrogen mustard and radiophosphorus in the 1940s.[13,14] In the 1950s, these were gradually replaced with busulfan and chlorambucil.

Many of the current concepts regarding the immunology and biology of CLL were proposed by Dameshek in 1967.[15] Over the past 20 years, a variety of lymphoid malignancies have been distinguished clinically, morphologically, and immunologically from CLL. These diseases are summarized in Table 28-1.

CLL is characterized by proliferation and accumulation of mature-appearing but biologically immature B lymphocytes. The National Cancer Institute–Sponsored Working Group[16] and the International Workshop on Chronic Lymphoid Leukemia[17] have proposed similar criteria for the diagnosis of CLL, which include:

- Lymphocytosis (higher than 5×10^9/L) sustained for 4 weeks
- Cells with κ or λ light-chain, low-density surface immunoglobulin (Ig) and CD5 antigen
- Mature lymphocytes with no more than 55% atypical and immature lymphoid cells
- Over 30% bone marrow involvement

Important advances have been made in our understanding of the complex immunology, cytogenetics, cell physiology, and biochemistry associated with CLL.

EPIDEMIOLOGY AND CAUSE

Typically, CLL occurs in people over 50 years of age (median age, 60 years). Less than 10% of cases occur in adults under 40 years of age; rare cases have been reported in children. CLL is acquired, and only rarely is there concordance in genetically identical twins. In one set of twins, Ig gene rearrangements in the twins were distinct.[18] No reproducible pattern of inheritance has been reported.[19]

The cause of CLL is unknown. Unlike CML and acute leukemias, CLL is not induced by radiation, chemicals, or alkylating agents.[20] CLL represents 30% of reported leukemia cases in the west. Ten thousand new cases are diagnosed annually in the United States. In contrast, CLL is rare in Asia, representing less than 5% of all leukemia cases.

Retroviruses are implicated in some rare forms of lymphoid leukemia. For example, human T-cell leukemia/lymphoma virus type I (HTLV-I) is implicated in the cause of adult T-cell leukemia/lymphoma (ATL)[21–23] (see Table 28-1). The mechanism whereby HTLV-I causes ATL is unknown. In addition to ATL, HTLV-I infection has been reported in a chronic form of ATL, persistent T lymphocytosis,[24] which resembles but is distinct from CLL.

Recently, HTLV-I infection was reported in 6 of 17 cases of CLL in Jamaica. The leukemia cells did not contain virus but, in some cases, synthesized antibody to a virus-related envelope protein designated p24. This led to the hypothesis that CLL might have arisen as a response to HTLV-I infection rather than through transformation of target cells.[25,26] A preliminary report described isolation of retroviral-like particles and reverse-transcriptase activity in cultured CLL cells.[27] A monoclonal antibody to the viral particles cross-reacted with HTLV-I. Additionally, antibody to the 19,000-dalton core protein of HTLV-I reacted with putative CLL virus. These findings are unconfirmed. A second related retrovirus, HTLV-II, was identified in T-cell prolymphocytic leukemia (PLL) and T-cell hairy-cell leukemia.[28,29]

The possible role of DNA viruses, such as Epstein-Barr virus (EBV) and cytomegalovirus, in CLL is unknown. Direct involvement of EBV seems unlikely. CLL cells can be infected by EBV as indicated by expression of Epstein-Barr nuclear antigen; this does not routinely lead to immortalization.[30] One EBV-infected cell line was shown to produce tumors in nude mice.[31]

TABLE 28-1. Clinical and Laboratory Features of the Chronic Lymphoid Leukemias

Disease	Median Age at Diagnosis (y)	Male/Female Ratio	Leukocyte Counts × 10^9/L	Lymph Nodes	Spleen (%)	Skin	Morphology (Figure)	Surface Immunoglobulin	Phenotype	Other
B LYMPHOCYTES										
Chronic lymphocytic leukemia	60	2:1	10–200	>50	50	<5	3	Weak	CD19, CD20, CD21, CD23, CD25, CD5	Autoimmunity, hypogammaglobulinemia
Prolymphocytic leukemia	65	4:1	100–500	<25	>90	<5	6	Strong	CD19, CD20, FMC7, CD22	
NHL follicular leukemia	50	2:1	50–200	>90	75	<5	8	Strong	CD10, CD19, CD20, CD21, FMC7, CD22	
Hairy-cell leukemia	50	5:1	1–100	<20	>75	<5	9	Strong	CD19, CD20, CD25, CD11c, B-ly7	Pancytopenia
Waldenström's macroglobulinemia	50	1:1	5–50	>30	30	<5	7	Strong	CD19, CD20, PCA-1	Elevated IgM
T LYMPHOCYTES										
Prolymphocytic leukemia	65	4:1	100–500	<25	>90	<10		Absent	CD2, CD3, CD4 and/or CD8	HTLV-2 (rare)
Adut T-cell leukemia/lymphoma	40	2:1	5–150	>90	>50	>50	14	Absent	CD2, CD3, CD4, CD25	HTLV-1, hypercalcemia, cutaneous disease
LGL leukemia	50	2:1	5–300	<10	30	<5	11	Absent	CD2, CD3, CD8, CD16, CD56	Granulocytopenia
Cutaneous T-cell lymphoma	55	2:1	5–150	50	10	100	17	Absent	CD2, CD3, CD4	Extensive cutaneous disease

NHL, non-Hodgkin's lymphoma; LGL, large granular lymphocytic; HTLV, human T-cell leukemia/lymphoma virus.

IMMUNOLOGY

Immune Features

Chronic lymphoid leukemia results from malignant transformation of a B lymphocyte; the small proportion of reported cases involving T lymphocytes most likely represent misdiagnosed cases of one of the chronic T-lymphoid leukemias presented in Table 28-1 or an unidentified T-cell malignancy. CLL is clonal; the cells express a single Ig light chain, either κ or λ, on the cell-surface membrane.[32,33] More sophisticated techniques confirm clonality by unique Ig idiotype,[34,35] a single pattern of glucose-6-phosphate dehydrogenase (G6PD) activity in heterozygotes,[36,37] clonal chromosomal abnormalities,[38] and clonal Ig gene rearrangement.[39,40]

CLL cells display low-density surface Ig, typically μ or μ and δ, less commonly γ, α, or no heavy chain. Surface Ig is estimated at about 9000 molecules per cell.[41] Cytoplasmic Ig is also present.[42] Distinct differences between cytoplasmic, surface, and secretory Ig are detected.[43] Cells from less than 5% of patients with CLL secrete sufficient levels of IgM to be detected by serum protein electrophoresis. Using high-resolution electrophoresis and immunofixation, circulating monoclonal IgM paraproteins are identified in one fourth to one half or more of patients.[44–46]

Additional surface features of CLL cells include the B-lymphocyte antigens CD19, CD20, CD21, CD23, and CD24.[47–57] The cells also express the nominal T-cell–associated antigen CD5, which is identified on a subpopulation of normal B cells.[57–59] CD5 B cells are also found in fetal liver and in the blood of bone marrow transplant recipients in the early recovery phase.[60,61] Cells from about half of patients with CLL express the CD25 activation antigen,[62] and most of these patients have soluble CD25 detected in their serum.[63] FMC7, CD22, and some myeloid antigens are identified in about one fourth of cases; CD10 and additional T-cell–associated antigens are not found.

The malignant B lymphocyte that is the usual target of transformation in CLL is an intermediate cell with some but not all morphologic features of mature B cells. This cell appears to be arrested in its normal differentiation scheme and does not normally progress to the final stages of B-cell development, although a small proportion of plasma cells from patients with CLL express the same Ig idiotype as the CLL cells, suggesting that they are a component of the malignant clone.[64] Incubation of CLL cells in vitro with tumor promoters, such as phorbol esters or B-cell mitogens, induces differentiation to activated cells similar to PLL cells,[65] hairy cells,[66] or mature plasma cells.[67–70] Under these conditions, the cells may begin to actively secrete Ig. Mitogen-induced switching from cell-surface IgM to secreted IgG is also reported.[71] These data confirm that the malignant B cells typical of CLL are not irreversibly frozen at an immature level of B-cell development.

Immune Function of Chronic Lymphoid Leukemia Cells

Many studies have been done on the immune function of CLL cells. Low levels of surface Ig and impaired Ig capping suggest abnormalities of membrane motility.[72] Despite the fact that CLL cells have Ia antigens, they show limited or no stimulatory activity in autologous and allogeneic mixed lymphocyte culture.[73,74] Other cell activities are also abnormal, including in vitro response to B-cell mitogens, such as pokeweed mitogen, lipopolysaccharide, and EBV, and decreased activity in antibody-dependent cellular cytotoxicity.[75–78] CLL cells have a decreased proliferative response to B-cell growth factor. This is likely to be secondary to the impaired expression of appropriate cell-surface receptors.[79] Cytochalasin B is a potent mitogen for CLL cells.[80] Several studies have used techniques to culture colonies of malignant B cells derived from patients with CLL in semisolid agar.[81–83] These techniques may help analyze details of immune function of CLL.

Immune Function of T Lymphocytes and Natural Killer Cells

Increased absolute numbers of T lymphocytes have been reported in untreated patients with CLL. These levels fluctuate during the course of the disease.[84] In general, patients with CLL show a marked inversion of the ratio of normal helper T cells (CD4) to suppressor T cells (CD8) in the blood[85–90] with increased suppressor T cells. Additional T-cell surface marker abnormalities include a decreased proportion of cells reactive with the pan-T anti-CD3 antibody and the presence of cells that simultaneously express helper T-cell–associated and suppressor T-cell–associated antigens,[91] a characteristic that is normally present on some thymocytes and in a minor population of circulating T lymphocytes.[92] These abnormalities of T-cell subsets or levels correlate with disease stage, therapy, or both in some studies.[93,94]

Some functional studies of T cells appear normal,[95] but proliferative responses to autologous or allogeneic B cells are impaired.[78,96] Progenitor T cells, assayed by colony growth in semisolid agar, have been reported decreased in some[97,98] studies.[99] Helper T-cell function is decreased,[100] and there may be abnormal suppressor T cells as well. It was recently reported that CLL cells secrete or shed an immune regulatory ganglioside suppressive for lymphocytes.[101]

Spontaneous and antibody-dependent cytotoxicity are also decreased in CLL, suggesting an abnormality in natural killer (NK) cells.[102,103] Numbers of NK cells detected by reactivity with CD56 and CD57 are increased in CLL; however, studies with CD16, which identifies the FcR III typical of NK cells, indicate that cells with this antigen are increased.[104,105] These data suggest increased numbers of functionally inactive NK cells in CLL. Some NK-cell functional abnormalities found in CLL are corrected by in vitro or in vivo exposure to interleukin-2 (IL-2), interferon (IFN), or synthetic thymic polypeptide.[106–108]

The origin of T-cell abnormalities in CLL is unknown; it is uncertain whether they are a cause or a consequence of the disease. T cells from patients with CLL are probably not part of the malignant clone. This notion is supported by the lack of chromosomal abnormalities typical of the CLL clone in T cells[109] and by heterozygosity for polymorphic X-linked genetic markers, such as G6PD.[110] Most of these studies, however, were performed in patients with CLL of relatively brief duration. The T cells tested may therefore have developed before the onset of leukemia. Consequently, it is not possible to exclude involvement of an immature stem cell with both T- and B-cell differentiation potential as the site of transformation in some cases of CLL. Consistent with this notion is the finding of clonal rearrangement of the T-cell β-receptor in the malignant B cells in about 10% of cases of CLL.[111] These data are also consistent with the origin of the disease in an immature B cell.

Hypogammaglobulinemia

Hypogammaglobulinemia occurs in patients with CLL. This incidence is time-dependent; eventually, almost all CLL patients develop hypogammaglobulinemia. Infections, particularly with encapsulated organisms, and more recently with gram-negative bacteria, are a frequent cause of morbidity and mortality.[112,113] Consistent with their abnormal B- and T-cell function, CLL patients have impaired antibody and cell-mediated immunity to recall antigens.[114–116]

The pathogenesis of hypogammaglobulinemia in CLL is controversial and likely reflects several factors. For example, decreased in vitro Ig synthesis to polyclonal mitogens or antigens has been reported.[117] Regulatory abnormalities of T cells may also be important,[88–90,118] including reversal of normal helper/suppressor T-cell ratios. NK cells (CD16+, CD3−) decrease Ig secretion by normal B cells in patients with CLL and hypogammaglobulinemia.[119]

Autoimmunity

Many patients with CLL may develop features of autoimmunity of the hematopoietic system. For example, autoimmune hemolytic anemia occurs in about 20% of cases sometime during the course of the disease.[120] This usually results from IgG antibodies against Rh blood group antigens. These autoantibodies are typically polyclonal and are therefore not produced by the malignant B-cell clone of CLL. Also, about 10% of patients with CLL develop thrombocytopenia or neutropenia from autoantibodies to platelets or neutrophils.[121,122] Rarely, patients develop a syndrome resembling pure red blood cell (RBC) aplasia.[123]

Why patients with CLL develop these autoimmune disorders with such high frequency, particularly in the face of seemingly diminished B-cell function, is unknown. As indicated, clinically important autoantibodies in CLL are directed predominantly to the hematopoietic system. Although there is no increased risk of nonhematologic autoimmune disease in patients with CLL, these seem to be increased in their relatives.[124]

Increased numbers of CD5 (Ly-1) B cells are seen in some mice prone to autoimmune disease,[125] and some display IgM autoantibodies.[126] In humans, CD5 B cells are increased in the human fetus[61] and in patients with rheumatoid arthritis and other autoimmune disorders.[127] In addition, mitogen-stimulated CLL cells secrete Ig that reacts with autoantigens (IgG, ssDNA, dsDNA, but not ANA).[127–129] All these data suggest that the CD5 B-cell plays a prominent role in autoimmune diseases. In a recent study,[130] a high proportion of patients with CLL reacted with an anti-idiotype antibody raised against an IgM rheumatoid κ light-chain cross-reacting idiotype. One fourth of CLL cases expressing κ light chain reacted with this antibody. This high frequency is related to a conserved variable region (V-gene) of the κ-IIIb sub-subgroup.[131] These investigators[132] further demonstrated that 20% of CLL cases studied reacted with an antiidiotype antibody that recognized an antibody heavy-chain–associated cross-reactive idiotype present on rheumatoid factor paraprotein.

CYTOGENETICS

Specific chromosomal abnormalities have been found to have clinical, prognostic, and pathogenic importance for a variety of hematologic malignancies. Most of this information has been focused on acute leukemias and CML. It has been considerably more difficult to study chromosomes in patients with CLL because of difficulty in obtaining sufficient metaphases for analysis. A new and exciting area of cytogenetics in CLL has emerged using a variety of B-cell mitogens, including pokeweed mitogen, cytochalasin B, lipopolysaccharide, phorbol esters, protein A, and EBV. An adequate number of metaphases to evaluate chromosomes is achieved in 50% to 90% of patients.[133–143] Among those metaphases that can be evaluated, half are consistently determined to be abnormal.

The most common chromosomal abnormality is trisomy 12 (Table 28-2; Fig. 28-1). About one third of patients have chromosome 12 as the only abnormality, and two thirds have additional aberrations. The next most common chromosomal abnormalities are probably equally divided among 14q+, 13q, and 11q abnormalities. The translocations most commonly involving chromosome 14 are at q32 (Ig heavy-chain gene locus), resulting in a 14q+ chromosome. The donor chromosome is typically from 11, although a variety of other donor chromosomes have been identified.[143] Deletions of chromosome 11 with breakpoints at 11q21, 11q22, and 11q14 have been identified.[143] Structural abnormalities of chromosome 13 typically involve bands 13q13 and 13q21.[151] Perhaps the next most common abnormality is a chromosome 6 deletion with a variety of breakpoint regions.[143] A high incidence of trisomy 12 has been reported in patients with small lymphocytic malignant lymphoma, which is the lymphoma counterpart of CLL.[144]

In a recently developed cytogenic method that allows simultaneous analysis of cell morphology, immune phenotype, and karyotype in the same cell, it was demonstrated that trisomy 12 occurs in the neoplastic B cells but not in the presumably normal T cells.[109] These investigators propose that this provides the explanation for the common finding of mitosis with normal karyotypes in patients with CLL. The presumed normal T cells have the normal karyotype, not the malignant B cells, where the karyotype would be expected to be found in all the clonally involved cells. One flaw to this argument is the possibility that the T cells studied were long-lived T cells that may have preceded the malignant clone. Investigators have used restriction fragment length polymorphism (RFLP) of genes located on the long arm of chromosome 12 to show that the trisomy consists of a duplication of one of the chromosomes 12, not a triplication of one chromosome 12 with the loss of the other. In addition, using RFLP technology, these investigators demonstrated that the trisomy 12 abnormality was found in all the malignant cells.[143]

TABLE 28-2. Common Chromosomal Abnormalities Reported in Patients With Chronic Lymphoid Leukemias

Chromosomal Abnormality	Comments
+12	Most common finding in chronic lymphocytic leukemia; may also be seen in Waldenström's macroglobulinemia, hairy-cell leukemia, and B-prolymphocytic leukemia
14q+	B-prolymphocytic leukemia, chronic lymphocytic leukemia, hairy-cell leukemia, adult T-cell leukemia
11q	Chronic lymphocytic leukemia
6q	Chronic lymphocytic leukemia, B-prolymphocytic leukemia, adult T-cell leukemia, cutaneous T-cell lymphoma
13q	Chronic lymphocytic leukemia
del(3)	B-prolymphocytic leukemia
+3	Adult T-cell leukemia
+7	Adult T-cell leukemia, cutaneous T-cell lymphoma
inv(14)	T-prolymphocytic leukemia, adult T-cell leukemia

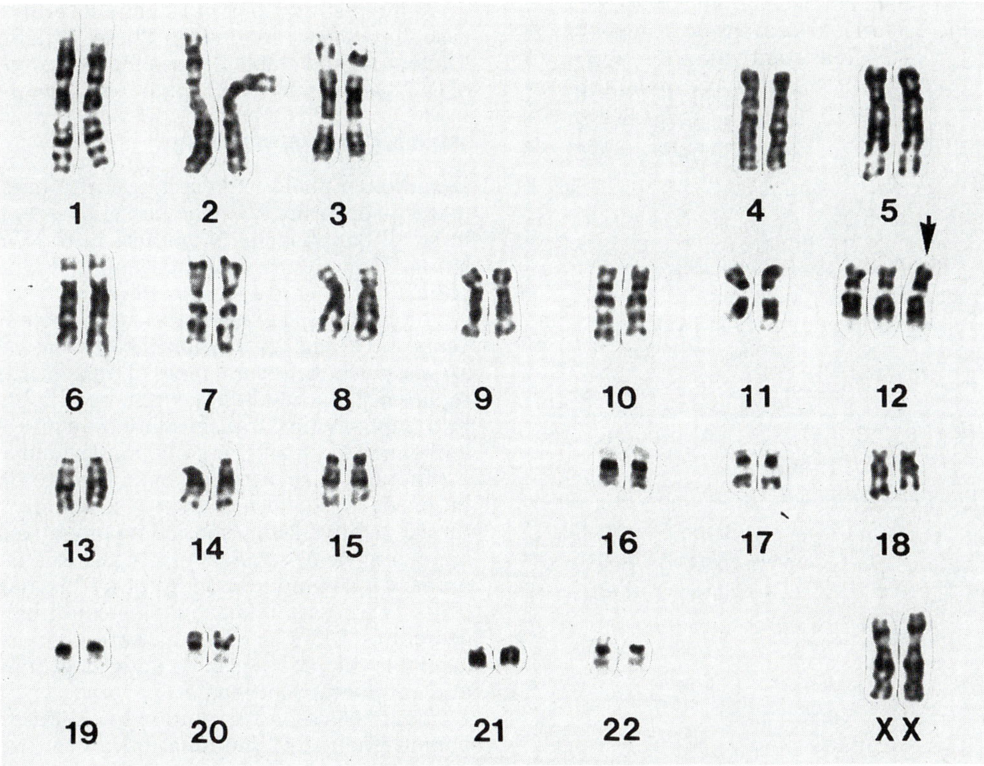

FIGURE 28-1. Trisomy 12 in a patient with chronic lymphocytic leukemia.

Important clinical correlations have been gleaned from recent studies. The first important correlation is that an abnormal karyotype is a poor prognostic sign[133,134,136] and that trisomy 12 and possibly 14q+ are the least favorable abnormalities.[143] In addition, patients with increasing numbers of chromosomal abnormalities do worse. One study reported that in most cases of CLL, the karyotype does not evolve in an individual patient.[142] Other studies have clearly demonstrated clonal evolution in selected patients with new chromosomal abnormalities.

ONCOGENES

Several studies have been done on protooncogenes in CLL and related diseases. Most show no specific abnormalities. Two cell lines derived from patients with PLL with the t(11;14)(q13;q32) translocation were studied.[145,146] In these cases, a break on chromosome 14 in the J region of the IgH locus was detected. The rearrangement on chromosome 11 involved a postulated protooncogene designated B-cell lymphoma/leukemia type 1 (*bcl-1*).

Cells from most cases of follicular B-cell lymphoma, a related disorder, have the t(14;18)(q32;q21) translocation.[147] Here, the genetic rearrangement on chromosome 18 involves another protooncogene, *bcl-2*. The mechanism of rearrangement between the IgH locus and *bcl-2* probably involves misrecognition of flanking heptamer–nonamer signal sequences by a normal recombinase involved in IgH recombination. Transgenic mice with a *bcl-2* IgH locus transgene demonstrate lymphadenopathy and abnormal B-lymphoid infiltrates and suggest a prospective role for the t(14;18) in B-cell growth.[148] The *bcl-2* oncogene controls apoptosis (programmed cell death). Overexpression of *bcl-2* inhibits apoptosis leading to a longer cell life.

The t(14;19)(q32;q13) translocation occurs rarely in cells from patients with CLL. The break on chromosome 14 occurs within one of the two α-switch regions in the Ig heavy-chain locus, and the break on chromosome 19 is upstream of the *bcl-3* gene.[149] The cDNA from *bcl-3* has been cloned and sequenced. Cells from patients with the t(14;19) have increased *bcl-3* RNA, suggesting a pathogenetic role.

CLINICAL FEATURES

One of the major challenges in CLL is to individualize therapy. The course of CLL is variable. Most patients are older (median age, 60 years) and may have only elevated lymphocytes, asymptomatic lymphadenopathy, or splenomegaly. Others have age-related medical complications. These older patients are unlikely to die from CLL and may require no specific treatment. In contrast, some patients with CLL present with severe bone marrow failure, including anemia and thrombocytopenia. They may have a rapid, progressive course, with a median survival of less than 2 years. Most patients with CLL have an intermediate prognosis and do reasonably well for several years without therapy but eventually require treatment. Rarely, spontaneous remissions are observed in patients with well-documented CLL.[150]

Ideally, one would use prognostic factors to select optimal therapy. Several staging systems that reflect grouping of prognostic variables are proposed. The Rai[151] classification (Fig. 28-2A) includes five stages based on lymphocyte levels, lymphadenopathy, splenomegaly or hepatomegaly, and non–immune-related anemia (less than 11 g/dL) and thrombocytopenia (less than 100×10^9/L). This system was simplified into three stages: low-risk (stage 0), intermediate-risk (stages I and II), and high-risk (stages III and IV).[152] These groups constitute about 30%, 60%, and 10% of patients, respectively (Table 28-3).

The Binet classification also has three stages[153] (see Table 28-3), which are distinguished based on bone marrow fail-

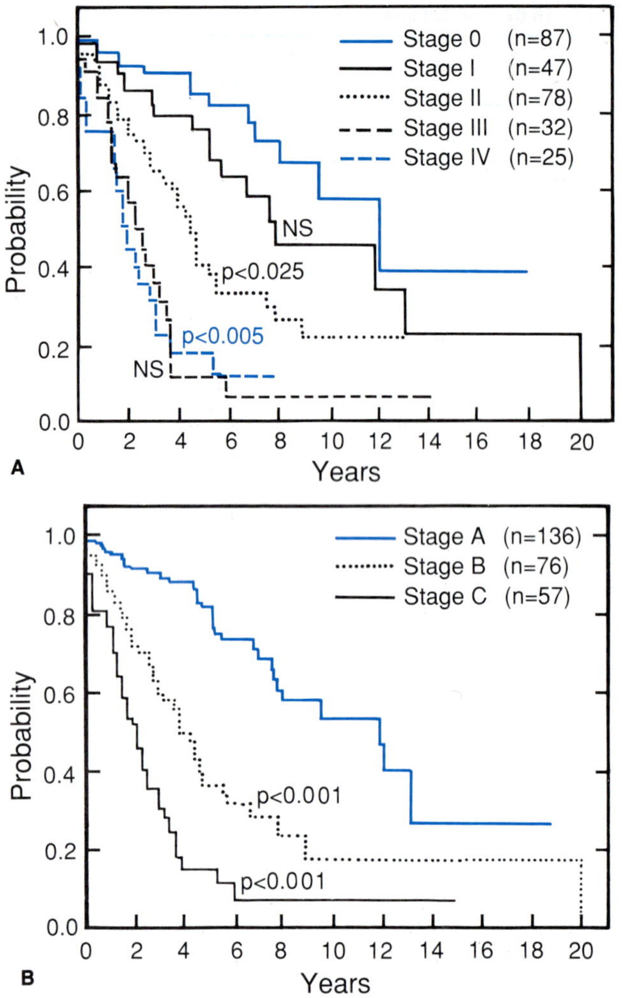

FIGURE 28-2. Actuarial survival curves of 269 patients classified by the Rai (**A**) and Binet (**B**) staging systems. (After Montserrat E, Rozman C. Prognostic factors in chronic lymphocytic leukemia. In: Polliak A, Catovsky D, eds. Chronic lymphocytic leukemia. Chur, Switzerland, Harwood Academic Publishers, 1988:111–122)

ure and the number of abnormal lymphoid areas. Groups A, B, and C account for 60%, 30%, and 10% of patients, respectively (see Fig. 28-2*B*).

Several investigators have tested numerous prognostic factors to determine if the course of CLL within a certain stage could be predicted accurately. A short list of these factors, which failed to consistently predict the clinical course of CLL, include the level of blood lymphocytosis,[154,155] proliferative index,[156–158] level of deoxythmidine kinase,[159] and phenotype.[160] Three factors (Table 28-4) stand out as most critical: (1) pattern of bone marrow infiltration,[161–164] (2) blood lymphocyte doubling time,[165] and (3) chromosome karyotype.[134,137,138]

Patients in whom the bone marrow shows diffuse lymphocyte infiltration are more likely to progress than those with a nondiffuse (nodular or interstitial) pattern of lymphocyte infiltration. Likewise, patients who are followed off therapy who have a blood lymphocyte doubling time of less than 12 months tend to do poorer than those with doubling times of greater than 12 months. This criteria cannot be determined at diagnosis. Chromosomal analysis is also useful but has limited availability, and most laboratories are successful in these analyses in only half of cases. However, an abnormal karyotype is an independent poor prognostic feature.

An interesting group of 20 patients with Rai stage 0 disease has been reported.[166] These patients had normal karyotypes and stable disease for 7 to 24 years. This form of CLL has been termed *benign monoclonal lymphocytosis*.

TRANSFORMATION

Chronic lymphoid leukemia typically involves relatively mature-appearing lymphocytes, similar to those observed in small lymphocytic lymphoma in the Working Formulation,[167] or diffuse well-differentiated lymphocytic lymphoma in the Rappaport classification.[168]

The phenotype of CLL is usually stable over months to years, but a small proportion of cases may evolve to a more aggressive form. Several types of transformation have been reported, including diffuse lymphoma (Richter's syndrome), prolymphocytoid transformation, acute lymphoblastic leukemia (ALL), and possibly, multiple myeloma.[169]

Whether transformation of CLL represents clonal evolution or a second malignancy is usually unknown. Although the two neoplastic cell types may express the same light- and heavy-chain Ig isotypes, this is not definitive proof of a common origin. In other instances, the heavy-chain Ig isotypes differ, but this could be due to isotype switching. More precise markers of clonality are now available, including cytogenetics, Ig gene rearrangement, and antiidiotype antibodies.

About 300 cases of evolution to a diffuse large cell lymphoma (Richter's syndrome) have been reported, with a projected incidence of 3% to 15% of cases.[170–174] Development of a diffuse large cell lymphoma in CLL is associated with clinical progression and increasing tumor mass. Whether Richter's syndrome is an independent disease or derived from the CLL clone is controversial since few cases are carefully studied; where studied, the data suggest some cases are clonal and others represent a second clone.[175–180]

PLL is a clinical entity distinct from CLL, with B- and T-cell variants.[181–184] A substantial proportion of patients with CLL, however, exhibit some cells that morphologically resemble prolymphocytes. When over 30% of the peripheral blood lymphocytes are prolymphocytes, this is referred to as prolymphocytic transformation of CLL and is distinct from de novo PLL.[185–189] Although some patients may develop more progressive disease states with resistance to therapy, this is not always the case. The blood usually contains two distinct populations: typical CLL cells and prolymphocytes. The latter have features similar to the CLL cells, including low-intensity cell-surface membrane Ig and the CD5 antigen. In contrast, cells from de novo PLL have high levels of surface Ig and do not express CD5 and CD23, but do express FMC7 and CD22. It is generally assumed that prolymphocytic transformation evolves from the CLL clone.

Another rare form of putative transformation in CLL is development of ALL.[190–192] This contrasts with the invariable progression to acute phase in CML. Most of these cases have the French–American–British classification L2 morphology, with clinical and laboratory features typical of adult ALL. Treatment with antileukemia therapy is usually ineffective perhaps owing to advanced disease or age. No definitive data indicate that the ALL is derived from the CLL clone. Another complication described in CLL is multiple myeloma. Several cases were studied; in most, the CLL and myeloma were not proved to be related,[193–197] and two cases appeared clonal.[198,199]

PATHOLOGY

The typical CLL cell is a mature, well-differentiated lymphocyte with a round, compact nucleus, clumped chromatin, and a distinct nucleolus (Fig. 28-3). These same cells

TABLE 28-3. Staging Systems for Chronic Lymphocytic Leukemia

	Criteria	Median Survival (y)
RAI STAGING SYSTEM		
Stage*		
0 (low-risk)	Lymphocytes >15 × 10^9/L Bone marrow >40% Lymphocytes	>10
I and II (intermediate-risk)	Blood and bone marrow lymphocytosis, lymphadenopathy, liver or spleen enlargement	6
III and IV (high-risk)	Blood and bone marrow lymphocytosis plus anemia (hemoglobin <11 g/dL) or thrombocytopenia (platelets <100 × 10^9/L)	2
BINET STAGING SYSTEM		
Group*		
A	No anemia or thrombocytopenia, less than three of the following five areas involved: axillary, inguinal, cervical (unilateral or bilateral), lymphadenopathy, liver, spleen	9
B	No anemia or thrombocytopenia; three or more involved areas	5
C	Anemia (hemoglobin <10 g/dL) or thrombocytopenia (platelets <100 × 10^9/L)	2

* Autoimmune hemolytic anemia and thrombocytopenia are independent of stage or group.

invade the lymph nodes in a diffuse pattern (malignant lymphoma, small lymphocytic), with effacement of the normal architecture (Fig. 28-4). The bone marrow involvement may be diffuse or focal, typically becoming more extensively replaced in advanced disease. Five patterns have been described: interstitial infiltration, nodular infiltration, diffuse involvement, mixed interstitial and nodular, and mixed nodular and diffuse (Fig. 28-5). As previously mentioned, some groups report a correlation between more extensive replacement of bone marrow or a diffuse pattern (or both) with a poor prognosis.

The spleen typically shows a replacement of normal architecture by CLL cells. The liver may be slightly enlarged due to lymphocytic infiltration of periportal tracts, with occasional nodular masses encroaching on the parenchyma. Virtually any other organ site may be infiltrated by CLL cells.

DIFFERENTIAL DIAGNOSIS

In contrast to the cell that appears morphologically mature, typical of CLL, B-cell–derived PLL is characterized by larger, less mature-appearing cells with condensed nuclear chromatin, prominent nucleoli[181,182,200] (Fig. 28-6), and surface markers distinct from CLL (Table 28-5). Most notable are, the presence of FMC7 and CD22[57,201] and high-density surface Ig and the absence of CD5. PLL cells typically have cytogenic abnormalities, particularly those involving chromosome 14,[202,203] which are not as common in CLL. Several clinical and laboratory features are also distinctive of B-cell PLL, including extreme leukocytosis (more than 100 × 10^9) and prominent splenomegaly, without substantial lymphadenopathy.

The relation between PLL and CLL is complex. At the extremes are classic CLL and classic PLL. The prolymphocytic variant of CLL has features of both diseases. Whereas the cells morphologically appear activated and look like classic PLL cells, they share most immunophenotypic features with CLL cells.[204] The clinical course follows the typical pattern of CLL.

Waldenström's macroglobulinemia is generally classified as a low-grade lymphoma. The malignant lymphocytes have plasmacytoid features,[205–208] often with abundant basophilic cytoplasm (Fig. 28-7). The periodic acid–Schiff (PAS) reaction is frequently positive, indicating the presence of polysaccharide; occasionally, this occurs in globules, leading to the term *grape cells.* Waldenström's cells typically have both surface and cytoplasmic IgM and secrete substantial amounts of IgM, resulting in a monoclonal peak on protein electrophoresis. Increased serum viscosity is found in about two thirds of patients; only half of these have symptoms associated with hyperviscosity. Waldenström's macroglobulinemia has a peak incidence in the sixth and seventh decades and is frequently an indolent disease with prolonged survival. Bone marrow involvement is invariably seen; most patients have circulating tumor cells, and some have high leukocyte counts. With disease progression, lymphadenopathy, splenomegaly, and hepatomegaly become prominent, and the clinical pattern resembles a lymphoma. In contrast to multiple myeloma, bone lesions are infrequent. Some investigators prefer to include Waldenström's macroglobulinemia under the

TABLE 28-4. Prognostic Factors in Chronic Lymphocytic Leukemia

Factor	Favorable	Unfavorable	References
Bone marrow pattern	Nodular, interstitial	Diffuse	161–164
Doubling time of peripheral blood cells	>12 mo	<12 mo	154, 155
Karyotype	Normal	Abnormal (trisomy 12)	134, 137, 138

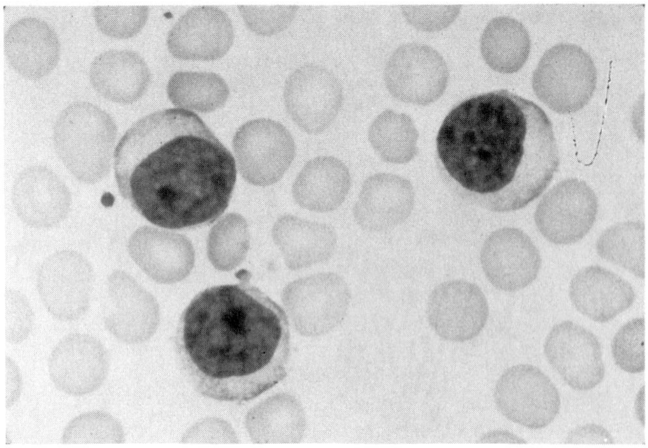

FIGURE 28-3. Peripheral blood, chronic lymphocytic leukemia (Wright-Giemsa stain, ×400). (See Color Fig. 28-3.)

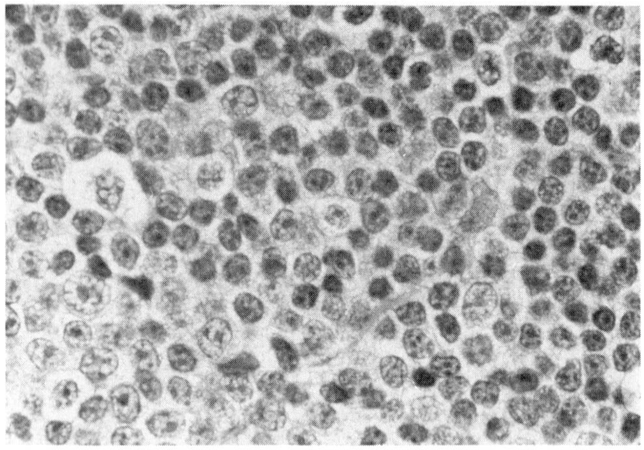

FIGURE 28-4. Lymph node of patient with malignant small-cell lymphocytic lymphoma (H&E, ×100). (See Color Fig. 28-4.)

broader heading of lymphoplasmacytic leukemias/lymphomas.[209] This would also include patients without a paraprotein, but with other similar morphologic and clinical features of Waldenström's macroglobulinemia.

A fourth type of chronic B-cell leukemia[210–212] typically represents the leukemia phase of a follicular small cleaved-cell lymphoma. The typical cells from follicular lymphomas are often pleomorphic, with small, prominent nucleoli (nuclear clefting), a finer chromatin pattern than typical CLL cells, and a high nuclear/cytoplasmic ratio (Fig. 28-8). This disorder typically presents as a lymphoma rather than as leukemia, but up to half of patients have bone marrow involvement at diagnosis. Some patients present with bone marrow and peripheral blood involvement without lymph node involvement; this may be difficult to distinguish from CLL. In the absence of a lymph node biopsy, the diagnosis should be made by morphologic features as well as immunologic features associated with follicular lymphomas, such as lack of mouse erythrocyte rosetting, normal capping, and bright surface membrane Ig fluorescence.[213,214] Unlike CLL, most cases of follicular lymphoma do not express the CD23 and CD5 antigens. Furthermore, most cases of follicular lymphoma express the CD10, CD22, and FMC7 antigens, which are absent in CLL.[215]

Two recently described leukemias/lymphomas are distinct from CLL. Splenic lymphoma with villous lymphocytes (SLVL) is a predominately splenic form of non-Hodgkin's lymphoma.[216,217] This tends to be an indolent

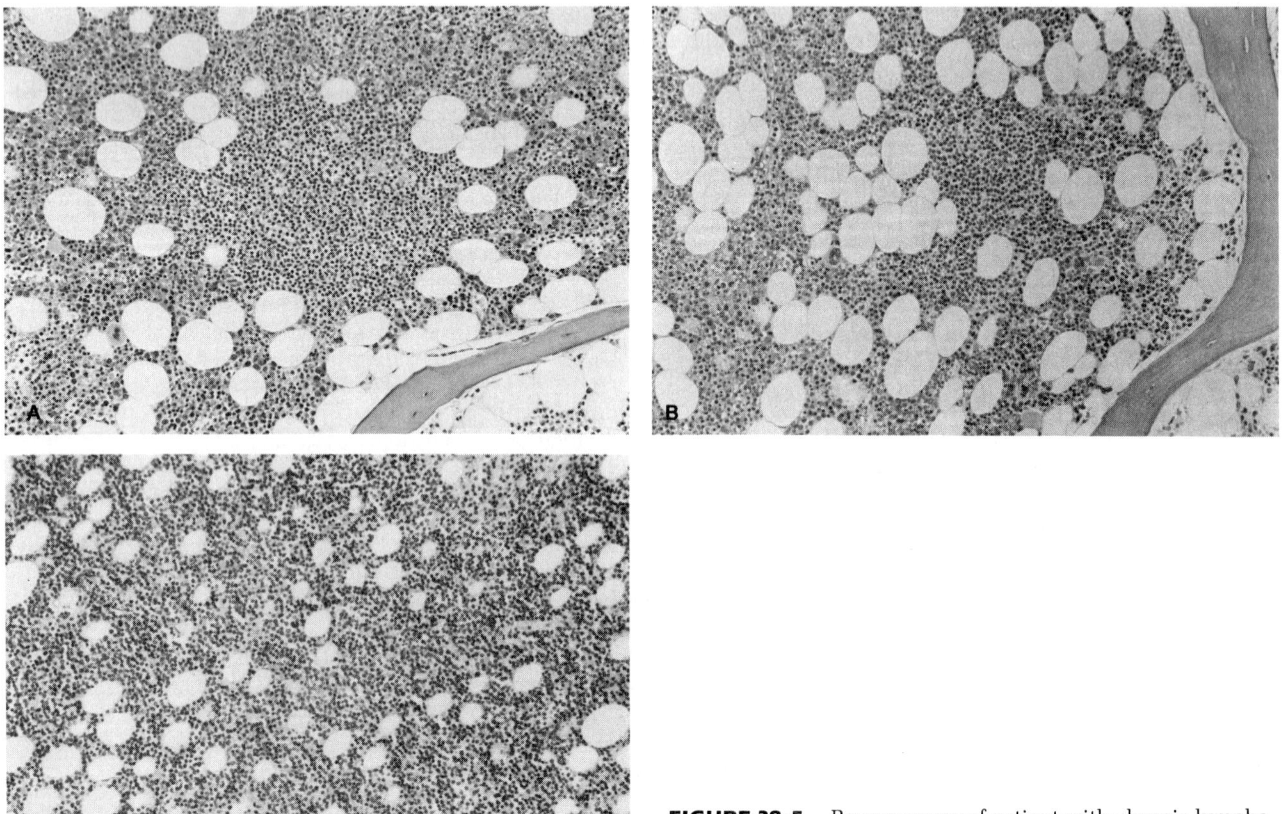

FIGURE 28-5. Bone marrow of patient with chronic lymphocytic leukemia: nodular (**A**), interstitial (**B**), diffuse (**C**) (H&E, ×160). (See Color Fig. 28-5).

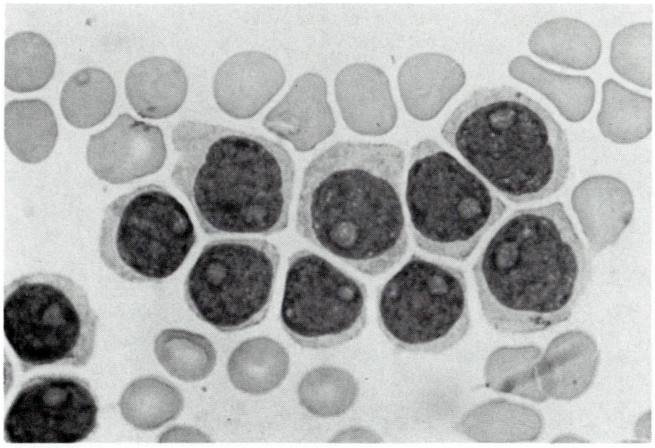

FIGURE 28-6. Peripheral blood of patient with prolymphocytic leukemia (Wright-Giemsa stain, ×400). (See Color Fig. 28-6.)

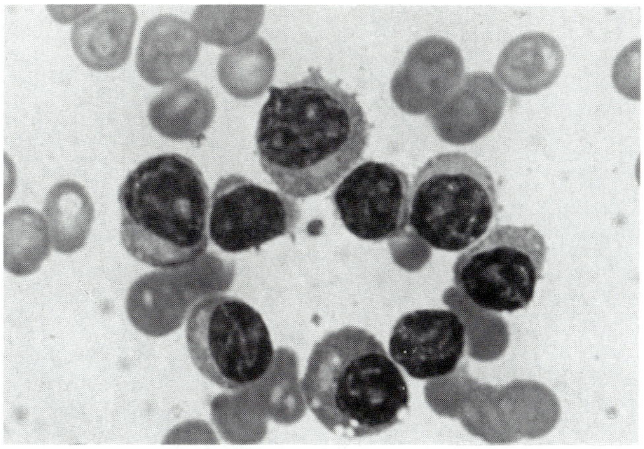

FIGURE 28-7. Peripheral blood of patient with Waldenström's macroglobulinemia (Wright-Giemsa stain, ×400). (See Color Fig. 28-7.)

disease. Two thirds of patients have a small monoclonal band. The leukocyte counts range from 5 to 40 × 10^9/L, and the circulating lymphocytes are larger than CLL cells and have short villi, often localized to one pole of the cell. In contrast to hairy-cell leukemia, the splenic infiltration is in the white pulp. Surface markers are similar to PLL.

The leukemic phase of mantle-zone lymphomas is characterized by an aggressive clinical course with a median survival of less than 2 years.[218] The blood films show a pleomorphic picture with medium-size lymphocytes with nuclear irregularities and clefts. The membrane phenotype shows intense surface membrane Ig and reactivity with CD5, CD19, CD20, FMC7, and CD22. CD10 is positive in half of cases. The lymph nodes show diffuse or a vaguely nodular pattern effacing the nodal architecture, and the bone marrow shows a diffuse pattern of infiltration. The t(11;14)(q13;q32) translocation with rearrangement of the *bcl-1* oncogene is commonly found in mantle-zone lymphomas.

Hairy-cell leukemia is another form of B-lymphocyte–derived chronic leukemia. The disease is so-termed because "hairy" cytoplasmic projections (Fig. 28-9) are sometimes visible by light, phase, or electron microscopy[219–221] (Fig. 28-10). Hairy-cell leukemia has a marked male predominance, with pancytopenia and prominent splenomegaly. Although most patients are leukopenic, some have a leukocytosis with a high percentage of hairy cells. This is discussed in a subsequent section.

A rare disorder termed *large granular lymphocytic* (LGL) *leukemia* or *chronic T-γ-lymphoproliferative disease* has been described.[222] The distinguishing morphologic feature is the presence of abundant cytoplasm, usually containing azurophilic granules[222–224] (Fig. 28- 11). Immune features include T-cell and NK-cell markers (CD2, CD3, CD8, CD56). Clinical features include relatively low levels of circulating leukocytes and granulocytopenia; recurrent infections are common, whereas lymphadenopathy and skin involvement are typically absent.

THERAPY

Immune Cytopenias and Infections

Immune-mediated hemolytic anemia, thrombocytopenia, and neutropenia are usually first treated with high-dose corticosteroid therapy (60 to 100 mg/m²/d). The underlying disease need not be treated (as described later) unless additional indications for therapy are present. Patients who do not respond to corticosteroid therapy may require splenectomy. Intravenous Ig may also be useful but is of unproven benefit for autoimmune complications of CLL.[225–229]

Patients with CLL have increased infections. Bacterial and viral infections are most common. The risk for infection correlates inversely with Ig levels. Consequently, several trials have evaluated the role of intravenous Ig in preventing infections in patients with CLL.

A double-blind, randomized study[230] in patients with CLL reported that intravenous Ig (400 mg/kg given every 3 weeks) reduced bacterial infections, particularly infections of moderate severity, by half. The actuarial probability of remaining infection-free and the time to first infection were

TABLE 28-5. Relation Between CLL, Prolymphocytic Transformation of CLL (CLL/PLL), and de novo PLL

	CLL	CLL/PLL	De Novo PLL
Age	60	60	70
Leukocyte count (×10^9/L)	50–120	>120	>150
PLL (%)	<30	30–80%	>50%
Spleen	++	+++	++++
Lymph nodes	++++	+++	+
CD5	>80%	>80%	<20%
FMC-7/CD22	<20%	<20%	>80%
Surface membrane immunoglobulin	Weak	Weak	Strong

CLL, chronic lymphoid leukemia; PLL, prolymphocytic leukemia; +, minimal; ++, moderate; +++, extensive.

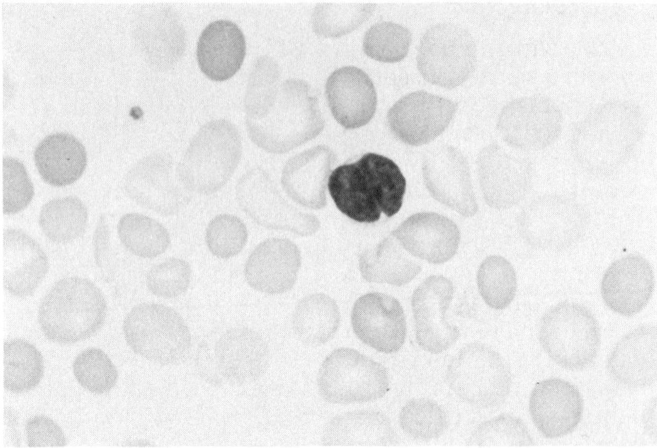

FIGURE 28-8. Peripheral blood of patient with small cleaved-cell lymphoma (Wright-Giemsa stain, ×400). (See Color Fig. 28-8.)

decreased. The incidence of minor and severe bacterial infections and of all viral infections remained unchanged. Twelve patients completing the trial entered a double-blind, cross-over study,[231] which confirmed the benefit of Ig. The major issue is determining who should receive this treatment. Patients who receive this treatment are likely to have severe hypogammaglobulinemia or a previous history of serious bacterial infections. Intravenous Ig should also be compared with alternative approaches such as prophylactic antibiotics.

Hyperleukocytosis

Rare patients with peripheral CLL counts exceeding 1000 $\times 10^9$/L may have hyperviscosity-related symptoms and would benefit from leukapheresis.[232,233]

Response Criteria

Evaluating therapy has been difficult in CLL because of the lack of uniform response criteria. Recently, the International Workshop[17] and the National Cancer Institute–Sponsored Working Group[16] (NCISWG) defined *complete remission* as the resolution of lymphadenopathy and organomegaly; lymphocytes less than 4×10^9/L; granulocytes more than 1.5×10^9/L; and platelet counts higher than 100×10^9/L. The International Workshop[17] includes the

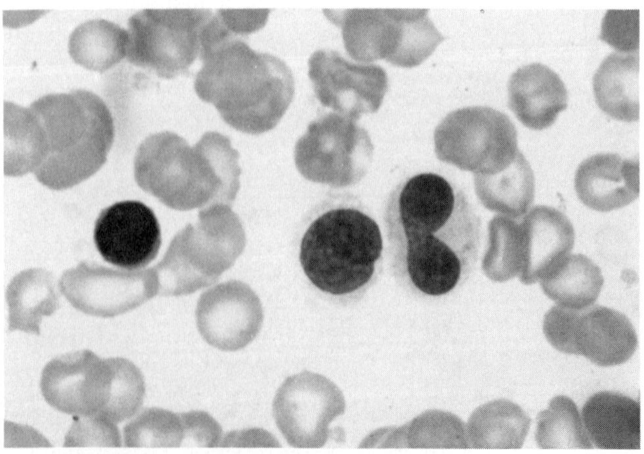

FIGURE 28-9. Peripheral blood of patient with hairy-cell leukemia (Wright-Giemsa stain, ×400). (See Color Fig. 28-9.)

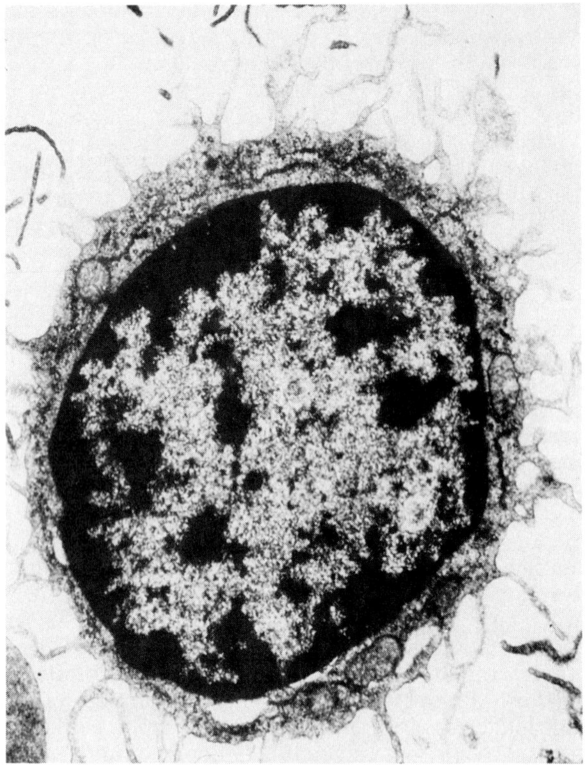

FIGURE 28-10. Peripheral blood of patient with hairy-cell leukemia seen by electron microscopy.

resolution of constitutional symptoms and a normal or nondiffuse pattern of bone marrow infiltration. The National Cancer Institute–sponsored Working Group[16] (NCIWG) requires fulfillment of the above criteria for longer than 2 months, after which a bone marrow aspiration and biopsy shows less than 30% lymphocytes. These criteria should provide a basis for comparing results of clinical trials. Their biologic impact has not been tested.

Additional tests to define complete remissions are used in some studies. These tests may indicate whether serum Ig levels, mouse rosette-forming cell levels, and the ratio of κ to λ light chains normalize and whether chromosomal abnormalities resolve. A more sensitive indicator of complete remission is the absence of cells expressing the Ig

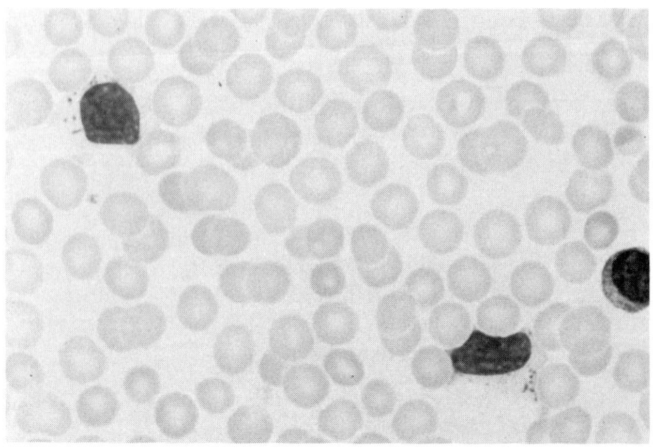

FIGURE 28-11. Peripheral blood of patient with large granular lymphocytic leukemia (Wright-Giemsa stain, ×400). (See Color Fig. 28-11.)

idiotype of the leukemia clone in the blood and bone marrow. Determining this absence requires developing anti-idiotype antibodies for each case of CLL. It also has its pitfalls, such as somatic mutation. Another approach is to study DNA from remission cells for clonal rearrangement of Ig heavy- or light-chain genes corresponding to the initial malignant clone by Southern blotting, but this technique is relatively insensitive. The polymerase chain reaction is more sensitive, but its use would require sequencing part of the uniquely rearranged Ig gene sequence for each patient. The ratio of κ to λ light chains (clonal excess) and dual staining for antigen combinations (eg, CD5 and CD20) are also used to document remission. The latter, however, may not differentiate the small percentage of normal circulating CD5 B cells from CLL cells. CLL cells are likely to persist in all patients considered to have complete remissions, even if these additional criteria are fulfilled.

Partial response, as defined by the International Workshop,[17] is a change from Binet stage C disease to stage A or B or from stage B to A. The NCIWG[16] defines a partial response as more than a 50% decrease in blood lymphocytes; a 50% decrease in enlarged lymph nodes, the spleen, and the liver; hemoglobin levels higher than 110 g/L (11 g/dL); platelet counts higher than 100×10^9/L; and granulocytes more than 1.5×10^9/L; or an improvement of 50% in these values from baseline. The analyses of most clinical studies are flawed by a lack of uniform response criteria. Future clinical trials should use these criteria.[16,17]

Approach to Therapy by Clinical Stage

At first examination, therapy of CLL appears straightforward, but this notion is far from correct, and controversies abound. This section considers several issues related to CLL treatment in the context of disease stage.

Low Risk

In planning strategy for each stage of CLL, it is necessary to consider median survival from diagnosis, likelihood of disease progression, and risk of death from leukemia. For example, patients with low-risk CLL have a median survival of longer than 10 years and are unlikely to die from leukemia. Consequently, the possibility of detecting a benefit of therapy is limited.

The first issue is whether therapy of low-risk CLL should be initiated at diagnosis or only on disease progression. This question has been addressed in a randomized trial comparing immediate versus delayed treatment with chlorambucil. These data suggest no advantage to early treatment.[234]

Several issues are unanswered. Would immediate treatment with another approach lead to a different conclusion? Alternative approaches include fludarabine, cladribine (2-chlorodeoxyadenosine), IFN-α, or multidrug chemotherapy, such as the CVP regimen—cyclophosphamide, vincristine, and prednisone—or the CHOP regimen—cyclophosphamide, hydroxydaunomycin (doxorubicin), vincristine (Oncovin), and prednisone. This has not been studied. However, the long survival, low likelihood of leukemia progression, and probability of death from leukemia make it unlikely that an impact of fludarabine, cladribine, or IFN-α could be detected. Furthermore, it is difficult to justify use of more intensive therapy under these conditions.

The sum of available data suggests a conservative approach in patients with low-risk CLL. Many affected patients may never need treatment. Others with progressive disease qualify for treatment approaches discussed for patients with intermediate- or advanced-stage CLL.

Intermediate Risk

Patients with intermediate-risk CLL have a median survival of about 5 years. Consequently, evaluating treatment strategies in this setting is easier than in low-stage CLL.

The first issue in therapy of intermediate-risk CLL is that of immediate versus delayed therapy. Patients with only modest symptoms, such as enlarged lymph nodes, may not require immediate therapy. In contrast, patients with severe symptoms or an extremely large tumor mass require immediate treatment. These two situations need to be considered separately.

Few data indicate whether it is better to delay treatment of patients with intermediate-risk CLL with a low tumor mass. The difference between this question and the seemingly similar issue discussed in patients with low-risk CLL is the greater likelihood of leukemia progression, briefer survival time, and death from leukemia. Treatments that might be considered in this setting include chlorambucil, fludarabine, cladribine, IFN-α, CVP, or CHOP[235–240] (Table 28-6). It is not possible to choose between delaying or initiating therapy. Because trials of more intensive treatment have not proved beneficial in intermediate-stage CLL, it seems reasonable to use chlorambucil therapy. Fludarabine, cladribine, and IFN-α are not tested in this setting. Whether they might prove equivalent or superior to chlorambucil is unknown.

Patients with intermediate-risk CLL and advanced tumor mass need immediate treatment. Considerable data suggest that chlorambucil and CVP produce equivalent results.[238,240] It is not clear whether more-intensive therapy with CHOP improves outcome or whether fludarabine and cladribine are as effective as chlorambucil.

High Risk

Patients with high-risk CLL have a median survival of 2 to 4 years, almost always progress, and are likely to die from leukemia. Because of these features, the issue in advanced-stage CLL is *how*, rather than *whether*, to treat affected patients.

Several trials have been conducted of alternative therapies for high-risk CLL. In one study,[241] CHOP resulted in better survival than CVP. Other studies[242] failed to confirm this. In another study,[243] survival of patients receiving chlorambucil or CVP was equivalent to the CHOP cohort of the CHOP versus CVP arm, suggesting that the better result with CHOP was due to inferior survival in the CVP arm rather than a benefit of CHOP. Fludarabine[244] and is active in previously untreated patients. Fludarabine is under investigation in an international radomized trial to de-

TABLE 28-6. Therapy for Chronic Lymphocytic Leukemia

PRIMARY THERAPY
Chlorambucil, 0.7 mg/kg PO in 1 day or divided over 2 days every 3 to 4 weeks (dose escalated by 0.1 mg/kg as tolerated).
SECOND-LINE THERAPY
Fludarabine, 25 to 30 mg/m²/d IV for 5 days every 4 weeks
Pentostatin, 4 mg/m² IV every 2 weeks (experimental)
Cladribine, 0.1 mg/kg/d for 7 days every 4 weeks by continuous IV infusion or 0.14 mg/kg/d IV over 2 hours for 5 consecutive days every 4 weeks (experimental)
Cyclophosphamide, 300 mg/m²/d PO for 5 days; vincristine, 1 mg/m² IV on day 1; prednisone, 40 mg/m²/d PO for 5 days, to be repeated monthly. Doxorubicin, 25 mg/m² IV on day 1 of each cycle, may be considered.

termine whether it is more active than chlorambucil as front-line therapy.

Summary

The lack of data from randomized trials precludes making definitive recommendations in many settings. In low-risk CLL, it seems reasonable to withhold therapy. A similar recommendation applies to intermediate-stage CLL with a low tumor mass, where therapy can be delayed.

Patients with intermediate-stage CLL who need treatment and patients with advanced-stage CLL benefit from chlorambucil. No data indicate that any alternative is better. Fludarabine is under investigation in this setting, as are combination chemotherapies and cladaribine. On initiating any new therapy, a 1-week course of 300 mg/d of allopurinal is recommended to prevent hyperuremia.

Second-Line Therapy

No standard approach has been established for patients with CLL who fail initial therapy. Many reports claim benefits for combination regimens,[245–251] but none have been confirmed.

Three new drugs (see Table 28-6) have been used as second-line therapy in CLL. One of the most promising is fludarabine monophosphate (2-floro, 5′-phosphate derivative of 9-β-D-arabinofuranosyl-adenine). In one study,[252] fludarabine, 25 to 30 mg/m^2/d intravenously for 5 days each month, was used in 74 previously treated patients with advanced CLL; there were 25 (33%) complete and 18 (24%) partial responses. In another study,[253] 22 of 42 (52%) patients responded. Side effects included myelosuppression, infections, and minor neurologic problems (peripheral neuropathy, muscle weakness, and decreased hearing).[198]

Pentostatin (2-deoxycoformycin), 4 mg/m^2 intravenously every 2 weeks, an adenosine-deaminase inhibitor, is also used in CLL, with responses in 13 of 48 patients with high-risk disease.[254] In two additional studies,[255,256] response rates of 26% and 34% were reported in 65 patients. Toxicities included infections, myelosuppression, nausea, vomiting, and pruritus.

A third new drug is cladribine, a halogenated purine analogue, given as 0.1 mg/kg/d by continuous intravenous infusion for 7 days each month or 0.14 mg/kg/d intravenously over 2 hours for 5 days each month. In one study,[257,258] 16 of 30 (53%) responses were reported in previously treated patients with advanced CLL.

In summary, patients who do not respond to chlorambucil, with or without prednisone, may require fludarabine therapy as second-line therapy. Alternatively, the patient may be encouraged to enter clinical research trials with pentostatin or cladribine. If these alternatives are not possible, combination chemotherapy, such as CHOP used in the French study[241] or other combination therapies,[190–196] are reasonable alternatives.

Radiation Therapy and Splenectomy

Total-body irradiation is not recommended for patients with CLL because it causes excessive myelosuppression. In contrast, radiation therapy to bulky lymph nodes or an enlarged spleen may be useful in symptomatic patients, especially when chemotherapy is ineffective. Splenectomy may be of benefit in hypersplenism unresponsive to radiation or chemotherapy.[259–261]

Bone Marrow Transplantation

Seventeen young patients (ranging from 32 to 49 years of age), predominately with advanced CLL, received high-dose chemotherapy and radiation followed by an HLA-matched bone marrow transplant. Fifteen achieved a complete remission. Nine patients are alive and disease-free, with a mean follow-up of 26 months after transplantation.[262] These data, albeit preliminary, are the first to suggest possible curability of CLL. This approach, however, applies to less than 5% of cases of CLL.

Biotherapy

Several studies used monoclonal antibodies to treat CLL and other chronic lymphoid leukemias.[263,264] Subjects with CLL received an anti-CD5 monoclonal antibody reactive with normal and malignant T lymphocytes and CLL cells.[265–271] This treatment transiently reduced levels of leukemia cells in the blood with no effect on the leukemia infiltration of bone marrow, lymph nodes, or organs. Side effects were minor. The use of human antibodies and antibodies conjugated to toxins[272,273] or isotopes may prove more effective and are under investigation.[274–276]

One interesting therapeutic approach is the use of monoclonal antibodies reactive with the idiotype of the Ig on malignant B cells (antiidiotype).[277,278] These antibodies are operationally *tumor-specific* in CLL. Reproducible responses to antiidiotype antibodies are reported in patients with non-Hodgkin's B-cell lymphomas. A major limitation of such therapy is that antiidiotype antibodies are custom-made for each patient. A recent study[279] reported that some antiidiotype antibodies identify isotypes common in patients with CLL. We studied these antiidiotype antibodies against more than 50 cases of CLL[280]; one fourth of the cases reacted with one or more of these antibodies, raising the possibility of using available antiidiotype antibodies for treatment.

IFN-α induces differentiation and proliferation of CLL cells in vitro.[281] Whether this occurs in vivo and whether it is clinically useful are unknown. IFN-α is not active in patients with intermediate- and high-risk CLL.[282,283] The low response rate to IFN-α in patients with advanced CLL contrasts with a 50% rate of response in patients with advanced, low-grade, non-Hodgkin's lymphoma[284–286]; a 50% rate of response in patients with cutaneous T-cell lymphoma (CTCL)[287]; and a 90% rate of response in patients with hairy-cell leukemia.[288,289] Recent studies reported greater than 50% responses in patients with previously untreated, low-risk CLL who were treated with low-dose (2 $\times 10^6$ IU/m^2 three times per week) recombinant IFN-α therapy.[290–292] Unfortunately, determining whether this treatment affects survival beneficially will take 10 to 15 years. A previously described study[180] showed no advantage of chlorambucil therapy over no therapy for patients with low-risk disease, despite the fact that most patients responded to chlorambucil.

PROLYMPHOCYTIC LEUKEMIA

Prolymphocytic leukemia was first described by Galton and coworkers in 1974.[181] The leukocyte count is typically greater than 100×10^9/L and consists predominately of prolymphocytes. Extensive spleen involvement is common, as are hepatomegaly and bone marrow infiltration; lymphadenopathy is usually absent or minimal. The disease is typically aggressive and responds poorly to therapy. PLL may be a disease of B or T cells.

Epidemiology and Cause

The median age of patients with PLL (both B- and T-cell types) is about 60 years, with a strong male predominance. The cause is unknown. Recent data suggest a possible association between HTLV-II and T-cell PLL.[28]

Immunology

Prolymphocytic leukemia cells resemble activated lymphocytes. The B-cell variety express strong surface Ig staining with either κ or λ light chain, Ia, CD19, CD20, CD21, and FMC7 and CD22. The cells exhibit heavy- and light-chain Ig gene rearrangements.[295] PLL cells do not have TdT; PAS staining is typically positive.

Most cases of T-cell PLL are CD4+ and CD8−. The CD8 antigen and combined CD4 and CD8 antigens are seen in a minority of cases.[209,296,297] The T-cell variant is typically acid phosphatase–positive and TdT-negative.

Cytogenetics

Several chromosomal abnormalities are described in B-cell PLL. Abnormalities of chromosome 14, particularly 14q+, are the most common.[202,203] The most common chromosome 14 abnormality is t(11;14)(q13;q32) associated with rearrangement of the *bcl*-1 protooncogene. Additional abnormalities include del(3), 6q−, trisomy 6, trisomy 12, and structural abnormalities of chromosome 1. Karyotypic evolution may be associated with disease progression.[203] In another study,[298] all five patients demonstrated a t(6;12)(q15;p13) translocation. T-cell PLL virtually always demonstrates inv(14)(q11;q32) or other 14q abnormalities.[297,299–301]

Clinical Features

Typical presenting features of B-cell PLL are fatigue, weakness, and weight loss.[181] Fever unassociated with infection is also common. Some patients experience abdominal pain and early satiety from massive splenomegaly. The outstanding physical sign is splenomegaly; hepatomegaly may also be prominent. Lymphadenopathy is absent or modest. Rare patients have petechiae and purpura from thrombocytopenia. T-cell PLL has similar features, with the addition of skin involvement in 25% of cases and lymphadenopathy in 50% of cases.

Leukocyte counts often exceed 100×10^9/L and are composed predominantly of prolymphocytes. The hemoglobin level is less than 12 g/dL, and platelet counts are less than 150×10^9/L; some patients have granulocytopenia.

Pathology

Prolymphocytic leukemia cells (see Fig. 28-6) appear more immature and have more cytoplasm than typical CLL cells and are thought to be *activated* lymphocytes.[200] The cells contain a large, vesicular nucleolus, condensed nuclear chromatin, and moderate cytoplasmic basophilia. PLL T cells may have nuclear irregularities and have been referred to as "knobby" cells.[209] Ultrastructural studies show coarse chromatin with a large nucleolus. Mitochondria are present, and some cells show strand-like projections (microvilli) from the cytoplasmic border.[181]

The bone marrow and spleen are typically diffusely infiltrated by prolymphocytes. Rarely, lymph nodes show diffuse infiltration with effacement of architecture. The liver often shows dense infiltration of the portal tracts and sinusoids.[302]

Differential Diagnosis

The distinction among PLL, CLL, SLVL, and the leukemic phase of mantle-zone and follicular lymphomas is discussed in the CLL section. PLL may be confused with ALL; however, patient age and the distinct morphologic features of the cells usually distinguish these diseases. The coarsely clumped nuclear chromatin characteristic of the PLL cell is unlike the typical finely reticulin nuclear chromatin and often inconspicuous nucleoli of the undifferentiated blasts of ALL. In ALL, massive enlargement of the liver and spleen is less common; leukocyte counts are typically higher in PLL than in ALL.

Therapy

Prolymphocytic leukemia typically exhibits a rapid downhill course, but some patients may have more indolent courses. Combination chemotherapy with cyclophosphamide, 750 mg/m^2 intravenously on day 1, doxorubicin, 50 mg/m^2 intravenously on day 1, vincristine, 2 mg intravenously on day 1, and prednisone, 100 mg/d by mouth on days 1 to 5, at 3- to 4-week intervals is often used.[303–305] Allopurinol, 300 mg/d, should be administered on the days of chemotherapy. Some complete remissions have been reported. Splenic irradiation is also used to treat PLL.[306] Twelve patients were treated with weekly doses of 1 Gy to a maximum of 10 Gy; there was little morbidity, and 7 patients responded. Splenectomy has been reported to be successful in some instances. When pentostatin was used to treat patients with PLL, a 50% response rate was reported.[297]

HAIRY-CELL LEUKEMIA

Hairy-cell leukemia, or leukemic reticuloendotheliosis, was first described by Borouncle and coworkers in 1958.[219] Remarkable progress in the diagnosis, biology, immunology, and therapy of this disease has occurred during the past 15 years. Hairy-cell leukemia is a B-cell disease; a rare T-cell variant has been reported and occurs in less than 1% of cases.

Epidemiology and Cause

Hairy-cell leukemia accounts for 1% to 2% of leukemia cases. It affects males predominantly in a ratio of 5:1. The median age of affected patients is about 50 years. In the United States, most patients are white.

HTLV-II has been isolated from cells of rare patients with T-cell hairy-cell leukemia.[28] The T-cell variant of hairy cell leukemia is so rare that many investigators question its existence. A viral cause for typical hairy-cell leukemia has not been implicated.

Immunology

Surface markers of hairy-cell leukemia are consistent with a clonal proliferation of B lymphocytes.[307] Surface membrane Ig with a single light chain confirms the clonality of the disease. B-cell–associated antigens, including CD19, CD20, CD21, FMC7, CD22, and sometimes CD23 and CD24, are also present.[308–310] The PCA-1 antigen,[311] typical of plasma cells, is present on some hairy cells. These data suggest that hairy cells may be preplasma cells.[312] Studies of Ig genes indicate clonal rearrangement of heavy-chain Ig genes and at least one light-chain Ig gene.[313,314]

Most cases of hairy-cell leukemia demonstrate the CD11c antigen as well as the CD25 antigen (IL-2 receptor) typically identified on malignant and activated T cells.[314] Several antigens appear to be restricted to hairy-cell leukemia cells, including the B-ly7 antigen.[315–317] Rare cases of hairy-cell leukemia with T-cell antigens have been reported.[318] Hairy-cell leukemia cells contain tartrate-resistant isoenzyme 5 of acid phosphatase (TRAP).[319] The PAS and α-naphthyl acetate esterase tests may be weakly positive, whereas naphthol AS-D-chloroacetate esterase and peroxidase reactions are negative.[320]

Some investigators have attempted to predict the course of hairy-cell leukemia by Ig light-chain involvement. In one study,[312] patients with λ light chains on the cell surface had a favorable prognosis; a second study[322] reached the opposite conclusion. With the new, effective therapies available today, such distinctions are probably unimportant.

Cytogenetics

The most common chromosomal abnormalities in hairy-cell leukemia involve chromosome 14.[323] In one study,[324] 5 of 12 cases had a 14q+ chromosome involving band q32. Additional abnormalities included trisomies 7, 12, 18, 22, 12p+, 12q−, monosomy 10 and 17, 6q−, and del(3p21).[323–325]

Clinical Features

The most common presenting complaints are weakness and fatigue.[220,326–328] One third of patients have a bleeding tendency and easy bruising; one third have recent recurrent infections. Abdominal discomfort from an enlarged spleen is present in one fourth of cases. A few patients have weight loss, fever, and night sweats. Splenomegaly is the most common physical finding at diagnosis and is found in virtually all patients, over 80% of patients having massive enlargement. About 10% of patients have lymphadenopathy and 20% hepatomegaly with abnormal liver function tests. The serum protein electrophoresis is abnormal in one fourth of cases, but a monoclonal pattern is rare. Recent data, however, suggest a monoclonal pattern is commonly detected by immunofixation.[329] Most patients present with mild to moderate normochromic normocytic anemia secondary to replacement of the bone marrow by leukemia cells and to hypersplenism. Although most patients have hairy cells identifiable on the peripheral smear, only 20% of patients have significantly elevated white blood cell counts. Eighty percent of affected patients have neutropenia; and 50% have platelet counts less than 100×10^9/L. Qualitative platelet abnormalities are common.[330]

One third of patients with hairy-cell leukemia develop infections during the course of their disease; over half of these involve gram-negative organisms.[326] Atypical mycobacteria is common and may require an open-lung biopsy. Disseminated fungal diseases may occur, whereas *Pneumocystis carinii* is rare.

Other complications of hairy-cell leukemia include vasculitis and bone lesions.[326] Systemic vasculitis is documented by biopsy of skin lesions. The management usually requires high-dose steroids. Long-bone involvement, usually of the femur, can result in lytic lesions and associated pain and pathologic fractures.

Pathology

The typical hairy-cell leukemia cell is an irregular cell with a serrated border (see Fig. 28-9). The cytoplasm is sky blue without granules. The nuclear membrane is distinct and the chromatin spongy. Occasionally, a single nucleolus is present. Electron micrographs show pseudopods and long cytoplasmic villi surface resembling hairs on the cell[327,328] (see Fig. 28-10). The cytoplasm contains abundant oval or round mitochondria with a well-developed Golgi apparatus and free ribosomes and rough endoplasmic reticulum.

The bone marrow cannot be aspirated in more than half of cases because of leukemia infiltration, fibrosis, or both. Core biopsies are usually diagnostic showing diffuse involvement with hairy cells and increased reticulin (Fig. 28-12). The spleen shows extensive diffuse infiltration of the red pulp, cords, and sinuses (Fig. 28-13). The lymph nodes usually demonstrate diffuse infiltration of the medulla with neoplastic cells that may extend into the surrounding fat. Obliteration of the lymph node architecture is not typically found. The liver may demonstrate portal infiltration and diffuse infiltration of the hepatic sinuses with hairy cells.

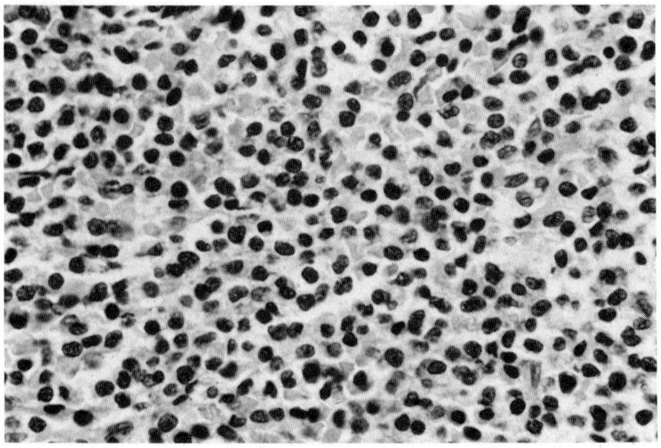

FIGURE 28-12. Bone marrow of patient with hairy-cell leukemia (H&E, ×100). (See Color Fig. 28-12.)

Differential Diagnosis

Diagnosis of hairy-cell leukemia is usually straightforward because of distinct morphologic features of the cells, the typical pattern of the bone marrow involvement, and clinical features. Pancytopenia may be confused with aplastic anemia, but the bone marrow biopsy should be diagnostic. SLVL may be confused with hairy-cell leukemia because of the primary splenic involvement, indolent course, and villi on the cells.[216,217] The nuclear/cytoplasmic ratio is higher than in hairy-cell leukemia, and the cells do not express CD25 and are TRAP-negative. Unlike in hairy-cell leukemia, the splenic infiltration in SLVL is in the white pulp. Waldenström's macroglobulinemia shares some features with hairy-cell leukemia, but the typical IgM monoclonal spike of Waldenström's is distinctive, as are morphologic features of the leukemia cells. The distinct features of CLL are discussed in the CLL section.

Histiocytic disorders, such as histiocytic medullary reticulosis, can resemble hairy-cell leukemia. Occasionally, hairy cells demonstrate erythrophagocytosis similar to

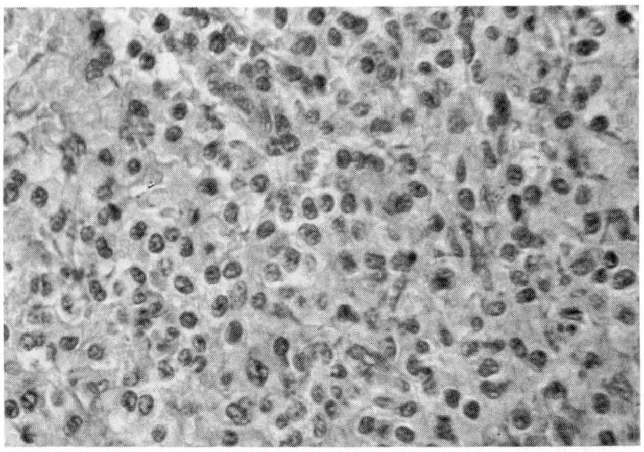

FIGURE 28-13. Spleen of patient with hairy-cell leukemia (H&E, ×400). (See Color Fig. 28-13.)

malignant histiocytes. Histiocytic medullary reticulosis is typically more aggressive than hairy-cell leukemia, rarely has marked splenomegaly, and has considerably less blood and bone marrow involvement.[328] The circulating cells in histiocytic disorders resemble monoblasts. These typically are nonspecific, esterase-positive, and TRAP-negative.

A rare variant of hairy-cell leukemia has been described.[331] The morphologic features of the hairy-cell variant are intermediate between hairy-cell leukemia and PLL, and the clinical course is chronic, with splenomegaly, leukocyte counts higher than 50×10^9/L, and no monocytopenia. Similar to hairy-cell leukemia, the variant cells infiltrate the red pulp of the spleen. The cells differ from classic hairy-cell leukemia in that they do not express the CD25 antigen.

Therapy

About 10% of patients with hairy-cell leukemia never require treatment. These patients are usually elderly, have only modest splenomegaly, and have granulocyte counts higher than 1×10^9/L.[326] The remainder ultimately require therapy. Historically, initial therapy for hairy-cell leukemia was splenectomy. Spleen size does not predict response to splenectomy.[326] About half of cases have normalization of blood counts; this response does not correlate with spleen size but rather with the degree of bone marrow replacement by hairy cells. Usually a low percentage of hairy cells persists in the peripheral blood. After splenectomy, most patients eventually show disease progression within months to years. About half develop a leukemia phase. In the remaining half of patients, bone marrow failure is the rule. In both groups, the bone marrow is densely infiltrated by hairy cells. Until recently, patients with progressive disease received chlorambucil. This improves erythrocytes and platelets but not granulocytes. Other putative therapies, such as oxymetholone, are not effective. Intensive combination chemotherapy is toxic and rarely effective.

Newer therapies are active in hairy-cell leukemia. IFN-α at low doses (2×10^6 IU/m^2 three times weekly with IFN-α_{2b}, or 3×10^6 IU/d with α_{2a}-IFN) induces complete or partial remissions in 90% of patients.[290,291,332] Because less than 5% of patients become resistant to IFN-α, and 90% have normalization or near normalization of blood counts, most live normal lives without transfusions, bleeding, or infections. Data suggest that about 5% of patients develop neutralizing antibody to IFN-α.[333] Toxicity is usually restricted to mild fatigue and malaise. Many patients with good partial remissions or complete remissions can discontinue IFN for periods of 1 to 3 years; they respond again when the disease progresses.[334] Interestingly, the variant form of hairy-cell leukemia is resistant to IFN-α.[335]

Also effective in treating hairy-cell leukemia is pentostatin, an adenosine deaminase inhibitor. Treatment with 4 mg/m^2 every 2 weeks produces complete and partial remissions in over 90% of cases.[336] In fact, pentostatin leads to more rapid and more complete responses than IFN-α. Toxicities include rash, diarrhea, nausea, and vomiting; these are generally mild at these doses. Data suggest that treatment with pentostatin causes a profound decrease in all lymphocyte subsets associated with a marked decrease in proliferative responses to mitogens and alloantigens. Six of 21 patients treated with pentostatin developed localized herpes infections.[337] A randomized trial of pentostatin versus IFN-α is underway.

2-Chlorodeoxyadenosine is a simple purine nucleoside that has activity in CLL and non-Hodgkin's lymphoma. Twelve patients were treated with 0.1 mg/kg/d by continuous intravenous infusion for 7 days. Seven had prior splenectomies, and five had been treated with IFN-α[338]; there were 11 complete and 1 partial responses lasting 7 to 46 months. No patient experienced relapse without maintenance therapy. Toxicity was limited to transient fever and neutropenia. To date, more than 500 patients have been treated with cladribine with similar results to those seen in the first 12 patients.

In summary, cladribine appears to be the most effective therapy with the least toxicity. Nearly all patients achieve a durable or complete response. This recently approved agent is the treatment of choice for hairy-cell leukemia.

ADULT T-CELL LEUKEMIA/LYMPHOMA

Adult T-cell leukemia/lymphoma is a T-cell lymphoproliferative syndrome first described in Japan in 1977[339] and later identified in the United States, the Caribbean, and other countries.[340–343] ATL is characterized by pleomorphic neoplastic cells with membrane features of mature helper T lymphocytes. Presenting features include lymphadenopathy, hepatomegaly, splenomegaly, cutaneous infiltration, hypercalcemia (with or without lytic bone lesions) and interstitial pulmonary infiltrates. Development of ATL is associated with infection by HTLV-I.[22,344,345]

Epidemiology and Cause

Epidemiologic studies of HTLV-I focus on serologic studies of normal populations that might elucidate the distribution of HTLV-I infection. Based on such studies, it is clear that ATL is correlated with HTLV-I infection. Additional data in the United States suggest that patients with the acquired immunodeficiency syndrome (AIDS) and hemophiliacs are often exposed to HTLV-I through blood or blood products. HTLV-I is also associated with a chronic progressive spastic paraparetic neurologic disease termed *HTLV-I–associated myelopathy and tropical spastic paraparesis.*[346] The disease onset is usually insidious, although in some cases, sudden events of illness similar to transverse myelitis occur. Spasticity is usually profound and may overshadow weakness. Motor strength is compromised more in the lower than upper extremities. Bladder and bowel dysfunction are frequent, as are dysesthesia and numbness. Histopathologic changes include mononuclear cell infiltration, lymphocytic perivascular cuffing, capillary proliferation, demyelination, and reactive astrocytosis. The epidemiologic patterns appear to parallel ATL.

When HTLV-I was first isolated from patients in the United States, it was thought that infection was related to mycosis fungoides. Serum specimens from Japanese patients with ATL, however, were positive for HTLV-I,[347,348] suggesting that the original US cases were incorrectly diagnosed. This led to testing in the Caribbean, where ATL was endemic; these patients also showed serologic and virologic evidence of infection with HTLV-I.[344] A low prevalence of HTLV-I infections has been found in normal individuals in populations where ATL is endemic. For instance, the highest prevalence of ATL in Japan is found in the southern island of Kyushi, where 10% to 15% of the population have antibody to HTLV-I.[347,348] On Japanese islands where ATL is rare, the rate is less than 1%. It is apparent from these and additional data from the Caribbean, southeastern United States, South American, and Africa that ATL clusters in regions where HTLV-I is prevalent.[347–349] It is not known how these regions are linked together, but one hypothesis is that HTLV-I was brought to the Americas from Africa by the slave trade and to the southern islands of Japan by trade with Japan and Africa.[347]

Several studies suggest that host susceptibility or a shared environmental exposure or both contribute to HTLV-I infection. The prevalence of HTLV-I antibodies in close family members is three to four times higher than in the corresponding normal population.[350] In some instances, cell cultures of antibody-positive, clinically normal patients yielded HTLV-I isolates.[351]

Retroviruses are a common cause of leukemia and lymphomas in many species; however, evidence of viral leukemogenesis in humans was slow to emerge. In the 1970s, major developments in two animal models rekindled interest in pursuing the search in humans. Retroviruses that cause leukemias in primates[352] and cattle[353] were isolated.

Retroviruses contain a single stranded RNA genome, usually consisting of three genes. The *gag* gene encodes a precursor peptide that is cleaved to form the major structural protein of the capsid as well as other core proteins. Protease is necessary for maturation of the *gag* polyprotein. The *pol* gene encodes the retroviral nucleic acid enzymatic gene and *env*, which encodes a single precursor peptide that is glycosylated and cleaved into a transmembrane protein and a spike protein.[347] The target of a retrovirus infection depends on interaction on the cell surface with the virus envelope. After entry to the cell, retroviral RNA is reverse-transcribed into a DNA provirus by reverse transcriptase; it then integrates into host DNA.

The first isolates of HTLV-I occurred after mature T cells were grown with T-cell growth factor or IL-2.[22] These first isolates contained reverse transcriptase, viral antigens, and high-molecular-weight RNA characteristic of type-C retroviruses. The major core protein, p24, was purified and sequenced.[354] Seroepidemiologic studies began using a radioimmunoprecipitate assay with purified p24 and assays using disrupted HTLV-I particles and a monoclonal antibody against another viral core protein, p19.[355] This led to the conclusion that the HTLV-I was endemic chiefly in Japan and the Caribbean. Worldwide isolates of HTLV-I proved similar to the first isolate.[347] This is a family of retroviruses in which the most frequently isolated strain is a member of the HTLV-I subgroup. Another subgroup, HTLV-II, with 60% homology to HTLV-I, was initially isolated from a rare case of T-cell–derived hairy-cell leukemia.[28]

HTLV-I isolates have four common features. These include isolation from and infection of mature T cells, reverse transcriptases with similar biochemical features, and cross-reacting internal core proteins. HTLV-I can infect and immortalize in vitro T cells from normal human umbilical cord, blood, and bone marrow.[23,356,357] The transfected cells express HTLV-I and resemble neoplastic T cells in that they develop lobulated nuclei, have unregulated growth, have a decreased requirement for IL-2, and express high levels of IL-2 receptors. Interestingly, the cells express foreign class 1 histocompatibility antigens similar to virus-infected tumor cells.

HTLV-I also exerts other biologic effects on T cells that may in turn modulate function of hematopoietic cells. HTLV-I–transformed T-cell lines produce several lymphokines, including colony-stimulating factors, IL-2, IL-6, and IFN-γ.[358] Some of these factors may be responsible for some secondary features of ATL. For example, hypercalcemia may result from increased osteoclast-activating factors. In addition, the observation that normal IL-2–dependent clones of functional cytotoxic and helper T cells sometimes lose immune function after infection with HTLV-I may explain why HTLV-I–infected patients are immunocompromised and prone to opportunistic infections.[359] Evidence also indicates that HTLV-I infection selectively kills self-tolerant cytotoxic T cells.[360] It is apparent that HTLV-I may exert profound effects on a spectrum of cells as well as the immediate target cell. Some seroepidemiologic data indicate that HTLV-I may be indirectly involved in the origin of rare B-cell leukemias in an endemic area of HTLV-I infection, such as Jamaica.[348]

Although the in vitro transformed cells provide a model for studying initiation of leukemogenesis by HTLV-I, a second event is likely required for progression to full disease.[347] This is suggested by the following observations. First, development of ATL requires long latency periods, whereas HTLV-I transforms cells rapidly (in 4 to 6 weeks). Second, although in vitro transformed cells usually retain a normal karyotype, ATL cells usually exhibit clonal chromosomal abnormalities. No consistent chromosomal abnormality, however, has been identified. Only a minor proportion of patients with HTLV-I infection develop ATL.

Immunology

The malignant cells from patients with ATL typically have the phenotype of mature helper T cells[361,362] and express the CD2, CD3, and CD4 antigens. They also express the CD25 antigen, which is the p55 subunit of the IL-2 receptor. Clonal rearrangements of the T-cell receptor β chain are present.[363–366] Leukemia cells have been reported to suppress B-cell Ig secretion by a complex mechanism involving induction of suppressor cells after activation of normal suppressor cell precursors.[361,362]

Cytogenetics

Several cytogenic abnormalities have been reported in patients with ATL.[367–374] Most common abnormalities include trisomy or partial trisomy 3q or 6q−, 14q, and inv(14). Others include loss of the X chromosome, t(9;21), 5p−, 2q+, 17q+, and trisomy 18. In some studies, survival correlates with karyotype abnormalities.[367]

Clinical Features

Adult T-cell leukemia/lymphoma has various clinical presentations, including an aggressive acute type with leukemia, a lymphoma without lymphocytosis, a chronic type with a modest leukemic phase, and a smoldering type.[374] The median age of patients with the aggressive acute type of ATL is about 40 years. They typically present with an elevated leukocyte count ranging from 5 to 100 $\times$ 10^9/L,[339,340,342] with circulating malignant lymphocytes in most cases. Anemia and thrombocytopenia are uncommon. Onset of symptoms is typically acute, with rapidly developing cutaneous lesions, hypercalcemia, or both. Skin lesions are variable. Some patients have discreet tumor nodules, and others have confluent smaller nodules. Some patients present with plaques, papules, and nonspecific erythematous patches and erythroderma. Patients with hypercalcemia typically have weakness, lethargy, confusion, polyuria, and polydipsia. Radionuclide bone scans show diffusely increased uptake throughout the skeleton, most prominent in the joints and skull. These scans are referred to as *super scans* and are unusual in other patients with malignant lymphomas. Isolated lytic bone lesions may also occur; alkaline phosphatase is typically elevated.

Lymph node enlargement occurs in all patients, although the nodes are initially small in some. Many have generalized lymphadenopathy, and most have retroperitoneal adenopathy. Hilar adenopathy is common, but a mediastinal mass is rare. Bone marrow may be infiltrated with leukemia cells. Additional sites of disease include the lung, liver, skin, gastrointestinal tract, and central nervous system.

Opportunistic infections are common in patients with ATL, even though most have normal serum Ig levels. *P carinii* infection is common, as is cryptococcal meningitis. Bacterial and fungal infections are also common. A variety of pulmonary problems develop, including infections and leukemic infiltrates.

Patients with the smoldering type of ATL have an indolent course, except for opportunistic infections.[340,375] They typically have a long survival without therapy and without hypercalcemia. Skin lesions are characteristic and occur as erythema, papules, or nodules. The proportion of ATL cells in the blood is low (less than 5%), with minimal lymphadenopathy, hepatosplenomegaly, and bone marrow infiltration. One patient developed aggressive ATL after more than 5 years of illness and another after 13 years. Patients with smoldering ATL are more likely to have a normal karyotype.

Pathology

An important feature is the presence of pleomorphic lymphoid cells in the blood[340] (Fig. 28-14). Although not all cases present with blood involvement, a leukemia phase develops in most at some point. ATL cells have moderately condensed nuclear chromatin, inconspicuous nucleoli, and a markedly irregular nuclear contour that divides the nucleus into several lobes. These cells are characteristic of HTLV-I–associated disease and are readily distinguished from Sézary cells and cells of other mature and immature T-cell malignancies. In about 20% of the cases, nuclear irregularities are less extreme; these cells may be difficult to distinguish from Sézary cells.

Pathologic features in lymph nodes and other tissues are more varied. ATL is associated with lymphomas of several histologic subtypes, including diffuse, poorly differentiated small cell; large, mixed small cell; and large cell immunoblastic.[343] No apparent correlation exists between clinical course and the histiologic cell type.

Cutaneous involvement occurs in about two thirds of patients with ATL. Focal epidermal infiltration with ATL cells or Pautrier microabscesses is seen in most patients with cutaneous involvement. These abscesses were thought to be pathognomonic of CTCL, and the retrovirus-associated disease was initially reported as CTCL. The acute course and absence of a chronic premycotic phase in most patients with ATL distinguishes it from typical CTCL. Furthermore, serologic studies in cases of CTCL show no association with HTLV-I infection. Rare patients with CTCL are HTLV-I–positive, but this is unusual.

Differential Diagnosis

Smoldering ATL could be confused with cutaneous T-cell lymphoma, since the skin lesions and clinical presentation may be similar. The aggressive form of ATL represents a rather unique constellation of clinical and pathologic findings that should be readily distinguished from other leukemias and lymphomas.

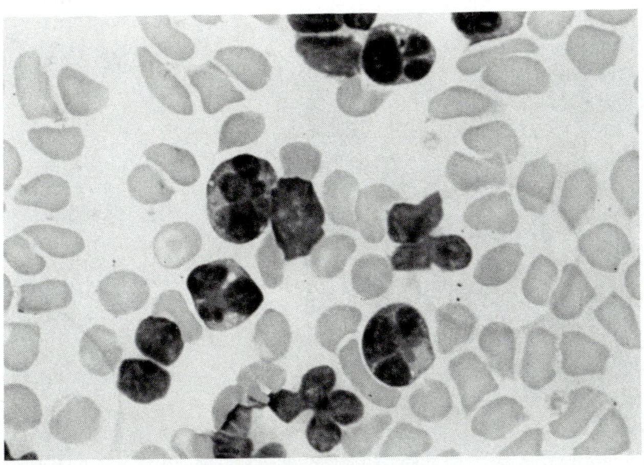

FIGURE 28-14. Peripheral blood of patient with adult T-cell leukemia (Wright-Giemsa stain, ×400). (See Color Fig. 28-14.)

Therapy

It is standard to treat patients with adult T-cell leukemia/lymphoma with combination chemotherapy using a regimen that includes doxorubicin, such as CHOP. Complete and partial responses are attained in most patients. However, most patients experience relapse within 6 to 12 months, and cures are not reported. Encouraging responses have been observed in patients who received passive immunotherapy or radioimmunotherapy using monoclonal antibodies specific for antigens expressed by the neoplastic T cells, such as CD25.[376] Other biologic agents, such as IFN-α, have had modest effects.[377,378] Therapy with the nucleoside pentostatin may benefit some patients with this disease.[379]

CUTANEOUS T-CELL LYMPHOMA

Cutaneous T-cell lymphoma consists of mycosis fungoides and the Sézary syndrome. These disorders are malignant proliferations of T lymphocytes of the helper phenotype in which the initial clinical presentation is in the epidermis.

Epidemiology and Cause

Cutaneous T-cell lymphoma is an uncommon malignancy in the United States, with about 1500 new cases reported per year.[380] The average annual adjusted mortality rate is about 400 to 500 deaths per year.[381] CTCL occurs most commonly in males, with a 2:1 ratio; it is less frequent in African Americans. The median age at diagnosis is 55 years. Initial skin lesions are clinically and histologically nonspecific and may take many years before the diagnosis is confirmed. Median survival after histologic diagnosis is about 10 years.

Although the cause is unknown, recent observations suggest that environmental, infectious, and genetic influences may be important. Exposure to toxic chemicals and physical agents and employment in manufacturing, particularly textiles, petrochemicals, and machinery, was reported to be associated with an increased incidence of CTCL, but this remains controversial.[380–382] As indicated, HTLV-I was originally isolated in the United States from patients thought to have CTCL.[22] Seroepidemiologic studies, however, have suggested that HTLV-I is associated with ATL; and serologic evidence of infection is found in less than 1% of patients with CTCL in the United States.[21] In a series of CD25-negative CTCL patients from Italy, a new retrovirus called HTLV-V was isolated.[383] The significance of this finding is not clear, and it requires confirmation. Evidence for genetic factors in the cause of CTCL is less impressive. Reports have been made of an increased incidence of lymphoma or leukemia in first-degree relatives of patients with CTCL.[380] Data conflict regarding whether there is an increased incidence of CTCL among family members.[383]

Immunology

In most cases, the cells express a phenotype associated with mature helper–inducer T lymphocytes that includes CD3, CD5, and CD4.[384–386] These cells can function as helper T lymphocytes in in vitro assays.[387] The CD7 antigen, which reacts with greater than 85% of normal circulating T lymphocytes, also reacts with mycosis fungoides cells in the skin, but not with circulating Sézary cells.[388] The cells are generally negative for markers of T-cell activation, which include Ia antigens and CD25 (IL-2 receptor). Like most malignant T cells, the CTCL cells stain for acid phosphatase, α-naphthyl acetate esterase, and β-glucoronidase. They are generally negative for peroxidase, alkaline phosphatase, and esterase. PAS-positive granules are present in some cases.

Cytogenetics

A wide range of chromosomal abnormalities are described in CTCL.[389] Chromosomes 1 and 6 are frequently involved in structural abnormalities, whereas chromosomes 7, 11, 21, and 22 are frequently involved in numeric abnormalities. Rearrangement of chromosome 10 was common in one study.[390] Chromosomal abnormalities often correlate with extent of disease and survival.

Clinical Features

Most cases of CTCL progress through distinct stages of skin involvement (Table 28-7). These stages begin with a premycotic, erythematous, or eczematoid stage, progress to an infiltrative plaque stage, and eventuate in the tumor stage.[380] Progression is variable but commonly occurs over several years.[391]

The premycotic or erythematous stage of CTCL is nonspecific; it is characterized by localized or widespread areas of erythema or dry eczema.[380] Lesions may be associated with pruritus. Histologic features are also nonspecific, and a definitive diagnosis is often not possible. This stage may last for months to years before progression. The plaque stage is distinguished by palpable, pruritic indurated lesions (Fig. 28-15). The tumor stage (Fig. 28-16) is characterized by large lesions; these may develop in previously normal skin or in premycotic lesions or plaques. The lesions occur most often on the face and in body folds, often in a "bathing trunk" distribution. Tumors are often generalized, and ulceration is common. Pruritus is absent.

The erythrodermic form of CTCL is manifested by generalized erythroderma and may precede appearance of other CTCL lesions by many years. It may also be preceded by premycotic lesions or may appear simultaneously with plaques or tumors. Two common types of erythroderma include exfoliative erythroderma, predominated by intense scaling and "1'-hoome-rouge," or "red man," syndrome, in which redness rather than scaling predominates. Transition between forms is common. Lymphadenopathy and alopecia are frequent manifestations.

In 1938, Sézary and Bouvrain[392] described a syndrome of pruritus, generalized exfoliative erythroderma, and abnormal hyperconvoluted lymphoid cells in the blood; this is referred to as *Sézary's syndrome*. Sézary's syndrome has biologic features similar to the other forms of mycosis fungoides. Most patients with generalized erythroderma have varying numbers of circulating Sézary cells (Fig. 28-17).

TABLE 28-7. Survival by Skin Stage of Cutaneous T-Cell Lymphoma Patients

Skin Stage	Mean Survival (y)	5-Year Survival (%)
Limited plaque (T1)	>9	90
Generalized plaque (T2)	>7	70
Cutaneous tumor (T3)	2.5	35
Generalized erythroderma (T4)	3.5	40

(Adapted from Winkler CF, Bunn PA. Cutaneous T-cell lymphoma: a review. CRC Crit Rev Oncol Hematol 1983;1:49)

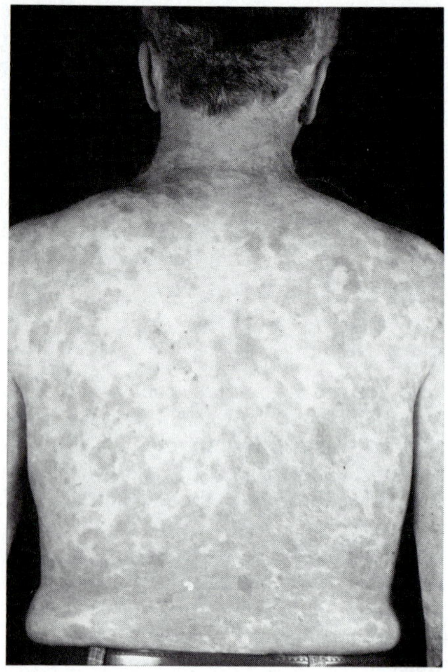

FIGURE 28-15. Multiple discrete and confluent plaques of cutaneous T-cell lymphoma. (See Color Fig. 28-15.)

One fourth of those with plaque or tumor stage also have circulating Sézary cells.

Autopsy studies of patients with advanced CTCL show extensive invasion of organs and tissues by malignant T cells. Pulmonary, cardiac, renal, and gastrointestinal involvement are infrequent clinically but are common autopsy findings.[391,393–395] Mediastinal and hilar adenopathy, pleural effusion, parenchymal nodules, and patchy infiltrates also occur. Bony abnormalities are rare despite bone marrow involvement in 30% to 40% of autopsy cases.[391,393] Bony lesions typically occur in long bones, are osteolytic, and may cause pathologic fractures.[396,397] CTCL of the cornea, sclera, and lacrimal glands has been reported.[398–400] Central and peripheral nervous system involvement by CTCL is documented in 10% of autopsy cases.[391,394] Leptomeningitis is common, but infiltrates have been reported in all areas of the neuroaxis.[401,402] Clinical manifestations reflect sites of involvement. Hematologic abnormalities in CTCL are often nonspecific, except for circulating Sézary cells. Bone marrow eosinophilia, monocytosis, and plas-

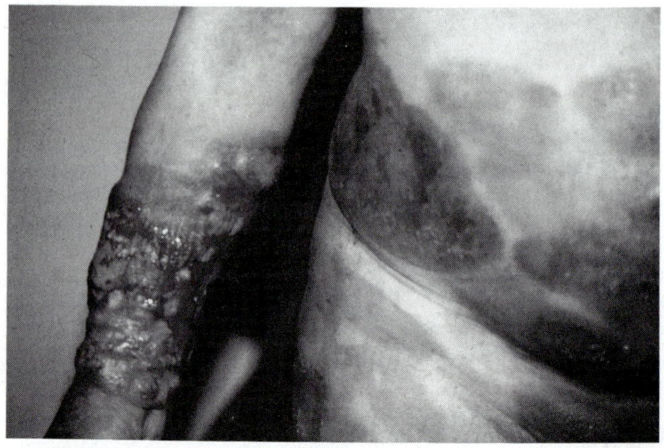

FIGURE 28-16. Multiple plaques of cutaneous T-cell lymphoma with tumor formation. (See Color Fig. 28-16.)

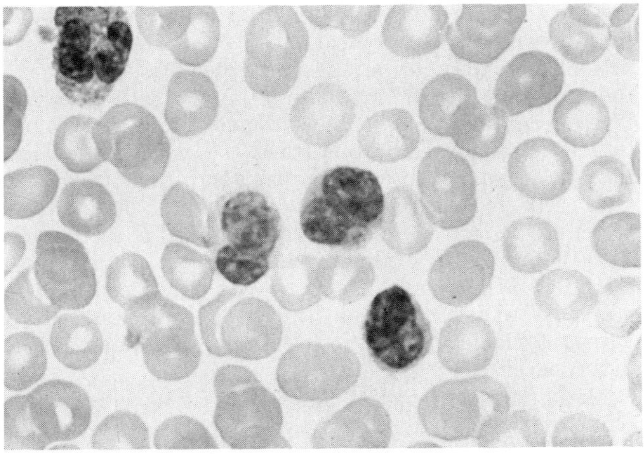

FIGURE 28-17. Peripheral blood of patient with cutaneous T-cell lymphoma, showing Sézary cells (Wright-Giemsa stain, ×400). (See Color Fig. 28-17.)

macytosis have been reported, as have elevations of serum Ig, usually IgA and IgE.[380]

Fifty percent of deaths of patients with CTCL result from infections. These are usually *Staphylococcus-* and *Pseudomonas*-related and develop from cutaneous lesions.[391,393,403] Septicemia and bacterial pneumonia are common. Herpes infections occur in up to 10% of patients with advanced CTCL.[404,405] Progressive CTCL with widespread visceral involvement is the next most common cause of death.[391]

Pathology

The initial clinical manifestations of CTCL are nearly always cutaneous, and the diagnosis is usually established by skin biopsy. Early lesions may show polymorphic infiltrations compatible with several benign diseases as well as CTCL. The malignant infiltrate in early CTCL is characteristically epidermotrophic, with exocytosis of single or clusters of convoluted CTCL cells. Epidermal clusters of these cells are termed *Pautrier microabscesses* (Fig. 28-18). The epidermis may also show parakeratosis and acanthosis. A band-like infiltrate in the upper dermis is composed of lymphocytes, neutrophils, eosinophils, plasma cells, blasts, and histiocytes in early lesions. The atypical, convoluted lymphocytes are present in clusters. In more advanced stages, the infiltrate is less polymorphic with a predominance of atypical cells extending deeper into the dermis; epidermotrophism may be lost.

Lymph nodes that drain affected areas show partial or complete effacement of normal architecture with a monomorphic infiltrate of CTCL cells. In most lymph nodes, the architecture is not effaced, and dermatopathic changes with varying numbers of atypical lymphocytes in the T-cell paracortical areas of the node are present. The cytologic appearance of the malignant cells in visceral organs is similar to the skin.[393,394] Lymph node involvement is associated with a poor prognosis.[406]

Staging

Cutaneous lesions are defined by using the T staging system. T1 (limited plaque stage) consists of erythematous patches and plaques covering less than 10% of the body. Plaques covering 10% or more of the skin surface are designated T2. Cutaneous tumors are designated T3 and generalized erythroderma, T4. Patients with limited plaque disease have the most favorable prognosis; those with generalized plaques have an intermediate prognosis; and those with tumors or erythroderma have the worst prognosis.[406]

As indicated, lymphadenopathy portends a poorer prognosis than disease limited to the skin.[391,406–411] Lymphadenopathy is present in about half of patients and increases with progressive cutaneous involvement.[410,412] Lymphangiograms were used to assess pretreatment involvement of intraabdominal lymph nodes. Computed axial tomographic scans are less invasive, however, and reveal similar information.[413,414]

Circulating Sézary cells also increase with advancing disease, which occurs in up to 90% of those with generalized erythroderma. Malignant cells can also be detected using sensitive techniques such as cytogenetics or T-cell receptor gene rearrangement studies. Patients with blood involvement have a higher likelihood of lymphadenopathy, visceral involvement, and shorter survival.[415,416] Bone marrow infiltration is infrequently detected by biopsy despite circulating malignant cells; it is identified at autopsy in 30% to 40% of cases.[397]

Patients with CTCL with visceral involvement that includes liver, spleen, pleura, and lung have the poorest prognosis; median survival is less than 1 year.[391,406,407] Visceral involvement does not appear until late.

Differential Diagnosis

The early diagnosis of CTCL is difficult and can be confused with several benign dermatologic diseases. Often, a definitive diagnosis is delayed for years.

Smoldering ATL has a number of clinical features similar to CTCL, but it can usually be distinguished by the presence of antibodies to HTLV-I and by its regional occurrence. Pagetoid reticulosis is a rare skin disorder consisting of solitary or localized cutaneous plaques. The involved areas show a prominent atypical mononuclear cell infiltrate with a hyperplastic epidermis.[418] Although this disease is usually indolent and localized, some patients present with a disseminated form referred to as the *Ketron-Goodman variant*.[419] Interestingly, recent studies have demonstrated that this is a disease of an activated T lymphocyte that only

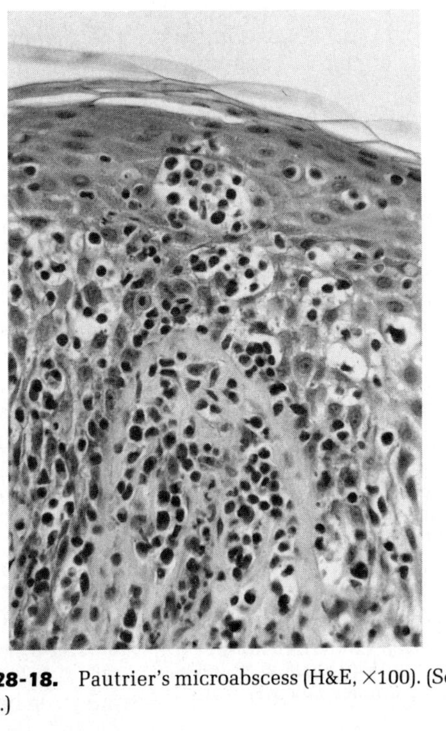

FIGURE 28-18. Pautrier's microabscess (H&E, ×100). (See Color Fig. 28-18.)

occasionally expresses the helper T-cell CD4 antigen.[420] Like CTCL, gene rearrangement for the β T-cell receptor is present.

Therapy

Four therapeutic modalities produce remissions in most patients with CTCL: topical nitrogen mustard, photochemotherapy with psoralen and ultraviolet A light (PUVA), radiation therapy (particularly total-body electron beam therapy), and systemic chemotherapy. Each induces remission, but cure is uncommon and possible only in early disease.

Topical nitrogen mustard is used predominantly in patients with early cutaneous stages of disease. In more advanced stages, this approach is used to supplement other therapies. The major advantage of topical therapy is that it is relatively nontoxic. Disadvantages include the inconvenience of daily application to large skin surfaces, the allergic reactions in up to half of cases,[421] the potential for development of skin cancer,[422] and the inability to cure the disease. Nitrogen mustard (10 mg diluted in 60 mL of tap water or 60 g of a water-misable cream or in an anhydrous ointment, which may have less allergic sensitization) is administered daily using a cotton swab or small paint brush. Therapy is continued for up to 12 months in responders. Frequency is then reduced to every other day for an additional 1 to 2 years. Therapy is discontinued after 3 years or when cutaneous lesions disappear completely.

Psoralen is a phototoxic furocoumarin activated by ultraviolet A light. In its active form, it binds covalently and irreversibly to DNA. Ultraviolet A light penetrates only the upper part of the dermis. Therefore, psoralen activated by ultraviolet A light affects cells primarily in the epidermis and papillary dermis. A 60% complete remission rate has been reported with psoralen; patients with generalized erythroderma and tumors have lower response rates than those with plaques.[423–425] Psoralen is usually given at a dose of 0.6 mg/kg orally 2 hours before the ultraviolet A light therapy. Treatments are initially given three times weekly. Maintenance therapy may be given every 2 to 4 weeks indefinitely. Adverse effects of PUVA therapy include mild nausea, pruritus, and sunburn-like changes with atrophy and dry skin. PUVA is not cross-resistant with other treatment modalities. Disadvantages are the inability to cure CTCL and expense. Long-term side effects are not yet reported.

Electron beam therapy penetrates only into the upper dermis, and there are minimal systemic effects and an 80% complete remission rate.[426] Twenty percent of patients remain relapse-free at 3 years. Typically, treatment is 4 Gy/wk to a total dose of 36 Gy in 8 to 9 weeks. The advantage of electron beam is a high frequency of durable complete responses without systemic toxicity. Disadvantages are alopecia, atrophy, edema, dermatitis, and high cost.[426,427]

The largest experience with single-agent chemotherapy is with alkylating agents, including nitrogen mustard, 0.4 mg/kg intravenously every 4 to 6 weeks, cyclophosphamide, and chlorambucil (see Table 28-6). Response rates of 60%, with 15% complete remissions, have been reported.[391,428–431] Similar results occur with methotrexate, 2.5 to 10 mg/d by mouth; bleomycin, 7.5 to 15 mg intramuscularly twice weekly; and doxorubicin.[391,432–438] Single-agent therapy does not cure CTCL. Combination therapy with these and other drugs produces objective responses in more than 80% of patients and complete responses in about one fourth of cases.[391,439–441] Duration of remission varies, with a median of about 1 year; no long-term disease-free survival has been reported.

Randomized trials with whole-body electron beam therapy as a single modality compared with electron beam therapy followed by topical nitrogen mustard suggest a benefit of combined therapy.[442] Studies of electron beam therapy combined with chemotherapy suggest an advantage over either alone,[443] but cutaneous and hematologic toxicity is increased. In one study,[443] combined modality therapy produced disease-free survival in some patients with early-stage disease; those with advanced disease failed to benefit. A report of patients randomized to early intensive therapy with cyclophosphamide, doxorubicin, vincristine, and etoposide combined with either topical nitrogen mustard or 30 Gy of electron beam radiation therapy, versus topical or radiation therapy only, showed no differences.[444]

Many therapeutic approaches to CTCL have been used. One study reported a 50% response with high-dose IFN-α.[445] In another study,[446] three of four patients receiving 13 *cis*-retinoic acid improved. Some studies[447,448] claimed success using leukopheresis to treat patients with CTCL. In other studies,[449] subjects receive oral psoralen followed by leukapheresis. The lymphocyte-enriched blood fraction was exposed to ultraviolet A light and returned. This approach decreased lymphocyte viability by 90%. Twenty-seven of 37 patients with otherwise resistant CTCL responded to the treatment. Treatment of four patients with advanced CTCL with pentostatin resulted in two complete and two partial responses.[450] Finally, therapy with monoclonal antibodies was also studied. Unlabeled monoclonal antibodies had only a minimal transient effect.[273–276] In one study,[285] iodine-131–labeled monoclonal antibody produced more prolonged and consistent responses.

LARGE GRANULAR LYMPHOCYTIC LEUKEMIA

Large granular lymphocytes are a heterogeneous group of thymus-independent cells that are largely responsible for most NK-cell activity and have an important role in antibody-dependent cell-mediated cytotoxicity.

Recently, a T-cell lymphoproliferative disorder—LGL leukemia, or chronic T-γ-lymphoproliferative disease[222,223,451]—was recognized. This disease typically follows a chronic course characterized by lymphocytosis with bone marrow infiltration, neutropenia, and recurrent infections.

Epidemiology and Cause

Median age of affected patients is 60 years; there is a 2:1 male/female ratio,[222] and virtually all patients are white. Attempts to isolate viruses from cases have been unsuccessful.

Immunology

Cells from patients with LGL leukemia usually contain acid phosphatase and β-glucoronidase. They may express the pan–T-cell antigens CD2, CD3, and CD5, and the suppressor T-cell–associated antigen CD8. They usually express NK-cell–associated antigens such as CD16 (Fc receptor for IgG), CD56, and CD57. Clonal rearrangement of the β T-cell receptor has been reported.[364,366] Some cases express only NK-cell–associated antigens, such as CD16, CD56, and CD57, without T-cell antigens and absence of rearrangement of the T-cell receptor gene.

The functions of cells from patients with LGL leukemia were studied. In most cases, there is a markedly decreased response to T-cell mitogens and to allogeneic lymphocytes in mixed lymphocyte culture.[222] Cells from most patients suppress normal T-cell mitogen responses and Ig production by pokeweed mitogen–stimulated normal B lymphocytes. Most cases studied were positive for antibody-dependent cellular cytotoxicity; only a small proportion showed NK-cell activity. NK-cell activity was induced in one study[452] by incubating leukemia cells overnight at 37°C or in the presence of IFN-β. Because of the granulocytopenia, some subjects were studied for the ability of their leukemia cells to suppress myeloid progenitor cells; no activity was detected. Cells from three patients with this disease and severe RBC aplasia and from one patient with anemia suppressed erythroid progenitor cells.[453–455]

Cytogenetics

Few reports have been made of cytogenic analyses in patients with this disorder. Chromosomal abnormalities are often not detected[456]; when detected, there are no consistent abnormalities. Trisomy 8 and 14, 6q−, and inv(14) have been reported.[457]

Clinical Features

The typical clinical presentation is that of recurrent bacterial infections, usually a consequence of granulocytopenia. Fatigue from anemia is also common. Bleeding is rare; platelet levels are usually normal. One half of cases have mild to moderate splenomegaly, about 20% have hepatomegaly, and less than 10% have lymphadenopathy. A small proportion have hypogammaglobulinemia, and about one third have hypergammaglobulinemia. Skin infiltration is rare.

In this disease, the malignant cells infiltrate the bone marrow, blood, spleen, and liver. In half of cases, lymphocyte counts are higher than 10×10^9/L. Bone marrow lymphocytosis ranges from 30% to 75%, and some patients have reduced myelopoiesis. About half of cases have severe granulocytopenia with levels less than 0.5×10^9/L. The mechanism underlying the neutropenia is not clear but could reflect decreased production, increased destruction, or both. Recent data suggest that normal large granular lymphocytes inhibit myeloid progenitor cells in vitro.[458,459] As indicated, this is uncommon in patients with LGL leukemia. Antineutrophil antibodies are rare but were reported in some cases.[457]

At least half of patients with this disorder have anemia with hemoglobin levels less than 12 g/dL. The underlying mechanism is unclear. Several mechanisms might operate: (1) bone marrow crowding due to lymphocyte infiltration; (2) direct suppression of erythropoiesis by LGL leukemia as suggested by in vitro inhibition of erythroid progenitor cells[452–454]; (3) reduced levels of erythropoietin; (4) autoantibodies that lyse RBCs by means of complement-dependent or complement-independent mechanisms[457]; or (5) erythrophagocytosis.[454] The Coombs' test is usually negative, suggesting that anemia is not antibody-mediated. Although the bone marrow of patients with LGL leukemia is usually infiltrated by large numbers of LGLs, this is probably insufficient to explain severe anemia. Several investigators suggested that LGLs may suppress erythroid progenitors. An interesting finding is the association with autoimmune diseases, including neutropenia, thrombocytopenia, hemolytic anemia, and rheumatoid arthritis.[457,460,461] It also has been suggested that patients with rheumatoid arthritis and severe granulocytopenia be evaluated for circulating LGLs.

This is typically a chronic disease. Patients often die from bacterial infections secondary to granulocytopenia. Some patients have been reported to develop high-grade lymphomas of LGLs.[462,463] Extensive liver and spleen involvement can occur, as can extensive lymphadenopathy. The course of the disease was rapidly progressive, and the patients were all treated with high-dose chemotherapy. Similar to LGL leukemia, the lymphocytes from these patients were morphologically and immunologically characterized as large granular lymphocytes. Whether this disorder is a variant or a phase of LGL leukemia remains to be determined. It may represent a less mature cell of the same lineage.

Pathology

The typical LGL cell is a large lymphocyte with a high cytoplasmic/nuclear ratio and coarse, azurophilic granules[222] (see Fig. 28-11). The cells are positive for acid phosphatase and β-glucoronidase and negative for esterase and terminal deoxynucleotidyl transferase. Leukemia cells are found in the peripheral blood and focally infiltrating the bone marrow. The spleen typically shows infiltration of the red pulp; the liver demonstrates sinusoidal infiltration with LGL cells.

Differential Diagnosis

This disease is commonly confused with CLL. In a review of the literature, many cases referred to as T-cell CLL were LGL leukemia.[222] This is an important distinction because the approach to therapy and disease course differ considerably. LGL leukemia is distinguished by its lack of lymph node involvement, limited bone marrow involvement, granulocytopenia disproportionate to lymphocytosis and extent of bone marrow involvement, and characteristic morphologic and immunologic features of the malignant cells.

Another diagnostic difficulty is hairy-cell leukemia. Both diseases present with splenomegaly and granulocytopenia, but the distinct morphologic and immunologic characteristics permit differential diagnosis.

Therapy

Most patients do not require therapy save for transfusions for anemia and antibiotics for infections. Chemotherapy with single alkylating agents, such as chlorambucil or cyclophosphamide, or combination chemotherapy with alkylating agents, vincristine, and prednisone are used to treat progressive disease. Although chemotherapy is usually not effective, some cases benefit.[222,223,464,465] Some patients were treated by splenectomy or by spleen irradiation without benefit. Because this disease appears to represent a spectrum from almost benign to a more aggressive malignancy, it is not possible to recommend a specific therapeutic approach. Clearly, many patients do not require chemotherapy and can be followed for many years.

We recently studied recombinant IFN-α in patients with LGL leukemia. No benefit was demonstrated. One patient with pure RBC aplasia associated with this disorder had normalization of hemoglobin without an apparent effect on the underlying disorder. Studies with pentostatin are in progress. Two patients treated with cyclosporine had dramatic increases in their absolute neutrophil count.[466] Hematopoietic growth factors, such as granulocyte colony-stimulating factor, have benefitted patients with granulocytopenia.

Acknowledgments

We express our appreciation to Dr. Neil Kay for reviewing this manuscript; to Irene Rakowski and Drs. Maurice Barcos, Steven Greenberg, and Howard Stoll for providing the pathology figures; to Drs. Tin Han and Ann Marie Block for providing the karyotype figures; and to Patricia Alvarado for typing the manuscript.

REFERENCES

1. Velpeau A. Sur la resorption du pusaet sur l'alteration du sang dans les maladies clinique de persection nenemant: premier observation. Rev Med 1827;2:216.
2. Donne A. Del' origine des glubules du sang, de leur mode de formation, de leur fin. Compt Red Acad De Sci 1842;14:366.
3. Fuller H. Particulars of a case in which enormous enlargement of the spleen and liver, together with dilation of all the blood vessels of the body, were found coincident with a peculiarly altered condition of the blood. Lancet 1846;2:32.
4. Bennett JH. Leucocythaemia or white cell blood. Edinburgh, Sutherland and Knox, 1852.
5. Virchow R. Weisses Blut und Milztumoren. II. Med Z 1847;16:9.
6. Virchow R. Zur pathologischen Physiologie des Bluts: die Bedeutung der nilz- und lymphdrusen-Krankheiten fur die Blutmischung (Leukaemie). Virchows Arch 1853;5:43.
7. Neumann E. Ein Fall von Leukamie mit Erkrankung des Knochenmarkes. Arch Heilk 1870;11:1.
8. Ehrlich P. Parbenanalytische Untersuchungen zur Histologie und Klinik des Blutes. Berlin, Hirschwald, 1891.
9. Osler W. Practice of medicine. New York, Appleton, 1906.
10. Ordway T. Remission in leukemia-produced radium in cases completely resistant to x-ray and benzol treatment. Boston Med Surg J 1917;176:490.
11. Pusey WA. Report of cases treated with roentgen rays. JAMA 1902;38:911.
12. Rénon D, Dreyfus L. Radium therapie de la leucemia myeloide. Arch Electric Med 1933;23:366.
13. Karnofsky DA. Chemotherapy of neoplastic disease. I. Methods of approach. N Engl J Med 1948;239:226.
14. Lawrence JH, Dobson RL, Low-Beer BVA, et al. Chronic myelocytic leukemia: study of 129 cases in which treatment was with radioactive phosphorus. JAMA 1948;136:672.
15. Dameshek W. Chronic lymphocytic leukemia: an accumulative disease of immunologically incompetent lymphocytes. Blood 1967;29:566.
16. Cheson BD, Bennett JM, Rai KR, et al. Guidelines for clinical protocols for chronic lymphocytic leukemia: recommendations of the National Cancer Institute–Sponsored Working Group. Am J Hematol 1988;29:152.
17. International Workshop on Chronic Lymphocytic Leukemia. Chronic lymphocytic leukemia: recommendations for diagnosis, staging and response criteria. Ann Intern Med 1989;110:236.
18. Brok-Simoni F, Rechavi G, Katzir N, et al. Chronic lymphocytic leukemia in twin sisters: monozygous but not identical. Lancet 1987;1:329.
19. Conley CL, Misiti, J, Laster AJ. Genetic factors predisposing to chronic lymphocytic leukemia and to autoimmune disease. Medicine 1980;5:323.
20. Bizzozero OJ Jr, Johnson KG, Ciocco A, et al. Radiation-related leukemia in Hiroshima and Nagasaki 1946 to 1964. II. Observations on type-specific leukemia survivorship, and clinical behavior. Ann Intern Med 1967;66:522.
21. Gallo RC, Kalyanaraman VS, Sarngadharan MG, et al. Association of the human type C retrovirus with a subset of adult T-cell cancers. Cancer Res 1983;43:3892.
22. Poiesz BJ, Ruscetti FW, Gazdar AF, et al. Detection and isolation of type-C retrovirus particles from fresh and cultured lymphocytes of a patient with cutaneous T-cell lymphoma. Proc Natl Acad Sci USA 1980;77:7415.
23. Popovic M, Sarin PS, Robert-Guroff M, et al. Isolation and transmission of human retrovirus (human T-cell leukemia virus). Science 1983;219:856.
24. Kinoshita K, Amagasaki P, Ikedas S, et al. Preleukemic state of adult T-cell leukemia: abnormal T-lymphocytosis induced by human T-cell leukemia-lymphoma virus. Blood 1985;66:120.
25. Mann DL, DeSantis P, Mark G. HTLV-I associated B-cell CLL: indirect role for retrovirus in leukemogenesis. Science 1987;263:1103.
26. Mann DL, LeSane F, Boumpas D, Dean M, Blattner WA. HTLV-I infection and chronic lymphocytic leukemia. Nouv Rev Fr Hematol 1988;30:267.
27. Garver FA, Kiefer CR, Moscoso H, et al. Characterization of a human retrovirus from cultured chronic lymphocytic leukemic B-cells. (Abstract) Blood 1984;64:202A.
28. Kalyanaraman VS, Sarnagadharan MG, Robert-Guroff M, et al. A new subtype of human T-cell leukemia virus (HTLV-2) associated with a T-cell variant of hairy cell leukemia. Science 1982;218:561.
29. Sohn CC, Blayney DW, Misset JL, et al. Leukopenic chronic T cell leukemia mimicking hairy cell leukemia: association with human retroviruses. Blood 1986;67:949.
30. Rickinson AB, Finerty S, Epstein MA. Interaction of Epstein-Barr virus with leukaemic B cells in vitro. I. Abortive infection and rare cell line establishment from chronic lymphocytic leukaemic cells. Clin Exp Immunol 1982;50:347.
31. Ghose T, Lee CL, Faulkner G, Fernandez LA, Lee SH. Progression of a human B cell chronic lymphocytic leukemia line in nude mide. Am J Hematol 1988;28:146.
32. Aisenberg AC, Bloch KJ. Immunoglobulins on the surface of neoplastic lymphocytes. N Engl J Med 1976;287:272.
33. Preud'Homme J, Seligmann M. Surface bound immunoglobulins as a cell marker in human lymphoproliferative disease. Blood 1972;40:777.
34. Godal T, Funderud S. Human B-cell neoplasms in relation to normal B-cell differentiation maturation processes. Adv Cancer Res 1982;36:211.
35. Hamblin TJ, Abdul-Ahad AK, Gordon J, et al. Preliminary experience in treating lymphocytic leukaemia with antibody to immunoglobulin idiotypes on the cell surfaces. Br J Cancer 1980;42:495.
36. Fialkow RJ, Najfeld V, Reddy A, et al. Chronic lymphocytic leukemia: clonal origin in a committed B lymphocyte progenitor. Lancet 1978;2:444.
37. Solanki DL, McCurdy PR, MacDermott RP. Chronic lymphocytic leukemia: a monoclonal disease. Am J Hematol 1982;13:159.
38. Gahrton G, Robert K-H, Friberg K, et al. Nonrandom chromosomal aberrations in chronic lymphocytic leukemia revealed by polyclonal B-cell mitogen stimulation. Blood 1980;56:640.
39. Korsmeyer SJ. Hierarchy of immunoglobulin gene rearrangements in B-cell leukemias. Ann Intern Med 1985;102:497.
40. Korsmeyer SJ, Heiter PA, Ravetch JV, et al. Developmental hierarchy of immunoglobulin gene rearrangements in human leukemic pre-B-cells. Proc Natl Acad Sci USA 1981;78:7096.
41. Ternynck T, Dighiero G, Follezou J, et al. Comparison of normal and CLL lymphocyte surface Ig determinants using peroxidase-labeled antibodies. I. Detection and quantitation of light chain determinant. Blood 1974;43:789.
42. Han T, Ozer H, Blood M, et al. The presence of monoclonal cytoplasmic immunoglobulins in leukemic B cells from patients with chronic lymphocytic leukemia. Blood 1982;59:435.
43. Rubartelli A, Sitia R, Zicca A, et al. Differentiation of chronic lymphocytic leukemia cells: correlation between the synthesis and secretion of immunoglobulins and the ultrastructure of the malignant cells. Blood 1983;62:495.
44. Deegan MJ, Abraham JP, Sawdy KM, et al. High incidence of monoclonal proteins in the serum and urine of chronic lymphocytic leukemia patients. Blood 1984;64:1207.
45. Fitzpatrick J, O'Donnell A, Diloro A, et al. Serum M-proteins in hairy cell leukemia (HCL), chronic lymphocytic leukemia (CLL) and free light chain (FLC) myeloma using high resolution electrophoresis/immunofixation (HRE/IFC). (Abstract) Blood 1986;68:208A.
46. Qian GX, Fu SM, Solanki DL, et al. Circulating monoclonal IgM proteins in B-cell chronic lymphocytic leukemia: their identification, characterization and relationship to membrane IgM. J Immunol 1984;133:3396.
47. Gupta S, Pahwa R, O'Reilly R, et al. Ontogeny of lymphocyte subpopulations in human fetal liver. Proc Natl Acad Sci USA 1976;73:919.
48. Ross GD, Polley MJ. Specificity of human lymphocyte complement receptors. J Exp Med 1975;141:1163.
49. Nadler IM, Anderson KC, Marti G, et al. B4, a human B lymphocyte-associated antigen expressed in normal, mitogen-activated, and malignant B lymphocytes. J Immunol 1983;131:244.
50. Stashenko P, Nadler RM, Hardy R, et al. Characterization of a human B lymphocyte specific antigen. J Immunol 1980;125:1678.
51. Nadler LM, Stashenko P, Hardy R, et al. Characterization of a human B-cell specific antigen (B2) distinct from B1. J Immunol 1981;126:1941.
52. Abramson CS, Kearsey JH, Lebien TW. A monoclonal antibody (BA-1) reactive with cells of human B lymphocyte lineage. J Immunol 1981;126:83.
53. Ritz J, Pesando JM, Notis-McConarty J, Lazarus H, Schlossman SH. A monoclonal antibody to human acute lymphoblastic leukemia antigen. Nature 1980;283:583.
54. LeBien TW, Bou DR, Bradley G, Kersey J. Antibody affinity may influence antigenic modulation of the common acute lymphoblastic leukemia antigen in vitro. J Immunol 1982;129:2287.
55. Faguet GB, Agee JF. Monoclonal antibodies against the chronic lymphatic leukemia antigen cCLLa: characterization and reactivity. Blood 1987;70:437.
56. Brooks DA, Beckman I, Bradley J, et al. Human lymphocyte markers defined by antibody derived from somatic cell hybrids. IV. A monoclonal antibody reacting specifically with a subpopulation of human B lymphocytes. J Immunol 1980;126:1373.
57. Foon KA, Todd RF III. Immunologic classification of leukemia and lymphoma. Blood 1986;68:1.
58. Caligaris-Cappio F, Gobbi M, Bofill M, et al. Infrequent normal B lymphocytes expressed features of B-chronic lymphocytic leukemia. J Exp Med 1982;155:623.
59. Gadol N, Ault RA. Phenotypic and functional characterization of human Leu 1 (CD5) B cells. Immunol Rev 1986;93:23.
60. Antin JH, Emerson SG, Martin P, et al. Leu 1+ (CD5+) B cells, a major lymphoid subpopulation in human fetal spleen: phenotype and functional studies. J Immunol 1986;136;505.
61. Freedman A, Horowitz J, Rosen K, et al. Subpopulations of activated B cells phenotypically resemble B-CLL cells. (Abstract) Blood 1986;68(Suppl 1):245.
62. Freedman AS, Boyd AW, Bieger FR, et al. Normal cellular counterparts of B-cell chronic lymphocytic leukemia. Blood 1987;70:418.

63. Kay NE, Burton J, Wagner D, Nelson DL. The malignant B cells from chronic lymphocytic leukemia patients release TAC-soluble interleukin-2 receptors.
64. Cooper MD, Bertoli LF, Borzillo GV, et al. Pathogenesis of B-cell malignancies. In: Gale RP, Golde DW, eds. Leukemia: recent advances in biology and treatment. New York, Alan R Liss, 1985:453.
65. Robert K-H, Juliusson G, Biberfeld P. Chronic lymphocytic leukemia cells activated in vitro reveal cellular changes that characterize B-prolymphocytic leukaemia and immunocytoma. Scand J Immunol 1983;17:397.
66. Caligaris-Cappio F, Pizzolo G, Chilosi M, et al. Phorbol ester induces abnormal chronic lymphocytic leukemia cells to express features of hairy cell leukemia. Blood 1985;66:1035.
67. Fu SM, Chiorazzi N, Kunkel HG, et al. Induction of in vitro differentiation and immunoglobulin synthesis of human leukemic B lymphocytes. J Exp Med 1978;148:1570.
68. Gordon J, Mellstedt H, Aman P, et al. Phenotypic modulation of chronic lymphocytic leukemia cells by phorbol ester: induction of IgM secretion and changes in the expression of B-cell associated surface antigens. J Immunol 1984;132:541.
69. Okamura J, Letarte M, Stein LD, et al. Modulation of chronic lymphocytic leukemia cells by phorbol ester: increase in Ia expression, IgM secretion and MLR stimulatory capacity. J Immunol 1982;128: 2276.
70. Totterman TH, Nilsson K, Sundstrom C. Phorbol ester–induced differentiation of chronic lymphocytic leukemia cells. Nature 1980;288: 176.
71. Juliusson G, Robert K-H, Hammerstrom L, et al. Mitogen-induced switching of heavy-chain class secretion in chronic B-lymphocytic leukaemia and immunocytoma cell populations. Scand J Immunol 1983;17:51.
72. Slease RB, Wistar R Jr, Scher I. Surface immunoglobulin density on human peripheral mononuclear cells. Blood 1979;54:72.
73. Halper JP, Fu SM, Gottlieb AB, et al. Poor mixed lymphocyte reactions stimulatory capacity of leukemic B cells of chronic lymphocytic leukemia patients despite the presence of Ia antigens. J Exp Med 1979;64: 1141.
74. Wolos JA, Davey FR. B lymphocyte function in B cell chronic lymphocytic leukaemia. Br J Haematol 1981;49:395.
75. Gale RP, Zighelboim J, Ossorio RC, et al. A comparison of human lymphoid cells in antibody-dependent cellular cytotoxicity (ADCC). Clin Immunol Immunopathol 1975;3:377.
76. Johnstone AP, Jensenius JC, Millard RE, et al. Mitogen-stimulated immunoglobulin production by chronic lymphocytic leukaemic lymphocytes. Clin Exp Immunol 1982;47:697.
77. Smith JL, Cowling DC, Barker C. Response of lymphocytes in chronic lymphocytic leukaemia to plant mitogens. Lancet 1972;1:229.
78. Smith JB, Knowlton RP, Koons LS. Immunologic studies in chronic lymphocytic leukemia: defective stimulation of T-cell proliferation in autologous mixed lymphocyte culture. JNCI 1977;58:579.
79. Perri RT. Impaired expression of cell surface receptors for B-cell growth factor by chronic lymphocytic leukemia cells. Blood 1986;67:943.
80. Larson RA, Yachnin S. Cytochalasin B is a potent mitogen for chronic lymphocytic leukemia cells in vitro. J Clin Invest 1983;72:1268.
81. Izaquirre ZA, Minden MD, Howatson AF, et al. Colony formation by normal and malignant human B lymphocytes. Br J Cancer 1980;42: 430.
82. Perri RT, Kay ME. Monoclonal CLL B-cells may be induced to grow in an in vitro B-cell colony assay system. Blood 1982;59:247.
83. Taetle R, Richardson D, To D, et al. Colony-forming assay for circulating chronic lymphocytic leukemia cells. Leuk Res 1982;6:335:344.
84. Kay NE, Johnson JD, Stanek R, et al. T-cell subpopulations in chronic lymphocytic leukemia: abnormalities in distribution and in in vitro receptor maturations. Blood 1979;54:540.
85. Chiorazzi N, Fu SM, Moutazen G, et al. T cell helper defect in patients with chronic lymphocytic leukemia. J Immunol 1979;122:1087.
86. Kay NE. Abnormal T-cell subpopulation function in CLL: excessive suppressor (T) and deficient helper (T) activity with respect to B-cell proliferation. Blood 1981;57:418.
87. Kay NE, Oken MM, Perri RT. The influential T cell in B-cell neoplasms. J Clin Oncol 1983;8:810.
88. Lauria F, Foa R, Catovsky D. Increase in T gamma lymphocytes in B-cell chronic lymphocytic leukemia. Scand J Haematol 1980;24:187.
89. Matutes E, Wechsler A, Gomez R, et al. Unusual T-cell phenotype in advanced B-chronic lymphocytic leukemia. Br J Haematol 1981;49: 635.
90. Platsoucas CD, Galiniski M, Kempin S, et al. Abnormal T lymphocyte subpopulations in patients with B cell chronic lymphocytic leukemia: an analysis by monoclonal antibody. J Immunol 1982;129:2305.
91. Kay NE, Kaplan ME. Defective expression of T cell antigens in chronic lymphocytic leukaemia: relationship to T cell dysfunction. Br J Haematol 1984;57:105.
92. Blue M-L, Daley JF, Levine H, Schlossman SF. Coexpression of T4 and T8 on peripheral blood T cells demonstrated by two-color fluorescence flow cytometry. J Immunol 1985;134:2281.
93. Catovsky D, Lauria F, Matutes E, et al. Increase in T gamma lymphocytes and B-cell chronic lymphocytic leukemia. II. Correlation with clinical stage and findings in B-prolymphocytic leukaemia. Br J Haematol 1981;47:539.
94. Kay NE, Howe RB, Douglas SD. Effect of therapy on T cell subpopulations in patients with chronic lymphocytic leukemia. Leuk Res 1982;6: 345.
95. Wybran J, Chantlet S, Fudenberg HH. Isolation of normal T-cells in chronic lymphocytic leukaemia. Lancet 1973;2:126.
96. Han T, Bloom ML, Dadly B, et al. Lack of autologous mixed lymphocyte reaction in patients with chronic lymphocytic leukemia: evidence for autoreactive T-cell dysfunction not correlated with phenotype, karyotype, or clinical status. Blood 1982;60:1075.
97. Foa R, Catovsky D, Lauria F, et al. Reduced T-colony forming capacity of T-lymphocytes and T-chronic lymphocytic leukemia. Br J Haematol 1980;46:623.
98. Foa R, Lauria F, Catovsky D, et al. Reduced T-colony forming capacity in B-chronic lymphocytic leukemia. II. Correlation with clinical stage and findings in B-prolymphocytic leukemia. Leuk Res 1982;6:329.
99. Fernandez LA, Macsween JM, Langley R. Normal T cell colony numbers in untreated patients with chronic lymphocytic leukaemia (CLL). Br J Haematol 1984;57:97.
100. Lauria F, Foa R, Mantovani B, et al. T-cell functional abnormality in B-chronic lymphocytic leukaemia: evidence of a defect of the T-helper subset. Br J Haematol 1983;54:277.
101. Burton JD, Kay NE. Evidence that malignant chronic lymphocytic leukemia (CLL) B-cells secrete immuno-suppressive ganglioside. (Abstract) Blood 1986;68:92A.
102. Platsoucas CD, Fernandes G, Gupta SL, et al. Defective spontaneous and antibody-dependent cytotoxicity mediated by E-rosette–positive and E-rosette–negative cells in untreated patients with chronic lymphocytic leukemia: augmentation by in vitro treatment with interferon. J Immunol 1980;125:1216.
103. Zeigler HW, Kay, NE, Zarling JM. Deficiency of natural killer cell activity in patients with chronic lymphocytic leukemia. Int J Cancer 1981;27:321.
104. Ziegler-Heitbrock HW, Rumpold H, Kraft D, et al. Patients with a deficiency of natural killer cell activity lack the VEP 13-positive lymphocyte subpopulation. Blood 1985;65:65.
105. Foa R, Fierro MT, Lusso P, et al. Reduced natural killer T-cells in B-cell chronic lymphocytic leukaemia identified by three monoclonal antibodies: Leu-11, A10, AB8.28. Br J Haematol 1986;62:151.
106. Kay NE, Zarling J. Restoration of impaired natural killer cell activity of B-chronic lymphocytic leukemia patients by recombinant interleukin-2. Am J Hematol 1987;24:161.
107. Hokland VP, Ellegaard J. Immunological studies in chronic lymphocytic leukemia. II. Natural killer- and antibody-dependent cellular cytotoxicity potentials of malignant and nonmalignant lymphocyte subsets and the effect of alpha-interferon. Leuk Res 1981;5:349.
108. Lauria F, Raspadore D, Tura D. Effect of a thymic factor on T lymphocytes in B cell chronic lymphocytic leukemia: in vitro and in vivo studies. Blood 1984;64:667.
109. Knuutila S, Elonen E, Teerenhovi L, et al. Trisomy 12 in B-cells of patients with B-cell chronic lymphocytic leukemia. N Engl J Med 1986;314:865.
110. Lucivero G, Prchal JT, Latwon AR, et al. Abnormal T-cell functions in B cell chronic lymphocytic leukemia do not imply T-lymphocyte involvement in the leukemic process: report of a case with demonstrated "polyclonality" of T lymphocytes. J Clin Immunol 1983;3:111.
111. O'Connor NTJ, Wainscoat TS, Weatherall DJ, et al. Rearrangement of the T-cell receptor beta-chain gene in the diagnosis of lymphoproliferative disorders. Lancet 1985;1:1295.
112. Chapel HM, Bunch C. Mechanisms of infection in chronic lymphocytic leukemia. Semin Hematol 1987;24:291.
113. Travade Ph, Dusart JD, Cavaroc M, Beytout J, Rey M. Les infections graves associees a la leucemie lymphoide chronique: 159 episodes infectieux observes chez 60 malades. Presse Med 1986;15:1715.
114. Cone L, Uhr JW. Immunologic deficiency disorders associated with chronic lymphocytic leukemia and multiple myeloma. J Clin Invest 1964;43:2241.
115. Shaw RK, Szwek C, Boggs DR, et al. Infection and immunity in CLL. Arch Intern Med 1960;106:467.
116. Miller DG, Karnofsky DA. Immunologic factors and resistance to infection in CLL. Am J Med 1961;31:748.
117. Fauci AS, Pratt KR, Whalen G. Intrinsic B cell defect in the immunoglobulin deficiency of chronic lymphocytic leukemia. (Abstract) Cancer Res 1977;25:482.
118. Fernandez LA, Macsween JM, Langley GR. Immunoglobulin secretory function of B cells from untreated patients with chronic lymphocytic leukemia and hypogammaglobulinemia: role of T cells. Blood 1983;62: 767.
119. Kay NE, Perri RT. Evidence that large granular lymphocytes from B-CLL patients with hypogammaglobulinemia down-regulate B-cell immunoglobulin synthesis. Blood 1989;73:1016.
120. Bergsagel DE. The chronic leukemias: a review of disease manifestations and the aims of therapy. Can Med Assoc J 1967;96:1615.
121. Ebbe S, Wittels B, Dameshek W. Autoimmune thrombocytopenic purpura ("ITP type") with chronic lymphocytic leukemia. Blood 1962;19: 23.

122. Rustagi P, Han T, Ziolkowski L, et al. Antigranulocyte antibodies in chronic lymphocytic leukemia and other chronic lymphoproliferative disorders. (Abstract) Blood 1983;62:106.
123. Abeloff MD, Waterbury L. Pure red cell aplasia and chronic lymphocytic leukemia. Arch Intern Med 1974;134:721.
124. Conley CL, Misiti J, Laster AJ. Genetic factors predisposing to chronic lymphocytic leukemia and to autoimmune disease. Medicine 1980;5:323.
125. Hayakawa K, Hardy RR, Parks DR, Herzenberg LA. The "Ly-1 B" cell subpopulation in normal, immunodefective and autoimmune mice. J Exp Med 1983;157:202.
126. Hayakawa K, Hardy RR, Honda M, Herzenberg LA, Steinberg AD, Herzenberg L. Ly-1 BN cells: functionally distinct lymphocytes that secrete IgM autoantibodies. Proc Natl Acad Sci USA 1984;81:2492.
127. Hardy RR, Hayakawa K, Shimizu M, Yamasaki K, Kishimoto T. Rheumatoid factor secretion from human Leu-1 + B cells. Science 1987;236:77.
128. Casali P, Burastero SE, Nakamura M, Inghirami G, Notkins AL. Human lymphocytes making rheumatoid factor and antibody to ssDNA belong to the Leu-1 + B-cell subset. Science 1987;236:75.
129. Sthoeger ZM, Wakai M, Tse DB, et al. Production of autoantibodies by CD5-expressing B lymphocytes from patients with chronic lymphocytic leukemia. J Exp Med 1989;169:255.
130. Kipps TJ, Fong S, Tomhave E, Goldfien RD, Chen PP, Carson DA. High-frequency expression of a conserved kappa light chain variable-region gene in chronic lymphocytic leukemia. Proc Natl Acad Sci USA 1987;84:2916.
131. Kipps TJ, Tomhave E, Chen PP, Carson DA. Autoantibody associated kappa light-chain variable-region gene expressed in chronic lymphocytic leukemia with little or no somatic mutation: implications for etiology and immunotherapy. J Exp Med 1988;167:840.
132. Kipps TJ, Robbin BA, Kustar P, Carson DA. Autoantibody associated cross-reactive idiotypes expressed at high frequency in chronic lymphocytic leukemia relative to B-cell lymphomas of follicular center cell origin. Blood 1988;72:422.
133. Gahrton G, Robert K-H, Friberg K, et al. Cytogenetic mapping of the duplicated segment of chromosome 12 and lymphoproliferative disorders. Nature 1982;297:513.
134. Han T, Ozer H, Sadamor N, et al. Prognostic importance of cytogenetic abnormalities in patients with chronic lymphocytic leukemia. N Engl J Med 1984;310:288.
135. Han T, Sadamori N, Ozer H, et al. Cytogenetic studies in 77 patients with chronic lymphocytic leukemia: correlations with clinical immunologic, and phenotypic data. J Clin Oncol 1984;2:1121.
136. Han T, Sadamori N, Takeuchi J, et al. Clonal chromosome abnormalities in patients with Waldenström's and CLL-associated macroglobulinemia: significance of trisomy 12. Blood 1983;62:525.
137. Juliusson G, Robert K-H, Ost A, et al. Prognostic information from cytogenetic analysis in chronic B-lymphocytic leukemia and leukemic immunocytoma. Blood 1985;65:134.
138. Pittman S, Catovsky D. Prognostic significance of chromosome abnormalities in chronic lymphocytic leukaemia. Br J Haematol 1984;58:649.
139. Robert K-H, Gahrton G, Friberg K, et al. Extra chromosome 12 and prognosis in chronic lymphocytic leukaemia. Scand J Haematol 1982;28:163.
140. Sonnier JA, Buchanan GR, Howard-Peebles PN, et al. Chromosomal translocation involving the immunoglobulin kappa-chain and heavy-chain loci in a child with chronic lymphocytic leukemia. N Engl J Med 1983;309:590.
141. Vahdati M, Graafland H, Emberger JM, Karyotype analysis of B-lymphocytes transformed by Epstein-Barr virus in 21 patients with B cell chronic lymphocytic leukemia. Hum Genet 1983;63:327.
142. Juliusson G, Friberg K, Gahrton G. Consistency of chromosomal aberrations in chronic B-lymphocytic leukemia: a longitudinal cytogenetic study of 41 patients. Cancer 1988;62:500.
143. Juliusson G, Gahrton G. Chromosome aberrations in B-cell chronic lymphocytic leukemia: pathogenic and clinical implications. Cancer Genet Cytogenet 1990;45:143.
144. Yunis JJ, Oken MM, Kaplan M, et al. Distinctive chromosomal abnormalities in histologic subtypes of non-Hodgkin's lymphoma. N Engl J Med 1982;307:1231.
145. Erikson J, Finan J, Tsujimoto Y, et al. The chromosome 14 breakpoint in neoplastic B cells with the t(11;14) translocation involves the immunoglobulin heavy chain locus. Proc Natl Acad Sci USA 1984;81:4144.
146. Tsujimoto Y, Yunis J, Onorato-Showe L, et al. Molecular cloning of the chromosomal breakpoint of B-cell lymphomas and leukemias with the t(11;14) translocation. Science 1984;224:1403.
147. Yunis JJ, Frizzera G, Oken MM, et al. Multiple recurrent genomic defects in follicular lymphoma: a possible model for cancer. N Engl J Med 1987;316:79.
148. McDonnell TJ, Deane N, Platt FM, et al. bcl-2-Immunoglobulin transgenic mice demonstrate extended B cell survival and follicular lymphoproliferation. Cell 1989;57:79.
149. Ohno H, Takimoto G, McKelthan TW. The candidate protooncogene bcl-3 is related to genes implicated in cell lineage determination and cell cycle control. Cell 1990;60:991.
150. Han T, Gomez GA, Henderson ES. Spontaneous remission in chronic lymphocytic leukemia. (Abstract) Blood 1986;68:199A.
151. Rai KR, Sawitsky A, Cronkite EP, et al. Clinical staging of chronic lymphocytic leukemia. Blood 1975;46:219.
152. Rai K. A critical analysis of staging in CLL in chronic lymphocytic leukemia. In: Gale RP, Rai K, eds. Recent progress and future directions. New York, Alan R Liss, 1987:253.
153. Binet JL, Auguier A, Dighiero G, et al. A new prognostic classification of chronic lymphocytic leukemia derived from a multivariate survival analysis. Cancer 1981;48:198.
154. Baccarani M, Gabol M, Gobbi M, et al. Staging of chronic lymphocytic leukemia. Blood 1982;59:1191.
155. Rozman C, Montserrat E, Feliu E, et al. Prognosis of chronic lymphocytic leukemia: a multivariate survival analysis of 150 cases. Blood 1982;59:1001.
156. Juliusson G, Robert K-H, Nilsson B, et al. Prognostic value of B-cell mitogen-induced and spontaneous thymidine uptake in vitro in chronic B-lymphocytic leukaemia cells. Br J Haematol 1985;60:429.
157. Moayeri H, Sokal JE. In vitro leukocyte thymidine uptake and prognosis in chronic lymphocytic leukemia. Am J Med 1979;66:773.
158. Simonsson B, Nilsson K. ^{3}H-thymidine uptake in chronic lymphocytic leukaemia cells. Scand J Haematol 1980;24:169.
159. Kallander CF, Simonsson B, Hagberg H, et al. Serum deoxthymidine kinase gives prognostic information in chronic lymphocytic leukemia. Cancer 1984;54:2450.
160. Baldini L, Mozzana R, Cortelezezzi A, et al. Prognostic significance of immunoglobulin phenotype in B cell chronic lymphocytic leukemia. Blood 1985;65:340.
161. Bartl R, Frisch B, Burkhardt R, et al. Assessment of marrow trephine in relation to staging in chronic lymphocytic leukaemia. Br J Haematol 1982;51:1.
162. Lipshutz MD, Mir R, Rai KR, et al. Bone marrow biopsy and clinical staging in chronic lymphocytic leukemia. Cancer 1980;46:1442.
163. Rozman C, Montserrat E, Rodrigues-Fernandez JM, et al. Bone marrow histological pattern: the best single prognostic multivariate survival analysis of 329 cases. Blood 1984;64:642.
164. Han T, Barcos M, Enrigh L, et al. Bone marrow infiltration patterns and their prognostic significance in chronic lymphocytic leukemia: correlations with clinical, immunologic, phenotypic, and cytogenetic data. J Clin Oncol 1984;2:562.
165. Montserrat E, Sanchez-Bisoni J, Vinolas N, Rozman C. Lymphocyte doubling time in chronic lymphocytic leukemia: analysis of its prognostic significance. Br J Haematol 1986;62:567.
166. Han T, Ozer H, Gavigan M, et al. Benign monoclonal B cell lymphocytosis: a benign variant of CLL—clinical, immunologic, phenotypic and cytogenetic studies in 20 patients. Blood 1984;64:244.
167. The Non-Hodgkin's Lymphoma Pathologic Classification Project. National Cancer Institute sponsored study of classification of non-Hodgkin's lymphomas: summary and description of a working formulation for clinical usage. Cancer 1982;49:2112.
168. Pangalis GA, Nathwani BN, Rappaport H. Malignant lymphoma, well differentiated lymphocytic: its relationship with chronic lymphocytic leukemia and macroglobulinemia of Waldenström. Cancer 1977;39:999.
169. Foon KA, Thiruvengadam R, Saven, et al. Genetic relatedness of lymphoid malignancies: transformation of chronic lymphocytic leukemias as a model. Ann Intern Med 1993;119:63.
170. Richter MN. Generalized reticular cell sarcoma of lymph nodes associated with lymphatic leukemia. Am J Pathol 1928;4:285.
171. Armitage JO, Dick FD, Corder MP. Diffuse histiocytic lymphoma complicating chronic lymphocytic leukemia. Cancer 1978;41:422.
172. Dick FR, Maca RD. The lymph node in chronic lymphocytic leukemia. Cancer 1978;41:283.
173. Long JC, Aisenberg AC. Richter's syndrome: a terminal complication of chronic lymphocytic leukemia with distinct clinical pathologic features. Am J Clin Pathol 1975;63:786.
174. Trump CL, Mann RB, Phelps R, Roberts H, Conley CL. Richter's syndrome: diffuse histiocytic lymphoma in patients with chronic lymphocytic leukemia. Am J Med 1980;68:539.
175. Bertoli LF, Kubagawa H, Borzillo GV, et al. Analysis with antiidiotype antibody of a patient with chronic lymphocytic leukemia and a large cell lymphoma (Richter's syndrome). Blood 1987;70:45.
176. Delsol G, Laurent G, Kuhlein E, Familiades J, Rigal F, Pris J. Case reports: Richter's syndrome—evidence for the clonal origin of the two proliferations. Am Soc Clin Pathol 1981;76:308.
177. Heslop HE, Fitzgerald PH, Beard MEJ. Sustained complete remission in Richter's syndrome. Cancer 1987;59:1036.
178. McDonnell JM, Beschorner WE, Staal S, Spivak JL, Mann RB. Richter's syndrome with two different B-cell clones. Cancer 1986;58:2031.
179. van Dongen JJM, Joojikaas H, Michiels JJ, et al. Richter's syndrome with different immunoglobulin light chains and different heavy chain gene rearrangements. Blood 1984;64:571.
180. Splinter TAW, Bom-van Noorloos A, van Heerde P. CLL and diffuse histiocytic lymphoma in one patient: clonal proliferation of two different B cells. Scand J Haematol 1978;10:29.
181. Galton DAG, Goldman JM, Wiltshaw E, Catovsky D, Henry K, Goldenberg GJ. Prolymphocytic leukemia. Br J Haematol 1974;27:7.
182. Katayama I, Aiba M, Pechet L, Sullivan JL, Roberts P, Humphreys RE.

B-lineage prolymphocytic leukemia as a distinct clinical pathological entity. Am J Pathol 1980;99:399.
183. Brouet JC, Flandrin G, Sasportes M, Preud'Homme JL, Seligmann M. Chronic lymphocytic leukaemia of T-cell origin: immunological and clinical evaluation in 11 patients. Lancet 1975;2:890.
184. Catovsky D, Galletto J, Okos A, Galton DAG, Wiltshaw E, Stathopoulos G. Prolymphocytic leukaemia of B and T cell type. Lancet 1973;2:232.
185. Enno A, Catovsky D, O'Brien M, Cherchi, M, Kumaran TO, Galton DAG. "Prolymphocytoid" transformation of chronic lymphocytic leukaemia. Br J Haematol 1979;41:9.
186. Stark AN, Limbert HJ, Roberts BE, Jones RA, Scott CS. Prolymphocytoid transformation of CLL: a clinical and immunological study of 22 cases. Leuk Res 1986;10:1225.
187. Kjeldsberg CR, Marty J. Prolymphocytic transformation of chronic lymphocytic leukemia. Cancer 1981;48:2447.
188. Ghani A, Krause JR, Brody JP. Prolymphocytic transformation of chronic lymphocytic leukemia: a report of three cases and review of the literature. Cancer 1986;57:75.
189. Melo JV, Wardle J, Chetty M, et al. The relationship between chronic lymphocytic leukaemia and prolymphocytic leukaemia. Br J Haematol 1986;64:469.
190. Miller ALC, Habershaw JA, Dhaliwhal HS, Lister TA. Chronic lymphocytic leukaemia presenting as a blast cell crisis. Leuk Res 1984;8: 905.
191. Frenkel EP, Ligler FS, Graham MS, Hernandez JA, Kettman JR Jr, Smith RG. Acute lymphocytic leukemic transformation of chronic lymphocytic leukemia: substantion by flow cytometry. Am J Hematol 1981;10: 381.
192. Laurent G, Gourdin MF, Flandrin G, Kuhlein E, Pris J, Reyes F. Acute blast crisis in a patient with chronic lymphocytic leukemia. Acta Haematol 1981;65:60.
193. Pines A, Ben-Bassat I, Selzer G, Ramot B. Transformation of chronic lymphocytic leukemia to plasmacytoma. Cancer 1984;54:1904.
194. Brouet JC, Germand JP, Laurent G, et al. The association of chronic lymphocytic leukaemia and multiple myeloma: a study of eleven patients. Br J Haematol 1985;59:55.
195. Hoffmann KD, Rudders RA. Multiple myeloma and chronic lymphocytic leukemia in a single individual. Arch Intern Med 1977;137:232.
196. Jeha MT, Hamblin J, Smith JL. Coincident chronic lymphocytic leukemia and osteosclerotic multiple myeloma. Blood 1981;57:617.
197. Pedersen-Bjergaard J, Petersen HD, Thomsen M, Wiik A, Wolff-Jensen J. Chronic lymphocytic leukemia with subsequent development of multiple myeloma. Scand J Haematol 1978;21:256.
198. Fermand JP, James JM, Herait P, Brouet JC. Associated chronic lymphocytic leukemia and multiple myeloma: origin from a single clone. Blood 1985;66:291.
199. Saltman DL, Ross JA, Banks RE, Ross FM, Ford AM, Mackie MJ. Molecular evidence for a single clonal origin in biphenotypic concomitant chronic lymphocytic leukemia and multiple myeloma. Blood 1989;74: 2062.
200. Lampert I, Catovsky D, Mersh GW, et al. Histopathology of prolymphocytic leukaemia with particular reference to the spleen: a comparison with chronic lymphocytic leukemia. Histopathology 1980;4:3.
201. Catovsky D, Cherchi M, Brooks D, et al. Heterogeneity of B-cell leukemias demonstrated by the monoclonal antibody FMC-7. Blood 1981;58:406.
202. Brito-Babapulle V, Pittman S, Melo JU, et al. Cytogenetic studies on prolymphocytic leukemia. 1. B-cell prolymphocytic leukemia. Hematol Pathol 1987;1:27.
203. Pittman S, Catovsky D. Chromosome studies in B-cell prolymphocytic leukemia: a study in nine cases. Cancer Genet Cytogenet 1983;9:355.
204. Melo JV, Catovsky P, Gregory CM, et al. The relationship between chronic lymphocytic leukemia and prolymphocytic leukemia. IV. Analysis of survival and prognostic factors. Br J Haematol 1987;65:23.
205. Krajny M, Pruzanski W. Waldenströms macroglobulinemia: review of 45 cases. Can Med Assoc J 1976;14:899.
206. Preud'Homme J, Seligmann M. Immunoglobulins on the surface of lymphoid cells in Waldenström macroglobulinemia. J Clin Invest 1972;551:701.
207. Waldenström J. Incipient myelomatosis or "essential" hyperglobulinemia with fibrinogenopenia: a new syndrome? Acta Med Scand 1974;117:216.
208. MacKenzie MR. Macroblogulinem. In: Wiernike PH, Canellos GP, Kyle RA, Schiffer CA, eds. Neoplastic disease of the blood. New York, Churchill Livingstone, 1991:501.
209. Bennett JM, Catovsky D, Daniel M-T, et al. Proposals for the classification of chronic (mature) B and T lymphoid leukemias. J Clin Pathol 1989;42:567.
210. Isaacs R. Lymphosarcoma cell leukemia. Ann Intern Med 1937;11:657.
211. Mintzer DM, Hauptman SP. Lymphosarcoma cell leukemia and other non-Hodgkin's lymphomas in leukemic phase. Am J Med 1983;75:110.
212. Zacharski LR, Linman JW. Chronic lymphocytic leukemia versus chronic lymphosarcoma cell leukemia: analysis of 496 cases. Am J Med 1969;47:75.
213. Aisenberg AC, Wilkes B. Lymphosarcoma cell leukemia: the contribution of cell surface study to diagnosis. Blood 1976;48:707.
214. Koziner B, Filippa DA, Mertelsmann R, et al. Characterization of malignant lymphoma in leukemia phase by multiple differentiation markers on leukemic cells: correlations with clinical features and conventional morphology. Am J Med 1977;63:556.
215. Ritz J, Nadler IM, Bhan AK, et al. Expression of common acute lymphoblastic leukemia antigen (CALLA) by lymphomas of B-cell and T-cell lineage. Blood 1981;58:648.
216. Melo JV, Hegde U, Parreira A, Thompson I, Lampert IA, Catovsky D. Splenic B cell lymphoma with circulating villous lymphocytes: differential diagnosis of B cell leukaemias with large spleens. J Clin Pathol 1987;40:642.
217. Neiman RS, Sullivan AL, Jaffe R. Malignant lymphoma simulating leukemia reticuloendotheliosis: a clinicopathologic study of ten cases. Cancer 1979;43:329.
218. DeOliveira MSP, Jaffe FS, Catovsky D. Leukaemic phase of mantle zone (intermediate) lymphoma: its characterization in 11 cases. J Clin Pathol 1989;42:962.
219. Bouroncle BA, Wiseman BK, Doan CA. Leukemic reticuloendotheliosis. Blood 1958;13:609.
220. Golomb HM, Catovsky D, Golde DW. Hairy cell leukemia: a clinical review based on 71 cases. Ann Intern Med 1978;89:677.
221. Golomb HM, Catovsky D, Golde DW. Hairy cell leukemia: a five-year update on seventy-one patients. Ann Intern Med 1983;99:485.
222. Reynold CW, Foon KA. T gamma-lymphoproliferative disorders in man and experimental animals: a review of the clinical, cellular and functional characteristics. Blood 1984;64:1146.
223. Newland AC, Catovsky D, Linch D, et al. Chronic T cell lymphocytosis: a review of 21 cases. Br J Haematol 1984;58:433.
224. Pandolfi F, Strong MD, Slease RB, et al. Characterization of a suppressor T-cell chronic lymphocytic leukemia with ADCC but not NK activity. Blood 1980;56:653.
225. Imbach P, Barandun S, d'Apuzzo V, et al. High-dose intravenous gamma globulin for idiopathic thrombocytopenic purpura in childhood. Lancet 1981;1:1228.
226. Carroll RR, Noyes WD, Rosse WF, Kitchens CS. Intravenous immunoglobulin administration in the treatment of severe chronic immune thrombocytopenic purpura. Am J Med 1984;76:181.
227. Bussell JB, Pham LC, Aledort L, Nachman R. Maintenance treatment of adults with chronic refractory immune thrombocytopenia purpura using repeated intravenous infusions of gamma globulin. Blood 1988;72: 121.
228. Bussell JB, Cunningham-Rundles C, Abraham C. Intravenous treatment of autoimmune hemolytic anemia with very high dose gamma globulin. Vox Sang 1986;51:264.
229. Besa EC. Use of intravenous immunoglobulin in chronic lymphocytic leukemia. Am J Med 1984;76:209.
230. Cooperative Group for the Study of Immunoglobulin in Chronic Lymphocytic Leukemia. Intravenous immunoglobulin for the prevention of infection in chronic lymphocytic leukemia: a randomized controlled clinical trial. N Engl J Med 1988;319:902.
231. Griffiths H, Brennan V, Lea J, Bunch C, Lee M, Chapel H. Crossover study of immunoglobulin replacement therapy in patients with low-grade B-cell tumors. Blood 1989;73:366.
232. Lichtman MA, Rowe JM. Hyperleukocytic leukemias: rheological, clinical, and therapeutic considerations. Blood 1982;60:279.
233. Baer MR, Stein RS, Dessypris EN. Chronic lymphocytic leukemia with hyperleukocytosis: the hyperviscosity syndrome. Cancer 1985;56:2865.
234. French Cooperative Group on Chronic Lymphocytic Leukemia. Effects of chlorambucil and therapeutic decision in initial forms of chronic lymphocytic leukemia (stage A): results of a randomized clinical trial on 612 patients. Blood 1990;75:1414.
235. Han T, Ezdinli EZ, Shimaoka KS, et al. Chlorambucil vs. combined chlorambucil-corticosteroid therapy in chronic lymphocytic leukemia. Cancer 1973;31:5021.
236. Knospe WH, Loeb V Jr, Huguley CM Jr. Bi-weekly chlorambucil treatment of chronic lymphocytic leukemia. Cancer 1974;33:555.
237. Sawitsky A, Rai KR, Glidewell O, et al. Comparison of daily versus intermittent chlorambucil and prednisone therapy in the treatment of patients with chronic lymphocytic leukemia. Blood 1977;50:1049.
238. French Cooperative Group on Chronic Lymphocytic Leukemia. A randomized clinical trial of chlorambucil versus COP in stage B chronic lymphocytic leukemia. Blood 1990;75:1422.
239. Montserrat E, Alcala A, Parody R, et al. Treatment of chronic lymphocytic leukemia in advanced stages: a randomized trial comparing chlorambucil plus prednisone versus cyclophosphamide, vincristine and prednisone. Cancer 1985;56:2369.
240. Raphael B, Andersen JW, Silber R, et al. Comparison of chlorambucil and prednisone versus cyclophosphamide, vincristine, and prednisone as initial treatment for chronic lymphocytic leukemia: long-term follow-up of an Eastern Cooperative Oncology Group randomized clinical trial. J Clin Oncol 1991;9:770.
241. French Cooperative Group on Chronic Lymphocytic Leukemia. Long-term results of the CHOP regimen in stage C chronic lymphocytic leukemia. Br J Haematol 1989;73:334.
242. Hansen MM, Andersen E, Christensen BE, et al. CHOP versus prednisone + chlorambucil in chronic lymphocytic leukemia: preliminary results of a randomized multicenter study. Nouv Rev Fr Hematol 1988;130:433.
243. Bennett JM. The use of "CHOP" in the treatment of CLL. (Letter) Br J Haematol 1990;74:546.

244. Keating MJ, Kantarjian H, O'Brien S, et al. Fludarabine: a new agent with marked cytoreductive activity in untreated chronic lymphocytic leukemia. J Clin Oncol 1991;9:44.
245. Liepman M, Votaw ML. The treatment of chronic lymphocytic leukemia with COP chemotherapy. Cancer 1978;41:1664.
246. Oken MM, Kaplan ME. Combination chemotherapy with cyclophosphamide, vincristine, and prednisone in the treatment of refractory chronic lymphocytic leukemia. Cancer Treat Rep 1979;63:441.
247. Kempin S, Lee BJ III, Koziner B, et al. Combination chemotherapy of advanced chronic lymphocytic leukemia: the M-2 protocol (vincristine, BCNU, cyclophosphamide, melphalan and prednisone). Blood 1982;60: 1110.
248. Keating MJ, Scouros M, Murphy S, et al. Multiple agent chemotherapy (POACH) in previously treated and untreated patients with chronic lymphocytic leukemia. Leukemia 1988;2:157.
249. Valesquez WS, McLaughlin P, Swan F, et al. Dexamethasone, high dose ara-C and cisplatin (DHAP): combination for progressive chronic lymphocytic leukemia. (Abstract) Blood 1986;68:234A.
250. Barton JH, Capizzi RL, Spurr CL, Brockschmidt J. High-dose ara-C (HIDAC) and asparaginase (A'ase) in refractory chronic lymphocytic leukemia. (Abstract) Proc Am Soc Clin Oncol 1990;9:205.
251. Friedenberg J, Andersen J, Oken M, Wolf B, Casseleth P. Modified VAD in the treatment of resistant or relapsing chronic lymphocytic leukemia (CLL): an ECOG Study. (Abstract) Proc Am Soc Clin Oncol 1990;9:210.
252. Keating MJ, Kantarjian H, Talpaz M, et al. Fludarabine: a new agent with major activity against chronic lymphocytic leukemia. Blood 1989;74:19.
253. Puccio C, Mittelman A, Lichtman S, et al. Phase II study of fludarabine phosphate (FAMP) in chronic lymphocytic leukemia (CLL). (Abstract) Proc Am Soc Clin Oncol 1990;9:206.
254. Grever M. Investigational chemotherapy of chronic lymphocytic leukemia. In: Gale RP, Rai K, eds. Chronic lymphocytic leukemia: recent progress and future directions. New York, Alan R Liss, 1987:399.
255. Dillman RO, Mick R, McIntyre OR. Pentostatin in chronic lymphocytic leukemia: a phase II trial of cancer and leukemia group B. J Clin Oncol 1989;7:433.
256. Ho AD, Thaler J, Stryckmans P, et al. Pentostatin in resistant chronic lymphocytic leukemia: a phase II trial of the European organization for research and treatment of cancer. (Abstract) Proc Am Soc Clin Oncol 1990;9:206.
257. Piro LD, Carrera CJ, Beutler E, Carson DA. Chlorodeoxyadenosine: an effective new agent for the treatment of chronic lymphocytic leukemia. Blood 1988;72:1069.
258. Saven A, Carrera CJ, Carson DA, Beutler E, Piro LD. Phase II trial update of 2-chlorodeoxyadenosine treatment of advanced chronic lymphocytic leukemia. (Abstract) Proc Am Soc Clin Oncol 1990;9:212.
259. Adler S, Stutzman L, Sokal JE, et al. Splenectomy for hematology depression in lymphocytic lymphoma and leukemia. Cancer 1975;35: 521.
260. Merl SA, Theodorakis ME, Goldbert J, et al. Splenectomy for thrombocytopenia in chronic lymphocytic leukemia. Am J Hematol 1983;15: 153.
261. Thiruvengadam R, Piedmonte M, Barcos M, Han T. Survival benefit of splenectomy in advanced chronic lymphocytic leukemia. (Abstract) Blood 1989;74:80A.
262. Michallet M, Corront B, Molina L, et al. Allogeneic bone marrow transplantation in chronic lymphocytic leukemia: 17 cases—report of the EBMT. Leukemia Lymphoma 1991;5:127.
263. Foon KA. Biological response modifiers: the new immunotherapy. Cancer Res 1989;49:1621.
264. Dillman RO. Monoclonal antibodies for treating cancer. Ann Intern Med 1989;111:592.
265. Dillman RO, Shawler DL, Sobol RE, et al. Murine monoclonal antibody therapy in two patients with chronic lymphocytic leukemia. Blood 1982;59:1036.
266. Foon KA, Schroff RW, Bunn RA, et al. Effects of monoclonal antibody therapy in patients with chronic lymphocytic leukemia. Blood 1984;64: 1085.
267. Miller RA, Maloney DG, McKillop J, et al. *In vivo* effect of murine hybridoma monoclonal antibody in a patient with T-CLL leukemia. Blood 1981;58:78.
268. Dillman RO, Shawler DL, Dillman JB, et al. Therapy of chronic lymphocytic leukemia and cutaneous T-cell lymphoma with T101 monoclonal antibody. J Clin Oncol 1984;8:881.
269. Foon KA, Bunn PA, Schroff RW, et al. Monoclonal antibody therapy of chronic lymphocytic leukemia and cutaneous T cell lymphoma: preliminary observations. In Boss BE, Langman RE, Trowbridge IS, et al, eds. Monoclonal antibodies and cancer. Orlando, Academic Press, 1983:39.
270. Miller RA, Levy R. Response of cutaneous T cell lymphoma to therapy with hybridoma monoclonal antibody. Lancet 1981;2:226.
271. Miller RA, Oseroff AR, Stratte PT, et al. Monoclonal antibody therapeutic trials in seven patients with T-cell lymphoma. Blood 1983;62: 988.
272. Hertler AA, Schlossman DM, Borowitz MJ, et al. A phase I study of T101-ricin A chain immunotoxin in refractory chronic lymphocytic leukemia. J Biol Response Mod 1988;7:97.
273. Laurent G, Pris J, Farcet JP, et al. Effects of therapy with T101 ricin A-chain immunotoxin in two leukemia patients. Blood 1986;67:1680.
274. DeNardo SJ, DeNardo GL, O'Grady LF, et al. Pilot study of radioimmunotherapy of B-cell lymphoma and leukemia using ^{131}I Lym-1 monoclonal antibody. Antibodies Immunoconjugates Radiopharm 1988;1:17.
275. Press OW, Eary JR, Badger CC, et al. Treatment of refractory non-Hodgkin's lymphoma with radiolabeled MB-1 (anti-CD37) antibody. J Clin Oncol 1989;7:1027.
276. Rosen S, Zimmer AM, Goldman-Neiken R, et al. Radioimmunodetection and radioimmunotherapy of cutaneous T-cell lymphomas using an ^{131}I-labeled monoclonal antibody: an Illinois Cancer Council Study. J Clin Oncol 1987;5:562.
277. Miller RA, Maloney DG, Warnke R, et al. Treatment of B-cell lymphoma with monoclonal anti-idiotype antibody. N Engl J Med 1982; 306:517.
278. Meeker TC, Lowder JN, Maloney DG, et al. A clinical trial of antiidiotype therapy for B-cell lymphocytic malignancies. Blood 1985;65:1349.
279. Miller RA, Hart S, Samoszuk M, et al. Shared idiotypes expressed by human B cell lymphomas. N Engl J Med 1989;321:851.
280. Chatterjee M, Barcos M, Han T, Liu X, Bernstein Z, Foon KA. Shared idiotype expression by chronic lymphocytic leukemia and B-cell lymphoma. Blood 1990;76:1825.
281. Ostlund L, Einhorn S, Robert KH, et al. Chronic B-lymphocytic leukemia cells proliferate and differentiate following exposure to interferon *in vitro*. Blood 1986;67:152.
282. Foon KA, Bottino GC, Abrams PG, et al. Phase II trials of recombinant leukocyte A interferon in patients with advanced chronic lymphocytic leukemia. Am J Med 1985;78:216.
283. Roth MS, Foon KA. Alpha interferon in the treatment of hematologic malignancies. Am J Med 1986;67:152.
284. Foon KA, Sherwin SA, Abrams PG, et al. Treatment of advanced non-Hodgkin's lymphoma with recombinant leukocyte A interferon. N Engl J Med 1984;311:1148.
285. Louie AC, Gallagher JG, Sikora K, et al. Follow-up observations on the effect of human leukocyte interferon on non-Hodgkin's lymphoma. Blood 1981;58:712.
286. Merigan TC, Sikora K, Breeden JH, Levy R, Rosenberg SA. Preliminary observations on the effect of human leukocyte interferon in non-Hodgkin's lymphoma. N Engl J Med 1978;299:1449.
287. Bunn PA Jr, Foon KA, Ihde DC, et al. Recombinant leukocyte A interferon: an active agent in advanced cutaneous T-cell lymphomas. Ann Intern Med 1984;101:484.
288. Foon KA, Maluish AE, Abrams PG, et al. Recombinant leukocyte A interferon therapy for advanced hairy cell leukemia: therapeutic and immunologic results. Am J Med 1986;80:351.
289. Quesada JR, Reuben J, Manning JR, et al. Alpha interferon for induction of remission in hairy-cell leukemia. N Engl J Med 1984;301:15.
290. Ratain MJ, Golomb HM, Vardiman JW, Vokes EE, Jacobs RH, Daly K. Treatment of hairy cell leukemia with recombinant alpha$_2$ interferon. Blood 1985;65:644.
291. Jacobs AD, Champlin RE, Golde DW. Recombinant alpha-2-interferon for hairy cell leukemia. Blood 1985;65:1017.
292. Rozman C, Montserrat E, Vinolas N, et al. Recombinant alpha-interferon in the treatment of B chronic lymphocytic leukemia in early stages. Blood 1988;71:1295.
293. Pangalis GA, Griva E. Recombinant alpha-2b-interferon in untreated stages A and B chronic lymphocytic leukemia: a preliminary report. Cancer 1988;61:869.
294. Ziegler-Heltbrock HW, Schlag F, Fleiger D, Thiel E. Favorable response of early stage B CLL patients to treatment with IFN-alpha. Blood 1989;73:1426.
295. Melo JV, Foroni L, Babapulle B, et al. Prolymphocytic leukemia of B cell type: rearranged immunoglobulin (Ig) genes with defective Ig production. Blood 1985;66:391.
296. Volk JR, Kjeldsberg CR, Eyre HJ, Marty J. T-cell prolymphocytic leukemia: clinical and immunologic characterization. Cancer 1983;52: 2049.
297. Matutes E, Brito-Babapulle V, Swansbury J, et al. Clinical and laboratory features of T-prolymphocytic leukemia. Blood 1991;78:3269.
298. Sadamori N, Han T, Minowada J, Bloom ML, Henderson ED, Sandberg AA. Possible specific chromosome change in prolymphocytic leukemia. Blood 1983;62:729.
299. Ueshima Y, Rowley JD, Variakojis D, et al. Cytogenetic studies in patients with chronic T-cell leukemia/lymphoma. Blood 1984;63:1028.
300. Zech L, Cahrton G, Hammarström L, et al. Inversion of chromosome 14 marks human T-cell chronic lymphocytic leukaemia. Nature 1984;308:858.
301. Croce CM, Isobe M, Polumbo A, et al. Gene for alpha chain of human T-cell receptor: location on chromosome 14 region involved in T-cell neoplasms. Science 1985;227:1044.
302. Polliack A, Leizerowitz R, Berrebi A, et al. Prolymphocytic leukaemia: surface morphology in 21 cases as seen by scanning electron microscopy and comparison with B-type CLL and CLL in prolymphocytoid transformation. Br J Haematol 1984;57:577.
303. Taylor HG, Butler WM, Rhoads J, Karcher DS, Detrick-Hooks B. Prolymphocytic leukemia: treatment with combination chemotherapy to include doxorubicin. Cancer 1982;49:1524.

304. Konig E, Meusers P, Brittinger G. Efficacy of doxorubicin in prolymphocytic leukaemia. Br J Haematol 1979;42:487.
305. Sibbald R, Catovsky D. Complete remission in prolymphocytic leukaemia with the combination chemotherapy CHOP. Br J Haematol 1979;42:488.
306. Oscier DG, Catovsky D, Errington RD, Goolden AWG, Roberts PD, Galton DAG. Splenic irradiation in B-prolymphocytic leukaemia. Br J Haematol 1981;48:577.
307. Catovsky D, Pettit JE, Galetto J, Okos A, Galton DAG. The B-lymphocyte nature of the hairy cell of leukemic reticuloendotheliosis. Br J Haematol 1974;26:29.
308. Jansen J, LeBien TW, Kersey JH. The phenotype of the neoplastic cells of hairy cell leukemia studies with monoclonal antibodies. Blood 1982;59:609.
309. Worman CP, Brooks DA, Hogg N, Zola H, Beverley PCL, Cawley JD. The nature of hairy cells: a study with a panel of monoclonal antibodies. Scand J Haematol 1983;30:223.
310. Divine M, Farcet JP, Gourdin MF, et al. Phenotype study of fresh and cultured hairy cells with the use of immunologic markers and electron microscopy. Blood 1984;64:547.
311. Anderson KC, Park EK, Bates MP, et al. Antigens on human plasma cells identified by monoclonal antibodies. J Immunol 1983;130:1132.
312. Anderson KA, Boyd AW, Fisher DC, et al. Hairy cell leukemia: a tumor of pre-plasma cells. Blood 1985;65:620.
313. Cleary ML, Woods GS, Warnke R, Chao J, Sklar J. Immunoglobulin gene rearrangements in hairy cell leukemia. Blood 1984;64:99.
314. Korsmeyer SJ, Greene WC, Cossman J, et al. Rearrangement and expression of immunoglobulin genes and expression of Tac antigen in hairy cell leukemia. Proc Natl Acad Sci USA 1983;80:4522.
315. Posnett DN, Chiorazzi N, Kunkel HG. Monoclonal antibodies with specificity for hairy cell leukemia cells. J Clin Invest 1982;70:254.
316. Foon KA, Robbins BA, Ellison DJ, Vaickus L. Immunodiagnosis of lymphoid malignancies. Adv Leukemia Lymphoma 1991;3:3.
317. Schwarting R, Stein H, Wang CY. The monoclonal antibodies alpha S-HCL1 (alpha Leu-M5) allow the diagnosis of hairy cell leukemia. Blood 1985;65:974.
318. Saxon A, Stevens RH, Golde DW. T-lymphocyte variant of hairy-cell leukemia. Ann Intern Med 1978;88:323.
319. Li CY, Yam LT, Lam KW. Studies of acid phosphatase isoenzymes in human leukocytes: demonstration of isoenzyme cell specificity. J Histochem Cytochem 1970;18:901.
320. Golomb H. Hairy cell leukemia: an unusual lymphoproliferative disease—a study of 24 patients. Cancer 1978;42:946.
321. Golomb H, Strehl S, Oleske D, Vardiman J. Prognostic significance of immunologic phenotype in hairy cell leukemia: does it exist? Blood 1985;66:1358.
322. Jansen J, Schuit HE, Hermans J, Hijmans W. Prognostic significance of immunologic phenotype in hairy cell leukemia. Blood 1984;63:1241.
323. Ohyashiki K, Ohyashiki JH, Takeuchi J, Han T, Henderson ES, Sandberg AA. Cytogenetic studies in hairy cell leukemia. Cancer Genet Cytogenet 1987;24:109.
324. Brito-Babapulle V, Pittman S, Melo JV, Parreira L, Catovsky D. The 14q+ marker in hairy cell leukaemia: a cytogenetic study of 15 cases. Leuk Res 1986;10:131.
325. Ueshima Y, Alimena G, Rowley JD, Golomb HM. Cytogenetic studies in patients with hairy cell leukemia. Hematol Oncol 1983;1:215.
326. Golomb HM. Hairy cell leukemia: lessons learned in twenty-five years. J Clin Oncol 1983;1:652.
327. Bouroncle BA. Leukemic reticuloendotheliosis (hairy cell leukemia). Blood 1979;53:3:412.
328. Catovsky D, Pettit JE, Galton DAG, Spiers SD, Harrison CV. Leukaemic reticuloendotheliosis ("hairy" cell leukaemia): a distinct clinicopathological entity. Br J Haematol 1974;26:9.
329. Fitzpatrick J, O'Donnell A, DiLoro A, Bhargava A. Serum M-proteins in hairy cell leukemia, chronic lymphocytic leukemia and free light chain myeloma causing high resolution electropheresis/immunofixation. Blood 1986;69:208A.
330. Rosove MH, Naeim F, Harwig S, Zighelboim J. Severe platelet dysfunction in hairy cell leukemia with improvement after splenectomy. Blood 1980;55:903.
331. Cawley JC, Burns GF, Hayhoe RGH. A chronic lymphoproliferative disorder with distinctive features: a distinct variant of hairy-cell leukemia. Leuk Res 1980;4:547.
332. Golomb HM, Jacobs A, Fefer A, et al. Alpha-2 interferon therapy of hairy-cell leukemia: a multicenter study of 64 patients. J Clin Oncol 1986:4:900.
333. Steis RG, Smith JW, Urba WJ, et al. Resistance to recombinant interferon alpha 2a in hairy cell leukemia associated with neutralizing anti-interferon antibodies. N Engl J Med 1988;318:1409.
334. Ratain MJ, Golomb HM, Bardawil RG, et al. Durability of responses to interferon alfa-2b in advanced hairy cell leukemia. Blood 1987;69:872.
335. Sainati L, Matutes E, Mulligan S, et al. A variant form of hairy cell leukemia resistant to alpha-interferon: clinical and phenotypic characteristics of 17 patients. Blood 1990;76:157.
336. Spiers SDC, Moore D, Cassileth PA, et al. Hairy cell leukemia: complete remission with pentostatin (2′deoxycoformycin). N Engl J Med 1987;316: 825.
337. Urba WJ, Baseler MW, Kopp WC, et al. Deoxycoformycin-induced immunosuppression in patients with hairy cell leukemia. Blood 1989;73: 38.
338. Piro LD, Carrera CJ, Carson DA, Beutler E. Lasting remissions in hairy cell leukemia induced by a single infusion of 2-chlorodeoxyadenosine. N Engl J Med 1990;322:117.
339. Uchiyama T, Yodoi J, Sagawa K, Takatsuki K, Uchino H. Adult T-cell leukemia: clinical and hematologic features of 16 cases. Blood 1977;50: 481.
340. Bunn PA, Schechter GP, Jaffe E, et al. Clinical course of retrovirus associated adult T-cell lymphoma in the United States: staging, evaluation and management. N Engl J Med 1983:309:257.
341. Catovsky D, Greaves MF, Rose M, et al. Adult T-cell lymphoma/leukaemia in blacks from the West Indies. Lancet 1982;1:639.
342. Bunn PA. Clinical features. In: Broder S, moderator: T-cell lymphoproliferative syndrome associated with human T-cell leukemia/lymphoma virus. Ann Intern Med 1984;100:543.
343. Blattner WA, Kalyanaraman VS, Robert-Guroff M, et al. The human type-C retrovirus HTLV, in blacks from the Caribbean region, and relationship to adult T-cell leukemia/lymphoma. Int J Cancer 1982;30: 257.
344. Posner LE, Robert-Guroff M, Kalyanaraman VS, et al. Natural antibodies to the human T-cell lymphoma virus in patients with T-cell lymphomas. J Exp Med 1981;154:333.
345. Kalyanaraman VS, Sarngadharan MG, Bunn PA, Minna JD, Gallo RC. Antibodies in human sera reactive against an internal structural protein of human T-cell lymphoma virus. Nature 1981:294:271.
346. Greenberg SJ, Tendler CL, Manns A, et al. Altered cellular gene expression in human retroviral-associated leukemogenesis. In: Blattner W, ed. Current issues in human retrovirology: HTLV-I. New York, Raven Press, 1990;87.
347. Wong-Staal F, Gallo RC. The family of human T-lymphotropic leukemia viruses: HTLV-I as the cause of adult T cell leukemia and HTLV-III as the cause of acquired immunodeficiency syndrome. Blood 1985;65: 253.
348. Blattner WA, Clark JW, Gibbs WN, et al. Human T cell leukemia/lymphoma virus: epidemiology and relationship to human malignancy. In: Gallo RC, Essex M, Gros L, eds. Human T-cell leukemia/lymphoma virus. Cold Spring Harbor, New York, Cold Spring Harbor Laboratory, 1984:267.
349. Saxinger W, Blattner WA, Levmett et al. Human T-cell leukemia virus (HTLV-1) antibodies in Africa. Science 1984;225:1473.
350. Robert-Guroff M, Kalyanaraman VS, Blattner WA, et al. Evidence for human T-cell lymphoma-leukemia virus infection of family members of human T cell lymphoma-leukemia virus positive T cell leukemia-lymphoma patients. J Exp Med 1983;157:248.
351. Sarin PS, Aoki T, Shibata A, et al. High incidence of human type-C retrovirus (HTLV) in family members of a HTLV-positive Japanese T cell leukemia patient. Proc Natl Acad Sci USA 1983;80:2370.
352. Homma T, Kanki PJ, King NW, et al. Lymphoma in macques: association with virus of human T lymphotropic family. Science 1984;225:716.
353. Ferrer JF, Abt DA, Bhatt DM, Marshak RR. Studies on the relationship between infection with bovine C-type virus, leukemia and persistent lymphocytes in cattle. Cancer Res 1974;34:893.
354. Kalyanaraman VS, Sarngadharan MG, Poiesz BJ, Ruscetti FW, Gallo RC. Immunological properties of a type C retrovirus isolated from cultured human T-lymphoma cells and comparison to other mamallian retroviruses. J Virol 1981;38:906.
355. Robert-Guroff M, Ruscetti FW, Posner LE, Poiesz BJ, Gallo RC. Dectection of the human T-cell lymphoma, virus p19 in cells of some patients with cutaneous T-cell lymphoma and leukemia using a monoclonal antibody. J Exp Med 1981;154:1957.
356. Miyoshi I, Kubonishi I, Yoshimoto S, et al. Type C virus particles in a cord T-cell line derived by co-cultivating normal human leukocytes and human leukaemic T cells. Nature 1981:294;770.
357. Popovic M, Lange-Wantzin G, Sarin PS, Mann D, Gallo RC. Transformation of human umbilical cord blood T cells by human T-cell leukemia/lymphoma virus. Proc Natl Acad Sci USA 1983;80:5402.
358. Salahuddin SZ, Markham PD, Lindner SG, et al. Lymphokine production by cultured human T-cells transformed by human T-cell leukemia-lymphoma virus-I. Science 1984;223:703.
359. Popovic M, Flomenberg N, Volkman DJ, et al. Alteration of T-helper cell functions by infection with HTLV-I and HTLV-II. Science 1984;226: 459.
360. Mitsuya H, Matis LA, Megson M, et al. Generation of the HLA-restricted cytotoxic T-cell line reactive against cultured tumor cells from a patient infected with human T-cell leukemia/lymphoma virus. J Exp Med 1983;158:994.
361. Morimoto C, Matsuyama T, Oshige C, et al. Functional and phenotypic studies of Japanese adult T-cell leukemia cells. J Clin Invest 1985;75: 836.
362. Waldmann TA, Greene WC, Sarin PS, et al. Functional and phenotypic comparison of human T cell leukemia/lymphoma virus positive adult T cell leukemia with human T cell leukemia/lymphoma virus negative Sézary leukemia, and their distinction using Anti-Tac. J Clin Invest 1984;73:1711.
363. Flug F, Pelicci P-G, Bonetti F, Knowles DM II, Dalla-Favera R. T-cell receptor gene rearrangements as markers of lineage and clonality in T cell neoplasms. Proc Natl Acad Sci 1985;82:3460.

364. Waldmann TA, David MM, Bongiovanni KF, Korsmeyer SJ. Rearrangements of genes for the antigen receptor on T cells as markers of lineage and clonality in human lymphoid neoplasms. N Engl J Med 1985;313:776.
365. Bertness V, Mirsch I, Hollis G, Johnson B, Bunn PA Jr. T-cell receptor gene rearrangements as clinical markers of human T-cell lymphomas. N Engl J Med 1985;313:534.
366. Aisenberg AC, Krontiris TG, Mak TW, Wilkes BM. Rearrangement of the gene for the beta chain of the T-cell receptor in T-cell chronic lymphocytic leukemia and related disorders. N Engl J Med 1985;313: 530.
367. Sanada I, Tanaka R, Kumagai E, et al. Chromosomal aberrations in adult T cell leukemia: relationship to the clinical severity. Blood 1985;65:649.
368. Verma RS, Macera MJ, Krishnamurthy M, Abramson J, Kapelner S, Dosik H. Chromosomal abnormalities in adult T-cell leukemia/lymphoma (ATL). J Cancer Res Clin Oncol 1987:113:2;892.
369. Miyamoto K, Tomita N, Ishii A, et al. Specific abnormalities of chromosome 14 in patients with acute type of adult T-cell leukemia/lymphoma. Int J Cancer 1987:40;461.
370. Shiraishi Y, Taguchi T, Kubonishi I, Taguchi H, Miyoshi I. Chromosome abnormalities, sister chromatid exchanges, and cell cycle analysis in phytohemagglutinin-stimulated adult T cell leukemia lymphocytes. Cancer Genet Cytogenet 1985:15;65.
371. Whang-Peng J, Bunn PA, Knutsen T, et al. Cytogenetic studies in human T-cell lymphoma virus (HTLV) positive leukemia-lymphoma in the United States. J Natl Cancer Inst 1985:74;357.
372. Shimoyama M, Abe T, Miyamoto K, et al. Chromosome aberrations and clinical features of adult T cell leukemia-lymphoma not associated with human T cell leukemia virus type I. Blood 1987:69;984.
373. Brito-Babapulle V, Matutes E, Parreira L, Catovsky D. Abnormalities of chromosome 7q and Tac expression in T cell leukemias. Blood 1986;67:516.
374. Shimoyama M. Diagnostic criteria and classification of clinical subtypes of adult T-cell leukemia–lymphoma: a report from the Lymphoma Study Group 1991;79:428.
375. Yamaguchi K, Nishimura H, Kohrogi H, Jono M, Miyamoto Y, Takatsuki K. A proposal for smoldering adult T-cell leukemia: a clinicopathologic study of five cases. Blood 1983;62:758.
376. Waldmann TA, Goldman CK, Bongiovanni KF, et al. Therapy of patients with human T-cell lymphotrophic virus I-induced adult T-cell leukemia with anti-Tac, a monoclonal antibody to the receptor for interleukin-2. Blood 1988;72:1805.
377. Tamura K, Makino S, Araki, Y, Imamura T, Seita M. Recombinant interferon beta and gamma in the treatment of adult T-cell leukemia. Cancer 1987;59:1069.
378. Saigo K, Shiozawa S, Shiozawa K, et al. Alpha-interferon treatment for adult T cell leukemia: low levels of circulating alpha-interferon and its clinical effectiveness. Blut 1988;56:83.
379. Daenen S, Rojer RA, Smit JW, Halie MR, Nieweg HO. Successful chemotherapy with deoxycoformycin in adult T-cell lymphoma-leukemia. Br J Haematol 1984;58:723.
380. Winkler CF, Bunn PA. Cutaneous T-cell lymphoma: a review. CRC Crit Rev Oncol Hematol 1983;1:49.
381. Fischmann AB, Bunn PA, Guccion JG, et al. Exposure to chemicals, physical agents and biologic agents in mycosis fungoides and Sézary syndrome. Cancer Treat Rep 1979;63:591.
382. Cohen SR. Mycosis fungoides: clinicopathologic relationships, survival and therapy in 59 patients with observations on occupation as a new prognostic factor. Cancer 1980;46:2654.
383. Manzari V, Gismondi A, Barillari G, et al. HTLV-V: a new human retrovirus isolated in a tac-negative T cell lymphoma/leukemia. Science 1987;238:1581.
384. Haynes BF, Metzgar RS, Minna JD, Bunn PA. Phenotypic characterization of cutaneous T cell lymphoma. N Engl J Med 1981;304:1319.
385. Kung PC, Berger CL, Goldstein G, LoGerfo P, Edelson RL. Cutaneous T-cell lymphoma: characterization by monoclonal antibodies. Blood 1981;57:261.
386. Schroff RW, Foon KA, Billing RJ, Fahey JL. Immunologic classification of lymphocytic leukemias based on monoclonal antibody-defined cell surface antigens. Blood 1982;59:207.
387. Broder S, Edelson RL, Lutzner M, et al. The Sézary syndrome: a malignant proliferation of helper T cells. J Clin Invest 1976;58:1297.
388. Haynes BF, Hensley LL, Jegasothy BV. Phenotypic characterization of skin-infiltrating T cells in cutaneous T-cell lymphoma: comparison with benign cutaneous T-cell infiltrates. Blood 1982;60:463.
389. Whang-Peng J, Bunn PA, Knutsen T, Matthews MJ, Schechter G, Minna JD. Clinical implications of cytogenetic studies in cutaneous T-cell lymphoma (CTCL). Cancer 1982;50:1139.
390. Shapiro PE, Warburton D, Berger CL, Edelson RL. Clonal chromosomal abnormalities in cutaneous T-cell lymphoma. Cancer Genet Cytogenet 1987;28:267.
391. Epstein EH Jr, Levin DL, Croft JD Jr, et al. Mycosis fungoides: survival, prognostic features, response to therapy, and autopsy findings. Medicine 1972;51:61.
392. Sézary A, Bouvrain Y. Etythodermic avec presence de cellules monstrueuses dan le derme et dans le lang circulant. Bull Soc Fr Dermatol Syph 1938;45:254.
393. Long JC, Mihm MC. Mycosis fungoides with extracutaneous dissemination: a distinct clinicopathologic entity. Cancer 1974;34:1745.
394. Rappaport H, Thomas LB. Mycosis fungoides: the pathology of extracutaneous involvement. Cancer 1974;34:1198.
395. Roberts WC, Glancy DL, DeVita VT Jr. Heart in malignant lymphoma (Hodgkin's disease, lymphosarcoma, reticulum cell sarcoma and mycosis fungoides): a study of 196 autopsy cases. Am J Cardiol 1968:22;85.
396. Greer KE, Legum LL, Hess CE. Multiple osteolytic lesions in a patient with mycosis fungoides. Arch Dermatol 1977;113:1242.
397. O'Reilly GV, Clark TM, Crum CP. Skeletal involvement in mycosis fungoides. Am J Roentgenol 1977;129:741.
398. Keltner JL, Fritsch E, Cykiert RC, Albert DM. Mycosis fungoides: intraocular and central nervous system involvement. Arch Ophthalmol 1977;95:545.
399. Kitchen CK. Mycosis fungoides keratitis. Am J Ophthalmol 1963;55: 758.
400. Wolter JR, Leenhouts TM, Hendricks RC. Corneal involvement in mycosis fungoides. Am J Ophthalmol 1963;55:317.
401. Lundberg WB, Cadman EC, Skeel RT. Leptomeningeal mycosis fungoides. Cancer 1976;38:2149.
402. Hauch TW, Shelbourne JD, Cohen HJ, et al. Meningeal mycosis fungoides: clinical and cellular characteristics. Ann Intern Med 1975;82: 499.
403. Posner LE, Fossieck BE, Eddy JL, Bunn PA Jr. Septicemic complications of the cutaneous T-cell lymphomas. Arch Dermatol 1981;71:210.
404. Vonderheid EC, Milstein HJ, Thompson KD, Wu BC. Chronic herpes simplex infection in cutaneous T-cell lymphomas. Arch Dermatol 1980: 116;1018.
405. Vonderheid EC, Vanvoorstvader PC. Herpes zoster-varicella in cutaneous T-cell lymphomas. Arch Dermatol 1980;116:408.
406. Bunn PA, Huberman MS, Whang-Peng J, et al. Prospective staging evaluation of patients with cutaneous T-cell lymphomas: demonstration of high frequency of extra-cutaneous dissemination. Ann Intern Med 1980;93:223.
407. Block JB, Edgcomb J, Eisen A, et al. Mycosis fungoides: natural history and aspects of its relationship to other malignant lyjphomas. Am J Med 1963:34:228.
408. Vonderheid EC, Van Scott EJ, Wallner PE, Johnson WC. A 10 year experience with topical mechlorethamine for mycosis fungoides: comparison with patients treated by total-skin electron beam radiation therapy. Cancer Treat Rep 1979;63:681.
409. Hoppe RT, Cox RS, Fuks Z, et al. Electron-beam therapy for mycosis fungoides: the Stanford University experience. Cancer Treat Rep 1979;63:691.
410. Lamberg SI, Green SB, Byar DP, et al. Status report of 376 mycosis fungoides patients at 4 years: Mycosis Fungoides Cooperative Group. Cancer Treat Rep 1979;63:701.
411. Winkelmann RK. Clinical studies of T-cell erythroderma in the Sézary syndrome. Mayo Clin Proc 1974;49:519.
412. Green SB, Byar DP, Lamberg SI. Prognostic variables in mycosis fungoides. Cancer 1981;47:2671.
413. Castellino RA, Hoppe RT, Blank N, et al. Experience with lymphography in patients with mycosis fungoides. Cancer Treat Rep 1979;63:581.
414. Hamminga L, Mulder JD, Evans C, et al. Staging lymphography with respect to lymph node histology, treatment, and follow-up in patients with mycosis fungoides. Cancer 1981;47:692.
415. Schechter GP, Bunn PA Jr, Fischmann AB, et al. Blood and lymph node T-lymphocyte in cutaneous T-cell lymphoma: evaluation by light microscopy. Cancer Treat Rep 1979;63:571.
416. Moran EM, Walher JR, Aronson IK, Variakojis D. Clinical significance of circulating Sézary cells in mycosis fungoides. Proc AACR ASCO 1977;18:276.
417. Fuks ZY, Bagshaw MA, Farber EM. Prognostic signs and the management of the mycosis fungoides. Cancer 1974;32:1385.
418. Deneau DG, Wood GS, Beckstead J, Hoppe RT, Price N. Woringer-Kolopp disease (Pagetoid reticulosis): four cases with histopathologic ultrastructural, and immunohistologic observations. Arch Dermatol 1984;120:1045.
419. Ketron LW, Goodman MH. Multiple lesions of skin apparently of epithelial origin resembling clinically mycosis fungoides: report of a case. Arch Dermatol Syph 1931;24:758.
420. Wood GS, Weiss LM, Hu C-H, et al. T-cell antigen deficiencies and clonal rearrangements of T-cell receptor genes in pagetoid recitulosis (Woringer-Kolopp disease). N Engl J Med 1988;318:164.
421. Vonderheid EC, Van Scott EJ, Johnson WC, et al. Topical chemotherapy and immunotherapy of mycosis fungoides: intermediate term results. Arch Dermatol 1977;113:454.
422. Devivier A, Vonderheid EC, Can Scott EJ, Urbach F. Mycosis fungoides, nitrogen mustard and skin cancer. Br J Dermatol 1978;99:61.
423. Gilchrest BA. Methoxsalen photochemotherapy for mycosis fungoides. Cancer Treat Rep 1979;63:633.
424. Roenigk HH. Photochemotherapy for mycosis fungoides: long-term follow-up study. Cancer Treat Rep 1979;63:699.
425. Briffa DV, Warin AP, Harrington CI, Bleehen SJ. Photochemotherapy in mycosis fungoides: a study of 73 patients. Lancet 1980;2:49.
426. Lo TCM, Salzman FA, Moschella SL, et al. Whole body surface electron irradiation in the treatment of mycosis fungoides: an evaluation of 200 patients. Radiology 1979;130:453.

427. Proctor MS, Porice NN, Cox AJ, Hoppe RT. Subcutaneous mycosis fungoides. Arch Dermatol 1978;114:1326.
428. Kierland RR, Watkins CH, Shullenberger CC. The use of nitrogen mustard in the treatment of mycosis fungoides. J Invest Dermatol 1947:9/10:195.
429. Van Scott EJ, Grekin DA, Kalmanson JD, et al. Frequent low doses of intravenous mechlorethamine for late-stage mycosis fungoides lymphoma. Cancer 1975;36:1613.
430. Van Scott EJ, Auerbach R, Clendenning WE. Treatment of mycosis fungoides with cyclophosphamide. Arch Dermatol 1962;85:107.
431. Wright JC, Lyons MM, Walker DB, et al. Observations on the use of cancer chemotherapeutic agents in patients with mycosis fungoides. Cancer 1964;17:1045.
432. Haynes HA, Van Scott EJ. Therapy of mycosis fungoides. Prog Dermatol 1968;3:1.
433. Wright JC, Gumport SL, Golomb FM. Remissions produced with the use of methotrexate in patients with mycosis fungoides. Cancer Chemother Rep 1960;9:11.
434. McDonald CJ, Bertino JR. Treatment of mycosis fungoides lymphomas: effectiveness of infusions of methotrexate followed by oral citovorum factor. Cancer Treat Rep 1979;62:1009.
435. Takeda K, Sagawa T, Arakawa T. Therapeutic effect of bleomycin for skin tumors. Cancer 1970;61:207.
436. Spigel SC, Coltman CA Jr. Therapy of mycosis fungoides with bleomycin. Cancer 1975;32:767.
437. Yogoda A, Mukherji B, Young C, et al. Bleomycin, an anti-tumor antibiotic. Ann Intern Med 1972;77:861.
438. Levi JA, Diggs CH, Wiernik PH. Adriamycin therapy in advanced mycosis fungoides. Cancer 1977;39:1967.
439. Grozea PN, Jones SE, McKelvey EM, et al. Combination chemotherapy for mycosis fungoides: a Southwest Oncology Group Study. Cancer Treat Rep 1979;63:647.
440. Leavell UW Jr, De Simone P. Combined chemotherapy (COP), in treatment of mycosis fungoides: report of four cases. South Med J 1976;69:915.
441. Tirelli W, Veronesi A, Galligiani E, et al. Clinical and immunological evaluation of 5 cases of mycosis fungoides in advanced stages. Tumori 1979;65:447.
442. Price NK, Hoppe RT, Constantine VS, et al. The treatment of mycosis fungoides: adjuvant topical mechlorethamine after electron beam therapy. Cancer 1977;40:2851.
443. Winkler CF, Sausville EA, Ihde DC, et al. Combined modality treatment of cutaneous T cell lymphoma: results of a 6 year follow up. J Clin Oncol 1986;4:1094.
444. Kaye F, Eddy J, Ihde DC, et al. Conservative vs aggressive therapy in mycosis fungoides. Proc ASCO 1989;8:257.
445. Bunn PA Jr, Ihde DC, Foon KA. The role of recombinant leukocyte A interferon in the therapy of cutaneous T-cell lymphomas. Cancer 1986;57:1315.
446. Kessler JF, Meyskens FL Jr, Levine N, Lynch PJ, Jones SE. Treatment of cutaneous T-cell lymphoma (mycosis fungoides) with 13-cis-retinoic acid. Lancet 1983;1:1345.
447. Pineda AA, Winkelmann RN. Leukapheresis in the treatment of Sézary syndrome. J Am Acad Dermatol 1981;5:544.
448. Edelson R, Facktor M, Andrews A, Lutzner M, Schein P. Successful management of the Sézary syndrome: mobilization and removal of extravascular neoplastic T-cells by leukapheresis. N Engl J Med 1974;291:293.
449. Edelson R, Berger C, Gasparro F, et al. Treatment of cutaneous T-cell lymphoma by extracorporeal photochemotherapy: preliminary results. N Engl J Med 1987;316:297.
450. Bisaccia ER, Grever MR, Scarborough DA, et al. 2'deoxycoformycin (CDF) induced remission in advanced cutaneous T-cell lymphomas (CTCL). Proc Am Soc Clin Oncol (Abstract) 1982;18:158.
451. Pandolfi F. T-CLL and allied diseases: new insights into classification and pathogenesis. Diagn Immunol 1986;4:61.
452. Itoh K, Tsuchikawa K, Awataguchi T, Shiiba K, Kumagai K. A case of chronic lymphocytic leukemia with properties characteristic of natural killer cells. Blood 1983;61:940.
453. Linch DC, Cawley JC, MacDonald SM, et al. Acquired pure red-cell aplasia associated with an increase of T cells bearing receptors for the Fc of IgG. Acta Haematol 1981;65:270.
454. Nagasawa T, Abe T, Nakagawa T. Pure red cell aplasia and hypogammaglobulinemia associated with Tr-cell chronic lymphocytic leukemia. Blood 1981;57:1025.
455. Hoffman R, Kopel S, Shu SD, Dainiak N, Zanjani ED. T cell chronic lymphocytic leukemia: presence in bone marrow and peripheral blood of cells that suppress erythropoiesis in vitro. Blood 1978;52:255.
456. Dallapicolla B, Alimena G, Chessa L, et al. Chromosome studies in patients with T-CLL chronic lymphocytic leukemia and expansions of granular lymphocytes. Int J Cancer 1984;34:171.
457. Loughran TP, Kadin ME, Starkebaum G, et al. Leukemia of large granular lymphocytes: association with clonal chromosomal abnormalities and autoimmune neutropenia, thrombocytopenia, and hemolytic anemia. Ann Intern Med 1985;102:169.
458. Moretta L, Loretta A, Canonica GW, Bacigalupo A, Mingari MC, Cerottini JC. Receptors for immunoglobulins on resting and activated human T cells. Immunol Rev 1981;56:141.
459. Spitzer G, Verma DS, Abramowitz S, Tomasovic B. Cells with Fc receptors from normal donors suppress granulocyte macrophage colony formation. Blood 1982;60:758.
460. Wallis WJ, Loughran TP, Kadin ME, Clark EA, Starkebaum GA. Polyarthritis and neutropenia associated with circulating large granular lymphocytes. Ann Intern Med 1985;103:357.
461. Barton JC, Prasthofer EF, Egan ML, Heck LW, Koopman WJ, Grossi CE. Rheumatoid arthritis associated with expanded populations of granular lymphocytes. Ann Intern Med 1986;104:314.
462. Kadin ME, Kamoun N, Lamberg J. Erythrophagocytic T lymphoma: a clinical pathologic entity resembling malignant histiocytosis. N Engl J Med 1981;304:648.
463. Pandolfi F, Pezzutto A, DeRossi G, et al. Characterization of two patients with lymphomas of large granular lymphocytes. Cancer 1984;53:445.
464. Palutke M, Eisenberg L, Kaplan J, et al. Natural killer and suppressor T-cell chronic lymphocytic leukemia. Blood 1983;62:627.
465. Hocking WG, Singh R, Schroff R, Golde DW. Cell mediated inhibition of erythropoiesis and megaloblastic anemia in T-cell chronic lymphocytic leukemia. Cancer 1983;51:631.
466. Baer MR, Martinez JY, Dadey B, Han T. Cyclosporin reverses agranulocytosis associated with large granular lymphocyte proliferation. (Abstract) Blood 1989;74:68A.

Blood: Principles and Practice of Hematology,
edited by Robert I. Handin, Thomas P. Stossel, and Samuel E. Lux.
J.B. Lippincott Company, Philadelphia © 1995.

29

Hodgkin's Disease

Alan C. Aisenberg

Hodgkin's disease is a neoplastic disorder of the lymphoid system characterized by the presence of diagnostic multinucleate giant cells, termed *Reed-Sternberg cells*, in an appropriate mixed inflammatory infiltrate. The enlarged lymph nodes of this condition must be distinguished from those of the other (non-Hodgkin's) malignant lymphomas. Without treatment, Hodgkin's disease evolves into a debilitating systemic illness, characterized by fever, night sweats, chills, weight loss, and itching; it leads to death in a few to many years. Radiation therapy and chemotherapy programs developed after World War II now cure most (two thirds) patients with this disorder[1] (Fig. 29-1). Thus, Hodgkin's disease represents an outstanding triumph of modern cancer management. Although constituting only 1% of the cancer incidence of developed countries, the disorder has played a pivotal role in the evolution of medical oncology. The youth of the affected patient population, the dramatic clinical picture, and, more recently, the success of treatment, have led to continuing interest within the medical profession and to an extensive literature.

HISTORY

In 1832, Thomas Hodgkin (Fig. 29-2) published a paper in the *Medical-Chirurgical Transactions*, entitled "On Some of the Morbid Appearances of the Absorbent Glands and Spleen."[2]

> ***Case 2***
> *September 24th, 1828. Ellenborough King [Fig. 29-3], aged ten years, was admitted to Luke's ward on the 6th of August 1828, under the care of Dr. Bright. He was the youngest of six children, of whom the first five were reported to be all healthy. This child had also been healthy till about thirteen months ago, when his strength, flesh, and healthy appearance began to fail. He was living at that time in the West of England. A tumour was observed in the left hypochondrium in the situation of the spleen, the glandulae concatenatae on the right side were observed to be considerably enlarged, but under the treatment used, these tumours, as well as that in the situation of the spleen, were at times very considerably reduced in size.*
>
> *It does not appear that he was ever subject to haemorrhage, nor till very lately to dropsical effusion; his appetite was generally good. After admission into the hospital the tumour on the left side was observed to extend considerably below the left hypochondrium, but was reported not to be as large as it had formerly been. The glands on the left side of the neck were swollen, as well as those on the right; the abdomen was somewhat distended, and there was considerable oedema of the scrotum. . . .*
>
> *The head was not opened.*
>
> *The glands in the neck had assumed the form of large ovoid masses, connected together merely by loose cellular membrane and minute vessels: when cut into they exhibited a firm cartilaginous structure of a light colour and very feeble vascularity, but with no appearance of softening or suppuration. Glands similarly affected accompanied the vessels into the chest, where the bronchial and mediastinal glands were in the same state and greatly enlarged. There were some old pleuritis adhesions. The substance of the lung was generally healthy. There was a good deal of clear serum in the pericardium, but this membrane, as well as the heart, was quite healthy.*
>
> *In the peritoneal cavity there was a considerable quantity of clear straw-coloured serum mixed with extensive, recent thin diaphanous films. The mucous membrane of the stomache and intestines was tolerably healthy.*
>
> *The mesenteric glands were but slightly enlarged, and but little if at all indurated; but those accompanying the aorta, the splenic artery, and the illiacs were in the same state as the glands of the neck.*
>
> *The liver contained no tubercles, and its structure was quite healthy. The pancreas was rather firm, and the glands situated along its upper edges were, as before stated, greatly enlarged. The spleen was enlarged to at least four times its natural size, its surface sprinkled with tubercles, presenting the same structure as the enlarged glands already described.*[2]

Hodgkin's astute observation was lost for a generation until Sir Samuel Wilks, working at Guy's Hospital with some of the same pathologic material, independently distinguished the condition from other causes of chronic lymphadenopathy (carcinoma, tuberculosis, amyloid). When Hodgkin's earlier study came belatedly to Wilks attention, Wilks generously credited the earlier observation and introduced the eponym by which the disorder is still known.[3] Histologic examination of Hodgkin's cases in the present century has verified the nature of three, possibly four, of the original seven cases, including case 2.

In the late 19th century, Greenfield,[4] among others, described characteristic giant cells in Hodgkin's disease. A full description of the diagnostic cell required Ehrlich's staining methods and awaited the publications of Sternberg[5] in 1898 and particularly of Dorothy Reed[6] in 1902 (Fig. 29-4). Reed clearly distinguished the process from tuberculosis, a condition that complicated Sternberg's cases.

The first modern approach to Hodgkin's disease can be found in the Jackson and Parker monograph published in 1947.[7] A conference held in Rye, New York, in 1966 provided a simplified version of the Lukes and Butler histologic classification, which remains in use today, and introduced

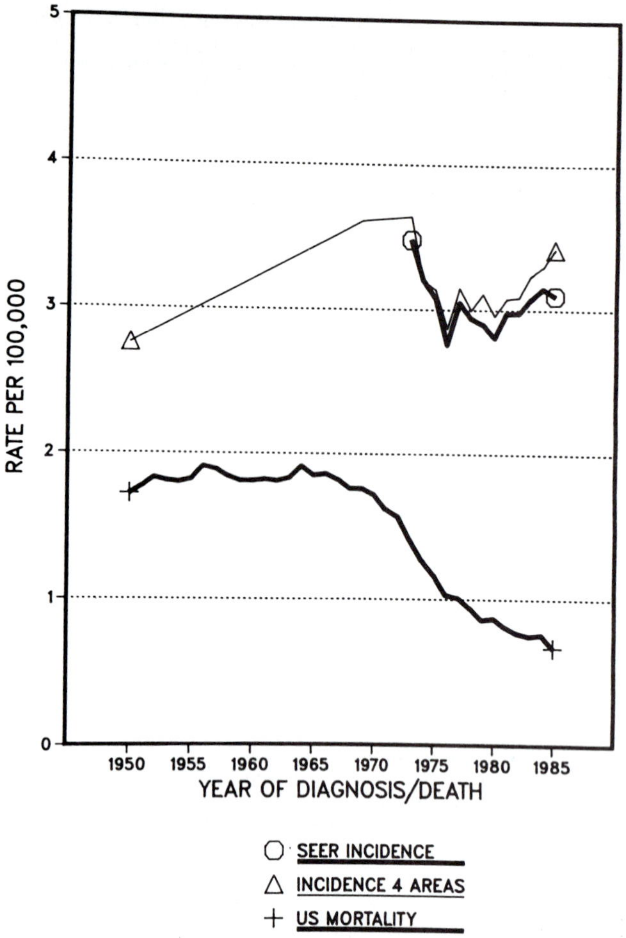

FIGURE 29-1. Hodgkin's disease incidence and mortality rate in white males and females. This chart documents the remarkable decrease in Hodgkin's disease mortality rate between 1967 and 1985, a period during which disease incidence was unchanged. (Annual Cancer Statistics Review. National Institutes of Health Publication 88-2789. Bethesda, MD, Department of Health and Human Services, National Cancer Institute 1987:II.153).

many modern ideas about staging, prognosis, and treatment.[8] Successive advances in radiation therapy can be attributed to René Gilbert,[9] Vera Peters and K.H.C. Middlemiss,[10] and Henry Kaplan.[11] Finally, the landmark use of the MOPP drug combination by Vincent DeVita and colleagues[12] at the National Cancer Institute was based on the earlier laboratory and clinical investigations of Frei, Freireich, Holland, Skipper, Carbone, and Pinkel. The late Henry Kaplan's monumental book on Hodgkin's disease remains an authoritative reference on many aspects of the disorder.[13]

EPIDEMIOLOGY

The epidemiology of Hodgkin's disease has been the subject of detailed investigation, although few conclusive facts have emerged.[13–15] The disorder accounts for about 1% of the malignant disease seen in developed countries, where an annual incidence of 2 to 3 per 100,000 and a male/female ratio of about 4:3, is reported. The bimodal age curve illustrated in Figure 29-5 is characteristic of developed countries: it features a low incidence in childhood, a rapid increase during the teens leading to a first peak at about age 25, a decreasing plateau through middle age, and a second peak in advanced age. MacMahon proposed that this bimodality results from the overlap of two disease distributions with differing age peaks.[16] Furthermore, he suggested that the young adult peak is the result of an infectious agent, whereas the cause of the peak in the elderly is similar to that of other lymphomas and malignant disease.

In economically disadvantaged countries, a different pattern is seen.[15–17] The initial peak is in childhood, particularly among boys; relatively low rates are seen among young adults; and the characteristic late peak of the elderly is preserved. The childhood peak seen in developing countries has been ascribed to a shift of the peak of early adulthood seen in the economically advantaged into childhood. As expected, marked differences exist in the occurrence of the various histologic subtypes of Hodgkin's disease between developed and developing counties (see section on histopathology). The nodular sclerosis subtype predominates in most affluent industrialized countries, but is uncommon among the economically disadvantaged, where the mixed-cellularity and lymphocyte depletion subtypes prevail. Furthermore, in developing countries, patients with Hodgkin's disease present much more frequently in the advanced clinical stage, and the disease pursues a more aggressive course.

Correa and O'Conor[17] applied the designation *type I* to the Hodgkin's disease pattern of economically disadvantaged countries, *type III* to the pattern of affluent nations, and *type II* to the pattern seen under intermediate economic conditions. African Americans exhibit the *same* type III pattern as whites in the United States, supporting an environmental explanation for the different disease patterns. Finally, an exceptional age incidence curve is exhibited in Japan, where Hodgkin's disease is extremely rare before the age of 50 years.

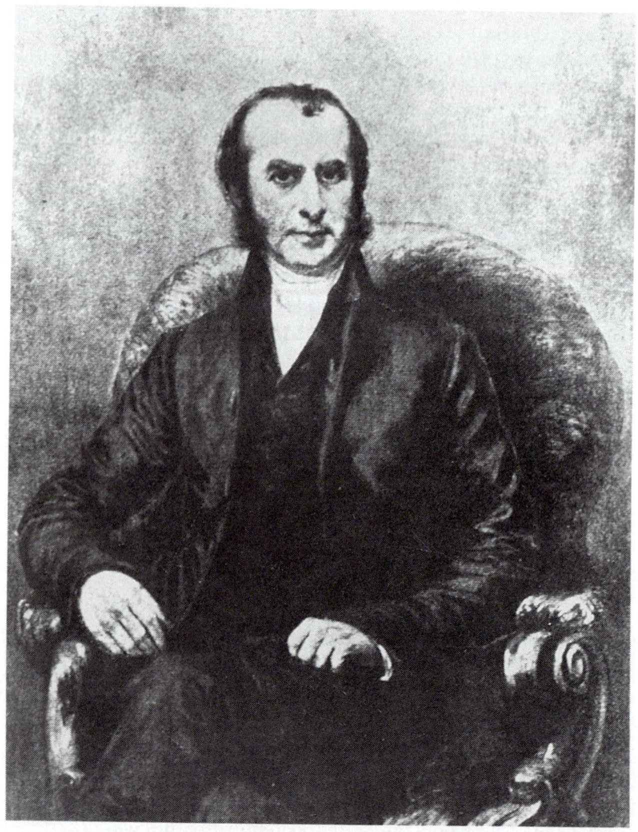

FIGURE 29-2. Thomas Hodgkin (1798 to 1866), "a man distinguished alike for scientific attainments, medical skill, and self-sacrificing philanthropy" (epitaph inscribed on Hodgkin's tomb in Jaffa).

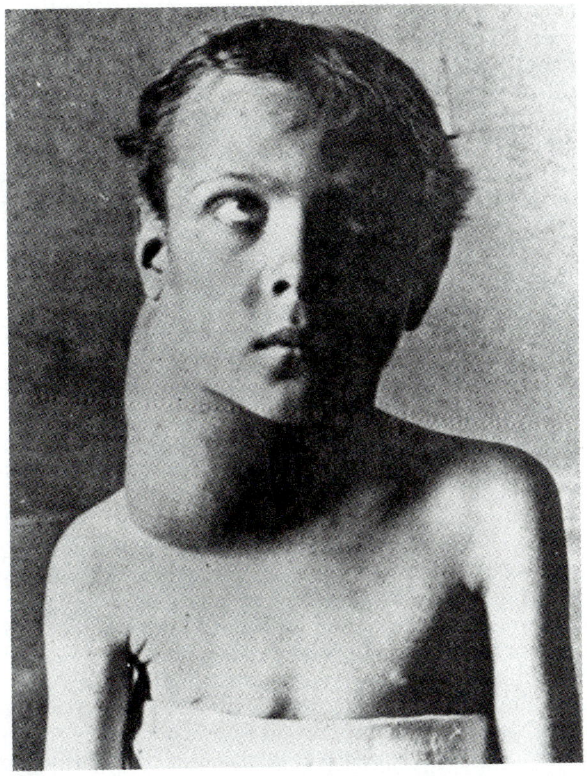

FIGURE 29-3. The picture is not that of Ellenborough King but a 7-year-old boy (WDM, case 7) in Dorothy Reed's classic paper. (Reed DM. On the pathological changes in Hodgkin's disease, with especial reference to the relation to tuberculosis. Johns Hopkins Hosp Rep 1902;10:Plate V)

Most experienced clinicians have observed one or more striking examples of the familial incidence of Hodgkin's disease. I observed two sisters, born 4 years apart, who developed similar presentations of Hodgkin's disease at almost the same chronologic age. Nevertheless, such occurrences are uncommon. A careful study of sibling pairs suggests a seven-fold higher incidence of Hodgkin's disease when a sibling is affected; sibling pairs of concordant sex have twice the risk of discordant pairs.[18] Given the low incidence of Hodgkin's disease, the risk even to concordant siblings is extremely small. Convincing evidence has never been obtained for increased risk to the parent, child, spouse, or physician of the patient with Hodgkin's disease.

Gutensohn[14,19] has proposed that Hodgkin's disease is the result of an uncommon host response to a common infectious agent. Her hypothesis, that economic advantage leads to late exposure and increased incidence, is based on certain parallels with poliomyelitis epidemiology. She reports that incidence of Hodgkin's disease increases with increasing maternal education and economic advantage, and decreases with increasing sibship size, multiple unit housing, and birth order. Not all observers can confirm these observations.

Other incidence factors have been studied. Vianna[20] has published extensively on the purported contagious aspect of Hodgkin's disease. Several meticulous studies failed to substantiate the claim, which is plausibly attributed to pitfalls in the statistical methods used. Tonsillectomy has also been raised as a risk factor, but this, too, has not survived rigorous statistical study.[21]

Epidemiology has produced a number of engaging hypotheses concerning the cause of Hodgkin's disease. Unfortunately, none is compelling, nor does the available epidemiologic evidence discriminate between alternate explanations involving putative etiologic and host factors.

IMMUNOLOGIC STATUS AND INFECTIONS

The immunologic status of the Hodgkin's disease patient is another aspect of the disorder that has been subject to close scrutiny.[22–27] The susceptibility of these patients to tuberculosis and other infections struck many early observers. In 1928, Ewing[28] observed infection in 20% of his Hodgkin's disease population and was led to write "tuberculosis follows Hodgkin's disease like a shadow." Surprisingly, Parker, Jackson, and associates[29] rarely found the tuberculin test to be positive in Hodgkin's disease, even in the presence of active tuberculosis. As the mechanism of cellular immunity emerged after World War II, it was possible to clarify this aspect of Hodgkin's disease. These patients exhibited impaired cellular immunity by (1) unresponsiveness when skin tested with delayed-type antigens to which a control population would regularly respond because of prior exposure (mumps, streptokinase or streptodornase, and fungal antigens)[30]; (2) inability to acquire

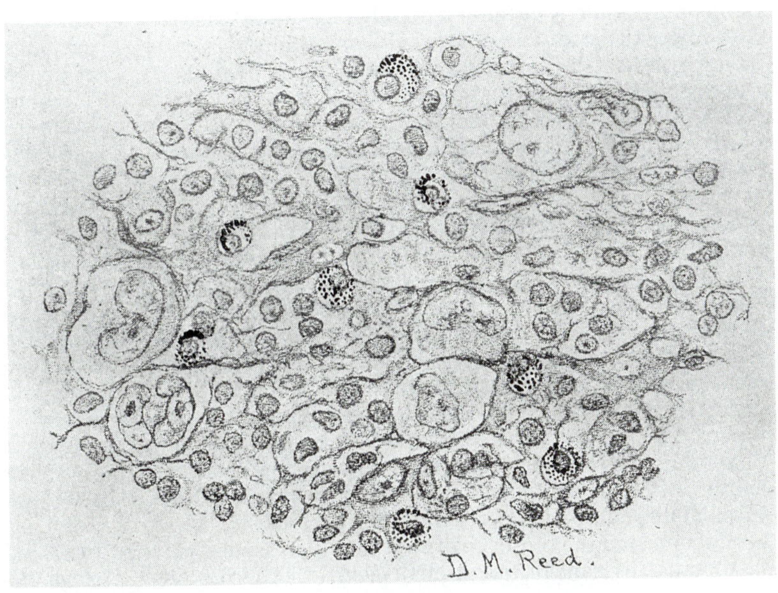

FIGURE 29-4. Reed-Sternberg cells drawn by Dorothy Reed's own hand. The mirror-image cell at the lower left is diagnostic. (Reed DM. On the pathological changes in Hodgkin's disease, with especial reference to the relation to tuberculosis. Johns Hopkins Hosp Rep 1902;10:Plate X)

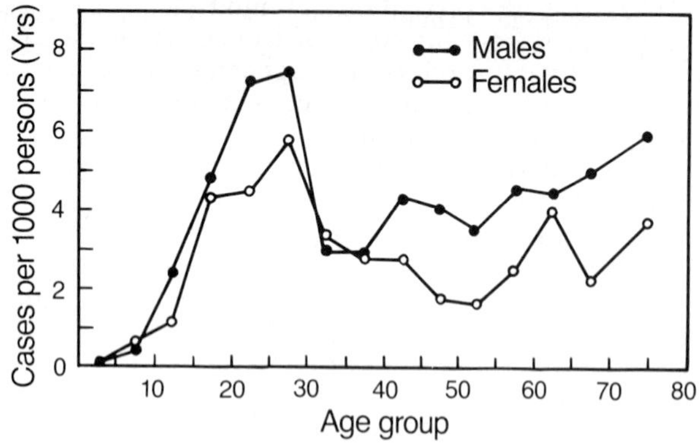

FIGURE 29-5. Age-specific incidence of Hodgkin's disease in the Boston and Worcester standard metropolitan statistical areas from mid-1973 through 1977, according to sex. (Gutensohn NE, Cole P. Childhood social environment and Hodgkin's disease. N Engl J Med 1981;304:135)

new sensitivities such as contact sensitivity to dinitrochlorobenzene[31]; and (3) impaired ability to reject skin homografts.[32] By contrast, humoral immunity (antibody formation) was essentially intact.

The introduction of aggressive treatment—first radiation therapy and later chemotherapy—confounded further study of the immune deficit because both treatment modalities impair immunity. Moreover, the term *anergy*, introduced to describe the defect in cell-mediated immunity,[30] was an unfortunate choice, being interpreted by some to mean the absence of cellular immunity[33] and by others to mean only a quantitative diminution in responsiveness.[22] Nonetheless, it is evident, on the basis of several meticulous studies, that a defect in delayed hypersensitivity (cellular immunity) can be demonstrated in untreated Hodgkin's disease patients, even those in whom early stage disease has been pathologically documented. Demonstration of the defect requires close attention to antigen dose when testing with recall antigens (antigens to which sensitivity was acquired by past exposure), and attention to both the sensitizing and testing concentrations of antigen when actively sensitizing with dinitrochlorobenzene.[34]

The time course of the in vitro lymphocyte response to graded doses of phytohemagglutinin is a particularly sensitive index of the defect.[35,36] Impaired cellular immunity can be observed in patients with early Hodgkin's disease but is more evident in those with advanced stage disease. Although existence of a deficit in cellular immunity in early Hodgkin's disease has been established, the specificity of the finding to that disease process has not been put to the test. Few patients with other disorders associated with impaired cellular immunity (sarcoidosis, measles, tuberculosis, leprosy) have been subject to the same rigorous investigation.

The mechanism of the defect of Hodgkin's disease remains under study.[26] Absolute lymphocytopenia is observed in only one third of those with untreated Hodgkin's disease, mostly those with advanced disease, and is therefore an unlikely explanation in most patients.[33] Similarly, the quantitative diminution in helper (T4) T lymphocytes is usually insufficient to explain the deficiency. Other parameters have been measured and explanations proposed[13,23,25–27]: deficiencies or intrinsic abnormalities of one or another T-lymphocyte subset, enhanced suppressor cell activity of T cells or of monocytes, enhanced prostaglandin E_2-mediated suppression, decreased interleukin-2 (IL-2) production, and the presence of immunosuppressive serum factors such as transforming growth factor-β (TGF-β). None has gained general acceptance. Sufficient numbers of appropriate patients are hard to assemble, experimental parameters are complex and difficult to measure, and the critical correlation of the level of the putative mediator with the in vivo level of cell-mediated immunity is usually neglected.

A second well-characterized immunologic defect observed in patients with Hodgkin's disease is a consequence of treatment.[25,36,37] Splenectomy (performed as part of staging laparotomy), radiation therapy, and chemotherapy all contribute to an impairment of humoral immunity (antibody formation). The unfortunate consequence of this confluence is the sporadic occurrence of fulminant, usually fatal, sepsis from encapsulated gram-positive (*Streptococcus pneumoniae*) and gram-negative (*Haemophilus influenzae*) bacteria.

In the Massachusetts General Hospital series, the complication has been restricted to patients who have undergone splenectomy and who received both total nodal irradiation and combination chemotherapy,[37] but other clinics have observed the distressing complication in patients who had undergone splenectomy and who were treated less aggressively.[38] Antibody levels to the two pathogens just mentioned, which are responsible for the major proportion of this sepsis, can be precisely related to the timing and extensiveness of prior Hodgkin's disease treatment, as can the patient's ability to respond to appropriate bacterial vaccines.[39] A minor risk of fulminant sepsis seems to be a consequence of splenectomy in any Hodgkin's disease patient, but this risk reaches a frightening level for several years in those who receive, in addition, both total nodal irradiation and combination chemotherapy. The excess risk of splenectomy in favorable Hodgkin's disease treated with radiation alone (over that of incidental splenectomy) remains to be determined.

The approach to treatment-induced fulminant sepsis remains a matter of contention. Some consider the risk of sepsis a reason to exclude staging laparotomy and splenectomy in Hodgkin's disease.[38] Others concentrate on avoiding total nodal irradiation plus combination chemotherapy in patients who underwent splenectomy and accept the small risk that splenectomy otherwise entails, with the view that the risk of sepsis must be weighed against the other risks of therapy and of Hodgkin's disease itself.[37] All Hodgkin's disease patients who have had splenectomy should receive pneumococcal and *H influenzae* vaccination as early after diagnosis as possible, and certainly before treatment is begun.[39] After therapy is underway, the Hodgkin's disease patient has limited ability to respond to these vaccines. The role of prophylactic antibiotics in patients at high risk of fulminant sepsis remains to be established. Whether or not this measure is used, vigilance is required in their follow-up.

As Hodgkin's disease is managed, most cases of herpes zoster occur within the first year after radiation therapy or chemotherapy, with a peak incidence in the few months that follow the completion of treatment.[40,41] In this clinical context, herpes zoster is usually segmental and follows the benign course that characterizes that disorder in patients who are immunologically intact. Herpes zoster in such persons should be sharply differentiated from that condition seen in individuals with advanced and uncontrolled Hodgkin's disease. The latter patients with a global immune deficit can be expected to experience severe local herpes zoster with more frequent dissemination. These patients should receive prompt treatment with intravenous acyclovir.

An extensive literature is available on infections in patients with Hodgkin's disease.[25,42–44] In the patient with end-stage Hodgkin's disease, the intrinsic Hodgkin's disease defect in cell-mediated immunity is compounded by the immune impairment from repeated courses of immunosuppressive drugs (particularly adrenal corticosteroids) and prior radiation. Such patients are susceptible to a variety of common types of infection with the usual gram-positive and gram-negative pathogens, as well as with the entire spectrum of opportunist pathogens listed in Table 29-1. Among the latter, central nervous system infection with *Cryptococcus neoformans* and pneumonia caused by *Pneumocystis carinii* are particularly significant. These patients with advanced disease exhibit an immune deficit and a susceptibility to infection that closely parallels that seen in patients with acquired immunodeficiency syndrome (AIDS). Fortunately, with present intermittent drug treatment schedules and with the restrained use of adrenal corticosteroids, global immune impairment is uncommon. Most Hodgkin's disease patients seen today are cured by modern chemotherapy or radiation; the small percentage who succumb to aggressive Hodgkin's disease usually do so rapidly. A clinically significant immunologic deficit, that is, one that leads to overt infection, is *unusual* in the present-day Hodgkin's disease population. Infection is rare prior to treatment, unless the condition is extraordinarily advanced or neglected. With the exceptions just noted, infection is also uncommon after judiciously administered combination chemotherapy or radiation, especially if the patient is in remission or has been cured.

ETIOLOGY

Few efforts in medical science have produced a more grudging return from the time and resource invested than the study of the causes of Hodgkin's disease. This can plausibly be attributed to the singular disadvantage of studying a neoplasm in which the neoplastic cell (Reed-Sternberg) seldom constitutes more than 1% of the tumor bulk and frequently constitutes less than one tenth of 1%. Few experimental techniques are successful against such odds. Perhaps techniques for Reed-Sternberg cell isolation will bear fruit.[45]

TABLE 29-1. Organisms Causing Infection in Hodgkin's Disease

GRAM-POSITIVE COCCI	**TUBERCULOSIS**
Streptococcus pneumoniae	*Mycobacterium tuberculosis*
Staphylococcus aureus	Atypical mycobacteria
Staphylococcus epidermidis	
Other streptococci	**FUNGI**
	Cryptococcus neoformans
GRAM-POSITIVE BACILLI	*Coccidioides immitus*
Listeria monocytogenes	*Histoplasma capsulatum*
Clostridium species	*Candida* species
Nocardia species	*Aspergillus* species
GRAM-NEGATIVE BACILLI	**PROTOZOA**
Escherichia coli	*Pneumocystis carinii*
Haemophilus influenzae	*Toxoplasma gondii*
Pseudomonas aeruginosa	
Klebsiella species	**VIRUSES**
Proteus species	Varicella
Salmonella species	Herpes zoster
Enterobacter species	Herpes simplex
Bacteriodes species	Cytomegalovirus
	Polyomavirus of multifocal leukoencephaplopathy

Also, most of the present insight into Hodgkin's disease etiology comes from the study of animal lymphoma and leukemia, the non-Hodgkin's lymphomas, and epithelial neoplasms. Although this subject is more appropriately considered elsewhere in this volume, a review is given here, followed by considerations specific to Hodgkin's disease. No attempt is made to describe the many "false hares" that have occupied scientists over the past half-century.

First, *viruses* play a causative role in the lymphomas and lymphocytic leukemias of mice, rats, hamsters, chickens, cats, dogs, cattle, and monkeys.[46] In human non-Hodgkin's lymphoma, the Epstein-Barr virus (EBV) plays a complex role in African Burkitt's lymphoma,[47,48] and the human T-cell leukemia virus I (HTLV-I) causes the adult T-cell leukemia-lymphoma first reported from Japan.[49,50] Second, specific *chromosomal abnormalities* are regularly observed in most subtypes of non-Hodgkin's lymphoma and lymphoid leukemia.[51,52] Third, *oncogenes* are increasingly implicated in non-Hodgkin's lymphoma and epithelial malignancy.[53] These genes, which regulate growth and cell division, may code for growth factors or their receptors. The oncogene defect may involve inappropriate activation of a regulatory gene or loss of an inhibitory factor. Oncogene activation may involve the juxtaposition of an extraneous DNA-controlling sequence, a point mutation of the oncogene, or oncogene duplication. Most recently, mechanisms involving transcription factors and cell cycle regulators termed cyclins have been increasingly implicated in oncogenesis.[54]

In non-Hodgkin's lymphoma, the commonly observed chromosome translocations may lead to oncogene dysregulation. This is well illustrated by the translocations [t(8;14), t(2;8), t(8;22)] of Burkitt's lymphoma, in which immunoglobulin gene sequences inappropriately regulate the *myc* oncogene, whose protein product is a DNA-binding transcription factor.[54,55] Neoplastic transformation probably requires the malfunction of at least two oncogenes. *Dysregulation, perhaps virus-induced, of two or more oncogenes is likely at the root of Hodgkin's disease.*

The preceding paragraph places current understanding of Hodgkin's disease etiology in the context of animal lymphomas and leukemias, and of other human lymphomas and epithelial neoplasms, and arrives at a likely conclusion about Hodgkin's disease from this context. On the other hand, the results of investigations applied directly to Hodgkin's disease have been disappointing, producing only a few findings of possible significance, a variety of artifacts, and one example of scientific fraud. Early studies using the electron microscope and efforts at direct virus isolation were unrevealing.

Cell Culture

The difficulty in establishing long-term cell cultures of Hodgkin's disease–derived cells was an obstacle to viral studies. As late as 1980, Henry Kaplan[13] could state, "no permanent cloned cell line unambiguously derived from the neoplastic giant cell population of a patient with a verifiable diagnosis of Hodgkin's disease has been established to the present time." Thereafter, at least 10 long-term Hodgkin's disease cell lines have been isolated and characterized.[56]

The cultured cells express surface markers that are similar to those of Reed-Sternberg cells in fresh Hodgkin's disease biopsy material; the Hodgkin's disease–associated activation antigen Ki-1 (CD30), the granulocyte-staining X-hapten (CD15), the IL-2 receptor (CD25), the transferrin receptor (CD71), and the major histocompatibility complex class IA (HLA-DR) antigen. The isolates are heterogeneous with respect to lineage—six appear to be of B-cell derivation and four of T-cell derivation—on the basis of immunophenotype and appropriately rearranged antigen receptor genes (immunoglobulin or T-cell receptor).[57] The Hodgkin's lines also display a heterogeneous assortment of nonrandom chromosomal abnormalities.[56] Finally, virus isolation from the cultured material has been unrewarding.

Therefore, cell culture has not established the etiology of Hodgkin's disease or the lineage of the Reed-Sternberg cell. The fact that 7 of the 10 lines are derived from effusions raises additional doubts about the applicability of the findings to the typical presentations of Hodgkin's disease.

Cytogenetics

Chromosome studies of Hodgkin's disease have been difficult because of the low mitotic yield of cells belonging to the malignant population.[13,58–62] Frequently, normal karyotypes derived from benign host cells predominate. Hodgkin's disease cells derived from pleural effusions yield more mitoses, but their karyotype may reflect karyotypic evolution. A multitude of marker chromosomes have been observed in more than half of cases in which chromosome analysis has been possible. In the small group of specimens exhibiting clearcut aneuploid lines, a small proportion of cases was near diploid, and slightly larger proportions were triploid to tetraploid and bimodal (with both near-diploid and triploid to tetraploid clones). Duplications of chromosomes 5, 2, 1, 12, and 21 have been noted frequently, whereas loss of chromosomes 22, 10, 13, and 17 occurs less often. Rearrangements, especially translocations and deletions, most often involve 1p, 1q, 2q, 6q, 8q, 11p, and 14q.[62] The breakpoints of some of the translocations seen in Hodgkin's disease are similar to those of non-Hodgkin's lymphomas (11q23, 14q32, 6q11-21, 8q22-24, 11q13).[60]

In summation, cytogenetic studies in Hodgkin's disease have been of limited value. The findings are consistent with a variable surplus of chromosomes in a neoplasm composed of variably polyploid and multinucleate tumor cells embedded in a milieu of normal host cells. Chromosomal abnormalities specific for Hodgkin's disease have not been reported so far.

Immunophenotype

The lineage of the multinucleate Reed-Sternberg cell and of the mononuclear variants encompassed by the rubric of Hodgkin's disease cells has been the subject of prolonged controversy.[13,56,63] Candidate progenitor cells include the B lymphocyte, the T lymphocyte, the histiocyte, and various interdigitating and dendritic (reticulum) cells.[56] Unfortunately, surface marker and histochemical studies have failed to resolve the controversy.[56,63] The initial finding of surface immunoglobulin associated with Reed-Sternberg cells was taken as evidence of B-cell lineage. Later investigation established the exogenous origin of the immunoglobulin from its polyclonal character (both κ and λ light chains were present).[64]

The generally agreed immunophenotype of the Reed-Sternberg cell is positive for CD30 (Ki-1), CD15 (Leu M1), HLA-DR, CD25 (IL-2 receptor), and CD71 (transferrin receptor), and negative for CD45 (leukocyte common antigen), T-cell antigens, B-cell antigens, and most monocyte–macrophage–histiocyte antigens.[56,63,65–71] The first two phenotype markers are the most useful and specific of these admittedly nonspecific determinants.

The Ki-1 antigen, detected by a monoclonal antibody raised against a Hodgkin's disease–derived cell line, is an activation antigen present in most but not all Reed-Sternberg and Hodgkin's cell populations.[69] It also reacts with many large cell lymphomas, particularly ones of T-cell lineage, and with a minor cellular constituent of benign proliferations. The monoclonal antibody Leu M1 reacts with a myeloid antigen present on neutrophils, some blood monocytes, some T cells, most but not all Hodgkin's disease cell populations, and some large cell lymphomas.[68]

The remaining determinants may help to identify Reed-Sternberg cells in certain morphologic contexts, but are subject to more frequent exceptions. Reed-Sternberg cells may occasionally exhibit the leukocyte common antigen, or one or another B-cell or T-cell lineage determinant. The IL-2 and transferrin receptors and HLA-DR are also widely distributed on activated lymphoid cells (of both B-cell and T-cell lineages) undergoing immunologic transformation and are not diagnostically reliable.

Reed-Sternberg cells in the nodular variant of lymphocyte-predominant Hodgkin's disease (lymphocytic and histiocytic cells) are exceptional in their surface marker characteristics, resembling B-lineage lymphoma cells much more closely than the Reed-Sternberg cells of other Hodgkin's disease subtypes.[70,71] Lymphocytic and histiocytic cells are usually unreactive with both the Ki-1 and Leu M1 reagents and exhibit some (B1 [CD20] and J chain) but not all (clonal immunoglobulin) B-cell lineage determinants.

Immunophenotypic study, particularly reactivity with Ki-1 and Leu M1 antisera, provides the pathologist with useful ancillary information, but does not serve as a final arbiter of diagnosis in Hodgkin's disease.[65–68,70,71]

Antigen Receptor Genes

Rearrangements of antigen receptor genes are used to determine lineage and clonality of both B-cell (immunoglobulin genes) and T-cell (T-cell receptor genes) proliferations (see Chap. 26). Unfortunately, a positive consensus has not emerged from the several studies performed with Hodgkin's disease tissue.[72–75] Some investigations have been negative; others report rearrangement of either an immunoglobulin or a T-cell receptor gene in a variable number of cases. Furthermore, the rearranged band is usually faint when compared with its germline counterpart: a coherent pattern of gene rearrangement (such as heavy plus light immunoglobulin chain genes) is rarely observed, and the percentage of positive samples is only in the 10% to 20% range. Attempts to select specimens rich in Reed-Sternberg cells or to concentrate these elements have sometimes, but not always, produced more encouraging results.[74,75] The inability to detect rearranged antigen receptor genes in Hodgkin's disease could result from the sparsity of tumor cells, but the published results are unimpressive.

Epstein-Barr Virus

Epstein-Barr virus has figured prominently as a putative causal agent of Hodgkin's disease.[13,14,76] Serologically confirmed infectious mononucleosis consistently confers a three-fold risk of subsequent Hodgkin's disease.[13,14] Although antibody to EBV capsid antigen is present in the same proportions in Hodgkin's disease patients and matched controls, the geometric mean titer is higher in those with Hodgkin's disease.

A concerted effort has been made to demonstrate EBV in Hodgkin's disease tissue. The EBV genome was detected in biopsy material by Southern blotting and localized to Reed-Sternberg cells by in situ hybridization in 25% to 30% of specimens.[77,78] With the aid of the polymerase chain reaction, the percentage of positive Hodgkin's disease specimens was increased to 58%, but only at the price of 36% EBV positivity in hyperplastic lymph nodes.[79] Most recently, EBV latent membrane protein expression was localized to Reed-Sternberg cells by in situ hybridization in almost half of the specimens studied.[80,81] During the past several years, evidence for the presence of EBV in a significant proportion of Hodgkin's disease patients has increased; unfortunately, the ubiquity of this agent in lymphoid tissue mandates a cautious interpretation of the findings.

Non-Hodgkin's lymphomas complicate many immunodeficiency states including AIDS,[82] a variety of congenital immunodeficiency disorders,[83,84] the X-linked immunodeficiency syndrome,[85] and organ transplantation.[86] Generally, the tumors are high-grade, large-cell lymphomas, and activation of the EBV can be readily demonstrated.[87] If Hodgkin's disease were observed to complicate these immunodeficiency states, this would be a strong argument for a viral role in pathogenesis, particularly for the EBV.

Hodgkin's disease occurs infrequently in organ transplant recipients and in those with the X-linked immunodeficiency syndrome.[86] It has been reported in patients with congenital immunodeficiency states,[83,84] but the incidence is no greater than would be expected in a population of the same age.[86] Cases of Hodgkin's disease have been recently reported in the AIDS population, but no statistical evidence has been presented that the incidence is greater than would be expected in a young, predominantly male population of the same size.[88,89]

In view of the frequency with which non-Hodgkin's lymphoma complicates immunodeficiency states, the incidence of Hodgkin's disease in immunodeficiency does not support a critical role of EBV in the pathogenesis of Hodgkin's disease. When Hodgkin's disease does occur in the immunodeficient person, both histologic subtype and prognosis are unfavorable, and response to treatment is usually poor.

The role of EBV in the pathogenesis of Hodgkin's disease remains unclear.

Miscellaneous

Both the systemic reaction of the host and the intense inflammatory tissue infiltrate could be mediated through cytokine production by Hodgkin's disease tumor cells. Some Hodgkin's disease cell lines have been found to produce interleukin-1 (IL-1).[90] Most lines express the IL-2 receptor α-chain antigen (CD25),[56] and a high serum IL-2 level is reported to have adverse prognostic significance in children with the disorder.[91] In addition, interleukin-5 messenger RNA has been regularly detected in the Reed-Sternberg cells of Hodgkin's disease patients with eosinophilia.[92] Finally, a unique TGF-β has been isolated from a Hodgkin's disease cell line.[93] Clearly, more than a few isolated observations are needed to clarify the role of cytokines in the pathogenesis of Hodgkin's disease.

Tumor-associated antigens, including ferritin, have been isolated from Hodgkin's disease tissue.[94] Recently, a novel treatment program using a yttrium-labeled antiferritin antibody has produced responses in patients with end-stage Hodgkin's disease.[95] Another abnormality that Hodgkin's disease shares with other neoplasms is the presence of circulating immune complexes.[96] Finally, the significance of the *bcl*-2 oncogene rearrangements reported in Hodgkin's disease tissue remains unclear.[97]

HISTOPATHOLOGY

The diagnosis of Hodgkin's disease is made with the microscope. Identification of diagnostic Reed-Sternberg cells in an appropriate histologic context is an absolute requirement.[70,71,98–100] Hodgkin's disease usually obliterates the normal architecture of the entire involved node; partial or focal involvement is less usual.

The surgeon should obtain a large intact lymph node from the center of the disease process, although mediastinoscopy specimens are usually satisfactory. Diagnosis can be made by needle biopsy, but most pathologists find a larger sample more satisfactory for both diagnosis and subclassification. Even an experienced hemopathologist, working with adequate tissue optimally fixed and stained, may have difficulty with the diagnosis. Occasionally, a second biopsy, performed immediately or after a suitable time interval, is needed to establish the diagnosis. Cells with the morphology of Reed-Sternberg cells have been described in infectious mononucleosis and other benign viral and hypersensitivity disorders; thus, premature or inappropriate biopsy of adenopathy in such conditions can lead to unnecessary confusion and anguish.

Usually, an unexplained lymph node should be more than 2 cm before biopsy is warranted; even then, nodes in the smaller size range should be present for at least 1 month. The author's adage holds that the initial diagnosis of Hodgkin's disease is unlikely to be made from a lymph node not externally visible. Trivial adenopathy is common; Hodgkin's disease is not.

Reed-Sternberg Cell

The diagnostic cell of Hodgkin's disease is a multinucleate giant cell with large eosinophilic inclusion-like nucleoli, a thick, well-defined nuclear membrane, and pale-staining chromatin.[98–100] The classic cell has two mirror-image nuclei, but cells with more than two nuclei are common and nuclear lobation may be prominent (Fig. 29-6). Reed-Sternberg cells must be identified to make the diagnosis of Hodgkin's disease; the variant mononuclear Hodgkin cells are insufficient.

Rye Classification

The goal of Hodgkin's disease pathologic classification is to provide a guide to prognosis and treatment in a disorder of extremely variable natural history. The system of Jackson and Parker,[7] the first modern classification, divided Hodgkin's disease into three categories: *Hodgkin's paragranuloma*, a benign process in which lymph nodes are largely composed of small lymphocytes; *Hodgkin's granuloma*, the major proportion of Hodgkin's disease; and *Hodgkin's sarcoma*, an aggressive condition in which the histology is dominated by pleomorphic Reed-Sternberg cells. The system was unsatisfactory because it did not discriminate among the 90% of Hodgkin's disease patients who fell within the granuloma subtype.

The Rye classification of Hodgkin's disease is a four-part system in wide use today.[8] It was developed in 1966 as a simplification of the more complex Lukes and Butler classification,[99] which, in turn, incorporated the earlier Jackson and Parker subdivisions.[7] The interrelations among the three systems are outlined in Table 29-2. The Jackson and Parker paragranuloma category was expanded into the *lymphocyte predominance* of the Rye classification, and the sarcoma category into *lymphocyte depletion*. The major novelty of the Rye system was the introduction of the *nodular sclerosis* subtype, which together with *mixed cellularity*, an ill-defined group, constitutes the major granuloma category of Jackson and Parker.

In most series from the United States and Europe, nodular sclerosis is responsible for 60% to 70% of cases of Hodgkin's disease, mixed cellularity for 20% to 30%, and lymphocyte predominance and depletion together for about 10%.[101] The major predictive value of the Rye system is the segregation of the favorable prognostic groups of nodular sclerosis and lymphocyte predominance.[99–103] A problem addressed be-

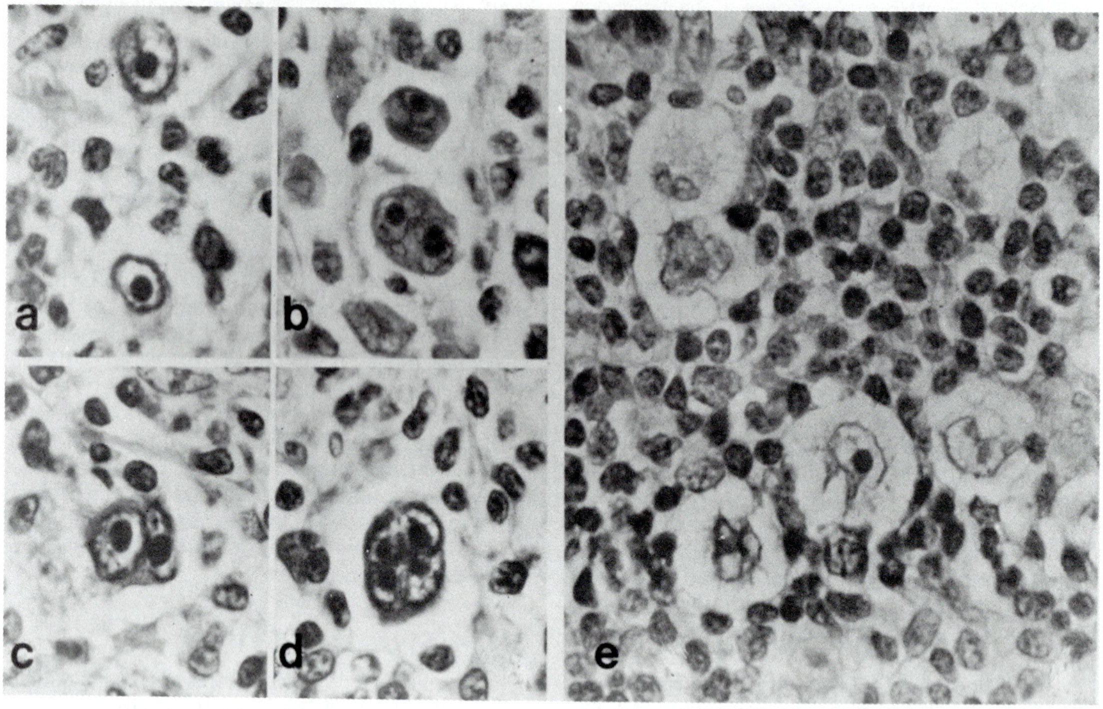

FIGURE 29-6. Typical diagnostic binucleate (**b** and **c**) and multinucleate (**d**) Reed-Sternberg cells with inclusion-like nucleoli and deeply staining cytoplasm compared with diagnostically unreliable mononuclear form (**a**) and with lacunar forms (**e**) seen in nodular sclerosis (hematoxylin and eosin, ×850). (Lukes RE. Criteria for involvement of lymph nodes, bone marrow, spleen and liver in Hodgkin's disease. Cancer Res 1971;31:1765)

low is the large proportion of cases still unfractionated within the nodular sclerosis category. As mentioned earlier, nodular sclerosis is much less common in economically disadvantaged populations.

Lymphocyte Predominance

The lymph node in this uncommon but most favorable category can be largely composed of benign lymphocytes, benign macrophages, or an admixture of the two[70,71,98–100,104] (Fig. 29-7*A*). The process can be diffuse or vaguely nodular. Characteristically, the histologic picture is bland for Hodgkin's disease; florid, diagnostic Reed-Sternberg cells are difficult to find, plasma cells and eosinophils are infrequent, and necrosis and fibrosis are minimal. Nodular lymphocyte predominance of Hodgkin's disease (NLPHD) is characterized by the lymphocytic and histiocytic or "popcorn" cell that differs from the classic Reed-Sternberg cell of other Hodgkin's disease subtypes. This cell is delicate with a multilobated nucleus, multiple small, usually basophilic nucleoli, and slightly basophilic cytoplasm.

Lymphocyte predominance in the Rye classification was born of a desire to simplify the Lukes and Butler system by combining the nodular and diffuse lymphocytic and histiocytic categories (see Table 29-2). A substantial amount of the recent pathologic literature on Hodgkin's disease questions the wisdom of this simplification.[70,71,104] The present consensus distinguishes NLPHD from other subtypes of the disorder and considers this variant an indolent non-Hodgkin's lymphoma of follicle center cell lineage that does not belong under the Hodgkin's disease rubric. As outlined in the earlier section on immunophenotype, the surface markers of the lymphocytic and histiocytic cell strongly support a B-cell derivation and contrast sharply with the usual Reed-Sternberg phenotype. NLPHD also contrasts with other Hodgkin's disease subtypes by its close relation to the benign disorder termed *progressive transformation of germinal centers*,[105] and by its propensity in

TABLE 29-2. Comparison of Hodgkin's Disease Classifications

Jackson and Parker[7]	Lukes and Butler[99]	Rye[8]
Paragranuloma	Lymphocytic or histiocytic	
	Nodular	Lymphocyte predominance
	Diffuse	
Granuloma	Nodular sclerosis	Nodular sclerosis
	Mixed cellularity	Mixed cellularity
	Diffuse fibrosis	Lymphocyte depletion
Sarcoma	Reticular	

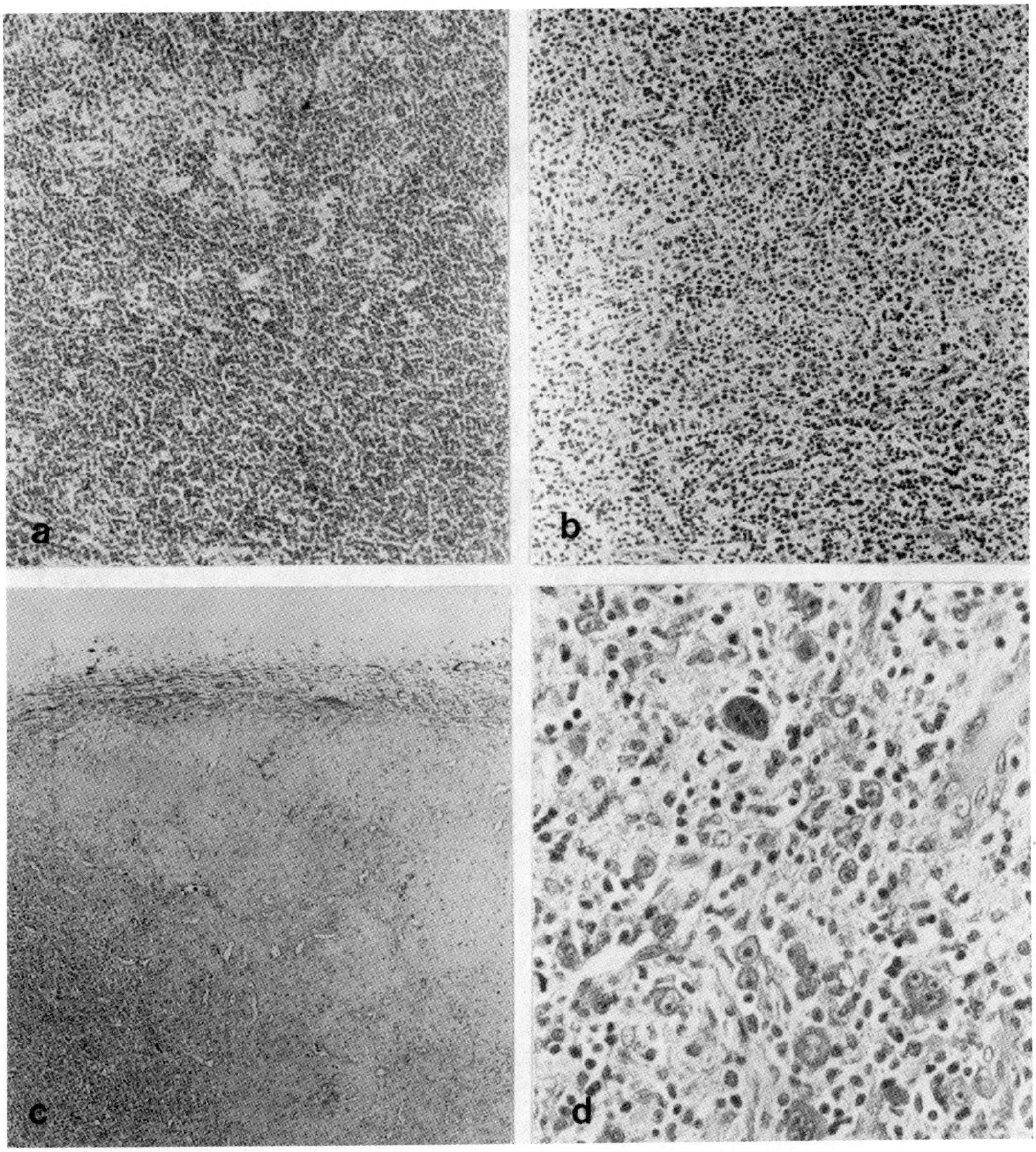

FIGURE 29-7. Histologic subtypes of Hodgkin's disease. (**a**) large histiocytes are scattered among a predominant population of small lymphocytes in this example of lymphocyte predominance (lymphocytic and histiocytic, diffuse). (**b**) Mixed population of normal and neoplastic cell components are seen in a mixed-cellularity specimen. (**c**) Hypocellular connective tissue with residual sinusoids typical of the diffuse fibrosis form of lymphocyte depletion. (**d**) Numerous pleomorphic Reed-Sternberg cells are found in the reticular variant of lymphocyte depletion (hematoxylin and eosin, ×150). (After Lukes RE, Butler JJ. The pathology and nomenclature of Hodgkin's disease. Cancer Res 1966;26:1061)

a small subset of patients to evolve into a high-grade B-cell lymphoma.[106]

Some authors report that the clinical behavior of NLPHD can be distinguished from other Hodgkin's disease subtypes by its indolent but relapsing course with little disease-related mortality.[107] Others find no difference between the clinical behavior of nodular and diffuse lymphocyte predominance Hodgkin's disease[108] or between NLPHD and other Hodgkin's disease subtypes.[109]

Nodular Sclerosis

The hallmarks of nodular sclerosis are bands of fibrosis (Fig. 29-8) and lacunar Reed-Sternberg cells[70,71,98–100] (see Fig. 29-6*E*). The interconnecting bands of birefringent connective tissue surround nodules of neoplastic and reactive cells. The amount of fibrosis is extremely variable from patient to patient, at different sites in the same patient, and even in different portions of the same specimen. The term *nodular sclerosis, cellular phase,* has been used to describe cases in which the fibrosis is limited in amount or distribution.

Lacunar cells are Reed-Sternberg variants with abundant clear cytoplasm and well-defined cell borders in which the nucleus appears to occupy a lacuna (see Fig. 29-6*E*). Cytoplasmic threads extending to the periphery may give the appearance of a spider's web, and the delicate nuclear chromatin and small nuclei differ from the classic Reed-Sternberg cell. Lacunar cells are characteristic of nodular sclerosis and can almost always be found in this subtype. Classic Reed-Sternberg cells, which may be sparse in nodular sclerosis, should always be identified.

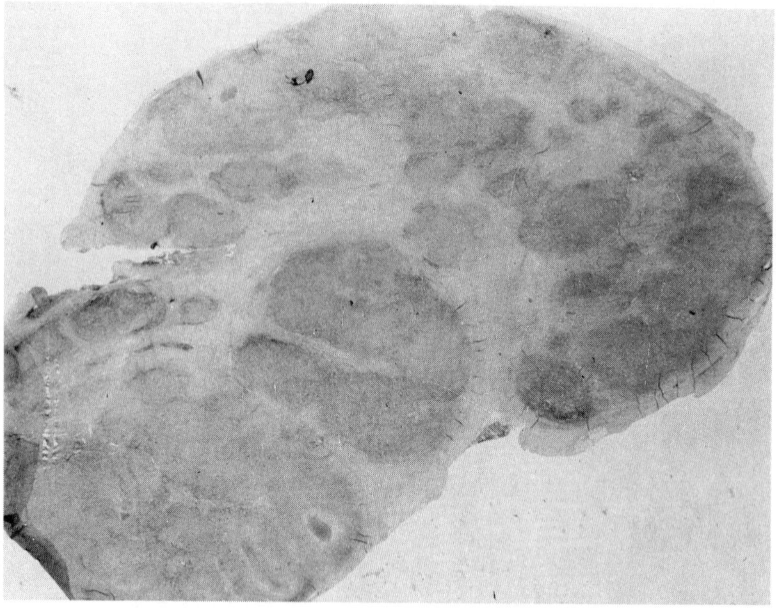

FIGURE 29-8. Nodular sclerosis. Broad bands of connective tissue and tumor nodules are evident (hematoxylin and eosin, ×8).

The variability of cell composition and the large size of the nodular sclerosis group has led to its subdivision into lymphocyte-predominant, mixed-cellularity, and lymphocyte-depletion variants. This has not proved to be prognostically useful, but a two-grade scheme devised by Bennett[110] has some prognostic significance. In the Bennett scheme, patients with marked lymphocyte depletion or numerous pleomorphic Hodgkin's disease cells make up the unfavorable grade 2; the remainder makes up grade 1.

Most patients who constitute the young adult peak of Hodgkin's disease exhibit the nodular sclerosis histopathology. Thus, most young persons with asymptomatic, localized disease, readily cured with radiation, fall into this subtype. The large, nodular sclerosis group also contains many patients with unfavorable clinical presentations of advanced disease. The diagnosis of nodular sclerosis should not be a reason for complacency.

Mixed Cellularity

The mixed-cellularity subgroup is a hodgepodge, consisting of specimens that lack sclerosis and that contain too many Reed-Sternberg cells for lymphocyte predominance and too few for lymphocyte depletion[71,98–100] (see Fig. 29-7*B*). Usually, an abundance of various nonneoplastic cells is present, including histiocytes, neutrophils, plasma cells, eosinophils, and lymphocytes. Diagnostic Reed-Sternberg cells can be easily identified, and foci of necrosis may be present. Patients with mixed cellularity are apt to be older than those with nodular sclerosis and are more likely to present with symptoms and in advanced stage; they have a less unfavorable prognosis since the introduction of modern drug regimens.

Lymphocyte Depletion

Lymphocyte depletion consisted of two groups of cases in the original Lukes and Butler system.[71,98–100] The diffuse fibrosis patients exhibit severe lymphocyte depletion (see Fig. 29-7*C*), disorderly fibrillar material and hypocellular areas composed of an eosinophilic amorphous, nonbirefringent material. Usually, areas with abundant Reed-Sternberg cells can be found. The reticular variant is dominated by a preponderance of pleomorphic Reed-Sternberg cells, a veritable Reed-Sternberg sarcoma (see Fig. 29-7*D*). Many cases that were designated the reticular variant of Hodgkin's disease in the past have been reassigned to various categories of pleomorphic non-Hodgkin's lymphoma, such as T-cell lymphoma and anaplastic large cell (Ki-1–positive) lymphoma.[71] Foci of necrosis are common in both variants of lymphocyte depletion. The lymphocyte depletion subtype is likely to present as symptomatic, advanced stage disease in older patients. Some of these patients have abdominal lymphoma in the absence of peripheral lymphadenopathy: they frequently do poorly, even with modern therapy.

Usefulness of the Rye Classification

How useful is the Rye classification in clinical management? Certainly, *stage* (extent of disease; see section on staging) is the major prognostic determinant in Hodgkin's disease, as opposed to the non-Hodgkin's lymphomas in which histopathologic subtype is paramount. Furthermore, the major contribution of histopathology, which is the difference in survival between those with the nodular sclerosis and the mixed-cellularity subtypes, has diminished as therapy has improved. Nonetheless, some recent critical studies (linear regression analyses) demonstrate that pathologic subtype influences prognosis independently of stage, age, sex, and other known variables (see section on prognostic factors; Tables 29-8 and 29-15).

Granulomas

Tuberculoid granulomas with Langerhans' giant cells are a common finding in patients with Hodgkin's disease, less common in non-Hodgkin's lymphomas.[111] Liver, spleen, lymph nodes, and bone marrow may be involved. These granulomas do *not* indicate involvement of that organ with Hodgkin's disease and have no adverse prognostic significance.

Contiguous Spread

Two mechanisms are involved in the spread of Hodgkin's disease. The first is contiguous spread by way of lymphatic channels. This mode of spread accounts for many of the

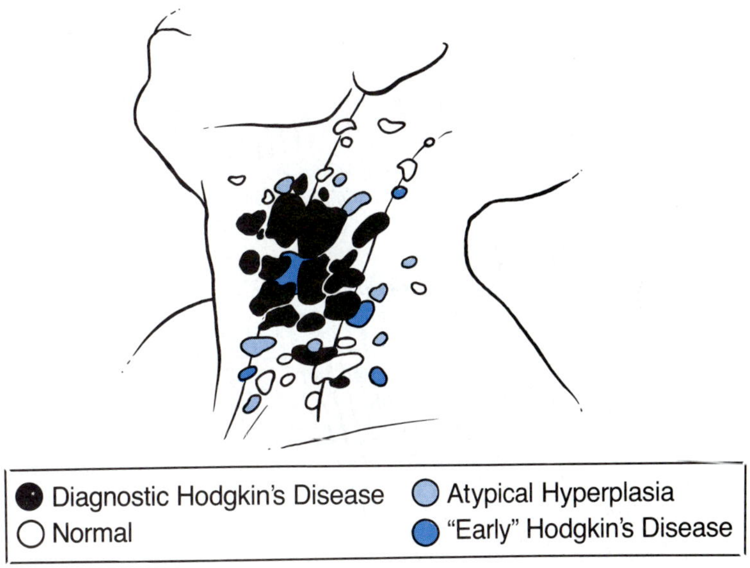

FIGURE 29-9. Schematic representation of nodal involvement from the neck dissection of a patient with Hodgkin's disease. (Slaughter DP, Economou SG, Southwick HW. The surgical management of Hodgkin's disease. Ann Surg 1958;148:705)

localized presentations of early Hodgkin's disease. Contiguous spread is also responsible for the asymmetric and localized distribution of peripheral, mediastinal, and abdominal lymph nodes, which is characteristic of Hodgkin's disease.

The multiplicity of lymphatic channels connecting the lymph nodes of the lower neck with those of the mediastinum explain the frequent occurrence of disease in those two areas in the same patient. Contiguous spread is obvious in Figure 29-9, a reconstruction of the neck findings in a patient with Hodgkin's disease. Less obvious but true is the fact that pulmonary involvement also follows the lymphatic pathways of the lung, with the process spreading from the nodes of the anterior mediastinum successively to the hilar and bronchopulmonary nodes, then through the lymphatic channels of the bronchovascular bundle into the lung substance and to the pleural surface. Similarly, Hodgkin's disease may enter the spinal canal via the lymphatic channels of abdominoaortic lymph nodes overlying the spine. Much can be learned of the spread of Hodgkin's disease from a detailed study of Rouvière's monograph[112] on the gross anatomy of the lymphoid system.

Hematogenous Spread

The second mechanism in Hodgkin's disease is hematogenous spread. Figure 29-10 is an example of such spread; numerous splenic nodules made up the only unanticipated intraabdominal lymphoma in a young woman who presented with Hodgkin's disease in the mediastinum and right neck. Bone and bone marrow involvement are other manifestations of hematogenous spread. Thus, a second route by which Hodgkin's disease may enter the spinal canal is from a diseased vertebral body.

Why hematogenous spread occurs early in one patient and late in another cannot be fully explained. Regardless of the reason, the occurrence is a central event in the evolution of each patient's Hodgkin's disease. After it has happened, systemic treatment with combination chemotherapy is needed. Radiation therapy can suffice only for localized Hodgkin's disease that has spread by contiguity alone.

CLINICAL PICTURE

Clinicians who did not observe Hodgkin's disease before the introduction of combination chemotherapy have difficulty appreciating the natural history of the disorder. Figure 29-11 depicts survival rate, with and without disease, in 340 patients treated at Freiburg i Br between 1948 and 1966.[113] The figure illustrates the chronicity of Hodgkin's disease in the era of orthovoltage radiation and primitive (alkylating agent) chemotherapy. A large proportion of patients exhibited a slow-paced disease with frequent recurrence into the sixth year and significant mortality rate into the 14th year after initial diagnosis. Unusual patients (not

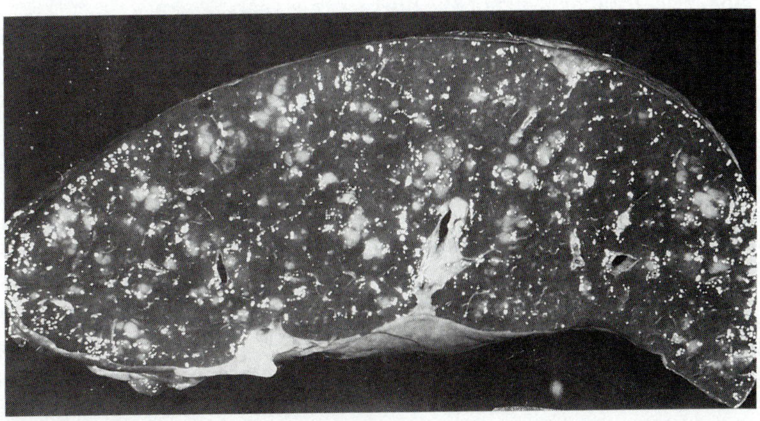

FIGURE 29-10. Cross section of the spleen obtained at staging laparotomy from an asymptomatic 19-year-old woman who presented with cervical and mediastinal adenopathy and a negative lymphangiogram.

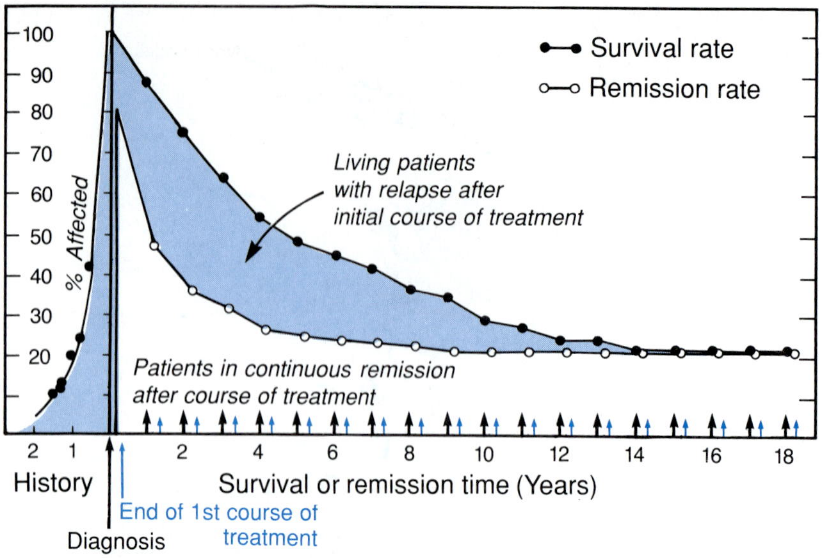

FIGURE 29-11. Natural history of 340 Hodgkin's disease patients treated at Freiburg i Br between 1945 and 1966. *History* refers to the percentage of patients with signs or symptoms of disease prior to treatment. *Survival rate* is the survival curve of the entire series. *Remission rate* is the survival curve of relapse-free patients. In this study, which predates curative combination chemotherapy, all patients with relapses died of Hodgkin's disease within 14 years. (Musshoff K, Boutis L. Therapy results in Hodgkin's disease, Freiburg i Br, 1948–1966. Cancer 1968;21:1100)

evident in the Freiburg experience) survive with active Hodgkin's disease into the third decade of disease. Long survival is associated with the absence of constitutional symptoms at presentation and their late development. A second group of patients, who exhibit much more aggressive disease, die within 2 or 3 years of diagnosis; these patients are likely to present with significant constitutional symptoms or to be more than 60 years of age, or both.

Although the manifestations of Hodgkin's disease are varied, the condition evolves in a highly predictable manner. The disorder is a creature of the lymphoid system. The primary sites of disease are the peripheral and mediastinal lymph nodes.[114–116] Abdominal lymph nodes and spleen are frequently diseased at the time of diagnosis, but infrequently the only sites of disease. Early involvement of the lung, liver, and bone marrow reflect the lymphoid component of these organs, and, in the case of lung and liver, the proximity to contiguous disease in the mediastinum and abdomen, respectively. Patients with Hodgkin's disease without lymph node involvement at the time of presentation deserve the closest scrutiny. Unlike the non-Hodgkin's lymphomas, Hodgkin's disease of extranodal origin is rare.

Spread of Hodgkin's disease to organs other than those just mentioned is infrequent and usually requires a protracted period of uncontrolled progression. With the aggressive application of radiation therapy and combination chemotherapy, many of the florid Hodgkin's disease manifestations described in the older literature are unusual today. Most deaths of patients with Hodgkin's disease are now found to be associated with rapidly progressive lymphoma; such patients do not live the requisite years. Today, patients with more indolent disease, who would have exhibited the full spectrum of tumor involvement before modern treatment, are usually cured of their disorder or, in some instances, die of a treatment complication. Spinal cord compression, obstruction of the superior vena cava or ureter, or invasion of the skin by Hodgkin's disease occur infrequently.[114] Even before the advent of effective therapy, involvement by Hodgkin's disease of the kidney, brain, endocrine glands, skeletal muscle, and male or female genitalia was rare.[13]

A second generalization can be made about the clinical evolution of Hodgkin's disease. In contrast to large-cell lymphomas and epithelial neoplasms, Hodgkin's disease is not usually an invasive process. It compresses rather than invades, and as a rule massive tumor is required before this compression compromises vital function. Therefore, a large mass of Hodgkin's disease in the mediastinum is much less likely to compromise the airway or circulatory function than a smaller pulmonary carcinoma or large-cell lymphoma would. This may reflect, in part, the resilient (rubbery) character of Hodgkin's disease tissue in contrast to the stony hard character of carcinoma.

Finally, our appreciation of the evolution of Hodgkin's disease has changed markedly and continues to change as a result of modern diagnostic studies. Lymphangiography, computed tomography (CT), magnetic resonance imaging (MRI), and, particularly, exploratory laparotomy and splenectomy have radically altered our knowledge of the initial spread of Hodgkin's disease, that is, its evolution before it reaches medical attention.

Initial Complaint

About 90% of patients with Hodgkin's disease present with painless enlargement of a superficial lymph node.[114–116] In about 75% of cases, the first node appreciated is in the neck (Fig. 29-12), whereas it is in the axilla or groin in the the remaining 25%. The enlarged node may be recently noticed or may have been present for a few to many months. It

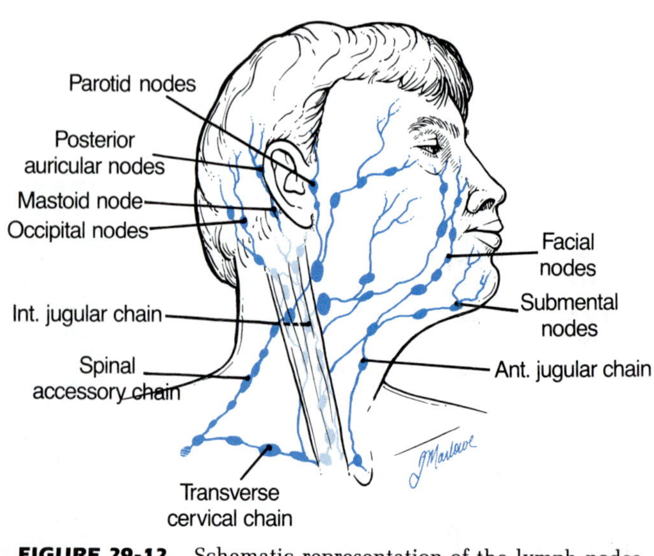

FIGURE 29-12. Schematic representation of the lymph nodes of the neck. (After Rouvière H. Anatomy of the human lymphatic system. Ann Arbor, Edwards Brothers, 1938:5)

may fluctuate in size in a deceptive manner and is usually nontender; on examination, it is firm and rubbery, not hard. Occasionally, the node is tender, or pain may occur after drinking alcohol; this complaint is infrequent, but is suggestive of Hodgkin's disease. Most who present without peripheral lymphadenopathy have a mediastinal tumor uncovered on chest x-ray examination that was performed routinely for pulmonary symptoms (usually cough), or, rarely, for intractable itching. Rarely also, Hodgkin's disease may be discovered in the abdominal or pelvic lymph nodes of a patient explored with fever or other systemic symptoms, or even as an incidental finding. About one third of Hodgkin's disease patients have systemic symptoms at time of diagnosis, with weight loss, night sweats, and fever each being present in about one fourth of the patient population, and itching in about one eighth.

Peripheral Lymphadenopathy

As just discussed, peripheral lymphadenopathy is the most prominent initial manifestation of active Hodgkin's disease. The incidence and distribution of enlargement of the various peripheral lymph nodes at the outset are indicated in Table 29-3 and Figure 29-13. When the disorder is not cured, relapse is frequently heralded by recurrent peripheral adenopathy, although areas that have received radiation in high dose are much less likely to be sites of recurrence.

Mediastinal Adenopathy

Intrathoracic lymphoma is a major manifestation of Hodgkin's disease, present in two thirds of patients at time of diagnosis.[114–117] The chest radiograph is as much a part of the examination of the patient as is palpation of the neck (Fig. 29-14). CT may help establish the presence of minimal disease (Fig. 29-15) and is needed to define the extent of known intrathoracic lymphoma (Fig. 29-16). The inability of radiation therapy to control CT-defined mediastinal lymphoma in some patients indicates that even CT does not always reveal the full extent of chest disease. MRI frequently provides the best definition of intrathoracic lymphoma (Fig. 29-17). Figure 29-18 is a diagrammatic representation of the anatomic relations of the various mediastinal and hilar (bronchopulmonary) lymph nodes.[118] Initially, Hodgkin's disease involves the anterior mediastinal, paratracheal, or tracheobronchial lymph node groups. Subtle widening of the superior mediastinum (widening of

TABLE 29-3. Anatomic Extent of Hodgkin's Disease at Presentation

Site	Involved at Onset (%)	Only Site Involved (%)	First Site Detected (%)
Right neck	55–60	5	55
Left neck	60–70	10	
Mediastinum	60–65	2	15
Axilla	20–25	5	10
Lung hilum	10–25	<1	
Paraaortic	25–35	<1	5
Illiac	10–15	<1	
Inguinal and femoral	5–15	<5	9
Mesenteric	1	<1	
Splenic hilum, celiac, portal	10–20	<1	
Spleen	30		
Liver	5–15		
Lung	10–20		
Bone	5–15		
Bone marrow	5–15		

(Modified from Selby P, McElwain TJ. Clinical features of Hodgkin's disease. In: Hodgkin's disease. Oxford, Blackwell Scientific, 1987:94)

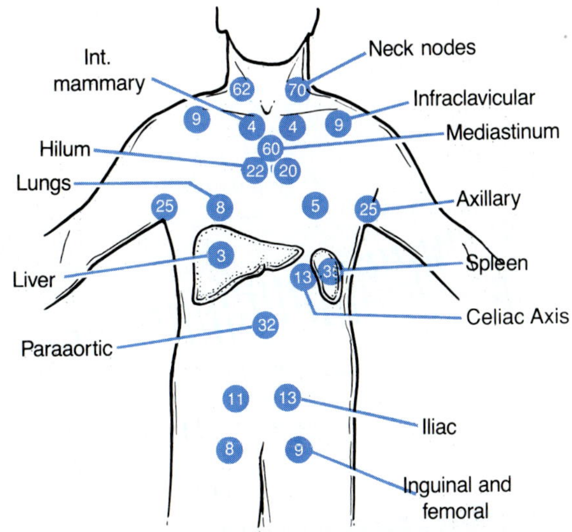

Mesenteric	1.0%	Bone	7.0%
Subcutaneous	2.0%	Bone marrow	3.0%
Epidural	0.4%	Other	4.0%

FIGURE 29-13. Distribution of Hodgkin's disease in 285 consecutive, untreated patients, 172 of whom had a staging laparotomy and splenectomy. The numbers indicate the percentage of patients with involvement at each site. (After Kaplan HS, Dorfman RF, Nelson TS, et al. Staging laparotomy and splenectomy in Hodgkin's disease: analysis of indications and patterns of involvement in 285 consecutive untreated patients. NCI Monogr 1973;36:291)

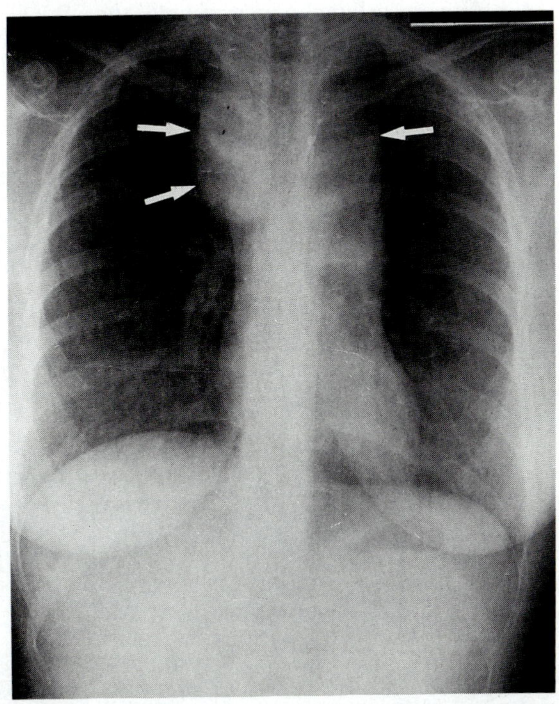

FIGURE 29-14. Pathologic stage IIA Hodgkin's disease of the nodular sclerosis type. This 11-cm asymptomatic mediastinal mass in a 28-year-old woman with cervical adenopathy measures more than one third of the maximum chest diameter (29 cm).

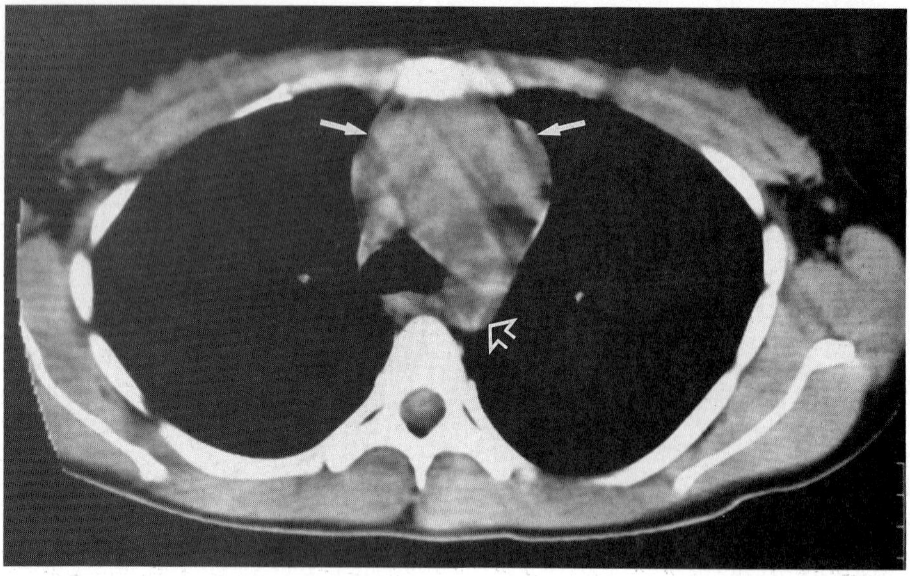

FIGURE 29-15. CT scan at the level of the aortic arch (*open arrow*) reveals a large anterior superior mediastinal mass (*solid arrows*). The abnormalities were subtle in this posteroanterior radiograph of a 23-year-old woman with pathologic stage IIA Hodgkin's disease of the nodular sclerosis type.

the tracheal stripe) detected on a routine chest radiograph may be the first evidence of Hodgkin's disease. The failure to recognize and act on this finding is a serious clinical error. More advanced mediastinal lymphoma may show spread to the hilum; in extreme instances, the tumor may reach the chest wall. Such advanced disease usually results in cough and other pulmonary complaints, although the process may be remarkably silent.

Lung and Pleura

Invasion of the lung or pleura can be demonstrated in 10% to 20% of patients at the time that the diagnosis of Hodgkin's disease is made.[114–117] A much larger proportion of those who are not cured experience this involvement. Occasionally, the pulmonary lymphoma dominates the clinical picture during the entire course of Hodgkin's disease, although this is much less common in this age of effective radiation and chemotherapy. Rarely, the lung condition may progress to cavity formation. Involvement of the lung parenchyma or the pleural surface by Hodgkin's disease is almost never seen without simultaneous or prior mediastinal lymphoma.[13] Involvement of a lung is usually associated with disease in the ipsilateral hilum; spread to the pleura is unusual without *massive* mediastinal adenopathy. All these findings are consistent with the previously mentioned view that spread to the lung and pleura are manifestations of contiguous spread from the mediastinal and hilar nodes by means of the lymphatics of the bronchovascular bundle. Hematogenous dissemination of Hodgkin's disease to the lung parenchyma is infrequently seen, particularly as an initial manifestation.

Pleural effusions in Hodgkin's disease are usually of intermediate specific gravity and cell count, and rarely yield diagnostic Reed-Sternberg cells on cytologic examination. If pathologic confirmation is considered essential, a pleural biopsy or thoracotomy is necessary.

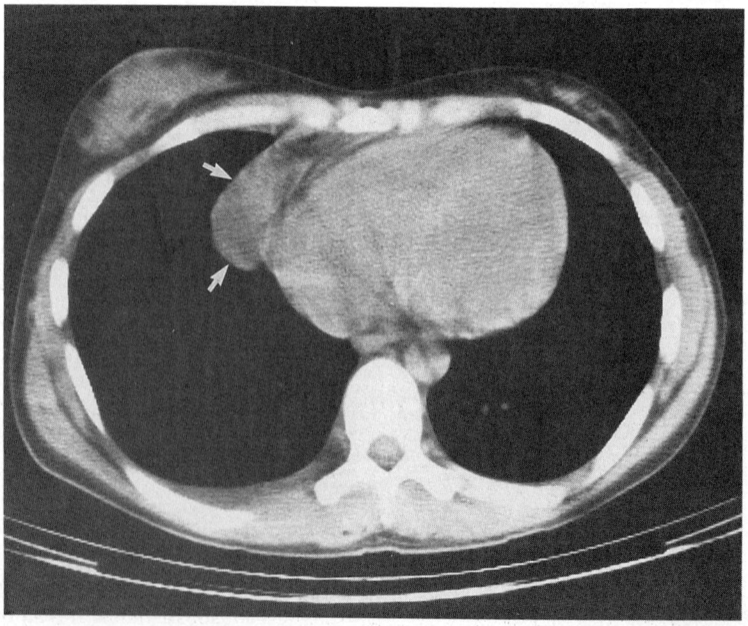

FIGURE 29-16. CT scan reveals that this mediastinal mass extends down the anterior and lateral aspects of the right side of the heart. The patient is a 25-year-old woman with pathologic stage IIA Hodgkin's disease of the nodular sclerosis type.

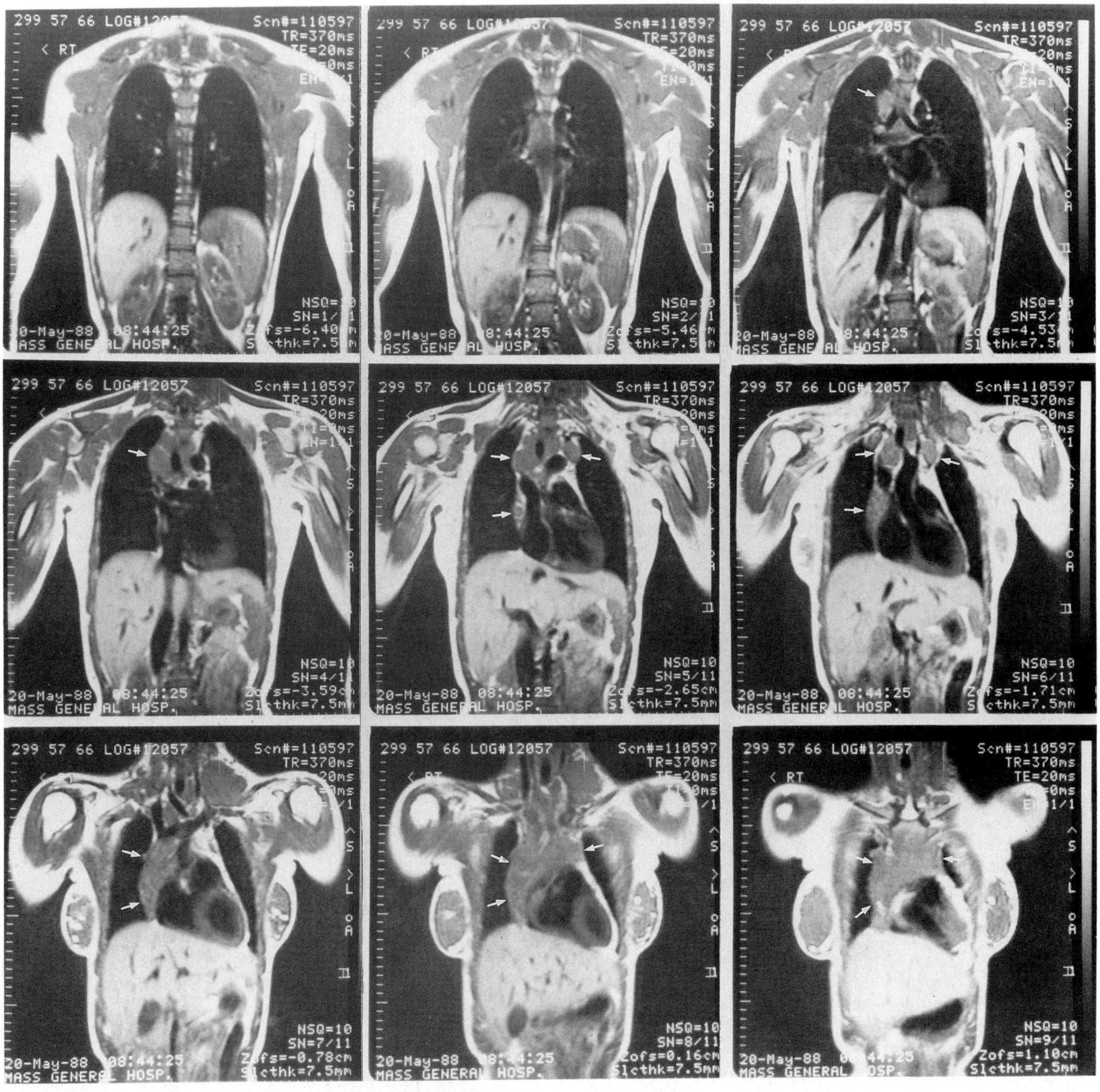

FIGURE 29-17. MRI scan in the same patient as depicted in Figure 29-16. Sagittal cuts proceeding from the vertebral column to the anterior surface of the heart graphically illustrate the full extent of this tumor.

Splenic Involvement

The spleen is the intraabdominal site most frequently involved at staging laparotomy; about one third of spleens are diseased at that time, and the splenic hilar lymph nodes are involved as well in half of these.[13,101,114–116] Except for the massively enlarged spleen, clinical appraisal of size correlates poorly with the presence of lymphoma. Only 60% to 65% of palpable or radiologically enlarged spleens reveal Hodgkin's disease, whereas 25% to 30% of normal-sized spleens are diseased.

Abdominal Adenopathy

Paraaortic lymphadenopathy, with or without enlargement of pelvic lymph nodes, is present in about 25% of Hodgkin's disease patients at the time of diagnosis.[13,101,114–116] Mesenteric nodes are diseased infrequently, only in about 1 in 100 cases. Abdominal lymph node involvement is almost always uncovered by a staging study, lymphangiography (Fig. 29-19), CT (Fig. 29-20), or laparotomy. Abdominal lymphadenopathy present at time of diagnosis is more likely to be associated with constitutional complaints, but is otherwise not a common source of symptoms. The abdominal lymph nodes are a common site of Hodgkin's disease relapse; such relapse, if advanced, is more likely to generate abdominal or even back pain.

Paraaortic lymph node disease, an important manifestation of Hodgkin's disease, is a result of contiguous spread from splenic hilar nodes and from the hematogenously involved spleen. The following evidence favors this reconstruction. First, the spleen is frequently diseased in the absence of paraaortic lymphoma, whereas paraaortic dis-

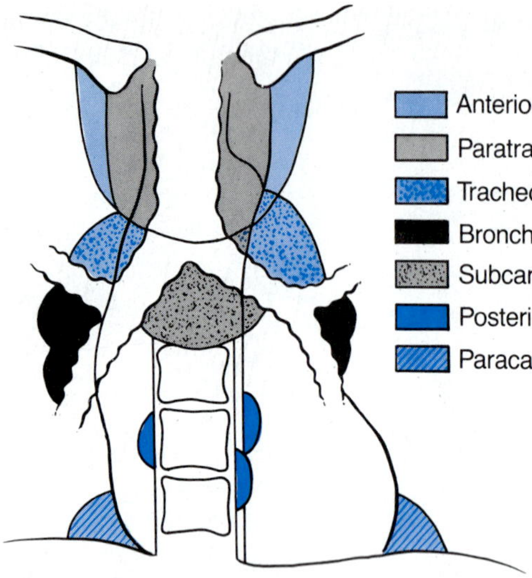

FIGURE 29-18. Diagrammatic representation of the major mediastinal and hilar (bronchopulmonary) lymph node groups. (Filly R, Blank N, Castellino RA. Radiographic distribution of intrathoracic disease in previously untreated patients with Hodgkin's disease and non-Hodgkin's lymphoma. Radiology 1976;120:277)

ease with a normal spleen is uncommon. Furthermore, half of patients with splenic lymphoma progress to hepatic lymphoma if they are not given systemic treatment, and almost all patients with bone marrow dissemination also have spread to the spleen. Finally, the absence of afferent splenic lymphatics argues against contiguous spread to the spleen.

Liver

At time of diagnosis, lymphoma in the liver is demonstrable in only 3% of Hodgkin's disease patients.[13,101,114–116] Neither abnormal liver function tests (elevated alkaline phosphatase and 5′-nucleotidase levels, the most useful liver function tests for this purpose) nor increased liver size reliably predicts hepatic involvement.[119] Abnormal liver function tests should be viewed as the functional counterpart of the nonspecific portal infiltrates frequently seen in liver biopsies.

The liver is almost never involved at staging laparotomy in the absence of lymphoma in the spleen. That finding, together with the observation that Hodgkin's disease is eventually demonstrable in the liver of half of those with spleen disease who do not receive chemotherapy, suggests that liver and spleen are involved together early in the course of hematogenous spread. The more thorough pathologic examination of the spleen could account for the higher rate of involvement of that organ demonstrated at the time of laparotomy.

Hodgkin's disease involves the liver of many persons who die of the disorder.[120] The picture is that of a focal intrahepatic obstructive process, characterized at first by a rise in alkaline phosphatase and 5′-nucleotidase levels, and later by a rise in bilirubin.[120] Less frequently, obstruction is caused by enlarged nodes in the porta hepatis. Finally, a rare intrahepatic obstructive picture without pathologic involvement of the liver has been described in patients with advanced Hodgkin's disease.[121]

Bone Marrow

Bone marrow dissemination is reported in 5% to 15% of patients with newly diagnosed Hodgkin's disease,[13,114–116,122,123] but the 3% figure for the Stanford laparotomy series is closer to the experience of referral centers, which see a more favorable patient population.[114] Spleen involvement almost always accompanies Hodgkin's disease in the marrow, and most patients are ill with constitutional symptoms. With advancing disease, the bone marrow becomes involved with increasing frequency. Bone marrow dissemination is usually a serious manifestation even with modern chemotherapy.

Bone

Dissemination to bone is also reported in 5% to 15% of newly diagnosed cases of Hodgkin's disease.[13,114–116] Two groups of patients can be distinguished, those in whom the involved bone is in direct contiguity to advanced lymph node disease and those in whom the spread is hematogenous. One or several lesions may be present, and the radiologic picture may be either lytic or blastic. Hodgkin's involvement of bone is usually preceded or accompanied by deep-seated bone pain. Bone lesions occur at any time in the course of the disorder and do not have the serious prognostic significance of bone marrow dissemination.

Central Nervous System (Spinal Cord Compression)

The remaining manifestations of Hodgkin's disease are encountered less frequently than those just described. Compression of the spinal cord was noted at time of diag-

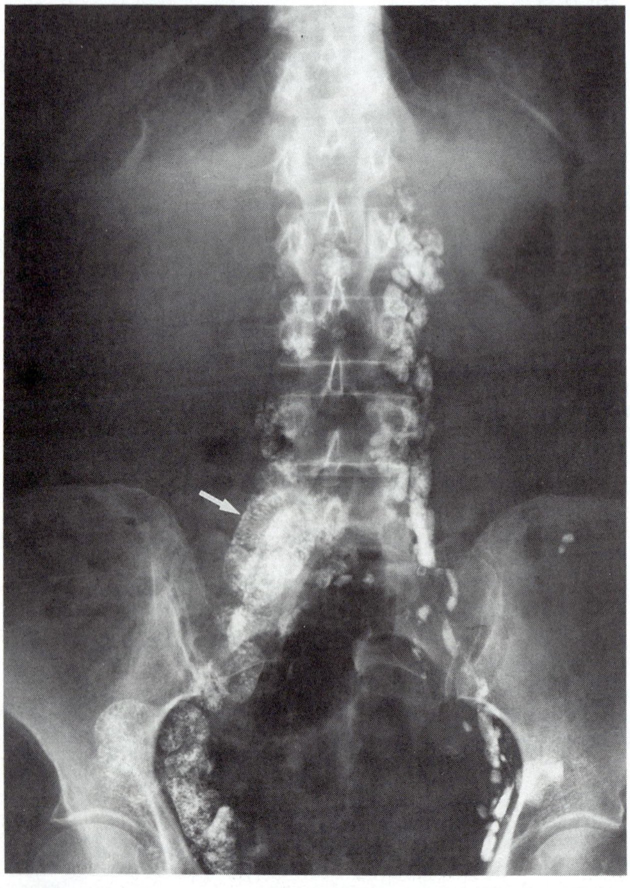

FIGURE 29-19. This 53-year-old woman presented with an asymptomatic node in the right groin. Lower extremity lymphangiogram shows enlarged and foamy (tumor-filled) inguinal, iliac, and paraaortic lymph nodes on the right, including the very large abnormal node indicated by the arrow. The abnormal nodes should be compared with normal-appearing iliac and inguinal nodes on the left. At laparotomy, the spleen was also involved by Hodgkin's disease.

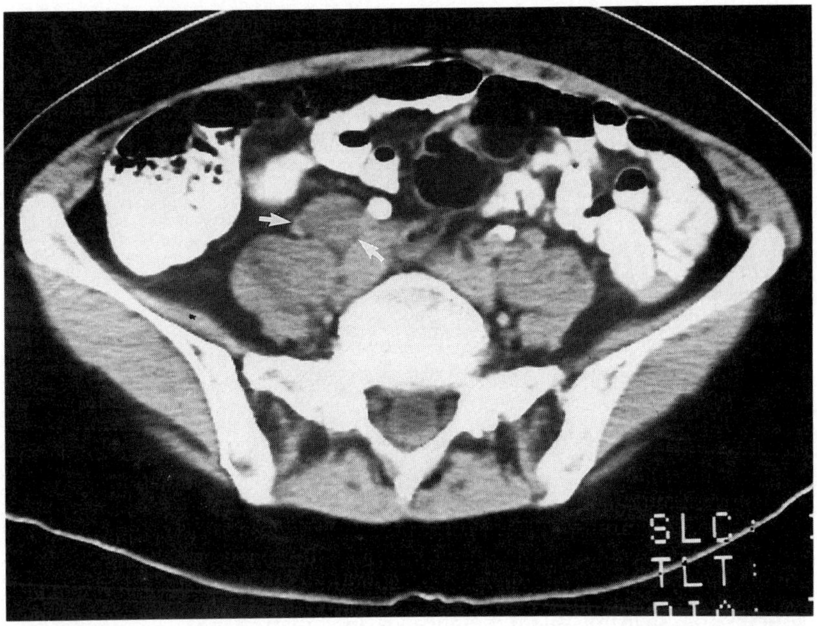

FIGURE 29-20. Abdominal CT scan at the level of the iliac crest reveals the large abnormal lymph node indicated in Figure 29-19 by the arrow.

nosis only once in the 285 consecutive cases reported from Stanford.[114] The complication occurred more frequently in the past and remains a significant risk in those with florid, uncontrolled Hodgkin's disease. Spinal compression is a rare occurrence in patients who have not been in relapse for several months or more and is usually heralded by a long period of back pain.[124,125] The thoracic spine is involved most frequently. Cord compression remains a difficult diagnosis to make before the onset of neurologic deficit (sensory loss, motor weakness, loss of bowel and bladder function), but diagnosis before the development of marked impairment is essential for a good functional result.[126,127] It is hoped that MRI, CT, and modern myelographic techniques will permit timely diagnosis in persons with back pain only. Hodgkin's disease can also compress nerve roots and plexuses outside the spinal canal.

Involvement of the brain or meninges is rare in patients with Hodgkin's disease; fewer than 50 cases of intracranial Hodgkin's disease have been reported in the world literature.[128] Alternate causes of symptomatology—infections such as progressive multifocal leukoencephalopathy and cryptococcal meningitis, still ill-defined paraneoplastic syndromes, and coincidental illness including Guillain-Barré syndrome—are more likely.[129]

Pericardium

Computed tomography and MRI allow detection of pericardial invasion. The same techniques disclose enlargement of the paracardiac lymph nodes. Hodgkin's disease infrequently causes symptomatic pericardial tamponade, nor does it otherwise cause clinically significant involvement of the heart.[13,114–116] Most cardiac problems are coincidental, or they are sequelae of mediastinal radiation.

Superior Vena Cava Obstruction

Hodgkin's disease patients may uncommonly present with superior vena cava compression,[13,114–116] but the complication is seen infrequently after aggressive modern treatment.

Skin and Subcutaneous Tissue

Another manifestation of advanced Hodgkin's disease, involvement of the skin and subcutaneous tissue, is also rare after modern therapy. It was present in 2% of the Stanford series at time of diagnosis.[13,114–116] The subcutaneous tissue is involved by extension from disease in the underlying lymph nodes and reflects advanced and uncontrolled lymphoma. Because of the frequent occurrence of pruritus, nonspecific cutaneous manifestations, particularly excoriations and prurigo-like papules, are common.

Genitourinary System

Obstruction of one or both ureters in patients with Hodgkin's disease was seen before techniques that readily detect paraaortic lymphadenopathy were available and before modern treatment.[130] A nephrotic syndrome on the basis of (immune complex) lipoid nephrosis remains a rare, well-documented manifestation of Hodgkin's disease.[131] It may precede the development of the lymphoma or accompany it. The renal problem remits with treatment of the primary disease and does not have separate prognostic significance. The nephrotic syndrome has also been reported in Hodgkin's disease on the basis of secondary amyloidosis and renal vein obstruction.[130] Clinically significant involvement of the kidney or of either the male or female genital systems by Hodgkin's disease is almost never seen.

Gastrointestinal and Endocrine Systems

Significant involvement of the gastrointestinal and endocrine systems is not well documented in patients with Hodgkin's disease, except for rare involvement of Waldeyer's tonsillar ring.

Constitutional Complaints

Fever is a hallmark of Hodgkin's disease.[13,114–116] Present in about 25% of persons at the outset, it develops in most of those who are not cured. Most frequently, the fever initially takes the form of an accentuated diurnal curve. This low-grade pyrexia, usually present in the late afternoon and evening, may be unnoticed at first, but progresses inevitably to high and debilitating fever when the disorder is unchecked. The pattern may be constant or remitting. Night sweats may be the earliest indication of the nocturnal defervescence of a low-grade fever and may become drenching and frequent as the fever mounts. Classic Pel-Ebstein fever, 1- to 2-week cycles of mounting and declining high fever separated by afebrile periods of similar length, is rarely seen. Hodgkin's disease patients frequently experience chilly sensations, and even frank chills associated with hectic fever charts that mimic bacterial sepsis. Spontaneous or drug-induced defervescence may be followed by a markedly subnormal body temperature. Infrequently, Hodgkin's disease patients report a period of fever at the time the initial adenopathy develops, which never recurs if the condition is cured. Occasionally, a fever spike follows the initiation of radiation or chemotherapy. The cause of fever in Hodgkin's disease remains obscure, but involvement of an interleukin mechanism, perhaps IL-1 production by the tumor tissue, is plausible.

Twenty-five percent of Hodgkin's disease patients have lost more than 10% of their body weight by the time the diagnosis is made, and almost all experience weight loss when progress of the disorder is not checked. Weight loss is associated with major fever but may also be seen in those who are afebrile.

Itching is present at the outset in about one in eight patients, but is experienced sometime during the course of the illness in most persons who are not cured. In the past, intractable pruritus dominated the course of Hodgkin's disease in some patients, but modern therapy has markedly reduced the severity and incidence of this distressing complaint.

Alcohol-induced pain is an uncommon but characteristic complaint. Although the symptom has been described in fractures and other benign bone lesions, alcohol-induced pain in lymph nodes is rarely caused by conditions other than Hodgkin's disease. Unlike pruritus, this complaint is infrequently a major source of distress.

Hematologic Parameters

The routine blood counts are normal in most untreated patients at time of diagnosis of Hodgkin's disease.[13,132] Nonetheless, they can provide useful information at the onset of disease and, more frequently, in advanced disease. Leukoctyosis is seen in 25% of patients at diagnosis, and its unexplained appearance may herald relapse. Rarely, leukemoid reactions, usually on the basis of marrow infiltration, are seen. An additional 5% of Hodgkin's disease patients present with leukopenia, another finding that can be on the basis of marrow infiltration. Absolute lymphopenia is seen in about 20% of patients at the time of onset, and is almost always present at the time of death. Hodgkin's disease is among the causes of eosinophilia and monocytosis, either of which may, rarely, be marked.

Anemia and thrombocytopenia are both infrequently seen in newly diagnosed Hodgkin's disease patients, although aggressive treatment contributes to their frequent occurrence later in the disorder.[13,132] The typical anemia of advanced disease is nondescript. Coombs-positive autoimmune hemolytic anemia is occasionally seen, most often with far-advanced disease where it may mirror disease activity.[133,134] This complication is less frequently seen after modern treatment. Autoimmune thrombocytopenia (secondary ITP) is another unusual, but well-recognized occurrence in Hodgkin's disease.[134,135] It is seen in various temporal relations to the primary disease, as the first manifestation, with active disease, or after remission or cure.

Acute-Phase Reactants

The erythrocyte sedimentation rate is a useful but highly nonspecific index of Hodgkin's disease activity.[136] It is elevated in about half of newly diagnosed patients, more frequently in those with constitutional symptoms or advanced stage disease.

Serum copper (ceruloplasmin) and zinc levels similarly mirror active Hodgkin's disease,[137] but suffer from similar nonspecificity.[13] Elevation of the serum copper was reported in 90% of newly diagnosed patients in one series and appeared to correlate with stage. Persistent elevation appeared to predict relapse.

STAGING

Stage, the extent of disease at time of diagnosis, is the most important guide to prognosis and treatment in Hodgkin's disease. Nevertheless, a few disclaimers are needed. First, dramatic advances in the treatment of Hodgkin's disease continually undermine the prognostic capability of any staging system. Second, a staging system should be recognized as an attempt to separate a continuum, the clinical picture of Hodgkin's disease at time of diagnosis, into discrete categories. Details are omitted and arbitrary boundaries are drawn to avoid making the system unworkably complex. This does not mean that the Ann Arbor Staging Classification is not an excellent first approximation of prognosis.[138] However, detailed clinical knowledge often supports more refined judgments than those based on this system (see section on prognostic features). It is an error to slavishly apply a staging system that may already be superseded by progress in diagnosis and treatment.

Ann Arbor Staging Classification

The four-part Ann Arbor Staging Classification remains in general use[138] (Table 29-4). The distinction between clinical staging and pathologic staging is a major one. Pathologic stage (PS) indicates that the extent of spread has been documented by histologic examination, in practice the result of a staging laparotomy and splenectomy. Clinical stage (CS) is based on all diagnostic procedures short of abdominal exploration.

Figure 29-21 illustrates the anatomic definition of separate lymph node regions adopted for staging at the Rye Symposium on Hodgkin's Disease.[8]

In 1988, a group of experts meeting in Cotswold, England, suggested that the Ann Arbor Staging Classification be modified by (1) the incorporation of the suffix *X* to denote

TABLE 29-4. The Ann Arbor Staging Classification*

Stage†	Involvement
Stage I	Involvement of a single lymph node region or of a single extranodal organ or site (I_E)
Stage II	Involvement of two or more lymph node regions on the same side of the diaphragm, or localized involvement of an extranodal organ or site (II_E) and of one or more lymph node regions on the same side of the diaphragm
Stage III	Involvement of lymph node regions on both sides of the diaphragm, which may also be accompanied by localized involvement of an extranodal organ or site (III_E) or spleen (III_S) or both (III_{SE})
Stage IV	Diffuse or disseminated involvement of one or more distant extranodal organs with or without associated lymph node involvement

* Clinical staging is based on all clinical and radiologic studies and the initial surgical biopsy. Pathologic staging includes the further surgical removal of tissue including staging laparotomy and splenectomy. Biopsy-documented involvement may be designated by the following symbols: N+, nodes; M+, marrow; H+, liver; L+, lung; P+, pleura; O+, bone; D+, skin.

† Fever over 38°C (100.5°F), night sweats, and weight loss of over 10% of body weight during the preceding 6 months are defined as systemic symptoms and denoted by the suffix *B*. Asymptomatic patients are denoted by the suffix *A*.

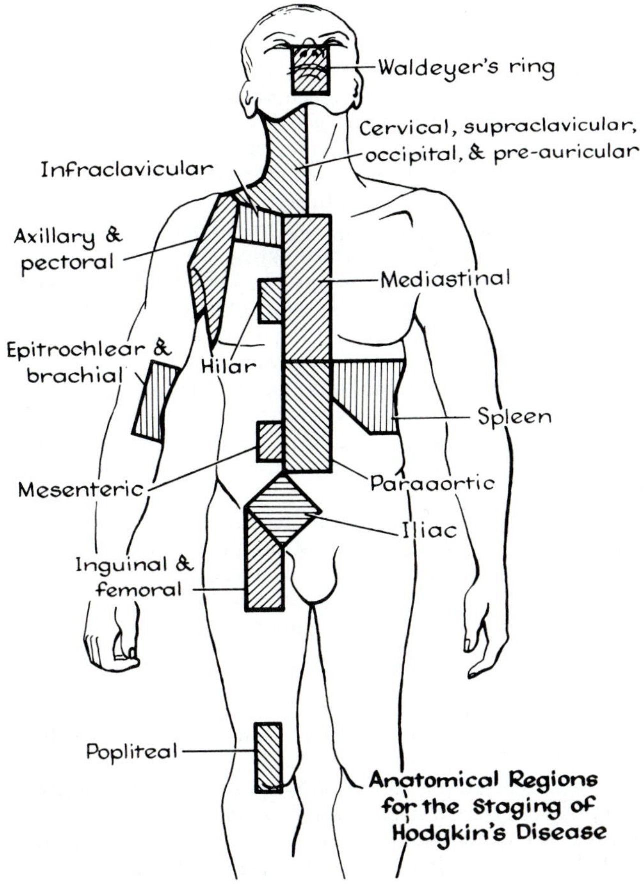

FIGURE 29-21. Diagram of the anatomic definition of separate lymph node regions adopted for staging purposes at the 1965 Rye Symposium on Hodgkin's Disease. (Kaplan HS, Rosenberg SA. The treatment of Hodgkin's disease. Med Clin North Am 1966;50:1591)

peripheral or abdominal adenopathy greater than 10 cm, or mediastinal adenopathy greater than one third of the chest diameter, and (2) the subdivision of pathologic stage IIIA into $IIIA_1$ (upper abdominal disease only) and $IIIA_2$ (lower abdominal disease with or without disease in the upper abdomen; see text that follows).[139] The group stressed the importance of recording the number of sites of involvement and also stressed the need to recognize how frequently the residual radiographic and tomographic findings constituted an isolated abnormality in patients cured of their disease.[140]

DIAGNOSTIC EVALUATION

Recommended Studies

Table 29-5 lists the diagnostic evaluation that I recommend for clinically staging the patient with Hodgkin's disease. This work-up differs substantially from the 1971 advice of the Ann Arbor Workshop.[141] The history, physical examination, and routine laboratory tests require no additional comment. Several points about the other staging procedures require more explanation.

Chest Radiography and Computed Tomography

Because the mediastinum is the major site of radiation failure, CT of the chest is mandatory for all patients with mediastinal disease who are destined to be treated with radiation therapy. As a logical extension of this principle,

TABLE 29-5. Recommended Diagnostic Studies in Staging Hodgkin's Disease

History with special attention to the presence or absence of fever, sweats, weight loss, and itching
Physical examination with attention to peripheral lymph nodes, liver, and spleen
Adequate surgical biopsy reviewed by an experienced hematopathologist
Routine laboratory tests: complete blood count, erythrocyte sedimentation rate, liver function tests
Radiography, CT scanning, and MRI of the chest for those in whom only radiation therapy is planned
Bilateral lower extremity lymphangiogram, CT scan of the abdomen and pelvis, or both
Core needle biopsy of the bone marrow of the posterior illiac crest for those with anemia or in clinical stage IIB and III
Staging laparotomy and splenectomy for patients in CS I and II except for those with large mediastinal masses, women in CS IA, and those in CS IA with groin or mediastinal presentations
Bone scan and radiographs if bone pain or tenderness is present

CT is indicated for all patients who are to be treated with radiation alone for cure; minimal mediastinal disease is easily missed with the chest radiograph. MRI has a role in defining pericardial or hilar invasion in patients with mediastinal lymphoma.

Bone Marrow Biopsy

Core needle biopsy of the bone marrow is unlikely to yield crucial staging information. I do not recommend the procedure in the patient with asymptomatic early disease (clinical stages IA and IIA). The yield is somewhat higher in those with symptomatic, advanced disease (clinical stage IIIB). In a consecutive series of 185 cases, a positive biopsy was obtained in 8 patients, all in clinical stage III or higher.[142] Some clinicians recommend bilateral biopsies in patients with advanced disease.

Lymphangiography and Computed Tomography of the Abdomen

Investigation of the abdomen and pelvis for clinical staging is accomplished with CT and bilateral lower extremity lymphangiogram. Of the two, the latter is superior when measured against the definitive findings of staging laparotomy.[143,144] Certainly, lymphangiography is more demanding of the radiologist's time and skill.[145] It is also invasive and time-consuming for the patient and is more expensive than CT. If excessive dye volume is avoided, and patients are screened for dye allergy and massive mediastinal lymphoma, serious reactions do not occur. The main argument for lymphangiography rather than CT is the greater accuracy of the former, both of positive and negative findings. Lymphangiography detected paraaortic adenopathy in 17 of 20 (85%) laparotomy-positive patients, whereas CT detected it in only 13 (65%).[143] Of 87 patients whose laparotomy was negative for paraaortic lymph nodes, lymphangiograms were correctly interpreted as negative in 85 (98%), whereas CT studies were correctly interpreted in only 80 (92%).

In a larger series, the lymphangiogram was interpreted correctly as positive in 93% of the 107 patients found to be positive at exploration, and it was correctly interpreted as negative in 92% of the 309 laparotomy-negative cases.[144] The ability of the lymphangiogram to detect gross defects in lymph node architecture provides the basis for its greater accuracy in detecting abdominal adenopathy. Theoretically, CT examination should be superior to lymphangiography in the upper abdomen, where nodes do not become opaque because lymphangiographic dye is shunted through the cisterna chyli and thoracic duct. In practice, involvement of mesenteric nodes is infrequently seen in patients with Hodgkin's disease, and almost never seen in the absence of paraaortic nodes. Furthermore, when mesenteric nodes are present, CT has not proved to be a sensitive measure of their involvement.[143] CT is also disappointing as a means of detecting splenic disease. Only 15 of 51 positive spleens (33%) were correctly identified, whereas 17 of 70 negative spleens (24%) were also considered positive. The minimal liver nodules presented at staging laparotomy are infrequently identified by CT. The ease and lesser expense of CT must be measured against the greater accuracy of lymphangiography for detecting paraaortic and pelvic lymphoma.[146,147]

Staging Laparotomy and Splenectomy

Staging laparotomy was introduced in 1969 by Glatstein and colleagues[148] to elucidate the cause of the high failure rate after radiation therapy and to provide a guide for improving radiation portals. The operation has provided major understanding of the evolution of Hodgkin's disease within the abdomen, particularly regarding the central role of the spleen.[13,114] Staging laparotomy has also provided the basis on which many clinics resolve the decision between radiation therapy and combination chemotherapy.[150–153] If the spleen is accepted as an index of hematogenous dissemination, cure of the patient with splenic Hodgkin's disease requires systemic treatment (combination chemotherapy).

The merits of staging laparotomy remain a source of controversy.[37,114,150–153] The swing of the pendulum, which strongly favored the operation in the 1970s, has, with the conservative political and medical climate of the late 1980s, swung against surgical staging. No consensus exists about the place of staging laparotomy in Hodgkin's disease management; all that can be offered is a choice of options and a coherent opinion. At the Massachusetts General Hospital, pathologic staging is still favored in a large proportion of Hodgkin's disease patients.

The operative procedure consists of splenectomy, more or less extensive biopsy of upper abdominal, paraaortic, and illiac lymph nodes, and wedge-and-needle biopsy of the liver. Oophoropexy is not often performed because the pelvis is infrequently irradiated and because moving the ovaries has been recognized as a threat to fertility. Major surgical complication of staging laparotomy are seen in about 10% of patients, but the operative mortality rate is less than 1% in the Hodgkin's disease population at centers devoted to the treatment of this condition. Our own experience of two deaths in more than 600 explorations is typical of large centers. One death occurred in a patient whose random liver biopsy unexpectedly revealed fulminant hepatitis; the other occurred in an obese alcoholic.

Splenectomy can also render patients with Hodgkin's disease susceptible to fulminant sepsis from encapsulated pathogens. As stated earlier, at the Massachusetts General Hospital,[37] this complication was restricted to patients who had undergone splenectomy and who had received both total nodal irradiation and combination chemotherapy (3 cases of sepsis—2 fatal—among 14 so treated), but the British National Lymphoma Investigation reported fatal sepsis in almost 2% of patients with splenectomy whose only treatment was extended-field irradiation.[38] Clearly, attitudes toward staging laparotomy are colored by the institutional experience with this catastrophic but fortunately uncommon complication.

Staging laparotomy often uncovers abdominal disease not appreciated by clinical study and less frequently reveals positive clinical findings to be false; that is, pathologic staging is far more accurate than clinical staging. Overall, about 30% of patients have their stage changed by laparotomy (32% of the Stanford series of 814 patients[13]; 28% of the Harvard Joint Radiotherapy Center series of 692 patients[154]). Figure 29-22 summarizes the results of the first 100 staging laparotomies at the Massachusetts General Hospital. In early clinical stages (I and II), abdominal disease was demonstrated in about 25% of those who were asymptomatic and 50% of those with symptoms. Because the splenic findings are the most frequent cause of revising stage, the importance of meticulous sectioning of the spleen specimen by the pathologist cannot be overemphasized. Table 29-6 analyzes the Harvard Joint Radiotherapy Center experience more closely. With a few exceptions (clinical stage IA females and clinical stage III and IV patients with constitutional symptoms and unfavorable histology), clinical staging proved inaccurate.

The British National Lymphoma Investigation has estimated the false-negative rate of staging laparotomy (rate at which abdominal lymphoma is missed at surgery) from the infradiaphragmatic relapse rate. About 4% of patients with negative explorations (pathologic stages I and II) relapsed below the diaphragm within 5 years of treatment, 6% within 7 years, and 10% within 10 years. In that study, the infradiaphragmatic relapse rate for *clinically* staged Hodgkin's disease patients (clinical stages I and II) was 30% at 7 years.[38,155]

Recommendations concerning the place of staging laparotomy vary from *almost never*,[38] to *sometimes*,[149] to *almost always*.[152] The almost-always position has been moderated over the past decade by an increasing list of exceptions.[156] Proponents of laparotomy argue that this procedure accurately defines the most important determinant of radiation therapy failure, that is, the presence and extent of intraabdominal spread. The almost-never group substitutes formulas based on a combination of clinical risk factors

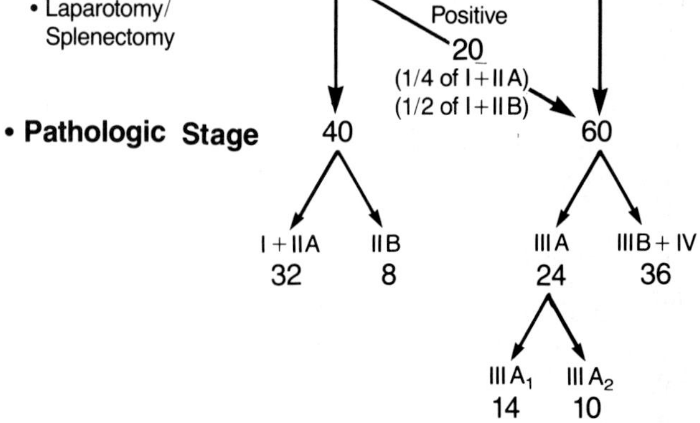

FIGURE 29-22. Distribution in 100 cases of Hodgkin's disease pathologically staged at Massachusetts General Hospital. Results are expressed in percentages and rounded to the nearest decile. Stage $IIIA_1$ designates disease restricted to the upper abdomen; stage $IIIA_2$ designates disease in the lower abdomen (with or without upper abdominal disease).

TABLE 29-6. Stage Change (Clinical Stage to Pathologic Stage) in 692 Patients Undergoing Laparotomy at the Harvard Joint Center for Radiation Therapy

Clinical Stage	Positive Laparotomy (Upstage) (%)	Negative Laparotomy (Downstage) (%)
I/II (552 CASES)	24	
A	21	
B	34	
Female	18	
Male	29	
1 site	17	
2 or more	27	
IA, female	6	
III/IV (140 CASES)		42
A		55
B		22
LP/NS		55
MC/LD		28
<40		48
>40		21
CS IIIA/IVA, NS/LP, <40		68
CS IIIB/IVB, MC/LD		12

CS, clinical stage; PS, pathologic stage; NS, nodular sclerosis; LP, lymphocyte predominance; MC, mixed cellularity; LD, lymphocyte depletion.
(Data from Mauch P, Larsen D, Osteen R, et al. Prognostic factors for positive surgical staging in patients with Hodgkin's disease. J Clin Oncol 1990;8:257)

(age, sex, histology, symptoms, sedimentation rate, bulky mediastinal disease or other bulk disease, and number of disease sites) to identify those patients who have an unacceptable failure rate with radiation alone and who should therefore receive adjuvant combination chemotherapy at the outset. The sometimes group also relies on formulas, but admits that even after the application of a formula, a significant proportion of patients remains whose disease is defined most accurately by staging laparotomy. Both the almost-never and the sometimes groups emphasize that patients who fail radiation therapy can be salvaged effectively by chemotherapy.

The crucial question is what, if anything, is lost by delaying chemotherapy until after relapse of Hodgkin's disease. The observation that 60% of radiation failures are salvaged by chemotherapy does not exclude the possibility of a higher cure rate if the same patients had received drugs at time of diagnosis.[157] Nor does the observation that 5% or even 10% of patients relapse within the abdomen despite a negative exploration[36,155] negate the usefulness of the operation for the 30% whose abdominal disease was detected.[13,154]

In view of the preceding considerations, we still recommend staging laparotomy for patients in whom the major treatment decision is influenced by surgery, that is, those who are not already committed to chemotherapy. Specifically, we recommend exploration of patients in clinical stages I and II with the following exclusions: patients with a mediastinal mass more than one third of the chest diameter, asymptomatic patients with stage IA mediastinal and groin presentations, and all women in clinical stage IA. We also continue to explore those in clinical stage IIIA in whom neither the lymphangiogram nor the CT scan is completely convincing. We consider exploration in similar stage IIIB patients with minor symptoms. Exploration is not indicated for the elderly or the very young, those with high fever or diminished performance status, and those with major complicating illness.

Bone Scans and Gallium Tomography

Bone scans are occasionally indicated in the work-up of patients in whom there is reason to anticipate bone involvement. High-dose gallium tomography, in appropriate hands, can be a sensitive indicator of Hodgkin's disease in the large proportion of patients whose tumor is gallium-avid.[158]

RADIATION THERAPY

Radiation therapists provided the first indication that Hodgkin's disease is not inevitably fatal. With strong convictions, but initially little data, first René Gilbert,[9] later Vera Peters,[10] and finally Henry Kaplan[11,13] published improving survival rates for patients presenting with localized (and defined by the primitive criteria of the time) Hodgkin's disease. In 1958, Peters and Middlemiss[10] concluded, "Thus, if a patient survives 10 years without recurrence, there is little risk of recurrence in the following 20 years." This was a dramatic statement to make at a time when few medical opinions conceded the possibility of cure in this disorder. The value of radiation therapy in Hodgkin's disease has *always* been demonstrated against historical controls, *never* against contemporaneous untreated patients.

Fields

Early workers established the need for large field size (Fig. 29-23) and adequate radiation dose to control Hodgkin's disease. Peters and Middlemiss[10] enunciated the principle of prophylactic treatment of apparently uninvolved lymph nodes one echelon removed from those diseased. With the development of megavoltage equipment, the treatment of large fields in continuity became feasible. Kaplan[11,13] introduced the linear accelerator into the therapy of these patients and established the now standard mantle, para-aortic, and inverted Y fields (Fig. 29-24).

Dose

Careful attention to recurrence patterns established a tumor dose curve for Hodgkin's disease[13,159] (Table 29-7). The commonly used schedules for wide-field megavoltage radiation are for 35 to 40 Gy to sites of bulk disease, and 30 to 35 Gy to clinically uninvolved areas, given at the rate 1.5 to 2 Gy/d 5 days per week.[157,160] This treatment schedule yields high control rates with minimal morbidity.

Indications for Radiation Therapy

From the data in Table 29-7, it is apparent that radiation would cure 95% of patients, if the disease were encompassed within the treatment portals. In fact, such cure rates are achieved in only small subsets of patients with localized Hodgkin's disease, mainly among those with pathologic stage IA presentations. Radiation of the entire group of *clinical* stages I and II patients with extended fields results in a relapse rate of 30% to 60%[157,161,162]; the transdiaphragmatic failure rate, by itself, is 30% to 40%. The question of treatment recommendations is covered later (see section on primary treatment recommendations).

Even among those in *pathologic* stages I and II, failure rates as high as 35% are seen after extended-field treatment.[159,161,163–167] Similarly, the presence of constitutional

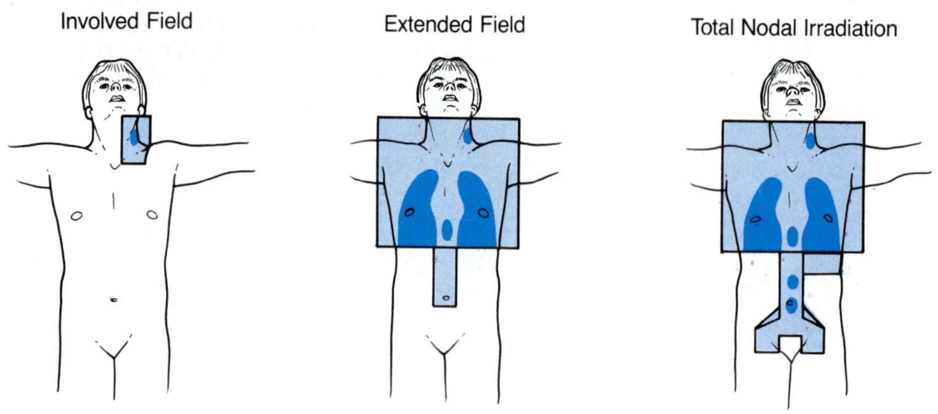

FIGURE 29-23. Involved-field, extended-field, and total nodal irradiation.

complaints requires more extensive treatment for satisfactory results, either total nodal irradiation or combined treatment with chemotherapy.[164,168] Most florid or unusual manifestations of Hodgkin's disease entail a high probability of radiation therapy failure; paracardiac, retrocrural, posterior mediastinal, or epitrochlear nodes, pericardial involvement, pleural fluid, caval obstruction, spinal cord compression, edema of a part from lymphatic obstruction, or local invasion of lung or bone. Only banal presentations of Hodgkin's disease are reliably contained by conventional radiation therapy portals. This does not mean that radiation is never indicated for these nonbanal manifestations but that high rates of cure cannot to be expected with this modality alone.

PROGNOSTIC FEATURES

The subject of prognosis logically follows the discussion on radiation therapy, since it deals largely with prognostic features that determine curability after irradiation. Some of these prognostic features also apply to patients treated with chemotherapy. Table 29-8 lists a variety of parameters that have been shown to influence cure or survival in patients with Hodgkin's disease. The effect of age, sex, histology, and clinical (Ann Arbor) stage are documented in Table 29-9 based on 1225 patients treated at Stanford with megavoltage radiation and combination chemotherapy.[13] The negative influence of male sex, advanced age, unfavorable histology, and advanced stage have been demonstrated in many other studies.

Several investigators have looked at constitutional symptoms more closely. Gobbi and associates[169] find the solitary complaint of *sweats* is without negative influence, whereas *severe pruritus* has the same unfavorable significance as fever and weight loss. Furthermore, they were able to demonstrate that minor degrees of fever (less than 100.5° F [38° C]) or weight loss (less than 10% of body weight in the preceding 6 months) were without prognostic significance. Another study has demonstrated that weight loss plus fever has more importance than either alone, at least in pathologic stage IIB disease.[170] Taken together, the two studies suggest that constitutional complaints contribute to poor prognosis in an incremental manner.

Tumor bulk is a second parameter that has been quantitatively linked to Hodgkin's disease prognosis. Tumor size was first shown to be prognostically important in the mediastinum. Although the presence of any mediastinal mass reduced radiation curability of early stage Hodgkin's disease (pathologic stages I and II) from 90% to 95% to about 80%, several centers reported that cure was reduced to about 50% when the tumor mass exceeded one third of the maximum chest diameter.[164,165,171,172] The Danish National Hodgkin's Disease Group has extended the study of the relation of tumor bulk to prognosis; they find that *total tumor burden* (a complex parameter obtained by summation of the tumor bulk of each involved site), not mediastinal mass alone, is by far the most important factor in predicting disease-free survival of patients in pathologic stages I and II.[173] In their complex multivariate analysis, histology and sex were the only other independent variables. Recently, it has been suggested that the Ann Arbor Staging Classification be modified by the addition of an X category to designate bulky disease (equal to or greater than 10 cm or one third the chest diameter).[174]

The European Organization for Research and Treatment of Cancer (EORTC) also undertook a multivariate analysis of survival in early (clinical stage I and II) Hodgkin's disease

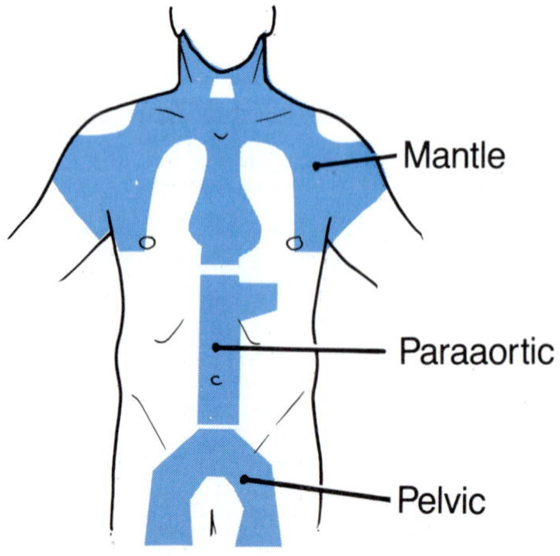

FIGURE 29-24. Mantle, paraaortic, and pelvic radiation fields.

TABLE 29-7. Relation of Dose to In-Field Recurrence in Hodgkin's Disease Patients

Dose (cGy)	Number of Node Areas	Percentage Control
<2500	9	89
2501–3000	16	94
3001–3500	78	99
3501–4000	317	96
4001–4500	402	96
>4500	37	84

(Hanks RE, Kinzie JJ, Herring DF, Kramer S. Patterns of care outcome studies in Hodgkin's disease: results of the national practice and implications for management. Cancer Treat Rep 1982;66:805)

TABLE 29-8. Unfavorable Prognostic Features

CLASSIC	
Advanced age (>60 y) and male sex	
Unfavorable histology (MC and LD versus LP and NS)	
Advanced stage (IIIB and IV)	
Symptoms; night sweats, fever, weight loss	
SYMPTOMS (REFINED)	
Severe pruritus; minor symptoms *not* significant: night sweats, fever <38°C (100.5°F), weight loss <10% body weight or mild pruritus	
Weight loss *plus* fever worse than either alone (PS IIB)	
CS I AND II	
Mediastinal disease	
Mediastinal mass diameter >⅓ chest diameter	
Bulky disease	
>2 Sites of disease	
Symptoms + ESR >30, or no symptoms and ESR >70	
<85% reduction (by CT) in mediastinal mass after radiation	
ESR (>30 mm/h 6 months after treatment) of disease	
PS IIIA	
Lower abdomen ($IIIA_2$) versus upper ($IIIA_1$)	
>4 Splenic nodules	

MC, mixed cellularity; LD, lymphocyte depletion; LP, lymphocyte predominance; NS, nodular sclerosis; PS, pathologic stage; CT, computed tomography; ESR, erythrocyte sedimentation rate.

treated solely with radiation.[175,176] They found that patients with three or more sites of involvement, or with systemic symptoms or a marked elevation of the erythrocyte sedimentation rate or both did poorly after irradiation.

Several attempts have been made to apply prognostic criteria to patients with abdominal Hodgkin's disease. The markedly unfavorable influence of constitutional complaints in these patients has long been recognized. In addition, several recent studies have demonstrated markedly inferior disease-free survival and somewhat inferior overall survival in Hodgkin's disease patients with disease in the lower abdomen (positive lymphangiogram) with or without disease in the upper abdomen, when compared with patients whose disease is restricted to the upper abdomen.[177,178] The patients in one study received only radiation as primary treatment, and the terms *stage* III_1 and *stage* III_2, respectively, were applied to those with disease in the upper abdomen only and to those with disease in the lower abdomen with or without involvement of the upper abdomen. Others failed to confirm the negative prognostic significance of spread to the lower abdomen, but found extensive splenic lymphoma (five or more nodules) to be the major negative variable in pathologic stage III disease.[179]

Finally, normalization of either the sedimentation rate or the chest CT after treatment is considered a highly favorable prognostic indicator. The EORTC stressed the importance of a normal sedimentation rate 6 months after completion of treatment,[180] and investigators at the Massachusetts General Hospital were impressed with the favorable significance of 85% reduction in the size of the mediastinal mass estimated from CT of the chest.[181]

CHEMOTHERAPY: THE BASICS

The chemotherapy of Hodgkin's disease, together with that of acute lymphocytic leukemia, provided the foundation of modern medical oncology. In addition, the drug treatments of these two diseases represent two of the most significant triumphs in the medical treatment of cancer.

During World War II, Gilman, Goodman, Lindskog, and Dougherty, in studies never published because of wartime security considerations, noted transient disease regression when patients with lymphomas and leukemias were given the mustard gas derivative tris-β-chloroethylamine hydrochloride (HN_3). In 1946, Goodman and associates[182] reported favorable responses to the closely related compound, nitrogen mustard (methyl-bis-β-chloroethylamine hydrochloride, HN_2), among 57 patients with advanced Hodgkin's disease. The era of modern cancer chemotherapy had begun.

The first attempts to combine drugs date to the early 1960s. Lacher and Durant[183] treated 16 Hodgkin's disease patients (many of whom had failed radiation therapy) with chlorambucil and vinblastine sulfate. A complete response rate of 63% was observed and a median duration of 7½ months, a result far exceeding that which could be achieved with either agent alone. The landmark study of DeVita, Serpick, and Carbone[12] was based on patients treated between 1964 and 1967 with the MOPP combination (HN_2, Oncovin [vincristine], prednisone, and procarbazine). An 81% complete response rate was obtained in 44 consecutive untreated Hodgkin's disease patients at the National Cancer Institute. When first reported, the minimum follow-up time was 32 months, the median survival rate of the 35 patients who achieved complete remission had not been reached, and 28 patients were still alive.

After 6 months of treatment with MOPP, 47% of patients with advanced Hodgkin's disease at risk for 4 years had been continuously free of disease. This achievement went an order of magnitude beyond prior experience.

TABLE 29-9. Survival of 1225 Hodgkin's Disease Patients Treated at Stanford Medical Center Between 1961 and 1977 With Megavoltage Radiation, Combination Chemotherapy, or Both

	Survival Rate (%)
Survival	
5 y	81
10 y	67
15 y	55
Clinical stage	
I	92
II	81
III	57
IV	<39
IIA	77
IIB	68
IIIA	66
IIIB	47
Histology	
LP	80
NS	71
MC	54
LD	<26
Sex	
Male	50
Female	61
Age	
<17	81
17–49	69
>49	30

LP, lymphocyte predominance; NS, nodular sclerosis; MC, mixed cellularity; LD, lymphocyte depletion.
(Kaplan HS. Hodgkin's disease, ed 2. Cambridge, MA, Harvard University Press, 1980:548)

Active Drugs

The ability to cure Hodgkin's disease with drug combinations is a consequence of the availability of many effective single agents.[13,184–186] Table 29-10 lists drugs whose effectiveness as single agents are well documented. The drugs listed in the lower half of the table became available after the MOPP combination; poorer response rates probably reflect the poor response of new drugs in patients who have already failed combination treatment rather than their lesser efficacy. The ineffectiveness of single agents compared with multidrug combinations restricts their use as such to clinical contexts in which therapy has limited goals.

MOPP and Its Variants

The treatment schedules for classic MOPP and MOPP variants are listed in Table 29-11. MOPP treatment usually consists of six cycles given every 28 days, with injections of HN_2 and vincristine on the first and eighth days of each cycle. Procarbazine and prednisone are given orally, the latter restricted to the first and fourth cycles only. Some clinics limit a single HN_2 dose to 10 mg, a single vincristine dose to 2 mg, and the daily oral procarbazine to 150 mg for 10 days, although these modifications have been criticized.[208] A complete blood count is required before each injection, and a dose reduction schedule such as that outlined in Table 29-12 must be used. Every effort should be made to give drugs at the scheduled time in the scheduled dose, although it is questionable that the administration of token amounts of drug improves the cure rate.

Prior radiation therapy or chemotherapy reduce bone marrow tolerance. The other important acute toxicities of the MOPP combination are HN_2-induced nausea and vomiting (which is ameliorated by antiemetic premedication), vincristine neurotoxicity, gastrointestinal toxicity and central nervous system depression from procarbazine (which abate with time), and the well-recognized side effects of high-dose corticosteroid administration. Procarbazine drug rashes may be the most frequent untoward reaction. Minor rashes can often be circumvented by omitting the offending drug for one cycle, but major febrile reactions usually require the substitution of another agent. Patients are usually treated for a minimum of six cycles and at least two cycles after complete remission is achieved. Patients should be completely reevaluated after four cycles and after the completion of treatment with all relevant diagnostic studies except a staging laparotomy.

Several regimens that are closely modeled after MOPP therapy are listed in Table 29-11. Although experience with these combinations is less extensive than that with MOPP, one or more large series has been reported with each of the listed programs. One variant of MOPP, MVPP (mustard, vinblastine, prednisone, and procarbazine), uses a 42-day cycle rather than the customary 28-day cycle.[202] Complete remission rates for MOPP and its variants in untreated patients with advanced stage Hodgkin's disease range from 70% to 80%, with 75% representing the average percentage (Table 29-13). Between 50% and 80% of complete responders (average, 65%) are relapse-free at 5 years by actuarial calculation.

The reported differences among results with the various MOPP variants are more likely to be related to differences in patient populations and to chance than to the particular drug regimen used. Thus, about 50% of patients (65% of 75%) can be expected to be alive and continuously free of disease 5 years after completing treatment. Response rates are lower in patients with constitutional symptoms and those with stage IV disease[201] (Table 29-14). Other negative factors are age over 40 years, bulky disease, and involvement of the bone marrow or multiple extranodal sites. Patients with the lymphocyte-depleted variant of nodular sclerosis have also been reported to do less well. Finally, those who have received significant prior chemotherapy do poorly, although patients who have failed radiation therapy are not at a disadvantage for subsequent MOPP treatment.

ABVD and Other MOPP Alternatives

In 1973, Bonnadonna and colleagues,[209–214] in Milan, introduced a new drug combination for the treatment of Hodgkin's disease. The ABVD regimen (Adriamycin, bleomycin, vinblastine, and DTIC [dacarbazine]), based on effective drugs not contained in MOPP, was initially used in patients who had failed with the latter combination. A later randomized trial of patients in stages IIB, III, and IV, revealed comparable complete remission rates for six cycles of MOPP (63%) and six cycles of ABVD (71%).[210,214] Although noncompliance may be higher with ABVD than with MOPP because of more severe nausea and vomiting, the incidence of leukemia and both male and female infertility is much lower. The toxicity problems of MOPP are discussed in the next section (see Complications of Treatment).

The Milan group next treated patients with pathologi-

TABLE 29-10. Single Agents Active in Hodgkin's Disease

Agent*	Response (%)	Complete Remission (%)	References
Nitrogen mustard (1948)	65	13	187, 188
Chlorambucil (1957)	60	16	184, 185
Cyclophosphamide (1959)	54	12	184, 185
Vinblastine (1961)	68	30	184, 185
Vincristine (1964)	58	36	184, 185
Procarbazine (1964)	69	38	184, 185
Prednisone (1953)	61	0	184, 185
BCNU† (1964)	44	5	189, 190
CCNU† (1969)	34	3	190, 192
Adriamycin† (1970)	30	5	193, 194
Bleomycin† (1970)	37	6	195–197
DTIC† (dacarbazine; 1971)	56	6	198
Etoposide† (1974)	27	6	199, 200

* Drugs tested in patients who had failed combination chemotherapy. Numbers in parentheses are the dates the drugs were introduced.

TABLE 29-11. Combination Chemotherapy for Hodgkin's Disease*

MOPP (NATIONAL CANCER INSTITUTE[201])
Nitrogen mustard 6 mg/m² IV, days 1, 8
Vincristine 1.4 mg/m² IV, days 1, 8
Procarbazine 100 mg/m² PO, days 1–14
Prednisone 40 mg/m² days 1–14 cycles 1 and 4
MVPP (ST BARTHOLOMEW'S HOSPITAL[202])
Nitrogen mustard 6 mg/m² IV, days 1, 8
Vinblastine 10 mg IV, days 1, 8
Procarbazine 100 mg/m² PO, days 1–14
Prednisolone 40 mg PO, days 1–14
ChlVPP (ROYAL MARDEN HOSPITAL[203])
Chlorambucil 6 mg/m² (maximum 10 mg) PO, days 1–14
Vinblastine 6 mg/m² (maximum 10 mg) IV, days 1, 8
Procarbazine 100 mg/m² PO, days 1–14
Prednisolone 40 mg PO, days 1–14
BCVPP (SOUTHWESTERN CANCER STUDY GROUP[204])
BCNU 100 mg/m² IV, day 1
Cyclophosphamide 600 mg/m² IV, day 1
Vinblastine 5 mg/m² IV, day 1
Procarbazine 50 mg day 1, 100 mg PO, days 2–10
Prednisone 60 mg PO, days 1–10
ABVD (MILAN[205])
Adriamycin 25 mg/m² IV, days 1, 15
Bleomycin 10 units/m² IV, days 1, 15
Vinblastine 6 mg/m² IV, days 1, 15
DTIC 375 mg/m² IV, days 1, 15
B-CAVe (STANFORD[206])
Bleomycin 5 units/m² IV, days 1, 28, 35
CCNU 100 mg/m² PO, day 1
Adriamycin 60 mg/m² IV, day 1
Vinblastine 5 mg/m² IV, day 1
MOPP/ABV HYBRID (VANCOUVER[207])
Nitrogen mustard 6 mg/m² IV, day 1
Vincristine 1.4 mg/m² (maximum 2 mg) IV, day 1
Procarbazine 100 mg/m² IV, days 1–7
Prednisone 40 mg/m² PO, days 1–14
Adriamycin 35 mg/m² IV, day 8
Bleomycin 10 units/m² IV, day 8
Vinblastine 6 mg/m² IV, day 8

* Treatment cycles are 28 days except for MVPP and B-CAVe, which are 42 days. Treatment is usually continued for six cycles and for at least two cycles after complete remission.

cally documented stage IV disease with alternating cycles of MOPP and ABVD over a 12-month period.[213] An extraordinary complete remission rate of 91% was reported in this unfavorable group of patients. At 5 years, freedom from progression was 77%, relapse-free survival rate was 83%, survival rate of those who achieved complete remission was 94%, and overall survival rate was 86%. It remains unclear whether equally good results can be readily obtained by others using alternating MOPP/ABVD. The MOPP/ABV hybrid represents a further evolution of Hodgkin's disease chemotherapy.[207] In the hybrid, each cycle includes all the drugs in MOPP and ABVD with the exception of DTIC. Seventy-three of 76 patients (96%) with advanced Hodgkin's disease experienced a complete remission, and 90% of the complete responders were relapse-free by actuarial calculation 5 years after completion of treatment.

Goldie-Coldman Hypothesis

The evolution of Hodgkin's disease chemotherapy is based, in part, on the Goldie-Coldman hypothesis that posits that the drug resistance of tumors results from the outgrowth of drug-resistant cells that arise through spontaneous mutation.[215] If this hypothesis is correct, cure is most likely when the tumor is exposed to the maximum number of drugs in the shortest time period. Based on this concept, the MOPP/ABV hybrid exposes Hodgkin's disease patients to seven drugs during the first 8 days of treatment. The hypothesis is consistent with the amply established observation that maintenance therapy—either single agent or additional cycles of combination treatment—is without benefit (see Table 29-14).

In Hodgkin's disease chemotherapy, cure has also been related to drug dose, but the available studies do not exclude the possibility that reduced drug dose was a consequence of disease-related unfavorable prognostic factors rather than a cause of treatment failure.[216–219] Drug dose should certainly not be reduced for trivial reasons, but the appropriate degree of life-threatening toxicity to be hazarded can be decided only by the treating clinician. The available evidence suggests that neither the choice of alkylating agent nor the particular periwinkle alkaloid (vinblastine or vincristine) makes much difference in the treatment results.

COMBINED CHEMOTHERAPY AND RADIATION

For the most part, combined-modality treatment has been used in early (stage I and II) and intermediate (stage IIIA) Hodgkin's disease patients. Several randomized studies of those with pathologic stages I and II agree that the addition of MOPP chemotherapy increases the relapse-free survival rate from the 70% figure seen with radiation therapy alone to about 90%.[163,165,167,220–222] Markedly increased disease-free survival rates were also seen in randomized, unfavorable clinical stages I and II disease and in those patients with bulky mediastinal tumors.[165] Overall survival rates were not significantly increased in patients in any of these studies, but it is too early to conclude that significant increases may not emerge in the future. The absence of proven benefit in overall survival combined with the demonstrated risks of chemotherapy (see text that follows) have led most clinicians to withhold drugs when radiation alone promises

TABLE 29-12. Dosage Reduction Schedules

WBCs/μL	Platelets/μL	Dose Adjustment
MOPP[24] (with modifications)		
>4000	>100,000	Full dosage
3000–4000	>100,000	50% nitrogen mustard and procarbazine
1000–3000	50,000–100,000	25% nitrogen mustard and procarbazine
<1000	<50,000	No therapy
ABVD[209]		
>3800	>120,000	Full dosage
2500–3800	75,000–120,000	50% Adriamycin and vinblastine
<2500	<75,000	No therapy

TABLE 29-13. Results of Combination Chemotherapy*

Agent†	Study	Complete Remissions (%)	Actuarial 4-Year Relapse-Free Survival of Complete Remissions (%)
MOPP	NCI[201]	80	68
	Milan[210]	74	50
	CALBG[211]	57–62	55–60
	ECOG[212]	73	55
MVPP	St Bart's[202]	82	70–75
	CALBG[211]	66	50
ChlVPP	Royal Marsden[203]	77	60–80
BCVPP	SCSG[204]	68–73	70
	ECOG[208]	76	70
ABVD	Milan[210]	71	
MOPP/ABVD*	Milan[213]	91	83
MOPP/ABV hybrid	Vancouver[207]	96	90

NCI, National Cancer Institute; CALBG, Cancer and Leukemia Group B; ECOG, Eastern Cooperative Ocology Group; St Bart's, St Bartholomew's; SCOG; Southeastern Cancer Oncology Group.
* Stage IV only.
† See Table 29-11 for drug regimens.

a relapse-free survival rate of more than 65% to 75%. This survival rate is easily achieved in pathologically staged patients by excluding those in whom a mediastinal mass exceeds one third of the chest diameter,[163,165,167,220–222] or it can be achieved without surgical staging by applying a variety of clinical criteria[161,162,220,223–225] (Table 29-15).

The place of combined-modality treatment is also an important issue in stage IIIA Hodgkin's disease. At least two studies demonstrate that both disease-free survival rate and overall survival rate are improved when chemotherapy is added to the radiation treatment of stage IIIA patients. Disease-free survival rates are 76% compared with 32% at Chicago,[226] and 90% compared with 43% at the Harvard Joint Radiotherapy Center,[227] whereas overall survival is 84% compared with 56% at Chicago (at 5 years) and 94% compared with 65% at Harvard (at 12 years). The Chicago data show that the statistically significant increase in overall survival rate is restricted to patients with involvement of lower abdominal nodes, whereas a Stanford study finds that the major proportion of patients with five or more tumor nodules in the spleen are at greatest risk.[228]

A recent randomized study failed to demonstrate the need for radiation for optimal treatment results in stage IIIA Hodgkin's disease.[229] A second randomized trial reported inferior disease-free survival rate in this stage for total nodal irradiation when compared with the MOPP variant MVPP.[230]

Combined-modality treatment is a less important issue in patients with advanced Hodgkin's disease in stage IIIB. It is generally agreed that chemotherapy is the primary treatment mode; the place of low-dose adjuvant radiation of bulk disease remains to be established.[231,232] A strong case has been made for combined treatment for advanced stage Hodgkin's disease with massive mediastinal involvement.[233]

COMPLICATIONS OF TREATMENT

During the past decade, concern about the grave complications of therapy has assumed a commanding role in planning Hodgkin's disease treatment.[234–241] In some series, deaths related to therapy have been nearly one third of the deaths from Hodgkin's disease itself, raising concern that overaggressive treatment may jeopardize the treatment gains of preceding decades. Since these complications are central to any treatment program, it is logical to consider them before making final recommendations. (Infectious complications have been discussed in an earlier section.)

Acute Nonlymphocytic Leukemia

The risk of acute nonlymphocytic leukemia (ANLL), the best-recognized grave complication of Hodgkin's disease treatment, has been defined with some precision.[241–246] These therapy-related leukemias present a characteristic picture within the spectrum of ANNL.[247] They are disorders of pleuripotent stem cells, involving myeloid, erythroid, and megakaryocytic lineages. The therapy-related leukemias are distinguished from de novo acute myelogenous leukemia by a high incidence of antecedent hematologic disorder (a preleukemic phase) and by frequent cytogenetic abnormalities involving the loss of part or all of chromosomes 5 or 7. Finally, although marrow transplantation may salvage patients in the preleukemic phase, patients who develop overt leukemia have a grave prognosis.

The incidence of leukemia in the Danish Lymphoma Study Group series has been carefully analyzed.[242,243,245] ANLL was restricted to Hodgkin's disease patients who received chemotherapy with alkylating agents. Cases of leukemia increased steadily from 1 year after the start of treatment and reached 13% at 10 years, with no additional cases thereafter.[245] When calculated from cessation of therapy (as opposed to the start of treatment), the risk curve increased sharply for the first 2 years, then gradually leveled off with no new cases observed beyond 7 years. The observation that leukemia risk was roughly proportional to the cumulative dose of alkylating agent and to the square of the patient's age is of importance when applying this data to other treatment regimens.

The shape of the age incidence curve of ANLL in treated Hodgkin's disease parallels the incidence of ANLL in the general Danish population. The leukemia risk in patients under the age of 40 years was only 5.6%. Furthermore, the extensive use of maintenance chlorambucil in Denmark resulted in a higher incidence of leukemia than would be expected after more conventional Hodgkin's disease chemotherapy. Finally, in the Danish study, leukemia was not seen in patients treated with radiation alone, nor was the incidence of leukemia in chemotherapy-treated patients increased by the addition of radiation. From other inves-

TABLE 29-14. **Results With MOPP in Patients With Advanced Hodgkin's Disease Treated at the National Cancer Institute**

PRIMARY THERAPY	
Complete remission (CR), total	80%
Histology	
Lymphocyte predominance	100%
Nodular sclerosis	84%
Mixed cellularity	81%
Lymphocyte depletion	70%
Stage	
CS II	93%
CSIII	84%
CS IV	76%
Symptoms	
A	100%
B	78%
Relapse-free survival	
5 years	68%
10 years	63%
Histology	
Nodular sclerosis	59%
Mixed cellularity	64%
Lymphocyte depletion	77%
Stage	
CS II and III	75%
CS IV	53%
Symptoms	
A	94%
B	58%
Maintenance chemotherapy	
No maintenance	60%
MOPP maintenance	66%
BCNU maintenance	73%
Overall survival	
5 years	65%
10 years	58%
TREATMENT OF RELAPSE	
CR in patients failing radiation	76%
CR after failing MOPP:	
Initial CR <12 mo	29%
Initial CR >12 mo	93%

(DeVita VT Jr, Simon RM, Hubbard SM, et al. Curability of advanced Hodgkin's disease with chemotherapy. Ann Intern Med 1980;92: 587)

tigations, it appears that a small risk of leukemia occurs from radiation alone, but that this risk, which is at most a tenth of the approximately 100-fold risk from alkylating agents, emerges only in large series.[239]

The results of the Danish study are consistent with several other investigations.[235–239] High leukemia risk after age 40,[235] limitation of the risk to the first decade after chemotherapy,[239,248] and low risk when radiation is the only treatment mode[235–239] all have been reported by others. The contribution of cumulative alkylating agent dose is seen in the high leukemia incidence in patients who received maintenance cycles and in those who require retreatment for relapse. The typical profile of the Hodgkin's disease patient who develops ANLL is that of an older person or one with moderately aggressive Hodgkin's disease requiring repeated courses of chemotherapy before eventual cure. The patient with very aggressive Hodgkin's disease is more likely to die of the underlying lymphoma before leukemia develops. Cumulative dose rather than the individual alkylating agent appears to be more important in leukemia induction.[244,245,249] Certainly, HN_2, chlorambucil, cyclophosphamide, melphalan, and the nitrosoureas all have been implicated.

The ABVD regimen has not been associated with ANLL,[238] although the experience with this program is less extensive than that with MOPP and its variants. It is puzzling that leukemia has not been reported with the PAVe regimen (procarbazine, HN_2, and vinblastine).[239] Finally, the suggestion that leukemia is increased in Hodgkin's disease patients who have undergone splenectomy requires further study.[250]

Leukemia risk is a central consideration in selecting a drug regimen for Hodgkin's disease patients. The greater experience with MOPP and its variants must be weighed against the lower leukemia risk of ABVD. From the available evidence, ABVD must take precedence over MOPP and its variants in those over the age of 40. Similarly, the MOPP/ABV hybrid that contains less alkylating agent is preferable to alternating MOPP/ABVD in older patients.

Solid Tumors

Knowledge of the risk of second solid tumors after Hodgkin's disease treatment is rudimentary compared with the knowledge about leukemia.[234–239] This is because the risk ratios for solid tumors are much smaller than those for leukemia, and a more extended period of observation is needed because risks extend at least through the second decade. The failure of some studies to detect an increased incidence of second solid tumors should not be a source of comfort. Because the tumors involved include common cancers and the risk period is protracted, the mortality from second solid neoplasms may ultimately exceed the leukemia mortality. Examining a composite series in the literature, a relative risk (RR) of 2.2 was found for all types of solid cancer.[240] The highest RRs are observed in neoplasms of the bones and joints (RR = 20), soft tissues (RR = 18), non-Hodgkin's lymphomas (RR = 8), and melanomas of the skin (RR = 7). RRs between 2 and 4 were seen for cancer of the buccal cavity and pharynx, brain and other nervous system, and respiratory and digestive systems.

TABLE 29-15. **Factors Adversely Influencing Survival in Clinical Stage Hodgkin's Disease That Can Be Used as Indications for Combined-Modality Treatment**

Institution	Criteria
European Organization for Research of Cancer[161]	Age >40 y; MC/LD histology; symptoms + ESR >30, or no symptoms and ESR >70; mediastinum negative; laparotomy positive
British National Lymphoma Investigation[223]	Older age; pathologic grade II (MC and unfavorable NS); mediastinum positive; higher ESR; male sex
Princess Margaret Hospital[162]	Age >50 y; stage II; systemic symptoms; MC/LD
Royal Marden Hospital[220,224]	LD histology; systemic symptoms; >3 sites involved; bulky mediastinal disease or At least two of: ESR >40; male sex; peripheral node mass >5 cm; >2 sites involved; MC histology

NS, nodular sclerosis; MC, mixed cellularity; LD, lymphocyte depletion; ESR, erythrocyte sedimentation rate.

Recently, an extraordinary risk of breast cancer has been noted in women irradiated for Hodgkin's disease before the age of 20.[250a,250b] The association of these second solid neoplasms was only with radiation therapy.[240] Thus, increased incidence was not seen after chemotherapy alone,[240] and from 60% to 80% of the tumors were confined to the radiation treatment fields.[239] The second solid tumors that follow therapy also differ from the treatment-induced leukemias in their curability; about 50% of the former are curable.[239] The incidence of aggressive secondary non-Hodgkin's lymphomas has been particularly high with the treatment programs used at Stanford.[239]

Toxicity of Mediastinal Radiation

Toxicity from mediastinal radiation has been markedly ameliorated by improved radiation therapy techniques.[13,24,157,251,252] The restrictive pericardial disease observed two decades ago after radiation therapy is not seen today. Changes in the chest radiograph and in pulmonary function are still common enough after full mantle treatment, but symptomatic radiation pneumonitis is recorded in less than 5% of patients and disabling pulmonary impairment is rare. Cardiac irradiation can result in coronary artery disease and cardiomyopathy, but these cardiac complications are less frequent with the portals and time–dose relations used today.[252]

Male and Female Fertility

Although not life-threatening, loss of fertility is of importance because of its regular occurrence after MOPP therapy and the young age of the Hodgkin's disease population.[13,253,254] Only 4 of 16 men treated with MOPP or MOPP variants had normal sperm counts when studied 6 months to 7 years after completion of chemotherapy.[255] The follicle-stimulating hormone level was elevated in 10 of 15 men, but libido was normal in all. Testicular biopsy revealed tubular damage with normal Sertoli and interstitial cells. A more extensive study of men treated with MVPP documented the return of spermatogenesis in only 4 of the 64 men studied from 15 to 51 months after cessation of therapy.[256] The remaining 60 were still azospermic, as was the entire group in the first 12 months after treatment. A decline in libido and sexual activity was noted in all men during that treatment; some recovery was experienced after treatment was stopped, but it remained incomplete in about 50%.

Although other MOPP variants have not been studied, it is best to assume that *permanent sterility* in males follows these drug regimens for Hodgkin's disease. Semen storage is indicated for those who still plan to have children, although about one third of patients with untreated Hodgkin's disease (predominantly those with fever) do not produce semen of adequate quality.[257] When fertility is a major concern, ABVD offers an attractive alternative because it causes much less testicular damage than MOPP; less azospermia immediately after treatment; and complete recovery in all cases.[258]

Although the ovary is less sensitive to alkylating agent treatment than the testes, most women do not experience normal menses after the completion of combination chemotherapy with MOPP or its variants.[259–262] Even those whose menses remain normal are likely to experience an early menopause. The younger the patient, the more likely that normal ovarian function will continue, but only women under the age of 30 have more than an even chance of retaining normal menses. Prolonged cessation of menses was not observed after ABVD. Pelvic irradiation also ablates ovarian function, although function is preserved in some patients if the ovaries are fixed in the midline and carefully shielded during treatment.[13,254] Temporary loss of ovarian function may even follow paraaortic radiation. Appropriate hormone replacement should be considered for all women and men with treatment-induced gonadal dysfunction.

Thyroid Function

Hypothyroidism is frequently observed after radiation therapy for supradiaphragmatic Hodgkin's disease.[254,263–266] Iodine from the lymphangiogram dye has been postulated to increase the thyroid gland's radiosensitivity. Overt hypothyroidism occurs in 5% to 10% of patients receiving mantle irradiation, whereas up to 50% of irradiated patients exhibit a rise in thyroid-stimulating hormone levels. Because both clinical and chemical hypothyroidism may first manifest themselves many years after treatment, thyroid function should be monitored once every 2 years for at least one decade. Replacement therapy is appropriate.

Osteonecrosis of the Femoral Head

An estimated 2% of patients treated with regimens that include high-dose intermittent adrenal corticosteroids develop aseptic necrosis of the femoral head, either unilateral or bilateral.[157,267,268] The complication may require hip replacement many years after the offending chemotherapy.

Bleomycin Lung Toxicity and Adriamycin Cardiotoxicity

Although susceptibility to bleomycin lung toxicity increases with age and total dose, a significant incidence of this grave treatment complication is observed even in young patients who receive total doses of less than 200 IU.[269,270] Moreover, the incidence of bleomycin lung toxicity is increased by prior mediastinal radiation, placing the Hodgkin's disease population at particular risk.[271] Finally, compromised lung function resulting from prior bleomycin could exclude patients with recurrent lymphoma from many marrow transplantation programs. For these reasons and because of the high mortality rate of this complication, the pulmonary function of patients receiving bleomycin should be carefully monitored. Chest radiographs and pulmonary function tests, including the diffusing capacity of the lung for carbon monoxide (DLco) should be obtained before treatment and after every other cycle of bleomycin-containing chemotherapy. Bleomycin should be discontinued if any radiographic findings or pulmonary signs or symptoms are compatible with bleomycin toxicity or if the DLco falls below 50% of the predicted value. Many experienced chemotherapists administer 100 mg of hydrocortisone intravenously before each bleomycin injection and strongly consider a trial of high-dose prednisone for clinically apparent lung toxicity.

Adriamycin does not frequently produce significant cardiotoxicity in the doses used in ABVD or the MOPP/ABV hybrid.[207,213,214] Nonetheless, it is prudent to obtain a gated blood pool scan before treatment with Adriamycin-containing regimens and to repeat the study after every third cycle. The drug should be stopped if the ejection fraction drops 10% or falls below 45%.

PRIMARY TREATMENT RECOMMENDATIONS

Early Disease (Stages I and II)

Table 29-16 is a summary of treatment recommendations for Hodgkin's disease patients assembled in 1992 on the basis of available data. Laparotomy has already been dis-

TABLE 29-16. Treatment Recommendations for Hodgkin's Disease

Stage	Large Mediastinal Mass*	Laparotomy	Extended-Field Radiation	Chemotherapy Under Age 40	Chemotherapy Over Age 40
PS IA and IIA	No	Yes†	Yes	No	No
PS IB and IIB	No	Yes	Yes	ABVD or MOPP	ABVD
CS IA and IIA	Yes	No	Yes	ABVD or MOPP	ABVD
CS IB and IIB	Yes	No	Yes	MOPP/ABV hybrid or MOPP/ABVD	MOPP/ABV hybrid
PS $IIIA_1$		For diagnosis	Yes	ABVD or MOPP	ABVD
CS $IIIA_2$		Only if LAG and CT equivocal	No	ABVD or MOPP MOPP/ABV hybrid or MOPP/ABVD	ABVD or MOPP/ABV hybrid
PS IIIB, CS IIIB, PS IV		No	No	MOPP/ABV or MOPP/ABVD hybrid	MOPP/ABV hybrid

CT, computed tomography; LAG, lymphangiogram; CS, clinical stage; PS, pathologic stage; MOPP/ABVD, alternating MOPP and ABVD.
* More than one third maximum chest diameter.
† Except mediastinal or groin, and all females with IA.

cussed in detail in this chapter under Diagnostic Evaluation. With the exception of patients with a mediastinal mass greater than one third of the chest diameter, those in clinical stage IA with primary mediastinal or groin presentations, and women in clinical stage IA, it is appropriate to explore all patients with early stage (I and II) disease. Patients in pathologic stages IA and IIA without large mediastinal masses are treated with extended-field irradiation. Similar symptomatic patients (pathologic stages IB and IIB) receive ABVD or MOPP followed by extended-field radiation if they are under the age of 40 years, and ABVD followed by radiation if they are over age 40. Asymptomatic patients with large mediastinal masses do not require surgical staging, but receive ABVD or MOPP followed by extended-field radiation if they are under age 40, and ABVD and radiation if over age 40.

Symptomatic patients with large mediastinal masses are treated more aggressively. Younger patients receive MOPP/ABV hybrid or alternating MOPP/ABVD followed by radiation; older patients receive the MOPP/ABV hybrid and radiation. (Excellent survival rates have been reported after MOPP treatment for early stage disease, but the late side effects of this option discourage its use[272,273].)

Intermediate Disease (Stage IIIA)

Patients in pathologic stage $IIIA_1$ (upper abdominal involvement only) will have been diagnosed by staging laparotomy. It is appropriate to use ABVD or MOPP followed by extended-field radiation for patients under the age of 40, and ABVD followed by radiation for older patients. We explore patients with positive lymphangiograms and abdominal CT scans (clinical stage $IIIA_2$) only when those studies are equivocal. Younger patients can be treated with ABVD or MOPP, MOPP/ABV hybrid, or alternating MOPP/ABVD. Older patients receive either ABVD or the hybrid.

Advanced Disease (Clinical and Pathologic Stages IIIB and IV)

Patients with advanced Hodgkin's disease are not explored. Younger patients receive the MOPP/ABV hybrid or alternating MOPP/ABVD, whereas older patients receive the hybrid to minimize the dose of alkylating agent.

TREATMENT OF RELAPSE

Conventional Chemotherapy

The shape of the Hodgkin's disease relapse curve is illustrated in Figure 29-25. Of 1360 patients treated in the Stanford University Department of Radiation Therapy and observed up to 20 years, 1312 entered complete remission and 424 of these (32%) subsequently had relapses.[274] Fifty-five cases, or 13% of the relapses, occurred more than 36 months after the completion of therapy (none after 15 years). Conversely, 87% of relapses occurred within the first 3 years after treatment, with the highest relapse rate in the first 2 years.

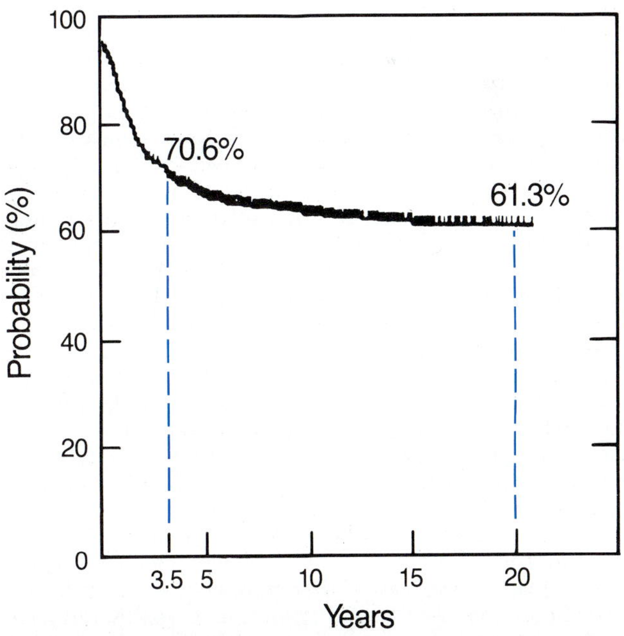

FIGURE 29-25. Relapse-free survival rate of 1360 patients treated at Stanford University between 1962 and 1979. Three years after completing 6 months of treatment, 70.6% were relapse-free. By 20 years after treatment, however, only 61.3% had not experienced relapse. The risk of late relapse in patients with an initial 3-year disease-free interval was 12.9%. (Herman TS, Hoppe RT, Donaldson SS, et al. Late relapses among patients treated for Hodgkin's disease. Ann Intern Med 1985;102:292)

MOPP chemotherapy cures about 60% of patients who relapse after radiation therapy for early stage Hodgkin's disease.[46–81,201,212,275–280] The extent of disease *at the time of relapse* is the main determinant of subsequent cure. Thus, nearly 90% of those in stages IA and IA_E were cured by subsequent MOPP chemotherapy, 60% of those in stages IIA, IIA_E, and IIIA, but only 34% of those with B symptoms or stage IV disease.[280] ABVD is at least as effective as MOPP in the treatment of relapse after radiation therapy.

Salvage of patients who relapse after MOPP is much less successful. Although the Milan group has reported complete remissions in 59% of MOPP-resistant patients treated with ABVD,[205] the average complete response rate with this combination for a group of clinics was only slightly more than 30%, no more than 50% of whom were long-term remissions.[187,206] The experience with combinations other than ABVD in patients who have failed MOPP is about the same.[187,206] In contrast to MOPP treatment of radiation failures, remissions after MOPP failure are not durable. The previous results can be compared with those with the use of MOPP itself in MOPP failures, in which the complete response rate was about 30% for those in whom the first remission was less than 1 year in duration and 93% for those with an initial remission of more than 1 year (see Table 29-14).

Complete remission rates with third-line (after the successive failure of MOPP and ABVD) salvage regimens, such as MIME (methyl-GAG, ifosfamide, methotrexate, etoposide)[281] or DHAP (cisplatin, cytosine arabinoside, dexamethasone),[282] are only 10% to 15%.[187,283] Finally, occasional patients who have failed combination chemotherapy can achieve prolonged disease-free survival with subsequent widefield irradiation.[284,285] The best candidates have experienced a long disease-free survival period from their initial chemotherapy and have relapsed in nodal sites.

Autologous Bone Marrow Transplantation

In the late 1950s, bone marrow transplantation was used in a few patients in an attempt to administer otherwise lethal doses of HN_2. Recently, the procedure has been used widely. Since few persons have appropriate sibling donors for allogeneic transplantation, autologous bone marrow transplantation (ABMT) was introduced to treat relapsed Hodgkin's disease patients who had failed two or more drug combinations. The chance of long-term survival for such patients is otherwise less than 10%; even in patients who have failed MOPP alone, less than 30% experience a prolonged remission. The numerous recent publications allow an early assessment of the place of ABMT in Hodgkin's disease management.[286–295]

Drug regimens containing cyclophosphamide, the nitrosourea carmustine, and etoposide are used most frequently for Hodgkin's disease marrow autografting. Other conditioning regimens include cytarabine, BCNU, melphalan, and total body irradiation. Marrow purging has not been necessary.

In early series, the preponderance of patients with Hodgkin's disease who had received transplants had recurrent and unresponsive disease after treatment with multiple-drug (more than two) combinations; many exhibited poor performance status as well. Forty to 50% of such patients experienced a complete remission after transplantation, but one third relapsed within 1 year.[286–292] Few patients achieved long-term disease-free survival—less than 25% of the original group. Furthermore, the mortality rate after ABMT was high (20% to 30%) in the patients with far-advanced Hodgkin's disease, higher than when the procedure is used in those with most other neoplasms who have received transplants. Extensive prior chemotherapy and radiation leave Hodgkin's disease patients fragile and susceptible to a variety of posttransplantation problems. Pulmonary complications are of particular concern in those who have had prior mediastinal radiation or chemotherapy regimens that included either bleomycin or a nitrosourea.[270] Transplantation regimens that include total body irradiation, the nitrosoureas, and, to a lesser degree, cyclophosphamide have been most frequently associated with grave pulmonary complications.

More recently, better results have been reported after ABMT in more favorable patients with modified treatment regimens. A 63% complete remission rate and a 77% projected 3-year survival rate were seen in patients with good performance status who had failed no more than two treatment regimens and whose Hodgkin's disease was still responding to conventional chemotherapy.[293] Another clinic reported a 50% complete remission rate in a heavily pretreated population of patients.[294] A third group has reported a 64% actuarial disease-free survival rate 3 years after transplantation of 16 patients treated after first relapse while still responsive to standard therapy.[295] Most recently, a 53% survival rate and a 47% event-free survival rate were reported after ABMT in 56 consecutive patients, 51 of whom had failed either the MOPP/ABV hybrid or both MOPP and ABVD.[296] Poor performance status and constitutional symptoms were negative risk factors.

ABMT offers a 50% chance of disease-free survival at 3 to 5 years if offered *promptly* to Hodgkin's disease patients who have failed MOPP/ABV(D), either as the hybrid or alternating regimens.[296–299] The treatment mortality rate should be less than 10% in such patients. Conventional treatment is to reduce bulk disease with radiation or chemotherapy before transplantation and to irradiate residual tumor after the procedure. Cytokine administration (G-CSF and GM-CSF) facilitates marrow recovery, and it appears likely that peripheral stem cell harvest will replace bone marrow as the source of hematopoietic precursors.[300]

ABMT is my first choice for the fit person under age 50 who has recurrence after MOPP and ABVD or after the MOPP/ABV hybrid. Marrow transplantation offers much less to the person with unresponsive residual disease or poor performance status, or who has failed more than two drug combinations.

SPECIAL TREATMENT CONSIDERATIONS

Children

Hodgkin's disease is uncommon in children in developed countries[13–16]; when it does occur in children, it presents special treatment-related problems because of infection and growth retardation. Except for these special treatment-related considerations, Hodgkin's disease in children is similar to that in adults, and the same prognostic factors apply.[301–309] The prognosis of childhood Hodgkin's disease is at least as favorable as that of the adult disorder, a well-established fact that corrects the earlier impression that children do less well. Most children present with early stage disease and favorable histology; constitutional symptoms are present in only 20% to 30%. The comments made here do not apply to developing countries where childhood Hodgkin's disease is more common.

Infection is an important consideration in the child with Hodgkin's disease. Postsplenectomy sepsis makes staging laparotomy a more hazardous undertaking in those under 5 years of age, particularly in the first 2 years of life.[310] Furthermore, surgical staging plays a less critical role in children because treatment has evolved more rapidly toward combined therapy.[302,308] Although radiation therapy is as curative in the child as in the adult, the cost in developmental abnormalities increases as bone age is reduced. Radiation therapists favor lower dose and smaller field size in children.[304,305,309,311] Except in very favorable presentations, adjuvant combination chemotherapy is used to avoid high recurrence rates.[301,302,304,308,309]

The leukemia risk from MOPP and its variants appears to be modest in children. Nonetheless, ABVD and other less leukemogenic combinations are being investigated. MOPP-like regimens markedly compromise male fertility, particularly in boys at the age of puberty. Hypothyroidism is seen in irradiated children, and, more significantly, second solid tumors, which continue to occur two decades after treatment.[312]

The Elderly

The elderly constitute the second peak of the bimodal incidence curve in Hodgkin's disease.[16] The survival rate of elderly patients with Hodgkin's disease is markedly lower than that of younger individuals.[313,314] Only 29% of patients over the age of 60 survived 5 years in a Stanford series, whereas 40% of those aged 50 to 59 survived, 77% of those aged 17 to 49, and 90% of those under the age of 17.[314] The poor survival rate partly reflects the less favorable natural history of this disease in the aged, that is, a preponderance of patients with advanced stage, constitutional symptoms, and unfavorable histology. It also reflects the poor tolerance of the elderly to aggressive management programs, particularly poor tolerance of their bone marrow to alkylating agents with their propensity for leukemogenesis. Finally, complicating disease exacts a toll. In one report of 47 elderly patients, the 33 who had died at the time of writing experienced a median survival of only 6 months.[313] Nonetheless, the prognosis was excellent in the small subgroup of aged patients at Stanford (86% of 15 patients survived 5 years), who presented with clinically localized disease and who were considered fit enough for a laparotomy, which was negative, and who subsequently received curative radiation therapy.[314]

In a recent multi-institution study, a comparison of 60- to 79-year-old Hodgkin's disease patients with those aged 40 to 59 showed that the older group experienced twice the risk of the younger group of dying of Hodgkin's disease and four times the risk of dying of other causes.[315] Nonetheless, Hodgkin's disease did not have a different natural history in older patients; the major risk factors were similar to those in younger patients and the disease was amenable to existing therapeutic approaches with similar complete remission rates.

The fit elderly should be staged with all measures except laparotomy. Those with asymptomatic early stage disease should be radiated with the understanding that the disorder is likely to recur. All others, and those that recur after irradiation, should receive combination chemotherapy. The aged are particularly sensitive to HN_2, and the high risk of leukemia from any alkylating agent in this age group has already been mentioned. The ABVD combination is an attractive alternative, but chemotherapeutic regimens for the elderly need further study.

Pregnancy

Since Hodgkin's disease is common during childbearing years, pregnancy may coincide with the initial diagnosis of Hodgkin's disease or with the presence of known or recurrent disease.[13,116,316,317] The solution to this complex problem depends on the duration of the pregnancy and the patient's attitude toward it and to the nature of the Hodgkin's disease insofar as it can be evaluated. If possible, the fetus, particularly in the first trimester, should not be exposed either to chemotherapy or to therapeutic or excessive diagnostic radiation. Usually, an early pregnancy must be terminated if the mother is to have optimal treatment, whereas a delay of 1 or 2 months is justifiable late in pregnancy to obtain a viable fetus.[13,116,316] Occasionally, a patient presenting with localized and favorable disease early in pregnancy can carry to term by judicious radiation therapy. Although chemotherapy during the first trimester is hazardous to the developing fetus, patients can be reassured that unfertilized germ cells do not experience occult genetic damage that could result in fetal deformity.[317]

Localized Infradiaphragmatic Presentations

Localized infradiaphragmatic presentations make up about 10% of clinical stage I and II Hodgkin's disease.[157,162] Although the reported survival rate of 80% (range, 70% to 90%) is similar to that for localized disease presenting above the diaphragm, patients who present with nodes in the inguinal, femoral, or superficial illiac regions constitute a special problem.[318–320] These patients with *external* presentations below the diaphragm should be distinguished from those in whom intraabdominal disease is first uncovered at laparotomy. The latter frequently have more extensive involvement and a less favorable prognosis.

Patients with infradiaphragmatic presentations of Hodgkin's disease fall into several groups on the basis of the presence or absence of constitutional symptoms and on the lymphangiographic (a crucial study) and laparotomy (useful in some subsets) findings. The Ann Arbor Staging Classification is unsatisfactory for localized infradiaphragmatic presentations because the presence of spleen involvement does not change the stage of stage II patients. From the available experience, patients in clinical stage IA do not require a staging laparotomy and do well when radiated to an inverted Y field (paraaortic and pelvic fields in continuity).[283] Patients in clinical stage II can be subdivided on the basis of the lymphangiogram, which is highly predictive of the presence of splenic involvement.[320] In a recent study, 52% of patients (14 of 27) with lymphangiographic evidence of involved paraaortic nodes were found to have splenic lymphoma at exploration, compared with only 14% (2 of 14: 0 of 6 in stage I; 2 of 8 in stage II) of those with negative paraaortic nodes by lymphangiogram.

Furthermore, a high relapse rate, including relapse above the diaphragm, is seen in patients in clinical and pathologic stage IIA treated with radiation to limited fields. Some recommend total nodal irradiation for such patients in stage IIA, but even this treatment is unsatisfactory for those with bulky splenic disease or bulky disease in the upper abdominal nodes.[318] Combined-modality therapy appears to be the preferred treatment here. Few subdiaphragmatic patients are in pathologic stage IB, but for those with symptoms in either pathologic or clinical stage II, combined-modality treatment is indicated also.

When to Treat

A strong case can be made for avoiding delay in the treatment of Hodgkin's disease. It is not a disorder in which untreated patients prosper. The early studies of Peters and Middlemiss[10] demonstrating an inverse relation between delay in diagnosis and survival should not be misinterpreted. The observation of improved survival with delayed diagnosis merely confirmed the importance of the aggressiveness of the disease process in an era when treatment was, for the most part, ineffective. Early treatment ensures less tumor bulk, a prognostic factor of demonstrated importance. Furthermore, even with modern treatment regimens, the agonal patient with Hodgkin's disease is rarely salvaged and the person with poor performance status is cured with difficulty.

With the increasing aggressiveness of modern treatment regimens, particularly ABMT, physicians may face the dilemma of instituting treatment at a time when the diagnosis of relapse is in doubt. Certainly, biopsy proof of recurrence is desirable, but it is arguable whether a formal thoracotomy is justified to confirm an obvious recurrence in the chest. Fortunately, modern diagnostic techniques such as CT, MRI, and lymphangiography usually permit early, accurate diagnosis of Hodgkin's disease. Moreover, the clinical context and the likelihood of recurrence, based on the pretreatment prognostic variables, often lead the experienced physician to a correct decision. Unfortunately, needle biopsy of chest or abdominal lesions is not usually helpful. Procrastination remains a serious error in this period of effective Hodgkin's disease treatment, perhaps more serious than it was before effective therapy was available.

When patients have relapsed after several drug regimens, little published information is available to guide the practitioner. Even at this stage, when cure or complete remission is ruled out, much can be done to prolong life and relieve suffering. Reference here is to specific treatment of lymphoma, not the wider issues of patient support, medical and psychological, which are equally applicable to other forms of malignant disease. Skillfully administered treatment can often prolong life in Hodgkin's disease, even after dramatic objective remissions are impossible. To obtain the most therapeutic benefit in the face of limited bone marrow reserve, the most myelotoxic drugs should be avoided, and those that are most likely to be effective in the individual patient should be used. Agents that were effective in the patient's remote past should be given preference to compounds recently proved ineffective. Patient response must be carefully monitored and ineffective drugs promptly discarded.

USEFUL PERCENTAGES

Table 29-17 is a compilation of useful percentages that have been introduced earlier in this chapter. Some of these percentages are secure; others are approximations. As the accuracy of these numbers is improved, treatment for Hodgkin's disease is refined.

TABLE 29-17. Useful Percentages in Treatment of Hodgkin's Disease

LAPAROTOMY	
Alteration of stage (CS to PS)	30
Abdominal disease after negative laparotomy	5–10
Mortality rate	<1
Postsplenectomy sepsis	2
CURE AFTER RADIATION THERAPY ALONE	
CS I and II (mantle and paraaortic)	65 (50–80)
PS I and II (mantle and paraaortic)	80 (70–85)
PS I and II, large mediastinal mass	50
PS IIIA	<50
CURE AFTER COMBINED-MODALITY TREATMENT	
CS I and II	90
PS I and II	90
PS I and II, large mediastinal mass	80
PS IIIA	90
PS IIIB	70
CURE AFTER CHEMOTHERAPY	
MOPP and variants (all stages)	50
MOPP for radiation failure	60 (45–80)
ABVD for radiation failure	75
MOPP/ABVD in stage IV	75
ABVD after MOPP failure	15–20
Third line (MOPP and ABVD failure)	<10
Autologous bone marrow transplant after MOPP/ABV(D) failure	40–50
TREATMENT TOXICITY	
Acute leukemia after MOPP and variants	
Under age 40	2–3
Age 40 and over	20–30
Solid cancers after radiation	2X*

CS, clinical stage; PS, pathologic stage.
* Age-adjusted risk expressed as multiple of normal risk.

FUTURE PROSPECTS

The exciting progress in Hodgkin's disease management came in the 1950s and 1960s. The 1970s and 1980s have witnessed a long period of consolidation and refinement of earlier discoveries. Although we have reached a satisfactory stage in which two out of three patients with the disorder are cured, we are impatient to know the reasons why the third patient eludes us. Probably, closely similar therapeutic results can be achieved by skilled clinicians using a variety of management plans: with or without staging laparotomy, with more or less radiation, with more or less chemotherapy, with more or less combined treatment. Results of therapy are sufficiently favorable that large numbers of patients are required to distinguish between the different treatment arms of acceptable (in that no treatment arm is clearly inferior at the time the protocol is devised) studies. Even with large studies, the mix of patients is likely to be more important in the final result than a minor modification of the treatment intervention.

Perhaps the most important avenue for progress is through minimizing treatment-related mortality. Figure 29-26 illustrates the increasing importance of deaths from therapy. Mortality from second solid neoplasms is a particular concern since the risk continues into the second decade. Furthermore, since significant second solid tumor mortality requires only modest increases in the relative risk of common neoplasms, it is more difficult to identify and quantitate the risk of solid tumors than that of leukemia. In this connection, the contribution of radiation to second neoplasms needs to be quantitated both in patients who receive combined-modality treatment and in those with pathologically staged supradiaphragmatic disease who receive abdominal radiation. Even with the limited information available, some secondary neoplastic consequences of Hodgkin's disease therapy have become a primary concern in treatment selection—that is, ANLL following alkylating agents in those above age 40, breast cancer following radiation of women below age 25, and lung cancer in irradiated smokers.

In the next decade, it should be possible to define the relative merits of MOPP, ABVD, alternating MOPP/ABVD, and the MOPP/ABV hybrid. Early results of cooperative studies suggest that MOPP is less satisfactory than either ABVD or alternating MOPP/ABVD,[321] and that MOPP/ABVD is inferior to the MOPP/ABV hybrid.[322] It appears likely that ABVD will replace MOPP as the combination of choice and that MOPP will be restricted to treatment of patients with advanced Hodgkin's disease, where it will be used only with ABVD. In the past, administration of in-

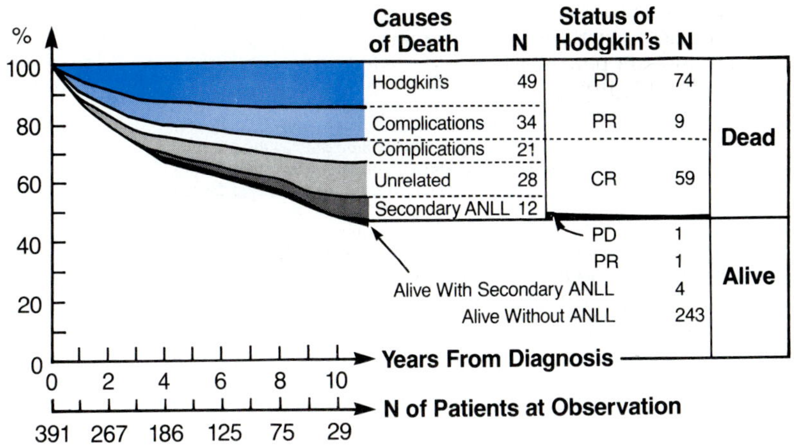

FIGURE 29-26. Survival after the start of treatment and causes of death in 391 Hodgkin's disease patients treated at the Finsen Institute in Denmark. ANLL, acute nonlymphocytic leukemia; CR, complete remission; N, number; PD, progressive disease; PR, partial remission. (Pedersen-Bjergaard J, Larsen SO. Incidence of acute nonlymphocytic leukemia, preleukemia, and myeloproliferative syndrome up to 20 years after treatment of Hodgkin's disease. N Engl J Med 1982;307:965)

creasing numbers of drugs over shorter periods of time have given superior results, suggesting that regimens similar to the MOPP/ABV hybrid will be increasingly favored for primary treatment in unfavorable clinical presentations. Third-line drug regimens (regimens using alternatives to those in MOPP and ABVD) appear best used in the context of ABMT, but much of the decade may be needed to establish the full potential of that technique.

The agent responsible for Hodgkin's disease and the nature of the Reed-Sternberg cell remain unknown, and it is hazardous to predict when these problems will be elucidated. It would not be surprising to find the elusive third Hodgkin's disease patient cured, but the nature of the disorder still unknown.

Yet, if the future is unclear, the past is a source of satisfaction.

REFERENCES

1. Annual cancer statistics review. National Institutes of Health Publication 88-2789. Bethesda, MD, Department of Health and Human Services, National Cancer Institute 1987:II.153.
2. Hodgkin T. On some morbid appearances of the absorbent glands and spleen. Med Chir Trans 1832;17:68.
3. Kass AM, Kass EH. Perfecting the world: the life and times of Dr. Thomas Hodgkins 1798. Boston, Harcourt Brace Jovanovich, 1988.
4. Greenfield WS. Specimens illustrative of the pathology of lymphadenoma and leucocythemia. Trans Pathol Soc Lond 1878;29:272.
5. Sternberg C. Uber eine eigenartige unter dem Bilde der Pseudoleukamie verlaufende Tuberculose des lymphatischen Apparates. Zeitschr Heilk 1898;19:21.
6. Reed DM. On the pathological changes in Hodgkin's disease, with especial reference to its relation to tuberculosis. John Hopkins Hosp Rep 1902;10:133.
7. Jackson H Jr, Parker F Jr. Hodgkin's disease and allied disorders. New York, Oxford University Press, 1947.
8. Obstacles to the control of Hodgkin's disease. Cancer Res 1966;26:1045.
9. Gilbert R. Radiotherapy in Hodgkin's disease maligant granulomatosis: anatomic and clinical foundations, governing principles, results. Am J Roentgenol 1939;41:198.
10. Peters MV, Middlemiss KCH. A study of Hodgkin's disease treated by irradiation. Am J Roentgenol 1956;79:114.
11. Kaplan HS. The radical radiotherapy of regionally localized Hodgkin's disease. Radiology 1962;78:553.
12. DeVita VT Jr, Serpick A, Carbone PP. Combination chemotherapy in the treatment of advanced Hodgkin's disease. Ann Intern Med 1970;73:881.
13. Kaplan HS. Hodgkin's disease, ed 2. Cambridge, MA, Harvard University Press, 1980.
14. Mueller (Gutensohn) NE. The epidemiology of Hodgkin's disease. In: Selby P, McElwain TJ, eds. Hodgkin's disease. Oxford, UK, Blackwell Scientific Publications, 1987:68.
15. Glaser SL. Hodgkin's disease in black populations: a review of the epidemiologic literature. Semin Hematol 1990;17:643.
16. MacMahon B. Epidemiology of Hodgkin's disease. Cancer Res 1966;26:1189.
17. Correa P, O'Conor GT. Epidemiologic patterns of Hodgkin's disease. Int J Cancer 1971;8:192.
18. Grufferman SG, Cole P, Smith PG, Lukes RJ. Hodgkin's disease in sibs. N Engl J Med 1977;296:248.
19. Gutensohn (Mueller) NE, Cole P. Childhood social environment and Hodgkin's disease. N Engl J Med 1981;304:135.
20. Vianna NJ, Greenwald P, Brady J, et al. Hodgkin's disease: cases with features of a community outbreak. Ann Intern Med 1972;77:169.
21. Gutensohn (Mueller) NE, Li FP, Johnson RE, Cole P. Hodgkin's disease, tonsillectomy and family size. N Engl J Med 1975;292:22.
22. Aisenberg AC. Manifestations of immunological unresponsiveness in Hodgkin's disease. Cancer Res 1966;26:1152.
23. Romagnani S, Ferrini PLR, Ricci M. The immune derangement in Hodgkin's disease. Semin Hematol 1985;22:41.
24. Hellman S, Jaffe ES, DeVita VT Jr. Hodgkin's disease. In: DeVita VT Jr, Hellman S, Rosenberg SA, eds. Cancer: principles and practice of oncology, ed 3. Philadelphia, JB Lippincott, 1989:1696.
25. Feld R, Sutcliffe SB. Immune deficiency and infectious complications of Hodgkin's disease. In: Selby P, McElwain TJ, eds. Hodgkin's disease. Oxford, UK, Blackwell Scientific Publications, 1987:301.
26. Bjorkholm M, Holm G, Mellstedt H. Immunocompetence in patients with Hodgkin's disease. In: Lacher MJ, Redman JR, eds. Hodgkin's disease: the consequences of survival. Philadelphia, Lea & Febiger, 1990:112.
27. Slivnick DJ, Ellis TM, Nawrocki JF, Fisher RI. The impact of Hodgkin's disease on the immune system. Semin Oncol 1990;17:673.
28. Ewing J. Neoplastic diseases: a treatise on tumors. Philadelphia, WB Saunders, 1940:416.
29. Parker F Jr, Jackson H Jr, Fitzhugh G, Spies TD. Studies of disease of the lymphoid and myeloid tissues. IV. Skin reactions to human and avian tuberculin. J Immunol 1932;22:272.
30. Schier WW. Cutaneous anergy in Hodgkin's disease. N Engl J Med 1954;250:353.
31. Aisenberg AC. Studies on delayed hypersensitivity in Hodgkin's disease. J Clin Invest 1962;41:1964.
32. Kelly WD, Lamb DL, Varco RL, Good RA. An investigation of Hodgkin's disease with respect to the problem of transplantation. Ann NY Acad Sci 1960;87:187.
33. Young RC, Corder MP, Haynes HH, DeVita VT Jr. Delayed hypersensitivity in Hodgkin's disease: a study of 103 untreated cases. Am J Med 1972;52:63.
34. Eltringham JR, Kaplan HS. Impaired delayed-hypersensitivity responses in 154 patients with untreated Hodgkin's disease. Natl Cancer Inst Monogr 1973;36:107.
35. Hersh EM, Oppenheim JJ. Impaired in vitro lymphocyte transformation in Hodgkin's disease. N Engl J Med 1965;273:1006.
36. Faguet G. Quantitation of immunocompetence in Hodgkin's disease. J Clin Invest 1975;56:951.
37. Weitzman S, Aisenberg AC. Fulminant sepsis after the successful treatment of Hodgkin's disease. Am J Med 1977;62:47.
38. Jeliffe AM, Hudson GV. Staging laparotomy in Hodgkin's disease. In: Selby P, McElwain TJ, eds. Hodgkin's disease. Oxford, UK, Blackwell Scientific Publications, 1987:160.
39. Siber GR, Weitzman SA, Aisenberg AC. Antibody response of patients with Hodgkin's disease to protein and polysaccharide antigens. Rev Infect Dis 1981;3(Suppl):S144S159.
40. Goffinet DR, Glatstein EJ, Merigan T. Herpes zoster-varicella infections and lymphoma. Ann Intern Med 1972;76:235.
41. Leyland-Jones B, Carr K, O'Dwyer P. Late infectious complications. In: Lacher MJ, Redman JR, eds. Hodgkin's disease: the consequences of survival. Philadelphia, Lea & Febiger, 1990:168.
42. Notter DT, Grossman PL, Rosenberg SA, Remington JS. Infections in

patients with Hodgkin's disease: a clinical study of 300 consecutive adult patients. Rev Infect Dis 1980;2:761.
43. Coker DD, Morris DM, Coleman JJ, et al. Infection among 210 patients with surgically staged Hodgkin's disease. Am J Med 1983;75:97.
44. Armstrong D, Minamoto GY. Infectious complications of Hodgkin's disease. In: Lacher MJ, Redman JR, eds. Hodgkin's disease: the consequences of survival. Philadelphia, Lea & Febiger, 1990:151.
45. Sitar G, Brusamolino E, Bernasconi C, Ascari J. Isolation of Reed-Sternberg cells from Hodgkin's disease lymph nodes. Blood 1989;73:222.
46. Hardy WD Jr. Epidemiology of primary neoplasms of lymphoid tissues in animals. In: Twomey JJ, Good RA, eds. Comprehensive immunology 4. The immunopathology of lymphoreticular neoplasms. New York, Plenum Press, 1978:129.
47. Magrath I. The pathogenesis of Burkitt's lymphoma. Adv Cancer Res 1990;55:133.
48. Miller G. Epstein-Barr virus: biology, pathogenesis and medical aspects. In: Fields BN, Knipe DM, et al, eds. Virology. ed 3. 1990:1921.
49. Cann AJ, Chen ISY. Human T-cell leukemia virus. In: Fields BN, Knipe DM, et al, eds. Virology, ed 3, 1990;1501.
50. Daefler S, Wong-Staal F. Molecular biology of human retroviruses and their relation to cancer. In: Broder S, ed. Molecular foundations of oncology. Baltimore, Williams & Wilkins, 1991:229.
51. Yunis JJ. The chromosomal basis of human neoplasia. Science 1983;221:227.
52. Rowley J. Cytogenetics: past present and future. In: Broder S, ed. Molecular foundations of oncology. Baltimore, Williams & Wilkins, 1991:3.
53. Reviews on oncogenic processes. Cell 1991;64:235.
54. Nichols J, Nimer SD. Transcription factors, translocations, and leukemia. Blood 1992;80:2953.
55. Taub R, Kirsch L, Morton C, et al. Translocation of the *c-myc* gene into the immunoglobulin heavy chain locus in human Burkitt's lymphoma and mouse plasmacytoma cells. Proc Natl Acad Sci USA 1982;79:7837.
56. Diehl V, vonKalle C, Fonatsch C, et al. The cell of origin of Hodgkin's disease. Semin Oncol 1990;17:660.
57. Drexler HG, Jones DB, Diehl V, et al. Is the Hodgkin's disease cell a T- or a B-lymphocyte? Recent evidence from geno- and immunophenotypic analysis and in vitro cell lines. Hematol Oncol 1989;7:95.
58. Rowley JD. Chromosomes in Hodgkin's disease. Cancer Treat Rep 1982;66:639.
59. Lawler SD, Swansbury GJ. Cytogenetic studies in Hodgkin's disease. In: Selby P, McElwain TJ, eds. Hodgkin's disease. Oxford, UK, Blackwell Scientific Publications, 1987:43.
60. Cabanillas F, Pathak S, Trujillo J, et al. Cytogenetic features of Hodgkin's disease suggest possible origin from a lymphocyte. Blood 1988;71:1615.
61. Schouten HC, Sanger WG, Duggan M. Chromosome abnormalities in Hodgkin's disease. Blood 1989;73:2149.
62. Thangavelu M, LeBeau MM. Chromosome abnormalities in Hodgkin's disease. Hematol Oncol Clin North Am 1989;3:221.
63. Foon KA, Todd RF III. Immunologic classification of leukemia and lymphoma. Blood 1986;68:1.
64. Kadin ME, Stites DP, Levy R, Warnke R. Exogenous immunoglobulin and the macrophage origin of Reed-Sternberg cells in Hodgkin's disease. N Engl J Med 1979;299:1208.
65. Picker LJ, Weiss LM, Medeiros LJ, et al. Immunophenotypic criteria for the diagnosis of non-Hodgkin's lymphoma. Am J Pathol 1987;128:181.
66. Jones DB. The histogenesis of the Reed-Sternberg cell and its mononuclear counterparts. J Pathol 1987;151:191.
67. Lee FD. Hodgkin's disease. Histopathology 1987;11:1211.
68. Hsu SM, Young K, Jaffe ES. Phenotypic expression of Hodgkin's and Reed-Sternberg cells in Hodgkin's disease. Am J Pathol 1985;118:209.
69. Stein H, Mason DY, Gerdes J, et al. The expression of the Hodgkin's disease associated antigen Ki-1 in reactive and neoplastic lymphoid tissue. Blood 1985;66:848.
70. Anastasi J, Bitter MA, Vardiman JW. The histopathological subclassification of Hodgkin's disease. Hematol Oncol Clin North Am 1989;3:187.
71. Banks PM. The pathology of Hodgkin's disease. Semin Oncol 1990;17:683.
72. Griesser H, Tkachuk D, Reis MD, Mak TW. Gene rearrangement in lymphoproliferative disease. Blood 1989;73:1402.
73. Reis MD, Griesser H, Mak TW. T cell receptor and immunoglobulin gene rearrangements in lymphoproliferative disease. Adv Cancer Res 1989;52:45.
74. Sundeen J, Lipford E, Uppenkamp M, et al. Rearranged antigen receptor genes in Hodgkin's disease. Blood 1987;70:96.
75. Brinker MGL, Poppema S, Buys CHCM, et al. Clonal immunoglobulin gene rearrangements in tissues involved by Hodgkin's disease. Blood 1987;70:186.
76. Mueller N, Evan A, Harris NL, et al. Hodgkin's disease and Epstein-Barr virus: altered antibody pattern before diagnosis. N Engl J Med 1989;320:689.
77. Weiss LM, Movahed LA, Warnke RA, Sklar J. Detection of Epstein-Barr viral genome in Reed-Sternberg cells of Hodgkin's disease. N Engl J Med 1989;320:502.
78. Agagnostopoulos I, Herbst H, Niedobitek G, Stein H. Demonstration of monoclonal EBV genome in Hodgkin's disease and Ki-1 positive anaplastic large cell lymphoma by combined Southern blot and in situ hybridization. Blood 1989;74:810.
79. Herbst H, Niedobitek G, Kneba M, et al. High incidence of Epstein-Barr virus genomes in Hodgkin's diseaser. Am J Pathol 1990;137:13.
80. Pallesen G, Hamilton-Dutoit SJ, Rowe M, Young LS. Expression of Epstein-Barr latent gene product in tumor cells of Hodgkin's disease. Lancet 1991;337:320.
81. Herbst H, Dallenbach F, Hummel M, et al. Epstein-Barr virus latent membrane protein expression in Hodgkin's disease Reed-Sternberg cells. Proc Natl Acad Sci USA 1991;88:4766.
82. Ziegler JL, Beckstead JA, Volberding PA, et al. Non-Hodgkin's lymphoma in 90 homosexual men. N Engl J Med 1984;311:565.
83. Filipovich AH, Heinitz KJ, Robison LL, Frizzera G. The Immunodeficiency Cancer Registry. Am J Pediatr Hematol Oncol 1987;9:183.
84. Spector BD, Perry GS III, Good RA, Kersey JH. Immunodeficiency diseases and malignancy. In: Twomey JJ, Good RA, eds. Comprehensive immunology 4. The immunopathology of lymphoreticular neoplasms. New York, Plenum Press, 1978:203.
85. Harrington DS, Weissenburger DD, Purtilo DT. Malignant lymphoma in the X-linked lymphoproliferative syndrome. Cancer 1987;59:1419.
86. Penn I. The occurrence of malignant tumors in immunosuppressed states. Progr Allergy 1986;37:259.
87. List AF, Greco FA, Vogler LB. Lymphoproliferative diseases in immunocompromized hosts: the role of the Epstein-Barr virus. J Clin Oncol 1987;5:1673.
88. Schoeppel SJ, Hoppe RT, Dorfman RF, et al. Hodgkin's disease in homosexual men with generalized lymphadenopathy. Ann Intern Med 1985;102:68.
89. Tirelli U, Vaccher E, Rezza G, et al. Hodgkin's disease and infection with the human immunodeficiency virus (HIV) in Italy. Ann Intern Med 1988;108:309.
90. Hsu S, Krupen K, Lachman LB. Heterogeneity of interleukin-1 production in cultured Reed-Sternberg cell lines HDLM-1, HDLM-1d and KM-H2. Am J Pathol 1989;135:33.
91. Pui Ching-Hon, Ip S, Thompson E, et al. High serum interleukin-2 levels correlate with a poor prognosis in children with Hodgkin's disease. Leukemia 1989;3:481.
92. Samoszuk M, Nansen L. Detection of interleukin-5 messenger RNA in Reed-Sternberg cells of Hodgkin's disease with eosinophilia. Blood 1990;75:13.
93. Newcom S, Kadin M, Ansari A, et al. L428 nodular sclerosing Hodgkin's cell secretes a unique transforming growth factor beta active at physiologic pH. J Clin Invest 1988;82:1915.
94. Esphar Z, Order SE, Katz DH. Ferritin, a Hodgkin's disease associated antigen. Proc Natl Acad Sci USA 1974;71:39.
95. Vriesendorp HM, Herpst JM, Germack MA, et al. Phase I-II study of yttrium-labelled antiferritin treatment for end-stage Hodgkin's disease, including Radiation Therapy Oncology Group 87. J Clin Oncol 1991;9:918.
96. Brown CA, Hall CL, Long JC, et al. Circulating immune complexes in Hodgkin's disease. Am J Med 1978;64:289.
97. Stetler-Stevenson M, Crush-Stanton S, Cossman J. Involvement of the *bcl2* gene in Hodgkin's disease. J Natl Cancer Inst 1990;82:855.
98. Lukes RJ. Criteria for involvement of lymph node, bone marrow, spleen and liver in Hodgkin's disease. Cancer Res 1971;31:1755.
99. Lukes RJ, Butler JJ. The pathology and nomenclature of Hodgkin's disease. Cancer Res 1966;26:1063.
100. Symmers WStC. Hodgkin's disease. In: Symmers WStC, ed. Systemic pathology, ed 2, vol 2. Edinburgh, Churchill Livingstone, 1978;784.
101. Keller AR, Kaplan HS, Lukes RJ, Rappaport H. Correlation of histopathology with other prognostic factors in Hodgkin's disease. Cancer 1968;22:487.
102. Butler JJ. Relationship of histological findings to survival in Hodgkin's disease. Cancer Res 1971;31:1770.
103. Berard CW, Thomas LB, Axtell LM, et al. The relationship of histopathological subtype to clinical stage of Hodgkin's disease at diagnosis. Cancer Res 1971;31:1776.
104. Wright DH. Pathology of Hodgkin's disease: anything new? Recent Results Cancer Res 1989;117:5.
105. Hansmann M-L, Fellbaum C, Hui PK, Moubayed P. Progressive transformation of germinal centers with and without association to Hodgkin's disease. Am J Clin Pathol 1990;93:219.
106. Chittal SM, Alard C, Rossi J-F, et al. Further phenotyypic evidence that nodular, lymphocyte-predominant Hodgkin's disease is a large B-cell lymphoma in evolution. Am J Surg Pathol 1990;14:1024.
107. Regula DP, Hoppe RT, Weiss LM. Nodular and diffuse types of lymphocyte predominance Hodgkin's disease. N Engl J Med 1988;318:214.
108. Boug-Grech A, Radford JA, Crowther D, et al. A comparative study of the nodular and diffuse variants of lymphocyte predominant Hodgkin's disease. J Clin Oncol 1989;7:1303.
109. Tefferi A, Zellers RA, Banks PM, et al. Clinical correlates of distinct immunophenotypic and histologic subcategories of lymphocyte-predominance Hodgkin's disease. J Clin Oncol 1990;8:1959.

110. MacLennan KA, Bennett MH, Tu A, et al. Relationship of histopathologic features to survival and relapse in nodular sclerosing Hodgkin's disease: a study of 1659 patients. Cancer 1989;64:1686.
111. Kadin ME, Donaldson SS, Dorfman RF. Isolated granulomas in Hodgkin's disease. N Engl J Med 1970;283:859.
112. Rouvière H. Anatomy of the human lymphatic system. Ann Arbor, Edwards Brothers, 1938.
113. Musshoff K, Boutis L. Therapy results in Hodgkin's disease, Freiburg i Br, 1948–1966. Cancer 1968;21:1100.
114. Kaplan HS, Dorfman RF, Nelson TS, Rosenberg SA. Staging laparotomy and splenectomy in Hodgkin's disease: analysis of indications and patterns of involvement in 285 consecutive, unselected patients. Natl Cancer Inst Monogr 1973;36:291.
115. Kennedy BJ, Loeb V, Peterson VM, et al. National survey patterns of care in Hodgkin's disease. Cancer 1985;56:2547.
116. Selby P. McElwain TJ. Clinical features of Hodgkin's disease. In: Selby P, McElwain TJ, eds. Hodgkin's disease. Oxford, UK, Blackwell Scientific Publications, 1987:94.
117. Diehl LF, Hopper KD, Giguere J, et al. The pattern of intrathoracic Hodgkin's disease assessed by computed tomography. J Clin Oncol 1991;9:438.
118. Filly R, Blank N, Castellino RA. Radiographic distribution of intrathoracic disease in previously untreated patients with Hodgkin's disease and non-Hodgkin's lymphoma. Radiology 1976;120:277.
119. Bagley CM Jr, Roth JA, Thomas LB, DeVita VT Jr. Liver biopsy in Hodgkin's disease. Ann Intern Med 1972;76:219.
120. Bouroncle BA, Old JW Jr, Vazques AG. Pathogenesis of jaundice in Hodgkin's disease. Arch Intern Med 1962;110:872.
121. Perera DR, Greene ML, Fenster F. Cholestasis associated with extrabiliary Hodgkin's disease. Gastroenterology 1974;67:680.
122. Myers CE, Chabner BA, DeVita VT, Gralnick HR. Bone marrow involvement in Hodgkin's disease. Blood 1974;44:197.
123. Rosenberg SA. Hodgkin's disease in the bone marrow. Cancer Res 1971;31:1733.
124. Friedman M, Kim TH, Panahon AM. Spinal cord compression in malignant lymphoma. Cancer 1976;37:1485.
125. Haddad P, Thaell JF, Kiely JM, et al. Lymphoma of the extradural space. Cancer 1976;38:1862.
126. Gilbert RW, Kim J-H, Posner JB. Epidural spinal cord compression from metastatic tumor: diagnosis and treatment. Ann Neurol 1978;3:40.
127. Posner JB. Back pain and epidural spinal cord compression. Med Clin North Am 1987;71:185.
128. Sapozink MD, Kaplan HS. Intracranial Hodgkin's disease. Cancer 1983;52:1301.
129. Posner JB. Secondary neoplastic diseases. In: Ashbury Ak, McKhann GM, McDonald WI, eds. Diseases of the nervous system. Philadelphia, WB Saunders, 1987.
130. Richmond J, Sherman RS, Diamond HD, Craver LF. Renal lesions associated with malignant lymphomas. Am J Med 1962;32:184.
131. Plager J, Stutzman L. Acute nephrotic syndrome as a manifestation of active Hodgkin's disease. Am J Med 1971;50:56.
132. Jandl JH. Blood: textbook of hematology. Boston, Little, Brown, 1987:853.
133. Levine AM, Thornton P, Forman SJ, et al. Positive Coombs test in Hodgkin's disease: significance and implications. Blood 1980;55:607.
134. Kempin S. Late hematologic complications of Hodgkin's disease. In: Lacher MJ, Redman JR, eds. Hodgkin's disease: the consequences of survival. Philadelphia, Lea & Febiger, 1990;63.
135. Waddell CC, Cimo PL. Idiopathic thrombocytopenic purpura occurring in Hodgkin's disease after splenectomy. Am J Hematol 1979;7:381.
136. Tubiana M, Henry-Amar M, Hayat M, et al. Prognostic significance of erythrocyte sedimentaion rate in clinical stages I-II of Hodgkin's disease. J Clin Oncol 1984;2:194.
137. Hrgovic MJ, Tessmer CF, Mumford DM, et al. Interpreting serum copper levels in Hodgkin's disease. Texas Med 1975;71:53.
138. Carbone PP, Kaplan HS, Musshoff K, et al. Report of the Committee on Hodgkin's Disease Staging Classification. Cancer Res 1971;31:1860.
139. Lister TA, Crowther D. Staging for Hodgkin's disease. Semin Oncol 1990;17:696.
140. Radford JA, Cowan RA, Flanagan M, et al. The significance of residual mediastinal abnormality on the chest radiograph following treatment for Hodgkin's disease. J Clin Oncol 1988;6:940.
141. Rosenberg SA, Boiron M, DeVita VT Jr, et al. Report of the Committee on Hodgkin's Disease Staging Procedures. Cancer Res 1971;31:1862.
142. Dorfman RE. Relationship of histology to site in Hodgkin's disease. Cancer Res 1971;31:1786.
143. Castellino RA, Hoppe RT, Blank N, et al. Computed tomography, lymphography, and staging laparotomy: correlations in initial staging of Hodgkin's disease. AJR 1984;143:37.
144. Marglin S, Castellino R. Lymphographic accuracy in 632 consecutive, previously untreated cases of Hodgkin's disease and non-Hodgkin's lymphoma. Radiology 1981;140:351.
145. Davidson JW. Malignant lymphoma. In: Fuchs WA, Davidson JW, Fischer HV. Lymphography in cancer, vol 23. Recent results in cancer research. New York, Springer-Verlag, 1969:176.
146. Blackledge G, Best JJK, Crowther D, Isherwood I. Computed tomography (CT) in the staging of patients with Hodgkin's disease: a report of 136 patients. Clin Radiol 1980;31:143.
147. Lee JKT, Balfe DM. Computed tomography evaluation of lymphoma patients. CRC Crit Rev Diagn Imaging 1982;18:1.
148. Glatstein E, Guernsey JM, Rosenberg SA, Kaplan HS. The value of laparotomy and splenectomy in the staging of Hodgkin's disease. Cancer 1969;24:709.
149. Bergsagel DE, Alison RE, Bean HA, et al. Results of treating Hodgkin's disease without a policy of laparotomy staging. Cancer Treat Rep 1982;66:717.
150. Kinsella TJ, Glatstein E. Staging laparotomy and splenectomy for Hodgkin's disease: current status. Cancer Invest 1983;1:87.
151. Scott JS, Dawson AA, et al. The place of staging laparotomy in the management of Hodgkin's disease. Clin Radiol 1984;35:261.
152. Rosenberg SA, Kaplan HS. The evolution and summary of the Stanford clinical trials of the management of Hodgkin's disease: 1962–1984. Int J Radiat Oncol Biol Phys 1985;11:5.
153. Rosenberg SA. Exploratory laparotomy and splenectomy for Hodgkin's disease: a commentary. J Clin Oncol 1988;6:574.
154. Mauch P, Larsen D, Osteen R, et al. Prognostic factors for positive surgical staging in patients with Hodgkin's disease. J Clin Oncol 1990;8:257.
155. Worthy TS. Evaluation of diagnostic laparotomy and splenectomy in Hodgkin's disease. Clin Radiol 1981;32:523.
156. Leibenhaut MH, Hoppe RT, Efron B, et al. Prognostic indicators of laparotomy findings in clinical stage I-II supradiaphragmatic Hodgkin's disease. J Clin Oncol 1989;7:81.
157. Timothy AR, Van Dyk J, Sutcliffe SB. Radiation therapy for Hodgkin's disease. In: Selby P, McElwain TJ, eds. Hodgkin's disease. Oxford, UK, Blackwell Scientific Publications, 1987:181.
158. Anderson KC, Leonard RCF, Canellos GP, et al. High-dose gallium imaging in lymphoma. Am J Med 1983;75:327.
159. Hanks RE, Kinzie JJ, Herring DF, Kramer S. Patterns of care outcome studies in Hodgkin's disease: results of the national practice and implications for management. Cancer Treat Rep 1982;66:805.
160. Hoppe RT. Radiation therapy management of Hodgkin's disease. Semin Oncol 1990;17:704.
161. Tubiana M, Henry-Amar M, Hayat M, et al. The EORTC treatment of early stages of Hodgkin's disease: the role of radiotherapy. Int J Radiat Oncol Biol Phys 1984;10:197.
162. Sutcliffe SB, Gospodarowicz MK, Bergsagel DE, et al. Prognostic groups for management of localized Hodgkin's disease. J Clin Oncol 1985;3:393.
163. Wiernik PH, Gustafson J, Schimpff SC, Diggs C. Combined modality treatment of Hodgkin's disease confined to lymph nodes. Am J Med 1979;67:183.
164. Hagermeister FB, Fuller LM, Velasquez WS, et al. Stage I and II Hodgkin's disease: involved-field radiotherapy versus extended-field radiotherapy versus involved-field radiotherapy followed by six cycles of MOPP. Cancer Treat Rep 1982;66:789.
165. Hoppe RT, Coleman NC, Cox RS, et al. The management of stage I-II Hodgkin's disease with irradiation alone or combined modality therapy: the Stanford experience. Blood 1982;59:455.
166. Mauch P, Lewin A, Hellman S. The role of radiation therapy in the treatment of stage I and II Hodgkin's disease. In: Rosenberg SA, Kaplan HS, eds. Malignant lymphomas: etiology, immunology, pathology, treatment. New York, Academic Press, 1982:453.
167. Nissen NI, Nordentoft AM. Radiotherapy versus combined modality treatment of stage I and II Hodgkin's diease. Cancer Treat Rep 1982;66:799.
168. Crnkovich MJ, Hoppe RT, Rosenberg SA. Stage IIB Hodgkin's disease: the Stanford experience. J Clin Oncol 1986;4:472.
169. Gobbi PG, Cavalli C, Gendarini A, et al. Reevaluation of prognostic significance of symptoms in Hodgkin's disease. Cancer 1985;56:2874.
170. Crnkovich MJ, Leopold K, Hoppe RT, Mauch PM. Stage I and IIB Hodgkin's disease: the combined experience at Stanford University and the Joint Center for Radiation Therapy. J Clin Oncol 1987;5:1041.
171. Mauch P, Garshein P, Cunningham J, Hellman S. Influence of mediastinal adenopathy on site and frequency of relapse in patients with Hodgkin's disease. Cancer Treat Rep 1982;66:809.
172. Liew KH, Easton D, Horwich A, et al. Bulky mediastinal Hodgkin's disease: management and prognosis. Hematol Oncol 1984;2:45.
173. Specht L, Nordentoft AM, Cold S, et al. Tumor burden as the most important prognostic factor in early stage Hodgkin's disease: relation to other prognostic factors and implications for choice of treatment. Cancer 1988;61:1719.
174. Lister TA, Crowther D, Sutcliffe SB, et al. Report of a committee convened to discuss the staging of patients with Hodgkin's disease: Cotswold Meeting. J Clin Oncol 1989;7:1630.
175. Tubiana M, Henry-Amar M, Hayat M, et al. Prognostic significance of the number of involved areas in the early stages of Hodgkin's disease. Cancer 1984;54:885.
176. Tubiana M, Henry-Amar M, van der Werf-Messing B, et al. A multivariate analysis of prognostic factors in early stage Hodgkin's disease. Int J Radiat Biol Phys 1985;11:23.
177. Stein RS, Golomb HM, Diggs CH, et al. Anatomic substages of stage IIIA Hodgkin's disease: a collaborative study. Ann Intern Med 1980;92:159.

178. Stein RS, Golomb HM, Wiernik PH, et al. Anatomic substages of stage IIIA Hodgkin's disease: followup of a collaborative study. Cancer Treat Rep 1982;66:733.
179. Hoppe RT, Cox RS, Rosenberg SA, Kaplan HS. Prognostic factors in pathologic stage III Hodgkin's disease. Cancer Treat Rep 1982;66:743.
180. Henry-Amar M, Friedman S, Hayat M, et al. Erythrocyte sedimentation rate predicts early relapse and survival in early-stage Hodgkin's disease. Ann Intern Med 1991;114:361.
181. Willett CG, Linggood RM, Leong JC, et al. Stage IA to IIB mediastinal Hodgkin's disease: three-dimensional volumetric assessment of response to treatment. J Clin Oncol 1988;6:819.
182. Goodman LS, Wintrobe MM, Dameshek W, et al. Nitrogen mustard therapy. Use of methyl-bis-(beta-chloroethyl) amine hydrochloride and tris-(beta-chloroethyl) amine hydrochloride for Hodgkin's disease, lymphosracoma, leukemia and certain allied and miscellaneous disorders. JAMA 1946;132:126.
183. Lacher MJ, Durant JR. Combined vinblastine and chlorambucil therapy of Hodgkin's disease. Ann Intern Med 1965;62:468.
184. Carter SK, Livingstone RB. Single-agent chemotherapy for Hodgkin's disease. Arch Intern Med 1973;131:377.
185. Desser RK, Ultmann JE. The sensitivity of Hodgkin's disease to single agents administered singly. Semin Haematol 1973;6:152.
186. Coltman CA Jr. Chemotherapy of advanced Hodgkin's disease. Semin Oncol 1980;7:155.
187. Selby P, McElwain TJ, Canellos G. Chemotherapy of Hodgkin's disease. In: Selby P, McElwain TJ, eds. Hodgkin's disease. Oxford, UK, Blackwell Scientific Publications, 1987:269.
188. Huguley CM, Durant JR, Moores RR, et al. A comparison of nitrogen mustard, vincristine, procarbazine and prednisone (MOPP) vs. nitrogen mustard in advanced Hodgkin's disease. Cancer 1975;36:1227.
189. Lessner HE. BCNU 1,3-bis(2-chloroethyl)-1-nitrosourea: effects on advanced Hodgkin's disease and other neoplasia. Cancer 1968;22:451.
190. Young RC, DeVita VT Jr, Serpick AA Jr, Canellos GP. Treatment of advanced Hodgkin's disease with (1,3-bis(2-chloroethyl)-1-nitrosourea) BCNU. N Engl J Med 1971;285:475.
191. Hoogstratten B, Gottlieb JA, Caoili E, et al. CCNU (1-(2-chloroethyl)-3-cyclohexyl-1-nitrosourea) in the treatment of cancer: phase II study. Cancer 1973;32:38.
192. Stolinsky DC, Solomon J, Weiner JM, Bateman JR. Results of CCNU in resistant Hodgkin's and non-Hodgkin's lymphoma. Oncology 1975;33:271.
193. Gottlieb JA, Gutterman JV, McCreedie KB, et al. Chemotherapy of malignant lymphoma with Adriamycin. Cancer Res 1973;33:3224.
194. Blum RH, Carter SK. Adriamycin: a new anticancer drug with significant clinical activity. Ann Intern Med 1974;80:249.
195. Blum RH, Carter SK, Agre K. A clinical review of bleomycin: a new antineoplastic agent. Cancer 1972;31:903.
196. Yagoda A, Mukherji B, Young C, et al. Bleomycin: an antitumor antibiotic. Ann Intern Med 1972;77:861.
197. Hass CD, Coltman CA Jr, Gottlieb JA, et al. Phase II evaluation of bleomycin. Cancer 1976;38:8.
198. Frei E III, Luce JK, Talley RW, et al. 5-(3,3-dimethyl-1-triazeno)imadazole-4-carbozamide in the treatment of lymphoma. Cancer Chemother Rep 1972;56:667.
199. Taylor RE, McElwain TJ, Barrett A, Peckham MJ. Etoposide as a single agent in relapsed advanced lymphoma. Cancer Chemother Pharmocol 1982;7:175.
200. Issell BF, Rudolph AR, Louie AC. In: Issell BF, Muggia FM, Carter SK, eds. Etoposide: current status and new developments. New York, Academic Press, 1984:1.
201. DeVita VT Jr, Simon RM, Hubbard SM, et al. Curability of advanced Hodgkin's disease with chemotherapy. Ann Intern Med 1980;92:587.
202. Sutcliffe SB, Wrigley PRM, Peto J, et al. MVPP chemotherapy in advanced Hodgkin's disease. Br J Med 1978;1:679.
203. Dady PJ, McElwain TJ, Austin DE, et al. Five years experience with ChlVPP: effective low-toxicity combination chemotherapy for Hodgkin's disease. Br J Cancer 1982;45:851.
204. Durant JR, Gams RA, Velez-Garcia E, et al. BCNU, velban, cyclophosphamide, procarbazine and prednisone (BCVPP) in advanced Hodgkin's disease. Cancer 1978;42:2102.
205. Santoro A, Bonfante V, Bonnadonna G. Salvage chemotherapy with ABVD in MOPP-resistant Hodgkin's disease. Ann Intern Med 1982;96:139.
206. Harker EG, Kushlan P, Rosenberg SA. Combination chemotherapy for advanced Hodgkin's disease after failure of MOPP: ABVD and B-CAVe. Ann Intern Med 1984;101:440.
207. Connors JM, Klimo P. MOPP/ABV hybrid chemotherapy for advanced Hodgkin's disease. Semin Hematol 1987;24(Suppl 1):35.
208. Longo DL, Young RC, Wesley M, et al. Twenty years of MOPP therapy for Hodgkin's disease. J Clin Oncol 1986;4:1295.
209. Santoro A, Bonnadonna G, Valagussa P, et al. Long-term results of combined chemotherapy-radiotherapy in Hodgkin's disease: superiority of ABVD plus radiotherapy versus MOPP plus radiotherapy. J Clin Oncol 1987;5:27.
210. Bonnadonna G, Santoro A, Valagussa P, et al. Current status of the Milan trials of Hodgkin's disease in adults. In: Cavelli F, Bonnadonna G, Rozencweig M, eds. Malignant lymphoma and Hodgkin's disease: experimental and therapeutic advances. The Hague, Martinus Nijhoff, 1985:299.
211. Cooper RM, Pajak TF, Nissen NI, et al. A new effective four-drug combination of CCNU, vinblastine, prednisone and procarbazine for the treatment of advanced Hodgkin's disease. Cancer 1980;46:654.
212. Bakemeier RF, Anderson JR, Costello W, et al. BCVPP chemotherapy for advanced Hodgkin's disease: evidence for greater duration of complete remission, greater survival and less toxicity than the MOPP regimen. Ann Intern Med 1984;101:447.
213. Bonnadonna G, Valagussa P, Santoro A. Alternating non-cross-resistant combination chemotherapy or MOPP in stage IV Hodgkin's disease. Ann Intern Med 1986;104:739.
214. Bonnadonna G. Chemotherapy strategies to improve the control of Hodgkin's disease: the Richard and Hilda Rosenthal Foundation Award Lecture. Cancer Res 1982;42:4309.
215. Goldie JH, Coldman AJ. A mathematical model for relating the drug sensitivity of tumors to their spontaneous mutation rate. Cancer Treat Rep 1979;63:1727.
216. Carde P, MacKintosh FR, Rosenberg SA. A dose time response analysis of the treatment of Hodgkin's disease with MOPP chemotherapy. J Clin Oncol 1983;1:146.
217. van Rijwijk REN, Haanen C, Dekker AW, deMeijer AJ, Verbeek J. Dose intensity of MOPP chemotherapy and survival in Hodgkin's disease. J Clin Oncol 1989;7:1776.
218. Longo DL. Chemotherapy for advanced aggresive lymphoma: more is better . . . or is it? J Clin Oncol 1990;8:952.
219. van Rijswijk REN, Haanen C, Dekker AW, et al. Dose intensity of MOPP chemotherapy and survival in Hodgkin's disease. J Clin Oncol 1989;7:1776.
220. Horwich A, Peckham MJ. Combined chemotherapy and radiotherapy in the management of adult Hodgkin's disease: indication and results. In: Selby P, McElwain TJ, eds. Hodgkin's disease. Oxford, UK, Blackwell Scientific Publications, 1987:250.
221. Anderson H, Deakin DP, Wagstaff J, et al. A randomized study of adjuvant chemotherapy after mantle radiotherapy in supradiaphragmatic Hodgkin's disease PS IA-IIB: a report from the Manchester lymphoma group. Br J Cancer 1984;49:695.
222. Coltman CA, Myers JW, Montague E, et al. The role of combined radiotherapy and chemotherapy in the primary management of Hodgkin's disease: Southwest Oncology Group studies. In: Rosenberg SA, Kaplan HS, eds. Malignant lymphomas. New York, Academic Press, 1982:523.
223. Haybrittle JL, Easterling MJ, Bennett MH, et al. Review of the British National Lymphoma Investigation studies of Hodgkin's disease and development of prognostic index. Lancet 1985;1:967.
224. Brada M, Easton DF, Horwich A, Peckham MJ. Clinical presentation as a predictor of laparotomy findings in supradiaphragmatic stage I and II Hodgkin's disease. Radiother Oncol 1986;5:15.
225. Tubiana M, Henry-Amar M, Carde P, et al. Toward comprehensive management tailored to prognostic factors of patients with clinical stages I and II in Hodgkin's disease: the EORTC Lymphoma Group controlled clinical trials: 1964–1987. Blood 1989;73:47.
226. Stein RS, Golomb HM, Diggs CH, et al. Anatomic substrates of stage IIIA Hodgkin's disease. Ann Intern Med 1980;92:159.
227. Mauch P, Goffman T, Rosenthal DS, et al. Stage III Hodgkin's disease: improved survival with combined modality therapy as compared with radiation therapy alone. J Clin Oncol 1985;3:1166.
228. Hoppe RT, Rosenberg SA, Kaplan HS, Cox RS. Prognostic factors in pathological stage IIIA Hodgkin's disease. Cancer 1980;46:1240.
229. Crowther D, Wagstaff J, Deakin D, et al. A randomized study comparing chemotherapy alone with chemotherapy followed by radiotherapy in patients with pathologically staged IIIA Hodgkin's disease. J Clin Oncol 1984;2:892.
230. Lister TA, Doreen MS, Faux M, et al. The treatment of stage IIIA Hodgkin's disease. J Clin Oncol 1983;1:745.
231. Prosnitz LR, Farber LR, Kapp DS, et al. Combined modality therapy for advanced Hodgkin's disease: 15 year follow-up data. J Clin Oncol 1988;6:603.
232. Straus DJ, Gaynor JJ, Myers J, et al. Prognostic factors among 185 adults with newly diagnosed Hodgkin's disease treated with alternating potentially non cross-resistant chemotherapy and intermediate-dose radiation therapy. J Clin Oncol 1990;8:1173.
233. Longo DL, Russo A, Duffey PL, et al. Treatment of advanced-stage massive mediastinal Hodgkin's disease: the case for combined modality treatment. J Clin Oncol 1991;9:227.
234. Canellos GP, DeVita VT, Arseneau JC, et al. Second malignancies complicating Hodgkin's disease in remission. Lancet 1975;1:947.
235. Coltman CA Jr, Dixon DO. Second malignancies complicating Hodgkin's disease: a Southwest Oncology Group 10-year followup. Cancer Treat Rep 1982;66:1023.
236. Glicksman AS, Pajak TF, Gottlieb A, et al. Second malignant neoplasms in patients successfully treated for Hodgkin's disease: a Cancer and Leukemia Group B study. Cancer Treat Rep 1982;66:1035.
237. Tetser WJ, Kinsella TJ, Waller B, et al. Second malignant neoplasms complicating Hodgkin's disease: the National Cancer Institute experience. J Clin Oncol 1984;2:762.
238. Valagussa P, Santoro A, Fossati-Bellani F, et al. Second acute leukemia

and other malignancies following treatment for Hodgkin's disease. J Clin Oncol 1986;4:830.
239. Tucker MA, Coleman CN, Cox RS, et al. Risk of second cancers after treatment for Hodgkin's disease. N Engl J Med 1988;318:76.
240. Boivin J-F, O'Brien K. Solid cancer risk after treatment of Hodgkin's disease. Cancer 1988;61:2541.
241. Lacher MJ, Redman JR. Hodgkin's disease: the consequences of survival. Philadelphia, Lea & Fegiger, 1990:447.
242. Pedersen-Bjergaard J, Larsen SO. Incidence of acute nonlymphocytic leukemia, preleukemia, and acute myeloproliferative syndrome up to 10 years after treatment of Hodgkin's disease. N Engl J Med 1982;307: 965.
243. Pederson-Bjergaard J, Erbsoll J, Sorensen HM, et al. Risk of acute nonlymphocytic leukemia and preleukemia in patients treated with cyclophosphamide for non-Hodgkin's lymphoma. Ann Intern Med 1985;103:195.
244. Coleman CN. Secondary malignancy after treatment of Hodgkin's disease: an evolving picture. J Clin Oncol 1986;4:821.
245. Pedersen-Bjergaard J, Larsen SO, Struck J, et al. Risk of therapy-related leukemia and preleukemia after Hodgkin's disease. Lancet 1987;2: 83.
246. Boivin J-F, Hutchison GB, Lyden M, et al. Second primary cancers following treatment of Hodgkin's disease. J Natl Cancer Inst 1984;72: 233.
247. Kantarjian HM, Keating MJ. Therapy-related leukemia and myelodysplastic syndrome. Semin Oncol 1987;14:435.
248. Blayney DW, Longo DL, Young RC, et al. Decreasing risk of leukemia with prolonged follow-up after chemotherapy and radiotherapy for Hodgkin's disease. N Engl J Med 1987;316:710.
249. Greene MH, Harris EL, Gershenson DM, et al. Melphalan may be a more potent leukemogen than cyclophosphamide. Ann Intern Med 1986;105:360.
250. Kaldor JM, Day NE, Clarke EA, et al. Leukemia following Hodgkin's disease. N Engl J Med 1990;322:7.
250a. Yahalom J, Petrak JA, Biddinger PW, et al. Breast cancer in patients irradiated for Hodgkin's disease: a clinical and pathologic analysis of events in 37 patients. J Clin Oncol 1992;10:1674.
250b. Hancock SL, Tucker MA, Hoppe RT. Breast cancer after Hodgkin's disease treatment. J Natl Cancer Inst 1993;85:25.
251. Glicksman AS, Pajak TS. Early and late effects of lymphoma treatment in the expectation of cure. In: Rosenberg SA, Kaplan HS, eds. Malignant lymphomas. New York, Academic Press, 1982:639.
252. Gerling B, Gottdiener J, Borer JS. Cardiovascular complications of the treatment of Hodgkin's disease. In: Lacher MJ, Redman JR, eds. Hodgkin's disease: the consequences of survival. Philadelphia, Lea & Febiger, 1990:267.
253. Chapman RM. Effect of cytotoxic therapy on sexuality and gonadal function. Semin Oncol 1982;9:84.
254. Sutcliffe SB. Infertility and gonadal function in Hodgkin's disease. In: Selby P, McElwain TJ, eds. Hodgkin's disease. Oxford, UK, Blackwell Scientific Publications, 1987:339.
255. Sherins RJ, DeVita VT Jr. Effect of drug treatment for lymphoma on male reproductive capacity. Ann Intern Med 1973;79:216.
256. Chapman RM, Sutcliffe SB, Rees LH, et al. Cyclical combination chemotherapy and gonadal function: retrospective study in males. Lancet 1979;1:285.
257. Chapman RM, Sutcliffe SB, Malpas JS. Male gonadal function in Hodgkin's disease: a prospective study. JAMA 1981;245:1323.
258. Viviani S, Santoro A, Ragni G, et al. Gonadal toxicity after combination chemotherapy for Hodgkin's disease. Eur J Cancer Clin Oncol 1985;21: 601.
259. Chapman RM, Sutcliffe SB, Malpas JS. Cytotoxic-induced ovarian failure in Hodgkin's disease. II. Effects on sexual function. JAMA 1979;242:1882.
260. Schilsky RL, Sherins RJ, Hubbard SM, et al. Long-term follow-up of ovarian function in women treated with MOPP chemotherapy for Hodgkin's disease. Am J Med 1981;71:552.
261. Horning SJ, Hoppe RT, Kaplan HS, Rosenberg SA. Female reproductive potential after treatment for Hodgkin's disease. N Engl J Med 1981;304: 1377.
262. Whitehead E, Shalet SM, Blackledge G, et al. The effect of combination chemotherapy on ovarian function in women treated for Hodgkin's disease. Cancer 1983;52:988.
263. Fuks Z, Glatstein E, Marsa GW, et al. Long term effects of external radiation on the pituitary and thyroid glands. Cancer 1976;37: 1152.
264. Schimpff SC, Diggs CH, Wiswell JG, et al. Radiation-related thyroid dysfunction: implications for the treatment of Hodgkin's disease. Ann Intern Med 1980;92:91.
265. Redman JR, Bajorunas DR. Therapy-related thyroid and parathyroid dysfunction in patients with Hodgkin's disease. In: Lacher MJ, Redman JR, eds. Hodgkin's disease: the consequences of survival. Philadelphia, Lea & Febiger, 1990:222.
266. Sutcliffe SB, Chapman R, Wrigley PFM. Cyclical combination chemotherapy and thyroid function in patients with advanced Hodgkin's disease. Med Pediatr Oncol 1981;9:439.
267. Ihde DC, DeVita VT Jr. Osteonecrosis of the femoral head in patients with lymphoma treated with intermittant combination chemotherapy (including corticosteroids). Cancer 1975;36:1585.
268. Mould JJ, Adam NM. The problem of avascular necrosis of bone in patients treated for Hodgkin's disease. Clin Radiol 1983;34:331.
269. Comis RL. Bleomycin pulmonary toxicity. In: Carter SK, Crooke ST, Umezawa H, eds. Bleomycin: current status and new developments. New York, Academic Press, 1978:279.
270. Ginsberg SJ, Comis RL. The pulmonary toxicity of antineoplastic agents. Semin Oncol 1982;9:34.
271. Samuels ML, Johnson DE, Holoye PY, et al. Large dose bleomycin pulmonary toxicity: a possible role of prior radiotherapy. JAMA 1976;235:1117.
272. Longo DL, Glatstein E, Duffey PL, et al. Radiation therapy versus combination chemotherapy in the treatment of early-stage Hodgkin's disease: seven-year results of a prospecive randomized trial. J Clin Oncol 1991;9:906.
273. Cimino G, Biti GP, Anselmo AP, et al. MOPP chemotherapy versus extended-field radiotherapy in the management of pathological stages I-IIA Hodgkin's disease. J Clin Oncol 1989;7:732.
274. Herman TS, Hoppe RT, Donaldson SS, et al. Late relapses among patients treated for Hodgkin's disease. Ann Intern Med 1985;102:292.
275. Canellos GP, Young RC, DeVita VT. Combination chemotherapy for Hodgkin's disease in relapse following extensive radiotherapy. Clin Pharmacol Ther 1972;13:750.
276. Portlock CS, Rosenberg SA, Glatstein E, et al. Impact of salvage treatment on initial relapses in patients with Hodgkin's disease stages I–III. Blood 1978;51:825.
277. Timothy AR, Sutcliffe SBJ, Wrigley PFM, et al. Hodgkin's disease: combination chemotherapy for relapse following radical radiotherapy. Int J Radiat Oncol Biol Phys 1979;5:165.
278. Cooper MR, Pajak TF, Gottlieb AJ, et al. The effects of prior radiation and age on the frequency and duration of complete remission among various four-drug regimens for advanced Hodgkin's disease. J Clin Oncol 1984;2:748.
279. Santoro A, Viviani S, Viilareal CJR, et al. Salvage chemotherapy in Hodgkin's disease irradiation failures: superiority of doxorubicin-containing regimens over MOPP. Cancer Treat Rep 1986;70:343.
280. Roach M III, Brophy IV, Cox R, Varghese A, Hoppe RT. Prognostic factors for patients relapsing after radiotherapy for early stage Hodgkin's disease. J Clin Oncol 1990;8:623,
281. Hagemeister FB, Tannir N, McLaughlin P, et al. MIME chemotherapy (methyl-GAG, ifosfamide, methotrexate, etoposide) as treatment for recurrent Hodgkin's diease. J Clin Oncol 1987;5:551.
282. Velasquez WS, Cabanillas F, Salvador P, et al. Effective salvage therapy for lymphoma with cisplatin in combination with high dose Ara- and dexamethasone (DHAP). Blood 1987;71:117.
283. Longo DL. The use of chemotherapy in the treatment of Hodgkin's disease. Semin Oncol 1990;17:716.
284. Mauch P, Tarbell N, Skarin A, et al. Wide-field radiation therapy alone and with chemotherapy for Hodgkin's disease in relapse after combination chemotherapy. J Clin Oncol 1987;5:544.
285. Roach M III, Kapp DS, Rosenberg SA, Hoppe RI. Radiotherapy with curative intent: an option for selected patients relapsing after chemotherapy for advanced Hodgkin's disease. J Clin Oncol 1987;5:550.
286. Canellos GP. Bone marrow transplantation as salvage therapy in advanced Hodgkin's disease: allogeneic or autologous. J Clin Oncol 1985;3:1451.
287. Applebaum FR, Sullivan KM, Thomas ED, et al. Allogeneic marrow transplantation in the treatment of MOPP-resistant Hodgkin's disease. J Clin Oncol 1985;3:1490.
288. Jagannath S, Dicke KA, Armitage JO, et al. High-dose cyclophosphamide, carmustine, etoposide and autologous bone marrow transplantation for relapsed Hodgkin's disease. Ann Intern Med 1986;104:163.
289. Phillips GL, Reece DE. Clinical studies of autologous bone marrow transplantation in Hodgkin's disease. Clin Hematol 1986;15:151.
290. Gribben JG, Vaughan Hudson B, Linch DC. The potential value of very intensive therapy with autologous bone marrow rescue in the treatment of malignant lymphomas. Hematol Oncol 1987;5:281.
291. Canellos GP, Armitage J, Ernst P, et al. Bone marrow transplantation in malignant lymphoma: report of a workshop at the Third International Conference in Lymphoma at Lugano, Switzerland, June 1987. Hematol Oncol 1987;5:295.
292. Canellos GP, Nadler L, Takvorian T. Autologous bone marrow transplantation in the treatment of malignant lymphoma and Hodgkin's diease. Semin Hematol 1988;25(Suppl 2):58.
293. Jagannath S, Armitage JO, Dicke KA, et al. Prognostic factors for response and survival after high-dose cyclophosphamide, Carmustine and etoposide with autologous bone marrow transplantation for relapsed Hodgkin's disease. J Clin Oncol 1989;7:179.
294. Gribben JG, Linch DC, Singer CRJ, et al. Successful treatment of refractory Hodgkin's disease by high-dose combination chemotherapy and autologous bone marrow transplantation. Blood 1989;73:340.
295. Jones RJ, Piantadosi S, Mann RB, et al. High-dose cytotoxic therapy and bone marrow transplantation for relapsed Hodgkin's disease. J Clin Oncol 1990;8:527.
296. Reece DE, Barnett MJ, Connors JM, et al. Intensive chemotherapy with cyclophosphamide, carmustine, and etoposide followed by au-

tologous bone marrow transplantation for relapsed Hodgkin's disease. J Clin Oncol 1991;9:1871.
297. Vose JM, Bierman PJ, Armitage JO. Hodgkin's disease: the role of bone marrow transplantation. Semin Oncol 1990;17:749.
298. Wheeler C, Antin JH, Churchill WH, et al. Cyclophosphamide, carmustine, and etoposide with autologous bone marrow transplantation in refractory Hodgkin's disease and non-Hodgkin's lymphoma: a dose finding study. J Clin Oncol 1990;8:648.
299. Armitage JO. Bone marrow transplantation of patients with lymphoma. Blood 1989;73:1749.
300. Cicco NA, Lubbert M, Oster W, Lindemann A, Mertelsmann R. Cytokines in the pathogenesis and management of non-Hodgkin's lymphoma. Hematol Oncol Clin North Am 1991;5:1053.
301. Wilmas J, Thompson E, Smith KL. Long term results of treatment of children and adolescents with Hodgkin's diease. Cancer 1980;46:2123.
302. Jenkin RTD, Berry MP. Hodgkin's disease in children. Semin Oncol 1980;7:202.
303. Donaldson SS, Kaplan HS. Complications of treatment of Hodgkin's disease in children. Cancer Treat Rep 1982;66:977.
304. Lange B, Littman P. Management of Hodgkin's diease in children and adolescents. Cancer 1983;51:1371.
305. Mauch PM, Weinstein H, et al. An evaluation of long-term survival and treatment complications in children with Hodgkin's disease. Cancer 1983;51:925.
306. Russell KJ, Donaldson SS, Cox RS, Kaplan HS. Childhood Hodgkin's disease: patterns of relapse. J Clin Oncol 1984;2:80.
307. Robinson R, Kingston JE, et al. Chemotherapy and irradiation in childhood Hodgkin's disease. Arch Dis Child 1985;59:1162.
308. Malpas JS. Hodgkin's disease in children. In: Selby P, McElwain TJ, eds. Hodgkin's disease. Oxford, UK, Blackwell Scientific Publications, 1987:386.
309. Donaldson SS. Hodgkin's disease in children. Semin Oncol 1990;17: 736.
310. Chilcote RR, Baehner RL, Hammond D. Septicemia and meningitis in children splenectomized for Hodgkin's diease. N Engl J Med 1976;295:798.
311. Donaldson SS, Link MP. Combined modality treatment with low-dose radiation and MOPP chemotherapy for children with Hodgkin's disease. J Clin Oncol 1987;5:742.
312. Meadows AT, Obringer AC, Marrero O, et al. Second malignant neoplasms following childhood Hodgkin's disease: treatment and splenectomy risk factors. Med Pediatr Oncol 1989;17:477.
313. Lokich JJ, Pinkus GS, Moloney WC. Hodgkin's disease in the elderly. Oncology 1974;29:484.
314. Austin-Seymour MM, Hoppe RT, Cox RS, et al. Hodgkin's disease in patients over sixty years old. Ann Intern Med 1984;100:13.
315. Guinee VF, Giacco GG, Durand M, et al. The prognosis of Hodgkin's disease in older adults. J Clin Oncol 1991;9:947.
316. Jacobs C, Donaldson SS, Rosenberg SA, Kaplan HS. Management of the pregnant patient with Hodgkin's disease. Ann Intern Med 1981;95: 669.
317. Redman JR, Bajorunas DR, Lacher MJ. Hodgkin's disease: pregnancy and progeny. In: Lacher MJ, Redman JR, eds. Hodgkin's disease: the consequences of survival. Philadelphia, Lea & Febiger, 1990:267.
318. Mauch P, Greenberg H, Lewin A, et al. Prognostic factors in patients with subdiaphragmatic Hodgkin's disease. Hematol Oncol 1983;1:205.
319. Krikorian JG, Portlock CS, Mauch PM. Hodgkin's diease presenting below the diaphragm: a review. J Clin Oncol 1986;4:1551.
320. Leibenhaut MH, Hoppe RT, Varghese A, Rosenberg SA. Subdiaphragmatic Hodgkin's disease: laparotomy and treatment results in 49 patients. J Clin Oncol 1987;5:1050.
321. Canellos GP, Anderson JR, Propert KJ, et al. Chemotherapy of advanced Hodgkin's disease with MOPP, ABVD, or MOPP alternating with ABVD. N Engl J Med 1992;327:1478.
322. Glick J, Tsiatis A, Schilsky R. A randomized phase III trial of MOPP/ ABV hybrid vs sequential MOPP-ABVD in advanced Hodgkin's disease: preliminary results of the intergroup trial. Proc Am Soc Clin Oncol 1991;10:271.

Blood: Principles and Practice of Hematology,
edited by Robert I. Handin, Samuel E. Lux, and Thomas P. Stossel.
J.B. Lippincott Company, Philadelphia © 1995.

30

Non-Hodgkin's Lymphoma

James O. Armitage

The diseases included in the category of non-Hodgkin's lymphoma (NHL) represent a diverse group of neoplasms. They range from some of the most indolent malignancies (small lymphocytic lymphoma and follicular small cleaved cell lymphoma) to the most rapidly growing and highly aggressive human tumors (small noncleaved cell or Burkitt's lymphoma). Until early in the 20th century, no distinction was made between NHL and Hodgkin's disease. By the 1950s, recognition of NHL as a separate subgroup of diseases, and recognizing specific subtypes of NHL became increasingly important. Burkitt's lymphoma was one of the first neoplasms shown to be curable with drugs. It was also first to be shown to have a consistent chromosomal abnormality and the first solid tumor known to be curable by means of autologous bone marrow transplantation. The more common large cell lymphomas were shown to be curable with combination chemotherapy in the 1970s. Studies of NHLs added greatly to our knowledge of the immune system, since these are the solid tumors of the immune system.

Any discussion of NHL is complicated by the complexity of histologic classification and nomenclature. Even though older terms such as *reticulum cell sarcoma* and *giant follicular lymphoma* have been discarded, a large number of recently proposed classification schemes remain in use in various countries around the world. Six of these schemes are listed in Table 30-1. A project was undertaken by the National Cancer Institute (NCI) to unify pathologic diagnosis of NHL. This led to the development of the Working Formulation for Non-Hodgkin's Lymphoma for Clinical Usage.[1,2] All these classification schemes attempt to group the NHLs in some clinically useful manner. Thus, they are naming the *same* diseases using *different* terms. The Working Formulation presents a method of translating the various classification schemes.

An accurate diagnosis is essential in making clinical decisions in the care of patients with malignancy. The histologic diagnosis of the NHL is among the most difficult tasks that surgical pathologists are asked to perform. Much disagreement occurs among pathologists when attempts are made to accurately classify NHLs. The results of several studies comparing diagnostic accuracy are listed in Table 30-2. These studies all reported results of concordance between institutional pathologists and an expert review panel of hematopathologists. The diagnosis of NHL compared with other malignancies was accurate 87% to 96% of the time. Also, the distinction between follicular and diffuse growth patterns was highly accurate.

Identification of the specific histologic subtype occurred slightly more than half of the time. Even when the expert pathologists who developed the Working Formulation were tested for consistency in their diagnoses, they reproduced the exact histologic subtype at a rate of 53% to 93%. Therefore, it must be recognized that a significant number of patients will not be diagnosed accurately and that treatment plans that vary widely for closely related subgroups of NHL probably do not make much sense.

Despite its shortcomings, the Working Formulation is the most useful way to subdivide patients with NHL. The remainder of this chapter uses the Working Formulation as the basis for distinction among the various types of NHL. Each major category in the Working Formulation is considered separately in the following sections according to clinically important characteristics and response to therapy. The various treatment regimens used in these patients and referred to throughout this chapter are presented in Table 30-3 and Figures 30-1 through 30-13.

LOW-GRADE LYMPHOMAS

Low-grade NHLs represent some of the more indolent neoplasms seen in man. Lymphomas classified under the category *small lymphocytic* have a diffuse growth pattern whereas the other two subgroups *follicular small cleaved cell* and *follicular mixed* have a follicular growth pattern. Distinction between the two subgroups is based on the number of admixed large transformed cells seen in the tumor. This is an arbitrary distinction. In the past, tumors were called follicular small cleaved cell when less than 20% of the cells within the nodule were large, and they were called follicular mixed when 20% to 50% of the cells within the nodules were large.[8] More recently, Mann and Berard[9] proposed that tumors should be called follicular small cleaved if they have fewer than 5 large cells per high-power field and follicular mixed if 5 to 15 large cells are present per high-power field. This is an increasingly popular method of making the distinction, which seems to have good clinical correlation.

The curability of low-grade NHL has been a point of debate. Although patients who present with truly localized disease can almost certainly be cured, after the disease has disseminated cure with cytotoxic chemotherapy is at best unusual. Patients with disseminated disease have highly responsive tumors and are regularly palliated by a variety of chemotherapeutic approaches.

(text continues on page 854)

TABLE 30-1. Working Formulation of Non-Hodgkin's Lymphomas for Clinical Usage*

WORKING FORMULATION

Low Grade

- Malignant lymphoma
  - Small lymphocytic
    - Consistent with CLL
    - Plasmacytoid
- Malignant lymphoma, follicular
  - Predominantly small cleaved cell
    - Diffuse areas
    - Sclerosis
- Malignant lymphoma, follicular
  - Mixed, small cleaved and large-cell
    - Diffuse areas
    - Sclerosis

Intermediate Grade

- Malignant lymphoma, follicular
  - Predominantly large cell
    - Diffuse areas
    - Sclerosis
- Malignant lymphoma, diffuse
  - Small cleaved cell
    - Sclerosis
- Malignant lymphoma, diffuse
  - Mixed, small and large cell
    - Sclerosis
    - Epithelioid cell component
- Malignant lymphoma, diffuse
  - Large cell
    - Cleaved cell
    - Noncleaved cell
    - Sclerosis

High Grade

- Malignant lymphoma
  - Large cell, immunoblastic
    - Plasmacytoid
    - Clear cell
    - Polymorphous
    - Epithelioid cell component
- Malignant lymphoma
  - Lymphoblastic
    - Convoluted cell
    - Nonconvoluted cell
- Malignant lymphoma
  - Small noncleaved cell
    - Burkitt's
    - Follicular areas

Miscellaneous

- Composite
- Mycosis fungoides
- Histiocytic
- Extramedullary plasmacytoma
- Unclassifiable
- Other

RAPPAPORT CLASSIFICATION

- Nodular
  - Lymphocytic, well differentiated
  - Lymphocytic, poorly differentiated
  - Mixed, lymphocytic and histiocytic
  - Histiocytic
- Diffuse
  - Lymphocytic, well differentiated without plasmacytoid features
  - Lymphocytic, well differentiated with plasmacytoid features
  - Lymphocytic, poorly differentated without plasmacytoid features
  - Lymphocytic, poorly differentiated with plasmacytoid features
  - Lymphoblastic, convoluted
  - Lymphoblastic, nonconvoluted
  - Mixed, lymphocytic and histiocytic
  - Histiocytic without sclerosis
  - Histiocytic with sclerosis
  - Burkitt's tumor
  - Undifferentiated
- Malignant lymphoma, unclassified
- Composite lymphoma

LUKES AND COLLINS CLASSIFICATION

- Undefined cell type
- T-cell type, small lymphocytic
- T-cell type, Sézary–mycosis fungoides (cerebriform)
- T-cell type, convoluted lymphocytic
- T-cell type, immunoblastic sarcoma (T cell)
- B-cell type, small lymphocytic
- B-cell type, plasmacytoid lymphocytic
- Follicular center cell, small cleaved
- Follicular center cell, large cleaved
- Follicular center cell, small noncleaved
- Follicular center cell, large noncleaved
- Immunoblastic sarcoma (B-cell)
  - Subtypes of follicular center cell lymphomas
    - Follicular
    - Follicular and diffuse
    - Diffuse
    - Sclerotic with follicles
    - Sclerotic without follicles
- Histiocytic
- Malignant lymphoma, unclassified

KIEL CLASSIFICATION

- Low-grade malignancy
  - Lymphocytic, chronic lymphocytic leukemia
  - Lymphocytic, other
  - Lymphoplasmacytoid
  - Centrocytic
  - Centroblastic–centrocytic, follicular, without sclerosis
  - Centroblastic–centrocytic, follicular, with sclerosis
  - Centroblastic–centrocytic, follicular and diffuse, without sclerosis
  - Centroblastic–centrocytic, follicular and diffuse, with sclerosis
  - Centroblastic–centrocytic, diffuse
  - Low-grade malignant lymphoma, unclassified
- High-grade malignancy
  - Centroblastic
  - Lymphoblastic, Burkitt's type
  - Lymphoblastic, convoluted cell type
  - Lymphoblastic, other (unclassified)
  - Immunoblastic
  - High-grade malignant lymphoma, unclassified
- Malignant lymphoma unclassified (unable to specify as high grade or low grade)
- Composite lymphoma

(continued)

TABLE 30-1. *(Continued)*

BRITISH NATIONAL LYMPHOMA INVESTIGATION CLASSIFICATION

Follicular lymphoma
- Follicle cells, predominantly small
- Follicle cells, mixed small and large
- Follicle cells, predominantly large

Diffuse lymphoma
- Lymphocytic, well differentiated
- (Small round lymphocyte)
- Lymphocytic, intermediately differentiated
- (Small follicle lymphocyte)
- Lymphocytic, poorly differentiated (lymphoblast)
  - Non-Burkitt's
  - Burkitt's tumors
  - Convoluted cell mediastinal lymphoma
- Lymphocytic/mixed small lymphoid and large cell (mixed follicle cells)
- Undifferentiated large cell (large lymphoid cell)
- Histiocytic cell (mononuclear phagocytic cell)
- Plasma cell (extramedullary plasma cell)
- Malignant lymphoma, unclassified
- Plasmacytoid differentiation
- Sclerosis, banded
- Sclerosis, fine

WHO CLASSIFICATION†

Nodular lymphosarcoma, prolymphocytic
Nodular lymphosarcoma, prolymphocytic–lymphoblastic
Diffuse lymphosarcoma, lymphocytic
Diffuse lymphosarcoma, lymphoplasmacytic
Diffuse lymphosarcoma, prolymphocytic
Diffuse lymphosarcoma, prolymphocytic–lymphoblastic
Diffuse lymphosarcoma, lymphoblastic
Diffuse lymphosarcoma, immunoblastic
Diffuse lymphosarcoma, Burkitt's tumor
Mycosis fungoides
Plasmacytoma
Reticulosarcoma
Malignant lymphoma, unclassified
Composite lymphoma

DORFMAN CLASSIFICATION

Follicular (or follicular and diffuse)
- Small lymphoid
- Mixed, small and large lymphoid
- Large lymphoid

Diffuse
- Small lymphocytic, without plasmacytoid differentiation
- Small lymphocytic, with plasmacytoid differentiation
- Atypical small lymphoid
- Lymphoblastic, convoluted
- Lymphoblastic, nonconvoluted
- Large lymphoid, without plasmacytoid differentiation
- Large lymphoid, with plasmacytoid differentiation
- Mixed small and large lymphoid
- Histiocytic Burkitt's lymphoma
- Lymphoepithelioid cellular (Lennert's lymphoma)
- Mycosis fungoides
- Undifferentiated
- Lymphoma associated with sclerosis
- Malignant lymphoma, unclassified
- Composite lymphoma

* Represents clinical characteristics of patients in the 10 subtypes of the Working Formulation of Non-Hodgkin's Lymphomas for Clinical Usage. Miscellaneous or composite lymphomas are not included.
† Adapted from the Non-Hodgkin's Lymphoma Pathologic Classification Project.

TABLE 30-2. Diagnostic Accuarcy in Non-Hodgkin's Lymphoma

	Diagnostic Concordance			
Reference	**NHL vs Other**	**Nodular vs Diffuse**	**Pattern and Cell Type**	**Specific Subtypes**
3	96%	85%	56%	DHL^{86} NPDL^{78} NM^{33} DPDL^{13}
4	87%	NA	56%	NPDL^{81} DHL^{71} DPDL^{46} NM^{41} DM^{35} DWDL^{33}
5	96%	NA	NA	NPDL^{84} DPDL^{64} DHL^{60} NM^{48} DWDL^{40} DM^{35}
6	NA	NA	55%	DHL^{59} NPDL^{52}
7	NA	90%–95%	53%–93% (ability to reproduce itself)	NA

DHL, diffuse histiocytic lymphoma; NPDL, nodular poorly differentiated lymphocytic; NM, nodular mixed; DM, diffuse mixed; DWDL, diffuse well-differentiated lymphocytic; DPDL, diffuse poorly differentiated lymphocytic.

TABLE 30-3. Chemotherapy Regimens Used for Patients With Non-Hodgkin's Lymphoma*

CHOP	MACOP-B
CNOP	ProMACE-CytaBOM
CVP (low-grade lymphomas)	LNH-80
C-MOPP	COPBLAM
DHAP (salvage regimen)	CAP-BOP
IMVP-16 (salvage regimen)	COPBLAM III
m-BACOD	

* Regimens are listed in order.

SMALL LYMPHOCYTIC LYMPHOMAS

The most salient features of small lymphocytic lymphomas are presented in Table 30-4. This tumor represents a neoplasm of small well-differentiated lymphocytes, usually of B-cell origin. In small lymphocytic lymphoma, the lymph node contains a diffuse proliferation of small to medium-sized round lymphocytes. Only slight variations occur in nuclear size and shape, and usually an absence or paucity of mitotic figures is found. A vague nodular pattern can be imparted by clusters of large cells with round vesicular nuclei and one or two prominent nucleoli. These clusters are known as *proliferation centers.*[10] The same morphologic features can be applied to tissue infiltration in cases of chronic lymphocytic leukemia. Small lymphocytic lymphoma and chronic lymphocytic leukemia probably represent two clinical manifestations of the same disease process in most cases. Plasmacytoid lymphocytes, occasionally with intracytoplasmic or intranuclear inclusions of immunoglobulins (so-called Russell or Dutcher bodies, respectively) may be prominent in the tumors of some patients. These patients are likely to have monoclonal immunoglobulins in the serum. When these features are present, the terms *plasmacytoid lymphocytic lymphoma* and *lymphoplasmacytic–lymphoplasmacytoid lymphoma* can be applied. When the monoclonal protein present is IgM, these lymphomas represent tissue manifestations of the disease, Waldenström's macroglobulinemia.

Small lymphocytic lymphoma made up about 4% of the lymphomas seen in the Working Formulation study. Because NHLs have increased in incidence to about 32,000 cases annually in the United States, this suggests that between 1000 to 2000 cases of small lymphocytic lymphoma are diagnosed each year.[11] The number would be signifi-

CNOP

	Days 1	5	22
Cyclophosphamide 750 mg/m² I.V.	x		
Mitoxantrone 12 mg/m² I.V.	x		
Vincristine 1.4 mg/m² I.V. (Maximum 2 mg)	x		
Prednisone 100 mg p.o.	xxxxx		
Repeat 21 Day Cycles			

FIGURE 30-2. The CNOP regimen.

CVP (Low Grade Lymphomas)

	Days 1	5	22
Cyclophosphamide 400 mg/m² p.o.	xxxxx		
1000 mg/m² I.V.	x		
Vincristine 1.4 mg/m² I.V. (Maximum 2 mg)	x		
Prednisone 100 mg/m² p.o.	xxxxx		
Repeat 21 Day Cycles			

FIGURE 30-3. The CVP or COP regimen.

CHOP

	Days 1	5	22
Cyclophosphamide 750 mg/m² I.V.	x		
Doxorubicin 50 mg/m² I.V.	x		
Vincristine 1.4 mg/m² I.V. (Maximum 2 mg)	x		
Prednisone 100 mg p.o.	xxxxx		
Repeat 21 Day Cycles			

FIGURE 30-1. The CHOP regimen.

C-MOPP

	Days 1	8	14	29
Cyclophosphamide 650 mg/m² I.V.	x	x		
Vincristine 1.4 mg/m² I.V. (Maximum 2 mg)	x	x		
Procarbazine 100 mg/m² p.o.	xxxxxxxxxxxxxx			
Prednisone 40 mg/m² p.o.	xxxxxxxxxxxxxx			
Repeat 28 Day Cycles				

FIGURE 30-4. The C-MOPP regimen.

DHAP (Salvage Regimen)

	Days 1	2	3	4	21	28
Dexamethasone 40 mg p.o. or I.V.	x	x	x	x		Repeat Cycle
Cisplatin 100 mg/m² I.V. continuous infusion/24 hrs.	x					
Cytarabine 2 g/m² I.V. X2 doses 12 hrs. apart		x				

Repeat 21-28 Day Cycles

FIGURE 30-5. The DHAP regimen.

IMVP-16 (Salvage Regimen)

	Days 1	3	5	10	29
Ifosfamide 1 gm/m² I.V.		x x x			
Mesna 200 mg/m² I.V. (In 3 Doses/Day)		x x x			
Methotrexate 30 mg/m² I.V.			x	x	
Etoposide 100 mg/m² I.V.	x				

Repeat 28 Day Cycle

FIGURE 30-6. The IMVP-16 regimen.

m-BACOD

	Days 1	5	8	15	22
Methotrexate 200 mg/m² I.V.			x	x	
Bleomycin 4 U/m² I.V.	x				
Doxorubicin 45 mg/m² I.V.	x				
Cyclophosphamide 600 mg/m² I.V.	x				
Vincristine 1 mg/m² I.V.	x				
Dexamethasone 6 mg/m² p.o.	xxxxx				

Repeat 21 Day Cycles

FIGURE 30-7. The m-BACOD regimen.

MACOP-B

	Weeks 1	2	3	4	5	6	7	8	9	10	11	12
Methotrexate 400 mg/m² I.V.		x				x				x		
Doxorubicin 50 mg/m² I.V.	x		x		x		x		x		x	
Cyclophosphamide 350 mg/m² I.V.	x		x		x		x		x		x	
Vincristine 1.4 mg/m² I.V. (Maximum 2 mg)		x		x		x		x		x		x
Bleomycin 10 U/m² I.V.				x				x				x
Prednisone 75 mg p.o. X1 daily	x ———											——— x
	Daily dose tapered over the last 15 days											
Co-trimoxazole 2 tablets p.o. X2 daily	x ———											——— x
Ketoconazole 200 mg p.o. X1 daily	x ———											——— x

FIGURE 30-8. The MACOP-B regimen.

ProMACE-CytaBOM

	Days 1	8	9	14
Cyclophosphamide 650 mg/m² I.V. push	x			
Doxorubicin 25 mg/m² I.V. push	x			
Etoposide (VP-16) 120 mg/m² I.V.	x			
Prednisone 60 mg/m² p.o. X14 days	x ———			——— x
Cytarabine 300 mg/m² I.V. push		x		
Bleomycin 5 U/m² I.V. push		x		
Vincristine 1.4 mg/m² I.V. push		x		
Methotrexate 120 mg/m² I.V. push		x		
Leucovorin Rescue 25 mg/m² p.o. q6h X6 doses			x	

FIGURE 30-9. The ProMACE-CytaBOM regimen.

LNH-80	Induction (Weeks)			Consolidation (Weeks)								Final Intensification (Weeks)		
	0	2	4	8	9	10	12	14	16	17	18	26	30	34
Cyclophosphamide 1200 mg/m² I.V.	x	x	x									x	x	
Doxorubicin 75 mg/m² I.V.	x	x	x											
Vindesine 2 mg/m² I.V.	x	x	x											
Bleomycin 5 U/m² I.V.	x	x	x									x	x	
Methylprednisolone 60 mg/m² I.V. X5 days	x	x	x									x	x	
Methotrexate 15 mg I.T.	x	x	x											
Cytarabine 100 mg/m²/day S.Q X4 days				x	x	x						x	x	
Methotrexate 3 g/m² I.V. plus leucovorin rescue 25 mg p.o. q6 hrs. X12 doses							x	x						
L-asparaginase 60,000 U/m² I.M.									x	x	x			
Teniposide 60 mg/m² I.V.												x	x	

FIGURE 30-10. The LNH-80 regimen.

COPBLAM	Days 1	10	14	22
Cyclophosphamide 400 mg/m² I.V.	x			Repeat Cycle
Vincristine 1 mg/m² I.V.	x			
Prednisone 40 mg/m² p.o. X 10 days	x———	———x		
Bleomycin 15 U			x	
Doxorubicin 40 mg/m² I.V.	x			
Procarbazine 100 mg/m² p.o. X 10 days	x———	———x		
Repeat 22 Day Cycles				

FIGURE 30-11. The COPBLAM regimen.

CAP-BOP	1	7	15	21
Cyclophosphamide 650 mg/m² I.V.	x			
Doxorubicin 50 mg/m² I.V.	x			
Procarbazine 100 mg/m² p.o.	x x x x x x x			
Bleomycin 10 U/m² S.Q. or I.V. Maximum 15 mg			x	
Vincristine 1.4 mg/m² I.V. Maximum 2 mg			x	
Prednisone 100 mg p.o.			x x x x x x x	
Repeat 21 Day Cycle				

FIGURE 30-12. The CAP-BOP regimen.

COPBLAM III

Week	1	4	7	10	13	16	19	22	25	28	31	34
Cycle	A	B	A	B	A	B	A	B	A	B	A	B

Cycle A	(Inpatient) Day 1	2	3	4	5	10	Cycle B	(Outpatient) Day 22	23	24	25	26
Vincristine 1 mg/m² I.V. infusion over 24 hrs. X2 days	x	x					**Vincristine** 1 mg/m² I.V.P.	x				
Bleomycin 4 U/m² I.V.P.- day 1 followed immediately by 4 U/m² continuous I.V. infusion over 24 hr. on days 1-5	x	x	x	x	x							
Cyclophosphamide 350 mg/m² I.V.P.	x						**Cyclophosphamide** 350 mg/m² I.V.P.	x				
Doxorubicin 35 mg/m² I.V.P.	x						**Doxorubicin** 35 mg/m² I.V.P.	x				
Prednisone 40 mg/m² p.o. q.d. X5 days	x	x	x	x	x		**Prednisone** 40 mg/m² p.o. q.d. X5 days	x	x	x	x	x
Procarbazine 100 mg/m² p.o. q.d. X5 days	x	x	x	x	x		**Procarbazine** 100 mg/m² p.o. q.d. X5 days	x	x	x	x	x

FIGURE 30-13. The COPBLAM III regimen.

cantly higher if all cases of chronic lymphocytic leukemia were included.

Biology and Differential Diagnosis

Clues to the cause of NHL, although not certain in any case, may come from the frequent occurrence of chromosomal abnormalities in these neoplasms. The most common chromosomal abnormalities found in patients with small lymphocytic lymphoma have involved breakpoints on chromosome 11 and 14 and the occurrence of an extra entire chromosome 12. These abnormalities have also been reported in patients with chronic lymphocytic leukemia.[12–15] The breakpoint on chromosome 11 most frequently is located at about q22 and on chromosome 14 at q32. The most common translocation reported involves these two breakpoints designated as t(11;14)(q22;q32). Chromosome studies are difficult to perform in well-differentiated lymphocytic proliferations and frequently are not successful when performed on lymph nodes. In patients with chronic lymphocytic leukemia, cytogenetic abnormalities have been suggested to be of prognostic significance. Patients with abnormal karyotypes,[13] particularly trisomy 12,[15] are seen to have a poorer survival rate.

Because NHLs are tumors of lymphocytes, it is not surprising that studies of the immunophenotype of the tumors often provide useful clinical information. Most small lymphocytic lymphomas are of B-cell derivation, although a small percentage (1% to 5%) are derived from T cells.[16] The most common immunophenotype seen in these tumors is listed in Table 30-4. In the most common type of small lymphocytic lymphoma, the pan–T-cell antibody CD5 (Leu-1) is positive. This can be a useful finding in identifying this histologic subtype. The existence of a monoclonal B-cell proliferation can be a key finding in making the differential diagnosis between a benign, well-differentiated lymphocytic infiltration and a small lymphocytic lymphoma. This presents a clinical problem when the infiltrate is in an extranodal site, which is likely in orbital lymphoid infiltrates.

Other immunologic studies have been suggested to be important in the evaluation of patients with small lymphocytic lymphoma. For example, antibodies that recognize the antigen, Ki-67, identify cells actively proliferating. A higher proportion of Ki-67–positive cells has been suggested to be associated with a poor prognosis.[17,18] In addition, the number of normal T cells infiltrating neoplastic B cells in a small lymphocytic lymphoma has been suggested to be inversely proportional to severity of disease; that is, patients with small numbers of infiltrating T cells have more aggressive disease.[18]

Some patients originally thought to have small lymphocytic lymphoma have tumor cells with different morphologic and immunologic characteristics, for which the term *intermediate lymphocytic lymphoma* or *mantle cell lymphoma* has been suggested.[19–21] These tumor cells appear to behave more aggressively than typical small lymphocytic lymphoma and are being increasingly diagnosed by pathologists. Small lymphocytic lymphoma can also be confused with diffuse small cleaved cell lymphoma and with the lymphocyte predominant subtype of Hodgkin's disease. The confusion of small lymphocytic lymphoma with lymphocyte-predominant Hodgkin's disease should be suspected whenever a young patient (under 30 years) is diagnosed as having small lymphocytic NHL.

The distinction between small lymphocytic lymphoma

TABLE 30-4. Small Lymphocytic Lymphoma

OTHER NAMES

Lymphocytic, well-differentiated (Rappaport classification)

Small lymphocytic and plasmacytoid lymphocytic (Lukes and Collins classification)

Lymphocytic, chronic lymphocytic leukemia, and lymphoplasmacytic/lymphoplasmacytoid (Kiel classification)

Diffuse, lymphocytic, well-differentiated (small round lymphocyte) (British National Lymphoma Investigation classification)

Lymphocytic (WHO classification)

Small lymphocytic (Dorfman classification)

IMMUNOPHENOTYPE

B-cell (95%–99%); T-cell (1%–5%)

MOST COMMON PHENOTYPE

Positive: CD19 (Leu-12), CD20 (Leu-16), CD22 (Leu-14), CD21 (B2), CD5 (Leu-1), HLA-DR, sIg (M/D)

Negative: CD10 (CALLA), pan–T-cell antigens except CD5 (Leu-1), TdT

Variable: CD14 (My-4)

Lymphoplasmacytoid variant of small lymphocytic lymphoma is consistently CD5 (Leu-1)-negative

ASSOCIATED CHROMOSOMAL ABNORMALITIES

Translocation (11;14) (q22;q32); trisomy 12

DIFFERENTIAL DIAGNOSIS

Reactive small lymphocytic infiltrates in extralymphatic sites

Chronic lymphocytic leukemia (ie, when more than 4000 circulating well-differentiated lymphocytes in bone marrow involvement are present)

Hairy-cell leukemia

PRESENTING FEATURES

Median age: 61 years (Working Formulation), 66 years (Nebraska)

Stage and Symptoms	Working Formulation	Nebraska
I	3%	22%
II	8%	11%
III	8%	11%
IV	81%	56%
A	80%	85%
B	20%	15%

CLINICAL EVOLUTION

Transformation to a diffuse, aggressive lymphoma with predominantly large cells (about 25% of the cases); more commonly progressive disease that becomes increasingly refractory to available therapies

TREATMENT APPROACHES

Observation without therapy in asymptomatic patients with advanced disease. For symptomatic, disseminated disease chlorambucil with or without prednisone or combination chemotherapy with cyclophosphamide, vincristine, and prednisone with or without doxorubicin with complete responses of about 50% reported.

SURVIVAL

Median survival, 6 years (Working Formulation); 5-year survival, 59% (Nebraska)

and chronic lymphocytic leukemia or, in tumors with a monoclonal IgM spike such as Waldenström's macroglobulinemia, is of little clinical value. The diagnosis of chronic lymphocytic leukemia rather than small lymphocytic lymphoma is usually made when patients have 4000 or more circulating, well-differentiated lymphocytes. No useful therapeutic distinction is made between the two diagnoses. In general, when patients present with lymphadenopathy and first undergo a lymph node biopsy, the diagnosis of small lymphocytic lymphoma is made. In contrast, the disease in patients who first have a peripheral lymphocytosis identified and then undergo a bone marrow biopsy is most likely to be called *chronic lymphocytic leukemia*.

Patients who were diagnosed in the past as having chronic lymphocytic leukemia were more frequently followed up without therapy or treated conservatively, whereas patients who were initially diagnosed as having small lymphocytic lymphoma received combination chemotherapy. This phenomenon placed pathologists in a position to choose the sort of therapy that the patient would receive, based on the diagnosis they issued. There is no reason to treat two patients with similar clinical characteristics differently depending on whether they have circulating lymphoma cells. A number of recently described staging systems for chronic lymphocytic leukemia have demonstrated that patients whose disease is confined to the bone marrow and blood with no bone marrow failure have the best prognosis, those with lymphadenopathy or hepatosplenomegaly have an intermediate prognosis, and those with bone marrow failure have the worse prognosis.[22]

Clinical Features

The presenting characteristics of patients with small lymphocytic lymphoma are listed in Table 30-4. The median age of the patients studied in the Working Formulation was 61 years. This probably is younger than the median age seen in the community, since patients from the Working Formulation study came from cancer centers or university teaching hospitals and probably reflect some referral bias. A slight male predominance was seen, as is true in most categories of NHL. Most patients presented with disease in lymph nodes, although bone marrow, liver, and spleen involvement were common. Seventy-one percent of patients in the Working Formulation had bone marrow involvement. The exact percentage with bone marrow involvement in a particular series depends on how the distinction between small lymphocytic lymphoma and chronic lymphocytic leukemia is made.

After the diagnosis of NHL is made, an appropriate staging evaluation needs to be performed to determine the extent of disease. Although this does not mean that every possible test must be done, at least a history and physical examination, white blood cell count and differential, hemoglobin, platelet count, screening chemistry studies including liver and kidney function tests, chest radiographs, bone marrow biopsy, and imaging studies directed at the abdomen such as computed tomography (CT) or sonography, should usually be performed.

In this chapter, stage is assigned based on the Ann Arbor Staging Classification unless otherwise recognized[23] (Table 30-5). The Ann Arbor Staging Classification was originally described for Hodgkin's disease. Its use in assigning extent of disease in patients with NHL is complicated because of the more frequent occurrence of extranodal disease. In this chapter, the stage IIE designation is used for organ involvement with lymphoma involving the regional lymph nodes. Multiple sites of extranodal organ involvement or a localized site of extranodal involvement but distant lymph nodes involved by the malignancy is designated as stage IV.

Small lymphocytic lymphoma usually presents with high stage disease. The incidence of stage IV disease in patients from the Working Formulation and in patients seen by oncologists in the Nebraska Lymphoma Study Group are pre-

TABLE 30-5. Ann Arbor Staging Classification

Stage I	
	Disease confined to one lymph node or one lymph node-bearing site
Stage II	
	Disease in two or more lymph node sites but confined to one side of the diaphragm
Stage III	
	Disease confined to lymph node or spleen but on both sides of the diaphragm
Stage IV	
	Bone marrow involvement, liver involvement, or other extensive extranodal disease
E	
	Designates sites of local extranodal involvement. For example, a tumor beginning in the stomach and confined to that organ would be Stage IE.
Symptom status A	
	Absence of fevers, night sweats, weight loss
Symptom status B	
	Unexplained fevers greater than 38°C, night sweats, or loss of more than 10% of body weight in the preceding 6 months

sented in Table 30-4. Unlike the more aggressive NHLs, small lymphocytic lymphoma generally does not present with systemic symptoms.

The natural history of small lymphocytic lymphoma is slow progression of the lymphadenopathy and a gradual increase in the number of involved sites. In the occasional patient with a large accumulation of IgM in the serum, hyperviscosity syndrome may be encountered. With extensive bone marrow involvement, thrombocytopenia and anemia may present clinical problems. Patients with small lymphocytic lymphoma often have hypogammaglobulinemia rather than a monoclonal appearing in their serum. All patients with small lymphocytic lymphoma and all patients with other NHLs have altered immune function and are at increased risk for infections even before the institution of therapy.[24] When the cellular immune defect associated with the occurrence of NHL is combined with hypogammaglobulinemia, affected patients develop both unusual infections such as *Pneumocystis carinii* and fungal infections and infections with encapsulated organisms such as *Streptococcus pneumoniae*. In such patients, periodic injections of γ-globulin may be appropriate.

Richter[25] described the occurrence of an aggressive reticulum cell sarcoma in a patient with chronic lymphocytic leukemia. The phenomenon of a high-grade, NHL developing in patients with indolent lymphoma or chronic lymphocytic leukemia is often termed *Richter's syndrome*. Most frequently, this means the development of a diffuse large cell or immunoblastic NHL. This syndrome occurs in as many as 25% of patients with small lymphocytic lymphoma seen at autopsy.[26] This phenomenon, also often called *histologic progression*, usually presents with rapid enlargement of one or more involved nodal sites and is frequently accompanied by the development of new symptoms. It probably represents a change in the original tumor (not a second lymphoma) and similar immunologic characteristics are frequently, but not always, shared by the two tumors.[27,28]

On some occasions, histologic progression may represent the occurrence of a new neoplasm, perhaps related to previous therapy. When histologic progression or conversion occurs, it is usually associated with a poor prognosis.[29–32] Even when patients have been previously treated, they can respond to subsequent chemotherapy and patients who have an excellent response to therapy seem to have prolonged survival. When patients with follicular low-grade lymphomas are followed up without therapy and treated after histologic conversion occurs, a particularly high incidence of complete remission seems to be achievable.[33] Whether this applies to patients with small lymphocytic lymphoma has not been tested.

Treatment and Prognosis

Because few patients with small lymphocytic lymphoma present with localized disease, little data are available about therapy for stage I disease. The patients who present with disease localized to one nodal or extranodal site seem to have excellent outlook with radiation therapy or, in a single extranodal site, surgery with or without subsequent radiation therapy.[34] The management of patients with more extensive disease is more controversial. Because many patients are asymptomatic at the time of presentation and the ability to cure disseminated disease is at best uncertain, close observation with no initial therapy has been proposed as the optimal treatment.[35] After a long follow-up, patients managed in this manner have not had a poorer outlook than patients who received therapy initially.[34] When patients receive chemotherapy initially, the most common treatment used has usually been oral chlorambucil or cyclophosphamide, with or without corticosteroids. In one series, no significant difference was found among patients who received a single alkylating agent or combination chemotherapy as their initial treatment.[34]

A few series of patients receiving combination chemotherapy are presented in Table 30-6. As can be seen, the complete response rate has been about 50%. It is not known

TABLE 30-6. Chemotherapy for Small Lymphocytic Non-Hodgkin's Lymphoma Patients

Reference	Regimen	Evaluable Patients	Complete Response	Frequency of Relapse*	Overall Survival Rate*
36	CHOP ± immunotherapy	52	2 (50%)	—	—
37	CHOP or HOP	45	26 (58%)	—	50% (3 y)
38	CVP	11	7 (64%)	71%	>50% (6 y)
39	CP	10	1 (10%)	—	—
	BP	7	1 (14%)	—	—
40	Interferon-α	6	0 (0%)	—	—
41	CVP	4	2 (50%)	—	—
	ABP	3	2 (67%)	—	—
42	COP	3	0 (0%)	—	33% (1 y)

* May be based on actuarial estimates of data.

whether there are long-term, disease-free survivors among those with extensive disease. The median period of survival of patients with small lymphocytic lymphoma has varied from 3 years to 10 years in various series.[43] This probably depends significantly on the way patients were selected for the various studies. An important prognostic factor for patients with this and most other NHLs is age. Younger patients survive longer.[43]

The management of patients with small lymphocytic lymphoma who progress after their initial therapy should be individualized. In many patients, supportive care and radiation to sites of symptomatic involvement are appropriate. Further use of single-agent or combination chemotherapy should be for manifestations of progressive disease that cannot be managed more simply. For the occasional young patient who has an HLA-matched sibling, allogeneic bone marrow transplantation may be an option.[44]

FOLLICULAR SMALL CLEAVED CELL LYMPHOMA

Follicular small cleaved cell NHL represents a tumor of follicular small cleaved center cells. This tumor is always a neoplasm of B-cell origin. The immunologic features and other key points are presented in Table 30-7. This form of lymphoma is characterized by follicles of relatively uniform size and shape, which lack a prominent and well-defined lymphoid cuff and which compress intervening lymphoid regions. Tingible body macrophages are generally absent, and usually no evidence of cellular polarization is seen within the follicles. Follicles are composed predominantly of small cells with scanty cytoplasm. These cells are usually larger than normal lymphocytes and have regular nuclei with prominent indentations and linear cleavage planes. The chromatin pattern is coarse, and nucleoli are small and inconspicuous. A small number of noncleaved cells are found, and a few large cells with basophilic cytoplasm (centroblasts) are always scattered among the small cells. Mitotic figures are uncommon.

By definition, the growth pattern of this neoplasm is partially or predominantly follicular. Some pathologists believe that *any* follicularity means that the tumor is a follicular small cleaved cell NHL rather than diffuse small cleaved cell lymphoma. Others designate tumors with a minor follicular component as *mixed follicular and diffuse small cleaved cell lymphoma.*

Follicular small cleaved cell NHL is the most common form of the indolent NHLs. Patients with this subtype made up 23% of those in the Working Formulation study. These tumors account for less than 10% of the NHLs seen in the Nebraska study.[45] Some evidence has been found that the incidence of follicular small cleaved cell NHL may be proportionally decreasing.[46] Because NHLs occur about 32,000 times annually in patients in the United States, between 3000 and 7000 cases of follicular small cleaved cell lymphoma are diagnosed each year.[11]

TABLE 30-7. Follicular Small Cleaved Cell Lymphoma

OTHER NAMES

Nodular, poorly differentiated lymphocytic (Rappaport classification)
Small cleaved follicular center cell (FCC), follicular or follicular and diffuse (Lukes and Collins classification)
Centroblastic enterocytic (small), follicular (Kiel classification)
Follicular lymphoma, follicle cells, predominantly small (British National Lymphoma Investigation classification)
Nodular prolymphocytic (WHO classification)
Follicular, small lymphoid (Dorfman classification)

IMMUNOPHENOTYPE

B-cell (100%)

MOST COMMON PHENOTYPE

Positive:	sIg (M, G, A), CD10 (CALLA), HLA-DR, CD19 (Leu-12), CD20 (Leu-16), CD22 (Leu-14)
Negative:	TdT, CD5 (Leu-1), pan–T-cell antigens
Variable:	DRC and CD21 (B2) outlying follicles

ASSOCIATED CHROMOSOMAL ABNORMALITIES

Translocation (14;18) (q32;q21)—often associated with numerous other abnormalities

DIFFERENTIAL DIAGNOSIS

Reactive follicular hyperplasia

PRESENTING FEATURES

Median age: 54 years (Working Formulation); 58 years (Nebraska)

Stage and Symptoms	Working Evaluation	Nebraska
I	8%	17%
II	10%	8%
III	16%	17%
IV	66%	58%
A	80%	83%
B	20%	17%

CLINICAL EVOLUTION

Transformation over time to a diffuse, aggressive lymphoma with an increasing proportion of large cells in most patients

TREATMENT APPROACHES

Observation without therapy in asymptomatic patients with advanced disease is an acceptable approach. The small proportion of patients who present with localized disease should receive radiation therapy with or without chemotherapy with the intent of cure. For symptomatic, disseminated disease, single-agent or combination chemotherapy regimens appear to produce about the same rate of survival. When a patient is treated, achievement of a complete remission is probably important.

SURVIVAL

Median, 7 years (Working Formulation); median 5-year survival, 70% (Nebraska)

Biology and Differential Diagnosis

Next to small noncleaved cell lymphomas, follicular small cleaved cell lymphomas have the most consistently occurring chromosomal abnormality, t(14;18)(q32;q21). This translocation has been reported to occur in 60% to 100% of patients with follicular small cleaved cell lymphoma.[47–50] This abnormality involves juxtaposition of the locus on chromosome 14 involved in immunoglobulin heavy-chain synthesis with the locus on chromosome 18, which includes the putative oncogene *bcl*-2. This probably has etiologic or pathogenetic significance. Even in patients in whom cytogenetic studies do not reveal the t(14;18)(q32;q21), molecular genetic studies show consistent structural abnormalities (the molecular features of the translocation) within the *bcl*-2 gene in virtually all cases.[51] A variety of other chromosomal abnormalities are often seen in association with the t(14;18)(q32;q31). These associated abnormalities have been thought to determine the histologic appearance and the clinical course of these tumors.[47,50]

Essentially all follicular small cleaved cell NHLs are of B-cell derivation. The most common immunologic phenotype seen is listed in Table 30-7. Occasionally, admixtures of normal T cells can infiltrate the tumor so as to obscure the B-cell origin.[52,53] This is particularly likely when immunophenotyping is done by flow cytometric analysis. The use of immunologic, cytogenetic, and molecular genetic studies can occasionally help resolve the major difficulty in differential diagnosis, which occurs in follicular small cleaved cell lymphoma.

The distinction between follicular small cleaved cell lymphoma and reactive hyperplasia is occasionally difficult. A variety of histologic features in the tumor can help to make this distinction.[54] In some cases, the distinction can be made only by documenting the monoclonal B-cell growth pattern, the existence of a t(14;18)(q32;q21), or rearrangements of the immunoglobulin genes or *bcl*-2.

Clinical Features

Patients with follicular small cleaved cell lymphoma commonly present with painless lymphadenopathy. The median age of these patients in the Working Formulation was 54 years, but this is probably less than the median age seen in the community and less than that seen in a state-wide study in Nebraska. A slight male predominance has been found. Most patients present with disseminated lymphadenopathy, although occasionally a patient's disease is confined to one lymph node-bearing area. Involvement of the bone marrow is seen in a high percentage of cases (51% of patients in the Working Formulation and 38% of patients seen in the Nebraska study). When the peripheral blood (circulating small cleaved cells) is also involved, the process is sometimes called *lymphosarcoma cell leukemia*. The liver and spleen are also frequently involved, but histologic examination of these tissues is less frequently performed than of the bone marrow. These patients are unlikely to present with systemic symptoms such as fever, night sweats, and weight loss.

As in other types of NHL, an appropriate staging evaluation should be performed to determine extent of disease after the diagnosis of follicular small cleaved cell lymphoma has been established. This generally includes a history and physical examination, hemogram, screening chemistry studies, chest radiographs, bone marrow biopsy, and imaging studies to identify occult disease in abdominal lymph nodes, liver, and spleen. Patients with follicular small cleaved cell lymphoma usually present with an advanced stage of disease. Only a small percentage of patients (about 10%) present with stage I disease. Over half of the patients are stage IV at diagnosis.

Treatment and Prognosis

The natural history of follicular small cleaved cell lymphoma involves slow progression until eventual death from infection or organ failure. The rate of progression is not always steady, and spontaneous regressions occasionally occur.[55–57] These spontaneous regressions can lead to complete remissions and can persist for prolonged periods of time. Their occurrence is one of the reasons why observation without initial therapy has become a popular management strategy for asymptomatic patients who present with follicular small cleaved NHL.[58] This treatment approach does not appear to compromise overall survival. On the other hand, it may not be the optimal treatment approach in younger patients. A recent trial contrasting aggressive therapy with the watch-and-wait approach showed no survival difference but a highly significant difference in the disease-free time, thus favoring early therapy.[59]

Arguments about the optimal treatment for follicular small cleaved cell lymphoma center on the issue of whether the disease is curable. It appears that the occasional patient who presents with truly localized disease can have long-term, disease-free survival with radiation therapy with or without chemotherapy.[60–62] Unfortunately, this accounts for only a small percentage of patients. Some evidence exists that patients with stage III disease who are treated with total lymph node irradiation can have prolonged, disease-free survival.[63] This again represents a small percentage of patients. The curability of advanced follicular small cleaved cell NHL with chemotherapy or combined chemotherapy and radiation has been proposed.[64,65] Most series have not found a high percentage of long-term disease-free survivors.

The results of several chemotherapy regimens in follicular small cleaved cell NHL are presented in Table 30-8. This tumor is highly responsive to chemotherapy. A variety of other treatment approaches have been tried in patients with follicular small cleaved cell lymphoma. This is one of the tumors that is responsive to interferon-α.[69] Low-dose total body radiation therapy can induce complete remissions about as frequently as combination chemotherapy.[70–72] Serious persistent thrombocytopenia has been a complication of low-dose total body radiation therapy. The use of a single alkylating agent such as chlorambucil or cyclophosphamide with or without prednisone has been a popular treatment approach in patients with follicular small cleaved cell lymphoma. In at least one randomized trial, this treatment approach was as effective as a more aggressive combination chemotherapy regimen.[73]

Most patients with follicular small cleaved cell lymphoma eventually fail their initial treatment. Although se-

TABLE 30-8. Chemotherapy for Follicular Small Cleaved Non-Hodgkin Lymphoma

Reference	Regimen	Evaluable Patients	Complete Response	Frequency of Relapse*	Overall Survival Rate*
36	CHOP ± immunotherapy	144	89 (62%)	—	—
37	CHOP, HOP	68	50 (74%)	—	85% (3 y)
38	CVP†	49	33 (67%)	64%	70% (3 y)
66	COP	23	10 (44%)	—	30% (3 y)
67	COPP	14	11 (79%)	—	—
68	CHOP-B	13	8 (62%)	13%	—
66	CHOP or HOP	12	10 (44%)	—	50% (3 y)
40	Interferon-α	9	1 (11%)	0%	—
42	COP	6	4 (67%)	—	67% (1 y)

* May be based on actuarial estimates of data.
† Patient received C-MOPP.

quential use of available chemotherapeutic agents or radiation therapy can palliate these patients (in many cases for extended periods of time), the disease is ultimately fatal. A recent approach has been to try to overcome treatment resistance by the use of high-dose chemotherapy and total body radiation therapy followed by autologous bone marrow transplantation.[74] Because of the long natural history of follicular small cleaved cell lymphoma, follow-up has not been long enough in patients treated with an autologous bone marrow transplant to know whether cure is achievable. A large percentage of patients achieve a complete remission and most patients remain in remission for follow-up periods of a few years.

The natural history of follicular small cleaved cell lymphoma involves histologic progression to a tumor with a diffuse growth pattern and increased numbers of large, transformed neoplastic lymphoid cells. This transformation occurs in 75% or more of patients.[26,75] After the patients undergo histologic progression, their prognosis is generally poor.[30–32] Histologic transformation does not always preclude a good response to therapy, particularly in patients who were followed up without initial therapy or minimally treated before progression. Patients who respond to therapy after histologic progression and achieve a complete remission have a superior survival.[29]

Factors that predict outcome in patients with follicular small cleaved cell lymphoma include age, systemic symptoms, and measurements of bulk of disease.[76,77] Unlike most other lymphomas, the prognostic value of achieving an initial complete remission has been a point of controversy.[58] The median survival period seen in patients with follicular small cleaved cell lymphoma was 7 years in the Working Formulation study and has been reported to be longer in patients treated in various prospective trials.[58] The survival is variable and some patients have an aggressive disease. As already noted, the time to histologic progression can have an important impact on total survival.

FOLLICULAR MIXED LYMPHOMA

Follicular mixed lymphomas differ from lymphomas classified as follicular small cleaved cell only in the proportion of admixed large transformed lymphoid cells. As described earlier in this chapter, how the distinction has been made between follicular mixed lymphomas and other follicular lymphomas with fewer large cells (follicular small cleaved cell) or more large cells (follicular large cell) is arbitrary and has varied over time. It has been proposed that tumors should be called follicular small cleaved cell if they have fewer than 5 large cells per high-power field, follicular mixed if they have 5 to 15 large cells per high-power field, and follicular large cell if they have more than 25 large cells per high-power field.[9] This comparatively simple and objective approach seems to have excellent clinical correlation and has become an increasingly popular way to classify these tumors. The fact that many rules have been followed to make this distinction may explain some of the controversy surrounding treatment outcome and natural history.

The names, immunologic characteristics, and typical chromosomal abnormalities for these tumors are listed in Table 30-9. They vary little from the findings for follicular small cleaved cell lymphoma. The major difference between the two tumors is the more aggressive natural history in follicular mixed cell lymphomas and the possibility of curability in follicular mixed cell but not in follicular small cleaved cell lymphoma. In most other ways, these two tumors resemble one another, and much of the data from the preceding section applies equally well to follicular mixed lymphoma.

TABLE 30-9. Follicular Mixed Lymphoma

OTHER NAMES

Nodular, mixed lymphocytic–histiocytic (Rappaport classification)
Small cleaved FCC, follicular; also, large cleaved FCC, follicular (Lukes and Collins classification)
Centroblastic–centrocytic (small), follicular (Kiel classification)
Follicular lymphoma, follicle cells, mixed small and large (British National Lymphoma Investigation classification)
Nodular, prolymphocytic–lymphoblastic (WHO classification)
Follicular, mixed small and large lymphoid (Dorfman classification)

IMMUNOPHENOTYPE

B-cell (100%)

MOST COMMON PHENOTYPE

Positive:	sIg (M, G, A), CD10 (CALLA), HLA-DR, CD19 (Leu-12), CD20 (Leu-16), CD22 (Leu-14)
Negative:	TdT, CD5 (Leu-1), pan–T-cell antigens
Variable:	DRC and CD21 (B2) outlying follicles

ASSOCIATED CHROMOSOMAL ABNORMALITIES

Translocation (14;18) (q32;q21)—often associated with numerous other abnormalities

DIFFERENTIAL DIAGNOSIS

Reactive follicular hyperplasia

PRESENTING FEATURES

Median age: 56 years (Working Formulation); 59 years (Nebraska)

Stage and Symptoms	Working Formulation	Nebraska
I	15%	14%
II	12%	14%
III	28%	22%
IV	46%	50%
A	80%	81%
B	20%	19%

CLINICAL EVOLUTION

The natural history involves gradual loss of follicular growth pattern and accumulation of more large cells. This occurs more quickly than in follicular small cleaved cell lymphoma.

TREATMENT APPROACHES

Observation without initial therapy is acceptable in asymptomatic patients with advanced disease. Time to progression tends to be shorter than in follicular small cleaved cell lymphoma. In all patients with localized disease, radiation therapy with or without chemotherapy should be used with curative intent. The curability of advanced follicular mixed lymphoma with aggressive combination chemotherapy regimens is a source of debate in the literature.

SURVIVAL

Median survival, 5 years (Working Formulation); 5-year survival, 50% (Working Formulation)

FCC, follicular center cell.

Whatever the histologic rules for distinguishing between follicular small cleaved cell and follicular mixed lymphoma, the tumors classified as follicular mixed—thus having more large cells—tend to follow a more aggressive clinical course. This is reflected in a shorter survival period, a lesser likelihood of spontaneous regression, and earlier histologic progression.[2,58] Because of this, patients with follicular mixed lymphomas are generally poorer candidates for initial observation without therapy than those with follicular small cleaved cell lymphoma. Observation without therapy can still be successful as an initial approach in a minority of patients.

Treatment and Prognosis

The major source of disagreement about the appropriate management of patients with follicular mixed lymphoma is whether these tumors can be cured with chemotherapy. Although patients with localized follicular mixed lymphoma can certainly be cured by radiation with or without chemotherapy,[60–62] patients with disseminated disease treated with chemotherapy have not been found to be curable in all series. Investigators from the NCI reported the results in 79 patients with follicular mixed lymphoma treated primarily with the C-MOPP regimen (cyclophosphamide substituted for nitrogen mustard in the MOPP regimen).[78] They found a complete response rate of 72% in patients with stage III or IV disease and an average remission of more than 6 years. They also found a striking difference in disease-free survival when these patients were contrasted with those treated in the same time period for follicular small cleaved cell lymphoma.

Subsequent to the NCI study, investigators from the Eastern Cooperative Oncology Group reported the results of a clinical trial in which 52 patients with stage III or IV follicular mixed lymphoma were treated with either cyclophosphamide and vincristine, the C-MOPP regimen, or a combination of carmustine, cyclophosphamide, vincristine, and prednisone.[79] Of the 18 patients treated with the C-MOPP regimen, 61% achieved a complete remission but only 27% remained disease-free with a median follow-up of 3 years. The differences between these studies may relate to the way the drugs were given, the pathologic definitions, or other factors.[80] The curability of disseminated follicular mixed lymphoma with chemotherapy remains a point of controversy. The fact that some patients seem to achieve durable complete remissions makes the use of combination chemotherapy in younger patients with this disease a reasonable treatment option. The results reported with several chemotherapy regimens in patients with follicular mixed lymphoma are listed in Table 30-10.

INTERMEDIATE- AND HIGH-GRADE NON-HODGKIN'S LYMPHOMAS

The intermediate- and high-grade NHLs are taken together here. Although these tumors vary considerably in their histologic appearance and clinical characteristics, they are all potentially curable with aggressive combination chemotherapy regimens. In general, these tumors are more likely to be localized, to present in an extranodal site, and to pursue an aggressive clinical course than the low-grade lymphomas. The tumors included here are uncommon tumors such as diffuse small cleaved cell lymphoma (with a comparatively indolent clinical course) and lymphoblastic and small noncleaved lymphomas (with a high growth fraction and rapid clinical evolution). The most common tumors in this subgroup (diffuse large cell and immunoblastic lymphomas) represent the prototype for aggressive, but chemotherapy-curable, NHLs.

FOLLICULAR LARGE CELL LYMPHOMA

The most salient characteristics of follicular large cell lymphoma and the various terms used to describe this tumor are presented in Table 30-11. All recognize the follicular growth pattern in the tumor and the existence of numerous large, or transformed, lymphoid cells in the follicles. The Working Formulation study found about 4% of NHLs to be follicular large cell in appearance. Thus, of the about 32,000 NHLs that occur annually in the United States, slightly more than 1000 are expected to be follicular large cell lymphomas.[11]

Biology and Differential Diagnosis

The most common specific immunophenotype seen in follicular large cell lymphoma is presented in Table 30-11. These tumors are essentially B cell in origin. Reactive T cells can represent a large percentage of cells in the tumor. When immunophenotyping is done by flow cytometry, this can lead to confusion regarding the immunophenotype of the tumor.[53]

As with other follicular lymphomas, the most common chromosomal abnormality seen in follicular large cell lymphoma is the t(14;18)(q32;q21). Using traditional cytogenetic techniques, this is found in about 50% of the tumors. Other cytogenetic abnormalities have been reported.[48,49] The existence of the 14;18 translocation on cytogenetic study of lymph nodes can occasionally be helpful in making the distinction between NHL and atypical reactive hyperplasia.

Clinical Features

Patients with follicular large cell lymphoma, as with most other follicular lymphomas, usually present with advanced stage and without systemic symptoms. The Working Formulation found that most patients present with stage IV disease. Other series have found stage III disease to be particularly common.[81] This may relate partly to the extent of the staging procedures performed. Follicular large cell

TABLE 30-10. Chemotherapy for Follicular Mixed Non-Hodgkin's Lymphoma Patients

Reference	Regimen	Evaluable Patients	Complete Response	Frequency of Relapse*	Overall Survival Rate*
36	CHOP ± immunotherapy	64	46 (72%)	—	—
78	C-MOPP	24	19 (79%)	43%†	—
37	CHOP or HOP	20	14 (70%)	—	30% (2 y)
79	CP	20	13 (65%)	—	95% (2 y)
	COPP	18	11 (61%)	73%‡	65% (2 y)
	BCVP	14	7 (50%)	—	70% (2 y)

* May be based on actuarial estimates of data.
† Incidence expected over a 5-year period.
‡ Of three patients with complete response continuing in remission, two have died with no evidence of recurrent disease.

TABLE 30-11. Follicular Large Cell Lymphoma

OTHER NAMES

Nodular histiocytic lymphoma (Rappaport classification)

Large cleaved or noncleaved follicular center cell lymphoma, follicular (Lukes and Collins classification)

Centroblastic–centrocytic (large) follicular (Kiel classification)

Follicular lymphoma, follicle cells, predominantly large (British National Lymphoma Investigation classification)

Nodular, prolymphocytic–lymphoblastic (WHO classification)

Follicular, large lymphoid (Dorfman classification)

IMMUNOPHENOTYPE

B-cell (100%)

MOST COMMON PHENOTYPE

Positive:	sIg (M, G, RA), CD10 (CALLA), HLA-DR, CD19 (Leu-12), CD20 (Leu-16), CD22 (Leu-14)
Negative:	TdT, CD5 (Leu-1), pan–T-cell antigens
Variable:	DRC and CD21 (B2) often outline follicles

ASSOCIATED CHROMOSOMAL ABNORMALITIES

t(14;18)(q21;q32) with or without other abnormalities

DIFFERENTIAL DIAGNOSIS

Benign follicular hyperplasia. The distinction between follicular and diffuse large cell lymphoma can be arbitrary in tumors with a minor follicular component

PRESENTING FEATURES

Median age: 55 years (Working Formulation); 64 years (Nebraska)

Stage and Symptoms	Working Formulation	Nebraska
I	15%	22%
II	12%	26%
III	15%	22%
IV	58%	28%
A	73%	80%
B	27%	20%

CLINICAL EVOLUTION

Unless a prolonged remission is achieved, the natural course of the illness is loss of follicular growth pattern and more aggressive clinical course with time.

TREATMENT APPROACHES

Radiation therapy or combined combination chemotherapy and radiation therapy for stage I; patients with stage II or greater should be treated with aggressive combination chemotherapy regimens (usually including doxorubicin).

SURVIVAL

5-year survival, about 50%. A survival plateau in patients treated with aggressive combination chemotherapy has been a point of disagreement in the literature.

lymphoma is a more aggressive neoplasm than the other follicular lymphomas. It has a shorter interval to progression when patients are followed after diagnosis without initial therapy; this approach is not the recommended course for patients with this subtype of lymphoma. As with other NHLs, the natural history involves steady progression and dissemination of the illness, with death of the patient due to organ malfunction or infectious complications unless therapeutic interventions are successful. Over time, follicular large cell lymphomas tend to lose the follicular growth pattern, and the tumors become both morphologically and clinically like those that present as diffuse large cell lymphoma.

Treatment and Prognosis

Patients who present with stage I disease can sometimes have durable remissions when treated with radiation therapy with or without combination chemotherapy. Stage I follicular large cell lymphoma is not common. For patients who present with more extensive disease, a variety of combination chemotherapy regimens have been employed. A sample of results is presented in Table 30-12. With an Adriamycin (doxorubicin)-containing combination chemotherapy regimen, the complete response rate was generally over 50%; less than 50% of patients achieving complete remission were reported to have suffered relapse by the time of the publication of the reports. Whether follicular large cell lymphomas are curable with combination chemotherapy has been a point of debate in the literature.

Table 30-13 lists results of four other series of patients treated for follicular large cell lymphoma. The 5-year survival rate was 50% or greater, and in two series the 10-year survival rate was at least 50%. Two of the series found an apparent plateau in the survival curve for complete responders after aggressive chemotherapy regimens. In one series, it was uncertain whether such a plateau existed, and one series definitely did not find a survival plateau. Thus, the curability of follicular large cell lymphoma remains uncertain. The fact that some patients can achieve durable remissions leaves little doubt about the appropriateness of aggressive therapy in these patients.

DIFFUSE SMALL CLEAVED CELL LYMPHOMA

Other names for diffuse small cleaved cell lymphoma are presented in Table 30-14. This tumor accounts for about 7% of all cases of NHL and thus affects between 2000 and 3000 patients each year in the United States. The tumor itself is composed of the same small cleaved follicular center cells seen in follicular small cleaved cell lymphoma. Although this is not generally a highly proliferative tumor, mitotic figures tend to be higher than those seen in the follicular subtype.

Biology and Differential Diagnosis

Diffuse small cleaved cell lymphoma usually represents a neoplasm of B cells. The most common immunologic phenotype is presented in Table 30-14. Although no predominant chromosomal abnormality has been described, the one most frequently found is the t(14;18)(q32;q21).

Diffuse small cleaved cell lymphoma is becoming less frequently diagnosed in the United States. Most of the patients in the Working Formulation study were from the Italian Center.[1] Whether the decreasing incidence of diagnosis of this histologic subtype represents a change in pathology and the attitudes of pathologists, or represents a real change in the incidence of the disease is unknown.

Clinical Features

The predominant presenting features, stage, and symptoms of patients with diffuse small cleaved cell lymphoma are presented in Table 30-14. The median age (58 years for Working Formulation; 62 for Nebraska study) is characteristic for patients with NHL and, as is found in patients

TABLE 30-12. **Chemotherapy for Follicular Large Cell Non-Hodgkin's Lymphoma Patients**

Reference	Regimen	Evaluable Patients	Complete Response	Frequency of Relapse*	Overall Survival Rate*
82	CHOP, CHOP-B, COP, COP-B, ± XRT‡	55	39 (71%)	—	—
36	CHOP ± immunotherapy	33	21 (64%)	—	—
81	CHOP	15	12 (80%)	20%	50% (5 y)
83	CHOP ± Bleo ± BCNU	14	(29%)	75%	—
66	COP	12	8 (67%)	—	—
84	MOPP, C-MOPP, CVP, BACOP	11	8 (73%)	13%†	50% (5 y)
85	CAP-BOP	10	5 (50%)	40%	50% (3 y)
86	BCOP	6	1 (17%)	—	—
83	CTX + Pred	6	(50%)	67%	—
	CHOP	4	(75%)	25%	
86	CHOP	4	1 (25%)	—	—
83	C-MOPP	1	(100%)	100%	—

XRT, radiation therapy.
* May be based on actuarial estimates of data.
† Only patients treated with either CVP or C-MOPP achieved long-term remission.
‡ CHOP-B was the regimen most commonly given.

with low-grade lymphoma, most patients have stage IV disease. Most patients present without systemic symptoms.

Treatment and Prognosis

Patients with diffuse small cleaved cell lymphoma represent an intermediate stage between the findings in patients with follicular small cleaved cell lymphoma and patients with diffuse large cell lymphoma in their clinical characteristics. Unfortunately, their response to therapy seems to take the worst aspects of both extremes. Patients with diffuse small cleaved cell lymphoma have a comparatively poor chance of achieving complete remission, and most complete responders eventually go into relapse. The results with a variety of chemotherapy regimens are listed in Table 30-15. Results from the Working Formulation study document that some patients with diffuse small cleaved cell lymphoma can be cured with combination chemotherapy.[1] This proportion is not large, and the subtype represents one of the most difficult to treat with available treatment approaches. Some oncologists feel that patients with disseminated diffuse small cleaved cell lymphoma should be managed like those with low-grade lymphoma using no initial therapy in asymptomatic patients and conservative approaches when treatment is initiated. This approach to management assumes that there is no real possibility for cure. Certainly, patients with localized disease at presentation should receive radiation therapy with or without chemotherapy with intent to cure.

DIFFUSE MIXED LYMPHOMA

The various names used to describe diffuse mixed lymphoma are presented in Table 30-16, along with the most common immunologic phenotype and cytogenetic abnormalities. Diffuse mixed lymphoma is the particular subtype of NHL that is proportionally most likely to have a T-cell immunophenotype. The special characteristics of these so-called peripheral T-cell lymphomas are dealt with in a subsequent section in this chapter. Diffuse mixed lymphomas make up about 7% of the NHLs; thus, 2000 to 3000 patients are diagnosed with this lymphoma each year in the United States.

Biology and Differential Diagnosis

Diffuse mixed lymphomas represent a heterogenous mixture of tumors with mixtures of large and small cells. Patients with B-cell immunophenotype usually have a mixture of small cleaved cells and large transformed cells. Patients with peripheral T-cell lymphoma more likely have mixtures of large and small cells with irregular but noncleaved nuclear contours.

The differential diagnosis of patients who have been diagnosed as having diffuse mixed lymphoma is important. This tumor can be confused with mixed-cellularity Hodgkin's disease. This confusion is a common problem with patients with diffuse mixed lymphoma of the peripheral T-cell variety. Patients with mixed-cellularity Hodgkin's

TABLE 30-13. **Follicular Large-Cell Lymphoma**

Reference	Patients	Stage IV	5-Y Survival	10-Y Survival	Apparent Survival Plateau in Complete Responders
82	62	27%	62%	—	No
81	50	10%	77%	63%	Yes (after CHOP or m-BACOD)
83	25	36%	<50%	—	Uncertain
84	16	56%	50%	50%	Yes

TABLE 30-14. Diffuse Small Cleaved Cell Lymphoma*

OTHER NAMES

Diffuse mixed lymphocytic–histiocytic (Rappaport classification)

Small cleaved, large cleaved, or large noncleaved FCC, diffuse; lymphoplasmacytoid polymorphic (Lukes and Collins classification)

Centroblastic–centrocytic, diffuse (Kiel classification)

Diffuse, mixed small lymphoid and large-cell (mixed follicle cells) (British National Lymphoma Investigation classification)

Diffuse prolymphocytic–lymphoblastic (WHO classification)

Diffuse mixed small and large lymphoid (Dorfman classification)

IMMUNOPHENOTYPE

B-cell (≥95%); T-cell (≤5%)

MOST COMMON PHENOTYPE

Positive:	sIg (M/D or G/M), CD5 (Leu-1), CD19 (Leu-19), CD20 (Leu-16), CD22 (Leu-14), HLA-DR
Negative:	TdT, pan–T-cell antigens
Variable:	CD9 (BA-2), CD21 (B2)

ASSOCIATED CHROMOSOMAL ABNORMALITIES

Most frequently the t(14;18)(q32;q21), although a wide variety of abnormalities are seen

DIFFERENTIAL DIAGNOSIS

Diffuse intermediate lymphoma, small lymphocytic lymphoid lymphoma, small noncleaved cell lymphoma and reactive infiltrate

PRESENTING FEATURES

Median age: 58 years (Working Formulation); 66 years (Nebraska)

Stage and Symptoms	Working Formulation	Nebraska
I	9%	8%
II	19%	5%
III	12%	10%
IV	60%	75%
A	82%	77%
B	18%	23%

CLINICAL EVOLUTION

Over time, an accumulation of more large cells in the tumor. Often progressive disease becomes increasingly refractory to available therapies.

TREATMENT APPROACHES

Some authors would propose observation without therapy in asymptomatic patients. This is less often possible in diffuse small cleaved cell lymphoma than in follicular small cleaved cell lymphoma. The occasional patient with localized disease should be treated with radiation therapy with or without chemotherapy. These patients respond less well to combination chemotherapy or single-agent chemotherapy than follicular small cleaved cell lymphoma patients. Long-term disease-free survival is possible in the minority of patients and is restricted to those who achieve a complete response to therapy.

SURVIVAL

Median survival, 3 years (Working Formulation); 5-year survival, 33% (Working Formulation)

FCC, follicular center cell.

* Diffuse small cleaved cell lymphoma is diagnosed more in some geographic locations than in others. In the Working Formulation study, most patients were from the Italian Center. This histologic subtype is diagnosed less and less frequently in the United States.

disease who don't respond to therapy as expected should be suspected of having an NHL. Diffuse mixed lymphoma is also one of the histologic subtypes that can be confused with reactive immunoblastic proliferations, as in infectious mononucleosis.

Clinical Features

Most of the clinical characteristics of diffuse mixed lymphoma are similar to those seen in diffuse large cell and immunoblastic lymphoma (see section that follows on diffuse large cell and immunoblastic NHL). One series of diffuse mixed lymphoma described a particularly high incidence of extranodal involvement.[94] Although most authors have not found a significant difference between the treatment outcome in diffuse large cell or immunoblastic lymphoma and diffuse mixed lymphoma, this is not always the case. In our experience, diffuse mixed lymphoma has exactly the same characteristics and response to therapy as diffuse large cell and immunoblastic lymphoma, when age, stage, and immunophenotype are taken into consideration.

Treatment and Prognosis

Results with a variety of chemotherapy regimens in diffuse mixed lymphoma are presented in Table 30-17. When an aggressive combination chemotherapy regimen including doxorubicin has been used, most patients achieve a complete remission and most complete remitters have durable remission. When patients suffer relapse, the only therapy with a significant likelihood for cure is autologous bone marrow transplantation. The discussion of therapeutic approaches in the following sections applies equally well to patients with diffuse mixed lymphoma.

DIFFUSE LARGE CELL AND IMMUNOBLASTIC NON-HODGKIN'S LYMPHOMA

Table 30-18 presents the salient features of diffuse large cell and immunoblastic lymphomas, along with their names in the other popular classifications. In this chapter, no distinction is made between immunoblastic and diffuse large cell lymphoma. The advantage in survival of patients with diffuse large cell lymphoma found in the Working Formulation study was slight. The distinction between immunoblastic and diffuse large cell lymphoma is not simple and is difficult to accomplish for most hematopathologists. The variation in the relative incidence of the two diagnoses suggests that all hematopathologists may not apply exactly the same criteria. Finally, most reports of combination chemotherapy regimens do not identify a difference in complete response rate or a significant survival difference between the two histologic subtypes.

Biology and Differential Diagnosis

Tumors in the diffuse large cell and immunoblastic categories can have either B-cell or T-cell immunophenotype. Although most series have identified a B-cell predominance,[98] one series reported 42% T-cell tumors.[99] The typical immunophenotype of B-cell tumors is presented in Table 30-18. T-cell lymphomas with predominant large cells fit into the category of peripheral T-cell lymphoma. These tumors are typically CD2+ (Leu-5), CD3+ (Leu-4), CD5+ (Leu-1), CD7+ (Leu-9), and CD4+ (Leu-3). CD8 (Leu-2) can be substituted for CD4 positivity in some cases. The tumors are negative for TdT (terminal deoxynucleotidyl transfer-

TABLE 30-15. Chemotherapy for Diffuse Small Cleaved Cell Non-Hodgkin's Lymphoma Patients

Reference	Regimen	Evaluable Patients	Complete Response	Frequency of Relapse*	Overall Survival Rates*
87	CP or BP	77	19 (25%)	—	47% (2 y)
37	CHOP	38	26 (68%)	20% (1 y)	75% (1 y)
	HOP	38	21 (55%)	20% (1 y)	75% (1 y)
88	(CTX-L2 or NHL-3 or NHL-5)† XRT‡	37	24 (65%)	42%	50% (3 y)
86	CHOP	28	4 (14%)	—	—
	BCOP	28	8 (29%)	—	—
89	CVP ± XRT	20	9 (45%)	80% (1 y)	—
90	MEV	16	7 (44%)	29%	—
91	BACOP	15	12 (80%)	—	60% (2 y)
42	COP	14	2 (14%)	—	29% (1 y)
92	CVP or MOPP	9	2 (22%)	—	30% (2 y)
93	Chlorambucil or cyclophosphamide	9	2 (22%)	—	20% (2 y)‡
41	ABP	6	2 (33%)	Median, 8 mo	—
	CVP	5	2 (40%)	Median, 14 mo	—

XRT, radiation therapy.
* May be based on actuarial estimates of data.
† Only three patients were treated with NHL-3.
‡ Includes two additional patients who received other single-agent therapy.

ase). A small percentage of cases do not mark as either T-cell or B-cell lymphoma. The percentage of such cases is decreasing as improved methods of immunophenotyping are increasingly available; these TdT-negative tumors should represent no more than 1% or 2% of large cell lymphomas. Molecular biologic studies for rearrangements of the immunoglobulin or T-cell receptor genes can further reduce the percentage of undiagnosable tumors.[100]

The most common cytogenetic abnormality in patients diagnosed as having diffuse large cell or immunoblastic lymphoma is the t(14;18)(q32;q21), seen in B-cell large cell lymphomas. Other abnormalities have been described, as noted in Table 30-18. The clinical significance of these abnormalities remains unclear beyond their usefulness in confirming the diagnosis of lymphoma. In many cases, the breakpoints are at sites of known oncogenes, and some pathogenetic significance of the abnormalities is likely. Patients with chromosome 7 trisomy in addition to the t(14;18)(q32;q21) are considered more likely to have a diffuse growth pattern than a follicular growth pattern.[47] Also, patients with abnormalities involving chromosome 17 or 7 are reported to have a shortened survival[101,102] and patients with breakpoints in the short arm of chromosome 2 to have an improved survival.[102]

Patients with diffuse large cell and immunoblastic lymphoma make up a large proportion of the patients with NHL. In the Working Formulation, these two subgroups accounted for 28% of the cases. In the Nebraska study, patients in these categories account for more than 40% of the diagnoses of NHL. Thus, of the 32,000 patients diagnosed each year in the United States with NHL, between 9000 and 14,000 fit into these subgroups.[11] Patients with diffuse large cell and immunoblastic lymphoma of both B-cell and T-cell immunophenotype often have a history of an immunologic disorder. One series described a previous disorder of the immune system in 31% of patients with B-cell immunoblastic sarcoma.[103] Of patients with aggressive T-cell lymphomas, 26% have been reported to have previous disorders of the immune system.[104] Even when other lymphoproliferative processes are excluded, a significant number of patients with a variety of autoimmune states subsequently develop large cell or immunoblastic lymphoma. An association has been noted between Sjögren's syndrome and the subsequent development of NHL.[105] A percentage of the aggressive lymphoproliferative disorders that occur in immunocompromised hosts (eg, status after organ transplantation) and are associated with the Epstein-Barr virus have the morphologic appearance of diffuse large cell or immunoblastic lymphoma.[106]

The differential diagnosis of diffuse large cell and immunoblastic lymphoma is listed in Table 30-18. Perhaps the most common confusion is between Hodgkin's disease and diffuse large cell or immunoblastic lymphoma. In particular, patients with the diagnosis of lymphocyte-depleted Hodgkin's disease frequently have been discovered to have large cell or immunoblastic lymphoma on more careful evaluation.[107] Also, patients with the peripheral T-cell variant of immunoblastic lymphoma can be easily confused with those with mixed-cellularity Hodgkin's disease. When acute nonlymphoblastic leukemia presents with extramedullary disease, it is frequently diagnosed as diffuse large cell lymphoma unless a stain for chloracetate esterase is performed.

Before immunologic studies were widely available, many patients with anaplastic large cell lymphomas would have been diagnosed as having epithelial neoplasms, anaplastic sarcomas, or malignant melanoma. Widely available stains for common leukocyte antigen and other antibodies marking B and T lymphocytes have reduced this possibility. A recent study suggests that patients who cannot be clearly diagnosed on morphologic criteria alone as having large cell lymphoma rather than an epithelial neoplasm, and whose tumor stains with the common leukocyte antigen, have a clinical outcome similar to those with easily diagnosable large cell or immunoblastic lymphoma.[108]

Plasmacytomas with numerous plasmablasts may be

TABLE 30-16. Diffuse Mixed Lymphoma

OTHER NAMES

Diffuse mixed lymphocytic–histiocytic (Rappaport classification)

Small cleaved, large cleaved, or large noncleaved FCC, diffuse; lymphoplasmacytoid polymorphic (Lukes and Collins classification)

Centroblastic–centrocytic, diffuse (Kiel classification)

Diffuse, mixed small lymphoid and large cell (mixed follicle cells) (British National Lymphoma Investigation classification)

Diffuse prolymphocytic–lymphoblastic (WHO classification)

Diffuse mixed small and large lymphoid (Dorfman classification)

IMMUNOPHENOTYPE

B-cell (~40%); T-cell (60%)

MOST COMMON PHENOTYPE

B-cell

Positive:	sIg, HLA-DR, CD19 (Leu-12), CD20 (Leu-16), CD22 (Leu-14), CD10 (CALLA)
Negative:	TdT, cytoplasmic immunoglobulin, and CD5 (Leu-1)

T-cell

Positive:	CD2 (Leu-5), CD3 (Leu-4), CD5 (Leu-1), CD7 (Leu-9), and CD4 (Leu-3) or CD8 (Leu-2)
Negative:	TdT and CD1 (Leu-6)
Variable:	HLA-DR and CD71 (OKT-9)

ASSOCIATED CHROMOSOMAL ABNORMALITIES

t(14;18)(q32;q31) in B-cell tumors. No consistent abnormalities in T-cell tumors.

DIFFERENTIAL DIAGNOSIS

Mixed-cellularity Hodgkin's disease, reactive immunoblastic proliferations as seen in infectious mononucleosis, small lymphocytic lymphoma with pseudoproliferation centers

PRESENTING FEATURES

Median age: 58 years (Working Formulation); 65 years (Nebraska)

Stage and Symptoms	Working Formulation	Nebraska
I	19%	15%
II	26%	23%
III	13%	10%
IV	42%	49%
A	79%	65%
B	21%	35%

CLINICAL EVALUATION

Natural history of both T- and B-cell neoplasms is aggressive with an increasing proportion of large cells seen in the tumor unless a durable complete remission is induced by therapy.

TREATMENT APPROACHES

Aggressive combination chemotherapy in the same manner for diffuse large cell and immunoblastic lymphoma. The eventual treatment outcome is similar to that seen in patients with diffuse large cell and immunoblastic lymphoma.

SURVIVAL

5-year survival, 40% (Working Formulation)

FCC, follicular center cell.

confused with immunoblastic lymphomas. Anaplastic tumors sometimes occur in the end stage of multiple myeloma, which may represent histologic transformation to B-cell immunoblastic sarcoma.[109] Finally, T-cell immunoblastic proliferations such as occur occasionally in infectious mononucleosis can be difficult to distinguish from T-cell immunoblastic lymphoma. Careful clinical correlation, viral serology, and molecular analysis in search of T-cell receptor gene rearrangements usually make this distinction possible. This can be difficult and can lead to a potentially disastrous clinical error. Note that cytogenetic abnormalities can occasionally occur in benign immunoblastic proliferations.[110]

Clinical Features

The pretreatment staging evaluation of patients with diffuse large cell or immunoblastic lymphoma is aimed at identification of those patients with stage I or minimal stage II disease in whom a reduced amount of chemotherapy can be used. The initial staging evaluation should include a history and physical examination, routine hematologic and chemical blood studies, chest radiographs, abdominal CT scan, and a bone marrow biopsy. Further imaging studies or biopsies should be performed, depending on the results of the tests. Because of the advanced stage of these patients, the staging laparotomy is rarely appropriate and is not necessary unless the intention is to use only radiation therapy for treatment. Staging evaluation should be performed expeditiously, since diffuse large cell or immunoblastic lymphoma can sometimes progress rapidly. This lymphoma frequently presents with extranodal sites of disease. The subtleties related to the specific site of involvement (described later in this chapter) should be taken into account in the staging evaluation.

Patients with diffuse large cell or immunoblastic lymphoma most frequently present with enlarging lymph nodes, signs of dysfunction of a particular internal organ, or systemic symptoms. Systemic symptoms are more common in patients with this histologic subtype than in those with low-grade lymphomas. Results of a staging evaluation are more likely to identify localized disease in patients with diffuse large cell and immunoblastic lymphoma than in low-grade lymphomas. About 40% of the patients have stage I or II disease and about 15% to 20% have stage I or IE. As with most other NHLs, a staging laparotomy is rarely appropriate in the evaluation of the patient. Many patients with diffuse large cell lymphoma are diagnosed at laparotomy.

Treatment and Prognosis

The therapy of patients with diffuse large cell and immunoblastic lymphoma should be determined based on stage, presenting symptoms, age, and performance status. The appropriate treatment of elderly patients with diffuse large cell and immunoblastic lymphoma has been a point of contention in the literature. Most large series describing the results with new chemotherapy regimens have predominantly treated patients much younger than those seen in the general population (median age under 64 years). Age has consistently been an important prognostic factor in the survival of patients treated for diffuse large cell and immunoblastic lymphoma.[111–114] Although the overall survival period is reduced in elderly patients, tumors may not be less responsive.[114] Thus, the decision on how to treat elderly patients with diffuse large cell lymphoma should be individualized. On the other hand, patients should not be denied a chance at curative therapy simply because of age.

When patients present with localized disease (stage I, IE, or minimal stage II or IIE), radiation therapy can be curative in 30% to 70% of patients. The achievable cure rate is dependent on the thoroughness of staging; that is, patients not carefully evaluated are more likely to have occult dissemination and thus fail local therapy.[115] Several trials have documented that initial radiation therapy followed by a

TABLE 30-17. Chemotherapy for Diffuse Mixed Cell Non-Hodgkin's Lymphoma Patients

Reference	Regimen	Evaluable Patients	Complete Response	Frequency of Relapse*	Overall Survival Rate*
94	CVP†	14	4 (29%)	50%	30% (3 y)
95	ProMACE-MOPP	13	11 (85%)	—	—
85	CAP-BOP	13	10 (77%)	40%	54% (3 y)
94	CHOP	13	9 (69%)	11%	62% (3 y)
86	CHOP	13	6 (46%)	—	—
	BCOP	9	4 (44%)	—	—
96	NHL-3	7	5 (72%)	—	—
91	BACOP	6	4 (67%)	—	35% (3 y)
97	HOP/AC	5	4 (80%)	0%	80% (3 y)

* May be based on actuarial estimates of data.
† Initial or second-line therapy; one patient received CVP plus radiation therapy.

course of moderately aggressive chemotherapy increases the durability of remission compared with that seen with radiation alone.[116–119] More recently, studies have demonstrated that initial, doxorubicin-based combination chemotherapy, with or without subsequent radiation therapy, yields a high disease-free survival rate.[120,121] Patients treated with the latter approach have an extremely high complete remission rate and a long-term survival rate of more than 80%. All patients with localized large cell lymphoma should receive chemotherapy as their initial treatment. Whether a reduced number of cycles of chemotherapy followed by adjuvant radiation therapy is better than, worse than, or the same as more cycles of chemotherapy is uncertain.

Disseminated diffuse large cell and immunoblastic lymphoma was one of the first neoplasms demonstrated to be curable with chemotherapy.[122,123] Patients were originally treated with regimens found to be curative in patients with Hodgkin's disease. The addition of an anthracycline to the therapeutic armamentarium made an important difference in the treatment results. The first and most popular regimen including doxorubicin was the CHOP (cyclophosphamide, hydroxydaunomycin, vincristine, and prednisone) regimen using cyclophosphamide, doxorubicin, vincristine, and prednisone. This regimen demonstrated a high complete response rate and an impressive durability of complete remission in patients with aggressive NHL. Subsequently, a plethora of other regimens have been developed. Table 30-19 lists those regimens that have been reported in series including at least 20 patients.

With the variety of regimens documented to be potentially curative in diffuse large cell and immunoblastic lymphoma, it is difficult to know which regimen is preferable. Guidelines can be developed to help in making this decision. For example, to effect a cure in patients with diffuse large cell lymphoma, it is necessary to achieve a complete remission, preferably rapidly.[124,132,143] Note that some patients who may actually be cured appear to have only a partial response because of persistent abnormal imaging studies.[144] Patients with residual fibrotic masses may be distinguished from those with persistent disease by the use of SPECT gallium scanning.[145] For this test to be useful, the tumor must be known to be gallium-avid at the outset of therapy.

The best available therapy must be administered initially because salvage regimens have been generally ineffective, curing no patients in most series and about 10% of those in the best reported results.[146] Also, the drugs must be delivered at optimal doses. In one study from the Southwest Oncology Group, initial dose reduction in poor-risk patients was associated with a much poorer ultimate survival than when similar patients received full doses of therapy.[112] Prolonged treatment clearly is not necessary to cure diffuse large cell and immunoblastic lymphoma, and patients need be treated only a few cycles after documentation of complete remission.

The MACOP-B regimen is administered for only 12 weeks and is capable of bringing about a cure of patients with these disorders.[128] Finally, remember that the toxicity of chemotherapy delivered at the intensity necessary to cure diffuse large cell and immunoblastic lymphoma is significant. Incidence of treatment-related deaths vary but average about 5%. Patients should be treated with these regimens only by physicians experienced in their use with adequate supportive care facilities available. A physician should probably not try to use different multiple regimens but adapt one for his or her use and become maximally experienced with its side effects.

A variety of studies have been aimed at identifying the important prognostic factors predicting therapeutic outcome in patients with diffuse large cell and immunoblastic lymphoma.[126,127,131,147–150] Although certain prognostic factors such as age have been reproducibly important, the significance of others has varied from study to study. Attempts have recently been made to develop prognostic indices to predict outcome and to allow stratification of patients in clinical trials.[126,127,148,151] Remember that the Ann Arbor Staging Classification represents such an attempt at predicting outcome. Whether any of the newer indices represent an advantage over the Ann Arbor Staging Classification has not been determined. The proliferative rate of the tumor appears to be an important prognostic factor in large cell lymphomas.[152,153] More rapidly proliferating tumors are less likely to be cured, presumably reflecting their ability to recover between cycles and to produce resistant clones more quickly.

As previously mentioned, salvage chemotherapy administered at the typical doses is rarely effective in curing patients with relapsed or refractory diffuse large cell immunoblastic lymphoma. High-dose chemotherapy or radiation therapy followed by autologous or allogeneic bone marrow transplantation can cure some patients.[74] In general, patients who go into relapse from complete remission but have chemotherapy-sensitive disease should be considered for either autologous or allogeneic transplantation before being exposed to multiple chemotherapy regimens. Patients who have been in complete remission and then

TABLE 30-18. Diffuse Large Cell and Immunoblastic Non-Hodgkin's Lymphoma

OTHER NAMES

Diffuse histiocytic (Rappaport classification)

Large cleaved or noncleaved follicular center cell, diffuse and immunoblastic sarcoma T- or B-cell type (Lukes and Collins classification)

Centroblastic–centrocytic (large), diffuse, centrocytic (large), centroblastic, diffuse, immunoblastic and T-zone lymphoma (Kiel classification)

Diffuse and differentiated large cell (lymphoid cell), plasma cell (extramedullary plasma cell) (British National Lymphoma Investigation classification)

Diffuse lymphosarcoma, prolymphocytic–lymphoblastic (WHO classification)

Diffuse large lymphoid (Dorfman classification)

IMMUNOPHENOTYPE

B-cell (~80%); T-cell (~15%); nonmarking <5%

ASSOCIATED CYTOGENETIC ABNORMALITIES

Most common is the t(14;18)(q32;21) in about 25%–30% of patients. Other abnormalities most frequently involving chromosomes 1, 2, 3, 6, and 17 are also seen.

DIFFERENTIAL DIAGNOSIS

True histiocytic malignancies; lymphocyte-depleted Hodgkin's disease; mixed-cellularity Hodgkin's disease; granulocytic sarcoma; epithelial neoplasms; sarcomas; malignant melanomas; plasmacytomas; infectious mononucleosis (benign immunoblastic proliferatives)

PRESENTING FEATURES

Age: 55 years (Working Formulation); 66 years (Nebraska)

Stage and Symptoms	Working Formulation	Nebraska
I	13%	16%
II	14%	19%
III	14%	15%
IV	59%	50%
A	71%	58%
B	29%	42%

CLINICAL EVOLUTION

Untreated, the natural history is rapidly progressive illness and death in a short time. Chemotherapy can induce durable complete remission.

TREATMENT APPROACHES

Chemotherapy with or without radiation therapy for stage I disease; multiagent doxorubicin-containing chemotherapy regimen for stages II through IV. For second-line therapies, a variety of combination regimens such as ifosfamide, methotrexate, and etoposide or dexamethasone, cytarabine, and cisplatin can induce second remissions, but the long-term, disease-free survival is less than 10%. Autologous bone marrow transplantation can cure 35% to 40% of patients with chemotherapy-sensitive, relapsed disease.

SURVIVAL

5-year survival, 30% to 40% (Working Formulation); results are stage dependent at greater than 50% of stage I and II patients surviving free of disease.

have a relapse can be cured 35% to 40% of the time if they undergo transplantation when the lymphoma is still sensitive to chemotherapy administered at the typical doses.[74]

The survival of patients with diffuse large cell lymphoma is age and stage dependent. Even in patients with advanced disease, about 30% to 60% may have prolonged survival with effective combination chemotherapy regimens. Up to 80% of patients who present with minimal disease can be long-term, disease-free survivors. The results from the Working Formulation study suggested that about 30% of patients achieve prolonged survival when treated with less aggressive treatment approaches. After patients achieve a complete remission with an aggressive combination chemotherapy regimen, 30% to 50% eventually suffer a relapse. Most relapses occur within the first 2 years after therapy is terminated. Patients who remain in complete remission for more than 2 years have a 70% to 90% probability of being cured.[154]

LYMPHOBLASTIC LYMPHOMA

Lymphoblastic lymphoma is one of the more distinctive subgroups of NHL. It occurs in a much younger age group than the types of NHL discussed thus far, and it pursues a more aggressive clinical course. Lymphoblastic lymphoma makes up about 4% of the NHLs, and thus is diagnosed about 1500 times each year in the United States. The various names applied to this tumor are listed in Table 30-20. A name that has been popular for a subset of patients with lymphoblastic lymphoma is *Sternberg's lymphoma* or *Sternberg's sarcoma*, denoting the association of a mediastinal mass in patients with a poorly differentiated lymphoma.[155] Lymphoblastic lymphoma is felt to occur most frequently in young men. Thus, Sternberg's lymphoma is a descriptive term for a subset of patients with lymphoblastic lymphoma.

Biology and Differential Diagnosis

The histologic appearance of lymphoblastic lymphoma is that of a diffuse effacement of the lymph node architecture by lymphoblasts of uniform size usually with prominent nucleoli. The tumor cells are generally smaller than those seen in diffuse large cell or immunoblastic lymphoma. Cytoplasm is scanty or indistinct. Occasionally, a "starry sky" pattern may be apparent as a result of macrophages being interspersed among the lymphoblasts. This finding can lead to confusion with small noncleaved cell lymphoma.

Most patients with lymphoblastic lymphoma have tumors with a T-cell immunophenotype. Occasionally, patients with B-cell lymphoblastic lymphoma or biphenotypic lymphoblastic lymphoma have been described.[156] The most common immunophenotype seen in lymphoblastic lymphoma is listed in Table 30-20. Considerable immunologic diversity is seen when lymphoblastic lymphomas are closely studied. Most patients have immature (or thymic) T-cell lymphomas. Subsets of patients with the pre–B-cell phenotype of typical acute lymphoblastic leukemia or with a more mature T-cell phenotype are frequently seen.[157–160] Although a variety of cytogenetic abnormalities have been seen in lymphoblastic lymphomas, no consistent abnormality has become apparent.

Lymphoblastic lymphoma is one of the histologic subtypes of NHL in which histologic diagnosis is sometimes difficult. The differential diagnosis of lymphoblastic lymphoma may include small noncleaved cell lymphoma, acute lymphoblastic leukemia, acute myeloid leukemia, diffuse small cleaved cell NHL, diffuse large cell lymphoma, and thymoma (in patients who present with a mediastinal mass). Because of the highly aggressive nature of this tumor, diagnostic decisions should be made quickly and appropriate staging evaluation and therapy accomplished promptly. This disease can progress rapidly, and affected patients should be given a high priority to complete their pretreatment evaluation and begin therapy as quickly as possible. The patient can go from a good prognostic category to a poor prognostic category during a leisurely evaluation.

TABLE 30-19. **Chemotherapy for Diffuse Large Cell and Immunoblastic Non-Hodgkin's Lymphoma**

Reference	Regimen	Evaluable Patients	Complete Response	Frequency of Relapse*	Overall Survival Rates*
124	LNH-84	452	(75%)	26%	60% (3 y)
125	CHOP ± Bleo or ± immunotherapy	418	222 (53%)	—	30% (7 y)
126	M-BACOD or m-BACOD	121	87 (72%)	—	62% (3 y)
127	CHOP-B ± XRT	105	74 (70%)	40%	50% (3 y)
128	MACOP-B	98	84 (86%)	30%	70% (2 y)
86	CHOP	90	49 (54%)	43%	48% (3 y)
	BCOP	80	27 (34%)	43%	35% (3 y)
129	COMLA	72	29 (40%)	28%	40% (3 y)
130	CHOP	65	38 (58%)	35%	43% (3 y)
131	BACOP	57	27 (47%)	—	38% (3 y)
95	ProMACE-MOPP	52	38 (73%)	—	—
132	CAP-BOP	51	37 (73%)	33%	54% (3 y)
133	CHOP/HOAP-Bleo/IMVP-16/OAP-Bleo	51	41 (80%)	—	—
124	LNH-80	48	41 (85%)	22%	—
96	NHL-3	44	22 (50%)	—	48% (3 y)
134	COPBLAM III	43	37 (86%)	—	—
135	ProMACE-CytaBOM	35	28 (80%)	—	80% (2 y)
136	F-MACHOP	32	26 (81%)	<20%	—
137	OPAL	32	16 (50%)	—	—
138	COPA	31	14 (45%)	80%	30% (3 y)
139	CTX-L2	30	7 (23%)	14%	45% (2 y)
122	C-MOPP or MOPP	27	11 (41%)	9%	37% (3 y)
140	CHOP ± P + XRT	26	23 (88%)	45%	55% (3 y)
97	HOP/AC	25	20 (80%)	15%	—
138	COPB	24	6 (25%)	100%	15% (3 y)
141	CHOP	23	9 (39%)	25%	—
138	CPOB	22	12 (55%)	50%	45% (3 y)
142	BACOP	22	11 (50%)	0%	40% (3 y)

XRT, radiation therapy.
* May be based on actuarial estimates of data.
† Rate of relapse was 20% in patients achieving a complete response in three cycles and 60% in patients requiring five cycles.

The distinction between lymphoblastic lymphoma and acute lymphoblastic leukemia can be arbitrary. This is especially true in children who present with mediastinal masses and with bone marrow and peripheral blood involvement. Because treatment approaches to patients labeled as having either T-cell acute lymphoblastic leukemia or lymphoblastic lymphoma are similar, the distinction is usually more of a semantic than a practical clinical problem.

Clinical Features

Patients with lymphoblastic lymphoma are often, but not always, children or young adults. They often present with symptoms referable to a mediastinal mass, with systemic symptoms, with peripheral lymphadenopathy, or with signs of bone marrow failure. Patients included in the Working Formulation study had a high rate of stage IV disease.[1] This has not been true from patients treated in the Nebraska Lymphoma Study Group as noted in Table 30-20. Patients in the Working Formulation study also had a higher incidence of systemic symptoms than we have observed in the Nebraska study. Patients with lymphoblastic lymphoma are particularly prone to bone marrow and central nervous system (CNS) involvement. In a large number of patients, these sites are involved at diagnosis. In patients who present without bone marrow or CNS involvement, rapid dissemination to these organs is common. Because patients with bone marrow or CNS involvement have a strikingly less favorable prognosis, therapy (including therapy to the CNS) should be initiated promptly to avoid dissemination. With aggressive chemotherapy regimens, investigators from St Jude's Hospital found no impact of histology on outcome when stage and serum lactate dehydrogenase were taken into account.[161]

The staging for children with lymphoblastic and small noncleaved lymphoma has often varied from the Ann Arbor system, which is most frequently used in adults.[161] In this system, stage I reflects a single site of involvement with the exclusion of the mediastinum and abdomen. Stage II disease can reflect two sites of involvement on one side of the diaphragm or an entirely resected primary gastrointestinal tumor. Stage III disease reflects two tumors on opposite sides of the diaphragm, all primary intrathoracic tumors, all unresectable intraabdominal disease, and any tumor with paraspinal or epidural tumors. Stage IV disease reflects CNS or bone marrow involvement.

Treatment and Prognosis

The treatment of lymphoblastic lymphoma involves the aggressive use of combination chemotherapy along with prophylactic (or therapeutic) treatment to the CNS. Children with lymphoblastic lymphoma generally fare better

TABLE 30-20. Lymphoblastic Lymphoma

OTHER NAMES

Lymphoblastic convoluted/nonconvoluted (Rappaport classification)

Convoluted T-cell (Lukes and Collins classification)

Lymphoblastic convoluted, or unclassified (Kiel classification)

Diffuse lymphocytic poorly differentiated (lymphoblast); convoluted cell mediastinal lymphoma (British National Lymphoma Investigation classification)

Diffuse lymphosarcoma, lymphoblastic (WHO classification)

Lymphoblastic, convoluted/nonconvoluted (Dorfman classification)

IMMUNOPHENOTYPE

T-cell (≥90%)

MOST COMMON IMMUNOPHENOTYPE

Positive:	TdT, CD1 (Leu-6), CD2 (Leu-5), CD7 (Leu-9)
Negative:	CD10 (CALLA), CD5 (Leu-1)
Variable:	CD4 (Leu-3), CD8 (Leu-2)

CYTOGENETICS

No consistent abnormality

DIFFERENTIAL DIAGNOSIS

Small noncleaved cell lymphoma; acute myeloid leukemia; diffuse small cleaved cell non-Hodgkin's lymphoma; thymoma; T-cell acute lymphoblastic leukemia

PRESENTING FEATURES

Median age: 17 years (Working Formulation); 22 years (Nebraska)

Stage and Symptoms	Working Formulation	Nebraska
I	7%	12%
II	20%	38%
III	2%	12%
IV	72%	38%
A	27%	75%
B	73%	25%

CLINICAL EVOLUTION

This tumor has an extremely high propensity to disseminate to the CNS and bone marrow. Distinction between lymphoblastic lymphoma and T-cell acute lymphoblastic leukemia can be arbitrary when the disease presents with bone marrow involvement.

TREATMENT APPROACHES

All patients with lymphoblastic lymphoma should be treated initially with an aggressive combination chemotherapy regimen. The most popular regimens are similar to those used for acute lymphoblastic leukemia.

SURVIVAL

5-year survival, 25% (Working Formulation)

Recent studies have demonstrated that patients who present with low levels of lactate dehydrogenase and minimal disease not involving the bone marrow or CNS have a greater than 50% survival rate with aggressive combination chemotherapy regimens. Patients without these characteristics have a survival rate below 20%.

than adults. A variety of treatment regimens has been proposed to be effective in childhood lymphoblastic lymphoma.[162–164] Recent studies by the Children's Cancer Study Group and the Pediatric Oncology Group have suggested that the 10-drug LSA2–L2 regimen may be superior to a CHOP-like regimen in childhood lymphoblastic lymphoma.[165,166] This is in contrast to superior results with a CHOP-like regimen in other subtypes of aggressive childhood NHL.[165]

The results of several chemotherapy regimens for lymphoblastic lymphoma in adults are listed in Table 30-21. This tumor is highly responsive to chemotherapy, and most patients achieve an apparent complete remission early in the course of therapy. Rapid relapse is common and frequently occurs during continuing therapy.

Several series have demonstrated the ability to predict outcome in adults with lymphoblastic lymphoma. Investigators at Memorial Sloan-Kettering showed that age was an important predictor; extremely poor results were seen in patients older than 30 years.[167] A recent report from Stanford University suggested that patients with lymphoblastic lymphoma could be subdivided into two major groups.[168] Patients with Ann Arbor stage I to III or stage IV disease without involvement of bone marrow or CNS, who also had a normal or minimally elevated serum LDH, had an excellent prognosis. About 90% of patients with these good characteristics achieved durable complete remissions with a treatment regimen including cyclophosphamide, doxorubicin, vincristine, prednisone, L-asparaginase, CNS prophylaxis, and maintenance treatment with methotrexate and 6-mercaptopurine. Patients with bone marrow or CNS involvement or a high LDH had a particularly poor outlook with less than 20% surviving free of disease.

Since the results of salvage therapy in patients with this and other types of NHL are poor, those patients who fit into the poor prognostic categories should be considered for alternate therapies early in the course of their disease. High-dose therapy and autologous or allogeneic bone marrow transplantation can induce durable remissions in patients with lymphoblastic lymphoma.[173] This treatment approach should be considered at best response in patients who present with poor-prognosis lymphoblastic lymphoma.

Lymphoblastic lymphoma is one of the histologic subtypes in which the initiation of therapy is often associated with tumor lysis syndrome (discussed in more detail in the following section). Its occurrence should be anticipated in patients with bulky, lymphoblastic lymphoma, and patients should be on allopurinol and well hydrated before therapy is instituted.

SMALL NONCLEAVED CELL LYMPHOMA

The category of small noncleaved cell lymphoma includes the neoplasms labeled as Burkitt's lymphoma and closely related tumors. The names used to describe this tumor in different classifications are presented in Table 30-22. This is perhaps the most homogenous category of NHL. Patients present with uniform clinical findings and follow a characteristic, rapid clinical course. Small noncleaved cell lymphomas make up about 5% of the NHLs and thus occur 1500 to 2000 times each year in the United States.

Small noncleaved cell lymphoma is historically important for epidemiologic, cytogenetic, and therapeutic reasons. The tumor was first described in the 1950s by Dr. Dennis Burkitt, a surgeon working in Uganda.[174] Subsequent reports documented distinctive clinical and histologic features of the tumor and its surprising response to chemotherapy.[175–177]

Biology and Differential Diagnosis

The histologic appearance of small noncleaved cell lymphoma is unusual in its uniformity. The neoplastic cell is termed *small* noncleaved in contrast to the larger noncleaved cells seen in diffuse large cell lymphoma. The nuclei of the tumor cells in small noncleaved cell lymphoma are larger than those of small lymphocytes. They are round or oval with a slight indentation. The nuclear membrane is prominent and several basophilic nucleoli are often ap-

TABLE 30-21. Chemotherapy for Lymphoblastic Non-Hodgkin's Lymphoma Patients

Reference	Regimen	Evaluable Patients	Complete Response	Frequency of Relapse*	Overall Survival Rate*
167	L2 or L10 or L10M or L17 or L17M	51	40 (78%)	25%	45% (5 y)
168	CHOP + L-asparaginase + methotrexate†	44	42 (95%)	44%	56% (5 y)
169	Variable	34	28 (74%)	60%	22% (5 y)
170	CHOP	25	11 (44%)	—	30% (3 y)
163	APO	21	20 (95%)	42%‡	—
171	Modified LSA^2-L2	15	11 (73%)	36%	42% (4 y)§
172	(CHOP-B or CVP) + XRT (bone marrow–negative)	15	7 (47%)	—	—
172	CODP/6-MP/methotrexate†	13	8 (62%)	—	—

XRT, radiation therapy.
* May be based on actuarial estimates of data.
† Intravenous and intrathecal.
‡ Estimated at 3 years.
§ Based on L10/L17 protocols.

parent. Each cell has a distinct rim of basophilic and intensely pyroninophilic cytoplasm. Numerous mytoses and a starry sky pattern are generally present. The latter is due to macrophages admixed with pale cytoplasm. Although the starry sky pattern is associated especially with small noncleaved cell or Burkitt's lymphoma, it can be seen in other diffuse aggressive lymphomas. These tumors are sometimes divided into Burkitt's and non-Burkitt's subtypes. The distinction between the two is based largely on the larger degree of nuclear variability seen in the non-Burkitt's subtype.

The epidemiology of small noncleaved cell lymphoma is unique in that cases can be divided into endemic or sporadic (American). These two subtypes of small noncleaved cell or Burkitt's lymphoma are said to differ in their association with the Epstein-Barr virus[178] and in their clinical characteristics.[179,180] Both types of small noncleaved cell lymphomas share common cytogenetic abnormalities. Essentially all patients display a translocation involving the site on chromosome 8 where the c-*myc* oncogene is found. The most characteristic translocation is between chromosome 8 and the site of the immunoglobulin heavy-chain locus on chromosome 14, t(8;14)(q24;q32), but translocations between the c-*myc* locus on chromosome 8 and the site of the immunoglobulin-κ light-chain locus on chromosome 2 or the locus coding for the λ light chain on chromosome 22 also occur. In tumors in which the translocation involves an immunoglobulin light-chain locus, it has been proposed that the corresponding immunoglobulin light chain will be displayed on the tumor surface.[181] Almost all tumors classified as small noncleaved cell lymphoma are neoplasms of B cells. Rare cases of T-cell small noncleaved cell lymphoma have been reported.[182] The most common immunophenotype seen in patients with small noncleaved cell lymphoma is listed in Table 30-22.

B-cell acute lymphoblastic leukemia classified in the FAB classification as the L3 subtype is a tumor of cells that closely resemble small noncleaved cell lymphoma. These tumors share the same cytogenetic abnormalities and immunologic characteristics. Although the L3 subtype of acute lymphoblastic leukemia is rare, it has an unusually poor prognosis. Patients with small noncleaved cell lymphoma often have dissemination to the bone marrow, and occasionally distinction between these two illnesses may be difficult and arbitrary.

Clinical Features

Patients with small noncleaved cell lymphoma can present with peripheral adenopathy but often present with sites of extranodal involvement. Patients are more likely to be male than female, and the typical involvement of the jaw seen in African patients is less common in the United States.[183] Patients are especially likely to present with gastrointestinal tract involvement or disease in other intraabdominal sites. Although bone marrow involvement is not seen in most patients at diagnosis, bone marrow is a frequent site of subsequent dissemination. The registry for American Burkitt's lymphoma exists to monitor the clinical characteristics of this illness.[184]

Small noncleaved cell lymphoma is most likely to be confused with other subtypes of aggressive lymphoma seen in young patients, for example, lymphoblastic lymphoma, diffuse large cell lymphoma, and, occasionally, acute lymphoblastic leukemia. The diagnostic difficulties that may be encountered can usually be resolved by consultation with an expert hematopathologist and by documentation of the characteristic chromosomal abnormalities seen in small noncleaved cell lymphoma.

The staging evaluation should be accomplished quickly. Small noncleaved cell lymphoma can progress extremely rapidly. A patient with apparently good prognostic features can quickly become one with a poor outlook. The results of staging evaluations are similar to the distribution seen in other types of diffuse aggressive lymphoma. That is, about half of the patients are predicted to have stage IV disease and another large group to have bulky stage II disease. Only occasional patients have stage I or stage III. Although the Working Formulation study found almost all patients to have systemic symptoms, a larger proportion of patients in the Nebraska study have not had fevers, night sweats, or weight loss.

Treatment and Prognosis

Because small noncleaved cell lymphoma can progress rapidly, with dissemination to the bone marrow and CNS in patients without these findings at diagnosis, prompt initiation of therapy is essential. As with other types of diffuse aggressive lymphoma, the results reported in children have been slightly better than those seen in adults.[185] The role

TABLE 30-22. Small Noncleaved Cell Lymphoma

OTHER NAMES

Undifferentiated, Burkitt's and non-Burkitt's (Rappaport classification)

Small noncleaved follicular center cell (Lukes and Collins classification)

Lymphoblastic, Burkitt's type and other B lymphoblastic (Kiel classification)

Diffuse lymphocytic, poorly differentiated (lymphoblast), non-Burkitt's and Burkitt's tumor (British National Lymphoma Investigation classification)

Burkitt's tumor (WHO classification)

Burkitt's lymphoma (Dorfman classification)

IMMUNOPHENOTYPE

B-cell (99%)

MOST COMMON PHENOTYPE

Positive: sIg, CD10 (CALLA), HLA-DR, CD19 (Leu-12), CD20 (Leu-16), CD22 (Leu-14)

Negative: Cytoplasmic immunoglobulin, TdT, CD25 (TAK)

ASSOCIATED CHROMOSOMAL ABNORMALITIES

t(8;14)(q24;q32); t(2;8)(;q24); t(8;22)(q24;)

DIFFERENTIAL DIAGNOSIS

Lymphoblastic lymphoma, diffuse large cell lymphoma, acute lymphoblastic leukemia

PRESENTING FEATURES

Median age: 30 years (Working Formulation); 34 years (Nebraska)

Stage and Symptoms	Working Formulation	Nebraska
I	13%	0%
II	21%	27%
III	9%	9%
IV	57%	55%
A	14%	45%
B	86%	55%

CLINICAL EVOLUTION

Fastest-growing human neoplasm; rapid dissemination to bone marrow and CNS. Prompt therapy is essential.

TREATMENT APPROACHES

Combination chemotherapy regimen should be used in all patients emphasizing high-dose cyclophosphamide. Initial treatment is frequently complicated by metabolic abnormalities associated with a tumor lysis syndrome.

SURVIVAL

5-year survival, 20% (Working Formulation)

Recent results have shown high rate of survival in children who present with localized disease, but the results remain poor in adults.

of debulking surgery preceding chemotherapy has been debated.[186] Short-term intensive chemotherapy can clearly be curative, and the treatment does not necessarily have to be extended over a long period of time.[186]

Aggressive combination chemotherapy regimens can cure patients with this type of lymphoma. A number of treatment regimens that have been used are listed in Table 30-23. Most regimens depend on comparatively high-dose cyclophosphamide administered early and include prophylactic intrathecal therapy for occult CNS disease. As with lymphoblastic lymphoma, it can be argued that patients with Burkitt's lymphoma present in two important prognostic categories. Patients with bulky tumor, high LDH, and bone marrow or CNS involvement have an especially poor outlook.[179,187,192] It has been proposed that these patients are especially likely to benefit from cytoreductive surgery, when possible, to remove large abdominal masses before the institution of chemotherapy.[193] Appropriately treated patients who present without these bad prognostic findings can be cured in most cases. A potential prognostic factor that does not seem to be important is the distinction between Burkitt's and non-Burkitt's subtypes of small noncleaved cell lymphoma.[185]

Patients with small noncleaved cell lymphoma who fail initial therapy can sometimes be cured with further aggressive chemotherapy. This was the first tumor shown to be curable with autologous bone marrow transplantation after high-dose chemotherapy.[194] Subsequent studies have documented that a significant number of patients can be cured with autologous bone marrow transplantation and that this treatment is more effective when administered early in the course of the disease.[195]

Patients with Burkitt's lymphoma are especially likely to display the acute tumor lysis syndrome with therapy.[196] In one series of 47 such patients, this complication was most likely to occur in patients with bulky tumor. Renal insufficiency, hyperuricemia, hyperkalemia, and hyperphosphatemia are important complications. Adequate pretreatment hydration and the administration of allopurinol are essential in these patients. Even when this is done appropriately, some patients develop life-threatening tumor lysis syndrome, which may require dialysis for control of the metabolic complications.

MISCELLANEOUS LYMPHOMAS

Intermediate Lymphocytic Lymphoma and Mantle Zone Lymphoma

Intermediate lymphocytic lymphoma and mantle zone lymphoma represent the diffuse and follicular growth patterns of neoplasms of the cells of the mantle zone surrounding B-cell follicles in normal lymph nodes. These tumors share characteristics of small lymphocytic lymphomas and lymphomas of the small cleaved cell variety. Patients with the more unusual mantle zone lymphoma tend to have an indolent clinical course,[197] whereas tumors of the diffuse intermediate lymphocytic type have a more aggressive clinical course.[20] The most common chromosomal abnormalities seen in these tumors are the t(11;14)(q22;q32) and trisomy 12, as frequently found in small lymphocytic lymphoma.[21] These tumors appear to have a course that is intermediate between that of small lymphocytic lymphoma and that of diffuse small cleaved cell lymphoma. Durable complete remissions are only rarely induced by chemotherapy. The optimal treatment approach is uncertain. A practical plan in younger patients is to try to induce a complete remission with an intensive chemotherapy regimen. If the patient fails to go into remission promptly (in three or four cycles of treatment) or is if the patient is old or has serious coexistent illnesses, a more cautious approach of judicious use of oral alkylating agents and local radiation therapy is reasonable.

Lennert's Lymphoma

Tumors classified as Lennert's lymphoma usually represent peripheral T-cell lymphomas with a high content of epithelioid histiocytes. This tumor was originally described by Karl Lennert as a variant of Hodgkin's disease.[198,199] Several investigators subsequently identified it as an NHL.[200–204] Lennert's lymphoma usually has been shown to be a variant of peripheral T-cell lymphoma.[205] Tumors

TABLE 30-23. Chemotherapy for Small Noncleaved Cell and Burkitt's Non-Hodgkin's Lymphoma Patients

Reference	Regimen	Evaluable Patients	Complete Response	Frequency of Relapse*	Overall Survival Rates*
187	CHOP + methotrexate†	51	44 (86%)	35%	56% (3 y)
188	Cyclophosphamide	42	34 (81%)	62%	33% (2 y)
189	MCOP + IMVP-16 + ara-C	41	32 (80%)	—	61% (5 y)
190	LNH-84	39	32 (82%)	38%	48% (3 y)
188	CVA + methotrexate‡	31	29 (94%)	31%	41% (2 y)
191	COP + methotrexate	24	22 (92%)	9%	75% (3 y)
192	CHOP + methotrexate + XRT	18	14 (78%)	7%	67% (5 y)

XRT, radiation therapy.
* May be based on actuarial estimates of data.
† Intravenous and intrathecal.
‡ Intrathecal.

classified as Lennert's lymphoma may also be neoplasms of B cells.[206]

The results of therapy in NHLs classified as Lennert's lymphoma probably do not vary from the results of therapy in other diffuse, aggressive NHLs. Patients should be evaluated with staging procedures in a manner analogous to patients with large cell lymphoma. Treatment regimens appropriate for large cell lymphoma should be applied, and if so, long-term, disease-free survival is a possibility.

Ki-1–Positive Lymphoma

Ki-1–positive (Ki-1+) lymphoma represents an unusual form of large cell lymphoma in which the neoplastic cells infiltrate the lymph node sinuses. It is not clear whether these tumors are derived from T cells, B cells, neither, or both. The tumors all have in common the expression of the Hodgkin's disease-related antigen Ki-1.[207] The first reports suggested that this lymphoma is a lymphoma of childhood.[208,209] Subsequent reports have documented that the tumor also occurs in adults.[210] A recent study of 19 patients found that most patients presented with peripheral lymphadenopathy or skin lesions. None had bone marrow involvement. Most cases appeared to be of T-cell origin. The clinical course and response to therapy of these patients are still uncertain. Durable complete remissions have been reported with combination chemotherapy.[209]

Composite Lymphoma

A small proportion of patients diagnosed as having NHL are predicted to have two lymph node biopsies from different sides demonstrating different histologic subtypes of lymphoma. Some cases of composite lymphoma may represent histologic progression of a low-grade lymphoma, whereas others probably are examples of two different lymphomas developing in the same patient. This phenomenon has been reported in from 6% to 9% of patients in large series.[211,212] In at least one case reported in the literature, immunophenotyping showed two different B-cell lymphomas with sufficiently different immunophenotypes (IgG-κ and IgM-λ) to apparently document the simultaneous occurrence of two separate monoclonal proliferations.[213]

The response to therapy and duration of survival in patients with composite lymphoma are potentially affected by the two different lymphomas being present. Patients in whom a low-grade lymphoma and an intermediate- or high-grade lymphoma are both present should probably be treated with an aggressive combination chemotherapy regimen with proven curative potential in large cell lymphomas. Late relapses can be seen, reflecting the natural history of low-grade lymphoma.

True Histiocytic Lymphoma

Diffuse large cell lymphomas in which the malignant cell is derived from histiocytes (macrophages) rather than lymphocytes is an extremely rare tumor.[214] Previous reports suggesting that these tumors occur frequently appear to have been incorrect since newer methods of immunophenotyping have identified many of these tumors as peripheral T-cell lymphomas.[215] These lymphomas need to be differentiated from the histiocytosis X syndromes seen in children,[216] and the hemophagocytic histiocytosis syndromes that are often not malignant.[217]

Peripheral T-Cell Lymphoma

Malignant lymphomas of T lymphocytes that display the immunophenotype of postthymic lymphocytes are often grouped together under the title peripheral T-cell lymphomas (as opposed to lymphoblastic or thymic lymphomas). These lymphomas, depending on one's definition, may include cutaneous T-cell lymphomas and represent about 10% of NHLs seen in the United States. They represent the largest group of T-cell lymphomas seen in the United States.

Peripheral T-cell lymphomas are usually classified in the immunoblastic, diffuse mixed, diffuse small cleaved, or small lymphocytic subcategories in the Working Formulation. They are especially likely to be classified as diffuse mixed cell lymphoma. In a recent study of 134 cases from three different centers in the United States, patients were found to have clinical characteristics much like other diffuse, aggressive NHLs.[104] This study did not find an especially high incidence of skin involvement as has been reported for peripheral T-cell lymphomas by other authors.[218,219] It should be emphasized that classification as a peripheral T-cell lymphoma requires immunophenotyping to have been performed on tumor tissue. Morphologic identification of immunophenotype is inaccurate when correlated with immunologic evaluation.[220]

Patients with peripheral T-cell lymphomas probably have a less favorable response to therapy and survival than patients from the same subgroup in the Working Formulation who have a B-cell immunologic subtype. Although series have been reported in which T-cell lymphomas did as well as B-cell lymphomas,[99,219] most recent reports have found a poorer outlook for patients with peripheral T-cell lymphoma.[221–223] Patients with peripheral T-cell lymphoma who present with stage IV disease have an especially poor outlook.[221]

Non-Hodgkin's Lymphomas in Immunodeficient Patients

A large number of NHLs occur in patients who are severely immunosuppressed. These neoplasms usually represent B-cell, diffuse large cell, or immunoblastic lymphomas and have been associated with a poor prognosis. NHLs have been reported in patients undergoing organ transplantation,[224] inherited immunodeficient states,[225] and the acquired immunodeficiency syndrome (AIDS).[226] These tumors are frequently associated with Epstein-Barr virus.[227] NHLs in the posttransplantation setting are sometimes preceded by polyclonal B-cell hyperplasia.[228] Patients with polyclonal B-cell hyperplasia sometimes improve when the immunosuppressive drugs are removed and acyclovir is administered.[229,230] On the other hand, in patients with established monoclonal lymphomas, the tumors rarely regress without combination chemotherapy. Even with chemotherapy, the outlook is poor.

NHLs in patients with AIDS are representing an increasingly important subgroup of the total group of patients with NHL. These tumors tend to present in extranodal sites and to follow a highly malignant clinical course. Therapy in such patients is often complicated by associated opportunistic infections. Patients in whom the only manifestation of AIDS other than infection by HIV is the development of an NHL should be offered combination chemotherapy. In those patients, durable complete remissions can be seen.[231,232]

Mediterranean Lymphoma

Mediterranean lymphoma manifested by diarrhea, malabsorption, weight loss, abdominal pain, and an extensive, predominantly plasmacytic infiltration involving the small bowel mucosa and mesenteric lymph nodes is probably best thought of as part of the syndrome called *immunoproliferative small intestinal disease.*[233] Affected patients represent a spectrum from those in whom no overt lymphoma can be diagnosed on biopsy to patients with a clear-cut large cell lymphoma in the intestine. Some of these patients have a circulating paraprotein consisting of incomplete α chains without attached light chains. Patients with Mediterranean lymphoma have been referred to as having α-chain disease. Patients with overt lymphoma often have a poor outlook. Treatments range from abdominal radiation and corticosteroids to aggressive combination chemotherapy. Because these patients often present in a debilitated state, the ability to deliver combination chemotherapy may be limited. Durable, complete remissions can be achieved with combination chemotherapy regimens.[233]

SPECIFIC SITES OF INVOLVEMENT BY LYMPHOMA

Gastrointestinal Tract

The most common site of extranodal involvement by NHL is the gastrointestinal tract (Table 30-24). Several reviews have been recently published on this subject.[234–238] When NHL involves the gastrointestinal tract, the most common histologic appearance is diffuse large cell or immunoblastic lymphoma. Nevertheless, any histologic abnormality may be seen. Note that small lymphocytic lymphoma involving the stomach in adults and small noncleaved cell lymphoma involving the small bowel in children are not rare. The most common site of involvement in the gastrointestinal tract is the stomach, with the small bowel and colon, respectively, next in order of incidence. The esophagus is rarely involved by the disease. The association between involvement of Waldeyer's ring and involvement of some more distal part of the gastrointestinal tract is well known. Patients with Waldeyer's ring involvement should be closely evaluated for another site of gastrointestinal lymphoma.[239,240] Conversely, patients who present with involvement of the stomach or small bowel should be evaluated for Waldeyer's ring involement by the same lymphoma.[241]

TABLE 30-24. Special Issues With Involvement of Specific Extranodal Sites by Lymphoma

Site of Involvement	Most Common Histologic Subtype	Special Considerations
Brain	Large cell	Primary brain lymphomas most common in severely immunosuppressed patients (eg, with AIDS after organ transplantation)
Meninges	Lymphoblastic, small noncleaved	With these histologies prophylactic therapy often indicated; with any histology meningeal spread seen with sinus or epidural lymphoma
Orbit	Small lymphocytic	Frequent difficult distinction between benign and malignant infiltrates
Sinus	Large cell	Frequent meningeal spread
Waldeyer's ring	Large cell	Frequent involvement of distal gastrointestinal tract
Lung	Large cell, small lymphocytic	Associated with Sjögren's syndrome
Gastrointestinal tract	Large cell	Frequent Waldeyer's ring involvement; important to resect primary tumor (particularly with small bowel and colon tumors) to avoid perforation or bleeding with initial chemotherapy
Testis	Large cell	Important to irradiate entire scrotal contents

The management of patients with lymphoma involving the gastrointestinal tract involves difficulties both in assigning stage and in choosing therapy. Patients with primary involvement of the gastrointestinal tract with no other sites of involvement would be stage IE, those with the primary site in the gastrointestinal tract and involvement of regional, draining lymph nodes would be stage IIE, but the assignment of stage to patients with involvement of the gastrointestinal tract and more distant lymph nodes is more controversial. I believe that patients with a primary site in the gastrointestinal tract and periaortic or supradiaphragmatic lymph nodes should probably be labeled stage IV rather than stage IIE, thus reflecting widely disseminated disease and bringing attention to the fact that systemic therapy is certainly required.

The initial choice of therapy in patients with involvement of the gastrointestinal tract must be made with the consideration that a rapid response to chemotherapy or radiation therapy may lead to severe hemorrhage or perforation or both. Because of this, it has been widely recommended that the primary tumor be removed surgically before systemic therapy is initiated. Whenever possible, this is a good approach. Some patients present prohibitive operative risks; for others, surgical resection is not technically possible. In patients with gastrointestinal tract involvement, fear of the early complications should not cause potentially curative therapy to be withheld. On the other hand, these patients need to be observed closely because perforation and hemorrhage are not theoretical risks.[237,242] The risk of serious morbidity and death may be greater with involvement of the small bowel and colon than with gastric lesions.

Patients with lymphoma confined to the gastrointestinal tract can theoretically be managed with surgery, radiation, chemotherapy, or a combination of these modalities. Although surgery alone can be curative, it is an unusual patient in whom this is the best initial treatment. For patients with diffuse large cell or immunoblastic lymphoma involving the gastrointestinal tract, a local treatment modality (surgery or radiation) should be combined with an effective combination chemotherapy regimen. In such patients, the likelihood of long-term, disease-free survival is great. The chemotherapy regimen selected should be based on the histologic subtype and not the site of involvement.

Bone

NHL can involve bone primarily through blood-borne metastases or direct extension. Lymphomas that originate in bone used to be called *reticulum cell sarcoma of bone.* A review of more recent literature documents that most patients with primary lymphomas in bone have diffuse large cell or immunoblastic lymphoma—usually of B-cell type.[243,244] The exact histologic appearance of the tumor in bone may have prognostic significance.[245]

The optimal management of patients with an aggressive NHL presenting in bone has been debated in the literature. It has been proposed that young patients with lymphoma in bone do well with chemotherapy only.[246] Also, radiation alone can clearly be curative.[247] After an adequate biopsy has documented the diagnosis of primary lymphoma in the bone, such patients should have an appropriate staging evaluation performed. Patients whose tumor is confined to the bone are candidates for any of the three approaches just listed. Combined-modality therapy seems to have the best results and minimizes the necessity of surgical staging. The chemotherapy regimen should generally be an intensive, multiagent regimen that results in a high cure rate for patients with diffuse large cell and immunoblastic lymphoma. This bone tumor is often seen initially by orthopedic surgeons and frequently reported in their literature.[248]

Heart

Non-Hodgkin's lymphoma is one of the few tumors that may involve the heart. In a recent study, 13 of 150 patients (9%) dying of malignant lymphoma and undergoing autopsy were found to have involvement of the heart or parietal pericardium.[249] Cardiac involvement by lymphoma can be silent clinically. When clinical symptoms are present, they may include dyspnea, chest pain, distended neck veins, other clinical findings of heart failure, and pericardial friction rub. Cardiac involvement generally is a terminal event, although patients with malignant pericardial infusion can be successfully managed. Patients presenting with primary lymphoma of the myocardium are often diagnosed only at autopsy. A recent report suggested that the incidence of cardiac involvement by lymphoma may be increasing and may be especially common in patients with AIDS-related lymphoma.[250]

Kidney

Renal involvement is not infrequent in diffuse NHLs but is rarely seen with follicular lymphoma. It may present as a primary lymphoma in the kidney or as secondary involvement from another primary site.[251] In a recent report, 5% of 175 patients with advanced, disseminated, diffuse aggressive NHL had renal involvement at diagnosis.[252] The diagnosis of renal lymphoma is usually suggested in a patient with renal insufficiency and kidneys found to be enlarged by imaging studies. Intravenous pyelograms should be approached cautiously in such patients; ultrasound examination is probably the preferable study. One study demonstrated that cytologic examination of the urine is frequently positive in patients with involvement of the kidney by lymphoma.[253] Patients with renal lymphoma can usually be managed with combination chemotherapy without resorting to radiation to the kidney. The selection of a treatment regimen should be based on the histologic subtype of lymphoma. In one series, all patients responded and none required hemodialysis, although the cure rate was not high.[252]

Renal failure can be seen in patients with lymphoma secondary to a number of causes. The cause of the renal insufficiency should be identified, since this may affect therapy. Causes include ureteral obstruction with an obstructive uropathy, direct involvement of the kidney by lymphoma,[254,255] nephrotic syndrome associated with a glomerulonephropathy,[256] and paraproteinic nephropathy (myeloma kidney).[257]

Testis

Testicular involvement by NHL is not rare (about 5% of testicular neoplasms) and can be either primary or secondary. Primary testicular lymphoma is most frequently a diffuse large cell or immunoblastic lymphoma with a median age at presentation of over 60 years.[258] In a high percentage of patients with primary testicular lymphoma, the disease apparently is confined to the testicle (stage IE); some of these patients can be cured with radiation therapy alone.[259] Most patients treated only with radiation therapy eventually experience relapse in other sites.[260] A recent report has suggested that the relapse rate can be markedly reduced in patients who receive a brief course of chemotherapy before the application of radiation therapy.[261] The survival was increased from 50% to 93% with three cycles of CHOP chemotherapy preceding radiation therapy. When this treatment approach is used, the extent of staging evaluation can be reduced, and staging laparotomy is definitely not necessary. Remember that radiation therapy fields should include the entire scrotal contents.

Although testicular lymphoma is much more common than involvement of the ovary, the latter can occur. A recent review identified several cases.[262]

Intrathoracic Lymphoma

Patients with NHL frequently present with or subsequently develop involvement of the mediastinum, lungs, or pleura. This occurs less frequently than with Hodgkin's disease.[263] In one series, 10% of the patients presented with primary mediastinal lymphoma.[264] This is especially likely to be seen in patients with lymphoblastic lymphoma but is also seen frequently in patients with diffuse large cell lymphoma. On biopsy, these tumors frequently display marked sclerosis that can obscure the correct diagnosis.[265] Patients who present with prominent mediastinal involvement may possibly develop the superior vena cava syndrome. These patients can be managed primarily with chemotherapy.[266] Although massive mediastinal involvement has been identified as a poor prognostic factor by some investigators, long-term disease-free survival is possible with chemotherapy, sometimes in combination with local radiation.[267]

The diagnosis of NHL primarily involving the lung has been difficult because of confusion among pseudolymphoma, lymphomatoid granulomatosis, and malignant lymphoma. Most patients previously diagnosed as having any of these conditions actually have NHL. Criteria for distinction among these entities continue to be developed.[268,269] One factor leading to confusion is that patients with pulmonary lymphoma have a disproportionately high incidence of small cell tumors when compared with other extranodal sites of lymphoma. Small lymphocytic lymphomas are especially common (sometimes with plasmacytoid differentiation),[270] whereas large cell lymphomas are rare.[271] The survival of patients with primary NHL in the lung is related to the histologic type of the lymphoma.

A rare site of lymphomatous involvement of the lung is endobronchial disease. Affected patients are likely to present with distal pneumonitis and can be recognized with bronchoscopy.[272] Pleural involvement by NHL is not unusual, particularly in patients with advanced disease. Cytologic evaluation can be especially difficult in patients with small lymphocytic lymphoma. The accuracy of diagnosis can sometimes be improved by the use of cytogenetics, molecular biologic studies, or pleural biopsy. Most pleural effusions in this disease are exudates.[273,274] A lymphomatous pleural effusion is best managed by the systemic administration of an effective combination chemotherapy regimen. Where the disease is chemotherapy resistant, the intrapleural instillation of tetracycline or bleomycin in combination with chest tube placement and drainage is often effective.

Thyroid

Although NHL involving the thyroid is not a common disorder, a number of large series have been collected. The disease presents in an older age group than does the more common thyroid carcinomas. Usually an enlarging thyroid mass is seen. Other symptoms such as a sensation of pressure in the neck, dysphagia, hoarseness, or pain may be noted along with enlarged lymph nodes. The most common histologic appearance is diffuse large cell lymphoma.[275] These tumors often occur in a setting of previous chronic lymphocytic thyroiditis.[275] The topic of thyroid lymphomas has been the subject of recent reviews.[276,277]

Management approaches to patients presenting with thyroid lymphoma include surgery, radiation therapy, chemotherapy, and combinations of these approaches. Excellent results have been reported with radiation therapy for localized disease.[278,279] Other investigators have seen poor results with radiation therapy and suggested adjuvant chemotherapy.[280] When combined-modality therapy has been used for localized thyroid lymphomas, results have been excellent except in patients with mediastinal extension.[281] The possibility of hypothyroidism as a late complication of therapy should not be overlooked.

Skin

Non-Hodgkin's lymphoma other than cutaneous T-cell lymphoma frequently involves the skin. Although skin involvement is especially common in peripheral T-cell lymphoma, it is also seen frequently in aggressive B-cell NHL.[221] The distinction among cutaneous T-cell lymphoma, benign lymphoid infiltrate, and other malignant lymphomas in the skin can pose a difficult problem for pathologists.[282] Sophisticated immunophenotyping and molecular biologic studies can sometimes help resolve this problem.[283] In this type of lymphoma with involvement of skin, the most common histologic type is large cell lymphoma.[284]

Unless the disease is localized to only one site in the skin, the primary therapy for patients with cutaneous involvement is likely to be chemotherapy. As with other sites of involvement, patients with apparently localized large cell lymphoma are probably best treated with combined-modality therapy. When aggressive lymphomas involve the skin, they seem to have a particularly good response to therapy.[149,285]

Eye and Orbit

Non-Hodgkin's lymphoma involving the orbit often presents a difficult diagnostic dilemma for the pathologist. These tumors are most commonly small lymphocytic lymphomas of B-cell origin, and the distinction between these and benign small lymphocytic infiltrates (so-called pseudolymphomas of the orbit) can be difficult. Both immunologic studies to document monoclonality and immunoglobulin gene rearrangement studies can be helpful in making this distinction.[286,287] Several large series of patients with these tumors document a generally indolent course.[288,289]

The most common therapy applied to lymphoid tumors of the orbit has been radiation treatment. Because these are usually low-grade lymphomas, cytotoxic chemotherapy regimens generally are not considered to be curative. Radiation therapy is highly effective in eliminating local tumor, but many patients suffer relapse with disseminated disease.[290–292]

Much less common than orbital lymphomas is involvement of the eye itself. This tumor has been called *ocular reticulum cell sarcoma*. The diagnosis is usually made on cytologic examination of cells aspirated from the vitreous. Patients with ocular involvement have a more aggressive course than those with orbital tumors. An important complication of ocular lymphoma is CNS dissemination.[293] It is possible to control intraocular lymphoma with chemotherapy alone when high-dose cytarabine is used.[294,295]

Central Nervous System

Lymphoma can involve the CNS as a solid tumor, in the meninges or an epidural tumor causing spinal cord compression. The latter has a high association with meningeal metastasis. In fact, patients who present with epidural compression should be considered for prophylactic intrathecal therapy.

Meningeal involvement by NHL is especially common in high-grade tumors. Patients with lymphoblastic and small noncleaved cell lymphoma should be considered for prophylactic intrathecal chemotherapy. Unfortunately, a significant number of patients with both histologic subtypes present with meningeal involvement. Meningeal involvement is significantly less likely (but not uncommon) with diffuse mixed, large cell, and immunoblastic lymphoma, and infrequent in the low-grade lymphomas.[296] Some evidence suggests that prophylactic therapy can reduce the incidence of meningeal relapse in high-grade lymphomas.[297,298] Treatment for established meningeal lymphoma is generally unsatisfactory, with most patients dying within 3 months of diagnosis.[299] The most commonly used therapy for meningeal lymphoma is intrathecal methotrexate twice weekly until the cerebrospinal fluid has cleared and then less frequently as maintenance therapy.

The incidence of NHL of the brain appears to be increasing and occurring particularly in patients with AIDS.[300] These patients present with symptoms of brain tumor characteristic for the specific site of involvement. A variety of treatments for these patients have been tried.[300] Although occasional patients are long survivors with cranial radiation therapy with or without associated chemotherapy, the long-term results have been poor with only a small percentage of disease-free survivors. Results have been particularly unsatisfactory in patients with AIDS.

Other Sites of Involvement

Malignant lymphoma has been reported to involve essentially every organ in the body. The most common site not yet dealt with is lymphoma involving the structures of the head and neck. Tumors in these sites, lumped together, make up one of the more common sites of extranodal involvement.[301] Other sites of reported involvement are bone marrow,[302] soft tissue,[303] breast,[304] liver,[305] pancreas,[306] adrenal gland,[307] ovary,[308] uterus and vagina,[309,310] bladder,[311] prostate,[312] and penis.[313]

REFERENCES

1. NCI-sponsored study of classifications of non-Hodgkin's lymphomas: summary and description of a working formulation for clinical usage. Cancer 1982;49:2112.
2. Simon R, Durrleman S, Hoppe RT, et al. The non-Hodgkin lymphoma pathologic classification project. Ann Intern Med 1988;109:939.
3. Jones SE, Butler JJ, Byrne GE, et al. Histopathologic review of lymphoma cases from the Southwest Oncology Group. Cancer 1977;39:1071.
4. Velez-Garcia E, Durant J, Gams R, et al. Results of a uniform histopathologic review system of lymphoma cases: a ten-year study from the Southeastern Cancer Study Group. Cancer 1983;52:675.
5. Ezdinli EZ, Costello W, Wasser LP, et al. Eastern Cooperative Oncology Group experience with the Rappaport classification of non-Hodgkin's lymphomas. Cancer 1979;43:544.
6. Bird CC, Lauder I, Kellett HS, et al. Yorkshire Regional Lymphoma Histopathology Panel: analysis of five years' experience. J Pathol 1984;143:249.
7. NCI Non-Hodgkin's Classification Project Writing Committee. Classification of non-Hodgkin's lymphomas: reproducibility of major classification systems. Cancer 1985;55:91.
8. Warnke RA, Kim H, Fuks Z, et al. The coexistence of nodular and diffuse patterns in nodular non-Hodgkin's lymphomas. Cancer 1977;40:1229.
9. Mann RB, Berard CW. Criteria for the cytologic subclassification of follicular lymphomas: a proposed alternative method. Hematol Oncol 1983;1:187.
10. Byrne GE Jr. Rappaport classification of non-Hodgkin's lymphoma: histologic features and clinical significance. Cancer Treat Rep 1977;61:935.
11. Silverberg E, Boring CC, Squires TS. Cancer statistics, 1990. CA 1990;40:9.
12. Hahn t, Sadamori N, Ozer H, et al. Cytogenetic studies in 77 patients with chronic lymphocytic leukemia: correlations with clinical, immunologic, and phenotypic data. J Clin Oncol 1984;2:1121.
13. Han T, Ozer H, Sadamori N, et al. Prognostic importance of cytogenetic abnormalities in patients with chronic lymphocytic leukemia. N Engl J Med 1984;310:288.
14. Juliusson G, Rober KH, Ost K, et al. Prognostic information from cytogenetic analysis in chronic B-lymphocyte leukemia and leukemic immunocytoma. Blood 1985;65:134.
15. Knuutila S, Elonen E, Teerenhovi L, et al. Trisomy 12 in B cells of patients with B-cell chronic lymphocytic leukemia. N Engl J Med 1986;314:865.
16. Grogan TM, Spier CM, Richter LC, et al. Immunologic approaches of the classification of non-Hodgkin lymphoma. In: Bennett JM, Foon KA, eds. Immunologic approaches to the classification and management of lymphomas and leukemias. New York, Kluwer Academic Publisher, 1988.
17. Hall PA, Richards MA, Gregory WM. The prognostic value of Ki 67 immunostaining in non-Hodgkins lymphoma. J Pathol 1988;154:223.
18. Medeiros LJ, Picker LJ, Gelb AB, et al. Numbers of host "helper" T cells and proliferating cells predict survival in diffuse small-cell lymphomas. J Clin Oncol 1989;7:1009.
19. Mann RB, Jaffe ES, Berard CW. Malignant lymphomas: a conceptual understanding of morphologic diversity. Am J Pathol 1989;94:105.
20. Weisenburger DD, Nathwani BN, Diamond LW, et al. Malignant lymphoma, intermediate lymphocytic type: a clinicopathologic study of 42 cases. Cancer 1981;48:1415.
21. Weisenburger DD, Sanger WG, Armitage JO, et al. Intermediate lymphocytic lymphoma: immunophenotypic and cytogenetic findings. Blood 1987;69:1617.
22. Rai KR, Sawitsky A, Cronkite EP, et al. Clinical staging of chronic lymphocytic leukemia. Blood 1975;46:219.
23. Carbone PP, Kaplan HS, Musshuff K, et al. Report of the Committee on Hodgkin's Disease Staging Classification. Cancer Res 1971;31:1860.
24. Jones SE, Griffith K, Dombrowski P, et al. Immunodeficiency in patients with non-Hodgkin lymphomas. Blood 1977;49:335.
25. Richter MN. Generalized reticular cell sarcoma of lymph nodes associated with lymphatic leukemia. Am J Pathol 1928;4:285.
26. Garvin AJ, Simon RM, Osborne CK, et al. An autopsy study of histologic progression in non-Hodgkin's lymphomas: 192 cases from the National Cancer Institute. Cancer 1983;52:393.
27. Michiels JJ, van Dongen JJM, Hagemeijer A, et al. Richter's syndrome with identical immunoglobulin gene rearrangements in the chronic lymphocytic leukemia and the supervening non-Hodgkin lymphoma. Leukemia 1989;3:819.
28. Van Dongen JJM, Hooijkaas H, Michiels JJ, et al. Richter's syndrome with different immunoglobulin light chains and different heavy chain gene rearrangements. Blood 1984;64:571.
29. Acker B, Hoppe RT, Colby TV, et al. Histologic conversion in the non-Hodgkin's lymphomas. J Clin Oncol 1983;1:11.
30. Armitage JO, Dick FR, Corder MP. Diffuse histiocytic lymphoma after histologic conversion: a poor prognostic variant. Can Treat Rep 1981;65:413.
31. Cullen MH, Lister TA, Brearley RL, et al. Histological transformation of non-Hodgkin's lymphoma: a prospective study. Cancer 1979;44:645.
32. Hubbard SM, Chabner BA, DeVita VT, et al. Histologic progression in non-Hodgkin's lymphoma. Blood 1982;59:258.
33. Young RC, Longo DL, Glatstein E, et al. Watchful-waiting vs aggressive combined modality therapy (Rx) in the treatment of stage III-IV indolent non-Hodgkin's lymphoma. Proc ASCO 1987;6:200.
34. Morrison WH, Hoppe RT, Weiss IM, et al. Small lymphocytic lymphoma. J Clin Oncol 1989;7:598.
35. Portlock CS, Rosenberg SA. No initial therapy for stage III and IV non-Hodgkin's lymphomas of favorable types. Ann Intern Med 1979;90:10.
36. Jones SE, Grozea PN, Miller TP, et al. Chemotherapy with cyclophosphamide, doxorubicin, vincristine, and prednisone alone or with levamisole or with levamisole plus BCG for malignant lymphoma: a Southwest Oncology Group study. J Clin Oncol 1985;3:1318.
37. McKelvey EM, Gottlieb JA, Wilson HE, et al. Hydroxyldaunomycin (Adriamycin) combination chemotherapy in malignant lymphoma. Cancer 1976;38:1484.
38. Anderson T, Bender RA, Fisher RI, et al. Combination chemotherapy in non-Hodgkin's lymphoma: results of long-term followup. Cancer Treat Rep 1977;61:1057.
39. Ezdinli EZ, Pocock S, Berard CW, et al. Comparison of intensive versus moderate chemotherapy of lymphocytic lymphomas: a progress report. Cancer 1976;38:1060.
40. O'Connell MJ, Colgan JP, Oken MM, et al. Clinical trial of recombinant leukocyte A interferon as initial therapy for favorable histology non-Hodgkin's lymphomas and chronic lymphocytic leukemia: an Eastern Cooperative Oncology Group pilot study. J Clin Oncol 1986;4:128.
41. Monfardini S, Tancini G, DeLena M, et al. Cyclophosphamide, vincristine, and prednisone (CVP) versus Adriamycin, bleomycin, and prednisone (ABP) in stage IV non-Hodgkin's lymphomas. Med Pediatr Oncol 1977;3:67.
42. Skarin AT, Pinkus GS, Myerowitz RL, et al. Combination chemotherapy of advanced lymphocytic lymphoma: importance of histologic classification in evaluating response. Cancer 1974;34:1023.
43. Ben-Ezra J, Burke JS, Swartz WG, et al. Small lymphocytic lymphoma: a clinicopathologic analysis of 268 cases. Blood 1989;73:579.

44. Bandini G, Rosti G, Albertazzi L, et al. Allogeneic bone marrow transplantation for chronic lymphocytic leukemia: UCLA Symposium. Mol Cell Biol 1990;137:387.
45. Harrington DS, Yuling Y, Weisenburger DD, et al. Malignant lymphoma in Nebraska and Guangzhou, China: a comparative study. Hum Pathol 1987;18:924.
46. Boring CC, Chan WC, Gregory HR, et al. Increase in high-grade lymphomas in young men. Lancet 1985;1:857.
47. Armitage JO, Sanger WG, Weisenburger DD, et al. Correlation of secondary cytogenetic abnormalities with histologic appearance in non-Hodgkin's lymphomas bearing t(14;18)(q32;q21). J Natl Cancer Inst 1988;80:576.
48. Koduru PRK, Filippa DA, Richardson ME, et al. Cytogenetic and histologic correlations in malignant lymphoma. Blood 1987;69:97:
49. Levine EG, Arthur DC, Frizzera G, et al. There are differences in cytogenetic abnormalities among histologic subtypes of the non-Hodgkin's lymphomas. Blood 1985;66:1414.
50. Yunis JJ, Frizzera G, Oken MM, et al. Multiple recurrent genomic defects in follicular lymphoma: a possible model for cancer. N Engl J Med 1987;316:79.
51. Weiss IM, Warnke RA, Sklar J, et al. Molecular analysis of the t(14;18) chromosomal translocation in malignant lymphomas. N Engl J Med 1987;317:1185.
52. Ramsay AD, Smith WJ, Isaacson PG. T-cell-rich B-cell lymphoma. Am J Surg Pathol 1988;12:433.
53. Winberg CD, Sheibani K, Burke JS, et al. T-cell-rich lymphoproliferative disorders: morphologic and immunologic differential diagnoses. Cancer 1988;62:1539.
54. Nathwani BN, Winberg CD, Diamond LW, et al. Morphologic criteria for the differentiation of follicular lymphoma from florid reactive follicular hyperplasia: a study of 80 cases. Cancer 1981;48:1794.
55. Gattiker HH, Wiltshaw E, Galton DAG. Spontaneous regression in non-Hodgkin's lymphoma. Cancer 1980;45:2627.
56. Horning SJ, Rosenberg SA. The natural history of initially untreated low-grade non-Hodgkin's lymphomas. N Engl J Med 1984;311:1471.
57. Krikorian JG, Portlock CS, Cooney DP, et al. Spontaneous regression of non-Hodgkin's lymphoma: a report of nine cases. Cancer 1980;46: 2093.
58. Rosenberg S. The low-grade non-Hodgkin's lymphomas: challenges and opportunities. J Clin Oncol 1985;3:299.
59. Young RC, Longo DL, Glatstein E, et al. The treatment of indolent lymphomas: watchful waiting V aggressive combined modality treatment. Semin Hematol 1988;25:11.
60. Lawrence TS, Urba WJ, Steinberg SM, et al. Retrospective analysis of stage I and II indolent lymphomas at the National Cancer Institute. Int J Radiat Oncol Biol Phys 1988;14:417.
61. McLaughlin P, Fuller IM, Velasquez WS, et al. Stage I–II follicular lymphoma: treatment results for 76 patients. Cancer 1986;58:1596.
62. Paryani SB, Hoppe RT, Cox RS, et al. Analysis of non-Hodgkin's lymphomas with nodular and favorable histologies, stages I and II. Cancer 1983;52:2300.
63. Paryani SB, Hoppe RT, Cox RS, et al. The role of radiation therapy in the management of stage III follicular lymphomas. J Clin Oncol 1984;2: 841.
64. Kalter S, Holmes L, Cabanillas F. Long-term results of treatment of patients with follicular lymphomas. Hematol Oncol 1987;5:127.
65. McLaughlin P, Fuller IM, Velasquez WS, et al. Stage III follicular lymphoma: durable remissions with a combined chemotherapy–radiotherapy regimen. J Clin Oncol 1987;5:867.
66. Cabanillas F, Rodriguez V, Freireich EJ. Improvement in complete response rate, duration of response and survival with Adriamycin combination chemotherapy for non-Hodgkin's lymphoma: a prognostic factor comparison of two regimens. Med Pediatr Oncol 1978;4:321.
67. Stein RD, Moran EM, Desser RK, et al. Combination chemotherapy of lymphomas other than Hodgkin's disease. Ann Intern Med 1974;81: 601.
68. Rodriguez V, Cabanillas F, Burgess MA, et al. Combination chemotherapy ("CHOP-Bleo") in advanced non-Hodgkin's malignant lymphoma. Blood 1977;49:325.
69. Gilewski TA, Richards JM. Biologic response modifiers in non-Hodgkin's lymphomas. Semin Oncol 1990;17:74.
70. Carabell SC, Chaffey JT, Rosenthal DS, et al. Results of total body irradiation in the treatment of advanced non-Hodgkin's lymphomas. Cancer 1979;43:994.
71. Choi NC, Timothy AR, Kaufman SD, et al. Low dose fractionated whole body irradiation in the treatment of advanced non-Hodgkin's lymphoma. Cancer 1979;43:1636.
72. Johnson RE, Canellos GP, Young RC, et al. Chemotherapy (Cyclophosphamide, vincristine, and prednisone) versus radiotherapy (total body irradiation) for stage III–IV poorly differentiated lymphocytic lymphoma. Cancer Treat Rep 1978;62:321.
73. Portlock CS, Rosenberg SA, Glatstein E, et al. Treatment of advanced non-Hodgkin's lymphomas with favorable histologies: preliminary results of a prospective trial. Blood 1976;47:747.
74. Armitage JO. Bone marrow transplantation in the treatment of patients with lymphoma. Blood 1989;73:1749.
75. Risdall R, Hoppe RT, Warnke R. Non-Hodgkin's lymphoma: a study of the evolution of the disease based upon 92 autopsied cases. Cancer 1979;44:529.
76. Gallagher CJ, Gregorgy WM, Jones AE, et al. Follicular lymphoma: prognostic factors for response and survival. J Clin Oncol 1986;4:1470.
77. Rudders RA, Kaddis M, DeLellis RA, et al. Nodular non-Hodgkin's lymphoma (NHL): factors influencing prognosis and indications for aggressive treatment. Cancer 1979;43:1643.
78. Longo DL, Young RC, Hubbard SM, et al. Prolonged initial remission in patients with nodular mixed lymphoma. Ann Intern Med 1984;100: 651.
79. Glick JH, Barnes JM, Ezdinli EZ. Nodular mixed lymphoma: results of a randomized trial failing to confirm prolonged disease-free survival with COPP chemotherapy. Blood 1981;58:920.
80. Cheson BD, Wittes RE, Friedman MA. Low grade non-Hodgkin lymphomas revisited. Cancer Treat Rep 1986;70:1051.
81. Horning SJ, Weiss LM, Nevitt JB, et al. Clinical and pathologic features of follicular large cell (nodular histiocytic) lymphoma. Cancer 1987;59: 1470.
82. Kantarjian HM, McLaughlin P, Fuller LM, et al. Follicular large cell lymphoma: analysis and prognostic factors in 62 patients. J Clin Oncol 1984;2:811.
83. Glick JH, McFadden E, Costello W, et al. Nodular histiocytic lymphoma: factors influencing prognosis and implications for aggressive chemotherapy. Cancer 1982;49:840.
84. Osborne CK, Norton L, Young RC, et al. Nodular histiocytic lymphoma: an aggressive nodular lymphoma with potential for prolonged disease-free survival. Blood 1980;56:98.
85. Armitage JO. Personal communication, 1986.
86. Gams RA, Rainey M, Dandy M, et al. Phase III study of BCOP v CHOP in unfavorable categories of malignant lymphoma: a Southeastern Cancer Study Group trial. J Clin Oncol 1985;3:1188.
87. Ezdinli EZ, Costello W, Lenhard RE Jr. Survival of nodular versus diffuse pattern lymphocytic poorly differentiated lymphoma. Cancer 1978;41:1990.
88. Al-Katib A, Koziner B, Kurland E, et al. Treatment of diffuse poorly differentiated lymphocytic lymphoma: an analysis of prognostic variables. Cancer 1984;53:2404.
89. Gorin NC, David R, Stachowiak J, et al. Combination of cyclophosphamide, vincristine, and prednisone, followed by maintenance chemotherapy, with and without radiotherapy, in the management of patients with non-Hodgkin's lymphomas. Med Pediatr Oncol 1977;3: 41.
90. Lauria F, Baccarani M, Fiacchini M, et al. Five-year survey of methotrexate, cyclophosphamide (Endoxan), and vincristine (MEV) therapy for advanced non-Hodgkin's lymphomas. Cancer Treat Rep 1978;62: 1193.
91. Skarin AT, Rosenthal DS, Moloney WC, et al. Combination chemotherapy of advanced non-Hodgkin's lymphoma with bleomycin, Adriamycin, cyclophosphamide, vincristine, and prednisone (BACOP). Blood 1977;49:759.
92. Schein PS, Chabner BA, Canellos GP, et al. Potential for prolonged disease-free survival following combination chemotherapy of non-Hodgkin's lymphoma. Blood 1974;43:181.
93. Jones SE, Rosenberg SA, Kaplan HS, et al. Non-Hodgkin's lymphomas. II. Single agent chemotherapy. Cancer 1972;30:31.
94. Foucar K, Armitage JO, Dick FR. Malignant lymphoma, diffuse mixed small and large cell: a clinicopathologic study of 47 cases. Cancer 1983;51:2090.
95. Fisher RI, DeVita VT Jr, Hubbard SM, et al. Diffuse aggressive lymphomas: increased survival after alternating flexible sequences of ProMACE and MOPP chemotherapy. Ann Intern Med 1983;98:304.
96. Koziner B, Sklaroff R, Little C, et al. NHL-3 protocol: six-drug combination chemotherapy for non-Hodgkin's lymphoma. Cancer 1984;53: 2592.
97. Dabich L, Ensminger WD, Zucherman KS, et al. High-dose Adriamycin combination chemotherapy for intermediate and high-grade non-Hodgkin's lymphomas. Semin Oncol 1985;12(Suppl 3):212.
98. Spier CM, Grogan TM, Lippman SM. The aberrancy of immunophenotype and immunoglobulin status as indicators of prognosis in B-cell diffuse large cell lymphoma. Am J Pathol 1988;133:118.
99. Cossman J, Jaffe ES, Fisher RI. Immunologic phenotypes of diffuse, aggressive, non-Hodgkin's lymphomas: correlation with clinical features. Cancer 1984;54:1310.
100. Weiss LM, et al. Large-cell hematolymphoid neoplasms of an uncertain linage. Hum Pathol 1988;19:976.
101. Cabanillas F, Pathak S, Grant G, et al. Refractoriness to chemotherapy and poor survival related to abnormalities of chromosomes 17 and 7 in lymphoma. Am J Med 1989;87:167.
102. Levine EG, Arthur DC, Frizzera G, et al. Cytogenetic Abnormalities predict clinical outcome in non-Hodgkin lymphoma. Ann Intern Med 1988;108:14.
103. Levine AM, Taylor CR, Schneider DR, et al. Immunoblastic sarcoma of T-cell versus B-cell origin. I. Clinical features. Blood 1981;58:52.
104. Armitage JO, Greer JP, Levine AM, et al. Peripheral T-cell lymphoma. Cancer 1989;63:158.
105. Kassan SS, Thomas TL, Moutsopoulos HM, et al. Increased risk of lymphoma in Sicca syndrome. Ann Intern Med 1978;89:888.

106. List AF, Greco FA, Vogler LB. Lymphoproliferative diseases in immunocompromised hosts: the role of Epstein-Barr virus. J Clin Oncol 1987;5:1673.
107. Kant JA, Hubbard SM, Longo DL, et al. The pathologic and clinical heterogeneity of lymphocyte-depleted Hodgkin disease. J Clin Oncol 1986;4:284.
108. Horning SJ, Carrier EK, Rouse RV, et al. Lymphomas presenting as histologically unclassified neoplasms: characteristics and response to treatment. J Clin Oncol 1989;7:1281.
109. Barlogie B, Smallwood L, Smith T, Alexanian R. High serum levels of lactic dehydrogenase identify a high-grade lymphoma-like myeloma. Ann Intern Med 1989;110:521.
110. Vose JM, Harrington D, Sanger W, et al. Cytogenetic abnormalities in Epstein-Barr virus (EBV) associated lymphoproliferative diseases (LDP) do not always signify lymphoma. Proc ASCO 1989;8:252.
111. Armitage JO, Potter JS. Aggressive chemotherapy for diffuse histiocytic lymphoma in the elderly: increased complications with advancing age. J Am Geriatr Soc 1984;32:269.
112. Dixon DO, Neilan B, Jones SE, et al. Effect of age on therapeutic outcome in advanced diffuse histiocytic lymphoma: the Southwest Oncology Group experience. J Clin Oncol 1986;4:295.
113. Solal-Celigny P, Chastang C, Herrera A, et al. Age as the main prognostic factor in adult aggressive non-Hodgkin's lymphoma. Am J Med 1987;83: 1075.
114. Vose JM, Armitage JO, Weisenburger DD, et al. The importance of age in survival of patients treated with chemotherapy for aggressive non-Hodgkin's lymphoma. J Clin Oncol 1988;6:1838.
115. Longo DL, Hapler NJ. Current therapy for diffuse large cell lymphoma. Progr Hematol 1987;14:115.
116. Carde P, Burgers JMV, van Glabbekem J, et al. Combined radiotherapy–chemotherapy for early stages non-Hodgkins lymphoma: the 1975–1980 EORTC controlled lymphoma trial. Radiother Oncol 1984;2:301.
117. Landberg TG, Hakansson LG, Moller TR, et al. CVP-remission maintenance in stage I or II non-Hodgkin's lymphomas: preliminary results of a randomized study. Cancer 1979;44:831.
118. Monfardini S, Banfi A, Bonadonna G, et al. Improved five year survival after combined radiotherapy-chemotherapy for stage I–II non-Hodgkin's lymphoma. Int J Radiat Oncol Biol Phys 1980;6:125.
119. Nissen NI, Ersboll J, Hansen HS, et al. A randomized study of radiotherapy versus radiotherapy plus chemotherapy in stage I–II non-Hodgkin's lymphomas. Cancer 1983;52:1.
120. Jones SE, Miller TP, Connors JM. Long term follow up and analysis for prognostic factors for patients with limited-stage diffuse large-cell lymphoma treated with initial chemotherapy with or without adjuvant radiotherapy. J Clin Oncol 1989;7:1186.
121. Longo DL, Glatstein E, Duffey PL, et al. Treatment of localized aggressive lymphomas with combination chemotherapy followed by involved-field radiation therapy. J Clin Oncol 1989;7:1295.
122. DeVita VT, Chabner B, Hubbard SP et al. Advanced diffuse histiocytic lymphoma, a potentially curable disease. Lancet 1975;1:248.
123. Levitt M, March JC, Conti R, et al. Combination sequential chemotherapy in advanced reticulum cell sarcoma. Cancer 1972;29:630.
124. Coiffier B, Lepage E. Prognosis of aggressive lymphomas: a study of five prognostic models with patients included in the LNH-84 regimen. Blood 1989;74:558.
125. Coltman CA Jr, Dahlberg S, Jones SE, et al. CHOP is curative in thirty percent of patients with large cell lymphoma: a twelve-year Southwest Oncology Group follow-up. In: Skarin AT, ed. Update on treatment for diffuse large cell lymphoma. New York, John Wiley & Sons, 1986: 71.
126. Shipp MA, Harrington DP, Klatt MM, et al. Identification of major prognostic subgroups of patients with large-cell lymphoma treated with m-BACOD or M-BACOD. Ann Intern Med 1986;104:757.
127. Jagannath S, Velasquez WS, Tucker SL. Tumor burden assessment and its implication for a prognostic model in advanced diffuse large-cell lymphoma. J Clin Oncol 1986;4:859.
128. Connors JM, Klimo P. MACOP-B chemotherapy for the treatment of diffuse large cell lymphoma: 1985 update. In: Skarin AT, ed. Update on treatment for diffuse large cell lymphoma. New York, John Wiley & Sons, 1986:37.
129. Gaynor ER, Ultman JE, Golomb HM, Sweet DL. Treatment of diffuse histiocytic lymphoma (DHL) with COMLA (cyclophosphamide, Oncovin, methotrexate, leucovorin, cytosine arabinoside): a 10-year experience in a single institution. J Clin Oncol 1985;3:1596.
130. Armitage JO, Fyfe MAE, Lewis J. Long-term remission durability and functional status of patients treated for diffuse histiocytic lymphoma with the CHOP regimen. J Clin Oncol 1984;2:898.
131. Levine AM, Goldstein M, Meyer PR, et al. Heterogeneity of response and survival in diffuse histiocytic lymphoma after BACOP therapy (bleomycin, doxorubicin, cyclophosphamide, vincristine, prednisone). Hematol Oncol 1985;3:87.
132. Armitage JO, Weisenburger DD, Hutchins M, et al. Chemotherapy for diffuse large-cell lymphoma: rapidly responding patients have more durable remissions. J Clin Oncol 1986;4:160.
133. Cabanillas F, Burgess MA, Bodey GP, Freireich EJ. Sequential chemotherapy and late intensification for malignant lymphomas of aggressive histologic type. Am J Med 1983;74:382.
134. Coleman M, Boyd DB, Beshevkin M, et al. COP-BLAM treatment of large cell lymphoma: a status report. In: Skarin AT, ed. Update on treatment for diffuse large cell lymphoma. New York, John Wiley & Sons, 1986:63.
135. Fisher RI. Personal communication, 1986.
136. Amadori S, Guglielmi C, Anselmo AP, et al. Treatment of diffuse aggressive non-Hodgkin's lymphomas with an intensive multi-drug regimen including high-dose cytosine arabinoside (F-MACHOP). Semin Oncol 1985;12(Suppl 3):218.
137. Gallagher CJ, Copplestone A, Meikle JD, Lister TA. The treatment of disseminated non-Hodgkin's lymphoma of unfavorable histology. Cancer Chemother Pharmacol 1982;8:237.
138. Johnson GJ, Costello WG, Oken MM, et al. Sequential cyclophosphamide-prednisone and vincristine-bleomycin (CPOB): an effective, schedule-dependent treatment for advanced diffuse histiocytic lymphoma. Cancer 1983;52:1133.
139. Garret TJ, Gee TS, Dowling MD, et al. Cyclophosphamide L2 protocol: a combination chemotherapeutic regimen for advanced non-Hodgkin's lymphoma. Cancer Treat Rep 1977;61:7.
140. Sullivan KM, Neiman PE, Kadin ME, et al. Combined modality therapy of advanced non-Hodgkin's lymphoma: an analysis of remission duration and survival in 95 patients. Blood 1983;62:51.
141. Elias L, Portlock CS, Rosenberg SA. Combination chemotherapy of diffuse histiocytic lymphoma with cyclophosphamide, Adriamycin, vincristine and prednisone (CHOP). Cancer 1978;42:1705.
142. Schein PS, DeVita VT Jr, Hubbard S, et al. Bleomycin, Adriamycin cyclophosphamide, vincristine, and prednisone (BACOP) combination chemotherapy in the treatment of advanced diffuse histiocytic lymphoma. Ann Intern Med 1976;85:417.
143. Guglielmi C, Amadori S, Ruco LP, et al. Combination chemotherapy for the treatment of diffuse aggressive lymphomas: F-MACHOP update. Semin Oncol 1987;14:104.
144. Surbone A, Long DL, DeVita VT, et al. Residual abdominal masses in aggressive non-Hodgkin's lymphoma after combination chemotherapy: significance and management. J Clin Oncol 1988;6:1832.
145. Anderson KC, Leonard RCF, Canellos GP, et al. High-dose gallium imaging in lymphoma. Am J Med 1983;75:327.
146. Cabanillas F, Hagemeister FB, McLaughlin P, et al. Results of MIME salvage regimen for recurrent or refractory lymphoma. J Clin Oncol 1987;5:407.
147. Armitage JO, Dick FR, Corder MP, et al. Predicting therapeutic outcome in patients with diffuse histiocytic lymphoma treated with cyclophosphamide, Adriamycin, vincristine, and prednisone (CHOP). Cancer 1982;50:1695.
148. Danieu L, Wong G, Koziner B, Clarkson B. Predictive model for prognosis in advanced diffuse histiocytic lymphoma. Cancer Res 1986;46: 5372.
149. Fisher RI, DeVita VT, Johnson BL, et al. Prognostic factors for advanced diffuse histiocytic lymphoma following treatment with combination chemotherapy. Am J Med 1977;63:177.
150. Todd MB, Portlock CS, Farber LR, et al. Prognostic indicators in diffuse large-cell (histiocytic) lymphoma. Int J Radiat Oncol Biol Phys 1986;12: 593.
151. Coiffier B, Gisselbrecht C, Vose JM, et al. Prognostic factors in aggressive malignant lymphomas: description and validation of a prognostic index that could identify patients requiring a more intensive therapy. J Clin Oncol 1991;9:211.
152. Grogan TM, Lippman SM, Spier CM, et al. Independent prognostic significance of a nuclear proliferation antigen in diffuse large cell lymphomas as determined by the monoclonal antibody Ki-67. Blood 1988;71:1157.
153. Wooldridge TN, Grierson HL, Weisenburger DD, et al. Association of DNA content and proliferative activity with clinical outcome in patients with diffuse mixed cell and large cell non-Hodgkin's lymphoma. Cancer Res 1988;48:6608.
154. Armitage JO, Cheson BD. Interpretation of clinical trials in diffuse large cell lymphoma. J Clin Oncol 1988;6:1335.
155. Starke ID, Wiltshaw E. Sternberg lymphoma: effect of treatment regimen upon prognosis in 38 cases. Br J Haematol 1980;46:351.
156. Childs CC, Chrystal GS, Strauchen JA. Biphenotypic lymphoblastic lymphoma. Cancer 1986;57:1019.
157. Cossman J, Chused TM, Fisher RI, et al. Diversity of immunological phenotypes of lymphoblastic lymphoma. Can Res 1983;43: 4486.
158. Grogan TM, Spier C, Wirt DP, et al. Immunologic complexity of lymphoblastic lymphoma. Diagn Imaging 1986;4:81.
159. Sheibani K, Nathwani BN, Winberg CD, et al. Antigenically defined subgroups of lymphoblastic lymphoma: relationship to clinical presentation and biologic behavior. Cancer 1987;60:183.
160. Weiss IM, Bindl JM, Picozzi VJ. Lymphoblastic lymphoma: an immunophenotype study of 26 cases with comparison to T cell acute lymphoblastic leukemia. Blood 1986;67:474.
161. Murphy SB, Fairclough DL, Hutchison RE, et al. Non-Hodgkin's lymphomas of childhood: an analysis of the histology, staging, and response to treatment of 338 cases at a single institution. J Clin Oncol 1989;7: 186.
162. Dahl GV, Rivera G, Pui C-H, et al. A novel treatment of childhood

lymphoblastic non-Hodgkin's lymphoma: early and intermittent use of teniposide plus cytarabine. Blood 1985;66:110.
163. Weinstein HJ, Cassady JR, Levey R. Long-term results of the AP protocol (vincristine, doxorubicin, [Adriamycin], and prednisone) for treatment of mediastinal lymphoblastic lymphoma. J Clin Oncol 1983;1:537.
164. Wollner N, Exelby PR, Lieberman PH. Non-Hodgkin's lymphoma in children: a progress report on the original patients treated with the LSA2-L2 protocol. Cancer 1979;44:1990.
165. Anderson JR, Wilson JF, Jenkin DT, et al. Childhood non-Hodgkin's lymphoma: the results of a randomized therapeutic trial comparing a 4-drug regimen (COMP) with a 10-drug regimen (LSA2-L2). N Engl J Med 1983;308:559.
166. Hvizdala EV, Berard C, Callihan T, et al. Lymphoblastic lymphoma in children-a randomized trial comparing LSA2-L2 with the A-COP+ therapeutic regimen: a pediatric oncology group study. J Clin Oncol 1988;6:26.
167. Slater DE, Mertelsmann R, Koziner B, et al. Lymphoblastic lymphoma in adults. J Clin Oncol 1986;4:57.
168. Coleman CN, Picozzi VJ, Cox RS, et al. Treatment of lymphoblastic lymphoma in adults. J Clin Oncol 1986;4:1628.
169. Salloum E, Henry-Amar M, Caillou B, et al. Lymphoblastic lymphoma in adults: a clinicopathological study of 34 cases treated at the Institut Gustave-Roussy. Eur J Cancer Clin Oncol 1988;24:1609.
170. Voakes JB, Jones SE, McKelvey EM. The chemotherapy of lymphoblastic lymphoma. Blood 1981;57:186.
171. Levine AM, Forman SJ, Meyer PR, et al. Successful therapy of convoluted T-lymphoblastic lymphoma in the adult. Blood 1983;61:92.
172. Bernasconi C, Brusamolino E, Lazzarino M, et al. Lymphoblastic lymphoma in adults: a study on 30 patients treated with two different programs according to bone marrow findings. Tumori 1984;70:355.
173. Santini G, Coser P, Chisesi T, et al. Autologous bone marrow transplantation for advanced stage adult lymphoblastic lymphoma in first complete remission: a pilot study of the Non-Hodgkin's Lymphoma Co-Operative Study Group (NHLCSG). Bone Marrow Transplant 1989;4: 399.
174. Burkitt D. A sarcoma involving the jaws in African children. Br J Surg 1958;46:218.
175. Burkitt D. Long-term remissions following one- and two-dose chemotherapy for African lymphoma. Cancer 1967;20:1756.
176. Burkitt D, O'Conor GT. Malignant lymphoma in african children. Cancer 1961;14:258.
177. O'Conor GT. Malignant lymphoma in African children. II. A pathological entity. Cancer 1961;14:270.
178. Ziegler JL. Burkitt's lymphoma. N Engl J Med 1981;305:735.
179. Arseneau JC, Canellos GP, Banks PM. American Burkitt lymphoma: a clinicopathologic study of 30 cases. Am J Med 1975;58:314.
180. Philip T, Lenoir GM, Bryan PA, et al. Burkitt-type lymphoma in France among non-Hodgkin malignant lymphomas in caucasian children. Br J Cancer 1982;45:670.
181. Lenoir GM, Preud-Homme JL, Bernheim A, et al. Correlation between immunoglobulin light chain expression and variant transplocation in Burkitt's lymphoma. Nature 1982;298:474.
182. Oliver JD, Grogan TM, Payne CM, et al. Burkitt's-like lymphoma of T-cell type. Mod Pathol 1988;1:15.
183. Saribin E, Donahue A, MacGrath IT. Jaw involvement in American Burkitt lymphoma. Cancer 1982;53:1777.
184. Levine PH, Kamaraju LS, Connelly RR, et al. The American Burkitt's Lymphoma Registry: eight years' experience. Cancer 1982;49:1016.
185. Hutchison RE, Murphy SB, Fairclough DL, et al. Diffuse small noncleaved cell lymphoma in children, Burkitt's versus non-Burkitt's types: results from the Pediatric Oncology Group and St Jude Children's Research Hospital. Cancer 1989;64:23.
186. Short-Term intensive therapy for childhood non-Hodgkin lymphoma. Lancet 1987;1:1410.
187. Magrath IT, Janus C, Edwards BD, et al. An effective therapy for both undifferentiated (including Burkitt's) lymphomas and lymphoblastic lymphomas in children and young adults. Blood 1984;63:1102.
188. Nkrumah FK, Perkins IV, Biggar RJ. Combination chemotherapy in abdominal Burkitt's lymphoma. Cancer 1977;40:1410.
189. Lopez T, Hagemeister F, Velasquez W, et al. Alternating chemotherapy regimens are effective in adult small noncleaved cell lymphoma (SNCCL) both HIV+ and HIV−. Proc ASCO 1989;8:274.
190. Herbrecht R, Coiffier B, Bosly A, et al. Small noncleaved cell lymphomas: clinical study of 39 cases treated with LNH 84 regimen. Proc ASCO 1989;8:261.
191. Sullivan MP, Ramirez I. Curability of Burkitt's lymphoma with high-dose cyclophosphamide: high-dose methotrexate therapy and intrathecal chemoprophylaxis. J Clin Oncol 1985;3:627.
192. Bernstein JI, Coleman CN, Strickler JG, et al. Combined modality therapy for adults with small noncleaved cell lymphoma (Burkitt's and non-Burkitt's type). J Clin Oncol 1986;4:847.
193. Kaufman BH, Burgert EO, Banks PM. Abdominal Burkitt's lymphoma: role of early aggressive surgery. J Pediatr Surg 1987;22:671.
194. Appelbaum FR, Deisseroth AB, Graw RG, et al. Prolonged complete remission following high dose chemotherapy of Burkitt's lymphoma in relapse. Cancer 1978;41:1059.
195. Philip T, Biron P, Philip I, et al. Massive therapy and autologous bone marrow transplantation in pediatric and young adults Burkitt's lymphoma (30 courses on 28 patients: a 5-year experience). Eur J Cancer Clin Oncol 1986;22:1015.
196. Cohen LF, Balow JE, Magrath IT, et al. Acute tumor lysis syndrome: a review of 37 patients with Burkitt lymphoma. Am J Med 1980;68: 46.
197. Weisenburger DD, Kim H, Rappaport H. Mantle-zone lymphoma: a follicular variant of intermediate lymphocytic lymphoma. Cancer 1982;49:1429.
198. Lennert K, Mestdeagh J. Hodgkins disease with a consistently high content of epithelioid histiocyte. Virchows Arch (A) 1968;344:1.
199. Lennert K. Zurhistologichen Diagnoze der Lymphogranulomatose. Frankfurt, Habil-Schraft, 1952.
200. Braylan RC, Long JC, Jaffe ES, et al. Malignant lymphoma obscured by concomitant extensive epithelioid granulomas: report of three cases with similar clinicopathologic features. Cancer 1977;39:1146.
201. Burke JS, Butler JJ. Malignant lymphoma with a high content of epithelioid histiocytes (Lennert's lymphoma). Am J Clin Pathol 1976;66: 1.
202. Hayes D, Robertson JH. Malignant lymphoma with a high content of epithelioid histiocytes. J Clin Pathol 1979;32:675.
203. Kim H, Jacobs C, Warnke RA, et al. Malignant lymphoma with a high content of epithelioid histiocytes: a distinct clinicopathologic entity and a form of so-called "Lennert's lymphoma." Cancer 1978;41:620.
204. Kim H, Nathwani BN, Rappaport H. So-called "Lennert's lymphoma": is it a clinicopathologic entity? Cancer 1980;45:1379.
205. Palutke T. Lennert's lymphoma: a T-cell neoplasm. Am J Clin Pathol 1978;69:643.
206. Spier CM, Lippman SM, Miller TP, et al. Lennert's lymphoma: a clinicopathologic study with emphasis on phenotype and its relationship to survival. Cancer 1988;61:517.
207. Stein H, Mason DY, Gerdes J, et al. The expression of the Hodgkin's disease associated antigen Ki-1 in reactive and neoplastic lymphoid tissue: evidence that Reed-Sternberg cells and histiocytic malignancies are derived from activated lymphoid cells. Blood 1985;66:848.
208. Kadin ME, Sako D, Berliner N, et al. Childhood Ki-1 lymphoma presenting with skin lesions and peripheral lymphadenopathy. Blood 1986;68:1042.
209. Schnitzer B, Roth MS, Hyder DM, et al. Ki-lymphomas in children. Cancer 1988;61:1213.
210. Agnarsson BA, Kadin ME. Ki-1 positive large cell lymphoma: a morphologic and immunologic study of 19 cases. Am J Surg Pathol 1988;12: 264.
211. Fisher RI, Jones RB, DeVita VT, et al. Natural history of malignant lymphomas with divergent histologies at staging evaluation. Cancer 1981;47:2022.
212. Mead GM, Kushlan P, O'Neil M, et al. Clinical aspects of non-Hodgkin's lymphomas presenting with discordant histologic subtypes. Cancer 1983;52:1496.
213. Wolfe JA, Borowitz MJ. Composite lymphoma: a unique case with two immunologically distinct B-cell neoplasms. Am J Clin Pathol 1984;81: 526.
214. Turner RR, Wood GS, Beckstead JH, et al. Histiocytic malignancies: morphologic, immunologic, and enzymatic heterogeneity. Am J Surg Pathol 1984;8:485.
215. Isaacson P, Wright DH, Jones DB. Malignant lymphoma of true histiocytic (monocyte/macrophage) origin. Cancer 1983;51:80.
216. Chu T, et al. Histiocytosis syndromes in children. Lancet 1987;1:208.
217. Reiner AP, Spivak JL. Hematophagic histiocytosis: a report of 23 new patients and a review of the literature. Medicine 1988;67:369.
218. Grogan TM, Fielder K, Rangel C, et al. Peripheral T-cell lymphoma: aggressive disease with heterogeneous immunotypes. Am J Clin Pathol 1985;83:279.
219. Horning SJ, Weiss LM, Crabtree GS, et al. Clinical and phenotypic diversity of T cell lymphomas. Blood 1986;67:1578.
220. Jaffe ES, Strauchen JA, Berard CW. Predictability of immunologic phenotype by morphologic criteria in diffuse aggressive non-Hodgkin's lymphomas. Am J Clin Pathol 1982;77:46.
221. Armitage JO, Vose JM, Linder J, et al. Clinical significance of immunophenotype in diffuse aggressive non-Hodgkin's lymphoma. J Clin Oncol 1989;7:1783.
222. Coiffier B, Berger F, Bryon PA, et al. T-cell lymphomas: immunologic, histologic, clinical, and therapeutic analysis of 63 cases. J Clin Oncol 1988;6:1584.
223. Lippman SM, Miller TP, Spier CM, et al. The prognostic significance of the immunotype in diffuse large-cell lymphoma: a comparative study of the T-cell and B-cell phenotype. Blood 1988;72:436.
224. Penn I. Lymphomas complicating organ transplantation. Transplant Proc 1983;15:2790.
225. Purtilo DT. Opportunistic non-Hodgkin's lymphoma in X-linked recessive immunodeficiency and lymphoproliferative syndromes. Semin Oncol 1977;4:335.
226. Levine AM. Lymphoma in acquired immunodeficiency syndrome. Semin Oncol 1990;17:104.
227. Purtilo DT, Sakamoto K, Saemundsen AK, et al. Documentation of

Epstein-Barr virus infection in immunodeficient patients with life-threatening lymphoproliferative diseases by clinical, virological, and immunopathological studies. Can Res 1981;41:4226.
228. Cleary ML, Warnke R, Sklar J. Monoclonality of lymphoproliferative lesions in cardiac-transplants recipients: clonal analysis based on immunoglobulin-gene rearrangements. N Engl J Med 1984;310:477.
229. Hanto DW, Frizzera G, Gajl-Peczalska KJ, et al. Epstein-Barr virus-induced B-cell lymphoma after renal transplantation. N Engl J Med 1982;306:913.
230. Starzl TE, Porter KA, Iwatsuki S, et al. Reversibility of lymphomas and lymphoproliferative lesions developing under cyclosporin-steroid therapy. Lancet 1984;1:583.
231. Knowles DM, Chamulak GA, Subar M, et al. Lymphoid neoplasia associated with the acquired immunodeficiency syndrome (AIDS). Ann Intern Med 1988;108:744.
232. Lowenthal DA, Straus DJ, Campbell SW, et al. AIDS-related lymphoid neoplasia: the Memorial Hospital experience. Cancer 1988;61:2325.
233. Gilinsky NH, Novis BH, Wright JP, et al. Immunoproliferative small-intestinal disease: clinical features and outcome in 30 cases. Medicine 1987;66:438.
234. Azab MB, Henry-Amar M, Rougier P, et al. Prognostic factors in primary gastrointestinal non-Hodgkin's lymphoma: a multivariate analysis, report of 106 cases, and review of the literature. Cancer 1989;64:1208.
235. Gray GM, Rosenberg SA, Cooper AD, et al. Lymphomas involving the gastrointestinal tract. Gastroenterology 1982;82:143.
236. Haber DA, Mayer RJ. Primary gastrointestinal lymphoma. Semin Oncol 1988;15:154.
237. List AF, Greer JP, Cousar JC, et al. Non-Hodgkin's lymphoma of the gastrointestinal tract: an analysis of clinical and pathologic features affecting outcome. J Clin Oncol 1988;6:1125.
238. Weingrad DN, Decosse JJ, Sherlock P, et al. Primary gastrointestinal lymphoma: a 30-year review. Cancer 1982;49:1258.
239. Hoppe RT, Burke JS, Glatstein E, et al. Non-Hodgkin's lymphoma: involvement of Waldeyer's ring. Cancer 1978;42:1096.
240. Rudders RA, Ross ME, DeLellis RA. Primary extranodal lymphoma: response to treatment and factors influencing prognosis. Cancer 1978;42:406.
241. Saul SH, Kapadia SB. Secondary lymphoma of Waldeyer's ring: natural history and association with prior extranodal disease. Am J Otolaryngol 1986;7:34.
242. Torosian MH, Turnbull ADM. Emergency laparotomy for spontaneous intestinal and colonic perforations in cancer patients receiving corticosteroids and chemotherapy. J Clin Oncol 1988;6:291.
243. Osrowski ML, Unni KK, Banks PM, et al. Malignant lymphoma of bone. Cancer 1986;58:2646.
244. Reimer RR, Chabner BA, Young RC, et al. Lymphoma presenting in bone: results of histopathology, staging and therapy. Ann Intern Med 1977;87:50.
245. Dosoretz DE, Raymond AK, Murphy GF, et al. Primary lymphoma of bone: the relationship of morphologic diversity to clinical behavior. Cancer 1982;50:1009.
246. Haddy TB, Keenan AM, Jaffe ES, et al. Bone involvement in young patients with non-Hodgkin's lymphoma: efficacy of chemotherapy without local radiotherapy. Blood 1988;72:1141.
247. Dosoretz DE, Murphy GF, Raymond AK, et al. Radiation therapy for primary lymphoma of bone. Cancer 1983;51:44.
248. Sweet DL, Mass DP, Simon MA, et al. Histiocytic lymphoma (reticulum-cell sarcoma) of bone: current strategy for orthopaedic surgeons. J Bone Joint Surg 1981;63A:79.
249. McDonnell PJ, Mann RB, Bulkley BH. Involvement of the heart by malignant lymphoma. Cancer 1982;49:944.
250. Gill PS, Chandraratna AN, Meyer BR, et al. Malignant lymphoma: cardiac involvement at initial presentation. J Clin Oncol 1987;5:216.
251. Kandel LB, McCullough DL, Harrison LH, et al. Primary renal lymphoma. Cancer 1987;60:386.
252. Geffen DB, Fisher RI, Long DL, et al. Renal involvement in diffuse aggressive lymphomas: results of treatment with combination chemotherapy. J Clin Oncol 1985;3:646.
253. Cheson BD, Schumann JL, Schumann GB. Urinary cytodiagnostic abnormalities in 50 patients with non-Hodgkin lymphomas. Cancer 1984;54:1914.
254. Glicklich D, Sung MW, Frey M. Renal failure due to lymphomatous infiltration of the kidneys: report of 3 new cases in review of the literature. Cancer 1986;58:748.
255. Trung LD, Sorok AS, Satth AV, et al. Primary renal lymphoma presenting as acute renal failure. Am J Kidney Dis 1987;9:502.
256. Belghit ID, Vernant JP, Hirbec G, et al. A nephrotic syndrome associated with T-cell lymphoma. Cancer 1981;48:1878.
257. Burke JF, Flis R, Lasker N, Simenhoff M. Malignant lymphoma with "myeloma kidney" acute renal failure. Am J Med 1976;60:1055.
258. Doll DC, Wiss RB. Malignant lymphoma of the testis. Am J Med 1986;81:515.
259. Turner RR, Colby TV, Mackintosh FR. Testicular lymphomas: clinical pathologic study of 35 cases. Cancer 1981;48:2095.
260. Martenson JA, Buskirk SJ, Ilstrup DM, et al. Patterns of failure in primary testicular non-Hodgkins lymphoma. J Clin Oncol 1988;6:297.
261. Connors JM, Klimo P, Foss N, et al. Testicular lymphoma: improved outcome with early brief chemotherapy. J Clin Oncol 1988;6:776.
262. Pail AD, Ugu RR, Beraman RM, et al. Malignant lymphoma with primary manifestation in the gonad. Cancer 1980;45:561.
263. Filly R, Blank N, Castellino RA. Radiographic distribution of intrathoracic disease in previously untreated patients with Hodgkin disease and non-Hodgkin lymphoma. Radiology 1976;120:277.
264. Lichtenstein AK, Levine A, Taylor CR, et al. Primary mediastinal lymphoma in adults. Am J Med 1980;68:509.
265. Perrone T, Frizzera AG, Rosa IJ. Mediastinal diffuse large cell lymphoma with sclerosis. Am J Surg Pathol 1986;10:176.
266. Perez-Soler R, McLaughlin P, Valesquez WS, et al. Clinical futures and results from management of superior vena cava syndrome secondary to lymphoma. J Clin Oncol 1984;2:216.
267. Jacobson JO, Eisenberg AC, Lamarre L, et al. Mediastinal large cell lymphoma: an uncommon subset of adult lymphoma curable with combined modality therapy. Cancer 1988;62:1893.
268. Colby TV, Carrington CV. Pulmonary lymphomas: current concepts. Hum Pathol 1983;14:884.
269. Kennedy JL, Nathwani BN, Burke JS, et al. Pulmonary lymphomas and other pulmonary lymphoid lesions. Cancer 1985;56:539.
270. Turner RR, Colby TV, Doggett RS. Well differentiated lymphocytic lymphoma: the study of 47 patients with primary manifestations in the lung. Cancer 1984;54:2088.
271. Koss MN, Hochholzer L, Nichols PW, et al. Primary non-Hodgkin lymphoma and pseudolymphoma of the lung. Hum Pathol 1983;14:1024.
272. Ros RM, Grigas D, Strattemeir E, et al. Endobronchial involvement with non-Hodgkin lymphoma. Cancer 1986;57:1750.
273. Weick JK, Keilly JM, Harrison EG, et al. Pleural effusions in lymphoma. Cancer 1973;31:848.
274. Xaube TA, Diumenjo MC, Montserrat E, et al. Characteristics in prognostic value of pleural effusions in non-Hodgkin lymphomas. Eur J Respir Dis 1985;66:135.
275. Burke JS, Butler JJ, Fuller IM. Malignant lymphomas of the thyroid. Cancer 1977;38:1587.
276. Hamburger JI, Miller JM, Kini SR. Lymphoma of the thyroid. Ann Intern Med 1983;99:685.
277. Oertel JE, Heffess CS. Lymphoma of the thyroid and related disorders. Semin Oncol 1987;14:333.
278. Blair TJ, Evans RG, Buskirk SJ, et al. Radiotherapeutic management of primary thyroid lymphoma. Int J Radiat Oncol Biol Phys 1985;11:365.
279. Chak LY, Hoppe RT, Burke JS, Kaplan HS. Non-Hodgkin lymphoma presenting as thyroid enlargement. Cancer 1981;48:2712.
280. Tupchong L, Hughes F, Harmar CL. Primary lymphoma of the thyroid: clinical features, prognostic factors, and results of treatment. Int J Radiat Oncol Biol Physics 1986;12:1813.
281. Vigliotti A, Fuller LM, Valasquez WS, et al. Thyroid lymphomas stages IE and IIE: comparative results for radiotherapy only, combination chemotherapy only, and multimodality treatment. Int J Radiat Oncol Biol Phys 1986;12:1807.
282. Evan HL, Winklemann RK, Banks PM. Differential diagnosis of malignant and benign cutaneous lymphoid infiltrates. Cancer 1979;44:699.
283. Wood GS, Burke JS, Horning S, et al. The immunologic and clinicopathologic heterogeneity of cutaneous lymphomas other than mycosis fungoides. Blood 1983;62:464.
284. Burke JS, Hoppe RT, Cibull ML, Dorfman RF. A cutaneous malignant lymphoma: a pathologic study of 50 cases with clinical analysis of 37. Cancer 1981;47:300.
285. Willemzer, Meijercj IM, Scheffer E, et al. Diffuse large cell lymphomas of follicular center cell origin presenting in the skin. Am J Pathol 1987;126:325.
286. Neri A, Jakobiec FA, Pelicci PG, et al. Immunoglobulin T-cell receptor beta chain rearrangement analysis of ocular adnexal lymphoid neoplasms: clinical and biologic implications. Blood 1987;70:1519.
287. Turner RR, Egbert TP, Warnke RA. Lymphocytic infiltrates with a conjunctiva and orbit: immunohistochemical standing of 16 cases. Am J Clin Pathol 1984;81:477.
288. Ellis JH, Banks PM, Campbell RJ, Liesegang TJ. Lymphoid tumors of the ocular adnexa. Ophthalmology 1985;92:1311.
289. Harris ML, Harmon DC, Pilch BZ et al. Immunohistological diagnosis of orbital lymphoid infiltrates. Am J Surg Pathol 1984;8:83.
290. Austin-Seymour MM, Donaldson SS, Egbert PR, et al. Radiotherapy of lymphoid diseases of the orbit. Int J Radiat Oncol Biol Phys 1985;11:371.
291. Barthold HJ, Harvey A, Marcoe AM, et al. Treatment of orbital pseudotumors and lymphoma. Am J Clin Oncol 1986;9:527.
292. Fitzpatrick PJ, Mack OS. Lymphoid tumors of the orbit. Int J Radiat Oncol Biol Phys 1984;10:333.
293. Char DH, Ljung BM, Miller T, Philips T. Primary interocular lymphoma (ocular reticulum cell sarcoma) diagnosis and management. Ophthalmology 1988;95:625.
294. Baumann MA, Ritch PS, Hande KR, et al. Treatment of intraocular lymphoma with high-dose ara-C. Cancer 1986;57:1273.
295. Strauchen JA, Dalton J, Friedman AH. Chemotherapy in the management of intraocular lymphoma. Cancer 1989;63:1918.

296. Ersboll LJ, Schultz HB, Thomsen BLR, et al. Meningeal involvement in non-Hodgkin lymphoma: symptoms, incidence, risk factors and treatment. Scand J Haematol 1985;35:487.
297. Nkrumah FK, Neequaye JE, Biggar R. Intrathecal chemoprophylaxis in the prevention of central nervous system relapse in Burkitt lymphoma. Cancer 1985;56:239.
298. Perez-Soler R, Smith TL, Cabanillas S. Central nervous system prophylaxis with combined intravenous intrathecal methotrexate in diffuse lymphoma of aggressive histologic type. Cancer 1986;57:971.
299. Young RC, Howser DM, Anderson T, et al. Central nervous system complications of non-Hodgkin lymphoma. Am J Med 1979;66:435.
300. Deangelis LM, Yahalom J, Rosenblum M, Posner JB. Primary CNS lymphoma: managing patients with spontaneous and AIDS-related disease. Oncology 1987;1:52.
301. Jacobs C. Lymphomas of extranodal head and neck sites. In: Jacobs C, ed. Cancers of the head and neck. Boston, Martinus Nijhoff, 1987.
302. McKenna RW, Hernandez JA. Bone marrow and malignant lymphoma. Hematol Oncol Clin North Am 1988;2:617.
303. Lanham GR, Weiss SW, Ensinjenzinger FM. Malignant lymphoma: a study of 75 cases presenting in soft tissue. Am J Surg Pathol 1989;13:1.
304. Brustein S, Kimmel M, Lieberman, et al. Malignant lymphoma of the breast: study of 53 patients. Ann Surg 1987;205:144.
305. Osborne BM, Butler JJ, Guarda LA. Primary lymphoma of the liver. Cancer 1985;56:2902.
306. Webb TH, Lillemoe KD, Pitt HA, et al. Pancreatic lymphoma. Ann Surg 1989;209:25.
307. Harris GJ, To FO, VonHoff DD. Primary adrenal lymphoma. Cancer 1989;63:799.
308. Fox H, Langley FA, Govan ADT, et al. Malignant lymphoma presenting as an ovarian tumor: a clinicopathological analysis of 34 cases. Br J Obstet Gynecol 1988;95:386.
309. Harris NL, Scully RE. Malignant lymphoma and granulocytic sarcoma of the uterus and vagina. Cancer 1984;52:2530.
310. Komaki R, Cox JD, Hanson RM, et al. Malignant lymphoma of the uterine cervix. Cancer 1984;54:1699.
311. Forrest JB, Saypol DC, Mills SE, Gillenwater JY. Immunoblastic sarcoma of the bladder. J Urol 1983;130:350.
312. Bostwick DG, Mann RB. Malignant lymphoma involving a prostate. Cancer 1985;56:2932.
313. Marks D, Crosthwit EA, Vairogos G, et al. Therapy of primary diffuse large cell lymphoma of the penis with preservation of function. J Urol 1988;139:1057.

Blood: Principles and Practice of Hematology,
edited by Robert I. Handin, Thomas P. Stossel, and Samuel E. Lux.
J.B. Lippincott Company, Philadelphia © 1995.

31

Plasma Cell Diseases and Related Disorders

Lawrence N. Shulman

This chapter deals with three diseases that are characterized by the production of monoclonal immunoglobulins. Two of these diseases, multiple myeloma and Waldenström's macroglobulinemia, are clearly malignant diseases of clonal lymphocytes that have destructive effects on host organs and frequently cause death. In *multiple myeloma,* the malignant cell resembles a plasma cell, and immunoglobulins of the IgG, IgA, or IgD class are usually produced; occasionally, only free light chains are produced. *Waldenström's macroglobulinemia* is a clonal malignancy in which cells described as "plasmacytoid lymphocytes" produce IgM immunoglobulins. The clinical manifestations of these diseases are discussed later in this chapter.

In the third disease, *benign monoclonal gammopathy,* a monoclonal immunoglobulin is produced without clinical manifestations of either multiple myeloma or macroglobulinemia. In some instances, benign monoclonal gammopathy is an early stage of either multiple myeloma or macroglobulinemia, and the evolution into one of these diseases occurs with time. In other circumstances, no progression to a clearly malignant disease is apparent, and the significance of the monoclonal gammopathy is not known.

EVALUATION OF A MONOCLONAL IMMUNOGLOBULIN

When a monoclonal gammopathy is suspected, the first test to be performed is the serum protein electrophoresis (see Chap. 15). This must be performed on serum rather than plasma, because the peak from free unclotted fibrinogen can confuse the interpretation of the electrophoresis. When serum is run on an electrophoretic gel, a sharp peak occurs at the anodal end representing albumin, as shown in Figure 31-1. Moving toward the cathode, albumin is followed by the α_1-globulin peak, the α_2-globulin region, the β-globulin region, and finally the γ-globulin region. Most immunoglobulins travel in the γ-globulin region, but some travel in the β-globulin region. Other major serum components accounting for the various peaks are also shown in Figure 31-1. In the normal state, a low broad band is seen in the γ-globulin region representing normal amounts of polyclonal immunoglobulin. In inflammatory conditions such as hepatitis and other chronic infections, a polyclonal increase in immunoglobulins can occur, as shown in Figure 31-2. The γ-globulin peak is increased but is diffuse and broad. In a patient with a monoclonal immunoglobulin, a sharp peak occurs in the γ-globulin region, as shown in Figure 31-3. This result indicates that a monoclonal immunoglobulin is present but does not characterize the type or quantity of monoclonal immunoglobulin.

The techniques commonly used to characterize monoclonal immunoglobulins are immunoelectrophoresis and immunofixation. Both methods rely on the use of monospecific antibodies directed against either the heavy chain that determines the class of immunoglobulin (IgG, IgA, IgD, IgM, IgE) or against the light chains (κ and λ). With these techniques, the specific type of immunoglobulin (for instance, IgG-κ or IgM-λ) can be identified. Figure 31-4 shows immunofixation demonstrating monoclonal immunoglobulin. The monoclonal protein can also be quantitated, which becomes essential in evaluating the monoclonal gammopathies (as will be discussed later).

In some cases of benign monoclonal gammopathy and myeloma, only light chains are produced and no heavy chains can be detected. Light chains are small and readily filtered by the renal glomerulus. As a result, they are rarely found in the serum in significant amounts. Since the quantity of normal polyclonal immunoglobulins is often reduced in the serum in myeloma, when light-chain monoclonal gammopathy is present, the γ-globulin peak of the serum protein electrophoresis is reduced and flat, as shown in Figure 31-5. In this case, the urine should be analyzed and the monoclonal light chain confirmed on protein electrophoresis. Characterization can be carried out as in the serum with either an immunoelectrophoresis or immunofixation.

BENIGN MONOCLONAL GAMMOPATHY

As early as the 1950s, it was recognized that some patients had monoclonal immunoglobulins in their serum without any manifestations of either multiple myeloma or macroglobulinemia. The significance of these immunoglobulins was not known. In the 1960s and 1970s, a more systematic study of these patients was presented.[1] Monoclonal immunoglobulins can be found incidentally in about 3% of a randomly chosen, apparently healthy population.[2] With increasing age, the incidence of unsuspected monoclonal immunoglobulins in the population increases. A study of unselected retirement home residents showed a greater than 10% incidence of monoclonal immunoglobulin in patients 80 years and older.[3]

Initially, it was not clear whether the incidentally discovered monoclonal immunoglobulin was an insignificant finding or whether myeloma or macroglobulinemia would develop with time. In 1978, Kyle[4] reported a follow-up of

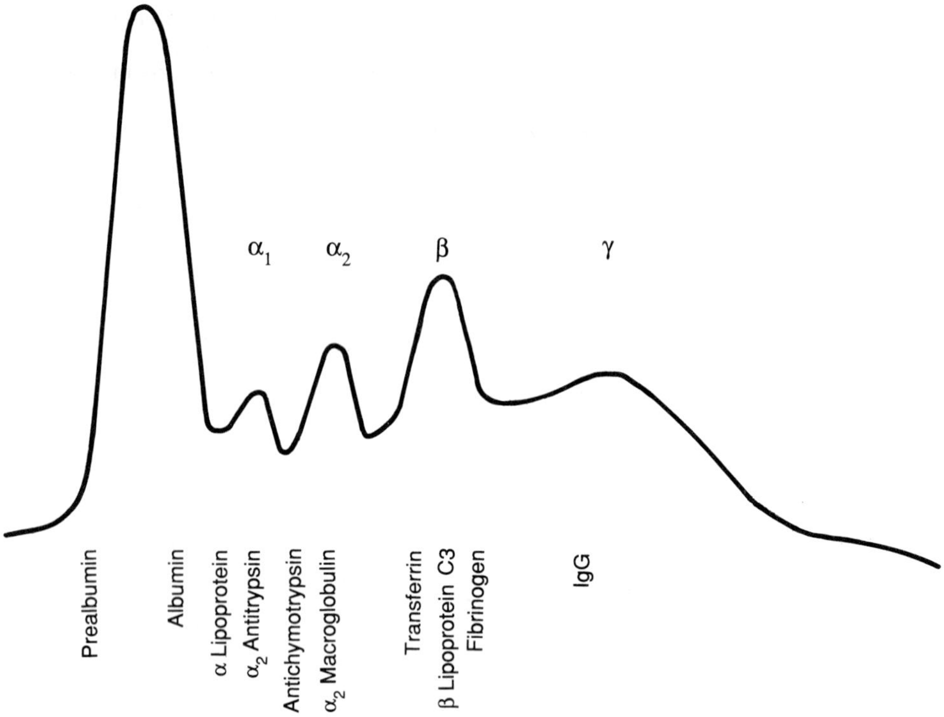

FIGURE 31-1. The normal serum protein electrophoresis. Constituents of the different peaks are listed below them. Immunoglobulins generally travel in the γ-globulin peak but occasionally occur in the β-globulin peak.

241 patients who were initially thought to have a benign monoclonal gammopathy. He demonstrated that these monoclonal gammopathies were not always benign and sometimes developed into overt myeloma or macroglobulinemia. *Monoclonal gammopathy of undetermined significance* was suggested as a better term to describe the clinical implications of these immunoglobulins. In this group of patients, 75% had IgG monoclonal proteins, 10% IgA, and 15% IgM. The mean level of immunoglobulin was 1.8 g/dL. When followed up for a minimum of 5 years and a median of 19 years, 24% of patients had no significant increase in immunoglobulin level and remained alive and well.[5] In 22%, myeloma or macroglobulinemia was found. Three percent of the patients had more than a 50% increase in their immunoglobulins without evidence of malignancy. An additional 51% of patients died from other causes without developing a malignant disease related to their monoclonal gammopathy. As shown in Figure 31-6, a slow and progressive conversion to overt malignant disease occurs, but most patients do not develop myeloma or macroglobulinemia, possibly because many are elderly and die of comorbid disease before the development of these diseases and possibly because their disease is truly benign.

Kyle[6] updated the status of these 241 patients in 1993, and little had changed from the original report. With a minimum of 20 and a maximum of 35 years of follow-up, 19% had no significant increase in the serum or urine monoclonal protein, 10% had increases in the monoclonal protein to 3 g/dL or higher without evidence of clinical disease, 47% had died of unrelated causes, and 24% (as compared with 22% in the original report) developed myeloma, macroglobulinemia, amyloidosis, or related disease.

Blade and colleagues[7] reported on 128 patients with monoclonal gammopathy of undetermined significance

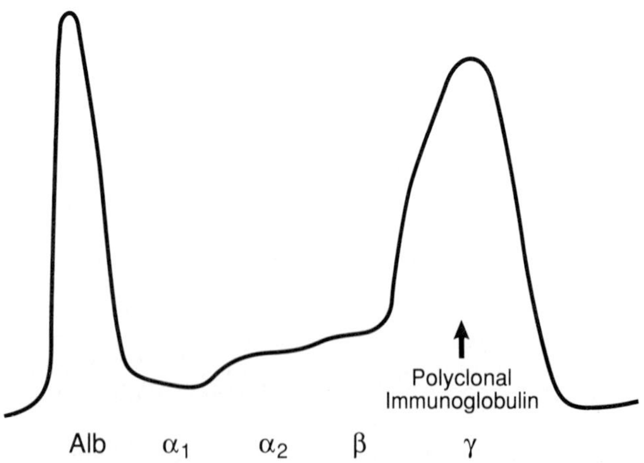

FIGURE 31-2. Serum protein electrophoresis with a polyclonal increase in immunoglobulins as might occur with chronic inflammatory diseases such as chronic hepatitis.

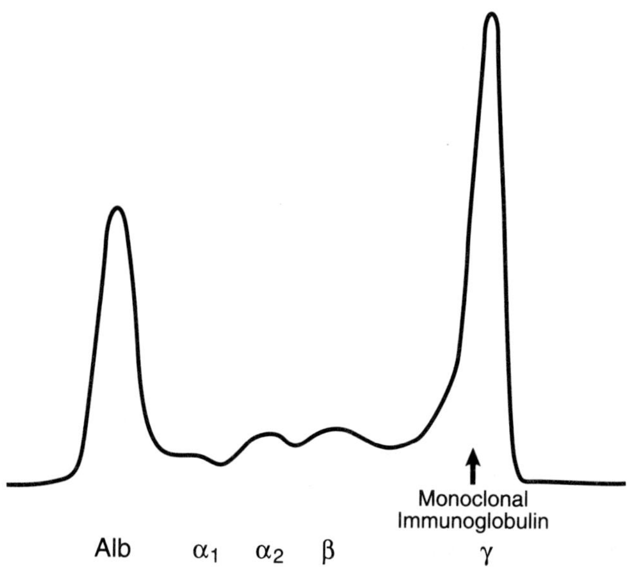

FIGURE 31-3. Serum protein electrophoresis with a monoclonal immunoglobulin. The sharp peak in the γ-globulin region denotes the presence of the monoclonal immunoglobulin but does not identify the type (eg, IgG, IgM), the light-chain specificity (κ or λ), or serum concentration of the immunoglobulin.

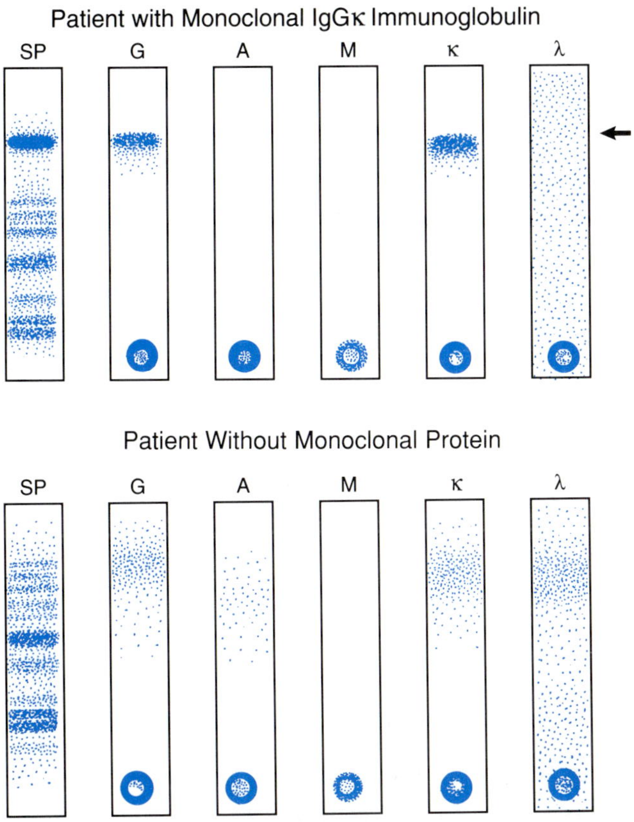

FIGURE 31-4. Immunofixation performed on serum from a patient with a monoclonal IgG κ immunoglobulin and a patient without a monoclonal protein.

observed for a median of 56 months. In this series, the monoclonal protein remained unchanged in 79% of patients, 11% died of unrelated causes, and 10% progressed to myeloma, amyloidosis, or macroglobulinemia. The actuarial risk of developing a malignant disease at 10 years was 19% in this series, similar to the data reported by Kyle.

Evaluation of the Patient With Suspected Benign Monoclonal Gammopathy

Patients who are incidentally found to have monoclonal immunoglobulins should be carefully evaluated for myeloma or macroglobulinemia. The basic approach is to look for indications of malignancy with involvement of visceral organs, electrolyte disturbances, or histologic confirmation. The specific approach depends on whether the monoclonal immunoglobulin is IgG, IgA, IgD (in which case multiple myeloma should be ruled out), or IgM (in which case macroglobulinemia should be ruled out). Clinical features that should be investigated are listed in Table 31-1.

In an IgG, IgA, or IgD monoclonal gammopathy, the patient should be investigated for signs of myeloma. The actual level of the immunoglobulin is important in the evaluation. In the Mayo Clinic series, the average level of monoclonal immunoglobulin in patients with monoclonal gammopathy of undetermined significance was less than 2 g/dL.[4] The higher the monoclonal immunoglobulin, the more likely it represents a manifestation of malignancy. The presence of hypercalcemia or lytic bone lesions is suggestive of myeloma and is not usually compatible with monoclonal gammopathy of undetermined significance. Renal impairment without other known cause may also indicate that the patient has myeloma, although reports exist of patients whose renal failure probably resulted from their monoclonal immunoglobulin (or light chain) but who had no other manifestations of myeloma.

In myeloma patients, although an increased level of monoclonal immunoglobulin is present, generally a reduction in the level of the normal polyclonal immunoglobulins is found. The levels of normal immunoglobulins were once thought to be a good indication of whether the patient has benign monoclonal gammopathy or true myeloma and patients with benign monoclonal gammopathy were thought to have normal levels of the normal polyclonal immunoglobulins. In the Mayo Clinic series, about 20% of patients with apparent monoclonal gammopathy of undetermined significance had reduced levels of normal immunoglobulins. In addition, the presence of reduced levels of normal immunoglobulins did not predict whether the patient would develop overt myeloma during the follow-up period.[4]

Evaluation of histologic findings of the bone marrow for plasma cells can sometimes help the clinician to distinguish between benign monoclonal gammopathy and myeloma, but findings can often be difficult to interpret and the aid of an experienced hematopathologist is helpful in difficult cases. Plasma cells are present in small numbers in the normal bone marrow and increase in number with the increasing age of the patient. The actual number of plasma cells found in the bone marrow is not always indicative of the presence or absence of myeloma. Reactive plasmacy-

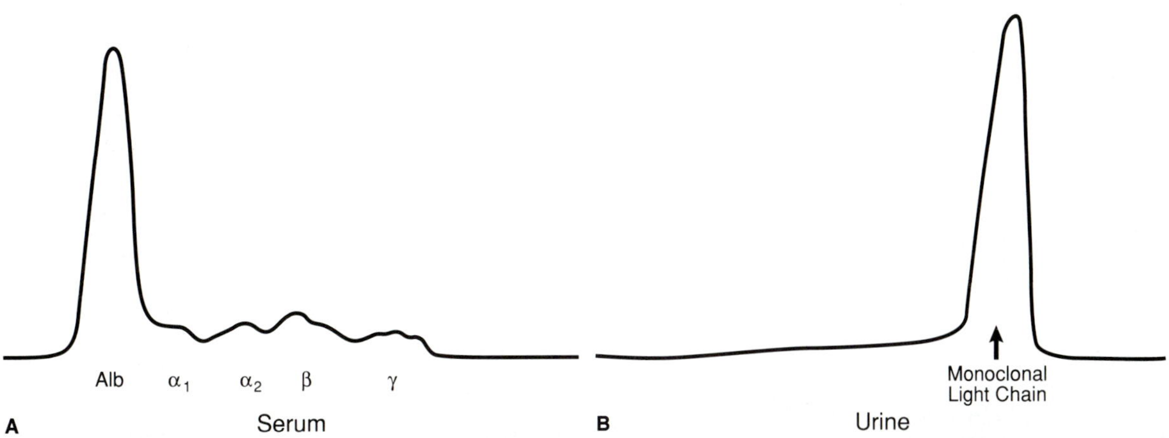

FIGURE 31-5. (**A**) Serum protein electrophoresis from a patient with light-chain myeloma. No monoclonal peak is seen, and a decrease has occurred in the normal immunoglobulins, leading to a flattening of the γ-globulin peak. (**B**) Protein electrophoresis performed on urine from the same patient shows a peak representing the monoclonal light chain produced by the myeloma cells.

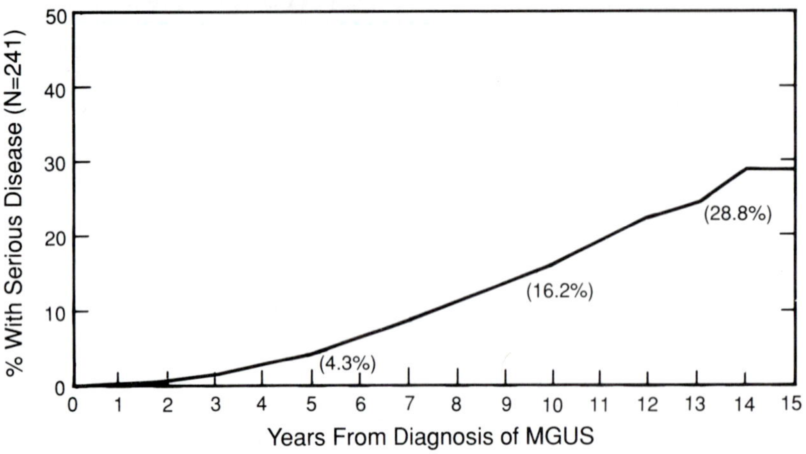

FIGURE 31-6. For patients with monoclonal gammopathy of undetermined significance (MGUS), the likelihood of developing multiple myeloma, macroglobulinemia, amyloidosis, or lymphoproliferative disease after the discovery of the monoclonal protein is shown. Actuarial analysis percentages for conversion to one of these diseases are given for 5, 10, and 15 years. (After Kyle RA. Benign monoclonal gammopathy: a misnomer. JAMA 1984;251:1849)

tosis can occur in response to chronic infections and inflammatory diseases. In reactive plasmacytosis, the plasma cells are dispersed throughout the normal hematopoietic elements and are polyclonal for expression of λ and κ light chains. Aggregates of plasma cells in the bone marrow core biopsy are suggestive of myeloma, even if the percentage of plasma cells of the total bone marrow cellularity is not great. In addition, if the plasma cells are undifferentiated or plasmablastic, myeloma is likely. Reactive and benign plasma cells appear mature and well differentiated. Examples of these morphologies are shown in the section on multiple myeloma.

In a patient with monoclonal IgM immunoglobulin, macroglobulinemia must be ruled in or out. Hypercalcemia and lytic bone lesions are usually not present in this disease, and renal disease is uncommon. Lymphadenopathy and splenomegaly are often present and can be diagnostic. Lymph node findings (described in detail later in the chapter) usually show effacement of the normal architecture with monoclonal B cells of the lymphoplasmacytic type. A bone marrow biopsy may show the same findings.

TABLE 31-1. Evaluation of the Patient With Monoclonal Gammopathy of Undetermined Significance (MGUS)

FOR IgG, IgA, IgD: RULE OUT MULTIPLE MYELOMA
Serum or urine monoclonal protein—high levels of either, suggestive of myeloma
Radiographs—osteolytic lesions or severe osteopenia suggestive of myeloma
Hematocrit and platelet count—usually normal in MGUS; anemia and thrombocytopenia suggestive of myeloma
Serum calcium level—normal in MGUS, possibly elevated in myeloma
Serum creatinine level—almost always normal in MGUS, possibly normal or elevated in myeloma
Bone marrow aspirate and biopsy—plasmacytosis over 20%, plasmablast morphology or plasma cells occurring in aggregates on core biopsy sample suggestive of myeloma
FOR IgM: RULE OUT WALDENSTRÖM'S MACROGLOBULINEMIA
Serum IgM—levels higher than 3 g/dL suggestive of macroglobulinemia
Lymphadenopathy and splenomegaly—presence suggestive of macroglobulinemia. Lymph node biopsy—lymphoplasmacytic lymphoma diagnostic of macroglobulinemia
Bone marrow biopsy—presence of aggregates of lymphoplasmacytic lymphoma cells diagnostic of macroglobulinemia

Even after the evaluations just recommended are performed, it is often difficult to be sure of the patient's present status and future prognosis. Therefore, counseling patients with apparent benign monoclonal gammopathy is often difficult. Most patients remain well, particularly the elderly, who have only a few years at risk for the development of malignancy. Patients are forced to live with an uncertainty, however, knowing that they are at risk for the development of a serious and potentially fatal disease.

Follow-up of Patients With Benign Monoclonal Gammopathy

Because of the uncertain prognosis of patients with benign monoclonal gammopathy, every patient should be considered at risk for developing myeloma or macroglobulinemia. Close follow-up is essential to diagnose progression to malignancy before serious organ compromise develops such as renal failure and pathologic fractures.

MULTIPLE MYELOMA

History

In 1845, a 45-year-old man from London named Thomas Alexander McBean was seen in consultation by Dr. William MacIntyre.[8] Dr. MacIntyre was immediately struck by the fact that severe bone pain was a cardinal feature of this patient's disease, and he was later able to show that pathologic fractures were also present. MacIntyre was also the first to discover the unusual properties of the urinary protein excreted by this patient. On heating the urine, protein was seen initially to precipitate then to redissolve at higher temperatures. On cooling, the protein again precipitated. MacIntyre sent specimens of the urine to Dr. Henry Bence Jones, who confirmed his observations and received credit for the description. When the patient died, the cause of death was listed as "atrophy from albuminuria." This was not entirely misleading because at the time *albuminuria* was a term used to describe any proteinuric syndrome. The autopsy revealed that the bone marrow had been replaced by a gelatinous material, leaving the bones weak and brittle. Microscopic examination by Dr. John Dalrymple was remarkable for a description of what was certainly single and multinucleate plasma cells. They wondered why the tumor was confined to the bones without extraosseous extension.

Definition

Multiple myeloma is a malignant proliferation of clonal plasma cells, usually associated with the production of a complete or incomplete monoclonal immunoglobulin. As described in the previous section, clonal plasma cell proliferation can be present with production of monoclonal immunoglobulin characterized as benign monoclonal gammopathy and not myeloma. Therefore, both clonal plasma cell proliferation and manifestations of malignant behavior of the plasma cells need to be seen to verify that myeloma is present.

The National Cancer Institute published a proposed set of diagnostic criteria in 1973 in an attempt to standardize eligibility criteria for the entry of patients into chemotherapy trials for myeloma. These criteria are outlined in Table 31-2. Some areas are still open to interpretation, such as what constitutes a chronic inflammatory disease. Patients who have early myeloma may not meet these criteria. The authors state, "A few patients who do not meet these criteria may eventually prove to have myeloma: however, until these criteria are satisfied the diagnosis will be uncertain. They should not be entered into therapeutic trials."[9]

The cardinal features of multiple myeloma are listed in Table 31-3, although frequently only some of these features are present. The diagnosis can be made with certainty in most circumstances, particularly when a constellation of these findings is present. In a patient with anemia, a high level of monoclonal IgG, IgA, or IgD, hypercalcemia, lytic bone lesions, and extensive replacement of the bone marrow with plasma cells, the diagnosis is not in doubt.

In the upcoming sections, the characteristics of myeloma are outlined. An understanding of these features will aid in the evaluation and diagnosis of patients presenting with findings suggestive of myeloma.

Epidemiology

Myeloma is clearly an age-dependent disease. As shown in Figure 31-7, it is rare in young persons and its incidence increases dramatically with age.[10] The incidence values are expressed on a logarithmic scale, making the increasing incidence with age even more dramatic than it appears.

For several decades, it has been speculated whether the incidence of myeloma is increasing in the United States and elsewhere in the world.[11-13] Some authors think that myeloma has increased in incidence in all age groups in the last several decades, possibly because of increased antigenic stimulation from increased pollution, whereas others believe that the increased incidence reflects increased detection. The truth may lie somewhere between the two theories.

Rare cases are reported of myeloma or benign monoclonal gammopathy or both occurring in families. One series reported eight families in whom multiple siblings were affected.[14] Familial myeloma is rare and myeloma shows no familial tendency in most cases.

TABLE 31-2. Task Force Criteria for the Diagnosis of Multiple Myeloma

For patients with a detectable monoclonal immunoglobulin, one of the followng must be present:
Bone marrow plasmacytosis over 5% in the absence of chronic inflammatory disease
Biopsy tissue demonstrating replacement and distortion of normal tissue by plasma cells
More than 500 plasma cells/μL in the peripheral blood
Osteolytic lesions unexplained by other causes
For patients without a detectable monoclonal immunoglobulin, an osteolytic lesion or palpable tumor plus one of the following must be present
Bone marrow plasmacytosis over 20% in two separate sites in the absence of chronic inflammatory disease
Tissue biopsy showing replacement and distortion of normal tissue by plasma cells

(Adapted from Chronic Leukemia-Myeloma Task Force. Proposed guidelines for protocol studies: plasma cell myeloma. Cancer Chemother Rep 1973;4:145)

TABLE 31-3. Characteristics of Multiple Myeloma

Monoclonal immunoglobulin
IgG—60%
IgA—22%
IgD–2%
Light chains only—15%
No immunoglobulin—1%
Anemia—often present, thrombocytopenia sometimes present
Bone marrow—plasmacytosis often over 20% and occurring in aggregates
Bone disease—osteolytic lesions or generalized osteopenia or both, rarely osteosclerosis
Hypercalcemia
Renal disease
Immune compromise with decreased production of normal immunoglobulins
Hyperviscosity—rare, usually with IgG3 or IgA

Pathogenesis

The pathogenesis of myeloma in humans is not known. Since the incidence of myeloma increases dramatically with increasing age, it has been suggested that myeloma develops because of repeated antigenic stimulation over many years, but this has not been demonstrated in humans.

Considerable experience exists in the experimental development of a myeloma syndrome in mice. It was discov-

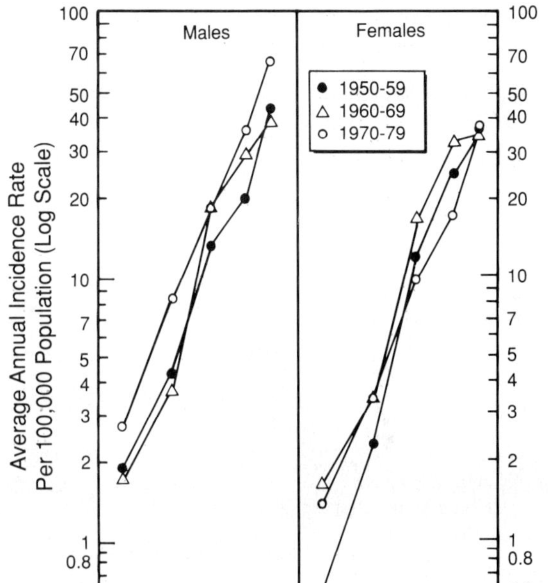

FIGURE 31-7. Annual incidence of multiple myeloma (Malmo, Sweden, 1950 to 1979) according to age and sex. (After Turesson I, Zettervall O, Cuzick J, et al. Comparison of trends in the incidence of multiple myeloma in Malmo, Sweden, and other countries, 1950–1979. N Engl J Med 1984;310:421)

ered by chance that some strains of mice (initially the BALB/c mouse) developed plasma cell tumors in their peritoneal cavity when foreign bodies were implanted there for long periods of time.[15] It also became clear that many agents that cause chronic inflammation could be administered intraperitoneally and cause the formation of plasmacytomas. The inflammatory response characterized by the infiltration of macrophages could be inhibited by indomethacin.[16] The generation of oxygen free radicals as part of the inflammatory response has been suggested as being involved in the carcinogenic process and that this generation was inhibited by indomethacin.

Plasmacytomas can be induced only in certain mouse strains, suggesting that a genetic predisposition must accompany the chronic inflammatory response. In many of the susceptible mouse strains, nonrandom translocations involving the c-*myc* gene are found in the plasmacytoma cells, and the gene appears to be deregulated.[17] Elevations of c-*myc* messenger RNA has also been found in humans with myeloma but only in a minority of those studied, leaving its significance uncertain.[18] Although the mouse model for the development of plasmacytomas is an extremely important one, its relevance to humans in not clear.

Myeloma Cell Morphology

Myeloma cell morphology can be extremely variable. Myeloma cells may appear identical with well-differentiated normal plasma cells; in other circumstances, they may appear much less well differentiated and are often referred to as *plasmablasts.*

Well-differentiated myeloma cells are shown in Figure 31-8. They have eccentrically placed nuclei with chromatin strands radiating from a central core to the rim that gives the appearance of the spokes of a wheel. A perinuclear clear zone contains the Golgi apparatus that processes synthesized immunoglobulin. Normal plasma cells can be found in a binucleate form, so that binuclearity itself is not diagnostic of myeloma. The presence of three or more nuclei per cell makes it more likely that the cell represents a myeloma cell.

Less well-differentiated cells, so-called plasmablasts, are shown in Figure 31-9. The nuclear chromatin is more open, nucleoli are often present, and the nuclear/cytoplasmic ratio is higher than that of typical plasma cells. The nucleus is also usually eccentric. In the extreme, plasmablasts can be difficult to distinguish from the immunoblasts seen in immunoblastic lymphoma.

When bone marrow core biopsies are examined in myeloma, the plasma cells tend to occur in clusters, as shown in Figure 31-10. This finding can be extremely helpful when the bone marrow plasmacytosis is only modest on the bone marrow aspirate and when the plasma cells are well differentiated. In reactive plasmacytosis, the plasma cells are evenly distributed throughout the bone marrow, compared with the clustering often seen in myeloma.

Terpstra and associates[19] analyzed bone marrow aspirate samples and biopsy specimens from 54 patients with myeloma and found that biopsy was more helpful overall. Aspiration and biopsy gave concordant results in 48% of patients; in 20% of patients, however, aspirate samples demonstrated less than 20% plasma cells, whereas biopsy specimens showed over 50% plasma cells. In these patients, plasma cells tended to occur in clusters in the biopsy specimen, and bone marrow fibrosis was often present as well. In only 2 of the 54 patients were more plasma cells seen in aspirate samples than in biopsy specimens.

Multiple attempts have been made to correlate morphology with prognosis. The Mayo Clinic found that patients whose myeloma cells had plasmablast morphology had a shorter survival than patients whose myeloma cells had more well-differentiated morphologies.[20] Carter and coworkers[21] found that all grades of morphologic immaturity are prognostic for survival, patients with well-differentiated myeloma having a median survival of 60 months; those with immature myeloma, 32.2 months; those with plasmablastic myeloma, 10.9 months.

Immunologic Features and the Origin of Myeloma Cells

Plasma cells are the final product of normal B-cell differentiation. Myeloma cells phenotypically are also representative of the final stage of B-cell differentiation. In most cases, these cells produce IgG, IgA, or IgD and have the expected immunologic features of mature plasma cells. In almost all patients, monotypic expression of either κ or λ is found, but rarely of both, as is seen in biclonal myeloma. In addition, about 90% of patients show expression of heavy chain of either the γ, α, or δ type; in 10%, only light-chain production is seen. Myeloma cells usually do not express early B-cell antigens such as CD19, CD20, and CD10 (com-

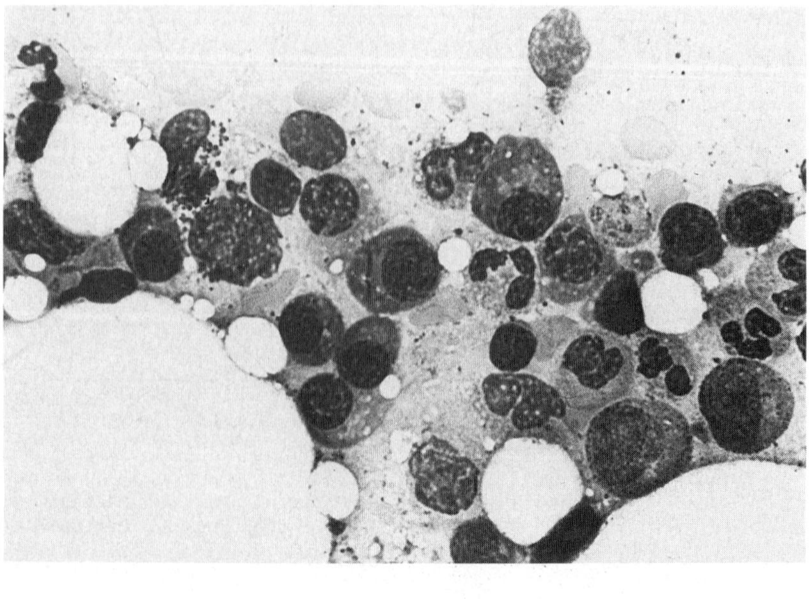

FIGURE 31-8. Well-differentiated myeloma cells are shown in the bone marrow aspirate smear of a patient with myeloma. The nuclei are relatively small with condensed chromatin. They are eccentrically placed, and a perinuclear clear zone is present.

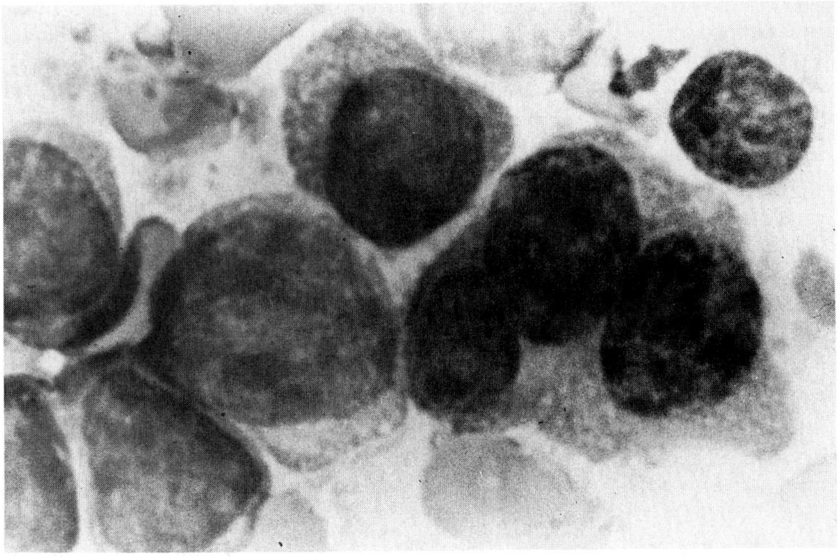

FIGURE 31-9. Plasmablasts (undifferentiated myeloma cells) are shown on a bone marrow aspirate smear of a patient with myeloma. The nuclei are large, and the nuclear/cytoplasmic ratio is high. The nuclear chromatin is dispersed and fine, and nucleoli are often present.

mon acute lymphocytic leukemia antigen), although in rare circumstances these antigens may be present.[22] Antigens specific to plasma cells such as PCA-1 and MM4 are present on myeloma cells.[23]

Morphologic features of plasmablastic myeloma can be confused with immunoblastic lymphoma. In some cases of myeloma, immunoblastic lymphoma evolves, presumably as a transformation to a more undifferentiated and aggressive disease.[24] Other investigators have demonstrated that with the exception of cases that appear to represent a transformation, myeloma and immunoblastic lymphoma are two distinct entities.[22] Immunoblastic lymphoma cells are more likely to contain IgM than IgG or IgA and are more likely to express κ than λ light chains.[25] The clinical manifestations of immunoblastic lymphoma are those of high-grade non-Hodgkin's lymphoma rather than of myeloma.

Patients with myeloma have rare B cells from early in the B-cell differentiation pathway in their peripheral blood, which are phenotypically identical with the malignant clonal myeloma plasma cells.[26,27] In some cases, these cells also express the pre–B-cell antigen, CALLA, as well as myelomonocytic antigens and erythroid antigens.[28] This has raised the question as to whether the clonal cell of origin in multiple myeloma is an early hematopoietic progenitor and whether the morphologically recognizable myeloma cells are the maturing phenotypic progeny of these primitive clonal cells. Jensen and coworkers[29] studied monoclonal B-lineage cells from the peripheral blood of 42 patients with myeloma and of 13 patients with monoclonal gammopathy of undetermined significance and found that most circulating clonal cells were CD10+ and PCA-1+. In addition, the cells strongly expressed CD45RO and weakly expressed CD45RA, suggesting that these clonal cells were at a late stage of B-cell differentiation, close to the plasma cell stage. More work needs to be done to further clarify the relation between these early progenitor cells and the mature myeloma cells.

Shared Idiotypes by Immunoglobulins in Patients With Myeloma

Each immunoglobulin has a specific protein sequence in the variable regions of the light and heavy chains, which gives it a unique structure and is referred to as its *idiotype.*

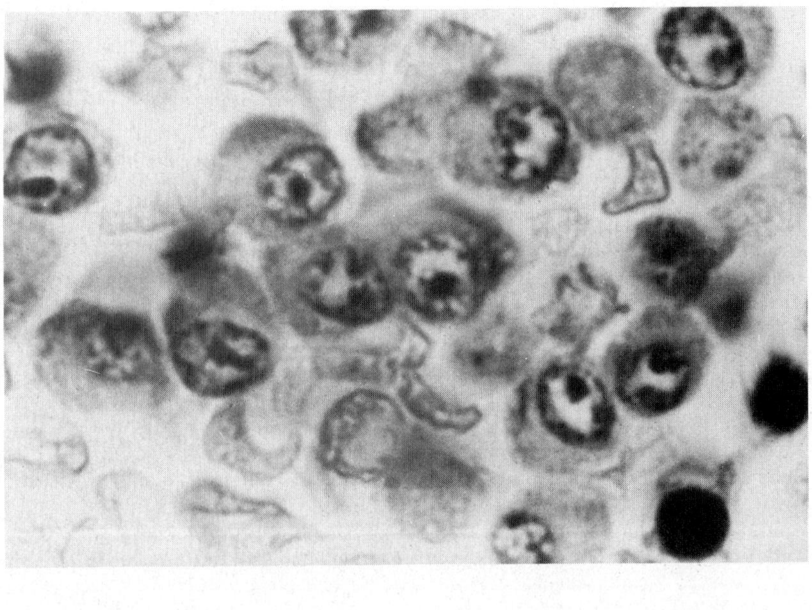

FIGURE 31-10. Bone marrow biopsy specimen from a patient with myeloma. The myeloma cells occur in aggregates.

Because of the observed diversity and multitude of idiotypes expressed by normal B cells, the number of idiotypes expressed by B-cell malignancies might be expected to be large. These malignant lymphomas appear to express a relatively limited number of idiotypes, and these commonly appearing idiotypes are now referred to as shared idiotypes.[30] The same has been shown for myeloma when shared idiotypes by immunoglobulins from patients with myeloma have been found.[31] In all cases studied, the idiotype found on bone marrow myeloma cells was identical with that of the serum monoclonal immunoglobulin. One particular idiotype, S30-47, was found frequently in myeloma patients and also in a patient with monoclonal gammopathy of undetermined significance. Other shared idiotypes were also found in the immunoglobulin samples from patients with monoclonal gammopathy of undetermined significance, suggesting that, as suspected, these diseases are closely related.[31] The predominance of certain idiotypes may reflect an abnormal distribution in normal lymphocytes.

Association of Myeloma and Chronic Lymphocytic Leukemia

Occasional cases have been reported of either the coexistence of or the sequential development of chronic lymphocytic leukemia (CLL) and myeloma.[32,33] Whether these entities represent different manifestations of the same malignant clone or two separate and distinct malignant transformations has been the subject of considerable speculation. Early analyses were indeterminate, since they were based on expression of either κ or λ light chains and since both diseases had a 50% probability of expressing the same light chain even if the lights chains were not related. Rare patients with CLL of long-standing duration developed myeloma as a terminal event.[34] In these patients, it was not clear whether the two were phenotypically the same.

Phenotypic expression of heavy- and light-chain specificity may ultimately be inadequate to determine whether two clonal populations of cells arise from the same malignant cell. One patient who had CLL expressing IgM-κ and myeloma expressing IgA-λ had extensive evaluation of the immunoglobulin heavy-chain gene.[35] In both CLL cells and myeloma cells, an identical heavy-chain rearrangement was present and suggested that these two phenotypically distinct malignancies arose from a common precursor cell. In this patient, the CLL cells may have had successful rearrangement of the κ light-chain gene; in the development of the myeloma clone from the same precursor, however, failure to successfully rearrange the κ gene occurred and therefore λ rearrangement occurred. It would also have to be hypothesized that during the progression from CLL phenotype to the myeloma phenotype, heavy-chain switching from μ to α was found.

Examples such as this have brought to light the complexities of cell development, particularly in the setting of malignant transformation. Coexisting diseases previously thought to be unrelated may arise from common primitive malignant clones even when the mature phenotypes are different.

Karyotypic Abnormalities in Myeloma Cells

Karyotypic analysis can be difficult to perform on myeloma cells because of their slow rate of proliferation (see section on myeloma tumor cell kinetics). In addition, physicians do not attempt to perform karyotypic analysis on myeloma cells on a routine basis as has been increasingly the practice in the acute leukemias. In one series, karyotypic analyses of myeloma cells from 115 patients showed evaluable metaphases. Forty-six percent of the patients were found to have karyotypic abnormalities.[36] The specific abnormalities were highly variable including trisomies of chromosomes 3, 5, 7, 9, 11, 15, 18, 19, and 21 and monosomies of chromosomes 8, 13, 16, 20, and 22. Also, translocations involving chromosomes 8, 11, and 14 were found as might be expected in a B-cell neoplasm. No characteristic chromosomal abnormalities were identified.

In the study of malignancy in general, considerable attention has been paid to the p53 suppressor gene, which has been mapped to the short arm of chromosome 17. This gene appears to be important in carcinogenesis in a number of tumors, including colon cancer, breast cancer, chronic myelogenous leukemia, and others. It has been sought in myeloma cells and found to be a rare chromosomal event, appearing in only 1 of 37 patients in one series.[37] When patients with advanced or particularly virulent forms of myeloma were studied, it was found more frequently, in 7 of 52 patients studied by Neri and associates.[38] These data suggest that mutations of the p53 gene are not important for the initial development of myeloma but may occasionally be associated with tumor progression.

Myeloma Tumor Cell Kinetics

Myeloma is a tumor that generally has a low percentage of cells undergoing DNA synthesis. When ^{3}H-thymidine is used to determine the labeling index of myeloma cells, usually less than 5% of cells are found to be actively synthesizing DNA. A labeling index of 3% was used as the cutoff point to distinguish between high and low proliferative myeloma; this has been useful in assessing prognosis, as shown in Figure 31-11.[39] The same investigators also

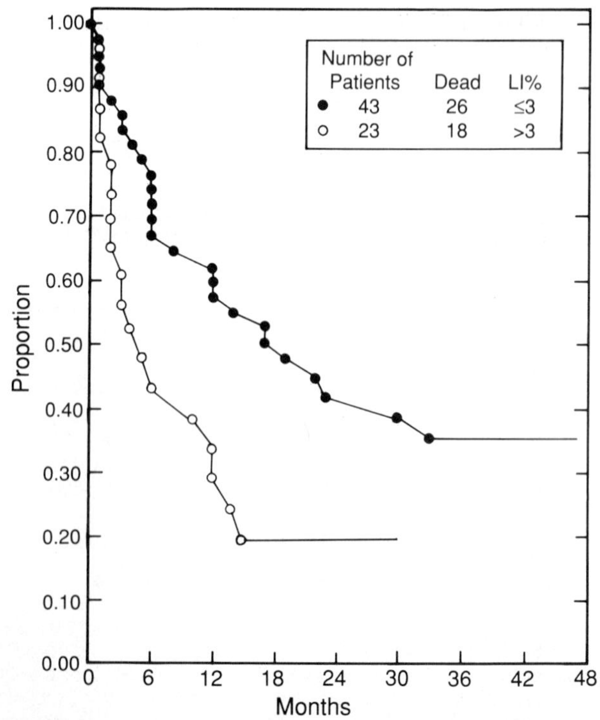

FIGURE 31-11. Kaplan-Meier survival curves for patients with myeloma whose myeloma cells have low and high labeling index values (LI%). The difference between the curves is significant ($P < .02$). (After Hofmann V, Salmon SE, Durie BGM. Drug resistance in multiple myeloma associated with high in vitro incorporation of ^{3}H-thymidine. Blood 1981;58:471)

measured grain counts over the nuclei of myeloma cells to determine the amount of DNA synthesis occurring in individual cells. They found that prognosis was poor for patients with high grain counts, even if the labeling index was low, suggesting that this is an additional independent prognostic variable.[39]

The labeling index has been used to distinguish myeloma from monoclonal gammopathy of undetermined significance. Although myeloma cells may have a low labeling index, plasma cells obtained in a study of patients with monoclonal gammopathy of undetermined significance invariably had low labeling indices, as shown in Figure 31-12.[40] As can be seen, patients with benign monoclonal gammopathy generally had a labeling index of less than 0.8%. Some patients with myeloma also often have labeling indices that are in this same range, whereas others have higher labeling indices.

Labeling index studies using ^{3}H-thymidine are difficult to perform. New techniques using 5-bromo-2-deoxyuridine may be simpler and more generally applicable; in most cases, they are well correlated with standard ^{3}H-thymidine studies.[40] This technique has been shown in one study to be predictive of the patient's response to chemotherapy.[41]

The labeling index may also be predictive of the ability to grow myeloma cells in vitro.[42] Myeloma cells with a high labeling index are more likely to grow in in vitro culture systems; this phenomenon may be indicative of increased numbers of clonogenic cells.

Myeloma Cell Immunoglobulin Production

The fact that myeloma cells produce a monoclonal immunoglobulin in over 95% of patients has proved to be a valuable tool for the study of tumor cell synthetic rates and for the determination of total body tumor cell burden. Immunoglobulin production varies among myeloma cells from different patients. In one series, immunoglobulin synthesis rates varied from 2.5 to 35 pg per myeloma cell per day.[43] Using these calculations, it is possible to estimate that myeloma becomes detectable when about 10 g of myeloma cells are present, representing about 10^{10} cells, as shown in Figure 31-13. Clinical diagnosis is not likely to be made before there are more than 10^{11} cells, and death results from one more log of cell growth, at a tumor burden of about 5×10^{12} cells.

Biclonal Immunoglobulin Production

In less than 10% of patients with myeloma, two monoclonal immunoglobulins are found. The significance of these cases has been debated, but several pathophysiologic explanations are possible. In a series reported from the Mayo Clinic, biclonal gammopathy was recognized in 57 patients, representing 1.5% of the total number of gammopathies diagnosed during the period studied.[44] In this series, biclonal gammopathy of undetermined significance represented 65% of the cases, whereas myeloma represented only 16% of the cases. Fifty percent of the patients had IgG and IgA components, and 26% had IgG and IgM immunoglobulins. Three percent had two distinct IgG immunoglobulins.

Several potential explanations account for the occurrence of biclonal gammopathies. In the Mayo Clinic series, the incidence of biclonal gammopathies approximates that of incidentally found monoclonal proteins and could represent just that. In several cases in which the patients' myeloma progressed, only one of the monoclonal immunoglobulins increased in amount, suggesting that only that single monoclonal immunoglobulin was being produced from the malignant myeloma and that the other monoclonal immunoglobulin may have been produced by a second clone representing a benign monoclonal gammopathy. In support of this theory, several demonstrations of the divergence of the histologic origin of the biclonal immunoglobulins in bone marrow samples have been noted in these cases. One plasma cell population clearly expressed one monoclonal immunoglobulin, and another plasma cell or

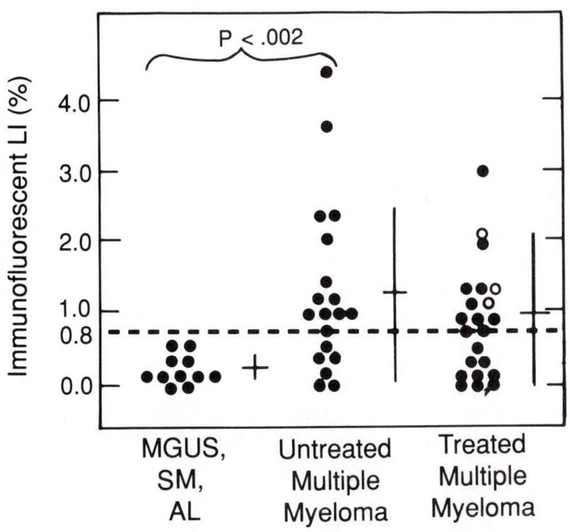

FIGURE 31-12. Immunofluorescence labeling index values (LI) for patients with monoclonal gammopathy of undetermined significance (MGUS), smoldering myeloma (SM), amyloidosis (AL), and untreated and treated multiple myeloma. The cutoff value for distinguishing patients with stable disease from those with active disease was 0.8%. In the group of patients with treated myeloma, the open circles represent patients in relapse. (After Greipp PR, Witzig TE, Gonchoroff NJ, et al. Immunofluorescence labeling indices in myeloma and related monoclonal gammopathies. Mayo Clin Proc 1987;62:969)

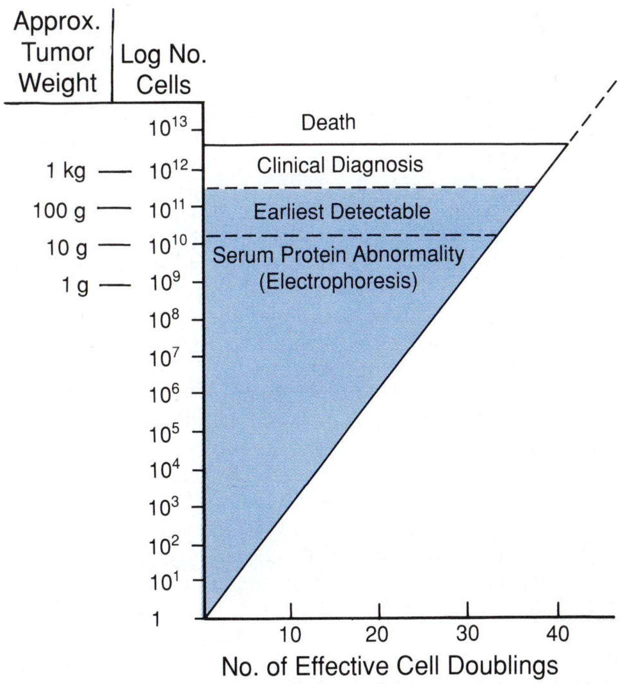

FIGURE 31-13. Relation of tumor weight and cell number to the number of effective cell doublings from the initiation of a malignant monoclone. The figure is designed to show the "iceberg" of preclinical doublings that go on before potential detection of an M component on serum electrophoresis. Clinical diagnosis is generally at least 1 log above that point. (After Salmon SE. Immunoglobulin synthesis and tumor kinetics of multiple myeloma. Semin Hematol 1973;10:135)

lymphocytic population expressed the other monoclonal immunoglobulin.[45,46]

In other circumstances, a single myeloma cell has been shown to produce two distinct immunoglobulins.[47,48] In these cases, immunoglobulin synthesis has been altered in such a way as to allow expression of either two heavy chains or two light chains in the same cell. It has become increasingly clear that myeloma cells are more heterogeneous and complex genetically than previously appreciated and that the production of two monoclonal proteins from a single myeloma cell may be a result of this complexity.[49]

Nonsecretory Myeloma

In 1% to 5% of patients with myeloma, no detectable immunoglobulin is found in either the serum or the urine. These cases have always been referred to as nonsecretory myeloma but probably include two entities. Most affected patients have truly nonsecretory myeloma with monoclonal immunoglobulin identified in the cytoplasm of their cells but not in the serum. Some cases represent plasma cell tumors that do not produce immunoglobulins at all. In these myeloma cells, no monoclonal immunoglobulin can be found in the cytoplasm or serum.[50–52]

Growth Factors and Myeloma Cells

Normal plasma cells are the end product of B-cell differentiation, and multiple growth factors are now linked to B-cell growth and differentiation. In particular, interleukin-6 (IL-6) has been shown to be important for the terminal stages of normal B-cell differentiation.[53] The effects of IL-6 on myeloma cells have also been studied and shown to be variably stimulatory in vitro, sometimes active only to cells with high labeling indices in vivo as shown by bromodeoxyuridine techniques.[54] In addition, some myeloma cells produce Il-6, leading to autocrine stimulation.[55] In one such cell line, U266, Schwab and coworkers[56] demonstrated production of IL-6 and inhibition of proliferation by the addition of IL-6 antisense oligonucleotides. Proliferation could be restored by the addition of exogenous IL-6, and it appeared that IL-6 released a block in the G1 phase of the cell cycle.

Other cytokines have been shown to affect the IL-6 pathway in myeloma cell lines. Kobayashi and colleagues[57] demonstrated that IL-6 upregulates the number of Il-6 receptors on the surface of cells from the HSM-2.3 myeloma cell line. GM-CSF has been shown to increase the in vitro responsiveness of some myeloma cells to IL-6 and to increase their proliferation.[58] This effect did not appear to result from increased autocrine production of IL-6 but was blocked by anti–IL-6 antibodies. In other studies, IL-1α, IL-1β, and tumor necrosis factor—all of which can be produced by myeloma cells—have been shown to stimulate freshly isolated myeloma cells to produce IL-6.[59] This may lead to enhanced autocrine growth.

Another important B-cell growth factor is interleukin-4 (IL-4), which not only stimulates B-cell growth and differentiation but also increases the expression of the Ia antigen and Fc receptor on resting B cells.[60–62] The effects of IL-4 on myeloma cells have been less predictable. Growth of myeloma cells was inhibited by IL-4 in about 50% of cases studied, in 40% IL-4 had no effect on growth, and it was stimulatory in less than 10% of cases.[63] Herrmann and associates[64] demonstrated that in vitro exposure of myeloma cell lines to IL-4 inhibited the synthesis of IL-6, thereby inhibiting the autocrine stimulatory pathway for IL-6. The resultant inhibition of growth could be reversed by the addition of exogenous IL-6.

IL-1β produced by myeloma cells is probably the osteoclast-stimulating activity of myeloma cells responsible for lytic bone lesions and hypercalcemia,[65] as discussed later in this chapter. Bone marrow stromal cells, obtained from patients with myeloma and found to consist primarily of fibroblasts and macrophages, produce high levels of IL-6 and measurable amounts of IL-1β.[66] Secretion of these cytokines by the marrow stromal elements may be important in supporting myeloma cell growth and may in part explain the propensity for myeloma to grow primarily in the bone marrow.

Clinical Presentation and Differential Diagnosis

The primary clinical manifestations of myeloma are shown in Table 31-3. When many or all of the manifestations are present, the diagnosis is easy to make. No single test is in itself diagnostic of myeloma; a constellation of findings is necessary to be sure of the diagnosis. Differentiation of myeloma from monoclonal gammopathy of undetermined significance is important, since many patients with that entity do not progress to overt myeloma and therefore do not require therapy.

The Monoclonal Protein

The presence of the monoclonal protein often first leads a physician to a diagnosis of myeloma. Characterization of the monoclonal protein as IgG, IgA, or IgD or free light chains is one of the first priorities. The immunoglobulin must be determined to be monoclonal, and its concentration must be determined. Low levels of monoclonal immunoglobulin, whether complete immunoglobulin or free light chain, are more suggestive of monoclonal gammopathy of undetermined significance, and high levels are more suggestive of myeloma, but no specific value separates the two entities. As described earlier, immunoglobulin levels below 2 g/dL are consistent with, but not diagnostic of, monoclonal gammopathy of undetermined significance. Details of the evaluation of the monoclonal immunoglobulin were described earlier in this chapter.

Anemia and Thrombocytopenia

There are laboratory values that are often available early in the evaluation of the patient with suspected myeloma, since they are routinely obtained in most patients. Patients with myeloma are usually anemic and sometimes thrombocytopenic. The presence of both findings are consistent with myeloma but are obviously nonspecific and could be indicative of many other diseases. Myeloma can be present in the absence of anemia or thrombocytopenia.

Anemia and thrombocytopenia are primarily due to the replacement of the bone marrow space by myeloma cells, but the degree of anemia in particular is thought to be out of proportion to the degree of marrow replacement with myeloma cells. No strong evidence supports a humoral suppression of normal hematopoiesis, but some patients with myeloma and anemia have inappropriately low levels of endogenous erythropoietin.[67] In one study, erythropoietin production was inordinately low in many patients with myeloma and anemia, and the likelihood of having a low erythropoietin level was directly related to stage of disease. This low level was responsible for suboptimal red cell production.[68] The reason for this is not known, but when some of these patients are given exogenous erythropoietin, their hemoglobin and hematocrit levels rise.

Bone Marrow Plasmacytosis

In patients with myeloma, a plasmacytosis in the bone marrow is almost always seen. The degree of plasmacytosis can be extremely variable, with plasma cells accounting for only 5% to 10% of the bone marrow elements, or the bone marrow can be almost entirely replaced with plasma cells. In patients with chronic inflammatory diseases, such as chronic infections or collagen-vascular diseases, reactive plasma cells can account for 10% to 20% of the bone marrow cellularity. In patients with 30% to 40% or more of plasma cells, it is extremely unlikely that these cells represent anything other than myeloma, especially when they are present together with a monoclonal immunoglobulin.

The morphology of the plasma cells may also be helpful. The plasma cells in a reactive plasmacytosis are mature, well-differentiated plasma cells. Binucleate forms are rare, and it is unusual to find plasma cells with three or more nuclei in patients with reactive plasmacytosis. When the plasma cells are more immature or resemble plasmablasts, they are diagnostic of myeloma and cannot represent a benign process. The major disease in the differential diagnosis when plasmablasts are present is immunoblastic lymphoma, which is immunologically different as described earlier in this chapter.

When only a modest plasmacytosis is present in the bone marrow, the core biopsy can sometimes be particularly helpful. In reactive plasmacytosis, the plasma cells are polyclonal and interspersed throughout the normal hematopoietic elements. In myeloma, often a clustering of the plasma cells is present, which can be distinct on the core biopsy. In addition, myeloma cells stain with a monoclonal pattern for either κ or λ light chains.

Bone Disease

Bone disease is a hallmark of myeloma. Over 75% of patients have significant bone disease, and this gives the patients their most troublesome symptoms. Vertebral body compression fractures, rib fractures, and fractures of the long bones of the legs can cause considerable morbidity, particularly pain. Osteopenia, with general loss of bone mass, is a common finding in patients with myeloma along with the classic lytic bone lesions without surrounding osteosclerotic reaction.

For many years, secretion of one or more cytokines originally named *osteoclast-activating factor* has been thought to account for these findings.[69] Lymphotoxin has been implicated as a humoral cause of bone resorption in myeloma patients.[70] When lymphotoxin is injected subcutaneously into normal mice, their serum calcium level rises, and evidence shows that it stimulates bone resorption in vitro. It has been suggested that not lymphotoxin but IL-1β is the putative osteoclast-activating factor.[65] The in vitro osteolytic activity of IL-1β can be neutralized by specific antibodies. IL-1β appears to lead to unbalanced bone resorption in myeloma, and not only is increased osteoclastic activity almost always present, but suppression of osteoblastic activity also appears prominent. Bone destruction is most pronounced when osteoblastic activity is also reduced,[71] which may help to explain why so little osteosclerotic reaction surrounds lytic bone lesions in myeloma.

Osteopenia and lytic bone lesions are most obvious on plain radiographs of the skull, vertebral bodies, and long bones of the extremities (Fig. 31-14). Radiographs of all these bones should be performed when a diagnosis of myeloma is suspected or made. They can help to confirm the diagnosis and can also identify weight-bearing bones that

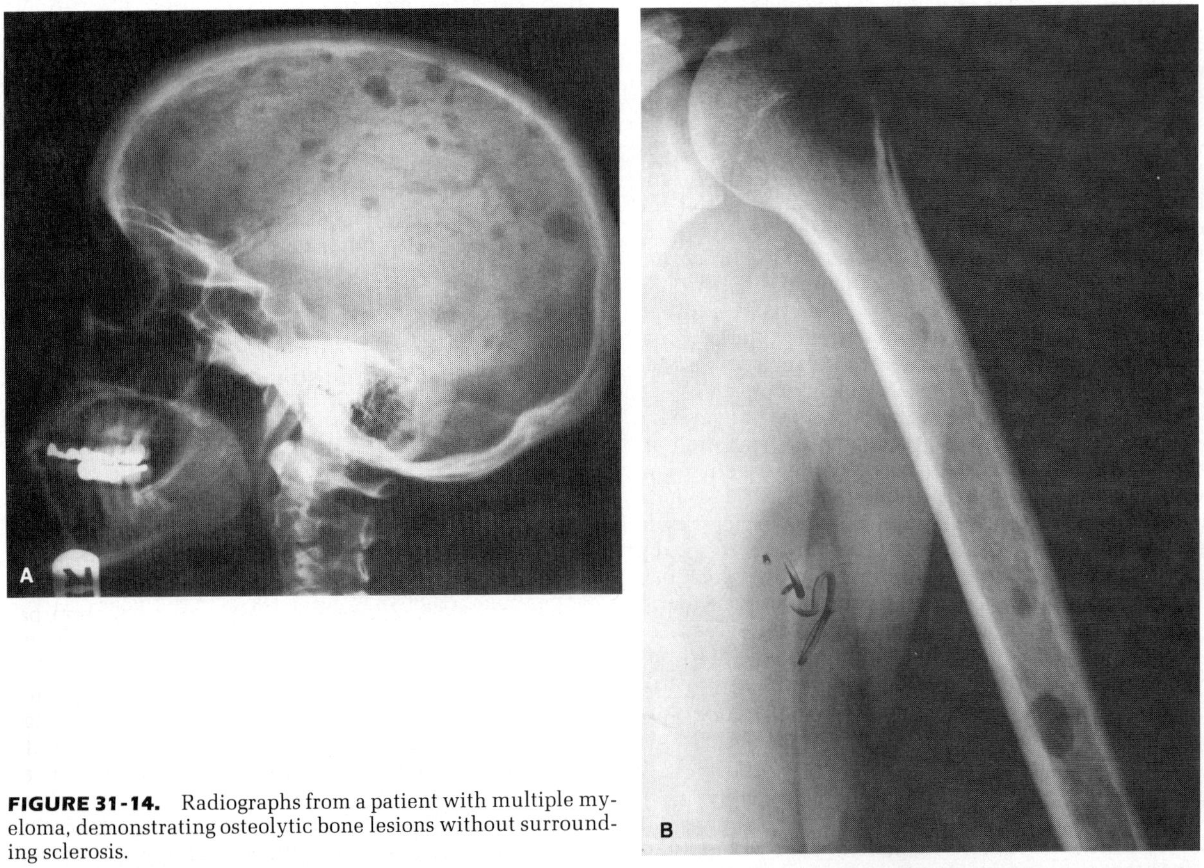

FIGURE 31-14. Radiographs from a patient with multiple myeloma, demonstrating osteolytic bone lesions without surrounding sclerosis.

may be at risk for fracture, thus requiring urgent radiation therapy or surgical fixation. The evaluation of osteopenic lesions can be difficult. Myeloma usually occurs in the elderly, who often have osteoporosis (particularly women). It becomes a professional judgment as to whether the degree of osteopenia is consistent with the patient's age or is so severe that it represents a pathologic state such as myeloma. Lytic bone lesions are clearly pathologic. The main differential diagnosis of lytic lesions is that of other tumors metastasizing to the bone. Many carcinomas can give largely lytic bone disease, although usually but not always, there is surrounding sclerosis.

Bone scans are usually not helpful in the evaluation of patients with myeloma. Bone scans are generally abnormal in areas of new bone formation and osteoblastic activity. Since myeloma is generally associated with osteoclastic activity with little or no surrounding osteoblastic activity, the bone scan is usually negative. Occasionally, an osteolytic lesion can be so large that it gives subtle changes in a bone scan showing decreased activity rather than increased activity in the area of the lytic lesion. In the rare cases of osteosclerotic myeloma, the bone scan is positive. For the same reason, serum alkaline phosphatase activity is usually normal in patients with bone involvement secondary to myeloma, since the alkaline phosphatase activity in the serum is a reflection of osteoblastic activity.

In generalized osteopenia secondary to myeloma, when the bone density falls below 11%, an increased risk for the development of pathologic fractures exists. Discrete osteolytic lesions are not necessary for the development of pathologic fractures.[71] The most common site of pathologic fractures secondary to osteopenia is the vertebral bodies, and back pain is the initial complaint in many patients with myeloma. The vertebral compression fractures can be so severe and extensive that patients lose significant height. Osteopenia in the long bones of the leg, particularly the proximal femur, can lead to pathologic fractures.

Plasmacytomas growing out of osteolytic lesions can result in compression of the spinal cord or nerve roots in vertebral lesions or of cranial nerve roots in osteolytic lesions of the base of the skull. Local radiation therapy may be indicated in these cases.

Control of the osteopenia or osteolytic bone lesions of myeloma is largely dependent on the ability to control the myeloma. If the myeloma progresses, it is likely that the bone disease will also progress. Therefore, an attempt to control the myeloma is the first therapeutic maneuver that should be made. Even when the myeloma is controlled, often poor or no recalcification of involved bone is found. Attempts to improve bone repair and prevent the progression of pathologic fractures have been disappointing. Fluoride compounds, vitamin D, calcium preparations, and corticosteroids all have been tried without proven success.[72] In some studies, an increase in bone mass was demonstrated, but no clinical benefit was routinely seen.[73] The diphosphonate compound etidronate disodium has been studied in a randomized double-blind trial to determine whether administration of this agent in patients receiving melphalan and prednisone chemotherapy would reduce bony complications of myeloma.[74] No difference was found between treatment groups for height loss, pathologic fractures, bone pain, or hypercalcemia, suggesting that etidronate disodium is ineffectual in limiting progression of bone disease in patients with myeloma. No agents are currently recommended to increase bone repair in patients with myeloma.

POEMS Syndrome and Osteosclerotic Myeloma

An osteosclerotic form of bone disease occurs in less than 5% of patients with myeloma. It is often associated with polyneuropathy, organomegaly, endocrinopathy, and skin changes, a constellation given the acronym *POEMS syndrome*.[75] Of 2714 patients seen at the Mayo Clinic with plasma cell dyscrasias, 1.4% were classified as having POEMS syndrome.[76] All had polyneuropathy, with 37 of 38 patients demonstrating combined sensorimotor deficits and 1 patient having primary motor neuropathy. Osteosclerotic bone lesions were present in 82% of patients, skin abnormalities in 58%, lymphadenopathy in 42%, papilledema in 37%, peripheral edema in 29%, hepatomegaly in 24%, splenomegaly in 21%, and ascites in 11%. Monoclonal proteins, primarily of the IgA-λ or IgG-λ type, were present in the serum or urine of 87% of patients. Five-year survival rate was estimated to be 60%, better than for myeloma patients in general.

Hypercalcemia

The mechanisms of hypercalcemia in myeloma are complex and not fully understood. Hypercalcemia is clearly related to the increased bone resorption seen in myeloma patients, but not all patients with significant bone disease have hypercalcemia. Only 20% to 40% of patients with myeloma develop hypercalcemia, whereas more than 75% have significant bone disease.[77] Although a good correlation exists between bone resorption activity in vitro with cultured myeloma cells and bone disease in vivo, no good correlation is found between bone resorption in vitro and hypercalcemia.[78]

It has been suggested that hypercalcemia is more common in patients with myeloma who have renal impairment, but hypercalcemia often contributes to the renal impairment in myeloma patients. Therefore, it is not clear whether a causal relation exists.[79]

The rapid treatment of hypercalcemia in the patient with myeloma is essential. As is typical of patients with hypercalcemia, these patients tend to be dehydrated. Dehydration is a particularly important concern in this patient population, because it can lead to a precipitous and sometimes irreversible worsening of renal function. Therefore, adequate hydration, often administering saline intravenously at 150 to 200 mL/h, is initial therapy. Furosemide is used as needed to keep the fluid balance even. This saline diuresis causes urinary calcium loss and usually improves the degree of hypercalcemia substantially but not always completely. Reduction of the myeloma tumor burden is the best long-term method to control the hypercalcemia, but immediate control of the myeloma is not often possible because of a delay in the effect from chemotherapy or because the patient is refractory to chemotherapy. Other methods used to control hypercalcemia are shown in Table 31-4 and include administration of mithramycin, diphos-

TABLE 31-4. Therapy for Hypercalcemia*

Drug and Schedule	Toxicities
Saline diuresis, 150—200 mL/h IV (furosemide to maintain urine output and prevent fluid overload)	Fluid overload
Mithramycin, 25 μg/kg IV every 2–3 d	Thrombocytopenia; tissue vesicant
Pamidronate, 60–90 mg by continuous IV infusion of 24 h × 1	
Etidronate, 7.5 mg/kg/d IV for 3 d, then 20 mg/kg d PO	Renal dysfunction
Calcitonin, 4 IU/kg SC every 12 h (may be more effective if given with corticosteroids)	Nausea and vomiting; allergic reactions

* Doses and toxicities listed are merely guidelines; more complete information should be obtained before using these agents.

phonates, and calcitonin. The choice and number of agents must be tailored to the individual clinical scenario.

Renal Disease and Amyloidosis in Myeloma

Many potential causes of renal disease exist in patients with myeloma, and renal failure is a common consequence of the disease. Renal dysfunction at presentation has a significant impact on survival. In one study, patients who presented with serum creatinine levels lower than 2 mg/dL had a median survival of 41 months, whereas those presenting with creatinine levels of 2 mg/dL or above had a median survival of only 14 months.[80] Causes of renal failure in patients with myeloma include the following:

Myeloma kidney—precipitation of light chains in the renal tubules
Deposition disease—reabsorption of light chains into the renal tubular cells with deposition along their basement membranes
Amyloid kidney—formation of amyloid in the renal tubules, arterioles, and glomeruli
Hypercalcemia

Each is an important potential cause of renal failure, and often several are present.

Patients whose myeloma produces primarily free light chains are particularly prone to renal failure. These patients often present with renal failure as their initial manifestation of myeloma. In one series, the mean creatinine level of patients presenting with light-chain myeloma was 4.1 mg/dL with a range of 0.8 to 15 mg/dL; these patients presented with an average 24-hour urine protein excretion rate of 8 g.[81] Free immunoglobulin light chains cause renal failure by three mechanisms: tubular precipitation, renal tubular cell reabsorption with basement membrane deposition, and amyloidosis.

Myeloma kidney is a term used to describe the precipitation of light chains in the renal tubules. Renal biopsy of myeloma kidney demonstrates proteinaceous tubular casts. Light-chain deposition disease is caused by a reabsorption of free light chains into the tubular cells, glomerular cells, and mesangium.[82] These deposits usually occur along the basement membrane of the renal tubular or glomerular cells and lead to progressive renal dysfunction. It is not understood why some light chains precipitate in the renal tubules and why some are reabsorbed leading to light-chain deposition disease. Possibly, electrostatic charge or other specific properties of the individual light chains involved are responsible for the propensity to develop tubular precipitation or tubular cell deposition. To further study this problem, Solomon and colleagues[83] obtained Bence Jones protein samples from 40 patients with myeloma and injected them into the peritoneal cavities of mice, killing them 48 hours later for renal analysis. An excellent correlation was found between renal disease in the patients and renal involvement in the mice, suggesting that properties of the free light chains determined their propensity to cause renal damage.

Amyloidosis is found in about 5% of all patients with myeloma and 20% of patients with light-chain disease. Some light chains, particularly those of the $V_{\lambda VI}$ group, are more likely than others to lead to the deposition of amyloid deposits.[84] Amyloid kidneys are generally large, and amyloid substance is deposited in the arterial walls, interstitial tissue, and glomeruli. Amyloid deposits are accumulations of the light chain that are produced by the myeloma cells. The deposits show a typical apple green birefringence when stained with Congo red. When the glomerulus is involved, nephrotic syndrome often is present. Renal failure usually results from the arterial and tubular damage. In these instances, other organs are also generally involved, with amyloid deposition leading to considerable morbidity and mortality. The median survival for patients with myeloma and amyloidosis is about 20 months.[85] Cardiac involvement with amyloid carries the worst prognosis with a median survival of only 7 months.

A renal biopsy is often necessary to definitively distinguish among the various causes of kidney dysfunction in myeloma patients. In reality, the biopsy is rarely performed, since it usually does not affect therapeutic decisions and is not without risk. The management of chronic renal disease due to light-chain production, regardless of the mechanism, revolves around control of the myeloma and its continued production of light chains. As previously mentioned, patients presenting with renal failure have a poor prognosis. This may reflect the present inability to control light-chain production adequately in these patients and to stop or reverse the chronic renal failure. Even when the myeloma is well controlled for a period of time, the renal function does not always improve.

In patients with *acute* renal failure from light-chain disease, renal failure may be reversed by the rapid institution of plasmapheresis.[86] Patients who present for the first time with renal failure and light-chain disease should be given the benefit of doubt, assuming that their renal failure is acute and potentially reversible by plasmapheresis. Hydration, diuresis, and dialysis, although necessary in individual patients according to the clinical scenario, are not likely to reverse acute renal failure and should not be substituted for plasmapheresis. How frequently plasmapheresis should be performed in this setting has not been established, but it should initially be used every 2 to 3 days, observing the serum creatinine level to monitor progress.

Hypercalcemia can also lead to renal dysfunction. Dehydration exacerbates this effect, making rapid rehydration imperative when a patient with myeloma presents with hypercalcemia. Worsening dehydration that can result from continued osmotic diuresis from hypercalcemia or other osmotic stresses such as the administration of intravenous contrast dye can lead to progressive and irreversible renal failure.

Immune Competence and Infection in Myeloma

Although most patients with myeloma make large amounts of monoclonal immunoglobulin, they make reduced amounts of normal polyclonal immunoglobulin. In the 1950s, Zinneman and Hall[87] described an association between this finding and an increased risk of serious infection, particularly pneumonia. Infection was and continues to be the most common cause of death in patients with myeloma, accounting for 20% to 50% of deaths.[88] Bacterial pneumonias are particularly troubling and common infections in these patients, accounting for 49% of serious infections in one series, and are caused by both gram-positive and gram-negative organisms. Urinary tract infections accounted for 22% of infections and 10% of the patients had sepsis. Organisms responsible for these infections included *Pneumococcus* sp (26%), *Staphylococcus* sp (10%), *Escherichia coli* (13%), *Pseudomonas* sp (6%), and *Haemophilus influenzae* (5%).

For myeloma patients, the risk of developing an infection is related to the level of the normal polyclonal immunoglobulins and the serum creatinine at presentation.[89] Patients with depressed levels of normal immunoglobulins had a 49% infection rate during the first 2 months of therapy, whereas patients with normal polyclonal immunoglobulins had a 25% likelihood of infection in this time period. Similarly, 73% of patients with a creatinine level higher than 2 mg/dL became infected, and only 39% of patients with creatinine levels of less than 2 mg/dL became infected. As shown in Figure 31-15, the highest risk of infection was shortly after diagnosis and institution of chemotherapy, but the risk continued with time. For patients who responded to chemotherapy, the risk of infection was still present but decreased.

Patients with myeloma have reduced amounts of *Pneumococcus*-specific antibodies specific for all polysaccharide types and respond poorly to the administration of polyvalent pneumococcal polysaccharide capsular vaccine.[90] The response varies considerably from patient to patient, and some patients may have a significant response to vaccination. It is therefore reasonable to vaccinate myeloma patients, but it should be recognized that the response may be poor.

Other immunologic defects are probably present in patients with myeloma but have been more difficult to elucidate. Fewer T cells of the CD4 class may be present in the blood of patients with myeloma, although a causal relation between this finding and the reduced levels of normal polyclonal immunoglobulins has not been established.[91] In addition, opsonization appears to be depressed in patients with myeloma and may relate to decreased complement levels.[92] Defective opsonization has not been correlated with a predisposition toward clinical infection. Defective opsonization may be due to impaired activation of the complement component C3.[93] Multiple defects may contribute to this dysfunction, and multiple components of the complement pathway were decreased in patients studied.

Another potential cause of increased susceptibility to infection is granulocytopenia. Rarely, this is caused merely by replacement of the normal hematopoietic elements of the bone marrow by myeloma cells; granulocytopenia from this cause is usually not as pronounced as is the degree of anemia and thrombocytopenia. More frequently, granulocytopenia is caused by bone marrow suppression from chemotherapeutic agents. In this circumstance, the bone marrow involvement with myeloma cells can result in patients being exceptionally sensitive to the suppressive effects of these agents.

Hyperviscosity

Hyperviscosity is a lesser clinical problem in patients with myeloma than in those with macroglobulinemia (IgM), but it does occur. (The clinical aspects of hyperviscosity syndrome are outlined in the section on macroglobulinemia.) Hyperviscosity is found in 3% to 4% of patients with IgG myeloma and in 5% to 10% of patients with IgA myeloma.[94]

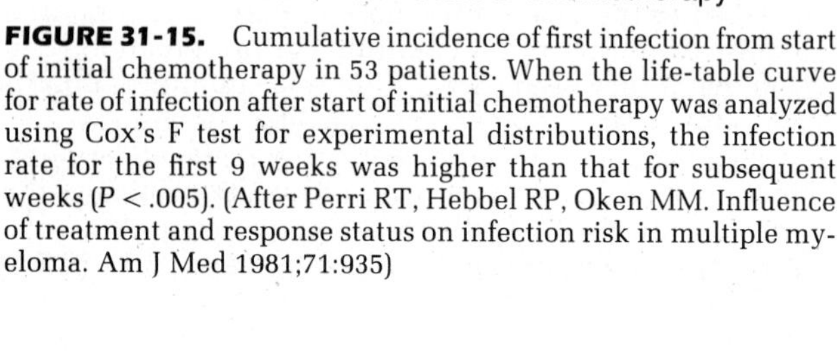

FIGURE 31-15. Cumulative incidence of first infection from start of initial chemotherapy in 53 patients. When the life-table curve for rate of infection after start of initial chemotherapy was analyzed using Cox's F test for experimental distributions, the infection rate for the first 9 weeks was higher than that for subsequent weeks ($P < .005$). (After Perri RT, Hebbel RP, Oken MM. Influence of treatment and response status on infection risk in multiple myeloma. Am J Med 1981;71:935)

IgG immunoglobulin is a monomer, and IgA occurs as a monomer or polymer but most frequently as a dimer. With any given level of IgG or IgA, hyperviscosity is extremely variable.[95] The IgG3 subclass is particularly prone to hyperviscosity; this finding has led to the realization that further polymerization in vivo may play a role in hyperviscosity.[96] With IgG3 immunoglobulins, hyperviscosity is often a problem when the paraprotein concentration reaches 4 to 5 g/dL. The other IgG immunoglobulins usually do not cause hyperviscosity until the concentration is over 15 g/dL. Hyperviscosity is also highly variable in IgA myeloma, suggesting that molecular interactions probably occur in vivo, which are important in determining true viscosity.[97] With monomeric IgA immunoglobulin, paraprotein levels generally are above 10 to 11 g/dL before hyperviscosity becomes clinically significant, whereas in the polymeric form hyperviscosity can become evident at concentrations of 6 to 7 g/dL.

Light-Chain Disease

In the normal plasma cell, heavy-chain and light-chain production is balanced. Myeloma cells sometimes produce both heavy and light chains, with an excess of light chains. This leads to complete monoclonal immunoglobulin in the serum and free light chains in the urine. In about 10% to 20% of patients with myeloma, the malignant cells produce no heavy chain but do produce monoclonal light chain.[98] In patients with light-chain disease, usually no identifiable monoclonal immunoglobulin is found in the serum, but monoclonal light chains can be found in the urine. Serum protein electrophoresis often shows reduced amounts of the normal polyclonal immunoglobulins, and since no monoclonal immunoglobulin is present in the serum, the γ-globulin region of the electrophoresis is flat (see Fig. 31-5). Electrophoresis of the urine demonstrates the monoclonal protein.

The finding of free monoclonal light chains in the urine is not necessarily indicative of myeloma. Patients with non-Hodgkin's lymphoma, CLL, and monoclonal gammopathy of undetermined significance may have monoclonal light chains in the urine.[81] Quantitation of the 24-hour excretion of monoclonal light chains is useful in distinguishing myeloma from the other disorders. Myeloma patients had a mean excretion of 8.54 g/24 h, whereas patients with non-Hodgkin's lymphoma had a mean excretion of 0.67 g/24 h, those with CLL, 0.16 g/24 h, and those with monoclonal gammopathy of undetermined significance, 0.05 g/24 h.[81] Normal polyclonal immunoglobulins were reduced in 100% of the patients with myeloma, in about 60% of the patients with non-Hodgkin's lymphoma or CLL, and in none of the patients with monoclonal gammopathy of undetermined significance in this series.

Renal failure is a predominant characteristic of patients with light-chain disease. More than one third of patients present with renal failure, and the mean creatinine level of the entire group averages between 3 and 4 mg/dL.[99] As previously mentioned, the cause of renal failure in patients with light-chain disease is myeloma kidney with precipitation of the light chains in the renal tubules, tubular dysfunction with reabsorption of the light chain into the renal tubular cells with disruption of the cellular basement membrane, or amyloid deposition in the kidney. About 20% of patients with light-chain disease have amyloidosis.[99] Specific properties of the light chains appear to determine the occurrence of amyloid formation, tubular cell damage, or precipitation of light chain in the tubules.

Over 50% of patients with light-chain disease have lytic bone lesions, and the myeloma cells account for over 50% of the bone marrow cellularity. Median survival is poor.

Patients without amyloid have a median survival duration of 19 months, and those with amyloid have a median survival of 7 months.

γ Heavy-Chain Disease

In 1964, Franklin and associates[100] described a patient whose myeloma cells produced only γ heavy chains without producing light chains. Since then, this syndrome has become a recognized but rare entity with several characteristics that are distinct from the typical cases of myeloma.[101] The morphology of the malignant cell is often variable. Classic plasma cells may be present, although sometimes the cells appear more as a plasmacytoid lymphocyte or a small well-differentiated lymphocyte. These variable morphologies also occur in combination. Lymphadenopathy and splenomegaly, which are uncommon in classic myeloma, are often present in this disease.

Survival in heavy-chain disease is variable, but the median survival is only 12 months. Because of the rarity of γ heavy-chain disease, little can be said about the ideal treatment methods for this group of patients. Patients are usually treated in the same fashion as other myeloma patients.

α Heavy-Chain Disease

Rarely have malignant lymphomas been associated with the production of free α heavy chains. α Heavy-chain diseases are probably not closely related to myeloma other than for the production of a monoclonal incomplete immunoglobulin. These diseases appear to consist primarily of non-Hodgkin's lymphomas, which have a propensity to occur in the gastrointestinal tract. Progression of disease may occur, beginning with plasma cells that produce α heavy chain and aggregate in the intestinal tract with subsequent transformation into a malignant non-Hodgkin's lymphoma of the immunoblastic type, probably arising from the more mature plasma cells.[102] The ideal therapy for α heavy-chain disease is not known because of its rarity, but intensive chemotherapy often including intravenous cyclophosphamide, doxorubicin, vincristine, and oral prednisone appears to offer some patients long-term remissions.

IgD Myeloma

IgD myeloma is a rare disease, accounting for about 2% of all cases of myeloma.[103] The monoclonal protein is usually present in small amounts and can be easily missed because it is hidden in the β-globulin region of the serum protein electrophoresis. Often excess production of light chains occurs leading to Bence Jones proteinuria, and renal failure is seen at diagnosis in about two thirds of patients. About 90% of IgD monoclonal immunoglobulins bear λ light-chain specificity. IgD myeloma has a predilection for men (3:1), whereas other myeloma subtypes have an equal distribution between the sexes. The average age of patients with IgD myeloma is 56 years compared with 63 years for IgG myeloma patients. Osteolytic lesions are seen in 79% of patients. Survival is poor and averages a little over 1 year.

IgE Myeloma

Rare cases of IgE-producing myeloma have been reported.[104,105] Because of the small number of reported cases, firm conclusions cannot be drawn about the clinical picture of these patients. Sex distribution is similar to myeloma, and slightly more young patients are affected. Osteolytic lesions, osteoporosis, and osteosclerosis all have been reported. The monoclonal immunoglobulin appears to be nonfunctional; therefore, symptoms associated with the allergic response related to normal IgE are generally not present.

Solitary Plasmacytoma

Rarely, patients present with a solitary lesion, either a bony abnormality or a soft tissue mass, which on biopsy reveals a plasma cell tumor.[106] These plasma cell tumors are monoclonal in nature as determined by heavy-chain and light-chain analysis. Careful evaluation of random iliac crest bone marrow samples show no evidence of myeloma, and further radiographic studies show only the solitary lesion that was initially seen. The clinical behavior of solitary bone plasmacytomas and extramedullary plasmacytomas appears to be the same,[107] although Holland and coworkers[108] have suggested that patients with extramedullary solitary plasmacytomas may have a lower incidence of conversion to myeloma than do patients with solitary plasmacytomas of bone.

If after careful evaluation, no systemic disease is found, it is common practice to treat the solitary lesion with local radiation therapy. If the monoclonal protein persists after treatment, the rapid development of myeloma is inevitable.[107] In patients whose monoclonal protein becomes undetectable after local radiation therapy, a steady progression occurs to overt multiple myeloma with time.[109] The probability of developing disseminated myeloma is 55% at 5 years, 77% at 10 years, and 77% at 15 years. Nuclear immaturity in the malignant plasma cells of the solitary plasmacytoma is more highly associated with early conversion to myeloma. Patients with well-differentiated tumors also develop disseminated disease, although less frequently and at a later time.[110] Because some patients do not develop disseminated myeloma, it is prudent to treat patients with local radiation therapy only, followed by close observation. Once there is evidence of dissemination the survival is identical with that of other patients with stage I myeloma, with a median survival of about 4 years.

Smoldering Myeloma

Most patients with overt myeloma have a poor prognosis with progression of disease and death in 1 to 4 years, depending on the stage of disease at diagnosis. A subgroup of patients appears to have a more indolent course of myeloma.[111] They are considered to have myeloma on the basis of monoclonal immunoglobulin levels higher than 3 g/dL and plasma cells accounting for more than 10% of the bone marrow cellularity. These patients have myeloma cells with labeling indices of 0%. None has developed bone lesions or hypercalcemia after follow-up of 5 to 16 years.

Although progressive disease is a rare phenomenon, patients who present with the findings of a monoclonal protein of greater than 3 g/dL and 10% or more plasma cells in the bone marrow, but without other signs of myeloma, should be closely observed for indications of progressive disease before initiation of chemotherapy. If the patient does not develop progressive disease over many years, clearly early treatment with chemotherapy would not be indicated.

Myeloma in Young Men

Myeloma is uncommon in young people, but on rare occasions it occurs in patients—usually men—between the ages of 15 and 25 years.[112,113] These patients have long, indolent disease courses. Even when the disease begins to progress and a response is obtained with chemotherapy, the response can be long-lasting.

Plasma Cell Leukemia

In rare circumstances, myeloma cells are found in the peripheral blood in sufficient numbers to be recognized morphologically. This clinical finding is referred to as plasma cell leukemia and represents two distinct entities. In primary plasma cell leukemia, circulating myeloma cells are present at the time of diagnosis. In secondary plasma cell leukemia, myeloma is present for some period of time without a leukemic phase; then, in the advanced stage of disease, a leukemic picture develops.[114] Among patients with plasma cell leukemia, about 50% have primary plasma cell leukemia and 50% have the secondary variety.

Patients with primary plasma cell leukemia often have different clinical characteristics than patients with myeloma in general.[115] Lytic bone lesions are present frequently (66%) but less frequently than in myeloma patients. Patients with plasma cell leukemia are more likely to be severely anemic and thrombocytopenic. They are also more likely to be hypercalcemic and uremic than myeloma patients in general. In addition, hepatosplenomegaly is seen in 50% to 70% of patients with plasma cell leukemia but in only 5% to 15% of patients with myeloma. Lymphadenopathy is seen in 40% of patients with plasma cell leukemia and in only 8% of patients with myeloma.

The prognosis of patients with primary plasma cell leukemia is poor, with median survivals of 2 to 6 months.[114,115] Intensive chemotherapy protocols using multiple alkylating agents have shown a slightly increased response rate but have not resulted in improved survival.

Secondary plasma cell leukemia occurs as a terminal event in about 1% to 5% of patients with myeloma. These patients have far-advanced bone disease and high levels of monoclonal immunoglobulin. In contrast to that which occurs in patients with primary plasma cell leukemia, hepatosplenomegaly and lymphadenopathy are rare. The bone marrow is usually almost entirely replaced by plasma cells. When this occurs, prognosis is poor, with a median survival of about 1 month.

Staging of Patients With Myeloma

Several staging systems have been proposed for patients with myeloma. Because, with the exception of solitary plasmacytomas, the disease is always disseminated, myeloma is not staged like the lymphomas. Staging does not distinguish sites of disease but attempts to reflect total body tumor burden. Tumor burden has been shown to correlate well with survival.

The most widely used staging system was proposed by Durie and Salmon[116] in 1975. This system is based on estimates of tumor cell mass and systemic effects of myeloma (Table 31-5). The main criteria used to distinguish one stage from another are hemoglobin level, hypercalcemia, bone lesions, and immunoglobulin levels. In addition, patients are classified as A or B, depending on renal function. This staging system readily predicts clinical outcome in response to chemotherapy and is therefore useful as a prognosticator. Although stage does not determine which type of therapy to use, it is useful in standardizing and evaluating chemotherapy trials.

Many other staging systems have been proposed for patients with myeloma. One of the simplest and most popular systems is based on serum levels of β_2-microglobulin. Pretreatment serum levels of β_2-microglobulin are roughly correlated with tumor burden and well correlated with survival.[117] The addition of other parameters, such as serum albumin and calcium level, also contributes to prognosis. A high β_2-microglobulin (more than 6 μg/mL is considered the cutoff value) and a serum albumin of less than 3 g/dL identify a very poor prognostic group. As shown in Table 31-6, the combination of serum albumin and β_2-microglobulin can divide myeloma patients into good-, intermediate-, and poor-risk groups with survival figures as shown.

TABLE 31-5. Staging of Multiple Myeloma: The Durie-Salmon Staging System

STAGE I
All of the following:
Hemoglobin >10 g/dL
Serum calcium <12 mg/dL
One or no lytic bone lesions
Low monoclonal protein level:
IgG <5 g/dL
IgA <3 g/dL
Urine light-chain excretion <4 g/24 h
STAGE II
Fitting neither stage I nor stage III
STAGE III
Any one of the following:
Hemoglobin <8.5 g/dL
Serum calcium >12 mg/dL
Advanced lytic bone lesions
High monoclonal protein level:
IgG >7 g/dL
IgA >5 g/dL
Urine light-chain excretion >12 g/24 h
SUBCLASSIFICATION
A—serum creatinine <2 mg/dL
B—serum creatinine ≥2 mg/dL

(Adapted from Durie BGM, Salmon SE. A clinical staging system for multiple myeloma: correlation of measured myeloma cell mass with presenting clinical features, response to treatment, and survival. Cancer 1975;36:842)

It is now known that IL-6 stimulates the synthesis of some acute-phase–reactant proteins, including C-reactive protein, and the serum concentration of C-reactive protein reflects IL-6 activity.[119] Serum C-reactive protein concentration has been shown to be predictive, independent of β_2-microglobulin, of survival for patients with myeloma. When C-reactive protein is considered together with β_2-microglobulin, patients can be divided into three prognostic groups—those with low serum levels of both, those with elevation of one protein, and those with elevations of both. Survivals for the groups were 54, 27, and 6 months, respectively.

Therapy of Myeloma

The evaluation of any treatment program for patients with myeloma requires an understanding of several important factors. The first is the response criteria that are used. Most studies use the objective response criteria developed by the Chronic Leukemia-Myeloma Task Force in 1973.[9] A response is defined as a 50% or greater reduction in the serum monoclonal immunoglobulin concentration, a 50% or greater reduction in urinary monoclonal protein excretion, a 50% or greater reduction in the cross-sectional area of a plasmacytoma, or recalcification of bone lesions without the appearance of new lesions. This is a straightforward

TABLE 31-6. Median Survival of Patients With Myeloma Stratified by Serum β_2-Microglobulin (Sβ_2M) and Serum Albumin (SAlb) Levels

Stratification (Staging)	No. Patients	No. Alive	Median Survival (mo)
I. LOW RISK			
Sβ_2M < 6 μg/mL SAlb > 3 g/dL	254	182 (72%)	38
II. INTERMEDIATE RISK			
Sβ_2M < 6 μg/mL SAlb ≤ 3 g/dL	59	29 (49%)	27
or			
Sβ_2M ≥ 6 μg/mL SAlb > 3 g/dL	160	81 (51%)	24
III. HIGH RISK			
Sβ_2M ≥ 6 μg/mL SAlb ≤ 3 g/dL	61	22 (36%)	14

(Durie BGM, Stock-Novack D, Salmon SE, et al. Prognostic value of pretreatment serum β2-microglobulin in myeloma: a Southwest Oncology Group study. Blood 1990;75:823)

and simple system and has been accepted by most investigators. Because catabolism of IgG immunoglobulin varies according to serum concentration and because increased catabolism is seen with higher serum levels, the Southwest Oncology Group proposed a system in which an objective response was based on a 75% reduction in the production of myeloma protein.[118] In practical terms, these two systems yielded similar results when applied to the same cohort of patients.[120] Because of this similarity, the simpler guidelines of the Task Force are generally preferred.

When the literature is analyzed, similar treatment protocols may have vastly different results in different studies. Aspects of patient selection play an important role in the generation of these differences. A significant number of myeloma patients present with advanced disease; these patients may have a short survival. They are often omitted from chemotherapy trials because of the advanced nature of their disease, which creates a favorable bias in results. Patients with renal failure have a particularly poor prognosis and are sometimes also excluded from clinical trials. When comparing two trials, it is important to understand the stated eligibility criteria as well as the stage distribution of patients, although many unwritten selection biases may still be present.

In myeloma as with any other neoplasm, considerable variability has been used in the scheduling of similar drugs. Many melphalan and prednisone schedules are radically different and yield different results. Because of this and the previously mentioned considerations, evaluation of the treatment programs in myeloma has been difficult, and some controversy remains concerning optimal therapy for each stage of disease.

Therapy of Previously Untreated Patients

With the exception of solitary plasmacytomas, myeloma is a systemic disease and the mainstay of therapy is systemic chemotherapy. In 1958, Blokhin and colleagues[121] reported the use of melphalan (L-phenylalanine mustard) in the treatment of patients with myeloma. In the 1960s, many institutions began to use melphalan with and without prednisone in the treatment of patients with myeloma. Today, melphalan and prednisone remain the mainstay of previously untreated patients with myeloma. Some chemotherapy regimens used in the treatment of myeloma patients are shown in Table 31-7.

TABLE 31-7. Selected Chemotherapy Regimens in the Treatment of Multiple Myeloma*

Regimen	Drug Dose	Frequency	Reference
M-P	Melphalan, 0.25 mg/kg/d × 4 d PO Prednisone, 2 mg/kg/d × 4 d PO	Every 6 wk	122
BCMP	BCNU, 100 mg/m² × 1 IV, day 1 Cyclophosphamide, 300 mg/m² × 1 IV, day 1 Melphalan, 8 mg/m² × 1 IV, day 1 Prednisone, 1.2 mg/kg PO every day (10-wk taper)	Every 6 wk	125
VMCP	Vincristine, 1 mg/m² (max 1.5 mg) × 1 IV, day 1 Melphalan, 6 mg/m² PO × 4, days 1–4 Cyclophosphamide, 125 mg/m² PO × 4, days 1–4 Prednisone, 60 mg/m² PO × 4, days 1–4	Every 3 wk	126
VCAP	Vincristine, 1 mg/m² (max 1.5 mg) × 1 IV, day 1 Cyclophosphamide, 125 mg/m² PO × 4, days 1–4 Doxorubicin, 30 mg/m² IV × 1, day 1 Prednisone, 60 mg/m² PO × 4, days 1–4	Every 3 wk	126
VBAP	Vincristine, 1 mg/m² (max 1.5 mg) × 1, day 1 BCNU, 30 mg/m² IV × 1, day 1 Doxorubicin, 30 mg/m² IV × 1, day 1 Prednisone, 60 mg/m² PO × 4, days 1–4	Every 3 wk	126
M2	Vincristine, 0.03 mg/kg IV × 1, day 1 BCNU, 0.5 mg/kg IV × 1, day 1 Cyclophosphamide, 10 mg/kg IV × 1, day 1 Melphalan, 0.25 mg/kg PO × 4 d, or 0.1 mg/kg PO × 7–10 d Prednisone, 1 mg/kg/d PO, taper	Every 5 wk	129
VAD	Vincristine, 0.4 mg/d IV by continuous infusion × 4 d Doxorubicin, 9 mg/m²/d IV by continuous infusion × 4 d Dexamethasone, 40 mg/d PO × 4 d, days 1, 9, 17	Every 4 wk	148

* These chemotherapy regimens are merely outlined; physicians should refer to references cited before administering them.

In 1969, the Southwest Cancer Chemotherapy Study Group showed that intermittent melphalan was superior to continuous daily melphalan and that intermittent melphalan with concurrent prednisone was superior therapy to melphalan alone.[122] Daily melphalan alone had a response rate of 19%, whereas intermittent melphalan alone had a response rate of 35%. Addition of concurrent prednisone increased the response rate to 73%, proving the usefulness of prednisone in the treatment of this disease. The melphalan dose in this last regimen was 0.25 mg/kg/d for 4 days every 6 weeks. It was also noted that the addition of prednisone did not increase the incidence of serious infection. This was a well-formulated, randomized study with patient characteristics being similar in all treatment groups. About 25% of patients had renal failure at presentation, and the response criteria of the Task Force were used.

Several factors have caused investigators to study new chemotherapy regimens with multiple agents. First and foremost, although the response rates are reasonable with oral melphalan and prednisone, the response is short and most patients die in 2 to 3 years. Essentially no patients are cured with this regimen. In the middle to late 1960s, chemotherapy trials in patients with Hodgkin's disease demonstrated that when effective single agents are combined, patients with advanced disease can be cured (MOPP). These results cannot be obtained with single agents, and the particulars of the combination are essential, since many combinations are not curative. In myeloma patients, evidence shows that many alkylating agents are active and that cross-resistance between alkylating agents is not always present.[123] Another concern is apparent erratic intestinal absorption of oral melphalan. This might lead to suboptimal results, since some patients may never achieve adequate drug levels. Another issue (discussed later in the chapter) is the occurrence of acute myelogenous leukemia in a significant number of patients. Melphalan may have a role in leukemogenesis in this situation. A summary of some chemotherapy trials is listed in Table 31-8.

In 1970, the Southeastern Cancer Study Group began a trial using BCNU, cyclophosphamide, and prednisone in one of the first of many efforts combining multiple alkylating agents in an attempt to improve response rates and survival.[124] This produced a response rate of about 50% in previously untreated patients and a median survival of 2 years. These data were similar to those obtained when melphalan and prednisone were given concurrently in an intermittent schedule.

The Cancer and Leukemia Group B compared oral melphalan and prednisone with intravenous melphalan, cyclophosphamide, BCNU, and prednisone.[125] Using the Task Force response criteria, they found that in good-risk patients response was better with the multiagent regimen (70% compared with 57%), but that survival was the same (30 months compared with 38 months in the melphalan and prednisone arm). In the bad-risk patients, survival was improved in the multiagent arm, 24 months compared with 12 months in the melphalan and prednisone arm.

A highly controversial trial was conducted by the Southwest Oncology Group (SWOG) in which oral melphalan and prednisone administered every 3 weeks was compared with vincristine, melphalan, cyclophosphamide, and prednisone (VMCP) alternating with vincristine, cyclophosphamide, doxorubicin, and prednisone, or a regimen of three cycles of VMCP followed by three cycles of vincristine, BCNU, doxorubicin, and prednisone (VBAP).[126] The response rate was 32% for the melphalan and prednisone arm and 54% for the combination arms. In addition, survival was improved in the multiagent chemotherapy arm (43 months compared with 23 months for the melphalan and prednisone arm). This study has been cited extensively to support the use of intensive therapy in this disease. It has also been heavily criticized because of the scheduling of the melphalan and prednisone arm and because of its apparent inferior response and survival rates compared with those of other melphalan studies. In this study, melphalan was administered at 8 mg/m² orally for 4 days every 21 days, and concurrent prednisone was given at 60 mg/

TABLE 31-8. Chemotherapy for Patients With Previously Untreated Multiple Myeloma

Treatment Regimen	Patient Stratification	Response Rate (%)	Median Survival (mo)	Reference
Melph, daily oral	None	19†	18	122
Melph, intermittent oral	None	35†	18	122
Melph-pred, intermittent oral	None	73†	24	122
BCNU, CTX, Pred	None	53†	28	124
	Good risk	55†	42	124
	Bad risk	51†	21	124
Melph, CTX, BCNU, pred*	Good risk	70†	30	125
Melph-pred*	Good risk	57†	38	125
Melph, CTX, BCNU, pred*	Bad risk	64†	24	125
Melph-pred*	Bad risk	55†	12	125
Melph-pred*	None	32‡	23	126
VMCP, VCAP, VBAP*	None	54‡	43	126
Melph-pred*	None	62†	32	128
VMCP, VBAP*	None	56†	28	128
M2 (VCR, BCNU, CTX, pred)*	None	74†	33	130
Melph-pred*	None	53†	29	130

Melph-pred, oral melphalan and prednisone; CTX, cyclophosphamide; VCR, vincristine; VMCP, vincristine, melphalan, cyclophosphamide, prednisone; VCAP, vincristine, cyclophosphamide, doxorubicin, prednisone; VBAP, vincristine, BCNU, doxorubicin, prednisone.

* Randomized studies.

† Myeloma Task Force response criteria.

‡ Southwest Oncology Group response criteria.

m^2 orally also for 4 days. In addition, 15% of patients treated with the multidrug regimens had life-threatening hematologic toxicity, whereas only 2% of the patients treated with melphalan and prednisone had similar toxicity. Because of these criticisms, the superiority of multiple alkylating agent therapy in these patients has not been universally accepted.

Alexanian and Dreicer[127] reported a study using regimens similar to those used by SWOG and found no difference in response rates or survival. In a more recent study reported from Sweden, the standard regimen of melphalan and prednisone was compared in patients with Durie stage II and III; the SWOG VMCP was given for stage II patients and alternating VMCP and VBAP for stage III patients.[128] In this well-conducted, randomized study, melphalan and prednisone achieved equal response and survival rates compared with those with the multidrug SWOG regimens. The response rate of melphalan and prednisone was 69% in stage II patients and 58% in stage III patients, suggesting that the much lower response rates obtained in the SWOG study may have resulted from suboptimal scheduling.

Memorial Sloan-Kettering Cancer Center reported results of a nonrandomized multiagent intensive regimen consisting of vincristine, BCNU, melphalan, cyclophosphamide, and prednisone (M2 regimen), suggesting a response rate of 87% and an improved median survival of 50 months.[129] The Eastern Cooperative Oncology Group compared the M2 regimen with melphalan and prednisone, and although the response rate was higher with the M2 protocol (74% compared with 53%), the median survival times were no different (33 months compared with 29 months), respectively.[130]

The Italian Multiple Myeloma Study Group[131] reported on a trial comparing a VMCP/VBAP alternating regimen with mephalan and prednisone and found no response of survival advantage to the multidrug combination over melphalan and prednisone. This was true in all patient subgroups, including those patients with poor-prognosis disease. Gregory and colleagues[132] performed an overview of published trials comparing combination chemotherapy with melphalan and prednisone and suggested that melphalan and prednisone was superior therapy for patients with good-risk myeloma and combination chemotherapy was advantageous for patients with poor-risk myeloma. This conclusion has not been universally accepted, however.

α-Interferon (IFN-α) has demonstrated activity against myeloma and has been incorporated into primary treatment regimens by a number of groups. Osterborg and associates[133] conducted a study for the Myeloma Group of Central Sweden, randomly assigning patients to receive oral melphalan and prednisone every 6 weeks, with or without IFN-α for 5 days every 3 weeks. Treatment was continued until tumor progression, but the IFN-α dose was reduced at the time of maximum response. Responses were more frequent in patients receiving IFN-α together with melphalan and prednisone as compared with those receiving melphalan and prednisone alone (68% versus 42%), but survival was not different between the two groups. Only the subset of patients with IgA myeloma or light chain disease appeared to benefit from the addition of IFN-α to melphalan and prednisone. The Cancer and Leukemia Group B also compared melphalan and prednisone with and without IFN-α in the treatment of previously untreated patients with myeloma.[134] In contrast to the findings reported by the Swedish group, the response rate of patients receiving only melphalan and prednisone was 44%; for those patients receiving IFN-α with melphalan and prednisone, the response rate was only 33%. There was no difference in survival between the two treatment groups. The IFN-α dose in this study was lower, and it was administered less intensively than in the Swedish study, which could account for the differences.

Because the results of therapy for myeloma have been so poor, other investigators have explored dose-intensive therapy in previously untreated patients with myeloma. The Cancer and Leukemia Group B treated patients with cyclophosphamide followed by escalating doses of high-dose intravenous melphalan.[135] This regimen proved to be extremely toxic, with only 2 of 28 patients (7%) achieving a complete remission and 12 of 28 (43%) attaining a partial remission. The French reported on a trial in which previously untreated patients received either VAD—vincristine, doxorubicin (Adriamycin), and dexamethasone (Decadron)—or VMCP, followed by high-dose melphalan and total body irradiation with autologous bone marrow transplantation and maintenance IFN-α.[136] Of 35 patients treated, 15 (43%) achieved a complete response and 14 (40%) had a partial response; of those attaining a complete response, 13 (85%) remained progression-free at 33 months. At 42 months, the probability of survival was 81%. The therapy appeared to be most beneficial for patients with low β_2-microglobulin levels, a group with a more favorable prognosis. The Northern California Oncology Group added hemibody radiation therapy to induction chemotherapy but found no additional benefit in this circumstance.[137]

Multiple other studies have been conducted in an attempt to design a combination chemotherapy protocol that is superior to melphalan and prednisone. No conclusive evidence exists that multiagent therapy is superior to melphalan and prednisone, and it is certainly more toxic and more cumbersome to administer. Although controversy remains, most physicians still consider melphalan and prednisone to be the optimal initial therapy for patients with myeloma.

Kinetics of the Cellular Response to Chemotherapy

In patients who respond to initial chemotherapy, the cellular response follows the Gompertzian law of kinetics.[138] An initial, rapid fall-off in tumor cell number (and immunoglobulin level) occurs for the first three or four treatment cycles. A slowing of response and a plateau phase with little additional tumor cell decline then occur. Almost all patients follow this pattern of response, and therapy leads to only a 1- to 2-log cell kill. Although this degree of tumor cell reduction is important to decrease symptoms and increase survival, it is clearly inadequate as a long-term goal. The meaning of this limited response and subsequent plateau is not completely understood but is highly significant, since the end result is an inability to totally eradicate the tumor clone.

To understand this phenomenon, tumor cell kinetics have been assessed before and during chemotherapy. As tumor cell number decreases in response to therapy, labeling index rises progressively.[139] It is hypothesized that the plateau phase seen after the initial several cycles of chemotherapy represents the effect of increased myeloma cell turnover balanced with decreasing cell kill from the therapy. In an attempt to take advantage of this finding, patients were treated with cycle-specific agents such as vincristine and cytosine arabinoside during the period when they would be expected to have a high labeling index. Neither of these agents has significant antitumor effect in this circumstance. Other investigators have suggested that there is a small nonproliferating myeloma cell compartment during this plateau phase and that this compartment is responsible for the maintenance of the active tumor burden and is unaffected by cycle-specific agents.[140]

Further attempts to modulate myeloma cell kinetics have

yielded mixed results. Patients who had become resistant to standard doses of cyclophosphamide were treated with high doses of intravenous cyclophosphamide, and labeling index was assessed.[141] Maximum labeling index values were obtained 9 days after cyclophosphamide administration, and an additional agent, doxorubicin, was therefore administered at that time. The investigators describe improved response rates and survival in an uncontrolled group of patients. Other studies have failed to show important improvements using analogous treatment plans.

Initial labeling index values may also be important in analyzing results of therapy. Patients who responded rapidly to chemotherapy but had labeling index of 2% or more at the time of therapy had an unusually poor survival.[41] The importance of this finding is unknown, and these data have not been used to design a different, potentially more effective therapy for this subgroup of patients.

Role of Maintenance Therapy

Gompertzian response kinetics demonstrate that a significant residual tumor burden remains after initial therapy with melphalan and prednisone or similar agents. The suggestion that this plateau may be the result of increased myeloma cell turnover makes the issue of maintenance chemotherapy especially important. In patients who respond to initial therapy, the amount of reduction of monoclonal immunoglobulin is predictive of the rapidity of rise after the cessation of therapy.[142] After an initial year of chemotherapy, patients who attained at least a partial remission (by SWOG criteria) were randomized to receive no maintenance therapy, continued melphalan and prednisone, or BCNU and prednisone. The addition of maintenance therapy did not improve survival when compared with the no-treatment control group. Therefore, in spite of the finding that myeloma tumor mass would grow after cessation of therapy, continued therapy was of no benefit.

IFN-α, when used at an initial dose of 12×10^6 IU/m^2, induces a response rate of about 50% in previously untreated patients. In patients who have received prior chemotherapy and failed, IFN-α has a response rate of about 15%.[143] All patients required dose reduction by 24 weeks in this study. A randomized trial using IFN-α_{2b} as maintenance therapy showed statistically significant improvement in survival for patients treated with IFN compared with that of patients receiving no maintenance therapy.[144] In this study, IFN was administered at a much lower dose, 3 $\times 10^6$ IU/m^2 three times per week, with much less toxicity. Patients were initially treated for 1 year with either melphalan and prednisone or VMCP or VBAP. If the patients attained a response or had stable disease, they were randomized to either receive IFN or to be followed without therapy. In patients who achieved a response (by Task Force criteria), maintenance therapy with IFN showed a significant survival advantage. Patients with stable disease tended toward improved survival with IFN, but this difference was not statistically significant.

Therapy of Relapsed or Resistant Myeloma

About half of newly diagnosed patients respond to therapy. Therefore, half of patients demonstrate primary resistant disease to initial therapy. Even patients who do respond to initial therapy rapidly develop relapsed or resistant disease. In these circumstances, many treatment approaches have been tried, and although success is variable, the overall outcome is usually poor.[145] When possible, studies that evaluate patients in this situation should distinguish between patients who were responders to initial therapy and those who had primary resistant disease.

Corticosteroids alone have produced responses in patients with progressive myeloma. Prednisone, used at a dose of 60 mg/m^2/d for 5 days produced true responses (by SWOG criteria) in 3 of 16 patients and overall responses (over 50% tumor mass reduction) in 31% of patients.[146] These responses were seen in both initially responsive and nonresponsive patients. The median duration of myeloma control for responding patients was only 7 months. High-dose dexamethasone, 40 mg orally for 4 days beginning on days 1, 9, and 17 of a 5-week cycle, produced a response rate of 27% in patients with previously unresponsive disease and 21% in patients with previously responsive disease.[147] In patients with previously unresponsive disease, the addition of doxorubicin and vincristine did not improve the response rate, whereas patients who previously responded to therapy showed an increase in response rate to 65% with the addition of these agents. This finding suggests that patients who were initially sensitive to one chemotherapy regimen were more likely to be sensitive to a second-line regimen, and those with initial resistance were likely to be resistant to other chemotherapy agents.

An innovative regimen using continuous intravenous infusions of vincristine and doxorubicin over 4 days together with dexamethasone (VAD) was reported in 1984.[148] Eleven of 13 patients with previously responsive disease and 3 of 7 with primary resistant disease responded to this regimen for a total response rate of 70%. The major toxicity of this regimen is hematologic but is mild and tolerable. Etoposide, dexamethasone, cytarabine, and cisplatin have also been used successfully in relapsed or refractory patients.[149] In patients previously treated with melphalan or VAD, a 40% response rate was seen. Despite this response rate in a poor prognostic group of patients, the median survival was only 6.5 months in the responding patients and 1.5 months in the nonresponding patients.

High doses of intravenous melphalan (70 to 90 mg/m^2) are successful in attaining responses in patients who failed on oral melphalan or VAD.[150] In patients who had been previously sensitive to chemotherapy or those who had less than 12 months of resistant disease, the response rate is over 50%. Three of 43 patients attained complete remissions, but hematologic toxicity is universally severe. Pneumonia or sepsis occurred in 63% of the patients, and 19% died as a result of bone marrow suppression. Barlogie and associates[151] treated a subsequent group of patients with high-dose melphalan, 100 mg/m^2, followed by the hematopoietic growth factor GM-CSF. Of 23 patients treated, 9 (39%) achieved partial remission and only 2 died of infectious complications during the period of postchemotherapy neutropenia. A regimen of high-dose cyclophosphamide (3 g/m^2) and etoposide (900 mg/m^2) followed by GM-CSF was administered to patients who had failed on VAD, resulting in a response rate of 42%.[152]

Bone Marrow Transplantation

Bone marrow transplantation remains an experimental and controversial procedure for multiple myeloma. Both allogeneic and autologous transplants have been performed. Most patients with myeloma are too old to be safely offered transplantation of either kind and often suffer from comorbid disease that would make transplantation more hazardous than usual. In addition, since standard chemotherapy results in only a 1- to 2-log cell kill, even when doses of chemotherapy or radiation are raised to transplant levels, concern remains that cell kill will not be sufficient to completely eradicate the disease.

Autologous bone marrow transplantation has the advantage of being safer than allogeneic transplantation in older patients, particularly in relation to graft-versus-host disease. In addition, an acceptable HLA-matched donor is not required. The fact that the bone marrow of most patients remains significantly involved with myeloma cells, even after initial induction therapy, is a major negative factor in autologous bone marrow transplantation. Because of this, considerable effort has been expended on attempting to develop monoclonal antibodies specific for myeloma cells and efficient enough to adequately purge involved marrow of all clonogenic tumor cells. Antibodies such as PCA-1 and MM4 have been developed but may not be sufficiently effective to render an involved marrow free of clonogenic tumor cells.[153,154]

In one study, seven patients underwent autologous transplantation without marrow purging.[155] High-dose melphalan and total body irradiation were used as a conditioning regimen. The patients ranged from 45 to 63 years in age. Two transplant deaths occurred, and three of the patients remained disease-free for 2 to 21 months. Anderson and coworkers[156] performed autologous transplantations on 11 patients using high-dose melphalan and total body irradiation. All patients had less than 10% plasma cells in the bone marrow at the time of transplantation, and the harvested marrow was treated in vitro with antibodies against CD10, CD20, and PCA-1. Eight patients achieved complete remission, but only three remained disease-free with short follow-up. Mansi and associates[157] treated 13 patients with high-dose busulfan and autologous bone marrow transplantation. Many of the patients had previously been treated with high-dose melphalan. Four achieved complete remission, and two others attained partial remission—for an overall response rate of 46%—but three patients died of treatment-related toxicity.

One way to avoid potential problems due to bone marrow involvement with myeloma is to reconstitute the patient with peripheral blood stem cells. Eight patients were treated in this fashion after conditioning with carmustine, etoposide, melphalan, and total body irradiation. One patient had an early death, and engraftment was successful in all other patients. Two patients attained complete remission and remain disease-free at 15 and 16 months. The follow-up in these studies is still short, and a major concern is continued late relapses. Since myeloma cells can be found in the peripheral blood by immunologic techniques, doubts about this strategy remain.

Allogeneic transplantation has also been attempted. This has the potential advantage of not requiring minimal bone marrow involvement or purging of the bone marrow. The disadvantages of this approach include age restrictions, the need for an HLA-matched donor, and graft-versus-host disease. The European Group for Bone Marrow Transplantation reported their experience with allogeneic bone marrow transplantion performed on 90 patients with myeloma at various institutions.[158] Patients received different conditioning regimens, including total body irradiation plus high-dose chemotherapy in 81 patients and high-dose chemotherapy alone in 9 patients. Thirty-nine patients (43%) achieved complete remission after transplantation, and 11 (12%) remained in complete remission at 24 to 68 months of follow-up. With longer follow-up, it is possible that additional patients would have experienced relapse. Survival depended on attaining complete remission after transplantation, the number of previous chemotherapy regimens given, and the stage of disease at presentation, with patients with stage I disease surviving longer. Therefore, it appears that allogeneic transplantation benefits only a small fraction of patients with myeloma since most are not eligible because of age, lack of an acceptable donor, comorbid disease, or disease resistant to initial therapy. In addition, of those patients who receive transplants, only a small minority experience durable remission.

Radiation Therapy

Radiation therapy is a valuable tool in treating local plasmacytomas that are symptomatic, especially when impingement of local structures such as the spinal cord or nerve root is present. It is also helpful in arresting local bone disease before the point of fracture. Radiation therapy works by reducing local myeloma tumor burden and diminishing effects on surrounding structures but does not in itself lead to bone healing. After extensive bone loss with or without fracture, often little or no restructuring or recalcification of the bone occurs. Radiation therapy may not relieve pain once fractures occur, particularly in vertebral bodies or ribs, but it may slow disease progression and prevent future fractures. When the myeloma is under good control from systemic chemotherapy, radiation therapy is less likely to be helpful in pain control.

The weight-bearing bones most often require radiation therapy for pain relief and to prevent fracture. In one series, the most common sites of radiation were the femur, spine, ribs, pelvis, and humerus.[159] This retrospective study also looked at the doses of radiation therapy and subsequent need for radiation as an index of lasting effectiveness. Most frequently used doses were between 1500 and 2500 rad, and no relation was found between dose delivered and lasting effectiveness.

Systemic radiation therapy has also been used as palliative therapy in patients with advanced disease resistant to chemotherapy. A variety of techniques have been used; most have resulted in some palliation and considerable toxicity. One technique involved an attempt to irradiate most of the bone marrow in a segmental fashion, not dissimilar to that attempted with total nodal irradiation for patients with Hodgkin's disease, with the addition of electron beam therapy to the ribs and skull.[160] The axial skeleton received 1900 rad and the ribs and skull 2000 rad. Neutropenia and thrombocytopenia were severe. Seven of nine patients experienced pain relief and four of nine patients had an objective response (Task Force criteria) to therapy. In some patients, the number of myeloma cells decreased in the bone marrow.

Hemibody irradiation has also been used in patients with refractory myeloma. In one series, patients received either hemibody radiation only (usually from the xiphoid process to the knees) or sequential lower and upper body hemibody radiation.[161] A dose of 850 rad was delivered in each hemibody treatment. Seventeen of the 19 patients in this series reported subjective improvement in pain, usually within the first 24 hours. Hematologic toxicity was severe when both upper body and lower body were irradiated. Objective responses using Task Force criteria were observed in 6 of 19 patients, and the median survival of all patients was 6 months.

Novel Therapies in Myeloma

With the failure to achieve sufficient success in the treatment of myeloma with the standard therapies described, new and innovative therapies are being explored, in part based on our new understanding of lymphoid development. Because it is apparent that IL-6 is important for the growth of some myeloma cell lines, investigators have attempted to exploit this finding to inhibit tumor growth in vivo. Klein and colleagues[162] adminstered anti–IL-6 antibody to a patient with myeloma and noted a transient stabilization of disease. Bone marrow myeloma cell kinetics were analyzed and demonstrated a marked decrease in the percentage of myeloma cells undergoing DNA synthesis during the antibody therapy. Although the benefits were minimal and transient, this experiment may lead to more productive approaches in the future. Other investigators treated human myeloma cells in vitro with IL-6 linked to a mutant form of *Psudomonas* exotoxin and found killing of myeloma cells without significant effects on bone marrow progenitor cells.[163] It is possible this technique would be useful for purging bone marrow used for autologous marrow transplantation and could be useful in vivo. Chimeric mouse–human antibodies to CD38 have been prepared and tested in vitro against human myeloma cells, and preliminary results are encouraging.[164] Between 79% and 97% of plasma cells were found to bear the CD38 antigen, and other serious immunologic effects were not noted in these preliminary studies.

Myeloma and the Risk of Acute Myelogenous Leukemia

An association between myeloma and acute myelogenous leukemia was noted by several investigators in the early 1970s. In 1974, the Cancer and Leukemia Group B reported additional cases and reviewed a total of 46 cases.[165] Twenty-two of the cases were described as myeloblastic, 21 as myelomonocytic, 2 as promyelocytic, and 1 as erythroleukemic. Although the authors implicated melphalan as a possible causative agent, most of the patients received melphalan, which made it difficult to know whether melphalan truly played a role in the development of the leukemias. In addition, 11 of the 46 cases of leukemia appeared to occur simultaneously with the myeloma, suggesting that the association may be inherent rather than therapy related. Another study suggested that the actuarial risk of developing acute myelogenous leukemia in myeloma patients was 17% at 50 months.[166] In this series, the leukemias were also predominantly myeloblastic and monocytic. The risk was independent of the chemotherapy regimen that the patients received, although all treatment groups received melphalan.

WALDENSTRÖM'S MACROGLOBULINEMIA

Definition and Differential Diagnosis

In the 1930s and 1940s, Waldenström described a syndrome of hypergammaglobulinemia, hyperviscosity, and hemorrhage. We now know Waldenström's macroglobulinemia to be a disease characterized by a clonal malignant lymphoplasmacytic proliferation and production of monoclonal IgM from the malignant cell. In the Working Formulation Classification of non-Hodgkin's lymphomas, this disease is referred to as *malignant lymphoma, small lymphocytic, plasmacytoid*.[167] It is grouped with malignant lymphoma, small lymphocytic, consistent with CLL and is included in the group of low-grade lymphomas. In this chapter, the term *macroglobulinemia* refers to the malignant disease Waldenström's macroglobulinemia, or lymphoplasmacytic lymphoma with IgM monoclonal gammopathy.

Macroglobulinemia is not the only cause of monoclonal IgM production. About half of patients found to have monoclonal IgM do not have an apparent malignant process and are classified as having monoclonal gammopathy of undetermined significance as outlined earlier in the chapter.[168] Of patients who have monoclonal IgM associated with a malignancy, most have macroglobulinemia and a small number have other non-Hodgkin's lymphomas or CLL.

About 17% of patients who present with elevated IgM levels without other manifestations of macroglobulinemia or other malignancy (monoclonal gammopathy of undetermined significance) develop a malignant lymphoid disease with a median of 4 years from the time of discovery of the monoclonal protein to diagnosis of malignancy. About 10% of patients have a modest increase in IgM levels without developing other signs of malignancy. Of those patients who have apparent monoclonal gammopathy of undetermined significance, 40% have light-chain excretion in the urine.

The manifestations of macroglobulinemia are distinct from those of myeloma. Bone disease and renal disease, two of the hallmarks of myeloma, are much less common in patients with macroglobulinemia. The monoclonal IgM causes problems directly, particularly hyperviscosity and neurologic symptoms. A major factor in the pathogenesis of these problems is that the IgM immunoglobulin produced is a pentamer and because of its size is largely intravascular and has a higher viscosity per gram of protein in the serum.

Histologic Features

Macroglobulinemia is a malignant non-Hodgkin's lymphoma of small lymphocytes, often referred to as plasmacytoid lymphocytes or lymphoplasmacytic cells, as shown in Figure 31-16. These cells have less cytoplasm than plasma cells but retain a slightly eccentric nucleus. They are slightly larger than well-differentiated lymphocytes (normal or those seen in CLL). Being intermediate in size between plasma cells and well-differentiated lymphocytes and retaining an eccentric nucleus make the cells appear as a hybrid between the two; thus, the term *lymphoplasmacytic lymphocytes*. In a given bone marrow or lymph node sample, morphologic variation is often present. Most cells appear to be typical lymphoplasmacytes, but classic plasma cells and well-differentiated lymphocytes also may be present. These are monoclonal, with the malignant cell bearing the same immunoglobulin subtype as the plasmacytoid lymphocytes. The cells are always B cells and produce the monoclonal IgM, and their characteristics can be confirmed by immunochemistry demonstrating presence of μ heavy chain and either λ or κ light chain, but not both. The light- and heavy-chain specificity is the same as that found on the circulating monoclonal immunoglobulin.

Histologic confirmation of the malignant cell is necessary for diagnosis of macroglobulinemia. This confirmation can often be obtained from bone marrow or lymph node biopsy. Since bone marrow is often involved and more easily obtained than lymph node tissue, bone marrow biopsy is usually the diagnostic technique chosen. The aspirate of the bone marrow shows the typical plasmacytoid lymphocytes. As just described, increased numbers of well-differentiated lymphocytes and plasma cells are also present, and these cells are part of the malignant clone. The concentration of these cells in the bone marrow aspirate or biopsy is variable. Some areas may contain many of these cells and other areas may contain few. The malignant cells tend to occur in aggregates, although they often stream out into the surrounding normal marrow. The aggregates are sometimes paratrabecular. The lymph node pathology demonstrates a diffuse effacement of normal lymph node architecture with the lymphoplasmacytic cells. Again, immunochemistry can demonstrate monoclonality with the same immunoglobulin subtype as the circulating immunoglobulin. An increase in mast cells is also often seen, but the significance of this finding is not clear.

Clinical Features

The clinical features of macroglobulinemia are listed below:

- Monoclonal IgM
- Hyperviscosity
- Visual disturbances—fundus paraproteinaemicus

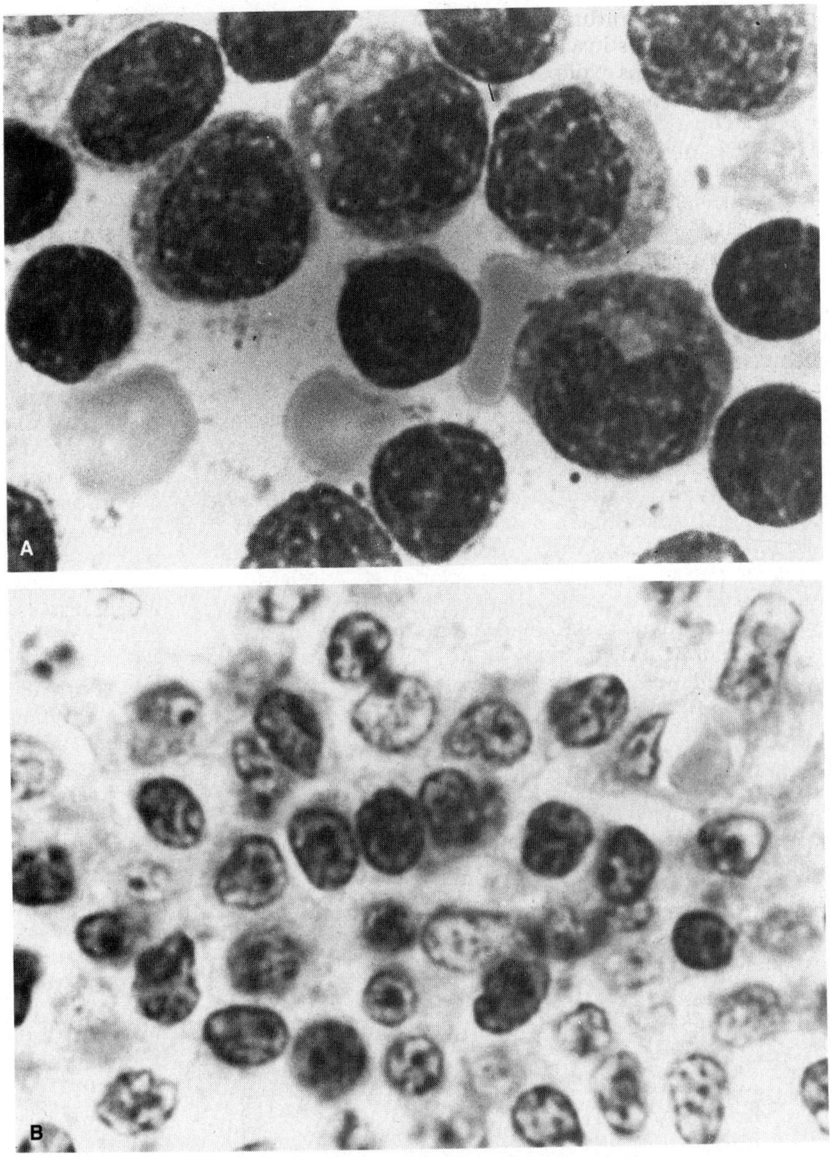

FIGURE 31-16. Lymphoplasmacytic lymphoma cells of Waldenström's macroglobulinemia. (**A**) Cells on the bone marrow aspirate. (**B**) Aggregates of lymphoma cells on the bone marrow core biopsy. The cells are intermediate in size between small lymphocytes and plasma cells, and the placement of the nucleus in the cells is slightly eccentric.

- Neurologic defects—central from hyperviscosity, peripheral
- Hemorrhage syndrome—binding of several coagulation proteins
- Cutaneous lesions—infiltration by lymphoma cells, monoclonal protein, or purpura
- Lymphadenopathy and splenomegaly
- Cryoglobulinemia and cold agglutinin disease
- Bone disease and renal disease (uncommon)

They are different from the features seen in myeloma and, in general, are more closely related to those seen in low-grade lymphomas, as well as those specifically attributable to the monoclonal IgM immunoglobulin. Complications usually arise as a result of the IgM immunoglobulin before other effects of the lymphoma so that many of the features described in the literature deal with these findings.

Hyperviscosity

Waldenström[170] described the syndrome of hypergammaglobulinemia and hyperviscosity in one of his original manuscripts. Subsequently, it was determined that IgM immunoglobulins were particularly prone to hyperviscosity. In most cases, when IgG is increased in the serum, the increase in viscosity is directly proportional to the immunoglobulin concentration.[171] By contrast, when IgM is increased in the serum, the increase in viscosity is directly proportional to IgM only at low concentrations. When concentrations reach about 3 g/dL, the viscosity rises more rapidly. Viscosity measurements should be performed on serum since viscosity in whole blood is more complicated because of the interaction of the IgM immunoglobulin with the red blood cells and fibrinogen. Some investigators have measured viscosity using plasma rather than serum so that the fibrinogen interaction is present. Measurements performed with serum probably underestimate the real increase in viscosity, but they are easy to perform and standardize and correlate well with clinical symptoms.

Measurement of serum viscosity is a simple and straightforward procedure that merely requires a glass viscometer to measure the speed with which the serum passes through a small-bore hole. The normal serum viscosity is between 1.4 and 1.8 times that of water. It is recommended that the test be performed with the serum at 37°C. When a viscometer is not available, crude determinations can be made using standard pipettes and observing the time required for the water or serum to drop from one mark to another and computing the ratio. A simple screening test using a red cell pipette has been shown to give accurate and reproducible results when compared with viscometer measurements.[172] The measurements seemed to be reliable when performed at room temperature with either serum or plasma.

Symptoms of hyperviscosity when the serum viscosity is below 4 cp are uncommonly seen. Symptoms are often present when viscosity reaches values of 6 and 7 cp. This generally occurs when the serum IgM concentrations reach 3.5 to 4 g/dL. The serum viscosity can vary for different IgM proteins, as shown in Figure 31-17.[173] Because of this variability and because of other poorly defined factors, symptoms occur at different levels of IgM in different patients. The physician needs to ascertain the threshold for each patient and to keep the IgM concentration below this level. The factors that contribute to these variations from patient to patient are not always clear but sometimes relate to hematocrit and arterial vascular patency. After it is determined what level of IgM symptoms become significant for the individual patient, it is possible to use this known value of IgM level in management of the patient.

In one study of carefully performed viscosity measurements on patients with both monoclonal IgG and IgM immunoglobulins, out of 118 patients with plasma viscosities of less than 3 cp, no patient had symptoms of hyperviscosity.[173] One of 21 patients with values between 3 and 4 cp, 6 of 6 patients with values between 4 and 5 cp, and 6 of 8 with values over 5 cp had symptoms.

Visual Disturbances

Patients with hyperviscosity often complain of nonspecific visual disturbances such as decreased visual acuity, blurred vision, and diplopia. A funduscopic examination reveals a classic and essentially pathognomonic constellation of findings in patients with hyperviscosity known as fundus paraproteinaemicus. The retinal veins are distended and tortuous, taking on a boxcar or sausage appearance. When a patient presents with mental status changes or other neurologic findings (described in the next section), or visual

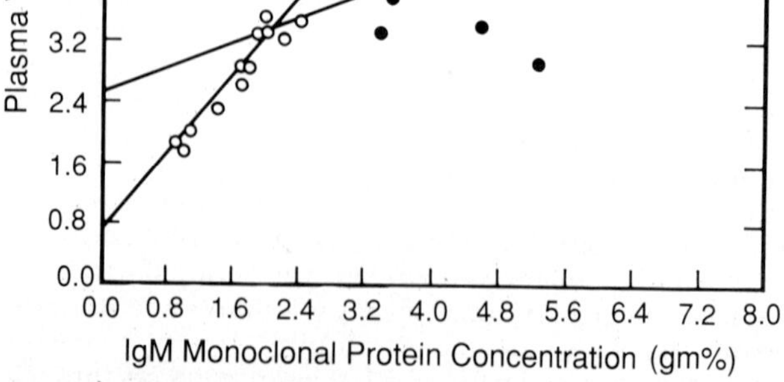

FIGURE 31-17. Correlation of plasma viscosity with monoclonal IgM concentration is shown in two patients. In both patients, a relatively linear relation between IgM concentration and viscosity is seen, but the increase in viscosity with increasing concentration of IgM is different, demonstrating the variability of hyperviscosity from patient to patient. (After Crawford J, Cox EB, Cohen HJ. Evaluation of hyperviscosity in monoclonal gammopathies. Am J Med 1985;79:13)

disturbances and funduscopic changes, hyperviscosity should be suspected and must be evaluated promptly. Retinal hemorrhages are also common and may be a manifestation of a systemic hemorrhagic syndrome.

Neurologic Syndromes

Neurologic syndromes in macroglobulinemia can be separated into two distinct categories: those due specifically to hyperviscosity and those due to involvement of peripheral nerves by the monoclonal protein.

Neurologic symptoms due to hyperviscosity are generally nonfocal and include headache, lethargy, coma, dizziness, vertigo, and seizures.[174] The clinical constellation of these findings varies from patient to patient and is often gradual in onset. Left untreated, these findings progress with increasing IgM concentrations, and the reversibility of the neurologic deficits depends on early recognition of the condition and reversal of the hyperviscosity.

Peripheral neuropathies are seen in about 5% of patients with macroglobulinemia. They are usually mixed motor and sensory neuropathies and probably occur by several mechanisms. Most intriguing is the finding that the monoclonal IgM immunoglobulin reacts directly with myelin in some of these patients.[175] In 40% of patients studied, the IgM Fab reacted with primate myelin and many of these IgM immunoglobulins shared idiotypes. In this subset of patients, the neurologic symptoms occur early in the course of illness, when the IgM levels are still low and no other significant manifestations of disease are present. This observation suggests that the specific antibody–myelin interaction was important enough to cause the neuropathy. In the 60% of cases in which the direct interaction was not found, the peripheral neuropathy tended to occur at a more advanced stage of disease with higher levels of immunoglobulin and greater systemic manifestations of the lymphoma. Although the cause is not known, peripheral neuropathy in these patients may be due to infiltration of the nerves with the malignant lymphocytes, amyloid deposits in the nerve fibers, or vascular compromise due to hyperviscosity. These associations are correlative findings only, and causality has not been firmly established.

Reversal of the peripheral neuropathy is possible when the IgM level is reduced. This is true even when the neuropathy has been present for long periods. Since the group of patients just described with direct reactivity of IgM with peripheral nerve myelin had symptoms early and had low levels of IgM, it follows that the patient with peripheral neuropathy and minimal elevation of monoclonal IgM should be aggressively treated.

Hemorrhagic Manifestations

Hemorrhagic complications are a common presenting sign of macroglobulinemia. The mechanisms that cause hemorrhage are complex and not always clear. Monoclonal IgM interacts with several coagulation proteins including factors V, VII, VIII, and the prothrombin complex.[94] In some cases, the monoclonal protein binds to fibrinogen causing poor fibrin formation, clot retraction, and prolonged thrombin time. When amyloid is present, factor X can bind directly to the amyloid causing an acquired factor deficiency. Platelets can become coated with the monoclonal immunoglobulin causing abnormal platelet aggregation and adhesion.[176] Clinical manifestations of macroglobulinemic coagulopathy are epistaxis, retinal hemorrhage, and mucous membrane bleeding. These complications can be reversed with plasmapheresis and reduction of the monoclonal IgM immunoglobulin.

Cutaneous Manifestations

Cutaneous manifestations of macroglobulinemia are uncommon, but when seen they often appear as one or both of two patterns.[177] One lesion appears as a violaceous plaque or tumor, and histologically the lesions are composed of an infiltrate of the malignant lymphocytes. The other lesion is a shiny pink papule composed of hyaline deposits of the IgM monoclonal protein. Occasionally, these lesions are the first manifestation of disease. They tend to regress when chemotherapeutic treatment is successful.

Another rare cutaneous manifestation of macroglobulinemia is benign hypergammaglobulinemic purpura of Waldenström. These lesions most frequently occur in females and are associated with other causes of hypergammaglobulinemia, particularly rheumatologic diseases. The lesions appear to represent a vasculitis and may reflect antibody–antigen complex disease or complement activation in the skin.[178]

Cryoglobulinemia

Cryoglobulins can be formed when the monoclonal IgM reacts with IgG to form a complex. This occurs in 5% to 10% of patients with macroglobulinemia.[168] These complexes cause the typical symptoms associated with cryoglobulins, including Raynaud's phenomenon and digital ischemia.

Cold Agglutinin Disease

In about one third of patients with macroglobulinemia, the IgM immunoglobulins have cold reactive properties. Symptoms of hemolytic anemia and cold-induced digital ischemia may be present if the IgM is around or above 3 g/dL. The actual value of IgM that gives rise to symptoms is related to the thermal amplitude of the protein and other less well-defined properties of an individual protein.

Urinary Light-Chain Excretion

Urinary light-chain excretion is found in about 80% of patients with macroglobulinemia.[168] κ Light chains are found twice as frequently as λ light chains. The amount of light chain excreted is small, averaging 1 g/24 h with a range of 0.2 to 4.4 g/24 h. Renal dysfunction is uncommon in macroglobulinemia and may reflect the modest amount of light chain excreted or the different physical properties of the light chains.

Systemic Amyloidosis

Systemic amyloidosis is a rare development in patients with IgM monoclonal gammopathy. Of patients who have monoclonal IgM associated with macroglobulinemia, monoclonal gammopathy of undetermined significance, and other lymphoproliferative disorders seen at the Mayo Clinic, 2.2% also had systemic amyloidosis.[169] Cardiac amyloid was present in 44% of patients, and of those who died, 53% succumbed to cardiac disease. Of those who presented with amyloid cardiomyopathy, the median survival was only 11 months, whereas it was 27 months in those patients without cardiomyopathy. Renal, hepatic, and pulmonary amyloid was present in 32%, 14%, and 10% of patients, respectively.

Intravascular Plasma Expansion

Because about 80% of the monoclonal IgM protein is intravascular owing to its size, osmotic forces associated with increased levels of IgM cause an increase in intravascular volume in some cases, and this can precipitate congestive heart failure. It also spuriously lowers the hematocrit in relation to red cell mass because of the dilutional aspects of increased plasma volume.

Lymphadenopathy and Splenomegaly

Malignant plasmacytic lymphocytes often infiltrate lymph nodes and the spleen, accounting for enlargement of these organs in about 40% of patients with macroglobulinemia. As a rule, the adenopathy is generalized and modest in degree at presentation, with nodes between 2 and 5 cm. Splenomegaly is also usually not severe, with spleens felt 3 to 5 fingerbreadths below the left costal margin.

Bone Disease

A minority of patients with macroglobulinemia develop overt lytic or osteopenic bone disease. Since almost all patients have involvement of the bone marrow with malignant plasmalymphocytic lymphoma cells, this indicates that these malignant cells usually do not produce osteoclast-activating factors as seen in myeloma. In one series, only 3 of 40 patients demonstrated osteolytic bone lesions.[179]

Circulating Lymphoma Cells

Malignant cells are not usually recognizable in peripheral blood smears from patients with macroglobulinemia, but rare malignant cells can be detected in the blood by immunologic techniques (as in many low-grade non-Hodgkin's lymphomas).[180] The number of circulating cells closely reflects the clinical course in these patients.

Lymphoplasmacytic Lymphoma Associated With Monoclonal IgG and IgA Rather Than IgM

Well-documented case reports exist of patients with lymphoma histologically identical to macroglobulinemia but with production of IgG or IgA monoclonal protein.[181] The monoclonal protein found in the blood is the same type as that found in the malignant cells. Some of these patients have adenopathy and hepatosplenomegaly, but bone disease is rare. The clinical course is that of macroglobulinemia rather than myeloma. The reason why the malignant cells from these patients produce IgA or IgG rather than IgM is not known.

Prognosis

Like the other low-grade non-Hodgkin's lymphomas, macroglobulinemia is not a curable disease. Intensive chemotherapy, although effective at inducing remissions, does not appear to be curative. Also, like the other low-grade non-Hodgkin's lymphomas, early in the disease when IgM levels are low and there are no symptoms related to the disease, therapy may not be necessary. When chemotherapy is indicated, generally oral alkylating agents should be used, as described in the section on chemotherapy. Survival is variable but has been improved because of the benefit of plasmapheresis in maintaining the IgM level below that which causes problems and because monoclonal protein production and lymphomatous manifestations of disease can often be controlled with the judicious use of chemotherapy. Although reported survivals in the literature may be only 3 to 5 years, many patients are now living longer. This improved survival may be due partly to improved therapy and supportive care. It may also represent a lead-time bias, since commonly performed chemistry evaluations so frequently performed with modern-day routine examinations often detect monoclonal proteins before the onset of symptoms.

Seventeen percent of patients with elevated IgM without other clinical evidence of macroglobulinemia (monoclonal gammopathy of undetermined significance) developed overt macroglobulinemia in a median of 4 years.[168] After patients develop overt macroglobulinemia, their median survival is $6\frac{1}{2}$ years. Patients who present with overt macroglobulinemia have a median survival of 5 years.

Therapy for Macroglobulinemia

Therapy for macroglobulinemia focuses on the removal of the monoclonal IgM from the plasma (since this protein causes so many of the complications of the disease) and on suppression of the malignant clone of lymphocytes that produce this protein. Because patients often present with acute complications directly related to their increased IgM protein and because suppression of the malignant lymphoid clone by chemotherapy is often slow, urgent therapy is frequently centered around physical removal of the protein.

Plasmapheresis

In the 1950s, it was discovered that the intravascular concentration of the monoclonal IgM could be significantly reduced by removal of plasma. It was immediately appreciated that this reduction could dramatically reverse the symptoms caused by the immunoglobulin when levels of IgM were reduced below the threshold concentration, as already described.[182,183] As plasmapheresis machines became available in the 1970s, a prolonged and cumbersome procedure became easier and more efficient to perform. The level of immunoglobulin can now be reduced and critical symptoms can be reversed rapidly in most patients. This ability to reverse symptoms and potentially avoid permanent neurologic damage makes recognition of macroglobulinemia with hyperviscosity a medical emergency. Since no large tissue compartment exists for IgM, recurrent increases in plasma IgM concentrations are derived from the malignant lymphoplasmacytic clone. To avoid the need for repeated plasmaphereses, it is usually wise to initiate antineoplastic therapy directed at the malignant clone to suppress further production of the IgM protein.

Chemotherapy

Oral alkylating agents have been and remain the mainstay of therapy for patients with macroglobulinemia. Chlorambucil, cyclophosphamide, and melphalan all have been used, but the first two are used most often. Cyclophosphamide is sometimes used in daily oral doses of 50 to 150 mg or in pulse oral doses of 150 to 300 mg/m^2 for 5 days every 3 to 4 weeks. Chlorambucil may be given orally at doses of 8 mg/m^2 for 5 days every 3 to 6 weeks. Generally, these agents are administered without prednisone, but there is no clearcut evidence for or against its role in this disease. Response rates with single oral alkylating agents have been about 40%.[179] Responders lived about 4 years and nonresponders about 2 years.

Patients have also been treated with more intensive chemotherapy programs including the M2 protocol originally designed for treatment of patients with myeloma, using BCNU, cyclophosphamide, vincristine, melphalan, and prednisone (for dosages, see section on myeloma).[184] Of 14 patients treated, all responded, including 3 who had been previously treated. There were two complete responses and all patients were alive 2 to 35 months after initiation of therapy. Nevertheless, no evidence exists that intensive multiagent chemotherapy should be first-line therapy in macroglobulinemia patients, and oral alkylating agents should be the first therapy used. More intensive regimens should be reserved for patients with disease resistant to oral alkylating agents.

The deoxyadenosine analogue 2-chlorodeoxyadenosine (2CDA) has been used in the therapy of previously untreated and previously treated patients with macroglobulinemia.[185] All 9 of the previously untreated patients in one series responded to therapy. Eight of the 20 previously treated patients responded, and only 1 of the responding patients demonstrated disease progression with short follow-up.

Eventually, the lymphoma cells become resistant to chemotherapy, and plasmapheresis must be used more frequently to keep the IgM protein below the threshold that gives a patient symptoms. Uncontrolled hyperviscosity, lymphadenopathy, and pancytopenia secondary to bone marrow replacement with lymphoma are manifestations of the terminal phase of the disease.

REFERENCES

1. Hallen J. Discrete gammaglobulin (M-) components in serum: clinical study of 150 subjects without myelomatosis. Acta Med Scand 1966;462(Suppl):1.
2. Kyle RA, Finkelstein S, Elveback LR, et al. Incidence of monoclonal proteins in a Minnesota community with a cluster of multiple myeloma. Blood 1972;40:719.
3. Crawford J, Eye MK, Cohen HJ. Evaluation of monoclonal gammopathies in the "well" elderly. Am J Med 1987;82:39.
4. Kyle RA. Monoclonal gammopathy of undetermined significance: natural history in 241 cases. Am J Med 1978;64:814.
5. Kyle RA, Lust JA. Monoclonal gammopathies of undetermined significance. Semin Hematol 1989;26:176.
6. Kyle RA. "Benign" monoclonal gammopathy: after 20 to 35 years of follow-up. mayo Clin Proc 1993;68:26.
7. Blade J, Lopez-Guillermo A, Rozman C, et al. Malignant transformation and life expectancy in monoclonal gammopathy of undetermined significance. Br J Haematol 1992;81:391.
8. Clamp JR. Some aspects of the first recorded case of multiple myeloma. Lancet 1967;2:1354.
9. Chronic Leukemia-Myeloma Task Force: proposed guidelines for protocol studies: plasma cell myeloma. Cancer Chemother Rep 1973;4:145.
10. Turesson I, Zettervall O, Cuzick J, et al. Comparison of trends in the incidence of multiple myeloma in Malmo, Sweden, and other countries, 1950–1979. N Engl J Med 1984;310:421.
11. Blattner WA, Blair A, Mason TJ. Multiple myeloma in the United States, 1950–1975. Cancer 1981;48:2547.
12. Linos A, Kyle RA, O'Fallon WM, Kurland LT. Incidence and secular trend of multiple myeloma in Olmsted County, Minnesota. 1965–77. J Natl Cancer Inst 1981;66:17.
13. Dawson AA, Ogston D. High incidence of myelomatosis in northeast Scotland. Scott Med J 1973;18:75.
14. Maldonado JE, Kyle RA. Familial myeloma: report of eight families and a study of serum proteins in their relatives. Am J Med 1974;57:875.
15. Potter M. Plasmacytomas in mice. Semin Oncol 1986;13:275.
16. Potter M, Wax JS, Anderson AL, et al. Inhibition of plasmacytoma development in BALB/c mice by indomethacin. J Exp Med 1985;161:996.
17. Fahrlander PD, Sumegi J, Yang J-Q, et al. Activation of the c-*myc* oncogene by the immunoglobulin gene enhancer after multiple switch region-mediated chromosomal rearrangements in a murine plasmacytoma. Proc Natl Acad Sci USA 1985;82:3746.
18. Selvanayagam P, Blick M, Narni F, et al. Alternation and abnormal expression of the c-*myc* oncogene in human multiple myeloma. Blood 1988;71:30.
19. Terpstra WE, Lokhorst HM, Blomjous F, et al. Comparison of plasma cell infiltration in bone marrow biopsies and aspirates in patients with multiple myeloma. Br J Haematol 1992;82:46.
20. Greipp PR, Raymond NM, Kyle RA, O'Fallon WM. Multiple myeloma: significance of plasmablastic subtype in morphological classification. Blood 1985;65:305.
21. Carter A, Hocherman I, Linn S, Cohen Y, Tatarshy I. Prognostic significance of plasma cell morphology in multiple myeloma. Cancer 1987;60:1060.
22. Strickler JG, Audeh W, Copenhaver CM, Warnke RA. Immunophe-

notypic differences between plasmacytoma/multiple myeloma and immunoblastic lymphoma. Cancer 1988;61:1782.
23. Tong AW, Lee JC, Stone MJ. Characterization of a monoclonal antibody having selective reactivity with normal and neoplastic plasma cells. Blood 1987;69:238.
24. Falini B, De Solas I, Levine AM, et al. Emergence of B-immunoblastic sarcoma in patients with multiple myeloma: a clinicopathologic study of 10 cases. Blood 1982;59:923.
25. Strand WR, Banks PM, Kyle RA. Anaplastic plasma cell myeloma and immunoblastic lymphoma: clinical, pathologic, and immunologic comparison. Am J Med 1984;76:861.
26. Ruiz-Arguelles GJ, Katzmann JA, Greipp PR, et al. Multiple myeloma: circulating lymphocytes that express plasma cell antigens. Blood 1984;64:352.
27. King MA, Nelson DS. Tumor cell hetergeneity in multiple myeloma: antigenic, morphologic, and functional studies of cells from blood and bone marrow. Blood 1989;73:1925.
28. Epstein J, Xiao H, He X-Y. Markers of multiple hematopoietic-cell lineages in multiple myeloma. N Engl J Med 1990;322:664.
29. Jensen GS, Mant MJ, Belch AJ, et al. Selective expression of CD45 isoforms defines CALLA+ monoclonal B-lineage cells in peripheral blood from myeloma patients as late stage B cells. Blood 1991;78:711.
30. Miller RA, Hart S, Samoszuk M, et al. Shared idiotypes expressed by human B-cell lymphomas. N Engl J Med 1989;321:851.
31. Berenson JR, Lichtenstein A, Hart S, et al. Expression of shared idiotypes by paraproteins from patients with multiple myeloma and monoclonal gammopathy of undetermined significance. Blood 1990;75:2107.
32. Vander JB, Johnson HA. Chronic lymphatic leukemia and multiple myeloma in the same patient. Ann Intern Med 1960;53:1052.
33. Naidu RT, Rosner F. Combined multiple myeloma and chronic lymphatic leukemia. N Engl J Med 1971;284:108.
34. Kough RH, Makary AZ. Chronic lymphocytic leukemia (CLL) terminating in multiple myeloma: report of two cases. Blood 1978;52:532.
35. Saltman DL, Ross JA, Banks RE, et al. Molecular evidence for a single clonal origin in biphenotypic concomitant chronic lymphocytic leukemia and multiple myeloma. Blood 1989;74:2062.
36. Gould J, Alexanian R, Goodacre A, Pathak S, Hecht B, Barlogie B. Plasma cell karyotype in multiple myeloma. Blood 1988;71:453.
37. Preudhomme C, Facon T, Zandecki M et al. Rare occurrence of p53 gene mutations in multiple myeloma. Br J Haematol 1992;81:440.
38. Neri A, Baldini L, Trecca D, et al. p53 gene mutations in multiple myeloma are associated with advanced forms of malignancy. Blood 1993;81:128.
39. Hofmann V, Salmon SE, Durie BGM. Drug resistance in multiple myeloma associated with high in vitro incorporation of 3H-thymidine. Blood 1981;58:471.
40. Greipp PR, Witzig TE, Gonchoroff NJ, et al. Immunofluorescence labeling indices in myeloma and related monoclonal gammopathies. Mayo Clin Proc 1987;62:969.
41. Boccadoro M, Marmont F, Tribalto M, et al. Early responder myeloma: kinetic studies identify a patient subgroup characterized by very poor prognosis. J Clin Oncol 1989;7:119.
42. Durie BGM, Young LA, Salmon SE. Human myeloma in vitro colony growth: interrelationships between drug sensitivity, cell kinetics, and patient survival duration. Blood 1983;61:929.
43. Salmon SE. Immunoglobulin synthesis and tumor kinetics of multiple myeloma. Semin Hematol 1973;10:135.
44. Kyle RA, Robinson RA, Katzmann JA. The clinical aspects of biclonal gammopathies: review of 57 Cases. Am J Med 1981;71:999.
45. Rosen BJ, Smith TW, Bloch KJ. Multiple myeloma associated with two serum M components: gG type κ and gA type I. N Engl J Med 1967;277: 902.
46. Bjerrum OJ, Weeke B. Two M components (gGK and gML) in different cells of the same patient. Scand J Haematol 1968;5:215.
47. Bouvet JP, Buffe D, Oriol R, Liacopoulos P. Two myeloma globulins IgG1-κ and IgG1-I, from a single patient. Immunology 1974;27:1095.
48. Hopper JE. Comparative studies on monotypic IgM and IgG from an individual patient. IV. Immunofluorescent evidence for a common clonal synthesis. Blood 1977;50:203.
49. Smith L, Barlogie B, Alexanian R. Biclonal and hypodiploid multiple myeloma. Am J Med 1986;80:841.
50. Rubio-Felix D, Giralt M, Giraldo P, et al. Nonsecretory multiple myeloma. Cancer 1987;59:1847.
51. Mancilla R, Davis GL. Nonsecretory multiple myeloma: immunohistologic and ultrastructural observations on two patients. Am J Med 1977;63:1015.
52. Dreicer R, Alexanian R. Non-secretory multiple myeloma. Am J Hematol 1982;13:313.
53. Muraguchi A, Hirano T, Tang B, et al. The essential role of B cell stimulatory factor 2 (BSF-2/IL-6) for the terminal differentiation of B cells. J Exp Med 1988;167:332.
54. Zhang, XG, Klein B, Bataille R. Interleukin-6 is a potent myeloma-cell growth factor in patients with aggressive multiple myeloma. Blood 1989;74:11.
55. Hitzler JK, Martinez-Valdez H, Bergsagel DB, et al. Role of interleukin-6 in the proliferation of human multiple myeloma cell lines OBI-My 1 to 7 established from patients with advanced stage of the disease. Blood 1991;78:1996.
56. Schwab G, Siegall CB, Aarden LA, et al. Characterization of an interleukin-6–mediated autocrine growth loop in the human multiple myeloma cell line, U266. Blood 1991;77:587.
57. Kobayashi M, Tanaka J, Imamura M, et al. Up-regulation of IL-6–receptors by IL-3 on a plasma cell leukaemia cell line which proliferates dependently on both IL-3 and Il-6. Br J Haematol 1993;83:535.
58. Zhang X-G, Bataille R, Jourdan M, et al. Granulocyte-macrophage colony-stimulating factor synergizes with interleukin-6 in supporting proliferation of human myeloma cells. Bllod 1990;76:2599.
59. Carter A, Merchav S, Silvian-Draxler I, Tatarsky I. The role of interleukin-1 and tumour necrosis factor-α in human multiple myeloma. Br J Haematol 1990;74:424.
60. Defrance T, Vandervliet B, Aubry JP, et al. B cell growth-promoting activity of recombinant human interleukin 4. J Immunol 1987;4:1135.
61. Noelle R, Krammer PH, Ohara J, Uhr JW, Vitetta ES. Increased expression of la antigens on resting B cells: an additional role for B-cell growth factor. Proc Natl Acad Sci USA 1984;81:6149.
62. Defrance T, Aubry JP, Rousset F, et al. Human recombinant interleukin 4 induces Fc receptors (CD23) on normal human B lymphocytes. J Exp Med 1987;165:1459.
63. Taylor CW, Grogan TM, Salmon SE. Effects of interleukin-4 on the in vitro growth of human lymphoid and plasma cell neoplasms. Blood 1990;75:1114.
64. Herrmann F, Andreeff M, Gruss H-J, et al. Interleukin-4 inhibits growth of multiple myelomas by suppressing interleukin-6 expression. Blood 1991;78:2070.
65. Kawano M, Yamamoto I, Iwato K, et al. Interleukin-1 beta rather than lymphotoxin as the major bone resorbing activity in human multiple myeloma. Blood 1989;73:1646.
66. Caligaris-Cappio F, Mergui L, Gregoretti MG, et al. Role of bone marrow stromal cells in the growth of human multiple myeloma. Blood 1991;77: 2688.
67. Ludwig H, Fritz E, Kotzmann H, et al. Erythropoietin treatment of anemia associated with multiple myeloma. N Engl J Med 1990;322: 1693.
68. Beguin Y, Yerna M, Loo M, et al. Erythropoiesis in multiple myeloma: defective red cell production due to inappropriate erythropoietin production. Br J Haematol 1992;82:648.
69. Mundy GR, Raisz LG, Cooper RA, et al. Evidence for the secretion of an osteoclast stimulating factor in myeloma. N Engl J Med 1974;291: 1041.
70. Garrett IR, Durie BGM, Nedwin GE, et al. Production of lymphotoxin, a bone-resorbing cytokine, by cultured human myeloma cells. N Engl J Med 1987;317:526.
71. Bataille R, Chappard D, Marcelli C, et al. Mechanisms of bone destruction in multiple myeloma: the importance of an unbalanced process in determining the severity of lytic bone disease. J Clin Oncol 1989;7: 1909.
72. Cohen HJ, Silberman HR, Tornyos K, Bartolucci AA. Southeastern Cancer Study Group (SECSG): comparison of two long-term chemotherapy regimens, with or without agents to modify skeletal repair, in multiple myeloma. Blood 1984;63:639.
73. Kyle RA, Jowsey J, Kelly PJ, Taves DR. Multiple myeloma bone disease: the comparative effect of sodium fluoride and calcium carbonate or placebo. N Engl J Med 1975;293:1334.
74. Belch AR, Bergsagel DE, Wilson K, et al. Effect of daily etidronate on the osteolysis of multiple myeloma. J Clin Oncol 1991;9:1397.
75. Bardwick PA, Zvaifler NJ, Gill GN, et al. Plasma cell dyscrasia with polyneuropathy, organomegaly, endocrinopathy, M protein, and skin changes: the POEMS syndrome. Medicine 1980;59:311.
76. Miralles DG, O'Fallon JR, Talley NJ. Plasma-cell dyscrasia with polyneuropathy: the spectrum of POEMS syndrome. N Engl J Med 1992;327: 1919.
77. Mundy JR, Bertolini DR. Bone destruction and hypercalcemia in plasma cell myeloma. Semin Oncol 1986;13:291.
78. Durie BGM, Salmon SE, Mundy GR. Relation of osteoclast-activating factor production to the extent of bone disease in multiple myeloma. Br J Haematol 1981;47:21.
79. Snapper I, Kahn A. Myelomatosis. Basel, Switzerland, S Karger, 1971.
80. Corrado C, Santarelli MT, Pavlovsky S, et al. Prognostic factors in multiple myeloma: definition of risk groups in 410 previously untreated patients: a grupo Argentino de Tratamiento de la Leucemia Aguda study. J Clin Oncol 1989;7:1839.
81. Pascali E, Pezzoli A. The clinical spectrum of pure Bence Jones proteinuria: a study of 66 patients. Cancer 1988;62:2408.
82. Solomon A. Clinical implications of monoclonal light chains. Semin Oncol 1986;13:341.
83. Solomon A, Weiss DT, Kattine AA. Nephrotoxic potential of Bence Jones proteins. N Engl J Med 1991;324:1845.
84. Solomon A, Fangione B, Franklin EC. Bence Jones proteins and light chains of immunoglobulins: preferential association of the VIVI subgroup of human light chains with amyloidosis AL(I). J Clin Invest 1982;70:453.
85. Gertz MA, Kyle RA. Primary systemic amyloidosis: a diagnostic primer. Mayo Clin Proc 1989;64:1505.

86. Misiani R, Remuzzi G, Bertani T, et al. Plasmapheresis in the treatment of acute renal failure in multiple myeloma. Am J Med 1979;66:684.
87. Zinneman HH, Hall WH. Recurrent pneumonia in multiple myeloma and some observations on immunologic response. Ann Intern Med 1954;41:1152.
88. Twomey JT. Infections complicating multiple myeloma and chronic lymphocytic leukemia. Arch Intern Med 1973;132:562.
89. Perri RT, Hebbel RP, Oken MM. Influence of treatment and response status on infection risk in multiple myeloma. Am J Med 1981;71:935.
90. Lazarus HM, Lederman M, Lubin A, et al. Pneumococcal vaccination: the response of patients with multiple myeloma. Am J Med 1980;69: 419.
91. Oken MM, Kay NE. T-cell subpopulations in multiple myeloma: correlation with clinical disease status. Br J Haematol 1981;49:629.
92. Cheson BD, Plass RR, Rothstein G. Defective opsonization in multiple myeloma. Blood 1980;55:602.
93. Zurlo JJ, Schechter GP, Fries LF. Complement abnormalities in multiple myeloma. Am J Med 1989;87:411.
94. Patterson WP, Caldwell CW, Doll DC. Hyperviscosity syndromes and coagulopathies. Semin Oncol 1990;17:210.
95. Pruzanski W, Watt JG. Serum viscosity and hyperviscosity syndrome in IgG multiple myeloma: report of 10 cases and a review of the literature. Ann Intern Med 1972;77:853.
96. Capra JD, Kunkel HG. Aggregation of gG3 proteins: relevance to the hyperviscosity syndrome. J Clin Invest 1970;49:610.
97. Chandy KG, Stockley RA, Leonard RCF, et al. Relationship between serum viscosity and intravascular IgA polymer concentration in IgA myeloma. Clin Exp Immunol 1981;46:653.
98. Kyle RA. Multiple myeloma: review of 869 cases. Mayo Clin Proc 1975;50:29.
99. Stone MJ, Frenkel EP. The clinical spectrum of light chain myeloma: a study of 35 patients with special reference to the occurrence of amyloidosis. Am J Med 1975;58:601.
100. Franklin EC, Lowenstein J, Bigelow B, Meltzer M. Heavy chain disease: a new disorder of serum γ-globulins: report of the first case. Am J Med 1964;37:332.
101. Kyle RA, Greipp PR, Banks PM. The diverse picture of gamma heavy-chain disease: report of seven cases and review of the literature. Mayo Clin Proc 1981;56:439.
102. Guardia J, Rubies-Prat J, Gallart MT, et al. The evolution of alpha heavy chain disease. Am J Med 1976;60:596.
103. Jancelewicz Z, Takatsuki K, Sugai S, Pruzanski W. IgD multiple myeloma: review of 133 cases. Arch Intern Med 1975;135:87.
104. Ogawa M, Kochwa S, Smith C, et al. Clinical aspects of IgE myeloma. N Engl J Med 1969;281:1217.
105. Endo T, Okumura H, Kikuchi K, et al. Immunoglobulin E (IgE) multiple myeloma: a case report and review of the literature. Am J Med 1981;70: 1127.
106. Knowling MA, Harwood AR, Bergsagel DE. Comparison of extramedullary plasmacytomas with solitary and multiple plasma cell tumors of bone. J Clin Oncol 1983;1:255.
107. Bataille R, Sany J. Solitary myeloma: clinical and prognostic features of a review of 114 cases. Cancer 1981;48:845.
108. Holland J, Trenkner DA, Wasserman TH, Fineberg B. Plasmacytoma: treatment results and conversion of myeloma. Cancer 1992;69:1513.
109. Chak LY, Cox RS, Bostwick DG, Hoppe RT. Solitary plasmacytoma of bone: treatment, progression, and survival. J Clin Oncol 1987;5:1811.
110. Meis JM, Butler JJ, Osborne BM, Ordonez NG. Solitary plasmacytomas of bone and extramedullary plasmacytomas: a clinicopathologic and immunohistochemical study. Cancer 1987;59:1475.
111. Kyle RA, Greipp PR. Smoldering multiple myeloma. N Engl J Med 1980;302:1347.
112. Hewell GM, Alexanian R. Multiple myeloma in young persons. Ann Intern Med 1976;84:441.
113. Lazarus HM, Kellermeyer RW, Aikawa M, Herzig RH. Multiple myeloma in young men: clinical course and electron microscopic studies of bone marrow plasma cells. Cancer 1980;46:1397.
114. Noel P, Kyle RA, Plasma cell leukemia: an evaluation of response to therapy. Am J Med 1987;83:1062.
115. Woodruff RK, Malpas JS, Paxton AM, Lister TA. Plasma cell leukemia (PCL): a report on 15 patients. Blood 1978;52:839.
116. Durie BGM, Salmon SE. A clinical staging system for multiple myeloma: correlation of measured myeloma cell mass with presenting clinical features, response to treatment and survival. Cancer 1975;36:842.
117. Durie BGM, Stock-Novack D, Salmon SE, et al. Prognostic value of pretreatment serum β_2-microglobulin in myeloma: a Southwest Oncology Group study. Blood 1990;75:823.
118. Alexanian R, Gehan E, Bonnet J, et al. Combination chemotherapy for multiple myeloma. Cancer 1972;30:382.
119. Bataille R, Boccadoro M, Klein B, et al. C-reactive protein and β_2-microglobulin produce a simple and powerful myeloma staging system. Blood 1992;80:733.
120. Bergsagel DE. Controversies in the treatment of plasma cell myeloma. Postgrad Med J 1985;61:109.
121. Blokhin H, Larionov LF, Perevodchikova NI, et al. Clinical experiences with sarcolysin in neoplastic disease. Ann NY Acad Sci 1958;68:1128.
122. Alexanian R, Haut A, Khan AU, et al. Treatment for multiple myeloma: combination chemotherapy with different melphalan dose regimens. JAMA 1969;208:1680.
123. Bergsagel DE, Cowan DH, Hasselback R. Plasma cell myeloma: response of melphalan resistant patients to high-dose cyclophosphamide. Can Med Assoc J 1072;107:851.
124. Cohen HJ, Silberman HR, Larsen WE, et al. Combination chemotherapy with intermittent BCNU, cyclophosphamide, and prednisone for multiple myeloma. Blood 1979;54:824.
125. Harley JB, Pajak TF, McIntyre OR, et al. Improved survival of increased-risk myeloma patients on combined triple alkylating agent therapy: a study of the CALGB. Blood 1979;54:13.
126. Salmon SE, Haut A, Bonnet JD, et al. Alternating combination chemotherapy and levamisole improves survival in multiple myeloma: a SWOG study. J Clin Oncol 1983;1:453.
127. Alexanian R, Dreicer R. Chemotherapy for multiple myeloma. Cancer 1984;53:583.
128. Hjorth M, Hellquist L, Holmberg E, et al. Initial treatment in multiple myeloma: no advantage of multidrug chemotherapy over melphalan prednisone. Br J Haematol 1990;74:185.
129. Case DC, Lee BJ III, Clarkson BD. Improved survival times in multiple myeloma treated with melphalan, prednisone, cyclophosphamide, vincristine and BCNU: M2 protocol. Am J Med 1977;63:897.
130. Oken MM, Tsiatis A, Abramson N, Glick J. Comparison of standard MP with intensive VBMCP therapy for the treatment of multiple myeloma (MM). (Abstract) Proc Am Soc Clin Oncol 1984;3:270.
131. Boccadoro M, Marmot F, Tribalto M, et al. Multiple myeloma: VMCP/VBAP alternating combination chemotherapy is not superior to melphalan and prednisone even in high-risk patients. J Clin Oncol 1991;9: 444.
132. Gregory WM, Richards MA, Malpas JS. Combination chemotherapy versus melphalan and prednisolone in the treatment of multiple myeloma: an overview of published trials. J Clin Oncol 1992;10:334.
133. Osterborg A, Björkholm M, Björeman M, et al. Natural interferon-α in combination with melphalan/prednisone in the treatment of multiple myeloma stages II and III: a randomized study from Myeloma Group of Central Sweden. Blood 1993;81:1428.
134. Cooper MR, Dear K, McINtyre OR, et al. A randomized clinical trial comparing melphalan/prednisone with or without interferon alfa-2b in newly diagnosed patients with multiple myeloma: a Cancer and Leukemia Group B study. J Clin Oncol 1993;11:155.
135. Case DC, Coleman M, Gottlieb A, McCarroll K. Phase I-II trial of high-dose melphalan in previously untreated stage III multiple myeloma: Cancer and Leukemia Group B study 8512. Cancer Invest 1992;10:11.
136. Attal M, Huguet F, Schlaifer D, et al. Intensive combined therapy for previously untreated aggressive myeloma. Blood 1992;79:1130.
137. MacKenzie MR, Wold H, Gandara GD, et al. Consolidation hemibody radiotherapy following induction combination chemotherapy in high–tumor-burden multiple myeloma. J Clin Oncol 1992;10:1769.
138. Sullivan PW, Salmon SE. Kinetics of growth and regression in IgG multiple myeloma. J Clin Invest 1972;41:1697.
139. Salmon SE. Expansion of the growth fraction in multiple myeloma with alkylating agents. Blood 1975;45:119.
140. Drewinko B, Alexanian R, Boyer H, et al. The growth fraction of human myeloma cells. Blood 1981;57:333.
141. Karp JE, Humphrey RL, Burke PJ. Timed sequential chemotherapy of cytoxan-refractory multiple myeloma with cytoxan and adriamycin based on induced tumor cell proliferation. Blood 1981;57:468.
142. Alexanian R, Gehan E, Haut A, et al. Unmaintained remissions in multiple myeloma. Blood 1978;51:1005.
143. Quesada JR, Alexanian R, Hawkins M, et al. Treatment of multiple myeloma with recombinant α-interferon. Blood 1986;67:275.
144. Manelli F, Avvisati G, Amadori S, et al. Maintenance treatment with recombinant interferon alpha-2b in patients with multiple myeloma responding to conventional induction chemotherapy. N Engl J Med 1990;322:1430.
145. Buzaid AC, Durie BGM. Management of refractory myeloma: a review. J Clin Oncol 1988;6:889.
146. Alexanian R, Yap BS, Bodey GP. Prednisone pulse therapy for refractory myeloma. Blood 1983;62:572.
147. Alexanian R, Barlogie B, Dixon D. High-dose glucocorticoid treatment of resistant myeloma. Ann Intern Med 1986;105:8.
148. Barlogie B, Smith L, Alexanian R. Effective treatment of advanced multiple myeloma refractory to alkylating agents. N Engl J Med 1984;310:1353.
149. Barlogie B, Velasquez WS, Alexanian R, Cabanillas F. Etoposide, dexamethasone, cytarabine, and cisplatin in vincristine, doxorubicin, and dexamethasone-refractory myeloma. J Clin Oncol 1989;7:1514.
150. Barlogie B, Alexanian R, Smallwood L, et al. Prognostic factors with high-dose melphalan for refractory multiple myeloma. Blood 1988;72: 2015.
151. Barlogie B, Jagannath S, Dixon DO, et al. High-dose melphalan and granulocyte-macrophage colony-stimulating factor for refractory myeloma. Blood 1990;76:677.
152. Dimopoulos MA, Delasalle KB, Champlin R, Alexanian R. Cyclophosphamide and etoposide therapy with GM-CSF for VAD-resistant multiple myeloma. Br J Haematol 1993;83:240.
153. Tong AW, Lee JC, Fay JW, Stone MJ. Elimination of clonogenic stem

cells from human multiple myeloma cell lines by a plasma cell-reactive monoclonal antibody and complement. Blood 1987;70:1482.
154. Anderson KC, Park EK, Bates MP, et al. Antigens on human plasma cells identified by monoclonal antibodies. J Immunol 1983;130:1132.
155. Barlogie B, Alexanian R, Dicke KA, et al. High-dose chemoradiotherapy and autologous bone marrow transplantation for resistant multiple myeloma. Blood 1987;70:869.
156. Anderson KC, Barut BA, Ritz J, et al. Monoclonal antibody–purged autologous bone marrow transplantation therapy for multiple myeloma. Blood 1991;77:712.
157. Mansi J, da Costa F, Viner C, et al. High-dose busulfan in patients with myeloma. J Clin Oncol 1992;10:1569.
158. Gahrton G, Tura S, Ljungman P, et al. Allogeneic bone marrow transplantation in multiple myeloma. N Engl J Med 1991;325:1267.
159. Mill WB, Griffith R. The role of radiation therapy in the management of plasma cell tumors. Cancer 1980;45:647.
160. Coleman M, Saletan S, Wolf D, et al. Whole bone marrow irradiation for the treatment of multiple myeloma. Cancer 1982;49:1328.
161. Rostom AY, O'Cathail SM, Folkes A. Systemic irradiation in multiple myeloma: a report on nineteen cases. Br J Haematol 1984;58:423.
162. Klein B, Wijdenes J, Zhang X-G, et al. Murine anti–interleukin-6 monoclonal antibody therapy for a patient with plasma cell leukemia. Blood 1991;78:1198.
163. Kreitman RJ, Siegall CB, FitzGerald DJP, et al. Interleukin-6 fused to a mutant form of *Pseudomonas* exotoxin kills malignant cells from patients with multiple myeloma. Blood 1992;79:1775.
164. Stevenson FK, Bell AJ, Cusack R, et al. Preliminary studies for an immunotherapeutic approach to the treatment of human myeloma using chimeric anti-CD38 antibody. Blood 1991;77:1071.
165. Rosner F, Grunwald H. Multiple myeloma terminating in acute leukemia. Am J Med 1974;57:927.
166. Bergsagel DE, Bailey AJ, Langley GR, et al. The chemotherapy of plasma-cell myeloma and the incidence of acute leukemia. N Engl J Med 1979;301:743.
167. Non-Hodgkin's Lymphoma Pathologic Classification Project. National Cancer Institute sponsored study of classifications of non-Hodgkin's lymphomas. Cancer 1982;49:2112.
168. Kyle RA, Garton JP. The spectrum of IgM monoclonal gammopathy in 430 cases. Mayo Clin Proc 1987;62:719.
169. Gertz MA, Kyle RA, Noel P. Primary Systemic amyloidosis: a rare complication of immunoglobulin M monoclonal gammopathies and Waldenström's macroglobulinema. J Clin Oncol 1993;11:914.
170. Waldenström J. Incipient myelomatosis or "essential" hyperglobulinemia with fibrinogenopenia: a new syndrome? Acta Med Scand 1944;117:216.
171. Fahey JL, Barth WF, Solomon A. Serum hyperviscosity syndrome. JAMA 1965;192:464.
172. Wright DJ, Jenkins DE. Simplified method for estimation of serum and plasma viscosity in multiple myeloma and related disorders. Blood 1970;36:516.
173. Crawford J, Cox EB, Cohen HJ. Evaluation of hyperviscosity in monoclonal gammopathies. Am J Med 1985;79:13.
174. Somer T. Rheology of paraproteinaemias and the plasma hyperviscosity syndrome. Baillieres Clin Haematol 1987;1:695.
175. Dellagi K, Dupouey P, Brouet JC, et al. Waldenström's macroglobulinemia and peripheral neuropathy: a clinical and immunologic study of 25 patients. Blood 1983;62:280.
176. Godal HC, Borchgrevink CF. The effect of plasmapheresis on the hemostatic function in patients with macroglobulinemia Waldenström and multiple myeloma. Scand J Clin Lab Invest 1965;17(Suppl 84):133.
177. Mascaro JM, Montserrat E, Estrach T, et al. Specific cutaneous manifestations of Waldenström's macroglobulinemia: a report of two cases. Br J Dermatol 1982;106:217.
178. Ferreiro JE, Pasarin G, Quesada R, Gould E. Benign hypergammaglobulinemic purpura of Waldenström associated with Sjogren's syndrome: case report and review of immunologic aspects. Am J Med 1986;81: 734.
179. MacKenzie MR, Fudenberg HH. Macroglobulinemia: an analysis for forty patients. Blood 1972;39:874.
180. Smith BR, Robert NJ, Ault KA. In Waldenström's macroglobulinemia the quantity of detectable circulating monoclonal B lymphocytes correlates with clinical course. Blood 1983;61:911.
181. Tursz T, Brouet J-C, Flandrin G, et al. Clinical and pathologic features of Waldenström's macroglobulinemia in seven patients with serum monoclonal IgG or IgA. Am J Med 1977;63:499.
182. Skoog WA, Adams WS. Plasmapheresis in case of Waldenström's macroglobulinemia. Clin Res 1959;7:96.
183. Schwab PJ, Fahey JL. Treatment of Waldenström's macroglobulinemia by plasmapheresis. N Engl J Med 1960;263:574.
184. Case DC. Combination chemotherapy (M-2) protocol (BCNU, cyclophosphamide, vincristine, melphalan, and prednisone) for Waldenström's macroglobulinemia: preliminary report. Blood 1982;59:934.
185. Dimopoulos MA, Kantarjian H, Estey E, et al. Treatment of Waldenström macroglobulinemia with 2-chlorodeoxyadenosine. Ann Intern Med 1993;118:195.

32

Blood: Principles and Practice of Hematology,
edited by Robert I. Handin, Thomas P. Stossel, and Samuel E. Lux.
J.B. Lippincott Company, Philadelphia © 1995.

Histiocytoses and Disorders of the Reticuloendothelial System

Robert J. Arceci

Disorders referred to as histiocytoses or lymphohistiocytoses represent one of the most heterogeneous collections of disease states. Often when description of clinical syndromes precedes understanding of the biology of disease, nomenclature and classification schemes are based on anecdotal descriptions associated with historical eponyms. This has been especially true of histiocytoses. Nevertheless, much progress has recently been made in furthering our understanding of the origin, heterogeneity, and function of the histiocyte and also in the classification and treatment of histiocytic and lymphohistiocytic disorders. This chapter focuses on the primary histiocytic disorders but includes lymphohistiocytic syndromes that are related by virtue of their clinical presentation or histopathology.

THE HISTIOCYTE AND THE MONONUCLEAR PHAGOCYTIC SYSTEM

The histiocyte is not a single cell type but represents a group of anatomically and functionally distinct cell types that make up part of the phagocytic and antigen-presenting arm of the host's immune system. The histiocyte, which is involved in most histiocytic disorders, is actually the mononuclear phagocyte. These cells represent cells derived from bone marrow hematopoietic precursors and probably arise from circulating monocytes when they take up residence in tissues. Depending on the microenvironment in which they then find themselves, histiocytes or macrophages take on many different forms such as hepatic and splenic sinusoidal macrophages, pulmonary alveolar macrophages, pleural, synovial, and peritoneal macrophages, osteoclasts, and central nervous system (CNS) microglia.

The primary function of macrophages is phagocytosis, antigen processing, and antigen presentation to lymphocytes during an immune response. Another class of histiocytes called *dendritic cells* (also referred to as dendritic reticulum cells) includes the dendritic cell located in lymphoid follicles, the interdigitating dendritic cell (also called interdigitating reticulum cell) found in the paracortical regions of lymph nodes, and Langerhans cells found primarily in the skin and other organs. Also belonging to this class of histiocytes is the indeterminate cell, which is found primarily in the skin. The indeterminate cell has been considered a precursor to the Langerhans cell. Dendritic cells are only weakly phagocytic compared with macrophages but play an essential role in antigen presentation. The follicular dendritic cell presents antigen primarily to B lymphocytes, whereas the paracortical interdigitating cell and the Langerhans cell present antigen to T lymphocytes. Although dendritic cells are derived from bone marrow hematopoietic precursors, it is not clear what the cell of origin is.

All these cell types belong to the mononuclear phagocytic system or reticuloendothelial system. The concept of such a system is based partly on anatomic localization of its component cells and similarity of shared cell type markers as well as an essential role played in host defense. Critical functions are phagocytosis of invading microorganisms, processing of foreign antigens followed by their presentation to other cells of the immune system such as lymphocytes, and the ability to secrete and respond to a diverse range of cytokines important in an immune response.

IMPORTANT CELL TYPES AND DISTINGUISHING MARKERS

The two major groups of cells involved in the histiocytic disorders are tissue macrophages and dendritic cells, particularly the Langerhans cell. Although these two groups of cells share many biochemical, immunologic, and functional features, they also express enough significant differences to warrant a more detailed comparison. Such a comparison is not purely academic in that it forms the basis for a pathologic diagnosis and classification of the diverse proliferative histiocytic disorders.

Monocytes and their tissue counterparts, macrophages, are large mononuclear cells with gray-blue cytoplasm characterized by many vacuoles representing their intense lysosomal activity. Langerhans cells are also large mononuclear cells but usually display a slightly eosinophilic to clear cytoplasm, which contains little vacuolization. They display long cytoplasmic extensions or processes from which the term *dendritic cell* derives. The nucleus of Langerhans cells is often folded and indented, and has an irregular, fine chromatin pattern. These monocytes were discovered in 1868 by Paul Langerhans, then a medical student at the Berlin Pathological Institute. Langerhans cells are located primarily in the skin and buccal, gingival, esophageal, and vaginal mucosa as well as in bone marrow, spleen, thymus, lymph nodes, and other organs.

Ultrastructural analysis of Langerhans cells has revealed characteristic intracytoplasmic organelles called *Birbeck granules* or *X bodies*.[1,2] These organelles are rarely found in the nucleus. Birbeck granules are rod-shaped structures with a central, striated line; they occasionally terminate in a vesicular dilation, giving them a racquet shape (Fig. 32-1). They are variable in length (190 to 360 nm) with a uniform width of about 33 nm. The Birbeck granule may arise secondary to the process of receptor-mediated endocytosis, since cell surface antigens have been localized within them. Monocytes and non-Langerhans macrophages lack Birbeck granules. Thus, ultrastructural analysis of biopsy specimens is particularly useful in distinguishing the type of histiocyte present in a lesion.

Unlike other tissue macrophages, Langerhans cells are negative for lysozyme, α_1-antitrypsin, α_1-antichymotrypsin, aminopeptidase, peroxidase, alkaline phosphatase, α-naphthol-chloroacetate esterase and β-glucuronidase. Langerhans cells are positive for adenosine triphosphatase and strongly express α-mannosidase, which is expressed to a much lesser degree by other tissue macrophages.[2]

Several other cell markers aid in distinguishing Langerhans cells from other tissue macrophages when studied in formalin-fixed, paraffin-embedded specimens. The staining pattern for peanut agglutinin in Langerhans cells shows a unique pattern of paranuclear and cell surface deposition of reaction products, whereas other tissue macrophages show a diffuse reaction.[1] Langerhans cells also show a positive reaction when stained with anti–S-100 antibodies, whereas other tissue macrophages are usually negative.[1,2] The Langerhans cell contains the S-100 β-subunit. Monocytes and macrophages may express the S-100 α-subunit but not the β-subunit.[2] S-100 is a calcium-binding complex that was initially identified in brain tissue. Most Langerhans cells are CD1a antigen–positive (best detected on frozen tissue sections), which is a marker also found on early T lymphocytes in the thymus. Macrophages are negative for CD1a.[3–5]

Conversely, monocytes and macrophages are positive for the nonspecific carcinoembryonic cross-reacting antigen, whereas Langerhans cells are negative.[1,2] Most macrophages stain positive for the CD4 antigen, whereas Langerhans cells are negative or show variable expression.[1,2] Macrophages are strongly positive for nonspecific esterase and the cell surface marker, CD11c (Leu-M5). Both the Langerhans cell and the macrophage usually express class II major histocompatibility molecules, which are involved in the presentation of foreign antigens during an immune response. A comparison of some of the distinguishing features of these different cell types is shown in Table 32-1.

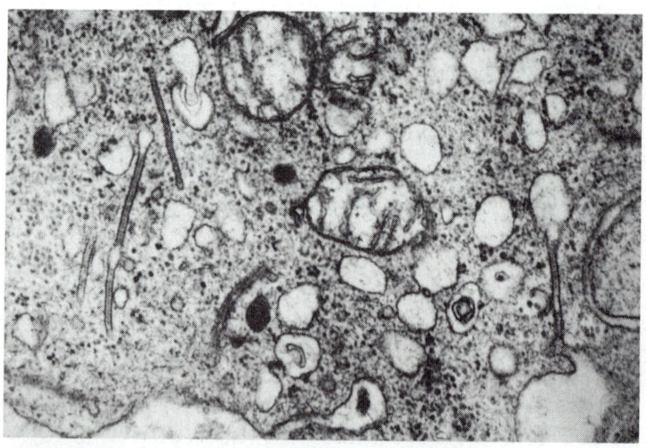

FIGURE 32-1. Birbeck granules in the cytoplasm of a Langerhans cell observed at the electron microscopic level. (Courtesy of Dr. Antonio Perez, Department of Pathology, Children's Hospital, Boston)

Thus, the suitable handling of biopsy specimens for both electron microscopic and immunocytochemistry analysis, including frozen tissue sections, is critical in the evaluation of lesions that may represent disorders of the histiocyte. Through a combination of these techniques by experienced pathology laboratory professionals, it is usually possible to discriminate which type of histiocyte is predominantly involved in the disease process.

PATHOPHYSIOLOGY AND CLASSIFICATION OF HISTIOCYTIC DISORDERS

Several important pathophysiologic consequences of the presentation of foreign antigens to lymphocytes are known. If this finely orchestrated interaction of activation, proliferation, recruitment, and suppression is defective at any point, this process, which is normally designed to protect the organism, can result in deleterious consequences.

The activation and recruitment of monocytes and macrophages as well as lymphocytes and granulocytes result in a mixture of reactive cells, that is, granuloma formation. Evidence of phagocytosis of microorganisms may be found as well as hemophagocytosis resulting from the interaction of the macrophage Fc receptor for IgG present on hematopoietic cells. Fever may result from released endogenous pyrogens. Dermal infiltrations may give rise to various types of rash and nodular infiltrates. Bone lesions, usually osteolytic, may result from the secretion of interleukin-1 and prostaglandin E_2 by macrophages.[6] Finally, infiltration of any organ may affect its function because of disruption of normal histologic architecture, such as occurs in the liver, or because of replacement of normal tissue elements, such as in the bone marrow.

The proliferative histiocytoses may be the result of the dysregulated response to some as yet unknown inciting agent or antigen. All are characterized by the reactive proliferation of histiocytes as well as other cell types involved in the immune response. The type of histiocyte may depend on the inciting agent or on where it enters the body, or it may possibly be a result of a cell type–specific lesion in the histiocyte itself or in the helper or suppressor T lymphocytes regulating its biologic behavior. These proliferative histiocytic disorders thus are not malignant diseases histologically.[7,8]

The proliferative histiocytoses have been grouped or classified according to the type of histiocyte presumed to be primarily involved.[9] For example, *Langerhans cell histiocytoses* refers to histiocytic disorders involving Langerhans or Langerhans-like histiocytes. These disorders have historically been referred to as *histiocytosis X*, eosinophilic granuloma, Hand-Schüller-Christian disease and Letterer-Siwe disease. Now separated from this group are the so-called non–Langerhans cell histiocytoses, which include such disorders as familial erythrophagocytic lymphohistiocytosis, hemophagocytic syndromes, and sinus histiocytosis.

Flow cytometry studies of the cells from Langerhans cell histiocytosis infiltrates have demonstrated a diploid DNA content, normal proliferative index, and no evidence of a clonal population.[10] Another report has observed aneuploidy from lesions of disseminated forms of Langerhans cell histiocytoses.[11] Recent data demonstrate that the CD1a-positive histiocytes in involved sites from three patients with Langerhans cell histiocytosis are clonal in origin.[11a] Further data also demonstrated that Langerhans cells from both unifocal lesions and from patients with more extensive and disseminated disease are clonally derived.[11b] These data strongly suggest that Langerhans cell histiocytosis is a neoplastic disorder that arises from somatic genetic

TABLE 32-1. Distinguishing Characteristics of Histiocyte Cell Types*

Feature	Macrophage	Follicular Dendritic Cell†	Paracortical Interdigitating Cell‡	Indeterminate Dendritic Cell	Langerhans Cell
CYTOPLASMIC MARKERS					
Nonspecific esterase	+	±	±	±	±
Acid phosphatase	+	±	±	±	±
ATPase	−	+	+	+	+
ATPase-1-antichymotrypsin	+	−	−	−	−
ATPase-1-antitrypsin	+	−	−	±	−
S-100	±	−	+	+	+
Lysozyme	±	−	−	−	−
Peanut lectin staining	Diffuse, cytoplasmic	?	Plasma membrane & paranuclear dot	?	Plasma membrane & paranuclear dot
Birbeck granules	−	−	−	−	+
SURFACE ANTIGENS					
IgG Fc receptor (C3b)	+	+	+	+	+
Ia antigen	+	+	+	+	+
CD1a (T6)	−	±	±	+	+
CD4 (T4)	+	−	±	±	±
CD25 (IL-2R)	+	−	−	?	−
CD11c (Leu-M5)	+	−	−	−	−
CD21 (C3d)	+	+	−	?	−
CD14 (MY4)	+	−	−	?	−
PHYSIOLOGY					
Phagocytic activity	Strong	Weak	Weak	?	Weak
Antigen presentation	+	+	+	?	+
Cytokine secretion	+	+	+	?	+

±, low-level or variable expression.
* This table is not intended to be all-inclusive but rather to demonstrate some of the more important features that can help to distinguish the different subsets of histiocytes discussed in this chapter. See text for details and references.
† Referred to as the dendritic reticulum cell in Farber.[13]
‡ Referred to as the interdigitating reticulum cell in Farber.[13]

changes and has variable clinical behavior. These important findings also provide the basis for the identification of the genetic changes that lead to the clonal proliferation of Langerhans cells in these disorders. This issue needs further experimental clarification. Malignant histiocytosis, histiocytic sarcoma, and monocytic leukemia represent true histologically malignant conditions of the monocyte lineage (Table 32-2).

In rare instances, the normal phagocytic function of the macrophage is disrupted as a result of an inherited enzymatic defect resulting in abnormal intracellular accumulation of undegraded lysosomal substrates. Such macrophages function poorly and accumulate in multiple organ systems, resulting in displacement of normal organ architecture with subsequent enlargement and dysfunction. These inherited disorders of the histiocyte are referred to as *lysosomal storage disease* and represent a separate class.

Occasionally, similar overloading of macrophages with lipid can occur in patients with chronic myelogenous leukemia or hemolytic disorders caused by the excessive turnover of hematopoietic precursors and their progeny. This acquired form of lipoidosis results when the ability of the macrophage to metabolize normal phagocytized material is exceeded and not caused by an inherent defect of the macrophage.

Thus, inherited and acquired storage disorders are not primary proliferative histiocytoses secondary to immune dysregulation. Nevertheless, they result in organ dysfunction caused by the malfunction of the macrophage as well as the disruption of organ architecture and function.

CLASS I: LANGERHANS CELL HISTIOCYTOSES

The Langerhans cell histiocytoses represent a group of disorders with diverse clinical manifestations. Based on the clinical presentations, a wide variety of names have been used to describe these disorders. Historically they include eosinophilic granuloma, Hand-Schüller-Christian disease and Letterer-Siwe disease, which have been referred to as different forms of histiocytosis X. An excellent historical review has been written and should be referred to for more detail.[12]

In 1941, Sidney Farber[13] first noted the pathologic similarity among the diverse class I histiocytoses, thereby questioning their separation as distinct diseases. Lichtenstein[14] subsequently introduced a unifying classification that brought the many different eponyms under the generic term *histiocytosis X*. The X was used to signify the still unknown cause of these disorders. Other syndromes such as familial erythrophagocytic lymphohistiocytosis, and infection-associated hemophagocytic syndrome have often been erroneously included under histiocytosis X.

TABLE 32-2. Lymphohistiocytic Disorders of the Reticuloendothelial System

PROLIFERATIVE DISORDERS
Class I. Langerhans Cell Histiocytosis
Eosinophilic granuloma
Hand-Schüller-Christian disease
Letterer-Siwe disease
Hashimoto-Pritzker disease
Indeterminate cell proliferative disorder*
Class II. Non-Langerhans Cell Disorders
Familial erythrophagocytic lymphohistiocytosis
Infection-associated hemophagocytic syndrome
Histiocytic medullary reticulosis
X-linked lymphoproliferative syndrome
Lymphomatoid granulomatous disease
Sinus histiocytosis with massive lymphadenopathy
Xanthogranuloma
Benign cephalic histiocytosis
Histiocytic necrotizing lymphadenitis
Miscellaneous and unclassified
Class III. Malignant Histiocytic Disorders
Malignant histiocytosis
Histiocytic sarcoma (true histiocytic lymphoma)
Langerhans cell type
Malignant fibrous histiocytoma
Monocytic leukemia
LYSOSOMAL STORAGE DISORDERS
Inherited
Sphingolipidoses
Mucopolysaccharidoses
Mucolipidoses
Miscellaneous
Acquired

* The indeterminate cell has been postulated to represent a precursor to the Langerhans cell. See text and Harrist and colleagues[84] and Wood and associates.[85]

(Adapted in part from the classification system proposed by the Histiocyte Society)

The term *Langerhans cell histiocytoses* has replaced many names, including histiocytosis X, in an attempt to reduce the confusion and to be more consistent with what is now known concerning the pathology of these disorders.[9] Thus, Langerhans cell histiocytosis is a pathologic diagnosis, and the extent of disease or systemic involvement is added to clarify the clinical presentation.

The diagnosis of Langerhans cell histiocytosis should be based on several pathologic criteria.[1,7,15] First, as noted, a biopsy specimen of a lesion should have the characteristic reactive infiltrate (Fig. 32-2). In addition, the histiocytes within the lesion should have two or more of the following features: positive staining for ATPase, S-100 protein, α-D-mannosidase, and characteristic binding of peanut lectin. Finally, the documentation of Birbeck granules by electron microscopy or positive immunostaining for CD1a antigenic determinants on the surface of the histiocytes makes the diagnosis definitive.

Although the Langerhans cell of histiocytosis is generally believed to represent an abnormally proliferating Langerhans cell, some controversy still exists because of the similarity of the two cell types.[2] Both share many functional and phenotypic similarities, although some differences have been reported. For example, Harrist and coworkers[16] have reported that Langerhans cells of histiocytosis react with anti-CD4 antibodies, whereas normal Langerhans cells do not. In addition, other investigators have reported that Langerhans cells of histiocytosis express C3b receptors, which are usually not present on Langerhans cells.[17] Such differences may represent different physiologic or pathophysiologic characteristics. Most evidence points to the Langerhans cell of histiocytosis being an abnormal Langerhans cell that is intrinsically involved in this type of histiocytosis.[11a]

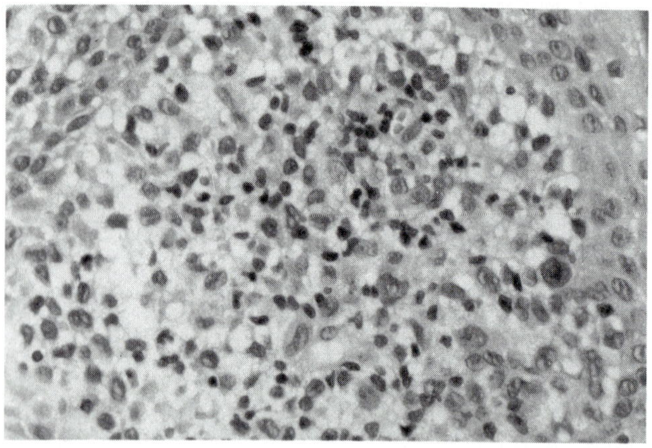

FIGURE 32-2. Photomicrograph showing a typical reactive infiltrate involving the epidermis observed in Langerhans cell histiocytosis. Numerous dendritic cells and eosinophils can be seen.

Clinical Manifestations

Langerhans cell histiocytoses can occur at any age, although it occurs most frequently in children between 1 and 15 years old. The disease is most often found in patients of northern European descent and rarely in blacks. An association of Langerhans cell histiocytosis with the development of various malignant disorders has been suggested.[17a–17c] A variety of tissues and organs may be affected by the disorder. The signs and symptoms vary according to the site of the lesions. Considerable variability may occur in any one patient during the course of the disease. Historically, Langerhans cell histiocytoses have been clinically described as three separate entities: eosinophilic granuloma, Hand-Schüller-Christian disease, and Letterer-Siwe disease.

Eosinophilic Granuloma

Eosinophilic granuloma is characterized by solitary or multiple bone lesions. Solitary lesions are more common than multifocal disease. Eosinophilic granuloma usually occurs in older children and adults. Prognosis is excellent. The most common site of involvement is the calvaria.[18,19] Other commonly involved bones are the femur, scapula, rib, mandible, vertebra, and ilium.[18–25] Cervical vertebrae are most frequently affected followed by thoracic and lumbar sites.[25] Vertebral planar is a characteristically observed abnormality and usually represents old lesions that are asymptomatic. Although any bone in the body may be affected, the small bones of the hands and feet are rarely involved.

The patient usually presents with a complaint of pain, often associated with soft tissue swelling over the involved site. Limp due to pain associated with weight bearing may occur with vertebral and lower extremity lesions. Young children may refuse to walk. Lesions of the mandible may be associated with pain on chewing. Spinal cord compression can occur with extension of a lesion into the epidural space, resulting in paralysis.[26–28] Systemic symptoms are rare.

The bone lesions are usually lytic and give rise to a "punched-out" appearance on radiographs, although some lesions may also show a blastic component (Fig. 32-3). A radiographic skeletal survey is believed to be the best way to detect other nonsymptomatic lesions, since most radionuclide isotopes are usually taken up poorly by the lesions. Occasionally, a bone scan may demonstrate involvement in the absence of other radiographic findings.[29–31]

Hematologic manifestations may be a mild leukocytosis and an elevated sedimentation rate. No significant alterations in biochemical parameters are observed.

Hand-Schüller-Christian Disease

Hand-Schüller-Christian disease is classically characterized by the triad of lytic skull lesions, exophthalmos, and diabetes insipidus, but it often refers to a subset of multifocal Langerhans cell disease. Young children, usually between 2 to 5 years, are most commonly affected, although this type of disease involvement has been described in all age groups. Hand-Schüller-Christian disease is often chronic, and the patient is likely to suffer relapse. Prognosis for survival is good. Long-term sequelae are not uncommon, however.[23,25]

The lytic skull lesions are often associated with tender swelling. Exophthalmos develops secondary to orbital bone involvement with soft tissue extension of the reactive infiltrates.[18] In addition, involvement of the sphenoid bone, sella turcica, mandible, mastoid, and the extremity long bones may be present. Mandibular involvement usually presents as a painful, swollen mass and may lead to eventual diminished height of the mandibular rami as well as displacement and loss of teeth. Maxillary involvement is less common. Temporal and mastoid bone involvement may lead to chronic otitis media with resultant formation of cholesteatomas.[32,33] Long-term sequelae include deafness.[34]

In addition to the involvement of the osseous aspects of the head, oral cavity disease is frequently present in Hand-Schüller-Christian disease (Fig. 32-4). It is associated with swollen, often hemorrhagic gums and mucosal ulceration.[35] The periapical region of teeth commonly shows the first signs of involvement, with subsequent erosion of the lamina dura eventually giving rise to the characteristic radiographic picture of teeth floating in their sockets (Fig. 32-5). Careful oral examination is therefore critical in evaluating any patient with suspected histiocytosis. Biopsy specimens are easily obtained for diagnosis, thus obviating the need for biopsy of more difficult sites. Cervical adenopathy usually accompanies such oral involvement. The diagnosis of histiocytosis has been made in infants manifesting gingival involvement and premature eruption of teeth.[35,36] The course of the disease may often be monitored by following the status of oral involvement, even when other physical signs have regressed.

Diabetes insipidus with polyuria, dehydration, and polydipsia occurs in as much as 20% to 50% of children with multifocal histiocytosis.[18,37–41] It probably results from cellular infiltration of the posterior pituitary fossa.[42] Diabetes insipidus usually occurs in patients after the diagnosis of histiocytosis has already been made, often during or after the cessation of treatment.[23,38] In adults, diabetes insipidus may precede other evidence of disease. Laboratory findings establish the diagnosis and reveal hypernatremia and low urine osmolality. After a fluid restriction of several hours, a relative increased serum osmolality and a persistent decreased urine osmolality are observed. In infants and young children, this period of fluid restriction should be done under medical supervision. Radiographic examination by routine film or by computed tomography (CT) may often be negative, although magnetic resonance imaging may reveal hypothalamic or pituitary involvement.[43–47a]

Involvement of the hypothalamus may result in growth hormone deficiency,[37,48] which may subsequently result in decreased stature. Affected children may also develop hypogonadism and delayed puberty.[34,40] Thyroid involvement with histiocytosis has also been reported.[18,34,49]

Histiocytosis may involve the brain as an eosinophilic granuloma in the multifocal form of the disease or even more rarely as an isolated lesion.[50] Isolated brain involvement occurs more frequently in older children and adults.[34,51] Neurologic signs and symptoms are headache, vertigo, ataxia, paresis, seizures, dysphagia, nystagmus, and clonus. Focal cranial nerve involvement rarely occurs. Cognitive deficits have also been reported.[26] Cerebellar involvement may result in ataxia, dysdiadochokinesia, and dysmetria.[25,34,51a]

In addition to problems with otitis media, chronic external otitis media is frequently observed in children with Hand-Schüller-Christian disease. This is often accompanied by a seborrheic rash of the external ear canal, the posterior auricular region, and the scalp. Adenopathy in nodal groups draining these anatomic areas is common. Occasionally, skin involvement may be limited to intertriginous areas, the penis, or the vulva. Hepatosplenomegaly may be present and associated with mild abnormalities of liver-derived transaminases.[18,34]

Pulmonary involvement may occur in multifocal or disseminated histiocytosis. Isolated pulmonary involvement is more frequently seen in adolescents and young adults.[25,52,53] There is a strong male predominance.[53] Findings include cough, dyspnea, pain, hemoptysis, and pneumothoraces. Chest radiograph reveals micronodular opacities (Fig. 32-6). Pulmonary function tests demonstrate decreased lung compliance and oxygenation. A lung biopsy should be done to confirm pulmonary involvement with histiocytosis. Because the respiratory tract normally contains Langerhans cells, increased numbers of these cells should be observed to make the diagnosis of histiocytosis involvement.[54] Liver involvement may become chronic and result in cirrhosis and sclerosing cholangitis.[55,56]

Laboratory tests frequently reveal an elevated sedimentation rate and increased platelet count. Immunologic analysis has not revealed any consistent defect, with most children exhibiting normal B- and T-lymphocyte function.[57–59] Some children have been described as having a deficiency of a suppressor T-lymphocyte population associated with increased numbers of autoreactive cytotoxic T lymphocytes.[60,61] These defects resolved with improvement of the disease status. Other studies have not demonstrated such observations, and they remain controversial.[62–64]

Letterer-Siwe Disease

Letterer-Siwe disease represents the most severe form of Langerhans cell histiocytoses. Infants less than 2 years of age are most frequently afflicted, although cases in adults have been reported.[65] The disease may be apparent at birth. There is no obvious genetic predisposition, although anecdotal familial cases have been reported.[66,67] Prognosis is poor; mortality rate is over 50%.[18,23,38,39,68]

Letterer-Siwe disease was first described in 1924 by Dr. Erich Letterer[69] in a 6-month-old infant with fever, purpura, otitis media, lymphadenopathy, and hepatosplenomegaly. In 1933, Dr. Sture Siwe reported another case and noted the similarities between his patient, that of Dr. Letterer's, and two other patients.[70] Abt[71] first referred to the syndrome

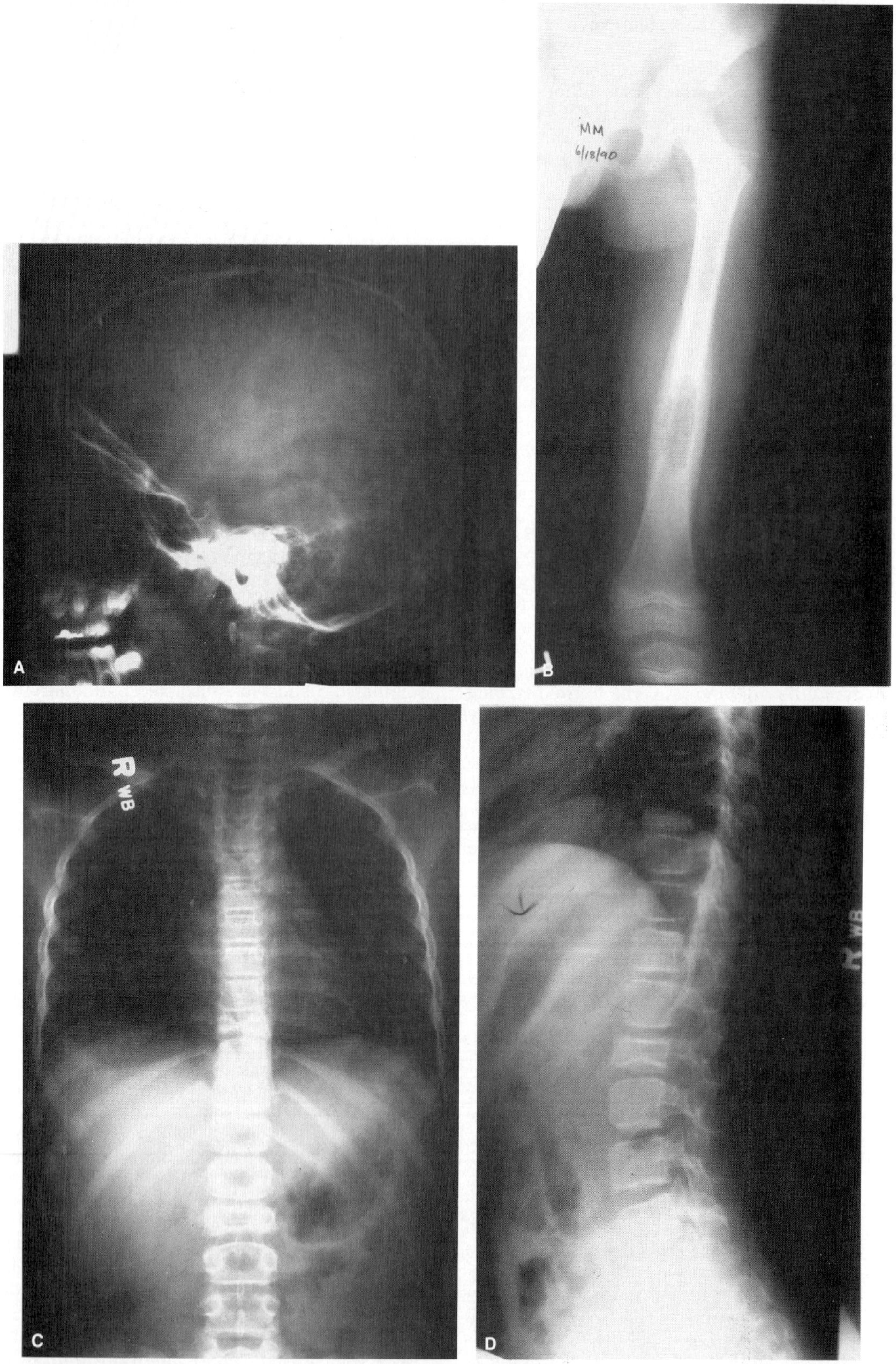

FIGURE 32-3. Radiographs of some bone lesions seen in Langerhans cell histiocytosis. (**A**) Lateral view of skull, showing a large lytic lesion superiorly. (**B**) Lytic lesion of distal left femur. (**C** and **D**) Anteroposterior and lateral views of spine, demonstrating vertebral planar defect. (Courtesy of Children's Hospital Radiology Library Collection, Boston)

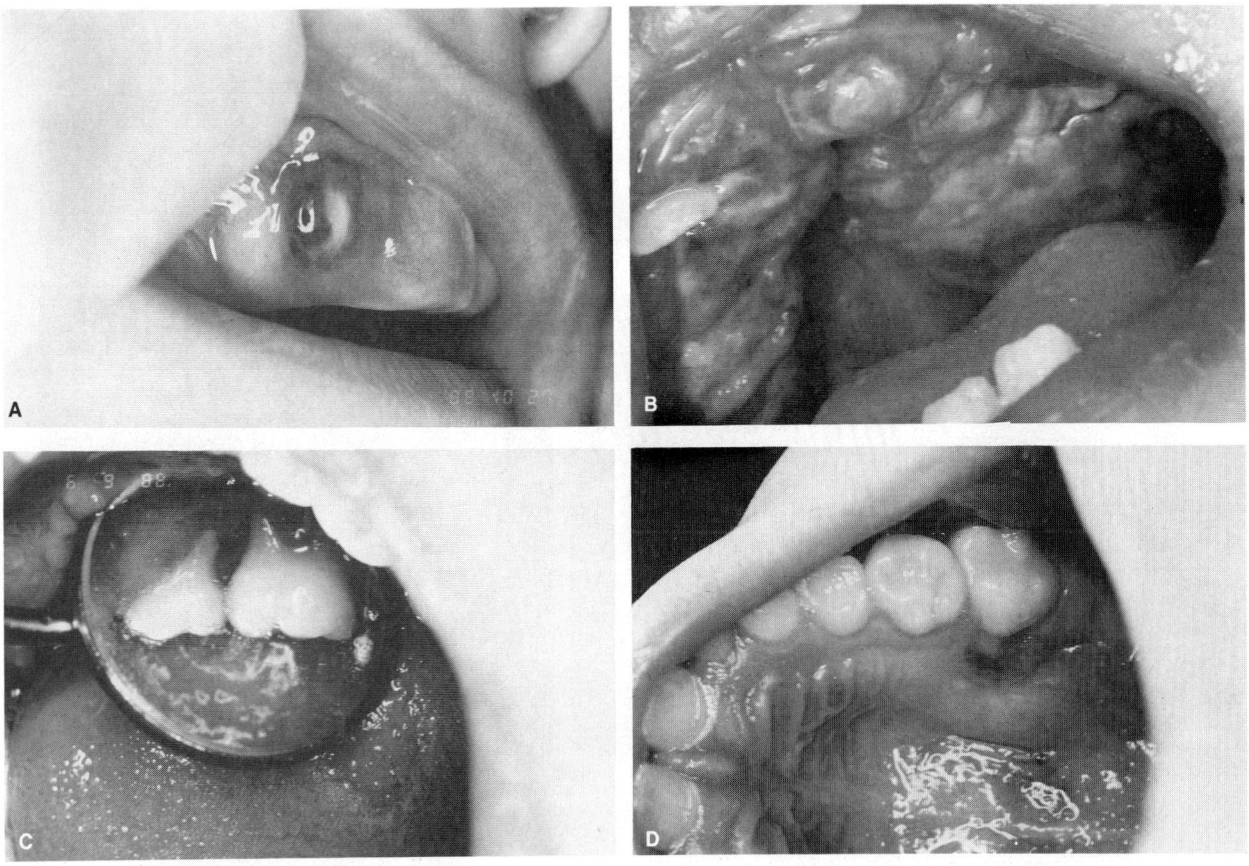

FIGURE 32-4. Oral lesions observed in Langerhans cell histiocytosis. (**A**) Predentate anterior gum infiltrative lesion. (**B**) Severe infiltrative disease of palate in infancy. (**C**) Localized bony destruction exposing roots of primary posterior mandibular molars. (**D**) Localized palatal lesion in an older child. (See Color Fig. 32-4.) (Courtesy of Dr. Howard Needleman, Department of Dentistry, Children's Hospital, Boston)

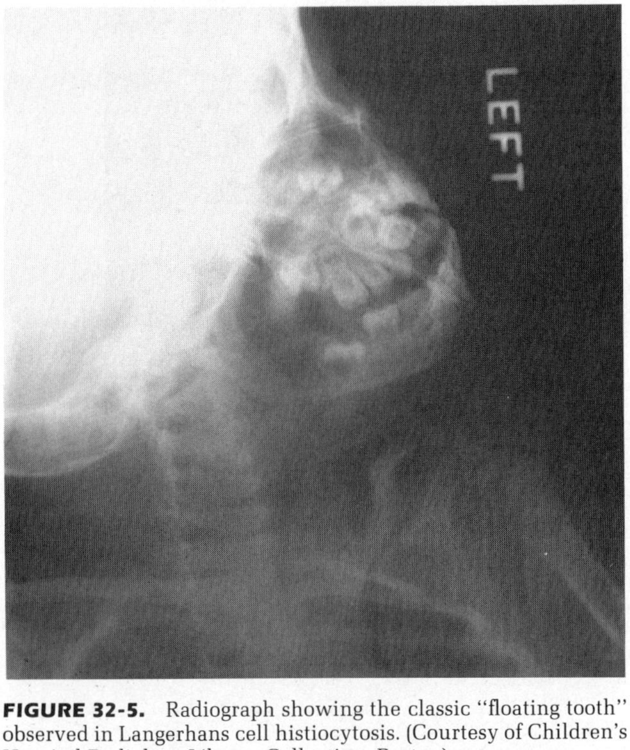

FIGURE 32-5. Radiograph showing the classic "floating tooth" observed in Langerhans cell histiocytosis. (Courtesy of Children's Hospital Radiology Library Collection, Boston)

as Letterer-Siwe disease in 1939. Diffuse histiocytic infiltration of involved tissues was observed in all cases.

Patients with Letterer-Siwe disease usually present with intractable fever and a maculopapular or eczematoid, often purpuric rash (Fig. 32-7). The rash is often most severe in its involvement of the scalp, ear canals, and face, but it extends to the trunk and intertriginous areas. Oral involvement is common. The rash frequently becomes denuded and ulcerated, leading to superinfection with microorganisms. The patient has extreme irritability, anorexia, and failure to thrive.

Purulent otitis media and lymphadenopathy are usually present in patients with Letterer-Siwe disease. Hepatosplenomegaly is prominent. Liver involvement may eventually result in extensive fibrosis with associated cholestasis, jaundice, portal hypertension, and esophageal varices.[72,73] Liver failure in progressive cases may lead to hypoproteinemia, severe coagulopathy, and hemorrhage. Diarrhea is often secondary to liver disease or histiocytic infiltration of the intestinal lamina propria.

Pulmonary involvement may produce cough, dyspnea, tachypnea, pneumothorax, hemoptysis, and poor gas exchange.[74–76] Chest radiograph reveals a micronodular and reticular pattern, which may lead to a honeycomb appearance.

Bone marrow involvement is common in patients with Letterer-Siwe disease and may result in pancytopenia. Decreased blood counts may be secondary to hypersplenism and hemophagocytosis as well as extensive replacement of

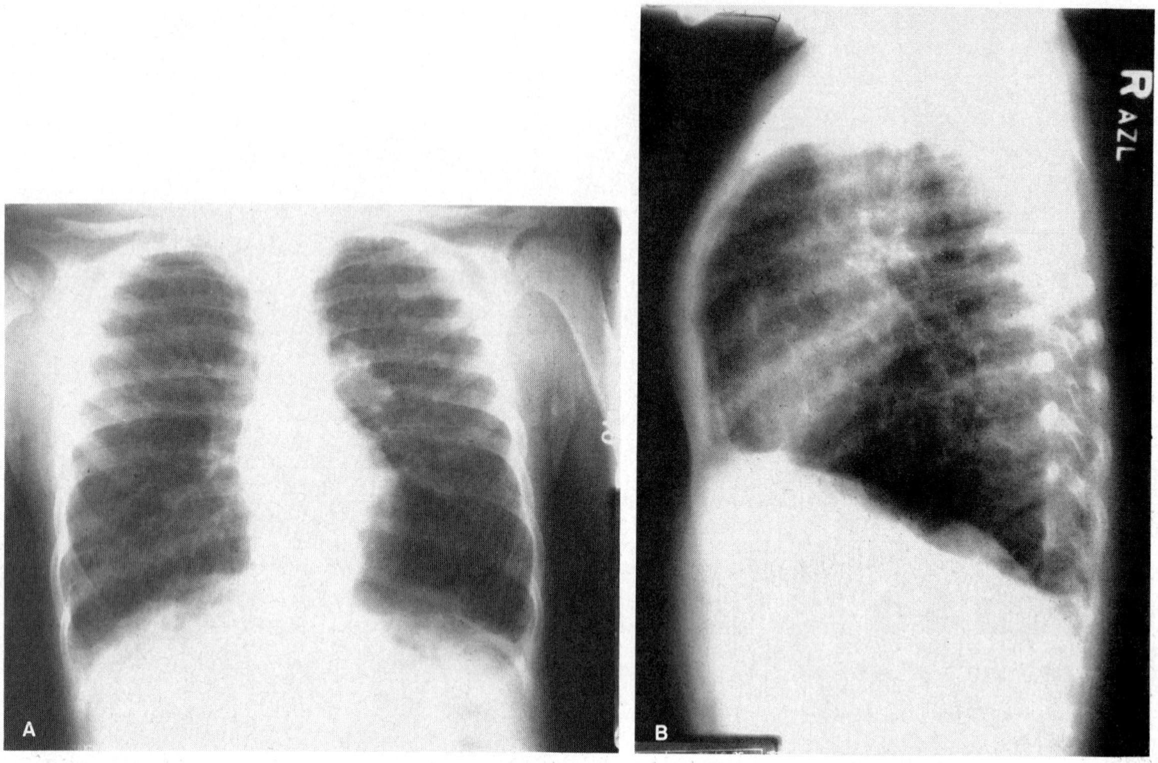

FIGURE 32-6. Pulmonary involvement in Langerhans cell histiocytosis. (Courtesy of Children's Hospital Radiology Library Collection, Boston)

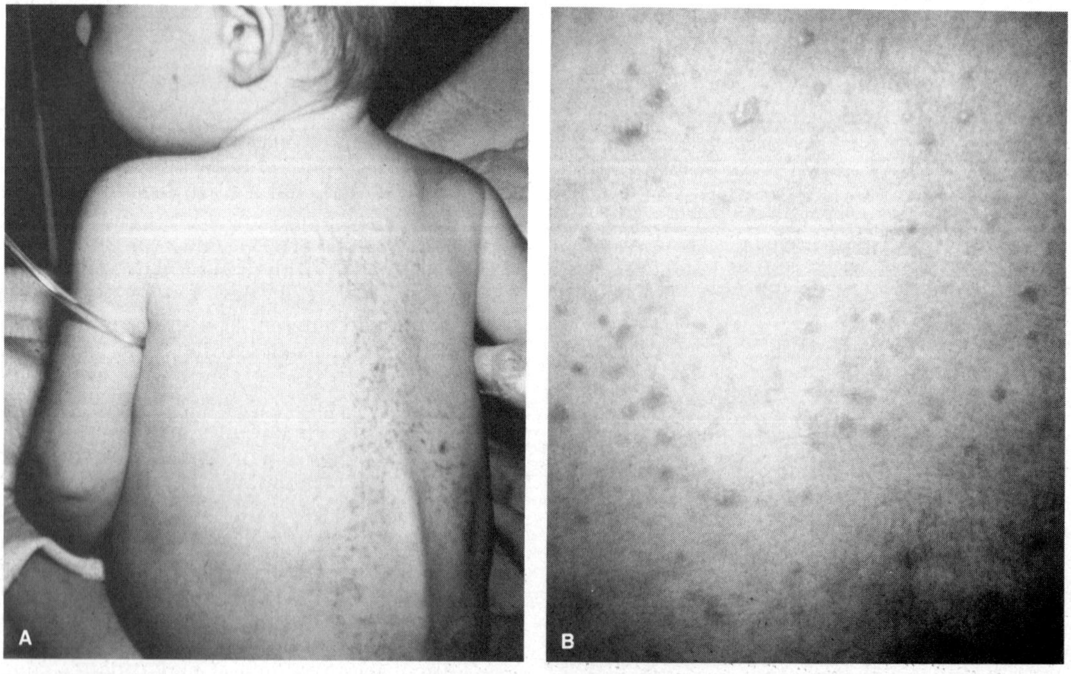

FIGURE 32-7. The maculopapular rash often observed in patients with Letterer-Siwe disease. (See Color Fig. 32-7.) (Courtesy of Steven Gellis, MD, Department of Dermatology, Children's Hospital, Boston)

normal bone marrow hematopoietic elements by histiocytic infiltration. Sepsis and hemorrhage frequently result. Severe hematopoietic compromise is associated with an extremely poor prognosis.[18,20,38,39,68,77]

In all cases of suspected Letterer-Siwe disease, an extensive work-up of the immune system should be undertaken to rule out a primary or acquired immunodeficiency.[58] In addition, an extensive search for infectious agents, particularly viral, should be accomplished (see below).

Hashimoto-Pritzker Disease

Hashimoto-Pritzker disease, also referred to as *congenital self-healing histiocytosis*, presents in early infancy, usually in the newborn period.[78,79] Infants show multiple reddish purple nodular lesions, which primarily involve the scalp and face but which may extend to other parts of the body. Patients appear healthy otherwise. The nodules tend to involve the deeper portions of the dermis with sparing of the epidermis. Over a period of several months, the lesions spontaneously regress, sometimes leaving areas of residual hyperpigmentation. Therefore, no treatment is indicated. The nodular lesions are histologically characterized by accumulations of large multinucleated histiocytes. Although the histiocytes within these lesions have been shown to share a similar immunohistochemical phenotype to Langerhans cells, the two cell types have been demonstrated to differ at the ultrastructural level.[80] These differences as well as the unique clinical course of the disorder have raised the question of whether to include Hashimoto-Pritzker disease among the Langerhans cell histiocytoses.[80]

Indeterminate Cell Proliferative Disorder

The indeterminate cell is a histiocyte that is similar to the Langerhans cell in its morphology and its histochemical and surface antigen phenotype.[81–84] The two cell types differ in that the indeterminate cell lacks Birbeck granules. It has been suggested that the epidermal, indeterminate cell is a precursor to the Langerhans cell.[81]

Indeterminate cell proliferative disorder is characterized by erythematous cutaneous papules that can enlarge to form disfiguring nodules.[85] These lesions involve the face, extensor surfaces of the forearms and legs, and the lateral aspects of the thighs, buttocks, and torso. Spontaneous involution is observed in some of the nodules, whereas others persist. The lesions may become encrusted and infected with resident skin bacteria. For patients whose disease does not spontaneously regress, treatment with vinblastine has been reported to be efficacious.[85]

Natural History and Prognostic Factors

Assessment of prognostic factors is particularly valuable for guiding therapeutic interventions, counseling patients, and evaluating clinical trials. This is especially true for patients with Langerhans cell histiocytoses because of the wide spectrum of disease manifestations and the high incidence of spontaneous remissions and exacerbations. In addition, the disease may wax and wane for several years, thus making the response to any initial therapeutic interventions difficult to interpret in terms of long-term outcome.

Lahey[68,86] first proposed a scoring or staging system that was predictive of eventual outcome for patients with Langerhans cell histiocytoses. Based on both clinical assessment and laboratory data, the most significant prognostic factors were considered to be age of onset, number of organs involved, and, most important, the presence or absence of dysfunction of the liver, lung, and hematopoietic system. Subsequently, other reports have confirmed and extended these observations, resulting in several staging or grouping systems.[38,39,87–91] One such system is represented in Table 32-3. In this system, points are assigned to a patient based on age, number of organs involved, and the presence of organ dysfunction.

Patients under 2 years old with Langerhans cell histiocytoses tend to have a poorer prognosis, whereas those over 2 years have a better prognosis. Patients with localized disease involving four or fewer organ systems have a better prognosis than those with involvement of more than four organ systems. The presence of dysfunction in the hepatic, pulmonary, or hematopoietic system appears to be the most important prognostic variable. Organ dysfunction is defined as described in Table 32-3. Prognosis correlates with the number of points assigned to an individual patient; that is, patients with more total points may be expected to do worse. Thus, a young adult with a solitary bone lesion has the best prognosis, whereas an infant with disseminated disease and organ dysfunction has the worst prognosis. Patients with intermediate scores may be predicted to lie between these two extremes but should ultimately do well.

The initial clinical evaluation of patients with biopsy-proven Langerhans cell histiocytoses should include a thorough history and physical examination as well as appropriate laboratory investigations to evaluate the different organ systems. The extent of the laboratory studies should be tailored to more detailed examination of those organ systems with suspected involvement from the results of more routine tests.

Therapy

The grouping systems for the Langerhans cell histiocytoses are particularly useful for the physician in deciding whether to initiate treatment and in deciding what inter-

TABLE 32-3. Clinical Grouping System for Langerhans Cell Histiocytosis

Factor	Points
AGE	
>2	0
<2	1
EXTENT OF DISEASE	
<4 organs	0
>4 organs	1
ORGAN DYSFUNCTION* (1, 2, or 3 systems)	
No	0
Yes	1
GROUP	**TOTAL POINTS**
0	Monostotic eosinophilic granuloma
I	0
II	1
III	2
IV	3

* Hepatic, pulmonary, or hematopoietic as defined by Lahey[68,86]:
Hepatic dysfunction: hypoproteinemia, (total protein < 5.5 g/dL), albumin < 2.4, or both; edema; ascites; hyperbilirubinemia (<1.5 mg/dL).
Pulmonary dysfunction: tachypnea, dyspnea, cyanosis, cough, pneumothorax, pleural effusion.
Hematopoietic dysfunction: anemia (hemoglobin < 10 g/dL), leukopenia (leukocytes < 4000/μL), thrombocytopenia (<1,000,000).
(Data from Lahey[68,86] and Lipton[39])

vention should be used. The goal of any therapy should be to control, not necessarily eradicate, the disease while at the same time carefully minimizing both the short-term and long-term adverse consequences of that therapy. This is particularly true in patients with Langerhans cell histiocytosis, which has a high incidence of spontaneous remission and displays a tendency to eventually burn itself out.

Evaluating the response to a therapy has also been difficult in patients with these disorders because of the often spontaneously remitting and relapsing course. In addition, the patient may appear to respond well in one site or organ system, while simultaneously worsening in another. Therefore, any evaluation of response should include an assessment of each involved site.

The primary physician caring for a patient with Langerhans cell histiocytosis should be involved in coordinating many subspecialty services such as dermatology, orthopedics, dentistry, radiation therapy, endocrinology, ophthalmology, otolaryngology, and oncology. This is especially true for patients with multifocal or disseminated disease.[39,59]

The first decision to be made in treating patients with Langerhans cell histiocytoses is whether any therapeutic intervention is needed. An initial reasonable approach is to observe patients without symptomatic lesions for spontaneous improvement. Treatment is then reserved for patients with symptomatic lesions or those with more advanced and disseminated disease.

Patients with single bone lesions, and sometimes with multifocal bone lesions, can usually be treated with surgical curettage of a symptomatic and surgically accessible lesion. The surgeon should not necessarily attempt to perform a wide excision or remove a lesion completely as in a cancer operation. Thus, there is no need to put a patient at risk for an orthopedic or cosmetic deformity to remove any residual disease. Simple curettage is sufficient in most cases to effect regression of a symptomatic lesion. In addition, curettage of multiple sites is not indicated.

If a lesion recurs after curettage, other local measures are often effective, such as intralesional injections with corticosteroids or low-dose radiation therapy.[91–97] It is not clear which approach is more efficacious in easily accessible lesions since no comparative trials have been performed. The dose of radiation used is usually between 600 and 1000 rad delivered in 200-rad daily fractions. In the young child, doses between 450 and 600 rad have proved effective.[36,82,83] In older patients, the lower dose schedule may sometimes result in subsequent local failure. For such patients, an initial dose of 1500 to 2000 rad has been recommended.[94] Radiation therapy is especially indicated when the potential for serious consequences appears imminent, such as in vertebral involvement with signs or symptoms of impending spinal cord compression or in severe exophthalmus. Care should be taken to avoid irradiation of radiosensitive sites such as the lens of the eye and the thyroid gland.[94,95]

The role of radiation therapy in the pituitary in the treatment of new-onset diabetes insipidus remains controversial. Greenberger and associates[38] reported improvement in 8 of 21 such cases treated with radiation therapy. The diagnosis of diabetes insipidus in this report was based on clinical findings. Without simultaneous support for the diagnosis from laboratory investigations, it is difficult to interpret these data and thus to recommend such treatment to larger groups of patients.[96] In addition, the use of magnetic resonance imaging to document hypothalamic or pituitary involvement may prove to be helpful in these cases.[47,98–101] Many physicians caring for patients with Langerhans cell histiocytoses have observed transient episodes of polyuria and polydipsia without frank diabetes insipidus.[41]

Treatment for severe skin disease has been accomplished with topical therapy without systemic agents. The first principle in treating areas of involved skin, auditory canals, and gums should be good hygiene. In addition, judicious topical application of nitrogen mustard or corticosteroid creams to limited areas has been successfully used.[102,103] Ultraviolet light treatment has been used in older patients.[104] Both mustine creams and ultraviolet light therapy may predispose the patient to developing cutaneous malignancy.

For more advanced disease (severe multifocal or disseminated forms), systemic therapy with a variety of agents has been used. Over the past 50 years, treatment of advanced histiocytosis with systemic agents has been what might be called a "shotgun" approach to treatment. Patients have been treated with dietary manipulations, arsenic, glycoprotein, and corticosteroids, antibiotics, heliotherapy, and a variety of cytotoxic agents to treat malignancies.[12] Many of these approaches have by themselves produced significant morbidity and at times have precipitated fatalities. Within the past 20 years, treatment for advanced disease has primarily included a variety of cytotoxic agents. Response rates vary widely, between 25% and 90%, and may reflect the difficulties in discerning true responses from spontaneous regression.[39] The emphasis on using chemotherapeutic agents has resulted in the referral of these patients to oncologists.

The major controversy regarding systemic chemotherapeutic agents has centered on "how many and how much." In other words, how aggressive should one be with a treatment regimen? Most evidence supports a more conservative approach to treatment, guided by the philosophy that the therapy should not be worse than the disease and that the intensity of the treatment should be tailored to the severity of the disease.[39,59,105–109]

Many groups initiate systemic treatment for Langerhans cell histiocytoses with moderate doses and schedules of single cytotoxic agents. Vinblastine, given weekly at 0.45 $mg/m^2/wk$ intravenously has proved to be both efficacious and safe. The major side effect is myelosuppression, but this can usually be avoided with judicious administration. Patients do not experience nausea or vomiting, have little or no problem with constipation, and seldom develop alopecia. For patients who experience only a partial response to vinblastine, the addition of a short course of oral prednisone, 40 $mg/m^2/d$ orally for about 2 weeks, followed by a dose tapering over the course of 1 week, often effects a desired response. Although no evidence proves that vinblastine is more efficacious than vincristine, vinblastine is usually preferred because of fewer problems with neurotoxicity. Other groups begin treatment with moderately high doses of prednisone, although significant problems may occur with hypertension, growth, emotional changes, hyperphagia, and body image. Methotrexate, 10 $mg/m^2/wk$ intramuscularly or intravenously, and 6-mercaptopurine, 20 $mg/m^2/d$ orally for 14 days of a 21-day cycle, either alone or in combination, have been used effectively, although the potential for hepatic toxicity must be considered.

Some evidence exists that the epipodophyllotoxin, VP-16, is an effective agent, particularly in patients who have failed treatment with other agents.[59,110–116] This agent has been used intravenously at a dose of 150 $mg/m^2/d$ for 3 days for a total of 3 to 6 courses. The major side effects are hypotensive episodes during administration, allergic reactions, alopecia, and myelosuppression.[105] Some concern over the possibility of VP-16 being involved in the development of myeloid neoplasia has been raised.[117,118] Table 32-4 presents a treatment program in use at the Dana Farber Cancer Institute, Boston.

Little evidence supports the role of aggressive combination chemotherapy in Langerhans cell histiocytoses.[59] Such approaches have been associated with significant morbidity and mortality. The use of chemotherapeutic agents such as procarbazine and various alkylating agents such as chlorambucil should be avoided because of the higher risk of treatment-induced malignancies.[39,59,105,119] In one report, 5 of 84 patients treated with chemotherapy, including chlorambucil or nitrogen mustard with or without radiation, developed late malignancies.[38] Three patients who received such chemotherapy plus radiation developed acute leukemia. One patient developed thyroid carcinoma. Another patient who received chemotherapy alone developed hepatocellular carcinoma. A sixth patient who received only radiation therapy developed a thyroid carcinoma. The time to development of these malignancies varied from 2 to 28 years. Other neoplasms such as astrocytoma, medulloblastoma, meningioma, and osteogenic sarcoma have been reported as late complications of treatment in Langerhans cell histiocytoses.[34]

The duration of treatment may be variable, although most patients with Langerhans cell histiocytoses are treated for at least 3 months to 1 year. On resolution of disease, which may be expected within the first several months of therapy, most physicians extend the treatment for several more weeks. It does not appear to be beneficial to put patients on a type of maintenance therapy because of the potential risks and lack of clear-cut benefit.[59,107] If symptomatic disease recurs after cessation of treatment, therapy should be reinstituted. The patient almost invariably responds again to the treatment regimen used initially. A recurrence does not necessarily mean that the disease will be more difficult to control or that it will return in a more aggressive form.

Attempts to manipulate the immune response as a form of therapy in patients with Langerhans cell histiocytoses have been made.[60,90,120,121] Such strategies have been based on the hypothesis that patients lack a specific subset of suppressor T cells. Osband and associates[60] reported that intramuscular injection of calf thymus extract was as effective as chemotherapy in patients with multifocal disease but not any better in patients with disseminated disease. In addition to the clinical response, these investigators observed an improvement in immunologic abnormalities. The use of historic controls, that is, patients treated with chemotherapy, as well as the small numbers of patients evaluated, prevent this report from being definitive.

In addition, at least two other studies—one involving a crossover with a chemotherapy regimen—have demonstrated no significant efficacy for such an approach.[120] Nevertheless, more extensive multicenter trials may be useful in further evaluating such therapeutic approaches with immunomodulators.[90] Anecdotal experience has been gathered with the use of cyclosporine and α-interferon, and larger trials are underway.[122–124] Anecdotal responses have also been observed with the use of 2-chlorodeoxyadenosine.[124a]

For patients who have aggressive, disseminated disease that is refractory to conventional therapies, allogeneic bone marrow transplantation has been successfully used.[125–128] The use of autologous bone marrow transplantation is hindered by the lack of any means of eradicating the extensive bone marrow involvement commonly observed in severely affected children.

TABLE 32-4. Chemotherapeutic Treatment Program for Histiocytosis*

PROGRAM I

Vinblastine, 5 mg/m^2/wk intravenously as a single weekly dose. If patient is not improved after 2 weeks, increase dose by 20%. Vinblastine is tapered from weekly to every other week to every 3 weeks; then dosage is reduced to 5 mg/m^2 every 3 weeks before discontinuation. Reinstitute lowest dose for disease rebound. The highest nonmyelosuppressive dose is used. Patients should be treated initially with vinblastine only. If no or slow improvement, add:

Prednisone, 40 mg/m^2/d orally or methylprednisolone, 32 mg/m^2/d intravenously. With improvement, taper to the smallest effective dose on an alternate day schedule. With continued improvement or satisfactory control, a slow taper of prednisone is undertaken but should be discontinued prior to the vinblastine taper.

PROGRAM II (IF PROGRAM I FAILS)†

Methotrexate, 10 mg/m^2/wk intramuscularly or intravenously and 6-mercaptopurine (6-MP), 20 mg/m^2/d orally for 14 days of 21-day cycle. The highest nontoxic dose is used (toxicity: myelosuppression, mouth sores, hepatotoxicity). On improvement, both drugs are slowly tapered. Methotrexate is tapered from weekly to every other week to every 3 weeks. The 6-MP schedule is maintained while the dose is reduced 10% to 15% per cycle. Reinstitute lowest effective dose for disease rebound.

PROGRAM III (IF PROGRAMS I AND II FAIL)†

VP-16, 150 mg/m^2/d, for 3 days for each cycle of therapy. Cycles are separated by 3- to 4-week intervals, depending on the time of bone marrow recovery. Corticosteroids may be given concomitantly as described under Program I. Usually four to six courses are given.

* This program is being used at the Dana Farber Cancer Institute. See text for details regarding indications for initiating chemotherapeutic treatment.

† A therapeutic regimen is considered to have failed if disease and symptoms progress as assessed by laboratory data (eg, liver function deterioration, progressive thrombocytopenia), radiographic evaluation (eg, worsening chest radiograph, progression of intracranial lesion), or clinical assessment by history and physical examination (eg, failure to thrive, worsening rash, progressively enlarging liver and spleen) while patient is being treated. Patient should have been on maximum therapy of a particular program for at least 4 weeks.

CLASS II: NON–LANGERHANS CELL HISTIOCYTOSES

Non–Langerhans cell histiocytoses represent a group of disorders characterized by immunoreactive infiltrates consisting of cells of the mononuclear phagocytic system and lymphocytes without Langerhans cell involvement.[9] The two major types are familial erythrophagocytic lymphohistiocytosis and infection-associated hemophagocytic syndrome. Discriminating between these two disorders is clinically important because of their differing treatments and prognoses.

Familial Erythrophagocytic Lymphohistiocytosis

Familial erythrophagocytic lymphohistiocytosis (FEL) was first described by Farquhar and Clairveaux[129] and thought to be a rapidly fatal familial form of Letterer-Siwe disease, which they termed *familial hemophagocytic reticulosis.* Subsequent reports have demonstrated that FEL is different from Letterer-Siwe disease in its histopathology, biochemical features, inheritance, clinical course, and treat-

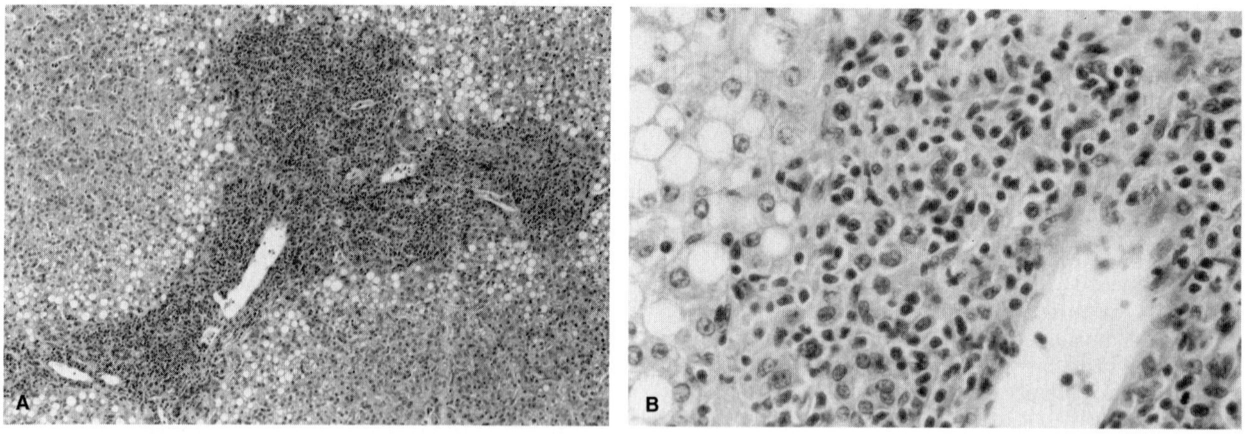

FIGURE 32-8. Pathologic biopsy specimen of liver, demonstrating the lymphohistiocytic infiltrate in portal areas in a patient with familial erythrophagocytic lymphohistiocytosis. (See Color Fig. 32-8.)

ment.[130–135] The diagnosis is made by considering the clinical presentation, histopathology of biopsies, and several biochemical findings.

FEL is an autosomal recessive disorder, which presents during infancy (up to 4 years of age) with fever, failure to thrive, hepatosplenomegaly, pancytopenia, hepatic dysfunction, a bleeding diathesis, and frequently neurologic manifestations characterized by seizures, disorientation, and stupor.[133] Bone lesions are usually absent. A maculopapular rash is occasionally observed with predilection for the scalp. This rash is red to purple in color and often shows areas of skin breakdown. Lymphadenopathy may occur early in the disease, but eventually lymphoid depletion results. Patients with FEL are acutely ill with multiorgan involvement and require hospitalization, expedient evaluation, and treatment. Although occasional chromosomal abnormalities have been reported in patients with FEL, no consistent finding has been demonstrated.[133a]

Diagnostic biopsies can be obtained from several tissue sources including lymph nodes, skin, liver, spleen, lungs, and bone marrow. Because of associated coagulopathy, the least invasive biopsy should be attempted. This is often from an involved lymph node, skin, and bone marrow. With proper precautions, a liver biopsy is often useful. Examination reveals a lymphohistiocytic infiltration of portal areas. Langerhans cells are absent in such biopsies[131] (Fig. 32-8).

Biochemical features include a marked hyperlipidemia (particularly a hypertriglyceridemia), a profound hypofibrinogenemia, elevated hepatic transaminases, and increased bilirubin.[133–137] The presence of a plasma inhibitor of lymphocyte mitogenic stimulation has been observed in patients with FEL.[138] Many different defects in both cellular and humoral immunity have been described in such patients, but no consistent etiologic abnormality has been confirmed.[138–145]

Hematologically, patients with FEL have pancytopenia secondary to both hepatosplenomegaly and bone marrow involvement. Splenectomy has not had any significant, sustained benefit. In addition to a bone marrow aspirate, a bone marrow biopsy is also useful in establishing cellularity since normal marrow constituents may occasionally be replaced by sheets of invading histiocytes.

CNS involvement is common and is characterized by both meningeal infiltration and focal masses.[146,147] A lumbar puncture often reveals a pleocytosis, sometimes with evidence of erythrophagocytosis (Fig. 32-9), and increased protein. A CT scan of the head frequently shows single or multiple foci of parenchyma destruction. Lung involvement may be manifested by increased oxygen requirement secondary to pulmonary infiltrates or pleural effusions. Pulmonary hemorrhage may occur and be fatal.

The presence of a positive family history is often lacking. In the face of a negative family history, it may be difficult to differentiate FEL from infection-associated hemophagocytic syndrome (discussed in the following section). Thus, in all cases, an exhaustive search for potential infectious agents, particularly viral, should be performed.

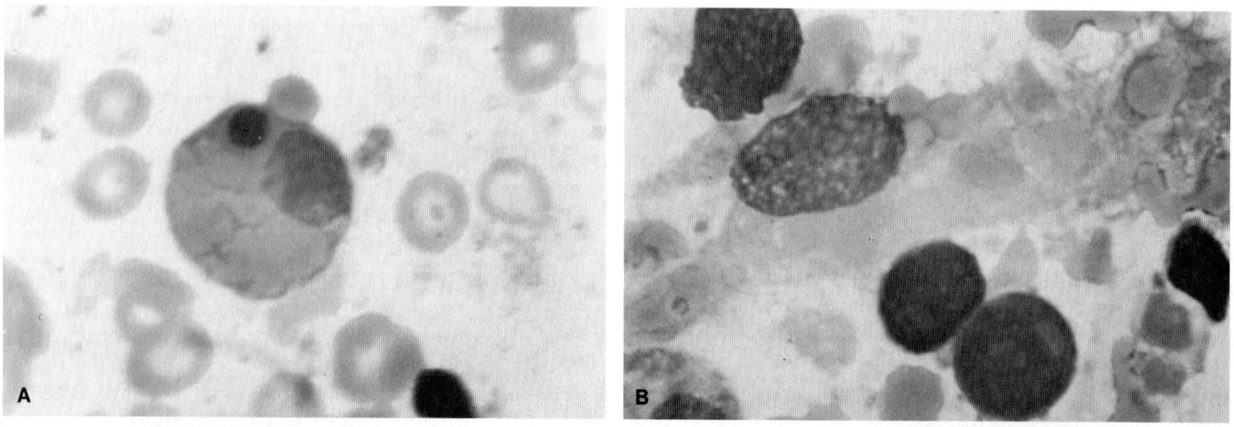

FIGURE 32-9. Examples of erythrophagocytosis in a patient with histiocytic medullary reticulosis. (See Color Fig. 32-9.) (Courtesy of Pearl Levitt, Department of Hematology, Dana Farber Cancer Institute)

Up until the past several years, FEL has uniformly followed a rapidly fatal course, usually as a result of overwhelming infection or hemorrhagic complications. Several different chemotherapeutic regimens, usually including vinblastine and prednisone, have not resulted in a significantly improved prognosis. The introduction of VP-16 has, however, proved effective in many patients in inducing complete remissions.[148–153] Prednisone is usually included in treatment, although its benefit remains unclear. In addition, reports have stressed the importance of treating the meningeal involvement with intrathecal methotrexate or cytarabine. For severe brain parenchymal involvement, cranial irradiation may be indicated, in which case intrathecal methotrexate should be avoided. Plasmapheresis has been used, the rationale being to reduce the plasma inhibitory activity. Occasionally, clinical improvement has been reported with repeated plasmapheresis, but this effect is usually transient.[138] Complete remissions have also been obtained using antithymocyte globulins, steroids, and cyclosporin A.[138a] Allogeneic bone marrow transplantation has been used successfully in anecdotal cases.[154] Experience indicates the initial use of VP-16 with or without prednisone along with treatment of the CNS to obtain an initial remission. Allogeneic bone marrow transplantation should then be performed.[154a–154c]

Infection-Associated Hemophagocytic Syndrome

Infection-associated hemophagocytic syndrome (IAHS) presents with a clinical picture essentially indistinguishable from FEL, although FEL is rare in children over 4 years old. These two disorders may also be similar in terms of laboratory findings, although elevated serum triglycerides are more characteristic of FEL.[138–140] Biopsy specimens in both disorders reveal reactive lymphohistiocytic infiltrates with erythrophagocytosis and hemophagocytosis.[155,156] These two disorders may in reality represent overlapping disease groups and be best characterized as hemophagocytic lymphohistiocytoses (HLHs). Nevertheless, a positive family history of the identification of an infectious agent may be helpful in distinguishing between the two disorders. The most definitive way to distinguish these two disorders is by the identification of an infectious agent or a positive family history.

IAHS is most often observed in an immunocompromised patient in association with a variety of infections due to viral, bacterial, fungal, and parasitic agents.[155] The immununodeficiency in these patients may be inherited or acquired.[156] The most commonly encountered viruses are those of the herpes group, such as cytomegalovirus, Epstein-Barr virus (EBV), and varicella zoster, as well as parainfluenza virus and adenovirus.[155,157,158] Bacterial infections associated with IAHS have included both gram-negative and gram-positive bacteria, *Mycobacterium tuberculosis*, syphilis, mycoplasma, listeriosis, typhoid fever, and leprosy.[155,159–164] A number of anecdotal cases have also been reported in association with fungal infections such as histoplasmosis, cryptococcosis, and candidiasis in addition to parasitic infections including brucellosis, malaria, toxoplasmosis, leishmaniasis, and babesiosis.[155,165] In rare instances, IAHS has been associated with exposure to certain drugs such as beryllium, zirconium, and diphenylhydantoin.[155] Several reports have observed the development of IAHS in association with various types of malignancies.[155,166–171] Thus, an exhaustive search for any of these conditions along with a thorough work-up of any underlying immunodeficiency is critical in patients suspected of having IAHS.

The importance of distinguishing IAHS from FEL and other histiocytic disorders is crucial, albeit difficult, because the use of cytotoxic and immunosuppressive agents may be contraindicated in patients with IAHS. If possible, therapies directed at treating any infectious cause should be used first. Some cases of IAHS may be self-limited, although the disorder is often progressive and fatal. New therapeutic modalities are clearly needed.

Histiocytic Medullary Reticulosis

Scott and Robb-Smith[172] first described a rapidly progressive and fatal disorder characterized by fever, wasting, hepatosplenomegaly, jaundice, and lymphadenopathy associated with tissue infiltration of histiocytes. They termed this condition histiocytic medullary reticulosis (HMR) based on the finding of histiocytic infiltration of the medullary zone of lymph nodes. Although this syndrome has been viewed as a malignant disorder, it is now considered more likely to represent a fulminant form of a reactive hemophagocytic syndrome.[15,172–177]

HMR has been reported to affect all age groups. No sex predilection has been observed in childhood cases, although males appear to be affected more frequently in adulthood. A high incidence of HMR has been reported in areas of Africa and Asia, suggesting the possible contribution of an infectious agent in the cause of HMR in these areas.[177]

Lymphadenopathy may develop late in the course in adult HMR patients. Cervical and axillary nodes are commonly involved and often painful and show evidence of ulceration. Mediastinal adenopathy and pericardial involvement may be observed. In children, abdominal pain and distention often accompany intraabdominal lymphadenopathy. Enlarged pelvic lymph nodes may result in ureteral obstruction and hydronephrosis. Cutaneous involvement is evident in over 50% of cases, most frequently presenting as indurated, dermal infiltrative lesions. A purpuric, maculopapular rash involving the trunk has also been reported. Pulmonary involvement may occur with interstitial infiltration as well as pleural effusions. Involvement of the CNS and gastrointestinal tract and lytic bone lesions have been observed.[173]

A normochromic anemia has been observed in over two thirds of patients. Thrombocytopenia is observed in about one third of patients. Leukocytosis associated with neutrophilia is common. Pancytopenia frequently develops in advanced disease. Bone marrow aspiration and biopsy may show infiltration with histiocytes, although it is rare to observe high percentages of these cells and total marrow replacement. Hemophagocytosis is commonly seen and may contribute to pancytopenia (see Fig. 32-9).

Hepatic involvement is manifested by elevated hepatocellular transaminases and increased serum bilirubin. Coagulopathy may also develop and be exacerbated by thrombocytopenia. Increased levels of serum lysozyme and ferritin have been reported.[176,178]

Histopathologic examination of a biopsy is essential for diagnosis. This is best achieved by lymph node biopsy, although liver biopsy may also be diagnostic. Lymph node involvement early in the course of the disease is characterized by the infiltration of histiocytes into the subcapsular and medullary sinuses. Eventually, total replacement of the nodal architecture occurs. Usually a spectrum of morphologic stages is observed among the histiocytes.[176,179] The more differentiated histiocytes are more likely to show hemophagocytosis. It is thus essential to correlate the morphologic appearance of the histiocytes with both histochemical and immunophenotypic markers of the histiocytic lineage.[179]

The differential diagnosis of HMR includes several other

disorders, such as monocytic leukemia and true malignant histiocytosis. In monocytic leukemia, bone marrow replacement by immature monoblasts is observed, whereas bone marrow involvement in patients with HMR is often minimal with extramedullary sites more extensively affected. In malignant histiocytosis, a proliferation of malignant histiocytes appears to be at an intermediate stage of differentiation between the monoblasts of acute monocytic leukemia and the malignant tissue macrophage of histiocytic sarcoma or lymphoma.[15,176,179] In addition, the histiocytes characteristic of HMR include a range of differentiated forms unlike the uniform population observed in true leukemia. Letterer-Siwe disease can be distinguished from HMR by the demonstration of reactive infiltrates characterized by the presence of Langerhans dendritic cells. FEL may also present with a similar clinical picture but differs from HMR by virtue of age, familial nature, lipid abnormalities, severe hypofibrinogenemia, and pathology of the infiltrates. Sinus histiocytosis (see section on sinus histiocytosis with massive lymphadenopathy) represents a more limited disorder; the patients usually do not appear ill, and the tissue infiltrates are cytologically benign. Histiocytic lymphoma and sarcoma usually present with less fulminant courses than HMR and represent more localized malignant processes. The distinction between the lesions observed in HMR patients and those with non-Hodgkin's lymphomas rests on pathologic, histochemical, and immunophenotypic criteria.

The prognosis for patients with HMR remains guarded. Because past reports of HMR may have included cases of true malignant histiocytosis, it is difficult to unequivocally make conclusions regarding the use of chemotherapeutic regimens.

X-Linked Lymphoproliferative Syndrome

X-linked lymphoproliferative syndrome (XLPS) may also be confused with both FEL and IAHS. This disorder was originally described in the early 1970s, and more than 100 cases have now been described.[180–184] The most common presentation is in the young male child with a severe, often fatal, EBV infection. The course of XLPS is progressive and characterized by hepatitis followed by massive hepatic necrosis. High fevers, maculopapular rash, and leukocytosis associated with a marked increase in atypical lymphocytes are observed. Not infrequently, pancytopenia, hypogammaglobulinemia, and a severe coagulopathy develop. About 15% of patients develop lymphoma.

XLPS may involve any organ system with infiltration by both T- and B-cell immunoblasts. In the liver, infiltration is primarily periportal. Early in the course of the disease, lymph nodes may be enlarged secondary to the proliferation of these immunoblastic infiltrates, although lymphoid depletion is observed in the terminal phases with associated histiocytic infiltration. The extent of histiocytic proliferation observed in XLPS is usually not as great as that observed in FEL or IAHS.

The diagnosis of XLPS should be considered in young male children with the above clinical and pathologic characteristics associated with evidence of EBV infection as documented by IgM antibody directed against viral capsid antigen as well as early EBV antigens. As noted previously, the histopathology of XLPS may not show the extensive histiocytic proliferation as observed in FEL and IAHS. Although not necessarily definitive, immunologic studies may be useful in discriminating these syndromes.[185] For example, in FEL, decreased responses to lymphocyte mitogen stimulation are often observed as well as decreased natural killer cell activity.[185] IAHS, even when caused by EBV infection, does not usually show the degree of atypical lymphocytes observed in XLPS. Finally, the finding of infectious agents other than EBV makes the diagnosis of IAHS more probable.

A number of different treatments have been used to attempt to reverse the often fatal course of XLPS. Acyclovir, a potent antiviral agent, has been used but without apparent success.[186] Similarly, the use of γ-globulin preparations with high titers of anti-EBV reactivity has been disappointing.[184–186] Interferons, which are antiviral compounds made by the host in response to viral infections, may prove useful, but definitive studies have not been reported.[186,187] The best approach may be to determine means by which predisposed males can be identified and subsequently given immunoprophylaxis before experiencing exposure to EBV infection.[186,187]

Lymphomatoid Granulomatosis

Lymphomatoid granulomatosis is a distinctive disorder characterized by angiocentric, destructive granulomatous lesions with a predilection for pulmonary involvement.[188,189] It is usually included among granulomatous disorders of unknown cause such as sarcoidosis, Wegener's granulomatosis, and giant cell arteritis. Lymphomatoid granulomatosis most commonly occurs in adults, but cases have been reported in children.[190–192] Lymphomatoid granulomatosis often occurs in patients with chronic inflammatory disorders and underlying malignancy. Lymphoma, frequently involving the brain, may develop in up to half of lymphomatoid granulomatosis patients.[191–194]

Patients usually present with fever of unknown origin, weight loss, and cough. Skin involvement manifested by infiltrative plaques is common and offers an easily accessible site for diagnostic biopsy. The disease has a strong predilection for the lungs; chest radiograph and CT scans reveal multiple, bilateral nodules and micronodular disease. CNS involvement frequently manifests as seizures.[190–193]

Pathologic examination of lesions of lymphomatoid granulomatosis patients demonstrates infiltrates of primarily atypical lymphocytes and plasmacytoid cells. These infiltrates are characteristically angiocentric and destructive. Vasculitis is evident. There are no characteristic laboratory findings, although patients are usually anergic to hypersensitivity skin tests.[192–194]

Prognosis remains poor with mortality reported in up to 60% of patients with lymphomatoid granulomatosis. Corticosteroids and cyclophosphamide have been used with some success in controlling the underlying malignancy.

Sinus Histiocytosis With Massive Lymphadenopathy

Sinus histiocytosis with massive lymphadenopathy (SHML) was first described by Rosai and Dorfman in 1969.[196] SHML usually is seen during the first decade of life, although cases have been reported in patients over age 60. It occurs in all parts of the world but is observed more frequently in young black patients.

SHML is characterized by massive, painless, cervical lymphadenopathy, although other lymph nodes may also be involved. Bilateral cervical enlargement is typical. Occasionally, extranodal involvement includes the upper respiratory tract, salivary glands, orbit, bone, testis, and skin. A rare finding of epidural involvement resulting in paraplegia has been reported.[197] Usually chronic, low-grade fevers are present. Laboratory data include leukocytosis with increased granulocytes and a concomitant decreased lymphocyte count. A normochromic anemia may be present. The sedimentation rate is markedly elevated, and a polyclonal hypergammaglobulinemia is frequently observed.[198] Several reports have also demonstrated increased titers to EBV as well as to *Klebsiella* antigens.[198,199] An exaggerated immune response to rubella virus has been reported.[200] Herpesvirus 6 has been detected in involved tissues from several patients.[200a] In spite of such associations, the cause of SHML remains unknown.

Biopsy of an involved lymph node in SHML reveals sinusoidal dilatation with benign-appearing histiocytes and reactive lymphocytes. The histiocytes may be multinucleated and demonstrate a large amount of foamy cytoplasm (referred to as *Mikulicz cells*). Leukophagocytosis is extensive, and erythrophagocytosis may be present. S100-positive histiocytosis demonstrating extensive lymphophagocytosis is pathologically diagnostic of SHML.[200b]

SHML usually follows a relatively benign course with gradual resolution over several months to years. In rare cases, upper respiratory tract involvement may result in airway compromise.[201] In addition, orbital involvement may cause proptosis. Such cases may require a brief course of therapy, either with agents such as prednisone and vinblastine or low-dose radiation therapy.[198,199,201,202] A response to acyclovir has been reported in a single case.[202a] Because SHML is self-limited and self-resolving, therapeutic interventions are usually not indicated.

Miscellaneous Forms of Non–Langerhans Cell Histiocytoses

A number of cutaneous non–Langerhans cell histiocytic disorders have also been described. *Juvenile xanthogranuloma*, first described in 1954 by Helwig and Hackney,[203] is a disorder that occurs primarily in infants and young children, who present with cutaneous nodular lesions involving the head, extremities, and sometimes the trunk. Noncutaneous involvement is rare. The lesions require no treatment and usually resolve over the course of several months to years.

Benign cephalic histiocytosis usually presents within the first 2 years of life with the development of numerous, small, reddish-brown macules, which primarily involve the scalp but may extend to the shoulders and upper extremities.[204–208] The lesions are usually less than 5 mm in diameter and do not display seborrheic or hemorrhagic manifestations observed in Letterer-Siwe disease. The disease slowly regresses over the course of several months to years often with residual pigmented macules. No treatment is required.

Histiocytic necrotizing lymphadenitis (*Kikuchi's disease*) represents a reactive lymphadenopathy.[209–212] An inciting agent has not been identified. It appears to be more common in Asian populations and particularly in young females. Subsequent development of systemic lupus erythematosus may be associated.[212] Presentation is usually in the form of painless, enlarging cervical and axillary lymph nodes, sometimes associated with low-grade fever and malaise. Lymph node biopsy reveals infiltration with reactive histiocytes and lymphocytes accompanied by areas of focal necrosis. The disorder is self-limited and therapeutic interventions are not required.

CLASS III: MALIGNANT HISTIOCYTOSES

Malignant histiocytosis is a rare and fulminant disorder affecting mostly older children and young adults, although it has been reported during infancy.[213–216] As previously mentioned, some cases of true malignant histiocytosis have been diagnosed as hemophagocytic disorders; the reverse has also occurred.[169–172,176]

Patients usually present with intractable fevers, wasting, lymphadenopathy, and hepatosplenomegaly. Skin infiltration is common. Bone marrow involvement may result in pancytopenia. Diagnosis can be made by lymph node biopsy, which demonstrates infiltration with cytologically malignant histiocytes.[13,173,176,179] Immunocytochemical and immunohistochemical identification of the malignant cells as belonging to the histiocytic lineage is important to establish an accurate diagnosis and distinguish malignant histiocytosis from lymphomas.[176,217–221] Circulating malignant cells are rare but have been observed.[176]

Cytogenetic analysis of malignant histiocytosis has not definitively delineated a characteristic chromosomal aberration. Several cases have been reported, including hyperdiploid karyotypes, extra C group chromosomes, and a variety of translocations.[215,221] Of particular note are reports of translocations involving a breakpoint at 5q35, particularly t(2;5)(p23;q35).[223] Located in this distal region of chromosome 5 are the genes encoding macrophage–monocyte colony-stimulating factor and its receptor c-*fms*, which are known to influence the growth and function of specific mononuclear phagocytic cells. This observation of a common chromosomal breakpoint is still controversial in that other reports have presented evidence that this translocation is observed in patients with Ki-1 antigen-positive T-cell lymphoma presenting with a clinical picture similar to that of malignant histiocytosis.[179,224] Continued cytogenetic and molecular analyses involving cases of malignant histiocytosis rigorously diagnosed according to clinical, pathologic, and immunophenotypic criteria are needed.[225]

The prognosis for patients with malignant histiocytosis has improved significantly over the past decade. Initially a uniformly fatal disease, long-term remissions can be achieved in up to 40% to 50% of cases. Several combination chemotherapeutic regimens have been successfully used. They usually involve the use of cyclophosphamide, vincristine, prednisone, methotrexate, and doxorubicin.[214,226–228] After an intensive induction period to achieve remission, most treatment regimens continue for 1 to 2 years with a maintenance phase of therapy. The need for CNS prophylaxis with intrathecal methotrexate is still controversial. Excellent responses have also been reported with VP-16 in combination with cytosine arabinoside.[229] This particular regimen may be especially useful in the patient who has significant hepatic involvement and increased serum bilirubin and in whom the use of doxorubicin might be contraindicated because of its hepatic excretion. Allogeneic bone marrow transplantation after ablative therapy with high-dose VP-16 and cyclophosphamide along with total body irradiation has also been used to treat malignant histiocytosis successfully.[230–232]

Histiocytic sarcomas, also referred to as *true histiocytic lymphoma*, are rare malignancies of adulthood. They represent more localized disease than observed in malignant histiocytosis. Patients usually present with lymphadenopathy although involvement of bone, skin, and gastrointestinal tract has been reported.[13,233,234] An unusual cutaneous form of histiocytic sarcoma that has a more indolent course has been described.[233–235] Malignant transformation of Langerhans cells is exceedingly rare.[236,237]

Acute monocytic leukemia and malignant fibrous histiocytoma also represent malignant transformation of cells belonging to the mononuclear phagocytic lineage. In addition, several reports have described neoplastic proliferations of dendritic and interdigitating cells resulting in localized lymphadenopathy.[238–241] Lymph node biopsy demonstrates primarily parafollicular involvement of large, S-100–positive, cytologically malignant cells with areas of focal necrosis. Success with chemotherapy has been limited.

LYSOSOMAL STORAGE DISEASES

Lysosomes normally function partly to catabolize the complex biosynthetic products of cells and their breakdown products including lipids, carbohydrates, proteins, and nucleotides. The lysosomal storage diseases represent a group of disorders in which an inherited defect in one of the genes encoding a lysosomal hydrolytic enzyme results in the abnormal accumulation of a specific substance. The progressive accumulation of nonmetabolized material eventually leads to a disruption of normal cell function and tissue architecture. Occasionally, during clinical situations of increased catabolism, such as in myeloproliferative disorders and hemolytic anemias, even normal degradative pathways can be exceeded, resulting in excessive accumulation of cellular breakdown products within lysosomal compartments.

The organ systems that are most frequently affected in lysosomal storage diseases reflect the normal sites of metabolism or utilization of the nondegradable substance. Organs with active reticuloendothelial components, such as the liver and spleen, frequently become enlarged and structurally disrupted because of the active role of tissue macrophages in the elimination of cell breakdown products. Disorders of ganglioside metabolism have a predilection for affecting CNS, resulting in a variety of symptoms including seizures, blindness, and mental retardation. Because of the ubiquitous presence of complex carbohydrates, defects in enzymes involved in their metabolism may affect many different organ systems as well as particular extracellular compartments. Dysmorphic facial features, corneal clouding, and skeletal defects are common findings. Excessive accumulation of certain products may be demonstrable in the cytoplasm of peripheral blood leukocytes including monocytes, polymorphonucleocytes, and lymphocytes. This may serve as an early diagnostic clue, suggesting a particular storage disorder. Pancytopenia may develop secondary to hypersplenism as well as bone marrow failure due to replacement of normal hematopoietic precursors with storage cells.

The primary laboratory features of lysosomal storage disease are both morphologic and biochemical. The presence of foam cells in biopsy specimens can be interpreted as evidence for a lysosomal storage disorder (Fig. 32-10). Foam cells are abnormally enlarged macrophages caused by excessive cytoplasmic accumulation of lysosomal storage material. They may be up to 100 μm in diameter. Multinuclearity may occur. Their large size and relatively clear cytoplasm easily distinguish them from other cell types, particularly on microscopic darkfield illumination. The staining characteristics of foam cells differ according to the undegraded substance that accumulates. Because many of these substances dissolve in organic solvents, special caution should be used in handling biopsy specimens of patients suspected of having a storage disease. Differences also are seen in the ultrastructural analysis of the foam cells in patients with different storage diseases. Thus, portions of each biopsy should be frozen for cryosectioning and biochemical analysis and fixed in glutaraldehyde for electron microscopic evaluation.

Although specific staining reactions of histologic material are useful in categorizing what type of compound is accumulated, definitive biochemical identification is difficult because of limited quantities of biopsy material. Both the urine and the plasma are often found to contain sufficient quantities of the undegraded, accumulating substance. The storage material can be identified using a variety of chromatographic separation methods.

Final diagnosis of lysosomal storage disease is usually made by the identification of a specific enzyme deficiency.

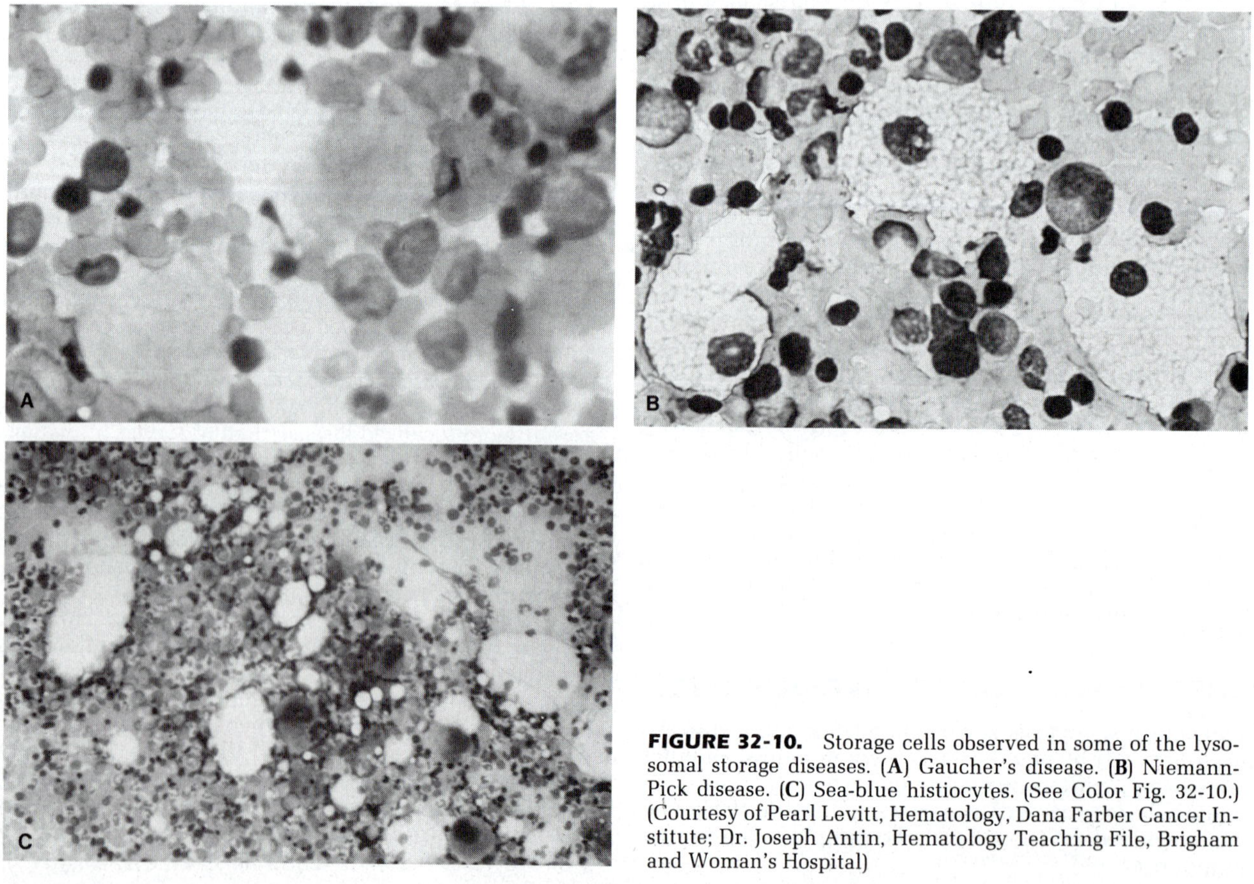

FIGURE 32-10. Storage cells observed in some of the lysosomal storage diseases. (**A**) Gaucher's disease. (**B**) Niemann-Pick disease. (**C**) Sea-blue histiocytes. (See Color Fig. 32-10.) (Courtesy of Pearl Levitt, Hematology, Dana Farber Cancer Institute; Dr. Joseph Antin, Hematology Teaching File, Brigham and Woman's Hospital)

A variety of substrates are used, which form colored derivatives when acted on by a specific enzyme. These byproducts of enzymatic action can then be assayed using simple colorimetric methods. Such assays can be performed on small amounts of serum, plasma, peripheral blood leukocytes, and biopsy specimens including those from skin or liver. Measurement of specific enzyme activities also allows for the identification of persons with intermediate levels of enzyme activity, and thus, persons who are heterozygotic for the abnormal gene. Because most of the lysosomal storage disorders are inherited in an autosomal recessive manner, the identification of such persons becomes extremely important in genetic counseling. The enzymatic assays can furthermore be used in prenatal diagnosis.

Prognosis is highly dependent on the specific lysosomal disorder affecting the patient. Significant heterogeneity exists in the presenting signs, symptoms, and clinical course of these disorders. In general, the earlier in a person's life that the signs and symptoms arise, the more rapid the course of the disease will be, whereas milder clinical courses are often observed when onset occurs later in life.

The approach to treatment of affected patients is best accomplished with a multidisciplinary team, including medical, social, psychology, and educational services. Most treatment is directed at anticipating potential complications and providing supportive care. Based on the premise that extracellular lysosomal enzymes can be taken up by cells through pinocytosis, the prospect of using infusions of enzyme preparations in patients has been under extensive investigation. Initially, infusion of fresh frozen plasma from normal donors into patients affected with mucopolysaccharidosis produced minimal and transient clinical improvement.[242–244] In 1974, Brady and colleagues[245] infused purified enzyme in patients with Gaucher's disease, again with transient clinical and biochemical improvement. Beutler and Dale[246] similarly treated such patients with mixed results. Others studies have used infusion of enzyme-loaded liposomes or erythrocyte ghosts, but these preparations have not been effective.[247,248] Improved success has been reported using purified enzyme infusion therapy in patients with Gaucher's disease.[249,250]

An alternative to enzyme infusion has been organ transplantation of kidney, spleen, and liver.[248,251–253] This approach has not produced any sustained clinical improvement. The use of bone marrow transplantation has been attempted with some success in limited numbers of patients.[254] In a growing number of the storage disorders, the genes for the deficient enzyme have been cloned, offering the future possibility of attempting gene replacement strategies. A major problem with these therapeutic interventions is the failure to reverse or prevent CNS disease.

Prevention continues to remain an important form of intervention in storage disorders. Most storage disorders are inherited in an autosomal recessive manner. Heterozygotic carriers of the abnormal gene can often be identified by either biochemical or genetic analyses. When both parents carry the defective gene, a 25% probability exists that a child will be affected. The availability of prenatal detection of the homozygous fetus offers the possibility of pregnancy termination. On the other hand, determining that a fetus will not be affected provides a means of avoiding unnecessary termination of a pregnancy. Mass screening for heterozygotic carriers has been carried out in specific groups of people with a known high incidence of the defective gene, such as those with Tay-Sachs and Gaucher's disease in the Ashkenazi Jewish population. Screening the general population for carriers of many storage diseases has been felt to be impractical because of the rarity of the conditions.

Discussed in this chapter are the more common forms of lysosomal disorders that make an impact on the reticuloendothelial system. These and some less common disorders are listed in Table 32-5.

Gaucher's Disease

Three distinct forms of Gaucher's disease can be distinguished, which are based on genetic heterogeneity, clinical onset, course, and organ system involvement.[255] Gaucher's disease is particularly prevalent among Ashkenazi Jews, in whom the gene incidence may be as high as 1 in 12 persons. This disorder is usually inherited as an autosomal recessive condition. It is caused by a defective gene encoding the glucocerebroside β-glucosidase lysosomal enzyme. The type 1 form of Gaucher's disease is referred to as *chronic adult nonneuropathic Gaucher's disease.*[256] This form represents most of the cases.

Onset of clinical signs and symptoms in patients with Gaucher's disease may occur in early childhood or any time thereafter. Hepatosplenomegaly is marked and present in nearly all patients, resulting in abdominal distention. Skin involvement may be manifest by yellow to brown areas of pigmentation most noticeable on exposed body surfaces.[257] Conjunctival pingueculae may be present, particularly in adults. Occasionally, diffuse pulmonary involvement may develop. Skeletal involvement is common and characterized by leg pain, joint swelling, and deformities.[258,259] These features are secondary to the infiltration of the medullary cavity by Gaucher's cells, which leads to thinning of the cortical bone, pathologic fractures, infarction, and osteonecrosis. Most patients show an Erlenmeyer flask deformity of the long bones, characterized by cortical thinning of the midshaft with widening of the distal ends (Fig. 32-11).

The hematologic picture of Gaucher's disease may initially be that of a mild normochromic, normocytic anemia secondary to hypersplenism. As the disease progresses, severe pancytopenia develops, resulting from both hypersplenism and bone marrow infiltration with Gaucher's cells. Severe episodes of bleeding may develop caused by the thrombocytopenia. Factor IX deficiency has also been reported in Gaucher's disease and may contribute to the bleeding diathesis.[260] Bleeding may occur during the menstrual cycle or may be caused by ruptured esophageal varices secondary to portal hypertension. A leukoerythroblastic blood smear is indicative of marrow infiltration with Gaucher's cells. Increased serum levels of nontartrate-inhibitable acid phosphatase, angiotensin-converting enzyme, and transcobalamin may be present in homozygotes.[261,262]

Diagnosis of Gaucher's disease is made by documenting the presence of Gaucher's cells in the bone marrow and by demonstrating a deficiency of β-glucosidase activity in peripheral blood leukocytes or cultured skin fibroblasts. The latter approach is less invasive and can be done on small volumes of blood.[263] Heterozygotic carriers may be identified by demonstrating decreased levels of β-glucosidase. Gaucher's cells are not present in heterozygotes. Prenatal diagnosis is available by examining β-glucosidase levels from amniocentesis specimens both in terms of β-glucosidase levels as well as with molecular genetic approaches.

The clinical course of Gaucher's disease is variable, even within members of the same family.[264] Some patients may demonstrate mild hypersplenism, whereas others may develop severe hematologic and bone involvement. Splenectomy may be beneficial to relieve thrombocytopenia and bleeding.[265–267] It has been argued that the absence of the spleen may worsen the involvement of the liver and bones

TABLE 32-5. Lysosomal Storage Diseases

Disease	Stored Material	Enzyme Deficiency	Inheritance	Hematologic Findings	Clinical Features
SPHINGOLIPIDOSES					
Gaucher's disease	Glucocerebroside	Glucocerebroside, β-glucosidase	AR	Gaucher cells in bone marrow, anemia, thrombocytopenia	Infantile—hepatosplenomegaly, progressive CNS degeneration, death by age 2 y Juvenile—hepatosplenomegaly, CNS degeneration, mixed seizure disorders Adult—hepatosplenomegaly, skeletal changes, bleeding, nonneuronopathic
Niemann-Pick disease	Sphingomyelin	Sphingomyelinase	AR	Foam cells in bone marrow, lymphocyte vacuolization (especially in type E)	Type A (Acute neuronopathic)—hepatosplenomegaly, cherry red macula, developmental delay, death by age 2–3 Type B—chronic, nonneuronopathic, osteoporosis Type C—onset at age 1–3 y, hepatosplenomegaly, CNS degeneration Type D—Nova Scotia variant, signs similar to type C Type E—adult onset, nonneuronopathic, few clinical signs/symptoms
Fabry's disease	Globotriaosylceramide and glycolipids	α-Galactosidase	X	Foam cells in bone marrow	Onset in young adult males, angiokeratomas, corneal and lens opacities, heart, kidney, brain and intestine infarction
GM_1 gangliosidosis	GM_1-ganglioside	GM_1-ganglioside, β-galactosidase	AR	Foam cells in bone marrow, vacuolated lymphocytes	Type 1—onset in infancy, hepatosplenomegaly, coarse facies, cherry red macula; CNS degeneration Type 2—onset within first 2 y, hepatosplenomegaly, CNS degeneration Type 3—onset late childhood to young adulthood, progressive pyramidal and extrapyramidal signs
Tay-Sachs disease	GM_2-ganglioside	Hexosaminidase A	AR	Bone marrow lacks foam cells	Onset during first year of life, CNS degeneration, cherry red macula, blindness
GM_2-gangliosidosis, Sandhoff variant	GM_2-ganglioside, globoside	Hexosaminidases A and B	AR	Foam cells in bone marrow, vacuolated lymphocytes	Similar to Tay-Sachs
Farber's disease	Ceramide	Ceramide	AR	Foam cells in bone marrow	Onset in infancy; painful, swollen joints; swallowing and respiratory difficulties; death by age 2 y
MUCOPOLYSACCHARIDOSES					
Hurler's disease	Dermatan sulfate, heparin sulfate	α-L-Iduronidase	AR	Leukocyte granulations, vacuolated leukocytes	Onset during first year; coarse facies, hepatosplenomegaly, corneal clouding, gingival hyperplasia, skeletal deformities, psychomotor and mental retardation, heart failure; death before puberty
Hunter's disease	Dermatan sulfate, heparin sulfate	Iduronosulfate sulfatase	X	Leukocyte granulations, vacuolated leukocytes	Mild to severe mental retardation, hirsutism, skeletal malformations, white skin nodules, coarse facies, atypical retinitis pigmentosa, deafness, no corneal opacification; death before age 15 or possible survival into adulthood with milder form
Sanfilippo's disease					
Type A	Heparin sulfate	Sulfamidases	AR	Leukocyte granulations, vacuolated leukocytes	Onset in early childhood; developmental delay and severe mental retardation, hepatosplenomegaly, skeletal deformities, corneal opacities rare; death in childhood

Type B	Heparin sulfate	*N*-Acetyl-α-glucosaminidase	AR		
Type C	Heparin sulfate	Heparin *N*-acetyl transferase	AR		
Type D	Heparin sulfate	Heparin-6-sulfate sulfatase	AR		
Morquio's syndrome					
Type A	Keratin sulfate	*N*-Acetyl galactosamine 6-SO_4 sulfatase	AR	Leukocyte granulations	Onset age 1 to 2 y; skeletal deformities, including short neck and trunk, bowed knees, vertebral subluxation; normal intellect
Type B	Keratin sulfate	B-Galactosidase	AR	Leukocyte granulations	Hyperflexible joints, coarse facies, deafness, corneal clouding, valvular heart disease, mild hepatosplenomegaly, survival into adulthood
Scheie's syndrome	Dermatan sulfate, heparin sulfate	α-L-Iduronidase	AR		Onset in school age; joint stiffness, claw-hand deformity, corneal opacifications, normal intellect, coarse facies, decreased hearing, hepatosplenomegaly, heart valve problems; survival into adulthood
Maroteaux-Lamy syndrome	Dermatan sulfate	Arylsulfatase B	AR	Leukocyte granulations	Onset in early childhood; normal intellect, severe skeletal deformities including short stature, claw-hand deformity, joint contraction and facies; corneal opacification, deafness, hepatosplenomegaly, heart valve involvement, much clinical heterogeneity
Sly's disease	Dermatan sulfate, heparin sulfate	β-Glucuronidase	AR	Leukocyte granulations	Onset usually in early childhood; coarse facies, hepatosplenomegaly, inguinal hernias, anterior chest wall deformity, normal intellect to mild retardation, no corneal opacification; course variable
Mucosulfatidosis	Sulfatides, mucopolysaccharides	Multiple sulfatases	AR	Leukocyte granulations, vacuolated leukocytes	Onset during first year of life; developmental delay, spastic tetraparesis, blindness, seizures, hepatosplenomegaly variable, skeletal deformities, ichthyosis; progressive, fatal course
MUCOLIPIDOSES					
Sialidoses I	Sialyloligosaccharides, glycoproteins	α-Neuramidase	AR	Lymphocyte vacuolation, bone marrow foam cell	Onset late childhood to adolescence; normal to mildly decreased intellect, decreased vision, cherry red macula, lenticular opacities, pronounced myoclonus, seizures
Sialidoses II	Sialyloligosaccharides	α-Neuramidase, β-galactosidase	AR	Leukocyte fine granulations, lymphocyte vacuolation, bone marrow foam cells	Congenital: hydrops fetalis, hepatosplenomegaly, skeletal deformities Infantile: coarse facies, delayed development, mental retardation, cherry red macula; lenticular opacities, decreased hearing, myoclonus, hepatosplenomegaly, skeletal deformities Juvenile: onset in mid to late childhood; coarse facies, spine deformities, mild decrease in intellect

(continued)

TABLE 32-5. *(Continued)*

Disease	Stored Material	Enzyme Deficiency	Inheritance	Hematologic Findings	Clinical Features
MUCOLIPIDOSES (Continued)					
Type II (I-cell disease)	Sialyloligosaccharides, glycoproteins, glycolipids	*N*-Acetylglucosamine-1-phosphate transferase	AR	Lymphocyte vacuolation	Onset at birth; coarse dysmorphic facies, developmental delay, mental retardation, inguinal hernias, thickened skin, hepatosplenomegaly, corneal opacification, gingival hyperplasia, skeletal deformities, valvular heart disease, no mucopolysacchariduria, dense inclusions in fibroblasts (I cells); death by age 8 y
Type III (Pseudo-Hurler polydystrophy)	Glycoproteins, glycolipids	*N*-Acetylglucosamine-1-phosphate transferase	AR	Vacuolated plasma cells in bone marrow	Onset in early childhood; coarse facies, restricted joint mobility, carpal tunnel syndrome, claw-hand deformity, skeletal deformities and short stature, mild mental retardation, corneal opacification, retinal degeneration, valvular heart disease, I cells present; survival into adulthood
Type IV	Glycoproteins, glycolipids	Ganglioside neuramidase	AR	Variable presence of bone marrow foam cells, vacuolated plasma cells	Onset at birth and early infancy; corneal opacification, psychomotor retardation, retinal degeneration
MISCELLANEOUS					
Fucosidoses	Fucoglycolipids, fucosyloligosaccharides	α-Fucosidase	AR	Lymphocyte vacuolation	Onset and course variable; psychomotor delay, coarse facies, skeletal deformities, hepatosplenomegaly, corneal opacification, gallbladder dysfunction and hyperhidrosis in early-onset type
Mannosidosis	Mannosyloligosaccharides	α-Mannosidase	AR	Leukocyte granulations, lymphocyte vacuolation	Onset in first year of life; coarse facies, psychomotor retardation, skeletal deformities, mild hepatosplenomegaly; survival into adulthood
Aspartylglucosaminuria	Aspartylglucosamine	Aspartylglucosaminidase	AR	Lymphocyte vacuolation	Onset in early childhood; psychomotor retardation, coarse facies, skeletal deformities, skin changes including large nevi and photosensitivity; course variable, survival possible into adulthood
Wolman's disease	Cholesterol esters, triglycerides	Acid lipase	AR	Leukocyte (sudanophilic) vacuoles; vacuolate histiocytes in bone marrow	Onset during first year of life; vomiting, abdominal distention, foul-smelling stools, wasting, adrenal calcifications; death by age 1 y
Cholesterol ester storage disease	Cholesterol esters, tryglycerides	Hepatic acid esterase	AR	Leukocyte vacuolation, bone marrow foam cells	Onset in early childhood; marked hepatomegaly that may progress to fibrosis; splenomegaly and esophageal varices may develop; survival possible beyond childhood
Neuronal ceroid lipofucinosis	Ceroid-lipofuscin pigments	Unknown	AR	Lymphocyte vacuolation, leukocyte azurophilic granulations, bone marrow foam cells	Onset from infancy to adulthood; psychomotor abnormalities, retinal degeneration and optic nerve atrophy, seizures, cerebellar disturbances

AR, autosomal recessive; X, X-linked.

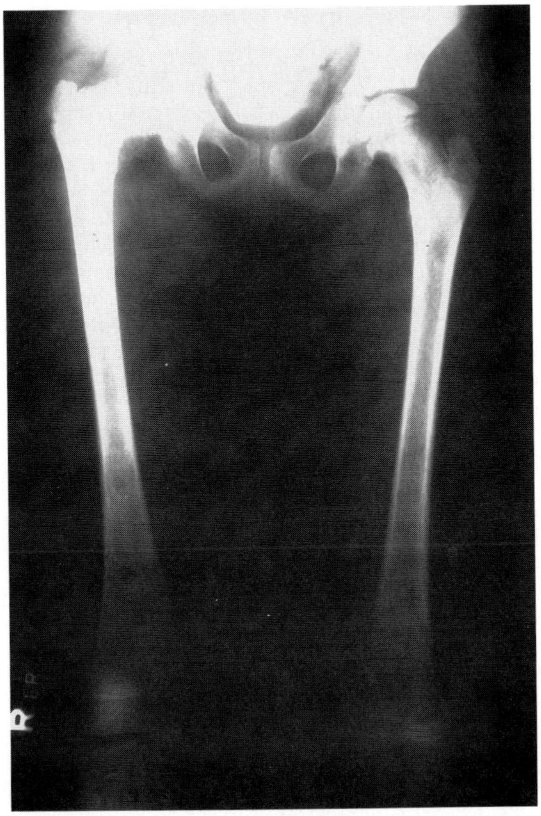

FIGURE 32-11. Erlenmeyer flask deformity of femur observed in Gaucher's disease. (Courtesy of Children's Hospital Radiology Library Collection, Boston)

by diverting the accumulating sphingolipid to these sites.[268] As already noted, enzyme infusions are now demonstrating improved efficacy.[250] Bone marrow transplantation may offer a reasonable choice for severe cases, because type 1 disease does not involve the CNS and is primarily a disorder of the reticuloendothelial system, which can be transplanted from a normal bone marrow donor.[250,254,269]

Type 2 Gaucher's disease is referred to as *acute neuropathic infantile Gaucher's disease.*[255] Although normal at birth, infants usually develop symptoms before age 6 months. Marked hepatosplenomegaly, failure to thrive, and progressive neurologic deterioration including hypertonia, spasticity, strabismus, dysphagia, laryngeal spasm, and opisthotonic positioning are seen. Pulmonary involvement causes cough and may lead to cyanosis. The hematologic and laboratory features are similar to those of type 1 disease. Death usually occurs before age 2 years. Inheritance is autosomal recessive and both carrier status and prenatal diagnosis can be determined. Because of the CNS involvement and the rapidly fatal clinical course, prevention should be stressed to families at risk.

Type 3 Gaucher's disease is called *subacute neuropathic juvenile Gaucher's disease.* Signs of neurologic deterioration and hepatosplenomegaly are seen in older children and adults.[255] Also, considerable variation in severity is found among different patients. There is no predilection for the Ashkenazi Jewish population. In addition to the neurologic symptoms described for type 2 disease, a number of patients with type 3 Gaucher's disease may present with a seizure disorder, deteriorating mentation, and loss of control of voluntary movement. The course is progressive and becomes dominated by the neurologic deterioration. Other than supportive care, no definitive treatment exists. It is not clear whether bone marrow transplantation is beneficial for such patients.[254,270,271]

At least some of the clinical heterogeneity in Gaucher's disease can be explained from recent molecular analyses. Both the genomic and cDNA sequences encoding glucocerebrosidase have been identified.[272–276] The gene has been mapped to chromosome 1.[277,278] Nucleotide sequence analyses have documented specific mutations leading to amino acid changes in the glucocerebrosidase enzyme. Of particular importance are the observations that certain mutations appear to be specific for either type 1 or type 2 disease and predictive of severity of disease.[279–284] As more sequence information becomes available, the clinical course of Gaucher's disease will be able to be predicted more accurately. This information aids in genetic counseling and prenatal diagnosis as well as in planning potential therapeutic interventions such as bone marrow transplantation.

Niemann-Pick Disease

Niemann-Pick disease represents a group of rare disorders characterized by the infiltration of organs, particularly the reticuloendothelial system with foam cells containing excess sphingomyelin and to a lesser extent cholesterol and other phospholipids. The enzyme, sphingomyelinase, is deficient in those with most types of Niemann-Pick disease, but in some forms normal enzyme activity is shown even though excess sphingomyelin still accumulates. The existence of affected patients with normal sphingomyelinase activity suggests a genetic heterogeneity leading to a similar phenotype.[268,285,286] Isolation of complementary DNA clones encoding sphingomyelinase has been accomplished.[287] With these nucleic acid probes, it is now possible to better understand the genetic basis of Niemann-Pick disease and possibly to determine more predictive markers for known and yet-to-be described subtypes. Most forms are inherited in an autosomal recessive manner. Although a relatively high incidence of Niemann-Pick disease is found among Ashkenazi Jews, it is about five times less common than Gaucher's disease.

Scattered foam cells are found in affected tissues in patients with Niemann-Pick disease. Hepatocytes and Kupffer cells can be similarly affected. These foam cells have a pale yellow to yellow-brown cytoplasm when stained with hematoxylin and eosin. Giemsa staining produces a sea blue cytoplasm, giving rise to the term *sea blue histiocyte.* Because no absolutely specific stains exist for sphingomyelin, chemical or enzymatic analyses are critical in making a definitive diagnosis. In addition, vacuolated cytoplasm in circulating lymphocytes and monocytes may sometimes be observed, particularly in the Nova Scotia variants.

Type A Niemann-Pick disease is referred to as *acute neuropathic Niemann-Pick disease.* Patients usually present during the first few months of life with failure to thrive, feeding difficulties, massive hepatosplenomegaly, lymphadenopathy, and neurologic and developmental deterioration. About half of the patients have a cherry red spot observable in the macula (Fig. 32-12). Nervous system involvement includes spasticity, blindness, deafness, and impaired mental development.[288] No effective treatment is known and death usually occurs before the patient is 3 years of age. Preventive measures through genetic counseling and prenatal diagnosis offer means to avoid having an affected child. Sphingomyelinase activity is usually measured in skin fibroblasts and amniotic fluid or trophoblast samples obtained prenatally.[289]

Type B Niemann-Pick disease represents a more chronic form of progressive reticuloendotheliosis but without nervous system involvement. Patients usually present in childhood with an enlarging abdomen associated with hepatosplenomegaly, which is secondary to foam cell infiltration. Although bone deformities may occur, the in-

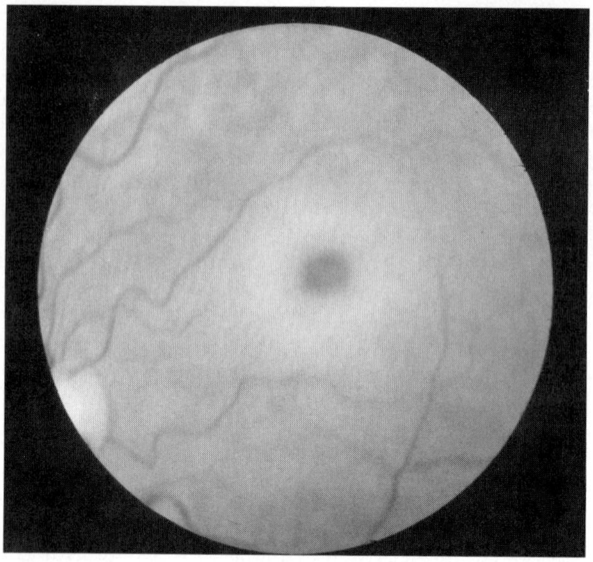

FIGURE 32-12. Cherry red macula of Niemann-Pick disease. (See Color Fig. 32-12.) (Courtesy of Dr. Robert Peterson, Department of Ophthalmology, Children's Hospital, Boston)

volvement is significantly less than in Gaucher's disease. Involvement of bone marrow and lungs may become extensive and contribute to death in the second to fourth decades of life. Because this form of Niemann-Pick disease does not involve the CNS, allogeneic bone marrow transplantation or exogenous enzyme replacement offers potentially effective modes of therapy. Preliminary findings with bone marrow transplantation are encouraging with evidence of decreased accumulation of sphingomyelin from liver and bone marrow.[290]

Types C and D Niemann-Pick disease represent more chronic forms of the disorder with neurologic involvement.[291,292] The type D form occurs mainly in patients of Nova Scotian descent, although biochemical and clinical parameters are similar to those in type C patients. This group of disorders is often referred to as *juvenile neuropathic Niemann-Pick disease.* Although onset is in early childhood, organ involvement and time to progression may be variable. The patient usually develops normally for 1 to 3 years, followed by neurologic deterioration in the form of diminishing cognitive ability, weakness, ataxia, and loss of speech. Patients may also develop seizures, dysphagia, cranial nerve palsies, and incoordination. Hepatomegaly is common. Death usually occurs by the second or third decade.[268,293]

No effective treatment for types C and D Niemann-Pick disease is yet known, and prenatal diagnosis is complicated by the fact that sphingomyelinase activities are variable. For example, some patients may show partial deficiency in some tissues but not in others. Normal levels of sphingomyelinase activity have frequently been observed, both in tissues and in cultured skin fibroblasts. A major focus for future research is to ascertain predictive genetic markers for this variable form of the disease.

Type E Niemann-Pick disease is referred to as the *adult nonneuropathic Niemann-Pick disease.* Affected patients have increased storage of sphingomyelin in their viscera and few clinical symptoms, and they often survive until old age. Sphingomyelinase levels may vary from low to normal.[294,295] Treatment is based on anticipating possible complications and symptomatic measures, although exogenous enzyme replacement may ultimately prove beneficial in such patients.

Sea-Blue Histiocyte Syndrome

In 1970, Silverstein and colleagues[296] described sea-blue histiocyte syndrome as a disorder of adulthood characterized by hepatosplenomegaly, thrombocytopenia, and sea-blue histiocytes in the bone marrow. Although the course of this syndrome is usually mild, progressive hepatic cirrhosis can develop.

The sea-blue histiocyte is a large (up to 60 μm in diameter), foam cell with an abundant cytoplasm containing blue-green granules when treated with Giemsa or Wright stain. This type of staining is believed to be due to the storage of ceroid, which is partly defined by its insolubility in hydrocarbon lipid solvents as well as its reactivity with fat stains such as Oil red O and Sudan black.[297]

The syndrome of the sea-blue histiocyte has been described as either a primary or an acquired disorder.[297–303] The primary form has been noted with more than one offspring being affected within a family; it is believed to be inherited as an autosomal recessive condition.[301,302] All patients should be suspected of having the primary form and should be extensively tested to exclude other causes. For example, other disorders leading to the accumulation of sea-blue histiocytes are inherited disorders such as Niemann-Pick disease, Tay-Sachs disease, Wolman's disease, generalized gangliosidoses, Fabry's disease, cholesterol ester storage disease, and type I hyperlipoproteinemia. In addition, the accumulation of sea-blue histiocytes has been observed in association with chronic granulomatous disease, chronic myelogenous leukemia, idiopathic thrombocytopenic purpura, dyserythropoietic anemia, sickle cell anemia, and thalassemia.[297,304,305] It is not clear whether such acquired forms of sea-blue histiocyte accumulation reflect an underlying deficiency in a lysosomal enzyme present in affected patients or whether excess cell turnover and lysosomal overloading are solely responsible.

Fabry's Disease

Fabry's disease is an X-linked, recessive sphingolipidosis caused by a deficiency in the activity of the lysosomal enzyme, α-galactosidase. This deficiency results in excess accumulation of globotriaosylceramide and related glycolipids in the serum and tissues. One of the primary sites of deposition of these substrates is the vascular endothelium, which leads to the major complications of this disorder.

Onset of Fabry's disease usually occurs in adolescent boys. They present with episodes of painful hands and feet as well as with angiokeratoma.[306] The vascular endothelium is usually severely affected, leading to ischemia and infarction involving the heart, kidney, brain, and intestine. Corneal and lenticular opacities observable by slit lamp examination are common.[307,308] Death occurs during the third to fifth decades secondary to renal, cardiac, or cerebral complications.[306,309,310] Curative treatments have not been found for patients with Fabry's disease, although enzyme replacement therapies are being attempted.[311]

Most patients severely affected with Fabry's disease have no measurable α-galactosidase activity, although immunoreactive enzyme may be present.[312,313] Some patients have mild clinical courses and have been shown to have some residual enzyme activity, suggesting that genetic heterogeneity exists. The diagnosis is made by the clinical presentation and a demonstrated defect in α-galactosidase activity as well as by increased serum or urine levels of the excess glycolipids.[312–315]

The identification of female carriers has been complicated by the random X-chromosome inactivation that occurs during embryogenesis and results in chimeric persons with varying enzyme levels. Thus, female carriers may have enzyme activities that vary from essentially zero to normal.[316] In addition, some recent evidence suggests that with aging, genes located on previously inactivated X chromosomes may become reexpressed.[317,318] Despite these reservations, many female carriers can be identified by intermediate enzyme levels as well as by the presence of the characteristic corneal opacities.

Both the cDNA and the gene for α-galactosidase have been cloned, and the gene has been mapped to Xq21.33-Xq22.[319–324] In addition, a variety of mutations have been described in patients with Fabry's disease including DNA deletions, partial duplications, point mutation, and altered α-galactosidase mRNA size and amounts.[322–324] The identification of such structural alterations in the α-galactosidase gene has allowed the unequivocal identification of heterozygotes as well as extensive pedigree analyses. Such analyses should be instrumental in prenatal diagnosis and eventually in the prediction of the course of atypical cases of Fabry's disease.

GM_1 Gangliosidosis

The GM_1 gangliosidoses represent a spectrum of disorders caused by decreased activity of the lysosomal enzyme, β-galactosidase, resulting in excess accumulation of ganglioside GM_1 in the reticuloendothelial system and the CNS. Regardless of the patient's age, signs and symptoms involving the CNS predominate. The lysosomal accumulation of ganglioside GM_1 is evident by the presence of enlarged, foamy histiocytes and abnormal storage in hepatocytes, renal tubular cells, and the epidermis. In addition, increased levels of the storage products are found in the serum and urine.[268] Diagnosis is made by clinical and pathologic criteria as well as the demonstration of decreased β-galactosidase activity in the plasma, leukocytes, or cultured fibroblasts.[325]

Type 1 GM_1 gangliosidosis is referred to as *severe infantile GM_1 gangliosidosis*. The disease may be evident in the newborn period, with patients presenting with poor feeding, weak sucking ability, slow weight gain, edema, hypotonia, an exaggerated startle response, and hepatosplenomegaly. The facies are coarse with frontal bossing and a depressed nasal bridge. Delayed developmental milestones soon become evident. A cherry red spot in the macula is present in over 50% of the cases. Skeletal deformities include short and thickened fingers, broad long bones, and flattened ribs as well as fractures of the lumbar vertebrae. The neurologic involvement progresses rapidly, leading to tonic–clonic seizures, rigidity, deafness, blindness, and eventually quadriplegia. Patients usually die before age 2 years.

Type 2 GM_1 gangliosidosis refers to a mild infantile or juvenile form of the disorder with the onset of symptoms occurring by age 1 year or early childhood. The first signs and symptoms usually appear as decreased motor and developmental milestones. A macular cherry red spot is not observed, although corneal clouding may develop. Convulsions occur along with rotary nystagmus and a positive Babinski's sign. Hepatosplenomegaly usually does not occur. Patients usually do not survive beyond the age of 10 years.

Type 3 GM_1 gangliosidosis usually has its onset in late childhood or early adulthood. Skeletal changes, hepatosplenomegaly, and macular cherry red spot are not observed. The major symptoms are the development and progression of pyramidal and extrapyramidal signs and symptoms.

The gene for β-galactosidase has been localized to chromosome 3.[326] In addition, cDNAs encoding this enzyme have been cloned and sequenced.[327] This work has further demonstrated that in some cases of infantile GM_1 gangliosidosis, total absence of mRNA for β-galactosidase has occurred. In other cases, reduced mRNA levels or abnormal-sized mRNAs are present. In an adult patient, β-galactosidase mRNA was present in normal amounts and was the appropriate size, suggesting a different type of mutational event affecting the enzyme structure and activity.[327] These studies confirm the genetic heterogeneity of the mutations leading to GM_1 gangliosidosis and should further help in predicting which form of the disease a patient will develop as well as provide help in prenatal diagnosis for this disorder. Diagnosis becomes especially important in light of no known effective therapy.

GM_2 Gangliosidosis

The GM_2 gangliosidoses are autosomal recessive disorders resulting from mutations affecting any of the three genes involved in the lysosomal degradation of ganglioside GM_2. The three genes encode the α- and β-subunits of the β-hexosaminidase enzyme as well as the GM_2 activator protein.[328] The result of a defect in any of these components is the excess accumulation of ganglioside GM_2, particularly in the brain and to a lesser extent in other visceral organs according to the type of mutation involved.[328]

The historically classic and most common form of GM_2 gangliosidosis is Tay-Sachs disease. A brief discussion of this disorder is relevant because of its historic importance and similar clinical presentation to GM_2 gangliosidosis, Sandhoff variant. Only the latter disorder significantly involves the reticuloendothelial system. This disorder is especially prevalent among Ashkenazi Jews, in whom the incidence of carriers has been estimated at about 1 in 27. The infantile form of Tay-Sachs disease may be noted within the first few months of life when hypotonia and an exaggerated startle response can be observed. During the next several months, increasing weakness develops as well as wandering eye movements. A cherry red spot can usually be observed in the fundus of the eye. Progressive neurologic deterioration ensues and is characterized by seizures, abnormal cranial enlargement, spasticity, drooling, blindness, and abnormalities in autonomic function such as unexplained fevers and irregular breathing. Death usually occurs by age 4 years.

Patients with Tay-Sachs disease have a lack of β-hexosaminidase activity due to mutations affecting the α-subunit of this enzyme complex.[329–335] About 30% of these patients demonstrate a splice junction mutation of intron 12, and the remaining 70% have a mutation involving a 4-base pair insertion into exon 11 of the α-subunit gene.[329–332] These mutations result in the lack of α-subunit mRNA and protein.[331,333–337] The identification of the gene and its mutations has allowed more definitive methods to be used for the identification of carriers compared with traditional enzyme activity measurement.[338,339] Because no effective treatment for Tay-Sachs disease is known, prevention remains an important alternative for parents who are carriers.

Juvenile GM_2 gangliosidosis is characterized by a similar clinical course but with onset of symptoms in early childhood and a more protracted course. Several mutations in the coding regions of the α-subunit have been reported to be correlated with this form of GM_2 gangliosidosis.[339,340] Some mutations appear to produce a defective α-subunit. This results in retention of the α-subunit in the endoplasmic reticulum of the cell, preventing it from properly associating with the β-subunit.[341–343]

The adult onset form of GM_2 gangliosidosis usually begins to become evident during the second and third decades of life. Symptoms include lower motor neuron and pyramidal tract disease and cerebellar signs resulting in ataxia and psychomotor retardation. Megalocephaly and fundal cherry red spots are not observed. Optic atrophy may develop. In addition, psychosis may develop and in some patients precedes the other neurologic signs and symptoms. In these adult patients, the α chain mRNA and protein of β-hexosaminidase A complex are usually readily detectable.[339,344,345] Decreased activity of β-hexosaminidase is observed, suggesting that the α chain is unable to associate properly with the β chain to form a functionally normal enzyme complex. Molecular analysis has documented a mutation leading to the substitution of glycine[291] with a serine.[339] This substitution leads to an α chain that is defective in forming a normal hexosaminidase complex. Affected patients have been further shown to have compound heterozygotes for this mutation and one of the two infantile Tay-Sachs alleles just described.[339] This type of molecular analysis should prove to be extremely valuable in predicting the clinical course and inheritance of the these GM_2 gangliosidoses.

The Sandhoff variants (also referred to as *O variants*) of the GM_2 gangliosidoses result from a defect in the β-subunit of the β-hexosaminidase enzyme complex.[346] These variants do not have a predilection for the Ashkenazi Jewish population. Onset of the infantile form of this variant is within the first few months of life; initially it is indistinguishable from Tay-Sachs disease. In the juvenile form, clinical signs and symptoms usually begin when the child is between the ages of 3 and 11 years, and patients may survive into adulthood. Patients with the Sandhoff variant may display more marked accumulation of GM_2 ganglioside in the reticuloendothelial system than do patients with Tay-Sachs disease.[328] This may result from the decreased activities of both hexosaminidase A and B, since the β-subunit is shared by both enzyme complexes.[346] Thus, unlike in Tay-Sachs disease, patients with the Sandhoff variant have detectable foam cells in the bone marrow and other involved organs.

When enzyme activities are measured in patients with infantile and juvenile forms of Sandhoff's disease, no activity is detectable in the former and some residual activity is found in the latter.[346] These results provide evidence that the residual enzyme activity in the juvenile form is sufficient to delay the onset of juvenile Sandhoff's disease. In some cases of infantile Sandhoff's disease, molecular studies have shown partial gene deletions at the 5′ end of the β-subunit encoding gene, thus accounting for the absence of its mRNA.[346]

The AB variant of the GM_2 gangliosidoses has been shown to be the result of a defect in the GM_2 activator protein.[328] This subunit of the hexosaminidase enzyme complex is responsible for stimulating the catalysis of the ganglioside GM_2. As in the other GM_2 gangliosidoses, the AB variant primarily involves the CNS and displays significant clinical heterogeneity. cDNA sequences encoding this activator protein have been cloned, and work is being directed toward further understanding mutations that may affect its expression and function.[347]

Other variants of the GM_2 gangliosidoses affect patients of different ethnic backgrounds and involve point mutations in the α-subunit gene.[328] Probably the best described is the B1 variant, which represents an enzymatically unique β-hexosaminidase.[268,328] Affected patients synthesize hexosaminidase A, which appears to have normal activity when tested against certain laboratory substrates such as 4-methylumbelliferyl N-acetylglucosaminide. This substrate is acted on by the active site of the β-subunit. The B1 variant hexosaminidase does not cleave naturally occurring ganglioside GM_2 or the artificial substrate 4-methylumbelliferyl N-acetylglucosamine-6-sulfate; both of these substrates are acted on by the catalytic site of the α-subunit.[348–351] Single point mutations in exon 5 of the α-subunit gene have been demonstrated in such patients leading to variable levels of the α-subunit mRNA and the characteristic defective features of the β-hexosaminidase enzyme complex.[352]

Farber's Disease

Farber's disease is a rare autosomal recessive disorder caused by a deficiency of the enzyme acid ceramidase leading to the increased accumulation of ceramide.[353–355] Onset occurs during early infancy with painful, swollen joints, particularly of the hands and feet. Granulomatous nodules may enlarge to such an extent as to cause flexion contractures. In addition, swelling of the epiglottis results in difficulty in swallowing. Laryngeal involvement can lead to severe respiratory problems requiring tracheostomy. Treatment is palliative, and death usually occurs before the patient is 2 years old.

Mucopolysaccharidoses and Mucolipidoses

The mucopolysaccharidoses represent a group of rare inherited disorders characterized by excessive accumulation of mucopolysaccharides and glycolipids within lysosomes as well as by an increase in urinary excretion of these metabolic products. Mucopolysaccharidoses are caused by enzyme deficiencies affecting the metabolism of the complex carbohydrate moieties of glycoproteins. The type of stored material depends on the specific enzyme deficiency. Such deficiencies have been described for a large number of enzymes.[268,328,356–360]

The clinical features associated with these enzyme deficiencies are variable, and the classification of mucopolysaccharidoses and mucolipidoses is now based on the specific defective enzyme, although historic eponyms are often used (see Table 32-5). All of these syndromes are inherited as autosomal recessive conditions with the exception of Hunter's disease, which is inherited as an X-linked recessive. They can all be diagnosed prenatally based on assessment of specific enzyme activities. The mucolipidoses are also caused by lysosomal enzyme deficiencies, but they do not display the same mucopolysacchariduria and more accumulation of lipids products is observed.

Although the mucopolysaccharidoses result in many of the same clinical features seen in the lipidoses, they also produce several unique manifestations as a result of the ubiquitous presence of the stored substrates in the connective tissue of the body. For example, these disorders result in a phenotype characterized by coarse facial features, skeletal abnormalities including bone dysplasias, dwarfism, and restriction of joint movement. In addition, neurologic involvement may result in psychomotor retardation, deafness, thickening of the leptomeninges, arachnoid cyst formation, hydrocephalus, ataxia, mental status disturbances with psychosis, hyperactivity, and sleep apnea. Corneal clouding is commonly observed. Pathologic changes in the myocardium may lead to congestive heart failure, whereas valvular disease often leads to aortic regurgitation. Renal parenchymal involvement results in tubular dysfunction. Patients have a tendency to develop both inguinal and umbilical hernias. Gum hypertrophy is often seen, and teeth are widely spaced. Persistent rhinorrhea, middle ear infections, stertorous breathing, and apnea may result from enlargement of tonsillar and adenoidal tissues. Hepatosplenomegaly is frequently observed. Increased susceptibility to infections is common. Death usually occurs during childhood or early adolescence, but some patients survive into adulthood.

The increased storage of mucopolysaccharide results in characteristic hematologic findings in both the bone marrow and the peripheral blood cells.[361] In most patients, azurophilic granulations (Alder-Reilly bodies) can be observed in polymorphonuclear cells and their bone marrow precursors as well as in lymphocytes.[362] In some patients, circulating lymphocytes may contain metachromatic vacuoles referred to as Mittwoch bodies.[363] In other cases, vacuoles containing basophilic granules are found in lymphocytes and bone marrow plasma cells and reticulocytes.[361] The reticuloendothelial system may display foam cell infiltration.

This clinical picture in conjunction with the hematologic and biochemical findings suggests the proper diagnosis, which can be confirmed by demonstration of decreased activity of a specific enzyme in cultured fibroblasts or leukocytes.[357,358] Such enzyme assays are also useful in diagnosing heterozygotes and in prenatal detection of the autosomal recessive conditions but less so in Hunter's disease, which is inherited as an X-chromosome recessive. The genes and cDNAs for these various enzyme deficiencies are being cloned and should prove instrumental in genetic counseling.

Although exogenous enzyme replacement in vitro has been accomplished with promising results, attempts to treat mucopolysaccharidoses with enzyme or leukocyte infusion have not resulted in complete resolution of signs and symptoms.[242–244,360,364] Attempts at using fibroblast transplantation have resulted in minimal biochemical changes but no significant clinical improvement.[365,366] Allogeneic bone marrow transplantation has been the most successful.[360,367–370] The possible role of gene replacement therapy awaits demonstration of successful long-term expression of the normal genes in transplantable stem cells.[360]

REFERENCES

1. Favara BE, Jaffe R. Pathology of Langerhans cell histiocytosis. Hematol Oncol Clin North Am 1987;1:75.
2. Ishii E, Watanabe S. Biochemistry and biology of the Langerhans cell. Hematol Oncol Clin North Am 1987;1:99.
3. Murphy GF, Bhan AK, Sato S, et al. A new immunologic marker for human Langerhans cells. N Engl J Med 1981;304:791.
4. Murphy GF, Bhan AK, Sato S, et al. Characterization of Langerhans cells by the use of monoclonal antibodies. Lab Invest 1981;45:465.
5. Fithian E, Kung P, Goldstein G, et al. Reactivity of Langerhans cells with hybridoma antibody. Proc Natl Acad Sci USA 1981;78:2541.
6. Arenzana-Seisdedos F, Barbey S, Virelizier JL, Kornprobst M, Nezelof C. Histiocytosis X: purified (T6+) cells from bone granuloma produce interleukin-1 in prostaglandin E2 in culture. J Clin Invest 1986;77:326.
7. Favara BE, McCarthy RC, Mireau GW. Histiocytosis X. Hum Pathol 1983;14:663.
8. Groopman JE, Golde DW. The histiocytic disorders: a pathophysiologic analysis. Ann Intern Med 1981;94:95.
9. Chu T, D'Angio GJ, Favara B, Ladisch S. Histiocytosis syndromes in children. Lancet 1987;1:208.
10. McLelland J, Newton J, Malone M, et al. A flow cytometric study of Langerhans cell histiocytosis. Br J Dermatol 1989;120:485.
11. Ornvold K, Carstensen H, Larsen JK, et al. Flow cytometric DNA analysis of lesions from 18 children with Langerhans cells histiocytosis (histiocytosis X). Am J Pathol 1990;136:1301.
11a. Yu RC, Chu C, Buluwela L, Chu AC. Clonal proliferation of Langerhans cells in Langerhans cell histiocytosis. Lancet 1994;343:767.
11b. Willman CL, Busque L, Griffith BB, et al. Langerhans cell histiocytosis (histiocytosis X): a clonal proliferative disease. N Engl J Med 1994 (in press)
12. Komp DM. Historical perspectives of Langerhans cell histiocytosis. Hematol Oncol Clin North Am 1987;1:9.
13. Farber S. The nature of "solitary or eosiniphilic granuloma" of bone. Am J Pathol 1941;17:625.
14. Lichtenstein L. Histiocytosis X: integration of eosiniphilic granuloma of the bone: Letterer-Siwe disease and Schuller-Christian disease as related manifestations of a single nosologic entity. Arch Pathol 1953;56:84.
15. Gonzalez CL, Jaffe ES. The histiocytoses: clinical presentation and differential diagnosis. Oncology 1990;4:47.
16. Harrist TJ, Bhan AK, Murphy GF, et al. Histiocytosis-X: in situ characterization of cutaneous infiltrates with monoclonal antibodies. Am J Clin Pathol 1983;79:294.
17. Bieber T, Nanau D, Heid E, et al. Histiocytosis-X cells express C3b, C3d, and 3bi receptor (CR1, CR2, and CR3) antigens. Arch Dermatol Res 1985;277:496.
17a. Mandel M, Toren A, Kende G, et al. Familial clustering of malignant germ cell tumors and Langerhans histiocytosis. Cancer 1994;73:1980.
17b. Camargo B, Alves AC, Gorender EF, Bianchi A. Association of malignancy and Langerhans cell histiocytosis: report of three cases. Med Pediatr Oncol 1993;21:451.
17c. Egeler RM, Meglia JP, Puccetti DM, et al. Association of Langerhans cell histiocytosis with malignant neoplasms. Cancer 1993;71:865.
18. Avery ME, McAfee JG, Guild HC, et al. The course and prognosis of reticuloendotheliosis (eosinophilic granuloma), Schuller-Christian disease and Letterer-Siwe disease: a study of 40 cases. Am J Med 1957;636.
19. Bartholdy N, Thommesen P. Histiocytosis-X. VIII. Prognostic significance of skull lesions. Acta Radiol (Oncol) 1983;22:125.
20. Lieberman PH, Jones CR, Dargeon HWK, et al. A reappraisal of eosinophilic granuloma of bone, Hand-Schuller-Christian syndrome and Letterer-Siwe syndrome. Medicine 1969;48:375.
21. Lucaya J. Histiocytosis-X. Am J Dis Child 1971;121:289.
22. Oberman HA. Idiopathic histiocytosis: a clinicopathologic study of 40 cases and review of the literature on eosinophilic granuloma of bone, Hand-Schuller-Christian disease and Letterer-Siwe disease. Pediatrics 1961;28:307.
23. Berry DH, Gresik MV, Humphrey GB, et al. Natural history of histiocytosis-X: a Pediatric Oncology Group study. Med Pediatr Oncol 1986;14:1.
24. McGavran MH, Spady HA. Eosinophilic granuloma of bone: a study of 28 cases. J Bone Joint Surg 1960;42A:979.
25. Berry DH, Becton DL. Natural history of histiocytosis-X. Hematol Oncol Clin North Am 1987;1:23.
26. Cardozo LJ, Bailey IC, Billinghurst JR, et al. Non-osseous eosinophilic granuloma presenting as acute transverse myelitis. Br J Surg 1974;61:747.
27. Carlson RA, Hattery RR, O'Connel EJ, et al. Pulmonary involvement by histiocytosis-X in the pediatric age group. Mayo Clin Proc 1976;51:542.
28. Esterly NB, Maurer HS, Ganzalez-Crussi F. Histiocytosis-X: a seven year experience at a children's hospital. J Am Acad Dermatol 1985;13:481.
29. Crone-Munzebrock W, Brassow F. A comparison of radiographic and bone scan findings in histiocytosis-X. Skeletal Radiol 1983;9:170.
30. Parker BR, Pinckney L, Etcubanas E. Relative efficacy of radiographic and radionuclide bone surveys in the detection of skeletal lesions of histiocytosis-X. Radiology 1980;134:377.
31. Siddiqui AR, Tashjlan JH, Lazarus K, et al. Nuclear medicine studies in evaluation of skeletal lesions in children with histiocytosis-X. Radiology 1981;140:787.
32. Coutte A, Brache CP, Bartholdy N, et al. Histiocytosis-X: recurrent otitis media as a presenting symptom in children with special reference to cholesteatoma. Clin Otolaryngol 1984;9:111.
33. Van Baarle PWC. Positive "fistula sign" with intact ear drum in a patient with eosinophil granuloma of the mastoid. J Laryngol Otol 1976;90:801.
34. Komp DM. Long-term sequelae of histiocytosis-X. Am J Pediatr Hematol Oncol 1981;3:163.
35. McDonald JS, Miller RL, Bernstein ML, et al. Histiocytosis-X: a clinical presentation. J Oral Pathol 1980;9:342.
36. Rapidis AD, Langdon JD, Harvey PW, et al. Histiocytosis-X: an analysis of 50 cases. Int J Oral Surg 1978;7:76.
37. Braunstein GD, Kohler PO. Endocrine manifestations of histiocytosis. Am J Pediatr Hematol Oncol 1981;3:67.
38. Greenberger JS, Cassady JR, Jaffe N, et al. Radiation therapy in patients with histiocytosis: management of diabetes insipidus and bone lesions. Int J Radiat Oncol Biol Phys 1979;5:1749.
39. Lipton JM. The pathogenesis, diagnosis and treatment of histiocytosis syndromes. Pediatr Dermatol 1983;1:112.
40. Sims DG. Histiocytosis-X: followup of 43 cases. Arch Dis Child 1977;52:433.
41. Dunger BD, Broadbent V, Yeoman E, et al. The frequency and natural history of diabetes insipidus in children with Langerhans-cell histiocytosis. N Engl J Med 1989;321:1157.
42. Vawter GF, Greenberger JS, Crocker AC. A retrospective clinicopathologic analysis of diabetes insipidus in dendritic cell disease. Med Pediatr Oncol 1986;14:112.
43. Kaufman A, Bukberg PR, Werlin S, et al. Multifocal eosinophilic granuloma ("Hand-Schuller-Christian disease"): report illustrating H-S-C chronicity and diagnostic challenge. Am J Med 1976;60:541.
44. Ober KP, Alexander E Jr, Challa VR, et al. Histiocytosis X of the hypothalamus. Neurosurgery 1989;24:93.
45. Graif M, Pennock JM. MR imaging of histiocytosis-X in the central nervous system. AJNR 1986;7:21.
46. Jinkins JR. Histiocytosis-X of the hypothalamus: case report and literature review. Comput Radiol 1987;11:181.

47. Chiumello G, di Natale B, Pellini C, et al. Magnetic resonance imaging in diabetes insipidus. Lancet 1989;4:901.
47a. Rosenfield NS, Abrahams J, Komp D. Brain MR in patients with Langerhans cell histiocytosis: findings and enhancement with Gd-DTPA. Pediatr Radiol 1990;20:433.
48. Latorre H, Kenney FM, Lahey ME, et al. Short stature and growth hormone deficiency in histiocytosis-X. J Pediatr 1974;85:813.
49. Zinkham WH. Multifocal eosinophilic granuloma: natural history, etiology and management. Am J Med 1976;60:457.
50. Burn DJ, Watson JD, Roddie M, et al. Langerhans cell histiocytosis and the nervous system. J Neurol 1992;239:345.
51. Geoffray A. Case of the season: diagnosis: histiocytosis-X of the central nervous system. Semin Roentgenol 1984;19:257.
51a. Grois N, Barkovich AJ, Rosenau W, Ablin AR. Central nervous system disease associated with Langerhans cell histiocytosis. Am J Pediatr Hematol Oncol 1993;15:245.
52. Marcy TW, Reynolds HY. Pulmonary histiocytosis-X. Lung 1985;163:129.
53. Basset F, Corrin B, Spencer H, et al. Pulmonary histiocytosis-X. Am Rev Respir Dis 1978;118:811.
54. Favara BE. The histiocytoses: clinical presentation and differential diagnosis: a review. Oncology 1990;4:60.
55. Rand EB, Whitington PF. Successful orthotopic liver transplantation in two patients with liver failure due to sclerosing cholangitis with Langerhans cell histiocytosis. J Pediatr Gastoenterol Nutr 1992;15:202.
56. Mahmoud H, Gaber O, Wang W, et al. Successful orthotopic liver transplantation in a child with Langerhans cell histiocytosis. Transplantation 1991;51:278.
57. Newton WA Jr, Hamoudi AB, Shannon BT. Role of the thymus in histiocytosis-X. Hematol Oncol Clin North Am 1987;1:63.
58. Nesbit ME, O'Leary M, Dehner LP, et al. Histiocytosis continued: the immune system and histiocytosis syndrome. Am J Pediatr Hematol Oncol 1981;3:141.
59. McLelland J, Pritchard J, Chu AC. Current controversies. Hematol Oncol Clin North Am 1987;1:147.
60. Osband ME, Lipton JM, Lavin P, et al. Histiocytosis-X: demonstration of abnormal immunity, T cell histamine H_2-receptor deficiency, and successful treatment with thymic extract. N Engl J Med 1981;304:146.
61. Broadbent V, Davies EG, Heaf D, et al. Spontaneous remission of multisystem histiocytosis-X. Lancet 1984;1:253.
62. Shannon B, Newton W, Jacobs D. Lack of suppressor cell activity in children with active histiocytosis-X. Med Pediatr Oncol 1986;14:111.
63. Ceci A. Clinical prognostic factors in Langerhans histiocytosis: comparison of retrospective and prospective studies. (Abstract) Histiocytosis Society, European Meeting, 1986.
64. Zaizov R, Stark B, Friedman I, et al. Cell mediated immunity and activation of macrophages in childhood histiocytoses. Med Pediatr Oncol 1986;14:110.
65. Wolfson WL, Gossett T, Pagani J. Systemic giant-cell histiocytosis: report of a case and a review of the adult form of Letterer-Siwe disease. Cancer 1976;38:2529.
66. Glass AG, Miller RW. US mortality from Letterer-Siwe disease 1900–1964. Pediatrics 1968;42:364.
67. Jugberg RC, Kloepfer HW, Oberman HA. Genetic determination of acute disseminated histiocytosis X (Letterer-Siwe syndrome). J Pediatr 1974;85:466.
68. Lahey ME. Histiocytosis-X: an analysis of prognostic factors. J Pediatr 1975;87:184.
69. Letterer E. Aleukamische Retikulose (ein Beitrag zu den proliferativen Erkankungen des Retikuloendothelialapparates). Frank Z Pathol 1924;30:377.
70. Siwe SA. Die Reticuloendotheliose: ein neues Krankheitsbild unter den Hepatosplenomegalien. Z Kinderheilk 1933;55:212.
71. Abt AF, Denenholz EJ. Letterer-Siwe's disease. Splenomegaly associated with wide-spread hyperplasia of nonlipoid-storing macrophages. Am J Dis Child 1936;51:499.
72. Leblanc A, Hadchouel M, Jehan M, et al. Obstructive jaundice in children with histiocytosis-X. Gastroenterology 1981;80:134.
73. Thompson HH, Pitt HA, Lewin KJ, et al. Sclerosing cholangitis and histiocytosis-X. Gut 1984;25:526.
74. Smith M, McCormack LJ, Van Ordstrand HS, et al. "Primary" pulmonary histiocytosis-X. Chest 1974;65:176.
75. Carlson RA, Hattery RR, O'Connel EJ, et al. Non-osseous eosinophilic granuloma presenting as acute transverse myelitis. Br J Surg 1974;61:747.
76. Stanford W, Spivey C, Lindberg EF, et al. Eosinophilic granuloma of the lung. Ann Thorac Surg 1971;11:299.
77. Matus-Ridley M, Raney RB Jr, Thawerani H, et al. Histiocytosis-X in children: patterns of disease and results of treatment. Med Pediatr Oncol 1983;11:99.
78. Hashimoto K, Pritzker MS. Electron microscopic study of reticulohistiocytoma: an unusual case of congenital, self-healing reticulohistiocytosis. Arch Dermatol 1983;107:263.
79. Hashimoto K, Griffin D, Kohsbaki M. Self-healing reticulohistiocytosis: a clinical, histiologic, and ultrastructural study of the fourth case in the literature. Cancer 1982;49:2236.
80. Kanitakis J, Zambruno G, Schmitt D, et al. Congenital self-healing histiocytosis (Hashimoto-Pritzker): an ultrastructural and immunohistochemical study. Cancer 1988;61:508.
81. Murphy GF, Bhan AK, Harrist TJ, Mihn MC Jr. In situ identification of T6-positive cells in normal human dermis by immunoelectron microscopy. Br J Dermatol 1983;108:423.
82. Chu A, Eisinger M, Lee JS, et al. Immunoelectron microscopic identification of Langerhans cells using a new antigenic marker. J Invest Dermatol 1982;78:177.
83. Cocchia D, Mitchetti F, Donato R. Immunochemical and immunocytochemical localization of S-100 antigen in normal human skin. Nature 1981;294:85.
84. Harrist TJ, Muhlbauer JE, Murphy GF et al. T6 is superior to Ia (HLA-DR) as a marker for Langerhans cells and indeterminate cells in normal epidermis: a monoclonal antibody study. J Invest Dermatol 1983;80:100.
85. Wood GS, Hu C-H, Beckstead JH, et al. The indeterminate cell proliferative disorder: report of a case manifesting as an unusual cutaneous histiocytosis. J Dermatol Surg Oncol 1985;11:11.
86. Lahey ME. Prognosis in reticuloendotheliosis in children. J Pediatr 1962;60:664.
87. Slater JM, Swarm OJ. Eosinophilic granuloma of bone. Med Pediatr Oncol 1980;8:151.
88. Komp DM, Herson J, Starling KA, et al. A staging system for histiocytosis-X: a Southwest Oncology Group study. Cancer 1981;47:798.
89. Nezelof C, Frileux-Herbet F, Cronier-Sachot J. Disseminated histiocytosis-X: analysis of prognostic factors based on a retrospective study of 50 cases. Cancer 1979;44:1824.
90. Lavin PT, Osband ME. Evaluating the role of therapy in histiocytosis-X: clinical studies, staging, and scoring. Hematol Oncol Clin North Am 1987;1:35.
91. Broadbent V, Pritchard J. Histiocytosis-X: current controversies. Arch Dis Child 1985;60:605.
92. Wirtschafter JD, Nesbit M, Anderson P, McClain K. Intralesional methylprednisolone for Langerhans cell histiocytosis of the orbit and cranium. J Pediatr Ophthalmol Strabismus 1987;24:194.
93. Bokkerink JPM, Cluitmans JJM, Holland R, de Vaan GAM. Histiocytosis-X: retrospective study of 28 cases. Eur Paediatr Haematol Oncol 1984;1:89.
94. Cassady, JR. Current role of radiation therapy in the management of histiocytosis-X. Hematol Oncol Clin North Am 1987;1:123.
95. Richter MP, D'Angio GJ. The role of radiation therapy in the management of children with histiocytosis X. Am J Pediatr Hematol Oncol 1981;3:161.
96. Minehan KJ, Chen MG, Zimmerman D, et al. Radiation therapy for diabetes insipidus caused by Langerhans cell histiocytosis. Int J Radiat Oncol Biol Phys 1992;23:519.
97. Egeler RM, Thompson RC Jr., Voute PA, Nesbit ME Jr. Intralesional infiltration of corticosteroids in localized Langerhans cell histiocytosis. J Pediatr Orthop 1992;12:811.
98. Maghnie M, Arico M, Villa A, et al. MR of the hypothalamic-pituitary axis in Langerhans cell histiocytosis. AJNR 1992:13:1365.
99. Maghnie M, Villa A, Arico M, et al. Correlation between magnetic resonance imaging of posterior pituitary and neurohypophyseal function in children with diabetes insipidus. J Clin Endocrinol Metab 1992;74:795.
100. Rosenfield NS, Abrahams J, Komp D. Brain MR in patients with Langerhans cell histiocytosis: findings and enhancement with Gd-DTPA. Pediatr Radiol 1990;20:433.
101. Tien RD, Newton TH, McDermott MW, et al. Thickened pituitary stalls on MR images in patients with diabetes insipidus and Langerhans cell histiocytosis. AJNR 1990;11:703.
102. Atherton DJ, Broadbent V, Pritchard J. Topical use of mustine hydrochloride in cutaneous histiocytosis-X. Med Pediatr Oncol 1986;14:112.
103. Sheehan MP, Atherton DJ, Broadbent V, Pritchard J. Topical nitrogen mustard: an effective treatment for cutaneous Langerhans cell histiocytosis. J Pediatr 1991;119:317.
104. Iwatsuki K, Tsugiki M, Yoshizawa N, et al. The effect of phototherapies on cutaneous lesions of histiocytosis-X in the elderly. Cancer 1986;57:1931.
105. Starling KA. Chemotherapy of histiocytosis-X. Hematol Oncol Clin North Am 1987;1:119.
106. Lahey ME. Comparison of three treatment regimens in histiocytosis-X in children: Proceedings of the International Cancer Congress, Houston, May 1970.
107. Jones B, Kung F, Chevalier L, et al. Chemotherapy of reticuloendotheliosis: comparison of methotrexate plus prednisolone vs vincristine plus prednisolone. Cancer 1974;34:1011.
108. Starling KA. Chemotherapy of histiocytosis. Am J Pediatr Hematol Oncol 1981;3:157.
109. Komp DM. Therapeutic strategies for Langerhans cell histiocytosis. J Pediatr 1991;119:274.
110. Ceci A, de Terlizzi M, Colella R, et al. Etoposide in recurrent childhood Langerhans cell histiocytosis: an Italian Cooperative Study. Cancer 1988;62:2528.
111. Urbano-Marquez A, Estruch R, Fernandez-Huerta JM, et al. Etoposide in the treatment of multifocal eosinophilic granuloma. Cancer Treat Rep 1985;69:238.

112. Ishii E, Matsuzaki A, Okamura J, Inoue T, et al. Treatment of Langerhans cell histiocytosis in children with etoposide. Am J Clin Oncol 1992;15:515.
113. Tsele E, Thomas DM, Chu AC. Treatment of adult Langerhans cell histiocytosis with etoposide. J Am Acad Dermatol 1992;27:61.
114. Pedrol E, Estruch R, Marrades RM, Ingelmo M. Etoposide (VP16) treatment of Langerhans cell histiocytosis. Rev Clin Esp 1991;188:319.
115. Viana MB, Oliveira BM, Silva CM, Rios Leite VH. Etoposide in the treatment of six children with Langerhans cell histiocytosis (histiocytosis X). Med Pediatr Oncol 1991;19:289.
116. Broadbent V, Pritchard J, Yeomans E. Etoposide (VP16) in the treatment of multisystem Langerhans cell histiocytosis (histiocytosis X). Med Pediatr Oncol 1989;17:97.
117. Puy CH, Hancock ML, Raimondi SC, et al. Myeloid neoplasia in children treated for solid tumours. Lancet 1991;336:417.
118. Pui CH, Ribeiro RC, Hancock ML, et al. Acute myeloid leukemia in children treated with epipodophyllotoxins for acute lymphoblastic leukemia. N Engl J Med 1991;325:1682.
119. Pritchard J. Histiocytosis-X: natural history and management in childhood. Clin Exp Dermatol 1979;4:421.
120. Davies EG, Levinsky RJ, Butler M, et al. Thymic hormone therapy for histiocytosis-X. N Engl J Med 1983;309:493.
121. Eckstein R, Huhn D, Schneider D, et al. Influence on immune function parameters in histiocytosis-X of thymostimulin. Arzneimittelforschung 1984;125:2611.
122. Jakobson AM, Kreuger A, Hagberg H, Sundstrom C. Treatment of Langerhans cell histiocytosis with alpha-interferon. Lancet 1987;2:1520.
123. Mahmoud HH, Wang WC, Murphy S. Cyclosporine therapy for advanced Langerhans cell histiocytosis. Blood 1991;77:721.
124. Bellmont J, Albanell J, Salud A, et al. Interferon and disseminated Langerhans cell histiocytosis. Med Pediatr Oncol 1992;20:336.
124a. Saven A, Figueroa ML, Piro LD, Rosenblatt JD. 2-Chlorodeoxyadenosine to treat refractory histiocytosis X. N Engl J Med 1994;329:734.
125. Ringden O, Ahstrom L, Lonnqvist B, et al. Allogeneic bone marrow transplantation in a patient with chemotherapy-resistant progressive histiocytosis X. N Engl J Med 1987;316:733.
126. Dehner LP. Allogeneic bone marrow transplantation in a patient with chemotherapy resistant progressive histiocytosis X. (Letter) N Engl J Med 1987;317:773.
127. Stoll M, Freund M, Schmid H, et al. Allogeneic bone marrow transplantation for Langerhans cell histiocytosis. Cancer 1990;66:284.
128. Greinix HT, Storb R, Sanders JE, Petersen FB. Marrow transplantation for treatment of multisystem progressive Langerhans cell histiocytosis. Bone Marrow Transplant 1992;10:39.
129. Farquhar J, Clairveaux A. Familial haemophagocytic reticulosis. Arch Dis Chld 1952;27:519.
130. MacMahon HE, Bedizel M, Ellis CA. Familial erythrophagocytic lymphohistiocytosis. Pediatrics 1963;32:868.
131. Goldberg JC, Nezelof C. Familial lymphohistiocytosis: the pathologist's view. Pediatr Hematol Oncol 1989;6:199.
132. Perry MC, Harrison EG Jr, Burgert EO Jr, Gilchrist GS. Familial erythrophagocytic lymphohistiocytosis: report of two cases and clinicopathologic review. Cancer 1976;38:209.
133. Hsu Ts, Komp DM. Clinical features of familial histiocytosis. Am J Pediatr Hematol Oncol 1981;1:61.
133a. Kletzel M, Gollin SM, Gloster ES, et al. Chromosomal abnormalities in familial hemophagocytic lymphohistiocytosis. Cancer 1986;57:2153.
134. Wieczorek R, Greco A, McCarthy K, et al. Familial erythrophagocytic lymphohistiocytosis: immunophenotypic, immunohistochemical, and ultrastructural demonstration of the relation to sinus histiocytes. Hum Pathol 1986;17:55.
135. Kletzel M, Gollin SM, Gloster ES, et al. Chromosome abnormalities in familial hemophagocytic lymphohistiocytosis. Cancer 1986;57:2153.
136. Ishii E, Hara T, Ohga S. Familial erythrophagocytic lymphohistiocytosis: surface marker analysis using monoclonal antibodies. Eur J Haematol 1987;38:63.
137. Ansbacher LE, Singsen BH, Hosler MW, et al. Familial erythrophagocytic lymphohistiocytosis: an association with serum lipid abnormalities. J Pediatr 1983;102:270.
138. Ladisch S, Ho W, Matheson D, et al. Immunologic and clinical effects of repeated blood exchange in familial erythrophagocytic lymphohistiocytosis. Blood 1982;60:814.
138a. Stephan JL, Donadieu J, Ledeist F, et al. Treatment of familial hemophagocytic lymphohistiocytosis with antithymocyte globulins, steroids, and cyclosporin A. Blood 1993;82:2319.
139. Ladisch S, Poplack DG, Holiman B, Blaese RM. Immunodeficiency in familial erythrophagocytic lymphohistiocytosis. Lancet 1978;1:581.
140. Ammann AJ, Addiego J, Ladisch S, et al. Immunodeficiency in familial erythrophagocytic lymphohistiocytosis. Lancet 1978;2:789.
141. Nespoli ML, Maccario R, Montagna D, et al. Natural cytotoxicity impairment in familial haemophagocytic lymphohistiocytosis. Dis Child 1988;63:292.
142. Kawai H, Komiymama A, Aoyama K, et al. Absence of circulating natural killer (NK) cells in a child with erythrophagocytic lymphohistiocytosis lacking NK cell activity. Am J Hematol 1988;28:107.
143. Stark B, Cohen IJ, Pecht M, et al. Immunologic dysregulation in a patient with familial hemophagocytic lymphohistiocytosis. Cancer 1987;60:2629.
144. Komp DM, McNamara J, Buckley P. Elevated soluble interleukin-2 receptor in childhood hemophagocytic histiocytic syndromes. Blood 1989;73:2128.
145. Perez N, Virelizier JL, Arenzana-Seisdedos F, et al. Impaired natural killer activity in lymphohistiocytosis syndrome. J Pediatr 1984;104:569.
146. Price DL, Woolsey JE, Rosman NP, Richard EP JR. Familial lymphohistiocytosis of the nervous system. Arch Neurol 1971;24:270.
147. Akima M, Sumi SM. Neuropathology of familial erythrophagocytic lymphohistiocytosis: six cases and review of the literature. Hum Pathol 1984;15:161.
148. Lilleyman JS. The treatment of familial erythrophagocytic lymphohistiocytosis. Cancer 1980;46:468.
149. Ambruso DR, Hays T, Zwartjes WJ, et al. Successful treatment of lymphohistiocytic reticulosis with phagocytosis with epipodophyllotoxin VP-16-213. Cancer 1980;45:2516.
150. Alvarado CS, Buchanan GR, Kim TH, et al. Use of VP-16-213 in the treatment of familial erythrophagocytic lymphohistiocytosis. Cancer 1986;57:1097.
151. Henter J-I, Elinder G, Finkel Y, Soder O. Successful induction with chemotherapy including teniposide in familial erythrophagocytic lymphohistiocytosis. Lancet 1986;1:1402.
152. Fischer A, Virelizier JL, Arenzana-Seisedos F, et al. Treatment of four patients with erythrophagocytic lymphohistiocytosis by a combination of epipodophyllotoxin, steroid, intrathecal methotrexate, and cranial irradiation. Pediatrics 1985;76:263.
153. Brown RE, Bowman WP, D'Cruz CA, et al. Endoperoxidation, hyperprostaglandinemia, and hyperlipidemia in a case of erythrophagocytic lymphohistiocytosis: reversal with VP-16 and indomethacin. Cancer 1987;60:2388.
154. Fischer A, Cerf-Bensussan N, Blanche S, et al. Allogeneic bone marrow transplantation for erythrophagocytic lymphohistiocytosis. J Pediatr 1986;108:267.
154a. Ware R, Friedman HS, Kinney TR, et al. Familial erythrophagocytic lymphohistiocytosis: late relapse despite continuous high-dose VP-16 chemotherapy. Med Pediatr Oncol 1990;18:27.
154b. Blanche S, Caniglia M, Fischer A, Griscelli C. Treatment of familial lymphohistiocytosis: chemotherapy or bone marrow transplant? Pediatr Hematol Oncol 1989;6:273.
154c. Nespoli L, Locatelli F, Bonetti F, et al. Familial haemophagocytic lymphohistiocytosis treated with allogenic bone marrow transplantation. Bone Marrow Transplant 1991;7:139.
155. Risdall RJ, McKenna RW, Nesbit ME, et al. Virus-associated hemophagocytic syndrome: a benign histiocytic proliferation distinct from malignant histiocytosis. Cancer 1979;44:993.
156. Ezdinli EZ, Kucuk O, Chedid A, et al. Hypogammaglobulinemia and hemophagocytic syndrome associated with lymphoproliferative disorders. Cancer 1986;57:1024.
157. Wilson ER, Malluh A, Stagno S, Crist WM. Fatal Epstein-Barr virus–associated hemophagocytic syndrome. J Pediatr 1981;98:260.
158. Daum GS, Sullivan JL, Ansell J, et al. Virus-associated hemophagocytic syndrome: identification of an immunoproliferative precursor lesion. Hum Path 1987;18:1071.
159. Campo E, Condom E, Miro M-J, et al. Tuberculosis-associated hemophagocytic syndrome: a systemic process. Cancer 1986;58:2640.
160. Risdall RJ, Brunning RD, Hernandez JI, Gordon DH. Bacteria-associated hemophagocytic syndrome. Cancer 1984;54:2968.
161. Mallou AA, Saadi AR. Hemophagocytosis with typhoid fever. Pediatr Infect Dis 1986;5:720.
162. Fame TM, Engelhard D, Riley HD Jr. Hemophagocytosis accompanying typhoid fever. Pediatr Infect Dis 1986;5:367.
163. Udden MM, Banez E, Sears DA. Bone marrow histiocytic hyperplasia and hemophagocytosis with pancytopenia in typhoid fever. Am J Med Sci 1986;291:396.
164. Weintraub M, Siegman-Igra Y, Josiphov J, et al. Histiocytic hemophagocytosis in miliary tuberculosis. Arch Intern Med 1984;144:2055.
165. Auerbach M, Haubenstock A, Soloman G. Systemic babesiosis. Another cause of the hemophagocytic syndrome. Am J Med 1986;80:301.
166. Yin JAL, Kumaran TO, Marsh GW, et al. Complete recovery of histiocytic medullary reticulosis-like syndrome in a child with acute lymphobalstic leukemia. Cancer 1983;51:200.
167. Chen T, Nesbit M, McKenna R, et al. Histiocytic medullary reticulosis in acute lymphocytic leukemia of T-cell origin. Am J Dis Child 1976;130:1262.
168. Rubin M, Rothenberg SP, Panchacharam P. A histiocytic medually reticulosis-like syndrome as the terminal event in lymphocytic lymphoma. Am J Med Sci 1984;287:60.
169. Theodorakis ME, Zamkoff KW, Davey FR, et al. Acute nonlymphocytic leukemia complicated by severe cytophagocytosis of formed blood elements by nonmalignant histiocytes: cause of significant clinical morbidity. Med Pediatr Oncol 1983;11:20.
170. Liang DC, Chu ML, Shih CC. Reactive histiocytosis in acute lymphoblastic leukemia and non-Hodgkin's lymphoma. Cancer 1986;58:1289.
171. Takasaki N, Kaneko Y, Maseki N, et al. Hemophagocytic syndrome

complicating T-cell acute lymphoblastic leukemia with a novel t(11;14)(p15;q11) chromosome translocation. Cancer 1987;59:424.
172. Scott RB, Robb-Smith AHT. Histiocytic medullary reticulosis. Lancet 1939;2:194.
173. Warnke RA, Kim H, Dorfman RF. Malignant histiocytosis (histiocytic medullary reticulosis). I. Clinicopathologic study of 29 cases. Cancer 1975;35:215.
174. Reiner AP, Spivak JL. Hematophagic histiocytosis: a report of 23 new patients and a review of the literature. Medicine 1988;67:369.
175. Rappaport H. Tumors of the hematopoietic system. In: Atlas of tumor pathology, fascicle 8, series 1. Washington, DC, Armed Forces Institute of Pathology, 1966:49.
176. Lampert IA, Catovsky D, Bergier N. Malignant histiocytosis: a clinicopathological study of 12 cases. Br J Haematol 1978;40:65.
177. Molyneux ME, Tozer RA, Hutt MSR. Histiocytic medullary reticulosis in Africa. Lancet 1978;2:1202.
178. Esumi N, Ikushima S, Hibi S, et al. High serum ferritin level as a marker of malignant histiocytosis and virus-associated hemophagocytic syndrome. Cancer 1988;61:2071.
179. Wilson MS, Weiss LM, Gatter KC, et al. Malignant histiocytosis: a reassessment of cases previously reported in 1975 based on paraffin section immunophenotyping studies. Cancer 1990;66:530.
180. Bar RS, Delor RS, Clausen KP, et al. Fatal infectious mononucleosis in a family. N Engl J Med 1974;290:363.
181. Provisor AJ, Iacuone JJ, Chilcote RR, et al. Acquired agammaglobulinemia after a life-threatening illness with clinical and laboratory features of infectious mononucleosis in three related male children. N Engl J Med 1975;293:62.
182. Purtilo DT, Cassel CK, Yang JP, Harper R. X-linked recessive progressive combined variable immunodeficiency. Lancet 1975;1:935.
183. Purtilo DT, Sakamoto K, Barnabei V, et al. Epstein-Barr virus-induced diseases in boys with the X-linked lymphoproliferative syndrome XLP. Am J Med 1982;73:49.
184. Sullivan JL, Byron KS, Brewster FE, et al. X-linked lymphoproliferative syndrome. J Clin Invest 1983;83:1765.
185. Sullivan JL. Epstein-Barr virus and the X-linked lymphoproliferative syndrome. In: Roizman B, ed. The herpesviruses, vol 4. New York, Plenum Press, 1985:229.
186. Sullivan JL, Byron KS, Brewster FE, et al. Treatment of life-threatening Epstein-Barr virus infectious with acyclovir. Am J Med 1982;73:262.
187. Sullivan JL, Medveczky P, Forman SJ, et al. Epstein-Barr virus induced lymphoproliferation: implications for anti-viral chemotherapy. N Engl J Med 1984;311:1163.
188. Leibow AA, Carrington CRB, Friedman PJ. Lymphomatoid granulomatosis. Hum Pathol 1972;3:457.
189. Lee SC, Roth LM, Brashear RE. Lymphomatoid granulomatosis: a clinicopathologic study of four cases. Cancer 1976;38:846.
190. Fauci AS, Haynes BF, Costa J, et al. Lymphomatoid granulomatosis: prospective clinical and therapeutic experience over 10 years. N Engl J Med 1982;306:68.
191. Patton WF, Lynch JP. Lymphomatoid granulomatosis: clinicopathologic study of four cases and literature review. Medicine 1982;61:1.
192. Sordillo PP, Epremian B, Koziner B, et al. Lymphomatoid granulomatosis: an analysis of clinical and immunologic characteristics. Cancer 1982;49:2070.
193. Katzenstein AL, Carrington CB, Yiebow AA. Lymphomatoid granulomatosis: a clinicopathologic study of 152 cases. Cancer 1979;43:360.
194. Conn DL, McDuffie FC, Holley KE, Schroeter AL. Immunologic mechanisms in systemic vasculitis. Mayo Clin Proc 1976;51:511.
195. Israel HL, Patchefsky AS, Saldana MJ. Wegener's granulomatosis, lymphomatoid granulomatosis and benign lymphocytic angiitis and granulomatosis of lung: recognition and treatment. Ann Intern Med 1977;87:691.
196. Rosai J, Dorfman RF. Sinus histiocytosis with massive lymphadenopathy: a pseudolymphomatous benign disorder: analysis of 34 cases. Cancer 1972;30:1174.
197. Kessler E, Srulijes C, Toledo E, Shalit M. Sinus histiocytosis with massive lymphadenopathy and spinal epidural involvement: a case report and review of the literature. Cancer 1976;38:1614.
198. Foucar E, Rosai J, Dorfman RF, et al. Immunologic abnormalities and their significance in sinus histiocytosis with massive lymphadenopathy. Am J Clin Pathol 1984;5:515.
199. Lampert F, Lennert K. Sinus histiocytosis with massive lymphadenopathy: fifteen new cases. Cancer 1976;37:783.
200. Sumaya CV, Cherry JD, Gohd R. Exaggerated antibody response following rubella vaccination in a child with sinus histiocytosis with massive lymphadenopathy. J Pediatr 1976;89:81.
200a. Levine PH, Jahan N, Murari P, Manak M, Jaffe ES. Detection of human herpesvirus 6 in tissues involved by sinus histiocytosis with massive lymphadenopathy (Rosai-Dorfman disease). J Infect Dis 1992;166:291.
200b. McAlister WH, Herman T, Dehner LP. Sinus histiocytosis with massive lymphadenopathy (Rosai-Dorfman disease). Pediatr Radiaol 1990;20:425.
201. Suarez CR, Zeller WP, Silberman S, et al. Sinus histiocytosis with massive lymphadenopathy: remission with chemotherapy. Am J Pediatr Hematol Oncol 1983;5:235.
202. Komp DM. The treatment of sinus histiocytosis with massive lymphadenopathy (Rosai-Dorfman disease). Semin Diagn Pathol 1990;7:83.
202a. Baildam EM, D'Souza SW, Stevens RF, Ewing CI. Sinus histiocytosis with massive lymphadenopathy (Rosai-Dorfman disease): response to acyclovir. R Soc Med 1992;85:179.
203. Helwig EB, Hackney VC. Juvenile xanthogranuloma (nevoxanthoendothelioma). Am J Pathol 1954;30:625.
204. Gianotti F, Caputo R, Ermacora E. Singulière histiocytose infantile à cellules avec particules vermiformes intracytoplasmiques. Bull Soc Fr Dermatol Syphiligr 1971;78:232.
205. Gianotti F. Histiocytose à cellules avec particules vermiformes intracytoplasmiques: deuxième cas infantile. Bull Soc Fr Dermatol Syphiligr 1972;79:244.
206. Gianotti F, Caputo R. Unknown histiocytoses with intracytoplasmic worm-like particles in two children. 14th International Congress of Dermatology, Amsterdam, Holland, 1974:47.
207. Gianotti F. Cutaneous proliferative histiocytoses in children. G Ital Dermatol Venereol 1980;115:59.
208. Eisenberg EL, Bronson DM, Barsky S. Benign cephalic histiocytosis: a case report and ultrastructural study. J Am Acad Dermatol 1985;12:328.
209. Kikuchi M. Lymphadenitis showing focal reticulum cell hyperplasia with nuclear debris and phagocytes: a clinicopathological study. Nippon Ketsueki Gakkai Zasshi 1972;35:379.
210. Pileri S, Kikuchi M, Helbron D, et al. Histiocytic necrotizing lymphadenitis without granulocytic infiltration. A Pathol Anat Histopathol 1982;395:257.
211. Turner RR, Martin J, Dorfman RF. Necrotizing lymphadenitis: a study of 30 cases. Am J Surg Pathol 1983;7:115.
212. Dorfman RF, Berry GJ. Kikuchi's histiocytic necrotizing lymphadenitis: an analysis of 108 cases with emphasis on differential diagnosis. Semin Diagn Pathol 1988;5:329.
213. Esseltine DW, Leeuw NKM, Berry GR. Malignant histiocytosis. Cancer 1983;52:1904.
214. Zucker JM, Caillaux JM, Vanel D, Gerard-Marchant R. Malignant histiocytosis in childhood: clinical study and therapeutic results in 22 cases. Cancer 1980;45:2821.
215. Schouten TJ, Hustinx TWJ, Scheres MJC, et al. Malignant histiocytosis: clinical and cytogenetic studies in a newborn and a child. Cancer 1983;52:1229.
216. Warnke R, Kim H, Dorfman R. Malignant histiocytosis: clinicopathologic study of 29 cases. Cancer 1975;35:215.
217. Weiss LM, Trela MJ, Cleary ML, et al. Frequent immunoglobulin tne T-cell receptor gene rearrangements in "histiocytic neoplasms." Am J Pathol 1985;121:369.
218. Franchino C, Reuh C, Dutenfeld A, et al. A clinicopathologically distinctive primary histiocytic neoplasm: demonstration of its histiocytic derivation by immunophenotypic and molecular genetic analysis. Am J Surg Pathol 1988;12:398.
219. Kadin ME, Kamoun M, Lamberg J. Erythrophagocytic T_μ lymphoma: a clinicopathologic entity resembling malignant histiocytosis. N Engl J Med 1981;304:648.
220. O'Connor NTJ, Stein H, Gatter KC, et al. Genotypic analysis of large cell lymphomas which express the Ki-1 antigen. Histopathology 1987;11:733.
221. Ishii E, Hara T, Okamura J, et al. Malignant histiocytosis in infants: surface marker analysis of malignant cells in two cases. Med Pediatr Oncol 1987;15:102.
222. Abe R, Akaike Y, Yokoyama A, et al. High incidence of 17p13 chromosomal abnormalities in malignant histiocytosis. Cancer 1990;65:2689.
223. Benz-Lemoine E, Brizard A, Huret J-L, et al. Malignant histiocytosis: a specific t(2;5)(p23;q35) translocation: review of the literature. Blood 1988;72:1045.
224. Kaneko Y, Frizzera G, Edamura S, et al. A novel translocation, t(2;5)(p23;q35), in childhood phagocytic large T-cell lymphoma mimicking malignant histiocytosis. Blood 1989;73:806.
225. Kamesaki H, Koya M, Miwa H, et al. Malignant histiocytosis with rearrangement of the heavy chain gene and evidence of monocyte-macrophage lineage. Cancer 1988;62:1306.
226. Simon JH, Tebbi CK, Freeman AI, et al. Malignant histiocytosis: complete remission in two pediatric patients. Cancer 1987;59:1566.
227. Ducaman BS, Wick MR, Morgan TW, et al. Malignant histiocytosis: a clinical, histologic and immunohistochemical study of 20 cases. Hum Pathol 1984;15:368.
228. Cabanillas F, Rodriguez V, Valdivieso M, et al. Effective combination chemotherapy of adult malignant histiocytosis (histiocytic medullary reticulosis). Med Pediatr Oncol 1978;4:29.
229. Vera R Jr, Bertino JR, Cadman E, Waldron JA. Malignant histiocytosis: response to VP-16-213 and cytosine arabinoside. Cancer 1984;54:991.
230. Vowels MR, Lam-Po-Tang R, Mameghan H, et al. Bone marrow transplantation for malignant histiocytosis in childhood. Cancer 1985;56:2786.
231. Cazin B, Gorin NC, Jouet JP, et al. Successful autologous bone marrow transplantation in second remission of malignant histiocytosis. Bone Marrow Transplant 1990;6:431.
232. Kao WY, Hwang WS. Bone marrow transplantation for malignant histiocytosis. Transplant Proc 1992;24:1524.

233. Jaffe ES. Malignant histiocytosis and true histiocytic lymphomas. In: Jaffe ES, ed. Surgical pathology of lymph nodes and related organs. Philadelphia, WB Saunders, 1985:381.
234. Willemze R, Rinter DJ, Willem A, et al. Reticulum cell sarcomas (large cell lymphomas) presenting in the skin: high frequency of true histiocytic lymphoma. Cancer 1982;50:1367.
235. Barron DR, Davis BR, Pomeranz JR, et al. Cytophagic histiocytic panniculitis: a variant of malignant histiocytosis. Cancer 1985;55:2538.
236. Goldberg NS, Bauer K, Rosen ST, et al. Histiocytosis-X. Arch Dermatol 1986;122:446.
237. Tani M, Ishii N, Kumagai M, et al. Malignant Langerhans cell tumor. Br J Dermatol 1992;126:398.
238. Monda I, Warnke R, Rosai J. A primary lymph node malignancy with features suggestive of dendritic reticulum cell differentiation: a report of 4 cases. Am J Pathol 1986;122:562.
239. Feltkamp CA, van Heerde P, Feltkamp-Vroom TM, et al. A malignant tumor arising from interdigitating cells: light microscopical, ultrastructural, immuno- and enzyme-histochemical characteristics. Virchows Arch 1981;393:183.
240. Chan W, Zaatari G. Lymph node interdigitating reticulum cell sarcoma. Am J Clin Pathol 1986;85:739.
241. Nakamura S, Hara K, Suchi T, et al. Interdigitating cell sarcoma: a morphologic, immunohistologic and enzyme histochemical study. Cancer 1988;61:562.
242. DiFerrante N, Nichols BL, et al. Induced degradation of glycosaminoglycans in Hurler's and Hunter's syndromes by plasma infusion. Proc Natl Acad Sci USA 1971;68:303.
243. Dekaban AS, Holden KR, et al. Effects of fresh plasma or whole blood transfusions on patients with various types of mucopolysaccharidoses. Pediatrics 1972;50:688.
244. Danes BS, Degnan M, et al. Intravenous injection of purified hexosaminidase A into a patient with Tay-Sachs disease. In: Bergsma D, ed. Enzyme therapy in genetic diseases. Baltimore, Williams & Wilkins, 1973:120.
245. Brady RO, Pentchev PC, et al. Replacement therapy for inherited enzyme deficiency: use of purified glucocerebrosidase in Gaucher's disease. N Engl J Med 1974;291:989.
246. Beutler E, Dale GL. Enzyme replacement therapy: model and clinical studies. In: Desnick RJ, Gatt S, Grabowski GA, eds. Gaucher disease: a century of delineation and research. New York, Alan R Liss, 1982: 703.
247. Finkelstein M, Weissmann G. The introduction of enzymes into cells by means of liposomes. J Lipid Res 1978;19:289.
248. Ihler GM, Glew RH, et al. Enzyme loading of erythrocytes. Proc Natl Acad Sci USA 1973;70:2663.
249. Barton NW, Furbish FS, Murray GJ, et al. Therapeutic response to intravenous infusions of glucocerebrosidase in a patient with Gaucher disease. Proc Natl Acad Sci USA 1990;87:1913.
250. Beutler E. Gaucher's disease. N Engl J Med 1991;325:1354.
251. Groth CG, Blomstrand R, et al. Metabolic changes following splenic transplantation in a case of Gaucher's disease. In: Volk BW, Aronson SM, eds. Sphingolipids, sphingolipidoses and allied disorders. New York, Plenum Press, 1972:633.
252. Desnick SJ, Desnick RJ, et al. Renal transplantation in type II Gaucher disease. In: Bergsma D, ed. Enzyme therapy in genetic diseases. Baltimore, Williams & Wilkins, 1973:109.
253. Daloze P, Delvin EE, et al. Replacement therapy for inhertied enzyme deficiency: liver orthotopic transplantation in Niemann-Pick disease type A. Am J Med Genet 1977;1:229.
254. Groth CG, Ringden O. Transplantation in relation to the treatment of inherited disease. Transplantation 1984;38:319.
255. Desnick RJ, Gatt S, Grabowski GA, eds. Gaucher disease: a century of delineation and research. New York, Alan R Liss, 1982:1.
256. Goldblatt J. Type I Gaucher disease. J Med Genet 1988;25:415.
257. Goldblatt J, Beighton P. Cutaneous manifestations of Gaucher disease. Br J Dermatol 1984;111:331.
258. Stowens DW, Teitelbaum SL, Kahn AJ, Barranger, JA. Skeletal complications of Gaucher disease. Medicine 1985;64:310.
259. Beighton P, Goldbatt J, Sacks S. Bone involvement in Gaucher disease: a century of delineation and research. New York, Alan R Liss, 1982: 107.
260. Boklan BF, Sawitsky A. Factor IX deficiency in Gaucher disease. Arch Intern Med 1976;136:489.
261. Lieberman I, Beutler E. Elevation of serum angiostensin converting enzyme in Gaucher's disease. N Engl J Med 1976;294:1442.
262. Gilbert HS, Weinreb N. Increased circulating levels of transcobalamin II in Gaucher's disease. N Engl J med 1976;294:1442.
263. Beutler E, Saven A. Misuse of marrow examination in the diagnosis of Gaucher disease. Blood 1990;76:646.
264. Erikson A. Gaucher disease: Norrbottnian type (III)— neuropaediatric and neurobiological aspects of clinical patterns and treatment. Acta Paediatr Scand 1986;326(Suppl):1.
265. Shiloni E, Bitran D, Rachmilewitz E, Durst AL. The role of splenectomy in Gaucher's disease. Arch Surg 1983;118:929.
266. Thanopoulos BD, Frimas CA, Mantagos SP, Beratis NG. Gaucher disease: treatment of hypersplenism with splenic embolization. Acta Paediatr Scand 1987;76:1003.
267. Rubin M, Yampolski I, Lambrozo R, et al. Partial splenectomy in Gaucher's disease. J Pediatr Surg 1986;21:125.
268. Kolodny EH, Boustany R-M. Storage diseases of the reticuloendothelial system. In: Nathan D, Oskieds F, eds. Hematology of infancy and childhood. Philadelphia, WB Saunders, 1987:1212.
269. Starer F, Sargent JD, Hobbs JR. Regression of the radiological changes of Gaucher's disease following bone marrow transplantation. Br J Radiol 1987;60:1189.
270. Bayever E, Ladisch S, et al. Bone-marrow transplantation for metachromatic leukodystrophy. Lancet 1985;2:471.
271. Rappeport JM, Ginns EI. Bone-marrow transplantation in severe Gaucher's disease. N Engl J Med 1984;311:84.
272. Reiner O, Wigderson M, Horowtiz M. Structural analysis of the human glucocerebrosidase genes. DNA 1988;7:107.
273. Sorge J, West C, Westwood B, Beutler E. Molecular cloning and nucleotide sequence of human glucocerebrosidase cDNA. Proc Natl Acad Sci USA 1985;82:7289.
274. Graves PN, Grabowski GA, Eisner R, et al. Gaucher disease type 1: cloning and characterization of a cDNA encoding acid β-glucosidase from an Ashkenazi Jewish patient. DNA 1988;7:521.
275. Reiner O, Wigderon M, Horowitz M. Structural analysis of the human glucocerebrosidase genes. DNA 1988;7:107.
276. Horowitz M, Wilder SY, Horowitz Z, et al. The human glucocerebrosidase gene and pseudogene: structure and evolution. Genomics 1989;4: 87.
277. Devine EA, Smith M, Arredondo-Vega FX, et al. Chromosomal localization of the gene for Gaucher disease. In: Desnick RJ, Gatt S, Grabowski GA, eds. Gaucher disease: a century of delineation and research. New York, Alan R Liss 1982:511.
278. Ginns EI, Choudary PV, Tsuji S, et al. Gene mapping and leader polypeptide sequence of human glucocerebrosidase: implications for Gaucher disease. Proc Natl Acad Sci USA 1985;82:7101.
279. Tsuji S, Choudary PV, Martin BM, et al. A mutation in the human glucocerebrosidase gene in neuronopathic Gaucher's disease. N Engl J Med 1987;316:570.
280. Tsuji S, Martin BM, Barranger JA, et al. Genetic heterogeneity in type 1 Gaucher disease: multiple genotypes in Ashkenazic and non-Ashkenazic individuals. Proc Natl Acad Sci USA 1988;85:2349.
281. Zimran A, Gross E, West C, et al. Prediction of severity of Gaucher's disease by identification of mutations at DNA level. Lancet 1989;2: 349.
282. Zimran A, Kuhl WC, Beutler E. Detection of the 1226 (Jewish) mutation for Gaucher's disease by color PCR. Am J Clin Pathol 1990;93:788.
283. Zimran A, Sorge J, Gross E, et al. A glucocerebrosidase fusion gene in Gaucher disease: implications for the molecular anatomy, pathogenesis, and diagnosis of this disorder. J Clin Invest 1990;85:219.
284. Firon N, Eyal N, Kolodny EH, Horowitz M. Genotype assignment in Gaucher disease by selective amplification of the active glucocerebrosidase gene. Am J Hum Genet 1990;46:527.
285. Besley GTN, Elleder M. Enzyme activities and phospholipid storage patterns in brain and spleen samples from Niemann-Pick disease variants: a comparison of neuropathic and non-neuropathic forms. J Inherit Metab Dis 1986;9:59.
286. Wenger DA, Wharton C, Sattler M, Clark C. Niemann-Pick disease: prenatal diagnoses and studies of sphingomyelinase activities. Am J Med Genet 1978;2:345.
287. Quintern LE, Schuchman EH, Levran O, et al. Isolation of cDNA clones encoding human acid sphingomyelinase: occurrence of alternatively processed transcripts. EMBO J 1989;8:2469.
288. Walton DS, et al. Ocular manifestations of Group A Niemann-Pick disease. Am J Ophthalmol 1978;85:174.
289. Simoni G, Brambati B, Danesino C, et al. Diagnostic application of first trimester trophoblast sampling in 100 pregnancies. Hum Genet 1984;66: 252.
290. Vellodi A, Hobbs JR, O'Donnell NM, et al. Treatment of Niemann-Pick disease type B by allogeneic bone marrow transplantation. Br Med J 1987;295:1375.
291. Yatziv S, Gershon ZL, Ornoy A, Bach G. Clinical heterogeneity in a sibship with Niemann-Pick disease type C. Clinical Genet 1983;23: 125.
292. Vanier MT, Wenger DA, Comly ME, et al. Niemann-Pick disease group C: clinical variability and diagnosis based on defective cholesterol esterification—a collaboration study on 70 patients. Clin Genet 1988;33: 331.
293. Breen L, Morris HH, et al. Juvenile Niemann-Pick disease with vertical supranuclear ophthalmoplegia. Arch Neurol 1981;38:388.
294. Chan WC et al. Adult Niemann-Pick disease: a case report. J Pathol 1977;121:177.
295. Callahan JW, Khalil M. Sphingomyelinases in human tissues. III. Expression of Niemann-Pick disease in cultured skin fibroblasts. Pediatr Res 1975;9:914.
296. Silverstein MN, Ellefson RD, Ahern EJ. The syndrome of the sea-blue histiocyte. N Engl J Med 1970;282:1.
297. Dawson PJ, Dawson G, Adult Niemann-Pick disease with sea-blue histiocytes in the spleen. Hum Pathol 1982;13:1115.
298. Tachibana F, et al. Syndrome of the sea-blue histiocyote: the first case

report in Japan and review of the literature. Acta Pathol Jpn 1979;29: 73.
299. Quattrin N, et al. Sea-blue histiocytosis: a clinical cytologic and nosographic study on 23 cases. Klin Wochenschr 1978;56:17.
300. Dewhurst N, Besley GT, Finlayson ND, Parker AC. Sea blue histiocytosis in a patient with chronic non-neuropathic Niemann-Pick disease. J Clin Pathol 1979;32:1121.
301. Silverstein MN, Ellefson Rd. The syndrome of the sea-blue histiocyte. Semin Hematol 1972;9:299.
302. Sawitsky A, et al. The sea-blue histiocyte syndrome, a review: genetic and biochemical studies. Semin Hematol 1971;9:285.
303. Vacher-Lavenu MC, Baron-Selme V, Abelanet R, et al. Le syndrome des histiocytes bleus: revue de la littérature à propos d'une observation de splénomegalie idiopathique chez l'adulte. Sem Hop Paris 1984;60: 1333.
304. Dosik H, et al. Acquired lipidosis: Gaucher-like cells and "blue cells" in chronic granulocytic leukemia. Semin Hematol 1972;9:309.
305. Tanaka T, Takahashi K, Morita H, et al. Chronic granulomatous disease of childhood and sea-blue histiocytosis: a pathologic study of an autopsy case. Acta Pathol Jpn 1984;34:1385.
306. Columbi A, et al. Angiokeratoma corporis diffusum: Fabry's disease. Helv Med Acta 1967;34:67.
307. Avila JL, et al. Fabry's disease: normal α-galactosidase activity and urinary-sediment glycosphingolipid levels in two obligate heterozygotes. Br J Dermatol 1973;89:149.
308. Weingeist JA, Blodi FC. Fabry's disease: ocular findings in a female carrier: a light and electron microscopic study. Arch Ophthalmol 1973;85:169.
309. Donati D, Novario R, Gastaldi L. Natural history and treatment of uremia secondary to Fabry's disease: an European experience. Nephron 1987;46:353.
310. Sakuraba H, Yanagawa Y, Igarashi T, et al. Cardiovascular manifestations in Fabry's disease: a high incidence of mitral valve prolapse in hemizygotes and heterozygotes. Clin Genet 1986;29:276.
311. Desnick RJ, Dean KJ, Grabowski G, et al. Enzyme therapy XII: enzyme therapy in Fabry's disease: differential enzyme and substrate clearance kinetics of plasma and splenic α-galactosidase isozymes. Proc Natl Acad Sci USA 1979;76:5326.
312. Beutler E, Kuhl W, Matsumoto F, et al. Acid hydrolases in leukocytes and platelets of normal subjects and in patients with Gaucher and Fabry's disease. J Exp Med 1976;143:975.
313. Galjaard H, Niermeijer MF, Hahnemann N, et al. An example of rapid prenatal diagnosis of Fabry's disease using microtechniques. Clin Genet 1974;5:368.
314. Kleijer WJ, Hussaarts-Odijk LM, Sachs ES, et al. Prenatal diagnosis of Fabry's disease by direct analysis of chorionic villi. Prenatal Diagn 1987;7:283.
315. Cable WJL, McCluer RH, Kolodny EH, Ullman MD. Fabry disease: detection of heterozygotes by examination of glycoplipids in urinary sediment. Neurology 1982;32:1139.
316. Desnick RJ, Bernstein HS, Astrin KH, Bishop DF. Fabry disease: molecular diagnosis of hemizygotes and heterozygotes. Enzyme 1987;38: 54.
317. Wareham KA, Lyon MF, Glenisler PH, et al. Age related reactivation of an X-linked gene. Nature 1987;327:725.
318. Wilson VL, Smith RA, Ma S, et al. Genomic 5-methyldeoxycytidine decreases with age. J Biol Chem 1987;262:9948.
319. Calhoun DH, Bishop DF, Bernstein HS, et al. Fabry disease: isolation of a cDNA clone encoding human α-galactosidase A. Proc Natl Acad Sci USA 1985;82:7364,
320. Quinn M, Hantzopoulos P, Fidanza V, Calhoun DH. A genomic clone containing the promoter for the gene encoding the human lysosomal enzyme, α-galactosidase A. Gene 1987;58:177.
321. MacDermot D, Morgan SH, Cheshire JK, Wilson TM. Anderson Fabry disease: a close linkage with highly polymorphic DNA markers DXS17, DXS87 and DXS88. Hum Genet 1987;77:263.
322. Bernstein HS, Bishop DF, Astrin KH, et al. Fabry disease: six gene rearrangements and an exonic point mutation in the α-galactosidase gene. J Clin Invest 1989;83:1390.
323. Bishop DF, Kornreich R, Desnick RJ. Structural organization of the human α-galactosidase A gene: further evidence for the absence of a 3′ untranslated region. Proc Natl Acad Sci USA 1988;85:3903.
324. Kornreich R, Bishop DF, Desnick RJ. α-Galactosidase A gene rearrangements casuing Fabry disease: identification of short direct repeats at breakpoints in an *Alu*-rich gene. J Biol Chem 1990;265:9319.
325. Raghavan S, Gajewski A, Kolodny EH. G_{M1}-ganglioside β-galactosidase in leukocytes and cultured fibroblasts. Clin Chim Acta 1977;81:47.
326. Shows TB, Scrafford-Wolff LR, Brown JA, Meisler M. Assignment of a beta-galactosidase gene (beta GALA) to chromosome 3 in man. Cytogenet Cell Genet 1978;22:219.
327. Morreau H, Galjart NJ, Gillemans N, et al. Alternative splicing of β-galactosidase mRNA generates the classic lysosomal enzyme and a β-galactosidase–related protein. J Biol Chem 1989;264:20655.
328. Sandhoff K, Conzelmann E, Neufeld EF, et al. In: Scriver CR, Beaudet AL, Sly WS, Valle D, eds. The metabolic basis of inherited disease. New York, McGraw-Hill, 1989:1807.
329. Myerowitz R. Splice junction mutation in some Ashkenazi Jews with Tay-Sachs disease: evidence against a single defect within this ethnic group. Proc Natl Acad Sci USA 1988;85:3955.
330. Arpaia E, Dumbrille-Ross A, Maler T, et al. Identification of an altered splice site in Ashkenazi Tay-Sachs disease. Nature 1988;333:85.
331. Ohno K, Suzuki K. A splicing defect due to an exon–intron junctional mutation results in abnormal β-hexosaminidase α-chain mRNA in Ashkenazi Tay-Sachs fibroblasts. Biochem Biophys Res Commun 1988;153:463.
332. Myerowitz R, Costigan FC. The major defect in Ashkenazi Jews with Tay-Sachs disease is an insertion in the gene for the α-chain of β-hexosaminidase. J Biol Chem 1988;263:18587.
333. Myerowitz R, Proia RL. cDNA clone for the α-chain of human β-hexosaminidase: deficiency of α-chain mRNA in Ashkenazi Tay-Sachs fibroblasts. Proc Natl Acad Sci USA 1984;81:5394.
334. Myerowtiz R, Piekarz R, Neufeld EF, et al. Human β-hexosaminidase α-chain: coding sequence and homology with the B-chain. Proc Natl Acad Sci USA 1985;82:7830.
335. Korneluk RG, Mahuran DJ, Neote K, et al. Isolation of cDNA clones coding for the α-subunit of human β-hexosaminidase: extensive homology between the α and β-subunits and studies on Tay-Sachs disease. J Biol Chem 1986;261:8401.
336. Hasilik A, Neufeld EF. Biosynthesis of lysosomal enzymes in fibroblasts: synthesis as precursors of higher molecular weight. J Biol Chem 1980;255:4937.
337. Proia RL, Neufeld EF. Synthesis of β-hexosaminidase in cell-free translation and in intact fibroblasts: an insoluble precursor α chain in a rare form of Tay-Sachs disease. Proc Natl Acad Sci USA 1982;79: 6360.
338. Triggs-Raine BL, Feigenbaum ASJ, Natowicz M, et al. Screening for carriers of Tay-Sachs disease among Ashkenazi Jews: a comparison of DNA-based and enzyme-based tests. N Engl J Med 1990;323:6.
339. Navon R, Proia RL. The mutations in Ashkenazi Jews with adult G_{M2} gangliosidosis: the adult form of Tay-Sachs disease. Science 1989;243: 1471.
340. Paw BH, Moskowitz SM, Uhrhammer N, et al. Juvenile G_{m2} gangliosidosis caused by substitution of histidine for arginine at position 499 or 504 of the α-subunit of β-hexosaminidine. J Biol Chem 1990;265: 9452.
341. Lau MMH, Neufeld EF. A frameshift mutation in a patient with Tay-Sachs disease causes premature termination and defective intracellular transport of the α-subunit of β-hexosaminidase. J Biol Chem 1989;264: 21376.
342. Zokaeem G, Bayleran J, Kaplan P, et al. A shortened β-hexosaminidase α-chain in an Italian patient with infantile Tay-Sachs disease. Am J Hum Genet 1987;40:537.
343. Nakano T, Muscillo M, Ohno K, et al. A point mutation in the coding sequence of the β-hexosaminidase α gene results in defective processing of the enzyme protein in an unusual GM2-gangliosidosis variant. J Neurochem 1988;51:984.
344. Frisch A, Baram D, Nabon R. Hexosaminidase A deficient adults: presence of α-chain precursor in cultured skin fibroblasts. Biochem Biophys Res Commun 1984;119:101.
345. d'Azzo A, Prois RL, Kolodny EH, et al. Faulty association of α- and β-subunits in some forms of β-hexosaminidase A deficiency. J Biol Chem 1984;259:110070.
346. O'Dowd BF, Klavins MH, Willard HF, et al. Molecular heterogeneity in the infantile and juvenile forms of Sandhoff disease (O-variant GM_2 gangliosidosis). J Biol Chem 1986;261:12680.
347. Schroder M, Klima H, Nakano T, et al. Isolation of a cDNA encoding the human G_{M2} activator protein. FEBS Lett 1989;251:197.
348. Goldman JE, Yamanaka T, Rapin I, et al. The AB variant of GM2-gangliosidosis: clinical, biochemical and pathological studies of two patients. Acta Neuropathol (Berl) 1980;52:189.
349. Li Y-T, Hirabayashi Y, Li S-C. A new variant of type-AB GM2-gangliosidosis. Biochem Biophys Res Commun 1981;101:479.
350. Kytzia H-J, hinrichs U, Maire I, et al. Variant of GM2-gangliosidosis with hexosaminidase A having a severely changed substrate specificity. EMBO J 1983;2:1201.
351. Kytzia H-J, Sandhoff K. Evidence for two different active sites on human hexosaminidase A: interaction of GM2 activator protein with hexosaminidase A. J Biol Chem 1985;260:7568.
352. Tanaka A, Ohno K, Sandhoff K, et al. GM2-gangliosidosis B1 variant: analysis of β-hexosaminidase α gene abnormalities in seven patients. Am J Hum Genet 1990;46:329.
353. Farber S, Cohen J, et al. Lipogranulomatosis: a new lipoglycoprotein "storage" disease. J Mt Sinai Hosp 1957;24:816.
354. Antonarakis SE, Valle D, Moser HW, et al. Phenotypic variability in siblings with Farber disease. J Pediatr 1984;104:496.
355. Ng Ying Kin NMK, Wolfe LS. Characterization of oligosaccharides and glycopeptides excreted in the urine of G_{M1}-gangliosidosis patients. Biochem Biophys Res Commun 1975;66:123.
356. Wraith JE, Rogers JG, Danks DM. The mucopolysaccharidoses. Aust Paediatr J 1987;23:329.
357. Van Hoof F. Mucopolysaccharidoses and mucolipidoses. J Clin Pathol 1974;8:64.
358. Muenzer J. Mucopolysaccharidoses. Adv Pediatr 1986;33:269.

359. Crocker AC. Histiocytoses and lipidoses. Lecture 25 in hematology. In: Beck WS, ed. Cambridge, MA, MIT Press, 1981.

360. Hopwood JJ, Morris CP. The mucopolysaccharidoses: diagnosis, molecular genetics and treatment. Mol Biol Med 1990;7:381.

361. Hansen HG. Hematologic studies in mucopolysaccharidoses and mucolipidoses. Birth Defects 1972;8:115.

362. Reilly WA. The granules in the leukocytes in gargoylism. Am J Dis Child 1941;62:489.

363. Mittwoch U. Inclusions of mucopolysaccharides in the lymphocytes of patients with gargoylism. Nature 1961;191:1315.

364. Adinolfi M, Brown S. Strategies for the correction of enzymatic deficiencies in patients with mucopolysaccharidoses. Develop Med Child Neurol 1874;26:401.

365. Crow J, Gibbs DA, Cozens W, et al. Biochemical and histopathological studies on patients with mucopolysaccharidoses, two of whom had been treated by fibroblast transplantation. J Clin Pathol 1983;36:415.

366. Gibbs DA, Spellacy E, Tompkins R, Watts RWE. A clinical trial of fibroblast transplantation for the treatment of mucopolysaccharidoses. J Inherit Metab Dis 1983;6:62.

367. Hobbs JR. Bone marrow transplantation for inborn errors. Lancet 1981;2: 735.

368. O'Reilly RJ, et al. Marrow transplantation for congenital disorders. Semin Hematol 1984;21:188.

369. Krivit W, et al. Bone-marrow transplantation in the Maroteaux-Lamy syndrome (mucopolysaccharidosis type VI): biochemical and clinical status 24 months after transplantation. N Engl J Med 1984;311:1606.

370. Hobbs JR, Hugh Jones K, et al. Reversal of clinical features of Hurler's disease and biochemical improvement after treatment by bone marrow transplantation. J Inherit Metab Dis 1982;5(Suppl):59.

5

Hemostasis

Blood: Principles and Practice of Hematology,
edited by Robert I. Handin, Thomas P. Stossel, and Samuel E. Lux.
J.B. Lippincott Company, Philadelphia © 1995.

33

The Hemostatic System

Stuart E. Lind

Blood is a remarkable organ. Like a gas or liquid, it assumes the shape of the vessel that holds it. Unlike either, blood is able to stem its own loss when the integrity of its physiologic container is breached. A multitude of theories of hemostasis have been proposed by a great many scientists and physicians, who have labored over several centuries to understand just how this process occurs. Because blood clotting in a patent vessel results in ischemia and necrosis of the tissues that it serves, it is important for the host to have the hemostatic system carefully regulated and coagulation initiated only when necessary and terminated as soon as hemorrhage is brought under control. Study of the hemostatic system has helped to establish many important ideas about physiologic homeostasis, some of which are helpful during the clinical evaluation and treatment of patients. The following are some general principles that should be borne in mind:

1. Hemostasis and thrombosis are opposite sides of the same biologic coin. In general, thrombosis involves the same processes as does coagulation but in a different environment. The same principles that govern the activation of platelets, endothelial cells, coagulation, and fibrinolytic proteins are involved in both processes. The major difference between hemorrhage and thrombosis is that in hemorrhage, the inciting stimuli are usually evident, whereas in thrombosis, they often are not.
2. The well-functioning hemostatic system is like a good government: checks and balances are essential for proper functioning and an imbalance may result in a gradual slide into chaos (Table 33-1).
3. Coagulation proteins and platelets are present in greater concentrations in the normal person than are needed for effective hemostasis. Thus, laboratory abnormalities must be evaluated with knowledge of the natural history of each disorder. The need for prophylactic blood product administration should not be based simply on the desire to generate a normal laboratory value for a particular test. For example, although marked prolongations of bleeding or clotting times are often associated with bleeding, less pronounced abnormalities may not be associated with either spontaneous or procedure-related bleeding.
4. Blood coagulation is a complex process involving many participants (platelets, red blood cells [RBCs], white blood cells [WBCs], endothelial cells, coagulation factors, fibrinolytic proteins, and protease inhibitors), whose contributions wax and wane with time. Readily available clinical assays do not provide a complete picture of the functioning of many of these components.
5. Each of the three major participants in the hemostatic process (platelets, fibrinolytic proteins, coagulation proteins) interacts with and influences the others.

Because concepts of hemostasis have focused either on platelet activation or blood coagulation, focus traditionally has been on primary (platelet-mediated) and secondary (fibrin-mediated) phases of hemostasis. Clinicians have therefore been taught to obtain a history using a two-component classification system in which defects in primary hemostasis result in immediate bleeding and defects in secondary hemostasis cause delayed bleeding (Table 33-2). Although effective in analyzing most hemorrhagic events, this formulation tends to downplay the role of late events in hemostasis, such as clot maturation, the action of factor XIII, and the involvement of the fibrinolytic system. Because these components are also difficult to analyze in the clinical laboratory, they can be overlooked unless specifically considered. In some instances, this results in giving too much importance to minor abnormalities in laboratory test results that are not truly linked to clinical events.

The discussion that follows emphasizes three phases of the hemostatic process (Fig. 33-1). Although it is useful to divide this complex system for the sake of discussion and analysis, the temporal involvement described is approximate and based on observations of normal subjects. Pathologic conditions or surgical intervention may alter the relative timing or importance of each phase, with resulting clinical consequences.

PRIMARY HEMOSTASIS: PLATELET AND ENDOTHELIAL CELL ACTIVATION

Although the hemostatic system evolved to prevent blood loss after injury to a blood vessel, it can be partially or wholly activated under other circumstances, commonly as a result of trauma, preeclampsia, or the entry of bacteria into the bloodstream. Understanding of these latter events also evolved from an understanding of the hemostatic mechanisms that are activated after physical injury to a blood vessel. Although much of the following discussion of hemostasis is based on biochemical observations, microscopy has played an important role in understanding the sequence of events that accompanies such injury.[1]

TABLE 33-1. Mechanisms of Control of the Hemostatic System

PLATELETS	
Endothelial prostacyclin Production	
Endothelial and leukocyte membrane ADPase activity	
Endothelial nitric oxide Production	
Protease inhibitors that limit thrombin action	
Endothelial cell tissue plasminogen activator release	
COAGULATION SYSTEM	
Protein C System	
Protein C	
Protein S	
Thrombomodulin	
C_{4b}-binding protein	
CIRCULATING ANTIPROTEASES	
Antiproteases	**Proteases**
Primary inhibitors	
TFPI	Factor Xa, factor VIIa/ tissue factor
Antithrombin III and heparin-like molecules	Thrombin, factors Xa, IXa, XIa, XIIa, kallikrein
C1-esterase inhibitor	Kallikrein, C1, factor XIIa, plasmin
α_2-Macroglobulin	Plasmin, kallikrein, thrombin, factor Xa, protein C_a
Protein C inhibitor	Protein C_a, kallikrein
Secondary inhibitors, or antiproteases of uncertain significance	
α_1-Antitrypsin	Factor XIa, trypsin
Pregnancy zone protein	Plasmin
Heparin cofactor II	Thrombin
Platelet factor XIa inhibitor	Factor XIa
Protease nexin-1	Thrombin
Protease nexin-2/amyloid β-protein precursor	Factor XIa
FIBRINOLYTIC SYSTEM	
α_2-Antiplasmin	
Plasminogen activator inhibitor-1	
Plasminogen activator inhibitor-2	

After injury to the blood vessel, a *hemostatic plug* is formed, which is composed predominantly of platelets. Investigation of platelet function has been directed at determining the sequence of events that is responsible for hemostatic plug formation. Three phases of platelet activation have been described, each of which is associated with one or more clinical bleeding disorders (Fig. 33-2).

Platelet Adhesion

Platelet adhesion is the initial phase of platelet activation whereby a one-cell-thick "carpet" is formed in response to exposure of an appropriate surface. The relevant natural surface in vivo is believed to be the subendothelial matrix, which is rich in collagen, fibronectin, von Willebrand factor (vWF), and other potentially relevant molecules. Artificial surfaces such as vascular grafts also initiate platelet adherence. Adherence depends largely on the presence of platelet surface glycoproteins that bind vWF as well as adequate plasma or subendothelial concentrations of vWF polymers. Deficiencies in either the glycoprotein platelet receptor for vWF, the gpIb/IX complex, or vWF itself, as seen in von Willebrand's disease (vWD), are most often responsible for defects in platelet adhesion. Direct measurements of platelet adhesion are not available in the clinical laboratory, although the ristocetin cofactor test is a surrogate for testing the interaction of vWF with glycoprotein Ib.

Platelet Aggregation

Platelet aggregation is the term used to describe the self-association of platelets into a platelet plug. Platelet aggregation is easily studied clinically and is thus familiar to many clinicians. Platelet aggregation is mediated by the interaction of fibrinogen with glycoprotein receptors on the platelet surface (gpIIb/IIIa complex). The two glycoprotein components of the fibrinogen receptor are held together by the presence of micromolar concentrations of calcium. Removal of calcium by strong chelating agents such as ethylenediamintetraacetic acid ([EDTA], which is found in purple top blood drawing tubes) irreversibly dissociates the complex. Platelet aggregation is usually performed in blood anticoagulated with citrate (found in blue top tubes) because it allows micromolar concentrations of calcium to remain associated with the gpIIb/IIIa complex, thereby maintaining its functional integrity.

TABLE 33-2. Clinical Bleeding Syndromes

	Immediate (Minutes)	Delayed (Hours to Days)
Etiology	Platelet defect	Coagulation or fibrinolytic system defect
Common anatomic sites	Skin, mucosal surfaces, including gums, oral mucosa, nose, gastrointestinal tract, endometrium	Skin, muscles, joints
Type of skin bleeding	Petechiae or multiple ecchymoses; after shaving	Large ecchymoses
Common diseases	von Willebrand's disease; drug-induced platelet dysfunction, paraproteins, uremia	Hemophilia A or B, other factor deficiencies; fibrinolytic overactivity
Clinical history	Easy bruising; prolonged menses; excessive bleeding after dental extraction or tonsillectomy	Bleeding after circumcision, surgery, deep hematoma disproportionate to trauma, hemarthroses

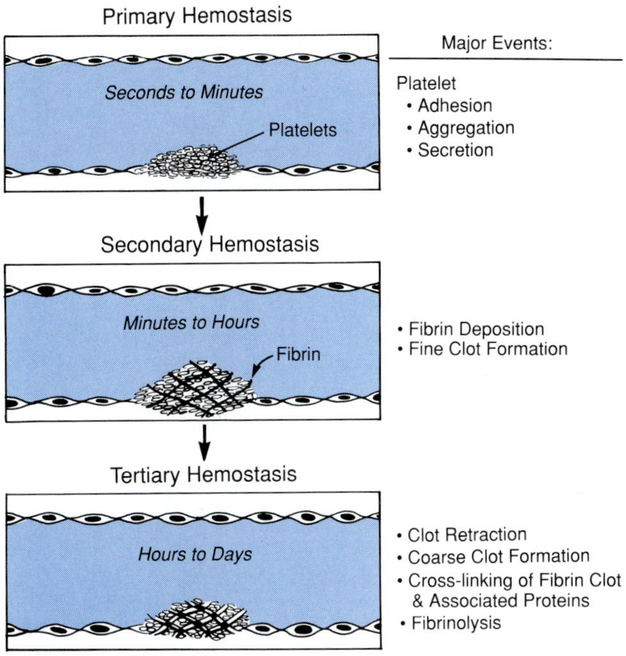

FIGURE 33-1. Temporal phases of the hemostatic process. The division of this complex process into distinct phases is useful for the sake of illustration and analysis of patient's problems, but it is not physiologically correct insofar as there is significant temporal overlap in the phases. Depending on the anatomic site of the thrombus, there may be ongoing accretion of platelets, fibrin, or both onto the clot (which accounts for clot extension), even as the fibrinolytic system is actively digesting certain of its parts. Not illustrated here is the infiltration of the clot by macrophages and fibroblasts, each of which may release compounds that modify the clot's life-span.

Platelet Secretion

Platelet secretion describes the process whereby platelet granules release their contents into the extracellular space. This results in high local concentrations of the contents of the platelets' two major types of granules, many of which contribute to the formation of the stable platelet plug. The platelet dense granules contain adenosine diphosphate (ADP), serotonin, and Ca^{2+}, whereas the α granules contain proteins. Two of these proteins, platelet factor 4 and β-thromboglobulin, are found only in platelets and megakaryocytes. Unlike other α-granule proteins, such as vWF and fibrinogen, which play a role in hemostasis, platelet factor 4 and β-thromboglobulin are not recognized to have a specific hemostatic function. Tests of platelet secretion are generally performed only in specialized hemostasis laboratories.

Platelets also provide a specialized surface on which coagulation and fibrinolytic proteins are activated, a property shared with other cell surfaces (such as those of endothelial cells and monocytes). The importance of the ability of these other membranes to substitute for the platelet surface is evident when one considers that thrombocytopenic patients do not have the same bleeding manifestations as do hemophiliacs. This clinical observation suggests that other membrane surfaces are able to support the formation of a fibrin clot. The ability of phosphatidylserine exposed on the platelet membrane to accelerate coagulation is the basis of the platelet factor 3 availability test, which is no longer performed but may be found in the older literature.

Roles of Endothelial Cells

Endothelial cells play a number of roles in the hemostatic process in addition to binding coagulation factors that lead to thrombin generation and function to prevent, minimize, or terminate the action of platelets and activated coagulation factors. Endothelial cells alter platelet function in several ways. They contain an ADPase, which destroys ADP and limits platelet activation,[2] and they produce two potent antiplatelet compounds, prostacyclin (PGI_2) and nitric oxide (NO).

Endothelial cells also modulate the coagulation system and the life-span of fibrin clots in several ways. First, they contain on their surface a thrombin-binding glycoprotein, thrombomodulin, which keeps thrombin from cleaving fibrinogen and allows it to activate the important anticoagulant protein, protein C. Second, the Weibel-Palade bodies of the endothelial cells are the source of plasma vWF multimers. Endothelial cells in culture secrete large vWF multimers, which are more active than the multimers usually found in plasma, and the appearance of large multimers in plasma may explain aspects of some disease processes such as thrombotic thrombocytopenic purpura[3] and sickle cell anemia.[4] Third, they release the major intravascular activator of the fibrinolytic system, tissue plasminogen activator (tPA), and are likely an important source of its major regulatory protein, plasminogen activator inhibitor (PAI-1).

Endothelial cells exposed to compounds such as thrombin, endotoxin, interleukin-1, and tumor necrosis factor are known to exhibit alterations in hemostatic properties, as evidenced by their ability to express tissue factor, promote protein C activation, or release fibrinolytic system proteins. Depending on the stimulus involved, endothelial cells may acquire an increased or decreased propensity for promoting or supporting platelet activation and clot formation.[5] Although tests of endothelial function are not available in routine hospital laboratories, they may move into clinical use during the next decade.

SECONDARY HEMOSTASIS: COAGULATION AND FORMATION OF THE FIBRIN CLOT

Early Studies

Blood coagulation has been the object of study by a large number of physicians and scientists. Despite many years of study, information continues to emerge that changes our view of how coagulation occurs. In 1905, Morawitz[5a] presented an integrated theory of blood coagulation that was based on the work performed up to that time, as shown in Figure 33-3. This view postulated that coagulation was initiated after plasma was exposed to tissue thromboplastin, which is now recognized as being a phospholipid-bearing membrane surface containing the membrane-bound glycoprotein, tissue factor. Only two plasma proteins, prothrombin and fibrinogen, and calcium were believed to be necessary for clot formation. The prothrombin time (PT), which we understand to depend on adequate amounts of factors VII, X, V, and II, was based on this model. Because studies showed adequate levels of fibrinogen in most bleeding patients, it was thought that by adding thromboplastin and calcium to plasma one could assay for the only other factor required for hemostasis, prothrombin (hence its name).[6] It was not until the 1950s that all the other components of what is now called the *extrinsic pathway* (factors V, VII, and X) were discovered. Thus, for the first half of this century, the initiation of blood coagulation was believed to require the addition of a substance not

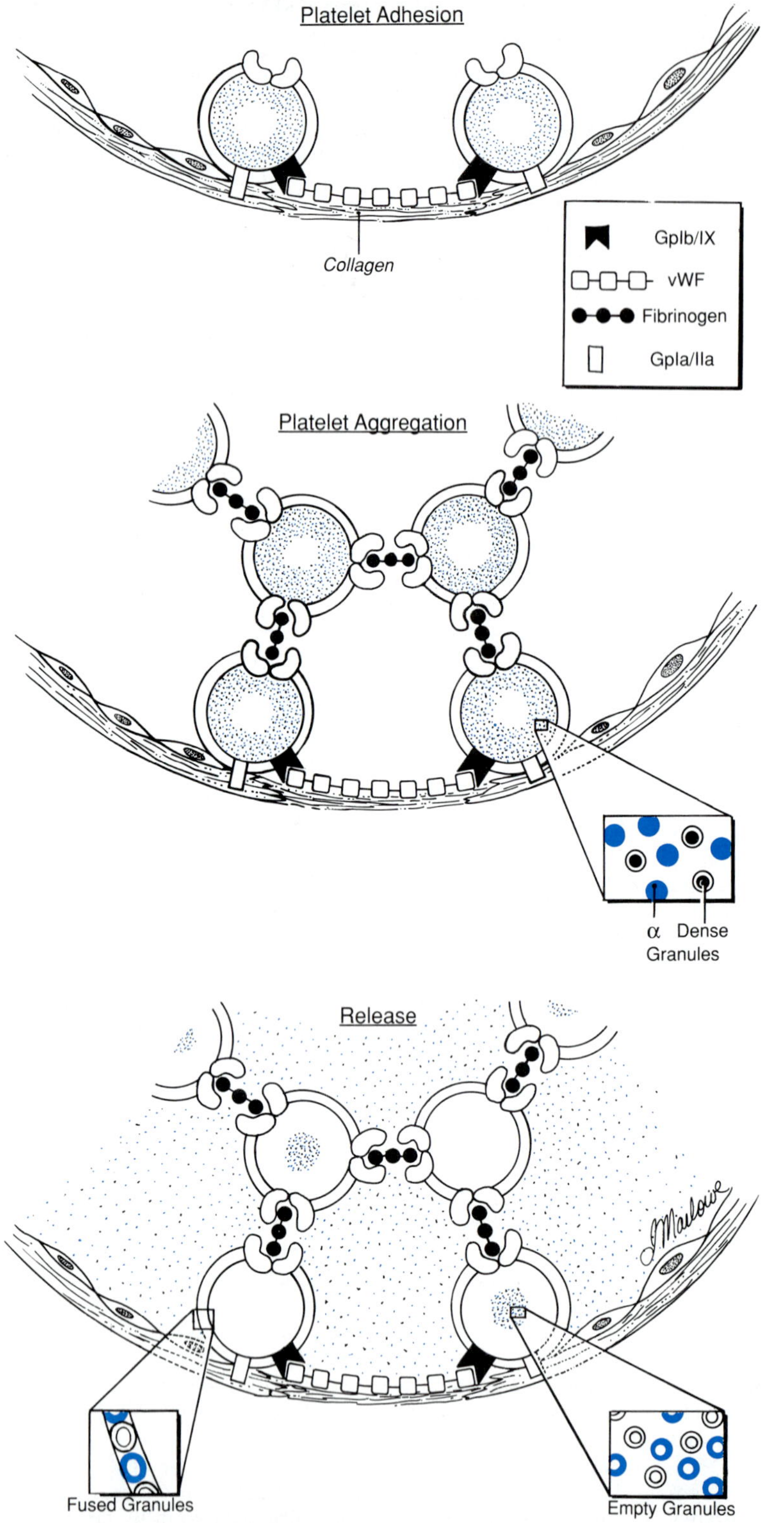

FIGURE 33-2. Platelet function. *Platelet adhesion* is the process whereby platelets form a one-cell-thick carpet-like monolayer on a blood vessel wall at the site of injury and exposure of the subendothelium because of the interaction of plasma membrane glycoproteins with constituents of the subendothelial matrix. The most important interactions are between the gpIb/IX complex and von Willebrand factor (vWF) and between the gpIa/IIa complex and collagen. *Platelet aggregation* results when platelet surface receptors for fibrinogen (gpIIb/IIIa complex) become activated, allowing platelet aggregation formation to occur. The *platelet release reaction* results from a series of intracellular signaling events that cause platelet granule membranes to fuse with the invaginations of the plasma membrane known as the surface-connected canalicular system, leading to discharge of the granule contents into the extracellular space. The added membrane allows the cell to swell, and allows antibodies to bind to proteins originally present in the membranes of the platelet's granules. Some of these proteins (such as P-selectin) allow platelets to interact with other cells.

normally found in blood; thus grew the idea of an extrinsic pathway.

Experiments performed in the late 1940s helped to change thinking about how coagulation was initiated.[7] By showing that blood does not clot when placed in a silicone-coated container but does clot when allowed to come into contact with glass, Conley and associates[7] helped to shift the focus of coagulation theories from the extrinsic pathway to one that was intrinsic to the blood itself. Thus, rather than postulate that coagulation resulted from the addition of a tissue factor, it was thought that alterations in the surface at which blood came into contact with its container led to clotting. Recognition of these hemostatic surfaces was found to be mediated by complex interactions of four proteins (factors XI and XII, high-molecular-weight [HMW] kininogen, and prekallikrein) known collectively as the *contact system*.

The rediscovery[8] that blood can clot in vitro in the absence of tissue factor suggested to some that it was not necessary to postulate the need for tissue factor to explain clotting in vivo, and the intrinsic pathway was viewed as the major physiologic pathway for blood coagulation. This

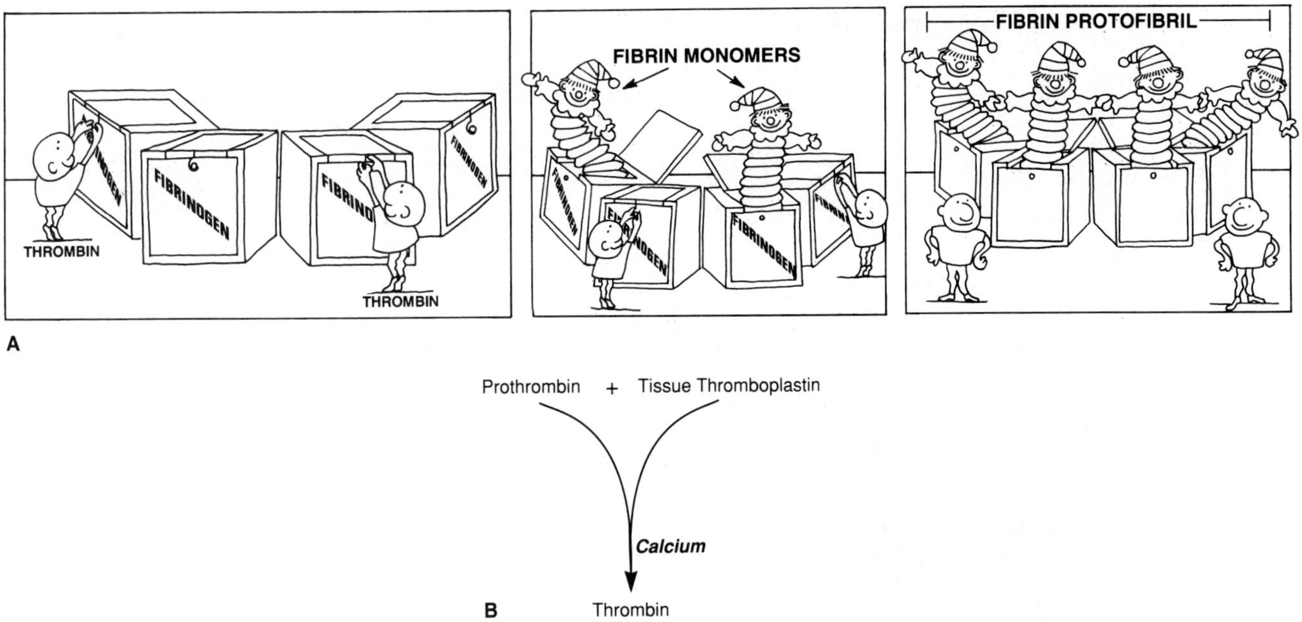

FIGURE 33-3. Coagulation at the beginning of the 20th century. **(A)** Early theories of blood coagulation are thought to have been based on the writings of Plato, who postulated that fibrin was a circulating substance that formed a clot at sites when it left the body and became cooled. By the mid-1800s, it was recognized that blood clotted at physiologic temperatures and resulted from the action of thrombin on fibrinogen. **(B)** Morawitz integrated the work of a number of investigators in his theory of coagulation published in 1905. The extract known as *tissue thromboplastin* is now understood to be composed of anionic phospholipids and the membrane-bound glycoprotein, tissue factor. Phospholipids form the surface on which coagulation reactions take place, while tissue factor is the physiologic activator of factor VII. All theories of coagulation recognized the ability of thrombin to clot fibrinogen.

view was reinforced by the fact that in vitro clotting of plasma through the addition of tissue factor (as measured by the PT) is normal in patients with hemophilia, whereas clotting initiated by surface activation (as measured by the partial thromboplastin time [PTT]) is prolonged.

Several lessons are worth remembering in this story. First, theories that overlook sound observations can be accepted only as temporary bridges to a more complete understanding. Second, laboratory tests of coagulation are often developed to distinguish a particular group of patients from normal persons. Although the tests are performed in a manner that makes them most effective in this regard, it is not uncommon for physicians to extrapolate from these results to other groups of patients, or normal physiology, reaching inappropriate conclusions that may take decades to rectify. An example of this is found in the older literature concerning the PT and hemophilia.

The PT was developed in 1935 by Quick,[6] who reported that when an excess of thromboplastin is used (conditions still used today in all clinical laboratories), the PT of hemophiliac patients is normal. Five years later, Dam and Venndt[9] noted that when less thromboplastin is added, hemophiliac plasma takes longer to coagulate than does normal plasma. Despite this and later confirmatory observations,[10] it was believed for many years that coagulation initiated by tissue factor resulted from a biochemical flow down the extrinsic pathway. Theories of coagulation have since expanded to account for these observations, as discussed in the text that follows. Third, the failure of blood to clot in a silicone container serves to point out that stasis by itself is not a physiologic explanation for thrombosis.[7]

Others have gone on to establish animal models that clearly demonstrate that thrombosis occurs only when stasis is accompanied by a significant change in the biochemical milieu and not simply when blood flow is stopped in a normal vasculature.[11]

That the intrinsic pathway was the subject of most thought and attention is evident in the two independent concepts of blood coagulation published in 1964,[12,13] which stressed the sequential nature of blood protein activation. Both the formulation of the "waterfall"[12] and the "cascade"[13] contained diagrams of the intrinsic pathway. In neither paper was the extrinsic pathway specifically shown, although it was later integrated into the coagulation scheme that has been reproduced in many articles, chapters, and lectures about blood coagulation (Fig. 33-4).

Because factor VII deficiency results in a bleeding disorder, activation of the extrinsic pathway was taken to occur under some circumstances. The discovery that the two pathways can interact brought into question the idea that blood coagulation results from activation of one or the other pathway. Since factor VIIa can activate factor IX[14] and factor IXa can activate factor VII,[15] many began to think that coagulation could occur through a combination of the two pathways, and a crossover pathway was added to diagrams of the coagulation system (Fig. 33-5).

The Tissue Factor Pathway

This development led to a reconsideration of the importance of tissue thromboplastin (or more properly, tissue factor), which was spurred on by several independent lines of thought and investigation. First, the fact that patients lacking proteins found in the initial part of the intrinsic coagulation pathway (factor XII, prekallikrein, and HMW kininogen) do not have a bleeding disorder raised questions about the physiologic importance of this mode of activation (contact pathway). Second, isolation[16] and immunochemical localization[17] of tissue factor caused it to be reconsidered as an initiator of coagulation, as did studies showing that it could be induced to appear on the surface of vascular cells by physiologically relevant stimuli.[5] Third, the de-

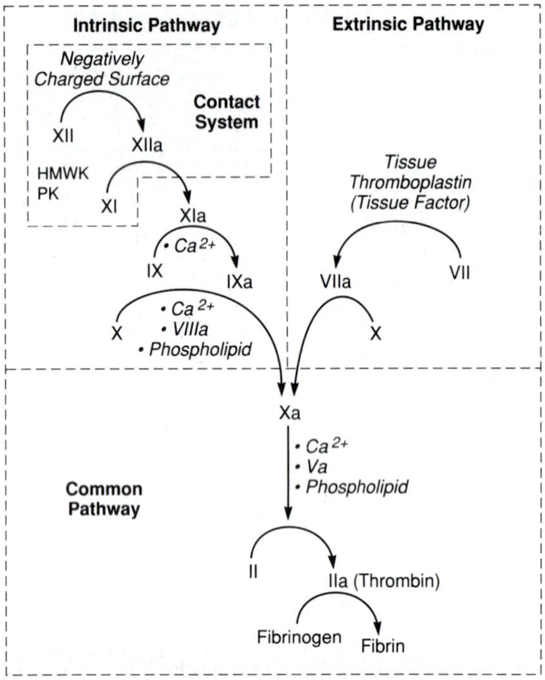

FIGURE 33-4. Waterfall or cascade scheme of coagulation. Coagulation was viewed in 1964 as a sequence of proteolytic cleavages. Because the intrinsic pathway was believed to be the physiologically important pathway, the extrinsic pathway was not included in the original formulation, although it was added over subsequent years.

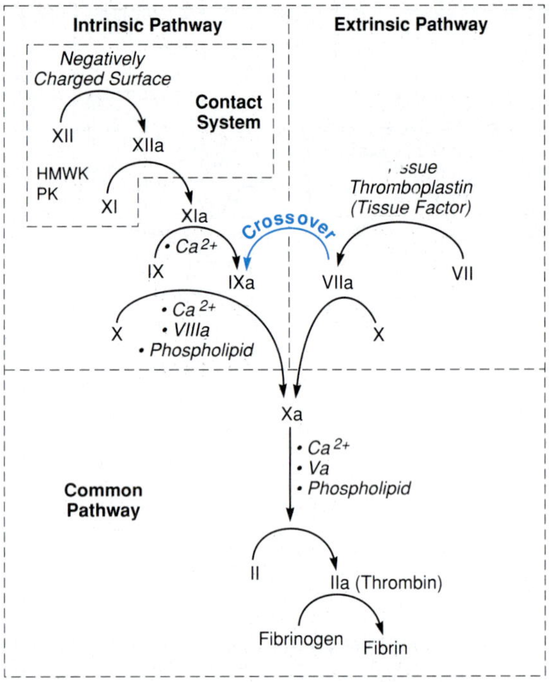

FIGURE 33-5. Crossover scheme of coagulation. After it was recognized that factor VIIa could activate factor IX, a crossover pathway was added to the coagulation scheme. This pathway allowed physicians to consider how proteins of both the intrinsic and extrinsic pathways might work together to promote physiologic hemostasis and provided a rationale for trials of factor VIIa infusions as therapy for patients with anti–factor VIII antibodies.

velopment of immunoassays[18] allowed coagulation system activation to be monitored directly. These assays can detect small peptides released while clotting factors (or fibrinogen) are activated or complexes of a protease and its regulatory antiprotease such as thrombin and antithrombin III. By monitoring the pathways of coagulation activation with these assays, it has become clear that the coagulation system is continually being activated in a controlled manner through the tissue factor (extrinsic) pathway.[19] Fourth, the ability of thrombin to activate clotting factors other than fibrinogen (such as factors V, VIII, and XI), stimulated consideration of coagulation pathways in which thrombin could provide a positive feedback signal and a degree of amplification not proposed in the classic cascade/waterfall hypothesis. Finally, the isolation and characterization of a lipoprotein-associated inhibitor of the extrinsic pathway (tissue factor pathway inhibitor [TFPI]), helped to focus attention on tissue factor-initiated hemostasis.

The history of TFPI illustrates how biochemical investigation may be driven by observations that have been made many years previously.[20] TFPI activity was first detected in plasma in 1947, when it was shown that preincubation of serum with tissue thromboplastin prevented the lethal reaction that occurs if thromboplastin is injected directly into animals.[21,22] It was not until the 1980s that TFPI was isolated,[23] its cDNA cloned,[24] and its mechanism of action defined.[25,26]

Unlike other antiproteases, TFPI circulates in plasma bound to lipoproteins (and was therefore previously called the lipoprotein-associated coagulation inhibitor) and is released in significant quantities by activated platelets. TFPI is different from other antiproteases, which bind only one protease molecule at a time, insofar as it contains three separate regions capable of binding serine proteases, known as Kunitz-type domains. One Kunitz domain binds factor Xa, one binds the tissue factor–factor VIIa complex, and the function of the third domain is unknown. TFPI is itself under a novel form of regulation. Because it must bind factor Xa before it can bind and inhibit the tissue factor–factor VIIa complex, TFPI's inhibitory activity is not expressed at the first exposure of plasma to tissue factor but only after factor Xa is produced. This ensures that coagulation is initiated before the tissue factor pathway is turned off. If TFPI were able to neutralize tissue factor–factor VIIa complex directly (that is, in the absence of factor Xa), coagulation would not occur until all the TFPI in the microenvironment were saturated, thereby prolonging the onset of clot formation and increasing blood loss. The inability of TFPI to bind factor VIIa in the absence of factor Xa probably explains why activated factor VII is able to circulate in an active form for a relatively long period of time[27] and may explain part of its success as a therapy for patients with factor VIII inhibitors.

Because the tissue factor–VIIa complex is inactivated by TFPI after coagulation has begun, a second mechanism must be responsible for the ongoing generation of factor Xa that is required to ensure complete clot formation. Two theories have been proposed to explain how this may occur, based on recently discovered biochemical interactions (Fig. 33-6). Both postulate that coagulation is initiated by the exposure of plasma to tissue factor, which leads to the generation of factors VIIa and Xa and thrombin. The two theories also agree that additional factor Xa depends on the activation of factors IXa and VIIIa. They differ only with regard to the mechanism responsible for factor IX activation.

One theory is based on a detailed analysis of factor IX activation. Factor IX must be cleaved at two points to become the fully activated protease (factor IXa) capable of cleaving factor X. Contrary to previous conceptions, factor

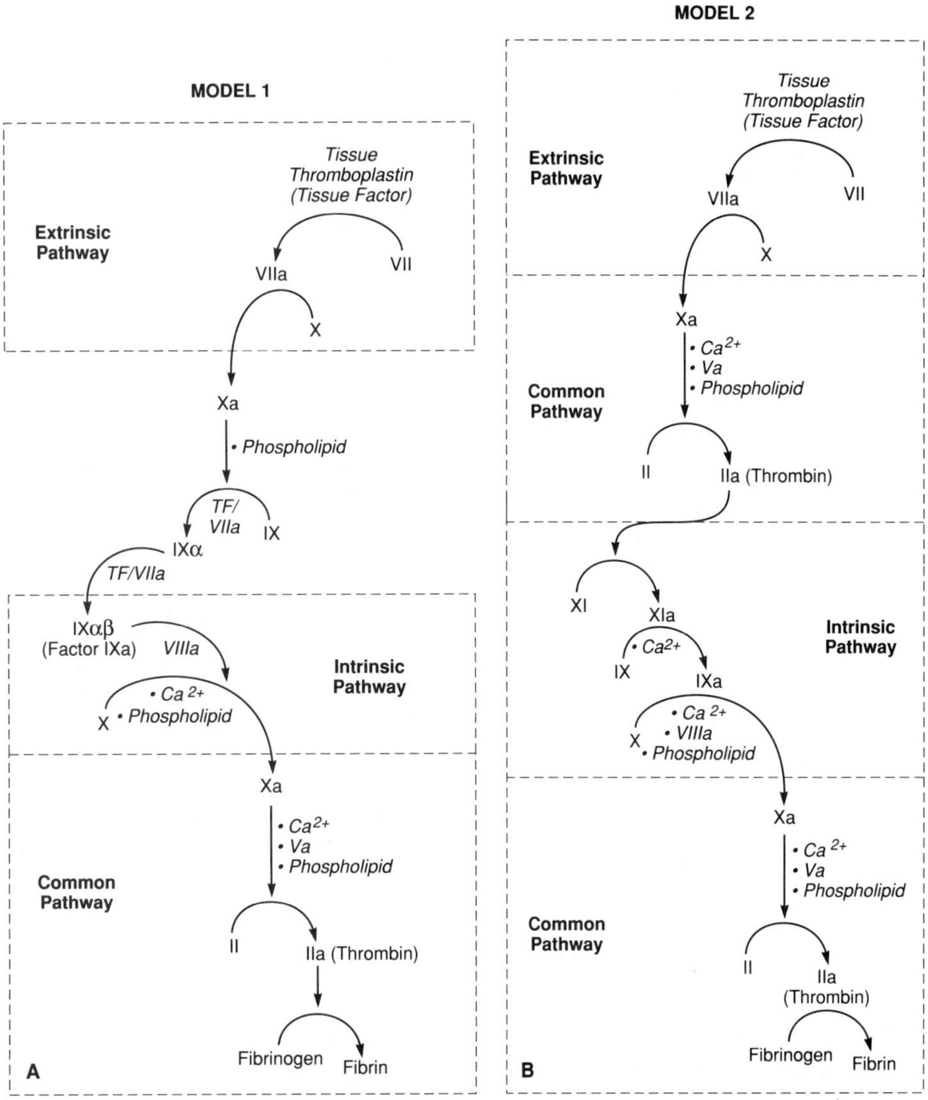

FIGURE 33-6. Current schemes of coagulation. The use of molecular markers of coagulation system activation and the delineation of tissue factor (TF) have led to new concepts of how the coagulation system functions. Both models are based on the idea that activation of coagulation follows exposure of blood to TF and the generation of factor VII. **(A)** Model 1 postulates that membrane-bound factor Xa makes the first of the two cleavages required to activate factor IX, generating the inactive species factor IX_α, which then undergoes further cleavage by the TF–factor VIIa complex to form factor $IX_{\alpha\beta}$ (also known as factor IXa), which is able to activate factor X in the presence of factor VIIIa. The overall flow, using the terminology of previous schemata, is extrinsic pathway → intrinsic pathway → common pathway → fibrin clot. **(B)** Model 2 is based on the observation that thrombin, in the presence of a negatively charged surface, can activate factor XI, thereby leading to activation of factor IX. The flow of reactions in this model is extrinsic pathway → common pathway → intrinsic pathway → common pathway → fibrin clot. Although differing in how factor IX becomes activated, the models are similar in their emphasis on the importance of TF-mediated factor VII activation in the initiation of coagulation and the obligatory involvement of factors VIII and IX in the generation of a fibrin clot. (**A** after Mann KG, Krishnaswamy S, Lawson JH. Surface-dependent hemostasis. Semin Hematol 1992;29:213; **B** after Broze GJJ. The role of tissue factor pathway inhibitor in a revised coagulation cascade. Semin Hematol 1992;29:159)

Xa can make the first of these cuts if exposed to factor IX in the presence of a membrane surface.[28] It has therefore been postulated that factor Xa generated by the tissue factor–factor VIIa complex makes the first cut in factor IX, generating the inactive precursor, factor IXα. The tissue factor–factor VIIa complex makes the second, generating active factor IXa, which in turn activates factor X. The resulting "pulse" of factor Xa is postulated to overcome the local concentrations of TFPI, allowing additional thrombin generation.[28,29]

The second theory is based on observations that factor XI can be activated by thrombin in the presence of a negatively charged surface.[30,31] It postulates that thrombin's activation of factor XI leads to factor IX activation, as conceived by the waterfall/cascade model. In this model, thrombin is not the last of the proteases generated by the coagulation system but an active participant in an active feed-forward loop. This model can account for activation of factor IX in the presence of uncomplexed TFPI.[20]

These models both postulate that coagulation is initiated by the extrinsic pathway, maintained by involvement of factors VIII and IX, and differ only with respect to how factor IX becomes activated. One theory emphasizes the importance of factor XI in blood coagulation; the other theory tries to account for coagulation without implicating it. Neither theory is able to fully explain why some patients with factor XI deficiency bleed and some do not, so neither is a wholly adequate explanation. Both theories may turn out to be true, depending on the circumstances. Because it has not been determined exactly what negatively charged surface is required physiologically for factor XI to be activated by thrombin, it is possible that this surface is not exposed to plasma under all conditions in which coagulation is required. When such a surface is present, coagulation may proceed via factor XI, and when it is not, via activation of factor IX by membrane-bound factor Xa.

Most important, both theories place tissue factor in a primary position with regard to the initiation of hemostasis and view the involvement of factors VIII and IX as obligatory for promoting clot formation. Thus, coagulation is the result of a carefully regulated sequence of events that involves elements of both the intrinsic and extrinsic pathways.

Mechanisms of Control of the Coagulation System

Although activation of the coagulation cascade is crucial, uncontrolled generation of thrombin can lead to disaster. Two major mechanisms are responsible for terminating the generation of fibrin: limited proteolysis of factors Va and

VIIIa by activated protein C (protein C_a) and neutralization of activated coagulation proteases by circulating antiproteases (Fig. 33-7).

The protein C system operates in two stages. First, thrombin binds to the endothelial surface protein, thrombomodulin, with a resulting loss of its ability to activate platelets and clot fibrinogen. This is not due to a simple quenching of its proteolytic activity, since thrombin bound to thrombomodulin is able to cleave protein C, a vitamin K–dependent protein. This mechanism represents an unusual example of how a protease's substrate specificity may be changed. The second stage of the protein C system requires the interaction of activated protein C with protein S, another vitamin K–dependent protein, and a cell surface. Under these conditions, activated protein C is able to make proteolytic cleavages in factors Va and VIIIa, which inactivates them and stops thrombin generation.

Several antiproteases are involved in the control of the coagulation system, all of which function by binding to or sterically interfering with the enzymatically active site of the relevant protease (see Table 33-1). The resulting protease–antiprotease complex can be detected by ELISA, using antibodies that bind to each component of the complex. Antithrombin III, the best-known antiprotease, is unusual insofar as it binds poorly to proteases in the absence of a cofactor (heparin or related molecules). Because antithrombin III–heparin complexes are unable to neutralize thrombin[32] or factor Xa[32,33] that are bound to a clot's surface, interest has developed in the clinical use of anticoagulant compounds that can neutralize proteases that are free in solution or bound to a clot surface. Two such compounds under clinical investigation are the thrombin inhibitor hirudin (and various derivatives)[34] and a tick-derived anticoagulant peptide capable of inhibiting factor Xa.[33,35]

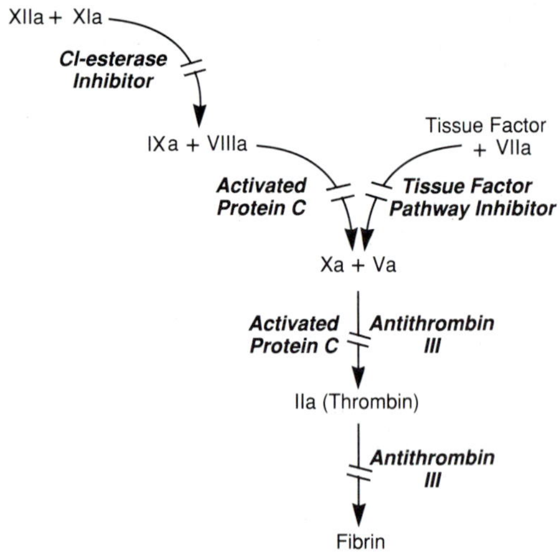

FIGURE 33-7. Major mechanisms of control of hemostasis. Regulation of the coagulation system is accomplished by the action of plasma proteins that either inhibit activation or terminate ongoing thrombin generation. One means of regulation is through the binding of inhibitors (tissue factor pathway inhibitor, C1-esterase inhibitor, and antithrombin III) to active serine proteases; another means is the proteolysis of required cofactors (factors Va and VIIIa) by activated protein C. Other plasma and endothelial proteins may also play an important role in regulating coagulation reactions. Different control mechanisms operate to regulate the activation and function of platelets and the fibrinolytic system.

TERTIARY HEMOSTASIS: CONSOLIDATION AND GRADUAL DISSOLUTION OF THE FIBRIN CLOT

Maturation of the Fibrin Clot

The study of bleeding problems experienced by patients with absent or abnormal plasma proteins has made it clear that clotting tests are not able to account for all abnormalities in clinical hemostasis and thrombosis. Increasing attention is therefore being paid to the molecular events that follow the initial formation of a fibrin clot, since, in some cases, these events are important in determining whether delayed bleeding or thrombosis emerges as a clinical problem. This phase of the hemostatic process is important in determining the life-span of a clot and therefore the natural history of an injured or occluded vessel, a thrombus, or an embolus. This period, here called tertiary hemostasis, may be broken down into several components: formation of a mature clot; cross-linking of fibrin monomers within the clot; cross-linking of auxiliary proteins to the clot; and controlled activation of the fibrinolytic system (Fig. 33-8).

The life-span of a clot may also be influenced by its cellular composition, which varies with the clinical circumstances. Different cell types may influence the natural history of a clot, including neutrophils, which can release elastase, a protease capable of cleaving fibrinogen and lysing fibrin clots[36]; platelets, whose granules release PAI-1, which inhibits plasmin generation,[37] and thrombospondin, which inhibits plasmin[38]; and fibroblasts, which can infiltrate clots and deposit collagen, thereby inhibiting fibrinolysis.[39]

The process of clot formation begins with the linear association of fibrin monomers first into protofibrils and then into long fibrils. The initial result of this process is the formation of a *fine clot*. The fibrils in the clot are flexible, rather than rigid, and are able to move, much as spaghetti moves in boiling water. When the fibrils come into contact with each other, they tend to self-associate, forming thick bundles. The resulting clot is called a *coarse clot*. The bundles scatter light and thereby change the optical properties of the clot. Clotted plasma is transparent initially and gradually becomes opaque over the next 10 to 30 minutes, well after clot formation has occurred. In addition to having different optical properties, fine clots are brittle and are easily fractured. This may be of clinical significance, particularly in regions in which the physical demands on the clot are great, such as the alveoli of mechanically ventilated patients.

Two lines of investigation indicate that clot structure is important in determining the clot's susceptibility to lysis, hence its life-span. First, clots formed in the presence of the radiocontrast agent iopamidol do not exhibit the usual fine-to-coarse transition and are resistant to lysis.[40] Second, abnormal fibrinogen molecules have been isolated from patients suffering from recurrent thrombosis that form fine plasmin-resistant clots.[41,42] Together, these studies suggest that clot structure may be clinically important in determining susceptibility to lysis.

Although the clot's structure may undergo significant change immediately after it is formed, it is soon locked into a fixed configuration by the action of factor XIIIa, which forms new covalent bonds between adjacent fibrin monomers, thereby cross-linking the clot. The first bonds are formed between two γ chains of adjacent fibrin molecules, whereas later bonds involve the long extensions of α chains. Electrophoretic analysis shows that HMW complexes are formed, indicating the fusion of many α chains. Cross-linking of fibrin clots is important because it enhances their rigidity and increases their resistance to plasmin-induced fibrinolysis. A failure to cross-link fibrin clots, or unusually rapid activation of the fibrinolytic system that exposes clots to plasmin before factor XIIIa has cross-linked the clot, results in clinically significant delayed bleeding. A number

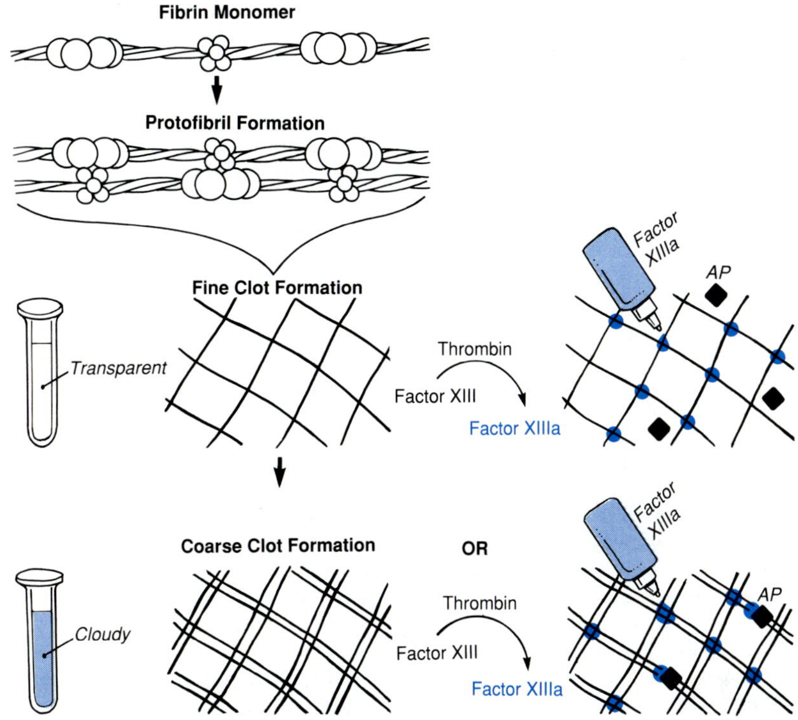

FIGURE 33-8. Tertiary hemostasis. The fibrin clot is initially transparent because its fibrils are randomly distributed in a fine meshwork. Until the clot becomes cross-linked by factor XIIIa (which takes place over several hours), the fibrils are able to diffuse within the clot and form stable side-to-side associations. The resulting thick fibrin bundles scatter light, rendering the coarse clot opaque or cloudy. Factor XIIIa, a molecular glue, cross-links fibrils to each other and forms covalent bonds between fibrin and key regulatory proteins, such as α_2-antiplasmin. Also part of this phase (not illustrated here) is the initiation of fibrinolysis by tissue plasminogen activator (tPA), which is released from endothelial cells in the vicinity of a thrombus.

of proteins are also cross-linked to fibrin's α chains, the most important of which is α_2-antiplasmin, because its absence is associated with premature clot lysis and clinically significant bleeding.[43]

Activation of the Fibrinolytic System

The fibrinolytic system is generally believed to be activated in concert with the coagulation system, although patients are occasionally seen who have clear evidence of an activated fibrinolytic system in the absence of the usual laboratory markers of coagulation system activation (Fig. 33-9).

There are two physiologic activators of plasminogen, tPA and urokinase. tPA is the major activator of the intravascular space and is released from stimulated endothelial cells. Urokinase is the major activator of the extravascular space and is synthesized by a number of cell types. Also found in neutrophil precursors, urokinase appears to be responsible for bleeding in some patients with acute leukemia, especially promyelocytic leukemia.[44] Although activation of the fibrinolytic system is commonly envisioned as taking place on the surface of a clot or in the plasma, fibrinolytic system activation is increasingly recognized as being a cell surface–associated event. For example, a variety of cell types can bind the components of the fibrinolytic system, including plasminogen,[45] plasmin,[46] urokinase,[47] and tPA.[48] A cellular receptor for plasmin has also been found on the surface of certain group A streptococci,[49] which is an evolutionary testimony to the importance of cell surface binding of fibrinolytic proteins.

Both plasminogen and plasmin bind to other proteins through specialized domains known as *kringles*, a configuration formed by three disulfide bonds within an 80-amino acid structure. Plasminogen and plasmin have five kringle domains, which bind to certain lysine residues of potential substrates (such as fibrin or fibrinogen) or cellular binding sites. The lysine-binding sites of the kringles serve as a site of action of two antifibrinolytic drugs, ε-aminocaproic acid and tranexamic acid. These compounds are lysine ana-

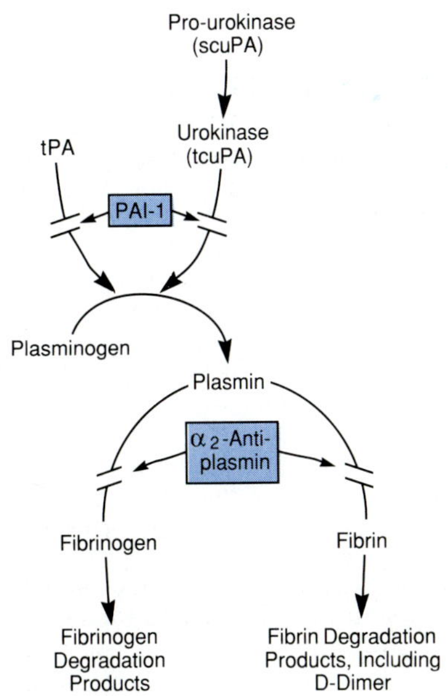

FIGURE 33-9. Fibrinolytic system pathways. The two major activators of the fibrinolytic system are tissue-type and urokinase-type plasminogen activators (tPA and uPA, respectively). tPA is fully active when secreted and is inhibited by plasminogen activator-1 (PAI-1), an acute phase reactant. uPA is secreted as a single-chain protein (scuPA or prourokinase) that is cleaved by plasmin to the two-chain form (tcuPA), which is used clinically as urokinase. Although both tPA and scuPA are much more effective plasminogen activators in the presence of a fibrin clot, their mechanism of action is different. tcuPA, on the other hand, quickly cleaves plasminogen in the absence of a clot, and its injection quickly leads to the generation of plasmin and fibrinogen degradation products. α_2-Antiplasmin is the major inhibitor of plasmin and can become depleted in states where there is ongoing fibrinolytic system activation.

logues and are able to bind the kringle regions. Given in sufficient amounts, ε-aminocaproic acid and tranexamic acid are also able to displace plasmin and plasminogen from fibrin clots, thereby preventing fibrinolysis. Thus, they inhibit proteolysis in an indirect manner.

Another class of plasmin inhibitors, typified by the drug aprotinin (also known as bovine pancreatic trypsin inhibitor or its European trade name, Trasylol), binds directly to plasmin's enzymatically active site, and thereby directly inhibits its enzymatic activity. α_2-Antiplasmin, the major circulating plasmin inhibitor, binds to both the kringle and active site regions of plasmin.

Each of the two major plasminogen activators differs from each other and from other serine protease zymogens in important ways. tPA is released by endothelial cells after injury or stimulation. Unlike most serine proteases, it is an active enzyme when secreted and does not require activation by another protease. Its affinity for plasminogen is low, and in the absence of a cofactor protein capable of binding tPA and plasminogen, little plasmin is formed, as when tPA is simply added to plasma. In the presence of an appropriate cofactor, tPA is brought into close contact with plasminogen and is able to make the single cleavage that converts plasminogen to plasmin. Fibrin is the most important of such cofactors, although similar effects are brought about by intracellular and extracellular proteins not normally considered to be part of the fibrinolytic system but that may be present in certain pathologic conditions.[50,51]

Urokinase is secreted as a single-chain molecule (called *prourokinase* or *scu-PA*), which is also relatively inactive in the absence of a fibrin clot. Prourokinase is susceptible to cleavage by plasmin, which generates two-chain urokinase, a fully active plasminogen activator, even in the absence of a fibrin clot. Two-chain urokinase is the species found in urine and the form used clinically for several decades. It had been thought that prourokinase is active only after it is cleaved to two-chain urokinase, but evidence indicates that prourokinase itself is active in the presence of a fibrin clot, indicating a unique mechanism of action.[52,53]

Two bacterial plasminogen activators, streptokinase and staphylokinase, have been studied in great detail, and used clinically. They differ from tPA and urokinase in their mechanism of action insofar as they are not serine proteases and do not directly cleave plasminogen. Instead, each binds to plasminogen, forming an activator complex that becomes capable of cleaving other plasminogen molecules, generating plasmin. Research suggests that staphylokinase may be more fibrin specific than streptokinase.[54]

Like coagulation proteins, fibrinolytic proteins are subject to regulation by specialized circulating antiproteases. The major inhibitor that neutralizes free plasmin is α_2-antiplasmin, whereas the major tPA inhibitor is PAI-1. PAI-1 is released from endotoxin-treated endothelial cells[55] and from the granules of stimulated platelets.[56]

Clinically significant bleeding may be associated with the excessive release of plasminogen activators, as occurs during liver transplantation,[57] or with the absence of the inhibitors of the fibrinolytic system (such as PAI-1[58–60] or α_2-antiplasmin[61,62]). Although some reports have correlated subnormal release of tPA with thrombotic events in certain families,[63] this type of measurement does has not provide a general approach for the clinical evaluation of patients with thrombotic disorders.[64]

High levels of fibrinolytic inhibitors such as PAI-1 have been associated with thrombotic states, such as acute myocardial infarction in some case-control studies.[65] Care must be exercised in studies of this sort because some plasma proteins (including PAI-1) are acute-phase reactants and their plasma levels may change soon after a clinical event and not correlate with plasma levels drawn in the basal state. These studies are valuable in making initial observations and generating hypotheses that can be tested in prospective studies, which are more rigorous methodologically. Prospective monitoring trials have contributed important information with regard to the relation between plasma levels of coagulation and fibrinolytic proteins and vascular disease. Examples include the confirmation of previously suspected correlations between low plasma fibrinolytic activity[66] or elevations in plasma fibrinogen concentration[67] and myocardial infarction; the failure to confirm observations made by case-control studies that PAI-1 levels are related to the subsequent risk of developing deep venous thrombosis[68]; the stimulation of new lines of investigation by revealing important associations not previously well appreciated, such as the relation between the risk of heart disease and plasma levels of tPA[69] or factor VII.[70]

In addition to modifying our concepts of risk factors, prospective trials may provide a basis for understanding clinical events. For example, a relation has been described between postoperative levels of plasma PAI-1, postoperative arterial thrombosis, and the type of anesthesia used (general or local) during lower-extremity vascular surgery.[71] Additional studies of this sort may lead to an increased understanding of the "fibrinolytic shutdown" that follows surgery and suggest ways that the shutdown might be ameliorated.

CHECKS AND BALANCES IN THE HEMOSTATIC SYSTEM

Although clinical thinking about hemostasis tends to focus on visible initiating events (surgery, trauma, bacteremia) or clinical endpoints (bleeding, embolism, thrombosis), hemostatic homeostasis depends on the appropriate function of relatively invisible control mechanisms (see Table 33-1). These controls effectively define thresholds of activation that must be surpassed for cellular or biochemical cascades to begin and define their physical and temporal limitations. If all goes well, they are unseen and unappreciated as they operate behind the clinical scene. Only relatively recently have deficiencies of some of these regulatory proteins been appreciated to cause bleeding or thrombosis. Unfortunately, tests of many of these regulatory proteins are not clinically available on short notice and therefore cannot rapidly influence clinical decision making.

When measuring plasma antiprotease concentrations, be certain of the type of assay (immunologic versus functional) that is being used. Immunologic measurements may not distinguish protease–antiprotease complexes from uncomplexed (free) antiprotease molecules, whereas functional assays measure only the free species. Newer immunoassays have been developed to measure specific protease antiprotease complexes.

INTERACTIONS AMONG MAJOR MEMBERS OF THE HEMOSTATIC SYSTEM

The frequent division of textbooks into separate chapters discussing coagulation, platelets, or the fibrinolytic system might suggest that these are independent entities, both clinically and academically. Based on both clinical and laboratory observations, it is becoming increasingly clear that this is not true. Three examples are offered to illustrate this point.

Generation of Thrombin at the Cell Surface

Phospholipids have long been known as being necessary for the rapid generation of thrombin. They are not free-floating but are incorporated into the plasma membranes of cells, particularly platelets, endothelial cells, and monocytes, all of which can bind activated clotting factors, most important, factors Va and Xa. Thrombin is thus generated on a surface and not simply in the fluid phase of plasma. This is important not only from the standpoint of how and where clot formation is initiated, but also because thrombin has potent effects on cells and can activate both platelets and endothelial cells to change their shape and release their granules into the extracellular space.

Generation of Plasmin at the Cell Surface

Although hematologic discussions of plasmin focus on its function as a fibrinolytic protein, it actually serves a more fundamental role physiologically and is a major protease of the extracellular space.[72] As such, it is able to regulate or influence a number of biologic events. For example, plasmin can cleave procollagenase into collagenase and convert latent transforming growth factor β (TGF_β) to an active form. It plays a major role in such diverse biologic processes as tumor cell migration, inflammation, ovulation, and trophoblast invasion.[72,73] As previously noted, cellular receptors are recognized for plasminogen, prourokinase, and tPA. Interaction of these proteins with their cellular receptors increases the rate at which plasminogen activators generate plasmin, while binding of plasmin to cellular receptors protects it from inactivation by α_2-antiplasmin.

Effects of Fibrinolytic Proteins on Platelet Function

An interaction of plasmin with platelets was first noted 20 years ago[74] and has since been recognized to be of clinical importance. The effects of plasmin on platelets are complex and seemingly paradoxical, for both platelet activation and inhibition has been reported. These disparate findings have been reconciled by following platelet function over time, which reveals that the augmentation and inhibition of platelet function are a function of the plasmin dose and time of exposure to platelets.[75] The effects of plasmin are also temperature dependent,[76] which may be clinically relevant in explaining differences in blood loss observed when cardiac surgery is conducted at different temperatures.[77,78]

Interest in the interaction between plasmin and platelets has been spurred on largely by the renewed interest in thrombolytic therapy for myocardial infarction that developed in the early 1980s and by the observation in the late 1980s that prophylactic administration of aprotinin reduced blood loss after cardiac surgery. The finding that thrombolytic therapy increased plasma levels of fibrinopeptide A, a marker of thrombin generation,[79] led to studies that have documented a previously unsuspected interaction of platelets with the coagulation and fibrinolytic systems.[80,81] Similarly, efforts to understand why aprotinin reduces blood loss during cardiac surgery[82] have led investigators to consider whether the platelet defect of cardiac surgery might result from the interaction of plasmin with platelets.[78,83]

INFLUENCE OF OTHER CELLS OF THE VASCULAR SPACE ON HEMOSTASIS

As the foregoing has emphasized, hemostasis is a complex process that involves the cooperative interactions of many components. Although platelets and proteins of the coagulation and fibrinolytic systems are the most important members of the hemostatic system, they are subject to influence by other cells found in the vascular space, as well as by cells and proteins of the extravascular space. The following are three examples of the multiple interactions that take place between the main members of the hemostatic system and other cell types.

Endothelial Cells

Endothelial cells interact with all three major components of the hemostatic system. They provide a surface to which factors IXa and Xa may bind, thereby promoting thrombin generation, and have receptors for tPA and plasminogen and thereby promote plasmin formation. Endothelial cells help to regulate the duration of coagulation system activation by virtue of the plasma membrane protein, thrombomodulin, which binds thrombin and allows it to activate protein C. As previously noted, endothelial cells produce substances (PGI_2, NO, ADPase) that directly affect platelet function and can also metabolize prostanoids released by other cells to form prostacyclin.[84] Finally, the endothelial cell synthesizes and releases both vWF and tPA when stimulated with agonists such as thrombin or histamine, and thus plays an active role in both clot formation and lysis.

Red Blood Cells

Long considered to be hemostatically inert, RBCs are increasingly recognized as playing a role in the hemostatic process. In 1910, Duke[85] noted that anemia resulted in the prolongation of the bleeding time. The idea that RBCs and platelets interact was strengthened by studies that showed that RBC transfusions shorten the prolonged bleeding time of many uremic patients.[86] More than 80 years after Duke's observations, laboratory investigations are beginning to provide explanations for these clinical findings.[87,88] Finally, many clinicians have noted that patients with severe anemia have retinal hemorrhages, which is commonly ascribed to tissue hypoxia. It is interesting to speculate that retinal hemorrhage in anemia is due partly to a diminished interaction of erythrocytes and platelets in a particularly vulnerable vasculature.

Although the outer surface of the normal RBC does not support the development of the prothrombinase complex, exposure of plasma to the phospholipids (notably phosphatidylserine) normally found on the inner surface of the RBC membrane accelerates coagulation.[89] Exposure of these phospholipids during major transfusions when cells are lysed in the intravascular space may at least partly explain the disseminated intravascular coagulation (DIC) that often accompanies this event. Their presence on the external surface of erythrocytes obtained from patients with sickle cell anemia[90] may explain observations of coagulation system activation in patients with sickle cell disease.[91,92]

White Blood Cells

White blood cells are able to influence platelets as well as some plasma proteins of importance for hemostasis. They down-regulate platelet function by virtue of an ADPase on their surface[93] as well as by their ability to produce NO, a platelet inhibitory substance.[94] Neutrophils release potent proteases such as elastase, which can alter the function of platelets,[95] endothelial cells,[96] TFPI,[97] and plasminogen.[98] Neutrophils can also metabolize icosanoids derived from platelets.[99] DIC is a well-known complication of acute leukemia and results from several distinct effects of immature neoplastic leukocytes on the hemostatic system.[100]

LABORATORY TESTS OF HEMOSTASIS

The time it takes for a fibrin clot to form or a bleeding time wound to stop bleeding are commonly used endpoints in the laboratory. These endpoints are not readily appreciated as being biologically meaningful values, since the normal values of bleeding and clotting time tests may be dramatically changed by alterations in the way the tests are performed. Normal values thus acquire meaning as a result of repeated correlations with clinical events, and errors in clinical judgment are made when seemingly reasonable extrapolations are made.

Many hemostatic tests were either devised for specific groups of patients or initially performed in an arbitrary, rather than clinically significant, manner. For example, the PT performed in the usual manner has long been recognized as being normal in patients with hemophilia.[6] It would be understandable to conclude on the basis of this information that tissue factor–initiated coagulation proceeds normally in hemophiliacs, but doing so would be premature. Instead, the conditions of the test should be varied, to determine whether the same conclusion can always be reached. (This point is of practical benefit when dealing with a lupus anticoagulant, as discussed in section on detection of circulating inhibitors.) In fact, when dilute thromboplastin is used to initiate coagulation, the PT of hemophiliacs is prolonged, a finding taken today to be compatible with the idea that coagulation is initiated by the tissue factor pathway but requires participation of factors IX and VIII.[10,101] It is appropriate to exclude hemophilia in a patient with a normal PT because the test as currently performed has been validated by clinical observation and experience. The clinician should keep in mind that many tests, especially functional tests such as bleeding and clotting times, which depend on incompletely defined interactions may be misinterpreted because of explicit or implicit assumptions that have been forgotten or overlooked.

The PTT was developed[102] and subsequently modified[103] to detect patients with deficiencies of factors VIII, IX, XI, or XII and not to detect those who might bleed during or after surgery. Since the prevalence of these hereditary deficiencies in unselected persons is low (less than 1%), the predictive value of a positive test also is low. It is not surprising that many abnormal preoperative activated PTT (aPTT) determinations are false-positives with regard to this endpoint.[104] (The aPTT may have value as a predictor of bleeding, if performed in high-risk patients,[105] emphasizing the importance of the pretest likelihood of disease in test utilization.)

The desire to avoid operative hemorrhage has resulted in the routine use of bleeding and clotting times that were never clinically validated for this purpose, despite longstanding pleas to the contrary.[106] For example, it has been known for some time that an abnormal PT does not predict bleeding after surgery or invasive procedures such as thoracentesis or liver biopsy, and some clinicians proceed under these circumstances on the basis of clinical experience. Others are unwilling to do so and give patients plasma transfusions in an attempt to lower the PT, assuming that they will reduce the risk of hemorrhage. The conflict between these views can be resolved only by analyzing clinical outcomes, so that the need for transfusion can be assessed objectively. Efforts in this area have documented the inadequacy of tests such as the PT in predicting bleeding.[107,108] This is not surprising because, although a mild depression of a single clotting factor does not prolong the clotting time, the simultaneous depression of several factors does prolong it.[109] This is unlikely to be of clinical significance. In addition, the normal range of the thrombin time is determined by the mean and standard deviation of the test performed on a given number of healthy people and is not a reflection of the normal range associated with good postprocedure hemostasis.

The history and use of the bleeding time are similar in many ways. The Ivy bleeding time, forerunner of the method used today, was developed because investigators wanted to develop a laboratory test that would be abnormal in a clinically defined patient population, much as the developers of the PTT sought to identify hemophiliacs by a laboratory test. Ivy wrote, "some way should be found to make a patients with a hypothetical latent bleeding tendency in jaundice bleed excessively from an ordinary skin puncture, and thus possibly make it manifest."[110]

None of the modifications made over the intervening years was designed specifically to aid in the preoperative evaluation of healthy patients but rather only to improve the reproducibility of the test or its sensitivity to aspirin ingestion. Given this history, it is not surprising that the bleeding time has not been found to be a valid predictor of bleeding when used as a screening test,[111–113] although many continue to use it for this purpose.

Commonly Used Tests of the Coagulation System

Prothrombin Time

The PT test is performed essentially as described by Quick[6] in 1935. It involves the addition of calcium and thromboplastin (a human or rabbit brain extract that provides both a phospholipid surface as well as tissue factor) to the patient's citrated plasma (Fig. 33-10). The amount of thromboplastin used in the test results in a normal value of about 11 to 13 seconds and causes a clot to form via the extrinsic pathway. It is sensitive to deficiencies of factors VII, X, V, II, and fibrinogen, as well as circulating inhibitors.

Thromboplastin preparations are widely recognized to differ in their ability to activate coagulation. A strong activator results in a normal PT, even with some degree of depletion of clotting factors. A weak activator is more sensitive to clotting factor depletion, such as that induced by warfarin ingestion, even though it may give the same result as the strong activator when tested with normal plasma. Different PTs can thus be obtained from the same plasma, depending on the thromboplastin preparation being used. Testing in different laboratories may lead to divergent conclusions regarding the adequacy of a patient's anticoagulation therapy, with attendant risks if the therapy is inappropriately modified.

Thus, the PT index (ratio of a patient's PT to a control PT) of different patients cannot be compared unless the same thromboplastin was used for all tests, making clinical trials and reports originating from different centers in Europe and America difficult to compare. As a result, efforts have been undertaken to develop a means whereby the degree of anticoagulation brought about by warfarin therapy may be compared, which depends on a mathematical formulation to correct for differences in thromboplastin

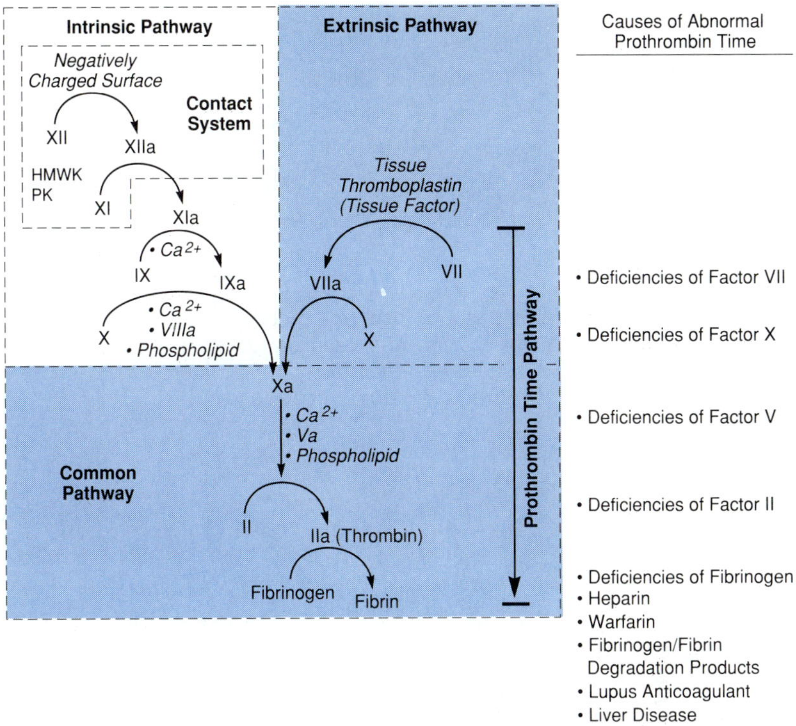

FIGURE 33-10. The prothrombin time (PT) of plasma was developed by Quick in 1935 and is based on Morawitz's model of coagulation (see Fig. 33-3*B*). Clotting is initiated by the addition of calcium and tissue thromboplastin, an extract containing both phospholipid and the glycoprotein now known as tissue factor. Because acquired fibrinogen deficiency was thought to be uncommon, and factors V, VII, and X had not been discovered, Quick concluded that a prolongation of PT was due to prothrombin deficiency. It is now recognized that this test depends on the functional integrity of the entire extrinsic pathway.

preparations. The use of this index, the International Normalized Ratio (INR), is hoped to lead to more uniform (hence, better) patient care. The INR is calculated from the formula:

$$\text{INR} = \left(\frac{\text{PT}_{\text{patient}}}{\text{mean PT}_{\text{normals}}}\right)^{\text{ISI}}$$

where:

$\text{PT}_{\text{patient}}$ = patient's PT (in seconds)

mean $\text{PT}_{\text{normals}}$ = mean PT determined in each laboratory using that particular thromboplastin

ISI = International Sensitivity Index, a value assigned to each thromboplastin by its manufacturer after it is calibrated against a World Health Association reference thromboplastin

The INR was devised to aid in the monitoring of patients taking oral anticoagulants.[114] The INR should not be used to assess the hemostatic system or thrombotic tendency of patients whose PTs are prolonged for other reasons.

Partial Thromboplastin Time

The PTT was originally performed by measuring the time required (usually 80 to 90 seconds) for a clot to form after phospholipid and calcium are added to citrated plasma. Greater sensitivity and reproducibility are obtained when a particulate activator of the intrinsic pathway (which uses factors XII, XI, IX, VIII, X, V, and II, fibrinogen, HMW kininogen, and prekallikrein) is used to initiate coagulation (Fig. 33-11). The resulting aPTT is used in almost all laboratories today and is especially sensitive to heparin and levels of factors VIII and IX below 25%. False-normal aPPTs may be seen in patients who are deficient in one clotting factor or have elevated levels of another (often factor VIII, an acute-phase reactant).[115]

Thrombin Time

The test for thrombin time is performed by measuring the time required for a citrated plasma sample to clot after the addition of thrombin (Fig. 33-12). The amount of thrombin used—hence the thrombin time—may differ among laboratories, and there is no standard normal value. The thrombin time may be prolonged by low levels of fibrinogen, abnormal fibrinogen molecules (dysfibrinogenemia), heparin, antibodies, or elevated levels of fibrin degradation products. The *reptilase time* is performed by substituting a snake venom for thrombin in the assay. Because reptilase is not inhibited by heparin, it may be used to confirm the presence of heparin in suspected samples, such as those drawn from intensive care patients with indwelling catheters. Prolonged thrombin times (usually performed using bovine thrombin) have been reported in patients exposed to topical (bovine) thrombin during surgery,[116] presumably because of immunization and formation of antibodies.[117] In most cases, this is of no clinical importance. There are reports of such patients developing a clinically significant antibody to factor V (human), presumably as the result of cross-reactivity with bovine factor V present in topical thrombin preparations, which may cause significant hemorrhage.[118,119]

Fibrinogen

A variety of methods are available for measuring plasma concentrations of fibrinogen, including immunologic techniques that detect the intact molecule as well as degradation products; salt precipitation methods; determination by chemical means of the amount of protein that is clotted by the addition of large doses of thrombin; and measurement of the rate of clotting of diluted plasma treated with thrombin (in quantities sufficient to overcome typical doses of heparin). The latter method (named after its inventor, Clauss) is commonly used but may be affected by the presence of high concentrations of fibrinogen degrada-

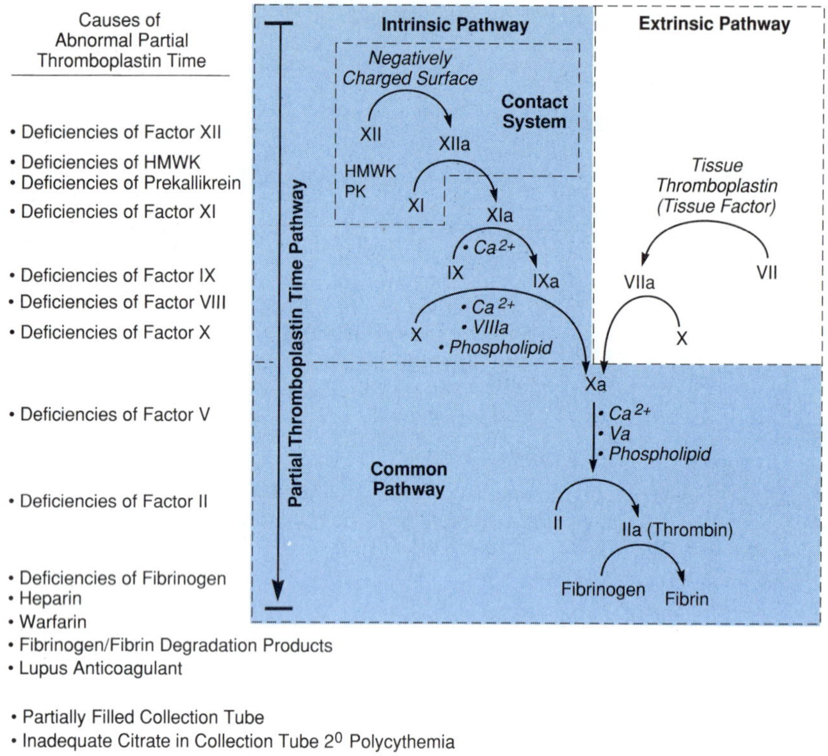

FIGURE 33-11. The partial thromboplastin time (PTT) of plasma was developed in 1953, as a way of differentiating normal subjects from patients with hemophilia. Coagulation is initiated by the addition of calcium and partial thromboplastin, which lacks the tissue factor found in complete tissue thromboplastin. The normal value for the original PTT was 80 to 90 seconds. The test was modified in 1961 to generate what is now known as the activated partial thromboplastin time (aPTT) by the addition of an exogenous negatively charged surface (such as kaolin, a porcelain clay). This results in more rapid activation of the contact system, whose members include prekallikrein (PK), high-molecular-weight kininogen (HMWK), and factors XII and XI, resulting in a normal value of about 30 seconds.

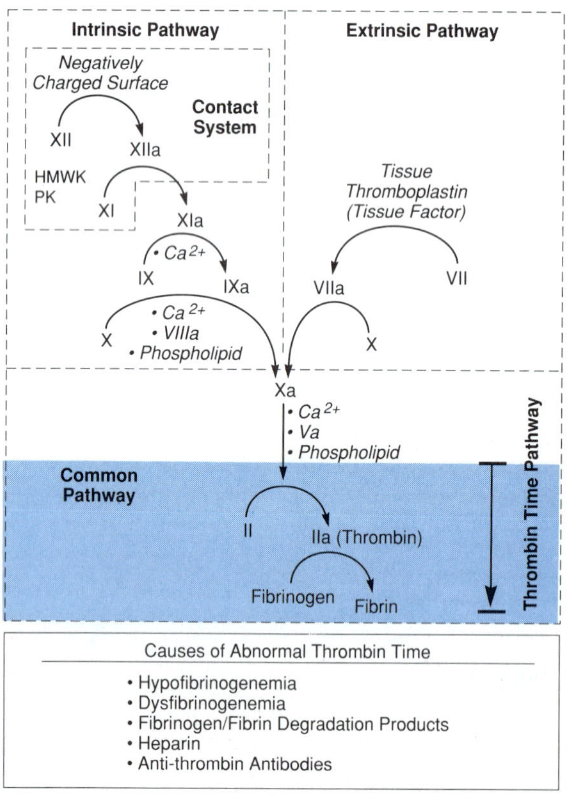

FIGURE 33-12. Thrombin time. The addition of thrombin (usually of bovine origin) to plasma results in cleavage of fibrinogen and clot formation. The normal value depends on the amount of thrombin added and varies from one laboratory to another. It has been recognized that some patients exposed to topical bovine thrombin during surgery may develop antibodies that prolong the thrombin time. Less frequently, these patients also develop antibodies to factor V and may also have prolonged prothrombin times and activated partial thromboplastin times.

tion products that can inhibit fibrin fibril polymerization, leading to an underestimation of the true fibrinogen concentration.

Tests of Fibrin and Fibrinogen Degradation Products

Several methods have been developed to detect proteolytic degradation products of fibrin or fibrinogen. These tests cannot distinguish fragments derived from fibrin from those derived from fibrinogen and are therefore said to measure FDP/fdp. (FDP refers to those species derived from fibrinogen; fdp refers to those from fibrin.) A commonly used assay for FDP/fdp uses an antibody to fibrinogen to detect fragments that are not removed when the patient's plasma is clotted by measuring the titer of the specimen able to agglutinate latex beads coated with antifibrinogen antibody. Some tests are calibrated so that the reciprocal of the least reacting dilution (titer) is equal to the plasma concentration (in micrograms per milliliter) of FDP/fdp.

A more recently developed test, which is being used increasingly more frequently, is the D-dimer assay. This test uses a monoclonal antibody that recognizes the new epitope formed when fibrin is cross-linked by factor XIIIa (see Fig. 33-8). Its detection in the circulation is thus taken to indicate the prior production of both thrombin and plasmin in the vascular space. It may be best used in conjunction with other assays for FDP for seeking to make the diagnosis of DIC.[120]

Coagulation Factor Assays

Coagulation factor assays are functional assays performed by determining how well a patient's plasma corrects the clotting deficiency of someone known to be lacking a specific coagulation factor. Although these assays are basically variants of the PT and aPTT, they require precision in their performance and specialized reagents to perform. Immunologic measurements of clotting factors are not generally available.

Detection of Circulating Inhibitors

One of the first steps taken by the clinician confronted by a patient with a prolonged clotting time, especially the aPTT, is to determine whether the abnormality is due to the lack of one or more clotting factors or to the presence of a circulating inhibitor, which slows coagulation. In some hospitals, the key test in making this determination is called the *1:1 plasma mix*; in others, it is simply known as an *inhibitor screen*. The test is based on the observations that clotting times are not prolonged when the level of any one clotting factor is greater than 25% to 30% of normal, and that circulating inhibitors are present in sufficient amounts that they retain their ability to slow coagulation when diluted. The test is performed by mixing equal volumes of the patient's plasma with plasma from a normal donor and then measuring the clotting time (aPTT or PT) of the mixture (Fig. 33-13). In some cases, it is useful to measure the clotting time at various time points after the mixture is prepared (0, 30, 60, 120 min). If the clotting time of the 1:1 mix is normal, the patient's defect is said to have been corrected by the addition of normal plasma, implying a lack of clotting factor as the explanation for the initial abnormally long clotting time. If the clotting time of the mixture is prolonged, the test is interpreted to indicate the presence of a circulating inhibitor able to affect the normal plasma, as well as the patients.

The four major types of circulating inhibitors are heparin (or other anticoagulants such as dermatan sulfate or hirudin); high levels of fibrinogen/fibrin degradation products; antibodies to coagulation factors; and antibodies that react with the phospholipid surface required for coagulation, which is called the *lupus anticoagulant*.

The first two causes of an abnormal inhibitor screen, heparin and elevated levels of fibrinogen/fibrin degradation products may be determined with routine clotting tests. As previously mentioned, it can be concluded that heparin is present if the thrombin time is abnormal and the simultaneous Reptilase time is normal. Antibodies that interfere with specific clotting factors are detected by finding depression of the plasma levels of only one factor. If multiple clotting factors appear to be depressed, the presence

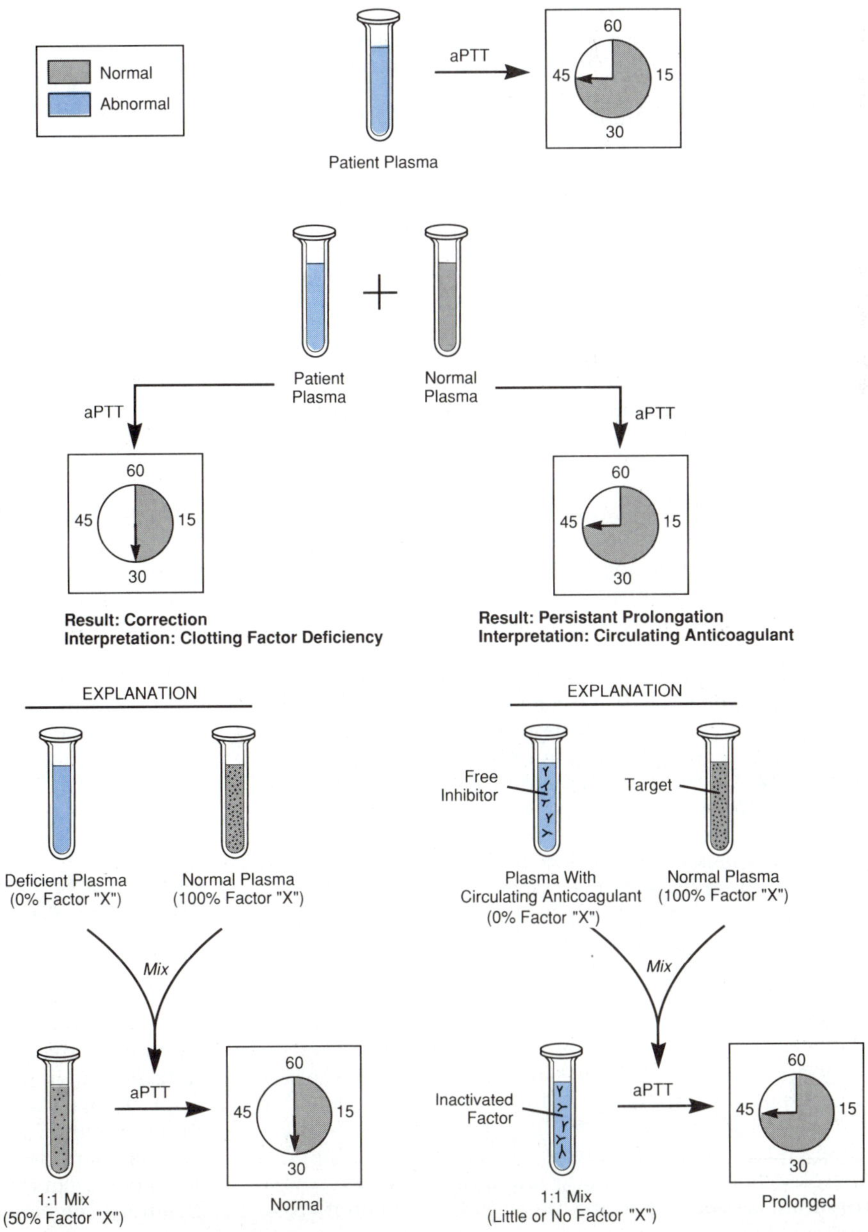

FIGURE 33-13. Screening for a circulating anticoagulant. Normal plasma contains at least a two-fold excess of all coagulation factors, and dilution of plasma with an equal volume of saline does not result in a significantly prolonged clotting time. Thus, if a patient has a long clotting time because of a factor deficiency, the clotting time will correct when a 1:1 mix of patient and normal plasma is tested. Additional testing to identify the missing coagulation factor should be performed. If the patient's plasma contains a circulating anticoagulant (eg, heparin, fibrin degradation products, a lupus anticoagulant, or a neutralizing antibody that reacts with a specific coagulation protein), the clotting time of the mixture remains prolonged because the inhibitor also inactivates the relevant factor or factors contributed by the normal plasma, and additional tests to identify the circulating anticoagulant should be performed.

of an antibody to a substance (phospholipid) common to all the clotting factor tests must be considered, that is, the lupus anticoagulant.

Lupus anticoagulants are antibodies, usually of the IgG class, which interfere with coagulation by binding to phospholipids and thereby inhibiting thrombin generation. Despite its name, the lupus anticoagulant is found in many patients who do not have autoimmune diseases and should be considered in everyone with characteristic laboratory tests results, regardless of their clinical status. The as-yet unexplained paradox of the lupus anticoagulant is that although the coagulation times are prolonged, most patients with a lupus anticoagulant do not have excessive spontaneous or postsurgical bleeding. This provides another example of the poor predictive ability of abnormal clotting tests for surgical bleeding. Furthermore, patients with lupus anticoagulants appear to have a greater than average risk of suffering from thrombotic disorders, another finding that has not been satisfactorily explained.

A number of coagulation tests may be used to look for the lupus anticoagulant in the patient with an abnormal inhibitor screen, including the tissue thromboplastin inhibition test, the kaolin clotting time, the dilute Russell viper venom test, and the aPTT.[121,122] Neutralization of the antibody's effects by the addition of excess phospholipid is advocated as a means of confirming the diagnosis. This may be accomplished by adding high doses of rabbit brain thromboplastin to the kaolin clotting time[123] or lyophilized platelets (platelet neutralization procedure).[124] The relation of lupus anticoagulants to antiphospholipid or anticardiolipin antibodies is confusing. Strictly speaking, lupus anticoagulants are defined by their property of affecting clotting tests. Because some patients with the lupus anticoagulant have anticardiolipin antibodies and others do not, it seems most appropriate at this time to consider them to be distinct but probably related, especially since many questions remain about their chemistry and mode of action in vivo.[125]

Antibodies to coagulation factor proteins are rare but clinically important and are usually associated with clinically significant bleeding. These antibodies most often arise in patients with moderate or severe hemophilia as a result of receiving replacement therapy, but they can develop in any patient with a severe plasma protein deficiency exposed to sufficient amounts of that protein. Because factor VIII deficiency is the most common congenital clotting factor deficiency state, antifactor VIII antibodies are the most common antibodies of this class detected in the laboratory. For reasons that have yet to be explained, factor VIII is also the most common antigenic target in nonhemophilic persons who spontaneously develop an antibody to a specific clotting factor. Although anti–factor VIII antibodies have spontaneously developed in normal persons as well as in patients with a variety of autoimmune diseases, they are most commonly present either in the elderly or in women in the postpartum period. These patients usually present with spontaneous, often severe bleeding. Surprisingly, the plasma of these patients may have measurable factor VIII levels (1% to 5%), even though they have moderate or high titer inhibitors.[126] Simple modifications of the aPTT allow factor VIII inhibitors to be detected in routine laboratories that are not able to perform the specialized Bethesda inhibitor assays used to quantify factor VIII inhibitors.[127]

Use of bovine thrombin as a hemostatic agent during surgery has been associated with the development of antithrombin and anti–factor V antibodies, as mentioned in the previous discussion regarding thrombin time. If the antibody reacts only with bovine thrombin, the patient has an isolated prolongation of thrombin time, because bovine thrombin is used to perform this test. Only when it cross-reacts also with human thrombin are the PT and aPTT be prolonged.

In some cases, it may be difficult to distinguish true anticoagulation factor antibodies from the lupus anticoagulant, a situation that may be worsened if decisions must be made at a time when specialized laboratory tests cannot be easily obtained. At such times, the clinician should analyze the situation in terms of the known natural history and associated clinical features that accompany these disorders and arrive at a working diagnosis. Even when the laboratory assistance required to measure clotting factor levels is available, uncertainty about the correct diagnosis may remain, especially if several factors appear to be depressed. Because factor level measurements are based on the same clotting tests that may be affected by the lupus anticoagulant, the clinician must consider whether one mechanism is responsible for all the abnormal tests, whether there are multiple antibodies to different clotting factors, or whether the patient has both a lupus anticoagulant and a specific anticlotting factor antibody.

Several points should be borne in mind that may help in considering this differential diagnosis:

1. Lupus anticoagulant antibodies are common.
2. True antifactor antibodies are rare.
3. The lupus anticoagulant is usually not present in very high concentrations, and its effects are more likely to be affected by diluting the plasma than are most antibodies to clotting factors. Therefore, if multiple clotting factors appear to be depressed, the clinician should call the laboratory and determine whether the levels were determined with relatively low (1:10) dilutions of the patient's plasma and, if so, request that they be determined with plasma diluted at 1:20 or greater. Thus, the effect of the lupus anticoagulant is such that levels of multiple clotting factors appear to increase (in relation to normal persons) as increasingly diluted plasma is assayed.
4. Acquired antifactor VIII antibodies, especially in nonhemophiliacs, do not alter the 1:1 mixing test if it is performed immediately after mixing, but they do prolong the aPTT if tested after a 1- to 2-hour incubation period at 37 °C.

Factor XIII cross-links fibrin monomers to each other after a clot has formed. Because clot formation, rather than cross-linking, is the endpoint of PT, aPTT, and thrombin time, a lack of factor XIII is not detected by these tests, and the clinician must specifically request a test of factor XIII function. The most frequently used tests are performed by placing a clot formed from the patient's plasma in a concentrated salt solution (5 mol/L urea or 1 mol/L monochloroacetic acid). In the absence of cross-linking (covalent bond formation), the fibrin monomers dissociate from each other and the clot is not visible after 24 hours, whereas a cross-linked clot is stable under such conditions.

Commonly Used Platelet Function Tests[128]

Bleeding Time

The test for bleeding time has the longest history of use of any hemostatic test.[129] Because it is the only test of platelet function in vivo, it is frequently said to be the best test of platelet function. Unfortunately, this idea has kept physicians from critically evaluating its performance in various clinical conditions. Research suggests that it should not be used as a screening test for asymptomatic persons who do not have a personal or family history of bleeding.[111–113] Bleeding time may be useful in examining patients whose personal or family history suggests a defect of platelet function (ie, immediate bleeding). A variety of drugs may affect the bleeding time, but many more drugs affect platelet aggregation studies but not the bleeding time.[130] Also, drug combinations may have unique effects on bleeding time. Unfortunately, relatively little information exists to help the clinician faced with patients using specific drug combinations.[131]

Platelet Aggregation Studies

Platelet aggregation studies have become a mainstay of the clinical coagulation laboratory, but their usefulness has also been called into question.[132] Platelet aggregation has traditionally been performed by examining the behavior of platelets in platelet-rich plasma. Whole blood aggregometers have also been developed that examine platelet aggregation without removing RBCs and WBCs. A consensus has not been reached as to which method is better for clinical use.

Platelet Release Reaction

Platelet release reaction may be studied in several ways. After radioactive serotonin (5-HT) is added to platelets, it is taken up and stored in the cells' dense granules. If the cells are then stimulated, the serotonin is released into the surrounding medium, where it can be assayed. Tests using this observation have been developed to identify patients with storage pool disease and to detect heparin-dependent antibodies. Dense granule secretion can also be monitored by measuring ATP release after the addition of an activating agent. α-Granule secretion results in the release of proteins such as platelet factor 4 and β-thromboglobulin, which can be measured by immunoassays.

Tests of the Fibrinolytic System

The euglobulin lysis time (ELT) determines how quickly a person's fibrin clot dissolves in autologous plasma. The plasma is first treated in a manner that removes fibrinolytic inhibitors and is then clotted. The time required for the resulting clot to lyse (usually 60 to 300 min) is proportionate to the concentration of plasminogen activators present in the sample (if there are normal levels of plasminogen and fibrinogen). The test is usually performed with the aim of determining whether a hyperfibrinolytic state is present (ie, the euglobulin lysis time is short). Hypofibrinogenemia may also result in a short ELT, and the fibrinogen level should be obtained near the time of the test's performance. An alternate evaluation of the fibrinolytic system may be performed by measuring how long a dilute clot takes to lyse.

Activation of the fibrinolytic system results in the production of FDP/fdp or D-dimers. Because activation of the fibrinolytic system is considered to be a physiologic response to fibrin deposition (which occurs normally in many inflammatory states), it may be difficult to differentiate normal from pathologic fibrinolysis with these tests.

An alternative way of assessing the activation of the fibrinolytic system is by performing a functional measurement of α_2-antiplasmin. Depletion of this antiprotease has been documented in diseases known to result in a hyperfibrinolytic state[62] and is used in some centers to guide the administration of antifibrinolytic therapy to patients with acute promyelocytic leukemia. Thromboelastography is used to detect excessive fibrinolysis during liver transplantation and to guide the administration of antifibrinolytic agents,[133] although it is not widely used in hemostasis laboratories.

CLINICAL BLEEDING SYNDROMES

Immediate Bleeding

Bleeding occurring immediately after a vascular insult suggests a failure of hemostatic plug formation. This is most frequently due to a failure of platelet function but may also be seen in patients with rare disorders in which the ability of the vasculature to support hemostasis is compromised because of a quantitative or qualitative platelet defect.

Delayed Bleeding

Bleeding that becomes evident hours to days after an injury indicates an inability to form a stable clot. The formation of the stable clot requires that (1) clot formation occurs in a timely manner; (2) continued accretion of fibrin into the clot occurs; and (3) the clot is able to resist (appropriately) the action of the fibrinolytic system to dissolve it. This last point is determined by several factors, including cross-linking of fibrin monomers within the clot by factor XIII; the amount of plasminogen activator released in the vicinity of the clot; and the local concentrations of the antiproteases that regulate the fibrinolytic system (α_2-antiplasmin and PAI-1). Thus, delayed bleeding may be due to one or more of the following five conditions: low levels of clotting factors, circulating anticoagulants, decreased amounts of factor XIII, increasing plasminogen activators, or deficiencies of α_2-antiplasmin or PAI-1.

Combined Immediate and Delayed Bleeding

Immediate and delayed bleeding implies the presence of both platelet function defects (or thrombocytopenia) and another factor that promotes bleeding. The clinician should consider vWD as a single cause in patients with a history compatible with a congenital disorder, and liver disease, DIC, or a paraproteinemia as possible acquired causes of this constellation of findings.

PATIENT WORK-UP

History

The hemostatic history is a key element of the clinical evaluation of the patient because its findings determine which laboratory tests are ordered by the clinician; it often requires careful interpretation of many subjective impressions or poorly documented clinical events. The areas to be covered may be grouped into several major categories, as shown in Table 33-3.

Many normal persons describe themselves as having suffered from excessive bleeding, whereas many persons with defined bleeding disorders have benign histories, particularly if they have not been exposed to a significant hemostatic stress. Because a hemostatic questionnaire alone is rarely adequate for determining a valid hemostatic history, the patient must be questioned personally by the physician. After the history, the physician can decide whether there is a high, low, or indeterminate probability that the patient has a bleeding disorder. This estimation can then be used in deciding which, if any, laboratory tests to obtain.

Physical Examination

The physical examination is usually not helpful in evaluating patients in the preoperative setting, especially if they are asymptomatic. Although bruises are of concern to many patients, extensive work-ups usually fail to reveal a defined

TABLE 33-3. The Hemostatic History

EVENTS ASSOCIATED WITH HEMOSTATIC STRESSES OF DAILY LIVING
Easy brusing, no recognized precipitating events
Easy brusing in response to minor trauma (Note if purpura or ecchymoses)
Hematoma formation or joint bleeding, no recognized precipitating events
Hematoma formation or joint bleeding in response to trauma
Bleeding after shaving
Excessive menstrual bleeding
Epistaxis
Gum bleeding (especially if not associated with gum disease)
Gastrointestinal tract bleeding (with or without telantiectasias)
Urinary tract bleeding
HEMOSTATIC STRESSES ASSOCIATED WITH MEDICAL PROCEDURES OR TRAUMA
Procedures associated with good surgical hemostasis
Most types of surgery
Procedures in which surgical hemostasis may be incomplete
Childbirth
Dental extractions
Abortions
Tonsillectomy
Needle biopsies
Trauma or fractures
Cardiac surgery
Circumcision
ASSOCIATED FACTORS TO INQUIRE ABOUT IF BLEEDING HISTORY IS POSITIVE
Transfusion history
Medications
Medical history, with particular attention paid to signs, symptoms, and laboratory data suggestive of diseases associated with bleeding
Acute or chronic liver disease
Renal insufficiency
Myeloma or paraproteinemia
Amyloidosis
Hypercortisolism
Myelodysplasia
Myeloproliferative disorders
Leukemia
Scurvy
Connective tissue disorders
Vasculitis
FAMILY HISTORY
Family members believed to be (or to have been) bleeders
Sex and age of affected and unaffected members
Evidence for defining a hemorrhagic tendency
Transfusion history
Cause of death (if applicable)

hematologic condition, especially if the patient is female.[134] Persons who are seen because of complaints related to skin hemorrhage should be evaluated for signs of vasculitis (palpable purpura); evidence of a coagulation factor, rather than platelet, disorder (as may be suggested by the presence of ecchymoses and not purpura); perifollicular hemorrhage (a sign of scurvy); and bleeding in areas not usually subject to overt or occult trauma. Physical findings of splenic enlargement or hepatic disease may help to focus the subsequent work-up.

Evidence of a coagulopathy may be sought in the hospitalized patient by examining the skin overlying the back, flanks, buttocks, and thighs for discoloration, which could suggest a deep site of bleeding, and by examining surgical or traumatic wounds, dressings, sites of catheter insertion, the sputum or stomach suction bottles, and urinary drainage bags.

Laboratory Evaluation

Evaluation of Patient Without History of Bleeding

Testing the category of patients with no history of bleeding is appropriately called *screening*. The term *screening test* has acquired two meanings with regard to the hemostatic system. The first indicates that the test itself is a screen for a hemostatic defect but is not specific for a given disorder. Thus, the aPTT is a good screening test for hemophilia because it is able to detect most patients who have the disorder, but it is nonspecific because its prolongation could also be due to poor collection technique, a lupus anticoagulant, or vitamin K deficiency. The term screening is more commonly used by physicians to indicate that one is testing patients who are judged to have a low risk of the disorder in question. A common example is the routine performance of mammography examinations for asymptomatic women.

Use of the expression, *screening tests of hemostasis*, means one thing to hematologists, who understand the limitations of the tests, but something else to other physicians, surgeons, and anesthesiologists, who are more often dealing with asymptomatic, nonbleeding patients. As a result, discussions by hematologists of screening tests of hemostasis may lead these physicians to conclude that it is appropriate to use these tests in asymptomatic persons. Discussion of this issue often provokes emotional responses, in large part because of the fear of catastrophic bleeding and a failure to consider the relevant clinical epidemiologic issues.

The performance of such routine tests in low-risk patients is to be discouraged for several reasons. First, if the probability of a patient's having a disease is low, then a positive test result has relatively little effect on the probability that the patient has the disease and is more likely to be a false-positive than a true-positive, even if the test has a high sensitivity and specificity (Fig. 33-14). An abnormal PT, aPTT, or bleeding time result obtained from a patient who has previously undergone surgery uneventfully and has no recent bleeding history or new medical problems is much more likely to be a falsely abnormal result than a sign of a true hemostatic defect.

Although there is usually an explanation for a prolonged clotting time—if only poor blood drawing technique[135]—the same cannot be said for a prolonged bleeding time, since it is not uncommon to find a prolonged bleeding time on one day and a normal one on the next without obvious cause. Many physicians are surprised to learn that the bleeding time has not proved itself as a predictor of surgical bleeding.[111–113] This is not surprising when it is realized that the bleeding time is frequently normal in patients with vWD,[136] the most prevalent and carefully studied platelet disorder, and that normal values are simply derived from the mean and standard deviations found in healthy ambulatory persons and not from the study of patients undergoing surgery.

After an abnormal screening test result is obtained, there is inevitably a delay of surgery, worry on the patient's part, and additional expense while consultations and additional

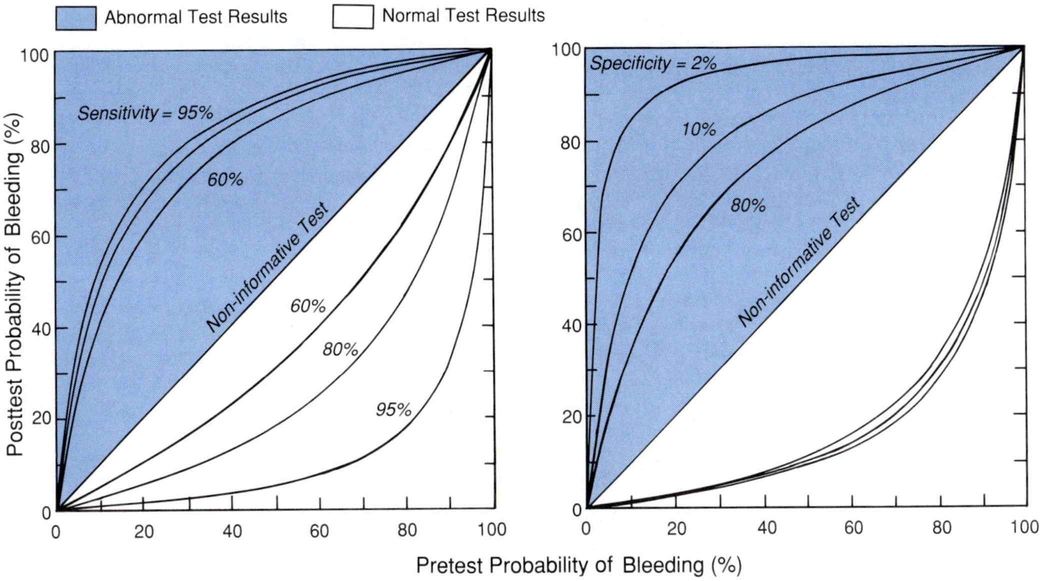

FIGURE 33-14. Application of Bayes' theorem to the assessment of the likelihood of bleeding in patients with abnormal coagulation test results. Bayes' theorem states that the probability that a disease is present when an abnormal result is obtained depends on the likelihood that the disease (here, excessive bleeding) is present in the patient before the test is performed. Thus, if the physician concludes on the basis of the history and physical examination that the patient has a low probability of having a hemorrhagic tendency, an abnormal result will not raise the probability of such a disorder to greater than 50% unless the test is highly sensitive and specific. The graphs show that the information gained from a test varies with the pretest probability that the disease is present as well as the sensitivity and specificity of the test. The curves above the line of identity (denoting a test that conveys no meaningful information) show the results of abnormal (positive) tests, and those below this line indicate the posttest probabilities if the results are normal (negative). (After Sox HC. Probability theory in the use of diagnostic tests. Ann Intern Med 1986;104:60)

laboratory tests are obtained. In some instances, physicians may administer transfusions of blood products in an attempt to correct the abnormal laboratory value. This exposes the patient to the risk of transfusion-transmitted diseases without necessarily decreasing the risk of perioperative hemorrhage.

In general, excessive surgical bleeding is uncommon. Although everyone fears a disastrous, potentially life-threatening hemorrhage, these low-incidence events cannot be avoided simply by ordering enough screening tests. Tonsillectomy, for example, is a procedure that is of concern to physicians because it usually involves children and a mucosal surface where surgical hemostasis may be difficult to attain. One study shows that even when screening tests are used, bleeding occurs in 2% to 3% of patients, comparable to that seen in other published series.[137] Thus, screening tests of hemostasis have little overall effect on eliminating operative hemorrhage in the setting in which there is little operative bleeding. Even less usefulness would be anticipated when applied to operations in which all patients lose significant amounts of blood. The importance of detecting mild defects in the hemostatic system is also minimized in operations in which good surgical hemostasis is possible, since one suture is equivalent to many tens of thousands of platelets.

Evaluation of Patient With Family History of Bleeding

Several hemostatic disorders with genetic components warrant specialized evaluation. The most common is vWD, estimated to affect about 1 in 1000 persons (although estimates range widely, from 1 in 100 to 1 in 10,000). Most persons have type I vWD, have only a mild bleeding disorder, and inherit the disease in an autosomal dominant pattern. Rarely, vWD may be inherited in an autosomal recessive manner.

Hemophilia A (factor VIII deficiency) accounts for about 85% of the congenital clotting factor deficiencies and affects 1 in 10,000 males. It is generally inherited in a sex-linked manner, and women who are carriers generally (but not invariably) have no symptoms. Hemophilia B (factor IX) deficiency accounts for about 10% of the hereditary coagulopathies and is inherited in a sex-linked manner. It is clinically indistinguishable from factor VIII deficiency. Persons with mild hemophilia (A or B) have levels that are 5% to 25% of normal levels and may not experience any bleeding until they experience surgical or traumatic stresses. Rare cases of apparent autosomal hemophilia have been recognized as well, which appear to be due to a mutation in the vWF gene, which leads to a failure of vWF to bind to factor VIII and protect it from rapid degradation in the circulation.

Factor XI deficiency is usually thought to affect mainly Ashkenazi Jews (whose calculated gene frequency for factor XI deficiency ranges from 2% to 12%, depending on location). Many factor XI–deficient patients are not of Jewish origin,[138] and a different ethnic background should not preclude testing for this disorder under appropriate circumstances.

Evaluation of Patient With Clear or Questionable Bleeding History

The history may clearly indicate a bleeding tendency (clinical estimate of the probability of a bleeding disorder of more than 90%) or may simply raise the probability above the baseline level that one has for previously unstressed patients (less than 5%). In this intermediate range of probabilities, clinical test results have their greatest effects (see Fig. 33-14). The same initial laboratory approach should be taken for evaluating both groups of patients. The tests usually obtained include a complete blood count and platelet count, aPTT, PT, thrombin time, and fibrinogen level. If the patient is known to have a disorder associated with DIC, a test for fibrinogen/fibrin degradation products or D-dimer may be useful. If the history is suggestive of a disorder of primary hemostasis, a bleeding time test may be useful as well. If these tests are normal, the clinician must decide whether the history warrants additional testing. Table 33-4 suggests additional testing that may be performed. Referral of the patient or the patient's plasma to a specialized laboratory for additional testing may be advisable.

WORK-UP OF COMMON ABNORMALITIES OF HEMOSTATIC SCREENING TESTS

Abnormal Platelet Count

There are many causes of a low platelet count, some of which are shown in Table 33-5. Because platelet counts are no longer obtained only on physician request, many asymptomatic patients are incidentally discovered to have thrombocytopenia when screening complete blood counts are obtained. No cause is usually found, and patients are thus accurately classified as having idiopathic thrombocytopenia. Although not well documented, clinical observation suggests that the natural history of patients with low platelet counts is benign. The usefulness of the Coombs' test in diagnosing autoimmune hemolytic anemia has led many to assume that a positive test for antiplatelet antibodies should be obtained before making the diagnosis of idiopathic thrombocytopenia, but there are many reasons for not accepting this as a necessary criterion for making this diagnosis. First, a variety of tests are used in different centers, and cross-center validation of assays is not possible. Second, as many as 15% of clinically diagnosed patients with idiopathic thrombocytopenia may have negative tests, depending on the assay. Third, all platelet-associated IgG is not necessarily antiplatelet antibody, since IgG may be found in the platelet α granules, in the surface-connected canalicular system, or on the plasma membrane, and care must be taken in interpreting these tests.[139] This may explain why the positive predictive value of one test measuring platelet-associated IgG was only 46%.[140] Furthermore, immune complexes bind to platelet surfaces during viral and bacterial infections[141,142] and may be mistaken for true antiplatelet antibodies.

TABLE 33-4. Unusual Causes of Bleeding

PLATELET DEFECTS

- Plasma membrane receptor defects
  - gpIb/IX—Bernard-Soulier syndrome, pseudo-von Willebrand's disease
  - gpIIb/IIIa—Glanzmann's thrombasthenia
- Platelet granule deficiencies (storage pool disease)
- Hereditary thrombocytopenias, including Alport's syndrome, Fanconi's syndrome, thrombocytopenia with absent radius syndrome
- Platelet function defects associated with other congenital abnormalities, including Wiskott-Aldrich syndrome, Hermansky-Pudlak syndrome (albinism), Chediak-Higashi syndrome, May-Hegglin anomaly, Ehlers-Danlos syndrome
- Snake venoms

COAGULATION PROTEIN DEFECTS

- Deficiencies of factors II, V, X, VII, XIII
- Dysfibrinogenemia
- Antibodies to coagulation factors
- Amyloidosis
- Snake venoms

EXCESSIVE FIBRINOLYTIC SYSTEM ACTIVATION

- α_2-Antiplasmin deficiency
- Plasminogen activator inhibitor deficiency
- Thrombolytic agents
- Acute promyelocytic leukemia
- Cardiopulmonary bypass
- Amyloidosis
- Liver disease, liver transplantation

TABLE 33-5. Common Causes of Thrombocytopenia

IMMUNE

- Primary
  - Idiopathic (autoimmune)
- Secondary (immune complex mediated)
  - Collagen vascular diseases, especially systemic lupus erythematosus
  - Infections, including viruses such as human immunodeficiency virus, parasites, bacteria
  - Malignancies
  - Drugs
- Posttransfusion purpura
- Alloimmune thrombocytopenia (in newborns)

NONIMMUNE

- Marrow suppression due to infection
- Drugs, including alcohol
- Disseminated intravascular coagulation
- Thrombotic thrombocytopenic purpura
- Hemolytic–uremic syndrome
- Hypersplenism
- Pregnancy
  - Benign thrombocytopenia of pregnancy
  - Preeclampsia
  - HELLP syndrome (hemolysis, elevated liver enzymes, and low platelet counts)
  - Eclampsia
- Aplastic anemia
- Marrow infilatration (tuberculosis, granulomas, myelofibrosis, leukemia, myeloma, carcinoma)
- Myelodysplastic syndrome
- Vitamin B_{12} or folate deficiency, rarely iron deficiency
- Radiation therapy
- Renal transplant rejection
- Massive transfusion (dilutional)
- Intravascular devices

PSEUDOTHROMBOCYTOPENIA

- Clotting of blood specimen
- Platelet-reactive cold agglutinins
- Clumping due to antibodies reacting with chelating anticoagulants

Abnormal Bleeding Time

There are many reported causes of a prolonged bleeding time (Table 33-6). In many cases, the abnormal test result cannot be duplicated. This may be due to variations in technique, cessation of drugs (or combinations of drugs) that affect the bleeding time, or otherwise unexplained bi-

TABLE 33-6. Common Causes of a Prolonged Bleeding Time

Thrombocytopenia
von Willebrand's disease
Drugs
Aspirin
Nonsteroidal antiinflammatory agents
High-dose penicillins
Drug combinations
Uremia
Cirrhosis
Myeloproliferative disorders
Myelodysplastic disorders
Paraproteinemia
Platelet dysfunction syndromes
Chronic disseminated intravascular coagulation

ologic variability of the sort that has been documented to occur in patients with vWD. Although normal upper limits for this test usually range from 9 to 10 minutes, many clinicians believe that minor prolongations (up to 15 minutes) are not associated with a significant bleeding risk. A minor prolongation of the bleeding time should not overshadow a patient's history of successful surgical hemostasis, especially if the surgery involved the creation of irregular mucosal surfaces (as follows tonsillectomy or dental extraction) that are known to be associated with excessive bleeding in patients with vWD.

Persistent or extreme abnormalities in the bleeding time may justify platelet aggregation studies and other specialized tests to determine whether the patient has vWD. Although platelet aggregation studies are frequently ordered, their overall benefit is unclear. Because vWD, renal or liver disease, drug ingestion, and unexplained variability in the bleeding time all are more common causes of a prolonged bleeding time than primary platelet disorders (storage pool disease, Bernard-Soulier disease, thrombasthenia), a stepped approach to the evaluation of platelet function is warranted.[132]

Abnormal Coagulation Tests

Causes of abnormal coagulation tests are shown in Table 33-7. The clinician should know that some plasma protein deficiencies are not associated with an increased risk of bleeding, even though they cause a prolonged clotting time, typically the aPTT.

If the history suggests that the probability of a bleeding disorder is moderate to high, the clinician should consider further testing to determine whether the patient has a factor XIII deficiency or an abnormality affecting proteins of the fibrinolytic system (see Table 33-4). Also, patients with mild hemophilia may have clotting factor levels as high as 25% of normal and may exhibit minimal elevations of aPTT. Such patients frequently report that they have experienced little or no bleeding until challenged with surgery, after which they suffer from delayed bleeding. For this reason, a minimally prolonged aPTT in a male patient who has not previously undergone surgery should be followed by measurements of factor VIII and IX levels, even if he has no family history of bleeding.

SUMMARY

Despite many years of study, and establishment of the basic principles that define the workings of the hemostatic system, an ongoing rapid evolution is occurring in knowledge

TABLE 33-7. Abnormal Coagulation Tests

CAUSES OF PROLONGED CLOTTING TESTS
Partial thromboplastin time (aPTT)
Clotting factor deficiencies (except factor VII)
Antibodies to clotting factors
Lupus anticoagulant
Heparin
Elevated fibrin degradation products
Warfarin or related compounds
Prothrombin time (PT)
Deficiencies of factors VII, X, V, II, fibrinogen
Antibodies to clotting factors
Elevated fibrin degradation products
Occasionally lupus anticoagulant
Heparin
Warfarin or related compounds
Thrombin time (TT)
Low or absent fibrinogen
Dysfibrinogenemia
Heparin
Elevated fibrin degradation products
Hyperfibrinogenemia
Antibodies to thrombin
COAGULATION ABNORMALITIES ASSOCIATED WITH INCREASED RISK OF HEMORRHAGE
Prolonged aPTT (other tests normal)
Factor VIII deficiency
Factor IX deficiency
Factor XI deficiency (in some patients)
von Willebrand's disease
Prolonged PT (other tests normal)
Warfarin or related compounds
Vitamin K deficiency (particularly intensive care patients)
Liver disease
Factor VII deficiency
Combined prolongation of PT and PTT
Warfarin or related compounds
Vitamin K deficiency (particularly intensvie care patients)
Liver disease
Disseminated intravascular coagulation or excessive fibrinolysis
Factor X deficiency
Factor V deficiency
Factor II (prothrombin) deficiency
Hypofibrinogenemia
Heparin
Abnormal inhibitor screening test (1:1 plasma mix)
Antibody to clotting factor
Most common: anti–factor VIII, see both in patients with hemophilia A and in previously healthy persons
Antibodies to factor V in surgical patients exposed to topical thrombin
Heparin
Fibrin degradation products
Lupus anticoagulant in a patient with thrombocytopenia or low factor II
LABORATORY ABNORMALITIES NOT ASSOCIATED WITH INCREASED RISK OF BLEEDING
Lupus anticoagulant (unless associated with thrombocytopenia or low factor II)
Factor XII deficiency
Prekallikrein deficiency
High-molecular-weight kininogen deficiency
Some patients with prolonged bleeding times

concerning this system, which has direct bearing on the clinical management of patients. The ability to evaluate and treat patients with congenital hemostatic defects is relatively well developed. Unfortunately, available laboratory tests are not able to predict with a high degree of accuracy which apparently normal patients will bleed with surgical stress. For this reason, the history, as imperfect as it may be, remains the best tool for determining which patients may be at increased risk for hemorrhage. Extra efforts aimed at obtaining a good history through questioning by the physician and at ensuring good surgical hemostasis are more likely to prevent excessive bleeding than adopting a rigid schedule of screening laboratory tests.

REFERENCES

1. Sixma JJ, Wester J. The hemostatic plug. Semin Hematol 1977;14:265.
2. Marcus AJ, Safier LB, Hajjar KA, et al. Inhibition of platelet function by an aspirin-insensitive endothelial cell ADPase: thromboregulation by endothelial cells. J Clin Invest 1991;88:1690.
3. Moake JL, McPherson PD. von Willebrand factor in thrombotic thrombocytopenic purpura and the hemolytic-uremic syndrome. Transfus Med Rev 1990;4:163.
4. Wick TM, Moake JL, Udden MM, Eskin SG, Sears DA, McIntire LV. Unusually large von Willebrand factor multimers increase adhesion of sickle erythrocytes to human endothelial cells under controlled flow conditions. J Clin Invest 1987;80:905.
5. Rodgers GM. Hemostatic properties of normal and perturbed vascular cells. FASEB J 1988;2:116.
5a. Morawitz P. Die Chemie der Blutgerinnung. Ergebn Physiol 1905: 307.
6. Quick AJ, Stanley-Brown M, Bancroft FW. A study of the coagulation defect in hemophilia and in jaundice. Am J Med Sci 1935;190:501.
7. Conley CL, Hartmann RC, Worse WI. The clotting behavior of human "platelet-free" plasma: evidence for the existence of a "plasma thromboplastin." J Clin Invest 1949;28:340.
8. Lister J. On the coagulation of the blood. Proc R Soc Lond 1863;12: 580.
9. Dam H, Venndt H. Observations on the coagulation of blood plasma in haemophilia. Lancet 1940;238:70.
10. Biggs R, Nossel HL. Tissue extract and the contact reaction in blood coagulation. Thromb Diath Haemorrh 1961;6:1.
11. Wessler S, Reimer SM, Sheps MC. Biologic assay of a thrombosis-inducing activity in human serum. J Appl Physiol 1959;14:943.
12. Davie EW, Ratnoff OD. Waterfall sequence for intrinsic blood clotting. Science 1964;145:1210.
13. Macfarlane RG. An enzyme cascade in the blood clotting mechanism, and its function as a biochemical amplifier. Nature 1964;202:498.
14. Østerud B, Rapaport SI. Activation of factor IX by the reaction product of tissue factor and factor VII: additional pathway for initiating blood coagulation. Proc Natl Acad Sci USA 1977;74:5260.
15. Seligsohn U, Østerud B, Brown SF, Griffin JH, Rapaport SI. Activation of human factor VII in plasma and in purified systems: roles of activated factor IX, kallikrein, and activated factor XII. J Clin Invest 1979;64:1056.
16. Bach R, Nemerson Y, Konigsberg W. Purification and characterization of bovine tissue factor. J Biol Chem 1981;256:8324.
17. Drake TA, Morrissey JH, Edgington TS. Selective cellular expression of tissue factor in human tissues. Am J Pathol 1989;134:1087.
18. Bauer KA. Laboratory markers of coagulation activation. Arch Pathol Lab Med 1993;117:71.
19. Bauer KA, Mannucci PM, Gringeri A, et al. Factor IXa–factor VIIIa–cell surface complex does not contribute to the basal activation of the coagulation mechanism in vivo. Blood 1992;79:2039.
20. Broze GJJ. The role of tissue factor pathway inhibitor in a revised coagulation cascade. Semin Hematol 1992;29:159.
21. Schneider C. The active principle of placental toxin: thromboplastin; its inactivator in blood: antithromboplastin. Am J Physiol 1947;149: 123.
22. Thomas L. Studies on the intravascular thromboplastin effect of tissue suspensions in mice. II. A factor in normal rabbit serum which inhibits the thromboplastin effect of the sedimentable tissue component. Bull Johns Hopkins Hosp 1947;81:26.
23. Broze GJJ, Miletich JP. Isolation of the tissue factor inhibitor produced by HepG2 hepatoma cells. Proc Natl Acad Sci USA 1987;84:1886.
24. Wun T-C, Kretzmer KK, Girard TJ, Miletich JP, Broze GJJ. Cloning and characterization of a cDNA coding for the lipoprotein-associated coagulation inhibitor shows that it consists of three tandem Kunitz-type inhibitory domains. J Biol Chem 1988;263:6001.
25. Rao LVM, Rapoport SI. Studies of a mechanism inhibiting the initiation of the extrinsic pathway of coagulation. Blood 1987;69:645.
26. Broze GJJ, Warren LA, Novotny WF, Higuchi DA, Girard JJ, Miletich JP. The lipoprotein inhibitor that inhibits the factor VII-tissue factor complex also inhibits factor Xa: insight into its possible mechanism of action. Blood 1988;71:335.
27. Seligsohn U, Kasper CK, Østerud B, Rapaport SI. Activated factor VII: presence in factor IX concentrates and persistence in the circulation after infusion. Blood 1979;53:828.
28. Lawson JH, Mann KG. The cooperative activation of human factor IX by the human extrinsic pathway of blood coagulation. J Biol Chem 1991;266:11317.
29. Mann KG, Krishnaswamy S, Lawson JH. Surface-dependent hemostasis. Semin Hematol 1992;29:213.
30. Gailani D, Broze GJJ. Factor XI activation in a revised model of blood coagulation. Science 1991;253:909.
31. Naito K, Fujikawa K. Activation of human blood coagulation factor XI independent of factor XII: factor XI is activated by thrombin and factor XIa in the presence of negatively charged surfaces. J Biol Chem 1991;266:7353.
32. Hogg PJ, Jackson CM. Fibrin monomer protects thrombin from inactivation by heparin-antithrombin III: implications for heparin efficacy. Proc Natl Acad Sci USA 1989;86:3619.
33. Eisenberg PR, Siegel JE, Abendschein DR, Miletich JP. Importance of factor Xa in determining the procoagulant activity of whole-blood clots. J Clin Invest 1993;91:1877.
34. Weitz JI, Hudoba M, Massel D, Maraganore J, Hirsh J. Clot-bound thrombin is protected from inhibition by heparin-antithrombin III but is susceptible to inactivation by antithrombin III-independent inhibitors. J Clin Invest 1990;86:385.
35. Sitko GR, Ramjit DR II, Lehman D, Lynch JJ, Vlasuk GP. Conjunctive enhancement of enzymatic thrombolysis and prevention of thrombotic reocculsion with the selective factor Xa inhibitor, tick anticoagulant peptide. Circulation 1992;85:805.
36. Plow EF, Edgington TS. An alternative pathway for fibrinolysis. I. The cleavage of fibrinogen by leukocyte proteases at physiologic pH. J Clin Invest 1975;56:30.
37. Braaten JV, Handt S, Jerome WG, Kirkpatrick J, Lewis JC, Hantgan RR. Regulation of fibrinolysis by platelet-released plasminogen activator inhibitor 1: light scattering and ultrastructural examination of lysis of a model platelet-fibrin thrombus. Blood 1993;81:1290.
38. Hogg PJ, Stenflo J, Mosher DF. Thrombospondin is a slow tight-binding inhibitor of plasmin. Biochemistry 1992;31:265.
39. Mirashahi M, Azzarone B, Soria J, Mirshahi F, Soria C. The role of fibroblasts in organization and degradation of a fibrin clot. J Lab Clin Med 1991;117:274.
40. Gabriel DA, Muga K, Boothroyd EM. The effect of fibrin structure on fibrinolysis. J Biol Chem 1992;267:24259.
41. Carrell N, Gabriel DA, Blatt PM, Carr ME, McDonagh J. Hereditary dysfibrinogenemia in a patient with thrombotic disease. Blood 1983;62: 439.
42. Soria J, Soria C, Caen JP. A new type of congenital dysfibrinogenaemia with defective fibrin lysis—Dusard syndrome: possible relation to thrombosis. Br J Haematol 1983;53:575.
43. Sakata Y, Aoki N. Significance of cross-linking of α_2-plasmin inhibitor to fibrin in inhibition of fibrinolysis and in hemostasis. J Clin Invest 1982;69:536.
44. Bennett B, Booth NA, Croll A, Dawson AA. The bleeding disorder in acute promyelocytic leukemia: fibrinolysis due to u-PA rather than defibrination. Br J Haematol 1989;71:511.
45. Miles LA, Plow EF. Binding and activation of plasminogen on the platelet surface. J Biol Chem 1985;260:4303.
46. Correc P, Fondaneche M-C, Bracke M, Burtin P. The presence of plasmin receptors on three mammary carcinoma MCF-7 sublines. Int J Cancer 1990;46:745.
47. Vassalli J-D, Baccino D, Belin D. A cellular binding site for the M_r 55,000 form of the human plasminogen activator, urokinase. J Cell Biol 1985;100:86.
48. Hajjar KA, Hamel NM, Harpel PC, Nachman RL. Binding of tissue plasminogen activator to cultured human endothelial cells. J Clin Invest 1987;80:1712.
49. Broder CC, Lottenberg R, von Mering GO, Johnston KH, Boyle MDP. Isolation of a prokaryotic plasmin receptor. J Biol Chem 1991;266: 4922.
50. Stack S, Gonzalez-Gronow M, Pizzo SV. Regulation of plasminogen activation by components of the extracellular matrix. Biochemistry 1990;29:4966.
51. Lind SE, Smith CJ. Actin accelerates plasmin generation by tissue plasminogen activator. J Biol Chem 1991;266:17673.
52. Fleury V, Lijnen HR, Anglés-Cano E. Mechanism of the enhanced intrinsic activity of single-chain urokinase-type plasminogen activator during ongoing fibrinolysis. J Biol Chem 1993;268:18554.
53. Liu J, Pannell R, Gurewich V. A transitional state of prourokinase that has a higher catalytic efficiency against Glu-plasminogen than urokinase. J Biol Chem 1993;267:15289.
54. Matsuo O, Okada K, Fukao H, et al. Thrombolytic properties of staphylokinase. Blood 1990;76:925.
55. Keeton M, Eguchi Y, Sawdey M, Ahn C, Loskutoff DJ. Cellular localization of type 1 plasminogen activator inhibitor messenger RNA and protein in murine renal tissue. Am J Pathol 1993;142:59.
56. Erickson LA, Ginsberg MH, Loskutoff DJ. Detection and partial char-

acterization of an inhibitor of plasminogen activation in human platelets. J Clin Invest 1984;74:1465.

57. Dzik WH, Arkin CF, Jenkins RL, Stump DC. Fibrinolysis during liver transplantation in humans: role of tissue-type plasminogen activator. Blood 1988;71:1090.
58. Schleef RR, Higgins DL, Pillemer E, Levitt LJ. Bleeding diathesis due to decreased functional activity of type 1 plasminogen activator inhibitor. J Clin Invest 1989;83:1747.
59. Fay WP, Shapiro AD, Shih JL, Schleef RR, Ginsburg D. Complete deficiency of plasminogen-activator inhibitor type 1 due to a frameshift mutation. N Engl J Med 1992;327:1729.
60. Lee MH, Vosburgh E, Anderson K, McDonagh J. Deficiency of plasma plasminogen activator inhibitor 1 results in hyperfibrinolytic bleeding. Blood 1993;81:2357.
61. Saito H. α_2-Plasmin inhibitor and its deficiency states. J Lab Clin Med 1988;112:671.
62. Williams EC. Plasma α_2-antiplasmin activity: role in the evaluation and management of fibrinolytic states and other bleeding disorders. Arch Intern Med 1989;149:1769.
63. Stead NW, Bauer KA, Kinney TR, et al. Venous thrombosis in a family with defective release of vascular plasminogen activator and elevated plasma factor VIII/von Willebrand's factor. Am J Med 1983;74:33.
64. Prins MH, Hirsh J. A critical review of the evidence supporting a relationship between impaired fibrinolytic activity and venous thromboembolism. Arch Int Med 1991;151:1721.
65. Hamsten A, Wiman B, De Faire U, Blombäck M. Increased plasma levels of a rapid inhibitor of tissue plasminogen activator in young survivors of myocardial infarction. N Engl J Med 1985;313:1557.
66. Meade TW, Ruddock V, Chakrabarti R, Miller GJ. Fibrinolytic activity, clotting factors, and long-term incidence of ischaemic heart disease in the Northwick Park Heart Study. Lancet 1993;342:1076.
67. Wilhelmsen L, Svärdsudd K, Korsan-Bengtsen K, Larrson B, Welin L, Tibblin G. Fibrinogen as a risk factor for stroke and myocardial infarction. N Engl J Med 1984;311:501.
68. Ridker PM, Vaughan DE, Stampfer MJ, et al. Baseline fibrinolytic state and the risk of future venous thrombosis: a prospective study of endogenous tissue-type plasminogen activator and plasminogen activator inhibitor. Circulation 1992;85:1822.
69. Ridker PM, Vaughan DE, Stampfer MJ, Manson JE, Hennekens CH. Endogenous tissue-type plasminogen activator and risk of myocardial infarction. Lancet 1993;341:1165.
70. Meade TW, North WRS, Chakrabarti R, Stirling Y, Haines AP, Thompson SG. Haemostatic function and cardiovascular death: early results of a prospective study. Lancet 1980;1:1050.
71. Rosenfeld BA, Beattie C, Christopherson R, et al. The effects of different anesthetic regimens on fibrinolysis and the development of postoperative arterial thrombosis. Anesthesiology 1993;79:435.
72. Vassalli J-D, Sappino A-P, Belin D. The plasminogen activator/plasmin system. J Clin Invest 1991;88:1067.
73. Danø K, Andreasen PA, Grøndahl-Hansen J, Kristensen P, Nielsen LS, Skriver L. Plasminogen activators, tissue degradation, and cancer. Adv Can Res 1985;44:139.
74. Niewiarowski S, Senyi AF, Gillies P. Plasmin-induced platelet aggregation and platelet release reaction. J Clin Invest 1973;52:1647.
75. Penny WF, Ware JA. Platelet activation and subsequent inhibition by plasmin and recombinant tissue-type plasminogen activator. Blood 1992;79:91.
76. Lu H, Soria C, Cramer EM, et al. Temperature dependence of plasmin-induced activation or inhibition of human platelets. Blood 1991;77:996.
77. Valeri CR, Khabbaz K, Khuri SF, et al. Effect of skin temperature on platelet function in patients undergoing extracorporeal bypass. J Thorac Cardiovasc Surg 1992;104:108.
78. Boldt J, Knothe C, Zickmann B, Bill S, Dapper F, Hempelmann G. Platelet function in cardiac surgery: influence of temperature and aprotinin. Ann Thorac Surg 1993;55:652.
79. Eisenberg PR, Sherman LA, Jaffe AS. Paradoxic elevation of fibrinopeptide A after streptokinase: evidence for continued thrombosis despite intense fibrinolysis. J Am Coll Cardiol 1987;10:527.
80. Winters KJ, Santoro SA, Miletich JP, Eisenberg PR. Relative importance of thrombin compared with plasmin-mediated platelet activation in response to plasminogen activation with streptokinase. Circulation 1991;84:1552.
81. Aronson DL, Chang P, Kessler CM. Platelet-dependent thrombin generation after in vitro fibrinolytic treatment. Circulation 1992;85:1706.
82. Bidstrup BP, Royston D, Sapsford RN, Taylor KM. Reduction in blood loss and blood use after cardiopulmonary bypass with high dose aprotinin (Trasylol). J Thorac Cardiovasc Surg 1989;97:364.
83. van Oeveren W, Harder MP, Roozendaal KJ, Eijsman L, Wildevuur CRH. Aprotinin protects platelets against the initial effect of cardiopulmonary bypass. J Thorac Cardiovasc Surg 1990;99:788.
84. Marcus AJ, Safier LB. Thromboregulation: multicellular modulation of platelet reactivity in hemostasis and thrombosis. FASEB J 1993;7:516.
85. Duke WW. The relation of blood platelets to hemorrhagic disease: description of a method for determining the bleeding time and coagulation time and report of three cases of hemorrhagic disease relieved by transfusion. JAMA 1910;55:1185.
86. Livio M, Gotti E, Marchesi D, Mecca G, Remuzzi G, de Gaetoma G. Uraemic bleeding: role of anaemia and beneficial effect of red cell transfusions. Lancet 1982;2:1013.
87. Lüthje J. Extracellular adenine compounds, red blood cells and haemostasis: facts and hypotheses. Blut 1989;59:367.
88. Santos MT, Valles J, Marcus AJ, et al. Enhancement of platelet reactivity and modulation of eicosanoid production by intact erythrocytes. J Clin Invest 1991;87:571.
89. Zwaal RFA, Comfurius P, van Deenen LLM. Membrane asymmetry and blood coagulation. Nature 1977;268:358.
90. Chiu D, Lubin B, Roelofsen B, van Deenen LLM. Sickled erythrocytes accelerate clotting in vitro: an effect of abnormal membrane lipid symmetry. Blood 1981;58:398.
91. Rickles FR, O'Leary DS. Role of coagulation system in pathophysiology of sickle cell disease. Arch Intern Med 1974;133:635.
92. Devine DV, Kinney TR, Thomas PF, Rosse WF, Greenberg CS. Fragment D-dimer levels: an objective marker of vaso-occlusive crisis and other complications of sickle cell disease. Blood 1986;68:317.
93. Smith GP, Peters TJ. Subcellular localization and properties of adenosine diphosphatase activity in human polymorphonuclear leukocytes. Biochim Biophys Acta 1981;673:234.
94. Wright CD, Mülsch A, Busse R, Osswald H. Generation of nitric oxide by human neutrophils. Biochem Biophys Res Commun 1989;160:813.
95. Kornecki E, Ehrlich YH, De Mars DD, Lenox RH. Exposure of fibrinogen receptors in human platelets by surface proteolysis with elastase. J Clin Invest 1986;77:750.
96. LeRoy EC, Ager A, Gordon JL. Effects of neutrophil elastase and other proteases on porcine aortic endothelial prostaglandin I_2 production, adenine nucleotide release, and responses to vasoactive substances. J Clin Invest 1984;74:1003.
97. Higuchi DA, Wun T-C, Likert KM, Broze GJJ. The effect of leukocyte elastase on tissue factor pathway inhibitor. Blood 1992;79:1712.
98. Machovich R, Owen WG. An elastase-dependent pathway of plasminogen activation. Biochemistry 1989;28:4517.
99. Valles J, Santos MT, Marcus AJ, et al. Downregulation of human platelet reactivity by neutrophils. Participation of lipoxygenase derivatives and adhesive proteins. J Clin Invest 1993;92:1357.
100. Tallman MS, Kwaan HC. Reassessing the hemostatic disorder associated with acute promyelocytic leukemia. Blood 1992;79:543.
101. Dam H, Venndt H. Observations on the coagulation of blood plasma in hemophilia. Lancet 1940;238:70.
102. Langdell RD, Wagner RH, Brinkhous KM. Effect of antihemophilic factor on one-stage clotting tests: a presumptive test for hemophilia and a simple one-stage antihemophilic factor assay procedure. J Lab Clin Med 1953;41:637.
103. Proctor RR, Rapaport SI. The partial thromboplastin time with kaolin: a simple screening test for the first stage plasma clotting factor deficiencies. Am J Clin Pathol 1961;36:212.
104. Eisenberg JM, Clarke JR, Sussman SA. Prothrombin and partial thromboplastin times as preoperative screening tests. Arch Surg 1982;117:48.
105. Suchman AL, Mushlin AI. How well does the activated partial thromboplastin time predict postoperative hemorrhage? JAMA 1986;256:750.
106. Diamond LK, Porter FS. The inadequacies of routine bleeding and clotting times. N Engl J Med 1958;259:1025.
107. McVay PA, Toy PTCY. Lack of increased bleeding after liver biopsy in patients with mild hemostatic abnormalities. Am J Clin Pathol 1990;94:747.
108. McVay PA, Toy PTCY. Lack of increased bleeding after paracentesis and thoracentesis in patients with mild coagulation abnormalities. Transfusion 1991;31:164.
109. Burns ER, Goldberg SN, Wenz B. Paradoxic effect of multiple mild coagulation factor deficiencies on the prothrombin time and activated partial thromboplastin time. Am J Clin Pathol 1993;100:94.
110. Ivy A, Shapiro PF, Melnick P. The bleeding tendency in jaundice. Surg Gynecol Obstet 1935;60:781.
111. Burns ER, Lawrence C. Bleeding time: a guide to its diagnostic and clinical utility. Arch Pathol Lab Med 1989;113:1219.
112. Rodgers RPC, Levin J. A critical reappraisal of the bleeding time. Semin Thromb Hemostas 1990;16:1.
113. Lind SE. The bleeding time does not predict surgical bleeding. Blood 1991;77:2547.
114. Nichols WL, Bowie EJW. Standardization of the prothrombin time for monitoring orally administered anticoagulant therapy with use of the international normalized ratio. Mayo Clin Proc 1993;68:897.
115. Edson JR, Krivit W, White JG. Kaolin partial thromboplastin time: high levels of procoagulants producing short clotting times or masking deficiencies of other procoagulants or low concentrations of anticoagulants. J Lab Clin Med 1967;70:463.
116. Stricker RB, Lane PK, Leffert JD, Rogers GM, Shuman MA, Corash L. Development of antithrombin antibodies following surgery in patients with prosthetic cardiac valves. Blood 1988;72:1375.
117. Flaherty MJ, Henderson R, Wener MH. Iatrogenic immunization with

bovine thrombin: a mechanism for prolonged thrombin times after surgery. Ann Intern Med 1989;111:631.
118. Berruyer M, Amiral J, Ffrench P, et al. Immunization by bovine thrombin used with fibrin glue during cardiovascular operations: development of thrombin and factor V inhibitors. J Thorac Cardiovasc Surg 1993;105:892.
119. Cmolik BL, Spero JA, Magovern GJ, Clark RE. Redo cardiac surgery: late bleeding complications from topical thrombin-induced factor V deficiency. J Thorac Cardiovasc Surg 1993;105:222.
120. Carr JM, McKinney M, McDonagh J. Diagnosis of disseminated intravascular coagulation. Am J Clin Pathol 1989;91:280.
121. Lazarchick J, Kizer J. The laboratory diagnosis of lupus anticoagulants. Arch Pathol Lab Med 1989;113:177.
122. Triplett DA. Coagulation assays for the lupus anticoagulant: review and critique of current methodology. Stroke 1992;23(Suppl I):I-11.
123. Rosove MH, Ismail M, Koziol BJ, Runge A, Kasper CK. Lupus anticoagulants: improved diagnosis with a kaolin clotting time using rabbit brain phospholipid in standard and high concentrations. Blood 1986;68:472.
124. Triplett DA, Brandt JT, Kaczor D, Schaeffer J. Laboratory diagnosis of lupus inhibitors: a comparison of the tissue thromboplastin inhibition procedure with a new platelet neutralization procedure. Am J Clin Pathol 1983;79:678.
125. Feinstein DI. Lupus anticoagulant, anticardiolipin antibodies, fetal loss, and systemic lupus erythematosus. Blood 1992;80:859.
126. Herbst KD, Rapaport SI, Kenoyer DG, Stanton W, Feinstein DI. Syndrome of an acquired inhibitor of factor VIII responsive to cyclophosphamide and prednisone. Ann Intern Med 1981;95:575.
127. Lossing TS, Kasper CK, Feinstein DI. Detection of factor VIII inhibitors with the partial thromboplastin time. Blood 1977;49:793.
128. The British Society for Haematology BCSH Haemostasis and Thrombosis Task Force. Guidelines on platelet function testing. J Clin Pathol 1988;41:1322.
129. Bowie EJW, Owen CAJ. The bleeding time. Prog Hemost Thromb 1974;2:249.
130. Lind SE. The prolonged bleeding time. Am J Med 1984;77:305.
131. Deykin D, Janson P, McMahon L. Ethanol potentiation of aspirin-induced prolongation of the bleeding time. N Engl J Med 1982;306:852.
132. Remaley AT, Kennedy JM, Laposata M. Evaluation of the clinical utility of platelet aggregation studies. Am J Hematol 1989;31:188.
133. Kang Y, Lewis JH, Navalgund A, et al. Epsilon-aminocaproic acid for treatment of fibrinolysis during liver transplantation. Anesthesiology 1987;66:766.
134. Lackner H, Karpatkin S. On the "easy bruising" syndrome with normal platelet count. Ann Intern Med 1975;83:190.
135. Peterson P, Gottfried EL. The effects of inaccurate blood sample volume on prothrombin time (PT) and activated partial thromboplastin time (aPTT). Thromb Haemostas 1982;47:101.
136. Abildgaard CF, Suzucki Z, Harrison J, Jefcoat K, Zimmerman TS. Serial studies in von Willebrand's disease: variability versus "variants." Blood 1980;56:712.
137. Burk CD, Miller L, Handler SD, Cohen AR. Preoperative history and coagulation screening in children undergoing tonsillectomy. Pediatrics 1992;89:691.
138. Ragi MV, Sinha D, Seaman F, Lewis JH, Spero JA, Walsh PN. Comparison of bleeding tendency, factor XI coagulant activity, and factor XI antigen in 25 factor XI–deficient kindreds. Blood 1985;65:719.
139. George JN. Platelet immunoglobulin G: its significance for the evaluation of thrombocytopenia and for understanding the origin of the alpha-granule proteins. Blood 1990;76:859.
140. Kelton JG, Powers PJ, Carter CJ. A prospective study of the usefulness of the measurement of platelet-associated IgG for the diagnosis of idiopathic thrombocytopenic purpura. Blood 1982;60:1050.
141. Kelton JG, Neame PB, Gauldie J, Hirsh J. Elevated platelet-associated IgG in the thrombocytopenia of septicemia. N Engl J Med 1979;300:760.
142. Walsh CM, Nardi MA, Karpatkin S. On the mechanism of thrombocytopenic purpura in sexually active homosexual men. N Engl J Med 1984;311:635.

Blood: Principles and Practice of Hematology,
edited by Robert I. Handin, Samuel E. Lux, and Thomas P. Stossel.
J.B. Lippincott Company, Philadelphia © 1995.

34

The Platelet Life Cycle: Quantitative Disorders

Theodore E. Warkentin
John G. Kelton

PLATELET PRODUCTION, DISTRIBUTION, AND CONSUMPTION

Platelet Production

The Megakaryocyte

The megakaryocyte is the cell of origin of the platelet. Although platelets constitute about 5% of circulating blood cells, megakaryocytes are relatively infrequent in the bone marrow, making up only 0.05% of the nucleated marrow cells.[1,2] The explanation is that each megakaryocyte produces thousands of platelets. The normal human marrow contains about 40 million megakaryocytes.[2]

Megakaryocytes undergo a unique biologic process known as *endomitosis*, which is defined as repeated nuclear replication in the absence of cytoplasmic division. Thus, megakaryocytes possess 2^n polyploid nuclei, with 4 to 64 times the amount of haploid nuclear material (4N to 64N). The modal ploidy for human megakaryocytes is 16N.[3–5]

Megakaryocytes are the largest marrow cells, with an average diameter of 35 μm.[4,6] Although present in greatest numbers within the bone marrow, megakaryocytes are also found in extravascular sites within the spleen.[7] Megakaryocytes can also circulate and have been identified in intravascular sites within the lung, liver, heart, and other organs.[7]

Megakaryocyte Development

Megakaryocytes develop in several stages.[8–11] The earliest committed megakaryocyte precursor is the burst-forming unit–megakaryocyte (BFU-meg), which is characterized in vitro by high proliferative capacity, relatively delayed colony formation (21 days), absolute requirement for interleukin-3 (IL-3) or granulocyte-macrophage colony-stimulating factor (GM-CSF), and resistance to 5-fluorouracil.[12,13] The subsequent stage in megakaryocyte development is the colony-forming unit–megakaryocyte (CFU-meg). In contrast, these cells demonstrate lower proliferative capacity, more rapid colony formation (12 days), responsiveness to several hematopoietic growth factors, and decreased colony formation after pretreatment with 5-fluorouracil.[11–13] Both cells express human progenitor cell antigen 1, whereas only the CFU-meg express HLA-DR antigens.[13] These progenitor cells, which cannot be recognized morphologically, represent intermediate stages between the multipotential stem cell and morphologically recognizable megakaryocytes.

The first visually identifiable megakaryocyte precursor is the promegakaryoblast (transitional immature megakaryocyte). This cell morphologically resembles a lymphoid cell and therefore can only be distinguished by antibodies against specific platelet membrane components (eg, gpIIb/IIIa, gpIb)[4,14,15] or cytoplasmic (eg, von Willebrand factor [vWF])[15,16] proteins. In rodents, a similar lymphoid-like megakaryocyte precursor cell exists that, unlike its human counterpart, possesses acetylcholinesterase activity.[14,17]

The megakaryoblast represents the next stage of megakaryocyte development. This is the first cell of megakaryocyte lineage that can be recognized morphologically using routine stains. The subsequent stages of megakaryocyte differentiation—basophilic megakaryocyte, granular megakaryocyte, and platelet-releasing megakaryocyte—are identified by characteristic morphologic features.

Endomitosis is completed early in megakaryocyte differentiation, usually by the megakaryoblast stage.[18] Most nuclear lobulation and cytoplasmic differentiation begin after the final polyploid state of the cell has been attained.[18,19]

Complex cytoplasmic changes occur during megakaryocyte development. The most unique and dramatic is the formation of extensive tubular, membrane-like organelles, termed the *demarcating membrane system*, which are involved in platelet formation. Other cytoplasmic constituents that are synthesized include rough endoplasmic reticulum and polyribosomes, which are important for protein synthesis, as well as platelet-specific granules (α granules, dense granules), which become increasingly evident with progressive megakaryocyte maturation.

Platelet Formation

Megakaryocytes, like other hematopoietic precursor cells, are located in the extravascular marrow space. Their position is not random but adjacent to the abluminal side of sinus endothelial cells.[20,21] The megakaryocytes are anchored to the endothelium by multiple, organelle-free cytoplasm projections, which protrude through the sinus endothelium (transendothelial penetration). It has been speculated that these projections monitor circulating hormone levels and platelet numbers.[21]

A second type of megakaryocyte projection is involved in platelet formation. These are lengthy (up to 120 μm), organelle-containing cytoplasmic projections, termed *proplatelets*, which also traverse the sinus epithelium into the sinus cavity.[21,22] The proplatelets are released into the sinus and fragment intravascularly into about 1000 platelets. It is estimated that each megakaryocyte is capable of synthesizing six to eight proplatelets.[22]

Once, it was postulated that the megakaryocyte demarcation membranes delineate future platelets, that is, that platelet membrane and cytoplasmic apposition is established early within the megakaryocyte. It has been proposed, however, that the demarcation membrane serves a reservoir function, continuously providing membrane for the growing cytoplasmic proplatelet projections.[23] This tubular invagination of the megakaryocyte membrane appears to contribute ultimately to the platelet membrane as well as the open canalicular system.[24]

Megakaryocytes can enter the peripheral blood through the marrow sinuses, as evidenced by the finding of circulating megakaryocytes in normal people.[25,26] Platelets can be released from these ectopic megakaryocytes lodged within the lungs.[27]

Platelet Heterogeneity

One of the most remarkable features of the platelet is its marked size heterogeneity. Electronic particle counting and sizing instruments reveal the normal platelet size histogram to be right-skewed; that is, there is a prominent "tail" of large-sized platelets. The size distribution can be normalized statistically by converting the platelet volume determinations to corresponding log values[28] (log-normal distribution).

Two hypotheses have been proposed to account for platelet heterogeneity. The first is that as platelets age, they become smaller and less dense, possibly due to fragmentation or loss of granule or membrane proteins.[29] Considerable debate have been generated regarding this proposal. Some investigators,[30–32] but not others,[33,34] have shown a correlation between platelet size and density. Furthermore, platelet density may actually increase with age.[33,35,36] Quantitation of platelet class I HLA antigens may be useful in determining platelet age.[37]

Platelet size heterogeneity is determined at the megakaryocyte level either because of heterogeneity of proplatelet fragmentation[38] or because of the formation of larger platelets by larger megakaryocytes with greater ploidy.[31,39,40] The positive correlation, however, between platelet and megakaryocyte size and ploidy can be dissociated. For instance, animal models of acute thrombocytopenia demonstrate that rapid increases in mean platelet volume (MPV) precede increases in megakaryocyte ploidy by many hours.[41,42] The ability to increase platelet size rapidly supports the hypothesis that megakaryocyte demarcation membranes serve as a readily available membrane reserve.

Platelet Distribution

After release from the marrow or ectopic sites like the lungs, a large number of platelets are reversibly pooled within the spleen.[43,44] Although the spleen receives about 5% of the cardiac output and contains only 2% of the blood volume, about 30% of the platelets are present in the spleen.[43,45,46] In pathologic states associated with splenomegaly, the platelet pool can contain up to 90% of the platelet mass (hypersplenism).

Studies[46–52] using radionuclide-labeled platelet localization techniques have characterized certain features of splenic platelet pooling. The average time the platelet spends in the spleen (splenic transit time) is about 10 minutes.[46,47] Two factors determine the extent of splenic pooling[47]: splenic blood flow and splenic transit time. The most important determinant of splenic blood flow is the size of the spleen,[47,52] and the most important determinant of splenic transit time is perfusion pressure (spleen blood flow/spleen size).[49,52] Disorders associated with alterations in splenic transit time, however, such as congestive heart failure or rheumatologic disorders, usually have counterbalancing effects on splenic blood flow.[48,49] Thus, in practical and clinical terms, the size of the spleen correlates with splenic platelet pooling.

It is not known why platelets spend about a third of their 9-day life-span in the spleen. Granulocytes are pooled in the spleen to a similar extent as platelets.[53] The splenic transit time of red blood cells, however, is considerably shorter. Since platelets are much smaller than RBCs, a simple mechanical explanation is untenable. Splenic platelet pooling is not increased appreciably in idiopathic thrombocytopenic purpura (ITP),[50] suggesting that platelet-bound immunoglobulin (Ig) is not responsible. Furthermore, platelet survival is usually normal or only slightly decreased in patients with hypersplenism.[43]

Infusion of isoprenaline (isoproterenol), a β-adrenergic agonist, into normal volunteers causes a drop in the platelet count. This is caused by increased splenic blood flow resulting in increased splenic platelet pooling.[51] Infusion of epinephrine, however, a mixed α- and β-adrenergic agonist, mobilizes platelets from the splenic pool and increases the platelet count in human volunteers.[43] This suggests that α-adrenergic stimulation causes changes in the splenic microvasculature that result in an earlier return of the platelets to the systemic circulation.

Physiologic Platelet Consumption

Determinants

The normal platelet life-span is about 9 days.[54,55] Three factors appear to determine the length of platelet survival: platelet age (senescence),[56,57] a fixed platelet requirement,[58] and random loss.[59,60]

Platelet Senescence. The age of the platelet probably is the most important factor that determines when it will be removed from the circulation.[56] Age-related changes in surface glycoprotein composition[59,61] and amounts of surface Ig[62,63] could be involved in determination of senescence. It has been proposed that specific sialylated proteins present on all circulating blood cells, such as glycophorin on red blood cells and sialophorin on platelets and leukocytes, block access to cryptic senescence antigens located on the cell surface.[64]

Fixed Platelet Requirement. Radioisotope platelet life-span studies demonstrate a reduced platelet life-span in all thrombocytopenic patients or animals. To account for this observation, it has been proposed that a minimal, fixed number of platelets (7×10^9/L, about 20% of normal platelet turnover) is removed from the circulation daily independent of the platelet count.[58] The function of these platelets is unknown, although they may be involved in platelet–endothelial interactions.

Random Platelet Loss. Although platelet senescence is the primary factor determining physiologic platelet consumption, experimental evidence suggests that random events can contribute to the loss of senescent platelets.[59] It is likely that random platelet loss becomes increasingly important in destructive thrombocytopenic disorders.[60]

Sites

Studies[65,66] using the radioisotope indium-111 (^{111}In) have shown that, in normal people, about 30% of platelet destruction occurs in the liver and spleen each, about 20% occurs in the bone marrow, and the remainder occurs in unknown sites.

Platelet Life-Span Studies

Platelet life-span studies can provide definitive information useful for classifying the mechanism of thrombocytopenia in a particular patient. Several types of platelet life-span measurements are available, which can be divided into two general groups: nonradioactive and radioactive.

Measurements Using Nonradioactive Techniques

The anuclear platelet cannot regenerate irreversibly inactivated enzymes, a fact that is exploited in nonradioactive platelet life-span techniques.[67–70] For example, the test subject can be given aspirin to inactivate platelet cyclooxygenase, the rate-limiting enzyme of the prostaglandin pathway. Assuming a steady state of platelet turnover, the time to recovery of platelet prostaglandin metabolism, as measured by malondialdehyde or thromboxane B_2 generation, correlates with the mean platelet survival. Nonradioactive techniques are less accurate than measurements using radiolabeled platelets, however, and therefore are used by few centers.

Measurements Using Radiolabels

The most accurate and widely used tests for determining the platelet life-span employ radioisotopes. Two general types of platelet-labeling techniques have been used—cohort labels and random labels.

Cohort Radiolabeling. Cohort radiolabeling means that a single age of platelets (eg, young platelets) is labeled by the radiolabel. The radioactivity of these platelets is then followed in the circulation with the time required for the radioactivity to appear and then disappear, defining the platelet life-span. The cohort labels have included ^{75}Se-selenomethionine,[35] ^{35}S-sulphate,[71] and ^{3}H-amino acids.[72] Although these techniques have proved useful for research purposes, their potential hazards have prevented routine use.

Random Radiolabeling. Random radiolabeling means that platelets of all ages are labeled to an equal extent by the radiolabel. Hence, during the radiolabeling process, platelets of all ages must be radiolabeled to a similar extent, or an erroneous result is obtained. Normally, since platelets leave the circulation predominantly by an age-dependent process, a linear decline in the radioactivity from the circulation is observed.

Certain characteristics are necessary for a radiolabel to be useful for platelet labeling:

1. The label must bind to proteins within the platelets that are not released during platelet activation. Otherwise, a falsely shortened platelet survival might be obtained.
2. The radiolabel must not damage the platelets or otherwise affect their function. For example, if a radiolabel impairs platelet function, then the platelets theoretically might live longer should platelet destruction be platelet function–dependent (platelet interaction with an abnormal vessel wall or prosthetic heart valve).
3. The radiolabel must be taken up by the platelet efficiently so that the amount of radioactivity per platelet (specific activity) permits measurement.
4. The half-life of the radiolabel should be appropriate for the life-span of the cell of interest. For example, if one is interested in measuring the life-span of an RBC (normal, 120 days), a radiolabel with a life-span of only a few days cannot be used because the radioisotope will have decayed to undetectable levels before the survival study has been completed. Conversely, a radioisotope with a long life-span cannot be used to measure the life-span of a cell with a much shorter life-span.
5. All the platelets should be radiolabeled equally. If young or old platelets were preferentially labeled, then the apparent life-span would be falsely increased or decreased, respectively. Or, if radiolabeling is performed to study platelet viability (eg, techniques for platelet storage), then both viable and nonviable platelets should be labeled equally.

Selection of Radioisotopes. The two main radiolabels used for platelet radiolabeling are ^{51}Cr-sodium chromate and ^{111}In.[73] ^{111}In is the preferred radiolabel, for the following reasons:

1. The labeling efficiency of ^{111}In is superior to ^{51}Cr. Only 10% to 20% of ^{51}Cr is taken up by platelets (low specific activity). Therefore, large numbers of platelets must be radiolabeled with ^{51}Cr to ensure adequate radioactivity for counting, which precludes the possibility of performing an autologous platelet life-span study in a severely thrombocytopenic patient. In contrast, most (80% to 95%) of the ^{111}In is incorporated into platelets, and therefore autologous platelet life-span studies usually can be performed in severely thrombocytopenic patients.
2. Although both radiolabels bind to cytoplasmic proteins within the platelets, platelet release is associated with loss of ^{51}Cr but not ^{111}In from the platelets. Hence, if there is in vivo platelet activation and release during the platelet life-span study, a falsely shortened life-span could result using ^{51}Cr-labeled platelets.
3. The half-life of ^{111}In is 2.8 days, compared with 21 days for ^{51}Cr. This makes ^{111}In an ideal label for platelets because its decay parallels the normal platelet life-span. To ensure that decay of ^{111}In does not affect the results, all blood samples are saved, and the radioactivity is counted after completion of the test.
4. The superior gamma-ray emission profile of ^{111}In compared with ^{51}Cr allows for improved imaging of platelet-sequestering organs, such as the spleen or splenic remnants (accessory spleens).

Performance of a Platelet Life-Span. The optimal method for the performance of a platelet life-span has been published.[73] In brief, blood is collected, preferably from the patient (autologous study) or a healthy donor (homologous study). The platelets are isolated by differential centrifugation and washed, and the radiolabel is added. After sufficient time to permit incorporation of the radiolabel into the platelets, the platelets are pelleted, and any unbound label is washed away. Several quality control maneuvers are performed, including measurement of platelet, RBC, and plasma radioactivity. The platelets are infused intravenously into the subject, and blood is collected after the platelets have had enough time to equilibrate (typically 30 to 60 minutes). An anticoagulated blood sample is collected daily for the next 7 to 10 days. Subsequently, the samples are measured for radioactivity.

The percentage of platelet recovery is determined by measuring the percentage of radiolabeled platelets in the circulation at 30 to 60 minutes after administration. This measured amount is compared with the predicted platelet recovery, which is based on the patient's blood volume, the number of radiolabeled platelets given, and the physiologic splenic sequestration.

Interpretation of the Platelet Life-Span Study. The result of a platelet life-span study has one of three general patterns:

Normal recovery and survival. This is characterized by a 60% to 80% platelet recovery and a life-span of about 7 to 10 days. This is observed in normal people and in most patients with thrombocytopenia due to decreased platelet production. Apparent reduced platelet survival in this latter situation could reflect the relative increased importance of the fixed platelet requirement with severe thrombocytopenia.[58]

Hypersplenism. This is characterized by a markedly reduced percentage of platelet recovery (typically, 20% to 40%) and a normal or near-normal platelet life-span.

Shortened platelet survival. A shortened platelet survival occurs in destructive thrombocytopenic states. Patients with a rapid rate of platelet destruction can have an apparent reduced platelet recovery, although it is uncertain whether platelet sequestration is truly increased or whether the apparent sequestration is caused by an artifact of the rapid rate of destruction.

Ideally, the result of the platelet life-span study is either normal or markedly reduced, but sometimes it can be difficult to be certain into which group the results fall. To avoid potential errors of subjective analysis, several approaches have been used for data analysis. The best is to use a computer model that determines the best fit of the data points. This technique, known as the *gamma function analysis,* removes any potential observer bias from the analysis of the results. Another approach is to measure the time required for loss of one half of the radioactivity from the circulation, the half-life.

Indirect Determination of Platelet Life-Span

Plasma Glycocalicin

At many hospitals, it is not possible to perform a platelet life-span measurement. The report of plasma glycocalicin measurements in thrombocytopenic patients may allow this test to replace the platelet life-span test.[74] Glycocalicin is a soluble proteolytic product of gpIb. Elevated plasma glycocalicin levels are seen in disorders of increased platelet destruction (eg, active ITP), whereas normal levels are generally found in patients with decreased platelet production (eg, aplastic anemia). However, elevated levels have also been found in some patients with uremia, cirrhosis, and acute myeloid leukemia,[75] and further experience is required to determine whether glycocalicin measurements will permit accurate classification of the mechanism of thrombocytopenia.

Platelet RNA

The number of platelets with residual amounts of RNA can be quantitated using flow cytometric analysis of thiazole orange uptake by platelets. In one study,[76] this technique was helpful in the evaluation of thrombocytopenic patients with an increased percentage of RNA-containing platelets ("stress platelets") found in patients with destructive thrombocytopenia.

APPROACH TO THE THROMBOCYTOPENIC PATIENT

When assessing a thrombocytopenic patient, the clinician simultaneously must estimate the bleeding risk and determine the cause of the thrombocytopenia.

Many thrombocytopenic patients are not bleeding. The clinician must identify those patients at risk for serious bleeding, however, so that appropriate therapy can be started. Similarly, avoiding inappropriate interventions for the asymptomatic, thrombocytopenic patient prevents treatment-related morbidity.

Unless mimicked by a spurious laboratory result, such as pseudothrombocytopenia, thrombocytopenia is always abnormal. The greatest threat to the patient usually is not the thrombocytopenia itself, but the underlying pathologic process, which must be identified and treated.

Estimation of the Bleeding Risk

Clinical Features

Petechiae and Ecchymoses. Petechiae are the hallmark of thrombocytopenia. These are small (less than 2 mm) purpura and represent tiny cutaneous or mucosal collections of RBCs that have leaked from the blood vessels. Petechiae are nonpalpable and typically occur on the dependent regions of the body, especially the legs. Larger subcutaneous collections of blood are called ecchymoses. These can be painful and palpable and at times mimic vasculitic lesions.

Clinicians have attempted to estimate the bleeding risk according to the location and extent of petechiae and ecchymoses. In general, the more extensive the purpura, the greater the bleeding risk.

Other types of nonthrombocytopenic purpura must be identified since these are not associated with bleeding. These lesions include vasculitic purpura, which are frequently palpable, sometimes painful, located on dependent regions, and associated with characteristic histopathologic features; senile purpura, which are caused by subcutaneous fat atrophy and typically occur on the lax skin on the dorsum of the hands; and various pigmented purpuric eruptions.[77]

Mucosal and Internal Bleeding. Severe thrombocytopenia can be associated with mucosal bleeding, including bleeding from the mouth, nose, gastrointestinal tract, uterus and vagina, and bladder. Mucous membrane bleeding signifies an even higher risk for serious bleeding than purpura. Although uncommon, some patients with severe thrombocytopenia can develop spontaneous life-threatening intracranial or visceral hemorrhage.

Coexisting Hemostatic Dysfunction. The clinician also should determine if the patient has other hemostatic defects, such as damage to blood vessels (operative procedures), platelet dysfunction (antiplatelet drugs, alcohol, uremia), and coagulopathy (liver disease, vitamin K deficiency, hyperfibrinolysis).

Laboratory Tests

The hemostatic risk depends on many factors in addition to the absolute value of the platelet count. Different patients with the identical platelet count may or may not bleed when challenged hemostatically (ie, in surgery). Nevertheless, it is important to estimate bleeding risk so that preventive measures (platelet transfusions) can be considered.

Platelet Count. In general, a very low platelet count (below $20 \times 10^9/L$) indicates that the patient has an increased risk of bleeding. The hemostatic risk tends to be even higher for thrombocytopenic disorders characterized by a low platelet volume. Patients with mild thrombocytopenia (platelet count above $80 \times 10^9/L$) have a minimal hemostatic risk of bleeding. For patients with intermediate severity of thrombocytopenia who are asymptomatic, however, it may be difficult to estimate the risk of bleeding. In these patients, a bleeding-time test may be helpful.

Bleeding Time. The bleeding-time test usually is performed using a template-guided blade to make a longitudinal incision on the patient's volar forearm. The time to cessation of bleeding is recorded. Many factors affect the bleeding time, including operator-dependent and operator-independent differences in technique and patient-related factors. Hence, like many tests, the bleeding-time test is neither completely sensitive nor specific for platelet-mediated bleeding disorders.[78-80] Indeed, the test has never been shown to predict bleeding at surgery.[80]

We sometimes use the bleeding-time test to help identify those thrombocytopenic patients who require treatment. For example, we do not treat patients with no or only mild symptoms who have stable, moderately severe thrombocytopenia if a normal bleeding time has been documented on different occasions. However, some investigators have questioned the role of the bleeding-time test in therapeutic decisions.[79,80]

Diagnostic Approach to Thrombocytopenia

Thrombocytopenic disorders are classified into three general groups: increased platelet destruction, platelet sequestration, and decreased platelet production. Although the definitive classification of a patient requires a platelet survival study, in most circumstances, a patient can be appropriately classified using other information, including history and physical examination, MPV, and blood film and bone marrow examination. Although these investigations sometimes provide the diagnosis, more often they suggest one or more diagnostic possibilities, which can be confirmed by specific tests.

History and Physical Examination

Many patients with thrombocytopenia are identified during routine laboratory investigation or during the investigation of another disorder. In these patients, a meticulous history that probes every possible disease association is less fruitful than a few carefully chosen laboratory tests.

The focus of the history requires knowing the probable cause of the thrombocytopenia. Consequently, it is helpful to consider the results of the complete blood count. For example, isolated thrombocytopenia is usually caused by increased platelet destruction, whereas pancytopenia is usually associated with disorders of decreased platelet production or sequestration.

Identification of Thrombocytopenic Risk Factors. Although many thrombocytopenic disorders can affect patients of all ages, several are restricted to certain age groups. For example, many disorders only occur in the neonate (eg, passive autoimmune thrombocytopenia, neonatal alloimmune thrombocytopenia). Infants and young children often develop a severe but self-limited thrombocytopenia (acute ITP).

Potentially serious thrombocytopenic disorders that typically begin during late pregnancy or the puerperium include preeclampsia-associated thrombocytopenia; thrombotic microangiopathy; disseminated intravascular coagulation (DIC), which can be secondary to amniotic fluid embolism, abruptio placentae, dead fetus syndrome, retained placenta, or preeclampsia; and puerperal septicemia. However, the most common explanation for mild thrombocytopenia (75 to $150 \times 10^9/L$ during pregnancy is an entirely benign condition known as *incidental thrombocytopenia of pregnancy.*[81,82] This occurs in about 7% of pregnant women and is characterized by an absence of a history of maternal thrombocytopenia or bleeding.[81,82] The thrombocytopenia may be related to increased plasma volume in pregancy without a compensatory thrombopoietic response (hemodilution).[83] Infants born to these mothers do not develop thrombocytopenia or bleeding complications.[81,82] Accordingly, no special obstetric maneuvers are indicated for women with incidentally detected thrombocytopenia.[84]

Thrombocytopenia that occurs in a postoperative patient is frequently caused by septicemia or drug-induced thrombocytopenia (most frequently heparin) but rarely also by posttransfusion purpura (PTP) or a hemolytic transfusion reaction.

A meticulous drug history should be taken that includes agents purchased without prescription. Particularly for patients with episodic thrombocytopenia of abrupt onset, the physician should inquire about possible exposure to quinine, which is found in many beverages (eg, gin and tonic) and can cause quinine-induced thrombocytopenia.

The presence of certain medical disorders, including systemic lupus erythematosus (SLE) and other rheumatic disorders, lymphoproliferative neoplasms, and infection by the human immunodeficiency virus (HIV), suggest an immune destructive thrombocytopenia.

A family history of thrombocytopenia, bleeding tendency, or immune disorders should be sought; it suggests hereditary thrombocytopenia.

Temporal Profile of Symptoms. The insidius onset of easy bruising and epistaxis of several months' or years' duration typically occurs in patients with chronic ITP. The abrupt onset of bleeding symptoms characterizes acute ITP and immune drug-induced thrombocytopenia.

Physical Examination. The physician should look for be physical signs (eg, fever, lymphadenopathy, splenomegaly, hepatomegaly, rash) suggestive of underlying disorders that can associated with thrombocytopenia. The presence of intravascular catheters could indicate septicemia or heparin-induced thrombocytopenia. Arterial or venous thrombotic events that occur in thrombocytopenic patients suggest heparin-induced thrombocytopenia, antiphospholipid antibody (lupus anticoagulant) syndrome, neoplasia-associated DIC, or paroxysmal nocturnal hemoglobinuria.

Platelet Size

Blood count determinations are obtained using electronic particle counters, which provide the platelet count, MPV, and platelet distribution width (PDW; a marker of platelet heterogeneity). The normal platelet count typically ranges from 150 to $450 \times 10^9/L$. There is no normal range for the MPV because the MPV must be interpreted with the platelet count.[85,86] As shown in Figure 34-1, the MPV bears a nonlinear, inverse relation to the platelet count. Thus, the normal MPV for a platelet count of $150 \times 10^9/L$ is 9 to 12 fL, whereas for a platelet count of $400 \times 10^9/L$, it is 7.5 to 10 fL.[85]

By correlating the platelet count with the MPV, the clinician can obtain data that help in the classification of the platelet disorder[85,86] (see Fig. 34-1). Thrombocytopenia caused by increased platelet destruction with a normal megakaryocyte response is characterized by a larger MPV and more hemostatically effective platelets than disorders characterized by thrombocytopenia due to impaired platelet production or hypersplenism. There is an exception to this generalization: some myeloproliferative and myelo-

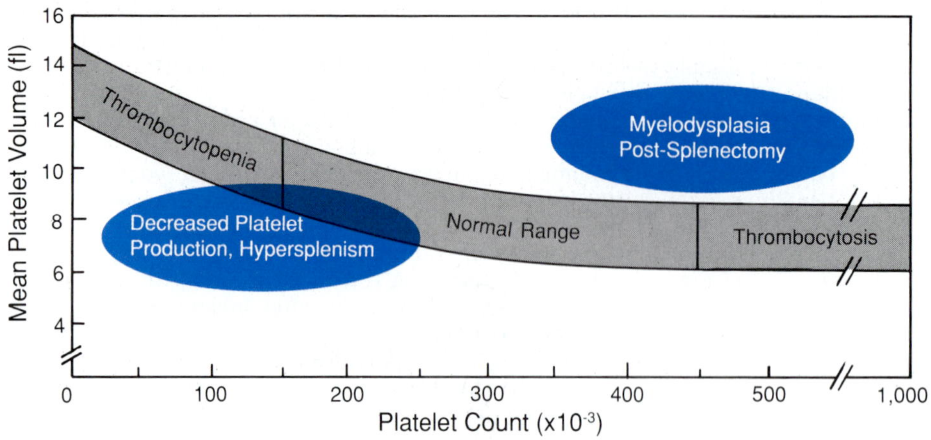

FIGURE 34-1. Mean platelet volume–platelet count relation in various platelet disorders. (After Bessman JD. Platelets. In: Bessman JD. Automated blood counts and differentials: a practical guide. Baltimore, Johns Hopkins University Press, 1986:57; and Bessman JD, Gilmer PR, Gardner FH. Use of mean platelet volume improves detection of platelet disorders. Blood Cells 1985;11:127)

dysplastic conditions can have large platelets with impaired function.

Increased platelet heterogeneity, measured as increased PDW, has been observed in myeloproliferative disease with both normal and increased platelet counts.[87] The diagnostic value of abnormal PDW in thrombocytopenic disorders has not been established, however.

Peripheral Blood Film and Marrow Examination

Peripheral Blood Film. Examination of the peripheral blood film can be helpful in elucidating the cause of unexplained thrombocytopenia. Paradoxically, inspection of the RBCs and leukocytes is usually more helpful than the platelets in determining the cause of the thrombocytopenia. RBC fragments suggest thrombocytopenia due to microangiopathy. Thrombocytopenia can occur with infiltrating marrow disorders ("tear-drop" and nucleated RBCs), megaloblastic anemia (macrocytes), immune hemolysis (spherocytes), and malaria (protozoal inclusions). Toxic granules, vacuolation, and pale blue cytoplasmic inclusions (Döhle bodies) in leukocytes suggest thrombocytopenia associated with septicemia. Reactive, atypical lymphocytes occur in viral infections, many of which can be complicated by thrombocytopenia. Neoplastic leukocytes suggest thrombocytopenia due to decreased platelet production. Dysplastic leukocytes (eg, hypogranular, Pelger-Huët anomaly) suggest myelodysplasia. Abnormal leukocyte inclusions are characteristic of some hereditary thrombocytopenic disorders, such as May-Hegglin and Fechtner syndromes.

It is important to verify by microscopy an apparent low platelet count since electronic particle counters can give erroneous platelet counts in certain situations. For instance, the presence of platelet clumps or platelets adherent to neutrophils and monocytes suggests pseudothrombocytopenia (discussed subsequently). It is preferable to use the electronic determination of the MPV rather than to attempt to judge platelet size morphologically. This is because platelet heterogeneity ensures that occasional large platelets are present even in the blood films of patients with a small MPV.[85] Circulating megakaryocyte fragments can be identified in the blood films of some patients with myeloid neoplastic disorders. Extremely large platelets are observed in some patients with myelodysplasia or myeloid leukemia, and are characteristic of the hereditary macrothrombocytopenic disorders.

Marrow Examination. Megakaryocytes are usually present in normal or increased numbers in thrombocytopenic disorders caused by platelet destruction or sequestration. Depending on the specific pathologic process, megakaryocytes are often reduced or absent (and may be morphologically abnormal) in disorders characterized by decreased platelet production. Sometimes, the bone marrow examination is diagnostic, as in acute leukemia or marrow infiltration by malignancy.

Megakaryocyte ploidy measurements using flow cytometry have been shown to correlate with the mechanism of thrombocytopenia.[5] For example, increased megakaryocyte ploidy was a feature of destructive thrombocytopenia in one study.[5]

Spurious Thrombocytosis and Pseudothrombocytopenia

Although platelet count measurements by electronic particle counters are more accurate and less expensive than conventional manual techniques, there is a potential for spurious overestimation or underestimation of the platelet count. For example, abnormal particles similar in size to platelets, such as schistocytes, microspherocytes, leukemic cell fragments, Pappenheimer bodies, and bacteria, can be counted erroneously as platelets and falsely suggest thrombocytosis.[85,88–91]

More important is spurious thrombocytopenia, which, if unrecognized, can lead to unnecessary tests or inappropriate therapy. Termed *pseudothrombocytopenia,* this artifact is caused by in vitro platelet clumping or platelet adherence to leukocytes, which result in failure of the electronic particle counter to recognize the platelets (Fig. 34-2). Therefore, it is essential that the blood film be examined in every patient with purported thrombocytopenia.[92]

EDTA-Dependent Pseudothrombocytopenia. Ethylenediaminetetraacetic acid (EDTA) is the anticoagulant used most commonly for determination of the complete blood count. Pseudothrombocytopenia occurs in up to 0.1% of all complete blood counts and is usually caused by an EDTA-dependent platelet-agglutinating antibody.[93,94] Platelet clumps usually are seen throughout the blood film, although occasionally the clumps are most prominent at the tail of the blood smear. These agglutinins are of no pathologic significance, and in vivo platelet levels are normal.

This in vitro artifact is caused by EDTA-dependent antibodies that are directed against a cryptic antigen on the platelet gpIIb/IIIa complex that becomes exposed in the presence of EDTA.[95,96] The agglutinins are usually IgG but can be IgM or IgA.[95,97] These EDTA-dependent agglutinins usually are most reactive below room temperature.[95]

Platelet Satellitism. Platelet satellitism is a rare cause of pseudothrombocytopenia characterized by EDTA-dependent rosetting of platelets around neutrophils or monocytes.[98–102] This in vitro phenomenon is probably

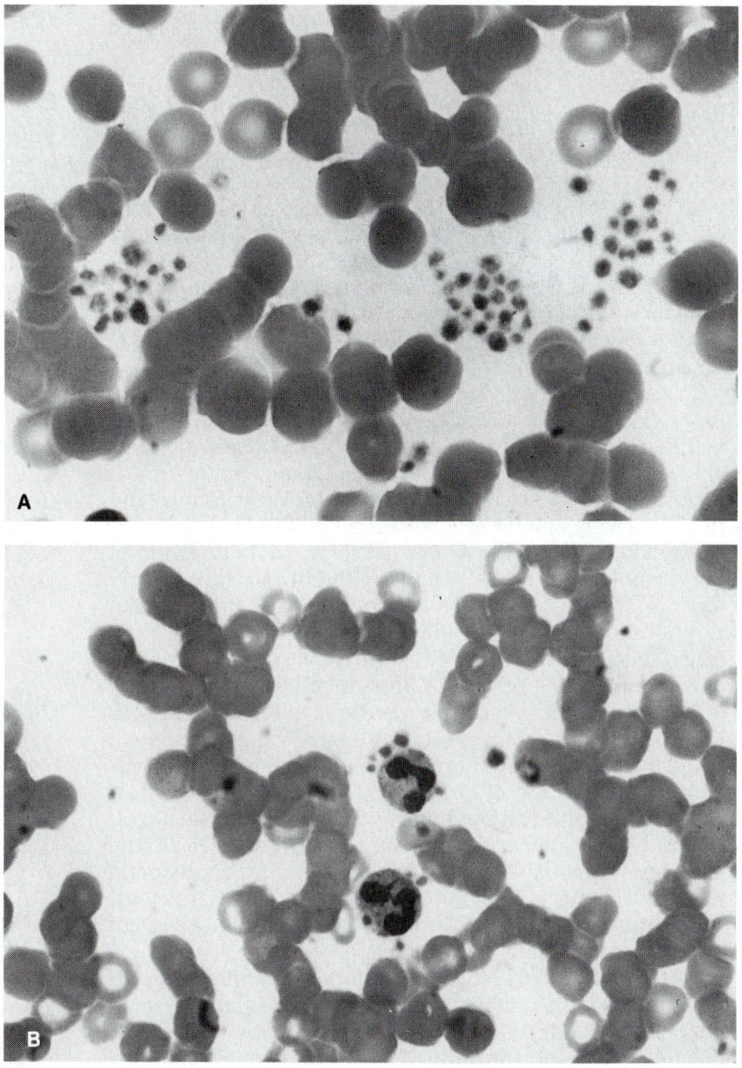

FIGURE 34-2. Photomicrograph of two types of pseudothrombocytopenia. (**A**) EDTA-dependent platelet clumping. (**B**) Platelet satellitism.

caused by antibodies in most cases, but EDTA-dependent interactions of cryofibrinogen with platelet and leukocyte surfaces have also been implicated.[101]

Platelet Cold Agglutinin. Much less commonly, pseudothrombocytopenia is caused by platelet-reactive cold agglutinins that cause platelet clumping in all anticoagulants.[103,104]

Monoclonal Platelet Agglutinin. A patient with anticoagulant- and temperature-independent pseudothrombocytopenia caused by a monoclonal IgM paraprotein was described.[105] It was impossible to obtain an accurate platelet count in this patient.

Artifacts of Blood Collection. Spurious thrombocytopenia can be caused by technically inadequate blood collection. This is usually obvious because clots are seen in the anticoagulated sample. Thrombocytopenia is not present when the platelet count is measured using another blood sample. Overfilling of the vacuum tube can also result in spurious thrombocytopenia.[106]

Platelet Count Determination in Pseudothrombocytopenia

Although these agglutinins cause in vitro artifacts and are without in vivo significance, they can prevent accurate determination of the platelet count. It is possible that pseudothrombocytopenia can complicate accurate platelet count determinations in a patient with a coexisting thrombocytopenic disorder.[107]

Several methods can be tried to obtain an accurate platelet count, including the following:

- Collecting the blood sample into different anticoagulants, such as sodium citrate or heparin
- Collecting the blood sample into an anticoagulant with a lower pH[108]
- Collecting the blood sample into a prewarmed tube that is maintained at 37°C until testing
- Determining the platelet count by phase-contrast microscopy using a sample obtained by finger-prick

General Approach to the Treatment of Thrombocytopenic Patients

Who Should Receive Treatment?

The most important issue is whether the patient requires treatment. For example, many patients with chronic ITP and moderate thrombocytopenia (platelet count, 20 to 80 $\times 10^9/L$) do not bleed except under exceptional circumstances. For these patients, the treatment (eg, corticosteroids) carries a higher morbidity than no treatment at all. Thus, factors such as the estimated bleeding risk and natural history of the illness influence whether specific treatment is required.

Prevention of Bleeding

General Measures. Thrombocytopenic patients should not receive intramuscular injections or drugs that interfere with platelet function. We specify these contraindications on the patient's chart to minimize their inadvertent application.

Prophylactic Platelet Transfusions. The use of platelet transfusion therapy is described in detail elsewhere in this book, and we discuss only the general use of platelet transfusions in thrombocytopenic patients here.

Two considerations influence the decision to administer *prophylactic* platelet transfusions. The first is the general mechanism of the thrombocytopenia. Transfused platelets are usually destroyed rapidly if the thrombocytopenia is caused by an increased rate of platelet destruction, and therefore little benefit is achieved by prophylactic platelet transfusions. The other factor is the probable duration of the thrombocytopenia. Patients with chronic thrombocytopenia (hereditary platelet disorders, aplastic anemia) should not receive prophylactic platelet transfusions because the short-term benefit is outweighed by the risk of developing platelet-reactive alloantibodies, which could jeopardize future use of *therapeutic* platelet transfusions. For these reasons, the best candidates for prophylactic platelet transfusion therapy are patients who have thrombocytopenia caused by underproduction and in whom it is likely that the platelet count will rise to normal levels in a relatively short period of time (eg, patients receiving chemotherapeutic agents for leukemia). Prophylactic platelet transfusions sometimes are given to patients with self-limited, destructive thrombocytopenia if the risk of bleeding on clinical grounds appears to be high (eg, bacteremia-associated thrombocytopenia, immune drug-induced thrombocytopenia).[109] Prophylactic platelet transfusions are contraindicated in patients with thrombotic thrombocytopenic purpura (TTP) or heparin-induced thrombocytopenia, since acute platelet-mediated thrombosis can occur after the platelet transfusion.

Treatment of Bleeding. Platelet transfusions should be given to all patients with serious or potentially life-threatening bleeding, even if the bleeding is caused by increased platelet destruction. This is because a transient improvement in hemostasis can be achieved during this critical interval before attaining therapeutic efficacy of other specific therapy.

Antifibrinolytic therapy (ϵ-aminocaproic acid or tranexamic acid) has been given to control bleeding in patients with chronic thrombocytopenia refractory to specific therapy and platelet transfusions. Two retrospective studies[110,111] have described benefit for both prevention and control of bleeding. However, a small, randomized, controlled trial did not show benefit using tranexamic acid in thrombocytopenic patients.[112]

DESTRUCTIVE THROMBOCYTOPENIA CAUSED BY IMMUNE MECHANISMS

Immune mechanisms usually cause isolated thrombocytopenia. In some disorders, such as chronic ITP, the pathogenic role of the platelet-reactive IgG autoantibodies is well established. In other disorders, such as acute ITP, HIV-associated thrombocytopenia, idiosyncratic drug-induced thrombocytopenia, and PTP, the role of immune platelet destruction is established, but the nature of the platelet–antibody interaction is less well understood.

Platelet–Antibody Interactions

Overview

IgG can bind to platelets in a number of different ways, as illustrated in Figure 34-3.

Autoantibody. The antigen-combining Fab regions of IgG can bind to platelet-specific glycoprotein alloantigenic or glycolipid determinants on autologous platelets (eg, chronic ITP).

Alloantibody. The Fab regions of IgG can bind to platelet-specific glycoprotein determinants on homologous platelets (eg, neonatal alloimmune thrombocytopenia, PTP, passive alloimmune thrombocytopenia). Alloantigens are genetically determined structural differences in proteins or carbohydrates that can be recognized immunologically by certain individuals who are exposed to these antigens through pregnancy or transfusion. It is possible that adsorbed platelet-nonspecific alloantigens can be implicated in some disorders (eg, platelet-adsorbed RBC antigens as a cause of refractoriness to platelet transfusion therapy).

Antibody-Recognizing Foreign Antigen. The Fab region of IgG can bind to nonplatelet foreign antigens (eg,

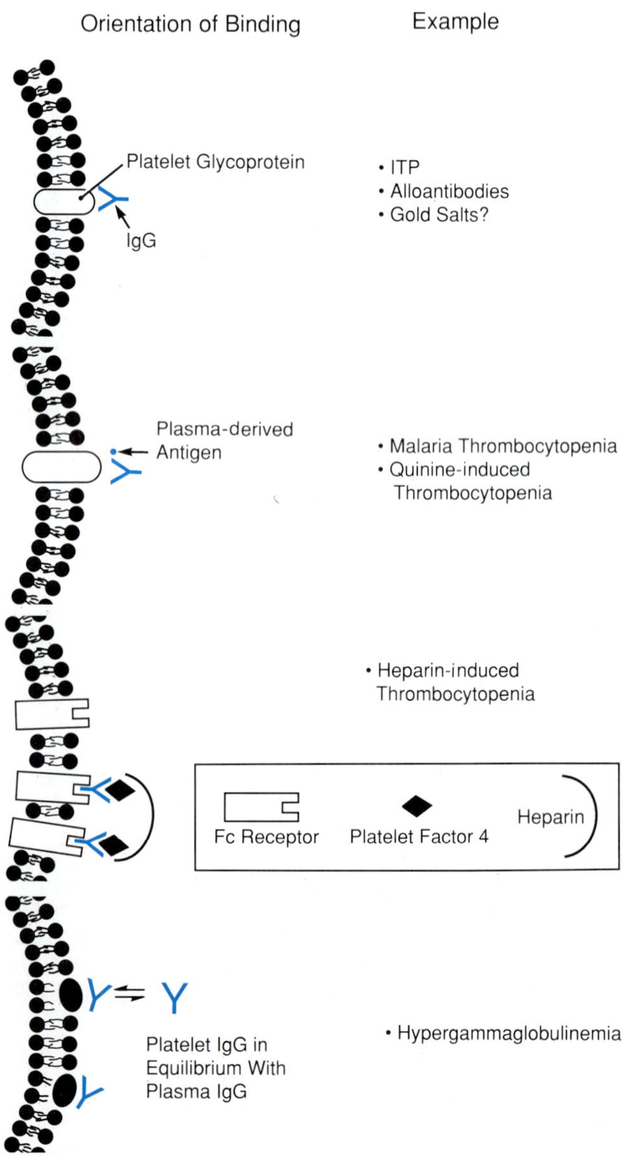

FIGURE 34-3. Schematic representation of how IgG can bind to platelet surfaces.

drugs, microbes) that adsorb to the platelet surface (eg, quinidine-induced thrombocytopenia, malaria-associated thrombocytopenia).

Immune Complex. The Fab region of IgG can bind to certain antigens (heparin/platelet factor 4 complex), and the resulting immune complex interacts with and activates the platelet by means of the platelet Fc II receptors (heparin-induced thrombocytopenia).

Nonspecific Antibody. IgG can bind to platelets nonspecifically through a poorly defined mechanism (hypergammaglobulinemia).

Platelet-Specific Glycoproteins

Several glycoproteins occur predominantly on platelets, such as various members of the integrin family (eg, gpIIb/IIIa, gpIa/IIa) or leucine-rich glycoprotein family (gpIb/IX/V complex). Although not always unique to platelets (eg, gpIb can be detected on cultured human endothelial cells[113]), they are often called platelet-specific. In contrast, there are other glycoproteins (eg, HLA) and glycolipids (eg, blood group ABH antigens) that are relatively ubiquitous or that are found in much larger quantities on certain cells other than platelets (eg, Fc receptors on leukocytes and platelets). These are platelet-nonspecific molecules.

Glycoprotein Ib/IX Complex and Glycoprotein V. The gpIb/IX complex is important for the initial contact (adhesion) of the platelet to the damaged vessel wall.[114] The contact between platelet gpIb and the vessel wall is mediated by a large, multimeric protein, known as *von Willebrand factor*, which acts as the platelet–vessel wall "glue."[115] Deficiency of gpV and gpIb/IX in the Bernard-Soulier syndrome[116,117] indicates that all three glycoproteins may exist together in a macromolecular complex (Fig. 34-4).

Glycoprotein Ib can be an autoantigen in ITP.[118–123] The gpIb/IX complex is also involved in the binding of drugs, such as quinidine and quinine, in drug-induced immune thrombocytopenia.[124,125] The amino acid polymorphism that defines the Ko alloantigen system has been localized to the α subunit of gpIb[126] (see Fig. 34-4).

Acquired structural modification of RBC carbohydrates is encountered in some neoplastic myeloid states and results in the exposure of the Tn antigen (N-acetylgalactosamine) to naturally occurring anti-Tn antibodies.[127,128] Similar structural modifications occur in the glycocalicin region of gpIb,[129] and it is possible that immune mechanisms can contribute to thrombocytopenia in the Tn syndrome.

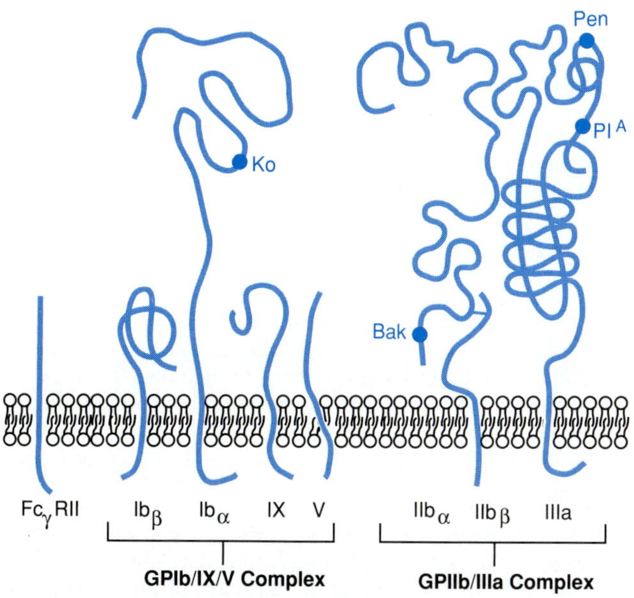

FIGURE 34-4. Schematic representation of selected platelet alloantigens located on various platelet glycoproteins.

Platelet Integrins. These constitute a superfamily of integral membrane proteins involved in cell–vessel wall and cell–cell contact.[130–132] The integrins are characterized by the noncovalent association of two different proteins (heterodimer) consisting of a larger α (sometimes consisting of two covalently linked peptide chains (eg, gpIIb; see Fig. 34-4) and a smaller β subunit. The integrins are subclassified on the basis of common β chains. Members of the β_3 and β_1 families are present on platelets.

The platelet β_3-integrins, which are involved in cytoadhesion, are gpIIb/IIIa (also known as $\alpha_{IIb}\beta_3$) and the vitronectin receptor ($\alpha_v\beta_3$).[131–136] The platelet β_1-integrins, which are involved in platelet interactions with extracellular matrix proteins, consist of gpIa/IIa ($\alpha_2\beta_1$), gpIc/IIa ($\alpha_5\beta_1$), and gpIc′/IIa ($\alpha_6\beta_1$).[131,137–143]

Several platelet integrins are implicated in clinical disorders. For example, the gpIIb/IIIa complex is the most important target autoantigen in chronic ITP.[120,144–147] It can also bind drug, thereby contributing to the antigenic target complex in quinine- or quinidine-dependent immune thrombocytopenia.[148] Many of the platelet alloantigen systems are located on gpIIb/IIIa (see Fig. 34-4). Glycoprotein IIIa is the site of the $Pl^{A1/A2}$ ($Zw^{a/b}$)* and $Pen^{a/b}$ alloantigen systems. Glycoprotein IIb_α is the site for $Bak^{a/b}$ ($Lek^{a/b}$). Several more recently described "private" alloantigens (eg, Sr^a, Tu^a, Mo^a) are also found on gpIIIa. The $Br^{a/b}$ ($Zav^{a/b}$) system is located on gpIa of the collagen receptor integrin gpIa/IIa. Table 34-3, which appears in the section on alloimmune thrombocytopenic disorders, summarizes the platelet alloantigen systems.

Molecular Biology of the Pl^{A1} System. The $Pl^{A1/A2}$ alloantigen system was first characterized at the molecular level. Initial work showed that the alloantigen site was not on a carbohydrate but rather on a 17-kd peptide fragment of gpIIIa.[149] The amino acid sequence of the Pl^{A1} phenotype of gpIIIa was deduced by the sequencing of relevant cDNA clones.[150–152] The Pl^{A2} phenotype is defined by a single amino acid substitution of proline for leucine at residue 33 of the mature gpIIIa molecule.[153] The ability to detect the associated DNA polymorphism using the polymerase chain reaction provides a means to identify a patient's Pl^A alloantigen status without the requirement for platelet samples or serologic techniques.[153]

Platelet-Nonspecific Glycoproteins

HLA antigens are a highly polymorphic multiallelic system important in the immunologic distinction between self and nonself. HLA antigens are subdivided into class I (HLA-A, -B, -C) and class II (HLA-DR, -DQ, -DP) antigens. Genes coding for HLA specificity are closely linked on the short arm of chromosome 6 and are inherited in a unit termed the *haplotype*.

HLA class I antigens are located on most cells, including lymphocytes, granulocytes, and platelets, but not RBCs. They are important for the recognition of self by cytotoxic T cells. HLA class II antigens are important in the presentation of antigens by macrophages and B lymphocytes to helper T cells.

HLA class I, but not class II, antigens are expressed on

* Most of the alloantigen systems have more than one designation. In this chapter, we use the names that are most widely accepted; we also indicate alternate names in Table 34-3.

platelets. HLA class I antigens are intrinsic membrane constituents[154] present in higher densities on platelets compared with lymphocytes.[155] HLA-A and -B antigens are strongly, although variably, expressed[37,155–157] whereas HLA-C antigens are weakly expressed.[158]

Alloantibodies frequently form against HLA antigens; about 20% to 30% of multiparous women, and many polytransfused patients, have identifiable antibodies against HLA antigens. HLA alloantibodies are thought to be important in the development of refractoriness to platelet transfusions. Although some physicians have claimed that HLA antibodies were responsible for cases of neonatal alloimmune thrombocytopenia,[159,160] this remains unproved, and it is likely that in many instances a platelet-specific alloantibody was present but not detected.

Platelet-Nonspecific Glycolipids and Phospholipids

RBC Antigens. The RBC alloantigens ABH, Lewis, Ii, and P are found on platelets.[161–167] The ABH and Lewis antigens are glycosphingolipids that are adsorbed to platelets from the plasma.[161,164] Additionally, ABH antigens are constitutive platelet membrane components carried on certain glycoproteins[163] and are intrinsic antigens that are made by megakaryocytes.[162,168] These antigens are variably expressed.[169]

The importance of group A and B antigens in platelet transfusion incompatibility is debated but can account for a reduced posttransfusion platelet recovery in some patients.[170–176] The Lewis, Ii, and P alloantigen systems have no clinical relevance to platelet transfusion.

Other Glycolipids. Glycolipids consist of three basic units—sphingosine, fatty acid, and sugar—and are either neutral or acidic.[177] Acidic glycolipids can be either gangliosides or sulfatides, depending on whether the acidic component is sialic acid or sulfate, respectively. Investigations suggest that these glycolipids may play an important role in platelet activation.[177]

Glycolipids are known to be immunogenic[178] and have been implicated as target autoantigens in some patients with chronic ITP.[179–181]

Phospholipids. Many different phospholipids constitute the platelet lipid bilayer membrane, with the most plentiful being phosphatidylcholine, phosphatidylethanolamine, phosphatidylserine, and sphingomyelin.[182] These molecules are asymmetrically distributed; most of the sphingomyelin is present in the outer membrane layer, whereas most of the phosphotidylserine is present on the inner membrane layer.[183] Phosphatidylethanolamine and phosphatidylinositol are also more plentiful in the inner membrane layer. These inner membrane phospholipids become exposed during platelet activation.[184]

Autoantibodies against phospholipid or phospholipid–protein structures prolong certain clotting tests. These autoantibodies have been called *lupus anticoagulants,* and patients with these autoantibodies can have recurrent arterial and venous thrombosis and recurrent fetal loss (lupus anticoagulant or antiphospholipid syndrome). Some studies suggest that thrombocytopenia occurs commonly in these patients. In one study,[185] anticardiolipin antibodies (cardiolipin is a target antigen in the antiphospholipid syndrome) were detected in 30% of patients with apparent chronic ITP.

Cryptic Antigens and Neoantigens. *Cryptic antigens* are hidden antigens that could become exposed under certain circumstances. *Neoantigens* are antigens that are formed only after changes in molecular conformation (eg, after platelet activation). It can be difficult to distinguish these two types of antigen.

It is possible that autoantibodies against senescent cryptic antigens or neoantigens are involved in senescent platelet clearance.

Pseudothrombocytopenia caused by EDTA-dependent autoantibodies could be caused by EDTA-induced formation of either cryptic antigens or neoantigens.[186]

A human monoclonal antibody has been described that reacts with gpIIb/IIIa only after platelet activation or storage, suggesting involvement of an activation-dependent neoantigen.[187]

Adsorbed Nonplatelet Antigens. The platelet has been characterized as a sponge that is capable of adsorbing nonplatelet molecules. For example, both Ig and albumin are present on normal platelets.[188,189] Indeed, the quantities of the Ig classes and subclasses on the platelet parallel their plasma concentrations. Ig and albumin are also found within the platelet α granules,[190,191] although it remains uncertain whether incorporation occurs primarily at the megakaryocyte or platelet level. Evidence suggests that endocytosis of fibrinogen occurs with both megakaryocytes[192–194] and platelets.[194] Other endogenous molecules, such as DNA, can bind to receptors on the platelet surface.[195] Finally, foreign substances, such as microbes and drugs, can be adsorbed to the platelet surface.

Nonspecific adsorption of Ig can be caused by the initial binding of platelet-reactive autoantibody and may contribute to platelet destruction.[196,197]

Adsorbed autoantigens, such as DNA, can be involved in the pathogenesis of thrombocytopenia in some autoimmune disorders.[198–200]

The thrombocytopenia associated with malaria[201] and drugs such as quinidine[124,125] is caused by the binding of IgG to these foreign antigens adsorbed to platelets.

Platelet Immunoglobulin Fc Receptors. The platelet IgG Fc receptor is a 40-kd, transmembrane receptor that binds with a low affinity to the Cγ2 region of IgG.[202–204] The platelet Fc receptor is identical to the type II (FcγRII) IgG receptor found on phagocytic cells. The platelet carries about 1500 to 3000 copies of these receptors. The binding of IgG complexes to the platelet FcγII receptors initiates platelet aggregation and release. Platelets also possess IgE Fc receptors that resemble the type II (FcϵRII) receptors found on eosinophils.[204]

Involvement of the FcγII receptors has been implicated in the pathogenesis of heparin-induced thrombocytopenia.[205] It is possible that thrombocytopenia results from interaction of immune complexes (either antibody–antigen or antibody–anti-antibody) with platelet Fc receptors in SLE and other immune thrombocytopenic disorders, but this remains unproved. It is unkown whether platelet IgE Fc receptors play any role in the pathogenesis of thrombocytopenia in IgE-mediated allergic disorders.

Platelet Antibody Testing

Advances in the understanding of immune platelet disorders have in large part resulted from the increasing sophistication and widespread application of in vitro platelet antibody tests. Literally hundreds of these tests have been described. To simplify the discussion, these assays have been classified into three groups termed phase I, II, and III assays according to the time of introduction and general technique. In brief, phase I assays, which were first developed in the 1950s, measure a functional platelet-dependent endpoint, usually platelet activation. Phase II assays detect the presence of Ig or complement on or within the platelet; these assays, first developed in 1975, are often referred to as tests for platelet-associated IgG (PAIgG). In 1984, assays that measure the binding of Ig to specific platelet proteins were developed, which we refer to as phase III assays.

Although most of these assays were developed to detect platelet antibodies in ITP patients, modifications permit their use in other clinical situations. For example, platelets of known alloantigen specificity can be used in the identification of alloantibodies. Platelet antibody testing in the presence and absence of certain drugs and their metabolites can be useful for confirming the diagnosis of drug-induced immune thrombocytopenia.

Phase I Assays

In all phase I assays, patient plasma or serum is added to normal platelets, and a platelet-dependent endpoint, such as platelet activation, is measured. Platelet activation can be detected by several methods, including aggregation,[206,207] ^{14}C- or ^{3}H-serotonin release from platelet granules,[208,209] release of cytoplasmic ^{51}Cr, increased availability of platelet factor 3 (procoagulant activity),[210,211] and inhibition of a platelet function (eg, migration inhibition, clot retraction).[212]

Generally speaking, phase I assays have low sensitivity and specificity for detecting platelet–antibody interactions. The sensitivity is low because not all test samples contain sufficiently reactive antibody to result in platelet activation. The specificity is low because platelet activation is not specific for IgG; small amounts of thrombin or immune complexes in the test sample can produce a false-positive result. An exception to these generalizations is the platelet ^{14}C-serotonin release assay for heparin-induced thrombocytopenia.[205,213,214] This test has high sensitivity for heparin-induced thrombocytopenia because it exploits the potent platelet-activating properties of the pathogenic IgG. The specificity is high because various control maneuvers (eg, high heparin concentrations, platelet Fc receptor blocking monoclonal antibody) have been incorporated to distinguish heparin-induced thrombocytopenia IgG from thrombin or immune complexes.

Phase II Assays

Phase II assays are the dominant type of assay used. Phase II assays are superior to phase I assays because they detect Ig or complement on the platelet rather than infer its presence through an endpoint such as platelet activation.

All phase II assays use an immunologic probe to detect surface-bound Ig or complement. Usually, these probes are antibodies (polyclonal or monoclonal anti-Ig or anticomplement probes), although staphylococcal protein A can be used to detect IgG subtypes 1, 2, and 4. The probes are usually labeled with a radioisotope, fluorescent marker or are enzyme-linked. The labeled probe is mixed with the test platelets, which can be intact or lysed, and then the amount of probe that binds to the test platelets is measured. Amplification of the signal can be achieved by using a polyclonal, labeled second antibody (anti–anti-IgG) or a biotin–avidin detection system. The IgG that is detected using these phase II assays is termed PAIgG. The designation of PAIgG is used because these assays measure all platelet IgG irrespective of the type of binding to the platelet.

The three general categories of phase II assays are direct-binding assays, two-stage (consumption) assays, and assays for total PAIgG.

Direct-Binding Assays. In these assays, the binding of a labeled anti-Ig probe to the platelet surface is quantitated (Fig. 34-5).

These assays are performed by incubating the washed test platelets with the labeled anti-Ig probe. After equilibrium is reached, the unbound probe is washed away, and the amount bound to the platelets is measured (radioactivity, fluorescence, enzyme activity).[215–222] The assays are semiquantitative because although the specific activity of the labeled probes can be determined, theoretic binding ratios must be used (eg, assumption of 1:1 binding of monoclonal probe to platelet-bound Ig). Alternatively, the binding of the probe to known amounts of IgG on another cell (eg, anti-D on an RBC) can be used for assay calibration. Flow cytometry has been used to determine PAIgG levels using antiglobulin probes linked to fluorescent markers.[223–225]

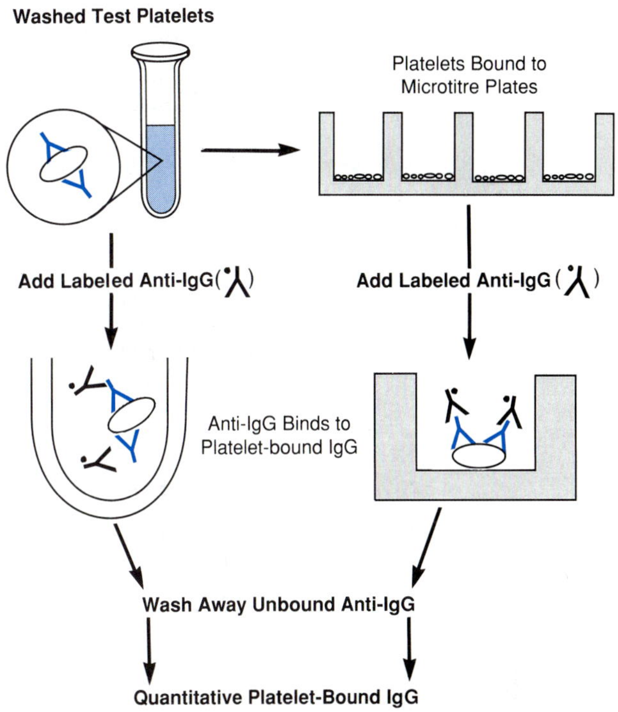

FIGURE 34-5. Schematic representation of a direct-binding assay for platelet-associated IgG.

A problem for the direct-binding assays is nonspecific binding of the labeled probe to the platelets. Nonspecific binding is the amount of probe bound in the presence of supersaturating amounts of unlabeled probe. Nonspecific binding of the anti-Ig probe to the platelets can be reduced by the use of protein-containing media (blocking buffer). Because monoclonal antibodies can be used at extremely low concentrations, and because nonspecific binding is concentration-dependent, the high purity of monoclonal probes dramatically reduces nonspecific binding.[219,220]

Two-Stage Assays (Consumption Assays). These assays are performed in two stages (Fig. 34-6). In the first stage, varying numbers of test platelets are incubated with the probe (anti-IgG). Known amounts of IgG in solution are substituted for the test platelets in a separate test to generate a standard curve. The anti-IgG probe must be in excess of the amount of IgG on the test platelets (or IgG standard). In the second stage, the anti-IgG that is not consumed by the platelet-bound IgG (or IgG standard) is quantitated by measuring its binding to IgG fixed to a solid phase. The solid-phase IgG can be bound to a bead, cell (eg, sheep red blood cells), or microtiter well.[226–229] The anti-IgG probe can be labeled with radioisotope, fluorescein, or with an enzyme, or it can be unlabeled and quantitated using a labeled anti–anti-Ig (probe amplification). A biologic endpoint (eg, complement-mediated lysis of sheep red blood cells) also has been used.[226]

An advantage of the two-stage assays is that quantitation is simplified because known amounts of IgG (the standard)

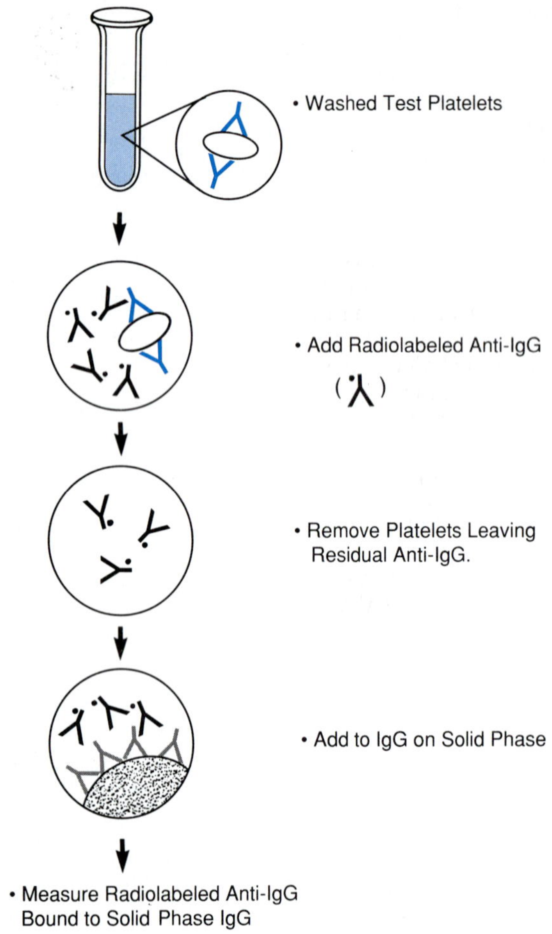

FIGURE 34-6. Schematic representation of a two-stage assay (consumption assay) for platelet-associated IgG.

can substitute for the test platelets. The problem of nonspecific binding of the probe to the platelets is overcome using the second stage. A disadvantage is that these assays are more complex than the other phase II assays. Another disadvantage is theoretic: it has been suggested that these assays give an incorrectly high estimate of the amount of platelet-bound Ig.[230,231] Although the actual amounts of IgG on the surface of normal and abnormal platelets remain unresolved, no type of phase II assay demonstrates superior specificity in the diagnosis of immune thrombocytopenia.[232] These issues are discussed in a later section.

Assays for Total PAIgG. The total amount of IgG, from both the interior and the surface of the platelet, is measured in these assays[233–237] (Fig. 34-7).

The test platelets are washed and counted, and then the bilipid platelet membranes are lysed by detergent (eg, Triton X-100), sonication, or repeated freezing and thawing. The total IgG, which is released from the membrane, cytosol, and α granules, can be measured by any technique that quantitates small amounts of fluid-phase IgG, including nephelometry or immunoradiometric assay. There is general agreement that the total PAIgG of normal platelets is 10,000 to 20,000 molecules (2.5 to 5 fg) per platelet.[235–237]

These assays are simple to perform, and because the platelet membrane is dissolved, there is no nonspecific binding of the anti-IgG to the membrane. A further advantage is that the platelet lysates can be stored frozen, allowing the tests to be batched. A disadvantage is the theoretic possibility that changes in total PAIgG might correlate poorly with pathophysiologically important changes in surface-bound PAIgG. In practice, however, assays for total PAIgG correlate well with other phase II assays.[232,236] The biologic basis for the correlation between surface-bound and total PAIgG is uncertain.

Technical Considerations. Processing of the platelets for testing requires isolation from anticoagulated whole blood, followed by washing to remove loosely bound plasma protein from the platelets. The best anticoagulant is acid citrate dextrose since platelets can be stored for up to 5 days at room temperature before testing.[238] EDTA causes platelet swelling and a spurious increase in the PAIgG.[239,240] Washing can be accomplished either by use of large-pore gels or by repetitive aqueous washing followed by centrifugation.

Use. These assays are used most frequently to assist in the diagnosis of immune thrombocytopenic disorders such as ITP. All these assays have similar sensitivity and specificity for immune thrombocytopenia.[232] Additionally, they may be used for other purposes, such as for platelet typing and crossmatching.

Phase III Assays

Phase III assays measure the binding of antibody to specific platelet proteins. The phase III assays differ in the way the platelet proteins are presented to the antiplatelet antibodies. These assays have been developed only during the past decade, and questions about sensitivity and specificity in immune thrombocytopenic disorders remain.

Immunoblotting (Western Blotting). Patient serum is allowed to interact with platelet proteins that have been separated electrophoretically and immobilized on nitrocellulose.[145,147,241]

The test platelets are washed, and the bilipid layer is dissolved by detergent (Fig. 34-8). The platelet proteins are separated according to size using sodium dodecylsulfate polyacrylamide gel electrophoresis (SDS-PAGE). The platelet proteins are transferred to nitrocellulose paper (blotting). The test serum is added to the nitrocellulose,

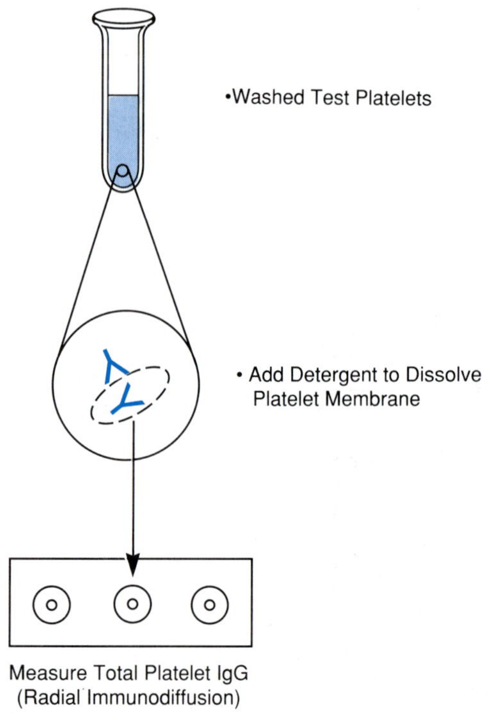

FIGURE 34-7. Schematic representation of an assay for total platelet-associated IgG.

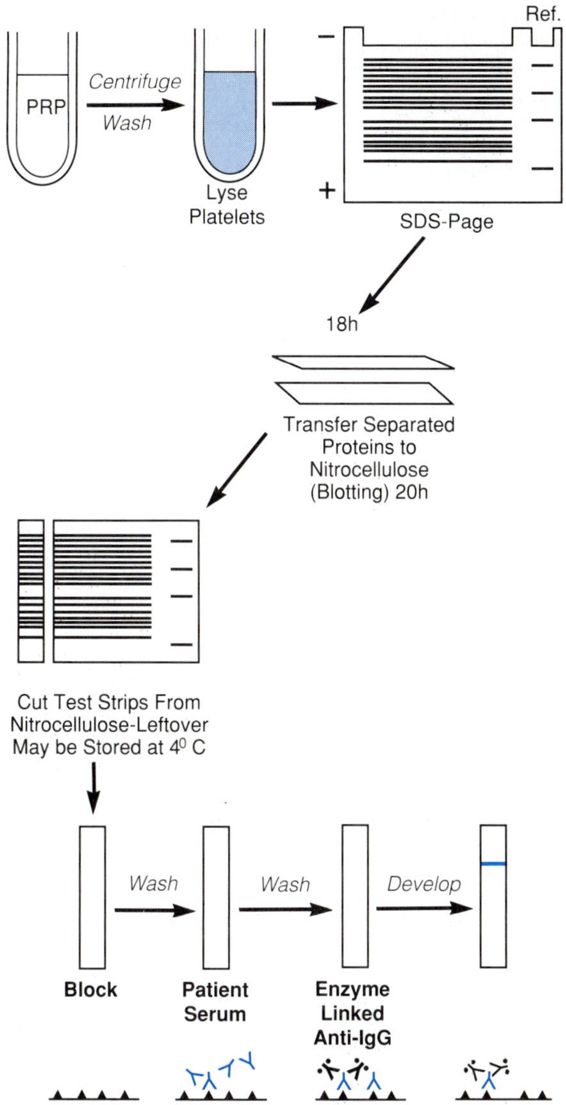

FIGURE 34-8. Immunoblotting to detect IgG reactive with specific platelet glycoproteins.

and after a wash step, binding of patient antibody to specific protein bands is detected using a labeled anti-Ig.

Western blotting offers the advantages of simplicity and ability to store the immobilized platelet proteins for long periods of time. A disadvantage is that some of the protein antigens may be altered or lost during blotting. Most importantly, IgG from normal sera frequently react in immunoblot assays with platelet glycoproteins, some of which have been identified as the internal platelet proteins vinculin and talin, suggesting that caution should be used in interpreting the results of immunoblots.[242,243]

Radioimmunoprecipitation. In this assay, patient serum is allowed to interact with radiolabeled platelet membrane proteins. In a subsequent step, the antibody-sensitized radiolabeled platelet membrane proteins are separated and identified[244] (Fig. 34-9).

After washing the test platelets, the surface proteins are radiolabeled. The test serum is then incubated with the radiolabeled platelets. After the binding by specific antiplatelet antibody, detergent is added to solubilize the protein–antibody complexes, which are subsequently precipitated by the addition of an anti-Ig bound to a solid phase (often immobilized staphylococcal protein A). The radiolabeled protein–antibody complexes are washed, and the platelet proteins are separated by SDS-PAGE with detection by autoradiography. The target protein antigen can be identified by its characteristic electrophoretic mobility (see Fig. 34-9). In a modification of this assay, platelet-reactive autoantibodies have been demonstrated directly by radiolabeling washed patient and control platelets without any serum incubation step (direct radioimmunoprecipitation).[245,246]

Radioimmunoprecipitation offers advantages over immunoblotting because the antibody binds to native platelet proteins. The major disadvantages of radioimmunoprecipitation are the requirement for radioactive tracers and the possibility that not all the platelet proteins of interest are radiolabeled. These disadvantages can be overcome using the nonradioactive label biotin, which also labels more glycoproteins than radioactive iodine.[247] These assays are technically demanding.

Protein-Capture Assays. In these assays, monoclonal antibodies are used to capture a certain platelet glycoprotein so that specific IgG–platelet protein interactions can be detected.[118,120,146,248]

In the initially described method, solid-phase, immobilized monoclonal antibodies that recognized a specific platelet protein (eg, gpIIb/IIIa complex) were used to capture the platelet proteins from lysed platelets. Patient serum was subsequently added, and after a wash step, labeled anti-Ig was used to detect patient IgG that had bound to immobilized platelet proteins.[118,146] In subsequently reported methods, patient serum was incubated with intact platelets before lysis[120,248,249] (Fig. 34-10). Because this modification avoids sodium dodecyl sulfate (SDS) denaturation until after the serum has reacted with the intact platelets, test sensitivity is improved.[120,248,249] Moreover, background is markedly reduced because direct contact betwen the test serum and microtiter plates is avoided.

Protein-capture assays are much simpler to perform than the other phase III assays. The requirement for specific monoclonal antibodies is a disadvantage because these monoclonal reagents are not universally available. These assays also give falsely negative results if the patient antibody binds to the same epitope that is recognized by the monoclonal antibody.[248,250] False-positive results can be caused by naturally occurring human anti–mouse IgG antibodies.[251] However, this problem is avoided by preincubating target platelets with test serum, followed by washing, before addition of mouse monoclonal antibody, as described using the modified monoclonal antibody immobilization of platelet antigens assay.

Use. It is unlikely that phase III assays will offer greater sensitivity for the diagnosis of immune thrombocytopenic disorders compared with phase II assays. Because phase III assays permit the characterization of antibody interaction with specific platelet proteins, however, these assays allow the direct identification of glycoprotein specificity of autoantibodies and alloantibodies. Thus, diagnostic specificity of immune thrombocytopenic disorders is enhanced.

Controversies in Platelet Antibody Testing

Several issues concerning platelet antibody testing remain unresolved.

Amount of IgG on Washed Platelets From Normal Donors. Most agree that the amount of IgG detected from lysed platelets (total PAIgG) ranges from 10,000 to 20,000 molecules of IgG per platelet.[252,253] There is controversy, however, regarding the amount of IgG on the surface of washed platelets from normal subjects. Using a two-stage assay, the amount of IgG is about 3000 to 8000 molecules

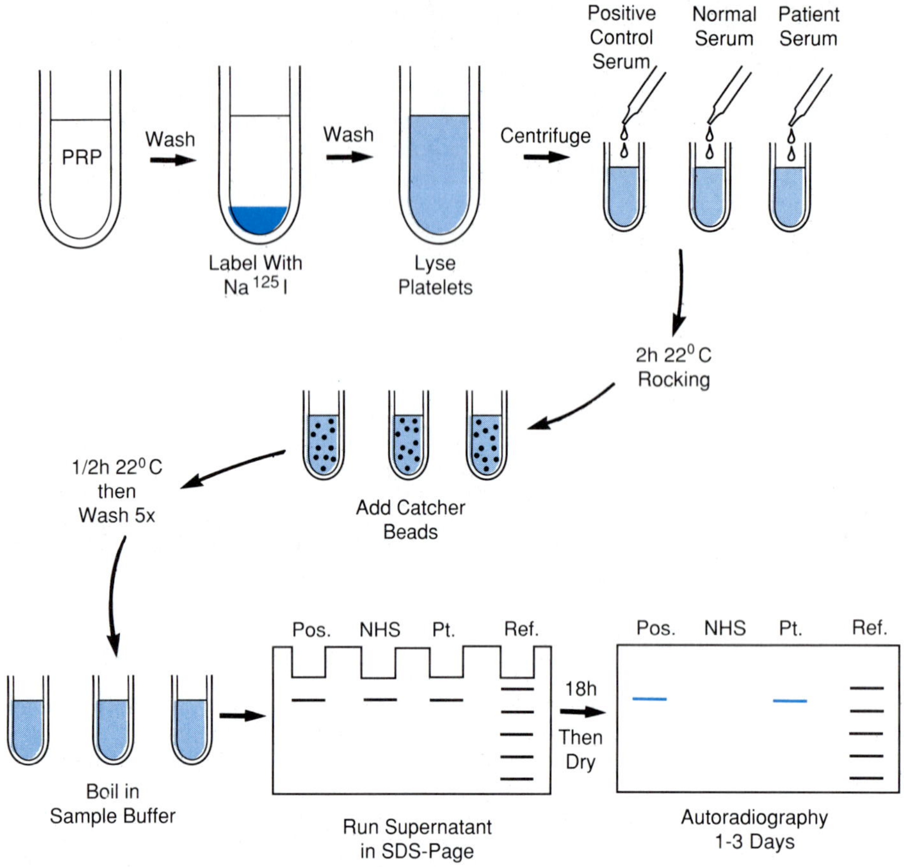

FIGURE 34-9. Radioimmunoprecipitation to detect IgG reactive with specific platelet glycoproteins.

per platelet.[252,253] Similar results have been reported with direct-binding assays employing polyclonal anti-Ig reagents.[221,222,252,253] When a monoclonal anti-IgG is used, a far lower value for IgG is obtained on normal platelets, usually 100 to 200 molecules of IgG per platelet.[189,219,220,232]

The reason for the differences in the amount of PAIgG almost certainly is due to a systematic calibration error for one of the assays. Two groups of investigators have suggested that two-stage PAIgG assays overestimate the true amount of PAIgG.[230,231] Another group has demonstrated essentially identical binding characteristics of the antibody to IgG, whether the test IgG is present in the solid phase (ie, on platelets) or in the fluid phase.[227] Further evidence supporting the validity of the higher estimate of normal PAIgG comes from other investigators. Kiefel and associates[254] used both polyclonal and monoclonal anti-IgG reagents in a two-stage assay. Identical results were obtained with either reagent, and a normal surface PAIgG of about 5500 molecules of IgG per platelet was shown. These workers suggested that direct-binding assays using monoclonal reagents or staphylococcal protein A underestimates the amount of surface PAIgG.[254] Hotchkiss and associates[255] used another approach. They eluted IgG from the test platelets and measured it in a fluid-phase assay to overcome the problems of calibration. They reported similarly high levels of IgG per platelet (5200 molecules per platelet).

Sensitivity and Specificity of Platelet Antibody Testing

Phase I Assays. Phase I assays are no longer used for the diagnosis of ITP because of low sensitivity and specificity.

Phase II Assays. The sensitivity of phase II assays for ITP ranges from 60% to 90%.[219,220,226,232,233,256,257] The severity of the thrombocytopenia can affect the determination of test sensitivity; the test sensitivity of PAIgG is higher for ITP patients with severe than with mild to moderate thrombocytopenia. A study[232] comparing four major assays for PAIgG (direct-binding assay using staphylococcal protein A or monoclonal anti-IgG; two-stage assay using polyclonal anti-IgG; assay for total PAIgG) showed that they all had a similar sensitivity for ITP.

There is disagreement about the specificity of phase II assays for ITP. In most initial reports, the results were reported as negative in patients with nonimmune thrombocytopenic disorders (ie, high specificity). However, several studies have demonstrated that PAIgG frequently is elevated in "nonimmune" thrombocytopenic disorders such as acute leukemia, thrombotic thrombocytopenic purpura, preeclampsia, and septicemia.[256,257] Some investigators have claimed that diagnostic specificity for immune thrombocytopenia is increased using direct binding assays employing a radiolabeled monoclonal anti-IgG or staphylococcal protein A.[219,220] However, a prospective study demonstrated that these assays did not have different specificity for ITP compared with two-stage assays or assays for total PAIgG.[232]

Theoretically, the elevated PAIgG found in nonimmune disorders could be related to the thrombocytopenia itself. However, results from an animal model of thrombocytopenia do not support this view.[258] In these studies, thrombocytopenia was induced in rabbits using guinea pig anti–rabbit platelet antiserum (immune destructive thrombocytopenia), administration of adenosine diphosphate (nonimmune destructive thrombocytopenia), and total body irradiation (thrombocytopenia due to decreased platelet production). Rabbit PAIgG was measured using a direct binding assay employing radiolabeled staphylococcal protein A. Only the rabbits with immune thrombocytopenia had elevated PAIgG levels, suggesting that thrombocytopenia per se does not result in elevated PAIgG.[258] If the elevated surface PAIgG contributes to increased platelet destruction in some nonimmune thrombocytopenic dis-

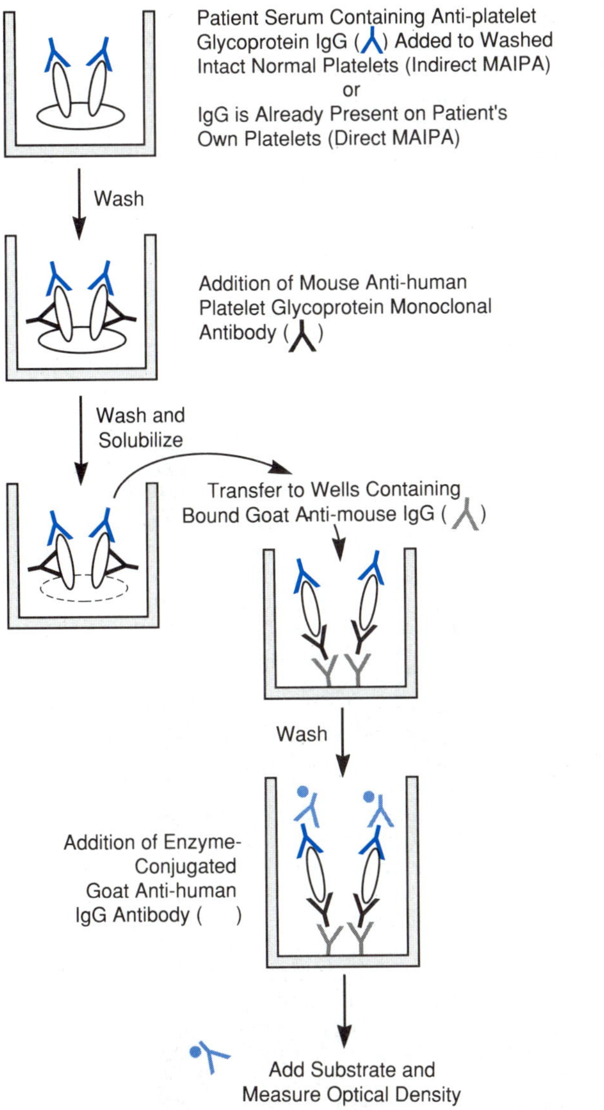

FIGURE 34-10. Modified monoclonal antibody immobilization of platelet antigens (MAIPA) assay to detect IgG reactive with platelet glycoproteins.

orders, it would indicate that immune mechanisms contribute to the pathogenesis of many more thrombocytopenic disorders that was once thought likely.

It has also been suggested that elevated total PAIgG in both immune and nonimmune thrombocytopenic disorders is the result of IgG incorporation into platelet α granules at the megakaryocyte level and that the elevated total PAIgG reflects the lower mean platelet age of younger platelets, which contain higher amounts of PAIgG.[189,259] However, this proposal does not account for the elevated total PAIgG level seen in some disorders of decreased platelet production, nor does it account for the elevated surface PAIgG seen in nonimmune thrombocytopenic disorders.[232] It is also possible that elevated total PAIgG reflects internalization of antibody or immune complexes that become bound to the platelet surface.[260,261]

Phase III Assays. Although it is unlikely that sensitivity for ITP will be increased by the phase III assays, it is anticipated that specificity for autoimmune thrombocytopenic disorders such as ITP will be increased because a positive test outcome depends on demonstrating the specific interaction of antibody with platelet-specific proteins.

Specific Versus Nonspecific PAIgG in ITP. Platelets from patients with ITP can carry large amounts of IgG on their surfaces, up to hundreds of thousands of molecules of IgG per platelet.[196,232] It remains uncertain what proportion of this IgG represents specifically bound autoantibody and how much represents IgG bound nonspecifically. The proportions of the platelet surface–bound immunoglobulin classes and subclasses resemble their respective plasma concentrations,[217,262,263] which suggests that most of the PAIgG could be nonspecific IgG. It has also been observed that platelet-bound albumin is increased in parallel with PAIgG.[188] A possible explanation for these observations is that the initial binding of autoantibodies to the platelet membrane results in membrane changes promoting the nonspecific adherence of many plasma proteins, including nonspecific IgG and albumin.[196,197] Although the observation of increased platelet-bound albumin on ITP platelets has been confirmed by other groups of investigators,[224,225,255] the explanation remains unknown.

Idiopathic Thrombocytopenic Purpura

Idiopathic thrombocytopenic purpura is a common disorder characterized by autoimmune platelet destruction. ITP is diagnosed by demonstrating an immune destructive thrombocytopenia and excluding other causes. Positive phase III assays may be helpful diagnostically by confirming the autoimmune nature of the disorder.

Pathogenesis and Cause

Idiopathic thrombocytopenic purpura is caused by the binding of autoantibodies to platelet antigens. Thrombocytopenia is a consequence of the premature destruction of the platelets by the reticuloendothelial system.

Platelet-Reactive Autoantibodies. About 40 years ago, Harrington and colleagues[264] performed a series of experiments that defined the basic pathogenesis of ITP. They infused plasma from ITP patients into healthy volunteers and documented the development of acute and severe thrombocytopenia. These dramatic experiments demonstrated that ITP is caused by a plasma factor that results in platelet destruction. Subsequent investigators demonstrated that the plasma factor is usually IgG, although in some patients, IgM and IgA platelet-reactive antibodies were identified.[217,265–267]

In 1972, McMillan and associates[268] showed that lymphocytes from ITP splenic tissue produced antiplatelet autoantibodies. Subsequent investigations from this group demonstrated that antiplatelet antibody binds to platelets through its Fab terminus[241,269] and that the antibody is capable of depositing complement on the platelets.[270] It remains uncertain whether completion of the complement sequence in vivo leads to platelet destruction in ITP patients. β-Thromboglobulin, which is released from activated platelets, is normal in the plasma of ITP patients, arguing against in vivo platelet lysis.[271]

As discussed previously in the section on controversies in platelet antibody testing, it is probable that much of the PAIgG detected on ITP platelets is not autoantibody. Although the explanation for this finding is unknown, it is possible that such nonspecifically bound IgG contributes to the enhanced platelet clearance in ITP.

Platelet Autoantigens. Some of the target platelet autoantigens in ITP patients have been identified. Indirect evidence that autoantibodies could recognize platelet glycoproteins was first provided by Van Leeuwen and colleagues.[272] They showed that antiplatelet antibody from patients with ITP failed to bind to platelets from patients with Glanzmann's thrombasthenia (lacking gpIIb/IIIa). IgG binding to gpIIb-IIIa was proved directly a short time later by two other groups using different phase III assays.[145,146] gpIIb/IIIa is the most frequent target autoantigen, but the gpIb/IX complex also has been implicated in many patients.[118–123] Further work using several different monoclonal antibodies against the gpIIb/IIIa complex has shown that the anti–gpIIb/IIIa autoantibodies from different ITP patients react with different epitopes.[250] Evidence suggests that platelet glycolipids also can be autoantigen targets in chronic ITP.[179–181]

Platelet Kinetics. Initial studies,[273–275] which often employed ^{51}Cr-labeled homologous platelets, suggested that the platelet life-span in ITP patients was uniformly reduced and that platelet turnover was increased. Studies by several groups of investigators[276–280] using ^{111}In-labeled autologous platelets showed considerable heterogeneity in platelet turnover in chronic ITP. Although the platelet life-span is often markedly decreased, in some patients, the life-span is only mildly reduced; furthermore, platelet turnover (a measure of platelet production) is frequently subnormal.[308–313] In one large study,[280] about 40% of ITP patients had a reduced platelet turnover. Low platelet turnover might be the result of megakaryocyte damage by autoantibodies[281] or intramedullary destruction of platelets by marrow monocytes and macrophages. Alternatively, the apparent low platelet turnover could reflect the measurement of a subpopulation of longer-lived platelets.

Both in vitro and clinical studies have shown that the spleen is an important site of antibody production[268,281] and is also the dominant organ for the clearance of IgG-coated platelets.[280,282] In a minority of patients, hepatic clearance predominates.[280]

Cause. The fundamental disturbance leading to autoantibody formation in ITP is not known. Several studies[283–285] investigating HLA phenotypes in patients with ITP have not revealed consistent associations. Several quantitative lymphocyte abnormalities have been reported in chronic ITP, including decreased T4-positive/T8-positive ratios,[286] increased numbers of T4-positive, T8-positive lymphocytes,[287] and increased Ia-positive T-lymphocyte numbers.[288] Decreased T-lymphocyte responsiveness to mitogens and antigens also has been reported.[289,290] These abnormalities might indicate an intrinsic immune regulatory defect in patients with chronic ITP. It is uncertain whether the autoimmune defect occurs de novo or whether an antecedent event (eg, viral infection) is required. Sequence analysis of a human lymphoblastoid cell line VH gene sequences derived from an ITP patient with anti-gpIb IgG identified multiple base substitutions (compared with germline sequence), suggesting that the autoantibodies were generated by antigen-driven, mature B cells.[291]

Clinical and Laboratory Features

Although chronic ITP can occur at any age and in both sexes, women between 20 and 50 years of age are most commonly affected. The female/male ratio is about 3:1.

The onset of bleeding typically is insidious. Recent aspirin ingestion, however, can cause a patient with asymptomatic chronic ITP to bleed. Most of the bleeding is mucocutaneous and consists of purpura (petechiae and ecchymoses), epistaxis, menorrhagia, oral mucosal bleeding, and gastrointestinal bleeding. Rarely, severe thrombocytopenia can be complicated by spontaneous intracranial hemorrhage. Except for the bleeding symptoms, the patients are asymptomatic.

The complete blood count reveals isolated thrombocytopenia, although anemia of iron deficiency can occur with chronic bleeding. The MPV usually is increased, although in our experience, patients with severe thrombocytopenia may have a normal or even reduced MPV. The bone marrow examination shows normal or increased numbers of megakaryocytes. We do not always perform a bone marrow aspirate if the patient presents with typical ITP, but many hematologists routinely perform a marrow examination in this clinical situation.

The bleeding time tends to be long if there is marked thrombocytopenia (below 20×10^9/L),[292] although some patients have abnormal platelet function and a prolonged bleeding time despite mild or moderate thrombocytopenia (50 to 150×10^9/L).[293]

Many patients with otherwise typical ITP have positive antinuclear antibody (ANA) tests,[294–298] usually of low titer. It is controversial whether the presence of a high-titer ANA or antibodies against soluble ribonucleoprotein antigens (SS-A/Ro, nuclear RNP) help to identify the minority of ITP patients who subsequently develop SLE.[295–297] It is also uncertain whether the prognosis for ANA-positive ITP patients differs from that for those who lack this antibody. Other laboratory tests that should be performed in ITP patients include thyroid function studies because of the association between ITP and immune thyroid dysfunction. Patients with clinical evidence suggesting infectious mononucleosis or HIV infection should have the appropriate serologic tests performed.

Cyclic Thrombocytopenia. Cyclic thrombocytopenia is characterized by regular fluctuations in the platelet count, ranging from severe, symptomatic thrombocytopenia to thrombocytosis. In some women with cyclic thrombocytopenia, platelet count fluctuations parallel the menstrual cycle, with the platelet count nadir coinciding with menstruation.[299] Intermittent increased platelet destruction by platelet-reactive autoantibodies may be causative in some instances,[299,300] with the platelet count variability attributable to fluctuations either in levels of platelet-reactive autoantibody[300] or in reticuloendothelial function.[299] In other reports, normal platelet survival and reduced megakaryocyte numbers[301,302] and evolution to persisting amegakaryocytic thrombocytopenia[303] suggest a disorder of platelet production.

Overview of Treatment

The principles of treatment of ITP in adults are predicated on the following characteristics of the disorder:

1. Most patients with immune thrombocytopenia have hyperfunctional platelets associated with an increased MPV.[292,304] Thus, many patients do not need treatment despite moderate or even severe thrombocytopenia.
2. The goal of treatment is to achieve a safe platelet count, not necessarily a normal platelet count. In the absence of bleeding symptoms, a bleeding-time test may be helpful in determining whether treatment is required.
3. Most adults have chronic ITP. Therefore, the long-term risks of treatment must be balanced against the long-term risk of life-threatening bleeding in patients with chronic hemostatic impairment. Most adult patients are not cured by prednisone. Splenectomy is the preferred treatment of adults with chronic ITP because it offers the best chance for a cure of the thrombocytopenia and avoids the toxicity of medical therapies.
4. About 10% to 15% of patients fail corticosteroid therapy and splenectomy, and for them, the treatment options are less satisfactory. It is important to exclude an accessory spleen in these patients. Many treatments have been used, including danazol, vinca alkaloids, cyclophosphamide, azathioprine, intravenous Ig, Rh immune globulin (anti-D), and plasmapheresis.

5. Patients should avoid drugs that interfere with platelet function, particularly aspirin, other nonsteroidal antiinflammatory agents, and alcohol.[305,306]

Corticosteroids

Mechanism of Action. Corticosteroids increase platelet life-span in ITP,[307] possibly by inhibiting both phagocytic activity[282,308] and autoantibody synthesis.[309] Reduction or disappearance of anti-gpIIb/IIIa antibodies has been shown in patients who respond clinically to corticosteroids.[310] Investigators[311] employing ^{111}In-labeled autologous platelet survival studies concluded that corticosteroids improve marrow platelet production, possibly by inhibiting intramedullary platelet destruction by marrow phagocytic cells. Corticosteroids also reduce capillary leaks, an observation that could explain the reduction in bleeding symptoms that sometimes precedes the rise in the platelet count.[312]

Dosage. Prednisone is usually given at an initial dose of 1 to 1.5 mg/kg/d. As soon as the platelet count has risen to safe levels (judged clinically, but usually a minimum of 50 × 10^9/L), the prednisone is tapered over a few weeks. We administer prednisone on alternate days during tapering to minimize side effects. The prednisone should not be continued in large doses for more than 4 weeks in nonresponders because delayed response is unlikely and the risk of adverse effects increases.

Two prospective trials[294,313] compared standard with lower doses of prednisone as induction therapy for acute ITP (1 versus 0.25 mg/kg/d, and 1.5 versus 0.5 mg/kg/d). There was no difference in the likelihood of remission at 6 months follow-up in either study. The larger study, however, observed a trend toward an increased frequency of complete remission (46% versus 35%) in the group given the larger dose of prednisone. Moreover, a faster rise in the platelet count was observed in the group receiving the larger dose of prednisone (77% versus 51% having a platelet count above 50 × 10^9/L after 14 days of prednisone).[313]

Very large doses of corticosteroids ("pulse" methylprednisolone) have been reported to raise the platelet count rapidly in adults with ITP.[314,315] Controlled comparative trials with standard-dose prednisone have not been described.

Results of Treatment. ITP in adults is usually a chronic disorder. Most patients have a relapse of the thrombocytopenia as the prednisone dose is decreased or during subsequent follow-up observation. Hence, response to prednisone therapy must be related to length of follow-up.

Initial Response. About two-thirds of patients attain a safe platelet count (minimum, 50 × 10^9/L) while receiving corticosteroids, and most achieve a high platelet count (above 100 to 150 × 10^9/L).[294,313,316–319]

Early Follow-up. Several studies[294,313,316–318,320–322] provide information about the likelihood of remission after discontinuation of corticosteroids. The number of patients in complete remission (platelet count greater than 150 × 10^9/L) after discontinuation of prednisone therapy is about 30%. An additional 20% of patients are in partial remission (platelet count 50 to 150 × 10^9/L). Thus, about half of patients who receive corticosteroids have a safe platelet count after discontinuation of corticosteroid therapy during a relatively brief follow-up period (several months).

Patients with a shorter duration of bleeding symptoms are more likely to respond favorably.[317,318,321,322] In one study,[322] 94 of 241 (39%) ITP patients who had symptoms for 6 months or less attained a complete remission, compared with only 19 of 132 (14%) patients who were symptomatic for longer than 6 months. For patients who relapse after an initial complete remission, a repeat course of prednisone can be effective.[321]

Late Follow-up. Studies[317,319,321] describing longer follow-up (minimum, 2 years for all patients) indicate that there is continuing risk of relapse in adult patients after initial complete remission with corticosteroid therapy. In one study,[321] only 29% of adult patients who had a complete remission remained in remission at 4 years. In summary, only about 10% to 15% of all adult ITP patients who receive prednisone therapy have a durable remission. Consequently, most require either further medical therapy or splenectomy.

Adverse Effects. Two studies[318,322] described the frequency of complications of corticosteroid therapy given to adult patients with ITP. Common adverse effects (5% to 20% of patients treated) included cushingoid facies, weight gain, nonspecific abdominal symptoms, and acne. Less common (1% to 5%) but important complications included infection, myopathy, diabetes, psychosis, hypertension, and hypokalemia. Osteonecrosis, usually affecting the hips or shoulders, occurs in about 5% of patients receiving prolonged corticosteroid treatment, although some patients experience this serious complication after intensive, short-term treatment.[323]

Splenectomy

Mechanism of Action. Splenectomy is frequently successful because in most patients, the spleen is both the major site of autoantibody production and platelet destruction.[268] Platelet survival studies indicate improved platelet life-span after splenectomy.[311]

Perioperative Management. All patients should receive polyvalent pneumococcal and meningococcal vaccines at least 2 weeks before surgery.[324,325] *Haemophilus influenzae* type b vaccination should be given to children, and some physicians also recommend this vaccine for adults.[324,325] Because most patients who undergo splenectomy have been treated previously with prednisone, perioperative administration of parenteral corticosteroids is usually advised.

Adequate hemostasis usually can be obtained by raising the platelet count perioperatively with corticosteroids, high-dose intravenous γ-globulin, or Rh immune globulin. Despite these maneuvers, many patients are thrombocytopenic at the time of splenectomy; however, most do not have excess bleeding. Accordingly, platelet transfusions should not be given prophylactically but should be reserved for those patients with intraoperative bleeding. In one study in which platelets were administered only to patients with "marked oozing" at the end of the procedure,[319] only 10 of 55 (18%) patients required platelet transfusions.

Because thromboembolic complications have been described in these patients after splenectomy,[326–329] we administer prophylactic antithrombotic treatment with heparin as the platelet count rises to normal level, if the patient remains immobilized.

Results of Treatment. About 75% of patients enter a complete remission within 4 to 6 weeks after splenectomy.[319,322–331] In the complete responders, normal platelet counts are reached within 7 days in 90% of patients and within 6 weeks in 98%[330]; spontaneous remission rarely occurs thereafter.[331]

A partial remission is achieved for about 5% to 10% of patients,[319,322,326,329] and these patients are asymptomatic. Of the remaining nonresponders, some benefit from low doses of prednisone.

Certain features are associated with a higher probability of response to splenectomy. These include a prior response to corticosteroids[328,332,333] and younger age.[321,327,328,331,334] Some investigators have reported that a predominant splenic clearance of platelets, as shown by radionuclide platelet imaging techniques[311,326,329,331] or normal to increased platelet turnover,[280] also predicts a good response to splenectomy; however, not all investigators have reached these conclusions.[278,280,311,335] Measurement of PAIgG levels does not predict response to splenectomy.[280,327,331,334] In contrast to results of corticosteroid therapy, patients with a longer duration of thrombocytopenia are not less likely to respond to splenectomy.[322]

The risk for a relapse of thrombocytopenia after complete remission postsplenectomy is low (about 10% to 15% at 10 years).[329,331]

Accessory Spleens. It is important to search for an accessory spleen both at surgery and in patients who relapse after splenectomy. Accessory spleens are identified at the time of primary splenectomy in about 20% of patients.[327,330,333] A history that suggests the possibility of an accessory spleen is one in which the patient has an initial response to splenectomy that is later followed by a relapse of the ITP. About 40% to 50% of these patients have a residual accessory spleen, demonstrated with sensitive imaging techniques.[321,336,337] About 65% of these patients achieve complete remission after removal of the accessory spleen.[321,327,336,337]

It is less certain whether residual accessory splenic tissue accounts for *early* postsplenectomy failure (ie, persisting or recurrent thrombocytopenia within 6 weeks after splenectomy). In this situation, children often do not respond to the removal of the accessory splenic tissue.[338] The results are better for adults; early splenectomy failures can achieve complete remission after removal of an accessory spleen.[327,337]

A number of methods can be used to look for an accessory spleen. The presence of typical postsplenectomy changes in the blood film (eg, Howell-Jolly bodies) does not rule out the possibility of an accessory spleen.[321,337] CT scan, ultrasound, and radionuclide imaging methods have been used successfully. The radionuclide methods include ^{99m}Tc sulfur colloid scans, ^{111}In platelet localization studies, and radiolabeled heat-aggregated RBC studies. We look for accessory splenic tissue by nuclear imaging during the performance of a platelet survival study using ^{111}In. The intraoperative use of a hand-held isotope detector probe can help locate an accessory spleen during surgery.[327]

Adverse Effects. Perioperative mortality is less than 1%, with most deaths due to thromboembolic complications.[319,322–330] Morbidity is under 10%, and the most frequent complications are pleuropulmonary (pneumonia, subphrenic abscess, pleural effusion in 4%), followed by major bleeding in 1.5% and thromboembolic complications in 1%.[319,322–330]

No late deaths due to overwhelming bacterial septicemia occurred in any of these studies. In one study[340] of 256 adults who underwent splenectomy for a variety of indications, however, 2.7% died of fulminant septicemia (mean follow-up, almost 4 years). This study was completed before vaccination against pneumococcus became routine. In addition, the risk may be lower in patients undergoing splenectomy for ITP.

Second-Line Therapy

About 10% to 15% of patients with ITP cannot be controlled by corticosteroid therapy and splenectomy. The large number of therapies that have been used for these treatment failures attests to the difficulty in managing this patient group.

Danazol

Mechanism of Action. Danazol is an attenuated androgen with mild virilizing effects, which can be used in men and nonpregnant women. It is possible that danazol works by counteracting the effects of estrogens on phagocytic cells. Estrogens increase Fc receptor numbers and increase the rate of clearance of IgG-sensitized RBCs,[341] while danazol reduces the number of phagocytic cell Fc receptors.[342] Danazol also corrects the abnormal T-cell subpopulations found in patients with ITP.[343]

Dosage. Usually 300 to 900 mg are administered daily, although a report described effectiveness using low doses (50 mg).[344] Response is usually seen within 2 months, although it may take up to 6 months when low doses are used.[344]

Results of Treatment. Danazol has been used in over 100 adult patients with refractory chronic ITP.[342–355] Pooling these studies, danazol—when used in standard doses for a minimum of 2 months—produces a sustained increase in the platelet count above 100×10^9/L in 30% of patients. An additional 10% of patients have a rise in platelet count to 50 to 100×10^9/L. Three of these trials[346,350,353] had essentially negative results, with sustained benefit demonstrated in less than 10% of patients. One study[355] suggested that older women were most likely to respond to treatment. Often, the danazol must be continued to maintain the platelet count, although the clinician periodically should attempt to reduce the dose.

Adverse Effects. Danazol is generally well tolerated. The most frequent adverse effects are fluid retention, persistent nausea, oligo- and amenorrhea, headache, and hepatitis.[345,347,348,350–355] Rarely encountered side effects include peliosis of liver and spleen,[356,357] increased fibrinolysis,[351,358] and mild virilization. Concerns about fetal damage precludes the use of danazol during pregnancy.[359,360] Rarely, idiosyncratic thrombocytopenia has been described.[361,362]

Vinca Alkaloids

Mechanism of Action. The mechanism of action of vinca alkaloids is uncertain, but it could be related to inhibition of phagocytic cell function. The vinca alkaloids (vincristine and vinblastine) bind to platelet microtubules,[363] which theoretically could help localize the drugs to the platelet-destroying phagocytic cells.

Dosage and Methods of Administration. In adults, the usual dose of vincristine is 1 to 2 mg, and for vinblastine it is 5 to 10 mg. The treatment can be repeated at 5- to 10-day intervals until response or toxicity is encountered. No more than three doses should be given if a response is not seen because subsequent benefit is unlikely and side effects become increasingly problematic.

Usually, the vinca alkaloids are given by rapid intravenous infusion; however, different methods have been used in an attempt to increase delivery to the phagocytic cells. One method consists of administering the vinca alkaloids by slow infusion (over 4 to 8 hours).[364–369] Another method whereby platelets are incubated in vinblastine or vincristine ("vinca-loaded" platelets)[363,365,370] is seldom used because of toxicity and a lack of evidence of superior efficacy.[371,372]

Results of Treatment. The use of vincristine in ITP was first reported in 1974.[373] Several studies[373–378] described the efficacy of vincristine in eight or more patients. Summarizing these studies, about 65% of patients respond to treatment with a rise in the platelet count to greater than 50×10^9/L. In about half of responders, the platelet count entered the normal range. Only a few patients, however, had a sustained remission,[373,375,377] and most required maintenance injections. In one study,[322] none of 19 patients who received vincristine for refractory, chronic ITP had a sustained remission. Concomitant treatment with azathioprine may increase the likelihood of long-term response to vincristine.[378,379]

In 1984, Ahn and colleagues[364] reported the use of vincristine or vinblastine given by slow infusion for chronic ITP. The platelet count rose to greater than $50 \times 10^9/L$ in 17 of 26 patients (65%), and sustained responses (minimum, 2 years) were seen in 6 patients. Three other groups subsequently reported their results with slow infusions of vincristine[366,368] or vinblastine.[367] Summarizing the results of these three studies in patients with chronic ITP, response was seen in 67% of patients, but sustained complete remission (greater than 6-months duration) was seen in only 2 of 21 patients. A randomized trial did not show greater benefit giving vinblastine by slow, rather than rapid, infusion.[369]

Three studies[366–368] reported the response of adult patients with acute ITP (duration less than 6 months) to slow infusion of vinca alkaloids. All 13 patients responded favorably to treatment, and 10 continued in sustained complete remission during a median follow-up of 6 months (range, 2 to 29 months).

Adverse Effects. Peripheral neuropathy is a common complication of vincristine or vinblastine. Leukopenia and alopecia can complicate vinblastine therapy.[364] Fever can occur after repeated injections of vinca by slow infusion.[364] Vinca alkaloids are not leukemogenic.

Cyclophosphamide and Azathioprine

Mechanism of Action. Cyclophosphamide and azathioprine are considered together in this section because of their similar immunosuppressive activity, clinical efficacy, and toxicities. Cyclophosphamide is an alkylating agent, whereas azathioprine is metabolized to 6-mercaptopurine, a purine antimetabolite.

Dosage. The usual dosage of both azathioprine and cyclophosphamide is between 50 and 200 mg/d, with the dose reduced if the patient becomes leukopenic. It usually takes a minimum of 2 to 4 weeks before response to either agent occurs, and sometimes 3 to 6 months of treatment must be given before a response is seen. Cyclophosphamide has also been given by intermittent bolus.[380]

Results of Treatment. In 1976, Caplan and Berkman[381] reviewed 28 published reports on the use of immunosuppressive treatments for ITP. Overall, 33% of patients had complete remission after treatment with cyclophosphamide and 21% after treatment with azathioprine. Including patients who had partial benefit from these treatments, about two thirds of all patients responded to cyclophosphamide or azathioprine. Subsequently, the results of a large, multicenter study were reported.[322] Sustained complete remissions occurred in about 20% of the patients receiving cyclophosphamide or azathioprine.[322] Including lesser responses (temporary complete remission, partial remission), between 50% and 60% of patients benefited from these agents.[322]

Adverse Effects. Toxicities from these drugs are considerable. The most important side effects include leukemogenesis (cyclophosphamide, azathioprine), hemorrhagic cystitis (cyclophosphamide), and marrow suppression (cyclophosphamide, azathioprine). Cases of acute leukemia after the use of cyclophosphamide for ITP have been described[382] but are rare.

High-Dose Intravenous Immunoglobulin G

Large doses of intravenous IgG (IVIgG) have been used to treat ITP since 1981.[383] IVIgG is prepared by ethanol precipitation of pooled plasma, followed by techniques to minimize IgG self-aggregation.[384] Immune serum globulin cannot be given by the intravenous route because of severe adverse reactions, including anaphylactoid reactions, caused by the large amounts of IgG aggregates within the preparation.[385]

At least 90% to 95% of the IV IgG preparation is composed of monomeric IgG. The IgG retains normal Fab and Fc functions required for antigen binding and phagocytic cell interaction, respectively. IgG aggregates, IgA, and other contaminants constitute a negligible fraction. IVIgG has a normal IgG half-life in vivo, with a physiologic subclass distribution.[384]

Mechanism of Action. A number of models have been proposed to explain the efficacy of IVIgG in ITP.[386–390] The two most widely accepted explanations are impairment of phagocytic cell function and suppression of autoantibody synthesis.

Most clinicians think that IVIgG works by reticuloendothelial cell blockade ("medical splenectomy"; Fig 34-11). The usual total dose of IVIgG (2 g/kg) raises the serum IgG concentration by two- to four-fold, a level that has been shown to block the clearance of radiolabeled, IgG-sensitized RBCs.[391,392] Consistent with this view is the observation that disease-related polyclonal hypergammaglobulinemia also is associated with impaired reticuloendothelial cell function.[393] We believe that the monomeric IgG is in equilibrium with the Fc receptor on the phagocytic cells. Even though the binding affinity of Fc receptors for monomeric IgG is low, the high plasma concentration of IgG results in these receptors being occupied.[393] It is possible that minor amounts of contaminating Ig aggregates could contribute to phagocytic cell receptor blockade.[389] One group[390] has proposed that phagocytic cell inhibition is related to anti-HLA antibodies contained within the Ig preparations.

The phagocytic cell blockade theory, however, cannot explain the occasional long-term responses that follow treatment with IVIgG, nor the observation that Fc-depleted preparations sometimes are effective in ITP.[394,395] Thus, immune suppression has been invoked as a mechanism of action. In support of this concept is the observation that PAIgG and anti-gpIIb/IIIa levels decline after successful treatment with IVIgG.[310,396] The immune suppression could be related to nonspecific effects of large amounts of IgG to reduce antibody synthesis, or by specific interaction of certain IgG molecules within the IVIgG preparation with the pathogenic autoantibodies (antiidiotype interactions), thereby blocking autoantibody binding to platelets.[397–399] Alterations in lymphocyte subpopulations and reductions in mitogen-stimulated Ig synthesis occur following IVIgG treatment.[400–402]

Dosage and Preparations. The usual dose of IVIgG is 2 g/kg given over 2 to 5 days (1 g/kg for 2 days, or 0.4 g/kg for 5 days). The 2-day regimen is becoming increasingly popular. To minimize side effects, the infusion is given over 6 to 8 hours. Three preparations are available in the United States: Gamimune-N (Cutter Laboratories, Berkeley, CA), Gammagard (Hyland-Travenol, Glendale, CA), and Sandoglobulin (Sandoz Inc, East Hanover, NJ). There is no evidence that any one of these products offers a major advantage over the others.[384]

Results of Treatment. The administration of IVIgG to adults with chronic ITP raises the platelet count above $50 \times 10^9/L$ in about 80% of patients. In more than half of responders, the platelet count becomes normal.[384,403] Unfortunately, the response is usually transient. The platelet count begins to rise within 1 to 3 days of commencing treatment, peaking at 5 to 10 days, and returning to baseline level by 2 to 6 weeks.

Although long-lasting complete remissions in adults with chronic ITP are rare after IVIgG, a report notes that repeated treatment with IVIgG (maintenance therapy) sometimes is associated with complete or partial remission. Bussel and

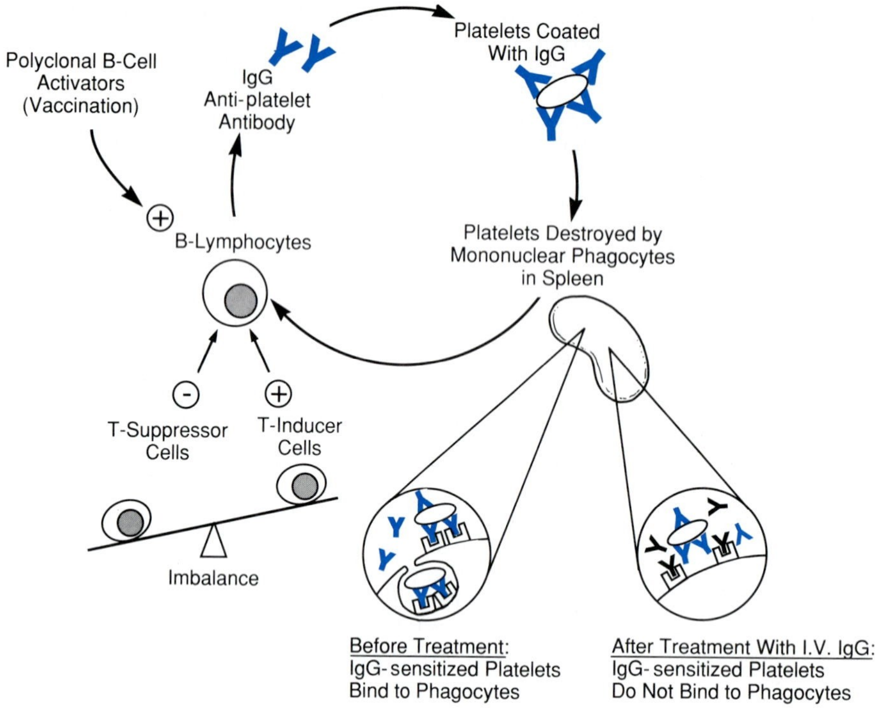

FIGURE 34-11. Schematic representation of one mechanism of action of high-dose intravenous immunoglobulin (IVIgG): occupancy of macrophage Fc receptors by IgG.

associates[404] treated 40 adult patients with chronic ITP with repeated courses of IVIgG. Five patients entered a complete remission, and 11 were classified as "stable without therapy," defined as persisting thrombocytopenia that is asymptomatic or with minor bruising. Thirteen patients required continued maintenance treatment, and the remaining 11 patients became refractory to treatment.

Adverse Effects. IVIgG is remarkable for its safety. Side effects are infrequent and usually mild.[384] Most common are headache, local phlebitis, flushing, and fever at a frequency of 3% to 20%. These symptoms are controlled by briefly stopping or reducing the rate of infusion. Chest pain, hypertension, hypotension, bronchospasm, and laryngeal edema have been described[405] but are uncommon. These adverse reactions occur with increased frequency in patients with congenital IgA deficiency.

Rare side effects include overwhelming septicemia, hemolysis due to ABO hemolysins contained within the IVIgG,[406] acute cryoglobulinemic nephropathy in rheumatoid factor–positive recipients,[407] and fatal thrombotic events in elderly patients.[408]

Because IVIgG is prepared from the pooled plasma of thousands of donors, there is potential risk of infection, but the risk is extremely low.[409,410] Transmission of HIV has not been documented, but several cases of non-A, non-B hepatitis have followed the administration of certain lots of IVIgG.[411–414]

Other Uses. Although IVIgG is seldom used as a maintenance therapy for adults with chronic ITP, it is used more frequently in other clinical situations involving immune thrombocytopenic disorders (Table 34-1). These are discussed later in this chapter.

Rh Immune Globulin

Mechanism of Action. Rh immune globulin (anti-D) has been used to treat Rh(D)-positive ITP patients.[415,416] The mechanism of action probably is by means of phagocytic cell blockade due to occupancy of the phagocytic cell Fc receptors by the IgG-sensitized RBCs. This prevents the platelets from binding to these receptors. Since a 100-μg dose of anti-D contains only 5 to 200 mg of additional nonspecific IgG,[417,418] there is not enough IgG to invoke phagocytic cell blockade by monomeric IgG as with IVIgG. Furthermore, anti-D is not effective in Rh(D)-negative patients, although plasma containing high-titer anti-c has been shown to be effective in patients carrying this antigen.[419]

Dosage. The probability of response increases with the dose administered.[420] Successful doses have ranged from 100 μg given as a single intravenous dose (insufficient to cause a positive direct antiglobulin test)[420] to almost 20 mg administered over 14 days.[421] Usually, 25 to 75 μg/kg (total dose) given in divided doses over 2 to 5 days is used.[419,422–425] The most common regimen is to administer 25 μg/kg of anti-D intravenously and repeat the same dose 2 days later if no or minimal response is evident.[425] Anti-D can be given safely by intravenous injection over a few minutes. Some groups administer RBCs that have been sensitized with anti-D in vitro.[426,427] Patients who respond to anti-D often can be maintained with small intermittent maintenance doses of anti-D.[424]

Results of Treatment. The frequency of response using optimal, individualized doses of anti-D is similar to that using IVIgG and, like IVIgG, the increase in the platelet count usually is transient (2 to 6 weeks).[419,422–425] Occasional long-term responses can occur.[420,426,428] Compared with IVIgG, the peak platelet count tends to be lower, and the time to reach the peak platelet count often is longer. Therefore, a greater interval between maintenance injections may be possible using anti-D. Some patients who fail to respond to IVIgG can still benefit from anti-D, and vice versa; however, patients who have undergone splenectomies have a lower probability of response to anti-D.[425]

Adverse Effects. A positive, direct antiglobulin test and laboratory evidence of hemolysis are present in most patients.[416,423] The decline in hemoglobin ranges from 0 to 20 g/L, and most patients do not have to discontinue treatment because of anemia. Response to treatment does not correlate with the degree of hemolysis.[423]

Other Treatments

α-Interferon,[429] cyclosporine,[430–432] colchicine,[433,434] plasma perfusion over staphylococcal protein A columns,[435,436]

TABLE 34-1. Indications for the Use of Intravenous Immunoglobulin in Patients With Immune Thrombocytopenia

DEFINITE INDICATIONS	
Immune thrombocytopenia at risk for life-threatening bleeding*	
ITP	
Secondary ITP (collagen disease, neoplasia, HIV infection)	
Drug-induced immune thrombocytopenia	
Posttransfusion purpura	
Neonatal alloimmune thrombocytopenia	
Neonatal passive autoimmune thrombocytopenia	
Preparation for urgent surgery in patients with immune thrombocytopenia	
Acute ITP of childhood	
POSSIBLE INDICATIONS	
Chronic ITP of childhood to avoid splenectomy, or for refractory disease	
Pregnant women with a history of an infant affected by neonatal alloimmune thrombocytopenia or with a fetus proved to have in utero alloimmune thrombocytopenia	
Pregnant women with ITP not controlled adequately by low doses of corticosteroids	
UNCERTAIN INDICATIONS	
Maintenance therapy for chronic ITP in adults	
Maintenance therapy for chronic secondary immune thrombocytopenia (eg, HIV-associated thrombocytopenia)	
NOT INDICATED	
Treatment of refractoriness to platelet transfusions	

ITP, idiopathic thrombocytopenic purpura; HIV, human immunodeficiency virus.

* For patients with the indications listed in this category, use of intravenous immunoglobulin should be reserved for those patients with symptoms or signs of hemostatic dysfunction, or in whom the risk of progressive thrombocytopenia (eg, neonatal alloimmune thrombocytopenia) is high.

combination chemotherapy,[437] and repeated courses of high-dose dexamethasone[438] have been used in refractory ITP, but experience is minimal.

Elderly and High-Risk Patients

Elderly patients may have a lower probability of benefit from splenectomy.[327,331] Particularly in poor surgical candidates, we[439] have used splenic irradiation rather than splenectomy for some patients. Evidence suggests that danazol may be more effective in older patients than in younger female patients,[355] and we sometimes try danazol before splenectomy. Dapsone produces oxidant hemolysis and has been used to treat ITP in elderly patients who have not had splenectomies,[440] in whom it may work by blocking phagocytic cell function nonimmunologically.

Emergency Treatment of a Bleeding Patient

IVIgG and Platelet Transfusions. It is uncommon for ITP patients to develop life-threatening bleeding. These patients should immediately receive platelet transfusions (10 to 20 units). The patient then should receive IVIgG, 1 g/kg over 6 to 8 hours, to block the phagocytic system. Some clinicians also administer high doses of corticosteroids. The IVIgG should be followed by further platelet transfusions. This approach almost always raises the platelet count.[441] Other treatments to achieve longer-term control of the thrombocytopenia should be commenced simultaneously.

Routine Platelet Transfusions. Platelet transfusions in ITP patients often produce a transient rise in the platelet count.[442] Consequently, although platelet transfusions are acceptable in certain clinical situations, such as life-threatening or perioperative bleeding, they are not indicated prophylactically. This is because the hazards of platelet transfusion (eg, risk of alloimmunization and non-A, non-B hepatitis) outweigh the benefits of a short-lived increase in the platelet count in a chronic disorder.

Plasmapheresis. Plasma exchange has been used successfully in some adult patients with severe acute or chronic ITP.[443,444] In some patients with acute ITP, long-lasting remissions have been obtained, and splenectomy could be avoided; however, it is possible that the remission was unrelated to the plasma exchange. In chronic ITP, the response is almost always transient.

Some investigators have reported the use of plasma exchange as an emergency maneuver for bleeding ITP patients, but we believe that equal or better efficacy can be achieved more rapidly in most patients by administering IVIgG. Plasmapheresis alone or in conjunction with IVIgG can be effective in patients refractory to IVIgG alone.[445,446]

Monoclonal Antibody Against Fcγ Receptor. A murine monoclonal antibody with specificity for monocyte and macrophage Fc receptors that can block the reticuloendothelial system has been used in patients with severe, refractory ITP.[447,448] Unfortunately, because the monoclonal antibody is murine, it cannot be given repeatedly. This approach must be considered experimental.

Idiopathic Thrombocytopenic Purpura in Pregnancy

Overview. ITP in pregnancy is a common clinical event. Our understanding of this disorder and its impact on both mother and fetus has changed dramatically over the past several years. Previously, it was estimated that a large proportion of mothers with ITP in pregnancy and their neonates would have serious bleeding.[449] This led to recommendations for cesarean section delivery for all thrombocytopenic mothers. This approach is flawed in several ways. First, no study has demonstrated that delivery by cesarean section represents a reduced risk for the fetus compared with a vaginal delivery. Second, although many neonates with passively acquired antiplatelet autoantibodies are thrombocytopenic at birth, severe thrombocytopenia and morbidity are uncommon.[450–453] Third, some women with thrombocytopenia detected incidentally during pregnancy—a common clinical event that is not associated with an increased risk of neonatal thrombocytopenia or bleeding,[81,82,84]—might also undergo unnecessary intervention.

The risk of neonatal hemorrhage has been overestimated by case reports and small patient series. Reviewing the largest 11 informative studies (288 neonates),[451] the risk of a platelet count (umbilical cord sample taken at birth) below $50 \times 10^9/L$ was only 10%, and below $20 \times 10^9/L$, it was about 4%. No neonatal deaths or intracranial hemorrhage occurred in these 11 reports.

Management. Many pregnant ITP patients do not require specific treatment. We treat the mother if the platelet count falls to low levels (less than 20 to $50 \times 10^9/L$) or if the patient has evidence of a hemostatic defect. Treatment includes corticosteroids, which should be avoided during the first trimester because of teratogenicity, or IVIgG. IVIgG seldom produces a long-lasting remission in a patient with ITP, but we believe it is indicated for the management of a relatively short-term event such as pregnancy. At the time of delivery, we are cautious not to subject the patient to a potentially dangerous hemostatic insult, such as an epidural analgesic. If the patient has received corticosteroids, the dose is boosted. Otherwise, no special steps are taken.

The other patient who must be managed is the fetus. Unfortunately, the fetal platelet count cannot easily be obtained until delivery. A number of maneuvers have been suggested to manage these patients:

Prediction of neonatal thrombocytopenia. The maternal platelet count cannot be used to predict which infants will be thrombocytopenic.[454] Indeed, women cured of ITP by splenectomy can have thrombocytopenic babies. It is possible that ITP mothers who have had a previous thrombocytopenic infant are at higher risk for subsequent similar outcomes. Although both elevated maternal PAIgG[450] and serum platelet-bindable IgG[455,456] are correlated with increased risk of thrombocytopenia in the neonate, the predictive value of these tests is too low to allow a role in the management of pregnant ITP patients.

Antepartum maneuvers to raise the fetal platelet count. One study[457] suggested that the administration of low doses of corticosteroids (20 mg/d) to ITP mothers results in their infants having a higher platelet count. Although this is a simple therapy, it has not yet been confirmed by other investigators, and its precise usefulness is uncertain.

Several investigators have proposed that, by giving IVIgG to pregnant ITP patients, their infants will not be severely affected.[458–461] It is possible that the administration of IVIgG to the mother could block the transplacental passage of pathogenic autoantibodies, or that the fetal reticuloendothelial system could be blocked by the IgG that enters the fetal circulation.[462] We do not think this approach is justified as a prenatal treatment for the infants because most infants born to these mothers are not thrombocytopenic, nor do they often suffer morbidity as a result of the thrombocytopenia.

Determination of the fetal platelet count by fetal cord sampling (cordocentesis). It is possible to measure the platelet count in the fetus by sampling umbilical vein blood under ultrasound guidance.[463,464] Since this procedure has risks of fetal morbidity and mortality, however, we do not think it is justified.

Determination of the fetal platelet count by fetal scalp sampling. Several years ago, fetal scalp platelet count measurements were advocated.[465,466] The fetal scalp platelet count is obtained after the fetal head is engaged and after a spontaneous or an elective rupture of the membranes. The scalp is wiped clean and a small incision is made using a lancet. A sample of fetal scalp blood is collected and the count is determined using phase microscopy or a particle counter or by examining a stained blood film. We used this approach on a number of patients but found that it frequently fails for technical reasons, and a falsely low platelet count is obtained that results in an unnecessary cesarean section. We no longer use this test in ITP patients.

Recommended Approach. We follow pregnant ITP patients with platelet counts every 1 to 2 weeks. We also screen these mothers for the presence of a lupus anticoagulant because this abnormality may be an indication for treatment with corticosteroids and aspirin.[467] If treatment for the thrombocytopenia is indicated, we start prednisone after the third month of gestation. If a safe platelet count can be maintained by a low dose of prednisone (20 mg/d), the treatment can be continued for the duration of the pregnancy. Larger doses of corticosteroids place the mother at risk for complications, including hypertension. If prednisone is contraindicated, or if the patient cannot be maintained on low doses of corticosteroids, we administer IVIgG to maintain the patient at a safe platelet count.

The optimal management of the infant remains uncertain. It is becoming increasingly clear that, except for mothers with lupus anticoagulant, the actual risk to the infant is low.[450,451] If the mother has had previous uncomplicated deliveries and the obstetrician anticipates no problems, we recommend a spontaneous vaginal delivery. Infants for whom a difficult delivery is anticipated may be delivered by cesarean section, but there is no evidence that this approach reduces the risk of bleeding.

The platelet count of the newborn infant with passive autoimmune thrombocytopenia falls after delivery and reaches a nadir within 2 to 5 days.[450] Therefore, daily platelet counts should be obtained in these neonates.

For infants who develop significant thrombocytopenia (less than 50×10^9/L), treatment with IVIgG, sometimes combined with corticosteroids or platelet transfusions, raises the platelet count.[468]

Acute Idiopathic Thrombocytopenic Purpura of Childhood

Acute ITP is a relatively common disorder, with an annual incidence of about 1 in 10,000 children. The peak incidence occurs between 2 and 6 years of age, with boys and girls affected equally. About 80% of the children with acute ITP recover completely, usually within 6 months.[469] The remainder, who have persistent thrombocytopenia, have chronic ITP, a disorder that probably differs in cause and pathogenesis.

Pathogenesis and Cause

Immune mechanisms are responsible for acute ITP of childhood. Although initial work[469,470] using phase I assays suggested that children with ITP differed from adults by having negative assays for serum platelet-bindable IgG, studies[471,472] employing phase II assays demonstrated circulating antiplatelet antibodies in at least half of children with acute ITP. Furthermore, phase II assays detect elevated platelet-associated Ig in at least 85% of children.[471,473–475] In some children, only platelet-associated IgM is found.[471] Some,[473,474] but not other,[475] investigators reported higher levels of PAIgG in patients with acute compared with chronic ITP. PAIgG levels return to normal after resolution of thrombocytopenia and remain normal.[474]

The cause of increased IgG binding to platelets is uncertain. Since acute ITP often follows viral infections, the thrombocytopenia could be related to adsorption of virus to platelets, deposition of virus-containing immune complexes onto platelets, or exposure of cryptic autoantigens on virus-damaged platelets. Thrombocytopenia often occurs weeks after infection, however, when viremia is no longer apparent. Furthermore, the high incidence of elevated PAIgG and PAIgM, as well as the antiplatelet reactivity of Ig eluted from platelets,[471,476] is consistent with an autoimmune process, perhaps resulting from an aberrant immune response to a viral trigger. Evidence implicating autoantibodies against the gpIIb/IIIa complex and gpIb in acute ITP has been presented.[472,476]

Clinical and Laboratory Features

The typical clinical presentation of acute ITP is the abrupt onset of bleeding and bruising in a healthy child weeks after a viral infection. Physical examination usually reveals purpura in the absence of lymphadenopathy or organomegaly. Mortality, which is less than 0.5%, usually is due to intracranial hemorrhage.

Laboratory features include thrombocytopenia with elevated MPV and normal RBC and leukocyte counts. The thrombocytopenia usually is severe, and the platelet count can be less than $10 \times 10^9/L$. Many pediatricians perform a bone marrow aspiration.[477] This test, however, is seldom helpful diagnostically and more frequently is performed to reassure the physician and parents. Bone marrow examination reveals normal or increased numbers of megakaryocytes in ITP. Sometimes, morphologically distinct lymphoid cells, originally termed *hematogones*, constitute up to half of the marrow cells and may cause confusion with acute leukemia.[478] These nonneoplastic cells are characterized by scant, agranular cytoplasm; homogeneous, condensed nuclei lacking nucleoli; and the surface immunophenotypic profile of immature lymphocytes.[478] Increased marrow lymphocytosis may be associated with longer duration of thrombocytopenia.[469]

Treatment

Fatalities are rare in acute ITP; however, the low incidence of poor outcomes has made it impossible to perform a clinical trial to assess whether treatment may prevent deaths. Therefore, clinical trials have focused on the time required to raise the platelet count to safe levels.

Corticosteroids. Three prospective, randomized clinical trials[479–481] (two double-blind) compared prednisone (2 mg/kg/d or 60 mg/m^2/d) to no therapy in acute ITP of childhood. Two of the trials[480,481] demonstrated a more rapid increase in platelet count in the corticosteroid-treated group than in the control group, and the third[479] demonstrated a similar trend, which was not significant.

Larger initial doses of corticosteroids have also been used for these children, such as prednisone (4 to 8 mg/kg/d)[482] or intravenous methylprednisolone (5 to 30 mg/kg/d).[483–486] Almost all the children achieved a platelet count greater than $20 \times 10^9/L$ within 72 hours of commencing treatment. Side effects, including glycosuria, hypertension, and transient weight gain, were uncommonly encountered during the brief treatment periods.

IVIgG. In 1981, Imbach and colleagues[383] reported that IVIgG raised the platelet count in children with acute or chronic ITP. Subsequently, these workers reported the results of a prospective, randomized, multicenter trial comparing prednisone (60 mg/m^2/d for 3 weeks) with IVIgG (0.4 g/kg/d for 5 days) as alternate treatment for children with acute ITP (platelet counts less than $30 \times 10^9/L$).[487] The study demonstrated that for about 60% of the children, either treatment produced a rapid rise in the platelet count to safe levels. For the remainder who were less responsive to treatment, the IVIgG resulted in a faster rise in the platelet count.[487]

A dose of 1 g/kg/d for 2 consecutive days has also been used successfully. Response to treatment is sufficiently rapid in half the children that only a single dose of IVIgG is required.[488]

Recommended Treatment. The risk of life-threatening bleeding is highest within the first few weeks, so affected children should avoid trauma and restrict physical activity as much as possible. Most children with acute ITP have a benign clinical course and recover without therapy. Unfortunately, it is impossible to identify those who will develop life-threatening bleeding. The available evidence suggests that either corticosteroids or IVIgG reduces the duration of severe thrombocytopenia and that, in some children, IVIgG is of greater benefit than corticosteroids. Therefore, for children with clinical hemostatic dysfunction or severe thrombocytopenia (platelet count less than $20 \times 10^9/L$), we recommend treatment with IVIgG. Some pediatricians favor corticosteroids primarily because of the lower cost. For patients with more severe hemorrhage (eg, intracranial or mucosal bleeding), the combined use of IVIgG and high-dose corticosteroids may be more effective.[489,490] Emergency splenectomy should be considered for the rare patient with life-threatening bleeding who does not respond to platelet transfusions, IVIgG, and high-dose corticosteroid therapy.

Chronic Idiopathic Thrombocytopenic Purpura of Childhood

Thrombocytopenia persists for longer than 6 months (chronic ITP) in about 10% to 20% of children with ITP. As many as one third of children with chronic ITP, however, can have a spontaneous remission months or years later.[469] About 5% of children with ITP have recurrent ITP, characterized by intermittent episodes of thrombocytopenia followed by lengthy periods of remission.

Pathogenesis

Chronic ITP in children resembles the adult form of ITP. About two thirds of children have elevated serum platelet-bindable IgG[472]; 85% of children have elevated PAIgG[471]; and autoantibodies against the gpIIb/IIIa complex have been implicated.[472,491] Thus, it appears that chronic ITP in children is caused by antiplatelet autoantibodies that lead to platelet destruction by the reticuloendothelial system.

Clinical and Laboratory Features

Several clinical and laboratory features are seen more frequently in children with chronic than with acute ITP, although these features are not sufficiently distinctive to be useful in individual patients. Children who develop chronic ITP are likely to be more than 10 years old and female[492]; have an insidious onset of bleeding symptoms; lack a viral prodrome; have less severe thrombocytopenia (platelet count often greater than $20 \times 10^9/L$); have less marked elevation of the PAIgG[473,474]; and have an increased frequency of other immune abnormalities,[493] including selective hypogammaglobulinemia, positive ANA, and decreased lymphocyte responsiveness to mitogen stimulation.[494]

Treatment

For many children with chronic ITP, the thrombocytopenia is only moderate, and the symptoms are absent or minimal. For these children, specific treatment is not required. For symptomatic children, the treatment options include maintenance IVIgG or anti-D injections, chronic or intermittent administration of corticosteroids, splenectomy, vinca alkaloids, or immunosuppressive agents.

Corticosteroids. Most children with chronic ITP achieve a safe platelet count on corticosteroid therapy, but the long-term toxicity of this treatment does not justify its prolonged use, except for the rare patient who responds to small doses of alternate-day prednisone. Short courses of corticosteroids can be useful for patients with exacerbations of symptomatic thrombocytopenia or in whom surgical procedures are considered.

Pulse methylprednisolone has been used in patients with chronic ITP.[483,489,495,496] In the largest series,[496] about half the children maintained a platelet count above $50 \times 10^9/L$ for a minimum of 1 month after a 3-day course of methylprednisolone (15 mg/kg/d).

IVIgG. IVIgG (2 g/kg total dose administered over 2 to 5 days) raises the platelet count in most children with chronic ITP.[383,392,497–500] Repeated courses of IVIgG have been used to defer or avoid splenectomy in children with chronic ITP.[498,500] The intervals between the treatment with IVIgG are dictated by symptoms or the platelet count. Most children respond favorably to such maintenance therapy. Some enter a long-term complete or partial remission and require no further therapy. Other children remain asymptomatic but require intermittent injections of IVIgG.[498,500] About one fourth of children become refractory to treatment.[498] Cost-effectiveness analysis demonstrates a lower cost for young children treated with maintenance IVIgG than with splenectomy.[501] Low-dose alternate-day prednisone therapy may improve the results achieved with maintenance IVIgG.

Anti-D. Anti-D also is effective in raising the platelet count in most children with chronic ITP, and some children have a long-term response. Benefit is usually transient, with a median duration of 3 weeks in one study.[502] Anti-D also can be effective as maintenance therapy.[502,503]

Splenectomy. About 75% of children have a complete remission after splenectomy.[469,492,504] The long-term risk of postsplenectomy septicemia in children with ITP is about 8%, with a case-mortality rate of 15% (overall, 1% mortality).[505] This risk appears to be even greater in the subgroup of children under 3 years of age.[505] Because of the risks of postsplenectomy septicemia, the possibility of late spontaneous remission of the ITP, and the frequent efficacy of intermittent maintenance therapy with IVIgG or anti-D, splenectomy should not be performed in very young children with chronic ITP. Children should receive polyvalent pneumococcal and *Haemophilus* vaccination, and possibly meningococcal vaccination, before the elective splenectomy.

Vinca Alkaloids and Immunosuppressive Agents. Treatment results with vinca alkaloids and immunosuppressive agents are variable, but generally poor,[504,506] and this form of treatment should be restricted to the most severely affected patients.

Systemic Lupus Erythematosus

Thrombocytopenia occurs at some time in 15% to 40% of patients with SLE.[507–511] Platelet antibodies can be detected in most SLE patients using phase I and phase II assays.[210,257] Not infrequently, patients with SLE have elevated PAIgG but are not thrombocytopenic. Since most nonthrombocytopenic SLE patients have normal platelet life-spans,[512] it is possible that the hypergammaglobulinemia that often complicates SLE impairs phagocytic cell function, preventing the destruction of the IgG-sensitized platelets.[393,513]

The nature of the platelet-reactive antibodies in SLE is uncertain. Both autoantibodies[246,514,515] and complement-binding immune complexes[516,517] have been implicated. Additionally, the presence of antiphospholipid antibodies, which frequently are found in the sera of SLE patients, has been correlated with thrombocytopenia.[518–521] Antiphospholipid antibodies can bind to platelets after perturbation of their membranes, suggesting that these antibodies may bind preferentially to activated platelets.[522] Antibodies reactive against platelet-bound but nonspecific antigens, such as DNA, are also possible.[200]

Thrombocytopenia is encountered in two clinical settings in SLE.[523] In some patients, thrombocytopenia is chronic, mimicking ITP. In other patients, acute thrombocytopenia complicates systemic flares of the SLE.

Treatment of Thrombocytopenia

Thrombocytopenia complicating SLE is treated similarly to ITP but with one major difference—we use danazol before splenectomy (discussed subsequently).

Corticosteroids are the initial therapy. Prednisone usually is effective, but tapering with a view to discontinuing the drug is complicated by the high rate of thrombocytopenic relapse. Long-term use of low doses of corticosteroids may be justified, however, particularly if the drug also achieves control of other symptoms of the SLE.

Controversy has surrounded the role of splenectomy in thrombocytopenic SLE patients since Dameshek[524] suggested in 1956 that splenectomy can worsen the course of SLE. This postulate probably is not correct.[525] Nevertheless, controversy persists: some physicians[526–528] report that splenectomy in SLE results in as good a rate of response as occurs in ITP, whereas others[529] report that benefit is much less likely. Because of the possible reduced likelihood of success and the increased risk of postsplenectomy infections in this immunocompromised population,[530] we prefer a trial of danazol before splenectomy. Three small series have reported benefit—sometimes dramatic—after administration of danazol for the thrombocytopenia of SLE.[531–533] In most patients, the danazol must be continued to maintain the platelet count at safe levels.

Other treatments that have been used in thrombocytopenic patients with SLE include vinca alkaloids,[373] immunosuppressive agents, IVIgG,[534] cyclosporine,[432] and plasmapheresis.[535] The use of synchronized plasmapheresis and cyclophosphamide for severe exacerbations of SLE (including thrombocytopenia) was reported.[536] These investigators postulated that the removal of the autoantibody by means of plasmapheresis stimulated autoreactive clones, which were then destroyed by the cyclophosphamide.

Antiphospholipid Antibody Syndrome

Thrombocytopenia can occur as part of the antiphospholipid antibody syndrome, which also has been termed the *lupus anticoagulant syndrome* and the *anticardiolipin syndrome*. These patients often suffer from recurrent arterial or venous thrombotic complications[518,519] rather than from bleeding. Other associated abnormalities include recurrent miscarriages, thromboembolic pulmonary hypertension, cardiac valvulitis or cardiomyopathy, adrenal failure, and neurologic disturbances, including strokes and transient ischemic attacks, migraine, and chorea.[520,537–542] Associated dermatologic manifestations include livedo reticularis, Raynaud's phenomenon, leg ulcers, symmetric gangrene of the fingers and toes, and acral microlivedo (nonblanching erythematous or cyanotic macules located on the palms, soles, fingertips, or toes).[543–545] In one prospective study,[511] 43% of patients with SLE had positive anticardiolipin antibodies. These autoantibodies also have been associated with other connective tissue diseases; ITP; malignancies; infections, including HIV; and certain drugs, such as chlorpromazine and procainamide.[546] The antiphospholipid syndrome also can occur as a primary disorder without associated SLE or other immune disturbance.[546,547] It is possible that the thrombocytopenia is caused by other platelet-reactive IgG[548] rather than the antiphospholipid antibodies per se.

The sine qua non of the syndrome is the laboratory demonstration of antiphospholipid antibodies. These polyclonal antibodies can often be detected by their ability to prolong phospholipid-dependent clotting tests (lupus anticoagulant), or by using solid-phase assays employing negatively charged phospholipid target antigens (eg, anticardiolipin antibody assay), or sometimes by causing a biologic false-positive VDRL result.[537] These antiphospholipid antibodies have been shown to react with negatively charged phospholipids such as cardiolipin or phosphatidylserine in the presence of a plasma protein cofactor, β_2-glycoprotein I.[549,550] The protein cofactor antigen target for antibodies with lupus anticoagulant activity has been identified as prothrombin.[551,552]

A cross-sectional study showed evidence of elevated baseline thrombin generation in SLE patients with anticardiolipin antibodies.[553] It is possible that enhancement of platelet activation by antiphospholipid antibodies contributes to this prothrombotic state.[554,555]

No laboratory features of the antiphospholipid antibody syndrome reliably predict thrombosis. Thus, long-term antiplatelet or anticoagulant therapy is recommended for patients who have already developed an arterial or venous thrombotic event, respectively. Corticosteroid therapy may worsen clinical manifestations in some patients.[556]

Thrombocytopenia Complicating Other Immune Disorders

Immune thrombocytopenia can complicate other disorders of immune dysregulation, including autoimmune hemolysis (Evans's syndrome),[557,558] rheumatoid arthritis,[558] dermatomyositis,[559] progressive systemic sclerosis,[560] localized scleroderma,[561] Sjögren's syndrome,[562] Graves's disease,[563–565] Hashimoto's thyroiditis,[564,566,567] pernicious anemia,[558] sarcoidosis,[568–570] myasthenia gravis,[567,571,572] inflammatory bowel disease,[573,574] celiac disease,[575] primary biliary cirrhosis,[576] autoimmune hyperchylomicronemia,[577] and bullous pemphigoid.[578] Although an autoimmune pathogenesis is suspected for some of these disorders, proof has only rarely been provided using phase III platelet antibody tests.[571,579]

The approach to treatment should parallel considerations given for the treatment of primary ITP. It is possible that for some of these conditions, such as Evans's syndrome, the thrombocytopenia is less responsive to first-line treatment (corticosteroids and splenectomy).[557]

Neoplasia-Associated Immune Thrombocytopenia

Immune thrombocytopenia can precede, accompany, or follow neoplastic disease,[580–582] particularly the chronic lymphoproliferative syndromes.[558,583–601] Immune thrombocytopenia occurs in 2% to 3% of patients with chronic lymphocytic leukemia.[587–589] Conversely, in a series of more than 500 patients with clinical and laboratory evidence for immune thrombocytopenia, 15% had associated neoplastic lymphoproliferative disorders.[558]

Decreased platelet survival[597] and elevated PAIgG[232,256,590] have been demonstrated in several studies of patients with thrombocytopenia complicating lymphoproliferative neoplasms. Autoantibodies against the gpIIb/IIIa complex have been demonstrated in patients with lymphoma.[146,579,598]

Immune thrombocytopenia has been estimated to occur in 1% to 2% of patients with Hodgkin's disease.[583,596] The immune thrombocytopenia is often not related to the neoplastic disease activity, and the occurrence of immune thrombocytopenia in a patient who is thought to be cured of the Hodgkin's disease does not necessarily mean that the illness has relapsed.

Thrombocytopenia occurs in about half of patients with rheumatoid arthritis and clonal proliferation of large granular lymphocytes (T_γ-lymphoproliferative disease).[599] In this rare disorder, hypersplenism and elevated PAIgG[600,601] may interact to produce the high frequency of thrombocytopenia.

Often, the thrombocytopenia represents less of a risk to the patient than the underlying malignancy, and the first step in the management of these patients is to treat the underlying disorder. In some patients, the thrombocytopenia resolves as the malignancy responds to therapy, while in others, the thrombocytopenia requires specific treatment. The approach to treatment is similar to the treatment of patients with chronic ITP (ie, corticosteroids followed by splenectomy). One study[594] that reviewed the literature on immune thrombocytopenia complicating Hodgkin's disease concluded that 30% of patients responded to corticosteroids, whereas 75% benefited from splenectomy.

Thrombocytopenia complicating chronic lymphoproliferative disease can also be caused by marrow infiltration with tumor or by effects of therapy. Sometimes, all these processes coexist. A bone marrow examination is often required to determine treatment. Thrombocytopenia that occurs in the setting of a nonlymphoproliferative malignancy is much more likely to be caused by nonimmune mechanisms, such as marrow replacement by tumor, marrow suppression by chemotherapy, or DIC.

Human Immunodeficiency Virus–Associated Immune Thrombocytopenia

Immune thrombocytopenia is part of the spectrum of HIV infection and has been described in homosexual men,[602–605] intravenous drug abusers,[606] patients with hemophilia,[607] and people infected by heterosexual contact.[608] Immune thrombocytopenia occurs in about 10% to 15% of asymptomatic HIV carriers and in 30% to 40% of patients with the acquired immunodeficiency syndrome (AIDS).[609–611] A case of severe thrombocytopenia occurring in a woman with human T-cell leukemia virus type I in fection was described.[612]

Increased levels of PAIgG, PAIgM, and platelet-bound complement are present in most cases of HIV-associated thrombocytopenia.[602,604,606,613,614] These levels are often higher than in classic ITP. Two types of platelet antibody have been described: (1) immune complexes consisting of anti-HIV antibodies and anti-F(ab')$_2$ antibodies (anti-antibodies),[614,615] and (2) platelet-reactive autoantibodies.[616,617] A recent report[618] suggests a unifying explanation for these observations—some anti-HIV antibodies cross-react with gpIIb/IIIa.

Although a reduction in T-helper cells is usually observed, patients with normal lymphocyte numbers and thrombocytopenia have been described.[608,619,620] The finding of reduced numbers of T-helper cells is more frequent in adults than in children with HIV-associated thrombocytopenia.[621]

The occurrence of thrombocytopenia does not increase the risk for progression to more advanced stage of HIV infection,[622] and in some cases, the thrombocytopenia spontaneously disappears.[603,604]

The results of treatment of HIV-associated thrombocytopenia are similar to those in classic ITP. About 75% of patients have a response to corticosteroids, given at a dose of 1 mg/kg/d. In almost half of the responses, the platelet count is more than 100×10^9/L. Only 20% of the patients maintain an adequate platelet count after tapering or discontinuation of the corticosteroid.[603–605,623] Complications of treatment include oral candidiasis and reactivation of oral and genital herpes.[604,605] Some physicians do not use corticosteroids because of the potential risk of infectious complications in this patient population.[624]

Splenectomy results in complete or partial remission in about 80% of patients.[603–606,623,625–630] Humoral immunity is impaired in HIV patients,[631] and some physicians administer long-term penicillin prophylaxis in addition to routine preoperative pneumococcal vaccination for HIV patients who undergo splenectomy.[627,629] Splenectomy does not appear to increase the rate of progression to AIDS.[630]

Baseline reticuloendothelial function is impaired in patients with HIV infection,[632,633] Nevertheless, about 80% of patients who receive the reticuloendothelial-blocking treatment, high dose IVIgG, have a transient rise in the platelet count to above 50×10^9/L.[623,625,627,634] Particularly in children, HIV-associated thrombocytopenia has been successfully managed for lengthy periods with repeated injections of IVIgG.[620]

Anti-D can also transiently raise the platelet count in about 80% of Rh-positive patients with HIV-associated thrombocytopenia who have not undergo splenectomy.[419,424,635] Hemolysis caused by anti-D is usually mild and well tolerated, and therefore repeated-dose maintenance therapy is often possible.[424,635] An advantage of anti-D is that it can be given at home.[424]

The antiretroviral agent zidovudine (also known as azidothymidine or AZT) increases the platelet count in patients with HIV-associated thrombocytopenia, often within the first 2 weeks of therapy.[636,637] Anemia and granulocytopenia can complicate this treatment.

α-Interferon raises the platelet count in some patients with HIV-associated thrombocytopenia,[638–640] possibly by improving platelet survival.[640] Other treatments with reported benefit in these patients include danazol[623] and dapsone,[641] extracorporeal immunoadsorption,[642] and splenic irradiation.[643]

In summary, for patients with mild or no bleeding symptoms, it is acceptable to follow the patient without specific treatment.[611] Ziduvidine can elevate the platelet count and may be helpful in preventing the progression of AIDS; however, some patients cannot receive this agent because of anemia or neutropenia. Benefit from prednisone is usually temporary and can contribute to infectious complications. Splenectomy offers a high probability of sustained complete or partial remission and appears to be safe in this patient population. Acute or chronic bleeding symptoms can usually be controlled with reticuloendothelial blockade (IVIgG or anti-D), with the decreased costs favoring the use of anti-D in Rh-positive patients.

Bone Marrow Transplantation–Associated Immune Thrombocytopenia

Early, severe thrombocytopenia caused by marrow ablative therapy is a universal consequence of bone marrow transplantation. Several syndromes of isolated thrombocytopenia that occur later in the posttransplantation course of allogeneic or autologous bone marrow transplantation have been described, including transient benign thrombocytopenia[644,645]; chronic, persistent thrombocytopenia[644,646]; and late-onset thrombocytopenia.[647–649]

Transient Benign Thrombocytopenia

In transient benign thrombocytopenia, the platelet count recovery after transplantation is initially normal, with a rise in the platelet count to above 100×10^9/L. These patients then become thrombocytopenic before day 50, with subsequent platelet count recovery before day 70.[644] The incidence of transient benign thrombocytopenia is about 15%, and it usually is not serious.

Chronic Persistent Thrombocytopenia

Patients with chronic persistent thrombocytopenia do not develop a platelet count greater than 100×10^9/L during the first 2 to 4 months after transplantation.[644,646] This complication, which has an incidence of about 25%,[644] is frequently associated with acute chronic graft-versus-host disease and has a poor prognosis.[644,646] Persistent thrombocytopenia has also been associated with hepatic veno-occlusive disease.[650]

Late-Onset Immune Thrombocytopenia

Rarely, isolated thrombocytopenia secondary to immune mechanisms can develop several months after transplantation.[647–649]

Pathogenesis

Sometimes, isolated thrombocytopenia occurring after transplantation is caused by drugs (eg, sulfamethoxazole, trimethoprim),[644] graft rejection,[646] leukemic relapse,[646] or a complicating infection.[646] Furthermore, the marrow response to thrombocytopenia is impaired in the early post-transplantation setting.[646] In many patients, however, immune mechanisms are implicated, as shown by platelet antibody tests[644–646,649] and markedly reduced platelet lifespan.[644,646,649] It has been suggested that most cases are caused by autoantibodies produced by donor lymphocytes reacting to donor platelets.[645,646,651] Pathogenic factors could include transient immune system dysregulation accompanying donor immune engraftment[645] or graft-versus-host disease[644,646] as well as an altered expression of self caused by viral infections.[648] Other reported mechanisms include autoimmune thrombocytopenia caused by lymphocytes derived from a donor with compensated ITP[652] and alloimmune thrombocytopenia (anti-Pl^{A1}) caused by residual recipient lymphocytes producing alloantibodies against Pl^{A1}-positive platelets from the donor.[649]

Treatment

Drug toxicity, infection, and other treatable causes should be sought. The immune thrombocytopenia in some patients is self-limited (transient benign thrombocytopenia). Chronic, persistent thrombocytopenia associated with graft-versus-host disease sometimes responds favorably to increased immunosuppressive maneuvers, but most therapy is ineffective.[646] Late-onset thrombocytopenia responds to corticosteroids, IVIgG, and splenectomy.[647,649]

Drug-Induced Thrombocytopenia

Thrombocytopenia is a common and potentially serious complication of drug therapy.[653] Drugs usually cause thrombocytopenia by impaired platelet production or immune platelet destruction. Much less common causes of drug-induced thrombocytopenia include drug-induced platelet activation (hematin)[654,655] or agglutination (ristocetin, porcine factor VIII),[656,657] drug-induced reticuloendothelial sequestration of platelets (protamine sulfate),[658] or drug-induced liver disease with secondary hypersplenism (α-methyldopa, methotrexate).

Impaired platelet production most frequently is caused by drugs with predictable, dose-dependent cytotoxicity, such as anti-cancer chemotherapy. Some drugs, however, such as chloramphenicol, phenylbutazone, and gold, cause aplastic anemia only in susceptible people. Although most drugs that cause thrombocytopenia through marrow suppression damage the hematopoietic stem cell and produce pancytopenia, some agents, such as alcohol, primarily inhibit megakaryocyte production and cause isolated thrombocytopenia. The combination of cimetidine and phenytoin has been implicated as a cause of isolated thrombocytopenia with decreased marrow megakaryocytes.[659] Cimetidine has been shown to be myelotoxic in vitro.[660]

Drug-induced thrombocytopenia characterized by increased platelet destruction is almost always caused by immune mechanisms. Immune drug-induced thrombocytopenia is important in clinical medicine for several reasons:

1. Many drugs can cause immune thrombocytopenia, including commonly used agents, such as heparin, quinine, and sulfonamides (Table 34-2).
2. The thrombocytopenia occurs unexpectedly and unpredictably in susceptible people (idiosyncratic).
3. Complications, such as life-threatening bleeding

(many drugs) or arterial or venous thrombosis (heparin), can occur.

Immune Drug-Induced Destructive Thrombocytopenia

A drug can be implicated definitively as causing idiosyncratic thrombocytopenia only if all the following criteria are met[653]: (1) the thrombocytopenia develops while the patient is receiving the drug and resolves after the drug is stopped, (2) other causes of thrombocytopenia are excluded, and (3) the thrombocytopenia recurs after readministration of the drug (in vivo challenge). Readministration is potentially dangerous, however, and confirmation of the diagnosis is best achieved by (4) in vitro techniques. The platelet antibody tests previously discussed can be performed in the presence or absence of the drug. As shown in Table 34-2, confirmatory data are not available for many drugs suspected of causing immune thrombocytopenia. In some cases, it may be necessary to test drug metabolites when investigating a patient with suspected drug-induced thrombocytopenia.[663,795]

Clinical Importance of Drug-Induced Immune Thrombocytopenia

The clinical importance of drugs causing immune thrombocytopenia depends on how frequently the drug is prescribed, the risk for idiosyncratic thrombocytopenia associated with the drug, and the clinical impact of the thrombocytopenic syndrome, including the temporal course, severity, and complications.

Although many drugs have been implicated as causing immune thrombocytopenia (see Table 34-2), in most instances, the risk associated with any drug is low. Some drugs, however, cause thrombocytopenia much more commonly than others. For instance, heparin causes thrombocytopenia in 1% to 3% of patients.[727,728] This is especially remarkable because heparin is usually administered for less than 10 days. The high incidence in conjunction with its widespread use means that many patients develop this complication. In addition, although it rarely causes bleeding, heparin-induced thrombocytopenia can be associated with life-threatening arterial or venous thrombosis.[727,728] Furthermore, it is difficult to find an acceptable replacement antithrombotic agent when heparin-induced thrombocytopenia or thrombosis occurs. For these reasons, heparin is the most important cause of immune drug-induced thrombocytopenia.

Another important cause of drug-induced thrombocytopenia is gold. Although use of gold is restricted to patients with rheumatoid arthritis, gold causes thrombocytopenia in about 2% to 3% of patients exposed. Bleeding symptoms are frequent. Furthermore, the thrombocytopenia can persist for many weeks or months after stopping the gold.

Although quinidine causes thrombocytopenia in about 1 in 1000 people,[802] the thrombocytopenia is often severe and can be life-threatening. Exposure to quinine (found in tonic water) is ubiquitous, but it can be difficult to establish exposure by history. Thus, these agents are important causes of drug-induced thrombocytopenia.

Most of the agents listed in Table 34-2 rarely cause thrombocytopenia, and the clinical importance approximates the frequency of use. Thus, thrombocytopenia is seen mostly frequently with heparin, gold, quinidine and quinine, sulfonamides, and penicillin.

Valproic acid and amrinone are other drugs associated with a high incidence of thrombocytopenia (about 20% to 30% in prospective studies). An immune pathogenesis is suggested by the finding of elevated PAIgG in several patients. The clinical importance is small, however, because the thrombocytopenia is mild and self-limited.[676–678,799]

Immune drug-induced platelet destruction can be caused by several mechanisms: formation of drug–platelet protein–IgG immune complexes that bind to platelets by means of the platelet Fc receptors (heparin); IgG Fab binding to drug–platelet complex (quinidine and quinine); and Fab binding of IgG autoantibodies to platelet autoantigens (possibly procainamide).

Drug-Dependent Fc Binding of IgG to Platelets: Heparin-Induced Thrombocytopenia and Thrombosis

Heparin is a heterogeneous and polydispersed glycosaminoglycan composed of alternating substituted uronic acid and glucosamine saccharide units. Standard preparations are extracted from bovine lung or porcine intestinal mucosa and have a molecular weight ranging from 10 to 20 kd. Low-molecular-weight (LMW) preparations usually are prepared by chemical or physical manipulations of the standard preparations.

Heparin is useful as an antithrombotic agent because it catalyzes the inactivation by antithrombin III of thrombin, Xa, and IXa. It also binds binds to platelets in a specific and saturable fashion[803] and can cause platelet aggregation.[804–806] Heparin also can prolong the bleeding time.[807] These nonidiosyncratic interactions of heparin with platelets are of uncertain clinical relevance.

In contrast, a minority of patients (about 1% to 3%) who receive heparin develop a syndrome characterized by in vivo platelet activation that usually begins 5 to 10 days afer beginning heparin therapy. [727,728,806] Despite a low (or falling) platelet count and the administration of heparin, many of these patients develop paradoxical arterial or venous thrombosis. Heparin-induced thrombocytopenia is caused by a platelet-activating IgG that is triggered by treatment with heparin. A similar prothrombotic syndrome can be caused by the heparinoid pentosan polysulphate[808,809] or a polysulfated chondroitin sulfate (Arteparon)[810] used to treat arthritis. In contrast, a mixture of glycosaminoglycans known as Org 10172 (Orgaran) is useful in the treatment of heparin-induced thrombocytopenia.[811,812]

Clinical Features. The risk for heparin-induced thrombocytopenia (defined as platelet count lower than 100 $\times 10^9$/L) in patients receiving therapeutic doses of bovine lung heparin is about 5% and for porcine mucosal heparin is about 1%.[727,728,806] However, heparin-induced thrombocytopenia also can occur in patients receiving low (prophylactic) doses of heparin[806,813] or even lower doses used to maintain the patency of intravascular catheters. The use of heparin-coated pulmonary artery catheters has also been implicated in some patients with heparin-induced thrombocytopenia.[814] The thrombocytopenia usually begins between 5 and 10 days after starting heparin therapy; however, thrombocytopenia and thrombosis can occur within hours if the patient previously received heparin.[815]

In contrast to drug-induced thrombocytopenia caused by quinine, quinidine, or sulfa drugs, very severe thrombocytopenia (platelet count below 10 $\times 10^9$/L) is rare in heparin-induced thrombocytopenia. Typically, platelet counts range from 20 to 150 $\times 10^9$/L, with a median of 50 $\times 10^9$/L in many patient series.[728] Occasionally, thrombotic complications accompany a heparin-induced fall in the platelet count that does not reach thrombocytopenic levels.[816,817]

As many as 30% of patients who develop heparin-induced thrombocytopenia also have thrombotic complications.[728,806] Arterial complications are most characteristic and include aortic or iliofemoral artery thrombosis (often leading to amputation), thrombotic cerebrovascular occlusion, and myocardial infarction. Less frequent

TABLE 34-2. Drugs Implicated in Immune Thrombocytopenia*

Drug	In Vivo Challenge	In Vitro Phase I Assay	In Vitro Phase II Assay	References
Acetaminophen	+	+	−	661–663
Acetazolamide	−	+	−	664–666
Acetylsalicylic acid	−	+	−	666, 667
Actinomycin D	−	−	−	668
Allylisopropylcarbamide (Sedormid)	+	+	−	669
Alprenolol	+	−	−	670
Aminoglutethimide	+	−	−	671, 672
Amiodarone	+	−	−	673
Ampicillin	−	+	+	666, 674, 675
Amrinone	+	−	+†	676–678
Antazoline	−	+	−	679
Apalcillin	−	−	−	680
Butobarbitone	+	−	−	681
Captopril	−	−	−	682, 683
Carbamazepine	−	+	−	666, 684, 685
Cefotetan	−	−	+	686
Cephalexin	−	+	−	666
Cephalothin	+	+	−	687, 688
Cephamandole	−	−	+	689
Chlordiazepoxide–clidinium bromide	−	−	−	693
Chlorpheniramine	−	+	−	690
Chlorpropamide	−	−	−	694
Chlorthalidone	−	+	−	666
Chlorthiazide	+	+	−	666, 691, 692
Cimetidine	+	+	+	675, 695–698
Clinoril	−	−	−	699, 700
Clonazepam	−	−	−	701
Cocaine	−	−	−	702
Danazol	−	+	−	361, 362
Desferrioxamine	+	−	−	703
Desipramine	−	+	−	704
Diatrizoate	−	−	−	705
Diazepam	+	+	+	706, 707
Diazoxide	−	−	−	708, 709
Diclofenac	−	−	−	710
Difluoromethylornithine	+	−	−	711
Diflunisal	−	+	−	712
Digitoxin	+	+	−	713–715
Digoxin	+	+	+	675, 716, 717
Diphenylhydantoin	+	−	−	666, 707, 718
Etretinate	−	−	−	719
Ethchlorvynol	−	+	−	720
Fenoprofen	−	−	−	721
Furosemide	+	+	−	722
Gentamicin	−	+	−	723
Gold	+	−	+	675, 724, 725
Glibenclamide	−	−	−	726
Heparin	+	+	+	727, 728
Heroin	−	−	−	729–731
Hydrochlorthiazide	−	+	−	675, 692, 732
Imipramine	−	+	−	666
Indomethacin	−	−	−	733
Insecticide	−	−	−	734
α-Interferon	+	−	+†	735–737
β-Interferon	−	−	+†	736

(continued)

TABLE 34-2. *(Continued)*

Drug	In Vivo Challenge	In Vitro Phase I Assay	In Vitro Phase II Assay	References
Iopanoic acid	+	+	−	738
Isoniazid	−	−	−	739
Isotretinoin	+	−	−	740
Levamisole	+	−	−	741
Levodopa	−	−	−	742
Lidocaine	+	+	−	743
Lincomycin	−	−	−	744
Meprobamate	−	+	−	666
Methicillin	+	+	−	745
Methyldopa	+	+	−	666, 746–748
Mexiletine	−	−	−	749
Mianserin	−	−	+	750
Minoxidil	−	+	−	751
Morphine	−	+	−	752
Nalidixic acid	+	−	−	753
Nimesulide	+	−	−	754
Nitroprusside	−	−	−	755
Nomifensine	−	+	−	756
Novobiocin	+	+	−	757
Oxyphenbutazone	−	−	−	758
Oxprenolol	+	−	−	759–761
Oxytetracycline	−	−	−	762
Paraaminosalicylic acid	+	−	−	763
Penicillin	+	+	+	675, 764, 765
Pentagastrin	+	−	−	766
Pentamidine	−	−	−	767, 768
Phenylbutazone	−	+	−	769
Pirenzepine	−	−	−	770
Piroxicam	−	−	−	771
Primidone	−	−	−	772
Procainamide	+	+	−	666, 773–775
Quinidine	+	+	+	666, 675, 776
Quinine	+	+	+	666, 675, 729, 776
Ranitidine	−	−	+	777, 778
Rifampin	+	+	−	779–781
Salicylate	−	−	−	782
Spironolactone	−	+	−	666
Stibophen	+	+	−	783, 784
Sulfamezathine	−	+	−	776
Sulfamethoxypyridazine	−	−	−	785
Sulfasalazine	+	−	−	787, 788
Sulfisoxazole	+	+	+	675, 707, 789
Sulindac	−	−	−	786
Thioguanine	−	+	−	666
Tobramycin	−	−	−	790
Tolbutamide	−	−	−	791
Tolmetin	−	−	−	793
Toluene diisocyanate	−	−	−	792
Trimethoprim-sulfamethoxazole	+	+	+	675, 794–797
Turpentine	−	−	−	798
Valproic acid	−	−	+†	799
Vancomycin	+	−	+	800, 801

* Evidence supporting immune drug-induced platelet destruction is indicated by + if the following were demonstrated: in vivo rechallenge, drug-dependent platelet-antibody test using phase I tests, or drug-dependent platelet-antibody test using phase II tests.

† Elevated PAIgG was found in these patients with thrombocytopenia, but in vitro drug-dependent platelet-associated immunoglobulin G increase was not reported.

thrombotic complications include upper limb arterial thrombosis and thrombosis of the mesenteric, renal, or spinal arteries.[727,728,806]

The risk and type of thrombotic complications depend on the type of patient population receiving heparin.[818] For example, deep venous thrombosis and pulmonary embolism are more commonly seen in postoperative patients who develop heparin-induced thrombocytopenia while receiving postoperative heparin prophylaxis. Dural sinus thrombosis has occurred in several pregnant women who developed heparin-induced thrombocytopenia.[819,820]

We have also observed limb loss secondary to severe phlegmasia cerulea dolens, progressing to venous gangrene, in some patients who received aggressive warfarin anticoagulation for deep venous thrombosis complicating heparin-induced thrombocytopenia; we believe that this devastating thrombotic complication represents the adverse interaction of two anticoagulants: warfarin-induced limb gangrene complicating heparin-induced thrombocytopenia.

Thrombosis complicates heparin-induced thrombocytopenia much more commonly than does bleeding. Indeed, there is only one characteristic hemorrhagic manifestation of heparin-induced thrombocytopenia: adrenal hemorrhage.[728,821–824] However, this sequela probably results from adrenal hemorrhagic infarction secondary to adrenal vein thrombosis.[821] The adrenal infarction can be bilateral or unilateral and can present as severe abdominal or flank pain, with or without symptoms and signs of acute or chronic adrenal insufficiency.

Some patients experience painful skin reactions beginning 5 days or more after commencing subcutaneous heparin injections.[825–828] Ranging from small erythematous papules to large areas of dermal necrosis, these skin reactions may not necessarily be accompanied by thrombocytopenia; in our experience, however, heparin-dependent IgG can be detected in the sera of these patients.

Administration of intravenous bolus heparin to patients who have formed heparin-dependent IgG can be complicated within 30 minutes by the onset of an acute systemic inflammatory reaction accompanied by an abrupt fall in the platelet count.[829] Characteristic symptoms and signs include fever, chills, hypertension and tachycardia, dyspnea, flushing, nausea, and vomiting. Sudden death has also been described.[830] Some patients have also developed severe but transient anterograde amnesia (transient global amnesia) following bolus heparin administration.[831]

Heparin resistance (ie, increasing heparin doses required to maintain therapeutic levels of anticoagulation) often occurs in heparin-induced thrombocytopenia.[832] However, this is a nonspecific finding observed commonly in patients who receive heparin.

Although susceptible patients can develop recurrent thrombocytopenia on reexposure to heparin, this is not universal.[832,833] Furthermore, in some patients, the thrombocytopenia resolves despite continued administration of heparin.[806,834] These atypical features are not seen with other immune drug-induced thrombocytopenic disorders and remain unexplained.

Pathogenesis. The heparin-dependent platelet-activating factor is IgG.[205,835] In recent years, insights into both the mechanism of platelet activation and the nature of the target antigen, have been gained.

Platelet activation occurs via binding of the IgG Fc moiety to the platelet FcγII receptors.[205,836,837] Heparin-dependent IgG is a potent platelet activation stimulus, as shown by its ability to aggregate and cause granule release from washed platelets (ie, lacking exogenous fibrinogen)[213,838] and to produce platelet thromboxane generation.[835] In addition, platelet activation by heparin-dependent IgG stimulates the generation of platelet-derived microparticles with procoagulant activity.[839]

Several groups of investigators were unable to demonstrate that heparin alone was the target antigen. In 1978, it was first suggested that a platelet factor might interact with heparin to form the target antigen.[840] It remained until the 1990s, however, that the platelet component of the antigen complex was identified as an α-granule constituent, *platelet factor 4*.[841–844] It appears that a macromolecular complex of heparin and platelet factor 4 is formed on the platelet surface[844]; interaction of patient IgG with this complex and the platelet FcγII receptors results in platelet activation.

It is uncertain why only some patients develop devastating thrombotic complications. Clinical factors[818] appear to play an important role: for example, thrombosis occurred frequently in large arteries or veins that had recently been punctured for placement of intravascular catheters in one study.[845] Variability in patient platelet FcγII receptor number[846] or function[847] could also explain differences in severity of thrombocytopenia and clinical outcome. In addition, some patients can form heparin-dependent IgG without developing thrombocytopenia.[848] It is also possible that the thrombosis is related to endothelial activation, by means of endogenous heparan sulfate on endothelium, by the heparin-dependent IgG,[843,844,849] Figure 34-12 depicts our model for how various pathogenic factors interact with the IgG that causes heparin-induced thrombocytopenia to produce the various laboratory and clinical manifestations of this syndrome.

Diagnostic Test. Heparin-dependent platelet aggregation using platelet-rich plasma is probably the most common test used to diagnose heparin-induced thrombocytopenia. This assay has poor sensitivity and specificity for heparin-induced thrombocytopenia, however.[834,838,850] Selecting reactive platelet donors can improve test sensitivity.[851]

In 1986, a highly sensitive and specific assay for heparin-induced thrombocytopenia was reported.[213] This assay exploits the ability of IgG contained within patient serum to cause ^{14}C-serotonin release from washed donor platelets in the presence of low (0.1 to 0.3 U/mL) heparin concentrations. A characteristic feature is that platelet activation by positive sera is inhibited in the presence of high heparin (100 U/mL) concentrations (Fig. 34-13). We also use a monoclonal antibody (IV.3) that blocks the platelet FcγII receptor to maximize diagnostic specificity. Thus, a positive test is defined as platelet activation (high serotonin release) in the presence of 0.1 U/mL heparin and patient serum, with background (low) serotonin release in the presence of patient serum and 100 U/mL heparin, or in the presence of patient serum, 0.1 U/mL heparin, and Fc receptor blocking monoclonal antibody. To optimize test sensitivity, we use both weak and strong positive control heparin-induced thrombocytopenia sera, to ascertain that the washed donor platelets (obtained from selected donors) are optimally reactive to heparin-induced thrombocytopenia IgG.[847] The test has also been modified to use alternate platelet endpoints such as platelet aggregation[838] or generation of platelet-derived microparticles[852] rather than ^{14}C-serotonin release.

An enzyme-linked immunosorbent assay (ELISA) using heparin–platelet factor 4 as the target antigen has been developed.[841] It appears that this assay has similar, but not identically overlapping, sensitivity and specificity for heparin-induced thrombocytopenia as assays using functional assays using washed donor platelets.[853]

Prevention. The risk for thrombocytopenia and thrombosis can be reduced by minimizing the duration of heparin exposure[815]; by using porcine instead of bovine heparin[806]; and, possibly, by daily monitoring of the platelet count with early institution of alternate anticoagulation when a heparin-induced platelet count reduction is recognized. A drop

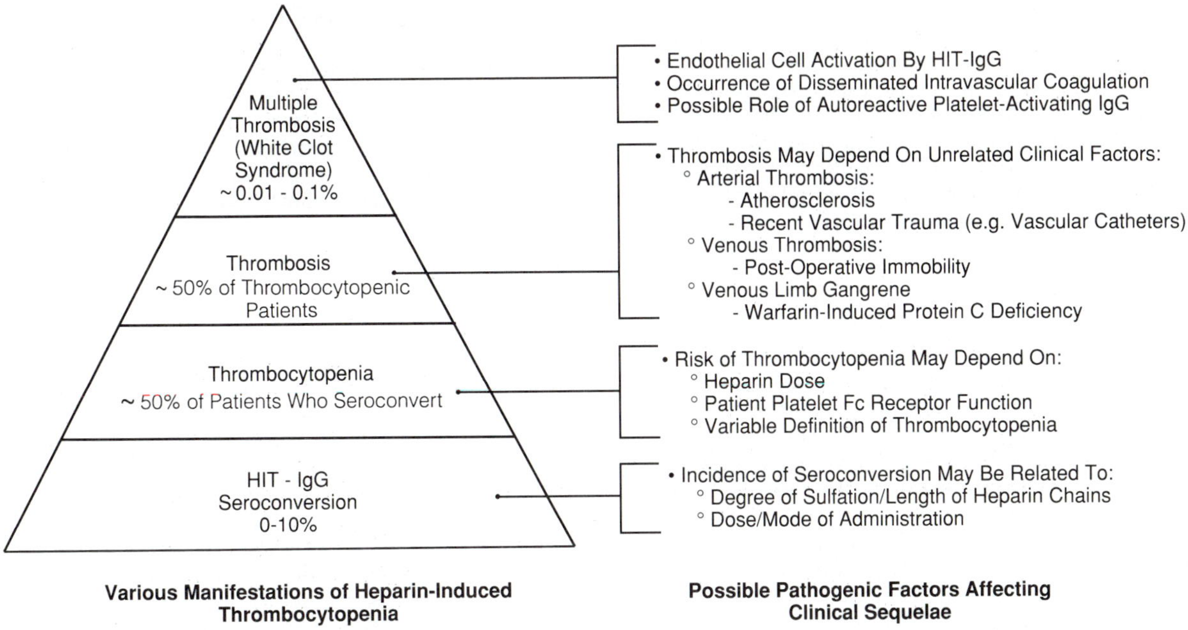

FIGURE 34-12. "Iceberg" model of heparin-induced thrombocytopenia. (After Warkentin TE, Kelton JG. Interaction of heparin with platelets, including heparin-induced thrombocytopenia. In: Bounameaux H, ed. Low-molecular-weight heparins in prophylaxis and therapy of thromboembolic diseases. New York, Marcel Dekker, 1994:75)

in the platelet count of 30% or more, even in the absence of thrombocytopenia, can be associated with thrombotic complications.[816,817]

Treatment of Heparin-Induced Thrombocytopenia. Prophylactic platelet transfusions should be avoided, even in severely thrombocytopenic patients, because bleeding is uncommon and transfusion therapy can precipitate arterial thrombosis.[854,855] Although thrombosis occurs in a minority of patients, this complication can be devastating, and heparin must be discontinued immediately. If the patient requires ongoing anticoagulant therapy, the clinician has several options, outlined in the following sections.

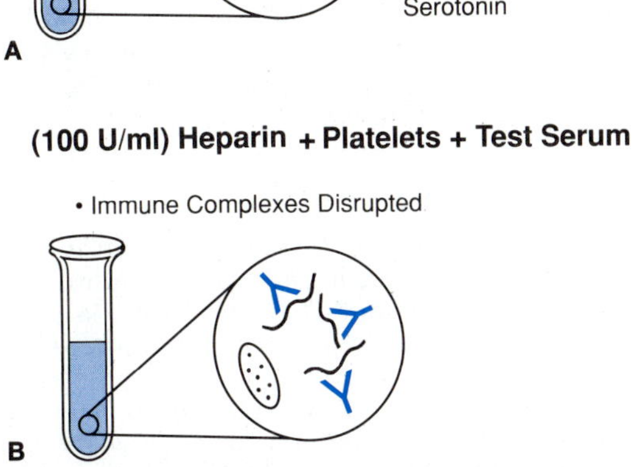

FIGURE 34-13. Schematic representation of the technique for testing for the presence of heparin-induced thrombocytopenia IgG. (**A**) The platelet release of radiolabeled serotonin is triggered by the binding of heparin–platelet factor 4–IgG complexes to platelet Fc receptors. (**B**) High heparin concentrations displace the platelet factor 4 and IgG from the platelet surface, preventing platelet Fc receptor occupancy and platelet activation.

Ancrod. Ancrod (Arvin) is a defibrinogenating agent derived from Malayan pit viper venom[856] that has been used to maintain anticoagulation in patients who developed heparin-induced thrombocytopenia.[857,858] We administer ancrod intravenously, giving 70 units over 8 to 12 hours for an average-sized adult. After the target fibrinogen level (approximately 0.5 g/L) is achieved, further ancrod doses are based on follow-up fibrinogen levels. Potential disadvantages of ancrod include difficulties in laboratory monitoring (eg, the need to measure fibrinogen using the Clauss assay; difficulty in using the prothrombin time to monitor warfarin anticoagulation) and the inability of this drug to inhibit thrombin generation.

LMW Heparinoid Org 10172. The heparinoid Org 10172 (Orgaran) is a mixture of glycosaminoglycans (predominantly low-sulfated heparan sulfate) with anticoagulant properties.[859] In vitro and in vivo evidence suggests that Org 10172 is a safe substitute for most patients with heparin-induced thrombocytopenia.[811,812,845,860] For a few patients (probably less than 5%), there appears to be persisting thrombocytopenia and risk of thrombosis that may be caused by cross-reactivity of the heparin-dependent IgG for sulfated glycosaminoglycans contained within the Org 10172. We usually give Org 10172 intravenously: an initial loading regimen (400 U/h for 4 hours, then 300 U/h for 4 hours), followed by a maintenance dose (150 to 200 U/h). Dose adjustments are made on the basis of anti-Xa anticoagulant levels.

LMW Heparin. Some patients with heparin-induced thrombocytopenia have been reported on who were successfully treated with LMW heparin substituted for unfractionated heparin; unfavorable outcomes, however, such as persisting thrombocytopenia, new thrombosis, and death, have also been described.[806] In laboratory testing, there is virtual 100% cross-reactivity between LMW heparin and unfractionated heparin for the heparin-dependent

IgG.[728,848] We do not recommend LMW heparin as treatment for heparin-induced thrombocytopenia.

Other Treatments. Plasmapheresis has been reported to benefit patients with heparin-induced thrombocytopenia,[861,862] possibly by removing pathogenic IgG as well as correcting coagulation disturbances. Some high-dose IVIgG preparations are effective in vitro in inhibiting platelet activation by heparin-dependent IgG[863]; rapid platelet count increases have been reported after treatment with IVIgG.[728,864] Recently, thrombin inhibitors such as Hirulog have been used to treat patients with heparin-induced thrombocytopenia.[865] We believe that antiplatelet agents such as aspirin[866] and dextran are relatively ineffective treatment for heparin-induced thrombocytopenia.

Warfarin Treatment. Although many patients with heparin-induced thrombocytopenia and thrombotic complications should receive warfarin for several weeks or months after discharge from hospital, we recommend caution in the use of warfarin during acute heparin-induced thrombocytopenia. This is because we have observed several patients who have lost limbs secondary to venous gangrene following warfarin administration. We recommend initiating warfarin anticoagulation only after the platelet count has recovered to normal after discontinuation of heparin, and only after adequate anticoagulation has been reached with an alternate anticoagulant such as Org 10172 or ancrod.

Treatment of Heparin-Induced Thrombosis. For some patients with heparin-induced arterial thrombi (eg, iliofemoral thrombosis), it is possible to salvage the limb by thromboembolectomy.[867] Selected thromboses may benefit from fibrinolytic therapy.[868,869]

Situations Usually Mandating Heparin Reexposure. Some patients with histories of heparin-induced thrombocytopenia require surgery that necessitates repeated exposure to heparin (eg, heart operations requiring cardiopulmonary bypass). Anecdotal reports suggest awaiting the loss of the heparin-dependent antibody from the circulation, at which time brief exposure to heparin is possible (ie, during the cardiopulmonary bypass),[870] or using alternate anticoagulants during extracorporeal circulation, such as Org 10172[871] or ancrod.[872]

Heparin-induced thrombocytopenia, sometimes accompanied by extracorporeal circuit thrombosis, has been described in patients in chronic hemodialysis.[873–876] Heparin-free dialysis, using prostacyclin[874] or a synthetic thrombin inhibitor,[876] has been used. Recurrent heparin-induced thrombocytopenia was prevented in one patient by aspirin.[873]

Drug-Dependent Fab Binding of Immunoglobulin G to Platelets: Quinidine- and Quinine-Induced Thrombocytopenia

The stereoisomers quinidine and quinine are important causes of immune destructive thrombocytopenia. Quinidine- and quinine-induced thrombocytopenia have been well characterized at the molecular level and are discussed here as a paradigm for drug-dependent, Fab-mediated IgG binding to platelet-specific proteins.

Clinical Features. Abrupt onset of severe thrombocytopenia with purpura and mucosal hemorrhage characterizes quinidine- and quinine-induced thrombocytopenia. It can be difficult to establish a history of drug ingestion[877] because quinine is present in many tonics and beverages and can contaminate illicit heroin preparations.[729] Usually, the platelet count returns to normal within several days of discontinuing the drug, although thrombocytopenia persisting for several weeks is sometimes observed.[675] Rarely, there is concomitant immune hemolysis or neutropenia. Different drug-dependent antibody populations are responsible for the different cytopenias observed.[878,879]

Pathogenesis. Although IgG mediates quinidine- and quinine-induced thrombocytopenia, the specific interaction of drug, IgG, and platelets is heterogeneous. Different patient sera demonstrate variability both in the affinity and saturability of IgG for drug and platelet[675,880]; furthermore, the drug epitopes differ: some sera recognize both quinidine and quinine, and other sera recognize only one drug.[881]

The details of the molecular basis of IgG, drug, and platelet interaction were described. The IgG–drug interaction often involves the platelet gpIb/IX complex.[882] For example, there usually is no drug-dependent binding of IgG to Bernard-Soulier platelets, which lack this glycoprotein complex.[878,880,883] Furthermore, immunoprecipitation of gpIb and gpIX by drug-dependent IgG[124,878] and inhibition of drug-dependent IgG binding by monoclonal antibodies directed against the membrane-associated region of the gpIb/IX complex[124] have been shown. The orientation of binding of the IgG to the platelet is mediated by the Fab region of the IgG molecule, as shown by two observations: the drug-dependent binding of $(Fab')_2$ is similar to that observed using intact IgG,[884] and staphylococcal protein A beads can bind to platelets containing IgG–drug complexes.[881]

These data indicate that the drug-dependent IgG binds by means of its antigen-recognizing Fab region to quinidine or quinine, which is bound to the membrane-associated region of the gpIb/IX complex. The initial event appears to be formation of a labile drug–IgG complex that is stabilized by binding to the platelet surface.[881] Other platelet glycoproteins may also be involved in some instances.[148,885,886]

In some patients, the thrombocytopenia persists for several weeks after discontinuation of the drug. Drug-independent antibodies have been demonstrated in some of these patients, suggesting that formation of an antiplatelet autoantibody can follow drug-induced thrombocytopenia.[675] Reports[125,887] of drug-independent antibodies associated with quinidine-induced thrombocytopenia have appeared.

Diagnostic Test. Many in vitro assays are suitable for the diagnosis of quinidine- or quinine-induced thrombocytopenia, including phase I (eg, ^{51}Cr-release assay),[883] phase II (eg, direct-binding assay using radiolabeled assays),[147] and phase III assays. None of these assays has been prospectively evaluated, so their clinical usefulness remains unknown.

Treatment. The responsible drug should be discontinued. For bleeding patients or those judged, on clinical grounds, to be at high risk of life-threatening hemorrhage, treatment should include platelet transfusions and IVIgG. Corticosteroids are often given, but their efficacy has not been proved. Drug sensitivity is usually lifelong, and patients should avoid reexposure.

Gold-Induced Thrombocytopenia

About 2% to 3% of patients who receive gold injections develop immune thrombocytopenia, usually within the first 20 weeks of administration. Thrombocytopenia has also been described with the newer orally administered preparations.[724,725] There are two unique temporal features of gold-induced thrombocytopenia. The thrombocytopenia persists for several weeks, months, or even years despite discontinuation of gold therapy.[888] Rarely, gold-induced thrombocytopenia can occur as many as 18 months after the gold injections were discontinued.[889,890] It is possible that both of these unusual temporal features are caused by otherwise typical drug-dependent platelet-reactive antibodies[675,725] that destroy platelets long after discontinuation of the drug because of the prolonged mobilization of gold from tissue storage sites. Alternatively, other investigators have proposed that gold causes autoimmune thrombocytopenia.[891]

Decreased platelet survival[892] and elevated PAIgG[675,893] have been demonstrated, and megakaryocytes are either normal or increased in number. In the less common and more serious syndrome of idiosyncratic gold-induced aplastic anemia, marrow examination reveals reduced megakaryocytes with generalized hypoplasia.

As many as 85% of patients with gold-induced thrombocytopenia carry the HLA-DR3 alloantigen,[894] whereas the prevalence of this HLA antigen in the general population is about 22%. Because most patients who possess this HLA phenotype gene do not develop gold-induced thrombocytopenia, however, the practical value of this marker is uncertain.

The risk for severe gold-induced thrombocytopenia or pancytopenia can be reduced by monitoring the complete blood count before each injection to ensure that there has been no drop in the platelet count or other cellular elements. If cytopenia develops, the gold must be discontinued immediately. For patients with symptomatic thrombocytopenia, additional treatment is required. Corticosteroids are frequently effective[893] and are the first-line treatment. For patients with persisting symptomatic thrombocytopenia inadequately controlled with corticosteroids, other treatments include IVIgG,[895] immunosuppressive drugs,[896,897] and splenectomy.[893] Chelating agents (eg, dimercaprol, N-acetylcysteine) may be useful to promote gold excretion.[890,898,899]

Drug-Induced Autoimmune Thrombocytopenia

Some drugs may induce the generation of platelet-reactive autoantibodies, analogous to the generation of RBC autoantibodies by α-methyldopa. For example, this mechanism was ascribed to procainamide in one patient who was shown to have antibodies reactive with gpIb and gpV.[773] It is not possible, however, to distinguish serologically between true drug-induced autoantibodies and drug-independent platelet-reactive antibodies that have formed because of drug-induced alteration of platelet glycoproteins.

Alloimmune Thrombocytopenic Disorders

Platelet-specific alloantibodies can cause thrombocytopenia in two uncommon but important clinical disorders: neonatal alloimmune thrombocytopenia and PTP. Although refractoriness to platelet transfusions is usually caused by HLA alloantibodies, platelet-specific alloantibodies may be important in some patients. Table 34-3 lists the platelet-specific alloantibody systems that have been described.

Neonatal Alloimmune Thrombocytopenia

Neonatal alloimmune thrombocytopenia is a transient but potentially life-threatening thrombocytopenic disorder limited to fetal and neonatal life. It is caused by maternal IgG alloantibodies that cross the placenta and result in the premature destruction of platelets bearing paternally derived platelet alloantigens (analogous to hemolytic disease of the newborn). Neonatal alloimmune thrombocytopenia occurs in about 1 in every 2000 newborns.[962,963]

Pathogenesis

Most cases of neonatal alloimmune thrombocytopenia are caused by anti-Pl^{A1} (anti-Zw^a) and anti-Br^a (anti-Zav^a) alloantibodies.[963] Other alloantigens that have been implicated in the syndrome include Pl^{A2},[905] Bak^a,[919] Bak^b,[924] Pen^a,[931,933] Pen^b,[932] Pl^{E2},[902] Ko^a,[916] and Br^b.[944] More recently, several low-incidence or "private" alloantigens have been found to cause neonatal alloimmune thrombocytopenia (Tu^a[948] or Ca,[949] Mo^a,[951] Sr^a,[952] Va^a[956]). In the largest series of serologically confirmed cases, anti-Pl^{A1} was found in 75% of the cases, anti-Br^a in about 20%, and remaining specificities in less than 5%.[963] Serologic evidence for alloantibodies is lacking in about 60% of possible cases that were identified with clinical criteria.[963] Although HLA or ABO alloantibodies have been claimed to cause thrombocytopenia in some neonates, it remains possible that undetected platelet-specific alloantibodies were responsible for the thrombocytopenia. HLA alloantibodies were shown not to influence cord platelet counts in one study.[964]

Because the frequency of the Pl^{A1}-negative phenotype is about 2%, about 1 in 50 newborns is theoretically at risk for neonatal alloimmune thrombocytopenia. The actual risk for neonatal alloimmune thrombocytopenia is much lower, however, since only a minority of susceptible women exposed to heterologous platelets during pregnancy form antiplatelet antibodies.[962] There is strong evidence that one or more immune-response genes determines the formation of anti-Pl^{A1} alloantibodies. In several studies, women possessing the HLA-DR3 alloantigen constituted from 70% to 95% of affected patients, which corresponded to a 10- to 30-fold increased risk of forming anti-Pl^{A1} alloantibodies.[907–910] Alloimmunization against the Br^a alloantigen is associated with HLA-DRw6.[943] Both HLA-DR3 and HLA-Dw6 are part of the supertypic determinant DRw52.[909]

Clinical and Laboratory Features

Neonatal alloimmune thrombocytopenia typically presents with unexpected isolated, severe thrombocytopenia in an otherwise healthy neonate. Petechiae are found in 90%, gastrointestinal tract hemorrhage in 30%, and hemoptysis, hematuria, and retinal bleeding in less than 10% of patients.[963] About 15% of affected neonates have intracranial hemorrhage.[963] Serious sequelae of fetal and neonatal intracranial bleeding include hydrocephalus,[963] porencephalic cysts,[931,965] and epilepsy. First-born offspring constitute about half of cases, suggesting that, unlike hemolytic disease of the newborn, sensitization can occur early during the first pregnancy.[902,963] Subsequent affected siblings are usually thrombocytopenic to a similar or greater extent.

The thrombocytopenia usually is severe, with the platelet count falling to 10×10^9/L or lower, but is transient, and the platelet count returns to normal within several weeks after birth. Bone marrow examination reveals normal or increased megakaryocyte numbers. Anemia and hyperbilirubinemias can occur from extravasation and resorption of blood.[963]

Serologic Investigation

The evaluation of possible neonatal alloimmune thrombocytopenia involves three steps. The first is to have a high index of suspicion in any thrombocytopenic infant. Isolated thrombocytopenia in an otherwise well infant must be assumed to be neonatal alloimmune thrombocytopenia until proved otherwise. The second step is to type maternal platelets to see if the mother lacks certain platelet alloantigens that often are associated with alloimmune thrombocytopenia. The third step is to determine whether the mother has antiplatelet alloantibodies in her serum. Not infrequently, no alloantibodies can be detected in the mother's serum despite severe neonatal thrombocytopenia. About one fourth of Pl^{A1}-negative mothers suspected to

TABLE 34-3. Platelet-Specific Alloantigen Systems*

New HPA Nomenclature	Original Designations	Caucasian Genotype Frequency	Caucasian Phenotype Frequency	Japanese Genotype Frequency	Japanese Phenotype Frequency	Clinical Alloimmune Syndromes Described	Glycoprotein Localization and Identification of Amino Acid Polymorphism	Comments	References
HPA-1a	Zw^a, Pl^{A1}	0.85	0.98	0.98	>0.999	NAT, PTP, PTR, PAT, TAT	IIIa	Anti–HPA-1a is most frequent cause of severe alloimmune syndromes in caucasians; alloimmunization associated with HLA-DRw52a (HLA-DR3 locus)	149–153, 649, 900–913
-1b	Zw^b, Pl^{A2}	0.15	0.27	0.02	0.04	NAT, PTP, PTR	Leu 33/Pro 33		
HPA-2a	Ko^b	0.911	0.992	0.864	0.982		Ib_α	Usually IgM antibodies; only a single report of NAT caused by IgG anti–HPA-2b—this patient had transient amegakaryocytosis; anti–HPA has been reported to cause PTR in Japan	126, 914–918
-2b	Ko^a, Sib^a	0.089	0.169	0.136	0.254	NAT, PTR	Thr 145/Met 145		
HPA-3a	Bak^a, Lek^a	0.61	0.85	0.54	0.79	NAT, PTP	IIb_α	Although alloantigenic determinant due to amino acid polymorphism, serologic studies indicate that sialic acid residues could contribute to epitopic heterogeneity	903, 912, 919–930
-3b	Bak^b, Lek^b	0.39	0.66	0.46	0.71	NAT, PTP, PTR	Ile 843/Ser 843		
HPA-4a	Pen^a, Yuk^b	>0.99	>0.999	0.9917	>0.999	NAT, PTP	IIIa	More frequent alloimmune syndromes in Japanese than caucasians because of higher frequency of homozygous HPA-4b phenotype	931–937
-4b	Pen^b, Yuk^a	<0.01	<0.0001	0.0083	0.017	NAT	Arg 143/Gln 143		
HPA-5a	Br^b, Zav^b	0.89	0.99	—	—	NAT	Ia	Can only be detected by sensitive methods; alloimmunization associated with HLA-DRw6; first and second most common cause of NAT in Japanese and caucasian populations, respectively	938–947
-5b	Br^a, Zav^a, Hc^a	0.11	0.21	—	—	NAT, PTP, PTR, PAT	Glu 505/Lys 505		

HPA-6b	Tu[a], Ca	~0.003	~0.007	—	—	NAT	IIIa Arg 489/Gln 489	Low-incidence antigen found in several unrelated families	948–950
HPA-7b	Mo[a]	~0.001	~0.002	—	—	NAT	IIIa Pro 407/Ala 407	"Private" alloantigen system, since Mo[a] antigen so far only identified in proband's family	951
HPA-8b	Sr[a]	<0.003	<0.01	—	—	NAT	IIIa Arg 636/Cys 636	"Private" alloantigen system, since Sr[a] antigen so far only identified in proband's family	952, 953
	Pl[E1] Pl[E2]	0.975 0.025	0.999 0.05	— —	— —	— NAT	Ibα	Alloantigen system not well established, since only one example of each alloantiserum has been identified in past 25 years; it is possible that anti-Pl[E1] represented an isoantibody	902, 954
	Gov[a] Gov[b]	0.53 0.47	0.81 0.74	— —	— —	PTP?	p175	Can be identified only by using sensitive techniques; no clinical effects of the alloantibodies have been established	955
	Va[a]	<0.002	<0.004	—	—	NAT	IIb/IIIa	"Private" alloantigen system, since Va[a] antigen so far only identified in proband's family	956
	Nak[a] GPIV isoantibody	0.94	0.9966	0.70	0.96	PTR	IV (CD36)	Anti-Nak[a] isoantibodies can form in polytransfused GPIV-deficient patients; *Nak*[a] phenotype is common in Japan (3%–4%)	957–959

NAT, neonatal alloimmune thrombocytopenia; PTP, posttransfusion purpura; PTR, platelet transfusion refractoriness; PAT, passive alloimmune thrombocytopenia; TAT, transplantation-associated thrombocytopenia.

* Platelet alloantigen systems implicated in platelet alloimmune syndromes. The human platelet antigen (HPA) system was proposed to systemize platelet alloantigen nomenclature.[960] A drawback of this system, however, is that apparently different alloantigens named in the HPA system (eg, HPA-1a, HPA-4a, HPA-6a, HPA-7a, HPA-8a) are identical at the molecular level.[961] Anti-Nak[a] are isoantibodies rather than alloantibodies, since anti-Nak[a] are formed by individuals deficient in gpIV.

have had infants with neonatal alloimmune thrombocytopenia cannot be shown to have anti-Pl^{A1} alloantibodies.[963] It is possible that the inability to detect maternal alloantibody may predict a more benign outcome.[966] The potential role of low-incidence platelet-specific alloantigens indicates the importance of testing maternal serum against paternal platelets whenever possible.

Differential Diagnosis of Neonatal Thrombocytopenia

This is discussed elsewhere in this chapter.

Treatment

Neonatal thrombocytopenia is much more severe, and the bleeding symptoms more prominent, than the thrombocytopenia in neonates with passive autoimmune thrombocytopenia caused by maternal ITP. For this reason, we manage mothers with ITP conservatively and do not favor invasive procedures such as percutaneous umbilical blood sampling. In contrast, the frequently unfavorable outcome of infants with alloimmune neonatal thrombocytopenia supports a more aggressive approach to diagnosis and intervention. The explanation for the increased risk is not known but may be related to the more severe thrombocytopenia that characterizes alloimmune thrombocytopenia. It is even possible that some alloantibodies cause platelet dysfunction by binding to functional sites on platelet glycoproteins. Evidence suggests that severe thrombocytopenia and serious bleeding is less frequently caused by the anti-Br^a alloantibody.[963] The $Br^{a/b}$ alloantigen system resides on gpIa/IIa, which is present in far smaller numbers than gpIIb/IIIa.

Prenatal Management. In about half of cases, neonatal alloimmune thrombocytopenia is suspected during the prenatal period. Usually, this is because the mother previously had an affected infant. The risk of intracranial hemorrhage during the fetal period has led to attempts to prevent in utero bleeding. Ultrasound examination beginning at 20 weeks gestation is recommended to look for evidence of intracranial hemorrhage. In some centers, cordocentesis (umbilical vein blood sampling) permits detection of thrombocytopenia as early as 20 weeks of gestation and allows for transfusion of compatible platelets to thrombocytopenic fetuses.[463,967–969] A fetus should be considered to be at high risk for bleeding if there is a history of a severely affected sibling or if the fetus has been shown to be thrombocytopenic in utero by umbilical vein sampling. These infants should receive in utero platelet transfusions, usually commencing between the 26th and 30th gestational weeks, with elective cesarean section performed when fetal maturity is documented.[970] Alternatively, the weekly administration of high-dose IVIgG (with or without dexamethasone) to the mother during the latter part of the pregnancy has been described to be successful in these patients.[971] This approach awaits confirmation, however, and has not been uniformly successful.[972] The benefit, if any, of dexamethasone remains uncertain.

Delivery of infants at risk should be by cesarean section. Cesarean section has never been shown to protect thrombocytopenic neonates; however, it allows for an organized approach to the peripartum care of the newborn.

Postnatal Management. The cornerstone of treatment is the immediate administration of washed, irradiated maternal platelets to the thrombocytopenic neonate.[973,974] The platelets are obtained using pheresis and should be washed to remove the maternal alloantibody and irradiated to prevent graft-versus-host disease, which could be caused by maternal lymphocytes. Frozen maternal platelets collected earlier during the pregnancy have also been used successfully.[975] Although platelets lacking the implicated alloantigen (such as Pl^{A1}) from an unrelated donor could be used, maternal platelets are preferred since they are readily available, certain to be compatible with the neonate, and provide less risk of infection. In an emergency, immediate administration of random donor platelets may be of some benefit to a bleeding infant. Administration of IVIgG to the infant is effective in raising the platelet count[976,977] and should be given with the maternal platelets. Corticosteroids are not effective in this disorder.[902]

Posttransfusion Purpura

Posttransfusion purpura is a rare disorder characterized by the abrupt onset of severe thrombocytopenia that begins about 1 week after receiving a blood transfusion. Invariably, high-titer, platelet-specific alloantibodies are found in the patient's serum or plasma.[978] Although the platelet-specific alloantibodies are causative, the pathogenesis remains obscure, and the conundrum is why autologous platelets are destroyed.

Pathogenesis

Four hypotheses have been developed that relate to the pathogenesis of PTP:[979]

Immune-complex platelet destruction. Autologous platelets are destroyed by immune complexes consisting of alloantibodies interacting with allogeneic platelet antigens.[978]

Conversion of antigen-negative to antigen-positive platelets. Allogeneic platelet antigens are absorbed onto autologous platelets, rendering them susceptible to alloimmune destruction.[980]

Alloantibodies cross-reactive with antigen-positive and antigen-negative platelets. The pathogenic alloantibody recognizes the autologous allele in addition to the foreign alloantigen.[981]

Concurrent production of autoantibody. An antiplatelet autoantibody is produced concurrently with the alloantibodies.[982]

Although Pl^{A1} (Zw^a) is the alloantigen most frequently implicated in PTP, other alloantigens have been described in PTP, including Pl^{A2},[904] Bak^a,[920,921] Bak^b,[923] Pen^a,[934] and Br^a.[945] Sometimes, more than one type of platelet-specific alloantibody can be identified in the patient's serum.[941,983]

As in neonatal alloimmune thrombocytopenia, the HLA-DR3 antigen is found in most Pl^{A1}-negative patients with PTP.[909] This HLA antigen was also found in two sisters who developed PTP.[984]

Clinical and Laboratory Features

The disease usually occurs in middle-aged or older women who have been pregnant. A literature survey of PTP demonstrated that 95% of patients are women, and 85% were between the ages of 40 and 80.[979] Almost always, there is a history of previous pregnancy, although in a few patients, the initial sensitization is believed to have occurred through previous blood transfusion.[985,986]

Typically, the onset of bleeding and thrombocytopenia occurs 5 to 10 days after the transfusion of RBCs, which presumably results in resensitization by contaminating platelets. Rarely, plasma transfusions cause the syndrome.[987] Although the thrombocytopenia usually lasts from 1 to 4 weeks, the duration can be as short as 3 days to as long as 4 months or more.[988–990] The thrombocytopenia is severe, usually less than $10 \times 10^9/L$.[979] Cutaneous, mucosal, and postoperative wound bleeding are encountered frequently, and fatal outcome has been reported.

Passive alloimmune thrombocytopenia can result from transfusion of a blood product (usually plasma) that contains platelet-specific alloantibodies.[991–994] This syndrome is clinically distinct from PTP, however, since the thrombocytopenia immediately follows the transfusion, and the duration of thrombocytopenia is shorter (several hours to a few days).

Treatment

Exchange transfusion or plasmapheresis can raise the platelet count promptly in most cases, although recurrent thrombocytopenia may mandate further treatments.[979] Benefit from high-dose IVIgG for PTP was first reported in 1983.[995] A review indicates that more than 90% of patients respond favorably, with an average of 4 days before attaining a platelet count above 100×10^9/L.[996] The high probability and rapidity of response, as well as the relative ease of administration compared with plasmapheresis, suggest that IVIgG should be considered the treatment of choice for PTP.[996]

Corticosteroids are frequently administered but probably do not influence the natural history and should be considered as possible adjunct but not primary therapy.

Random donor platelets should not be administered since they are ineffective and can cause severe febrile and anaphylactoid reactions.[997] The experience with Pl^{A1}-negative platelet transfusions is limited. Some[998] but not other[999] reports indicate lack of benefit. RBC products should be washed before administration to remove contaminating platelet antigens.

Splenectomy has been used successfully for a patient refractory to corticosteroids, plasmapheresis, IVIgG, and matched platelet transfusions.[1000]

Future Precautions

Posttransfusion purpura can recur if the patient receives future blood products containing the incriminated platelet alloantigen. Not every patient will have a recurrence,[1001] however, and it has been suggested that residual high-titer alloantibodies can protect against recurrence by destroying the transfused incompatible platelet antigens. Regardless, patients with a history of PTP should only receive washed or autologous red blood cells and platelet alloantigen-compatible plasma or platelet products.[979]

Affected patients should not donate blood because their plasma contains potentially pathogenic platelet-specific alloantibodies.[991,992]

Alloimmune Platelet Transfusion Refractoriness

Refractoriness to platelet transfusions is defined by a less than expected rise in the platelet count after a platelet transfusion. This problem is encountered frequently in multitransfused patients and has multiple causes, both alloimmune and nonalloimmune. Alloimmune platelet destruction is caused most commonly by HLA alloantibodies,[1002] although in rare patients, platelet-specific alloantibodies may play a role.[913,917,1003] A poor response to platelet transfusions can also be caused by other factors, such as fever, septicemia, medications, hypersplenism, DIC, and bleeding.[1004,1005] In our experience, these factors are more important than alloantibodies in determining the response to the transfused platelets.

Uniformly poor platelet count increments at 10 minutes, 60 minutes, and 24 hours after platelet transfusion characterize alloimmune platelet destruction. Adequate 10-minute and 60-minute increments, but a poor increment at 24 hours, are more frequently observed in patients with refractoriness due to nonalloimmune factors.[1006,1007]

Patients with aplastic anemia are at the highest risk for forming alloantibodies after multiple transfusions. The risk is less (25% to 50%) for polytransfused acute leukemia patients, possibly because of immune suppression by chemotherapy.[1008] Alloantibodies also can disappear in some patients.[1009]

Measurement of lymphocytotoxic antibodies usually is used in the serologic assessment of platelet alloimmunization. Most clinically stable patients with a negative lymphocytotoxicity assay have a good posttransfusion increment, whereas only about 10% with a positive test for these HLA antibodies have a good increment.[1008,1010]

Approaches to prevent alloimmunization against platelet alloantigens have been summarized[1008,1011] and include single-donor platelet transfusions, which can be matched or unmatched for HLA alloantigens,[1012,1013] and leukocyte-depleted RBC and platelet products.[1003,1014–1018] The latter approach is based on experimental evidence suggesting that leukocytes contaminating RBC and platelet preparations are responsible for alloimmunization against HLA alloantigens.[1019] The efficacy of either approach is not proved, and in most centers, leukemic patients are treated with random donor platelets.

The treatment of patients who are refractory to platelet transfusions is debated. The approaches that have been used include the following:

- Transfusion with larger numbers of platelets,
- Use of single-donor, HLA-matched platelets,[1005]
- In vitro platelet crossmatch to select compatible platelets,[1005,1020,1021]
- Plasmapheresis to remove the alloantibodies,
- Use of high-dose IVIgG to block reticuloendothelial-mediate alloimmune platelet destruction,[1022,1023]
- Use of immunosuppressive drugs, such as cyclosporine.[1024]

The practical benefit of these different maneuvers is difficult to ascertain because of role of nonalloimmune factors in many of these patients.

THROMBOCYTOPENIA CAUSED BY THROMBIN (DISSEMINATED INTRAVASCULAR COAGULATION)

Disseminated intravascular coagulation is defined as excess of thrombin generation within the vasculature, resulting in generalized derangement of the hemostatic mechanism. The excess thrombin results in increased consumption of coagulation factors, especially fibrinogen and factors V and VIII. There is often increased consumption of inhibitors of coagulation, such as antithrombin and protein C, which if sufficiently depleted leads to exacerbation of DIC. Usually, there is a parallel generation of plasmin and formation of products of fibrinolysis, including fibrin and fibrinogen degradation products. In addition, increased platelet turnover is a universal feature of DIC, resulting in thrombocytopenia in almost all patients. Platelet destruction may be related to direct activation by thrombin, which is the most potent of all physiologic platelet agonists. Indeed, concentrations of α-thrombin as low as 0.15 nmol/L can activate platelets without any effect on fibrin generation.[1025] Thrombin-induced platelet activation is associated with generation of procoagulant platelet-derived microparticles,[1026] suggesting that platelet activation plays an important role in promoting the consumption of the coagulation factors in DIC.

The clinical spectrum of DIC is wide and ranges from laboratory abnormalities without clinical sequelae to severe bleeding caused by depletion of coagulation factors and platelets. Some patients have evidence of organ ischemia and infarction resulting from microvascular thrombosis. The course of DIC can be acute, fulminant, and rapidly fatal. Alternatively, the process can be chronic and compensated, with increased factor production leading to maintenance of adequate levels of coagulation factors and platelets.[1027–1029]

DESTRUCTIVE THROMBOCYTOPENIA OF NONIMMUNE, POSSIBLE IMMUNE, OR UNCERTAIN PATHOGENESIS

Several thrombocytopenic disorders, such as the thrombocytopenia of infections (viral, bacterial, fungal, protozoal), TTP and hemolytic-uremic syndrome (HUS), and preeclampsia-associated thrombocytopenia are discussed together. Although these disorders have different inciting events and disease associations, they all are characterized by thrombocytopenia caused by increased platelet destruction. These disorders usually are not accompanied by DIC. Ironically, there is a common historical thread for all of these illnesses: in each disorder, it was once assumed that either clinical or subclinical DIC mediates the thrombocytopenia. Indeed, in some of these disorders, it is still suggested that thrombin is responsible for the thrombocytopenia. Prospective studies, however, using sensitive markers for thrombin action (eg, fibrinopeptide A assay), as well as other tests for thrombin action on fibrinogen (eg, protamine sulfate paracoagulation assay), indicate that DIC is uncommon.

The pathogenesis of the platelet destruction remains unresolved for these disorders. In the thrombocytopenia of infection, the evidence indicates that immune mechanisms may be responsible for the thrombocytopenia. Although elevated PAIgG is sometimes found in TTP, HUS, and preeclampsia, it remains uncertain whether the increased PAIgG is causal or coincidental.

Other thrombocytopenic disorders have been identified in which the pathogenesis is poorly understood, although it is probable that increased platelet destruction occurs. These include thrombocytopenia associated with allergy and anaphylaxis, glomerulonephritis, renal transplantation rejection, extracorporeal circulation, intravascular catheters and prostheses, cardiopulmonary bypass surgery, cardiovascular disease, severe bleeding requiring massive transfusion support, and administration of fatty acids. All these syndromes are reviewed briefly.

Thrombocytopenia of Infection

Thrombocytopenia Complicating Bacteremia and Fungemia

Thrombocytopenia is a frequent and sometimes early sign of systemic bacterial or fungal infections. The frequency of thrombocytopenia ranges from 15% to 35% for patients with clinical evidence for infection,[1030,1031] to 45% to 75% for patients with positive blood cultures,[1032–1036] to 90% to 95% for patients with evidence of septic shock or DIC.[1037–1039]

Usually, the thrombocytopenia is moderately severe, with the platelet counts averaging from 50 to 100 × 10^9/L. Occasionally, it can be severe, with platelet counts falling below 10 × 10^9/L. Blood cultures should be performed in patients in whom the diagnosis is suspected. Coagulation tests also should be performed, although DIC is relatively uncommon.

Thrombocytopenia complicating infections is usually caused by increased platelet destruction, but the precise pathogenesis remains unclear. There are a number of possible ways in which bacteria or fungi could cause platelet destruction: immune mechanisms; thrombin generation (DIC); microbe-induced platelet activation; endothelial damage, resulting in platelet interaction with subendothelial tissues; and hypersplenism or reticuloendothelial cell proliferation secondary to the infection.

Immune Thrombocytopenia of Septicemia. Elevated PAIgG is a frequent finding in septicemic, thrombocytopenic patients.[1034,1040,1041] Furthermore, higher levels of PAIgG correlate with a more severe degree of thrombocytopenia.[1034] It is uncertain whether the platelet–antibody interaction in most cases is due to specific IgG against platelet-adsorbed microbial antigens, as occurs in malaria-associated thrombocytopenia[201]; binding of immune complexes, consisting of bacterial antigens and IgG to platelet Fc receptors[1042]; microbial damage to platelets, resulting in expression of cryptic autoantigens[1043]; or nonspecific binding of IgG to damaged platelets.

Disseminated Intravascular Coagulation. In a prospective study using sensitive and specific markers for thrombin activation, including fibrinopeptide A levels and fibrinogen gel chromatography for detection of fibrin and fibrinogen multimers, most patients with mild to moderate thrombocytopenia complicating bacteremia had no evidence of DIC. DIC was found, however, in most patients with a platelet count below 50 × 10^9/L.[1035] A large retrospective study found evidence for DIC in only 20% of thrombocytopenic patients with gram-negative bacteremia.[1036]

Severe DIC with life-threatening systemic thrombosis (purpura fulminans) occurs most frequently with bacteremia caused by certain organisms, including *Neisseria meningitidis*, *H influenzae*, and *Streptococcus pneumoniae*,[1044] particularly in the postsplenectomy patient. Thrombocytopenia, purpuric rash, and multiorgan dysfunction are common in Rocky Mountain spotted fever. This is the result of endothelial invasion by the pathogenic *Rickettsia rickettsii*,[1045] probably generating procoagulant tissue factor on endothelium.[1046]

Microbe-Induced Platelet Activation. Some bacteria cause platelet activation by means of endotoxin[1047–1049] or other toxins,[1050,1051] although it is possible that thrombocytopenia results from endotoxin-induced release of endogenous mediators, such as platelet-activating factor.[1052,1053]

Endothelial Damage. Microbe-induced endothelial damage may cause thrombocytopenia by exposing subendothelial tissues to the flowing blood.[1054]

Hypersplenism. Reticuloendothelial cell hyperplasia can contribute to thrombocytopenia in some chronic infections, such as subacute bacterial endocarditis and malaria.

Thrombocytopenia Complicating Viral Infections

Acute ITP can develop weeks after infection with rubella, rubeola, varicella, live virus vaccines,[1055] or, most frequently, an unidentified viral upper respiratory tract infection.[1056] Thrombocytopenia also occurs during the active phase of viral infections, especially infections caused by the herpesviruses (Epstein-Barr virus, cytomegalovirus, herpes simplex virus),[1057–1060] but also with varicella,[1061] mumps,[1062] rubella,[1063] measles,[1064] and parvovirus[1065] infection. Although the frequency of thrombocytopenia with acute viral infection is not known, it may be high. For example, in one study, about 75% of patients with Epstein-Barr virus–induced infectious mononucleosis developed mild to moderate thrombocytopenia during the second week of illness.[1057] Severe thrombocytopenia (platelet count less than $25 \times 10^9/L$) occurred in about 1%.[1058]

Although viral infections can be associated with reduced numbers of marrow megakaryocytes or hypersplenism, almost always the thrombocytopenia is caused by an increased rate of platelet destruction. Destruction is probably mediated by immune mechanisms since elevated levels of PAIgG typically occur in thrombocytopenic patients.[1058,1066,1067]

Pancytopenia can occur in immunocompromised patients as part of the virus-associated hemophagocytic syndrome. This is characterized by constitutional symptoms, lymphadenopathy, hepatomegaly, splenomegaly, and coagulopathy.[1068–1071] Histologically benign histiocytes exhibiting erythrophagocytosis can be demonstrated in marrow aspirates, liver, or lymph node biopsy specimens. The syndrome occurs most frequently in association with Epstein-Barr virus, cytomegalovirus, herpes simplex virus, or adenovirus infections. This syndrome may represent an aberrant T-cell response to infection.

Thrombocytopenia Complicating Protozoal Infections

Malaria is a common and well-studied parasitic infection that often causes thrombocytopenia. Indeed, two prospective studies have shown that thrombocytopenia complicates virtually every case of malaria.[1072,1073] Thrombocytopenia is caused by increased platelet destruction[1074,1075] secondary to immune mechanisms.[201,1076] In vitro studies have shown that specific antimalaria IgG binds to malarial antigens adsorbed to the platelet membrane[201] (Fig. 34-14).

Management

The general approach to all infection-induced thrombocytopenia is the same: treat the underlying infection, evaluate the hemostatic risk, and treat the hemostatic dysfunction.

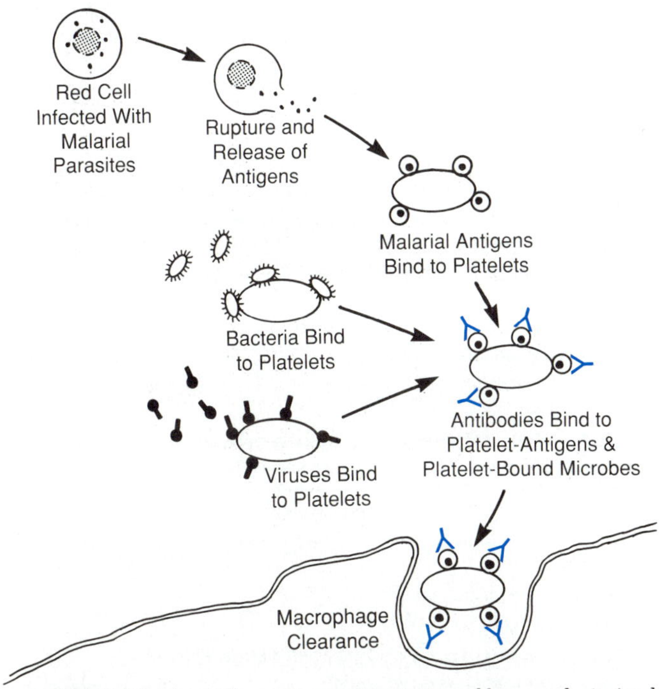

FIGURE 34-14. Schematic representation of how malaria (and possibly other types of infection) can cause thrombocytopenia.

The diagnosis of thrombocytopenia complicating bacteremia or fungemia requires a high index of suspicion. Often, the thrombocytopenia precedes other evidence for infection, including fever and leukocytosis. Hence, we consider isolated thrombocytopenia in a patient at risk as presumptive evidence of an infection.

The most important treatment is to start appropriate antimicrobial treatment. For patients with severe thrombocytopenia (platelet count less than $20 \times 10^9/L$), we administer prophylactic platelet transfusions.[109] Even though the transfused platelets are cleared rapidly, they can prevent life-threatening bleeding during the short period of risk before onset of antibiotic efficacy. Furthermore, there is the theoretic benefit that they will help clear microbial particles. Platelet transfusions also are given to patients with higher platelet counts if bleeding occurs.

The role of anticoagulant therapy in DIC complicating septicemia is debated. Heparin can improve the coagulation indices, although no impact on survival has been demonstrated.[1037] For patients with clinical evidence of microvascular thrombosis, including acral ischemia, livedo reticularis, or purpura fulminans, heparin therapy should be considered because of the prospect of ongoing thrombin generation and microvascular fibrin deposition in multiple organs before the onset of antibiotic efficacy.

Thrombotic Microangiopathic Disorders

Thrombotic microangiopathy (also known as microangiopathic hemolytic anemia) is defined as the triad of microangiopathic hemolytic anemia, destructive thrombocytopenia, and microvascular platelet thrombi. Patients with the syndrome have laboratory evidence of schistocytic hemolysis and thrombocytopenia. Often, but not always, there is organ dysfunction caused by microvascular thrombosis.

The prototypic illness is TTP. Patients with TTP always have thrombocytopenia and schistocytic hemolysis and often central nervous system and renal impairment presumably caused by ischemia. HUS is a related condition in which the microangiopathic process is usually limited to the kidneys. Sometimes, the distinction between the syndromes is blurred. Renal dysfunction can be prominent in TTP, and focal neurologic deficits can occur in otherwise typical HUS.[1077–1080]

TTP usually is a primary illness, although secondary disease associations have been described (Table 34-4). In contrast, many episodes of HUS are accompanied by secondary disorders, such as concomitant gastrointestinal infection by verotoxin-producing *Escherichia coli* (see Table 34-4). About 5% to 10% of patients with *E coli* O157:H7 infection develop HUS; children and elderly patients are at the highest risk.

Although TTP and HUS share the common pathologic feature of intraluminal platelet thrombus formation, it remains uncertain whether a common pathogenesis exists. These disorders can also be confused with other illnesses that can produce schistocytic hemolysis and thrombocytopenia (Table 34-5).

Thrombotic Thrombocytopenic Purpura

Pathogenesis. Although the cause of TTP is unknown, the pathogenesis is becoming better understood. Interest has centered around two laboratory abnormalities found in many patients with TTP: the presence of platelet-aggregating factor and the role of high-molecular-weight (HMW) multimeric forms of vWF.

In 1979, Lian and colleagues[1140] described a platelet-aggregating factor in the plasma of TTP patients. Later in-

TABLE 34-4. Secondary Causes of Thrombotic Microangiopathy

THROMBOTIC THROMBOCYTOPENIC PURPURA

Infections
- Viral[1081–1083]
- Mycoplasma[1084]
- Rickettsia[1085]
- Bacterial[1086,1087]

Pregnancy and the postpartum period[1088–1090]
Drugs and toxins[1091–1095]
Rheumatic disorders[1096–1099]
Human immunodeficiency virus infection[1100–1102]
Human T-lymphotropic virus, type 1[1103]
Familial[1104,1105]

HEMOLYTIC-UREMIC SYNDROME

Infections
- Enteric pathogens
  - Verotoxin-producing *Escherichia coli*[1106–1109]
  - *Shigella dysenteriae*[1110,1111]
  - *Salmonella typhi*[1112]
  - Nontyphoidal *Salmonella*[1113]
  - *Campylobacter*[1114,1115]
  - *Yersinia* sp[1116]
- *Streptococcus pneumoniae*[1117,1118]
- *Rickettsia* sp[1085]

Pregnancy and the postpartum period[1090,1119,1120]
Drugs and toxins[1094,1095,1121–1125]
Allogeneic bone marrow transplant recipients[1126,1127]
Human immunodeficiency virus infection[1128]
Familial[1104,1129–1131]

vestigations by this group[1141] indicated that the platelet-aggregating factor was a 37-kd protein whose activity could be inhibited by IgG. In 1982, Moake and coworkers[1142] described abnormalities in the HMW multimeric forms of vWF in patients with chronic relapsing TTP. Another group[1143] of investigators found that the activity of the platelet-aggregating factor in the serum of TTP patients could be enhanced by adding a preparation rich in the large multimers of vWF. They suggested that the platelet-aggregating factor played a synergistic role with the vWF. Further investigations by this group[1144–1147] have identified the aggregating factor as a proteolytic enzyme termed *calcium-dependent cysteine protease* (calpain). This enzyme is a normal constituent of RBCs, leukocytes, and platelets and is inhibited by kininogens.[1148] Other workers have identified a cathepsin-like cysteine protease activity in blood from TTP patients.[1149]

The putative pathogenic role of immune complexes,[1150] elevated platelet-associated Ig,[1151] primary endothelial injury,[1152,1153] prostacyclin deficiency,[1154,1155] diminished fibrinolytic capacity,[1156] and DIC[1157] remains uncertain.

Clinical and Laboratory Features. TTP is a rare disease with an annual incidence of about 1 in 1,000,000 people.[1158,1159] There is a slight female preponderance (3:2), and most patients are young or middle-aged adults, although patients of all ages have been affected.

Symptoms and signs of organ dysfunction are frequent, with neurologic dysfunction (confusion, headache, focal neurologic defects, coma) relatively common. Dramatic recovery from profound neurologic dysfunction, including coma, is possible with treatment. Other clinical features that have been described include abdominal pain, visual complaints, heart failure, cardiac arrhythmia, and pulmonary edema. Nonspecific symptoms, including fever, can be prominent. Although hematuria, proteinuria, and mild renal dysfunction are frequent, oliguria and severe renal failure are uncommon.

Thrombocytopenia caused by increased platelet destruction characterizes TTP. Although the thrombocytopenia can be severe and accompanied by platelet dysfunction,[1160] bleeding symptoms are uncommon. Anemia due to microangiopathic hemolysis is common, although severe anemia is rare. Schistocytes and polychromatophilia are observed in the stained blood film, and nucleated red blood cells can be seen. Laboratory signs of hemolysis include reticulocytosis, free plasma hemoglobin, decreased plasma haptoglobin, elevated lactate dehydrogenase of RBC origin, and unconjugated hyperbilirubinemia. The direct antiglobulin test is negative. Coagulation changes of DIC are rarely encountered, but azotemia and hyperamylasemia are noted in some patients.

The characteristic pathologic lesions are disseminated arteriolar and capillary hyaline thrombi made of platelet aggregates enmeshed in fibrinogen and vWF. Adjacent endothelial swelling is often observed.

Treatment. Without therapy, TTP often is fulminant and fatal, with a mortality rate as high as 95%.[1161] At least 50% to 80% of patients recover with plasma therapy delivered by infusion or exchange.[1162–1164] The efficacy of exchange transfusion with whole blood was first reported in 1959,[1165] and at least half of patients benefit from this treatment.[1166] Subsequently, fresh frozen plasma administered by infusion[1166–1168] or apheresis[1169,1170] became commonly used. A randomized trial reported showed that plasma is most effective for TTP when given by exchange.[1163]

Antiplatelet agents, including aspirin (325 to 1300 mg/d) and dipyridamole (200 to 600 mg/d), often are used as an adjunct to plasma therapy.[1082,1171] Many physicians administer high-dose corticosteroid therapy (eg, prednisone 200 mg/d) for TTP patients.[1172] Case reports[1084] indicate possible who benefit from splenectomy for refractory patients, but this has not been the experience of all investigators.[1173]

Platelet transfusions are contraindicated because they can result in clinical deterioration.[1174] Similarly, patients can die suddenly after an initial response to treatment, suggesting that increased platelet numbers are hazardous if the platelet-aggregating process remains unchecked.[1174]

The recommended treatment is fresh frozen plasma administered by apheresis. Patients who do not respond within a few days to plasmapheresis should receive larger volume plasma exchanges or have (vWF-depleted) cryosupernatant substituted for fresh frozen plasma.[1175,1176] Splenectomy[1084,1177–1179] or vincristine[1180] should also be considered for refractory patients. High-dose IVIgG appears to be ineffective for TTP and may even exacerbate the illness.[1181]

Early or late relapse is relatively common in patients who have recovered from TTP.[1164,1179] Some physicians give

TABLE 34-5. Differential Diagnosis of Schistocytic Hemolysis and Thrombocytopenia

Disseminated intravascular coagulation[1027]
Vasculitis, including systemic lupus erythematosus and polyarteritis nodosa[1132,1133]
Preeclampsia or eclampsia[1090]
Disseminated carcinoma[1134–1136]
Malignant hypertension (including sclerodermal kidney)[1137]
Primary pulmonary hypertension[1138]
Dysfunctional prosthetic heart valves or infectious endocarditis[1139]

antiplatelet drugs for several months after remission, but it is unknown whether this reduces the risk of relapse.

Hemolytic-Uremic Syndrome

Hemolytic-uremic syndrome occurs most frequently in infants and young children and represents the most common cause of acute renal failure in this age group. The annual incidence of HUS in children under the age of 5 years is about 1 in 100,000 and may be increasing.[1182,1183] HUS can also occur in adults, particularly in the aged, suggesting that susceptibility to HUS is greatest at the extremes of age.

Pathogenesis. It was first recognized in 1977 that certain strains of *E coli* produce a toxin active on Vero cells, a cell line derived from African green monkey kidney cells.[1184] In 1983, Karmali and associates[1106] described a striking association between HUS and evidence of infection by this organism. These workers[1107] found that 75% of Canadian children with HUS had been infected by verotoxin-producing *E coli*. In another investigation, about one third of children with HUS in the United Kingdom were found to have had an infection with verotoxin-producing organisms.[1185]

Two distinct verotoxins (Shiga-like toxins) have been described. Both are similar to the Shiga toxin,[1186,1187] which also has been implicated in HUS. The toxin consists of two distinct subunits: subunit A is homologous to ricin and is cytotoxic because it inhibits protein synthesis; subunit B binds to endothelial receptors.[1186,1188] Several strains of *E coli* have been implicated as producing one or both verotoxins,[1186] most frequently *E coli* O157:H7.[1185,1189]

It is uncertain how these bacterial cytotoxins produce HUS, although damage to endothelium probably is important, possibly with resulting secondary platelet activation. Lytic antiendothelial antibodies have been described in patients with HUS.[1190] Impaired endothelial prostacyclin (PGI_2) production caused by deficiency of a prostacyclin regulatory factor has been postulated to participate in the disorder.[1191] A circulating inhibitor of prostacyclin synthetase also has been implicated.[1192] No convincing clinical or laboratory evidence, however, indicates that alterations in PGI_2 alone can cause the disease. Oxidant damage of cell membranes has been proposed,[1193] and deficiency of the antioxidant vitamin E has been described in some patients with HUS.[1194] An HUS-like illness has been described in vitamin E–deficient neonates.[1195] A platelet-aggregating factor also has been found in HUS.[1196]

Clinical and Laboratory Features. HUS commonly follows an acute diarrheal episode. Hemorrhagic colitis, usually caused by verotoxin-producing *E coli*, is frequent, but HUS has been associated with other dysenteric syndromes, including those caused by *Shigella*, *Salmonella*, and *Campylobacter jejuni* (see Table 34-4). The gastrointestinal symptoms can range from mild and nonspecific to severe and life-threatening. Abdominal pain and vomiting are common. Less commonly, the prodrome consists of upper or lower respiratory tract symptoms (atypical HUS). The prognosis may be worse for patients with atypical HUS. HUS can occur as an inheritable form beginning in early childhood.[1129–1131]

Anemia and thrombocytopenia tend to be less severe than in TTP. At presentation, the platelet count is greater than $100 \times 10^9/L$ in half of patients.[1197] Like TTP, bleeding is uncommon. Nonspecific neurologic symptoms attributable to the metabolic effects of azotemia are frequent. On rare occasions, focal neurologic symptoms and signs indicative of thrombosis are seen.[1077–1080]

Oliguria or anuria usually is present. Hyperkalemia secondary to hemolysis and renal impairment also is commonly encountered. Laboratory evidence for DIC is usually not present but can occur.[1198] HUS associated with *Shigella* infections may be more likely to lead to DIC.[1111,1199]

Stool cultures may be positive for the pathogenic organism. Other diagnostic techniques include demonstration of verotoxin or specific bacterial DNA in stool extracts and a rise in the titer of specific antibodies.[1107]

Renal histopathology reveals a preglomerular and glomerular thrombotic microangiopathy. The colon in verotoxin-associated HUS is hemorrhagic and edematous, without inflammation or ulceration.[1200]

Treatment. Despite appropriate treatment, as many as 10% of children with HUS die from the disease. A further 10% have severe, irreparable renal damage, and 10% are left with some degree of renal impairment.[1201] The mortality rate is greater in the elderly.[1189]

Supportive care, including attention to fluid and electrolyte balance, control of hypertension, transfusion for anemia, and dialysis when necessary for renal failure, is the mainstay of treatment.[1193,1202]

Two controlled trials[1203,1204] were unable to demonstrate improved survival using infusion therapy with fresh frozen plasma; however, in one study,[1204] the number of children with impaired renal function was less (about 25% versus 55%) in the group that received plasma infusion. Controlled trials of plasma exchange have not been done. We think that plasma infusion or exchange plays a role in the treatment of severe, typical HUS. There is no question that plasma therapy is highly beneficial in atypical or familial HUS.

Other treatments have been tried without obvious benefit; these include heparin,[1205,1206] thrombolytic agents,[1207,1208] prostacyclin (PGI_2),[1209] antiplatelet agents, IVIgG, and vitamin E.[1202] Immunopheresis using staphylococcal protein A columns has been used to treat cancer-associated HUS.[1210]

Renal transplantation has been effective for many patients with chronic renal failure after HUS, but recurrence of the HUS after transplantation has been described in some recipients.[1211,1212]

Preeclampsia

Preeclampsia is a common hypertensive disorder of pregnancy defined by hypertension and proteinuria that begins between 20 weeks of gestation and 4 weeks postpartum. Preeclampsia complicates about 7% of pregnancies and is most common in primigravida women. Thrombocytopenia occurs in about 10% to 20% of preeclamptic women and in about half of women with severe preeclampsia or eclampsia.[1213–1215] A subgroup of thrombocytopenic, preeclamptic women with associated microangiopathic hemolysis and elevated liver enzymes, termed the *HELLP syndrome* (hemolysis, elevated liver enzymes, low platelets), has been described,[1216] but the distinctive nature of this entity has been questioned.[1217]

The thrombocytopenia is caused by increased platelet destruction.[1213,1218–1220] Furthermore, in some patients, platelet dysfunction is evidenced by a bleeding time that is disproportionately prolonged[1213,1221] as well as by defective in vitro thromboxane synthesis in preeclamptic patients' platelets.[1213] Elevated plasma β-thromboglobulin[1222,1223] and urinary thromboxane B_2[1224] levels in preeclampsia suggest that in vivo platelet activation may contribute to the impaired platelet function.

The pathogenesis of the thrombocytopenia in preeclampsia is unknown. Different investigators have postulated different causes for the destructive thrombocytopenia, including abnormal prostacyclin production,[1225] immune mechanisms,[1213,1226] and subclinical DIC.[1227–1229] Perhaps the greatest debate has involved the role of thrombin (DIC) in the thrombocytopenia. In one study,[1229] almost

40% of preeclamptic women had elevated D-dimer levels. Many of these patients also had a positive protamine sulfate test. Elevated D-dimer levels in preeclampsia also have been observed by other investigators.[1228] Other groups[1228,1230–1232] have identified reduced antithrombin levels in preeclamptic women. Studies measuring specific markers of thrombin activation, such as fibrinopeptide A, have demonstrated slight increases in preeclampsia.[1230,1233] Although these data are consistent with the hypothesis that coagulation system activation could be the cause of the thrombocytopenia in preeclampsia, it also has been proposed that primary platelet activation results in fibrin generation.[1230] A prospective study by another group of investigators,[1213] however, did not find elevated fibrinopeptide A levels or positive protamine sulfate assays in preeclamptic patients. The coexistence of overt DIC and preeclampsia can also indicate underlying abruptio placentae complicating preeclampsia.[1234]

An important question for the clinician is whether the presence of maternal thrombocytopenia with or without microangiopathic hemolysis or liver dysfunction indicates a worse prognosis or a different treatment approach for preeclamptic women. Many physicians regard isolated thrombocytopenia or elevated liver enzymes as evidence of severe preeclampsia regardless of the degree of hypertension and advise aggressive treatment, usually prompt delivery.[1216,1235] Thrombocytopenic preeclamptic or eclamptic women usually do not have serious bleeding at the time of delivery, and routine platelet transfusions are not recommended.

The possibility that platelet activation and release of vasoactive substances plays a primary role in the pathogenesis of preeclampsia[1236] has led to clinical trials investigating the role of antiplatelet agents in the prevention and treatment of preeclampsia. Low doses of aspirin, with or without dipyridamole, appear to prevent or ameliorate preeclampsia.[1237–1239]

Allergy and Anaphylaxis

Allergic and anaphylactic reactions in people sensitized to various allergens, including foods, can be accompanied by thrombocytopenia.[1240–1244] Food antigen–containing immune complexes can be demonstrated after ingestion,[1245] and it is possible that platelet destruction is caused by platelet IgG Fc receptors interacting with the circulating immune complexes. The role of the platelet IgE Fc receptors in this regard is unknown. Inflammatory mediators, such as platelet-activating factor, may play a role in the thrombocytopenia of anaphylaxis.[1052]

Glomerulonephritis

Rarely, poststreptococcal glomerulonephritis is complicated by severe, transient thrombocytopenia.[1246,1247] Decreased platelet survival in the absence of thrombocytopenia has been observed in glomerulonephritis.[1248] Histopathologic evidence of platelet thrombi[1249] and clinical benefit from antiplatelet agents[1250] indicate that platelets participate in the pathogenesis of membranoproliferative glomerulonephritis type I.

Thrombocytopenia Associated With Renal Transplantation

Intermittent thrombocytopenia can occur with normally functioning renal allografts[1251] and during rejection episodes.[1252,1253] It is possible that platelet activation and deposition in the renal vessels contributes to the rejection process.[1254] Destructive thrombocytopenia probably of immune pathogenesis can also complicate the administration of antithymocyte globulin for the treatment of renal transplant rejection.[1255,1256]

Platelets in Contact With Foreign Materials

Extracorporeal Perfusion

Cardiopulmonary Bypass. During cardiopulmonary bypass, there is extensive contact between heparin-anticoagulated blood and the synthetic surfaces of the extracorporeal perfusion device (blood oxygenator). Excess bleeding is a frequent problem in these patients. The hemostatic defect is multifactorial, and bleeding can be caused by thrombocytopenia,[1257–1259] platelet dysfunction,[1258,1259] increased fibrinolysis,[1259–1262] dilutional coagulopathy,[1258,1260] and residual effects of heparin.[1263–1265] In addition, some patients undergoing heart surgery are taking antiplatelet agents.

Thrombocytopenia. Although hemodilution by priming fluids is the major cause of the thrombocytopenia that begins immediately after initiation of the bypass procedure, the magnitude of the fall in the platelet count cannot be explained fully by dilutional factors.[1257,1266,1267] Furthermore, thrombocytopenia sometimes persists for several days after surgery. A study of ^{111}In-labeled platelet kinetics during cardiopulmonary bypass demonstrated that about one third of the platelet mass is lost during surgery in the extracorporeal device and from intraoperative bleeding.[1266] Platelet membrane glycoproteins are lost to the surface of the extracorporeal circuit.[1268,1269] The use of protamine sulfate to reverse heparin anticoagulation at the end of cardiopulmonary bypass causes a further transient reduction in the platelet count.[1259,1266]

Platelet Dysfunction. Marked prolongation of the bleeding time to greater than 30 to 40 minutes[1258,1266] despite only moderate thrombocytopenia demonstrates that platelet dysfunction is a regular feature of cardiopulmonary bypass. The bleeding time usually returns to normal within 24 hours of surgery.[1266] Numerous types of platelet defects have been documented by several investigators, including decreased platelet aggregation to several agonists[1258,1259,1267,1270,1271]; decreased platelet membrane proteins, including α_2-adrenergic receptors[1272] and gpIIb/IIIa[1269,1273,1274]; and selective depletion of α granules.[1258,1270] Elevated plasma fibrinopeptide A, thromboxane B_2, β-thromboglobulin, and platelet factor 4 levels suggest that in vivo platelet activation occurs.[1258,1275,1276] A recent study indicated that the large doses of heparin given to patients undergoing heart surgery plays a major role in the platelet dysfunction.[1277]

Treatment and Prevention of Bleeding. The first step when faced with a patient who has excessive bleeding after cardiopulmonary bypass is to determine whether there is a surgical cause for the bleeding. Support should include platelet transfusions and possible coagulation factor replacement if a dilutional coagulopathy is suspected.[1278] Other treatments to consider include antifibrinolytic therapy and additional protamine sulfate for inadequate heparin neutralization. Some patients benefit from cryoprecipitate, possibly because of replacement of HMW multimers of vWF.

Although many prophylactic methods to prevent cardiopulmonary bypass–associated bleeding have been reported, no method is universally accepted. Desmopressin acetate, also known as 1-desamino-8-*D*-arginine vasopressin (DDAVP), may reduce blood losses in some patients undergoing cardiopulmonary bypass,[1279,1280] possibly by increasing vWF,[1281] although other workers[1282,1283] have not shown benefit. The use of the platelet activation inhibitors prostacyclin and prostaglandin E_1 to limit platelet activation and thrombocytopenia has met with variable results[1284–1288]; furthermore, these agents can cause hypotension. The platelet inhibitor dipyridamole preserved platelet counts and reduced blood losses in one study.[1289] Blood loss can be reduced by about 50% using the serine protease inhibitor aprotinin.[1290,1291] Aprotinin does not reduce platelet losses, but platelet function is better preserved.[1290,1292] Prophylactic use of ϵ-aminocaproic acid may have a slight benefit in reducing blood losses.[1293,1294]

Hemodialysis. Uremic patients often have mild thrombocytopenia due to decreased platelet production.[1295] Thrombocytopenia can also be caused by hemodialysis, probably because of platelet consumption in the dialyzer membrane.[1296–1298] This rarely causes significant bleeding.[1299] Idiosyncratic heparin-induced thrombocytopenia and extracorporeal circuit thrombosis can also occur in some uremic patients exposed to heparin during hemodialysis.[873–876]

Apheresis. Thrombocytopenia occurs frequently in patients undergoing apheresis procedures, especially with continuous flow systems.[1278] In vitro platelet dysfunction has also been demonstrated.[1300] Bleeding is uncommon.

Catheters and Prostheses

The platelet life-span is reduced in patients with prosthetic heart valves, arterial catheters, Dacron vascular grafts, arteriovenous Silastic cannulas, balloon-tipped pulmonary artery (Swan-Ganz) catheters, and ventriculojugular shunts.[1301–1305] Thrombocytopenia is rare, however, because of compensatory increases in platelet production. Decreased platelet adenine nucleotide and β-thromboglobulin levels suggest that in vivo platelet activation occurs, with release of granule constituents.[1306,1307] The platelet life-span improves over time, presumably because of progressive endothelialization of the implanted foreign material.[1303,1308] Persistence of heparin-induced thrombocytopenia in some cases has been attributed to continued exposure to heparin from heparin-coated pulmonary artery catheters.[814]

Thrombocytopenia Associated With Cardiovascular Disease

Congenital Cyanotic Heart Disease

Thrombocytopenia caused by a decrease in platelet life-span occurs in many patients with cyanotic congenital heart disease, particularly when there is marked arterial hypoxemia (oxygen saturation less than 60%) and polycythemia (hematocrit greater than 0.6).[1309–1315] Increased platelet destruction could be caused by DIC triggered by hyperviscosity and venous stasis. Although there is laboratory evidence of DIC in some patients,[1314,1315] in most patients, there is no evidence of DIC.[1310,1316] Bleeding in these patients can be related to the thrombocytopenia, platelet function defects,[1311,1317,1318] coagulopathy,[1319,1320] and hyperfibrinolysis.[1321–1323] Some of the hemostatic defects described, however, could be secondary to in vitro artifacts,[1324,1325] and care should be taken to adjust the amount of anticoagulant for the hematocrit to reduce the likelihood of spurious results. Reduction in the hematocrit by combining phlebotomy with plasma infusion can improve the hemostatic defects.[1320,1326]

Valvular Heart Disease

Mild thrombocytopenia occurs in some patients with valvular heart disease.[1327,1328] Concomitant microangiopathic hemolysis is often present. Increased platelet destruction may be related to increased consumption on a diseased valve. HMW multimers of vWF are reduced in some of these patients,[1329] suggesting their participation in the platelet destruction.

Pulmonary Hypertension

Primary pulmonary hypertension can be accompanied by thrombocytopenia.[1330,1331] Platelet survival is diminished in most patients with pulmonary hypertension, but the pathogenesis is uncertain.[1328] Thrombocytopenia occurs in infants with elevated pulmonary artery pressures related to aortopulmonary transposition with an intact ventricular septum. Improvement in the platelet count after corrective surgery despite persisting pulmonary hypertension suggests that hypoxemia and polycythemia are more important in the pathogenesis of thrombocytopenia than the degree of pulmonary hypertension.[1313]

Pulmonary Embolism

Thrombocytopenia has been reported to occur in association with occult pulmonary embolism. It is possible that this is related to DIC.[1332,1333] Heparin-induced thrombocytopenia should always be considered in patients who develop thrombocytopenia and pulmonary embolism during or shortly following a course of heparin prophylaxis or treatment.

Bleeding and Hemodilution

Bleeding patients who require massive transfusion support often develop thrombocytopenia. Thrombocytopenia occurs because of platelet losses at sites of tissue injury and by hemodilution resulting from administration of blood products. Sometimes, DIC occurs because of trauma and shock. Platelet counts typically fall to about 100×10^9/L after replacement of one blood volume by packed RBCs and plasma, and platelet count recovery can be delayed for a few days.[1334,1335] Furthermore, platelet dysfunction can be associated with tissue injury independent of the thrombocytopenia.[1336,1337] A prospective, randomized, double-blind trial did not demonstrate a benefit for prophylactic platelet transfusions in massive transfusion.[1338] However, prophylactic platelet transfusions are often given to patients at high risk for bleeding (eg, trauma, postoperative) if the platelet count has fallen below 50×10^9/L.

Fatty Acid–Induced Thrombocytopenia

Intravenous administration of fat emulsions over several weeks can cause thrombocytopenia. In one study, decreased platelet life-span was documented, and sea-blue histiocytes exhibiting hemophagocytosis were evident on marrow examination. It was proposed that increased platelet destruction occurs as a result of fat emulsion–induced reticuloendothelial system hyperactivation.[1339] Dietary therapy of adrenoleukodystrophy with Lorenzo's oil (contains glycerol trierucate) often produces a mild to moderate thrombocytopenia.[1340]

Thrombocytopenia Occurring in the Neonatal Period

Healthy, full-term and premature infants have the same normal platelet count range as do adults (150 to 450×10^9/L).[1341] Thrombocytopenia is frequently encountered in the sick neonate. In one prospective study,[1342] 22% of 807 consecutive infants admitted to a neonatal intensive care unit developed thrombocytopenia within the first week of life.

Radionuclide platelet survival studies indicated that platelet destruction was the predominant mechanism for the thrombocytopenia, with platelet sequestration playing a contributory role in some neonates.[1342,1343] DIC was identified in 20% of thrombocytopenic neonates, and poorly defined immune mechanisms, identified by elevated PAIgG, were operative in about half of the neonates. In 12%, thrombocytopenia was ascribed to exchange transfusions, and in the remaining 20%, the pathogenesis remained undefined[1342] (Fig. 34-15). However, increased thrombin generation indicative of DIC may occur in newborns without abnormalities in the platelet count or screening coagulation assays.[1344]

Almost all the causes of neonatal thrombocytopenia are due to increased platelet destruction. For convenience, however, neonatal thrombocytopenic disorders caused by hemodilution (exchange transfusion) and decreased platelet production (eythroblastosis fetalis, some congenital infections, congenital infiltrative marrow disorders) are discussed here as well.

Asphyxia

Birth asphyxia, as assessed by 5-minute Apgar scores, was found in 70% of neonates with thrombocytopenia, compared with 32% of a control group of sick, nonthrombocytopenic neonates.[1342] The etiologic role for this thrombocytopenic risk factor remains uncertain. Thrombocytopenia is frequently encountered in infants with intrauterine growth retardation, which could reflect increased platelet consumption associated with placental dysfunction and chronic hypoxia.[1345]

Fetal and Neonatal Infections

Infection is a common cause of thrombocytopenia in the newborn and can be related to infections acquired in utero or during the neonatal period (eg, cytomegalovirus, rubella, herpesvirus, echovirus, toxoplasmosis, syphilis).[1346–1351] Purpura accompanied by jaundice, hepatosplenomegaly, intracranial calcifications, neurologic defects, and congenital heart disease suggests the possibility of a congenital infection.

In many septicemic infants, the platelet count is markedly reduced.[1351,1352] Although increased platelet destruction is the most frequent mechanism of thrombocytopenia,[1342,1343] in some infections, such as the congenital rubella syndrome, decreased numbers of megakaryocytes suggest decreased platelet production.[1346] Evidence for immune mechanisms in the pathogenesis of thrombocytopenia accompanying neonatal infections has been seen.[1040,1342]

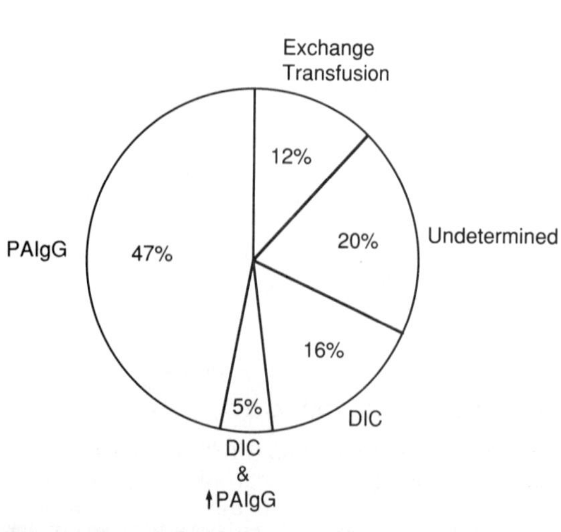

FIGURE 34-15. Mechanisms responsible for thrombocytopenia in 97 consecutive infants with platelet counts lower than 100 $\times 10^9$/L. The mechanism can be identified in 80% of infants.

Disorders Associated With Prematurity

Thrombocytopenia occurs frequently in premature infants and may be secondary to respiratory distress syndrome, perinatal aspiration, necrotizing enterocolitis, and hyperbilirubinemia requiring phototherapy.[1353]

Thrombocytopenia is frequently encountered in the newborn with respiratory distress syndrome. One group has identified mechanical ventilation as an independent factor in contributing to thrombocytopenia in these infants.[1354] Persistent pulmonary hypertension can be a sequela of both respiratory distress syndrome or perinatal aspiration.[1355–1357] Of interest, intrapulmonary platelet aggregation and the release of platelet-derived vasoactive substances, such as thromboxane A_2, have been implicated in the pathogenesis of persistent pulmonary hypertension.[1357] One group[1358] noted the presence at necropsy of platelet microthrombi on cardiac valves and in pulmonary arteries in neonates with thrombocytopenia and severe respiratory distress.

Necrotizing enterocolitis occurs in premature infants and is associated with gastrointestinal bleeding in most patients. About half of affected infants have thrombocytopenia, which could contribute to the bleeding.[1359,1360]

Phototherapy given for neonatal hyperbilirubinemia may also cause mild thrombocytopenia. Phototherapy reduces platelet survival in rabbits.[1361]

Exchange Transfusions

Exchange transfusion therapy, which is used in the management of alloimmune hemolytic disease of the newborn, is a common cause of thrombocytopenia in the neonatal intensive care unit.[1342] Dilutional thrombocytopenia occurs because the transfused RBCs and plasma do not contain viable platelets. The platelet count begins to rise in affected infants within 3 days and reaches preexchange levels by day 7.[1341]

Maternal Preeclampsia

Transient neonatal thrombocytopenia is sometimes encountered in the offspring of preeclamptic mothers.[1362–1365] It is likely that the thrombocytopenia reflects prematurity and comorbid illnesses in these infants.

Thrombocytopenia Associated With Hemangiomas (Kasabach-Merritt Syndrome)

Kasabach-Merritt syndrome is the association between giant cavernous hemangiomas in infancy and thrombocytopenia.[1366] The syndrome is congenital, and the hemangiomas and thrombocytopenia are discovered within the first few days or weeks of life.[1367] Sometimes, the syndrome begins later in childhood as the hemangioma increases in size. The hemangiomas usually are solitary and superficial, involving the proximal extremities, trunk, and neck. A similar syndrome also can be caused by acquired benign or malignant vascular neoplasms during later life.[1368] Placental vascular tumors can also be responsible for transient neonatal thrombocytopenia.[1369,1370]

Laboratory studies usually reveal a platelet count below 50 $\times 10^9$/L, with schistocytic RBCs. Coagulation abnormalities are the rule and include hypofibrinogenemia, elevated fibrin and fibrinogen degradation products, and other tests indicative of DIC. These laboratory findings relate to the underlying pathogenesis, which is localized consumption of platelets and fibrinogen within the abnormal tumor vasculature.[1371–1375]

Many children have no or minimal bleeding symptoms, and eventual spontaneous tumor regression usually occurs. For symptomatic lesions, several treatment options can be considered, including corticosteroids,[1367,1376–1379] tumor excision,[1380] local irradiation,[1381,1382] and tumor embolization.[1383] Treatment of the coagulopathy has included antifibrinolytic treatment,[1384–1386] heparin, and blood product replacement with platelet, plasma, and cryoprecipitate transfusions. In one report,[1387] platelet destruction decreased after use of aspirin and dipyridamole. Treatment decisions are based on considerations of bleeding risk, tumor location and size, and natural history.

Neonatal Alloimmune Thrombocytopenia

Neonatal alloimmune thrombocytopenia was discussed in the section on alloimmune thrombocytopenic disorders.

Transient Passive Autoimmune Thrombocytopenia

Transient neonatal immune thrombocytopenia can also be caused by the transplacental passage of maternal autoantibodies, as found in ITP and SLE.[1388,1389] This is discussed in the section on ITP in pregnancy.

Maternal Drugs

Rarely, transplacental passage of drug and drug-dependent antibodies can result in both maternal and neonatal thrombocytopenia, as has been documented for quinine.[1390] Maternal ingestion of thiazide diuretics,[1391] hydralazine,[1392] and tolbutamide[1393] has been implicated in neonatal thrombocytopenia, but the evidence is circumstantial and sometimes disputed.[1394,1395] Neonatal platelet dysfunction can occur secondary to maternal ingestion of aspirin.[1396]

Neonatal Thrombosis

Thrombocytopenia in some neonates has been attributed to platelet consumption secondary to thrombosis at the site of an indwelling plastic catheter.[1397,1398] Thrombocytopenia is frequently encountered in sick neonates with umbilical catheters (76% in one study),[1342] so an association with catheter-related thrombosis remains speculative. Thrombocytopenia can also occur in neonates developing renal vein or inferior vena caval thrombosis.[1399–1401] One study suggested the intriguing possibility that thrombosis and thrombocytopenia occurring in certain neonates might be secondary to an immune-mediated drug reaction (heparin-induced thrombocytopenia).[1402]

Polycythemia

Polycythemic neonates with a hematocrit greater than 0.70 are commonly thrombocytopenic, particularly if they have associated cyanotic heart disease.[1310,1404] The platelet count rises after phlebotomy.[1320]

Congenital Thrombocytopenia and Microangiopathic Hemolysis

Several patients have been described with recurrent thrombocytopenia and microangiopathic hemolysis beginning in early childhood that responds to plasma infusion.[1145,1405–1407] Studies indicate that some of these patients have abnormal vWF and the presence of calpain in their plasma, similar to the abnormalities of TTP.[1145]

Homozygous Protein C Deficiency

Thrombocytopenia can be a prominent feature of homozygous protein C deficiency, which can present as neonatal purpura fulminans syndrome.[1408,1409]

Fatty Acid–Induced Thrombocytopenia

Thrombocytopenia temporally related to the parenteral administration of lipid emulsions has been described in the neonate.[1410] Platelet activation by administered fatty acids[1411] may be responsible for the thrombocytopenia as well as for the intimal vascular lesions that neonates receiving parenteral lipid preparations can develop.[1412,1413] Alternatively, enhanced platelet destruction by reticuloendothelial cells has been described.[1339]

Inherited Metabolic Disorders

Inherited metabolic disorders associated with thrombocytopenia include methylmalonic acidemia,[1414] ketotic glycinemia,[1414] mevalonic aciduria,[1415] holocarboxylase synthetase deficiency,[1416] and isovaleric acidemia.[1417] Pancytopenia associated with isovaleric acidemia was attributed to marrow progenitor cell maturation defects caused by the elevated isovaleric acid levels.[1417]

Erythroblastosis Fetalis

Thrombocytopenia and neutropenia can complicate Rh hemolytic disease of the newborn. The thrombocytopenia, which can persist for as long as 1 week after birth, is associated with increased risk of hemorrhage. The findings of a low MPV and reduced numbers of megakaryocyte progeny generated in vitro from circulating multipotent progenitor cells suggest reduced platelet production.[1418] Other potential contributory factors include hypersplenism in hydropic infants and exchange transfusion using platelet-poor concentrated RBC preparations.

Hereditary Thrombocytopenic Disorders

Both the hereditary hypomegakaryocytic (eg, thrombocytopenia and absent radii syndrome, Fanconi's anemia) and hereditary ineffective thrombopoiesis disorders (eg, Wiskott-Aldrich syndrome) are discussed in the section on decreased platelet production.

Congenital Infiltrative Marrow Disorders

Thrombocytopenia, in association with depression of both myeloid and erythroid elements during the neonatal period, can be the consequence of congenital infiltrative marrow disorders such as acute leukemia,[1419,1420] stage IV congenital neuroblastoma,[1421] osteopetrosis, and histiocytosis X.[1422,1423] Sometimes, children with trisomy 21 (Down's syndrome) present with marked leukocytosis mimicking acute leukemia (leukemoid reaction), which spontaneously resolves.[1424]

THROMBOCYTOPENIA CAUSED BY PLATELET SEQUESTRATION

Hypersplenism

Hypersplenism is defined as a reduction in one or more of the peripheral blood counts caused by increased blood cell sequestration by the spleen. The spleen is enlarged and almost always palpable. Table 34-6 lists the causes of hypersplenism. The hematologic cytopenias of hypersplenism can be cured by splenectomy, although this procedure is rarely indicated.

Pathogenesis

The spleen normally pools about one third of the platelets (see section on platelet distribution). This physiologic splenic pooling (sequestration) is related to the splenic blood flow and the comparatively lengthy transit time of the blood cells through the spleen, which is about 10 minutes for platelets and leukocytes and 2 minutes for RBCs.

The pathogenesis of the hematologic cytopenias in hypersplenism is multifactorial[1425] but predominantly is related to increased pooling within an enlarged spleen. Increased blood flow to a larger spleen results in increased pooling of blood cells within the spleen, even if the transit time is unchanged.[52] Increased cell destruction also contributes to the thrombocytopenia of hypersplenism. This may be the result of the longer splenic transit time, allowing the cells to interact with phagocytic cells. In addition, patients with hypersplenism typically have an increased plasma volume,[1426] which contributes to the cytopenia by a dilutional effect. Finally, it is also possible that some patients with hypersplenism underproduce one or more of the cellular elements.

Diagnosis

The diagnosis of hypersplenism is usually one of exclusion. Typically, the patient has thrombocytopenia and leukopenia, with anemia being less severe, although a disproportionate reduction in any single cell line can occur. The patient has an enlarged spleen, which is almost always sufficiently enlarged to be palpable. In patients in whom it is technically difficult to palpate the spleen, an accurate determination of spleen size can be obtained using radionuclide scanning techniques.

The diagnosis of hypersplenic thrombocytopenia can be confirmed by a radiolabeled platelet life-span study. Patients with hypersplenism have a dramatically reduced platelet recovery. The normal percentage of recovery of autologous platelets is about 70%, whereas the percentage of platelet recovery in a hypersplenic patient is often much less than 50%. Platelet survival is normal or only mildly reduced.[1427,1428]

Treatment

It is rare for a patient with cytopenia caused by hypersplenism to require treatment for the cytopenia. Although the platelets are reduced in patients with hypersplenism, the thrombocytopenia is not severe, and the platelet count typically ranges from 50 to 100 $\times$ 10^9/L. Consequently, these patients do not bleed because of the thrombocytopenia. Similarly, the leukopenia and anemia tend to be mild and asymptomatic. The definitive treatment of hypersplenism is splenectomy, and although splenectomy can be performed as a treatment for hypersplenism, it is more frequently performed for other reasons.

Sometimes, a procedure other than a splenectomy has therapeutic benefit. For example, the most common cause of hypersplenism in North America and Europe is alcoholic cirrhosis. In these patients, the hypersplenism is caused by portal hypertension, and death is much more likely to result from variceal hemorrhage than from complications of the hypersplenic cytopenias. Decompressive procedures, such as the distal splenorenal shunt, which have been used to prevent variceal hemorrhage due to portal hypertension, can improve the cytopenias.[1429]

TABLE 34-6. Causes of Hypersplenism

CONGESTIVE SPLENOMEGALY
Cirrhosis
Budd-Chiari syndrome (hepatic vein thrombosis)
Portal vein obstruction
Chronic passive congestion secondary to cardiac failure or constrictive pericarditis
Hepatic schistosomiasis
ACUTE AND CHRONIC INFECTIONS
Viral illnesses* (especially infectious mononucleosis and acute hepatitis)
Malaria*
Tuberculosis
Typhoid fever
Bacterial endocarditis*
Leishmaniasis
Brucellosis
Trypanosomiasis
Echinococcosis
Leprosy
INFLAMMATORY CONDITIONS
Sarcoidosis*
Systemic lupus erythematosus*
Felty's syndrome
Rheumatoid arthritis associated with proliferation of large granular lymphocytes
Vasculitis
CHRONIC HEMOLYTIC DISORDERS
Congenital hemolytic disorders
Acute splenic sequestration crises
HEMATOLOGIC NEOPLASMS
Myeloproliferative syndromes (polycythemia rubra vera, chronic myeloid leukemia, agnogenic myeloid metaplasia)
Lymphoproliferative disorders* (Hodgkin's and nonHodgkin's lymphoma, chronic lymphocytic leukemia, hairy-cell leukemia)
Histiocytosis X
NONHEMATOLOGIC NEOPLASMS
Metastatic carcinoma
Sarcoma
Hemangiomas
Lymphangiomas
STORAGE DISORDERS
Gaucher's disease
Niemann-Pick disease
Amyloidosis
Sea-blue histiocytosis
Diabetic lipemia
Tangier disease
Hurler's syndrome
Hunter's syndrome
MISCELLANEOUS
Primary splenic hyperplasia (tropical and nontropical)
Thyrotoxicosis
Splenic cysts
Hamartoma
Amyloidosis
Hereditary hemorrhagic telangiectasia

* Thrombocytopenia in these disorders may be more frequently caused by immune platelet destruction than by hypersplenism.

Investigators[1430,1431] have described the deliberate infarction of a proportion of the spleen by splenic arterial embolization. Although long-term benefit can result, more frequently, efficacy is relatively transient, and the procedure has many complications. For this reason, except in highly selected patients in whom the procedure is performed by skilled physicians, we do not believe that partial splenic infarction is appropriate.

Splenectomy is frequently effective in treating the cytopenias associated with hairy-cell leukemia. In addition to correction of hypersplenism, splenectomy removes a large tumor burden and reduces the neoplastic cell–associated humoral suppression of normal hematopoiesis.[1432] Patients with agnogenic myeloid metaplasia frequently benefit from splenectomy not only because of improvement in the cytopenias but also because of control of pain and discomfort caused by the enlarged spleen.[1433,1434]

Gaucher's disease is a storage disease caused by deficiency in glucocerebrosidase. Deposition of glucocerebroside occurs in the reticuloendothelial organs. Splenectomy is effective for the massive splenomegaly and hypersplenism, but bone destruction and liver failure due to increased deposition of glucocerebroside in those organs can occur after splenectomy. Partial splenectomy may be the treatment of choice because it allows the deposition of glucocerebroside in the splenic remnant.[1435] Partial splenic embolization also has been used.[1436]

Idiopathic splenomegaly (primary splenic hyperplasia) is a rare cause of hypersplenism that is associated with an increased risk of lymphoma.[1437] Splenectomy sometimes reveals lymphoma in patients in whom the cause of splenomegaly cannot be identified using noninvasive techniques.[1438]

Complications of Splenectomy

The complications of splenectomy were discussed in the section on ITP and consist of early postoperative complications (pleuropulmonary, infections, embolism) and late risk of overwhelming postsplenectomy septicemia. The complication rate is reported to be highest in patients with myeloproliferative syndromes.[1439]

Hypothermia

Observations in experimental and hibernating animals, as well as in humans being cooled for surgery, indicate that hypothermia is frequently accompanied by mild to moderate thrombocytopenia.[1440–1443] Thrombocytopenia has also been observed in accidental hypothermia both in infants and in the elderly[1444–1447] as well as in infants suffering from hypothalamic dysfunction and temperature dysregulation.[1448] The thrombocytopenia is transient and corrects with rewarming. In some patients, bleeding symptoms were attributed to the thrombocytopenia.[1444,1448] Platelet kinetic studies in cooled dogs demonstrated reversible hepatic and splenic platelet sequestration.[1440,1449,1450] Indirect evidence suggests that decreased platelet production may play a contributory role.[1444,1448]

Red Blood Cell Transfusions

It has been observed[1451] that platelet count reductions averaging 33% occur in patients receiving three to five units of packed RBCs. Radionuclide studies revealed that this phenomenon was associated with increased splenic platelet sequestration. Removal of microaggregate debris by filtration or washing of the packed RBCs markedly reduced the extent of platelet count decrease.

THROMBOCYTOPENIA CAUSED BY DECREASED PLATELET PRODUCTION

Thrombocytopenia often is caused by decreased platelet production, which can be divided into three categories: acquired, generalized marrow disorders; acquired, isolated megakaryocytic disorders; and hereditary thrombocytopenic disorders.

By far the most common cause of decreased platelet production is acquired, generalized marrow disorders. The pathologic process disturbs all cell lines, and pancytopenia typically results. Occasionally, however, isolated thrombocytopenia is the first abnormality detected during the early stages of a panmyelopathy.

Except for alcohol-induced thrombocytopenia, acquired disorders restricted to megakaryocytes are uncommon.

The hereditary thrombocytopenic disorders also are rare. They can broadly be considered in two categories: hypomegakaryocytic thrombocytopenia and ineffective thrombopoiesis. The hypomegakaryocytic thrombocytopenic disorders are characterized by absent or markedly reduced megakaryocyte numbers. They usually present in infancy, and associated nonhematologic phenotypic abnormalities are frequent. The hereditary disorders of ineffective thrombopoiesis are a heterogeneous group ranging from isolated, clinically insignificant thrombocytopenia to severe, symptomatic thrombocytopenia associated with nonhematologic abnormalities, such as immune deficiency (Wiscott-Aldrich syndrome). Megakaryocyte numbers are usually normal.

Acquired, Generalized Marrow Disorders

Acquired, generalized marrow disorders are discussed in detail elsewhere in this book, and except for myelodysplasia-associated thrombocytopenia, are summarized here in outline form only.

Nonneoplastic Hypoproliferative Stem Cell Disorders

Thrombocytopenia accompanies aplastic anemia, chemotherapy-induced pancytopenia, and idiosyncratic drug-induced aplastic anemia. Sometimes, isolated thrombocytopenia is a precursor of aplastic anemia.

Neoplastic Stem Cell Disorders (Including Myelodysplasia)

Thrombocytopenia is common with primary neoplastic disorders of the bone marrow. These include neoplasms of the myeloid series, such as acute myeloid leukemia, myelodysplasia, myeloproliferative syndromes, and paroxysmal nocturnal hemoglobinuria. Lymphoid neoplasms include acute lymphoid leukemia and many chronic lymphoproliferative disorders, such as chronic lymphoid leukemia, hairy-cell leukemia, non-Hodgkin's lymphoma, adult T-cell leukemia and lymphoma, multiple myeloma, and Waldenström's macroglobulinemia.

Isolated thrombocytopenia can be a presenting feature of the myelodysplastic disorders.[1452,1453] The thrombocytopenia can be of sufficient severity that death from bleeding is a relatively common event. Bleeding symptoms are often a prominent problem, especially since many patients have a coexisting defect in platelet function.[1454,1455]

Peripheral blood examination often reveals giant platelets, sometimes with prominent granules. Marrow examination reveals dysmegakaryocytopoiesis in half of cases. Typically, the megakaryocytes are abnormally small, but large mononuclear and multilobed nuclear forms are found in some patients.[1456] Megakaryocyte numbers are usually normal, but amegakaryocytic thrombocytopenia has been described as a presenting feature.[1453]

Treatment includes supportive care and, in selected cases, chemotherapy. Recombinant granulocyte-macrophage colony-stimulating factor may help raise the platelet count in some patients.[1457] In a minority of patients, danazol administration results in improvement in the thrombocytopenia.[1458–1460]

Infiltrative Marrow Disorders

Thrombocytopenia can be secondary to infiltration of the bone marrow by nonhematologic metastatic malignancies, infectious organisms, storage-cell disorders, myelofibrosis, and osteopetrosis.

Megaloblastic Anemia

Megaloblastic anemia, which usually is caused by vitamin B_{12} or folic acid deficiency, is often associated with thrombocytopenia. Vitamin deficiency–induced defective DNA synthesis results in megakaryocytes of low ploidy, which produce small platelets.[40] Thus, the combination of large, heterogeneous red cells together with small platelets (low MPV) suggests megaloblastic anemia, although it also can be seen in some patients with primary marrow disorders.

Acquired Megakaryocytic Disorders

Alcohol-Induced Thrombocytopenia

Thrombocytopenia is a common complication of alcohol abuse, occurring in about one fourth of alcoholic patients admitted to the hospital.[1461] Severe thrombocytopenia and bleeding are uncommon, although platelet counts as low as $10 \times 10^9/L$ have been described.[1462] Consequently, a bleeding patient should be investigated for local causes of bleeding (esophageal varices, gastritis, peptic ulcers) and other causes of hemostatic impairment (coagulopathy, platelet dysfunction of cirrhosis). Other causes of thrombocytopenia, including hypersplenism and folate deficiency, should also be considered. Alcohol itself causes platelet dysfunction.[305,306,1463,1464]

Alcohol-induced thrombocytopenia can occur in the absence of liver disease or nutrient deficiency.[1465–1468] In one study,[1466] administration of alcohol and normal calorie and nutrient supplementation caused an isolated fall in the platelet count in half of the volunteers after 3 to 5 weeks of daily alcohol consumption. In two other studies,[1467,1468] in which hospitalized patients were allowed alcohol ad libitum, thrombocytopenia developed within 11 to 15 days. The platelet count begins to rise 2 to 3 days after cessation of alcohol consumption and reaches normal values usually within 1 week. The maximal platelet count, which often reaches supernormal values, usually occurs 10 to 18 days after stopping alcohol.[1465–1468] Rebound thrombocytosis after alcohol cessation can occur in the absence of preceding thrombocytopenia.[1469]

The bone marrow examination usually shows normal megakaryocyte morphology, although normoblast and promyelocyte vacuolations frequently are evident.[1465,1466] Reduced megakaryocyte numbers can occur and may be associated with slower recovery of platelet counts.[1470]

Platelet kinetic data,[1471] recovery patterns from plateletpheresis,[1472] MPV studies,[1473] and marrow culture studies[1470,1474] all indicate that the platelet production is impaired by alcohol. The in vitro studies, both in humans[1470] and rodents,[1474] suggest that alcohol decreases platelet production by suppressing the maturing megakaryocytes, with little effect on the progenitor CFU-meg cells. Other effects of alcohol include moderate reduction in platelet life-span[1471] and platelet ultrastructural alterations.[1463]

Acquired Amegakaryocytic Thrombocytopenia

Acquired amegakaryocytic thrombocytopenia is a rare, acquired disorder characterized by isolated thrombocytopenia associated with a total or marked reduction in megakaryocytes. Sometimes, there is associated RBC macrocytosis, and progression to aplastic anemia or myelodysplasia can occur.[1453,1475–1477] The disorder also has been described in association with SLE[1478] and idiosyncratic drug reaction.[1479] Cyclic amegakaryocytic thrombocytopenia also has been observed in two patients.[1480,1481]

The pathogenesis is heterogeneous, and four different mechanisms have been implicated: an intrinsic stem cell defect, as evidenced by defective growth of megakaryocyte precursors[1476]; cytotoxic IgG autoantibody against megakaryocyte precursors[1476,1482]; T-cell–mediated suppression of megakaryocyte development[1478]; and IgG autoantibody inhibiting the responsiveness of megakaryocyte progenitor cells to granulocyte-macrophage colony-stimulating factor.[1480]

Standard-dose corticosteroids, androgens, lithium, 6-mercaptopurine, vincristine, and splenectomy are generally ineffective.[1475,1476] Partial or complete responses to antithymocyte globulin,[1483,1484] high-dose corticosteroids,[1478,1485] or both[1477] have been reported. Case reports have described benefit from cyclosporine,[1481,1486] danazol,[1487] vinblastine,[1482] and cyclophosphamide.[1488]

Iron Depletion and Repletion

Although iron deficiency is usually associated with normal or increased numbers of platelets,[1489] thrombocytopenia can accompany severe iron deficiency anemia.[1490–1498] Marrow megakaryocytes were reduced in some reported patients.[1491,1495,1497,1498] Some patients with iron deficiency anemia and normal or elevated platelet counts developed transient thrombocytopenia after iron replacement therapy, with platelet count nadirs noted 6 to 12 days after institution of iron repletion.[1499,1500] The cause of thrombocytopenia in iron depletion or after repletion is unknown, although impaired platelet production has been postulated. Iron may have a dual role in the production and regulation of platelet production.[1501]

Hereditary Thrombocytopenic Disorders

Hereditary thrombocytopenic disorders are rare. When they occur, they can sometimes be recognized by characteristic nonhematologic phenotypic features. If the thrombocytopenia is an isolated finding that is first identified later in life, the disorder can be misdiagnosed as ITP. Inherited thrombocytopenic platelet disorders can be divided into two major groups: hypomegakaryocytic thrombocytopenia and ineffective thrombopoiesis with adequate megakaryocyte numbers.

Hereditary Hypomegakaryocytic Thrombocytopenia

Multiple congenital malformations, most frequently absent radii, can accompany hereditary hypomegakaryocytic thrombocytopenic disorders. Sometimes, isolated thrombocytopenia heralds the onset of pancytopenia in patients with a hereditary aplastic anemia, such as Fanconi's anemia or dyskeratosis congenita.

Thrombocytopenia With Absent Radii

The autosomal recessive syndrome of hypomegakaryocytic thrombocytopenia with bilateral absent radii (TAR) usually presents with thrombocytopenia or bleeding during the first weeks or months of life. Rarely, patients do not develop thrombocytopenia until adult age.[1502–1504] For most patients, the thrombocytopenia is most severe during the first year of life and gradually improves, so that most patients become asymptomatic.[1503] Bone marrow examination shows absent or markedly reduced numbers of megakaryocytes that appear immature. The thrombocytopenia is probably due to a disorder of committed megakaryocytic progenitors since the virtual absence of CFU-meg has been described in an affected patient, with substantial megakaryocyte colony-stimulating activity present in the serum.[1505]

Skeletal defects involving intercalary (nonterminal) bones of the upper and lower extremities are common.[1502,1503] Thus, in contrast to Fanconi's anemia, the thumb and fingers are present, but they may be hypoplastic. About 20% of patients also have cardiac anomalies. Some affected infants demonstrate failure to thrive and milk intolerance.[1505,1506] A leukemoid reaction, sometimes accompanied by eosinophilia, is common during the neonatal period and usually subsides spontaneously within a few months. Chromosomal abnormalities have not been described.

Although the syndrome of thrombocytopenia and absent radii is an autosomal recessive disorder, consanguinity is uncommon, suggesting that affected patients may be heterozygous for two distinct genetic defects.[1507] These patients have about a 25% risk for future affected offspring. Prenatal diagnosis is possible by radiography or ultrasonography[1508,1509] together with fetal blood sampling.[1510]

Corticosteroids and splenectomy are not usually effective. Bone marrow transplantation is not indicated because of the favorable natural history. Patients with bleeding may require platelet transfusions and fibrinolytic inhibitors.[1503] Orthopedic procedures to improve upper-limb function or appearance are best postponed until after infancy when the platelet counts are improved.

Other Hereditary Hypomegakaryocytic Disorders

Two unrelated families have been reported with an autosomal dominant disorder characterized by upper-limb abnormalities, thrombocytopenia, hearing impairment, and strabismus. Severely affected patients can have asymmetric hypoplasia of the radii and hand bones.[1511,1512]

Although congenital hypomegakaryocytic thrombocytopenia usually occurs with bilateral absent radii, it can be associated with other congenital abnormalities. These include trisomy 18,[1513–1515] microcephaly,[1516,1517] multiple malformations and neurologic dysfunction,[1518] and elevated fetal hemoglobin.[1519]

Alloimmune megakaryocyte damage is a rare cause of transient neonatal thrombocytopenia.[159,160,916]

Hereditary Aplastic Anemia

Fanconi's Anemia. Fanconi's anemia is an autosomal recessive disorder characterized by aplastic anemia, usually beginning between the ages of 5 and 10 years. The anemia occurs in association with various extrahematologic abnormalities, which include growth retardation, skeletal malformations (especially dysplasia or absence of the thumbs, sometimes with absent radii), neurologic abnormalities (microcephaly, microophthalmia, strabismus, mental retardation in 20%), skin pigment abnormalities (hyperpigmentation, café-au-lait spots, and areas of depigmentation), renal abnormalities, and genital abnormalities (genital hypoplasia and cryptorchism in males).[1520,1521] These patients are at increased risk for developing acute myeloid leukemia.[1521] Elevated fetal hemoglobin and multiple chromosomal breaks are characteristic.

Isolated thrombocytopenia usually precedes the pancytopenia. Thus, a patient with Fanconi's anemia and absent radii who presents with thrombocytopenia during infancy may be thought to have the syndrome of thrombocytopenia with absent radii.[1522] In distinction to thrombocytopenia with absent radii, however, the thumbs are lacking in Fanconi's anemia if the radii are absent. The chromosomal and hemoglobin findings characteristic of Fanconi's anemia also aid in differentiating these disorders.

Although blood counts (including platelets) improve with anabolic steroid treatment,[1521] there is considerable toxicity with this treatment. Bone marrow transplantation can be curative.[1523]

Other Hereditary Aplastic Anemias. Patients with congenital hypomegakaryocytic thrombocytopenia without stigmata of thrombocytopenia with absent radii, congenital infection, or alloimmune thrombocytopenia, are at high risk for subsequently developing aplastic anemia.[1524,1525]

For example, male infants with congenital thrombocytopenia, microcephaly, cerebellar hypoplasia, and growth failure progressing to aplastic anemia have been described.[1517,1526]

Isolated thrombocytopenia can precede or accompany the development of dyskeratosis congenita (reticular skin pigmentation, nail dystrophy, mucosal leukokeratosis), a hereditary disorder frequently associated with onset of aplastic anemia in childhood.[1527,1528]

A syndrome of X-linked congenital amegakaryocytic thrombocytopenia with elevated fetal hemoglobin progressing to aplastic anemia has been described.[1529]

A syndrome of bone marrow failure occurring in adulthood associated with proximal fusion of the radius and ulna was described in two unrelated families.[1530] Thrombocytopenia and macrocytosis preceded the development of pancytopenia in some of the patients. Inheritance is autosomal dominant, and the chromosomes are normal.

Hereditary Thrombocytopenia With Ineffective Thrombopoiesis

Hereditary thrombocytopenia with ineffective thrombopoiesis is characterized by thrombocytopenia with normal or increased numbers of megakaryocytes and normal RBC and leukocyte counts. Although decreased platelet survival is found in some patients, reduced platelet turnover suggesting ineffective thrombopoiesis is the predominant abnormality.[1531]

Ineffective Thrombopoiesis With Macrothrombocytes

Most patients with hereditary ineffective thrombopoiesis have large platelets, and the mode of inheritance is autosomal dominant.[1532–1534] Sometimes, only a minority of the platelets are large, and the MPV can be within the normal range.[1535,1536] Platelet survival is reduced in some patients[1536,1537] but usually is normal.[1534,1538] Defective thrombopoiesis in an animal model of congenital macrothrombocytopenia (Wistar Furth rat) has been described.[1539,1540]

Several distinct clinical syndromes are recognized:

Macrothrombocytopenia With Leukocyte Inclusions (May-Hegglin Anomaly). This autosomal dominant disorder is characterized by giant platelets and blue, spindle-shaped inclusions within granulocytes and monocytes.[1541,1542] By ultrastructural analysis, these inclusions consist of rough endoplasmic reticulum, ribosomes, and parallel filaments.[1542] Many patients have mild to moderate thrombocytopenia, although bleeding symptoms are uncommon.[1542,1543] Platelet function can be normal[1543,1544] or impaired.[1545]

Macrothrombocytopenia, Glomerulonephritis, and Deafness. In 1972, a family with thrombocytopenia, large platelets, glomerulonephritis, and sensorineural deafness inherited as an autosomal dominant trait was described (Epstein's syndrome).[1546] Similar reports followed,[1547–1550] although platelet aggregation abnormalities were noted in some other families.[1547,1548] Thrombocytopenia occurs in infancy, but progressive albuminuria, hematuria, and renal insufficiency, as well as sensorineural hearing impairment predominantly affecting high-pitched tones, develops in childhood or early adulthood.

Patients with the triad of thrombocytopenia, glomerulonephritis, and deafness also can have blue-staining leukocyte inclusions (Fechtner's syndrome).[1551–1553] Cataracts have been described in affected members of two families.[1551,1553] The leukocyte inclusions (Fechtner's inclusions) are composed of dispersed filament, ribosomes, and endoplasmic reticulum in a pattern ultrastructurally distinct from Döhle bodies and May-Hegglin inclusions.[1542,1551,1552] Megakaryocytes demonstrate abnormal patterns of cytoplasmic fragmentation.[1552] Other families with macrothrombocytopenia and leukocyte inclusions, but lacking one or more features of Alport's syndrome (deafness, glomerulonephritis), have been described.[1542,1554]

Macrothrombocytopenia With Platelet Procoagulant Defect. Several families have been described with macrothrombocytopenia and bleeding with in vitro evidence of impaired platelet procoagulant activity (decreased platelet factor 3).[1537,1538,1555] A family with a severe bleeding disorder caused by qualitative platelet factor V deficiency (factor V Quebec) has been described.[1556] However, the platelet size is normal in this family.

Pseudo von Willebrand's Disease and Type IIB von Willebrand's Disease. Pseudo von Willebrand's disease (platelet-type von Willebrand's disease) is an autosomal dominant disorder characterized by mild intermittent thrombocytopenia, mild bleeding, absence of HMW vWF multimers, and increased ristocetin-induced platelet aggregation. The defect resides not within the vWF molecule, but within the platelet membrane, which has enhanced reactivity to vWF.[1557,1558]

Type IIB von Willebrand's disease is similar clinically. In this disorder, an abnormal vWF with increased platelet reactivity causes intermittent thrombocytopenia, particularly during pregnancy[1559,1560] and the postoperative state.[1561] The usual mode of inheritance is autosomal dominant, but patients with an autosomal recessive inheritance have been described.[1562] Abnormal vWF within platelets can cause platelet aggregation in the absence of platelet agonists.[1563] DDAVP treatment is contraindicated in these von Willebrand's disease variants because it can provoke or exacerbate thrombocytopenia.[1564] A family has been described with chronic thrombocytopenia and spontaneous platelet aggregation in vitro (type IIB Tampa).[1565] Another variant disorder has been described that is characterized by thrombocytopenia after DDAVP administration but normal in vitro platelet responsiveness to ristocetin (type IIB Buffalo).[1566]

Gray-Platelet Syndrome. The gray-platelet syndrome is an inherited disorder characterized by large, agranular, gray-appearing platelets on the stained blood film.[1567,1568] Usually, the thrombocytopenia and bleeding symptoms are mild. There is a virtual absence of α granules in platelets and megakaryocytes.[1569] It is possible that the defect is due to abnormal incorporation of proteins into the megakaryocyte granules.[1570]

Bernard-Soulier Syndrome. Bernard-Soulier syndrome is an autosomal recessive disorder characterized by thrombocytopenia, giant platelets, and prolonged bleeding time.[1571] The platelets cannot be agglutinated by ristocetin and have markedly impaired in vivo adhesion due to the complete or partial absence of the gpIb/IX membrane complex.[114,116,1572] Desmopressin infusion can correct the prolonged bleeding times in these patients.[1573,1574] A variant disorder characterized by macrothrombocytopenia and reduced sialic acid on gpIb has also been described.[1575]

Other Macrothrombocytopenic Disorders. An autosomal dominant bleeding disorder characterized by thrombocytopenia, giant platelets, abnormal platelet aggregation, normal platelet factor 3 activity, and abnormal megakaryocyte ploidy has been described.[1535] These patients also had a deficiency of arachidonic acid in their platelets.

A family with asymptomatic chronic macrothrombocytopenia and autosomal dominant inheritance has been described in whom decreased glycosylation of platelet gpIV was detected.[1576]

A hereditary giant-platelet syndrome (Montreal platelet syndrome), characterized by bleeding, thrombocytopenia, spontaneous platelet aggregation, and hypervolumetric shape change on platelet activation, has been described in a family.[1577,1578] The abnormal platelet aggregation is not mediated by fibrinogen and calcium. A defect in platelet calpain has been identified in this syndrome.[1579]

One family has been reported with thrombocytopenia and bleeding of moderate severity with reduced platelet survival that was inherited in an autosomal dominant fashion.[1580] Their platelets survived normally when administered to normal people, while normal platelets given to these patients had reduced survival. All six affected members of the family had normal PAIgG levels. Infusion of filtered platelet-poor plasma into an affected member caused transient elevation of the platelet count and correction of the bleeding-time prolongation.[1581] It was postulated that this family lacks a humoral factor necessary for normal platelet survival.

Two unrelated families have been described with thrombocytopenia and myopathy inherited in an autosomal dominant fashion.[1582,1583] In one family, the platelets appeared to be larger than normal, and RBC abnormalities suggesting hyposplenism were evident.[1582]

The platelets from a patient with a mild bleeding tendency, macrothrombocytopenia, abnormal platelet aggregation, and reduced platelet survival demonstrated dilated canaliculi ultrastructurally.[1584] Similar "Swiss-cheese platelets" also have been identified in patients with myelodysplasia and pernicious anemia,[1585] and it is unclear whether these changes are characteristic of a hereditary platelet disorder.

Mild thrombocytopenia and elevated MPV can be found in healthy people of Mediterranean ancestry.[1586,1587]

Ineffective Thrombopoiesis With Normal-Sized Platelets

Several families with hereditary thrombocytopenia and normal-sized platelets have been described. Bleeding is mild, and the inheritance usually is autosomal dominant.[1588–1593] Although some patients have normal in vitro platelet function,[1588,1590] others have defective platelet aggregation.[1591–1593] The platelet life-span was normal in some families[1588,1589] and reduced in others.[1588,1590] In one family, an apparent increase in the incidence of hematologic malignancies was observed.[1593]

Ineffective Thrombopoiesis With Microthrombocytes

Wiskott-Aldrich Syndrome. Wiskott-Aldrich syndrome consists of eczema, thrombocytopenia (platelet count usually below 50×10^9/L), and an impaired immune system manifest as an increased susceptibility to viral and bacterial infections.[1594] The illness is often fatal by 10 years of age due to bleeding, infection, or lymphoreticular malignancy.[1595] The immune defects can be profound, with impairment of both cellular and humoral immunity. There is progressive decline in lymphocyte number during early childhood and reduced lymphocyte response to mitogens, allogeneic cells, and polysaccharide antigens.[1596] Allergy to cow milk and other foods is common. The disorder is inherited in a X-linked recessive fashion, and the defective gene has been localized to the short arm of the X chromosome.[1597]

Platelet survival is reduced by about half[1596,1598] and is caused by an intrinsic platelet abnormality since survival of homologous platelets is normal in patients with Wiskott-Aldrich syndrome.[1598–1600] Platelet production is decreased, however, despite adequate megakaryocyte numbers (ineffective thrombopoiesis).[1596]

The platelets are reduced in size by one half to two thirds of normal.[1596,1598,1601,1602] Indeed, the reduced MPV is sufficiently unique that electronic platelet sizing of fetoscopically obtained blood can be used for the prenatal diagnosis of the syndrome.[1601] Despite the small platelets, the level of platelet-associated IgG is strikingly elevated.[1602] The platelets also demonstrate morphologic and functional evidence of a storage-pool disorder.[1598] Platelet dysfunction may be caused by a defect in regulation of energy generation.[1603]

In contrast to the other hereditary thrombocytopenic disorders, splenectomy usually raises the platelet count to normal.[1604,1605] Splenectomy also appears to improve survival and is therefore the recommended treatment for most children with Wiskott-Aldrich syndrome.[1605] However, allogeneic bone marrow transplantation is preferred over splenectomy for those children who have an available HLA-matched sibling donor.[1605,1606]

Both platelet size and PAIgG levels normalize after splenectomy.[1602] To account for the normalization of platelet number, size, and PAIgG after splenectomy, one investigator[1607] related the Wiskott-Aldrich syndrome to hereditary spherocytosis and hypothesized that a platelet cytoskeletal abnormality could result in platelet remodeling by the spleen, with resulting platelet membrane and volume reduction and increased platelet destruction. A heavily sialylated 115-kd membrane glycoprotein termed *sialophorin* is defective in Wiskott-Aldrich lymphocytes.[64,1608] The putative role of sialophorin, which is found on all circulating non-erythroid cells, is to shield cellular senescent antigens.[64]

The cellular immune deficiency makes these patients susceptible to graft-versus-host disease caused by transfused lymphocytes, and platelets and other blood products should be irradiated before administration. These children must receive antibiotic prophylaxis after splenectomy in addition to vaccination before.[1605]

X-Linked Thrombocytopenia (Variant Wiskott-Aldrich Syndrome). Hereditary thrombocytopenia inherited in an X-linked recessive fashion has been described in several families.[1609–1618] Atopic symptoms,[1610,1611,1614–1618] laboratory immunologic abnormalities,[1610,1612,1615,1616,1618] reduced MPV,[1614,1617,1618] and elevated PAIgG[1617,1618] in some affected thrombocytopenic patients suggest a forme fruste relation to the Wiskott-Aldrich syndrome. In contrast to patients with hereditary thrombocytopenia of autosomal dominant inheritance and like patients with the Wiskott-Aldrich syndrome, these patients respond to splenectomy.[1609–1616] In one family with X-linked thrombocytopenia, linkage studies indicated that the abnormal gene was located in the same region as the Wiskott-Aldrich gene.[1618] A family has also been described with apparent X-linked thrombocytopenia in which the platelet size appeared to be normal or increased.[1619]

REFERENCES

1. Pizzolato P. Sternal marrow megakaryocytes in health and disease. Am J Clin Pathol 1948;18:891.
2. Harker L. Megakaryocyte quantitation. J Clin Invest 1968;47:452.
3. Queisser U, Queisser W, Spiertz B. Polyploidization of megakaryocytes in normal humans, in patients with idiopathic thrombocytopenia and with pernicious anaemia. Br J Haematol 1971;20:489.
4. Tomer A, Harker LA, Burstein SA. Purification of human megakaryocytes by fluorescence-activated cell sorting. Blood 1987;70:1735.
5. Tomer A, Friese P, Conklin R, et al. Flow cytometric analysis of megakaryocytes from patients with abnormal platelet counts. Blood 1989;74:594.
6. Berkow RL, Straneva JE, Bruno E, et al. Isolation of human megakaryocytes by density centrifugation and counterflow centrifugal elutriation. J Lab Clin Med 1984;103:811.
7. Smith EB, Butcher J. The incidence, distribution and significance of megakaryocytes in normal and diseased human tissues. Blood 1952; 7:214.
8. Bessis M. The thrombocytic series. In: Bessis M, translated by Weed RI. Living blood cells and their ultrastructure. Berlin, Springer-Verlag, 1973:367.
9. Bessis M. Thrombocytic series. In: Bessis M, translated by Brecher G. Blood smears reinterpreted. Berlin, Springer-Verlag, 1977:129.
10. Penington DG, Streatfield K, Weste SM. Megakaryocyte ploidy and ultrastructure in stimulated thrombopoiesis. In: Baldini MG, Ebbe S, eds. New York, Grune & Stratton, 1974:115.
11. Hoffman R. Regulation of megakaryocytopoiesis. Blood 1989;74:1196.
12. Long MW, Gragowski LL, Heffner CH, Boxer LA. Phorbol diesters stimulate the development of an early murine progenitor cell: the burst-forming unit–megakaryocyte. J Clin Invest 1985;76:431.
13. Briddell RA, Brandt JE, Straneva JE et al. Characterization of the human burst-forming unit–megakaryocyte. Blood 1989;74:145.
14. Mazur EM, Hoffman R, Chasis J, et al. Immunofluorescent identification of human megakaryocyte colonies using an antiplatelet glycoprotein antiserum. Blood 1981;57:277.
15. Levene RB, Williams NT, Lamaziere JMD, Rabellino EM. Human megakaryocytes. IV. Growth and characterization of clonable megakaryocyte progenitors in agar. Exp Hematol 1987;15:181.
16. Piovella F, Nalli G, Malamani GD, et al. The ultrastructural localization of factor VIII–antigen in human platelets, megakaryocytes and endothelial cells utilizing a ferritin-labelled antibody. Br J Haematol 1978;39:209.
17. Jackson CW. Cholinesterase as a possible marker for early cells of the megakaryocyte series. Blood 1973;42:413.
18. Feinendegen LE, Odartchenko N, Cottier H, Bond VP. Kinetics of megacaryocyte proliferation. Proc Soc Exp Biol Med 1962;111:177.
19. Paulus JM. DNA metabolism and development of organelles in guinea-pig megakaryocytes: a combined ultrastructural, autoradiographic and cytophotometric study. Blood 1970;35:298.
20. Lichtman MA, Chamberlain JK, Simon W, Santillo PA. Parasinusoidal location of megakaryocytes in marrow: a determinant of platelet release. Am J Hematol 1978;4:303.
21. Tavassoli M, Aoki M. Localization of megakaryocytes in the bone marrow. Blood Cells 1989;15:3.
22. Becker RP, De Bruyn PPH. The transmural passage of blood cells into myeloid sinusoids and the entry of platelets into the sinusoidal circulation: a scanning electron microscopic investigation. Am J Anat 1976;145:183.
23. Radley JM, Haller CJ. The demarcation membrane system of the megakaryocyte: a misnomer? Blood 1982;60:213.
24. Behnke O, Pedersen TN. Ultrastructural aspects of megakaryocyte maturation and platelet release. In: Baldini GM, Ebbe S, eds. Platelet: production, function, transfusion and storage. New York, Grune & Stratton, 1974:21.
25. Melamed MR, Clifton EE, Mercer C, Koss LG. The megakaryocyte blood count. Am J Med Sci 1966;252:301.
26. Jackson JF. Histochemical identification of megakaryocytes from peripheral blood examined for tumor cells. Cancer 1962;15:259.
27. Kaufman RM, Airo R, Pollack S, et al. Origin of pulmonary megakaryocytes. Blood 1965;25:767.
28. Paulus JM. Platelet size in man. Blood 1975;46:321.
29. Amorosi E, Garg SK, Karpatkin S. Heterogeneity of human platelets. IV. Identification of a young platelet population with [^{75}Se] selenomethionine. Br J Haematol 1971;21:227.
30. Karpatkin S. Heterogeneity of human platelets. I. Metabolic and kinetic evidence suggestive of young and old platelets. J Clin Invest 1969;48: 1073.
31. Penington DG, Lee NLY, Roxburgh AE, McGready JR. Platelet density and size: the interpretation of heterogeneity. Br J Haematol 1976; 34:365.
32. Corash L, Tan H, Gralnick HR. Heterogeneity of human whole blood platelet subpopulations. I. Relationship between buoyant density, cell volume, and ultrastructure. Blood 1977;49:71.
33. Mezzano D, Hwang K, Catalano P, Aster RH. Evidence that platelet buoyant density, but not size, correlates with platelet age in man. Am J Hematol 1981;11:61.
34. Levin J, Bessman JD. The inverse relation between platelet volume and platelet number. J Lab Clin Med 1983;101:295.
35. Martin JF, Penington DG. The relationship between the age and density of circulating ^{51}-Cr labelled platelets in the sub-human primate. Thromb Res 1983;30:157.
36. Savage B, McFadden PR, Hanson SR, Harker LA. The relation of

platelet density to platelet age: survival of low-and high-density ^{111}indium-labeled platelets in baboons. Blood 1986;68:386.
37. Pereira J, Cretney C, Aster RH. Variation of class I HLA antigen expression among platelet density cohorts: a possible index of platelet age? Blood 1988;71:516.
38. Paulus JM, Bury J, Grosdent JC. Control of platelet territory development in megakaryocytes. Blood Cells 1979;5:59.
39. Martin JF, Trowbridge EA, Salmon G, Plumb J. The biological significance of platelet volume: its relationship to bleeding time, platelet thromboxane B_2 production and megakaryocyte nuclear DNA concentration. Thromb Res 1983;32:443.
40. Bessman JD. The relation of megakaryocyte ploidy to platelet volume. Am J Hematol 1984;16:161.
41. Odell TT, Murphy JR, Jackson CW. Stimulation of megakaryocytopoiesis by acute thrombocytopenia in rats. Blood 1976;48:765.
42. Corash L, Chen HY, Levin J, et al. Regulation of thrombopoiesis: effects of the degree of thrombocytopenia on megakaryocyte ploidy and platelet volume. Blood 1987;70:177.
43. Aster RH. Pooling of platelets in the spleen: role in the pathogenesis of "hypersplenic" thrombocytopenia. J Clin Invest 1966;45:645.
44. Penny R, Rozenberg MC, Firkin BG. The splenic platelet pool. Blood 1966;27:1.
45. Harker LA, Finch CA. Thrombokinetics in man. J Clin Invest 1969;48: 963.
46. Wadenvik H, Jacobsson S, Kutti J, Syrjala M. In vitro and in vivo behavior of ^{111}In-labelled platelets: an experimental study of healthy male volunteers. Eur J Haematol 1987;38:415.
47. Peters AM, Klonizakis I, Lavender JP, Lewis SM. Use of ^{111}indium-labelled platelets to measure spleen function. Br J Haematol 1980; 46:587.
48. Peters AM, Lavender JP. Factors controlling the intrasplenic transit of platelets. Eur J Clin Invest 1982;12:191.
49. Peters AM, Saverymuttu SH, Wonke B, et al. The interpretation of platelet kinetic studies for the identification of sites of abnormal platelet destruction. Br J Haematol 1984;57:637.
50. Peters AM, Saverymuttu SH, Bell RN, Lavender JP. The kinetics of short-lived indium-^{111} radiolabelled platelets. Scand J Haematol 1985;34:137.
51. Wadenvik H, Kutti J. The effect of an isoprenaline infusion on the splenic blood flow and intrasplenic platelet kinetics. Eur J Haematol 1987;39:7.
52. Wadenvik H, Denfors I, Kutti J. Splenic blood flow and intrasplenic platelet kinetics in relation to spleen volume. Br J Haematol 1987; 67:181.
53. Peters AM, Saverymuttu SH, Keshavarzian A, et al. Splenic pooling of granulocytes. Clin Sci 1985;68:283.
54. Aas KA, Gardner FH. Survival of blood platelets labeled with chromium^{51}. J Clin Invest 1958;37:1257.
55. Heaton WA, Davis HH, Welch MJ, et al. Indium-111: a new radionuclide label for studying human platelet kinetics. Br J Haematol 1979;42:613.
56. Ginsburg AD, Aster RH. Kinetic studies with ^{51}chromium-labeled platelet cohorts in rats. J Lab Clin Med 1969;74:138.
57. Harker LA. Platelet survival time: its measurement and use. Prog Hemost Thromb 1978;4:321.
58. Hanson SR, Slichter SJ. Platelet kinetics in patients with bone marrow hypoplasia: evidence for a fixed platelet requirement. Blood 1985;66: 1105.
59. Blajchman MA, Senyi AF, Hirsh J, et al. Hemostatic function, survival, and membrane glycoprotein changes in young versus old rabbit platelets. J Clin Invest 1981;68:1289.
60. Meuleman DG, Vogel GMT, Stulemeyer SM, Moelker HCT. Analysis of platelet survival curves in an arterial thrombosis model in rats. Thromb Res 1980;20:31.
61. Steiner M, Vancura S. Asymmetrical loss of sialic acid from membrane glycoproteins during platelet aging. Thromb Res 1985;40:465.
62. Kelton JG, Denomme G. The quantitation of platelet-associated IgG on cohorts of platelets separated from healthy individuals by buoyant density centrifugation. Blood 1982;60:136.
63. Kay MMB. Isolation of the phagocytosis-inducing IgG-binding antigen on senescent somatic cells. Nature 1981;289:491.
64. Remold-O'Donnell E, Zimmerman C, Kenney D, Rosen FS. Expression on blood cells of sialophorin, the surface glycoprotein that is defective in Wiskott-Aldrich syndrome. Blood 1987;70:104.
65. Heyns A du P, Lotter MG, Badenhorst PN, et al. Kinetics, distribution and sites of destruction of ^{111}indium-labelled human platelets. Br J Haematol 1980;44:269.
66. Heyns A du P, Lotter MG, Kotze HF, et al. Quantification of in vivo distribution of platelets labeled with indium-111 oxine. (Letter) J Nucl Med 1982;23:943.
67. Stuart MJ, Murphy S, Oski FA. A simple nonradioisotope technic for determination of platelet life-span. N Engl J Med 1975;292:1310.
68. Boneu A, Sie P, Caranobe C, et al. Platelet regeneration time after aspirin ingestion and platelet survival time after labelling with ^{51}chromium or ^{111}indium oxine: a comparative study. Thromb Haemost 1985;53:260.
69. Boneu B, Sie P, Caranobe C, et al. Malondialdehyde (MDA) reappearance in human platelet density subpopulations after a single intake of aspirin. Thromb Res 1980;19:609.
70. Chamberlain KG, Tong M, Chiu E, Penington DG. The relationship of human platelet density to platelet age: platelet population labeling by monoamine oxidase inhibition. Blood 1989;73:1218.
71. Rand ML, Greenberg JP, Packham MA, Mustard JF. Density subpopulations of rabbit platelets: size, protein, and sialic acid content, and specific radioactivity changes following labeling with ^{35}S-sulphate in vivo. Blood 1981;57:741.
72. Corash L, Shafer B. Use of asplenic rabbits to demonstrate that platelet age and density are related. Blood 1982;60:166.
73. Snyder EL, Moroff G, Simon T, et al. Recommended methods for conducting radiolabeled platelet survival studies. Transfusion 1986; 26:37.
74. Steinberg MH, Kelton JG, Coller BS. Plasma glycocalicin: an aid in the classification of thrombocytopenic disorders. N Engl J Med 1987;317:1037.
75. Beer JH, Büchi L, Steiner B. Glycocalicin: a new assay—the normal plasma levels and its potential usefulness in selected diseases. Blood 1994;83:691.
76. Kienast J, Schmitz G. Flow cytometric analysis of thiazole orange uptake by platelets: a diagnostic aid in the evaluation of thrombocytopenic disorders. Blood 1990;75:116.
77. Sherertz EF. Pigmented purpuric eruptions. Semin Thromb Hemost 1984;10:90.
78. Koster T, Caekebeke-Peerlinck KMJ, Briet E. A randomized and blinded comparison of the sensitivity and the reproducibility of the Ivy and Simplate II® bleeding time techniques. Am J Clin Pathol 1989;92:315.
79. Rodgers RPC, Levin J. A critical reappraisal of the bleeding time. Semin Thromb Hemost 1990;16:1.
80. Lind SE. The bleeding time does not predict surgical bleeding. Blood 1991;77:2547.
81. Burrows RF, Kelton JG. Incidentally detected thrombocytopenia in healthy mothers and their infants. N Engl J Med 1988;319:142.
82. Burrows RF, Kelton JG. Thrombocytopenia at delivery: a prospective survey of 6715 deliveries. Am J Obstet Gynecol 1990;162:731.
83. Rinder HM, Bonan JL, Anandan S, Rinder CS, Rodrigues PA, Smith BR. Noninvasive measurement of platelet kinetics in normal and hypertensive pregnancies. Am J Obstet Gynecol 1994;170:117.
84. Aster RH. Gestational thrombocytopenia. A plea for conservative management. N Engl J Med 1990;323:264.
85. Bessman JD. Platelets. In: Bessman JD. Automated blood counts and differentials: a practical guide. Baltimore, Johns Hopkins University Press, 1986:57.
86. Bessman JD, Gilmer PR, Gardner FH. Use of mean platelet volume improves detection of platelet disorders. Blood Cells 1985;11:127.
87. Van der Lelie J, Von dem Borne AEGK. Platelet volume analysis for differential diagnosis of thrombocytosis. J Clin Pathol 1986;39:129.
88. Gloster ES, Strauss RA, Jiminez JF, et al. Spurious elevated platelet counts associated with bacteremia. Am J Hematol 1985;18:329.
89. Akwari AM, Ross DW, Stass SA. Spuriously elevated platelet counts due to microspherocytosis. Am J Clin Pathol 1982;77:220.
90. Morton BD, Orringer EP, Lattart LA, Stass SA. Pappenheimer bodies: an additional cause for a spurious platelet count. Am J Clin Pathol 1980;74:310.
91. Stass SA, Holloway ML, Peterson V, et al. Cytoplasmic fragments causing spurious platelet counts in the leukemic phase of poorly differentiated lymphocytic leukemia. Am J Clin Pathol 1979;71:125.
92. Nilsson T, Norberg B. Thrombocytopenia and pseudothrombocytopenia: a clinical and laboratory problem. Scand J Haematol 1986; 37:341.
93. Payne BA, Pierre RV. Pseudothrombocytopenia: a laboratory artifact with potentially serious consequences. Mayo Clin Proc 1984;59: 123.
94. Berkman N, Michaeli Y, Or R, Eldor A. EDTA-dependent pseudothrombocytopenia: a clinical study of 18 patients and a review of the literature. Am J Hematol 1991;36:195.
95. Pegels JG, Bruynes ECE, Engelfriet CP, Von dem Borne AEGK. Pseudothrombocytopenia: an immunologic study on platelet antibodies dependent on ethylene diamine tetra-acetate. Blood 1982;59:157.
96. Van Vliet HH, Kappers-Klunne MC, Abels J. Pseudothrombocytopenia: a cold antibody against platelet glycoprotein GP IIb. Br J Haematol 1986;62:501.
97. Veenhoven WA, Van der Schans GS, Huiges W, et al. Pseudothrombocytopenia due to agglutinins. Am J Clin Pathol 1979;72:1005.
98. Prchal JT, Blakely J. Granulocyte platelet rosettes. (Letter) N Engl J Med 1973;289:1146.
99. Greipp PR, Gralnick HR. Platelet to leukocyte adherence phenomena associated with thrombocytopenia. Blood 1976;47:513.
100. Cohen AM, Lewinski UH, Klein B, Djaldetti M. Satellitism of platelets to monocytes. Acta Hematol 1980;64:61.
101. McGregor DH, Davis JW, Liu PI, et al. Platelet satellitism: experimental studies. Lab Invest 1980;42:343.
102. Bizzaro N. Platelet satellitosis to polymorphonuclears: cytochemical, immunological, and ultrastructural characterization of eight cases. Am J Hematol 1991;36:235.

103. Watkins SP Jr, Shulman NR. Platelet cold agglutinins. Blood 1970; 36:153.
104. Cunningham VL, Brandt JT. Spurious thrombocytopenia due to EDTA-independent cold-reactive agglutinins. Am J Clin Pathol 1992;97:359.
105. Hoyt RH, Durie BGM. Pseudothrombocytopenia induced by a monoclonal IgM kappa platelet agglutinin. Am J Hematol 1989;31:50.
106. Pewarchuk W, VanderBoom J, Blajchman MA. Pseudopolycythemia, pseudothrombocytopenia, and pseudoleukopenia due to overfilling of blood collection vacuum tubes. Arch Pathol Lab Med 1992;116:90.
107. Forscher CA, Sussman II, Friedman EW, et al. Pseudothrombocytopenia masking true thrombocytopenia. Am J Hematol 1985;18:313.
108. Berning H, Stilbo I. Pseudothrombocytopenia and the haematology laboratory. (Letter) Lancet 1982;2:1469.
109. Kelton JG, Ali AM. Platelet transfusions: a critical appraisal. Clin Oncol 1983;2:549.
110. Gardner FH, Helmer RE III. Aminocaproic acid: use in control of hemorrhage in patients with amegakaryocytic thrombocytopenia. JAMA 1980;243:35.
111. Garewal HS, Durie BGM. Anti-fibrinolytic therapy with aminocaproic acid for the control of bleeding in thrombocytopenic patients. Scand J Haematol 1985;35:497.
112. Fricke W, Alling D, Kimball J. Lack of efficacy of tranexamic acid in thrombocytopenic bleeding. Transfusion 1991;31:345.
113. Konkle BA, Shapiro SS, Asch AS, Nachman RL. Cytokine-enhanced expression of glycoprotein Ib_α in human endothelium. J Biol Chem 1990;265:19833.
114. George JN, Nurden AT, Phillips DR. Molecular defects in interactions of platelets with the vessel wall. N Engl J Med 1984;311:1084.
115. Houdijk WPM, Sakariassen KS, Nievelstein PFEM, Sixma JJ. Role of factor VIII–von Willebrand factor and fibronectin in the interaction of platelets in flowing blood with monomeric and fibrillar human collagen types I and III. J Clin Invest 1985;75:531.
116. Clemetson KJ, McGregor JL, James E, et al. Characterization of the platelet membrane glycoprotein abnormalities in Bernard-Soulier syndrome and comparison with normal by surface-labeling techniques and high-resolution two-dimensional gel electrophoresis. J Clin Invest 1982;70:304.
117. Berndt MC, Phillips DR. Purification and preliminary physicochemical characterization of human platelet membrane glycoprotein V. J Biol Chem 1981;256:59.
118. Woods VL Jr, Kurata Y, Montgomery RR, et al. Autoantibodies against platelet glycoprotein Ib in patients with chronic immune thrombocytopenic purpura. Blood 1984;64:156.
119. Szatkowski NS, Kunicki TJ, Aster RH. Identification of glycoprotein Ib as a target for autoantibody in idiopathic (autoimmune) thrombocytopenic purpura. Blood 1986;67:310.
120. McMillan R, Tani P, Millard F, et al. Platelet-associated and plasma anti-glycoprotein autoantibodies in chronic ITP. Blood 1987;70:1040.
121. Kiefel V, Santoso S, Katzmann E, Mueller-Eckhardt C. Autoantibodies against platelet glycoprotein Ib/IX: a frequent finding in autoimmune thrombocytopenic purpura. Br J Haematol 1991;79:256.
122. Kunicki TJ, Newman PJ. The molecular immunology of human platelet proteins. Blood 1992;80:1386.
123. Nugent DJ. Autoimmune thrombocytopenic purpura. In: Bona CA, Siminovitch KA, Zanetti M, Theofilopoulos AN, eds. The Molecular Pathology of Autoimmune Diseases. Switzerland, Harwood Publishers, 1993:471.
124. Berndt MC, Chong BH, Bull HA, et al. Molecular characterization of quinine/quinidine drug-dependent antibody platelet interaction using monoclonal antibodies. Blood 1985;66:1292.
125. Nieminen U, Kekomäki R. Quinidine-induced thrombocytopenic purpura: clinical presentation in relation to drug-dependent and drug-independent platelet antibodies. Br J Haematol 1992;80:77
126. Murata M, Furihata K, Ishida F, et al. Genetic and structural characterization of an amino acid dimorphism in glycoprotein Ibα involved in platelet transfusion refractoriness. Blood 1992;79:3086.
127. Bird GWG, Wingham J, Pippard, et al. Erythrocyte membrane modification in malignant diseases of myeloid and lymphoreticular tissue. I. Tn-polyagglutination in acute myeloid leukeamia. Br J Haematol 1976;33:289.
128. Ness PM, Garraty G, Morel PA, Perkins HA. Tn polyagglutination preceding acute leukemia. Blood 1979;54:30.
129. Blanchard D, Kieffer N, Nurden AT, Cartron JP. Structural modifications of platelet membrane glycoprotein GPIb in the Tn syndrome. Curr Stud Hematol Blood Transfus 1988;55:45.
130. Hynes RO. Integrins: a family of cell surface receptors. Cell 1987;48: 549.
131. Kunicki TJ. The molecular biology of platelet membrane glycoproteins. Transfus Med Rev 1990;4:91.
132. Ruoslahti E. Integrins. J Clin Invest 1991;87:1.
133. Plow EF, Pierschbacher MD, Ruoslahti E, et al. The effect of Arg-Gly-Asp-containing peptides on fibrinogen and von Willebrand factor binding to platelets. Proc Natl Acad Sci USA 1985;82:8057.
134. Pidard D, Montgomery RR, Bennett JS, Kunicki TJ. Interaction of AP-2, a monoclonal antibody specific for the human platelet glycoprotein IIb–IIIa complex, with intact platelets. J Biol Chem 1983;258: 12582.
135. Charo IF, Bekeart LS, Phillips DR. Platelet glycoprotein IIb-IIIa–like proteins mediate endothelial cell attachment to adhesive proteins and the extracellular matrix. J Biol Chem 1987;262:9935.
136. Lam SCT, Plow EF, D'Souza SE, et al. Isolation and characterization of a platelet membrane protein related to the vitronectin receptor. J Biol Chem 1989;264:3742.
137. Pischel KD, Bluestein HG, Woods VL Jr. Platelet glycoproteins Ia, Ic, and IIa are physicochemically indistinguishable from the very late activation antigens adhesion-related proteins of lymphocytes and other cell types. J Clin Invest 1988;81:505.
138. Nieuwenhuis HK, Akkerman JWN, Houdijk WPM, Sixma JJ. Human blood platelets showing no response to collagen fail to express surface glycoprotein Ia. Nature 1985;318:470.
139. Nieuwenhuis HK, Sakariassen KS, Houdijk WPM, et al. Deficiency of platelet membrane glycoprotein Ia associated with a decreased platelet adhesion to subendothelium: a defect in platelet spreading. Blood 1986;68:692.
140. Santoro SA. Identification of a 160,000 dalton platelet membrane protein that mediates the initial divalent cation–dependent adhesion of platelets to collagen. Cell 1986;46:913.
141. Kunicki TJ, Nugent DJ, Staats S, et al. The human fibroblast class II extracellular matrix receptor mediates platelet adhesion to collagen and is identical to the platelet glycoprotein Ia-IIa complex. J Biol Chem 1988;263:4516.
142. Piotrowicz RS, Orchekowski RP, Nugent DJ, et al. Glycoprotein Ic–IIa functions as an activation-independent fibronectin receptor on human platelets. J Cell Biol 1988;106:1359.
143. Sonnenberg A, Modderman PW, Hogervorst F. Laminin receptor on platelets is the integrin VLA-6. Nature 1988;336:487.
144. Van Leeuwen EF, Van der Ven JTM, Engelfriet CP, Von dem Borne AEGK. Specificity of autoantibodies in autoimmune thrombocytopenia. Blood 1982;59:23.
145. Beardsley DS, Spiegel JE, Jacobs MM, et al. Platelet membrane glycoprotein IIIa contains target antigens that bind anti-platelet antibodies in immune thrombocytopenias. J Clin Invest 1984;74:1701.
146. Woods VL Jr, Oh EH, Mason D, McMillan R. Autoantibodies against the platelet glycoprotein IIb/IIIa complex in patients with chronic ITP. Blood 1984;63:368.
147. Devine DV, Rosse WF. Identification of platelet proteins that bind alloantibodies and autoantibodies. Blood 1984;64:1240.
148. Christie DJ, Mullen PC, Aster RH. Quinine- and quinidine platelet antibodies can react with GPIIb/IIIa. Br J Haematol 1987;67:213.
149. Newman PJ, Martin LS, Knipp MA, Kahn RA. Studies on the nature of the human platelet alloantigen, Pl^{A1}: localization to a 17,000-dalton polypeptide. Mol Immunol 1985;22:719.
150. Fitzgerald LA, Steiner B, Rall SC Jr, et al. Protein sequence of endothelial glycoprotein IIIa derived from a cDNA clone: identity with platelet glycoprotein IIIa and similarity to "integrin." J Biol Chem 1987;262:3936.
151. Zimrin AB, Eisman R, Vilaire G, et al. Structure of platelet glycoprotein IIIa: a common subunit for two different membrane receptors. J Clin Invest 1988;81:1470.
152. Rosa JP, Bray PF, Gayet O, et al. Cloning of glycoprotein IIIa cDNA from human erythroleukemia cells and localization of the gene to chromosome 17. Blood 1988;72:593.
153. Newman PJ, Derbes RS, Aster RH. The human platelet alloantigens, Pl^{A1} and Pl^{A2}, are associated with a $leucine^{33}/proline^{33}$ amino acid polymorphism in membrane glycoprotein IIIa, and are distinguishable by DNA typing. J Clin Invest 1989;83:1778.
154. Santoso S, Mueller-Eckhardt G, Santoso S, et al. HLA antigens on platelet membranes: in vitro and in vivo studies. Vox Sang 1986; 51:327.
155. Haynes WDG, Jones JV, Cumming JCO. HL-A antigens on circulating platelets: ultrastructural demonstration. Transplantation 1974;18:81.
156. Aster RH, Szatkowski N, Liebert M, Duquesnoy RJ. Expression of HLA-B12, HLA-B8, w4 and w6 on platelets. Transplant Proc 1977;9: 1695.
157. Liebert M, Aster RH. Expression of HLA-B12 on platelets, on lymphocytes and in serum: a quantitative study. Tissue Antigens 1977; 9:199.
158. Mueller-Eckhardt G, Hauck M, Kayser W, Mueller-Eckhardt C. HLA-C antigens on platelets. Tissue Antigens 1980;16:91.
159. Pearson HA, Shulman NR, Marder VJ, Cone TE Jr. Isoimmune neonatal thrombocytopenic purpura: clinical and therapeutic considerations. Blood 1964;23:154.
160. Evans D. Immune amegakaryocytic thrombocytopenia of the newborn: association with anti-HLA-A2. J Clin Pathol 1987;40:258.
161. Kelton JG, Hamid C, Aker S, Blajchman MA. The amount of blood group A substance on platelets is proportional to the amount in the plasma. Blood 1982;59:980.
162. Dunstan RA, Simpson MB, Knowles RW, Rosse WF. The origin of ABH antigens on human platelets. Blood 1985;65:615.
163. Santoso S, Kiefel V, Mueller-Eckhardt C. Blood groups A and B determinants are expressed on platelet glycoproteins IIa, IIIa and Ib. Thromb Haemost 1991;65:196.
164. Dunstan RA, Simpson MB, Rosse WF. Le^a blood group antigen on human platelets. Am J Clin Pathol 1985;83:90.

165. Dunstan RA, Simpson MB, Rosse WF. The presence of the Ii blood group system on human platelets. Am J Clin Pathol 1984;82:74.
166. Dunstan RA, Simpson MB, Rosse WF. Presence of P blood group antigens on human platelets. Am J Clin Pathol 1985;83:731.
167. Dunstan RA, Simpson MB, Rosse WF. Erythrocyte antigens on human platelets: absence of Rh, Duffy, Kell, Kidd and Lutheran antigens. Transfusion 1984;24:243.
168. Mollicone R, Caillard T, Le Pendu J, et al. Expression of ABH and X (Le^X) antigens on platelets and lymphocytes. Blood 1988;71:1113.
169. Dunstan RA, Simpson MB. Heterogeneous distribution of antigens on human platelets demonstrated by fluorescence flow cytometry. Br J Haematol 1985;61:603.
170. Aster RH. Effect of anticoagulant and ABO incompatibility on recovery of transfused human platelets. Blood 1965;26:732.
171. Duquesnoy RJ, Anderson AJ, Tomasulo PA, Aster RH. ABO compatibility and platelet transfusions of alloimmunized thrombocytopenic patients. Blood 1979;54:595.
172. Brand A, Sintnicolaas K, Claas FHJ, Eernisse JG. ABH antibodies causing platelet transfusion refractoriness. Transfusion 1986;26:463.
173. Heal JM, Blumberg N, Masel D. An evaluation of crossmatching, HLA, and ABO matching for platelet transfusions to refractory patients. Blood 1987;70:23.
174. Murphy S. ABO blood groups and platelet transfusion. Transfusion 1988;28:401.
175. Skogen B, Rossebo Hansen B, Husebekk A, et al. Minimal expression of blood group A antigen on thrombocytes from A_2 individuals. Transfusion 1988;28:456.
176. Lee EJ, Schiffer CA. ABO compatibility can influence the results of platelet transfusions: results of a randomized trial. Transfusion 1989;29:384.
177. Schick PK. Platelet glycolipids. In: Kunicki TJ, George JN, eds. Platelet immunobiology. Philadelphia, JB Lippincott, 1989:31.
178. Marcus DM, Schwarting GA. Immunolochemical properties of glycolipids and phospholipids. Adv Immunol 1976;23:203.
179. Van Vliet HHDM, Kappers-Klunne MC, Van der Hel JWB, Abels J. Antibodies against glycosphingolipids in sera of patients with idiopathic thrombocytopenic purpura. Br J Haematol 1987;67:103.
180. Koerner TAW, Weinfeld HM, Bullard LSB, Williams LCJ. Antibodies against platelet glycosphingolipids: detection in serum by quantitative HPTLC-autoradiography and association with autoimmune and alloimmune processes. Blood 1989;74:274.
181. Murakami H, Lam Z, Furie BC, et al. Sulfated glycolipids are the platelet autoantigens for human platelet-binding monoclonal anti-DNA autoantibodies. J Biol Chem 1991;266:15414.
182. Marcus AJ, Ullman HL, Safier LB. Lipid composition of subcellular particles of human blood platelets. J Lipid Res 1969;10:108.
183. Chap HJ, Zwaal RFA, Van Deenen LLM. Action of highly purified phospholipases on blood platelets: evidence for an asymmetric distribution of phospholipids in the surface membrane. Biochim Biophys Acta 1977;467:146.
184. Zwaal RFA. Membrane and lipid involvement in blood coagulation. Biochim Biophys Acta 1978;515:163.
185. Harris EN, Gharavi AE, Hegde U, et al. Anticardiolipin antibodies in autoimmune thrombocytopenic purpura. Br J Haematol 1985;59:231.
186. Von dem Borne AEGK, Van der Lelie H, Vos JJE, et al. Antibodies against cryptantigens of platelets: characterization and significance for the serologist. Curr Stud Hematol Blood Transfus 1986;52:33.
187. Nugent DJ, Kunicki TJ, Berglund C, Bernstein ID. A human monoclonal autoantibody recognizes a neoantigen on glycoprotein IIIa expressed on stored and activated platelets. Blood 1987;70:16.
188. Kelton JG, Steeves K. The amount of platelet-bound albumin parallels the amount of IgG on washed platelets from patients with immune thrombocytopenia. Blood 1983;62:924.
189. George JN, Saucerman S. Platelet IgG, IgM, and albumin: correlation of platelet and plasma concentrations in normal subjects and in patients with ITP or dysproteinemia. Blood 1988;72:362.
190. George JN, Saucerman S, Levine SP, et al. Immunoglobulin G is a platelet alpha granule-secreted protein. J Clin Invest 1985;76:2020.
191. Sixma JJ, Van den Berg A, Schiphorst M, et al. Immunocytochemical localization of albumin and factor XIII in thin cryo sections of human blood platelets. Thromb Haemost 1984;51:388.
192. Cramer EM, Debili N, Martin JF et al. Uncoordinated expression of fibrinogen compared with thrombospondin and von Willebrand factor in maturing human megakaryocytes. Blood 1989;73:1123.
193. Handagama PJ, Shuman MA, Bainton DF. Incorporation of intravenously injected albumin, immunoglobulin G, and fibrinogen in guinea pig megakaryocyte granules. J Clin Invest 1989;84:73.
194. Harrison P, Wilbourn B, Debili N et al. Uptake of plasma fibrinogen into the alpha granules of human megakaryocytes and platelets. J Clin Invest 1989;84:1320.
195. Clejan L, Menahem M. Binding of deoxyribonucleic acid to the surface of human platelets. Acta Haematol 1977;58:84.
196. Kelton JG. The measurement of platelet-bound immunoglobulins: an overview of the methods and the biological relevance of platelet-associated IgG. Progr Hematol 1983;13:163.
197. Sinha RK, Horsewood P, Warkentin TE, Hayward CPM, Kelton JG. Nonimmune and immune binding of IgG to platelets in immune thrombocytopenia. Blood 1994, in press.
198. Asano T, Furie BC, Furie B. Platelet binding properties of monoclonal lupus autoantibodies produced by human hybridomas. Blood 1985;66:1254.
199. Jacob L, Lety MA, Louvard D, Bach JF. Binding of a monoclonal anti-DNA autoantibody to identical protein(s) present at the surface of several human cell types involved in lupus pathogenesis. J Clin Invest 1985;75:315.
200. Rauch J, Meng QH, Tannenbaum H. Lupus anticoagulant and anti-platelet properties of human hybridoma autoantibodies. J Immunol 1987;139:2598.
201. Kelton JG, Keystone J, Moore J, et al. Immune-mediated thrombocytopenia of malaria. J Clin Invest 1983;71:832.
202. Rosenfeld SI, Looney RJ, Leddy JP, et al. Human platelet Fc receptor for immunoglobulin G: identification as a 40,000 molecular-weight membrane protein shared by monocytes. J Clin Invest 1985;76:2317.
203. Kelton JG, Smith JW, Santos AV, et al. Platelet IgG Fc receptor. Am J Hematol 1987;25:299.
204. Rosenfeld SI, Anderson CL. Fc receptors of human platelets. In: Kunicki TJ, George JN, eds. Platelet immunobiology. Philadelphia, JB Lippincott, 1989:337.
205. Kelton JG, Sheridan D, Santos A, et al. Heparin-induced thrombocytopenia: laboratory studies. Blood 1988;72:925.
206. Deykin D, Hellerstein LJ. The assessment of drug-dependent and isoimmune antiplatelet antibodies by the use of platelet aggregometry. J Clin Invest 1972;51:3142.
207. Pogliani E, Lambertenghi Deliliers G, Ferrari R, et al. Platelet aggregometry and anti-platelet isoantibodies. Haemostasis 1975;4:23.
208. Hirschman RJ, Shulman NR. The use of platelet serotonin release as a sensitive method for detecting anti-platelet antibodies and a plasma anti-platelet factor in patients with idiopathic thrombocytopenic purpura. Br J Haematol 1973;24:793.
209. Gockerman JP, Bowman RP, Conrad ME. Detection of platelet isoantibodies by [^{3}H] serotonin platelet release and its clinical application to the problem of platelet matching. J Clin Invest 1975;55:75.
210. Karpatkin S, Strick N, Karpatkin MB, Siskind GW. Cumulative experience in the detection of antiplatelet antibody in 234 patients with idiopathic thrombocytopenic purpura, systemic lupus erythematosus and other clinical disorders. Am J Med 1972;52:776.
211. Mueller-Eckhardt C, Mersch-Baumert K. The problem of platelet autoantibodies. I. Evaluation of the platelet factor 3 availability test for their detection. Vox Sang 1977;33:221.
212. Duquesnoy RJ, Lorentsen DF, Aster RH. Platelet migration inhibition: A new method for detection of platelet antibodies. Blood 1975; 45:741.
213. Sheridan D, Carter C, Kelton JG. A diagnostic test for heparin-induced thrombocytopenia. Blood 1986;67:27.
214. Warkentin TE, Hayward CPM, Smith CA, et al. Determinants of donor platelet variability when testing for heparin-induced thrombocytopenia. J Lab Clin Med 1992;120:371.
215. Mueller-Eckhardt C, Mahn I, Schulz G, Mueller-Eckhardt G. Detection of platelet autoantibodies by a radioactive anti-immunoglobulin test. Vox Sang 1978;35:357.
216. Boonpucknavig S, Vuttivirojana O, Srichaikul T. Immunofluorescent staining of platelet suspensions and detection of antiplatelet antibody in patients with idiopathic thrombocytopenic purpura. Vox Sang 1979;36:115.
217. Von dem Borne AEGK, Helmerhorst FM, Van Leeuwen EF, et al. Autoimmune thrombocytopenia: detection of platelet autoantibodies with the suspension immunofluorescence test. Br J Haematol 1980; 45:319.
218. Gudino M, Miller WV. Application of the enzyme linked immunospecific assay (ELISA) for the detection of platelet antibodies. Blood 1981;57:32.
219. LoBuglio AF, Court WS, Vinocur L, et al. Immune thrombocytopenic purpura: use of a ^{125}I-labeled antihuman IgG monoclonal antibody to quantify platelet-bound IgG. N Engl J Med 1983;309:459.
220. Shaw GM, Axelson J, Maglott JG, LoBuglio AF. Quantification of platelet-bound IgG by ^{125}I-staphylococcal protein A in immune thrombocytopenic purpura and other thrombocytopenic disorders. Blood 1984;63:154.
221. Cines DB, Schreiber AD. Immune thrombocytopenia: use of a Coombs antiglobulin test to detect IgG and C3 on platelets. N Engl J Med 1979;300:106.
222. Sugiura K, Steiner M, Baldini MG. Platelet antibody in idiopathic thrombocytopenic purpura and other thrombocytopenias: a quantitative, sensitive, and rapid assay. J Lab Clin Med 1980;96:640.
223. Lazarchick J, Hall SA. Platelet-associated IgG assay using flow cytometric analysis. J Immunol Methods 1986;87:257.
224. Rosenfeld CS, Nichols G, Bodensteiner DC. Flow cytometric measurement of antiplatelet antibodies. Am J Clin Pathol 1987;87:518.
225. Heaton WA, Holme S, Hartman P. Elevated levels of PA IgG in thrombocytopenic patients are not related to the presence of microthrombocytes or megathrombocytes. Am J Clin Pathol 1988;89:88.
226. Dixon R, Rosse W, Ebbert L. Quantitative determination of antibody in idiopathic thrombocytopenic purpura: correlation of serum and platelet-bound antibody in clinical response. N Engl J Med 1975; 292:230.
227. Kelton JG, Denomme G, Walker C, et al. The measurement of platelet-

associated IgG using an immunoradiometric assay. J Immunoassay 1983;4:65.
228. Hegde UM, Gordon-Smith EC, Worlledge S. Platelet antibodies in thrombocytopenic patients. Br J Haematol 1977;35:113.
229. Vos JJE, Huisman JG, Van der Lelie J, Von dem Borne AEGK. Platelet-associated IgG in thrombocytopenia: a comparison of two techniques. Vox Sang 1987;53:162.
230. Rosse WF, Devine DV, Ware R. Reactions of immunoglobulin G-binding ligands with platelets and platelet-associated immunoglobulin G. J Clin Invest 1984;73:489.
231. Blumberg N, Masel D, Stoler M. Disparities in estimates of IgG bound to normal platelets. Blood 1986;67:200.
232. Kelton JG, Murphy WG, Lucarelli A, et al. A prospective comparison of four techniques for measuring platelet-associated IgG. Br J Haematol 1989;71:97.
233. Luiken GA, McMillan R, Lightsey AL, et al. Platelet-associated IgG in immune thrombocytopenic purpura. Blood 1977;50:317.
234. Morse BS, Giuliani D, Nussbaum M. Quantitation of platelet-associated IgG by radial immunodiffusion. Blood 1981;57:809.
235. Morse BS, Giuliani D, Nussbaum M. A rapid quantitation of platelet-associated IgG by nephelometry. Am J Hematol 1982;12:271.
236. Kelton JG, Denomme G, Lucarelli A, et al. Comparison of the measurement of surface or total platelet-associated IgG in the diagnosis of immune thrombocytopenia. Am J Hematol 1985;18:1.
237. Cheung NKV, McFall P, Schulman I. A microtiter solid-phase radioimmunoassay for platelet-associated immunoglobulin G. J Lab Clin Med 1983;101:392.
238. Gibbons S, Kelton JG. Assessment of the optimal anticoagulant solution for storage of whole blood samples prior to measurement of platelet-associated IgG. Transfusion 1982;22:295.
239. Lippi U, Schinella M, Modena N, Nicoli M. Unpredictable effects of K_3 EDTA on mean platelet volume. Am J Clin Pathol 1987;87: 391.
240. Lucas GF, Holburn AM. The effect of anticoagulant on platelet associated IgG. Br J Haematol 1987;65:111.
241. McMillan R, Mason D, Tani P, Schmidt GM. Evaluation of platelet surface antigens: localization of the Pl^{A1} alloantigen. Br J Haematol 1982;51:297.
242. Reid DM, Jones CE, Vostal JG, Shulman NR. Western blot identification of platelet proteins that bind normal serum immunoglobulins: characteristics of a 95-Kd reactive protein. Blood 1990;75:2194.
243. Reid DM, Jones CE, Luo CY, Shulman NR. Immunoglobulins from normal sera bind platelet vinculin and talin and their proteolytic fragments. Blood 1993;81:745.
244. Degos L, Tobelem G, Lethielleux P, et al. Molecular defect in platelets from patients with Bernard-Soulier syndrome. Blood 1977;50:899.
245. Tomiyama Y, Take H, Honda S, et al. Demonstration of platelet antigens that bind platelet-associated autoantibodies in chronic ITP by direct immunoprecipitation procedure. Br J Haematol 1990;75:92.
246. Kurata Y, Hayashi S, Kosugi S, et al. Elevated platelet-associated IgG in SLE patients due to anti-platelet autoantibody: differentiation between autoantibodies and immune complexes by ether elution. Br J Haematol 1993;85:723.
247. Smith JW, Hayward CPM, Warkentin TE, et al. Investigation of human platelet alloantigens and glycoproteins using non-radioactive immunoprecipitation. J Immunol Methods 1993;158:77.
248. Kiefel V, Santoso S, Weisheit M, Mueller-Eckhardt C. Monoclonal antibody-specific immobilization of platelet antigens (MAIPA): a new tool for the identification of platelet-reactive antibodies. Blood 1987;70: 1722.
249. Kiefel V. The MAIPA assay and its applications in immunohaematology. Transfus Med 1992;2:181.
250. Tsubakio T, Tani P, Woods VL Jr, McMillan R. Autoantibodies against platelet GPIIb/IIIa in chronic ITP react with different epitopes. Br J Haematol 1987;67:345.
251. Hewitt J, Burton IE. Incidence of autoantibodies to GPIIb/IIIa in chronic autoimmune thrombocytopenic purpura may be overestimated by the MAIPA. Br J Haematol 1994;86:418.
252. Kelton JG, Murphy WG. Techniques used to measure immunoglobulins on platelets. In: Dutcher JP, ed. Modern transfusion therapy II. Boca Raton, CRC Press, 1989:97.
253. Sinha RK, Kelton JG. Current controversies concerning the measurement of platelet-associated IgG. Transfus Med Rev 1990;4:121.
254. Kiefel V, Jager S, Mueller-Eckhardt C. Competitive enzyme-linked immunoassay for the quantitation of platelet-associated immunoglobulins (IgG, IgM, IgA) and complement (C3c, C3d) with polyclonal and monoclonal reagents. Vox Sang 1987;53:151.
255. Hotchkiss AJ, Leissinger CA, Smith ME, et al. Evaluation by quantitative acid elution and radioimmunoassay of multiple classes of immunoglobulins and serum albumin associated with platelets in idiopathic thrombocytopenic purpura. Blood 1986;67:1126.
256. Kelton JG, Powers PJ, Carter CJ. A prospective study of the usefulness of the measurement of platelet-associated IgG for the diagnosis of idiopathic thrombocytopenic purpura. Blood 1982;60:1050.
257. Mueller-Eckhardt C, Kayser W, Mersch-Baumert K, et al. The clinical significance of platelet associated IgG: a study on 298 patients with various disorders. Br J Haematol 1980;46:123.
258. Arnott J, Horsewood P, Kelton JG. Measurement of platelet-associated IgG in animal models of immune and nonimmune thrombocytopenia. Blood 1987;69:1294.
259. Geroge JN. Platelet immunoglobulin G: its significance for the evaluation of thrombocytopenia and for understanding the origin of α-granules proteins. Blood 1990;76:859.
260. Behnke O. Surface membrane clearing of receptor-ligand complexes in human blood platelets. J Cell Sci 1987;87:465.
261. Spycher MO, Nydegger UE. Part of the activating cross-linked immunoglobulin G is internalized by human platelets to sites not accessible for enzymatic digestion. Blood 1986;67:12.
262. Hymes K, Schur PH, Karpatkin S. Heavy chain subclass of bound antiplatelet IgG in autoimmune thrombocytopenic purpura. Blood 1980;56:84.
263. Rosse WF, Adams JP, Yount WJ. Subclasses of IgG antibodies in immune thrombocytopenic purpura (ITP). Br J Haematol 1980;46:109.
264. Harrington WJ, Minnich V, Hollingsworth JW, Moore CV. Demonstration of a thrombocytopenic factor in the blood of patients with thrombocytopenic purpura. J Lab Clin Med 1951;38:1.
265. Nel JD, Stevens K, Mouton A, Pretorius FJ. Platelet-bound IgM in autoimmune thrombocytopenia. Blood 1983;61:119.
266. Hegde UM, Ball S, Zuiable A, Roter BLT. Platelet associated immunoglobulins (PAIgG and PAIgM) in autoimmune thrombocytopenia. Br J Haematol 1985;59:221.
267. Cines DB, Wilson SB, Tomaski A, Schreiber AD. Platelet antibodies of the IgM class in immune thrombocytopenic purpura. J Clin Invest 1985;75:1183.
268. McMillan R, Longmire RL, Yelenosky R, et al. Immunoglobulin synthesis in vitro by splenic tissue in idiopathic thrombocytopenic purpura. N Engl J Med 1972;286:681.
269. Mason D, McMillan R. Platelet antigens in chronic idiopathic thrombocytopenic purpura. Br J Haematol 1984;56:529.
270. McMillan R, Martin M. Fixation of C3 to platelets in vitro by antiplatelet antibody from patients with immune thrombocytopenic purpura. Br J Haematol 1981;47:251.
271. Han P, Turpie AGG, Genton E. Plasma β-thromboglobulin: differentiation between intravascular and extravascular platelet destruction. Blood 1979;54:1192.
272. Van Leeuwen EF, Van der Ven JTH, Engelfriet CP, Von dem Borne AEG. Specificity of autoantibodies in autoimmune thrombocytopenia. Blood 1982;59:23.
273. Aster RH, Keene WR. Sites of platelet destruction in idiopathic thrombocytopenic purpura. Br J Haematol 1969;16:61.
274. Harker LA. Thrombokinetics in idiopathic thrombocytopenic purpura. Br J Haematol 1970;19:95.
275. Branehog I, Kutti J, Weinfeld A. Platelet survival and platelet production in idiopathic thrombocytopenic purpura (ITP). Br J Haematol 1974;27:127.
276. Grossi A, Vannucchi AM, Casprini P, et al. Different patterns of platelet turnover in chronic idiopathic thrombocytopenic purpura. Scand J Haematol 1983;31:206.
277. Schmidt KG, Rasmussen JW. Kinetics and distribution in vivo of ^{111}In-labelled autologous platelets in idiopathic thrombocytopenic purpura. Scand J Haematol 1985;34:47.
278. Heyns A du P, Lotter MG, Badenhorst PN, et al. Kinetics and sites of destruction of 111-indium-oxine–labeled platelets in idiopathic thrombocytopenic purpura: a quantitative study. Am J Hematol 1982;12:167.
279. Ballem PJ, Segal GM, Stratton JR, et al. Mechanisms of thrombocytopenia in chronic autoimmune thrombocytopenic purpura: evidence of both impaired platelet production and increased platelet clearance. J Clin Invest 1987;80:33.
280. Siegel RS, Rae JL, Barth S, et al. Platelet survival and turnover: important factors in predicting response to splenectomy in immune thrombocytopenic purpura. Am J Hematol 1989;30:206.
281. McMillan R, Luiken GA, Levy R, et al. Antibody against megakaryocytes in idiopathic thrombocytopenic purpura. JAMA 1978;239:2460.
282. McMillan R, Longmire RL, Tavassoli M, et al. In vitro platelet phagocytosis by splenic leucocytes in idiopathic thrombocytopenic purpura. N Engl J Med 1974;290:249.
283. Karpatkin S, Fotino M, Gibofsky A, Winchester RJ. Association of HLA-DRw2 with autoimmune thrombocytopenic purpura. J Clin Invest 1979;63:1085.
284. Mayr WR, Mueller-Eckhardt G, Kruger M, et al. HLA-DR in chronic idiopathic thrombocytopenic purpura (ITP). Tissue Antigens 1981; 18:56.
285. McMillan R, Pellegrino MA, Ferrone S. Letter. Blood 1980;55:709.
286. Mylvaganam R, Ahn YS, Harrington WJ, et al. Differences in T cell subsets between men and women with idiopathic thrombocytopenic purpura. Blood 1985;66:967.
287. Mizutani H, Katagiri S, Uejima K, et al. T-cell abnormalities in patients with idiopathic thrombocytopenic purpura: the presence of OKT4+8+ cells. Scand J Haematol 1985;35:233.
288. Mizutani H, Tsubakio T, Tomiyama Y, et al. Increased circulating Ia-positive T cells in patients with idiopathic thrombocytopenic purpura. Clin Exp Immunol 1987;67:191.
289. Zinberg M, Francus T, Weksler ME, et al. Abnormal autologous mixed lymphocyte reaction in autoimmune thrombocytopenic purpura. Blood 1982;59:148.

290. Mylvaganam R, Garcia RO, Ahn YS, et al. Depressed functional and phenotypic properties of T but not B lymphocytes in idiopathic thrombocytopenic purpura. Blood 1988;71:1455.
291. Hiraiwa A, Nugent DJ, Milner EB. Sequence analysis of monoclonal antibodies derived from a patient with idiopathic thrombocytopenic purpura. Autoimmunity 1990;8:107.
292. Harker LA, Slichter SJ. The bleeding time as a screening test for evaluation of platelet function. N Engl J Med 1972;287:155.
293. Stuart MJ, Kelton JG, Allen JB. Abnormal platelet function and arachidonate metabolism in chronic idiopathic thrombocytopenic purpura. Blood 1981;58:326.
294. Mazzucconi MG, Francesconi M, Fidani P, et al. Treatment of idiopathic thrombocytopenic purpura (ITP): results of a multicentric protocol. Haematologica (Pavia) 1985;70:329.
295. Anderson MJ, Peebles CL, McMillan R, Curd JG. Fluorescent antinuclear antibodies and anti-SS-A/Ro in patients with immune thrombocytopenia subsequently developing systemic lupus erythematosus. Ann Intern Med 1985;103:548.
296. Perez HD, Katler E, Embury S. Idiopathic thrombocytopenic purpura with high-titer, speckled pattern antinuclear antibodies: possible marker for systemic lupus erythematosus. Arthritis Rheum 1985; 28:596.
297. Kurata Y, Miyagawa S, Kosugi S, et al. High-titer antinuclear antibodies, anti-SSA/Ro antibodies and anti-nuclear RNP antibodies in patients with idiopathic thrombocytopenic purpura. Thromb Haemost 1994;71:184.
298. Panzer S, Penner E, Graninger W, et al. Antinuclear antibodies in patients with chronic idiopathic autoimmune thrombocytopenia followed 2–30 years. Am J Hematol 1989;32:100.
299. Tomer A, Schreiber AD, McMillan R, et al. Menstrual cyclic thrombocytopenia. Br J Haematol 1989;71:519.
300. Menitove JE, Pereira J, Hoffman R, et al. Cyclic thrombocytopenia of apparent autoimmune etiology. Blood 1989;73:1561.
301. Engstrom K, Lindquist A, Soderstrom N. Periodic thrombocytopenia or tidal platelet dysgenesis occurring in a man. Scand J Haematol 1966;3:290.
302. Cohen T, Cooney DP. Cyclic thrombocytopenia: case report and review of literature. Scand J Haematol 1974;12:9.
303. Balduini CL, Stella CC, Rosti V, Bertolino G, Noris P, Ascari E. Acquired cyclic thrombocytopenia-thrombocytosis with periodic defect of platelet function. Br J Haematol 1993;85:718.
304. Thompson CB, Jakubowski JA, Quinn PG, et al. Platelet size as a determinant of platelet function. J Lab Clin Med 1983;101:205.
305. Haut MJ, Cowan DH. The effect of ethanol on hemostatic properties of human blood platelets. Am J Med 1974;56:22.
306. Rand ML, Packham MA, Kinlough-Rathbone RL, Mustard JF. Effects of ethanol on pathways of platelet aggregation in vitro. Thromb Haemost 1988;59:383.
307. Branehog I, Weinfeld A. Platelet survival and platelet production in idiopathic thrombocytopenic purpura (ITP) before and during treatment with corticosteroids. Scand J Haematol 1974;12:69.
308. Handin RI, Stossel TP. Effect of corticosteroid therapy on the phagocytosis of antibody-coated platelets by human leukocytes. Blood 1978;51:771.
309. McMillan R, Longmire R, Yelenosky R. The effect of corticosteroids on human IgG synthesis. J Immunol 1976;116:1592.
310. Berchtold P, Wenger M. Autoantibodies against platelet glycoproteins in autoimmune thrombocytopenic purpura: their clinical significance and response to treatment. Blood 1993;81:1246.
311. Gernsheimer T, Stratton J, Ballem PJ, Slichter SJ. Mechanisms of response to treatment in autoimmune thrombocytopenic purpura. N Engl J Med 1989;320:974.
312. Kitchens CS. Amelioration of endothelial abnormalities by prednisone in experimental thrombocytopenia in the rabbit. J Clin Invest 1977;60: 1129.
313. Bellucci S, Charpak Y, Chastang C, et al. Low doses v conventional doses of corticoids in immune thrombocytopenic purpura (ITP): results of a randomized clinical trial in 160 children, 223 adults. Blood 1988;71:1165.
314. Yoshida K, Wakui H, Mamiya S, et al. Bolus methylprednisolone therapy in adult idiopathic thrombocytopenic purpura. Jpn J Med 1987;26:172.
315. von dem Borne AEGK, Vos JJE, Pegels JG, et al. High dose intravenous methylprednisolone or high dose intravenous gammaglobulin for autoimmune thrombocytopenia. Br Med J 1988;296:249.
316. Thompson RL, Moore RA, Hess CE, et al. Idiopathic thrombocytopenic purpura: long-term results of treatment and the prognostic significance of response to corticosteroids. Arch Intern Med 1972;130:730.
317. Ikkala E, Kivilaakso E, Kotilainen M, Hastbacka J. Treatment of idiopathic thrombocytopenic purpura in adults: long-term results in a series of 41 patients. Ann Clin Res 1978;10:83.
318. Kochupillai V, Nundy S, Sharma S. Idiopathic thrombocytopenic purpura in adults: response to corticosteroids and splenectomy. J Assoc Physicians India 1986;34:555.
319. Jacobs P, Wood L, Dent DM. Results of treatment in immune thrombocytopenia. Q J Med 1986;58:153.
320. Jiji RM, Firozvi T, Spurling CL. Chronic idiopathic thrombocytopenic purpura: treatment with steroids and splenectomy. Arch Intern Med 1973;132:380.
321. DiFino SM, Lachant NA, Kirshner JJ, Gottlieb AJ. Adult idiopathic thrombocytopenic purpura: clinical findings and response to therapy. Am J Med 1980;69:430.
322. Pizzuto J, Ambriz R. Therapeutic experience on 934 adults with idiopathic thrombocytopenic purpura: multicentric trial of the Cooperative Latin American Group on Hemostasis and Thrombosis. Blood 1984;64:1179.
323. Mankin HJ. Nontraumatic necrosis of bone (osteonecrosis). N Engl J Med 1992;326:1473.
324. Gardner P, Schaffner W. Immunization of adults. N Engl J Med 1993;328:1252.
325. Centers for Disease Control and Prevention. Recommendations of the Advisory Committee on Immunization Practices (ACIP). Use of vaccines and immune globulins in patients with altered immunocompetence. MMWR 1993;42:1.
326. Cola B, Tonielli E, Sacco S, et al. Surgical treatment of chronic idiopathic thrombocytopenic purpura: results in 107 cases. Int Surg 1986;71:195.
327. Akwari OE, Itani KM, Coleman RE, Rosse WF. Splenectomy for primary and recurrent immune thrombocytopenic purpura (ITP): current criteria for patient selection and results. Ann Surg 1987;206:529.
328. Coon WW. Splenectomy for idiopathic thrombocytopenic purpura. Surg Gynecol Obstet 1987;164:225.
329. Russo D, Gugliotta L, Mazzucconi MG, et al. Long-term results of splenectomy in adult chronic idiopathic thrombocytopenic purpura. Haematologica 1987;72:445.
330. Schwartz SI, Hoepp LM, Sachs S. Splenectomy for thrombocytopenia. Surgery 1980;88:497.
331. Fenaux P, Caulier MT, Hirschauer MC, et al. Reevaluation of the prognostic factors for splenectomy in chronic idiopathic thrombocytopenic purpura (ITP): a report on 181 cases. Eur J Haematol 1989; 42:259.
332. Brennan MF, Rappeport JM, Moloney WC, Wilson RE. Correlation between response to corticosteroids and splenectomy for adult idiopathic thrombocytopenic purpura. Am J Surg 1975;129:490.
333. Mintz SJ, Petersen SR, Cheson B, et al. Splenectomy for immune thrombocytopenic purpura. Arch Surg 1981;116:645.
334. Fabris F, Zanatta N, Casonato A, et al. Response to splenectomy in idiopathic thrombocytopenic purpura: prognostic value of the clinical and laboratory evaluation. Acta Haematol 1989;30:206.
335. Aster RH. Platelet sequestration studies in man. Br J Haematol 1972; 22:259.
336. Ambriz P, Munoz R, Quintanar E, et al. Accessory spleen compromising response to splenectomy for idiopathic thrombocytopenic purpura. Radiology 1985;155:793.
337. Gibson J, Rickard KA, Bautovich G, et al. Management of splenectomy failures in chronic immune thrombocytopenic purpura: role of accessory splenectomy. Aust NZ J Med 1986;16:695.
338. Reid MM, Saunders PWG, Fenwick JD, Walker W. Splenunculectomy in thrombocytopenic purpura. Arch Dis Child 1986;61:192.
339. Warkentin TE, Kelton JG. Immune thrombocytopenia. Medicine 1989;30:5495.
340. O'Neal BJ, McDonald JC. The risk of sepsis in the asplenic adult. Ann Surg 1981;194:775.
341. Friedman D, Netti F, Schreiber AD. Effect of estradiol and steroid analogues on the clearance of immunoglobulin G-coated erythrocytes. J Clin Invest 1985;75:162.
342. Schreiber AD, Chien P, Tomaski A, Cines DB. Effect of danazol in immune thrombocytopenic purpura. N Engl J Med 1987;316:503.
343. Mylvaganam R, Ahn YS, Harrington WJ, Kim CI. Immune modulation by danazol in autoimmune thrombocytopenia. Clin Immunol Immunopathol 1987;42:281.
344. Ahn YS, Mylvaganam R, Garcia RO, et al. Low-dose danazol therapy in idiopathic thrombocytopenic purpura. Ann Intern Med 1987; 107:177.
345. Ahn YS, Harrington WJ, Simon SR, et al. Danazol for the treatment of idiopathic thrombocytopenic purpura. N Engl J Med 1983;308:1396.
346. Almagro D. Danazol in idiopathic thrombocytopenic purpura. (Letter) Acta Haematol 1985;74:120.
347. Ambriz-Fernandez R, Chavez-Sanchez G, Pizzuto-Chavez J, et al. Danazol in refractory autoimmune thrombocytopenic purpura (ATP): a new therapeutic sequence. Arch Invest Med (Mex) 1985;16:295.
348. Buelli M, Cortelazzo S, Viero P, et al. Danazol for the treatment of idiopathic thrombocytopenic purpura. Acta Haematol 1985;74:97.
349. Heyd J, Hershko C. Use of danazol in the management of chronic idiopathic thrombocytopenic purpura. Isr J Med Sci 1985;21:418.
350. McVerry BA, Auger M, Bellingham AJ. The use of danazol in the management of chronic immune thrombocytopenic purpura. Br J Haematol 1985;61:145.
351. Ambriz R, Pizzuto J, Morales M, et al. Therapeutic effect of danazol on metrorrhagia in patients with idiopathic thrombocytopenic purpura (ITP). Nouv Rev Fr Hematol 1986;28:275.
352. Kotlarek-Haus S, Podolak-Dawidziak M. Danazol in chronic idiopathic thrombocytopenic purpura resistant to corticosteroids. Folia Haematol (Leipz) 1987;114:768.

353. Mazzucconi MG, Francesconi M, Falcione E, et al. Danazol therapy in refractory chronic immune thrombocytopenic purpura. Acta Haematol 1987;77:45.
354. Nalli G, Sajeva MR, Maffe GC, Ascari E. Danazol therapy for idiopathic thrombocytopenic purpura (ITP). Haematologica (Pavia) 1988;73:55.
355. Ahn YS, Rocha R, Mylvaganam R, Garcia R, et al. Long-term danazol therapy in autoimmune thrombocytopenia: unmaintained remission and age-dependent response in women. Ann Intern Med 1989; 111:723.
356. Cassi E, De' Paoli A, Tosi A. Splenic peliosis after danazol therapy for idiopathic thrombocytopenic purpura (ITP). Haematologica (Pavia) 1985;70:549.
357. Nesher G, Dollberg L, Zimran A, Hershko C. Hepatosplenic peliosis after danazol and glucocorticoids for ITP. N Engl J Med 1985;312: 242.
358. Rizzo SC, Grignani G, Gamba G, Nalli G. Fibrinolysis induced by danazol. (Letter) Blut 1986;53:351.
359. Wentz AC. Adverse effects of danazol in pregnancy. Ann Intern Med 1982;96:672.
360. Brunskill PJ. The effects of fetal exposure to danazol. Br J Obstet Gynaecol 1992;99:212.
361. Arrowsmith JB, Dreis M. Thrombocytopenia after treatment with danazol. (Letter) N Engl J Med 1986;315:585.
362. Rabinowe SN, Miller KB. Danazol-induced thrombocytopenia. (Letter) Br J Haematol 1987;65:383.
363. Ahn YS, Harrington WJ, Mylvaganam R. Use of platelets as drug carriers for the treatment of hematologic diseases. Methods Enzymol 1987;149:312.
364. Ahn YS, Harrington WJ, Mylvaganam R, et al. Slow infusion of vinca alkaloids in the treatment of idiopathic thrombocytopenic purpura. Ann Intern Med 1984;100:192.
365. Ahn YS, Harrington WJ. Clinical uses of macrophage inhibitors. Adv Intern Med 1980;25:453.
366. Manoharan A. Slow infusion of vincristine in the treatment of idiopathic thrombocytopenic purpura. Am J Hematol 1986;21:135.
367. Simon M, Jouet JP, Fenaux P, et al. The treatment of adult idiopathic thrombocytopenic purpura: infusion of vinblastine in ITP. Eur J Haematol 1987;39:193.
368. Linares M, Cervero A, Sanchez M, et al. Slow infusion of vincristine in the treatment of refractory thrombocytopenic purpura. Acta Haematol 1988;80:173.
369. Facon T, Caulier MT, Wattel E, Jouet JP, Bauters F, Fenaux P. A randomized trial comparing vinblastine in slow infusion and by bolus i.v. injection in idiopathic thrombocytopenic purpura: a report on 42 patients. Br J Haematol 1994;86:678.
370. Ahn YS, Byrnes JJ, Harrington WJ, et al. The treatment of idiopathic thrombocytopenia with vinblastine-loaded platelets. N Engl J Med 1978;298:1101.
371. Kelton JG, McDonald JWD, Barr RM, et al. The reversible binding of vinblastine to platelets: implications for therapy. Blood 1981;57:431.
372. Rosse WF. Whatever happened to vinca-loaded platelets? N Engl J Med 1984;310:1051.
373. Ahn YS, Harrington WJ, Seelman RC, Eytel CS. Vincristine therapy of idiopathic and secondary thrombocytopenias. N Engl J Med 1974;291:376.
374. Burton IE, Roberts BE, Child JA, et al. Responses to vincristine in refractory idiopathic thrombocytopenic purpura. (Letter) Br Med J 1976;2:918.
375. Tangun Y, Atamer T. More on vincristine in treatment of ITP. (Letter) N Engl J Med 1977;297:894.
376. Cervantes F, Montserrat E, Rozman C, et al. Low-dose vincristine in the treatment of corticosteroid-refractory idiopathic thrombocytopenic purpura (ITP) in non-splenectomized patients. Postgrad Med J 1980; 56:711.
377. Cervantes F, Montserrat E, Rozman C. Treatment of idiopathic thrombocytopenic purpura. (Letter) N Engl J Med 1981;305:830.
378. Kueh YK. Vincristine therapy in refractory chronic idiopathic thrombocytopenic purpura. Ann Acad Med Singapore 1982;11:290.
379. Van Zyl-Smit R, Jacobs P. The use of vincristine in refractory autoimmune thrombocytopenic purpura. S Afr Med J 1974;48:2039.
380. Weinerman B, Maxwell I, Hryniuk W. Intermittent cyclophosphamide treatment of autoimmune thrombocytopenia. Can Med Assoc J 1974;111:1100.
381. Caplan SN, Berkman EM. Immunosuppressive therapy of idiopathic thrombocytopenic purpura. Med Clin North Am 1976;60:971.
382. Krause JR. Chronic idiopathic thrombocytopenic purpura (ITP): development of acute non-lymphocytic leukemia subsequent to treatment with cyclophosphamide. Med Pediatr Oncol 1982;10:61.
383. Imbach P, Barandun S, d'Appuzo V, et al. High-dose intravenous gammaglobulin for idiopathic thrombocytopenic purpura in childhood. Lancet 1981;1:1228.
384. Boshkov LK, Kelton JG. Use of intravenous gammaglobulin as an immune replacement and an immune suppressant. Transfus Med Rev 1989;3:82.
385. Barandun S, Kistler P, Jeunet F, Isliker H. Intravenous administration of human γ-globin. Vox Sang 1962;7:157.
386. Imbach P, Jungi TW. Possible mechanisms of intravenous immunoglobulin treatment in childhood idiopathic thrombocytopenic purpura (ITP). Blut 1983;46:117.
387. Bussel JB, Hilgartner MW. The use and mechanism of action of intravenous immunoglobulin in the treatment of immune haematologic disease. Br J Haematol 1984;56:1.
388. Kelton JG. The interaction of IgG with reticuloendothelial cells: biological and therapeutic implications. In: Garratty G, ed. Current concepts in transfusion therapy. Arlington, VA, American Association of Blood Banks, 1985:51.
389. Saleh M, Court W, Huster W, et al. Effect of commercial immunoglobulin G preparation on human monocyte Fc-receptor dependent binding of antibody coated platelets. Br J Haematol 1988;68:47.
390. Neppert J, Clemens M, Mueller-Eckhardt C. Immune phagocytosis inhibition by commercial immunoglobulins. Blut 1986;52:67.
391. Fehr J, Hofmann V, Kappeler U. Transient reversal of thrombocytopenia in idiopathic thrombocytopenic purpura by high-dose intravenous gammaglobulin. N Engl J Med 1982;306:1254.
392. Bussel JB, Kimberly RP, Inman RD, et al. Intravenous gammaglobulin treatment of chronic idiopathic thrombocytopenic purpura. Blood 1983;62:480.
393. Kelton JG, Singer J, Rodger C, et al. The concentration of IgG in the serum is a major determinant of Fc-dependent reticuloendothelial function. Blood 1985;66:490.
394. Emilia G, Sacchi S, Torelli G, et al. Low-dose intravenous pepsin-treated gammaglobulin for idiopathic thrombocytopenic purpura in adults. (Letter) Br J Haematol 1984;58:761.
395. Burdach SEG, Evers KG, Geursen RG. Treatment of acute idiopathic thrombocytopenic purpura of childhood with intravenous immunoglobulin G: comparative efficacy of 7S and 5S preparations. J Pediatr 1986;109:770.
396. Winiarski J, Kreuger A, Ejderhamn J, Holm G. High dose intravenous IgG reduces platelet associated immunoglobulins and complement in idiopathic thrombocytopenic purpura. Scand J Haematol 1983; 31:342.
397. Sultan Y, Kazatchkine MD, Maisonneuve P, Nydegger UE. Anti-idiotypic suppression of autoantibodies to factor VIII (antihaemophilic factor) by high-dose intravenous gammaglobulin. Lancet 1984;2:765.
398. Tankersley DL, Preston MS, Finlayson JS. Immunoglobulin G dimer: an idiotype-anti-idiotype complex. Mol Immunol 1988;25:41.
399. Berchtold P, Dale GL, Tani P, McMillan R. Inhibition of autoantibody binding to platelet glycoprotein IIb/IIIa by anti-idiotypic antibodies in intravenous gammaglobulin. Blood 1989;74:2414.
400. Macey MG, Newland AC. The modulation of T and B cells during IVIgG treatment. Plasma Ther Transfus Technol 1988;9:139.
401. Macey MG, Newland AC. CD4 and CD8 subpopulation changes during high dose intravenous immunoglobulin treatment. Br J Haematol 1990;76:513.
402. Tsubakio T, Kurato Y, Katageri S, et al. Alteration of T cell subsets and immunoglobulin synthesis in vitro during high dose gammaglobulin therapy in patients with idiopathic thrombocytopenic purpura. Clin Exp Immunol 1983;53:607.
403. Bussel JB, Pham LC. Intravenous treatment with gammaglobulin in adults with immune thrombocytopenic purpura: review of the literature. Vox Sang 1987;52:206.
404. Bussel JB, Pham LC, Aledort L, Nachman R. Maintenance treatment of adults with chronic refractory immune thrombocytopenic purpura using repeated intravenous infusions of gammaglobulin. Blood 1988;72:121.
405. Lederman HM, Roifman CM, Lavi S, Gelfand EW. Corticosteroids for prevention of adverse reactions to intravenous immune serum globulin infusions in hypogammaglobulinemic patients. Am J Med 1986; 81:443.
406. Kim HC, Park CL, Cowan JH III, et al. Massive intravascular hemolysis associated with intravenous immunoglobulin in bone marrow transplant recipients. Am J Pediatr Hematol Oncol 1988;10:69.
407. Barton JC, Herrera GA, Galla JH, Bertoli LF, Work J, Koopman WJ. Acute cryoglobulinemic renal failure after intravenous infusion of gamma globulin. Am J Med 1987;82:624.
408. Woodruff RK, Grigg AP, Firkin FC, Smith IL. Fatal thrombotic events during treatment of autoimmune thrombocytopenia with intravenous immunoglobulin in elderly patients. (Letter) Lancet 1986;2:217.
409. Imbach P, Perret BA, Babinton R, et al. Safety of intravenous immunoglobulin preparation: a prospective multicenter study to exclude the risk of non-A, non-B hepatitis. Vox Sang 1991;61:240.
410. Rousell RH, Budinger MD, Pirofsky B, Schiff RI. Prospective study on the hepatitis safety of intravenous immunoglobulin, pH 4.25. Vox Sang 1991;60:65.
411. Lever AML, Webster ADB, Brown D, Thomas HC. Non-A, non-B hepatitis occurring in agammaglobulinaemic patients after intravenous immunoglobulin. Lancet 1984;2:1062.
412. Ochs HD, Fischer SH, Virant FS, et al. Non-A, non-B hepatitis and intravenous immunoglobulin. (Letter) Lancet 1985;1:404.
413. Weiland O, Mattsson L, Glaumann H. Non-A, non-B hepatitis after intravenous gammaglobulin. (Letter) Lancet 1986;1:976.
414. Williams PE, Yap PL, Gillon J, et al. Transmission of non-A, non-B hepatitis by pH4-treated intravenous immunoglobulin. Vox Sang 1989;57:15.

415. Salama A, Mueller-Eckhardt C, Kiefel V. Effect of intravenous immunoglobulin in immune thrombocytopenia: competitive inhibition of reticuloendothelial system function by sequestration of autologous red blood cells? Lancet 1983;2:193.
416. Salama A, Kiefel V, Amberg R, Mueller-Eckhardt C. Treatment of autoimmune thrombocytopenic purpura with rhesus antibodies (anti-Rh_o [D]). Blut 1984;49:29.
417. Friesen AD, Bowman JM, Price HW. Column ion exchange preparation and characteristics of an Rh immune globulin (WinRho) for intravenous use. J Appl Biochem 1981;3:164.
418. Contreras M, Mollison PL. Anti-Rh(D) immunoglobulin for immune thrombocytopenic purpura. (Letter) Lancet 1986;2:49.
419. Oksenhendler E, Bierling P, Brossard Y, et al. Anti-RH immunoglobulin therapy for human immunodeficiency virus–related immune thrombocytopenic purpura. Blood 1988;71:1499.
420. Boughton BJ, Chakraverty R, Baglin TP, et al. The treatment of chronic idiopathic thrombocytopenia with anti-D (Rho) immunoglobulin: its effectiveness, safety and mechanism of action. Clin Lab Haematol 1988;10:275.
421. Durand JM, Harle JR, Verdot JJ, et al. Anti-Rh(D) immunoglobulin for immune thrombocytopenic purpura. Lancet 1986;2:49.
422. Mueller-Eckhardt C, Salama A. Anti-Rh(D) immunoglobulin for immune thrombocytopenic purpura. (Letter) Lancet 1986;2:50.
423. Panzer S, Grumayer ER, Haas OA, et al. Efficacy of rhesus antibodies (anti-Rh_o[D]) in autoimmune thrombocytopenia: correlation with response to high dose IgG and the degree of haemolysis. Blut 1986; 52:117.
424. Cattaneo M, Gringeri A, Capitanio AM, et al. Anti-D immunoglobulin for treatment of HIV-related immune thrombocytopenic purpura. (Letter) Blood 1989;73:357.
425. Bussel JB, Graziano JN, Kimberly RP, et al. Intravenous anti-D treatment of immune thrombocytopenic purpura: analysis of efficacy, toxicity, and mechanism of effect. Blood 1991;77:1884.
426. Ambriz R, Munoz R, Pizzuto J, et al. Low-dose autologous in vitro opsonized erythrocytes: radioimmune method and autologous opsonized erythrocytes for refractory autoimmune thrombocytopenic purpura in adults. Arch Intern Med 1987;147:105.
427. Ruiz-Argüelles GJ, Apreza-Molina MG, Pérez-Romano B, Ruiz-Argüelles A. The infusion of anti-Rh_o-(D) opsonized erythrocytes may be useful in the treatment of patients, splenectomized or not, with chronic, refractory autoimmune thrombocytopenic purpura: a prospective study. Am J Hematol 1993;43:72.
428. Salama A, Kiefel V, Mueller-Eckhardt C. Effect of IgG anti-Rh_o(D) in adult patients with chronic autoimmune thrombocytopenia. Am J Hematol 1986;22:241.
429. Proctor SJ, Jackson G, Carey P, et al. Improvement of platelet counts in steroid-unresponsive idiopathic immune thrombocytopenic purpura after short-course therapy with recombinant α2b interferon. Blood 1989;74:1894.
430. Kelsey PR, Schofield KP, Geary CG. Refractory idiopathic thrombocytopenic purpura (ITP) treated with cyclosporine. Br J Haematol 1985;60:197.
431. Velu TJ, Debusscher L, Stryckmans PA. Ciclosporine for the treatment of refractory idiopathic thrombocytopenic purpura. (Letter) Eur J Haematol 1987;38:95.
432. Matsumura O, Kawashima Y, Kato S, et al. Therapeutic effect of cyclosporine in thrombocytopenia associated with autoimmune disease. Transplant Proc 1988;20:317.
433. Strother SV, Zuckerman KS, LoBuglio AF. Colchicine therapy for refractory idiopathic thrombocytopenic purpura. Arch Intern Med 1984;144:2198.
434. Jim RTS. Therapeutic use of colchicine in thrombocytopenia. Hawaii Med J 1986;45:221.
435. Guthrie TH Jr, Oral A. Immune thrombocytopenia purpura: a pilot study of staphylococcal protein A immunomodulation in refractory patients. Semin Hematol 1989;26:3.
436. Snyder HW Jr, Cochran SK, Balint JP Jr, et al. Experience with protein A-immunoadsorption in treatment-resistant adult immune thrombocytopenic purpura. Blood 1992;79:2237.
437. Figueroa M, Gehlsen J, Hammond D, et al. Combination chemotherapy in refractory immune thrombocytopenic purpura. N Engl J Med 1993;328:1226.
438. Andersen JC. Response of resistant idiopathic thrombocytopenic purpura to pulsed high-dose dexamethasone therapy. N Engl J Med 1994;330:1560.
439. Calverley DG, Jones GW, Kelton JG. Splenic irradiation as a potential treatment for corticosteroid resistant immune thrombocytopenia. Ann Intern Med 1992;116:977.
440. Durand JM, Lefevre P, Hovette P, et al. Dapsone for idiopathic autoimmune thrombocytopenic purpura in elderly patients. Br J Haematol 1991;78:459.
441. Baumann MA, Menitove JE, Aster RH, Anderson T. Urgent treatment of idiopathic thrombocytopenic purpura with single-dose gammaglobulin infusion followed by platelet transfusion. Ann Intern Med 1986;104:808.
442. Carr JM, Kruskall MS, Kaye JA, Robinson SH. Efficacy of platelet transfusions in immune thrombocytopenia. Am J Med 1986;80:1051.
443. Marder VJ, Nusbacher J, Anderson FW. One-year follow-up of plasma exchange therapy in 14 patients with idiopathic thrombocytopenic purpura. Transfusion 1981;21:291.
444. Blanchette VS, Hogan VA, McCombie NE, et al. Intensive plasma exchange in ten patients with idiopathic thrombocytopenic purpura. Transfusion 1984;24:388.
445. Pettersson T, Riska H, Nordstrom D, Honkanen E. Plasmapheresis for idiopathic thrombocytopenic purpura unresponsive to intravenous immunoglobulin. (Letter) Eur J Haematol 1987;39:92.
446. Bussel JB, Saal S, Gordon B. Combined plasma exchange and intravenous gammaglobulin in the treatment of patients with refractory immune thrombocytopenic purpura. Transfusion 1988;28:38.
447. Clarkson SB, Bussel JB, Kimberly RP, et al. Treatment of refractory immune thrombocytopenic purpura with an anti-Fc_γ-receptor antibody. N Engl J Med 1986;314:1236.
448. Soubrane C, Tourani JM, Andrieu JM, et al. Biologic response to anti-CD16 monoclonal antibody therapy in a human immunodeficiency virus–related immune thrombocytopenic purpura patient. Blood 1993;81:15.
449. Territo M, Finklestein J, Oh W, et al. Management of autoimmune thrombocytopenia in pregnancy and in the neonate. Obstet Gynecol 1973;41:579.
450. Kelton JG, Inwood MJ, Barr RM, et al. The prenatal prediction of thrombocytopenia in infants of mothers with clinically diagnosed immune thrombocytopenia. Am J Obstet Gynecol 1982;144:449.
451. Burrows RF, Kelton JG. Pregnancy in patients with idiopathic thrombocytopenic purpura: assessing the risks for the infant at delivery. Obstet Gynecol Surv 1993;48:781.
452. Burrows RF, Kelton JG. Low fetal risks in pregnancies associated with idiopathic thrombocytopenic purpura. Am J Obstet Gynecol 1990;163: 1147.
453. Burrows RF, Kelton JG. Fetal thrombocytopenia and its relation to maternal thrombocytopenia. N Engl J Med 1993;329:1463.
454. Barbui T, Cortelazzo S, Viero P, et al. Idiopathic thrombocytopenic purpura and pregnancy: maternal platelet count and antiplatelet antibodies do not predict the risk of neonatal thrombocytopenia. La Ricerca Clin Lab 1985;15:139.
455. Cines DB, Dusak B, Tomaski A, et al. Immune thrombocytopenic purpura and pregnancy. N Engl J Med 1982;306:826.
456. Mazzucconi MG, Francesconi M, Fidani P, et al. Pregnancy, delivery and detection of antiplatelet antibodies in women with idiopathic thrombocytopenic purpura. Haematologica (Pavia) 1985;70:506.
457. Karpatkin M, Porges RF, Karpatkin S. Platelet counts in infants of women with autoimmune thrombocytopenia: effects of steroid administration to the mother. N Engl J Med 1981;305:936.
458. Newland AC, Boots MA, Patterson KG. Intravenous IgG for autoimmune thrombocytopenia in pregnancy. (Letter) N Engl J Med 1984; 310:261.
459. Wenske G, Gaedicke G, Heyes H. Idiopathic thrombocytopenic purpura in pregnancy and neonatal period. Blut 1984;48:377.
460. Davidson BN, Rayburn WF, Bishop RC, et al. Immunoglobulin therapy for autoimmune thrombocytopenic purpura during pregnancy: a report of two cases. J Reprod Med 1987;32:107.
461. Barton JC, Saleh MN, Stedman CM, Lobuglio AF. Case report. Immune thrombocytopenia: effects of maternal gamma globulin infusion on maternal and fetal serum, platelet, and monocyte IgG. Am J Med Sci 1987;293:112.
462. Sacher RA, King JC. Intravenous gamma-globulin in pregnancy: a review. Obstet Gynecol Surv 1989;44:25.
463. Daffos F, Forestier F, Kaplan C, Cox W. Prenatal diagnosis and management of bleeding disorders with fetal blood sampling. Am J Obstet Gynecol 1988;158:939.
464. Daffos F, Capella-Pavlovsky M, Forestier F. Fetal blood sampling during pregnancy with use of a needle guided by ultrasound: a study of 606 consecutive cases. Am J Obstet Gynecol 1985;153:655.
465. Ayromlooi J. A new approach to the management of immunologic thrombocytopenic purpura in pregnancy. Am J Obstet Gynecol 1978;130:235.
466. Scott JR, Cruikshank DP, Kochenour NK, et al. Fetal platelet counts in the obstetric management of immunologic thrombocytopenic purpura. Am J Obstet Gynecol 1980;136:495.
467. Branch DW, Scott JR, Kochenour NK, Hershgold E. Obstetric complications associated with the lupus anticoagulant. N Engl J Med 1985;313:1322.
468. Ballin A, Andrew M, Ling E, et al. High-dose intravenous gammaglobulin therapy for neonatal autoimmune thrombocytopenia. J Pediatr 1988;112:789.
469. Hoyle C, Darbyshire P, Eden OB. Idiopathic thrombocytopenia in childhood: Edinburgh experience 1962–82. Scott Med J 1986;31:174.
470. Karpatkin M, Karpatkin S. Immune thrombocytopenia in children. Am J Pediatr Hematol Oncol 1981;3:213.
471. Van Leeuwen EF, Von dem Borne AEGK, Van der Plas-Van Dalen C, Engelfriet CP. Idiopathic thrombocytopenic purpura in children: detection of platelet autoantibodies by immunofluorescence. Scand J Haematol 1981;26:285.
472. Winiarski J, Ekelund E. Antibody binding to platelet antigens in acute and chronic idiopathic thrombocytopenic purpura: a platelet mem-

brane ELISA for the detection of antiplatelet antibodies in serum. Clin Exp Immunol 1986;63:459.
473. Lightsey AL Jr, Koenig HM, McMillan R, Stone JR Jr. Platelet-associated immunoglobulin G in childhood idiopathic thrombocytopenic purpura. J Pediatr 1979;94:201.
474. Ware R, Kinney TR, Friedman HS, et al. Prognostic implications for direct platelet-associated IgG in childhood idiopathic thrombocytopenic purpura. Am J Pediatr Hematol Oncol 1986;8:32.
475. Cheung NKV, Hilgartner MW, Schulman I, et al. Platelet-associated immunoglobulin G in childhood idiopathic thrombocytopenic purpura. J Pediatr 1983;102:366.
476. Winiarski J. IgG and IgM antibodies to platelet membrane glycoprotein antigens in acute childhood idiopathic thrombocytopenic purpura. Br J Haematol 1989;73:88.
477. Dubansky AS, Oski FA. Controversies in the management of acute idiopathic thrombocytopenic purpura: a survey of specialists. Pediatr 1986;77:49.
478. Longacre TA, Foucar K, Crago S, et al. Hematogones: a multiparameter analysis of bone marrow precursor cells. Blood 1989;73:543.
479. Buchanan GR, Holtkamp CA. Prednisone therapy for children with newly diagnosed idiopathic thrombocytopenic purpura: a randomized clinical trial. Am J Pediatr Hematol Oncol 1984;6:355.
480. Dunn NL, Maurer HM. Prednisone treatment of acute idiopathic thrombocytopenic purpura of childhood. Am J Pediatr Hematol Oncol 1984;6:159.
481. Sartorius JA. Steroid treatment of idiopathic thrombocytopenic purpura in children: preliminary results of a randomized cooperative study. Am J Pediatr Hematol Oncol 1984;6:165.
482. Suarez CR, Rademaker D, Hasson A, Mangogna L. High-dose steroids in childhood acute idiopathic thrombocytopenia purpura. Am J Pediatr Hematol Oncol 1986;8:111.
483. Ohya M, Kishida K, Nakamura E, et al. "Pulse" methylprednisolone therapy in children with idiopathic thrombocytopenic purpura. Rinsho Ketsueki 1985;26:1600.
484. Jayabose S, Patel P, Inamdar S, et al. Use of intravenous methylprednisolone in acute idiopathic thrombocytopenic purpura. Am J Pediatr Hematol Oncol 1987;9:133.
485. Van Hoff J, Ritchey AK. Pulse methylprednisolone therapy for acute childhood idiopathic thrombocytopenic purpura. J Pediatr 1988; 113:563.
486. Ozsoylu S, Irken G, Karabent A. High-dose intravenous methylprednisolone for acute childhood idiopathic thrombocytopenic purpura. Eur J Haematol 1989;42:431.
487. Imbach P, Wagner HP, Berchtold W, et al. Intravenous immunoglobulin versus oral corticosteroids in acute immune thrombocytopenic purpura in childhood. Lancet 1985;2:464.
488. Bussel JB, Goldman A, Imbach P, et al. Treatment of acute idiopathic thrombocytopenic purpura of childhood with intravenous infusions of gammaglobulin. J Pediatr 1985;106:886.
489. Hara T, Miyazaki S, Yoshida N, Goya N. High doses of gamma globulin and methylprednisolone therapy for idiopathic thrombocytopenic purpura in children. Eur J Pediatr 1985;144:240.
490. Bussel JB, Hilgartner MW. Intravenous immunoglobulin therapy of idiopathic thrombocytopenic purpura in childhood and adolescence. Hematol Oncol Clin North Am 1987;1:465.
491. Berchtold P, McMillan R, Tani P, Sommerville-Nielsen S, Blanchette VS. Autoantibodies against platelet membrane glycoproteins in children with acute and chronic immune thrombocytopenic purpura. Blood 1989;74:1600.
492. Simons SM, Main CA, Yaish HM, Rutzky J. Idiopathic thrombocytopenic purpura in children. J Pediatr 1975;87:16.
493. McIntosh S, Johnson C, Hartigan P, et al. Immunoregulatory abnormalities in children with thrombocytopenic purpura. J Pediatr 1981; 99:525.
494. Tomar RH, Stuart MJ. Predicting acute vs chronic childhood idiopathic thrombocytopenic purpura. Am J Dis Child 1981;135:446.
495. Menichelli A, Del Principe D, Rezza E. Intravenous pulse methylprednisolone in chronic idiopathic thrombocytopenia. Arch Dis Child 1984;59:777.
496. Del Principe D, Menichelli A, Mori PG, et al. Phase II trial of methylprednisolone pulse therapy in childhood chronic thrombocytopenia. Acta Haematol 1987;77:226.
497. Mori PG, Mancuso G, Del Principe D, et al. Chronic idiopathic thrombocytopenia treated with immunoglobulin. Arch Dis Child 1983; 58:851.
498. Bussel JB, Schulman I, Hilgartner MW, Barandun S. Intravenous use of gammaglobulin in the treatment of chronic immune thrombocytopenic purpura as a means to defer splenectomy. J Pediatr 1983; 103:651.
499. Warrier I, Lusher JM. Intravenous gamma globulin treatment for chronic idiopathic thrombocytopenic purpura in children. Am J Med 1984;76:193.
500. Imholz B, Imbach P, Baumgartner C, et al. Intravenous immunoglobulin (i.v. IgG) for previously treated acute or for chronic idiopathic thrombocytopenic purpura (ITP) in childhood: a prospective multicenter study. Blut 1988;56:63.
501. Hollenberg JP, Subak LL, Ferry JJ Jr, Bussel JB. Cost-effectiveness of splenectomy versus intravenous gamma globulin in treatment of chronic immune thrombocytopenic purpura in childhood. J Pediatr 1988;112:530.
502. Becker T, Kuenzlen E, Salama A, et al. Treatment of childhood idiopathic thrombocytopenic purpura with rhesus antibodies (anti-D). Eur J Pediatr 1986;145:166.
503. Andrew M, Blanchette VS, Adams M, et al. A multicenter study of the treatment of childhood chronic idiopathic thrombocytopenic purpura with anti-D. J Pediatr 1992;120:522.
504. Den Ottolander GJ, Gratama JW, De Konig J, Brand A. Long-term follow-up study of 168 patients with immune thrombocytopenia: implications for therapy. Scand J Haematol 1984;32:101.
505. Konigswieser H. Incidence of serious infections after splenectomy in children. Prog Pediatr Surg 1985;18:173.
506. Joseph A, Evans DI. Immunosuppressive treatment of idiopathic thrombocytopenic purpura in children. Acta Paediatr Scand 1982; 71:467.
507. Budman DR, Steinberg AD. Hematologic aspects of systemic lupus erythematosus: current concepts. Ann Intern Med 1977;86:220.
508. Tan EM, Cohen AS, Fries JF, et al. The 1982 revised criteria for the classification of systemic lupus erythematosus. Arthritis Rheum 1982;25:1271.
509. Smolen JS, Morimoto C, Steinberg AD, et al. Systemic lupus erythematosus: delineation of subpopulations by clinical, serologic, and T cell subset analysis. Am J Med Sci 1985;289:139.
510. Kaufman LD, Gomez-Reino JJ, Heinicke MH, Gorevic PD. Male lupus: retrospective analysis of the clinical and laboratory features of 52 patients, with a review of the literature. Semin Arthritis Rheum 1989;18:189.
511. Jonsson H, Nived O, Sturfelt G. Outcome in systemic lupus erythematosus: a prospective study of patients from a defined population. Medicine 1989;68:141.
512. Bergstrom AL, Olsson LB, Kutti J. Platelet survival and platelet production in systemic lupus erythematosus (SLE). Scand J Rheum 1980; 9:209.
513. Kelton JG, Carter CJ, Rodger C, et al. The relationship among platelet-associated IgG, platelet lifespan, and reticuloendothelial cell function. Blood 1984;63:1434.
514. Kaplan C, Champeix P, Blanchard D, et al. Platelet antibodies in systemic lupus erythematosus. Br J Haematol 1987;67:89.
515. Howe SE, Lynch DM. Platelet antibody binding in systemic lupus erythematosus. J Rheumatol 1987;14:482.
516. Dixon RH, Rosse WF. Platelet antibody in autoimmune thrombocytopenia. Br J Haematol 1975;31:129.
517. Pfueller SL, Firkin BG, McGrath KM, Logan D. Analysis of immunoglobulins that bind to platelets from serum of patients with immune thrombocytopenia: molecular weight distribution. Thromb Res 1987;47:305.
518. Harris EN, Gharavi AE, Boey ML, et al. Anticardiolipin antibodies: detection by radioimmunoassay and association with thrombosis in systemic lupus erythematosus. Lancet 1983;2:1211.
519. Averbuch M, Koifman B, Levo Y. Lupus anticoagulant, thrombosis and thrombocytopenia in systemic lupus erythematosus. Am J Med Sci 1987;293:1.
520. Deleze M, Oria CV, Alarcon-Segovia D. Occurrence of both hemolytic anemia and thrombocytopenic purpura (Evans' syndrome) in systemic lupus erythematosus: relationship to antiphospholipid antibodies. J Rheumatol 1988;15:611.
521. Kalunian KC, Peter JB, Middlekauff HR, et al. Clinical significance of a single test for anti-cardiolipin antibodies in patients with systemic lupus erythematosus. Am J Med 1988;85:602.
522. Khamashta MA, Harris EN, Sharavi AE, et al. Immune mediated mechanism for thrombosis: antiphospholipid antibody binding to platelet membranes. Ann Rheum Dis 1988;47:849.
523. Miller MA, Urowitz MB, Gladman DD. The significance of thrombocytopenia in systemic lupus erythematosus. Arthritis Rheum 1983;26:1181.
524. Dameshek W, Reeves WH. Exacerbation of lupus erythematosus following splenectomy in "idiopathic" thrombocytopenic purpura and autoimmune hemolytic anemia. Am J Med 1956;21:560.
525. Best WR, Darling DR. A critical look at the splenectomy-SLE controversy. Med Clin North Am 1962;46:19.
526. Homan WP, Dineen P. The role of splenectomy in the treatment of thrombocytopenic purpura due to systemic lupus erythematosus. Ann Surg 1978;187:52.
527. Jacobs P, Wood L, Dent DM. Splenectomy and the thrombocytopenia of systemic lupus erythematosus. (Letter) Ann Intern Med 1986; 105:971.
528. Coon WW. Splenectomy for cytopenias associated with systemic lupus erythematosus. Am J Surg 1988;155:391.
529. Hall S, McCormick JL Jr, Greipp PR, et al. Splenectomy does not cure the thrombocytopenia of systemic lupus erythematosus. Ann Intern Med 1985;102:325.
530. Rivero SJ, Alger M, Alarcon-Segovia D. Splenectomy for hemocytopenia in systemic lupus erythematosus: a controlled appraisal. Arch Intern Med 1979;139:773.
531. Agnello V, Pariser K, Gell J, et al. Preliminary observations on danazol

therapy of systemic lupus erythematosus: effects on DNA antibodies, thrombocytopenia and complement. J Rheumatol 1983;10:682.
532. Marino C, Cook P. Danazol for lupus thrombocytopenia. Arch Intern Med 1985;145:2251.
533. West SG, Johnson SC. Danazol for the treatment of refractory autoimmune thrombocytopenia in systemic lupus erythematosus. Ann Intern Med 1988;108:703.
534. Gaedicke G, Teller WM, Kohne E, et al. IgG therapy in systemic lupus erythematosus: two case reports. Blut 1984;48:387.
535. Wall BA, Weinblatt ME, Agudelo CA. Plasmapheresis in the treatment of resistant thrombocytopenia in systemic lupus erythematosus. South Med J 1982;75:1277.
536. Schroeder JO, Euler HH, Loffler H. Synchronization of plasmapheresis and pulse cyclophosphamide in severe systemic lupus erythematosus. Ann Intern Med 1987;107:344.
537. Harris EN, Asherson RA, Hughes GRV. Antiphospholipid antibodies: autoantibodies with a difference. Annu Rev Med 1988;39:261.
538. Levine SR, Welch KM. The spectrum of neurologic disease associated with antiphospholipid antibodies. Arch Neurol 1987;44:876.
539. Chartash EK, Lans DM, Paget SA, et al. Aortic insufficiency and mitral regurgitation in patients with systemic lupus erythematosus and the antiphospholipid syndrome. Am J Med 1989;86:407.
540. Conley CL, Savarese DM. Biologic false-positive serologic tests for syphilis and other serologic abnormalities in autoimmune hemolytic anemia and thrombocytopenic purpura. Medicine 1989;68:67.
541. Alperin N, Babu S, Weinstein A. Acute adrenal insufficiency and the antiphospholipid syndrome. Ann Intern Med 1989;111:950.
542. McCroskey RD, Phillips A, Mott F, Williams EC. Antiphospholipid antibodies and adrenal hemorrhage. Am J Hematol 1991;36:60.
543. Asherson RA, Mavou SC, Merry P, et al. The spectrum of livedo reticularis and anticardiolipin antibodies. Br J Dermatol 1989; 120:215.
544. Grob JJ, Bonerandi JJ. Thrombotic skin disease as a marker of the anticardiolipin syndrome: livedo vasculitis and distal gangrene associated with abnormal antiphospholipid activity. J Am Acad Dermatol 1989;20:1063.
545. Grob JJ, San Marco M, Aillaud MF, et al. Unfading acral microlivedo: a discrete marker of thrombotic skin disease associated with antiphospholipid antibody syndrome. J Am Acad Dermatol 1991;24:53.
546. Asherson RA. A "primary" antiphospholipid syndrome? J Rheumatol 1988;15:1742.
547. Asherson RA, Khamashta MA, Gil A, et al. Cerebrovascular disease and antiphospholipid antibodies in systemic lupus erythematosus, lupus-like disease, and the primary antiphospholipid syndrome. Am J Med 1989;86:391.
548. Galli M, Daldossi M, Barbui T. Anti-glycoprotein Ib/IX and IIb/IIIa antibodies in patients with antiphospholipid antibodies. Thromb Haemost 1994;71:571.
549. McNeil HP, Simpson RJ, Chesterman CN, Krilis SA. Antiphospholipid antibodies are directed against a complex antigen that includes a lipid-binding inhibitor of coagulation: β_2-glycoprotein I (apolipoprotein H). Proc Natl Acad Sci USA 1990;87:4120.
550. Galli M, Comfurius P, Maassen C, et al. Anticardiolipin antibodies (ACA) are directed not to cardiolipin but to a plasma protein cofactor. Lancet 1990;335:1544.
551. Bevers EM, Galli M, Barbui T, Comfurius P, Zwaal RF. Lupus anticoagulant IgG's (LA) are not directed to phospholipids only, but to a complex of lipid-bound human prothrombin. Thromb Haemost 1991;66:629.
552. Permpikul P, Rao LV, Rapaport SI. Functional and binding studies of the roles of prothrombin and beta 2-glycoprotein I in the expression of lupus anticoagulant activity. Blood 1994;83:2878.
553. Ginsberg JS, Demers C, Brill-Edwards P, et al. Increased thrombin generation and activity in patients with systemic lupus erythematosus and anticardiolipin antibodies: evidence for a prothrombotic state. Blood 1993;81:2958.
554. Lellouche F, Martinuzzo M, Said P, Maclouf J, Carreras LO. Imbalance of thromboxane/prostacyclin biosynthesis in patients with lupus anticoagulant. Blood 1991;78:2894.
555. Martinuzzo ME, Maclouf J, Carreras LO, Lévy-Toledano S. Antiphospholipid antibodies enhance thrombin-induced platelet activation and thromboxane formation. Thromb Haemost 1993;70:667.
556. Davies GE, Triplett DA. Corticosteroid-associated blue toe syndrome: role of antiphospholipid antibodies. Ann Intern Med 1990;113:893.
557. Wang WC. Evans syndrome in childhood: pathophysiology, clinical course, and treatment. Am J Pediatr Hematol Oncol 1988;10:330.
558. Hegde UM, Zuiable A, Ball S, Roter BLT. The relative incidence of idiopathic and secondary autoimmune thrombocytopenia: a clinical and serological evaluation in 508 patients. Clin Lab Haematol 1985;7:7.
559. Cooper C, Fairris G, Cotton DWK, et al. Dermatomyositis associated with idiopathic thrombocytopenia. Dermatologica 1986;172:173.
560. Pettersson T, Von Bonsdorff M. Auto-immune haemolytic anaemia and thrombocytopenia in scleroderma. Acta Haematol 1988;80:179.
561. Neucks SH, Moore TL, Lichtenstein JR, et al. Localised scleroderma and idiopathic thrombocytopenia. J Rheumatol 1980;7:741.
562. Sugai S, Tachibana J, Shimizu S, Konda S. Thrombocytopenia in patients with Sjögren's syndrome. (Letter) Arthritis Rheum 1989; 32:234.
563. Dunlap DB, McFarland KF, Lutcher CL. Graves' disease and idiopathic thrombocytopenic purpura. Am J Med Sci 1974;268:107.
564. Hymes K, Blum M, Lackner H, Karpatkin S. Easy bruising, thrombocytopenia, and elevated platelet immunoglobulin G in Graves' disease and Hashimoto's thyroiditis. Ann Intern Med 1981;94:27.
565. Valenta LJ, Treadwell T, Berry R, Elias AN. Idiopathic thrombocytopenic purpura and Graves disease. Am J Hematol 1982;12:69.
566. Crabtree GR, Lee JC, Cornwell GG III. Autoimmune thrombocytopenic purpura and Hashimoto's thyroiditis. (Letter) Ann Intern Med 1975; 83:371.
567. Segal BM, Weintraub MI. Hashimoto's thyroiditis, myasthenia gravis, idiopathic thrombocytopenic purpura. (Letter) Ann Intern Med 1976;85:761.
568. Thomas LLM, Alberts C, Pegels JG, et al. Sarcoidosis associated with autoimmune thrombocytopenia and selective IgA deficiency. Scand J Haematol 1982;28:357.
569. Lawrence HJ, Greenberg BR. Autoimmune thrombocytopenia in sarcoidosis. Am J Med 1985;79:761.
570. Field SK, Poon MC. Sarcoidosis presenting as chronic thrombocytopenia. West J Med 1987;146:481.
571. Anderson MJ, Woods VL Jr, Tani P, et al. Autoantibodies to platelet glycoprotein IIb/IIIa and to the acetylcholine receptor in a patient with chronic idiopathic thrombocytopenic purpura and myasthenia gravis. Ann Intern Med 1984;100:829.
572. Jansen PHP, Renier WO, De Vaan G, et al. Effect of thymectomy on myasthenia gravis and autoimmune thrombocytopenic purpura in a 13-year-old girl. Eur J Pediatr 1987;146:587.
573. Kosmo MA, Bordin G, Tani P, McMillan R. Immune thrombocytopenia and Crohn's disease. (Letter) Ann Intern Med 1986;104:136.
574. Gupta S, Saverymuttu SH, Marsh JCW, et al. Immune thrombocytopenic purpura, neutropenia and sclerosing cholangitis associated with ulcerative colitis in an adult. Clin Lab Haematol 1986;8:67.
575. Stenhammar L, Ljunggren CG. Thrombocytopenic purpura and coeliac disease. Acta Paediatr Scand 1988;77:764.
576. Chalmers EA, Chan Lam D, Holden RJ, Fitzimons EJ. Familial primary biliary cirrhosis and autoimmune thrombocytopenia. Scott Med J 1987;32:152.
577. Kihara S, Matsuzawa Y, Kubo M, et al. Autoimmune hyperchylomicronemia. N Engl J Med 1989;320:1255.
578. Taylor G, Venning V, Wojnarowska F. Bullous pemphigoid and associated autoimmune thrombocytopenia: two case reports. J Am Acad Dermatol 1993;29:900.
579. Berchtold P, Harris JP, Tani P, et al. Autoantibodies to platelet glycoproteins in patients with disease-related immune thrombocytopenia. Br J Haematol 1989;73:365.
580. Schwartz KA, Slichter SJ, Harker LA. Immune-mediated platelet destruction and thrombocytopenia in patients with solid tumors. Br J Haematol 1982;51:17.
581. Amylon MD, Link MP, Glader BE. Immune thrombocytopenia associated with acute nonlymphocytic leukemia. J Pediatr 1984;105:776.
582. Rao S, Pang EJM. Idiopathic thrombocytopenic purpura in acute lymphoblastic leukemia. J Pediatr 1979;94:408.
583. Rudders RA, Aisenberg AC, Schiller AL. Hodgkin's disease presenting as "idiopathic" thrombocytopenic purpura. Cancer 1972;30:220.
584. Grossbard ML, Harris NL, Boland GW, Carey RW. A 37-year-old woman with thrombocytopenia and a paragastric mass after treatment for Hodgkin's disease: Hodgkin's disease, recurrent, involving stomach and paragastric lymph nodes. N Engl J Med 1994;330:698.
585. Jones SE. Autoimmune disorders and malignant lymphoma. Cancer 1973;31:1092.
586. Carey RW, McGinnis A, Jacobson BM, Carvalho A. Idiopathic thrombocytopenic purpura complicating chronic lymphocytic leukemia: management with sequential splenectomy and chemotherapy. Arch Intern Med 1976;136:62.
587. Hamblin TJ, Oscier DG, Young BJ. Autoimmunity in chronic lymphocytic leukaemia. J Clin Pathol 1986;39:713.
588. Duhrsen U, Augener W, Zwingers T, Brittinger G. Spectrum and frequency of autoimmune derangements in lymphoproliferative disorders: analysis of 637 cases and comparison with myeloproliferative diseases. Br J Haematol 1987;67:235
589. Kipps TJ, Carson DA. Autoantibodies in chronic lymphocytic leukemia and related systemic autoimmune diseases. Blood 1993;81:2475.
590. Kaden BR, Rosse WF, Hauch TW. Immune thrombocytopenia in lymphoproliferative diseases. Blood 1979;53:545.
591. Murphy WG, Allan NC, Perry DJ, Stockdill G. Hodgkin's disease presenting as idiopathic thrombocytopenic purpura. Postgrad Med J 1984;60:614.
592. Verdirame JD, Feagler JR, Commers JR. Multiple myeloma associated with immune thrombocytopenic purpura. Cancer 1985;56:1199.
593. Yasuda K, Yatomi Y, Matsushima T, et al. A case of POEMS syndrome with thrombocytopenia and biliverdinaemia. Br J Haematol 1994; 86:389.
594. Sonnenblick M, Kramer MR, Hershko C. Corticosteroid responsive immune thrombocytopenia in Hodgkin's disease. Oncology 1986; 43:349.

595. Pedro-Botet J, Estruch R, Montserrat E, et al. Thrombocytopenic purpura as first manifestation of an inapparent Hodgkin's disease. Scand J Haematol 1986;36:408.
596. Xiros N, Binder T, Anger B, et al. Idiopathic thrombocytopenic purpura and autoimmune hemolytic anemia in Hodgkin's disease. Eur J Haematol 1988;40:437.
597. Hassidim K, McMillan R, Conjalka MS, Morrison J. Immune thrombocytopenic purpura in Hodgkin disease. Am J Hematol 1979;6:149.
598. Kubota T, Tanoue K, Murohashi I, et al. Autoantibody against platelet glycoprotein IIb/IIIa in a patient with non-Hodgkin's lymphoma. Thromb Res 1989;53:379.
599. Barton JC, Prasthofer EF, Egan ML, et al. Rheumatoid arthritis associated with expanded populations of granular lymphocytes. Ann Intern Med 1986;104:314.
600. Linch DC, Newland AC, Turnbull AL, et al. Unusual T cell proliferations and neutropenia in rheumatoid arthritis: comparison with classical Felty's syndrome. Scand J Haematol 1984;33:342.
601. Loughran TP Jr, Kadin ME, Starkebaum G, et al. Leukemia of large granular lymphocytes: association with clonal chromosomal abnormalities and autoimmune neutropenia, thrombocytopenia, and hemolytic anemia. Ann Intern Med 1985;102:169.
602. Morris L, Distenfeld A, Amorosi E, Karpatkin S. Autoimmune thrombocytopenic purpura in homosexual men. Ann Intern Med 1982; 96:714.
603. Goldsweig HG, Grossman R, William D. Thrombocytopenia in homosexual men. Am J Hematol 1986;21:243.
604. Walsh CM, Krigel R, Lennette E, Karpatkin S. Thrombocytopenia in homosexual patients: prognosis, response to therapy, and prevalence of antibody to the retrovirus associated with the acquired immunodeficiency syndrome. Ann Intern Med 1985;103:542.
605. Abrams DI, Kiprov DD, Goedert JJ, et al. Antibodies to human T-lymphotropic virus type III and development of the acquired immunodeficiency syndrome in homosexual men presenting with immune thrombocytopenia. Ann Intern Med 1986;104:47.
606. Savona S, Nardi MA, Lennette ET, Karpatkin S. Thrombocytopenic purpura in narcotics addicts. Ann Intern Med 1985;102:737.
607. Ratnoff OD, Menitove JE, Aster RH, Lederman MM. Coincident classic hemophilia and "idiopathic" thrombocytopenic purpura in patients under treatment with concentrates of antihemophilic factor (factor VIII). N Engl J Med 1983;308:439.
608. Karpatkin S, Nardi MA, Hymes KB. Immunologic thrombocytopenic purpura after heterosexual transmission of human immunodeficiency virus (HIV). Ann Intern Med 1988;109:190.
609. Murphy MF, Metcalfe P, Waters AH, et al. Incidence and mechanism of neutropenia and thrombocytopenia in patients with human immunodeficiency virus infection. Br J Haematol 1987;66:337.
610. Zon LI, Arkin C, Groopman JE. Haematologic manifestations of the human immune deficiency virus (HIV). Br J Haematol 1987;66:251.
611. Goldsmith JC, Kisker CT. Successful conservative management of thrombocytopenia in adult hemophiliacs. Transfusion 1988;28:68.
612. Matsuoka T, Tamura H, Fujishita M, et al. Thrombocytopenic purpura in a carrier of human T-cell leukemia virus type I. Am J Hematol 1988;27:142.
613. Walsh CM, Nardi MA, Karpatkin S. On the mechanism of thrombocytopenic purpura in sexually active homosexual men. N Engl J Med 1984;311:635.
614. Karpatkin S, Nardi M, Lennette ET, et al. Anti-human immunodeficiency virus type 1 antibody complexes on platelets of seropositive thrombocytopenic homosexuals and narcotic addicts. Proc Natl Acad Sci USA 1988;85:9763.
615. Yu J-R, Lennette ET, Karpatkin S. Anti-F(ab')$_2$ antibodies in thrombocytopenic patients at risk for acquired immunodeficiency syndrome. J Clin Invest 1986;77:1756.
616. van der Lelie J, Lange JMA, Vos JJE, van Dalen CM, Danner SA, von dem Borne AEGK. Autoimmunity against blood cells in human immunodeficiency-virus (HIV) infection. Br J Haematol 1987;67:109.
617. Bettaieb A, Oksenhendler E, Fromont P, Duedari N, Bierling P. Immunochemical analysis of platelet autoantibodies in HIV-related thrombocytopenic purpura: a study of 68 patients. Blood 1989;73:241.
618. Bettaieb A, Fromont P, Louache F, et al. Presence of cross-reactive antibody between human immunodeficiency virus (HIV) and platelet glycoproteins in HIV-related immune thrombocytopenic purpura. Blood 1992;80:162.
619. Shannon KM, Ammann AJ. Acquired immune deficiency syndrome in childhood. J Pediatr 1985;106:332.
620. Kurtzberg J, Friedman HS, Kinney TR, et al. Management of human immunodeficiency virus–associated thrombocytopenia with intravenous gamma globulin. Am J Pediatr Hematol Oncol 1987;9:299.
621. Falloon J, Eddy J, Wiener L, Pizzo PA. Human immunodeficiency virus infection in children. J Pediatr 1989;114:1.
622. Holzman RS, Walsh CM, Karpatkin S. Risk for the acquired immunodeficiency syndrome among thrombocytopenic and nonthrombocytopenic homosexual men seropositive for the human immunodeficiency virus. Ann Intern Med 1987;106:383.
623. Oksenhendler E, Bierling P, Farcet JP, et al. Response to therapy in 37 patients with HIV-related thrombocytopenic purpura. Br J Haematol 1987;66:491.
624. Shafer RW, Offit K, Macris NT, et al. Possible risk of steroid administration in patients at risk for AIDS. (Letter) Lancet 1985;1:934.
625. Panzer S, Zeitelhuber U, Hach V, et al. Immune thrombocytopenia in severe hemophilia A treated with high-dose intravenous immunoglobulin. Transfusion 1986;26:69.
626. Schneider PA, Abrams DI, Rayner AA, Hohn DC. Immunodeficiency-associated thrombocytopenic purpura (IDTP). Arch Surg 1987;122: 1175.
627. Beard J, Savidge GF. High-dose intravenous immunoglobulin and splenectomy for the treatment of HIV-related immune thrombocytopenia in patients with severe haemophilia. Br J Haematol 1988; 68:303.
628. Tyler DS, Shaunak S, Bartlett JA, Iglehart JD. HIV-1–associated thrombocytopenia: the role of splenectomy. Ann Surg 1990;211211.
629. Alonso M, Gossot D, Bourstyn E, et al. Splenectomy in human immunodeficiency virus–related thrombocytopenia. Br J Surg 1993; 80:330.
630. Oksenhendler E, Bierling P, Chevret S, et al. Splenectomy is safe and effective in human immunodeficiency virus–related immune thrombocytopenia. Blood 1993;82:29.
631. Ballet JJ, Sulcebe G, Couderc LJ, et al. Impaired anti-pneumococcal antibody response in patients with AIDS-related persistent generalized lymphadenopathy. Clin Exp Immunol 1987;68:479.
632. Bender BS, Quinn TC, Spivak JL. Homosexual men with thrombocytopenia have impaired reticuloendothelial system Fc receptor–specific clearance. Blood 1987;70:392.
633. Bender BS, Frank MM, Lawley TJ, et al. Defective reticuloendothelial system Fc-receptor function in patients with acquired immunodeficiency syndrome. J Infect Dis 1985;152:409.
634. Pollak AN, Janinis J, Green D. Successful intravenous immune globulin therapy for human immunodeficiency virus–associated thrombocytopenia. Arch Intern Med 1988;148:695.
635. Rossi E, Vimercati AR, Damasio EE, et al. Treatment of idiopathic thrombocytopenic purpura in HIV-positive patients with rhesus antibodies (anti-D). Haematologica (Pavia) 1987;72:529.
636. Swiss Group for Clinical Studies on the Acquired Immunodeficiency Syndrome (AIDS). Zidovudine for the treatment of thrombocytopenia associated with human immunodeficiency virus (HIV): a prospective study. Ann Intern Med 1988;109:718.
637. Rarick MU, Espina B, Montgomery T, et al. The long-term use of zidovudine in patients with severe immune-mediated thrombocytopenia secondary to infection with HIV. AIDS 1991;5:1357.
638. Lee CA, Kernoff PBA, Karayiannis P, Thomas HC. Interferon therapy for chronic non-A non-B and chronic delta liver disease in haemophilia. Br J Haematol 1989;72:235.
639. Northfelt DW, Kaplan LD, Abrams DI. Continuous, low-dose therapy with interferon-α for human immunodeficiency virus (HIV)-related immune thrombocytopenic purpura. Am J Hematol 1991;38:238.
640. Vianelli N, Catani L, Gugliotta L, et al. Recombinant α-interferon 2b in the treatment of HIV-related thrombocytopenia. AIDS 1993;7:823.
641. Godeau B, Oksenhendler E, Bierling P. Dapsone for autoimmune thrombocytopenic purpura. Am J Hematol 1993;44:70.
642. Snyder HW Jr, Bertram JH, Henry DH, et al. Use of protein A immunoadsorption as a treatment for thrombocytopenia in HIV-infected homosexual men: a retrospective evaluation of 37 cases. AIDS 1991;5: 1257.
643. Needleman SW, Sorace J, Poussin-Rosillo H. Low-dose splenic irradiation in the treatment of autoimmune thrombocytopenia in HIV-infected patients. Ann Intern Med 1992;116:310.
644. First LR, Smith BR, Lipton J, et al. Isolated thrombocytopenia after allogeneic bone marrow transplantation: existence of transient and chronic thrombocytopenic syndromes. Blood 1985;65:368.
645. Minchinton RM, Waters AH, Malpas JS, et al. Platelet-and granulocyte-specific antibodies after allogeneic and autologous bone marrow grafts. Vox Sang 1984;46:125.
646. Anasetti C, Rybka W, Sullivan KM, et al. Graft-v-host disease is associated with autoimmune-like thrombocytopenia. Blood 1989;73: 1054.
647. Spruce W, Forman S, McMillan R, et al. Idiopathic thrombocytopenic purpura following bone marrow transplantation. Acta Haematol 1983;69:47.
648. Minchinton RM, Waters AH. Autoimmune thrombocytopenia and neutropenia after bone marrow transplantation. (Letter) Blood 1985; 66:752.
649. Panzer S, Kiefel V, Bartram CR, et al. Immune thrombocytopenia more than a year after allogeneic marrow transplantation due to antibodies against donor platelets with anti-Pl^{A1} specificity: evidence for a host-derived immune reaction. Br J Haematol 1989;71:259.
650. Rio B, Andreu G, Nicod A, et al. Thrombocytopenia in venoclusive disease after bone marrow transplantation or chemotherapy. Blood 1986;67:1773.
651. Bierling P, Cordonnier C, Fromont P, et al. Acquired autoimmune thrombocytopenia after allogeneic bone marrow transplantation. Br J Haematol 1985;59:643.
652. Minchinton RM, Waters AH, Kendra J, Barrett AJ. Autoimmune thrombocytopenia acquired from an allogeneic bone-marrow graft. Lancet 1982;2:627.

653. Hackett T, Kelton JG, Powers P. Drug-induced platelet destruction. Semin Thromb Hemost 1982;8:116.
654. Glueck R, Green D, Cohen I, Ts'Ao CH. Hematin: unique effects on hemostasis. Blood 1983;61:243.
655. Neely SM, Gardner DV, Reynolds N, et al. Mechanism and characteristics of platelet activation by haematin. Br J Haematol 1984; 58:305.
656. Gangarosa EJ, Johnson TR, Ramos HS. Ristocetin-induced thrombocytopenia: site and mechanism of action. Arch Intern Med 1960; 105:83.
657. Green D, Tuite GF Jr. Declining platelet counts and platelet aggregation during porcine VIII:C infusions. Am J Med 1989;86:222.
658. Heyns A du P, Lotter MG, Badenhorst PN, et al. Kinetics and in vivo redistribution of ^{111}indium-labelled human platelets after intravenous protamine sulphate. Thromb Haemost 1980;44:65.
659. Yue CP, Mann KS, Chan KW. Severe thrombocytopenia due to combined cimetidine and phenytoin therapy. Neurosurgery 1987;20:963.
660. Gross S, Worthington-White DA. Cimetidine suppression of CFU-C in males. Am J Hematol 1984;17:279.
661. Kornberg A, Polliack A. Paracetamol-induced thrombocytopenia and haemolytic anaemia. (Letter) Lancet 1978;2:1159.
662. Schoenfeld Y, Shaklai M, Livni E, Pinkhas J. Thrombocytopenia from acetaminophen. (Letter) N Engl J Med 1980;303:47.
663. Eisner EV, Shahidi NT. Immune thrombocytopenia due to a drug metabolite. N Engl J Med 1972;287:376.
664. Bertino JR, Rodman T, Myerson RM. Thrombocytopenia and renal lesions associated with acetazoleamide (Diamox) therapy. Arch Intern Med 1957;99:1006.
665. Reisner EH, Morgan MC. Thrombocytopenia following acetazolamide (Diamox) therapy. JAMA 1956;160:206.
666. Karpatkin M, Siskind GW, Karpatkin S. The platelet factor 3 immunoinjury technique re-evaluated: development of a rapid test for antiplatelet antibody—detection in various clinical disorders, including immunologic drug-induced and neonatal thrombocytopenias. J Lab Clin Med 1977;89:400.
667. Garg SK, Sarker CR. Aspirin-induced thrombocytopenia on an immune basis. Am J Med Sci 1974;267:129.
668. Hodder FS, Kempert P, McCormack S, et al. Immune thrombocytopenia following actinomycin-D therapy. J Pediatr 1985;107:611.
669. Ackroyd JF. The pathogenesis of thrombocytopenic purpura due to hypersensitivity to sedormid (allyl-isopropyl-acetyl-carbamide). Clin Sci 1949;7:249.
670. Magnusson B, Rodjer S. Alprenolol-induced thrombocytopenia. Acta Med Scand 1980;207:231.
671. Ardman B, Rudders R. Aminoglutethimide-induced thrombocytopenia. (Letter) Cancer Treat Rep 1982;66:1785.
672. Ragaz J, Buskard N, Manji M. Thrombocytopenia after combination therapy with aminoglutethimide and tamoxifen: which drug is to blame? Cancer Treat Rep 1984;68:1015.
673. Weinberger I, Rotenberg Z, Fuchs J, et al. Amiodarone-induced thrombocytopenia. Arch Intern Med 1987;147:735.
674. Brooks AP. Thrombocytopenia during treatment with ampicillin. (Letter) Lancet 1974;2:723.
675. Kelton JG, Meltzer D, Moore J, et al. Drug-induced thrombocytopenia is associated with increased binding of IgG to platelets both in vivo and in vitro. Blood 1981;58:524.
676. Rubin SA, Lee S, O'Connor L, et al. Thrombocytopenia and fever in a patient taking amrinone. (Letter) N Engl J Med 1979;301:1185.
677. Ansell J, Tiarks C, McCue J, et al. Amrinone-induced thrombocytopenia. Arch Intern Med 1984;144:949.
678. Kinney EL, Ballard JO, Carlin B, Zelis R. Amrinone-mediated thrombocytopenia. Scand J Haematol 1983;31:376.
679. Ackroyd JF. The immunological basis of purpura due to drug hypersensitivity. Proc R Soc Med 1962;55:30.
680. Lee M, Sharifi R. Severe thrombocytopenia due to apalcillin. Urol Int 1987;42:313.
681. Young F. Severe post-operative thrombocytopenic purpura. Br Med J 1957;2:919.
682. Walsh KP, Walsh MJ, Branagan JP. Reversible severe thrombocytopaenia associated with captopril therapy. Irish Med J 1986;79:43.
683. Pujol M, Durán-Suárez JR, Martín Vega C, et al. Autoimmune thrombocytopenia in three patients treated with captopril. (Letter) Vox Sang 1989;57:218.
684. Pearce J, Ron MA. Thrombocytopenia after carbamazepine. (Letter) Lancet 1968;2:223.
685. Kornberg A, Kobrin I. IgG antiplatelet antibodies due to carbamazepine. Acta Haematol 1982;68:68.
686. Christie DJ, Lennon SS, Drew RL, Swinehart CD. Cefotetan-induced immunologic thrombocytopenia. Br J Haematol 1988;70:423.
687. Gralnick HR, McGinnis M, Hatterman R. Thrombocytopenia with sodium cephalothin therapy. Ann Intern Med 1972;77:401.
688. Sheiman L, Spielvogel AR, Horowitz HI. Thrombocytopenia caused by cephalothin sodium: occurrence in a penicillin-sensitive individual. JAMA 1968;203:601.
689. Lown J, Barr A. Immune thrombocytopenia induced by cephalosporins specific for thiomethyltetrazole side chain. (Letter) J Clin Pathol 1987;40:700.
690. Eisner EV, LaBocki NL, Pinckney L. Chlorpheniramine-dependent thrombocytopenia. JAMA 1975;231:735.
691. Nordqvist P, Cramer G, Bjorntorp P. Thrombocytopenia during chlorothiazide treatment. Lancet 1959;1:271.
692. Ball P. Thrombocytopenia and purpura in patients receiving chlorothiazide and hydrochlorothiazide. JAMA 1960;173:663.
693. Celada A, Herreros V, Rudolf H. Thrombocytopenic purpura during treatment with Librax. Br Med J 1977;1:268.
694. FitzPatrick WJ. Thrombocytopenia occurring during chlorpropamide therapy. Diabetes 1963;12:457.
695. Isaacs AJ. Cimetidine and thrombocytopenia. Br Med J 1980;280:294.
696. Yates VM, Kerr REI. Cimetidine and thrombocytopenia. (Letter) Br Med J 1980;280:1453.
697. McDaniel JL, Stein JJ. Thrombocytopenia with cimetidine therapy. (Letter) N Engl J Med 1979;300:864.
698. Mar DD, Brandstetter RD, Miskowvitz PF, Fotino M. Cimetidine-induced, immune-mediated leukopenia and thrombocytopenia. South Med J 1982;75:1283.
699. Stambaugh JE Jr, Gordon RL, Geller R. Leukopenia and thrombocytopenia secondary to clinoril therapy. (Letter) Lancet 1980;2:594.
700. Rosenbaum JT, O'Connor M. Thrombocytopenia associated with sulindac. (Letter) Arthritis Rheum 1981;24:753.
701. Veall RM, Hogarth HC. Thrombocytopenia during treatment with clonazepam. (Letter) Br Med J 1975;4:462.
702. Leissinger CA. Severe thrombocytopenia associated with cocaine use. Ann Intern Med 1990;112:708.
703. Walker JA, Sherman RA, Eisinger RP. Thrombocytopenia associated with intravenous desferrioxamine. Am J Kid Dis 1985;6:254.
704. Rachmilewitz EA, Dawson RB Jr, Rachmilewitz B. Serum antibodies against desipramine as a possible cause for thrombocytopenia. Blood 1968;32:525.
705. Shojania AM. Immune-mediated thrombocytopenia due to an iodinated contrast medium (diatrizoate). Can Med Assoc J 1985;133:123.
706. Conti L, Gandolfo GM. Benzodiazepine-induced thrombocytopenia: demonstration of drug-dependent platelet antibodies in two cases. Acta Haematol 1983;70:386.
707. Cimo PL, Pisciotta AV, Desai AG, et al. Detection of drug-dependent antibodies by the ^{51}Cr platelet lysis test: documentation of immune thrombocytopenia induced by diphenylhydantoin, diazepam, and sulfixoxazole. Am J Hematol 1977;2:65.
708. Combs JT, Grunt JA, Brant IK. Hematologic reactions to diazoxide. Pediatrics 1967;40:90.
709. Wales J, Wolff F. Haematologic side-effects of diazoxide. (Letter) Lancet 1967;1:53.
710. Kramer MR, Levene C, Hershko C. Severe reversible autoimmune haemolytic anaemia and thrombocytopenia associated with diclofenac therapy. Scand J Haematol 1986;36:118.
711. Tietze KJ, Gaska JA, Cosgrove EM. Thrombocytopenia and vomiting due to difluoromethylornithine. Drug Intell Clin Pharm 1987;21:627.
712. Bobrove AM. Diflunisal-associated thrombocytopenia in a patient with rheumatoid arthritis. (Letter) Arthritis Rheum 1988;31:148.
713. Berger H. Thrombopenic purpura following use of digitoxin. JAMA 1952;148:282.
714. Young RC, Nachman RL, Horowitz HI. Thrombocytopenia due to digitoxin: demonstration of antibody and mechanisms of action. Am J Med 1966;41:605.
715. Hess T, Riesen W, Scholtysik G, Stucki P. Digitoxin intoxication with severe thrombocytopenia: reversal by digoxin-specific antibodies. Eur J Clin Invest 1983;13:159.
716. Pirovino M, Ohnhaus EE, Von Felten A. Digoxin-associated thrombocytopenia. Eur J Clin Pharmacol 1981;19:205.
717. Lahav M, Arav R. Diltiazem and thrombocytopenia. (Letter) Ann Intern Med 1989;110:327.
718. Fincham RW, Hamilton HE, Schottelius DD. Late-onset thrombocytopenia with phenytoin therapy. Ann Neurol 1979;6:370.
719. Liang R. Thrombocytopenia associated with etretinate therapy. Acta Haematol 1988;79:112.
720. Jacobson ES. Fatal immune thrombocytopenia induced by ethchlorvynol. Ann Intern Med 1972;77:73.
721. Simpson RE, Goldstein DJ, Hjette GS, Evans ER. Acute thrombocytopenia associated with fenoprofen. (Letter) N Engl J Med 1978; 298:629.
722. Duncan A, Moore SB, Barker P. Thrombocytopenia caused by frusemide-induced platelet antibody. (Letter) Lancet 1981;1:1210.
723. Chen JH, Wiener L, Distenfeld A. Immunologic thrombocytopenia induced by gentamicin. NY State J Med 1980;80:1134.
724. Cicuttini FM, Wiley JS, Fraser KJ. Immune thrombocytopenia in association with oral gold treatment. (Letter) Arthritis Rheum 1988; 31:299.
725. Kosty MP, Hench PK, Tani P, McMillan R. Thrombocytopenia associated with auranofin therapy: evidence for a gold-dependent immunologic mechanism. Am J Hematol 1989;30:236.
726. Israeli A, Matzner Y, Or R, Raz I. Glibenclamide causing thrombocytopenia and bleeding tendency: case reports and a review of the literature. Klin Wochenschr 1988;66:223.
727. Warkentin TE, Kelton JG. Heparin and platelets. Hematol Oncol Clin North Am 1990;4:243.

728. Warkentin TE, Kelton JG. Interaction of heparin with platelets, including heparin-induced thrombocytopenia. In: Bounameaux H, ed. Low-molecular-weight heparins in prophylaxis and therapy of thromboembolic diseases. New York, Marcel Dekker, 1994:75.
729. Christie DJ, Walker RH, Kolins MD, et al. Quinine-induced thrombocytopenia following intravenous use of heroin. Arch Intern Med 1983;143:1174.
730. Moss RA, Okun DB. Heroin-induced thrombocytopenia. Arch Intern Med 1979;139:752.
731. Fishman AJ. Thrombocytopenia and heroin. (Letter) Ann Intern Med 1981;94:280.
732. Eisner EV, Crowell EB. Hydrochlorothiazide-dependent thrombocytopenia due to IgM antibody. JAMA 1971;215:480.
733. Camba L, Joyner MV. Acute thrombocytopenia following ingestion of indomethacin. Acta Haematol 1984;71:350.
734. Kulis JC. Chemically induced, selective thrombocytopenic purpura. Arch Intern Med 1965;116:559.
735. McLaughlin P, Talpaz M, Quesada JR, et al. Immune thrombocytopenia following α-interferon therapy in patients with cancer. JAMA 1985;254:1353.
736. Kanfer EJ, McCarthy DM. Immune thrombocytopenia and interferon alfa. Br Med J 1988;297:1613.
737. Abdi EA, Brien W, Venner PM. Auto-immune thrombocytopenia related to interferon therapy. Scand J Haematol 1986;36:515.
738. Hysell JK, Hysell JW, Gray JM. Thrombocytopenic purpura following iopanoid acid ingestion. JAMA 1977;237:361.
739. Hansen JE. Hypersensitivity to isoniazid with neutropenia and thrombocytopenia. Am Rev Resp Dis 1961;83:744.
740. Johnson TM, Rapini RP. Isotretinoin-induced thrombocytopenia. (Letter) J Am Acad Dermatol 1987;17:838.
741. El-Ghobarey AF, Capell HA. Levamisole-induced thrombocytopenia. Br Med J 1977;2:555.
742. Wanamaker WM, Wanamaker SJ, Celesia GG, Koeller AA. Thrombocytopenia associated with long-term levodopa therapy. JAMA 1976;235:2217.
743. Stefanini M, Hoffman MN. Studies on platelet. XXVIII. Acute thrombocytopenic purpura due to lidocaine (Xylocaine) mediated antibody. Report of a case. Am J Med Sci 1978;275:365.
744. Raff MJ. Lincomycin: thrombocytopenia? Ann Intern Med 1973; 78:779.
745. Schiffer CA, Weinstein HJ, Wiernik PH. Methicillin-associated thrombocytopenia. (Letter) Ann Intern Med 1973;85:338.
746. Manohitharajah SM, Jenkins WJ, Roberts PD, Clarke RC. Methyldopa and associated thrombocytopenia. Br Med J 1971;1:494.
747. Pai RG, Pai SM. Methyldopa-induced reversible immune thrombocytopenia. Am J Med 1988;85:123.
748. Polk OD, Kletter GG, Smith J, Castro O. Impaired clot retraction in thrombocytopenia due to methyldopa. South Med J 1982;75:374.
749. Fasola GP, D'Osualdo F, De Pangher V, Barducci E. Thrombocytopenia and mexiletine. (Letter) Ann Intern Med 1984;100:162.
750. Stricker BHC, Barendregt JNM, Claas FHJ. Thrombocytopenia and leucopenia with mianserin-dependent antibodies. Br J Clin Pharmacol 1985;19:102.
751. Peitzman SJ, Martin C. Thrombocytopenia and minoxidil. (Letter) Ann Intern Med 1980;92:874.
752. Cimo PL, Hammond JJ, Moake JL. Morphine-induced immune thrombocytopenia associated with a platelet antibody cross-reactive with other opiates. (Abstract) Clin Res 1979;27:744A.
753. Meyboom RHB. Thrombocytopenia induced by nalidixic acid. Br Med J 1984;289:962.
754. Pasticci MB, Menichetti F, Di Candilo F. Nimesulide, thrombocytopenic purpura, and human immunodeficiency virus (HIV) infection. (Letter) Ann Intern Med 1990;112:233.
755. Mehta P, Mehta J, Miale TD. Nitroprusside lowers platelet count. (Letter) N Engl J Med 1978;299:1134.
756. Green PJ, Naorose-Abidi SMH. Nomifensine and thrombocytopenia. Br Med J 1984;288:830.
757. Day HJ, Conrad FG, Moore JE. Immunothrombocytopenia induced by novobiocin. Am J Med Sci 1958;236:475.
758. Armstrong FB, Scherbel AL. Review of toxicity of oxyphenebutazone: report of a case of thrombocytopenic purpura. JAMA 1961;175: 614.
759. Hare DL, Hicks BH. Thrombocytopenia due to oxprenolol. (Letter) Med J Aust 1979;2:259.
760. Dodds WN, Davidson RJL. Thrombocytopenia due to slow-release oxprenolol. (Letter) Lancet 1978;2:683.
761. Patrassi GM, Casonato A, Fabris F, Girolami A. Thrombocytopenia secondary to oxprenolol, a β-blocking agent. Acta Haematol 1982; 68:75.
762. Kounis NG. Oxytetracycline-induced thrombocytopenic purpura. JAMA 1975;231:734.
763. Wurzel HA, Mayock RL. Thrombocytopenia induced by sodium para-aminosalicyclic acid: report of a case. JAMA 1953;153:1094.
764. Murphy MF, Riordan T, Minchinton RM, et al. Demonstration of an immune-mediated mechanism of penicillin-induced neutropenia and thrombocytopenia. Br J Haematol 1983;55:155.
765. Salamon DJ, Nusbacher J, Stroupe T, et al. Red cell and platelet-bound IgG penicillin antibodies in a patient with thrombocytopenia. Transfusion 1984;24:395.
766. Arnved J, Skov PS, Winter K. Pentagastrin-induced thrombocytopenia. (Letter) Lancet 1985;2:1068.
767. Levy MA, Senior RM, Sneider RE. Severe thrombocytopenic purpura complicating pentamidine therapy for *Pneumocystis carinii* pneumonia. Cancer 1974;34:441.
768. Christie DJ, Sauro SC, Cavanaugh AL, Kaplan ME. Severe thrombocytopenia in an acquired immunodeficiency syndrome patient associated with pentamidine-dependent antibodies specific for glycoprotein IIb/IIIa. Blood 1993;82:3075.
769. Davidson C, Manohitharajah SM. Drug-induced antiplatelet antibodies. (Letter) Br Med J 1973;3:545.
770. Stricker BHC, Meyboom RHB, Bleeker PA, Van Wieringen K. Blood disorders associated with pirenzepine. Br Med J 1986;293:1074.
771. Bjornstad H, Vik O. Thrombocytopenic purpura associated with piroxicam. Br J Clin Pract 1986;40:42.
772. Parker WA. Primidone thrombocytopenia. (Letter) Ann Intern Med 1974;81:559.
773. Devine DV, Currie MS, Rosse WF, Greenberg CS. Pseudo–Bernard-Soulier syndrome: thrombocytopenia caused by autoantibody to platelet glycoprotein Ib. Blood 1987;70:428.
774. Rosenstein R, Kosfeld RE, Leight L, Liu YK. Procainamide-induced thrombocytopenia. Am J Hematol 1984;16:181.
775. Meisner DJ, Carlson RJ, Gottlieb AJ. Thrombocytopenia following sustained-release procainamide. Arch Intern Med 1985;145:700.
776. Bolton FG, Young RV. Observations on cases of thrombocytopenic purpura due to quinine, suphamezathine, and quinidine. J Clin Pathol 1953;6:320.
777. Spychal RT, Wickham NWR. Thrombocytopenia associated with ranitidine. Br Med J 1985;291:1687.
778. Gibson PR, Pidcock ME. Immune-mediated thrombocytopenia associated with ranitidine therapy. Med J Aust 1986;145:661.
779. Blajchman MA, Lowry RC, Pettit JE, Stradling P. Rifampicin-induced immune thrombocytopenia. Br Med J 1970;3:24.
780. Pau AK, Fisher MA. Severe thrombocytopenia associated with once-daily rifampin therapy. Drug Intell Clin Pharm 1987;21:882.
781. Kakaiya RM, Dehertogh D, Walker FJ, et al. Rifampin-induced thrombocytopenia: a case report. Vox Sang 1989;57:185.
782. Rappaport AE, Nixon CE, Barker WA. Fatal secondary, toxic thrombocytopenic purpura due to sodium salicylate: report of a case. J Lab Clin Med 1945;30:916.
783. Kahn HR, Brod RC. Thrombocytopenia due to stibophen. Arch Intern Med 1961;108:496.
784. Rivera JV, Rodriguez HF, et al. Thrombocytopenic purpura due to faudin (Stibophen). Am J Trop Med Hyg 1956;5:863.
785. Thomas TF. Thrombocytopenic purpura secondary to sulfamethoxypyridazine. NY State J Med 1963;63:2554.
786. Karachalios GN, Parigorakis JG. Thrombocytopenia and sulindac. (Letter) Ann Intern Med 1986;104:128.
787. Farr M, Tunn E, Bacon PA, Smith DH. Hypogammaglobulinemia and thrombocytopenia associated with sulphasalazine therapy in rheumatoid arthritis. Ann Rheum Dis 1985;44:723.
788. Pena JM, Gonzalez-Garcia JJ, Garcia-Alegria J, et al. Thrombocytopenia and sulfasalazine. (Letter) Ann Intern Med 1985;102:277.
789. Hamilton HE, Sheets RF. Sulfisoxazole-induced thrombocytopenic purpura: immunologic mechanism as cause. JAMA 1978;239:2586.
790. Greenlaw CW, Stolley SN, Henrietta GC. Tobramycin-induced thrombocytopenia. (Letter) Drug Intell Clin Pharmacol 1978;12:682.
791. Balodimos MC, Camerini-Davalos RA, Marble A. Nine years' experience with tolbutamide in the treatment of diabetes. Metabolism 1966;15:957.
792. Jennings GH, Gower ND. Thrombocytopenic purpura in toluene diisocyanate workers. Lancet 1963;1:406.
793. Lockhart JM. Tolmetin-induced thrombocytopenia. (Letter) Arthritis Rheum 1982;25:1144.
794. Schwartz RH, Rodriguez WJ, Luban NLC. Thrombocytopenia associated with PF_3 antiplatelet activity against the sulfa component of trimethoprim-sulfamethoxazole. South Med J 1981;74:640.
795. Kiefel V, Santoso S, Schmidt S, et al. Metabolite-specific (IgG) and drug-specific antibodies (IgG, IgM) in two cases of trimethoprim-sulfamethoxazole–induced immune thrombocytopenia. Transfusion 1987;27:262.
796. Barr AL, Whineray M. Immune thrombocytopenia induced by cotrimoxazole. Aust NZ J Med 1980;10:54.
797. Claas FHJ, Van der Meer JWM, Langerak J. Immunological effect of co-trimoxazole on platelets. Br Med J 1979;2:898.
798. Wahlberg P, Nyman D. Turpentine and thrombocytopenic purpura. (Letter) Lancet 1969;2:215.
799. Barr RD, Copeland SA, Stockwell ML, et al. Valproic acid and immune thrombocytopenia. Arch Dis Child 1982;57:681.
800. Walker RW, Heaton A. Thrombocytopenia due to vancomycin. (Letter) Lancet 1985;1:932.
801. Christie DJ, van Buren N, Lennon SS, Putnam JL. Vancomycin-dependent antibodies associated with thrombocytopenia and refractoriness to platelet transfusion in patients with leukemia. Blood 1990;75:518.

802. Danielson DA, Douglas SW III, Herzog P, et al. Drug-induced blood disorders. JAMA 1984;252:3257.
803. Sobel M, Adelman B. Characterization of platelet binding of heparins and other glycosaminoglycans. Thromb Res 1988;50:815.
804. Brace LD, Fareed J. An objective assessment of the interaction of heparin and its fractions with human platelets. Semin Thromb Hemost 1985;11:190.
805. Salzman EW, Rosenberg RD, Smith MH, et al. Effect of heparin and heparin fractions on platelet aggregation. J Clin Invest 1980;65:64.
806. Warkentin TE, Kelton JG. Heparin-induced thrombocytopenia. In: Coller BS, ed. Progress in hemostasis and thrombosis, vol 10. Philadelphia, WB Saunders, 1990.
807. Kelton JG. Heparin-induced thrombocytopenia. Haemostasis 1986;16:173.
808. Follea G, Hamandjian I, Trzeciak MC, et al. Pentosane polysulphate associated thrombocytopenia. Thromb Res 1986;42:413.
809. Tardy-Poncet B, Tardy B, Grelac F, et al. Pentosan polysulfate-induced thrombocytopenia and thrombosis. Am J Hematol 1994;45:252.
810. Greinacher A, Michels I, Schafer M, Kiefel V, Mueller-Eckhardt C. Heparin-associated thrombocytopenia in a patient treated with polysulphated chondroitin sulphate: evidence for immunological crossreactivity between heparin and polysulphated glycosaminoglycans. Br J Haematol 1992;81:252.
811. Chong BH, Ismail F, Cade J, et al. Heparin-induced thrombocytopenia: studies with a new low molecular weight heparinoid, Org 10172. Blood 1989;73:1592.
812. Magnani HN. Heparin-induced thrombocytopenia (HIT): an overview of 230 patients treated with Orgaran (Org 10172). Thromb Haemost 1993;70:554.
813. Hrushesky WJ. Subcutaneous heparin–induced thrombocytopenia. Arch Intern Med 1978;138:1489.
814. Laster J, Silver D. Heparin-coated catheters and heparin-induced thrombocytopenia. J Vasc Surg 1988;7:667.
815. King DJ, Kelton JG. Heparin-associated thrombocytopenia. Ann Intern Med 1984;100:535.
816. Phelan BK. Heparin-associated thrombosis with thrombocytopenia. Ann Intern Med 1983;99:637.
817. Ramirez-Lassepas M, Cipolle RJ, Rodvold KA, et al. Heparin-induced thrombocytopenia in patients with cerebrovascular disease. Neurology 1984;34:736.
818. Boshkov LK, Warkentin TE, Hayward CPM, Andrew M, Kelton JG. Heparin-induced thrombocytopenia and thrombosis: clinical and laboratory studies. Br J Haematol 1993;84:322.
819. Calhoun BC, Hesser JW. Heparin-associated antibody with pregnancy: discussion of two cases. Am J Obstet Gynecol 1987;156:964.
820. van der Weyden MB, Hunt H, McGrath K, et al. Delayed-onset heparin-induced thrombocytopenia: a potentially malignant syndrome. Med J Aust 1983;2:132.
821. Arthur CK, Grant SJB, Murray WK, et al. Heparin-associated acute adrenal insufficiency. Aust NZ J Med 1985;15:454.
822. Findling JW, Korducki JM, Lahiri PK, et al. Bilateral adrenal hemorrhage associated with heparin-induced thrombocytopenia. Wisc Med J 1987;86:2.
823. Ernest D, Fisher MM. Heparin-induced thrombocytopaenia complicated by bilateral adrenal haemorrhage. Intens Care Med 1991; 17:238.
824. Bleasel JF, Rasko JEJ, Rickard KA, Richards G. Acute adrenal insufficiency secondary to heparin-induced thrombocytopenia-thrombosis syndrome. Med J Aust 1992;157:192.
825. Stricker H, Lämmle B, Furlan M, Sulzer I. Heparin-dependent in vitro aggregation of normal platelets by plasma of a patient with heparin-induced skin necrosis: specific diagnosis for a rare side effect. Am J Med 1988;85:721.
826. White PW, Sadd JR, Nensel RE. Thrombotic complications of heparin therapy. Including six cases of heparin-induced skin necrosis. Ann Surg 1979;190:595.
827. Platell CFE, Tan EGC. Hypersensitivity reactions to heparin: delayed onset thrombocytopenia and necrotizing skin lesions. Aust NZ J Surg 1986;56:621.
828. Ojeda E, del Carmen Perez M, Mataix R, et al. Skin necrosis with a low molecular weight heparin. Br J Haematol 1992;82:620.
829. Warkentin TE, Soutar RL, Panju A, Ginsberg JS. Acute systemic reactions to intravenous bolus heparin therapy: characterization and relationship to heparin-induced thrombocytopenia. (Abstract) Blood 1992;80(Suppl 1):160a.
830. Ansell JE, Clark WP Jr, Compton CC. Fatal reactions associated with intravenous heparin. Drug Intell Clin Pharm 1986;20:74.
831. Warkentin TE, Hirte HW, Anderson DR, O'Connell GJ, Lo RC. Transient global amnesia associated with acute heparin-induced thrombocytopenia. Am J Med 1994, in press.
832. Rhodes GR, Dixon RH, Silver D. Heparin induced thrombocytopenia: eight cases with thrombotic-hemorrhagic complications. Ann Surg 1977;186:752.
833. Laster J, Cikrit D, Walker N, Silver D. The heparin-induced thrombocytopenia syndrome: an update. Surgery 1987;102:763.
834. Kelton JG, Sheridan D, Brain H, et al. Clinical usefulness of testing for a heparin-dependent platelet-aggregating factor in patients with suspected heparin-associated thrombocytopenia. J Lab Clin Med 1984;103:606.
835. Chong BH, Pitney WR, Castaldi PA. Heparin-induced thrombocytopenia: association of thrombotic complications with heparin-dependent IgG antibody that induces thromboxane synthesis and platelet aggregation. Lancet 1982;2:1246.
836. Chong BH, Fawaz I, Chesterman CN, Berndt MC. Heparin-induced thrombocytopenia: mechanism of interaction of the heparin-dependent antibody with platelets. Br J Haematol 1989;73:235.
837. Adelman B, Sobel M, Fujimura T, Ruggeri ZM, Zimmerman TS. Heparin-associated thrombocytopenia: observations on the mechanism of platelet aggregation. J Lab Clin Med 1989;113:204.
838. Greinacher A, Michels I, Kiefel V, Mueller-Eckhardt C. A rapid and sensitive test for diagnosing heparin-associated thrombocytopenia. Thromb Haemost 1991;66:734.
839. Warkentin TE, Hayward CPM, Boshkov LK, et al. Sera from patients with heparin-induced thrombocytopenia generate platelet-derived microparticles with procoagulant activity: an explanation for the thrombotic complications of heparin-induced thrombocytopenia. Blood 1994; in press.
840. Green D, Harris K, Reynolds N, Roberts M, Patterson R. Heparin immune thrombocytopenia: evidence for a heparin-platelet complex as the antigenic determinant. J Lab Clin Med 1978;91:167.
841. Amiral J, Bridey F, Dreyfus M, et al. Platelet factor 4 complexed to heparin is the target for antibodies generated in heparin-induced thrombocytopenia. (Letter) Thromb Haemost 1992;68:95.
842. Kelton JG, Smith JW, Warkentin TE, et al. Immunoglobulin G from patients with heparin-induced thrombocytopenia binds to a complex of heparin and platelet factor 4. Blood 1994; 83: 3232-3239.
843. Visentin GP, Ford SE, Scott JP, Aster RH. Antibodies from patients with heparin-induced thrombocytopenia/thrombosis are specific for platelet factor 4 complexed with heparin or bound to endothelial cells. J Clin Invest 1994;93:81.
844. Greinacher A, Pötzsch B, Amiral J, Dummel V, Eichner A, Mueller-Eckhardt C. Heparin-associated thrombocytopenia: isolation of the antibody and characterization of a multimolecular PF4-heparin complex as the major antigen. Thromb Haemost 1994;71:247.
845. Makhoul RG, Greenberg CS, McCann RL. Heparin-associated thrombocytopenia and thrombosis: a serious clinical problem and potential solution. J Vasc Surg 1986;4:522.
846. Chong BH, Pilgrim RL, Cooley MA, Chesterman CN. Increased expression of platelet IgG Fc receptors in immune heparin-induced thrombocytopenia. Blood 1993;81:988.
847. Warkentin TE, Hayward CPM, Smith CA, Kelly PM, Kelton JG. Determinants of donor platelet variability when testing for heparin-induced thrombocytopenia. J Lab Clin Med 1992;120:371.
848. Warkentin TE, Levine MN, Roberts RS, et al. Heparin-induced thrombocytopenia is more common with unfractionated heparin than with low molecular weight heparin. (Abstract) Thromb Haemost 1993;69:911.
849. Cines DB, Tomaski A, Tannenbaum S. Immune endothelial-cell injury in heparin-associated thrombocytopenia. N Engl J Med 1987;316:581.
850. Favaloro EJ, Bernal-Hoyos E, Exner T, Koutts J. Heparin-induced thrombocytopenia: laboratory investigation and confirmation of diagnosis. Pathology 1992;24:177.
851. Chong BH, Burgess J, Ismail F. The clinical usefulness of the platelet aggregation test for the diagnosis of heparin-induced thrombocytopenia. Thromb Haemost 1993;69:344.
852. Warkentin TE, Santos AV, Hayward CPM, et al. Importance of platelet preparation in diagnostic testing for heparin-induced thrombocytopenia. (Abstract) Blood 1991;78(Suppl 1):344a.
853. Greinacher A, Amiral J, Dummel V, et al. Laboratory diagnosis of heparin-associated thrombocytopenia and comparison of platelet aggregation test, heparin-induced platelet activation test, and platelet factor 4/heparin enzyme-linked immunosorbent assay. Transfusion 1994;34:381.
854. Babcock RB, Dumper CW, Scharfman WB. Heparin-induced immune thrombocytopenia. N Engl J Med 1976;295:237.
855. Cimo PL, Moake JL, Weinger RS, et al. Heparin-induced thrombocytopenia: association with a platelet-aggregating factor and arterial thromboses. Am J Hematol 1979;6:125.
856. Bell WR. Defibrinogenating enzymes. In: Colman RW, Hirsh J, Marder VJ, Salzman EW, eds. Hemostasis and thrombosis: basic principles and clinical practice, ed 2. Philadelphia, JB Lippincott, 1987:886.
857. Cole CW, Bormanis J. Ancrod: a practical alternative to heparin. J Vasc Surg 1988;8:59.
858. Demers C, Ginsberg JS, Brill-Edwards P, et al. Rapid anticoagulation using ancrod for heparin-induced thrombocytopenia. Blood 1991:78:2194.
859. Meuleman DG. Orgaran (Org 10172): its pharmacological profile in experimental models. Haemostasis 1992;22:58.
860. Harenberg J, Zimmermann R, Schwarz F, et al. Treatment of heparin-induced thrombocytopenia with thrombosis by new heparinoid. Lancet 1983;1:986.
861. Bouvier JL, Lefevre P, Villain P, et al. Treatment of serious heparin-induced thrombocytopenia by plasma exchange: report on 4 cases. (Letter) Thromb Res 1988;51:335.

862. Brady J, Riccio JA, Yumen OH, et al. Plasmapheresis. A therapeutic option in the management of heparin-associated thrombocytopenia with thrombosis. Am J Clin Pathol 1991;96:394.
863. Greinacher A, Liebenhoff U, Kiefel V, et al. Heparin-associated thrombocytopenia: the effects of various intravenous IgG preparations on antibody mediated platelet activation—a possible new indication for high dose i.v. IgG. Thromb Haemost 1994;71:641.
864. Frame JN, Mulvey KP, Phares JC, Anderson MJ. Correction of severe heparin-associated thrombocytopenia with intravenous immunoglobulin. Ann Intern Med 1989;111:946.
865. Nand S. Hirudin therapy for heparin-associated thrombocytopenia and deep vein thrombosis. Am J Hematol 1993;43:310.
866. Gruel Y, Lermusiaux P, Lang M, et al. Usefulness of antiplatelet drugs in the management of heparin-associated thrombocytopenia and thrombosis. Ann Vasc Surg 1991;5:552.
867. Sobel M, Adelman B, Szentpetery S, et al. Surgical management of heparin-associated thrombocytopenia: strategies in the treatment of venous and arterial thromboembolism. J Vasc Surg 1988;8:395.
868. Cohen JI, Cooper MR, Greenberg CS. Streptokinase therapy of pulmonary emboli with heparin-associated thrombocytopenia. Arch Intern Med 1985;145:1725.
869. Cummings JM, Mason TJ, Chomka EV, et al. Fibrinolytic therapy of acute myocardial infarction in the heparin thrombosis syndrome. Am Heart J 1986;112:407.
870. Olinger GN, Hussey CV, Olive JA, Malik MI. Cardiopulmonary bypass for patients with previously documented heparin-induced platelet aggregation. J Thorac Cardiovasc Surg 1984;87:673.
871. Doherty DC, Ortel TL, De Bruijn N, Greenberg CS, Van Trigt P III. "Heparin-free" cardiopulmonary bypass: first reported use of heparinoid (Org 10172) to provide anticoagulation for cardiopulmonary bypass. Anesthesiology 1990;73:562.
872. Zulys VJ, Teasdale SJ, Michel ER, et al. Ancrod (Arvin) as an alternative to heparin anticoagulation for cardiopulmonary bypass. Anesthesiology 1989;71:870.
873. Janson PA, Moake JL, Carpinito G. Aspirin prevents heparin-induced platelet aggregation *in vivo*. Br J Haematol 1983;53:166.
874. Miller LC, Hall JC, Crow JW, et al. Hemodialysis in heparin-associated thrombocytopenia: epoprostenol (PGI_2) as sole anticoagulant. Dial Transplant 1985;14:579.
875. Leehey DJ, Kanak RJ, Messmore HL, et al. Heparin-associated thrombocytopenia in maintenance hemodialysis patients. Int J Artif Organs 1987;10:390.
876. Matsuo T, Chikahira Y, Yamada T, et al. Effect of synthetic thrombin inhibitor (MD805) as an alternative drug on heparin induced thrombocytopenia during hemodialysis. Thromb Res 1988;52:165.
877. Reid DM, Shulman NR. Drug purpura due to surreptitious quinidine intake. Ann Intern Med 1988;108:206.
878. Chong BH, Berndt MC, Koutts J, Castaldi PA. Quinidine-induced thrombocytopenia and leukopenia: demonstration and characterization of distinct antiplatelet and antileukocyte antibodies. Blood 1983;62:1218.
879. Zeigler Z, Shadduck RK, Winkelstein A, Stroupe TK. Immune hemolytic anemia and thrombocytopenia secondary to quinidine: in vitro studies of the quinidine-dependent red cell and platelet antibodies. Blood 1979;53:396.
880. Christie DJ, Aster RH. Drug-antibody-platelet interaction in quinine and quinidine-induced thrombocytopenia. J Clin Invest 1982;70:989.
881. Christie DJ, Weber RW, Mullen PC, et al. Structural features of the quinidine and quinine molecules necessary for binding of drug-induced antibodies to human platelets. J Lab Clin Med 1984;104:730.
882. Kunicki TJ, Russel N, Nurden AT, et al. Further studies of the human platelet receptor for quinine- and quinidine-dependent antibodies. J Immunol 1981;126:398.
883. Kunicki TJ, Johnson MM, Aster RH. Absence of the platelet receptor for drug-dependent antibodies in the Bernard-Soulier syndrome. J Clin Invest 1978;62:716.
884. Smith ME, Reid DM, Jones CE, et al. Binding of quinine-and quinidine-dependent drug antibodies to platelets is mediated by the Fab domain of the immunoglobulin G and is not Fc dependent. J Clin Invest 1987;79:912.
885. Visentin GP, Newman PJ, Aster RH. Characteristics of quinine- and quinidine-induced antibodies specific for platelet glycoproteins IIb and IIIa. Blood 1991;77:2668.
886. Pfueller SL, Bilston RA, Logan D, et al. Heterogeneity of drug-dependent platelet antigens and their antibodies in quinine- and quinidine-induced thrombocytopenia: involvement of glycoproteins Ib, IIb, IIIa, and IX. Blood 1988;72:1155.
887. Lerner W, Caruso R, Faig D, Karpatkin S. Drug-dependent and non–drug-dependent antiplatelet antibody in drug-induced immunologic thrombocytopenic purpura. Blood 1985;66:306.
888. Herbst KD, Stone WH, Flannery EP. Chronic thrombocytopenia following gold therapy. (Letter) Arch Intern Med 1975;135:1622.
889. Barton JJ, Burke JP, Casey EB, McCann SR. Observations on the clinical and therapeutic aspects of gold induced thrombocytopenia. Irish Med J 1985;78:167.
890. Stafford BT, Crosby WH. Late onset of gold-induced thrombocytopenia: with a practical note on the injections of dimercaprol. JAMA 1978;239:50.
891. Von dem Borne AEGK, Pegels JG, Van der Stadt RJ, et al. Thrombocytopenia associated with gold therapy: a drug-induced autoimmune disease? Br J Haematol 1986;63:509.
892. Levin HA, McMillan R, Tavassoli M, et al. Thrombocytopenia associated with gold therapy: observations on the mechanism of platelet destruction. Am J Med 1975;59:274.
893. Coblyn JS, Weinblatt M, Holdsworth D, Glass D. Gold-induced thrombocytopenia: a clinical and immunogenetic study of twenty-three patients. Ann Intern Med 1981;95:178.
894. Adachi JD, Bensen WG, Kassam Y, et al. Gold-induced thrombocytopenia: 12 cases and a review of the literature. Semin Arthritis Rheum 1987;16:287.
895. Goldstein R, Blanchette VS, Huebsch LB, McKendry RJR. Treatment of gold-induced thrombocytopenia by high-dose intravenous gamma globulin. Arthritis Rheum 1986;29:426.
896. Ball GV. Gold-induced thrombocytopenia: response to vincristine? (Letter) Arthritis Rheum 1977;20:1288.
897. Kozloff M, Votaw M, Penner JA. Gold-induced thrombocytopenia responsive to cyclophosphamide. South Med J 1979;72:1490.
898. England JM, Smith DS. Gold-induced thrombocytopenia and response to dimercaprol. Br Med J 1972;2:748.
899. Godfrey NF, Peter A, Simon TM, Lorber A. IV N-acetylcysteine treatment of hematologic reactions to chrysotherapy. J Rheumatol 1982;9:519.
900. Van Loghem JJ Jr, Dorfmeijer H, Van der Hart M, Schreuder F. Serological and genetical studies on a platelet antigen (Zw). Vox Sang 1959;4:161.
901. Van der Weerdt CM, Veenhoven-von Riesz LE, Nijenhuis LE, Van Loghem JJ. The Zw blood group system in platelets. Vox Sang 1963;8:513.
902. Shulman NR, Marder VJ, Hiller MC, Collier EM. Platelet and leukocyte isoantigens and their antibodies: serologic, physiologic and clinical studies. Prog Hematol 1964;4:222.
903. Langenscheidt F, Kiefel V, Santoso S, Mueller-Eckhardt C. Platelet transfusion refractoriness associated with two rare platelet-specific alloantibodies (anti-Bak^a and anti-Pl^{A2}) and multiple HLA antibodies. Transfusion 1988;28:597.
904. Taaning E, Morling N, Ovesen H, Svejgaard A. Posttransfusion purpura and anti-Zw^b (-Pl^{A2}). Tissue Antigens 1985;26:143.
905. Mueller-Eckhardt C, Becker T, Weisheit M, et al. Neonatal alloimmune thrombocytopenia due to fetomaternal Zw^b incompatibility. Vox Sang 1986;50:94.
906. Kunicki TJ, Aster RH. Isolation and immunologic characterization of the human platelet alloantigen, Pl^{A1}. Mol Immunol 1979;16:353.
907. Reznikoff-Etievant MF, Dangu C, Lobet R. HLA-B8 antigens and anti-PL^{a1} allo-immunization. Tissue Antigens 1981;18:66.
908. Mueller-Eckhardt C, Mueller-Eckhardt G, Willen-Ohff H, et al. Immunogenicity of and immune response to the human platelet antigen Zw^a is strongly associated with HLA-B8 and DR3. Tissue Antigens 1985;26:71.
909. De Waal LP, Van Dalen CM, Engelfriet CP, Von dem Borne AEGK. Alloimmunization against the platelet-specific Zw^a antigen, resulting in neonatal thrombocytopenia or posttransfusion purpura, is associated with the supertypic DRw52 antigen including DR3 and DRw6. Hum Immunol 1986;17:45.
910. Reznikoff-Etievant MF, Kaplan C, Muller JY, et al. Allo-immune thrombocytopenias, definition of a group at risk: a prospective study. Curr Stud Hematol Blood Transfus 1988;55:119.
911. Cobos E, Gandara DR, Geier LJ, Kirmani S. Post-transfusion purpura and isoimmune neonatal thrombocytopenia in the same family. Am J Hematol 1989;32:235.
912. Letellier SJ, Hunter JB, Aster RH. Probable genetic linkage between genes coding for platelet-specific antigens of the Pl^A and Bak systems. Am J Hematol 1988;29:139.
913. Kickler T, Kennedy SD, Braine HG. Alloimmunization to platelet-specific antigens on glycoproteins IIb-IIIa and Ib/IX in multiply transfused thrombocytopenic patients. Transfusion 1990;30:622.
914. Van der Weerdt CM, Van den Wiel-Dorfmeyer H, Engelfriet CP, Van Loghem JJ. A new platelet antigen. Basel, Switzerland, Karger, 1962:379.
915. Marcelli-Barge A, Poirier JC, Dausset J. Allo-antigens and allo-antibodies of the Ko system, serological and genetic study. Vox Sang 1973;24:1.
916. Bizzaro N, Dianese G. Neonatal alloimmune amegakaryocytosis: case report. Vox Sang 1988;54:112.
917. Saji H, Maruya E, Fujii H, et al. New platelet antigen, Sib^a, involved in platelet transfusion refractoriness in a Japanese man. Vox Sang 1989;56:283.
918. Kuijpers RWAM, Ouwehand WH, Bleeker PMM, et al. Localisation of the platelet-specific HPA-2 (Ko) alloantigens on the N-terminal globular fragment of platelet glycoprotein Ibα. Blood 1992;79:283.
919. Von dem Borne AEGK, Von Riesz E, Verheugt FWA, et al. Bak^a, a new platelet-specific antigen involved in neonatal allo-immune thrombocytopenia. Vox Sang 1980;39:113.

920. Boizard B, Wautier JL. Lek[a], a new platelet antigen absent in Glanzmann's thrombasthenia. Vox Sang 1984;46:47.
921. Kiemowitz RM, Collins J, Davis K, Aster RH. Post-transfusion purpura associated with alloimmunization against the platelet-specific antigen, Bak[a]. Am J Hematol 1986;21:79.
922. Von dem Borne AEGK, Van der Plas-van Dalen CM. Bak[a] and Lek[a] are identical antigens. (Letter) Br J Haematol 1986;62:404.
923. Kickler TS, Herman JH, Furihata K, et al. Identification of Bak[b], a new platelet-specific antigen associated with posttransfusion purpura. Blood 1988;71:894.
924. McGrath K, Minchinton R, Cunningham I, Ayberk H. Platelet anti-Bak[b] antibody associated with neonatal alloimmune thrombocytopenia. Vox Sang 1989;57:182.
925. Kiefel V, Santoso S, Glockner WM, et al. Posttransfusion purpura associated with an anti-Bak[b]. Vox Sang 1989;56:93.
926. Kieffer N, Boizard B, Didry D, et al. Immunochemical characterization of the platelet-specific alloantigen Lek[a]: a comparative study with the Pl[A1] alloantigen. Blood 1984;64:1212.
927. Mulder A, van Leeuwen EF, Veenboer GJM, et al. Immunochemical characterization of platelet-specific alloantigens. Scand J Haematol 1984;33:267.
928. Lyman S, Aster RH, Visentin GP, Newman PJ. Polymorphism of human platelet membrane glycoprotein IIb associated with the Bak[a]/Bak[b] alloantigen system. Blood 1990;75:2343.
929. Take H, Tomiyama Y, Shibata Y, et al. Demonstration of the heterogeneity of epitopes of the platelet-specific alloantigen, Bak[a]. Br J Haematol 1990;76:395.
930. Goldberger A, Kolodziej M, Poncz M, et al. Effect of single amino acid substitutions on the formation of the Pl[A] and Bak alloantigenic epitopes. Blood 1991;78:681.
931. Friedman JM, Aster RH. Neonatal alloimmune thrombocytopenic purpura and congenital porencephaly in two siblings associated with a "new" maternal antiplatelet antibody. Blood 1985;65:1412.
932. Shibata Y, Matsuda I, Miyaji T, Ichikawa Y. Yuk[a], a new platelet antigen involved in two cases of neonatal alloimmune thrombocytopenia. Vox Sang 1986;50:177.
933. Shibata Y, Miyaji T, Ichikawa Y, Matsuda I. A new platelet antigen system, Yuk[a]/Yuk[b]. Vox Sang 1986;51:334.
934. Simon TL, Collins J, Kunicki TJ, et al. Posttransfusion purpura associated with alloantibody specific for the platelet antigen, Pen[a]. Am J Hematol 1988;29:38.
935. Santoso S, Shibata Y, Kiefel V, Mueller-Eckhardt C. Identification of the Yuk[b] allo-antigen on platelet glycoprotein IIIa. Vox Sang 1987; 53:48.
936. Furihata K, Nugent DJ, Bissonette A, et al. On the association of the platelet-specific alloantigen, Pen[a], with glycoprotein IIIa: evidence for heterogeneity of glycoprotein IIIa. J Clin Invest 1987;80:1624.
937. Wang R, Furihata K, McFarland JG, et al. An amino acid polymorphism within the RGD binding domain of platelet membrane glycoprotein IIIa is responsible for the formation of the Pen[a]/Pen[b] alloantigen system. J Clin Invest 1992;90:2038.
938. Kiefel V, Santoso S, Katzmann B, Mueller-Eckhardt C. A new platelet-specific alloantigen Br[a]: report of 4 cases with neonatal alloimmune thrombocytopenia. Vox Sang 1988;54:101.
939. Santoso S, Kiefel V, Mueller-Eckhardt C. Immunochemical characterization of the new platelet alloantigen system Br[a]/Br[b]. Br J Haematol 1989;72:191.
940. Kiefel V, Santoso S, Katzmann B, Mueller-Eckhardt C. The Br[a]/Br[b] alloantigen system on human platelets. Blood 1989;73:2219.
941. Smith JW, Kelton JG, Horsewood P, et al. Platelet specific alloantigens on the platelet glycoprotein Ia/IIa complex. Br J Haematol 1989; 72:534.
942. Woods VL Jr, Pischel KD, Avery ED, Bluestein HG. Antigenic polymorphism of human very late activation protein-2 (platelet glycoprotein Ia-IIa): platelet alloantigen Hc[a]. J Clin Invest 1989;83:978.
943. Mueller-Eckhardt C, Kiefel V, Kroll H, Mueller-Eckhardt G. HLA-DRw6, a new immune response marker for immunization against the platelet alloantigen Br[a]. Vox Sang 1989;57:90.
944. Bettaieb A, Fromont P, Rodet M, et al. Br[b], a platelet alloantigen involved in neonatal alloimmune thrombocytopenia. Vox Sang 1991; 60:230.
945. Christie DJ, Pulkrabek S, Putnam JL, et al. Posttransfusion purpura due to an alloantibody reactive with glycoprotein Ia/IIa (anti-HPA-5b). Blood 1991;77:2785.
946. Santoso S, Kalb R, Walka M, et al. The human platelet alloantigens Br[a] and Br[b] are associated with a single amino acid polymorphism on glycoprotein Ia (integrin subunit $\alpha 2$). J Clin Invest 1993;92:2427.
947. Kalb R, Santoso S, Unkelbach K, et al. Localization of the Br polymorphism on a 144 bp exon of the GPIa gene and its application in platelet DNA typing. Thromb Haemost 1994;71:651.
948. Kekomäki R, Jouhikainen T, Ollikainen J, et al. A new platelet alloantigen, Tu[a], on glycoprotein IIIa associated with neonatal alloimmune thrombocytopenia in two families. Br J Haematol 1993;83:306.
949. McFarland JG, Blanchette V, Collins J, et al. Neonatal alloimmune thrombocytopenia due to a new platelet-specific alloantibody. Blood 1993;81:3318.
950. Wang R, McFarland JG, Kekomaki R, Newman PJ. Amino acid 489 is a mutational "hot spot" on the $\beta 3$ integrin chain. The CA/Tu human platelet alloantigen system. Blood 1993;82:3386.
951. Kuijpers RWAM, Simsek S, Faber NM, et al. Single point mutation in human glycoprotein IIIa is associated with a new platelet-specific alloantigen (Mo) involved in neonatal alloimmune thrombocytopenia. Blood 1993;81:70.
952. Kroll H, Kiefel V, Santoso S, Mueller-Eckhardt C. Sr[a], a private platelet antigen on glycoprotein IIIa associated with neonatal alloimmune thrombocytopenia. Blood 1990;76:2296.
953. Santoso S, Kalb R, Kroll H, et al. A point mutation leads to an unpaired cysteine residue and a molecular weight polymorphism of a functional platelet β_3 integrin subunit. The Sr[a] alloantigen system of GPIIIa. J Biol Chem 1994;269:8439.
954. Furihata K, Hunter J, Aster RH, et al. Human anti-Pl[E1] antibody recognizes epitopes associated with the alpha subunit of platelet glycoprotein Ib. Br J Haematol 1988;68:103.
955. Kelton JG, Smith JW, Horsewood P, et al. The Gov[a/b] alloantigen system on human platelets. Blood 1990;75:2172.
956. Kekomäki R, Raivio P, Kero P. A new low-frequency platelet alloantigen, Va[a], on glycoprotein IIb/IIIa associated with neonatal alloimmune thrombocytopenia. Transfus Med 1992;2:27.
957. Ikeda H, Mitani T, Ohnuma M, et al. A new platelet-specific antigen Nak[a] involved in the refractoriness of HLA-matched platelet transfusion. Vox Sang 1989;57:212.
958. Tomiyama Y, Take H, Ikeda H, et al. Identification of the platelet-specific alloantigen, Nak[a], on platelet membrane glycoprotein IV. Blood 1990;75:684.
959. Yamamoto N, Ikeda H, Tandon NN, et al. A platelet membrane glycoprotein (GP) deficiency in healthy blood donors: Nak[a-] platelets lack detectable GPIV (CD36). Blood 1990;76:1698.
960. Von dem Borne AEG, Décary F, and the ICSH/ISBT Expert Panel on Serology Working Party on Platelet Serology. Nomenclature of platelet specific antigens. Br J Haematol 1990;74:239.
961. Newman PJ. Nomenclature of human platelet alloantigens: a problem with the HPA system? Blood 1994;83:1447.
962. Blanchette VS, Chen L, Salomon de Friedber Z, et al. Alloimmunization to the Pl[A1] platelet antigen: results of a prospective study. Br J Haematol 1990;74:209.
963. Mueller-Eckhardt C, Kiefel V, Grubert A, et al. 348 cases of suspected neonatal alloimmune thrombocytopenia. Lancet 1989;1:363.
964. Skacel PO, Stacey TE, Tidmarsh EF, Contreras M. Maternal alloimmunization to HLA, platelet and granulocyte-specific antigens during pregnancy: its influence on cord blood granulocyte and platelet counts. Br J Haematol 1989;71:119.
965. Burrows RF, Caco CC, Kelton JG. Neonatal alloimmune thrombocytopenia: spontaneous in utero intracranial hemorrhage. Am J Hematol 1988;28:98.
966. McFarland JG, Frenzke M, Aster RH. Testing of maternal sera in pregnancies at risk for neonatal alloimmune thrombocytopenia. Transfusion 1989;29:128.
967. Nicolini U, Rodeck CH, Kochenour NK, et al. In-utero platelet transfusion for alloimmune thrombocytopenia. Lancet 1988;2:506.
968. Kaplan C, Daffos F, Forestier F, et al. Management of alloimmune thrombocytopenia: antenatal diagnosis and in utero transfusion of maternal platelets. Blood 1988;72:340.
969. Murphy MF, Pullon HWH, Metcalfe P, et al. Management of fetal alloimmune thrombocytopenia by weekly in utero platelet transfusions. Vox Sang 1990;58:45.
970. Management of alloimmune neonatal thrombocytopenia. (Editorial) Lancet 1989;1:137.
971. Bussel JP, Berkowitz RL, McFarland JG, et al. Antenatal treatment of neonatal alloimmune thrombocytopenia. N Engl J Med 1988;319: 1374.
972. Mir N, Samson D, House MJ, Kovar IZ. Failure of antenatal high-dose immunoglobulin to improve fetal platelet count in neonatal alloimmune thrombocytopenia. Vox Sang 1988;55:188.
973. Kelton JG, Blanchette VS, Wilson WE, et al. Neonatal thrombocytopenia due to passive immunization: prenatal diagnosis and distinction between maternal platelet alloantibodies and autoantibodies. N Engl J Med 1980;302:1401.
974. Adner MM, Fisch GR, Starobin SG, Aster RH. Use of "compatible" platelet transfusions in treatment of congenital isoimmune thrombocytopenic purpura. N Engl J Med 1969;280:244.
975. McGill M, Mayhaus C, Hoff R, Carey P. Frozen maternal platelets for neonatal thrombocytopenia. Transfusion 1987;27:347.
976. Sidiropoulos D, Straume B. The treatment of neonatal isoimmune thrombocytopenia with intravenous immunoglobulin (IgG i.v.). Blut 1984;48:383.
977. Massey GV, McWilliams NB, Mueller DG, et al. Intravenous immunoglobulin in treatment of neonatal alloimmune thrombocytopenia. J Pediatr 1987;111:133.
978. Shulman NR, Aster RH, Leitner A, Hiller MC. Immunoreactions involving platelets. V. Post-transfusion purpura due to a complement-fixing antibody against a genetically controlled platelet antigen: a proposed mechanism for thrombocytopenia and its relevance in "autoimmunity." J Clin Invest 1961;40:1597.
979. Kunicki TJ, Beardsley DS. The alloimmune thrombocytopenias: neo-

natal alloimmune thrombocytopenic purpura and post-transfusion purpura. Prog Hematol 1989;9:203.
980. Kickler TS, Ness PM, Herman JH, Bell WR. Studies on the pathophysiology of posttransfusion purpura. Blood 1986;68:347.
981. Mueller-Eckhardt C. Post-transfusion purpura. Br J Haematol 1986; 64:419.
982. Morrison FS, Mollison PL. Post-transfusion purpura. N Engl J Med 1966;275:243.
983. Chapman JF, Murphy MF, Berney SI, et al. Post-transfusion purpura associated with anti-Bak^{a} and anti-Pl^{A2} platelet antibodies and delayed haemolytic transfusion reaction. Vox Sang 1987;52:313.
984. Chaplin H, Aster RH, Morgan LK, et al. First example of familial posttransfusion purpura in two Pl^{A1}-negative sisters. Transfusion 1988;28:326.
985. Zeigler Z, Murphy S, Gardner FH. Post-transfusion purpura: a heterogeneous syndrome. Blood 1975;45:529.
986. Slichter SJ. Post-transfusion purpura: response to steroids and association with red blood cell and lymphocytotoxic antibodies. Br J Haematol 1982;50:599.
987. Cimo PL, Aster RH. Post-transfusion purpura: successful treatment by exchange transfusion. N Engl J Med 1972;287:290.
988. Soulier JP, Patereau C, Gobert N, et al. Posttransfusional immunologic thrombocytopenia: a case report. Vox Sang 1979;37:21.
989. Lillicrap DP, Ford PM, Giles AR. Prolonged thrombocytopenia in post-transfusion purpura (PTP) associated with changes in the crossed immunoelectrophoretic pattern of von Willebrand factor (vWF), circulating immune complexes and endothelial cell cytotoxicity. Br J Haematol 1986;62:37.
990. Chong BH, Cade J, Smith JA, Tatoulis J. An unusual case of post-transfusion purpura: good transient response to high-dose immunoglobulin. Vox Sang 1986;51:182.
991. Ballem PJ, Buskard NA, Decary F, Doubroff P. Post-transfusion purpura secondary to passive transfer of anti-Pl^{A1} by blood transfusion. Br J Haematol 1987;66:113.
992. Scott EP, Moilan-Bergeland J, Dalmasso AP. Posttransfusion thrombocytopenia associated with passive transfusion of a platelet-specific antibody. Transfusion 1988;28:73.
993. Nijjar TS, Bonacosa IA, Israels LG. Severe acute thrombocytopenia following infusion of plasma containing anti Pl^{A1}. Am J Hematol 1987;25:219.
994. Warkentin TE, Smith JW, Hayward CPM, et al. Thrombocytopenia caused by passive transfusion of anti-glycoprotein Ia/IIa alloantibody (anti-HPA-5b). Blood 1992;79:2480.
995. Mueller-Eckhardt C, Kuenzlen E, Thilo-Korner D, Pralle H. High-dose intravenous immunoglobulin for post-transfusion purpura. (Letter) N Engl J Med 1983;308:287.
996. Mueller-Eckhardt C, Kiefel V. High-dose IgG for post-transfusion purpura: revisited. Blut 1988;57:163.
997. Walker WS, Yap PL, Kilpatrick DC, et al. Post-transfusion purpura following open heart surgery: management by high dose intravenous immunoglobulin infusion. Blut 1988;57:323.
998. Gerstner JB, Smith MJ, Davis KD, et al. Posttransfusion purpura: therapeutic failure of Pl^{A1}-negative platelet transfusion. Am J Hematol 1979;6:71.
999. Lippman SM, Lizak GE, Foung SKH, Grumet FC. The efficacy of Pl^{A1}-negative platelet transfusion therapy in posttransfusion purpura. West J Med 1988;148:86.
1000. Cunningham CC, Lind SE. Apparent response of refractory post-transfusion purpura to splenectomy. Am J Hematol 1989;30:112.
1001. Lau P, Sholtis CM, Aster RH. Post-transfusion purpura: an enigma of alloimmunization. Am J Hematol 1980;9:331.
1002. Yankee RA, Grumet FC, Rogentine GN. Platelet transfusion: the selection of compatible platelet donors for refractory patients by lymphocyte HL-A typing. N Engl J Med 1969;281:1208.
1003. Brand A, Claas FHJ, Voogt PJ, et al. Alloimmunization after leukocyte-depleted multiple random donor platelet transfusions. Vox Sang 1988;54:160.
1004. Bishop JF, McGrath K, Wolf MM, et al. Clinical factors influencing the efficacy of pooled platelet transfusions. Blood 1988;71:383.
1005. McFarland JG, Anderson AJ, Slichter SJ. Factors influencing the transfusion response to HLA-selected apheresis donor platelets in patients refractory to random platelet concentrates. Br J Haematol 1989;73:380.
1006. Daly PA, Schiffer CA, Aisner J, Wiernik PA. Platelet transfusion therapy. One-hour posttransfusion increments are valuable in predicting the need for HLA-matched preparations. JAMA 1980;243:435.
1007. O'Connell B, Lee EJ, Schiffer CA. The value of 10-minute posttransfusion platelet counts. Transfusion 1988;28:66.
1008. Schiffer CA. Prevention of alloimmunization in platelet transfusion recipients. In: Kunicki TJ, George JN, eds. Platelet immunobiology: molecular and clinical aspects. Philadelphia, JB Lippincott, 1989:454.
1009. Murphy MF, Metcalfe P, Ord J, et al. Disappearance of HLA and platelet-specific antibodies in acute leukaemia patients alloimmunized by multiple transfusions. Br J Haematol 1987;67:255.
1010. Hogge DE, Dutcher JP, Aisner J, Schiffer CA. Lymphocytotoxic antibody is a predictor of response to random donor platelet transfusions. Am J Hematol 1983;14:363.
1011. Aster RH. New approaches to an old problem: refractoriness to platelet transfusions. Transfusion 1988;28:95.
1012. Gmur J, Von Felten A, Osterwalder B, et al. Delayed alloimmunization using random donor platelet transfusions: a prospective study in thrombocytopenic patients with acute leukemia. Blood 1983;62:473.
1013. Messerschmidt GL, Makuch R, Appelbaum F, et al. A prospective randomized trial of HLA-matched versus mismatched single-donor platelet transfusions in cancer patients. Cancer 1988;62:795.
1014. Eernisse JG, Brand A. Prevention of platelet refractoriness due to HLA antibodies by administration of leukocyte-poor blood components. Exp Hematol 1981;9:77.
1015. Schiffer CA, Dutcher JP, Aisner J, et al. A randomized trial of leukocyte-depleted platelet transfusion to modify alloimmunization in patients with leukemia. Blood 1983;62:815.
1016. Murphy MF, Metcalfe P, Thomas H, et al. Use of leucocyte-poor blood components and HLA-matched-platelet donors to prevent HLA alloimmunization. Br J Haematol 1986;62:529.
1017. Sniecinski I, O'Donnell MR, Nowicki B, Hill LR. Prevention of refractoriness and HLA-alloimmunization using filtered blood products. Blood 1988;71:1402.
1018. Andreu G, Dewailly J, Leberre C, et al. Prevention of HLA immunization with leukocyte-poor packed red cells and platelet concentrates obtained by filtration. Blood 1988;72:964.
1019. Claas FHJ, Smeenk RJT, Schmidt R, et al. Alloimmunization against the MHC antigens after platelet transfusions is due to contaminating leukocytes in the platelet suspension. Exp Hematol 1981;9:84.
1020. Kickler TS, Ness PM, Braine HG. Platelet crossmatching: a direct approach to the selection of platelet transfusions for the alloimmunized thrombocytopenic patient. Am J Clin Pathol 1988;90:69.
1021. Freedman J, Garvey MB, Saloman de Friedberg Z, et al. Random donor platelet crossmatching: comparison of four platelet antibody detection methods. Am J Hematol 1988;28:1.
1022. Kurtzberg J, Friedman HS, Kinney TR, et al. Treatment of platelet alloimmunization with intravenous immunoglobulin: two case reports and review of the literature. Am J Med 1987;83:30.
1023. Kickler T, Braine HG, Piantadosi S, et al. A randomized, placebo-controlled trial of intravenous gammaglobulin in alloimmunized thrombocytopenic patients. Blood 1990;75:313.
1024. Yamamoto M, Ideguchi H, Nishimura J, et al. Treatment of platelet-alloimmunization with cyclosporin A in a patient with aplastic anemia. Am J Hematol 1990;33:220.
1025. Jamieson GA. The activation of platelets by thrombin: a model for activation by high and moderate affinity receptor pathways. In: Jamieson GA, ed. Platelet membrane receptors: molecular biology, immunology, biochemistry, and pathology. Prog Clin Biol Res 1988;283:137.
1026. Sims PJ, Wiedmer T, Esmon CT, et al. Assembly of the platelet prothrombinase complex is linked to vesiculation of the platelet plasma membrane: studies in Scott syndrome—an isolated defect in platelet procoagulant activity. J Biol Chem 1989;264:17049.
1027. Bick RL. Disseminated intravascular coagulation and related syndromes. Semin Thromb Hemost 1988;14:299.
1028. Baker WF Jr. Clinical aspects of disseminated intravascular coagulation: a clinician's point of view. Semin Thromb Hemost 1989;15:1.
1029. Muller-Berghaus G. Pathophysiologic and biochemical events in disseminated intravascular coagulation: dysregulation of procoagulant and anticoagulant pathways. Semin Thromb Hemost 1989;15:58.
1030. Goldenfarb PB, Zucker S, Corrigan JJ Jr, Cathey MH. The coagulation mechanism in acute bacterial infection. Br J Haematol 1970;18:643.
1031. Svanbom M. A prospective study on septicemia. II. Clinical manifestations and complications, results of antimicrobial treatment and a report of a follow-up study. Scand J Infect Dis 1980;12:189.
1032. Riedler GF, Straub PW, Frick PG. Thrombocytopenia in septicemia: a clinical study for the evaluation of its incidence and diagnostic value. Helv Med Acta 1971;36:23.
1033. Corrigan JJ Jr. Thrombocytopenia: a laboratory sign of septicemia in infants and children. J Pediatr 1974;85:219.
1034. Kelton JG, Neame PB, Gauldie J, Hirsh J. Elevated platelet-associated IgG in the thrombocytopenia of septicemia. N Engl J Med 1979; 300:760.
1035. Neame PB, Kelton JG, Walker IR, et al. Thrombocytopenia in septicemia: the role of disseminated intravascular coagulation. Blood 1980;56:88.
1036. Kreger BE, Craven DE, McCabe WR. Gram-negative bacteremia. IV. Re-evaluation of clinical features and treatment in 612 patients. Am J Med 1980;68:344.
1037. Corrigan JJ Jr, Jordan CM. Heparin therapy in septicemia with disseminated intravascular coagulation: effect on mortality and on correction of hemostatic defects. N Engl J Med 1970;283:778.
1038. Milligan GF, MacDonald JAE, Mellon A, Ledingham IM. Pulmonary and hematologic disturbances during septic shock. Surg Gynecol Obstet 1974;138:43.
1039. Oppenheimer L, Hryniuk WM, Bishop AJ. Thrombocytopenia in severe bacterial infections. J Surg Res 1976;20:211.
1040. Tate D, Carlton GT, Johnson D, et al. Immune thrombocytopenia in severe neonatal infections. J Pediatr 1981;98:449.
1041. Davenport A, Rugman FP, Desmond MJ, Ganta R. Is thrombocytopenia

seen in patients with leptospirosis immunologically mediated? (Letter) J Clin Pathol 1989;42:439.
1042. Poskitt TR, Poskitt PK. Thrombocytopenia of sepsis: the role of circulating IgG-containing immune complexes. Arch Intern Med 1985;145:891.
1043. Van der Lelie J, Van der Plas-Van Dalen CM, Von dem Borne AEGK. Platelet autoantibodies in septicaemia. Br J Haematol 1984;58:755.
1044. Levin S, Goodman LJ, Fuhrer J. Fulminant community-acquired infectious diseases: diagnostic problems. Med Clin North Am 1986;70:967.
1045. Helmick CG, Bernard KW, D'Angelo LJ. Rocky Mountain spotted fever: clinical, laboratory, and epidemiological features of 262 cases. J Infect Dis 1984;150:480.
1046. Sporn LA, Haidaris PJ, Shi RJ, et al. *Rickettsia rickettsii* infection of cultured human endothelial cells induces tissue factor expression. Blood 1994;83:1527.
1047. Clawson CC, White JG. Platelet interaction with bacteria. I. Reaction phases and effects of inhibitors. Am J Pathol 1971;65:367.
1048. MacIntyre DE, Allen AP, Thorne KJI, et al. Endotoxin-induced platelet aggregation and secretion. I. Morphological changes and pharmacological effects. J Cell Sci 1977;28:211.
1049. Hawiger J, Hawiger A, Steckley S, et al. Membrane changes in human platelets induced by lipopolysaccharide endotoxin. Br J Haematol 1977;35:285.
1050. Hawiger J, Steckley S, Hammond D, et al. Staphylococci-induced human platelet injury mediated by protein A and immunoglobulin G Fc fragment receptor. J Clin Invest 1979;64:931.
1051. Arvand M, Bhakdi S, Dahlbäck B, Preissner KT. *Staphylococcus aureus* α-toxin attack on human platelets promotes assembly of the prothrombinase complex. J Biol Chem 1990;265:14377.
1052. Feuerstein G, Siren AL. Platelet-activating factor and shock. Prog Biochem Pharmacol 1988;22:181.
1053. Lopez Diez F, Nieto ML, Fernandez-Gallardo S, et al. Occupancy of platelet receptors for platelet-activating factor in patients with septicemia. J Clin Invest 1989;83:1733.
1054. McGrath JM, Stewart GJ. The effect of endotoxin on vascular endothelium. J Exp Med 1969;129:833.
1055. Nieminen U, Peltola H, Syrjälä MT, et al. Acute thrombocytopenic purpura following measles, mumps and rubella vaccination. A report on 23 patients. Acta Pædiatr 1993;82:267.
1056. McClure PD. Idiopathic thrombocytopenic purpura in children: diagnosis and management. Pediatrics 1975;55:68.
1057. Carter RL. Platelet levels in infectious mononucleosis. Blood 1965;25:817.
1058. Steeper TA, Horwitz CA, Moore SB, et al. Severe thrombocytopenia in Epstein-Barr virus–induced mononucleosis. West J Med 1989;150:170.
1059. Chanarin I, Walford DM. Thrombocytopenic purpura in cytomegalovirus mononucleosis. Lancet 1973;2:238.
1060. Whitaker JA III, Hardison JE. Severe thrombocytopenia after generalized herpes simplex virus-2 (HSV-2) infection. South Med J 1978;71:864.
1061. Brook I. Disseminated varicella with pneumonia, meningoencephalitis, thrombocytopenia, and fatal intracranial hemorrhage. South Med J 1979;72:756.
1062. Graham DY, Brown CH III, Benry J, Butel JS. Thrombocytopenia: a complication of mumps. JAMA 1974;227:1162.
1063. Bayer WL, Sherman FE, Michaels RH, et al. Purpura in congenital and acquired rubella. N Engl J Med 1965;273:1362.
1064. Ackerman Z, Ackerman E, Shouval D. Measles: clinical and laboratory observations in young adults during an epidemic. South Med J 1988;81:1396.
1065. Yoto Y, Kudoh T, Suzuki N, et al. Thrombocytopenia induced by human parvovirus B19 infections. Eur J Haematol 1993;50:255.
1066. Ellman L, Carvalho A, Jacobson BM, Colman RW. Platelet autoantibody in a case of infectious mononucleosis presenting as thrombocytopenic purpura. Am J Med 1973;55:723.
1067. Kernoff LM. Demonstration of increased platelet-bound IgG in infectious mononucleosis complicated by severe thrombocytopenia. Scand J Infect Dis 1980;12:67.
1068. Risdall RJ, McKenna RW, Nesbit ME, et al. Virus-associated hemophagocytic syndrome: a benign histiocytic proliferation distinct from malignant histiocytosis. Cancer 1979;44:993.
1069. Sullivan JL. Hematologic consequences of Epstein-Barr virus infection. Hematol Oncol Clin North Am 1987;1:397.
1070. Watson HG, Goulden NJ, Manson LM, et al. Virus-associated haemophagocytic syndrome: further evidence for a T-cell mediated disorder. Br J Haematol 1994;86:213.
1071. Kikuta H, Sakiyama Y, Matsumoto S, et al. Fatal Epstein-Barr virus–associated hemophagocytic syndrome. Blood 1993;82:3259.
1072. Hill GJ II, Knight V, Jeffery GM. Thrombocytopenia in vivax malaria. Lancet 1964;1:240.
1073. Beale PJ, Cormack JD, Oldrey TBN. Thrombocytopenia in malaria with immunoglobulin (IgM) changes. Br Med J 1972;1:345.
1074. Skudowitz RB, Katz J, Lurie A, et al. Mechanisms of thrombocytopenia in malignant tertial malaria. Br Med J 1973;2:515.
1075. Horstmann RD, Dietrich M, Bienzle U, Rasche H. Malaria-induced thrombocytopenia. Blut 1981;42:157.
1076. Grau GE, Piguet PF, Greterner D, et al. Immunopathology of thrombocytopenia in experimental malaria. Immunology 1988;65:501.
1077. Balc JR, Brasher C, Siegler RL. CNS manifestations of the hemolytic-uremic syndrome: relationship to metabolic alterations and prognosis. Am J Dis Child 1980;134:869.
1078. DiMario FJ, Bronte-Stewart H, Sherbotie J, Turner ME. Lacunar infarction of the basal ganglia as a complication of hemolytic-uremic syndrome. Clin Pediatr 1987;26:586.
1079. Trevathan E, Dooling EC. Large thrombotic strokes in hemolytic-uremic syndrome. J Pediatr 1987;111:863.
1080. Siegler RL, Brewer ED, Swartz M. Ocular involvement in hemolytic-uremic syndrome. J Pediatr 1988;112:594.
1081. Wasserstein A, Hill G, Goldfarb S, Goldberg M. Recurrent thrombotic thrombocytopenic purpura after viral infection: clinical and histologic simulation of chronic glomerulonephritis. Arch Intern Med 1981;141:685.
1082. Myers TJ, Wakem CJ, Ball ED, Tremont SJ. Thrombotic thrombocytopenic purpura: combined treatment with plasmapheresis and antiplatelet agents. Ann Intern Med 1980;92:149.
1083. Satoh K, Takahashi H, Nagai K, Shibata A. Thrombotic thrombocytopenic purpura and herpes zoster infection. (Letter) Ann Intern Med 1988;108:154.
1084. Reynolds PM, Jackson JM, Brine JAS, Vivian AB. Thrombotic thrombocytopenic purpura: remission following splenectomy—report of a case and review of the literature. Am J Med 1976;61:439.
1085. Mettler NE. Isolation of a microtatobiote from patients with hemolytic-uremic syndrome and thrombotic thrombocytopenic purpura and from mites in the United States. N Engl J Med 1969;281:1023.
1086. Jaeschke R, Irvine EJ, Moore J, Kelton J. *Campylobacter jejuni* and thrombotic thrombocytopenic purpura. Can J Gastroenterol 1990;4:154.
1087. Kovacs MJ, Roddy J, Grégoire S, et al. Thrombotic thrombocytopenic purpura following hemorrhagic colitis due to *Escherichia coli* 0157:H7. Am J Med 1990;88:177.
1088. Upshaw JD Jr, Reidy TJ, Groshart K. Thrombotic thrombocytopenic purpura in pregnancy: response to plasma manipulations. South Med J 1985;78:677.
1089. Vanderkerckhove F, Noens L, Colardyn F, et al. Thrombotic thrombocytopenic purpura mimicking toxemia of pregnancy. Am J Obstet Gynecol 1984;150:320.
1090. Weiner CP. Thrombotic microangiopathy in pregnancy and the postpartum period. Semin Hematol 1987;24:119.
1091. McShane PM, Bern MM, Schiff I. Thrombotic thrombocytopenic purpura associated with oral contraceptives: a case report. Am J Obstet Gynecol 1983;145:762.
1092. Ahmed F, Sumalnop V, Spain DM, Tobin MS. Thrombohemolytic thrombocytopenic purpura during penicillamine therapy. Arch Intern Med 1978;138:1292.
1093. Stonesifer LD, Bone RC, Hiller FC. Thrombotic thrombocytopenic purpura in carbon monoxide poisoning. Arch Intern Med 1980;140:104.
1094. Kwaan HC. Miscellaneous secondary thrombotic microangiopathy. Semin Hematol 1987;24:141.
1095. Murgo AJ. Thrombotic microangiopathy in the cancer patient including those induced by chemotherapeutic agents. Semin Hematol 1987;24:161.
1096. Ridolfi RL, Bell WR. Thrombotic thrombocytopenic purpura: report of 25 cases and review of the literature. Medicine 1981;60:413.
1097. Steinberg AD, Green WT Jr, Talal N. Thrombotic thrombocytopenic purpura complicating Sjögren's syndrome. JAMA 1971;215:257.
1098. Ter Borg EJ, Houtman PM, Kallenberg CGM, et al. Thrombocytopenia and hemolytic anemia in a patient with MCTD due to thrombotic thrombocytopenic purpura. J Rheumatol 1988;15:1174.
1099. Fox DA, Faix JD, Coblyn J, et al. Thrombotic thrombocytopenic purpura and systemic lupus erythematosus. Ann Rheum Dis 1986;45:319.
1100. Nair JMG, Bellevue R, Bertoni M, Dosik H. Thrombotic thrombocytopenic purpura in patients with the acquired immunodeficiency syndrome (AIDS)–related complex: a report of two cases. Ann Intern Med 1988;109:209.
1101. Meisenberg BR, Robinson WL, Mosley CA, et al. Thrombotic thrombocytopenic purpura in human immunodeficiency (HIV)–seropositive males. Am J Hematol 1988;27:212.
1102. Leaf AN, Laubenstein LJ, Raphael B, et al. Thrombotic thrombocytopenic purpura associated with human immunodeficiency virus type 1 (HIV-1) infection. Ann Intern Med 1988;109:194.
1103. Dixon AC, Kwock DW, Nakamura JM, et al. Thrombotic thrombocytopenic purpura and human T-lymphotropic virus, type 1 (HTLV-1). (Letter) Ann Intern Med 1989;110:93.
1104. Elias M, Horowitz J, Tal I, et al. Thrombotic thrombocytopenic purpura and haemolytic uraemic syndrome in three siblings. Arch Dis Child 1988;63:644.
1105. Waage A, Siegel J, Thorstensen K, Lamvik J. Thrombotic thrombocytopenic purpura in 2 siblings: defective platelet function and platelet

factor deficiency occurring simultaneously. Scand J Haematol 1986; 36:55.
1106. Karmali MA, Steele BT, Petric M, Lim C. Sporadic cases of haemolytic-uraemic syndrome associated with faecal cytotoxin and cytotoxin-producing *Escherichia coli* in stools. Lancet 1983;1:619.
1107. Karmali MA, Petric M, Lim C, et al. The association between idiopathic hemolytic uremic syndrome and infection by verotoxin-producing *Eschericia coli*. J Infect Dis 1985;151:775.
1108. Chart H, Smith HR, Scotland SM, et al. Serological identification of *Escherichia coli* O157:H7 infection in haemolytic uraemic syndrome. Lancet 1991;337:138.
1109. Griffin PM, Tauxe RV. The epidemiology of infections caused by *Escherichia coli* O157:H7, other enterhemorrhagic *E. coli*, and the associated hemolytic uremic syndrome. Epidemiol Rev 1991;13:60.
1110. Raghupathy P, Date A, Shastry JCM, et al. Haemolytic-uraemic syndrome complicating Shigella dysentery in South Indian children. Br Med J 1978;1:1518.
1111. Badami KG, Srivastava RN, Kumar R, Saraya AK. Disseminated intravascular coagulation in post-dysenteric haemolytic uraemic syndrome. Acta Paediatr Scand 1987;76:919.
1112. Baker NM, Mills AE, Rachman I, Thomas JEP. Haemolytic-uraemic syndrome in typhoid fever. Br Med J 1974;2:84.
1113. Khoshoo V, Moudgil A, Vasudev AS, et al. Haemolytic uraemic syndrome associated with *Salmonella* dysentery. Acta Paediatr Scand 1988;77:604.
1114. Denneberg T, Friedberg M, Holmberg L, et al. Combined plasmapheresis and hemodialysis treatment for severe hemolytic-uremic syndrome following *Campylobacter* colitis. Acta Pediatr Scand 1982;71:243.
1115. Delans RJ, Biuso JD, Saba SR, Ramirez G. Hemolytic uremic syndrome after *Campylobacter*-induced diarrhea in an adult. Arch Intern Med 1984;144:1074.
1116. Davenport A, O'Connor B, Finn R. Acute renal failure following *Yersinia pseudotuberculosis* septicaemia. Postgrad Med J 1987;63:815.
1117. Alon U, Adler SP, Chan JC. Hemolytic-uremic syndrome associated with *Streptococcus pneumoniae*: report of a case and review of the literature. Am J Dis Child 1984;138:496.
1118. Klein PJ, Bulla M, Newman RA, et al. Thomsen-Friedenreich antigen in haemolytic-uraemic syndrome. (Letter) Lancet 1977;2:1024.
1119. Lazebnik N, Jaffa AJ, Peyeser MR. Hemolytic-uremic syndrome in pregnancy: review of the literature and report of a case. Obstet Gynecol Surv 1985;40:618.
1120. Hayslett JP. Current concepts: postpartum renal failure. N Engl J Med 1985;312:1556.
1121. Jackson AM, Rose BD, Graff LG, et al. Thrombotic microangiopathy and renal failure associated with antineoplastic chemotherapy. Ann Intern Med 1984;101:41.
1122. Verwey J, De Vries J, Pinedo HM. Mitomycin C–induced renal toxicity: a dose-dependent side effect? Eur J Cancer Clin Oncol 1987;23:195.
1123. Weinblatt ME, Kahn E, Scimeca PG, Kochen JA. Hemolytic uremic syndrome associated with cisplatin therapy. Am J Pediatr Hematol Oncol 1987;9:295.
1124. Hauglustaine D, Van Damme B, Vanrenterghem Y, et al. Recurrent hemolytic uremic syndrome during oral contraception. Clin Nephrol 1981;15:148.
1125. Van Buren D, Van Buren CT, Flechner SM, et al. De novo hemolytic uremic syndrome in renal transplant recipients immunosuppressed with cyclosporine. Surgery 1985;98:54.
1126. Marshall RJ, Sweny P. Haemolytic-uraemic syndrome in recipients of bone marrow transplants not treated with cyclosporin A. Histopathology 1986;10:953.
1127. Craig JIO, Sheehan T, Bell K. The haemolytic uraemic syndrome and bone marrow transplantation. Br Med J 1987;295:887.
1128. Boccia RV, Gelmann EP, Baker CC, et al. A hemolytic-uremic syndrome with the acquired immunodeficiency syndrome. (Letter) Ann Intern Med 1984;101:716.
1129. Carreras L, Romero R, Requesens C, et al. Familial hypocomplementemic hemolytic uremic syndrome with HLA-A3, B7 haplotype. JAMA 1981;245:602.
1130. Kaplan BS, Chesney RW, Drummond KN. Hemolytic uremic syndrome in families. N Engl J Med 1975;292:1090.
1131. Karlsberg RP, Lacher JW, Bartecchi CE. Adult hemolytic-uremic syndrome: familial variant. Arch Intern Med 1977;137:1155.
1132. Benitez L, Mathews M, Mallory GK. Platelet thrombosis with polyarteritis nodosa: report of a case. Arch Pathol 1964;77:116.
1133. Magil AB, McFadden D, Rae A. Lupus glomerulonephritis with thrombotic microangiopathy. Hum Pathol 1986;17:192.
1134. Sennesael JJ, Vanden Houte KM, Spapen HD, et al. Recurrent hemolytic uremic syndrome and metastatic malignancy. Am J Nephrol 1987;7:60.
1135. Hales CA, Mark EJ. A 43-year-old woman with breast cancer and the abrupt onset of respiratory failure. N Engl J Med 1987;317:225.
1136. Antman KH, Skarin AT, Mayer RJ, et al. Microangiopathic hemolytic anemia and cancer: a review. Medicine 1979;58:377.
1137. Dumas R, Baldet P, Rolin B, Jean R. Hypertension and segmental renal hypoplasia causing a syndrome of haemolysis and uraemia. Arch Dis Child 1981;56:403.
1138. Stuard ID, Huesinkveld RS, Moss AJ. Microangiopathic hemolytic anemia and thrombocytopenia in primary pulmonary hypertension. N Engl J Med 1972;287:869.
1139. Bayer AS, Theofilopoulos AN, Eisenberg R, et al. Thrombotic thrombocytopenic purpura–like syndrome associated with infective endocarditis: a possible immune complex disorder. JAMA 1977;238:408.
1140. Lian EC, Harkness DR, Byrnes JJ. Presence of a platelet aggregating factor in the plasma of patients with thrombotic thrombocytopenic purpura (TTP) and its inhibition by normal plasma. Blood 1979; 53:333.
1141. Siddiqui FA, Lian ECY. Novel platelet-agglutinating protein from a thrombotic thrombocytopenic purpura plasma. J Clin Invest 1985;76: 1330.
1142. Moake JL, Rudy CK, Troll JH, et al. Unusually large plasma factor VIII: von Willebrand factor multimers in chronic relapsing thrombotic thrombocytopenic purpura. N Engl J Med 1982;307:1432.
1143. Kelton JG, Moore J, Santos A, Sheridan D. Detection of a platelet-agglutinating factor in thrombotic thrombocytopenic purpura. Ann Intern Med 1984;101:589.
1144. Kelton JG, Moore JC, Murphy WG. Studies investigating platelet aggregation and release initiated by sera from patients with thrombotic thrombocytopenic purpura. Blood 1987;69:924.
1145. Murphy WG, Moore JC, Kelton JG. Calcium-dependent cysteine protease activity in the sera of patients with thrombotic thrombocytopenic purpura. Blood 1987;70:1683.
1146. Moore JC, Murphy WG, Kelton JG. Calpain proteolysis of von Willebrand factor enhances its binding to platelet membrane glycoprotein IIb/IIIa: an explanation for platelet aggregation in thrombotic thrombocytopenic purpura. Br J Haematol 1990;74:457.
1147. Kelton JG, Warkentin TE, Hayward CPM, Murphy WG, Moore JC. The calpain activity in patients with thrombotic thrombocytopenic purpura is associated with platelet microparticles. Blood 1992;80:2246.
1148. Muller-Esterl W. Novel functions of the kininogens. Semin Thromb Hemost 1987;13:115.
1149. Falanga A, Consonni R, Ruggenenti P, Barbui T. A cathepsin-like cysteine proteinase proaggregating activity in thrombotic thrombocytopenic purpura. Br J Haematol 1991;79:474.
1150. Brain MC, Neame PB. Thrombotic thrombocytopenic purpura and the hemolytic uremic syndrome. Semin Thromb Hemost 1982;8: 186.
1151. Bodensteiner D, Rosenfeld C. Elevated platelet-surface–bound IgM in thrombotic thrombocytopenic purpura. South Med J 1988;81:81.
1152. Brain MC, Dacie JC, Hourihane DO. Microangiopathic haemolytic anaemia: the possible role of vascular lesions in pathogenesis. Br J Haematol 1962;8:358.
1153. Burns ER, Zucker-Franklin D. Pathologic effects of plasma from patients with thrombotic thrombocytopenic purpura on platelets and cultured endothelial cells. Blood 1982;60:1030.
1154. Remuzzi G, Zoja C, Rossi EC. Prostacyclin in thrombotic microangiopathy. Semin Hematol 1987;24:110.
1155. Hensby CN, Lewis PJ, Hilgard P, et al. Prostacyclin deficiency in thrombotic thrombocytopenic purpura. (Letter) Lancet 1979;2:748.
1156. Kwaan HC. Role of fibrinolysis in thrombotic thrombocytopenic purpura. Semin Thromb Hemost 1987;24:101.
1157. Takahashi H, Tatewaki W, Wada K, Shibata A. Thrombin generation in patients with thrombotic thrombocytopenic purpura. Am J Hematol 1989;32:255.
1158. Kwaan HC. Clinicopathologic features of thrombotic thrombocytopenic purpura. Semin Hematol 1987;24:71.
1159. Petitt RM. Thrombotic thrombocytopenic purpura: a thirty-year review. Semin Thromb Hemost 1980;6:350.
1160. Kitchens CS. Studies of a patient with recurring thrombotic thrombocytopenic purpura. Am J Hematol 1982;13:259.
1161. Amorosi EL, Ultmann JE. Thrombotic thrombocytopenic purpura: report of 16 cases and review of the literature. Medicine 1966;45:139.
1162. Shepard KV, Bukowski RM. The treatment of thrombotic thrombocytopenic purpura with exchange transfusions, plasma infusions, and plasma exchange. Semin Hematol 1987;24:178.
1163. Rock GA, Shumak KH, Buskard NA, et al. Comparison of plasma exchange with plasma infusion in the treatment of thrombotic thrombocytopenic purpura. N Engl J Med 1991;325:393.
1164. Hayward CPM, Sutton DMC, Carter WH Jr, et al. Treatment outcomes in patients with adult thrombotic thrombocytopenic purpura-hemolytic uremic syndrome. Arch Intern Med 1994;154:982.
1165. Rubinstein MA, Kagan BM, MacGillviray MH, et al. Unusual remission in a case of thrombotic thrombocytopenic purpura syndrome following fresh blood exchange transfusions. Ann Intern Med 1959;51:1409.
1166. Bukowski RM, Hewlett JS, Reimer RR, et al. Therapy of thrombotic thrombocytopenic purpura: an overview. Semin Thromb Hemost 1981;7:1.
1167. Byrnes JJ, Khurana M. Treatment of thrombotic thrombocytopenic purpura with plasma. N Engl J Med 1977;297:1386.
1168. Byrnes JJ, Lian ECY. Recent therapeutic advances in thrombotic thrombocytopenic purpura. Semin Thromb Hemost 1979;5:199.
1169. Bukowski RM. Thrombotic thrombocytopenic purpura: a review. Prog Hemost Thromb 1982;6:287.
1170. Blitzer JB, Granfortuna JM, Gottlieb AJ, et al. Thrombotic thrombo-

cytopenic purpura: treatment with plasmapheresis. Am J Hematol 1987;24:329.
1171. Del Zoppo GJ. Antiplatelet therapy in thrombotic thrombocytopenic purpura. Semin Hematol 1987;24:130.
1172. Bell WR, Braine HG, Ness PM, Kickler TS. Improved survival in thrombotic thrombocytopenic purpura-hemolytic uremic syndrome. Clinical experience in 108 patients. N Engl J Med 1991;325:398.
1173. Kennedy SS, Zacharski LR, Beck JR. Thrombotic thrombocytopenic purpura: analysis of 48 unselected cases. Semin Thromb Hemost 1980;6:341.
1174. Gordon LI, Kwaan HC, Rossi EC. Deleterious effects of platelet transfusions and recovery thrombocytosis in patients with thrombotic microangiopathy. Semin Hematol 1987;24:184.
1175. Byrnes JJ, Moake JL, Klug P, Periman P. Effectiveness of the cryosupernatant fraction of plasma in the treatment of refractory thrombotic thrombocytopenic purpura. Am J Hematol 1990;34:169.
1176. Molinari E, Costamagna L, Perotti C, et al. Refractory thrombotic thrombocytopenic purpura: successful treatment by plasmapheresis with plasma cryosupernatant. Haematologica 1993;78:389.
1177. Rutkow IM. Thrombotic thrombocytopenic purpura (TTP) and splenectomy: a current appraisal. Ann Surg 1978;188:701.
1178. Rosove MH, Bhuta S. Splenectomy and extravascular platelet destruction in thrombotic thrombocytopenic purpura. Arch Intern Med 1985;145:937.
1179. Onundarson PT, Rowe JM, Heal JM, Francis CW. Response to plasma exchange and splenectomy in thrombotic thrombocytopenic purpura. A 10-year experience at a single institution. Arch Intern Med 1992;152: 791.
1180. O'Connor NT, Bruce-Jones P, Hill LF. Vincristine therapy for thrombotic thrombocytopenic purpura. Am J Hematol 1992;39:234.
1181. Durand JM, Lefevre P, Kaplanski G, et al. Deleterious effects of intravenous immunoglobulin in a patient with thrombotic thrombocytopenic purpura. (Letter) Am J Hematol 1993;44:214.
1182. Kinney JS, Gross TP, Porter CC, et al. Hemolytic-uremic syndrome: a population-based study in Washington, DC and Baltimore, Maryland. Am J Public Health 1988;78:64.
1183. Tarr PI, Neill MA, Allen J, et al. The increasing incidence of the hemolytic-uremic syndrome in King county, Washington: lack of evidence for ascertainment bias. Am J Epidemiol 1989;129:582.
1184. Konowalchuk J, Speirs JI, Stavric S. Vero response to a cytotoxin of *Escherichia coli*. Infect Immunol 1977;18:775.
1185. Scotland SM, Rowe B, Smith HR, et al. Vero cytotoxin-producing strains of *Escherichia coli* from children with haemolytic uraemic syndrome and their detection by specific DNA probes. J Med Microbiol 1988;25:237.
1186. Smith HR, Scotland SM. Vero cytotoxin-producing strains of *Escherichia coli*. J Med Microbiol 1988;26:77.
1187. Calderwood SB, Auclair F, Donohue-Rolfe A, et al. Nucleotide sequence of the Shiga-like toxin genes of *Escherichia coli*. Proc Natl Acad Sci USA 1987;84:4364.
1188. Obrig TG, Del Vecchio PJ, Karmali MA, et al. Pathogenesis of haemolytic uraemic syndrome. (Letter) Lancet 1987;2:687.
1189. Carter AO, Borczyk AA, Carlson JAK, et al. A severe outbreak of *Escherichia coli* 0157:H7-associated hemorrhagic colitis in a nursing home. N Engl J Med 1987;317:1496.
1190. Leung DYM, Moake JL, Havens PL, et al. Lytic anti-endothelial cell antibodies in haemolytic-uraemic syndrome. Lancet 1988;2:183.
1191. Remuzzi G, Misiani R, Marchesi D, et al. Haemolytic uraemic syndrome: deficiency of plasma factor(s) regulating prostacyclin activity? Lancet 1978;2:871.
1192. Levin M, Elkon KB, Nokes TJ, et al. Inhibitor of prostacyclin production in sporadic haemolytic uraemic syndrome. Arch Dis Child 1983; 58:703.
1193. Powell HR. Haemolytic uraemic syndrome: new perspectives. Aust Paediatr J 1987;23:213.
1194. O'Regan S, Chesney RW, Kaplan BS, Drummond KN. Red cell membrane phospholipid abnormalities in the hemolytic uremic syndrome. Clin Nephrol 1981;15:14.
1195. Stuart MJ. Deficiency of plasma PGI2-like regenerating activity in neonatal plasma: reversal by vitamin E *in vitro*. Pediatr Res 1981; 15:971.
1196. Monnens L, Van de Meer W, Langenhuysen C, et al. Platelet aggregating factor in the epidemic form of hemolytic uremic syndrome. Clin Nephrol 1985;24:135.
1197. Neild G. The haemolytic uraemic syndrome: a review. Q J Med 1987;63:367.
1198. Kaplan BS, Thomson PD, de Chadarevian JP. The hemolytic uremic syndrome. Pediatr Clin North Am 1976;23:761.
1199. Koster F, Levin J, Walker L, et al. Hemolytic-uremic syndrome after shigellosis: relation to endotoxemia and circulating immune complexes. N Engl J Med 1978;298:927.
1200. Richardson SE, Karmali MA, Becker LE, Smith CR. The histopathology of the hemolytic uremic syndrome associated with verocytotoxin-producing *Escherichia coli* infections. Hum Pathol 1988;19:1102.
1201. Van Dyck M, Proesmans W, Depraetere M. Hemolytic uremic syndrome in childhood: renal function ten years later. Clin Nephrol 1988;29:109.
1202. Siegler RL. Management of hemolytic-uremic syndrome. J Pediatr 1988;112:1014.
1203. Rizzoni G, Claris-Appiani A, Edefonti A, et al. Plasma infusion for hemolytic-uremic syndrome in children: results of a multicenter controlled trial. J Pediatr 1988;112:284.
1204. Loirat C, Sonsino E, Hinglais N, et al. Treatment of hemolytic uremic syndrome (HUS) with fresh frozen plasma (FFP): a prospective trial from the French Society of Pediatric Nephrology. (Abstract) Pediatr Nephrol 1987;1:C52.
1205. Vitacco M, Sanchez Avalos J, Gianantonio CA. Heparin therapy in the hemolytic-uremic syndrome. J Pediatr 1973;83:271.
1206. Proesmans W, Eeckels R, Van Damme B, et al. Antithrombotic therapy in childhood haemolytic uraemic syndrome: a randomised prospective study. In: Brodehl J, Ehrich JHH, eds. Paediatric nephrology. Berlin, Springer-Verlag, 1984:285.
1207. Diekmann L. Streptokinase- und Heparinbehandlung beim hamolytisch-uramischen Syndrom. Klin Paediatr 1980;192:430.
1208. Jones RWA, Morris MC, Maisey MN, et al. Endarterial urokinase in childhood hemolytic uremic syndrome. Kidney Int 1981;20:723.
1209. Beattie TJ, Murphy AV, Willoughby MLN. Prostacyclin infusion in haemolytic-uraemic syndrome of children. Br Med J 1981;283:470.
1210. Lesesne JB, Rothschild N, Erickson B, et al. Cancer-associated hemolytic-uremic syndrome: analysis of 85 cases from a national registry. J Clin Oncol 1989;7:781.
1211. Van Den Berg-Wolf MG, Kootte AMM, Weening JJ, Paul LC. Recurrent hemolytic uremic syndrome in a renal transplant recipient and review of the Leiden experience. Transplantation 1988;45:248.
1212. Springate J, Fildes R, Anthone S, et al. Recurrent hemolytic syndrome after renal transplantation. Transplant Proc 1988;20:559.
1213. Burrows RF, Hunter DJS, Andrew M, Kelton JG. A prospective study investigating the mechanism of thrombocytopenia in preeclampsia. Obstet Gynecol 1987;70:334.
1214. Gibson B, Hunter D, Neame PB, Kelton JG. Thrombocytopenia in preeclampsia and eclampsia. Semin Thromb Hemost 1982;8:234.
1215. Romero R, Mazor M, Lockwood CJ, Emamian M, et al. Clinical significance, prevalence, and natural history of thrombocytopenia in pregnancy-induced hypertension. Am J Perinatol 1980;6:32.
1216. Weinstein L. Syndrome of hemolysis, elevated liver enzymes, and low platelet count: a severe consequence of hypertension in pregnancy. Am J Obstet Gynecol 1982;142:159.
1217. Stubbs TM, Lazarchick J, Horger EO III, Loadholt CB. Schistocytosis, aminotransferase elevation and thrombocytopenia in preeclampsia/eclampsia. J Reprod Med 1987;32:777.
1218. Giles C, Inglis TCM. Thrombocytopenia and macrothrombocytosis in gestational hypertension. Br J Obstet Gynaecol 1981;88:1115.
1219. Rakoczi I, Tallian F, Bagdany S, Gati I. Platelet life-span in normal pregnancy and pre-eclampsia as determined by a non-radioisotope technique. Thromb Res 1979;15:553.
1220. Stubbs TM, Lazarchick J, Van Dorsten JP, et al. Evidence of accelerated platelet production and consumption in nonthrombocytopenic preeclampsia. Am J Obstet Gynecol 1986;155:263.
1221. Kelton JG, Hunter DJS, Neame PB. A platelet function defect in preeclampsia. Obstet Gynecol 1985;65:107.
1222. Borok Z, Weitz J, Owen J, et al. Fibrinogen proteolysis and platelet alpha-granule release in preeclampsia/eclampsia. Blood 1984;63: 525.
1223. Socol ML, Weiner CP, Louis G, et al. Platelet activation in preeclampsia. Am J Obstet Gynecol 1985;151:494.
1224. Fitzgerald DJ, Rocki W, Murray, et al. Thromboxane A_2 synthesis in pregnancy-induced hypertension. Lancet 335:751.
1225. Remuzzi G, Marchesi D, Zoja C, et al. Reduced umbilical and placental vascular prostacyclin in severe pre-eclampsia. Prostaglandins 1980; 20:105.
1226. Samuels P, Main EK, Tomaski A, et al. Abnormalities in platelet antiglobulin tests in preeclamptic mothers and their neonates. Am J Obstet Gynecol 1987;157:109.
1227. McKay DG. Hematologic evidence of disseminated intravascular coagulation in eclampsia. Obstet Gynecol Surv 1972;27:399.
1228. Kobayashi T, Terao T. Preeclampsia as chronic disseminated intravascular coagulation. Study of two parameters: thrombin–antithrombin III complex and D-dimers. Gynecol Obstet Invest 1987;24:170.
1229. Trofatter KF Jr, Howell ML, Greenberg CS, Hage ML. Use of the fibrin D-dimer in screening for coagulation abnormalities in preeclampsia. Obstet Gynecol 1989;73:435.
1230. Weiner CP. The mechanism of reduced antithrombin III activity in women with preeclampsia. Obstet Gynecol 1988;72:847.
1231. Weiner CP, Brandt J. Plasma antithrombin III activity: an aid in the diagnosis of preeclampsia–eclampsia. Am J Obstet Gynecol 1982;142: 275.
1232. Weenink GH, Borm JJJ, Ten Cate JW, Treffers PE. Antithrombin III levels in normotensive and hypertensive pregnancy. Gynecol Obstet Invest 1983;16:230.
1233. Douglas JT, Shah M, Lowe GDO, et al. Plasma fibrinopeptide A and beta-thromboglobulin in pre-eclampsia and pregnancy hypertension. Thromb Haemost 1982;47:54.
1234. Sibai BM, Spinnato JA, Watson DL, et al. Pregnancy outcome in 303 cases with severe preeclampsia. Obstet Gynecol 1984;64:319.

1235. Worley RJ. Pathophysiology of pregnancy-induced hypertension. Clin Obstet Gynecol 1984;27:821.
1236. Redman CWG, Bonnar J, Beilin L. Early platelet consumption in pre-eclampsia. Br Med J 1978;1:467.
1237. Beaufils M, Uzan S, Donsimoni R, Colau JC. Prevention of pre-eclampsia by early antiplatelet therapy. Lancet 1985;1:840.
1238. Wallenburg HCS, Dekker GA, Makovitz JW, Rotmans P. Low-dose aspirin prevents pregnancy-induced hypertension and pre-eclampsia in angiotensin-sensitive primigravidae. Lancet 1986;1:1.
1239. Schiff E, Peleg E, Goldenberg M, et al. The use of aspirin to prevent pregnancy-induced hypertension and lower the ratio of thromboxane A_2 to prostacyclin in relatively high risk pregnancies. N Engl J Med 1989;321:351.
1240. Storck H, Hoigne R, Koller F. Thrombocytes in allergic reactions. Int Arch Allergy Appl Immunol 1955;6:372.
1241. Johansson SA, Lundberg A, Sjoberg HE. Influence of heparin on thrombocytopenia in allergic reactions. Acta Med Scand 1960;168: 165.
1242. Caffrey EA, Sladen GE, Isaacs PET, Clark KGA. Thrombocytopenia caused by cow's milk. (Letter) Lancet 1981;2:316.
1243. Mueller-Eckhardt C. Immune reactions of platelets and their clinical significance. Klin Wochenschr 1975;53:889.
1244. Bousquet J, Huchard G, Michel FB. Toxic reactions induced by Hymenoptera venom. Ann Allergy 1984;52:371.
1245. Paganelli R, Levinsky RJ, Atherton DJ. Detection of specific antigen within circulating immune complexes: validation of the assay and its application to food antigen–antibody complexes formed in healthy and food-allergic subjects. Clin Exp Immunol 1981;46:44.
1246. Kaplan BS, Esseltine D. Thrombocytopenia in patients with acute poststreptococcal glomerulonephritis. J Pediatr 1978;93:974.
1247. Medani CR, Pearl PL, Hall-Craggs M. Acute renal failure, hemolytic anemia, and thrombocytopenia in poststreptococcal glomerulonephritis. South Med J 1987;80:370.
1248. George CRP, Slichter SJ, Quadracci LJ, et al. A kinetic evaluation of hemostasis in renal disease. N Engl J Med 1974;291:1111.
1249. Miller K, Dresner IG, Michael AF. Localization of platelet antigens in human kidney disease. Kidney Int 1980;18:472.
1250. Donadio JV Jr, Anderson CF, Mitchell JC III, et al. Membranoproliferative glomerulonephritis: a prospective clinical trial of platelet inhibitor therapy. N Engl J Med 1984;310:1421.
1251. Landis TF, Von Felten A, Berchtold H. Thrombocytopenic episodes in patients with well-functioning renal allografts: inverse relationship between platelet count and platelet size pointing to intermittent platelet destruction. Acta Haematol 1979;61:2.
1252. Pillay VKG, Kurtzman NA, Manaligod JR, Jonasson O. Selective thrombocytopenia due to localised microangiopathy of renal allografts. Lancet 1973;2:988.
1253. Bunting RW, Quay SC. Case records of the Massachusetts General Hospital. N Engl J Med 1979;300:1262.
1254. Leithner C, Sinzinger H, Schwarz M. Treatment of chronic kidney transplant rejection with prostacyclin: reduction of platelet deposition in the transplant; prolongation of platelet survival and improvement of transplant function. Prostaglandins 1981;22:783.
1255. Lawley TJ, Bielory L, Gascon P, et al. A prospective clinical and immunologic analysis of patients with serum sickness. N Engl J Med 1984;311:1407.
1256. Madaio MP, Spiegel JE, Levey AS. Life-threatening thrombocytopenia complicating antithymocyte globulin therapy for acute kidney transplant rejection: evidence of in situ immune complex formation on the platelet surface. Transplantation 1988;45:647.
1257. Pike OM, Marquiss JE, Weiner RS, Brechenridge RT. A study of platelet counts during cardiopulmonary bypass. Transfusion 1972;12: 119.
1258. Harker LA, Malpass TW, Branson HE, et al. Mechanism of abnormal bleeding in patients undergoing cardiopulmonary bypass: acquired transient platelet dysfunction associated with selective α-granule release. Blood 1980;56:824.
1259. Holloway DS, Summaria L, Sandesara J, et al. Decreased platelet number and function and increased fibrinolysis contribute to postoperative bleeding in cardiopulmonary bypass patients. Thromb Haemost 1988;59:62.
1260. Muller N, Popov-Cenic S, Buttner W, et al. Studies of fibrinolytic and coagulation factors during open heart surgery. II. Postoperative bleeding tendency and changes in the coagulation system. Thromb Res 1975;7:589.
1261. Lambert CJ, Marengo-Rowe AJ, Leveson JE, et al. The treatment of postperfusion bleeding using epsilon-aminocaproic acid, cryoprecipitate, fresh-frozen plasma, and protamine sulfate. Ann Thorac Surg 1978;28:440.
1262. Kucuk O, Kwaan HC, Frederickson J, et al. Increased fibrinolytic activity in patients undergoing cardiopulmonary bypass operation. Am J Hematol 1986;23:223.
1263. Soloway HB, Cornett BM, Donahoo JV, Cox SP. Differentiation of bleeding diatheses which occur following protamine correction of heparin anticoagulation. Am J Clin Pathol 1973;60:188.
1264. Lambert CJ, Marengo-Rowe AJ, Leveson J, et al. The tri-F titer: a rapid test for estimation of plasma fibrinogen and detection of fibrinolysis, fibrin(ogen) split products, and heparin. Ann Thorac Surg 1974; 18:357.
1265. Gundry SR, Drongowski RA, Klein MD, Coran AG. Postoperative bleeding in cardiovascular surgery: does heparin rebound really exist? Am Surg 1989;55:162.
1266. Hope AF, Heyns A du P, Lotter MG, et al. Kinetics and sites of sequestration of indium 111–labeled human platelets during cardiopulmonary bypass. J Thorac Cardiovasc Surg 1981;81:880.
1267. Mammen EF, Koets MH, Washington BC, et al. Hemostasis changes during cardiopulmonary bypass surgery. Semin Thromb Hemost 1985;11:281.
1268. Gluszko P, Rucinski B, Musial J, et al. Fibrinogen receptors in platelet adhesion to surfaces of extracorporeal circuit. Am J Physiol 1987;252: H615.
1269. Wenger RK, Lukasiewicz H, Mikuta BS, et al. Loss of platelet fibrinogen receptors during clinical cardiopulmonary bypass. J Thorac Cardiovasc Surg 1989;97:235.
1270. Edmunds LH Jr, Ellison N, Colman RW, et al. Platelet function during cardiac operation: comparison of membrane and bubble oxygenators. J Thorac Cardiovasc Surg 1982;83:805.
1271. Hennessy VL Jr, Hicks RE, Niewiarowski S, et al. Function of human platelets during extracorporeal circulation. Am J Physiol 1977;232: H622.
1272. Wachtfogel YT, Musial J, Jenkin B, et al. Loss of platelet α_2-adrenergic receptors during simulated extracorporeal circulation: prevention with prostaglandin E_1. J Lab Clin Med 1985;105:601.
1273. Musial J, Niewiarowski S, Hershock D, et al. Loss of fibrinogen receptors from the platelet surface during similated extracorporeal circulation. J Lab Clin Med 1985;105:514.
1274. Dechavanne M, Ffrench M, Pages J, et al. Significant reduction in the binding of a monoclonal antibody (LYP 18) directed against the IIb/IIIa glycoprotein complex to platelets of patients having undergone extracorporeal circulation. Thromb Haemost 1987;57:106.
1275. Addonizio VP Jr, Smith JB, Strauss JF III, et al. Thromboxane synthesis and platelet secretion during cardiopulmonary bypass with bubble oxygenator. J Thorac Cardiovasc Surg 1980;79:91.
1276. Davies GC, Sobel M, Salzman EW. Elevated plasma fibrinopeptide A and thromboxane B_2 levels during cardiopulmonary bypass. Circulation 1980;61:808.
1277. Kestin AS, Valeri CR, Khuri SF, et al. The platelet function defect of cardiopulmonary bypass. Blood 1993;82:107.
1278. Bick RL. Hemostasis defects associated with cardiac surgery, prosthetic devices, and other extracorporeal circuits. Semin Thromb Hemost 1985;11:249.
1279. Salzman EW, Weinstein MJ, Weintraub RM, et al. Treatment with desmopressin acetate to reduce blood loss after cardiac surgery: a double-blind randomized trial. N Engl J Med 1986;314:1402.
1280. Czer LS, Bateman TM, Gray RJ, et al. Treatment of severe platelet dysfunction and hemorrhage after cardiopulmonary bypass: reduction in blood product usage with desmopressin. J Am Coll Cardiol 1987;9: 1139.
1281. Weinstein M, Ware JA, Troll J, Salzman E. Changes in von Willebrand factor during cardiac surgery: effect of desmopressin acetate. Blood 1988;71:1648.
1282. Hackmann T, Gascoyne RD, Naiman SC et al. A trial of desmopressin (1-desamino-8-D-arginine vasopressin) to reduce blood loss in uncomplicated cardiac surgery. N Engl J Med 1989;321:1437.
1283. Rocha E, Llorens R, Paramo JA, et al. Does desmopressin acetate reduce blood loss after surgery in patients on cardiopulmonary bypass? Circulation 1988;77:1319.
1284. Longmore DB, Bennett JG, Hoyle PM, et al. Prostacyclin administration during cardiopulmonary bypass in man. Lancet 1981;1:800.
1285. Aren C, Feddersen K, Radegran K. Effects of prostacyclin infusion on platelet activation and postoperative blood loss in coronary bypass. Ann Thorac Surg 1983;36:49.
1286. Malpass TW, Amory DW, Harker LA, et al. The effect of prostacyclin infusion on platelet hemostatic function in patients undergoing cardiopulmonary bypass. J Thorac Cardiovasc Surg 1984;87:550.
1287. Van den Dungen JJAM, Karliczek GF, Brenken U, et al. The effect of prostaglandin E_1 in patients undergoing clinical cardiopulmonary bypass. Ann Thorac Surg 1983;35:406.
1288. Fish KJ, Sarnquist FH, Van Steennis C, et al. A prospective, randomized study of the effects of prostacyclin on platelets and blood loss during coronary bypass operations. J Thorac Cardiovasc Surg 1986;91:436.
1289. Teoh KH, Christakis GT, Weisel RD, et al. Dipyridamole preserved platelets and reduced blood loss after cardiopulmonary bypass. J Thorac Cardiovasc Surg 1988;96:332.
1290. Bidstrup BP, Royston D, Sapsford RN, et al. Reduction in blood loss and blood use after cardiopulmonary bypass with high-dose aprotinin (Trasylol). J Thorac Cardiovasc Surg 1989;97:364.
1291. Harder MP, Eijsman L, Roozendaal KJ, et al. Aprotinin reduces intraoperative and postoperative blood loss in membrane oxygenator cardiopulmonary bypass. Ann Thorac Surg 1991;51:936.
1292. Van Oeveren W, Eijsman L, Roozendaal KJ, Wildevuur CRH. Platelet preservation by aprotinin during cardiopulmonary bypass. (Letter) Lancet 1988;1:644.
1293. Vander Salm TJ, Ansell JE, Okike ON, et al. The role of epsilon-

aminocaproic acid in reducing bleeding after cardiac operation: a double-blind randomized study. J Thorac Cardiovasc Surg 1988; 95:538.
1294. DelRossi AJ, Cernaianu AC, Botros S, et al. Prophylactic treatment of postperfusion bleeding using EACA. Chest 1989;96:27.
1295. Gafter U, Bessler H, Malachi T, et al. Platelet count and thrombopoietic activity in patients with chronic renal failure. Nephron 1987;45:207.
1296. Docci D, Turci F, Del Vecchio C, et al. Hemodialysis-associated platelet loss: study of the relative contribution of dialyzer membrane composition and geometry. Int J Artif Organs 1984;7:337.
1297. Hakim RM, Schafer AI. Hemodialysis-associated platelet activation and thrombocytopenia. Am J Med 1985;78:575.
1298. Schmitt GW, Moake JL, Rudy CK, et al. Alterations in hemostatic parameters during hemodialysis with dialyzers of different membrane composition and flow design: platelet activation and factor VIII–related von Willebrand factor during hemodialysis. Am J Med 1987;83:411.
1299. Vicks SL, Gross ML, Schmitt GW. Massive hemorrhage due to hemodialysis-associated thrombocytopenia. Am J Nephrol 1983; 3:30.
1300. Smith DA, Monaghan WP, Hann WD, Schumacher H. Evaluation of in vivo platelet adhesiveness during discontinuous-flow centrifugal thrombocytapheresis. Plasma Ther Transfus Technol 1983;4:37.
1301. Harker LA, Slichter SJ. Studies of platelet and fibrinogen kinetics in patients with prosthetic heart valves. N Engl J Med 1970;283:1302.
1302. Harker LA, Slichter SJ. Platelet and fibrinogen consumption in man. N Engl J Med 1972;287:999.
1303. Harker LA, Slichter SJ, Sauvage LR. Platelet consumption by arterial prostheses: the effects of endothelialization and pharmacologic inhibition of platelet function. Ann Surg 1977;186:594.
1304. Stuart M, Stockman J, Scott M, et al. Shortened platelet life span in patients with hydrocephalus and ventriculojugular shunts: results of preliminary attempts at correction. J Pediatr 1972;80:21.
1305. Meuleman DG, Vogel GMT, VAN Delft AML. Effects of intraarterial cannulation on blood platelet consumption in rats. Thromb Res 1980;20:45.
1306. Savage B, Malpass TW, Stratton JR, Harker LA. Platelet adenine nucleotide levels in patients with Dacron vascular prostheses. Thromb Res 1983;32:365.
1307. Pumphrey CW, Dawes J. Platelet alpha-granule depletion: findings in patients with prosthetic heart valves and following cardiopulmonary bypass surgery. Thromb Res 1983;30:257.
1308. Stratton JR, Thiele BL, Ritchie JL. Natural history of platelet deposition on Dacron aortic bifurcation grafts in the first year after implantation. Am J Cardiol 1983;52:371.
1309. Gross S, Keefer V, Liebman J. The platelets in cyanotic congenital heart disease. Pediatrics 1968;42:651.
1310. Wedemeyer AL, Edson JR, Krivit W. Coagulation in cyanotic congenital heart disease. Am J Dis Child 1972;124:656.
1311. Goldschmidt B. Platelet functions in children with congenital heart disease. Acta Paediatr Scand 1974;63:271.
1312. Waldman JD, Czapek EE, Paul MH, et al. Shortened platelet survival in cyanotic heart disease. J Pediatr 1975;87:77.
1313. Terai M, Nakazawa M, Takao A, Imai Y. Thrombocytopenia in patients with aortopulmonary transposition and an intact ventricular septum. Br Heart J 1987;57:371.
1314. Komp DM, Sparrow AW. Polycythemia in cyanotic heart disease: a study of altered coagulation. J Pediatr 1970;76:231.
1315. Ihenacho HN, Fletcher DJ, Breeze GR, et al. Consumption coagulopathy in congenital heart disease. Lancet 1973;1:231.
1316. Ekert H, Gilchrist GS, Stanton R, et al. Hemostasis in cyanotic congenital heart disease. J Pediatr 1970;76:221.
1317. Maurer HM, McCue CM, Caul J, Still WJS. Impairment in platelet aggregation in congenital heart disease. Blood 1972;40:207.
1318. Ekert H, Dowling SV. Platelet release abnormality and reduced prothrombin levels in children with cyanotic congenital heart disease. Aust Paediatr J 1977;13:17.
1319. Henriksson P, Värendh G, Lundstrom NR. Haemostatic defects in cyanotic congenital heart disease. Br Heart J 1979;41:23.
1320. Wedemeyer AL, Lewis JH. Improvement in hemostasis following phlebotomy in cyanotic patients with heart disease. J Pediatr 1973; 83:46.
1321. Brodsky I, Gill DN, Lusch CJ. Fibrinolysis in congenital heart disease: preoperative treatment with epsilon amincaproic acid. Am J Clin Pathol 1969;51:51.
1322. Gralnick HR. Epsilon aminocaproic acid in preoperative correction of haemostatic defects in cyanotic congenital heart disease. Lancet 1970;1:1204.
1323. Ekert H, Sheers M. Pre and postoperative studies of fibrinolysis and prothrombin in cyanotic congenital heart disease. Haemostasis 1974; 3:158.
1324. Naiman JL. Clotting and bleeding in cyanotic congenital heart disease. J Pediatr 1970;76:333.
1325. Kelton JG, Powers P, Julian J, et al. Sex-related differences in platelet aggregation: influence of hematocrit. Blood 1980;56:38.
1326. Maurer HM, McCue CM, Robertson LW, et al. Correction of platelet dysfunction and bleeding in cyanotic congenital heart disease by simple red cell volume reduction. Am J Cardiol 1975;35:831.
1327. Jacobson RJ, Rath CE, Perloff JK. Intravascular haemolysis and thrombocytopenia in left ventricular outflow obstruction. Br Heart J 1973;35:849.
1328. Steele PP, Weily HS, Davies H, et al. Platelet survival in patients with rheumatic heart disease. N Engl J Med 1974;290:537.
1329. Gill JC, Wilson AD, Endres-Brooks J, Montgomery RR. Loss of the largest von Willebrand factor multimers from the plasma of patients with congenital cardiac defects. Blood 1986;67:758.
1330. Wang Y, From AHL, Krivit W, et al. Disseminated pulmonary arterial thrombosis associated with thrombocytopenia: occurrence in identical twins. Circulation 1965;31:215.
1331. Edwards BS, Weir EK, Edwards WD, et al. Coexistent pulmonary and portal hypertension: morphologic and clinical features. J Am Coll Cardiol 1987;10:1233.
1332. Stahl RL, Javid JP, Lackner H. Unrecognized pulmonary embolism presenting as disseminated intravascular coagulation. Am J Med 1984;76:772.
1333. Mustafa MH, Mispireta LA, Pierce LE. Occult pulmonary embolism presenting with thrombocytopenia and elevated fibrin split products. Am J Med 1989;86:490.
1334. Noe DA, Graham SM, Luff R, Sohmer P. Platelet counts during rapid massive transfusion. Transfusion 1982;22:392.
1335. Hewson JR, Neame PB, Kumar N, et al. Coagulopathy related to dilution and hypotension during massive transfusion. Crit Care Med 1985;13:387.
1336. Harrigan C, Lucas CE, Ledgerwood AM, Mammen EF. Primary hemostasis after massive transfusion for injury. Am Surg 1982;48:393.
1337. Lim RC Jr, Olcott C IV, Robinson AJ, Blaisdell FW. Platelet response and coagulation changes following massive blood replacement. J Trauma 1973;18:577.
1338. Reed RL II, Heimbach DM, Counts RB, et al. Prophylactic platelet administration during massive transfusion: a prospective, randomized, double-blind clinical study. Ann Surg 1986;203:40.
1339. Goulet O, Girot R, Maier-Redelsperger M, et al. Hematologic disorders following prolonged use of intravenous fat emulsions in children. J Parenter Enteral Nutr 1986;10:284.
1340. Zierz S, Schröder R, Unkrig CJ. Thrombocytopenia induced by erucic acid therapy in patients with X-linked adrenoleukodystrophy. Clin Invest 1993;71:802.
1341. Andrew M, Kelton J. Neonatal thrombocytopenia. Clin Perinatol 1984;11:359.
1342. Castle V, Andrew M, Kelton J, et al. Frequency and mechanism of neonatal thrombocytopenia. J Pediatr 1986;108:749.
1343. Castle V, Coates G, Kelton JG, Andrew M. ^{111}In-oxine platelet survivals in thrombocytopenic infants. Blood 1987;70:652.
1344. Schmidt B, Vegh P, Johnston M, et al. Do coagulation screening tests detect increased generation of thrombin and plasmin in sick newborn infants? Thromb Haemost 1993;69:418.
1345. Perlman M, Dvilansky A. Blood coagulation status of small-for-dates and postmature infants. Arch Dis Child 1975;50:424.
1346. Cooper LZ, Green RH, Krugman S, et al. Neonatal thrombocytopenic purpura and other manifestations of rubella contracted in utero. Am J Dis Child 1965;110:416.
1347. Vossaugh P, Leikin S, Avery G, et al. Neonatal thrombocytopenia in association with rubella. Acta Haematol 1966;35:158.
1348. Hanshaw JB. Congenital and acquired cytomegalovirus infection. Pediatr Clin North Am 1966;13:279.
1349. Whitaker JA, Sartain P, Shaheedy M. Hematological aspects of congenital syphilis. J Pediatr 1965;66:629.
1350. Jones MJ, Kolb M, Votava JH, et al. Intrauterine echo-virus type 11 infection. Mayo Clin Proc 1980;55:509.
1351. Zipursky A, Jaber HM. The haematology of bacterial infections in newborn infants. Clin Haematol 1978;7:175.
1352. Modanlou HD, Ortiz OB. Thrombocytopenia in neonatal infection. Clin Pediatr 1981;20:402.
1353. Mehta P, Vasa R, Neumann L, Karpatkin, M. Thrombocytopenia in the high risk infant. J Pediatr 1980;97:791.
1354. Ballin A, Koren G, Kohelet D, et al. Reduction of platelet counts induced by mechanical ventilation in newborn infants. J Pediatr 1987;111:445.
1355. Segall ML, Goetzman BW, Schick JB. Thrombocytopenia and pulmonary hypertension in the perinatal aspiration syndromes. J Pediatr 1980;96:727.
1356. Levin DL, Weinberg AG, Perkin RM. Pulmonary microthrombi syndrome in newborn infants with unresponsive persistent pulmonary hypertension. J Pediatr 1983;102:299.
1357. Hammerman C, Lass N, Strates E, et al. Prostanoids in neonates with persistent pulmonary hypertension. J Pediatr 1987;110:470.
1358. Favara BE, Franciosi RA, Butterfield LJ. Disseminated intravascular and cardiac thrombosis of the neonate. Am J Dis Child 1974;127:197.
1359. Tudehope Dl, Yu VYH. The haematology of neonatal necrotizing enterocolitis. Aust Paediatr J 1977;13:193.
1360. Stein H, Beck J, Solomon A, et al. Gastroenteritis with necrotizing enterocolitis in premature babies. Br Med J 1972;2:616.
1361. Maurer HM, Frakin M, McWilliams MB. Effects of phototherapy on platelet counts in low-birthweight infants and on platelet production and life span in rabbits. Pediatr 1976;57:506.

1362. Nielsen NC. Influence of pre-eclampsia upon coagulation and fibrinolysis in women and their newborn infants immediately after delivery. Acta Obstet Gynecol Scand 1969;48:523.
1363. Kleckner HB, Giles HR, Corrigan JJ Jr. The association of maternal and neonatal thrombocytopenia in high-risk pregnancies. Am J Obstet Gynecol 1977;128:235.
1364. Brazy JE, Grimm JK, Little VA. Neonatal manifestations of severe maternal hypertension occurring before the thirty-sixth week of pregnancy. J Pediatr 1982;100:265.
1365. Pritchard JA, Cunningham FG, Pritchard SA, Mason RA. How often does maternal preeclampsia–eclampsia incite thrombocytopenia in the fetus? Obstet Gynecol 1987;69:292.
1366. Kasabach HH, Merritt KK. Capillary hemangioma with extensive purpura: report of case. Am J Dis Child 1940;59:1063.
1367. Shim WKT. Hemangiomas of infancy complicated by thrombocytopenia. Am J Surg 1968;116:896.
1368. Banks PA, Rosenberg AE. A 27-year-old Greek woman with portal-vein thrombosis and an epigastric mass. N Engl J Med 1989;320:301.
1369. Froehlich LA, Housler M. Neonatal thrombocytopenia and chorangioma. J Pediatr 1971;78:516.
1370. Bauer CR, Fojaco RM, Bancalar E, Fernandez-Rocha L. Microangiopathic hemolytic anemia and thrombocytopenia in a neonate associated with a large placental chorioangioma. Pediatrics 1978;62:574.
1371. Propp RP, Scharfman WB. Hemangioma–thrombocytopenia syndrome associated with microangiopathic hemolytic anemia. Blood 1966; 28:623.
1372. Brizel HE, Raccuglia G. Giant hemangioma with thrombocytopenia: radioisotypic demonstration of platelet sequestration. Blood 1965; 26:751.
1373. Inceman S, Tangun Y. Chronic defibrination syndrome due to a giant hemangioma associated with microangiopathic hemolytic anemia. Am J Med 1969;46:997.
1374. Schmidt RP, Lentle BC. Hemangioma with consumptive coagulopathy (Kasabach-Merritt syndrome): detection by indium-111–oxine labeled platelets. Clin Nucl Med 1984;9:389.
1375. Sondel PM, Ritter MW, Wilson DG, Lieberman LM. Use of ^{111}In platelet scans in the detection and treatment of Kasabach-Merritt syndrome. J Pediatr 1984;104:87.
1376. Fost NC, Esterly NB. Successful treatment of juvenile hemangiomas with prednisone. J Pediatr 1968;72:351.
1377. Brown SH Jr, Neerhout RC, Fonkalsrud EW. Prednisone therapy in the management of large hemangiomas in infants and children. Surgery 1972;71:168.
1378. Folkman J. Toward a new understanding of vascular proliferative disease in children. Pediatr 1984;74:850.
1379. Folkman J, Langer R, Linhardt RJ, et al. Angiogenesis inhibition and tumor regression caused by heparin or a heparin fragment in the presence of cortisone. Science 1983;221:719.
1380. Linderkamp O, Hopner F, Klose H, et al. Solitary hepatic hemangioma in a newborn infant complicated by cardiac failure, consumption coagulopathy, microangiopathic hemolytic anemia, and obstructive jaundice: case report and review of the literature. Eur J Pediatr 1976;124:23.
1381. Nordberg UB, Sundberg J. Indications and methods for radiotherapy of cavernous haemangiomas: a study of 1191 haemangiomas following radiotherapy. Acta Radiol Therap 1963;1:257.
1382. Williams OK, Van Buskirk FW, Burns S, Mellish RWP. Giant hemangioendothelioma with thrombocytopenia and hypofibrinogenemia. AJR 1969;106:204.
1383. Argenta LC, Bishop E, Cho KJ, et al. Complete resolution of life-threatening hemangioma by embolization and corticosteroids. Plast Reconstr Surg 1982;70:739.
1384. Astedt B, Henriksson P, Nilsson IM, Svanberg L. Regression of hemangioma–thrombocytopenia syndrome. Acta Obstet Gynecol Scand 1982;61:479.
1385. Neidhart JA, Roach RW. Successful treatment of skeletal hemangioma and Kasabach-Merritt syndrome with aminocaproic acid: is fibrinolysis "defensive"? Am J Med 1982;73:434.
1386. Ortel TL, Onorato JJ, Bedrosian CL, Kaufman RE. Antifibrinolytic therapy in the management of the Kasabach Merritt syndrome. Am J Hematol 1988;29:44.
1387. Koerper MA, Addiego JE, deLorimier AA, et al. Use of aspirin and dipyridamole in children with platelet-trapping syndromes. J Pediatr 1983;102:311.
1388. Hanada T, Saito K, Nagasawa T, et al. Intravenous gammaglobulin therapy for thromboneutropenic neonates of mothers with systemic lupus erythematosus. Eur J Haematol 1987;38:400.
1389. Watson R, Kang JE, May M, et al. Thrombocytopenia in the neonatal lupus syndrome. Arch Dermatol 1988;124:560.
1390. Mauer AM, DeVaux LO, Lahey MD. Neonatal and maternal thrombocytopenic purpura due to quinine. Pediatrics 1957;19:84.
1391. Rodriguez SU, Leikin SL, Hiller MC. Neonatal thrombocytopenia associated with ante-partum administration of thiazide drugs. N Engl J Med 1964;270:881.
1392. Widerlov E, Karlman I, Storsater J. Hydralazine-induced neonatal thrombocytopenia. (Letter) N Engl J Med 1980;303:1235.
1393. Schiff D, Aranda JV, Stern L. Neonatal thrombocytopenia and congenital malformations associated with administration of tolbutamide to the mother. J Pediatr 1970;77:457.
1394. Merenstein GB, O'Loughlin EP, Plunket DC. Effects of maternal thiazides on platelet counts of newborn infants. J Pediatr 1970;76:766.
1395. Jerkner K, Kutti J, Victorin L. Platelet counts in mothers and their newborn infants with respect to ante-partum administration of oral diuretics. Acta Med Scand 1973;194:473.
1396. Stuart MJ, Gross SJ, Elrad H, Graeber JE. Effects of acetylsalicylic-acid ingestion on maternal and neonatal hemostasis. N Engl J Med 1982;307:909.
1397. Wigger HJ, Bransilver BR, Blanc WA. Thromboses due to catheterization in infants and children. J Pediatr 1970;76:1.
1398. Nachman RL, Thomas M, Patel D, Gottbrath E. Thrombocytopenia as evidence of local thrombus: the umbilical arterial catheter. (Letter) Pediatrics 1972;50:825.
1399. Jones JE, Reed JF Jr. Renal vein thrombosis and thrombocytopenia in a newborn infant. J Pediatr 1965;67:681.
1400. Renfield ML, Kraybill EN. Consumptive coagulopathy with renal vein thrombosis. J Pediatr 1973;82:1054.
1401. Hawker RE, Celermajer JM, Cartmill TB, et al. Thrombosis of the inferior vena cava following balloon septostomy in transposition of the great arteries. Am Heart J 1971;82:593.
1402. Spadone D, Clark F, James E, et al. Heparin-induced thrombocytopenia in the newborn. J Vasc Surg 1992;15:306.
1403. Rivers RPA. Coagulation changes associated with a high haematocrit in the newborn infant. Acta Paediatr Scand 1975;64:449.
1404. Katz J, Rodriguez E, Mandani G, Branson HE. Normal coagulation findings, thrombocytopenia, and peripheral hemoconcentration in neonatal polycythemia. J Pediatr 1982;101:99.
1405. Schulman I, Pierce M, Lukens A, Currimbhoy Z. Studies on thrombopoiesis. I. A factor in normal human plasma required for platelet production: chronic thrombocytopenia due to its deficiency. Blood 1960;16:943.
1406. Monnens LAH, Retera RJM. Thrombotic thrombocytopenic purpura in a neonatal infant. J Pediatr 1967;71:118.
1407. Upshaw JD Jr. Congenital deficiency of a factor in normal plasma that reverses microangiopathic hemolysis and thrombocytopenia. N Engl J Med 1978;298:1350.
1408. Peters C, Casella JF, Marlar RA, et al. Homozygous protein C deficiency: observations on the nature of the molecular abnormality and the effectiveness of warfarin therapy. Pediatrics 1988;81:272.
1409. Pegelow CH, Curless R, Bradford B. Severe protein C deficiency in a newborn. Am J Pediatr Hematol Oncol 1988;10:326.
1410. Lipson AH, Pritchard J, Thomas G. Thrombocytopenia after intralipid infusion in a neonate. (Letter) Lancet 1974;2:1462.
1411. Spragg RG, Abraham JL, Loomis WH. Pulmonary platelet deposition accompanying acute oleic acid-induced pulmonary injury. Am Rev Resp Dis 1982;126:553.
1412. Dahms BB, Halpin TC Jr. Pulmonary arterial lipid deposit in newborn infants receiving intravenous lipid infusion. J Pediatr 1980;97:800.
1413. Wakely PE, Hug G. Intralipid vasculopathy. (Letter) Lancet 1981;2: 1416.
1414. Morrow G III, Barness LA, Auerbach VH, et al. Observations on the coexistence of methylmalonic acidemia and glycinemia. J Pediatr 1969;74:680.
1415. De Klerk JB, Duran M, Dorland L, et al. A patient with mevalonic acidura presenting with hepatosplenomegaly, congenital anaemia, thrombocytopenia and leukocytosis. J Inherited Metab Dis 1988; 11:233.
1416. Roth KS, Yang W, Foreman JW, et al. Holocarboxylase synthetase deficiency: a biotin-responsive organic acidemia. J Pediatr 1980; 96:845.
1417. Kelleher JF Jr, Yudkoff M, Hutchinson R, et al. The pancytopenia of isovaleric acidemia. Pediatrics 1980;65:1023.
1418. Koenig JM, Christensen RD. Neutropenia and thrombocytopenia in infants with Rh hemolytic disease. J Pediatr 1989;114:625.
1419. Wagner HP, Tonz O, Von Greyerz-Gloor RD. Congenital lymphoid leukemia: case report with chromosomal studies. Helv Paediatr Acta 1968;23:591.
1420. Wolk JA, Stuart MJ, Davey FR, Nelson DA. Congenital and neonatal leukemia: lymphocytic or myelocytic? Am J Dis Child 1974;128:864.
1421. Shown TE, Durfee MF. Blueberry muffin baby: neonatal neuroblastoma with subcutaneous metastases. J Urol 1970;104:193.
1422. Cohen DM, Mitchell CB, Alexander JW. Letterer-Siwe disease in a newborn. Arch Pathol 1966;81:347.
1423. Hertz CG, Hambrick GW Jr. Congenital Letterer-Siwe disease: a case treated with vincristine and corticosteroids. Am J Dis Child 1968; 116:553.
1424. Weinstein HI. Congenital leukemia and the neonatal myeloproliferative disorders associated with Down's syndrome. Clin Haematol 1978;7:147.
1425. Sills RH. Hypersplenism. In: Pochedly C, Sills RH, Schwartz AD, eds. Disorders of the spleen: pathophysiology and management. New York: Marcel Dekker, 1989:167.
1426. Todd D, Chan TK. Abnormalities of blood volume in disorders of the spleen. In: Bowdler AJ, ed. The spleen: structure, function and clinical significance. London, Chapman and Hall, 1990:191.

1427. Schmidt KG, Rasmussen JW, Bekker C, Modsen PER. Kinetics and *in vivo* distribution of ^{111}In-labelled autologous platelets in chronic hepatic disease: mechanisms of thrombocytopenia. Scand J Haematol 1985;34:39.
1428. Hill-Zobel RL, McCandless B, Kang SA, et al. Organ distribution and fate of human platelets: studies of asplenic and splenomegalic patients. Am J Hematol 1986;23:231.
1429. Henderson JM, Warren WD. Selective variceal decompression: current status and recent advances. Adv Surg 1984;18:81.
1430. Yoshioka H, Kuroda C, Hon S, et al. Splenic embolization for hypersplenism using steel coils. AJR 1985;144:1269.
1431. Kumpe DA, Rumack CM, Pretorius DH, et al. Partial splenic embolization in children with hypersplenism. Radiology 1985;155:357.
1432. Lindemann A, Ludwig WD, Oster W, et al. High-level secretion of tumor necrosis factor-alpha contributes to hematopoietic failure in hairy cell leukemia. Blood 1989;73:880.
1433. Benbasset J, Penchas S, Ligumski M. Splenectomy in patients with agnogenic myeloid metaplasia: an analysis of 321 published cases. Br J Haematol 1979;42:207.
1434. Brenner B, Nagler A, Tatarsky I, Hashmonai M. Splenectomy in agnogenic myeloid metaplasia and postpolycythemic myeloid metaplasia: a study of 34 cases. Arch Intern Med 1988;148:2501.
1435. Rubin M, Yampolski I, Lambrozo R, et al. Partial splenectomy in Gaucher's disease. J Pediatr Surg 1986;21:125.
1436. Thanopoulos BD, Frimas CA, Mantagos SP, Beratis NG. Gaucher disease: treatment of hypersplenism with splenic embolization. Acta Paediatr Scand 1987;76:1003.
1437. Dacie JV, Brain MC, Harrison CV, et al. "Non-tropical idiopathic splenomegaly" ("primary hypersplenism"): a review of ten cases and their relationship to malignant lymphomas. Br J Haematol 1969;17:317.
1438. Hermann RE, DeHaven KE, Hawk WA. Splenectomy for the diagnosis of splenomegaly. Ann Surg 1968;168:896.
1439. Malmaeus J, Akre T, Adami HO, Hagberg H. Early postoperative course following elective splenectomy in haematological disease: a high complication rate in patients with myeloproliferative disorders. Br J Surg 1986;73:720.
1440. Villalobos TJ, Adelson E, Riley PA Jr, Crosby WH. A cause of thrombocytopenia and leucopenia that occurs in dogs during deep hypothermia. J Clin Invest 1958;37:1.
1441. Bjork VO, Hultquist G. Brain damage in children after deep hypothermia for open-heart surgery. Thorax 1960;15:284.
1442. Reddick RL, Poole BL, Penick GD. Thrombocytopenia of hibernation: mechanism of induction and recovery. Lab Invest 1973;28:270.
1443. Shenaq SA, Yawn DH, Saleem A, et al. Effect of profound hypothermia on leukocytes and platelets. Ann Clin Lab Sci 1986;16:130.
1444. O'Brien H, Amess JA, Mollin DL. Recurrent thrombocytopenia, erythroid hypoplasia and sideroblastic anaemia associated with hypothermia. Br J Haematol 1982;51:451.
1445. Cohen IJ, Amir J, Gedaliah A, et al. Thrombocytopenia of neonatal cold injury. J Pediatr 1984;104:620.
1446. Easterbrook PJ, Davis HP. Thrombocytopenia in hypothermia: a common but poorly recognized complication. Br Med J 1985;291:23.
1447. Vella MA, Jenner C, Betteridge DJ, Jowett NI. Hypothermia-induced thrombocytopenia. J Roy Soc Med 1988;81:228.
1448. Holm IA, McLaughlin JF, Feldman K, Stone EF. Recurrent hypothermia and thrombocytopenia after severe neonatal brain infection. Clin Pediatr 1988;27:326.
1449. Pina-Cabral JM, Amaral I, Pinto MM, Gerra LH. Hepatic and splenic platelet sequestration during deep hypothermia in the dog. Haemostasis 1974;2:235.
1450. Hessel EA II, Schmer G, Dillard DH. Platelet kinetics during deep hypothermia. J Surg Res 1980;28:23.
1451. Bareford D, Chandler ST, Hawker RJ, et al. Splenic platelet-sequestration following routine blood transfusion is reduced by filtered/washed blood products. Br J Haematol 1987;67:177.
1452. Tricot G, Criel A, Verwilghen RL. Thrombocytopenia as presenting symptom of preleukaemia in 3 patients. Scand J Haematol 1982;28:243.
1453. Hallett JM, Martell RW, Sher C, Jacobs P. Amegakaryocytic thrombocytopenia with duplication of part of the long arm of chromosome 3. Br J Haematol 1989;71:291.
1454. Rai V, Lintula R. Platelet function in the myelodysplastic syndromes. Scand J Haematol 1986;36:71.
1455. Berndt MC, Kabral A, Grimsley P, et al. An acquired Bernard-Soulier-like platelet defect associated with juvenile myelodysplastic syndrome. Br J Haematol 1988;68:97.
1456. Bennett JM. Classification of the myelodysplastic syndromes. Clin Haematol 1986;15:909.
1457. Vadhan-Raj S, Keating M, LeMaistre A, et al. Effects of recombinant human granulocyte-macrophage colony–stimulating factor in patients with myelodysplastic syndromes. N Engl J Med 1987;317:1545.
1458. Buzaid AC, Garewal HS, Lippman SM, et al. Danazol in the treatment of myelodysplastic syndromes. Eur J Haematol 1987;39:346.
1459. Cines DB, Cassileth PA, Kiss JE. Danazol therapy in myelodysplasia. Ann Intern Med 1985;103:58.
1460. Catalano L, Selleri C, Montuori N, et al. Danazol for myelodysplastic syndromes. (Letter.) Br J Haematol 1993;85:230.
1461. Cowan DH. Effect of alcoholism on hemostasis. Semin Hematol 1980;17:137.
1462. Post RM, Desforges JF. Thrombocytopenia and alcoholism. Ann Intern Med 1968;68:1230.
1463. Cowan DH, Graham RC Jr. Studies on the platelet defect in alcoholism. Thromb Diath Haemorrh 1975;33:310.
1464. Haut MJ, Cowan DH. The effect of ethanol on hemostatic properties of human blood platelets. Am J Med 1974;56:22.
1465. Lindenbaum J, Hargrove RL. Thrombocytopenia in alcoholics. Ann Intern Med 1968;68:526.
1466. Lindenbaum J, Lieber CS. Hematologic effects of alcohol in man in the absence of nutritional deficiency. N Engl J Med 1969;281:333.
1467. Ryback R, Desforges J. Alcoholic thrombocytopenia in three inpatient drinking alcoholics. Arch Intern Med 1970;125:475.
1468. Cowan DH, Hines JD. Thrombocytopenia of severe alcoholism. Ann Intern Med 1971;74:37.
1469. Haselager EM, Vreeken J. Rebound thrombocytosis after alcohol abuse: a possible factor in the pathogenesis of thromboembolic disease. Lancet 1977;1:774.
1470. Gewirtz AM, Hoffman R. Transitory hypomegakaryocytic thrombocytopenia: aetiological association with ethanol abuse and implications regarding regulation of human megakaryocytopoiesis. Br J Haematol 1986;62:333.
1471. Cowan DH. Thrombokinetic studies in alcohol-related thrombocytopenia. J Lab Clin Med 1973;81:64.
1472. Sullivan LW, Adams WH, Liu YK. Induction of thrombocytopenia by thrombopheresis in man: patterns of recovery in normal subjects during ethanol ingestion and abstinence. Blood 1977;49:197.
1473. Sahud MA. Platelet size and number in alcoholic thrombocytopenia. N Engl J Med 1972;286:355.
1474. Levine RF, Spivak JL, Meagher RC, Sieber F. Effect of ethanol on thrombopoiesis. Br J Haematol 1986;62:345.
1475. Stoll DB, Blum S, Pasquale D, Murphy S. Thrombocytopenia with decreased megakaryocytes: evaluation and prognosis. Ann Intern Med 1981;94:170.
1476. Hoffman R, Bruno E, Elwell J, et al. Acquired amegakaryocytic thrombocytopenic purpura: a syndrome of diverse etiologies. Blood 1982;60:1173.
1477. Chan DKY, O'Neill B. Successful trial of antithymocyte globulin therapy in amegakaryocytic thrombocytopenic purpura. (Letter) Med J Aust 1988;148:602.
1478. Nagasawa T, Sakurai T, Kashiwagi H, Abe T. Cell-mediated amegakaryocytic thrombocytopenia associated with systemic lupus erythematosus. Blood 1986;67:479.
1479. Font J, Nomdedeu B, Martinez-Orozco F, et al. Amegakaryocytic thrombocytopenia and an analgesic. (Letter) Ann Intern Med 1981;95:783.
1480. Hoffman R, Briddell RA, Van Besien K, et al. Acquired cyclic amegakaryocytic thrombocytopenia associated with an immunoglobulin blocking the action of granulocyte-macrophage colony–stimulating factor. N Engl J Med 1989;321:97.
1481. Telek B, Kiss A, Pecze K, et al. Cyclic idiopathic pure acquired amegakaryocytic thrombocytopenic purpura: a patient treated with cyclosporin A. Br J Haematol 1989;73:128.
1482. Hoffman R, Zaknoen S, Yang HH, et al. An antibody cytotoxic to megakaryocyte progenitor cells in a patient with immune thrombocytopenic purpura. N Engl J Med 1985;312:1170.
1483. Faldt R. Remission of amegakaryocytic thrombocytopenia induced by antilymphocyte globulin (ALG). Br J Haematol 1986;63:205.
1484. Khelif A, Ffrench M, Follea G, et al. Amegakaryocytic thrombocytopenic purpura treated with antithymocyte globulin. (Letter) Ann Intern Med 1985;102:720.
1485. Smeets REH, Hillen HFP. Acquired amegakaryocytic thrombocytopenic purpura: treatment with high-dose dexamethasone pulse therapy and review of the literature. Neth J Med 1988;32:27.
1486. Hill W, Landgraf R. Successful treatment of amegakaryocytic thrombocytopenic purpura with cyclosporine. (Letter) N Engl J Med 1985;312:1060.
1487. Kayser W, Euler HH, Schmitz N, et al. Danazol in acquired amegakaryocytic thrombocytopenic purpura: a case report. Blut 1985;51:401.
1488. El Saghir NS, Geltman RL. Treatment of acquired amegakaryocytic thrombocytopenic purpura with cyclophosphamide. Am J Med 1986;81:139.
1489. Schloesser LL, Kipp MA, Wenzel FJ. Thrombocytosis in iron deficiency anemia. J Lab Clin Med 1967;66:107.
1490. Gross S, Keefer V, Newman AJ. The platelets in iron-deficiency anemia. I. The response to oral and parenteral iron. Pediatrics 1964;34:315.
1491. Lopas H, Rabiner SF. Thrombocytopenia associated with iron deficiency anemia: a report of five cases. Clin Pediatr 1966;5:609.
1492. Dincol K, Aksoy M. On the platelet levels in chronic iron deficiency anemia. Acta Haematol 1969;41:135.
1493. Sonneborn D. Thrombocytopenia and iron deficiency. (Letter) Ann Intern Med 1974;80:111.

1494. Sahud MA, Olsen H, Pedemont L. Thrombocytopenia and iron deficiency. (Letter) Ann Intern Med 1974;81:132.
1495. Scher H, Silber R. Iron responsive thrombocytopenia. (Letter) Ann Intern Med 1976;84:571.
1496. Beard MEJ, Johnson SAN. Thrombocytopenia and iron deficiency anemia in a patient with a_1-thalassaemia trait: response to iron therapy. Acta Haematol 1978;59:114.
1497. Michaeli J, Admon D, Lugassy G, Matzner Y. Idiopathic thrombocytopenic purpura presenting as iron-responsive thrombocytopenia. Haemostasis 1987;7:105.
1498. Berger M, Brass LF. Severe thrombocytopenia in iron deficiency anemia. Am J Haematol 1987;24:425.
1499. Knizley H Jr, Noyes WD. Iron deficiency anemia, papilledema, thrombocytosis, and transient hemiparesis. Arch Intern Med 1972; 129:483.
1500. Soff GA, Levin J. Thrombocytopenia associated with repletion of iron in iron deficiency anemia. Am J Med Sci 1988;295:35.
1501. Karpatkin S, Garg SK, Freedman ML. Role of iron as a regulator of thrombopoiesis. Am J Med 1974;57:521.
1502. Hall JG, Levin J, Kuhn JP, et al. Thrombocytopenia with absent radius (TAR). Medicine 1969;48:411.
1503. Hedberg VA, Lipton JM. Thrombocytopenia with absent radii: a review of 100 cases. Am J Pediatr Hematol Oncol 1988;10:51.
1504. Fayen WT, Harris JW. Case report: thrombocytopenia with absent radii. Am J Med Sci 1980;280:95.
1505. Homans AC, Cohen JL, Mazur EM. Defective megakaryocytopoiesis in the syndrome of thrombocytopenia with absent radii. Br J Haematol 1988;70:205.
1506. Whitefield MF, Barr DGD. Cow's milk allergy in the syndrome of thrombocytopenia with absent radius. Arch Dis Child 1976;51:337.
1507. Aldenhoff P, von Muhlendahl KE, Waldenmaier C. Das EEC-Syndrom: Fallbericht und Uberlegungen zur pathogenese. Monatsschr Kinderheilkd 1978;126:575.
1508. Luthy DA, Mack L, Hirsch J, Cheng E. Prenatal ultrasound diagnosis of thrombocytopenia with absent radii. Am J Obstet Gynecol 1981; 141:350.
1509. Donnenfeld AE, Wiseman B, Lavi E, Weiner S. Prenatal diagnosis of thrombocytopenia absent radius syndrome by ultrasound and cordocentesis. Prenat Diagn 1990;10:29.
1510. Labrune P, Pons JC, Khalil M, et al. Antenatal thrombocytopenia in three patients with TAR (thrombocytopenia with absent radii) syndrome. Prenat Diagn 1993;13:463.
1511. Arias S, Penchaszadeh VB, Pinto-Cisternas J, Larrauri S. The IVIC syndrome: a new autosomal dominant complex pleiotropic syndrome with radial ray hypoplasia, hearing impairment, external ophthalmoplegia, and thrombocytopenia. Am J Med Genet 1980;6:25.
1512. Sammito V, Motta D, Capodieci G, et al. IVIC syndrome: report of a second family. Am J Med Genet 1988;29:875.
1513. Christodoulou C, Werner B. A girl with 18-trisomy and thrombocytopenia. Acta Genet 1967;17:77.
1514. Rabinowitz JG, Moseley JE, Mitty HA, et al. Trisomy 18, esophageal atresia, anomalies of the radius and congenital hypoplastic thrombocytopenia. Radiology 1967;89:488.
1515. Markenson AL, Hilgartner MW, Miller DR. Transient thrombocytopenia in 18-trisomy. J Pediatr 1975;87:834.
1516. Eisenstein EM. Congenital amegakaryocytic thrombocytopenic purpura. Clin Pediatr 1966;5:143.
1517. Hoyeraal HM, Lamvik J, Moe PJ. Congenital hypoplastic thrombocytopenia and cerebral malformations in two brothers. Acta Paediatr Scand 1970;59:185.
1518. Gardner RJM, Morrison PS, Abbott GD. A syndrome of congenital thrombocytopenia with multiple malformations and neurologic dysfunction. J Pediatr 1983;102:600.
1519. Van Oostrom CG, Wilms RHH. Congenital thrombocytopenia, associated with raised concentrations of haemoglobin F. Helv Paediatr Acta 1978;33:59.
1520. Fanconi G. Familial constitutional panmyelocytopathy, Fanconi's anemia (F.A.). Semin Hematol 1967;4:233.
1521. Gordon-Smith EC, Rutherford TR. Fanconi anaemia: constitutional, familial aplastic anaemia. Baillieres Clin Haematol 1989;2:139.
1522. McIntosh S, Breg WR, Lubiniecki AS. Fanconi's anemia: the preanemic phase. Am J Pediatr Hematol Oncol 1979;1:107.
1523. Gluckman E. Bone marrow transplantation for Fanconi's anaemia. Baillieres Clin Haematol 1989;2:153.
1524. O'Gorman-Hughes DW. Aplastic anaemia in childhood. III. Constitutional aplastic anaemia and related cytopenias. Med J Aust 1974;1:51.
1525. Alter BP, Potter NU, Li FP. Classification and aetiology of the aplastic anaemias. Clin Haematol 1978;7:431.
1526. Hreidarsson S, Kristjansson K, Johannesson G, Johannsson JH. A syndrome of progressive pancytopenia with microcephaly, cerebellar hypoplasia and growth failure. Acta Paediatr Scand 1988;77:773.
1527. De Boeck K, Degreef H, Verwilghen R, et al. Thrombocytopenia: first symptom in a patient with dyskeratosis congenita. Pediatrics 1981; 67:898.
1528. Juneja HS, Elder FFB, Gardner FH. Abnormality of platelet size and T-lymphocyte proliferation in an autosomal recessive form of dyskeratosis congenita. Eur J Haematol 1987;39:306.
1529. Griffiths AD. Constitutional aplastic anemia: a family with a new X linked variety of amegakaryocytic thrombocytopenia. J Med Genet 1983;20:361.
1530. Dokal I, Ganly P, Riebero I, et al. Late onset bone marrow failure associated with proximal fusion of radius and ulna: a new syndrome. Br J Haematol 1989;71:277.
1531. Slichter SJ, Harker LA. Thrombocytopenia: mechanisms and management of defects in platelet production. Clin Haematol 1978;7:523.
1532. Lecompte T. Hereditary thrombocytopenias. Curr Stud Hematol Blood Transfus 1988;55:162.
1533. Guerois G, Gruel Y, Petit A, et al. Familial macrothrombocytopenia: clinical, ultrastructural and biochemical study. Curr Stud Hematol Blood Transfus 1988;55:153.
1534. Najean Y, Lecompte T. Genetic thrombocytopenia with autosomal dominant transmission: a review of 54 cases. Br J Haematol 1990; 74:203.
1535. Greaves M, Pickering C, Martin J, et al. A new familial "giant platelet syndrome" with structural, metabolic and functional abnormalities of platelets due to a primary megakaryocyte defect. Br J Haematol 1987;65:429.
1536. Law IP, Deveny A, Meiser RJ. Case report: familial thrombocytopenia in seven members of three generations. Postgrad Med 1978;63:136.
1537. Cullum C, Cooney DP, Schrier SL. Familial thrombocytopenia thrombocytopathy. Br J Haematol 1967;13:147.
1538. Kurstjens R, Bolt C, Vossen M, Haanen C. Familial thrombopathic thrombocytopenia. Br J Haematol 1968;15:305.
1539. Jackson CW, Hutson NK, Steward SA, et al. The Wistar Furth rat: an animal model of hereditary macrothrombocytopenia. Blood 1988;71: 1676.
1540. Leven RM, Tablin F. Megakaryocyte and platelet ultrastructure in the Wistar Furth rat. Am J Pathol 1988;132:417.
1541. Hegglin R. Gleichzeitige konstitutionelle Veranderungen an Neutrophilen und Thrombozyten. Helv Med Acta 1945;12:439.
1542. Greinacher A, Mueller-Eckhardt C. Hereditary types of thrombocytopenia with giant platelets and inclusion bodies in the leukocytes. Blut 1990;60:53.
1543. Godwin HA, Ginsburg AD. May-Hegglin anomaly: a defect in megakaryocyte fragmentation? Br J Haematol 1974;26:117.
1544. Hamilton RW, Shaikh BS, Ottie JN, et al. Platelet function, ultrastructure, and survival in the May-Hegglin anomaly. Am J Clin Pathol 1980;74:663.
1545. Davis JW, Wilson SJ. Platelet survival in the May-Hegglin anomaly. Br J Haematol 1966;12:61.
1546. Epstein CJ, Sahud MA, Piel CF, et al. Hereditary macrothrombocytopathia, nephritis and deafness. Am J Med 1972;52:299.
1547. Eckstein JD, Filip DJ, Watts JC. Hereditary thrombocytopenia, deafness, and renal disease. Ann Intern Med 1975;82:639.
1548. Catarini M. Hereditary macrothrombocytopenia, deafness, nephropathy. Haematologica (Pavia) 1988;73:43.
1549. Hansen MS, Behnke O, Tinggaard Pedersen N, Videbaek A. Megathrombocytopenia associated with glomerulonephritis, deafness and aortic cystic medianecrosis. Scand J Haematol 1978;21:197.
1550. Standen GR, Saunders J, Michael J, Bloom AL. Epstein's syndrome: case report and survey of the literature. Postgrad Med J 1987;63:573.
1551. Peterson LC, Rao VK, Crosson JT, White JG. Fechtner syndrome: a variant of Alport's syndrome with leukocyte inclusions and macrothrombocytopenia. Blood 1985;65:397.
1552. Heynen MJ, Blockmans D, Verwilghen RL, Vermylen J. Congenital macrothrombocytopenia, leucocyte inclusions, deafness and proteinuria: functional and electron microscopic observations on platelets and megakaryocytes. Br J Haematol 1988;70:441.
1553. Gershoni-Baruch R, Baruch Y, Viener A, Lichtig C. Fechtner syndrome: clinical and genetic aspects. Am J Med Genet 1988;31:357.
1554. Brivet F, Girot R, Barbanel C, et al. Hereditary nephritis associated with May-Hegglin anomaly. Nephron 1981;29:59.
1555. Ardlie NG, Coupland WW, Schoefl GI. Hereditary thrombocytopathy: a familial bleeding disorder due to impaired platelet coagulant activity. Aust NZ J Med 1976;6:37.
1556. Tracy PB, Giles AR, Mann KG, et al. Factor V (Quebec): a bleeding diathesis associated with a qualitative platelet factor V deficiency. J Clin Invest 1984;74:1221.
1557. Weiss HJ, Meyer D, Rabinowitz R, et al. Pseudo-von Willebrand's disease: an intrinsic platelet defect with aggregation by unmodified human factor VIII/von Willebrand factor and enhanced adsorption of its high-molecular-weight multimers. N Engl J Med 1982;306:326.
1558. Gralnick HR, Williams SB, Shafer BC, Corash L. Factor VIII/von Willebrand factor binding to von Willebrand's disease platelets. Blood 1982;60:328.
1559. Giles AR, Hoogendoorn H, Benford K. Type IIB von Willebrand's disease presenting as thrombocytopenia during pregnancy. Br J Haematol 1987;67:349.
1560. Lopez-Fernandez MF, Lopez-Berges C, Martin-Bernal JA, et al. Type IIB von Willebrand's disease associated with a complex thrombocytopenic thrombocytopathy. Am J Hematol 1988;27:291.

1561. Hultin MB, Sussman II. Postoperative thrombocytopenia in type IIB von Willebrand disease. Am J Hematol 1990;33:64.
1562. Donner M, Holmberg L, Nilsson IM. Type IIB von Willebrand's disease with probable autosomal recessive inheritance and presenting as thrombocytopenia in infancy. Br J Haematol 1987;66:349.
1563. Gralnick HR, McKeown LP, Williams S, et al. Platelet aggregation induced by type IIb platelet von Willebrand factor. Br J Haematol 1989;71:253.
1564. Holmberg L, Nilsson IM, Borge L, et al. Platelet aggregation induced by 1-desamino-8-D-arginine vasopressin (DDAVP) in type IIB von Willebrand's disease. N Engl J Med 1983;309:816.
1565. Saba HI, Saba SR, Dent J, et al. Type IIB Tampa: a variant of von Willebrand disease with chronic thrombocytopenia, circulating platelet aggregates, and spontaneous platelet aggregation. Blood 1985;66:282.
1566. Sweeney JD, Hoernig LA, Behrens AN, et al. Von Willebrand's variant (type II Buffalo): thrombocytopenia after desmopressin but absence of in vitro hpersensitivity to ristocetin. Am J Clin Pathol 1990;93:522.
1567. Raccuglia G. Gray platelet syndrome: a variety of qualitative platelet disorder. Am J Med 1971;51:818.
1568. Berndt MC, Castaldi PA, Gordon S, et al. Morphological and biochemical confirmation of gray platelet syndrome in two siblings. Aust NZ J Med 1983;13:387.
1569. White JG. Ultrastructural studies of the gray platelet syndrome. Am J Pathol 1979;95:445.
1570. Breton-Gorius J, Vainchenker W, Nurden A, et al. Defective α granule production in megakaryocytes from gray platelet syndrome ultrastructural studies of bone marrow cells and megakaryocytes growing in culture from blood precursors. Am J Pathol 1981;102:10.
1571. Bernard J, Soulier JP. Sur une nouvelle variete de dystrophie thrombocytaire hemorrhagique congenitale. Semin Hop Paris 1948;24:3217.
1572. Drouin J, McGregor JL, Parmentier S, et al. Residual amounts of glycoprotein Ib concomitant with near-absence of glycoprotein IX in platelets of Bernard-Soulier patients. Blood 1988;72:1086.
1573. Greinacher A, Potzsch B, Kiefel V, et al. Evidence that DDAVP transiently improves hemostasis in Bernard-Soulier syndrome independent of von Willebrand factor. Ann Hematol 1993;67:149.
1574. Kamahli S, Canatan D, Uysal Z, et al. DDAVP shortens bleeding time in Bernard-Soulier syndrome. (Letter) Thromb Haemost 1994;71:675.
1575. Aakhus AM, Stavem P, Hovig T, et al. Studies on patient with thrombocytopenia, giant platelets and a platelet membrane glycoprotein Ib with reduced amount of sialic acid. Br J Haematol 1990;74:320.
1576. Yufu Y, Ideguchi H, Narishige T, et al. Familial macrothrombocytopenia associated with decreased glycosylation of platelet membrane glycoprotein IV. Am J Hematol 1990;33:271.
1577. Milton JG, Frojmovic MM. Shape-changing agents produce abnormally large platelets in a hereditary "giant platelets syndrome (MPS)." J Lab Clin Med 1979;93:154.
1578. Milton JG, Frojmovic MM, Tang SS, Whith JG. Spontaneous platelet aggregation in a hereditary giant platelet syndrome (MPS). Am J Pathol 1984;114:336.
1579. Okita JR, Frojmovic MM, Kristopeit S et al. Montreal platelet syndrome: a defect in calcium-activated neutral proteinase (calpain). Blood 1989;74:715.
1580. Stavem P, Abrahamsen AF, Vartdal F, et al. Hereditary thrombocytopenia with excessively prolonged bleeding time, corrected by infusions of platelet poor plasma. Scand J Haematol 1986;37:210.
1581. Stavem P, Jeremic M, Hjort PF, et al. Hereditary thrombocytopenia with excessively prolonged bleeding time. Scand J Haematol 1969; 6:250.
1582. Stormorken H, Sjaastad O, Langslet A, et al. A new syndrome: thrombocytopathia, muscle fatigue, asplenia, miosis, migraine, dyslexia and ichthyosis. Clin Genet 1985;28:367.
1583. Mahon M, Cumming WJK, Kristmundsdottir F, et al. Familial myopathy associated with thrombocytopenia: a clinical and histomorphometric study. J Neurol Sci 1988;88:55.
1584. Smith TP, Dodds WJ, Tartaglia AP. Thrombasthenic-thrombopathic thrombocytopenia with giant, "Swiss-cheese" platelets: a case report. Ann Intern Med 1973;79:828.
1585. Maldonado JE. "Swiss-chesse" platelets. Ann Intern Med 1974; 81:860.
1586. Von Behrens WE. Mediterranean macrothrombocytopenia. Blood 1975;46:199.
1587. Paulus JM, Casals FJ. Platelet formation in Mediterranean macrothrombocytosis. Nouv Rev Fr Hematol 1978;20:151.
1588. Myllyla G, Pelkonen R, Ikkala E, Apajalahti J. Hereditary thrombocytopenia: report of three families. Scand J Haematol 1967;4:441.
1589. Gutenberger J, Trygstad CW, Stiehm ER, et al. Familial thrombocytopenia, elevated serum IgA levels and renal disease: a report of a kindred. Am J Med 1970;49:729.
1590. Murphy S, Oski FA, Gardner FH. Hereditary thrombocytopenia with an intrinsic platelet defect. N Engl J Med 1969;281:857.
1591. Sheth NK, Prankerd TAJ. Inherited thrombocytopenia with thromasthenia. J Clin Pathol 1968;21:154.
1592. Danielsson L, Jelf E, Lundkvist L. A new family with inherited thrombocytopenia. Scand J Haematol 1980;24:427.
1593. Dowton SB, Beardsley D, Jamison D, et al. Studies of a familial platelet disorder. Blood 1985;65:557.
1594. Aldrich RA, Steinberg AG, Campbell DC. Pedigree demonstrating a sex-linked recessive condition characterized by draining ears, eczematoid dermatitis and bloody diarrhea. Pediatrics 1954;13:133.
1595. Ten Bensel RW, Stadlan EM, Krivit W. The development of malignancy in the course of the Aldrich syndrome. J Pediatr 1966;68:761.
1596. Ochs HD, Slichter SJ, Harker LA, et al. The Wiskott-Aldrich syndrome: studies of lymphocytes, granulocytes, and platelets. Blood 1980; 55:243.
1597. Peacocke M, Siminovitch KA. Linkage of the Wiskott-Aldrich syndrome with polymorphic DNA sequences from the human X chromosome. Proc Natl Acad Sci USA 1987;84:3430.
1598. Grottum KA, Hovig T, Holmsen H, et al. Wiskott-Aldrich syndrome: qualitative platelet defects and short platelet survival. Br J Haematol 1969;17:373.
1599. Krivit W, Yunis E, White JG. Platelet survival studies in Aldrich syndrome. Pediatrics 1966;37:339.
1600. Pearson HA, Shulman NR, Oski FA, Eitzman DV. Platelet survival in Wiskott-Aldrich syndrome. J Pediatr 1966;68:754.
1601. Holmberg L, Gustavii B, Jonsson A. A prenatal study of fetal platelet count and size with application to fetus at risk for Wiskott-Aldrich syndrome. J Pediatr 1983;102:773.
1602. Corash L, Shafer B, Blaese M. Platelet-associated immunoglobulin, platelet size, and the effect of splenectomy in the Wiscott-Aldrich syndrome. Blood 1985;65:1439.
1603. Verhoeven AJM, Van Oostrum IEA, Van Haarlem H, Akkerman JWN. Impaired energy metabolism in platelets from patients with Wiskott-Aldrich syndrome. Thromb Haemost 1989;61:10.
1604. Lum LG, Tubergen DG, Corash L, Blaese RM. Splenectomy in the management of the thrombocytopenia of the Wiskott-Aldrich syndrome. N Engl J Med 1980;302:892.
1605. Mullen CA, Anderson KD, Blaese RM. Splenectomy and/or bone marrow transplantation in the management of the Wiskott-Aldrich syndrome: long-term follow-up of 62 cases. Blood 1993;82:2961.
1606. Parkman R, Rappeport J, Geha R, et al. Complete correction of the Wiskott-Aldrich syndrome by allogeneic bone-marrow transplantation. N Engl J Med 1978;298:921.
1607. Nathan DG. Splenectomy in the Wiskott-Aldrich syndrome. N Engl J Med 1980;302:916.
1608. Remold-O'Donnell E, Kenney DM, Parkman R, et al. Characterization of a human lymphocyte surface sialoglycoprotein that is defective in Wiskott-Aldrich syndrome. J Exp Med 1984;159:1705.
1609. Schaar FE. Familial idiopathic thrombocytopenic purpura. J Pediatr 1963;62:546.
1610. Vestermark B, Vestermark S. Familial sex-linked thrombocytopenia. Acta Paediatr Scand 1964;53:365.
1611. Ata M, Fisher OD, Holman CA. Inherited thrombocytopenia. Lancet 1965;1:119.
1612. Canales L, Mauer AM. Sex-linked hereditary thrombocytopenia as a variant of Wiskott-Aldrich syndrome. N Engl J Med 1967;277:899.
1613. Chiaro JJ, Dharmkrong-at, Bloom GE. X-linked thrombocytopenic purpura. Am J Dis Child 1972;123:565.
1614. Murphy S, Oski FA, Naiman JL, et al. Platelet size and kinetics in hereditary and acquired thrombocytopenia. N Engl J Med 1972; 286:499.
1615. Weiden PL, Blaese RM. Hereditary thrombocytopenia: relation to Wiskott-Aldrich syndrome with special reference to splenectomy. J Pediatr 1972;80:226.
1616. Cohn J, Hauge M, Andersen V, et al. Sex-linked hereditary thrombocytopenia with immunological defects. Hum Hered 1975;25:309.
1617. Standen GR, Lillicrap DP, Matthews N, Bloom AL. Inherited thrombocytopenia, elevated serum IgA and renal disease: identification as a variant of the Wiskott-Aldrich syndrome. Q J Med 1986;59:401.
1618. Donner M, Schwartz M, Carlsson KU, Holmberg L. Hereditary X-linked thrombocytopenia maps to the same chromosomal region as the Wiskott-Aldrich syndrome. Blood 1988;72:1849.
1619. Knox-Macaulay HHM, Bashawri L, Davies KE. X linked recessive thrombocytopenia. J Med Genet 1993;30:968.

Blood: Principles and Practice of Hematology,
edited by Robert I. Handin, Samuel E. Lux, and Thomas P. Stossel.
J.B. Lippincott Company, Philadelphia © 1995.

35

Platelet Membrane Proteins and Their Disorders

Robert I. Handin

Platelets play an important role in the process of hemostasis by interacting with components of the blood vessel wall and linking together to form multicellular aggregates. The formation of platelet plugs rapidly stops the flow of blood from damaged vessels. Platelets also generate and secrete a diverse group of biologic mediators that help regulate hemostasis, fibrinolysis, and wound repair. Finally, platelets bind coagulation proteins and increase the rate of plasma coagulation reactions. All these events are regulated, to a large degree, by specific platelet membrane proteins. Although the structural features of the platelet membrane—a series of glycoproteins embedded in a phospholipid bilayer—are not unique, the large repertoire of receptor proteins, the diversity of potential platelet-mediated interactions, and the dramatic consequences of receptor-mediated platelet activation are impressive. Thus, platelets have become a subject of intense study by hematologists interested in understanding why patients bleed, by cardiologists and other clinicians who wish to prevent arterial thrombosis, as well as by a diverse group of scientists interested in cell–cell interactions, lipid metabolism, signal transduction, and cytoskeletal organization. This chapter reviews the structure and function of the principal platelet membrane proteins and the disorders caused by their loss or dysfunction. The role of membrane protein antigens in the pathogenesis of thrombocytopenia is covered in Chapter 34; platelet signal transduction and qualitative platelet disorders that do not involve membrane proteins directly are discussed in Chapter 37. In addition, the structure and function of the two most important plasma proteins that interact with platelet receptors to mediate adhesion and aggregation, the von Willebrand's factor (vWF) and fibrinogen, are discussed in separate chapters (see Chaps. 36 and 41).

CLASSIFICATION OF THE PLATELET MEMBRANE GLYCOPROTEINS

As in many other areas of medicine, the nomenclature used to classify the platelet membrane glycoproteins is confusing and somewhat arcane (Table 35-1). Platelet membrane proteins were first classified on the basis of their electrophoretic mobility and molecular mass. Originally, three broad groups (gpI, II, and III) were described.[1] With improvements in electrophoretic techniques, additional proteins were identified within these original groups (eg, gpIa, IIb, IIIa).[2,3] Unfortunately, this classification gives little insight into protein function and does not take into account the polypeptide composition of multisubunit proteins. Moreover, this classification only includes those proteins that can be resolved by polyacrylamide gel electrophoresis (SDS-PAGE) and are sufficiently abundant to be detected by protein staining. There are several important platelet receptors, which are discussed here, that are present in low copy number and must be identified by other techniques. Despite its limitations, the nomenclature derived from SDS-PAGE is widely used, firmly entrenched in the medical literature, and unlikely to be supplanted rapidly.

Two additional systems of nomenclature need to be understood. With the proliferation of monoclonal antibodies recognizing epitopes on cell surfaces, a system of cluster differentiation antigens (CD nomenclature) has appeared. Although usually thought of as a way to define lymphocyte antigens (eg, CD4, CD8), the system has been extended to include platelets and other hematopoietic cells. Finally, several of the platelet membrane glycoproteins are members of large protein families with their own nomenclature. For example, several platelet proteins are members of the integrin family.[4,5] All the integrins are heterodimeric molecules in which there is a unique α chain that is noncovalently linked to a common β chain shared by other integrins. The α chains may be designated either by a specific number or by the receptor from which they are derived. To illustrate the complexity caused by multiple names for the same protein, the platelet *fibrinogen receptor*, referred to by people working in the platelet field as the glycoprotein IIb/IIIa complex (gpIIb/IIIa), is also designated the $\alpha_{IIb}\beta_3$-integrin and has been assigned the cluster differentiation antigen number CD41a (see Table 35-1). Throughout this chapter, the functional property, when known, and the glycoprotein number based on SDS-PAGE are be used because these are most often used in the literature. Either the CD number or the integrin nomenclature also is given, in parentheses, if the protein is frequently referred to by these names in the published literature.

MEMBRANE PROTEINS THAT REGULATE PLATELET ADHESION

The initial event in hemostasis, the attachment or adhesion of platelets to vascular subendothelium, as well as the subsequent spreading of adherent platelets, is mediated by the

TABLE 35-1. Classification of Platelet Membrane Proteins

Function	Electrophoretic Classification	Cluster Differentiation Classification	Integrin Classification
Collagen receptor	gpIa/IIa	CD49b	$\alpha_2\beta_1$
Fibronectin receptor	gpIc/IIa	CD49e	$\alpha_5\beta_1$
Vitronectin receptor			$\alpha_V\beta_3$
Fibrinogen receptor	gpIIb/IIIa	CD41	$\alpha_{IIb}\beta_3$
Laminin receptor	gpIc′/IIa	CD49f	$\alpha_6\beta_1$
von Willebrand's receptor	gpIb/IX	CD42a,b,c	Not an integrin
?Collagen or thrombospondin receptor	gpIV	CD36	Not an integrin

platelet collagen receptors and the gpIb/IX and gpIIb/IIIa complexes. Collagen receptors interact directly with collagen subtypes present in vascular subendothelium, while gpIb/IX and gpIIb/IIIa bind immobilized forms of two adhesive glycoproteins—vWf and fibronectin. These two proteins, in turn, are bound to collagen and other components of vascular subendothelium.

Platelet Collagen Receptors

The adhesion of platelets to the collagenous components of the vascular subendothelium is one of the first events in the process of hemostasis. Although the platelet–collagen interaction has been the subject of intense study, its mechanism remains unclear. The critical collagen subtypes involved have not been determined, and there are a large number of candidate collagen receptors (Fig. 35-1). Several platelet proteins, such as fibronectin, vWf, thrombospondin, and the platelet transglutaminase factor XIII, have been proposed as collagen receptors.[6–9] Three different proteins have also been identified in detergent extracts of platelet membranes that can bind to insolubilized human collagens. Chiang and Kang first identified a 65-kd protein in human platelet membrane extracts that bound to a cyanogen bromide fragment derived from chick skin collagen.[10] They subsequently identified a 90-kd membrane protein that also bound to collagen and showed that antibodies to this protein inhibited collagen-induced platelet aggregation.[11] Kotite and Cunningham then reported that a 61-kd glycoprotein, identified by surface labeling of human platelets, bound to collagen[12]. At the same time, Lahav isolated an 80-kd membrane protein from rabbit platelets that bound to fibrillar type I bovine collagen.[13] Although each observation is of considerable interest, the clinical relevance of these three proteins has not been determined, and no patients have yet been identified with hemostatic defects that can be traced to these proteins.

Additional collagen receptor candidates have emerged from clinical studies of patients with defective collagen-induced aggregation. Nieuwenhuis and colleagues, in 1985, described a patient who had a mild bleeding disorder and platelets that did not aggregate in response to collagen and who was missing platelet gpIa.[14] Subsequently, a second patient with a similar defect was reported by another group.[15] In this case, however, the deficiency in gpIa was accompanied by a decrease in platelet thrombospondin content and remitted spontaneously. These additional features suggested that the deficiency may have been an acquired abnormality or part of another syndrome. The possible role of the gpIa/IIa complex as a platelet collagen receptor is also supported by in vitro studies. First, there is good evidence that the fibroblast class II extracellular matrix receptor, a member of the integrin family ($\alpha_2\beta_1$), is identical to platelet gpIa/IIa and that this protein mediates adhesion to collagen in many different cell types.[16] The gpIa/IIa complex, for example, binds to collagen-coated surfaces and to a cyanogen bromide fragment (α_1[i]-CB3) derived from type I collagen.[17] A second platelet membrane protein has been implicated as a collagen receptor from clinical studies. Moroi and colleagues described a patient whose platelets lacked glycoprotein VI and did not aggregate or adhere to fibrillar types I and III collagen.[18]

There has been a great deal of interest in another platelet protein, gpIV (also known in some classifications as gpIIIb and as CD36) which binds to type I collagen fibrils. The Fab fragments of antibodies raised against purified gpIV

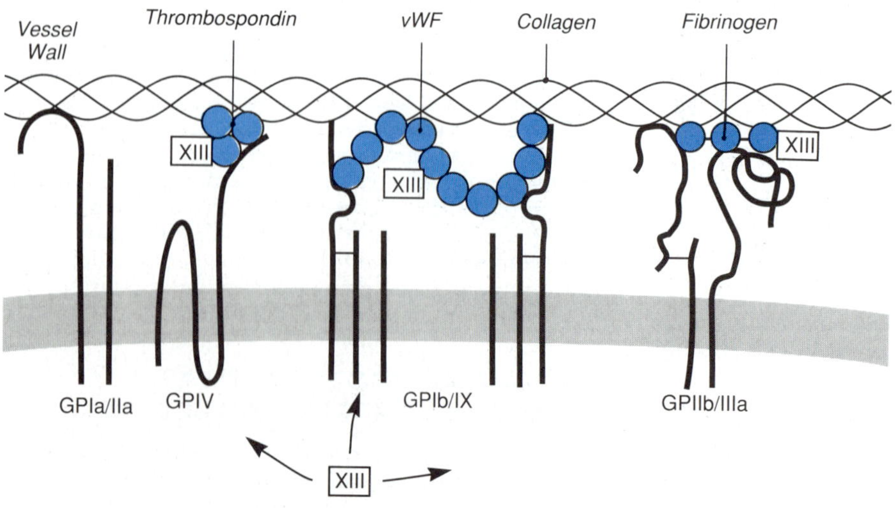

FIGURE 35-1. Candidate collagen receptors on the platelet surface are depicted. The integrin protein gpIa/IIa, which is the most well-characterized collagen receptor, binds to collagen directly. Platelet gpIV may either bind directly or bind to collagen by means of thrombospondin. The von Willebrand's factor (vWF) and fibrinogen may also link platelets to collagen after their interactions with gpIb/IX or gpIIb/IIIa. Finally, factor XIII, which is present in plasma, and the platelet cytosol may cross-link thrombospondin, vWF, and fibrinogen in situ collagen fibrils.

and soluble gpIV itself inhibit platelet activation and aggregation in response to type I collagen.[19,20] The domains responsible for CD36 binding to collagen and thrombospondin have been identified.[21] It is of interest that gpIV (CD36) is not detected on platelets obtained from large numbers of apparently healthy Japanese blood donors.[22] This finding raises some questions about the role of this protein in hemostasis. Because gpIV (CD36) is expressed in several other cell types, including erythrocytes and monocytes, it is possible that it may have other functions that are more important than its proposed role in hemostasis. There is evidence that CD36 mediates the entry of malarial parasites into red cells.[23,24] It also binds the adhesive protein thrombospondin and may promote monocyte interactions with tumor cells.[25]

In conclusion, there may be more than one platelet membrane protein capable of interacting with collagen. Rather than a single platelet collagen receptor, it is possible that several of the candidate receptors that have been identified mediate platelet adhesion and that individual receptors may recognize specific collagen subtypes. Alternately, the interactions detected with in vitro tests and purified receptor proteins may not reflect in vivo interactions. No animal models in which individual candidate receptors have been inactivated are available to help determine the physiologic relevance of some of the potential receptors. The extensive clinical and laboratory evidence that is available, however, suggests a major role for the gpIa/IIa complex in platelet adhesion. An additional role for gpIV, gpVI, or possibly, for some of the other less well-characterized proteins can certainly not be excluded.

Platelet gpIb/IX Complex

Although platelet binding to collagen is the initial step in hemostasis, stable adhesion under the high-flow, high-shear conditions encountered in the vasculature requires a second interaction. The platelet gpIb/IX complex plays this particularly important role in platelet adhesion as it binds to vWF deposited onto vascular subendothelium and, thereby, strengthens the linkage between adherent platelets and the vessel wall. The vWF receptor, gpIb/IX (CD42), is one of the most abundant platelet membrane glycoproteins, with about 25,000 copies of the complex present on the platelet surface.[26]

Glycoprotein Ib is a heterodimer made up of a larger α-polypeptide, (gpIbα, 143 kd) covalently linked to a smaller β subunit (gpIbβ, 22 kd)[27,28] (Fig. 35-2). The gpIbα/Ibβ complex then forms a noncovalent complex with a third protein, glycoprotein IX (gpIX, 20 kd).[29] The receptor was originally thought to be made up solely of the gpIbα/Ibβ heterodimer. However, analysis of patients with Bernard-Soulier syndrome, who are missing gpIb, revealed deficiencies in two other membrane proteins, gpIX and gpV.[30] In addition, when platelet membranes are solubilized in nonionic detergents and undergo affinity chromatography with an antibody directed against gpIbα, stoichiometric amounts of a third protein, gpIX, copurify with the gpIbα/Ibβ complex. Studies in which the gpIbα/Ibβ and gpIX cDNAs were cotransfected and coexpressed in heterologous cells have confirmed that all three polypeptides are needed for the assembly and surface expression of a functional gpIb/IX complex.[31] Cotransfection of gpV was not needed for expression of the complex, even though it is deficient in some patients with Bernard-Soulier syndrome. Although gpV may not be part of the functional gpIb/IX complex, gpIb/IX may be needed for stable expression of gpV. The recent molecular cloning of gpV should permit cotransfection studies, which may help resolve this issue.[32,33]

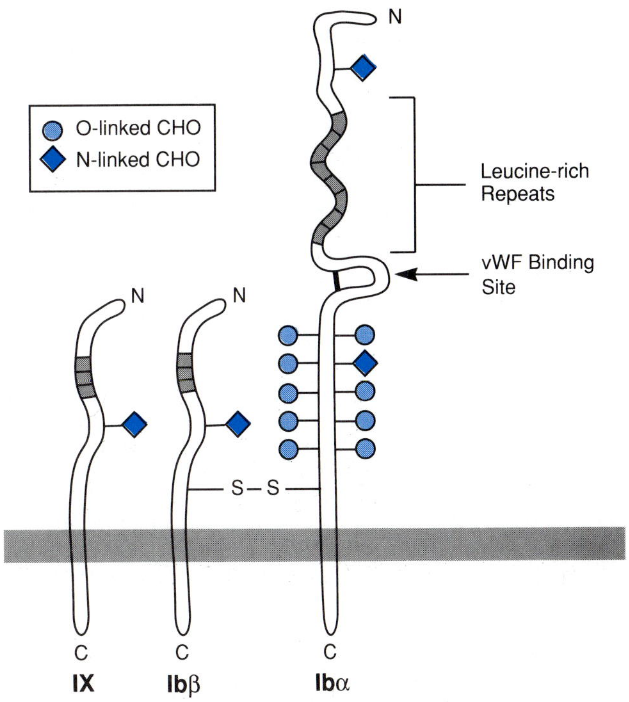

FIGURE 35-2. The structure and polypeptide composition of the platelet gpIb/IX complex is depicted. The gpIbα and gpIbβ polypeptides are covalently linked by a single disulfide bond. gpIX is noncovalently bound to the gpIbα/gpIbβ complex. The location of O-linked and N-linked carbohydrate, the leucine-rich repeats, and the von Willebrand's factor binding sites are also depicted. The gpIbα polypeptide contains over 50 identical O-linked oligosaccharides, which comprise half the mass of the protein. The biologic function of the leucine-rich repeats that are present in all three polypeptides has not yet been determined.

The gpIb/IX complex is a major constituent of the platelet surface glycocalyx—a carbohydrate-rich zone surrounding the plasma membrane of many cells.[34,35] Although all three of the subunit polypeptides contain carbohydrate, gpIbα is the most heavily glycosylated with a series of 50 identical O-linked hexasaccharide chains concentrated in a serine-threonine–rich region just proximal to the transmembrane domain.[36,37] In fact, half the molecular mass of gpIbα can be attributed to carbohydrate, and this single polypeptide is the major repository of platelet surface sialic acid.

The structure of the gpIb/IX complex has been partially defined by electron microscopy and probing with proteolytic enzymes.[38] Using electron microscopic examination, the complex appears as an elongated, 60-nm rod. The extracellular, amino-terminal portion of the rod-shaped molecule extends about 50 nm from the plasma membrane. The shorter, globular carboxy terminus of the molecule contains the transmembrane and intracellular extensions of the subunit polypeptides. gpIbα is cleaved by platelet calpain at a site that is just proximal to the transmembrane domain to yield the 120-kd soluble receptor fragment: glycocalicin.[35,39] Small quantities of glycocalicin have been detected in the circulation,[40] and exposure of platelets to a variety of proteolytic enzymes, including plasmin, generates large quantities of glycocalicin. The digestion of glycocalicin with trypsin yields two smaller polypeptides: an NH_2-terminal 45-kd fragment, which contains vWF and thrombin-binding sites, and a heavily glycosylated carboxyl-terminal macroglycopeptide.[41–43]

Primary Structure and Molecular Cloning of gpIb/IX

The cDNAs encoding the three polypeptide chains have been cloned, and the primary structure of each polypeptide has been determined (Fig. 35-3). They each have a hydrophobic signal sequence, which targets the protein for secretion and is subsequently cleaved, and a hydrophobic transmembrane domain, which anchors the protein in the platelet membrane. The mature gpIbα, Ibβ, and IX polypeptides contain 610, 181, and 160 amino acids, respectively, with large extracellular and smaller intracellular domains.[44–47] As first pointed out by Roth, each of the three polypeptides in the gpIb/IX complex contains varying numbers of a 24 amino acid sequence rich in the amino acid leucine that has been noted in a number of otherwise unrelated proteins with diverse functions.[48] Glycoprotein Ibα contains seven tandem copies of the leucine-rich glycoprotein (LRG) repeat located between amino acids 36 and 200, while gpIbβ and gpIX each contain a single LRG repeat. The LRG repeats are, in turn, flanked by a highly conserved 22 amino acid sequence, producing a flank–LRG–flank motif.

The gene that encodes the gpIbα polypeptide has been localized to the distal end of the short arm of chromosome 17 (17p12ter).[49] The gene has only a single 233-base intron located just upstream of the initiator methionine codon that marks the start of translation and divides the gene into two exons.[49] The first exon contains a short 5′ untranslated sequence, and the entire coding sequence of gpIbα is contained in the large second exon of the gene. gpIX has been located on chromosome 3.[47] The chromosomal localization of gpIbβ has not been reported. All three genes are intron depleted and organized similar to gpIbα. Expression of the gpIb/IX complex is restricted, with most of the protein found in megakaryocytes and platelets. There is accumulating evidence that endothelial cells express low levels of the gpIb/IX complex and that gpIb/IX expression is substantially increased when endothelial cells are exposed to tumor necrosis factor and other combinations of cytokines.[50,51] The physiologic role of endothelial gpIb/IX is still being debated.

The gpIbα polypeptide contains the binding site for vWF, its principal ligand, as well as a high-affinity binding site for thrombin (Fig. 35-4). As reviewed in Chapter 36, each vWF subunit contains homologous repeated sequences—the A and D repeats. The first A repeat, amino acid residues 449 through 705, contains the information needed to bind to the gpIb/IX complex.[52–54] The vWF binding site on gpIb/IX has also been localized to a discrete segment of the gpIbα polypeptide. Studies using peptide inhibitors, as well as experiments with recombinant gpIbα polypeptides, have localized the vWF binding site to a disulfide bonded loop structure between residues 220 and 310 of the gpIbα chain.[55–57] This "hinge region" lies between the LRG repeats and the serine-threonine–rich region that contains sites for O-linked oligosaccharides. This loop contains a high proportion of charged amino acid residues, which may explain, in part, its binding properties. Between residues 269 and 287, there are 10 negatively charged amino acids, followed by 5 positively charged amino acids within the next 13 residues.

Studies with recombinant gpIbα polypeptides suggest that this region alone is sufficient to account for vWF binding. The mechanism for regulating vWF binding when the sequence is placed in the context of the entire gpIb/IX complex is not well understood. The synthetic peptides or recombinant gpIbα polypeptides that have been studied bind directly to the vWF A1 domain. In contrast, vWF in plasma does not bind to platelet gpIb/IX. However, the adsorption

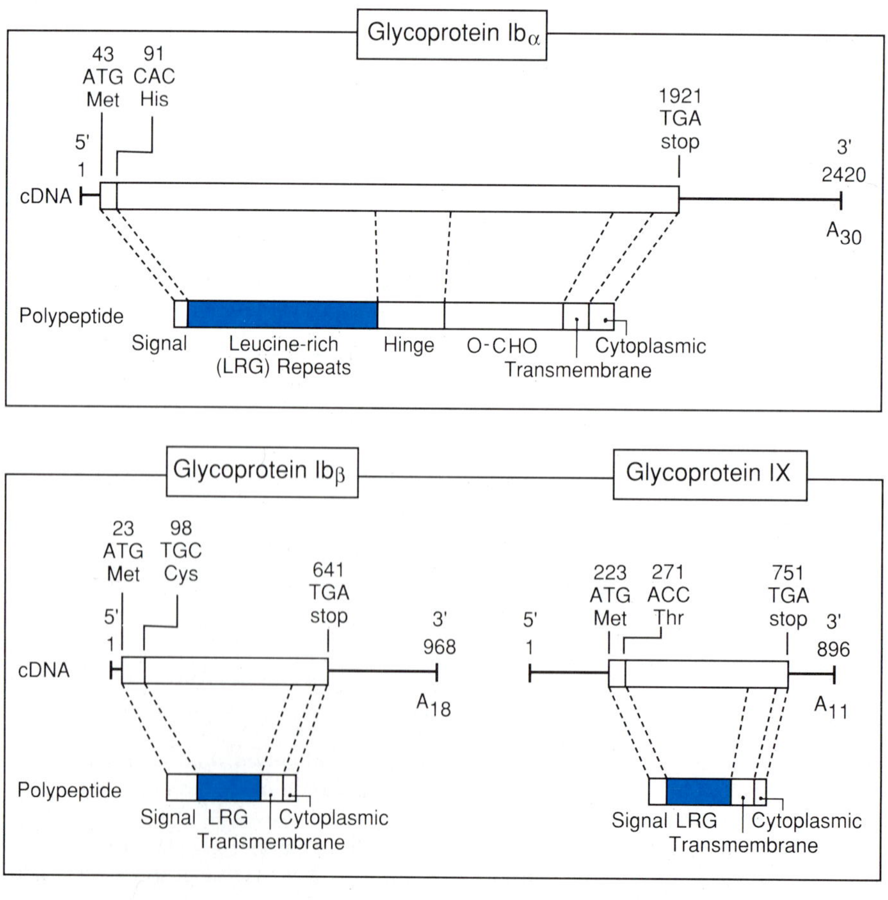

FIGURE 35-3. The structure of the gpIbα/Ibβ and gpIX cDNAs and the polypeptides they encode is depicted. Each contains a conventional signal sequence, leucine-rich repeats, and a single transmembrane domain. They each also have a short cytoplasmic extension.

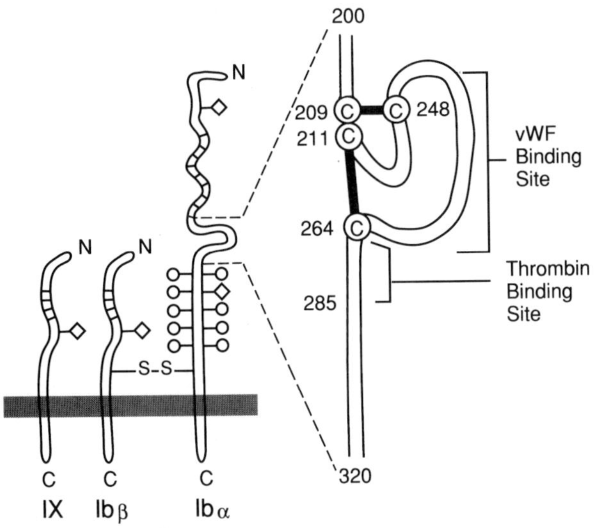

FIGURE 35-4. The location of the von Willebrand factor (vWF) and thrombin-binding sites in the gpIb/IX complex is depicted. Both binding sites are in a discrete region of the gpIbα polypeptide between amino acids 209 and 285. The vWF binding site is located in a disulfide-bonded loop structure and the thrombin site just carboxy terminal to this loop.

of vWF onto a surface, the subjecting of platelet–vWF suspensions to shear stress in a cone plate viscometer, and the addition of the cationic antibiotic Ristocetin or the snake venom Botrocetin to platelet suspensions all induce vWF binding to platelet gpIb/IX.[58–61] The in vivo counterparts of these experimental maneuvers are, most likely, the shear forces induced by blood flow and the binding of vWF to vascular subendothelium.

The thrombin-binding site has been localized, with peptide inhibitors to a sequence spanning residues 271 to 284 of gpIbα.[62] The binding of thrombin to this site is of high affinity with a reported affinity of less than 10 nM. Although the relation between this high-affinity binding site and the recently identified platelet thrombin receptor, discussed below, remains unclear, thrombin binding to gpIb/IX can affect platelet function. Platelets from patients with Bernard-Soulier syndrome, which do not express gpIb/IX, require higher than normal concentrations of thrombin to get full activation and aggregation.[63]

Each of the three polypeptides in the gpIb/IX complex contains sequences that can interact with cytoskeletal proteins or other cytoplasmic components. There is good evidence that gpIb/IX interacts with the actin cytoskeletal by means of actin-binding protein (ABP).[64,65] Glycoprotein Ibβ contains a cyclic AMP–dependent phosphorylation site at tyrosine 166, and phosphorylation at this residue affects the interaction between gpIb/IX and the actin–ABP complex.[66] There is also an unpaired cysteine in the cytoplasmic extension of the gpIbβ polypeptide that could form mixed disulfide linkages with cytosol constituents.[45] In addition, there is an unpaired cysteine in the transmembrane domain of gpIX that could be a site for fatty acid acylation.[46]

The interaction between gpb/IX and the platelet cytoskeleton plays an important role in determining platelet size and shape. Patients with Bernard-Soulier syndrome who lack functional gpIb/IX are known to have unusually large platelets.[67,68] Studies have shown that this increase in platelet size may be due to the lack of normal linkage between gpIb/IX and the actin cytoskeleton, which produces a "relaxed" redundant platelet membrane.[69]

After the binding of ligands like vWF to the gpIb/IX complex, there is evidence for signal transduction. vWF binding produces a transient calcium flux, hydrolysis of phospholipid, and the generation of thromboxane A_2.[70] Similar signals can be induced by the addition of Ristocetin or by subjecting platelet–vWF suspensions to shear stress in a cone plate viscometer.[71] Signal transduction can be abolished by preincubation with aspirin or indomethacin, suggesting that vWF functions as a weak agonist. Although vWF is not a potent activator by itself, in conjunction with collagen, it may induce early platelet activation before significant thrombin generation. (For a more detailed discussion of platelet signal transduction mechanisms refer to Chap. 37).

Bernard-Soulier Syndrome

Molecular Basis

Although there is some heterogeneity among various kindreds, most Bernard-Soulier platelets are deficient in four membrane glycoproteins—the gpIbα and Ibβ polypeptides, gpIX, and gpV.[30] The availability of cDNAs for $gpIb_{\alpha,\beta}$ and gbIX has provided a means to detect the mutations responsible for the Bernard-Soulier syndrome and to analyze the biosynthesis and assembly of the gpIb/IX complex. As previously discussed, simultaneous transfection of heterologous cells with gpIbα/Ibβ and gpIX cDNAs permits the assembly of a functional gpIb/IX complex on the cell surface. Thus, gpV is not critical for gpIb/IX assembly. On the other hand, the absence of gpV from Bernard-Soulier platelets implies that expression of the gpIb/IX complex may be necessary for the stable expression of gpV. By analogy with other systems, mutations in either the gpIbα or Ibβ polypeptides or in gpIX would be expected to cause the Bernard-Soulier phenotype, while mutations in gpV should not. In addition, because all three of the polypeptides have been mapped to autosomal chromosomes, the complete absence of the gpIb/IX complex would require patients to be either homozygous for a single mutation or compound heterozygotes. Relatively few mutations have been characterized to date (Table 35-2). There was one published study of a heterozygous point mutation in the gpIbα polypeptide that causes the synthesis of truncated gpIbα chains that remain in the platelet cytosol.[72] There was another report of a family with the Bernard-Soulier syndrome that is not linked to polymorphisms in the gpIbα gene.[73] In support of this, a family has been reported with mutations in both alleles of the gpIX gene.[74] One allele had an Asp 261 → Gly substitution, and the second had an Asp 45 → Ser. These two gpIV missense mutations prevent assembly of the gpIb/IX complex. There are also two families with missense mutations in the gpIbα polypeptide.[75,76] These mutations (Ala 156 → Val and Leu 57 → Phe) impaired vWF binding to the gpIb/IX complex.

Clinical Features

Two distinct hemostatic abnormalities can be traced to defects in the gpIb/IX complex. The first is platelet-type or pseudo–von Willebrand's disease. In this entity, point mutations in gpIbα permit the spontaneous binding of plasma vWF to platelets. This results in thrombocytopenia and depletion of high-molecular-weight multimers from plasma and is covered in Chapter 36.

The most well known entity is the Bernard-Soulier syndrome, which is usually inherited as an autosomal recessive trait. It is characterized by moderate to severe bleeding, a marked decrease in shear-dependent platelet adhesion to vascular subendothelium, thrombocytopenia, and giant platelets (Table 35-3). The syndrome was first described by two French physicians, Bernard and Soulier, in 1948.[68]

TABLE 35-2. Molecular Basis of the Bernard-Soulier Syndrome

Inheritance	Phenotype	Chain	Mutation	Reference
Autosomal recessive	Abnormal band on SDS-Page	α	Trp 343 Stop (Allele 2 unknown)	Ware et al, 1990[72]
Autosomal recessive	gpIb/IX present	α	Ala 156 → Val (pt. homozygous)	Ware et al, 1993[75]
Autosomal recessive	No detectable gpIb/IX	IX IX	1-Asp 216 → Gly 2-Asn 45 → Ser	Wright et al, 1993[74]
Autosomal dominant	gpIb/IX present N1 vWF binding Absent RIPA	α	Leu 57 → Phe Allele 2-N1	Miller et al, 1992[76]

RIPA, ristocetin-induced platelet agglutination.

They reported on a young patient whom they had encountered with thrombocytopenia, giant platelets, and a severe bleeding disorder. Subsequently, additional families were discovered with a similar clinical picture. The common feature of all these patients is a lack of gpIb/IX complex on their platelets.

Patients with the Bernard-Soulier syndrome usually present during infancy or as young children. They have fairly severe mucous membrane bleeding and skin bleeding with prominent ecchymoses, epistaxis, and gingival bleeding.[77] Older patients may develop severe menorrhagia, gastrointestinal bleeding, and extensive hemorrhage after surgery or trauma. The bleeding in these patients is usually sufficiently severe to require platelet transfusions and suppression of menses.[77,78] In fact, in one large series with 59 cases, there were 10 deaths from the complications of bleeding.[78] Paradoxically, there are also occasional patients who experience less severe bleeding as they grow older.[78]

The critical defect in Bernard-Soulier platelets is an inability to adhere to vascular subendothelium despite normal quantities of plasma vWF. This leads to characteristic laboratory abnormalities. The bleeding time is invariably prolonged and often is longer than 20 minutes.[79,80] Virtually all patients are moderately thrombocytopenic, and platelet counts as low as 20,000/μL have been reported. When stained films of peripheral blood are examined, the platelets are larger than normal (Fig. 35-5). Most Bernard-Soulier platelets have a mean diameter greater than 3.5 μm, and occasional platelets as large as 20 to 30 μm are seen.[81–83] These giant platelets approximate the size of mature lymphocytes. Other blood cells are normal, as are bone marrow megakaryocytes.

The diagnostic laboratory abnormality is the failure of Bernard-Soulier platelets to agglutinate when incubated with ristocetin (decreased RIPA).[80] Furthermore, unlike patients with von Willebrand's disease, this defect cannot be corrected by the addition of vWF. In contrast, aggregation with other agonists, including adenosine diphosphate (ADP), collagen, and epinephrine, is normal. As previously discussed, platelet aggregation with thrombin is partially impaired, requiring higher than normal concentrations of thrombin to induce complete aggregation and granule secretion. An abnormality in prothrombin consumption has been reported and is reflected by a shortened serum prothrombin time.[84,85] The mechanism for this abnormality is unclear because platelet coagulant activity (PF-3) and platelet support of prothrombinase activity are actually increased on Bernard-Soulier platelets.[85,86] The increased coagulant activity may be due, simply, to an increase in membrane surface area or, perhaps, is secondary to changes in the distribution of anionic phospholipids in the plasma membrane.

TABLE 35-3. Clinical Criteria for the Diagnosis of the Bernard-Soulier Syndrome

Autosomal recessive inheritance (usually)
Epistaxis, ecchymoses, gingival bleeding beginning in infancy
Menorrhagia, gastrointestinal bleeding, posttraumatic hemorrhage
Prolonged bleeding time
Variable, moderate to severe thrombocytopenia
Large (lymphocytoid) platelets
Failure of platelets to agglutinate with Ristocetin
No correction with added von Willebrand's factor
Absence of the gpIb/IX complex by electrophoresis, flow cytometry or presence of a dysfunctional complex

Differential Diagnosis

Several other syndromes are characterized by large platelets and thrombocytopenia, but the Bernard-Soulier syndrome is the only disorder in which Ristocetin-induced platelet agglutination is defective. For example, giant platelets, thrombocytopenia, and Döhle bodies in leukocytes are the classic findings in May-Hegglin anomaly. May-Hegglin platelets, however, function normally, and there is no abnormality in any of the identified membrane proteins.[87,88] Bleeding is unusual in May-Hegglin patients and has been observed, only occasionally, in patients with marked thrombocytopenia.[89] Patients with Epstein's syndrome—autosomal dominant hereditary nephritis and sensorineural deafness—may also have thrombocytopenia and large platelets.[87] There are some reports of a functional abnormality in these patients characterized by decreased aggregation and secretion in response to ADP, collagen, and epinephrine.[90–92] The Montreal platelet syndrome is a disorder with giant platelets, thrombocytopenia, a prolonged bleeding time, normal aggregation in response to agonists, but spontaneous aggregation when platelets are stirred at 37°C.[93–96] In contrast to Bernard-Soulier syndrome, it is inherited as an autosomal dominant trait. Membrane glycoprotein patterns are normal, but calcium-activated protease activity is reduced.[97] Finally, patients with the gray platelet syndrome, a rare form of storage pool disease (see Chap. 37), in which there is a deficiency in α granules, may have thrombocytopenia and giant platelets.[98,99] On close examination of Wright-Giemsa–stained smears, the platelets are pale because they lack α-granule staining. The platelets agglutinate normally with Ristocetin. There are also a few poorly characterized cases of giant platelets and thrombocytopenia that do not have any of the previously described clinical features.[100,101]

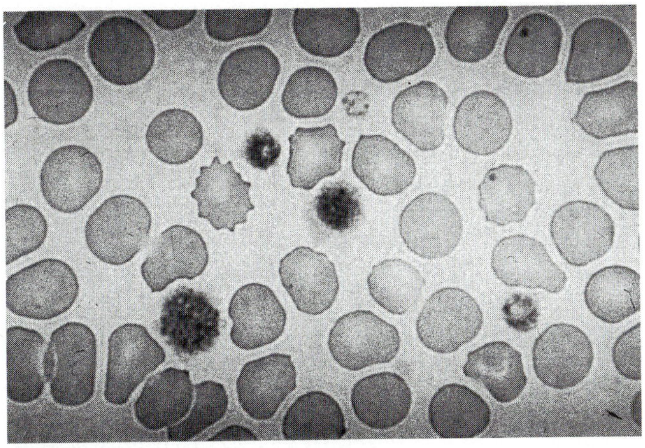

FIGURE 35-5. The peripheral blood smear of a patient with Bernard-Soulier syndrome is shown. While reduced in number, platelets are large and can approach the size of mature lymphocytes.

Treatment

The treatment of bleeding episodes in Bernard-Soulier syndrome is straightforward. The only option available is platelet transfusion. Unfortunately, after multiple transfusions, patients may become alloimmunized and refractory to subsequent transfusions. In addition, Bernard-Soulier patients can develop antibodies to the gpIb/IX complex, which is present in normal platelets but lacking in their platelets. These antibodies inhibit vWF binding to transfused normal platelets and can become a major source of morbidity by increasing the likelihood and severity of bleeding episodes.

Various nonspecific treatments have been tried with little success. Because of the thrombocytopenia, physicians have been tempted to try splenectomy, which has not been of any long-term benefit.[79] Corticosteroids are also ineffective. The administration of desmopressin acetate (DDAVP) shortened the bleeding time in one of two patients with Bernard-Soulier syndrome.[102,103] Its effect on clinical bleeding is unknown. Because DDAVP works, in part, by increasing plasma vWF concentration, and because Bernard-Soulier platelets do not bind vWF, its potential therapeutic role appears limited.

Acquired Forms of Bernard-Soulier Syndrome

Acquired forms of this relatively rare inherited disorder are even more infrequent. A small number of patients with idiopathic or autoimmune thrombocytopenia have antibodies that recognize epitopes on the gpIb/IX complex. In a few cases, binding of these antibodies to the platelet has produced a syndrome that resembles Bernard-Soulier syndrome.[104,105] These patients had thrombocytopenia and platelets that did not agglutinate with Ristocetin; however, the platelets were of normal size, and there was no family history of the disease. In addition, the antibody can be detected in plasma or eluted from the patient's platelets. A patient with a lymphoproliferative disorder was reported who had an immunoglobulin G antibody that inhibited Ristocetin-dependent platelet agglutination.[106] The patient had a prolonged bleeding time, normal platelet morphology, and a normal platelet count. The antibody appeared to interact with a 210-kd platelet protein, which is larger than any of the components of the gpIb/IX complex. There was also one case of childhood myelodysplasia with bleeding, in which there was a population of large platelets that did not react with Ristocetin.[107] Further examination showed that the platelets lacked the gpIb/IX complex.

MEMBRANE PROTEINS THAT REGULATE PLATELET ACTIVATION AND SIGNAL TRANSDUCTION

Platelet Thrombin Receptor

Thrombin, which has multiple roles in blood coagulation, is one of the most potent platelet agonists. Until recently, it was difficult to explain how thrombin activates platelets, despite detailed knowledge of its proteolytic action on fibrinogen and other coagulation proteins (see Chap. 41). Conversely, models of thrombin activation based on the occupancy of a classic type of platelet receptor, with thrombin behaving like a conventional ligand, do not explain the need for proteolytically active thrombin to get agonist activity. Studies using thrombin as a ligand have also identified proteins, like gpIb/IX, which bind thrombin with high affinity but do not transduce a sufficiently potent activating signal to explain thrombin's agonist activity.[108–111] Furthermore, modified thrombins, which are no longer proteolytically active, bind to these proteins with the same affinity and kinetics as proteolytically active thrombin, even though they no longer trigger platelet activation.[112–116] To reconcile these paradoxes, theories have been proposed that combine both mechanisms of action—a classic receptor ligand interaction followed by proteolysis of a specific substrate.

The puzzle was partially solved by Vu and colleagues, who cloned a platelet thrombin receptor cDNA and showed that it encoded a polypeptide that is a novel member of the seven-membrane–spanning family of G-protein–coupled receptors[117] (Fig. 35-6). This rapidly growing family of receptor proteins includes a number of important signaling molecules, such as the α- and β-adrenergic receptors, and receptors for small neural peptides, such as substance P and substance K. A potential thrombin cleavage site is located at the amino terminus of the thrombin receptor at arginine 41 (R41; see Fig. 35-6). Just beyond the R41 cleavage site, the thrombin receptor contains a sequence that is identical to one seen at the carboxy terminus of the leech anticoagulant peptide hirudin, which is known to bind thrombin with high affinity. The thrombin receptor's hirudin-like sequence was then shown to bind thrombin, which facilitates receptor cleavage at R41.[118,119] The cleaved receptor's new amino terminus can then interact with the membrane-bound portion of the thrombin receptor to induce platelet signal transduction (Fig. 35-7), functioning, in the authors' words, as a "tethered ligand."[117]

Three lines of evidence support this model for thrombin-induced platelet activation. First, mutations that abolish the thrombin cleavage site at R41 inactivate the thrombin receptor.[117] Second, substitution of a sequence recognized by another proteolytic enzyme, enterokinase, for the native sequence changes receptor specificity.[118] Third, a peptide containing the sequence present in the receptor's amino terminal tethered ligand exposed by thrombin cleavage can substitute for thrombin and activates the recombinant thrombin receptor when expressed in frog oocytes as well as the native receptor expressed in platelets and endothelial cells.[119] This peptide, which contains the sequence SFLLNPNDK, is referred to as the thrombin receptor–activating peptide (TRAP).

The events that follow receptor cleavage and production of the tethered ligand are less well defined. It is thought that the active form of the thrombin receptor transduces a signal by means of a G-protein–linked transduction

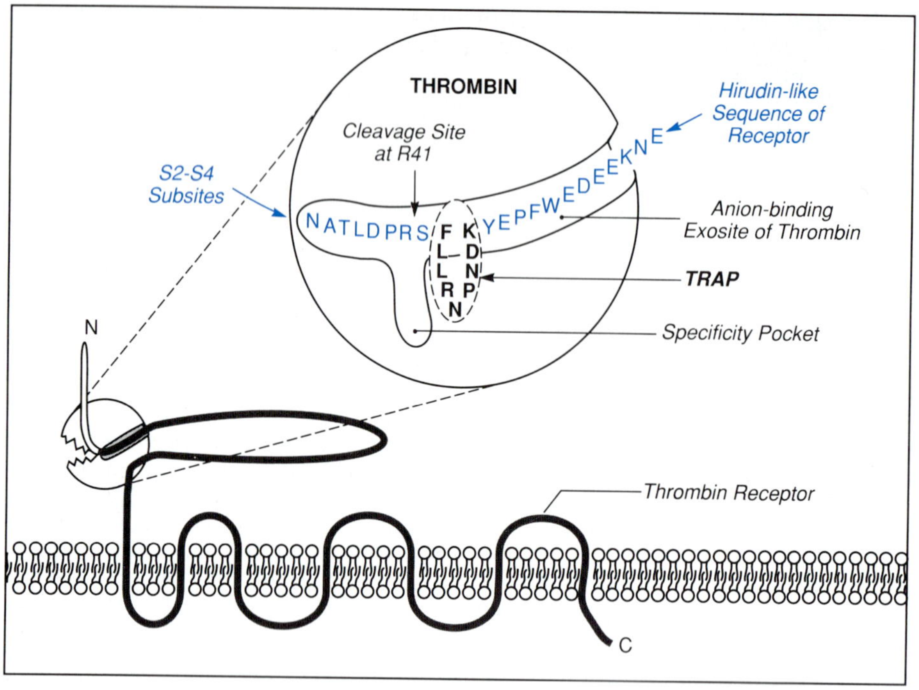

FIGURE 35-6. The interactions between thrombin and the platelet thrombin receptor are depicted. Thrombin binds to the receptor and activates it by a specific proteolytic cleavage at arg 41 (R41). The thrombin receptor contains an amino terminal sequence that binds to the S2-S4 subsite of thrombin and a hirudin-like sequence that fits into the anion exosite of thrombin.

mechanism and that this, in turn, leads to a calcium transient, phospholipid hydrolysis, changes in platelet cytoskeleton organization, and eventually, global platelet activation and granule secretion. Identifying the site in the thrombin receptor that actually interacts with the tethered ligand and investigating the possibility that there are additional thrombin cleavage sites in the receptor are problems that are under active investigation.

The relation between the seven-membrane–spanning thrombin receptor and the other known thrombin-binding proteins, particularly the gpIb/IX complex, is unclear. As previously discussed, thrombin binds to gpIb/IX with high affinity. It binds to a specific sequence on the gpIbα polypeptide adjacent to the vWF interaction site (see Fig. 35-4). The potential relevance of this interaction is underscored by studies carried out with platelets obtained from patients with Bernard-Soulier syndrome who do not express the gpIb/IX complex. Their platelets, in addition to adhering poorly to vascular subendothelium, have a blunted response to thrombin, and higher concentrations of thrombin are needed to activate platelets. This raises the interesting possibility that binding to the gpIb/IX complex facilitates thrombin's agonist action by increasing its effective concentration at the cell surface. An alternative, proposed by Coughlin and colleagues, is that gpIb/IX serves as a thrombin "sink" and at low ambient thrombin concentrations may sequester thrombin and prevent it from chronically activating and, eventually, desensitizing the thrombin receptor.[120] It is also possible that thrombin binding to gpIb/IX subserves a novel and as yet undefined function in hemostasis.

Direct evidence is accumulating for an important role for this receptor in platelet activation. For example, antibodies directed against the tethered ligand sequence of the thrombin receptor completely abolish thrombin-induced platelet activation.[121] The discovery of thrombin receptor expression in many other cell types suggests that it may play an important role in signal transduction in other tissues as well. No patients have been described, to date, whose platelet dysfunction can be ascribed to a defect in

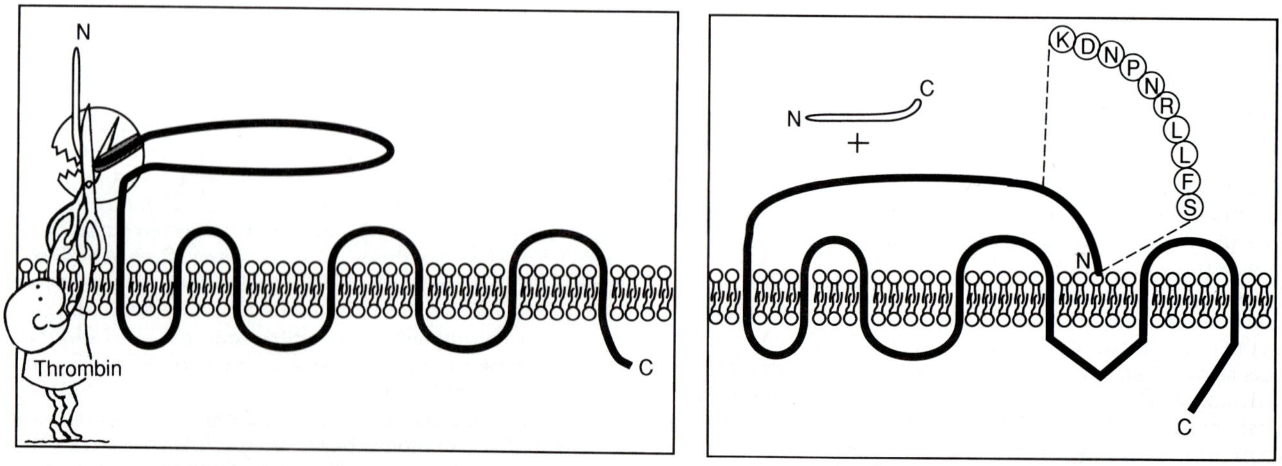

FIGURE 35-7. The mechanism of thrombin activation of the thrombin receptor is depicted. Cleavage at arginine 41 of the receptor produces a new amino terminal sequence, which can fold over and activate the receptor. The sequence acts as a "tethered ligand."

the thrombin receptor, and genetically engineered mice lacking the thrombin receptor are not yet available. Given its ubiquitous expression, a thrombin receptor mutation could have far-reaching consequences and might produce a phenotype with multiple defects.

Platelet Adenosine Diphosphate Receptor

Adenosine diphosphate is of considerable historical importance because it was the first agent shown to aggregate platelets in vitro.[122] ADP induces both platelet shape change and aggregation. Under certain conditions (ie, a slightly reduced plasma calcium concentration, platelet production of thromboxane A_2, and subsequent platelet–platelet interactions), ADP also stimulates the release of platelet granule contents. ADP also induces a rapid and transient influx of calcium with little or no phospholipid hydrolysis. By these criteria, ADP has been classified as a "weak" platelet agonist. In contrast, thrombin, a "strong" agonist, induces a more sustained calcium elevation, which is accompanied by phosphatidyl inositol hydrolysis and the generation of large quantities of inositol tris-triphosphate. In addition, thrombin-induced granule secretion does not require either platelet aggregation or thromboxane generation. This distinction between strong and weak agonists is somewhat arbitrary and is based on in vitro criteria that may not be completely relevant. Although not a potent inducer of thromboxane production or granule secretion, ADP does induce rapid and complete platelet aggregation.

The evidence that ADP plays an important role in hemostasis remains largely indirect. Damaged red cells and tissues are thought to be the most likely source of the ADP that promotes hemostasis. In support of this, the infusion of enzymes into experimental animals, which metabolize ADP, prolongs the bleeding time.[123] In addition, the infusion of stable ATP analogues, which are competitive inhibitors of ADP, has a similar effect.[124–126] Moreover, there is evidence that local instillation of ADP into an uninjured vessel by iontophoresis induces rapid and reversible platelet aggregation at the site of ADP entry into the microcirculation.

Despite intense interest in the effects of ADP on the platelet, its cognate receptor has not yet been identified, and its mode of action is not well understood. The molecular cloning of two other purinergic receptors, which bind adenosine and adenosine triphosphate (ATP), respectively, has provided some new insights into the biochemical mechanism of action of purines on cells.[127] The ATP and adenosine receptors are both seven-membrane–spanning, G-protein–linked molecules. By analogy, it appears likely that the platelet ADP receptor is also a member of this receptor family.

The purinergic receptors have been subdivided, based on their pharmacologic characteristics, into the P_1 subclass, which binds adenosine, and the P_2, subclass which bind ADP and ATP.[128,129] The P_2 purinoreceptors have been further subdivided into those that mediate smooth muscle contraction (P_{2X}) and those that mediate relaxation (P_{2Y}). The platelet receptor does not fit into any of the known P_2 subclasses and has been denoted as a separate and unique P_{2T} receptor subclass.[129] In all other tissues studied, ATP and ADP are both agonists and have similar dose–response curves. In the platelet, ADP alone is an agonist, and ATP acts as a competitive antagonist. Second, the structural requirements for agonist activity that were outlined previously are much more stringent for the platelet P_{2T} receptor than for the P_{2X} and P_{2Y} receptors present in other tissues.

Other nucleoside diphosphates cannot substitute for ADP, and most modifications to the adenosine base portion of ADP impair its activity.[130–135] Substitutions at the second position of the purine ring, however, are well tolerated, and the two analogues 2-chloro-ADP and 2-methylthio-ADP have increased agonist activity. The number of phosphate groups attached to the adenosine moiety is also important because hydrolysis of the terminal 5′ phosphate to produce AMP or the addition of a third phosphate to yield ATP converts the agonist into competitive antagonists.[136–138] Modification of the oxygen molecule bridging the two phosphates in ADP also reduces its agonist activity.[139,140]

Direct-binding studies using radiolabeled ADP or its analogues to identify the platelet ADP receptor have yielded conflicting and uninterpretable results. In most cases, these studies have reported unrealistically high numbers of ADP-binding sites[141] or have identified enzymes, such as nucleoside diphosphokinase, that can transiently bind and metabolize added ADP[142] rather than the receptor itself. One potential problem with these studies is uncertainty regarding the final form of the added radioligand. After its addition to platelet suspensions, the ligand (ADP) may be phosphorylated or dephosphorylated by platelet surface or plasma enzymes. To circumvent some of these earlier problems that used metabolically active platelets, investigators reported ligand-binding studies with formalin-fixed platelets.[143,144] Again, the number of apparent binding sites far exceeded the density of any of the known purinergic receptors on other cells.

An adenosine analogue that covalently modifies nucleotide-binding proteins, fluorosulfonyl benzoyl adenosine (FSBA), has been shown to inhibit ADP-induced aggregation[145–148] and was thought to have promise as a ligand for identifying the ADP receptor. Unfortunately, FSBA breaks down to adenosine in aqueous media. Because adenosine is a potent inhibitor of platelet aggregation, this may explain its inhibitory role.[149] In addition, FSBA is nonselective and not only inhibits ADP-induced aggregation but also inhibits platelet aggregation by other agonists.[147] These observations suggest that FSBA is unlikely to bind directly to the ADP receptor. Colman and colleagues, however, using FSBA as an affinity ligand, identified a 100-kd platelet membrane protein, which they have called "aggregin," and suggest that it is the ADP receptor.[145–150] The protein has not been purified, and its primary structure and biochemical properties are unknown. MacFarlane and colleagues developed an ADP analogue, 2-methylthio-ADP, which binds reversibly to several hundred sites in the platelet membrane with high affinity and appropriate kinetics.[151,152] This ligand is most promising because it identifies an appropriate number of sites. It can also be radiolabeled to high specific activity and may help to identify and, eventually, clone the actual ADP receptor.

A number of additional platelet membrane receptors regulate platelet activation and signal transduction and are also members of the large family of seven-membrane–spanning proteins. Human platelets, but not platelets derived from most other species, express α_2-adrenergic receptors.[153,154] They are coupled, by means of a G protein, to adenylate cyclase. Although their role in hemostasis is not entirely clear, submicromolar concentrations of epinephrine synergize with other aggregating agents, while higher concentrations can induce platelet aggregation. Many patients with myeloproliferative disorders, especially essential thrombocytosis, selectively lose their ability to aggregate with epinephrine.[155] Their platelets are also missing α_2-adrenergic receptors when assessed by radioligand-binding assays and coupling to adenylate cyclase.[156,157] The clinical significance of this abnormality is unclear. In addition, platelets from up to 10% of apparently normal people may fail to aggregate when challenged with epinephrine.[158]

Platelets also contain receptors for several of the important biologically active eicosanoids.[159] Platelets, which are a major source of thromboxane A_2, contain a seven-membrane–spanning thromboxane receptor[160] through which thromboxane exerts its biochemical action—inhibition of adenylate cyclase and platelet activation. Platelets also contain a receptor for prostacyclin (PGI_2), an endothelial cell prostaglandin that is a potent platelet inhibitor. Binding of PGI_2 to this receptor stimulates adenylate cyclase activity and inhibits platelet function.[161] A few patients have been described who have a mild bleeding disorder due to congenital absence of a receptor for thromboxane A_2. This is discussed in Chapter 37. There are as yet no known clinical disorders ascribed to the PGI_2 receptor.

Platelets contain several receptors, which are expressed on other target tissues as well, that are of uncertain significance. For example, platelets contain a receptor for vasopressin[162] and both a membrane transporter and a type II receptor for serotonin.[163] The clinical relevance of the vasopressin and serotonin receptors is unclear, although high quantities of both agonists can induce platelet aggregation in vitro.

PLATELET MEMBRANE RECEPTORS THAT REGULATE PLATELET AGGREGATION

Platelet Fibrinogen Receptor (gpIIb/IIIa)

One of the most dramatic events in hemostasis is the rapid linkage of individual platelets to form hemostatic plugs. This phenomenon, termed *platelet aggregation,* is absolutely dependent on the binding of the plasma glycoprotein fibrinogen to the activated form of the gpIIb/IIIa complex (Figs. 35-8 and 35-9). As previously discussed, the platelet fibrinogen receptor is a member of the integrin family of adhesion protein receptors and is referred to as the $\alpha_{IIb}\beta_3$-integrin or, in the CD nomenclature, as CD41a. The platelet actually expresses four additional integrins—the collagen receptor gpIa/IIa ($\alpha_2\beta_1$), the fibronectin receptor gpIc/IIa ($\alpha_5\beta_1$), the vitronectin receptor or VnR ($\alpha_v\beta_3$), and the laminin receptor gpIc′/IIa ($\alpha_6\beta_1$). The fibrinogen and VnRs share a common β_3 chain, and the other three integrins share the β_1-polypeptide (see Table 35-1). In each case, receptor specificity is determined by unique determinants on the α-polypeptide chain.

The complete amino acid sequences of gpIIb and gpIIIa have been deduced from sequencing their cDNAs.[164–167] The amino acid sequence in gpIIb is 40% identical to sequence in the α-chain polypeptides of the fibronectin and VnRs.[168,169] There is also substantial (25%) sequence similarity with the α subunit on the leukocyte integrins Mac-1 and gp150,95.[170–173] The amino acid sequence of gpIIIa, in turn, is about 40% identical to the sequence of the β-polypeptides of the other integrins.

The genes encoding gpIIb and IIIa are closely linked and reside on a portion of the long arm of chromosome 17 (q21-23).[174,175] This close physical linkage raises the possibility that gpIIb/IIIa expression is coordinately regulated, like the globin gene cluster. Thus, some forms of Glanzmann's thrombasthenia, like thalassemia, might be caused by defects in coordinate regulation. This hypothesis is probably incorrect because it is possible to dissociate expression of the two genes. Endothelial cells, for example, produce gpIIIa, which is used to assemble the VnR, but do not ex-

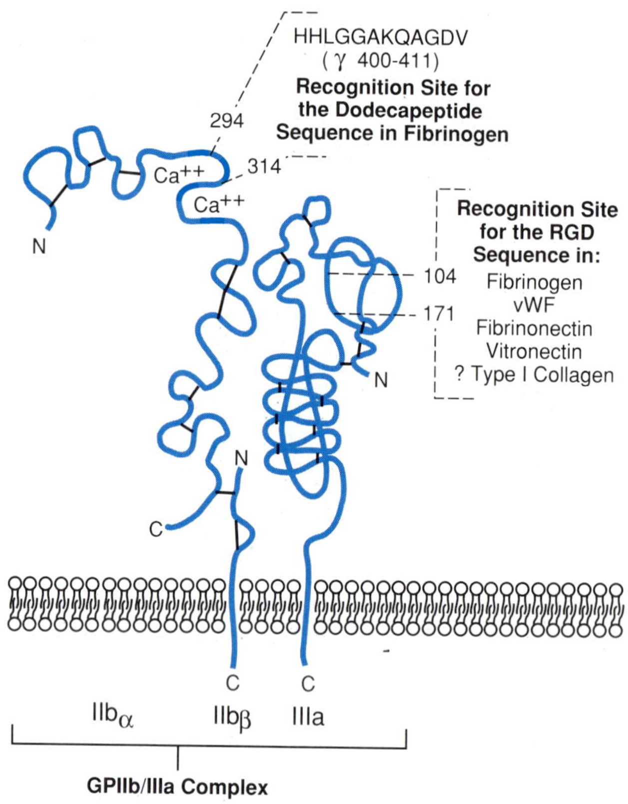

FIGURE 35-9. The fibrinogen-binding sites on gpIIIb/IIIa are depicted. There are two sequences in fibrinogen that are known to bind to gpIIb/IIIa—a γ chain dodecapeptide (HHLGGAKQAGDV) and an α RGD sequence. Residues 294 through 314 of gpIIbβ interact with the dodecapeptide of fibrinogen. The RGD recognition site is located between amino acids 109 and 171 of gpIIIa and interacts with RGD sequences present in a variety of proteins as well as fibrinogen.

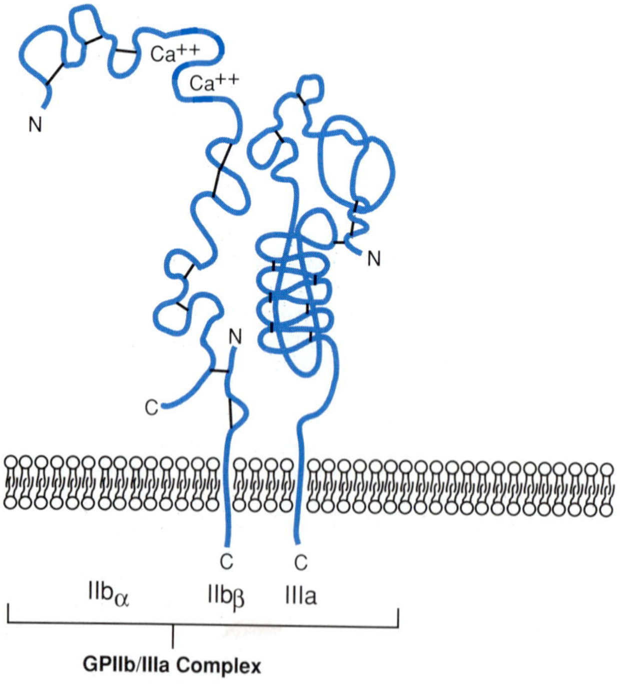

FIGURE 35-8. The structure of the gpIb/IIIa complex is shown here. gpIIb is synthesized as a single precursor, which is cleaved to produce gpIIbα and gpIIbβ. gpIIbβ anchors the protein in the lipid bilayer of the membrane and is disulfide-bonded to gpIIbα. gpIIb contains four calcium-binding domains. gpIIIa is a single-chain polypeptide that contains a cysteine-rich sequence just distal to the plasma membrane.

press gpIIb. This differential expression suggests that there are tissue-specific factors within specific cell types that regulate independent expression of the two genes. There is evidence that the gpIIb promoter element has a GATA 1-binding site, a GATA1-binding protein is present in erythroid, and megakaryocytic cells may regulate megakaryocyte-specific expression of gpIIb.[176,177]

Biosynthesis and Assembly

Each of the two subunits of the fibrinogen receptor is derived from a separate mRNA transcript; therefore, regulation of biosynthesis is likely to be a posttranslational event.[178] The gpIIIa polypeptide is about 90-kd and is synthesized as a single-chain precursor. Fifteen percent of its molecular mass is composed of unmodified N-linked carbohydrate chains with high mannose content. Like other β-integrins, gpIIIa contains multiple cysteine residues that are organized into several cysteine-rich domains (see Fig. 35-8). There are a total of five domains in gpIIIa, a unique cysteine-rich sequence at the amino terminus of the polypeptide, and four homologous repeated sequences that precede the hydrophobic membrane insertion sequence.

Glycoprotein IIb, in turn, is a typical α-integrin subunit with a molecular mass of 145-kd. It consists of two covalently linked subunits and has only nine disulfide bonds, which are distributed evenly along the subunit. Mature gpIIb is derived from a precursor pro-IIb molecule, which associates with gpIIIa in the endoplasmic reticulum.[179,180] The pro-IIb/IIIa complex then enters the Golgi apparatus where the pro-IIb moiety is cleaved to produce the heavy and light chains of the mature polypeptide. The two chains remain covalently linked by means of a disulfide bond between Cys 826 and Cys 880. The smaller gpIIbβ chain provides the membrane-anchoring sequence, and the larger gpIIbα polypeptide, which is entirely extracellular, remains linked only by the single disulfide and by noncovalent interactions with gpIIIa (see Fig. 35-8). After modification of N-linked carbohydrate and the addition of O-linked carbohydrate in the Golgi apparatus, the mature gpIIb/IIIa complex is transported to the cell surface.

Ligand Binding

The mechanism by which the gpIIb/IIIa complex interacts with its adhesive ligands has been intensively studied but is not completely understood. Several important characteristics of gpIIb/IIIa–ligand interactions remain enigmatic. First, unlike many other integrin-receptor interactions, the binding of adhesive ligands to gpIIb/IIIa requires prior activation of the platelet.[181–186] The nature of this activation, at the receptor level, remains only partially understood. Second, although the principal ligand is fibrinogen, gpIIb/IIIa is a "promiscuous" receptor and will, under certain conditions, also bind fibronectin, vitronectin, and vWF.[187,188] Because the plasma concentration of fibrinogen is far higher than any of the other potential ligands, it is most likely the major plasma protein binding to the gpIIb/IIIa complex. Third, although the consensus adhesion sequence Arg-Gly-Asp (RGD) is clearly important in fibrinogen binding, it is not the sole determinant, and a second site on the fibrinogen α chain is also involved.[187] Finally, the fibrinogen-binding site on gpIIb/IIIa, unlike the vWF interaction site on gpIb/IX, is made up of sequences on both the gpIIb and IIIa subunit polypeptides (see Fig. 35-9).

As mentioned previously, the RGD consensus adhesion sequence, which is present in a large number of the adhesive glycoproteins, occurs twice in the Aα chain of fibrinogen as well as in the other potential gpIIb/IIIa ligands—fibronectin, vitronectin and vWF. The dodecapeptide sequence HHLGAKQAGDV, at the carboxy terminus of the γ chain of fibrinogen (residues 400 through 411), also binds to gpIIb/IIIa.[189] The γ-chain sequence, however, is unique to fibrinogen and is not found in the other adhesive ligands.

Several different approaches have been used to localize the adhesive interaction sites on the gpIIb/IIIa complex. Given the complexity of the interactions, the results are still incomplete and somewhat confusing. Two different groups have used chemical cross-linking approaches to define the RGD peptide recognition sites of gpIIb/IIIa. Although the RGD peptide makes contact with sequences on both gpIIb and IIIa, platelet activation markedly increases binding of the RGD peptide to one or more gpIIIa sites.[190–192] An RGD recognition site has also been located on a polypeptide fragment spanning residues 109 to 171 of gpIIIa (see Fig. 35-9). This polypeptide was derived by limited proteolytic digestion of gpIIIa with Staph V8 protease. The relevance of this site was confirmed by the finding of a patient with a variant form of Glanzmann's thrombasthenia who had a single base substitution, Arg for Tyr, at residue 119 of gpIIIa.[191] Platelets from this patient expressed normal quantities of the gpIIb/IIIa complex but would not bind fibrinogen.[192] In contrast, the γ-chain dodecapeptide preferentially associates with sequences on gpIIb.[193] A tentative dodecapeptide recognition sequence has been localized to residues 294 through 314 on gpIIb.

Platelet aggregation does not occur until there is agonist-induced exposure or rearrangement of critical sequences within gpIIb/IIIa complex that are needed for binding fibrinogen or vWF. Although fibrinogen is the preferred ligand, under certain circumstances, when fibrinogen concentration is reduced, vWF and fibronectin may bind to gpIIb/IIIa. There is increasing evidence that optimal adhesion and thrombus formation on vascular subendothelium requires interactions of vWF with both the gpIb/IX and gpIIb/IIIa receptor sites. Although vitronectin and fibronectin can also interact with gpIIb/IIIa, their role in normal platelet physiology is not well defined. As previously discussed, there are separate receptors on the platelet for these two ligands. The two critical agonists for gpIIb/IIIa activation are ADP and thrombin, whose cognate receptors were discussed earlier in this chapter.

After ligand binding and platelet aggregation, there is an interaction between the cytoplasmic portions of gpIIb/IIIa and the platelet cytoskeleton.[194] This interaction, which involves coupling to the submembranous actin cytoskeleton, involves the cytoskeletal protein talin.[195] In addition, this interaction is thought to provide the contractile force that regulates clot retraction. In addition to the 50-kd gpIIb/IIIa molecules present on the platelet surface, there are additional copies of the complex present in the membranes of the surface-connected canalicular system of the platelet and on the membranes that delimit platelet α granules. These additional gpIIb/IIIa molecules may become available after platelet activation. Although the major focus has been on the interaction of gpIIb/IIIa with fibrinogen, the complex, after suitable activation, also binds fibrin an interaction that may stabilize platelet aggregates and mediate clot retraction.

Glanzmann's Thrombasthenia

The clinical entity thrombasthenia, literally "weak platelets," was first described by the German physician Glanzmann in 1918.[196] Glanzmann described a hereditary bleeding disorder characterized by a normal platelet count, normal platelet morphology, and abnormal clot retraction (Table 35-4). It was recognized, subsequently, that platelets

TABLE 35-4. Clinical Criteria for the Diagnosis of Thrombasthenia

Autosomal recessive inheritance
Epistaxis, ecchymoses, gingival bleeding beginning in infancy
Menorrhagia, gastrointestinal bleeding, posttraumatic hemorrhage
Prolonged bleeding time
Normal platelet count and size
Platelets fail to aggregate with any agonists and do not bind fibrinogen
Agglutination with Ristocetin and binding of the von Willebrand factor is normal
Absence (type I) or reduction (type II) of the gpIIb/IIIa complex or presence of dysfunctional proteins that cannot bind fibrinogen

from patients with thrombasthenia also failed to aggregate when exposed to the usual agonists.[197] As the critical role of the platelet gpIIb/IIIa complex in mediating aggregation was appreciated, it was anticipated that mutations in the gpIIb/IIIa gene complex would cause thrombasthenia. This prediction has been confirmed by reports from several laboratories of mutations in either the gpIIb or gpIIIa genes that cause thrombasthenia.

Molecular Basis

The disorder is inherited as an autosomal recessive trait, and clusters of the disease have been observed in populations in which there is a high degree of consanguinity.[198–200] Patients can have either a complete absence or a marked reduction in the gpIIb/IIIa complex because of a mutation in either the gpIIb or IIIa. Based on the molecular genetic analysis of other inherited disorders, a failure to express the gpIIb/IIIa complex would most likely be due to a nonsense mutation that terminated transcription prematurely, a deletion or insertion in the gene that caused a shift in the reading frame, or an abnormality in RNA splicing due to loss or mutation of a splice donor or acceptor site. Missense mutations, in which there is a substitution of an amino acid at a critical position in either the gpIIb or IIIa gene, could also impair the biosynthesis and assembly of gpIIb/IIIa or result in the expression of a normal amount of a nonfunctional gpIIb/IIIa complex. Although mutations can occur in either allele of either of the two genes, obligate heterozygotes, who have 50% to 60% of the normal platelet content of gpIIb/IIIa (ie, about 25,000 receptor sites/platelet) have normal hemostasis.[198–201] Symptomatic patients are either homozygous for a single mutation or compound heterozygotes carrying two independent mutations.

The kindreds examined to date display a spectrum of different mutations (Table 35-5). Seven independent gpIIb mutations have been identified, all of which result in the classic thrombasthenia phenotype—absence of the platelet gpIIb/IIIa complex. One kindred had a 4.5-kb deletion in the gpIIb gene, which eliminated exons 2 through 9.[202] Two families had aberrant splicing, which produced an abnormal mRNA,[203,204] and two families had nonsense mutations, which produced premature termination of translation.[205,206] One patient had a missense mutation (Gly 273 → Asp) in the fourth calcium-binding domain of gpIIb, which impaired the biosynthesis and assembly of the gpIIb/IIIa complex.[207] There is a preliminary report of another patient with a similar phenotype who had a Gly 418 → Asp mutation.[208]

Seven kindreds have been identified with mutations in the gpIIIa gene. Three pedigrees had classic thrombasthenia, and four had the variant phenotype with normal or near-normal expression of a nonfunctional protein (see Table 35-5). The mutations causing the classic phenotype included a 15-kb inversion and 1-kb deletion.[209,210] A second

TABLE 35-5. Molecular Basis of Glanzmann's Thrombasthenia

Inheritance	Phenotype	Mutation	Reference
MUTATIONS IN THE gpIIb POLYPEPTIDE			
AR	gpIIb/IIIa absent	Deletion exons 2–9; allele 2 unknown	Burk et al, 1991[202]
AR	gpIIb/IIIa absent	13 base pairs deletion in exon 4 and in exon 12 causing abnormal splicing and 6 amino acid deletion (patients homozygous)	Newman et al, 1991[203]
AR	gpIIb/IIIa absent	1. Stop in exon 17 2. Splice mutation in exon 26; deletion of exons 25–27; 43 base pairs deletion in protein	Kato et al, 1992[204]
AR	gpIIb/IIIa absent	Gly 418 → Asp	Wilcox et al, 1992[208]
AR	gpIIb/IIIa absent	Arg 584 Stop; allele 2 unknown	Gu et al, 1993[206]
AR	gpIIb/IIIa absent	Gly 273 → Asp; allele 2 unknown	Poncz et al, 1994[207]
AR	gpIIb/IIIa absent	Deletion exon 28 (Gln 948 → Stop); allele 2 unknown	Iwamoto et al, 1994[205]
MUTATIONS IN THE gpIIIa POLYPEPTIDE			
AR	gpIIb/IIIa absent	15-kb inversion; 1-kb deletion; allele 2 unknown	Li & Bray, 1993[210]
AR	gpIIb/IIa absent	Splice donor site loss; exon 1/intron 1 boundary causing 86 base pairs deletion and premature termination (patients homozygous)	Simsek et al, 1993[211]
AR	gpIIb/IIIa present No fibrinogen binding	Arg 214 → Trp; allele 2 unknown	Lanza et al, 1992[214]
AR	gpIIb/IIa absent	11 base pairs deletion in exon 12 causing premature termination (patients homozygous)	Newman et al, 1991[203]
AR	gpIIb/IIIa present No fibrinogen binding	Ser 752 → Pro; allele 2 unknown	Chen et al, 1992[212]
AR	gpIIb/IIIa present No fibrinogen binding	Asp 119 → Tyr	Loftus et al, 1990[213]
AR	gpIIb/IIIa present No fibrinogen binding	Arg 214 → Gln	Bajt et al, 1992[215]

AR, autosomal recessive.

case had an 11 base pair deletion, which caused a shifted reading frame and premature termination of translation.[203] A third patient had an 86 base pair deletion due to loss of a splice sequence.[211] The missense mutations included point mutations at residues 119, 214, and 752 (Asp 119 → Tyr, Arg 214 → Trp/Gln, and Ser 752 → Pro). All these mutations caused defective fibrinogen binding.[212–215] As expected, patients with mutations in gpIIIa have a parallel defect in VnR expression because the VnR shares the gpIIIa subunit. In fact, parallel measurement of the platelet VnR level can determine whether a thrombasthenic patient has a gpIIb or IIIa mutation.[216]

Diagnosis and Treatment

Thrombasthenic patients, like patients with other abnormalities in primary hemostasis, usually present with mucocutaneous bleeding.[198,199,217–219] Epistaxis and gingival bleeding are common, and some patients may present during the neonatal period with bleeding after circumcision or bleeding from the umbilical cord stump. In women, menorrhagia and bleeding after childbirth are common events. In addition, many patients have episodes of gastrointestinal or genitourinary bleeding. Patients with thrombasthenia have a high likelihood of bleeding after surgery or trauma and must receive platelet transfusions.

There is considerable variability in the severity of bleeding among thrombasthenic patients. Some patients are plagued with lifelong, recurrent severe bleeding, while others have only mild bruising or occasional epistaxis. The severity of bleeding can vary among members of the same kindred and does not correlate with the number of gpIIb/IIIa molecules expressed on the platelet.[219]

The diagnosis of thrombasthenia is usually straightforward. The typical patient has a markedly prolonged bleeding time with a normal platelet count and normal platelet morphology. Platelet aggregation is usually diagnostic because platelets from patients with Glanzmann's disease do not aggregate in response to the usual panel of agonists—epinephrine, collagen suspensions, thrombin, ADP, or arachidonic acid. The platelets secrete their granule contents after challenge with a strong agonist like thrombin, but do not secrete with the weaker agonists ADP or epinephrine, which require platelet–platelet interactions and aggregate formation to induce secretion. Platelets from thrombasthenic patients, however, agglutinate when incubated with Ristocetin because this agent induces vWF binding to gpIb/IX—a pathway that is not impaired in Glanzmann's disease. Clot retraction, which is not usually measured, is either completely absent or markedly impaired.[217,218] Tests of plasma coagulation, including the prothrombin time and partial thromboplastin time, are normal.

Quantitation of the number of gpIIb/IIIa sites per platelet using monoclonal antibody probes and flow cytometry is a simple diagnostic test.[220,221] This can be carried out on small quantities of whole blood and is useful for neonatal or even prenatal diagnosis. Flow cytometry can also differentiate between the classic form of thrombasthenia, in which protein expression is reduced, and variants with dysfunctional molecules. As discussed previously, parallel flow cytometry with anti-VnR antibodies helps to pinpoint the affected gene.

As discussed previously, most thrombasthenic patients have a quantitative disorder with either a reduction or a complete absence of the gpIIb/IIIa complex. Patients have been divided into two categories—type I and type II—on the basis of the severity of their defect.[222] Type I patients, who have less than 5% of the normal count of gpIIb/IIIa, have absent clot retraction and an absence of fibrinogen from their α granules.[223] Type II thrombasthenic patients have 10% to 20% of the normal gpIIb/IIIa molecules on their platelets, which may function, although imperfectly. After agonist challenge, their platelets may bind some fibrinogen and display minimal amounts of aggregation. In addition, their platelets may support clot retraction and contain α-granule fibrinogen. This observation is not surprising because platelet α-granule fibrinogen is not synthesized de novo but is endocytosed by megakaryocytes.[224–226] The receptor site for adsorptive endocytosis is the gpIIb/IIIa complex. Clot retraction is partially corrected in type II patients. As previously discussed, clot retraction requires the transmission of a contractile force by means of platelet gpIIb/IIIa to the cytoskeleton after it has attached to clot-bound fibrin strands.

A lifelong history of bleeding, coupled with the diagnostic laboratory finding of absent platelet aggregation, is characteristic of Glanzmann's thrombasthenia and few other disorders. Patients have been described who have an acquired disorder that closely resembles Glanzmann's disease owing to an antibody directed against fibrinogen-binding sites on the gpIIb/IIIa complex.[227,228] This syndrome has been seen in patients with multiple myeloma, other immune disorders, and rarely, idiopathic or immunologic thrombocytopenia. In most cases of acquired thrombasthenia, there is little or no circulating antibody in plasma, and it is necessary to elute the antibody from the affected platelets to verify its biologic properties. The antiplatelet agent ticlopidine also blocks platelet aggregation and induces a thrombasthenic picture.[229]

The only effective treatment of bleeding episodes in patients with thrombasthenia is transfusion with normal platelets. DDAVP, corticosteroids, and ε-aminocaproic acid (EACA) have all been tried and are ineffective.[217,230,231] Oral contraceptives can be used to suppress menses in patients with severe menorrhagia. Because patients may require repeated transfusion, the use of single-donor platelets and, if readily available, human leukocyte antigen–matched platelets should be considered. The development of alloimmunization will limit the effectiveness of future transfusions. In addition, several patients have been described who have developed alloantibodies that bind to epitopes on gpIIb/IIIa and that inhibit fibrinogen binding to normal platelets.[232,233] There was one report of a severely affected child with thrombasthenia who was cured after bone marrow transplantation using a heterozygous sibling as a donor.[234]

PLATELET REGULATION OF COAGULATION REACTIONS

In addition to their important role in primary hemostasis, platelets are one of the principal sites for plasma coagulation reactions. The plasma membrane of activated platelets provides a surface on which coagulation factor complexes assemble. There is evidence that both the "Xase" complex (factors IXa, VIIIa, and X) and the "prothrombinase" complex (factors Xa and Va and prothrombin) assemble on the platelet surface.[235] The platelet surface accelerates these important reactions several thousand-fold by increasing the proximity and concentration of the reactants and providing the appropriate phospholipid moieties needed for both reactions. This property of activated platelets was formerly referred to as *platelet factor 3 activity*. The Xase and prothrombinase complexes also bind to artificial micelles made up of anionic phospholipids[235,236] (Fig. 35-10). Although there is little anionic phospholipid in the outer leaflet of the unactivated platelet, activation by agonists like thrombin or collagen is thought to reorient membrane phospholipids and bring the appropriate anionic phospho-

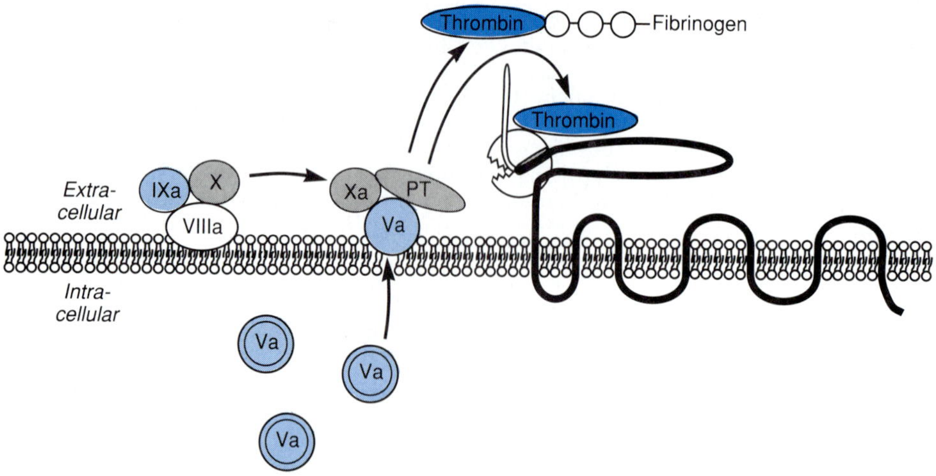

FIGURE 35-10. The role of the platelet in accelerating plasma coagulation reactions is depicted. The assembly of the "Xase" and the "prothrombinase" complexes both require phospholipid that is supplied by the platelet membrane. Factor VIIIa, derived from plasma, binds to platelet membrane phospholipids and then binds factors IXa and X. Factor Xa generated from the complex then assembles with prothrombin and factor Va to form the prothrombinase complex. Factor Va is derived from plasma and from platelet granules. Thrombin generated from the complex can bind to the platelet thrombin receptor, other cells, or generate fibrin from fibrinogen.

lipid to the outer leaflet. Alternately, activation may induce membrane vesiculation and the production of platelet microparticles with procoagulant activity[237] (Fig. 35-11).

A selective deficiency in platelet coagulant activity is a rare clinical event but has been described.[237–241] This phenomenon has been referred to as *Scott's syndrome* after the propositus of one well-studied family. The patient had prolonged bleeding after dental extractions, bleeding after surgical procedures, and a spontaneous retroperitoneal hematoma[238] (Table 35-6). The patient has been carefully studied and is the subject of several papers. The patient secreted a normal quantity of factor Va, a platelet α-granule constituent, but had only 20% to 25% of the normal number of factor Xa binding sites on activated platelets.[240] Moreover, when platelets were challenged with the agonists thrombin and collagen, fewer anionic phospholipid-binding sites were translocated to the platelet surface[241] (see Fig. 35-11). In addition, the formation of microparticles is defective in patients with Scott's syndrome.[237] This is important because platelet-binding sites for factor Va appear on the microparticles generated after platelet activation.

These fairly well-defined biochemical abnormalities produce a distinct set of laboratory abnormalities. Although this is a platelet defect, patients with Scott's syndrome have a normal bleeding time and normal platelet aggregation and secretion. In addition, standard screening tests for plasma coagulation such as the prothrombin time and partial thromboplastin time, which use artificial lipid micelles, are normal. The diagnostic abnormality is a shortened serum prothrombin time owing to reduced prothrombin consumption. This is due to the inability to generate normal platelet procoagulant activity. Patients can be readily treated with platelet transfusions, which will improve hemostasis and reduce postoperative blood loss.

CONCLUSION

During the past few years, there has been an explosion of new information about the structure and function of platelet membrane proteins and their role in hemostasis. With this information, the molecular basis of platelet membrane disorders like Bernard-Soulier syndrome, Glanzmann's thrombasthenia, and Scott's syndrome have been defined. In addition, low copy number receptors, which bind important ligands like thrombin, catecholamines, DDAVP, and

TABLE 35-6. Clinical Criteria for the Diagnosis of Scott's Syndrome

History of mild to moderate bleeding
Normal bleeding time and platelet aggregation
Autosomal recessive inheritance
Reduced prothrombin consumption and short *serum* prothrombin time
Platelet procoagulant activity decreased
Reduced factor Xa binding to platelets

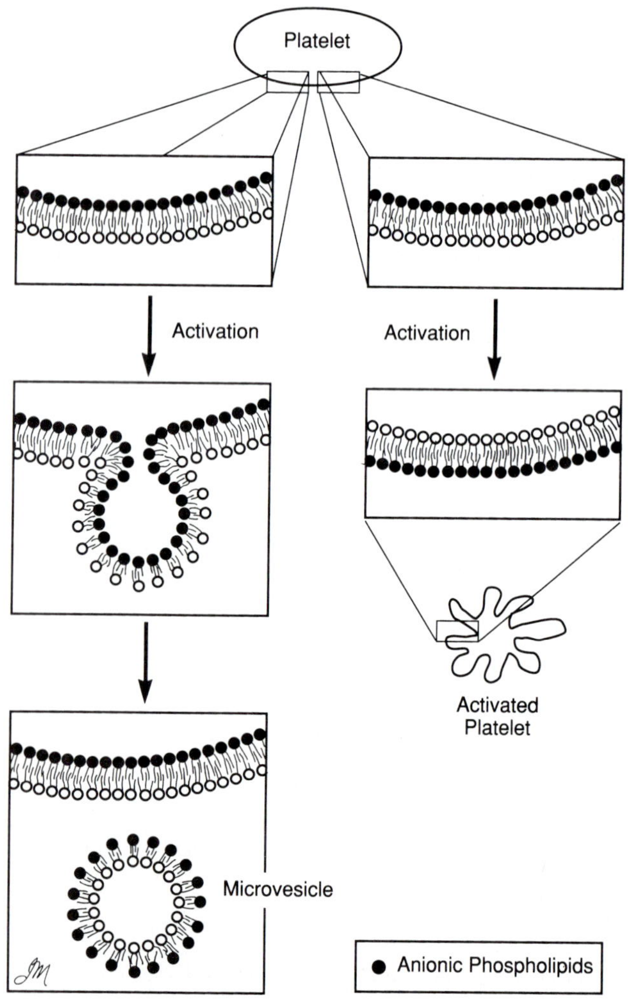

FIGURE 35-11. The generation of a platelet membrane surface that supports coagulation reactions, and potential defects in Scott's syndrome are depicted. The platelet membrane alters its natural phospholipid asymmetry by redistributing anionic phospholipids to the outer leaflet of the plasma membrane or to buds of microvesicles that have anionic phospholipids on their outer surface. Inability to carry out either function may result in defective platelet procoagulant activity (Scott's syndrome).

serotonin, have been identified and characterized. In some cases, like the identification of cellular thrombin receptors and the analysis of adhesive protein–integrin interactions, the platelet has played a crucial role in helping to define general cellular processes.

In the future, additional receptors like that which binds ADP should be fully characterized and help to define its role in hemostasis. Moreover, the information gained from studying protein function in normal hemostasis is being used to design new generations of antithrombotic agents. Receptor-level antagonists of platelet adhesion and aggregation or agents that block platelet thrombin or ADP receptor function may be useful in this regard and will supplement the limited number of antiplatelet agents with antithrombotic activity. The power of combining insights from clinical medicine with the techniques of modern genetics and molecular and cellular biology is nicely demonstrated by the progress that has been made in understanding the platelet membrane and its disorders.

REFERENCES

1. Nachman RL, Ferris B. Studies on the proteins of human platelet membranes. J Biol Chem 1972;247:4468..
2. Phillips DR. Effect of trypsin on the exposed polypeptides and glycoproteins in the human platelet membrane. Biochemistry 1972;11:4582.
3. Phillips DR, Agin PP. Platelet plasma membrane glycoproteins: evidence for the presence of nonequivalent disulfide bonds using nonreduced-reduced two-dimensional gel electrophoresis. J Biol Chem 1977;252: 2121.
4. Hynes RO. Integrins: a family of cell surface receptors. Cell 1987;48: 549.
5. Ruoslahti E, Pierschbacher MD. New perspectives in cell adhesion: RGD and integrins. Science 1987;238:491.
6. Ruoslahti E, Haymannn EG, Kuusela P, et al. Isolation of a tryptic fragment containing the collagen-binding site of plasma fibronectin. J Biol Chem 1978;254:6054.
7. Santoro SA, Cowan JF. Adsorption of von Willebrand factor by fibrillar collagen: implications concerning the adhesion of platelets to collagen. Collagen Relat Res 1982;2:31.
8. Lahav J, Schwartz MA, Hynes RO. Analyses of platelet adhesion using radioactive chemical crosslinking reagent: interaction of thrombospondin with fibronectin and collagen. Cell 1982;31:253.
9. Saito Y, Imada T, Takagi J, et al. Platelet factor XIII, the collagen receptor. J Biol Chem 1986;2261:1355.
10. Chiang TM, Kang AH. Isolation and purification of collagen α1(1) receptor from human platelet membrane. J Biol Chem 1982;257:7581.
11. Chiang TM, Jin A, Kang AH. Platelet-collagen interaction: inhibition by a monoclonal antibody which binds a 90,000 dalton platelet glycoprotein. Thromb Res 1989;53:129.
12. Kotite NJ, Cunningham LW. Specific adsorption of a platelet membrane glycoprotein to human insoluble collagen. J Biol Chem 1986;261:8342.
13. Lahav J. Identification of a surface protein of the rabbit blood platelet with high affinity for collagen. Exp Cell Res 1987;168:447.
14. Nieuwenhuis HK, Akkermann JWN, Houdjik WPM, Sixma JJ. Human blood platelets showing no response to collagen fail to express surface glycoprotein Ia. Nature 1985;318:470.
15. Kehrel B, Balleisen L, Kokott R, et al. Deficiency of thrombospondin and platelet glycoprotein Ia in platelets with defective collagen-induiced aggregation and spontaneous loss of disorder. Blood 1988;71:1074.
16. Kunicki TJ, Nugent DF, Staats S, et al. The human fibroblast class II extracellular matrix receptor mediates platelet adhesion to collagen and is identical to the platelet GpIa–IIa complex. J Biol Chem 1988;263: 4516.
17. Staatz WD, Walsh JJ, Pexton JJ, et al. The alpha2 1 integrin cell surface collagen receptor binds to the alpha1(i)-CB3 peptide of collagen. J Biol Chem 1990;265:4778.
18. Moroi M, Jung SM, Okuma M, Shinmyozu K. A patient with platelets deficient in glycoprotein VI that lack both collagen-induced platelet aggregation and adhesion. J Clin Invest 1989;84:1440.
19. Tandon NN, Kralisz U, Jamieson GA. Identification of glycoprotein IV (CD36) as a primary receptor for platelet-collagen adhesion. J Biol Chem 1989;264:7376.
20. Tandon NN, Jamieson GA. Role of GpIV as a platelet receptor for collagen adhesion. In: Jamieson GA, ed. Platelet membrane receptors. New York, Liss, 1988:315.
21. Asch AS, Liu I, Briccetti FM, et al. Analysis of CD36 binding domains: ligand specificity controlled by dephosphorylation of an ectodomain. Science 1993;262:1436.
22. Yamamoto N, Ikeda H, Tandon NN, et al. A platelet membrane glycoprotein (GP) deficiency in healthy blood donors: NaKa-platelets lack detectable GpIV (CD36). Blood 1988;76:1698.
23. Barnwell JW, Asch AS, Nachman RL, et al. A human 88-kd membrane glycoprotein (CD36) functions in vitro as a receptor for a cytoadherence ligand on *Plasmodium falciparum*–infected erythrocytes. J Clin Invest 1989;84:765.
24. Ockenhouse CF, Klotz PW, Tandon NN, et al. Sequestrin, a CD36 recognition protein on *Plasmodium falciparum* malaria–infected erythrocytes identified by anti-idiotype antibodies. Proc Natl Acad Sci USA 1991;88:3175.
25. McGregor JL, Catimel B, Parmentier S, et al. Rapid purification and partial characterizatiion of human platelet glycoprotein IIIb: interaction with thrombospondin and its role in platelet aggregation. J Biol Chem 1989;264:501.
26. Coller BS, Peerschke EI, Scudder IE, Sullivan CA. Studies with a murine monoclonal antibody that abolished the ristocetin induced binding of von Willebrand factor to platelets: additional evidence in support of GP Ib as a platelet receptor for von Willebrand factor. Blood 1983;61: 99.
27. Wicki AN, Clemetson KJ. Structure and function of platelet membrane glycoproteins Ib and V: effects of leucocyte elastase and other proteases on platelet response to von Willebrand factor and thrombin. Eur J Biochem 1985;153:1.
28. Berndt MC, Gregory C, Kabral A, Zola H, Fournier D, Castaldi PA. Purification and preliminary characterization of the GP Ib complex on the human platelet membrane. Eur J Biochem 1985;151:637.
29. Du X, Beutler L, Ruan C, Castaldi PA, Berndt MC. Glycoprotein Ib and glycoprotein IX are fully complexed in the intact platelet membrane. Blood 1987;69:1524.
30. Clemetson KI, McGregor JL, James E, Dechavanne M, Luscher EF. Characterization of the platelet membrane glycoprotein abnormalities in Bernard-Soulier syndrome and comparison with normal by surface-labeling techniques and high-resolution two-dimensional electrophoresis. J Clin Invest 1982;70:304.
31. Lopez JA, Lears B, Reynolds CC, et al. Efficient plasma membrane expression of a platelet glycoprotein Ib-IX complex requires the presence of its three subunits. J Biol Chem 1992;267:12851.
32. Hickey MJ, Hagen FS, Yasi M, et al. Human platelet glycoprotein V: characterization of the polypeptide and the related Gp IB-V-IX receptor system of adhesive leucine-rich glycoproteins. Proc Natl Acad Sci USA 1993;90:8327.
33. Lanza F, Morales M, de la Salle C, et al. Cloning and characterization of the gene encoding the human platelet glycoprotein V: a member of the leucine-rich glycoprotein family cleaved during thrombin activation. J Biol Chem 1993;268:20801.
34. Behnke O. Electron microscopical observations on the surface coating of blood platelets. J Ultrastruct Res 1968;24:51.
35. Okumura T, Lombart C, Jamieson GA. Platelet glycocalicin II: purification and characterization. J Biol Chem 1976;251:5950.
36. Judson PA, Anstee DJ, Clamp JR. Isolation and characterization of the major oligosaccharide of human platelet membrane glycoprotein Ib. Biochem J 1982;205:81.
37. Tsuji T, Tsunehisa S, Watanabe Y, Yamamoto K, Tohyama H, Osawa T. The carbohydrate moiety of human platelet glycocalicin. J Biol Chem 1983;258:6335.
38. Fox JEB, Aggerbeck LP, Berndt MC. Structure of the glycoprotein Ib-IX complex from platelet membranes. J Biol Chem 1988;263:4882.
39. Phillips DR, Jakabova M. Ca2+-dependent protease in human platelets. J Biol Chem 1977;252:5602.
40. Coller BS, Kalomiris E, Steinberg M, et al. Evidence that glycocalicin circulates in normal plasma. J Clin Invest 1984;73:794.
41. Okumura T, Hasitz M, Jamieson GA. Platelet glycocalicin: interaction with thrombin and role as a thrombin receptor on the platelet surface. J Biol Chem 1978;253:3435.
42. Yamamoto K, Yamamoto N, Kitagawa H, Tanoue K, Kosaki G, Yamazaki H. Localization of a thrombin-binding site on human platelet membrane glycoprotein Ib determined by a monoclonal antibody. Thromb Haemost 1986;55:162.
43. Pepper DS, Jamieson GA. Isolation of a macroglycopeptide from human platelets. Biochemistry 1970;9:3706.
44. Lopez JA, Chung DW, Fujikawa K, Hagen FS, Papayannopoulou T, Roth GJ. Cloning of the alpha chain of human platelet glycoprotein Ib: a transmembrane protein with homology to leucine-rich alpha2 glycoprotein. Proc Natl Acad Sci USA 1987;84:5616.
45. Lopez JA, Chung DW, Fujikawa K, Hagen FS, Davie EW, Roth GJ. The alpha and beta chains of human platelet glycoprotein Ib are both transmembrane proteins containing a leucine-rich amino acid sequence. Proc Natl Acad Sci USA 1988;85:2135.
46. Hickey MJ, Williams SA, Roth GJ. Human platelet glycoprotein IX: an adhesive prototype of leucine-rich glycoproteins with flank-center-flank structures. Proc Natl Acad Sci USA 1989;86:6773.
47. Hickey MJ, Deaven LL, Roth GJ. Human platelet glycoprotein IX: characterization of "full-length" cDNA and localization to chromosome 3. FEBS Lett 1990;274:189.
48. Roth GJ. Developing relationships: arterial platelet adhesion, glycoprotein Ib and leucine-rich glycoproteins. Blood 1991;77:5.
49. Wenger RH, Wieki AN, Kieffer N, Adolph S, Hameister H, Clemetson KJ. The 5′ flanking region and chromosomal localization of the gene encoding human platelet membrane glycoprotein Ib alpha. Gene 1989;85:517.

50. Sprandio JD, Shapiro SS, Thiagarajan P, McCord S. Cultured human umbilical vein endothelial cells contain a membrane glycoprotein immunologically related to platelet glycoprotein Ib. Blood 1988;71:234.
51. Asch AS, Adelman B, Fujimoto M, Nachman RL. Identification and isolation of a platelet GP Ib–like protein in human umbilical vein endothelial cells and bovine aortic smooth muscle cells. J Clin Invest 1988;81:1600.
52. Sixma JJ, Sakariassen KS, Stel HV, et al. Functional domains on von Willebrand factor: recognition of discrete tryptic fragments by monoclonal antibodies that inhibit interaction of von Willebrand factor with platelets and with collagen. J Clin Invest 1984;74:736.
53. Girma JP, Kalafatis M, Pietu G, et al. Mapping of distinct von Willebrand factor domains interacting with platelet GpIb and GpIIb/IIIa and with collagen using monoclonal antibodies. Blood 1986;67:1356.
54. Cruz MA, Handin RI, Wise RJ. The interaction of the von Willebrand factor-A1 domain with platelet glycoprotein Ib/IX: the role of glycosylation and disulfide bonding in a monomeric recombinant A1 domain protein. J Biol Chem 1993;268:21238.
55. Vicente V, Kostel PJ, Ruggeri ZM. Isolation and functional characterization of the von Willebrand factor-binding domain located in residues His1-Arg 293 of the alpha chain of glycoprotein Ib. J Biol Chem 1988;263: 8473.
56. Vicente V, Houghton RA, Ruggeri ZM. Identification of a site in the alpha chain of platelet glycoprotein Ib that participates in von Willebrand factor binding. J Biol Chem 1990;265:274.
57. Cruz MA, Petersen E, Turci SM, Handin RI. Functional analysis of a recombinant glycoprotein Ib alpha polypeptide which inhibits von Willebrand factor binding to the platelet glycoprotein Ib/IX complex and to collagen. J Biol Chem 1992;267:1303.
58. Howard MA, Firkin BG. Ristocetin: a new tool in the investigation of platelet aggregation. Thromb Diath Haemmorrh 1971;26:362.
59. Moake JL, Turner NA, Stathopoulos NA, Nolasco L, Hellems JD. Shear-induced platelet aggregation can be mediated by vWf released from platelets, as well as by exogenous large or unusually large vWf multimers, requires adenosine diphosphate, and is resistant to aspirin. Blood 1988;71:1366.
60. Chow TW, Hellums JD, Moake JL, et al. Shear stress-induced von Willebrand factor binding to platelet glycoprotein Ib initiates calcium influx in association with aggregation. Blood 1992;80:113.
61. Read MS, Smith SV, Lamb MA, et al. Role of botrocetin in platelet agglutination: formation of an activated complex of botrocetin and von Willebrand factor. Blood 1989;74:1031.
62. DeMarco L, Mazzucato M, Masotti A, et al. Localization and characterization of a thrombin-binding site on platelet glycoprotein Ib. J Biol Chem 1994;269:6478.
63. Garguly P. Binding of thrombin to functionally defective platelets: a hypothesis on the nature of the thrombin receptor. Br J Haematol 1977;37:47.
64. Fox JEB. Identification of actin-binding protein as the protein linking the membrane skeleton to glycoproteins on platelet plasma membranes. J Biol Chem 1985;260:11970.
65. Okita JR, Pidard D, Newman PJ, Montgomery RR, Kunicki TJ. On the association of glycoprotein Ib and actin-binding protein in human platelets. J Cell Biol 100:317, 1985.
66. Wyler B, Bienz D, Clemetson KJ, Luscher EF. Glycoprotein Ib-beta is the only phosphorylated major membrane glycoprotein in human platelets. Biochem J 1986;234:373.
67. Grottum KA, Solum NO. Congenital thrombocytopenia with giant platelets: a defect in the platelet membrane. Br J Haematol 1969;16: 277.
68. Bernard J, Soulier J-P. Sur une nouvelle variete de dystrophie thrombocytaire-hemorragipare congenitale. Semin Hop Paris 1948; 24:3217.
69. White JG, Burris SM, Hasegawa D, Johnson MM. Micropipette aspiration of human blood platelets: a defect in Bernard-Soulier syndrome. Blood 1984;63:1249.
70. Nurden AT, Dupuis D, Kunicki TJ, Caen JP. Analysis of the I glycoprotein and protein composition of Bernard-Soulier platelets by single and two-dimensional sodium dodecyl sulfate-polyacrylamide gel electrophoresis. J Clin Invest 1981;67:1431.
71. Kroll MH, Harris TS, Moake JL, Handin RI, Schafer AI. Von Willebrand factor binding to platelet GpIb initiates signals for platelet activation. J Clin Invest 1991;88:1568.
72. Ware J, Russell SR, Vicente V, et al. Nonsense mutation in the glycoprotein Ib coding sequence associated with Bernard-Soulier syndrome. Proc Natl Acad Sci USA 1990;87:2026.
73. Finch CN, Miller JL, Lyle VA, Handin RL. Evidence that an abnormality in the glycoprotein Ib alpha gene is not the cause of abnormal platelet function in a family with classic Bernard-Soulier disease. Blood 1990;75: 2357.
74. Wright SD, Michaelides K, West NC, et al. Double heterozygosity for mutations in the platelet glycoprotein IX gene in three siblings with Bernard-Soulier syndrome. Blood 1993;81:2339.
75. Ware J, Russell SR, Marchese P, et al. Point mutation in a leucine-rich repeat of platelet glycoprotein Ib resulting in the Bernard-Soulier syndrome. J Clin Invest 1993;92:1213.
76. Miller JL, Lyle VA, Cunningham D. Mutation of leucine-57 to phenylalanine in a platelet glycoprotein Ib alpha leucine tandem repeat occurring in patients with an autosomal dominant variant of Bernard-Soulier disease. Blood 1992;79:439.
77. Bernard J. History of congenital hemorrhagic thrombocytopathic dystrophy. Blood Cells 1983;9:179.
78. Belluci S, Tobelem G, Caen JP. Inherited platelet disorders. Prog Hematol 1983;13:223.
79. Grottum KA, Solum NO. Congenital thrombocytopenia with giant platelets: a defect in the platelet membrane. Br J Haematol 1969;16: 277.
80. Howard MA, Hutton RA, Hardisty RM. Hereditary giant platelet syndrome: a disorder of a new aspect of platelet function. Br Med J 1973;4: 586.
81. Evensen SA, Solum NO, Grottum KA, Hovig T. Familial bleeding disorder with a moderate thrombocytopenia and giant blood platelets. Eur J Haematol 1974;13:203.
82. George JN, Nurden AT, Phillips DR. Molecular defects in interactions of platelets with the vessel wall. N Engl J Med 1984;311:1084.
83. McGill M, Jamieson GA, Drouin J, et al. Morphometric analysis of platelets in Bernard-Soulier syndrome: size and configuration in patients and carriers. Thromb Haemost 1984;52:37.
84. Caen J, Bellucci S. The defective prothrombin consumption in Bernard-Soulier syndrome: hypotheses from 1948 to 1982. Blood Cells 1983;9: 389.
85. Bitmell TC, Parekh SJ, Strong RR. Platelet-function studies in the Bernard-Soulier syndrome. Ann NY Acad Sci 1972;201:145.
86. Walsh PN, Mills DCB, Pareti FL, et al. Hereditary giant platelet syndrome: absence of collagen-induced coagulant activity and deficiency of factor-XI binding to platelets. Br J Haematol 1975;29:639.
87. Coller BS, Zarrabi MH. Platelet membrane studies in the May-Hegglin anomaly. Blood 1981;58:279.
88. Epstein CJ, Sahud MA, Piel CF, et al. Hereditary macrothrombocytopathia, nephritis, deafness. Am J Med 1972;52:299.
89. Godwin HA, Ginsburg AD. May-Hegglin anomaly: a defect in megakaryocyte fragmentation? Br J Haematol 1974;26:117.
90. Eckstein JD, Filip DJ, Watts JC. Hereditary thrombocytopenia, deafness, and renal disease. Ann Intern Med 1975;82:639.
91. Peterson LC, Rao KV, Crosson JT, et al. Fechtmer syndrome: a variant of Alport's syndrome with leukocyte inclusions and macrothrombocytopathia. Blood 1985;65:397.
92. Bernheim J, Dechavanne M, Bryon PA, et al. Thrombocytopenia, macrothrombocytopathia, nephritis and deafness. Am J Med 1976;61:145.
93. Milton JG, Frojmovic MM. Shape-changing agents produce abnormally large platelets in a hereditary "giant platelet syndrome (MPS)." J Lab Clin Med 1979;93:154.
94. Frojmovic MM, Milton JG. Physical, chemical and functional changes following platelet activation in normal and "giant" platelets. Blood Cells 1983;9:359.
95. Milton JG, Frojmovic MM, Tang SS, et al. Spontaneous platelet aggregation in a hereditary giant platelet syndrome (MPS). Am J Pathol 1984;114:336.
96. Milton JG, Hutton RA, Tuddenham EGD, et al. Platelet size and shape in hereditary giant platelet syndromes on blood smear and in suspension: evidence for two types of abnormalities. J Lab Clin Med 1985;106: 326.
97. Okita JR, Frojmovic MM, Fristopeit S, et al. Montreal platelet syndrome: a defect in calcium-activated protease (Calpain). Blood 1989;74:715.
98. Raccuglia G. Gray platelet syndrome. Am J Med 1971;51:818.
99. Gerrard JM, Phillips DR, Rao GHR, et al. Biochemical studies of two patients with the gray platelet syndrome. J Clin Invest 1980;66:102.
100. Greaves M, Pickering C, Martin J, et al. A new familial "giant platelet syndrome" with structural, metabolic and functional abnormalities of platelets due to a primary megakaryocyte defect. Br J Haematol 1987;65: 429.
101. Beck EA. Idiopathic thrombocytopenia with giant platelets. Johns Hopkins Med J 1980;146:281.
102. Cuthbert RJG, Heather HK, Watson SL, et al. DDAVP shortens the bleeding time in Bernard-Soulier syndrome. Thromb Res 1988;49:649.
103. Mant W. DDAVP in Bernard-Soulier syndrome. Thromb Res 1988;52: 77.
104. Stricker RB, Wong D, Saks SR, et al. Acquired Bernard-Soulier syndrome: evidence for the role of a 210,000-molecular weight protein in the interaction of platelets with von Willebrand factor. J Clin Invest 1985;76:1274.
105. Szatkowski NS, Kunicki TJ, Aster RH. Identification of glycoprotein Ib as a target for auto antibody (autoimmune) thrombocytopenic purpura. Blood 1986;67:310.
106. Devine DV, Currie MS, Rosse WF, et al. Pseudo-Bernard Soulier syndrome: thrombocytopenia caused by autoantibody to platelet glycoprotein Ib. Blood 1987;70:428.
107. Berndt MC, Kabral A, Grimsley P, et al. An acquired Bernard-Soulier-like platelet defect associated with juvenile myelodysplastic syndrome. Br J Haematol 1988;68:97.
108. Shuman MA. Thrombin-cellular interactions. Ann NY Acad Sci 1986;485:228.
109. Berndt MC, Gregory C, Dowden G, Castaldi PA. Thrombin interactions with platelet membrane proteins. Ann NY Acad Sci 1985;483:374.

110. Gronke RS, Bergman RS, Bakers JB. Thrombin interaction with platelets: influence of a platelet proease nexin. J Biol Chem 1978;262:3030.
111. Okamura T, Hasitz M, Jamieson GA. Platelet glycocalicin interaction with thrombin and role as thrombin receptor on the platelet surface. J Biol Chem 1978;253:3435.
112. Davey MG, Lüscher EF. Actions of thrombin and other coagulant and proteolytic enzymes on blood platelets. Nature 1967;216:857.
113. Phillips DR. Thrombin interaction with human platelets: potentiation of thrombin-induced aggregation and release by inactivation thrombin. Thromb Diath Haemorrh 1974;32:207.
114. Martin BM, Feinman RD, Detwiler TC. Platelet stimulation by thrombin and other proteases. Biochemistry 1975;14:1308.
115. Tollefson DM, Feagler JR, Majerus PW. The binding of thrombin to the surface of platelets. J Biol Chem 1974;249:2645.
116. Workman EF, White II GC, Lundblad RL. Structure-function relationships in the interaction of alpha-thrombin and blood platelets. J Biol Chem 1977;252:7118.
117. Vu T-KH, Hung DT, Wheaton VI, Coughlin SR. Molecular cloning of a functional thrombin receptor reveals a novel proteolytic mechanism of receptor activation. Cell 1991;64:1057.
118. Vu T-KH, Wheaton VI, Hung DT, Charo I, Coughlin SR. Domains defining thrombin-receptor interaction. Nature 1991;353:674.
119. Liu L-W, Vu T-KH, Esomn CT, Coughlin SR. The region of the thrombin receptor resembling hirudin binds to thrombin and alters enzyme specificity. J Biol Chem 1991;266:16977.
120. Coughlin SR, Vu T-KH, Hung DT, Wheaton VI. Characterization of a functional thrombin receptor: issues and opportunities. J Clin Invest 1992;89:351.
121. Hung DT, Vu TK, Wheaton VI, Ishii K, Coughlin SR. Cloned platelet thrombin receptor is necessary for thrombin-induced platelet activation. J Clin Invest 1992;89:1350.
122. Born GVR. Aggregation of blood platelets by adenosine diphosphate and its reversal. Nature 1962;194:927.
123. Zawilska KM, Born GVR, Begent NA. Effect of ADP-utilizing enzymes on the arterial bleeding time in rats and rabbits. Br J Haematol 1982;50: 317.
124. Born GVR, Cusack NJ, Darwin C, McClure M. Prolongation of bleeding time in rats by ADP receptor antagonists. J Physiol Lond 1986;381: 22.
125. McClure MO, Kakker A, Cusack NJ, Born GVR. Evidence for dependence of arterial haemostasis on ADP. Proc R Soc Lond [Biol] 1988;234: 255.
126. Kim BK, Blackburn GM, Zamecnik PC. Antithrombotic effects of beta, beta-monochloromethylene diadenosine 5′,5‴-P1,P4-tetraphosphate (CHCI-APA4A). Thromb Haemost 1989;62:269.
127. Dubyak GR, El-Moatassim C. Signal transduction via P2-purinergic receptors for extracellular ATP and other nucleotides. Am J Physiol 1993;265:577c.
128. Burnstock G. A basis for distinguishing two types of purinergic receptor. In: Straub RW, Bolis L, eds. Cell membrane receptors for drugs and hormones: a multidisciplinary approach. New York, Raven Press, 1978: 107.
129. Gordon JL. Extracellular ATP: effects, sources and fate. Biochem J 1986;233:309.
130. Haslam RJ, Cusack NJ. Blood platelet receptors for ADP and for adenosine. In: Burnstock G, ed. Purinergic receptors: receptors and recognition series B, vol 12. London, Chapman & Hall, 1981:221.
131. Hourani SMO, Cusack NJ. Actions and structure-activity relationships of purines on platelets. In: Stone TW, ed. Purines: pharmacology and physiological roles. London, Macmillan, 1985:163.
132. Cusack NJ, Hourani SMO, Welford LA. Characterisation of ADP receptors. Adv Exp Med Biol 1985;192:29.
133. Cusack NJ, Hourani SMO. Adenosine, adenine nucleotides and platelet function. In: Phillis J, ed. Purinergic regulation of cell function. New York, CRC Press, 1991:121.
134. Gaardner A, Laland S. Hypothesis for the aggregation of platelets by nucleotides. Nature 1964;202:909.
135. Stone JV, Singh RK, Horak H, Barton PG. Sulfhydryl analogues of adenosine diphosphate: chemical synthesis and activity as platelet aggregating agents. Can J Biochem 1976;54:529.
136. Packham MA, Ardlie NG, Mustard JF. Effect of adenine compounds on platelet aggregation. Am J Physiol 1969;217:1009.
137. Packham MA, Guccione MA, Perry DW, Kinlough-Rathbone RL, Mustard JF. AMP inhibition of reactions of ADP with washed platelets from humans and rabbits. Am J Physiol 1972;223:419.
138. MacFarlane DE, Mills DCB. The effects of ATP on platelets: evidence against the central role of released ADP in primary aggregation. Blood 1975;46:309.
139. Cusack NJ, Hourani SMO. Partial agonist behaviour of adenosine 5′-O-(2-thiodiphosphate) on human platelets. Br J Pharmacol 1981;73: 405.
140. Cusack NJ, Hourani SMO. Effects of Rp and Sp diastereoisomers of adenosine 5′-O-(1-thiodiphosphate) on human platelets. Br J Pharmacol 1981;73:409.
141. Jefferson JR, Harmon JT, Jamieson GG. Identification of high affinity and low affinity platelet binding sites for ADP and competition by ADP analogues. Blood 1988;71:110.
142. Adler JR, Handin RI. Solubilization and characterization of a platelet membrane ADP-binding protein. J Biol Chem 1979;254:3866.
143. Greco N, Tandon NN, Jackson BW, et al. Low structural specificity for nucleoside triphosphates as antagonists of ADP-induced platelet activation. J Biol Chem 1992;267:2966.
144. Jefferson JR, Harmon JT, Jamieson GA. Identification of high-affinity and low-affinity platelet binding sites for ADP and competition with ADP analogues. Blood 1988;71:110.
145. Figures WR, Niewiarowski S, Morinelli TA, Colman RF, Colman RW. Affinity labeling of a human platelet membrane protein with 5-p-fluorosulphonylbenzoyl adenosine. J Biol Chem 1981;256:7789.
146. Colman RW, Figures WR, Colman RF, Morinelli TA, Niewiarowski S, Mills DCB. Identification of two distinct adenosine diphosphate receptors in human platelets. Trans Assoc Am Physicians 1980;93:305.
147. Colman RW. Platelet activation: role of an ADP receptor. Semin Haematol 1986;23:119.
148. Colman RW. Aggregin: a platelet ADP receptor mediating activation. FASEB J 1990;4:1425.
149. Mills DCB, Figures WR, Scearce LM, Stewart GJ, Colman RF, Colman RW. Two mechanisms for inhibition of ADP-induced platelet shape change by 5-p-fluoro-sulfonyl-benzoyladenosine. J Biol Chem 1985;260: 8078.
150. Bennett JS, Colman RF, Colman RW. Identification of adenine nucleotide binding proteins in human platelet membranes by affinity labelling with 5-p-fluorosulfonylbenzoyl adenosine. J Biol Chem 1978;253:7346.
151. MacFarlane DE, Mills DCB, Shrivasta PC. Binding of 2-azidoadenosine [B-32P] diphosphate to the receptor on intact human blood platelets which inhibits adenylate cyclase. Biochemistry 1982;21:544.
152. MacFarlane DE, Srivastava PC, Mills DCB. 2-Methylthioadenosine [B-32P] diphosphate: an agonist and radioligand for the receptor that inhibits the accumulation of cyclic AMP in intact blood platelets. J Clin Invest 1983;71:420.
153. Lanza F, Cazenave JP. Recepteurs adrenergiques des plaquettes sanguines. Nouv Rev Fr Hematol 1987;29:407.
154. Kerry R, Scrutton MC, Platelet adrenoceptors. In: Longnecker GL, ed, Platelets: physiology and pharmacology. Orlando, Academic Press, 1985:113.
155. Spaet TH, Lejnieks I. Studies on the mechanism whereby platelets are clumped by adenosine diphosphate. Thromb Diath Haemorrh 1966;15: 36.
156. Cooper B, Handin RJ, Young LH, Alexander RW. Agonist regulation of the human platelet alpha-adrenergic receptor. Nature 1978;271:703.
157. Cooper B, Shafer AI, Puchalsky D, Handin RJ. Platelet resistance to PGD2 in patients with myeloproliferative disorders. Blood 1978;52: 618.
158. Scrutton MC, Clare KA, Hutton RA, Bruckdorfer KR. Depressed responsiveness to adrenaline in platelets from apparently normal human donors: a familial trait. Br J Haematol 1981;49:303.
159. Narumiya S, Hirata N, Namba T, et al. Structure and function of prostanoid receptors. J Lipid Mediat 1993;6:155.
160. Nusing RM, Hirata M, Kakizuka A, et al. Characterization and chromosomal mapping of the human thromboxane A2 receptor gene. J Biol Chem 1993;268:25253.
161. Schafer AI, Cooper B, O'Hara D, Handin RI. Identification of platelet receptors for prostaglandin I2 and D2. J Biol Chem 1979;254:2914.
162. Thibonnier M, Roberts JM. Characterization of human platelet vasopressin receptors. J Clin Invest 1985;76:1857.
163. DeClerck F, Xhonneux B, Leysen J, Janssen PAJ. Evidence for functional 5-HT2 receptor sites on human blood platelets. Biochem Pharmacol 1984;33:2807.
164. Fitzgerald LA, Steiner B, Rafl SC Jr, et al. Protein sequence of endothelial glycoprotein IIIa derived from a cDNA clone. J Biol Chem 1987;262: 3936.
165. Zimrin A, Eisman R, Vilaire G, et al. The structure of platelet glycoprotein IIIa: a common subunit for two different membrane receptors. J Clin Invest 1988;81:1470.
166. Rosa J-P, Bray PF, Gayet O, et al. Cloning of glycoprotein IIIa from human erythroleukemia cells and localization of the gene to chromosome 17. Blood 1988;72:593.
167. Poncz M, Eisman R, Heidenreich R, et al. Structure of the platelet membrane glycoprotein IIb. J Biol Chem 1987;262:8476.
168. Ginsberg MH, Loftus J, Ryckwaert J-J, et al. Immunochemical and amino-terminal sequence comparison of two cytoadhesions indicates they contain similar or identical beta subunits and distinct alpha subunits. J Biol Chem 1987;262:5437.
169. Lam SC-T, Plow EF, D'Souza SE, et al. Isolation and characterization of a platelet membrane protein related to the vitronectin receptor. J Biol Chem 1989;264:3742.
170. Anderson DC. Leukocyte adhesion deficiency: an inherited defect in the Mac1, LFA-I, and pl50,95 glycoproteins. Annu Rev Med 1987;38: 175.
171. Fischer A, Losowska-Crospierre B, Anderson DC, et al. Leukocyte adhesion deficiency: molecular basis and functional consequences. Immunodeficiency Rev 1988;1:39.
172. Kishimoto TK, O'Connor K, Lee A, et al. Cloning of the β subunit of the leukocyte adhesion proteins: homology to an extracellular matrix receptor defines a novel supergene family. Cell 1987;48:681.

173. Law SKA, Gagnon J, Hildreth JEK, et al. The primary structure of the β-subunit of the cell surface adhesion glycoproteins LFA-I, CR3, and pl50,95 and its relationship to the fibronectin receptor. Embo J 1987;6: 915.
174. Sosnoski DM, Emanuel BS, Hawkins AL, et al. Chromosomal localization of the genes for the vitronectin and fibronectin receptor subunits and for platelet glycoproteins IIb and IIIa. J Clin Invest 1988;81:1993.
175. Bray PF, Barsh G, Rosa J-P, et al. Physical linkage of the genes for platelet membrane glycoproteins IIb and IIIa. Proc Natl Acad Sci USA 1988;85:8683.
176. Martin F, Frandini MH, Thevenon D, et al. The transcription factor GATA-1 regulates the promoter activity of the platelet glycoprotein IIb gene. J Biol Chem 1993;268:21606.
177. Lemarchandel V, Kghysdael J, Mignotte V, et al. GATA and Ets cis-acting sequences mediate megakaryocyte-specific expression. Mol Cell Biol 1993;13:668.
178. O'Toole TE, Lomis JC, Plow EF, et al. Efficient surface expression of platelet GP IIb-IIIa requires both subunits. Blood 1989;74:14.
179. Rosa J-P, McEver RP. Processing and assembly of the integrin, glycoprotein IIb-IIIa by HEL cells. J Biol Chem 1989;264:12596.
180. Russell ME, Seligsohn U, Coller BS, et al. Structural integrity of the glycoprotein IIb and IIIa genes in Glanzmann thrombasthenia patients from Israel. Blood 1908;72:1833.
181. Bennett JS, Hoxie JA, Leitman SF, et al. Inhibition of fibrinogen binding to stimulated human platelets by a monoclonal antibody. Proc Natl Acad Sci USA 1983;80:2417.
182. Pidard D, Montgomery RR, Bennett JS, et al. Interaction of AP-2, a monoclonal antibody specific for the human platelet glycoprotein IIb-IIIa complex, with intact platelets. J Biol Chem 1983;258:12582.
183. Coller BS, Peerschke EL, Scudder LE, et al. Murine monoclonal antibody that completely blocks the binding of fibrinogen to platelets produces a thrombasthenia-like state in normal platelets and binds to glycoproteins IIb and or IIIa. J Clin Invest 1983;72:1.
184. McEver RP, Bennett EM, Martin MN. Identification of two structurally and functionally distinct sites on human platelet membrane glycoprotein IIb-IIIa using monoclonal antibodies. J Biol Chem 1983;258: 5269.
185. Bennett JS, Vilaire G, Cines DB. Identification of the fibrinogen receptor on human platelets by photoaffinity labeling. J Biol Chem 1982;257: 8049.
186. Plow EF, Ginsberg MH. Specific and saturable binding of plasma fibronectin to thrombin-stimulated human platelets. J Biol Chem 1981;268:9477.
187. Pytela R, Pierschbacher MD, Ginsberg MH, et al. Platelet membrane glycoprotein IIb-IIIa: member of a family of Arg-Gly-Asp-specific adhesion receptors. Science 1986;231:1559.
188. Pietu G, Cherel G, Marguerie G, et al. Inhibition of von Willebrand factor-platelet interaction by fibrinogen. Nature (Lond) 1984;308: 648.
189. Kloczewiak M, Timmons S, Lukas TJ, Hawiger J. Platelet receptor recognition site on human fibrinogen: synthesis and structure-function relationship of peptides corresponding to the carboxy-terminal segment of the gamma chain. Biochemistry 1984;23:1767.
190. Santoro SA, Lawig WJ. Competition for related but non-identical binding sites on the glycoprotein IIb-IIIa complex by peptides derived from platelet adhesive proteins. Cell 1987;48:867.
191. D'Souza S, Ginsberg MH, Burke TA, Lam SC-T, Plow EF. Localization of an Arg-Gly-Asp recognition site within an integrin adhesion receptor. Science 1988;242:91.
192. Loftus JC, O'Toole TE, Plow EF, Glass A, Frelinger AL, Ginsberg MH. A beta 3 integrin mutation abolishes ligand binding and alters divalent cation-dependent conformation. Science 1990;249:915.
193. D'Souza SE, Ginsberg MH, Burke TA, Plow EF. The ligand binding site of the platelet integrin receptor GPIIb-IIIa is proximal to the second calcium binding domain of its alpha subunit. J Biol Chem 1990;265: 3440.
194. Phillips DR, Jennings LJ, Edwards HH. Identification of membrane proteins mediating the interaction of human platelets. J Cell Biol 1980;86: 77.
195. Horwitz A, Duggan K, Buck C, Beckerle MC, Burridge K. Interaction of plasma membrane fibronectin receptor with talin: a transmembrane linkage. Nature 1986;320:531.
196. Glanzmann E. Hereditare hamorrhagische Thrombasthenie: ein Beitrag zur Plattchen. J Kinderkr 1918;88:1.
197. Nurden AT. Glycoprotein defects responsible for abnormal platelet function in inherited platelet disorders. In: George JN, Nurden AT, Philips DR, eds. Platelet membrane glycoproteins. New York, Plenum Press, 1985:357.
198. Reichert N, Seligsohn U, Ramot B. Clinical and genetic aspects of Glanzmann's thrombasthenia in Israel. Thromb Diath Haemorrh 1975;34:806.
199. Khanduri U, Pulimood R, Sudarsanam A, et al. Glanzmann's thrombasthenia: a review and report of 42 cases from South India. Thromb Haemost 1981;46:717.
200. Seligsohn U, Rososhansky S. A Glanzmann's thrombasthenia cluster among Iraqi Jews in Israel. Thromb Haemost 1984;52:230.
201. McEver RP, Baenziger NL, Majerus PW. Isolation and quantitation of the platelet membrane glycoprotein deficient in thrombasthenia using a monoclonal antibody. J Clin Invest 1980;66:1311.
202. Burk CD, Newman PJ, Lyman G, et al. A deletion in the gene for glycoprotein IIb associated with Glanzmann's thrombasthenia. J Clin Invest 1991;87:270.
203. Newman PJ, Seligsohn U, Lyman S, et al. The molecular genetic basis of Glanzmann thrombasthenia in the Iraqi-Jewish and Arab populations in Israel. Proc Natl Acad Sci USA 1991;88:3160.
204. Kato A, Yamamoto K, Miyazaki S, et al. Molecular basis for Glanzmann's thombasthenia (GT) in a compound heterozygote with glycoprotein IIb gene defects: a proposal for the classification of GT based on the biosynthetic pathway of glycoprotein IIb-IIIa complex. Blood 1992;79: 3212.
205. Iwamaoto S, Nishiumi E, Kajii LA, et al. An exon 28 mutation resulting in alternative splicing of the glycoprotein IIb transcript and Glanzmann's thrombasthenia. Blood 1994;83:1017.
206. Gu JM, Xu WF, Wang XD, et al. Identification of a nonsense mutation at amino acid 584-arginine of platelet glycoprotein IIb in patients with type I Glanzmann thrombasthenia. Br J Haematol 1993;83:442.
207. Poncz M, Rifat S, Coller BS, et al. Glanzmann thrombasthenia secondary to a Gly273-Asp mutation adjacent to the first calcium-binding domain of platelet glycoprotein IIb. J Clin Invest 1994;93:172.
208. Wilcox DA, Wautier J-C, Pidard D, et al. An amino acid substitution within the fourth calcium binding domain of GPIIb results in degradation of the integrin GPIIb-IIIa and Type I Glanzmann thrombasthenia. Circulation 1992;86:682a.
209. Bray PF, Shuman MA. Identification of an abnormal gene for the GpIIIa subunit of the platelet fibrinogen receptor resulting in Glanzmann's thrombasthenia. Blood 1990;75:881.
210. Li L, Bray PF. Homologous recombination among three intragene Alu sequences causes an inversion-deletion resulting in the hereditary bleeding disorder Glanzmann thrombasthenia. Am J Hum Genet 1993;53:140.
211. Simsek S, Heyboer H, De Bruijne-Admiraal LG, et al. Glanzmann's thrombasthenia caused by homozygosity for a splice defect that leads to deletion of the first coding exon of the glycoprotein IIIa mRNA. Blood 1993;81:2044.
212. Chen YP, Djaffar I, Pidard D, et al. Ser-752-Pro mutation in the cytoplasmic domain of the integrin 3 subunit and defective activation of platelet intregrin αIIb 3 (glycoprotein IIb-IIIa) in a variant of Glanzmann thrombasthenia. Proc Natl Acad Sci USA 1992;89:10169.
213. Loftus JC, O'Toole TE, Plow EF, et al. A β integrin mutation abolishes ligand binding and alters divalent cation-dependent conformation. Science 1990;249:915.
214. Lanza F, Stierle A, Fournier D, et al. A new variant of Glanzmann's thrombasthenia (Strasbourg I): platelets with functionally defective glycoprotein IIb-IIIa complexes and a glycoprotein IIIa 214Arg-214Trp mutation. J Clin Invest 1992;89:1995.
215. Bajt ML, Ginsberg MH, Frelinger AL III, et al. A spontaneous mutation of integrin αIIb 3 (platelet glycoprotein IIb-IIIa) helps define a ligand binding site. J Biol Chem 1992;267:3789.
216. Coller BS, Cheresh DA, Asch E, et al. Platelet vitronectin receptor expression differentiates Iraqi-Jewish from Arab patients with Glanzmann thrombasthenia in Israel. Blood 1991;77:75.
217. Caen JP, Castaldi PA, Leclerc JC, et al. Congenital bleeding disorders with long bleeding time and normal platelet count. Am J Med 1966;41:4.
218. Hardisty RM, Dormand KM, Hutton RA. Thrombasthenia: studies on three cases. Br J Haematol 1964;10:371.
219. George FN, Nurden AT, Caen JP. Glanzmann's thrombasthenia: the spectrum of clinical disease. Blood 1990;75:1383.
220. Jennings LK, Ashmun RA, Wang WC, et al. Analysis of human platelet glycoproteins IIb-IIIa and Glanzmann's thrombasthenia in whole blood by flow cytometry. Blood 1986;68:173.
221. Michelson AD. Flow cytometric analysis of platelet surface glycoproteins: phenotypically distinct subpopulations of platelets in children with chronic myeloid leukemia. J Lab Clin Med 1987;110:346.
222. Caen J. Glanzmann thrombasthenia. Clin Haematol 1972;1:383.
223. Nurden AT, Didry D, Kieffer N, et al. Residual amounts of glycoproteins IIb and IIIa may be present in the platelets of most patients with Glanzmann's thrombasthenia. Blood 1985;65:1021.
224. Handagama PJ, Shuman MA, Bainton DF. Incorporation of intravenously injected albumin, immunoglobulin G, and fibrinogen in guinea pig megakaryocyte granules. J Clin Invest 1989;84:73.
225. Handagama PJ, Scarborough RM, Shuman MA, et al. Endocytosis of fibrinogen into megakaryocyte and platelet alpha-granules is mediated by alpha-IIb 3 (glycoprotein IIb-IIIa). Blood 1993;82:135.
226. Handagama P, Bainton DF, Jackques Y, et al. Kistrin, an integrin antagonist, blocks endocytosis of fibrinogen into guinea pig megakaroycyte and platelet alpha-graunles. J Clin Invest 1993;91:193.
227. Niessner H, Clemetson KJ, Panzer S, et al. Acquired thrombasthenia due to GPIIB-IIIa-specific platelet autoantibodies. Blood 1986;68:571.
228. DiMinno G, Coraggio F, Cerbone AM. A myeloma paraprotein with specificity for platelet glycoprotein IIIa in a patient with a fatal bleeding disorder. J Clin Invest 1986;77:157.
229. DiMinno C, Cerbone AM, Mattioli PL, et al. Functional thrombasthenia state in normal platelets following the administration of ticlopidine. J Clin Invest 1985;75:328.

230. Kobrinsky NL, Israels ED, Genard JM, et al. Shortening of bleeding time by 1-Deamino-8-arginine vasopressin in various bleeding disorders. Lancet 1984;1:1145.
231. Schulman S, Johnsson H, Egberg N, et al. DDAVP-induced correction of prolonged bleeding time in patients with congenital platelet function defects. Thromb Res 1987;45:165.
232. Levy-Toledano S, Tobelem C, Legrand C, et al. Acquired IgG antibody occurring in a thrombasthenia patient: its effect on human platelet function. Blood 1978;51:1065.
233. Bierling P, Fromont P, Elbez A, et al. Early immunization against platelet glycoprotein IIIa in a newborn Glanzmann Type I patient. Vox Sang 1988;55:109.
234. Bellucci S, Devergie A, Gluckman E, et al. Complete correction of Glanzmann's thrombasthenia by allogeneic bone-marrow transplantation. Br J Haematol 1985;59:635.
235. Rosing J, van Rijn JLML, Bevers EM, et al. The role of activated human platelets in prothrombin and factor X activation. Blood 1985;65:319.
236. Zwall RFA, Comfurius P, van Deenen LLM. Membrane asymmetry and blood coagulation. Nature (Lond) 1977;268:358.
237. Sims PJ, Wiedmer T, Esmon CT, et al. Assembly of the platelet prothrombinase complex is linked to vesiculation of the platelet plasma membrane. Studies in Scott syndrome: an isolated defect in platelet procoagulant activity. J Biol Chem 1989;264:17049.
238. Weiss HJ, Vicic WJ, Lages BA, et al. Isolated deficiency of platelet procoagulant activity. Am J Med 67:206, 1979.
239. Minkoff M, Wu KK, Walasek J, et al. Bleeding disorder due to an isolated platelet factor 3 deficiency. Arch Intern Med 1980;140:366.
240. Miletich JP, Kane WH, Hofmann SL, et al. Deficiency of factor Xa-factor V binding sites on the platelets of a patient with a bleeding disorder. Blood 1979;54:1015.
241. Rosing J, Bevers EM, Comfurius P, et al. Impaired factor X and prothrombin activation associated with decreased phospholipid exposure in platelets from a patient with a bleeding disorder. Blood 1985;65:1557.

Blood: Principles and Practice of Hematology,
edited by Robert I. Handin, Samuel E. Lux, and Thomas P. Stossel.
J.B. Lippincott Company, Philadelphia © 1995.

36

Von Willebrand's Disease

Bruce M. Ewenstein
Robert I. Handin

Von Willebrand's disease (vWD), the most common inherited coagulopathy, is best defined as a group of autosomally inherited bleeding disorders caused by quantitative or qualitative abnormalities in von Willebrand factor (vWF). vWF has two roles in normal hemostasis. First, vWF provides a molecular bridge between platelets and the exposed subendothelium in damaged blood vessels[1] (Fig. 36-1). Second, vWF serves as an intravascular carrier for factor VIII, the procoagulant protein with which it is noncovalently complexed in the plasma.[2] Thus, abnormalities in vWF may produce defects in both primary and secondary hemostasis.

The definition of von Willebrand's disease as a clinical entity dates back to 1924, when Professor Eric von Willebrand evaluated a 5-year-old girl who was brought to a Helsinki hospital from her native Föglö Island in the Åland archipelago of Finland. She and many of her siblings had severe bleeding symptoms and four had died of hemorrhagic complications. After studying a total of 66 family members, Dr. von Willebrand concluded that the affected patients were suffering from a previously undescribed disorder, which now bears his name.

PATHOGENESIS

Von Willebrand's disease was shown to differ from classic hemophilia in three important ways.[3,4] First, the inheritance pattern was autosomal dominant and not X-linked. Second, the bleeding primarily involved mucous membranes, and hemarthroses—common in classic hemophilia—were absent in this family. Third, unlike hemophiliacs, patients with vWD had prolonged bleeding times. Descriptions of similar patients appeared in the late 1920s in the American clinical literature.[5,6] In 1953, several reports appeared of a bleeding disorder characterized by an increased bleeding time and decreased factor VIII coagulant activity.[7–9] The similarity between this disorder and the condition uncovered almost three decades earlier was made when the original Åland archipelago pedigree was reinvestigated and these patients also were shown to have diminished levels of plasma factor VIII.[10,11]

The pathophysiology of vWD was first suggested by the early studies of von Willebrand. Prompted by his clinical observations, von Willebrand developed a glass capillary apparatus to measure platelet function in vitro and found a delay in thrombus formation in blood from the affected members of this pedigree but not in blood from patients with hemophilia.[12] Modified forms of this test, using glass beads, were reintroduced in the 1960s and were found to be sensitive ways to detect vWD.[13,14] Later, model systems were developed to evaluate the role of vWF in platelet–subendothelial matrix interactions in flowing blood.[15] Rabbit blood vessels denuded of subendothelium were perfused with blood under varying flow rates and shear stresses. Under conditions of high shear stress, the interactions between platelets and subendothelium required the plasma factor missing in vWD.

The common feature of diminished plasma factor VIII levels in both vWD and classic hemophilia suggested a relation between these disorders despite differences in their clinical presentation and mode of inheritance. In the late 1950s and early 1960s, a series of publications confirmed that the defect in vWD resided in the plasma.[16–21] The prolonged bleeding time in vWD patients could be corrected by plasma and plasma-derived concentrates but not by platelets from normal donors.[16,22–24] Conversely, platelets from patients with vWD improved hemostasis in patients with severe thrombocytopenia secondary to aplastic anemia. Plasma infusion had different effects in these two conditions. The infusion of plasma into a patient with hemophilia A resulted in an immediate peak in factor VIII levels followed by a rapid decline. In contrast, infusion of hemophilic plasma into a patient with vWD produced a delayed but sustained increase in factor VIII levels.[24,25] Finally, after infusion of the more highly purified concentrates of factor VIII that became available in the 1970s, there was a clear dissociation between the elevation of factor VIII, the correction of the bleeding time, and the control of clinical bleeding.[26,27]

Further elucidation of the relation between factor VIII and vWD was achieved following the development of immunologic reagents.[28,29] Using the immunoelectrophoretic technique of Laurell,[30] Zimmerman and associates[28] observed a diminished quantity of "factor VIII–related antigen" in patients with vWD but not in those with hemophilia A. In the same year, Howard and Firkin[31] observed that the previously described agglutination of normal platelets by the antibiotic ristocetin was absent in some patients with vWD.[32] Later it was shown that the reduced ristocetin-induced platelet agglutination could be corrected by plasma or purified vWF.[33]

vWF is synthesized by endothelial cells and megakaryocytes and circulates in plasma as a heterogenous series of multimers that are assembled from a 220-kd subunit polypeptide. Plasma vWF multimers vary in size from 440 to

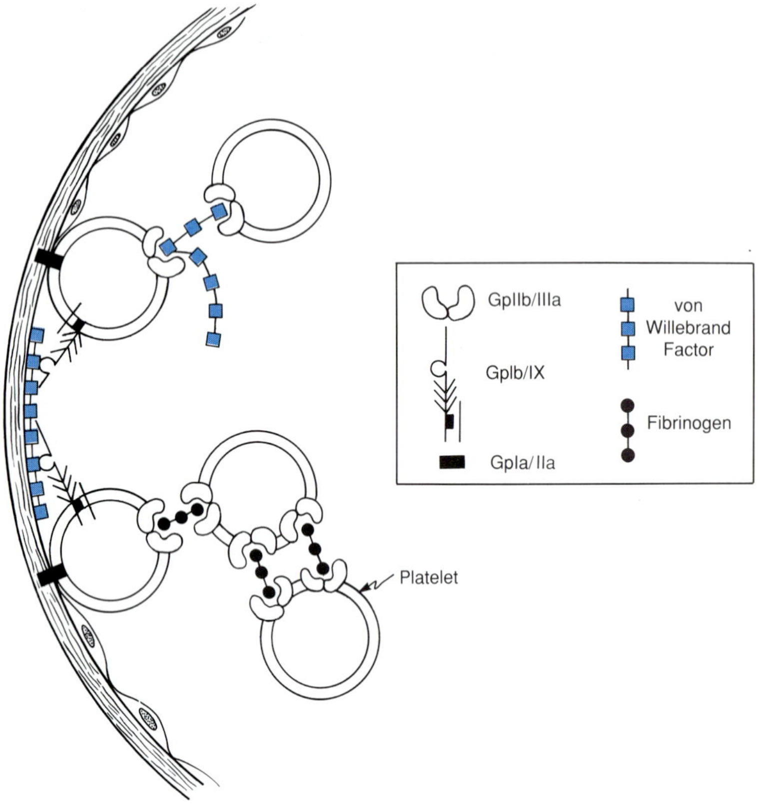

FIGURE 36-1. Role of vWF in platelet adhesion and aggregation. Platelets adhere directly to collagen via a specific collagen receptor on the gpIa/IIa complex. vWF adheres to constituents in vascular subendothelium, primarily collagen, and to the platelet gpIb/IX compex. This interaction stabilizes adherent platelets and prevents their detachment during high-flow or high-shear stress. Adherent activated platelets then bind fibrinogen to the gpIIb/IIIa complex and form aggregates. In addition, some component of adhesion is due to an interaction between vWF and gpIIb/IIIa (not shown).

10 × 10,000 kd, with even larger multimers noted within endothelial cell storage organelles. Studies from multiple laboratories have demonstrated a close relation between multimer size and the hemostatic effectiveness of vWF.[34,35] The ability of vWF to support shear-induced platelet aggregation is dependent on multimer size.[36] As further proof of this relation, in disorders like thrombotic thrombocytopenic purpura, in which there is unregulated secretion of very large vWF multimers from endothelial cells, patients develop thrombocytopenia and platelet thrombi.[37] Conversely, in some forms of vWD in which a selective loss of high-molecular-weight (HMW) vWF multimers and a normal plasma level of vWF are seen, patients have defective hemostasis and clinical bleeding.

vWF has been purified to homogeneity and its complete amino acid sequence determined by both classic protein chemistry[38] and molecular cloning techniques.[39–42] The defects that cause vWD are beginning to be defined at the molecular level, producing some unifying theories and at the same time raising new issues.[43] Despite the rapidity of recent progress, our knowledge of the molecular and cellular basis of most cases of vWD remains imperfect. Moreover, the wide variety of defects, which together are termed vWD, and the variable expression of vWD phenotypes, have made it difficult to establish clearcut diagnostic criteria.

STRUCTURE OF VON WILLEBRAND FACTOR

The primary vWF translation product is protein containing 2813 amino acids with a predicted molecular weight of 309 kd.[44–48] Based on direct protein sequencing, the amino terminal of the mature vWF subunit can be located at codon 764.[38] The first 763 amino acids consist of a 22–amino acid hydrophobic signal peptide and a large propeptide that is identical with a protein found in plasma called vW antigen II.[49,50] The vWF propeptide is cleaved from the mature subunit between codons 763 and 764 after a pair of basic amino acids (Lys-Arg). Cleavage is presumed to be mediated by a member of a newly discovered enzyme family, with specificity for pairs of basic amino acids amd thus given the acronym *PACE* (*p*aired *a*mino acid *c*leaving *e*nzyme).[51] They are members of a subtilisin-related family of endoproteases and are homologous to the yeast enzyme Kex2.[52,53] Site specific mutagenesis of the vWF Lys-Arg sequence abolishes cleavage of the propolypeptide without disrupting vWF multimer assembly or function.[54,55] Persons have been described whose circulating vWF multimers are made up of an approximately equal mix of cleaved and uncleaved pro-vWF subunits.[56] It is presumed, but not proved, that they have mutations in the PACE recognition sequence. Despite the retention of the prosequence, hemostatic function is completely normal. In contrast, removal of the propeptide sequence from the vWF cDNA abolishes multimer formation, suggesting that at least one important function of the propeptide is to direct the assembly of vWF dimers into multimers.[54,55]

vWF is almost entirely composed of four types of homologous repeated sequences (Fig. 36-2). The D repeats, which contain most of the 233 cysteine residues found in each subunit, is repeated twice in the propeptide and again in the amino- and carboxy-terminal portions of each mature subunit. These cysteine-rich D repeats form large globular domains that are readily visible by molecular level electron microscopy.[57] The A repeats, which contain relatively few cysteine residues, are located in an extended filamentous region in the central third of each subunit.

The ligand interaction sites in vWF have been localized to specific repeats in the vWF polypeptide. The vWF A1 repeat, which extends from residues 449 to 728 of the mature vWF subunit, mediates vWF binding to the platelet gpIb/IX receptor[58,59] as well as to sulfated glycosaminoglycans, including heparin,[60–62] and to sulfatides.[63] Data derived from competitive inhibition binding studies with

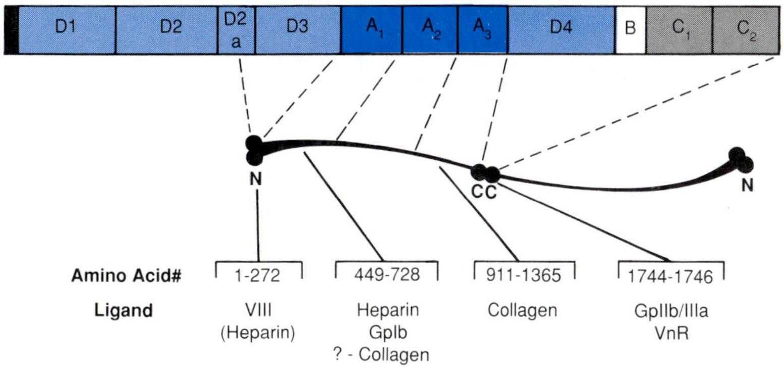

FIGURE 36-2. Organization of vWF cDNA and subunit polypeptide. The vWF cDNA encodes a series of homologous repeats. The D repeats encode much of the propolypeptide and the globular amino- and carboxy-terminal domains of the mature vWF subunit polypeptide. The triplicated A domains encode a filamentous extended region in the central third of each subunit. The A1 and A3 domains contain ligand binding sites of vWF interactions with collagen and heparin, as depicted. The binding site for factor VIII is located at the amino terminal of each subunit, and the gpIIb/IIIa interaction site is located near the carboxy terminal.

tryptic fragments of polymeric vWF and chemically synthesized peptides suggested, initially, that collagen binding sites were in both the A1 and A3 repeats.[64–67] More recent studies using purified recombinant proteins encoding the A1 and A3 domains have shown the principal collagen binding site in the mature vWF subunit is in the A3 domain between amino acids 911 and 1365.[68] The A2 repeat, made up of residues 729 to 910, has no known binding function, although, as discussed in the text that follows, it contains a protease-sensitive region important in the pathogenesis of some forms of type IIA vWD. The factor VIII binding site of vWF has been localized to the amino terminal 272 amino acid residues of the mature vWF subunit. Although the sequence spanning residues Thr78 to Thr96 was originally proposed as the entire factor VIII binding site,[69,70] subsequent experience with mutant forms of vWF that cannot bind factor VIII suggests that additional sites are important for the regulation of factor VIII binding outside this sequence.

The binding of factor VIII to vWF prevents its interaction with phospholipids.[71] Infusion of vWF into patients with severe vWD results in a prolonged supranormal elevation of factor VIII levels,[72] suggesting that vWF influences factor VIII biosynthesis or secretion.[73] This contention is supported by more recent experiments demonstrating that vWF promotes the association of the light and heavy chains of factor VIII[74,75] and enhances recombinant factor VIII production by transfected mammalian cells.[76]

Two RGD consensus adhesion recognition sequences are in the primary pro-vWF transcript. The RGD sequence is present in a number of adhesive glycoproteins and mediates their binding to cellular integrin receptors.[77] The importance of the RGD in the vWF propeptide is unclear. The second RGD sequence, at residues 1744 to 1746, is critically important for vWF binding to platelet gpIIb/IIIa.[78,79] Monoclonal antibodies recognizing epitopes in this region as well as high concentrations of the tetrapeptide RGDs inhibit vWF binding to activated platelets.[80,81] In addition, point mutations in the vWF RGD sequence selectively abolishes vWF binding to platelet gpIIb/IIIa.[82] Thus, each vWF subunit contains the information necessary to mediate all known vWF interactions. Despite the presence of functional binding sites in the vWF polypeptide subunit, the ability of vWF to mediate platelet adhesion depends on the assembly of multiple subunits into a large multimeric structure.[83]

The vWF gene contains 52 exons that span 178 kb of DNA on chromosome 12[84] (Fig. 36-3). The gene is so large that it encompasses 0.1% of the chromosome 12 DNA. Individual exons vary considerably in size, ranging from 40 bp to 1.4 kb. In general, little correlation exists between intron/exon boundaries and the homologous repeats previously noted in the vWF subunit polypeptide. Exon 28, the largest, encodes the entire A1 and A2 domains. This is of particular interest, since the mutations causing type IIA and IIB vWD are located in this segment of the vWF gene. In contrast, the A3 repeat, which is highly homologous, is encoded by five separate exons.

The human vWF gene has been localized to chromosome 12p12→pter.[85,86] The original gene localization studies were carried out with probes encoding the most 5′ regions of the vWF cDNA. When probes encoding sequence in the middle of the cDNA were used, a second vWF locus was identified, which was subsequently shown to be an incomplete pseudogene.[87] The pseudogene is located on chromosome 22q11.22-q11.23 and represents a nonprocessed duplication of exons 23 through 34.[88] It shares 97% sequence identity with the corresponding region of the authentic gene, although it also contains multiple translational stop signals and does not encode any protein product.[89] The human vWF pseudogene appears to be of relatively recent origin because it is not present in the genome of a number of

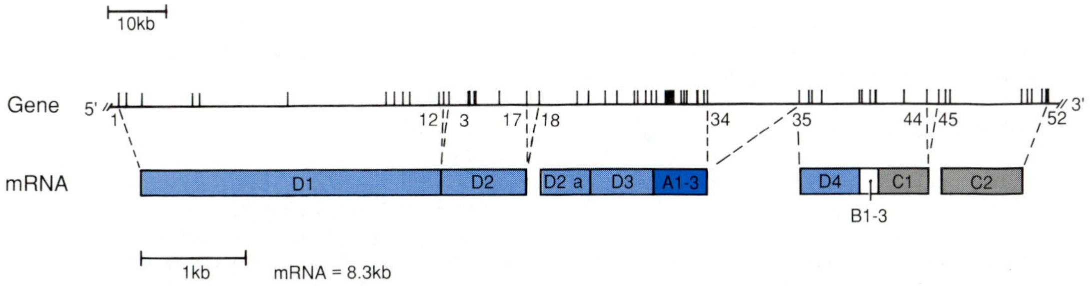

FIGURE 36-3. Organization of the vWF gene and its primary translation product. The gene is composed of 52 exons, which vary in size from 40 to 1400 bp. The single large exon of 28 encodes the entire A1 and A2 repeats and is the location of mutations causing type IIA and IIB vWD. The vWF gene is located on chromosome 12, and the incomplete pseudogene, which encompasses exons 23 to 34, is located on chromosome 22.

other mammalian species.[90,91] The presence of the pseudogene and the high degree of sequence identity between it and the authentic gene have complicated the analysis of vWF mutations, particularly in patients with type IIA and IIB vWD.

A large number of polymorphisms have been discovered in the vWD gene that have been used to study linkage between various vWD phenotypes and the vWF gene.[92–102] In addition, a useful variable number tandem repeat, with at least eight allelic forms, has been identified in intron 40.[103] The high degree of heterozygosity at this marker has made it informative in the study of families with various forms of vWD.

Little information is available on potential regulatory elements in the vWF gene. The translational start site has been mapped. Although there is a typical TATA box at position −30, no CCAAT or GC box elements have been described to date.[84,91,104] The paucity of information regarding vWF promoter elements may be due to the difficulty of transfecting the two relevant cell types, endothelial cells and megakaryocytes.

BIOSYNTHESIS, STORAGE, AND SECRETION OF VON WILLEBRAND FACTOR

Although vWF is usually thought of as a plasma protein, four distinct pools of vWF exist. Endothelial cell–derived vWF is secreted into the plasma, where it circulates in a complex with factor VIII and can bind to exposed subendothelium. Endothelial cells can also secrete vWF directly into subendothelium and contain a secretory pool of vWF, sequestered in Weibel-Palade bodies, which may be released during primary and secondary hemostasis. Megakaryocyte-derived vWF, which is localized in platelet α granules, is secreted by platelets during the formation of hemostatic plugs.

Endothelial Cells

Von Willebrand factor can be localized to endothelial cells within vascular tissue sections[105,106] and is readily detected in cultured endothelial cells.[107–111] The ability to establish and passage endothelial cells in culture has permitted a detailed understanding of vWF biosynthesis.[107,112] Although these processes have been chiefly characterized in human umbilical vein endothelial cells, more limited studies of endothelial cells derived from a number of adult vessels[113] and megakaryocytes[114] indicate that the umbilical vein is a representative model of vWF biosynthesis.

The precursor pro-vWF subunits first form covalently linked dimers in the endoplasmic reticulum through an unknown number of disulfide bonds in the COOH-terminal regions of adjacent subunits.[115,116] The addition of high-mannose carbohydrate is required for dimerization of vWF, since inhibition of Asn-linked glycosylation by pretreatment with tunicamycin prevents dimer formation and subsequent secretion.[117] The high-mannose carbohydrate is then processed to a more complex form in the Golgi apparatus yielding an approximately 600-kd dimer. Each subunit has 12 Asn-linked glycosylation sites, all but one of which contains the consensus Asn-X-Thr/Ser sequence.[38] A limited number of these Asn-linked oligosaccharides are also sulfated.[118,119] Complex carbohydrate formation is apparently not critical for subsequent molecular processing because inhibition of the Golgi enzyme mannosidase II by swainsonine does not prevent secretion of vWF.[120] Ten O-linked glycosylation sites (eight threonine and two serine residues) are also present in the vWF sequence,[38] and it may be presumed that these amino acids are glycosylated in the Golgi apparatus. Eight of these sites are clustered in the A1 domain, flanking a disulfide loop created by cysteines 509 and 695. Mature vWF contains 18.7% carbohydrate.[121]

The formation of larger multimers from pro-vWF dimers begins in the trans-Golgi and is completed in secretory vesicles. In this process, dimeric units are linked in a head-to-head fashion through disulfide bonds located within the D region (D3) of the NH_2 terminal to form expanding multimeric complexes.[115,116] Strong evidence suggests that the vWF propeptide mediates N-terminal polymerization of dimers into multimers. First, a truncated form of recombinant vWF lacking the propeptide sequence fails to form large multimers when expressed in heterologous cells.[54,55] Multimerization is restored by the coexpression of the vWF propeptide even when it is not expressed *cis* to the mature vWF subunit.[55] This suggests that free propeptide may transiently link to the mature vWF subunit and provide proper alignment of adjacent provWf dimers.[122] Recent evidence suggests that the presence of vicinal cysteines in each of the D domains in the propolypeptide is also needed for proper multimer assembly.[123] Cleavage of the 741 amino acid propolypeptide is one of the last steps in vWF biosynthesis and the cleaved pro sequence is colocalized and secreted along with mature vWF in both platelets[124] and endothelial cells.[125,126] In plasma, the propeptide circulates independently of vWF as a noncovalently linked homodimer of 100-kd subunits. Although it binds to collagen and inhibits platelet-collagen interactions, no specific biologic function has been ascribed to the circulating vWF propeptide.[127,128]

Storage Pools

Weibel-Palade Bodies. The endothelial cell vWF storage organelle is the Weibel-Palade body, a rod-shaped structure unique to endothelium. First described in large blood vessels, Weibel-Palade bodies have since been found in virtually all vascular and lymphatic endothelial cells.[129] Their abundance appears to be proportional to the diameter of the blood vessel[130] and may be increased in neovascular tissue surrounding certain tumors.[131–133] In the electron microscope, Weibel-Palade bodies are 0.1 μm in diameter and up to 4 μm in length and are surrounded by a unit membrane. Within the organelle are longitudinally arranged tubules, 150 Å in diameter, embedded in an electron-dense matrix. From electron microscopic studies, Weibel-Palade bodies appear to originate from the trans-Golgi apparatus and eventually distribute throughout the endothelial cytoplasm.[134,135]

The presence of vWF within the Weibel-Palade body was first demonstrated by immunoelectron microscopy[108–111] and later confirmed by cell fractionation techniques.[126,136] Fully processed vWF (subunit of 220 kd) and its propeptide (vW AgII) are the only secreted proteins identified within the organelle so far.[126,136,137] SDS-agarose analysis of Weibel-Palade body vWF has shown that it consists of an unusually large size distribution of multimeric forms.[126] The unique morphology of the Weibel-Palade body most likely is a result of the highly polymerized state of its principal secretory product. The precise conditions within the organelle that facilitate multimerization are not known, but both high protein concentration[138] and acidic conditions[139] promote vWF polymerization in vitro and are likely to contribute to the process. This contention is supported by the finding that multimer formation is inhibited by weak bases such as ammonium chloride or chloroquine, which disrupt the normally acidic conditions present within secretory organelles.[117]

Clinical Relevance. Clinical evidence shows that a sizable portion of the body stores of vWF exists in a rapidly mobilized storage pool. This accounts for the rapid rise in plasma vWF levels after exercise,[140] or the injection of agents, such as adrenalin,[140] vasopressin, nicotinic, acid and a vasopressin analogue, 1-deamino-8-D-arginine-vasopressin (DDAVP).[141] Vascular endothelium is thought to be the principal source of the increased plasma vWF observed under these conditions. vWF is also secreted by platelets stimulated by a variety of physiologic agonists, including thrombin, collagen, adenosine diphosphate, and epinephrine, although much of this protein remains associated with the platelet surface.[142]

Secretion

Endothelial cells, in culture, secrete vWF along both constitutive and regulated pathways.[143] The constitutive pathway is responsible for the basal secretion of smaller multimers. This pathway is directly linked to protein synthesis, since basal secretion can be blocked by cycloheximide, an inhibitor of protein synthesis.[144] In contrast, secretion by the regulated pathway, which requires exogenous stimulation of the endothelium, results in the release of unusually large vWF multimers and is unaffected by cycloheximide. In cultured endothelial cells, 5% of newly synthesized vWF is targeted for the regulated pathway, whereas the remainder is constitutively secreted.[145] The relative contribution of these two pathways to the plasma and subendothelial pools of vWF is unknown.

The basal rate of vWF secretion in cultured endothelial cells is regulated by both genetic and extragenic factors. Endothelial cells cultured from the umbilical vein of neonates subsequently diagnosed with type I vWD endothelial cells constitutively secrete less vWF and contain less vWF messenger RNA (mRNA) than their normal counterparts.[146–148] Harrison and McKee[149] demonstrated a significant increase in constitutive secretion of vWF in cultured endothelial cells in response to 17β-estradiol, a finding that mirrors the elevation of vWF plasma levels observed in pregnancy and in response to oral contraceptive medications.[150–152] Plasma vWF levels are also elevated during the course of bacterial, viral, and parasitic infections. It has been proposed that these acute, transient elevations are mediated by circulating mediators of the acute phase response such as interleukin-1 and tumor necrosis factor.[153] There have been conflicting reports on the effects of these cytokines on vWF secretion in vitro.[154–158]

Cultured endothelial cells rapidly secrete vWF in response to a number of naturally occurring agonists, including thrombin,[159,160] histamine,[161] leukotriene D4,[162] platelet-activating factor, vascular permeability factor, fibrin[163,164] and the terminal components of complement[165] (Fig. 36-4). In contrast, vasopressin analogues such as DDAVP, which cause rapid and marked elevations of vWF in vivo (see earlier discussion), do not directly stimulate vWF secretion in cultured endothelial cells.[166,167] Rather, they appear to act independently, by stimulating monocyte production of one or more endothelial cell agonists.[168]

Elevation of $[Ca^{2+}]_i$, in response to agonist is thought to be the critical second messenger regulating vWF secretion in endothelial cells.[107,144,161,169–171] In contrast to that which occurs in platelets, elevation of intracellular cAMP levels in endothelial cells does not inhibit thrombin- or calcium ionophore–induced vWF secretion.[144]

After agonist stimulation, Weibel-Palade bodies are rapidly translocated to the cell surface.[172] Fusion of organelle and plasma membranes occurs rapidly after agonist addition and is maximal within 10 minutes.[165] Release of vWF within the granules takes longer, and "release patches" of vWF, noted by immunofluorescence, can persist for several hours.[145,163] In contrast, vW AgII, which colocalizes with vWF in the Weibel-Palade body, does not remain associated with the cells after release.[122] The association of vWF with the external surface of the endothelial cell may be mediated by the endothelial vitronectin receptor,[173,174] by the gpIb receptor,[175,176] or by an as yet unidentified constituent of the Weibel-Palade body itself.

Plasma Von Willebrand Factor

Origin and Physical Characteristics

The plasma concentration of vWF is about 10 μg/mL. Although vWF is synthesized in both endothlial cells and megakaryocytes, both clinical observations and animal models suggest that most of the plasma vWF is derived from vascular endothelial cells. First, patients with severe thrombocytopenia secondary to bone marrow failure (aplastic anemia, congenital amegakaryocytosis) have normal plasma vWF levels. Second, transplantation of normal bone marrow into a pig with severe vWD fails to elevate

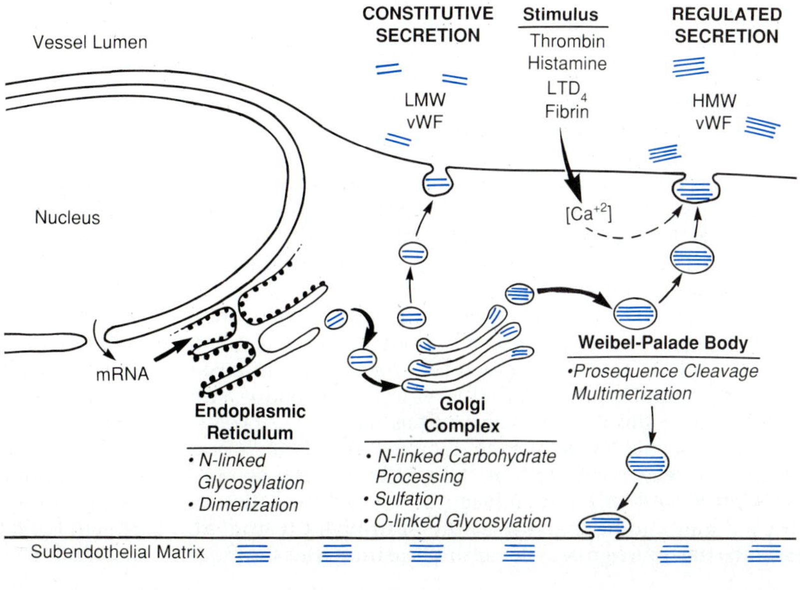

FIGURE 36-4. Biosynthesis and secretion of vWF in endothelial cells (see text for details). This model is based principally on in vitro data, and the relative contributions of the constitutive and regulated pathway in the formation of plasma vWF multimeric pattern are not known.

the plasma vWF levels, despite normalization of platelet vWF content.[177]

One of the hallmarks of vWF is its propensity to form extremely large polymers (multimers) made up of integral numbers of dimeric units each of which in turn contain two identical 220-kd subunits. A series of such multimers is normally found in plasma ranging in size from 450 to 20,000 kd.[178,179] The relative contribution of the constitutive and regulated pathways of endothelial cell secretion to the spectrum of plasma multimers remains controversial.[145,180,181] Even under normal circumstances, a small fraction of subunits consists of uncleaved precursor or proteolytically degraded forms that give rise to satellite bands on high-resolution SDS-agarose gels.

In plasma, vWF circulates in a noncovalent complex with factor VIII with a stoichiometry of about 50:1 (vWF to factor VIII) by weight. This association serves to stabilize plasma factor VIII activity that is otherwise lost because of proteolysis[2,182,183] and to facilitate factor VIII activation by thrombin.[184]

Extragenic Modulation of Plasma Levels

Influence of Blood Type. The influence of the ABO blood group locus on plasma levels of the VIII/vWF complex was first noted by Preston and Barr[185] and has been confirmed and extended in several subsequent studies. Blood type O has been universally associated with lower factor VIII[186–190] and vWF[187–192] levels, although some disagreement exists on possible differences among individuals with the A, B, and AB blood group types. In one carefully performed study of 158 monozygotic and dizygotic twin pairs, Ørstavik and associates[188] concluded that the effect on factor VIII was secondary to the effect on vWF and that 30% of the genetic variance of the level of vWF was due to the ABO blood type. Moreover, these investigators determined that the level of vWF varied inversely with the amount of plasma H substance, being lowest in group O, intermediate in group A_2 and highest in group A_1, B, and AB individuals. This conclusion was further supported by the finding that among persons belonging to blood group O, those found to be secretors (Lewis phenotype [Le(a−b+)]), and thus known to have the highest levels of plasma H substance,[193] also had the lowest levels of vWF and factor VIII.[194]

The mechanism by which the ABO locus influences vWF levels is unknown. The association is clearly not the result of genetic linkage between ABO and vWF genes since the gene for ABO is on chromosome 9,[195] whereas the gene for vWF is on chromosome 12.[39] Blood group antigens A, B, and H are present on vWF.[196,197] It has been postulated that these oligosaccharide structures influence the biosynthesis, secretion, or catabolism of the protein. Since removal of terminal sialic acid residues from vWF oligosaccharides shortens its survival, the catabolism of the protein may be influenced by ABO-related carbohydrate moieties.[196]

Age. Both factor VIII and vWF levels are moderately low in preterm infants then rise above adult norms at term.[198] The stress of the delivery itself may be at least partially responsible for the elevation of the factor VIII/vWF complex. For this reason, the diagnosis of vWD may be missed in the newborn period.[199] Both fetal and neonatal plasma contain unusually large vWF multimers similar to those seen found in endothelial Weibel-Palade bodies and platelet α granules.[200–202] Among persons aged 10 to 70 years, plasma concentrations of both factor VIII[186,188,203,204] and vWF[188] increase with age. Although both Graham and associates[189]and Gill and colleagues[190] found the increase in vWF levels to be linear over the entire period studied, Jeremic and colleagues[186] noted that the increase was more marked in the later years. As is true for the effects of blood group antigens, the effect of age on factor VIII is due to its primary effect on vWF levels.[188]

Hormonal Influences. Increased levels of vWF have been reported in healthy pregnant women and in women taking oral contraceptives.[152,205,206] Similar findings have been reported in most[150,151,207–210] but not all[207,211] patients with vWD. vWF levels rise incrementally throughout pregnancy and, in type I vWD patients, often reach normal at term.[210] This spontaneous correction in vWF during pregnancy obviates the need for specific therapy in the normal delivery of most patients, although postpartum hemorrhage may occur caused by the rapid fall of vWF and factor VIII levels that follow delivery.[207,209,212] Pregnancy-associated increases in plasma levels of abnormal vWF with hyperaffinity to platelets in patients with type IIB vWD (see later discussion) may lead to profound thrombocytopenia.[213,214]

Thyroid hormone also influences vWF levels,[215] and hypothyroidism may induce mild acquired vWD with clinical bleeding.[216–219] In all reported cases, plasma vWF returned to normal after correction of the hormonal deficiency. Moreover, both hyperthyroidism and the administration of thyroxine to euthyroid subjects increase vWF levels.[215,220] The mechanism by which thyroid hormone controls vWF plasma levels is not known but has been postulated to result from nonspecific effects on mRNA and protein synthesis.[217]

Physical Activity. A rapid increase in plasma factor VIII activity after exercise was first noted by Rizza[221] and later confirmed in a number of independent studies.[222,223] Exercise also induces a rapid but slightly smaller increase in both plasma vWF:Ag and vWF:RCoF activity.[223–226] It is not known whether the disproportionate increase in factor VIII activity is due to preferential release of factor VIII from a separate storage site, enhancement of factor VIII activity,[224] or an increase in factor VIII binding to vWF after exercise. Prior treatment with the calcium channel blocker verapamil (but not nicardipine) blunts the rise in exercise-induced vWF:Ag release.[227]

Extracellular Matrix

The vWF present in vascular subendothelium is predominantly derived from the overlying endothelial cell layer.[228,229] vWF binds to the subendothelium in an unsaturable manner that does not require calcium.[230,231] Binding is principally to types I, III, and VI collagen,[232–236] although binding to fibronectin[237] and heparin[238] may also be important. vWF can bind to both fibrillar and nonfibrillar type III collagen, whereas nonfibrillar type I collagen binds vWF poorly.[234] All three chains of type VI collagen, which is abundant in extracellular matrices,[239] contain regions homologous to the vWF A domains and to platelet gpIb, which could play a role in binding.[240] The binding of vWF to immobilized collagen fibrils is saturable and reversible and of moderately high affinity.[241]

vWF in the extracellular cellular matrix consists of extremely HMW multimers containing fully processed 225-kd subunits.[242] Although HMW forms of vWF bind most avidly to subendothelium,[235,243,244] lower-molecular-weight forms of vWF are also capable of supporting platelet adhesion.[245]

The role of subendothelial matrix–vWF interactions in primary hemostasis has been inferred, chiefly from perfusion experiments. In 1973, Baumgartner[15] described a technique performed with blood in which an annular device with a central core containing an everted segment of rabbit aorta that had been previously denuded of endothelial cells by balloon catheterization. Experiments have used everted segments of human renal or umbilical artery.[230,246] Blood is passed over the vessel segments under controlled conditions of temperature and flow, permitting detailed rheologic analysis.[247,248] After perfusion, the number of platelets bound, or bound to and spread on the subendothelial surface, as well as any platelet thrombi, can be determined using standard histologic methods. A modification of this technique permits perfusion of unanticoagulated venous blood.[249]

In these perfusion models, performed at high shear rates corresponding to those encountered in small arteries and capillaries, platelet–subendothelial matrix interactions depend on the vWF bound to the subendothelial matrix.[249] Thus, when plasma vWF is bound to subendothelium and the subendothelium subsequently exposed to reconstituted blood, platelet adherence correlates with the amount of prebound vWF.[230] Preincubation of vessel segments or extracellular matrix with antibodies to vWF reduces platelet adhesion.[250–252] The adhesion of platelets to subendothelium at arterial shear rates (500 to 1000 s^{-1}) is reduced after perfusion with citrated blood from patients with vWD[253] or from normal persons who had been depleted of vWF by adsorption with anti-vWF antibodies.[254] The adhesion of platelets to subendothelium at arterial shear rates (500 to 1000 s^{-1}) is reduced after perfusion with citrated blood from patients with vWD[253] or from normal persons who had been depleted of vWF by adsorption with anti-vWF antibodies.[254] Immobilized fractions of purified vWF have also been shown to support platelet adhesion in parallel plate perfusion chambers.[255–257]

Adhesion of platelets to native vWF occurs only when the vWF is bound to a surface. It has been proposed that the binding of vWF to subendothelial proteins, or to other substrates, induces a change in confirmation that supports platelet adhesion,[258] but the molecular nature of this alteration is unknown.

Megakaryocytes and Platelets

Von Willebrand factor is also synthesized by megakaryocytes[259] and stored within the α granules of mature platelets.[260–265] The complex steps of vWF biosynthesis in the megakaryocyte appear to be similar to those previously noted in the endothelial cells.[114] Platelet α granules are membrane-limited, spherical bodies (0.3 to 0.5 μm in diameter) that contain numerous other proteins in addition to vWF. In contrast to other α-granule proteins, vWF is eccentrically localized within the organelle and forms tubular structures reminiscent of those seen in Weibel-Palade bodies.[266] Many α-granule constituent proteins are not synthesized by the megakaryocyte or the platelet but enter the megakaryocyte endocytosis and are then transported to the α granule.[267] Although megakaryocytes synthesize vWF in culture,[259] the possibility that some fraction of the platelet-associated vWF might be derived from the plasma pool cannot be excluded.

Platelet vWF content is between 0.25 and 0.8 U/10^9 platelets as measured by electroimmunoassay (EIA) and immunoradiometric assay (IRMA) and accounts for about 20% of the blood pool of vWF.[28,268,269] Platelet-associated vWF, like the Weibel-Palade body pool of endothelial cell vWF, contains an increased proportion of large multimeric species and an increased ratio of vWF:RCoF activity to vWF:Ag when compared with that contained in plasma.[269,270] On stimulation, vWF is secreted along with the other granule contents. About 65% of the α-granule pool of vWF remains associated with the platelet.[142,270–272]

The physiologic relevance of platelet vWF is underscored by a number of clinical and experimental observations. First, the prolonged bleeding time in subsets of patients with type I vWD (see text that follows) can be best correlated with the amount of platelet-associated vWF.[273,274] Second, platelets obtained from type III vWD patients, when resuspended in normal plasma, adhere less well to collagen fibrils or rabbit subendothelium than do normal platelets.[275,276] Third, patients with severe vWD treated with both normal platelets and cryoprecipitate have a more pronounced shortening of the bleeding time than those treated with cryoprecipitate alone.[277]

Heterologous Expression

Although vWF biosynthesis is normally restricted to endothelial cells and megakaryocytes, vWF cDNA can be transfected into a variety of heterologous cells to produce functional vWF multimers. The original transfections were carried out in COS and CHO cells but have been extended to a variety of other cultured cell lines.[44,54,123,278–281] In each case, vWF multimers are constitutively secreted into the conditioned medium. In contrast, in endothelial cells and megakaryocytes, much or all of the vWF is packaged into secretory organelles like the Weibel-Palade body and the α granule. Packaging of vWF for secretion has also been achieved in a heterologous cell model. The transfection of vWF cDNA into AtT20 cells, a pituitary cell line that secretes ACTH, results in the assembly and packaging of vWF multimers in granules.[278,281] These studies suggest that all the information needed for both the assembly of multimeric vWF and its sorting into granules is derived from its primary sequence. In addition, they suggest that the tissue-specific expression is regulated by *cis* and *trans* regulatory elements in the vWF promoter region.

CLINICAL DESCRIPTION

Presentation

Most patients with vWD have clinical symptoms consistent with a primary hemostatic defect. Mucocutaneous bleeding, including epistaxis, easy bruising, and gingival bleeding, was reported in 35% to 60% of patients observed in two large studies.[24,282] Menorrhagia, often severe, is reported in about one third of women with vWD. Postsurgical bleeding, especially after dental extraction or tonsillectomy, is common and is often the event that leads to the initial diagnosis. Gastrointestinal bleeding, sometimes associated with colonic angiodysplasia or telangiectasia, is seen in about 10% of patients. Hemarthroses and muscle bleeding are decidedly rare, except in severely affected patients with factor VIII levels of less than 5%.

Prevalence

Generally vWD is claimed to be the most common inherited bleeding disorder. Previously cited incidences, of between 4 and 7 per 100,000 population, are likely to be underestimates.[283,284] In a recent epidemiologic investigation of more than 1200 schoolchildren in northern Italy, vWD as defined by a low vWF level in combination with either a family history of low vWF levels or a personal or family history of clinically significant bleeding, was diagnosed in 1% of children studied.[285] The incidence of severe type III vWD varies from 0.11 to 0.55 per million persons in most of Europe to about 3.1 per million persons in Sweden and 5.3 per million persons in Israel.[286–288] Overall, mild type I vWD accounts for 75% to 80% of all cases, with the remainder classified principally to one of the type II varieties.[289,290]

LABORATORY EVALUATION

In severe cases, with unequivocal quantitative or qualitative vWF abnormalities, the diagnosis of vWD is straightforward. In contrast, the diagnosis in mild cases can be problematic. The bleeding time, factor VIII, vWF antigen and vWF:RCoF activity have become the standard screening tests for vWD. Based on these conventional laboratory tests, it has been estimated that the penetrance of the vWD genotype varies from 60% to 90%.[291,292] Yet, in a study of affected persons from two extended families, only 15% had abnormal results on all four tests and 50% of patients carrying a vWD allele by pedigree analysis had only one abnormal test result.[291,292] Thus, the sensitivity and specificity of laboratory tests for the vWD phenotype are lower than those observed in other common disorders. In light of the pronounced intraindividual variability of different hemostatic variables, most clinicians recommend repeated testing of a person who is at risk before excluding the diagnosis of vWD.[293,294] Although the use of discriminant analysis improves the diagnosis of the heterozygous vWD phenotype, this approach is not commonly used.[292]

Bleeding Time

Bleeding time is regarded by many clinicians as the most reliable in vivo indicator of primary hemostatic function. Although, when carefully analyzed, measurement of bleeding time is not generally useful for the preoperative screening of patients without a personal or family bleeding history,[295–297] bleeding time remains an important tool in the diagnosis of vWD. The method of Duke (1910), which measures the duration of bleeding from small incisions in the ear lobe, was the technique used in the earliest descriptions of vWD.[298] This method is relatively insensitive and difficult to quantitate and may induce uncontrollable hemorrhage and hematomas in patients with severe vWD.

In most hospitals, bleeding times are performed using a modification[299,300] of the Ivy technique.[301] This involves making an incision on the volar aspect of the forearm while venous pressure is maintained at 40 mm Hg with a blood pressure cuff. Tests based on Ivy methodology are more sensitive than those based on the older Duke ear lobe method for detecting vWD.[302,303] Tests for bleeding time remain difficult to standardize, are notoriously dependent on the experience of the person administering the test, and may be produce normal results in a large percentage of mildly affected patients.[291,292,304,305] It had been suggested that the sensitivity of bleeding time for the diagnosis of vWD could be increased by first treating patients with low doses of aspirin.[306,307] A third technique, involving the puncture of the tip of a finger with a surgical blade, was shown to be as sensitive as the Ivy method.[308] Although this method enjoys the advantage of not producing a scar at the site of incision, it is not widely used.

Despite these limitations, the judicious use of the bleeding time in patients with an established diagnosis of vWD provides some measure of the severity of the bleeding diathesis. Similarly, the bleeding time can be used, in certain circumstances, to help judge the effectiveness of treatment.

Factor VIII

As discussed, factor VIII biosynthesis, secretion, and plasma stability are regulated by vWF. Thus, a diminution of plasma vWF:Ag levels is usually accompanied by a parallel reduction in factor VIII.[289] However, reduction of factor VIII is not a universal finding in mild vWD, and increased factor VIII/vWF:Ag ratios are not uncommon.[305,309] Because factor VIII levels are only moderately reduced in most forms of vWD, the activated partial thromboplastin time may remain in the normal range. Thus, a normal aPTT does not exclude the diagnosis of vWD.

In Vitro Assays of Von Willebrand Factor

Immunologic Measurements

Immunologic measurements of vWF (vWF:Ag) may be performed by EIA,[28] IRMA,[310–314] or enzyme-linked immunoassay (ELISA).[315–318] In EIA,[30] plasma samples undergo electrophoresis through agarose gels containing polyspecific anti-vWF antibodies. The resulting precipitin line appears as a rocket, whose height depends on the concentration of vWF present in the original plasma sample. Increased sensitivity can be achieved by using radiolabeled anti-vWF antibodies in the agarose gel.[319] IRMA and ELISA of vWF offer greater sensitivity. Important methodologic differences exist between EIA, which measures the number of vWF molecules, and both IRMA and ELISA, which measure the number of antigenic sites on vWF. Thus, vWF:Ag levels appear higher in vWD subtypes with a reduced concentration of large multimers when measured by EIA than when analyzed by IRMA or ELISA methods. This discrepancy is often so pronounced that it has been suggested as a means of identifying subtypes of vWD that lack the HMW vWF multimers in the plasma.[320]

Multimeric Analysis

Crossed Immunoelectrophoresis. One of the earliest methods devised to analyze the multimeric composition of vWF was crossed immunoelectrophoresis. vWF multimers are first separated by electrophoresis in agarose, then subjected to immunoelectrophoresis in a second direction through agarose containing anti-vWF antibodies. The resultant precipitin line reflects the partial separation of vWF multimers in the first dimension. Thus, samples deficient in the multimers with the highest molecular weights, like those found in the plasma of patients with type II vWD, lack the most cathodal portion of the normal protein arc.

SDS-Agarose Electrophoresis. More recently, electrophoretic methods have been developed, which more clearly separate each of the many multimeric forms of vWF. In this method, vWF multimers are separated on agarose gels in the presence sodium dodecyl sulfate. Resolution in the regions of the multimeric spectrum with the highest or lowest molecular weights can be optimized by varying the concentration and gelling characteristics of the agarose and the length of the gel.[179,268,321] The multimers are then visualized by incubation of the gel with ^{125}I-labeled[268] or enzyme-linked antibodies[322] to vWF. Alternatively, the separated multimers of vWF may be transferred to nitrocellulose and detected with one of several enzyme-linked antibody systems.[323–327] Each of these electrophoretic methods permits a direct and clear comparison among several samples in a single run and has provided potentially important insights into the molecular basis of the abnormalities underlying type II vWD. For example, in the regions of the gel with the lowest molecular weight, high-resolution SDS-agarose electrophoresis has demonstrated that each multimeric band is actually composed of a predominant species accompanied by two to four satellite components with slightly different electrophoretic mobilities.[179,328] The satellite components are thought to represent proteolytic fragments of the predominant species. Several of the type II vWD subtypes (see text that follows) have been defined based on differences in the electrophoretic patterns produced by these fragments. Typical electrophoretic patterns are shown in Figures 36-5 through 36-8.

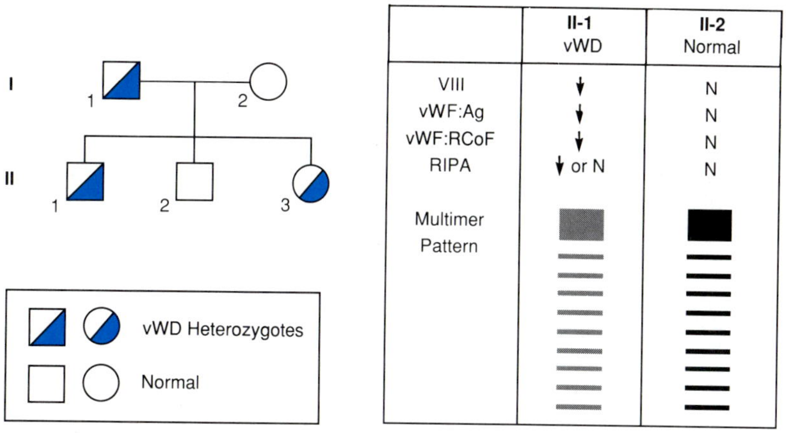

FIGURE 36-5. Inheritance and laboratory abnormalities in type I vWD. Typically, there is a proportional decrease in factor VIII, vWF:Ag, and vWF:RCoF activity. RIPA is most often normal. All multimeric forms are present, albeit in reduced abundance. Incomplete penetrance of the vWD phenotype is common, and direct linkage of type I vWD to the vWF gene has been established in only a few pedigrees.

Functional Assays of Von Willebrand Factor

Background

Early studies of von Willebrand and Jurgens[12] demonstrated that, in contrast to platelets derived from normal persons or from patients with classic hemophilia, platelets from patients with vWD did not agglutinate normally in a "capillary thrombometer." A number of laboratory techniques are available to demonstrate abnormal vWF-platelet interactions in vWD. Perhaps the most relevant are those that analyze platelet–subendothelial matrix interactions under defined conditions of temperature and flow rate.[253] Although such studies have provided valuable insights into vWF physiology, they require highly sophisticated equipment and are technically difficult to perform. Similarly, assays based on the retention of platelets on glass beads[13,329,330] are sensitive indicators of vWF dysfunction even when other laboratory tests are equivocal.[24] Some investigators have found this test inconsistent and nonspecific and it is rarely used today.[331] In contrast, assays based on the interaction of the antibiotic ristocetin with vWF and platelets are relatively simple to perform and have become the predominant clinical laboratory test of vWF function.

Ristocetin-Based Assays

Ristocetin is an antibiotic isolated from *Nocardia lurida*, which has a molecular structure and spectrum of activity similar to those of vancomycin. It was withdrawn soon after its introduction in the 1950s because it caused thrombocytopenia and macroscopic aggregation of platelets in vitro.[32] The link between this deleterious side effect and vWF was made by Howard and Firkin,[31] who observed that ristocetin induced platelet aggregation in platelet-rich plasma from normal persons but not in that from vWD patients.

The molecular basis of the ristocetin-mediated binding of vWF to the platelets has been partially elucidated. Ristocetin-induced platelet aggregation is known to be mediated by the passive binding of vWF to platelet gpIb/IX and subsequent platelet activation through a poorly defined signal transduction pathway.[332,333] The essential role of gpIb/IX in the process is demonstrated by the fact that ristocetin fails to induce the aggregation of platelets from patients with Bernard-Soulier syndrome, who lack the gpIb/IX receptor complex.[33,334,335] Platelets treated with proteolytic enzymes that partially degrade gpIb and platelets that have been treated with monoclonal antibodies to gpIb do not agglutinate with ristocetin.[336,337] Although, in the presence of vWF, appropriate concentrations of ristocetin can induce metabolically active platelets to aggregate with activation of the gpIIb/IIIa receptor, the binding of vWF to gpIb/IX and the initial wave of agglutination constitute a passive process and occur even with formalin-fixed platelets.

The mechanism by which ristocetin induces vWF-mediated platelet agglutination is complex and incompletely understood. Ristocetin binds to platelets and reduces their electrostatic surface charge, which could promote the binding of vWF to gpIb/IX.[338] Other cationic compounds, such as Polybrene, can also promote vWF-dependent platelet agglutination.[339–341] Ristocetin can also bind to vWF and may reduce its net negative charge and alter its confirmation. Similarly, modified vWF, in which

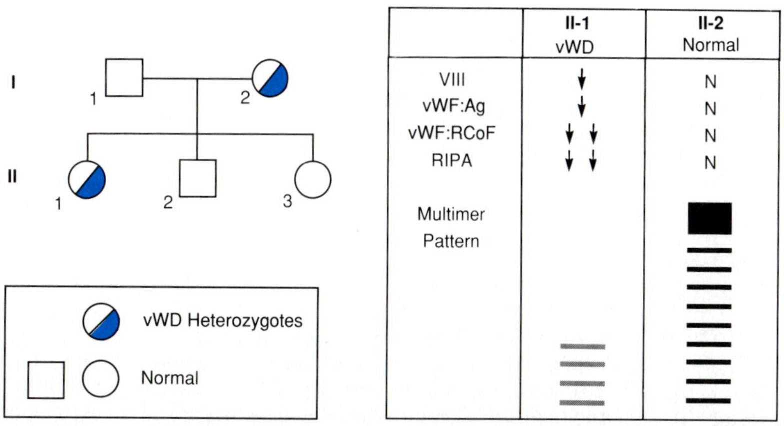

FIGURE 36-6. Inheritance pattern and expected laboratory abnormalities in type IIA vWD. A disproportionate reduction in vWF:RCoF activity is typical, and vWF:Ag and factor VIII levels may be in the low-normal range. Both large and intermediate-sized multimers are absent in the plasma but may be present in the platelet. Similar laboratory abnormalities are seen in other forms of type II vWD and can be distinguished only by high-resolution agarose gel electrophoretic patterns.

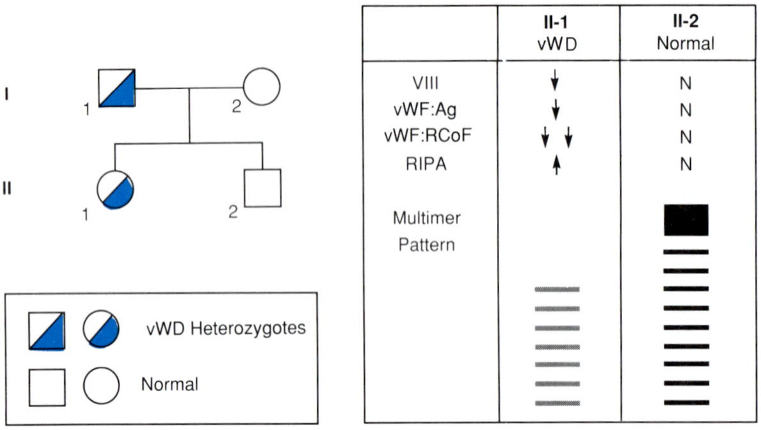

FIGURE 36-7. Inheritance pattern and laboratory abnormalities in type IIB vWD. Hypersensitivity to ristocetin in the RIPA assay is diagnostic of this (or related) subtype. The largest multimer species are typically lacking in plasma but present in the platelet pool.

negatively charged sialic acid residues have been enzymatically removed (asialo vWF), induces platelet aggregation in the absence of ristocetin.[342–344]

Evidence also exists that ristocetin-mediated platelet agglutination depends most heavily on the largest multimeric forms of vWF. First, ristocetin-mediated platelet agglutination is diminished out of proportion to vWF:Ag in those vWD subtypes in which high molecular vWF multimers are missing.[268,345,346] Second, pools of HMW vWF show enhanced binding to gpIb/IX and increased ristocetin-dependent platelet agglutination.[34,347,348] Whether the requirement of HMW weight forms of vWF for optimal ristocetin-dependent platelet-vWF interactions is related to the increased number of potential platelet receptor binding sites, or simply to an increase in the size of the vWF molecule, is unknown.

Ristocetin-Induced Platelet Aggregation

In the ristocetin-induced platelet aggregation (RIPA) assay, final concentrations of 0.3 to 1.2 mg/mL of ristocetin are added to platelet-rich plasma in an aggregometer. Despite attempts to make the test semiquantitative by careful titration of pH and standardization of mixing conditions, the test remains qualitative.[349] Most clinical laboratories simply report the minimum concentration of ristocetin capable of inducing a preestablished degree of aggregation, usually a 30% increase in light transmission. The RIPA test is relatively insensitive, is not abnormal until the vWF:Ag level falls below 30%, and thus fails to detect many patients with mild to moderate vWD.[33,350] The RIPA test is easy to perform in conjunction with other platelet aggregation studies and is essential in diagnosing those vWD variants with enhanced responsiveness to ristocetin such as type I (*New York*),[351] type IIB[352] and pseudo-vWD.[353] Patients whose defects reside in the vWF molecule (eg, vWD type IIB) can also be distinguished from those with abnormal platelets (pseudo-vWD) by comparing the response of washed normal platelets in the presence of patient plasma with that of washed patient platelets in the presence of normal plasma.

Ristocetin Cofactor Activity

Ristocetin cofactor (RCof) activity assays are designed to obtain information about the function of the plasma vWF. Dilutions of patient plasma are tested for their ability to induce the agglutination of either washed normal platelets[25] or paraformaldehyde-fixed platelets[332] in the presence of a fixed concentration of ristocetin (usually 1 mg/mL). The availability of lyophilized fixed platelets has allowed standardization among clinical laboratories.[354] The vWF:RCoF activity can be quantified by measuring the maximal rate of agglutination or the time to visible agglutination.[355] In type I vWD, the reduction in vWF:RCoF activity parallels that of vWF:Ag. In many of the subtypes in which HMW multimers are absent or reduced in the plasma, vWF:RCoF

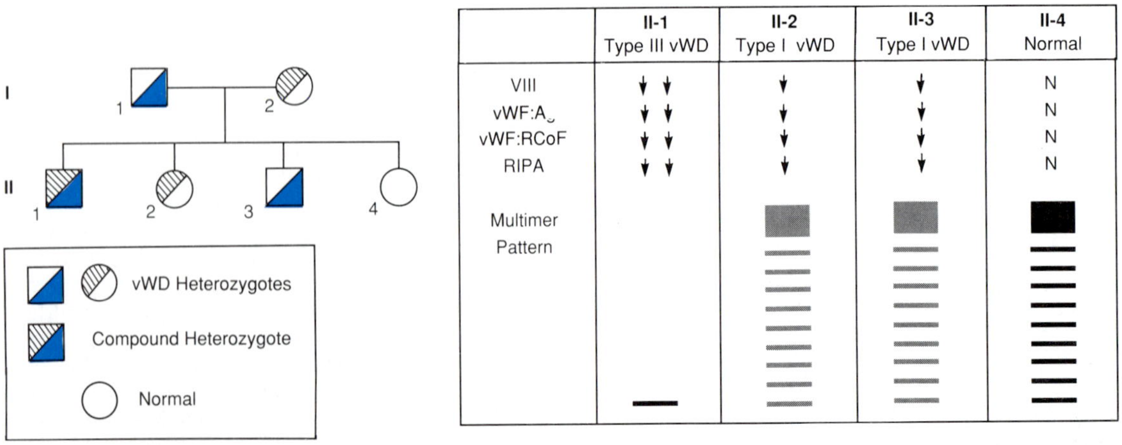

FIGURE 36-8. The inheritance pattern and expected laboratory abnormalities in type III vWD. Typically, vWF:Ag and vWF:RCoF are undetectable and factor VIII levels are measureable but low (below 5 U/dL) in type III vWD patients. Obligate heterozygotes often appear as type I vWD patients but are sometimes clinically normal and may even exhibit normal laboratory parameters.

activity may be decreased disproportionately. This test correlates moderately well with both the bleeding time and clinical bleeding.[25,289,356]

Platelet Retention on Glass Beads

In this assay, citrated blood is passed over a column of glass beads, and the difference between the afferent and efferent platelet count is recorded to calculate platelet adhesiveness or retention.[13,329,330,357] Net retention on the column is dependent on initial adhesion of platelets to the beads, which is largely dependent on fibrinogen, and subsequent platelet–platelet interactions and aggregate formation, which are dependent on both vWF and released adenosine diphosphate. A number of important variables that can affect the assay have been identified, including presence or absence of red cells, temperature, contact time of blood with the glass beads, type of anticoagulant and type of plastic used in the column.[358] The assay is technically difficult and has been supplanted by the ristocetin-based tests.

CLASSIFICATION

More than 20 distinct variants of vWD have been described.[359] Although a complete classification of vWD requires a fuller understanding of the molecular basis of the disease, it has been possible to establish a working classification system based on clinical and laboratory criteria. As in other genetic disorders, the present classification seeks to first differentiate between quantitative and qualitative abnormalities (Table 36-1).

Quantitative Disorders of Von Willebrand Factor

The quantitative group includes subtypes with a reduction in plasma vWF but, with few exceptions, no obvious abnormalities in vWF structure or function. This group may be broadly divided on the basis of vWF:Ag levels into mild (5 to 35 U/dL) and severe (less than 5 U/dL) categories. Characteristically, there is a concordant reduction of vWF: Ag levels, vWF:RCoF activity, and factor VIII levels.

Type I

Mild or type I vWD accounts for 60% to 70% of all cases of vWD.[346,360] Affected patients manifest highly variable clinical symptoms, but the bleeding diathesis is rarely life-threatening. Characteristically, there is a concordant reduction of vWF:Ag, vWF:RCoF activity, and factor VIII levels (see Fig. 34-5). A full range of vWF multimers is exhibited on SDS-agarose gels, although the intensities of high-, intermediate-, and low-molecular-weight forms may not always be normal.

The molecular basis of most forms of type I vWD has not been elucidated. Perhaps most perplexing is the fact that the phenotypic expression of the severe vWD genotype is variable. Thus, gene deletions or nonsense mutations, when present in the homozygous form, markedly reduce vWF levels and cause severe clinical disease, and may produce mild bleeding, modest laboratory abnormalities, or a totally normal phenotype in heterozygotes.[87,286,361–363] This variability in the phenotypic expression in heterozygotes is probably due to the influences of factors both intrinsic to the vWD gene and to a variety of extragenic influences that may affect the biosynthesis, intracellular storage, and secretion of vWF. Many patients with autosomal dominant type I vWD are likely to carry alleles that function in a "dominant-negative" manner and interfere with the expression of the normal vWF allele.[43]

Platelet-Associated vWF. Patients with type I vWD can be subdivided on the basis of the platelet vWF content. By comparing platelet and plasma vWF levels, Weiss and associates[320] identified three distinct vWD subgroups. In patients classified as having type I-1, a parallel reduction was found in both plasma and platelet vWF:Ag content. In contrast, five unrelated patients classified as having type I-2 had moderately decreased plasma vWF levels (33 to 57 U/dL), but normal levels of platelet vWF (58 to 130 U/dL). Finally, two patients, classified as having type I-3, were described in whom platelet vWF, but not plasma vWF, was reduced. One of these patients was the asymptomatic father of a severely affected vWD patient.

An alternative subdivision of type I vWD patients on the basis of platelet vWF content was proposed by Mannucci and associates,[273] who described six patients from four kindred with severe reductions in plasma vWF:Ag (4 to 11 U/dL) and vWF:RCoF (below 7 U/dL) levels and normal platelet levels of vWF. These patients were classified as "platelet-normal" to distinguish them from "platelet-low" patients in whom similar reductions in plasma and platelet vWF:Ag and vWF:RCoF activity were noted. It has been hypothesized that platelet-low vWD results from defective production of vWF, whereas platelet-normal vWD arises from the impaired release of vWF from cellular compartments. Importantly, the bleeding time in platelet-normal patients is either normal or modestly prolonged despite the striking reduction in plasma vWF levels.[273] A highly significant inverse relation between bleeding time and the level of platelet (but not plasma) vWF in type I vWD patients was also noted by Gralnick and colleagues.[274] Moreover, platelet-normal patients have a better response to DDAVP infusions when judged by the increase in plasma vWF levels and reduction in bleeding time. The molecular and cellular basis of the discordance between plasma and platelet vWF has not been established.

vWD Vicenza. Two kindreds have been identified in which plasma vWF contains a set of larger-than-normal (supranormal) vWF multimers, similar to those present in plasma after desmopressin infusion (see later discussion).[364] In this subtype, termed vWD *Vicenza*, although plasma factor VIII, vWF:Ag, and vWF:RCoF activity levels are low, the bleeding time is slightly prolonged and bleeding manifestations are mild. The relatively mild clinical symptoms associated with this subtype are thought to be due to normal levels of platelet vWF.[365] The gentic defect has been localized close to or within the vWF gene.[366]

Type III

Type III vWD is characterized by marked reductions in vWF:Ag (less than 4 U/dL), vWF:RCoF (less than 5 U/dL) and factor VIII (less than 20 U/dL) levels[286,367] (see Fig. 36-8). In some patients, plasma vWF:Ag is undetectable by sensitive radioimmunoassays, with sensitivity down to 0.01 U/dL.[312] vWF is also markedly decreased or absent in platelets[368] and in vascular endothelial cells.[369] Factor VIII levels are always depressed although still measurable (1 to 5 U/dL) even in patients in whom the vWF:Ag activity is undetectable.[361,367] Clinically, patients are severely affected and experience frequent mucocutaneous bleeding episodes. Because factor VIII is also severely diminished, patients may experience classic hemophilic symptoms, including hemarthroses and deep hematomas.

The inheritance of type III vWD is usually recessive and carriers (identified by restriction fragment length polymorphism [RFLP] or gene deletion analysis) of the type III vWD trait may be asymptomatic and have normal laboratory tests. In a number of cases, carriers have subnormal vWF:Ag or vWF:RCoF activity levels, similar to type I vWD

TABLE 36-1. Summary of Inherited von Willebrand's Disease Phenotypes

Subtype	Clinical Features	Mode of Inheritance	Laboratory Diagnosis	Comments
QUANTITATIVE				
Type I (classic)	Mild to moderate bleeding	Autosomal dominant (incomplete penetrance ≈60%)	Concordant reduction of plasma vWF:Ag, vWF:RCoF, FVIII (5–40 U/dL)	Subtypes may be defined based on analysis of platelet vWF; represents 60%–70% of all vWD
Type III	Moderate to severe bleeding, including both mucosal and deep tissues	Autosomal recessive (usually compound heterozygotes)	Marked reduction in vWF:Ag, vWF:RCoF and FVIII (<5 U/dL)	
QUALITATIVE				
Diminished RIPA Activity				
Type I variants	Mild to moderate bleeding	Autosomal dominant	Plasma studies similar to type I but with decreased vWF:RCoF/Ag ratio; all multimers present; relative abundance of high-molecular-weight multimers may be abnormal; abnormal satellite subbands may be present	Subtypes include type IB ("platelet discordant"), IC; patients often exhibit a poor response to DDAVP
Type IIA	Mild to moderate bleeding	Autosomal dominant	Variable reduction in vWF:Ag, FVIII; marked reduction in vWF:RCoF; large and intermediate-sized multimers are absent; prominent satellite bands	Subdivision possible based on in vitro studies; large multimers may be present in the platelet
Type IIC	Mild to moderate bleeding	Autosomal recessive	Similar to type IIa, except satellite bands are absent	May represent compound heterozygotes
Type IID-I Type II *Buffalo* Type B	Mild to moderate bleeding	Autosomal dominant	Similar to type IIA, but with unique electrophoretic patterns on high-resolution gels	Type IID described in several independent pedigrees; other subtypes represent single families
Enhanced RIPA Activity				
Type I *New York* and other variants	Mild to moderate bleeding	Autosomal dominant	Similar to type I (classic), but with increased sensitivity to ristocetin in RIPA	Described in three pedigrees
Type IIB (and variants)	Mild to moderate bleeding	Autosomal dominant (a few exceptions)	Plasma studies similar to type IIA; hypersensitivity in RIPA (aggregation at ristocetin ≤0.5 mg/mL); high-molecular-weight multimers absent in the plasma; all multimers present in the platelet	Patients usually exhibit mild to moderate thrombocytopenia that is exacerbated by stresses such as pregnancy or surgery
Platelet-type vWD (pseudo-vWD)	Mild to moderate bleeding	Autosomal dominant	Similar to type IIB	Defect lies within the platelet gpIb receptor; laboratory differentiation from type IIB by mixing studies with normal platelets and plasma
Other				
Factor VIII binding defects	Variable bleeding of the hemophilic type	Autosomal recessive (heterozygotes may be mildly affected)	Marked reduction in FVIII/vWF:Ag ratio	Distinguished from mild hemophilia A by specialized binding studies and mode of inheritance

patients.[286,361] Patients with type III vWD with consanguineous parents have been identified as being homozygous for either complete[87,361] or partial gene deletions.[362] This subset of patients appears to be at greatest risk of developing inhibitors to vWF after exposure to blood products. Other patients have been described who are heterozygous for a vWF gene deletion[87,361] or in whom no gross genetic alteration could be detected.[370] Recently, Nichols and associates[363] demonstrated defective vWF mRNA expression from both maternal and paternal alleles in one type III VWD pedigree by comparing genomic DNA and platelet vWF mRNA (using the polymerase chain reaction technique).

Qualitative Disorders of Von Willebrand Factor

There are a large number of vWD subtypes with a structural or functional abnormality in vWF. Affected patients have a reduced ratio of vWF:RCoF/vWF:Ag and either a reduction or a complete loss of HMW and intermediate-molecular-weight plasma multimers. These qualitative disorders may be further subdivided into two clinically important subgroups. The first subgroup comprises those subtypes (IB, IC, IIA, IIC through II-I) in which the characteristic plasma findings are also reflected in platelet vWF and the RIPA response is either lost or markedly reduced. The second subgroup comprises those subtypes (IIB, IIB *Tampa*, type I [*New York*]) in which HMW forms of vWF are present in platelets and a heightened RIPA response is present. As described in the following section, these two different responses in the RIPA assay have important clinical implications for both diagnosis and treatment.

More recently, patients have been identified in whom vWF levels are modestly reduced but who exhibit a disproportionate reduction in factor VIII levels as a result of abnormal binding of the factor VIII molecule to its vWF carrier.[371,372] Finally, there is a rare platelet disorder, platelet-type vWD (pseudo-vWD), which is clinically indistinguishable from most forms of type IIB vWD.

Subtypes With Diminished RIPA Activity

Type I Variants. Two type I variants have been described in which there is the full range of vWF multimers but functional abnormalities. The inheritance pattern in each of these subtypes is autosomal dominant.

Type IB (Platelet Discordant). In 1983, Hoyer and associates[346] characterized a variant of vWD, which they termed *type IB*. Although all multimeric species were present, a relative reduction in the largest forms was seen. This variant was not uncommon and was detected in 15 of 47 families studied. The patients had clinical bleeding, moderately prolonged bleeding times, and reduced vWF:RCoF activity. A similar variant was described in four patients from three kindreds by Mannucci and associates[273] and termed *platelet discordant* to reflect the discordance between vWF:RCoF and vWF:Ag levels in the platelet. They also noted a decreased ratio of plasma vWF:RCoF/vWF:Ag that was accentuated after treatment with DDAVP. Type IB patients had markedly prolonged bleeding times and poor clinical responses to DDAVP.

Type IC. Five persons from two unrelated families have been described with mild bleeding symptoms in whom all plasma multimers are present but in whom an abnormal satellite pattern is seen by high resolution SDS-agarose electrophoresis.[321] Despite normal vWF antigen levels, most affected members of these families had a prolonged bleeding time and reduced vWF:RCoF activity. This disorder is transmitted as an autosomal dominant trait.

Type II Variants. These variants are characterized by the absence of the large and intermediate-sized multimers in the plasma and a decreased vWF:RCoF/vWF:Ag ratio. They are a heterogenous group with both autosomal dominant and recessive inheritance patterns, variable clinical manifestations, and a variety of electrophoretic abnormalities. In some variants, a reproducible increase of a 176 kd proteolytic fragment (type IIA) is found, and in others, proteolytic fragments of vWF are either reduced (types IIE, IIF, IIH, II-I) or undetectable (types IIC and IID).

Type IIA. Type IIA vWD may be defined as a group of molecular defects producing markedly reduced vWF:RCoF and RIPA activity and a characteristic electrophoretic pattern consisting chiefly of the five smallest oligomers of vWF with an increased abundance of the fastest migrating band in the triplet structure[268] (see Fig. 36-6). Clinical symptoms range from mild to severe bleeding. The structural abnormalities were first suggested by increased anodal mobility in cross-immunoelectrophesis and are thought to arise in some kindreds from enhanced proteolysis of circulating vWF (see following text).[86,345,373] In this variant, plasma vWF:Ag levels may be normal or reduced, with values obtained by Laurell EIA consistently higher than those determined by IRMA.[320] Factor VIII levels vWF:Ag levels are usually concordant. Platelet vWF also lacks the large forms of vWF, although intermediate-sized forms are present and a few patients (termed *type II-3*) have been described in which the platelet vWF electrophoretic pattern appears normal.[320]

Heterogeneity within the IIA subtype was first suggested by a variable degree of susceptibility to in vitro proteolysis[374,375] and a variable response to DDAVP as judged by the appearance of large multimeric forms in the plasma and correction of the bleeding time.[375–377] The inheritance pattern has been reported to be autosomal dominant in all[268,346,378,379] but one[380] of the large number of kindreds that have been studied.

Compelling evidence suggests that either decreased secretion or increased proteolysis of the HMW forms of vWF may give rise to the type IIA variants.[381,382] In the first instance, it has been suggested that point mutations lead to defects in intracellular transport or degradation within the endothelial cell, resulting in the preferential retention of the largest forms of vWF. In the second mechanism, vWF with a normal multimeric distribution is secreted but is unusually susceptible to subsequent proteolysis.[383] The collection of blood from patients carrying these mutations into protease inhibitors results in a variable and incomplete restoration of the larger vWF multimers, suggesting that the proteolysis is an in vivo phenomenon.[374,375] The enzyme or enzymes responsible for the proteolysis of vWF in vivo is not known. Although a number of proteases, including calpain I,[384] elastase,[385] and plasmin,[386,387] can cleave vWF in vitro, epitope mapping of the resultant fragments have shown that these are derived from different regions of the vWF subunit than the 176-kd fragment present in either normal persons or patients with type IIA vWD.[388,389]

Genetic linkage studies first established that the type IIA phenotype was tightly linked to the vWD gene.[390] Subsequently, point mutations were identified in the vWF gene in a number of type IIA patients. Fourteen missense mutations have been identified in 17 families[43,359,381,382,391] (Fig. 36-9). All but two of these mutations fall within the vWF A2 domain between residues 742 and 875, and at least three are close to the previously identified site of proteolysis within vWF, which produces the normally observed 176 Kd fragment.[392] It is interesting that one of these mutations (Arg 834 → Trp) has been identified in six unrelated type IIA patients.[43] Expression of recombinant vWF containing several of the identified type IIA mutations in heterologous cells has resulted in the production of mutant vWF devoid of the largest multimers.[381,382] In addition, an endothelial cell culture derived from the umbilical vein of a patient carrying the Ser 850 → Pro mutation produced vWF with decreased amounts of large multimers and an increase in rapidly migrating satellite species.[393,394]

Type IIC. The type IIC variant is characterized by a unique electrophoretic pattern showing the loss of large and intermediate sized multimers from both plasma and platelets. There is a relative increase in the smallest oligomer and an absence of satellite bands and triplet structure.[346,395–397] When analyzed under reducing conditions by SDS-PAGE, the normal 176- and 140-kd proteolytic fragments are missing, suggesting markedly decreased or absent proteolysis of circulating vWF.[383] However, the addition of protease inhibitors during blood collection enhanced the structural differences noted between plasma and platelet pools of vWF in one family.[375,398] vWF:RCoF activity is markedly reduced and the bleeding time is significantly prolonged. Clinical symptoms range from mild to severe, and the response to DDAVP is poor.

Although the inheritance of type IIC variant was classically described as autosomal recessive,[395,397] an increased

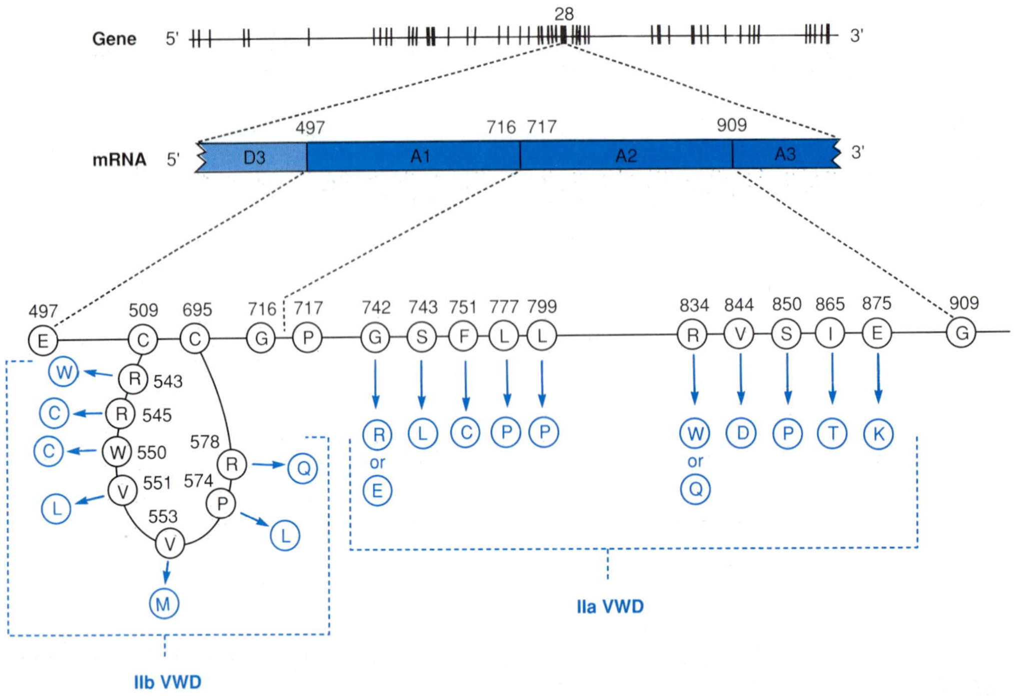

FIGURE 36-9. Schematic representation of some of the known mutations in the A1 and A2 domains of vWF causing, respectively, types IIB and IIA vWD. Both the A1 and A2 domains are encoded by exon 28 in the vWF gene.[359]

bleeding time and mild clinical symptoms have been described in heterozygotes in several kindreds.[399,400] Moreover, unaffected members of these families may have crossed immunoelectrophoretic or SDS-agarose multimer patterns that are intermediate between normal and type IIC individuals. vWD type IIC patients probably are compound heterozygotes.[397,399,400]

Type IID. In the type IID subtype, the normal satellite pattern observed on high percentage agarose gels is replaced by a unique complex of bands. Similar electrophoretic patterns have been reported in four unrelated families from Japan, Sweden, England, and Scotland,[273,401–403] suggesting that this variant may not be rare. vWF:Ag and VIII:C levels are unusually normal but the vWF:RCoF is moderately or severely reduced. Ristocetin-induced platelet aggregation is reduced and the response to DDAVP appears to be modest.[403] As in type IIC, the normal triplet structure is absent in type IID plasma.[383]

Other Variants. Several variants of type II vWD, types IIE through II-I, have been reported in which there is a selective loss of the large multimeric forms of plasma vWF and unique electrophoretic abnormalities on high resolution SDS-agarose gels. In general, they are associated with mild to moderate bleeding and decreased vWF:RCoF/vWF:Ag ratios.

The type IIE variant was described in two members of a single family.[383] The multimeric pattern appears similar to type IIC except that the dominance of the smallest oligomer is not seen and the inheritance pattern is autosomal dominant. Similar to types IIC and IID, there is a reduction in the circulating 176-kd proteolytic fragment although not to the same extent as in these other variants.

Type IIF was described in a single patient with a lifelong bleeding tendency and a markedly prolonged bleeding time.[328] Plasma vWF from this variant is characterized by the absence of large multimers and the presence of a unique satellite banding pattern. In contrast, platelet vWF levels are not reduced and the electrophoretic pattern of this vWF pool is indistinguishable from that seen in normal platelets. Although DDAVP was found to elevate both vWF:Ag and vWF:RCoF activity, the bleeding time remained prolonged and the clinical response was poor. The inheritance pattern could not be formally evaluated but appeared to be recessive.

Type IIG was likewise described in a single patient with moderate clinical symptoms and a markedly prolonged bleeding time. A uniquely abnormal multimeric organization was found in vWF from both plasma and platelets.[374] It is interesting that the electrophoretic pattern found in the platelet pool, but not in the plasma pool of vWF, could be corrected by collection of blood directly into EDTA or protease inhibitors.

Type IIH was discovered in a patient with a lifelong history of bleeding whose initial diagnosis was obscured by normal measurements of vWF:Ag and borderline normal vWF:RCoF activity in the presence of a prolonged bleeding time.[348] RIPA was abnormal, and an electrophoretic pattern similar to, but distinct from, type IIC was noted on high resolution agarose gels. A short-lived correction of the bleeding time occurred after DDAVP infusion.

Type II-I vWD was described in two family members with lifelong histories of severe bleeding and a unique electropheretic pattern on high-resolution gels. Similar to that which occurs in some type IIA variants, the platelet vWF multimeric structure was normal. However, unlike that seen in previously reported type IIA patients, no increase in the quantity of proteolytic fragments of vWF in the plasma was seen. Unlike type IIF, the inheritance pattern of type II-I appears to be dominant.[404]

Type II *Buffalo* was described in three members of a single family and is characterized by a very low vWF:RCoF/vWF:Ag ratio and a multimeric pattern similar to type IIA vWD. Administration of DDAVP induced platelet agglutination and thrombocytopenia similar to that observed in type IIB patients. However, unlike type IIB vWD, there was no hypersensitivity to ristocetin.[405]

Type B vWD was described in a single patient with undetectable vWF:RCoF activity despite normal levels of vWF:Ag and factor VIII. It is of interest that normal platelet aggregation was observed with botrocetin, which also induces vWF binding to gpIb.[406] Multimer analysis revealed a unique electrophoretic pattern. A single amino acid substitution, Gly 561 → Ser in the A1 domain of vWF is responsible for this unique phenotype.[407]

Subtypes With Heightened Responsiveness to Ristocetin

The vWD variants considered in this section are characterized by a heightened interaction between platelets and vWF manifesting as hyperresponsiveness to ristocetin in RIPA assays or spontaneous platelet aggregation.

Type I *New York*. Three independent kindreds have been reported in whom there is a mild to moderate bleeding diathesis with increased RIPA and a normal distribution of vWF multimers.[351,408,409] Mixing studies using washed platelets and platelet-poor plasma from affected patients and normal persons distinguish this condition from pseudo-vWD, whereas the normal multimeric pattern distinguishes this from type IIB vWD (see next section). vWF binds to platelet gpIb/IX and gpIIb/IIIa in an abnormal manner, and the sialic content of the vWF appears normal.[351] Note that DDAVP shortens the prolonged bleeding time found in some of these patients without inducing the thrombocytopenia that is usually associated with the use of this drug in type IIB patients.[408]

Type IIB. The type IIB vWD variant was first recognized in a study of 20 patients from 5 unrelated families who, in contrast to other vWD patients studied at that time, demonstrated platelet aggregation in the presence of reduced concentrations of ristocetin (less than 0.6 mg/mL).[352] Most of these patients had elevated bleeding times (some greater than 30 minutes) despite normal or moderately reduced levels of vWF:Ag. When analyzed by SDS-agarose gel electrophoresis, the largest vWF multimers were missing from plasma although platelet multimers were normal (see Fig. 36-7). As in type IIA vWF, plasma vWF from type IIB variants has an abnormal triplet structure on SDS-agarose gels with an enhancement of the fastest migrating band in each oligomeric group and an increased quantity of the 176-kd proteolytic fragment.[383]

Administration of DDAVP to patients with type IIB produces a rapid appearance of larger multimers in the plasma which are then quickly cleared from the circulation.[376] This process is due to the release of an abnormal vWF molecule and its subsequent adsorption on platelet surfaces.[376,410] The splenic clearance of the resultant platelet aggregates produces a transient but often profound thrombocytopenia.[161,411] Similarly, transient or even chronic thrombocytopenia has been found in subsets of type IIB vWD patients, termed *type IIB Tampa*[213,343,412–417] and may worsen with the physiologic increase in circulating vWF seen in pregnancy,[213,214] normal aging,[418] or after surgery.[419]

In most pedigrees type IIB vWD is dominantly inherited, although a few cases have been reported with a recessive phenotype.[420,421] A total of nine amino acid substitutions and one insertion have been identified in patients with type IIB vWD[359,422–426] and four of these mutations account for 90% of the families studied to date.[43] Several of these mutations have been reported in more than one pedigree as a result of what is presumed to be independent genetic events.[422] All but three of these mutations are located between amino acid residues 540 and 578 in the A1 domain (see Fig. 36-9). This region of vWF, between amino acid residues Val 449 and Lys 728, had previously been demonstrated to contain the platelet gpIb binding site.[427,428] Normally, vWF binding to this receptor requires prior activation of vWF, which may be produced by binding of vWF to collagen, or a reduction in net negative charge by agents such as ristocetin. The single amino acid substitutions, which have been described in type IIB patients, are presumed to facilitate vWF binding to platelet gpIb/IX by introducing conformational changes that either mimic the effects of collagen or ristocetin. Full-length recombinant vWF containing some of the described mutations has been expressed and has been shown to bind spontaneously to platelets[422,429–433]

Variants With Defective Factor VIII Binding

In most vWD variants, the level of plasma factor VIII is decreased in rough proportion to the decreased level of plasma vWF. Pedigrees have been described, however, in which factor VIII deficiency was autosomally inherited without a proportionate reduction in plasma vWF levels.[434–436] This led to the hypothesis that mutations in vWF could reduce factor VIII binding capacity. Recently, three mutations within the N-terminal region of vWF have been described in eight apparently unrelated families, which reduce or eliminate factor VIII binding in vitro and decrease factor VIII/vWF ratios in the plasma of affected persons[371,372,437–444] (Fig. 36-10). The most frequently observed mutation is Arg 91 → Gln. This mutation lies within the region of vWF (residues 78 to 96) that was previously shown to be critical for factor VIII binding using monoclonal antibodies.[69,70] At least three of the four affected individuals are compound heterozygotes and carry both the Arg 91 → Gln mutation and a type I vWD allele. Since recombinant vWF containing this mutation has a markedly decreased capacity for factor VIII binding,[440,442] there may be partial compensation by the incorporation of low levels of the other allelic product into vWF multimers. A second mutation, Thr 28 → Met, has been identified in two families and produces severe factor VIII deficiency with variable vWF protein levels in the homozygous state.[438,445] A substitution of Arg 53 → Trp has been detected in two persons with low factor VIII levels and normal vWF protein levels. One of these persons also carried the Arg 91 → Gln mutation.[439] A second double mutation, Arg 19 → Trp and His 54 → Gln, has also been described.[441] The frequency of these mutations is unknown, but they may account for a significant proportion of patients previously diagnosed with mild hemophilia A.

Acquired Von Willebrand's Disease

Acquired vWD comprises a heterogenous group of disorders in which previously normal individuals develop a mucosal

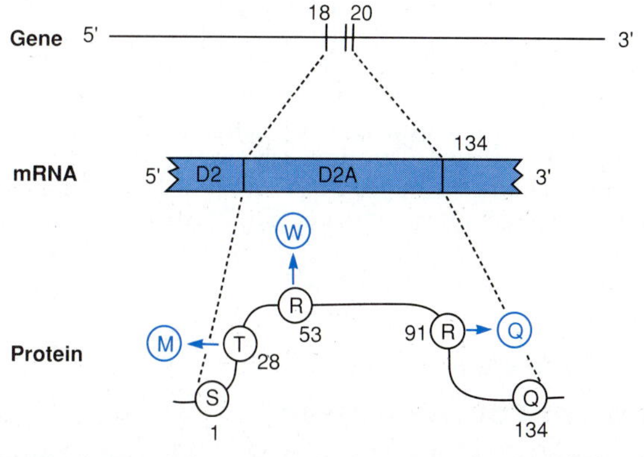

FIGURE 36-10. Schematic representation of some of the mutations causing autosomal hemophilia, the variant form of vWD in which factor VIII binding to vWF is perturbed. All mutations described to date arose in exons 18 to 20 of the vWF gene.[359]

bleeding disorder and decreased levels of vWF. The clinical presentation is similar to that seen in other vWD patients except that the patients are generally elderly and have no family or previous personal history of bleeding. Epistaxis and easy bruising are the most common presenting complaints. Laboratory features of acquired vWD are identical with those seen in congenital vWD and include reduced plasma levels of factor VIII, vWF:Ag, and vWF:RCoF. In some cases, selective depletion of the largest forms of vWF occurs, resulting in a plasma multimeric distribution similar to that seen in congenital type II vWD.[446,447]

At least three distinct mechanisms that cause acquired vWD have been described. In some patients, diminished vWF levels result from the presence of a circulating inhibitor, usually an antibody of the IgG or IgM class.[448] These inhibitors may be associated with monoclonal gammopathies,[449] multiple myeloma,[449] lymphoproliferative diseases such as chronic lymphocytic leukemia,[448] poorly differentiated lymphocytic lymphoma,[450] hairy cell leukemia,[451] and autoimmune diseases such as systemic lupus erythematosus[452] and mixed connective tissue disease.[453] The presence of the circulating inhibitor can sometimes be detected by the loss of vWF:RCoF activity, and sometimes decreased factor VIII activity, in mixtures of normal and patient plasmas.[448,454–456] In other cases, nonneutralizing antibodies may form immune complexes with vWF leading to increased clearance in the reticuloendothelial cells.[457,458]

Acquired vWD may also result from the absorption of vWF onto the surface of malignant cells such as lymphoid tumors,[450] Waldenström's macroglobulinemia,[82,459] multiple myeloma,[460] Wilms' tumor,[121,461,462] and other solid tumors.[463–465] In such cases, there is often a selective loss of the largest vWF multimers with a consequent loss of ristocetin cofactor activity that is out of proportion to the vWF antigen. In some cases, internalization of vWF by the tumor cells could be demonstrated.[460,465] Acquired vWD may also be seen in patients with myeloproliferative diseases.[466,467] In such patients, selective loss of the largest multimeric forms of vWF may result from increased proteolysis, which is suggested by abnormal satellite banding patterns on SDS-agarose gels.[467]

Platelet-Type Von Willebrand's Disease

Platelet-type vWD, or pseudo-vWD, is a rare autosomal disorder with a clinical phenotype that most closely resembles type IIB vWD.[353,468,469] Large vWF multimers are absent in the plasma but are present in platelet lysates. Plasma vWF:RCoF activity is decreased, but responsiveness to ristocetin in RIPA assays is heightened. In contrast to other variants of vWD with hyperresponsiveness to ristocetin, the defect responsible for platelet-type vWD lies within the platelet itself, within the gpIb/IX complex. To date, two point mutations with the α-chain of gpIb have been described.[470,471] Laboratory differentiation between platelet-type vWD and type IIB and similar variants involves the addition of normal cryoprecipitate or purified vWF to washed patient platelets.[353,469,472] A less cumbersome assay taking advantage of the hyperaffinity of type IIB vWF, but not vWF from platelet-type vWD patients, for formalin-fixed platelets has been described.[473]

TREATMENT

General Considerations

Few controlled studies are available to guide the clinician with respect to intensity or duration of treatment in vWD. In most vWD patients, factor VIII levels are high enough to support normal thrombin generation and bleeding is primarily of the mucosal type. Because laboratory tests are often imprecise measures of the hemostatic defect in vWD, treatment is often empiric with the efficacy judged by clinical endpoints. In certain situations, such as high-risk surgery, therapy should be monitored by measuring the bleeding time. While the Duke bleeding time is more easily corrected than the template modification of the Ivy bleeding time, correction of the Duke bleeding time correlates with improved hemostasis.[303,474]

In patients with severe vWD, who can develop hemophilic-type bleeding, the aim of therapy is to increase plasma factor VIII levels to 30 to 50 U/dL, as well as correct the defect in primary hemostasis. The duration of treatment is determined by the severity of hemorrhage and clinical response. Life-threatening hemorrhage (eg, intracranial bleeding), which is exceedingly rare in vWD, may raise the factor VIII level to 100 U/dL. When patients with vWD are treated with vWF-containing products, the elevation in plasma factor VIII levels lasts longer than in hemophilia A patients.[19]

Therapeutic Modalities

Desmopressin

Desmopressin acetate (1-deamino-8-D-arginine; DDAVP) is a synthetic analogue of the antidiuretic hormone L-arginine vasopressin with enhanced antidiuretic potency but little pressor activity. Infusion of a standard dose of 0.3 μg/kg desmopressin into healthy volunteers results in a two- to three-fold increase in vWF antigenic levels and a five- to six-fold increase in factor VIII levels.[141,475,476] Peak responses are usually seen 30 to 60 minutes after infusion and persist for up to 6 hours. Desmopressin is almost always administered intravenously, although subcutaneous[477–479] or intranasal[480,481] administration of more concentrated forms of the drug are equally effective.

Desmopressin is effective for only 6 to 12 hours, and tachyphylaxis may be observed after as few as two or three doses.[482] In such cases, effective hemostasis may require infusion of an exogenous source of vWF. The duration of responsiveness to DDAVP varies, and repeated responses have been documented over several days.[483] A single daily dose, which may be sufficient in some clinical settings, reduces the likelihood of tachyphylaxis.[484]

Desmopressin generally causes only minor side effects, which include facial flushing and, less frequently, nausea and headache. Reducing the rate of infusion usually obviates these difficulties. More serious side effects have also been reported. First, through its antidiuretic effect, desmopressin may produce clinically significant water intoxication and hyponatremia, which may be profound enough to precipitate seizures.[485–487] Infancy, frequent dosing, and the concomitant use of narcotics appear to be additional risk factors for hyponatremia. Frequent monitoring of serum sodium and careful fluid management may be necessary in high-risk patients. Second, desmopressin has been associated with thrombosis and myocardial infarction in anecdotal reports.[488,489]

However, a statistical examination of these reports failed to establish causality.[490] Finally, it is widely believed that the use of DDAVP in patients with type IIB vWD is contraindicated because the release of high-molecular-weight forms of the abnormal vWF found in these patients may worsen the often present thrombocytopenia.[410,411] Although more recent reports suggest some type IIB patients are clinically improved by treatment with DDAVP and that at least some instances of decreased platelet counts may be a blood collection artefact (pseudothrombocytopenia), the routine use of DDAVP in type IIB vWD cannot be advocated at this time. Similarly, the use of DDAVP is not recommended in patients with platelet-type vWD.

Exogenous Sources of von Willebrand Factor

The treatment of vWD patients who not respond to desmopressin, or who have experienced tachyphylaxis to the drug, depends on exogenous sources of vWF. In the past, cryoprecipitate has been the preferred blood product because it contains the full range of vWF multimers. Typically used doses of cryoprecipitate are 1 U/10 kg every 12 to 24 hours. The duration of therapy depends on the clinical circumstances but is usually 48 to 72 hours. Although most factor VIII concentrates contain significant quantities of vWF, they are typically deficient in the HMW multimers normally found in plasma and are not effective in correcting the primary hemostatic defect present in vWD patients.[491] At least one such concentrate, Humate-P (Behringwerke; Armour), has a significant fraction of the higher-molecular-weight forms of vWF normally found in plasma,[492,493] can correct the laboratory abnormalities, and improve hemostasis in patients with type I, type II, and severe (type III) vWD.[85,492–495] Because Humate-P is produced by a process that includes viral inactivation by heat treatment in the wet state (pasteurization), the risk of HIV and viral hepatitis transmission is low.[495,496] Typically, empiric doses of 40 U factor VIII per kilogram are given every 12 to 24 hours. A high-purity, virally attenuated, vWF concentrate has been introduced in Europe, which contains HMW vWF multimers and a high specific activity of ristocetin cofactor activity. The clinical efficacy of this product is still under investigation but appears to show promising results in a limited number of patients.[493,497,498] The use of this product in severe vWD patients may be limited by the expected delay in achieving therapeutic factor VIII levels. Other intermediate- and high-purity factor VIII concentrates are under investigation for the treatment of vWD.

Adjunctive Therapy

In addition to specific therapy aimed at increasing plasma vWF levels, a number of adjunctive measures are often useful in the treatment of vWD. Oral cavity bleeding is effectively treated with the antifibrinolytic drugs, ε-aminocaproic acid (EACA) or tranexamic acid, which block plasminogen activation.[499] Each drug may be given intravenously, orally, or topically as an oral rinse; they are particularly useful in preventing bleeding after dental surgery and tonsillectomy.[500] Severe menorrhagia may require hormonal therapy with oral contraceptives, which reduces menstrual blood loss and increases vWF levels in mildly affected patients. High doses of conjugated estrogens may be required in unusually severe cases. The use of brief courses of conjugated estrogens has been proposed as treatment for women undergoing elective surgery.[501]

Treatment Strategies

The choice of the therapeutic strategy depends primarily on the subtype of vWD and the nature of the bleeding diathesis (Table 36-2).

TABLE 36-2. Treatment Strategies in von Willebrand's Disease

vWD Variant	Primary Therapy	Secondary Therapy
Type I	Desmopressin	Factor concentrate* Cryoprecipitate
Type IIA (and related subtypes)	Desmopressin	Factor concentrate* Cryoprecipitate
Type IIB	Factor concentrate* Cryoprecipitate	?? Desmopressin
Type III	Factor concentrate* Cryoprecipitate	Platelet transfusion Desmopressin
Autosomal hemophilia (vWD Normandy)	Factor concentrate*	Desmopressin
Acquired vWD†	Desmopressin	Platelet transfusion Factor concentrate*

* Refers to intermediate purity factor VIII concentrates (see text). These products are not yet licensed in the United States for the treatment of vWD.
† Refers to therapy of acute bleeding manifestations. Long-term management is best achieved by treatment of the underlying disease.

Subtypes

Type I. Most patients with type I vWD respond to desmopressin with a marked rise in all components of the vWF:factor VIII complex and a shortening or normalization of the bleeding time. DDAVP has become the mainstay of treatment for most of these patients. Aa small subset of patients with diminished levels of platelet-associated vWF either do not have a significant rise in vWF or fail to show any improvement in hemostasis.[273] Responses to desmopressin among type I patients are inconsistent enough to warrant a test infusion to help predict the likelihood of a response.[502] After the response to DDAVP has been demonstrated, treatment can usually be instituted when needed at a later date.

As discussed, the goal of treatment in type I vWD patients in the postoperative period requires adequate primary hemostasis for 48 to 72 hours. Although this may be achieved with DDAVP alone, it is advisable to have exogenous sources of vWF available, especially for patients undergoing high-risk surgical procedures or in whom rapid tachyphylaxis has been observed.

Type II. Highly variable responses to desmopressin have been observed in patients with type II vWD. Thus, although most type II patients have a significant increase in vWF antigen and factor VIII,[503,504] normalization of the vWF multimeric pattern and improvement in bleeding time are not consistently observed.[376,377] Infusion of desmopressin in patients with type IIB vWD results in the transient appearance of HMW forms of the vWF, which are then rapidly cleared from the plasma.[376,410] Desmopressin is said to be contraindicated in type IIB patients because it exacerbates the thrombocytopenia seen in this subtype.[410] Two reports[505,506] suggest that the decrease in platelet count after DDAVP administration to type IIB vWD patients is artifactual (pseudothrombocytopenia) and that the drug has clinical benefit.

Type III. Patients with type III vWD do not increase either vWF antigen or factor VIII levels after DDAVP infusion. The use of desmopressin in conjunction with cryoprecipitate shortens the bleeding time more effectively than cryoprecipitate, suggesting an additional action of desmopressin independent of its effect on vWF secretion.[507] In addition, platelet transfusion may provide an important additional source of vWF for severe vWD patients who fail to respond to exogenous vWF alone.[277,508] Platelet transfusion may be especially helpful in treating type III vWD patients who have developed alloantibodies to vWF as a result of previous treatment with exogenous vWF preparations.

Autosomal Hemophilia. Treatment of patients with autosomal hemophilia requires an exogenous source of vWF. The infusion of intermediate purity factor VIII concentrates produces an immediate correction of factor VIII levels and a prolonged elevation of factor VIII due to the stimulation of endogenous biosynthesis and enhanced plasma stability.[437,509]

Acquired Disease. The treatment of acquired vWD is often problematic. Treatment of the underlying condition, if possible, often leads to the disappearance of the vWD manifestations.[451,452,462,465,467] Amelioration of acute bleeding manifestations can sometimes be achieved with DDAVP or large amounts of exogenous vWF. Platelet transfusions may also be useful in patients who fail to respond to other measures.

Special Considerations

Surgery. In preoperative patients, it is necessary to ensure a factor VIII level over 50 U/dL, as well as to raise the ristocetin cofactor activity and shorten the bleeding time. Although little specific evidence supports this point, most clinicians attempt to achieve ristocetin cofactor activity levels of at least 50 U/dL and to partially correct the template Ivy bleeding time.[484] For patients with more severe defects or when surgery results in mucosal bleeding, more careful attention to both the bleeding time and the ristocetin cofactor levels is recommended. For the typical vWD patient with an adequate level of factor VIII, the defect is predominantly one of primary hemostasis. Thus, treatment can often be limited to the first 48 to 72 hours after surgery. Although this may be achievable in some patients with DDAVP alone, it is generally advisable to consider the use of exogenous sources of vWF, especially in patients undergoing high-risk surgical procedures or in whom rapid tachyphylaxis has been observed. In unusually severe type I vWD patients, further therapy may be required to maintain the factor VIII levels above 30 U/dL for an additional 4 to 7 days. When appropriate therapy is instituted, the operative risk in vWD is not increased.[510] As in other patients with bleeding disorders, antiplatelet drugs, particularly aspirin, should be avoided.

Pregnancy. The management of vWD in pregnancy is a commonly encountered clinical problem that deserves special consideration. Pregnancy induces a significant increase in factor VIII, vWF:Ag, and vWF:RCoF in most type I vWD patients, although the Ivy bleeding time may remain prolonged.[205] The likelihood of hemorrhage at the time of delivery is acceptably small so long as the factor VIII level is over 50 U/dL, as is true in most vWD patients at the time of delivery.[212,511] Although there is less evidence on this point, it appears that even cesarean section can be safely performed without specific therapy in most vWD patients.[416] Because plasma vWF may rapidly return to baseline levels in the postpartum period, careful monitoring for excessive mucosal bleeding is warranted. Special consideration should also be given to those women with other subtypes of vWD in whom correction of the hemostatic defects is less predictable. In women with type IIB and similar vWD variants, thrombocytopenia may result from increased plasma levels of the abnormal vWF protein.[214,414] When treatment is required, first consideration should be given to the use of DDAVP, especially in patients with a previously documented history of a favorable response. Documentation of the efficacy of DDAVP in the peripartum period is highly limited and the need for exogenous vWF replacement must be individually evaluated.

REFERENCES

1. Meyer D, Baumgartner HR. Role of von Willebrand factor in platelet adhesion to the subendothelium. Br J Haematol 1983;54:1.
2. Weiss HJ, Sussman II, Hoyer LW. Stabilization of factor VIII in plasma by the von Willebrand factor: studies on posttransfusion and dissociated factor VIII and in patients with von Willebrand's disease. J Clin Invest 1977;60:390.
3. Von Willebrand EA. Hereditär pseudohemofili. Finska Läkaresällskapets Handlingar 1926;67:7.
4. Von Willebrand EA. Ueber hereditaere pseudohaemophilie. Acta Med Scand 1931;76:521.
5. Minot GR. A familial hemorrhagic condition associated with prolongation of bleeding times. Am J Med Sci 1928;175:301.
6. Buckman TE. Atypical pathologic hemorrhage in early life. Am J Med Sci 1928;175:307.
7. Alexander B, Goldstein R. Dual hemostatic defect in pseudohemophilia. J Clin Invest 1953;32:551.
8. Quick AJ, Hussey CV. Hemophilic condition in the female. J Lab Clin Med 1953;42:929.
9. Larrieu MJ, Soulier JP. Deficit en facteur antihémophilique A chez une fille associé a un trouble saignement. Rev Hematol 1953;8:361.
10. Nilsson IM, Blombäck M, von Francken I. On an inherited autosomal hemorrhagic diathesis with antihemophilic globulin (AHG) deficiency and prolonged bleeding time. Acta Med Scand 1957;159:35.
11. Juergens R, Lehmann W, Wegelius O, et al. Antihemophilic globulin factor (factor VIII) deficiency in Aland (Willebrand-Juergens) thrombopathy. Thromb Diath Haemorrh 1957;1:257.
12. Von Willebrand EA, Juergens R. Ueber ein neue Bluterkrankheit, die konstitutionelle Thrombopathie. Klin Wochenschr 1933;12:414.
13. Salzman EW. Measurement of platelet adhesiveness: a simple in vitro technique demonstrating an abnormality in von Willebrand's disease. J Lab Clin Med 1963;62:724.
14. Bowie EJW, Owen CA Jr, Thompson JH Jr, Didisheim P. Platelet adhesiveness in von Willebrand's disease. Am J Clin Pathol 1969;52:69.
15. Baumgartner HR. The role of blood flow in platelet adhesion, fibrin deposition and formation of mural thrombi. Microvasc Res 1973;5:167.
16. Nilsson IM, Blomback M, Jorpes E, et al. Von Willebrand's disease and its correction with human plasma fraction I-0. Acta Med Scand 1957;159:179.
17. Nilsson IM, Blombäck M, Blombäck B. Von Willebrand's disease in Sweden: its pathogenesis and treatment. Acta Med Scand 1959;164:263.
18. Weiss HJ. The use of plasma and plasma fractions in the treatment of a patient with von Willebrand's disease. Vox Sang 1962;7:267.
19. Biggs R, Matthews JM. The treatment of haemorrhage in von Willebrand's disease and the blood level of factor VIII (AHG). Br J Haematol 1963;9:203.
20. Cornu P, Larrieu MJ, Caen JP, Bernard J. Transfusion studies in von Willebrand's disease: effect on bleeding time and factor VIII. Br J Haematol 1963;9:189.
21. Perkins HA. Correction of the hemostatic defects in von Willebrand's disease. Blood 1967;30:375.
22. Bennett E, Dormandy K. Pool's cryoprecipitate and exhausted plasma in the treatment of von Willebrand's disease and factor XI deficiency. Lancet 1966;2:731.
23. Weiss HJ, Rogers J. Correction of the platelet abnormality in von Willebrand's disease by cryoprecipitate. Am J Med 1972;53:734.
24. Larrieu MJ, Caen JP, Meyer DO, et al. Congenital bleeding disorders with long bleeding time and normal platelet count II von Willebrand's disease (report of thirty-seven patients). Am J Med 1968;45:354.
25. Weiss HJ, Rogers J, Brand H. Defective ristocetin-induced platelet aggregation in von Willebrand's disease and its correction by factor VIII. J Clin Invest 1973;52:2697.
26. Green D, Potter EV. Failure of AHF concentrate to control bleeding in von Willebrand's disease. Am J Med 1976;60:357.
27. Blatt PM, Brinkhous KM, Culp HR, et al. Antihemophilic factor concentrates therapy in von Willebrand's disease: dissociation of bleeding-time factor and ristocetin-cofactor activities. JAMA 1976;236:2770.
28. Zimmerman TS, Ratnoff OD, Powell AE. Immunologic differentiation of classic hemophilia (factor VIII deficiency) and von Willebrand's disease, with observations on combined deficiencies of antihemophilic factor and proaccelerin (factor V) and an acquired circulating anticoagulant against antihemophlic factor. J Clin Invest 1971;50:244.
29. Stites DP, Hershgold EJ, Perlman JD, Fudenberg HH. Factor VIII detection by hemagglutination inhibition: hemophilia A and von Willebrand's disease. Science 1971;171:196.
30. Laurell CB. Quantitative estimation of proteins by electrophoresis in agarose gel containing antibodies. Anal Biochem 1966;15:45.
31. Howard MA, Firkin BG. Ristocetin: a new look in the investigation of platelet aggregation. Thromb Haemost 1971;26:362.
32. Gangarosa EJ, Johnson TR, Ramos HS. Ristocetin-induced thrombocytopenia: site and mechanism of action. Arch Intern Med 1960;105:83.
33. Howard MA, Sawers RJ, Firkin BG. Ristocetin: a means of differentiating von Willebrand's disease into two groups. Blood 1973;41:687.
34. Doucet-deBruine MHM, Sixma JJ, Over J, Beeser-Visser NH. Heterogeneity of human factor VIII. II. Characterization of forms of factor VIII binding to platelets in the presence of ristocetin. J Lab Clin Med 1978;92:96.
35. Martin SE, Marder VJ, Francis CW, Barlow GH. Structural studies on the functional heterogeneity of von Willebrand protein polymers. Blood 1981;57:313.

36. Moake JL, Turner MA, Stathopoulos NA, Nolasco LH, Jellums JD. Involvement of large plasma von Willebrand factor (vWF) multimers and unusually large vWF forms derived from endothelial cells in shear stress-induced platelet aggregation. J Clin Invest 1986;78:1456.
37. Moake JL. Von Willebrand factor and the pathophysiology of thrombotic thrombocytopenia: from human studies to a new animal model. Lab Invest 1988;59:415.
38. Titani K, Kumar S, Takio K, et al. Amino acid sequence of human von Willebrand factor. Biochemistry 1986;25:3171.
39. Ginsburg D, Handin RI, Bonthron DT, et al. Human von Willebrand factor (vWF): isolation of complementary DNA (cDNA) clones and chromosomal localization. Science 1985;228:1401.
40. Lynch DC, Zimmerman TS, Collins CJ, et al. Molecular cloning of cDNA for human von Willebrand factor: authentication by a new method. Cell 1985;41:49.
41. Sadler JE, Shelton-Inloes BB, Sorace JM, et al. Cloning and characterization of two cDNAs coding for human von Willebrand factor. Proc Natl Acad Sci USA 1985;82:6394.
42. Verweij CL, de Vries CJM, Distel B, et al. Construction of cDNA coding from Human von Willebrand factor using antibody probes from colonly-screening and mapping of the chromosomal gene. Nucleic Acids Res 1985;13:4699.
43. Ginsburg D, Bowie EJW. Molecular genetics of von Willebrand disease. Blood 1992;79:2507.
44. Bonthron DT, Handin RI, Kaufman RJ, et al. Structure of pre-pro-von Willebrand factor and its expression in heterologous cells. Nature 1986;324:270.
45. Bonthron DT, Orr EC, Mitsock LM, Ginsburg D, Handin RI, Orkin SH. Nucleotide sequence of pre–pro-von Willebrand factor cDNA. Nucleic Acids Res 1986;14:7125.
46. Shelton-Inloes BB, Broze GR Jr, Miletich JP, Sadler JE. Evoluation of human von Willebrand factor: cDNA sequence polymorphisms, repeated domains, and relationship to von Willebrand antigen II. Biochem Biophys Res Commun 1987;144:657.
47. Shelton-Inloes BB, Titani K, Sadler JE. cDNA sequences for human von Willebrand factor reveal five types of repeated domains and five possible protein sequence polymorphisms. Biochemistry 1986;25: 3164.
48. Verweij CL, Diergaarde PJ, Hart M, Pannekoek H. Full length von Willebrand factor (vWF) cDNA encodes a highly repetitive protein considerably larger than the mature vWF subunit. EMBO J 1986;5: 1839.
49. Fay PJ, Kawai Y, Wagner DD, et al. Propolypeptide of von Willebrand factor circulates in blood and is identical to von Willebrand antigen II. Science 1986;232:995.
50. Montgomery RR, Zimmerman TS. Von Willebrand's disease antigen II. J Clin Invest 1978;61:1498.
51. Wise RJ, Barr PJ, Wong PA, Kiefer MC, Brake AJ, Kaufman RJ. Expression of a human proprotein processing enzyme: correct cleavage of the von Willebrand factor precursor at a paired basic amino acid site. Proc Natl Acad Sci USA 1990;87:9378.
52. Barr PJ. Mammalian Subtilisins: the long-sought dibasic processing endoproteases. Cell 1991;66:1.
53. Smeekens SP. Processing of protein precursors by a novel family of subtilisin-related mammalian endoproteases. Bio/Technology 1993;11: 182.
54. Verweij CL, Hart M, Pannekoek H. Expression of variant von Willebrand factor (vWF) cDNA in heterologous cells: requirement of the pro-polypeptide in vWF multimer formation. Embo J 1987;6:2885.
55. Wise RJ, Pittman DD, Handin RI, Kaufman RJ, Orkin SH. The propeptide of von Willebrand factor independently mediates the assembly of von Willebrand multimers. Cell 1988;52:229.
56. Montgomery RR, Dent J, Schmidt W, et al. Hereditary persistence of circulating pro von Willebrand factor (pro-vWF). Circulation 1986;74(Suppl II):406.
57. Slayter H, Loscalzo J, Bockenstedt PL, Handin RI. Native conformation of human von Willebrand protein: analysis by electron microscopy and quasielastic light scattering. J Biol Chem 1985;260:8559.
58. Mohri H, Fujimura Y, Shima M, et al. Structure of the von Willebrand factor domain interacting with glycoprotein Ib. J Biol Chem 1988;263: 17901.
59. Berndt MC, Ward CM, Booth WJ, et al. Identification of aspartic acid 514 through glutamic acid 542 as a glycoprotein Ib-IX complex receptor recognition sequence in von Willebrand factor: mechanism of modulation of von Willebrand factor by ristocetin and botrocetin. Biochemistry 1992;31:11144.
60. Mohri H, Yoshioka A, Zimmerman TS, et al. Isolation of the von Willebrand factor domain interacting with platelet glycoprotein Ib, heparin, and collagen and characterization of its three distinct functional sites. J Biol Chem 1989;264:17361.
61. Fujimura Y, Titani K, Holland LZ, et al. A heparin-binding domain of human von Willebrand factor: characterization and localization of a tryptic fragment extending from amino acid residue Val449 to Lys728. J Biol Chem 1987;262:1734.
62. Sixma JJ, Schiphorst ME, Verweij CL, et al. Effect of deletion of the A1 domain of von Willebrand factor on its binding to heparin, collagen and platelets in the presence of ristocetin. Eur J Biochem 1991;196: 369.
63. Christophe O, Obert B, Meyer D, et al. The binding domain of von Willebrand factor to sulfatides is distinct from those interacting with glycoprotein Ib, heparin, and collagen and resides between amino acid residues Leu512 and Lys673. Blood 1991;78:2310.
64. Pareti FI, Niiya K, McPherson JM, Ruggeri ZM. Isolation and characterization of two domains of human von Willebrand factor that interact with fibrillar collagen types I and III. J Biol Chem 1987;262:13835.
65. Mohri H, Fujimura Y, Shima M, et al. Isolation of the von Willebrand factor domain interacting with platelet glycoprotein Ib, herparin, and collagen and characterization of its three distinct functional sites. J Biol Chem 1989;264:17361.
66. Roth GJ, Titani K, Hoyer LW, Hickey MJ. Localization of binding sites within human von Willebrand factor for monomeric type III collagen. Biochemistry 1986;25:8357.
67. Kalafatis M, Takahashi Y, Girma JP, Meyer D. Localization of a collagen-interactive domain of human von Willebrand factor between amino acid residues Gly 911 and Glu 1365. Blood 1987;70:1577.
68. Cruz MA, Handin RI, Wise RJ. The interaction of the von Willebrand factor–A1 domain with platelet glycoprotein Ib/IX: the role of glycosylation and disulfide bonding in a monomeric recombinant A1 domain protein. J Biol Chem 1993;268:21238.
69. Bahou WF, Ginsburg D, Sikkink R, Litwiller R, Fass DN. A monoclonal antibody to von Willebrand factor (vWF) inhibits factor VIII binding. J Clin Invest 1989;84:56.
70. Ginsburg D, Bockenstedt PL, Allen EA, et al. Fine mapping of monoclonal antibody epitopes on human von Willebrand factor using a recombinant peptide library. Thromb Haemost 1991;67:166.
71. Fay PJ, Coumans JV, Walker FJ. von Willebrand factor mediates protection of factor VIII from activated protein C–catalyzed inactivation. J Biol Chem 1991;266:2172.
72. Tuddenham EGD, Lane RS, Rotblat F, et al. Response to infusions of polyelectrolyte fractionated human factor VIII concentrate in human hemophilia A and von Willebrand disease. Br J Haematol 1982;52: 259.
73. Kaufman RJ. Biological regulation of factor VIII activity. Annu Rev Med 1992;43:325.
74. Fay PJ. Reconstitution of human factor VIII from isolated subunits. Arch Biochem Biophys 1988;262:525.
75. Wise RJ, Dorner AJ, Krane M, et al. The role of von Willebrand factor multimers and propeptide cleavage in binding and stabilization of factor VIII. J Biol Chem 1991;266:21948.
76. Kaufman RJ, Wasley LC, Dorner AJ. Synthesis, processing and secretion of recombinant human factor VIII expressed in mammalian cells. J Biol Chem 1988;263:6352.
77. Ruoslahti E, Pierschbacher MD. New perspectives in cell adhesion: RGD and integrins. Science 1987;238:491.
78. Ruggeri ZM, DeMarco L, Gatti L, Bader R, Montgomery RR. Platelets have more than one binding site of von Willebrand factor that mediates platelet adhesion on subendothelium is not collagen. J Clin Invest 1983;72:1.
79. Sakariassen KS, Nievelstein PFEM, Coller BS, Sixma JJ. The role of platelet membrane glycoproteins Ib and IIb-IIIa in platelet adherence to human artery subendothelium. Br J Haematol 1986;63:681.
80. Berliner S, Niiya K, Roberts Jr, Houghten RA, Ruggeri ZM. Generation and characterization of peptide-specific antibodies that inhibit von Willebrand factor binding to glycoprotein IIb-IIIa without interacting with other adhesive molecules. J Biol Chem 1988;263:7500.
81. Parker RI, Gralnick HR. Inhibition of platelet-von Willebrand factor binding to platelets by adhesion site peptides. Blood 1989;74:1226.
82. Brody JI, Haidar ME, Rossman RE. A hemorrhagic syndrome in Waldenstrom's macroglobulinemia secondary to immunoadsorption of factor VIII: recovery after splenectomy. N Engl J Med 1979;300:408.
83. Sixma JJ, Sakariassen KS, Beeser-Visser NH, et al. Adhesion of platelets to human artery subendothelium: effect of factor VIII–von Willebrand factor of various multimeric composition. Blood 1984;63:128.
84. Mancuso DJ, Tuley EA, Westfield LA, et al. Structure of the gene for human von Willebrand factor. J Biol Chem 1989;264:19514.
85. Fukui H, Nishino M, Terada S, et al. Hemostatic effect of a heat-treated factor VIII concentrate (Haemate P) in von Willebrand's disease. Blut 1988;56:171.
86. Peake IR, Bloom AL, Giddings JC. Inherited variants of factor VIII-related protein in von Willebrand's disease. N Engl J Med 1974;291: 113.
87. Shelton-Inloes BB, Chelab FF, Mannucci PM, et al. Gene deletions correlate with the development of alloantibodies in von Willebrand disease. J Clin Invest 1987;79:1459.
88. Patracchini P, Calzolari E, Aiello V, Palazzi P, Banin P, Marchetti GB. Sublocalization of von Willebrand factor pseudogene to 22q11.22-q11.23 by in situ hybridization. Hum Genet 1989;83:264.
89. Mancuso DJ, Tuley EA, Westfield LA, et al. Human von Willebrand factor gene and pseudogene: structural analysis and differentiation by polymerase chain reaction. Biochemistry 1991;30:253.
90. Bahou WF, Bowie EJW, Fass DN, Ginsburg D. Molecular genetic analysis of porcine von Willebrand disease: tight linkage to the von Willebrand factor locus. Blood 1988;72:308.
91. Collins CJ, Underdahl JP, Levene RB, et al. Molecular cloning of the human gene for von Willebrand factor and identification of the transcription initiation site. Proc Natl Acad Sci USA 1987;84:4393.

92. Verweij CL, Hofker M, Quadt R, Briet E, Pannekoek H. RFLP for a human von Willebrand factor cDNA clone, pvWF1100. Nucleic Acids Res 1985;13:8289.
93. Nishino K, Lynch DC. A polymorphism of the human von Willebrand factor gene with BamHI. Nucleic Acids Res 1986;14:4697.
94. Quadt R, Verweij CL, DeVries CJM, Briët E, Pannekoek H. A polymorphic Xba I site within the human von Willebrand factor gene identified by a vWF cDNA clone. Nucleic Acids Res 1986;14:7139.
95. Bernardi J, Marchetti G, Bertagnolo V, Faggioli L, Del Senno L. Two TaqI RFLPs in the human von Willebrand factor gene. Nucleic Acids Res 1987;15:1347.
96. Iannuzzi MC, Konkle BA, Ginsburg D, Collins FS. RsaI RFLP in the human von Willebrand factor gene. Nucleic Acids Res 1987;15:5909.
97. Konkle BA, Kim S, Iannuzzi MC, Alani R, Collins FS, Ginsburg D. SacI RFLP in the human von Willebrand factor gene. Nucleic Acids Res 1987;15:6766.
98. Lavergen JM, Bahnak BR, Verweij CL, Pannekoek H, Meyer D. A second Xba I polymorphic site within the human von Willebrand factor gene. Nucleic Acids Res 1987;15:9099.
99. Lavergen JM, Bahnak BR, Assouline Z, et al. A Taq I polymorphism in the 5′ region of the von Willebrand factor gene. Nucleic Acids Res 1988;16:2742.
100. Lindstedt M, Anvret M. An EcoRI polymorphism of the human von Willebrand factor cDNA. Nucleic Acids Res 1989;17:2882.
101. Inbal A, Handin RI. Two TaqI polymorphisms in the 5′ region of the von Willebrand factor gene. Nucleic Acids Res 1989;17:10143.
102. Sadler JE, Ginsburg D. A database of polymorphisms in the von Willebrand factor gene and pseudogene. Thromb Haemost 1993;69:185.
103. Peake IR, Bowen D, Bignell P, et al. Family studies and prenatal diagnosis is severe von Willebrands disease by polymerase chain reaction amplification of a variable repeat region of the von Willebrand factor gene. Blood 1990;76:555.
104. Bonthron D, Orkin SH. The human von Willebrand factor gene: structure of the 5′ region. Eur J Biochem 1988;171:51.
105. Bloom AL, Giddings JC, Wilk CJ. Factor VIII on the vascular intima: possible importance in hemostasis and thrombosis. Nat New Biol 1973;241:217.
106. Hoyer LW, de los Santo RP, Hoyer JR. Antihemophilic factor antigen. Localization in endothelial cells by immunofluorescent microscopy. J Clin Invest 1973;52:2737.
107. Jaffe EA, Hoyer LW, Nachman RL. Synthesis of antihemophilic factor antigen by cultured human endothelial cells. J Clin Invest 1973;52:2757.
108. Wagner DD, Olmsted JB, Marder VJ. Immunolocalization of von Willebrand protein in Weibel-Palade bodies of human endothelial cells. J Cell Biol 1982;95:355.
109. Hormia M, Lehto VP, Virtanen I. Factor VIII-related antigen: a pericellular matrix component of culture human endothelial cells. Exp Cell Res 1983;149:483.
110. Kagawa H, Fujimoto S, Ueda H, Hamasaki K. Immunocytochemical localization of factor VIII-related antigen in human umbilical vein. J Voeh 1985;7:365.
111. Warhol MJ, Sweet JM. The ultrastructural localization of von Willebrand factor in endothelial cells. Am J Pathol 1984;117:310.
112. Gimbrone MA Jr. Culture of Vascular Endothelium. In: Spaet TH, ed. Progress in hemostasis and thrombosis, vol 3. New York, Grune & Stratton, 1973:1.
113. van Wachem PB, Reinders JH, van Buul-Wortelboer MF, et al. Von Willebrand factor in cultured human vascular endothelial cells from adult and umbilical cord arteries and veins. Thromb Haemost 1986;56:189.
114. Sporn LA, Chavin SI, Marder VJ, Wagner DD. Biosynthesis of von Willebrand protein by human megakaryocytes. J Clin Invest 1985;76:1102.
115. Fretto LJ, Fowler WE, Darrell DR, et al. Substructure of human von Willebrand factor: proteolysis by V8 and characterization of two functional domains. J Biol Chem 1986;261:15679.
116. Wagner DD, Lawrence SO, Ohlsson-Wilhelm BM, et al. Topology and order of formation of interchain disulfide bonds in von Willebrand factor. Blood 1987;69:27.
117. Wagner DD, Mayadas T, Marder VJ. Initial glycosylation and acidic pH in the Golgi apparatus are required for multimerization of von Willebrand factor. J Cell Biol 1986;102:1320.
118. Browning PJ, Ling EH, Zimmerman TS, Lynch DC. Sulfation of von Willebrand factor by human umbilical vein endothelial cells. Blood 1983;62:281a.
119. Carew JA, Browning PJ, Lynch DC. Sulfation of von Willebrand factor. Blood 1990;76:2530.
120. Wagner DD, Mayadas T, Urban-Pickering M, et al. Inhibition of disulfide bonding of vW protein by monensin results in small, functionally defective multimers. J Cell Biol 1985;101:112.
121. Chopek MW, Girma J-P, Fujikawa K, et al. Human von Willebrand factor: a multivalent protein composed of identical subunits. Biochemistry 1986;25:3146.
122. Wagner DD, Fay PJ, Sporn LA, Sinha S, Lawrence SO, Marder VJ. Divergent fates of von Willebrand factor and its propolypeptide (von Willebrand antigen II) after secretion from endothelial cells. Proc Natl Acad Sci USA 1987;84:1955.
123. Mayadas TN, Wagner DD. Vicinal cysteines in the prosequence play a role in von Willebrand factor multimer assembly. Proc Natl Acad Sci USA 1992;89:3531.
124. Scott JP, Montogomery RR. Platelet von Willebrand's antigen II: active release by aggregating agents and a marker of platelet release in vivo. Blood 1981;58:1075.
125. McCarroll DR, Levin EG, Montgomery RR. Endothelial cell synthesis of von Willebrand antigen II, von Willebrand factor, and von Willebrand factor/von Willebrand antigen II complex. J Clin Invest 1985;75:1089.
126. Ewenstein BM, Warhol MJ, Handin RI, Pober JS. Composition of the vWF storage organelle (Weibel-Palade body) isolated from cultured human umbilical vein endothelial cells. J Cell Biol 1987;104:1423.
127. Takagi J, Sekiya F, Kasahara K, Inada Y, Saito Y. Inhibition of platelet-collagen interaction by propolypeptide of von Willebrand factor. J Biol Chem 1989;264:6017.
128. Takagi J, Kasahara K, Sekiya F, Inada Y, Saito Y. A collagen-binding glycoprotein from bovine platelets is indentical to the propolypeptide of von Willebrand factor. J Biol Chem 1989;264:10425.
129. Weibel ER, Palade GC. New cytoplasmic components in arterial endothelia. J Cell Biol 1964;23:101.
130. Fuchs A, Weibel ER. Morphometrische untersuchung der verterlung liner spezifischen cytoplasmatischen organelle in endothelzellen der ratte. Z Zellforsch 1966;73:1.
131. Kumar P, Kumar S, Marsden HB, et al. Weibel-Palade bodies in endothelial cells as a marker for angiogenesis in brain tumors. Cancer Res 1980;40:2010.
132. Kumar P, Erroi A, Sattar A, Kumar S. Weibel-Palade bodies as a marker for neovascularization induced by tumor and rheumatoid angiogenesis factors. Cancer Res 1985;45:4339.
133. Ho KL. Ultrastructure of cerebellar cappillary hemangioblastoma. 1. Weibel-Palade bodies and stroma cell histogenesis. J Neuropathol Exp Neurol 1984;43:592.
134. Matsuda H, Sugiura S. Ultrastructure of "tubular body" in endothelial cells of the the ocular blood vessels. Invest Ophthalmol 1970;9:919.
135. Sengel A, Stoebner P. Golgi origin of tubular inclusions in endothelial cells. J Cell Biol 1970;44:223.
136. Reinders JH, deGroot PG, Gonsalves MD, et al. Isolation of a storage and secretory organelle containing vW protein from cultured human endothelial cells. Biochim Biophys Acta 1984;844:306.
137. Reinders JH, de Groot PG, Dawes J, et al. Comparison of secretion and subcellular localization of von Willebrand protein with that of thrombospondin and fibronectin in cultured human vascular endothelial cells. Biochim Biophys Acta 1985;884:306.
138. Loscalzo J, Fisch M, Handin RI. Solution studies of the quaternary structure and assembly of human von Willebrand factor. Biochemistry 1985;24:4468.
139. Mayadas TN, Wagner DD. In vitro multimerization of von Willebrand factor is triggered by low pH. Importance of the propolypeptide and free sulfhydryls. J Biol Chem 1989;264:13497.
140. Prentice CRM, Forbes CD, Smith SM. Rise of factor VIII after exercise and adrenalin infusion measured by immunolgical and biological techniques. Thromb Res 1972;1:493.
141. Mannucci PM, Åberg M, Nilsson IL, Robertson B. Mechanism of plasminogen activator and factor VIII increase after vasoactive drugs. Br J Haematol 1975;30:81.
142. Koutts J, Walsh PN, Plow EF, et al. Active release of human platelet factor VIII-related antigen by adenosine diphosphate, collagen and thrombin. J Clin Invest 1978;62:1255.
143. Kelly RB. Pathways of protein secretion in eukaryotes. Science 1985;230:25.
144. Loesberg C, Gonsalves MD, Zanderbergen J, et al. The effect of calcium on the secretion of factor VIII-related antigen by cultured human endothelial cells. Biochim Biophys Acta 1983;763:160.
145. Sporn LA, Marder VJ, Wagner DD. Inducible secretion of large, biologically potent von Willebrand factor multimers. Cell 1986;46:185.
146. Booyse FM, Quarfoot AJ, Chediak J, Stemerman MB, Magiac T. Characterization and properties of cultured human von Willebrand umbilical vein endothelial cells. Blood 1981;58:788.
147. Ewenstein BM, Inbal A, Pober JS, Handin RI. Molecular studies of von Willebrand's disease: reduced von Willebrand factor biosynthesis, storage and release in endothelial cells derived from patients with type I von Willebrand's disease. Blood 1990;75:1466.
148. Federici AB, DeGroot PG, Moia M, Ijsseldijk JW, Sixma JJ, Mannucci PM. Type I von Willebrand disease, subtype "platelet low": decreased platelet adhesion can be explained by low synthesis of von Willebrand factor in endothelial cells. Br J Haematol 1992;83:88.
149. Harrison RL, McKee PA. Estrogen stimulates von Willebrand factor production by cultured endothelial cells. Blood 1984;63:657.
150. Strauss HS, Diamond LK. Elevation of factor VIII (antihemophilic factor) during pregnancy in normal persons and in a patient with von Willebrand's disease. N Engl J Med 1963;269:1251.
151. Leone G, Moneta E, Paparatti G, Boni P. Von Willebrand's disease in pregnancy. N Engl J Med 1975;293:456.
152. Crowell EB, Clatanoff DV, Kiekhofer W. The effect of oral contraceptive on factor VIII levels. J Lab Clin Med 1971;77:551.
153. Pottinger BE, Read RC, Paleolog EM, Pearson JD. Von Willebrand factor is an acute phase reactant in man. Thromb Res 1989;53:389.
154. Schorer AE, Moldow CF, Rick ME. Interleukin 1 or endotoxin increases

the release of von Willebrand factor from human endothelial cells. Br J Haematol 1987;67:193.
155. Giddings JC, Shall L. Enhanced release of von Willebrand factor by human endothelial cells in culture in the presence of phorbol myristate acetate and interleukin 1. Thromb Res 1987;47:259.
156. de Groot PG, Verweij CL, Nawrath PP, et al. Interleukin 1 inhibits the synthesis of von Willebrand factor in endothelial cells which results in a decreased reactivity of their matrix towards platelets. Arterioscl 1987;7:605.
157. Zavoico GB, Ewenstein BM, Schafer AI, Pober JS. IL-1 and related cytokines enhance thrombin stimulated PGI2 production in cultured endothelial cells without affecting thrombin-stimulated von Willebrand factor secretion or platelet-activating factor biosynthesis. J Immunol 1989;142:3993.
158. Paleolog EM, Crossman DC, McVey JH, Pearson JD. Differential regulation by cytokines of constitutive and stimulated secretion of von Willebrand factor from endothelial cells. Blood 1989;75:688.
159. Levine JD, Harlan JM, Harker LA, et al. Thrombin-mediated release of factor VIII antigen from human umbilical vein endothelial cells in culture. Blood 1982;60:531.
160. de Groot PG, Gonsalves MD, Loesberg C, et al. Thrombin-induced release of von Willebrand factor from endothelial cells is mediated by phospholipid methylation. Prostacyclin synthesis is independent of phosphilipid methylation. J Biol Chem 1984;259:13329.
161. Hamilton KK, Sims PJ. Changes in cytosolic Ca2+ associated with von Willebrand factor release in endothelial cells exposed to histamine. J Clin Invest 1987;79:600.
162. Ewenstein BM, Jacobson BC, Romano M, Serhan CN. Peptido-leukotrienes stimulate von Willebrand factor release from human endothelial cells. Blood 1991;78:69a.
163. Ribes JA, Francis CW, Wagner DD. Fibrin induces release of von Willebrand factor from endothelial cells. J Clin Invest 1987;79:117.
164. Ribes JA, Ni F, Wagner DD, Francis CW. Mediation of fibrin-induced release of von Willebrand factor from cultured endothelial cells by the fibrin beta chain. J Clin Invest 1989;84:435.
165. Hattori R, Hamilton KK, McEver RP, Sims PJ. Complement proteins C5b-9 induce secretion of high molecular weight multimers of endothelial von Willebrand factor and translocation of granule membrane protein GMP140 to the cell surface. J Biol Chem 1989;264:9053.
166. Booyse FM, Osilowicz G, Feder S. Effects of various agents on ristocetin-Willebrand factor activity in long term cultures of vWF and normal human umbilical vein endothelial cells. Thromb Haemost 1981;46:668.
167. Tuddenham EGD, Lazarchich J, Hoyer LW. Synthesis and release of factor VIII by cultured human endothelial cells. Br J Haematol 1981;47:617.
168. Hashemi S, Tackaberry ES, Palmer DS, Rock G, Ganz RP. DDAVP-induced release of von Willebrand factor from endothelial cells in vitro: the effect of plasma and blood cells. Biochim Biophys Acta 1990;1052:63.
169. Hallam TJ, Jacob R, Merritt JE. Evidence that agonists stimulate bivalent-cation influx into human endothelial cells. Biochem J 1988;255:179.
170. Rotrosen D, Gallin JI. Histamine type I receptor occupancy increases endothelial cytosolic calcium, reduces F-actin, and promotes albumin diffusion across cultured endothelial monolayers. J Cell Biol 1986;130:2379.
171. Birch KA, Pober JS, Zavoico GB, et al. Calcium/calmodulin transduced thrombin-stimulated secretion: studies in intact and minimally permeabilized human umbilical vein endothelial cells. J Cell Biol 1992;118:1501.
172. McNiff JM, Gil J. Secretion of Weibel-Palade bodies observed in extraalveolar vessels of rabbit lung. J Appl Physiol 1983;54:1284.
173. Fitzgerald LA, Charo IF, Philips DR. Human and bovine endothelial cells synthesize membrane proteins similar to human platelet glycoproteins IIb and IIIa. J Biol Chem 1985;260:10893.
174. Beacham DA, Wise RJ, Turci SM, Handin RI. Selective inactivation of the Arg-Gly-Asp-Ser (RGDS) binding site in von Willebrand factor by site-directed mutagenesis. J Biol Chem 1992;267:3409.
175. Sprandio JD, Shapiro SS, Thiagarjan P, McCord. Cultured human vein endothelial cells contain a membrane glycoprotein immunologically related to platelet glycoprotein Ib. Blood 1988;71:234.
176. Konkle BA, Shapiro SS, Asch AS, Nachman RL. Cytokine-enhanced expression of glycoprotein Ib in human endothelium. J Biol Chem 1990;265:19838.
177. Bowie EJW, Solberg LA, Fass DN, et al. Transplantation of normal bone marrow into a pig with severe von Willebrand's disease. J Clin Invest 1986;78:26.
178. Hoyer LW, Shainoff JR. 1980. Factor VIII-related protein circulates in normal human plasma as high molecular weight multimers. Blood 1980;55:1056.
179. Ruggeri ZM, Zimmerman TS. The complex multimeric composition of factor VIII/von Willebrand factor. Blood 1981;57:1140.
180. Sporn LA, Marder VJ, Wagner. Differing polarity of the constitutive and regulated secretory pathways for von Willebrand factor in endothelial cells. J Cell Biol 1989;108:1283.
181. Tsai H-M, Nagel RL, Hatcher VB, et al. The high molecular weight form of endothelial cell von Willebrand factor is released by the regulated pathway. Br J Haematol 1991;79:239.
182. Koedam JA, Meijers JCM, Sixma JJ, et al. Inactivation of human factor VIII by activated protein C. Cofactor activity of protein S and protective effect of von Willebrand factor. J Clin Invest 1988;82:1236.
183. Fay PJ, Coumans JV, Walker FJ. Von Willebrand factor mediates protection of factor VIII from activated protein C-catalyzed inactivation. J Biol Chem 1991;266:2172.
184. Hamer RJ, Koedam JA, Beeser-Visser NH, Sixma JJ. The effect of thrombin on the complex between factor VIII and von Willebrand factor. Eur J Biochem 1987;167:253.
185. Preston AE, Barr A. The plasma concentration of factor VIII in the normal population: the effects of age, sex and blood groups. Br J Haematol 1964;10:238.
186. Jeremic M, Weisert O, Gedde-Dahl TW. Factor VIII (AHG) levels in 1016 regular blood donors: the effects of age, sex and ABO blood groups. Scand J Clin Lab Invest 1976;36:461.
187. McCallum CJ, Peake IR, Newcombe RG, Bloom AL. Factor VIII levels in blood group antigens. Thrombosis Haemostas (Stuttg) 1983;50:757.
188. Ørstavik KH, Magnus P, Reisner H, Berg K, Graham JB, Nance W. Factor VIII and factor IX in a twin population: evidence for a major effect of ABO locus on factor VIII level. Am J Hum Genet 1985;37:89.
189. Graham JB, Rizza CR, Chediak J, et al. Carrier detection in hemophilia A: a cooperative international study. I. The carrier phenotype. Blood 1986;67:1554.
190. Gill JC, Endres-Brooks J, Bauer PJ, et al. The effect of ABO blood group on the diagnosis of von Willebrand disease. Blood 1987;69:1691.
191. Stormorken H, Erikssen J. Plasma antithrombin III and factor VIII antigen in relation to angiographic findings, angina and blood groups in middle-aged men. Thrombosis Haemostas (Stuttg) 1977;38:874.
192. Wahlberg TB, Savidge GF, Blombäck M, Wiechel B. Influence of age, sex and blood groups on 15 blood coagulation laboratory variables in a reference material composed of 80 blood donors. Vox Sang 1980;39:301.
193. Rouger P, Riveau D, Salmon C. Detection of the H and I blood group antigens in normal plasma. Vox Sang 1979;37:78.
194. Ørstavik KH, Kornstad L, Reisner H, Berg K. Possible effect of secretor locus on plasma concentrations of factor VIII and von Willebrand factor. Blood 1989;73:990.
195. Van Cong N, Weil D, Finaz C, et al. Assignment of the ABO-Np-Akl linkage group to chromosome 9 in man-hamster hybrids. Cytogenet Cell Genet 1976;16:241.
196. Sodetz JM, Paulson JC, McKee PA. Carbohydrate composition and identification of blood groups A, B and H oligo-saccharide structures of human factor VIII/von Willebrand factor. J Biol Chem 1979;254:10754.
197. Mazurier C, Samor B, Mannessier L, et al. Blood group A and B activity associated with factor VIII/von Willebrand factor. Blood Transfus Immunohaematol 1981;24:289.
198. Johnson SS, Montgomery RR, Hathaway WE. Newborn factor VIII complex: elevated activities in term infants and alterations in electrophoretic mobility related to illness and activated coagulation. Br J Haematol 1981;47:597.
199. Weinger RS, Cecalupo AJ, Olson JD, Frankel L. Neonatal von Willebrand's disease: diagnostic difficulty at birth. Am J Dis Child 1980;134:793.
200. Weinstein MJ, Blanchard R, Moake JL, Vosburgh E, Moise K. Fetal and neonatal von Willebrand factor (vWF) is unusually large and similar to the vWF in patients with thrombotic thrombocytopenic purpura. Br J Haematol 1989;72:68.
201. Katz JA, Moake JL, McPherson PD, et al. Relationship between human development and disappearance of unusually large von Willebrand factor multimers from plasma. Blood 1989;73:1851.
202. Maruzier C, Daffos F, Forestier F. Electrophoretic and functional characteristics of the von Willebrand factor in human fetal plasma. Br J Haematol 1992;81:263.
203. Cooperberg AA, Teitelbaum J. The concentration of antihemophilic globulin (AHG) related to age. Br J Haematol 1960;6:281.
204. Pitney WR, Kvik RL, Arnold BJ, Stenhouse NS. Plasma antihaemophilic factor (factor VIII) concentrations in normal families. Br J Haematol 1962;8:421.
205. Kasper CK, Hoag MS, Aggeler PM, Stove S. Blood clotting factor in pregnancy: factor VIII concentrates in normal and AHF-deficient women. Obstet Gynecol 1964;24:242.
206. Bennett B, Ratnoff OD. Changes in antihemophilic factor (AHF, factor VIII) procoagulant activity and AHF-like antigen in normal pregnancy, and following exercise and pneumoencephalography. J Lab Clin Med 1972;80:256.
207. Noller KL, Bowie EJW, Kempers RD, Owen CA. von Willebrand's disease in pregnancy. Obstet Gynecol 1973;41:865.
208. Bennett B, Oxnard SC, Douglas AS, Ratnoff OD. Studies on antihemophilic factor (AHF, factor VIII) during labor in normal women, in patients with premature separation of the placenta, and in a patient with von Willebrand's disease. J Lab Clin Med 1974;84:851.
209. Krishnamurthy M, Miotti AB. Von Willebrand's disease and pregnancy. Obstet Gynecol 1977;49:244.
210. Chediak JR, Alban GM, Maxey B. Von Willebrand's disease and pregnancy: management during delivery and outcome of offspring. Am J Obstet Gynecol 1986;155:618.

211. Adashi EY. Lack of improvement in von Willebrand's disease during pregnancy. N Engl J Med 1980;303:1178.
212. Punnonen R, Nyman D, Grönroos M, Wallén O. Von Willebrand's disease and pregnancy. Acta Obstet Gynecol Scand 1981;60:507.
213. Rick ME, Williams SB, Sacher RA, McKeown LP. Thrombocytopenia associated with pregnancy in a patient with type IIB von Willebrand's disease. Blood 1987;69:786.
214. Giles AR, Hoogendoorn H, Benford K. Type IIB von Willebrand's disease presenting as thrombocytopenia during pregnancy. Br J Haematol 1987;67:349.
215. Rogers JS II, Shane SR, Jencks FS. Factor VIII activity and thyroid function. Ann Intern Med 1982;97:713.
216. Egeberg O. Influence of thyroid function on the blood clotting system. Scand J Clin Lab Invest 1963;15:1.
217. Dalton RG, Dewar MS, Savidge GF, et al. Hypothyroidism and von Willebrand's disease. Lancet 1987;1:1007.
218. MacCallum PK, Rodgers M, Taberner DA. Hypothyroidism and von Willebrand's disease. Lancet 1987;1:1314.
219. Smith SR, Auger MJ. Hypothyroidism and von Willebrand's disease. Lancet 1987;1:1314.
220. Rogers JS II, Shane SR. Factor VIII activity in normal volunteers receiving oral thryroid hormone. J Lab Clin Med 1983;102:444.
221. Rizza CR. Effect of exercise on the level of antihaemophilic globulin in human blood. J Physiol Lond 1961;156:128.
222. Egeberg O. On the nature of blood and antihemophilic A factor (AHA-FVIII) increase associated with muscular excercise. Scand J Clin Lab Invest 1963;15:202.
223. Stibbe J. Effect of exercise on FVIII complexes: proportional increase of ristocetin cofactor (von Willebrand factor) and FVIII-AGN, but disproportional increase of FVIII-AHF. Thromb Res 1977;10:163.
224. Brown JE, Baugh RF, Hougie C. Effector of exercise on the factor VIII complex: correlation of the von Willebrand antigen and factor VIII coagulant antigen increase. Thromb Res 1979;15:61.
225. Wheeler ME, Davis GL, Gillespie WJ, Bern MM. Physiological changes in hemostasis associated with acute exercise. J Appl Physiol 1986;60:986.
226. Andrew M, Carter C, O'Brodovich H, Heigenhauser G. Increases in factor VIII complex and fibrinolytic activity are dependent on exercise intensity. J Appl Physiol 1986;60:1917.
227. Musemeci V, Cardillo C, Baroni S, et al. Effects of calcium channel blockers on the endothelial release of von Willebrand factor after exercise in healthy subjects. J Lab Clin Med 1989;113:525.
228. Rand JH, Sussman II, Gordon RE, Chu SSV, Solomon V. Localization of factor VIII-related antigen in human vascular subendothelium. Blood 1980;55:752.
229. Sussman II, Rand JR. Subendothelial deposition of von Willebrand factor requires the presence of endothelial cells. J Lab Clin Med 1982;100:526.
230. Sakariassen KS, Bolhuis PA, Sixma JJ. Human blood platelet adhesion to artery subendothelium is mediated by factor VIII-von Willebrand factor bound to the subendothelium. Nature 1979;279:636.
231. Sakariassen KS, Ottenhof-Rovers M, Sixma JJ. Factor VIII-von Willebrand factor requires calcium for facilitation of platelet adherence. Blood 1984;63:996.
232. Scott DM, Griffin B, Pepper DS, Barnes MJ. The binding of purified factor VIII/von Willebrand factor to collagens of different type and forms. Thromb Res 1981;24:467.
233. Santoro SA. Adsorption of von Willebrand factor/VIII by the genetically distinct interstitial collagens. Thromb Res 1981;21:689.
234. Morton LF, Griffin B, Pepper DS, Barnes MJ. The interaction between collagens and factor VIII/von Willebrand factor: investigation of the structural requirements for interaction. Thromb Res 1983;32:545.
235. Kessler CM, Floyd CM, Rick ME, et al. Collagen-factor VIII/von Willebrand factor protein interaction. Blood 1984;63:1291.
236. Rand JH, Patel ND, Schwartz E, Zhou SL, Potter BJ. 150-kD von Willebrand factor binding protein extracted from human vascular subendothelium is type VI collagen. J Clin Invest 1991;88:253.
237. Wagner DD, Urban-Pickering M, Marder VJ. Von Willebrand protein binds to extracellular matrices independently of collagen. Proc Natl Acad Sci USA 1984;81:471.
238. Madaras F, Bell WR, Castaldi PA. Isolation and insolubilisation of human F-VIII by affinity chromatography. Haemostasis 1978;7:321.
239. Trueb B, Schreier T, Bruckner P, Winterhalter KH. Type VI collagen represents a major fraction of connective tissue collagens. Eur J Biochem 1987;166:699.
240. Bonaldo P, Colombatti A. The carboxyl terminus of the chicken alpha 3 chain of collagen VI is a unique mosaic structure with glycoprotein Ib-like, fibronectin type III, and Kunitz modules. J Biol Chem 1989;264:20235.
241. Bockenstedt P, McDonagh J, Handin RI. Binding and covalent cross-linking of purified von Willebrand factor to native monomeric collagen. J Clin Invest 1986;78:551.
242. Tannenbaum SH, Rick ME, Shafer B, Gralnick HR. Subendothelial matrix of cultured endothelial cells contains fully processed high molecular weight von Willebrand factor. J Lab Clin Med 1989;113:372.
243. Santoro SA. Preferential binding of high molecular weight forms of von Willebrand factor to fibrillar collagen. Biochim Biophys Acta 1983;756:123.
244. Sporn LA, Marder VJ, Wagner DD. Von Willebrand factor released from Weibel-Palade bodies binds more avidly to extracellular matrix than that secreted constitutively. Blood 1987;69:1531.
245. Sixma JJ, Sakariassen KS, Beeser-Visser NH, et al. Adhesion of platelets to human artery subendothelium: effect of factor VIII-von Willebrand factor of various multimeric composition. Blood 1984;63:128.
246. Tschopp TB, Baumgartner HR, Silberbauer K, Sinzinger H. Platelet adhesion and platelet thrombus formation on subendothelium of human arteries and veins exposed to flowing blood in vitro. A comparison with rabbit aorta. Haemostasis 1979;8:19.
247. Turitto VT, Baumgartner HR. Platelet deposition on subendothelium exposed to flowing blood: mathematical analysis of physical parameters. Trans Am Soc Artif Intern Organs 1975;21:593.
248. Turitto VT, Baumgartner HR. Rheological factors influencing platelet interaction with vessel surfaces. J Rheology 1979;23:735.
249. Weiss HJ, Turitto VT, Baumgartner HR. Effect of shear rate on platelet interaction with subendothelium in citrated and native blood. Shear-rate dependent decrease of adhesion in von Willebrand's disease and the Bernard-Soulier syndrome. J Lab Clin Med 1978;92:750.
250. Stel HV, Sakariassen KS, deGroot PG, et al. Von Willebrand factor in the vessel wall mediates platelet adherence. Blood 1985;65:85.
251. Turitto VT, Weiss HJ, Zimmerman TS, Sussman II. Factor VIII/von Willebrand factor in subendothelium mediates platelet adhesion. Blood 1985;65:823.
252. Baruch D, Denis C, Mareaux C, Schoevaert D, Coulombel L, Meyer D. Role of von Willebrand factor associated to extraceliular matrices in platelet adhesion. Blood 1991;77:519.
253. Tschopp TB, Weiss HJ, Baumgartner HR. Decreased adhesion of platelets to subendothelium in von Willebrand's disease. J Lab Clin Med 1974;83:296.
254. Baumgartner HR, Turitto VT, Weiss HJ. Effect of shear rate on platelet interaction with subendothelium in citrated and native blood. II. Relationships among platelet adhesion, thrombus dimensions and fibrin formation. J Lab Clin Med 1980;95:208.
255. Sakariassen KS, Aarts PAMM, deGroot PD, Houdijk WPM, Sixma JJ. A perfusion chamber to investigate platelet interaction in flowing blood with human vessel wall cells, their extracellular matrix and purified components. J Lab Clin Med 1983;102:522.
256. Sixma JJ, Nievelstein PFEM, Houdijk WPM, van Breugel H, Hindriks G, deGroot PG. Adhesion of blood platelets to isolated components of the vessel walls. Ann NY Acad Sci 1987;509:103.
257. Olson JD, Zaleski A, Herrman D, Flood PA. Adhesion of platelets to purified solid-phase von Willebrand factor: effects of walls shear rate, ADP, thrombin and ristocetin. J Lab Clin Med 1989;114:6.
258. Furlan M. Factor VIII/von Willebrand factor: a multivalent ligand binding to platelets and collagen. Blut 1986;52:329.
259. Nachman RL, Levine R, Jaffe EA. Synthesis of factor VIII antigen by cultured guinea pig megakaryocytes. J Clin Invest 1977;60:914.
260. Howard MA, Montgomery DC, Hardisty RM. Factor VIII related antigen in platelets. Thromb Res 1974;4:617.
261. Nachman RL, Jaffe EA. Subcellular platelet factor VIII antigen and von Willebrand factor. J Exp Med 1975;141:1101.
262. Slot JW, Bouma BN, Montgomery R, Zimmerman TS. Platelet factor VIII-related antigen: immunofluorescent localization. Thromb Res 1978;13:871.
263. Zucker MB, Broekman MJ, Kaplan KL. Factor VIII-related antigen in human blood platelets. J Lab Clin Med 1979;94:675.
264. Wencel-Drake JD, Painter RG, Zimmerman TS, Ginsburg MH. Ultrastructural localization of human platelet thrombospondin, fibrinogen and fibronectin and vW factor in frozen thin section. Blood 1985;65:929.
265. Jeanneau C, Avner P, Sultan Y. Use of monoclonal antibody and colloidal gold in E.M. localization of von Willebrand factor in megacytes and platelets. Cell Biol Int Rep 1984;8:841.
266. Cramer EM, Meyer D, le Menn R, Breton-Gorius J. Eccentric localization of vW factor in an internal structure of platelet-granule resembling that of Weibel-Palade bodies. Blood 1985;66:710.
267. Harrison P, Savidge GF, Cramer EM. The origin and pysiologic relevance of granules adhesive proteins. Br J Haematol 1990;74:125.
268. Ruggeri ZM, Zimmerman TS. Variant von Willegrand's disease: characterization of two subtypes by analysis of multimeric composition of factor VIII/von Willebrand factor in plasma and platelets. J Clin Invest 1980;65:1318[a].
269. Gralnick HR, Williams SB, McKeown LP, et al. Platelet von Willebrand factor: comparison with plasma von Willebrand factor. Thromb Res 1985;38:623.
270. Fernandez MFL, Ginsburg MH, Ruggeri ZM, et al. Multimeric structure of platelet factor VIII/von Willebrand factor: the presence of larger multimers and their reassociation with thrombin-stimulated platelets. Blood 1982;60:1132.
271. George JN, Onofre AR. Human platelet surface binding of endogenous secreted factor VIII-von Willebrand factor and platelet factor 4. Blood 1982;59:194.
272. Parker RI, Rick ME, Gralnick HR. Effect of calcium on the availability of platelet von Willebrand factor. J Lab Clin Med 1985;106:336.
273. Mannucci PM, Lombardi R, Bader R, et al. Heterogeneity of type I von Willebrand disease: evidence for a subgroup with an abnormal von Willebrand factor. Blood 1985;66:796.

274. Gralnick HR, Rick ME, McKeown LP, et al. Platelet von Willebrand factor: an important determinant of the bleeding time in type I von Willebrand's disease. Blood 1986;68:58.
275. Fressinaud E, Baruch D, Rothschild C, et al. Platelet von Willebrand factor: evidence for its involvement in platelet adhesion to collagen. Blood 1987;70:1214.
276. Castillo R, Escolar G, Monteagudo J, et al. Role for platelet von Willebrand factor in supporting platelet-vessel wall interactions in von Willebrand disease. Am J Hematol 1989;31:153.
277. Castillo R, Monteagudo J, Escolar G, et al. Hemostatic effect of normal platelet transfusion in severe von Willebrand disease patients. Blood 1991;77:1901.
278. Voorberg J, Fonjijn R, Calafat J, Janssen H, Mourik JA, Pannekoek H. Biogenesis of von Willebrand factor-containing organelles in heterologous transfected CV-1 cells. 1993:749.
279. Kramer W, Drutsa V, Jansen HW, Kramer B, Pfugleder M, Fritz HJ. The gapped duplex DNA approach to oligonucleotide-directed mutation construction. Nucleic Acids Res 1984;12:9441.
280. Meulien P, Nishino M, Mazurier C, et al. Processing and characterization of recombinant von Willebrand factor expressed in different cell types using a vaccinia virus vector. Thromb Haemost 1992;67:154.
281. Wagner DD, Saffaripour S, Bonfanti R, et al. Induction of specific organelles by von Willebrand factor propolypeptide. Cell 1991;64:403.
282. Silwer J, Nilsson IM. On a Swedish family with 51 members affected by von Willebrand's disease. Acta Med Scand 1964;175:627.
283. Bloom AL. The von Willebrand syndrome. Semin Hematol 1980;17: 215.
284. Bachman F. Diagnostic approach to mild bleeding disorders. Semin Hematol 1980;17:292.
285. Rodeghiero F, Castman G, Dini E. Epidemiological investigation of the prevalence of von Willebrand's disease. Blood 1987;69:454.
286. Berliner SA, Seligsohn U, Zivelin A, et al. A relatively high frequency of severe (type III) von Willebrand's disease in Israel. Br J Haematol 1986;62:535.
287. Weiss HJ, Ball AP, Mannucci PM. Incidence of severe von Willebrand's disease. N Engl J Med 1982;307:127.
288. Mannucci PM, Bloom AL, Larrieu MJ, Nilsson IM, West RR. Atherosclerosis and von Willebrand factor: prevalence of severe von Willebrand's disease in western Europe and Israel. Br J Haematol 1984;57: 163.
289. Italian Working Group. Spectrum of von Willebrand's disease: a study of 100 cases. Br J Haematol 1977;35:101.
290. Holmber L, Nilsson IM. Von Willebrand's disease. Eur J Haematol 1992;48:127.
291. Miller CH, Graham JB, Goldin LR, Elston RC. Genetics of classic von Willebrand's disease. I. Phenotypic variation within families. Blood 1979;54:117.
292. Miller CH, Graham JB, Goldin LR, Elston RC. Genetics of classic von Willebrand's disease. II. Optimal assignment of the heterozygous genotype (diagnosis) by discriminant analysis. Blood 1979;54:137.
293. Blombäck M, Eneroth P, Landgren BM, Lagerström M, Andersson O. On the intraindividual and gender variability of haemostatic components. Thromb Haemost 1992;67:70.
294. Blombäck m, Eneroth P, Andersson O, Anvret M. On laboratory problems in diagnosing mild von Willebrand's disease. Am J Hematol 1992;40:117.
295. Lind SE. Prolonged bleeding time. Am J Med 1984;77:305.
296. Burns ER, Lawrence C. Bleeding time. A guide to its diagnostic and clinical utility. Arch Pathol Lab Med 1989;113:1219.
297. Rodgers RPC, Levin J. A critical reappraisal of the bleeding time. Semin Thromb Hemostas 1990;16:1.
298. Bowie EJW, Didisheim P, Thompson JH, Owen CA Jr. Von Willebrand's disease: a critical review. Hematol Rev 1968;1:1.
299. Mielke CH, Kaneshiro MM, Maher IA, et al. The standardized normal Ivy bleeding time and its prolongation by aspirin. Blood 1969;34:204.
300. Kumar R, Ansell JE, Canoso RT, Deykin D. Clinical trials of a new bleeding time device. Am J Clin Pathol 1978;70:642.
301. Ivy AC, Shapiro PF, Melnich P. The bleeding tendency in jaundice. Surg Gynecol Obstet 1935;60:357.
302. Nilsson IM, Magnusson S, Borchgrevink C. The Duke and Ivy methods for determination of the bleeding time. Thromb Diath Haemorrh 1963;10:223.
303. Borchgrevink CF, Egeberg O, Godal HC, et al. The effect of plasma and Cohn's fraction I on the Duke and Ivy bleeding times in von Willebrand's disease. Acta Med Scand 1963;173:235.
304. Pitney WR, Arnold BJ. Laboratory findings in families of patients suffering from von Willebrand's disease. Br J Haematol 1960;6:81.
305. Abildgaard CF, Suzuki Z, Harrison J, et al. Serial studies in von Willebrand's disease: variability versus "variants." Blood 1980;56:712.
306. Quick AJ. Salicylates and bleeding: the aspirin tolerance test. Am J Med Sci 1967;252:265.[a].
307. Quick AJ. The Minot-von Willebrand syndrome. Am J Med Sci 1967;253: 520.
308. Ratnoff OD, Bennett B. Clues to the pathogenesis of bleeding in von Willebrand's disease. N Engl J Med 1973;289:1182.
309. Lian EC, Deykin D. In vivo dissociation of factor VIII (AHF) activity and factor VIII-related antigen in von Willebrand's disease. Am J Hematol 1976;1:71.
310. Hoyer LW. Immunological studies on antihemophilia factor (AHF, factor VIII). IV. Radioimmunoassay of AHF antigen. J Lab Clin Med 1972;80: 822.
311. Counts RB. Solid-phase immunoradiometric assay of factor-VIII protein. Br J Haematol 1975;31:429.
312. Ruggeri ZM, Mannucci PM, Jeffcoate SL, Ingram GIC. Immunoradiometric assay of Factor VIII related antigen, with observations in 32 patients with von Willebrand's disease. Br J Haematol 1976;33:221.
313. Green D, Reynolds N. Double-antibody radioimmunassay for factor VIII-related antigen. Clin Chem 1977;23:1648.
314. Girma J-P, Ardaillou N, Meyer D, et al. Fluid-phase immunoradiometric assay for the detection of qualitative abnormalities of factor VIII/von Willebrand factor in variants of von Willebrand's disease. J Lab Clin Med 1979;93:926.
315. Bartlett A, Dormandy KM, Hawkey CM, et al. Factor VIII-related antigen: measurement by enzyme immuno-assay. Br Med J 1976;1: 994.
316. Mazurier C, Parquet-Gernez A, Goudemand M. Dosage de l'antigène lié au facteur VIII par la technique ELISA: interêt dans l'étude de la maladie de Willebrand. Pathol Biol 1977;25(Suppl):18.
317. Yorde LD, Hussey CV, Yorde DE, Sasse EA. Competitive enzyme-linked immunoassay for factor VIII antigen. Clin Chem 1979;25:1924.
318. Short PE, Williams CE, Picken AM, Hill FGH. Factor VIII related antigen: an improved enzyme immunoassay. Med Lab Sci 1982;39:351.
319. Batlle J, Lopez-Fernandez MF. Laboratory assays for von Willebrand factor. In: Zimmerman TS, Ruggeri ZM, eds. Coagulation and bleeding disorders. New York and Basel: Marcel Dekker, 1989:325.
320. Weiss HJ, Pietu G, Rabinowitz R, et al. Heterogenous abnormalities in the multimeric structure, antigenic properties, and plasma-platelet content of factor VIII/von Willebrand factor in subtypes of classic (type I) and variant (type IIA) von Willebrand's disease. J Lab Clin Med 1983;101:411.
321. Ciavarella G, Ciavarella N, Antoncecchi S, et al. High-resolution analysis of von Willebrand factor multimeric composition defines a new variant of type I von Willebrand disease with aberrant structure but presence of all size multimers (type IC). Blood 1985;66:1423.
322. Aihara M, Sawada Y, Ueno K, et al. Visualization of von Willebrand factor multimers by immunoenzymatic stain using avidin-biotin peroxidase complex. Thromb Haemost 1986;55:263.
323. Miller MA, Pascak JE, Thompson MR, Martelo OJ. A modified SDS agarose gel method for determining factor VIII von Willebrand factor multimers using commercially available reagents. Thromb Res 1983;39: 777.
324. Chow R, Savidge GF. Enzyme linked antibody system for the visualization of FVIII multimers. Thromb Haemost 1985;54:75a.
325. Bukh A, Ingerslev J, Stenbjerg S, et al. The multimeric structure of plasma FVIII: Ag studies by electroelution and immunoperoxiadase detection. Thromb Res 1986;43:579.
326. Lombardi R, Gelfi C, Righetti P, et al. Electroblot and immunoperoxidase staining for rapid screening of the abnormalities of the multimeric structure of von Willebrand factor in von Willebrand's disease. Thromb Haemost 1986;55:246.
327. Brosstad F, Kjoennisksen I, Roenning B, et al. Visualization of von Willebrand factor multimers by enzyme-conjugated secondary antibodies. Thromb Haemost 1986;55:276.
328. Mannucci PM, Lombardi R, Federici AB, et al. A new variant of type II von Willebrand disease with aberrant multimeric structure of plasma but not platelet von Willebrand factor (type IIF). Blood 1986;68:269.
329. Zucker MB. In vitro abnormality of the blood in von Willebrand's disease correctable by normal plasma. Nature (Lond) 1963;197:601.
330. O'Brien JR, Heywood JB. Some interactions between human platelets and glass: von Willebrand's disease compared with normal. J Clin Pathol 1967;20:56.
331. Weiss HJ. Von Willebrand's disease: diagnostic criteria. Blood 1968;32: 668.
332. Allain JP, Cooper HA, Wagner RH, Brinkhous KM. Platelets fixed with paraformaldehyde: a new reagent for assay of von Willebrand factor and platelet aggregating factor. J Lab Clin Med 1975;85:318.
333. Kroll MH, Harris TS, Moake JL, Handin RI, Schafer AI. Von Willebrand factor binding to platelet GpIb initiates signals for platelet activation. J Clin Invest 1991;88:1568.
334. Jenkins CSP, Phillips DR, Clemetson KJ, et al. Platelet membrane glycoproteins implicated in ristocetin-induced aggretation. J Clin Invest 1976;57:112.
335. Moake JL, Olson JD, Troll JH, et al. Binding of radioiodinated human von Willebrand factor to Bernard-Soulier, thrombasthenic and von Willebrand's disease platelets. Thromb Res 1980;19:21.
336. Ruan C, Tobelem G, McMichael AJ, et al. Monoclonal antibody to human platelet glycoprotein I. II. Effects on human platelet function. Br J Haematol 1981;49:511.
337. Coller BS, Peerschke EI, Scudder LE, Sullivan CA. Studies with a murine monoclonal antibody that abolished ristocetin-induced binding of von Willebrand factor to platelets: additional evidence in support of Gp Ib as a platelet receptor for von Willebrand factor. Blood 1983;61:99.
338. Coller BS. The effects of ristocetin and von Willebrand factor on platelet electrophoretic mobility. J Clin Invest 1977;61:1168.
339. Rosborough TK, Swaim WR. Abnormal Polybrene-induced platelet agglutination in von Willebrand's disease. Thromb Res 1978;12:937.

340. Rosborough TK. Von Willebrand factor, polycations, and platelet aggregation. Thromb Res 1980;17:481.
341. Coller BS. Polybrene-induced agglutination and reduction in electrophoretic mobility: enhancement by von Willebrand factor and inhibition by vancomycin. Blood 1980;55:276.
342. De Marco L, Shapiro SS. Properties of human asialo-factor VIII: a ristocetin-independent platelet-aggregating agent. J Clin Invest 1981;68: 321.
343. Gralnick HR, Williams SB, McKeown LP, et al. Von Willebrand's disease with spontaneous platelet aggregation induced by an abnormal plasma von Willebrand factor. J Clin Invest 1985;76:1522.
344. De Marco L, Grolami A, Russell S, Ruggeri ZM. Interaction of asialo von Willebrand factor with glycoprotein Ib induces fibrinogen binding to the glycoprotein IIb/IIIa complex and mediates platelet aggregation. J Clin Invest 1985;75:1198.
345. Gralnick HR, Sultan Y, Coller BS. Von Willebrand's disease: combined qualitative and quantitative abnormalities. N Engl J Med 1977;296: 1024.
346. Hoyer LW, Rizza CR, Tuddenham EGD, et al. Von Willebrand factor multimer patterns in von Willebrand's disease. Br J Haematol 1983;55: 493.
347. Gralnick HR, Williams SB, Morisato DK. Effect of the multimeric structure of the factor VIII/von Willebrand factor protein on binding to platelets. Blood 1981;58:387.
348. Federici AB, Mannucci PM, Lombardi R, et al. Type IIH von Willebrand disease: new structural abnormality of plasma and platelet von Willebrand factor in a patient with prolonged bleeding time and borderline levels of ristocetin cofactor activity. Am J Hematol 1989;32:287.
349. Coller BS, Franza B Jr, Gralnick HR. The pH dependence of quantitative ristocetin-induced platelet aggregation: theoretical and practical implications: a new device for maintenance of platelet-rich plasma pH. Blood 1976;47:841.
350. Weiss HJ. Abnormalities of factor VIII and platelet aggregation-use of ristocetin in diagnosiing the von Willebrand syndrome. Blood 1975;45: 403.
351. Weiss HJ, Sussman II. A new von Willebrand factor variant (type I, New York): increased ristocetin-induced platelet aggregation and plasma von Willebrand factor containing all vWF multimers. Blood 1986;68:149.
352. Ruggeri ZM, Pareti FI, Mannucci PM, et al. Heightened interaction between platelets and factor VIII/von Willebrand factor in a new subtype of von Willebrand's disease. N Engl J Med 1980;302:1047b.
353. Weiss HJ, Meyer D, Rabinowitz R, et al. Pseudo-von Willebrand's disease: an intrinsic platelet defect with aggregation by unmodified factor VIII/von Willebrand factor and enhanced adsorption of its high-molecular-weight multimers. N Engl J Med 1982;306:326.
354. Brinkhous KM, Read MS. Preservation of platelet receptors for platelet aggregating factor/von Willebrand factor by air drying, freezing or lyophilization: new stable platelet preparations for von Willebrand factor assays. Thromb Res 1978;13:591.
355. Sarji KE, Stratton RD, Wagner RH, Brinkhous KM. Nature of von Willebrand factor: a new assay and a specific inhibitor. Proc Natl Acad Sci USA 1974;71:2937.
356. Weiss HJ. Relation of von Willebrand factor to bleeding time. (Letter) N Engl J Med 1974;291:420.
357. Hellem AJ. Platelet adhesiveness in von Willebrand disease: a study with a new modification of the glass bead filter method. Scand J Haematol 1970;7:374.
358. Bowie EJW, Owen CA Jr. Some factors influencing platelet retention in glass bead columns, including the influence of plastics. Am J Clin Pathol 1971;56:479.
359. Ginsburg D, Sadler JE. von Willebrand disease: a database of point mutations, insertions, and deletions. Thromb Haemost 1993;69:177.
360. Nilsson IM. Von Willebrand's disease from 1926. Scand J Haematol 1984;33:21.
361. Ngo KY, Glotz VT, Koziol JA, et al. Homozygous and heterozygous deletions of the von Willebrand factor gene in patients and carriers of severe von Willebrand disease. Proc Natl Acad Sci USA 1988;85:2753.
362. Peake IR, Liddell MB, Moodie P, et al. Severe type III von Willebrand's disease caused by deletion of exon 42 of the von Willebrand factor gene: family studies that identify carriers of the condition and a compound heterozygois individual. Blood 1990;75:654.
363. Nichols WC, Lyons SE, Harrison JS, et al. Severe von Willebrand disease due to a defect at the level of von Willebrand factor mRNA expression: detection by exonic PCR-restriction fragment length polymorphism analysis. Proc Natl Acad Sci USA 1991;88:3857.
364. Mannucci PM, Lombardi R, Castaman G, et al. Von Willebrand disease "Vicenza" with larger-than-normal (supranormal) von Willebrand factor multimers. Blood 1988;71:65.
365. D'Alessio PA, Castaman G, Rodeghiero F, et al. In vivo experiments indicate that relatively high platelet deposition in von Willebrand's disease "Vicenza" is caused by normal platelet-VWF levels rather than by high VWF-multimers in plasma. Thromb Res 1992;65:221.
366. Randi AM, Sacchi E, Castaman GC, et al. The genetic defect of type I von Willebrand disease "Vicenza" is linked to the von Willebrand factor gene. Thromb Haemost 1993;69:173.
367. Zimmerman TS, Ruggeri ZM, Fulcher CA. Factor VIII/von Willebrand factor. Prog Hematol 1983;13:279.
368. Ruggeri ZM, Mannucci PM, Bader R, Barbui T. Factor VIII-related properties in platelets from patients with von Willebrand's disease. J Lab Clin Med 1978;91:132.
369. Holmberg L, Mannucci PM, Turesson I, et al. Factor VIII antigen in the vessel walls in von Willebrand's disease and haemophilia A. Scand J Haematol 1974;13:33.
370. Bernardi F, Guerra S, Paracchini P, et al. Von Willebrand disease investigated by two novel RFLPs. Br J Haematol 1988;68:243.
371. Nishino M, Girma J-P, Rothschild C, Fressinaud E, Meyer D. New variant of von Willebrand disease with defective binding to factor VIII. Blood 1989;74:1591.
372. Mazurier C, Dieval J, Jorieux S, Delobel J, Goudemand M. A new von Willebrand factor (vWF) defect in a patient with factor VIII (FVIII) deficiency but with normal levels and multimeric patterns of both plasma and platelet vWF: characterization of abnormal vWF/FVIII interaction. Blood 1990;75:20.
373. Kernoff PBA, Gruson R, Rizza CR. A variant of factor VIII related antigen. Br J Haematol 1974;26:435.
374. Gralnick HR, Williams SB, McKeown LP, et al. A variant of type II von Willebrand disease with an abnormal triplet structure and discordant effects of protease inhibitors on plasma and platelet von Willebrand factor structure. Am J Hematol 1987;24:259.
375. Batlle J, Lopez-Fernandez MF, Campos M, et al. The heterogeneity of type IIA von Willebrand's disease: studies with protease inhibitors. Blood 1986;68:1207.
376. Ruggeri ZM, Mannucci PM, Lombardi R, et al. Multimeric composition of factor VIII/von Willebrand factor following administration of DDAVP: implications for pathophysiology and therapy of von Willebrand's disease subtypes. Blood 1982;59:1272.
377. Gralnick HR, Williams SB, McKeown LP, et al. DDAVP in type IIA von Willebrand's disease. Blood 1986;67:465.
378. Sultan Y, Simeon J, Caen JP. Electrophoretic heterogeneity of normal factor VIII/von Willebrand protein and abnormal electrophoretic mobility in patients with von Willebrand disease. J Lab Clin Med 1976;87: 185.
379. Hill FGH, Enayat MS, George AJ. Investigation including VIII R:Ag multimeric analysis of a large kindred with type II A von Willebrand's disease showing a dominant inheritance and a similar gene expression in four generations. Thromb Haemost 1983;50:735.
380. Asakura A, Harrison J, Gomperts E, Abildgaard C. Type IIA von Willebrand disease with apparent recessive inheritance. Blood 1987;69: 1419.
381. Ginsburg D, Konkle BA, Gill JC, et al. Molecular basis of human von Willebrand disease: analysis of platelet von Willebrand factor mRNA. Proc Natl Acad Sci USA 1989;86:3723.
382. Lyons SE, Bruck ME, Bowie EJW, Ginsburg D. Impaired intracellular transport produced by a subset of type IIA von Willebrand mutations. J Biol Chem 1992;267:4424.
383. Zimmerman TS, Dent JA, Ruggeri ZM, Nannini LH. Subunit composition of plasma von Willebrand factor: cleavage is present in normal individuals, increased in IIA and IIB von Willebrand disease, but minimal in variants with aberrant structure of individual oligomers (types IIC, IID, and IIE). J Clin Invest 1986;77:947.
384. Kunicki TJ, Montgomery RR, Shullek J. Cleavage of human von Willebrand factor by platelet calcium-activated protease. Blood 1985;66: 352.
385. Thompson EA, Howard MA. Proteolytic cleavage of human von Willebrand factor induced by enzyme(s) released from polymorphonuclear cells. Blood 1986;67:1281.
386. Federici AB, Elder JH, De Marco L, et al. Carbohydrate moiety of von Willebrand factor is not necessary for maintaining multimeric structure and ristocetin cofactor activity but protects from proteolytic degradation. J Clin Invest 1984;74:2049.
387. Hamilton KK, Fretto LJ, Grierson DS, McKee PA. Effects of plasmin on von Willebrand multimers: degradation in vitro and stimulation of release in vivo. J Clin Invest 1985;76:261.
388. Berkowitz SD, Dent J, Roberts J, et al. Epitope mapping of the von Willebrand factor subunit distinguishes fragments present in normal and type IIA von Willebrand disease from those generated by plasmin. J Clin Invest 1987;79:524.
389. Berkowitz SD, Nozaki H, Titani K, et al. Evidence that calpains and elastase do not produce the von Willebrand factor fragments present in normal plasma and IIA von Willebrand disease. Blood 1988;72:721.
390. Verweij CL, Quadt R, Briet E, et al. Genetic linkage of two intragenic restriction fragment length polymorphisms with von Willebrand's disease type IIA. Evidence for a defect in the von Willebrand factor gene. J Clin Invest 1988;81:1116.
391. Iannuzzi MC, Hidaka N, Boehnke ML, et al. Analysis of the relationship of von Willebrand disease (vWD) and hereditary hemorrhagic telangiectsia and identification of a potential type IIAvWD mutation. Am J Hum Genet 1991;48:757.
392. Dent JA, Berkowitz SD, Ware J, et al. Identification of a cleavage site directing the immunochemical detection of molecular abnormalities in type IIA von Willebrand factor. Proc Natl Acad Sci USA 1990;87: 6306.
393. Levene RB, Booyse FM, Chediak J, et al. Expression of abnormal von Willebrand factor by endothelial cells from a patient with type IIA von Willebrand disease. Proc Natl Acad Sci USA 1987;84:6550.

394. Chang H-Y, Chen Y-P, Chediak JR, et al. Molecular analysis of von Willebrand factor produced by endothelial cell strains from patients with type IIA von Willebrand disease [abstract]. Blood 1989;74:131a.
395. Ruggeri ZM, Nilsson IM, Lombardi R, et al. Aberrant multimeric structure of von Willebrand factor in a new variant of von Willebrand's disease (type IIC). J Clin Invest 1982;70:1124.
396. Armitage H, Rizza CR. Two populations of factor VIII-related antigen in a family with von Willebrand's disease. Br J Haematol 1979;55: 493.
397. Mannucci PM, Lombardi R, Pareti FI, et al. A variant of von Willebrand's disease characterized by recessive inheritance and missing triplet structure of von Willebrand factor multimers. Blood 1983;62:1000.
398. Batlle J, Lopez-Fernandez MF, Fernandez Villamor A, et al. Multimeric pattern discrepancy between platelet and plasma von Willebrand factor in type IIC von Willebrand disease. Am J Hematol 1986;22:87.
399. Batlle J, Lopez-Fernandez MF, Lasierra J, et al. Von Willebrand disease type IIC with different abnormalities of von Willebrand factor in the same sibship. Am J Hematol 1986;21:177.
400. Mazurier C, Mannucci PM, Parquet-Gernez A, et al. Investigation of a case of subtype IIC von Willebrand disease: characterization of the variability of this subtypes. Am J Hematol 1986;22:301.
401. Lamme S, Wallmark A, Holmberg L, et al. The use of monoclonal antibodies in measuring factor VIII/von Willebrand factor. Scand J Clin Lab Invest 1985;15:17.
402. Hill FGH, Enayat MS, George AJ. Investigation of a kindred with a new autosomal dominantly inherited variant type von Willebrand's disease (possibly type IID). J Clin Pathol 1985;38:665.
403. Thomas N, O'Callaghan U, Lowe GDO, et al. Response to desmopressin in type IID von Willebrand's disease. Clin Lab Haemat 1989;11:189.
404. Castaman G, Rodeghiero F, Lattuada A, Mannucci PM. A new variant of von Willebrand disease (type II I) with a normal degree of proteolytic cleavage of von Willebrand factor. Thromb Res 1991;65:343.
405. Sweeney JD, Hoernig LA, Behrens AN, et al. Von Willebrand's variant (type II Buffalo). Am J Clin Pathol 1990;93:522.
406. Fujimura Y, Holland LZ, Ruggeri ZM, et al. The von Willebrand factor domain-mediating botrocetin-induced binding to glycoprotein Ib lies between Val449 and Lys728. Blood 1987;70:985.
407. Rabinowitz I, Tuley EA, Mancuso DJ, et al. von Willebrand disease type B: a missense mutation selectively abolishes ristocetin-induced von Willebrand factor binding to platelet glycoprotein Ib. Proc Natl Acad Sci USA 1992;89:9846.
408. Holmberg L, Berntorp E, Donnér M, Nilsson IM. Von Willebrand's disease characterized by increased ristocetin sensitivity and the presence of all von Willebrand factor multimers in plasma. Blood 1986;68:668.
409. Wylie B, Gibson J, Urh E, Kronenberg H. Von Willebrand's disease characterized by increased ristocetin sensitivity and the presence of all von Willebrand factor multimers in plasma: a new subtype. Pathology 1988;62:63.
410. Holmberg L, Nilsson IM, Borge L, et al. Platelet aggregation induced by 1-desamino-8-D-arginine vasopressin (DDAVP) in type IIB von Willebrand's disease. N Engl J Med 1983;309:816.
411. Kyrle PA, Niessner H, Dent J. IIB von Willebrand's disease: pathogenetic and therapeutic studies. Br J Haematol 1988;69:55.
412. Rivard GE, Daviault M, Brault N, et al. Von Willebrand's disease associated with thrombocytopenia and a fast migrating factor VIII related antigen. Thromb Res 1977;11:507.
413. Andes A. Thrombocytopenia in von Willebrand's disease. Thromb Res 1983;30:391.
414. Giles AR. Type IIB von Willebrand's disease presenting as a lifelong bleeding diathasis associated with chronic thrombocytopenia and spontaneous platelet aggregation. Thromb Haemost 1985;54:1126.
415. Saba HI, Saba SR, Dent J, et al. Type IIB Tampa: a variant of von Willebrand disease with chronic thrombocytopenia, circulating platelet aggregates, and spontaneous platelet aggregation. Blood 1985;66:282.
416. Conti M, Mari D, Conti E, et al. Pregnancy in women with different types of von Willebrand disease. Obstet Gynecol 1986;68:282.
417. De Marco L, Mazzuccato M, Del Ben MG, et al. Type IIb von Willebrand factor with normal sialic content induces platelet aggregation in the absence of ristocetin. J Clin Invest 1987;80:475.
418. Mazurier C, Parquet-Gernez A, Goudemand J, et al. Investigation of a large kindred with type IIB von Willebrand's disease, dominant inheritance and age-dependent thrombocytopenia. Br J Haematol 1988;69: 499.
419. Hultin MB, Sussman II. Postoperative thrombocytopenia in type IIB von Willebrand disease. Am J Hematol 1990;33:64.
420. Federici AB, Mannucci PM, Bader R, et al. Heterogeneity in type IIB von Willebrand disease: two unrelated cases with no family history and mild abnormalities of ristocetin-induced interaction between von Willebrand factor and platelets. Am J Hematol 1986;23:381.
421. Donnér M, Holmberg L, Nilsson IM. Type IIB von Willebrand's disease with probable autosomal recessive inheritance and presenting as thrombocytopenia in infancy. Br J Haematol 1987;66:349.
422. Cooney KA, Nichols WC, Bruck ME, et al. The molecular defect in type IIB von Willebrand disease: identification of four potential missense mutations within the putative GpIb binding domain. J Clin Invest 1991;87:1227.
423. Randi AM, Rabinowitz I, Mancuso DJ, et al. Molecular basis of von Willebrand disease type IIb. Candidate mutation cluster in one disulfide loop between proposed platelet glycoprotein Ib binding sequences. J Clin Invest 1991;87:1220.
424. Ware J, Dent JA, Azuma H, et al. Identification of a point mutation in type IIB von Willebrand disease illustrating the regulation of von Willebrand factor affinity for the platelet membrane glycoprotein Ib-IX receptor. Proc Natl Acad Sci USA 1991;88:2946.
425. Cooney KA, Lyons SE, Ginsburg D. Functional analysis of a type IIB von Willebrand disease missense mutation: increased binding of large von Willebrand factor multimers to platelets. Proc Natl Acad Sci USA 1992;89:2869.
426. Murray EW, Giles AR, Lillicrap D. Germ-line mosaicism for a valine-to-methionine substitution at residue 553 in the glycoprotein Ib-binding domain of von Willebrand factor, causing type IIB von Willebrand disease. Am J Hum Genet 1992;50:199.
427. Fujimura Y, Titani K, Holland LZ, et al. Von Willebrand factor: a reduced and alkylated 52/48-kDa fragment beginning at amino acid residue 449 contains the domain interacting with platelet glycoprotein Ib. J Biol Chem 1986;261:381.
428. Mohri H, Fujimura Y, Shima M, et al. Structure of the von Willebrand factor domain interacting with glycoprotein Ib. J Biol Chem 1988;263: 17901.
429. Rabinowitz I, Randi AM, Shindler KS, et al. Type IIB mutation His-505 → Asp implicates a new segment in the control of von Willebrand factor binding to platelet glycoprotein Ib. J Biol Chem 1993;268:20497.
430. Hilbert L, Gaucher C, deRomeuf C, et al. Leu697→Val mutation in mature von Willebrand factor is responsible for type IIB von Willebrand disease. Blood 1994;83:1542.
431. Kroner PA, Kluessendorf ML, Scott JP, et al. Expressed full-length von Willebrand factor containing missense mutations linked to type IIB von Willebrand disease shows enhanced binding to platelets. Blood 1991;79:2048.
432. Randi AM, Jorieux S, Tuley EA, et al. Recombinant von Willebrand factor Arg578→Gln. J Biol Chem 1992;267:21187.
433. Ribba A-S, Voorberg J, Meyer D, et al. Characterization of recombinant von Willebrand factor corresponding to mutations in type IIA and type IIB von Willebrand disease. J Biol Chem 1992;267:23209.
434. Veltkamp JJ, van Tilburg NH. Autosomal hemophilia: a variant of von Willebrand's disease. Br J Haematol 1974;26:141.
435. Graham JB, Barrow ES, Roberts HR, et al. Dominant inheritance of hemophilia A in three generations of women. Blood 1975;46:175.
436. Montgomery RR, Hathaway WE, Johnson J, et al. A variant of von Willebrand's disease with abnormal expression of factor VIII procoagulant activity. Blood 1982;60:201.
437. Mazurier C, Gaucher C, Jorieux S, Parquet-Gernez A, Goudemand M. Evidence for a von Willebrand factor defect in factor VIII binding in three members of a family previously misdiagnosed as mild haemophilia A and haemophilia A carriers: consequences for therapy and genetic functional sites. Br J Haematol 1990;76:372.
438. Gaucher C, Jorieux S, Mercier B, Oufkir D, Mazurier C. The "Normandy" variant of von Willebrand disease: characterization of a point mutation in the von Willebrand factor gene. Blood 1991;77:1937.
439. Gaucher C, Mercier B, Jorieux S, Oufkir D, Mazurier C. Identification of two point mutations in the von Willebrand factor gene of three families with the "Normandy" variant of von Willebrand disease. Br J Haematol 1991;78:506.
440. Kroner PA, Friedman KD, Fahs SA, Scott JP, Montgomery RR. Abnormal binding of factor VIII is linked with the substitution of glutamine for arginine 91 in von Willebrand factor in a variant form of von Willebrand disease. J Biol Chem 1991;266:19146.
441. Kroner PA, Fahs SA, Vokac EA, et al. Novel missense mutations in von Willebrand factor (vWF) associated with defective vWF/factor VIII interaction in a patient with type I von Willebrand disease. Blood 1991;78:178a.
442. Cacheris PM, Nichols WC, Ginsburg D. Molecular characterization of a unique von Willebrand disease variant: a novel mutation affecting von Willebrand factor/factor VIII interaction. J Biol Chem 1991;266: 13499.
443. Tuley EA, Gaucher C, Jorieux S, Worrall NK, Sadler JE, Mazurier C. Expression of von Willebrand factor "Normandy," an autosomal mutation that mimics hemophilia A. Proc Natl Acad Sci USA 1991;88: 6377.
444. Jorieux S, Tuley EA, Gaucher C, Mazurier C, Sadler JE. The mutation Arg(53) → Trp causes von Willebrand disease Normandy by abolishing binding to factor VIII: studies with recombinant von Willebrand factor. Blood 1992;79:563.
445. Wise RJ, Ewenstein BM, Gorlin J, Narins SC, Jesson M, Handin RI. Autosomal recessive transmission of hemophilia A due to a von Willebrand factor mutation. Hum Genet 1993;91:367.
446. Meyer D, Frommel D, Larrieu MJ, Zimmerman TS. Selective absence of large forms of factor VIII/von Willebrand factor in acquired von Willebrand's syndrome: response to transfusion. Blood 1979;54:600.
447. Ball J, Malia RG, Greaves M, Preston FE. Demonstration of abnormal factor VIII multimers in acquired von Willebrand's disease associated with a circulating inhibitor. Br J Haematol 1987;65:95.
448. Handin RI, Martin V, Moloney WC. Antibody-induced von Willebrand's disease: a newly defined inhibitor syndrome. Blood 1976;48:393.
449. Mannucci PM, Lombardi R, Bader R, et al. Studies of the pathophysiology of acquired von Willebrand's disease in seven patients with

lymphoproliferative disorders or benign monoclonal gammopathies. Blood 1984;64:614.
450. Joist JH, Cowan JF, Zimmerman TS. Acquired von Willebrand's disease: evidence for a quantitative and qualitative factor VIII disorder. N Engl J Med 1978;298:988.
451. Roussi JH, Houbouyan LL, Alterescu R, et al. Acquired von Willebrand's syndrome associated with hairy cell leukaemia. Br J Haematol 1980;46: 503.
452. Simone JV, Cornet JA, Abildgaard CF. Acquired von Willebrand's syndrome in systemic lupus erythematosus. Blood 1968;31:806.
453. Yoshida H, Arai K, Wakashin M. Development of acquired von Willebrand's disease after mixed connective tissue disease. Am J Med 1988;85:445.
454. Stableforth P, Tamagnini GL, Dormandy KM. Acquired von Willebrand's syndrome and thrombopathy in patient with chronic lymphocytic leukemia. Scand J Haematol 1970;16:128.
455. Gazengel C, Prieur AM, Jacques C, Buriot D, Nedellec J, Josso F. Antibody induced von Willebrand's syndrome: inhibition of VIII-vWF and VIII-Agn with sparing of VIII-Ahf by the autoantibody. Am J Hematol 1978;5:355.
456. Gouault-Heilmann M, Dumont MD, Intrator L, Chenal C, Lejon JL. Acquired von Willebrand's syndrome with IgM inhibitor against von Willebrand factor. J Clin Pathol 1979;32:1030.
457. Zettervall O, Nilsson IM. Acquired von Willebrand's disease caused by a monoclonal antibody. Acta Med Scand 1978;204:521.
458. Gan TE, Sawers RJ, Koutts J. Pathogenesis of antibody induced acquired von Willebrand syndrome. Am J Hematol 1980;9:363.
459. Bovill EG, Ershler WB, Golden EA, et al. A human myeloma-produced monoclonal protein directed against the active subpopulation of von Willebrand factor. Am J Clin Pathol 1986;85:115.
460. Richard C, Cuadrado MA, Prieto M, et al. Acquired von Willebrand disease in multiple myeloma secondary to absorption of von Willebrand factor by plasma cells. Am J Hematol 1990;35:114.
461. Noronha PA, Hruby MA, Maurer HS. Acquired von Willebrand disease in a patient with Wilms' tumor. J Pediatr 1979;95:997.
462. Scott JP, Montgomery RR, Tubergen DG, Hays T. Acquired von Willebrand's disease in association with Wilms' tumor: regression following treatment. Blood 1981;58:665.
463. Holland L, Adamson A, Ingram GIC, Chalmers DG. Acquired von Willebrand syndrome. Br J Haematol 1980;45:161.
464. Sampson BM, Greaves M, Malia RG, Preston FE. Acquired von Willebrand's disease: demonstration of a circulating inhibitor to the factor VIII complex in four cases. Br J Haematol 1983;54:233.
465. Facon T, Caron C, Courtin P, et al. Acquired type II von Willebrand's disease associated with adrenal cortical carcinoma. Blood 1992;80:488.
466. Budde U, Schaefer G, Mueller N, et al. Acquired von Willebrand's disease in the myeloproliferative syndrome. Blood 1984;64:981.
467. Budde V, Dent JA, Berkowitz SC, Ruggeri ZM, Zimmerman TS. Subunit composition of plasma von Willebrand factor in patients with the myeloproliferative syndrome. Blood 1986;68:1213.
468. Takahasi H. Studies on the pathophysiology and treatment of von Willebrand's disease. IV. Mechanism of increased ristocetin-induced platelet aggregation in von Willebrand's disease. Thromb Res 1980;19: 857.
469. Miller JL, Castella A. Platelet-type von Willebrand's disease: characterization of a new bleeding disorder. Blood 1982;60:790.
470. Miller JL, Cunningham D, Lyle VA, Finch CN. Mutation in the gene encoding the α chain of platelet glycoprotein Ib in platelet-type von Willebrand disease. Proc Natl Acad Sci USA 1991;88:4761.
471. Russell SD, Roth GJ. A mutation in the platelet glycoprotein (GP) Ib alpha gene associated with pseudo–von Willebrand disease. Blood 1991;78:281.
472. Miller JL, Kupinski JM, Castella A, Ruggeri ZM. Von Willebrand factor binds to platelets and induces aggregation in platelet-type but not type IIb von Willebrand disease. J Clin Invest 1983;72:1532.
473. Scott JP, Montgomery RR. The rapid differentiation of type IIb von Willebrand's disease from platelet-type (pseudo-) von Willebrand's disease by the "neutral" monoclonal antibody binding assay. Am J Clin Pathol 1991;96:723.
474. Bowie EJW, Owen CA Jr. The bleeding time. Prog Hemost Thromb 1974;2:249.
475. Cash JD, Gader AMA, Da Costa J. Release of plasminogen activator and factor VIII in response to LVP, AVP, DDAVP, angiotensin II and oxytocin in man. Br J Haematol 1974;27:363.
476. Mannucci PM, Canciani MT, Rota L, Donovan BS. Response of factor VIII/von Willebrand factor to DDAVP in healthy subjects and patients with haemophilia A and von Willebrand's disease. Br J Haematol 1981;47:283.
477. Köhler M, Hellstern P, Reiter B, et al. The subcutaneous administration of the vasopressin analogue 1-desamino-8-D-arginine vasopressin in patients with von Willebrand's disease and hemophilia. Klin Wochenschr 1984;62:543.
478. de Sio L, Mariani G, Muzzucconi MG, et al. Comparison between subcutaneous and intravenous DDAVP in mild and moderate hemophilia. Thromb Haemost 1985;54:387.
479. Mannucci PM, Vicente V, Alberca I, et al. Intravenous and subcutaneous administration of desmopressin (DDAVP) to hemophiliacs: pharmacokinetics and factor VIII responses. Thromb Haemost 1987;58:1037.
480. Lethagen S, Harris AS, Nilsson IM. Intranasal desmopressin (DDAV) by spray in mild hemophilia A and von Willebrand's disease type I. Blut 1990;60:187.
481. Rose EH, Aledort LM. Nasal spray desmopressin (DDAVP) for mild hemophilia A and von Willebrand disease. Ann Intern Med 1991;114: 563.
482. Theiss W, Schmidt G. DDAVP in von Willebrand's disease: repeated administration and the behaviour of the bleeding time. Thromb Res 1978;13:1119.
483. Isola L, Forster A, Aledort LM. Desamino-D-arginine vasopressin and bleeding time in von Willebrand's disease. Ann Intern Med 1984;101: 719.
484. Aledort LM. Treatment of von Willebrand's disease. Mayo Clin Proc 1991;66:841.
485. Smith TJ, Gill JC, Ambruso DR, Hathaway WE. Hyponatremia and seizures in young children given DDAVP. Am J Hematol 1989;31:199.
486. Sheperd LL, Hutchinson RJ, Worden EK, Koopmann CF, Coran A. Hyponatremia and seizures after intravenous administration of desmopressin acetate for surgical hemostasis. J Pediatr 1989;144:470.
487. Weinstein RE, Bona RD, Altman AJ, et al. Severe hyponatremia after repeated intravenous administration of desmopressin. Am J Hematol 1989;32:258.
488. O'Brien JR, Green PJ, Salmon G, et al. Desmopressin and myocardial infarction. Lancet 1989;1:664.
489. Byrnes JJ, Larcada A, Moake JL. Thrombosis following desmopressin for uremic bleeding. Am J Hematol 1988;28:63.
490. Mannucci PM, Lusher JM. Desmopressin and thrombosis. Lancet 1989;2: 675.
491. Nilsson IM, Hedner U. Characteristics of various factor VIII concentrates used in treatment of hemophilia. Br J Haematol 1977;37:543.
492. Berntorp E, Nilsson IM. Biochemical, in vivo properties of commercial virus-inactivated factor VIII concentrates. Eur J Haematol 1988;48:205.
493. Mannucci PM, Tenconi PM, Castaman G, Rodeghiero F. Comparison of four virus-inactivated plasma concentrates for treatment of severe von Willebrand disease: a cross-over randomized trial. Blood 1992;79: 3130.
494. Köhler M, Hellstern P, Wenzel E. The use of heat-treated factor VIII-concentrates in von Willebrand's disease. Blut 1985;50:25.
495. Schimpf K, Mannucci PM, Kreutz W, et al. Absence of hepatitis after treatment with a pasteurized factor VIII concentrate in patients with hemophilia and no previous transfusions. N Engl J Med 1987;316:918.
496. Fukui H, Nishino M, Terada S, et al. Hemostatic effect of a heat-treated factor VIII concentrate (Haemate-P) in von Willebrand's disease. Blut 1988;56:171.
497. Mazurier C, Jorieux S, de Romeuf C, et al. In vitro evaluation of a very-high-purity solvent/detergent-treated, von Willebrand factor concentrate. Vox Sang 1991;61:1.
498. Rothschild C, Fressinaud E, Wolf M, et al. Unexpected results following treatment of patients with von Willebrand disease with a new highly purified von Willebrand factor concentrate. Thromb Haemost 1991;65: 1126.
499. Ogston D. Antifibrinolytic drugs: chemistry, pharmacology and clinical usage. Chichester, UK, John Wiley & Sons, 1984.
500. Sindet-Pedersen S, Ramstrom G, Bernvil S, Blombäck M. Hemostatic effect of tranexamic acid mouthwash in anticoagulant-treated patients undergoing oral surgery. N Engl J Med 1989;320:840.
501. Alperin JB. Estrogens and surgery in women with von Willebrand's disease. Am J Med 1982;73:367.
502. Rodeghiero F, Castaman G, diBona E, Ruggeri M. Consistency of responses to repeated DDAVP infusions in patients with von Willebrand's disease and hemophilia A. Blood 1989;74:1997.
503. De la Fuente B, Kasper CK, Rickles FR, Hoyer LW. Response of patients with mild and moderate hemophilia A and von Willebrand's disease to treatment with desmopressin. Ann Intern Med 1985;103:6.
504. Mannucci PM. Desmopressin (DDAVP) for treatment of disorders of hemostasis. In: Coller BS, ed. Progress in hemostasis and thrombosis, vol 8. Philadelphia, Grune & Stratton, 1986:19.
505. Casonato A, Sartori T, deMarco L, et al. 1-Desamino-8-D-arginine vasopressin (DDAVP) infusion in type IIB von Willebrand's disease: shortening of bleeding time and induction of a variable pseudothrombocytopenia. Thromb Haemost 1990;64:117.
506. Feigert JM, Wolf DJ, Schleider MA. Porcine factor (PF) VIII controls severe bleeding in acquired von Willebrand's disease (AVWD) by supplying von Willebrand's factor (vWF). Blood 1987;58:371.
507. Cattaneo M, Moia M, Valle PD, et al. DDAVP shortens the prolonged bleeding times of patients with severe von Willebrand disease treated with cryoprecipitate: evidence for a mechanism of action independent of released von Willebrand factor. Blood 1989;74:1972.
508. Boda Z, Pfliegler G, Harsfalvi J, et al. Successful treatment of a severe bleeding episode in type III von Willebrand's disease by simultaneous administration of cryoprecipitate and platelet concentrate. Thromb Haemost 1991;65:1125.
509. Lopez-Fernandez MF, Blanco-Lopez MJ, Castiñeira MP, Batlle J. Further evidence for recessive inheritance of von Willebrand disease with abnormal binding of von Willebrand factor to factor VIII. Am J Hematol 1992;40:20.
510. Blombäck M, Johansson G, Johnsson H, et al. Surgery in patients with von Willebrand's disease. Br J Surg 1989;76:398.
511. Telfer MC, Checiak J. Factor VIII–related disorders and their relationship to pregnancy. J Reprod Med 1977;19:211.

Blood: Principles and Practice of Hematology,
edited by Robert I. Handin, Samuel E. Lux, and Thomas P. Stossel.
J.B. Lippincott Company, Philadelphia © 1995.

37

The Platelet Life Cycle: Normal Function and Qualitative Disorders

Andrew I. Schafer

It is not difficult to understand how platelets were once mistaken for particles of dust when examined under the light microscope. These terminally differentiated pieces of cytoplasm, fragmented from their megakaryocyte precursors in the bone marrow, devoid of nuclei and all but trace amounts of nucleic acids,[1] and capable of only vestigial protein synthesis,[2] do indeed appear innocuous and impotent compared with their more imposing circulating blood cell companions, the leukocytes and erythrocytes. Yet, electron microscopic and biochemical analyses reveal platelets to be complex cells that are equipped to respond in a highly organized and coordinated manner to a wide variety of external signals. Platelets respond explosively to focal demands for hemostasis by instantaneously forming occlusive aggregates in injured vessels, by supporting and accelerating localized fibrin formation, and by releasing potent vasoactive substances. The extraordinary sensitivity of platelets to extracellular stimuli normally serves the purposes of hemostasis well, but at the same time makes these cells highly vulnerable to a variety of structural and functional defects. These qualitative abnormalities may render platelets incapable of normal participation in the hemostatic process, resulting in clinical bleeding problems or, at the other end of the spectrum, causing them to be hyperreactive and to either initiate or fuel thrombosis and vascular disease.

PLATELET MORPHOLOGY

The average dimensions of circulating platelets, as determined by electron microscopy, are about 1.5 μm in diameter and 0.5 to 1 μm in thickness.[3] Average platelet volumes range from 5 to 7 μL[4]; however, there is considerable heterogeneity of platelet size in the circulation.[5] Since the peripheral platelet count varies over a wide range in normal subjects, and there is normally an inverse correlation between the platelet count and the mean platelet volume (MPV),[6,7] it has been hypothesized that platelet production is regulated to maintain a constant circulating "platelet mass" (the product of the platelet count and the MPV).[8] There is, likewise, considerable normal heterogeneity in circulating platelet density, which depends primarily on the concentration of intracellular storage granules.[9] The relation between platelet aging and platelet density in the circulation remains an issue of controversy.[10]

White[11,12] divided the morphology of the platelet into distinct functional regions subserving different platelet activities. The *cytoskeleton* or *peripheral zone* consists of the membranes and the walls of the surface-connected open canalicular system (OCS). The *sol-gel zone* is the matrix of the platelet cytoplasm, including the contractile system. The *organelle zone* consists of the storage granules, including α granules, electron-dense bodies, lysosomes and microperoxisomes, as well as the mitochondria, which are randomly dispersed throughout the cytoplasm. Finally, the *membrane systems* of the platelet include the dense tubular system (DTS) and the surface-connected OCS. This concept of functional zones has facilitated understanding of structure–function relations in platelet activation.

After the stimulation of platelets by a variety of activators, the normally discoid shape of platelets rapidly changes to round and swollen forms with extensions of long pseudopods. At the same time, the randomly dispersed storage granules within the platelets move to the center of the cells and become surrounded by a ring of microfilaments and microtubules. The release reaction then occurs by fusion of the centralized granules with the surface-connected OCS, leading to the selective discharge of granule constituents to the exterior.

Peripheral Zone

The platelet surface and the OCS are considered together as a single unit since the channels of the latter represent continuous invaginations of the cell wall. Thus, conventional cell-sizing measurements greatly underestimate the total sponge-like surface area of platelets that is actually exposed to plasma. The *glycocalyx* is the net negatively charged, carbohydrate-rich *exterior coat* of the platelet. Within the platelet exterior coat are several major classes of membrane glycoproteins, including gpIa-IIa, gpIb-IX, gpIIb-IIIa, gpIV, and gpV,[13,14] as discussed in detail in Chapter 32. Specific membrane glycoproteins serve as receptors for the adhesive macromolecules involved in critical platelet-surface reactions, including platelet attachment to injured vascular intima (adhesion) and platelet–platelet interactions (aggregation). Other, less well-characterized membrane glycoproteins represent the sites for a variety of other platelet-surface receptors for both positive extracellular signals (agonists) and negative extracellular signals (inhibitors) that modulate the state of platelet activation.

The platelet *unit membrane* is generally similar to the trilaminar membrane of other blood cells. Buried within the lipid constituents of the split lipid bilayer of platelet membranes are the transmembrane proteins. The major phospholipid classes are distributed asymmetrically in the lipid bilayer.[15] The structure and organization of the platelet unit membrane support a number of important physiologic processes. The transmission of extracellular signals occurs through membrane-associated G proteins and enzymes that act to generate membrane phospholipid-derived intracellular mediators (vide infra). Another important property of the platelet unit membrane is the maintenance of transmembrane ionic gradients.[16] Blood coagulation is also supported by platelet membranes since thrombin generation is greatly accelerated on activated platelet surfaces compared with the same reactions proceeding in fluid phase.[17,18]

Sol-Gel Zone

The sol-gel zone represents the matrix of the platelet cytoplasm and consists primarily of the *circumferential microtubule band* and the *microfilaments*. The prominent circumferential band, which consists of a single, continuous, coiled microtubule,[19] lies just beneath the cell surface and is separated from the cell wall by submembrane filaments. The microtubule participates in cytoskeletal support and maintenance of the normal discoid shape of platelets. Platelet shape change and loss of the normal discoid form are accompanied by disappearance of the circumferential band of microtubules, which is subsequently reformed if the discoid shape is recovered.[20] The other major constituents of the sol-gel zone are the microfilaments, which are the structural elements of the platelet contractile system.

The maintenance of the normal discoid shape of unstimulated platelets and the physicochemical responses of platelets to activation (including shape change, degranulation, and platelet-mediated clot retraction) are regulated by the coordinated actions of several *platelet contractile proteins*.[21] Although many of the properties of these contractile proteins are indistinguishable from those of muscle cells, some important structural and functional differences have been identified.

Actin is the most abundant protein in platelets, constituting about 15% of total platelet protein.[22–24] Rapidly following platelet activation, actin monomers polymerize into long, double-helical filaments (termed *F-actin*). Unstimulated platelets contain about 40% of their total actin in the filamentous F-actin form, and this increases to 70% to 80% of total actin in activated platelets.[25,26] The rate-limiting step in polymerization is the formation of nuclei (nucleation), which is followed by the rapid addition of monomers to either end of the growing filament by the process of elongation. After platelet activation, actin filaments reorganize from loose, random arrays to tightly structured bundles and rings surrounding the intracellular granules. Then, the granules (vide infra) are forced into the center of the platelets, and their contents are discharged into the OCS. As noted later, the submembranous actin filaments are released from gpIb and become attached to the gpIIb-IIIa complex. These changes in actin are mediated by various other contractile proteins that bind to actin filaments, and the association with or dissociation from actin of these other contractile proteins is initiated at least in part by changes in cytosolic free Ca^{2+}.[27,28]

Myosin[29,30] constitutes only about 1% to 2% of platelet protein. It resembles muscle myosin but occurs in much smaller amounts relative to actin in platelets. Myosin filaments form during platelet activation when they are required for contractile events. Actin–myosin interactions in platelets (as well as in smooth muscle and other nonmuscle cells) are initiated by phosphorylation of the light chain of myosin,[31] which has actin-activatable adenosine triphosphatase (ATPase) activity. The specific kinase that catalyzes the phosphorylation of myosin light chain[32,33] is absolutely dependent on calmodulin and Ca^{2+} for activity, and therefore, the entire process of actin–myosin interaction must be initiated by the rise in cytosolic free Ca^{2+} that occurs on platelet activation. Thus, the release of free Ca^{2+} into the cytosol after platelet stimulation induces binding of calmodulin to myosin light-chain kinase, leading to activation of the kinase, phosphorylation of the 20-kd light chain of myosin, and the interaction of myosin with actin filaments, a sequence of reactions that results in the generation of force within the platelet.

Actin-binding protein,[34] which may be identical to filamin, is composed of long subunits[35,36] that associate to form head-to-head dimers. Actin-binding protein may have an important role in regulating actin polymerization, and actin-binding protein dimers can bind to F-actin to mediate the cross-linking of actin filaments into networks. Actin-binding protein also is associated with membrane gpIb-IX and thereby links gpIb-IX to the submembranous actin filaments in unstimulated platelets.[37–39] The linkage of gpIb-IX to the membrane skeleton appears to maintain the glycoprotein in a uniform distribution on the unstimulated platelet surface, thus maximizing the chances of an interaction with von Willebrand factor (vWF) since disruption of the membrane skeleton causes clustering of this glycoprotein complex.[40] These actions of actin-binding protein are terminated when the protein becomes hydrolyzed by calcium-dependent proteases in the platelet, leading to loss of the ability of the actin-binding protein to cross-link actin filaments into networks[41,42] and to disruption of its ability to link actin filaments to gpIb-IX. Since the activation of Ca^{2+}-dependent proteases in platelets is a delayed event that follows cell stimulation, the loss of these actin-binding, protein-dependent effects (eg, the disruption of actin filament networks formed early in platelet activation) has been considered to play a role in promoting clot retraction.[43] Actin-binding protein is stabilized against proteolysis in response to cyclic adenosine monophosphate (cAMP) elevating agents (through its phosphorylation by cAMP–dependent protein kinase), and this blocks cytoskeleton reorganization.[44]

Platelet *α-actin* is structurally similar to the muscle protein.[45] It is partly membrane-associated[46] and may serve as a membrane attachment site for actin filaments. Unlike muscle α-actin, the platelet protein binds to actin filaments and induces the formation of actin filament networks only in the absence of Ca^{2+}. In the presence of Ca^{2+}, while α-actin dissociates from actin filaments, *gelsolin* binds to actin filaments[47,48] and disrupts actin filament networks. Gelsolin is one of a group of F-actin severing (disrupting) proteins that has been described in platelets and other nonmuscle cells[49] that affect the reorganization of actin filaments during platelet activation. In the process of platelet activation, gelsolin subsequently attaches to membrane polyphosphoinositides, thus releasing gelsolin from actin oligomers to permit rapid actin filament assembly.[50,51]

A number of other, less prominent platelet contractile proteins have been identified, but their functions are less well understood. These include *profilin*[52]; *p235* or band 2[53]; *vinculin*[54]; *spectrin*,[55] which is the major protein involved in maintaining the submembranous network of proteins in red cells[56]; *ankyrin*[57]; protein 4.1[58]; and tropomyosin.[59] In platelets, many of these proteins may provide attachment sites for actin filaments to the inner surface of the plasma membrane in addition to the previously described linkage of actin filaments to gpIb by actin-binding protein. In general, it appears that actin-binding protein serves the same functions in platelets as does spectrin in red cells: these are the major proteins in their respective cells that cross-link actin filaments of the membrane skeleton and link the actin filaments to plasma membrane glycoproteins.[40] Some of the proteins (profilin and possibly p235 and α-actin) may also bind to the ends of F-actin and serve as capping proteins to prevent polymerization of the actin filaments in unstimulated platelets.[46,52,53]

Organelle Zone

The platelet interior contains a variety of formed elements. These include mitochondria, which are easily distinguished on electron microscopy by the plication of their internal membranes into cristae,[11] and glycogen. The most abundant of the intracellular organelles are storage granules, which contain various substances that are secreted during the platelet-release reaction. Based on ultrastructural appearance, density, and content, using electron microscopy and subcellular fractionation studies, the storage granules of platelets can be divided into four populations: α granules, dense granules, lysosomes, and microperoxisomes.[60] The distinctions among the different types of granules have been further defined by immunofluorescence studies and experiments of nature involving patients with specific platelet granule defects, the so-called storage-pool diseases that are discussed later.

The *α granules* are the most numerous of the platelet storage organelles. They appear to be formed in the later stages of megakaryocyte development.[61,62] α-Granule constituents include the platelet-specific proteins platelet factor 4 (PF4) and β-thromboglobulin (β-TG), as well as platelet-derived growth factor (PDGF), fibrinogen, vWF, thrombospondin (TSP), and fibronectin.[63] The *dense granules* (or δ granules or dense bodies) are the most electron-dense and most clearly distinguishable organelles on electron microscopy. The major contents of dense granules are adenosine triphosphate (ATP), adenosine diphosphate (ADP), calcium, pyrophosphate, and serotonin.[64] Although serotonin uptake and concentration into megakaryocytes have been observed, dense granules are not prominently visualized in megakaryocytes. It is possible that megakaryocytes contain unidentified organelles that are precursors of the dense granules.

Unlike α granules and dense granules, which can be identified within platelets morphologically, *lysosomes* and *microperoxisomes* are recognizable only by specific cytochemical staining techniques. Lysosomes (or λ-granules) are small vesicles that are much less abundant in the platelet than α granules. These organelles are found even in the most immature megakaryocytes. They are the storage site for many enzymes, including acid phosphatases, aryl sulfatase, β-glucuronidase, cathepsin, and β-galactosidase.[65–67] Like lysosomes, microperoxisomes form early in megakaryocyte differentiation. These storage organelles are few in number in the platelet and contain primarily catalase.[68]

The mechanism of exocytosis in platelets and the resultant selective release of granule constituents differ from the process in neutrophils and other cells.[60] The secretory pathway in platelets is best characterized for α granules. The work of White and colleagues has convincingly demonstrated that secretion occurs through fusion of the storage granules with the surface-connected OCS. The microtubules of activated platelets constrict to squeeze storage granules toward the cell center. The centralized granules of activated platelets then fuse with other granules and the OCS to form large vacuoles, and as these vacuoles form, the openings to the exterior widen to permit the rapid discharge of granule contents to the external milieu.[69,70]

Membrane Systems

As noted previously, the surface-connected OCS consists of tortuous invaginations of the platelet surface that tunnel throughout the cytoplasm of the cell in a serpentine fashion.[11] These channels serve as the conduits for the extrusion of platelet granule constituents during the release reaction. The DTS is also randomly dispersed throughout the platelet cytoplasm. It has been considered to represent residual smooth endoplasmic reticulum from the parent megakaryocyte.[71] The DTS serves as the major intracellular Ca^{2+}-sequestering system, with an active Ca^{2+}/Mg^{2+} ATPase that pumps Ca^{2+} out of the cytoplasm into the DTS to maintain a low, cytosolic free Ca^{2+} concentration in resting platelets.[72] The DTS is also the major site of platelet prostaglandin and thromboxane biosynthesis.[73] Consistent with this role, the DTS membrane is enriched in phospholipid-bound arachidonic acid, arachidonic acid mobilizing enzymes (phospholipase A_2, diglyceride lipase), and arachidonic acid–metabolizing enzymes (cyclooxygenase, thromboxane synthase).[74] A close physical relation exists between the OCS and DTS in the platelet. The striking structural and functional similarities of the platelet OCS and DTS to the transverse tubules and sarcotubules of skeletal muscle strongly suggest that these two platelet membrane systems are the equivalent of the sarcoplasmic reticulum of muscle cells.[75]

GENERAL OUTLINE OF PLATELET–VESSEL WALL INTERACTIONS AND PLATELET ACTIVATION

Under normal circumstances, the monolayer of endothelial cells that lines the intimal surfaces of all blood vessels acts as an extraordinarily effective thromboresistant surface to maintain blood fluidity (Fig. 37-1). In fact, no artificial surface has been designed that can mimic the antithrombotic efficacy of normal endothelium. This is not surprising when one considers that healthy endothelial cells not only serve a barrier function to prevent access of blood to thrombogenic subendothelial connective tissue but also possess exquisitely regulated, multifaceted, and metabolically interrelated thromboresistant activities (Table 37-1). In addition to the fibrin inhibitory properties of heparan sulfates (to activate antithrombin III), thrombomodulin (to activate protein C), and plasminogen activators (to digest fibrin), normal endothelial cells are also equipped with a number of platelet-inhibitory properties. The negative surface charge of endothelial cells may repel negatively charged platelets. Prostacyclin (PGI_2) is a potent vasodilator and antiplatelet eicosanoid that is released by endothelial cells and inhibits platelet activation by raising platelet cAMP. Endothelium-derived relaxing factor (EDRF) is another endothelial product, at least one major component of which is nitric oxide.[76,77] EDRF, in addition to its vasoactive actions, also inhibits platelet activation through cyclic guanosine monophosphate (cGMP).[78] Finally, an ADPase ectoenzyme on endothelial cell surfaces exerts its antiplatelet actions by destroying platelet-activating ADP.[79]

When endothelial cells are perturbed by certain activators (eg, exposure to cytokines), the net antithrombotic properties of resting endothelium may shift to a net thrombogenic state. Disruption of endothelial contiguity by focal vascular injury initiates primary hemostasis not only through the loss of thromboresistant endothelium but also by exposure of subendothelial structures to flowing blood.

In response to intimal vascular damage, platelets initially adhere and spread in a monolayer to replace and cover exposed subendothelium (platelet adhesion). The subendothelial components to which platelets adhere have not

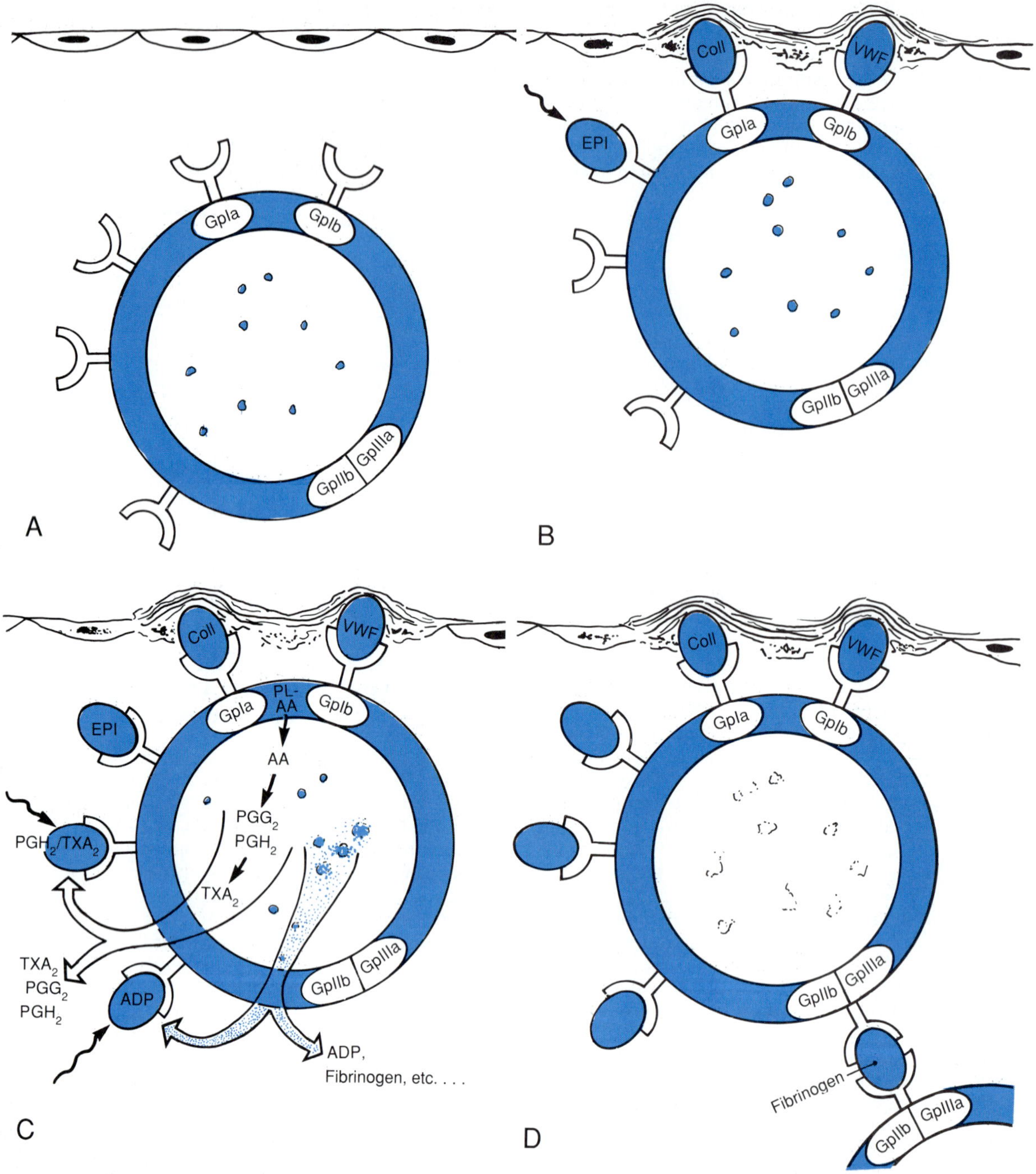

FIGURE 37-1. General scheme of platelet–vessel wall interactions and platelet activation. (**A**) The thromboresistant properties of intact vascular endothelial cells promote blood fluidity and prevent the activation of circulating platelets. (**B**) Focal vascular injury exposes subendothelial connective tissue. Platelet adhesion (platelet–vessel wall interaction) is mediated by collagen (Coll) binding directly to platelet receptors localized to membrane gpIa (at lower shear rates) or by vWF bridging of connective tissue to platelet membrane vWF receptors localized to gpIb (at higher shear rates). Other agonists, such as epinephrine (EPI), may also bind to specific platelet-surface receptors to initiate or amplify platelet activation. (**C**) Adherent platelets undergo the release reaction, during which prepackaged storage granule constituents (eg, ADP) are secreted and arachidonic acid (AA) is hydrolyzed from phospholipid (PL) pools and metabolized to biologically active eicosanoids (eg, PGG_2, PGH_2, TXA_2). Released ADP, PGH_2, and TXA_2 are platelet stimulants that bind to specific platelet receptors to amplify the activation process and to activate neighboring platelets. (**D**) The process of platelet aggregation (platelet–platelet interaction) is mediated by fibrinogen binding to specific receptors that are exposed on the platelet surface with the formation of the Ca^{2+}-dependent GpIIb–IIIa heterodimer complex. Fibrinogen links aggregating platelets by binding to GpIIb–IIIa on opposing membranes of neighboring platelets. At high shear levels, vWF substitutes for fibrinogen as the ligand mediating platelet aggregation. This scheme does not illustrate various other platelet receptors that are exposed during the process of platelet activation, such as the binding sites for coagulation factor Xa, which confer procoagulant properties on the platelet surface, or receptors for inhibitors (eg, prostaglandins) that tend to offset activating signals.

TABLE 37-1. Thromboresistant Activities of Normal Endothelium*

FIBRIN-INHIBITORY PROPERTIES
Heparan sulfate
Thrombomodulin
Plasminogen activator
PLATELET-INHIBITORY PROPERTIES
Negative surface charge
Prostacyclin (PGI_2)
Endothelium-derived relaxing factor or nitric oxide
ADPase

* Normal, unperturbed vascular endothelial cells provide a thromboresistant surface to maintain blood fluidity by means of a number of antifibrin and antiplatelet activities. Fibrin accumulation is inhibited by (1) *heparan sulfates* on intimal surfaces that activate antithrombin III and accelerate the neutralization of thrombin; (2) *thrombomodulin,* which activates protein C; and (3) *plasminogen activator* that is released to lyse fibrin. Platelet accumulation is inhibited by (1) the *negative surface charge* of endothelial cells, which repels negatively charged platelets; (2) *prostacyclin,* a vasodilator and inhibitor of platelets acting through cAMP; (3) *endothelium-derived relaxing factor or nitric oxide,* a vasodilator and inhibitor of platelets acting through cGMP; and (4) *ADPase,* an endothelial cell ectoenzyme that destroys platelet-activating ADP.

been definitively identified[80] but appear to involve types I and III collagen[81,82] and noncollagenous microfibrils.[83,84] At the high shear rates (more than 800 s^{-1}) that are found in small arteries and the microvasculature, the adhesive macromolecule vWF is required to attach platelets to subendothelial connective tissue.[85,86] At lower shear rates (eg, in aorta and large vessels), vWF has much less importance, and platelets may directly adhere to fibrils of collagen.[87] Platelet membrane gpIb, which is associated with the minor membrane gpIX, is the primary receptor for vWF on the surfaces of unstimulated platelets. In vitro, the interaction between gpIb and vWF requires a cofactor (typically ristocetin); the endogenous, physiologic "ristocetin equivalent" has not been identified for this cofactor requirement, although mechanical shear stress may serve this function (vide infra). Unstimulated platelets have completely functional receptors for vWF since platelets fixed in paraformaldehyde can still be agglutinated by vWF in the presence of ristocetin.[88] In fact, platelet activation may actually block vWF binding to platelets.[89–91]

After adhesion, platelets are activated to undergo the "release reaction." Multiple potential agonists may act on platelets, probably simultaneously and in synergy, to trigger the release reaction. The tertiary structure of subendothelial collagen fibrils may activate adherent platelets.[87] Also, vWF may serve as a platelet agonist and as the major adhesive protein.[92–94] Large or unusually large vWF multimers produced within endothelial cells and stored in platelet α granules can induce platelet activation even in the absence of ristocetin under conditions of high shear stress.[95,96] Platelets may also respond to a variety of other positive signals (eg, epinephrine, ADP, thrombin, prostaglandin endoperoxides), as described in detail later.

Agonist-induced platelet activation stimulates the release reaction, during which platelets degranulate to secrete storage granule constituents and also generate biologically active metabolites of arachidonic acid, such as thromboxane A_2 (TXA_2). These released substances then recruit additional platelets from the circulation and promote the formation of a hemostatic platelet plug (platelet aggregation) at the site of vascular injury. The process of platelet aggregation is mediated primarily by fibrinogen, which binds to specific platelet-surface receptors localized to the membrane gpIIb-IIIa complex[97] and thus provides a bridge between neighboring platelets within an aggregate. After Ca^{2+} mobilization in activated platelets, the Ca^{2+}-dependent heterodimer complex of gpIIb-IIIa undergoes a conformational change to provide binding sites for fibrinogen[98–105] that are unavailable on the surfaces of resting platelets. The activated platelet surface not only exposes binding sites for fibrinogen but also permits interactions with coagulation proteins to accelerate localized thrombin generation. Glycoprotein IIb-IIIa is one member of an adhesion receptor superfamily, termed *integrins*,[106] and serves as a promiscuous receptor for fibrinogen as well as for vWF, fibronectin, and vitronectin, all of which can bind to gpIIb-IIIa by means of a common recognition sequence of amino acid residues on these ligands that is composed of Arg-Gly-Asp (RGD sequence).[107–109] Although fibrinogen has been considered to be the primary protein that mediates the aggregation of activated platelets after its binding to gpIIb-IIIa, other adhesive proteins (particularly vWF and vitronectin) may substitute for fibrinogen as the major ligands that bind to gpIIb-IIIa and mediate platelet aggregation under conditions of high shear stress in the circulation.[110] Finally, TSP, which originates in platelet α granules and vascular cells, further promotes platelet aggregation through TSP receptors localized to gpIV[111] and enhances agonist-induced platelet aggregation through gpIIb-IIIa.[112] TSP also increases the size of platelet aggregates, and it has been proposed that TSP cross-links platelet–fibrinogen aggregates[113] or acts synergistically with fibrinogen through gpIIb-IIIa on the platelet surface.[112] Platelet membrane glycoproteins are discussed in more detail in Chapter 32.

BIOCHEMICAL MECHANISMS OF PLATELET ACTIVATION

General Scheme of Platelet Signal–Response Coupling (Fig. 37-2)

Two major signal transduction pathways have been described in platelets as well as in most other cell types.[114–116] The major stimulatory pathway in platelets uses two intracellular second messengers, inositol 1,4,5-triphosphate (IP_3) and sn-1,2-diacylglycerol (DG), which are simultaneously formed from the phospholipase C–stimulated hydrolysis of membrane inositol phospholipids after extracellular agonist binding to membrane receptors.[117–119] The major inhibitory pathway in platelets uses the intracellular second messenger cAMP, which is produced by the action of adenylate cyclase on ATP after the binding of extracellular antagonists (inhibitors) to membrane receptors.[120] The second messengers of both the excitatory and inhibitory pathways are generated internally by the activation of membrane-associated amplifier enzymes (phospholipase C and adenylate cyclase, respectively) through receptor-linked changes in a family of signal-transducing guanosine triphosphate (GTP) binding regulatory proteins (G proteins) in the platelet membrane. The second messengers formed by these reactions exert their intracellular actions by inducing conformational changes in target proteins either directly or indirectly through the activation of specific protein kinases: IP_3 releases Ca^{2+} into the cytosol, which binds calmodulin and leads to the activation of Ca^{2+}- and calmodulin-dependent protein kinase[119]; DG activates protein kinase C[117–119]; and cAMP activates a cAMP-dependent protein kinase.[120]

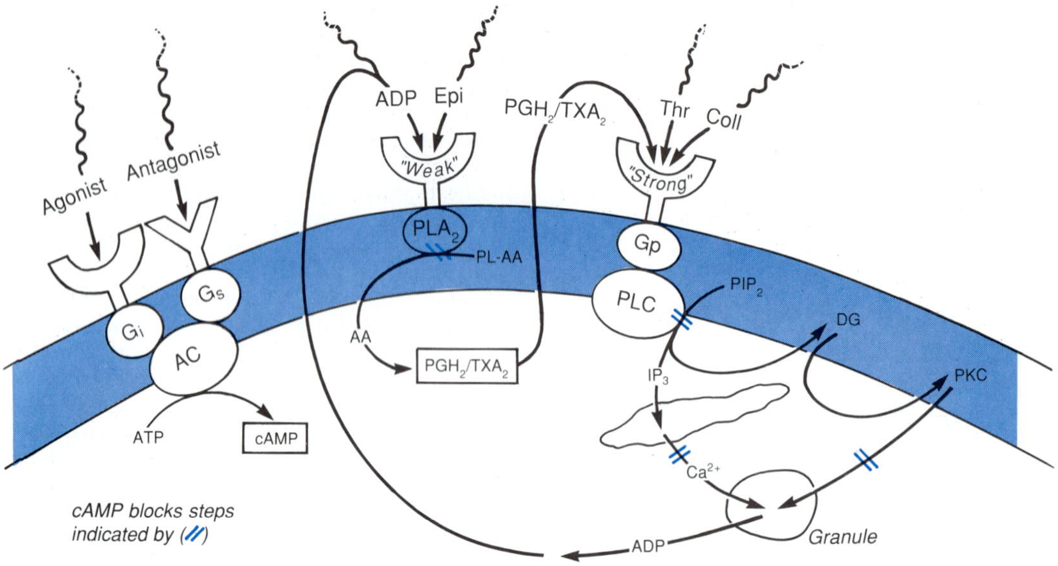

FIGURE 37-2. Outline of signal–response coupling in platelets. Weak agonists (eg, ADP, epinephrine) stimulate phospholipase A_2 (PLA_2) mediated hydrolysis of free arachidonic acid (AA) from membrane phospholipid (PL) pools. AA is converted by means of the cyclooxygenase pathway to endoperoxides PGG_2 and PGH_2 and to TXA_2. PGG_2, PGH_2, TXA_2, and other strong agonists (eg, thrombin, collagen) stimulate phospholipase C (PLC) through a G protein (Gp). PLC cleaves phosphatidylinositol 4,5-bisphosphate (PIP_2) to generate two second messengers: diacylglycerol (DG), which activates protein kinase C (PKC), and inositol 1,4,5-triphosphate (IP_3), which translocates Ca^{2+} from intracellular storage sites to the cytosol. Strong agonists also activate PLA_2, either directly or by mobilizing free cytosolic Ca^{2+} to activate PLA_2. PKC activation and Ca^{2+} mobilization act synergistically to induce secretion; ADP released from storage granules during secretion amplifies functional platelet responses by acting as a weak agonist. These activation pathways are modulated by cAMP, the major inhibitory second messenger in platelets. cAMP is generated from ATP by adenylyl cyclase (AC), which is under dual control by an inhibitory G protein (G_i) that is linked to agonists and a stimulatory G protein (G_s) that is linked to antagonists (eg, PGI_2). cAMP, directly or indirectly, inhibits a number of processes in platelet activation, including PLA_2, PLC, PKC, and Ca^{2+} mobilization. cGMP (not shown) is also an inhibitory second messenger in platelets.

Ligand–Receptor Interactions

Platelets may be exposed to stimulatory and inhibitory extracellular signals that are derived from a variety of sources. The signals may be plasma constituents (eg, catecholamines or coagulation proteases such as thrombin or plasmin), products of blood vessels (eg, PGI_2, EDRF or nitric oxide, or collagen), or products of platelets (eg, ADP, TXA_2, or PGD_2) or they may originate from multiple blood cell and vascular sources (eg, platelet-activating factor, PAF, or vWF). In general, platelet signals have been divided into three groups according to mechanisms of action: (1) strong agonists (eg, thrombin, collagen, PAF, prostaglandin endoperoxides, and TXA_2); (2) weak agonists, which depend on the platelet-release reaction (including endogenous ADP secretion and TXA_2 production) to effect a full response (eg, ADP, epinephrine); and (3) antagonists (eg, PGI_2, EDRF or nitric oxide). The platelet receptors for many of these ligands have been characterized.[121–138]

G Proteins

In platelets, there are three functionally distinct, but not necessarily structurally unique, guanine nucleotide-binding regulatory (G) proteins.[139,140] One of these, G_p, serves to couple agonist-occupied receptors to the stimulation of phosphoinositide-specific phospholipase C. The other two G proteins couple receptors to adenylate cyclase: G_i links agonist-occupied receptors to the inhibition of adenylate cyclase, while G_s links antagonist-occupied receptors to the activation of adenylate cyclase. Each of these G proteins is a heterotrimeric complex composed of α, β, and γ subunits. In the basal unstimulated state, guanosine diphosphate (GDP) is tightly bound to the α subunit, as shown in Figure 37-3. After receptor-ligand coupling, GDP dissociates, and GTP becomes bound to the now available guanine nucleotide–binding site of the α subunit. The binding of GTP to the α subunit results in the dissociation of the α subunit from the $\alpha\beta\gamma$ complex. The dissociated $G_\alpha \cdot GTP$ then interacts with the appropriate signal-amplifier enzyme (phospholipase C or adenylate cyclase) in the plasma membrane to convert phosphorylated precursors (ATP or phosphatidylinositol bisphosphate) into intracellular second messengers (cAMP or IP_3 and DG). The G protein signal is finally terminated when the intrinsic GTPase activity of the α subunit autohydrolyzes GTP to GDP, thus permitting the GDP-bound α subunit to reassociate with the $\beta\gamma$ component to restore the basal G-protein complex.

Platelet-Activation Pathways

Phospholipase C

As in other cell types, a major pathway of platelet activation involves phospholipase C. As a consequence of receptor occupancy by agonists, this enzyme breaks down a highly phosphorylated inositol phospholipid species, phosphatidylinositol bisphosphate (PIP_2), to create the two potent intracellular second messengers, IP_3 and DG.[141–143] These molecules affect divergent but complementary pathways

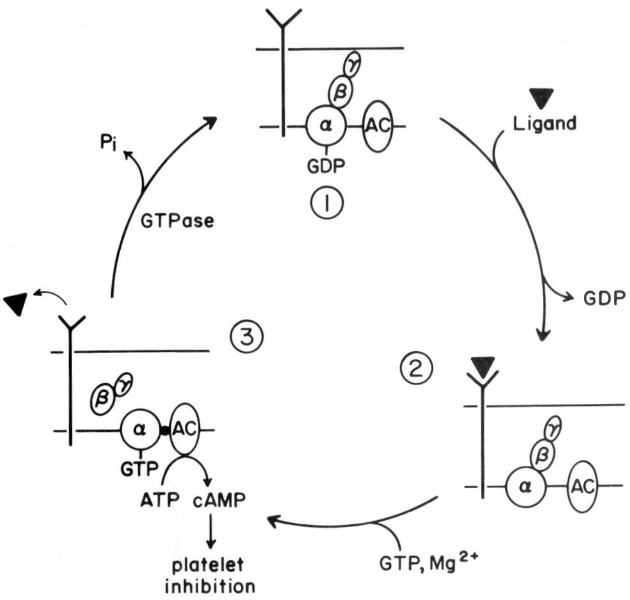

FIGURE 37-3. General model by which G proteins transmit extracellular signals into intracellular responses. (Kroll MH, Schafer AI. Biochemical mechanisms of platelet activation. Blood 1989;74:1181)

of platelet activation. IP_3 releases calcium from its internal storage organelles[144–147] and thereby induces a rise in cytosolic free calcium levels. At the same time, DG causes the activation of protein kinase C. Both calcium mobilization and protein kinase C activation can independently mediate platelet activation, but together they act synergistically to stimulate the full biologic responses of secretion and aggregation.[148,149]

Changes in intracellular calcium levels regulate the activation of platelets and other cell types through several possible mechanisms.[150] These may include the activation of the Ca^{2+}- and calmodulin-dependent protein kinase, which initiates platelet shape change; Ca^{2+}-dependent proteases; phospholipase A_2 (vide infra); and phospholipase C. The mechanisms by which protein kinase C activation stimulates platelets are incompletely understood. This enzyme induces the phosphorylation of a cloned 47-kd platelet protein,[151] the function of which is unknown.

Phospholipase A_2

In addition to the activating events described previously, the stimulation of platelets by various agonists also induces phospholipase A_2 activity.[152] Phospholipase A_2 is the major route of mobilization of free arachidonic acid from platelet membrane phospholipids. The enzyme directly cleaves the free fatty acid from the second carbon (C2) position of phospholipids. Whereas the preferred phospholipid substrate for phospholipase C in signal transduction is PIP_2, phospholipase A_2 acts primarily on phosphatidylcholine to liberate free arachidonic acid. Free arachidonic acid can also be produced through the phospholipase C system by means of lipases that act on DG or its phosphorylated metabolite, phosphatidic acid, but these pathways of arachidonic acid hydrolysis in platelets are relatively minor compared to the phospholipase A_2 pathway.

After deacylation, free arachidonic acid in the platelet is rapidly metabolized to various biologically active products (termed *eicosanoids*) through the actions of the oxygenating enzymes cyclooxygenase and lipoxygenase.[153,154] Cyclooxygenase, which is irreversibly acetylated by aspirin and reversibly blocked by nonsteroidal antiinflammatory agents, converts arachidonic acid to the labile prostaglandin endoperoxides PGG_2 and PGH_2, which are then further transformed by thromboxane synthase to TXA_2. PGG_2, PGH_2, and TXA_2 are potent platelet agonists that bind to specific platelet receptors and, through the G-protein signal transduction system described previously, directly activate phospholipase C.

Synergy in Platelet Activation

The magnitude of response of platelets to two different agonists may be greater than the arithmetic sum of each response to the individual agonists separately, and this constitutes *synergy*. Synergism has been observed with several different pairs of platelet agonists. Epinephrine in particular has been found to stimulate platelets synergistically with most other agonists that have been tested. Since platelets in the circulation are undoubtedly exposed simultaneously to more than one agonist at any given moment, this may represent an in vivo amplification system to fully activate platelets. The precise mechanism of platelet synergism is unknown, but there is evidence that functionally trivial rises in intracellular free calcium in response to below-threshold stimuli may prime the platelet aggregation response to subsequent excitation by various agonists.[155,156]

Platelet Inhibition

The activation of platelets is counterregulated by biochemical processes that attenuate or prevent agonist-induced responses.[114] Under normal circumstances, these inhibitory influences prevail in the circulation to maintain platelets in their unactivated state. The most important inhibitory second messenger in platelets is cAMP, the intracellular levels of which are raised when adenylate cyclase is activated in response to negative extracellular signals. Vascular PGI_2 acts as a potent platelet inhibitor by binding to specific platelet receptors, activating adenylate cyclase through its G protein, G_s, and thereby raising the level of cAMP within the platelet. cAMP has pleiotropic inhibitory effects in platelets, blocking both the initiation and the maintenance of stimulatory responses. This inhibitory second messenger may block agonist binding to platelet surfaces,[157,158] inhibit phospholipase C–mediated IP_3 and DG formation,[141,159] indirectly and directly block protein kinase C,[160] and antagonize calcium-mediated responses, including the mobilization of arachidonic acid by phospholipase A_2,[161] cytoskeletal assembly,[162] and the phosphorylation of myosin light chain.[163]

The role of cGMP as an inhibitory second messenger in platelets is not as well established. Increasing platelet cGMP (eg, by organic nitrates) inhibits agonist-induced responses such as phospholipase C activation.[164–166] EDRF or nitric oxide inhibits platelet function through the selective activation of platelet guanylate cyclase,[167,168] and this inhibitory signal acts synergistically with cAMP to block platelet activation.[169]

Thus, the state of activation of platelets in the circulation is dynamically determined from moment to moment by a delicate balance between multiple excitatory and inhibitory influences. These extracellular signals may work in an antagonistic or a synergistic relation with each other. It is the task of the interrelated network of signal-transducing and intracellular second messenger systems described in this section (summarized in Fig. 37-2) to organize these extracellular signals and to coordinate the platelet response.

CLINICAL EVALUATION OF PATIENTS WITH DISORDERS OF PLATELET FUNCTION

The clinical history of a patient with a suspected disorder of platelet function, or any other coagulopathy, is of primary importance. Laboratory testing is only ancillary and complementary to the history and examination of such patients. For example, a patient who has withstood recent surgery without excessive bleeding has had a better test of hemostasis than any laboratory examination can provide. In fact, some laboratory tests of hemostasis may actually be misleading without a knowledge of the patient's bleeding history.

Several aspects of the clinical history of patients with suspected functional platelet disorders should be specifically probed. A positive family history of bleeding suggests a hereditary cause but, as with other coagulopathies, including hemophilia, a negative family history should not exclude this possibility. A history of recent systemic illnesses may provide important information about the cause of the platelet dysfunction. A careful history of drug ingestion is critical since numerous medications (including components of many nonprescription remedies) may interfere with platelet function; these may include aspirin, most nonsteroidal antiinflammatory drugs, various antibiotics, β-blockers, alcohol (exacerbating the bleeding tendency associated with aspirin), and ω-3 fatty acid fish oil supplements. Finally, patients should be asked about previous responses to major surgery, trauma, and various commonly experienced challenges to the integrity of the hemostatic system, including menses, tonsillectomy, dental extractions, inoculations, and so forth. The determination of a lack of bleeding complications after these events is at least as important as the finding of excessive hemorrhage. This aspect of the history may provide important clues to the duration and clinical significance of the bleeding tendency.

Patients with functional platelet disorders exhibit characteristic clinical patterns of bleeding problems. Whereas coagulation factor deficiencies typically cause deep tissue hemorrhage (eg, hemarthrosis, deep muscle hematomas, retroperitoneal bleeding) that is often delayed in onset after trauma or surgery, qualitative platelet abnormalities are usually associated with superficial hemorrhage that is either spontaneous or occurs immediately after injury. Superficial bleeding complications in these patients most commonly include ecchymoses (common bruises), purpura, or mucosal hemorrhage (eg, epistaxis; oropharyngeal, gastrointestinal, or genitourinary bleeding; and menorrhagia). Petechiae are more characteristic manifestations of severe thrombocytopenia. In general, patients with specific defects of platelet adhesion (eg, von Willebrand's disease) and platelet aggregation (eg, thrombasthenia) tend to have more serious bleeding complications than patients with platelet-release defects (eg, storage-pool deficiency [SPD] or aspirin ingestion). In fact, a number of studies have demonstrated a significant but usually not clinically critical increase in perioperative bleeding complications in patients undergoing various surgical procedures shortly after the ingestion of aspirin[170–172] or nonsteroidal antiinflammatory drugs.[173]

LABORATORY EVALUATION OF PLATELET FUNCTION

A wide array of laboratory tests have been devised to assess platelet function and to diagnose clinical disorders of primary hemostasis.[174,175] Most of these assays are seriously flawed in specificity, sensitivity, reproducibility, or clinical applicability, and only a few have withstood the test of time. Although most of the classic tests of platelet function were designed to investigate the role of platelets in bleeding disorders, attention has also been focused on tests of platelet hyperreactivity that may contribute to the pathogenesis of thrombosis and vascular disease. A critical shortcoming of our present laboratory armamentarium is the almost complete lack of any useful tests to evaluate platelet–vessel wall interactions, primary vascular defects, and endothelial cell dysfunction, which undoubtedly contribute to a considerable number of undefined bleeding (and thrombotic) disorders.

Bleeding Time

Since its initial description in 1910,[176] the bleeding time has remained the single best clinically applicable test of in vivo platelet function. This test simply measures the time to cessation of bleeding from a small, standardized puncture or incision in a specific area of skin. The bleeding time thus reflects the time to formation of a hemostatic platelet plug at the site of microvascular injury. The original Duke[176] and Ivy[177] methods used puncture wounds in the earlobe and forearm. These techniques suffered problems of reproducibility and have been largely supplanted by various template modifications. The method of Mielke[178] employs a scalpel incision on the volar aspect of the forearm, using a template with a slit to produce a wound of standard length and depth. To minimize variability in blood pressure in the small vessels, a blood pressure cuff on the arm is inflated to 40 mmHg to occlude venous return before the incision. Based on this technique, several commercial devices using disposable spring-loaded blades are available. It is important for each institution to establish a normal range for the exact method used[175] since considerable variability in normal values has been found between laboratories, even with a template method.[179] Although the bleeding time can be an extremely useful screening test of in vivo platelet function and platelet–vessel wall interactions, it is still prone to falsely normal and falsely abnormal results due to improper technique and therefore should be performed by experienced laboratory personnel.[180] A number of variables, including venous pressure, length, direction, pressure, depth and number of incisions, skin temperature, and sex and age of the subject may all affect bleeding time determinations.[174,181] Using standardized template techniques, bleeding times in infants and children have been found to be similar to those in adults.[182]

In general, the normal bleeding time depends on the three variables of primary hemostasis: (1) platelet count, (2) platelet function (including platelet–vessel wall interactions), and (3) vascular integrity. The bleeding time is prolonged when the platelet count is less than 100,000/μL; below this level, there is a direct correlation between the degree of thrombocytopenia and the extent of prolongation of the bleeding time (Fig. 37-4). A disproportionately prolonged bleeding time is found when a qualitative platelet defect coexists with thrombocytopenia (eg, in Wiskott-Aldrich syndrome). Conversely, in patients with thrombocytopenia due to peripheral destruction and high turnover of platelets (eg, immune thrombocytopenic purpura), the circulating platelet pool is enriched with a population of young, hemostatically more effective platelets that may produce bleeding times that are disproportionately short for that predicted for the degree of thrombocytopenia. A prolonged bleeding time associated with a normal platelet count is indicative of some abnormality in platelet function or platelet–vascular interactions, including defects in platelet adhesion, platelet release, or platelet aggregation. Primary vascular disorders, including vascular purpura, may also cause prolongation of the bleeding time. Although

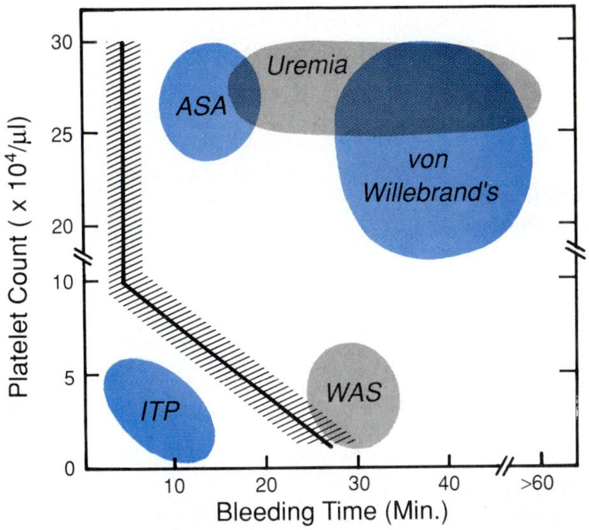

FIGURE 37-4. Inverse relation of bleeding time to platelet count in patients with thrombocytopenia resulting from impaired platelet production. When thrombocytopenia is due to increased platelet turnover (eg, ITP), the bleeding time may be disproportionately short for the degree of thrombocytopenia. In thrombocytopenic states associated with a coexisting functional platelet disorder (eg, Wiskott-Aldrich syndrome [WAS]), the bleeding time is disproportionately prolonged for the degree of thrombocytopenia. Examples of clinical situations associated with variably prolonged bleeding times in the absence of thrombocytopenia include aspirin ingestion (ASA), uremia, and von Willebrand's disease. (After Harker LA, Slichter SJ. The bleeding time as a screening test for evaluation of platelet function. N Engl J Med 1972;287:155)

the bleeding time characteristically tests the integrity of primary hemostasis and does not reflect the components of the coagulation cascade and fibrin formation, prolonged bleeding times have been found in some patients with factor V deficiency[183] and severe hemophilia.[184,185] Severe anemia may also be associated with a prolonged bleeding time, and this can be corrected by red cell transfusion.[186]

Because the bleeding time is a pivotal screening test of hemostasis, a clinical approach to its further work-up is presented in Figure 37-5. The flow and extent of this evaluation must be individualized, however, depending on the urgency and the clinical implications of a precise diagnosis. The utility of the bleeding time as a routine preoperative screening test of hemostasis has been debated.[187–190] Studies[191–193] have led to the recommendation that it is an unnecessary preoperative test in the absence of bleeding risk factors (including aspirin use) as determined by a careful history. Unfortunately, many cases of prolonged bleeding times remain unsolved even after an exhaustive investigation; these patients may have undefined primary vascular disorders. In many such instances, when an abnormality in the test is detected in anticipation of a surgical procedure, empiric therapeutic trials may be indicated in an attempt to temporarily normalize the prolonged bleeding time (vide infra).[194]

Platelet Adhesion

No clinically applicable assays are available that specifically test this initial step in platelet activation. The glass-bead–column platelet retention test[195–198] measures the percentage of platelets retained by a single passage of whole blood through a column of glass beads, calculated from the precolumn and postcolumn infusion platelet counts. This test is difficult to standardize and is relatively nonspecific for adhesion since the retention of platelets in the column also depends on the formation of platelet aggregates. Because of these limitations, the platelet retention test is no longer widely used. Several variations on the basic method developed by Baumgartner[199] involve the direct microscopic assessment of platelet adhesion to a denuded endothelial surface during the continuous passage of whole blood over an everted segment of rabbit aorta. The extent of platelet adhesion in this system can be further quantitated by using platelets radiolabeled with indium-111. The Baumgartner method has the additional advantage of being able to reproduce physiologic shear rates over the vessel surface. Although this approach may represent a true test of platelet adhesion, its expense and technical difficulty have restricted it to research studies.

Platelet-Release Reaction: Secretion of Granule Constituents and Arachidonic Acid Metabolism

Abnormalities of the platelet-release reaction may involve defects in secretion (degranulation) or arachidonic acid metabolism (TXA_2 formation), platelet products that act in concert to mediate the process of aggregation (vide infra). A number of laboratory tests have been developed to assess the integrity of these components of the platelet-release reaction.

The most direct approach to determining whether there is an anatomic deficiency of platelet storage granules is to study the platelet ultrastructure by transmission electron microscopy. Electron microscopy is useful in making a definitive diagnosis of platelet storage-pool disease, including the gray-platelet syndrome variant, which involves a selective deficiency of α granules. The finding of normal platelet ultrastructure by electron microscopy, however, does not indicate that the platelets are functionally capable of degranulating and secreting their stored constituents when stimulated.

Therefore, to test platelet secretion, various techniques have been developed to measure the appearance of released products into the extracellular fluid after platelet activation. A widely used, relatively simple screening test is to measure the release of serotonin. In this method, platelets are incubated with ^{14}C-serotonin, which should be preferentially taken up into the dense granules, and then stimulated with various agonists to provoke the release of the ^{14}C-serotonin, which can be measured in the supernatant.[200] The anatomic deficiency of storage granules (storage-pool disease) causes an abnormal pattern of serotonin uptake, while a functional release defect is associated with normal uptake but defective release of the radiolabeled serotonin. A simple, semiquantitative assay of adenine nucleotide release from dense granules has also been developed. Using the firefly reagents luciferin and luciferase, ATP released from the dense granules of activated platelets into the medium produces measurable luminescence. Like the serotonin-release assay, this technique is useful for the diagnosis of storage-pool disease involving a deficiency of dense granules. It has been made more convenient by the introduction of the lumiaggregometer,[201] an instrument which permits continuous and simultaneous monitoring of both platelet aggregation (vide infra) and ATP secretion. In general, the diagnosis of a platelet-release defect is most easily made using either the serotonin or ATP secretion assays. It is usually unnecessary, for strictly clinical purposes, to perform electron microscopy of the platelets to further define the defect.

The release of platelet α-granule contents can be measured using commercially available kits for radioimmunoassays of the α-granule platelet-specific proteins, PF4 or

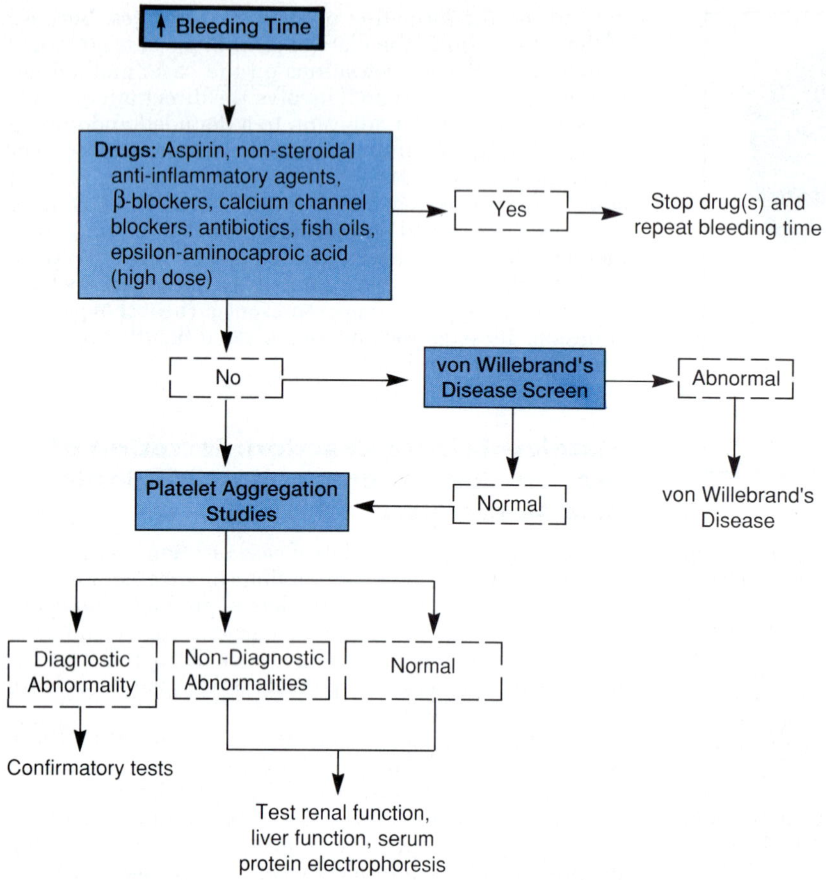

FIGURE 37-5. A clinical approach to the evaluation of a prolonged bleeding time.

βTG. In addition to their use in the diagnosis of α-granule deficiency,[202] these assays have also been extensively applied to detect in vivo platelet activation (and secretion) in thrombotic and vascular disorders by measuring the ambient levels of PF4 or βTG in plasma samples. Considerable caution must be used in interpreting plasma concentrations of these platelet-specific proteins since improper methods of blood sample collection and processing can cause ex vivo platelet release and thereby produce artifactually elevated plasma levels. Furthermore, plasma concentrations of PF4 may be falsely increased in patients receiving heparin due to the displacement of PF4 from endothelial-binding sites.[203] Plasma levels of βTG, which is cleared by the kidneys, may also be elevated in the absence of in vivo platelet activation in patients with renal failure.[204]

Platelet-release defects due to abnormalities of arachidonic acid metabolism can be assessed by a variety of techniques. Acquired cyclooxygenase blockade by drugs (most notably aspirin and nonsteroidal antiinflammatory agents) is the most common defect of this metabolic pathway, but congenital cyclooxygenase deficiency, thromboxane synthase deficiency, loss of platelet endoperoxide and thromboxane receptors, and acquired lipoxygenase deficiency in the myeloproliferative disorders may all contribute to platelet dysfunction and a clinical bleeding tendency. Although seldom indicated for clinical purposes, specific abnormalities of arachidonic acid metabolism are most easily tested by radioimmunoassay of TXB_2 (the stable breakdown product of TXA_2) generated by platelets activated in vitro. More detailed analysis of platelet arachidonic acid metabolism can be performed by labeling platelet membrane phospholipid pools with radioactive arachidonic acid, and then measuring the radiolabeled products formed after platelet activation using thin-layer or high-performance liquid chromatography. The determination of peripheral plasma levels of TXB_2 is prone to the same serious potential problems of artifactual elevations caused by ex vivo platelet activation that complicate assays of PF4 and βTG. To circumvent this problem, the physiologic in vivo dinor metabolite of TXA_2 (or vascular endothelial PGI_2) can be measured in urine or plasma by gas chromatography and mass spectroscopy.[205] This approach has been used in a number of studies of the role of platelet hyperreactivity in various types of thrombotic and vascular disorders.[206] These technically difficult assays remain largely restricted to research laboratories.

Platelet Aggregation

The ability of platelets to aggregate in vitro in response to a variety of stimuli is usually studied by the turbidimetric method of Born.[207] Platelet-rich plasma (PRP) is prepared from citrated whole blood by centrifugation and then continuously stirred at 37°C in a cuvette placed in an aggregometer. Unactivated platelets uniformly suspended in plasma impart a characteristic turbidity to PRP. When platelets aggregate after the injection of an agonist, the turbidity of PRP falls, and light transmission through it increases proportionally. Continuous changes in the transmission of a light beam directed through the cuvette containing PRP can thus be monitored, producing an aggregation tracing on the recorder of the aggregometer.

Clinical coagulation laboratories generally use a battery of aggregating agents to test platelet responsiveness, and each of these stimuli normally produces a characteristic pattern of aggregation, as shown in the top panel of Figure 37-6. ADP, at concentrations of 2.5 to 5 μmol/L, typically induces a biphasic aggregation tracing. The first wave corresponds to initial, reversible aggregation, and the second wave corresponds to irreversible aggregation that is me-

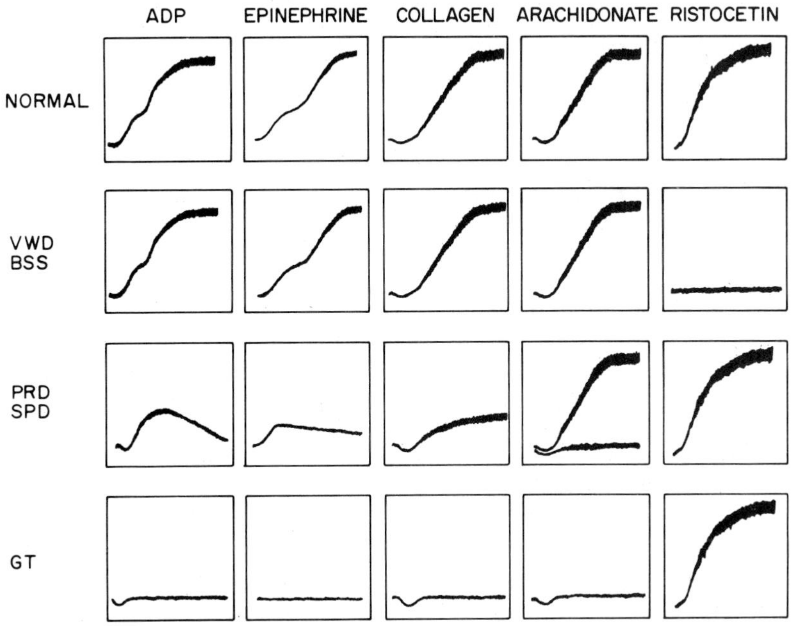

FIGURE 37-6. Typical patterns of platelet aggregation in response to ADP, epinephrine, collagen, arachidonate, and ristocetin in (1) normal subjects; (2) patients with disorders of adhesion, including von Willebrand's disease (VWD) and Bernard-Soulier syndrome (BSS); (3) patients with disorders of platelet secretion, including platelet-release defects (PRD) and storage-pool deficiency (SPD); and (4) patients with disorders of aggregation, including Glanzmann's thrombasthenia (GS). Platelet aggregation induced by arachidonate in patients with disorders of secretion may be normal or absent. (Schafer AI. Thrombocytopenia and disorders of platelet function. In: Stein JH, ed. Internal medicine, ed 3. Boston, Little, Brown, 1990:1041)

diated by products of the release reaction (including endogenous platelet ADP); the release reaction occurs during the plateau phase between the two waves of aggregation. Lower concentrations of ADP normally stimulate only first-wave, reversible aggregation, while at higher concentrations of ADP, only a single irreversible aggregation curve is detectable. Epinephrine likewise stimulates a biphasic aggregation pattern in this in vitro test. More potent agents, such as collagen, arachidonic acid, thrombin, calcium ionophore, or PAF, induce a single wave of irreversible aggregation. A small decrease in light transmission preceding the onset of aggregation reflects the initial platelet shape change that follows the addition of different stimuli except epinephrine. The aggregation of platelets by the antibiotic ristocetin (which is usually included in the battery of aggregating agents used in clinical laboratories) actually involves agglutination since it can be reproduced even with metabolically inert, formalin-fixed platelets. Defective ristocetin-induced platelet aggregation is characteristic of von Willebrand's disease and the Bernard-Soulier syndrome, although it has also been found in some healthy black subjects.[208] In type IIb von Willebrand's disease, platelets actually demonstrate heightened (rather than absent) responsiveness to ristocetin, and this can be detected by performing a ristocetin titration.

A number of variables can affect platelet aggregation studies, even in normal subjects. The responsiveness of platelets to different agonists may vary somewhat with the anticoagulant used (usually sodium citrate), PRP platelet count, platelet size distribution, time of day, temporal relation to meals and physical activity, and the time elapsed between blood collection and study. These problems of reproducibility make precise quantitation of platelet aggregability difficult. Characteristic patterns of abnormalities of platelet aggregation are summarized in Table 37-2 and Figure 37-6 and are discussed in more detail with specific platelet disorders later.

Platelet aggregation in whole blood rather than in plasma has been investigated using either a whole-blood platelet counter[209] or impedance aggregometry.[210] The impedance technique monitors the continuous increase in electrical impedance between two electrodes as platelets adhere to and aggregate on these electrodes in stirred whole blood.[175] Despite certain theoretical advantages to whole-blood ag-

TABLE 37-2. Functional Platelet Disorders Associated With Abnormalities of Platelet Aggregation

Response to Aggregating Agents						
Epinephrine	**Collagen**	**ADP**	**Arachidonate**	**Ristocetin**	**Other**	**Associated Disorder**
Absent	Normal	Normal	Normal	Normal		Loss of α_2-adrenergic receptors: congenital or acquired (myeloproliferative disorders)
Normal	Absent	Normal	Normal	Normal		Gpla deficiency
Normal	Normal	Normal	Normal	Absent		von Willebrand's disease; Bernard-Soulier syndrome; normal variant in blacks
Absent	Absent	Absent	Absent	Normal		Glanzmann's thrombasthenia
Second-wave absent	Normal or ↓	Second-wave absent	Absent	Normal		Storage-pool deficiency; aspirin
Second-wave absent	Normal or ↓	Second-wave absent	Normal	Normal		Storage-pool deficiency
Normal or absent	Normal	Normal	Normal	Normal	Spontaneous aggregation	Myeloproliferative disorders

gregometry, including the inclusion of other blood cells to provide a more physiologic milieu for platelets and the lack of a need to centrifuge blood samples that may selectively remove larger platelets, this method is not adequately standardized and validated for routine clinical use.

Other Specialized Tests of Platelet Function

A number of other specialized tests of platelet function have been used to describe or confirm specific qualitative platelet abnormalities. These methods remain largely confined to research laboratories. *Platelet coagulant activity* assays[211,212] have been developed to assess the contribution of platelets to prothrombin activation by providing a surface for the support of proteolytic activation of coagulation proteins. This property of activated platelet membranes was previously referred to as *platelet factor 3 activity*, a term that has been largely abandoned. A routine screening test for platelet coagulant activity measures the prothrombin time in serum compared with that in citrated, platelet-poor plasma.[213] Changes in platelet coagulant activity have been described in patients with a variety of hereditary or acquired bleeding or thrombotic problems.[212–218] In patients suspected of having abnormalities of platelet surface membrane glycoproteins, various techniques have been developed to directly identify the defects. Surface membrane glycoproteins are generally radiolabeled, and after solubilization of cell membranes in sodium dodecyl sulfate, they are separated, identified, and quantitated by polyacrylamide gel electrophoresis. "Activation-dependent" monoclonal antibodies have been developed to permit the direct detection of activated platelets in whole blood by flow cytometry.[219] Methods have also been developed to measure changes in platelet *cytosolic free calcium* levels. These techniques employ cytosol-trapped fluorophores (eg, Quin-2, Indo-1, Fura-2) or photoproteins (aequorin), which may detect different pools and distributions of cytosolic free calcium.[220–222]

DISORDERS OF PLATELET ADHESION

Bernard-Soulier Syndrome

Bernard-Soulier syndrome (see Chap. 32) is a rare, autosomal recessive disorder that can cause serious and occasionally fatal platelet-type bleeding complications.[223–225] The homozygous state is characterized by a prolonged bleeding time, thrombocytopenia, and giant platelets on the peripheral blood smear. The heterozygous form of the syndrome is clinically silent, although large platelets are occasionally found on the peripheral smear, and partial deficiencies of platelet membrane glycoproteins (vide infra) have been noted.[226] Functional studies of homozygous Bernard-Soulier platelets have been hampered by the low platelet counts and the difficulty of isolating large platelets from other blood cells. The characteristic abnormality of platelet aggregation studies in this disorder is a loss of response to ristocetin, as in classic von Willebrand's disease (see Fig. 37-6 and Table 37-2). Thrombin-induced aggregation is also diminished in most cases,[227] but the platelet responses to other agonists, such as ADP, epinephrine, and collagen, are entirely normal.[228] As in von Willebrand's disease, the platelets of patients with Bernard-Soulier syndrome exhibit impaired adhesion to deendothelialized vessel segments under conditions of rapid blood flow.[229–231]

Although the clinical and laboratory manifestations of the Bernard-Soulier syndrome mimic those of classic von Willebrand's disease, the addition of exogenous vWF in vitro does not correct the ristocetin agglutination defect, and the transfusion of plasma or cryoprecipitate does not correct the clinical hemostatic defect of the Bernard-Soulier syndrome. Thus, the major abnormality of this syndrome is the loss of binding of vWF to intrinsically defective platelets in the presence of ristocetin.[232,233] The molecular basis of this platelet disorder was identified by Nurden and Caen,[234] who demonstrated the absence of the vWF-binding sites on membrane gpIb in platelets of Bernard-Soulier patients. The absence of platelet membrane gpIb in this disorder has been confirmed by crossed immunoelectrophoretic analysis of membrane glycoproteins[235,236] and by failure of the platelets to bind polyclonal or monoclonal anti-gpIb antibodies.[237–239] Additional abnormalities of platelet membrane glycoproteins have been demonstrated in patients with Bernard-Soulier syndrome. Glycoprotein IX, a protein that coisolates with gpIb by immunochemical methods and is associated with gpIb as a native heterodimer complex in the intact platelet membrane,[240] is also absent in this disorder.[241,242] Bernard-Soulier platelets also exhibit a loss of gpV. Since both gpIb and gpV may be involved in the normal interaction of platelets with thrombin,[243–245] these membrane glycoprotein defects may explain the blunted responsiveness of Bernard-Soulier platelets to thrombin.[227]

Detectable but reduced amounts of gpIb, gpIX, and gpV have been found in some patients with Bernard-Soulier syndrome,[241,242,246] and the molecular heterogeneity of this hereditary disorder is being increasingly recognized.[247] An acquired form of the Bernard-Soulier syndrome associated with a myelodysplastic syndrome has also been described.[248]

von Willebrand's Disease and Pseudo–von Willebrand's Disease

Von Willebrand's disease, unlike Bernard-Soulier syndrome, is an autosomal dominant disorder. Heterozygous patients are typically affected clinically; a rare, severe form of the disease afflicts homozygous or double heterozygous patients. The disease is caused by one of several quantitative or qualitative abnormalities in the vWF protein. In contrast to the Bernard-Soulier syndrome, therefore, the adhesion defect of von Willebrand's disease is due to an abnormality of plasma vWF rather than an intrinsic deficiency of platelets to bind the protein. Thus, the rational therapy for von Willebrand's disease is to transfuse a source of the normal protein (eg, cryoprecipitate) rather than platelets.

A familial bleeding disorder that resembles type II von Willebrand's disease has been found to be caused, not by an abnormality in the plasma vWF, but by an intrinsic platelet defect in binding the protein. It has been termed *pseudo–* or *platelet-type* von Willebrand's disease.[249–251] In these cases, increased selective absorption of higher-molecular-weight multimers of vWF by the abnormal platelets apparently leads to depletion of these multimers from plasma, thus producing a plasma multimer analysis that mimics type II von Willebrand's disease. Unlike type IIB von Willebrand's disease, in which the selective depletion of plasma vWF is attributable to a defect in the protein itself, pseudo–von Willebrand's disease is caused by a defect in the platelet vWF receptor localized to membrane gpIb.[252] In contrast to the Bernard-Soulier syndrome, in which vWF binding to platelet gpIb is absent or deficient, in pseudo–von Willebrand's disease, plasma vWF has a higher-than-normal affinity for its receptor on platelet gpIb.[250,251,253] Thus, the platelet abnormalities are in many ways the opposite of those observed in the Bernard-Soulier syndrome.[249] Also, vWF can bind to and directly induce the agglutination of platelets from patients with pseudo–von Willebrand's disease without the addition of ristocetin, which is a cofactor required by normal platelets. Although pseudo–von Willebrand's disease characteristically involves an abnormality of the platelet gpIb receptor complex, little is known about the precise underlying structural defects in the platelet membrane.

Patients with pseudo–von Willebrand's disease characteristically have a mild, platelet-type bleeding disorder, intermittent and mild thrombocytopenia, and plasma vWF levels and multimer analysis that are similar to those described in patients with type IIB von Willebrand's disease. There is a theoretic but undocumented risk of precipitating thrombosis associated with in vivo platelet aggregation and increased thrombocytopenia by infusing cryoprecipitate in these patients.[224,254]

DISORDERS OF AGONIST-INDUCED PLATELET ACTIVATION

Collagen Receptor Defect

A variety of proteins have been proposed as the platelet receptors for collagen, including fibronectin,[255,256] vWF,[257] TSP,[258] complement component C1s,[259] and platelet factor XIII.[260] In addition, specific integral platelet membrane proteins have been identified that bind to soluble or insoluble collagen.[261,262] A patient with a hemorrhagic disorder and a markedly prolonged bleeding time was found to have a selective and complete loss of platelet responsiveness to collagen with platelet aggregation studies.[263] The platelets of this patient failed to undergo shape change or aggregate in response to several types of fibrillar collagen, even at high concentrations, either in plasma or in washed suspension, while ADP, epinephrine, ionophore A23187, arachidonic acid, PAF, and ristocetin-induced aggregation responses were preserved (see Table 37-2). Platelet adhesion to collagen and the spreading of platelets on a subendothelial vascular surface in a perfusion chamber[264] were also impaired. Analysis of the platelet proteins of this patient with one- and two-dimensional gel electrophoresis showed an isolated deficiency of the membrane gpIa. Another patient with a severe, lifelong platelet-type bleeding tendency, who also had a selective loss of collagen-induced platelet aggregation, was deficient in membrane gpIa and platelet TSP.[265] Collagen-induced aggregation in this patient could be restored by the addition of TSP, suggesting that both TSP and gpIa are normally required for collagen-stimulated platelet aggregation. Interestingly, both the clinical bleeding problems and the platelet membrane abnormalities of this latter patient spontaneously remitted at menopause.

Epinephrine (α_2-Adrenergic) Receptor Defect

Functional and biochemical responses of platelets to epinephrine (including aggregation, secretion, and inhibition of adenylate cyclase activity) are mediated by surface α_2-adrenergic receptors. The expression of platelet α_2-adrenergic receptors and epinephrine responsiveness varies somewhat even among normal subjects[266] and may be under genetic control.[267,268] Furthermore, platelet α_2-adrenergic receptors may be modulated by variations in levels of endogenous catecholamines,[269–272] although this regulatory influence has been disputed.[273–275]

Selective and complete loss of epinephrine-induced platelet aggregation has been found in patients with myeloproliferative disorders, a group of patients who are prone to bleeding and thrombotic complications (vide infra). The platelets of these patients exhibit loss of even first-wave aggregation in response to high concentrations of epinephrine, while the aggregation responses to other agonists may remain entirely normal. Patients with essential thrombocythemia (ET) and absent epinephrine-stimulated platelet aggregation have been found to have a nearly 50% reduction in α_2-adrenergic receptors.[276,277] A family with a mild platelet-type bleeding tendency associated with prolonged bleeding times has been characterized, in which impaired platelet aggregation and secretion responses to epinephrine, with normal responses to other agonists, has been found (see Table 37-2).[278] Platelet α_2-adrenergic receptors were reduced by more than half in the clinically affected members of this family.

Defect of Responsiveness to Thromboxane A_2

Several patients with bleeding disorders have been reported whose platelets fail to aggregate or secrete normally in response to TXA_2 but can convert exogenous arachidonic acid to TXA_2. These cases probably represent heterogeneous defects in platelet TXA_2 responsiveness.

Wu and colleagues[279] described a mild familial bleeding disorder associated with a prolonged bleeding time and aspirin-type platelet aggregation abnormalities, in which platelets failed to respond to TXA_2 but synthesized normal amounts of TXA_2. A specific platelet TXA_2 and PGH_2 receptor abnormality was proposed as the mechanism. Other cases of platelet refractoriness to TXA_2 have been described in association with a lifelong bleeding tendency[280–282] or acquired secondary to a myeloproliferative disorder.[283] These studies suggested a defect in TXA_2- and PGH_2-mediated intracellular calcium mobilization or use rather than a loss of TXA_2 and PGH_2 receptors. Subnormal platelet responses to TXA_2 in another patient with a myeloproliferative disorder were found to be associated with normal TXA_2 receptors by direct radioligand-binding studies.[284] Despite normal affinity and concentration of platelet TXA_2-binding sites, TXA_2 mimetics failed to stimulate intracellular postreceptor reactions, suggesting that the patient's platelets had defective TXA_2-mediated signal transduction. Rao and Holmsen[285] suggested that, in many of these cases, the abnormalities could be attributed to a general platelet secretion defect rather than a specific impairment in the platelet response to TXA_2.

Other Agonist-Induced Activation Defects

A patient with systemic lupus erythematosus was reported to have a selective loss of platelet aggregation induced by PAF, with normal responses to other agonists.[286] This patient had a normal bleeding time and no history of clinical bleeding problems. A group of patients with mild bleeding disorders and normal or slightly prolonged bleeding times was described, with weak platelet agonist response defects.[287] In these cases, platelet aggregation studies revealed impaired initial platelet responses to one or more weak agonists (ADP, epinephrine, and low concentrations of collagen), and it was proposed that the platelets of these patients were defective in some early postreceptor process of platelet activation common to a variety of agonists.

DISORDERS OF PLATELET SECRETION (RELEASE)

Platelet adhesion and the initial events in agonist-induced platelet activation are followed by platelet secretion when the cells degranulate and release the contents of their storage organelles. Disorders of platelet secretion can be broadly classified into two categories. First, the platelets of patients with SPD are unable to undergo the release reaction because of an ultrastructural absence or deficiency of one or more types of storage granules. Second, the platelets of patients with functional release defects are equipped with normal storage granules that are incapable of secreting their constituents because of some metabolic abnormality, most commonly impaired synthesis of TXA_2 (ie, aspirin-like defect). Both types of platelet secretion disorders can be either congenital or acquired, although SPD tends to be more frequently congenital, while functional release defects are usually acquired.

As noted previously, patients with disorders of platelet secretion typically exhibit mild platelet-type bleeding or bruising. In fact, many patients are entirely asymptomatic and are discovered to have a platelet secretion abnormality only because of the finding of a slightly prolonged bleeding time during preoperative screening.

Platelet aggregation studies usually show normal first-wave but absent second-wave responses to epinephrine and ADP, diminished response to collagen, and normal response to ristocetin. Platelet aggregation induced by arachidonic acid is variable in SPD and invariably absent in functional release defects caused by the ingestion of aspirin or nonsteroidal antiinflammatory drugs (see Fig. 37-6 and Table 37-2). Although these patterns of platelet aggregation abnormalities have been considered to be characteristic of disorders of platelet secretion, it is now recognized that some patients with prolonged bleeding times due to congenital or acquired SPD (vide infra) may have other or even entirely normal platelet aggregation results.[288,289]

Storage-Pool Deficiency

Early studies that distinguished this type of qualitative abnormality of platelets attributed the abnormal aggregation induced by epinephrine, ADP, and collagen to a defect in the secretion of ADP.[290,291] The familial platelet disorder of deficiency in the storage pool of ADP was subsequently defined.[292–294] The mode of inheritance of SPD has not been clearly established, although an autosomal dominant pattern has been found in some cases.[292,295] SPD is a heterogeneous group of disorders of storage organelles, representing a spectrum of abnormalities of platelet granule morphogenesis. The storage-pool diseases have been classified[296] as involving: (1) deficiency of only dense granules and dense-granule substances (δ-SPD); (2) deficiency of only α granules (α-SPD), also referred to as the "gray-platelet syndrome"; or (3) deficiencies of both types of granules (αδ-SPD).

δ-SPD and αδ-SPD

These are the prototypes of congenital platelet SPD, in which a mild bleeding disorder is associated with the platelet aggregation abnormalities described previously. Electron microscopy directly demonstrates a marked loss or complete absence of dense granules, with or without some loss of α granules,[296–298] as shown in Figure 37-7. Dense-granule contents, including ADP, calcium, pyrophosphate, and serotonin, are decreased in the platelets of these patients.[293,294,296] There is an inverse correlation between dense-granule ADP content and the bleeding time in these patients.[299] Incubation of the platelets with ^{14}C-serotonin results in normal initial uptake followed by rapid loss of the radiolabel from the platelets due to the deficiency of serotonin-storage organelles and the susceptibility of the amine to degradation by platelet monoamine oxidases if it cannot be sequestered.[285]

The variable aggregation responses to arachidonic acid seen in δ-SPD platelets may be due to abnormalities of arachidonic acid mobilization and metabolism, which have been reported to coexist in some cases.[300–303] Another metabolic abnormality in severe δ-SPD is impaired secretion of lysosomal acid hydrolases, despite a normal platelet content of these enzymes. It has been shown that the addition of ADP corrects this secretory defect, suggesting that it is secondary to the dense-granule deficiency in SPD platelets.[304]

Although SPD usually occurs as an isolated finding, the platelet abnormality has been found in association with other congenital disorders in some cases.[305] Patients with the autosomal recessive Hermansky-Pudlak syndrome have tyrosinase-positive oculocutaneous albinism and progressive pulmonary disease, with deposition of a ceroid-like pigment throughout the reticuloendothelial system and the bone marrow. A mild bleeding tendency and a prolonged bleeding time in these families have been found to be due to platelet SPD.[306–309] Patients with the autosomal recessive Chédiak-Higashi syndrome, who likewise have albinism as well as defective leukocyte function, can also have platelet SPD.[310–313] In patients with the Hermansky-Pudlak and Chédiak-Higashi syndromes, the platelet SPD may be part of a more generalized cellular defect of storage organelle morphogenesis that can also involve melanocytes and phagocytes as well as platelets. Congenital platelet SPD has been found in patients with the syndrome of thrombocytopenia with absent radii[314] and with Wiskott-Aldrich syndrome.[315] Wiskott-Aldrich syndrome is an X-linked recessive immunodeficiency disease characterized clinically by eczema, susceptibility to infections, and thrombocytopenia. In addition to being reduced in number, platelets in this syndrome are smaller than normal in size. Ultrastructurally, these platelets are deficient in storage granules and mitochondria. Splenectomy often results in correction of the thrombocytopenia and normalization of platelet size, ultrastructure, and function of the platelets in Wiskott-Aldrich syndrome,[316] suggesting that the defects observed in this syndrome are not intrinsic to the platelets. An autoimmune process has been proposed to explain the thrombocytopenia.[316] White[305] speculated that Wiskott-Aldrich syndrome may represent a disorder of delayed platelet maturation due to prolonged membrane development of the megakaryocytes.

α-SPD (Gray-Platelet Syndrome)

Rare cases of SPD have been reported in which there is an isolated loss of α granules with preservation of dense granules and lysosomes.[317–322] This form of SPD has been referred to as the gray-platelet syndrome because of the light gray, agranular appearance of the platelets on Wright-stained blood smears. Patients with gray-platelet syndrome have a congenital bleeding disorder usually associated with mild thrombocytopenia and a prolonged bleeding time. The clinical bleeding problems are generally superficial cutaneous and mucosal hemorrhage, typical of other platelet disorders. Episodes of recurrent hemarthrosis[317,319] and spontaneous hematomas[320] that are more consistent with coagulation factor deficiencies have also been reported in patients with this form of SPD. In contrast to the characteristic pattern of platelet aggregation abnormalities found in δ-SPD, patients with α-SPD exhibit highly variable and sometimes essentially normal platelet aggregation responses.[317,319,320]

In α-SPD, platelets and megakaryocytes are selectively deficient in all α-granule proteins, including PF4, βTG, PDGF, vWF, TSP, and fibronectin.[319–321,323] The plasma levels of these proteins are elevated,[319,320] however, suggesting

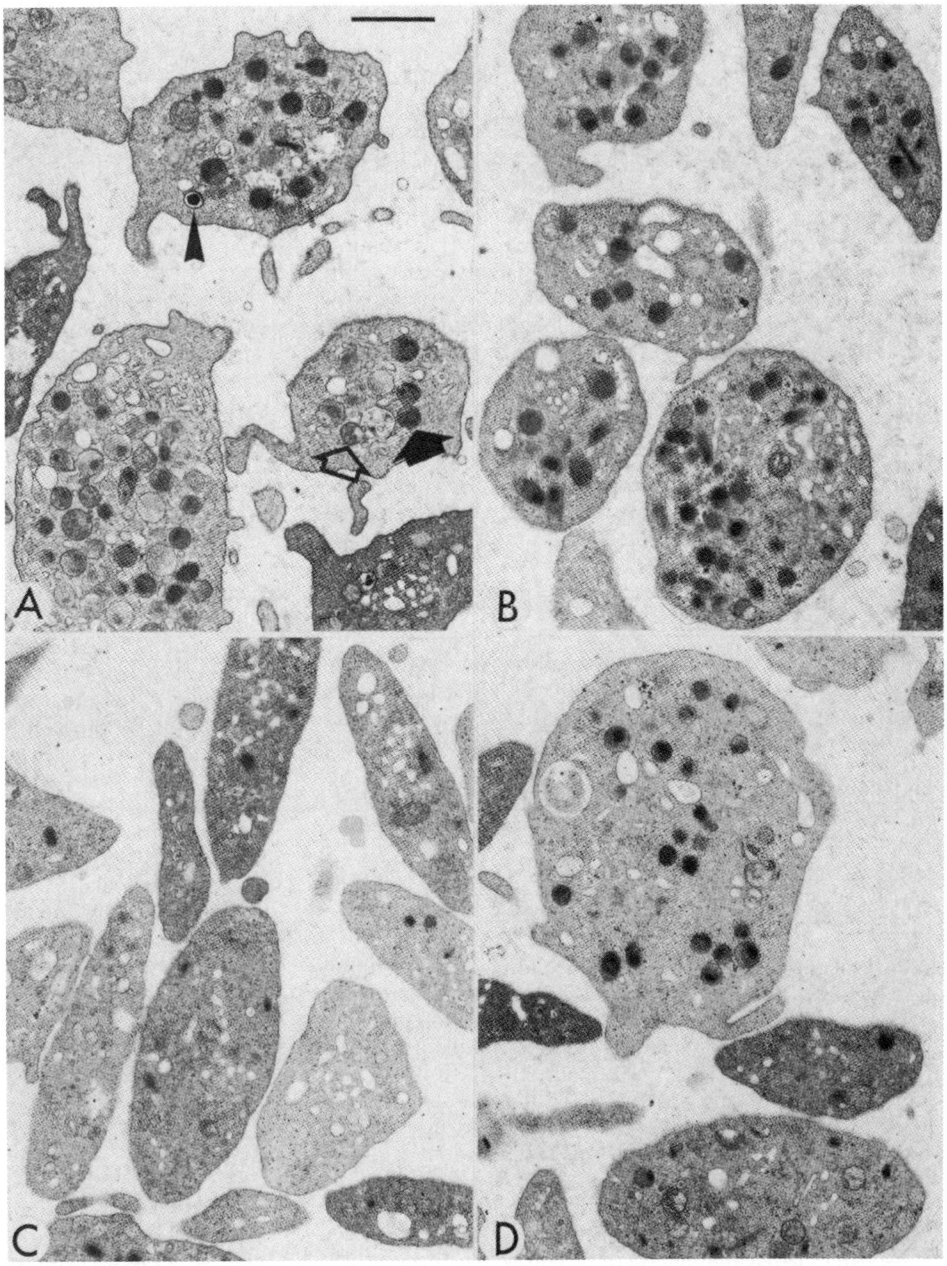

FIGURE 37-7. Electron micrographs of platelets. (**A**) Normal patient. (**B**) Patient with dense-granule deficiency. (**C**) Patient with α-granule deficiency (gray-platelet syndrome) whose platelets had greatly reduced α granules. (**D**) Patient with α-granule deficiency whose platelets had normal numbers of granules. Open arrow, mitochondrion; black arrow, α granule; arrowhead, dense granule. (Weiss HJ, Witte LD, Kaplan KL, et al. Heterogeneity in storage pool deficiency: studies on granule-bound substances in 18 patients including variants deficient in α-granules, platelet factor 4, β-thromboglobulin, and platelet-derived growth factor. Blood 1979;54: 1296)

that the defect in α-SPD may involve a problem of packaging of the proteins into abnormally matured megakaryocyte α granules.[323] The premature discharge of PDGF, along with other α-granule proteins, from the abnormal megakaryocytes into the bone marrow of α-SPD patients may explain the finding of myelofibrosis that has been observed in some of these cases.[320,323]

The cause of bleeding in the gray-platelet syndrome is not clearly understood. Defective release of fibrinogen from the deficient α granules may impair fibrinogen-mediated cell contact during the process of aggregation, and the deficiency of other α-granule proteins (vWF, TSP, fibronectin) may interfere with normal platelet adhesion and cohesion of the platelet aggregate. Platelets from patients with the gray-platelet syndrome are also probably deficient in coagulation factor V stored in α granules. This may contribute to impaired thrombin generation and fibrin formation, possibly causing the clinical bleeding complications that suggest a coagulation factor abnormality rather than a platelet disorder, as noted previously.[224]

Acquired Storage-Pool Deficiency

A variety of clinical disorders have been associated with acquired SPD. Immune thrombocytopenias, both of the idiopathic type and secondary to collagen vascular disease, are sometimes complicated by the coexisting qualitative platelet abnormality of SPD.[324,325] This functional platelet defect may be corrected by treatment with corticosteroids.[324] Platelets can degranulate during the passage of blood across abnormal vascular surfaces, leading to the circulation of spent or "exhausted" platelets and producing a picture of acquired SPD. This may be the mechanism in cases of SPD associated with thrombotic thrombocytopenic purpura, hemolytic–uremic syndrome, renal transplant rejection,[326] disseminated intravascular coagulation,[327] and multiple congenital cavernous hemangiomas.[328] Acquired SPD has been identified as one of many possible functional disorders of platelets in patients with myeloproliferative disorders (vide infra). Release of both α- and dense-granule contents during the storage of platelets for more than 72 hours has also been shown to lead to an acquired storage-pool deficit in banked platelet concentrates.[329]

A number of hemostatic abnormalities contribute to the bleeding complications observed in some patients during open heart surgery and cardiopulmonary bypass. These include decreased levels of coagulation factors, heparin anticoagulation with inadequate reversal, increased fibrinolytic activity, and thrombocytopenia. In addition, a characteristic platelet abnormality of cardiopulmonary bypass is an acquired and transient form of the gray-platelet syndrome.[330] α-Granule proteins are selectively discharged during the passage of platelets through the extracorporeal circuit, leaving recirculating platelets depleted of their α granules. The degree of platelet function impairment correlates with the duration of cardiopulmonary bypass as well as with the level of hypothermia and other factors.[330] In general, the platelet abnormality is rapidly reversible after termination of the bypass, although persistent clinical hemorrhage and prolongation of the bleeding time in occasional patients may indicate additional defects of platelet function, such as abnormal membrane binding of fibrinogen and vWF.[331,332]

Functional Release (Secretion) Defects

Patients with primary defects in platelet release (or secretion) exhibit clinical and laboratory manifestations, including platelet aggregation abnormalities, that are similar to those of δ-SPD. In contrast to SPD, however, platelet storage organelles are intact, and the platelets contain normal levels of all granule constituents. The cause of the functional release defect in these cases is most commonly impaired platelet TXA_2 formation.

Drug- and Diet-Induced Inhibition of Platelet Cyclooxygenase Activity

Aspirin (acetylsalicylic acid) blocks platelet TXA_2 production by inactivating cyclooxygenase. This enzyme normally converts free arachidonic acid mobilized from membrane phospholipids to prostaglandin endoperoxides (PGG_2 and PGH_2), which then serve as substrates for thromboxane synthase in the formation of TXA_2. After the absorption of aspirin from the gastrointestinal tract, the drug is hydrolyzed to liberate free acetyl groups that covalently bind to various proteins, including the cyclooxygenase enzyme. The covalent acetylation of cyclooxygenase irreversibly inhibits the enzyme and accounts for the antiplatelet effects of aspirin.[333] Since platelets cannot synthesize new enzyme, this effect lasts for the lifetime of the platelet. Within 12 hours of the ingestion of 325 mg (1 tablet) of aspirin, the bleeding times of normal subjects become prolonged to about twice baseline values and then return to normal after 24 to 48 hours. The correction of the bleeding time within 2 days reflects the release into the circulation of a sufficiently large cohort of newly formed and unaffected platelets to permit restoration of this laboratory test of primary hemostasis. The typical platelet aggregation abnormalities caused by aspirin (absent arachidonate and blunted collagen responses and loss of second-wave aggregation with ADP and epinephrine) persist for 4 to 7 days after a single oral dose.[334]

The consumption of alcohol, which by itself does not significantly affect the bleeding time, potentiates the aspirin-induced prolongation of the bleeding time.[335] In occasional patients, the use of aspirin results in an exaggerated prolongation of the bleeding time. This finding has been considered to occur in patients with underlying mild functional platelet disorders or von Willebrand's disease in whom aspirin presumably unmasks a subclinical hemostatic defect.[336]

The inhibitory effect of aspirin on vascular cyclooxygenase, which is required for PGI_2 production, would tend to offset its antiplatelet effect in blocking platelet cyclooxygenase and TXA_2 production, thus creating an "aspirin dilemma." This has prompted attempts to find a low, platelet-selective dose of aspirin that spares vascular endothelial cyclooxygenase.[337] A single low dose of aspirin (40 to 80 mg) can inhibit platelet aggregation and block TXA_2 production while largely sparing endothelial PGI_2 synthetic capacity.[338] The issue of differences in sensitivity of platelet and vascular cyclooxygenase to aspirin remains unsettled.[339–342]

Nonsteroidal antiinflammatory drugs, such as indomethacin, phenylbutazone, meclofenamic acid, ibuprofen, and sulindac, interfere with platelet function at the same metabolic site as aspirin.[343–345] These drugs, however, are reversible rather than irreversible inhibitors of cyclooxygenase, and therefore their antiplatelet actions are terminated with the clearance of the drugs from the circulation, generally within 6 hours.

ω-3 Polyunsaturated fatty acids, primarily eicosapentaenoic acid (EPA) and docosahexaenoic acid, contained in cold-water fish or in medicinal supplements, may protect against atherosclerotic cardiovascular disease through a number of possible mechanisms.[346–351] The antithrombotic alterations in platelet–vascular interactions promoted by these fish oils are due, at least in part, to competition between EPA and arachidonic acid for cyclooxygenase (Fig. 37-8). In contrast to arachidonic acid–derived TXA_2, EPA-derived TXA_3 produced by platelets has no platelet-activating or vasoconstrictor properties. EPA-derived PGI_3 produced by vascular cells has the same platelet inhibitory and vasodilatory properties as arachidonic acid–derived PGI_2.[352–356] Thus, diets rich in ω-3 fatty acids or large doses of medicinal fish oil supplements have the net effect of favorably shifting the balance of these platelet and vascular eicosanoids to produce an antithrombotic effect. Ingestion of ω-3 fatty acids, therefore, may cause a clinical bleeding diathesis, with prolongation of the bleeding time, aspirin-like platelet aggregation abnormalities, and impaired platelet adhesion,[357] although these manifestations depend on a number of factors, including the dose and bioavailability of the fish oils.

Other Defects of Platelet Thromboxane A_2 Production

A number of patients have been described with an apparently congenital deficiency of platelet cyclooxygenase.[358–364] Platelet functional abnormalities mimic those of normal subjects after aspirin ingestion, including failure of platelets to aggregate and produce TXA_2 after the addition of arachidonic acid, while retaining a normal response to exogenously added endoperoxides (which bypass the cyclooxygenase reaction). In one case, vascular cyclooxygenase was also deficient, resulting in impaired synthesis of PGI_2 as well as platelet TXA_2.[360] The net clinical consequence of cyclooxygenase deficiency in most of the reported cases has been a mild bleeding tendency, although one patient had thrombotic and vascular complications.[361] In two studies, immunoreactive platelet cyclooxygenase protein was normal, suggesting the presence of a functionally abnormal enzyme.[362,364]

Some patients with platelet-release defects have impaired TXA_2 production due to a defect in the mobilization of endogenous free arachidonic acid from membrane phospholipid pools,[302,365] although a specific biochemical abnormality in phospholipase activity has not been identified. Congenital deficiency of thromboxane synthase, the enzyme that converts endoperoxides to TXA_2, has also been described in patients with a bleeding tendency.[366,367] Patients with defects in the platelet response to TXA_2 were described previously.

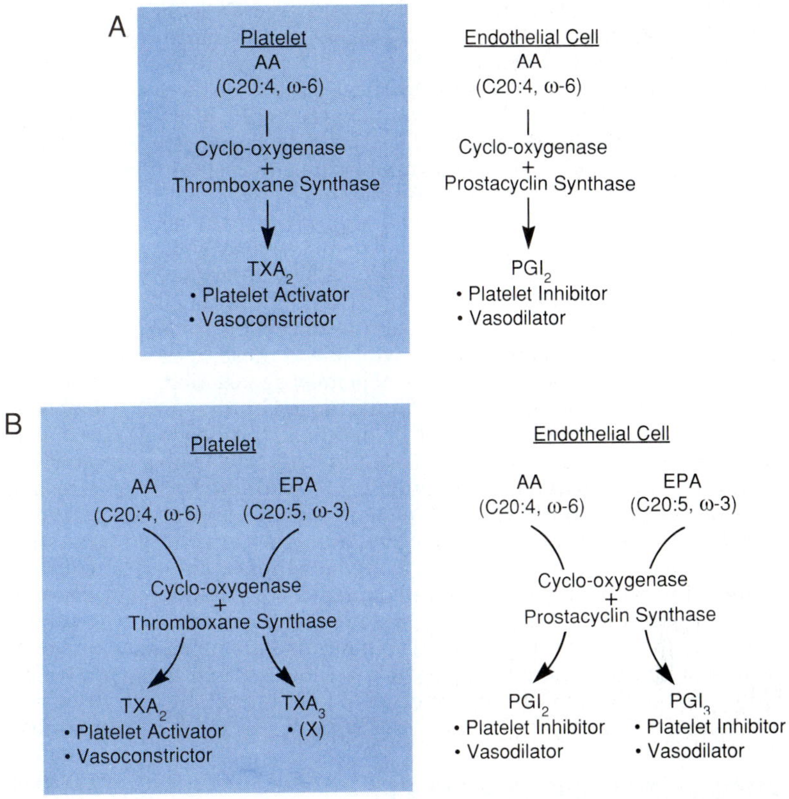

FIGURE 37-8. Effects of ω-3 fatty acids on platelet–vessel wall interactions. (**A**) The predominant substrate for cyclooxygenase in platelets and vascular endothelial cells of subjects ingesting a western diet is arachidonic acid (AA), an ω-6 fatty acid. AA oxygenation in platelets leads to the formation of the potent platelet aggregator and vasoconstrictor TXA_2; the biologic actions of platelet TXA_2 tend to be offset by the production of the platelet inhibitor and vasodilator PGI_2 by oxygenation of AA in endothelial cells. (**B**) In subjects ingesting an Eskimo diet, or in those supplementing their diets with medicinal fish oil, eicosapentaenoic acid (EPA), an ω-3 fatty acid, competes with AA for cyclooxygenase in both platelets and endothelial cells. In platelets, EPA is converted to the biologically inactive TXA_3; in endothelial cells, it is converted to PGI_3, which retains the antithrombotic properties of PGI_2.

Unclassified Disorders of Platelet Secretion

The disorders of platelet secretion discussed previously can usually be attributed to either SPD or impaired TXA_2 synthesis. Some patients, however, have a mild bleeding diathesis caused by secretion defects, but their platelets have normal granule stores and generate TXA_2 normally in response to stimuli. These unclassified disorders of platelet secretion may actually constitute a large fraction of patients with congenital functional release defects.[285] Some of these patients have been postulated to have an abnormality in the translocation or response to intracellular calcium after exposure of the platelets to various activators.

Some patients with attention deficit disorder, a behavioral disorder, have easy bruising and impaired platelet aggregability and dense-granule secretion, particularly in response to the calcium ionophore A23187 and thrombin.[285,368] An abnormality in calcium mobilization has been considered to be the mechanism of platelet dysfunction in a number of other cases.[280,369–370] In another patient whose platelets exhibited a normal rise in cytosolic Ca^{2+} after platelet activation, a defect in calcium-mediated intracellular processes (eg, myosin phosphorylation) was considered to be the mechanism of the disorder of platelet secretion.[282] The specific site of the abnormality in platelet signal–response coupling has not been clearly defined in any of these studies.

DISORDERS OF PLATELET AGGREGATION

Glanzmann's Thrombasthenia

Glanzmann's thrombasthenia (see Chap. 32) is a rare, autosomal recessive disorder[371] that causes serious platelet-type bleeding complications clinically indistinguishable from those of the Bernard-Soulier syndrome,[224] even though the defect in platelet function involves an abnormality in aggregation rather than adhesion. In contrast to the Bernard-Soulier syndrome, platelet count and morphology are normal in thrombasthenia. Heterozygous patients have a normal bleeding time, no abnormalities in platelet function, and usually no significant clinical bleeding problems.[372,373]

The platelets of homozygous patients undergo normal adhesion to vascular subendothelium[374] and secrete[375] and synthesize TXA_2[376] normally in response to all agonists. The external surface of the platelets, however, is not transformed to the state required for aggregation. Therefore, although platelets undergo normal shape change,[377] their ability to aggregate in response to any physiologic agonist is completely lost, leading to absence of even first-wave aggregation (see Fig. 37-6 and Table 37-2).

Fibrinogen is required for normal platelet aggregation. Although thrombasthenic platelets bind physiologic agonists such as ADP[378] and thrombin[379] normally, their activated surfaces are unable to bind fibrinogen, which is necessary for platelet–platelet interaction.[380,381] The molecular basis of this platelet disorder has been demonstrated to be the loss of membrane gpIIb and gpIIIa,[382,383] the heterodimeric complex of which serves as the platelet fibrinogen receptor on the activated platelet surface. In some variants of thrombasthenia, apparently normal amounts of platelet membrane gpIIb and gpIIIa are qualitatively defective for normal fibrinogen binding, leading to the characteristic clinical and platelet function abnormalities of thrombasthenia.[374,384] Thus, it appears that, as in the Bernard-Soulier syndrome, heterogeneous molecular defects produce the phenotypic manifestations of thrombasthenia.[385]

Afibrinogenemia

As von Willebrand's disease is the defective extracellular plasma protein counterpart of the Bernard-Soulier syndrome in disorders of platelet adhesion, so afibrinogenemia would be expected to be the counterpart of Glanzmann's thrombasthenia in disorders of platelet aggregation. Patients with the rare disorder of autosomal recessive afibrinogenemia have a clinical bleeding diathesis of both platelet-type cutaneous and mucosal hemorrhage as well as deep muscle hematomas and hemarthroses characteristic of coagulation factor deficiencies.[386] In these patients, fibrinogen levels in plasma and in platelet α granules are either absent or extremely low,[386,387] and the bleeding time is characteristically prolonged. Although platelet aggregation patterns in afibrinogenemia would be expected to mirror the severe abnormalities of thrombasthenia, in fact, ADP-induced aggregation is only mildly abnormal, and thrombin-induced aggregation is normal.[386,387] It is possible that even trace amounts of fibrinogen that may be available in these cases are sufficient to support some degree of platelet aggregation. The normal dissociation constant for fibrinogen binding to platelets still permits about half of maximal fibrinogen binding even at the very low plasma fibrinogen concentrations of these patients, thus providing an explanation for the relatively mild defects in platelet function in this disease.[389] Alternatively, adhesive proteins other than fibrinogen (eg, vWF) may substitute to mediate the platelet–platelet interactions, particularly under conditions of high shear stress in the circulation.[110] Mutant fibrinogen molecules in patients with dysfibrinogenemias may be defective in supporting platelet aggregation as does normal fibrinogen, but the clinical consequences of this abnormality are unclear.[390]

DISORDERS OF PLATELET PROCOAGULANT ACTIVITY

Although a number of patients have been described with a defect in platelet-surface procoagulant activity, many of these patients have had other abnormalities of platelet function.[285] In the patients studied with an isolated deficiency of procoagulant activity (*platelet factor 3 deficiency*, according to older nomenclature), bleeding times, platelet aggregation, and secretion studies have been generally normal.[391–393] The specific biochemical defect in one case is the decreased binding of factor Xa to the activated platelet surface due to a deficiency in platelet factor Va–binding sites.[394] This abnormality leads to defective assembly of the prothrombinase complex on activated platelet surfaces. Further studies in this case have also demonstrated an impaired ability of the platelets to promote the activation of factor X and prothrombin associated with decreased exposure of phospholipids at the outer surface of the activated platelets.[395]

OTHER ACQUIRED DISORDERS OF PLATELET FUNCTION

Uremia

Bleeding of varying degrees of severity frequently occur in patients with either acute or chronic renal failure.[396] Mucocutaneous sites of hemorrhage are most characteristic, including ecchymoses, purpura, epistaxis, and gingival and gastrointestinal bleeding. Gastrointestinal bleeding is usually associated with ulceration[397] or telangiectasia.[398] It occurs in 10% to 40% of patients with acute renal failure and represents the leading cause of death in this group.[399] Remuzzi[400] reviewed the more unusual clinical bleeding manifestations of uremia. Retroperitoneal bleeding, manifested by abdominal, flank, or back pain and abdominal distention, may develop spontaneously in various types of renal disease[401–404] or may occur as a complication of percutaneous femoral catheterization for hemodialysis.[405] Hemorrhagic pericarditis (sometimes associated with tamponade) and pleural effusion were seen more frequently in the predialysis era.[406,407] Right upper quadrant or epigastric abdominal pain, tenderness over the liver, fever, and progressive anemia may be signs of spontaneous subcapsular hematoma of the liver.[408] Unilateral or bilateral subdural hematomas may occur in uremic patients spontaneously or in association with head trauma, anticoagulation, or hypertension.[409–411]

Despite considerable work to develop tests of primary hemostasis that would be predictive of uremic bleeding, the template bleeding time remains the most reproducible and consistent laboratory abnormality of hemostasis in these patients. Aspirin ingestion causes an exaggerated prolongation of the bleeding time in uremic patients,[412] although the mechanism of action of aspirin in this situation may be unrelated to its inhibition of platelet cyclooxygenase.[413] The results of platelet aggregation studies are highly variable and unpredictable. They range from global defects in response to all agonists to entirely normal or even hyperreactive responses.[414–416] The finding of reduced platelet granule stores of ADP and serotonin has suggested that an acquired SPD (vide supra) may be the basis of uremic bleeding in some cases.[417]

The management of uremic bleeding is more advanced than our understanding of its pathophysiology. The section on treatment of platelet disorders includes more detailed discussion of therapeutic modalities such as cryoprecipitate, desmopressin, conjugated estrogens, and raising of the hematocrit by either red cell transfusions or recombinant erythropoietin. The efficacy of these interventions in many patients with uremic bleeding has provided important leads to elucidating the causes of hemorrhage in renal failure. Because the bleeding diathesis of uremia is characterized by a prolonged bleeding time, without significant thrombocytopenia or coagulation factor abnormalities (typically with a normal prothrombin time and partial thromboplastin time), the pathophysiology most likely involves an impairment of platelet function or platelet–vessel wall interactions.[330,396,400,418,419]

Various uremic toxins, such as urea, phenolic acids, and guanidosuccinic acid, were previously considered to cause the defect in primary hemostasis in renal failure.[419] Attempts, however, to correlate the bleeding time or other platelet function studies with various biochemical parameters of uremia have yielded conflicting results.[420–422] Furthermore, although the prolongation in bleeding time, abnormalities in platelet function, and the clinical bleeding tendency can be fully corrected by peritoneal dialysis and at least partially corrected by hemodialysis,[330,423] such improvements are not always achieved.[419,422] These observations suggest that uremic bleeding is not directly or exclusively caused by dialyzable toxins accumulating in this disorder.[419]

Several lines of investigation have provided promising information about the pathophysiology of uremic bleeding, although no direct causal relations have been clearly established. Studies have focused primarily on abnormalities in three aspects of hemostasis. First, a shift in the balance of production of vascular PGI_2 and platelet TXA_2 has been found to favor an antiplatelet effect in some studies of renal failure. Uremic platelets generate less TXA_2 than normal platelets in response to thrombin or arachidonic acid.[417,424–427] Furthermore, the vessel walls of patients with advanced renal failure[428] and of rats after bilateral nephrectomy[429] produce increased amounts of PGI_2. Uremic plasma has been reported to stimulate increased release of PGI_2 by cultured endothelial cells.[430] The lack of correlation between the bleeding time and vascular PGI_2, however, suggests that this abnormality is unlikely to be the sole determinant of uremic bleeding.[400]

A second area of investigation involves a possible abnormality of vWF. This line of studies has been based largely on the clinical observations of the therapeutic efficacy of cryoprecipitate, desmopressin, and estrogens, agents that also ameliorate the bleeding tendency of von Willebrand's disease. Although one study reported a decrease in ristocetin cofactor activity in uremia,[431] others have consistently shown an actual increase in vWF antigen.[432,433] It was suggested that the high vWF levels in uremic plasma compensate for a relative adhesion defect of unknown cause.[434] Furthermore, the multimeric structure of the vWF molecule[435] and vWF or fibrinogen binding to platelets[436,437] are normal in renal failure. One study[437] reported an absence of the largest multimers of vWF in uremic plasma and a reduction in platelet vWF. Deykin[418] discussed possible explanations for the apparent discrepancy between the lack of any consistently demonstrable and significant structural abnormality of the vWF molecule and the clinical observations that various maneuvers that increase plasma levels of the factor VIII–vWF complex cause shortening of the bleeding time in uremia. These include: (1) lack of sufficiently sensitive assays to detect a defect in vWF multimers; (2) a more critical role of abnormalities in the processing of large multimers released from endothelial cells than the circulating plasma multimer distribution; (3) alterations in other components of the factor VIII–vWF complex; or (4) a nonspecific shortening of the bleeding time produced by raising the concentration of vWF to supernormal levels.[418]

A third potentially important pathophysiologic factor in uremic bleeding is related to the moderately severe anemia that is characteristic of advanced renal failure. This is supported by several clinical observations. There is an inverse correlation between the bleeding time and the hematocrit in uremic patients on dialysis.[438] Treatment of the anemia of renal failure with either red cell transfusions[426,438] or recombinant erythropoietin[439,440] tends to normalize the bleeding time. The role of red cells in hemostasis was noted previously, particularly under the high shear rate flow conditions of the microcirculation.[441] Red cells promote platelet–vessel wall interactions by causing radial diffusion of platelets in flowing blood, thus enhancing platelet collisions with the injured vessel wall.[441,442] The loss of this hemostatic factor in anemic patients with renal failure may contribute to the impairment of primary hemostasis in these patients. In fact, the bleeding time was found to be reversibly prolonged in nonuremic patients with anemia, although to a lesser extent than in uremic patients with anemia.[186]

It is unlikely that any of the abnormalities of hemostasis described previously will provide an exclusive and definitive explanation of the pathophysiology of uremic bleeding. These patients have a complex and multifaceted defect in primary hemostasis for which effective but largely empiric therapeutic modalities are available (vide infra).

Liver Disease

Patients with liver failure have numerous, potentially complex causes for bleeding complications. These include anatomic abnormalities that predispose to gastrointestinal hemorrhage (eg, esophageal varices, gastritis), thrombocytopenia secondary to hypersplenism, and various derangements of the coagulation and fibrinolytic systems that may produce a state of disseminated intravascular coagulation. Disorders of platelet function may also contribute to the bleeding diathesis of liver disease,[443] and prolongation of the bleeding time is not uncommon in these patients.[444,445] As in uremia, platelet aggregation results are highly variable, and no characteristic pattern of abnormalities is found. A possible cause of platelet dysfunction in liver failure is the frequently increased level of fibrin (or fibrinogen) degradation products (FDP) that can theoretically inhibit platelet aggregation,[446,447] although no correlation between platelet aggregation defects and plasma levels of FDP has been found in these patients.[445] Another potential factor in some cases is the presence of an acquired dysfibrinogenemia,[448] which may prevent normal platelet–platelet interactions.

Dysproteinemias

Patients with Waldenström's macroglobulinemia and multiple myeloma are predisposed to serious bleeding complications. The coagulopathy of dysproteinemias is multifactorial, including problems of rheology (hyperviscosity), fibrin polymerization, and thrombocytopenia. Qualitative platelet defects may also be involved, and prolongation of the bleeding time and abnormalities of platelet aggregation, adhesion, and procoagulant activity have been found.[449,450] The mechanism of platelet dysfunction has not been clearly elucidated, but it has been proposed that paraproteins nonspecifically coat the platelet surface and thereby interfere with agonist receptor occupancy. In some cases, the bleeding that occurs in dysproteinemias may be the result of a specific interaction of monoclonal paraproteins with platelets.[451] The ineffectiveness of platelet transfusions in these patients is consistent with either of these models, while treatment of the underlying dysproteinemia by plasmapheresis usually improves the bleeding tendency.[330]

Myeloproliferative Disorders

Bleeding and thrombosis are major causes of morbidity and mortality in patients with chronic myeloproliferative disorders,[452] the group of related diseases of the pluripotent hematopoietic stem cell that includes polycythemia vera (PV), chronic myelogenous leukemia, ET, and myelofibrosis and myeloid metaplasia. Functionally impaired or hyperreactive platelets are thought to play an important role in the hemostatic complications of these patients.

Sites of bleeding in the myeloproliferative disorders reflect a defect in primary hemostasis and involve predominantly mucocutaneous surfaces. Deep-seated hemorrhage (eg, into joints or retroperitoneum) is rare. Thrombotic complications may involve both the arterial and venous systems. Deep vein thrombosis and pulmonary embolism are the most common thrombotic manifestations. Some distinct types of thrombosis, however, are characteristic of the myeloproliferative disorders. Budd-Chiari syndrome (hepatic vein thrombosis) and portal vein thrombosis may develop in the course of or even antedate the clinical diagnosis of a myeloproliferative syndrome, particularly PV.[453–455] Various nonspecific or focal neurologic manifestations may occur as the result of cerebrovascular ischemia; these complications can be caused by increased whole-blood viscosity in patients with uncontrolled PV or by platelet thrombi, particularly in patients with ET.[456] Finally, digital microvascular ischemia may develop, especially in patients with ET, causing severe throbbing, aching, and burning pain in the extremities, sometimes accompanied by pregangrenous or even gangrenous changes in the involved areas. Erythromelalgia,[457] characterized by localized pain, warmth, duskiness, and mottled erythema of the extremities, in association with histologic evidence of arteriolar platelet thrombi and inflammatory changes,[458] is a characteristic syndrome in the myeloproliferative disorders.[459] Bleeding and thrombotic complications occur in a largely unpredictable manner in these patients. Some symptomatic patients may exhibit a pattern of exclusively recurrent bleeding or recurrent thrombosis, while others may have both types of hemostatic problems.

Several factors may be involved in the pathogenesis of bleeding and thrombosis in the myeloproliferative disorders. Increased whole-blood viscosity due to erythrocytosis can contribute to thrombosis in uncontrolled PV. Patients with comparable degrees of erythrocytosis caused by secondary polycythemias are much less prone to thrombosis, and therefore increased blood viscosity is unlikely to be the sole determinant in patients with PV. Considerable controversy surrounds the relation between bleeding and thrombotic complications and thrombocytosis, which may occur not only in ET but also in any of the myeloproliferative disorders. No clear causal association has been established between thrombocytosis, however extreme, and clinical hemostatic problems in these patients.[452]

A variety of qualitative platelet abnormalities have been described in patients with myeloproliferative disorders[452,460] (Fig. 37-9). Abnormalities of platelet morphology are common. Platelets are often hypogranular, imparting a clear blue appearance on routine Wright's stain of the peripheral smear. They may be heterogeneous in size, with giant, bizarre-shaped forms and, occasionally, megakaryocyte fragments circulating in the peripheral blood. The bleeding time is usually normal; when prolonged, it does not correlate with an increased risk of hemorrhage.[461–463] Platelet aggregation studies may reveal highly variable results. In some cases, platelets are hyperaggregable or may even spontaneously aggregate,[464,465] although these findings are not diagnostic of a myeloproliferative syndrome. The most characteristic defect in platelet function, particularly in patients with ET, is the complete loss of both first- and second-wave aggregation with epinephrine, which is associated with a loss of membrane α_2-adrenergic receptors[466] (see Table 37-2). Although the finding of an isolated loss of epinephrine responsiveness is highly suggestive of a myeloproliferative disorder (and can be useful in discriminating ET from secondary thrombocytosis), it is not a diagnostic abnormality (vide supra). Platelet aggregation responses to ADP and collagen are more variable.[452]

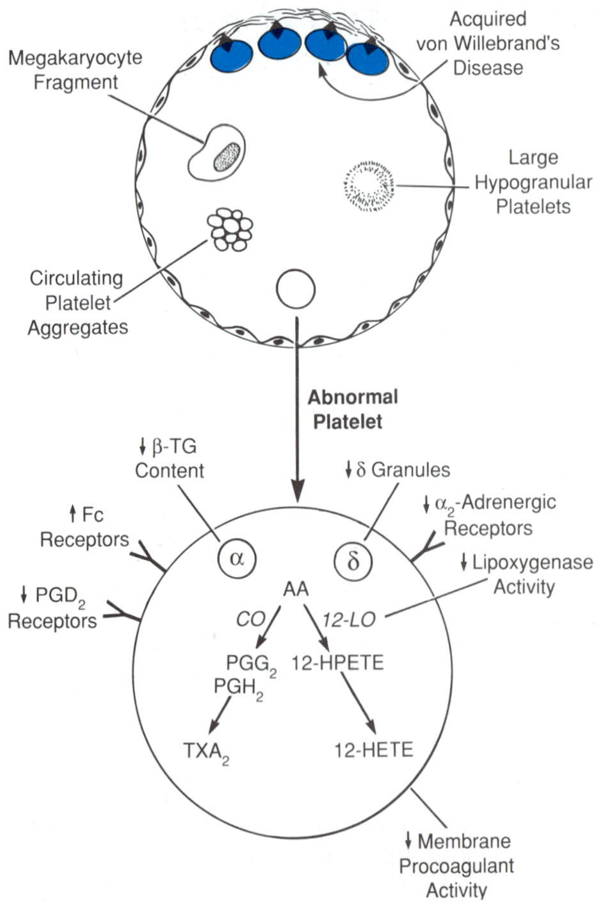

FIGURE 37-9. Morphologic, metabolic, and biochemical abnormalities of platelets that may be found in patients with myeloproliferative disorders. (After Mitus AJ, Schafer AI. Thrombocytosis and thrombocythemia. Hematol Oncol Clin North Am 1990;4:157)

Specific biochemical defects of platelets found in some patients with myeloproliferative disorders are depicted schematically in Figure 37-9. In addition to loss of α_2-adrenergic receptors,[466] a decreased number of prostaglandin D_2 receptors[467] and increased expression of Fc receptors[468] have been noted. Other platelet-surface abnormalities that have been reported are changes in membrane glycoproteins[469] and platelet procoagulant activity.[470] Acquired SPD has been associated with the myeloproliferative syndromes,[471–473] although it is not known if this is intrinsic to the abnormal megakaryocyte clone or if it is acquired by degranulation of platelets in the circulation.[474] Abnormalities of platelet lipoxygenase activity have been described.[475,476] The myeloproliferative disorders have also been associated with acquired von Willebrand's disease,[477] resembling the congenital type II form of this disease with a reduction in the large multimers of the vWF protein and disproportionately reduced levels of ristocetin cofactor activity.[478,479] Abnormal platelets in these disorders have been postulated to adsorb vWF onto their surfaces, resulting in deficiency of the protein in plasma.

Although multiple platelet defects have been described in patients with myeloproliferative syndromes, none of these findings clearly correlates with or predicts clinical patterns of bleeding or thrombosis. The reason for these discrepancies is unclear, but it is possible that multiple defects exist simultaneously in the circulating population of platelets, platelet abnormalities change with the natural history or the treatment of the disease,[480] or disorders of other components of hemostasis are also causally related to clinical complications.

Some special considerations apply to the prevention and treatment of hemostatic complications in the myeloproliferative disorders. While the efficacy of maintaining a normal hematocrit in PV is clearly established, controversy persists regarding the role of lowering the platelet count in asymptomatic patients with thrombocytosis associated with myeloproliferative disorders.[481,482] There is sufficient anecdotal evidence, however, to support reduction of the platelet count in symptomatic patients with thrombocytosis who have recurrent bleeding or thrombosis, particularly those with digital or cerebrovascular ischemia.[452,460] The use of antiplatelet agents such as aspirin in these patients is controversial. The indiscriminate use of aspirin to prevent thrombosis in patients with myeloproliferative disorders cannot be advocated because of its lack of proven efficacy and its potential to increase the predilection to hemorrhage.[483,484] In selected patients with thrombotic complications, however, especially those with digital or cerebrovascular ischemia, the use of aspirin, with or without maneuvers to reduce the platelet count, may offer dramatic clinical benefit.[452]

Drugs

Antiplatelet Agents

A number of drugs are specifically designed to interfere with platelet function for use as antithrombotic agents. A more detailed discussion of the clinical use of these drugs appears elsewhere.

Aspirin and nonsteroidal antiinflammatory drugs inhibit platelet (and vascular) cyclooxygenase, cause prolongations of the bleeding time, and produce platelet aggregation changes that reflect a release defect. ω-3 Fatty acids (fish oils) cause similar antiplatelet effects, at least in part by competing with arachidonic acid for cyclooxygenase. These agents were described in greater detail earlier.

Dipyridamole,[485] unlike aspirin, does not prolong the bleeding time[486] and inhibits platelet aggregation in vitro only at concentrations that are considerably higher than those attained in blood with clinical use.[487,488] Dipyridamole has been found to inhibit platelet adhesion in some studies.[489–492] The in vivo antiplatelet effects of dipyridamole are most clearly demonstrated by the ability of the drug to prolong platelet survival and reduce platelet turnover in various thrombotic and vascular disorders.[493–495] The mechanism of action of dipyridamole is probably multifactorial[485,496] and possibly includes stimulation of PGI_2 production by vascular endothelium,[497–499] potentiation of the platelet inhibitory effects of PGI_2,[500] inhibition of platelet phosphodiesterase to raise platelet levels of cAMP,[501,502] and blockade of the uptake of adenosine into endothelial cells, red cells, and leukocytes to cause local accumulation of this platelet-inhibitory and vasodilating compound in the thrombotic microenvironment.[485,503,504]

Sulfinpyrazone, a uricosuric drug with structural similarity to phenylbutazone,[339,505] acts like dipyridamole (and unlike aspirin) to normalize the increased platelet turnover in various clinical vascular disorders.[506,507] Sulfinpyrazone is an incomplete and reversible inhibitor of platelet cyclooxygenase,[508,509] although this effect is unlikely to account entirely for the antiplatelet actions of the drug. As a cyclooxygenase inhibitor, sulfinpyrazone inhibits ex vivo platelet aggregation and release in response to weak agonists.[510]

Ticlopidine is a thienopyridine derivative with potent antiplatelet effects. It appears to act by blocking fibrinogen binding to the platelet membrane gpIIb–IIIa complex,[511] thus causing a thrombasthenic-like defect with complete inhibition of even first-wave platelet aggregation ex vivo, similar to the effects of agents that elevate platelet cAMP (eg, PGI_2). Ticlopidine and its potent analogue, clopidogrel, have also been found to block ADP receptor–mediated platelet activation.[512,513]

Antimicrobial Agents

Antibiotic-induced platelet dysfunction may cause serious bleeding complications, particularly in the setting of severe systemic illness, renal insufficiency, and coexisting thrombocytopenia. A number of penicillins, including penicillin G,[514–516] carbenicillin,[517,518] ticarcillin,[519] and ampicillin,[514] have been shown to inhibit platelet function and to cause a clinically significant hemorrhagic diathesis when administered in high doses.[517] Some of the newer semisynthetic penicillins like piperacillin have less potent antiplatelet effects.[520] Cephalosporins, such as moxalactam,[521,522] nitrofurantoin,[523] and hydroxychloroquine,[524] can interfere with platelet function.

Antimicrobial agents cause prolongation of the bleeding time, inhibition of platelet aggregation and secretion in response to several agonists, decreased ristocetin-induced platelet agglutination, and impaired platelet adhesion to subendothelial and collagen-coated surfaces.[50,525] Platelet dysfunction is typically noted within hours of starting the offending antibiotic, is maximal after 3 to 4 days of continuous administration, and resolves within days of discontinuation of the drug.[526] The mechanism of the antiplatelet actions of the drugs is not completely understood, but high doses of the penicillins interfere with the binding of different agonists (epinephrine, ADP, vWF) to the platelet surface,[527] thereby presumably blocking the initiation of platelet signal transduction. Other studies of platelet inhibition by these antibiotics suggest an irreversible mechanism involving postreceptor impairment of signal transduction in response to various agonists.[528]

β-Adrenergic Blocking Agents

Propranolol reduces the hyperreactivity of platelets from patients with coronary artery disease, raising the abnormally low thresholds for aggregation induced by different agonists to normal.[529] Propranolol is only a weak direct inhibitor of platelet function, however, and not all subjects taking the drug have impaired in vitro platelet function.[530] It inhibits second-wave aggregation in response to ADP and epinephrine only at relatively high concentrations in vitro.[531] The mechanism of the antiplatelet effects of propranolol is not clear. It is unlikely to act through its β-blocking effects since platelets do not have β-adrenergic receptors, its actions are not stereospecific, and nonlipophilic β-adrenergic blocking agents do not exert these effects on platelet function.[531] Propranolol probably binds to platelet membrane phospholipids[532] and may interfere with the phospholipase A_2–mediated release of free arachidonic acid from phospholipid pools.[533,534]

Miscellaneous Agents

Dextrans cause prolongation of the bleeding time and inhibition of platelet aggregation within hours after initiating an intravenous infusion.[535,536] The mechanism of antiplatelet action of dextrans is not clearly understood, although these polysaccharides adsorb to platelets and possibly cause in vivo platelet activation, resulting in the circulation of spent platelets that are refractory to subsequent stimulation.[537]

In addition to the idiosyncratic, immune-mediated severe thrombocytopenia associated with the use of heparin in some patients, heparin also has direct actions on platelet function. The higher-molecular-weight, nonanticoagulant fractions of commercial heparin preparation may cause in vivo platelet activation, resulting in impaired in vitro platelet responsiveness due to the induced refractory state.[538,539]

Local and general anesthetics may inhibit platelet responses in vitro by acting as membrane-stabilizing agents, and general anesthesia with halothane has been associated with prolongation of the bleeding time.[540] Likewise, tricyclic antidepressants (eg, imipramine, amitriptyline) and phenothiazines (eg, chlorpromazine, trifluoperazine) may exert membrane-stabilizing actions to interfere with platelet function in vitro, although the effect of these drugs on clinical hemostasis is questionable.[541–543]

The antifibrinolytic agent, epsilon-aminocaproic acid (EACA), causes prolongation of the bleeding time when administered at a dose of 24 g/d or more. The effect on the bleeding time correlates with the duration of EACA therapy and returns to normal within 72 hours of discontinuation of the drug.[544] The in vitro actions of EACA on inhibition of ADP and collagen-induced platelet aggregation and secretion and impairment of fibrinogen binding are not observed in platelets isolated from patients receiving the drug, suggesting that its in vivo effects are exerted on platelet–vascular interactions.[544]

Alcohol,[545] the consumption of which potentiates aspirin-induced prolongation of the bleeding time, and dietary constituents such as onion,[546,547] garlic,[548] black tree fungus

(Szechwan purpura),[549] and vitamin E[550] have been reported to cause inhibition of platelet function in vitro, but the clinical significance of these observations has not been established.

TREATMENT OF DISORDERS OF PLATELET FUNCTION

Platelet Transfusions

In principle, platelet transfusions[551] should correct the hemostatic defect of patients with intrinsic abnormalities of platelet function (Table 37-3); however, surprisingly little systematic information is available regarding their utility in these disorders.[552] In Glanzmann's thrombasthenia[553–555] and in the Bernard-Soulier syndrome,[556,557] the development of antibodies against the deficient platelet membrane glycoprotein may, in some cases, mitigate the efficacy of the transfusion of normal platelets. Anecdotal evidence supports the utility of platelet transfusions in platelet storage-pool disease.[558–560] In view of the risk of alloimmunization and transmission of blood-borne viral infections from platelet transfusions, however, alternate therapeutic or prophylactic treatments (vide infra) should be considered in patients with less serious disorders of platelet function.

Corticosteroids

A short course of prednisone (20 to 60 mg/d) can correct the prolonged bleeding time of some patients with qualitative platelet disorders[561,562] (see Table 37-3). In one study of 14 preoperative patients with platelet aspirin-like release defects,[562] the prolonged bleeding times corrected after 3 days of prednisone therapy in all cases, and none of the patients suffered postoperative bleeding complications. Despite these effects on the bleeding time, corticosteroids do not reverse the abnormal platelet aggregation pattern.[561,562] The mechanism of action in these cases may involve nonspecific vasoactive effects that provide short-term improvement in microvascular integrity. Not all patients with disorders of platelet function predictably respond to prednisone in this manner, however, and this treatment has been found to be ineffective in normalizing the bleeding time in Glanzmann's thrombasthenia[563] or in normal subjects after aspirin ingestion.[564]

Cryoprecipitate

Cryoprecipitate is effective in some patients with uremic bleeding. In the original study, Janson and colleagues[565] infused 10 bags of cryoprecipitate into each of 6 patients with renal failure and found shortening or complete correction of the prolonged bleeding times in all cases within 1 to 12 hours, returning to pretreatment levels after 24 to 36 hours. Cryoprecipitate controlled major bleeding complications and permitted major surgical or invasive procedures to be performed with effective hemostasis. Since platelet aggregation abnormalities persisted despite correction of the bleeding time and the patients did not initially exhibit abnormalities of plasma vWF, the mechanism of action of cryoprecipitate in this clinical setting is unclear. The efficacy of cryoprecipitate in uremia has been confirmed by some[566] but not other[567] studies.

Cryoprecipitate infusion also shortens the bleeding time in patients with platelet SPD, permitting uncomplicated surgery with a prophylactic, twice-daily infusion regimen.[568] There is preliminary evidence for the efficacy of cryoprecipitate in some patients with an abnormal bleeding time associated with liver disease.[569]

Desmopressin

Desmopressin (1-desamino-8-D-arginine vasopressin) is a synthetic analogue of the antidiuretic hormone, which has little or no effect on vascular, uterine, or gastrointestinal smooth muscle.[570] The hemostatic effect of desmopressin was originally noted in patients with von Willebrand's disease and mild to moderate hemophilia in whom, as in healthy subjects, infusion of the drug increases plasma factor VIII and vWF concentrations.[571–573] Prophylactic intravenous infusion of desmopressin in patients with these disorders has permitted the performance of uncomplicated surgical procedures without the need to transfuse blood products.[573–576]

Desmopressin has also been found to be effective in patients with other defects in primary hemostasis, including uremia, various qualitative platelet abnormalities, and cirrhosis.[570] Desmopressin infusion shortens or normalizes the bleeding time in most patients with renal failure.[577,578] Peak improvement in the bleeding time typically occurs within 1 to 4 hours of administration and terminates after 8 hours. Desmopressin prevents postoperative bleeding and arrests spontaneous hemorrhage in some patients with ure-

TABLE 37-3. Treatment of Disorders of Platelet Function

Treatment	Disorders Where Effective
Platelet transfusions	Most disorders of platelet function; possibly development of antibodies against abnormal membrane protein in Bernard-Soulier syndrome and thrombasthenia
Corticosteroids (prednisone, 20–60 mg/d)	Shortens bleeding time in aspirin-like release defects; not effective in thrombasthenia or normal subjects taking aspirin
Cryoprecipitate	Shortens bleeding time in von Willebrand's disease, storage-pool deficiency, liver disease
Desmopressin (DDAVP, 0.3–0.4 μg/kg IV q 12–24 h)	Shortens bleeding time in von Willebrand's disease, uremia, liver disease, most disorders of platelet function (including normal subjects taking aspirin); may reduce operative blood loss in scoliosis and heart surgery
Conjugated estrogens	Shortens bleeding time in uremia
Red cell transfusions or recombinant erythropoietin	Shortens bleeding time in uremia

mia.[579,580] Patients with a prolonged bleeding time due to various acquired or congenital functional platelet disorders like SPD, as well as healthy subjects who have ingested aspirin, respond to desmopressin with significant shortening of the bleeding time, usually without any improvement in the intrinsic platelet dysfunction.[581–585] Desmopressin has also been reported to be effective in correcting the prolonged bleeding time associated with hepatic cirrhosis,[582,586] but its ability to reduce the risk of bleeding in this complex coagulopathy remains to be established. Finally, desmopressin has been found to reduce postoperative blood loss in patients who have apparently normal preoperative hemostasis, including scoliosis patients undergoing spinal fusion[587] and patients having heart surgery using cardiopulmonary bypass.[588–590] Reports have failed to confirm the efficacy of desmopressin in reducing blood loss or transfusion requirements with coronary artery bypass surgery.[591–593]

The mechanism of action of desmopressin in improving hemostasis in patients with von Willebrand's disease primarily involves its ability to transiently raise plasma levels of vWF, presumably by inducing its release from vascular endothelial storage sites. Reasons for its efficacy in other disorders of primary hemostasis and in reducing surgical blood loss in patients who are hemostatically normal before surgery are unclear.

Desmopressin is usually administered by intravenous infusion at a dose of 0.3 to 0.4 μg/kg. The infusion can be repeated at intervals of 12 to 24 hours, depending on the risk of bleeding and the clinical response in the individual patient. Subcutaneous desmopressin was shown to be as effective as the intravenous regimen at the same dose, and it is more practical for self-administration.[594,595] Intranasal desmopressin may prove to be the most practical route of self-administration in emergencies, but current preparations require more than 10 times the recommended intravenous or subcutaneous dose to achieve an equivalent hemostatic effect.[596,597]

In general, desmopressin has no serious adverse effects.[570] An important limitation of its usefulness is the rapid development of tachyphylaxis in some patients.[573,598,599] Although this does not always occur, when it does occur, an effective response can usually be reestablished after 3 to 4 days.[570,600] Transient flushing, headache, and a slight increase in heart rate and blood pressure can be avoided by slowing the rate of infusion, and severe water retention with hyponatremia is rare.[601,602] Isolated cases of acute myocardial infarction and stroke have been reported in patients receiving desmopressin,[603,604] and although a causal association cannot be proved, it has been recommended that the drug be administered with caution to elderly patients with severe underlying vascular disease.

Other Therapeutic Modalities for Uremic Bleeding

A randomized, double-blind, cross-over trial comparing the effect of conjugated estrogens with that of placebo in patients with uremic bleeding has been reported.[605] Patients received a conjugated estrogen preparation at a dose of 0.6 mg/kg/d by intravenous infusion for 5 consecutive days, and the bleeding times shortened in all subjects. The effect was detectable 6 hours after the first infusion, reached its maximum between days 5 and 7, and lasted for 14 days. The mechanism of action of estrogens is not clear since plasma levels of vWF and platelet dysfunction were unchanged despite improvement in the bleeding times. This treatment, however, may offer a more sustained effect than desmopressin or cryoprecipitate in renal failure.

As noted previously, there is an inverse correlation between the hematocrit and the bleeding time in uremic patients.[438] Transfusion of red cells into patients with renal failure can shorten the bleeding time and reduce clinical bleeding.[426,438] The progressive rise in hematocrit that occurs in response to the administration of recombinant human erythropoietin was found to be paralleled by a pronounced shortening of the bleeding time[439,440] in uremic patients.

REFERENCES

1. Newman PJ, Gorski J, White GC, et al. Enzymatic amplification of platelet-specific messenger RNA using the polymerase chain reaction. J Clin Invest 1988;82:739.
2. Kieffer N, Guichard J, Farcet J-P, et al. Biosynthesis of major platelet proteins in human platelets. Eur J Biochem 1987;164:189.
3. Hovig T. The ultrastructure of blood platelets in normal and abnormal states. Series Haematol 1968;1:3.
4. Karpatkin S. Heterogeneity of human platelets. I. Metabolic and kinetic evidence suggestive of young and old platelets. J Clin Invest 1969;47:1073.
5. Thompson CB, Jakubowski JA. The pathophysiology and clinical relevance of platelet heterogeneity. Blood 1988;72:1.
6. O'Brien JR, Jamieson S. A relationship between platelet volume and platelet number. Thromb Diath Haemorrh 1974;31:363.
7. Levin J, Bessman JD. The inverse relationship between platelet volume and platelet number: abnormalities in hematologic disease and evidence that platelet size does not correlate with platelet age. J Lab Clin Med 1983;101:295.
8. Frojmovic MM, Milton JG. Human platelets size, shape, and related functions in health and disease. Physiol Rev 1982;62:185.
9. Corash L, Costa JL, Shafer B, et al. Heterogeneity of human whole blood platelet subpopulations. III. Density-dependent differences in subcellular constituents. Blood 1984;64:185.
10. Corash L. Platelet density heterogeneity. Blood 1985;65:779.
11. White JG. The ultrastructure and regulatory mechanisms of blood platelets. In: Lasslo A, ed. Blood platelet function and medicinal chemistry. New York, Elsevier Science Publishing, 1984:15.
12. White JG. Platelet morphology. In: Johnson SA, ed. The circulating platelet. New York, Academic Press, 1971:45.
13. George JN, Nurden AT, Phillips DR. Molecular defects in interactions of platelets with the vessel wall. N Engl J Med 1984;311:1084.
14. Nurden AT, George JN, Phillips DR. Platelet membrane glycoproteins: their structure, function, and modification in disease. In: Phillips DR, Shuman MA, eds. Biochemistry of platelets. Orlando, Academic Press, 1986:160.
15. Shick PK, Kurica KB, Chacko GK. Localization of phosphatidylethanolamine and phosphatidylserine in human platelet plasma membrane. J Clin Invest 1976;57:1221.
16. Horne WC, Norman NE, Schwartz DB, Simons ER. Changes in cytoplasmic pH and in membrane potential in thrombin stimulated platelets. Eur J Biochem 1981;120:295.
17. Marcus AJ, Zucker-Franklin D. Studies on subcellular platelet particles. Blood 1964;23:389.
18. Miletich JP, Jackson CM, Majerus PW. Properties of the factor Xa binding site on human platelets. J Biol Chem 1978;253:6908.
19. Kenney DM, Linck RW. The cytoskeleton of unstimulated blood platelets: structure and composition of the isolated marginal microtubular band. J Cell Sci 1985;78:1.
20. White JG. Fine structural alterations induced in platelets by adenosine diphosphate. Blood 1968;31:604.
21. Fox JEB. Platelet contractile proteins. In: Phillips DR, Shuman MA, eds. Biochemistry of platelets. Orlando, Academic Press, 1986:115.
22. Gordon DJ, Boyer JL, Korn ED. Comparative biochemistry of non-muscle actins. J Biol Chem 1977;252:8300.
23. Landon F, Huc C, Thomé F, et al. Human platelet actin: evidence of β and γ forms and similarity of properties with sarcomeric actin. Eur J Biochem 1977;81:571.
24. Rosenberg S, Stracher A, Lucas RC. Isolation and characterization of actin and actin-binding protein from human platelets. J Cell Biol 1981;91:201.
25. Fox JEB, Phillips DR. Inhibition of actin polymerization in blood platelets by cytochalasins. Nature (London) 1981;292:650.
26. Jennings LK, Fox JEB, Edwards HH, Phillips DR. Changes in the cytoskeletal structure of human platelets following thrombin activation. J Biol Chem 1981;256:6927.
27. Feinstein MB. Release of intracellular membrane-bound calcium precedes the onset of stimulus-induced exocytosis in platelets. Biochem Biophys Res Commun 1980;93:593.
28. Rink TJ, Smith SW, Tsien RY. Cytoplasmic free Ca^{2+} in human platelets: Ca^{2+} thresholds and Ca-independent activation for shape-change and secretion. FEBS Lett 1982;148:21.

29. Adelstein RS, Conti MA. The characterization of contractile proteins from platelets and fibroblasts. Cold Spring Harbor Symp Quant Biol 1972;37:599.
30. Pollard TD, Thomas SM, Niederman R. Human platelet myosin. I. Purification by a rapid method applicable to other nonmuscle cells. Anal Biochem 1974;60:258.
31. Adelstein RS, Pollard TD, Kuehl WM. Isolation and characterization of myosin and two myosin fragments from human blood platelets. Proc Natl Acad Sci USA 1971;68:2703.
32. Dabrowska R, Hartshorne DJ. A Ca^{2+}-and modulator-dependent myosin light chain kinase from non-muscle cells. Biochem Biophys Res Commun 1978;85:1352.
33. Hathaway DR, Adelstein RS. Human platelet myosin light chain kinase requires the calcium-binding protein calmodulin for activity. Proc Natl Acad Sci USA 1979;76:1653.
34. Hartwig JH, Stossel TP. Isolation and properties of actin, myosin, and a new actin-binding protein in rabbit alveolar macrophages. J Biol Chem 1975;250:5696.
35. Hartwig JH, Stossel TP. Structure of macrophage actin-binding protein molecules in solution and interacting with actin filaments. J Mol Biol 1981;145:563.
36. Fox JEB, Goll DE, Reynolds CC, Phillips DR. Identification of two proteins (actin-binding protein and P235) that are hydrolyzed by endogenous Ca^{2+}-dependent protease during platelet aggregation. J Biol Chem 1985;260:1060.
37. Fox JEB. Identification of actin binding protein as the protein linking the membrane skeleton to glycoproteins on platelet plasma membranes. J Biol Chem 1985;260:11970.
38. Fox JEB. Linkage of a membrane skeleton to integral membrane glycoproteins in human platelets: identification of one of the glycoproteins as glycoprotein Ib. J Clin Invest 1985;76:1673.
39. Ezzell RM, Kenney DM, Egan S, et al. Localization of the domain of actin-binding protein that binds to membrane glycoprotein Ib and actin in human platelets. J Biol Chem 1988;263:13303.
40. Fox JEB, Boyles JK. The membrane skeleton: a distinct structure that regulates the function of cells. BioEssays 1988;8:14.
41. Truglia JA, Stracher A. Purification and characterization of a calcium-dependent sulfhydryl protease from human platelets. Biochem Biophys Res Commun 1981;100:814.
42. Davies PJA, Wallach D, Willingham MC, et al. Filamin-actin interaction: dissociation of binding from gelation by Ca^{2+}-activated proteolysis. J Biol Chem 1978;253:4036.
43. Cohen I, Gerrard JM, White JG. Ultrastructure of clots during isometric contraction. J Cell Biol 1982;93:775.
44. Chen M, Stracher A. In situ phosphorylation of platelet actin-binding protein by cAMP-dependent protein kinase stabilizes it against proteolysis by calpain. J Biol Chem 1989;264:14282.
45. Landon F, Olomucki A. Isolation and physico-chemical properties of blood platelet α-actin. Biochim Biophys Acta 1983;742:129.
46. Sixma JJ, Schiphorst ME, Verhoeckx C, Jockusch BM. Peripheral and integral proteins of human blood platelet membranes: α-actin is not identical to glycoprotein III. Biochim Biophys Acta 1982;704:333.
47. Kurth MC, Bryan J. Platelet activation induces the formation of a stable gelsolin-actin complex from monomeric gelsolin. J Biol Chem 1984;259:7473.
48. Lind SE, Janmey PA, Chaponnier C, Herbert TJ, Stossel TP. Reversible binding of actin to gelsolin and profilin in human platelet extracts. J Cell Biol 1987;105:833.
49. Lind SE, Yin HL, Stossel TP. Human platelets contain gelsolin, a regulator of actin filament length. J Clin Invest 1982;69:1384.
50. Janmey PA, Iida K, Yin HL, Stossel TP. Polyphosphoinositide micelles and polyphosphoinositide-containing vesicles dissociate endogenous gelsolin-actin complexes and promote actin assembly from the fast-growing end of actin filaments blocked by gelsolin. J Biol Chem 1987;262:12228.
51. Hartwig JH, Chambers KA, Stossel TP. Association of gelsolin with actin filaments and cell membranes of macrophages and platelets. J Cell Biol 1989;108:467.
52. Markey F, Persson T, Lindberg U. Characterization of platelet extracts before and after stimulation with respect to the possible role of profilactin as microfilament precursor. Cell 1981;23:145.
53. Collier NC, Wang K. Human platelet P235: a high Mr protein which restricts the length of actin filaments. FEBS Lett 1982;143:205.
54. Rosenfeld GC, Hou DC, Dingus J, et al. Isolation and partial characterization of human platelet vinculin. J Cell Biol 1985;100:669.
55. Davies GE, Cohen CM. Platelets contain proteins immunologically related to red cell spectrin and protein 4.1. Blood 1985;65:52.
56. Lux SE. Dissecting the red cell membrane skeleton. Nature (London) 1979;281:426.
57. Bennett V. Immunoreactive forms of human erythrocyte ankyrin are present in diverse cells and tissues. Nature (London) 1979;281:597.
58. Spiegel JE, Beardsley DS, Southwick FS, Lux SE. An analogue of the erythroid membrane skeletal protein 4.1 in nonerythroid cells. J Cell Biol 1984;99:886.
59. Coté GP, Smillie LB. Preparation and some properties of equine platelet tropomyosin. J Biol Chem 1981;256:11004.
60. Stenberg PE, Bainton DF. Storage organelles in platelets and megakaryocytes. In: Phillips DR, Shuman MA, eds. Biochemistry of platelets. Orlando, Academic Press, 1986:257.
61. Bentfeld ME, Bainton DF. Cytochemical localization of lysosomal enzymes in rat megakaryocytes and platelets. J Clin Invest 1975;56:1635.
62. Bentfeld-Barker ME, Bainton DF. Identification of primary lysosomes in human megakaryocytes and platelets. Blood 1982;59:472.
63. Kaplan KL. Platelet granule proteins: localization and secretion. In: Gordon AS, ed. Platelet in biology and pathology, vol. 5. Amsterdam, Elsevier/North-Holland Biomedical Press, 1981:77.
64. Holmsen H. Platelet secretion. In: Colman RW, Hirsh J, Marder VJ, Salzman EW, eds. Hemostasis and thrombosis. Philadelphia, JB Lippincott, 1987:606.
65. Marcus AJ, Zucker-Franklin D, Safier LB, Ullman HL. Studies on human platelet granules and membranes. J Clin Invest 1966;45:14.
66. Holmsen H, Day HJ. The selectivity of the thrombin-induced platelet release reaction: subcellular localization of released and retained constituents. J Lab Clin Med 1970;75:840.
67. Niewiarowski S. Proteins secreted by the platelet. Thromb Haemost 1977;38:924.
68. Breton-Gorius J, Guichard J. Two different types of granules in megakaryocytes and platelets as revealed by the diaminobenzidine method. J Microsc Biol Cell 1975;23:197.
69. White JG, Estensen RD. Degranulation of discoid platelets. Am J Pathol 1972;68:289.
70. Stenberg PE, Shuman MA, Levine SP, Bainton DF. Redistribution of alpha-granules and their contents in thrombin-stimulated platelets. J Cell Biol 1984;98:748.
71. White JG. Interaction of membrane systems in blood platelets. Am J Pathol 1972;66:295.
72. Cutler L, Rodan G, Feinstein MB. Cytochemical localization of adenylate cyclase and of calcium ion, magnesium ion-activated ATP-ases in the dense tubular system of human blood platelets. Biochim Biophys Acta 1978;542:357.
73. Carey F, Menashi S, Crawford N. Localization of cyclooxygenase and thromboxane synthetase in human platelet intracellular membranes. Biochem J 1982;204:847.
74. Gerrard JM. Platelet aggregation: cellular regulation and physiologic role. Hosp Pract 1988;23:89.
75. White JG. Is the canalicular system the equivalent of the muscle sarcoplasmic reticulum? Hemostasis 1975;4:185.
76. Palmer RM, Ferrige AG, Moncada S. Nitric oxide release accounts for the biological activity of endothelium-derived relaxing factor. Nature 1987;327:524.
77. Furchgott RF, Zawadzki JV. The obligatory role of endothelial cells in the relaxation of arterial smooth muscle by acetylcholine. Nature 1980;288:373.
78. Moncada S, Radomski MW, Palmer RMJ. Endothelium-derived relaxing factor. Biochem Pharmacol 1988;37:2495.
79. Wilson PD, Lieberman GE, Peters TJ. Ultrastructural localization of adenosine diphosphatase activity in cultured aortic endothelial cells. Histochem J 1982;14:215.
80. Chesterman CN, Berndt MC. Platelet and vessel wall interaction and the genesis of atherosclerosis. Clin Hematol 1986;15:323.
81. Baumgartner HR, Tschopp TB, Meyer D. Shear rate dependent inhibition of platelet adhesion and aggregation on collagenous surfaces by antibodies to human factor VIII/von Willebrand factor. Br J Haematol 1980;44:127.
82. Houdijk WP, Sakariassen KS, Nievelstein PFEM, Sixma JJ. Role of von Willebrand factor and fibronectin in the interaction of platelets in flowing blood with monomeric and fibrillar human collagen types I and III. J Clin Invest 1985;75:531.
83. Legrand YJ, Fauvel F, Gutman N, et al. Microfibrils (MF) platelet interaction: requirement of von Willebrand factor. Thromb Res 1980;19:737.
84. Fauvel F, Grant ME, Legrand YJ, et al. Interaction of blood platelets with a microfibrillar extract from adult bovine aorta: requirement of von Willebrand factor. Proc Natl Acad Sci USA 1983;80:551.
85. Weiss HJ, Turitto VT, Baumgartner HR. Effect of shear rate on platelet interaction with subendothelium in citrated and native blood. I. Shear rate-dependent decrease of adhesion in von Willebrand's disease and the Bernard-Soulier syndrome. J Lab Clin Med 1978;92:750.
86. Sakariassen KS, Bolhuis PA, Sixma JJ. Human blood platelet adhesion to artery subendothelium is mediated by factor VIII-von Willebrand factor bound to the subendothelium. Nature 1979;279:636.
87. Packham MA, Mustard JF. Platelet adhesion. Prog Hemost Thromb 1984;7:211.
88. Allain JP, Cooper HA, Wagner RH, Brinkhous KM. Platelets fixed with paraformaldehyde: a new reagent for assay of von Willebrand factor and platelet aggregating factor. J Lab Clin Med 1975;85:318.
89. Grant RA, Zucker MB, McPherson J. ADP-induced inhibition of von Willebrand factor-mediated platelet agglutination. Am J Physiol 1976;230:1406.
90. Kunicki TJ. Organization of glycoproteins within the platelet plasma membrane. In: George JN, Nurden AT, Phillips DR, eds. Platelet membrane glycoproteins. New York, Plenum, 1985:87.
91. George JN, Torres MM. Thrombin decreases von Willebrand factor binding to platelet glycoprotein Ib. Blood 1988;71:1253.

92. de Marco L, Girolami A, Russell S, Ruggeri ZM. Interaction of asialo von Willebrand factor with glycoprotein Ib induces fibrinogen binding to the glycoprotein IIb/IIIa complex and mediates platelet aggregation. J Clin Invest 1985;75:1198.
93. Gralnick HR, Williams SB, Coller BS. Asialo von Willebrand factor interactions with platelets: interdependence of glycoproteins Ib and IIb/IIIa for binding and aggregation. J Clin Invest 1985;75:19.
94. Kroll MH, Harris TS, Moake JL, Handin RI, Schafer AI. Von Willebrand factor binding to platelet GpIb initiates signals for platelet activation. J Clin Invest 1991;88:1568.
95. Moake JL, Turner NA, Stathopoulos NA, et al. Involvement of large plasma von Willebrand factor (vWF) multimers and unusually large vWF forms derived from endothelial cells in shear stress-induced platelet aggregation. J Clin Invest 1986;78:1456.
96. Moake JL, Turner NA, Stathopoulos NA, et al. Shear-induced platelet aggregation can be mediated by vWF released from platelets, as well as by exogenous large or unusually large vWF multimers, requires adenosine diphosphate, and is resistant to aspirin. Blood 1988;71:1366.
97. Phillips DR, Charo IF, Parise LV, Fitzgerald LA. The platelet membrane glycoprotein IIb-IIIa complex. Blood 1988;71:831.
98. Kunicki TJ, Pidard D, Rosa J-P, Nurden AT. The formation of Ca^{2+}-dependent complexes of platelet membrane glycoprotein IIb and IIIa in solution as determined by crossed immunoelectrophoresis. Blood 1981;58:268.
99. Howard L, Shulman S, Sadanandan S, Karpatkin S. Crossed immunoelectrophoresis of human platelet membranes: the major antigen consists of a complex of glycoproteins, GP IIb and GP IIIa, held together by Ca^{2+} and missing in Glanzmann's thrombasthenia. J Biol Chem 1982;257:8331.
100. Jennings LK, Phillips DR. Purification of glycoproteins IIb and III from human platelet plasma membranes and characterization of a calcium-dependent glycoprotein IIb-III complex. J Biol Chem 1982;257:10458.
101. McEver RP, Bennett EM, Martin MN. Identification of two structurally and functionally distinct sites on human platelet membrane glycoprotein IIb-IIIa using monoclonal antibodies. J Biol Chem 1983;258:5269.
102. Fujimura K, Phillips DR. Calcium cation regulation of glycoprotein IIb-IIIa complex formation in platelet plasma membranes. J Biol Chem 1983;258:10247.
103. Coller BS, Peerschke EI, Scudder LE, Sullivan CA. A murine monoclonal antibody that completely blocks the binding of fibrinogen to platelets produces a thrombasthenic-like state in normal platelets and binds to glycoproteins IIb and/or IIIa. J Clin Invest 1983;72:325.
104. Fitzgerald LA, Phillips DR. Calcium regulation of the platelet membrane glycoprotein IIb-IIIa complex. J Biol Chem 1985;260:11366.
105. Pidard D, Montgomery RR, Bennett JS, Kunicki TJ. Interaction of AP-2, a monoclonal antibody specific for the human platelet glycoprotein IIb-IIIa complex, with intact platelets. J Biol Chem 1983;258:12582.
106. Hynes RO. Integrins: a family of cell surface receptors. Cell 1987;48:549.
107. Ginsberg MH, Loftus JC, Plow EF. Cytoadhesins, integrins, and platelets. Thromb Haemost 1988;59:1.
108. Pierschbacher MD, Ruoslahti E. Variants of the cell recognition site of fibronectin that retain attachment-promoting activity. Proc Natl Acad Sci USA 1984;81:5985.
109. Asch E, Podack E. Vitronectin binds to activated human platelets and plays a role in platelet aggregation. J Clin Invest 1990;85:1372.
110. Weiss HJ, Hawiger J, Ruggeri ZM, et al. Fibrinogen-independent platelet adhesion and thrombus formation on subendothelium mediated by glycoprotein IIb-IIIa complex at high shear rate. J Clin Invest 1989;83:288.
111. Ash AS, Barnwell J, Silverstein RL, Nachman RL. Isolation of the thrombospondin membrane receptor. J Clin Invest 1987;79:1054.
112. Tuszynski GP, Rothman VL, Murphy A, et al. Thrombospondin promotes platelet aggregation. Blood 1988;72:109.
113. Leung LLK. Role of thrombospondin in platelet aggregation. J Clin Invest 1984;74:1764.
114. Kroll MH, Schafer AI. Biochemical mechanisms of platelet activation. Blood 1989;74:1181.
115. Berridge MJ. The molecular basis of communication within the cell. Sci Am 1985;253:142.
116. Ashby B, Daniel JL, Smith JB. Mechanisms of platelet activation and inhibition. Hematol Oncol Clin North Am 1990;4:1.
117. Berridge MJ. Inositol trisphosphate and diacylglycerol: two interacting second messengers. Annu Rev Biochem 1987;56:159.
118. Nomura H, Nakanishi H, Ase K, et al. Inositol phospholipid turnover in Otimulus-response coupling. In: Coller BS, ed. Progress in hemostasis and thrombosis, vol. 8. Orlando, Grune and Stratton, 1986:143.
119. Majerus PW, Connolly TM, Deckmyn H, et al. The metabolism of phosphoinositide-derived messenger molecules. Science 1986;234:1519.
120. Feinstein MB, Zavoico GB, Halenda SP. Calcium and cyclic AMP: antagonistic modulators of platelet function. In: Longenecker GL, ed. The platelets: physiology and pharmacology. Orlando, Academic Press, 1985:237.
121. Santoro SA. Identification of a 160,000 dalton platelet membrane protein that mediates the initial divalent cation-dependent adhesion of platelets to collagen. Cell 1986;46:913.
122. Halushka PV, Mais DE, Saussy DL Jr. Platelet and vascular smooth muscle thromboxane A_2/prostaglandin H_2 receptors. Fed Proc 1987;46:149.
123. Hwang SB, Lee CSC, Cheah MJ, Shen TY. Specific receptor sites for 1-O-alkyl-2-O-acetyl-sn-glycero-3-phosphocholine (platelet activating factor) on rabbit platelet and guinea pig smooth muscle membranes. Biochemistry 1983;22:4756.
124. Siess W, Stifel M, Binder H, Weber PC. Activation of V_1-receptors by vasopressin stimulates inositol phospholipid hydrolysis and arachidonate metabolism in human platelets. Biochem J 1986;233:83.
125. de Chaffoy de Courcelles D, Leysen JE, de Clerck F, et al. Evidence that phospholipid turnover is the signal transducing system coupled to serotonin-S_2 receptor sites. J Biol Chem 1985;260:7603.
126. Bennett JS, Colman RF, Colman RW. Identification of adenine nucleotide binding proteins in human platelet membranes by affinity labeling with 5'-p-fluorosulfonylbenzoyl adenosine. J Biol Chem 1978;253:7346.
127. Adler JR, Handin RI. Solubilization and characterization of a platelet membrane ADP-binding protein. J Biol Chem 1979;254:3866.
128. Alexander RW, Cooper B, Handin RI. Characterization of the human platelet α-adrenergic receptor. J Clin Invest 1978;78:1136.
129. Schafer AI, Cooper B, O'Hara D, Handin RI. Identification of platelet receptors for prostaglandin I_2 and D_2. J Biol Chem 1979;254:2914.
130. Dutta-Roy AK, Sinha AK. Purification and properties of prostaglandin E_1/prostacyclin receptor of human blood platelets. J Biol Chem 1987;262:12685.
131. Colman RW. Platelet receptors. Hematol Oncol Clin North Am 1990;4:27.
132. Shuman MA. Thrombin-cellular interactions. Ann NY Acad Sci 1986;485:228.
133. Okumura T, Hasitz M, Jamieson GA. Platelet glycocalicin: interaction with thrombin and role as thrombin receptor of the platelet surface. J Biol Chem 1978;253:3435.
134. Jamieson GA, Okumura T. Reduced thrombin binding and aggregation in Bernard-Soulier platelets. J Clin Invest 1978;61:861.
135. Harmon JT, Jamieson GA. Activation of platelets by α-thrombin is a receptor-mediated event. J Biol Chem 1986;261:15928.
136. Tollefsen DM, Feagler JR, Majerus PW. The binding of thrombin to the surface of human platelets. J Biol Chem 1974;249:2646.
137. Phillips DR, Agin PP. Platelet plasma membrane glycoproteins: identification of a proteolytic substrate for thrombin. Biochem Biophys Res Commun 1977;75:940.
138. McGowan EB, Duig A, Detwiler TC. Correlation between thrombin-induced glycoprotein V hydrolysis and platelet activation. J Biol Chem 1983;258:11243.
139. Casey PJ, Gilman AG. G protein involvement in receptor-effector coupling. J Biol Chem 1988;263:2577.
140. Neer EJ, Clapham DE. Roles of G protein subunits in transmembrane signalling. Nature 1988;333:129.
141. Rittenhouse-Simmons S. Production of diglyceride from phosphatidylinositol in activated human platelets. J Clin Invest 1979;63:580.
142. Bell RL, Majerus PW. Thrombin-induced hydrolysis of phosphatidylinositol in human platelets. J Biol Chem 1980;255:1790.
143. Agranoff BW, Murphy P, Seguin EB. Thrombin-induced phosphodiesteratic cleavage of phosphatidylinositol bisphosphate in human platelets. J Biol Chem 1983;258:2076.
144. Brass LF, Joseph SK. A role for inositol trisphosphate in intracellular Ca^{2+} mobilization and granule secretion in platelets. J Biol Chem 1985;260:15172.
145. Lapetina EG, Watson SP, Cuatrecasas P. myo-Inositol 1,4,5-trisphosphate stimulates protein phosphorylation in saponin-permeabilized human platelets. Proc Natl Acad Sci USA 1984;81:7431.
146. O'Rourke FA, Halenda SP, Zavoico GB, Feinstein MB. Inositol 1,4,5-trisphosphate releases Ca^{2+} from a Ca^{2+}-transporting membrane vesicle fraction derived from human platelets. J Biol Chem 1985;260:956.
147. Authi KS, Crawford N. Inositol 1,4,5-trisphosphate-induced release of sequestered Ca^{2+} from highly purified human platelet intracellular membranes. Biochem J 1985;230:247.
148. Yamanishi J, Takai Y, Kaibuchi K, et al. Synergistic functions of phorbol ester and calcium in serotonin release from human platelets. Biochem Biophys Res Commun 1983;112:778.
149. Nishizuka Y. Studies and perspectives of protein kinase C. Science 1986;233:305.
150. Rasmussen H. The calcium messenger system. N Engl J Med 1986;314:1094.
151. Tyers M, Rachubinski RA, Steward MI, et al. Molecular cloning and expression of the major protein kinase C substrate of platelets. Nature 1988;333:470.
152. Chang J, Musse JH, McGregor H. Phospholipase A_2: function and pharmacological regulation. Biochem Pharmacol 1987;36:2429.
153. Lagarde M. Metabolism of fatty acids by platelets and the functions of various metabolites in mediating platelet function. Prog Lipid Res 1988;27:135.
154. Needleman P, Turk J, Jakschik BA, et al. Arachidonic acid metabolism. Annu Rev Biochem 1986;55:69.
155. Kroll MH, Zavoico GB, Schafer AI. Second messenger function of phosphatidic acid in platelet activation. J Cell Physiol, in press.
156. Ware JA, Smith M, Salzman EW. Synergism of platelet aggregating

agents: role of elevation of cytoplasmic calcium. J Clin Invest 1987;80: 267.
157. Lerea KM, Glomset JA, Krebs EG. Agents that elevate cAMP levels in platelets decrease thrombin binding. J Biol Chem 1987;262:282.
158. Lerea KM, Glomset JA. Agents that elevate the concentration of cAMP in platelets inhibit the formation of a $NaDodSO_4$-resistant complex between thrombin and a 40-kDa protein. Proc Natl Acad Sci USA 1987;84:5620.
159. Knight DE, Scrutton MC. Cyclic nucleotides control a system which regulates Ca^{2+} sensitivity of platelet secretion. Nature 1984;309:66.
160. Kroll MH, Zavoico GB, Schafer AI. Control of platelet protein kinase C activation by cyclic AMP. Biochim Biophys Acta 1988;970:61.
161. Panocchia A, Hardisty RM. Cyclic AMP inhibits platelet activation independently of its effect on cytosolic free calcium. Biochem Biophys Res Commun 1985;127:339.
162. Cox AC, Carroll RC, White JG, Rao GHR. Recycling of platelet phosphorylation and cytoskeletal assembly. J Cell Biol 1984;98:8.
163. Feinstein MB, Egan JJ, Opas EE. Reversal of thrombin-induced myosin phosphorylation and the assembly of cytoskeletal structures in platelets by the adenylate cyclase stimulants prostaglandin D_2 and forskolin. J Biol Chem 1983;258:1260.
164. Mellion BT, Ignarro LJ, Ohlstein EH, et al. Evidence for the inhibitory role of guanosine 3',5'-monophosphate in ADP-induced human platelet aggregation in the presence of nitric oxide and related vasodilators. Blood 1981;57:946.
165. Nakashima S, Tohmatsu T, Hattori H, et al. Inhibitory action of cyclic GMP on secretion, polyphosphoinositide hydrolysis, and calcium mobilization in thrombin-stimulated human platelets. Biochem Biophys Res Commun 1986;135:1099.
166. Durante W, Kroll MH, Vanhoutte PM, Schafer AI. Endothelium-derived relaxing factor inhibits thrombin-induced platelet aggregation by inhibiting platelet phospholipase C. Blood 1992;79:110.
167. Furlong B, Henderson AH, Lewis MJ, Smith JA. Endothelium-derived relaxing factor inhibits in vitro platelet aggregation. Br J Pharmacol 1987;90:687.
168. Alheid U, Frölich JC, Förstermann U. Endothelium-derived relaxing factor from cultured human endothelial cells inhibits aggregation of human platelets. Thromb Res 1987;47:561.
169. MacDonald PS, Read MA, Dusting GJ. Synergistic inhibition of platelet aggregation by endothelium-derived relaxing factor and prostacyclin. Thromb Res 1988;49:437.
170. Kitchen L, Erichson RB, Sideropoulos H. Effect of drug-induced platelet dysfunction on surgical bleeding. Am J Surg 1982;143:215.
171. Amrein PC, Ellman L, Harris WH. Aspirin-induced prolongation of bleeding time and perioperative blood loss. JAMA 1981;245:1825.
172. Ferraris VA, Ferraris SP, Lough FC, Berry WR. Preoperative aspirin ingestion increases operative blood loss after coronary artery bypass grafting. Ann Thorac Surg 1988;45:71.
173. Halonen P, Lindo K, Wirtavuori K, et al. Evaluation of risk factors in intraoperative bleeding tendency. Ann Chir Gynaecol 1987;76:298.
174. Day HJ, Rao AK. Evaluation of platelet function. Semin Hematol 1986;23: 89.
175. Yardumian DA, Mackie IJ, Machin SJ. Laboratory investigation of platelet function: a review of methodology. J Clin Pathol 1986;39:701.
176. Duke W. The relation of blood platelets in hemorrhagic disease: description of method for determining the bleeding time and coagulation time and report of three cases of hemorrhagic diseases relieved by transfusions. JAMA 1910;55:1185.
177. Ivy AC, Shapiro PF, Melnick G. The bleeding time in jaundice. Surg Gynecol Obstet 1935;66:781.
178. Mielke CH, Konashro MM, Maher JD, et al. The standardized normal Ivy bleeding time and its prolongation by aspirin. Blood 1969:34:204.
179. Poller L, Thompson JM, Tanenson JA. The bleeding time: current practice in the UK. Clin Lab Haematol 1984;6:369.
180. Gobel V, Van Hoss H, Jurgen H, et al. The reproductiveness of bleeding time tests. Minerva Pediatr 1978;30:1391.
181. Nieuwenhuis HK, Sixma JJ. Bleeding time measurements. In: Harker LA, Zimmerman TS, eds. Measurement of platelet function. New York, Churchill Livingstone, 1983:26.
182. Feusner JH. Normal and abnormal bleeding times in neonates and young children utilizing a fully standardized template technique. Am J Clin Pathol 1980;74:73.
183. Borchgrevink CF, Owren PA. The hemostatic effect of normal platelets on hemophilia and factor V deficiency. Acta Med Scand 1961;170:375.
184. Buchanan GR, Holthamp CA. Prolonged bleeding time in children and young adults with hemophilia. Pediatrics 1980;66:951.
185. Eyster ME, Gordon RA, Bullard JO. The bleeding time is longer than normal in hemophilia. Blood 1981;58:719.
186. Hellem AJ, Borchgrevink CF, Ames SB. The role of red cells in hemostasis: the relationship between hematocrit, bleeding time and platelet adhesiveness. Br J Haematol 1961;76:42.
187. Bowie EJW, Owen CA. The significance of abnormal preoperative hemostatic tests. Prog Hemost Thromb 1980;5:179.
188. Lind SE. The bleeding time does not predict surgical bleeding. Blood 1991;77:2547.
189. Rodgers RPC, Levin J. A critical reappraisal of the bleeding time. Semin Thromb Hemost 1990;16:1.
190. Burns ER, Lawrence C. Bleeding time: a guide to its diagnostic and clinical utility. Arch Pathol Lab Med 1989;113:1219.
191. Rapaport SI. Preoperative hemostatic evaluation: which tests, if any? Blood 1983;61:229.
192. Barber A, Green D, Galluzzo T, Ts'ao C-H. The bleeding time as a preoperative screening test. Am J Med 1985;78:761.
193. Rohrer MJ, Michelotti MC, Nahrwold DL. A prospective evaluation of the efficacy of preoperative coagulation testing. Ann Surg 1988;208: 554.
194. Lind SE. Prolonged bleeding time. Am J Med 1984;77:305.
195. Hellem AJ. The adhesiveness of human blood platelets in vitro. Scand J Clin Lab Invest 1980;12:12.
196. Hellem AJ. Platelet adhesiveness. Series Haematol 1968;2:99.
197. Salzman EW. Measurement of platelet adhesiveness: a simple in vitro technique demonstrating an abnormality of von Willbrand's disease. J Lab Clin Med 1963;62:724.
198. Zucker MB, Rifkin PL, Friedburg NM, Coller BS. Mechanism of platelet function as revealed by the retention of platelets in glass bead columns. Ann NY Acad Sci 1972;201:138.
199. Turitto VT, Baumgartner HR. Platelet adhesion. In: Harker LA, Zimmerman TS, eds. Measurement of platelet function. Edinburgh, Churchill Livingstone, 1983:46.
200. Holmsen H, Ostvold AC, Day HJ. Behaviour of endogenous and newly absorbed serotonin in the platelet release reaction. Biochem Pharmacol 1981;22:2599.
201. Feinman RD, Lubowsky J, Charo IF, et al. The lumiaggregometer: a new instrument for simultaneous measurement of secretion and aggregation. J Lab Clin Med 1977;90:125.
202. Gerrard JM, Phillips DR, Rao GH, et al. Biochemical studies of two patients with the gray platelet syndrome. J Clin Invest 1980;66:102.
203. Rao AK, Niewiarowski S, James P, et al. Effect of heparin on the in vivo release and clearance of human platelet factor 4. Blood 1983;61: 1208.
204. Guzzo J, Niewiarowski S, Musial J, et al. Secreted platelet proteins with anti-heparin and mitogenic activities in chronic renal failure. J Lab Clin Med 1980;96:102.
205. FitzGerald GA, Lawson JA, Blair IA, Brash AR. Analysis of urinary metabolites of thromboxane and prostacyclin by negative-ion chemical-ionization gas chromatography/mass spectrometry. Adv Prostaglandin Thromboxane Leukotriene Res 1986;15:87.
206. Oates JA, FitzGerald GA, Branch RA, et al. Clinical implications of prostaglandin and thromboxane A_2 formation. N Engl J Med 1988;319: 689.
207. Born GVR. Quantitative investigations into the aggregation of blood platelets. J Physiol 1962;162:67.
208. Buchanan GR, Holtkamp CA, Levy EN. Racial differences in ristocetin-induced platelet aggregation. Br J Haematol 1981;49:455.
209. Lumley P, Humphrey PPA. A method for quantitating platelet aggregation and analysing drug receptor interactions on platelets in whole blood in vitro. J Pharmacol Methods 1981;6:153.
210. Ingerman CM, Smith JB, Silver MJ. Evaluation of electrical aggregometry: comparison with optical aggregometry, secretion of ATP and accumulation of radiolabeled platelets. J Lab Clin Med 1983;101:42.
211. Walsh PN. The effect of dilution of plasma on coagulation. The significance of dilution-activation phenomenon for the study of platelet coagulant activities. Br J Haematol 1972;22:219.
212. Walsh PN, Pareti FI, Corbett JJ. Platelet coagulant activities and serum lipids in transient cerebral ischemia. N Engl J Med 1976;295:854.
213. Parry DH, Giddings JC, Bloom AL. Familial haemostatic defect associated with reduced prothrombin consumption. Br J Haematol 1980;44: 323.
214. Weiss HJ, Vicic WJ, Lages BA. Isolated deficiency of platelet procoagulant activity. Am J Med 1979;67:206.
215. Walsh PN, Mills DCB, Pareti FI, et al. Hereditary giant platelet syndrome: absence of collagen-induced coagulant activity and deficiency of factor XI binding to platelets. Br J Haematol 1975;29:639.
216. Semararo N, Corellazzo S, Colucci M, et al. A hitherto undescribed defect of platelet coagulant activity in polycythemia vera and essential thrombocythemia. Thromb Res 1979;16:795.
217. Rao AK, Mintz PD, Levine SJ, et al. Coagulant activities of platelets in coronary artery disease. Circulation 1984;69:16.
218. Rao AK, Goldberg RE, Walsh PN. Platelet coagulant activities in diabetes mellitus. J Lab Clin Med 1984;103:82.
219. Abrams C, Shattil SJ. Immunological detection of activated platelets in clinical disorders. Thromb Haemostas 1991;65:467.
220. Grynkiewicz G, Poenie M, Tsien RY. A new generation of Ca^{2+} indicators with greatly improved fluorescence properties. J Biol Chem 1985;260:3440.
221. Tsien RY, Rink TJ, Poenie M. Measurement of cytosolic free Ca^{2+} in individual small cells using fluorescence microscopy with dual excitation wavelengths. Cell Calcium 1985;6:145.
222. Johnson PC, Ware JA, Cliveden PB, et al. Measurement of ionized calcium in blood platelets with the photoprotein aequorin. J Biol Chem 1985;260:2069.
223. Bernard J, Soulier JP. Sur une nouvelle variété de dystrophie thrombocytaire hémorragipare congénitale. Semin Hop Paris 1948;24: 3217.

224. George JN, Nurden AT, Phillips DR. Molecular defects in interactions of platelets with the vessel wall. N Engl J Med 1984;311:1084.
225. Weiss HJ. Congenital disorders of platelet function. Semin Hematol 1980;17:228.
226. George JN, Reimann TA, Moake JL, et al. Bernard-Soulier disease: a study of four patients and their parents. Br J Haematol 1981;48:459.
227. Jamieson GA, Okumura T. Reduced thrombin binding and aggregation in Bernard-Soulier platelets. J Clin Invest 1978;61:861.
228. Howard MA, Hutton RA, Hardisty RM. Hereditary giant platelet syndrome: a disorder of a new aspect of platelet function. Br Med J 1973;2:586.
229. Weiss HJ, Tschopp TB, Baumgartner HR, et al. Decreased adhesion of giant (Bernard-Soulier) platelets to subendothelium: further implications on the role of the von Willebrand factor in hemostasis. Am J Med 1974;57:920.
230. Weiss HJ, Turitto VT, Baumgartner HR. Effect of shear rate on platelet interaction with subendothelium in citrated and native blood. I. Shear rate-dependent decrease of adhesion in von Willebrand's disease and the Bernard-Soulier syndrome. J Lab Clin Med 1978;92:750.
231. Meyer D, Baumgartner HR. Role of von Willebrand factor in platelet adhesion to the subendothelium. Br J Haematol 1983;54:1.
232. Zucker MB, Kim S-J, McPherson J, Grant RA. Binding of factor VIII to platelets in the presence of ristocetin. Br J Haematol 1977;35:535.
233. Moake JL, Olson JD, Troll JH, et al. Binding of radioiodinated human von Willebrand factor to Bernard-Soulier, thrombasthenic and von Willebrand's disease platelets. Thromb Res 1980;19:21.
234. Nurden AT, Caen JP. Specific roles for platelet surface glycoproteins in platelet function. Nature 1975;255:720.
235. Hagen I, Nurden A, Bjerrum OJ, et al. Immunochemical evidence for protein abnormalities in platelets from patients with Glanzmann's thrombasthenia and Bernard-Soulier syndrome. J Clin Invest 1980;65:722.
236. Kunicki TJ, Nurden AT, Pidard D, et al. Characterization of human platelet glycoprotein antigens giving rise to individual immunoprecipitates in crossed-immunoelectrophoresis. Blood 1981;58:1190.
237. Degos L, Tobelem G, Lethielleux P, et al. Molecular defects in platelets from patients with Bernard-Soulier syndrome. Blood 1977;50:899.
238. Coller BS, Peerschke EI, Scudder LE, Sullivan CA. Studies with a murine monoclonal antibody that abolishes ristocetin-induced binding of von Willebrand factor to platelets: additional evidence in support of GPIb as platelet receptor for von Willebrand factor. Blood 1983;61:99.
239. Montgomery RR, Kunicki TJ, Taves C, et al. Diagnosis of Bernard-Soulier syndrome and Glanzmann's thrombasthenia with a monoclonal assay on whole blood. J Clin Invest 1983;71:385.
240. Du X, Beutler L, Ruan C, et al. Glycoprotein Ib and glycoprotein IX are fully complexed in the intact platelet membrane. Blood 1987;69:1524.
241. Clemetson KJ, McGregor JL, James E, et al. Characterization of the platelet membrane glycoprotein abnormalities in Bernard-Soulier syndrome and comparison with normal by surface-labeling techniques and high-resolution two-dimensional gel electrophoresis. J Clin Invest 1982;70:304.
242. Berndt MC, Gregory C, Chong BH, et al. Additional glycoprotein defects in Bernard-Soulier's syndrome: confirmation of genetic basis by parental analysis. Blood 1983;62:800.
243. Okumura T, Hasitz M, Jamieson GA. Platelet glycocalicin: interaction with thrombin and role as thrombin receptor of the platelet surface. J Biol Chem 1978;253:3435.
244. Berndt MC, Phillips DR. Purification and physicochemical characterization of human platelet membrane glycoprotein V. J Biol Chem 1981;256:59.
245. McGowan EB, Ding A, Detwiler TC. Correlation of thrombin-induced glycoprotein V hydrolysis and platelet activation. J Biol Chem 1983;258:11243.
246. Nurden AT, Didry-Dupuis D, Rosa JP. Molecular defect of platelets in the Bernard-Soulier syndrome. Blood Cells 1983;9:333.
247. Drouin J, McGregor JL, Parmentier S, et al. Residual amounts of glycoprotein Ib concomitant with near-absence of glycoprotein IX in platelets of Bernard-Soulier patients. Blood 1988;72:1086.
248. Berndt MC, Kabral A, Grimsley P, et al. An acquired Bernard-Soulier-like platelet defect associated with juvenile myelodysplastic syndrome. Br J Haematol 1988;68:97.
249. Weiss HJ, Meyer D, Rabinowitz R, et al. Pseudo–von Willebrand's disease: an intrinsic platelet defect with aggregation by unmodified human factor VIII/von Willebrand factor and enhanced adsorption of its high-molecular-weight multimers. N Engl J Med 1982;306:326.
250. Miller JL, Castella A. Platelet-type von Willebrand's disease: characterization of a new bleeding disorder. Blood 1982;60:790.
251. Miller JL, Kupinsi JM, Castella A, Ruggeri ZM. Von Willebrand factor binds to platelets and induces aggregation in platelet-type but not type IIB von Willebrand disease. J Clin Invest 1983;72:1532.
252. Miller JL, Ruggeri ZM, Lyle VA. Unique interactions of asialo von Willebrand factor with platelets in platelet-type von Willebrand disease. Blood 1987;70:1804.
253. Gralnick HR, Williams SB, Shafer BC, Corash L. Factor VIII/von Willebrand factor binding to von Willebrand's disease platelets. Blood 1982;60:328.
254. Takahashi H, Okada K, Abe S, et al. Platelet aggregation induced by cryoprecipitate infusion in platelet-type von Willebrand's disease. Thromb Res 1987;46:255.
255. Ruoslahti E, Haymann EG, Kuusela P, et al. Isolation of a tryptic fragment containing the collagen-binding site of plasma fibronectin. J Biol Chem 1978;254:6054.
256. Bensusan HB, Koh TL, Henry KG, et al. Evidence that fibronectin is the collagen receptor on platelet membranes. Proc Natl Acad Sci USA 1978;75:5864.
257. Santoro SA, Cowan JF. Adsorption of von Willebrand factor by fibrillar collagen: implications concerning the adhesion of platelets to collagen. Coll Relat Res 1982;2:31.
258. Lahav J, Schwartz MA, Hynes RO. Analyses of platelet adhesion using a radioactive chemical crosslinking reagent: interaction of thrombospondin with fibronectin and collagen. Cell 1982;31:253.
259. Tiffany ML, Penner JA. Effect of complement on collagen-induced platelet aggregation. J Lab Clin Med 1980;96:796.
260. Saito Y, Imada T, Takagi J, et al. Platelet factor XIII, the collagen receptor? J Biol Chem 1986;261:1355.
261. Chiang TM, Kang AH. Isolation and purification of collagen α1(I) receptor from human platelet membrane. J Biol Chem 1982;257:7581.
262. Kotite NJ, Cunningham LW. Specific adsorption of a platelet membrane glycoprotein by human insoluble collagen. J Biol Chem 1986;261:8342.
263. Nieuwenhuis HK, Akkerman JWN, Houdijk WPM, Sixma JJ. Human blood platelets showing no response to collagen fail to express surface glycoprotein Ia. Nature 1985;318:470.
264. Nieuwenhuis HK, Sakariassen KS, Houdijk WPM, et al. Deficiency of platelet membrane glycoprotein Ia associated with a decreased platelet adhesion to subendothelium: a defect in platelet spreading. Blood 1986;68:692.
265. Kehrel B, Balleisen L, Kokott R, et al. Deficiency of intact thrombospondin and membrane glycoprotein Ia in platelets with defective collagen-induced aggregation and spontaneous loss of disorder. Blood 1988;71:1074.
266. O'Brien JR. Variability in the aggregation of human platelets by adrenaline. Nature 1964;202:1188.
267. Scrutton MC, Clare KA, Hutton RA, Bruckdorfer KR. Depressed responsiveness to adrenaline in platelets from apparently normal human donors: a familial trait. Br J Haematol 1981;49:303.
268. Propping P, Friedl W. Genetic control of adrenergic receptors on human platelets: a twin study. Hum Genet 1983;64:105.
269. Davies IB, Sudera D, Sever PS. Endogenous agonist regulation of α_2-adrenoreceptors in man. Clin Sci 1981;61:207S.
270. Hollister AS, Fitzgerald GA, Naudeau HJ, Robertson D. Acute reduction in human platelet α_2-adrenoreceptor affinity for agonist by endogenous and exogenous catecholamines. J Clin Invest 1983;72:1498.
271. Hollister AS, Onrot J, Lonce S, et al. Plasma catecholamine modulation of alpha$_2$ adrenoreceptor agonist affinity and sensitivity in normotensive and hypertensive human platelets. J Clin Invest 1986;77:1416.
272. Brodde OE, Bock KD. Changes in platelet alpha$_2$ adrenoreceptors in human phaeochromocytoma. Eur J Clin Pharmacol 1984;26:265.
273. Pfeifer MA, Ward K, Malpass T, et al. Variations in circulating catecholamines fail to alter human platelet alpha$_2$-adrenergic receptor number or affinity for ^{3}H-yohimbine or ^{3}H-dihydroergocryptine. J Clin Invest 1984;74:1063.
274. Snavely MD, Motulsky HJ, O'Connor DT, et al. Adrenergic receptors in human and experimental pheochromocytoma. Clin Exp Hypertens 1982;A4:829.
275. Willich SN, Tofler GH, Brezinski D, et al. Platelet alpha-2 adrenoreceptor characteristics during morning increase in platelet aggregability. Eur Heart J 1992;13:550.
276. Kaywin P, McDonough M, Insel PA, Shattil SJ. Platelet function in essential thrombocythemia: decreased epinephrine responsiveness associated with a deficiency of platelet α_2-adrenergic receptors. N Engl J Med 1978;299:505.
277. Swart SS, Pearson D, Wood JK, Barnett DB. Functional significance of the platelet alpha$_2$-adrenoreceptor studies in patients with myeloproliferative disorders. Thromb Res 1984;33:531.
278. Rao AK, Willis J, Kowalska MA, et al. Differential requirements for platelet aggregation and inhibition of adenylate cyclase by epinephrine: studies of a familial platelet alpha$_2$-adrenergic receptor defect. Blood 1988;71:494.
279. Wu KK, Le Breton GC, Tai H-H, Chen Y-C. Abnormal platelet response to thromboxane A_2. J Clin Invest 1981;67:1801.
280. Lages B, Malmsten C, Weiss HJ, Samuelsson B. Impaired platelet response to thromboxane A_2 and defective calcium mobilization in a patient with a bleeding disorder. Blood 1981;57:545.
281. Samama M, Lecrubier C, Conrad J, et al. Constitutional thrombocytopathy with subnormal response to thromboxane A_2. Br J Haematol 1981;48:293.
282. Hardisty RM, Machin SJ, Nokes TJC, et al. A new congenital defect of platelet secretion: impaired responsiveness of the platelets to cytoplasmic free calcium. Br J Haematol 1983;53:543.
283. Okuma M, Takayama H, Uchino H. Subnormal platelet response to thromboxane A_2 in a patient with chronic myeloid leukaemia. Br J Haematol 1982;51:469.
284. Ushikubi F, Okuma M, Kanaji K, et al. Hemorrhagic thrombocytopathy

with platelet thromboxane A_2 receptor abnormality: defective signal transduction with normal binding activity. Thromb Haemost 1987;57:158.
285. Rao AK, Holmsen H. Congenital disorders of platelet function. Semin Hematol 1986;23:102.
286. Pelczar-Wissner CJ, McDonald EG, Sussman II. Absence of platelet activating factor (PAF) mediated platelet aggregation: a new platelet defect. Am J Hematol 1984;16:419.
287. Lages B, Weiss HJ. Heterogeneous defects of platelet secretion and responses to weak agonists in patients with bleeding disorders. Br J Haematol 1988;68:53.
288. Nieuwenhuis HK, Akkerman JN, Sixma JJ. Patients with a prolonged bleeding time and normal aggregation tests may have storage pool deficiency: studies on one hundred six patients. Blood 1987;70:620.
289. Israels SJ, McNicol A, Robertson C, Gerrard JM. Platelet storage pool deficiency: diagnosis in patients with prolonged bleeding times and normal platelet aggregation. Br J Haematol 1990;75:118.
290. Weiss HJ. Platelet aggregation, adhesion and ADP release in thrombopathia (platelet factor 3 deficiency): a comparison with Glanzmann's thrombasthenia and von Willebrand's disease. Am J Med 1967;43:570.
291. Hardisty RM, Hutton RA. Bleeding tendency associated with "new" abnormality of platelet behavior. Lancet 1967;1:983.
292. Weiss HJ, Chervenick PA, Zalusky R, Factor A. A familial defect in platelet function associated with impaired release of adenosine diphosphate. N Engl J Med 1969;281:1264.
293. Holmsen H, Weiss HJ. Hereditary defect in the release reaction caused by a deficiency in the storage pool of platelet adenine nucleotides. Br J Haematol 1970;19:643.
294. Holmsen H, Weiss HJ. Further evidence for a deficient storage pool of adenine nucleotides in platelets from some patients with thrombocytopathia: "storage pool disease." Blood 1972;39:197.
295. Maurer HM, Still WJS, Caul J, et al. Familial bleeding tendency associated with microcytic platelets and impaired release of adenosine diphosphate. J Pediatr 1971;78:86.
296. Weiss HJ, Witte LD, Kaplan KL, et al. Heterogeneity in storage pool deficiency: studies of granule-bound substances in 18 patients including variants deficient in α-granules, platelet factor 4, β-thromboglobulin, and platelet-derived growth factor. Blood 1979;54:1296.
297. White JG, Edson JR, Desnick SJ, Witkop CJ. Studies of platelets in a variant of the Hermansky-Pudlak syndrome. Am J Pathol 1971;63:319.
298. Weiss HJ, Ames RP. Ultrastructural findings in storage-pool disease and aspirin-like defects of platelets. Am J Pathol 1973;71:447.
299. Akkerman JWN, Nieuwenhuis HK, Mommersteeg-Leautaud ME, et al. ATP-ADP compartmentation in storage pool deficient platelets: correlation between granule-bound ADP and the bleeding time. Br J Haematol 1983;55:135.
300. Willis AI, Weiss HJ. A congenital defect in platelet prostaglandin production associated with impaired hemostasis in storage pool disease. Prostaglandins 1972;4:783.
301. Malmsten C, Kindahl H, Samuelsson B, et al. Thromboxane synthesis and the platelet release reaction in Bernard-Soulier syndrome, thrombasthenia, Glanzmann and Hermansky-Pudlak syndrome. Br J Haematol 1977;35:511.
302. Rendu F, Breton-Gorius J, Trugnan G, et al. Studies on a new variant of the Hermansky-Pudlak syndrome: qualitative, ultrastructural, and functional abnormalities of the platelet-dense bodies associated with a phospholipase A defect. Am J Hematol 1978;4:387.
303. Weiss HJ, Lages B. Platelet malondialdehyde production and aggregation responses induced by arachidonate, prostaglandin G_2, collagen and epinephrine in 12 patients with storage pool deficiency. Blood 1981;58:27.
304. Lages B, Dangelmaier CA, Holmsen H, Weiss HJ. Specific correction of impaired acid hydrolase secretion in storage pool-deficient platelets by adenosine diphosphate. J Clin Invest 1988;81:1865.
305. White JG. Inherited abnormalities of the platelet membrane and secretory granules. Hum Pathol 1987;18:123.
306. Hermansky F, Pudlak P. Albinism associated with hemorrhagic diathesis and unusual pigmented reticular cells in the bone marrow: report of two cases with histochemical studies. Blood 1959;14:162.
307. Logan LJ, Rapaport SI, Mather I. Albinism and abnormal platelet function. N Engl J Med 1971;284:1340.
308. Hardisty RM, Mills DCB, Ketsa-Ard K. The platelet defect associated with albinism. Br J Haematol 1972;23:679.
309. White JG, Witkop CJ. Effects of normal and aspirin platelets on defective secondary aggregation in the Hermansky-Pudlak syndrome: a test for storage pool-deficient platelets. Am J Pathol 1972;68:57.
310. Buchanan GR, Handin RI. Platelet function in the Chediak-Higashi syndrome. Blood 1976;47:941.
311. Costa JL, Fauci AS, Wolff SM. A platelet abnormality in the Chediak-Higashi syndrome of man. Blood 1976;48:517.
312. Boxer GJ, Holmsen H, Robkin L, et al. Abnormal platelet function in Chediak-Higashi syndrome. Br J Haematol 1977;35:521.
313. Apitz-Castro R, Cruz MR, Ledezma C, et al. The storage pool deficiency in platelets from humans with the Chediak-Higashi syndrome: study of six patients. Br J Haematol 1985;59:471.
314. Day HJ, Holmsen H. Platelet adenine nucleotide "storage pool deficiency" in thrombocytopenic absent radius syndrome. JAMA 1972;221:1053.
315. Grottum KA, Hovig T, Holmsen H. Wiskott-Aldrich syndrome: qualitative platelet defects and short platelet survival. Br J Haematol 1969;17:373.
316. Lum LG, Tubergen DG, Corash L, Blaese RM. Splenectomy in the management of the thrombocytopenia of the Wiskott-Aldrich syndrome. N Engl J Med 1980;302:892.
317. Raccuglia G. Gray platelet syndrome: a variety of qualitative platelet disorder. Am J Med 1971;51:818.
318. White JG. Ultrastructural studies of the gray platelet syndrome. Am J Pathol 1979;95:445.
319. Gerrard JM, Phillips DR, Rao GHR, et al. Biochemical studies of two patients with the gray platelet syndrome: selective deficiency of platelet alpha granules. J Clin Invest 1980;66:102.
320. Levy-Toledano S, Caen JP, Breton-Gorius J, et al. Gray platelet syndrome: α-granule deficiency—its influence on platelet function. J Lab Clin Med 1981;98:831.
321. Nurden AT, Kunicki TJ, Dupuis D, et al. Specific protein and glycoprotein deficiencies in platelets isolated from two patients with the gray platelet syndrome. Blood 1982;59:709.
322. Mori K, Suzuki S, Sugai K. Electron microscopic and functional studies on platelets in gray platelet syndrome. Tohoku J Exp Med 1984;153:261.
323. Breton-Gorius J, Vainchenker W, Nurden A, et al. Defective α-granule production in megakaryocytes from gray platelet syndrome: ultrastructural studies of bone marrow cells and megakaryocytes growing in culture from blood precursors. Am J Pathol 1981;102:10.
324. Zahari J, Marder VJ. Acquired storage pool disease of platelets associated with circulating anti-platelet antibodies. Am J Med 1974;56:883.
325. Weiss HJ, Rosove MH, Lages BA, Kaplan KL. Acquired storage pool deficiency with increased platelet-associated IgG: report of five cases. Am J Med 1980;69:711.
326. Pareti FI, Capitanio A, Mannucci C, et al. Acquired dysfunction due to the circulation of "exhausted" platelets. Am J Med 1980;69:235.
327. Pareti FI, Capitanio A, Mannucci PM. Acquired storage pool disease in platelets during disseminated intravascular coagulation. Blood 1976;48:511.
328. Khurana MS, Lian ECY, Harkness DR. Storage pool disease of platelets associated with multiple congenital cavernous hemangiomas. JAMA 1980;244:169.
329. Rao AK, Niewiarowski S, Murphy S. Acquired granular pool defect in stored platelets. Blood 1981;57:203.
330. Harker LA. Acquired disorders of platelet function. Ann NY Acad Sci 1987;509:188.
331. Musial J, Niewiarowski S, Hershock D, et al. Loss of fibrinogen receptors from the platelet surface during simulated extracorporeal circulation. J Lab Clin Med 1985;105:514.
332. Mammen EF, Koets MH, Washington BC, et al. Hemostasis changes during cardiopulmonary bypass surgery. Semin Thromb Hemost 1985;11:281.
333. Roth GJ, Majerus PW. The mechanism of the effect of aspirin on human platelets. I. Acetylation of a particulate fraction protein. J Clin Invest 1975;56:624.
334. Weiss HJ, Aledort LM, Kochwa S. The effect of salicylates on the hemostatic properties of platelets in man. J Clin Invest 1968;47:2169.
335. Deykin D, Janson P, McMahon L. Ethanol potentiation of aspirin-induced prolongation of the bleeding time. N Engl J Med 1982;306:852.
336. Czapek EE, Deykin D, Salzman E, et al. Intermediate syndrome of platelet dysfunction. Blood 1978;52:103.
337. Loscalzo J, Schafer AI. Anticoagulants, antiplatelet agents, and fibrinolytics. In: Loscalzo J, Dzau VJ, Creager MA, eds. Textbook of vascular medicine. Boston, Little, Brown, 1992:659.
338. Weksler BB, Pett SB, Alonso D, et al. Differential inhibition by aspirin of vascular and platelet prostaglandin synthesis in atherosclerotic patients. N Engl J Med 1983;308:800.
339. Pedersen AK, FitzGerald GA. The human pharmacology of platelet inhibition: pharmacokinetics relevant to drug action. Circulation 1985;112:1164.
340. Baenziger NL, Dillenden MJ, Majerus PW. Cultured human skin fibroblasts and arterial cells produce a labile platelet inhibiting prostaglandin. Biochem Biophys Res Commun 1977;78:294.
341. Jaffe EA, Weksler BB. Recovery of endothelial cell prostacyclin production after low doses of aspirin. J Clin Invest 1979;63:532.
342. Preston FE, Shipps S, Jackson C, et al. Inhibition of prostacyclin and platelet thromboxane A_2 after low-dose aspirin. N Engl J Med 1981;304:76.
343. Simon LS, Mills JA. Non-steroidal anti-inflammatory drugs. N Engl J Med 1980;302:1179.
344. Weiss HJ. Platelets: pathophysiology and antiplatelet drug therapy. New York, Alan R Liss, 1982.
345. Patrono C, Ciabattoni G, Patrignani P, et al. Clinical pharmacology of platelet cyclooxygenase inhibition. Circulation 1985;72:1177.
346. Bang HO, Dyerberg J, Nielsen AB. Plasma lipid and lipoprotein pattern in Greenlandic West-Coast Eskimos. Lancet 1971;1:1143.
347. Bang HO, Dyerberg J. The bleeding tendency in Greenland Eskimos. Dan Med Bull 1980;27:202.
348. Kromhout D, Bosscheiter EB, de Lezenne Coulander C. The inverse

relation between fish consumption and 20-year mortality from coronary heart disease. N Engl J Med 1985;312:1205.
349. Shekelle RB, Missell LV, Paul O, et al. Fish consumption and mortality from coronary heart disease. N Engl J Med 1985;313:820.
350. Fish oil for the heart. Med Lett 1987;29:7.
351. Kantha SS. Dietary effects of fish oils on human health: a review of recent studies. Yale J Biol Med 1987;60:37.
352. Hamberg M, Svensson J, Samuelsson B. Thromboxanes: a new group of biologically active compounds derived from prostaglandin endoperoxides. Proc Natl Acad Sci USA 1975;72:2994.
353. Needleman P, Raz A, Minkes MS, et al. Triene prostaglandins: prostacyclin and thromboxane biosynthesis and unique biological properties. Proc Natl Acad Sci USA 1979;176:944.
354. Knapp HR, Reilly IAG, Alessandrini P, FitzGerald GA. In vivo indexes of platelet and vascular function during fish-oil administration in patients with atherosclerosis. N Engl J Med 1986;314:937.
355. Fischer S, Weber PC. Prostaglandin I_2 is formed in vivo in man after dietary eicosapentaenoic acid. Nature 1984;307:165.
356. von Schacky C, Fischer S, Weber PC. Long-term effects of dietary marine omega-3 fatty acids upon plasma and cellular lipids, platelet function, and eicosanoid formation in humans. J Clin Invest 1985;76:1626.
357. Li X, Steiner M. Fish oil: a potent inhibitor of platelet adhesiveness. Blood 1990;76:938.
358. Malmsten C, Hamberg M, Svensson J, Samuelsson B. Physiological role of an endoperoxide in human platelets: hemostatic defect due to platelet cyclooxygenase deficiency. Proc Natl Acad Sci USA 1975;72:1446.
359. Lagarde M, Byron PA, Vargaftig BB, Dechavanne M. Impairment of platelet thromboxane A_2 generation and of the platelet release reaction in two patients with congenital deficiency of platelet cyclooxygenase. Br J Haematol 1978;38:251.
360. Pareti FI, Mannucci PM, D'Angelo A, et al. Congenital deficiency of thromboxane and prostacyclin. Lancet 1980;1:898.
361. Rak K, Boda Z. Hemostatic balance in congenital deficiency of platelet cyclooxygenase. Lancet 1980;2:44.
362. Roth GJ, Machuga ET. Radioimmune assay of human platelet prostaglandin synthetase. J Lab Clin Med 1982;99:187.
363. Horellou MH, Lecompte T, Lecrubier C, et al. Familial and constitutional bleeding disorder due to platelet cyclooxygenase deficiency. Am J Hematol 1983;14:1.
364. Ehara H, Yoshimoto T, Yamamoto S, Hattori A. Enzymological and immunological studies on a clinical case of platelet cyclooxygenase abnormality. Biochim Biophys Acta 1988;960:35.
365. Rao AK, Koike K, Willis J, et al. Platelet secretion defect associated with impaired liberation of arachidonic acid and normal myosin light chain phosphorylation. Blood 1984;64:914.
366. Mestel F, Oetilker O, Beck E, et al. Severe bleeding associated with defective thromboxane synthetase. Lancet 1980;1:157.
367. Defryn G, Machin SJ, Carreras LO, et al. Familial bleeding tendency with partial platelet thromboxane synthetase deficiency: reorientation of cyclic endoperoxide metabolism. Br J Haematol 1981;49:29.
368. Koike K, Rao AK, Holmsen H, et al. Platelet secretion defect in patients with the attention deficit disorder and easy bruising. Blood 1984;63:427.
369. Hattori A, Takahashi H, Takahashi M, et al. A new familial defect of platelet release mechanism (the intracellular Ca^{2+} transport defect?) Acta Haematol Jap 1981;44:969.
370. Takahashi H, Hattori A, Ihzumi T, et al. A family of platelet release mechanism abnormality with normal arachidonate metabolism and defective response to ionophore A23187. Blood Vessels 1981;12:223.
371. Glanzmann E. Hereditare hemorrhagische Thrombasthenie: Ein Beitrag zur pathologic der Blutplattchen. Jahrb Kinderheilk 1918;88:1.
372. Reichert N, Seligsohn U, Ramot B. Clinical and genetic aspects of Glanzmann's thrombasthenia in Israel: report of 22 cases. Thromb Diath Haemorrh 1975;34:806.
373. Stormorken H, Gogstad GO, Solum NO, Pande H. Diagnosis of heterozygotes in Glanzmann's thrombasthenia. Thromb Haemost 1982;48:217.
374. Tschopp TB, Weiss HJ, Baumgartner HR. Interaction of platelets with subendothelium in thrombasthenia: normal adhesion, impaired aggregation. Experientia 1975;31:113.
375. Levy-Toledano S, Maclouf J, Rendu F, et al. Ionophore A23187 and thrombasthenic platelets: a model of disassociating serotonin release and thromboxane formation from the aggregation. Thromb Res 1979;16:453.
376. Malmsten C, Kindahl H, Samuelsson B, et al. Thromboxane synthesis and the platelet release reaction in Bernard-Soulier syndrome, thrombasthenia, Glanzmann and Hermansky-Pudlak syndrome. Br J Haematol 1977;35:511.
377. Caen JP, Castaldi PA, Leclerc JC, et al. Congenital bleeding disorders with long bleeding time and normal platelet count. I. Glanzmann's thrombasthenia (report of fifteen patients). Am J Med 1966;41:4.
378. Legrand C, Caen JP. Binding of ^{14}C-ADP by thrombasthenic platelet membranes. Haemostasis 1976;5:231.
379. White GC II, Workman EF Jr, Lundblad RL. Thrombin binding to thrombasthenic platelets. J Lab Clin Med 1978;91:76.
380. Mustard JF, Kinlough-Rathbone RE, Packham MA, et al. Comparison of fibrinogen association with normal and thrombasthenic platelets on exposure to ADP or chymotrypsin. Blood 1979;54:987.
381. Bennett JS, Vilaire G. Exposure of platelet fibrinogen receptors by ADP and epinephrine. J Clin Invest 1979;64:1393.
382. Nurden AT, Caen JP. Specific roles for platelet surface glycoproteins in platelet function. Nature 1975;225:720.
383. Phillips DR, Jenkins CSP, Luscher EF, Larrieu M-J. Molecular differences of exposed surface proteins on thrombasthenic platelet plasma membranes. Nature 1975;257:559.
384. Ginsberg MH, Forsyth J, Lightsey A, et al. Reduced surface expression and binding of fibronectin by thrombin-stimulated thrombasthenic platelets. J Clin Invest 1983;71:619.
385. Bray PF, Shuman MA. Identification of an abnormal gene for the GpIIIa subunit of the platelet fibrinogen receptor resulting in Glanzmann's thrombasthenia. Blood 1990;75:881.
386. Weiss HJ, Rogers J. Fibrinogen and platelets in the primary arrest of bleeding: studies in two patients with congenital afibrinogenemia. N Engl J Med 1971;285:369.
387. Gugler E, Luscher EF. Platelet function in congenital afibrinogenemia. Thromb Diath Haemorrh 1965;14:361.
388. Marguerie GA, Thomas-Maison N, Larrieu M-J, Plow EF. The interaction of fibrinogen with human platelets in a plasma milieu. Blood 1982;49:91.
389. Bennett JS, Vilaire G. Exposure of platelet fibrinogen receptors by ADP and epinephrine. J Clin Invest 1979;64:1393.
390. Galanakis DK, Henschen A, Peerschke EIB, Kehl M. Fibrinogen Stony Brook, a heterozygous $A\sigma 16Arg \rightarrow Cys$ dysfibrinogenemia: evaluation of diminished platelet aggregation support and enhanced inhibition of fibrin assembly. J Clin Invest 1989;84:295.
391. Girolami A, Brunetti A, Fioretti D, et al. Congenital thrombocytopathy (platelet factor 3 defect) with prolonged bleeding but normal platelet adhesiveness and aggregation. Acta Haematol (Basel) 1973;50:116.
392. Sultan Y, Brouet JC, Divergie A. Isolated platelet factor 3 deficiency. N Engl J Med 1976;294:1121.
393. Weiss HJ, Vicic WJ, Lages BA, et al. Isolated deficiency of platelet procoagulant activity. Am J Med 1979;67:206.
394. Miletich JP, Kane WH, Hofman SL, et al. Deficiency of factor Xa-factor Va binding sites on platelets of a patient with a bleeding disorder. Blood 1979;54:1015.
395. Rosing EM, Bevers P, Confurius P, et al. Impaired factor X and prothrombin activation associated with decreased phospholipid exposure in platelets from a patient with a bleeding disorder. Blood 1985;65:1557.
396. Carvalho AC. Acquired platelet dysfunction in patients with uremia. Hematol Oncol Clin North Am 1990;4:129.
397. Margolis DM, Saylor JL, Geisse G, et al. Upper gastrointestinal disease in chronic renal failure: a prospective evaluation. Arch Intern Med 1978;138:1214.
398. Zuckerman GR, Cornette GL, Clouse RE, Harter HR. Upper gastrointestinal bleeding in patients with chronic renal failure. Ann Intern Med 1985;102:588.
399. Balsov JT, Jorgensen NE. A survey of 499 patients with acute anuric renal insufficiency: causes, treatment, complications and mortality. Am J Med 1963;34:754.
400. Remuzzi G. Bleeding in renal failure. Lancet 1988;1:1205.
401. Shaw RE. Spontaneous rupture of the kidney. Br J Surg 1957;45:68.
402. Horner BA, Hunt JC, Kincaid OW, et al. Perirenal hematoma secondary to intrarenal microaneurysms of periarteritis nodosa demonstrated radiographically. Mayo Clin Proc 1966;41:169.
403. Link GS. Spontaneous bilateral perirenal hematoma. J Urol 1953;69:13.
404. Howalt JS, Squires JW. Spontaneous rupture of the kidney: a cause of atraumatic retroperitoneal bleeding. Am J Surg 1972;123:484.
405. Kjellstrand CM, Merino CE, Mauer SM, et al. Complications of percutaneous femoral vein catheterization for hemodialysis. Clin Nephrol 1975;4:37.
406. Symons HS, Wrong OM. Uremic pericarditis with cardiac tamponade: a report of four cases. Br Med J 1964;1:605.
407. Berger HW, Rammohan G, Neff MS, Buhain WJ. Uremic pleural effusion: a study in 14 patients on chronic dialysis. Ann Intern Med 1975;82:362.
408. Borra S, Kleinfield M. Subcapsular liver hematomas in a patient on chronic hemodialysis. Ann Intern Med 1980;93:574.
409. Pan A, Rogers AG, Pearlman D. Subdural hematoma complicating anticoagulant therapy. Can Med Assoc J 1960;82:1162.
410. Maher JF, Schreiner GE. Hazards and complications of dialysis. N Engl J Med 1966;272:370.
411. Bechar M, Lakke JP, Hem GK, et al. Subdural hematoma during long-term hemodialysis. Arch Neurol 1972;26:513.
412. Livio M, Benigni A, Vigano G, et al. Moderate doses of aspirin and risk of bleeding in renal failure. Lancet 1986;1:414.
413. Gaspari F, Vigano G, Orisio S, et al. Aspirin prolongs bleeding time in uremia by a mechanism distinct from platelet cyclooxygenase inhibition. J Clin Invest 1987;79:1788.
414. Lindsay RM, Moorthy AV, Koens F, Linton AL. Platelet function in dialyzed and non-dialyzed patients with chronic renal failure. Clin Nephrol 1975;4:52.
415. Evans EP, Branch RA, Bloom AL. A clinical and experimental study of platelet function in chronic renal failure. J Clin Pathol 1987;25:745.

416. Moosa A, Greaves M, Brown CB, MacNeil S. Elevated platelet-free calcium in uraemia. Br J Haematol 1990;74:300.
417. DiMinno G, Martinez J, McKean M-L, et al. Platelet dysfunction in uremia: multifaceted defect partially corrected by dialysis. Am J Med 1985;79:552.
418. Deykin D. Uremic bleeding. Kidney Int 1983;24:698.
419. Livio M, Benigni A, Remuzzi G. Coagulation abnormalities in uremia. Semin Nephrol 1985;5:82.
420. Horowitz HI. Uremic toxins and platelet function. Arch Intern Med 1970;126:823.
421. Rabiner SF. Bleeding in uremia. Med Clin North Am 1972;56:221.
422. Remuzzi G, Livio M, Marchiaro G, et al. Bleeding in renal failure: altered platelet function in chronic uraemia only partially corrected by haemodialysis. Nephron 1978;22:347.
423. Rao AK, Walsh PN. Acquired qualitative platelet disorders. Clin Haematol 1983;12:201.
424. Smith MC, Dunn MJ. Impaired platelet thromboxane production in renal failure. Nephron 1981;29:133.
425. Remuzzi G, Benigni A, Dodesini P, et al. Reduced platelet thromboxane formation in uremia: evidence for a functional cyclooxygenase defect. J Clin Invest 1983;71:762.
426. Fernandez F, Goudable C, Sie P, et al. Low hematocrit and prolonged bleeding time in uraemic patients: effect of red cell transfusions. Br J Haematol 1985;59:139.
427. Bloom A, Greaves M, Preston FE, Brown CB. Evidence against a platelet cyclooxygenase defect in uraemic subjects on chronic haemodialysis. Br J Haematol 1986;62:143.
428. Remuzzi G, Cavenaghi AE, Mecca G, et al. Prostacyclin-like activity and bleeding in renal failure. Lancet 1977;2:1195.
429. Leithner CH, Winter M, Silbauer K, et al. Enhanced prostacyclin availability of blood vessels in uraemic humans and rats. In: Robinson RHB, Hawkins JB, eds. Dialysis transplantation nephrology. Proceedings of the 15th Congress of European Dialysis and Transplant Association. Tunbridge Wells, Pitman Medical, 1978:418.
430. Defreyn G, Vergara Dauden M, Machin SJ, et al. A plasma factor in uraemia which stimulates prostacyclin release from cultured endothelial cells. Thromb Res 1980;19:695.
431. Kazatchikne M, Sultan Y, Caen JP, Bariety J. Bleeding in renal failure: a possible cause. Br Med J 1976;2:612.
432. Remuzzi G, Livio M, Roncaglioni MC, et al. Bleeding in renal failure: is von Willebrand factor implicated? Br Med J 1977;2:359.
433. Warrell RP, Hultin MB, Coller BS. Increased factor VIII/von Willebrand factor antigen and von Willebrand factor activity in renal failure. Am J Med 1979;66:226.
434. Zwaginga JJ, Ijsseldijk MJW, Beeser-Visser N, et al. High von Willebrand factor concentration compensates a relative adhesion defect in uremic blood. Blood 1990;75:1498.
435. Mannucci PM, Remuzzi G, Pusineri F, et al. Deamino-8-D-arginine vasopressin shortens the bleeding time in uremia. N Engl J Med 1983;308:8.
436. Gralnick HR, McKeown L, Williams S, et al. Plasma and platelet von Willebrand factor in uremia. Blood 1987;70:374A.
437. Gralnick HR, McKeown LP, Williams SB, et al. Plasma and platelet von Willebrand factor defects in uremia. Am J Med 1988;85:806.
438. Livio M, Marchesi D, Remuzzi G, et al. Uraemic bleeding: role of anaemia and beneficial effect of red cell transfusions. Lancet 1982;2:1013.
439. Moia M, Vizzotto L, Cattaneo M, et al. Improvement in the haemostatic defect on uraemia after treatment with recombinant human erythropoietin. Lancet 1987;2:1227.
440. Gordge MP, Leaker B, Patel A, et al. Recombinant human erythropoietin shortens the uraemic bleeding time without causing intravascular haemostatic activation. Thromb Res 1990;57:171.
441. Turitto VT, Weiss HJ. Red blood cells: their dual role in thrombus formation. Science 1980;207:541.
442. Turitto VT, Baumgartner HR. Platelet interaction with subendothelium in flowing rabbit blood: effects of blood shear rate. Microvasc Res 1979;17:38.
443. Glassman AB. Platelet abnormalities in hepatobiliary diseases. Ann Clin Lab Sci 1990;20:119.
444. Thomas DP. Abnormalities of platelet aggregation in patients with alcoholic cirrhosis. Ann NY Acad Sci 1972;201:243.
445. Ballard HS, Marcus AJ. Platelet aggregation in portal cirrhosis. Arch Intern Med 1976;136:316.
446. Jerushalmy Z, Zucker MB. Some effects of fibrinogen degradation products (FDP) on blood platelets. Thromb Diath Haemorrh 1966;15:413.
447. Stachurska J, Latallo Z, Kopec M. Inhibition of platelet aggregation by dialysable fibrinogen degradation products (FDP). Thromb Diath Haemorrh 1970;23:91.
448. Martinez J, Palascak JE, Kwasniak D. Abnormal sialic acid content of the dysfibrinogenemia associated with liver disease. J Clin Invest 1978;61:535.
449. Perkins HA, McKenzie MR, Fudenberg HH. Hemostatic defects in dysproteinemias. Blood 1970;35:695.
450. Saraya AK, Kasturi J, Kishan R. A study of haemostasis in macroglobulinaemia. Acta Haematol 1972;47:33.
451. DiMinno G, Coraggio F, Cerbone AM, et al. A myeloma paraprotein with specificity for platelet glycoprotein IIIa in a patient with a fatal bleeding disorder. J Clin Invest 1986;77:157.
452. Schafer AI. Bleeding and thrombosis in the myeloproliferative disorders. Blood 1984;64:1.
453. Mitchell MC, Boitnott JK, Kaufman S, et al. Budd-Chiari syndrome: etiology, diagnosis and management. Medicine 1982;61:199.
454. Valla D, Casadevall N, Lacombe C, et al. Primary myeloproliferative disorder and hepatic vein thrombosis: a prospective study of erythroid colony formation in vitro in 20 patients with Budd-Chiari syndrome. Ann Intern Med 1985;103:329.
455. Valla D, Casadevall N, Huisse MG, et al. Etiology of portal vein thrombosis in adults: a prospective evaluation of primary myeloproliferative disorders. Gastroenterology 1988;94:1063.
456. Jabaily J, Iland HJ, Laszlo J, et al. Neurologic manifestations of essential thrombocythemia. Ann Intern Med 1983;99:513.
457. Mitchell SW. On a rare vaso-motor neurosis of the extremities, and on the maladies with which it may be confounded. Am J Med Sci 1878;76:2.
458. Michiels JJ, ten Kate FWJ, Vuzevski VD, et al. Histopathology of erythromelalgia in thrombocythaemia. Histopathology 1984;8:669.
459. Michiels JJ, Abels J, Steketee J, et al. Erythromelalgia caused by platelet-mediated arteriolar inflammation and thrombosis in thrombocythemia. Ann Intern Med 1985;102:466.
460. Mitus AJ, Schafer AI. Thrombocytosis and thrombocythemia. Hematol Oncol Clin North Am, 1990;4:157.
461. Murphy S, Davis JL, Walsh PN, et al. Template bleeding time and clinical hemorrhage in myeloproliferative disease. Arch Intern Med 1978;138:1251.
462. Boneu B, Nouvel C, Sie P, et al. Platelets in myeloproliferative disorders. I. A comparative evaluation with certain platelet function tests. Scand J Haematol 1980;25:214.
463. Barbui T, Cortelazzo S, Viero P, et al. Thrombohaemorrhagic complications in 101 cases of myeloproliferative disorders: relationship to platelet number and function. Eur J Cancer Clin Oncol 1983;19:1593.
464. Waddell CC, Brown JA, Repinecz YA. Abnormal platelet function in myeloproliferative disorders. Arch Pathol Lab Med 1981;105:432.
465. Wu KK-Y. Platelet hyperaggregability and thrombosis in patients with thrombocythemia. Ann Intern Med 1978;88:7.
466. Kaywin P, McDonough M, Insel PA, et al. Platelet function in essential thrombocythemia: decreased epinephrine responsiveness associated with a deficiency of platelet α-adrenergic receptors. N Engl J Med 1978;299:505.
467. Cooper B, Ahern D. Characterization of the platelet prostaglandin D_2 receptors in platelets of patients with myeloproliferative disorder. J Clin Invest 1979;64:586.
468. Moore A, Nachman RL. Platelet Fc receptor: increased expression in myeloproliferative disease. J Clin Invest 1981;67:1064.
469. Bolin RB, Okumura T, Jamieson GA. Changes in distribution of platelet membrane glycoproteins in patients with myeloproliferative disorders. Am J Hematol 1977;3:63.
470. Semeraro N, Cortellazzo S, Colucci M, et al. A hitherto undescribed defect of platelet coagulant activity in polycythaemia vera and essential thrombocythaemia. Thromb Res 1979;16:795.
471. Russell NH, Salmon J, Keenan JP, et al. Platelet adenine nucleotides and arachidonic acid metabolism in the myeloproliferative disorders. Thromb Res 1981;22:389.
472. Pareti FI, Gugliotta L, Mannucci L, et al. Biochemical and metabolic aspects of platelet dysfunction in chronic myeloproliferative disorders. Thromb Haemost 1982;47:84.
473. Luzzatto G, Fabris F, Mazzucato M, Girolami A. PF_4 versus βTG as evidence of platelet activation in myeloproliferative disorders. Scand J Haematol 1985;35:299.
474. Boughton BJ, Corbett WEN, Ginsburg AD. Myeloproliferative disorders: a paradox of *in-vivo* and *in-vitro* platelet function. J Clin Pathol 1977;30:228.
475. Okuma M, Uchino H. Altered arachidonate metabolism by platelets in patients with myeloproliferative disorders. Blood 1979;54:1258.
476. Schafer AI. Deficiency of platelet lipoxygenase activity in myeloproliferative disorders. N Engl J Med 1982;306:381.
477. Budde V, Schaefer G, Mueller N, et al. Acquired von Willebrand's disease in the myeloproliferative syndrome. Blood 1984;64:981.
478. Raman BKS, Sawdyk M, Saeed SM. Essential thrombocythemia with acquired von Willebrand's disease. Am J Clin Pathol 1987;88:102.
479. Sato K. Plasma von Willebrand factor abnormalities in patients with essential thrombocythemia. Keio J Med 1988;37:54.
480. Baker RI, Manoharan A. Platelet function in myeloproliferative disorders: characterization and sequential studies show multiple platelet abnormalities, and change with time. Eur J Haematol 1988;40:267.
481. Kessler CM, Klein HG, Havlik RJ. Uncontrolled thrombocytosis in chronic myeloproliferative disorders. Br J Haematol 1982;50:157.
482. Lahuerta-Palacios JJ, Bornstein R, Fernandez-Debora FJ, et al. Controlled and uncontrolled thrombocytosis: its clinical role in essential thrombocythemia. Cancer 1988;61:1207.
483. Tartaglia AP, Goldberg JD, Berk PD, et al. Adverse effects of antiaggregating platelet therapy in the treatment of polycythemia vera. Semin Hematol 1986;23:172.

484. Barbui T, Buelli M, Cortelazzo S, et al. Aspirin and risk of bleeding in patients with thrombocythemia. Am J Med 1987;83:265.
485. FitzGerald GA. Dipyridamole. N Engl J Med 1987;316:1247.
486. Dale J, Myhre E, Rostwelt K. Effects of dipyridamole and acetylsalicylic acid on platelet functions in patients with aortic ball-valve prosthesis. Am Heart J 1975;89:613.
487. Weiss HJ. Platelets: pathophysiology and antiplatelet drug therapy. New York, Alan R Liss, 1982.
488. Emmons PR, Harrison MJG, Honour AJ, Mitchell JRA. Effect of dipyridamole on human platelet behaviour. Lancet 1965;2:603.
489. Sullivan JM, Kagnoff MF, Gorlin R. Reduction of platelet-adhesiveness in patients with coronary artery disease. Am J Med Sci 1968;255: 292.
490. Rajah SM, Crow MJ, Perry AF, et al. The effects of dipyridamole on platelet function: correlation with blood levels in man. Br J Clin Pharmacol 1979;4:129.
491. Weiss HJ, Turitto FT, Vicic WJ, Baumgartner HR. Effect of aspirin and dipyridamole on the interaction of human platelets with subendothelium: studies using citrated and native blood. Thromb Haemost 1981;45: 136.
492. Graves HM, Kinlough-Rathbone RL, Cazenave J-P, et al. Effect of dipyridamole and prostacyclin on rabbit platelet adherence in vitro and in vivo. J Lab Clin Med 1982;99:548.
493. Ritchie JL, Harker LA. Platelet and fibrinogen survival in coronary atherosclerosis: response to medial and surgical therapy. Am J Cardiol 1977;39:595.
494. Harker LA, Slichter SJ. Platelet and fibrinogen consumption in man. N Engl J Med 1972;287:999.
495. Genton E, Ellis J, Steele P. Comparative effects of platelet suppressant drugs on platelet survival time. Thromb Diath 1975;34:522.
496. Webster J, Douglas AS. Aspirin and other antiplatelet drugs in the prophylaxis of thrombosis. Blood Reviews 1987;1:9.
497. Masotti G, Poggesi L, Galanti G, Neri Serneri GG. Stimulation of prostacyclin by dipyridamole. Lancet 1979;1:1412.
498. Blass K-E, Block H-U, Forster W, Ponicke K. Dipyridamole: a potent stimulator of prostacyclin (PGI_2) biosynthesis. Br J Pharmacol 1980;68: 71.
499. Boeynaems JM, Van Coevorden A, Demolle D. Dipyridamole and vascular prostacyclin production. Biochem Pharmacol 1986;35:2897.
500. Moncada S, Korbut R. Dipyridamole and other phosphodiesterase inhibitors act as anti-thrombotic agents by potentiating endogenous prostacyclin. Lancet 1978;1:1286.
501. Mills DCB, Smith JB. The influence on platelet aggregation of drugs that affect the accumulation of adenosine 3′:5′-cyclic monophosphate in platelets. Biochem J 1971;121:185.
502. Tsien W-H, Sheppard H. The lack of correlation between inhibition of platelet aggregation and cAMP levels. Fed Proc 1981;40:809.
503. Gresele P, Arnout J, Deckmyn H, Vermylen J. Mechanism of the antiplatelet action of dipyridamole in whole blood: modulation of adenosine concentration and activity. Thromb Haemost 1986;55:12.
504. Crutchley DJ, Ryan US, Ryan JW. Effects of aspirin and dipyridamole on the degradation of adenosine diphosphate by cultured cells derived from bovine pulmonary artery. J Clin Invest 1980;66:29.
505. Margulies EH, White AM, Sherry S. Sulfinpyrazone: a review of its pharmacological properties and therapeutic use. Drugs 1980;20:179.
506. Steele P, Carrol J, Overfield D, Genton E. Effect of sulfinpyrazone on platelet survival time in patients with transient cerebral ischemic attacks. Stroke 1977;8:396.
507. Steele P, Weily HS, Davies H, Genton E. Platelet survival in patients with rheumatic disease. N Engl J Med 1974;290:537.
508. Ali M, McDonald JWD. Effects of sulphinpyrazone on platelet prostaglandin synthesis and platelet release of serotonin. J Lab Clin Med 1977;89:868.
509. FitzGerald GA, Oates JA, Hawiger J, et al. Endogenous biosynthesis of prostacyclin and thromboxane and platelet function during chronic administration of aspirin in man. J Clin Invest 1983;71:676.
510. Chignard M, Wal F, Lefort J, Vargaftig BB. Inhibition by sulphinpyrazone of the platelet-dependent bronchoconstriction due to platelet-activating factor (PAF-acether) in the guinea-pig. Eur J Pharmacol 1982;78:71.
511. Di Minno G, Cerbone AM, Mattioli PL. Functionally thrombasthenic state in normal platelets following the administration of ticlopidine. J Clin Invest 1985;75:328.
512. Gachet C, Savi P, Ohlmann P, Maffrand JP, Jakobs KH, Cazenave JP. ADP receptor–induced activation of guanine nucleotide binding proteins in rat platelet membranes: an effect selectively blocked by the thienopyridine clopidogrel. Thromb Hemost 1992;68:79.
513. Mills DC, Puri R, Hu CJ, et al. Clopidogrel inhibits the binding of ADP analogues to the receptor, mediating inhibition of adenylate cyclase. Arterioscler Thromb 1992;12:430.
514. Brown CH III, Bradshaw MW, Natelson EA, et al. Defective platelet function following the administration of penicillin compounds. Blood 1976;47:949.
515. Andrassy K, Ritz E, Hasper B, et al. Penicillin-induced coagulation disorder. Lancet 1976;2:1039.
516. Cazenave JP, Guccione MA, Packham MA, Mustard JF. Effects of cephalothin and penicillin G on platelet function in vitro. Br J Haematol 1977;35:135.
517. Brown CH III, Natelson EA, Bradshaw MW, et al. The hemostatic defect produced by carbenicillin. N Engl J Med 1974;291:265.
518. Haburchak DR, Head DR, Everett ED. Postoperative hemorrhage associated with carbenicillin administration: report of two cases and review of the literature. Am J Surg 1977;134:630.
519. Brown CH III, Natelson EA, Bradshaw MW. A study of the effects of ticarcillin on blood coagulation and platelet function. Antimicrob Agents Chemother 1975;7:652.
520. Gentry LO, Jemsek JG, Natelson EA. Effects of sodium piperacillin on platelet function in normal volunteers. Antimicrob Agents Chemother 1981;19:532.
521. Pakter RL, Russell TR, Mielke CH, West D. Coagulopathy associated with the use of moxalactam. JAMA 1982;248:1100.
522. Weitekamp MR, Aber RC. Prolonged bleeding times and bleeding diathesis associated with moxalactam administration. JAMA 1983;1:249.
523. Rossi EC, Levin NW. Inhibition of primary ADP-induced platelet aggregation in normal subjects after administration of nitrofurantoin (Furadantin). J Clin Invest 1973;52:2457.
524. Carter AE, Eban R, Perrett RD. Prevention of postoperative deep venous thrombosis and pulmonary embolism. Br Med J 1971;1:312.
525. Cazenave JP, Packham MA, Guccione MA, Mustard JF. Effects of penicillin G on platelet aggregation, release and adherence to collagen. Proc Soc Exp Biol Med 1973;142:159.
526. Johnson GJ, Rao GHR. Platelet dysfunction induced by parenteral carbenicillin and ticarcillin. Am J Pathol 1978;91:85.
527. Shattil SJ, Bennett JS, McDonough M, Turnbull J. Carbenicillin and penicillin G inhibit platelet function in vitro by impairing the interaction of agonists with the platelet surface. J Clin Invest 1980;65:329.
528. Burroughs SF, Johnson GJ. β-Lactam antibiotic-induced platelet dysfunction: evidence for irreversible inhibition of platelet activation in vitro and in vivo after prolonged exposure to penicillin. Blood 1990;75: 1473.
529. Frishman WH, Weksler B, Christodoulo JB, et al. Reversal of abnormal platelet aggregability and change in exercise tolerance in patients with angina pectoris. Circulation 1974;50:887.
530. Leon R, Tiarks CY, Pechet L. Some observations on the *in vitro* effect of propranolol on platelet aggregation and release. Am J Hematol 1978;5: 117.
531. Weksler BB, Gillik M, Pink J. Effect of propranolol on platelet function. Blood 1977;49:185.
532. Dachary-Prugent J, Dufourcq J, Lusson C, Boisseau M. Propranolol, chlorpromazine and platelet membrane: a fluorescence study of the drug-membrane interaction. Thromb Res 1979;14:15.
533. Hawiger J, White RB. Propranolol and prostacyclin inhibit human platelet phospholipase A-induced release of arachidonic acid. Circulation 1978;58:II-138.
534. Vanderhoek JY, Feinstein MB. Local anesthetics, chlorpromazine and propranolol inhibit stimulus-activation of phospholipase A_2 in human platelets. Mol Pharmacol 1979;16:171.
535. Langdell RD, Adelson EA, Furth FW. Dextran and prolonged bleeding time. JAMA 1958;166:346.
536. Weiss HJ. The effect of clinical dextran on platelet aggregation, adhesion and ADP release in man: in vivo and in vitro studies. J Lab Clin Med 1967;69:37.
537. Evans RJ, Gordon JL. Mechanism of the antithrombotic action of dextran. N Engl J Med 1974;290:748.
538. Zucker MB. Heparin and platelet function. Fed Proc 1977;36:47.
539. Salzman EW, Rosenberg RD, Smith MH, et al. Effect of heparin and heparin fractions on platelet aggregation. J Clin Invest 1980;65:64.
540. Dalsgaard-Nielsen J, Risbo A, Simmelkjaer P, Gormsen J. Impaired platelet aggregation and increased bleeding time during general anaesthesia with halsthane. Br J Anaesth 1981;53:1039.
541. Jain MF, Eskow E, Kuchibhotla J, Colman RW. Correlation of inhibition of platelet aggregation by phenothiazines and local anesthetics with their effects on a phospholipid bilayer. Thromb Res 1978;13:1067.
542. White GC, Raynor ST. The effects of trifluoroperazine, an inhibitor of calmodulin on platelet function. Thromb Res 1980;18:279.
543. Warlow C, Ogston D, Douglas AS. Platelet function after administration of chlorpromazine to human subjects. Haemostasis 1976;5:21.
544. Green D, Tsao CH, Cerullo L, et al. Clinical and laboratory investigation of the effects of epsilon-aminocaproic acid on hemostasis. J Lab Clin Med 1985;105:321.
545. Bengmark S, Elmer O, Garansson G, Zoucas E. In vitro effect of ethanol on ADP and collagen-induced platelet aggregation. Thromb Haemost 1981;46:673.
546. Baghurst KI, Raj MJ, Truswell AS. Onions and platelet aggregation. Lancet 1977;1:101.
547. Phillips C, Poyser NL. Inhibition of platelet aggregation by onion extracts. Lancet 1978;1:1051.
548. Makheja AN, Vanderhoek JY, Bailey JM. Inhibition of platelet aggregation and thromboxane synthesis by onion and garlic. Lancet 1979;1: 781.
549. Hammerschmidt DE. Szechwan purpura. N Engl J Med 1980;302:1191.
550. Steiner M, Anastasi J. Vitamin E: an inhibitor of the platelet release reaction. J Clin Invest 1976;57:732.
551. Slichter SJ. Platelet transfusion therapy. Hematol Oncol Clin North Am 1990;4:291.

552. Ratnoff OD. Some therapeutic agents influencing hemostasis. In: Colman RW, Hirsh J, Marder VJ, Salzman EW, eds. Hemostasis and thrombosis. Philadelphia, JB Lippincott, 1987:1026.
553. Degos L, Dautigny A, Brouet JC, et al. A molecular defect in thrombasthenic platelets. J Clin Invest 1975;56:236.
554. Brown CH, Weisberg RJ, Natelson EA, Alfrey CP Jr. Glanzmann's thrombasthenia: assessment of the response to platelet transfusions. Transfusion 1975;15:124.
555. Sundqvist S-B, Nilsson IM, Svanberg L, Cronberg S. Pregnancy and parturition in a patient with severe Glanzmann's thrombasthenia. Scand J Haematol 1981;27:159.
556. Degos L, Tobelem G, Lethielleaux P, et al. Molecular defect in platelets from patients with Bernard-Soulier syndrome. Blood 1977;50:899.
557. Tobelem G, Levy-Toledano S, Nurden AT, et al. Further studies on a specific platelet antibody found in Bernard-Soulier syndrome and its effects on normal platelet function. Br J Haematol 1979;41:427.
558. Sahud MA, Aggeler PM. Platelet dysfunction: differentiation of a newly recognized primary type from that produced by aspirin. N Engl J Med 1969;280:453.
559. Locke HR, Hathaway WE, Feiler F, Dawson DL. Preoperative correction of a platelet functional disorder. Ann Intern Med 1973;78:972.
560. Khurana MS, Lian EC-Y, Harkness DR. "Storage pool disease" of platelets: association with multiple congenital cavernous hemangiomas. JAMA 1980;244:169.
561. Zucker S, Mielke CH, Durocher JR, Crosby WH. Oozing and bruising due to abnormal platelet function (thrombocytopathia). Ann Intern Med 1972;76:725.
562. Mielke CH, Levine PH, Zucker S. Preoperative prednisone therapy in platelet function disorders. Thromb Res 1981;21:655.
563. Caen JP, Castaldi PA, Leclerc JC. Congenital bleeding disorders with long bleeding time and normal platelet count. I. Glanzmann's thrombasthenia: report of fifteen patients. Am J Med 1966;41:4.
564. Thong KK, Mant MJ, Grace MG. Lack of effect of prednisone administration on bleeding time and platelet function of normal subjects. Br J Haematol 1978;38:373.
565. Janson PA, Jubelirer SJ, Weinstein MJ, Deykin D. Treatment of the bleeding tendency in uremia with cryoprecipitate. N Engl J Med 1980;303:1318.
566. Maierhoter W, Adams MB, Kleinman JG, Roth DA. Treatment of the bleeding tendency in uremia with cryoprecipitate. N Engl J Med 1981;305:645.
567. Liu YK, Kosfeld RE, Marcum SG. Treatment of uraemic bleeding with conjugated oestrogen. Lancet 1984;2:887.
568. Gerritsen SW, Akkerman J-WN, Sixma JJ. Correction of the bleeding time in patients with storage pool deficiency by infusion of cryoprecipitate. Br J Haematol 1978;40:153.
569. Scialla S, Kachline D, Decker P. Shortening of the bleeding time with cryoprecipitate in patients with liver dysfunction. (Abstract) Clin Res 1982;30:691A.
570. Mannucci PM. Desmopressin: a nontransfusional form of treatment for congenital and acquired bleeding disorders. Blood 1988;72:1449.
571. Cash JD, Gader AMA, DaCosta J. The release of plasminogen activator and factor VIII by LVP, AVP, DDAVP, AT III, and OT in man. Br J Haematol 1974;27:363.
572. Mannucci PM, Pareti FI, Holmberg L, et al. Studies on the prolonged bleeding time in von Willebrand disease. J Lab Clin Med 1976;88:662.
573. Mannucci PM, Ruggeri ZM, Pareti FI, Capitanio A. DDAVP: a new pharmacological approach to the management of hemophilia and von Willebrand disease. Lancet 1977;1:689.
574. Warrier I, Lusher JM. DDAVP: a useful alternative to blood components in moderate hemophilia A and von Willebrand's disease. J Pediatr 1983;102:228.
575. Mariani C, Ciaverella N, Mazzucconi MG, et al. Evaluation of the effectiveness of DDAVP in surgery and bleeding episodes in hemophilia and von Willebrand's disease: a study of 43 patients. Clin Lab Haematol 1984;6:229.
576. De La Fuente B, Kasper CK, Rickles FR, Hoyer LW. Response of patients with mild and moderate hemophilia A and von Willebrand disease to treatment with desmopressin. Ann Intern Med 1985;103:6.
577. Watson AJS, Koegh JAB. Effect of l-deamino-8-D-arginine vasopressin on the prolonged bleeding time in chronic renal failure. Nephron 1982;32:49.
578. Mannucci PM, Remuzzi G, Pusineri F, et al. Deamino-8-D-arginine vasopressin shortens the bleeding time in uremia. N Engl J Med 1983;308:8.
579. Gotti E, Mecca G, Valentino C, et al. Renal biopsy in patients with acute renal failure and prolonged bleeding time. Lancet 1984;2:978.
580. Canavese C, Salomone M, Pacitti A, et al. Reduced response of uremic bleeding time to repeated doses of desmopressin. Lancet 1985;1:867.
581. Kobrinsky NL, Israel ED, Gerrard JM, et al. Shortening of bleeding time by 1-deamino-8-D-arginine vasopressin in various bleeding disorders. Lancet 1984;1:1145.
582. Mannucci PM, Vicente V, Vianello L, et al. Controlled trial of desmopressin (DDAVP) in liver cirrhosis and other conditions associated with a prolonged bleeding time. Blood 1986;67:1148.
583. Schulman S, Johnsson H, Egberg N, Blomback M. DDAVP-induced correction of prolonged bleeding time in patients with congenital platelet function defects. Thromb Res 1987;45:165.
584. Nieuwenhuis HK, Sixma JJ. 1-Deamino-8-D-arginine vasopressin (desmopressin) shortens the bleeding time in storage pool deficiency. Ann Intern Med 1988;108:65.
585. Kentro TB, Lottenberg R, Kitchens CS. Clinical efficacy of desmopressin acetate for hemostatic control in patients with primary platelet disorders undergoing surgery. Am J Hematol 1987;24:215.
586. Burroughs AK, Matthews K, Qadiri M, et al. Desmopressin and bleeding time in patients with cirrhosis. Br Med J 1985;291:1377.
587. Kobrinsky NL, Letts RP, Patel RL, et al. DDAVP shortens the bleeding time and decreases the blood loss in hemostatically normal subjects undergoing spinal fusion surgery. Ann Intern Med 1987;107:446.
588. Salzman EW, Weinstein MJ, Weintraub RM, et al. Treatment with desmopressin acetate to reduce blood loss after cardiac surgery. N Engl J Med 1986;314:1402.
589. Rocha E, Llorens R, Paramo JA, et al. Does desmopressin acetate reduce blood loss after surgery in patients on cardiopulmonary bypass? Circulation 1988;77:1319.
590. Czer LSC, Bateman TM, Gray RJ, et al. Treatment of severe platelet dysfunction and hemorrhage after cardiopulmonary bypass: reduction in blood product usage with desmopressin. J Am Coll Cardiol 1987;9:1139.
591. Hackmann T, Gascoyne RD, Naiman SC, et al. A trial of desmopressin (1-desamino-8-D-arginine vasporessin) to reduce blood loss in uncomplicated cardiac surgery. N Engl J Med 1989;321:1437.
592. Anderson TL, Solem JD, Tengborn L, Vinge E. Effects of desmopressin on platelet aggregation, von Willebrand factor, and blood loss after cardiac surgery with extracorporeal circulation. Circulation 1990;81:872.
593. Hedderich GS, Petsikas DJ, Cooper BA, et al. Desmopressin acetate in uncomplicated coronary artery bypass surgery: a prospective randomized clinical trial. Can J Surg 1990;33:33.
594. De Sio L, Mariani G, Mazzucconi MG, et al. Comparison between subcutaneous and intravenous DDAVP in mild and moderate hemophilia A. Thromb Haemost 1985;54:387.
595. Mannucci PM, Vicente V, Alberca I, et al. Intravenous and subcutaneous administration of desmopressin (DDAVP) to hemophiliacs: pharmacokinetics and factor VIII responses. Thromb Haemost 1987;58:1037.
596. Mannucci PM, Canciani MT, Rota L, Donovan BS. Response of factor VIII/von Willebrand factor to DDAVP in healthy subjects and patients with hemophilia A and von Willebrand's disease. Br J Haematol 1981;47:283.
597. Lethagen S, Harris AS, Sjorin E, Nilsson IM. Intranasal and intravenous administration of desmopressin: effect of F VIII/VWF pharmacokinetics and reproducibility. Thromb Haemost 1987;58:1033.
598. Mannucci PM. Desmopressin (DDAVP) for treatment of disorders of hemostasis. Prog Hemost Thromb 1986;8:19.
599. Canavese C, Salomone M, Pacitti A, et al. Reduced response of uremic bleeding time to repeated doses of desmopressin. Lancet 1985;1:867.
600. Mannucci PM, Ruggeri ZM, Pareti FI, Capitanio AM. DDAVP in hemophilia. Lancet 1977;2:1171.
601. Lowe J, Pettigrew A, Middleton S, et al. DDAVP in hemophilia. Lancet 1977;2:614.
602. Mathias CJ, Fosbraey P, da Costa DF, et al. The effect of desmopressin on nocturnal polyuria, overnight weight loss and morning postural hypotension in patients with autonomic failure. Br Med J 1986;293:353.
603. Bond L, Bevan D. Myocardial infarction in a patient with hemophilia treated with DDAVP. N Engl J Med 1988;318:121.
604. Byrnes JJ, Larcada A, Moake JL. Thrombosis following desmopressin for uremic bleeding. Am J Hematol 1988;28:63.
605. Livio M, Mannucci PM, Vigano G, et al. Conjugated estrogens for the management of bleeding associated with renal failure. N Engl J Med 1986;315:731.

Blood: Principles and Practice of Hematology,
edited by Robert I. Handin, Samuel E. Lux, and Thomas P. Stossel.
J.B. Lippincott Company, Philadelphia © 1995.

38

The Contact System and Its Disorders

Michael Silverberg
Sesha R. Reddigari
Allen P. Kaplan

When blood is drawn into a clean glass tube, it rapidly clots. If the tube is coated with silicone or is made of plastic, clotting is delayed. This interaction of a group of plasma proteins with the negatively charged surface of clean glass to initiate blood coagulation is known as *contact activation*. The coagulation pathway activated by this mechanism is termed *intrinsic* because all the protein factors required for clotting are found in the plasma; this is in contrast to the *extrinsic* pathway, which requires the exposure of plasma to cell-surface tissue factor for clotting to occur. Factor X activation is conventionally depicted as the site of the branch point between the intrinsic and extrinsic coagulation pathways.

The protein components of the contact system have been identified through the discovery of persons with abnormal clotting times that resulted from a deficiency of one of the components. The pathway has been shown to consist of a complex loop of interactions in which two zymogens—factor XII (Hageman factor) and prekallikrein (Fletcher factor)—become activated to trypsin-like proteases in the presence of the nonenzymatic cofactor high-molecular-weight (HMW) kininogen and an appropriate surface (Fig. 38-1). This complex trimolecular reaction is the first step in the intrinsic coagulation cascade, and all three proteins are clotting factors. The intrinsic coagulation pathway is then activated through the action of activated factor XII on factor XI. As a result, factor XI becomes activated and a series of additional conversions of proenzyme to enzyme leads to the formation of thrombin and the conversion of fibrinogen to fibrin to form a clot.

In addition, kallikrein, which is also formed during the contact phase, generates bradykinin by digestion of HMW kininogen; bradykinin is a nine–amino acid vasoactive peptide, which is an important component of the body's inflammatory response. Other activities that are dependent on the activation of factor XII have also been identified. These are weak fibrinolytic activity, the activation of prorenin to renin, and interactions with the complement system and cellular components of the blood.

Although all these pathways have been described and characterized in vitro, the physiologic functioning of the contact activation system remains obscure in several aspects. Thus, despite profound prolongation of the activated partial thromboplastin time (APTT), none of the persons described with deficiencies has a bleeding diathesis except those with a deficiency of factor XI. This deficit causes a varying and usually mild form of hemophilia. Similarly, the role of bradykinin in the inflammatory process has not been clearly defined. This may change now that kinin antagonists are available for experimental studies.

The application of the methods of modern molecular biology has resulted in the determination of the amino acid sequences of all of the proteins of the contact system as well as in the elucidation of their gene structures. The most surprising aspect of these results has been the close evolutionary relationship between the enzymes of the contact system and the fibrinolytic enzymes, urokinase and tissue plasminogen activator (tPA).

FACTOR XII

Biochemistry

Properties of Zymogen

Factor XII (Hageman factor) circulates as a single-chain zymogen with no detectable enzymatic activity. The zymogen migrates as a β-globulin, and its apparent molecular weight is 80 kd on SDS gel electrophoresis.[1] When a reducing agent is omitted, the apparent molecular weight is lower, implying that the intact disulfide bonds maintain the protein in a more compact, possibly globular, structure. Hageman factor is synthesized in the liver and circulates in normal plasma at a concentration of 30 to 35 μg/mL.[1] This number implies that the specific clotting activity of purified factor XII, referred to normal plasma defined as having one unit per milliliter, should be about 28 to 35 U/mg. In practice, investigators have reported values ranging from 40 to as high as 80 U/mg. The reason for this discrepancy is not known. Other physical and chemical data are listed in Table 38-1.

Mechanism of Activation

Factor XII zymogen has no enzymatic activity against synthetic oligopeptide substrates, nor does it react with specific inhibitors.[2] During contact activation of normal human plasma, it is converted into a functional serine protease by kallikrein in the presence of HMW kininogen.[3–5] This reaction is contingent on the introduction of a polyanionic substance (see section on HMW kininogen). Purified factor

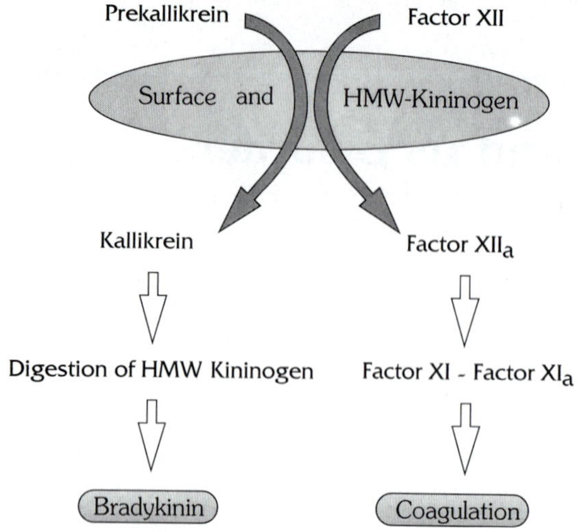

FIGURE 38-1. The factor XII–dependent pathways of contact activation.

XII can be activated by kallikrein in vitro in the absence of HMW kininogen.[6] The rate of this reaction is accelerated by polyanionic substances, apparently through the induction of a favorable conformation for cleavage by the binding of the factor XII zymogen to the polyanion.[7,8]

A second reaction observed in vitro is the autoactivation of factor XII, which occurs as the polyanion-catalyzed activation of factor XII zymogen by factor XIIa.[9] This reaction is much slower than the activation by kallikrein, but may be responsible for the increase in the clotting activity of prekallikrein-deficient plasma when the contact time is prolonged.[8]

Activation of factor XII by kallikrein gives a series of active enzymes formed by successive cleavages. The first cleavage to produce factor XIIa from factor XII[5] occurs within a disulfide bond and thus yields a two-chain disulfide-linked molecule with the new amino-terminal sequence of Val-Val-Gly.[10] The newly formed factor XIIa retains the 80 kd of the zymogen, but on reduced SDS gels is seen to be composed of a heavy chain of 50 kd and a light chain of 28 kd. The light chain contains the catalytic domain and is derived from the carboxy-terminal region of the zymogen, whereas the heavy chain, which contains the surface binding region, is derived from the amino-terminal region.[11] Further cleavage can occur in the heavy chain to produce a series of fragments of activated factor XII, all of which retain enzymatic activity.[12,13]

The most prominent cleavage product of factor XIIa is the 30-kd species termed *factor XIIf*. Careful examination of the bands obtained on SDS gel electrophoresis in the absence of reducing agent indicated that a doublet is seen and that the band of higher molecular weight is converted to one of lower molecular weight at about 28.5 kd.[13] Reduced gels of high acrylamide content show that these species are made up of the light chain of factor XIIa and a small fragment of the original heavy chain.

A minor cleavage product formed from factor XIIa is a 40 kd species, which represents cleavage of factor XIIa into two half-molecules. The C-terminal half is composed of the 28-kd serine protease moiety linked by a disulfide bridge to a portion of 12 to 15 kd. When the activation is accomplished by factor XIIa (autoactivation), the 40-kd fragments are produced in much greater proportion than when factor XII is digested by kallikrein.[13]

Function of Activated Molecule

The activated forms of factor XII are trypsin-like serine proteases. When assayed with low molecular weight substrates, they show a strong preference for cleavage at the carboxy terminal of arginine residues. Kinetic data have been obtained with a number of tripeptide and tetrapeptide substrates and inhibitors.[14] In all cases, factor XIIa and factor XIIf show identical kinetics with low molecular weight compounds.

The major macromolecular substrates for factor XIIa are prekallikrein and factor XI. In addition, factor XII is a substrate in the autoactivation reaction,[9] and since prolonged incubation gives rise to the series of fragments described above,[12] factor XIIa must be able to further cleave the heavy chain. Factor XIIf cleaves prekallikrein in the fluid phase,[16–18] but does not readily cleave factor XI and so is not a procoagulant enzyme.[19] Thus, in clotting assays, factor XIIf has only 2% to 4% of the activity of factor XIIa.[20] Similarly, factor XIIf does not activate factor XII zymogen.[9] The lack of activity against these two substrates must reflect the absence of the surface-binding site that is found in the heavy chain. We can envisage, therefore, that during contact activation, surface-bound factor XIIa becomes cleaved to factor XIIf, which, free of the surface-binding domain, can diffuse away and promote kinin generation by activation of prekallikrein at sites distant from the original activation site.[11] Perhaps the heavy chain is left to compete for binding to the surface and could serve to limit further activation.

Factor XIIf can also activate the first component of complement[21] and factor VII, a critical component of the intrinsic pathway.[22] In addition, factor XIIa has been reported to aggregate neutrophils and cause degranulation.[23] The physiologic significance, if any, of these activities is not known.

The role of plasma inhibitors in regulating the activity of activated factor XII is discussed in the section on initiation and regulation of the contact activation system. Several inhibitors are useful for in vitro studies; these are listed in Table 38-2.

TABLE 38-1. Physical and Chemical Data

Protein	Factor XII	Prekallikrein	Factor XI	High-Molecular-Weight Kininogen
Molecular weight (daltons; calculated)	80,427	79,545	140,000	116,643
Carbohydrate (w/w)	16.8%	15%	5%	40%
Isoelectric point	6.3	8.7	8.6	4.7
Extinction coefficient ($E^{1\%}_{280/nm}$)	14.2	11.7	13.4	7.0
Plasma concentration				
μg/mL	30–45	35–50	4–6	70–90
nmol/L (average)	400	534	36	686

TABLE 38-2. **Inhibitors Useful in Studies of Contact Activation***

Inhibitor	Factor XIIa	Kallikrein
Pancreatic or lung trypsin inhibitor (aprotinin)	−	+
Soybean trypsin inhibitor	−	+
Lima bean trypsin inhibitor	+	−
Corn inhibitor	+	−
Peptide chloromethyl ketones†		
phe-phe-arg	+	+++
phe-pro-arg	+	+
pro-phe-arg	+	++
dansyl-glu-gly-arg	+	−
p-Amidino phenylmethylsulfonyl fluoride	+	+
Diisopropyl fluorophosphate	+	+

* Kinetic constants are not given since, even when known, they depend on conditions of buffer, ionic strength, pH, and so on.
† Chloromethyl ketones are listed in order of reactivity with factor XIIa.[14] Where quantitative measurements[14,15] have indicated that kallikrein is much more reactive than factor XIIa, it is indicated by ++ or +++.

Structure

The Protein

The primary structure of factor XII is known from analysis of complementary DNA isolated from human liver cDNA libraries[24,25] and from direct protein sequence data.[10,26] The mature protein has a sequence of 596 amino acids; the molecular weight is 66,915 daltons excluding carbohydrate. Together with the measured carbohydrate content of 16.8%, the total predicted molecular weight is 80,427 daltons.

The amino-terminal heavy-chain region of the protein shows extensive homologies with other proteins. In particular, distinct domains bear strong homology with characteristic domains of fibronectin, plasminogen, and plasminogen activators (Fig. 38-2). The immediate amino-terminal region is homologous with the type II "finger" region of fibronectin; residues 13 to 69 share about 40% homology with the two fibronectin sequences. These sequences in fibronectin are probably involved in collagen binding. Two regions (residues 79 to 111 and 159 to 190) of the sequence are homologous with epidermal growth factor sequences found in a number of proteins including tPA and several other clotting factors. These regions are separated by a region (residues 116 to 151) bearing limited homology with the type I finger region of fibronectin. The final recognizable domain of the heavy-chain region is an 83-residue "kringle" (193 to 276) as found in prothrombin, plasminogen, and the plasminogen activators. This structure is characterized by six invariant half-cystines giving a characteristic pattern of three disulfide bridges. The kringle region of the sequence is followed by a region (residues 279 to 330), which connects the heavy chain with the catalytic serine protease domain. This connecting region has 17 prolines in 52 residues and also bears the proposed attachment sites of six *O*-linked carbohydrate chains.

The C-terminal residues from 354 to 596 make up the catalytic domain of the factor XII sequence. This light-chain region is homologous with the pancreatic serine proteases: trypsin, chymotrypsin, and elastase. The cleavage by kallikrein to form factor XIIa occurs at Arg^{353}—Val^{354} (Figs. 38-2 and 38-3).[24,26] The sequence data also account for the observations of two forms of factors XIIf.[13] Thus, cleavage at Arg^{334} produces a disulfide-linked two-chain molecule composed of the serine protease moiety linked to a 19-

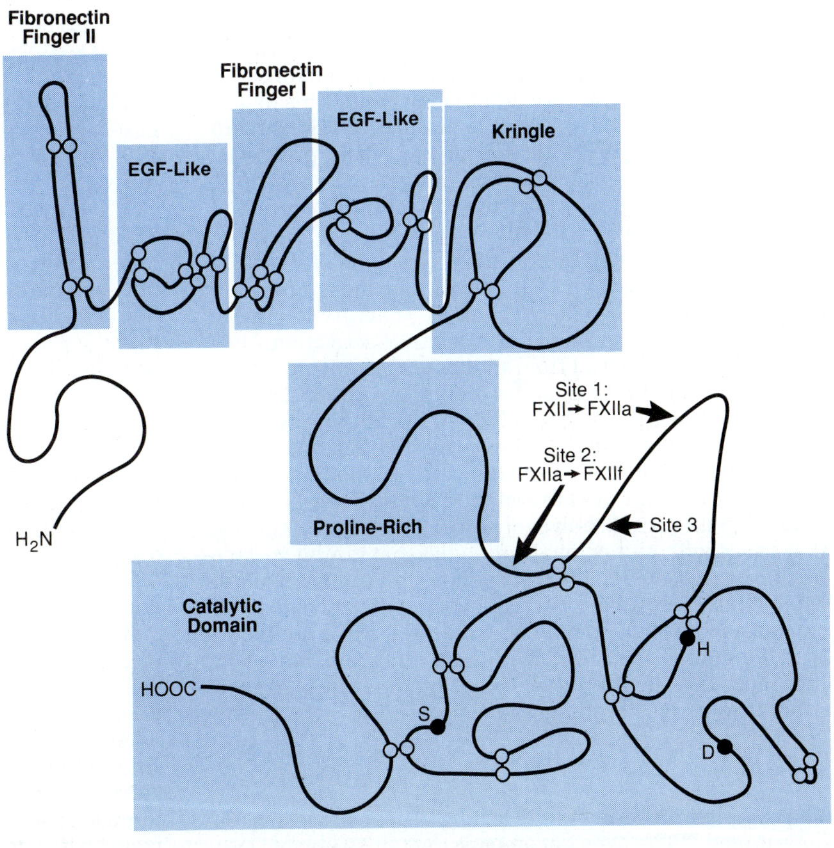

FIGURE 38-2. Schematic diagram of the protein chain of factor XII, showing the structural domains inferred from sequence homologies. The catalytic triad residues are shown by solid circles, half-cystines are indicated by open circles, and the cleavage sites leading to activation (site 1) and the two forms of factor XIIf (sites 2 and 3) are marked with arrows. The domains are fibronectin type II, growth factor–like (EGF-like), fibronectin type I, kringle, and proline-rich. (After Cool DE, Edgell CS, Louie GV, et al. Characterization of human blood coagulation factor XII cDNA. J Biol Chem 1985;25:13666)

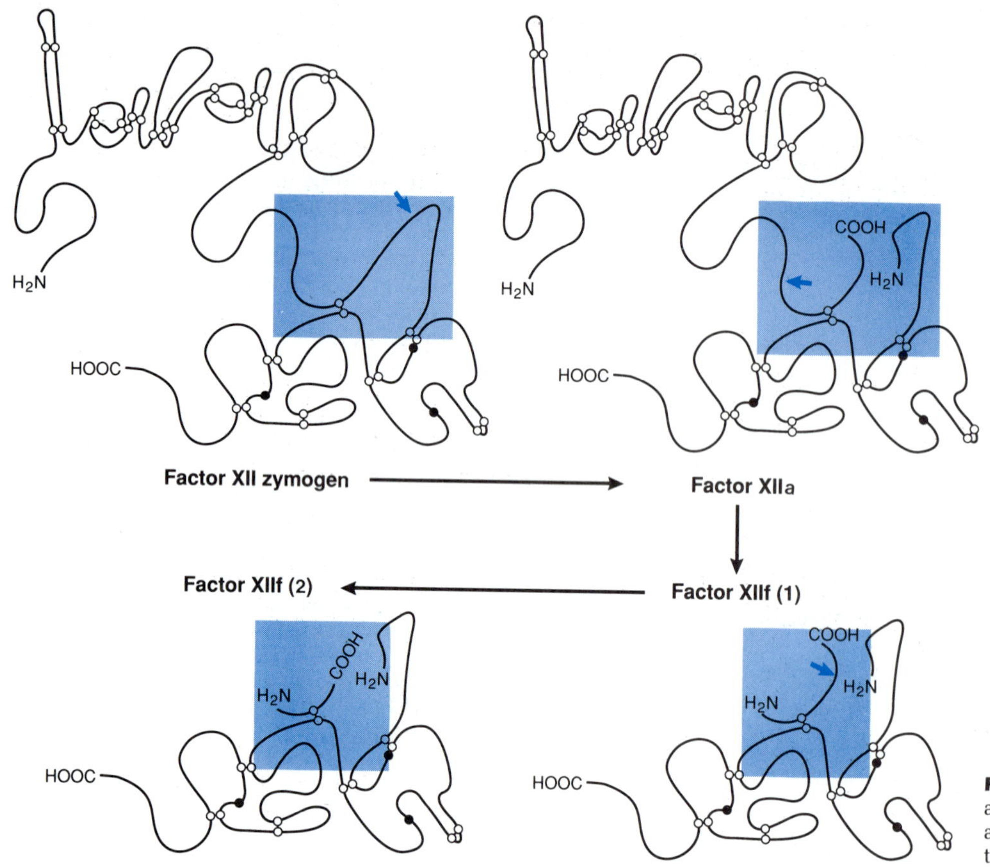

FIGURE 38-3. Diagram of the activation of factor XII to factor XIIa and the sequential production of the two forms of factor XIIf.

amino acid peptide. A second cleavage occurs at Arg^{343} to leave a nine-residue peptide linked through the disulfide bond to the serine protease (see Fig. 38-3). The catalytic domain bears an average 36% homology with the pancreatic serine proteases, which is similar to the 41% figure for their homology among themselves. In addition, five of the seven disulfide bridges of the factor XII light chain occur in similar positions in trypsin or chymotrypsin. This makes it likely that the tertiary structure of the catalytic domain is closely homologous with that of the serine proteases. The members of the catalytic triad of factor XIIa are His^{40}, Asp^{89} and Ser^{191}, numbering from the amino terminus of the light chain (residue 354 of the zymogen).

Apart from the catalytic domain, the relation of structure to function remains largely unknown. The most important known property of the heavy chain is its ability to bind to negatively charged surfaces during contact activation. Data in the literature derived from studies with monoclonal antibodies amd synthetic peptides identified two separate regions that appeared to be involved in the binding of factor XII to the surface. Initial studies suggested that an epitope comprising residues 134 to 153, located in the fibronectin type I–like domain, was the surface binding site.[27] A subsequent publication, however, reported that the epitope that reacts with monoclonal antibodies that inhibit surface binding was located in the first amino acid residues of factor XII.[28] Thus, the primary surface-binding site appears to be located in the first domain of factor XII, the fibronectin type II domain. The initial results may indicate, however, that there is at least one secondary binding site that contributes to surface binding.

The Gene

The complete structure of the factor XII gene has also been determined.[29] The gene encompasses about 12 kbp of DNA consisting of 14 exons and 13 introns (Fig. 38-4). Twelve exons are located within a stretch of 4.2 kb. The first exon at the 5′ end codes for a putative 19-residue signal peptide. Subsequent exons code for the discrete domains described in the preceding section. The kringle and the proline-rich region are together encoded by the eighth and ninth exons. The catalytic domain is encoded by five exons, with the catalytic histidine, aspartate, and serine residues all located in separate exons. The final exon is the largest and includes 150 bp corresponding to the untranslated 3′ end of the mRNA.

The human factor XII gene had been tentatively located to either chromosome 6 or 7, based on correlations between other observable abnormalities and factor XII deficiency, but each of these assignments was subsequently disputed. Studies with cDNA hybridization probes[30,31] have shown that the gene is in fact found on chromosome 5, and it has been localized to the 5q33-qter region of the chromosome.[31]

Homologies With Other Proteins

As previously described, the domain structure of factor XII has been defined on the basis of sequence homologies with corresponding domains of fibronectin, plasmin, plasminogen inhibitors, and pancreatic serine proteases. For some of the domains like the kringle and catalytic domains, it has been possible to extend the analysis of homologies.

A detailed study of the homologies of the kringles in plasmin, prothrombin, tPA, urokinase, and factor XII has been made.[32] The factor XII sequence shows the closest homologies with tPA kringle 2; 41 residues are conserved when one gap of three residues is inserted into the factor XII sequence. Other close homologies are with urokinase (39 residues) and tPA kringle 1 (35 residues). In contrast, the widest separation in sequence homology was between factor XII and prothrombin kringle S, which still had 27

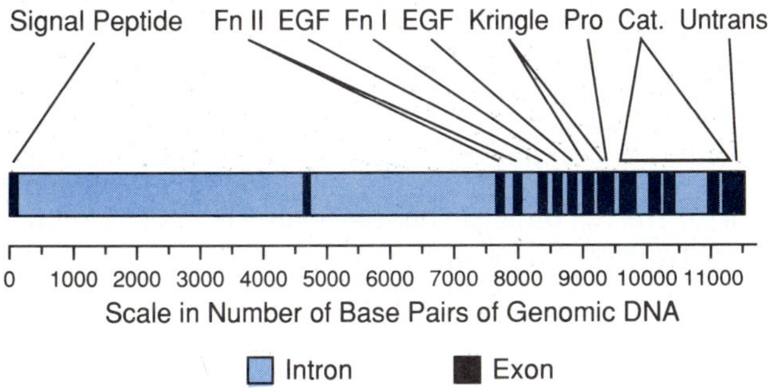

FIGURE 38-4. Structure of the factor XII gene, showing introns and the exons coding for the domains shown in Figure 38-2. (Data from Cool DE, MacGillivray RT. Characterization of the human blood coagulation factor XII gene: intron/exon gene organization and analysis of the 5′-flanking region. J Biol Chem 1987;262:13662)

residues conserved. This high degree of sequence homology between the kringles of factor XII and other proteins does not necessarily translate into close structural homology. Secondary structure prediction showed a marked difference between the predicted structures of the factor XII and urokinase kringles despite their close sequence homologies. These differences arise from significant single amino acid substitutions.

In the case of the catalytic domain, however, there is good reason for proposing close structural homologies with other serine proteases. The 36% sequence homology with the pancreatic serine proteases is similar to the 41% average homology among themselves. The latter homology translates to highly homologous (about 85%) tertiary structures. Thus, a tentative tertiary structure of the catalytic domain has been proposed, which allows the insertions in the sequence relative to the pancreatic enzymes to be accommodated at the surface of the molecule.[24]

Having the sequence of the factor XII gene also allows the analysis of homology in terms of intron and exon structure.[29] The exons coding for the fibronectin type I, the growth factor domain, and the kringle in factor XII are also all found in tPA and urokinase, but the proline-rich region of factor XII is unique. In the serine protease region, the factor XII gene is also much more closely related to the plasminogen activators than to the clotting factors or the pancreatic enzymes.

Overall, the results of analysis of both the DNA and protein sequences show that tPA is the protein most closely related to factor XII. Other close homologies are with urokinase and plasmin. The clotting factors such as prothrombin show relatively little homology in either sequence or gene structure.

PREKALLIKREIN

Biochemistry

Like factor XII, prekallikrein is a zymogen without detectable activity, which is converted to a functional serine protease during contact activation.[17] On SDS gel electrophoresis, purified prekallikrein yields two bands at 85 and 88 kd, regardless of the source. Activation is accomplished in plasma by either factor XIIa or factor XIIf and results in a disulfide-linked two-chain form composed of a heavy chain of 56 kd and a light chain bearing the catalytic center. The heterogeneity shown by the zymogen is reflected in the light chain; on reduction, a pair of bands at 33 and 36 kd is seen, each of which contains a diisopropylfluorophosphate (DFP)-inhibitable active site.[17,33] Physical and chemical data for human plasma prekallikrein are found in Table 38-1.

Prekallikrein binds to HMW kininogen through a site on its heavy chain with a dissociation constant of 12 to 15 nmol/L.[34,35] This value, which is unchanged by conversion to kallikrein, is such that at plasma concentrations of HMW kininogen and prekallikrein about 80% to 90% of the prekallikrein circulates bound to HMW kininogen in a 1:1 complex. Thus, it is the prekallikrein–HMW kininogen complex that participates in surface-induced contact activation and the binding of prekallikrein to the surface is probably mediated through the HMW kininogen. The dissociation of 10% to 20% of the kallikrein into the fluid phase may serve to propagate both the activation of factor XII and the generation of bradykinin.[36,37]

Most of the measurable proteolytic activity evolved in normal human plasma as a result of contact activation is due to kallikrein. It is responsible for most of the factor XII activation that takes place in plasma, and it converts factor XIIa to factor XIIf.[12,13] Kallikrein also digests HMW kininogen to liberate the vasoactive peptide bradykinin. Kallikrein shows preference for cleaving peptide bonds on the carboxy side of arginine residues, and it cleaves HMW kininogen and factor XII at a number of different arginine-containing sequences. In the case of the liberation of bradykinin, however, the second cleavage to liberate the bradykinin from the carboxy-terminal end of the kininogen heavy chain occurs at the sequence Leu-Met-Lys. Apparently, the quaternary structure of the substrate HMW kininogen must be present to induce kallikrein to cleave this bond.[38] Kallikrein is active in the factor XII–dependent fibrinolytic pathway in two ways. It can directly convert plasminogen to plasmin,[39,40] and it also converts plasma prourokinase to urokinase.[41–43]

Kallikrein possesses other functions that may have a role in inflammation. It is chemotactic for human neutrophils[44] and monocytes,[45] and it causes neutrophil aggregation[46] and secretion of elastase.[47] However, controversy exists regarding these functions among different laboratories.[48] Kallikrein also can destroy the first component of complement,[49] and activate factor B of the alternative complement pathway.[50] Finally, kallikrein can convert plasma prorenin to renin, and it is responsible for the neutral phase of acid-induced prorenin activation.[51,52]

Kallikrein is inhibited in plasma mainly by C1 inhibitor and by α_2-macroglobulin.[53–55] The role of these inhibitors in regulating contact activation is described in the section on initiation and regulation of the contact activation system. Table 38-2 indicates nonphysiologic inhibitors that are of experimental importance.

Structure

The entire amino acid sequence of the protein has been determined by a combination of direct protein sequence and amino acid sequence prediction from cDNAs isolated from a λgt-11 expression library.[56] The structure of the gene has not been reported. The signal peptide of 19 residues is followed by the sequence of the mature plasma prekallikrein molecule, which has 619 amino acids with a calculated molecular weight of 69,710 daltons; together with 15% carbohydrate the total molecular weight is predicted as 79,545 daltons. Five asparagine residues have been identified as attachment sites for carbohydrate— three in the light chain and two in the heavy chain; all are Asn residues. The molecular weight heterogeneity seen on SDS gel electrophoresis is not explained by any sequence heterogeneity and may therefore be due to variations in glycosylation.

The site of the cleavage that generates kallikrein from prekallikrein is at Arg^{371}-Ile^{372}, generating a light chain of 248 amino acid residues with the new amino-terminal sequence Ile-Val-Gly. The catalytic triad is composed of

His[415], Asp,[464] and Ser[559]. The amino acid sequence of the heavy chain is unusual and has little homology with other serine proteases of the coagulation cascade with the exception of factor XI. In place of the heterogeneous domain structure found in factor XII, the heavy-chain sequence of prekallikrein comprises four tandem repeats, each of which contains about 90 to 91 amino acids (Fig. 38-5). The presence of six conserved half-cystines per repeat suggests a repeating structure with three disulfide loops. The two carbohydrate sites in the heavy chain are found in the second and fourth repeats. It is postulated that a gene segment coding for the ancestor of the repeat sequence duplicated and then the entire segment duplicated again to give the present structure.

FACTOR XI

Biochemistry

Like factor XII and prekallikrein, factor XI is a zymogen that is activated to a serine protease during contact activation. Factor XI is unique among the clotting factors in that the circulating zymogen consists of two identical subunits that are linked by disulfide bonds; the dimer has an apparent molecular weight of 160 kd on SDS gel electrophoresis.[57,58] The major activator of factor XI is factor XIIa; other enzymes produced during contact activation, including the low molecular weight forms of activated factor XII, are not efficient activators of factor XI. The activation of factor XI follows the familiar pattern of cleavage of a peptide bond within a disulfide linkage to yield an amino-terminal heavy chain and a disulfide-linked light chain. Since both precursor subunits can be cleaved and each resulting light chain bears a functional active site, factor XIa is a four-chain protein with two active sites. Physical and chemical data for human factor XI are found in Table 38-1.

Factor XI circulates with a plasma concentration of only 4 to 6 μg/mL. The heavy chain of factor XIa, like that of kallikrein, binds to the light chain of HMW kininogen. Thus, factor XI and HMW kininogen also circulate as a complex[59]; the dissociation constant is about 70 nmol/L, which is high enough to ensure that about 90% of the factor XI is complexed.[60] The molar ratio of the complex can vary from one to two molecules of HMW kininogen per factor XI because of the dimeric nature of factor XI.[61] The binding site for HMW kininogen on the factor XI heavy chain has been localized to the first (amino-terminal) tandem repeat.[62]

Although prekallikrein can be activated in the fluid phase by factor XIIf—bound or not bound to HMW kininogen—factor XI activation requires interaction with the surface[19] and HMW kininogen is an obligate cofactor.[4,63,64] Thus, both factor XII and HMW kininogen interact with the initiating surface, and HMW kininogen facilitates factor XI cleavage by factor XII.

The primary function of factor XIa is to activate the next protein in the intrinsic coagulation cascade, that is, to convert factor IX to IXa. This next step is the first one involving a vitamin K–dependent clotting factor, and the reaction is accelerated by calcium ions. In the later reactions of the clotting pathway, the vitamin K–dependent factors, factor X and prothrombin, are activated by calcium-dependent surface assemblies of enzyme (factor IXa or Xa, respectively) and a protein cofactor (factor VIII or V, respectively). By contrast, the activation of factor IX by factor XIa does not require a protein cofactor. The presence of a binding site on the heavy chain of factor XI for factor IXa has been inferred from studies with monoclonal antibodies.[65] This site is distinct from the catalytic center on the light chain and appears to interact with factor IX only in the presence of calcium ions.[66] Thus, in a sense, the heavy chain of factor XIa may function as an intrinsic "protein cofactor." The binding of HMW kininogen to factor XIa does not affect the reaction with factor IX. Thus, the HMW kininogen–factor XIa complex activates factor IX, and activation may take place on the contact surface.

Factor XIa also makes a small contribution to factor XII–dependent fibrinolysis by its ability to directly convert plasminogen to plasmin.[17] Its potency is about equal to that of kallikrein,[40] but it makes a lesser contribution because

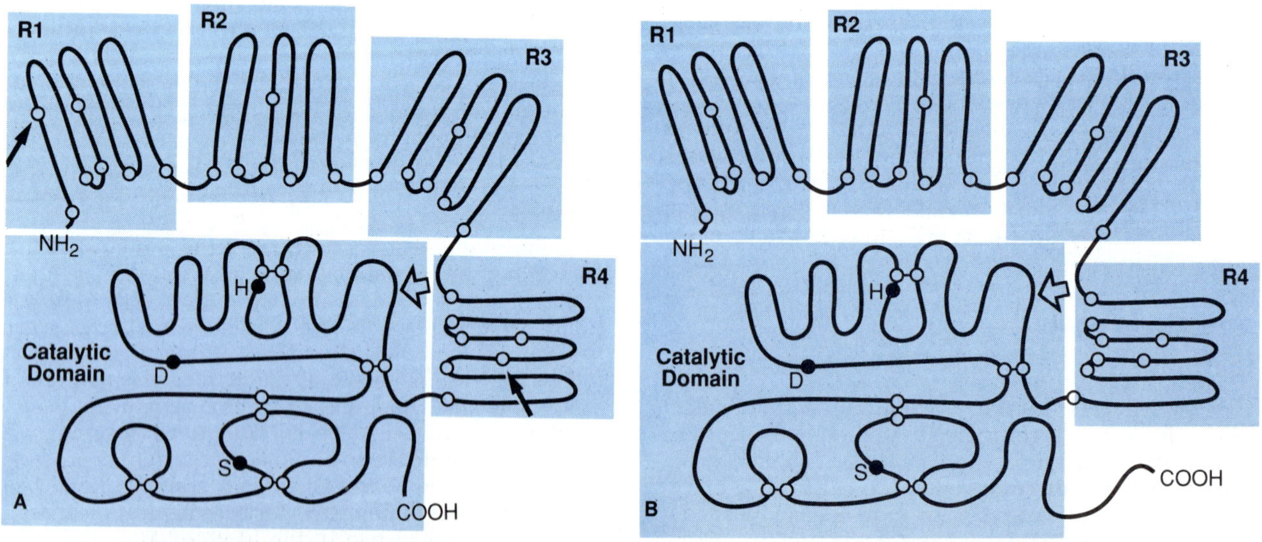

FIGURE 38-5. Schematic diagram of the protein chains of factor XI (**A**) and prekallikrein (**B**), showing the structural domains inferred from sequence homologies. The catalytic triad residues are shown by solid circles, half-cystines are indicated by open circles, and the cleavage sites leading to activation by activated factor XII are marked with open arrows. The solid arrows indicate the unmatched half-cystines that might be involved in interchain disulfide bonds. (After Fujikawa K, Chung DW, Hendrickson LE, Davie EW. Amino acid sequence of human factor XI: a blood coagulation factor with four tandem repeats that are highly homologous with plasma prekallikrein. Biochemistry 1986;25: 2417)

kallikrein is generated in greater quantities. Receptors for factor XI and factor XIa are found on platelets,[67,68] and these may be involved in a platelet-dependent but factor XII–independent pathway for factor XI activation.[69] Whether such binding is relevant to physiologic factor IX activation is not clear.

Structure

The Protein

The amino acid sequence of human factor XI has been determined by translation of a cDNA insert obtained from a λgt-11 cDNA library prepared from human liver poly(A) RNA.[70] An 18-amino acid leader peptide is followed by a 607 amino acid sequence for each of the two subunits of the mature protein. The calculated molecular weight of the two polypeptide chains totals 135,979 daltons; with the addition of 5% carbohydrate, the total molecular weight would be about 140 kd. Five potential N-glycosylation sites have been identified in each subunit: three in the heavy-chain and two in the light-chain portion of the sequence.

Conversion of factor XI to factor XIa occurs by cleavage between Arg^{369} and Ile^{370}, giving a light chain of 238 amino acids with a new N-terminal sequence of Ile-Val-Gly-Gly. The light chain has the characteristic features of the trypsin-like serine proteases, the catalytic triad being made up of His^{44}, Asp^{93}, and Ser^{188}. The sequence of the heavy chain of factor XIa, like that of kallikrein, contains four tandem repeats of about 90 amino acids including 6 conserved half-cystines. This suggests that each repeat forms a domain containing three internal disulfide bridges (see Fig. 38-5). Unpaired half-cystines in the first and fourth repeats are postulated to form the interchain disulfide bridges between monomers to produce the factor XI homodimer. The presence of two interchain disulfide bonds in factor XI allows for either a parallel or an antiparallel structure.

The Gene

The gene for factor XI spans 23 kbp and is divided into 15 exons and 14 introns.[71] Each tandem repeat found in the protein heavy-chain sequence is demarcated by an intron at its amino-terminal end, and each contains one intron in essentially the same position. The catalytic domain is coded for by five exons arranged identically with the exon structure of tPA and urokinase.

Homologies With Other Proteins

The amino acid sequence of factor XI shows a striking degree of homology with prekallikrein. Thus, the complete sequence of factor XI has 58% identity with that of prekallikrein and, if homologous amino acids are included, the degree of homology is 67%.[70] Thirty-four of 36 half-cystines are in matching positions; the remaining two are believed to be involved in the interchain disulfide bonds as described earlier. The carboxy-terminal sequence of 88 amino acids, which includes the active site serine residue and the substrate binding pocket, has 81% identity. These data show that both proteins are likely to have evolved from a common ancestor.

Both prekallikrein and factor XI have five potential sites for Asn-linked carbohydrate. Three sites are identical in the two proteins. One is in the heavy chain and two are in the light chain, but the carbohydrate content of factor XI is only 5% compared with about 15% in prekallikrein. Whether the difference is accounted for by fewer attached chains or shorter ones is undetermined.

The structure of the gene for the active site domain of factor XI is very similar to those for tPA, urokinase, and factor XII. The heavy-chain region, however, is quite different from the strings of kringles and growth factor-like regions described for factor XII. The structure of the gene for prekallikrein has not been reported and cannot be compared with that for factor XI.

HIGH-MOLECULAR-WEIGHT KININOGEN

Biochemistry

High-molecular-weight kininogen (also abbreviated HK[72]) circulates as a single-chain glycoprotein with an apparent molecular weight of 200 kd by gel filtration[34] and 115 kd by SDS gel electrophoresis under reducing conditions.[73] HMW kininogen circulates at a plasma concentration of 70 to 90 $\mu g/mL$[74–77] and forms a noncovalent complex with prekallikrein[34] with a dissociation constant of 15 nmol/L[35,78] and a similar complex with factor XI[59] with a dissociation constant of 70 nmol/L.[60] Other physical and chemical data are given in Table 38-1.

During contact activation, plasma kallikrein digests HMW kininogen and leaves a disulfide-linked heterodimer, consisting of an amino-terminal heavy chain (65 kd) and initially a carboxy-terminal light chain of 56 to 62 kd. A subsequent cleavage reduces the light chain to 45 to 49 kd.[78–82] The digestion of HMW kininogen by kallikrein releases bradykinin (NH_2-Arg-Pro-Pro-Gly-Phe-Ser-Pro-Phe-Arg-COOH), which is a potent vasoactive peptide with multiple effects in inflammation.[73,83,84] (Bradykinin is discussed in more detail in the section on inactivation of bradykinin.) HMW kininogen is also cleaved by tissue kallikrein* to form the heterodimer of the heavy chain and the 56- to 62-kd light chain; the additional cleavage made by plasma kallikrein in the light chain is not made by the tissue enzyme.[81,82,85]

The complexes of HMW kininogen with prekallikrein and factor XI are formed with the light chain region, and the isolated reduced and alkylated light chain of HMW kininogen forms these complexes with the same dissociation constants as the whole molecule.[35,60,78,86] Calculations of the proportion of plasma HMW kininogen that circulates as complexes with prekallikrein and factor XI give results in the range of 80% to 90%.

Secondary structure prediction from the sequence of the light chain suggests a low degree of α-helix and a highly flexible structure.[87] This is in accord with the experimental observation that light chain isolated after reduction, alkylation, and gel filtration in guanidine hydrochloride retains full functional activity.[84]

Kallikrein first cleaves HMW kininogen at the carboxy terminal of the bradykinin sequence, leaving the bradykinin attached to the carboxy-terminal end of the heavy chain of cleaved HMW kininogen.[38,80,81] The sequence Leu-Met-Lys-Arg is cleaved at the Lys-Arg bond to liberate bradykinin from the heavy chain (Fig. 38-6).

---

* Tissue kallikrein is another enzyme that is a kallikrein; that is, it can release kinin from kininogen. This enzyme is released from tissue as an active enzyme, not a zymogen, and is also found in urine. Tissue or urinary kallikrein is not related to plasma kallikrein immunologically and has a different substrate specificity when assayed with peptide substrates. Tissue kallikrein digests HMW kininogen to liberate bradykinin, but its primary substrate is low-molecular-weight kininogen (LMW kininogen). Tissue kallikrein cleaves LMW kininogen to release lysyl-bradykinin (kallidin). The pharmacologic properties of kallidin are similar to those of bradykinin; a plasma aminopeptidase converts kallidin to bradykinin.

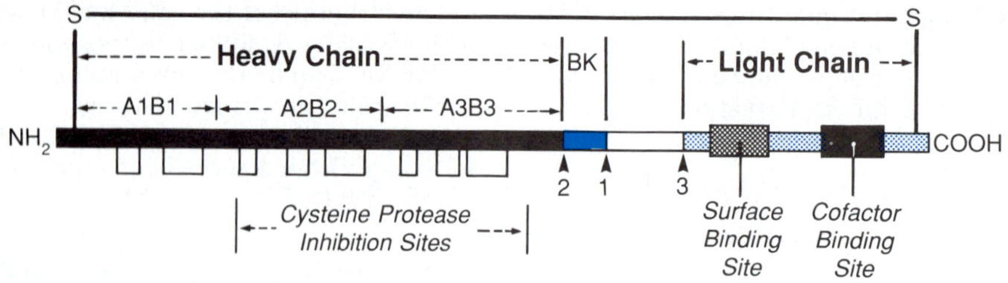

FIGURE 38-6. The structure of high-molecular-weight (HMW) kininogen. The heavy-chain region consists of three homologous domains—A1B1, A2B2, and A3B3—of which the latter two are sulfhydryl protease inhibition sites. The small rectangles under the heavy-chain region represent the eight intra–heavy-chain disulfide bonds. The light-chain region of HMW kininogen, which contains the binding sites for surface and prekallikrein or factor XI, is located toward the C-terminal end of the protein. The heavy and light chains are held together by the ninth disulfide bond. The arrowheads labeled 1, 2, and 3 indicate the sites and the order in which plasma kallikrein cleaves HMW kininogen. BK, bradykinin.

As described above, HMW kininogen binds to negatively charged surfaces through the histidine-rich region of the light chain. The ability to bind to a surface and simultaneously complex factor XI or prekallikrein is responsible for its cofactor activity in contact activation.[36] When a surface such as a glass slide is introduced into plasma, it is first coated with fibrinogen that is rapidly displaced by HMW kininogen.[88–90] The mechanism of this effect is not fully understood. HMW kininogen also binds to heparin and may influence thereby the inhibition of clotting by antithrombin III in heparinized plasma.[91] The manner in which HMW kininogen functions as a cofactor in contact activation is discussed in detail in the section on the role of HMW kininogen.

Structure

The Protein

The complete amino acid sequence of HMW kininogen has been determined from cDNA as well as from direct sequence analysis of purified protein.[92–95] HMW kininogen contains a total of 626 amino acid residues with a calculated molecular weight of 69,896 daltons, which, together with 40% carbohydrate, gives a total molecular weight close to that observed. The heavy chain of 362 residues, which is derived from the N terminus, is followed by the 9-residue bradykinin sequence, then by the light-chain sequence of 255 residues (see Fig. 38-6). The mature protein has a blocked N-terminal amino acid (pyroglutamic acid). Three glycosidic linkage sites are on the heavy chain and 9 are on the light chain. All the glycosidic bonds on the heavy chain are N-linked, and those on the light chain are O-linked. The relevance of this unique glycosidic linkage distribution is unknown.

The heavy chain contains three contiguous sequences that are homologous with each other: domain 1 comprises residues 1 to 116, domain 2 residues 117 to 238, and domain 3 residues 239 to 360 (see Fig. 38-6). Of the 17 half-cystines, one is near the N terminal and forms a disulfide bond with the light chain; the others form a linear arrangement of eight consecutive disulfide loops aligned with the sequence repeats.[92] These three domains share considerable homology with a family of small (12 to 13 kd) cysteine protease inhibitors called *cystatins*; domains 2 and 3, not 1, exhibit cysteine protease inhibitor activity.[96–99] It has been shown by limited proteolytic digestion that protease-sensitive sites on the heavy-chain map to its interdomain junctions. Possibly, cleavage at these sites may occur in plasma to release the inhibitory domains under certain pathologic conditions. The isolated heavy chain has greater cysteine protease inhibitor activity than native HMW kininogen and is able to bind two molecules of papain.[98]

The procoagulant properties of HMW kininogen are all resident in the light-chain portion of HMW kininogen.[84,86] The light chain is divided into a basic amino-terminal portion that binds to activating surfaces[84,86,100] and an acidic carboxy-terminal portion that bears the binding sites for prekallikrein and factor XI.[60,101] The surface-binding region spanning residues 91 to 121 of the light chain is called the *histidine-rich region*, since 24 out of 91 residues are histidines and an additional 11 residues are lysine. This histidine-rich region also exhibits three internally homologous sequences of about 30 residues each, and each in turn contains further internally homologous sequences. The entire histidine-rich region is suggested to have evolved by repeated duplication of the sequence Gly-His (or His-Gly).[94] The sole half-cystine found in the light chain forms a disulfide bond with the heavy chain. No homologies with any protein except for other kininogens have been recognized.

The prekallikrein binding site of HMW kininogen maps to residues 194 to 224 of the light chain (31 amino acids).[60,101] A corresponding synthetically prepared peptide has been shown to bind prekallikrein with the same affinity as that of the intact light chain. Factor XI also bound to the same region of HMW kininogen but, in this case, optimal binding required a 58–amino acid peptide spanning residues 185 to 242 of the light chain.[60]

Relation to Low-Molecular-Weight Kininogen

Another circulating protein is found to be a kininogen; at only 68 kd, it is called *low-molecular-weight (LMK) kininogen.* Like HMW kininogen, LMW kininogen is digested by tissue kallikrein to a two-chain form from which bradykinin has been excised.[102,103] This digestion yields a 65-kd amino-terminal heavy-chain disulfide linked to a light chain of 4 kd.[92,104,105] In contrast to HMW kininogen, LMW kininogen is not cleaved by plasma kallikrein. The sequences of LMW kininogen and HMW kininogen are identical from the amino terminal through the bradykinin sequence and the next 12 amino acids.[104] Studies of the cDNAs show that the identity persists through the 18-residue signal peptide and the 5′ untranslated region of the mRNA.[93]

Kininogen Genes

Both HMW kininogen and LMW kininogen are produced from a single gene (27 kbp) that is thought to have originated by two successive duplications of a primordial kininogen gene.[93] As schematically represented in Figure 37-7, this gene consists of a total of 11 exons. Of these, the first nine exons code for the kininogen heavy chain; each of the three

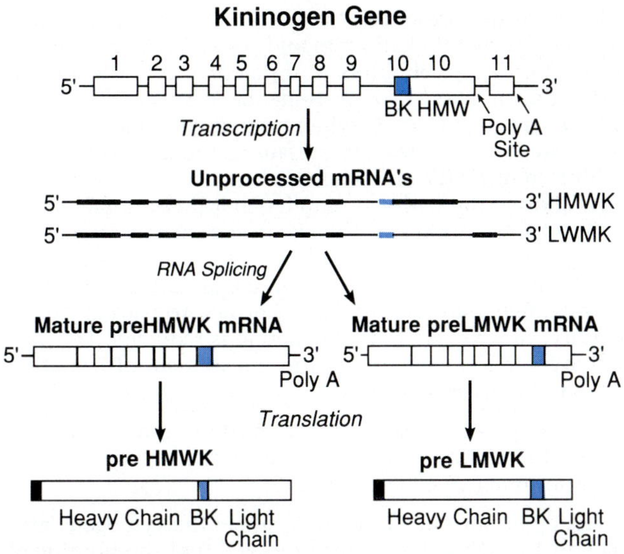

FIGURE 38-7. The gene for high-molecular-weight kininogen (HMWK). The boxes labeled 1 to 9 represent the exon coding for the heavy chain of both HMWK and low-molecular-weight kininogen (LMWK). Exon 10 codes for the bradykinin (BK) sequence and the light chain of HMWK, whereas exon 11 codes for the light chain of LMWK. The mature mRNAs are assembled by alternative splicing events in which the light-chain sequences are attached to the 3′ end of the 12–amino acid common sequence C terminal to BK.

domains indicated by the protein sequence is coded for by a set of three exons. The tenth exon codes for bradykinin and the light chain of HMW kininogen, whereas the light chain of LMW kininogen is coded for by exon 11. The mRNAs for HMW kininogen and LMW kininogen are produced from this single gene by alternative splicing, which includes the sequences for the heavy chain and bradykinin in both protein products but provides HMW kininogen and LMW kininogen with separate light-chain moieties.

INITIATION AND REGULATION OF THE CONTACT ACTIVATION SYSTEM

Initiation of the intrinsic coagulation pathway by the contact activation system occurs when a negatively charged surface is introduced into plasma containing the full complement of protease zymogens (factor XII, prekallikrein[6,16]) and protein cofactors (HMW kininogen[3]). Contact with the surface induces the formation of the active enzymes, factor XIIa and kallikrein, as depicted in Figure 38-1. The second step, separated arbitrarily, can be viewed as the activation of factor XI by factor XIIa (Fig. 38-8; see also Fig. 38-1); the roles of prekallikrein and HMW kininogen, viewed from a coagulation point of view, are to accelerate conversion of factor XII to factor XIIa. To explain initiation and regulation of contact activation, we need to understand how the activation of factor XII is triggered by the introduction of a surface and why it does not occur before then. The first question concerns the interactions of the proteins with the surface and with each other; the second involves the influence of other plasma proteins, notably the various protease inhibitors.

Interactions of Proteins and Surfaces in the Initiation of Contact Activation

Character of the Surface

Contact activation was originally observed by the interaction of blood with glass surfaces[106]; subsequently, finely divided kaolin was used extensively as an experimental surface and for coagulation assays.[107] Both materials are ill-defined in terms of their interactions with plasma proteins, and neither bears any obvious relation to physiologic

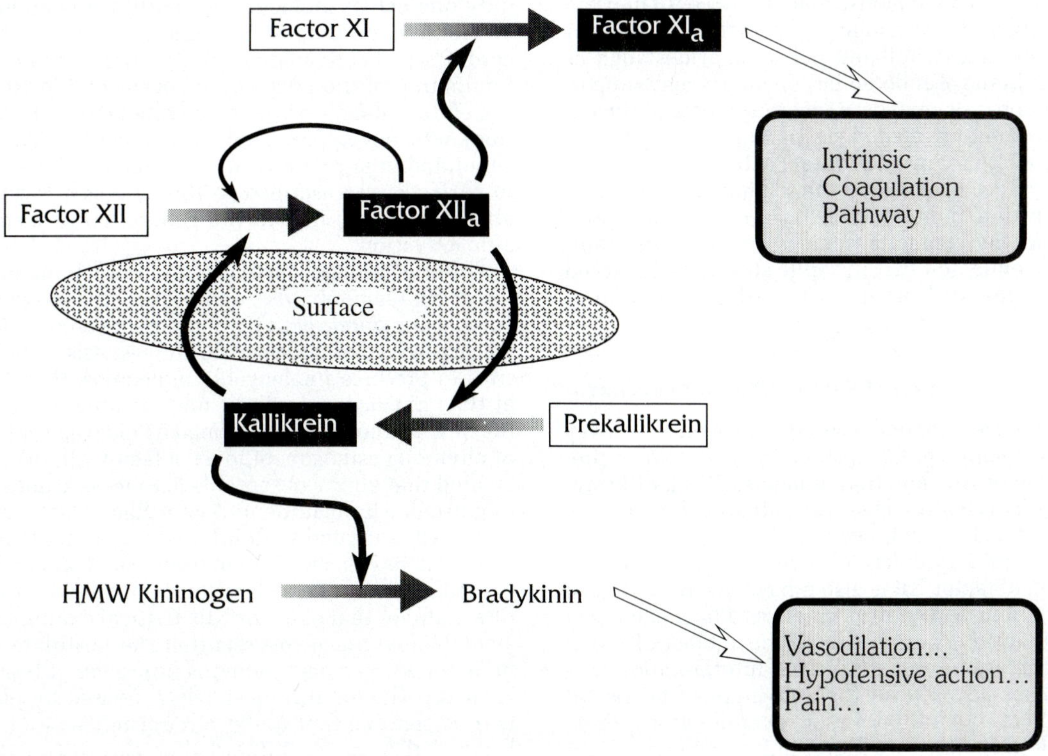

FIGURE 38-8. The pathways of contact activation. Open boxes, zymogens; black boxes, proteases; graded arrows, activation reactions; solid arrows, catalytic activities.

substances. The first apparently soluble activator of contact activation was the tannin-like substance *ellagic acid*,[108] which has also been used as a component of commercial assay systems. Ellagic acid has been since shown to be effective only when it can form large sedimentable aggregates in the presence of traces of contaminant heavy metal ions[109]; ellagic acid must therefore also be considered a particulate activator.

Dextran sulfate[110,111] and sulfatide[111] are now commonly used for studies of contact activation. Sulfatide is a naturally occurring sphingolipid bearing a galactose sulfate group. Normally found in small quantities in nerve tissue, it is too diluted by other lipids to be a likely physiologic activator. Purified sulfatide can form micelles with a highly charged surface of sulfate groups; such micelles are efficient activators of the contact system.[112,113]

Dextran sulfate is a truly soluble activator and a close homologue of naturally occurring sulfated polysaccharides. Initially, high-molecular-weight preparations (500 kd nominal) were found to support the activation of factor XII and prekallikrein.[2,8,111] In a study of factor XII autoactivation, much smaller fractions were found to be capable of supporting the reaction.[114] When the dependence of the rate of autoactivation on the size of the dextran sulfate was examined, a low but definite reaction was seen with molecular weights as low as 5 kd. The rate increased markedly above 10 kd, in which range the theoretical number of binding sites per particle increased from one to two.

Similar results were obtained with heparin,[114] indicating that this naturally occurring polysaccharide could support contact activation by a similar mechanism to dextran sulfate. Other studies of naturally occurring sulfated polysaccharides have found that only highly sulfated species such as heparin or chondroitin sulfate E were active.[115] This requirement for a high density of strong negative charges was also suggested by the finding of a relationship between the rate of factor XII autoactivation and the sulfate content of a series of dextran sulfate preparations.[116]

Although naturally occurring sulfated polysaccharides can support contact activation reactions in vitro, contact activation has not been demonstrated in vivo with heparin or similar compounds. Although it is attractive to consider that substances rich in sulfated polysaccharides such as basement membrane of endothelial cell matrix may support contact activation, this remains a theoretical possibility and has not been demonstrated. One pathophysiologic substance that is likely to initiate contact activation in vivo is endotoxin.[117–119] As discussed in the section on assessment of contact activation in human disease, there is good reason to believe that the contact system is activated in gram-negative septicemia and that in septic shock the observed symptoms are due, at least in part, to the generation of bradykinin.

Surface-Induced Activation of Factor XII and Prekallikrein

The most striking feature of the contact activation pathway is its cyclic or reciprocal form, since the activator of prekallikrein is factor XIIa and that of factor XII is kallikrein[6] (see Fig. 38-8). This feature gives the pathway the property of positive feedback, which ensures that the reaction accelerates after initiation has occurred.[2,8] Similarly, the autoactivation of factor XII is also a mechanism with positive feedback,[9] but with slower kinetics.[8] The mechanism by which initiation occurs has been the subject of much research, speculation, and conflicting interpretation. Attention has been focused on the activation of factor XII rather than on that of kallikrein for several reasons. First, the longest clotting times are found in factor XII–deficient plasma, whereas prekallikrein-deficient plasma is able to activate in the presence of a surface at a lower rate than normal plasma.[4] Prekallikrein and HMW kininogen appear to function as accelerators of the activation of factor XII rather than as absolute requirements.[5] Also, purified factor XII preparations activate when treated with a surface or a polyanion such as dextran sulfate in the absence of prekallikrein or HMW kininogen.[8,9,120]

As shown, the pathway implies that if two unactivated zymogens or pure factor XII are present, no reactions will take place unless some outside stimulus is applied. Negatively charged surfaces or other polyanionic substances provide such a stimulus but do not have intrinsic enzymatic activity. Clearly, further explanation is required. The various hypotheses concerning the mechanism of initiation resolve into three categories:

- Presence of a functional active site in the zymogen
- Participation of an extraneous enzyme
- Maintenance of a steady state

The hypothesis of a functional site in the zymogen dates back to 1974,[121] when it was proposed that the binding of factor XII to an activating surface induced a functional active site into the zymogen. In this hypothesis, the induction of a low level of enzymatic activity precedes the cleavage of factor XII.[122] Others have later suggested that the macromolecular substrates, prekallikrein and factor XI, are able to induce an active conformation in surface-bound factor XII that has similar activity to factor XIIa.[123]

These hypotheses are attractive in their simplicity, but proof requires that a clear distinction be made between intrinsic enzymatic activity in the bulk of the uncleaved zymogen molecules and contaminating traces of activated factor XII. This is difficult to do experimentally, and often the presence of a low percentage (2%) of active enzyme has been ignored. Under such conditions, the positive feedback inherent in the mechanism of reciprocal activations results in rapid acceleration of the rate of generation of active enzyme, thus obscuring the kinetics of the initiation. For example, it has been shown that mixing plasma concentrations of factor XII and prekallikrein containing only one active molecule per milliliter is enough to give 50% activation of both proteins in 13 seconds.[8] This concentration of activated enzymes represents a level of contamination of the purified zymogens of 5×10^{-13}%. Also, the ability of factor XIIa to activate factor XII (autoactivation) was not appreciated until recently. Thus, activity generated in pure preparations of factor XII after exposure to surfaces was ascribed to the zymogen[122] when it was almost certainly due to the generation of factor XIIa by autoactivation.

The plasminogen activators closely homologous with factor XII—namely, tPA and prourokinase—possess measurable enzymatic activity in their single-chain forms. This was confirmed by site-specific mutagenesis at their cleavage sites to produce uncleavable molecules.[124–127] In the case of tPA, fibrinogen or fibrin may be able to substitute for the new amino terminus formed by cleavage of trypsinogen or chymotrypsinogen. Studies of factor XII, in contrast, indicated that all the observable activity is kinetically indistinguishable from authentic factor XIIa or factor XIIf.[2] When factor XII is treated with inhibitors to remove most of the active factor XIIa and is then used to activate prekallikrein, a distinct phase of acceleration occurs before the reaction rate matches that of factor XIIf. Critical examination of the available evidence suggests that the postulate of activity in factor XII zymogen remains unproven at best.

Factor XII can also be slowly activated by plasmin.[20] It is thus possible that under circumstances such as the release of tPA, factor XII and then the rest of the contact system could become activated. This hypothesis has received little attention in the literature although the activation of factor XII by cell-derived proteases might be a potent inflammatory mechanism. Clearly, in cell-free plasma in contact with surfaces, cell-derived proteases are not responsible for contact activation.

The final hypothesis is that the contact activation reactions are proceeding continuously at a low rate in plasma, thereby maintaining low steady-state concentrations of the enzymes factor XIIa and kallikrein.[2,116] Acceleration would be prevented by the reaction of the enzymes with the plasma inhibitors. In experiments in which purified factor XII was incubated with C1 inhibitor (C1 INH) for prolonged periods,[128] the C1 INH failed to prevent slow conversion of factor XII to factor XIIa and factor XIIf. No enzymatic activity was detected since the inhibitor stoichiometrically binds factor XIIa and XIIf and inactivates them. Thus, slow turnover of factor XII may always be present, and the presence of only a few molecules per milliliter of factor XIIa that are not inhibited may be sufficient to initiate contact activation when an appropriate surface is added. The introduction of a surface or other polyanionic substance would then induce "activation" by accelerating many thousand-fold the baseline turnover of factor XII and prekallikrein, rapidly generating significant quantities of factor XIIa and kallikrein.

Contact with a surface accelerates activation by two mechanisms. The first is a localization effect that comes from the two zymogens and their enzymes all being able to bind reversibly to the surface.[36,37,63,113,116] This creates a local milieu in the fluid phase contiguous to the surface where the local concentrations of the zymogens and their activated forms are greater than in the bulk fluid phase. This greatly increases the rates of the reciprocal activations, since they are critically dependent on the product of the respective concentrations of the two reactants. The second effect is a conformational change in factor XII such that, when bound to the surface, it becomes more susceptible to cleavage and activation by various proteases.[7] Although the reactants of the contact system are bound to the surface, the inhibitors, especially C1 INH, are not; therefore, surface binding offers some protection against inactivation.[129] Thus, the balance between the rates of the activation reactions and the inactivation reactions is profoundly changed at the fluid–surface interface.

Whether the surface-bound zymogens are activated by neighboring surface-bound enzyme molecules or by fluid phase enzymes is not clear. In a study of the effect of molecular size of dextran sulfate on the rate of factor XII autoactivation,[114] the maximum rate varied with the size of the polyanion but it always occurred at the same relative concentrations of factor XII and factor XII binding sites, implying an optimal ratio of free to bound factor XII. Also, activation occurred with molecular weights of dextran sulfate that probably had only one binding site for factor XII per particle, implying that activation of bound factor XII by fluid-phase factor XIIa was occurring. In studies of the activation of factor XII by kallikrein, enhancements of 3000- to 12,000-fold have been found when surface was added.[8,130] This enhancement must include a component ascribable to the binding of factor XII to the surface and also a component ascribable to the binding to the surface by kallikrein. The isolated, active, light chain of kallikrein (which lacks the surface-binding site) is far less effective than intact kallikrein; in the presence of surface, it digested factor XII only 30 times faster than it did in the fluid phase.[130] Thus, the kallikrein–surface interaction may have a 100-fold kinetic effect. This could be the result of localization effects or of a requirement for bound enzyme to cleave bound substrate. In a different study, the authors concluded that surface-bound factor XII was activated by fluid-phase kallikrein so that the localization effect may be the prime mechanism by which the surface enhances the rate of factor XII activation by kallikrein.[113]

In the reciprocal reaction (the activation of prekallikrein by activated factor XII), the surface appears to play a smaller role. Thus, the effect of dextran sulfate was to increase by 70-fold the rate of prekallikrein activation by factor XIIa.[8] Factor XIIf, the final cleavage product of factor XII activation, cleaved prekallikrein at a similar rate to that of factor XIIa in solution, but since factor XIIf does not have surface-binding sites, its activation of prekallikrein is unaffected by the presence of surface. This result indicates that, in contrast to factor XII, the binding of prekallikrein to the surface does not cause a change in its properties as a substrate. In the presence of HMW kininogen, the situation may be different, as described later.

Whatever the mechanism by which factor XII activation is initiated, after some kallikrein has been formed by the action of factor XIIa on prekallikrein, it rapidly digests surface-bound factor XII, creating the positive feedback kinetics characteristic of the contact activation pathway. The activation of surface-bound factor XII by kallikrein is about 2000-fold more rapid than the rate of factor XII autoactivation, so that when factor XII activation is considered quantitatively, the major activator is kallikrein.[8] This kinetic dominance of kallikrein in the activation of factor XII indicates that prekallikrein must be considered to be a coagulation factor. Plasma that is congenitally deficient in prekallikrein (Fletcher trait plasma) has been shown to have a clotting defect that is unique. Its partial thromboplastin time is abnormal, but it autocorrects as the time of incubation with the surface is increased from 2 to 10 minutes before the addition of calcium.[4,131–133] During this time, sufficient factor XIIa is formed to activate factor XI normally. We believe this autocorrection results from the factor XII autoactivation pathway.

Role of High-Molecular-Weight Kininogen

If purified factor XII and prekallikrein are mixed in the presence of a substance such as dextran sulfate or sulfatide, the reciprocal activations previously described generate the active forms of both proteins. In plasma, the involvement of a third protein was indicated by the discovery of persons who were not deficient in either prekallikrein or factor XII but whose plasma had long APTTs and who generated no bradykinin.[134] This phenomenon was explained by the identification of HMW kininogen as a nonenzymatic cofactor in contact activation.[3,135,136] Initial observations suggested that HMW kininogen accelerated the activations of both factor XII and prekallikrein as well as that of factor XI.[4,5,63,64]

It was subsequently demonstrated that both prekallikrein[34] and factor XI[59] form specific complexes with HMW kininogen. By analogy with the mechanism for cofactor activity in the activation of factor X and prothrombin, HMW kininogen might be predicted to also interact with factor XII, thus forming a ternary activation complex on the surface. In fact, no evidence has been adduced for such a complex, and as we have described previously in buffer systems, when dextran sulfate or sulfatides are used as initiators of contact activation, both factor XII and prekallikrein can be rapidly activated even in the absence of HMW kininogen. Under some experimental conditions, high concentrations of HMW kininogen relative to the surface cause inhibition of contact activation reactions.[137] This is almost certainly due to competition between HMW kininogen and factor XII for the same binding sites on the surface.[138]

As described in preceding sections, the magnitudes of

the dissociation constants and the plasma concentrations of the three proteins are such that about 90% of the factor XI and prekallikrein circulate bound to HMW kininogen. Thus, the substrates for factor XIIa during contact activation are prekallikrein and factor XI bound to the surface by HMW kininogen[36,64] (Fig. 38-9). It appears that the function of the HMW kininogen is to present the substrates for factor XIIa in a conformation that facilitates their activation.[36] Thus, prekallikrein was found to bind to kaolin in the absence of HMW kininogen but was not subsequently activated by factor XII. Peptides bearing the carboxy-terminal sequence of the HMW kininogen light chain inhibited HMW kininogen–dependent coagulant activity of normal plasma by competitively interfering with the binding of prekallikrein to the light chain of HMW kininogen, thereby preventing its activation by activated factor XII.[60] Similarly, a monoclonal antibody directed against the prekallikrein binding site of HMW kininogen inhibited coagulation and the activation of prekallikrein in plasma.[139] Thus, HMW kininogen appears to catalyze conversion of prekallikrein to kallikrein either by altering the conformation of prekallikrein or by preventing the formation of an unfavorable conformation when prekallikrein binds directly to the surface. For some surfaces, the presence of HMW kininogen also increases the amount of prekallikrein that is bound,[36,64] although this may be of lesser importance. Factor XI activation is almost totally dependent on the formation of surface-binding complexes with HMW kininogen.[63,64]

HMW kininogen can augment the rate of factor XII activation in plasma,[5,64] although it does not augment the activity of kallikrein directly against synthetic substrates or fluid phase factor XII; rather, its effects appear to be largely indirect. First, HMW kininogen is required for efficient generation of kallikrein in surface-activated plasma. Furthermore, since the kallikrein–HMW kininogen complex has a dissociation constant of 15 nmol/L,[35] at plasma concentrations about 10% of the kallikrein dissociates; kallikrein formed on the surface can thereby dissociate and interact with surface-bound factor XII on other particles, thus disseminating the reaction.[36,37] As a result, the effective concentration ratio of kallikrein to factor XII is increased in the presence of HMW kininogen and may account for the augmentation seen. Finally, in plasma, HMW kininogen is able to displace other adhesive glycoproteins, such as fibrinogen, from the surface.[89]

These data indicate that HMW kininogen must also be considered to be a coagulation cofactor, because it is required for normal generation of kallikrein and factor XIa. Plasma that lacks HMW kininogen is found to have a relative absence of prekallikrein; thus factor XII activation is slow and dependent largely on autoactivation. The factor XIIa generated then does not convert factor XI to XIa because factor XI binding to HMW kininogen and attachment of the complex to surfaces are also required for normal factor XI activation[4,64] (see Fig. 38-9). Consequently, the plasma has a profoundly prolonged APTT that is almost as abnormal as that of factor XII deficiency.

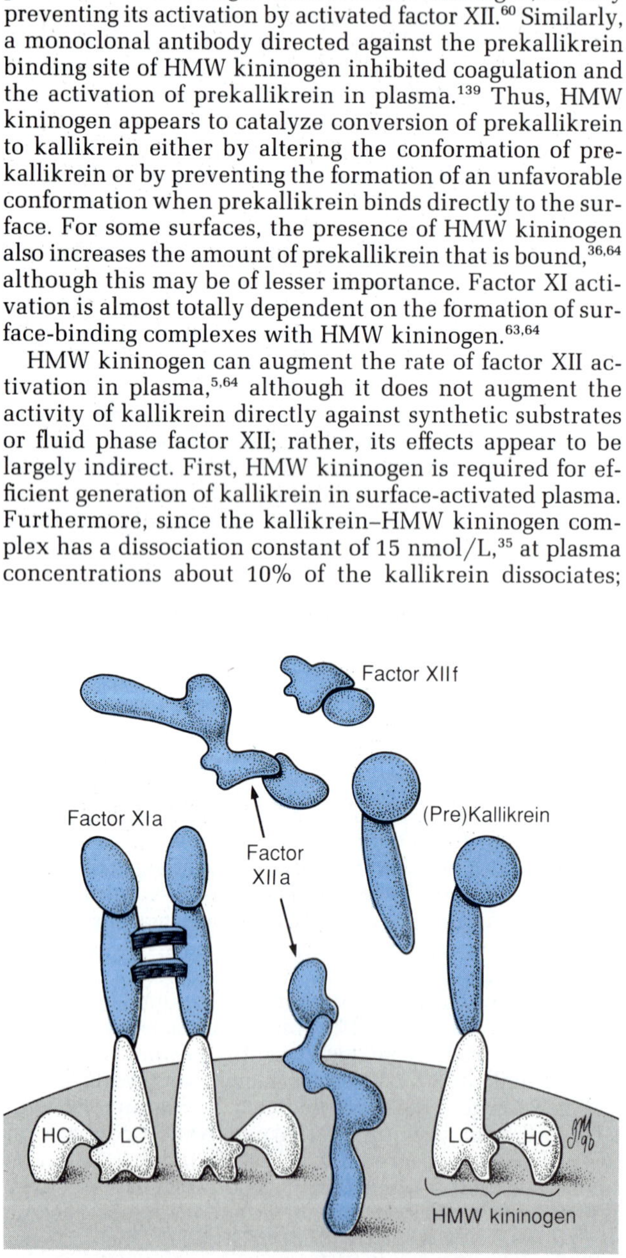

FIGURE 38-9. Illustration of the interactions between the proteins and the surface in contact activation. Prekallikrein and factor XI are shown bound to the surface by the light chain of high-molecular-weight (HMW) kininogen. Factor XII binds directly to the surface. (No distinction is made in the figure between the zymogens and their disulfide-linked two-chain activated forms.) Factor XII, prekallikrein, and factor XIIf are also found in the fluid phase.

Regulation of Contact Activation

Inhibition of Contact Activation

Regulation of factor XII–dependent pathways occurs by both intrinsic and extrinsic controls. Cleavage of factor XIIa to factor XIIf is one example of an intrinsic control. The factor XIIf produced is not surface bound and is a very poor activator of factor XIa. At the same time, the heavy-chain moiety, which has no enzymatic activity, retains the surface-binding site and can compete with factor XII and HMW kininogen for the surface. Thus, the conversion of factor XIIa to factor XIIf reduces the rate of the surface-dependent reactions of coagulation, whereas bradykinin generation by means of fluid-phase activation of prekallikrein continues. Similarly, digestion of kinin-free HMW kininogen by factor XIa has been reported to limit its coagulant activity,[140] although in this case the kinetics appear to be too slow to be of physiologic importance.[82]

Extrinsic controls are provided by plasma inhibitors for each enzyme. Table 38-3 indicates the major inhibitors of each active enzyme and, where known, their relative contributions to the total inhibition in plasma. Inhibition of the contact activation proteases is clearly different from that of the rest of the coagulation pathways in that antithrombin III (ATIII) appears to play only a minor role. Instead, contact activation appears to be limited mainly by C1 inhibitor (C1 INH), which is not active against any other of the clotting factors except for a weak inhibition of factor XI. C1 INH is a monovalent inhibitor that is cleaved by the protease it inhibits, but remains at the active site in a covalent complex. It may remain in a stable form of the acyl enzyme intermediate found in the normal serine protease mechanism.[141] Thus, after a protease has reacted with C1 INH, it cannot digest protein substrates or hydrolyze small synthetic substrates, and the reaction of the active site serine with DFP is abolished.

C1 INH is the only major plasma inhibitor of factor XIIa and factor XIIf.[142–145] Although ATIII can inhibit activated factor XII,[144,146,147] its contribution to factor XIIa inhibition in plasma is apparently only a few percent of that due to C1 INH.[144,145] Some disagreement exists over the effect of heparin on the inhibition of factor XIIa by ATIII. Some investigators have observed little enhancement of the rate of factor XIIa inhibition,[148] whereas others have observed a significant increase.[146,147] Heparin can act as an activating surface for contact activation and factor XII and factor XIIa can bind to it.[114,115] This binding is a factor in the inhibition by ATIII as the inhibition of factor XIIf, which lacks the

TABLE 38-3. Plasma Inhibitors of Enzymes of Contact Activation: Relative Contributions to Inhibition in Normal Human Plasma

	Enzyme			
Inhibitor	**Factors XIIa and XIIf**		**Kallikrein**	**Factor XIa**
C1 inhibitor	91.3	93	52 (84)*	8
Antithrombin III†	1.5	4	nd	16
α_2-Macroglobulin	4.3	—	35 (16)*	—
α_1-Protease inhibitor	—	—	nd	68
α_2-Antiplasmin	3.0	3	nd	8

nd, not determined separately.
* Data obtained from generation of kallikrein in situ.
† Data are for results obtained in the absence of added heparin.

surface-binding site, is not augmented in the presence of heparin as much as that of factor XIIa.[147] Curiously, α_2-macroglobulin, although thought of as a universal protease inhibitor,[149] does not significantly inhibit either form of activated factor XII.

The two major inhibitors of plasma kallikrein are C1 INH and α_2-macroglobulin.[53,150,151] Together, they account for over 90% of the kallikrein inhibitory activity of plasma, with the remainder contributed by ATIII.[54,55] When kallikrein is added to plasma, about 50% is bound to C1 INH and 50% to α_2-macroglobulin.[54,55,152] α_2-Macroglobulin does not bind to the active site of kallikrein but appears to trap the protease within its structure so as to sterically interfere with its ability to cleave large protein substrates.[149] The degree of inhibition is over 95%, but the residual activity is detectable when assayed for lengthy incubation periods. (In contrast, digestion of small synthetic substrates is much less affected and about one third of the starting activity is retained.) When a surface such as kaolin is added to plasma, so that kallikrein is generated in situ, close to 70% or 80% is bound to C1 INH.[152] The reason for the difference between the patterns of inhibition of added kallikrein and of endogenously produced kallikrein is unknown. At low temperatures, most of the inhibition of added kallikrein is accounted for by α_2-macroglobulin[152]; C1 INH appears to be ineffective in the cold, which may underlie the phenomenon of cold activation.[147] The inhibition of kallikrein by ATIII is also enhanced by heparin and may become significant in heparinized plasma.[153]

The major inhibitor of factor XIa is α_1-antiproteinase inhibitor (α_1-antitrypsin).[154,155] This is unusual and is the only major role for this inhibitor in the coagulation cascade (see Table 38-3). Other factor XIa inhibitors are C1 INH[156] and ATIII.[155] Again, the importance of heparin as a cofactor in ATIII inhibition has been disputed.[157,158]

The predominant role of C1 INH in the regulation of contact activation in human plasma is underscored by the fact that it alone is an efficient inhibitor of both activated factor XII and kallikrein and contributes to the inhibition of factor XIa. In plasma from patients with hereditary angioedema, in which C1 INH is absent, the amount of dextran sulfate required to produce activation is reduced 10-fold compared with that for normal plasma[147]; similar results are obtained in cold plasma. Because some surface was still required for activation under these conditions, we may surmise that the other inhibitors that are active against the contact factors also serve to limit their reactions; in normal plasma, however, we conclude that inhibition by C1 INH must mostly be overcome before contact activation can proceed. The plasma concentration of C1 INH is about 2 μmol/L, and it is remarkable that its inhibition is ever overcome. That surfaces are able to induce activation must reflect the protection of the proteases at the surface from inhibition. It has also been proposed that kallikrein bound to HMW kininogen is protected from inactivation by C1 INH[159,160] and α_2-macroglobulin[160,161] and that factor XIa is similarly protected from α_1-antiproteinase inhibitor.[155] This mechanism has been disputed for kallikrein and C1 INH[55,162] and may not be an important factor.

Inactivation of Bradykinin

Bradykinin is an exceedingly potent vasoactive peptide that can cause venular dilatation, activation of arterial endothelial cells, increased vascular permeability, hypotension, constriction of uterine and gastrointestinal smooth muscle, constriction of the coronary and pulmonary vasculature, bronchoconstriction, and activation of phospholipase A_2 to augment arachidonic acid metabolism. Its regulation is of prime importance, and a variety of enzymes in plasma contribute to kinin degradation. The first cleavage (Fig. 38-10) by carboxypeptidase N[163] removes the C-terminal Arg to leave an octapeptide, des-Arg^9 bradykinin.[164] Next, the octapeptide is digested by angiotensin-converting enzyme (ACE) to form the pentapeptide Arg-Pro-Pro-Gly-Phe, plus the tripeptide, Ser-Pro-Phe. This is a recently described tripeptidase activity of the enzyme.[165] Enzymes have not been characterized that rapidly digest Ser-Pro-Phe to individual amino acids and more slowly convert the pentapeptide to Arg-Pro-Pro plus Gly, and Phe. The final products of bradykinin degradation are the peptide Arg-Pro-Pro, plus one mole each of Gly, Ser, Pro, and Arg, and two moles of Phe[166] (see Fig. 38-10). The initial change of bradykinin to des-Arg^9 bradykinin by carboxypeptidase N is fast, whereas the other steps are slower when assessed in vitro. It is interesting that the product of this initial cleavage may retain activities in some instances.[167] For example, des-Arg^9 bradykinin can interact with B_1 receptors in the vasculature and cause hypotension, but its activities on the skin and the contraction of other smooth muscles are abolished. Bradykinin interacts with B_2 receptors to mediate all its functions, and a selective B_2 receptor antagonist has been synthesized.[168,169]

When blood is clotted and serum is studied, all the reactions for bradykinin degradation occur as described; the rate of the initial Arg removal is accelerated five-fold.[166] It has been suggested that small quantities of a carboxypeptidase-B–like activity may be secreted from platelets or perhaps neutrophils or that carboxypeptidase N can be cleaved and further activated or that a cofactor is provided that augments bradykinin degradation. It should also be noted that bradykinin degradation in vivo occurs largely along the pulmonary vasculature and that endothelial cells have carboxypeptidase as well as ACE activities. In the pulmonary circulation, the initial cleavage may occur by

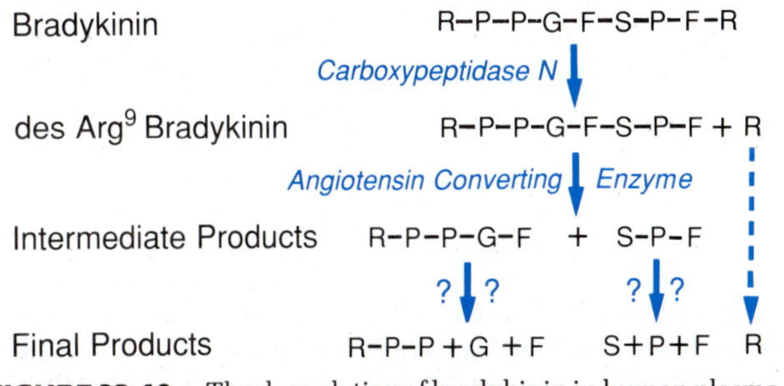

FIGURE 38-10. The degradation of bradykinin in human plasma. Proteolytic cleavages are denoted by the solid arrows, which are labeled with the name of the enzyme if known.

ACE acting as a dipeptidase to first remove Phe-Arg, then Ser-Pro (each of which is next cleaved to free amino acids) leaving the pentapeptide Arg-Pro-Pro-Gly-Phe. This is then metabolized further as described. The cough, wheeze, and angioedema sometimes associated with the use of ACE inhibitors for treatment of hypertension or heart failure may be due to inhibition of kinin metabolism leading to increased levels of bradykinin. Since bradykinin is a peripheral vasodilator, it has been considered to be a counterbalance to the vasopressor effects of angiotensin II. The two peptides are also clearly related in terms of metabolism, since ACE cleaves His-Leu from the C terminal of angiotensin I, a decapeptide, to leave the octapeptide, angiotensin II. Thus, ACE creates a vasoconstrictor and inactivates a vasodilator.

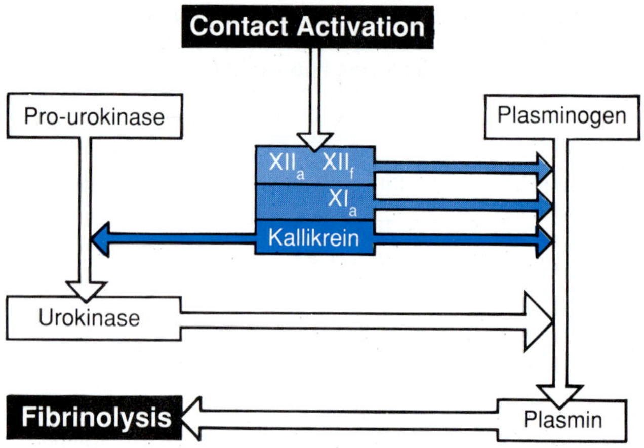

FIGURE 38-11. Pathways of factor XII–dependent fibrinolysis.

RELATION OF CONTACT FACTORS TO OTHER SYSTEMS

The Intrinsic Fibrinolytic Cascade

A factor XII–dependent pathway leading to the conversion of plasminogen to plasmin was described in the 1960s and early 1970s,[170–172] and a defect in this pathway has been observed in plasmas deficient in factor XII, prekallikrein, or HMW kininogen.[3,131–133,135,136] The factor XII–dependent fibrinolytic activity is relatively weak and difficult to demonstrate in whole plasma because large quantities of a potent plasminogen activator are not formed. Relatively little plasmin is generated, and this is rapidly inactivated by plasma inhibitors (α_2-antiplasmin, α_2-macroglobulin). Most studies have therefore used diluted, acidified plasma[173] or chloroform-treated plasma[171] in which inhibition of contact activation and plasmin is minimized or have studied a euglobulin preparation that concentrates the plasma enzymes and cofactors but limits inhibition,[174] or they have added organic compounds that destroy α_2-antiplasmin and C1 INH.[41,175,176] In comparison, such measures are not needed to study blood coagulation or the liberation of bradykinin.

Factor XII–dependent activation of plasminogen is accomplished primarily by kallikrein[39] and factor XIa.[17,40] When purified preparations are compared, kallikrein and factor XIa are equipotent as direct plasminogen activators.[40] The plasma concentration of prekallikrein is about 10-fold higher than that of factor XI; in addition, factor XIIf can readily convert prekallikrein to kallikrein in the fluid phase,[16,18] whereas it has minimal activity on factor XI.[20] Additional kallikrein can dissociate from surfaces and act in the fluid phase, whereas factor XIa cannot. For these reasons, kallikrein is more important in this pathway. Nevertheless, it is possible to demonstrate a fibrinolytic abnormality in factor XI-deficient plasma.[177]

Activated factor XII (XIIa or XIIf) can also convert plasminogen to plasmin,[178] but its activity is only 5% of that of kallikrein. These are all weak reactions in that the potencies of kallikrein and factor XIa as plasminogen activators are thousands of times lower than that of urokinase.[40,179,180] Thus, it can be argued that plasminogen is not a significant substrate for any of them. Although each of these proteins is capable of converting plasminogen to plasmin, the other blood-clotting enzymes—factors IXa, Xa, VIIa, and thrombin—have no such activity, which argues against this activity's being an unspecified epiphenomenon.

The most recent studies of contact-activated fibrinolysis suggest that kallikrein activates the trace quantity of prourokinase in plasma[181] and that urokinase is the main plasminogen activator of plasma[182] (Fig. 38-11). Inhibition by antiurokinase antisera supports this notion as do zymographic gel studies using plasma euglobulin preparations.[41,43] Other investigators have suggested a role for plasma urokinase in factor XII–independent fibrinolysis.[183] Although urokinase is clearly a much more potent plasminogen activator than any of the enzymes associated with contact activation, the quantities of urokinase generated are small. If the effects of α_2-antiplasmin and C1 INH are abrogated by addition of flufenamic acid derivatives, contact activation results in the formation of about 35 ng/mL of plasmin,[176] which represents activation of 0.05% of plasma plasminogen. Thus, the role in vivo of this cascade as a pathway for fibrinolysis is questionable. The close sequence homologies with the fibrinolytic proteins, described in previous sections, are thus not matched by functional relationship with them.

An alternative interaction between the kallikrein–kinin system and in vivo fibrinolysis is suggested by the observation that bradykinin is a potent stimulator of the release of tPA from endothelial cells.[184]

Regulation of Blood Pressure

The possible relation of the contact system to blood pressure regulation is an intriguing question. As already seen, ACE creates the hypertensive peptide, angiotensin II, and plays a major role in inactivating the hypotensive product of contact activation, bradykinin. An unfortunate circumstance has dramatized the kinin-forming capacity of factor XIIf; trauma patients given plasma protein fractions as plasma expanders that were contaminated with factor XIIf showed profound hypotension.[185,186] The mechanism by which infused factor XIIf causes hypotension has been demonstrated to involve bradykinin formation rather than prostaglandins.[187]

Also, a much more tenuous connection exists between blood pressure regulation and the contact system in the factor XII–dependent activation of plasma prorenin. Prorenin is activated to renin by cold treatment of plasma or acidification to pH 3.3. With acid treatment, most of the renin activity is produced after reneutralization; this alkaline phase activation is mediated by kallikrein,[51,52] as is the cold-induced activation.[188] Kallikrein is able to activate purified prorenin, but when added to plasma, it does not cause prorenin activation without an acidification step.[189] Although the acid treatment is supposed to destroy kallikrein inhibitors, prorenin is not activated in plasma deficient in C1 INH or α_2-macroglobulin.[190] Thus, some other unknown event must occur on acidification. The physiologic significance of this reaction is uncertain.

Interaction With Other Plasma Proteases

Factor XIIf has been reported to activate factor VII[22,191] and thereby initiate the extrinsic coagulation pathway. This reaction contributes minimally to the kaolin-APTT as usually performed, but it is responsible for the shortened clotting time seen when plasma is exposed to the cold.[192,193] This is accentuated in women who use oral contraceptives containing estrogen, apparently due to an increased concentration of factor XII.[194–196] This pathway might contribute to the increased incidence of thrombosis reported as a complication of oral contraceptive use.

Factor XIIf (but not factor XIIa) can enzymatically activate the first component of complement when it is incubated with purified C1 or added to plasma[197] (see Fig. 38-7). C1 activation is due to cleavage of the C1r subcomponent[21] by factor XIIf. Little complement activation is seen when kaolin is incubated with whole plasma, and significant complement activation may be seen only in conditions that result in substantial conversion of factor XIIa to factor XIIf. One such circumstance is C1 INH deficiency (hereditary angioedema) in which factor XII activation may contribute to complement consumption.[198,199] Kallikrein can also cleave C1 subcomponents, but the net result is destruction rather than activation. On the other hand, kallikrein can activate factor B of the alternative complement pathway and thereby substitute for factor D.[50]

Interactions With Cells

Kallikrein has been reported to interact with human leukocytes in a variety of ways. It is a chemotactic factor for neutrophils[44] and monocytes,[45] and it has been shown to cause neutrophil aggregation[46] and release of elastase.[47] In a rabbit model, kallikrein stimulation of chemotaxis appeared to require cleavage of C5 and release of C5a chemotactic factor.[48] Therefore, C5 bound to the surface of neutrophils can possibly be cleaved in the aforementioned reactions. Antikallikrein serum was inhibitory, whereas anti-C5 serum had no effect. The authors therefore concluded that the effect of kallikrein on human neutrophils is independent of complement. Furthermore, a degraded form of kallikrein (β-kallikrein), in which the heavy chain is partially digested, is enzymatically active on kininogen to form kinin, but its reactivity with neutrophils is markedly attenuated.[200] Factor XIIa has also been shown to stimulate neutrophils; since factor XIIf did not do this, a requirement for a binding site in the heavy chain was inferred.[23] No studies have demonstrated either a cell surface receptor for these enzymes or required cleavage of surface components. In each instance, the active site of the enzyme is required so that the proenzyme or DFP-treated enzyme is inactive.[44,46]

The components of the contact activation system also appear to interact with platelets. Apparently, plasma factor XI and factor XIa have separate platelet receptors.[67] Platelets also have an intrinsic protein with factor XI activity, which cross-reacts with plasma factor XI immunologically but differs from it in molecular weight and isoelectric point. This activity is present in patients who are deficient in plasma factor XI.[201,202] Platelet-associated factor XI can be activated by factor XII–dependent and factor XII–independent mechanisms.[69] The membrane of activated platelets may also provide a surface on which factor XII can be activated in the presence of prekallikrein and HMW kininogen,[69] so that bound factor XI is then activated. HMW kininogen has been shown to be present within the α granules of platelets[203] and to become available during platelet activation.[204] HMW kininogen exhibits zinc-dependent[205] binding to the platelet surface[203,206] and augments binding of factor XIa.[67]

Despite the demonstrated interactions of contact factors with platelets, platelets clearly are not requisite for contact activation as they are for later steps in coagulation. Thus, contact activation proceeds normally in platelet-poor plasma and the addition of platelets provides little or no augmentation. In fact, evidence exists that platelets may actually inhibit prekallikrein and factor XII activation by secretion of β-thromboglobulin.[207,208] Nevertheless, platelet activation in peripheral tissues due to injury or localized thrombosis may possibly contribute to contact activation and local kinin formation. In some circumstances, the platelets may also provide a factor XII bypass in contact activation.[209]

A promising area of study is the relation of the contact activation system to endothelium. Bradykinin has been shown to stimulate the release of prostaglandin I_2 and thromboxane A_2 from cultured endothelial cells,[210,211] and bradykinin has been identified as a powerful stimulant of the release of tPA from endothelial cells.[184] Recent studies have shown that HMW kininogen can directly bind to vascular endothelial cells by its heavy- and light-chain moieties.[212–214] Endothelial cell–bound HMW kininogen was able to bind factor XI and promoted the activation of factor IX, suggesting that the interaction of HMW kininogen with endothelial cells may participate in the initiation of blood coagulation at sites of vascular injury.[215] Interaction of HMW kininogen with endothelial cells and subsequent generation of bradykinin from cell-bound HMW kininogen[216] may also be physiologically significant, since bradykinin stimulates the production of endothelium-derived relaxing factor (chemically related to nitric oxide) in these cells, which has profound effects on the vascular tone.[217,218]

DEFICIENCIES OF PROTEINS OF THE CONTACT ACTIVATION SYSTEM

Historically, the proteins of the contact system, like other coagulation proteins, each have been discovered as a consequence of the identification of persons whose plasma was found to give abnormal clotting times in in vitro assays. Deficiencies of each of the proteins of the contact system are well recognized and are characterized by abnormal results in tests of the intrinsic coagulation pathway and in some cases by clinical bleeding.

Deficiency of any of the contact factors may be suspected when a coagulation profile reveals prolongation of the APTT with a normal prothrombin time. It is most important to rule out the possibility of factor VIII or factor IX deficiency, since these deficiencies result in serious defects of hemostasis. Generally, patients with these deficiencies present with a major bleeding diathesis, and often they or their male relatives (they are X-linked traits) have a history of repeated bleeding. If these factors are specifically assayed and found to be normal, a defect in one of the early components (factor XII, prekallikrein, HMW kininogen, or factor XI) would be likely. The plasma in question can be assayed for each of these by testing its ability to correct the APTT of plasmas that are selectively deficient in each component; such plasmas are commercially available. If a functional defect of any of the components is seen, it can be determined whether the protein is absent or whether a defective protein has been synthesized. This is done by quantitative immunoassays using monospecific antisera.

The degree of prolongation of clotting time varies with the particular protein deficiency. No correlation is seen in the severity of any of the defects of in vitro coagulation and clinical sequelae. So far, no contact factor deficiencies, except factor XI deficiency, has been associated with a bleeding diathesis. Conversely, plasmas deficient in factor XII, prekallikrein, or HMW kininogen do not generate any bradykinin on the addition of a surface. Thus, we will consider factor XI deficiency, in which kinin formation is normal, separately from that of the proteins of the kinin-forming pathways, namely, factor XII, prekallikrein, and HMW kininogen.

Deficiency of Factor XI

Clinical Manifestations

Of all the contact system proteins, factor XI is the only one for which a deficiency is associated with a hemophiliac syndrome.[219,220] It is characterized in this case by the variability in its clinical picture. About half of identified factor XI–deficient patients have experienced postoperative or posttrauma bleeding. Other patients are frequently identified by abnormal APTTs with no history of bleeding. When APTTs were not a standard preoperative procedure, the deficiency was not always recognized until excessive postoperative hemorrhage occurred.[221] Even with routine APTT screens, no close correlation is found between the severity of bleeding, if any, and the measured level of factor XI activity or factor XI antigen. Even the distinction of heterozygotes (with 15% to 62% factor XI activity) from homozygotes (with less than 15% activity) does not divide bleeders from nonbleeders, since equal frequencies of bleeding are found in each group.[222]

Although no cases of bleeding into joints have been reported, reports of mild spontaneous bleeding have been made in the form of nosebleeds, hematuria, menorrhagia, and retinal hemorrhage (one).[223] Little or no spontaneous bruising and little abnormal bruising even in response to severe trauma have occurred.[224] Some women have reported episodes of spontaneous bruising, sometimes associated with heavy menstrual bleeding for up to 2 weeks.[225]

A characteristic of factor XI deficiency is that the same patient seems to show great variability in the tendency to bleed in response to different surgical procedures at different times.[225,226] The reason for this variability is not known; suggestions of fluctuation with time of the residual plasma levels of factor XI[223] have not been supported by long-term studies, and the apparent variation may in fact be a response to varying degrees of hemostatic challenge. To the extent that major surgery is often accompanied by transfusions of whole blood or plasma, normal hemostasis may be attained. In minor surgery, abnormal bleeding often occurs. This is especially the case with tooth extractions and tonsillectomies, which leave open surfaces in the oral cavity where high levels of plasminogen activator have been found in the subendothelial areas of the oral mucosa.[227] Vigorous bleeding requiring transfusion has been reported, although a slow ooze beginning 3 to 4 days after extraction seems to be more common.[223,224,226] Surgical procedures of the urologic system have also been found to cause problems for factor XI–deficient patients.[221,228]

Deficiencies of factor XI in the form of circulating anticoagulant antibodies have been reported, which were acquired either spontaneously[229] or after replacement therapy.[230–232] In several cases, the antibodies described blocked the binding of factor XI to surfaces[231,233] or to HMW kininogen.[232]

Genetics

Factor XI deficiency was originally described as a rare autosomal dominant trait[220] occurring in 1 of 100,000 persons. Subsequent work indicated that factor XI deficiency is transmitted by an incompletely recessive autosomal gene so that heterozygotes may have factor XI levels of 20% to 60% of normal levels.[223,224]

Factor XI deficiency is largely found in the Ashkenazi Jewish population with an incidence of 0.15% to 0.3%[234]; the incidence of heterozygotes ranges from 5% to 11%. Among the Ashkenazi population, no evidence exists of a regional localization in eastern Europe but the gene appears to be distributed throughout the whole Ashkenazi population. Initially, only a handful of cases of factor XI deficiency were described in which Jewish descent was improbable. More recently, two studies,[222,235] consisting of a total of 105 factor XI-deficient kindreds, found that 82 were Jewish and the remaining kindreds included members of a variety of ethnic groups. Some statistically significant difference appears to exist between the "Jewish" factor XI deficiency and the non-Jewish syndrome. Thus, a larger proportion of Jewish propositi have factor XI levels below 15% and are classified as homozygotes.[235] Within the respective homozygote and heterozygote populations, however, Jewish propositi have higher mean factor XI : c levels.[222] The significance, if any, of these observations remains unknown.

One study found that the likelihood of bleeding or not bleeding, although not correlated with factor XI levels, was consistent within families.[235] Thus, in 12 families in which the propositus was a nonbleeder, no other factor XI–deficient family member was found to bleed. On the other hand, in 13 families in which the propositus was a bleeder, other family members were also bleeders.

In all studies of multiple kindreds, the level of cross-reacting antigen (cross-reacting material [CRM]) was closely correlated with the level of factor XI activity, although a very few persons have been found to be CRM-positive. In this respect, factor XI deficiency differs from deficiencies of other clotting factors, in which CRM-positive variants are commonly found.

Therapy

The absence of significant spontaneous bleeding or bruising in factor XI deficiency means that maintenance therapy is not usually required. Surgical patients with factor XI deficiency, however, need careful management to reduce the risk of postoperative hemorrhage. Generally, the circulating level of factor XI needs to be raised to 20% to 30% of normal,[221,236] using fresh whole blood or plasma or fresh-frozen plasma (banked whole blood loses 80% of its factor XI content during the first week of storage[237]). If cryoprecipitate supernatant is available, it may also be used because it retains most of the factor XI activity.[238] The half-life of infused factor XI is 60 to 80 hours,[236] and hemostasis is normally achieved with plasma administration of 10 to 20 mL/kg/d.[221,226] The progress of the treatment can be monitored with APTT or specific factor XI assays.

Deficiencies of Proteins Involved in Kinin Formation

Factor XII

Several hundred cases of factor XII deficiency (Hageman trait) have been identified. The APTT is markedly prolonged in patients with factor XII deficiency. In a manual assay using kaolin, clotting times of 200 to 300 seconds are found compared with less than 50 seconds for controls. If the second stage is performed at room temperature, a clot may not form for 20 minutes. Automated commercial APTT systems give clotting times of about 100 seconds.

Despite the profound defect of in vitro functioning of the intrinsic pathway, no bleeding disorder is seen in factor XII deficiency, nor is there protection against thrombotic disease. In fact, Mr. Hageman, the propositus case of factor XII deficiency, died of a pulmonary embolus,[239] and several other patients have suffered myocardial infarction.[240–242]

The gene for factor XII has been localized to chromosome 5.[30,31] Most cases have no antigenic material in circulation, although at least one CRM+ person has been described. In one study of factor XII deficiency, a mutation frequently occurred in the second intron of the gene such that homozygotes were markedly deficient and heterozygotes had a partial deficiency.[243] This was seen in four of five unrelated Italian subjects with factor XII deficiency from different regions of the country. No deletions were identified.

Prekallikrein

Prekallikrein deficiency[131] (Fletcher trait) is known to occur in about 30 families. The APTT of prekallikrein-deficient plasma is unique because the final clotting time after recalcification shortens as the length of the activation step is prolonged.[4,131–133] This autocorrection implies that the role of kallikrein in the activation of the intrinsic clotting pathway is to accelerate the activation of factor XII. Without kallikrein, factor XII becomes activated much more slowly, but eventually enough factor XIIa accumulates to activate factor XI at a normal rate. The slow activation of factor XII in prekallikrein-deficient plasma may be achieved through the autoactivation reaction and possibly a positive feedback by factor XIa. Prekallikrein-deficient plasma does not generate bradykinin on activation.[132]

Like Hageman trait, Fletcher trait is not characterized by any observable hemostatic abnormalities,[244] and cases of prekallikrein deficiency with myocardial infarction[245] and multiple episodes of cerebral thrombosis[246] have been reported.

Nonfunctional antigenic species of prekallikrein have been found in several cases of Fletcher trait.[247] In one family,[248] three children had 35% antigen and no function; others had twice as much antigenic content as functional activity. A nonfunctional variant protein that had no clotting activity was isolated; it was cleaved by activated factor XII at 0% to 5% of the normal rate, but the product was functionless. The protein at 80 kd was immunologically undistinguishable from normal protein, and it complexed normally with HMW kininogen. Isoelectric focusing suggested a unit charge difference; thus, a single amino acid substitution is implied.

High-Molecular-Weight Kininogen

High-molecular-weight kininogen deficiency was discovered almost simultaneously in three different patients, Fitzgerald,[249] Williams,[3] and Flaujeac[135] and has been named after all three. Other cases have since been reported, although the total number known remains small, probably fewer than 20. The APTT is markedly prolonged but not so much as in factor XII deficiency. Manual clotting times with kaolin range from 100 to 200 seconds, and automated instruments can give times less than 100 seconds (compared with less than 40 seconds for controls). As with factor XII or prekallikrein deficiency, deficiencies of HMW kininogen do not cause apparent defects in normal hemostasis.

HMW kininogen deficiency can occur as a complete absence of HMW kininogen and LMW kininogen (Williams) or lack only the HMW kininogen species (Fitzgerald). Because the mRNAs for the two proteins are transcribed from the same gene (see Fig. 38-7), these phenotypic variants might represent defects in either the heavy-chain sequence or the sequence coding for the light chain of HMW kininogen, respectively.

Relation of Contact Factor Deficiencies to Hemostasis

The contrast between the role of contact activation in in vitro clotting assays and its apparent irrelevance in vivo is a striking enigma. The only known pathway for factor XI activation is through factor XIIa, and the participation of prekallikrein and HMW kininogen is required for efficient activation of factor XII. Thus, the longest clotting times are found in factor XII deficiency followed by deficiency of HMW kininogen, whereas the clotting times of factor XI–deficient plasmas are much shorter. The relatively high in vitro clotting ability of factor XI–deficient plasma could be explained by the ability of factor XIIf to activate factor VII of the extrinsic pathway, thereby bypassing the activation of factor IX by factor XIa. This pathway does not account for the contrary clinical data that deficiency of factor XI causes a hemostatic abnormality, whereas deficiencies of the other proteins of the contact system do not. This suggests that in vivo hemostasis does not depend on an intact contact activation system. A further paradox is that, in marked contrast to the deficiencies of factors VIII and IX, the hemophilia associated with factor XI deficiency is both mild and variable, and no apparent correlation exists between the measured factor XI clotting activity and the degree of clinical hemophilia.

A possible explanation for these observations is the existence of alternative pathways for the activation of factor XI and for the factor XI–independent activation of factor IX. Such pathways would be independent of factor XII, prekallikrein, and HMW kininogen and therefore bypass defects in the latter proteins. The activation of factor IX by factor VIIa of the extrinsic pathway is clearly a significant physiologic pathway that might be of greater hemostatic significance than the activation by factor XI, although the observed kinetics of the two pathways are similar. Also of importance might be factor XI or a factor XI–like molecule on the platelet, which could be present even when plasma factor XI is absent and which can be activated in the absence of factor XII. The precise mechanism has not been defined, nor is it certain that its contribution to local hemostasis is sufficient to act as an effective bypass. No systematic study has been reported in which the levels of platelet factor XI have been determined in plasma factor XI deficiency.

More recently, two reports have described the activation of purified factor XI by thrombin or by autoactivation, both in the presence of negatively charged surfaces.[250,251] The demonstration of a thrombin feedback to activate factor XI appears to offer a solution to the enigma posed by the requirement for factor XI, but not factor XII, for normal hemostasis. Other reports have disputed this finding, however. In one case, the activation of factor XI by thrombin and its autoactivation on surfaces using purified proteins was confirmed, but the addition of purified fibrinogen of HMW kininogen to the mixture abrogated the reaction.[252] In the other report, the generation of factor XIa in plasma was contingent on the presence of factor XII and a surface; in the absence of either, factor XI was not cleaved.[253] Thus, the activation of the extrinsic pathway and the consequent activation of endogenous prothrombin did not cause the cleavage of factor XI in factor XII–deficient plasma. At this time, we have to conclude that the description of the intrinsic coagulation pathway being initiated by thrombin activation of factor XI, without a role for factor XII, is premature and may not be correct.

Clearly, defects in in vitro clotting assays do not necessarily imply clinical bleeding. The properties of coagulation factors that determine whether bleeding results possibly have more to do with interactions with platelets or with endothelial cells and are distinct from their contribution to thrombin formation in plasma. The interactions of the contact factors with cells are not well understood; these proteins may behave differently from the clotting factors in this regard. A final speculation is that the presence of bradykinin or the ability to generate bradykinin is necessary for bleeding to occur and that patients deficient in factor XII, prekallikrein, or HMW kininogen, who are unable to generate bradykinin in plasma, are somehow protected.

ASSESSMENT OF CONTACT ACTIVATION IN HUMAN DISEASE

The factor XII–dependent pathways described herein do not appear to contribute to thrombosis and hemostasis in a major way. Thus, although activation of factor XII leads to in vitro coagulation, in most thrombotic disorders the effects of activation of the extrinsic (tissue factor) pathway predominate. Certainly, no thrombosis is associated with hereditary angioedema, a disorder in which contact activation is prominent. Similarly, patients deficient in factor XII, prekallikrein, and HMW kininogen have no obvious bleeding diathesis, and the bleeding disorder in factor XI–deficient patients is highly variable and often mild (see section on deficiency of factor XI). Most evidence suggests that the importance of the cascade relates to the pathogenesis of inflammatory reactions, the local control of blood flow (in which bradykinin functions as a hormone), and perhaps control of blood pressure.

Hereditary angioedema has received considerable attention because C1 INH is absent and because activation of the factor XII–dependent pathways and the classic complement pathways occurs simultaneously. Aside from hereditary angioedema, a relatively large literature describes activation of the factor XII–dependent pathways in plasma or serum in a wide variety of inflammatory disorders. In some disorders, activation is coincident with the patients' symptoms. No data prove that the consequences of such activation lead to disease manifestations or, conversely, that inhibition of the pathway ameliorates symptoms. These should be viewed as promising associations and are important areas for future investigation. The reader is referred to Table 38-4 for a list of these disorders; some are briefly described in the next section.

TABLE 38-4. Disorders Associated With Contact Activation

Disease	Reference
Adult respiratory distress syndrome	254
Carcinoid syndrome	255, 256
Cirrhosis	See text
Disseminated intravascular coagulation	See text
Hereditary angioedema	See text
Nephrotic syndrome	See text
Postgastrectomy dumping syndrome	257
Polycythemia vera	258
Rocky Mountain spotted fever	259
Sepsis (septic shock)	See text
Transfusion reactions	See text
Typhoid fever	260
Type II hyperlipidemia	261

Assay Methods

To assess the factor XII–dependent pathways in human disease, ideally the concentrations of each active enzyme should be measured, the extent of HMW kininogen cleavage should be determined, and bradykinin should be assayed. These measurements are difficult because the enzymes are rapidly inactivated and bradykinin is rapidly degraded. Thus, often only the level of residual proenzyme can be determined. Factor XII, prekallikrein, and HMW kininogen in plasma can be quantitated by coagulant assay,[107] by immunologic determination of antigen levels,[262–264] or by in vitro activation and assay of evolved enzymatic activity.[110,265–268] Shifts in electrophoretic mobility indicate complex formation between enzymes and their inhibitors and provide qualitative evidence that activation has occurred. Thus far, monoclonal antibodies that react solely with the active site of enzymes have not been developed, although monoclonal antibodies have been described, which react with neoantigens in C1 INH that has formed complexes with plasma enzymes.[269,270]

The previously described assays are useful when sufficient activation has occurred to cause significant depletion of substrate. When only a small amount of each factor is converted, it may be missed. Assays have been developed for enzyme–inhibitor complexes based on the assay for plasmin-α_2 antiplasmin complexes by Harpel.[271] These include double-antibody, enzyme-linked immunosorbent assay methods for factor XIIa–C1 INH,[272] kallikrein–C1 INH,[273] and kallikrein–α_2-macroglobulin complexes,[152] which can detect as little as 1% activation of any of the components. A radioimmunoassay based on a monoclonal antibody to a neodeterminant in complexed or cleaved C1 INH has been reported to detect 0.05% activation of factor XII or prekallikrein.[274] Bradykinin[275] and des-Arg^9 bradykinin[276] can also be determined by radioimmunoassay.

Finally, assays using immunoblotting (Western blot) can detect cleaved HMW kininogen in plasma[82]; immunoblotting can be used to develop a quantitative assay.[77] The latter assays have begun to be applied to disease states. Most of the literature refers to results obtained with earlier methods describing depletion of contact factors, particularly prekallikrein, associated with particular conditions.

Hereditary Angioedema

Hereditary angioedema is the disease state associated with a deficiency of C1 INH. Patients present with episodic swelling occurring virtually anywhere in the body, attacks of severe abdominal pain due to edema of the bowel wall, and laryngeal edema. Although a kinin derived from a cleavage product of the second complement component was thought to be responsible for the edema,[277] other studies suggest that bradykinin is the critical peptide.[199,278] On the other hand, a kinin-like vasoactive substance may yet be shown to be a complement derivative, as noted in recent reports.[279] During attacks of angioedema, depletion of prekallikrein and HMW kininogen[280] occurs, and blisters induced in the skin of patients are found to contain elevated plasma kallikrein levels.[281] The formation of bradykinin[282] and cleaved HMW kininogen[283] has been detected. The complement activation appears to be due to autoactivation of C1 (specifically C1r) in the absence of C1 INH,[284,285] but this may be augmented by factor XIIf,[21,197] particularly during acute attacks of swelling.

Sepsis and Disseminated Intravascular Coagulation

Severe infections with gram-negative organisms leading to septic shock carry a poor prognosis and a high mortality rate. The pooling of fluid into body cavities, the intravascular volume depletion, and the hypotension may be caused by release of bradykinin. Activation of factor XII can be induced by the lipid A component of endotoxin,[117,118,286] and contact activation proteins are depleted in endotoxic shock.[287–290] In patients hospitalized because of trauma, onset of sepsis has been shown to be associated with kininogen depletion. Determination of serial kininogen levels had prognostic value,[288] since a drop in the kininogen level to near zero usually indicated a lethal outcome as did lower prekallikrein levels.[291] Enzyme–C1 INH complexes may be difficult to detect in sepsis, even when factor XII and prekallikrein levels are reduced, because of rapid clearance.[274]

In patients with disseminated intravascular coagulation due to endothelial injury or endotoxemia (including gram-negative sepsis, gram-positive sepsis, and viremia), decreased levels of plasma factor XII and prekallikrein and kallikrein inhibitory activity are seen.[292,293] These changes were not observed in disseminated intravascular coagulation associated with leukemia, carcinoma, or abortion. The data suggest activation of the factor XII–dependent pathways. A case has also been reported of disseminated intravascular coagulation in preeclampsia in which activation of the contact system was seen.[294]

Other Disorders With Associated Contact Activation

Contact activation may occur during allergic diseases; for example, nasal washings of patients with allergic rhinitis who have been challenged with antigen contain lysyl bradykinin, bradykinin, kininogen, and kallikreins derived from mast cells and plasma.[295–298] The latter may represent contact activation on a surface altered by the initial inflammation. Other possibilities for activation include negatively charged macromolecules in mucosal secretions and mast cell heparin.[115] Although we routinely use dextran sulfates as model compounds on which factor XII activation can occur, other sulfated mucopolysaccharides may serve similar functions in vivo.[299]

The synovial fluid of patients with rheumatoid arthritis has been shown to contain plasma kallikrein, which has been shown to activate procollagenase to collagenase.[300] Uric acid and pyrophosphate crystals can act as surfaces for contact activation and may contribute to the inflammation of gout and pseudogout.[301,302] A role for the contact activation system in inflammatory arthritis is therefore possible and may involve other functions of the enzymes in addition to any effects of kinins. Note that at least one case of gout[242] and one case of rheumatoid arthritis[303] associated with factor XII deficiency have been reported.

In some patients with nephrotic syndrome, a diminution of factor XII has been reported, which could not be explained simply by a loss of proteins in the urine.[304,305] Immunoreactive but nonfunctional factor XII was found in the plasma, which suggested that activation of factor XII in the nephrotic kidney might be occurring.[306,307] Disagreement exists over whether prekallikrein is also diminished in nephrotic syndrome.

Cirrhosis, as might be anticipated, is associated with diminished levels of plasma prekallikrein, HMW kininogen, and, to a lesser degree, factor XII, which seems to be caused by a diminished rate of protein synthesis.[265,308,309] A similar depression of prekallikrein level apparently related to liver dysfunction has been noted in dengue fever.[310]

Other associations of contact activation with disease states are listed in Table 38-4.

SUMMARY AND CONCLUSIONS

The contact system is unusual among proteolytic pathways because of its self-contained cyclic nature. Rather than being activated by an extrinsic activity, it is able to switch itself on, converting two zymogens to proteases—factor XIIa and kallikrein. The process is initiated by surface activation and characterized by extreme positive feedback. After they are formed, the proteases can participate in the initiation of a number of pathways, especially blood coagulation, fibrinolysis, and bradykinin formation. It is a paradox that despite these multiple activities, deficiencies of contact activation do not have any obvious clinical consequences. This may reflect the observed parallelism in the pathways that maintain homeostasis. A number of disease states are associated with activation of the contact system, including endotoxic shock and allergic and inflammatory reactions, but no unequivocal attribution of symptoms to the products of contact activation is known. Nevertheless, if mutations leading to deficiencies of contact system proteins were truly neutral, one would expect them to be common, whereas they have been found relatively infrequently. Taken together, these observations suggest that the role of the contact system may be more critical in host defense mechanisms and the pathogenesis of inflammation than in hemostasis. These questions will be more amenable to study as clinically useful antagonists to bradykinin and to the contact system enzymes become available.

REFERENCES

1. Revak SD, Cochrane CG, Johnston AR, Hugli TE. Structural changes accompanying enzymatic activation of human Hageman factor. J Clin Invest 1974;54:619.
2. Silverberg M, Kaplan AP. Enzymatic activities of activated and zymogen forms of human Hageman factor (factor XII). Blood 1982;60:64.
3. Colman RW, Bagdasarian A, Talamo RC, et al. Williams trait: human kininogen deficiency with diminished levels of plasminogen proactivator and prekallikrein associated with abnormalities of the Hageman factor–dependent pathways. J Clin Invest 1975;56:1650.
4. Meier HL, Pierce JV, Colman RW, Kaplan AP. Activation and function of human Hageman factor: the role of high molecular kininogen and prekallikrein. J Clin Invest 1977;60:18.
5. Revak SD, Cochrane CG, Griffin JH. The binding and cleavage characteristics of human Hageman factor during contact activation: a comparison of normal plasma with plasma deficient in factor XI, prekallikrein or high molecular weight kininogen. J Clin Invest 1977;58:1167.
6. Cochrane CG, Revak SD, Wuepper KD. Activation of Hageman factor in solid and fluid phases. J Exp Med 1973;138:1564.
7. Griffin JH. Role of surface in surface-dependent activation of Hageman factor (blood coagulation factor XII). Proc Natl Acad Sci 1978;75:1998.
8. Tankersley DL, Finlayson JS. Kinetics of activation and autoactivation of human factor XII biochemistry. 1984;23:273.
9. Silverberg M, Dunn JT, Garen L, Kaplan AP. Autoactivation of human Hageman factor. J Biol Chem 1980;255:7281.
10. Fujikawa K, McMullen BA. Amino acid sequence of human b-factor XIIa. J Biol Chem 1983;258:10924.
11. Revak SD, Cochrane CG. The relationship of structure and function in human Hageman factor. J Clin Invest 1977;57:852.
12. Dunn JT, Silverberg M, Kaplan AP. The cleavage and formation of activated Hageman factor by autodigestion and by kallikrein. J Biol Chem 1982;275:1779.
13. Dunn JT, Kaplan AP. Formation and structure of human Hageman factor fragments. J Clin Invest 1982;70:627.
14. Silverberg M, Kaplan AP. Human Hageman factor and its fragments. Methods Enzymol 1988;163:68.
15. Kettner C, Shaw E. Inactivation of trypsin-like enzymes with peptides of arginine chloromethyl ketone. Methods Enzymol 1981;80:826.
16. Kaplan AP, Austen KF. A pre-albumin activator of prekallikrein. J Immunol 1970;105:802.
17. Mandle RJJ, Kaplan AP. Hageman factor substrates. II. Human plasma prekallikrein: mechanism of activation by Hageman factor and par-

ticipation in Hageman factor–dependent fibrinolysis. J Biol Chem 1977;252:6097.
18. Tankersley DL, Fournel MA, Schroeder DD. Kinetics of activation of prekallikrein by prekallikrein activator. Biochemistry 1980;19:3121.
19. Revak SD, Cochrane CG, Bouma BN, Griffin JH. Surface and fluid phase activities of two forms of activated Hageman factor produced during contact activation of plasma. J Exp Med 1978;147:719.
20. Kaplan AP, Austen KF. A prealbumin activator of prekallikrein. II. Derivation of activators of prekallikrein from active Hageman factor by digestion with plasmin. J Exp Med 1971;133:696.
21. Ghebrehiwet B, Randazzo BP, Dunn JT, et al. Mechanism of activation of the classical pathway of complement by Hageman factor fragment. J Clin Invest 1983;71:1450.
22. Radcliffe R, Bagdassarian B, Colman RW, Nemerson YN. Activation of factor VII by Hageman factor fragments. Blood 1977;59:611.
23. Wachtfogel YT, Pixley RA, Kucich U, et al. Purified plasma factor XIIa aggregates human neutrophils and causes degranulation. Blood 1986;67:1731.
24. Cool DE, Edgell CS, Louie GV, et al. Characterization of human blood coagulation factor XII cDNA. J Biol Chem 1985;25:13666.
25. Que BG, Davie EW. Characterization of a cDNA coding for human factor XII (Hageman factor). Biochemistry 1986;8:1525.
26. McMullen BA, Fujikawa K. Amino acid sequence of the heavy chain of human a-factor XIIa (activated Hageman factor). J Biol Chem 1985;260:5328.
27. Pixley RA, Stumpo LG, Birkmeyer K, et al. A monoclonal antibody recognizing an icosapeptide sequence in the heavy chain of human factor XII inhibits surface-catalyzed activation. J Biol Chem 1987;262:10140.
28. Clarke BJ, Côté HCF, Cool DE, et al. Mapping of a putative surface-binding site of human coagulation factor XII. J Biol Chem 1989;264:11497.
29. Cool DE, MacGillivray RT. Characterization of the human blood coagulation factor XII gene: intron/exon gene organization and analysis of the 5′-flanking region. J Biol Chem 1987;262:13662.
30. Citarella F, Tripodi M, Fantoni A, et al. Assignment of human coagulation factor XII (fXII) to chromosome 5 by cDNA hybridization to DNA from somatic cell hybrids. Hum Genet 1988;80:397.
31. Royle NJ, Nigli M, Cool D, et al. Structural gene encoding human factor XII is located at 5q33-qter. Somat Cell Mol Genet 1988;14:217.
32. Castellino FJ, Beals JM. The genetic relationships between the kringle domains of human plasminogen, prothrombin, tissue plasminogen activator, urokinase, and coagulation factor XII. J Mol Evol 1987;26:358.
33. Bouma BN, Miles LA, Barretta G, Griffin JH. Human plasma prekallikrein: studies of its activation by activated factor XII and of its inactivation by diisopropyl phosphofluoridate. Biochemistry 1980;19:1151.
34. Mandle RJ, Colman RW, Kaplan AP. Identification of prekallikrein and high molecular weight kininogen as a complex in plasma. Proc Natl Acad Sci USA 1976;73:4179.
35. Bock PE, Shore JD, Tans G, Griffin JH. Protein-protein interactions in contact activation of blood coagulation: binding of high molecular weight kininogen and the 5-(iodoacetamido) fluorescein-labeled kininogen light chain to prekallikrein, kallikrein, and the separated kallikrein heavy and light chains. J Biol Chem 1985;260:12434.
36. Silverberg M, Nicoll JE, Kaplan AP. The mechanism by which the light chain of cleaved HMW-kininogen augments the activation of prekallikrein, factor XI, and Hageman factor. Thromb Res 1980;70:173.
37. Cochrane CG, Revak SD. Dissemination of contact activation in plasma by plasma kallikrein. J Exp Med 1980;152:608.
38. Bouma BN, Easton E, van Iwaarden F. Thromb Haemost 1985;54:228.
39. Colman RW. Activation of plasminogen by plasma kallikrein. Biochem. Biophys Res Commun 1969;351:273.
40. Mandle RJJ, Kaplan AP. Hageman factor dependent fibrinolysis: generation of fibrinolytic activity by the interaction of human activated factor XI and plasminogen. 1979;54:850.
41. Miles LA, Rothschild Z, Griffin JH. Dextran sulfate stimulated fibrinolytic activity in whole human plasma: dependence on the contact activation system and a urokinase-related antigen. Thromb Haemost 1981;46:211.
42. Ichinose A, Fujikawa K, Suyama T. The activation of pro-urokinase by plasma kallikrein and its inactivation by thrombin. J Biol Chem 1986;261:3486.
43. Hauert J, Nicoloso G, Schleuning WD, et al. Plasminogen activators in dextran sulfate-activated euglobulin fractions: a molecular analysis of factor XII- and prekallikrein-dependent fibrinolysis. Blood 1989;73:994.
44. Kaplan AP, Kay AB, Austen KF. A prealbumin activator of prekallikrein. III. Appearance of chemotactic activity for human neutrophils by the conversion of human prekallikrein to kallikrein. J Exp Med 1972;135:81.
45. Gallin JI, Kaplan AP. Mononuclear cell chemotactic activity of kallikrein and plasminogen activator and its inhibition by C1 INH and α_2 macroglobulin. J Immunol 1974;113:1928.
46. Schapira M, Despland E, Scott CF, et al. Purified human plasma kallikrein aggregates human blood neutrophils. J Clin Invest 1982;69:1199.
47. Wachtfogel YT, Kucich U, James HL, et al. Human plasma kallikrein releases neutrophil elastase activity during blood coagulation. J Clin Invest 1983;22:1672.
48. Wiggins RC, Giglas RC, Henson PM. Chemotactic activator generated from the fifth component of complement by plasma kallikrein of the rabbit. J Exp Med 1981;153:1391.
49. Cooper NR, Miles LA, Griffin JH. Effects of plasma kallikrein and plasmin on the first complement component. J Immunol 1980;124:1517.
50. DiScipis RG. The activation of the alternative pathway C3 convertase by human plasma kallikrein. 1982;45:587.
51. Derkx FHM, Bouma BN, Schalekamp MPA, Schalekamp MADH. An intrinsic factor XII–prekallikrein–dependent pathway activates the human plasma renin-angiotensin system. 1979;280:315.
52. Sealey JE, Atlas SA, Laragh JH, Silverberg M, Kaplan AP. Initiation of plasma prorenin activation by Hageman factor–dependent conversion of plasma prekallikrein to kallikrein. Proc Natl Acad Sci USA 1979;76:5914.
53. Harpel PC. Circulatory inhibitors of human plasma kallikrein. In: Pisano JJ, Austen KF, eds. Chemistry and biology of the kallikrein-kinin system in health and disease. Washington, DC, US Government Printing Office, 1974:169.
54. Schapira M, Scott CF, Colman RW. Contribution of plasma protease inhibitors to the inactivation of kallikrein in plasma. J Clin Invest 1982;69:462.
55. van der Graaf F, Koedam JA, Bouma BN. Inactivation of kallikrein in human plasma. J Clin Invest 1983;71:149.
56. Chung DW, Fujikawa K, McMullen BA, Davie EW. Human plasma prekallikrein: a zymogen to a serine protease that contains four tandem repeats. Biochemistry 1986;25:2410.
57. Bouma BN, Griffin JH. Human blood coagulation factor XI: purification, properties, and mechanism of activation by factor XII. J Biol Chem 1977;252:6432.
58. Kurachi K, Davie EW. Activation of human factor XI (plasma thromboplastin antecedent) by factor XII (activated Hageman factor). Biochemistry 1977;16:5831.
59. Thompson RE, Mandle RJ, Kaplan AP. Association of factor XI and high molecular weight kininogen in human plasma. J Clin Invest 1977;60:1376.
60. Tait J, Fujikawa K. Primary structure requirements for the binding of human high molecular weight kininogen to plasma prekallikrein and factor XI. J Biol Chem 1987;262:11651.
61. Warn-Cramer BJ, Bajaj SP. Stoichiometry of binding of high molecular weight kininogen to factor XI/XIa. Biochem Biophys Res Commun 1985;133:417.
62. Baglia FA, Sinha D, Walsh PN. Functional domains in the heavy-chain region of factor XI: a high molecular weight kininogen-binding site and a substrate binding site for factor IX. Blood 1989;74:244.
63. Griffin JH, Cochrane CG. Mechanisms for the involvement of high molecular weight kininogen in surface-dependent reactions of Hageman factor. Proc Natl Acad Sci USA 1976;73:2554.
64. Wiggins RC, Bouma BN, Cochrane CG, Griffin JH. Role of high molecular weight kininogen in surface binding and activation of coagulation factor XI and prekallikrein. Proc Natl Acad Sci USA 1977;77:4636.
65. Sinha D, Koshy A, Seaman FS, Walsh PN. Functional characterization of human blood coagulation factor XIa using hybridoma antibodies. J Biol Chem 1985;260:10714.
66. Sinha D, Seaman FS, Walsh PN. Role of calcium ions and the heavy chain of factor XIa in the activation of human coagulation factor IX. Biochemistry 1987;26:3768.
67. Sinha D, Seaman FS, Koshy A, et al. Blood coagulation factor XIa binds specifically to a site on activated human platelets distinct from that for factor XI. J Clin Invest 1984;73:1550.
68. Greengard JS, Heeb MJ, Ersdal E, et al. Binding of coagulation factor XI to washed human platelets. Biochemistry 1986;25:3884.
69. Walsh PN, Griffin JH. Contributions of human platelets to the proteolytic activation of blood coagulation factors XII and XI. Blood 1981;57:106.
70. Fujikawa K, Chung DW, Hendrickson LE, Davie EW. Amino acid sequence of human factor XI: a blood coagulation factor with four tandem repeats that are highly homologous with plasma prekallikrein. Biochemistry 1986;25:2417.
71. Asakai R, Davie EW, Chung DW. Organization of the gene for human factor XI. Biochemistry 1987;26:7221.
72. Colman RW, Muller-Esterl W. Nomenclature of kininogens. Thromb Haemost 1988;60:340.
73. Keribiriou DM, Griffin JH. Human high molecular weight kininogen: studies of structure–function relationships and of proteolysis of the molecule occurring during contact activation of plasma. J Biol Chem 1979;245:12020.
74. Proud D, Pierce JV, Pisano JJ. Radioimmunoassay of human high molecular weight kininogen in normal and deficient plasma. J Lab Clin Med 1980;95:563.
75. Adam A, Albert A, Calay G, et al. Human kininogens of low and high molecular mass: quantification by radioimmunoassay and determination of reference values. Clin Chem 1985;31:423.
76. Berrettini M, Lammle B, White T, et al. Detection of in vitro and in vivo cleavage of high molecular weight kininogen in human plasma by immunoblotting with monoclonal antibodies Blood 1986;68:455.
77. Reddigari SR, Kaplan AP. Quantification of human high molecular weight kininogen by immunoblotting with a monoclonal anti–light chain antibody. J Immunol Methods 1989;19.
78. Bock PE, Shore JD. Protein-protein interaction of blood coagulation:

characterization of a fluoroscein-labeled human high molecular weight kininogen light chain as a probe. J Biol Chem 1983;258:15079.
79. Schiffman S, Mannhalter C, Tynerk D. Human high molecular weight kininogen: effects of cleavage by kallikrein on protein structure and procoagulant activity. J Biol Chem 1980;255:6433.
80. Mori K, Nagasawa S. Studies on human high molecular weight (HMW) kininogen. II. Structural change in HMW kininogen by the action of human plasma kallikrein. J Biochem 1981;89:1465.
81. Mori K, Sakamoto W, Nagasawa S. Studies on human high molecular weight (HMW) kininogen. III. Cleavage of HMW kininogen by the action human salivary kallikrein. J Biochem 1981;90:503.
82. Reddigari SR, Kaplan AP. Cleavage of high molecular weight kininogen by purified kallikreins and upon contact activation of plasma. Blood 1988;71:1334.
83. Nakayasa T, Nagasawa S. Studies on human kininogen. I. Isolation, characterization, and cleavage by plasma kallikrein of high molecular weight kininogen. J Biochem 1979;85:249.
84. Thompson RE, Mandle RJ, Kaplan AP. Characterization of human high molecular weight kininogens: procoagulant activity associated with the light chain of kinin-free high molecular weight kininogen. J Exp Med 1978;147:488.
85. Maier M, Austen KF, Spragg J. Characterization of the procoagulant chain derived from high molecular weight kininogen (Fitzgerald factor) by tissue kallikrein. Blood 1983;62:457.
86. Thompson RE, Mandle RJ, Kaplan AP. Studies of the binding of prekallikrein and factor XI to high molecular weight kininogen and its light chain. Proc Natl Acad Sci USA 1979;79:4862.
87. Villanueva GB, Leung L, Bradford H, Colman RW. Conformation of high molecular weight kininogen: effects of kallikrein and factor XIa cleavage. Biochem Biophys Res Commun 1989;158:72.
88. Vroman L, Adams AL, Fischer GC, Munoz PC. Interaction of high molecular weight kininogen, factor XII and fibrinogen in plasma at interfaces. Blood 1980;55:
89. Schmaier AH, Silver L, Adams AL, et al. The effects of high molecular weight kininogen on surface-adsorbed fibrinogen. Thromb Res 1984;33:51.
90. Brash JL, Scott CF, ten Hove P, et al. Mechanism of transient adsorption of fibrinogen from plasma to solid surfaces: role of the contact and fibrinolytic systems. Blood 1988;71:932.
91. Bjork I, Olson ST, Sheffer RG, Shore JD. Binding of heparin to human high molecular weight kininogen. Biochemistry 1989;28:1213.
92. Kellermann J, Lottspeich F, Henschen A, Muller-Esterl W. Completion of the primary structure of human high molecular weight kininogen: the amino acid sequence of the entire heavy chain and evidence for its evolution by gene triplication. Eur J Biochem 1986;154:471.
93. Kitamura N, Kitagawa H, Fukushima D, et al. Structural organization of the human kininogen gene and a model for its evolution. J Biol Chem 1985;260:8610.
94. Lottspeich F, Kellermann J, Henschen A, et al. The amino acid sequence of the light chain of human high molecular mass kininogen. Eur J Biochem 1985;152:307.
95. Takagaki Y, Kitamura N, Nakanishi S. Cloning and sequence analysis of cDNAs for high molecular weight and low molecular weight prekininogens. J Biol Chem 1985;260:8601.
96. Gounaris AD, Brown MA, Barrett AJ. Human plasma α_1-cysteine proteinase inhibitor: purification by affinity chromatography, characterization, and isolation of an active fragment. Biochem J 1984;221:445.
97. Muller-Esterl W, Fritz H, Machleidt IW, et al. Human plasma kininogens are identical with α_2-cysteine protease inhibitors: evidence from immunological, enzymological, and sequence data. FEBS Lett 1985;182:310.
98. Higashiyama S, Ohkubo I, Ishiguro H, et al. Human high molecular weight kininogen as a thiol protease inhibitor: presence of the entire inhibition capacity in the native form of heavy chain Biochemistry 1986;25:1669.
99. Ishiguro H, Higashiyama S, Ohkubo I, Sasaki M. Mapping of functional domains of human high molecular weight and high molecular weight and high molecular weight kininogens using murine monoclonal antibodies. Biochemistry 1987;26:7021.
100. Ikari N, Sugo T, Fujii S, Kato H, Iwanaga S. The role of bovine high molecular weight kininogen in contact-mediated activation of bovine factor XII: interaction of HMW kininogen with kaolin and plasma prekallikrein. J Biochem 1981;89:1699.
101. Tait J, Fujikawa K. Identification of the binding site plasma prekallikrein in human high molecular weight kininogen. J Biol Chem 1986;261:15396.
102. Jacobsen S, Kritz M. Some data on two purified kininogens from human plasma. Br J Pharmacol 1967;29:25.
103. Lottspeich F, Kellermann J, Henschen A, et al. Human Low-molecular-mass kininogen: amino acid sequence of the light chain; homology with other protein sequences. Eur J Biochem 1984;142:227.
104. Muller-Esterl W, Rauth G, Lottspeich F, et al. Limited proteolysis of human low-molecular mass kininogen by tissue kallikrein: isolation and characterization of the heavy and light chains. Eur J Biochem 1985;149:15.
105. Johnson DA, Salveson G, Brown M, Barrett AJ. Rapid isolation of human kininogens. Thromb Res 1987;48:187.
106. Margolis J. Activation of plasma by contact with glass: evidence for a common reaction which releases plasma kinin and initiates coagulation. J Physiol 1958;144:1.
107. Proctor RR, Rapaport SI. The partial thromboplastin time with kaolin: a simple screening test for first stage clotting deficiencies. Am J Clin Pathol 1961;35:212.
108. Ratnoff OD, Crum JD. Activation of Hageman factor by solutions of ellagic acid. J Lab Clin Med 1964;63:359.
109. Bock PE, Srinivasan KR, Shore JD. Activation of intrinsic blood coagulation by ellagic acid: insoluble ellagic acid metal ion complexes are the activating species. Biochemistry 1981;20:7258.
110. Kluft C. Determination of prekallikrein in human plasma: optimal conditions for activating prekallikrein. J Lab Clin Med 1978;91:83.
111. Fujikawa K, Heimark RL, Kurachi K, Davie EW. Activation of bovine factor XII (Hageman factor) by plasma kallikrein. Biochemistry 1980;19:1322.
112. Tans G, Griffin JH. Properties of sulfatides in factor XII dependent contact activation. Blood 1982;59:69.
113. Griep MA, Fujikawa K, Nelsestuen GL. Binding and activation properties of human factor XII, prekallikrein and derived peptides with acidic lipid vesicles. Biochemistry 1985;24:4124.
114. Silverberg M, Diehl SV. The autoactivation of factor XII (Hageman factor) induced by low Mr heparin and dextran sulphate. Biochem J 1987;248:715.
115. Hojima Y, Cochrane CG, Wiggins RC, et al. In vitro activation of the contact (Hageman factor) system of plasma by heparin and chondroitin sulfate E. Blood 1984;63:1453.
116. Silverberg M, Diehl SV. The activation of the contact system of human plasma by polysaccharide sulfates. Ann NY Acad Sci 1987;516:268.
117. Morrison DC, Cochrane CG. Direct evidence for Hageman factor (factor XII) activation by bacterial lipopolysaccharides (endotoxins). J Exp Med 1974;140:787.
118. Pettinger MA, Young R. Endotoxin-induced kinin (bradykinin) formation: activation of Hageman factor and plasma kallikrein in human plasma. Life Sci 1970;9:313.
119. Roeise O, Bouma BN Stadaas JO, Aasen AO. Dose dependence of endotoxin-induced activation of the plasma contact system: an in vitro study. Circ Shock 1988;26:419.
120. Tans G, Rosing J, Griffin JD. Sulfatide dependent autoactivation of human blood coagulation factor XII (Hageman factor) J Biol Chem 1983;258:8215.
121. McMillin CR Saito H, Ratnoff OD, Walton AG. The secondary structure of human Hageman factor (factor XII) and its alteration by activating agents. J Clin Invest 1974;54:1312.
122. Ratnoff OD, Saito H. Amidolytic properties of single chain activated Hageman factor. Proc Natl Acad Sci USA 1979;76:1411.
123. Kurachi K, Fujikawa K, Davie EW. Mechanism of activation of bovine factor XI by factor XII and factor XII_a. Biochemistry 1980;19:1330.
124. Tate KM, Higgins DL, Holmes WE, et al. Functional role of proteolytic cleavage at arginine-275 of human tissue plasminogen activator as assessed by site-directed mutagenesis. Biochemistry 1987;26:338.
125. Petersen LC, Johannessen M, Foster D, et al. The effect of polymerised fibrin on the catalytic activities of one-chain tissue-type plasminogen activator as revealed by an analogue resistant to plasmin cleavage. Biochim Biophys Acta 1988;952:245.
126. Nelles L, Lijnen HR, Collen D, Holmes WE. Characterization of recombinant human single chain urokinase-type plasminogen activator mutants produced by site-specific mutagenesis of lysine 158. J Biol Chem 1987;262:5682.
127. Lijnen HR, Gheysen D, de Foresta F, et al. Characterization of a mutant recombinant human single chain urokinase-type plasminogen activator (scu-PA), obtained by substitution of arginine 156 and lysine 158 with threonine. Fibrinolysis 1988;2:85.
128. Weiss R, Silverberg M, Kaplan AP. The effect of C1 inhibitor upon Hageman factor autoactivation. Blood 1986;68:239.
129. Pixley RA, Schmaier A, Colman RW. Effect of negatively charged activating compounds on inactivation of factor XIIa by C1 inhibitor. Arch Biochem Biophys 1987;256:490.
130. Rosing J, Tans G, Griffin JH. Surface-dependent activation of human factor XII by kallikrein, and its light chain. Eur J Biochem 1985;151.
131. Wuepper KD. Prekallikrein deficiency in man. J Exp Med 1973;138:1345.
132. Weiss AS, Gallin JI, Kaplan AP. Fletcher factor deficiency: a diminished rate of Hageman factor activation caused by absence of prekallikrein with abnormalities of coagulation, fibrinolysis, chemotactic activity and kinin generation. J Clin Invest 1974;53:622.
133. Saito H, Ratnoff OD, Donaldson VH. Defective activation of clotting, fibrinolytic and permeability-enhancing systems in human Fletcher trait. Circ Res 1974;34:641.
134. Schiffman S, Lee P. Preparation, characterization and activation of a highly purified factor XI: evidence that hitherto unrecognised plasma activating factor participates in the interaction of factors XI and XII. Br J Haematol 1974;27:101.
135. Wuepper KD, Miller DR, LaCombe MJ. Flaujeac trait: deficiency of human plasma kininogen. J Clin Invest 1975;56:1663.
136. Donaldson VH, Glueck HI, Miller MA. Kininogen deficiency in Fitzgerald trait: role of high molecular weight kininogen in clotting and fibrinolysis. J Lab Clin Med 1976;89:327.
137. Espana F, Ratnoff OD. The role of prekallikrein and high molecular

weight kininogen in the contact activation of Hageman factor (factor XII) by sulfatides and other agents. J Lab Clin Med 1983;102:487.
138. Shimada T, Kato H, Maeda H, Iwanaga S. Interaction of factor XII, high molecular weight kininogen and prekallikrein with sulfatide: analysis by fluorescence polarization. J Biochem 1985;97:1637.
139. Reddigari SR, Kaplan AP. Monoclonal antibody to human high molecular weight kininogen recognizes its prekallikrein binding site and inhibits its coagulant activity. Blood 1989;74:695.
140. Scott CF, Silver LD, Purdon D, Colman RW. Cleavage of human high molecular weight kininogen by factor XIa in vitro: effect on structure and function. J Biol Chem 1985;260:10856.
141. Travis J, Salvesen GS. Human plasma proteinase inhibitors. Annu Rev Biochem 1983;52:655.
142. Forbes CO, Pensky J, Ratnoff OD. Inhibition of activated Hageman factor and activated plasma thromboplastin antecedent by purified Cl inactivator. J Lab Clin Med 1970;76:809.
143. Schreiber AD, Kaplan AP, Austen KF. Inhibition by C 1 INH of Hageman factor fragment activation of coagulation, fibrinolysis, and kinin generation. J Clin Invest 1973;52:1402.
144. de Agostini A, Lijnen HR, Pixley RA, et al. Inactivation of factor XII active fragment in normal plasma: predominant role of Cl-inhibitor. J Clin Invest 1984;73:1542.
145. Pixley RA, Schapira M, Colman RW. The regulation of human factor XII by plasma proteinase inhibitors. J Biol Chem 1985;260:1723.
146. Stead N, Kaplan AP, Rosenberg RD. Inhibition of activated factor XII by antithrombin–heparin cofactor. J Biol Chem 1976;251:6481.
147. Cameron CL, Fisslthaler B, Sherman A, et al. Studies on contact activation: effects of surfaces and inhibitors. Med Progr Technol 1989;15:53.
148. Pixley RA, Colman RW. Effect of heparin in the inactivation of human factor XIIa by antithrombin III. Blood 1985;66:198.
149. Barrett AJ Starkey PM. The interaction of α_2-macroglobulin with proteinases. Biochem J 1973;133:709.
150. Gigli I, Mason JW, Colman RW, Austen KF. Interaction of plasma kallikrein with C1 inhibitor. J Immunol 1970;104:574.
151. McConnell DJ. Inhibitors of kallikrein in human plasma. J Clin Invest 1972;51:1611.
152. Harpel RC, Lewin MF, Kaplan AP. Distribution of plasma kallikrein between C1 inactivator and α_2-macroglobulin–kallikrein complexes. J Biol Chem 1985;4257.
153. Vennerod AM, Laake K, Solberg AK, Stromland S. Inactivation and binding of human plasma kallikrein by antithrombin III. Thromb Res 1976;9:457.
154. Heck LW, Kaplan AP. Substrates of Hageman factor. I. Isolation and characterization of human factor XI (PTA) and inhibition of the activated enzyme by α_1-antitrypsin. J Exp Med 1974;140:1615.
155. Scott CF, Schapira M, James HL, et al. Inactivation of factor XIa by plasma protease inhibitors: predominant role of α_1-protease inhibitor and protective effect of high molecular weight kininogen. J Clin Invest 1982;69:844.
156. Meijers JC, Vlooswijk RAA, Bouma BN. Inhibition of human blood coagulation factor XIa by C1 Inhibitor. Biochemistry 1988;27:959.
157. Scott CF, Schapira M, Colman RW. Effect of heparin on the inactivation of human factor XIa by antithrombin III. Blood 1982;60:940.
158. Beeler DL, Marcum JA, Schiffman S, Rosenberg RD. Interaction of factor XIa and antithrombin in the presence and absence of heparin. Blood 1985;67:1488.
159. Schapira M, Scott CF, Colman RW. Protection of human plasma kallikrein from inactivation by C1 Inhibitor and other protease inhibitors: the role of high molecular weight kininogen Biochemistry 1981;20:2738.
160. Schapira M, Scott CF, James A, et al. High molecular weight kininogen or its light chain protects human plasma kallikrein from inactivation by plasma protease inhibitors. Biochemistry 1982;21:567.
161. van der Graaf F, Rietveld A, Keus FJA, Bouma BN. Interaction of human plasma kallikrein and its light chain with α_2-macroglobulin. Biochemistry 1984;23:1760.
162. Silverberg M, Longo J, Kaplan AP. Study of the effect of high molecular weight kininogen upon the fluid phase inactivation of kallikrein by C1-inhibitor. J Biol Chem 1986;261:14965.
163. Erdos EG, Sloane GM. An enzyme in human plasma that inactivates bradykinin and kallidins. Biochem Pharmacol 1962;11:585.
164. Sheikh IA, Kaplan AP. Studies of the digestion of bradykinin, lysylbradykinin and kinin degradation products by carboxypeptidases A, B and N. Biochem Pharmacol 1986;35:1957.
165. Sheikh IA, Kaplan AP. Studies of the digestion of bradykinin, lysylbradykinin and des-arg[9] bradykinin by angiotensin converting enzyme. Biochem Pharmacol 1986;35:1951.
166. Sheikh IA, Kaplan AP. The mechanism of digestion of bradykinin and lysylbradykinin (kallidin) in human serum: the role of carboxypeptidase, angiotensin converting enzyme, and determination of final degradation products. Biochem Pharmacol 1989;38:993.
167. Marceau F, Lussier A, Regoli D, Girond PJ. Pharmacology of kinins: their relevance to tissue injury and inflammation. Gen Pharmacol 1983;14:209.
168. Vavrek RJ, Stewart JM. Competitive antagonists of bradykinin. Peptides 1985;6:1610164.
169. Beierwaltes WH, Carretero OA, Scicli AG. et al. Competitive analog antagonist of bradykinin in the canine hindlimb. Proc Soc Exp Biol Med 1987;186:79.
170. Iatridis PG, Ferguson JH. Active Hageman factor: a plasma lysokinase of the human fibrinolytic system. J Clin Invest 1962;41:1277.
171. Ogston D, Ogston LM, Ratnoff OD, Forbes CO. Studies on a complex mechanism for the activation of plasminogen by kaolin and by chloroform: the participation of Hageman factor and additional cofactors. J Clin Invest 1967;48:1786.
172. McDonagh JS, Ferguson JH. Studies on the participation of Hageman factor in fibrinolysis. Thromb Haemost 1970;24:1.
173. Ogston D, Bennett NB, Ogston CM, Ratnoff OD. The assay of a plasma component necessary for the generation of a plasminogen activator in the presence of Hageman factor (Hageman factor cofactor). Br J Haematol 1971;20:209.
174. Kluft C. Occurrence of C1-Inhibitor and other proteinase inhibitors in euglobulin fractions and their influence on fibrinolytic activity. Haemostasis 1976;5:136.
175. Kluft C. Elimination of inhibition of euglobulin fibrinolysis by use of flufenamate: involvement of C1-inactivator. Haemostasis 1977;6:351.
176. Miles LA, Rothschild Z, Griffin JH. Dextran sulfate dependent fibrinolysis in whole human plasma. J Lab Clin Med 1983;101:214.
177. Saito H. The participation of plasma thromboplastin antecedent (factor XI) in contact-activated fibrinolysis. Proc Soc Exp Biol Med 1980;164:153.
178. Goldsmith G, Saito H, Ratnoff OD. The activation of plasminogen by Hageman factor (factor XII) and Hageman factor fragments. J Clin Invest 1978;12:54.
179. Miles LA, Greengard JS, Griffin JH. A comparison of the abilities of plasma kallikrein, factor XIIa, factor XIa, and urokinase to activate plasminogen. Thromb Res 1983;29:407.
180. Jorg M, Binder BR. Kinetic analysis of plasminogen activation by purified plasma kallikrein. Thromb Res 1985;39:323.
181. Hauert J, Bachmann F. Prourokinase activation in euglobulin fractions. Thromb Haemost 1985;54:122.
182. Huisveld IA, Haspers H, Van Heeswijk GM, et al. Contribution of contact activation factors to urokinase-related fibrinolytic activator in whole plasma. Thromb Haemost 1985;54:102.
183. Kluft C, Wijngaards G, Jie, AFH. Intrinsic plasma fibrinolysis: involvement of urokinase-related activity in the factor XII independent plasminogen proactivator pathway. J Lab Clin Med 1984;103:408.
184. Smith D, Gilbert M, Owen WG. Tissue plasminogen activator release in vivo in response to vasoactive agents. Blood 1985;66:835.
185. Alving BM, Hojima Y, Pisano JJ, et al. Hypotension associated with prekallikrein activator (Hageman factor fragments) in plasma protein fraction. N Engl J Med 1978;229:66.
186. Alving BM, Tankersley DL, Mason BL, et al. Contact activation factors: contaminants of immunoglobulin preparations with coagulant and vasoactive properties. J Lab Clin Med 1980;96:334.
187. Waeber G, Schapira M, Waeber B, Aubert JF, Nussberger J, Brunner HR. Hypotensive effect of the active fragment derived from factor XII is mediated by an activation of the plasma kallikrein-kinin system. Circ Shock 1988;26:375.
188. Brown CF, Osmond DH. Factor XII and prekallikrein-kallikrein-kinin in the cryoactivation of human plasma prorenin. Clin Sci 1984;66:533.
189. Yokosawa N, Takahashi N, Inagami T, Page DL. Isolation of completely inactive plasma prorenin and its activation by kallikreins. Biochim Biophys Acta 1979;569:211.
190. Purdon AD, Schapira M, de Agostini A, Colman RW. Prorenin activation by plasma kallikrein in inhibitor deficient plasma. J Lab Clin Med 1985;105:694.
191. Seligsohn U, Osterud B, Brown JF, Griffin JH, Rapaport SI. Activation of human factor VII by Hageman factor fragments. J Clin Invest 1979;64:1056.
192. Gjonnaess H. Cold promoting activation of factor VII. III. Relation to the kallikrein system. Thromb Diath Haemorrh 1972;28:182.
193. Laake K, Vennerod AM, Hargen G, Gjonnaess H. Cold-promoted activation of factor VII in human plasma: studies on the associated acylarginine esterase activity. Thromb Res 1974;4:769.
194. Gordon EM, Ratnoff OD, Saito H, Donaldson VH, Pensky J, Jones PK. Rapid fibrinolysis, augmented Hageman factor (factor XII) titers and decreased C1 esterase inhibitor titers in women using oral contraceptives. J Lab Clin Med 1980;96:762.
195. Gordon EM, Douglas J, Ratnoff OD. Influence of augmented Hageman factor (factor XII) titers on the cryoactivation of plasma prorenin in women using oral contraceptives. J Clin Invest 1983;72:1833.
196. Jesperson J, Kluft C. Increased euglobulin potential in women on oral contraceptives low in oestrogen-levels of extrinsic and intrinsic plasminogen activators, prekallikrein, factor XII and C1-inactivator. Thromb Haemost 1985;54:454.
197. Ghebrehiwet B, Silverberg M, Kaplan AP. Activation of the classical pathway of complement by Hageman factor fragment. J Exp Med 1981;153:665.
198. Donaldson VH. Mechanism of activation of C1 esterase in hereditary angioneurotic edema *in vitro*: the role of Hageman factor, a clot promoting agent. J Exp Med 1967;127:411.
199. Fields T, Ghebrehiwet B, Kaplan AP. Kinin formation in hereditary

angioedema plasma: evidence against kinin derivation from C2 and in support of spontaneous formation of bradykinin. J Allergy Clin Immunol 1983;72:54.
200. Colman RW, Wachtfogel YT, Kucich V, et al. Effect of cleavage of the heavy chain of human plasma kallikrein on its functional properties. Blood 1985;65:311.
201. Lipscomb MS, Walsh PN. Human platelets and factor XI: localization in platelet membranes of factor XI–like activity and its functional distinction from that of factor XI. J Clin Invest 1979;63:1006.
202. Tuszynski GP, Bevacona SJ, Schmaier AH, Colman RW, Walsh PN. Factor XI antigen and activity in human platelets. Blood 1982;59:1148.
203. Schmaier AH, Zuckerberg A, Silverman C, Kuchibhotla J, Tuszynski GP, Colman RW. High molecular weight kininogen: a secreted platelet protein. J Clin Invest 1983;71:1477.
204. Schmaier AH, Smith PM, Purdon AD, White JG, Colman RW. High molecular weight kininogen: localization in unstimulated and activated platelets and activation by a platelet calpain(s). Blood 1986;67:119.
205. Gustafson EJ, Schutsky D, Knight LC Schmaier AH. High molecular weight kininogen binds to unstimulated platelets. J Clin Invest 1986;78: 310.
206. Greengard J, Griffin JH. Receptor for high molecular kininogen on stimulated washed human platelets. Biochemistry 1984;23:6863.
207. Scully MF, Weerasinghe K, Kakhar VV. Inhibition of contact activation by platelet factor 4. Thromb Res 1980;20:461.
208. Kodania K, Kato H, Iwanaga S. Isolation of bovine platelet cationic proteins which inhibit the surface-mediated activation of factor XII and prekallikrein. J Biochem 1985;97:139.
209. Walsh PN. The effects of collagen and kaolin on the intrinsic coagulant activity of platelets: evidence for an alternative pathway in intrinsic coagulation not requiring factor XII. Br J Haematol 1972;22:393.
210. Hong SL. Effect of bradykinin and thrombin on prostacyclin synthesis in endothelial cells from calf and pig aorta and human umbilical cord vein. Thromb Res 1980;18:787.
211. Crutchly DJ Ryan JW Ryan US, Fisher GH. Bradykinin induced release of prostacyclin and thromboxanes from bovine pulmonary artery endothelial cells. Biochim Biophys Acta 1983;751:99.
212. Schmaier AH, Kuo A, Lundberg D, Murray S, Cines DB. The expression of high molecular weight kininogen on human umbilical vein endothelial cells. J Biol Chem 1988;31:16327.
213. van iwaarden F, de Groot PG, Bouma BN. The binding of high molecular weight kininogen to cultures human endothelial cells. J biol Chem 1988;263:4698.
214. Reddigari SR, Kuna P, Miragliotta GF, Shibayama Y, Nishikawa K, Kaplan AP. Human high molecular weight kininogen binds to human umbilical vein endothelial cells via its heavy and light chains. Blood 1993;81:1306.
215. Berrettini M, Schleef RR, Heeb MJ, Hopmeier P, Griffin JH. Assembly and expression of an intrinsic factor IX activator complex on the surface of cultured human endothelial cells. J Biol Chem 1992;267:19833.
216. Nishikawa K, Shibayama Y, Kuna P, Calcaterra E, Kaplan AP, Reddigari SR. Generation of vasoactive peptide bradykinin from human umbilical vein endothelium–bound high molecular weight kininogen by plasm kallikrein. Blood 1992;80:1980.
217. Palmer RMJ, Ferrige AG, Moncada S. Nitric oxide release accounts for the biological activity of endothelium-derived relaxing factor. Nature 1987;327:524.
218. Pelc LR, Gross GJ, Warltier DC. Mechanism of coronary vasodilation produced by bradykinin. Circulation 1991;83:2048.
219. Rosenthal RH, Dreskin OH, Rosenthal N. New hemophiliac-like disease caused by a deficiency of a third plasma thromboplastin factor. Proc Soc Exp Biol Med 1953;82:171.
220. Rosenthal RL, Dreskin OH, Rosenthal N. Plasma thromboplastin antecedent (PTA) deficiency: clinical coagulation, therapeutic and hereditary aspects of a new hemophilia-like disease. Blood 1955;10:120.
221. Sidi A, Seligsohn U, Jonas P, Many M. Factor XI deficiency: detection and management during urological surgery. J Urol 1978;119:528.
222. Saito H, Ratnoff OD, Bouma BN, Seligsohn U. Failure to detect variant (CRM+) plasma thromboplastin antecedent (factor XI) molecules in hereditary plasma thromboplastin antecedent deficiency: a study of 125 patients of several ethnic backgrounds. J Lab Clin Med 1985;106: 718.
223. Leiba H, Ramot B, Many A. Hereditary and coagulation studies in ten families with factor XI (plasma thromboplastin antecedent) deficiency. Br J Haematol 1965;11:654.
224. Rapaport SI, Proctor RR, Patch MJ, Yettra M. The mode of inheritance of PTA deficiency: evidence for the existence of major PTA deficiency and minor PTA deficiency. Blood 1961;18:149.
225. Rimon A, Schiffman S, Feinstein DI, Rapaport SI. Factor XI activity and factor XI antigen in homozygous and heterozygous factor XI deficiency. Blood 1976;48:165.
226. Schwartz HC, Stone JD. Hereditary factor XI deficiency. J Oral Surg 1967;34:453.
227. Megquier RJ. Fibrinolytic activity in human dental sockets after extractions. J Oral Surg 1971;29:321.
228. Kaufmann JM. Prostatectomy in factor XI deficiency. J Urol 1977;117: 75.
229. Reece EA, Clyne LP, Romero R, Hobbins JC. Spontaneous factor XI inhibitors: seven additional cases and a review of the literature. Arch Intern Med 1984;144:525.
230. Stern DM, Nossel HL, Owen J. Acquired antibody to factor XI in a patient with congenital factor XI deficiency. J Clin Invest 1982;69:1270.
231. Morgan K Schiffman S, Feinstein D. Acquired factor XI inhibitors in two patients with hereditary factor XI deficiency. Thromb Haemost 1984;51:371.
232. De La Cadena RA, Baglia FA, Johnson CA, et al. Naturally occurring human antibodies against two distinct functional domains in the heavy chain of FXI/FXIa. Blood 1988;72:1748.
233. Chediak J, Madej ZP, Ratnoff OD, Goldsmith GJ, Everson B. Studies on a circulating anticoagulant inhibiting factor XI in a patient with congenital deficiency and carcinoma of the prostate. Br J Haematol 1986;63:123.
234. Seligsohn U. High gene frequency of factor XI (PTA) deficiency in Ashkenazi Jews. Blood 1978;51:1223.
235. Ragni MV, Sinha D, Seaman F, Lewis JH, Spero JA, Walsh PN. Comparison of bleeding tendency, factor XI coagulant activity, and factor XI antigen in 25 factor XI–deficient kindreds. Blood 1985;65:719.
236. Nossel HL, Niemetz J, Sawitsky A. Blood PTA (factor XI) levels following plasma infusion. Proc Soc Exp Biol Med 1964;115:896.
237. Horowitz HI, Fujimoto MM. Survival of factor XI *in vitro* and *in vivo*. Transfusion 1965;5:539.
238. Bennett E, Dormandy K. Pool's cryoprecipitate and exhausted plasma in the treatment of von Willebrand's disease and factor XI deficiency. Lancet 1966;2:731.
239. Ratnoff OD, Busce FJ, Sheon RP. The demise of John Hageman. N Engl J Med 1968;279:760.
240. Hoak JC, Swenson LW, Warner ED. Myocardial infarction associated with sever factor XII deficiency. Lancet 1966;2:884.
241. Goodnough LT, Saito H, Ratnoff OD. Thrombosis or myocardial infarction in congenital clotting factor abnormalities and chronic thrombocytopenia: a report of 21 patients and a review of 50 previously reported cases. Medicine 1983;62:248.
242. Londino A, Luparello FJ. Factor XII deficiency in a man with gout and angioimmunoblastic lymphadenopathy. Arch Intern Med 1984;144: 1497.
243. Bernardi F, Marchetti G, Volinia S, et al. A frequent factor XII gene mutation in Hageman trait. Hum Genet 1988;80:149.
244. Sollo DG, Saleem A. Prekallikrein (Fletcher factor) deficiency. Ann Clin Lab Sci 1985;15:279.
245. Currimbhoy Z, Vinciguerru V, Palakavongs P, Kuslansky P, Degnan TJ. Fletcher factor deficiency and myocardial infarction. Am J Clin Pathol 1976;65:970.
246. Harris MG, Exner T, Rickard KA, Kronenberg H. Multiple cerebral thrombosis in Fletcher factor (prekallikrein) deficiency: a case report. Am J Hematol 1985;19:387.
247. Saito H, Goodnough LT, Soria J, Soria C Aznar J, Espana F. Heterogeneity of human prekallikrein deficiency (Fletcher trait): evidence that 5 of 18 cases are positive for cross-reacting material. N Engl J Med 1981;305: 910.
248. Bouma BN, Kerbiriou DM, Baker J, Griffin JH. Characterization of a variant prekallikrein prekallikrein Long Beach, from a family with mixed cross-reacting material-positive and cross-reacting material-negative prekallikrein deficiency. J Clin Invest 1986;78:170.
249. Saito H, Ratnoff OD, Waldman R, Abraham JP. Fitzgerald trait: deficiency of a hitherto unrecognized agent, Fitzgerald factor, participating in surface-mediated reactions of clotting, fibrinolysis, generation of kinins, and the property of diluted plasma enhancing vascular permeability. J Clin Invest 1975;55:1082.
250. Gailani D, Broze GJ. Factor XI activation in a revised model of blood coagulation. Science 1991;253:909.
251. Naito K, Fujikawa K. Activation of human blood coagulation factor XI independent of factor XII: factor XI is activated by thrombin and factor XIa in the presence of negatively charged surfaces. J Biol Chem 1991;266:7353.
252. Scott CF, Colman RW. Fibrinogen blocks the autoactivation and thrombin-mediated activation of factor XI on dextran sulfate. Proc Natl Acad Sci USA 1992;89:11189.
253. Brunée TC, La Porta C, Reddigari SR, Salerno VM, Kaplan AP, Silverberg M. Activation of factor XI in plasma is dependent on factor XII. Blood 1993;81:580.
254. Carvalho AC, DeMarinis S, Scott CF, Silver LD, Schmaier AH, Colman RW. Activation of the contact system of plasma proteolysis in the adult respiratory distress syndrome. J Lab Clin Med 1988;112:270.
255. Oates JA, Pettinger WA, Doctor RB. Evidence for the release of bradykinin in carcinoid syndrome. J Clin Invest 1966;45:173.
256. Melmon KL, Lovenberg W, Sjoerdsma A. Characteristics of carcinoid tumor kallikrein: identification of lysyl-bradykinin as a peptide it produces *in vitro*. Clin Chim Acta 1965;12:292.
257. Wong PY, Talamo RC, Colman RW. Kallikrein-kinin system in postgastrectomy dumping syndrome. Ann Intern Med 1974;80:577.
258. Carvalho AC, Ellman L. Activation of the coagulation system in polycythemia vera. Blood 1976;47:669.
259. Yamada J, Herber P, Pettit GW, Wing DA, Oster CN. Activation of the kallikrein-kinin system in Rocky Mountain spotted fever. Ann Intern Med 1978;88:764.

260. Colman RW, Edelman R, Scott CF, Gilman RH. Plasma kallikrein activation and inhibition during typhoid fever. J Clin Invest 1978;61:287.
261. Carvalho AC, Lees RS, Vaillancourt RA, Cabral RB, Colman RW. Activation of the kallikrein system in hyperbetalipoproteinemia. J Lab Clin Med 1978;91:117.
262. Bouma BN, Keribiriou DM, Vluswijk RAA, Griffin JH. Immunological studies of prekallikrein, kallikrein and high molecular weight kininogen in normal and deficient plasmas and in normal plasma after cold dependent activation. J Lab Clin Med 1980;96:693.
263. Mancini G, Carbonara AO, Heremans JF. Immunochemical quantification of antigens by single radial immunodiffusion. Immunochemistry 1965;2:235.
264. Laurell CB. Quantitative estimate of proteins by electrophoresis in agarose gel containing antibodies. Anal Biochem 1966;15:45.
265. Fisher CA, Schmaier AH, Addonizio P, Colman RW. Assay of prekallikrein in human plasma: comparison of amidolytic, esterolytic, coagulation and immunochemical assays. Blood 1982;59:963.
266. Tankersley DL, Alving BM, Finlayson JS. Activation of factor XII by dextran sulfate: the basis for an assay of factor XII. Blood 1983;62:448.
267. Alving BM, Tankersley DL, Mason BL. Plasma prekallikrein: quantitative determination by direct activation with Hageman factor fragment (beta-XIIa). J Lab Clin Med 1983;101:226.
268. Gallimore MJ. Chromogenic substrate assays for studying components of the plasma kallikrein system in health and disease. In: Fritz HJ, Beck N, Dietze G, Haberland GL, eds. Kinins III. Part A. Advances in experimental medicine and biology. New York, Plenum Press, 1983: 225.
269. de Agostini A, Schapira M, Wachtfogel YT, Colman RW, Carrel S. Human plasma kallikrein and C I inhibitor form a complex possessing an epitope that is not detectable on the parent molecules: demonstration using a monoclonal antibody. Proc Natl Acad Sci USA 1985;82:5190.
270. de Agostini A, Patston PA, Marottoli V, Carrel S, Harpel RC, Schapira M. A common neoepitope is created when the reactive center of C1-inhibitor is cleaved by plasma kallikrein, activated factor XII fragment, C1 esterase, or neutrophil elastase. J Clin Invest 1988;82:700.
271. Harpel PC. α_2-Plasmin inhibitor and α_2-macroglobulin plasmin complexes in plasma: quantitation by an enzyme-linked differential antibody immunosorbent assay. J Clin Invest 1981;68:46.
272. Kaplan AP, Gruber B, Harpel PC. Assessment of Hageman factor activation in human plasma: quantification of activated Hageman factor-CI inactivator complexes by an enzyme-linked differential antibody immunosorbent assay. Blood 1985;66:636.
273. Lewin MF, Kaplan AP, Harpel PC. Studies of C1 inactivator-plasma kallikrein complexes in purified systems and in plasma: quantification by enzyme-linked differential antibody immunosorbent assay. J Biol Chem 1983;258:6415.
274. Nuijens JH, Huijbregts CC, Eerenberg-Belmer AJ, et al. Quantification of plasma factor XIIa-C1–inhibitor and kallikrein-C1–inhibitor complexes in sepsis. Blood 1988;72:1841.
275. Shimamoto K, Ando T, Nakao T, Tanaka S, Sakuma M, Miyahora M. A sensitive radioimmunoassay method for urinary kinins in man. J Lab Clin Med 1978;91:721.
276. Odya CE, Moreland P, Stewart JM, Barabe J, Regoli DC. Development of a radioimmunoassay for des-Arg^9-bradykinin. Biochem Pharmacol 1983;32:337.
277. Donaldson VH, Rosen FS, Bing DH. Role of the second component of complement (C2) and plasmin in kinin release in hereditary angioneurotic edema (HANE) plasma. Trans Assoc Am Phys 1977;40: 174.
278. Curd JG, Yelvington M, Burridge N, et al. Generation of bradykinin during incubation of hereditary angioedema plasma. Mol Immunol 1983;19:1365.
279. Strang CJ, Auerbach HS, Rosen FS. C1s-induced vascular permeability in C2-deficient guinea pigs. J Immunol 1986;137:631.
280. Schapira M, Silver LD, Scott CF, et al. Prekallikrein activation and high molecular weight kininogen consumption in hereditary angioedema. N Engl J Med 1985;3:1050.
281. Curd JG, Prograis LJJ, Cochrane CG. Detection of active kallikrein in induced blister fluids of hereditary angioedema patients. J Exp Med 1980;152:242.
282. Talamo RC, Haber E, Austen KF. A radioimmunoassay for bradykinin in plasma and synovial fluid. J Lab Clin Med 1969;74:816.
283. Lämmle B, Zuraw BL, Heeb MJ, et al. Detection and quantitation of cleaved and uncleaved high molecular weight kininogen in plasma by ligand blotting with radiolabeled plasma prekallikrein or factor XI. Thromb Haemost 1988;59:151.
284. Ziccardi RJ. Spontaneous activation of the first component of human complement (C1) by an intramolecular autocatalytic mechanism. J Immunol 1982;128:2500.
285. Cooper NR. Activation and regulation of the first component of complement. Fed Proc 1983;42:134.
286. Kimball HR, Melmon KL, Wolff SM. Endotoxin-induced kinin production in man. Proc Soc Exp Biol Med 1972;139:1078.
287. Mason JW, Kleeberg UR, Dolan P, Colman RW. Plasma kallikrein and Hageman factor in gram-negative bacteremia. Ann Intern Med 1970;73: 545.
288. Hirsch EF, Nakajima T, Oshima G, Erdos EG, Herman M. Kinin-system responses in sepsis after trauma in man. J Surg Res 1974;17:147.
289. Robinson JA, Klodynicky ML, Loeb HS, Recic MR, Gunnar RM. Endotoxin, prekallikrein, complement, and systemic vascular resistances: sequential measurement in man. Am J Med 1975;59:61.
290. O'Donnell TF, Clowes GHJ, Talamo RC, Colman RW. Kinin activation in the blood of patients with sepsis. Surg Gynecol Obstet 1976;143: 539.
291. Martinez-Brotóns F, Oncins JR, Mestres J, Amargos V, Reynaldo C. Plasma kallikrein-kinin system in patients with uncomplicated sepsis and septic shock: comparison with cardiogenic shock. Thromb Haemost 1987;4:709.
292. Mason JN, Colman RW. The role of Hageman factor in disseminated intravascular coagulation induced by sepsis, neoplasia, or liver disease. Thromb Diath Haemorrh 1971;26:325.
293. Lämmle B, Tran TH, Ritz R, Duckert F. Plasma prekallikrein, factor XII, antithrombin III, C_1-inhibitor and α_2-macroglobulin in critically ill patients with suspected disseminated intravascular coagulation (DIC). Am J Clin Pathol 1984;82:396.
294. Vaziri ND, Toohey J, Powers D, et al. Activation of intrinsic coagulation pathway in pre-eclampsia. Am J Med 1986;80:103.
295. Naclerio RM, Meier HL, Kagey-Sobotka A, et al. Mediator release after nasal airway challenge with allergen. Am Rev Respir Dis 1983;128: 597.
296. Proud D, Togias A, Naclerio RM, Crush SB, Norman PS, Lichtenstein LM. Kinins are generated in vivo following nasal airway challenge of allergic individuals with allergen. J Clin Invest 1983;72:1678.
297. Naclerio RM, Proud D, Togias AG, et al. Inflammatory mediators in late antigen-induced rhinitis. N Engl J Med 1985;313:65.
298. Baumgarten CR, Togias AG, Naclerio RM, Lichtenstein LM, Norman PS, Proud D. Influx of kininogens into nasal secretions after antigen challenge of allergic individuals. J Clin Invest 1985;76:191.
299. Moskowitz RW, Schwartz HJ, Michel B, Ratnoff OD, Astrup T. Generation of kinin-like agents by chondroitin sulfate, heparin, chitin sulfate, and human articular cartilage: possible pathophysiologic implications. J Lab Clin Med 1970;76:790.
300. Nagase H, Cawston JE, DeSilva M, Barrett AJ. Identification of plasma kallikrein as an activator of latent collagenase in rheumatoid synovial fluid. Biochim Biophys Acta 1982;707:133.
301. Kellermeyer RW, Breckenridge RT. The inflammatory process in acute gouty arthritis. I. Activation of Hageman factor by sodium urate crystals. J Lab Clin Med 1965;63:307.
302. Ginsberg M, Jaques B, Cochrane CG, Griffin JH. Urate crystal dependent cleavage of Hageman factor in human plasma and synovial fluid. J Lab Clin Med 1980;95:497.
303. Donaldson VH, Glueck HI, Fleming T. Rheumatoid arthritis in a patient with Hageman trait. N Engl J Med 1972;386:528.
304. Honig GR, Lindley A. Deficiency of Hageman factor (factor XII) in patients with the nephrotic syndrome. J Pediatr 1971;78:633.
305. Lange LGI, Carvalho A, Bagdasarian A, Lahiri B, Colman RW. Activation of Hageman factor in the nephrotic syndrome. Am J Med 1974;56:565.
306. Hruby MA, Honig GR, Shapira E. Immunoquantitation of Hageman factor in urine and plasma of children with nephrotic syndrome. J Lab Clin Med 1980;96:501.
307. Saito H, Goodnough LT, Makker SP, Kallen RJ. Urinary excretion of Hageman factor (factor XII) and the presence of nonfunctional factor in the nephrotic syndrome. Am J Med 1981;70:531.
308. Wong P, Colman RW, Talamo RC, Babior B. Kallikrein bradykinin system in chronic alcoholic liver disease. Ann Intern Med 1972;77: 205.
309. van Vliet ACM, van Vliet HHDM, Dzolijic-Danilovic G, Wilson JHP. Plasma prekallikrein and endotoxemia in liver cirrhosis. Thrombos Hemostas 1981;45:65.
310. Edelman R, Nimmannitya S, Colman RW, Talamo RC, Top FHJ. Evaluation of the plasma kinin system in dengue hemorrhagic fever. J Lab Clin Med 1975;86:410.

Blood: Principles and Practice of Hematology,
edited by Robert I. Handin, Thomas P. Stossel, and Samuel E. Lux.
J.B. Lippincott Company, Philadelphia © 1995.

39

Coagulation Factors V and VIII: Normal Function and Clinical Disorders

Gilbert C. White II

Coagulation factors V and VIII are structurally and functionally homologous plasma proteins that act as high molecular weight cofactors in the coagulation cascade. Analysis of the molecular organization of these proteins, made possible by cloning the genes for each, suggest that they are related in evolution. Despite the remarkable similarities between the two proteins, significant differences are found in the clinical deficiency syndromes and genetics associated with each protein. Thus, factor VIII deficiency (hemophilia A) is a severe X-linked hemorrhagic disorder, which was recognized clinically in antiquity. In contrast, factor V deficiency, an autosomal recessive trait, is a much milder disorder. The purpose of this chapter is to present what is known of the structure, function, and genetics of the two proteins and to describe and compare the associated clinical deficiency syndromes. The reader is also referred to several reviews.[1–4]

STRUCTURES OF FACTORS V AND VIII

The gene that codes for factor VIII is at the tip of the long arm of the X chromosome, near the genes for glucose-6-phosphate dehydrogenase and color vision (Fig. 39-1). It is made up of nearly 186,000 base pairs (bp) and constitutes about 0.1% of the X chromosome.[5,6] The gene is organized into 26 separate exons ranging in size from 69 to 3106 bp separated by 25 intervening regions (introns), which range in size from 207 to 32,400 bp. The complete gene consists of about 9 kb of exon and 177 kb of intron.

The factor VIII gene transcribes an mRNA that is 9029 bp in length.[5–7] A probable 5′ start site at position −170 is preceded in the genomic 5′ flank by the sequence GATAAA, which conforms with the ATA sequence required for initiation of transcription.[5] The mRNA consists of a short 5′ untranslated region, followed by a single, continuous open reading frame of 7053 bp that codes for a single polypeptide chain, and a 3′ untranslated region that is 1805 nucleotides in length and contains AATAAA and CATTG polyadenylation signals 19 bases upstream from the poly(A)+ tail.

The factor VIII mRNA encodes a precursor protein of 2351 amino acids, composed of a 19 amino acid hydrophobic signal peptide (removed during secretion) and the mature factor VIII protein. Analysis of the predicted amino acid sequence of mature human factor VIII reveals a complex protein with two types of internal homology[6,8] (Fig. 39-2). Three *A domain* repeats are present, each about 350 amino acids in length with about 30% amino acid homology between repeats. The first repeat begins at the amino terminus of the mature protein and is separated from the second repeat by 36 largely acidic amino acids. After the second A domain repeat and completing the heavy chain of mature plasma factor VIII is a stretch of 983 amino acids, which is rich in potential asparagine-linked glycosylation sites but, unlike the rest of factor VIII, contains few cysteines. This region, known as the *B domain*, is encoded entirely by a single large exon (which also encodes parts of the A2 and A3 repeats) and is presumed to be an ancient insertion into an existing gene. Of the 25 potential N-linked glycosylation sites (Asn-X-Thr/Ser) that are present in the mature protein, 19 are found in the B domain. The third A domain repeat is found at the amino terminus of the light chain of mature plasma factor VIII, immediately after another short segment of 41 predominantly acidic amino acids. This acidic region contains the putative binding site for von Willebrand's factor (vWF)[9,10] and is the site of tyrosine sulfation in factor VIII.[11]

The second internal homology is the *C domain*, which occurs as a contiguous tandem repeat at the carboxyl terminus of the molecule. Both copies are about 150 amino acids in length, with 37% homology between repeats. The third A domain and the two C-domain repeats make up the light chain of mature plasma factor VIII, whereas the A1, A2, and B domains make up the heavy chain.

The A domains show striking homology with similar repeats in ceruloplasmin, a blue copper-containing oxidase in human plasma. Like factor VIII, ceruloplasmin contains a triplicated repeat, each analogous to the A domain of factor VIII.[12] Copper binding occurs in the carboxyl terminal portion of each repeat. A total of six copper atoms are bound per mole of ceruloplasmin: four in the active site, each bound by different mechanisms (types I, II, III, and IV based on kinetic characteristics), and two elsewhere. The residues believed to be involved in binding copper atoms are also present in factor VIII. Since the role of factor VIII in factor X activation is divalent cation dependent, it is interesting to speculate that the binding of copper atoms, or the binding of calcium by the copper-binding sites, may be important

Supported in part by a grant from the Specialized Center for Research in Thrombosis from the National Heart, Lung, and Blood Institute (HL26309) and by a grant from the National Cancer Institute (CA43447).

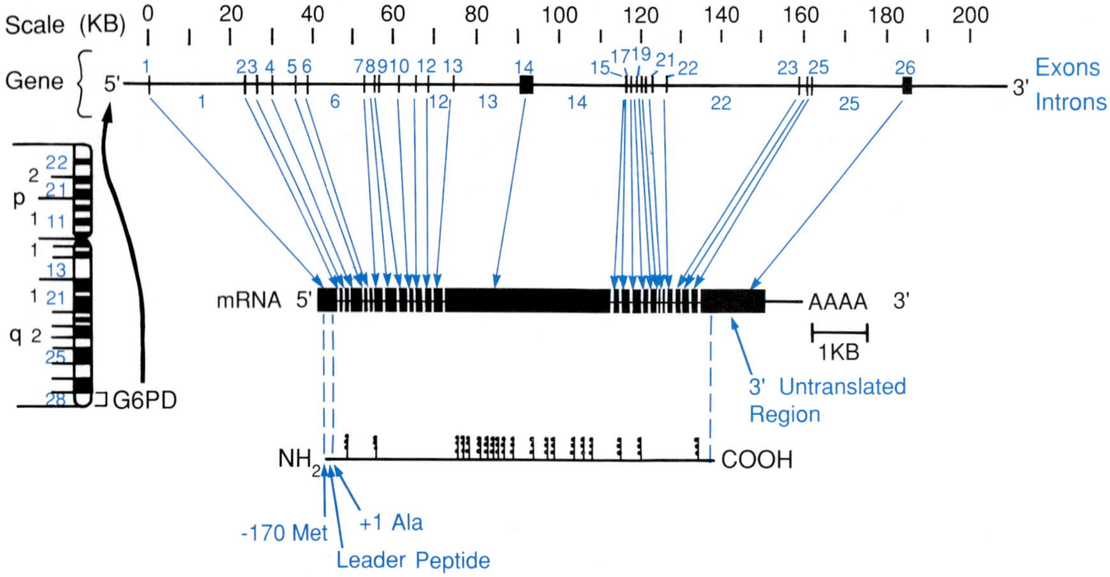

FIGURE 39-1. Map of human factor VIII gene. The factor VIII gene is at the tip of the long arm of the X chromosome near the gene for glucose-6-phosphate dehydrogenase. The gene (*top line*) spans 186 kb and consists of 26 exons or coding regions (*filled boxes*). The mRNA transcription product (*middle line*) is about 9 kb and codes for the 2351–amino acid factor VIII protein (*bottom line*). The curved lines on the protein indicate sites of potential N-linked glycosylation. (After White GC, Shoemaker CB. Factor VIII gene and hemophilia A. Blood 1989;73:1)

for factor VIII function. The C domain of factor VIII shares about 20% homology with discoidin I, a phospholipid- and galactose-binding lectin from the slime mold, *Dictyostelium discoideum*. The C domain may make up the phospholipid-binding domain of factor VIII.[13–15]

Although synthesized as a single polypeptide chain, factor VIII undergoes proteolytic processing before secretion such that plasma factor VIII circulates as a two-chain, metal ion-stabilized complex that consists of a variable heavy chain of 90 to 210 kd and a 80-kd light chain.[16–18] The role of metal ion in factor VIII structure is not clear, but chelation of calcium inhibits factor VIII activity and activity is not recovered on readdition of calcium.[17,19]

The factor V gene is located on chromosome 1 in humans[20] and contains 25 exons, which range in size from 72 to 2820 bp.[20a] The structure of the gene for factor V is similar to that for the gene for factor VIII. Of the 24 intron–exon boundaries in the factor V gene, 21 occur at the same location as in the factor VIII gene after the amino acid sequences of the two proteins are aligned.

The mRNA for factor V contains 6903 bp and consists of 76 nucleotides of 5′ untranslated sequence, 6672 nucleotides of coding sequence, and 155 nucleotides of 3′ untranslated sequence containing an AATAAA polyadenylation signal 9 bases upstream from the poly(A)+ tail.[21–23] The protein encoded by the factor V mRNA is composed of a hydrophobic leader peptide 28 amino acids in length, which is cleaved off during the secretion process, and a mature factor V protein 2196 amino acids in length.

Factor V contains triplicated A-domain repeats homologous with those of factor VIII and ceruloplasmin[21,24] (see Fig. 39-2). In contrast to factor VIII, factor V binds copper, but only two of the four residues necessary for type I copper binding to ceruloplasmin are conserved and factor V has been shown not to bind copper with type I kinetics.[25] The function, if any, of copper binding in factor V is unknown. The arrangement of A repeats in factor V is similar to the arrangement in factor VIII (A1–A2–connecting region–A3). One important difference between factor V and factor VIII is that the acidic regions between the A1 and A2 domains

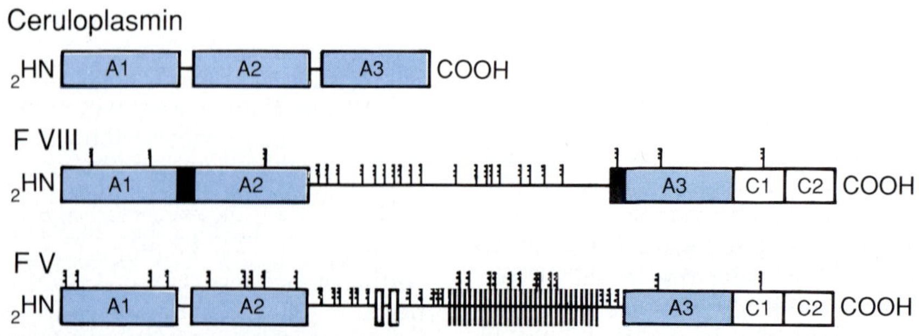

FIGURE 39-2. Domain structure of ceruloplasmin and human factors V and VIII. The colored boxes indicate the three A-domain repeats (A1, A2, A3) in each protein. The white boxes indicate the two C-domain repeats (C1 and C2) in factors V and VIII. The A2 and A3 domains of factors V and VIII are separated by nonhomologous connecting regions, which contain most of the potential N-linked glycosylation sites. The acidic regions between the A1 and A2 domains and between the B and A3 domains in factor VIII are shown as filled boxes. Potential N-linked glycosylation sites are indicated by the wavy line.

and B and A3 domains of factor VIII are not present in factor V. The connecting region of factor V is about 836 residues in length and bears no sequence homology with the B domain of factor VIII. The primary structural features of the connecting region of factor V are the presence of two tandem repeats of 17 amino acids with a consensus sequence of SQDTGSPSXMRPWEDXP followed by 31 tandem repeats of 9 amino acids with a consensus sequence of [T,N,P]LSPDLSQT. Like the B domain of factor VIII, the connecting region of factor V is a major site of potential carbohydrate attachment. Of the 37 potential N-linked oligosaccharide attachment sites (Asn-X-Ser/Thr) in factor V, 25 are in the connecting region. Also, like factor VIII, the connecting region is not needed for factor V coagulant activity. Factor V contains two segments that are homologous with the C-domain repeats of factor VIII. The overall amino acid sequences of factor V and factor VIII are about 30% homologous.

The mature factor V protein is a single-chain polypeptide with an estimated molecular weight of 286 kd.[26–28] It is about 13% carbohydrate by weight and contains both N-linked and O-linked carbohydrate chains.[29] Removal of sialic acid has little effect on factor V function, but removal of the penultimate galactose residues destroys factor V activity.[30,31] Physical characterization of the purified bovine protein indicates that it is highly asymmetric with a rod-like structure,[27,28,32] whereas electron microscopy of bovine and human factor V demonstrates a globular structure.[33]

BIOSYNTHESIS OF FACTORS V AND VIII

Both factors V and VIII are secretory proteins that are synthesized and glycosylated on membrane-bound polysomes in the rough endoplasmic reticulum, then transported by a GTP-dependent mechanism to the Golgi apparatus where sulfation occurs and where the oligosaccharides are further processed to complex type units containing sialic acid. From there, factors V and VIII are transported to secretory granules or vesicles from which the proteins are secreted. The signal peptide provides a crucial recognition site that targets the protein for secretion.

Early studies undertaken to identify the tissue of origin of factor VIII involved transplantation of selected organs into hemophilic animals.[34] These studies showed that transplantation of normal livers into hemophilic animals induced factor VIII production, whereas the transplantation of hemophilic livers into normal animals resulted in reduced, but adequate, factor VIII levels. These studies provided an early clue that factor VIII synthesis occurred in, but was not exclusive to, the liver. Recent reports of liver transplantation in hemophiliacs with end-stage liver disease have confirmed these animal studies and support the role of the liver in factor VIII synthesis.[35,36] With identification of the gene for factor VIII and the development of probes specific for mRNA coding for factor VIII, it has become possible to look for factor VIII expression in a variety of cell types. Wion and coworkers[37] have used such probes to identify factor VIII mRNA in liver, spleen, kidney, and lymphocytes, thus confirming the existence of multiple potential sites of factor VIII synthesis. Fractionation of liver revealed mRNA in the hepatocyte fraction and not in the sinusoidal fraction. At the same time, monoclonal antibodies to factor VIII have been used to localize factor VIII production.[38–40]

With the use of colloidal gold-labeled antibody to factor VIII, immunoreactive factor VIII has been demonstrated in normal hepatocytes, especially the rough endoplasmic reticulum and Golgi apparatus, but not in hemophilic hepatocytes nor in other cells in the liver. Based on the available studies, the major source of factor VIII appears to be the hepatocyte, but other sites of production exist and may play an important role in production of factor VIII in patients with liver disease. Endothelial cells, which synthesize vWF, do not synthesize factor VIII, but may provide a storage site for factor VIII.[40,41]

Control of factor VIII synthesis is poorly understood, although hormonal influences may be important. Vasopressin and its analogues can increase plasma levels of factor VIII in both normal persons and those with mild hemophilia[42,43] by a mechanism that can be blocked by propranolol suggesting involvement of β-adrenergic receptors.[44] Whether vasopressin acts at the level of transcription, translation, secretion, or sites of storage is unknown, but the rapidity of response to vasopressin suggests that the vasopressin effect is posttranslational. Like fibrinogen, factor VIII is an acute phase reactant, and levels of factor VIII increase in states of chronic infection and inflammation.[45] There also appears to be a relation between factor VIII levels and blood type with factor VIII levels decreased most in persons with blood group O.[46–49] Among persons belonging to blood group O, those who were secretors of ABH substances had the lowest factor VIII levels.[50]

An important question relates to how and where factor VIII, which is synthesized as a single polypeptide chain, is converted to the two-chain molecule found in plasma. Several lines of evidence suggest that the two-chain structure results from intracellular processing and not from plasma proteolysis. First, the structural heterogeneity of factor VIII persists when human plasma is collected in the presence of a variety of protease inhibitors. Under these conditions, factor VIII is a heterogeneous two-chain molecule with a variable heavy chain of 210 to 90 kd and a light chain of 80 kd similar to factor VIII isolated in the absence of inhibitors.[16–18] Second, multiple forms of active factor VIII, similar to those found in plasma, have been observed in the supernatants of cultured cells expressing recombinant factor VIII.[51,52] Third, pulse–chase studies in Chinese hamster ovary cells expressing recombinant factor VIII demonstrate immunoreactive 80-kd light chain in Golgi-enriched cellular fractions, but not in fractions enriched in rough endoplasmic reticulum, indicating that processing to a two-chain form had occurred within the Golgi apparatus.[52] This intracellular processing was not inhibited by the addition of serum as a source of vWF, although vWF may promote secretion of factor VIII.[52] The protease responsible for the intracellular processing of factor VIII has not been identified.

After it is secreted, factor VIII forms a noncovalent complex with plasma vWF and circulates bound in an approximate stoichiometry of one factor VIII molecule per vWF monomer.[53] The biologic half-life of factor VIII after transfusion into normal persons or patients with hemophilia is 8 to 12 hours (Table 39-1). In contrast, the half-life of purified factor VIII in patients with severe von Willebrand's disease is 1 to 2.4 hours, suggesting that the in vivo asso-

TABLE 39-1. Characteristics of Factors VIII and V

Parameter	Factor VIII	Factor V
Molecular weight (kd)	286	330
Specific activity (U/mg)	3500	2000
Site of synthesis	Liver, other	Liver, megakaryocyte
Plasma concentration (μg/mL)	0.05	7
Carrier protein	vWF	None
Biologic half-life (h)	8–12	12–15

ciation with vWF protects factor VIII from biologic degradation.[54,55]

Unlike factor VIII, factor V is found in both the plasma and the platelets.[56,57] Production of plasma factor V appears to occur primarily in the liver, although other cells have been shown to produce factor V, including bovine aortic, but not human umbilical vein, endothelial cells and rabbit alveolar macrophages.[58–60] Early studies implicating the liver as the source of plasma factor V consisted of whole organ perfusion experiments showing factor V production by the liver. Biosynthesis of factor V that is structurally, functionally, and immunologically indistinguishable from plasma factor V has been demonstrated in a human hepatocellular carcinoma cell line, HepG2, suggesting that the hepatocyte is the site of synthesis within the liver.[59] Factor V produced by HepG2 cells is a single-chain protein, and the rate of production of factor V by HepG2 cells in culture was about 5 ng/10^6 cells/h.

Another major site of factor V production is the megakaryocyte.[61,62] Human megakaryocytes cultured in factor V–deficient medium synthesize immunoreactive factor V. Despite inclusion of protease inhibitors, most of the factor V that was detected was a multichain form similar to the thrombin-activated form of plasma factor V. Immunoreactive factor V was also associated with small mononuclear cells that contained platelet membrane glycoproteins IIb and IIIa and platelet factor 4, suggesting that megakaryocyte precursors may also contain factor V. The subcellular localization of factor V within megakaryocytes is unknown, but its location in platelets has been the subject of several studies. By immunofluorescence microscopy, most of the platelet factor V colocalizes with platelet fibrinogen and is therefore believed to be in the α granules.[63,64] The concentration of factor V in platelets is about 1.1 μg/2.5 $\times$ 10^8 platelets, which constitutes almost 18% to 25% of the factor V in whole blood.[64]

Platelet factor V has been isolated and characterized. In contrast to plasma factor V, which is a single-chain protein, platelet factor V is present in multiple forms, ranging in size from 330 to 115 kd.[65] The mechanism of platelet factor V processing remains to be elucidated, but recent reports have suggested that factor V is a substrate for the platelet calcium-activated protease.[66,67]

BIOCHEMISTRY OF FACTORS V AND VIII

In contrast to other clotting factors that function as enzymatically active serine proteases, factors VIII and V are cofactors in the coagulation cascade. Neither protein is enzymatically active. Both act in a metal ion- and surface-dependent manner to accelerate coagulation, and both require proteolytic cleavage to become maximally active as cofactors. In the following sections, factors Va and VIIIa refer to the proteolytically activated forms of factors V and VIII.

Factor VIIIa is a cofactor in the activation of factor X to factor Xa by activated factor IX (Fig. 39-3). In the presence of ionic calcium and a phospholipid surface, the rate of factor X activation is increased over 10,000-fold by factor VIIIa.[68] Although mature factor VIII may have some activity, the catalytic efficiency of factor VIII is greatly increased by activation by thrombin or factor Xa.[16,18,68–73] Both the 90-kd heavy chain and 80-kd light chain are necessary for factor VIIIa activity. Although neither chain alone is active, factor VIIIa activity can be reconstituted from the isolated subchains by recombination in the presence of Mn^{2+} or Ca^{2+}.[74,75] Gene deletion studies have shown that the B domain is not needed for the procoagulant activity of factor VIII.[76–79] Factor VIIIa is inactivated by further exposure to thrombin or by activated protein C.[80]

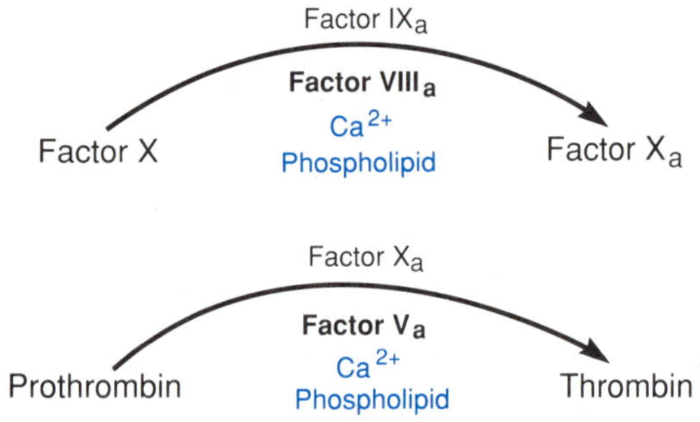

FIGURE 39-3. Factor V and factor VIII function. Factor VIII catalyzes the calcium- and phospholipid-dependent conversion of factor X to factor Xa by factor IXa. Factor V catalyzes the calcium- and phospholipid-dependent conversion of prothrombin to thrombin by factor Xa.

Activation and subsequent inactivation of factor VIII by thrombin has been correlated with a sequence of proteolytic cleavages.[6,8,17,52,81–83] Thrombin initially cleaves an Arg–Ser bond at position 740 of the mature protein, resulting in conversion of the variable-sized heavy chain to a uniform 90-kd heavy chain (Fig. 39-4). Subsequent processing by thrombin cleaves two bonds: the first at position 372, the junction between the first acidic region and the second A domain, and the second at position 1689, the junction between the second acidic region and the third A domain. As a result, the 90-kd heavy chain is converted to 50- and 43-kd polypeptides, and the 80-kd light chain is converted to a 73-kd polypeptide. When activated factor VIII is subjected to gel filtration chromatography, all three polypeptides comigrate, unless the activated factor VIII is treated with calcium chelating agents.[52]

To assess the relative importance of each proteolytic site in factor VIII activation, arginine residues at positions 740, 372, and 1689 were selectively mutated to isoleucine residues, and the procoagulant function of the altered factor VIII molecules was examined.[84] Modification of the arginine at position 740 inhibited cleavage at that site, but had little or no effect on in vitro procoagulant activity or activation of factor VIII by thrombin. In contrast, modification of the arginine at position 372 or 1689 inhibited thrombin cleavage at the modified site as well as activation by thrombin, although residual basal in vitro procoagulant activity was present. From this work, it appears that cleavage at both positions 372 and 1689 is required for activation of factor VIII, whereas the initial cleavage at position 740 is not. This conclusion is supported by two additional observations. The first is studies showing that monoclonal antibodies against the two acidic regions inhibit factor VIII cofactor activity.[85,86] The second is a report of a patient with severe hemophilia and a mutation of the thrombin cleavage site at position 1689.[87] The patient had normal antigenic levels of factor VIII in plasma, but the factor VIII was functionally inactive.

On longer exposure to thrombin, factor VIII is inactivated.[16,52,68–73] Inactivation correlates with cleavage within the heavy chain of an Arg–Ser bond at position 336 between the first A domain and the first acidic region. As a result, the 50-kd fragment is converted to a 45-kd fragment. Modification of the Arg at position 336 results in enhanced activity of factor VIII under basal conditions.[84] Activation of the modified factor VIII by thrombin occurs normally.

Thrombin-activated factor VIII is also susceptible to inactivation through proteolytic cleavage by activated protein C. The proposed site of cleavage by activated protein C is also at the Arg–Ser bond at position 336 and results in the release of the 36-residue acidic peptide separating the first two A domain repeats.[80,83,84] Thus, activation of factor VIII appears to involve release of the acidic peptide at the amino

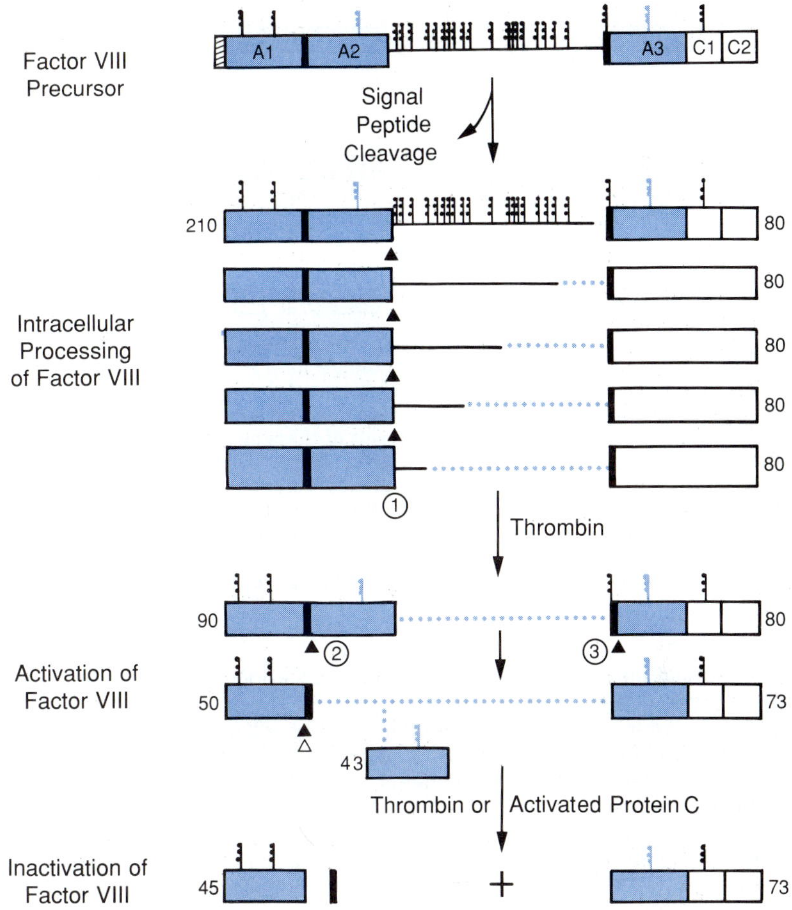

FIGURE 39-4. Factor VIII processing. Factor VIII is processed intracellularly and circulates in multiple active forms with variable heavy chains of between 90 and 210 kd and a light chain of 80 kd. Activation of factor VIII by thrombin occurs through a series of proteolytic cleavages. The factor VIII heavy chain is cleaved at the junction of the A2 and B domains to form a uniform 90-kd heavy chain. A second cleavage occurs in the heavy chain at the junction of the acidic region and the A2 domain to convert the heavy chain to 50- and 45-kd polypeptides. The light chain is cleaved at the junction of the acidic region and the A3 domain to form a 73-kd light chain. Activated factor VIII is inactivated by further processing by thrombin or activated protein C through cleavage of the heavy chain between the A1 domain and the acidic region. Solid arrowheads, sites of thrombin cleavage; open arrowhead, site of protein C cleavage. (After White GC, Shoemaker CB. Factor VIII gene and hemophilia A. Blood 1989;73:1)

terminus of the light chain and separation of the first two A domain repeats while inactivation occurs with the subsequent release of the second acidic peptide.

Activated factor V is a cofactor in the conversion of prothrombin to thrombin by factor Xa in a reaction that is phospholipid and calcium dependent (see Fig. 39-3). The activator complex formed by factor Xa, activated factor V, phospholipid, and calcium is called the *prothrombinase complex*, and the activation of prothrombin by the fully formed complex is over 200,000 times faster than activation by factor Xa alone.[88–91]

Although the molecular architecture of the assembled prothrombinase complex is uncertain, several features are known from in vitro studies. First, activated factor V interacts with the phospholipid surface.[88–96] This interaction is through the 74-kd light chain of activated factor V, and acidic phospholipids are more active in binding factor V than neutral phospholipids.[95,96] In vivo, this phospholipid surface is thought to be provided by the platelet, and the same 74-kd light-chain fragment involved in binding of factor V to phospholipid surfaces is involved in binding of factor V to platelets.[97]

Second, activated factor V interacts with factor Xa with a molar stoichiometry of one mole of activated factor V per mole of factor Xa.[91–93,95,96,98–106] This interaction is calcium dependent and is enhanced by phospholipid.[107] The stimulation of factor Xa interaction with activated factor V by phospholipid requires an intact GLA domain in factor Xa.[107] In turn, the association with activated factor V promotes the binding of factor Xa to the negatively charged phospholipid surface. According to Rosing and colleagues,[91] the net effect of this is that more factor Xa is bound to phospholipid and participates in prothrombin activation. In the absence of activated factor V, activation of prothrombin by factor Xa is incomplete; prethrombin 2, rather than thrombin, is the main product.[108,109] The interaction of factor Xa with activated factor V can be inhibited by monoclonal antibodies to the 74-kd light chain,[103] although a direct interaction of factor Xa with the light chain of activated factor V cannot be demonstrated.[96,106]

Third, activated factor V binds to prothrombin.[106] The 94-kd heavy chain has been implicated in binding to prothrombin. This interaction appears to be calcium independent.[106]

Activation of factor V by thrombin is achieved through a series of proteolytic cleavages (Fig. 39-5). Cleavage sites for thrombin are present at position 709, between the A2 domain and the connecting peptide, position 1018 in the connecting peptide, and position 1545, between the connecting peptide and the A3 domain.[21–23] As a result of these cleavages, single-chain precursor factor V is converted to a two-chain, metal ion-linked molecule, activated factor V, which consists of a 115-kd heavy chain, and a 73-kd light chain.

Factor V can also be activated by a number of other enzymes, including factor Xa and an enzyme in Russell's viper venom.[29,110–112] Russell's viper venom cleaves factor V at only one site, position 1545, between the connecting peptide and the A3 domain, which is the same site cleaved by thrombin.[21] Since factor V activated by Russell's viper venom is functionally indistinguishable from thrombin-activated factor V, it can be concluded that cleavage of the Arg–Ser bond at position 1545, but not the cleavages at positions 709 and 1018, are required for activation of factor V by thrombin.

The relative roles of plasma and platelet factor V in formation of the prothrombinase complex remain to be determined. Studies in patients with congenital deficiency of plasma factor V have shown that the bleeding tendency correlates with the platelet levels of factor V, suggesting

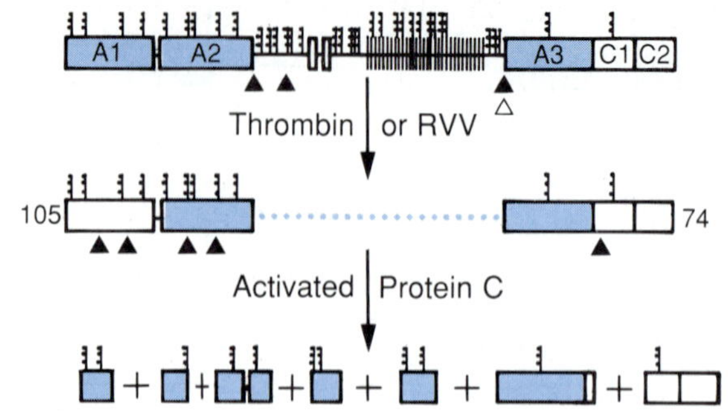

FIGURE 39-5. Factor V processing. Factor V circulates as a single polypeptide chain. On activation by thrombin, factor V is cleaved at the junction between the A2 and B domains and the junction between the B and A3 domains. A thrombin cleavage site is also present in the connecting region. As a result of these cleavages, factor V is converted to a two-chain–activated factor V consisting of a 105-kd heavy chain and a 74-kd light chain. Factor V can also be activated by Russell's viper venom through a single cleavage (*open arrowhead*) at the junction between the B and A3 domains. Factor V is inactivated by activated protein C. Multiple cleavage sites (*solid arrowheads*) for activated protein C are present in factor V.

that platelet factor V can be active in the formation of the prothrombin complex.[113] Further support for the importance of platelet factor V is provided by studies of a patient with a mild bleeding disorder who was found to have severely reduced levels of platelet factor V and only slightly reduced levels of plasma factor V and normal binding of exogenous plasma factor V to the patient's platelets.[114] The bleeding tendency in this defect, called *factor V Quebec*, was attributed to the abnormal platelet factor V. Finally, Nesheim[115] has reported a patient with an inhibitor to factor V who has less than 1% plasma factor V, but normal platelet factor V and no bleeding tendency.

Activated factor V is inactivated by activated protein C in a surface-dependent reaction that requires calcium ions and a nonenzymatic cofactor, protein S.[103,104,106,116,117] The initial cleavage by activated protein C is in the heavy chain and correlates with inactivation of factor Va. Several potential cleavage sites for activated protein C are present in human factor V. Based on the analogy with bovine factor V, the heavy chain of human factor Va appears to be cleaved at position 506, resulting in 70-kd and 20-kd fragments.[118] The light chain of activated factor V is cleaved more slowly than the heavy chain and results in 50-kd and 25-kd fragments. The probable site of human light-chain cleavage, based on the bovine model, is at position 1765.[118]

Factor V may also function as a cofactor for the degradation of factor VIIIa and factor Va by activated protein C.[118a] Abnormalities of factor V that interfere with this cofactor activity may result in resistance to activated protein C and a thrombotic tendency.

INCIDENCE AND MODE OF INHERITANCE OF FACTOR V AND VIII DEFICIENCY

Hemophilia A is one of the most common inherited bleeding disorders, occurring in about 20 of 100,000 males.[119,120] The disease is geographically dispersed and occurs about equally in all races. It is inherited in an X-linked recessive manner.[121,122] Thus, hemophilia is expressed in males, who inherit a hemophilic gene (X_h) from their mother and a male chromosome (Y) from their father; it is carried by females, who inherit a hemophilic gene (X_h) from one parent and a normal gene (X) from the other parent. As illustrated in Figure 39-6, all the daughters of a hemophilic male are obligate carriers, whereas the sons are normal. The sons of a carrier female have a 50:50 chance of having hemophilia and daughters have a 50:50 chance of being carriers.

In up to one third of cases, no family history of hemophilia is found. In some instances, this may be the result of a sporadic mutation in the factor VIII gene. A hemophilic gene is able to pass through several generations of females before becoming expressed in a male. Thus, in cases in which no family history of hemophilia exists, it can be difficult to determine whether hemophilia is the result of a spontaneous mutation or of inheritance, a distinction that may be of importance in genetic counseling. Previous estimates based on population genetics have suggested that sporadic mutations may account for the defect in up to 25% of hemophiliacs.[123] With the development of new genetic probes, it has become possible to estimate the mutation rate more accurately.[124]

Factor VIII deficiency may be expressed in females in certain situations, such as genetic mosaicism (46, XX/XO), testicular feminization, Turner's syndrome (45, XO), double heterozygotes (X_hX_h), lyonized carriers (see section on genetic counseling in hemophilia), and rare forms of autosomal inheritance, such as combined deficiency of factors V and VIII and Normandy-type von Willebrand's disease.[125–129]

The diagnosis of hemophilia A is based on the demonstration by specific assay of factor VIII deficiency. Screening coagulation tests typically reveal a prolonged partial thromboplastin time (PTT) and normal prothrombin time (PT) and thrombin time (TT). The prolongation of the PTT is proportional to the degree of factor VIII deficiency and may be normal in patients with mild hemophilia A. In general, the PTT is prolonged, with factor VIII levels of less than 20%, and normal with factor VIII levels of more than 30%. Assays for vWF and factor V should be performed in persons with mild to moderate factor VIII deficiency to rule out von Willebrand's disease and combined factor V–VIII deficiency (see following section).

Compared with hemophilia A, factor V deficiency or parahemophilia is an uncommon bleeding disorder with probably fewer than 500 patients affected worldwide and an incidence of less than 1 in 1 million. The inheritance of factor V deficiency is autosomal (see Fig. 39-6) and usually recessive, but both dominant and recessive forms have been described.[130]

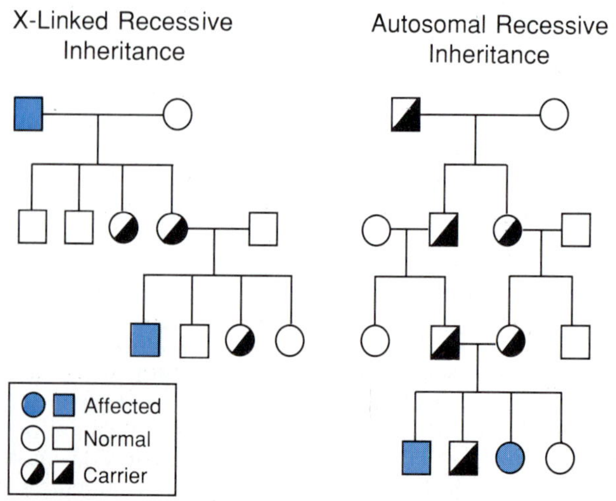

FIGURE 39-6. Genetic inheritance patterns of hemophilia A and factor V deficiency. Hemophilia A is inherited in a sex-linked recessive manner, whereas factor V deficiency is an autosomal recessive (or dominant) disorder.

Factor V deficiency is diagnosed by specific factor V assay. Since factor V acts as a cofactor in both intrinsic and extrinsic coagulation pathways, screening tests typically reveal a prolonged PTT and PT and a normal TT. The bleeding time has been prolonged in some patients with congenital factor V deficiency.

MOLECULAR GENETICS OF FACTOR V AND VIII DEFICIENCY

Phenotypically, patients with hemophilia are deficient in factor VIII. This deficiency is highly variable with levels of less than 1% to 60% (normal 60%). Some patients have no detectable factor VIII activity and normal levels of immunoreactive factor VIII. These patients have cross-reacting material and are said to be cross-reacting material (CRM)–positive. Others have reduced levels of immunoreactive factor VIII, but levels that are in excess of functional factor VIII. These patients are said to be CRM-reduced. Patients with levels of immunoreactive factor VIII that are similar to levels of functional protein are CRM-negative. The presence of cross-reacting material was first shown by Hoyer and Breckenridge[131] and by Denson and coworkers,[132] who found that some hemophilia A plasmas with no factor VIII activity were able to neutralize alloantibodies against factor VIII. This has been examined further by Reisner and coworkers[133] using an immunoradiometric

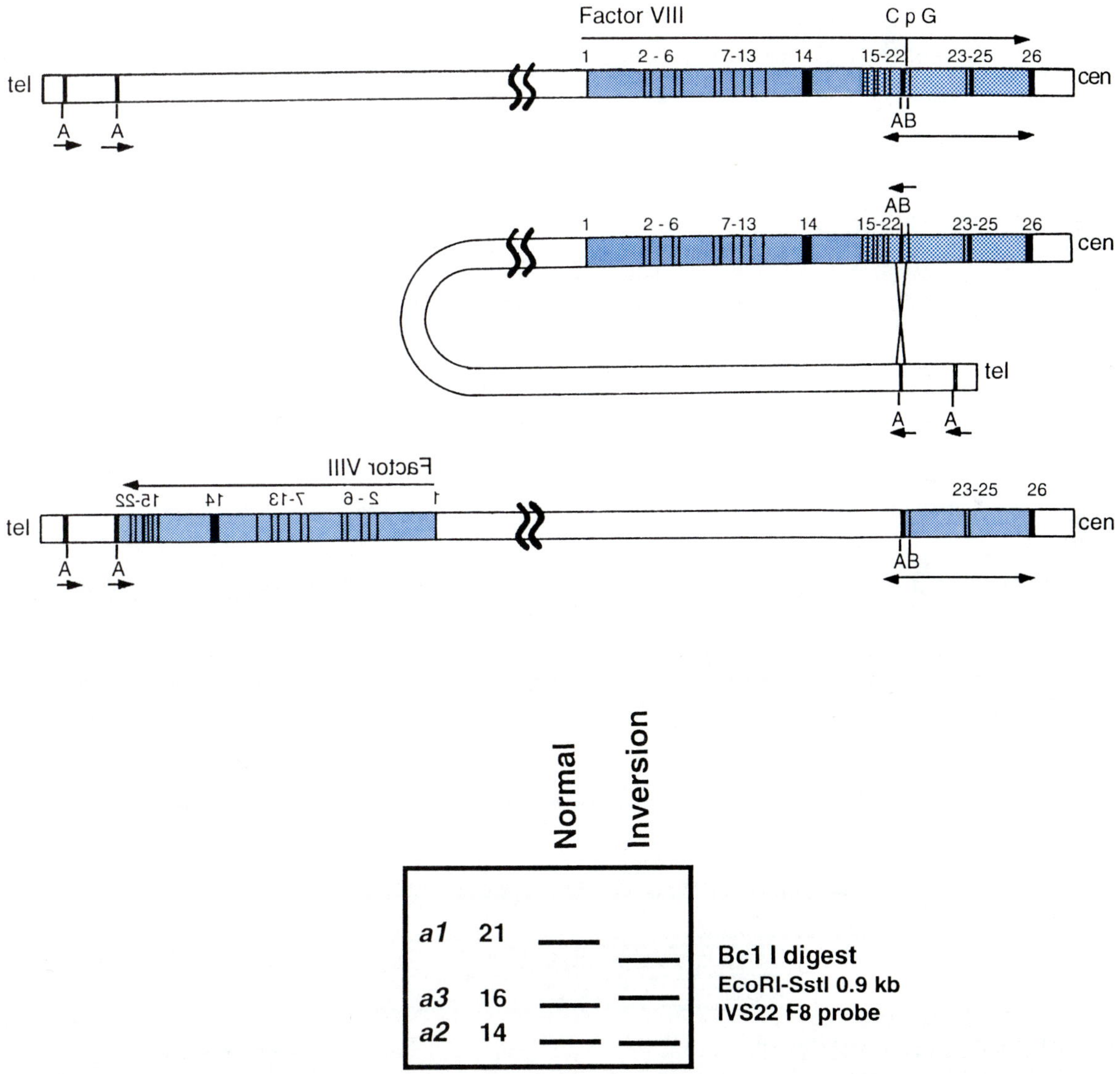

FIGURE 39-7. Diagram of the factor VIII gene and illustration of the inversion model. (**A**) Region of the q28 region of the X chromosome, with the telomere to the left and centromere to the right, showing the factor VIII gene and exons 1 to 26. Three copies of an intronless gene termed A are shown, one in intron 22 of the factor VIII gene and two upstream of factor VIII. A B gene is also shown in intron 22. The arrows indicate the direction of transcription of the factor VIII and internal A and B genes. The direction of the upstream A genes is hypothesized to be as shown. (**B**) Homologous recombination between the intron 22 copy of gene A and one of the two upstream copies. (**C**) A crossover between these two identical regions, oriented as shown, would result in an inversion of sequence between the two recombined A genes. Recombination could involve either of the upstream A genes, but only one is presented. The crossover could occur anywhere in the region of homology which includes the A genes. (Lakich D, Kazazian HH Jr, Antonarakis SE, et al. Inversions disrupting the factor VIII gene are a common cause of severe haemophilia A. Nature Genet 1993;5:236.)

assay to quantify factor VIII antigen (VIII:Ag) in hemophilic plasma. In a series of 43 arbitrarily chosen subjects studied by Reisner, 18 demonstrated VIII:Ag in excess of factor VIII activity; that is, 18 were CRM-positive or CRM-reduced.

Knowledge of the factor VIII gene and the availability of probes for the factor VIII gene have led to the identification of the molecular defects in a number of cases of hemophilia. More than 1000 patients with hemophilia A had been examined by recombinant DNA analysis to screen for the defects that cause factor VIII deficiency.[87,134–153] In moderate to mild hemophilia A, most defects are single amino acid missense mutations within functional regions of the factor VIII protein. The result is a reduction in factor VIII coagulant activity. In severe hemophilia A, a variety of molecular defects have been demonstrated. The most prevalent defect, accounting for nearly half of cases, is a partial inversion of the factor VIII gene due to homologous recombination between a small intronless "gene within a gene" in intron 22 of the factor VIII gene and one of two similar intronless genes at the tip of the X chromosome more than 400 kb distant.[153a,153b] As a result, the factor VIII gene up to and including exon 22 is inverted and separated from the 3′ end of factor VIII by 400 kb (Fig. 39-7). This disrupts factor VIII transcription, producing truncated, nonfunctional forms of the molecule. Along with deletions and insertions, point mutations resulting in nonsense defects, splice variants, or missense mutations account for most of the rest of the defects in patients with severe hemophilia.

A data base of known mutations in hemophilia has been compiled by Tuddenham and colleagues[153c] and is presented in Tables 39-2 and 39-3 and Figure 39-8. Several

(text continues on page 1164)

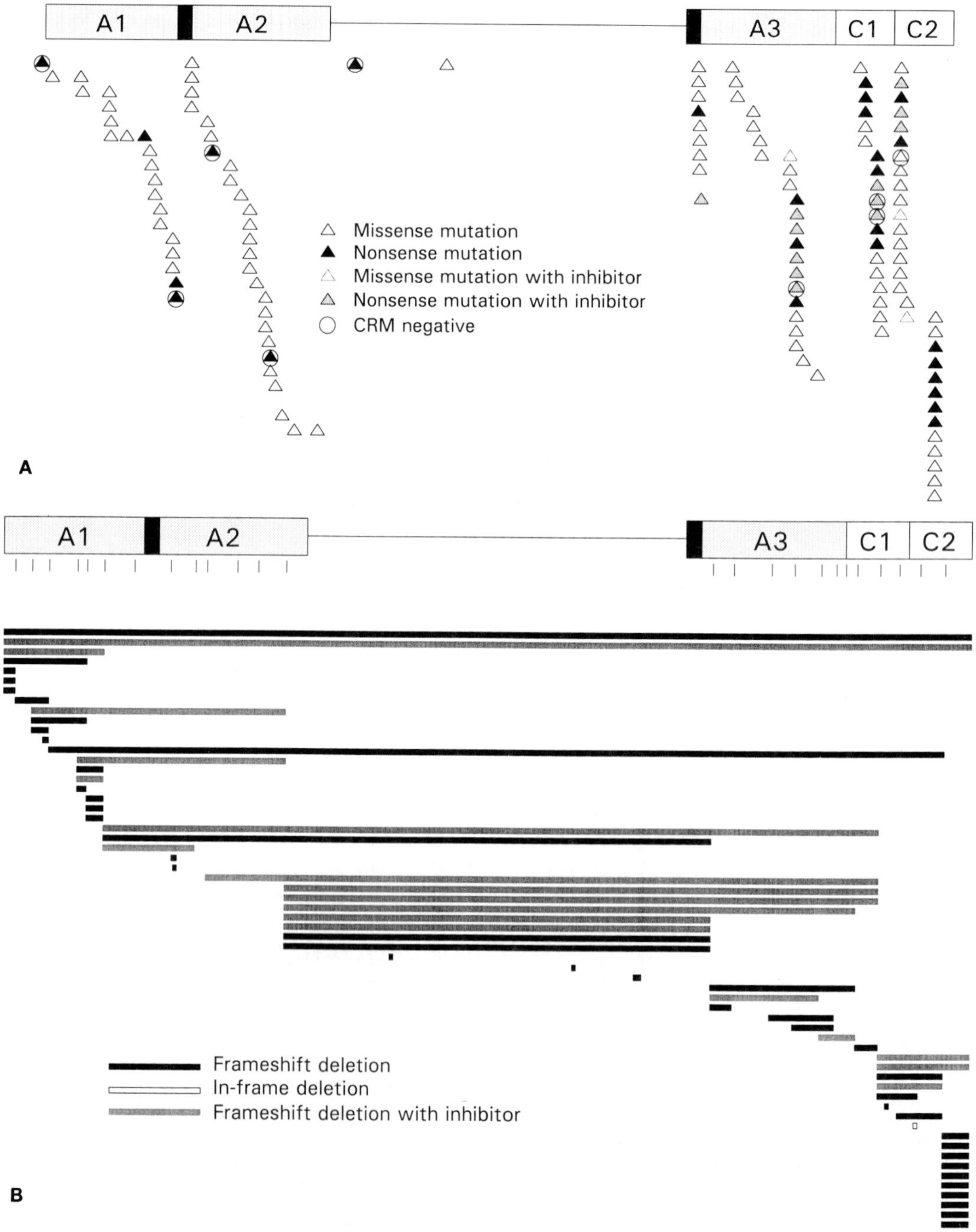

FIGURE 39-8. Gene defects in hemophilia. (**A**) Point mutations in the factor VIII protein. (**B**) Deletions in the factor VIII protein.

TABLE 39-2. Single Base Substitutions Found in the Factor VIII Gene of Patients With Hemophilia A

Exon/Intron	Codon*	Nucleotide Change	Codon Change	FVIII:C (U/dL)	FVIII:Ag (U/dL)	Severity	Inhibitors	Comments
Exon 1	−5	CGA → TGA†	Arg → Term	<1	<1	Severe	No	Signal peptide
Exon 1	11	GAA → GTA‡	Glu → Val	?	?	Mild	No	
Intron 2	—	CGA → TGA	—	<1	?	Severe	No	Probably a neutral change about 300 bp 3′ to exon 2
Exon 3	89	AAG → ACG‡	Lys → Thr	?	?	Mild	?	
Exon 3	91	ATG → GTG‡	Met → Val	?	?	Mild	?	
Exon 4	162	GTG → ATG‡	Val → Met	8	?	Moderate	No	
Exon 4	162	GTG → ATG‡	Val → Met	5	?	Mild	No	
Exon 4	166	AAA → ACA‡	Lys → Thr	19	?	Mild	?	
Exon 4	170	TCA → TTA‡	Ser → Leu	3.5	8.7	Moderate	No	
Intron 4	—	CGA → CAA	—	5–10	41	Mild	No	Proposed to activate cryptic splice site about 1 kb 3′ to exon 4
Exon 5	205	G/gt . . ag/GG → T/ gt . . ag/GG‡	Gly → Trp	3.2	?	Moderate	?	−1 IVS5 donor splice site
Intron 5		ag/→ gg/	—	<1	?	Severe	No	+1 IVS5 acceptor splice site
Intron 6	—	ag/→ ac/	—	?	?	Severe	?	+2 IVS6 acceptor splice site
Exon 7	255	TGG → TGA*	Trp → Term	?	?	Severe	?	
Exon 7	266	GTG → GGG‡	Val → Gly	?	?	Mild	?	
Exon 7	272	GAA → GGA‡	Glu → Gly	2	3.5	Moderate	No	
Exon 7	282	CGC → CAC‡	Arg → His	?	?	Severe	?	
Exon 7	282	CGC → CAC‡	Arg → His	?	?	Severe	?	
Exon 7	293	TTC → TCC‡	Phe → Ser	?	?	Mild	?	
Exon 7	295	ACT → GCT‡	Thr → Ala	14–16	?	Moderate	?	
Exon 8	326	GTA → CTA‡	Val → Leu	?	?	Severe	No	
Exon 8	326	GTA → CTA‡	Val → Leu	?	?	Moderate	?	
Exon 8	329	TGT → CGT‡	Cys → Arg	?	?	Severe	No	
Exon 8	336	CGA → TGA†	Arg → Term	0	?	Severe	?	Activated protein C cleavage site
Exon 8	336	CGA → TGA†	Arg → Term	<1	<1	Severe	No	Activated protein C cleavage site
Exon 8	372	CGC → TGC‡	Arg → Cys	3	80	Moderate	No	Thrombin activation site
Exon 8	372	CGC → TGC‡	Arg → Cys	3	74	Moderate	No	Thrombin activation site
Exon 8	372	CGC → TGC‡	Arg → Cys	3	?	Moderate	No	Thrombin activation site
Exon 8	372	CGC → CAC‡	Arg → His	5	325	Mild	No	Thrombin activation site
Exon 8	372	CGC → CAC‡	Arg → His	3	?	Moderate	No	Thrombin activation site
Exon 9	412	TTG → TTT‡	Leu → Phe	10.5	?	Mild	?	
Exon 9	425	AAA → AGA‡	Lys → Arg	?	?	Severe	?	
Exon 9	427	CGA → TGA†	Arg → Term	<1	<1	Severe	No	
Exon 10	473	TAT → CAT‡	Tyr → His	?	?	Mild	?	
Exon 10	473	TAT → TGT‡	Tyr → Cys	2.7/3.5	?	Moderate	?	
Exon 10	479	GGA → AGA‡	Gly → Arg	2	?	Moderate	No	
Exon 11	504	CTG → CTT‡	Leu → Leu	?	?	Mild	?	Potential new acceptor site (not proved to be causal)

(continued)

TABLE 39-2. *(Continued)*

Exon/Intron	Codon*	Nucleotide Change	Codon Change	FVIII:C (U/dL)	FVIII:Ag (U/dL)	Severity	Inhibitors	Comments
Exon 11	527	CGG → TGG‡	Arg → Trp	14.5/18/17–18	?	Mild	?	
Exon 11	527	CGG → TGG‡	Arg → Trp	?	?	?	?	
Exon 11	531	CGC → TGC‡	Arg → Cys	6.7/4.2	?	Moderate	?	
Exon 11	531	CGC → TGC‡	Arg → Cys	?	?	Moderate	?	
Exon 11	531	CGC → GGC‡	Arg → Gly	9.2	?	Moderate	?	
Exon 11	535	AGT → GGT‡	Ser → Gly	?	?	?	?	
Exon 11	542	GAT → GGT‡	Asp → Gly	?	?	Severe	?	
Exon 11	565	CAG/gt → AAG/gt‡	Gln → Lys	?	?	Mild/moderate	?	−3 IVS11 donor splice site
Exon 11	565	CAG/gt → AAG/gt‡	Glu → Lys	?	?	Moderate	?	−3 IVS11 donor splice site
Exon 12	566	ATA → ACA‡	Ile → Thr	?	?	Severe	?	New N-glycosylation site N564
Exon 12	577	TCT → CCT‡	Ser → Pro	?	?	?	?	
Exon 12	583	CGA → TGA†	Arg → Term	<1	<1	Severe	No	
Exon 12	584	AGC → ATC‡	Ser → Ile	?	?	?	?	Loss N-glycosylation site N58
Exon 12	593	CGC → TGC‡	Arg → Cys	?	?	Mild	?	
Exon 12	593	CGC → TGC‡	Arg → Cys	?	?	?	?	
Exon 12	612	AAC → AGC‡	Asn → Ser	?	?	?	?	
Intron 12	—	/gtgagt → gtgaat	—	?	?	Mild	?	+5 IVS12 donor splice site
Exon 13	644	GCA → GTA‡	Ala → Val	14	25	Mild/moderate	?	
Exon 14	704	[C]GCC → ACC‡	Ala → Thr	?	?	Mild	?	
Exon 14	795	CGA → TGA†	Arg → Term	<1	<1	Severe	No	
Exon 14	1038	GAG → AAG‡	Glu → Lys	2.4	?	Mild/moderate	?	
Exon 14	1680	TAT → TTT‡	Tyr → Phe	10	20	Mild	No	Tyrosine sulphation–vWF interaction
Exon 14	1680	TAT → TTT‡	Tyr → Phe	?	?	Mild	?	Tyrosine sulphation–vWF interaction
Exon 14	1680	TAT → TGT‡	Tyr → Cys	?	?	Severe	No	
Exon 14	1686	CAG → TAG†	Gln → Term	<1	?	Severe	?	
Exon 14	1689	CGC → TGC‡	Arg → Cys	4–5	100	Moderate	No	Thrombin activation site
Exon 14	1689	CGC → TGC‡	Arg → Cys	0	96	Severe	No	Thrombin activation site
Exon 14	1689	CGC → TGC‡	Arg → Cys	2–5	87–220	Mild/moderate	No	Thrombin activation site
Exon 14	1689	CGC → TGC‡	Arg → Cys	?	?	Moderate	No	Thrombin activation site
Exon 14	1689	CGC → TGC‡	Arg → Cys	<1	?	Severe	No	Thrombin activation site
Exon 14	1689	CGC → TGC‡	Arg → Cys	5	211	Moderate	No	Thrombin activation site
Exon 14	1689	CGC → CAC	Arg → His	7	165	Mild	No	Thrombin activation site
Exon 14	1696	CGA → TGA†	Arg → Term	<1	?	Severe	Yes	
Exon 14	1709	TAT → TGT	Tyr → Cys	18	?	Moderate	No	
Exon 15	1772	ATG → ACG‡	Met → Thr	?	?	Severe	?	New N-glycosylation site N177
Exon 16	1781	CGT → CAT‡	Arg → His	?	?	Mild/moderate	?	
Exon 16	1784	TCC → TAC‡	Ser → Tyr	?	?	Severe	?	
Exon 16	1825	CCC → TCC‡	Pro → Ser	15	?	Moderate	?	
Exon 16	1826	ACT → CCT‡	Thr → Pro	?	?	Mild	?	

Exon 16	1843	CTG/gt → CTA/gt	Leu → Leu	9–18	?	Moderate	?	−1 IVS16 donor splice site
Exam 17	1848	CAC → CGC‡	His → Arg	1–5	?	Mild/moderate	?	
Exon 18	1922	AAT → GAT‡	Asn → Asp	<1	?	Severe	Yes	
Exon 18	1922	AAT → GAT‡	Asn → Asp	?	?	Moderate	?	
Exon 18	1922	AAT → AGT‡	Asn → Ser	?	?	Moderate	?	
Exon 18	1941	CGA → TGA†	Arg → Term	<1	?	Severe	No	
Exon 18	1941	CGA → TGA†	Arg → Term	<1	?	Severe	Yes	
Exon 18	1941	CGA → TGA†	Arg → Term	<1	?	Severe	Yes	
Exon 18	1941	CGA → TGA†	Arg → Term	<1	?	Severe	No	
Exon 18	1941	CGA → TGA†	Arg → Term	<1	?	Severe	Yes	
Exon 18	1941	CGA → TGA†	Arg → Term	?	?	Severe	Yes	
Exon 18	1941	CGA → TGA†	Arg → Term	<1	<0.1	Severe	Yes	
Exon 18	1941	CGA → TGA†	Arg → Term	?	?	Severe	?	
Exon 18	1941	CGA → CAA‡	Arg → Gln	?	?	Mild	?	
Exon 18	1941	CGA → CAA‡	Arg → Gln	?	?	Mild	No	
Exon 18	1941	CGA → CAA‡	Arg → Gln	5	20	Moderate	No	
Exon 18	1941	CGA → CAA‡	Arg → Gln	2	?	Moderate	No	
Exon 18	1941	CGA → CTA‡	Arg → Leu	?	?	Moderate	?	
Exon 18	1966	CGA → TGA†	Arg → Term	0	?	Severe	Yes	
Exon 19	1997	CGG → TGG‡	Arg → Trp	3.4/2.6	?	Mild/moderate	?	
Exon 22	2101	TTT → TTG‡	Phe → Leu	11	?	Mild/moderate	?	
Exon 22	2105	TAT → TGT‡	Tyr → Cys	14	?	Mild	No	
Exon 22	2116	CGA → TGA†	Arg → Term	<1	?	Severe	No	
Exon 22	2116	CGA → TGA†	Arg → Term	0	?	Severe	No	
Exon 22	2116	CGA → TGA†	Arg → Term	<1	?	Severe	No	
Exon 22	2116	CGA → TGA†	Arg → Term	<1	?	Severe	No	
Exon 22	2116	CGA → CCA‡	Arg → Pro	<1	?	Severe	?	
Exon 22	2119	TCC → TAC‡	Ser → Tyr	5–8	?	Mild/moderate	?	
Exon 23	2147	CGA → TGA†	Arg → Term	<1	?	Severe	?	
Exon 23	2147	CGA → TGA†	Arg → Term	<1	?	Severe	No	
Exon 23	2147	CGA → TGA†	Arg → Term	<1	?	Severe	Yes	
Exon 23	2147	CGA → TGA†	Arg → Term	<1	<0.1	Severe	Yes	
Exon 23	2147	CGA → TGA†	Arg → Term	1	<0.1	Severe	Yes	
Exon 23	2147	CGA → TGA†	Arg → Term	<1	?	Severe	No	
Exon 23	2147	CGA → TGA†	Arg → Term	?	?	Severe	?	
Exon 23	2150	CGT → CAT‡	Arg → His	5–7	?	Mild/moderate	?	
Exon 23	2150	CGT → CAT‡	Arg → His	?	?	Mild/moderate	?	
Exon 23	2159	CGC → TGC‡	Arg → Cys	10	?	Mild	No	
Exon 23	2159	CGC → TGC‡	Arg → Cys	12	?	Mild	No	
Exon 23	2159	CGC → TGC‡	Arg → Cys	7.4	?	Moderate	?	
Exon 23	2163	CGC → CAC‡	Arg → His	?	?	Moderate	?	
Exon 23	2166	GTT → GCT‡	Leu → Ser	<1	?	Severe	No	

(continued)

TABLE 39-2. *(Continued)*

Exon/Intron	Codon*	Nucleotide Change	Codon Change	FVIII:C (U/dL)	FVIII:Ag (U/dL)	Severity	Inhibitors	Comments
Exon 24	2209	CGA → CTA‡	Arg → Leu	3	2.5	Moderate	No	
Exon 24	2209	CGA → TGA†	Arg → Term	0	?	Severe	Yes	
Exon 24	2209	CGA → TGA†	Arg → Term	<1	?	Severe	No	
Exon 24	2209	CGA → TGA†	Arg → Term	<1	?	Severe	Yes	
Exon 24	2209	CGA → TGA†	Arg → Term	<1	?	Severe	Yes	
Exon 24	2209	CGA → TGA†	Arg → Term	<1	?	Severe	No	
Exon 24	2209	CGA → TGA†	Arg → Term	?	?	Severe	?	
Exon 24	2209	CGA → CAA‡	Arg → Gln	<1	?	Severe	No	
Exon 24	2209	CGA → CAA†	Arg → Gln	<1	?	Severe	No	
Exon 24	2209	CGA → CAA‡	Arg → Gln	?	?	Severe	No	
Exon 24	2209	CGA → CAA‡	Arg → Gln	2–5	?	Moderate	No	
Exon 24	2209	CGA → CAA‡	Arg → Gln	7	130	Mild	Yes	
Exon 24	2209	CGA → CAA‡	Arg → Gln	<1	?	Severe	No	
Exon 24	2209	CGA → CAA‡	Arg → Gln	<1	?	Severe	No	
Exon 24	2209	CGA → CAA‡	Arg → Gln	<1	?	Severe	?	
Exon 24	2209	CGA → CAA‡	Arg → Gln	?	?	Severe	?	
Exon 24	2209	CGA → CAA‡	Arg → Gln	3	?	Moderate	?	
Exon 24	2209	CGA → CAA‡	Arg → Gln	3	?	Moderate	No	
Exon 25	2229	TGG → TGT‡	Trp → Cys	3	?	Mild/moderate	Yes	
Intron 25	—	CAA → CGA	—	<1	?	Severe	No	Probably a neutral change about 1.9 kb 5′ to exon 26
Exon 26	2300	CCG → CTG‡	Pro → Leu	7.5	?	Mild	?	
Exon 26	2304	CGC → TGC‡	Arg → Cys	?	?	Mild	?	
Exon 26	2307	CGA → TGA†	Arg → Term	0	?	Severe	No	
Exon 26	2307	CGA → TGA†	Arg → Term	<1	?	Severe	No	
Exon 26	2307	CGA → TGA†	Arg → Term	<1	?	Severe	No	
Exon 26	2307	CGA → TGA†	Arg → Term	<1	?	Severe	No	
Exon 26	2307	CGA → TGA†	Arg → Term	?	?	Severe	?	
Exon 26	2307	CGA → TGA†	Arg → Term	?	?	Severe	?	
Exon 26	2307	CGA → CTA‡	Arg → Leu	2	4	Mild	No	
Exon 26	2307	CGA → CTA‡	Arg → Leu	<1	?	Severe	No	
Exon 26	2307	CGA → CTA‡	Arg → Leu	?	?	Severe	?	
Exon 26	2307	CGA → CAA‡	Arg → Gln	10	6	Mild	No	
Exon 26	2307	CGA → CAA‡	Arg → Gln	2	?	Moderate	No	

* Codons numbered after the scheme of Wehar and colleagues (1984), which starts at mature N terminal and 19 signal peptide residues numbered negatively.
† Nonsense mutation.
‡ Missense mutation.

TABLE 39-3. Deletions Found in the Factor VIII Gene of Patients With Hemophilia A

Exon(s) Deleted	Codons	Size of Deletion	FVIII:C (U/dL)	FVIII:Ag (U/dL)	Severity	Inhibitors	Comments
LARGE DELETIONS							
1–26		>210 kb	?	?	Severe	No	
1–26		>210 kb	?	?	Severe	Yes	
1–6		>55 kb	<1%	?	Severe	Yes	
1–5		>35 kb	<1%	?	Severe	No	
1		>2 kb	<1%	<1%	Severe	No	
1		>1 kb	<1%	?	Severe	No	
1		?	?	?	Severe	?	
Intron 1*		7 kb	?	?	Severe	No	
2–3		9–12 kb	<1%	<1%	Severe	No	
3–13		60 kb	<1%	<1%	Severe	Yes	
3–5		11.7 kb	<1%	?	Severe	No	
3		1.7–2.0 kb	<1%	?	Severe	No	
4–25		133–145 kb	<1%	<1%	Severe	No	
5–13		57 kb	<1%	?	Severe	Yes	
5, 6		?	?	?	Severe	?	
5, 6		2.5–10 kb	?	?	Severe	Yes	
5		2 kb	?	?	Severe	No	
5 or 6		2 kb	?	?	Severe	?	
6		10 kb	?	?	Severe	No	
6		7 kb	<1%	<1%	Severe	No	
6		3–6 kb	?	?	Severe	No	
7–22		110 kb	?	?	Severe	Yes	
7–14		40–56 kb	<1%	<1%	Severe	No	
7–9		15–20 kb	<1%	?	Severe	Yes	
11–22		60 kb	?	?	Severe	Yes	
14–22		>36 kb	?	?	Severe	Yes	
14–22		?	?	?	Severe	Yes	
14–21		50 kb	<1%	?	Severe	Yes	
14		12–16 kb	<1%	?	Severe	Yes	
14		6 kb	<1%	<0.1%	Severe	Yes	
14		2.3–3.0 kb	<1%	?	Severe	No	
14		2.5 kb	<1%	<1%	Severe	No	
14		2.5 kb	?	?	Severe	?	
15–21		?	?	?	Severe	?	
15–18		13 kb	?	?	Severe	Yes	
15		?	?	?	Severe	?	
17–19		?	?	?	Severe	No	
18, 19†		?	?	?	Severe	?	
19–21		4.7 kb	<1%	?	Severe	Yes	
22		5.5 kb	2%–5%	?	Moderate	No	
Intron 22†		?	?	?	Severe	No	
Intron 22†		?	?	?	Moderate	No	
23–26		?	?	?	Severe	Yes	
23–26		?	?	?	Severe	Yes	
23–25		>16 kb	<1%	<1%	Severe	No	
23–25		39 kb	<1%	?	Severe	Yes	
23–24		?	?	?	Moderate	No	
24–25		>3.4 kb	<1%	<1%	Severe	No	
26		22	<1%	?	Severe	No	
26		>18 kb	<1%	?	Severe	No	
26		14 kb	<1%	<1%	Severe	No	
26		8.7 kb	?	?	Severe	?	
26		>2 kb	?	?	Severe	No	
26		>2 kb	?	?	Severe	No	
26		>2 kb	?	?	Severe	?	
26		?	?	?	Severe	?	
26		?	?	?	Severe	No	
26		?	?	?	Severe	No	
26		?	?	?	Severe	No	

(continued)

TABLE 39-3. *(Continued)*

Exon(s) Deleted	Codons	Size of Deletion	FVIII:C (U/dL)	FVIII:Ag (U/dL)	Severity	Inhibitors	Comments
SMALL DELETIONS							
	104–111	23 bp	?	?	Severe	?	Includes IVS3 donor splice site
	340–341	4 bp (AATG)	?	?	Severe	No	Frameshift in exon 8
	341	2 bp (GA)	?	?	Severe	?	Frameshift in exon 8
	1212	1 bp (C)	?	?	Severe	No	Frameshift in exon 14
	1439	1 bp (A)	?	?	Severe	?	A8 → A7, frameshift in exon 14
	1535–1536	2 bp (GA)	?	?	Severe	?	Frameshift in exon 14
	2136	2 bp (AA)	?	?	Severe	?	A4 → A2, frameshift in exon 23
	2204–2205	3 bp (CTC)	?	?	Moderate	?	Deletes 2205 Pro

* Not proved to be cause of disease phenotype but segregates with disease allele.
† Precise extent unknown but includes at least region indicated.

things are clear from the data presented. First, as with the thalassemias and hemophilia B, diverse defects give rise to the same clinical disorder recognized as hemophilia. Their distribution throughout the factor VIII gene indicates no evidence for a single mutational site causing hemophilia. Second, although it has been suggested that hemophilic patients with inhibitors may represent a subset of patients with significant deletions, the data suggest that patients with large deletions, even deletion of the entire factor VIII gene do not necessarily develop inhibitors. Furthermore, among patients with the same gene defect, some may develop an inhibitor and the others may not. Finally, many of the point mutations described to date in hemophilia have involved sites recognized by the restriction enzyme, *Taq* I. The recognition sequence for this nuclease, TCGA, contains the dinucleotide CpG, the most common site of methylation in human DNA and a possible site of increased mutation due to deamination of cytosine leading to C to T transitions.[154] Evidence for this as a mutational hot spot in hemophilia has been presented.[137]

Figures 39-9 and 38-10 show the molecular details of some of the defects that result in hemophilia. In Figure 39-9*A*, the defect is a 7-kb deletion that encompasses exons 24 and 25. This deletion results in a frame shift so that the normal translation reading frame is altered. As a result, not only are exons 24 and 25 lost, but exon 26 is either not translated or makes a nonsense protein. Thus, a large portion of the C domain (which constitutes most of the light chain of activated factor VIII) is abnormal. In Figure 39-9*B*, a 5.5-kb deletion encompasses exon 22. In contrast to the preceding example, this is an in-frame deletion; that is, the normal translation reading frame is not altered. In this case, amino acids encoded by exon 22 are not present, but exons 23 to 26 are translated and expressed. The result is production of a molecule with decreased but detectable clotting activity.

In Figure 39-9C, the defect is a point mutation at nucleotide 62 in exon 18. The nucleotide sequence AGGATTCGATGG is mutated to AGGATTTGATGG. As a result, CGA, which codes for an arginine residue in the mature protein, is changed to TGA, a signal to stop translation (called a *stop codon*). The result is premature termination of translation at amino acid 1940 and production of a shortened, nonfunctional factor VIII. In Figure 39-9*D*, the defect is a point mutation in exon 14. Instead of the normal nucleotide sequence CAGAGCCCCCGCAGCTTTC, the sequence is CAGAGCCCCTGCAGCTTTC. In this instance, codon 1689 is mutated from an arginine residue to a cysteine residue, resulting in the loss of the thrombin cleavage site between the second acidic region and the third A domain. Thus, in the patient, factor VIII antigenic levels are normal indicating that synthesis and secretion of factor VIII is normal, but the factor VIII cannot be activated by thrombin and is associated with a severe form of hemophilia.

Figure 39-10 shows how two distinct point mutations within a single codon can produce hemophilia of different severity. In Figure 39-10*A*, a CGA in exon 26, which codes for an arginine, is mutated to TGA, which is a stop codon. The resulting factor VIII molecule is significantly truncated and is associated with a severe hemorrhagic diathesis with less than 1% functional factor VIII. The defect illustrated in Figure 39-10*B* involves the same codon, but the mutation is CGA to CAA, which codes for a glutamine. The resulting factor VIII molecule is a full-length molecule with a single amino acid change; this is associated with a mild hemorrhagic diathesis with 9% functional factor VIII activity.

Kazazian and coworkers[155] have reported a novel mechanism for mutation of the factor VIII gene as a cause of hemophilia. They described two unrelated patients, both with severe hemophilia A, who had nonviral insertions of 3.8 and 2.3 kb, respectively, in exon 14. In both patients, the insertion contained the 3′ portion of the human *L1* sequence, a family of long, interspersed repeats that are present throughout the human genome and may function as retrotransposons. It was postulated that in both cases, the insertion of the *L1* sequence occurred through base-pairing of the poly(T) tail of *L1* cDNA with an A-rich region in exon 14 of factor VIII.

Much less is known about the molecular defects resulting in factor V deficiency. This is partly because factor V deficiency is an uncommon disorder and because the genomic sequence for factor V has not been determined. Most cases of factor V deficiency appear to be CRM-negative and were originally presumed to represent disorders in which synthesis of factor V was decreased.[156–159] Subsequent studies showed that in some CRM-negative patients, nonfunctional antigenic material was in their platelets, suggesting that a dysfunctional factor V molecule was produced. A series of CRM-positive patients has been described, with less than 10% coagulant activity and factor V antigen levels of 45% to 70%.[160] Thus, factor V deficiency, like factor VIII defi-

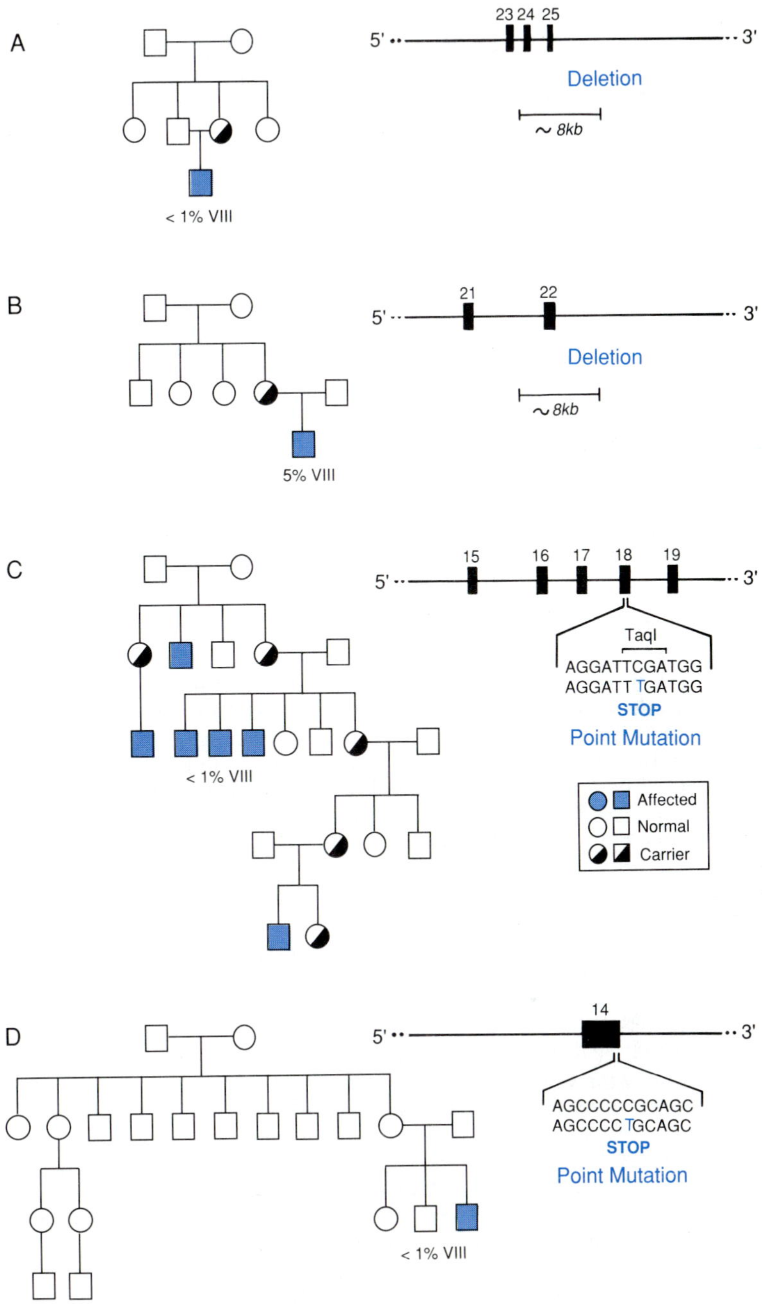

FIGURE 39-9. Genetic defects in hemophilia. (**A**) An 8-kb frameshift deletion encompassing exons 24 and 25, which results in severe hemophilia. (**B**) An 8-kb inframe deletion encompassing exon 22, which results in moderately severe hemophilia. (**C**) A nonsense mutation at a *Taq* I site in exon 18, which results in severe hemophilia. (**D**) A nonsense mutation in exon 14, which results in severe hemophilia.

ciency, appears to constitute a spectrum of genetic defects. Definition of these defects at the molecular level will provide important insight into the function of factor V.

Factor V Quebec is a variant form of factor V deficiency characterized by plasma factor V levels of 40% to 60%, plasma factor V antigen levels of 65% to 75%, platelet factor V activity of 2% to 4%, and platelet factor V antigen levels of 70% to 80%.[114] In the kindred reported, the factor V defect was inherited as an autosomal dominant trait. This appears to be the first description of a qualitative abnormality of platelet factor V.

Factor V deficiency may also be seen in association with factor VIII deficiency.[161–179] Combined factor V–VIII deficiency is inherited in an autosomal recessive manner. Levels of factor V and VIII are commensurately reduced and range from 5% to 25%. Antigenic levels of factors V and VIII may be normal or may be concordant with activity levels. The cause of combined factor V–VIII deficiency is uncertain. Because of the effect of activated protein C on factors V and VIII, deficiency of the inhibitor of activated protein C was originally considered to account for the autosomal inheritance pattern and for the deficiency of both factors V and VIII from a single gene defect.[180] Although this was an attractive and unifying hypothesis, subsequent studies have shown that both the activity and the antigenic levels of protein C inhibitor are normal in patients with combined factor V–VIII deficiency.[181–183]

Genetic Counseling in Hemophilia A

Standard methods of carrier detection in hemophilia A have been based on assays for factor VIII biologic activity. Although a female carrier possesses two X chromosomes (X_hX), only one of the X chromosomes is expressed in a

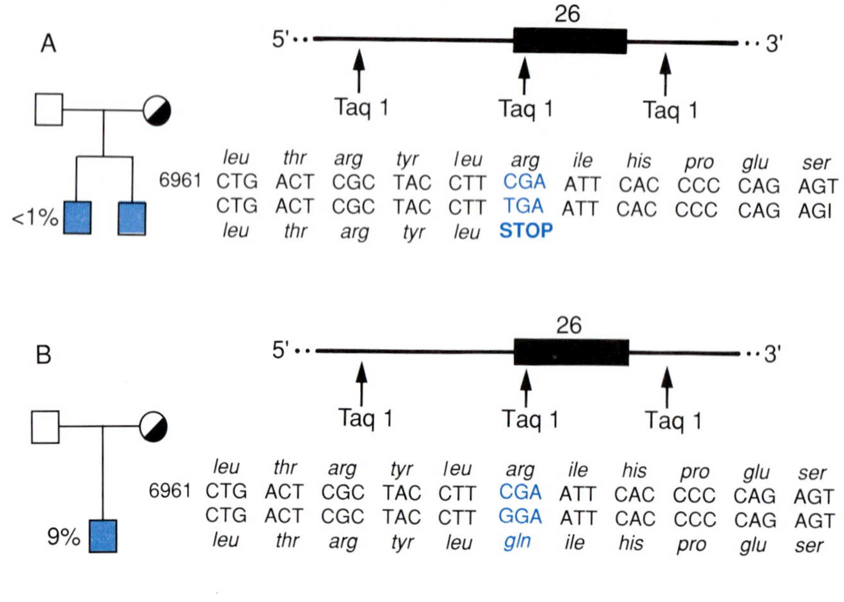

FIGURE 39-10. Genetic defects in hemophilia. Examples of point mutations within a single codon in exon 26 that cause hemophilia of different severity. The *Taq* I restriction sites are indicated by the letter *T* and an arrow. (**A**) Severe hemophilia resulting from a nonsense mutation. (**B**) Mild hemophilia resulting from a missense mutation.

given somatic cell. Inactivation of the second X chromosome occurs by a process known as *lyonization* (after Dr. Mary Lyon who first described the process) and is a random event. Thus, in a carrier, some factor VIII-producing cells (those with the X chromosome active) express normal amounts of factor VIII and other cells (those with the X_h chromosome active) express no factor VIII. Because of lyonization, only half of the potential factor VIII–producing cells in a carrier produce factor VIII. On the average, factor VIII levels in a carrier are half of the average level of factor VIII in normal females. Also, factor VIII activity in a large population of carrier females assumes a gaussian curve that overlaps with the gaussian curve obtained from a normal population. Because of this overlap, results of carrier testing based on factor VIII activity are always probabilistic.[184] The accuracy of carrier testing can be increased using bivariate analysis of factor VIII activity and von Willebrand antigen. With the use of both assays and statistical refinements, the error rate in carrier detection has been determined to be around 10%.[48,185]

The availability of genetic probes for factor VIII makes it possible to identify carriers with increased accuracy. In general, two approaches to carrier detection have been used. The first, which depends on the direct recognition of the specific genomic defect, is used when the gene defect in the pedigree under investigation is known. Detection of the defect may be by a labeled oligonucleotide probe specific for the defect or by restriction site analysis if the defect involves the recognition site for a restriction enzyme such as *Taq* I. This approach has the advantage of not requiring pedigree information if the precise defect has been established in the family under study. The second approach, called *RFLP analysis*, takes advantage of restriction fragment length polymorphisms (RFLP) linked to the factor VIII gene. The DNA probes used in this approach identify independently segregating restriction polymorphisms close to or in the factor VIII gene. With this technique, it is not necessary to know the specific genomic defect in a given family, but it requires an affected male to establish which allele contains the mutant X chromosome. It also requires that the mother be heterozygous for the polymorphism.

Numerous reports of DNA probes being used for carrier testing and prenatal diagnosis have appeared since 1984 when the factor VIII gene was cloned. Initial studies described a *Bgl* II RFLP detected with an X-chromosome–specific probe, DXS15 (DX13).[186] No crossovers between the hemophilia A locus and the DXS15 locus were observed. Oberle and coworkers[187] described a *Taq* I RFLP detected with DXS52 (St14), another X-chromosome–specific probe extragenic to the factor VIII gene. Reports of crossover between *Bgl* II–DXS15 or *Taq* I–DXS52 and the factor VIII gene have appeared.[188–191] Although this may limit the usefulness of these markers, they remain valuable probes for some patients.

RFLPs within the factor VIII gene provide more accurate carrier detection and prenatal diagnosis. To identify intragenic markers, Gitschier and coworkers[192] screened the factor VIII gene for polymorphisms with 37 restriction enzymes. One enzyme, *Bcl* I, revealed a polymorphic site that lies 3′ to exon 18; this has proved useful for carrier detection and antenatal diagnosis.[193,194] Additional intragenic polymorphisms with *Bgl* I, *Xba* I, *Msp* I, and *Hind* III have subsequently been described.[135,195–198] In addition to these polymorphic restriction sites, the factor VIII gene also contains a polymorphic hypervariable (CA)n dinucleotide repeat that can be used for carrier analysis.[198a] Table 39-4 summarizes polymorphic restriction sites that have been useful in the genetic diagnosis of hemophilia.

Carrier detection can be enhanced by using multiple DNA probes. Janco and coworkers[199] have compared the usefulness of three intragenic polymorphisms (*Bcl* I–F8IVS18,* *Xba* I–F8IVS22, and *Bgl* I–F8IVS25) and one extragenic polymorphism (*Taq* I–DXS52) for carrier detection. The intragenic polymorphisms alone were informative in 32% to 58% of women tested. *Bgl* I–F8IVS25 and *Bcl* I–F8IVS18 were in apparent linkage disequilibrium and provided no additional information. Using *Bcl* I–F8IVS18 and *Xba* I–F8IVS22, accurate information was obtained in 64% of women tested. The remaining women, who were uninformative with any intragenic probe, all were informative with the extragenic *Taq* I–DXS52 polymorphism. Because a significant risk of recombination between *Taq* I–DXS52 and the factor VIII gene exists, Janco and coworkers[199] recommended first testing with *Xba* I–F8IVS22 or *Xba* I–F8IVS22 and *Bcl* I–F8IVS18. In a similar study, Pecorara and coworkers[200] showed that the combination of *Bcl* I–

* The nomenclature used for polymorphisms specifies the restriction enzyme and the location of the polymorphic site. Thus, *Bcl* I–F8IVS18 denotes a polymorphic *Bcl* I site in intron (IVS) 18 of the factor VIII gene.

TABLE 39-4. DNA Polymorphisms for Diagnosis of Hemophilia

Probe	Enzyme	Number of Alleles	Heterozygosity	Polymorphic Site	Fragment Size (kb)	Allelic Incidence	Reference
EXTRAGENIC POLYMORPHISMS							
DXS15	*Bgl* II	2	50%	—	—	—	178
DXS52	*Taq* I	10	90%	—	—	—	179
	Msp I	3					
INTRAGENIC POLYMORPHISMS							
Factor VIII (p114.12)	*Bcl* I	—	—	Intron 18	1.2	29%	184
					0.8	71%	
Factor VIII (p114.12)	*Hind* III	—	—	Intron 19	2.7	82%	189, 190
					2.6	18%	
Factor VIII (p482.6)	*Xba* I	—	—	Intron 22	6.2	41%	187
					4.8	59%	
Factor VIII (C)	*Bgl* I	—	—	Intron 25	20	10%	126
					5	90%	
Factor VIII (p625.3)	*Msp* I	—	—	3′ flank	7.5	68%	188
					4.3	32%	
(CA)n	—	—	91%	Intron 13	—	—	198a

F8IVS18 and *Taq* I–DXS52 was informative in 91% of carriers whereas *Bcl* I–F8IVS18, *Taq* I–DXS52, and *Bgl* II–DXS15 were informative in 96% of carriers.

Genetic probes have also been used to estimate the rate of spontaneous mutations in hemophilia. In two recent studies, families with isolated or sporadic cases of hemophilia were studied by RFLP analysis.[124,200] The origin of the mutation was inferred from the RFLP pattern and coagulation studies. In 13 of 20 families, the mutation was derived from the normal maternal grandfather. Although both studies were small, the combined results indicate a higher mutation rate in males than in females and confirm previous studies based on segregation analysis and coagulation studies.[201]

A newer method that has proved to be useful in genetic diagnosis is the technique of gene amplification with the polymerase chain reaction method described by Saiki and coworkers.[202] This technique uses repeated cycles of DNA denaturation, primer reannealing, and DNA synthesis to amplify specific DNA sequences as much as several hundred thousand times. The advantages of this method are that it is rapid and it provides an alternate method to Southern blot, which is expensive. Instead of radioactive detection, amplified sequences can be restricted and visualized by ultraviolet fluorescence after staining with ethidium bromide. Kogan and colleagues[203] used this technique to successfully perform carrier detection and prenatal diagnosis in two families with hemophilia A.

Given the prevalence of the partial inversion, a rational approach to genetic counseling in families with severe hemophilia is to first screen for the inversion with simple Southern blotting procedures using F8IVS22 probes after digestion with *Bcl* I. If this is unrevealing and the molecular defect in the family is unknown, the next step is to analyze for polymorphic markers, perhaps starting with the hypervariable (CA)n repeat.

Prenatal Testing in Hemophilia A

Prenatal testing also has been based on factor VIII detection, but uses immunologic assays for VIII:Ag because of the small sample obtained. When a known or potential carrier female presents for prenatal evaluation, first discuss frankly and openly the goals of testing and her feelings and the family's feelings about termination of pregnancy. Why does she want prenatal testing? Does she understand the genetics of hemophilia? How strong are her feelings for or against abortion? The risks and accuracies of the procedures must be explained.

After these issues have been satisfactorily addressed, the first step in prenatal diagnosis is amniocentesis. This can be done between weeks 13 and 16 of pregnancy. Amniocentesis has a 0.5% morbidity rate, and it reveals the sex of the fetus. In addition, amniocentesis can provide DNA for analysis using the various techniques just described. DNA can be obtained earlier in the pregnancy (between 9 and 12 gestational weeks) by chorionic villus sampling. The risk of this procedure is also about 0.5%. If amniocentesis indicates that the fetus is a male and DNA studies fail to establish a diagnosis, the next step is fetal blood sampling, either by ultrasound guided-needle aspiration or by fetoscopy. In this procedure, umbilical vein blood is sampled and VIII:Ag determined. Obviously, measurement of VIII:Ag is diagnostic only in a CRM-negative family and cannot be used in CRM-positive families.

Often, sufficient fetal blood can be obtained by ultrasound guided-needle aspiration to permit measurement of factor VIII activity. This provides a useful alternative for CRM-positive families or families in whom no affected member is available. Fetal blood sampling is done between weeks 18 and 20 and has a 1% morbidity rate.

Graham and coworkers[184] and Lillicrap and coworkers[204] have reviewed the advantages of phenotypic and genotypic assays in carrier detection and prenatal diagnosis. Their conclusion is that genetic assays undoubtedly improve the accuracy of both carrier detection and prenatal diagnosis, but there are still many instances in which, because of the paucity of polymorphisms, DNA methods cannot be applied. Combining phenotypic and genotypic assays increases the certainty of diagnosis. The advantage of genotypic studies is that they are independent of lyonization and, when the marker is intragenic, the results are nonprobabilistic.

CLINICAL MANIFESTATIONS OF FACTOR VIII DEFICIENCY

The primary clinical manifestations of hemophilia patients result from bleeding and the complications of replacement therapy with plasma-derived blood products. The incidence

TABLE 39-5. Clinical Classification of Hemophilia A

Symptoms	Factor VIII
Severe	<1%
Moderate	1%–7%
Mild	>7%

and severity of bleeding are related to plasma levels of functional factor VIII (Table 39-5). Patients with less than 1% activity have a severe hemorrhagic tendency characterized by recurrent joint and soft tissue bleeding that may occur as often as two to four times per month. Hemorrhage after trauma may be life-threatening, and surgical bleeding, if not treated, is severe and may be complicated by delayed hemorrhage 7 to 14 days postoperatively. Patients with factor VIII levels of 2% to 7% have moderately severe hemophilia. Spontaneous hemorrhage may occur, especially in previously damaged joints, but it is much less common than in severe hemophilia. In contrast, bleeding after trauma or surgery is often severe and may be indistinguishable from that seen in patients with severe hemophilia. Patients with factor VIII levels higher than 7% have mild hemophilia. Spontaneous bleeding is rare. Surgery and other procedures may be performed with little or no bleeding on some occasions, but may be associated with excessive bleeding on other occasions. Many patients with mild hemophilia are completely asymptomatic and are diagnosed only incidentally.

Hemarthroses, which are joint hemorrhages, are the most characteristic and among the most disabling of the hemorrhages that occur in hemophilia.[205–207] They account for 75% to 85% of bleeding episodes in patients with severe disease. Two types of joint involvement are encountered: the acute manifestation of hemorrhage into the joint and the chronic changes in the joint that occur as a result of recurrent hemarthroses.

In acute hemarthroses, the initial observation as described by most patients is a "bubbling" or "tingling" sensation in the joint, which may last several hours. As bleeding into the joint continues, distention of the joint capsule and pain develop. If bleeding in the joint is allowed to persist, the joint may become swollen and visibly distended. Range of motion in the affected joint may become severely limited. Treatment with factor VIII generally stops the bleeding and relieves the symptoms. The earlier that treatment is started, the more rapidly the symptoms resolve. The proclivity for joint bleeding is characteristic of hemophilia and is not a feature of any blood-clotting factor deficiency other than factor IX and, possibly, factor VII deficiency. The reason for this peculiar distribution is unknown and is one of the great mysteries in the field.

With recurrent bleeding in the joint, damage to the synovial tissue occurs and progressive joint destruction produces the characteristic hemophilic arthropathy, which is the major disabling lesion in hemophilia. Initially, chronic synovitis with synovial hypertrophy develops. The joint becomes chronically swollen and boggy. A mild joint effusion may be present which, if tapped, is hemorrhagic. Arnold and Hilgartner[208] termed this stage "subacute hemarthropathy." Because of the vascularity of the hypertrophic synovium, such joints often bleed more frequently and become target joints. Later, more chronic changes occur. Loss of the synovium, erosion of cartilage, destruction of the joint space, and articulation of bone on bone occur. Severe limitation of motion results, which further stresses the joint and causes muscular atrophy. Deformities may further affect joint function. A vicious cycle ensues in which the damaged joint is more prone to bleeding, which further damages the joint. Chronic pain becomes more prominent. The changes that occur in the hemophilic joint can be visualized and graded radiologically (Fig. 39-11),[208–210] although the correlation between radiologic grade and joint function is only approximate. More modern imaging techniques such as nuclear magnetic resonance are being evaluated for correlation with joint function and surgical outcome.[211]

The pathophysiology of these destructive changes is uncertain but may involve mechanisms similar to those involved in the joint destruction seen in rheumatoid arthritis.[208,212–214] Blood breakdown products, including iron from erythrocytes and various proteases, growth factors, cytokines, and other inflammatory mediators from leukocytes and platelets, are released into the joint space. With repeated episodes of bleeding, the synovium becomes inflamed and thickened. Histologically, villous hypertrophy and a marked increase in vascularity are found. Iron particles are found in the synoviocytes along the villous processes, and foci of chronic inflammation are present throughout the synovium. Later in the course of joint damage, the synovium becomes replaced by fibrous tissue and disintegrates. This scarring is associated with a loss of joint motion.

In addition, after the protective synovium is lost, the articular cartilage becomes the target of attack. The chondrocyte is especially susceptible to damage by iron. Cartilaginous erosion occurs. Initially, the joint space is preserved, but as uneven wearing of the articular surface occurs, the joint space becomes narrowed and deformities begin to develop. Osteoporosis and bone cysts are prominent features later in the course of hemophilic arthropathy. In the advanced hemophilic joint, the joint space collapses and the joint range of motion becomes severely limited. At this stage, bleeding usually becomes infrequent because of limited joint motion and loss of vascular tissue in the joint.

In older hemophiliacs, arthritis is often a major complaint. Treatment with nonsteroidal antiinflammatory agents is beneficial in some patients, but impairment of platelet function may increase the incidence and severity of joint bleeding and other bleeding in the hemophiliac.[215,216] Peptic ulceration and gastritis with gastrointestinal bleeding secondary to nonsteroidal antiinflammatory agents may be especially dangerous in the hemophiliac. In patients in whom antiinflammatory agents either do not relieve pain or cannot be used because of complications, stronger, potentially addicting pain medications are frequently used. A major dilemma in hemophilia care is treading the fine line between pain relief and narcotic addiction. Psychological consultation, biofeedback, and transcutaneous nerve stimulators are part of the armamentarium of the physician caring for hemophiliacs with chronic pain.

Muscle hematomas occur less frequently than joint bleeds in patients with hemophilia, but the consequences may be more acute. Expansion of a hematoma in a muscle compartment may lead to vascular or neurologic compromise with acute and permanent loss of function. Retroperitoneal bleeding into the iliopsoas or iliacus muscles are especially prone to neurologic complications because the femoral nerve and iliopsoas traverse the ischial ramus together.[217–219] Extension of an iliopsoas or iliacus bleed inferiorly may result in compression of the femoral nerve. Clinically, patients with retroperitoneal hematomas present with lower abdominal and back pain that may mimic renal colic. The leg is typically held in flexion at the hip, and extension of the leg or rotation of the hip accentuates the pain. Dysesthesias in the distribution of the lateral cutaneous femoral nerve may be the first clue to incipient fem-

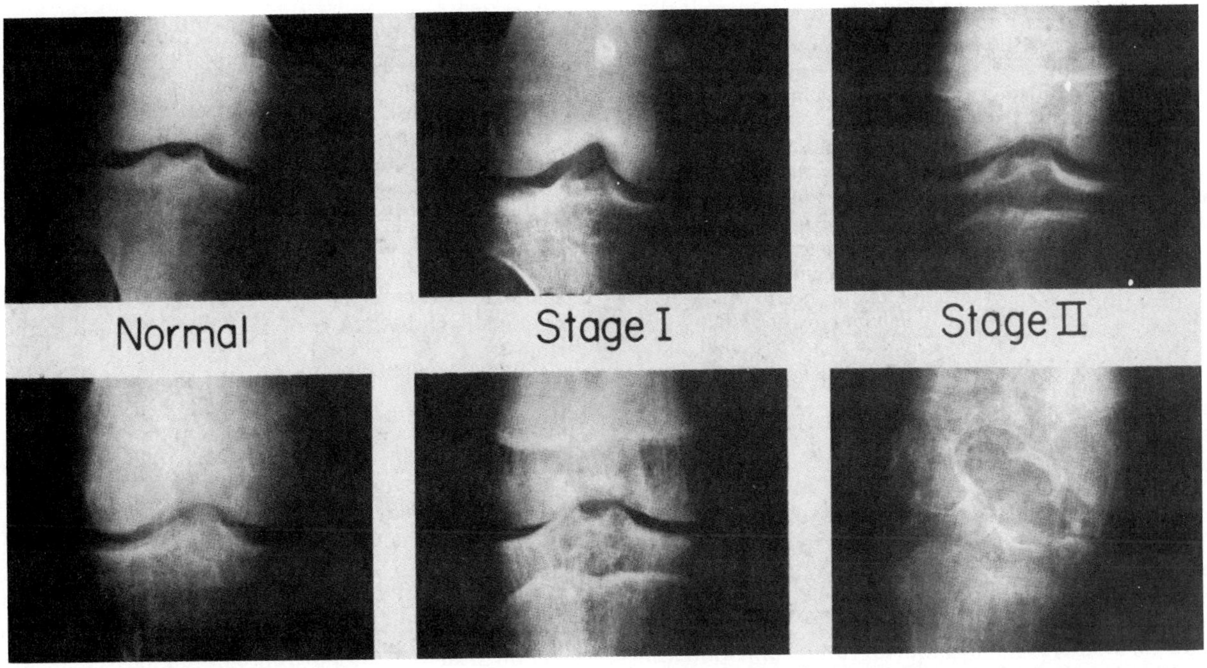

FIGURE 39-11. Radiologic knee joint changes in hemophilia A, illustrating the various changes of hemophilic arthropathy. *Stage I:* no skeletal abnormalities; soft tissue swelling due to bleeding in and around the joint. *Stage II:* osteoporosis and epiphyseal overgrowth; joint space intact; no bone cysts. *Stage III:* subchondral cysts, minor irregularities of the joint surface; joint space preserved. *Stage IV:* cysts and joint surface irregularities more prominent; joint space is narrowed as a result of cartilage damage. *Stage V:* loss of joint space; marked epiphyseal overgrowth. (White GC II. Disorders of blood coagulation. In: Stein JH. Internal medicine. Boston, Little, Brown, 1987:1012; courtesy of Bonner Guilford)

oral nerve damage. Hematuria is not present. Computed tomography (CT) of the abdomen usually reveals a characteristic mass lesion in the retroperitoneal tissues.

Hemophilic cysts or *pseudotumors* are tense, blood-filled cysts that can mimic osteogenic sarcomas radiologically.[220,221] Pseudotumors are found most frequently in the pelvis and thigh but have been reported in the calves, feet, arms, and hands. They usually occur in patients with severe hemophilia, but may also be seen in those with mild hemophilia. Aspiration of the cyst, which is fraught with danger, yields dark brown fluid. The wall of the pseudotumor is thick fibrous tissue. The origin of the pseudotumor is probably a hematoma with incomplete resolution. The encapsulated collection of blood breaks down and begins to expand from recurrent bleeds and increased oncotic pressure. As the encapsulated blood expands, it produces pressure on surrounding tissues and leads to pressure necrosis. The patient presents with a painless mass, 10 to 20 years after the initial bleeding episode. Destruction of bone may be evident radiologically.

Prior to AIDS, intracranial bleeds accounted for nearly 25% of the deaths in patients with hemophilia.[219,222,223] These include intracerebral, subarachnoid, subdural, and intraspinal bleeds. The symptoms are similar to intracranial bleeds in patients without hemophilia and include headache, nausea, seizures, nuchal rigidity, and progressive neurologic impairment. Although many patients have a history of significant trauma, almost half have no antecedent trauma.[223] A major goal of home treatment in hemophiliacs is early treatment after head trauma or after onset of a severe headache associated with a spontaneous intracranial bleed.

Hematuria occurs frequently in patients with hemophilia. Up to 83% of patients with severe hemophilia can expect to experience at least one episode of hematuria in their lifetime.[224] Most episodes are spontaneous, last 2 to 3 days, and resolve without treatment. Anemia due to hematuria in the hemophiliac is unusual. A careful history to exclude other causes of hematuria such as recent streptococcal infections, nephrolithiasis, urinary tract infection, and trauma must be obtained. Despite the bleeding tendency, extravasated blood in the urinary tract can clot and lead to obstructive symptoms. If hematuria persists, evaluation should include intravenous pyelography. This often shows abnormalities of the collecting system with filling defects due to clots. These may persist long after the hematuria has resolved.

Hemorrhage in other sites may also occur in hemophilia. Epistaxis may be prominent in children. Gastrointestinal bleeding is typically secondary to an intestinal lesion and should stimulate a complete gastrointestinal evaluation. Intramural hematomas in the intestine may occur in hemophiliacs and cause pain that can mimic acute appendicitis, acute cholecystitis, or other acute abdominal syndromes.

Inhibitors

Inhibitors are alloantibodies that specifically inhibit the procoagulant activity of factor VIII. Inhibitors occur in about 15% of persons with severe hemophilia. The first clue that a patient with hemophilia has developed an inhibitor is a failure to respond to replacement therapy with factor VIII. The diagnosis is confirmed by clotting assay. The inhibitor may be evident on a routine mixing assay, where equal parts of patient and normal plasma are mixed and then clotted. In the absence of an inhibitor, the level of factor VIII in the plasma mix is about 50%, which gives a normal PTT. In the presence of an inhibitor, the antibody is able to neutralize factor VIII in the normal plasma so that the level of factor VIII in the plasma mix is very low, 1% or 2%, and the PTT is prolonged. A prolonged PTT mix is seen in some patients with hemophilia A and an inhibitor, but in contrast to other inhibitors, the factor VIII inhibitor may be manifest only by incubation at 37°C for 2 hours. This curious property of factor VIII inhibitors forms the basis of the Bethesda assay, which is a standardized incubated PTT mix.[225] One Bethesda unit is defined as the amount of inhibitor that inactivates half of the factor VIII in 1 mL of normal plasma in 2 hours at 37°C.

Exposure to factor VIII is important for inhibitor development. A hemophiliac who does not receive transfusions rarely develops an inhibitor, and a hemophiliac treated on more than 250 occasions rarely develops an inhibitor.[226,227] The typical inhibitor is an IgG antibody, predominantly IgG4 or mixtures of IgG1 and IgG4.[228,229] Light-chain typing has revealed a single light-chain type, either κ or λ, in many cases. Thus, inhibitors to factor VIII appear to be restricted polyclonal antibodies.

Fulcher and coworkers[230] and Scandella and coworkers[230a,231] have analyzed the epitopes on factor VIII against which the inhibitor antibodies are directed. They found antibodies that reacted with the 69-kd light chain (carboxyl terminal or C-domain–derived part) of activated factor VIII, with the 90-kd heavy chain (amino terminal or A-domain–derived part), and with both chains. One hemophiliac with no clinical inhibitor was found to have an antibody directed against the factor VIII B domain. The reactivity with the 90-kd heavy chain was further localized to the 40-kd A2 domain part of the heavy chain; the reactivity with the light chain was further localized to the C2 domain (Fig. 39-12).

Preliminary studies in patients with hemophilia B have suggested that inhibitors occur in patients with gene deletions. As previously discussed in the section on molecular genetics of factor V and VIII deficiency, studies to date in hemophilia A do not support this association. Of a total of 20 hemophilia A subjects with gene deletions, only 8 have inhibitors (see Fig. 39-7*B*). Conversely, of 83 subjects with inhibitors, only 20 have detectable deletions. Why, then, do only 15% of hemophiliacs develop inhibitors? The location of the deletion may be important. A deletion involving some antigenic hot spot may be more likely to predispose to inhibitor formation. Correlation with CRM status may also be important. Further studies are needed to correlate the location of the deletion with the tendency to inhibitor formation.

In addition, other genetic host factors may be important in development of inhibitors. Several studies have reported an increased incidence of inhibitors in brother-pairs.[226,232] The first suggestion of a possible link between the immune response in hemophilia and HLA determinants was a report from Frommel and Allain.[233] Their study on a small number of brother-pairs indicated that HLA haplotypes tended to

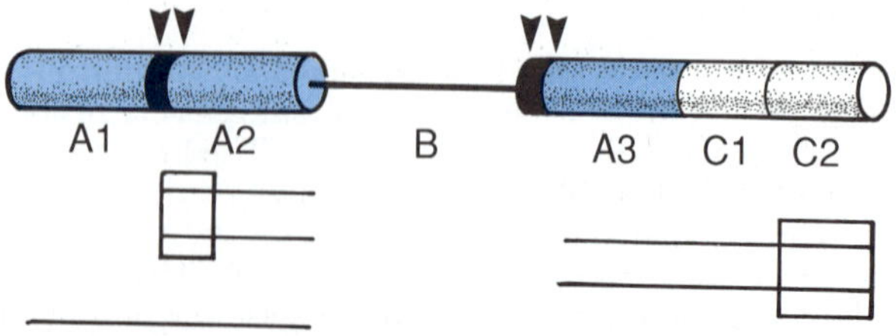

FIGURE 39-12. Factor VIII epitopes recognized by human alloantibodies. Horizontal lines show domains recognized by human factor VIII inhibitor antibodies. Boxes indicate antibodies that were studied further by synthesis of peptides and localized to the boxed regions. Arrowheads indicate thrombin cleavage sites.

be identical in brother-pairs with inhibitors and not identical in brother-pairs without inhibitors. This was followed by a large multicenter cooperative inhibitor study comparing the incidence of HLA-A and HLA-B alleles in hemophiliacs with and without inhibitors.[232] The results suggested a reduced incidence of HLA-A1 and HLA-B8 in inhibitor patients compared with that in noninhibitor patients, but the sample size was small and the HLA-DR locus, which has been shown to directly influence the antibody response to a variety of substances, was not analyzed.

The Gm series of γ-chain allotypes has also been associated with susceptibility to a variety of autoimmune disorders. In a series of 73 patients, including 37 inhibitor patients, Reisner and colleagues[234] showed a significant excess of Gm(a) in inhibitor patients compared with that in noninhibitor patients.

From a clinical perspective, two types of inhibitors are found.[235] *High-response inhibitors* are antibodies that exhibit an anamnestic response to administration of factor VIII. This response can be dramatic with increases from 1 or 2 Bethesda units up to more than 9000 Bethesda units. Several patterns of response may be seen. In the typical high-response person, the antibody rises to a level of 200 to 300 Bethesda units, beginning 4 to 7 days after administration of factor VIII. The inhibitor titer peaks, then begins to fall. If no further factor VIII is administered, the level may return to its original level after 3 to 5 months, only to increase after subsequent factor VIII infusion. In other hemophiliacs, the inhibitor may remain at high levels even in the absence of treatment. *Low-response inhibitors* are antibodies that do not exhibit anamnesis after factor VIII administration. Inhibitor levels remain below 10 Bethesda units despite repeated exposure to factor VIII. Patients with low-response inhibitors can be treated with factor VIII. Some low-response inhibitors in time convert to high-response inhibitors, and some go away.

Psychosocial Issues

Suicide is one of the leading causes of mortality in hemophilia. This is related partly to the high financial cost of hemophilia, to a poor self-image as a result of crippling hemarthropathy, to lifelong chronic pain and abuse of narcotic pain medications, and to family psychodynamics during childhood and adolescence.[236] The cost of care for a hemophilia patient can be staggering. The average hemophiliac uses about 50,000 U of factor VIII per year. At an average cost of $0.65/U, this can amount to $30,000 to $40,000 per year for replacement therapy alone. If hospitalization is required, the cost may soar to $40,000 to $50,000 per year. For patients with inhibitors, replacement therapy is even more expensive. Insurance caps are often reached and exceeded. Because of chronic joint disease, the hemophiliac is often unable to work and becomes dependent on social programs. Hemophilia assistance programs are active in some states but unavailable in others, and they fail to reflect the recent increases in the cost of replacement therapy in others. Comprehensive hemophilia clinics have been developed to deal partly with these complex issues.

CLINICAL MANIFESTATIONS OF FACTOR V DEFICIENCY

The clinical manifestations of factor V deficiency are variable but generally milder than those of factor VIII deficiency. The severity of symptoms depends in part on the plasma and platelet levels of factor V. Hemarthroses may occur in patients with severe factor V deficiency but are uncommon, and the chronic sequelae of hemarthroses that are typical of severe hemophilia are not seen in patients wtih factor V deficiency. The following are major clinical manifestations:

Ecchymoses: Patients with severe factor V deficiency bruise easily. Spontaneous and trauma-associated ecchymoses are common.

Epistaxis: Epistaxis is common in patients with factor V deficiency, but its rate of occurrence may decrease with age.

Menorrhagia: One of the most common symptoms in women with factor V deficiency, menorrhagia may be severe and cause anemia and iron deficiency. Usually, this can be controlled by administration of a progesterone preparation like Provera.

Inhibitors: Inhibitors to factor V may arise in patients with factor V deficiency. Like inhibitors to factor VIII, these are alloantibodies that specifically inhibit factor V clotting activity. The antibody is typically an IgG antibody. Antibodies to factor V neutralize factor V activity in a time- and temperature-dependent manner; therefore, diagnosis of a factor V inhibitor requires demonstration of an abnormal incubated PTT mix (see previous section on inhibitors).

TREATMENT FOR FACTOR VIII DEFICIENCY

Treatment for hemophilia consists of replacement of the deficient clotting factor with preparations of factor VIII. This is usually accomplished with commercial lyophilized concentrates of factor VIII or, in selected patients, blood-bank–prepared cryoprecipitate.[237] Both factor VIII concentrates and cryoprecipitate are prepared from donors screened for human immunodeficiency virus (HIV). In addition, all factor VIII concentrates are processed to reduce viral contaminants in the final product. Some concentrates are extracted with various solvents and detergents to lyse lipid-coated viruses. Others are pasteurized to destroy virus. Affinity chromatography with monoclonal antibodies to either factor VIII or vWF has been used to purify factor VIII and has also been shown to reduce viral contamination in factor VIII concentrates. Some of the products available are listed in Table 39-6. Because factor VIII concentrates are obtained from screened donors and have other viral reduction steps, their use is recommended over cryoprecipitate.

The normal level of factor VIII in plasma is one unit per milliliter (where a unit is defined as the amount of factor VIII present in 1 mL of normal plasma). Replacement with factor VIII is based on the following formula:

$$VIII_i = (VIII_f - VIII_s) \times P_V$$

where:

VIII_i = amount of factor VIII to be infused in units
VIII_f = desired peak VIII level in units per milliliter
VIII_s = initial VIII level in units per milliliter
P_V = plasma volume in milliliters

Plasma volume is estimated as 5% of the body weight in kilograms. Thus, a 60-kg person has a plasma volume of 60×0.05, or 3 L. To raise the factor VIII level in a 60-kg person with less than 1% (less than 0.01 U/mL) factor VIII to 30% (0.3 U/mL) would require infusion of $0.3 - 0.01 \times 3000$ or 900 U of factor VIII. Most manufacturers provide lyophilized factor VIII concentrates in vials containing about 250, 500, and 1000 U, which can be reconstituted in as little as 30 to 50 mL of diluent. To raise this theoretical 60-kg subject to 30%, a 1000-U vial could be reconstituted in 30 to 50 mL and infused as a bolus.

Most joint and simple muscle bleeds can be treated with a single bolus of factor VIII estimated to raise the factor VIII level to 30% (Table 39-7). Since the biologic half-life of factor VIII is 8 to 12 hours,[238] treatment with a single dose to 30% provides hemostatic levels of greater than 5% for more than 24 hours. Sometimes, a severe joint or muscle bleed may require a second treatment. In general, the faster a bleed is treated, the less factor is required to stabilize it. For this reason, early treatment is encouraged. Occasionally, bleeds recur in a single joint requiring treatment 2 to 4 times per month. Such a joint is called a *target joint.* Initial treatment of a target joint should be aimed at preventing bleeding by prophylactic use of factor VIII. A typical prophylactic regimen for target joints is treatment to 30% three times a week for 3 weeks, followed by treatment twice a week for 3 weeks. If this does not stop bleeding in the joint or if breakthrough bleeding occurs on prophylaxis, surgical intervention should be considered. In HIV-seropositive hemophiliacs, persistent joint pain may also be caused by septic arthritis.

For retroperitoneal, gastrointestinal, intracranial, neck, and muscle bleeding with incipient nerve compression, more prolonged treatment with factor VIII is needed (see Table 39-5). This can be done in one of two ways. One way is to infuse factor VIII at 12-hr intervals. For example, a

TABLE 39-6. Therapeutic Concentrates in Hemophilia A*

Concentrate	Volume to 100%	Ease of Use	Risk of Hepatitis	Risk of AIDS	Risk of Hemolysis
Plasma	3000	–	+	+	±
Cryoprecipitate	750	+	+	+	±
Concentrate					
Heated	50	4+	4+	±	4+
Solvent/detergent	50	4+	–	–	4+
Monoclonal	50	4+	–	–	–
Recombinant	50	4+	–	–	–

± to 4+, degree of increasing risk or ease of use with each product; –, no risk.

* Plasma and cryoprecipitate are usually obtained from the American Red Cross or blood banks, whereas factor VIII concentrates are obtained commercially or from the American Red Cross. Heated concentrate refers to product prepared from donors screened for HIV-1 antibodies and heated at 56–68° C during the manufacturing process to inactivate heat-sensitive viruses such as HIV-1. Solvent/detergent–extracted factor VIII concentrates are treated to remove coated viruses, including HIV-1 and hepatitis viruses. Monoclonal factor VIII concentrates are ultrapure products prepared using affinity chromatography and viral inactivation steps. Recombinant factor VIII is a synthetic product prepared in Chinese hamster ovary cells or baby hamster kidney cells.

TABLE 39-7. Treatment of Bleeding Episodes in Hemophilia A

Site	Level	Treatment Length
Joint	30%	1 dose
Muscle	30%	1 dose
Hematuria	30%	1 dose
Retroperitoneal	50%	5–7 d
Gastrointestinal	50%	5–7 d
Neck	100%	7–10 d
Intracranial	100%	10–14 d

60-kg person with retroperitoneal hemorrhage requires an initial infusion of 1500 U to raise the factor VIII level to 50%. Twelve hours later, when the level has fallen to 25%, a bolus of 750 U would raise the level to 50%. The disadvantage of this method is that although a level of 50% is achieved, at times the plasma factor VIII can drop to an unacceptably low level. It is also inconvenient to have to time a blood sample to check a factor VIII level. Another method to maintain treatment levels is to give a continuous infusion of factor VIII. In the same patient with retroperitoneal hemorrhage, an initial infusion of 1500 U is given and is immediately followed by 750 U that is infused over the next 12 hours. Blood for factor VIII levels can be drawn at any time, and no peaks and troughs should occur.

DDAVP

Following observations that epinephrine and stress increase levels of factor VIII in normal persons, studies were undertaken to evaluate the effect of a vasopressin analogue on factor VIII in patients with hemophilia.[42,43] The analogue, 1-deamino-8-D-arginine vasopressin (DDAVP, desmopressin acetate) has the same effect on factor VIII as vasopressin with less than 1% of the pressor effect of the parent compound.

DDAVP can be administered intravenously or subcutaneously with essentially equivalent results.[239] The response in hemophiliacs with factor VIII levels above 2% is a reproducible two- or three-fold increase in factor VIII activity. For hemophiliacs with a basal factor VIII level of 2% to 5%, this rise is generally not sufficient to permit invasive procedures, and factor VIII concentrates may be needed. For hemophiliacs with basal levels above 5% to 7%, the increase in response to DDAVP is sufficient for dental work and other minor procedures. The dose is 0.3 μg/kg administered intravenously in a volume of 100 mL over 30 minutes. For subcutaneous administration of DDAVP, the intravenous preparation is used at the same dose with subcutaneous injection of no more than 1.5 mL per site. (A single treatment may require three to four subcutaneous injections.) Intranasal preparations of DDAVP suitable for treating patients with hemophilia are available in Europe.

The response to DDAVP given on successive days diminishes (Fig. 39-13), presumably because of exhaustion of endothelial stores of vWf or factor VIII. For this reason, operative patients receiving DDAVP should be watched closely for signs of bleeding on the second to fourth postoperative days. The response returns to normal after several days. Water intoxication with hyponatremia is a rare complication of DDAVP use.

Home Therapy

Many patients with hemophilia treat themselves at home. Lyophilized concentrates can be stored at room temperature and transported on trips; they are easy to reconstitute.

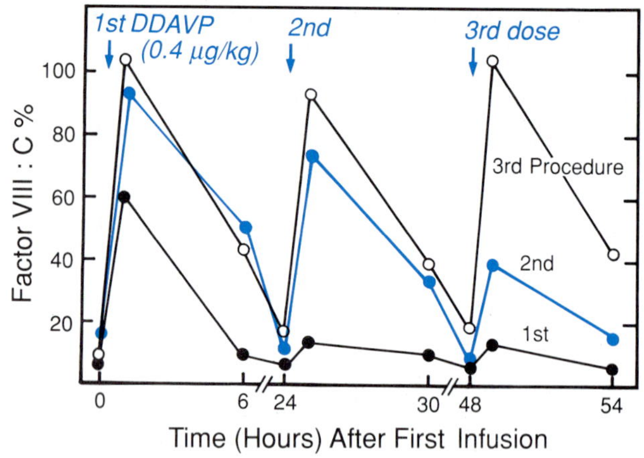

FIGURE 39-13. Response to repeated infusions of DDAVP. Repeated infusions of DDAVP were administered to a mild hemophiliac undergoing dental procedures several weeks apart. The doses used for procedure 4 were 0.3, 0.3, 0.2, 0.2, and 0.2 μg/kg. (Mannucci PM, Ruggeri ZM, Pareti FI, Capitanio A. 1-Deamino-8-D-arginine vasopressin: a new pharmacological approach to the management of hemophilia and von Willebrand's disease. Lancet 1977;1:869)

Home treatment may be life-saving in intracranial bleeding. Studies indicate that progression of joint deterioration may be retarded in patients on home treatment.[240–242]

Orthopedic Management

The indications for surgical treatment of joint disease in hemophilia are intractable bleeding that responds poorly to medical therapy and advanced joint destruction with disabling joint dysfunction. The decision to undertake surgery is a complicated one that must include a careful consideration of these indications but must also take into account the HIV status of the patient, his life expectancy, and his quality of life without surgery.

Initially, intractable bleeding should be treated medically with factor VIII and immobilization. Treatment to 30% levels with factor VIII two to three times per week for up to 6 weeks often stops the bleeding, and the patient can then resume normal demand therapy. In a number of patients, this fails to stop the bleeding or bleeding recurs after therapy is stopped. In such patients, when the bleeding appears to be caused by hypertrophied, vascularized synovium, synovectomy should be considered. Some centers, including our own, use radiologic staging to predict surgical response to synovectomy. In general, joints that are radiologic grade I or II appear to respond well to synovectomy, whereas joints that are grade III, IV, or V respond poorly if at all to synovectomy. Usually, synovectomy stops the recurrent bleeding in the joint, but loss of motion may occur in the joint after synovectomy, which may be as much as 45 to 50 degrees.[243,244] Radiation synovectomy, called *synoviorthesis*, is an alternative in some patients.[245]

Joint deformity may occur as a result of chronic arthropathy and may contribute to intractable bleeding and pain through biomechanical mechanisms. Osteotomy can lead to a more normal distribution of load, thereby relieving stress on the joint and resulting in symptomatic improvement.[246]

Joint replacement has been successfully performed in patients with hemophilia. Knee and hip replacements have been most frequently performed, but elbow and shoulder replacements have been described. Since the life-span of replaced joints is finite, these operations should be reserved for patients over 40 years with advanced joint disease as evidenced by chronic pain, significantly decreased joint range of motion, and advanced radiographic grade (stage IV, V, or VI). On the other hand, if the joint disease is sufficiently advanced that the joint is fixed and muscle atrophy has occurred, the long-term outcome of the replacement may be less favorable. Thus, the timing of joint replacement is important and requires orthopedic evaluation.

Finally, arthrodesis relieves symptoms of pain and bleeding, but may produce secondary changes in other joints.[247]

Inhibitors

The treatment of bleeding episodes in patients with inhibitors is determined by the titer of the antibody at the time treatment is required, the antibody response to administration of factor VIII, and the severity of the bleed. Patients with low-response inhibitors can be treated with factor VIII for all bleeding episodes, although doses of up to 4000 U or more may be needed to achieve factor VIII levels of 30%. Some patients with inhibitor titers of 1 to 2 Bethesda units can be maintained on home treatment after the appropriate dose of factor VIII is determined.

In patients with high-response, high-titer inhibitors, it is impossible to infuse sufficient factor VIII to achieve hemostasis. For these persons, several alternate treatment modalities are available, including porcine factor VIII, activated or nonactivated prothrombin complex concentrates, plasmapheresis, recombinant factor VIIa, and immunosuppressive agents, although none work as well as factor VIII in patients without inhibitors. The treatment of choice for a life- or limb-threatening bleed in patients with high-response, high-titer inhibitors is porcine factor VIII.[248,249] Porcine and human factor VIII are functionally similar but enough difference in primary structure is present that many alloantibodies do not recognize the porcine protein. By substituting porcine factor VIII for normal plasma in the Bethesda assay, the cross-reaction of the inhibitor for the porcine molecule can be determined. Doses of 5000 to 15,000 units are administered as a bolus. If an adequate level of factor VIII is achieved, treatment is continued. Complications of porcine factor VIII are allergic and pyrogenic reactions and mild thrombocytopenia. Anamnestic responses to porcine factor VIII may occur.

For a bleed that is not threatening to life or limb, the treatment of choice is more complicated and involves either doing nothing or using activated or nonactivated prothrombin complex concentrates (PCCs) or recombinant factor VIIa. Several studies have shown that nonactivated PCCs are clinically effective in 50% of patients with joint bleeds compared with a 25% placebo effect.[250,251] The 25% placebo effect observed in the Cooperative Inhibitor Study is interesting and illustrates the psychological effects of supportive care in the hemophiliac. Activated PCCs are control-activated by the addition of calcium to maximize the factor VIII inhibitor bypassing activity. Two products are available: Autoplex (Hyland) and FEIBA (Immuno). A double-blind, controlled trial comparing FEIBA with a nonactivated PCC in the treatment of joint and muscle bleeds showed FEIBA to be 64% effective compared with 52% response to the nonactivated PCC.[251] Subjective improvement as well as objective improvement in joint range of motion was observed. The active principle in PCCs may be activated factor VII or X.[252,253] Intravenous IgG has been used in acquired factor VIII inhibitors but is usually not efficacious in hemophilic inhibitors.

Patients with high-response, low-titer inhibitors can be treated with factor VIII, but this treatment is likely to result in an anamnestic increase in inhibitor titer. For this reason, use of factor VIII in these patients is often reserved for life-threatening bleeding episodes. For other hemorrhages like joint bleeds or hematuria, treatment with prothrombin complex concentrates is sometimes effective but is less likely to produce an anamnestic increase in inhibitor titer.[254]

CASE REPORT

A 21-year-old male hemophiliac with a high-response inhibitor presented to the emergency department with headache, lethargy, and early papilledema. His last inhibitor titer 1 month before was 4 Bethesda units. The last time he was treated with factor VIII, his inhibitor level rose from 10 to 349 Bethesda units. In the emergency department, the patient was given a bolus of 5000 U of factor VIII concentrate as soon as it was prepared, and he was sent for a CT scan of the head, which revealed an intracerebral hematoma. A postinfusion factor VIII level of 59% was obtained. He was given another 3000 U of factor VIII, and a continuous infusion of 250 U/h was started. His factor VIII level after the second bolus was 88%. He was seen by a neurosurgeon, and an angiogram revealed no aneurysm. The patient remained on factor VIII with levels between 90% and 130% until 5 days later, when his morning factor VIII was 16%. A second sample was obtained, and the factor VIII level was 2%. Another bolus of 5000 U was administered, after which the factor VIII level was 4%, indicating that anamnesis had occurred. To provide an additional 5 to 7 days of hemostasis for intracranial bleeding, the patient was given activated PCC, 75 U/kg every 8 hours. Recovery was uneventful and the patient was neurologically intact at discharge.

Three months later, the patient returned with spontaneous bleeding in the left knee. His inhibitor titer was 150 Bethesda units. He responded well to PCCs in the past and was admitted and treated with PCC, 75 U/kg every 8 hours, for a total of five doses. Joint pain resolved gradually, and range of motion improved. The patient's inhibitor level at the end of treatment was 135 Bethesda units.

The approaches outlined here are intended to treat acute hemorrhagic episodes. Several methods have been proposed to eradicate inhibitors. Many of these, like steroids, plasmapheresis, and cytotoxic agents, have not been uniformly successful. In 1977, Brackmann and Gormsen[255] described a protocol using high doses of factor VIII over prolonged periods of time. In their protocol, treatment with 100 U/kg is given twice a day for as long as 1 to 3 years. In the typical patient, the inhibitor titer rises over the first month, then starts to fall despite continued administration of factor VIII and continues to fall to undetectable levels. It has been suggested that treatment with large doses of factor VIII induces a state of immune tolerance. Although the average cost of this treatment may be as high as $1,000,000, it may be cost-effective in the inhibitor patient who is admitted many times a year.[256]

TREATMENT OF FACTOR V DEFICIENCY

Although factor V deficiency is a milder disorder than hemophilia A, patients with factor V deficiency may sometimes require replacement therapy. Treatment is usually with fresh frozen plasma, since no commercial concentrates of factor V are available. Recent studies indicate that platelet concentrates may also provide hemostasis in patients with factor V deficiency and in patients with inhibitors to factor V.

Plasma contains one unit of factor V per milliliter. Thus, replacement of factor V can be calculated as described for factor VIII replacement. For example, a 60-kg person with severe factor V deficiency with an estimated plasma volume of 3000 mL requires infusion of 900 U of factor V to raise the plasma factor V level to 30%. Because fresh frozen plasma is provided in bags of about 250 mL and plasma contains 1 U of factor V per milliliter, nearly 1000 mL (four bags) of fresh frozen plasma would be needed to achieve a factor V level of 30%. Estimation of replacement with platelet concentrates is more difficult because the number of platelets harvested may vary from donor to donor and from blood bank to blood bank. A gross rule of thumb based on the specific activity of factor V and the estimated concentration of factor V in platelets is 1500 to 3000 U per unit of apheresis platelets.

Because factor V deficiency is a milder bleeding disorder than hemophilia A and because large volumes of fresh frozen plasma are required to raise factor V levels above 40%, most bleeding episodes in patients with factor V deficiency can be treated with sufficient fresh frozen plasma to raise the plasma factor V level to 30%. Menorrhagia is best controlled hormonally.

COMPLICATIONS OF THERAPY

Hepatitis and Chronic Liver Disease

Transfusion-associated hepatitis occurs in a large percentage of hemophiliacs receiving replacement therapy. The incidence of acute hepatitis as manifested by jaundice and elevated liver enzymes is between 10% and 26% in most series.[257–260] Acute fulminant hepatitis in hemophilia is rare. When followed up for several years, nearly 80% of hemophiliacs who have multiple transfusions demonstrate at least intermittent abnormalities of liver function tests, and up to 30% demonstrate persistently abnormal liver function.

To evaluate the causes of liver dysfunction in hemophilia, several centers have performed liver biopsies in patients with persistently abnormal liver enzymes, defined as elevations of at least two times the normal for more than 6 months.[261–264] Of a total of 35 biopsies performed, 17 showed chronic active hepatitis and 16 showed chronic persistent hepatitis. These studies provided the first concrete evidence that severe forms of liver disease could occur in hemophilia. The patients who underwent biopsies in these studies were generally the most abnormal in each center. To more accurately gauge the liver disease that characterized most hemophiliacs, biopsies were performed on the livers of 18 randomly chosen hemophiliacs with mild or intermittent liver dysfunction.[265] Of the 18 patients, only 1 was found to have chronic active hepatitis. The remainder had chronic persistent hepatitis or mild portal inflammation. Thus, most hemophiliacs with multiple transfusions appear to have nonprogressive forms of liver disease.

All forms of transfusion-associated hepatitis have been reported in hemophilia. About 80% of hemophiliacs requiring replacement therapy have serologic evidence of exposure to hepatitis B virus. Antibody to HBV (HBsAb) is present in 60% to 80% and 10% to 15% are chronic carriers of HBsAg. Because most hemophiliacs have been immunized by exposure to HBV, acute HBV infection is rare in this population. Hepatitis C is now the most common cause of jaundice and acute liver disease in hemophiliacs. Delta hepatitis has also been reported in hemophiliacs.

Hepatitis B vaccine should be given to patients who have never been treated before or who demonstrate negative hepatitis B serology.

Hemolysis

Antibodies to red cell blood group substances may be present in intermediate purity preparations of factor VIII[266] and can cause red cell hemolysis in intensively treated patients with blood type A, B, or AB.[266,267] Newer ultrapure concentrates are generally free of these antibodies, and hemolysis has not been reported with these products.

Acquired Immunodeficiency Syndrome

Patients with hemophilia are also at risk to develop the acquired immunodeficiency syndrome (AIDS).[268–276] The source of infection is through the use of clotting factor concentrates that were contaminated with HIV. Retrospective studies suggest that concentrates were contaminated with HIV from about 1978 until 1984 to 1985,[272,273] when HIV antibody donor screening and viral inactivation steps during concentrate manufacture were instituted.[277–279] HIV infection is more prevalent in patients receiving factor VIII concentrates than in those receiving factor IX concentrates.[275,276] In the United States, 75% to 85% of severe hemophiliacs are infected with HIV.

AIDS in hemophilia is similar to AIDS in other risk groups except that Kaposi's sarcoma is extremely rare in hemophiliacs. Progression to AIDS in HIV-infected hemophiliacs occurs more rapidly in adults than in children.[280] Predictive markers for the development of AIDS are the percentage of CD4+ lymphocytes and viral antigenemia, as manifested by the presence of anti-p24 antibodies.[280–285] *Pneumocystis carinii* pneumonia, cryptococcal meningitis, toxoplasmosis, *Mycobacterium avium-intracellulare* infection, and disseminated cytomegalovirus infection are among the infections reported in HIV-infected hemophiliacs. In addition, septic arthritis, especially in hemophiliacs with joint replacements, and bacterial sinusitis occur more frequently.[286]

Recommendations for treatment of HIV-infected patients have been established. Seropositive persons with CD4+ counts below 200/μL should be started on prophylaxis for *P carinii* pneumonia with trimethoprim-sulfa, dapsone, or aerosolized pentamidine. Patients with AIDS or AIDS-related complex should be treated with zidovudine,[288] although recent studies suggest that resistance to zidovudine may develop in some patients.[289] Influenza vaccine should be administered to all HIV-seropositive persons. Safe sex precautions and routine use of condoms have been recommended for all hemophiliacs who have been treated with blood products during the risk period for infection. Since recent gene amplification techniques have shown HIV genetic sequence in some HIV-seronegative persons,[287] the recommendation regarding safe sex should extend to both seronegative and seropositive persons.

REFERENCES

1. Kane WH, Davie EW. Blood coagulation factors V and VIII: structural and functional similarities and their relationship to hemorrhagic and thrombotic disorders. Blood 1988;71:539.
2. Mann KG, Jenny RJ, Krishnaswamy S. Cofactor proteins in the assembly and expression of blood clotting enzyme complexes. Annu Rev Biochem 1988;57:915.
3. White GC, Shoemaker CB. Factor VIII gene and hemophilia A. Blood 1989;73:1.
4. Pittman DD, Kaufman RJ. Structure–function relationships of factor VIII elucidated through recombinant DNA technology. Thromb Haemost 1989;61:161.
5. Gitschier J, Wood WI, Goralka TM, et al. Characterization of the human factor VIII gene. Nature 1984;312:326.
6. Toole JJ, Knopf JL, Wozney JM, et al. Molecular cloning of a cDNA encoding human antihaemophilic factor. Nature 1984;312:342.
7. Truett MA, Blacher R, Burke RL, et al. Characterization of the polypeptide composition of human factor VIII:C and the nucleotide sequence and expression of the human cDNA. DNA 1986;4:333.
8. Vehar GA, Keyt B, Eaton D, et al. Structure of human factor VIII. Nature 1984;312:337.
9. Hamer RJ, Koedam JA, Beeser-Visser NH, et al. Factor VIII binds to von Willebrand factor via its Mr 80,000 light chain. Eur J Biochem 1987;166:37.
10. Foster PA, Fulcher CA, Houghten RA, Zimmerman TS. An immunogenic region within residues Val_{1670}–Glu_{1684} of factor VIII light chain

induces antibodies which inhibit binding of factor VIII to von Willebrand factor. J Biol Chem 1988;263:5230.

11. Pittman DD, Wasley LC, Murray BL, et al. Analysis of structural requirements for factor VIII function using site directed mutagenesis. Thromb Haemost 1987;58:344. Abstract.
12. Rydén L, Björk I. Reinvestigation of some physicochemical and chemical properties of human ceruloplasmin (ferroxidase). Biochemistry 1976;15:3411.
13. Bloom JW. The interaction of rDNA factor VIII, factor $VIII_{des979-1562}$ and factor $VIII_{des979-1562}$–derived peptides with phospholipid. Thromb Res 1987;48:439.
14. Arai M, Scandella D, Hoyer LW. Molecular basis of factor VIII inhibiting human antibodies: antibodies that bind to the factor VIII light chain prevent the interaction of factor VIII with phospholipid. J Clin Invest 1989;83:1978.
15. Foster PA, Fulcher CA, Houghten RA, Zimmerman TS. Synthetic factor VIII peptides with amino acid sequences contained within the C2 domain of factor VIII inhibit factor VIII binding to phosphatidylserine. (Abstract) Thromb Haemost 1989;62:34.
16. Vehar GA, Davie EW. Preparation and properties of bovine factor VIII. Biochemistry 1980;19:401.
17. Fass DN, Knutson GJ, Katzmann JA. Monoclonal antibodies to porcine factor VIII coagulant and their use in the isolation of active coagulant protein. Blood 1982;59:594.
18. Fulcher CA, Zimmerman TS. Characterization of the human factor VIII procoagulant protein with a heterologous precipitating antibody. Proc Natl Acad Sci USA 1982;79:1648.
19. Hultin MB. Modulation of thrombin-mediated activation of factor VIII:C by calcium ions, phospholipid, and platelets. Blood 1985;66: 53.
20. Dahlbäck B, Hansson C, Islam MQ, et al. Assignment of gene for coagulation factor V to chromosome 1 in man and chromosome 13 in rat. Somat Cell Mol Genet 1988;14:509.
20a. Cripe LD, Moore KD, Kane WH. Structure of the gene for human coagulation factor V. Biochemistry 1992;31:3777.
21. Kane WH, Davie EW. Cloning of a cDNA coding for human factor V: a blood coagulation factor homologous to factor VIII and ceruloplasmin. Proc Natl Acad Sci USA 1986;83:6800.
22. Jenny RJ, Pittman DD, Toole JJ, et al. Complete cDNA and amino acid sequence of human factor V. Proc Natl Acad Sci USA 1987;84:4846.
23. Kane WH, Ichinose A, Hagen FS, Davie EW. Cloning of cDNAs coding for the heavy chain region and connecting region of human factor V: a blood coagulation factor with four types of internal repeats. Biochemistry 1987;26:6508.
24. Fass DN, Hewick RM, Knutson GJ, et al. Internal duplication and sequence homology in factors V and VIII. Proc Natl Acad Sci USA 1985;82:1688.
25. Mann KG, Lawler CM, Vehar GA, Church WR. Coagulation factor V contains copper ions. J Biol Chem 1984;259:12949.
26. Saraswathi S, Rawala R, Colman RW. The subunit structure of bovine factor V: influence of proteolysis during blood coagulation. J Biol Chem 1978;253:1024.
27. Esmon CT. The subunit structure of thrombin-activated factor V. J Biol Chem 1979;254:964.
28. Nesheim ME, Myrmel KH, Hibbard L, et al. Isolation and characterization of single chain bovine factor V. J Biol Chem 1979;254:508.
29. Kane WH, Majerus PW. Isolation and characterization of human coagulation factor V. J Biol Chem 1981;256:1002.
30. Gumprecht JG, Colman RW. Roles of sialic acid in the function of bovine factor V. Arch Biochem Biophys 1975;169:278.
31. Saraswathi S, Colman RW. Role of galactose in bovine factor V. J Biol Chem 1975;250:8111.
32. Mann KG, Nesheim ME, Tracy PB. Molecular weight of undegraded factor V. Biochemistry 1981;20:28.
33. Dahlbäck B. Bovine coagulation factor V visualized with electron microscopy: ultrastructure of the isolated activated forms and of the activation fragments. J Biol Chem 1986;261:9495.
34. Webster WP, Zukoski CF, Hutchin P, et al. Plasma factor VIII synthesis and control as revealed by canine organ transplantation. Am J Physiol 1971;220:1147.
35. Bontempo FA, Lewis JH, Gorenc TJ, et al. Liver transplantation in hemophilia A. Blood 1987;69:1721.
36. Gibas A, Dienstag JL, Schafer AI. Cure of hemophilia A by orthotopic liver transplantation. Gastroenterology 1988;95:192.
37. Wion KL, Kelly D, Summerfield JA, et al. Distribution of factor VIII mRNA and antigen in human liver and other tissues. Nature 1985;317: 726.
38. Zelechowska MG, van Mourik JA, Brodniewicz-Proba T. Ultrastructural localization of factor VIII procoagulant antigen in human liver hepatocytes. Nature 1985;317:729.
39. van der Kwast TH, Stel HV, Cristen E, et al. Localization of factor VIII–procoagulant antigen: an immunohistochemical survey of the human body using monoclonal antibodies. Blood 1986;67:222.
40. Kadhom N, Wolfrom C, Gautier M, et al. Factor VIII procoagulant antigen in human tissues. Thromb Haemost 1988;59:289.
41. Wood WI, Capon DJ, Simonsen CC, et al. Expression of active human factor VIII from recombinant DNA clones. Nature 1984;312:330.
42. Mannucci PM, Ruggeri ZM, Pareti FI, Capitanio A. 1-Deamino-8-D-arginine vasopressin: a new pharmacological approach to the management of hemophilia and von Willebrand's disease. Lancet 1977;1: 869.
43. de la Fuente B, Kasper CK, Rickles FR, Hoyer LW. Response of patients with mild and moderate hemophilia A and von Willebrand's disease to treatment with desmopressin. Ann Intern Med 1985;103:6.
44. Ingram GIC, Vaughan-Jones R. The rise in clotting factor VIII induced in man by adrenaline: effect of α- and β-blockers. J Physiol 1966;187: 447.
45. Holmberg L, Nilsson IM. AHF related protein in clinical practice. Scand J Haematol 1974;12:221.
46. Preston AE, Barr A. The plasma concentration of factor VIII in the normal population: the effects of age, sex and ABO blood groups. Br J Haematol 1965;10:238.
47. McCallum CJ, Peake IR, Newcombe RG, Bloom AL. Factor VIII levels and blood group antigens. Thromb Haemost 1983;50:757.
48. Graham JB, Rizza CR, Chediak J, et al. Carrier detection in hemophilia A: a cooperative international study. I. The carrier phenotype. Blood 1986;67:1554.
49. Gill JC, Endress-Brooks J, Bauer PJ, Marks WJ Jr, Montgomery RR. The effect of ABO blood group on the diagnosis of von Willebrand disease. Blood 1987;69:1691.
50. Orstavik KH, Kornstad L, Reisner HM, et al. Possible effect of secretor locus on plasma concentrations of factor VIII and von Willebrand factor. Blood 1989;73:990.
51. Eaton DL, Hass PE, Riddle L, et al. Characterization of recombinant human factor VIII. J Biol Chem 1987;262:3285.
52. Kaufman RJ, Wasley LC, Dorner AJ. Synthesis, processing, and secretion of recombinant human factor VIII expressed in mammalian cells. J Biol Chem 1988;263:6352.
53. Lollar P, Parker CG. Stoichiometry of the porcine factor VIII-von Willebrand factor association. J Biol Chem 1987;262:17572.
54. Tuddenham EGD, Lane RS, Rotblat F, et al. Responses to infusions of polyelectrolyte fractionated human factor VIII concentrate in human haemophilia A and von Willebrand's disease. Br J Haematol 1982;52:259.
55. Brinkhous KM, Sandberg H, Garris JR, et al. Purified human factor VIII procoagulant protein: comparative hemostatic response after infusions into hemophilic and von Willebrand disease dogs. Proc Natl Acad Sci USA 1985;82:8752.
56. Tracy PB, Eide LL, Bowie EJW, et al. Radioimmunoassay of factor V in human plasma and platelets. Blood 1982;60:59.
57. Tracy PB, Eide LL, Mann KG. Human prothrombinase complex assembly and function on isolated peripheral blood cell populations. J Biol Chem 1985;260:2119.
58. Cerveny TJ, Fass DN, Mann KG. Synthesis of coagulation factor V by cultured aortic endothelium. Blood 1984;63:1467.
59. Wilson DB, Salem HH, Mruk JS, et al. Biosynthesis of coagulation factor V by a human hepatocellular carcinoma cell line. J Clin Invest 1984;73:654.
60. Rothberger H, McGee MP. Generation of coagulation factor V activity by cultured rabbit alveolar macrophages. J Exp Med 1984;160:1880.
61. Gewirtz AM, Keefer M, Doshi K, et al. Biology of megakaryocyte factor V. Blood 1986;67 1639.
62. Nichols WL, Hewick RM, Knutson GJ, et al. Identification of human megakaryocyte coagulation factor V. Blood 1985;65:1396.
63. Wencel-Drake JD, Dahlbäck B, White JG, et al. Ultrastructural localization of coagulation factor V in human platelets. Blood 1986;68:244.
64. Chesney CM, Pifer DD, Colman RW. Subcellular localization and secretion of factor V from human platelets. Thromb Res 1983;29:75.
65. Viskup RW, Tracy PB, Mann KG. The isolation of human platelet factor V. Blood 1987;69:1188.
66. Rodgers GM, Cong J, Goll DE, et al. Activation of coagulation factor V by calcium-dependent protease. Biochim Biophys Acta 1987;929: 263.
67. Bradford HN, Annamalai A, Doshi K, et al. Factor V is activated and cleaved by platelet calpain: comparison with thrombin proteolysis. Blood 1988;71:388.
68. van Dieijen G, Tans G, Rosing J, Hemker HC. The role of phospholipid and factor VIIIa in the activation of bovine factor X. J Biol Chem 1987;256:3433.
69. Rapaport SI, Shiffman S, Patch MJ, Ames SB. The importance of activation of antihemophilic globulin and proaccelerin by traces of thrombin in the generation of intrinsic prothrombinase activity. Blood 1963;21:221.
70. Knutson GJ, Fass DN. Porcine factor VIII:C prepared by affinity interaction with von Willebrand factor and heterologous antibodies: sodium dodecyl sulfate polyacrylamide gel analysis. Blood 1982;59: 615.
71. Hoyer LW, Trabold NC. The effect of thrombin on human factor VIII. Cleavage of the factor VIII procoagulant protein during activation. J Lab Clin Med 1981;97:50.
72. Griffith MJ, Reisner HM, Lundblad RL, Roberts HR. Measurement of human factor IXa activity in an isolated factor X activation system. Thromb Res 1982;27:289.
73. Hultin MB, Jesty J. The activation and inactivation of human factor VIII by thrombin: effect of inhibitors of thrombin. Blood 1981;57: 476.

74. Nordfang O, Ezban M. Generation of active coagulation factor VIII from isolated subunits. J Biol Chem 1988;263:1115.
75. Fay PJ. Reconstitution of human factor VIII from isolated subunits. Arch Biochem Biophys 1988;262:525.
76. Toole JJ, Pittman DD, Orr EC, et al. A large region (95 kDa) of human factor VIII is dispensible for *in vitro* procoagulant activity. Proc Natl Acad Sci USA 1986;83:5939.
77. Eaton DL, Wood WI, Eaton D, et al. Construction and characterization of an active factor VIII variant lacking the central one-third of the molecule. Biochemistry 1986;25:8343.
78. Pavirani A, Meulien P, Harrer H, et al. Two independent domains of factor VII co-expressed using recombinant vaccinia viruses have procoagulant activity. Biochem Biophys Res Commun 1987;145:234.
79. Burke RL, Pachl C, Quiroga M, et al. The functional domains of coagulation factor VIII:C. J Biol Chem 1986;261:12574.
80. Fulcher CA, Gardiner JE, Griffin JH, Zimmerman TS. Proteolytic inactivation of human factor VIII procoagulant protein by activated protein C and its analogy with factor V. Blood 1984;63:486.
81. Fulcher CA, Roberts JR, Zimmerman TS. Thrombin proteolysis of purified factor VIII procoagulant protein: correlation of activation with generation of a specific polypeptide. Blood 1983;61:807.
82. Fay P, Anderson MT, Chavin SI, Marder VJ. The size of human factor VIII heterodimers and the effects produced by thrombin. Biochim Biochem Acta 1986;871:268.
83. Eaton D, Rodriguez H, Vehar GA. Proteolytic processing of human factor VIII: correlation of specific cleavages by thrombin, factor Xa, and activated protein C with activation and inactivation of factor VIII coagulant activity. Biochemistry 1986;25:505.
84. Pittman DD, Kaufman RJ. Proteolytic requirements for thrombin activation of anti-hemophilic factor (factor VIII). Proc Natl Acad Sci USA 1988;85:2429.
85. Ware JA, Toomey JR, Stafford DW. Localization of a factor VIII–inhibiting antibody epitope to a region between residues 338 and 362 of factor VIII heavy chain. Proc Natl Acad Sci USA 1988;85:3165.
86. Shima M, Fulcher CA, de Graf Mahoney S, et al. Localization of the binding site for a factor VIII activity neutralizing antibody to amino acid residues Asp[1663]-Ser[1669]. J Biol Chem 1988;263:10198.
87. Gitschier J, Kogan S, Levinson B, et al. Mutations of the factor VIII cleavage sites in hemophilia A. Blood 1988;72:1022.
88. Jobin F, Esnouf MP. Studies on the formation of the prothrombin-converting complex. Biochem J 1967;102:666.
89. Esmon CT, Owen WG, Jackson CM. The conversion of prothrombin to thrombin. V. The activation of prothrombin by factor Xa in the presence of phospholipid. J Biol Chem 1974;249:7798.
90. Nesheim ME, Taswell JB, Mann KG. The contribution of bovine factor V and factor Va to the activity of prothrombinase. J Biol Chem 1979:254:10952.
91. Rosing J, Tans G, Govers-Riemslag JWP, et al. The role of phospholipids and factor Va in the prothrombinase complex. J Biol Chem 1980;255:274.
92. Papahadjopoulos D, Hanahan DJ. Observations on the interaction of phospholipids and certain clotting factors in prothrombin activator formation. Biochim Biophys Acta 1964;90:436.
93. Bloom JW, Nesheim ME, Mann KG. Phospholipid binding properties of bovine factor V and factor Va. Biochemistry 1979;18:4419.
94. Pusey ML, Mayer LD, Wei GJ, et al. Kinetic and hydrodynamic analysis of blood clotting factor V–membrane binding. Biochemistry 1982;21:5262.
95. Higgins DL, Mann KG. The interaction of bovine factor V and factor V-derived peptides with phospholipid vesicles. J Biol Chem 1983;258:6503.
96. van de Waart P, Bruls H, Hemker HC, et al. Interaction of bovine blood clotting factor Va and its subunits with phospholipid vesicles. Biochemistry 1983;22:2427.
97. Tracy PB, Mann KG. Prothrombinase complex assembly on the platelet surface is mediated through the 74,000-dalton component of factor Va. Proc Natl Acad Sci USA 1983;80:2380.
98. Nesheim ME, Eid S, Mann KG. Assembly of the prothrombinase complex in the absence of prothrombin. J Biol Chem 1981;256:9874.
99. Nesheim ME, Kettner C, Shaw C, et al. Cofactor dependence of factor Xa incorporation into the prothrombinase complex. J Biol Chem 1981;256:6537.
100. Tracy PB, Nesheim ME, Mann KG. Coordinate binding of factor Va and factor Xa to the unstimulated platelet. J Biol Chem 1981;256:743.
101. Kane WH, Majerus PW. The interaction of human coagulation factor Va with platelets. J Biol Chem 1982;257:3963.
102. Lindhout T, Govers-Riemslag JWP, van de Waart P, et al. Factor Va–factor Xa interaction: effects of phospholipid vesicles of varying composition. Biochemistry 1982;21:5494.
103. Tucker MM, Foster WB, Katzmann JA, et al. A monoclonal antibody which inhibits the factor Va:factor Xa interaction. J Biol Chem 1983;258:1210.
104. Tucker MM, Nesheim ME, Mann KG. Differentiation of enzyme and substrate binding in the prothrombinase complex. Biochemistry 1983;22:4540.
105. Morrison SA. Kinetics of activation of human prothrombin: use of a fluorescein-labeled derivative to obtain kinetic constants as a function of factor V concentration and activation state. Biochemistry 1983;22:4053.
106. Guinto ER, Esmon CT. Loss of prothrombin and of factor Xa–factor Va interactions upon inactivation of factor Va by activated protein C. J Biol Chem 1984;259:13986.
107. Skogen WF, Esmon CT, Cox AC. Comparison of coagulation factor Xa and des-(1-44) factor Xa in the assembly of prothrombinase. J Biol Chem 1984;259:2306.
108. Nesheim ME, Mann KG. The kinetics and cofactor dependence of the two cleavages involved in prothrombin activation. J Biol Chem 1983;258:5836.
109. Tans G, Rosing J. Multicomponent enzyme complexes of blood coagulation. In: Zwaal RFA, Hemker HC, eds. Blood coagulation. New York, Elsevier, 1986:59.
110. Smith CM, Hanahan DJ. The activation of factor V by factor Xa or alpha-chymotrypsin and comparison with thrombin and RVV-V action: an improved factor V isolation procedure. Biochemistry 1976;15:1830.
111. Esmon CT. The use of proteolytic enzymes in establishing the structure and activation pathways of factor V. In: Mann KG, Taylor FB, eds. The regulation of coagulation. New York, Elsevier, 1980:137.
112. Suzuki K, Dahlbäck B, Stenflo J. Thrombin-catalyzed activation of human coagulation factor V. J Biol Chem 1982;257:6556.
113. Miletich JP, Majerus DW, Majerus PW. Patients with congenital factor V deficiency have decreased factor Xa binding sites on their platelets. J Clin Invest 1978;62:824.
114. Tracy PB, Giles AR, Mann KG, et al. Factor V (Quebec): a bleeding diathesis associated with a qualitative platelet factor V deficiency. J Clin Invest 1984;74:1221.
115. Nesheim ME, Nichols WL, Cole TL, et al. Isolation and study of an acquired inhibitor of human coagulation factor V. J Clin Invest 1986;77:405.
116. Walker FJ, Sexton PW, Esmon CT. The inhibition of blood coagulation by activated protein C through the selective inactivation of activated factor V. Biochim Biophys Acta 1979;571:333.
117. Suzuki K, Stenflo J, Dahlbäck B, et al. Inactivation of human factor V by activated protein C. J Biol Chem 1983;258:1914.
118. Odegaard B, Mann KG. Proteolysis of factor Va by factor Xa and activated protein C. J Biol Chem 1987;262:11233.
118a. Dahlbäck B, Hildebrand B. Inherited resistance to activated protein C is corrected by anticoagulant cofactor activity found to be a property of factor V. Proc Natl Acad Sci 1994;91:1396.
119. Department of Health, Education and Welfare: National Heart, Lung and Blood Institute Study to Evaluate the Supply–Demand Relationships for AHF and PTC through 1980. Washington, DC, US Government Printing Office, 1977.
120. Ramgren O. A clinical and medico-social study of haemophilia in Sweden. Acta Med Scand 1962;171:759.
121. Graham JB. Biochemical genetics of blood coagulation. Am J Hum Genet 1956;8:63.
122. Kerr CB. Genetics of human blood coagulation. J Med Genet 1965;2:254.
123. Biggs R, Rizza CR. The sporadic case of hemophilia A. Lancet 1979;2:431.
124. Bernardi F, Marchetti G, Bertagnolo V, et al. RFLP analysis in families with sporadic hemophilia A: estimate of the mutation ratio in male and female gametes. Hum Genet 1987;76:253.
125. Holmberg L. Genetic studies in a family with testicular feminization, haemophilia and color blindness. Clin Genet 1972;3:253.
126. Andrejev YN, Korenevskaya MI, Rutbert RA, et al. Haemophilia A in a patient with testicular feminization. Thromb Diath Haemorrh 1965;14:332.
127. Bithell TC, Pizzaro A, Macdiarmid WD. Variant of factor IX deficiency in females with 45X Turner's syndrome. Blood 1970;36:169.
128. Gilchrist GS, Hammond D, Mecnyk J. Hemophilia A in a phenotypically normal female with XX/XO mosaicism. N Engl J Med 1965;273:1402.
129. Piétu G, Thomas-Maison N, Sié P, et al. Haemophilia A in a female: study of a family using intragenic and extragenic restriction site polymorphism. Thromb Haemost 1988;60:102.
130. Kingsley CS. Familial factor V deficiency: the pattern of heredity. Q J Med 1954;23:323.
131. Hoyer LW, Breckenridge RT. Immunologic studies of antihemophilic factor (AHF, factor VIII): cross-reacting material in a genetic variant of hemophilia A. Blood 1968;32:962.
132. Denson KWE, Biggs RG, Haddon ME, et al. Two types of haemophilia (A^+ and A^-): a study of 48 cases. Br J Haematol 1969;17:163.
133. Reisner HM, Price WA, Blatt PM, et al. Factor VIII coagulant antigen in hemophilic plasma: a comparison of five alloantibodies. Blood 1980;56:615.
134. Gitschier J, Wood WI, Tuddenham EGD, et al. Detection and sequence of mutations in the factor VIII gene of haemophiliacs. Nature 1985;315:425.
135. Antonarakis SE, Waber PG, Kittur SD, et al. Hemophilia A: detection of molecular defects and of carriers by DNA analysis. N Engl J Med 1985;313:842.
136. Gitschier J, Wood WI, Shuman MA, Lawn RM. Identification of a

missense mutation in the factor VIII gene of a mild hemophiliac. Science 1986;232:1415.

137. Youssoufian H, Kazazian HH Jr, Phillips DG, et al. Recurrent mutations in haemophilia A give evidence for CpG mutation hotspots. Nature 1986;324:380.

138. Youssoufian H, Antonarakis SE, Aronis S, et al. Characterization of five partial deletions of the factor VIII gene. Proc Natl Acad Sci USA 1987;84:3772.

139. Youssoufian H, Antonarakis SE, Bell W, et al. Nonsense and missense mutations in hemophilia A: estimation of the relative mutation rate at CG dinucleotides. Am J Hum Genet 1988;42:718.

140. Higuchi M, Kochhan L, Schwab R, et al. Detection of mutations of hemophilia A. Thromb Haemost 1987;58:336.

141. Levinson B, Janco RL, Phillips III J, Gitschier J. A novel missense mutation in the factor VIII gene identified by analysis of amplified hemophilia DNA sequences. Nucleic Acids Res 1987;15:9797.

142. Antonarakis SE. Hemophilia A persistence and gene mutational vulnerability. Hosp Pract 1987;22:93.

143. Youssoufian H, Wang C, Aronis S, et al. Moderately severe hemophilia A resulting from Glu→Gly substitution in exon 7 of the factor VIII gene. Am J Hum Genet 1988;42:867.

144. Mikami S, Nishimura T, Naka H, et al. Nonsense mutation in factor VIII gene of a severe hemophiliac patient with anti-factor VIII antibody. Jpn J Hum Genet 1988;33:409.

145. Inaba H, Fujimaki M, Kazazian HH. Mild hemophilia A resulting from Arg-to-Leu substitutions in exon 26 of the factor VIII gene. Hum Genet 1989;81:335.

146. Bernardi F, Volinia S, Patracchini P, et al. A recurrent missense mutation (Arg→Glu) and a partial deletion in factor VIII gene causing severe hemophilia A. Br J Haematol 1989;71:271.

147. Din N, Schwartz M, Kruse T, et al. Factor VIII gene-specific probes used to study heritage and molecular defects in hemophilia A. Res Clin Lab 1986;16:182.

148. Casarino L, Pecorara M, Mori PG, et al. Molecular basis for hemophilia A in Italians. Res Clin Lab 1986;16:227.

149. Bardoni B, Sampietro M, Romano M, et al. Characterization of a partial deletion of the factor VIII gene in a haemophiliac with inhibitor. Hum Genet 1988;79:86.

150. Lillicrap D, Taylor SAM, Grover H, et al. Genetic analysis in hemophilia A: identification of a large F. VIII gene deletion in a patient with high titre antibodies to human and porcine F. VIII. Blood 1986;68: 337a.

151. Youssoufian H, Patel A, Phillips D, et al. Hemophilia A: recurrent mutations and an unusual deletion. Pediatr Res 1987;21:296A.

152. Mikami S, Nishimura T, Naka H, et al. A deletion involving intron 13 and exon 14 of factor VIII gene in a haemophiliac with anti-factor VIII antibody. Jpn J Hum Genet 1988;33:401.

153. Youssoufian H, Kasper CK, Phillips DG, et al. Restriction endonuclease mapping of six novel deletions of the factor VIII gene in hemophilia A. Hum Genet 1988;80:143.

153a. Lakich D, Kazazian Jr HH, Antonarakis SE, et al. Inversions disrupting the factor VIII gene are a common cause of severe haemophilia A. Nature Genet 1993;5:236.

153b. Naylor J, Brinke A, Hassock S, et al. Characteristic mRNA abnormality found in half the patients with severe haemophilia A is due to large DNA inversions. Hum Mol Genet 1993;2:1773.

153c. Tuddenham EG, Cooper DN, Gitschier J, et al. Haemophilia A: database of nucleotide substitutions, deletions, insertions and rearrangements of the factor VIII gene. Nucleic Acids Res 1991;19:4821.

154. Barker D, Schafer M, White R. Restriction sites containing CpG show a higher frequency of polymorphism in human DNA. Cell 1984;36: 131.

155. Kazazian HH Jr, Wong C, Youssoufian H, et al. Haemophilia A resulting from *de novo* insertion of *L1* sequences represents a novel mechanism for mutation in man. Nature 1988;332:164.

156. Seeler RA. Parahemophilia: factor V deficiency. Med Clin North Am 1972;56:119.

157. Feinstein DI, Rapaport SI, McGehee WG, et al. Factor V anticoagulants: clinical, biochemical and immunological observations. J Clin Invest 1970;49:1578.

158. Fratantoni JW, Hilgartner MW, Nachman RL. Nature of the defect in congenital factor V deficiency: study in a patient with acquired circulating anticoagulant. Blood 1972;39:751.

159. Giddings JC, Shearn SAM, Bloom AL. The immunological localization of factor V in human tissue. Br J Haematol 1975;29:57.

160. Chiu HC, Whitaker E, Colman RW. Heterogeneity of human factor V deficiency: evidence for the existence of an antigen-positive variance. J Clin Invest 1983;72:493.

161. Hultin MD, Eyster ME. Combined factor V-VIII deficiency: a case report with studies of factor V and VIII activation by thrombin. Blood 1981;58:983.

162. Seligsohn U, Zivelin A, Zwang E. Combined factor V and factor VIII deficiency among non-Ashkenazi Jews. N Engl J Med 1982;307:1191.

163. Girolami A, Violante M, Cella G, et al. Combined deficiency of factor V and factor VIII: a report of another case. Blut 1976;32:415.

164. Girolami A, Brunetti A, de Mario L. Congenital combined factor V and factor VIII deficiency in a male born from brother-sister incest. Blut 1974;28:33.

165. Cimo PL, Moake JL, Gonzalez MF, et al. Inherited combined deficiency of factor V and factor VIII: report of a case with normal factor VIII antigen and ristocetin-induced platelet aggregation. Am J Hematol 1977;2:385.

166. Oeri J, Matter M, Isenschmid H. Angeborener mangel an Factor V (Parahemophilie) Verbunden mit echter Haemophilia A bie zwei brüdern. Bibl Pediatr 1954;58:575.

167. Iverson T, Bastrup-Madsen P. Congenital familial deficiency of factor V (parahemophilia) combined with deficiency of anti-hemophilic globulin. Br J Haematol 1956;2:265.

168. Seibert RH, Margolius A, Ratnoff OD. Observation on hemophilia, parahemophilia and co-existent hemophilia and parahemophilia. J Lab Clin Med 1958;52:449.

169. Jones JM, Rizza CR, Hardisty RM, et al. Combined deficiency of factor V and factor VIII (antihemophilic globulin): a report of three cases. Br J Haematol 1962;8:120.

170. Parr D, Egli H, Christians JM, et al. Kongenitaler mangel von faktor V and faktor VIII. Thromb Diath Haemorrh 1967;17:194.

171. Gobbi F, Ascari E, Barbieri U. Congenital combined deficiency of factor VIII (AHF) and factor V (proaccelerin) in two siblings. Thromb Diath Haemorrh 1967;17:194.

172. DeVries JT. Hemorragische diathese dorr tekort aan faktor V (proaccelerine). Ned Tijdschr Geneeskd 1968;12:741.

173. Ménaché D, Hakin S. Un nouveau cas de deficit associé en facteur VIII et V. Pathol Biol 1968;16:969.

174. Saito H, Shioya H, Koie K, et al. Congenital combined deficiency of factor V and factor VIII: a case report and the effect transfusion of normal plasma and hemophilic blood. Thromb Diath Haemorrh 1969;22:316.

175. Seligsohn U, Ramot B. Combined factor V and factor VIII deficiency: report of four cases. Br J Haematol 1969;16:475.

176. Smit-Sibinga CTH, Gökemeyer JDM, ten Kate LP, et al. Combined deficiency of factor V and factor VIII: report of a family and genetic analysis. Br J Haematol 1972;23:467.

177. Ciavarella H, Petronelli M, Wierdis T, et al. Su di un raro caso de deficit combinato de fattore V et di fattore VIII. Haematologica 1973;58: 778.

178. Kleinmans M, Kordich L. Vizcorguénga MI. Deficiencia congenita combinade de factores V y VIII. Sangre 1975;30:505.

179. Girolami A, Gastaldi G, Patrussi G, et al. Combined congenital deficiency of factor V and factor VIII: a report of a further case with some considerations on the hereditary transmission of this disorder. Acta Haematol 1976;55:234.

180. Marlar RA, Griffin JH. Deficiency of protein C inhibitor in combined factor V/VIII deficiency disease. J Clin Invest 1980;66:1186.

181. Canfield WM, Kisiel W. Evidence of normal functional levels of activated protein C inhibitor in combined factor V/VIII deficiency disease. J Clin Invest 1982;70:1260.

182. Giddings JC, Sugrue A, Bloom AL. Quantitation of coagulant antigens and inhibitor of activated protein C inhibitor in combined factor V-VIII deficiency. Br J Haematol 1982;52:495.

183. Suzuki K, Nishioka J, Hashimoto S, et al. Normal titer of functional and immunoreactive protein C inhibitor in plasma of patients with congenital combined deficiency of factor V and factor VIII. Blood 1983;62:1266.

184. Graham JB, Green PP, McGraw RA, Davis LM. Application of molecular genetics to prenatal diagnosis and carrier detection in the hemophilias: some limitations. Blood 1985;66:759.

185. Green PP, Mannucci PM, Briet E, et al. Carrier detection in hemophilia A: a cooperative international study. II. The efficiency of linear discriminants. Blood 1986;67:1560.

186. Harper K, Winter RM, Pembrey ME, et al. A clinically useful DNA probe closely linked to haemophilia A. Lancet 1984;2:6.

187. Oberle I, Camerino G, Heilig R, et al. Genetic screening for hemophilia A (classic hemophilia) with a polymorphic DNA probe. N Engl J Med 1985;312:682.

188. Winter RM, Harper K, Goldman E, et al. First trimester prenatal diagnosis and detection of carriers of haemophilia A using the linked DNA probe DX13. Br Med J 1985;291:765.

189. Peake IR, Lillicrap DP, Liddell MB, et al. Linked and intragenic probes for haemophilia A. Lancet 1985;2:1003.

190. Lehesjoki A-E, de la Chapelle A, Rasi V. Haemophilia A: two recombinations detected with probe St14. Lancet 1986;2:280.

191. Driscoll MC, Miller CH, Goldberg JD, et al. Recombination between factor VIII:C gene and St14 locus. Lancet 1986;2:279.

192. Gitschier J, Drayna D, Tuddenham EGD, et al. Genetic mapping and diagnosis of haemophilia A achieved through a *Bcl I* polymorphism in the factor VIII gene. Nature 1985;314:738.

193. Gitschier J, Lawn RM, Rotblat F, et al. Antenatal diagnosis and carrier detection of haemophilia A using factor VIII gene probe. Lancet 1985;1: 1093.

194. Din N, Schwartz M, Kruse T, et al. Factor VIII gene specific probe for prenatal diagnosis of haemophilia A. Lancet 1985;1:1446.

195. Wion KL, Tuddenham EGD, Lawn RM. A new polymorphism the

factor VIII gene for prenatal diagnosis of hemophilia A. Nucleic Acids Res 1986;14:4535.
196. Youssoufian H, Phillips DG, Kazazian HH Jr, Antonarakis SE. *Msp I* polymorphism in the 3′ flanking region of the human factor VIII gene. Nucleic Acids Res 1987;15:6312.
197. Ahrens P, Kruse TA, Schwartz M, et al. A new *Hind III* restriction fragment length polymorphism in the hemophilia A locus. Hum Genet 1987;26:127.
198. Bernardi F, Legnani C, Volinia S, et al. A Hind III RFLP and a gene lesion in the coagulation factor VIII gene. Hum Genet 1988;78:359.
198a. Lalloz MR, McVey JH, Pattinson JK, et al. Haemophilia A diagnosis by analysis of a hypervariable dinucleotide repeat within the factor VIII gene. Lancet 1991;338:207.
199. Janco RL, Phillips III JA, Orlando PJ, et al. Detection of hemophilia A carriers using intragenic factor VIII:C DNA polymorphisms. Blood 1987;69:1539.
200. Pecorara M, Casarino L, Mori PG, et al. Hemophilia A: carrier detection and prenatal diagnosis by DNA analysis. Blood 1987;70:531.
201. Vogel F, Rathenberg R. Spontaneous mutation in men. In: Harris H, Hirschhorn K, eds. Advances in human genetics. New York, Plenum Press, 1975:223.
202. Saiki RK, Scharf S, Faloona F. Enzymatic amplification of β-globin genomic sequences and restriction site analysis for diagnosis of sickle cell anemia. Science 1985;230:1350.
203. Kogan SC, Doherty M, Gitschier J. An improved method for prenatal diagnosis of genetic deseases by analysis of amplified DNA sequences: application to hemophilia A. N Engl J Med 1987;317:985.
204. Lillicrap D, Holden JJA, Giles AR, et al. Carrier detection strategy in haemophilia: the benefits of combined DNA marker analysis and coagulation testing in sporadic haemophilic families. Br J Haematol 1988;70:321.
205. Ahlberg A. Haemophilia in Sweden. VIII. Incidence, treatment and prophylaxis of arthropathy and other musculoskeletal manipulations of haemophilia A and B. Acta Orthop Scand 1965[ppl 77:5.
206. Gilbert MS. Musculoskeletal manifestations of hemophilia. Mt Sinai J Med 1977;44:339.
207. Hilgartner MW. Hemophilic arthropathy. Adv Pediatr 1975;21:139.
208. Arnold WD, Hilgartner MW. Hemophilic arthropathy. Current concepts of pathogenesis and management. J Bone Joint Surg 1975;59A:287.
209. Schreiber RR. Musculoskeletal system: radiologic findings. In: Brinkhous KM, Hemker HC, eds. Handbook of hemophilia. Part I. New York, American Elsevier, 1975:333.
210. Pettersson H, Ahlberg A, Nilsson IM. A radiologic classification of hemophilic arthropathy. Clin Orthop 1980;149:153.
211. Kulkarni MV, Drotshagen LE, Kaye JJ, et al. Imaging of hemophilic arthropathy. J Comput Assist Tomogr 1986;10:445.
212. Mainardi C, Levine PH, Werb Z, et al. Proliferative synovitis in hemophilia: biochemical and morphological observations. Arthritis Rheum 1978;21:137.
213. Harris ED Jr, Parker HG, Radin EL, et al. Effects of proteolytic enzymes on structural and mechanical properties of cartilage. Arthritis Rheum 1972;15:497.
214. Swanton MW. Hemophilic arthropathy in dogs. Lab Invest 1959;8:1269.
215. White II GC, Blatt PM, McMillan CW, Roberts HR. Use of analgesic and anti-inflammatory drugs in the haemophilias. In: Seligsohn U, Rimon A, Horoszowski H, eds. Haemophilia. Kent, England, Castle House, 1981:231.
216. Thomas P, Hepburn B, Kim HC, Saidi P. Nonsteroidal anti-inflammatory drugs in the treatment of hemophilic arthropathy. Am J Hematol 1982;12:131.
217. Tallroth A. Hemophilia with spontaneous hemorrhage in the iliopsoas muscle followed by injury to the femoral nerve. Acta Chir Scand 1941;84:124.
218. Silverstein A. Neuropathy in hemophilia. JAMA 1964;190:162.
219. van Trotsenburg L. Neurological complications of hemophilia. In: Brinkhous KM, Hemker HC. Handbook of hemophilia. Part I. New York, American Elsevier, 1975:389.
220. Gilbert MS. Characterizing the hemophilic pseudotumor. Ann NY Acad Sci 1975;240:311
221. Brant EE, Jordan HH. Radiologic aspects of hemophilic pseudotumors in bone. Am J Roentenol Radiat Ther 1972;115:525.
222. Silverstein A. Intracranial bleeding in hemophilia. Arch Neurol 1960;3:141.
223. Eyster ME, Gill FM, Blatt PM, et al. Central nervous system bleeding in hemophiliacs. Blood 1978;51:1179.
224. Prentice CR, Lindsay RD, Barr RD, et al. Renal complications in hemophilia and Christmas disease. Q J Med 1971;40:47.
225. Kasper CK, Aledort LM, Counts RB, et al. A more uniform measurement of factor VIII inhibitors. Thromb Diath Haemorrh 1975;34:869.
226. White II GC, McMillan CW, Blatt PM, et al. Factor VIII inhibitors: an overview. Am J Hematol 1982;13:335.
227. McMillan CW, Shapiro SS, Whitehurst D, et al. The natural history of factor VIII:C inhibitors in patients with hemophilia A: a national cooperative study. II. Observations on the initial development of factor VIII:C inhibitors. Blood 1988;71:344.
228. Hultin MB, London FS, Shapiro SS, et al. Heterogeneity of factor VIII antibodies: further immunochemical and biologic studies. Blood 1977;49:807.
229. Hoyer LW, Gawryl MS, de la Fuente B. Immunochemical characterization of factor VIII inhibitors. Prog Clin Biol Res 1984;150:73.
230. Fulcher CA, de Graf Mahoney S, Roberts JR, et al. Localization of human factor FVIII inhibitor epitopes to two polypeptide fragments. Proc Natl Acad Sci USA 1985;82:7728.
230a. Scandella D, Mattingly M, de Graf Mahoney S, et al. Localization of epitopes for human factor VIII inhibitor antibodies by immunoblotting and antibody neutralization. Blood 1989;74:1618.
231. Scandella D, de Graf Mahoney S, Mattingly M, et al. Epitope mapping of human factor VIII inhibitor antibodies by deletion analysis of factor VIII fragments expressed in *Escherichia coli*. Proc Natl Acad Sci USA 1988;85:6152.
232. Shapiro SS. Genetic predisposition to inhibitor formation. In: Hoyer LW, ed. Factor VIII inhibitors. New York, Alan R Liss, 1984:45.
233. Frommel D, Allain JP. Genetic predisposition to develop factor VIII antibody in chronic hemophilia. Clin Immunol Immunopathol 1977;8:34.
234. Reisner HM, Reisner EA, Kostyu DD, et al. Possible association of HLA and Gm with the alloimmune response to FVIII. Thromb Haemost 1987;58:338. Abstract.
235. Allain JP, Frommel D. Antibodies to factor VIII. V. Patterns of immune response to factor VIII in hemophilia. Blood 1976;47:973.
236. Hurt CH. Psychological and social aspects. In: Boone DC, ed. Comprehensive management of hemophilia. Philadelphia, FA Davis, 1977:117.
237. Brettler DB, Levine PH. Factor concentrates for treatment of hemophilia: which one to choose? Blood 1989;73:2067.
238. Biggs R, Denson KWE. The fate of prothrombin and factor VIII, IX, and X transfused to patients deficient in these factors. Br J Haematol 1963;9:532.
239. de Sio L, Mariani G, Muzzucconi MG, et al. Comparison between subcutaneous and intravenous DDAVP in mild and moderate hemophilia A. Thromb Haemost 1985;54:387.
240. Levine PH. Efficacy of home therapy in hemophilia: a study of 72 patients with hemophilia A and B. N Engl J Med 1974;291:1381.
241. Brettler D, Forsberg AD, O'Connell FD, et al. A long term study of hemophilic arthropathy of the knee joint in a program of factor VIII replacement at time of each hemarthrosis. Am J Hematol 1985;18:13.
242. Guenther EE, Hilgartner MW, Miller CH, Vienne G. Hemophilic arthropathy: effect of home care on treatment patterns and joint disease. J Pediatr 1980;97:378.
243. Storti E, Ascari E. Long-term evaluation of synovectomy in the treatment of recurrent hemophilic hemarthrosis. In: Brinkhous KM, Hemker HC, eds. Handbook of hemophilia. Part II. New York, American Elsevier, 1975:727.
244. Kay L, Stainsby D, Buzzard B, et al. The role of synovectomy in the management of recurrent haemarthroses in haemophilia. Br J Haematol 1981;49:53.
245. Gamba G, Grignani G, Ascari E. Synoviorthesis versus synovectomy in the treatment of recurrent haemophilic haemarthrosis: long-term evaluation. Thromb Haemost 1981;45:127.
246. Smith MS, Urqhuart DR, Savidge GF. The surgical management of varus deformity in haemophilia arthropathy of the knee. J Bone Joint Surg 1981;63B:261.
247. Houghten GR, Duthie B. Orthopaedic problems in haemophilia. Clin Orthop 1979;138:197.
248. Mayne EE, Madden M, Crothers IS, et al. Highly purified porcine factor VIII in haemophilia A with inhibitors to factor VIII. Br Med J 1981;282:318.
249. Kernoff PBA, Thomas ND, Lilley PA et al. Clinical experience with polyelectrolyte-fractionated porcine factor VIII concentrate in the treatment of hemophiliacs with antibodies to factor VIII. Blood 1984;63:31.
250. Lusher JM, Shapiro SS, Palascak JE, et al. Efficacy of prothrombin complex concentrates in hemophiliacs with antibodies to factor VIII: a multicenter therapeutic trial. N Engl J Med 1980;303:421.
251. Samsjoedin LJM, Heijnen L, Mauser-Bunschoten EP, et al. The effect of activated prothrombin complex concentrate (FEIBA) on joint and muscle bleeding in patients with hemophilia A and antibodies to factor VIII: a double-blind clinical trial. N Engl J Med 1981;305:717.
252. White II GC, Roberts HR, Kingdon HS, et al. Prothrombin complex concentrates: potentially thrombogenic materials and clues to the mechanism of thrombosis *in vivo*. Blood 1977;49:159.
253. Hultin MB. Studies of factor IX concentrate therapy in hemophilia. Blood 1983;62:677.
254. Kasper CK and the Hemophilia Study Group. Effect of prothrombin complex concentrates on factor VIII inhibitor levels. Blood 1979;54:1358.
255. Brackmann HH, Gormsen J. Massive factor-VIII infusion in haemophiliacs with factor-VIII inhibitor, high response. Lancet 1977;2:933.
256. White II GC, Taylor RE, Blatt PM, et al. Treatment of a high titer anti-factor VIII antibody by continuous factor VIII administration: report of a case. Blood 1983;62:141.

257. Mannucci PM, Capitanio A, del Ninno E, et al. Asymptomatic liver disease in haemophiliacs. J Clin Pathol 1974;28:620.
258. Hasiba UW, Spero JA, Lewis JH. Chronic liver dysfunction in multitransfused hemophiliacs. Transfusion 1977;17:490.
259. Cederbaum AI, Blatt PM, Levine PM. Abnormal serum transaminase levels in patients with hemophilia A. Arch Intern Med 1982;142:481.
260. Rizetto M, Morello C, Mannucci PM, et al. Delta infection and liver disease in hemophilic carriers of hepatitis B surface antigen. J Infect Dis 1982;145:18.
261. Lesesne HR, Morgan JE, Blatt PM, et al. Liver biopsy in hemophilia A. Ann Intern Med 1977;86:703.
262. Spero JA, Lewis JH, van Thiel DH, et al. Asymptomatic structural liver disease in hemophilia. N Engl J Med 1978;298:1373.
263. Preston FE, Triger DR, Underwood JCE, et al. Percutaneous liver biopsy and chronic liver disease in haemophiliacs. Lancet 1978;2:592.
264. Mannucci PM, Rhonchi G, Rota L, et al. A clinicopathologic study of liver disease in hemophilia. J Clin Pathol 1978;31:779.
265. White II GC, Zeitler KD, Lesesne HR, et al. Chronic hepatitis in patients with hemophilia A: histologic studies in patients with intermittently abnormal liver function tests. Blood 1982;60:1259.
266. Seeler RA, Telischi M, Langehennig PL, et al. Comparison of anti-A and anti-B titers in factor VIII and IX concentrates. J Pediatr 1976;89:87.
267. Orringer EO, Koury MJ, Blatt PM, et al. Hemolysis caused by factor VIII concentrates. Arch Intern Med 1976;136:1018.
268. Centers for Disease Control. *Pneumocystis carinii* pneumonia among persons with hemophilia. Morb Mortal Weekly Rep 1982;31:365.
269. Barre-Sinoussi F, Chermann JC, Rey F, et al. Isolation of a T-lymphotropic retrovirus from a patient at risk for acquired immunodeficiency syndrome. Science 1983;220:868.
270. Gallo RC, Salahuddin SZ, Popovic M, et al. Frequent detection and isolation of cytopathic retroviruses (HTLV-III) from patients with AIDS and at risk for AIDS. Science 1984;224:500.
270. Evatt BL, Ramsey RB, Lawrence MD, et al. The acquired immunodeficiency syndrome in patients with hemophilia. Ann Intern Med 1984;100:499.
271. Kitchen LW, Barin F, Sullivan JL, et al. Aetiology of AIDS: antibodies to human T-cell leukaemia virus (type III) in haemophiliacs. Nature 1984;312:367.
272. Geodert JJ, Sarngadharan MG, Eyster ME, et al. Antibodies reactive with human T-cell leukemia viruses (HTLV-III) in the sera of hemophiliacs receiving factor VIII concentrate. Blood 1985;65:492.
273. Evatt BL, Gomperts ED, McDougal JS, et al. Coincidental appearance of LAV1/HTLV-III antibodies in hemophiliacs and the onset of the AIDS epidemic. N Engl J Med 1985;312:483.
274. Levine PH. The acquired immunodeficiency syndrome in persons with hemophilia. Ann Intern Med 1985;103:723.
275. Ragni MV, Tegtmeier GE, Levy JA, et al. AIDS retrovirus antibodies in hemophiliacs treated with factor VIII or factor IX concentrates, cryoprecipitate, or fresh frozen plasma: prevalence, seroconversion, and clinical correlations. Blood 1986;67:592.
276. Jason J, McDougal JS, Holman RC, et al. Human T-lymphotropic retrovirus type III/lymphadenopathy–associated virus antibody. Association with hemophiliacs' immune status and blood component usage. JAMA 1985;253:3409.
277. McDougal JS, Martin LS, Cort SP, et al. Thermal inactivation of the acquired immunodeficiency syndrome virus, human T-lymphotropic virus-III/lymphadopathy–associated virus, with special reference to antihemophilic factor. J Clin Invest 1985;76:875.
278. Levy JA, Mitra GA, Wong MF, Mozen MM. Inactivation by wet and dry heat of AIDS-associated retroviruses during factor VIII purification from plasma. Lancet 1985;1:1456.
279. Piszkiewicz D, Bourret L, Lieu M, et al. Heat inactivation of human immunodeficiency virus in lyophilized factor VIII and factor IX concentrates. Thromb Res 1987;47:235.
280. Goedert JJ, Kessler CM, Aledort LM, et al. A prospective study of human immunodeficiency virus type I infection and the development of AIDS in subjects with hemophilia. N Engl J Med 1989;321:1141.
281. Jones P, Hamilton PJ, Bird G, et al. AIDS and haemophilia: morbidity and mortality in a well defined population. Br Med J 1985;291:695.
282. Kreiss JK, Kitchen LW, Prince EH, et al. Human T cell leukemia virus type III antibody, lymphadenopathy, and acquired immunodeficiency syndrome in hemophiliac subjects. Am J Med 1986;80:345.
283. Eyster ME, Gail MH, Ballard JO, et al. Natural history of human immunodeficiency virus infections in hemophiliacs: effects of T cell subsets, platelet counts, and age. Ann Intern Med 1987;107:1.
284. Allain JP, Laurian Y, Paul DA, et al. Long-term evaluation of HIV antigen and antibodies to p24 and gp41 in patients with hemophilia: potential clinical importance. N Engl J Med 1987;317:1114.
285. Eyster ME, Ballard JO, Gail MH, et al. Predictive markers for the acquired immunodeficiency syndrome (AIDS) in hemophiliacs: persistence of p24 antigen and low T4 cell count. Ann Intern Med 1989;110:963.
286. Pappo AS, Buchanan GR, Johnson A. Septic arthritis in children with hemophilia. Am J Dis Child 1989;143:1226.
287. Jackson JB, Sannerud KJ, Hopsicker JS, et al. Hemophiliacs with HIV antibody are actively infected. JAMA 1988;260:2236.
288. Fischl M, Richman D, Grieco MH, et al. The efficacy of azidothymidine (AZT) in the treatment of patients with AIDS and AIDS-related complex: a double-blind, placebo-controlled trial. N Engl J Med 1987;317:185.
289. Larder BA, Darby G, Richman DD. HIV with reduced sensitivity to zidovudine (AZT) isolated during prolonged therapy. Science 1989;243:1731.

Blood: Principles and Practice of Hematology,
edited by Robert I. Handin, Samuel E. Lux, and Thomas P. Stossel.
J.B. Lippincott Company, Philadelphia © 1995.

40

Vitamin K–Dependent Blood Coagulation Proteins: Normal Function and Clinical Disorders

Bruce Furie

Background and History

The vitamin K–dependent blood coagulation proteins were discovered sequentially over a 60-year period. The most abundant protein of this class, prothrombin, was identified almost 100 years ago by Alexander Schmidt,[1] who postulated that thrombin could not circulate free in the blood but must exist in a precursor form. Based on the classic theory of blood coagulation, Morawitz[2] proposed that prothrombin was converted to thrombin by a hypothetical enzyme, thrombokinase. Prothrombin was subsequently purified and extensively characterized, with the earliest work being dominated by Seegers.[3] As with many of the plasma proteins, the discovery of most of the vitamin K–dependent blood coagulation proteins was associated with the observation of "an experiment of nature"—a hereditary coagulation disorder due to a deficiency of an unknown clotting activity. Based on the observation that mixing of two hemophiliac plasmas from unrelated patients sometimes led to a correction of the clotting time of the mixed plasma, Aggeler and associates,[4] and Schulman and Smith[5] identified the protein known as factor IX in 1952. This protein is missing or defective in patients with hemophilia B, but it is distinct from factor VIII, the protein absent in hemophilia A. Factor VII was identified in 1951 after the evaluation of a patient with a hereditary clotting disorder.[6] Factor X was discovered simultaneously by Telfer and colleagues[7] and Hougie and associates[8] by detailed investigation of the plasma of patients with inherited hemorrhagic disorders due to absence of factor X. Proteins that require vitamin K for their synthesis are presented in Table 40-1. The positions of the vitamin K–dependent proteins in the coagulation cascade were proposed independently by Ratnoff and Davie[9] and by Macfarlane.[10] An updated version of the 1964 model of blood coagulation is presented in Figure 40-1. Considerable confusion arose from the original claim that the activities of "autoprothrombin III" (factor X), "cothromboplastin" (factor VII), and "autoprothrombin II" (factor IX) were derived from a single precursor "prothrombin" molecule.[11] Subsequent characterization of these plasma components led to their identification as distinct proteins derived as separate gene products but with structural homology to prothrombin.

As part of his investigation of cholesterol metabolism, Dam[12] observed in 1929 that chickens fed a diet depleted of fat-soluble components developed a hemorrhagic disorder. One of these components, Koagulations Vitamin, or vitamin K, was subsequently isolated from alfalfa.[13,14] The chemical structure of vitamin K was determined by Doisy and associates[15] (Fig. 40-2). Dam and Doisy shared the Nobel Prize in Medicine in 1943 for their pioneering work on vitamin K. The vitamin K antagonists, including warfarin, were discovered independently. A hemorrhagic disease of cattle plaguing farmers in the Great Plains in the 1920s was found to be associated with the ingestion of spoiled sweet-clover hay.[16,17] Campbell and Link[18] isolated bishydroxycoumarin (dicoumarol) from bacteria contaminating the hay and demonstrated that this material was the cause of hypoprothrombinemia in the cattle herds. This compound became the model for warfarin and for other coumarin compounds that are used as rodenticides and as anticoagulants for the treatment of human thrombotic disease.

Biosynthesis

The vitamin K–dependent plasma proteins required for normal blood clotting are synthesized in the liver.[19–21] The properties of these proteins are summarized in Table 40-2 and Figure 40-3. These proteins, including prothrombin and factors IX, X, and VII, circulate in the blood as trace components. Although the protein concentration of plasma is about 70 mg/mL, the concentrations of prothrombin and factors IX, X, and VII are 110, 5, 10, and 0.5 μg/mL, respectively. As with other secreted mammalian proteins, these proteins are synthesized in the hepatocyte in a precursor form and undergo extensive posttranslational modification during transit through the cell to the plasma.[22] All of the vitamin K–dependent proteins are synthesized with a signal peptide sequence and a propeptide sequence that are subsequently cleaved before the mature protein becomes extracellular.[22,23] The propeptide is positioned between the signal peptide and the mature form of the vitamin K–dependent proteins.[23] Posttranslational modifications of these proteins include glycosylation, signal peptide and propeptide cleavage, and disulfide bond formation. In ad-

TABLE 40-1. Vitamin K–Dependent Proteins

BLOOD COAGULATION PROTEINS
Prothrombin
Factor IX
Factor X
Factor VII
REGULATORY PROTEINS IN BLOOD COAGULATION
Protein C
Protein S
BONE PROTEINS
Osteocalcin (bone Gla protein)
Matrix Gla protein

dition, as members of a unique class of calcium-binding proteins that contain γ-carboxyglutamic acid,[24,25] the posttranslational synthesis of γ-carboxyglutamic acid from specific glutamic acid residues in these proteins occurs in the hepatocyte (Fig. 40-4). With the single exception of prothrombin, the vitamin K–dependent blood coagulation proteins also undergo β-hydroxylation of specific aspartic acid residues in certain epidermal growth factor (EGF)–like domains.[26,27]

Role of Vitamin K: Biosynthesis of γ-Carboxyglutamic Acid

Posttranslational modification of glutamic acid to γ-carboxyglutamic acid and regeneration of the active cofactor, vitamin KH_2, requires a series of linked enzyme reactions. The carboxylation reaction includes as substrates a reduced form of vitamin K (vitamin KH_2), molecular oxygen, carbon dioxide, and the protein precursor containing glutamic acid residues.[28] The vitamin K–dependent carboxylase, isolated in homogeneous form from bovine liver, has a molecular mass of about 80 kd.[29] This enzyme appears to be an integral membrane protein situated on the luminal side of the rough endoplasmic reticulum.[30–32]

The reaction catalyzed by the γ-carboxylase leads to the extraction of a hydrogen from the γ-carbon of glutamic acid residues on the protein and to the addition of a carboxyl group at this same position (Fig. 40-5). Carbon dioxide, not bicarbonate, is the probable substrate that is destined to form the new carboxyl group.[33] Unlike many other carboxylases, ATP and biotin are not required for this reaction.[34] The role of vitamin K, however, is unclear in this unique reaction. The vitamin K hydroquinone (vitamin KH_2) may activate a hydrogen at the γ-position of a glutamyl residue, facilitating carbon dioxide attack at this position.[35] It is likely that this hydrogen extraction generates a carbanion rather than a free radical at the γ-carbon.[36,37] The vitamin K epoxidase, an enzymatic activity closely linked to the vitamin K–dependent carboxylase, converts vitamin KH_2 to 2,3-vitamin K epoxide.[38–41]

Vitamin KH_2 is the active cofactor required for carboxylase activity.[42–44] Since vitamin K from dietary sources[15] or gut flora[45] is in the quinone form, liver microsomes contain quinone reductases to generate the vitamin K hydroquinone. Two different enzymes can reduce vitamin K to vitamin K hydroquinone. One of these is the microsomal equivalent of the NADPH-requiring oxidoreductase, DT-diaphorase.[46–48] Dithiothreitol reduces vitamin K to vitamin K hydroquinone in vitro.[49,50]

The vitamin K epoxide is recycled to vitamin K via the

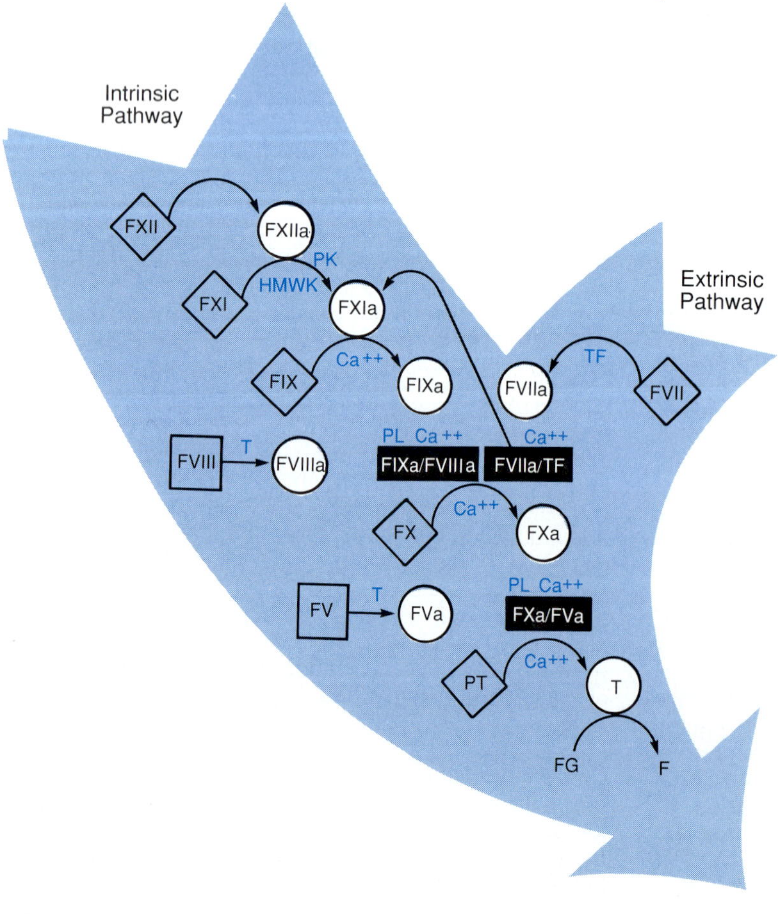

FIGURE 40-1. Role of the vitamin K–dependent proteins in blood coagulation. The blood coagulation cascade involves the intrinsic and the extrinsic pathways. The vitamin K–dependent proteins (*squares*) circulate in the blood in an inactive, proenzyme form. On activation of blood coagulation, they are converted to their active, procoagulant form (*circles*). These proteins have the special property of displaying maximal enzyme activity on membrane surfaces. (After Furie B, Furie BC. Molecular basis of blood coagulation. Cell 1988;53:505).

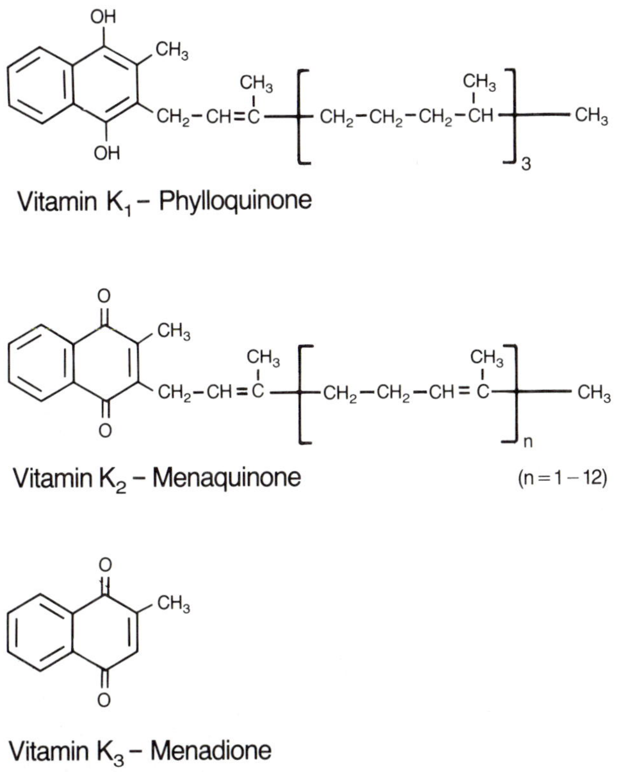

FIGURE 40-2. Chemical structure of vitamin K. Several forms of vitamin K are found in nature. Vitamin K_1 is a component of plants and vitamin K_2 is produced by bacteria. Vitamin K_3 contains the basic structure of vitamin K. The degree of fat solubility relates to the length of the terpine carbon chain.

vitamin K epoxide reductase. The vitamin K epoxide reductase uses a dithiol rather than a reduced pyridine nucleotide as a cofactor.[51,52] The product of the reaction catalyzed by the epoxide reductase is the quinone form of the vitamin.[53] This vitamin form is further reduced to the hydroquinone to provide active cofactor for the carboxylase reaction. A summary of the vitamin K cycle is shown in Figure 40-5.

Vitamin K antagonists used as oral anticoagulants, such as warfarin (Fig. 40-6), prevent the γ-carboxylation of the vitamin K–dependent proteins. The des-γ-carboxy (abnormal) forms of the vitamin K–dependent proteins are functionally inert and circulate in the blood in place of the active, carboxylated blood-clotting proteins. Warfarin inhibits the epoxide reductase and one quinone reductase, preventing recycling of the vitamin to its active form.[54] The NADPH-dependent reduction of vitamin K quinone to the hydroquinone is affected only minimally by warfarin and related compounds.[54]

Substrate Specificity

γ-Carboxyglutamic acid is synthesized by a vitamin K–dependent posttranslational carboxylation of specific glutamic acid residues in the intracellular precursor of the vitamin K–dependent proteins. These intracellular prothrombin precursors were first demonstrated in 1971 by Shah and Suttie.[55] When vitamin K was administered to vitamin K–deficient rats in the presence of an inhibitor of protein synthesis, cycloheximide, prothrombin activity increased rapidly despite the absence of de novo protein synthesis. The prothrombin released into the circulation on administration of vitamin K was derived from a precursor pool. This prothrombin precursor, like des-γ-carboxy (abnormal) prothrombin, contains an intact thrombin domain but cannot be activated by factor Xa. Presumably, this is because of the absence of γ-carboxyglutamic acid residues.[56] These observations demonstrate that the vitamin K-dependent step in the synthesis of prothrombin is the posttranslational modification of a hepatic prothrombin precursor.

Two prothrombin precursors have been isolated from rat liver,[57,58] and other forms have been observed.[59,60] These precursors are functionally distinct from des-γ-carboxy (abnormal) prothrombin,[61,62] the secreted form of prothrombin that is deficient in γ-carboxyglutamic acid, in that they are excellent substrates for the carboxylase. This observation indicates that there must be recognition sites on the prothrombin precursor that direct carboxylation in the liver; these sites are not present on the secreted forms of the protein.[63] In support of this hypothesis, the carboxylase activity in solubilized liver microsomes is bound to an endogenous precursor.[64] The carboxylase binds to a site on the protein substrate, the carboxylation-recognition site,[65] adjacent to the region that becomes carboxylated. This recognition element is located on the propeptide of the vitamin K–dependent proteins, a region of the precursor protein that is cleaved and discarded during the final stages of protein synthesis.[23]

Diuguid and associates[66] determined the size of the propeptide of factor IX by analysis of mutant factor IX, termed factor IX Cambridge. This mutant factor IX has an 18-residue NH_2-terminal extension due to the mutation of arginine −1 to a serine, thus precluding propeptide cleavage by a propeptidase with trypsin-like specificity. Factor IX Cambridge and factor IX San Dimas,[68] a mutant identical to factor IX Oxford 3,[67] are incompletely carboxylated, indicating a link between a propeptide point mutation and vitamin K-dependent carboxylation. These data and the marked sequence homology of this domain in γ-carboxyglutamic acid–containing proteins[69] (Fig. 40-7) led to the proposal that the propeptide targeted protein precursors for subsequent γ-carboxylation. Using site-specific mutagenesis and a heterologous mammalian expression system, Jorgensen and colleagues[65] and Rabiet and coworkers[70] demonstrated that factor IX lacking the 18-residue propeptide was not carboxylated in vivo. Similarly,

TABLE 40-2. **Properties of the Genes, mRNAs, and Gene Products of the Vitamin K–Dependent Blood Coagulation Proteins**

	Molecular Weight (kd)	Gene (kb)	Chromosome	mRNA (kb)	Exons	Plasma Conc (μg/mL)	Function
Prothrombin	72	21	11p11-q12	2.1	14	100	Protease zymogen
Factor X	56	22	13q34	1.5	8	10	Protease zymogen
Factor IX	56	34	Xq26-27.3	2.8	8	5	Protease zymogen
Factor VII	50	13	13q34	2.4	8	0.5	Protease zymogen

(Modified from Furie B, Furie BC. Molecular basis of blood coagulation. Cell 1988;53:505)

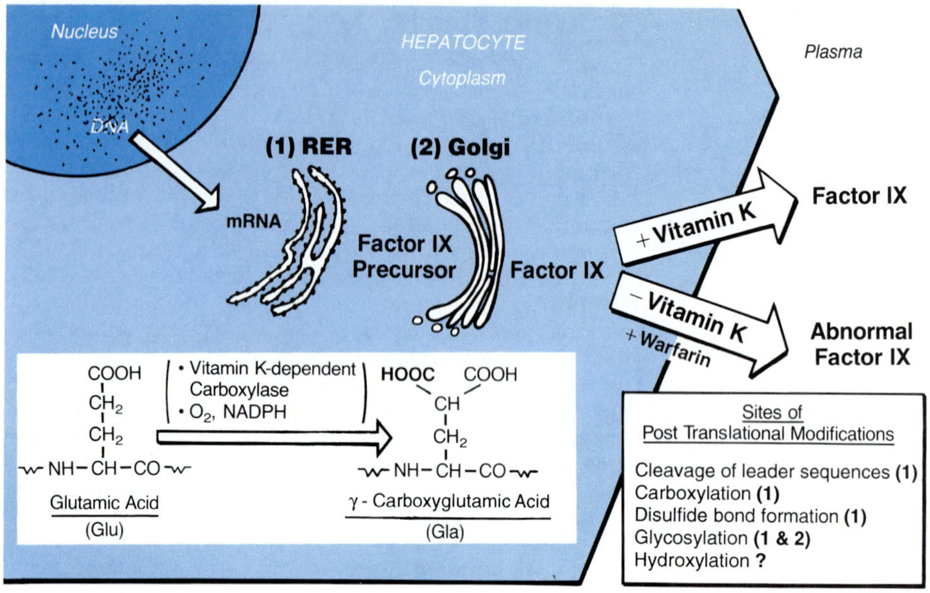

FIGURE 40-3. Biosynthesis of the vitamin K–dependent proteins. Factors IX, X, and VII and prothrombin are synthesized in the liver in a precursor, prozymogen form. The vitamin K–dependent carboxylase modifies this prozymogen posttranslationally, converting some N-terminal glutamic acid residues to γ-carboxyglutamic acid. This reaction requires vitamin K in its reduced form, carbon dioxide, and oxygen. After subsequent cleavage of the propeptide, the zymogen is secreted into the plasma.

point mutations at −16 (Phe → Ala) or −10 (Ala → Glu)—two positions highly conserved in the propeptides of the vitamin K–dependent proteins—inhibited γ-carboxylation. These results demonstrated that the propeptide contains a recognition element, designated the γ-carboxylation recognition site, which flags the vitamin K–dependent proteins during hepatic biosynthesis for γ-carboxylation. In related experiments, Foster and others[71] demonstrated that the expression of deletion mutants of proprotein C lacking residues in the −17 to −12 portion of the propeptide is associated with impaired γ-carboxylation.

A synthetic peptide comprising residues 5 to 9 of a carboxy bovine prothrombin (Phe-Leu-Glu-Glu-Val) serves as a substrate for ^{14}C-bicarbonate incorporation by a solubilized carboxylation system.[72] Studies of this substrate and related peptide substrates demonstrate that their carboxylation requires higher concentrations of vitamin K and that this pentapeptide has a much higher K_m than carboxylation of endogenous prothrombin precursors.[72–74] Also, only the first of two adjacent glutamic acid residues in these synthetic peptides is carboxylated.[75] These results suggest that substrate properties, other than the sequence immediately surrounding the glutamic acids that are destined to be carboxylated, are required for efficient carboxylation by the vitamin K–dependent carboxylase.

Ulrich and associates[76] have shown that the vitamin K–dependent carboxylase recognizes the γ-CRS. A 28-residue synthetic peptide based on residues −18 to +10 in prothrombin (the propeptide and the first 10 residues of the mature form of prothrombin) is efficiently carboxylated, with a K_m of 3 μmol/L. In contrast, synthetic peptides lacking the complete γ-CRS were not efficiently carboxylated. These peptides included the pentapeptide substrate FLEEL (K_m of 2200 μmol/L),[72] a 20-residue peptide analogous to residues −10 to +10 in prothrombin, and a 10-residue peptide analogous to residues +1 to +10 in prothrombin. Recombinant protein C expressed in *Escherichia coli* incorporated $^{14}CO_2$ into γ-carboxyglutamic acid only slightly better if the protein substrate also included a segment (residues −10 to −1) of the propeptide.[77] Given that the propeptide of protein C extends from −24 to −1,[71] these results and those of Ulrich and associates[76] indicate the importance of the intact γ-CRS for efficient carboxylation both in vivo and in vitro.

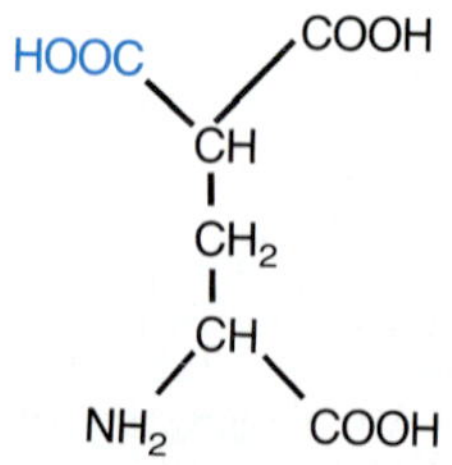

FIGURE 40-4. Chemical structure of γ-carboxyglutamic acid. γ-Carboxyglutamic acid is synthesized from glutamic acid residues in proteins. The additional carboxyl group is substituted for a γ-hydrogen in a reaction catalyzed by the vitamin K–dependent carboxylase.

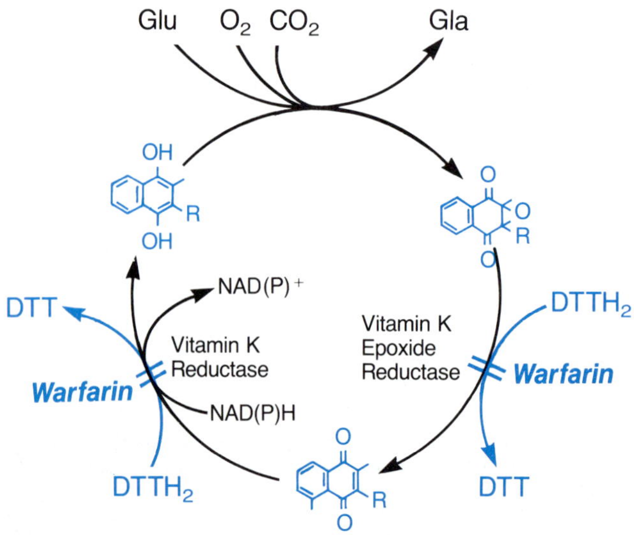

FIGURE 40-5. Vitamin K cycle. Vitamin K is an essential metabolite and can be considered a limited resource. Therefore, it is recovered in an altered form after carboxylation and recycled to its original chemical form. Vitamin K is reduced to vitamin KH_2. The vitamin K epoxide is formed by the vitamin K epoxidase that is closely linked to the vitamin K–dependent carboxylase. The vitamin K epoxide is then converted to vitamin K.

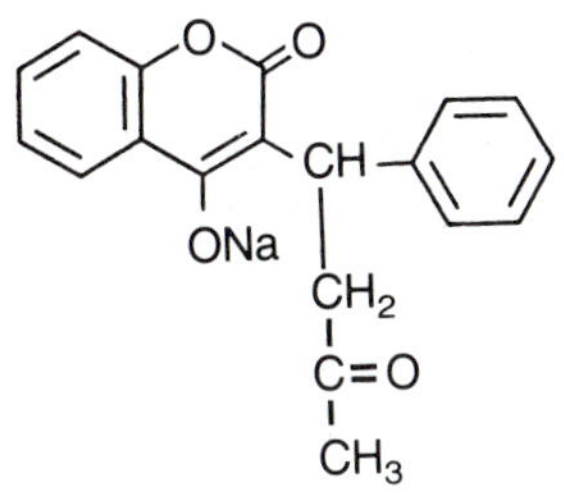

FIGURE 40-6. Chemical structure of warfarin. Warfarin sodium is a vitamin K antagonist that is employed as an anticoagulant. Its structure reassembles the essential elements of vitamin K.

Based on the predicted structure of the propeptide of factor X, Knobloch and Suttie[78] have proposed that an 18-residue peptide plays a regulatory role in carboxylation as an allosteric modifier of the vitamin K–dependent carboxylase. This peptide stimulates the carboxylation of a small synthetic substrate, but similar peptides inhibit the longer synthetic substrates that include the carboxylation recognition site.[76] These results raise the possibility that the propeptide may be an allosteric regulator of the carboxylase as well as a recognition element.

Except for the requirement that glutamic acid residues are in close proximity to the γ-carboxylation recognition site, there is no compelling evidence for a consensus sequence or a unique amino acid sequence adjacent to the glutamic acids that are to be carboxylated, although such a consensus sequence has been proposed.[79] Within the 28-residue synthetic peptide representing −18 to +10 of the proprothrombin sequence, substitution of alanine or aspartic acid for one of the two glutamic acids does not interfere with the carboxylation of the remaining glutamic acid.[80] Although the aspartic or alanine residues do not get carboxylated, their presence does not inhibit carboxylation of the adjacent glutamic acid. Furthermore, homologous synthetic peptides based on the primary structure of the propeptide and the first 10 residues of factor IX are also efficiently carboxylated. These results suggest similar chemical surfaces on the propeptides of prothrombin and on factor IX despite the absence of perfect sequence homology in these structures. Analysis of the propeptide's structure suggests that the polypeptide backbone assumes an α helical structure.[81] Propeptide models indicate that most of the hydrophobic amino acids are located on one side of the helix, whereas most of the hydrophilic amino acids are located on the other side—a characteristic of an amphipathic helix. The hydrophobic surface of the helix is assumed to be the carboxylation recognition site. The critical question of whether the presence of the carboxylation recognition site on the propeptide is sufficient to assure carboxylation of glutamic acid residues on the adjacent segment remains unanswered.

The vitamin K–dependent carboxylase is highly specific for glutamic acid residues. Using small synthetic peptides, aspartic acid residues can be β-carboxylated at about 10% of the rate of the γ-carboxylation of glutamic acids. Hubbard and colleagues,[80] however, have not observed β-carboxylation of aspartic acid in synthetic peptides that include the propeptide. When Glu-Glu sequences (homologous to residues 6 and 7 in prothrombin) in the 28-residue synthetic peptide (homologous to residues −18 to +10 in prothrombin) were altered to Glu-Ala, Glu-Asp, Ala-Glu, or Asp-Glu glutamyl residues at positions homologous to residues 6 and 7, both demonstrated equivalent kinetics of carboxylation. As previously discussed, these results confirm that, although not a carboxylation substrate, aspartic acid does not inhibit the carboxylation of an adjacent glutamic acid. Furthermore, glutamic acids at both positions can be carboxylated. The presence of two contiguous acidic amino acids is not necessary for efficient carboxylation.

The vitamin K–dependent carboxylase has been purified using a strategy based on its affinity to the propeptide.[81a] The enzyme has a molecular mass of 94 kd and exists as a single polypeptide chain. It would appear that the active site of the enzyme, which is responsible for carboxylation, and a domain that interacts with the carboxylation recognition site on the substrate are in close proximity. The availability of the purified carboxylase facilitates the definition of the mechanism of this enzyme and its cofactor, vitamin KH_2.

β-Hydroxylation. An unusual amino acid, erythro-β-hydroxyaspartic acid, is located in the EGF domains of protein C,[26] and factors IX, X, and VII[27,83,84] (Fig. 40-8). This amino acid is formed by posttranslational hydroxylation of aspartic acid. Recent evidence indicates that 2-oxoglutarate is a cofactor of the hydroxylase.[85] The function of this amino acid is not known, although the aspartic acid or its hydroxylated derivative may define a metal-binding site critical to protein function.[86,87]

In contrast to γ-carboxylation, β-hydroxylation of factor IX is not directed by the propeptide, nor does this reaction require vitamin K. Similarly, synthesis of factor IX in the presence of the vitamin K antagonists such as sodium warfarin impairs γ-carboxylation but not β-hydroxylation.[70] Factor IX mutants that have the propeptide deleted or contain point mutations that eliminate γ-carboxylation remain substrates for the β-hydroxylase.[70] β-Hydroxylation occurs in domains homologous to the EGF precursor in certain vitamin K–dependent proteins[88] as well as in proteins outside of this family, including the complement proteins C1r, C1s, thrombomodulin, uromodulin, and the low-density lipoprotein receptor.[89–91] A consensus sequence encom-

	−24						−18								−10									−1	+1
Factor IX							Thr	Val	Phe	Leu	Asp	His	Glu	Asn	Ala	Asn	Lys	Ile	Leu	Asn	Arg	Pro	Lys	Arg	Tyr
Prothrombin	Ser	Leu	Val	His	Ser	Gln	His	Val	Phe	Leu	Ala	Pro	Gln	Gln	Ala	Arg	Ser	Leu	Leu	Gln	Arg	Val	Arg	Arg	Ala
Factor X	Leu	Leu	Leu	Leu	Gly	Glu	Ser	Leu	Phe	Ile	Arg	Arg	Glu	Gln	Ala	Asn	Asn	Ile	Leu	Ala	Arg	Val	Thr	Arg	Ala
Protein C	Thr	Pro	Ala	Pro	Leu	Asp	Ser	Val	Phe	Ser	Ser	Ser	Glu	Arg	Ala	His	Gln	Val	Leu	Arg	Ile	Arg	Lys	Arg	Ala
Factor VII	Trp	Lys	Pro	Gly	Pro	His	Arg	Val	Phe	Val	Thr	Glu	Glu	Glu	Ala	His	Gly	Val	Leu	His	Arg	Arg	Arg	Arg	Ala
Protein S	Val	Leu	Pro	Val	Leu	Glu	Ala	Asn	Phe	Leu	Ser	Arg	Gln	His	Ala	Ser	Gln	Val	Leu	Ile	Arg	Arg	Arg	Arg	Ala
Bone Gla protein	Ser	Gly	Ala	Glu	Ser	Ser	Lys	Ala	Phe	Val	Ser	Lys	Gln	Glu	Gly	Ser	Glu	Val	Val	Lys	Arg	Pro	Arg	Arg	Tyr

FIGURE 40-7. Sequence homologies of the propeptide regions of the vitamin K–dependent proteins. The factor IX propeptide is 18 residues long and the protein propeptide is 24 residues long. The size of the other propeptides is not known. The γ-carboxylation recognition site is located on the propeptides of the vitamin K–dependent proteins. (After Furie B, Furie BC. Molecular basis of blood coagulation. Cell 1988;53:505)

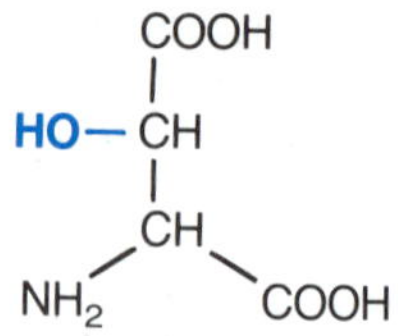

FIGURE 40-8. Chemical structure of β-hydroxyaspartic acid. This amino acid is observed in some epidermal growth factor domains of the vitamin K–dependent proteins. It is also observed in proteins that do not require vitamin K for their synthesis.

passing the β-hydroxylated Asp residue within a number of EGF domains—Cys-X-Asp/Asn-X-X-X-X-Phe/Tyr-X-Cys-X-Cys—has been noted by Stenflo and associates.[88] In some proteins, the presence of an asparagine in place of an aspartic acid leads to the hydroxylation of the asparagine.[88] EGF domains that lack the above consensus sequence do not undergo hydroxylation.

Cleavage of Prosequences. After γ-carboxylation and secretion, the propeptides of the vitamin K–dependent proteins are cleaved in the trans Golgi, and the mature proteins are secreted into the plasma. There are two contiguous basic amino acids on the N-terminal side of the propeptidase cleavage site in most of the vitamin K–dependent blood clotting proteins[23,92–96] (see Fig. 40-7). Although the propeptidases have not been identified, their specificity for arginine suggests a serine protease in the trypsin family. An Arg → Ser mutation at −1 in a naturally occurring mutant, factor IX Cambridge, inhibits propeptide cleavage.[66] The properties of naturally occurring factor IX mutants, factor IX Oxford and factor IX San Dimas, suggest that the propeptidase substrate specificity is not limited to the basic residues at −1 and −2,[67,68] since an Arg → Gln substitution at residue −4 in the propeptide completely inhibits propeptide cleavage. Deletion mutations in protein C further emphasize the role of the four COOH-terminal amino acids of the propeptide.[71]

Role of γ-Carboxyglutamic Acid

γ-Carboxyglutamic acid residues,[24,25] essential for biologic activity of these proteins, confer metal-binding properties on the vitamin K–dependent proteins and allow interaction with calcium ions and subsequent binding to phospholipid or membrane surfaces.[62,97–100] The N-terminal sequences of the vitamin K–dependent proteins, including the distribution and spacing of the γ-carboxyglutamic acid residues, are homologous across species (eg, bovine and human) and to each other.[101–107] Studies of the γ-carboxyglutamic acid–metal complex in solution using NMR paramagnetic relaxation techniques[108] suggest that the metal is bound by one or both of the γ-carboxyl groups. The γ-carboxyl oxygens are coordinated to half of the primary coordination sphere of the metal ion, leaving the other half available to interact with another γ-carboxyglutamic acid residue or with another metal ligand. The metal ion therefore serves as an intramolecular bridge to link a γ-carboxyglutamic acid in one region of a protein to a γ-carboxyglutamic acid in another region.[109] Indeed, the radiographic structure of the Gla domain reveals an internal core of calcium ions surrounded by chelating γ-carboxyglutamic acid residues.[109a]

The interaction of metal ions with γ-carboxyglutamic acid provides insight into the nature of the metal-binding sites of γ-carboxyglutamic acid–containing proteins like the vitamin K–dependent coagulation proteins. The proteins contain both high- and low-affinity metal–binding sites.[110–117] Occupancy of these sites by a variety of metal ions causes a conformational transition demonstrated by circular dichroism,[118] fluorescence spectroscopy,[119,120] and immunochemical studies using conformation-specific antibodies.[121–125] This conformational transition has been localized to the N terminal of prothrombin,[126] and it is required to obtain the functionally active conformer.

COMMON FEATURES OF VITAMIN K–DEPENDENT BLOOD CLOTTING PROTEINS

As previously discussed, the vitamin K–dependent plasma proteins involved in blood coagulation include the zymogens of four serine proteases: prothrombin, and factors X, IX, and VII. As determined by amino acid–sequence analysis[102–104,106,107,126–128] or by prediction of the amino acid sequence from the DNA sequence,[23,93,95,96] these four proteins show marked homology to each other. They are composed of structural units or domains that are common to many other proteins. One commonality is that these proteins are zymogens (proenzymes) of serine proteases, which use catalytic mechanisms that involve a serine in the active site.[130]

The N terminals of the vitamin K–dependent blood clotting proteins contain 10 to 12 γ-carboxyglutamic acid (Gla) residues within the first 42 amino acids.[101–107] Two, or possibly three, of these amino acids bind a single calcium ion,[108,109,131–133] thus forming a noncovalent intramolecular bridge between regions of the polypeptide backbone. This bond stabilizes the tertiary structure of this region of the protein.[126] On binding calcium, the proteins undergo two conformational changes that expose a membrane-binding site.[119,120,125,134,135] Although the *Gla domain* is required for these conformational transitions, it remains uncertain whether some of the γ-carboxyglutamic acids directly bind to membrane surfaces through calcium ion bridges[136] or whether metal binding to γ-carboxyglutamic acid in the Gla domain alters the structure of adjacent domains, exposing a membrane-binding surface.[125]

The *aromatic amino acid stack*, a short linking segment that contains the sequence Phe-Trp-X-X-Tyr, is present in all the prothrombin complex proteins. Although hydrophobic, this region is on the surface of prothrombin fragment 1 and may play a role in membrane binding.[137] There is speculation that this region plays a special role in heterodimer formation among various vitamin K–dependent proteins during protein assembly on membrane surfaces.[138] This is based on the formation of prothrombin fragment 1 dimers in the fragment 1 crystal and on the marked homology of the N-terminal domains in the vitamin K–dependent proteins.

With the exception of prothrombin, the vitamin K–dependent blood coagulation proteins contain two EGF domains that are homologous to a domain in the EGF precursor.[139] This domain is a 53–amino acid peptide containing three disulfide bonds that bind other proteins to specific cell surface receptors.[140,141] The role of the EGF domains in the vitamin K–dependent proteins is uncertain. In one instance, a mutation in factor IX at residue 47 (factor IX Alabama) is in the EGF domain and interferes with factor VIII binding.[142,143] Thus, the EGF domains may be responsible for the high-affinity interaction of some proteins with specific cell surfaces or, alternatively, with binding domains on other proteins, such as factors VIII and factor V.

There are two *kringle domains* on prothrombin, each about 100 amino acids long.[144] This domain contains three disulfide bonds. Its three-dimensional structure resembles an eccentric oblate ellipsoid, and its folding is defined by close contacts between the sulfur atoms of two of the disulfide bridges, which form a sulfur cluster in the center of the kringle.[137] Internal amino acids are well conserved among various proteins containing kringles. Differences in the molecular surfaces probably distinguish functional properties among proteins that contain kringle domains besides prothrombin, such as tissue plasminogen activator,[145] factor XII,[146] prourokinase,[147] and plasminogen.[148] The functions of these domains remain uncertain, but they likely contain recognition elements important for protein assembly on membrane surfaces.

The *serine protease domain* is common to all of the vitamin K–dependent blood coagulation proteins. The structure and organization of genes among the serine proteases emphasize that the evolution of new protein function occurs via gene duplication, gene modification, and exon shuffling.[149,150] Each of the exons may be considered a module coding for a homologous domain in each protein (Fig. 40-9). Evidence suggests that the three-dimensional structure of the polypeptide backbone of these domains is nearly identical. Substitutions in the amino acid side chains

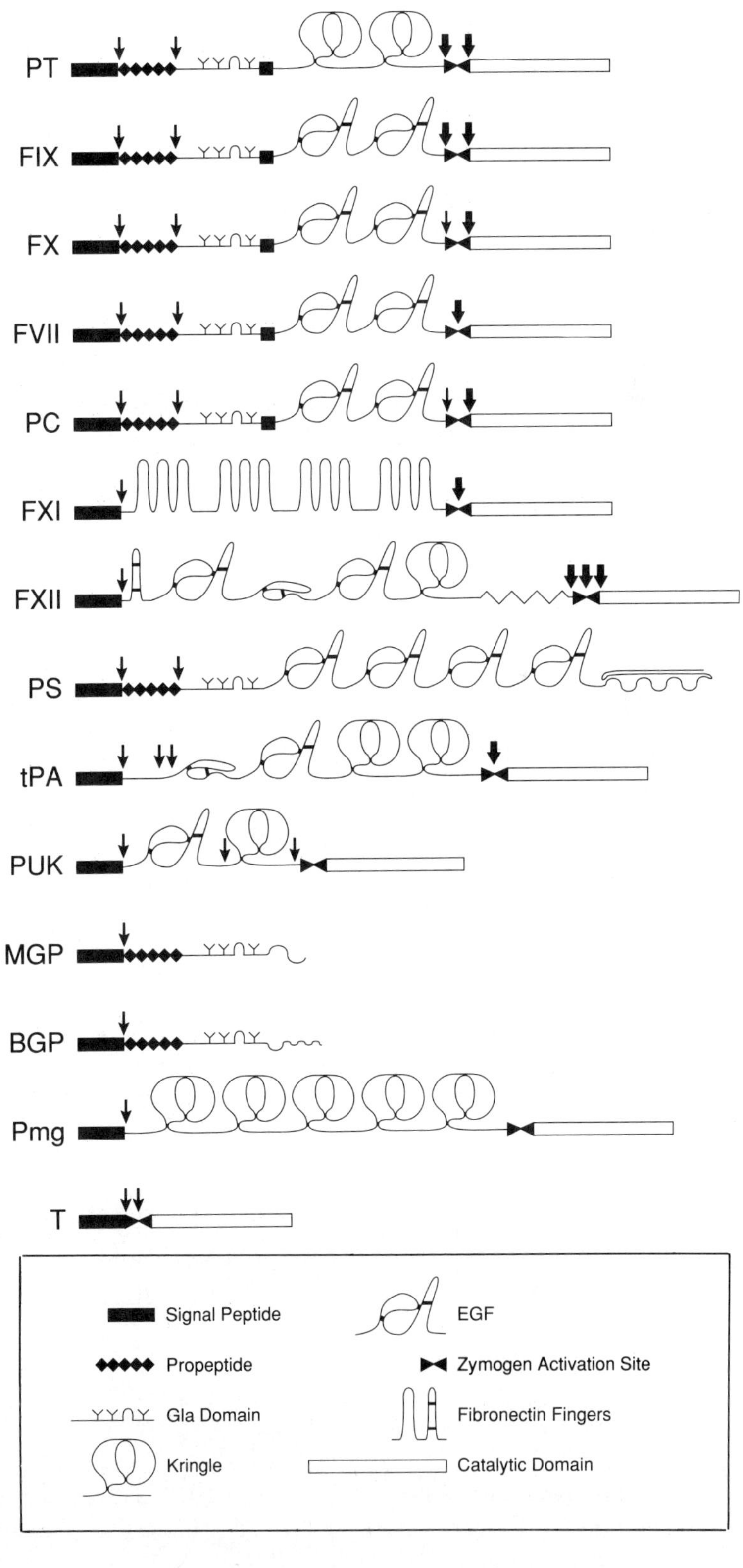

FIGURE 40-9. Domain structure of the vitamin K–dependent proteins and other proteins that are structurally or functionally related. Domains indicated include the signal peptide, the propeptide, the Gla domain, the epidermal growth factor domain, the repeat sequences, the kringle region, the fibronectin (type I and II) domains, the aromatic amino acid stack, the zymogen activation region, and the catalytic domain. The sites of proteolytic cleavage associated with synthesis of the mature protein are indicated by thin arrows. The sites of proteolytic cleavage associated with zymogen activation are indicated by the thick arrows. PT, prothrombin; FIX, factor IX; FX, factor X; FVII, factor VII; PC, protein C; FXI, factor XI; FXII, factor XII; PS, protein S; tPA, tissue-type plasminogen activator; PUK, prourokinase; MGP, matrix Gla protein; BGP, bone Gla protein; Pmg, plasminogen; T, trypsin. (After Furie B, Furie BC. Molecular basis of blood coagulation. Cell 1988;53:505)

on the protein surfaces define the unique properties of substrate recognition, cofactor binding, or membrane interaction.[151] The serine protease family as a whole, and the blood coagulation proteases in particular, remain a prime example of a family of proteins with diverse functional properties but common, unified structural elements.

The vitamin K–dependent blood clotting proteins circulate in the plasma in their proenzyme form.[9,10] Each of these proteins is converted to its active enzyme by the cleavage of one or two peptide bonds. Like trypsin and other serine proteases, they contain the catalytic triad of a serine, histidine, and aspartic acid in the active enzyme site. In the blood-clotting enzymes, the domain with marked sequence homology and presumed three-dimensional structural homology[151] with trypsin is known as the *catalytic domain*. The blood-clotting serine proteases have an active site and an internal core that is nearly identical to trypsin; however, the different molecular surfaces that surround the enzyme active site provide substrate-binding sites and are responsible for the unique substrate specificities of these enzymes.

PROTHROMBIN

Gene Structure

The human[130] and bovine[152] prothrombin genes are partially homologous to those encoding the other vitamin K–dependent proteins (Fig. 40-10). The human prothrombin gene is located in chromosome 11[153]; it includes about 24 kilobases (kb) of DNA and contains 14 exons. As shown in Figure 40-10, exon I encodes the signal peptide. Exon II encodes the propeptide (including the γ-carboxylation recognition site)[65,71] and the Gla domain. Exon III encodes the aromatic amino acid stack domain. Exons I, II, and III are homologous in structure and organization to the same exons in the factor IX gene family, which includes factors IX, X, and VII and protein C.[154–157] Exons IV, V, VI, and VII encode the two kringle regions. These domains are not parallel with structures in the factor IX family but are observed in other proteins involved in hemostasis including tissue plasminogen activator,[145] plasminogen,[148] prourokinase,[147] and factor XII.[146] Exons VIII and IX encode for the sites of proteolytic cleavage by factor Xa, which convert prothrombin to thrombin. The catalytic domain of thrombin is responsible for enzyme catalysis and substrate specificity; it is encoded by exons X, XI, XII, XIII, and XIV.

Despite the structural homologies of the catalytic domains in the vitamin K–dependent proteins, this portion of the gene's organization differs from the coding for the analogous domains in the factor IX gene family.[158] In prothrombin, the amino acids that form the catalytic triad of serine proteases are each on a separate exon, with histidine on exon X, aspartic acid on exon XI, and serine on exon XIII.

Protein Structure

The amino acid sequence of human prothrombin is diagrammed in Figure 40-11.[102,127] The sequences of the signal peptide and propeptide are also presented in this figure.[93,159] Human prothrombin is composed of a single polypeptide chain made up of 579 amino acids. Prothrombin is a glycoprotein; about 10% of its mass is carbohydrate. N-Asparagine–linked carbohydrate is attached to Asn 78, Asn 100, and Asn 373 in bovine prothrombin.[160] Human prothrombin likely contains carbohydrate in analogous positions since these asparagine residues are conserved in the bovine and human prothrombin sequences. Bovine prothrombin contains complex asparagine-linked oligosaccharides that include NeuAcα2 → 3Galβ1 → 3(NeuAcα2 → 6)GlcNAc components in the outer chain. The structure of these complex carbohydrates is known and includes Galβ1 → 3GlcNAc.[160] No specific role for the carbohydrate moieties has been elucidated.

The 10 γ-carboxyglutamic acid residues, located near the amino terminal of the protein, are found at positions 6, 7, 14, 16, 19, 20, 25, 26, 29, and 32 in human prothrombin.[102] This γ-carboxyglutamic acid–rich domain contains the calcium-binding sites of prothrombin.[110,126] Abnormal prothrombin lacks γ-carboxyglutamic acid residues and does not interact with calcium.[61,62,100,161] This interaction is critical for calcium-dependent prothrombin–membrane interaction.[99]

Prothrombin contains two kringle domains, each composed of 79 amino acid residues.[158] These structures have a characteristic distribution of cysteines that form a cluster of disulfide bonds in the center of each kringle. The three-dimensional structure of this region has been determined by x-ray crystallography.[137] The specific function of the kringles is unknown, however. There is speculation that the kringles play a role in protein assembly, by either interacting with membrane surfaces or with the cofactor, factor V. Alternately, as discussed, the aromatic acid stack sequence might bind factors V and VIII.

The serine protease domain stretches for about 250 amino acids, and is homologous to the prototypic serine protease, trypsin.[130] About 33% of this region, representing the enzyme thrombin, demonstrates marked sequence homology to trypsin.[127] The cleavage of two peptide bonds in the activation region of the serine protease domain converts the zymogen prothrombin to the enzyme thrombin. In the absence of crystallographic studies, a computer model of thrombin has provided a first approximation of the three-dimensional structure of this enzyme.[151] This model is based on the assumption that the marked sequence homology of trypsin to thrombin predicts homology of the tertiary structure. It also emphasizes the similarity of trypsin to thrombin in the internal core and in the complete preservation of the active site (Fig. 40-12). The differences lie in the unique molecular surface and clearly impart unique functional properties to these proteins. This surface

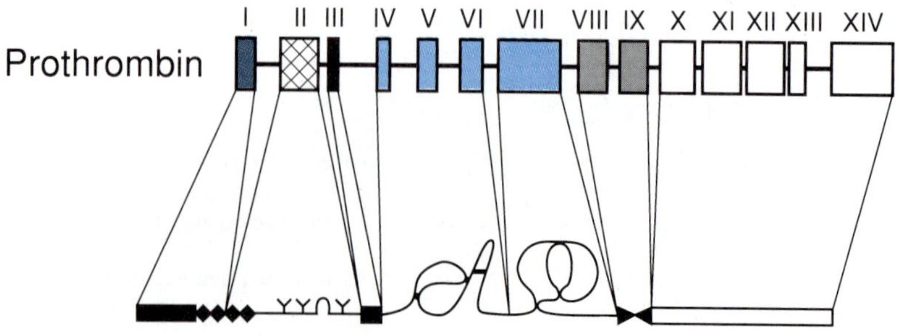

FIGURE 40-10. Gene structure of human prothrombin. Exons are shown schematically according to scale. Introns, indicated by double lines, are not drawn to scale. (After Furie B, Furie BC. Molecular basis of blood coagulation. Cell 1988;53:505)

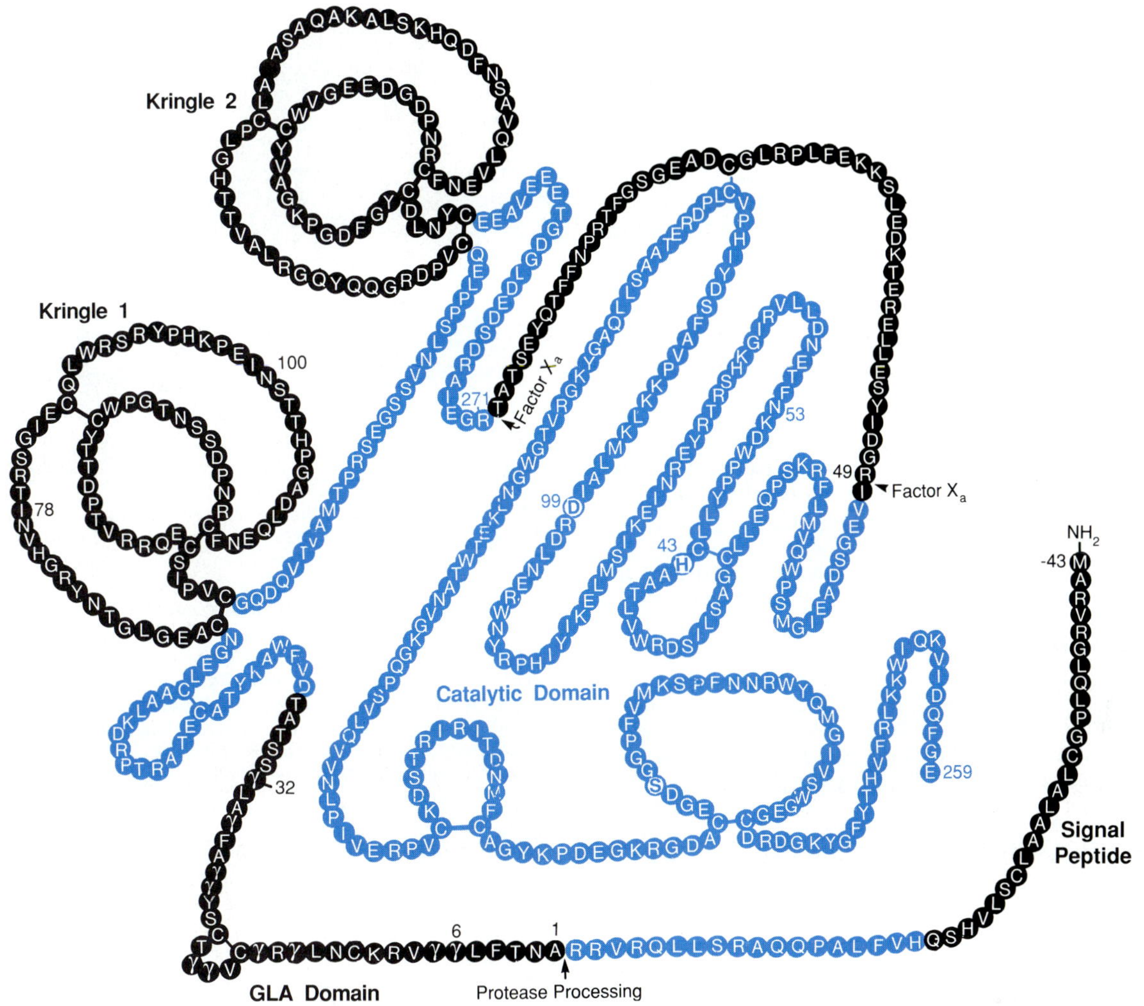

FIGURE 40-11. Amino acid sequence of human prothrombin.

defines unique substrate specificity for the macromolecular substrate by use of an extended substrate-binding site around the active site.

Calcium-Binding Properties

The metal-binding properties of prothrombin are confered by γ-carboxyglutamic acids. Although determining the precise number of binding sites is beyond current methodology, studies suggest that prothrombin has two or three high-affinity metal-binding sites and four to eight lower-affinity metal-binding sites.[110,111,113] A high-affinity metal-binding site in prothrombin has been shown to involve two or three γ-carboxyglutamic acid residues,[108,109,131,132] but only two γ-carboxyglutamic acid residues may define a magnesium ion binding site.[133] A model has been proposed where two nonadjacent γ-carboxyglutamic acid residues in the polypeptide chain chelate a single metal ion.[109] This structure is similar to that observed for the free γ-carboxyglutamic acid–metal complex.[108] There are multiple lower-affinity metal-binding sites that also contain γ-carboxyglutamic acid. The precise structure of these sites is not known but may comprise single γ-carboxyglutamic acid residues. Occupany of the high-affinity metal-binding sites facilitates binding of the lower-affinity sites. This phenomenon is known as positive cooperative binding.

Certain γ-carboxyglutamic acid residues that play a critical role in calcium binding and prothrombin function have been identified by indirect analysis. Analysis of a series of partially carboxylated prothrombins from a patient with a hereditary defect in carboxylation suggests that Gla 16 plays a special role in calcium binding and is the high-affinity metal-binding site in prothrombin.[161,162] This observation

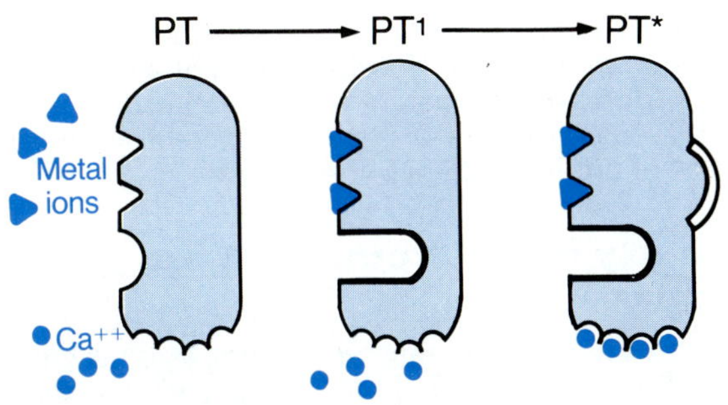

FIGURE 40-12. Metal-induced conformational transitions in human prothrombin. Prothrombin and the other vitamin K–dependent proteins undergo conformational changes that are induced by metal ions. Many metal ions, including calcium ions, occupy a first set of binding sites that leads to an initial conformational change, PT → P^1. A second conformational change, P^1 → P^*, is induced by the occupancy of a second set of metal-binding sites by calcium.

is consistent with earlier spectroscopic results that suggested that this residue might be involved in high-affinity metal binding.[109]

Metal-Induced Conformational Transitions

The addition of metal ions, including most divalent cations, induces an alteration in the conformation of prothrombin. This conformational change can be monitored by the quenching of the intrinsic fluoresence of the protein,[119,120] perturbation of the structure of the polypeptide backbone as monitored by circular dichroism measurements,[118] or by the expression of new antigenic determinants on the metal-stabilized conformer.[121–125] Only calcium ions, however, convert prothrombin to the active conformer that can bind to membrane surfaces. It appears that calcium also induces a second metal-dependent conformational transition, as has been observed by immunochemical techniques.[125] Both conformational transitions are induced by only calcium ions (see Fig. 40-12).

The second conformational change is associated with the expression of the phospholipid binding sites necessary for interaction of these proteins with phospholipid surfaces and for coagulant activity. Studies of a series of variant prothrombin molecules that are incompletely γ-carboxylated demonstrate that a full or nearly full complement of γ-carboxyglutamic acid residues is required for normal phospholipid binding and for full activity.[161] Similar results have been found for bovine prothrombin.[164]

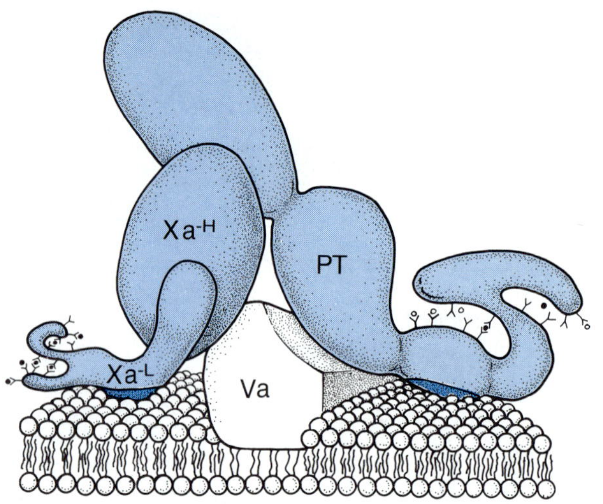

FIGURE 40-13. A model for protein complex formation associated with zymogen activation. The proteins involved in blood coagulation assemble on membrane surfaces. The interaction of calcium ions with the γ-carboxyglutamic acids on the vitamin K–dependent proteins stabilizes a conformer of the protein that expresses a membrane binding site. This assembly facilitates enzyme–substrate interaction. The protein cofactor may have a regulatory role in this complex. Xa^{-L}, light-chain enzyme; Xa^{-H} heavy-chain enzyme; PT, prothrombin substrate; Va, cofactor; open and filled circles, calcium ions; dark patch, lipid binding sites; Y, γ-carboxyglutamic acid. (After Furie B, Furie BC. Molecular basis of blood coagulation. Cell 1988;53:505)

Membrane-Binding Properties

In the presence of metal ions, prothrombin assumes a metal-stabilized conformation that interacts with phospholipid vesicles.[119,135] This conformational transition involves most, if not all, of the γ-carboxyglutamic acid residues.[161] Prothrombin has a strong preference for phospholipid vesicles composed of acidic phospholipids, specifically phosphatidylserine.[135] Interaction of prothrombin with phospholipid vesicles containing phosphatidylserine and phosphatidylcholine requires calcium ions; a binding constant, K_d, of 2.3 μmol/L describes this interaction.[165,168,169] The precise phospholipid binding site is not known, but it is contained within the fragment 1 (residues 1 to 155) region.[170] Kinetic studies suggest that the fragment 2 region of prothrombin (residues 156 to 271)[168,171] contains a site that interacts with the heavy chain of the factor Va cofactor.[172] Preliminary data indicate that the light chain of factor Xa interacts with the light chain of factor Va.[173,174]

Although artificial membranes can support the activation of prothrombin in vitro, the chemical nature of the membrane surfaces that support in vivo activation of prothrombin is not certain. There is no evidence of equilibrium binding of prothrombin to cell surfaces.

Assembly of the Prothrombinase Complex

The activation of prothrombin requires the assembly of the enzyme, factor Xa, and the active cofactor, factor Va, on phospholipid vesicles in the presence of calcium ions (Fig. 40-13). This macromolecular assembly—called the prothrombinase complex—efficiently cleaves prothrombin to thrombin.[175,176] A mathematical model of this process has been developed to simulate the kinetics of prothrombin activation by the prothrombinase complex.[177] If factor Va or if phospholipid membranes are deleted from the system, the relative rate of conversion of prothrombin decreases from 100% to 0.13% and 0.008%, respectively. If both factor Va and phospholipid membranes are removed from the activation mixture, the relative rate of prothrombin activation is decreased from 100% to 0.0007%. Factor Xa alone activates prothrombin at a relative rate of 0.0003%. Therefore, formation of the complete prothrombinase complex enhances the rate of factor Xa activation of prothrombin to thrombin about 300,000 times.

Although prothrombin alone does not bind to cells, the prothrombinase complex assembles on cell surfaces. Prothrombinase activity has been detected on platelets, endothelial cells,[182,183] monocytes, leukocytes[184,185] and diseased aorta.[187] Platelets bind about 1000 factor Va molecules with high affinity.[178] These high-affinity sites are not accessible to factor V, which binds to lower-affinity sites. Once bound, factor Va provides the receptor for factor Xa interaction.[179,180] Although the liver is the primary site of synthesis for factor V, factor V is also synthesized in megakaryocytes and stored in platelet α granules along with other proteins. On platelet stimulation and activation, platelet factor V is secreted and immediately binds to the plasma membrane in an active form (factor Va).[181]

Activation of Prothrombin

The proteolytic events leading to in vitro activation of prothrombin have been well characterized (Fig. 40-14). Prothrombin is converted to thrombin by the action of the enzyme, factor Xa, in a reaction that requires calcium ions and is greatly accelerated by factor Va and phospholipid vesicles.[175] Activation requires the sequential cleavage of at least two peptide bonds.[186–193] The cleavage of the Arg 271–Thr 272 bond yields prothrombin fragment 1·2 and prethrombin 2. The cleavage of the Arg 322–Ile 323 bond in prethrombin 2 then yields fully active thrombin that contains two chains, A and B, connected by a disulfide bond.[194] The precursor, prethrombin 2, has no enzymatic activity. Cleavage of prothrombin instead of prethrombin

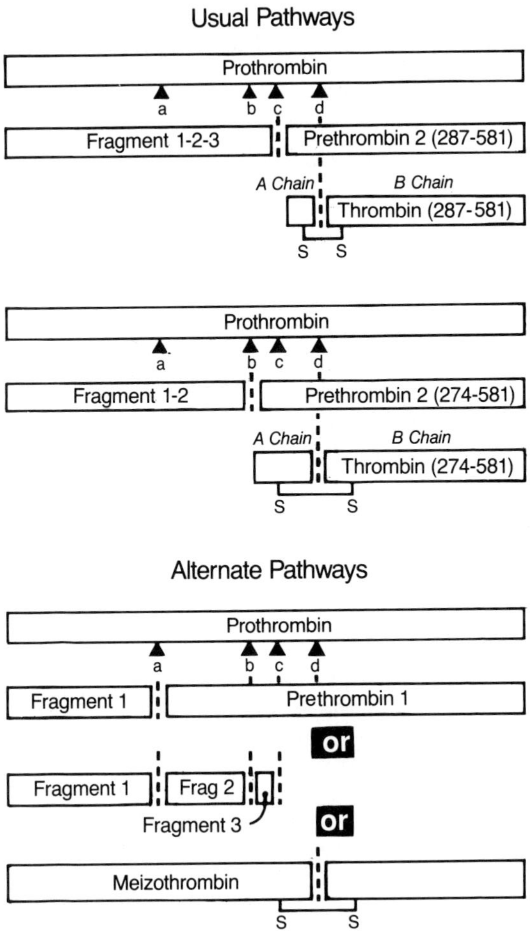

FIGURE 40-14. Activation pathways of human prothrombin. Prothrombin is cleaved at up to four sites (*arrowheads labeled a to d*) during activation to thrombin. Cleavage sites d and either b or c are required for thrombin formation. The intermediates that are generated depend on the conditions of the reaction. In plasma, it appears that the cleavage of bonds c and d occur without the cleavage at a and b.

2 at the Arg 322–Ile 323 bond generates meizothrombin, a form of thrombin that has enzymatic activity toward small synthetic substrates but that does not proteolyze macromolecular substrates.[195] Specifically, meizothrombin does not convert fibrinogen to fibrin. In vitro, thrombin generated during the activation of prothrombin can cleave the Arg 155–Ser 156 bond in prothrombin to yield fragment 1 (residues 1 to 155), and prethrombin 1 or the Arg 155–Ser 156 bond in fragment 1·2 to yield fragment 1 and fragment 2.[196]

During prothrombin activation in plasma, fragments 1 and 2 are not generated, indicating that the Arg 155–Ser 156 bond is not cleaved by thrombin under physiologic conditions.[197] When human prothrombin is activated in plasma, fragment 1·2·3 and a shortened form of prethrombin 2 are formed by the cleavage of Arg 284–Thr 286.[198] Under these conditions, cleavage of the Arg 271–Thr 272 bond observed in vitro is not seen. The precise activation pathway for the in vivo generation of thrombin is not certain. Antibodies that detect fragment 1·2 cross-react with fragment 1·2·3.[199] Therefore, of the four bonds in prothrombin that potentially could be cleaved during prothrombin activation, two (see Fig. 40-14, bonds c and d) are definitely cleaved, one (bond b) may be cleaved, and one (bond a) is not cleaved.

The in vivo activation of prothrombin can be monitored by the appearance of circulating fragment 1·2/fragment 1·2·3.[200] Given the pathways described above, the generation of each thrombin molecule generates either a fragment 1·2 or fragment 1·2·3 molecule. Thus, the plasma fragment 1·2 level accurately reflects the in vivo activation of prothrombin. The measurement of prothrombin activation by this methodology offers considerable insight into hypercoagulable states.[201] Studies with this technique have shown elevation of fragment 1·2 in patients with antithrombin III deficiency and protein C deficiency. These elevations may reflect low-grade subclinical clotting.

Structure and Function of Thrombin

As described earlier, α-thrombin (38 kd), the enzyme derived from the activation of prothrombin, contains two disulfide-linked polypeptide chains. The A chain has a molecular mass of 5 kd and the B chain has a molecular mass of 32 kd. The B chain shows remarkable sequence homology to trypsin, with about 70% of residues conserved.[158,127] It is possible to align the sequences of bovine trypsin and bovine thrombin and achieve maximum homology placing several small deletions and insertions in the thrombin molecule.[151] Thrombin contains the typical active site catalytic triad. Histidine 365, aspartic acid 419, and serine 527 correspond to residues 57, 102, and 195 in the chymotrypsin numbering system. These residues are in immediate proximity to each other in the active site, and are responsible for the *charge relay system* in all serine proteases. Thrombin is a trypsin-like serine protease, requiring an arginine or lysine in the substrate adjacent to the sessile bond. Thrombin specificity is defined by aspartic acid 521, which forms a salt bridge with the positively charged amino acid (lysine or arginine) in the substrate.

Although thrombin substrate specificity is similar to that of trypsin when cleaving small peptide or ester substrates,[203–205] the action of thrombin on proteins is highly selective.[202] Although all thrombin substrates contain an arginine or a lysine adjacent to the sessile bond, the extended binding site surrounding the active site of thrombin must be complementary to the protein substrate for efficient peptide bond hydrolysis.[151] A common cleavage site in thrombin substrates is X-Pro-Arg-↓-X.[202] Fibrinogen is an important natural substrate for thrombin.[202] Cleavage of the Arg 16–Gly 17 bond in the Aα chain leads to the release of fibrinopeptide A and the polymerization of fibrin. Cleavage of the Arg 14–Gly 15 bond in the Bβ chain leads to the release of fibrinopeptide B. Thrombin also cleaves two critical bonds in factor VIII, both adjacent to Arg 372 and to Arg 1689, that leads to the expression of factor VIIIa activity.[206] Similarly, thrombin cleaves two critical bonds in factor V, leading to the expression of the active cofactor, factor Va.[207,208] Other physiologically important substrates include factor XIII[209] and glycoprotein V on platelets cleared by thrombin.[210]

The platelet thrombin receptor has been identified and molecular clones have been obtained. Thrombin activates the receptor in a unique manner by hydrolyzing an N-terminal fragment, thereby producing a new amino terminal–activating peptide.[210a]

Thrombin also serves as a substrate. α-Thrombin undergoes limited autodigestion in vitro, with hydrolysis of the B chain from a molecular mass of 32 to 28 kd.[211] This produces β-thrombin, which cannot convert fibrinogen to fibrin but which retains hydrolytic activity toward small synthetic substrates. Autolysis of β-thrombin to γ-thrombin is associated with further reduction of the B chain to a molecular mass of 15 kd and total loss of enzymatic activity.

After activation, thrombin only circulates briefly in plasma. Several proteins inhibit thrombin function. Antithrombin III, also known as heparin cofactor, forms a complex with thrombin that completely inhibits coagulant activity.[212,213] The formation kinetics of this complex are greatly accelerated by heparin.[214] Antithrombin III plays a critical role in regulating blood coagulation by scavenging active thrombin molecules that have wandered from tissue injury and bleeding sites. Other plasma inhibitors of thrombin that are of possible physiologic importance include α_2-macroglobulin[215] and α_1-antiprotease.[216] Measurement of the thrombin–antithrombin complex may be a useful quantitative marker of thrombin generation.[201,223,224]

Hirudin is a potent anticoagulant found in leeches[217] that binds to thrombin and inhibits thrombin function. Although natural hirudin is not abundant, recombinant hirudin and analogues of hirudin may eventually prove useful as pharmacologic agents for anticoagulant therapy.

Physiology of Prothrombin

Prothrombin is synthesized exclusively in the liver within the hepatocyte.[19–21] Although the control mechanisms that regulate prothrombin gene expression and biosynthesis are unknown, the prothrombin level in plasma is tightly controlled at 100 μg/mL.[218,219] A biologic activity known as coagulopoetin II has been described.[220,221] This material increases the level of prothrombin. Under normal conditions, prothrombin does not form a complex with other plasma proteins but circulates free in the blood in its zymogen form. The basal conversion rate of prothrombin to thrombin is low in the absence of tissue injury. Even in the event of localized clot formation, the prothrombin level does not change measureably, indicating that minimal amounts of prothrombin are consumed while generating physiologically relevant quantities of thrombin.[222] The plasma half-life of prothrombin is about 3 days.

Warfarin sodium and other vitamin K antagonists inhibit the posttranslational γ-carboxylation of prothrombin.[61,62] Warfarin also inhibits synthesis of prothrombin antigen, as shown by a 30% decrease in total prothrombin antigen in the plasma of patients treated with warfarin.[219]

FACTOR X

Gene Structure

The factor X gene is 22 kb long and is located on the long arm of chromosome 13 at 13q34. As indicated in Figure 40-15, the coding region is found on eight separate exons.[154] Exon I encodes the signal peptide. Exon II encodes the propeptide and Gla domain. Exon III codes for the aromatic amino acid stack domain. Exons IV and V each code the EGF-like regions of factor X. Exon VI encodes the activation domain of factor X, whereas exons VII and VIII encode the catalytic domain. The organization of the factor X gene is nearly identical to that of factors IX and VII and protein C. After transcription, a factor X message is generated that is about 1.5 kb long.[96] This messenger RNA includes a short 3′ untranslated region of 10 nucleotides that follow the stop codon TGA. The polyadenylation site is embedded in the 3′ end of the coding sequence.

Protein Structure

Factor X (56 kd) is synthesized as a single chain[94,96] but is converted to a two-chain zymogen that circulates in the plasma. The heavy chain of bovine and human factor X has a molecular mass of about 38 kd[128,225,226]; the light chain

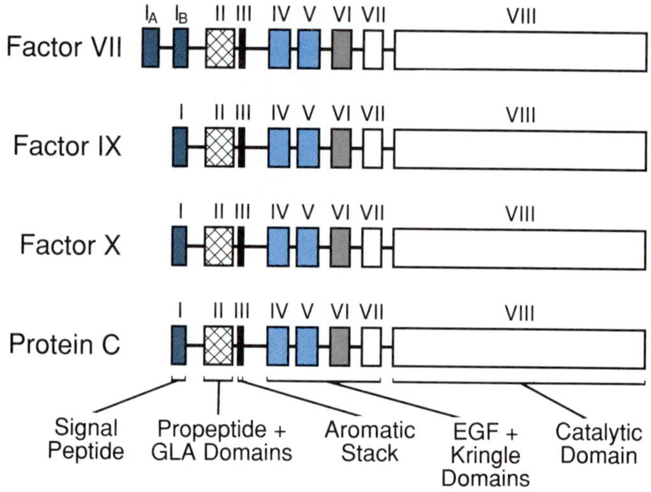

FIGURE 40-15. Gene structure of human factor X, factor VII, factor IX, and protein C. Exons are shown schematically according to scale. Introns, indicated by double lines, are not drawn to scale. (After Furie B, Furie BC. Molecular basis of blood coagulation. Cell 1988;53:505)

is about 18 kd.[103,104] The primary structure of human factor X, extrapolated from the cDNA of factor X,[94,96] is shown in Figure 40-16. The three amino acids Arg-Lys-Arg at residues 139 to 141 are removed from the single chain by cleavage of the Arg 139–Lys 140 bond and of the Arg 141–Ser 142 bond. This generates the light chain (residues 1 to 139) and the heavy chain (residues 142 to 445).[96] This segment may be removed within the cell, but the presence of some single-chain factor X circulating in the plasma suggests that cleavage is inefficient or that the process is also extracellular.

The light chain of human factor X includes 11 γ-carboxyglutamic acid residues, and the first EGF domain includes a single β-hydroxyaspartic acid at residue 63.[27,97] γ-Carboxyglutamic acid residues are found at positions 6, 7, 14, 16, 19, 20, 25, 26, 29, 32, and 39.[105] The activation peptide is cleaved from the heavy chain during activation of factor X by the factor IXa–factor VIIIa complex or by the factor VIIa–tissue factor complex to yield the enzyme, factor Xa.[227,228] It remains closely associated with factor Xa.[230] The remaining portion of the heavy chain contains the catalytic region homologous to trypsin. Nonphysiologic activation of factor X by the coagulant protein of Russell's viper venom yields the same reaction products.[229,230] The catalytic triad characteristic of the serine proteases includes Ser 233, His 93, and Asp 138 in bovine factor X.[231] The process of factor X activation involves functionally significant but structurally subtle conformational changes in factor X.[233]

Bovine factor X contains both asparagine-linked carbohydrate of Asp 36 and threonine-linked carbohydrate at Thr 300.[234] The complex asparagine-linked oligosaccharides have NeuAcα2 → 3Galβ1 → 3(NeuAcα2 → 6)GlcNAc components in the outer chain.

Assembly of Factor X on Membrane Surfaces

Factor X is a metal-binding protein that contains two or three high-affinity sites and multiple lower-affinity sites.[112,117] Factor X undergoes a conformational transition during metal binding that leads to the expression of both lipid-binding sites and new antigenic determinants.[135,165,166,169,235] The concentration of calcium that induces the half-maximal transition is about 200 μmol/L.

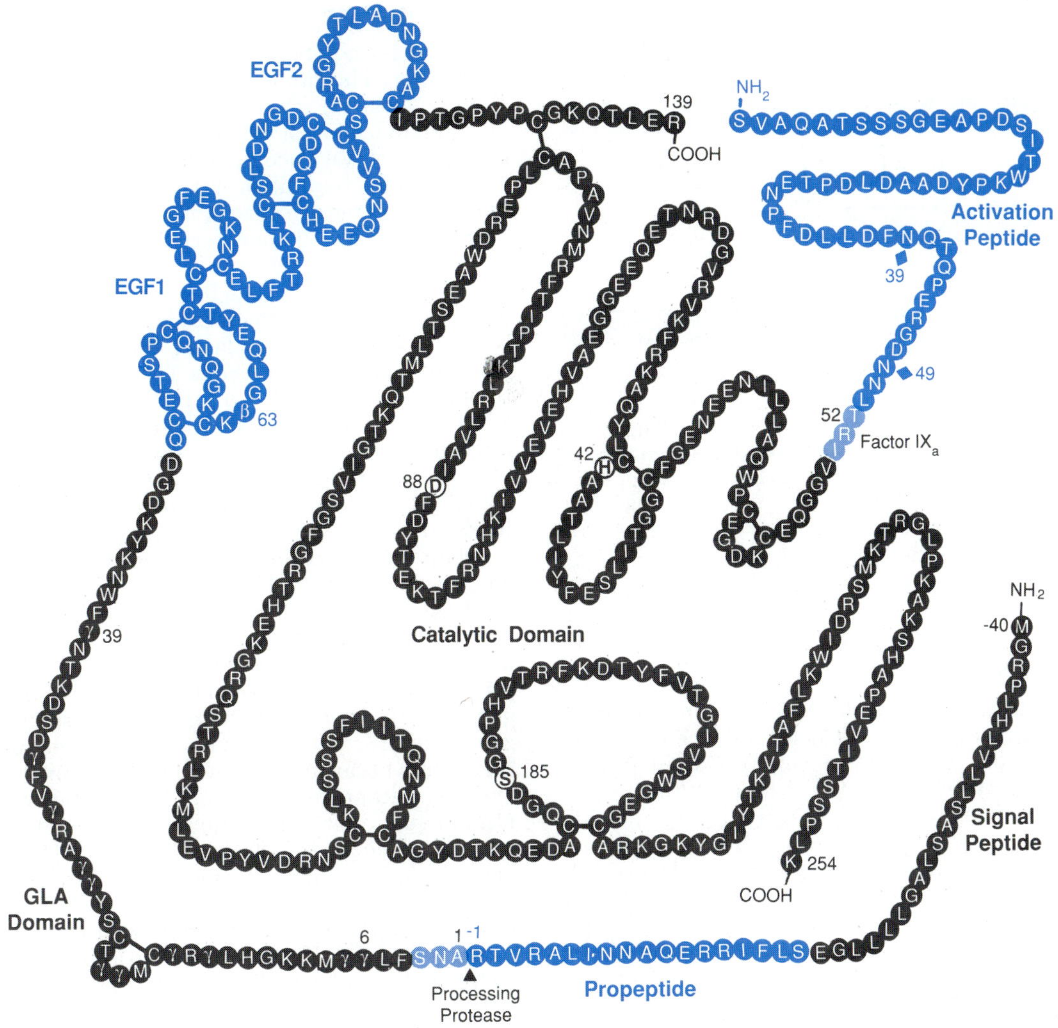

FIGURE 40-16. Amino acid sequence of human factor X.

Factor X binds to phospholipid vesicles in the presence of calcium ions with a preference for acidic phospholipids (eg, phosphatidylserine) that is characteristic of the vitamin K–dependent proteins.[169]

Factor Xa is the enzyme component of the prothrombinase complex. This complex includes factor Xa and factor Va and assembles on phospholipid surfaces in the presence of calcium ions. The characteristics of this complex, which catalyzes the conversion of prothrombin to thrombin,[136] are described in the section on prothrombin.

Factor Xa also binds tightly to platelet membranes in the presence of factor Va, catalyzing the conversion of prothrombin to thrombin.[180,236] Thrombin-activated platelets express about 300 factor Xa binding sites, whereas resting platelets do not bind to factor Xa. The interaction of factor Xa and activated platelets is of high affinity, with a binding constant of 3×10^{-11} mol/L determined.[180,236] The factor Xa binding site appears to be defined by factor V,[179,237] and activation of platelets leads to the secretion of factor Va from the α granules. Patients with factor V deficiency lack the expression of factor Xa binding sites.[181]

Activation of Factor X

Factor X is activated by the cleavage of a single peptide bond between Arg 51 and Ile 52 on the heavy chain[229,231] (Fig. 40-17). The activation peptide (1 to 51) remains noncovalently associated with factor Xa.[230] Cleavage of a peptide bond near the carboxy terminal is considered a side reaction with no functional consequences.[228] Several proteases are physiologically important activators of factor X, including factors IXa and VIIa. Other factor X activators play a pathologic role. For example, activation of factor X by trypsin may occur under pathologic conditions, as in severe pancreatitis. Factor X activator has been isolated from lung carcinoma tissue.[238,239] Furthermore, the coagulant protein in Russell's viper venom activates factor X.[230,231,240] This activity contributes to the bleeding syndrome that follows the bite of the Russell's viper.

Factor X is activated by a membrane complex composed of factors IXa and VIIIa that is generated by the intrinsic pathway of blood coagulation.[229,241] This reaction requires phospholipid vesicles and calcium, although cell surfaces may play an essential role in vivo. This complex is assembled on endothelial cell surfaces[242] and on artificial lipid membranes composed of acidic phospholipids.[243] Alternatively, factor X can be activated by the extrinsic pathway of blood coagulation by a membrane complex composed of factor VIIa and tissue factor.[244] The expression of tissue factor activity (a transmembrane protein found on many cell types) and the formation of a factor VIIa–tissue factor complex activates factor X. Factor X activated by either pathway is associated with the cleavage of the same peptide bond.

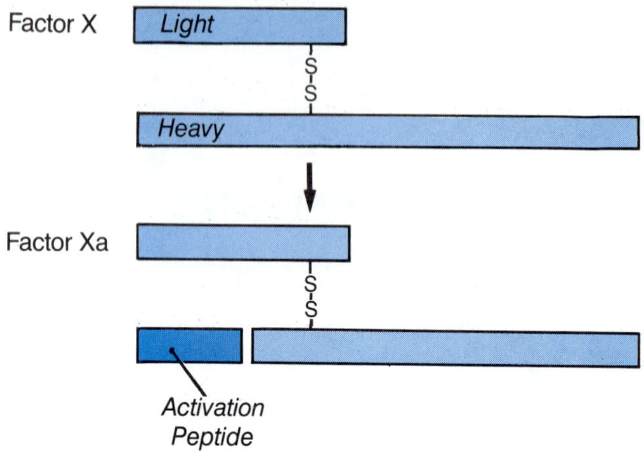

FIGURE 40-17. Activation of factor X. Factor X is activated to factor Xa by the factor IXa–factor VIII complex or the factor VIIa–tissue factor complex. A single bond is cleaved, generating an activation peptide.

Regulation of Factor X

The plasma concentration of factor X is maintained at about 10 μg/mL. The regulation of the factor X concentration is precise, but its molecular basis is uncertain. Coagulopoietin X, a heat stable material that is able to increase the plasma concentration of factor X, might play a role in this process.[245]

Factor Xa is inhibited by three of the major plasma protease inhibitors in the absence of heparin: antithrombin III, α_1-antitrypsin, and α_2-macroglobulin.[213,246,247] Although in vitro experiments have suggested that antithrombin III and α_1-proteinase inhibitor play a dominant role in the inhibition of factor Xa,[246] in vivo experiments suggest that α_2-macroglobulin is a major physiologic regulator of factor Xa.[247]

FACTOR VII

Gene Structure

The factor VII gene spans 13 kb[156] and is located on the long arm of chromosome 13 at 13q34, adjacent to the factor X gene.[248] The coding region is located on nine separate exons. Two alternate forms of preprofactor VII have been identified. One form, incorporating exon I, arises from a gene analogous to the factor X, factor IX, and protein C genes. The second form arises from a gene containing a ninth exon, exon Ia, which codes for a polypeptide extension of the NH_2 terminal that elongates the prepropeptide from 38 to 60 residues. The significance of these two preprofactor VII forms is unknown. Exon II encodes the propeptide and Gla domain. Exon III codes for the aromatic amino acid stack domain, a short linking segment common to all of the vitamin K–dependent proteins. Exons IV and V each code the EGF-like regions of factor VII. Exon VI encodes the activation domain of factor VII, whereas exons VII and VIII code the catalytic domain. The organization of the factor VII sere is nearly identical to that of factors IX and X and protein C. After transcription, a factor VII message is generated that is about 2.4 kb,[95] which contains a 3′ untranslated region of 1 kb and a poly(A) tail after the stop codon. This untranslated region also contains the polyadenylation sequence.

Protein Structure

Factor VII is a component of the extrinsic pathway of blood coagulation. This protein circulates in the blood as a single-chain zymogen,[249,250] with a molecular mass of about 50 kd. Human factor VII contains 406 amino acids,[95] whereas bovine factor VII is composed of 407 amino acids[107] (Fig. 40-18). These two factor VII forms show 71% sequence identity. Activation of factor VII occurs after the cleavage of an Arg 152–Ile 153 bond, leading to a two-chain form—factor VIIa, with a light chain and heavy chain linked by a disulfide bond.[251–253] The light chain contains 152 amino acids, and the heavy chain contains 254 amino acids. The NH_2-terminal domain of factor VII, identical to the light chain of factor VIIa, contains 11 γ-carboxyglutamic acid residues at positions 6, 7, 14, 16, 19, 20, 25, 26, 29, 34, and 35 in the bovine sequence.[107] As observed in factor IX, the aspartic acid in the first EGF domain, located at residue 63, is only 20% to 30% β-hydroxylated. The heavy chain contains the catalytic domain, homologous in structure and function to trypsin.

Factor VII, a glycoprotein, contains 13% carbohydrate by weight. One carbohydrate chain is linked to Asn 145 in the light chain. Another carbohydrate chain is linked to Asn 203 in the heavy chain.[107] The precise structure of the carbohydrate in factor VII is not known.

Unlike other blood coagulation proenzymes, the zymogen form of factor VII is thought to express significant enzyme activity.[254] It still remains to be demonstrated that this occurs because of the intrinsic enzyme activity of the zymogen rather than contamination of the zymogen with minute quantities of activated factor VII. To date, the observation of enzyme activity in the zymogen has been based on kinetic arguments rather than direct biochemical analysis.

Factor VII is activated to factor VIIa by thrombin, factor Xa or factor XIIa.[251,253] Factor VIIa, in a complex with tissue factor, activates factor X.

Assembly of Factor VII on Membranes

Tissue factor is a receptor protein, expressed on cell membranes, that is required for the activation of the extrinsic pathway of blood coagulation. Tissue factor is expressed constitutively on many extravascular cells; in addition, monocytes[264,265] and endothelial cells[242,266,267] can be induced to express tissue factor. Neoplastic cells can also express tissue factor.[268] This protein, which contains both lipid and carbohydrate, has an estimated molecular mass of 45 kd[255–257] and forms a calcium-dependent complex with factor VII on cell surfaces.[263] This tissue factor–factor VII complex then activates factor X to factor Xa, or factor IX to factor IXa.[258,259] The structure of tissue factor has recently been determined.[260,261] Tissue factor is a transmembrane protein composed of 263 amino acids. The largest domain, containing the NH_2 terminal, is extracellular and oriented toward the blood. A domain containing 23 amino acids, most with hydrophobic properties, spans the cell membrane. A small, 21–amino acid cytoplasmic domain includes the COOH terminal. This tail contains two fatty acids, palmitate and stearate, bound by a thioester bond to a free cysteine.[262]

Substrates of Tissue Factor–Factor VIIa Complex

Both factor VII and factor VIIa bind to tissue factor on cell surfaces, but the mechanism by which the initial factor VIIa is generated remains uncertain. One speculation is

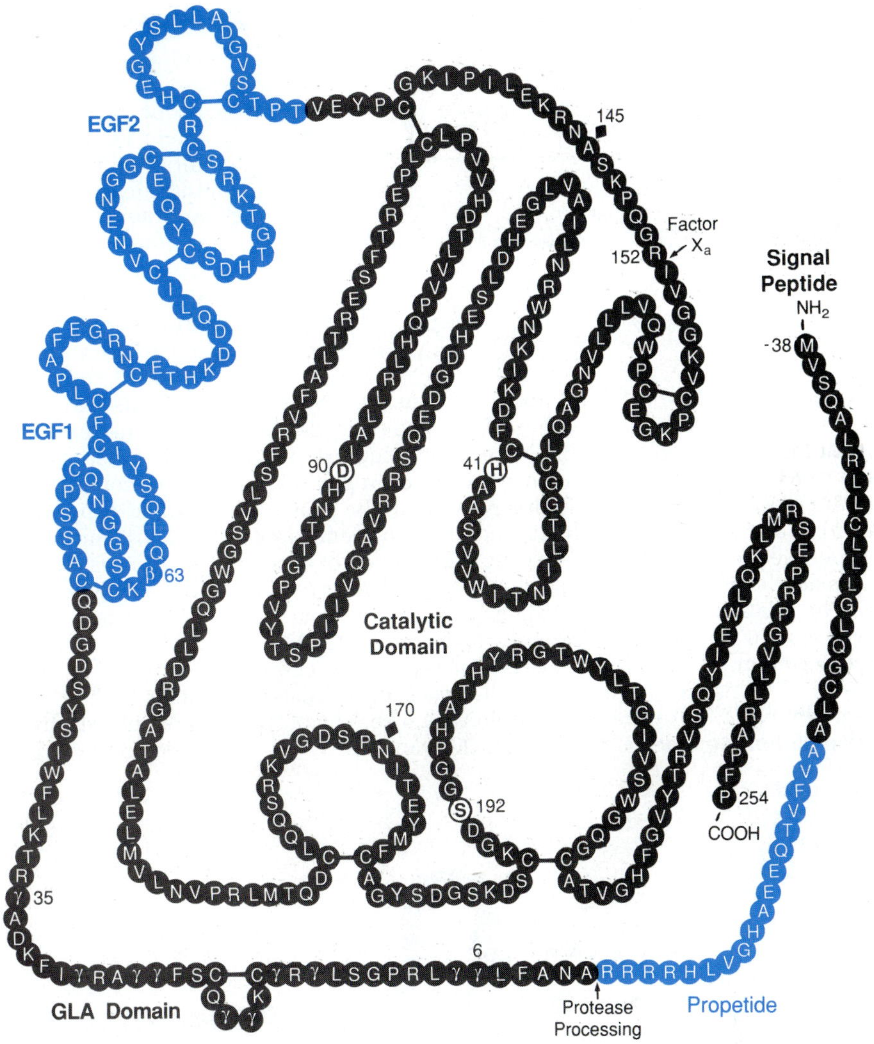

FIGURE 40-18. Amino acid sequence of human factor VII.

that factor VII is an active enzyme but considerably less active than factor VIIa.[254] The tissue factor–factor VII complex activates factor X to factor Xa. Factor Xa can then catalyze the conversion of factor VII to factor VIIa, increasing the efficiency of factor X activation.[269] Alternatively, perhaps another enzyme that is tissue associated converts factor VII to factor VIIa. The control of tissue factor–factor VII initiation of blood coagulation remains a major unresolved question.

The tissue factor–factor VII complex has two physiologically important substrates. Although this reaction has traditionally been viewed as a critical event in thrombin generation in the extrinsic pathway, the complex also activates factor IX in the intrinsic pathway to factor IXa[258,259] (Fig. 40-19). The rate of factor IX activation by this pathway is about six times slower than the rate of factor X activation by the tissue factor–factor VIIa complex.[270] Although activation is clearly demonstrated in vitro, the physiologic role of this alternate pathway remains unclear. Studies by Bauer and associates[224] suggest that the dominant basal mechanism in vivo is the activation of factor X by the factor VII complex.

Regulation of Factor VII

The plasma concentration of factor VII, 500 ng/mL, is the lowest of the vitamin K–dependent blood coagulation proteins. For this reason, less information is available about factor VII than about the other vitamin K–dependent proteins. Unlike the other serine proteases involved in blood coagulation, factor VIIa is not inhibited by antithrombin III.[271] The recent discovery of a lipoprotein-associated coagulation inhibitor that inhibits the tissue factor–factor VII complex suggests a regulatory role for this protein.[273–276] This protein, tissue factor inhibitor or LACI, first forms a complex with factor Xa, which in turn forms a complex with tissue factor–factor VII in the presence of calcium ions.[277]

FACTOR IX

Gene Structure

The factor IX gene is 34 kb, but only a limited amount of this DNA codes for the factor IX protein. The seven introns range in size from 188 nucleotides to almost 10 kb.[155] The gene is found on the tip of the long arm of the X chromosome, Xq26-27.3.[278] The coding region is found on eight separate exons (see Fig. 40-15). The first exon, exon I, codes for the signal peptide. The second exon, exon II, codes for the propeptide and Gla domain of factor IX. Exon III codes for a short linking segment common to all of the vitamin K–dependent proteins. Exons IV and V, separated by a large intron, each code the EGF-like regions of factor IX. Exon VI codes for the activation domain of factor IX, whereas exons VII and VIII code the catalytic domain. In the factor

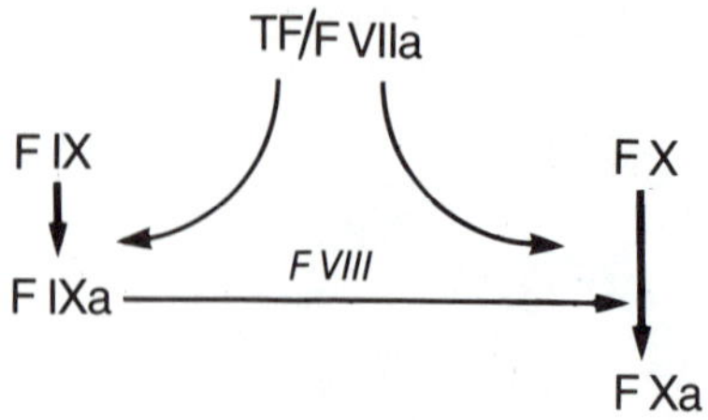

FIGURE 40-19. Alternate pathways of activation of blood coagulation by factor VIIa. The factor VIIa–tissue factor complex can activate factor X or factor IX.

IX gene, the entire catalytic domain is encoded by two exons, unlike prothrombin where five exons encode the homologous domain.[130,152] This observation suggests that the factor IX gene was derived ancestrally from a precursor of the prothrombin gene.[157] Reorganization of the gene by intron deletion led to consolidation of the exons encoding the serine protease domain. The gene organization of factor IX is nearly identical to that of factors X and VII and protein C. The relationship of this gene family to the prothrombin gene is shown by comparing Figures 40-10 and 40-15. After transcription, a factor IX message is generated that is about 2.8 kb.[23,92] This messenger RNA includes a 5′ untranslated region and a long 3′ untranslated region of 1.4 kb. The polyadenylation sequence is near the poly(A) tail.

Protein Structure

Human factor IX is a single-chain protein composed of 415 amino acids[23,92,106] (Fig. 40-20). It is a glycoprotein containing about 17% carbohydrate, and both bovine and human factor IX have a molecular mass of 56 kd.[279,280] The NH_2-terminal Gla domain includes 12 γ-carboxyglutamic acid residues at residues 7, 8, 15, 17, 20, 21, 26, 27, 30, 33, 36, and 40.[97,98] A small loop formed by cysteine residues at residues 18 and 23 is common to all of the vitamin K–dependent blood clotting proteins. As previously discussed, the Gla domain defines some of the metal-binding properties of factor IX, although the EGF domain also contains metal-binding sites.[281] Following a short linking segment, factor IX contains two adjacent EGF domains. These EGF domains are characterized by a segment of 53 amino acids and a pattern of disulfide-bonded cysteine residues, but their function is unknown. The first of the two EGF domains contains an unusual amino acid, β-hydroxyaspartic acid, at residue 64.[27] This modified amino acid is formed by posttranslational modification of aspartic acid. β-Hydroxyaspartic acid and β-hydroxyasparagine are found in the EGF domains of all of the vitamin K–dependent proteins except prothrombin, which lacks EGF domains, as well as in other proteins.[26,88] From the cDNA derived for factor IX,[23,92] factor X,[96] protein C,[282,283] protein S,[284] and factor VII,[95] it is apparent that specific aspartic acid or asparagine residues in precursor forms of these proteins undergo β-hydroxylation posttranslationally. The function

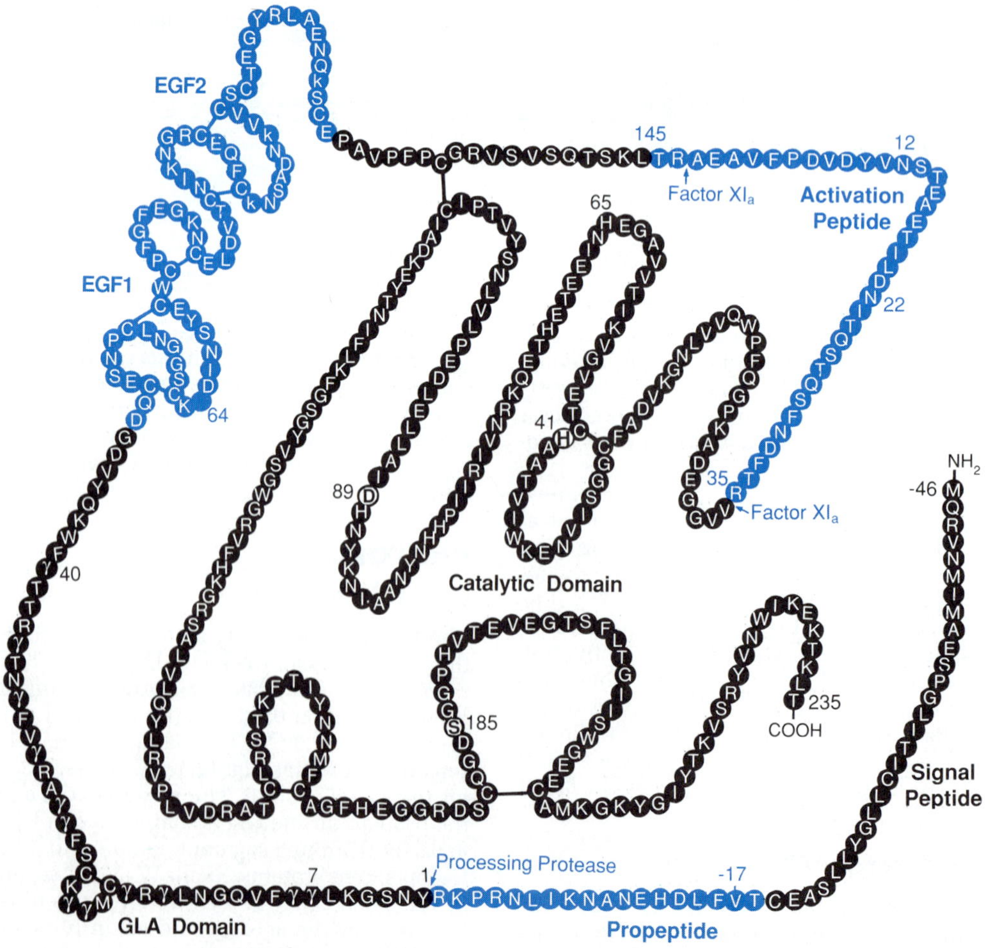

FIGURE 40-20. Amino acid sequence of human factor IX.

of β-hydroxyaspartic acid is unknown. Stern and coworkers[285] implicated this domain in the binding of factor IX and factor IXa to endothelial cells by demonstrating that a synthetic peptide (based on residues 47 to 54) inhibits protein–cell interaction. Furthermore, factor IX Alabama (Asp 47 → Gly), which binds to phospholipid vesicles,[286] does not bind to endothelial cells.[287] The remainder of factor IX demonstrates marked sequence homology to zymogens of serine proteases, such as trypsin. This region is almost 250 amino acids long and contains the enzymatic activity of factor IXa in latent form. The cleavage of two peptide bonds in factor IX leads to the generation of the enzyme, factor IXa.

Calcium-Binding Properties of Factor IX

Factor IX in its carboxylated form binds to metal ions. As with the other vitamin K–dependent proteins, there are two classes of metal-binding sites: one with high affinity for divalent cations and one with low affinity for divalent cations.[115] Although the Gla domain contains some of these metal-binding sites,[281] a highly conserved series of aspartic acid residues in the first EGF domain form another calcium-binding site.[87] For example, factor IX that is chemically modified by the removal of the Gla domain still retains calcium-binding properties.[281] The γ-carboxyglutamic acid–rich domain is responsible for the metal-dependent interaction of these proteins with membranes.[22] The β-hydroxyaspartic acid–containing EGF domain may also be important for cell membrane recognition. Rees and Brownlee have suggested that Asp 64 in factor IX may be part of a calcium-binding site and that mutation of Asp 64 inactivates factor IX.[87] These results suggest that Asp 64 in the EGF domain may define a metal-binding site and that the EGF domain may be critical for protein–cell membrane interaction.

Membrane-Binding Properties of Factor IX

The interaction of factor IX and factor IXa with phospholipid membranes has been studied using phosphatidylserine–phosphatidylcholine vesicles.[134,286] Factor IX binds to vesicles in the presence of Ca(II) but not in the presence of Mg(II) or EDTA. Furthermore, des-γ-carboxy factor IX, prepared from warfarinized plasma, does not interact with phospholipid vesicles even in the presence of Ca(II).[134] These results emphasize the importance of the γ-carboxyglutamic acid–rich region in defining the phospholipid binding properties. Furthermore, factor IX Alabama (Asp 47 → Gly), which can bind to artificial phospholipid vesicles, does not bind to cellular membranes.[286] The interaction of factor IX and factor IXa with cell membranes, however, is characterized by a different pattern. For example, factor IX and factor IXa bind to endothelial cells,[242] and a receptor protein of 140 kd has been identified.[289] Gla-domainless factor IX[281] can bind to endothelial cells. Therefore, the interaction of factor IX with phospholipid vesicles is independent of a protein cofactor, whereas the interaction of factor IX with endothelial cells involves a receptor protein. Activated platelets, but not resting platelets, bind factor IX and factor IXa.[290,291] Neither the nature of the platelet factor IX binding site nor the actual surfaces on factor IX that are required for interaction with cell membranes are known. Furthermore, the importance of factor VIII to the cell membrane (eg, as a receptor protein) remains uncertain.

Factor IX undergoes two conformational transitions that are metal induced and lead to the expression of a phospholipid binding site.[134] The first conformational transition is induced by a large number of divalent and trivalent metal ions and associated with quenching of the intrinsic fluorescence. The second conformational transition is induced primarily by calcium ions and is associated with the expression of the phospholipid binding site.

Activation of Factor IX

The activation of factor IX by factor IXa is highly metal selective,[115,288] with optimal activation achieved only in the presence of Ca(II); suboptimal activation occurs in the presence of Sr(II). Although the proteolytic activity of factor XIa is present on the light chain, the heavy chain of factor XIa may be necessary for the Ca(II)-dependent acceleration of factor IX activation.[292–294] Because the factor IX-phospholipid interaction is inhibited by anti-factor IX: Ca(II)-specific antibodies and the metal requirements parallel those for activation by factor XIa, a chemical similarity between a domain of factor XIa that interacts with factor IX and phospholipid vesicles in the presence of Ca(II) has been suggested.[134] On the basis of antibody inhibition studies using both antibodies to factor XIa[294] and to factor IX,[134] the heavy chain of factor XIa is implicated in the specific binding of the phospholipid binding site of factor IX in the presence of Ca(II).

Factor IX is converted to its enzyme form, factor IXa, by factor XIa (Fig. 40-21). This reaction requires calcium ions but takes place in solution. In contrast to the activation of other vitamin K–dependent blood clotting proteins, membrane surfaces (including phospholipid vesicles or cell surfaces) do not enhance factor IX activation. Activation of factor IX requires the cleavage of two peptide bonds, one located at Arg 145–Ala 146 and the other at Arg 180–Val 181.[295,296] With the release of the internal carbohydrate-rich activation fragment from residues 146 to 180, the factor IXa light chain (17 kd) and heavy chain (28 kd) remain bound by a single disulfide bond. The serine protease activity is associated with the heavy chain.

Once generated, factor IXa forms a complex with factor VIIIa on membrane surfaces in an interaction that is calcium dependent. This enzyme complex on the membrane

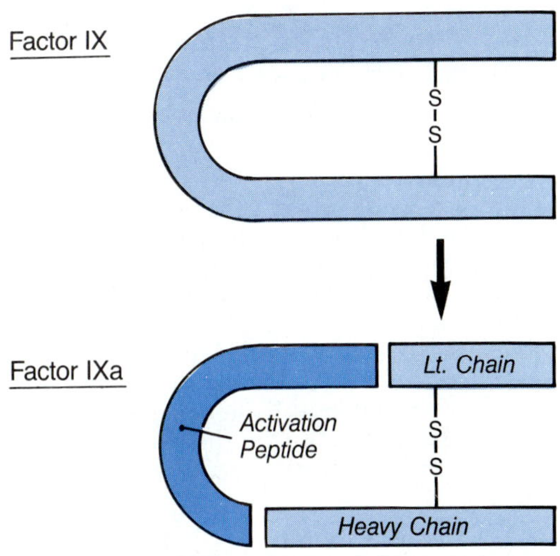

FIGURE 40-21. Activation of factor IX. Factor IX is activated by factor XIa or by the tissue factor–factor VIIa complex in a reaction that requires calcium ions. Factor IX requires the cleavage of two peptide bonds to generate factor IXa. An internal activation peptide is released during activation and a two-chain factor IXa results from proteolytic activation.

is required for activation of factor X at rates that are physiologically significant.[297] In contrast to the solution-phase activation of factor IX by factor XIa, factor X is converted to its enzyme form, factor Xa, by factor IXa in complex with factor VIIIa on membrane surfaces. This reaction also requires calcium ions. Either phospholipid vesicles or cell surfaces are required for significant factor X activation. Thus, factor IX is a membrane-binding protein, and the presence of γ-carboxyglutamic acid is thought to be intimately related to its membrane-binding properties. Whereas factor IX does not require membrane surface for activation, factor IXa requires a membrane surface to express its enzymatic activity. These proteins may have two distinct binding domains, one related to zymogen activation and the other to macromolecular assembly of the enzyme in complex with the specific cofactor.

Factor X is the physiologic substrate for factor IXa. Some evidence suggests, however, that factor IXa can activate factor VII and factor VIII.[298,299] As with all the trypsin-like serine proteases, factor IXa cleaves at peptide bonds adjacent to the arginine residues.

Regulation of Factor IX

The plasma concentration of factor IX is maintained at 5 μg/mL, but the molecular basis of regulation is not known. With the sequencing of the factor IX gene, several possible regulatory elements have been noted.[155] A TATA box, coded as TGTA, is located 27 nucleotides upstream from a proposed initiation site, which is located 29 nucleotides upstream from the initiator methionine. Other possible TATA sequences are located further upstream. Studying the transcription of factor IX following site-specific mutagenesis of these regions should lead to the identification of important regulatory elements. Recently, the promoter of the factor IX gene has been identified. Mutations in this promoter give rise to a curious form of hemophilia B in which males are born with a severe form of factor IX deficiency that corrects spontaneously during puberty.[300–302] These defects are detailed in the discussion of hemophilia B.

Plasma factor IXa is regulated by the protease inhibitors that modulate the other active blood clotting enzymes. For example, antithrombin III inhibits factor IXa activity.[303,304]

CLINICAL DISORDERS OF VITAMIN K–DEPENDENT PROTEINS

A bleeding tendency is associated with the decrease in biologic activities of the vitamin K–dependent blood coagulation proteins. The extent of this tendency correlates closely with the severity of the deficiency in these protein activities. Some deficiencies in the vitamin K–dependent blood clotting proteins are hereditary. That is, inherited genetic defects that interfere in the synthesis, processing, or normal life span of a protein can cause a bleeding disorder. Other disorders of the vitamin K–dependent proteins are acquired, not inherited. Diseases that interfere with the synthesis of the vitamin K–dependent blood clotting proteins in the liver or defects in the availability or utilization of vitamin K represent prime examples of these disorders.

INHERITED DISORDERS INVOLVING VITAMIN K–DEPENDENT BLOOD CLOTTING PROTEINS

A rare inherited defect in the synthesis of the vitamin K–dependent proteins was initially reported in four families, and additional examples of this defect continue to be observed.[305–307] Deficiency of factor IX, factor X, factor VII and prothrombin activities was observed in two patients.[305,306] These defects were associated with marked prolongation of the partial thromboplastin time, prothrombin time, and clinical bleeding manifestations. Partial correction of this coagulation defect was observed with high doses of vitamin K. Another patient, however, with mild combined deficiency of the vitamin K–dependent proteins did not correct on administration of high doses of vitamin K.[308] In these cases, a defect in vitamin K–dependent carboxylation could be associated with either a defect in vitamin K metabolism (eg, vitamin K absorption and transport, vitamin K reduction) or a defect in the vitamin K carboxylase itself. The discovery of two siblings with a combined carboxylation defect limited to prothrombin and factor X suggests a carboxylation abnormality and not a defect in vitamin K metabolism.[309] The mechanism for such a defect remains speculative, however.

Given the similarity of the carboxylation recognition site on the propeptides of the vitamin K–dependent proteins,[65,69] it remains unclear how a defect in the carboxylase can alter the posttranslational processing of some vitamin K–dependent proteins but not others. The possibility of a family of carboxylating enzymes has not been ruled out but appears unlikely. In the two siblings with combined prothrombin and factor X deficiency, the administration of large doses of vitamin K almost eliminated the synthesis of acarboxy (abnormal) prothrombin.

Disorders of Factor IX

Genetic defects in the vitamin K–dependent blood coagulation proteins may be associated with hemophilia, a disease characterized by increased bleeding connected with trauma or, in its most severe form, spontaneous bleeding. Defects in factor IX (hemophilia B) account for about 10% to 12% of the hereditary disorders of the blood clotting proteins. Correlation of the gene's structural defect to the protein's functional activity has contributed to our understanding of structure–function relation in these proteins and to our knowledge of the molecular basis of hemophilia B.

Hemophilia B is due to either a diminished factor IX antigen or functionally defective factor IX. In about a third of cases, the defective factor IX antigen includes a point mutation.[310] This mutant protein circulates in the blood, although its reduced biologic activity precludes normal participation in the blood clotting process. In other forms of hemophilia B, factor IX is not synthesized because of major defects in its gene structure, or an unstable factor IX is synthesized that is rapidly destroyed.

Point Mutations in Factor IX

As previously discussed, factor IX has a series of domains that carry out specific functions of the factor IX molecule. A point mutation in any of these domains may interfere with factor IX function. A priori, it is reasonable to assume one of the following:

1. A defect in the posttranslational process or a defect in the Gla domain may inhibit membrane binding.
2. A defect in the EGF domains may interfere with protein assembly on membrane surfaces and the interaction with factor VIII.
3. A defect in the activation domain may interfere in the zymogen activation of factor IX to factor IXa.
4. A defect in the active site or the extended substrate-binding site may alter the ability of the mutant factor IX to recognize or to cleave physiologically important substrates (Table 40-3).

TABLE 40-3. Molecular Defects Caused by Point Mutations Known to Cause Hemophilia B

Defect	Location	Phenotype	Reference
PROPEPTIDE POINT MUTATIONS			
FIX Cambridge	Arg −1 → Ser	Severe hemophilia B	Diuguid et al, 1986
FIX Oxford3	Arg −4 → Gln	Severe hemophilia B	Bentley et al, 1986
FIX San Dimas	Arg −4 → Gln	Severe hemophilia B	Ware et al, 1987
POINT MUTATIONS THAT INTERFERE WITH MACROMOLECULAR ASSEMBLY			
FIX Alabama	Asp 47 → Gly	Moderate hemophilia B	Davis et al, 1987
FIX Durham	Gly 60 → Ser	MIld hemophilia B	Denton et al, 1988
POINT MUTATIONS THAT INTERFERE WITH ZYMOGEN ACTIVATION			
FIX Chapel Hill	Arg 145 → His	Moderate hemophilia B	Noyes et al, 1983
FIX Hilo	Arg 180 → Gln	Hemophilia B_M	Huang et al, 1988
FIX Chicago II	Arg 145 → His	Severe hemophilia B	Diuguid et al, 1989
FIX Albuquerque	Arg 145 → Cys	Severe hemophilia B	Toomey et al, 1988
FIX Kashihara	Val 182 → Phe	Hemophilia B	Sakai et al, 1988
POINT MUTATIONS THAT ALTER ENZYME ACTIVITY AND SUBSTRATE BINDING			
FIX Angers	Gly 396 → Arg	Moderate hemophilia B	Vidaud et al, 1988
FIX Lake Elsinore	Ala 390 → Val	Severe hemophilia B_M	Spitzer et al, 1988
FIX Eagle Rock	Gly 363 → Val	Hemophilia B_M	Spitzer et al, 1988
FIX Vancouver	Ile 397 → Thr		
FIX Long Beach	Ile 397 → Thr		
FIX Los Angeles	Ile 397 → Thr	Hemophilia B	Ware et al, 1988

Factor IX Chapel Hill (Arg 145 → His) is the prototype for mutant zymogens that cannot be activated to their enzyme form because of mutation of the arginine adjacent to the sessile bond.[311,312] This mutant was the first hemophiliac factor IX to be characterized at the molecular level and the first identification of a specific point mutation. More recently, factor IX Chicago II and factor IX Albuquerque, discovered in unrelated patients, have the same molecular defect.[313,314] In this mutant form, the arginine adjacent to the cleavage site between the activation peptide and the light chain of factor IXa is substituted so that the sessile bond cannot be cleaved. Cleavage of this bond is necessary for the generation of activated factor IXa, which can act on factor X. In factor IX Hilo, the sessile bond between the activation peptide and the heavy chain cannot be cleaved because of mutation of arginine to glutamine.[315,316] In this mutant, the enzyme cannot be formed because this critical proteolytic event is analogous to the peptide bond cleaved to generate trypsin from trypsinogen. Similarly, factor IX Kashihara (Val 182 → Phe) has a substitution that interferes with the cleavage of the peptide bond between residues 180 and 181, yielding an inactive factor IX.[317]

Factor IX Cambridge (Arg −1 → Ser),[66] factor IX Oxford 3 (Arg −4 → Gln),[67] and factor IX San Dimas (Arg −4 → Gln)[68] contain point mutations in the propeptide domain of the factor IX precursor, profactor IX. In these factor IX mutants, a mutation at position −1 or −4 prevents proteolytic removal of the propeptide by a propeptidase. Failure to cleave the propeptide partially inhibits γ-carboxylation, leading to a protein that cannot bind to phospholipid vesicles or exhibit coagulant activity. Factor IX Cambridge does not undergo the metal-induced conformational change characteristic of factor IX, but factor IX San Dimas does undergo this conformational transition. These results suggest that the distribution of γ-carboxyglutamic acid residues differs in the partially carboxylated factor IX Cambridge and factor IX San Dimas.[68]

Factor IX Alabama (Asp 47 → Gly) probably lacks coagulant activity because it fails to bind to cell membrane surfaces.[142] This mutant, however, with its intact Gla region binds normally to phospholipid vesicles.[286] Alternatively, evidence suggests that this mutant does not bind to factor VIII.[143] Factor IX Durham (Gly 60 → Ser) has been isolated from two presumably unrelated patients with a mild form of hemophilia B.[318] These mutants represent defects in the first EGF domain, but a complete understanding of their functional implications is unavailable.

Point mutations in the catalytic domain have been described in mutant factor IXs isolated from patients with hemophilia B. Factor IX Vancouver (Ile 397 → Thr), factor IX Long Beach (Ile 397 → Thr), and factor IX Los Angeles (Ile 397 → Thr) share the same point mutation.[319–321] Residue 397 is near but not in the active site of factor IXa. The precise mechanism by which this substitution inhibits coagulant activity is unknown. Factor IX Lake Elsinore (Ala 390 → Val)[322] and factor IX Angers (Gly 396 → Arg)[323,324] disrupt enzymatic activity. Factor IX Eagle Rock (Gly 363 → Val) contains a substituted amino acid adjacent to the active site serine 365, thereby eliminating enzyme activity of the mutant factor IXa.[320] Factor IX London 2 includes a glutamine substituted for an arginine at position 333.[325] A summary of point mutations in hemophilia B is compiled in Figure 40-22.

Other factor IX mutants have been purified and characterized, but the precise point mutations are unknown. Factor IX Deventer cannot be activated by the coagulant protein of Russell's viper venom, suggesting a defect in zymogen activation.[326] Factor IX Zutphen contains an extra peptide of 33 kd that is cross-linked to the factor IX molecule through a disulfide bond.[327] This mutant factor IX has impaired calcium-binding properties.

Of the 11 factor IX mutants described, 3 groups have identical mutations: (1) factor IX Oxford 3 and factor IX San Dimas; (2) factor IX Chapel Hill, factor IX Chicago II and factor IX Albuquerque; and (3) factor IX Vancouver, factor IX Los Angeles and factor IX Long Beach. In patients

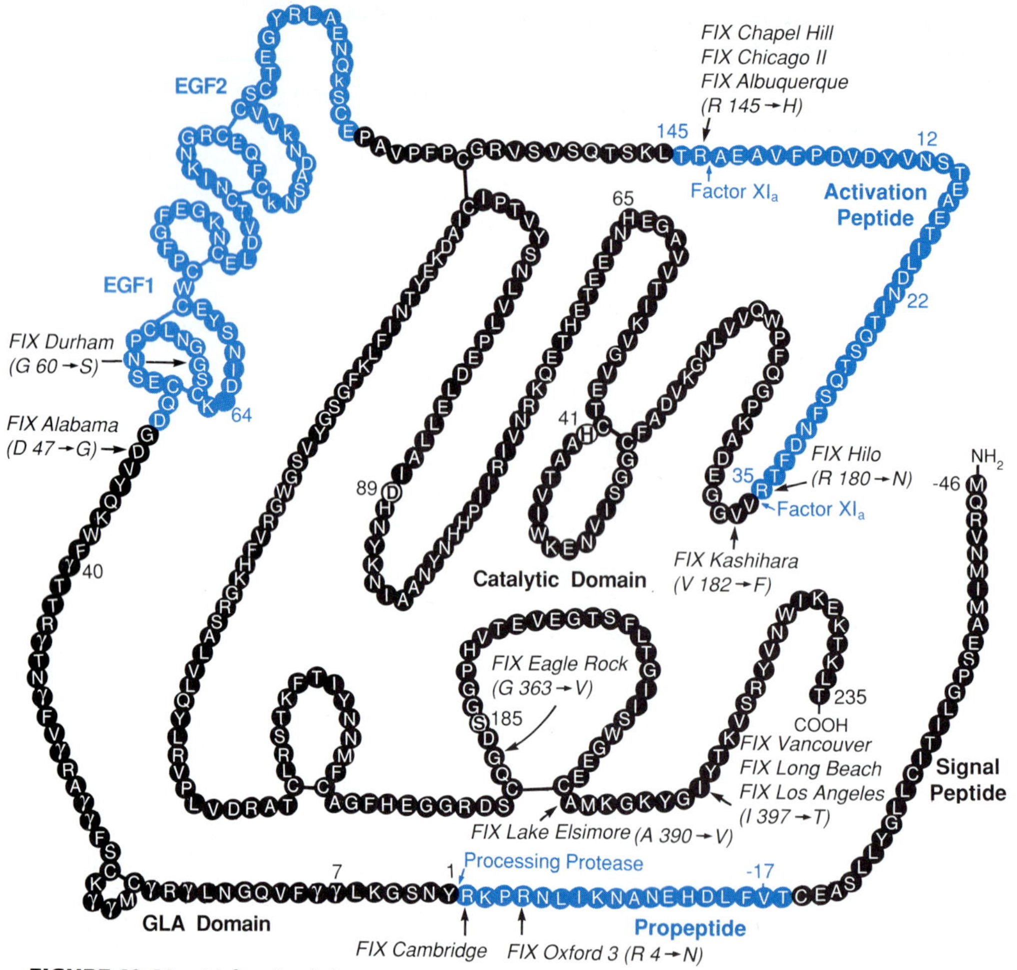

FIGURE 40-22. Molecular defects in mutant factor IX. The point mutations identified in factor IX are indicated by the solid circles. Mutations have been identified in the propeptide, epidermal growth factor domain, activation domain, and catalytic domain.

with mutant plasma proteins, the mutation of arginine to another amino acid appears to be a developing theme. The CG sequence, a component of four of the six arginine codons, as a mutational hot spot may represent an important cause for the development of spontaneous point mutations.[328,329] Since internal point mutations are likely to destabilize protein structure and lead to markedly diminished circulating protein levels, patients preselected for circulating mutant protein antigen are likely to contain amino acid substitutions on the protein surface. Arginines, located on the protein surface, are used by proteases of the trypsin family to hydrolyze adjacent bonds during protein processing and zymogen activation. Given the importance of arginines, it would appear that their mutation leads to phenotypically obvious defects in protein function.

Thus, as summarized in Figure 40-21, there are examples of factor IX mutants that interfere with posttranslational processing, factor IX cell interaction, factor IX zymogen activation, and enzyme activity or normal substrate-binding properties. In the past few years, 378 unique point mutations have been described.[329a]

Factor IX Gene Defects

Little or no factor IX antigen may circulate in the blood of some hemophiliacs. A particularly curious form of hemophilia B has been described in which male children are severely afflicted with factor IX deficiency, but factor IX approaches normal levels after puberty.[300] This form, factor IX Leyden, appears to involve alterations in the promoter region of the factor IX gene that are sensitive to sex hormones.[301,302] A mutation of adenosine for guanosine at position −6 relative to the transcription start site was found in a boy with factor IX deficiency and in his uncle, who had had factor IX deficiency before puberty.[301] In three additional cases, a T → A mutation at −20, an A deletion at +13, and an A → G at +13 is associated with the factor IX Leyden phenotype[330] (Table 40-4).

Hemophilia B can also result from gene deletions, abnormal splicing of the factor IX transcript, or nonsense mutations that terminate translation[331,332] (see Table 40-2). In the case of Chen and associates,[332] the 5′ end of the gene is intact and a truncated expression product of 36 kd is secreted but cleared from the blood into the urine.[333] In the abnormality described by Rees and others,[334] a point mutation (G → T) is located at base 21,165 within the obligatory GT of a splice junction at the 3′ site of exon VI. The change from GT to TT interferes with splicing, causing a severe defect in transcription. In factor IX Seattle,[335] an A at position 17,699 in the gene is deleted. This causes a frameshift, leading to the coding of a Val at residue 85 and a stop codon at position 86. Similarly, the factor IX Bordeaux gene codes for a stop sequence in place of lysine 411, terminating synthesis.[336] Deletion of the entire factor IX gene has been described by Peake[337] and Matthews,[338] and nearly complete factor IX gene deletions have been described by Hassan.[339]

TABLE 40-4. Point Mutations and Partial and Complete Factor IX Gene Deletions Associated With Hemophilia and Characterized by Decreased Factor IX Antigen in the Blood

Defect	Size (kb)	Location	Phenotype	Reference
DEFECTS IN SPLICING AND PROMOTOR (FACTOR IX LEYDEN)				
Point mutation		Splice 3′ of exon VI	Severe hemophilia B	Rees et al, 1985
Point mutation		Promoter (G −6 → A)	Severe prepuberty	Fahner, 1988
Point mutation		Promoter (T −20 → AP)	Severe hemophilia B	Reitsma et al, 1988
Point mutation		Promoter (A + 13 → G)	Severe prepuberty	Reitsma et al, 1988
Deletion		Promoter (A + 13)	Severe prepuberty	Reitsma et al, 1988
PARTIAL AND COMPLETE GENE DELETIONS				
Deletion	18	Exons I, II, III, IV–?	Severe hemophilia B	Giannelli et al, 1983
Deletion	18	Exons I, II, III, IV-?	Severe hemophilia B	Giannelli et al, 1983
Deletion	9	Exons III, IV–?	Severe hemophilia B	Giannelli et al, 1983
Deletion	10	Exons V, VI	Severe hemophilia B	Chen et al, 1985
Deletion/insertion		Intron between VI & VII	Severe hemophilia B	Trent, 1988
Deletion/frameshift	0.001	Exon V	Severe hemophilia B	Schach et al, 1987
Deletion	41	Exons I–VII	Severe hemophilia B	Hassan, 1985
Deletion	114	Exons I–VIII	Severe hemophilia B	Matthews, 1987
Deletion	??	Exons V, VII, VIII	Severe hemophilia B	Matthews, 1987
Deletion	2.8	Exon V	Severe hemophilia B	Vidaud, 1986
Deletion	120	Exons I–VIII	Severe hemophilia B	Peake, 1984
Nonsense		Lys 411 → Stop	Severe hemophilia B	Attree, 1988

A novel mechanism of hemophilia B involves the deletion and insertion of DNA between exons VI and VII.[340] Other partial and complete gene deletions have been identified and partially characterized.[341–347] These examples emphasize the heterogeneity of hemophilia B, particularly the form of hemophilia B in which defective factor IX does not circulate in the blood. A single base deletion and frameshift mutation, a point mutation in the splice junction, and partial or gross gene deletions have been described.

Laboratory Diagnosis of Hemophilia B

Hemophilia B is suspected when an isolated deficiency in plasma factor IX activity is observed by coagulation assay. This measurement, coupled with a history of life-long bleeding, a family history of hemophilia B, a documented life-long prolongation of the partial thromboplastin time, or previous documentation of deficient factor IX activity usually secures the diagnosis. In the factor IX activity assay, a partial thromboplastin time is used; known factor IX–deficient plasma is corrected with test plasma from the patient so that the factor IX activity of a patient sample can be compared directly with a normal plasma sample. Although this analysis is adequate to assess the factor IX activity level of a patient, other ancillary assays are of interest. For example, measurement of the plasma factor IX antigen distinguishes between patients that have improperly functioning circulating factor IX in their blood (eg, point mutations) and those who do not have circulating factor IX in their blood because of large gene deletions.

The evaluation of the factor IX level in family members gives insight into the pattern of inheritance and potential severity of hemophilia B. As a rule, the level of the factor IX deficiency in hemophilia B is consistent among members of a hemophilia family. Presumably, this is because the genetic defect is identical in all afflicted family members and each genetic defect is associated with a specific level of plasma factor IX activity. Stated otherwise, a specific genotype should manifest itself with a characteristic phenotype. Evaluation of the propositus often identifies other family members afflicted with this disorder and demonstrates transmission of the inherited defective factor IX gene from generation to generation. Carrier analysis of female members of hemophilia B families can be important for genetic counseling. Although the expression of excess factor IX antigen compared to activity (eg, ratio of factor IX activity to factor IX antigen in plasma) has been previously used to identify the carrier state,[348] these methods have limited predictive value because of random inactivation of the X chromosome in somatic cells and the variability of factor IX levels in normal individuals. For these reasons, direct genetic analysis using restriction fragment length polymorphisms has been used for accurate carrier state diagnosis and antenatal diagnosis.[349] Six intragenic and three closely linked extragenic polymorphisms have been described for factor IX in the white population.[278,349–353] On this basis, about 80% of families can be evaluated for a hemophilia B gene with about 99% accuracy.[351] The intragenic polymorphisms can be observed with a number of restriction enzymes. A BamH1 polymorphism, due to polymorphism at nucleotide −587, occurs in about 6% of subjects.[350] The DdeI polymorphism, due to a deletion at nucleotide position 5505 to 5554, is observed in 24% of subjects; the XmnI polymorphism, due to a G → C at 7076 has a frequency of 29%,[349] and the TaqI polymorphism, due to alteration at nucleotide 11,111, has a frequency of 35%.[278,353] MspI (altered near 16,000) and OP1 (due to G → A at 20,422) have frequencies of 22% and 33%, respectively.[352] Three closely linked extragenic polymorphisms have been observed with SstI and TaqI.[354–356] One of the factor IX polymorphisms, threonine or alanine at residue 148, can be detected immunochemically[357,358]; this method has also been explored for carrier detection.

Clinical Diagnosis of Hemophilia B. Hemophilia B is a sex-linked disease seen in males, with rare exception.[359,360] On the basis of symptoms and physical examination, hemophilia B is indistinguishable from hemophilia A, which is due to factor VIII deficiency. The clinical presentation of hemophilia is described in detail in Chapter 39. Ten percent of patients with hemophilia have factor IX deficiency. The severity of this disorder closely correlates with the level of factor IX activity in the plasma, although rare examples of a lack of concordance do exist. Patients with low levels of factor IX may be clinically normal; they may even proceed through surgery without special therapy or even the recognition of factor IX deficiency state. Other patients with factor IX levels that should correlate with mild hemophilia may have severe bleeding manifestations.

Patients with severe manifestations of hemophilia B usually have a factor IX activity that is less than 1% of the normal plasma level. These patients are characterized by recurrent, spontaneous bleeding episodes. Moderate hemophilia B is associated with plasma factor IX activity levels of 1% to 4%, and is less commonly associated with spontaneous bleeding. In the more mild forms of hemophilia B, the factor IX activity is above 4%. These patients often show little or no spontaneous bleeding and require attention only with surgery or after trauma.

Except in its most mild forms, hemophilia B is usually diagnosed in early childhood. If excessive bleeding from the umbilical cord or after circumcision goes unnoticed, ecchymoses during the minor trauma of the toddler phase may clue the parents to an underlying clotting disorder. Families with a history of hemophilia B are particularly alert to these bleeding abnormalities and request a plasma assay of factor IX during the first month or two after birth.

The laboratory diagnosis of factor IX requires measurement of the plasma factor IX activity. Because neonates have 50% of the adult level of the vitamin K–dependent proteins,[361] even when vitamin K replete, a low factor IX (eg, 30%) needs to be interpreted with caution before it is assumed that the child has hemophilia B. Because of the difficulties in sample handling and factor IX assay, clinical laboratories with considerable experience in the measurement of this protein should be used to obtain reliable results.

Clinical Manifestations of Hemophilia B. The clinical manifestations of hemophilia B and hemophilia A are indistinguishable. Depending on the severity of the disease, patients are characterized by spontaneous hemarthroses, hematomas, ecchymoses, and, rarely, spontaneous central nervous system bleeding. Hematuria is not uncommon, and gastrointestinal bleeding may also be observed. The most common problem by far involves hemarthroses, either spontaneous or associated with minor trauma. Hemorrhage into the ankle, knee, shoulder, or elbow is associated with severe pain, discomfort, or irritability. Long before there is clinical evidence for bleeding, patients easily identify the pain and inflammation of ongoing bleeding into the joint. The proper treatment is to stop the bleeding as soon as possible. If indicated, factor IX replacement therapy can be instituted. The joint is immobilized by bed rest or splinting. Some orthopedists advocate casting the limb for complete immobilization, but care must be exercised to assure that there is adequate room to accommodate tissue swelling associated with inflammation. As a compromise, a bivalve cast allows immobilization with the ease of routine observation of the joint. With effective therapy, the patient may observe the cessation of bleeding in 12 to 24 hours. Treatment should be continued for several days, then a physical therapy program should be instituted with factor IX coverage. Unlike other forms of arthritis, there is no need to tap the joint even if an effusion is present, unless a septic arthritis complicates the hemarthrosis.

Chronic debilitating arthritis remains a serious problem for the severe hemophiliac. Chronic pain, limitations of joint motion, and disfiguration of the joint are common problems in severe hemophilia. With chronic crippling hemarthroses, patients are often restricted in their abilities to perform certain tasks. Specifically, hemophiliacs with limited range of motion in their knees have difficulty in walking, standing from a seated position, and descending stairs.

In patients with the most crippling arthritis, orthopedic surgery, including joint fusion and joint replacement, may be considered. Chronic pain may be minimized with an ankle fusion, but movement in the joint is lost with the procedure. Prosthetic joints have been used successfully but are recommended only in instances where the patient is extremely disabled, and orthropedic surgery and hematology expertise is available to allow an ample repair without significant surgical risk. The patient must also be willing and able to participate in an extended, aggressive postsurgical physical rehabilitation program; otherwise, the patient risks an unfavorable outcome.

The onset of back or flank pain may be the initial presentation of retroperitoneal bleeding. Significant bleeding can usually be diagnosed radiographically by observation of the loss of the psoas shadow. With large hematoma formation, ureteral deviation or obstruction can occur. Bed rest and full factor IX replacement therapy are indicated.

Superficial hematomas, lacerations, and ecchymoses may not require more than conservative, supportive therapy. However, large hematomas, such as those that are formed in the closed space of the quadriceps, can significantly compromise the distal circulation. Urgent aggressive therapy is required.

Infection with or without abscess formation, a general complication of hematoma formation, is occasionally observed as a further complication of hemophilia B. Treatment with antibiotic therapy and surgical drainage are important considerations.

Treatment of Hemophilia B

Replacement therapy in hemophilia B includes the infusion of factor IX concentrate or fresh frozen plasma. Cryoprecipitate, factor VIII concentrate, and DDAVP have no role in the treatment of hemophilia B. Because blood products carry the risk of viral disease, specifically hepatitis, the indications for infusion must be weighed against the past exposure history of the patient. A severe hemophiliac who has been transfused multiple times with factor IX concentrate has been exposed to the hepatitis viruses, so hepatitis risk is of little concern. Such a patient can be treated with factor IX concentrate if there are appropriate clinical indications. Patients with mild hemophilia, however, may have had little or no exposure to blood products, and every effort should be made to reduce the risks of transmission of viral hepatitis. Factor IX concentrate should thus be avoided, since it is prepared from pooled plasma from thousands of donors. If conservative treatment measures are insufficient and replacement therapy is necessary, fresh frozen plasma may be used, since it carries a much lower risk of hepatitis transmission.

Factor IX has a plasma half-life of about 24 hours and rapidly equilibrates between the intravascular and extravascular space. Therefore, after an initial loading dose, factor IX can be administered once daily. The target level of plasma factor IX depends on the bleeding problem. For treatment of a mild hemarthrosis, a factor IX level of 30% to 40% is adequate. For major abdominal surgery, a central nervous system or retroperitoneal hemorrhage, normalization of the factor IX level is indicated. The factor IX dose using factor IX concentrate can be calculated from the body weight and the factor IX target level. For a 50-kg man in whom a 50% plasma factor IX level is desired, 2000 units of factor IX must be transfused (Fig. 40-23). This calculation is derived by multiplying the plasma volume of 2000 mL (50 kg × 40 mL/kg) by the desired factor IX level (0.5), then

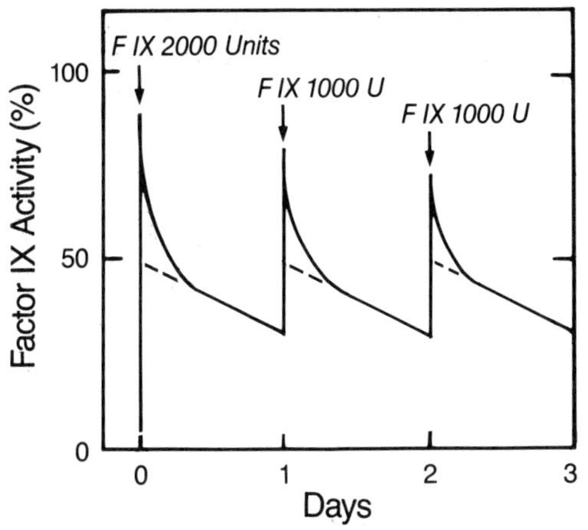

FIGURE 40-23. Factor IX infusion therapy in the treatment of hemophilia B. Factor IX, administered in the form of factor IX concentrate of intermediate purity, is infused initially at 2000 U. Because of equilibration between the intravascular and extravascular space over several hours, the factor IX level achieved is only about half that expected if all of the factor IX remains in the intravascular space. With a factor IX half-life of 24 hours, repeated infusions of factor IX are required on a daily basis. Evidence that a satisfactory factor IX level has been obtained should be established by the performance of a factor IX assay or, at a minimum, correction of the partial thromboplastin time.

multiplying by 2, given the dilution of factor IX equally between the intravascular and extravascular space. Because its half-life is 24 hours, infusion of 1000 units of factor IX every 24 hours should maintain a plasma factor IX level between 50% (after the infusion) and 25% (before the next infusion). These calculations provide useful predictions of the plasma factor IX level, but these estimates should be confirmed by direct monitoring of the factor IX level to assure adequate therapy.

Factor IX therapy is administered in three settings. Patients with severe hemophilia B are maintained in home treatment programs. In such programs, factor IX concentrate is refrigerated until needed, then infused by either the patient or a trained family member after the initiation of a bleeding episode. These programs have been highly successful in developing the medical independence of the patient and his family.[362] Furthermore, the cost of medical care has been significantly reduced. When hemophiliacs, including those on home treatment programs, develop significant bleeding problems that are beyond the scope of their training in routine care, outpatient care is sought in hospitals skilled in the treatment of hemophilia. Often, satisfactory treatment can be initiated in the emergency room or in the outpatient clinic, with follow-up care in the outpatient clinic. More serious problems, however, require inpatient admission for maintainance of replacement therapy.

Complications of Therapy

Factor IX concentrate carries attendant risks in addition to viral hepatitis.[363] Although the molecular basis cannot clear, the intermediate-purity factor IX concentrates cause a hypercoagulable state.[364–367] Hemophiliacs who receive an excessive quantity of the factor IX concentrates can develop deep venous thrombosis and pulmonary embolism.[364] This remains a particular problem in patients receiving considerable amounts of factor IX concentrate, as in those undergoing major surgery.[367] The quality of these factor IX concentrates has improved greatly, with highly purified factor IX currently available. The risk of human immunodeficiency virus (HIV) has been essentially eliminated since the introduction of a heat-treatment step to the production of factor IX concentrate.[368,369] All factor IX concentrates that are approved for human use in the United States are heat treated.

Some patients with hemophilia B develop antibodies to factor IX as an immunologic reaction to a foreign protein. The incidence of this complication is about 5% to 10% in all patients with hemophilia B, and it is most frequently observed in those with severe factor IX deficiency. Since many patients with severe hemophilia B have partial or complete gene deletions, it is suspected that the absence of factor IX antigen in the blood may predispose these patients to the production of anti-factor IX antibodies.[331] But many factor IX antigen-negative patients with gene deletions do not have circulating inhibitors against factor IX.[344] The development of factor IX antibodies has a significant consequence on the therapy of these patients. Factor IX replacement therapy is usually withheld to allow the titer of the anti-factor IX antibody to fall to low levels. Only conservative, supportive measures are taken to avoid reexposure to factor IX. When a life-threatening bleed develops, factor IX concentrate can be administered and the plasma factor IX level maintained transiently at normal levels before the amnestic response leads to a rise in factor IX antibody titer. During this brief period, bleeding can be controlled. Although immunosuppressive techniques have not in general been effective, a protocol for inducing tolerance has been suggested and is undergoing evaluation.[370]

Patients with hemophilia B that were treated with factor IX concentrate between 1979 and 1984 have a high risk of exposure to HIV.[371] About 60% to 70% of these patients have antibodies directed against HIV, and about 1% have developed acquired immunodeficiency syndrome (AIDS). This syndrome is clinically similar to that of patients who acquired AIDS by other routes. However, in hemophiliacs there appears to be a long latency period between exposure and development of AIDS. Furthermore, the number of HIV-positive patients who ultimately develop AIDS is unknown.

Immunoaffinity purification techniques have been applied to the purification of factor IX from plasma.[372–374] Recombinant factor IX has been expressed in active form in mammalian cells.[375–378] Improvements in the technology related to posttranslational processing, specifically γ-carboxylation, should ultimately make this source commercially feasible. Given the long half-life of factor IX, an inexpensive factor IX preparation could be administered prophylactically if it were not associated with complications or risks. The ultimate therapy, gene therapy, involves introduction of the normal factor IX gene into those patients with a defective gene. Transgenic mice that produce human factor IX have been developed.[379] The implantation of epithelial grafts expressing human factor IX shows some initial promise in animal studies.[380,381] An alternative form of therapy, liver transplantation, has been demonstrated to correct factor IX deficiency.[382] Because of both the costs and the attendant risks, however, this does not represent a practical therapeutic approach.

Disorders of Prothrombin

Mutant Prothrombins. Hereditary defects in the plasma prothrombin activity are rare; this is commensurate with the autosomal inheritance of mutant prothrombins and with the absence of clinical symptoms and signs in patients heterozygous for a mutant prothrombin. These patients have prothrombin levels about 50% of the normal level. Patients with hereditary prothrombin deficiency have a clinical bleeding disorder that is closely related to the quantity of prothrombin coagulant activity in the plasma and to the nature of the molecular defect. Therefore, only patients with homozygous prothrombin deficiency would be expected to be affected. Patients with heterozygous prothrombin deficiency have been identified, however.

As in factor IX deficiency, hereditary hypoprothrombinemia is a heterogeneous disorder. Some patients have low prothrombin activity levels despite normal prothrombin antigen levels. These patients are likely to have point mutations that give rise to dysprothrombinemias—mutant prothrombins with defective function circulating in the plasma. Other patients may not synthesize prothrombin and thus have a parallel deficiency of prothrombin activity and prothrombin antigen. These patients have aprothrombinemia.

In 1971, Josso and colleagues[383] reported one of the first cases of a congenital dysprothrombinemia, prothrombin Barcelona. This defect was characterized by the low level of thrombin generated from the mutant prothrombin during activation with factor Xa. The plasma prothrombin antigen level was normal, however. Family studies suggested that the propositus and three siblings were homozygous, and that the parents were heterozygous for mutant forms of prothrombin. Prothrombin Barcelona is characterized by a defect in zymogen activation where cleavage of the Arg 271-Thr 272 bond is precluded.[384] A second peptide bond is cleaved normally, however, generating an active enzyme with activity toward small synthetic substrates but not generating physiologically important substrates such as fibrinogen.[385] The defect in this protein is due to a mutation of arginine 271 to a cysteine.[386] Factor Xa is specific for peptide bonds adjacent to arginine; the conversion of this arginine to a cysteine precludes peptide bond hydrolysis and zymogen activation of prothrombin.

A second, unrelated patient with similar clinical symptoms had a mutant prothrombin known as prothrombin Madrid.[313,387] This mutant (Arg 271 → Cys) is identical to prothrombin Barcelona. From a functional point of view, these defects are analogous to those of factor IX Chapel Hill and factor IX Chicago II.

Two mutant prothrombins contain defects in the thrombin portion of the molecule. The defects interfere with the ability of these thrombins to convert fibrinogen to fibrin. Prothrombin Tokushima (Arg 418 → Trp) is defective at a site adjacent to the aspartic acid in the catalytic triad of the serine protease.[388,389] This enzyme is defective in catalytic activity against large and small substrates. The catalytic domain is also defective in prothrombin Quick I and prothrombin Quick II. Both proteins, isolated from the plasma of a single patient with severe hypoprothrombinemia (less than 2% prothrombin activity), represent gene products of two mutant prothrombin genes.[390] In prothrombin Quick I, a cysteine is substituted for an arginine at residue 382.[391] This enzyme is defective in the binding and conversion of fibrinogen. The molecular defect in prothrombin Quick II involves replacement of glycine 558 with valine. This mutant does not hydrolyze small substrates based on arginine but instead has substrate specificity resembling elastase.

Other prothrombin mutants have been purified and partially characterized, but prothrombin Barcelona, prothrombin Tokushima, prothrombin Quick I and prothrombin Quick II are the only mutant prothrombins to be characterized at the level of the molecular defect (Fig. 40-24 and Table 40-5). Prothrombin Cardeza[393] and prothrombin Clamart[394] cannot be converted to thrombin by factor Xa, indicating a defect in zymogen activation. Prothrombin Metz,[395] prothrombin Salakta[396,397] and prothrombin Molise[398] have defects in their catalytic domain.

TABLE 40-5. Molecular Defects Associated With Dysprothrombinemia

Defect	Location	Reference
POINT MUTATIONS THAT INTERFERE WITH ZYMOGEN ACTIVATION		
PT Barcelona	Arg 271 → Cys	Rabiet et al, 1986
PT Madrid	Arg 271 → Cys	Diuguid et al, 1989
POINT MUTATIONS THAT ALTER ENZYME ACTIVITY AND SUBSTRATE BINDING		
PT Quick I	Arg 382 → Cys	Henriksen & Mann, 1988
PT Takushima	Arg 418 → Trp	Miyata et al, 1987
PT Quick II	Gly 558 → Val	Henriksen & Mann, 1989

thrombin antigen are both low. The causes of hereditary aprothrombinemia are not known, but it is assumed that these cases are due to partial or complete deletions of the prothrombin gene or to structural alterations in the expressed prothrombin that lead to rapid clearance of the mutant prothrombin.

Clinical Aspects

As an autosomal recessive disorder, prothrombin deficiency in its heterozygous form is usually clinically silent. A careful family history may provide a clue to diagnosis. The prothrombin time and the partial thromboplastin time may be prolonged, but the extent of prolongation depends on the level of prothrombin activity deficiency. A direct prothrombin assay in prothrombin-deficient plasma allows determination of the plasma prothrombin coagulant activity. Immunoassay based on antiprothrombin antibodies permits the measurement of the plasma prothrombin antigen.

Even in the homozygous form, prothrombin deficiency causes only a moderate bleeding tendency because at least a small amount of this activity occurs. The clinical manifestations do not distinguish prothrombin deficiency from other hereditary clotting factor deficiencies. Hereditary prothrombin deficiency is treatable with the prothrombin contained in fresh frozen plasma or intermediate-purity factor IX concentrates, which contain prothrombin. As described, factor IX concentrates are associated with thromboembolic complications, hepatitis, and the transmission of other viral diseases. For patients without chronic need for replacement therapy, fresh frozen plasma offers therapy without a high risk of the transmission of viral diseases. The plasma half-life of prothrombin is about 3 days. Therefore, intermittent therapy is sufficient for the treatment of bleeding episodes. Vitamin K therapy has no role in the treatment of congenital prothrombin deficiency.

Disorders of Factor X

Mutant Factor X. Hereditary factor X deficiency is a rare autosomal recessive disorder. Mutant factor X molecules have not been isolated from patients with hereditary factor X deficiency and fully characterized with regard to point mutations, nor have genetic defects been defined. Therefore, the molecular basis of hereditary factor X deficiency is not known, but it is assumed that these disorders are heterogeneous and that they have the same pattern of defects associated with factor IX and prothrombin deficiency. Several mutant factor X molecules (including the two original families, Stuart & Prower) have been studied with biochemical and immunochemical techniques. Both

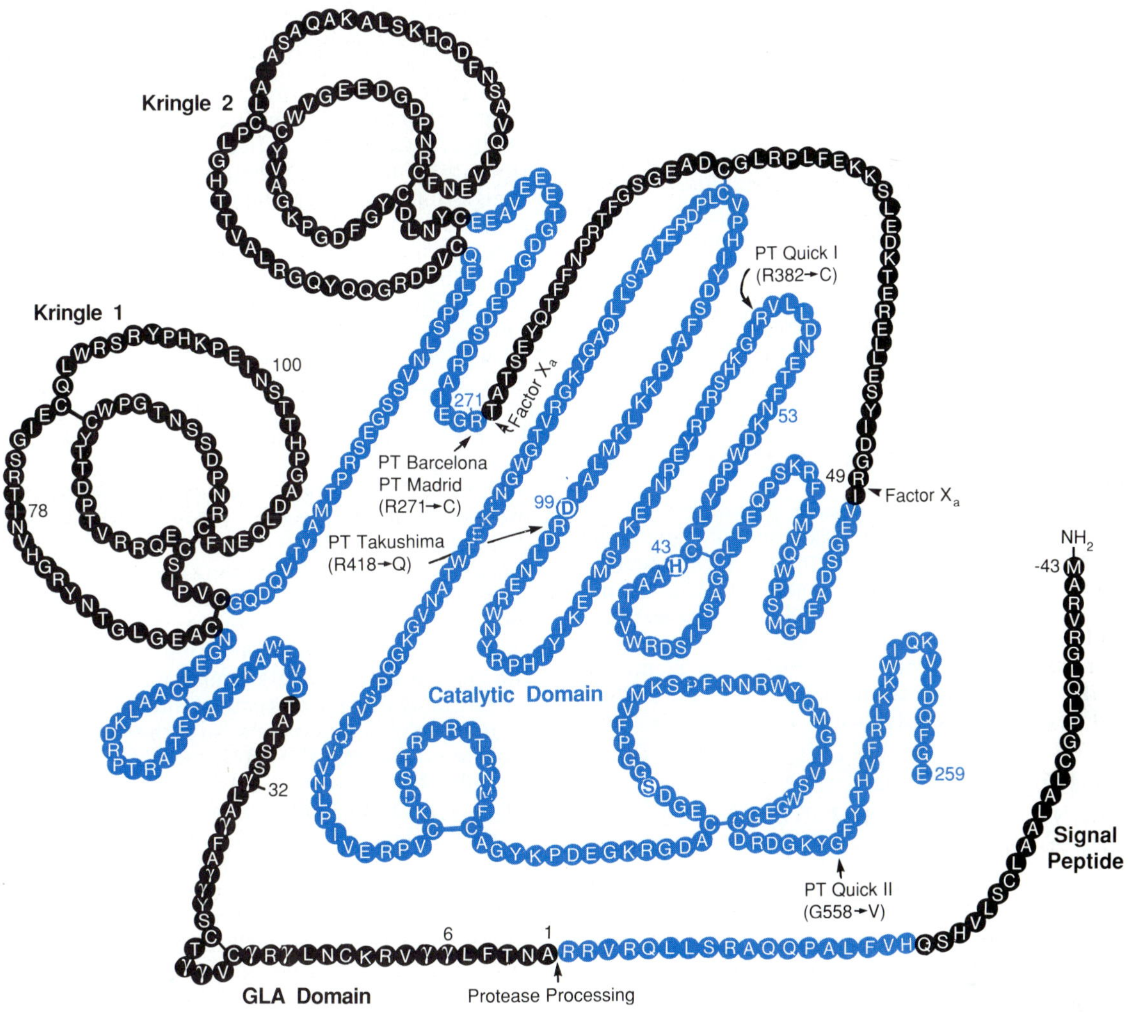

FIGURE 40-24. Molecular defects in mutant prothrombins. The point mutations identified in prothrombin are indicated by the solid circles. Mutations have been identified in the activation and catalytic domains.

factor X activity and antigen are low in Stuart plasma, whereas Prower plasma has low factor X activity and normal factor X antigen.[7,8] Factor X Friuli plasma is characterized by normal factor X antigen but a factor X activity of 5%.[399] The prothrombin time and partial thromboplastin time are abnormal, but activation of factor X Friuli by the coagulant protein in Russell's viper venom is normal. This defect is likely due to a point mutation. Approximately 50 cases of factor X deficiency have been described, but complete description of the biochemical defect is lacking.[400,401] Factor X Roma and factor X Padua are among these variant factor X molecules that have been partially characterized[402–404] and are likely to yield to detailed structural analyses.

The factor X gene is located on long arm of chromosome 13, closely linked to the factor VII gene.[248,405] Some patients with defects on chromosome 13 have associated factor X deficiency. Combined deficiency of factors X and VII also has been associated with deletion of chromosome 13.[406] Factor X deficiency associated with partial 4q duplication due to inherited der(13),t(4;13)(q26;q34)mat in a girl has been described.[407]

Clinical Characteristics. As discussed, hereditary factor X deficiency is inherited as an autosomal recessive disorder. About a third of these patients have a deficiency in factor X antigen and factor X activity; in the remaining patients, factor X activity is low despite normal antigen levels.[400,401] The severity of the clinical manifestations of factor X deficiency parallel the degree of factor X deficiency. Heterozygotes are usually asymptomatic and may go undetected. Their prothrombin times and partial thromboplastin times are usually marginally prolonged. In homozygotes, bleeding may be associated with surgery or trauma. Patients occasionally have sufficiently severe factor X deficiency to cause spontaneous bleeding. The pattern of the bleeding disorder does not distinguish it from any of the other forms of hemophilia.

Hereditary factor X deficiency is treated with fresh frozen plasma or intermediate-purity factor IX concentrate, which contains factor X. For patients who do not need chronic replacement therapy, fresh frozen plasma is a therapy without a high risk of transmitting viral diseases or inducing thromboembolic complications.

Disorders of Factor VII

Mutant Factor VII

Hereditary factor VII deficiency is an extremely rare, autosomal recessive disorder. Because of the low levels of factor VII in plasma, mutant factor VII molecules have not been isolated and their molecular defects determined. The study of factor VII deficiency has been limited to functional characterizations of these mutants, including the assay of factor VII activity and factor VII antigen.[408–411]

Clinical Characteristics

The clinical manifestations of factor VII deficiency are highly variable and do not correlate closely with the measured plasma factor VII activity using routinely available reagents. Some patients with severe deficiency have severe bleeding problems, including intracranial hemorrhage.[413] Other patients have typical musculoskeletal bleeding and hemarthroses.[414] Others are asymptomatic, even when subjected to surgical procedures.[415] Still others have disorders complicated by deep venous thrombosis and pulmonary embolism.[416] One study suggests that the major determinant of clinical bleeding in factor VII deficiency is racial origin, since none of nine evaluated black patients with factor VII deficiency had a history of bleeding whereas all of the whites in this study had bled.[408]

ACQUIRED DISORDERS OF VITAMIN K–DEPENDENT PROTEINS

Any process that interferes with protein synthesis in the liver or impairs the availability of vitamin K can alter the level of activity of the vitamin K–dependent blood coagulation proteins. Deficiency of these proteins may also occur by overutilization of the vitamin K–dependent proteins, as in intravascular coagulation, or by enhanced clearance mechanisms, as has been observed in the factor X deficiency associated with amyloidosis.

Impaired Protein Synthesis Run of Vitamin K–Dependent Proteins Due to Vitamin K Deficiency

As previously discussed, factor VII, factor IX, factor X, and prothrombin are part of a unique class of calcium-binding proteins that contain γ-carboxyglutamic acid.[24,25] A posttranslational processing step requires vitamin K. In its reduced form, vitamin K is an essential cofactor for a liver carboxylase.[28] In the absence of vitamin K or in the presence of vitamin K antagonists, γ-carboxylation of selected glutamic acid residues is blocked, and the resulting proteins have no or decreased amounts of γ-carboxyglutamic acid.[161,417,418] The γ-carboxyglutamic acid–deficient forms do not bind to phospholipid or calcium ions normally and have no biologic activity.[99,100] The sole known clinical manifestation of vitamin K deficiency in both children and adults is a reduction in the activity of the vitamin K–dependent proteins. Depending on the degree of vitamin K deficiency, the coagulant activities of these proteins may vary from only a laboratory abnormality to serious bleeding.

Food, especially fresh green leafy vegetables,[14] represents the primary nutritional source of vitamin K. Colonic bacteria produce vitamin K_2,[419] but it remains uncertain whether this source of vitamin K supplements the dietary intake, since bacteria are located in the large intestine and vitamin K absorption takes place in the ileum. Controversy remains regarding whether retrograde movement of vitamin K proximally to the ileum or whether passive absorption of vitamin K in the colon are important mechanisms. The daily dietary requirement for vitamin K is less than 1 μg/kg,[420] as measured by a prolongation of the prothrombin time. The daily vitamin K requirement may be closer to 2 to 3 μg/kg, however, if the appearance of abnormal (des-γ) carboxyprothrombin is used to monitor this requirement.[219]

Patients that are severely malnourished, especially those receiving antibiotics, are more prone to vitamin K deficiency. In these cases, both the dietary and bacterial sources of vitamin K are considerably reduced or eliminated.[421] Although vitamin K deficiency in the absence of antibiotics is unusual, bulimia can depress vitamin K–dependent protein activity.[422] Clinically, significant vitamin K deficiency can appear in a healthy individual in 1 or 2 weeks. In a typical example, a patient undergoes elective surgery and requires parenteral antibiotics and intravenous fluid. Within a week, the patient develops a prolonged prothrombin time. Patients with marginal vitamin K reserves, such as those with end-stage malignancy, may also develop severe vitamin K deficiency within a week. Vitamin K deficiency in the postsurgical patient is sufficiently common that this diagnosis is usually made by the surgical staff. Any medical or surgical patients who require parenteral nutrition should receive a vitamin K supplement. Patients with severe protracted vomiting may develop vitamin K deficiency, especially if they are treated with antibiotics. Vitamin K deficiency may also be a component of malabsorption syndromes such as sprue, kwashiorkor, or cholestasis.

Since both the intrinsic pathway and extrinsic pathway of blood coagulation involve vitamin K–dependent proteins, deficiency in the coagulation activity of these proteins prolongs both the prothrombin time and partial thromboplastin time. The diagnosis of vitamin K deficiency is confirmed by normalization of the prothrombin time 12 to 24 hours after the administration of 10 mg vitamin K_1. Vitamin K can be given by subcutaneous or intravenous injection. Partial or complete correction indicates a component of vitamin K deficiency as a cause of the prolonged prothrombin time. Although the prothrombin time and the partial thromboplastin time are both prolonged by vitamin K deficiency, the prothrombin time is routinely used to evaluate vitamin K deficiency. Since prolongation of the prothrombin time may be associated with numerous other disorders and is not specific for vitamin K deficiency, the diagnosis of vitamin K deficiency cannot be made unless vitamin K administration significantly reduces a prolonged prothrombin toward the normal value.

Specific immunoassay of plasma abnormal (des-γ-carboxy) prothrombin is about 1000 times more sensitive than the prothrombin time in the detection of vitamin K deficiency.[219,423] Since normal subjects do not have any circulating abnormal prothrombin in the plasma, the appearance of abnormal prothrombin in plasma can be readily detected by immunoassay. If the abnormal prothrombin appears because of a deficiency of vitamin K, administration of vitamin K leads to the disappearance of abnormal prothrombin in the plasma[424,425] (Fig. 40-25). A comparison of thrombin generation by factor Xa and by *Echis carinatus* venom also permits detection of vitamin K deficiency, but this approach is considerably less sensitive than the immunologic approach. Comparison of these assays before and after the administration of vitamin K allows the diagnosis of vitamin K deficiency over other conditions associated with a prolonged prothrombin time, such as liver disease.[426] Direct assay of vitamin K in serum, based on high performance liquid chromatography, has also been used to define vitamin K deficiency[427] but is a labor-intensive method that is not practical for general patient management.

Vitamin K deficiency is treated with vitamin K_1 (Aquamephyton), a water-soluble preparation. The absorption of oral vitamin K is variable and unpredictable, particularly in patients with cholestasis and malabsorption. For this reason, the diagnosis and treatment of vitamin K deficiency should involve the administration of parenteral vitamin K_1. Hematomas can form after intramuscular injection in a patient with severe vitamin K deficiency. Therefore, intramuscular injection should be avoided. The definitive treatment of vitamin K deficiency involves the infusion of 10 to 15 mg of vitamin K_1 intravenously. Because anaphy-

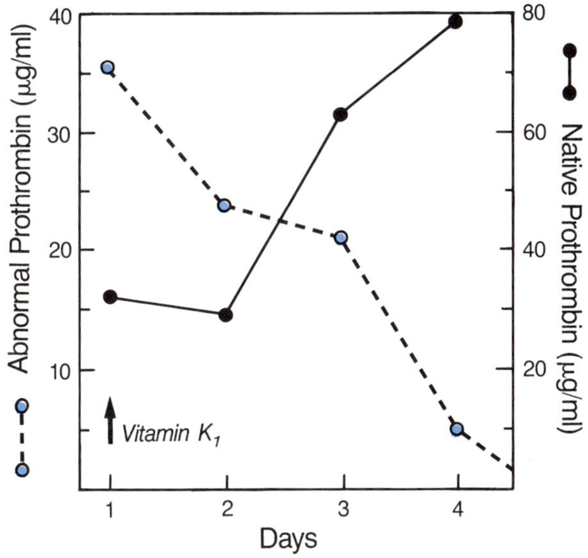

FIGURE 40-25. Vitamin K deficiency. Changes in the prothrombin time, native prothrombin antigen, and abnormal prothrombin antigen following treatment with vitamin K. (After Blanchard RA, Furie BC, Jorgensen MJ, et al. Acquired vitamin K-dependent carboxylation deficiency in liver disease. N Engl J Med 1981;305:242)

lactic reactions can be associated with intravenous vitamin K administration, albeit rarely, care should be taken when this route of administration is used. This therapy should be used only in a hospital setting, with epinephrine available for the treatment of emergent allergic reactions. The prothrombin time usually corrects in 12 to 24 hours after vitamin K infusion. Patients with a serious bleeding disorder, such as intraabdominal or intracranial hemorrhage, who require urgent treatment of their vitamin K deficiency should be treated with fresh frozen plasma to replace vitamin K–dependent proteins. Fresh frozen plasma carries the risk of viral infection, which must be balanced against the severity of the bleeding episode. Factor IX concentrates contain all of the vitamin K–dependent proteins. In available forms, however, they nearly guarantee the transmission of hepatitis to a patient without immunity to hepatitis. Therefore, these agents are contraindicated. Improvements in the large-scale preparation of purified vitamin K–dependent proteins may soon offer new agents that prove useful.[372–374]

Hemorrhagic Disease of the Newborn

Hemorrhagic disease of the newborn is a bleeding disorder arising immediately after birth because of vitamin K deficiency.[428–430] Bleeding usually begins between days 2 and 7 after birth and is clinically demonstrated by hematomas, bleeding from mucous membranes, hemorrhage following circumcision, and from venipuncture sites. In its most severe form, this disorder can cause internal bleeding, intracranial hemorrhage, and death.[431] Before the introduction of prophylactic vitamin K, about 1 of 100 neonates bled from this syndrome; about 25% of these infants died. As many as 25% of all untreated, asympmtomatic newborns have a prothrombin time and partial thromboplastin time consistent with hemorrhagic disease of the newborn.[432] Using the abnormal (des-γ-carboxy) prothrombin as a sensitive serum marker of vitamin K deficiency, essentially all newborns have evidence of vitamin K deficiency at birth, as do about 30% of their mothers.[433]

This hemorrhagic disorder is due to insufficient intake of vitamin K during the newborn period. This deficiency state is reversed on the colonization of the intestine with vitamin K–producing bacteria and the ingestion of vitamin K–containing food.[430] Breast-fed neonates are susceptible to vitamin K deficiency,[431,434,435] since human milk contains only 15 μg of vitamin K per liter.[430,436]

As in all vitamin K–deficient states, infants with hemorrhagic disease of the newborn have a prolonged partial thromboplastin time and prothrombin time. Because the synthesis of the vitamin K–dependent proteins is decreased in the neonate, and the levels of these proteins are only half of adult levels,[361] impaired carboxylation of these proteins due to concomitant vitamin K deficiency exaggerates the potential bleeding risk. The syndrome is reversed with the administration of vitamin K, but fresh frozen plasma, despite the risk of infection, is justified in patients with life-threatening hemorrhage. A single dose of vitamin K (100 μg) is sufficient to correct the bleeding tendency.

To prevent hemorrhagic disease of the newborn, all hospital-born infants in the United States are prophylactically treated with vitamin K at birth by the subcutaneous injection of vitamin K.[436] The usual dosage used is 100 μg to 1 mg.[436] Larger doses of vitamin K should be avoided, since it can interfere with the conjugation of bilirubin in the liver or cause hemolytic anemia.[437,438]

Deficiency of Vitamin K–Dependent Protein Due to Vitamin K Antagonists

Reduced vitamin K is required as a cofactor for vitamin K–dependent carboxylation. In the metabolic pathway that recovers and recycles vitamin K, reduced vitamin K is converted to the vitamin K epoxide in a reaction that is thought to be linked to the carboxylation process. Under the action of the vitamin K epoxide reductase, vitamin K epoxide is then converted to vitamin K. The vitamin K reductase converts vitamin K to reduced vitamin K, completing the vitamin K cycle. Sodium warfarin inhibits vitamin K–dependent carboxylation by inhibiting the vitamin K reductase and vitamin K epoxide reductase.[28] Since sodium warfarin is widely used clinically as an oral anticoagulant and is sold both as a pharmacologic agent and as a rodenticide, it is a frequent cause of reduced vitamin K–dependent protein activity. Some patients directed to take warfarin as an oral anticoagulant have bleeding complications despite careful monitoring of the prothrombin time.[439–445] With the introduction of lower intensity warfarin therapy,[439,441,446] the percentage of patients treated with warfarin who develop bleeding complications has decreased.

The accidental ingestion of warfarin or related agents can also lead to a deficiency of the vitamin K–dependent blood clotting proteins since rat poisons, or rodenticides, contain vitamin K antagonists. Children, particularly younger children, can come in contact with poorly placed bait and ingest the bait; severe bleeding can ensue within 48 hours to 1 week. Most of the first-generation rodenticides include warfarin as an active ingredient. The new superwarfarins, targeted at the warfarin-resistant rat populations, are fat-soluble and long-acting. These agents, such as brodifacoum, can cause prolongation of the prothrombin time for more than 6 months after a single ingestion.[447–449] Patients poisoned with these second-generation rodenticides require treatment with high doses of vitamin K_1 (100 mg/d) by the oral route. Therapy must be extended until the residual vitamin K antagonist is depleted.

The surreptitious ingestion of vitamin K antagonists can lead to a bleeding disorder, factitious purpura.[450–452] A severe psychologic disorder often leads to ingestion. Covert anticoagulant abuse is most often seen in individuals associated with the medical profession, such as medical students, nurses, and medical technologists. In addition, those with relatives of patients taking warfarin may use warfarin covertly. Treatment of covert warfarin ingestion or overdosage is identical in these patients and patients requiring anticoagulant therapy. Factitious superwarfarin ingestion, including brodifacoum, is particularly difficult to diagnose[453] (Fig. 40-26). The serum warfarin levels are undetectable despite a markedly prolonged prothrombin time and partial thromboplastin time. Patients who ingest these agents have marked prolongation of the prothrombin time for many months after a single exposure. Diagnosis is compounded inasmuch as serum assays for these agents are not readily available. High doses of vitamin K_1 (eg, 100 mg/d by the oral route) given chronically can titrate the effects of brodifacoum.

Acetylsalicylic acid in toxic doses is known to induce a vitamin K deficient–like state.[454] At high doses, acetylsalicylic acid likely oxidizes vitamin K so that it cannot be used in vitamin K–dependent carboxylation. This disorder responds to treatment with vitamin K. Certain antibiotics, including moxalactam, cause vitamin K deficiency.[455–457] The inhibition of the vitamin K–dependent carboxylase by moxalactam and other antibiotics has been proposed.[458] The precise structural moiety responsible for inhibition of vitamin K–dependent carboxylation is not known.

Treatment of warfarin toxicity or vitamin K inhibition depends on the severity of the clinical presentation. Furthermore, the clinical indication for oral anticoagulation must be weighed in the treatment plan. In the absence of clinically significant bleeding, warfarin may be discontinued, then restarted when the prothrombin time is in the therapeutic range. The prothrombin time gradually normalizes, particularly if a normal diet is continued. If necessary, the depletion of the vitamin K–dependent proteins can be reversed by the administration of vitamin K. These patients are refractory to further oral anticoagulant therapy for some time, however. When a bleeding disorder is serious and rapid replacement of the vitamin K–dependent proteins is indicated, fresh frozen plasma can be administered. Intermediate-purity factor IX concentrates should not be used because of the high incidence of viral infection.

Deficiency of Vitamin K–Dependent Protein Secondary to Liver Disease

The liver is the site of synthesis of the vitamin K–dependent blood coagulation proteins.[19–21] Parenchymal diseases of the liver (cirrhosis and hepatitis), infiltrative diseases involving the liver (metastatic neoplasms), and primary liver neoplasms (primary hepatocellular carcinoma) can all interfere with the normal synthesis of the vitamin K–dependent blood coagulation proteins.[459–461] Some patients may not demonstrate increased bleeding tendencies, but their prolonged prothrombin time is secondary to impaired synthesis of the vitamin K–dependent proteins. Prolongation of the prothrombin time is observed in moderate to severe cases of liver disease. Most often, the hemostatic abnormalities of liver disease are without overt clinical manifestations. Although des-γ-carboxy forms of prothrombin in the plasma of patients with liver disease serve as a diagnostic marker of impaired γ-carboxylation, the minor defect in the vitamin K–dependent carboxylation does not contribute significantly to the hemostatic disorder.[219] It is the generalized decreased synthesis of the vitamin K–dependent proteins, as measured by decreased plasma prothrombin antigen,[219,462] that causes the laboratory abnormalities.

These hemostatic abnormalities often are diagnosed when significant bleeding occurs in a patient with liver disease or when a preoperative bleeding evaluation is requested before liver biopsy. In liver disease patients with poor dietary intake and a history of alcohol abuse, the coagulation abnormalities may only partially arise from vitamin K deficiency. Therefore, the prothrombin time and partial thromboplastin time usually do not normalize with administration of vitamin K. The absence of at least partial correction of the prothrombin time 24 hours after administration of vitamin K_1 (10 to 15 mg) intravenously indicates a hemostatic abnormality other than vitamin K deficiency. Fresh frozen plasma, in adequate quantity, partially corrects the plasma levels of the vitamin K–dependent proteins and decreases the bleeding tendency during surgery.[463] Intermediate-purity factor IX concentrates, which are associated with the development of thromboembolic disease and transmission of hepatitis, are contraindicated in their current form in the treatment of severe liver disease.[364,464] This material induces a hypercoagulable state and is compounded by the acquired antithrombin III deficiency that characterizes severe liver disease.

Most patients with hepatitis and cirrhosis as well as those with primary hepatocellular carcinoma have a defect in vitamin K–dependent carboxylation.[219,465] In fact, abnormal (des-γ-carboxy) prothrombin can be used as a marker for hepatocellular carcinoma[465–467] and can supplement the α-fetoprotein assay (Fig. 40-27).

Acquired Factor X Deficiency and Amyloidosis

Rarely, primary amyloidosis is associated with an acquired coagulation disorder characterized by factor X deficiency.[468–470] These patients have bleeding complications in addition to the clinical manifestations of amyloidosis. This disorder is due to the removal of factor X from the plasma. Factor X is immobilized along the amyloid-

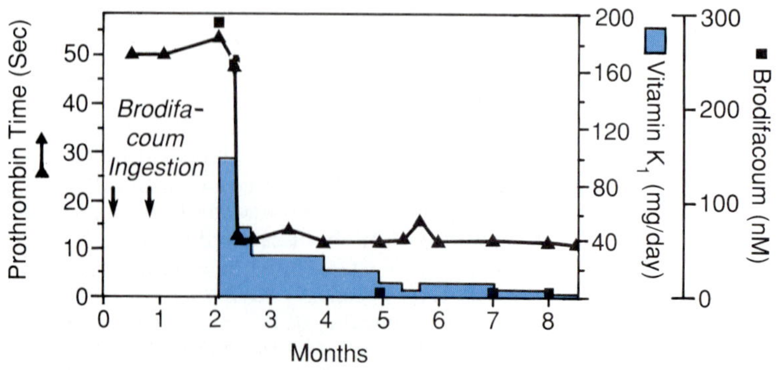

FIGURE 40-26. Deficiency of the vitamin K–dependent proteins due to ingestion of brodifacoum, a potent rodenticide. (After Weitzel JN, Sadowski JA, Furie BC, et al. Hemorrhagic disorder caused by surreptitious ingestion of a long-acting vitamin K antagonist/rodenticide, brodifacoum. Blood 1990;76:2555).

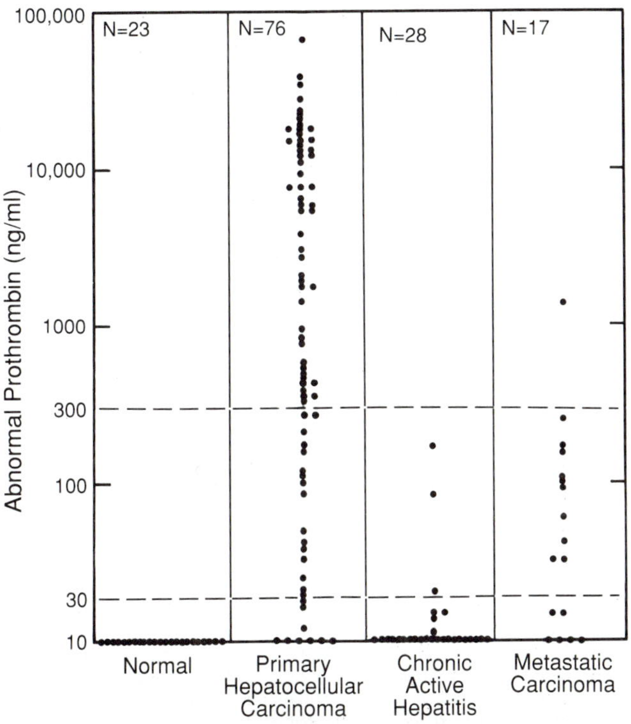

FIGURE 40-27. Impaired vitamin K–dependent carboxylation. Abnormal prothrombin as a marker of primary hepatocellular carcinoma. (After Liebman HA, Furie BC, Ting MJ, et al. Des-γ-carboxy (abnormal) prothrombin as a serum marker of primary hepatocellular carcinoma. N Engl J Med 1984;310:1427.)

infiltrated vasculature and distributed in the reticuloendothelial system.[470] Factor X has a curious affinity for amyloid fibrils.[471]

These patients do not respond to the infusion of factor X in fresh frozen plasma, intermediate-purity factor IX concentrates, or in large volume plasmapheresis and plasma exchange.[470,472] Splenectomy, with removal of a large burden of amyloid, has been associated with the rapid normalization of plasma factor X levels in two reported cases.[473,474] Unsuccessful treatments have not been reported in the literature, however. Chemotherapy with antimyeloma agents, such as cyclophosphamide and prednisone, has been successful in one case,[475] but most patients with amyloidosis that receive this therapy are not responsive.

Miscellaneous Acquired Defects of Vitamin K–Dependent Proteins

The lupus anticoagulant causes a prolongation of the partial thromboplastin time due to the inhibition of the assay by antiphospholipid antibodies. In a small percentage of cases, however, this antibody crossreacts with prothrombin and leads to the rapid clearance of prothrombin from the blood.[476] The induced hypoprothrombinemia can cause significant bleeding in contrast to the absence of bleeding problems associated with the lupus anticoagulant.

A deficiency of factor IX has been reported in association with the nephrotic syndrome.[477–479] This diagnosis is often made in patients under evaluation before renal biopsy. Although the presence of factor IX deficiency correlates with the extent of proteinuria, the mechanism of the factor IX deficiency is unknown.

REFERENCES

1. Schmidt A. Zur Blutlehre. Leipzig, Vogel, 1892.
2. Morawitz P. Die Chemie der Blutzgerinnung. Ergio Physiol 1905;4: 307.
3. Seegers WH. Prothrombin. Cambridge, MA, Harvard University Press, 1962.
4. Aggeler PM, White SG, Glendenning MB, et al. Plasma thromboplastin component (PTC) deficiency: a new disease resembling hemophilia. Proc Soc Exp Biol Med 1952;79:692.
5. Schulman I, Smith CH. Hemorrhagic disease in an infant due to deficiency of a previously undescribed clotting factor. Blood 1952;7:794.
6. Alexander B, Godstein R, Landwehr G, et al. Congenital SPCA deficiency: a hitherto unrecognized coagulation defect with hemorrhage rectified by serum and serum fractions. J Clin Invest 1951;30:596.
7. Telfer TP, Denson KW, Wright DR. A "new" coagulation defect. Br J Haematol 1956;2:308.
8. Hougie E, Barrow EM, Graham JB. Stuart clotting defect: I. segregation of an hereditary hemorrhagic state from the heterogeneous group heretofore called "stable factor" deficiency. J Clin Invest 1957;36:485.
9. Ratnoff OD, Davie EW. Waterfall sequence for intrinsic blood clotting. Science 1964;145:1310.
10. Macfarlane RG. An enzyme cascade in the blood clotting mechanism and its function as a biochemical amplifier. Nature 1964;202:498.
11. Seegers WH. Blood clotting mechanisms: three basic reactions. Annu Rev Physiol 1969;31:269.
12. Dam H. Cholesterinstoffwechsel in Huhnereiern und Huhnchen. Biochem Zeitschr 1929;215:475.
13. Dam H. The antihaemorrhagic vitamin of the chick: occurrence and chemical nature. Nature 1935;135:652.
14. Almquist HJ. Purification of the antihemorrhagic vitamin. J Biol Chem 1936;114:241.
15. Doisy EA, MacCorquodale DW, Thayer SA, et al. The isolation, constitution, and synthesis of vitamin K_1. Science 1939;90:407.
16. Schofield FW. A brief account of a disease in cattle simulating hemorrhagic septicemia due to feeding sweet clover. Can Vet Rec 1922;3: 74.
17. Roderick LM. A problem in the coagulation of the blood "sweet clover" disease of cattle. Am J Physiol 1931;96:413.
18. Campbell HA, Link KP. Studies on the hemorrhagic sweet clover disease: IV. the isolation and crystallization of the hemorrhagic agent. J Biol Chem 1941;138:21.
19. Mann FD, Shonyo ES, Mann FC. Effect of removal of the liver on blood coagulation. Am J Physiol 1951;164:111.
20. Pool J, Robinson J. In vitro synthesis of coagulation factors by rat liver slices. Am J Physiol 1959;196:423.
21. Olson JP, Miller LL, Troup SB. Synthesis of clotting factors by the isolated perfused rat liver. J Clin Invest 1966;45:690.
22. Furie B, Furie BC. Molecular basis of blood coagulation. Cell 1988;53: 505.
23. Kurachi K, Davie EW. Isolation and characterization of a cDNA coding for human factor IX. Proc Natl Acad Sci USA 1982;79:6461.
24. Stenflo J, Fernlund P, Egan W, et al. Vitamin K dependent modifications of glutamic acid residues in prothrombin. Proc Natl Acad Sci USA 1974;71:2730.
25. Nelsestuen GL, Zytkovicz TH, Howard JB. The mode of action of vitamin K. Identification of γ-carboxyglutamic acid as a component of prothrombin. J Biol Chem 1974;249:6347.
26. Drakenberg T, Fernlund P, Roepstorff P, et al. β-Hydroxyaspartic acid in vitamin K–dependent protein C. Proc Natl Acad Sci USA 1983;80: 1802.
27. McMullen BA, Fujikawa K, Kisiel W. The occurrence of β-hydroxyaspartic acid in the vitamin K–dependent blood coagulation zymogens. Biochem Biophys Res Commun 1983;115:8.
28. Suttie, JW. Mechanism of action of vitamin K: synthesis of gamma-carboxyglutamic acid. CRC Crit Rev Biochem 1980;8:191.
29. Hubbard B, Ulrich MMW, Jacobs M, et al. Vitamin K–dependent carboxylase: affinity purification from bovine liver using a synthetic propeptide containing the γ-carboxylation recognition site. Proc Natl Acad Sci 1989;86:6893.
30. Helgeland L. The submicrosomal site for the conversion of prothrombin precursor to biologically active prothrombin in rat liver. Biochim Biophys Acta 1977;499:181.
31. Wallin R, Prydz H. Studies on a subcellular system for vitamin K–dependent carboxylation. Thromb Haemost 1979;41:529.
32. Carlisle TL, Suttie JW. Vitamin K–dependent carboxylase: subcellular location of the carboxylase and enzymes involved in vitamin K metabolism in rat liver. Biochemistry 1980;19:1161.
33. Jones JP, Gardner EJ, Cooper TG, et al. Vitamin K–dependent carboxylation of peptide-bound glutamate: the active species of "CO_2" utilized by the membrane-bound preprothrombin carboxylase. J Biol Chem 1977;252:7738.
34. Friedman PA, Shia MA. The apparent absence of involvement of biotin in the vitamin K–dependent carboxylation of glutamic acid residues of proteins. Biochem J 1977;163:39.
35. Friedman PA, Shia MA, Gallop PM, et al. Vitamin K–dependent gamma-

carbon hydrogen bond cleavage and nonmandatory concurrent carboxylation of peptide-bound glutamic acid residues. Proc Natl Acad Sci USA 1979;76:3126.
36. Mctigue JJ, Suttie JW. Vitamin K–dependent carboxylase: demonstration of a vitamin K- and O_2-dependent exchange of ^3H from ^3H_2O into glutamic acid residues. J Biol Chem 1983;258:12129.
37. Anton DL, Friedman PA. Fate of the activated γ-carbon–hydrogen bond in the uncoupled vitamin K–dependent γ-glutamyl carboxylation reaction. J Biol Chem 1983;258:14084.
38. Wallin R, Suttie JW. Vitamin K–dependent carboxylase: evidence for cofractionation of carboxylase and epoxidase activities, and for carboxylation of a high molecular weight microsomal protein. Arch Biochem Biophys 1982;214:155.
39. Suttie JW, Larson AE, Canfield LM, et al. Relationship between vitamin K–dependent carboxylation and vitamin K epoxidation. Fed Proc 1978;37:2605.
40. Sadowski JA, Schnoes HK, Suttie JW. Vitamin K epoxidase: properties and relationship to prothrombin synthesis. Biochemistry 1977;16:3856.
41. Suttie JW, Geweke LO, Martin SL, et al. Vitamin K epoxidase: dependence of epoxidase activity on substrates of the vitamin K–dependent carboxylation reaction. FEBS Lett 1980;109:267.
42. Giradot J-M, Mack DO, Floyd RA, et al. Evidence for vitamin K semiquinone as the functional form of vitamin K in the liver vitamin K–dependent protein carboxylation reaction. Biochem Biophys Res Comm 1976;70:655.
43. Friedman PA, Shia M. Some characteristics of a vitamin K–dependent carboxylating system from rat liver microsomes. Biochem Biophys Res Comm 1976;70:647.
44. Esmon CT, Suttie JW. Vitamin K–dependent carboxylase: solubilization and properties. J Biol Chem 1976;251:6238.
45. Pennock JF. Occurrence of vitamin K and related quinones. Vitam Horm 1966;24:307.
46. Wallin R, Gabhardt O, Prydz H. NAD(P)H dehydrogenase and its role in the vitamin K (2-methyl-3-phytyl-1,4-napthaquinone)–dependent carboxylation reaction. Biochem J 1978;169:95.
47. Wallin R. No strict coupling of vitamin K_1 (2-methyl-3-phytyl-1,4-napthaquinone)–dependent carboxylation and vitamin K_1 epoxidation in detergent-solubilized microsomal fractions from rat liver. Biochem J 1979;178:513.
48. Wallin R, Hutson S. Vitamin K–dependent carboxylation: evidence that at least two microsomal dehydrogenases reduce vitamin K_1 to support carboxylation. J Biol Chem 1982;57:1583.
49. Whitlon DS, Sadowski JA, Suttie JW. Mechanism of coumarin action: significance of vitamin K epoxide reductase inhibition. Biochemistry 1978;17:1371.
50. Fasco MJ, Principe LM. Vitamin K_1 hydroquinone formation catalyzed by a microsomal reductase system. Biochem Biophys Res Comm 1980;97:1487.
51. Matschiner JT, Zimmerman A, Bell RG. The influence of warfarin on vitamin K epoxide reductase. Thromb Diath Haemorrh 1974;57 (Suppl): 45.
52. Zimmerman A, Matschiner JT. Biochemical basis of hereditary resistance to warfarin in the rat. Biochem Pharmacol 1974;23:1033.
53. Sherman PA, Sander EG. Vitamin K epoxide reductase: evidence that vitamin K dihydroquinone is a product of vitamin K epoxide reduction. Biochem Biophys Res Comm 1981;103:997.
54. Fasco MJ, Hildebrandt EF, Suttie JW. Evidence that warfarin anticoagulant action involves two distinct reduction activities. J Biol Chem 1982;257:11210.
55. Shah DV, Suttie JW. Mechanism of action of vitamin K: evidence for the conversion of a precursor protein to prothrombin in the rat liver. Proc Natl Acad Sci USA 1971;68:1653.
56. Suttie JW. Mechanism of action of vitamin K: demonstration of a liver precursor of prothrombin. Science 1973;179:192.
57. Esmon CT, Sadowski JA, Suttie JW. A new carboxylation reaction: the vitamin K–dependent incorporation of H_2CO_3 into prothrombin. J Biol Chem 1975;250:4744.
58. Grant GA, Suttie JW. Rat liver prothrombin precursors: purification of a second, more basic form. Biochemistry 1976;24:5387.
59. Graves GB, Brabau GG, Olson RE, et al. Immunochemical isolation and electrophoretic characterization of precursor prothrombins in H-35 rat hepatoma cells. Biochemistry 1980;19:266.
60. Swanson JC, Suttie JW. Prothrombin biosynthesis: characterization of processing events in rat liver microsomes. Biochemistry 1985;24:3890.
61. Ganrot PO, Nilehn JE. Plasma prothrombin during treatment with dicumarol: demonstration of an abnormal prothrombin fraction. Scand J Clin Invest 1968;22:23.
62. Nelsestuen GL, Suttie JW. The purification and properties of an abnormal prothrombin protein provided by dicumarol-treated cows. J Biol Chem 1972;247:8176.
63. Shah DV, Swanson JC, Suttie JW. Vitamin K–dependent carboxylase: effect of detergent concentrations, vitamin K status and added protein precursors on activity. Arch Biochem Biophys 1983;222:216.
64. DeMetz M, Vermeer C, Soute BAM, et al. Partial purification of bovine liver vitamin K–dependent carboxylase by immunospecific adsorption onto antifactor X. FEBS Lett 1981;123:215.
65. Jorgensen MJ, Cantor AB, Furie BC, et al. Recognition site directing vitamin K–dependent γ-carboxylation resides on the propeptide of factor IX. Cell 1987;48:185.
66. Diuguid DL, Rabiet M-J, Furie BC, et al. Molecular basis of hemophilia B: a defective enzyme due to an unprocessed propeptide is caused by a point mutation in the factor IX precursor. Proc Natl Acad Sci USA 1986;83:5803.
67. Bentley AK, Rees DJG, Rizza C, et al. Defective propeptide processing of blood clotting factor IX caused by mutation of arginine to glutamine at position −4. Cell 1986;45:343.
68. Ware J, Diuguid DL, Liebman HA, et al. Factor IX San Dimas: substitution of glutamine for arginine −4 in the propeptide leads to incomplete γ-carboxylation and altered phospholipid binding properties. J Biol Chem 1989;264:11401.
69. Pan LC, Price PA. The propeptide of rat bone gamma-carboxyglutamic acid protein shares homology with other vitamin K–dependent protein precursors. Proc Natl Acad Sci USA 1985;82: 6109.
70. Rabiet MJ, Jorgensen MJ, Furie B, et al. Effect of propeptide mutations on posttranslational processing of factor IX: evidence that β-hydroxylation and γ-carboxylation are independent events. J Biol Chem 1987;262:14895.
71. Foster DC, Rudinski MS, Schach BG, et al. Propeptide of human protein C is necessary for γ-carboxylation. Biochemistry 1987;26:7003.
72. Suttie JW, Hageman JM. Vitamin K–dependent carboxylase: development of a peptide substrate. J Biol Chem 1976;251:5827.
73. Suttie JW, Lehrman SR, Geweke LO, et al. Vitamin K–dependent carboxylase: requirement for carboxylation of soluble peptide substrates and substrate specificity. Biochem Biophys Res Comm 1979;86:500.
74. Rich DH, Lehrman SR, Kawai M, et al. Synthesis of peptide analogues of prothrombin precursor sequence 5–9: substrate specificity of vitamin K–dependent carboxylase. J Med Chem 1981;24:706.
75. Decottignies-Le Marechal P, Rikong-Adie H, Azerad R. Vitamin K–dependent carboxylation of synthetic substrates: nature of the products. Biochem Biophys Res Comm 1979;90:700.
76. Ulrich M, Furie B, Jacobs M, et al. Vitamin K–dependent carboxylation: a synthetic peptide based upon the γ-carboxylation recognition site sequence of the prothrombin propeptide is an active substrate for the carboxylase in vitro. J Biol Chem 1988;263:9697.
77. Suttie JW, Hoskins JA, Engelke J, et al. Vitamin K–dependent carboxylase: possible role of the substrate "propeptide" as an intracellular recognition site. Proc Natl Acad Sci USA 1987;84:2730.
78. Knobloch JE, Suttie JW. Vitamin K–dependent carboxylase: control of enzyme activity by the "propeptide" region of factor X. J Biol Chem 1987;262:15334.
79. Price PA, Fraser JD, Metz-Virca G. Molecular cloning of matrix Gla protein: implications for substrate recognition by the vitamin K–dependent γ-carboxylase. Proc Natl Acad Sci USA 1987;84:8335.
80. Hubbard B, Jacobs M, Ulrich M, et al. Vitamin K–dependent carboxylation: in vitro modification of synthetic peptides containing the γ-carboxylation recognition site. J Biol Chem 1989;264:14145.
81. Sanford DG, Kanagy C, Sudmeir JL, et al. Structure of the propeptide of prothrombin containing the γ-carboxylation recognition site determined by two-dimensional NMR spectroscopy. Biochemistry 1991;30: 9835.
81a. Wu SM, Morris DP, Stafford DW. Identification and purification to near homogeneity of the vitamin K–dependent carboxylase. Proc Natl Acad Sci USA 1991;88:2236.
82. McTigue JJ, Dhaon MK, Rich DH, et al. Vitamin K–dependent carboxylase: carboxylation of aspartyl residues to beta-carboxyaspartyl residues. J Biol Chem 1984;259:4272.
83. Fernlund P, Stenflo J. Beta-hydroxyaspartic acid in vitamin K–dependent proteins. J Biol Chem 1983;258:12509.
84. McMullen BA, Fujikawa K, Kisiel W, et al. Complete amino acid sequence of the light chain of human blood coagulation factor X: evidence for identification of residue 63 as β-hydroxyaspartic acid. Biochemistry 1983;22:2875.
85. Stenflo J, Holme E, Lindstedt S, et al. Hydroxylation of aspartic acid in domains homologous to the epidermal growth factor precursor is catalyzed by a 2-oxoglutarate-dependent dioxygenase. Proc Natl Acad Sci USA 1989;86:444.
86. Ohlin A-K, Landes G, Bourdon P, et al. β-Hydroxyaspartic acid in the first epidermal growth factor–like domain of protein C: its role in Ca^{2+} binding and biological activity. J Biol Chem 1988;263:19240.
87. Rees DJG, Jones IM, Handford PA, et al. The role of β-hydroxyaspartate and adjacent carboxylate residues in the first EGF domain of human factor IX. EMBO J 1988;7:2053.
88. Stenflo J, Lundwall A, Dahlback B. β-Hydroxyasparagine in domains homologous to the epidermal growth factor precursor in the vitamin K–dependent protein S. Proc Natl Acad Sci USA 1987;84:368.
89. Arlaud GJ, Van Dorsselaer A, Bell A, et al. Identification of erythro-β-hydroxyasparagine in the EGF-like domain of human Clr. FEBS Lett 1987;222:129.
90. Stenflo J, Onlin A-K, Owen WG, et al. β-Hydroxyaspartic acid or β-hydroxyasparagine in bovine low density lipoprotein receptor and in bovine thrombomodulin. J Biol Chem 1988;263:21.
91. Przysiecki CT, Staggers JE, Ramjit HG, et al. Occurrence of β-hydrox-

ylated asparagine residues in non-vitamin K–dependent proteins containing epidermal growth factor–like domains. Proc Natl Acad Sci USA 1987;84:7856.
92. Choo KH, Gould KG, Rees DJG, et al. Molecular cloning of the gene for human anti–haemophilic factor IX. Nature 1982;299:178.
93. Degen SJ, MacGillivrey RT, Davie EW. Characterization of the cDNA and gene coding for human prothrombin. Biochemistry 1983;22:2087.
94. Fung MR, Hay CW, MacGillivray RTA. Characterization of an almost full-length cDNA coding for human factor X. Proc Natl Acad Sci USA 1985;82:3591.
95. Hagen FS, Gray CL, O'Hara P, et al. Characterization of the cDNA coding for human factor VII. Proc Natl Acad Sci USA 1986;83:2412.
96. Leytus SP, Chung DW, Kisiel W, et al. Characterization of a cDNA coding for human factor X. Proc Natl Acad Sci USA 1984;81:3699.
97. Bucher D, Nebelin E, Thomsen J, et al. Identification of γ-carboxyglutamic acid residues in bovine factors IX and X, and in a new vitamin K–dependent protein. FEBS Lett 1976;68:293.
98. Fryklund L, Borg H, Andersson L-O. Amino terminal sequence of human factor IX: presence of γ-carboxyglutamic acid residues. FEBS Lett 1976;65:187.
99. Esmon CT, Suttie JW, Jackson CM. The functional significance of vitamin K action: difference in phospholipid binding between normal and abnormal prothrombin. J Biol Chem 1975;250:4095.
100. Stenflo J, Ganrot P-O. Vitamin K and the biosynthesis of prothrombin: identification and purification of a dicoumarol-induced abnormal prothrombin from bovine plasma. J Biol Chem 1972;247:8160.
101. Magnusson S, Sottrup-Jenssen L, Petersen TE, et al. Primary structure of the vitamin K–dependent part of prothrombin. FEBS Lett 1974;44:189.
102. Walz DA, Hewett-Emmett D, Seegers WH. Amino acid sequence of human prothrombin fragments 1 and 2. Proc Natl Acad Sci USA 1977;74:1969.
103. Enfield DL, Ericsson LE, Walsh KA, et al. Bovine factor X_1 (Stuart factor), primary structure of the light chain. Proc Natl Acad Sci USA 1975;72:16.
104. McMullen B, Fujikawa K, Kisiel W, et al. Complete amino acid sequence of the light chain of human blood coagulation factor X: evidence for identification of residue 63 as β-hydroxyaspartic acid. Biochemistry 1983;22:2875.
105. Morris HR, Dell A, Petersen TE, et al. Mass spectrometric identification and sequence location of the ten residues of the new amino acid (β-carboxyglutamic acid) in the N-terminal region of prothrombin. Biochem J 1976;153:663.
106. Katayama K, Ericsson L, Enfield D, et al. Comparison of amino acid sequence of bovine coagulation factor IX (Christmas factor) with that of other vitamin K–dependent proteins. Proc Natl Acad Sci USA 1979;76:4990.
107. Takeya H, Kawabata S-I, Nakagawa K, et al. Bovine factor VII: its purification and complete amino acid sequence. J Biol Chem 1988;263:14868.
108. Sperling R, Furie BC, Blumenstein M, et al. Metal binding properties of γ-carboxyglutamic acid. J Biol Chem 1978;253:3898.
109. Furie BC, Blumenstein M, Furie B. Metal binding sites of a γ-carboxyglutamic acid-rich fragment of bovine prothrombin. J Biol Chem 1979;254:12521.
109a. Soriano-Garcia M, Padmanabhan K, de Vos AM, Tulinsky A. The Ca^{2+} ion and membrane binding structure of the Gla domain of Ca-prothrombin fragment 1. Biochemistry 1992;31:2554.
110. Bajaj SP, Butkowski RJ, Mann KG. Prothrombin fragments, Ca^{2+} binding and activation kinetics. J Biol Chem 1975;250:2150.
111. Benarous R, Elion J, Labie D. Ca^{2+} binding properties of human prothrombin. Biochemistry 1976;38:391.
112. Furie BC, Furie B. Interaction of lanthanide ions with bovine factor X and their use in the affinity chromatography of the venom coagulant protein of *Vipera russelli*. J Biol Chem 1975;250:601.
113. Furie BC, Mann KG, Furie B. Substitution of lanthanide ions for calcium ions in the activation of bovine prothrombin by activated factor X: high affinity metal binding sites of prothrombin and the derivatives of prothrombin activation. J Biol Chem 1976;251:3235.
114. Nelsestuen GL, Broderius M, Zytkovicz TH, et al. On the role of γ-carboxyglutamic acid in calcium and phospholipid binding. Biochem Biophys Res Comm 1975;65:233.
115. Amphlett GW, Byrne R, Castellino FJ. The binding of metal ions to bovine factor IX. J Biol Chem 1978;253:6774.
116. Henriksen RA, Jackson CM. Cooperative calcium binding by the phospholipid binding region of prothrombin: a requirement for intact disulfide bridges. Arch Biochem Biophys 1975;170:149.
117. Robertson P Jr, Hiskey RG, Koehler KA. Calcium and magnesium binding to γ-carboxyglutamic acid-containing peptides via metal ion nuclear magnetic resonance. J Biol Chem 1978;253:5880.
118. Bloom JW, Mann KG. Metal ion-induced conformational transitions of prothrombin and prothrombin fragment 1. Biochemistry 1978;17:4430.
119. Nelsestuen GL. Role of gamma-carboxyglutamic acid: an unusual transition required for calcium-dependent binding of prothrombin to phospholipid. J Biol Chem 1976;251:5648.
120. Prendergast FG, Mann KG. Differentiation of metal ion-induced transitions of prothrombin fragment 1. J Biol Chem 1977;252:840.
121. Furie B, Provost K, Blanchard RA, et al. Antibodies directed against a γ-carboxyglutamic acid-rich region of bovine prothrombin: preparation, isolation and characterization. J Biol Chem 1978;253:8980.
122. Furie B, Furie BC. Conformation-specific antibodies as probes of the γ-carboxyglutamic acid-rich region of bovine prothrombin: studies of metal-induced structural changes. J Biol Chem 1979;254:9766.
123. Tai MM, Furie BC, Furie B. Conformation-specific antibodies directed against the bovine prothrombin-calcium complex. J Biol Chem 1980;255:2790.
124. Madar DA, Hall TJ, Reisner HM, et al. The interaction of bovine prothrombin fragment 1 with metal ions: an immunological approach to kinetic and equilibrium studies. J Biol Chem 1980;255:8599.
125. Borowski M, Furie BC, Bauminger S, et al. Prothrombin requires two sequential metal-dependent conformational transitions to bind phospholipid. J Biol Chem 1986;261:14969.
126. Tai MM, Furie BC, Furie B. Localization of the metal-induced conformational transition of bovine prothrombin. J Biol Chem 1984;259:4162.
127. Butkowski RJ, Elion J, Downing MR, et al. Primary structure of human prethrombin 2 and thrombin. J Biol Chem 1977;252:4942.
128. Titani K, Fujikawa K, Enfield DL, et al. Bovine factor X_1 (Stuart factor): amino acid sequence of heavy chain. Proc Natl Acad Sci USA 1975;72:3082.
129. Neurath H. Evolution of proteolytic enzymes. Science 1984;224:350.
130. Friezner Degen SJ, Davie EW. Nucleotide sequence of the gene for human prothrombin. Biochemistry 1987;26:6165.
131. Bajaj SP, Price PA, Russell WA. Decarboxylation of γ-carboxyglutamic acid residues in human prothrombin. J Biol Chem 1982;257:3726.
132. Bajaj SP, Saini R, Katz A, et al. Metal ion blockage of tritium incorporation into γ-carboxyglutamic acid of prothrombin. J Biol Chem 1988;263:9725.
133. Lewis MR, Deerfield DW II, Hoke RA, et al. Studies on Ca(II) binding to γ-carboxyglutamic acid. J Biol Chem 1988;263:1358.
134. Liebman HA, Furie BC, Furie B. The factor IX phospholipid-binding site is required for calcium-dependent activation of factor IX by factor XIa. J Biol Chem 1987;262:7605.
135. Nelsestuen GL, Broderius M, Martin G. Role of γ-carboxyglutamic acid: cation specificity of prothrombin and factor X–phospholipid interaction. J Biol Chem 1976;251:6886.
136. Mann KG, Nesheim ME, Tracy PB, et al. Assembly of the prothrombinase complex. Biophys J 1982;37:106.
137. Park CH, Tulinsky A. Three-dimensional structure of the kringle sequence: structure of prothrombin fragment 1. Biochemistry 1986;25:3977.
138. Harlos K, Holland SK, Boys CWG, et al. Vitamin K–dependent blood coagulation proteins form hetero-dimers. Nature 1987;330:82.
139. Cooke RM, Wilkinson AJ, Baron M, et al. The solution structure of human epidermal growth factor. Nature 1987:327:339.
140. Appella E, Robinson EA, Ullrich SJ, et al. The receptor-binding sequence of urokinase. J Biol Chem 1987;262:4437.
141. Heath WF, Merrifield RB. A synthetic approach to structure–function relationships in the murine epidermal growth factor molecule. Proc Natl Acad Sci USA 1986;83:6367.
142. Davis LM, McGraw RA, Ware JL, et al. Factor IX Alabama: a point mutation in a clotting protein results in hemophilia B. Blood 1987;69:140.
143. McCord DM, Monroe DM, Roberts HR. Characterization of the functional defect in factor IX Alabama: a mutation near the first EGF-like domain results in defective interaction with factor VIIIa. Blood 1988;72(Suppl):302a.
144. Magnusson S, Petersen TE, Sottrup-Jensen L, et al. Complete primary structure of prothrombin: isolation, structure and reactivity of ten carboxylated glutamic acid residues and regulation of prothrombin activation by thrombin. In: Reich E, Rifkin DB, Shaw E, eds. Proteases and Biological Control. Cold Spring Harbor, New York, Cold Spring Harbor Laboratory, 1973:123.
145. Ny T, Elgh F, Lund B. The structure of the human tissue-type plasminogen activator gene: correlation of intron and exon structures to functional and structural domains. Proc Natl Acad Sci USA 1984;81:5355.
146. Cool DE, Edgell CJS, Louie GV, et al. Characterization of human blood coagulation factor XII cDNA. J Biol Chem 1985;260:13666.
147. Holmes WE, Pennica D, Blaber M, et al. Cloning and expression of the gene for prourokinase in *E coli*. Biotechnology 1985;3:923.
148. Malinowski DP, Sadler JE, Davie EW. Characterization of a complementary deoxyribonucleic acid coding for human and bovine plasminogen. Biochemistry 1984;23:4243.
149. Gilbert W. Why genes in pieces? Nature 1978;271:501.
150. Patthy L. Evolution of the proteases of blood coagulation and fibrinolysis by assembly from modules. Cell 1985;41:657.
151. Furie B, Bing DH, Feldmann RJ, et al. Computer-generated models of blood coagulation factor Xa, factor IXa, and thrombin based upon structural homology with other serine proteases. J Biol Chem 1982;257:3875.

152. Irwin DM, Ahern KG, Pearson GD, et al. Characterization of the bovine prothrombin gene. Biochemistry 1985;24:6854.
153. Royle NJ, Irwin DM, Koschinsky ML, et al. Human genes encoding prothrombin and ceruloplasmin map to 11p11-q12 and 3q21-24 respectively. Somat Cell Mol Genet 1987;13:285.
154. Leytus SP, Foster DC, Kurachi K, et al. Gene for human factor X: a blood coagulation factor whose gene organization is essentially identical with that of factor IX and protein C. Biochemistry 1986;25:5098.
155. Yoshitake S, Schach BG, Foster DC, et al. Nucleotide sequence of the gene for human factor IX. Biochemistry 1985;24:3736.
156. O'Hara PJ, Grant FJ, Haldeman BA, et al. Nucleotide sequence of the gene coding for human factor VII, a vitamin K–dependent protein participating in blood coagulation. Proc Natl Acad Sci USA 1987;84:5158.
157. Foster DC, Yoshitake S, Davie EW. The nucleotide sequence of the gene for human protein C. Proc Natl Acad Sci USA 1985;82:4673.
158. Irwin DM, Robertson KA, MacGillivray RTA. Structure and evolution of the bovine prothrombin gene. J Mol Biol 1988;200:31.
159. Jorgensen MJ, Cantor AB, Furie BC, et al. Expression of completely γ-carboxylated recombinant human prothrombin. J Biol Chem 1987;262: 6729.
160. Mizuochi T, Yamashita K, Fujikawa K, et al. The carbohydrate of bovine prothrombin: occurrence of Gal-β 1-3GlcNAc grouping in asparagine-linked sugar chains. J Biol Chem 1979;254:6419.
161. Borowski M, Furie B, Goldsmith GH, et al. Metal and phospholipid binding properties of partially carboxylated variant prothrombins. J Biol Chem 1985;260:9258.
162. Borowski M, Furie BC, Furie B. Distribution of γ-carboxyglutamic acid residues in partially carboxylated prothrombins. J Biol Chem 1986;261: 1624.
163. Zapata GA, Berkowitz P, Noyes CM, et al. Chemical modification of bovine prothrombin fragment 1 in the presence of Tb^{+3} ions. J Biol Chem 1988;263:8150.
164. Wright SF, Berkowitz P, Deerfield DW II, et al. Chemical modification of bovine prothrombin fragment 1 in the presence of Tb^{3+} ions. J Biol Chem 1986;261:10598.
165. Nelsestuen GL, Lim TK. Equilibria involved in prothrombin- and blood clotting factor X–membrane binding. Biochemistry 1977;16:4164.
166. Lim TK, Bloomfield VA, Nelsestuen GL. Structure of the prothrombin- and blood clotting factor X–membrane complex. Biochemistry 1977;16: 4177.
167. Sommerville LE, Resnick RM, Thomas DD, et al. Terbium probe of calcium-binding sites on the prothrombin-membrane complex. J Biol Chem 1986;261:6222.
168. Bajaj SP, Butkowski RJ, Mann KG. Prothrombin fragments: calcium binding and activation kinetics. J Biol Chem 1975;250:2150.
169. Nelsestuen GL, Broderius M. Interaction of prothrombin and blood clotting factor X with membranes. Biochemistry 1977;16:4172.
170. Gitel SN, Owen WG, Esmon CT, et al. A polypeptide region of bovine prothrombin specific for binding to phospholipids. Proc Natl Acad Sci USA 1973;70:1344.
171. Esmon CT, Jackson CM. The conversion of prothrombin to thrombin: IV. the function of the fragment 2 region during activation in the presence of factor V. J Biol Chem 1974;249:7791.
172. Guinto ER, Esmon CT. Loss of prothrombin and of factor Xa–factor Va interactions upon inactivation of factor Va by activated protein C. J Biol Chem 1984;259:13986.
173. Tracy PB, Mann KG. Prothrombinase complex assembly on the platelet surface is mediated through the 74,000-dalton component of factor Va. Proc Natl Acad Sci USA 1983;80:2380.
174. Tucker MM, Foster WB, Katzmann JA, et al. A monoclonal antibody which inhibits the factor Va:factor Xa interaction. J Biol Chem 1983;258: 1210.
175. Mann KG, Jenny RJ, Krishnaswamy S. Cofactor proteins in the assembly and expression of blood clotting enzyme complexes. Annu Rev Biochem 198;57:915.
176. Rosing J, Tans G, Govers-Riemslag JWP, et al. The role of phospholipids and factor Va in the prothrombinase complex. J Biol Chem 1980;255: 274.
177. Nesheim ME, Tracy RP, Mann KG. Clotspeed, a mathematical simulation of the functional properties of prothrombinase. J Biol Chem 1984;259:1447.
178. Tracy PB, Peterson JM, Nesheim ME, et al. Interaction of coagulation factor V and factor Va with platelets. J Biol Chem 1979;254:10354.
179. Kane WH, Lindhout MJ, Jackson CM, et al. Factor Va–dependent binding of factor Xa to platelets. J Biol Chem 1980;255:1170.
180. Miletich JP, Jackson CM, Majerus PW. Interaction of coagulation factor Xa with human platelets. Proc Natl Acad Sci USA 1977;74:4033.
181. Miletich JP, Jackson CM, Majerus PW. Patients with congenital factor V deficiency have decreased factor Xa binding sites on their platelets. J Clin Invest 1978;62:824.
182. Maruyama I, Salem H, Majerus PW. Coagulation factor Va binds to human umbilical vein endothelial cells (HUVE) and accelerates protein C activation. J Clin Invest 1984;73:654.
183. Rodgers GM, Shuman MA. Prothrombin is activated on vascular endothelium by factor Xa and calcium. Proc Natl Acad Sci USA 1983;80: 7001.
184. Tracy P, Rohrbach MS, Mann KG. Functional prothrombinase complex assembly on isolated monocytes and lymphocytes. J Biol Chem 1983;258:7264.
185. Tracy P, Eide LL, Mann KG. Human prothrombinase complex assembly and function on isolated peripheral blood cell populations. J Biol Chem 1985;260:2119.
186. Stenn KS, Blout ER. Mechanism of bovine prothrombin activation by an insoluble preparation of bovine factor Xa (thrombokinase). Biochemistry 1972;11:4502.
187. Rodgers GM, Kane WH, Pitas RE. Formation of factor Va by atherosclerotic rabbit aorta mediates factor Xa–catalyzed prothrombin activation. J Clin Invest 1988;81:1911.
188. Rosenberg JS, Beeler DL, Rosenberg RD: Activation of human prothrombin by highly purified human factors V and Xa in the presence of human antithrombin. J Biol Chem 1975;250:1607.
189. Esmon CT, Jackson CM. The conversion of prothrombin to thrombin: V. the activation of prothrombin by factor Xa in the presence of phospholipid. J Biol Chem 1974;249:7798.
190. Esmon CT, Jackson CM. The conversion of prothrombin to thrombin: III. the factor Xa catalyzed activation of prothrombin. J Biol Chem 1974;249:7782.
191. Heldebrant CM, Butkowski RJ, Bajaj SP, et al. The activation of prothrombin. II. Partial reactions, physical and chemical characterization of the intermediates of activation. J Biol Chem 1973;248:7149.
192. Downing MR, Butkowski RJ, Clark MM, et al. Human prothrombin activation. J Biol Chem 1975;250:1607.
193. Nesheim ME, Mann KG. Kinetics and cofactor dependence of the two cleavages involved in prothrombin activation. J Biol Chem 1984;258: 5386.
194. Rosing J, Zwaal RFA, Tans G. Formation of meizothrombin as intermediate in factor Xa–catalyzed prothrombin activation. J Biol Chem 1986;261:4222.
195. van Rijn JLML, Govers-Riemslag JWP, Zwaal RFA, et al. Kinetic studies of prothrombin activation: effect of ractor Va and phospholipids on the formation of the enzyme-substrate complex. Biochemistry 1984;23: 4557.
196. Esmon CT, Owen WG, Jackson CM. The conversion of prothrombin to thrombin: II. differentiation between thrombin and factor Xa–catalyzed proteolysis. J Biol Chem 1974;249:606.
197. Aronson DL, Stevan L, Ball AP, et al. Generation of the combined prothrombin activation peptide (F1.2) during the clotting of blood and plasma. J Clin Invest 1977;60:1410.
198. Rabiet MJ, Blashill A, Furie B, et al. Prothrombin fragment 1.2.3, a major product of prothrombin activation in human plasma. J Biol Chem 1986;261:13210.
199. Teitel JM, Bauer KA, Lau HK, et al. Studies of the prothrombin activation pathway utilizing radioimmunoassays for the F2/F1+2 fragment and thrombin-antithrombin complex. Blood 1982;59:1086.
200. Lau HK, Rosenberg JS, Beeler DL, et al. The isolation and characterization of a specific antibody population directed against the prothrombin activation fragments F2 and F1+2. J Biol Chem 1979;254: 8751.
201. Bauer KA, Rosenberg RD. The pathophysiology of the prethrombotic state in humans: insights gained from studies using markers of hemostatic system activation. Blood 1987;70:343.
202. Blomback B, Blomback M, Hessel B, et al. Structure of N-terminal framents of fibrinogen and specificity of thrombin. Nature 1967;215: 1445.
203. Sherry S, Troll W. The action of thrombin on synthetic substrates. J Biol Chem 1954;208:95.
204. Chase T Jr, Shaw E. Comparison of the esterase activities of trypsin, plasmin and thrombin on guanidinobenzoate esters. Biochemistry 1969;8:2212.
205. Morita T, Kato H, Iwanaga S, et al. New fluorogenic substrates for α-thrombin, factor Xa, kallikreins and urokinase. J Biochem 1977;82: 1495.
206. Pittman D, Kaufman R. Proteolytic requirements for thrombin activation of anti–hemophilic factor (factor VIII). Proc Natl Acad Sci USA 1988;85:2429.
207. Esmon CT. The subunit structure of thrombin-activated factor V: isolation of activated factor V, separation of subunits and reconstitution of biological activity. J Biol Chem 1979;254:964.
208. Nesheim ME, Mann KG. Thrombin-catalyzed activation of single-chain bovine factor V. J Biol Chem 1979;254:10952.
209. Schwartz ML, Pizzo SV, Hill RL, et al. Human factor XIII from plasma and platelets. J Biol Chem 1973;248:1395.
210. McGowan EB, Ding A-H, Detwiler TC. Correlation of thrombin-induced glycoprotein V hydrolysis and platelet activation. J Biol Chem 1983;258: 11243.
210a. Vu TK, Hung DT, Wheaton VI, Conghlin SR. Molecular cloning of a functional thrombin receptor reveals a novel proteolytic mechanism of receptor activation. Cell 1991;64:1057.
211. Boissel JP, Le Bonnier B, Rabiet MJ, et al. Covalent structures of β and γ autolytic derivatives of human α-thrombin. J Biol Chem 1984;259: 5691.

212. Abildgaard U. Binding of thrombin to antithrombin III. Scand J Clin Lab Invest 1969;24:89.
213. Damus PS, Hicks M, Rosenberg RD. Anticoagulant action of heparin. Nature 1973;246:355.
214. Rosenberg RD, Damus PS. The purification and mechanism of action of human antithrombin–heparin cofactor. J Biol Chem 1973;248:6490.
215. Downing MR, Bloom JW, Mann KG. Comparison of the inhibition of thrombin by three plasma protease inhibitors. Biochemistry 1978;17: 2649.
216. Matheson NR, Travis J. Inactivation of human thrombin in the presence of human α_1-proteinase inhibitor. Biochem J 1976;159:495.
217. Markwardt F. Hirudin as an inhibitor. Methods Enzymol 1970;19:924.
218. Josso F, Lavergne JM, Weilland C, et al. Etude immunologique de la prothrombine et de la thrombine humaines. Thromb Diath Haemorrh 1967;18:311.
219. Blanchard RA, Furie BC, Jorgensen MJ, et al. Acquired vitamin K–dependent carboxylation deficiency in liver disease. N Engl J Med 1981;305:242.
220. Karpatkin M, Karpatkin S. Humoral factor that specifically regulates prothrombin (factor II) levels (coagulopoietin II). Proc Natl Acad Sci USA 1979;76:491.
221. Shah DV, Nyari LJ, Swanson JC, et al. Effect of a humoral factor on plasma prothrombin and vitamin K–dependent liver carboxylase levels in the rat. Thromb Res 1980;19:111.
222. Shapiro SS, Martinez J. Human prothrombin metabolism in normal man and in hypocoagulable subjects. J Clin Invest 1969;48, 1292.
223. Lau HK, Rosenberg RD. The isolation and characterization of a specific antibody population directed against the thrombin-antithrombin complex. J Biol Chem 1980;255:5885.
224. Bauer KA, Broekmans AW, Bertina RM, et al. Hemostatic enzyme generation in the blood of patients with hereditary protein C deficiency. Blood 1988;71:1418.
225. Jackson CM. Characterization of two glycoprotein variants of bovine factor X and demonstration that the factor X zymogen contains two polypeptide chains. Biochemistry 1972;11:4873.
226. Fujikawa K, Legaz ME, Davie EW. Bovine factors X_1 and X_2 (Stuart factor): isolation and characterization. Biochemistry 1972;11:4882.
227. Radcliffe RD, Barton PD. Comparisons of the molecular forms of activated bovine factor X. J Biol Chem 1973;248:6788.
228. Jesty J, Spencer AK, Nemerson Y. The mechanism of activation of factor X. J Biol Chem 1974;249:5614.
229. Fujikawa K, Coan MH, Legaz ME, et al. The mechanism of activation of bovine factor X (Stuart factor) by intrinsic and extrinsic pathways. Biochemistry 1974;13:5290.
230. Furie BC, Furie B, Gottlieb AJ, et al. Activation of bovine factor X by the venom coagulant protein of Vipera russelli: complex formation of the activation fragments. Biochim Biophys Acta 1974;365:121.
231. Fujikawa K, Legaz ME, Davie EW. Bovine factor X_1 (Stuart factor): mechanism of activation by protein from Russell's viper venom. Biochemistry 1972;11:4892.
232. Mizuochi T, Yamashita K, Fujikawa K, et al. The structures of the carbohydrate moieties of bovine blood coagulation factor X. J Biol Chem 1980;255:3526.
233. Furie B, Furie BC. Spectral changes in bovine factor X associated with activation by the venom coagulant protein of Vipera russelli. J Biol Chem 1976;251:6807.
234. Mizuochi T, Yamashita K, Fujikawa K, et al. The structures of the carbohydrate moieties of bovine blood coagulation factor X. J Biol Chem 1980;255:3526.
235. Keyt B, Furie BC, Furie B. Structural transitions in bovine factor X associated with metal binding and zymogen activation: studies using conformation-specific antibodies. J Biol Chem 1982;257:8687.
236. Dahlback B, Stenflo J: Binding of bovine coagulation factor Xa to platelets. Biochemistry 1978;17:4938.
237. Kane WH, Lindhout MJ, Jackson CM, et al. Factor Va–dependent binding of factor Xa to human platelets. J Biol Chem 1979;257:3963.
238. Gordon SG, Cross BA. A factor X–activating cysteine protease from malignant tissue. J Clin Invest 1981;67:1665.
239. Falanga A, Gordon SG. Isolation and characterization of cancer procoagulant: a cysteine proteinase from malignant tissue. Biochemistry 1985;24:5558.
240. Williams WJ, Esnouf MP. The fractionation of Russell's viper (Vipera russelli) venom with special reference to the coagulant protein. Biochem J 1962;84:52.
241. Hultin M, Nemerson Y. Activation of factor X by factors IXa and VIII: a specific assay for factor IXa in the presence of thrombin-activated factor VIII. Blood 1978;52:928.
242. Stern D, Nawroth P, Handley D, et al. An endothelial cell-dependent pathway of coagulation. Proc Natl Acad Sci USA 1985;82:2523.
243. Neuenschwander P, Jesty J. A comparison of phospholipid and platelets in the activation of human factor VIII by thrombin and factor Xa, and in the activation of factor X. Blood 1988;72:1761.
244. Silverberg SA, Nemerson Y, Zur M. Kinetics of the activation of bovine coagulation factor X by components of the extrinsic pathway: kinetic behavior of two-chain factor VII in the presence and absence of tissue factor. J Biol Chem 1977;252:8481.
245. Trauber D, Hawkins K, Karpatkin M, et al. Humoral factor that specifically regulates factor X levels in rabbits (coagulopoietin-X). J Clin Invest 1979;64:1713.
246. Gitel SN, Medina VM, Wessler S. Inhibition of human activated factor X by antithrombin III and alpha 1-proteinase inhibitor in human plasma. J Biol Chem 1984;259:6890.
247. Fuchs HE, Pizzo SV. Regulation of factor Xa in vitro in human and mouse plasma and in vivo in mouse: role of the endothelium and plasma proteinase inhibitors. J Clin Invest 1983;72:2041.
248. Gilgenkrantz S, Briquel ME, Andre E, et al. Structural genes of coagulation factors VII and X located on 13q34. Ann Genet 1986;29:32.
249. Broze GJ, Majerus PW. Purification and properties of human coagulation factor VII. J Biol Chem 1980;255:1242.
250. Radcliffe R, Nemerson Y. Activation and control of factor X and thrombin: isolation and characterization of a single chain form of factor VII. J Biol Chem 1974;250:388.
251. Kisiel W, Fujikawa K, Davie EW. Activation of bovine factor VII (Proconvertin) by factor XIIa (activated Hageman factor). Biochemistry 1977;16:4189.
252. Radcliffe R, Nemerson Y. Mechanism of action of bovine factor VII: products of cleavage of factor Xa. J Biol Chem 1976;251:4797.
253. Radcliffe R, Bagdassarian A, Colman R, et al. Activation of bovine factor VII by Hageman factor fragments. Blood 1977;50:611.
254. Zur M, Nemerson Y. The esterase activity of coagulation factor VII: evidence for intrinsic activity of the zymogen. J Biol Chem 1977;253: 2203.
255. Broze GJ, Leykam JE, Schwartz BD, et al. Purification of human brain tissue factor. J Biol Chem 1985;260:10917.
256. Guha A, Bach R, Konigsberg W, et al. Affinity purification of human tissue factor: interaction of factor VII and tissue factor in detergent micelles. Proc Natl Acad Sci USA 1986;83:299.
257. Bach R, Nemerson Y, Konigsberg W. Purification and characterization of bovine tissue factor. J Biol Chem 1981;256:8324.
258. Zur M, Nemerson Y. Kinetics of factor IX activation via the extrinsic pathway. J Biol Chem 1980;255:5703.
259. Osterud B, Rapaport SI. Activation of factor IX by the reaction product of tissue factor and factor VII: additional pathway for initiating blood coagulation. Proc Natl Acad Sci USA 1977;74:5260.
260. Spicer EK, Horton R, Bloem L, et al. Isolation of cDNA clones coding for human tissue factor: primary structure of the protein and cDNA. Proc Natl Acad Sci USA 1987;84:5148.
261. Morrissey JH, Fakhrai H, Edgington TS. Molecular cloning of the cDNA for tissue factor, the cellular receptor for the initiation of the coagulation protease cascade. Cell 1987;50:129.
262. Bach R, Konigsberg WH, Nemerson Y. Human tissue factor contains thioester-linked palmitate and stearate on the cytoplasmic half-cystine. Biochemistry 1988;27:4227.
263. Fair DS, MacDonald MJ. Cooperative interaction between factor VII and cell surface–expressed tissue factor. J Biol Chem 1987;262: 11692.
264. Niemetz J. Coagulant activity of leukocytes: tissue factor activity. J Clin Invest 1972;51:307.
265. Levy GA, Edgington TS. Lymphocyte cooperation is required for amplification of macrophage procoagulant activity. J Exp Med 1980;151: 1232.
266. Colucci M, Balconi G, Lounzet R, et al. Cultured human endothelial cells generate tissue factor in response to endotoxin. J Clin Invest 1983;71:1893.
267. Rodgers GM, Greenberg CS, Shuman MA. Characterization of the effects of cultured vascular cells on the activation of blood coagulation. Blood 1983;61:1155.
268. Ploplis VA, Edgington TS, Fair DS. Initiation of the extrinsic pathway of coagulation: association of factor VIIa with a cell line expressing tissue factor. J Biol Chem 1987;262:9503.
269. Zur M, Radcliffe RD, Oberdick J, et al. Dual role of factor VII in blood coagulation. J Biol Chem 1982;257, 5623.
270. Jesty J, Silverberg SA. Kinetics of the tissue factor–dependent activation of coagulation factors IX and X in a bovine plasma system. J Biol Chem 1979;254:12337.
271. Kondo S, Kisiel W. Regulation of factor VIIa activity in plasma: evidence that antithrombin III is the sole plasma protease inhibitor of human factor VIIa. Thromb Res 1987;46:325.
272. Fair DS. Quantitation of factor VII in the plasma of normal and warfarin-treated individuals by radioimmunoassay. Blood 1983;62:784.
273. Broze GJ Jr, Miletic JP. Isolation of the tissue factor inhibitor by HepG2 hepatoma cells. Proc Natl Acad Sci USA 1987;84:1886.
274. Sanders NL, Bajaj SP, Zivelin A, et al. Inhibition of tissue factor/factor VIIa activity in plasma requires factor X and an additional plasma factor. Blood 1985;66:204.
275. Rao LV, Rapaport SI. Studies of a mechanism inhibiting the initiation of the extrinsic pathway of coagulation. Blood 1987;69:645.
276. Rapaport SI. Inhibition of factor VIIa/tissue factor–induced blood coagulation: with particular emphasis upon a factor Xa–dependent inhibitory mechanism. Blood 1989;73:359.
277. Broze GJ Jr, Warren LA, Novotny WF, et al. The lipoprotein-associated coagulation inhibitor that inhibits the factor VII–tissue factor complex

also inhibits factor Xa: insight into its possible mechanism of action. Blood 1988;71:335.
278. Camerino G, Grzeschik KH, Jaye M, et al. Regional localization on the human X chromosome and polymorphism of the coagulation factor IX gene (hemophilia B locus). Proc Natl Acad Sci USA 1984;81:498.
279. Fujikawa K, Thompson AR, Legaz ME, et al: Isolation and characterization of bovine factor IX (Christmas factor). Biochemistry 1973;12: 4938.
280. DiScipio RG, Hermodson MA, Yates SG, et al. A comparison of human prothrombin, factor IX (Christmas factor), factor X (Stuart factor) and protein S. Biochemistry 1977;16:698.
281. Morita T, Isaacs BS, Esmon CT, et al. Derivatives of blood coagulation factor IX contain a high affinity Ca^{2+} binding site that lacks γ-carboxyglutamic acid. J Biol Chem 1984;259:5698.
282. Beckmann RJ, Schmidt RJ, Santerre RF, et al. The structure and evolution of a 461 amino acid human protein C precursor and its messenger RNA, based upon the DNA sequence of cloned human liver cDNAs. Nucleic Acids Res 1985;13:5233.
283. Long GL, Belagaje RM, MacGillivray RTA. Cloning and sequencing of liver cDNA coding for bovine protein C. Proc Natl Acad Sci USA 1984;81:5653.
284. Lundwall A, Dackowski W, Cohen E, et al. Isolation and sequence of the cDNA for human protein S, a regulator of blood coagulation. Proc Natl Acad Sci USA 1986;83, 6716.
285. Nawroth PP, Wilner GG, Stern DM. Circulation 1986;74(Suppl 2):232.
286. Jones ME, Griffity MJ, Monroe DM, et al. Comparison of lipid binding and kinetic proeprties of normal, variant, and γ-carboxyglutamic acid modified human factor IX and factor IXa. Biochemistry 1985;24:8064.
287. Ryan J, Wolitsky B, Heimer E, et al. Structural determinants of the factor IX molecule mediating interaction with the endothelial cell binding site are distinct from those involved in phospholipid binding. J Biol Chem 1989;264:20283.
288. Byrne R, Amphlett GW, Castellino FJ. Metal ion specificity of the conversion of bovine factors IX, IXα, and IXaα to bovine factor IXaβ. J Biol Chem 1980;255:1430.
289. Rimon S, Melamed R, Savion N, et al. Identification of a factor IX/IXa binding protein on the endothelial cell surface. J Biol Chem 1987;262: 6023.
290. Rawala R, Ahmad SS, Walsh PN. Factor IXa binding to activated human platelets promotes factor X activation. Blood 1987;70:393a.
291. Ahmad SS, Rawala-Sheikh RR, Walsh PN. Comparative interactions of factor IX and factor IXa with human platelets. J Biol Chem 1989;264: 3244.
292. van der Graaf F, Greengard JS, Bouma BN, et al. Isolation and functional characterization of the active light chain of activated human blood coagulation factor XI. J Biol Chem 1983;258:9669.
293. Sinha D, Koshy A, Seaman FS, et al. Functional characterization of human blood coagulation factor XIa using hybridoma antibodies. J Biol Chem 1985;260:10714.
294. Sinha D, Seaman FS, Walsh PN. Role of calcium ions and the heavy chain of factor IXa in the activation of human coagulation factor IX. Biochemistry 1987;26:3884.
295. DiScipio RG, Kurachi K, Davie EW. Activation of human factor IX (Christmas factor). J Clin Invest 1978;61:1528.
296. Lindquist PA, Fujikawa K, Davie EW. Activation of bovine factor IX (Christmas factor) by factor XIa (activated plasma thromboplastin antecedent) and a protease from Russell's viper venom. J Biol Chem 1978;254:1902.
297. van Dieigen G, Tans G, Rosing J, et al. The role of phospholipid and factor VIIIa in the activation of bovine factor X. J Biol Chem 1981;256: 3433.
298. Masys DR, Bajaj SP, Rapaport SI. Activation of factor VII by activated factors IX and X. Blood 1982;60:1143.
299. Rick ME. Activation of factor VIII by factor IXa. Blood 1982;60:744.
300. Briet E, Bertina RM, van Tilberg NH, et al. Hemophilia B Leyden. N Engl J Med 1982;306:788.
301. Fahner JB, Salier JP, Landa L, et al. Defective promoter structure in a human factor IX Leyden. Blood 1988;72(Suppl 1):295a.
302. Reitsma PH, Bertina RM, Ploos van Amstel JK, et al. The putative factor IX gene promoter in hemophilia Leyden. Blood 1988;72:1074.
303. Rosenberg J, McKenna P, Rosenberg RD. Inhibition of human factor IXa by human antithrombin. J Biol Chem 1975;250:8883.
304. Kurachi K, Fujikawa K, Schmer G, Davie EW. Inhibition of bovine factor IXa and factor Xa by antithrombin III. Biochemistry 1976;15: 373.
305. McMillan CW, Roberts HR. Congenital combined deficiency of coagulation factors II, VII, IX, X. N Engl J Med 1979;274:1313.
306. Chung KS, Bezeaud A, Goldsmith JC, et al. Congenital deficiency of blood clotting factors II, VII, IX and X. Blood 1979;53:776.
307. Vicente V, Maia R, Alberca I, et al. Congenital deficiency of vitamin K–dependent coagulation factors and protein C. Thromb Haemost 1984;51:343.
308. Johnson CA, Chung HS, McGrath KM, et al. Characterization of a variant prothrombin in a patient congenitally deficient in factor II, VII, IX and X. Br J Haematol 1980;44:461.
309. Goldsmith GH Jr, Pence RE, Ratnoff OD, et al. Studies on a family with combined functional deficiencies of vitamin K–dependent coagulation factors. J Clin Invest 1982;69:1253.
310. Kasper CK, Osterud B, Minami JY, et al. Hemophilia B: characterization of genetic variants and detection of carriers. Blood 1977;50:351.
311. Chung KS, Goldsmith JC, Roberts HR. Purification and characterization of factor IX Chapel Hill. Blood 1976;48:974.
312. Noyes CM, Griffith MJ, Roberts HR, et al. Identification of the molecular defect in factor IX Chapel Hill: substitution of histidine for arginine at position 145. Proc Natl Acad Sci USA 1983;80:4200.
313. Diuguid DL, Rabiet MJ, Furie BC, Furie B. Molecular defects of factor IX Chicago-2 (Arg 145 → His) and prothrombin Madrid (Arg 271 → Cys): arginine mutations that preclude zymogen activation. Blood 1989;74:193.
314. Toomey JR, Stafford D, Smith K. Factor IX Albuquerque (arginine 145 to cysteine) is cleaved slowly by factor XIa and has reduced coagulant activity. Blood 1988;72(Suppl 1):312a.
315. Huang MN, Kasper CK, Roberts HR, et al. Molecular defect in factor IX Hilo, a hemophilia B_M variant: Arg → Gln at the carboxy terminal cleavage site of the activation peptide. Blood 1988;72(Suppl 1):298a.
316. Monroe DM, McCord DM, High KA, et al. Functional consequences of an Arg 180 to Gln mutation in factor IX Hilo. Blood 1988;72(Suppl 1): 304a.
317. Sakai T, Fujimura Y, Yoshioka A, et al. Blood clotting factor IX Kasihara: amino acid substitution of valine 182 by phenylalanine. Blood 1988;72(Suppl 1):304a.
318. Denton PH, Fowlkes DM, Lord ST, et al. Hemophilia B Durham: a mutation in the first EGF-like domain of factor IX that is characterized by polymerase chain reaction. Blood 1988;72:1407.
319. Ware J, Davis L, Frazier D, et al. Genetic defect responsible for the dysfunctional protein: factor IX Long Beach. Blood 1988;72:820.
320. Spitzer SG, Warn-Cramer BJ, Kasper CC, et al. Mutations in the catalytic domain of factor IXa which prevent macromolecular catalysis. Circulation 1988;78(Suppl II):118.
321. Geddes VA, LeBonniec BF, Louie GV, et al. A moderate form of hemophilia B is caused by a novel mutation in the protease domain of factor IX Vancouver. J Biol Chem 1989;264:4689.
322. Spitzer SG, Pendurthi UR, Kasper CK, et al. Molecular defect in factor IX_{Bm} Lake Elsinore. J Biol Chem 1988;263:10545.
323. Vidaud M, Attree O, Schaad O, et al. Self-inhibition of factor IX by a Gly to Arg mutation at the substrate binding pocket is linked to severe hemophilia B. Blood 1988;72(Suppl 1):313a.
324. Attree O, Vidaud D, Vidaud M, et al. Rapid characterization of mutations in the catalytic domain of human coagulation factor IX. Blood 1988;72(Suppl 1):289a.
325. Tsang TC, Bentley DR, Mibashan RS, et al. A factor IX mutation, verified by direct genomic sequencing, causes haemophilia B by a novel mechanism. EMBO J 1988;7:3009.
326. Bertina RM, van der Linden IK. Factor IX Deventer: evidence for the heterogeneity of hemophilia B_M. Thromb Haemost 1985;54:120a.
327. Bertina RM, van der Linden IK. Factor IX Zutphen: a genetic variant of blood coagulation factor IX with an abnormally high molecular weight. J Lab Clin Med 1982;100:695–704, 1982.
328. Gitschier J, Wood WI, Shuman MA, et al. Identification of a missense mutation in the factor VIII gene of a mild hemophiliac. Science 1986;232: 1415.
329. Youssoufian H, Kazazian HH Jr, Phillips DG, et al. Recurrent mutations in haemophilia A give evidence for CpG mutation hotspots. Nature 1986;324:380.
329a. Gianelli F, Green PM, High KA, et al. Haemophilia B: database of point mutations and short additions and deletions. Nucleic Acids Res 1993;21: 3075.
330. Reitsma PH, Mandalaki T, Kasper CK, et al. Novel point mutations correlate with an altered developmental expression of blood coagulation factor IX (hemophilia B Leyden phenotype). Blood 1989;73:743.
331. Giannelli F, Choo KH, Rees DJG, et al. Gene deletions in patients with haemophilia B and anti–factor IX antibodies. Nature 1983;303:181.
332. Chen S-H, Yoshitake S, Chance PF, et al. An intragenic deletion of the factor IX gene in a family with hemophilia B. J Clin Invest 1985;76: 2161.
333. Bray GL, Thompson AR. Partial factor IX protein in a pedigree with hemophilia B due to a partial gene deletion. J Clin Invest 1986;77:1194.
334. Rees DJG, Rizza CR, Brownlee GG. Haemophilia B caused by a point mutation in a donor splice junction of the human factor IX gene. Nature 1985;316:643.
335. Schach BG, Yoshitake S, Davie EW. Hemophilia B factor IX (Seattle 2) due to a single nucleotide deletion in the gene for factor IX. J Clin Invest 1987;80:1023.
336. Attree O, Vidaud D, Vidaud M, et al. Mutations in the catalytic domain of human coagulation factor IX. Genomics 1989;4:266.
337. Peake IR, Furlong BL, Bloom AL. Carrier detection by direct gene analysis in a family with haemophilia B (factor IX deficiency). Lancet 1984;1: 242.
338. Matthews RJ, Anson DS, Peake IR, et al. Heterogeneity of the factor IX locus in nine hemophilia B inhibitor patients. J Clin Invest 1987;79: 746.
339. Hassan HJ, Leonardi JA, Guerriero R, et al. Hemophilia B with inhibitor:

molecular analysis of the subtotal deletion of the factor IX gene. Blood 1985;66:728.
340. Trent RJ, Wallace RC, Rickard KA. Deletion/insertion of DNA in an intron of the factor IX gene produces severe hemophilia B⁻. Blood 1988;72(Suppl 1):312a.
341. Poon MC, Chui DH, Patterson M, et al. Hemophilia B (Christmas disease) variants and carrier detection analyzed by DNA probes. J Clin Invest 1987;79:1204.
342. Vidaud M, Chabret C, Gazengel C, et al. A de novo intragenic deletion of the potential EGF domain of the factor IX gene in a family with severe hemophilia B. Blood 1986;68:961.
343. Bernard F, del Senno L, Barbieri R, et al. Gene deletion in an Italian hemophilia B subject. J Med Genet 1985;22:305.
344. Wadelius C, Blomback M, Pettersson U. Molecular studies of haemophilia B in Sweden: identification of patients with total deletion of the factor IX gene and without inhibitory antibodies. Hum Genet 1988;81:13.
345. Anson DS, Blake DJ, Winship PR, et al. Nullisomic deletion of the mcf.2 transforming gene in two haemophilia B patients. EMBO J 1988;7: 2795.
346. Tanimoto M, Kojima T, Kamiya T, et al. DNA analysis of seven patients with hemophilia B who have anti–factor IX antibodies: relationship to clinical manifestations and evidence that the abnormal gene was inherited. J Lab Clin Med 1988;112:307.
347. Taylor SA, Lillicrap DP, Blanchette V, et al. A complete deletion of the factor IX gene and new TaqI variant in a hemophilia B kindred. Hum Genet 1988;79:273.
348. Kasper CK, Osterud B, Minami JY, et al. Hemophilia B: characterization of genetic variants and detection of carriers. Blood 1977;50:351.
349. Winship PR, Anson DS, Rizza CR, et al. Carrier detection in hemophilia B using two further intragenic restriction fragment length polymorphisms. Nucleic Acids Res 1984;12:8861.
350. Hay CW, Robertson KA, Yong S-L, et al. Use of a BamHI polymorphism in the factor IX gene for the determination of hemophilia B carrier status. Blood 1986;67:1508.
351. Winship PR, Brownlee GG: Diagnosis of haemophilia B carriers using intragenic oligonucleotide probes. Lancet 1986;2:218.
352. Freedenberg DL, Chen S-H, Kurachi K, et al. MspI polymorphic site within the factor IX gene. Hum Genet 1987;76:262.
353. Giannelli F, Choo KH, Winship PR, et al. Characterization and use of an intragenic polymorphic marker for detection of carriers of haemophilia B (factor IX deficiency). Lancet 1984:1:239.
354. Mulligan L, Holden JJA, White BN. A DNA marker closely linked to the factor IX (haemophilia B) gene. Hum Genet 1987;75:381.
355. Drayna D, Davies K, Hartley D, et al. Genetic mapping of the human X chromosome by using restriction fragment length polymorphisms. Proc Natl Acad Sci USA 1984;81:2836.
356. Arveiler B, Oberle I, Vincent A, et al. Genetic mapping of the Xq27–q28 region: new RFPL markers useful for diagnostic applications in fragile-X and hemophilia B families. Am J Hum Genet 1988;42:380.
357. Thompson AR, Chen SH, Smith KJ. Diagnostic role of an immunoassay-detected polymorphism of factor IX for potential carriers of hemophilia B. Blood 1988;72:1633.
358. Smith KJ, Thompson AR, McMullen BA, et al. Carrier testing in hemophilia B with an immunoassay that distinguishes a prevalent factor IX dimorphism. Blood 1987;70:1006.
359. Lusher JM, McMillan CW. Hemophilia study group: severe factor VIII and factor IX deficiency in females. Am J Med 1978;65:637.
360. Nisen P, Stamberg J, Ehrenpreis R, et al. The molecular basis of severe hemophilia B in a girl. N Engl J Med 1986;315:1139.
361. Corrigan JJ Jr, Kryc JJ. Factor II (prothrombin) levels in cord blood: correlation of coagulant activity with immunoreactive protein. J Pediatr 1980;97:979.
362. Levine PH. Efficacy of self-therapy in hemophilia: a study of 72 patients with hemophilia A and B. N Engl J Med 1974;291:1381.
363. Faria R, Fiumara NJ. Hepatitis B associated with Konyne. N Engl J Med 1972;287:358.
364. Blatt PM, Lundblad RL, Kingdon HS, et al. Thrombogenic materials in prothrombin complex concentrates. Ann Intern Med 1974;81:766.
365. Cederbaum AI, Blatt PM, Roberts HR. Intravascular coagulation with use of human prothrombin complex concentrates. Ann Intern Med 1976;84:683.
366. Kasper CK. Clinical use of factor IX concentrates: report on thromboembolic complications. Thromb Diath Haemorrh 1975;33:642.
367. Kasper CK. Postoperative thrombosis in hemophilia B. N Engl J Med 1973;289:610.
368. Ragni MV, Winkelstein A, Kingsley L, et al. 1986 update of HIV seroprevalence, seroconversion, AIDS incidence and immunologic correlates of HIV infection in patients with hemophilia A and B. Blood 1987;70:786.
369. Brettler DB, Brewster F, Levine PH, et al. Immunologic aberrations, HIV seropositivity and seroconversion rates in patients with hemophilia B. Blood 1987;70:276.
370. Nilsson IM, Berntorp E, Zettervall O. Induction of split tolerance and clinical cure in high-responding hemophiliacs with factor IX antibodies. Proc Natl Acad Sci USA 1986;83:9169.
371. Stehr Green JK, Holman RC, Jason JM, et al. Hemophilia-associated AIDS in the United States, 1981 to September 1987. Am J Public Health 1988;78:439.
372. Liebman HA, Limentani SA, Furie BC, et al. Immunoaffinity purification of factor IX (Christmas factor) using conformation-specific antibodies directed against the factor IX–metal complex. Proc Natl Acad Sci USA 1985;82:3879.
373. Limentani SA, Furie BC, Poiesz BJ, et al. Separation of human plasma factor IX from HTLV-I or HIV by immunoaffinity chromatography using conformation-specific antibodies. Blood 1987;70:1312.
374. Smith KJ. Immunoaffinity purification of factor IX from commercial concentrates and infusion studies in animals. Blood 1988;72:1269.
375. Anson DS, Austen DEG, Brownlee GG. Expression of active human clotting factor IX from recombinant DNA clones in mammalian cells. Nature 1985;315:683.
376. Busby S, Kumar A, Joseph M, et al. Expression of active human factor IX in transfected cells. Nature 1985;316:271.
377. de la Salle H, Alterburger W, Elkaim R, et al. Active γ-carboxylated human factor IX expressed using recombinant DNA techniques. Nature 1985;316:268.
378. Kaufman R, Wasley L, Furie BC, et al. Expression, purification, and characterization of recombinant γ-carboxylated human factor IX. J Biol Chem 1986;261:9622.
379. Choo KH, Raphael K, McAdam W, et al. Expression of active human blood clotting factor IX in transgenic mice: use of a cDNA with complete mRNA sequence. Nucleic Acids Res 1987;15:871.
380. Anson DS, Hock RA, Austen D, et al. Toward gene therapy for hemophilia B. Mol Biol Med 1987;4:11.
381. Palmer TD, Thompson AR, Miller AD. Production of human factor IX in animals by genetically modified skin fibroblasts: potential therapy for hemophilia B. Blood 1989;73:438.
382. Merion RM, Delius RE, Campbell DA Jr, et al. Orthotopic liver transplantation totally corrects factor IX deficiency in hemophilia B. Surgery 1988;104:929.
383. Josso F, Monasterio de Sanchez J, Lavergne JM, et al. Congenital abnormality of the prothrombin molecule (factor II) in four siblings: prothrombin Barcelona. Blood 1971;38:9.
384. Rabiet MJ, Benarous R, Labie D, et al. Abnormal activation of a human prothrombin variant: prothrombin Barcelona. FEBS Lett 1978;87:132.
385. Rabiet MJ, Elion J, Benarous R, et al. Activation of prothrombin Barcelona: evidence for active high molecular weight intermediates. Biochim Biophys Acta 1979;584:66.
386. Rabiet MJ, Furie BC, Furie B. Molecular defect of prothrombin Barcelona. J Biol Chem 1986;261:15045.
387. Guillin M-C, Bezeaud A. Characterization of a variant of human prothrombin: prothrombin Madrid. Ann N Y Acad Sci 1981;370:414.
388. Inomoto T, Shirakami A, Kawauchi S, et al. Prothrombin Tokushima: characterization of dysfunctional thrombin derived from a variant of human prothrombin. Blood 1987;69:565.
389. Miyata T, Morita T, Inomoto T, et al. Prothrombin Tokushima, a replace of arginine 418 by tryptophan that impairs the fibrinogen clotting activity of derived thrombin Tokushima. Biochemistry 1987;26:1117.
390. Henriksen RA, Owen WG, Nesheim ME, et al. Identification of a congenital dysthrombin, thrombin Quick. J Clin Invest 1980;66:934.
391. Henriksen RA, Mann KG. Identification of the primary structural defect in the dysthrombin thrombin Quick I: substitution of cysteine for arginine 382. Biochemistry 1988;27:9160.
392. Henriksen RA, Mann KG. Substitution of valine for glycine 558 in the congenital dysthrombin Quick II alters primary substrate specificity. Biochemistry 1989;28:2078.
393. Shapiro SS, Martinez J, Holburn RR. Congenital dysprothrombinemia: an inherited structural disorder of human prothrombin. J Clin Invest 1969;48:2251.
394. Huisse M-G, Dreyfus M, Guillin M-C. Prothrombin Clamart: prothrombin variant with defective Arg 320–Ile cleavage by factor Xa. Thromb Res 1986;44:11.
395. Rabiet MJ, Jandrot-Perrus M, Boissel JP, et al. Thrombin Metz: characterization of the dysfunctional thrombin derived from a variant of human prothrombin. Blood 1984;63:927.
396. Bezeaud A, Drouet L, Soria C, et al. Prothrombin Salakta: an abnormal prothrombin characterized by a defect in the active site of thrombin. Thromb Res 1984;34:507.
397. Bezeaud A, Elion J, Guillin M-C. Functional characterization of thrombin Salakta: an abnormal thrombin derived from a human prothrombin variant. Blood 1988;71:556.
398. Girolami A, Coccheri G, Palaretti G, et al. Prothrombin Molise: a "new" congenital dysprothrombinemia, couble heterozygosis with an abnormal prothrombin and "true" prothrombin deficiency. Blood 1978;52: 115.
399. Girolami A, Molaro G, Lazzarin M, et al. A new congenital haemorrhagic condition due to the presence of an abnormal factor X (factor X Friuli): study of a large kindred. Br J Haematol 1970;19:179.
400. Fair DS, Plow EF, Edgington TS. Combined functional and immunochemical analysis of normal and abnormal human factor X. J Clin. Invest 1979;64:884.
401. Fair DS, Edgington TS. Heterogeneity of hereditary and acquired factor

X deficiencies by combined immunochemical and functional analyses. Br J Haematol 1985;59:235.
402. De Stefano V, Leone G, Ferrelli R, et al. Factor X Roma: a congenital factor X variant defective at different degrees in the intrinsic and extrinsic activation. Br J Haematol 1988;69:387.
403. Nora RE, Bell WR, Noe DA, et al. Novel factor X deficiency: normal partial thromboplastin time and associated spindle cell thymoma. Am J Med 1985;79:122.
404. Girolami A, Vicarioto M, Ruzza G, et al. Factor X Padua: a new congenital factor X abnormality with a defect only in the extrinsic system. Acta Haematol 1985;73:31.
405. Scamgler PJ, Williamson R. The structural gene for human coagulation factor X is located on chromosome 13q34. Cytogenet Cell Genet 1985;39:231.
406. Pfeiffer RA, Ott R, Gilgendrantz S, et al. Deficiency of coagulation factors VII and X associated with deletion of a chromosome 13 (q34). Hum Genet 1982;62:358.
407. Stoll C, Roth MP. Partial 4q duplication due to inherited der(13),t(4;13)(q26;q34) in a girl with a deficiency of factor X. Hum Genet 1980;53:303.
408. Triplett DA, Brandt JT, Batard MAM, et al. Hereditary factor VII deficiency: heterogeneity defined by combined functional and immunochemical analysis. Blood 1985;66:1284.
409. Girolami A, Fabris F, Zanon RDB, et al. Factor VII Padua: a congenital coagulation disorder due to an abnormal factor VII with a peculiar activation pattern. J Lab Clin Med 1978;91:387.
410. Briet E, Loeliger EA, van Tilberg NH, et al. Molecular variants of factor VII. Thromb Haemost 1976;42:289.
411. Mariani G, Mazzucconi MG, Hermans J, et al. Factor VII deficiency: immunological characterization of genetic variants and detection of carriers. Br J Haematol 1981;48:7.
412. Girolami A, Falezza G, Patrassi G, et al. Factor VII Verona coagulation disorder. Blood 1977;50:603.
413. Matthay KK, Koerper MA, Ablin AR. Intracranial hemorrhage in congenital factor VII deficiency. J Pediatr 1979;94:413.
414. Kuzel T, Green D, Stulberg SD, et al. Arthropathy and surgery in congenital factor VII deficiency. Am J Med 1988;84:771.
415. Yorke AJ, Mant MJ. Factor VII deficiency and surgery: is preoperative replacement therapy necessary? JAMA 1977;238:424.
416. Gershwin ME, Gude JK. Deep vein thrombosis and pulmonary embolism in congenital factor VII deficiency. N Engl J Med 1973;288:141.
417. Friedman PA, Rosenberg RD, Hauschka PV, et al. A spectrum of partially carboxylated prothrombin in the plasma of coumarin-treated patients. Biochim Biophys Acta 1977;494:271.
418. Esnouf MP, Prowse CV. The gamma-carboxyglutamic acid content of human and bovine prothrombin following warfarin treatment. Biochim Biophys Acta 1977;490:471.
419. McKee RW, Binkley SB, Thayer SA, et al. The isolation of vitamin K_2. J Biol Chem 1939;131:327.
420. Frick PG, Riedler G, Brogli H. Dose response and minimal daily requirement for vitamin K in man. J Appl Physiol 1967;23:387.
421. Ansell JE, Kumar R, Deykin D. The spectrum of vitamin K deficiency. JAMA 1977;237:40.
422. Niiya K, Kitagawa T, Fujishita M, et al. Bulemia nervosa complicated by deficiency of vitamin K–dependent coagulation factors. 1983;250:792.
423. Blanchard RA, Furie BC, Kruger SF, et al. Immunoassays of human prothrombin species which correlate with functional coagulant activities. J Lab Clin Med 1983;101:242.
424. Krasinski SD, Russell RM, Furie BC, et al. The prevalence of vitamin K deficiency in chronic gastrointestinal disorders. Am J Clin Nutr 1985;41:639.
425. Kaplan MM, Elta GH, Furie B, et al. Fat soluble vitamin nutriture in primary biliary cirrhosis. Gastroenterology 1988;95:787.
426. Bertina RM, Van der Marel-van Nieuwkoop W, Dubbeldam J, et al. New method for the rapid detection of vitamin K deficiency. Clin Chem Acta 1980;105:93.
427. Mummah-Schendel LL, Suttie JW. Serum phylloquinone concentrations in a normal adult population. Am J Clin Nutr 1986;44:686.
428. Brinkhous KM, Smith HP. Plasma prothrombin level in normal infancy and in hemorrhagic disease of the newborn. Am J Med Sci 1937;193:475.
429. Dam H, Tage-Hansen E. Vitamin K lack in normal and sick infants. Lancet 2;1157:1939.
430. Dam H, Dyggve H. Relation of vitamin K deficiency to hemorrhagic disease of the newborn. Adv Pediatr 1952;5:129.
431. Sutherland JM, Glueck HI, Glesser G. Hemorrhagic disease of the newborn. Am J Dis Child 1967;113:524.
432. Wefring KW. Hemorrhage in the newborn and vitamin K prophylaxis. J Pediatr 1962;61:686.
433. Shearer MJ, Rahim S, Stimmler L, et al. Plasma vitamin K_1 in mothers and their newborn babies. Lancet 1982;2:460.
434. Keenan WJ, Jewett T, Glueck HI. Role of feeding and vitamin K in hypoprothrombinemia of the newborn. Am J Dis Child 1971;121:271.
435. Schneider DL, Fluckiger HB, Manes JD. Vitamin K content of infants formula products. Pediatrics 1974;53:273.
436. Committee on Nutrition, American Academy of Pediatrics. Vitamin K supplementation for infants receiving milk substitute infant formulas and for those with fat malabsorption. Pediatrics 1972;48:483.
437. Bound JP, Telfer JP. Effect of vitamin K dosage on plasma bilirubin levels in premature infants. Lancet 1956;1:720.
438. Allison AC. Danger of vitamin K to newborn. Lancet 1955;1:669.
439. Hull R, Hirsh J, Jay R, et al. Different intensities of oral anticoagulant therapy in the treatment of proximal vein thrombosis. N Engl J Med 1982;307:1676.
440. Hull R, Delmore T, Carter C, et al. Adjusted subcutaneous heparin versus warfarin sodium in the long-term treatment of venous thrombosis. N Engl J Med 1982;306:189.
441. Turpie AGG, Gunstensen J, Hirsh J, et al. Randomised comparison of two intensities of oral anticoagulant therapy after tissue heart valve replacement. Lancet 1988;1:1242.
442. Forfar JC. Prediction of hemorrhage during long-term oral coumarin anticoagulation by excessive prothrombin ratio. Am Heart J 1982;103:445.
443. Coon WW, Willis PW. Hemorrhagic complications of anticoagulant therapy. Arch Intern Med 1974;133:386.
444. Coon WW, Willis PW. Thromboembolic complications during anticoagulant therapy. Arch Surg 1972;105:209.
445. Levine MN, Raskob G, Hirsh J. Hemorrhagic complications of long-term anticoagulant therapy. Chest 1986;89(Suppl 2):16.
446. Hirsh J, Deykin D, Poller L. "Therapeutic range" for oral anticoagulant therapy. Chest 1986;89(Suppl 2):11.
447. Lipton RA, Klass EM. Human ingestion of a "superwarfarin" rodenticide resulting in a prolonged anticoagulant effect. JAMA 1984;252:3004.
448. Jones EC, Growe GH, Naiman SC. Prolonged anticoagulation in rat poisoning. JAMA 1984;252:3005.
449. Chong LL, Chau WK, Ho CH. A case of "superwarfarin" poisoning. Scand J Haematol 1986;36:314.
450. O'Reilly RA, Aggeler PM. Covert anticoagulant ingestion: study of 25 patients and review of world literature. Medicine 1976;55:389.
451. O'Reilly RA, Aggeler PM, Gibbs JO. Hemorrhagic state due to surreptitious ingestion of bishydroxycoumarin. N Engl J Med 1962;267:19.
452. Bowie EJW, Todd M, Thompson JH Jr, et al. Anticoagulant malingerers ("the dicoumarol-eaters"). Am J Med 1965;39:855.
453. Weitzel JN, Sadowski JA, Furie BC, et al. Hemorrhagic disorder caused by surreptitious ingestion of a long-acting vitamin K antagonist/rodenticide, brodifacoum. Blood 1990;76:2555.
454. Goldsweig HG, Kapusta M, Schwartz J, et al. Bleeding, salicylates, and prolonged prothrombin time: three case reports and a review of the literature. J Rheumatol 1976;3:37.
455. Uotila L, Suttie JW. Inhibition of vitamin K–dependent carboxylase in vitro by cefamandole and its structural analogs. J Infect Dis 1983;148:571.
456. Bang NU, Tessler SS, Heidenreich RO, et al. Effects of moxalactam on blood coagulation and platelet function. Rev Infect Dis 1982;4:S546.
457. Barza M, Furie B, Brown AE, et al. Defects in vitamin K–dependent carboxylation associated with moxalactam treatment. J Infect Dis 1986;153:1166.
458. Lipksy JJ. Mechanism of the inhibition of the γ-carboxylation of glutamic acid by N-methylthiotetrazole-containing antibiotics. Proc Natl Acad Sci USA 1984;81:2893.
459. Ratnoff, OD. Hemostatic mechanisms in liver disease. Med Clin North Am 1963;47:721.
460. Rapaport SI, Ames SB, Mikkelsen S, et al. Plasma clotting factors in chronic hepatocellular disease. N Engl J Med 1960;263:278.
461. Donaldson GWK, Davies SH, Darg A, et al. Coagulation factors in chronic liver disease. J Clin Pathol 1969;22:199.
462. Corrigan JJ, Earnest DL. Factor II antigen in liver disease and warfarin-induced vitamin K deficiency. Am J Hematol 1980;8:249.
463. Spector I, Corn M, Ticktin HE. Effect of plasma transfusions on the prothrombin time and clotting factors in liver disease. N Engl J Med 1966;275:1032.
464. Green G, Dymock IW, Poller L, et al. Use of factor VII–rich prothrombin complex concentrate in liver disease. Lancet 1975;1:1311.
465. Liebman HA, Furie BC, Tong MJ, et al. Des-γ-carboxy (abnormal) prothrombin as a serum marker of primary hepatocellular carcinoma. N Engl J Med 1984;310:1427.
466. Fujiyama S, Morishita T, Hashiguichi O, et al. Plasma abnormal prothrombin (des-γ-carboxy prothrombin) as a marker of hepatocellular carcinoma. Cancer 1988;61:1621.
467. Fujiyama S, Morishita T, Sagara K, et al. Clinical evaluation of plasma abnormal prothrombin (PIVKA-II) in patients with hepatocellular carcinoma. Hepatogastroenterology 1986;33:201.
468. Howell M. Acquired factor X deficiency associated with systemic amyloidosis. Blood 1963;21:739.
469. Pechet L, Kastrul JJ. Amyloidosis associated with factor X (Stuart) deficiency. Ann Intern Med 1964;61:316.
470. Furie B, Greene E, Furie BC. Syndrome of acquired factor X deficiency and systemic amyloidosis. N Engl J Med 1977;297:81.
471. Furie B, Voo L, McAdam KPWJ, et al. Mechanism of factor X deficiency in systemic amyloidosis. N Engl J Med 1981;304:827.

472. Spero JA, Lewis JH, Hasiba V, et al. Treatment of amyloidosis associated factor X deficiency. Thromb Haemostis 1976;35:377.
473. Greipp PR, Kyle RA, Bowie EJW. Factor X deficiency in primary amyloidosis. N Engl J Med 1979;301:1018.
474. Rosenstein ED, Itzkowitz SH, Penziner AS, et al. Resolution of factor X deficiency in primary amyloidosis following splenectomy. Arch Intern Med 1983;143:597.
475. Camoriano JK, Greipp PR, Bayer GK, et al. Resolution of acquired factor X deficiency and amyloidosis with melphalan and prednisone therapy. N Engl J Med 1987;316:1133.
476. Bajaj SP, Rapaport SI, Barclay S, et al. Acquired hypoprothrombinemia due to non-neutralizing antibodies to prothrombin: mechanism and management. Blood 1985;65:1538.
477. Handley DA, Lawrence JR. Factor IX deficiency in the nephrotic syndrome. Lancet 1967;1:1079.
478. Natelson EA, Lynch EC, Hettig RA, et al. Acquired factor IX deficiency in the nephrotic syndrome. Ann Intern Med 1970;73:373.
479. Vaziri ND, Branson HE, Ness R. Changes in coagulation factors IX, VIII, VII, X and V in nephrotic syndrome. Am J Med Sci 1980;280:167.

Blood: Principles and Practice of Hematology, edited by Robert I. Handin, Samuel E. Lux, and Thomas P. Stossel. J.B. Lippincott Company, Philadelphia © 1995.

41

Fibrinogen and Factor XIII: Biology and Disorders of Fibrin Formation and Cross-Linking

Jan McDonagh
Elzbieta Kaczmarek
Myoung Hee Lee

Fibrinogen is a large glycoprotein, that is distributed primarily in plasma but is found also in platelets and in megakaryocytes. The normal plasma concentration is 1.5 to 3.5 g/L, or 4.4 to 10.3 μmol/L. Fibrinogen and its activated derivative, fibrin, are crucial to both the normal hemostatic and the fibrinolytic processes. The conversion of fibrinogen to fibrin is a seminal event in hemostasis that disrupts the fluidity of blood. This process must be carefully regulated, and fibrin plays a role in that regulation. Once fibrin is formed, it is a principal constituent for activation and assembly of the fibrinolytic system, ensuring that blood again becomes fluid. These two processes are vital for preventing the extravasation of blood when vessels become damaged and ensuring normal wound healing. Fibrinogen is also an acute-phase protein, which indicates its importance in the normal defense mechanisms.

The pathologic consequences of abnormally regulated conversion of fibrinogen to fibrin are arterial and venous thrombosis. Likewise, abnormal fibrinogens, which do not form fibrin normally, can cause hemorrhage or thrombosis. Fibrin is also associated with tumor cells and may play a role in metastasis.

Several comprehensive reviews on fibrinogen, fibrin formation and cross-linking, and factor XIII have been published during the last few years.[1–7] In this chapter, information concerning the structure and function of these proteins and the clinical disorders involving them is discussed, with emphasis on newer data.

STRUCTURE OF FIBRINOGEN

The formula for the structure of fibrinogen is $(A\alpha, B\beta, \gamma)_2$, indicating that it is composed of three pairs of nonidentical polypeptide chains and that the molecule is a dimer. The NH_2 terminals of all the peptides are arranged together in the middle of the molecule. The NH_2-terminal region of the Aα and Bβ chains contains the fibrinopeptides, A and B. Figure 41-1*A* is a molecular electron microscopic picture of fibrinogen, and Figure 41-1*B* is a model of this structure. Table 41-1 lists the important structural features of fibrinogen. Based on electron microscopic studies, Hall and Slayter[8] proposed in 1959 that the fibrinogen molecular structure was trinodular. Although a number of shapes were later proposed for the fibrinogen molecule, this original hypothesis is confirmed by a number of other methods, such as separation of chains by reduction of disulfide bridges, degradation of fibrinogen by plasmin, and cleavage at methionyl bonds by cyanogen bromide.[9–15] Examination with molecular electron microscopy shows the structure has two terminal D domains or nodules, and a central E domain. The D domain is frequently split into two parts. With later electron microscopic experiments, a small domain could be seen in each of the coiled-coil regions as well.[16,23]

The NH_2-terminal region of all six chains is tightly packed into a globular dimeric central nodule, the E domain. It is stabilized by disulfide bonds and contains fibrinopeptides A and B, which are released when thrombin acts on fibrinogen.[13,14] The D domains are located at the two ends of the trinodular fibrinogen molecule and primarily contain the COOH terminals of the β and γ chains, which are folded independently.[13–18] This accounts for the split in the D domains observed by electron microscopy. The two D domains are connected to the central E domain by a filamentous coiled-coil region. The carboxy-terminal region of the Aα chain, rich in hydrophilic residues, forms a separate folded domain that allows the COOH-terminal regions of two Aα chains to be joined together.[11,13,19–23] There is a twofold axis of symmetry for the molecule that passes through the middle of the central E domain.[24] Fibrinogen has the following dimensions: each D domain is 6.5 nm in diameter, the E domain is 5 nm in diameter, and each coiled-coil region is about 1 nm in diameter with a length of about 16 nm. The overall length is 45 to 47 nm.[25,26] The molecular weight of fibrinogen is 340 kd,[27,28] and its extinction coefficient is 15.1 to 15.5.[29]

Divalent calcium ions help maintain the structure and stability of fibrinogen molecules. Three high-affinity Ca^{2+}

Supported in part by grants HL 33014 and HL 29512 from the National Institutes of Health.

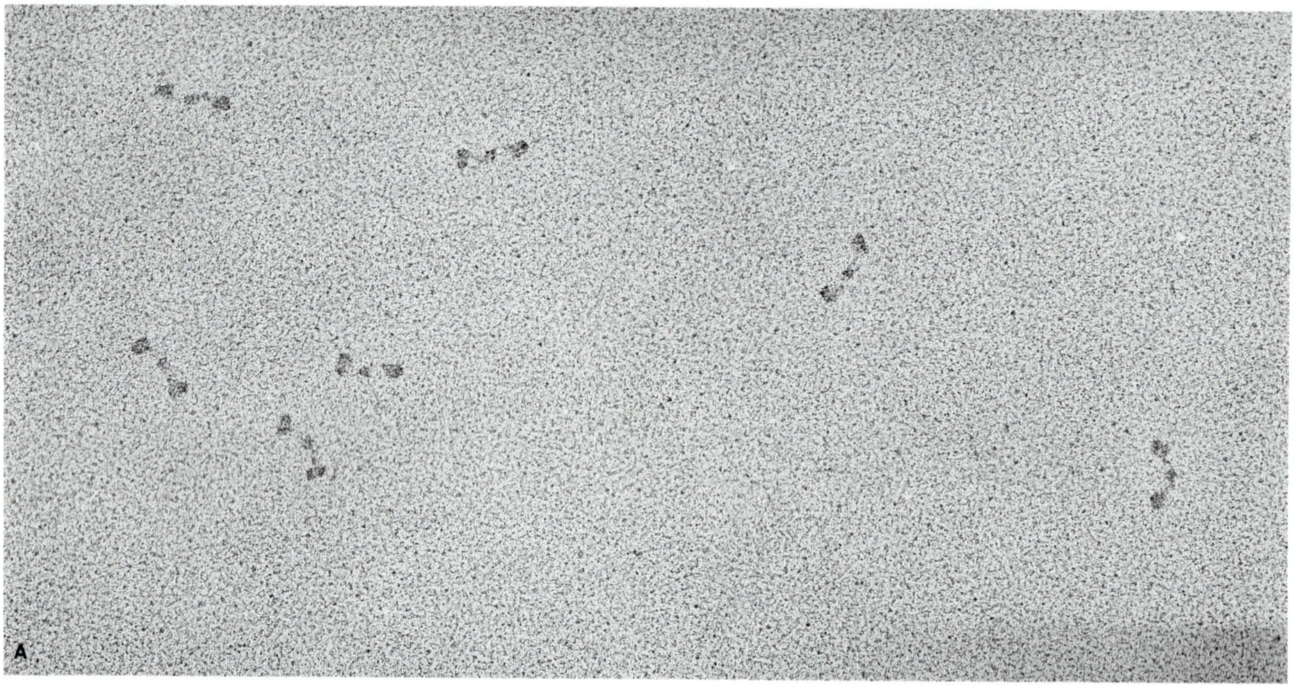

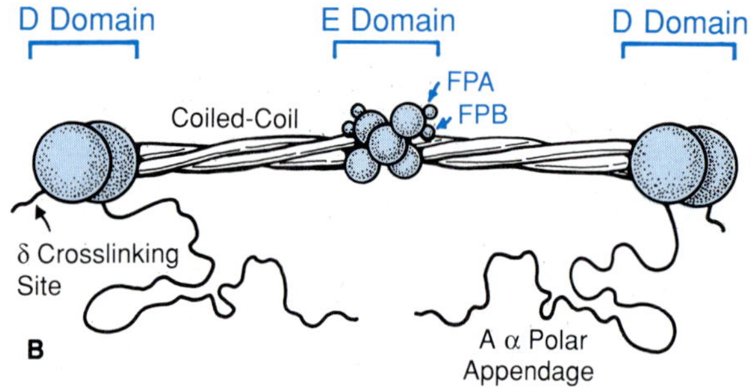

FIGURE 41-1. **(A)** Molecular electron microscopy of human rotary-shadowed fibrinogen (×223,529). Note the split in the D domains and the bend in some of the molecules. **(B)** Model of fibrinogen based on the dimensions from electron microscopy. (The α-chain extension is sometimes seen as a separate, smaller domain close to the E domain. The small γ-chain extension is not seen by microscopy.) (Courtesy of Dr. H. Slayter, Dana Farber Cancer Institute and Harvard Medical School, Boston)

binding sites are found in human fibrinogen.[30,31] Two are located in the D domains[30]—at γ-chain residues 303 to 356[32] or 311 to 336.[33] The third calcium-binding site is localized in the E domain.[34] Ca^{2+} protects fragment D from further degradation by plasmin[35] and also enhances fibrin polymerization and cross-linking.[36]

TABLE 41-1. Important Features of Fibrinogen Structure

	Polypeptide Chain		
	Aα	Bβ	γ
M_r	64 kd	56 kd	48 kd
Total number of amino acids	610	461	410
Terminal amino acids			
Amino	Ala	Glu	Tyr
Carboxyl	Val	Gln	Val
Domains			
Central, E	1–49	1–80	1–23
Coiled coil	50–160	81–192	24–134
Terminal, D	161–206	193–461	135–411
Polar appendage	207–610	—	—
Proximal S-S ring	45–49	76–80	19–23
Plasmin-sensitive region	96–119	130–150	70–93
Distal S-S ring	161–165	193–197	135–139
Number of cysteines	8	11	10
Carbohydrate cluster	—	364	52

Primary and Secondary Structural Analysis

The Aα, Bβ, and γ chains contain 625, 461, and 411 amino acids, respectively; their respective molecular weights are estimated to be 64, 56, and 48 kd.[33–39] Gene sequencing predicts that the α chain should be 15 amino acids longer. Removal of this fragment occurs as part of the normal specific processing events that occur intracellularly, and a small amount of this longer α chain is present in circulating plasmas.[44] Isolated fibrinogen chains have been sequenced in several laboratories.[37,42,45,46,49] Based on this work, the complete amino acid sequence of all three chains is presented in Figure 41-2. There is an excess of acidic amino acids (Asp + Glu = 382) over basic residues (Lys + Arg = 362), accounting for the acidic isoelectric point (pI = 5.1 to 6.3). There are no free sulfhydryl groups in fibrinogen.[47]

Human fibrinogen contains four carbohydrate side chains, one on each of the Bβ (Asn 364) and γ chains (Asn 52).[48,49] The oligosaccharide chains are biantennary and are composed of four residues of *N*-acetyl-glucosamine, three residues of mannose, two residues of galactose, and one or two residues of sialic acid. Carbohydrates constitute 2.6% of the mass of human fibrinogen.

The dimeric fibrinogen molecule is joined together by disulfide bridges. There are 58 half-cystine residues involved in the 29 disulfide bonds formed between all 6 chains.[47] Three bonds link the dimeric halves of the fibrinogen molecule together (interchains between the halves of the molecule).[50] These cysteine bonds are at α8–α8, α28–β65, and α9–α9. The first two are sufficient to hold the two halves of the molecule together.[51,56] The 7 interchain disulfide bonds connect individual polypeptides within each half of the molecule (14 altogether), and the remaining 12 disulfide bridges (6 per monomeric subunit set) are intrachain bonds.

Disulfide bridges are arranged in 5 domains called knots.[50–54] Eleven disulfides occur in the central (or E) domain, including the 3 bonds that hold the dimeric halves together. This region is called the N-DSK (N-terminal disulfide knot). Eight disulfides occur in each of the 2 D domains. The remaining 2 disulfides occur in the 2 Aα-chain extensions. There are 8, 11, and 10 cysteines in the Aα, Bβ and γ chains, respectively. Each chain has 2 sets of cysteines situated identically 111 or 112 amino acids apart with 3 residues between the cysteines. These encompass the coiled-coil region between the E and D domains and are referred to as the disulfide rings. Between the cysteines engaged in formation of the 2 disulfide rings, each of the fibrinogen chains is in an α-helix form. These helices interact via hydrogen bonds so that all three fibrinogen chains form a higher-order helix. This structure is designated the coiled-coil region, and it forms the interdomain-connecting region (see Table 41-1).[57] The secondary and tertiary structure of the γ chain has also been analyzed in detail.[58] The γ chain has multiple functions, including a polymerization domain, covalent binding sites, tPA and plasminogen binding domains, and sites for cellular interaction.

Heterogeneity

Under physiologic conditions, human plasma contains a population of fibrinogen molecules of varying molecular weights.[59,60] Sodium dodecyl sulfate electrophoresis under nonreducing conditions reveals that fibrinogen has three main bands of 340, 305, and 270 kd, described respectively as high-molecular-weight (HMW), low-molecular-weight (LMW), and LMW′. These bands are shown by immunoblotting of plasma with antibody to fibrinogen (Fig. 41-3). Normal plasma contains approximately 70% HMW fibrinogen, 26% LMW fibrinogen, and 4% LMW′ fibrinogen.[60] The HMW fibrinogen fraction (340 kd) contains intact Aα chain; LMW fibrinogen has one of the COOH terminals of the Aα chains proteolyzed, with release of a fragment of about 27 kd. The COOH terminals of both α chains have been proteolyzed in the LMW′.[60,61]

The heterogeneity of human fibrinogen is also caused by differences in the γ chain.[62,63] In addition to the most abundant γ chain, there is another normal γ-chain variant (γ′) that has an extended COOH-terminal sequence. The γ′ variant form has a more negative charge and larger size relative to the predominant γ chain, and this arises from alternative mRNA processing.[63,64] In human hepatocytes, the last intron of the γ gene remains unspliced in about 15% of transcripts, and a new COOH terminal is produced by translation on the last intron. The terminated polyadenylation signal from the last, ninth intron is used. Thus, in humans the mechanism for generation of γ′ chain mRNA is alternative polyadenylation.[63,64] Three forms of γ chain that differ in amino acid sequence at the COOH-terminal end have been found in plasma.[65,66] Two of these forms correspond to those previously described: γ, and γ′, and a third form of intermediate size. The smallest γ chain constitutes 93.5% of normal human plasma fibrinogen γ chain. The largest constitutes 5%, and the intermediate form is 1.5%. Their molecular weights have been estimated as 50, 57.5, and 55 kd, respectively. The biosynthetic mechanism that produces the intermediate human γ chain is not entirely clear, but the most likely explanation is proteolytic modification of the γ chain with cleavage of the final four amino acid residues. Thus, alternative splicing of mRNA accounts for two species of γ chains and the third minor γ chain arises from proteolytic modification of the longest γ chain. The γ chain will not support platelet aggregation, but it can be covalently cross-linked.[67]

Other causes of heterogeneity include the degree of phosphorylation on the Aα chain[68,69] and differences in the carbohydrate composition or in sialic acid content[70] of the Bβ and γ chains (see section on posttranslational modifications). Newly synthesized fibrinogen is secreted fully phosphorylated from hepatocytes. In normal plasma, however, only 20% to 25% of potential phosphorylation sites are phosphorylated. This indicates that fibrinogen is dephosphorylated in plasma.[69]

Heterogeneity of fibrinogen is also caused by genetic polymorphism. At least seven sites for normal fibrinogen variants have been identified in all three chains.[77–79] Several attempts have been made to correlate various phenotypes of fibrinogen with a thrombotic tendency, but this has not yet been proved.[84]

Fibrinogen from the cord blood of newborns is sometimes referred to as fetal fibrinogen. This fibrinogen has an increased amount of phosphorylation because cord fibrinogen is not dephosphorylated to the same extent as adult fibrinogen, or this represents newly synthesized fibrinogen.[84] It also has increased carbohydrate content with more sialic acid residues than adult fibrinogen, but the primary amino acid sequence between fetal and adult fibrinogen is identical.[69] Cord fibrinogen is more susceptible to proteolysis, and this, together with its extra negative charge, results in prolonged clotting times.

FUNCTIONAL ACTIVITIES

Fibrinopeptide Release

The final event of vertebrate blood coagulation is the conversion of the soluble protein, fibrinogen, to insoluble fibrin. This event can be divided into three general reactions: (1) fibrinopeptide release by thrombin; (2) polymerization, which is enzyme-independent; and (3) cross-linking by factor XIIIa. Thrombin cleaves fibrinopeptides A and B from the NH_2-terminal region of fibrinogen. This leads to formation of fibrin monomers, which spontaneously polymerize into a fibrin clot. Factor XIIIa stabilizes fibrin polymers by covalent cross-linking (Fig. 41-4).

Fibrin formation is initiated by limited proteolysis of fibrinogen by the serine protease, thrombin. Two small, negatively charged peptides are released from the amino-terminal ends of the Aα and Bβ chains by scission of an arginine-glycine bond.[80,85] Fibrinopeptide A contains 16 residues, and fibrinopeptide B has 14 residues.

The kinetic results of thrombin-catalyzed fibrinopeptide release indicate that fibrinopeptide A appears first, followed by fibrinopeptide B. Under normal circumstances, in the initial phase of the reaction, there is a lag before fibrinopeptide B is released. Two opposing mechanisms have been suggested as the cause. The sequential mechanism assumes that cleavage of fibrinopeptide A is necessary for fibrinopeptide B release, and that thrombin recognizes only the peptide A site in intact fibrinogen. Thrombin hydrolyzes peptide A, which initiates polymerization and results in a presumed conformational change in the molecule. Thrombin is then able to recognize the NH_2-terminal region of Bβ chain and release fibrinopeptide B.[86]

The competitive model assumes that thrombin releases both fibrinopeptides independently and that there is competition between them for thrombin.[87–89] The Aα chain is a better substrate for thrombin, so fibrinopeptide A is liberated first. The crystallization of thrombin and experiments with its substrates indicate that this is correct. Fur-

1 Ala Asp Ser Gly Glu Gly Asp Phe Leu Ala Glu Gly Gly Gly Val Arg↓Gly Pro Arg Val Val Glu Arg His Gln
26 Ser Ala Cys Lys Asp Ser Asp Trp Pro Phe Cys Ser Asp Glu Asp Trp Asn Tyr Lys Cys Pro Ser Gly Cys Arg
51 Met Lys Gly Leu Ile Asp Glu Val Asn Gln Asp Phe Thr Asn Arg Ile Asn Lys Leu Lys Asn Ser Leu Phe Glu
76 Tyr Gln Lys Asn Asn Lys Asp Ser His Ser Leu Thr Thr Asn Ile Met Glu Ile Leu Arg Gly Asp Phe Ser Ser
101 Ala Asn Asn Arg Asp Asn Thr Tyr Asn Arg Val Ser Glu Asp Leu Arg Ser Arg Ile Glu Val Leu Lys Arg Lys
126 Val Ile Glu Lys Val Gln His Ile Gln Leu Leu Gln Lys Asn Val Arg Ala Gln Leu Val Asp Met Lys Arg Leu
151 Glu Val Asp Ile Asp Ile Lys Ile Arg Ser Cys Arg Gly Ser Cys Ser Arg Ala Leu Ala Arg Glu Val Asp Leu
176 Lys Asp Tyr Glu Asp Gln Gln Lys Gln Leu Glu Gln Val Ile Ala Lys Asp Leu Leu Pro Ser Arg Asp Arg Gln
201 His Leu Pro Leu Ile Lys Met Lys Pro Val Pro Asp Leu Val Pro Gly Asn Phe Lys Ser Gln Leu Gln Lys Val
226 Pro Pro Glu Trp Lys Ala Leu Thr Asp Met Pro Gln Met Arg Met Glu Leu Glu Arg Pro Gly Gly Asn Glu Ile
251 Thr Arg Gly Gly Ser Thr Ser Tyr Gly Thr Gly Ser Glu Thr Glu Ser Pro Arg Asn Pro Ser Ser Ala Gly Ser
276 Trp Asn Ser Gly Ser Ser Gly Pro Gly Ser Thr Gly Asn Arg Asn Pro Gly Ser Ser Gly Thr Gly Gly Thr Ala
301 Thr Trp Lys Pro Gly Ser Ser Gly Pro Gly Ser Thr Gly Ser Trp Asn Ser Gly Ser Ser Gly Thr Gly Ser Thr
326 Gly Asn Gln Asn Pro Gly Ser Pro Arg Pro Gly Ser Thr Gly Thr Trp Asn Pro Gly Ser Ser Glu Arg Gly Ser
351 Ala Gly His Trp Thr Ser Glu Ser Ser Val Ser Gly Ser Thr Gly Gln Trp His Ser Glu Ser Gly Ser Phe Arg
376 Pro Asp Ser Pro Gly Ser Gly Asn Ala Arg Pro Asn Asn Pro Asp Trp Gly Thr Phe Glu Glu Val Ser Gly Asn
401 Val Ser Pro Gly Thr Arg Arg Glu Tyr His Thr Glu Lys Leu Val Thr Ser Lys Gly Asp Lys Glu Leu Arg Thr
426 Gly Lys Glu Lys Val Thr Ser Gly Ser Thr Thr Thr Thr Arg Arg Ser Cys Ser Lys Thr Val Thr Lys Thr Val
451 Ile Gly Pro Asp Gly His Lys Glu Val Thr Lys Glu Val Val Thr Ser Glu Asp Gly Ser Asp Cys Pro Glu Ala
476 Met Asp Leu Gly Thr Leu Ser Gly Ile Gly Thr Leu Asp Gly Phe Arg His Arg His Pro Asp Glu Ala Ala Phe
501 Phe Asp Thr Ala Ser Thr Gly Lys Thr Phe Pro Gly Phe Phe Ser Pro Met Leu Gly Glu Phe Val Ser Glu Thr
526 Glu Ser Arg Gly Ser Glu Ser Gly Ile Phe Thr Asn Thr Lys Glu Ser Ser Ser His His Pro Gly Ile Ala Glu
551 Phe Pro Ser Arg Gly Lys Ser Ser Ser Tyr Ser Lys Gln Phe Thr Ser Ser Thr Ser Tyr Asn Arg Gly Asp Ser
576 Thr Phe Glu Ser Lys Ser Tyr Lys Met Ala Asp Glu Ala Gly Ser Glu Ala Asp His Glu Gly Thr His Ser Thr
A 601 Lys Arg Gly His Ala Lys Ser Arg Pro Val

1 [Gln Gly Val Asn Asp Asn Glu Glu Gly Phe Phe Ser Ala Arg↓Gly His Arg Pro Leu Asp Lys Lys Arg Glu Glu
26 Ala Pro Ser Leu Arg Pro Ala Pro Pro Pro Ile Ser Gly Gly Gly Tyr Arg Ala Arg Pro Ala Lys Ala Ala Ala
51 Thr Gln Lys Lys Val Glu Arg Lys Ala Pro Asp Ala Gly Gly Cys Leu His Ala Asp Pro Asp Leu Gly Val Leu
76 Cys Pro Thr Gly Cys Gln Leu Gln Glu Ala Leu Leu Gln Gln Glu Arg Pro Ile Arg Asn Ser Val Asp Glu Leu
101 Asn Asn Asn Val Glu Ala Val Ser Gln Thr Ser Ser Ser Ser Phe Gln Tyr Met Tyr Leu Leu Lys Asp Leu Trp
126 Gln Lys Arg Gln Lys Gln Val Lys Asp Asn Glu Asn Val Val Asn Glu Tyr Ser Ser Glu Leu Glu Lys His Gln
151 Leu Tyr Ile Asp Glu Thr Val Asn Ser Asn Ile Pro Thr Asn Leu Arg Val Leu Arg Ser Ile Leu Glu Asn Leu
176 Arg Ser Lys Ile Gln Lys Leu Glu Ser Asp Val Ser Ala Gln Met Glu Tyr Cys Arg Thr Pro Cys Thr Val Ser
201 Cys Asn Ile Pro Val Val Ser Gly Lys Glu Cys Glu Glu Ile Ile Arg Lys Gly Gly Glu Thr Ser Glu Met Tyr
226 Leu Ile Gln Pro Asp Ser Ser Val Lys Pro Tyr Arg Val Tyr Cys Asp Met Asn Thr Glu Asn Gly Gly Trp Thr
251 Val Ile Gln Asn Arg Gln Asp Gly Ser Val Asp Phe Gly Arg Lys Trp Asp Pro Tyr Lys Gln Gly Phe Gly Asn
276 Val Ala Thr Asn Thr Asp Gly Lys Asn Tyr Cys Gly Leu Pro Gly Glu Tyr Trp Leu Gly Asn Asp Lys Ile Ser
301 Gln Leu Thr Arg Met Gly Pro Thr Glu Leu Leu Ile Glu Met Glu Asp Trp Lys Gly Asp Lys Val Lys Ala His
326 Tyr Gly Gly Phe Thr Val Gln Asn Glu Ala Asn Lys Tyr Gln Ile Ser Val Asn Lys Tyr Arg Gly Thr Ala Gly
351 Asn Ala Leu Met Asp Gly Ala Ser Gln Leu Met Gly Glu Asn Arg Thr Met Thr Ile His Asn Gly Met Phe Phe
376 Ser Thr Tyr Asp Arg Asp Asn Asp Gly Trp Leu Thr Ser Asp Pro Arg Lys Gln Cys Ser Lys Glu Asp Gly Gly
401 Gly Trp Trp Tyr Asn Arg Cys His Ala Ala Asn Pro Asn Gly Arg Tyr Tyr Trp Gly Gly Gln Tyr Thr Trp Asp
426 Met Ala Lys His Gly Thr Asp Asp Gly Val Val Trp Met Asn Trp Lys Gly Ser Trp Tyr Ser Met Arg Lys Met
B 451 Ser Met Lys Ile Arg Pro Phe Phe Pro Gln Gln

FIGURE 41-2. The complete amino acid sequence of the three chains of human fibrinogen: Aα chain **(A)**, Bβ chain **(B)**, and γ chain **(C)**. Arrows indicate the cleavage sites for fibrinopeptides A and B. (Data from references 37 to 42, 45, and 46)

thermore, experiments with trypsin, which cleaves both fibrinopeptides,[90] and with antibodies, which interact with both chains of native fibrinogen,[92,93] indicate that both peptide-cleavage sites are available on the surface of the intact molecule.

The most probable explanation for the observed lag in fibrinopeptide B release incorporates both theories. In the earlier stage, a mechanism of independent, competitive cleavage best fits the experimental data. The later stage of fibrinopeptide B release, however, is characterized by polymerization-dependent sequential cleavage.[94]

The interaction between thrombin and fibrinogen has been thoroughly studied, particularly for fibrinopeptide A cleavage.[95–97] Thrombin is a highly specific serine protease, cleaving only 4 of the 376 Arg/Lys-X bonds in fibrinogen. This specificity is confirmed by the mechanism of thrombin–fibrinogen interaction.[98] There is the cleavage or catalytic-binding site where the active site of thrombin binds to the substrate at the point of hydrolysis.[99] In the Aα chain, amino acids 7 to 16 contain the structural information necessary for thrombin binding.[100–103] Amino acids Asp 7, Phe 8, Gly 12, and Arg 16 are essential to this

```
  1 Tyr Val Ala Thr Arg Asp Asn Cys Cys Ile Leu Asp Glu Arg Phe Gly Ser Tyr Cys Pro Thr Thr Cys Gly Ile
 26 Ala Asp Phe Leu Ser Thr Tyr Gln Thr Lys Val Asp Lys Asp Leu Gln Ser Leu Glu Asp Ile Leu His Gln Val
 51 Glu Asn Lys Thr Ser Glu Val Lys Gln Leu Ile Lys Ala Ile Gln Leu Thr Tyr Asn Pro Asp Glu Ser Ser Lys
 76 Pro Asn Met Ile Asp Ala Ala Thr Leu Lys Ser Arg Lys Met Leu Glu Glu Ile Met Lys Tyr Glu Ala Ser Ile
101 Leu Thr His Asp Ser Ser Ile Arg Tyr Leu Gln Glu Ile Tyr Asn Ser Asn Asn Gln Lys Ile Val Asn Leu Lys
126 Glu Lys Val Ala Gln Leu Glu Ala Gln Cys Gln Glu Pro Cys Lys Asp Thr Val Gln Ile His Asp Ile Thr Gly
151 Lys Asp Cys Gln Asp Ile Ala Asn Lys Gly Ala Lys Gln Ser Gly Leu Tyr Phe Ile Lys Pro Leu Lys Ala Asn
176 Gln Gln Phe Leu Val Tyr Cys Glu Ile Asp Gly Ser Gly Asn Gly Trp Thr Val Phe Gln Lys Arg Leu Asp Gly
201 Ser Val Asp Phe Lys Lys Asn Trp Ile Gln Tyr Lys Glu Gly Phe Gly His Leu Ser Pro Thr Gly Thr Thr Glu
226 Phe Trp Leu Gly Asn Glu Lys Ile His Leu Ile Ser Thr Gln Ser Ala Ile Pro Tyr Ala Leu Arg Val Glu Leu
251 Glu Asp Trp Asn Gly Arg Thr Ser Thr Ala Asp Tyr Ala Met Phe Lys Val Gly Pro Glu Ala Asp Lys Tyr Arg
276 Leu Thr Tyr Ala Tyr Phe Ala Gly Gly Asp Ala Gly Asp Ala Phe Asp Gly Phe Asp Phe Gly Asp Asp Pro Ser
301 Asp Lys Phe Phe Thr Ser His Asn Gly Met Gln Phe Ser Thr Trp Asp Asn Asp Asn Asp Lys Phe Glu Gly Asn
326 Cys Ala Glu Gln Asp Gly Ser Gly Trp Trp Met Asn Lys Cys His Ala Gly His Leu Asn Gly Val Tyr Tyr Gln
351 Gly Gly Thr Tyr Ser Lys Ala Ser Thr Pro Asn Gly Tyr Asp Asn Gly Ile Ile Trp Ala Thr Trp Lys Thr Arg
376 Trp Tyr Ser Met Lys Lys Thr Thr Met Lys Ile Ile Pro Phe Asn Arg Leu Thr Ile Gly Glu Gly Gln Gln His
C 401 His Leu Gly Gly Ala Lys Gln Ala Gly Asp Val
```

FIGURE 41-2. (Continued)

binding.[104] Independent sites for apolar and anionic binding in thrombin are required for converting fibrinogen into fibrin, and fibrin interactions involve an anionic binding site.[105,106] In addition to the active site binding site, a second, extended substrate-binding site is important for stable interaction with thrombin.[91–93] This extended binding site for thrombin is localized in the E domain of fibrin(ogen),[106] and all three fragment E-chain remnants have extended binding sites.[107] It is not known whether these constitute a single extended binding site in vivo or whether they are three separate ones.

Human fibrinopeptides were isolated and partly sequenced for the first time by Blombäck and coworkers in 1966.[108] The peptides found in clot supernatant have several forms. Fibrinopeptide A occurs in three forms: (1) 70 % of the main variant, A; (2) 20% of the phosphorylated variant, AP; and (3) 10% of a shorter variant in which the NH_2-terminal amino acid is missing, AY.[108,109] Fibrinopeptide B occurs only in one form; however, after its release, it is digested by a carboxypeptidase in plasma, and a shorter form without COOH-terminal arginine appears. All the fibrinopeptide variants can be isolated by HPLC[109–111] (Fig. 41-5).

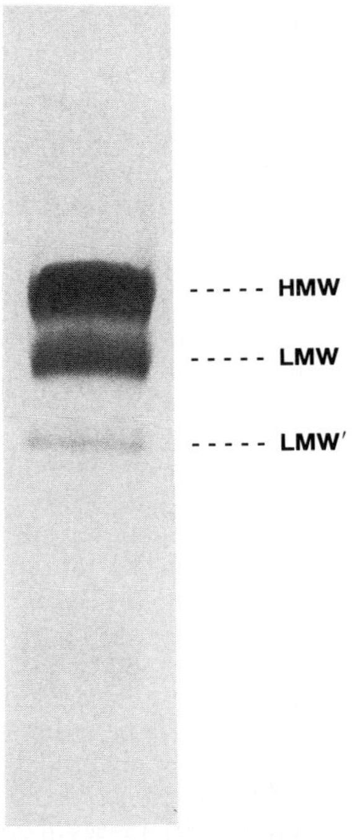

FIGURE 41-3. Immunoblotting of normal human plasma: gradient electrophoresis, blotting with a polyclonal antifibronogen antibody. (Data from J.M. Carr and J. McDonagh)

Fibrinopeptides A and B can be cleaved from fibrinogen by thrombin-like enzymes isolated from certain snakes. Reptilase (Batroxobin) purified from the venom of *Bothrops atrox* or *moojeni* and Ancrod (Arvin) from *Agkistrodon rhodostoma*; both selectively remove fibrinopeptide A,[90,112] while the venom from the southern copperhead snake (*Agkistrodon contortrix contortrix*) preferentially cleaves fibrinopeptide B, especially at lower temperature.[90,112,113] These venoms are particularly useful for studying the effect of selective removal of fibrinopeptides on fibrin polymerization and also for differentiating abnormal fibrinogens, since they have different substrate specificities than thrombin. Tissue plasminogen activator (tPA) is reported to release fibrinopeptides from fibrinogen but at a slower rate than thrombin.[114]

Fibrinopeptide release from bovine fibrinogen, catalyzed by thrombin, is accompanied by binding of Ca^{2+} to fibrin. The calcium uptake is coordinated with the release of fibrinopeptide B, while fibrinopeptide A is liberated mostly during the lag that precedes Ca^{2+} binding. Fibrinogen clotting with Ancrod is not followed by Ca^{2+} uptake. Thus, polymerization itself is not sufficient for Ca^{2+} binding, while fibrinopeptide B release appears to be obligatory.[115]

Polymer Assembly

Although the fibrinopeptides' molecular weight constitutes only about 1% to 2% of the total molecular weight of the fibrinogen molecule,[116] removal of these peptides leads to spontaneous polymerization of the newly formed fibrin monomers and a subtle reorientation of some domains in fibrin. With the electron microscope, the COOH terminal two thirds of the α chain may be seen as a nonstructured part or as a structured domain, folding back over the central domain; this depends on the environment.[23,119] This domain is dissociated when fibrin monomer is formed; it is important for fibrin polymerization, and a fragment of it inhibits polymerization.[23] There are also some new epitopes revealed in fibrin and hidden in fibrinogen, such as γ 312 to 324.[120] Removal of fibrinopeptide A is essential for poly-

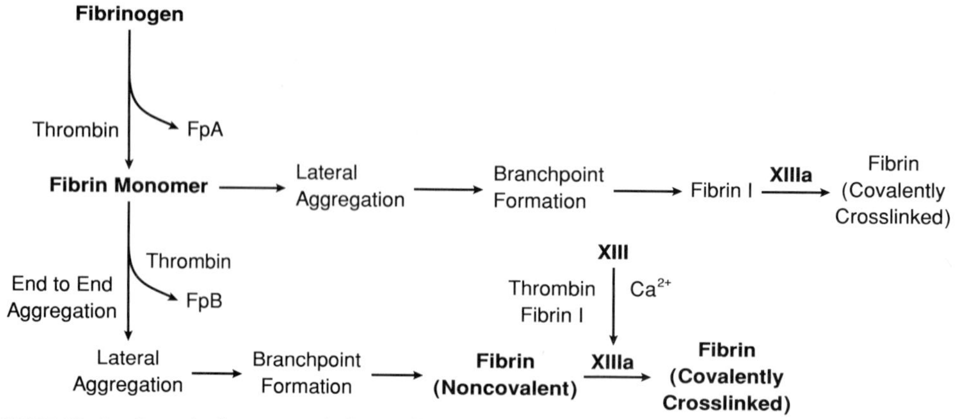

FIGURE 41-4. Steps in the terminal phase of blood clotting. The end products may be both fibrin I and fibrin II.

merization; removal of fibrinopeptide B makes the contacts between fibrin monomer units stronger.

Polymerization of fibrin monomers is kinetically regulated and occurs in ordered, sequential steps. Alignment of fibrin monomers is schematically shown in Figure 41-6. There are several complementary polymerization domains in fibrin, not all of which have been localized. Some of the polymerization domains are present in both fibrinogen and fibrin, whereas others are buried in fibrinogen and are made available only when fibrin monomer is formed. Removal of fibrinopeptide A makes available a polymerization domain, a site that begins with the first amino acids of the α chain, Gly-Pro-Arg-Val. This is the *A site.*[86,121] It interacts with a complementary, preformed domain in the COOH terminal of the γ chain, the *a site.* It has been variously suggested that this site corresponds to regions between γ 374 and 405.[126] Recently, the location of this polymerization site in the D domain has been narrowed to γ 356 to 375.[127] The tripeptide Gly-Pro-Arg, a potent inhibitor of polymerization,[128] bound to Tyr 363 in the γ chain; this indicates that this must be at or near the polymerization domain.[129] But results with abnormal fibrinogen molecules suggest that conformation of an extended γ-chain portion, rather than a short peptide, is crucial for proper fibrin polymerization.[130,131] Mutation of Asp 330 to Val in the abnormal fibrinogen Milano I causes a profound change in the microenvironment of γ Tyr 363.[132] Similarly, removal of fibrinopeptide B produces a polymerization domain beginning with Gly-His-Arg-Pro, the *B site,* which probably reacts with a complementary site in the β chain of the D domain, the *b site.* The Bb interaction is not so clearly known. The B domain begins with Gly-His-Pro-Arg, which can interact with the a site. A separate b site is probably conformationally dependent and is composed of noncontiguous amino acids on both the α and β chains in the D domain.[133] The Aa interaction, with or without the Bb interaction, is also called the DE staggered contact interaction, which refers to the interaction of nodular domains visualized by electron micrographs.[134] These may be the most important polymerization complementary domains, since the formation of a fibrin clot appears to be driven by this interaction. Fibrinolytic fragments X, Y, and early D and DD also inhibit polymerization, with dissociation constants in the nanomolar range.[135]

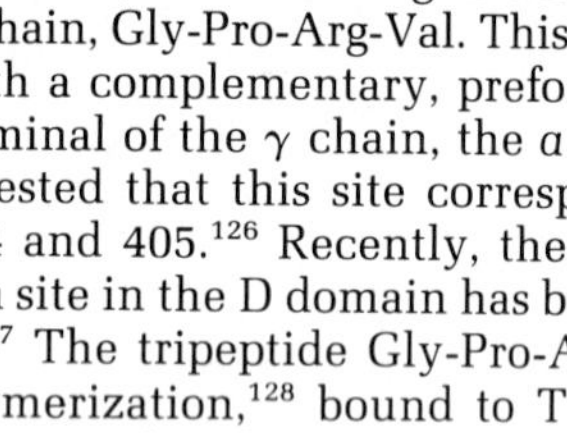

FIGURE 41-5. HPLC profile of fibrinopeptides. Elution was with 0.1% trifluoroaecetic acid in an H_2O/acetonitrile gradent. AP, phosphorylated fibrinopeptide A; A, fibrinopeptide A; B, fibrinopeptide B.

When the A site is exposed, it interacts with the complementary a site on another fibrin monomer in a half-staggered overlap manner. This is the first step in polymerization. The addition of monomer units continues in this fashion (see Fig. 41-6). Addition of the third monomer molecule to a dimer forms a new contact between the D domains of adjacent molecules in the same strand of the polymer (named DD-long) in addition to another two DE-stag contacts.[107] Each additional monomer to the growing, two-stranded polymer chain (protofibril) forms one DD-long and two DE-stag contacts. The DD-long contact is at or near the site of γ-chain cross-linking,[136] eventually forming fibrin protofibrils. Protofibrils are composed of two fibrin monomer chains, associated noncovalently, with a molecular diameter of two molecules (see Fig. 41-6). They are the building blocks for the three-dimensional gel, that is, protofibrils add to protofibrils.[134] Recently, a different mechanism was proposed, based on a single, interlocked strand,[142] but the weight of evidence, including recent electron micrographs,[137] favors the two-molecule, half-staggered overlap model. Lateral association occurs only between protofibrils and involves other additional noncovalent interactions known as DD-lateral contacts. Fibrin composed of monomer units with cleavage of only fibrinopeptide A is called fibrin I. Fibrin that has both the A and the B peptides cleaved is called fibrin II (see Fig. 41-4). When about 20% of fibrinopeptide A is cleaved, the fibrin monomers thus formed spontaneously polymerize to oligomers and ultimately to fibers (fibrin I).[137] At the same time, the cleavage rate of fibrinopeptide B increases greatly, and some fibrin II is formed. The rate of fibrinopeptide B release may also affect the thrombin clotting time.[138] Cleavage of fibrinopeptide B occurs preferentially from fibrin oligomers or protofibrils, and it contributes to the overall stability of the laterally associated protofibrils. There are differences in fibrin I and II that may be important physiologically. Fibrin II is mechanically stronger, so it should be less affected by rheologic forces in blood[140]; fibrin I is preferentially taken up by macrophages.[141]

Another model for fibrin polymerization is based on the observation that fibrin polymers formed in vivo still contain about 50% of fibrinopeptide A.[142] In this model, the half-

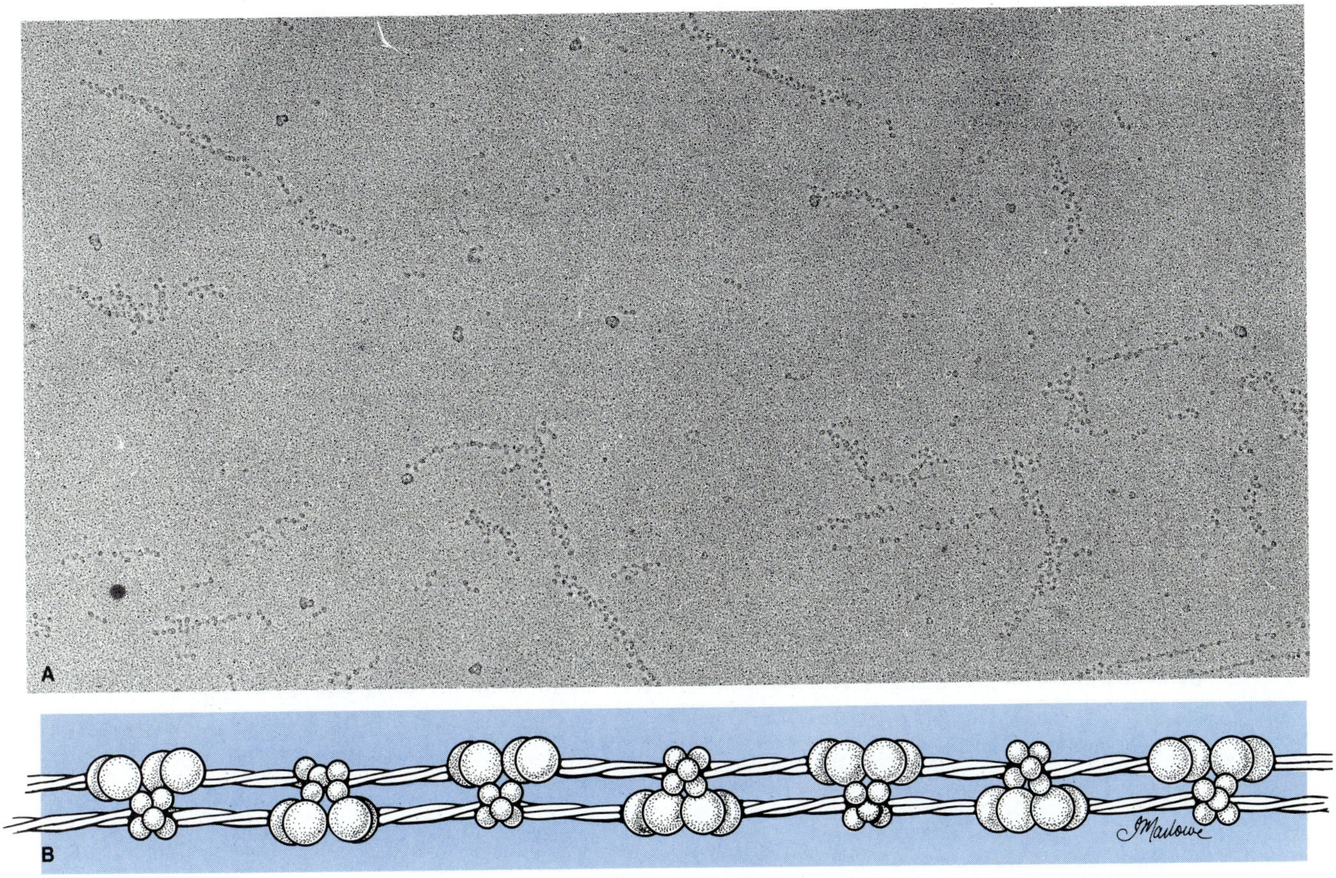

FIGURE 41-6. **(A)** Electron microscopic presentation of protofibrils. Samples were rotary shadowed (×51,200). **(B)** Model of a protofibril, indicating how fibrin monomers are aligned. (**A** courtesy of Dr. H. Slayter, Dana Farber Cancer Institute and Harvard Medical School, Boston; **B** adapted from Hermans J, McDonagh J. Fibrin: structure and interaction. Semin Thromb Hemost 1982;8:11)

molecule staggered overlap is stabilized by only one pair of complementary DE-contacts per fibrin monomer, compared with two pairs of contacts per monomer in the above models. These fibrinogen–fibrin complexes can disaggregate. There is evidence for formation of soluble fibrinogen–fibrin complexes in vivo.

It is shown clearly by electron microscopy that both thick and thin fibers branch, and branching must occur to form a three-dimensional fibrin mesh. Little is known, however, about this branching process. With rotary shadowed electron micrographs, it can be seen that protofibrils and fibers are twisted,[137] confirming a suggestion made some years ago on theoretical grounds.[134] Mass and length measurements from scanning electron micrographs have contributed new insights into the formation of a three-dimensional gel by showing two new types of branch points.[143] Tetramolecular junctions occur when two fibrils converge, creating a third branch with twice the mass and length of its constituents. Trimolecular junctions have three fibril branches of equal mass and length and may occur when an extraneous fibrin molecule initiates branching in a propagating fibril, by bridging across two unpaired complementary polymerization sites.[143] All of the interactions involving complementary domains in fibrin polymerization are noncovalent, and they are potentially reversible.

The final step in fibrin formation is covalent stabilization. This reaction is catalyzed by an enzyme, factor XIIIa, which covalently links ϵ-amino groups of lysine residues with γ-carboxyl groups of glutamine residues. This is a crucial step that makes a blood clot hemostatically effective. The positions of the covalent bonds are specific and they are located in COOH-terminal region of γ chains and are linked in an antiparallel arrangement.[144] The donor (Lys 406) and the acceptor (Glu 398) residues are engaged in the binding between γ chains of adjacent molecules. After cross-linking all of the γ chains in the fibrin clot, multiple cross-links between α chains are introduced. Each α chain has two glutamyl acceptor sites in positions 328 and 366, and five potential lysine donor sites, between positions 518 and 584.[145] Further studies suggest that Lys 508 and Lys 556 or 562 take part in α-chain cross-linking.[146] The α-chain cross-links probably stabilize the lateral association of protofibrils into thick fibers (see section on factor XIII).

Covalent cross-linking of α chains decreases the concentration of fibrin required for gel formation and also enhances the stiffness of the fibrin gel.[147] Studies have shown that cross-linking also increases the resistance of fibrin to plasmin degradation[148] through complex mechanisms. Cross-linking of γ chains is probably important for initial stabilization of the protofibril.

Fibrinolysis

As mentioned, fibrin is the major substrate of the fibrinolytic system and also a major cofactor in this system, where it is responsible for efficient fibrin clot dissolution. The primary fibrinolytic components are (1) the proenzyme plasminogen (which can be activated by limited proteolysis to the active enzyme, plasmin), (2) plasminogen activators (tPA and prourokinase), (3) inhibitors of plasmin (α_2-plasmin inhibitor and α_2-macroglobulin), and (4) inhibitors of plasminogen activation (PAI-1 and PAI-2 and others). The formation of fibrin signals the activation of the fibrinolytic system, and its activity ceases at the point of com-

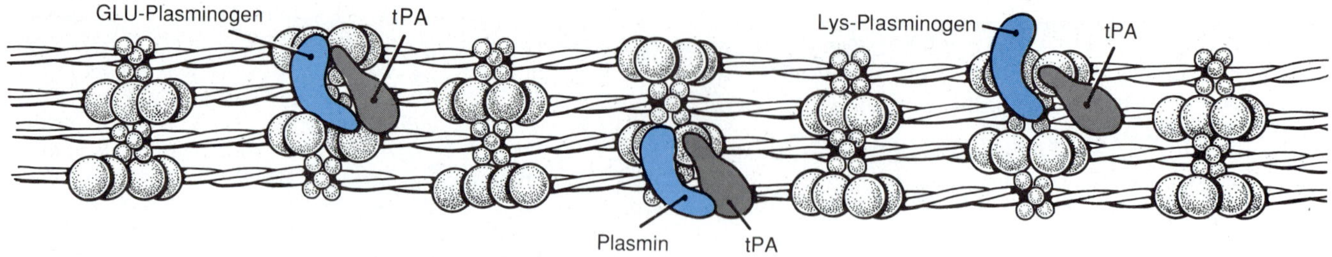

FIGURE 41-7. Model of the assembly of tPA and plasminogen on the fibrin surface.

plete degradation of fibrin. Fibrin formation is part of the homeostatic mechanism; physiologically, its purpose is to arrest bleeding and begin the wound-healing process. In some pathologic conditions, this mechanism is out of control, and thrombi result internally in a vessel or in the extracellular space surrounding tumor cells. These pathologic thrombi have dire consequences, producing myocardial infarction, deep venous thromboses and pulmonary emboli, strokes, thrombophlebitis, and protection of tumor cells. Fibrinolysis is the homeostatic mechanism to eliminate thrombi, and it is also carefully regulated. There is a delicate balance between the coagulation and the fibrinolytic systems. This results in a remarkably elegant homeostatic mechanism, which also can give rise to thrombosis or hemorrhage if the two systems are not precisely balanced. Discussion here is limited to the specific degradation products of fibrin(ogen) produced by activators of fibrinolysis. Plasmin is a serine protease that digests fibrin and fibrinogen at specific lysyl-x and arginyl-x bonds to produce small, soluble degradation products. In fibrin(ogen), twice as many Lys-x bonds are hydrolyzed by plasmin as arginine-x bonds.[150] Plasmin has broad specificity, but fibrin and fibrinogen are its principal targets in vivo. Plasminogen binds to fibrin through its lysine-binding sites; fibrin enhances the activation of plasminogen to the active enzyme plasmin by tPA, which also has a strong affinity for fibrin. In this manner, both plasminogen and tPA assemble on the surface of fibrin (Fig. 41-7). This as-

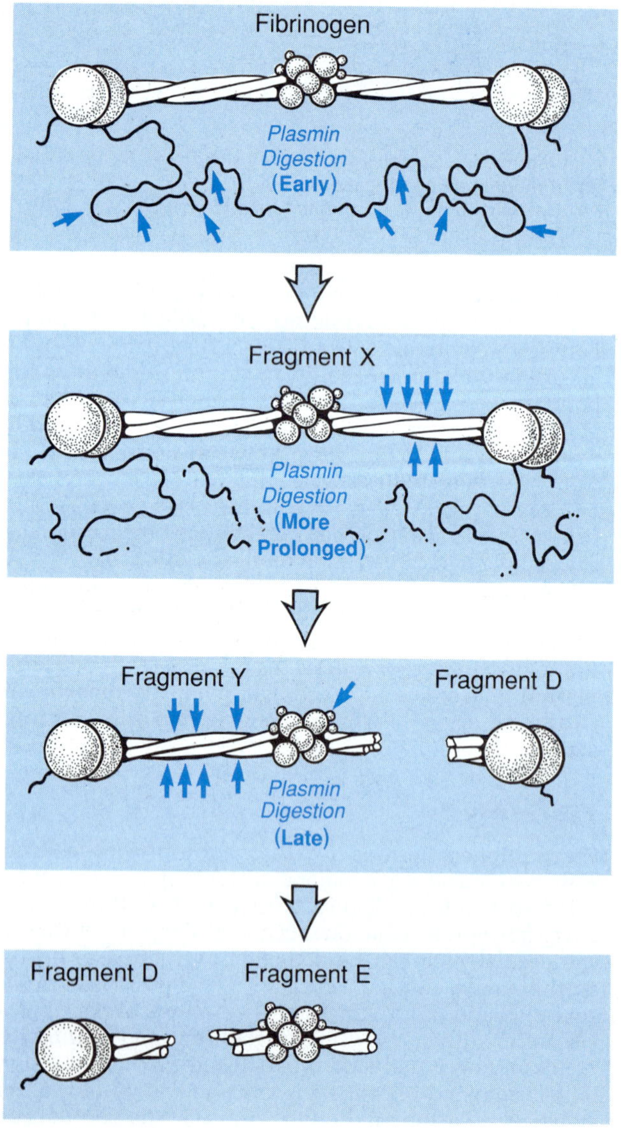

A

FIGURE 41-8. Model of the plasmin degradation products of fibrinogen **(A)** and fibrin **(B)**. Arrows indicate plasmin hydrolysis sites. White arrowheads indicate γ–γ cross-linking. All fragments from cross-linked fibrin have this cross-link. In the model, it is indicated only for the cross-linked polymer and for the terminal degradation product for clarity. (After Carr JM, McDonagh J. Fibrin(ogen) degradation products: analysis of measurement techniques, In: Dade Coagulation Technical Bulletin No. 20. American Dade, Miami, 1987) sembly promotes activation of plasminogen and makes the local concentration of plasmin higher within a fibrin clot. As plasmin digests fibrin, the stimulatory effect on plasminogen activation is decreased, providing an important step in regulation.

Plasmin cleaves the three chains of fibrin at selective sites, in an orderly manner, to release a variety of degradation products. The native fibrinogen molecule is hydrolyzed to smaller and more compact fragments. The first step involves the removal of the COOH-terminal Aα-chain segment by several orderly plasmin cleavages. The second step is the cleavage of a peptide from the NH_2 terminal end of the Bβ chain (Bβ 1 to 42).[151] In some abnormal fibrinogens, the first step is blocked, so there is no degradation of these abnormal fibrins.[152] Fragment X (240 kd) is then converted to an asymmetric intermediate, fragment Y (155 kd), and an equimolar amount of fragment D (83 kd). Fragment Y is further converted to fragment E (50 kd) and another fragment D. Terminally, a trinodular molecule of fibrinogen is digested to two fragments D and one fragment E, plus many small peptides.[153,154] All of these fragments actually represent families of fragments.[155] The γ and Bβ chains each have about a fourth of the plasmin cleavage points. The Aα has about half of the plasmin cleavage sites distributed in hydrophilic clusters. The Ca^{2+} protected cleavage site is at γ 302.[156]

The plasmin degradation scheme for fibrinogen is shown in Figure 41-8A. Non–cross-linked fibrin has the same

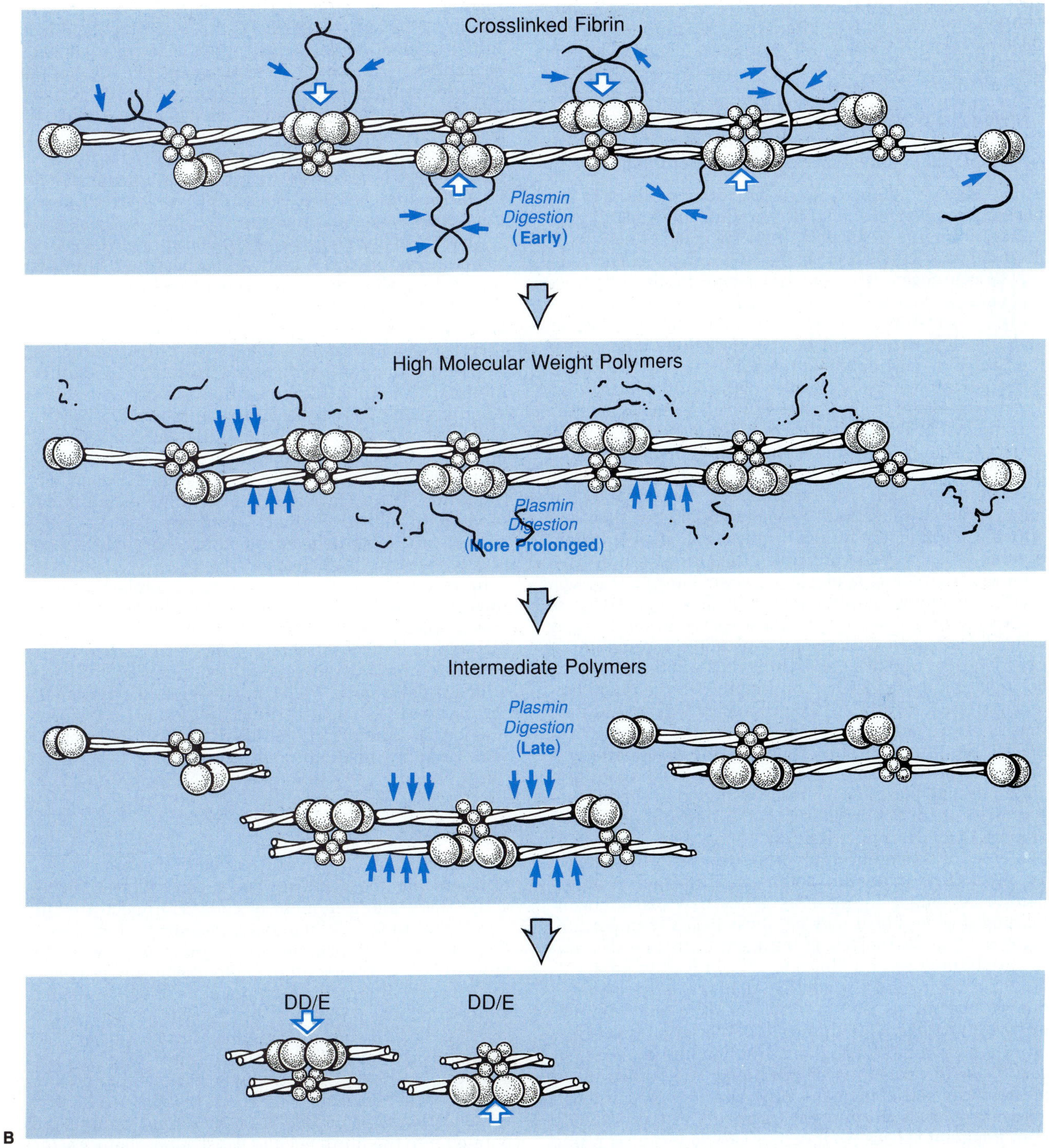

FIGURE 41-8. (Continued)

plasmin fragments, except that all of fragment E is missing fibrinopeptides, and in cross-linked fibrin, the plasmin-degradation fragments have covalent cross-links that are not degraded by plasmin. The fragments, derived from the same mechanism, include a family of HMW derivatives (eg, YXD-DXY, DXX-YY) and D dimer (DD) and E.[157] There is an affinity between DD and E, and a noncovalent complex is formed. The degradation products of cross-linked fibrin are shown in Figure 41-8*B*.

Interaction of Fibrin(ogen) With Other Macromolecules and Cells

Fibrinogen interacts with a number of proteins and cells, and many of these interactions are physiologically important. Fibrin(ogen) binds plasmin(ogen), tPA, α_2-antiplasmin, factor XIII/XIIIa and it interacts with fibronectin and thrombospondin (TSP) as well as with platelets and certain bacteria.

Components of the Fibrinolytic System: Plasminogen, Tissue Plasminogen Activator, Prourokinase, α_2-Antiplasmin, and Plasminogen Activator Inhibitor-1

This section is confined to the functions of fibrin in the fibrinolytic mechanism: (1) tPA binding to fibrin, (2) plasminogen binding to fibrin, and (3) the cofactor activity of fibrin in the conversion of plasminogen to plasmin by tPA. Plasminogen, tPA, and PAI-1 bind to fibrin, and α_2-antiplasmin binds to fibrin and is cross-linked to it. Because fibrin is a substrate, a cofactor for an enzymatic reaction, and a binding surface, the last two functions change over the course of degradation of the substrate. The formation of fibrin is the signal for activation of the fibrinolytic system, and the activity of this system stops when fibrin degradation is complete.[149] The activation of plasminogen on a fibrin surface is about 1000 times more efficient than in the fluid phase.

Plasminogen and tPA interact with fibrin COOH-terminal lysines through their strong lysine-binding sites, and with fibrin intrachain lysines through their weaker lysine-binding sites.[158,159] The principal circulating form of plasminogen is glutamic acid–plasminogen. Glu-plasminogen is converted to lysine-plasminogen by plasmin cleavage of an NH_2 terminal peptide, which exposes lysine binding site and change plasminogen polypeptide conformation.[160] Lys-plasminogen binds more readily to fibrin than glutamic acid–plasminogen, and lysine-plasminogen is a much better substrate for tPA.[161–164] Experimental evidence suggests that the two main domains of fibrin, D and E, both carry plasminogen-binding sites.[165] Intact fibrinogen interacts only with lysine-plasminogen because the binding sites for glutamic acid–plasminogen may be hidden in the fibrinogen molecule but exposed in fibrin through the formation of more COOH terminal lysines.[163] Thus there are at least two types of plasminogen-binding sites on fibrin—one on an intact fibrin clot, and another on fibrin that has been partially degraded by plasmin. These new plasminogen-binding sites on fibrin may be physiologically important, because once fibrinolysis is initiated, formation of additional plasminogen-binding sites would lead to an acceleration of the rate of fibrinolysis. All of the early cleavages during fibrinolysis are at lysyl bonds,[167] and new fibrin(ogen) fragments with the COOH-terminal lysine residues are essential for high-affinity binding to plasminogen.[168] With plasmin degradation, the amount of plasminogen bound increases nine-fold.[170,171] Plasminogen apparently binds fibrin(ogen) fragment E more strongly than fragment D because it carries COOH-terminal lysine residues on all three peptide chains. The family of fragments D may have 0-2 COOH-terminal lysine residues.[168] There is also electron microscopic evidence that lysine-plasminogen binds to fragment D or to the cleft formed by the two D domains in the fibrin polymer.[177] Although all of the precise binding mechanisms for plasminogen, tPA, and fibrin are unknown, it appears that plasminogen and tPA bind to fibrin in proximity.

tPA is a key enzyme in physiologic thrombolysis. It selectively binds fibrin, targeting plasminogen on the fibrin clot surface. The best cofactor for activity of tPA is fibrin II, then fibrin I; fibrinogen is a weak one. The newly formed plasmin is poised to act on the thrombus and is protected from circulating inhibitors in the blood.

The binding domain for tPA in fibrin(ogen) has not been identified with certainty, and the many reports are conflicting. The best evidence suggests that γ-chain residues 311 to 379, and especially γ Tyr 363 are involved in the initial interaction with tPA.[175] When fibrin is degraded, other sites in fragment D become available. Some of these γ-chain residues may be hidden in the native fibrinogen molecule and in early degradation products. It is also suggested that the Aα residues 154 to 159 of fibrinogen, especially Aα Lys 157, accelerate plasminogen activation by tPA.[173,174] It has also been suggested that fragment D binds both tPA and lysine-plasminogen, whereas fragment E binds only lysine-plasminogen.

The rate of fibrinolysis is controlled at many levels, other than the binding of tPA and plasminogen, and fibrin structure. Principally, the inhibitors of plasmin and tPA are extremely important. The primary, fast-acting plasmin inhibit is α_2-antiplasmin.[180] Under conditions of thrombolytic therapy, α_2-antiplasmin is totally consumed, and plasmin also forms complexes with α_2-macroglobulin and other inhibitors.[181] α_2-antiplasmin inhibits plasmin in solution. Approximately 20% of plasmin α_2-antiplasmin is covalently cross-linked to fibrin by factor XIIIa and is concentrated on the clot, where it still retains inhibitory activity, although plasmin bound to fibrin is relatively protected from inhibition.[182] α_2-Antiplasmin also inhibits plasminogen binding to fibrin. Patients who are deficient in α_2-antiplasmin have delayed bleeding syndromes, because plasmin activity is unchecked.[183]

In the control of fibrinolysis, PAI-1 is probably the most important inhibitor, since it inhibits the activity of both plasminogen activators, tPA, and urokinase. Many, but not all, studies indicate that high PAI-1 levels are associated with thrombotic disease and atherosclerosis.[186,187] Patients who are deficient in PAI-1 have bleeding syndromes resulting from unbalanced tPA activity and, therefore, increased plasmin formation.[184] PAI-1 is a complex molecule with complex functions; and it can bind to fibrin and the fibrin-bound PAI-1 can interact with tPA.[185]

Fibronectin

Fibronectin is an adhesive glycoprotein that binds a variety of ligands, including fibrin, fibrinogen, collagen, heparin, actin, DNA, and a number of cells. Fibronectin is incorporated into a fibrin clot under physiologic conditions, and the affinity of fibronectin for fibrin(ogen) is well documented.[189,190] Fibronectin binds to fibrinogen by means of noncovalent interactions through its finger domains,[190] which are located in a 27-kd NH_2-terminal fragment and in a 31-kd COOH-terminal region. Fibronectin can also be covalently cross-linked to fibrin by factor XIIIa via the Glu 3 residue in the 27-kd fragment of fibronectin and a lysyl residue in the COOH-terminal parts of the fibrin α chain.[191] Fibronectin is the second most abundant protein incorporated into the fibrin gel and constitutes about 3% to 4% of the mass. About half the fibronectin in plasma is cross-linked to the fibrin gel.[189] Under physiologic conditions, a gel formed with cross-linked fibronectin and fibrin is more elastic.[192] The cross-linking of fibrin to fibronectin may also be important in the process of wound healing.[193]

Other Proteins

Thrombospondin is an HMW adhesive glycoprotein secreted from α-granules of stimulated platelets. It interacts with platelets, heparin, and soluble plasma proteins such as fibronectin, plasminogen, histidine-rich glycoprotein, and fibrinogen. Platelet TSP interacts with fibrinogen in a specific and saturable manner.[194] Some studies show that TSP specifically binds to the Aα and Bβ chains of fibrinogen, and that this binding is not dependent on divalent ions.[195] But other experiments show that only the β-chain component of the D and DD plasmin-degradation fragment of fibrin is engaged in this interaction.[196]

It has been also reported that TSP was incorporated into fibrin clot and cross-linked by factor XIII.[200] In other experiments, however, there was no evidence of fibrin-TSP cross-linking.[201] TSP may preferentially bind non–cross-linked fibrin, which suggests that the TSP-fibrinogen–binding site is unavailable in cross-linked fibrin.[195] The TSP molecule is extremely adhesive, which may account for these conflicting results. In a model for the interaction of TSP with polymerizing fibrin, the three apparently identical subunits of TSP could interact with polymerizing fibrin intermediates and serve as a trifunctional branching unit. Because of this, TSP could be a factor in the formation of protofibrils.[202]

It is important in the coagulation system to localize a fibrin clot at the site of injury. Type IV collagen, which is a component of vascular basement membrane, interacts with fibrin and may provide the anchor site for a fibrin clot. It has been demonstrated that type IV collagen has a large effect on fibrin structure; thicker fibrin fibers are formed and the fiber mass/length ratio is increased.[203]

Fibrin(ogen) does not interact directly with plasma globulins. In patients with increased paraproteins (multiple myeloma, Waldenström's macroglobunemia), however, evidence suggests that the fibrin gel that forms is abnormal. Thin fibers with increased rigidity are formed; these abnormal fibrin gels are not correlated with viscosity.[204]

Cellular Interactions

The adhesion of platelets to the wall of an injured blood vessel, as well as the aggregation between platelets, is critical for normal hemostasis.[205] Fibrinogen plays a crucial role in platelet adhesion and aggregation. There are about 45,000 fibrinogen receptors per platelet. This receptor is a member of the integrin family with the two subunits GP IIb and IIIa. Platelets previously activated by agonists such as ADP, epinephrine, or thrombin, binds fibrinogen, and this binding requires extracellular Ca^{2+} or Mg^{2+}.[206,207] Fibrinogen binding to its platelet receptor is mediated by γ and Aα chains. The COOH-terminal end of the γ chain (located in the D domain) contains a 12-residue peptide (γ 400 to 411), which is responsible for binding to the platelet IIb/IIIa receptor.[208]

Two CNBr fragments of the human fibrinogen Aα chain also contain a platelet receptor factor-recognition domain. Residues 92 to 147 and 518 to 587 contain the cell-recognition sequence (RGD) present in many other adhesive proteins.[208,209] RGD of the Aα chain and the γ 400 to 411 fragment may share a common binding site on platelet glycoprotein IIb/IIIa.[210] It has also been proposed that another NH_2-terminal end of fibrinogen contains an additional platelet-binding site. Further studies localized this in the NH_2-terminal fragment of the Bβ chain (Bβ 15 to 42) and demonstrate that this fragment inhibits platelet aggregation and fibrinogen binding.[211]

Fibrin(ogen) binds to monocytes and macrophages,[141] and fibrin I is more readily taken up by the monocyte system than is fibrin II. This may be an important control mechanism for the elimination of fibrin, independent of fibrinolysis. This high-affinity binding can be inhibited by the thrombin-treated E domain and depends on the release of fibrinopeptide A. Gly-Pro-Arg-Pro and Gly-His-Arg-Pro (the tetrapeptides mimicking the newly exposed NH_2 terminals of the α and β chains after release of the fibrinopeptides) also are inhibitory. CD11c/CD18 on tumor necrosis factor–stimulated neutrophils is also a fibrin receptor, which recognizes Gly-Pro-Arg.[198] The binding sites on fibrinogen for platelets and gram-negative bacteria are localized in the COOH terminal of the γ chain (Glu 397—Val 411)[212] and in a region containing RGD sequence in the α chain (572 to 574).[213] Electron microscopy of fibrinogen binding to GP IIb/IIIa showed that it was highly specific and that the interaction was through the nodular head of GP IIb/IIIa and the D domains of fibrinogen. It was seen that one fibrinogen molecule would bridge two adjacent platelets with this interaction.[199]

Fibrinogen interacts with several other types of cells including certain bacteria (staphylococci, streptococci), monocytes, macrophages, fibroblasts, and some tumor cells.[214–216] Fibrinogen possesses cell agglutinating properties and interacts with a cell-wall component of certain staphylococci, inducing their clumping.[214] About 2100 fibrinogen molecules bind per bacterium. The staphylococcus-binding region has been identified in the COOH-terminal region of γ chain.[209,217] This is one of the sites in the γ chain (γ Glu 397 to Val 411) that also mediates platelet aggregation.[217]

STRUCTURE OF THE FIBRINOGEN GENES AND BIOSYNTHESIS

There are three separate genes that are transcribed into three mRNAs, which code for the three polypeptide chains of fibrinogen.[218,219] All the human fibrinogen genes are located in the long arm of chromosome 4, band 4q23–32.[191]

The cDNAs corresponding to the human and rat fibrinogen genes have been cloned and sequenced.[221] These results, electron microscopic heteroduplex mapping, and selective sequencing of intron–exon junction of genomic clones helped determine the structure of fibrinogen genes. The fibrinogen genes occur in single copies and are clustered in a region of approximately 50 kb. The Aα gene is located between Bβ and γ genes. γ and Aα genes have the same orientation and are transcribed towards the Bβ-chain gene, whereas the Bβ gene is transcribed toward Aα and γ genes from the opposite DNA strand.[223] There are two alternative mechanisms to explain this arrangement and the transcriptional orientation of the human fibrinogen genes. It may be either a three-step mechanism involving two duplications and inversion of the α/γ region, or a two-step mechanism with remote transposition and inversion. The Aα gene contains four introns, the Bβ gene at least seven, and the γ gene contains nine introns. Each gene is 6500 to 7500 bp in length.

Fibrinogen Genes, Domains, Organization, and Expression

The entire human fibrinogen can be assembled and expressed efficiently in Chinese hamster ovary cells. Fibrinopeptide A was found to be 22% phosphorylated, similar to the degree of phosphorylation in circulating plasma.[224] The original gene for fibrinogen probably was present in primitive organisms millions of years ago; there has been sufficient time for many mutations to occur. Some of the structural and functional domains in the fibrinogen molecule correspond to the exons in the fibrinogen genes. The location of several of the seven introns in the β gene is consistent with this hypothesis, even though all of the structural or functional domains of the β gene of fibrinogen are not known. The first exon contains the information for the signal peptide and a part of fibrinopeptide B. The second exon codes for the thrombin cleavage site and a fibrin polymerization domain. The third and fourth exons code for the coiled-coil region.[73] For the γ gene, the first exon codes for a signal peptide; exon 2 codes for the two cysteines involved in disulfide bridging of two γ chains. The first disulfide ring, some of the coiled-coil region, and the carbohydrate-attachment site at Asp 52 is contained in exon 3. Exon 4 codes for more of the coiled-coil region, and exon 5 has the COOH-terminal portion of the coiled-coil and the second disulfide ring. Exons 6, 7, and 8 all code for amino acids in the D domain. This region has the highest degree of homology compared with the β chain of fibrinogen.[225,226] Exon 9 codes for the residues involved in the covalent cross-linking of the γ chains. Exons 9 and 10 also code for amino acids involved in fibrin polymerization and platelet receptor recognition.[76]

The homology among the amino acid sequences of the human fibrinogen chains suggests that all three polypeptides derived from a common ancestral gene, which was duplicated and diverged because of separate mutations.[225,226] The three fibrinogen genes were separated during evolution before the appearance of vertebrates, since even the most primitive vertebrates have three different peptide chains.[227] The β and γ chains have more homology to each other than to the α chain,[228,229] so the divergence of the β and γ chains may have occurred about 500 million years ago. It has been postulated that the divergence of the α chain occurred earlier (about 1500 million years ago); however, the observation of the sixth exon in the α chain places this theory in doubt, since it makes the α chain more homologous with the β and γ chains. Sequences of mRNA and cDNA reveal that the human fibrinogen α chain should have 15 additional amino acid residues at the COOH terminal, compared with the α chain found in plasma fibrinogen, which has Val 610 as the last amino acid.[221] There are two hypotheses for this observation: RNA polymerase II may recognize more than one termination site, yielding mRNAs of different lengths on their 3′ ends, or some nuclease activity or processing event at the 3′ end may result in variation in the precise site of polyadenylation. These 15 residues at the COOH terminal (611 to 625) are removed during assembly or secretion, presumably by limited proteolysis inside the cell, or during the circulation of fibrinogen in plasma.[71,72] The Bβ a γ chains are degraded in the endoplasmic reticulum, but the Aα and Aα-γ complex are degraded by lysosomes.[74] The 5′ region that contains the signal peptide, the coding sequence for disulfide knot, and the region forming the α helix are the most variable portions of the three genes. In this region of the proteins, all amino acid substitutions that do not disrupt α helix formation and do not affect potential sites for plasmin hydrolysis are permitted. The β and γ chains show strong homology in certain portions of their chains that contribute to the D domain. Certain short regions have about 75% to 80% homology in cDNA.[40] Comparison of corresponding human and animal fibrinogen chains also provides information on the regions of the molecule that are essential for its function. Human and rat Aα chain have 53% identity,[76] human and bovine Bβ chains have 82% identity, human and rat γ chains have 83% identity,[223] and human and lamprey γ chains have 50% identity.[227] More critical functional areas, such as the Gly-Pro-Arg polymerization site and the γ–γ cross-linking sites have a low frequency of mutation.[226] Fibrinopeptides, which play a rather nonspecific screening role, are among the most variable parts of fibrinogen.[230] Also, the 3′ noncoding sequences of related genes diverge more rapidly than the protein-coding sequences and often have insertions and deletions in addition to base substitutions.[231] Introns also have been selectively lost or randomly inserted into the genes.[232]

cDNAs for all three fibrinogen chains were used as probes to characterize the size and levels of fibrinogen mRNAs. The Aα mRNA is about 2400 nucleotides, the Bβ mRNA is about 2000 nucleotides, and the γ mRNA is about 1800 nucleotides.[233] The expression of fibrinogen genes is limited to hepatocytes and megakaryocytes.[234,235] A nuclear protein that binds to the sequence required for hepatocyte-specific transcription of the Bβ gene was found in hepatocytes but not in other cell types. This protein, hepatocyte nuclear factor 1, also interacts with a homologous sequence necessary for optimal promoter function of the Aα gene. This factor is probably involved in the specific transcription of genes normally expressed selectively in the liver[234,236] (see section on biosynthesis of fibrinogen).

Because the mature fibrinogen molecule consists of two Aα, two Bβ and two γ chains, coordinate regulation of these three genes was expected. An increase in Bβ-chain synthesis specifically results in the production of the other two components in humans.[237,238] The sequences of the regions surrounding the points of transcriptional initiation of the three rat fibrinogen genes were determined, and two unique regions of homology in the 5′ flanking regions were located.[239] These areas of homology occur in sequences upstream from the sites of fibrinogen mRNA initiation of transcription and probably act as regulatory units of fibrinogen transcription. Sequences between 88 and 43 bp upstream of the γ transcription initiation site are responsible for initiation of transcription, and the two known and one putative transcriptional factors bind and modulate the activity of this promoter.[241] The adenovirus major, late-transcription factor specifically stimulates transcription of the rat γ gene through a high-affinity binding site, and it may be that one of the cellular functions of this factor is to control γ gene expression.[242]

For human fibrinogen, pre–Aα-, pre–Bβ-, and pre–γ-chain signal peptides have been found of 16 or 19,[72] 16, 27 or 30,[73] and 26[76,243] amino acid residues, respectively. These leader sequences are lost before fibrinogen leaves the hepatocyte. These prepeptides may play an important role in assembly of fibrinogen, since all six chains have amino terminals that are tightly gathered in the native molecule. Homology exists in the amino acid sequence between the rat and human signal peptides (52% for α chain and 66% for β chain), which suggests that there is strong selective pressure on this part of all three genes.[71,239] However, a natural product of a novel α-chain gene has been isolated; it is present in normal plasma in very small quantities. This α chain is extended at the COOH terminal by 35% and is due to a separate open reading frame that translates the sixth exon. This is highly homologous to the COOH terminals of the other two chains. Its synthesis is enhanced by interleukin-6, and it may be a marker for the acute-phase response.[209a]

Sequences of mRNA and cDNA reveal that the human fibrinogen α chain should have 15 additional amino acid residues at the COOH terminal, compared with the α chain found in plasma fibrinogen, which has Val 610 as the last amino acid.[221] There are two hypotheses for this observation. RNA polymerase II may recognize more than one termination site, yielding mRNAs of different lengths on their 3′ ends. Or some nuclease activity or processing event at the 3′ end may result in variation in the precise site of polyadenylation. These 15 residues at the COOH terminal (611 to 625) are removed during assembly or secretion, or during the circulation of fibrinogen in plasma, presumably by limited proteolysis inside the cell.[71,72]

Similar variations have also been observed in the 3′ region of the cDNA coding for the β chain of human fibrinogen.[73] Heterogeneity of these cDNAs indicates the presence of at least three different polyadenylated mRNA subpopulations, which differ in the length of their 3′ noncoding sequences. This could be from endonucleolytic processing of the mRNA before polyadenylation or from variations in transcription termination.[73]

Biosynthesis of Fibrinogen

Studies by Drury and McMaster in 1929 were the first to suggest that plasma fibrinogen was produced by the liver.[244] Ample evidence exists implicating hepatic parenchymal cells as the site of plasma fibrinogen biosynthesis,[244–246] although not all hepatocytes synthesize fibrinogen at any given time. The plasma half-life of fibrinogen in normal persons is 3 to 5 days.[247] The average half-life is 4 days. The steady-state synthetic rate is 1.7 to 5 g/d (30 mg/kg/d), and the fractional catabolic rate is 24% of the plasma protein per day.[248]

Studies on the biosynthesis of fibrinogen have shown that the three polypeptide chains, Aα, Bβ, and γ, are synthesized on separate polysomes by separate mRNAs,[71,72,218,230,243] and that subsequent assembly occurs in the rough endoplasmic reticulum (ER).[250,251] Synthesis, assembly, and secretion are complex, and there are species differences. For synthesis of human and rabbit fibrinogens, the signal event is synthesis of the Bβ chain. But for rat and chicken hepatocytes, the signal event is synthesis of the Aα chain.[252,253]

Once fibrinogen synthesis commences, assembly of the molecule involves a series of disulfide bond interactions between chains leading to the formation of a symmetric molecule. For secretion of fibrinogen, oligomeric assembly is usually necessary. However, assembly of fibrinogen is not obligatory for secretion. The conditioned media of hepatocytes or transfected COS cells also contained free α, free γ, A$\alpha\gamma_2$, and AαB$\beta\gamma_2$.[252]

Defibrination with Malayan pit viper (*Agkistrodon rhodostoma*) venom causes a rapid and substantial accumulation in rat liver of the three mRNAs for the Aα-, Bβ-, and γ-subunits of fibrinogen. The kinetics and extent of increase are nearly identical for each mRNA, resulting in an increase in fibrinogen synthesis.[255] Similar results can be obtained by treating an animal with turpentine, which creates a sterile abscess and chronic inflammation.[64] Corticosteroids also increase hepatocyte fibrinogen synthesis. This coordinate regulation of the three mRNAs suggests that fibrinogen assembly occurs cotranslationally, and no pool of individual subunits exists in the cell.[251]

Several observations, however, indicate that the three nascent subunits are not simultaneously assembled in a simple manner.[54,256,257] There is evidence that unequal synthesis of the fibrinogen chains occurs in the human hepatocarcinoma cell line, Hep G2.[257,259] Pulse-chase studies showed that the three chains are not immediately disulfide linked, and that there are partially assembled precursors as well as pools of unassembled Aα and γ chains.[257] Studies with Hep G2 cells also suggest that fibrinogen assembly commences with the independent attachment of preformed Aα or γ chains, drawn from an intracellular pool, to nascent Bβ chains that are still attached to membrane-bound polysomes. The two-chain Bβ–Aα and Bβ–γ complexes are released into the lumen of the rough ER. Each of these precursors gains an additional fibrinogen chain (again drawn from the intracellular pool) to form the fibrinogen half-molecule. The two half-molecules are then assembled into a dimeric fibrinogen molecule.[251] The final step probably involves the formation of two reciprocal disulfide bridges between γ8 and γ9, and a single disulfide bridge at Aα 28–Aα 28.[54] More is required to keep the two half-molecules together than just the disulfide bonds. The disulfide rings at the beginning and end of the coiled-coil region are also necessary. Their disruption causes nonsecretion of this fibrinogen.[55,56]

In contrast to human and rabbit fibrinogen where the synthesis of Bβ chain is the rate-limiting step,[256,257] the synthesis of Aα chain is the rate-limiting step in the production and secretion of fibrinogen by cultured rat hepatocytes.[259] There is nonstoichiometric synthesis of fibrinogen subunit chains by monolayer cultures of chick embryo hepatocytes cultured in the absence of added hormones.[260] Aα-chain synthesis is disproportionately low in these cells, and there is accumulation of relatively high intracellular levels of the Bβ and γ chains. Exposing the cells to serum differentially enhances fibrinogen chain synthesis, with the greatest increase in Aα-chain synthesis, making those levels equal to the previously excessive Bβ and γ chains. None of the individual subunits of fibrinogen is rate-limiting for canine hepatocyte fibrinogen formation.[250] It is not clear whether these discrepancies are due to species specificity or to different systems of analysis (ie, in vivo or culture).

Fibrinogen precursors do not appear to contain free sulfhydryl groups. This suggests that their sulfhydryl groups, which need further interaction to form a fibrinogen molecule, are blocked initially and are subsequently reduced during chain assembly.[259] Little is known about the enzymatic mechanism of the protein disulfide isomerase reaction, by which the fibrinogen chains may be assembled. This enzyme is present on the inner surface of the ER membrane in a large number of tissues and is particularly abundant in secretory tissues; it plays a critical role in the early stages of posttranslational protein processing.[261] The enzyme catalyzes the rearrangement of disulfide bonds, when in contact with an oxidized protein substrate, and it also catalyzes the formation of native disulfide bonds in reduced proteins.[261] Such an enzyme system can assemble fibrinogen precursors either in reduced or oxidized forms before further interactions with other fibrinogen chains.

About 3% of total blood fibrinogen exists in platelets. The biosynthetic origin of platelet fibrinogen has been controversial. Fibrinogen synthesis by megakaryocytes has been demonstrated,[232,233] and differences between platelet and plasma fibrinogen have been reported.[266,267,269,271] The structural differences[268] are in the extended γ chain, which is present in plasma fibrinogen but absent in platelet fibrinogen. Fibrinogen with γ' chains also does not bind to platelet fibrinogen receptors. γ' mRNA species are found in isolated rat megakaryocytes, however.[235] This suggests that the γ' mRNA is either not translated or the γ' chain is not incorporated to form a mature fibrinogen.

Congenital fibrinogen variants in the platelets of dysfibrinogenemic patients with fibrinogen Oslo I and Oslo III[269] suggest that plasma and platelet fibrinogen are products of the same gene. But the expression of fibrinogen in the megakaryocytes is not well understood, and there are conflicting observations as to whether megakaryocyte fibrinogen has a double origin, being partly synthesized and partly endocytosed.[272] In purified human megakaryocytes, fibrinogen was detected in the α granules of megakaryocytes grown only in normal plasma, not in the plasma of afibrinogenemic patients.[269] This suggested that while megakaryocytes synthesize fibrinogen, they can also endocytose it. The evidence that megakaryocytes can incorporate circulating proteins into α granules[273] makes the origin of fibrinogen in megakaryocytes complex, involving both synthesis and endocytosis.

Stimulation of Fibrinogen Synthesis in Hepatocytes

Induction of the acute-phase response genes in hepatocytes is mediated by cytokines. Synthesis may be stimulated 5 to 10 times and is regulated at the transcriptional level.[274] Interleukin-6 (IL-6), which may be identical to hepatocyte-stimulating factor (HSF), is the primary cytokine.[275] Interleukin-1 (IL-1) may also have a role in inducing fibrinogen biosynthesis. Interleukin-6 (HSF) apparently regulates hepatic plasma protein synthesis by changes in transcriptionally related events, since it increased and decreased, respectively, the mRNA of the positive and negative acute-phase reactants, fibrinogen and albumin.[274] Monocyte HSF may be regulated in part by the plasmin-derived fibrin(ogen) degradation products, D and E.[275] Fragments D and E both can stimulate hepatic fibrinogen synthesis via an indirect monocyte-mediated pathway, indicating fibrin(ogen) can function in an indirect feedback pathway that regulates the synthesis and secretion of HSF. However, other evidence indicates that these fibrinogen fragments have no effect on the synthesis of fibrinogen.[277]

Certain hormones (eg, glucocorticoids, thyroid hormones, and insulin) also stimulate fibrinogen synthesis in hepatocyte cultures,[276] and glucocorticoids may elevate fibrinogen mRNA levels in the liver.[255]

Maximal stimulation of fibrinogen biosynthesis requires both glucocorticoid and HSF in primary rat hepatocytes and in a rat hepatoma cell line.[274] HSF controls fibrinogen production by regulating the transcription of fibrinogen mRNAs; dexamethasone is not an essential component of this reaction but synergistically enhances the HSF effect. Thus, HSF may be exclusively a transcriptional regulator, and dexamethasone acts primarily by enhancing the HSF signal.[274]

In certain cultured, transformed rat hepatocytes, a third uncharacterized agent is responsible for the induction of fibrinogen during acute-phase response, which transduces its signal to the fibrinogen genes by a mechanism involving protein kinase C.[278]

Posttranslational Modifications

Fibrinogen undergoes several posttranslational modifications including glycosylation,[279] phosphorylation,[40] and sulfation.[280] The human γ chain is glycosylated at Asn 52 as an early cotranslational event. The β-chain carbohydrate is added to Asn 364 later in the elongation process, either at the time of polypeptide termination or soon after release from the ribosome into the cisternal space.[279,286]

Posttranslational modifications of canine fibrinogen during transit through the rough ER are well characterized.[250] The fibrinogen within the rough ER is already fully disulfide bonded and exists as a dimer. The nascent fibrinogen in the ER is not phosphorylated or sulfated. These modifications occur during a subsequent translocational event, but before secretion from the cell.

The site of sulfation has been identified in fibrinogen from many animal species, with sulfation on tyrosine residues in fibrinopeptide B in those species that contain tyrosine in fibrinopeptide B.[280,281] Fibrinogens that do not contain tyrosine in fibrinopeptide B (ie, rat and human) are sulfated as well,[280] suggesting that there are other sulfated residues.

Sulfation occurs on the tyrosine residue at the second position from its COOH terminal of the γ_B chain in primary cultures of rat hepatocytes.[282] Sulfotransferase activity is localized in the Golgi fraction, indicating that sulfation of fibrinogen takes place in the Golgi complex—especially in the trans-Golgi region—just before secretion.

FACTOR XIII

Factor XIII is essential for normal coagulation and fibrinolysis. Patients who are congenitally deficient or who have acquired inhibitors may have a severe hemorrhagic diathesis. Factor XIII also may have a more general role in the various processes involving cell proliferation, including wound healing and tissue repair, tumor growth and metastasis, and atherosclerosis. The existence of a factor that modified fibrin after it was formed was postulated in the 1940s,[283,284] and further work established this as factor XIII. The first case of congenital factor XIII deficiency was not reported until 1960.[285] Since its discovery, it has become clear that factor XIII has many unique biochemical and hematologic properties.

Factor XIII is the zymogen form of a blood coagulation factor present in plasma and cells. Factor XIIIa (plasma transglutaminase, fibrinoligase, fibrin-stabilizing factor) belongs to a group of Ca^{2+}-dependent enzymes called endo-γ-glutamine:ϵ-lysine transferases. The enzymes are more commonly referred to as transglutaminases,[286] although this name is not entirely correct. The Enzyme Commission (EC) nomenclature recommends RR:glutaminyl-peptide γ-glutamyl transferase (EC 2.3.2.13). In this chapter, factor XIII is used to designate proenzyme forms from both plasma and cells. Factor XIIIa similarly designates the active enzyme. The zymogen exists in two molecular forms, one of which is found intracellularly in platelets, megakaryocytes, monocytes, placenta, resident macrophages in uterus and prostate tissue and is a dimer of two identical A chains (A_2). The extracellular zymogen is found only in plasma; it has two A-subunits and two B-subunits (A_2B_2). The subunits in A_2 and A_2B_2 are complexed by noncovalent bonds only. Activation of factor XIII to XIIIa is a multistep process that results in exposure of an active center cysteine. Cysteine enzymes are principally intracellular, and plasma factor XIIIa is the only sulfhydryl enzyme known to function extracellularly. The function of factor XIIIa is catalysis of isopeptide bond formation between the γ-carbamoyl group of peptide-bound glutamine and the ϵ-amino group of lysine. This reaction occurs via intermediary acylation and deacylation steps in which glutamine functions as the electron acceptor and lysine as the electron donor. With this mechanism, two polypeptides can be covalently joined together.

Structure of the A and B Chains

The cDNA for the A chain has been cloned from placental libraries.[287,288] The amino acid sequence for A chain has also been determined.[289] A chain consists of 730 to 731 amino acids with an estimated molecular weight of about 82 kd. The cDNA consists of 2280 bp in an opening-reading frame, with 45 bp at the 5′ end open reading frame, with a 45-bp segment at the 5′ end, which is nontranslated. There is also a 1.6-kb segment as a 3′ nontranslated region. There is no amino-terminal hydrophobic leader sequence.[287,288] The gene for A subunit has been characterized also. It has about 71 kb and consists of 15 introns separated by 14 exons. The 5′ flanking region contains several TATA-like sequences and GC clusters as possible regulatory elements for transcription. The gene for A chain has been localized to chromosome 6p24-p25, linked to the major histocompatibility complex.[293]

From this work and biochemical characterization of the A protein, several important features are known about the structure of A protein. It is conclusively established that the extracellular and the intracellular A proteins are identical, and that all of the potential catalytic activity is in the A chain. There are nine cysteine residues, of which one (Cys 314) is in the active center (exon VII). There are six potential asparagine N-linked glycosylation sites, but there is no carbohydrate in A protein. Introns may separate the molecule into functional domains. The thrombin cleavage site, necessary for activation, is at Arg 37–Gly 38 (exon II). A second thrombin cleavage site, which inactivates the molecule, is at Lys 513–Ser or Arg 515–Ser[289] (exon XIII). There are several points of polymorphism: Leu 88–Phe, Ile 650–Val, Gln 651–Glu, Gly 77–Arg, and Lys 78–Arg. The cDNA sequence predicts Met 731 as the carboxy-terminal amino acid, but there is heterogeneity or degradation at the COOH-terminal end. Peptides ending in Gln 726, Pro 729, and Ser 730 have been found. A Ca^{2+}-binding site is in the A chain and may be at residues 468 to 479 on the basis of homology with calmodulin (exons VI and X). Otherwise, functional domains of the A protein have not been placed.

With electron microscopy, A appears as an asymmetric globular particle of 6×9 nm.[294] There are strong noncovalent interactions between the A proteins. The dimers are associated along their long axis, so the shape of A_2 is asymmetric.[294] The hydrodynamic properties of A_2 are in agreement with this shape.[5] The factor XIII A protein belongs to a superfamily of transglutaminases with an overall homology of about 30%.[295] The extended active site of factor XIII A contains about 10 amino acids around the active center, Cys 314, and His 373 is also essential for activity.[295] These two areas of the transglutaminases are highly homologous; this homology extends to red cell band 4.2, which is inactive because Cys 314 is converted to alanine and His 373 to glutamine.[295,296]

Furthermore, the transglutaminases are homologous at the active center with the cysteine proteases. This is a curious functional and structural relationship, since the proteases catalyze the hydrolysis of peptide bonds while the transglutaminases catalyze the formation of isopeptide bonds. Both involve formation of a covalent acyl intermediate, which results from the nucleophilic attack of an activated sulfhydryl group on the carbonyl of either a peptide bond or an amide group. It is not clear what factors activate the sulfhydryl group of cysteine, normally incapable of such a reaction, to become a strong nucleophile. These factors are probably to be found in the structure and interactions of the residues around this active cysteine. The sequence of A is unique. The active center (Tyr-Gly-Gln-Cys-Glu) is homologous to the active centers of other cysteine enzymes (cathepsins B and H, papain, calpain), but otherwise, the A chain does not show homology to any other protein. The secondary structure of A protein is predicted to be 36% β-pleated sheet, 35% β-turn, and 26% α-helix.[289] There is a nearly complete crystal structure of factor XIII A subunit.[299]

A partial cDNA for B protein was identified from a λGT11 expression library prepared from human liver mRNA. This cDNA has 2180 bp and encodes a partial leader sequence of 19 amino acids, the coding region for 641 amino acids for the mature B protein, and a 3′ noncoding sequence of 187 bp plus a poly$(A)^+$ tail.[298] There are no free sulfhydryl groups in the B chain. The protein has 10 repetitive, homologous segments, each with about 60 amino acids and 4 disulfide bonds. These repeated segments comprise amino acids 1 to 626 of the B protein. Based on homology to β_2-glycoprotein I, these domains are called B_2-glycoprotein I (GP-I) domains because they were first recognized in that protein[300,301]; they are also called sushi domains. A single exon codes for one GP-I structure in the B chain.[275] Thus, the B protein of factor XIII is a member of a superfamily of proteins that are composed of GP-I domains. Other members of this family include several complement-regulating proteins: complement factor Ba, complement receptors type I and II, C1r, C1s, C4b-binding protein, and decay accelerating factor and other noncomplement proteins, including haptoglobin α_1 chain and interleukin-2 receptor.[301,302]

There are three potential asparagine-linked carbohydrate sites.[298] There are about 5 mol of sialic acid per 1 mol of B.[303] The heterogeneity in B, observed with isoelectric focusing, is due in part to sialic acid.[303] With the carbohydrate, the molecular weight is estimated to be 76.5 kd. The amino-terminal amino acid is Glu, and the carboxy-terminal amino acid is Thr. There is an RGD sequence at Arg 596.[298]

Hydrodynamic properties indicate that B protein is highly elongated.[294] The image of B seen by electron microscopy is compatible with these data. B is a thin, flexible strand with random kinks, having a length of 30 nm and a diameter of about 2.5 nm. The repeat domain would have a mass of about 6.5 kd, which would be able to fold into a globular domain with a diameter of about 2.5 nm. Aligned linearly throughout the molecule, these small domains would impart flexibility.[298] One chain of C4b-binding protein has a similar shape, observed by electron microscopy,[304] and it is likely that all proteins composed of repeating GP-I domains have a similar shape.

B protein can be isolated as a monomer from $A_2'B_2$.[294] There are strong interactions between A protein and B protein in the zymogen complex. From a CNBr digest of B, a large fragment was isolated (about 48 kd) that contains disulfide bonds as well as about 50% of the B chain carbohydrate, and retains the ability to complex with A. Reduced and alkylated B also binds to A_2, but denatured B does not.[305] Recombinant A_2 associates with B to give a normal zymogen structure, rA_2B_2. If there is an excess of B, rA_2B_2 forms.[306]

The extracellular zymogen, A_2B_2, is formed through strong noncovalent bonds. There is a high affinity between A proteins and between A and B proteins, but there is no evidence for strong affinity between B proteins or between A_2' and B. These interactions are used to build the heterodimer. Precisely how the B protein is wrapped around A is not known. Because of the asymmetry of A_2B_2, B probably juts from the A proteins somewhat. The B protein must be more surface oriented than A, since B decreases the activation of A_2 and increases the Ca^{2+} concentration needed for activation. B also protects A from chemical modification. From these data, including electron microscopy images and hydrodynamic data, a model was constructed for A_2B_2[294] (Fig. 41-9). This model is consistent with all the data, but other models of how B wraps around A could be drawn.[294]

Biosynthesis of Homodimers (A_2) and Heterodimers (A_2B_2)

Much of the work on the biosynthesis of these proteins uses antibody identification, and there is some confusion in the literature because some of the antibodies are not monospecific. Some antibodies to A react against other plasma proteins. Nevertheless, many experiments lead to a consensus for the biosynthesis of intracellular and extracellular factor XIII.

Intracellular factor XIII is a homodimer of A proteins. It is synthesized as a zymogen, which can be easily activated intracellularly.[308,309] A_2 is widely distributed; it is present

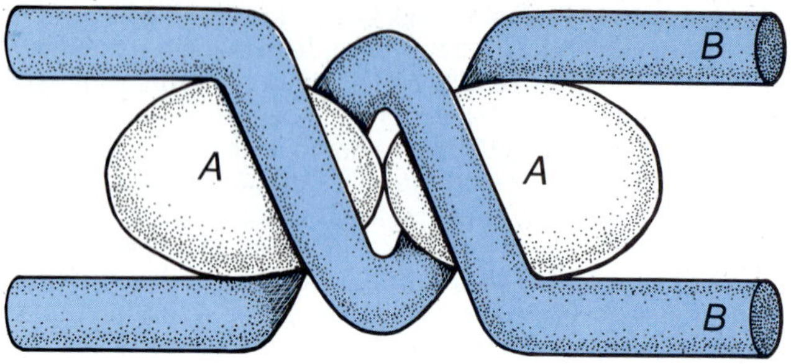

FIGURE 41-9. Model of the A and B polypeptides of factor XIII. (After Carrell NA, Crickson HP, McDonagh J. Electron microscopy and hydrodynamic properties of factor XII subunits. J Biol Chem 1989;264:551)

in certain bone marrow cells, monocytes, and megakaryocytes, but not in granulocytes or lymphocytes. Erythrocytes have a cellular transglutaminase activity unrelated to factor XIII (Fig. 41-10). Platelet factor XIII is probably synthesized in megakaryocytes. Megakaryocytes in the process of budding are positive for A_2, as observed under immunofluorescence.[311] Pericytes[312] and chondrocytes[313] are also positive for factor XIIIA. Additionally, factor XIII–deficient patients do not take up infused A_2B_2 from plasma into their platelets.[314] Placenta is a rich source of A, and a concentrate of factor XIII A (Fibrogammin) is made from placenta. mRNA from placenta is about 4000 bp[287,288] and, by Northern blot analysis of poly(A)$^+$ mRNA from placental cells, hybridization occurs.[291] mRNA for XIII A is also present in monocytes.

Much of the work on the biosynthesis of intracellular factor XIII has focused on monocytes (macrophages) and U937 cells (a monocyte-like transformed cell line). By use of various immunohistochemical techniques, A protein was found in peripheral blood monocytes, alveolar macrophages, peritoneal macrophages, tumor-associated macrophages, hystiocytes, and macrophages isolated from placenta and the uterus.[308,315,316] However, XIII A mRNA is not present in all resident macrophages. It is not in Kupffer cells of the liver or microglial cells of the brain.[292] ^{35}S-labeled A protein can be immunoprecipitated from cell lysates of U937 cells[309]; mRNA also has been identified in these cells and in unstimulated peripheral blood monocytes.[291] Monocytes from several plasma factor XIII–deficient patients were all deficient in A_2.[317] A_2 appears early in monocyte and megakaryocyte development and persists during differentiation.[318]

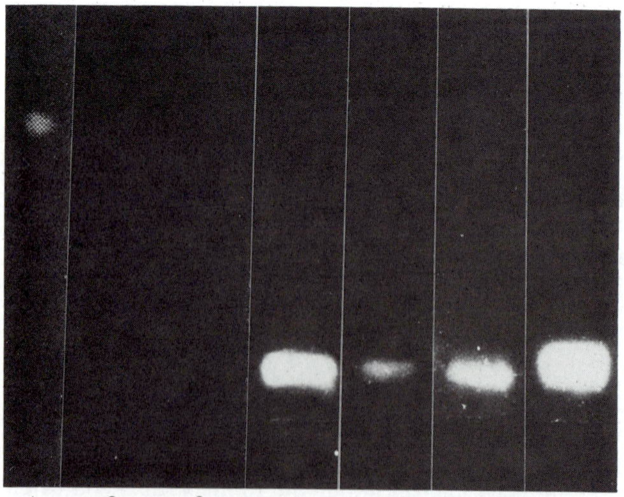

FIGURE 41-10. Blood cell distribution of factor XIII, demonstrated by electrophoresis and activity staining: (1) erthrocytes, (2) granulocytes, (3) lymphocytes, (4) monocytes, (5) platelets, (6) macrophages, and (7) plasma factor XIII (control). The cellular transglutaminase in erythrocytes is different from factor XIII. (Adapted from Henriksson P, Becker S, McDonagh J. Identification of intracellular factor XIII in human monocytes and macrophages. J Clin Invest 1985;76:528

It is clear that A_2 (but not B protein) is synthesized in monocytes and megakaryocytes and is present in peripheral blood monocytes, macrophages, and platelets, but there is little evidence that A_2 is secreted. Over 90% of A_2 is localized in the cytoplasm of resting platelets, and the rest is membrane associated.[319] Stimulation of platelets does not result in release of A_2.[320] Thrombin stimulation of platelets, however, results in translocation of endogenous A_2 to the surface of platelets.[321] Heat shock protein 27 (HSP 27) is colocalized with A_2 in platelets, is a substrate for cross-linking by factor XIII, and may serve as a molecular "chaperone" in the process of translocation of A_2 from the cytoplasm to the membrane. This is a reasonable hypothesis, but the precise mechanism for translocation is not known. In a similar manner, stimulating monocytes by lipopolysaccharide, phorbol myrisacetate, and interferon-γ also stimulated cell-surface expression of A_2.[309] The F(ab) fragment of anti-A_2 antibody aggregates platelets. It was postulated that A protein on the surface of platelets may serve as a collagen receptor,[324] but there is newer evidence that another platelet protein, the GP IIa/IIb complex, may serve as a collagen receptor. Clotting systems in which intracellular A_2 is the only source of factor XIII activity result in cross-linking of fibrin.[309] These experiments lead to several conclusions. There is little or no exchange between the intracellular and extracellular pools of A protein, although some A_2B_2 can be endocytosed with fibrinogen into the platelet and granule.[310] A protein, on the surface of cells, is effective in catalyzing cross-linking reactions. The concentration of available factor XIII activity may be higher at a local site of bleeding or wound healing because of the recruitment of platelets and macrophages to that area.

Extracellular factor XIII is a heterodimer (A_2B_2), and its biosynthesis is more complex and less well understood. B protein synthesis is confined to the liver; transformed liver cell lines (Hep G2 and PLC/PRF/5) synthesize and secrete ^{35}S-labeled B protein in vitro.[325] An estimate of secretion was 5 to 10 ng/mL in serum-free conditioned medium.[325] mRNA for XIII B has been found only in liver cells.[292]

Although B is bound to A tightly but reversibly in plasma, it is possible to dissociate the zymogen complex during purification[326] or activation.[327] In carefully prepared anticoagulated plasma, only half the total amount of B is in the complex, whereas the other half circulates as free B.[307] This amount of free B is relatively constant in normal persons, factor XIII–deficient patients, and their heterozygous relatives.[307] Regulation of the biosynthesis of B protein is not known. Infusion of deficient patients with placental factor XIII concentrate (A_2), however, results in rapid in vivo complex formation between the infused A_2 and the patients' plasma B protein (Ikematsu S, McDonagh J, unpublished data; Fig. 41-11*A* and *B*). There is an immediate rise in factor XIII activity due to A protein, which then slowly decreases. In addition, a delayed, apparent increase in the plasma concentration of B occurs, reaching a maximum about 5 days after transfusion[329,330] (see Fig. 41-11*C*). These occurrences are curious and indicate that the infusion of A_2 may result in increased biosynthesis or secretion of B, or in decreased degradation of B when it is complexed with A.

The biosynthesis of extracellular A protein is less well understood. After a few informative bone marrow trans-

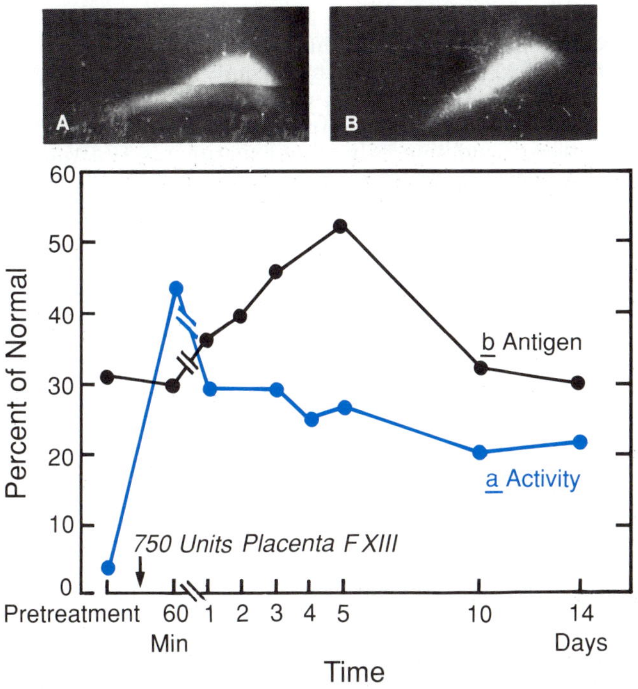

FIGURE 41-11. Effects of transfusion of A subunit in factor XIII–deficient patients. **(A** and **B)** Combination of A and B subunits in vivo, shown by superimposition of activity stainings and immunoprecipitate of B on crossed immunoelectrophoresis: normal plasma **(A)**; factor XIII–deficient plasma after infusion with A_2 concentrate **(B)**. **(C)** Rise in B subunit after infusion of A subunit. (**A** and **B** based on data from P. Henriksson, J. McDonagh J; **C** based on data from S. Ikematsu, J. McDonagh)

plantations, the polymorphism of A in A_2B_2 was the same as the donor's; after liver transplantation, the polymorphism of B in the recipient was the same as the donor's.[331] Monocytes or platelets cannot be the only source of plasma factor XIII A protein, but they could be a source. The hepatocyte is the most logical site for synthesis and secretion of A_2B_2. With Western blot analysis, there is evidence that A protein is synthesized in two hepatocyte cell lines, but the quantities are small.[325,332] mRNA experiments are somewhat conflicting. Three different cDNA probes have been used to probe for mRNA in liver cells and transformed liver cell lines. These studies identified mRNA for A in normal liver and two hepatocyte cell lines but the level of mRNA was found to be 10 to 20 times lower than that in placenta.[287] A fourth study did not detect this mRNA in liver with another probe type, however.[288] In tissue culture experiments, A protein was detected in small quantities in serum free conditioned medium of transformed hepatocyte cells.[332] Furthermore, when serum free conditioned medium from Hep G2 cells was used as the only source of factor XIII in a clotting experiment, γ dimers were formed, indicating that A protein was secreted from these cells in a potentially active form.[332]

Considerable evidence suggests that liver cells synthesize and secrete both proteins for extracellular factor XIII. Little is known about the formation of this heterodimer or about its regulation and degradation. Two ELISAs that are specific for the A_2B_2 complex have been developed.[307] Such tools are necessary to probe the formation of this heterodimer. Preliminary evidence indicates that these assays detect A_2B_2 in the cell lysate of transformed liver cell lines. As indicated, the gene for A protein does not have a hydrophobic leader sequence, which is usually necessary for secretion of proteins[287,288]; the gene for B protein has such a sequence.[298] Whether intracellular complex formation is the mechanism for the secretion of A protein is not known.

Activation of Intracellular and Extracellular Factor XIII

Both the intracellular and extracellular forms of factor XIII can be isolated as zymogens, and they require activation in a controlled, step-wise process. Most other forms of transglutaminases can be isolated as enzymes. The basic mechanism for full activation of A_2 requires (1) enzyme cleavage of an activation peptide from the NH_2 terminal of the A chain at Arg 37–Gly 38 to form A_2',[287,288] and (2) a conformational change induced by Ca^{2+}, which exposes the active center cysteine to form A_2^*.[327] This reaction can be diagramed simply:

$$A_2 \xrightarrow{\text{enzyme}} A_2' + \text{activation peptide} \tag{1}$$

$$A_2' \xrightarrow{Ca^{2+}} A_2^* \tag{2}$$

High concentrations of Ca^{2+} alone (without cleavage of the activation peptide) can generate some activity.[327] Purified intracellular factor XIII can readily be activated by thrombin and low concentrations of Ca^{2+}.[338] On the other hand, Ca^{2+} is not absolutely required for exposure of the active center from A_2', but with Ca^{2+} this reaction is faster.[338] No promoters are required for these reactions. Purified A_2 is sensitive to proteolysis by thrombin or trypsin, and Ca^{2+} protects A_2 somewhat.[339] A_2 within the cell can also be easily activated, but much less is known about this mechanism. Carboxy peptidase, cathepsin C,[340] and calpain I[341] have been implicated in the activation of A_2 inside platelets, and Cathepsin C also activates A_2 in vitro.[340] Aggregation of platelets by all agonists, except thrombin, does not seem to cause activation of A_2.[340] Activation by thrombin results in endogenous A_2^* on the platelet membrane.[321] Activation of monocytes may also result in A_2^* on the monocyte surface.[309] Studies to define the mechanism of intracellular A_2 activation in vivo are lacking. It seems unlikely that the small amount of prothrombin or factor Xa that is in platelets would have a role in activating A_2. Other possibilities include the lysosomal proteases released by the cell, mobilization of Ca^{2+} alone, and thrombin bound to the cell surfaces.[342] There are experiments showing enzyme-independent activation of factor XIII, which is regulated by Ca^{2+},[343] while calmodulin inhibits the activation of A_2 by sequestering Ca^{2+} in platelets.[342]

The activation of A_2B_2 is more complex, although the basic steps of enzyme activation and Ca^{2+}-dependent conformational changes are similar. For A_2B_2 activation, it is a requirement that 2 mol of Ca^{2+} be bound to the $A_2'B_2$ complex.[338] A few problems must be overcome for activation of A_2B_2 in plasma. First, the activation of coagulation and fibrinolytic zymogens does not occur readily in solution. Surface activation controls enzyme activation and serves to localize a higher concentration in the microenvironment of a clot or wound. Second, activation of A_2B_2 in vitro requires high, nonphysiologic concentrations of thrombin and Ca^{2+} to the physiologic range (1.5 mmol/L).[343] The binding of A_2B_2 to non–cross-linked fibrin I promotes A_2B_2 activation and obviates these problems. This promoter activity of fibrin makes activation of A_2B_2 more efficient by lowering the thrombin and Ca^{2+} concentrations needed for activation.[344–346] Binding to non–cross-linked fibrin also localizes A_2B_2 in the environment of clot formation. This promoter activity of fibrin is somewhat similar to its role in the activation of plasminogen by tPA. The observation that non–cross-linked, polymerized fibrin promotes release of the activation peptide from A_2B_2 is accounted for by complex formation with a concurrent reduction in $K_{m(app)}$.[345] About 80% to 90% of A_2B_2 binds to non–cross-linked polymers of fibrin.[346] The order of peptide release from fibrinogen and factor XIII by thrombin is fibrinopeptide A→activation peptide→fibrinopeptide B.[345] In vivo, there is probably a ternary complex formed, fibrin I—A_2B_2—thrombin.[344] This indicates that non–cross-linked fibrin I would be the physiologic promoter, although fibrin I, fibrin II, and fibrinogen polymerized by protamine sulfate are all good promoters in vitro. Cross-linked fibrin is not a good promoter, nor is fibrin monomer.[345,346] Thus, there is efficient control of activation of A_2B_2, which is limited to the time and location when substrate (polymerized non–cross-linked fibrin) is forming. The reaction for activation of A_2B_2 has three steps: proteolysis, dissociation of complex, and a Ca^{2+}-induced conformational change. It is diagrammed in these reactions:

$$A_2B_2 \xrightarrow{\text{thrombin}} \underset{\text{Fibrin I}}{\underset{|}{A_2'B_2}} + \text{activation peptide} \qquad (1)$$

$$\underset{\text{Fibrin I}}{\underset{|}{A_2'B_2}} \xrightarrow{Ca^{2+}} A_2' + 2B \qquad (2)$$

$$\underset{\text{Fibrin I}}{\underset{|}{A_2'}} \xrightarrow{Ca^{2+}} A_2^* \qquad (3)$$

Binding studies have been done to identify where the A protein binds to fibrin(ogen). In one report, this was considered to be in the middle region of the Aα chain of fibrinogen (residues 242 to 424).[348] In a separate report, it was found that A_2 binds to fibrin(ogen)-degradation fragments X, D_1 to D_3, and D-D, but not to E. A_2 also binds to the Aα and Bβ chains of fibrinogen and to the α and β chains of fibrin.[329a] In studies with recombinant A_2 and fibrin, fibrin binding was blocked by two peptides from the Aα chain (residues 389 to 402 and 241 to 476).[350] There are separate, noninteractive sites on fibrin for binding A_2B_2, A_2, and A_2'. A_2' binds more tightly than the others.[329c] Further studies will be useful to pinpoint the binding domains for A protein on fibrin and for fibrin, the A protein.

The A_2^* derived from intracellular and extracellular factor XIII molecules has the same enzymatic activity, although extracellular A_2B_2 is more difficult to activate than intracellular A_2. This implies that the B protein has a protective function, which might be necessary to avoid spontaneous activation in the plasma environment. When A_2 is reconstituted with purified B protein, it has the same activation kinetics as native A_2B_2.[344] The Ca^{2+} concentration for activation of A_2B_2 in purified systems is 10 times greater than that for A_2.[352]

Furthermore, A_2 activation is not enhanced by fibrin,[344] and A_2 can be more readily inactivated by thrombin to 51- and 24-kd fragments than can A_2B_2.[339] This inactivation reaction, cleaving at Lys 512,[288,289] points out the protective function of B protein. γ thrombin, which does not bind to fibrin, is not affected by fibrin as a promoter of A_2B_2 activation.[344] All of these experimental observations lead to the conclusion that A_2B_2 is more difficult to activate than is A_2 and that B chain protects A chain from activation in the extracellular zymogen complex. The problem of activation of A_2B_2 is overcome by binding $A_2'B_2$, the activation intermediate, and the active enzyme to nonpolymerized fibrin I.

Other functions of B protein (either dissociated from A_2 or free in plasma) should also be considered, particularly in regard to coagulation reactions. B protein inhibits contact activation of plasma by an ellagic acid-phospholipid suspension or by dextran sulfate, and B protein binds to the ellagic acid-phospholipid suspension.[353] In contrast, A_2B_2 has no inhibiting effect on contact activation of plasma. This may be important as a feedback inhibition mechanism in blood coagulation.[353] In other experiments, HMW kininogen (HMWK), important for contact activation of plasma, was found to be an effective inhibitor of A_2^*, but not of A_2B_2.[354] HMWK is thus far the only protein known to inhibit factor XIII activity. Since only A_2 is inhibited, B protein must interfere with A_2-HMWK complex formation. The B protein thus has a protective function against both activation and inhibition in plasma. These protective functions of B protein would be compatible with the structure of A_2B_2 derived from electron microscopy, where B is more surface oriented than A, and B is wound around A[294] (see Fig. 41-9).

The enzymatic action of A_2^* requires formation of a trimolecular complex between the enzyme and two protein substrates. The active center cysteine of the Ca^{2+}–A_2^* complex reacts first with a γ carbonyl of peptide-bound glutamine and results in formation of a γ-glutamyl-S-ester intermediate complex and aminolysis. This is a nucleophilic attack. It is thought that the enzyme–substrate complex is conformationally altered so that a functional site for interaction of a lysine ε-amino group with the active center is then formed.[355] This amino group reacts with the acylenzyme thioester bond, and formation of an ε-(γ-glutamyl)–lysyl bond occurs.

Substrates for Cross-Linking by A_2^*

A_2^* has a high degree of substrate specificity, so that only a few specific glutamine and lysine residues participate in the cross-linking reaction. Although the determinants of this specificity are not entirely clear, secondary interactions between the extended active site and the glutamine substrate are thought to be critical. The extended active site contains about 10 amino acids around the active center Cys 314.[355] Hydrophobic interactions between the active site and the amino acids around the reactive glutamine are important.[355] Examination of the linear sequences around known glutamine cross-linking sites shows little evidence for homology and also indicates that the tertiary conformation around a reactive glutamine is important in determining specificity (Table 41-2). Glutamine 167 in β-casein has been found to be highly reactive with factor XIIIa. Synthetic peptides modeled after the linear sequence around Gln 167 have been used to study the determinants of specificity. In model peptides, residues equivalent to Leu 163, Lys 169, Val 170, and Leu 171 were found to be important for specificity of A_2^*. However, β-casein was a significantly better substrate than the model peptide.[356] A tridecapeptide modeled after the sequence around Gln 398 in the γ chain of fibrinogen was found to be a poor substrate for A_2^*.[355] These studies all indicate that important determinants of specificity are provided by the tertiary structure of the substrates, as well as the active center residues of factor XIIIa. In contrast to the lack of homology around the substrate proteins, there is a high degree of homology around the active center Lys 314 and His 373, which is critical for activity.

Little information is available concerning specificity of the lysine substrates, and specific reactive lysines have been identified in only a few proteins (see Table 41-2). Studies with small synthetic peptides have shown that introduction of a hydrophobic residue on the amino-terminal side of the reactive lysine significantly enhances the reactivity of the small substrate.[355] This indicates that hydrophobic interactions between the acyl-enzyme and the ly-

TABLE 41-2. Sequence Around the Reactive Glutamines and Lysines for Known Substrates of Factor XIIIa

GLUTAMINE SITES				
Fibrinogen α chain	W N S G S S G T G S T G N	Q 328	N P G S P R P G S T G W	
Fibrinogen α chain	H W T S E S S U S G S T G	Q 366	W H S E S G S F R P D S P	
Fibrinogen γ chain	I I P F N R L T I G E G Q	Q 398	H H L G G A K Q A G D V −COOH	
Fibronectin	NH_2− E A	Q 3	Q I V Q P Q S P L T V S Q	
α_2-Macroglobulin	S K I R K P K M C P Q L Q	Q 670	Y E M H G P E G L R G F	
α_2–Plasmin inhibitor	NH_2− N	Q 2	E E V S P	
Vitronectin	T S D Q A Q S K G N P E	Q 93	T P V L P E E E A P A	
β-Casein	T V M F P P Q S V L S L S	Q 167	S K U L P V P E K A V P Y	
LYSINE SITES IN FIBRINOGEN				
α Chain	F D E A A F F D T A S T G	K 508	T F P G F F	S P M L G E
α Chain	S H H P G I A E F P S R G	K 556	S S S Y S K	Q F T S S T
α Chain	A E F P S R G K S S S Y S	K 562	Q F T S S T	S Y N R G D
γ Chain	T I G E G Q Q H H L G G A	K 406	Q A G D V −COOH	
α Chain site for α_2-plasmin inhibitor	N P G S S G T G G T A T W	K 303	P G S S G P	G S T G S W

sine substrate are important determinants. It has also been proposed that the glutamine substrate contributes to the specificity for the lysine substrate.[355] The turnover number for A_2^* on fibrin substrates is estimated to be 20 to 100 s^{-1}.

Factor XIII has stringent requirements for substrate specificity, yet there are numerous substrates for which covalent cross-linking may have physiologic or pathophysiologic importance (Table 41-3). Proteins are usually determined to be substrates for A_2^* if they can covalently incorporate a lysine analogue (such as putrescine or dansylcadaverine) in a concentration- and time-dependent manner, or if formation of a cross-linked complex can be demonstrated, usually by SDS gel electrophoresis under reducing conditions. Covalent complex formation has been observed for all of the plasma protein substrates. Although a specific protein could be a substrate by virtue of either a reactive glutamine or lysine, the plasma proteins designated thus far all contribute reactive glutamines, or both lysines and glutamines. These proteins also have several other features in common. Most of them are large, sticky proteins, plasma constituents, or α-granule components secreted by activated platelets. Some are also monocyte constituents. They all participate in assembly of a macromolecular protein complex on a surface, whether that surface is on a platelet, another cell membrane, a fibrin polymer, or the subendothelium.

TABLE 41-3. Cross-Linked Complexes Formed by Factor XIIIa

Fibrin–fibrin
Fibrin–fibrin(ogen)
Fibrin–α_2-plasmin inhibitor
Fibrin–fibronectin
Fibrin–von Willebrand factor
Factor V–fibrin or factor V
Thrombospondin–thrombospondin
Fibrin–actin
Fibronectin–collagen
Von Willebrand factor–collagen
Fibronectin–myosin
Actin–myosin
Tropomyosin
Gelsolin–fibrin or gelsolin
Vinculin–fibrin(ogen)
Vitronectin
Laminin–pro von Willebrand factor
Osteopontin
Heat shock protein 27
Glycoprotein IIb/IIIa (fibrinogen receptor)
Plasminogen activator inhibitor 2
Lipoprotein (a)
Factor XIIIa–factor XIIIa

Assembly of these macromolecular complexes would be greatly facilitated by formation of covalent bonds among the proteins. An important consequence of the cross-linking reaction is that equilibrium is shifted in favor of complex formation and the local concentration of a cross-linked protein is high. There are certain features that are common. For example, prolines are often found within a few residues following the substrate glutamine residues, and serine and threonine residues are heavily represented flanking the substrate lysine residues. It may be that a variety of factors, including accessibility and electrostatic and hydrophobic aspects, are important in substrate specificity for factor XIIIa. The relatively high specificity is probably related to characteristics of both the enzyme active site and the substrates themselves.

Fibrin

Fibrin is the most well-characterized cross-linking substrate and has the most obvious physiologic significance. The earliest observations on factor XIII indicated that fibrin formed from plasma in the presence of EDTA was more soluble than that formed without EDTA; this led ultimately to the discovery of factor XIII in plasma and also gave rise to the name *fibrin stabilizing factor*.[283,284] The cross-linking of fibrin is an orderly process. Six potential cross-linked bonds can be formed in purified fibrin—two in the γ chains and four in the α chains,[357] giving rise to γ-chain dimers and HMW α-chain polymers. There are other lysine residues in the α chain that can participate in heteropolymer cross-linking; or it may be that not all four of the lysine residues are involved in α-polymer formation.

Cross-linking of fibrin γ chains is very rapid and occurs at low enzyme concentration. It occurs at the stage of protofibril formation in the fibrin assembly process and is difficult to inhibit, possibly because of preassociation of the two substrate proteins. Electron microscopy and gel electrophoresis show that γ-dimer cross-links form linearly along the length of the protofibril. This results in the monomer units in each strand of the protofibril being covalently joined together. The two strands of the protofibril are not cross-linked to each other, however.[136,358] γ-Chain cross-linking alone does not make the fibrin gel insoluble in dilute acid; this requires the cross-linking of α chains.[359] γ-Chain cross-linking is the step in which the fibrin monomers in a protofibril are joined by covalent bonds.

One reactive glutamine (Gln 398) and one reactive lysine (Lys 406) are at the COOH-terminal end of each γ chain. Gln 398 in one γ chain forms a cross-link with Lys 406 in a second γ chain (see Table 41-2); Lys 406 in the first γ chain and Gln 398 in the second γ chain form another cross-link.[144] Cross-linking of γ chains is intermolecular and therefore results in a product composed of one γ chain from each of two fibrin molecules held together by two cross-linked bonds oriented in an antiparallel arrangement.[360]

Formation of these γ-chain cross-links results in a new epitope, and monoclonal antibodies have been produced against this epitope. Plasmin hydrolysis of cross-linked fibrin differs from non–cross-linked fibrin in that fragment D contains these γ-chain cross-links, resulting in the appearance of D-dimer as a terminal digestion fragment[361] (see Fig. 41-8). This is the basis of the fibrin-specific test for fibrin degradation products, since it tests only for the presence of D-dimer.[362] D-dimer can occur only by fibrin formation, fibrin cross-linking, and fibrin degradation, indicating that there has been coagulation and secondary fibrinolysis.

α-Chain cross-linking is slower, requires a higher A_2^* concentration, and is more complicated than γ-dimer formation. The cross-linked polymer contains five or more α chains per polymeric unit. Spatial organization of the polymer is difficult to study and has not been determined. The reactive glutamine and lysine residues, however, are in the COOH-terminal half of the α chain, which is hydrophilic and exposed on the surface of the molecule. Glutamine residues that participate in α polymer formation are at positions 328 and 366.[363] The reactive lysines have been tentatively assigned to positions 508 and 556 or 562.[146] There is an additional glutamine (residue 237) that incorporates lysine analogues, but this is thought not to be involved in α-polymer formation.[363] α Polymers have been found that have fibrinopeptide A, implying that some α polymers began with fibrinogen–fibrin complexes.

α Polymer is difficult to solubilize, and it conveys this insolubility to cross-linked fibrin. In cross-linked fibrin, the average number of cross-links is four to six per fibrin monomer unit. Other known proteins that cross-link to fibrin do so by having a reactive glutamine that participates in cross-linking to a lysine in the α chain of fibrin (see Tables 41-2 and 41-3). The specific lysine in fibrin has been identified except to α_2-plasmin inhibitor.[364] It is not known if the formation of heteropolymer can displace an α–α cross-link or always use another lysine in this reaction.

Fibrinogen

Both γ dimer and α polymer form readily in fibrin. There is no apparent difference in the cross-linking of fibrin I or fibrin II. By comparison, however, fibrinogen is a relatively poor substrate, even though the cross-linking residues are located at the same sites in fibrinogen and fibrin. Fibrinogen can be cross-linked to form γ dimers and α polymers, but the rates are much slower. Cross-linking is zero order with respect to fibrin and first order for fibrinogen; that is, the rate is independent of the fibrin concentration but dependent on the fibrinogen concentration. With high factor XIIIa concentration, however, fibrinogen can be covalently cross-linked to form a gel.[366] Two differences may account for this. Fibrin monomer does not promote activation of A_2B_2 as well as polymerized non–cross-linked fibrin I, and there is a difference in the spatial presentation of these substrates. Fibrin is a better cross-linking substrate, probably because the γ and α chains are appropriately aligned for cross-linking in fibrin monomer protofibrils, whereas the spatial arrangement of fibrinogen has no order per se. This is also supported by the observations that soluble fibrinogen–fibrin oligomers can be easily cross-linked and that fibrinogen in high concentration inhibits fibrin cross-linking.[366]

α_2-Plasmin Inhibitor

α_2-Plasmin inhibitor (α_2-antiplasmin) is the primary fast-acting inhibitor of plasmin activity in plasma. α_2-Plasmin inhibitor can complex with plasmin both in solution and when the inhibitor is cross-linked to fibrin. Plasmin activity is somewhat protected from inhibition when it is bound to fibrin,[365] but it is more efficient when the inhibitor is cross-linked to fibrin and a trimolecular fibrin–α_2-plasmin inhibitor–plasmin complex is formed. Covalent cross-linking occurs through a reactive glutamine (residue 2) in α_2-plasmin inhibitor and through a reactive lysine in the α chain of fibrin, Lys 303.[364] This cross-linking reaction occurs physiologically and is extremely important in regulating the lysis rate of blood clots.

Fibronectin

Fibronectin is the second most abundant protein in the normal fibrin gel and constitutes approximately 4% of the total protein in the gel.[189] Under normal circumstances, the fibronectin in the gel is covalently cross-linked to the α chain of fibrin.[368] This cross-linking reaction occurs principally through a glutamine at the NH_2 terminal of fibronectin (residue 3) and through a lysine in the fibrin α chain.[191] There are also other cross-linking sites in fibronectin. One is in the COOH-terminal region of the fibronectin chain.[335] Another site, which may become available in proteolyzed fibronectin, is in the cell-binding region.[369] This site is blocked in intact fibronectin. Fibronectin is not only cross-linked to fibrin but also to fibrinogen, with heteropolymers of very high molecular weight being formed,[370,371] but it can be cross-linked into the extracellular matrix[372] through its reactions with cells, von Willebrand protein, and collagen.

Cross-linking of fibronectin to itself can occur if the fibronectin dimer is first reduced.[189] This does not appear to be a significant reaction in the normal environment of fibrin gel formation, however. The cross-linking of fibronectin to fibrin alters the formation and structure of the fibrin clot; the cross-linking rate of α polymer formation is initially decreased. If the cross-linking reactions are allowed to proceed, all the fibronectin and α chains become cross-linked into HMW heteropolymers. Under certain in vitro conditions, a high concentration of fibronectin results in soluble fibrin.[373] Rapid cross-linking of fibronectin to α chain requires a higher factor XIIIa concentration than is needed for α polymer formation. By increasing the factor XIIIa level to twice the normal level in plasma, all the fibronectin in plasma is incorporated in a fibrin clot.[335] At the normal plasma concentration, about 30% to 50% of fibronectin is covalently bound to fibrin.[374] The cross-linking of fibronectin–fibrin increases the mass to length ratio of fibrin so the fibers are larger,[371,375] possibly because of alterations in the kinetics of fibrin gel formation (see Table 41-3). This may be partly because of a higher affinity of factor XIIIa for fibrin than for fibronectin. α-Chain fibronectin and α-chain–α_2-plasmin inhibitor cross-linking reactions are somewhat similar in that both proteins are covalently attached to lysine sites in α chains, and the reactive glutamines in both are at the NH_2-terminal end. These two cross-linking reactions do not compete with each other for the same α-chain lysine sites, however.[376] The concentration of α-chain sites is greatly in excess of both fibronectin and α_2-plasmin inhibitor in a physiologic fibrin gel. This makes it unlikely that both molecules could cross-link to a single α chain. Fibronectin can also be cross-linked to myosin and to collagen in vitro.

Von Willebrand Factor and Factor V

Plasma von Willebrand factor (vWF) is also a substrate for factor XIIIa and can be cross-linked to fibrin during gel formation.[377] This cross-linking reaction occurs in plasma when the clotting time is prolonged (ie, in hemophilic plasma) and can result in covalent cross-linking of 80% of plasma vWF to fibrin.[378] However, small amounts of vWF are cross-linked to fibrin under normal in vivo conditions. Polymeric vWF, either in plasma or in purified systems, does not cross-link to itself. vWF cross-links to fibrin through the α chain and decreases the initial rate of α-polymer formation. This raises the possibility that the fibrin structure that eventually form from hemophilic plasma is abnormal. vWF can be readily cross-linked to fibrin[378] and to collagen.[379] Thus, this protein, like fibronectin, has the potential to form a cross-linked bridge at the site of vessel injury. vWF and fibronectin do not compete for cross-linking to fibrin.

Human factor V and factor Va are substrates for covalent cross-linking.[380] The extent of cross-linking is the same for V and Va, but the rate is initially faster for Va. In both cases, the label indicating cross-linking (dansylcadaverine) appears in the largest activation fragment of factor V (150 kd). This is the first function observed for this large activation fragment, but its in vivo significance is not clear. This fragment can form HMW homopolymers or heteropolymers.

Other Proteins That Reside Primarily in Cells

Although platelet and monocyte A_2 is not secreted from resting cells, A_2 is translocated to the membrane when the cells are activated,[309,321] and there is sufficient factor XIII translocated to cross-link fibrin. Platelets and monocytes have substantial factor XIII activity.[309,333] With recruitment of platelets and monocytes to an area of hemorrhage or wound healing, the microenvironmental concentration of factor XIII activity may be high. This could strikingly alter the clot structure, since the amount of fibronectin cross-linked to fibrin is very sensitive to the factor XIII concentration.[335] Differences in fibrin cross-linking are also evident in normal persons in the coagulation of platelet-deficient plasma versus platelet-rich plasma.[336] With increasing platelet counts, there is more rapid and more complete formation of cross-linked α polymer.[336] This results in increased resistance to plasmin degradation.[337]

The α-granule protein, TSP, is a substrate for A_2^*,[382] and intact TSP readily incorporates 2 mol of amine-donor analogue in the presence of factor XIIIa.[200] Partial cleavage by thrombin of TSP (142 kd for each of three chains) results in a 116-kd fragment. This partially degraded TSP incorporates 3 mol of an amine donor analogue, and in this way is somewhat similar to factors V and Va.[380] These results indicate that the reactive glutamines are somewhat sterically hindered in intact TSP, and partial cleavage by thrombin makes them more accessible. Degradation by plasmin results in a core fragment of 50 to 53 kd. This fragment is in the central part of each chain, which is rich in disulfide bonds. The principal reactive glutamine involved in cross-linking is localized in this fragment.[201]

The cross-linking process of TSP to fibrin is unclear. Some studies have found evidence for TSP cross-linking to fibrin,[382] while others have not.[201]

Both exogenous and endogenous A_2^* molecules bind to thrombin-activated platelets.[383] The contractile system has several proteins that can be cross-linked into HMW polymers.[384] Actin, myosin, tropomyosin,[386] gelsolin,[381] and perhaps other proteins associated with the platelet (or muscle) contractile system are substrates for cross-linking. Tropomyosin also incorporates lysine analogues and is thought to be a substrate for factor XIIIa.[384] Actin cross-linking is inhibited by ATP.[386] Gelsolin is a protein in plasma and cells that binds actin and shortens actin filaments.[381] It also binds fibronectin and fibrin and is a substrate for cross-linking. Heteropolymers of gelsolin fibrin or homopolymers of gelsolin-gelsolin may form.[381] Because platelet factor XIII may be readily activated when the cytosolic Ca^{2+} concentration is raised (which might occur during platelet activation), it is thought that cross-linking of the platelet contractile system by platelet A_2^* may be a mechanism for irreversibly stabilizing an activated platelet aggregate. Covalent cross-linking of the membrane glycoproteins IIb and IIIa and other transmembrane proteins has also been observed.[384] It is not known if cross-linking substrates secreted from platelet α granules or distributed in the plasma milieu can be cross-linked to platelet-membrane proteins.

Proteins That Are Primarily in the Subendothelial Matrix

Osteopontin is an adhesive protein that is ubiquitous, but it is primarily in areas of rapid cell division.[387] It is synthesized in monocytes and can be cross-linked to itself or fibronectin. PAI-2 is in uterine cells[388] and synovial cells. It is not in plasma except during pregnancy. All of these cross-links may have physiologic or pathophysiologic significance; in some cases, they are correlated with disease, but the exact significance of each cross-link has not been fully proved.

Factor XIIIa cross-links fibronectin to collagen types I, II, III, and V, but not to type IV collagen.[389] There is also some evidence that vWF can be cross-linked to collagen.[379] Direct cross-linking of fibrin to collagen has not been substantiated. Both fibronectin and vWF could serve as covalent bridges between fibrin and collagen in a wound site, however. This is an interesting concept with respect to the role of factor XIII in wound healing and tissue repair, but direct evidence for such covalently cross-linked complexes is not yet available. Vinculin has been identified as a substrate for cross-linking. Cross-linked homopolymers of vinculin are not formed, but vinculin cross-links to fibrin(ogen).[390] Vitronectin[391] and possibly other structural proteins in the subendothelial matrix may be substrates for factor XIIIa. Many of the proteins distributed in plasma in the endothelial matrix have an RGD site and are often involved in cell spreading. There are other observations that make one think that factor XIIIa is involved in wound healing or inflammation. It decreases vascular permeability,[392] C5 is generated at the same time as factor XIII activation in monocytes and macrophages,[393] and cross-linking by factor XIIIa decreases the susceptibility of collagen precursors to proteolysis.[394]

FIBRINOGEN DYSFUNCTION

Congenital abnormalities of fibrinogen molecules have been reported in about 200 patients. These abnormalities are rare, and the true incidence in the population is unclear. *Afibrinogenemia* refers to the total absence of measurable fibrinogen, whereas *hypofibrinogenemia* and *hypodysfibrinogenemia* refer to decreased levels of normal and abnormal molecules, respectively. The term *dysfibrinogenemia* is reserved for the presence of abnormal molecules in plasma in normal or greater than normal amounts. Low fibrinogen values in functional assays, in combination with high values determined by immunochemical assays, are frequently found in abnormal fibrinogens and are diagnostic, particularly in combination with a long thrombin time or long clotting times with one of the snake venoms that cleave fibrinopeptide A, reptilase or ancrod. Biochemical studies of abnormal fibrinogens have demonstrated that base substitutions resulting in the functional defects are the result of alterations in amino acid sequence. These are frequently single amino acid substitutions, but segmental deletions or insertions are less common. Changes in carbohydrate composition have been found more frequently in acquired fibrinogen disorders.

Studies of abnormal fibrinogens often present interesting clinical problems and unique opportunities to examine the relation of structure and function. Comparisons between the abnormal and normal molecular structure and between the abnormal and normal biochemical properties allow detailed insight to the functional importance of single amino acid residues or regions in the molecule, but there are discrepancies in some patients with the same defect. This is probably due to many factors. Tests were not performed the same way and the concentration of fibrinogen is a large factor in some tests, so patients with the same mutation but different fibrinogen concentrations may give different results. Also, in many cases, the mutation introduces a new cysteine that can be symmetrically disulfide bonded within the same molecule or bonded to albumin in varying proportions or bonded to a free cysteine.

Congenital Dysfibrinogenemia

Congenital dysfibrinogenemia is an inherited functional defect of fibrinogen. The functional defect is caused by a structural abnormality of the variant molecule, although the particular abnormality may not be known. There are about 250 recorded cases of abnormal fibrinogens, and the specific mutation of more than 65 abnormal fibrinogens have been determined. Almost all of these are point mutations, although a deletion and an insertion have been observed. This section focuses on the fibrinogens in which the mutations are known. With time, the numbers of abnormal fibrinogens identified increase. Comprehensive reviews of this subject were published in 1991[432] and 1994.[132] Abnormal fibrinogens are, of course, discovered when they present abnormal test results. Not surprisingly, the most common test is for fibrinopeptide release and polymerization.

Analogous to abnormal hemoglobins, abnormal fibrinogens are named after the town of discovery (eg, fibrinogen Baltimore). Most abnormal fibrinogens were discovered when the patient presented, usually before surgery, with abnormal coagulation values; about half of these patients have no hemorrhagic or thrombotic tendencies. Approximately 25% have thrombosis, and about 25% have hemorrhagic problems. A few patients have abnormal wound healing and a tendency to abort spontaneously. A large number of mutations, affecting most of the known functional properties of fibrinogen, have been described.[395]

The mode of inheritance of congenital dysfibrinogenemia is autosomal codominant. Homozygous expression has been demonstrated in patients, fibrinogens Metz,[397] Bicêtre,[434] Charlottesville,[447] Detroit,[446,447] and Giessen I,[434] Giessen I,[401] Marburg,[402] Naples,[403] Lima, and Åarhus. Most patients are heterozygous for dysfibrinogenemia, having half normal and half variant chains. This is consistent with the observation that there are single copies of the genes coding for human Aα, Bβ, and γ chains closely linked on chromosome 4.[220,404]

Dysfibrinogenemias can be classed into five groups based on the physiologic steps of fibrin formation:

1. Abnormal fibrinopeptide release
2. Abnormal fibrin polymerization
3. Abnormal cross-linking of fibrin
4. Abnormal functions in fibrinolysis
5. Abnormal platelet aggregation function

The most commonly observed functional fibrinogen defects are abnormal fibrinopeptide release and abnormal fibrin polymerization. Essentially all abnormal fibrinogens are defective in peptide release, polymerization, or both. The most common mutation, accounting for about half of the mutation, is arginine to either histidine or cysteine. The DNA codon mutation is G → A for histidine and C → U for cysteine. Most of the point mutations determined in fibrinogen variants are in the fibrinopeptide A region or in the D domain of the γ chain, which encompasses one or more polymerization sites.

Abnormal Fibrinopeptide Release

Deficient fibrinopeptide release is usually demonstrated by kinetic studies in which fibrinopeptides are measured over time from plasma or purified fibrinogen by thrombin, reptilase, or both. Thrombin releases both fibrinopeptides A and B, and reptilase releases only fibrinopeptide A.[90,112] Reptilase fibrin, containing fibrinopeptide B, is therefore a marker for fibrin I. Because the substrate specificities for these enzymes are different, an abnormal fibrinogen may have defective release of peptide A with one or both enzymes. Some heterozygous abnormal fibrinogens release only half the normal amounts of fibrinopeptide (ie, Aα Arg 16 → Cys); others undergo slow, but ultimately complete, cleavage (ie, Aα Arg 16 → His).[433] As the fibrin-gel structure is kinetically determined, slow release of fibrinopeptide A influences the gel. Homozygous fibrinogens Metz,[434] Giessen,[435] and Bicêtre[434] release no fibrinopeptide A (Fig. 41-12).

The yields and properties of the fibrinopeptides released from abnormal fibrinogens by the action of thrombin or reptilase can be analyzed by high performance liquid chromatography (HPLC) procedures[69,110] (see Fig. 41-5). These HPLC methods allow the simultaneous, quantitative determination of all fibrinopeptides. Their qualitative abnormalities may be analyzed by observing retention times. Detailed amino acid sequencing studies demonstrate specific amino acid substitutions in the variant fibrinogens associated with disordered fibrinopeptide release.[395] Twelve different substitutions are reported in the Aα chain affecting release of fibrinopeptide A, all of which are in positions 7, 11, 12, 16, 17, 18, and 19 of the Aα chain, as shown in Figure 41-13. Glu 11 forms a salt bridge to Arg 173 in thrombin, so mutation of this residue to Gly breaks that bond.

Replacement of Arg 16 in the Aα chain—the thrombin cleavage bond—by histidine is the most commonly observed mutation. In fibrinogen Petoskey, thrombin cleavage of the His 16 bond is 200 times lower than that for Arg 16.[436] Reptilase does not cleave the abnormal His 16 bond.

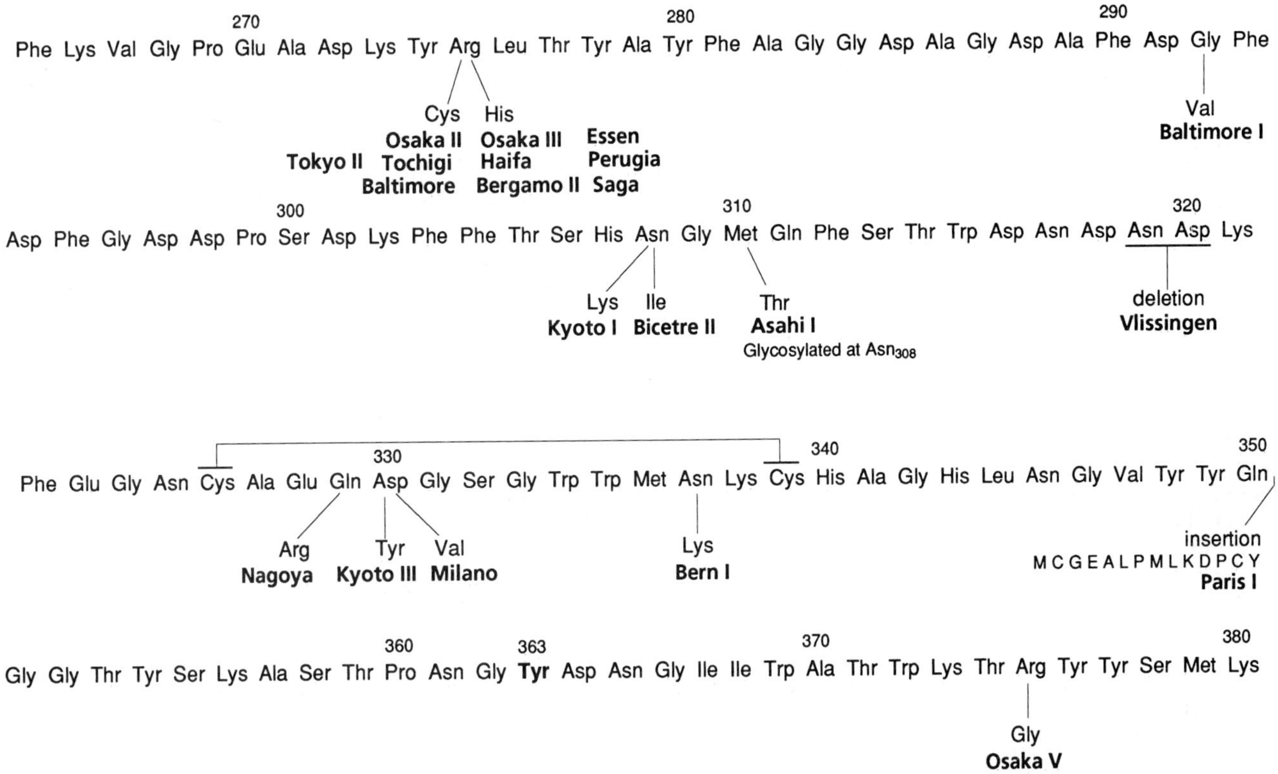

FIGURE 41-12. γ-Chain residues 265 to 380 (exons VII and VIII). Key for fibrinogens with Arg 16 → Cys: Bergamo I, Bern III, Frankfurt, Geneva, Kawaguchi, Ledyard, Lille, Osaka I, Schwarzach, Stony Brook I, Torino I, and Zurich. Key for fibrinogens with Arg 16 → His: Amiens I, Amiens II, Barcelona II, Bergamo III, Bern II, Bicêtre, Birmingham, Boston I, Boston II, Chapel Hill II, Clement-Ferrand, Giessen I, Louisville, Manchester, Milano IV, Milano VI, New Albany, Osaka III, Petofsky, Sapporo, Seattle II, Sheffield I, Sydney I, Sydney II, Stony Brook II, and White Marsh. (Data from references 130 and 472 to 482)

The ability of thrombin, but not reptilase, to cleave histidine slowly at position 16 could mean that when the substrate arginine is bound in the active-center pocket of thrombin, it assumes a histidine-like conformation. This apparently does not occur in the active-center binding of reptilase. Fibrinogens Bicêtre I[434] and Giessen I[401] are homozygous for this mutation, and these fibrinogens do not clot with reptilase.[437] All other patients known to have fibrinogens with Aα Arg 16 → His mutations are heterozygous, with approximately equal amounts of normal and abnormal molecules. These fibrinogens are characterized by long clotting times with both thrombin and reptilase. Heterozygous fibrinogen Birmingham contains heterodimeric species amounting to about half of the circulating fibrinogen molecules.[438] The existence of heterodimers is consistent with a nonselective intracellular process of constituent chain assembly of dimeric plasma fibrinogen molecules. Fibrinogen Louisville, however, exists only as a homodimeric mutant of normal and abnormal molecules, suggesting that the hepatic mechanism of intracellular fibrinogen assembly is different than that of fibrinogen Birmingham.[439]

Substitution of cystein for Arg 16 has also been detected in several fibrinogen variants. Fibrinogen Metz is homozygous for this mutation,[397,440] and the other known cases are heterozygous.[434,437] With cysteine in position 16, cleavage of abnormal fibrinopeptide A with either thrombin or reptilase does not occur. Homozygous fibrinogen Metz is interesting in that patients' whole blood clots, albeit slowly, even though no fibrinopeptide A is released. Fibrinopeptide

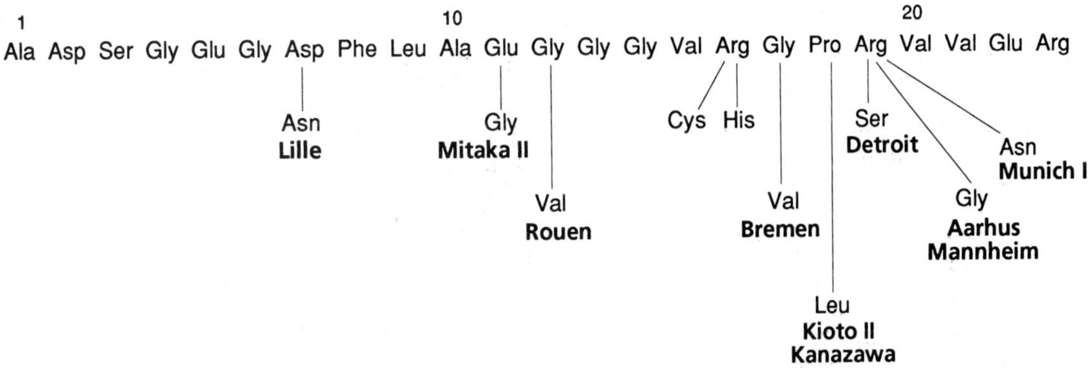

FIGURE 41-13. Aα-chain NH_2-terminal 23 residues. (Data from references 396, 405 to 417, and 419 to 432)

B release occurs normally or slightly faster than normal.[442] This is a special case where fibrin formation can occur in the absence of fibrinopeptide A cleavage, and fibrinogen Metz forms an abnormal gel structure. Fibrinogen Metz also provides evidence for the importance of the β-chain polymerization site. Fibrinopeptide A cannot be cleaved in this fibrinogen, and polymerization of this fibrinogen is greatly diminished by citrate.[397] The binding affinity of a tetrapeptide having the sequence of the amino-terminal β chain to the D domain is enhanced tenfold by Ca^{2-}. This leads to the hypothesis that in the absence of Ca^{2-}, the complementary binding domain for the β-chain site (the B site) in D (the b site) is much less accessible.[464] The functional characteristics of fibrinogen Metz appear to support this hypothesis. These patients have a history of moderate bleeding, with serious bleeding complications after surgery or dental extraction.[397] With this substitution, neither thrombin nor reptilase functions normally.

Fibrinogens Kawaguchi and Osaka I[441,442] exist as homodimeric molecules. The cysteine substitution at position 16 of one Aα chain forms an extra disulfide bridge with the cysteine of the other Aα chain.[442] Data on homozygous fibrinogen Metz molecules,[397,440,443] which have no free sulfhydryl groups and whose amino terminals are evidently close enough to undergo disulfide bridging,[443] support the formation of disulfide bonds at the Aα Cys 16. These observations on cysteine-substituted molecules do not necessarily contradict the theory that fibrinogen Aα-chain assembly in forming dimeric molecules is normally a nonselective process.[438]

In fibrinogen Rouen, glycine in position 12 is replaced by valine.[437] The thrombin clotting time is prolonged, but the reptilase clotting time is normal. The patient is heterozygous and asymptomatic. In fibrinogen Lille, aspartic acid in position 7 is replaced by asparagine.[444,445] The patient is also heterozygous and asymptomatic. Neither patients' plasma nor purified fibrinogen clots with reptilase. With thrombin, the normal fibrinopeptide A is released, but the abnormal one is not. The thrombin clotting time is greatly prolonged, as are the prothrombin time (PT) and the partial thromboplastin time (PTT). Addition of patients' plasma to normal plasma inhibits the thrombin-induced clotting of normal plasma.

Residues 17 to 20 are in the A polymerization domain, and all substitutions have caused abnormal polymerization as well as decreased release of fibrinopeptide A (see Fig. 41-13). Both the probands in Detroit and Åarhus are homozygous[376,379,381,394] (see Fig. 41-12). In fibrinogen Detroit, which was the first abnormal fibrinogen in which a sequence determination was made, Arg 19 Aα chain is replaced by serine.[400] All measurements of clotting in the patients' plasma are greatly prolonged, and the purified fibrinogen does not clot with thrombin, even though fibrinopeptide A cleavage from this fibrinogen is essentially normal with thrombin. Polymerization is markedly inhibited, however, and fibrinopeptide B cleavage is consequently slow. Only after sufficient B peptide is released by thrombin does a fibrin polymer slowly form. Reptilase also cleaves fibrinopeptide A normally; however, no fibrin polymer is formed.[86,400,446] The fibrin monomer prepared from fibrinogen Detroit will not bind normal fibrinogen. This is in contrast to normal fibrin monomer, which has a high affinity for fibrinogen. Normal fibrin monomer also binds fibrinogen Detroit.[447] These data indicate that a polymerization site (the A site) in the E domain is defective. The other mutations in the polymerization domain are heterozygous. For all of these, the rate of cleavage of fibrinopeptide A from fibrinogen is reduced, and unclotted fibrinogen can be found in serum. Fibrin polymerization is markedly abnormal, and clotting times are greatly prolonged.

Abnormal Fibrin Polymerization (With Normal Fibrinopeptide Release)

Fibrin polymerization should be studied by methods in which variations in fibrinopeptide release are controlled, because retarded or incomplete fibrinopeptide cleavage delays exposure of polymerization sites, which automatically results in delayed polymerization. One widely used technique is to measure the rate of repolymerization of preformed fibrin monomers prepared from the abnormal fibrinogen.[462] The time course, and degree of fibrin formation and polymerization may conveniently be evaluated by monitoring the increase in optical density of a solution containing fibrinogen and thrombin or separately prepared fibrin monomer. Abnormal polymerization can occur because of the mutation in the COOH-terminal regions of the D fragment, which makes the γ-chain polymerization sites defective. Mutation sites at γ 275, 308, and 330 are located near the Ca^{2-}-binding region of the γ chain of fibrinogen comprising residues γ 303 to 356[125] or γ 311 to 336.[33] Thus, a single amino acid substitution may well affect the Ca^{2-}-dependent conformer of the D domain of fibrinogen. The Aα and Bβ contacts are most important for protofibril formation, but other contacts in the fibrils are also important.

Gross abnormalities of the Bβ chain of fibrinogen Pontoise, evident on sodium dodecyl sulfate polyacrylamide gel electrophoresis, are the result of β-chain elongation; this results in abnormal polymerization.

The COOH-terminal region of the γ chain of fibrinogen contains the a site complementary to the A polymerization site, a tPA binding site,[175] a plasminogen binding site,[177] and a high-affinity Ca^{2+} binding site.[449] Mutations within this segment, residues 275 to 375 (exons VII and VIII) all have abnormal polymerization. Some mutants have abnormal Ca^{2+} binding, and some affect the fibrinolytic system. Tyr 363 is critical for polymerization,[448] and mutations near this residue have effects on the environment of this tyrosine. They all have normal release of fibrinopeptides A and B. This part of the molecule is retained in the largest subfragment of plasmic fragment D; that is, fragment D_1 prepared in the presence of Ca^{2+} but lost on further digestion by plasmin in the presence of chelating agents.[124,470,471] Several studies of several abnormal fibrinogens, all with impaired polymerization, demonstrated that γ Arg 275 was replaced by a cysteine[472,473] or by a histidine.[128,474] In fibrinogen Osaka II,[472] arginine in position 275 of the γ chain is replaced by cysteine, and an impaired fibrin-monomer polymerization was observed. This cysteine is linked to a free cysteine residue by a disulfide bond. This unique cysteine structure at the mutation site has not been reported in any abnormal protein, including fibrinogen. Isolated fragment D_1, with the cysteine substitution, failed to inhibit thrombin-mediated polymerization of normal fibrinogen and normal fibrin monomer, while normal fragment D_1 was strongly inhibitory.

These studies[472,473] seem to provide supporting evidence that the polymerization site or sites assigned to the D domain of fibrinogen may be dependent on tertiary structure, including the COOH-terminal segment of the γ chain as well as a contiguous region that contains the γ 275 residue.

Replacement of Arg 275 in the γ chain by histidine is a commonly observed mutation.[128,474] In all of these abnormal fibrinogens,[128] the rate of fibrinopeptide release by thrombin is normal, while fibrin polymerization reaction is strongly delayed. The abnormal fragment D_1 of fibrinogen Saga, separated from normal D_1, was devoid of the polymerization site or sites assigned to the D domain of fibrinogen. This abnormal fragment fails to inhibit thrombin clotting of normal fibrinogen and polymerization of normal fibrin monomer. The proposita from Bergamo II and several members of her family suffered from recurrent thromboembolism. Patients from two other families with the same mutation, Essen and Perugia, were asymptomatic.[129] However, the mechanism for this is not understood.

In fibrinogen Kyoto I,[484] asparagine in position 308 of the γ chain is replaced by a lysine with defective fibrin-monomer polymerization. These studies suggest that accelerated digestion of abnormal fragment D_1 in fibrinogen Kyoto is closely related to this new amino acid substitution, for which the generation of a new plasmin cleavage site is between lysine 307 and glycine 308. The calculated solution structures of residues for normal fibrinogen and fibrinogen Vlissingen are shown in Figure 41-14. It can be seen that the deletion of two amino acids at positions 319 and 320 resulted in substantial distortion of the whole segment, which is more compact, and the critical Tyr 363 is no longer accessible. This fibrinogen is characterized by delayed polymerization, and the patient had a thrombotic history.

Deficient Cross-Linking of Fibrin

Abnormalities in the stabilization of fibrin formation may result from some forms of dysfibrinogenemia. Fibrinogens Wiesbaden,[410] and Tokyo[411] are associated with the formation of urea-soluble fibrin, a finding that is presumptive for defective cross-linking.

Fibrinogen Paris I is characterized by an elongated γ chain, having an insert of 15 amino acids.[53,412,413] This could be caused by translation of a duplicated mRNA sequence arising from a pseudoexon,[55] and a likely mechanism producing the defect at reside 375 is abnormal splicing of mRNA transcripts. Paris I γ chains do not undergo covalent cross-linking catalyzed by factor XIIIa. In normal fibrinogen, the γ-chain amino acids involved in covalent cross-linking are Gln 397 and lysine 405. Paris I chains cannot incorporate a lysine analogue into the glutamine acceptor, further indicating an abnormality in this region. Plasmin digestion of fibrinogen Paris I produces an intermediate large fragment D containing the additional sequence.[414,415] The polymerization of Paris I is markedly disordered. It also inhibits polymerization of normal fibrin monomers.[416] Fibrinogen Baltimore I[478] also has markedly decreased cross-linking, possibly because the γ chains could not be aligned in the proper conformation, and in fibrinogen Chapel Hill II, the rate of α-polymer formation is decreased.[495] These mutations in the γ chain must act at a distance to produce environmental changes around Glu 397 and Lys 405 (see Fig. 41-14). Disordered apposition of cross-linking sites during early polymerization steps would be expected to produce a superimposed defect in fibrin stabilization. This is clearly shown in fibrinogen Paris I.[414,415]

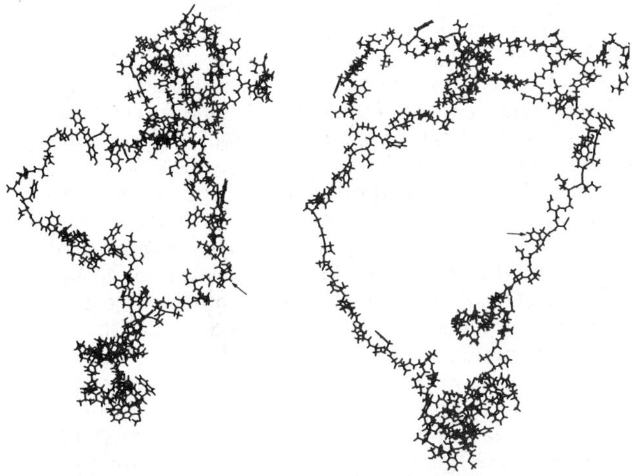

FIGURE 41-14. Calculated structures of fibrinogen γ-chain residues 240 to 411. The structure on the left is normal γ chain, and on the right is its mutant with residues 319 and 320 deleted (fibrinogen Wlissingen). Structures were calculated using a 50-ps molecular dynamics simulation. Arrows indicate Tyr 363.

Many reports of dysfibrinogenemia have described two or more functional defects in the same kindred. The most common combination is abnormalities of polymerization and disordered release of fibrinopeptides. These combined abnormalities may be attributable to extremely slow release of fibrinopeptides as in homozygous fibrinogen Detroit[392] and in fibrinogen Metz,[373] where fibrinopeptide A remains attached to the Aα chain after thrombin cleavage of fibrinopeptide B. Because fibrin polymerization is kinetically controlled, a delay in fibrinopeptide cleavages necessarily results in abnormal polymerization.

Abnormal thrombin binding of fibrinogen New York I, which also has defective binding sites, is due to Bβ 9–72 sequence deletion.

Fibrin(ogen) has several important functions in the fibrinolytic system. It binds tPA, plasminogen, PAI-1, and α_2-antiplasmin; it acts as a cofactor for tPA; and at the same time it is a substrate for plasmin. That way fibrin(ogen) is a key factor in balancing of coagulation and fibrinolysis. There are several mutated fibrinogens causing abnormal fibrinolysis, and localization of defects helps to understand structure–function relationship. For example, fibrinogen Dusart (Table 41-4), with Arg 554 substituted by Cys, has impaired plasminogen binding, since Cys is covalently bound to albumin.

Abnormal polymerization can occur because of the mutation in the COOH-terminal regions of the D fragment, which apparently make the β- or γ-chain polymerization sites defective. Gross abnormalities of the Bβ chain of fibrinogen Pontoise, evident on sodium dodecyl sulfate polyacrylamide gel electrophoresis, are the result of β-chain elongation; this results in abnormal polymerization.

Fibrinogen New York I[465] is heterozygous and missing the Bβ 9 to 72 sequence, which encompasses both the Bβ-thrombin cleavage bond and the β-chain polymerization site and the second degradation site. It also has defective cross-linking, probably as a result of the disordered apposition of the protofibril. The sequence deleted corresponds precisely to exon 2 of the fibrinogen gene.[466] Two moles of fibrinopeptide A, but only 0.6 to 1 mol of fibrinopeptide B are released per 1 mol of fibrinogen New York I. Although the Aα chain is structurally normal in this fibrinogen, fibrinopeptide A cleavage is markedly reduced with both thrombin and reptilase. The abnormal fibrinogen does not clot after the removal of fibrinopeptide A, but it does in the presence of Ca^{2-}. Since Cys 65 of the Bβ chain, which forms a disulfide bond with Cys 36 of the Aα chain,[467] is missing, fibrinogen New York I would be expected to have a free SH group at residue 36 of the Aα chain or a different arrangement of the disulfide bond. This would possibly result in a significant conformation change in the NH_2-terminal region of the abnormal fibrinogen. Thus, the deletion in the Bβ chain could lead to a structural change in the Aα chain, so that its binding affinity for thrombin is significantly diminished. Another interpretation would be that the NH_2-terminal region of the Bβ chain forms part of the primary thrombin-binding site necessary for fibrinopeptide A cleavage.

TABLE 41-4. Abnormal Fibrinogens With Mutations That Are Not Clustered in the NH_2 Terminal of the Aα Chain or in the COOH Terminal of γ Chain

Fibrinogen	Mutation
MUTATIONS IN THE Bβ CHAIN WITH ABNORMAL FIBRINOPEPTIDE A OR B RELEASE AND ABNORMAL POLYMERIZATION	
Seattle I	Bβ Arg 14 → Cys
Christchurch II	Bβ Arg 14 → Cys
IJmuiden	Bβ Arg 14 → Cys, disulfide-linked a
Ise	Bβ Gly 15 → Cys
New York	Bβ 1-72 deletion (exon II)
Naples	Bβ Ala 68 → Thr
MUTATIONS IN THE Aα AND Bβ CHAINS WITH ABNORMAL POLYMERIZATION	
Chapel Hill III	Aα Arg 554 → Cys, disulfide-bonded to albumin
Dusart	Aα Arg 554 → Cys, disulfide-bonded to albumin
Lima	Aα Arg 141 → Ser, carbohydrated at Asn 139
Marburg	Aα Lys 461 → stop codon TAA (461 to 610 deletion)
Nijmegen	Bβ Arg 44 → Cys
Pontoise	Bβ Ala 335 → Thr, new glycosylation site

(Data from references 401 to 403, 434, 448 to 461, 494, 495, 519, and 520)

Other mutations in the α and β chains that affect fibrinopeptide release and polymerization or only polymerization are shown in Table 41-4. Release of fibrinopeptides A and B was delayed in a homozygous patient with fibrinogen Naples.[448] It was found that thrombin binding to this fibrinogen is decreased to less than 10% of normal, since the mutation in fibrinogen Naples may affect its exosite binding for thrombin. The patient had a strong history of arterial and venous thrombosis, although his fibrinogen bound thrombin poorly.

Fibrinogen New York is associated clinically with thrombotic disease, including multiple episodes of venous thrombosis and pulmonary embolism. This presents an apparent paradox of a fibrinogen that clots poorly, with fibrinopeptide A release delayed, fibrinopeptide B release decreased, and fibrin polymerization disordered and yet there is thrombotic disease. This fibrin also fails to support enhanced activation of plasminogen by tPA. With this abnormal fibrin, the plasminogen activation rate is about 50 times less than that with normal fibrin.[468] It may be that although the variant fibrin forms slowly and is abnormal, fibrinolysis is also markedly slowed in vivo. Hence, the hemostatic balance may be tipped in favor of thrombosis.

In fibrinogen Dusard,[418] the abnormality presumably underlies the resistance of this fibrin to in vivo degradation by tPA-induced fibrinolysis. Normal fibrin enhances the activity of tPA, but in fibrinogen Dusard, the fibrin that is formed is less readily lysed by the tPA-activated fibrinolytic system.[419] This may explain the thromboembolic diathesis observed in these affected kindred.

Fibrinogen Chapel Hill III, which has the same structural defect, is highly resistant to lysis by plasmin.[495] This variant shows normal fibrinopeptide release with thrombin and defective polymerization in the formation of fibrin. The abnormal fibrin that forms is extremely rigid and is impervious to plasmin. The first plasmin cleavage is in the COOH terminal of the Aα, and since this step is blocked, all subsequent steps in plasmin cleavage are blocked. However with fibrinogen Dusart, the fibrinolytic abnormality can be corrected with dextran, while it cannot with fibrinogen Chapel Hill. Fibrinogen Marburg also demonstrates decreased plasminogen binding and thrombosis.

Several mutations in the γ chain lead to thrombosis, including fibrinogen Vlissingen, which is associated with decreased cofactor activity of fibrin for tPA (see Fig. 41-14). Fibrinogen Bicêtre II, Kyoto, and Bergamo II have thrombosis, but the mechanism is unknown. Fibrinogen Nijmegen, with albumin disulfide linked, is associated with a decrease in tPA binding (16% of normal). Fibrinogen Lima, with an extra carbohydrate at Asp 139, has thrombosis, which is presumably because of poor binding of plasminogen. Some other abnormal fibrinogens, such as Milano II (Naples) and Mitaka II, are associated with thrombosis, despite decreased thrombin binding. The precise mechanism for this is not known.

Synthetic Defects in Abnormal Fibrinogens

Plasma fibrinogen is synthesized in hepatocytes. Low levels of plasma fibrinogen could result from alterations in biosynthesis or catabolism. A number of patients have been described with congenitally low levels of fibrinogen, having ranges from undetectable to near normal.[496–499] In patients whose fibrinogen catabolism was measured, it was usually found to be normal. Fibrinogen genes were analyzed in two patients with congenital afibrinogenemia and found to be essentially normal by Southern blot analysis.[500] These observations imply that either partial or complete deficiency of fibrinogen is most likely due to defects in synthesis. Such defects could occur at several levels during synthesis, and the deficient patients may be a heterogeneous group. In several families, a hereditary defect in fibrinogen synthesis has been observed, characterized by immunochemically detectable deposits of fibrinogen-related material in hepatocytes, low levels of circulating fibrinogen, and slightly elevated serum transaminase levels. These findings have been interpreted as a defect in fibrinogen secretion.[501]

Platelet Fibrinogen in Congenital Dysfibrinogenemia

Platelet fibrinogen is synthesized in megakaryocytes[262]; exchange between the platelet pool and the plasma pool can occur by endocytosis, but the amounts are small. Studies demonstrate that normal fibrinogen within the platelet is structurally similar to plasma fibrinogen; the only difference is the absence of the normal γ′-chain variant within the platelet.[512,515] This normal variant of γ′ chain, which is slightly larger than γ chain and constitutes 15% of the total γ chain,[502] is produced from a single copy of the γ gene by alternative mRNA processing.[63,64,502] Platelet fibrinogen could be detected in one patient with congenital afibrinogenemia but not in another.[503] This and the absence of γ′-chain variant in platelets implies different regulatory mechanisms for fibrinogen synthesis in hepatocytes and megakaryocytes.

Platelet fibrinogen in congenital dysfibrinogenemia is of interest in this regard, and has been analyzed in several cases. In fibrinogen Paris I, the abnormal large γ chain was not observed in the platelet pool.[504] Similarly, the Aα-chain mutation in fibrinogen Metz was not found in the patients' platelet fibrinogen.[131] In fibrinogen Oslo I (which has a Bβ-chain alteration) and another variant termed FGG-2 (with a γ-chain mutation), however, platelet fibrinogen was found to contain the same abnormality as plasma fibrinogen.[269] These results are consistent with differential splicing in megakaryocytes and hepatocytes in the synthesis of fibrinogen from a single set of genes. The observation that platelet fibrinogen may be normal when plasma fibrinogen is defective may partly explain why some patients with dysfibrinogenemia are asymptomatic. However, fibrinogen Stony Brook I has abnormal ability to support platelet aggregation, while fibrinogen Ledyard, with the same mutation, supports platelet aggregation normally. Few of the abnormal fibrinogens have been tested for this function.

Acquired Dysfibrinogenemia

Acquired disorders of fibrinogen function are most often observed in association with liver disease. In one large study, 80% to 90% of patients with cirrhosis, chronic active liver disease, and liver failure had associated abnormalities of fibrinogen function.[505] Several abnormalities of fibrinogen function have been reported in patients with cirrhosis. Accelerated catabolism,[506] circulating fibrinogen derivatives missing the COOH-terminal segment of the Aα chain,[507] circulating intact fibrinogen molecules,[508] and the failure to form cross-linked α polymer[509] have all been observed in various patients with cirrhosis. Fibrinogen dysfunction is usually manifested by a prolongation of thrombin clotting time and reptilase clotting time, and by abnormal fibrin monomer polymerization. Fibrinogen concentration is variable and may be normal or high. Treatment with L-asparaginase may also result in synthesis of an abnormal fibrinogen.

The most clearly defined fibrinogen defect in patients with liver disease is increased carbohydrate content of the fibrinogen in some patients with cirrhosis or hepatoma.[510] Patients with cirrhosis have 1.5 to 3.5 additional residues of sialic acid per fibrinogen. These abnormal fibrinogens are characterized by prolonged thrombin clotting times, normal fibrinopeptide A cleavage, and delayed aggregation of fibrin monomers. Cleavage of the excess sialic acid with neuraminidase restored normal fibrinogen function.[510] The fibrinogen molecules also have increased β-galactose, but the presence of this excess neutral sugar does not affect the thrombin clotting time or the fibrin monomer polymerization rate.[510] The excess carbohydrate in abnormal fibrinogens is in the Bβ and γ chain and probably occurs because of an abnormality in the branching of the two oligosaccharides.

The mechanism for the abnormality in carbohydrate processing is unclear. Increased levels of sialyltransferase have been found in the plasma of patients with liver disease and hypersialylated fibrinogen. This leads to the hypothesis that hypersialylation of fibrinogen and other proteins occurs as a function of increased sialyltransferase activity in damaged liver undergoing hepatocellular regeneration.[511]

Removal of sialic acid from normal fibrinogen also results in a shorter thrombin clotting time and a faster polymerization rate.[512] Studies with abnormal monomers from patients[510] indicate that the defect is in the early phase of polymerization, probably at the protofibril stage. This implies that the negative charge of sialic acid has an effect on one or more of the polymerization domains involved in linear association of fibrin monomers.

Clinical Manifestations

Most patients with dysfibrinogenemia are asymptomatic, and the disorder is discovered during routine laboratory screening. As reviewed above, however, some patients have a marked bleeding history, and thrombosis is a major complication in others.[395,513] The seemingly paradoxical combination of bleeding and thrombosis is reported in only a few variants, as in fibrinogen Wiesbaden.[485] Because formation and degradation of fibrin clots are finely regulated and interrelated processes in vivo, a tendency toward hemorrhage or thrombosis results only when the overall balance between two processes is shifted.

Most patients with hereditary dysfibrinogenemia are heterozygous. This may be a principal reason for most patients being asymptomatic. If the concentration of normal fibrinogen is greater than approximately 100 mg/dL, there is a decreased tendency for hemorrhage. There are about nine patients who are homozygous for a fibrinogen abnormality.[400,440] All have no symptoms.

In afibrinogenemia and in severe dysfibrinogenemia where the fibrinogen concentration is low, there is a greater frequency of hemorrhage. If all measures of fibrinogen concentration, including immunochemical measurement, indicate 100 mg/dL or less, there is a high frequency of bleeding complications. Affected females in this group (fibrinogens Bethesda III and Chapel Hill VII) frequently experience spontaneous abortions or postpartum bleeding.[514,515]

Disorders of fibrinopeptide release and of fibrin crosslinking are most commonly associated with bleeding, and polymerization abnormalities appear to be more commonly associated with thrombosis.

The first reported abnormal fibrinogen with thrombotic complications was Oslo I. The fibrinogen is characterized by an abnormally short thrombin clotting time, abnormally fast polymerization, and enhanced support of platelet aggregation with ADP.[516] A few patients have deficient wound healing and wound dehiscence (eg, those with fibrinogen Paris I[62] or Cleveland I[521]).

Laboratory Diagnosis

Dysfunctional fibrinogen should be considered in any patient having an unusual history of hemorrhage or thrombosis for whom more common causes have been eliminated. The principles and practice of dysfibrinogenemia diagnosis are well established.[395] Initial screening tests for fibrinogen dysfunction should include fibrinogen concentration (measured functionally and immunochemically), thrombin clotting time, and clotting time with one or both of the venom enzymes, reptilase and ancrod.

A functional assay is based on the rate of fibrin formation and therefore measures the amount of clottable fibrinogen. Immunologically detectable fibrinogen is usually measured by radial immunodiffusion. Electroimmunoassay or other immunochemical assays can also be used. Most dysfunctional fibrinogens are also reflected in one or more abnormal clotting times. Either thrombin, snake venom, or both clotting times are usually prolonged. The PT and PTT may be normal. Fibrinogen Oslo[516,522] is an exception, since this variant has a short thrombin clotting time. Low or discordant fibrinogen levels combined with an abnormal clotting time are sufficient for a diagnosis of fibrinogen dysfunction. Determination of whether a fibrinogen abnormality is congenital or acquired may be difficult. The patient's history may be helpful. The simplest way to prove that an abnormality is hereditary is to determine the presence of the defect in a family member.

Additional studies to determine the precise nature of a fibrinogen defect involve purification of the abnormal fibrinogen. The cleavage rates of fibrinopeptides A and B can be readily determined by reverse-phase HPLC. A structural mutation in one of the peptides is also apparent from the chromatogram.[434,437] A point mutation in one of the three chains can be studied by a combination of (1) the purification of proteolytic degradation products by HPLC, and (2) analysis of these fragments by isoelectric focusing, two-dimensional electrophoresis, and amino acid sequence analysis.[130,472] Polymerization of fibrin monomers can be monitored by light scattering or by a change in turbidity with protofibril growth.[523,524] Detailed physical-chemical analyses of abnormal fibrinogen–fibrin and binding of functionally important ligands should be carried out.[525,526] Many structural alterations have now been determined by DNA analysis.

Therapy

Patients with afibrinogenemia or dysfibrinogenemia can be treated with fresh frozen plasma or cryoprecipitate when they have a life-threatening hemorrhage or surgery.[527] Normal hemostasis can be obtained in these patients by raising the fibrinogen levels to about 100 mg/dL plasma. The in vivo half-life of infused fibrinogen is about 4 days.[247,528–530] A patient with fibrinogen Detroit was treated with cryoprecipitate (with the clottable fibrinogen level slightly higher than 100 mg/dL) during surgery and postoperatively without hemorrhage.[531]

Doses of fibrinogen to be infused should be calculated, and fibrinogen assay should be followed to determine functional activity after infusion. The infusion of fibrinogen preparations can lead to allergic reactions[508] and, in rare instances, to the formation of fibrinogen antibodies. Antibodies to fibrinogen have been described in two afibrinogenemic patients after multiple transfusions.[532,533] The risk of hepatitis was a significant problem with the infusion of fibrinogen concentrates because hepatitis B surface antigen specifically binds to fibrinogen, and these concentrates are no longer licensed. This risk is significantly reduced with the use of cryoprecipitate or fresh frozen plasma. Pregnant patients with low fibrinogen (Bethesda III) are particularly at risk for spontaneous hemorrhage or postpartum bleeding.

Patients with thromboembolic disease should be treated accordingly.[395,484,534] Several therapeutic alternatives are available: thrombolytic therapy, anticoagulation with heparin or coumadin, or newer anticoagulant drugs. Another possibility is the administration of a thrombolytic agent,[534] which should be undertaken only if the abnormal fibrinogen acts normally in the fibrinolytic system. It may be that one of the plasminogen activators is preferable for a particular abnormal fibrinogen, depending on its characteristics. Ideally, to use thrombolytic therapy efficaciously in a patient with an abnormal fibrinogen and thrombosis, one should know the characteristics of the fibrinogen.

CROSS-LINKING DEFECTS

In Vivo Consequences of Cross-Linking Activity

Before describing various in vivo cross-linking defects, it is important to recall the in vivo consequences of cross-linking by A_2^* in the normal person. The cross-linking of fibrin is a principal catalytic function of A_2^* in blood coagulation, and patients who are deficient have bleeding diatheses. Analysis of fibrin clots, obtained at surgery, shows clearly that the fibrin cross-linking pattern observed in vitro also occurs in vivo. Clots formed in vivo contain cross-linked γ dimers and α polymers.[540] In vivo cross-linking of other proteins to fibrin has not been so precisely assessed. Based on decreased serum levels of plasma fibronectin and α_2-plasmin inhibitor versus normal plasma,[364,541] and on von Willebrand protein in hemophilic plasma,[378] it seems reasonable that these proteins are cross-linked to a fibrin clot in vivo. Soluble complexes of fibrinogen–fibrin and fibrinogen–fibronectin can be isolated from normal plasma in small quantities.[136] Fibrinogen–fibrin complexes can also be isolated from atheromatous plaques and may have a role in the etiology of plaque formation.[542]

An important consequence of fibrin cross-linking is that equilibrium is shifted in favor of gel formation, and presumably less fibrin monomer is required in vivo for formation of a stable hemostatic plug. Polymerization of fibrin monomers is reversible in the absence of factor XIIIa, but once cross-linking has occurred, depolymerization is effectively inhibited. This may be the function of γ-chain cross-linking, which cements fibrin monomers in place in protofibrils and has little other obvious effect on fibrin gel structure. Cross-linking of α chain alters the fibrin gel so that mechanical stability and resistance to plasmin degradation are increased.[147,148] When purified plasma factor XIII was added to factor XIII–deficient plasma, the elasticity of the fibrin gel that was subsequently formed increased five-fold.[543] Enhanced mechanical stability of fibrin gel should make it less susceptible to deformation by in vivo forces such as blood flow. The initial rate of plasmin cleavage is slower with a polymer than with a chain.[544] In summary, it is apparent that the net effect in vivo of factor XIIIa on fibrin is to promote the formation and maintenance of a fibrin network—by enhancing and stabilizing the network and by protecting it from mechanical and enzymatic disruption.

Factor XIII is also an essential component of the fibrinolytic system and functions as a regulator. Patients who are α_2 plasmin inhibitor–deficient have a bleeding diathesis due to uncontrolled plasmin activity,[545] which is similar to factor XIII–deficient patients. Factor XIII activity induces resistance of fibrin to lysis. This occurs in at least three ways. The cross-linking of α_2-plasmin inhibitor to the fibrin gel is a principal mechanism for increasing the resistance of cross-linked fibrin to plasmin degradation.[546] The average molar ratio of α_2-plasmin inhibitor to fibrin monomer in the fibrin gel is 45:1. Non–cross-linked fibrin accumulates more plasminogen than does cross-linked fibrin.[547] Some investigators find that cross-linking of α chains to form α polymer also increases resistance of the fibrin gel to plasmin.[544] Cross-linked α polymer is not as good a substrate for plasmin as non–cross-linked α chain.[544] Other investigators, however, find that the resistance of cross-linked clots to lysis is due only to α_2-plasmin inhibitor cross-linking to the clot.[546]

The in vivo significance of other cross-linking reactions is less firmly established. The plasma concentration of factor XIII is greatly in excess of that needed for fibrin cross-linking, and there is also a high intracellular concentration in platelets and monocytes. The availability and distribution of factor XIII coupled with experimental observations in vitro suggests that factor XIII has important roles in platelet reactions and wound healing. Demonstration of cross-linking of platelet membrane and contractile proteins, and A_2^* binding to platelets (together with the ready activation of A_2 in platelets) suggests the possible importance of these reactions. Several additional substrates are released during platelet activation and assemble in various complexes on the membrane where they could potentially be covalently cross-linked. There is suggestive, but not conclusive, evidence for factor XIII from platelets and monocytes having an in vivo function.

There is also evidence for factor XIII function in wound healing and tissue repair. Cross-linking of fibronectin to fibrin promotes fibroblast adhesion and spreading.[548] Fibroblast proliferation also occurs more readily on cross-linked plasma clots than on non–cross-linked clots.[549] The cross-linking of α chains enhances fibroblast migration and retards macrophage migration,[550] and there is A_2^* on the surface of macrophages.[332] Infusion of factor XIII concentrates is thought to promote tissue repair in experimental wounds and in surgical patients.[551] Although a specific mechanism for factor XIII in tissue repair (in addition to fibrin cross-linking) has not been delineated, there are several possibilities, particularly with regard to fibronectin cross-linking. There is additional general evidence for factor XIII function in cell proliferation.[552] Placenta is a rich source of intracellular factor XIII. A specific physiologic function for placental factor XIII has not been established, but in all reported cases of factor XIII–deficient women who became pregnant, however, spontaneous abortion occurred unless the patient was treated during the pregnancy.[553] The incidence of spontaneous abortion also may be higher than normal in women who are heterozygous for factor XIII. The role placental factor XIII may play in preventing spontaneous abortion is unknown. Both fetal and maternal cross-linking substrates are available, and cross-linking reactions may be necessary for placental adherence or to prevent uterine or placental hemorrhage.

Congenital Deficiency of Factor XIII

Congenital factor XIII deficiency is rare. The first patient congenitally deficient in factor XIII was described in 1960 in Switzerland,[285] and this family has been studied extensively.[554] Since then, about 200 cases have been recorded in various countries around the world, but more are known than have been published. The best guess for the incidence in the US population is 3 to 5 new cases per year. There seems to be no predilection for sex or ethnic group. This deficiency is inherited in an autosomal recessive manner, so there is a high incidence of consanguinity in families with factor XIII deficiency.[553,554] The gene locus for A protein is on chromosome 6ap,24-p25[480]; the gene locus for B protein is on chromosome 1. Pedigree analyses of families with congenital factor XIII deficiency also show autosomal transmission of factor XIII genes and indicate that phenotypic expression of a hemorrhagic disorder is recessive. Both proteins A and B are genetically polymorphic, as indicated by electrophoretic analyses.[555,556] This polymorphism, which may be due to polymorphisms in the gene for A and also to variation in carbohydrate for B protein, can be used to determine parentage.[557]

The most common form of congenital factor XIII deficiency is characterized biochemically by trace or undetectable levels of A protein in plasma, measured either by quantitative assays of A activity or immunochemically as A protein.[558] Over 97% of these patients have plasma A concentrations (by both methods) of less than 1%. There is no functional measurement of B protein; immunochemical analysis of B shows that most homozygous factor XIII–deficient patients have about 40% to 60% of the normal level of B protein in their plasma.[559] A few cases of deficiency have been reported in which the B protein level was also decreased, but there was not an absolute deficiency of A.[560] Whether patients who are factor XIII–deficient in their plasma are also deficient in cellular A protein has been studied in only a few cases, but in those patients there was a deficiency of both cellular and plasma factor XIII. Quantitation of A in the isolated platelets of a deficient patient showed that A was also absent in the platelets[314]; similar results were also found in monocytes from deficient patients.[317] This does not imply that all factor XIII–deficient patients are necessarily deficient in cellular A protein. However, there is one copy of each gene.

The phenotypic expression of factor XIII deficiency is variable and may result in mild to life-threatening hemorrhage. These patients all have the same low levels of plasma A protein (less than 1%). One explanation for the variability in symptoms might be that only some patients have intracellular A proteins, analogous to factor V deficiency. In the deficient state, there is no cross-linking of the patients' platelet-poor plasma, although this fibrin is not abnormal and cross-links normally if exogenous factor XIII is added. There is also no cross-linking of α_2-plasmin inhibitor to fibrin. In one study, plasma transfusion of a patient with no factor XIII in his platelets resulted in cross-linking of fibrin, but the overall assessment of coagulation and fibrinolysis was not normal.[314]

Obligate heterozygous members of factor XIII–deficiency kindred display decreased plasma levels of A and B proteins, with levels of A about 50% to 60% of normal and levels of B about 80% of normal.

In a few cases, the molecular defect is known for factor XIII deficiency. Two patients with factor XIII A protein deficiency have been described. In the first patient, the mutation is a G → A in the last base of exon 14, which results in Arg 681 → His, with no immunochemically measurable protein. In the second case, there is a deletion of AG at 211 to 212, at the intron B and exon III boundary. This causes a stop codon to be created and results in translation of a short, unstable protein. The third case is a deficiency of B protein, and the patient is a double heterozygote. There is an adenine 4161 deletion at the splice junction of intron A–exon II; and at guanosine 11499, there is a G → T substitution, resulting in a mutation of Cys 430 → Phe.

Clinical Manifestations

Factor XIII deficiency is characterized clinically by delayed bleeding after superficial trauma or skin abrasions. Typically, the clotting system is initially normal in these patients, as fibrin formation occurs normally. Between about 24 and 36 hours later, however, this initial clot is broken down and rebleeding occurs. Bleeding again stops, and delayed rebleeding recurs. This cycle continues until interrupted by treatment.[557] Most factor XIII–deficient patients present shortly after birth with delayed bleeding from the umbilical stump.[553,561] All forms of soft-tissue hemorrhage are common after minimal trauma; joint hemorrhage also occurs after trauma, but spontaneous joint hemorrhage is relatively rare in these patients. Hemorrhage in the central nervous system, either spontaneously or with only mild trauma, is relatively frequent and constitutes the most serious threat for these patients, requiring immediate, aggressive treatment.[553] This is documented in over 30% of patients and is the cause of death in about 50% of these.[561] Intracranial hemorrhage was reported in an infant at the age of two months.[562]

Factor XIII–deficient women who become pregnant always spontaneously abort if not treated throughout the pregnancy. These deficient women may carry to term with infusions of factor XIII.[563,564] It is not clear why the mother must have factor XIII for successful pregnancy. There are several fetal and maternal substrates for cross-linking that might be essential. Cross-linking reactions may be necessary for placental adherence or to prevent uterine or placental hemorrhage. Patients with very low fibrinogen (less than 50 to 75 mg/dL) also spontaneously abort.

The first reported case of factor XIII deficiency also had abnormal wound healing,[285] and fibroblasts would not grow normally in that patient's fibrin clots.[565] These observations, and much experimental data showing that factor XIII cross-links many substrates important for wound healing, lead to the postulation that factor XIII is necessary for normal wound healing. This could be true, but only about 14% of factor XIII–deficient patients have abnormalities in wound healing.[561] This may be because most patients are treated from an early age or because of inherent variability in clinical expression in these patients, or because the wound healing mechanism is inherently redundant. It has been demonstrated that administration of factor XIII concentrates to patients who have normal levels of factor XIII promotes wound healing after surgery in certain cases.[561,566,567]

Hemorrhage in factor XIII deficiency can be treated with relative ease. Treatment is facilitated by the relatively long half-life and the observation that low levels are sufficient to stop bleeding. The half-life of infused A_2 in factor XIII–deficient patients is on the order of 8 to 9 days[568] to 10 to 14 days.[561] Levels as low as 3% to 4% usually stop bleeding. Cryoprecipitate contains approximately the same concentration of factor XIII as does normal plasma. Factor XIII–deficient patients are usually treated with plasma or a concentrate from placenta that contains only A_2 (Fibrogammin). A new concentrate made from plasma is available, and limited clinical experience with this is encouraging.[569,570] There is, however, much clinical experience with the placental concentrate,[567] and this and plasma are the drugs of choice to treat hemorrhagic episodes in factor XIII–deficient patients. Clinical experience with placental concentrate is extensive outside the United States. There have been no reported cases of viral transmission. This drug can be obtained in the United States on a compassionate basis.

Initial levels of factor XIII after treatment should be in the range of about 50%, and for prophylaxis, this dose is usually given every 4 to 6 weeks. The factor XIII level should probably not fall below 5% to 10%. If one encounters a factor XIII–deficient patient (see section below for methods of diagnoses), the patient's plasma should be sent to a laboratory that does quantitative factor XIII assays. This often will confirm diagnosis and allow half-life studies. It is useful to document the half-life of the product used for treatment in a particular patient.

Phenotypic expression of factor XIII is variable, and there is no agreement as to whether treatment should be episodic or prophylactic. Because of the high frequency of intracranial hemorrhage, young children probably should be treated prophylactically. It is important that, after the mildest trauma to the head, the patient always be treated aggressively. Dental extractions pose a threat to factor XIII–deficient patients. These patients may be treated with factor XIII infusion or with fibrinolytic inhibitor drugs.[571]

After infusion of A_2 (placental concentrate) in factor XIII–deficient patients, the infused A protein immediately combines with B protein in the patients' plasma to form a complex similar or identical to the normal plasma complex. A protein in plasma rises to the expected value and then falls off. This has an unexpected effect on B protein. Infusion of A alone results in a delayed increase in B with a delayed falloff (see Fig. 41-11*B*). This observation has not been explained, but it may relate to the constant amount of free B in the plasma. Complex formation with infused A may be a signal for synthesis or mobilization of B into the circulation so that the level of free B is maintained.

Diagnosis

Patients who are factor XIII deficient have normal PT, PTT, thrombin clotting time, bleeding time, platelet aggregation, and α_2-plasmin inhibitor levels. The clinical screening test that is abnormal is clot solubility in 5 mol/L urea or 1% monochloroacetic acid. This test is based on the observation that solubility of fibrin in these solvents correlates with the degree of α-chain cross-linking in fibrin.[362,572] The clot solubility test is a widely used screen for factor XIII deficiency, and it differentiates those patients who have less than 1% A_2B_2. Test results may not be positive for those patients who have low factor XIII levels (4% to 10%), but this patient population represents about 3% of all factor XIII–deficient patients. Clot solubility testing also does not differentiate heterozygotes. The other disadvantage of the clot solubility test is that it is not entirely specific. Patients with low levels of fibrinogen, α_2-antiplasmin deficiency, or antibodies to factor XIII or to cross-linking sites on fibrin also have positive clot solubility tests. Nevertheless, this is a useful screening test and positive results are most helpful.

There are more quantitative and specific tests (performed in some research laboratories) that are useful for confirming the diagnosis of factor XIII deficiency and for measuring half-life of infused factor XIII in these patients. These quantitative assays, developed by Lorand and colleagues,[352,573] measure plasma factor XIII activity. They are based on the normal function of the enzyme—that is, covalent bond formation between a lysine and a peptide-bound glutamine. In the most widely used assays, a labeled lysine analogue (such as monodansylcadaverine or radiolabeled putrescine) is incorporated into a protein (such as casein); increased fluorescence or radioactivity of the protein is a direct measure of factor XIII activity. These assays are sensitive to about 1% of the normal A_2B_2 level. Gel filtration can be used to separate free and bound dansylcadaverine.[572,574]

Other assays quantitate factor XIII activity, including activity staining after gel electrophoresis,[575,576] quantitation of the amount of γ–γ dimer formed in fibrin,[577] release of NH_3 coupled to NADPH as an indicator,[578] and HPLC analysis.[579] A new activity assay uses a different approach. In this assay a biotinylated amine is used, and the biotin-avidin complex is monitored on ELISA plates.[580]

A and B proteins can also be measured immunochemically. Generally, measurements of A protein and factor XIII activity correlate well. Immunochemicial assays are the only assays for B protein. These measurements are most often done by electroimmunoassays,[581] but radioimmunoassays[556,557] and enzyme-linked immunoassays[307] (ELISAs) provide more quantitation. Some ELISAs directly measure the concentration of A_2B_2 in plasma.[307] A new immunochemical assay uses antibodies to the dansyl group in an ELISA to measure factor XIII activity.[582]

Other Cross-Linking Defects

Acquired Deficiencies

There are a number of reports that plasma factor XIII is decreased in various diseases, but significance of this with respect to hemorrhage is unclear. Diseases with activation of the clotting system (disseminated intravascular coagulation, deep vein thrombosis) result in decreased A_2B_2.[583–585] There are several reports of decreased A_2B_2 in leukemia; this may be associated with disseminated intravascular coagulation or with a release of circulating elastase.[583,585–587] In one controlled trial, treatment of leukemic patients with A_2 had no effect on bleeding.[561,588] A_2B_2 is also decreased in cirrhosis.[583,589] There also are some diseases (end-stage renal failure, obliterating atherosclerosis, and diabetic angiopathy) in which A_2B_2 may be elevated,[590,592] but whether this observation relates to the pathogenesis of these diseases is totally unclear.

There are anecdotal reports of treatment with factor XIII of patients with Henoch-Schönlein purpura with good results.[593,594] There are also a number of reports that treatment of patients with systemic scleroderma may result in improvement of cutaneous symptoms.[567,595,596] This might be because of the effects of factor XIII on wound healing and its interaction with collagen, but the specific reason is not known. There are also many anecdotal reports on the efficacy of treating inflammatory bowel disease (particularly ulcerative colitis and Crohn's disease) with factor XIII concentrates.[597] There are as yet no double-blinded clinical trials and also no unifying, accepted hypothesis.

Some abnormal fibrinogen molecules, which might not bind factor XIII well, may masquerade as a partial deficiency of factor XIII. Such was the case of fibrinogen Chapel Hill II.[598] Other similar defects will probably be described.

Antibodies to Factor XIII

Antibody inhibitors to fibrin cross-linking are extremely rare. About 12 cases have been reported,[599,600] and several more are known. Two were reported to be in factor XIII–deficient patients.[602,603] An unusual antibody to A_2' and A_2^* developed in an elderly woman who was taking procainamide. This antibody specifically inhibited a necessary binding site on A_2^* and A_2' for fibrin(ogen) and fibronectin. Thus, there was no cross-linking of fibrin or of fibrin–fibronectin. However, the antibody did not inhibit α_2–plasmin inhibitor cross-linking to fibrin α chains, implying that this molecule used at least one different binding site on A_2' and A_2^*.[601]

The other inhibitors were in patients who had previously normal A_2B_2 levels. These patients typically present with massive bleeding and no previous history of a coagulopathy. Like most coagulation inhibitors, these are difficult to treat. Frequently, the antibody titer is high. In about half of these patients, the inhibitor has regressed spontaneously; the other half have died from massive hemorrhage. The inhibitors are antibodies that may be directed at several epitopes. Antibodies to A_2B_2, $A_2'B_2$, A_2^*, and to cross-linking sites on fibrin have been found.[599–604] All of these antibodies result in defective cross-linking.

The reasons for a breakdown of immune tolerance are poorly understood. Several of the antibodies to factor XIII developed after patients had been treated with isoniazid. Isoniazid can be incorporated by factor XIIIa, and it is thought that this may be part of the mechanism for inducing antibodies in some patients.[604] Some of the patients had been treated with penicillin and diphenylhydantoin. Treatment with these drugs is associated with formation of other coagulation inhibitors by an unknown mechanism. Theoretically, it should be possible for any drug that is an analogue of lysine with a free NH_2 group off a carbon chain to be incorporated by factor XIII into fibrin. Thus far, the only one used clinically is isoniazid. Considering the large number of patients who take this drug, and the small number who develop antibodies to factor XIII, this abnormal metabolism is extremely rare. Drugs that inhibit cross-linking without provoking hemorrhage would make therapeutic lysis of clots easier. If one could design such an inhibitor drug, one might be able to lyse clots therapeutically with smaller dosages of fibrinolytic activators.

Acknowledgments

We thank Kristen Anderson for help in preparing this manuscript.

REFERENCES

1. Hantgan RR, Francis CW, Marder VJ. Fibrinogen, structure and physiology. In: Colman RV, Hirsh J, Marder VJ, Salzman EW, eds. Hemostasis and thrombosis: basic principles and clinical practice, ed 3. Philadelphia, JB Lippincott, 1994:277.
2. Doolittle RF. Evolution of the vertebrate plasma proteins. In: Putnam FW, ed. The plasma proteins: structure, function, and genetic control. Orlando, Academic Press, 1984:317.
3. Doolittle RF. Fibrinogen and fibrin. Annu Rev Biochem 1984;53:195.
4. Doolittle RF. Fibrinogen and fibrin. In: Bloom AL, Thomas DP, eds. Haemostasis and thrombosis, ed 2. London, Churchill Livingstone, 1987:192.
5. Henschen A, McDonagh J. Fibrinogen, fibrin and factor XIII. In: Zwaal RFA, Hemker HC, eds. Blood coagulation. Amsterdam, Elsevier Science Publishers, 1986:171.
6. Crabtree GR. The molecular biology of fibrinogen. In: Stamatoyannopoulos G, Nienhuis AW, Leder P, Majerus PW, eds. The molecular basis of blood diseases. Philadelphia, WB Saunders, 1987:631.
7. Furlan M. Structure of fibrinogen and fibrin. In: Francis JL, ed. Fibrinogen, fibrin stabilization, and fibrinolysis. Chichester, England, Ellis Horwood, 1988:17.
8. Hall CE, Slayter HS. The fibrinogen molecule: its size, shape and mode of polymerization. J Biophys Biochem Cytol 1959;5:11.
9. Fowler WE, Fretto LJ, Erickson HP, McKee PA. Electron microscopy of plasmic fragments of human fibrinogen as related to the trinodular structure of the intact molecule. J Clin Invest 1980;66:50.
10. Lucas MA, Fretto LJ, McKee PA. The relationship of fibrinogen structure to plasminogen activation and plasmin activity during fibrinolysis. Ann NY Acad Sci 1983;408:71.
11. Mosesson MW, Hainfeld J, Wall J, Haschemeyer RH. Identification and mass analysis of human fibrinogen molecules and their domains by scanning transmission electron microscopy. J Mol Biol 1981;153: 695.
12. Freyssinet JM, Torbet J, Hudry-Clergeon G, Maret G. Fibrinogen and fibrin structure and fibrin formation measured by using magnetic orientation. Proc Natl Acad Sci USA 1983;80:1616.
13. Telford JN, Nagy JA, Hatcher PA, Scheraga HA. Location of peptide fragments in the fibrinogen molecule by immunoelectron microscopy. Proc Natl Acad Sci USA 1980;77:2372.
14. Blömback B. Studies on the action of thrombatic enzymes on bovine fibrinogen as measured by N-terminal analysis. Arkiv Kemi 1958;12: 321.
15. Weisel JW, Stauffacher CV, Bullit E, Cohen C. A model for fibrinogen: domains and sequence. Science 1985;230:1388.
16. Erickson HP, Fowler WE. Electronmicroscopy of fibrinogen, its plasmic fragments and small polymers. Ann NY Acad Sci 1983;408:146.
17. Price T, Strong D, Rudee M, Doolittle R. Shadow-cast electron microscopy of fibrinogen with antibody fragments bound to specific regions. Proc Natl Acad Sci USA 1981;78:200.
18. Norton P, Slayter H. Immune labeling of the D and E regions of human fibrinogen by electron microscopy. Proc Natl Acad Sci USA 1981;78: 1661.
19. Rudee M, Price T. Observation of the α chain extensions of fibrinogen through a new electron microscope specimen preparation technique. Ultramicroscopy 1981;7:193.
20. Erickson HP, Fowler WE. Electron microscopy of fibrinogen and its plasmic fragments and small polymers. Ann NY Acad Sci 1983;408: 146.
21. Medved LV, Gorkun OV, Privalov PL. Structural organization of C-terminal parts of fibrinogen Aα-chains. FEBS Lett 1983;160:291.
22. Weisel JW, Phillips GN, Cohen C. A model from electron microscopy for the molecular structure of fibrinogen and fibrin. Nature 1981;289: 263.
23. Veklich YI, Garkun OV, Medved LV, et al. Carboxyl-terminal portions of the α chains of fibrinogen and fibrin: localizaiton by electron microscopy and the effects of isolated αC fragments on polymerization. J Biol Chem 1993;268:13577.
24. Cohen C, Weisel JW, Phillips GN, et al. The structure of fibrinogen and fibrin. I. Electron microscopy and x-ray crystallography of fibrinogen. Ann NY Acad Sci 1983;408:194.
25. Shulman S. The size and shape of bovine fibrinogen: studies of sedimentation, diffusion, and viscosity. J Am Chem Soc 1953;75:5846.
26. Tranqui L, Prandini MH, Suscillon M. Structure of fibrinogen and its derivatives: an electron microscope study. Thromb Haemost 1979;41: 655.
27. Hocking CS, Laskowski M, Scheraga HA. Size and shape of bovine fibrinogen. J Am Chem Soc 1952;74:775.
28. Katz S, Gutfreund K, Shulman S, Ferry JD. The conversion of fibrinogen to fibrin: X. light scattering studies of bovine fibrinogen. J Am Chem Soc 1952;74:5706.
29. Dellenback RJ, Chien S. The extinction coefficient of fibrinogen from man, dog, elephant, sheep, and goat at 280 μm. Proc Soc Exp Biol Med 1970;134:353.
30. Nieuwenhuizen W, van Ruijven-Vermeer IAM, Nooijen WJ, et al. Recalculation of calcium-binding properties of human and rat fibrin(ogen) and their degradation products. Thromb Res 1981;22: 653.
31. Mihalyi E, Donovan JW. Clotting of fibrinogen: 2. calorimetry of the reversal of the effect of calcium on clotting with thrombin and with ancrod. Biochemistry 1985;24:3443.
32. Nieuwenhuizen W, Haverkate F. Calcium binding regions in fibrinogen. Ann NY Acad Sci 1983;408:92.
33. Dang CV, Ebert RF, Bell WR. Localization of a fibrinogen calcium binding site between γ subunit positions 311 and 336 by terbium fluorescence. J Biol Chem 1985;260:9713.
34. Nieuwenhuizen W, Vermond A, Hermans J. Evidence for the local-

ization of a calcium-binding site in the amino-terminal disulphide knot of fibrin(ogen). Thromb Res 1983;31:81.
35. Haverkate F, Timan G. Protective effect of calcium in the plasmin degradation of fibrinogen and fibrin fragment D. Thromb Res 1977;10:803.
36. Hardy JJ, Correll NA, McDonagh J. Calcium ion functions in fibrinogen conversion to fibrin. Ann NY Acad Sci 1983;408:279.
37. Henschen A, Lottspeich F, Hessel B. Amino acid sequence of human fibrin: preliminary note on the completion of the intermediate part of the α-chain sequence. Hoppe-Seyler Z Physiol Chem 1979;360:1951.
38. Doolittle RF, Watt KWK, Cottrell BA, et al. The amino acid sequence of the α-chain of human fibrinogen. Nature 1979;280:464.
39. Watt KWK, Takagi T, Doolittle RF. Amino acid sequence of the β-chain of human fibrinogen. Biochemistry 1979;18:68.
40. Lottspeich F, Henschen A. Amino acid sequence of human fibrinogen: preliminary note on the completion of the N-terminal part of the α chain sequence. Hoppe-Seyler Z Physiol Chem 1978;359:1611.
41. Henschen A, Lottspeich F, Hessel B. Amino acid sequence of human fibrin: preliminary note on a disulfide-containing internal peptide of the α chain, obtained by plasmin digestion of fibrinogen. Hoppe-Seyler Z Physiol Chem 1978;359:1607.
42. Lottspeich F, Henschen A. Amino acid sequence of human fibrin: preliminary note on the completion of the C-terminal part of the α chain sequence. Hoppe-Seyler Z Physiol Chem 1978;359:1451.
43. McKee PA, Rogers LA, Marler E, Hill RL. The subunit polypeptides of human fibrinogen. Arch Biochem Biophys 1966;116:271.
44. Farrell DH, Huang S, Davie EW. Processing of the carboxyl 15 amino acids extension in the α-chain of fibrinogen. J Biol Chem 1993;268:10351.
45. Henschen A, Lottspeich F. Amino acid sequence of human fibrin: preliminary note on the completion of the β-chain sequence. Hoppe-Seyler Z Physiol Chem 1977;358:1646.
46. Lottspeich F, Henschen A. Amino acid sequence of human fibrin: preliminary note on the completion of the γ-chain sequence. Hoppe-Seyler Z Physiol Chem 1977;358:935.
47. Henschen A. Number and reactivity of disulfide bonds in fibrinogen and fibrin. Ark Kem 1964;22:355.
48. Topfer-Petersen E, Lottspeich F, Henschen A. Carbohydrate linkage site in the β chain of human fibrinogen. Hoppe-Seyler Z Physiol Chem 1976;357:1509.
49. Blombäck B, Grondahl NJ, Hessel B, et al. Primary structure of human fibrinogen and fibrin. II. Structural studies on the N-terminal part of the γ chain. J Biol Chem 1973;248:5806.
50. Blombäck B, Blombäck M, Henschen A, et al. The N-terminal disulphide knot of human fibrinogen. Nature 1968;218:130.
51. Huang S, Cao Z, Davie EW. The role of amino-terminal disulfide bonds in the structure and assembly of human fibrinogen. Biochem Biophys Res Comm 1993;190:488.
52. Bouma H, Takagi T, Doolittle RF. The arrangement of disulfide bonds in fragment D from human fibrinogen. Thromb Res 1978;13:557.
53. Henschen A. Disulfide bridges in the middle part of human fibrinogen. Hoppe-Seyler Z Physiol Chem 1978;359:1757.
54. Hoeprich PD Jr, Doolittle RF. Dimeric half-molecules of human fibrinogen are joined through disulfide bonds in an antiparallel orientation. Biochemistry 1983;22:2049.
55. Zhang J-Z, Redman CM. Identificaiton of Bβ chain domains involved in human fibrinogen assembly. J Biol Chem 1992;267:21727.
56. Zhang J-Z, Redman CM. Role of interchain disulfide bonds on the assembly and secretion of human fibrinogen. J Biol Chem 1994;269:652.
57. Doolittle RF, Goldbaum DM, Doolittle LR. Designation of sequences involved in the "coiled coil" interdomainal connector in fibrinogen: construction of an atomic scale model. J Mol Biol 1978;120:311.
58. Doolittle RF. A detailed consideration of principal domain of vertebrate fibrinogen and its relatives. Protein Sci 1992;1:1563.
59. Lipinska I, Lipinski B, Gurevich V. Fibrinogen heterogeneity in human plasma: electrophoretic demonstration and characterization of two major components. J Lab Clin Med 1974;84:509.
60. Holm B, Nilsen DWT, Kierulf P, Godal HC. Purification and characterization of 3 fibrinogens with different molecular weights obtained from normal human plasma. Thromb Res 1985;37:165.
61. Holm B, Nilsen DWT, Godal HC. Evidence that low molecular fibrinogen (LMW) is formed in man by degradation of high molecular weight fibrinogen (HMW). Thromb Res 1986;41:879.
62. Wolfenstein-Todel C, Mosesson MW. Carboxy-terminal amino acid sequence of a human fibrinogen γ chain variant (γ'). Biochemistry 1981;20:6146.
63. Chung DW, Davie EW. γ and γ' chains of human fibrinogen are produced by alternative mRNA processing. Biochemistry 1984;23:4232.
64. Fornance AJ, Cummings DE, Comeau CM, et al. Structure of the human γ fibrinogen gene. J Biol Chem 1984;259:12826.
65. Francis CW, Keele EM, Marder VJ. Purification of three γ-chains with different molecular weights from normal human plasma fibrinogen. Biochim Biophys Acta 1984;797:328.
66. Francis CW, Muller E, Henschen A, et al. Carboxyl-terminal amino acid sequences of two variant forms of the γ chain of human plasma fibrinogen. Proc Natl Acad Sci USA 1988;85:3358.
67. Adany R, Kiss A, Muszbek L. Factor XIII: a marker of mono- and megakaryocytopoiesis. J Clin Pathol 1988;41:49.
68. Southan C, Thompson E, Lane DA. Direct analysis of plasma fibrinogen-derived fibrinopeptides by high performance liquid chromatography: investigation of Aα chain N-terminal heterogeneity. Thromb Haemost 1986;56:193.
69. Seydewitz HH, Witt I. Increased phosphorylation of human fibrinopeptide A under acute phase conditions. Thromb Res 1985;40:29.
70. Straub PW, Kuyas C, Herbeli A. The plasma fibrinogen fraction with elevated sialic acid content and elongated γ chains. Ann NY Acad Sci 1983;408:114.
71. Kant JA, Lord ST, Crabtree GR. Partial mRNA sequence for human Aα, Bβ, and γ fibrinogen chains: evolutionary and functional implications. Proc Natl Acad Sci USA 1983;80:3953.
72. Rixon MW, Chan W-Y, Davie EW, Chung DW. Characterization of a complementary deoxyribonucleic acid coding for the α chain of human fibrinogen. Biochemistry 1983;22:3237.
73. Chung DW, Que BG, Rixon MW, et al. Characterization of complementary deoxyribonucleic acid and genomic deoxyribonucleic acid for the β chain of human fibrinogen. Biochemistry 1983;22:3244.
74. Roy S, Yu S, Banerjee D, et al. Assembly and secretion of fibrinogen: degradation of individual chains. J Biol Chem 1992;267:23151.
75. Humphries SE, Imam AMA, Robbins TP, et al. The identification of a DNA polymorphism of the α fibrinogen gene, and the regional assignment of the human fibrinogen genes to 4q26-qter. Hum Genet 1984;68:148.
76. Rixon MW, Chung DW, Davie EW. Nucleotide sequence of the gene for the γ chain of human fibrinogen. Biochemistry 1985;24:2077.
77. Mills KA, Even D, Murray JC. Tetranucleotide repeat polymorphism at the human alpha fibrinogen locus (FGA). Hum Mol Genet 1992;1:779.
78. Schmelzer CH, Ebert RF, Bell WR. A polymorphism at B beta 448 of fibrinogen identified during structural studies of fibrinogen Baltimore II. Thromb Res 1988;52:173.
79. Marchetti L, Zanelli T, Malcovati M, et al. Polymorphism of the human gamma chain fibrinogen gene. DNA Seq 1991;1:419.
80. Lorand L, Middlebrook WR. Studies on fibrino-peptide. Biochim Biophys Acta 1952;9:581.
81. Galanakis DK, Martinez J, McDevitt C, et al. Human fetal fibrinogen: its characteristics of delayed fibrin formation, high sialic acid and AP peptide content are more marked in preterm than in term infants. Ann NY Acad Sci 1983;408:640.
82. Galanakis DK, Mosesson MW. Evaluation of in vivo proteolysis (fibrinogenolysis) in prolonging the thrombin time of human umbilical cord fibrinogen. Blood 1976;48:109.
83. Dawson S, Hamsten A, Wiman B, et al. Genetic variation at the plasminogen activator inhibitor–1 locus is associated with altered levels of plasma plasminogen activator inhibitor–1 activity. Arteriosclerosis Thrombosis 1991;11:183.
84. Humphries SE, Cook M, Dubowitz, et al. Role of genetic variation at the fibrinogen locus in determination of plasma fibrinogen concentrations. Lancet 1987;1:1452.
85. Bettelheim FR. The clotting of fibrinogen. II. Fractionation of peptide material liberated. Biochim Biophys Acta 1956;19:121.
86. Blombäck B, Hessel B, Hogg D, Therkildsen L. A two-step fibrinogen–fibrin transition in blood coagulation. Nature 1978;275:501.
87. Nossel HL, Hurlet-Jensen A, Liu CY, et al. Fibrinopeptide release from fibrinogen. Ann NY Acad Sci 1983;408:269.
88. Martinelli RA, Scheraga HA. Steady-state kinetic study of the bovine thrombin-fibrinogen interaction. Biochemistry 1980;19:2343.
89. Higgins DL, Lewis SD, Shafer JA. Steady state kinetic parameters for the thrombin-catalyzed conversion of human fibrinogen to fibrin. J Biol Chem 1983;258:9276.
90. Bilezikian SB, Nossel HL, Butler VP Jr, Canfield RE. Radioimmunoassay of human fibrinopeptide B and kinetics of fibrinopeptide cleavage by different enzymes. J Clin Invest 1975;56:438.
91. Stubbs MT, Oschkinat H, Mayr I, et al. The interaction of thrombin with fibrinogen: a structural basis for its specificity. Eur J Biochem 1992;206:187.
92. Nagy JA, Meinwald YC, Scheraga HA. Immunochemical determination of conformational equilibria for fragments of the Aα chain of fibrinogen. Biochemistry 1982;21:1794.
93. Nagy JA, Meinwald YC, Scheraga HA. Immunochemical determination of conformational equilibria for fragments of the Bβ chain of fibrinogen. Biochemistry 1985;24:882.
94. Hanna LS, Scheraga HA, Francis CW, Marder VJ. Comparison of structures of various human fibrinogens and derivatives thereof by a study of the kinetics of release of fibrinopeptides. Biochemistry 1984;23:4681.
95. Landis WJ, Waugh DF. Interaction of bovine fibrinogen and thrombin. Arch Biochem Biophys 1975;168:498.
96. Liu CY, Nossel HL, Kaplan KL. The binding of thrombin by fibrin. J Biol Chem 1979;254:10421.
97. Kaminski M, McDonagh J. Studies on the mechanism of thrombin interaction with fibrin. J Biol Chem 1983;258:10530.
98. Stubbs MT, Bode W. A model for the specificity of fibrinogen cleavage by thrombin. Semin Thromb Hemost 1993;19:344.
99. Meinwald YC, Martinelli RA, van Nispen JW, Scheraga HA. Mech-

anism of action of thrombin on fibrinogen: size of the Aα fibrinogen-like peptide that contacts the active site thrombin. Biochemistry 1980;19:3820.
100. Vali Z, Scheraga HA. Localization of the binding site on fibrin for the secondary binding site of thrombin. Biochemistry 1988;27:1956.
101. Marsh HC, Meinwald YC, Lee S, Scheraga HA. Mechanism of action of thrombin on fibrinogen: direct evidence for the involvement of phenylalanine at position P9. Biochemistry 1982;21:6167.
102. Marsh HC, Meinwald YC, Thannhauser TW, Scheraga HA. Mechanism of action of thrombin on fibrinogen: kinetic evidence for involvement of aspartic acid at position P10. Biochemistry 1983;22:4170.
103. Hageman TC, Scheraga HA. Mechanism of action of thrombin on fibrinogen: reaction of the N-terminal CNBr fragment from the Aα chain of human fibrinogen with bovine thrombin. Arch Biochem Biophys 1974;164:707.
104. Martin PD, Robertson W, Turk D, et al. The structure of residues 7–16 of the Aα-chain of human fibrinogen bound to bovine thrombin at 2.3-A° resolution. J Biol Chem 1992;267:7911.
105. Berliner LJ, Shen YYL. Physical evidence for an apolar binding site near the catalytic center of human α-thrombin. Biochemistry 1977;16:4622.
106. Berliner LJ, Sugawara Y, Fenton JW II. Human α thrombin binding to non-polymerized fibrin-sepharose: evidence for an anionic binding region. Biochemistry 1985;24:7005.
107. Kaczmarek E, McDonagh J. Thrombin binding to the Aα, Bβ, and γ chains of fibrinogen and to their remnants contained in fragment E. J Biol Chem 1988;263:13896.
108. Blombäck B, Blombäck M, Edman P, Hessel B. Human fibrinopeptides: isolation, characterization and structure. Biochim Biophys Acta 1966;115:371.
109. Martinelli RA, Scheraga HA. Assay of bovine fibrinopeptides by high performance liquid chromatography. Anal Biochem 1979;96:246.
110. Kehl M, Lottspeich F, Henschen A. Analysis of human fibrinopeptides by high performance liquid chromatography. Hoppe-Seyler Z Physiol Chem 1981;362:1661.
111. Ebert RF, Bell WR. Assay of human fibrinopeptides by high performance liquid chromatography. Anal Biochem 1985;148:70.
112. Stocker K, Fischer H, Meier J. Thrombin-like snake venom proteinases. Toxicon 1982;20:265.
113. Shainoff JR, Dardik BN. Fibrinopeptide B and aggregation of fibrinogen. Science 1979;204:200.
114. Weitz JI, Cruickshank MK, Thong B, et al. Human tissue-plasminogen activator releases fibrinopeptides A and B from fibrinogen. J Clin Invest 1988;82:1700.
115. Mihalyi E. Clotting of bovine fibrinogen: calcium binding to fibrin during clotting and its dependence on release of fibrinopeptide B. Biochemistry 1988;27:967.
116. Lorand L. Fibrinopeptide: new aspects of the fibrinogen–fibrin transformation. Nature 1951;167:992.
117. Laurant TC, Blombäck B. On the significance of the release of two different peptides from fibrinogen during clotting. Acta Chem Scand 1958;12:1875.
118. Veklich YI, Gorkun OV, Medved LV, et al. Carboxyl-terminal portions of the α-chains of fibrinogen and fibrin: localization by electron microscopy and the effects of isolated α-C fragments on polymerization. J Biol Chem 1993;268:13577.
119. Mosesson MW, Hainfeld J, Wall J, Haschemeyer RH. J Mol Biol 1981;153:695.
120. Schielen WJG, Adams HPHM, van Leuven K, et al. The sequence γ(312-324) is a fibrin-specific epitope. Blood 1991;77:2169.
121. Olexa SA, Budzynski AZ. Evidence for four different polymerization sites involved in human fibrin formation. Proc Natl Acad Sci USA 1980;77:1374.
122. Olexa SA, Budzynski AZ. Localization of a fibrin polymerization site. J Biol Chem 1981;256:3544.
123. Horowitz BH, Varadi A, Scheraga HA. Localization of a fibrin γ chain polymerization site within segment Thr374 to Glu396 of human fibrinogen. Proc Natl Acad Sci USA 1984;81:5990.
124. Nieuwenhuizen W, Voskuilen M, Vermond A, et al. A fibrinogen fragment D (D intermediate) with calcium binding but without anticlotting properties. Biochim Biophys Acta 1982;707:190.
125. Varadi A, Scheraga HA. Localization of segments essential for polymerization and for calcium binding in the γ chain of human fibrinogen. Biochemistry 1986;25:519.
126. Southan C, Thompson E, Panico E, et al. Characterization of peptides cleaved by plasmin from the C-terminal polymerization domain of human fibrinogen. J Biol Chem 1985;260:13095.
127. Shimuru A, Nagel GM, Doolittle RF. Photoaffinity of the primary fibrin polymerization site: isolation and characterization of a labeled cyanogen bromide fragment corresponding to γ chain residues 337–379. Proc Natl Acad Sci 1992;89:2888.
128. Laudano AP, Doolittle RF. Studies on synthetic peptides that bind to fibrinogen and prevent fibrin polymerization: structural requirements, number of binding sites, and specific differences. Biochemistry 1980;19:1013.
129. Yamazumi K, Doolittle RF. Photoaffinity labeling of the primary fibrin polymerization site: localization of the label to gamma-chain Tyr-363. Proc Natl Acad Sci USA 1992;89:2893.
130. Reber P, Furlan M, Henschen A, et al. Three abnormal fibrinogen variants with the same amino acid substitution (γ 275Arg → His): fibrinogens Bergamo II, Essen and Perugia. Thromb Haemost 1986;56:401.
131. Reber P, Furlan M, Rupp C, et al. Characterization of fibrinogen Milano I: amino acid exchange γ 330Asp → Val impairs fibrin polymerization. Blood 1986;67:1751.
132. McDonagh J, Carrell N, Lee MH. Disfibrinogenemia and other disorders of fibrinogen structure and function. In: Colman RW, Hirsh J, Marder VJ, Slazman EM, eds. Hemostasis and thrombosis: basic principles and clinical practice, ed 3. Philadelphia, JB Lippincott, Philadelphia 1994;57.
133. Pandya BV, Gabriel JL, O'Brien J, Budzynski AZ. Polymerization site in the β chain of fibrin: mapping of the Bβ1-55 sequence. Biochemistry 1991;30:162.
134. Hermans J, McDonagh J. Fibrin: structure and interaction. Semin Thromb Hemost 1982;8:11.
135. Knoll D, Hantgan R, Williams J, et al. Characterization of soluble polymerized fibrin formed in the presence of excess fibrinogen fragment D. Biochemistry 1984;23:3708.
136. Fowler WE, Erickson HP, Hantgan RR, et al. Cross-linked fibrinogen dimers demonstrate a feature of the molecular packing in fibrin fibers. Science 1981;211:287.
137. Medved L, Ugarova T, Velklich Y, et al. Electron microscope investigation of the early stages of fibrin assembly: twisted protofibrils and dibers. J Mol Biol 1990;216:503.
138. Nawarawong W, Wyshock E, Meloni FJ, et al. The rate of fibrinopeptide B release modulates the rate of clot formation: a study with an acquired inhibitor to fibrinopeptide B release. Br J Haematol 1991;79:296.
139. Montejo JM, Raji Naqvi K, Pilar Lillo M, et al. Conformation of human fibrinogen in solution from polarized triplet spectroscopy. J Biol Chem 1992;31:7580.
140. Nelb GW, Kamykowski GW, Ferry JD. Rheology of fibrin clots. V. Shear modulus, creep, and creep recovery of fine unligated clots. Biophys Chem 1981;13:15.
141. Gonda SR, Shainoff JR. Adsorptive endocytosis of fibrin monomer by macrophages: evidence of a receptor for the amino terminus of the fibrin α chain. Proc Natl Acad Sci USA 1982;79:4565.
142. Dietler G, Kanzig W, Haberli A, Straub PW. Experimental tests of a geometrical abstraction of fibrin polymerization. Biopolymers 1986;25:905.
143. Mossesson MW, DiOrio JP, Siebenlist KR, et al. Evidence for a second type of fibril branch point in fibrin polymer networks, the trimolecular junction.
144. Chen R, Doolittle RF. γ–γ Cross-linking sites in human and bovine fibrin. Biochemistry 1971;10:4486.
145. Cottrell BA, Strong DD, Watt KWK, et al. Amino acid sequence studies of the α chain of human fibrinogen: exact location of crosslinking acceptors sites. Biochemistry 1979;18:5405.
146. Corcoran DH, Ferguson EW, Fretto LJ, McKee PA. Localization of a cross-link donor site in the α chain of human fibrin. Thromb Res 1980;19:883.
147. Shen LL, Hermans J, McDonagh J, et al. Effect of calcium ions and covalent crosslinking on formation and elasticity of fibrin gels. Thromb Res 1975;6:255.
148. Gaffney PJ, Whitaker AN. Fibrin crosslinks and lysis rates. Thromb Res 1979;14:85.
149. Nesheim M, Fredenburgh JC, Larsen GR. The dissociation constants and stoichiometries of the interactions of Lys-plasminogen and chloromethyl ketone derivatives of tissue plasminogen activator and the variant dFEIX with intact fibrin. J Biol Chem 1990;2165:21541.
150. Wilner GD, Danitz MP, Mudd MS, et al. Selective immobilization of α-thrombin by surface-bound fibrin. J Lab Clin Med 1981;97:403.
151. Pizzo SV, Schwartz ML, Hill RL, et al. The effect of plasmin on the subunit structure of human fibrinogen. J Biol Chem 1972;247:636.
152. Carrell NA, Gabriel DA, Blatt PM, et al. Hereditary dysfibrinogenemia in a patient with thrombotic disease. Blood 1983;62:439.
153. Marder VJ, Shulman NR, Carroll WR. High molecular weight derivatives of human fibrinogen produced by plasmin. J Biol Chem 1969;244:2111.
154. Dudek GA, Kloczewiak M, Budzynski AZ, et al. Characterization and comparison of macromolecular end products of fibrinogen and fibrin proteolysis by plasmin. Biochim Biophys Acta 1970;214:44.
155. Arnesen H. Characterization of fibrinogen and fibrin degradation products by isoelectric focusing in polyacrylamide gel. Thromb Res 1974;4:861.
156. Haverkate F, Timan G. Protective effect of calcium in the plasmin degradation of fibrinogen and fibrin fragments D. Thromb Res 1977;10:803.
157. Francis CW, Alkjaersig N, Galanakis DK, et al. Terminology for macromolecular plasmic derivatives of crosslinked fibrin. Thromb Haemost 1987;57:110.
158. Rakoczi I, Wiman B, Collen D. On the biological significance of the specific interaction between fibrin, plasminogen, and antiplasmin. Biochim Biophys Acta 1978;540:295.
159. Moroi M, Aoki N. Isolation and characterization of α_2-plasmin inhibitor from human plasma. J Biol Chem 1976;251:5956.
160. Mangel WF, Lin B, Ramakrishnan V. Characterization of an extremely

large, ligand-induced conformational change in plasminogen. Science 1990;248:69.
161. Markus G, Evers J, Hobika GH. Comparison of some properties of native (Glu) and modified (Lys) human plasminogen. J Biol Chem 1978;253:733.
162. Thorsen S, Mullertz S. Rate of activation and electrophoretic mobility of unmodified and partially degraded plasminogen: effects of 6-aminohexanoic acid and related compounds. Scand J Clin Lab Invest 1974;34:167.
163. Suenson E, Lutzen O, Thorsen S. Initial plasmin-degradation of fibrin as the basis of a positive feed-back mechanism in fibrinolysis. Eur J Biochem 1987;140:513.
164. Suenson E, Thorsen S. Secondary-site binding of Glu-plasmin, Lys-plasmin and miniplasmin to fibrin. Biochem J 1981;197:619.
165. Varadi A, Patthy L. Location of plasminogen-binding sites in human fibrin(ogen). Biochemistry 1983;22:2440.
166. Varadi A, Patthy L. β(Leu121-Lys122) segment of fibrinogen is in a region essential for plasminogen binding by fibrin fragment E. Biochemistry 1984;23:2108.
167. Rijken DC, Holyaerts M, Collen D. Fibrinolytic properties of one-chain and two-chain human extrinsic (tissue-type) plasminogen activator. Biochem J 1988;257:2920.
168. Christensen U. C-terminal lysine residues of fibrinogen fragments essential for binding to plasminogen. FEBS Lett 1985;182:43.
169. Henschen A, Lottspeich F. Fibrinogen structure and fibrinolysis. Haematologica 1980;65:535.
170. Fleury V, Angeles-Cano E. Characterization of the binding of plasminogen to fibrin surfaces: the role of carboxy-terminal lysines. Biochemistry 1991;30:7630.
171. Suenson E, Lutzen O, Thorsen S. Initial plasmin-degradation of fibrin as the basis of a positive feed-back mechanism in fibrinolysis. Eur J Biochem 1984;140:513.
172. Rijken DC, Hoylaerts M, Collen D. Fibrinolytic properties of one-chain and two-chain human extrinsic (tissue-type) plasminogen activator. J Biol Chem 1982;257:2920.
173. Schielen WJG, Adams HPHM, Voskuilen M, et al. Structural requirement of position Aa-157 in fibrinogen for the fibrin-induced rate enhancement of the activation of plasminogen by tissue-type plasminogen activator. Biochem J 1991;276:655.
174. Schielen WJG, Adams HPHM, Voskuilen M, et al. The sequence Aa-(154-159) of fibrinogen is capable of accelerating the t-PA catalyzed activation of plasminogen. Blood Coagul Fibrinolysis 1991;2:465.
175. Kaczmarek E, Lee MH, McDonagh J. Initial interaction between fibrin and tissue plasminogen activator (t-PA): the Gly-Pro-Arg-Pro binding site on fibrin(ogen) is important for t-PA activity.
176. Eastman D, Wurm RM, van Reis R, et al. A region of tissue plasminogen activator that affects plasminogen activation differentially with various fibrin(ogen)-related stimulators. Biochemistry 1992;31:419.
177. Weisel JW, Nagaswami C, Korsholm B, et al. Interactions of plasminogen with polymerizing fibrin and its derivatives, monitored with a photoaffinity cross-linker and electron microscopy. J Mol Biol 1994;235:1117.
178. Yonekawa O, Voskuilen M, Nieuwenhuizen W. Localization in the fibrinogen γ-chain of a new site that is involved in the acceleration on the tissue-type plasminogen activator-catalysed activation of plasminogen. Biochem J 1992;283:187.
179. Pannell R, Gurewich V. Activation of plasminogen by single-chain urokinase or by two-chain urokinase: a demonstration that single-chain urokinase has a low catalytic activity (pro-urokinase). Blood 1987;69:22.
180. Rakoczi, Wimona B, Collen D. On the biological significance of the specific interaction between fibrin, plasminogen, and antiplasmin. Biochim Biophys Acta 1978;540:295.
181. Carr JM, Bovill EG, Tracy RP, et al. Changes in fibrinogen after rt-PA administration. Submitted.
182. Thorsen S, Mullertrz S, Suenson E, et al. Sequence of formation of molecular forms of plasminogen and plasmin-inhibitor complexes in plasma activated by urokinase or tissue-type plasminogen activator. Biochem J 1984;223:179.
183. Saito H. α_2-Plasmin inhibitor and its deficiency state. J Lab Clin Med 1988;112:671.
184. Lee MH, Kaczmarek E, Chin DT, et al. Fibrinogen Ledyard (AαArg16 → Cys): biochemical and physical characterization. Blood 1991;78:1744.
185. Braaten JV, Handt WG, Jerome J, et al. Regulation of fibrinolysis by platelet-released plasminogen activator inhibitor 1: light scattering and ultrastructural examination of lysis of a model platelet-fibrin thrombus. Blood 1993;81:1290.
186. Dieval J, Nguyen G, Gross S, Delobel J, Kruithof EKO. A lifelong bleeding disorder associated with a deficiency of plasminogen activator inhibitor type 1. Blood 1991;77:528.
187. Schleef RR, Higgins DL, Pillemer E, Levitt LJ. Bleeding diathesis due to decreased functional activity of type 1 plasminogen activator inhibitor. J Clin Invest 1989;83:1747.
188. Stankiewicz AJ, Crowley JP, Steiner M. Increased levels of tissue plasminogen activator with a low plasminogen activator inhibitor-1 in a patient with postoperative bleeding. Am J Hemtol 1991;38:226.
189. Mosher DF, Johnson RB. Specificity of fibronectin–fibrin cross-linking. Ann NY Acad Sci 1983;408:583.
190. Petersen TE, Thøgersen HC, Skorstengaard K, et al. Partial primary structure of bovine plasma fibronectin: three types of internal homology. Proc Natl Acad Sci USA 1983;80:137.
191. McDonagh RP, McDonagh J, Peterson TE, et al. Amino acid sequence of the factor XIIIa acceptor site in bovine plasma fibronectin. FEBS Lett 1981;127:174.
192. Kamykowski GW, Mosher DF, Lorand L, Ferry JD. Modification of shear modulus and creep compliance of fibrin clots by fibronectin. Biophys Chem 1981;13:25.
193. Bevilacqua MP, Amrani D, Mosseson MW, Bianco C. Receptors for cold-insoluble globulin (plasma fibronectin) on human monocytes. J Exp Med 1981;153:42.
194. Leung LLK, Nachman RL. Complex formation of platelet thrombospondin with fibrinogen. J Clin Invest 1982;70:542.
195. Tuszynski GP, Srivastova S, Switalska HI, et al. The interaction of human platelet thrombospondin with fibrinogen. J Biol Chem 1987;260:12240.
196. Bacon-Baguley T, Kudryk BJ, Walz DA. Thrombospondin interaction with fibrinogen. J Biol Chem 1987;262:1927.
197. Shainoff JR, Stearns DJ, DiBello PM, et al. Characterization of a mode of specific binding of fibrin monomer through its amino-terminal domain by macrophages and macrophage cell-lines. Throm Haemost 1990;63:193.
198. Loike JD, Sodeik B, Cao L, et al. Cd 11c/CD18 on neutrophils recognizes a domain at the N terminus of the Aa chain of fibrinogen. Proc Natl Acad Sci USA 1991;88:1044.
199. Weisel JW, Nagaswami C, Vilaire G, et al. Examination of the platelet membrane glycoprotein IIb–IIIa complex and its interaction with fibrinogen and other ligands by electron microscopy. J Biol Chem 1992;267:16637.
200. Bale MD, Westrick LG, Mosher DF. Incorporation of thrombospondin into fibrin clots. J Biol Chem 1985;260:7502.
201. Lynch GW, Slayter HS, McDonagh J. Characterization of thrombospondin as a substrate for factor XIII transglutaminase. J Biol Chem 1987;262:1772.
202. Bale MD. Noncovalent and covalent interactions of thrombospondin with polymerizing fibrin. Semin Thromb Hemost 1987;13:326.
203. Jones M, Gabriel DA. Influence of the subendothelial basement membrane components on fibrin assembly: evidence for a fibrin binding site on type IV collagen. J Biol Chem 1988;263:7043.
204. Jones M, McDonagh J, Johnson CS, Gabriel DA. Paraprotein modified fibrin gels. In: Mosesson M, Amrani D, Siebenlist KR, et al, eds. Biochemistry, biologic function and gene regulation and expression of fibrinogen. Amsterdam, Excerpta Medica, 1988:117.
205. Sixma JJ, Webster J. The hemostatic plug. Semin Hematol 1977;14:265.
206. McEver RP, Baenziger NL, Majerus PW. Isolation and structural characterization of the polypeptide subunits of membrane glycoprotein IIb/IIIa from human platelets. Blood 1982;59:80.
207. Nachman RL, Leung LLK. Complex formation of platelet membrane glycoproteins IIb/IIIa with fibrinogen. J Clin Invest 1982;69:263.
208. Hawiger J, Timmons S, Kloczewiak M, et al. γ and α chains of human fibrinogen possess sites reactive with human platelet receptors. Proc Natl Acad Sci USA 1982;79:2068.
209. Hawiger J, Kloczewiak M, Bednarek MA, Timmon S. Platelet receptors recognition domains of the α chain of human fibrinogen: structure–function analysis. Biochemistry 1989;28:2909.
210. Lam SCT, Plow EF, Smith MA, et al. Evidence that arginyl-glycyl-aspartate peptides and fibrinogen γ chain peptides share a common binding site on platelets. J Biol Chem 1987;262:947.
211. Chen CS, Chou S-H, Thiagarajan P. Fibrin(ogen) peptide Bβ 15–42 inhibits platelet aggregation and fibrinogen binding to activated platelets. Biochemistry 1988;27:6121.
212. Kirschbaum NE, Mosesson MW, Amrani DL. Characterization of the γ chain platelet binding site on fibrinogen fragment D. Blood 1992;79:2643.
213. Hawiger J, Kloczewiak M, Bednarek MA, Timmons S. Platelet receptor recognition domains on the a chain of human fibrinogen: structure–function analysis. Biochemistry 1989;28:2909.
214. Strong DD, Laudano AP, Hawiger J, Doolittle RF. Isolation, characterization, and synthesis of peptides from human fibrinogen that block the staphylococcal clumping reaction and construction of a synthetic clumping particle. Biochemistry 1982;21:1414.
215. Hogg N. Human monocytes are associated with the formation of fibrin. J Exp Med 1983;157:473.
216. Colvin RB. Fibrinogen-fibrin interactions with fibroblasts and macrophages. Ann NY Acad Sci 1983;408:621.
217. Hawiger J, Timmons S, Strong DD, et al. Identification of a region of human fibrinogen interacting with staphylococcal clumping factor. Biochemistry 1982;21:1407.
218. Yu S, Redman CM, Goldstein J, Blombäck B. Biosynthesis of canine fibrinogen: in vitro synthesis of Aα, Bβ and γ precursor chains. Biochem Biophys Res Commun 1980;96:1032.
219. Uzan G, Besmond C, Kahn A, Marguerie G. Cell free translation of messenger RNA for human fibrinogen. Biochem Int 1982;4:271.

220. Olaisen B, Teisberg P, Gedde-Dahl T. Fibrinogen γ chain locus is on chromosome 4 in man. Hum Genet 1985;61:24.
221. Chung DW, Rixon MW, Que BG, Davie EW. Cloning of fibrinogen genes and their cDNA. Ann NY Acad Sci 1983;408:449.
222. Kant JA, Fornace AJ Jr, Saxe D, et al. Evolution and organization of the fibrinogen locus on chromosome 4: gene duplication accompanied by transposition and inversion. Proc Natl Acad Sci USA 1985;82:2344.
223. Kant JA, Crabtree GR. The rat fibrinogen genes: linkage of the Aα and γ chain genes. J Biol Chem 1983;258:4666.
224. Binnie CG, Hettasch JM, Strickland, et al. Characterization of purified recombinant fibrinogen: partial phosphorylation of fibrinopeptide A. Biochemistry 1993;32:107.
225. Henschen A, Lottspeich F, Kehl M, Southan C. Covalent structure of fibrinogen. Ann NY Acad Sci 1983;408:28.
226. Doolittle RF. Evolution of the vertebrate plasma proteins. In: Putnam FW, ed. The plasma proteins, vol 4. New York, Academic Press, 1984: 317.
227. Strong D, Moore M, Cottrel BA, et al. Lamprey fibrinogen γ chain: cloning, cDNA sequencing, and general characterization. Biochemistry 1985;24:92.
228. Henschen A, Lottspeich F. Sequence homology between β-chain and γ-chain human fibrin. Proc Natl Acad Sci USA 1979;76:1189.
229. Watt KWK, Takagi T, Doolittle RF. Amino acid sequence of the β-chain of human fibrinogen: homology with the γ-chain. Proc Natl Acad Sci USA 1978;75:1731.
230. Doolittle RF, Blombäck B. Amino acid sequence studies on fibrinopeptides from various mammals: evolutionary implications. Nature 1964;202:147.
231. Konkel DA, Maizel JV, Leder P. The evolution and sequence comparison of two recently diverged mouse chromosomal β-globin genes. Cell 1979;18:865.
232. Crabtree GR, Comeau CM, Fowlkes D, et al. Evolution and structure of the fibrinogen gene: random insertion of introns or selective loss? J Mol Biol 1985;185:1.
233. Crabtree GR, Kant JA, Fornace AJ Jr, et al. Regulation and characterization of the mRNAs for the Aα, Bβ and γ chains of fibrinogen. Ann NY Acad Sci USA 1983;408:457.
234. Courtois G, Morgan JG, Campbell LA, et al. Interaction of a liver-specific nuclear factor with the fibrinogen and α_1-antitrypsin promoters. Science 1987;238:688.
235. Uzan G, Courtois G, Stankovic Z, et al. Expression of the fibrinogen genes in rat megakaryocytes. Biochem Biophys Res Commun 1986;140: 543.
236. Kugler W, Wagner U, Ryffel GU. Tissue specificity of liver gene expression: a common liver-specific promoter element. Nucleic Acids Res 1988;16:3165.
237. Roy SN, Mukhopadhyay G, Redman CM. Regulation of fibrinogen assembly: transfection of HEP G2 cells with Bb cDNA specifically enhances synthesis of the component chains of fibrinogen. J Biol Chem 1990;265:6389.
238. Roy S, Overton O, Redman C. Overexpression of any fibrinogen chain by HEP G2 cells specifically elevates the expression of the other two chains. J Biol Chem 1994;269:691.
239. Fowlkes DM, Mullis NT, Comeau CM, Crabtree GR. Potential basis for regulation of the coordinately expressed fibrinogen genes: homology in the 5′ flanking regions. Proc Natl Acad Sci USA 1984;81: 2313.
240. Fu Y, Weissbach L, Plant PW, et al. Carboxy-terminal–extended variant of the human fibrinogen α subunit: a novel exon conferring marked homology to β and γ subunits. Biochemistry 1992;30:11968.
241. Morgan JG, Courtois G, Fourel G, et al. Sp1, a CAAT-binding factor, and adenovirus major late promoter transcription factor interact with functional regions of the γ-fibrinogen promoter. Mol Cell Biol 1988;8: 2628.
242. Chodosh LA, Carthew RW, Morgan JG, et al. The adenovirus major late transcription factor activates the rat γ-fibrinogen promoter. Science 1987;238:684.
243. Chung DW, Chan WY, Davie EW. Characterization of a complementary deoxyribonucleic acid coding for the γ chain of human fibrinogen. Biochemistry 1983;22:3250.
244. Drury DR, McMaster PD. The liver as the source of fibrinogen. J Exp Med 1929;50:569.
245. Grieninger G, Granick S. Synthesis and secretion of plasma proteins by embryonic chick hepatocytes. J Exp Med 1978;147:1806.
246. Rupp RG, Fuller GM. The effects of leukocytic and serum factors on fibrinogen biosynthesis in cultured hepatocytes. Exp Cell Res 1977;118: 23.
247. Collen D, Tytgat GN, Claeys H, et al. Metabolism and distribution of fibrinogen. I. Fibrinogen turnover in physiological conditions in humans. Br J Haematol 1972;22:681.
248. Takeda Y. Studies of the metabolism and distribution of fibrinogen in healthy men with autologous ^{125}I-labelled fibrinogen. J Clin Invest 1966;45:103.
249. Chung DW, MacGillivray RTA, Davie EW. The biosynthesis of bovine fibrinogen, prothrombin, and albumin in a cell-free system. Ann NY Acad Sci 1980;343:210.
250. Kudryk B, Okada M, Redman CM, Blombäch B. Biosynthesis of dog fibrinogen: characterization of nascent fibrinogen in the rough endoplasmic reticulum. Eur J Biochem 1982;125:673.
251. Bouma H, Kwan S-W, Fuller GM. Radioimmunological identification of polisomes synthesizing fibrinogen polypeptide chains. Biochemistry 1975;14:4787.
252. Hartwig R, Danishefsky KJ. Studies on the assembly and secretion of fibrinogen. J Biol Chem 1991;266:6578.
253. Grieninger G, Oddoux C, Diamond L, et al. Regulation of fibrinogen synthesis and secretion by the chicken hepatocyte. Ann NY Acad Sci 1989;557:257.
254. Oddoux C, Grieninger G. Fibrinogen assembly: insights from chicken hepatocytes. Hepatology 1994;19:688.
255. Crabtree GR, Kant JA. Coordinate accumulation of the mRNA for the α, β and γ chains of rat fibrinogen following defibrination. J Biol Chem 1982;257:7277.
256. Plant PW, Grieninger G. Noncoordinate synthesis of the fibrinogen subunits in hepatocytes cultured under hormone-deficient conditions. J Biol Chem 1986;261:2331.
257. Yu S, Sher B, Kudryk B, Redman CM. Fibrinogen precursors: order of assembly of fibrinogen chains. J Biol Chem 1984;259:10574.
258. Roy SN, Mukhopadhyay G, Redman CM. Regulation of fibrinogen assembly: transfection of HEP G2 cells with Bb cDNA specifically enhances synthesis of the component chains of fibrinogen. J Biol Chem 1990;265:6389.
259. Hirose S, Oda K, Ikehara Y. Biosynthesis, assembly and secretion of fibrinogen in cultured rat hepatocytes. Biochem J 1988;251:373.
260. Yu S, Kong V, Kudryk B, Redman CM. Endogenous forms of fibrinogen in HEP G2 cells. Thromb Res 1987;46:281.
261. Lambert N, Freedman RB. Kinetics and specificity of homogeneous protein disulphide-isomerase in protein disulphide isomerization and in thiol-protein-disulphide oxidoreduction. Biochem J 1983;213:235.
262. Leven RM, Shick PK, Budzynski AZ. Fibrinogen biosynthesis in isolated guinea pig megakaryocytes. Blood 1985;65:501.
263. Belloc F, Hourdille P, Fialon P, et al. Fibrinogen synthesis by megakaryocyte rich human marrow cell concentrates. Thromb Res 1985;38: 341.
264. Lange W, Luig A, Dolken G, et al. Fibrinogen γ-chain mRNA is not detected in human megakaryocytes. Blood 1991;78:20.
265. Louache F, Debili N, Cramer E, et al. Fibrinogen is not synthesized by human megakaryocytes. Blood 1991;77:311.
266. Kieffer N, Guichard J, Farcet JP, et al. Biosynthesis of major platelet proteins in human blood platelets. Eur J Biochem 1987;164:189.
267. Homandberg GA, Williams JE, Evans DB, Mosesson MW. Evidence that rat platelet fibrinogen molecules lack the γ chain variant found in plasma fibrinogen molecules. Thromb Res 1985;38:203.
268. Francis CW, Nachman RK, Marder VJ. Plasma and platelet fibrinogen differ in γ chain content. Thromb Haemost 1984;51:84.
269. Teige B, Gogstad G, Brosstad F, et al. Common structural genes for platelet and plasma fibrinogen. Blood 1985;65:120.
270. Ganguly P. Isolation and some properties of fibrinogen from human blood platelets. J Biol Chem 1972;247:1809.
271. Mosesson MW, Homandberg GA, Amrani DL. Human platelet fibrinogen γ chain structure. Blood 1984;63:990.
272. Cramer EM, Debili N, Martin JF, et al. Uncoordinated expression of fibrinogen compared with thrombospondin and von Willebrand factor in maturing human megakaryocytes. Blood 1989;73:1123.
273. Handagama PJ, Georges JN, Shuman MA, et al. Incorporation of circulating protein into megakaryocytes and platelet granules. Proc Natl Acad Sci USA 1987;84:861.
274. Otto JM, Grenett HE, Fuller GM. The coordinated regulation of fibrinogen gene transcription by hepatocyte-stimulating factor and dexamethazone. J Cell Biol 1987;105:1067.
275. Ritchie DG, Fuller GM. Hepatocyte-stimulating factor: a monocyte-derived acute phase regulatory protein. Ann NY Acad Sci 1983;408: 490.
276. Nham S-U, Fuller GM. Effect of fibrinogen degradation products on production of hepatocyte stimulating factor by macrophage cell line (P388D1). Thromb Res 1986;44:467.
277. Wang Y, Fuller GM. The putative role of fibrin fragments in the biosynthesis of fibrinogen by hepatoma cells. Biochem Biophys Res Comm 1991;175:562.
278. Evans E, Courtois GM, Kilian PL, et al. Induction of fibrinogen and a subset of acute phase response genes involves a novel monokine which is mimicked by phorbol esters. J Biol Chem 1987;262:10850.
279. Nickerson JM, Fuller GM. Modification of fibrinogen chains during synthesis: glycosylation of Bβ and γ chains. Biochemistry 1981;20: 2818.
280. Hille A, Rosa P, Huttner WB. Tyrosine sulfation: a post-translational modification of proteins destined for secretion? FEBS Lett 1984;177: 129.
281. Fuller GM, Nickerson JM, Adams MA. Translational and cotranslational events in fibrinogen synthesis. Ann NY Acad Sci 1983;408:440.
282. Hirose S, Oda K, Ikehara Y. Tyrosine O-sulfation of the fibrinogen γB chain in primary cultures of rat hepatocytes. J Biol Chem 1988;263: 7426.
283. Robbins KC. A study on the conversion of fibrinogen to fibrin. Am J Physiol 1944;142:581.

284. Laki K, Lorand L. On solubility of fibrin clots. Science 1948;108:280.
285. Duckert F, Jung E, Shmerling DH. A hitherto undescribed congenital hemorrhagic diathesis probably due to fibrin stabilizing factor deficiency. Thromb Diath Haemorrh 1960;5:179.
286. Clark DD, Mycek MJ, Neidle A, Waelsch H. The incorporation of amines into protein. Arch Biochem Biophys 1959;79:338.
287. Grundmann U, Amann E, Zettlmeissl G, Küpper HA. Characterization of a cDNA coding for human factor XIIIa. Proc Natl Acad Sci USA 1986;83:8024.
288. Ichinose A, Hendrickson LE, Fujikawa K, Davie EW. Amino acid sequence of the a subunit of human factor XIII. Biochemistry 1986;25:6900.
289. Takahashi N, Takahashi Y, Putnam FW. Primary structure of blood coagulation factor XIIIa (fibrinoligase, transglutaminase) from human placenta. Proc Natl Acad Sci USA 1986;83:8019.
290. Ichinose A, Kaetsu H. Molecular approach to structure–function relationship of human coagulation factor XIII. Methods Enzymol 1993;222:36.
291. Weisberg LJ, Shin DT, Greenberg CS, et al. Localization of the gene for coagulation factor XIII A-chain to chromosome 6 and identification of sites of synthesis. J Clin Invest 1987;79:649.
292. Liu Y, Kaczmarek E, Berse B. Biosynthesis of plasma factor XIII: evidence for transcription and translation in hepatoma cells. Submitted.
293. Board PG, Webb GC, McKee J, Ichinose A. Localization of the coagulation factor XIIIa subunit gene (F13A) to chromosome bands 6p24-p25. Cytogenet Cell Genet 1988;48:25.
294. Carrell NA, Erickson HP, McDonagh J. Electron microscopy and hydrodynamic properties of factor XIII subunits. J Biol Chem 1989;264:551.
295. Greenberg CS, Birckbichler PJ, Rice RH. Transglutaminases: multifunctional cross-linking enzymes that stabilize tissues. FASEB J 1991;5:3071.
296. Ichinose A, Bottenus RE, Davie EW. Structure of transglutaminases. J Biol Chem 1990;265:13411.
297. Micanovic R, Procyk R, Lin W, et al. Rolse of histidine 373 in the catalytic activity of coagulation factor XIII. FASEB J 1993;7:1190.
298. Ichinose A, McMullen BA, Fujikawa K, Davie EW. Amino acid sequence of the b subunit of human factor XIII, a protein composed of ten repetitive segments. Biochemistry 1986;25:4633.
299. Bishop PD, Lasser GW, Le Trong I, Stenkamp RE, et al. Human recombinant factor XIII from *Saccharomyces cerevisiae:* crystallization and preliminary x-ray data. J Biol Chem 1990;265:13888.
300. Lozier J, Takahashi N, Putnam FW. Complete amino acid sequence of human plasma β_2 glycoprotein I. Proc Natl Acad Sci USA 1984;81:3640.
301. Davie EW, Ichinose A, Leytus SP. Structural features of the proteins participating in blood coagulation and fibrinolysis: Cold Spring Harbor Symposium. Quant Biol 1986;51:509.
302. Nicholson-Weller A, Zaia J, Raum MG, Coligan J. Decay accelerating factor (DAF) peptide sequences share homology with a consensus sequence found in the super-family of structurally related complement proteins including haptoglobin, factor XIII, β 2-glycoprotein I, and IL-2 receptor. Immunol Lett 1987;14:307.
303. Bohn H. The human fibrin-stabilizing factors. Mol Cell Biochem 1978;20:67.
304. Dahlbäck B, Smith CA, Müller-Eberhard HJ. Visualization of human C4b-binding protein and its complexes with vitamin K–dependent protein S and complement protein C4b. Proc Natl Acad Sci USA 1983;80:3.
305. Seelig GF, Folk JE. Noncatalytic subunits of human blood plasma coagulation factor XIII. J Biol Chem 1980;255:8881.
306. Radek JT, Jeong JM, Wilson J, et al. Association of the A subunits of recombinant placental factor XIII with the native carrier B subunits from human plasma. Biochemistry 1993;32:3527.
307. Yorifugi H, Anderson K, Lynch GW, et al. B protein of factor XIII: differentiation between free B and complexed B. Blood 1988;72:1645.
308. Henriksson P, Becker S, McDonagh J. Identification of intracellular factor XIII in human monocytes and macrophages. J Clin Invest 1985;76:528.
309. Kradin RL, Lynch GW, Kurnick JT, et al. Factor XIIIa is synthesized and expressed on the surface of U937 cells and alveolar macrophages. Blood 1987;69:778.
310. Marx G, Korner G, Mou X, et al. Packaging zinc, fibrinogen, and factor XIII in platelet alpha-granules. J Cell Physiol 1993;156:437.
311. Kiesselbach TH, Wagner RH. Demonstration of factor XIII in human megakaryocytes by a fluorescent antibody technique. Ann NY Acad Sci 1972;202:318.
312. Nemes Z. Differentiation markers in hemangiopericytoma. Cancer 1992;69:133.
313. Morganroth GS, Chan LS, Winstein GD, et al. Proliferating cells in psoriatic dermis are comprised primarily of T cells, endothelial cells, and factor XIIIa+ perivascular dendritic cells. J Invest Dermatol 1991;96:333.
314. McDonagh J, McDonagh RP Jr, Delage JM, Wagner RH. Factor XIII in human plasma and platelets. J Clin Invest 1969;48:940.
315. Muszbek L, Adany R, Szegedi G, et al. Factor XIII of blood coagulation in human monocytes. Thromb Res 1985;37:401.
316. Nemes Z, Thomazy V. Factor XIIIa and the classic histiocytic markers in malignant fibrous histiocytoma: a comparative immunohistochemical study. Hum Pathol 1988;19:822.
317. Muszbek L, Adany R, Kavai M, et al. Monocytes of patients congenitally deficient in plasma factor XIII lack factor XIII subunit a antigen and transglutaminase activity. Thromb Haemost 1988;59:231.
318. Adany R, Kiss A, Muszbek L. Factor XIII: a marker of mono- and megakaryocytopoiesis. Br J Haematol 1987;67:167.
319. Lopaciuk S, Lovette KM, McDonagh J, et al. Subcellular distribution of fibrinogen and factor XIII in human blood platelets. Thromb Res 1976;8:453.
320. Broekman JJ, Handin RI, Cohen P. Distribution of fibrinogen and platelet factors IV and XIII in subcellular fractions of human platelets. Br J Haematol 1975;31:5.
321. Kreager JA, Devine DV, Greenberg CS. Cytofluorometric identification of plasmin-sensitive factor XIIIa binding to platelets. Thromb Haemost 1988;60:88.
322. Higgins D, Vehar G. Interaction of one-chain and two-chain tissue plasminogen activator with intact and plasmin-degraded fibrin. Biochemistry 1987;26:7786.
323. Ciocca DR, Oesterreich S, Chamness GC. Biological and clinical implications of heat shock protein 27000 (Hsp27): a review. J Natl Cancer Inst 1993;85:1558.
324. Kasahara K, Takagi J, Sekiya F, et al. "A" subunit of factor XIII is present on bovine platelet membrane and mediates collagen-induced platelet activation. Thromb Res 1988;50:253.
325. Nagy JA, Henriksson P, McDonagh J. Biosynthesis of factor XIII b subunit by human hepatoma cell lines. Blood 1986;68:1272.
326. Bohn H, Becker W, Trobish H. Die molekulare Struktur der fibrinstabilisierenden Faktoren des Menschen. II. Vergleichende immunologische Untersuchungen von Faktor-XIII Mangelplasma und normal Plasma. Blut 1973;36:303.
327. Curtis CG, Brown KL, Credo RB, et al. Calcium-dependent unmasking of active-center cysteine during activation of fibrin stabilizing factor. Biochemistry 1974;13:3774.
328. Hornyak TJ, Shafer JA. Role of calcium ion in the generation of factor XIII activity. Biochemistry 1991;30:6175.
329. Ikematsu S. An approach to the metabolism of factor XIII. Acta Haematol Jpn 1981;44:1499.
330. Rodeghiero F, Morbin M, Barbui T. Subunit A of factor XIII regulates subunit B plasma concentration. Thromb Haemost 1981;46:621.
331. Wolpl A, Lattke H, Board PG, et al. Coagulation factor XIII A and B subunits in bone marrow and liver transplantation. Transplantation 1987;43:151.
332. Nagy JA, Kradin RL, McDonagh J. Biosynthesis of factor XIII A and B subunits. In: Zappia V, Galletti P, Porta R, Wold F, eds. Advances in post-translational modifications of proteins and aging. New York, Plenum Press, 1987:29.
333. Weisberg LJ, Schiu PT, Conkling PK, Shuman MA. Identification of normal human peripheral blood monocytes and liver as sites of synthesis of coagulation factor XIII a-chain. Blood 1987;70:579.
334. McDevitt NB, McDonagh J, Taylor HL, Roberts HR. An acquired inhibitor to factor XIII. Arch Intern Med 1972;130:772.
335. McDonagh J, Hada M, Kaminski M. Plasma fibronectin and fibrin formation. In: McDonagh J ed. Plasma fibronectin: structure and function. New York, Marcel Dekker, 1985:121.
336. Francis CW, Marder VJ. Rapid formation of large molecular weight α-polymers in crosslinked fibrin induced by high factor XIII concentrations: role of platelet factor XIII. J Clin Invest 1987;80:1459.
337. Francis CW, Marder VJ. Increased resistance to plasmic degradation of fibrin with highly crosslinked α-polymer chains formed at high factor XIII concentrations. Blood 1988;71:1361.
338. Lorand L, Jeong J-M, Radek J, et al. Human plasma factor XIII: subunit interactions and activation of Zymogen. Methods Enzymol 1993;222:22.
339. Mary A, Achyuthan KE, Greenberg CS. B-chains prevent the proteolytic inactivation of the a-chains of plasma factor XIII. Biochim Biophys Acta 1988;966:328.
340. Lynch GW, Pfueller SL. Thrombin-independent activation of platelet factor XIII by endogenous platelet acid protease. Thromb Haemost 1988;59:372.
341. Ando Y, Imamura S, Yamagata Y, et al. Platelet factor XIII is activated by calpain. Biochem Biophys Res Commun 1987;144:484.
342. Cohen I, Kahn DR, Drisdel RC. Inhibition of platelet factor XIIIa–catalyzed reactions by calmodulin. Biochim Biophys Acta 1986;883:265.
343. Credo RB, Curtis CG, Lorand L. Ca^{2+}-related regulatory function of fibrinogen. Proc Natl Acad Sci USA 1978;75:4234.
344. Greenberg CS, Achyuthan KE, Fenton JW II. Factor XIIIa formation promoted by complexing of α-thrombin, fibrin, and plasma factor XIII. Blood 1987;69:867.
345. Lewis SD, Janus TJ, Lorand L, Shafer JA. Regulation of formation of factor XIIIa by its fibrin substrates. Biochemistry 1985;24:6772.
346. Greenberg CS, Miraglia CC. The effect of fibrin polymers on thrombin-catalyzed plasma factor XIIIa formation. Blood 1985;66:466.
347. Naski MC, Lorand L, Shafer JA. Characterization of the kinetic path-

way for fibrin promotion of alpha-thrombin–catalyzed activation of plasma factor XIII. Biochemistry 1991;30:934.

348. Credo RB, Curtis CG, Lorand L. α-Chain domain of fibrinogen controls generation of fibrinoligase (coagulation factor XIIIa): calcium ion regulatory aspects. Biochemistry 1981;20:3770.

349. Mary A, Achyuthan KE, Greenberg CS. Factor XIII binds to the Aα- and Bβ-chains in the D-domain of fibrinogen: an immunoblotting study. Biochem Biophys Res Comm 1987;147:608.

350. Procyk R, Bishop PD, Kudryk B. Fibrin–recombinant human factor XIII a-subunit association. Thromb Res 1993;71:127.

351. Hornyak TJ, Shafer JA. Interactions of factor XIII with fibrin as substrate and cofactor. 1992;31:423.

352. Curtis CG, Lorand L. Fibrin-stabilizing factor (factor XIII). Methods Enzymol 1976;45:177.

353. Halkier T, Magnusson S. Contact activation of blood coagulation is inhibited by plasma factor XIII b-chain. Thromb Res 1988;51:313.

354. McDonagh J, Kaminski M, Kaplan A. High molecular weight kininogen inhibits intracellular factor XIII. Circulation 1986(Suppl);74:II-92.

355. Folk JE. Mechanism and basis for specificity of transglutaminase-catalyzed ε-(γ-glutamyl) lysine bond formation. Adv Enzymol 1983; 54:1.

356. Gorman JJ, Folk JE. Structural features of glutamine substrates for transglutaminases. J Biol Chem 1984;259:9007.

357. Pisano JJ, Finlayson JS, Peyton MP. Chemical and enzymic detection of protein crosslinks: measurement of ε(γ-glutamyl) lysine in fibrin polymerized by factor XIII. Biochemistry 1969;8:871.

358. Bale MD, Janmey PA, Ferry JD, Lorand L. Kinetics of formation of fibrin oligimers. III. Ligation kinetics concurrent with and subsequent to oligimer assembly. Biopolymers 1984;23:127.

359. Schwartz ML, Pizzo SV, Hill RL, McKee PA. The effect of fibrin-stabilizing factor on the subunit structure of human fibrin. J Clin Invest 1971;50:1506.

360. Doolittle RF, Chen R, Lau F. Hybrid fibrin: proof of the intermolecular nature of crosslinking units. Biochem Biophys Res Commun 1971;44: 94.

361. Kopec M, Teisseyre E, Dudek-Wojciechowska G, et al. Studies on the "double D" fragment from stabilized bovine fibrin. Thromb Res 1973;2: 283.

362. Elms MJ, Bunce IH, Bundesen PG, et al. Rapid detection of crosslinked fibrin degradation products in plasma using monoclonal antibody-coated latex particles. Am J Clin Pathol 1986;85:360.

363. Doolittle RS, Cassman KG, Cottrell BA, Friezner SJ. Amino acid sequence studies on the α-chain of human fibrinogen: isolation and characterization of two linked α-chained cyanogen bromide fragments from fully crosslinked fibrin. Biochemistry 1977;16:1715.

364. Kimura S, Aoki N. Crosslinking site in fibrinogen for α_2-plasmin inhibitor. J Biol Chem 1986;261:15591.

365. Gron B, Filion-Myklebust C, Bennick, et al. Early cross-linked fibrin in human plasma contains alpha-polymers with intact fibrinopeptide. A. Blood Coagul Fibrinolysis 1992;3:731.

366. Kanaide H, Shainoff JR. Crosslinking of fibrinogen and fibrin by fibrin-stabilizing factor (factor XIIIa). J Lab Clin Med 1975;85:574.

367. Mimuro J, Kimura S, Aoki N. Release of α_2-plasmin inhibitor from plasma fibrin clots by activated coagulation factor XIII: its effect on fibrinolysis. J Clin Invest 1986;77:1006.

368. Iwanaga S, Suzuki K, Hashimoto S. Bovine plasma cold-insoluble globulin: gross structure and function. Ann NY Acad Sci 1978;312: 56.

369. Fesus L, Metsis ML, Muszbek L, Koteliansky VE. Transglutaminase-sensitive glutamine residues of human plasma fibronectin revealed by studying its proteolytic fragments. Eur J Biochem 1986;154:371.

370. Procyk R, Adamson L, Block M, Blombäck B. Factor XIII catalyzed formation of fibrinogen–fibronectin oligomers: a thiol-enhanced process. Thromb Res 1985;40:833.

371. Okada M, Blombäck B, Chang MD, Horowitz B. Fibronectin and fibrin gel structure. J Biol Chem 1985;260:1811.

372. Barry EL, Mosher DF. Factor XIII crosslinking of fibronectin at cellular matrix assembly sites. J Biol Chem 1988;263:10464.

373. Hörmann H, Stemberger A, Jilek F. Interaction of a soluble fibroblast surfact protein with fibrin. Thromb Haemost 1978(Suppl);63:379.

374. Mosesson MW, Umflect RA. The cold-insoluble globulin of human plasma. J Biol Chem 1970;245:5728.

375. Carr ME Jr, Gabriel DA, McDonagh J. Influence of factor XIII and fibronectin on fiber size and density in thrombin-induced fibrin gels. J Lab Clin Med 1987;110:747.

376. Tamaki T, Aoki N. Crosslinking of α_2-plasmin inhibitor and fibronectin to fibrin. Biochim Biophys Acta 1981;661:280.

377. Hada M, Katu M, Ikematsu S, et al. Possible crosslinking of factor VIII related antigen to fibrin by factor XIII in delayed coagulation process. Thromb Res 1982;25:163.

378. Hada M, Kaminski M, Bockenstedt P, McDonagh J. Covalent cross-linking of von Willebrand factor to fibrin. Blood 1986;68:95.

379. Bockenstedt P, McDonagh J, Handin RI. Binding and covalent cross-linking of purified von Willebrand factor to native monomeric collagen. J Clin Invest 1986;78:551.

380. Francis AT, McDonagh J, Mann KG. Factor V is a substrate for the transamidase factor XIII. J Biol Chem 1986;261:9787.

381. Smith DB, Janmey PA, Herbert TJ, Lind SE. Quantitative measurement of plasma gelsolin and its incorporation into fibrin clots. J Lab Clin Med 1987;110:189.

382. Bale MD, Mosher DF. Thrombospondin is a substrate for blood coagulation factor XIIIa. Biochemistry 1986;25:5667.

383. Greenberg CS, Shuman MA. Specific binding of blood coagulation factor XIIIa to thrombin-stimulated platelets. J Biol Chem 1984;259: 14721.

384. Cohen I, Glaser T, Veis A, Bruner-Lorand J. Ca^{2+}-dependent cross-linking processes in human platelets. Biochim Biophys Acta 1981;676: 137.

385. Zacharski LR, Brown FE, Memoli VA, et al. Pathways of coagulation activation in situ in rheumatoid synovial tissue. Clin Immunol Immunopathol 1992;63:155–62.

386. Cohen I, Blankenberg TA, Borden D, et al. Factor XIIIa–catalyzed crosslinking of platelet and muscle actin: regulation by nucleotides. Biochim Biophys Acta 1980;628:365.

387. Prince CW, Dickie D, Krwmdieck CL. Osteopontin, a substrate for transglutaminase and factor XIII activity. Biochem Biophys Res Comm 1991;177:1205.

388. Jensen PH, Lorand L, Ebbesen P. Type-2 plasminogen-activator inhibitor is a substrate for trophoblast transglutaminase and factor XIIIa: transglutaminase-catalyzed cross-linking to cellular and extracellular structures. Eur J Biochem 1993;214:141.

389. Mosher DF. Crosslinking of fibronectin to collagenous proteins. Mol Cell Biochem 1984;58:63.

390. Asijee GM, Muszbek L, Kappelmayer J, et al. Platelet vinculin: a substrate of activated factor XIII. Biochim Biophys Acta 1988;954:303.

391. Skorstengaard K, Halkier T, Hojrup P, et al. Sequence location of a putative transglutaminase cross-linking site in human vitronectin. FEBS Lett 1990;262:269.

392. Hirahara K, Shinbo K, Takahashi M. Suppressive effect of human blood coagulation factor XIII on the vascular permeability induced by anti–guinea pig endothelial cell antiserum in guinea pigs. Thromb Res 1993;71:139.

393. Okamoto M, Yamamoto T, Matsubara S. Factor XIII-dependent generation of 5th complement component (C5)-derived monocyte chemotactic factor coinciding with plasma clotting. Biochim Biophys Acta 1992;1138:53.

394. Paye M, Nusgens B, Lapier CM. Factor XIII of blood coagulation decreases the susceptibility of collagen precursors to proteolysis. Biochim Biophys Acta 1991;1073:437.

395. Rupp C, Beck EA. Congenital dysfibrinogenemia. In: Beck EA, Furlan M, eds. Current problems in clinical biochemistry: variants of human fibrinogen. Toronto, Hans Huber, 1984;14:65.

396. Yoshida N, Okuma M, Hirata H, et al. Fibrinogen Kyoto II, a new congenitally abnormal molecule, characterized by the replacement of A alpha proline-18 by leucine. Blood 1991;78:149.

397. Soria J, Soria C, Samama M, et al. Fibrinogen Troyes- fibrinogen Metz: two new cases of congenital dysfibrinogenemia. Thromb Diath Haemorrh 1972;27:619.

398. Henschen A, Kehl M, Southan C. Abnormal Fibrinogen: Beziehung zwischen Dysfunction und Strukturfehler. In: Van de Loo J, Asbeck F, eds. Haemostase, Thrombophilie und Arteriesklerose. Stuttgart, Schattauer Verlag, 1982:661.

399. Laugen RH, Bithell TC. Fibrinogen Charlottesville: hereditary dysfibrinogenemia characterized by slow fibrinopeptide release and competitive inhibition of thrombin. Blood 1977(Suppl);50:273.

400. Blombäck M, Blombäck B, Mammen EF, Prasad AS. Fibrinogen "Detroit": a molecular defect in the N-terminal disulfide knot of human fibrinogen? Nature 1968;218:134.

401. Alving BM, Henschen A. Fibrinogen Giessen I: a congenital homozygously expressed dysfibrinogenemia with Aα 16 Arg $\rightarrow$ His substitution. Am J Hematol 1987;25:479.

402. Koopman J, Haverkate F, Grimbergen J, et al. Fibrinogen Marburg: a homozygous case of dysfibrinogenemia, lacking amino acids A alpha 461-610 (Lys 461 AAA $\rightarrow$ stop TAA). Blood 1992;80:1972.

403. Koopman J, Haverkate F, Grimbergen J, et al. Molecular basis for fibrinogen Dusart (A alpha 554 Arg $\rightarrow$ Cys) and its association with abnormal fibrin polymerization and thrombophilia.

403a. Lee MH, Tullis JL, Mankowski M, McDonagh L. Dysfibrinogenemia (fibrinogen Boston) associated with thrombosis: a possible mechanism of plasminogen binding to fibrin. Fibrinolysis 1992;6:70A.

404. Henry I, Uzan G, Wei D, et al. The genes coding for Aα, Bβ and γ chains of fibrinogen map to 4q2. Am J Hum Genet 1984;36:760.

405. Niwa K, Yaginuma A, Nakanishi M, et al. Fibrinogen Mitaka II: a hereditary dysfibrinogen with defective thrombin binding caused by an A alpha Glu-11 to Gly substitution. Blood 1993;82:3658.

406. Carr ME, Jr, Qureshi GD. The impact of delayed fibrinopeptide: a release on fibrin structure. J Biol Chem 1987;262:15568.

407. Wada Y, Niwa K, Maekawa, Asakura S, et al. A new type of congenital dysfibrinogen, fibrinogen Bremen, with an A alpha Gly-17 to Val substitution associated with hemorrhagic diathesis and delayed wound healing. Thromb Haemost 1993;70:397.

408. Uotani C, Miyata T, Kumabashiri I, et al. Fibrinogen Kanazawa: a congenital dysfibrinogenaemia with delayed polymerization having

a replacement of proline-18 by leucine in the A alpha-chain. Blood Coagul Fibrinolysis 1991;2:413.
409. Asakura S, Terukina S, Yamazumi K, et al. Fibrinogen Sapporo: dysfibrinogenemia characterized by the replacement of Aα arginine-16 by histidine resulting in the delayed release of fibrinopeptide A by thrombin. Nippon Ketsueki Gakkai Zasshi 1989;52:1094.
410. Matsuda M, Yoshida N, Terukina S, et al. Molecular abnormalities of fibrinogen: the present status of structure elucidation. In: Matsuda M, Iwanaga S, Takada A, Henschen A, eds. Fibrinogen 4. Current basic and clinical aspects. Amsterdam, Elsevier, 1990:139.
411. Dempfle CEH, Henschen A. Fibrinogen Mannheim I: identification of an Aα19Arg → Gly substitution in dysfibrinogenaemia associated with bleeding tendency. In: Matsuda M, Iwanaga S, Takada A, Henschen A, eds. Fibrinogen 4. Current basic and clinical aspects. Amsterdam, Elsevier, 1990:159.
412. Soria J, Soria C, Bertrand O, et al. Molecular basis for the Aα-chain substitutions in dysfibrinogenemia with a description of two new cases of the disorder: fibrinogen Amiens I and fibrinogen Amiens II. In: Lowe GDO, Douglas CD, Forbes CD, et al, eds. Fibrinogen 2. Biochemistry, physiology and clinical relevance. Amsterdam, Elsevier, 1987:57.
413. Seydewitz HH, Gram J, Bruhn HD. Fibrinogen Kiel: a congenital dysfibrinogenaemia with (A alpha-16 Arg → His) substitution characterized by HPLC without prior isolation of fibrinogen. Blood Coagul Fibrinolysis 1991;2:501.
414. Furlan M, Leupin L, Biasiutti FD, et al. Fibrinogen Bern III: a further case of hereditary fibrinogen variants with substitution A alpha 16 Arg → Cys. Schweiz Med Wochenschr 1991;121:1068.
415. Reber P, Furlan M, Beck EA. Fibrinogen "Bergamo I" (Aα-16 Arg → Cys): alternative methods for structure elucidation. In: Lane DA, Henschen A, Jasani MK, eds. Fibrinogen, fibrin formation and fibrinolysis. Berlin, Walter de Gruyter, 1986:103.
416. Galanakis D, Spitzer S, Scharrer I. Unusual A alpha 16 Arg → Cys dysfibrinogenaemic family: absence of normal A alpha-chains in fibrinogen from two of four heterozygous siblings. Blood Coagul Fibrinolysis 1993;4:67.
417. Lee MH, Tullis JL, Mankowski M, et al. Dysfibrinogenemia (fibrinogen Boston) associated with thrombosis: a possible mechanism of plasminogen binding to fibrin. Fibrinolysis 1992;6:70a.
418. Furlan M, Bogli C, Hofer A, et al. Fibrinogen Geneva, a new case of A alpha 16 Arg → Cys dysfibrinogenaemia. Blood Coagul Fibrinolysis 1990;1:139.
419. Lee MH, Kaczmarek E, Chin DT, et al. Fibrinogen Ledyard (AαArg16 → Cys): biochemical and physiologic characterizaiton. Blood 1991;78:1744.
420. Henschen A, Kehl M, Deutsch E. Novel structure elucidation strategy for genetically abnormal fibrinogens with incomplete fibrinopeptide release as applied to fibrinogen Schwarzack. Hoppe Seylers Z Physiol Chem 1983;364:1747.
421. Henschen A, Kehl M, Southan C, et al. Genetically abnormal fibrinogens: some current characterization strategies. In: Haverkate F, Henschen A, Nieuwenhuizen W, Straub PW, eds. Fibrinogen: structure, functional aspects, metabolism. Berlin, Walter de Gruyter, 1983: 125.
422. Borrell M, Vila L, Sola J, et al. Fibronigen Barcelona II: a new case of A alpha 16 Arg → His substitution. Haemostasis 1990;20:1.
423. Rupp C, Sievi R, Furlan M, et al. Fibrinogen Bern II: hereditary fibrinogen variant with amino acid substitution of arginine replaced by histidine in position 16 of the Aα-chain. Schweiz Med Wochenschr 1983;113:1460.
424. Soria J, Soria C, Samama M, et al. Study of ten cases of congenital dysfibrinogenemia. Clinical and molecular biological aspects. In: Henschen A, Hessel B, McDonagh J, et al, eds. Fibrinogen: structural variants and interactions. Berlin, Walter de Gruyter, 1985:165.
425. Galanakis DK, Hultin M. Fibrinogen Stony Brook II: partial characterization of a heterozygously transmitted peptide A anomaly. Blood Coagul Fibrinolysis 1990;1:567.
426. Southan C, Henschen A, Lane DA. Fibrinogens Sydney I and II: a kinetic study of (His-16) FPA Cleavage and its effect of FPB cleavage. In: Henschen A, Hessel B, McDonagh J, Saldeen T, eds. Fibrinogen: structural variants and interactions. Berlin, Walter de Gruyter, 1985: 125.
427. Bogli C, Cofrancesco E, Cortellaro M, et al. Fibrinogen Milano VI: a heterozygous dysfibrinogenemia (A alpha 16 Arg → His) with bleeding tendency.
428. Bogli C, Hofer A, Baudo F, et al. Fibrinogen Milano IV another case of congenital dysfibrinogenemia with an abnormal fibrinopeptide A release (A alpha 16 Arg → His). Haemostasis 1992;22:7.
429. Yamazumi K, Terukina S, Matsuda M, et al. Fibrinogen Osaka IV: a congenital dysfibrinogenemia found in a patient originally reported in relation to surgery, now defined to have an A alpha arginine-16 to histidine substitution. Surg Today 1993;23:45.
430. Ebert RF, Schreiber WE, Bell WR. Fibrinogen Seattle II: congenital dysfibrinogenemia with an Arg (Aα-16) → His substitution. Thromb Res 1986;43:17.
431. Southan C, Thompson E, Lane DA. Direct analysis of plasma fibrinogen-derived fibrinopeptides by high-performance liquid chromatography: investigation of the nine congenital fibrinogen abnormalities. Br J Haematol 1987;65:469.
432. Ebert RF. Index of variant human fibrinogens. Boca Raton, CRC Press, 1991:1.
433. Crum E. Abnormal fibrinogens. In: Ogston D, Bennett B, eds. Haemostasis: biochemistry, physiology and pathology. London, Wiley, 1977:424.
434. Southan C, Henschen A, Lottspeich F. The search for molecular defects in abnormal fibrinogens. In: Henschen A, Graeff H, Lottspeich F, eds. Fibrinogen: recent biochemical and medical aspects. Berlin, Walter de Gruyter, 1982:153.
435. Krause WH, Heene DL, Lasch HG. Congenital dysfibrinogenemia (fibrinogen Giessen). Thromb Diath Haemorrh 1973;29:547.
436. Higgins DL, Shafer JA. Fibrinogen Petosky: a dysfibrinogenemia characterized by replacement of Arg Aα 16 by a histidyl residue: evidence for thrombin-catalyzed hydrolysis at a histidyl residue. J Biol Chem 1981;256:12013.
437. Kehl M, Lottspeich F, Henschen A. Genetically abnormal fibrinogens releasing abnormal fibrinopeptides as characterized by high-performance liquid chromatography. In: Haverkate F, Henschen A, Nieuwenhuizen W, Straub PW, eds. Fibrinogen: structure, functional aspects, metabolism. Berlin, Walter de Gruyter, 1983:183.
438. Siebenlist KR, Prchal JT, Mosesson MW. Fibrinogen Birmingham: a heterozygous dysfibrinogenemia (Aα 16 Arg → His) containing heterozygous molecules. Blood 1988;71:613.
439. Galanakis DK, Henschen A, Keeling M, et al. Fibrinogen Louisville: an Aα 16 Arg → His defect that forms no hybrid molecules in heterozygous individuals and inhibits aggregation of normal fibrin monomers. Ann NY Acad Sci 1983;408:644.
440. Soria J, Soria C, Samama M, et al. Detection of fibrinogen abnormality in dysfibrinogenemia: special report on fibrinogen Metz characterized by an amino acid substitution located at the peptide bond cleaved by thrombin. In: Henschen A, Graeff H, Lottspeich F, eds. Fibrinogen: recent biochemical and medical aspects. Berlin, Walter de Gruyter, 1982:129.
441. Matsuda M, Terukina S, Miyata T, Iwanaga S. Defective release of fibrinopeptide A due to substitution of Aα arginine-16 by cysteine in two abnormal fibrinogens Kawaguchi and Osaka. In: Müller-Berghaus G, Scheefers-Borchel U, et al, eds. Fibrinogen and its derivatives: biochemistry, physiology and pathophysiology. Proceedings of the Fibrinogen Workshop. New York, Elsevier, 1972;27:619.
442. Miyata T, Terukina S, Matsuda M, et al. Fibrinogens Kawaguchi and Osaka: an amino acid substitution of Aα arginine to cysteine which forms an extra interchain disulfide between the two Aα chains. J Biochem (Tokyo) 1987;102:93.
443. Mosesson MW, Siebenlist KR, DiOrio JP, et al. Evidence that proximal NH_2-terminal portions of fibrinogen Metz (Aα 16 Arg → Cys) Aα chains are oriented in the same direction. In: Müller-Berghaus G, Scheefers-Borchel U, et al, eds. Fibrinogen and its derivatives: biochemistry, physiology and pathophysiology. Proceedings of the Fibrinogen Workshop. New York, Elsevier, 1986:3.
444. Denninger MH, Finlayson JS, Reamer LA, et al. Congenital dysfibrinogenemia: fibrinogen Lille. Thromb Res 1978;13:453.
445. Morris S, Denninger MH, Finlayson JS, Menache D. Fibrinogen Lille: Aα 7 Asp → Asn. Thromb Haemost 1981;46:104.
446. Mammen EF, Prasad AS, Barnhart MI, Au CC. Congenital dysfibrinogenemia: fibrinogen Detroit. J Clin Invest 1969;48:235.
447. Kudryk B, Blombäck B, Blombäck M. Fibrinogen Detroit: an abnormal fibrinogen with non-functional NH_2-terminal polymerization domain. Thromb Res 1976;9:25.
448. Koopman J, Haverkate F, Lord ST, et al. Molecular basis of fibrinogen Naples associated with defective thrombin binding and thrombophilia: homozygous substitution of B beta 68 Ala → Thr. J Clin Invest 1992;90: 238.
449. Pirkle H, Kaudewitz H, Henschen A, et al. Substitution of Bβ-14 arginine by cyst(e)ine in fibrinogen Seattle I. In: Lowe GDO, Douglas JT, Forbes CD, Henschen A, eds. Fibrinogen 2. Biochemistry, physiology and clinical relevance. Amsterdam, Elsevier, 1987:49.
450. Kaudewitz H, Henschen A, Soria A, et al. The molecular defect of the genetically abnormal fibrinogen Christchurch II. In: Muller-Berghaus G, Scheefers-Borchel V, Selmayr E, Henschen A, eds. Fibrinogen and its derivatives. Amsterdam, Elsevier, 1986:31.
451. Koopman J, Haverkate F, Grimbergen J, et al. Abnormal fibrinogens IJmuiden (B beta Arg 14 → Cys) and Nijmegen (B beta Arg 44 → Cys) form disulfide-linked fibrinogen-albumin complexes. Proc Natl Acad Sci USA 1992;89:3478.
452. Yoshida N, Wada H, Morita K, et al. A new congenital abnormal fibrinogen Ise characterized by the replacement of B beta glycine-15 cystine. Blood 1991;77:1958.
453. Liu CY, Wallen P, Handley DA. Fibrinogen New York I: the structural, functional, and genetic defects and an hypothesis of the role of fibrin in the regulation of coagulation and fibrinolysis. In: Lane DA, Henschen A, Jasani MK, eds. Fibrinogen: fibrin formation and fibrinolysis. Berlin, Walter de Gruyter, 1986:79.
454. Maekawa H, Yamazumi K, Muramatsu W, et al. Fibrinogen Lima: a homozygous dysfibrinogen with an A alpha-arginine-141 to serine substitution associated with extra N-glycosylation at A alpha-

asparagine-130: impaired fibrin gel formation but normal fibrin-facilitated plasminogen activation catalyzed by tissue-type plasminogen activator. J Clin Invest 1992;90:67.
456. Arocha-Pinango CL, Rodriguez S, Nagy H, et al. Fibrinogen Lima. A new dysfibrinogenaemia with a high-molecular-weight alpha-chain and effective polymerization. Blood Coagul Fibrinolysis 1990;1:561.
457. Personal communication, S. Lord
458. Collet JP, Soria J, Mirshahi M, et al. Dusart syndrome: a new concept of the relationship between fibrin clot architecture and fibrin clot degradability: hypofibrinolysis related to an abnormal clot structure. Blood 1993:82:2462.
459. Koopman J, Haverkate F, Grimbergen J, et al. Molecular basis for fibrinogen Dusart (A alpha 554 Arg → Cys) and its association with abnormal fibrin polymerization and thrombophilia. J Clin Invest 1993;91:1637.
460. Henschen A, Kehl M, Southan C, et al. Genetically abnormal fibrinogens—some current characterization strategies. In: Haverkate F, Henschen A, Nieuwenhuizen W, Straub PW, eds. Fibrinogen: structure, functional aspects, metabolism. Berlin, Walter de Gruyter, 1983: 125.
461. Liu CY, Koehn JA, Morgan FJ. Characterization of fibrinogen New York I. A dysfunctional fibrinogen with a deletion of Bβ (9-72) corresponding exactly to exon 2 of the gene. J Biol Chem 1985;260:4390: 395A.
462. Lane DA, Southan C, Ireland H, et al. Delayed release of an abnormal fibrinopeptide A from fibrinogen Manchester. Br J Haematol 1983;53: 587.
463. Haverkate F, Timan G, Soria J, et al. Studies on the structure of the fragment D moiety of abnormal fibrinogens: influence of calcium ions. Thromb Res 1978;13:689.
464. Laudano AP, Cottrell BA, Doolittle RF. Synthetic peptides modeled on fibrin polymerization sites. Ann NY Acad Sci 1983;408:315.
465. Liu CY, Koehn JA, Morgan FJ. Characterization of fibrinogen New York I: a dysfunctional fibrinogen with a deletion of Bβ(9–72) corresponding exactly to exon 2 of the gene. J Biol Chem 1985;260:4390.
466. Liu CY, Morgan FJ. Fibrinogen New York I: a deletion in the Bβ chain corresponding to exon 2 of the gene. Circulation 1984;70:II-351.
467. Blombäck B, Hessel B, Hogg D. Disulfide bridges in NH_2-terminal part of human fibrinogen. Thromb Res 1976;8:639.
468. Liu CY, Wallen P. Fibrinogen New York I: defective fibrin potentiation of plasminogen activation by tissue plasminogen activator. Circulation 1983;70:II-366.
469. Kudryk BJ, Collen D, Woods KR, Blombäck B. Evidence for localization of polymerization sites in fibrinogen. J Biol Chem 1974;249:3322.
470. Haverkate F, Timan G, Nieuwenhuizen W. Anticlotting properties of fragments D from human fibrinogen and fibrin. Eur J Clin Invest 1979;9: 253.
471. Nieuwenhuizen W, Gravesen M. Anticoagulant and calcium-binding properties high molecular weight derivatives of human fibrinogen produced by plasmin (fragments X). Biochim Biophys Acta 1981;668: 81.
472. Terukina S, Matsuda M, Hirata H, et al. Substitution of γ Arg-275 by Cys in an abnormal fibrinogen, "fibrinogen Osaka II". Evidence for a unique solitary cystine structure at the mutation site. J Biol Chem 1988;263:13579.
473. Yoshida N, Ota K, Moroi M, Matsuda M. An apparently higher molecular weight in a new congenital abnormal fibrinogen Tochigi characterized by the replacement of γ arginine-275 by cysteine. Blood 1988;71:480.
474. Yamazumi K, Terukina S, Onohara S, Matsuda M. Normal plasmic cleavage of the γ-chain variant of "fibrinogen Saga" with an Arg-275 to His substitution. Thromb Haemost 1988;60:476.
475. Grailhe P, Boyer-Neumann C, Haverkate F, et al. The mutation in fibrinogen Bicêtre II (gamma Asn 308 → Lys) does not affect the binding of t-PA and plasminogen to fibrin. Blood Coagul Fibrinolysis 1993;4P: 679.
476. Schmelzer CH, Ebert RF, Bell WR. Fibrinogen Baltimore IV: congenital dysfibrinogenemia with a γ(275) (Arg → Cys) substitution.
477. Siebenlist KR, Mosesson MW, DiOrio JP, et al. The polymerization of fibrin prepared from fibrinogen Haifa (γ_{275} Arg → His). Thromb Haemost 1989;62:875.
478. Bantia S, Mane SM, Bell WR, et al. Fibrinogen Baltimore I: polymerization defect associated with a gamma 292Gly → Val (GGC → GTC) mutation. Blood 1990;76:2279.
479. Koopman J, Haverkate F, Briet E, et al. A congenitally abnormal fibrinogen (Vlissingen) with a 6-base deletion in the gamma-chain gene, causing defective calcium binding an impaired fibrin polymerization. J Biol Chem 1991;266:13256.
480. Matsuda M, Nakamikawa C, Bab M, et al. Fibrinogen Tokyo II: And abnormal fibrinogen with an impaired polymerization site on the aligned DD domain of fibrin molecules. In: Henschen A, Hessel B, McDonagh J, Saldeen T, eds. Fibrinogen: structural variants and interactions. Berlin, Walter de Gruyter, 1985:213.
481. Steinmann C, Reber P, Jungo M, et al. Fibrinogen Bern I: substitution gamma 337 Asn → Lys is responsible for defective fibrin monomer polymerization. Blood 1993;82:2104.
482. Rosenberg JB, Newman PJ, Mosesson MW, et al. Paris I dysfibrinogenemia: a point mutation in intron 8 results in insertion of a 15 amino acid sequence in the fibrinogen gamma-chain. Thromb Haemost 1993;69:217.
483. Yoshida N, Hirata H, Morigami Y, et al. Characterization of an abnormal fibrinogen Osaka V with the replacement of gamma-arginine 375 by glycine: the lack of high affinity calcium binding to D-domains and the lack of protective effect of calcium on fibrinolysis. J Biol Chem 1992;267:2753.
484. Yoshida N, Terukina S, Okuma M, et al. Characterization of apparently lower molecular weight γ-chain variant in fibrinogen Kyoto I. J Biol Chem 1988;263:13848.
485. Wickelman G. Kongenitale Dysfibrinogenamie: Bericht über eine neue Familie (Fibrinogen "Wiesbaden"). Thromb Diath Haemorrh 1973(Suppl);55:345.
486. Samori T, Yatabe M, Ukita M, et al. A new type of congenital dysfibrinogenemia (fibrinogen Tokyo) with defective stabilization of fibrin polymers. Thromb Diath Haemorrh 1975;35:329.
487. Menache D. Constitutional and familial abnormal fibrinogen. Thromb Diath Haemorrh 1984(Suppl);10:173.
488. Budzynski AZ, Marder VJ, Menache D, Guillin MC. Defect in the γ polypeptide chain of congenital abnormal fibrinogen Paris I. Nature 1974;252:66.
489. Mosesson MW, Denninger MH, Menache D. Hydrolysis of fibrinogen Paris I by plasmin. Thromb Res 1976;9:115.
490. Budzynski AZ, Marder VJ. Plasmic degradation of fibrinogen Paris I. J Lab Clin Med 1976;88:817.
491. Finlayson JS, Reamer LA, Mosesson MW, Menache D. Fibrinopeptide release from fibrinogen Paris I. Thromb Res 1980;17:577.
492. Lane D, Allen A, Markwick J, et al. Carbohydrate in abnormal fibrinogens. In: Henschen A, Graeff H, Lottspeich F, eds. Fibrinogen: recent biochemical and medical aspects. Berlin, Walter de Gruyter, 1982:183.
493. Soria J, Soria C, Caen JP. A new type of congenital dysfibrinogenemia with defective fibrin lysis, Dusard syndrome: possible relation to thrombosis. Br Haematol 1983;53:575.
494. Lijnen HR, Soria J, Soria C, et al. Dysfibrinogenemia (fibrinogen Dusard) associated with impaired fibrin-enhancing plasminogen activation. Thromb Haemost 1984;51:108.
495. Carrell N, Gabriel DM, Carr ME, et al. Hereditary dysfibrinogenemia in a patient with thrombotic disease. Blood 1983;62:439.
496. Werder E. Kongenitale Afibrinogenamie. Helv Paediatr Acta 1963;118: 208.
497. Yamagata S, Mori K, Kayaba T, et al. A case of congenital afibrinogenemia and review of reported cases in Japan. J Exp Med 1968;96: 15.
498. Egbring R, Andrassy K, Egli H, Meyer-Lindenberg J. Diagnostische und therapeutische Probleme bei kongenitale Afibrinogenamie. Blut 1971;22:175.
499. Hahn L, Lunberg PA, Teger-Nilsson AC. Congenital hypofibrinogenaemia and recurrent abortion. Br J Obstet Gynaecol 1978;85:790.
500. Uzan G, Courtois G, Besmond C, et al. Analysis of fibrinogen genes in patients with congenital afibrinogenemia. Biochem Biophys Res Commun 1984;120:376.
501. Wehinger H, Klinge O, Alexandrakis E, et al. Hereditary hypofibrinogenemia with fibrinogen storage in the liver. Eur J Pediatr 1983; 141:109.
502. Crabtree GR, Kant JA. Organization of the rat γ-fibrinogen gene: alternative mRNA splice patterns produce the γA and the γB (γ') chains of fibrinogen. Cell 1982;31:159.
503. Gross R, Schwick G, Lang N, et al. Untersuchungen einer angeborenen Afibrinogenamie (zur Rolle der Blutgerinnung bei der Blutstillung). Klin Wochenscher 1963;41:695.
504. Jandrot-Perrus M, Mosesson MW, Denninger MH, Menache D. Studies on platelet fibrinogen from a subject with a congenital plasma fibrinogen abnormality (fibrinogen Paris I). Blood 1979;54:1109.
505. Francis JL, Armstrong DJ. Acquired dysfibrinogenemia in liver disease. J Clin Pathol 1982;35:667.
506. Clark RD, Gazzard BG, Lewis ML, et al. Fibrinogen metabolism in acute hepatitis and active chronic hepatitis. Br J Haematol 1975;30: 95.
507. Weinstein MJ, Deykin D. Quantitative abnormality of an Aα chain molecular weight form in the fibrinogen of cirrhotic patients. Br J Haematol 1978;40:617.
508. Lane DA, Scully MF, Thomas DP, et al. Acquired dysfibrinogenemia in acute and chronic liver disease. Br J Haematol 1977;35:301.
509. Klingemann HG, Egbring R, Havemann K. Structure of fibrin and fibrin monomer in renal and hepatic failure. Klin Wochenschr 1980;58: 533.
510. Martinez J, MacDonald KA, Palascal JE. The role of sialic acid in the dysfibrinogenemia associated with liver disease: distribution of sialic acid on the constituent chains. Blood 1983;61:1196.
511. Francis JL, Armstrong DJ. Sialic acid and sialyltransferase in the pathogenesis of acquired dysfibrinogenemia. In: Haverkate F, Henschen A, Nieuwenhuizen W, Straub PW, eds. Fibrinogen: structure, functional aspects, metabolism. Berlin, Walter de Gruyter, 1982: 195.

512. Martinez J, Keane PM, Gilmon PB, Palascak JE. The abnormal carbohydrate composition of the dysfibrinogenemia associated with liver disease. Ann NY Acad Sci 1983;408:388.
513. Menache D. Congenital fibrinogen abnormalities. Ann NY Acad Sci 1983;408:121.
514. Gralnick HR, Coller BS, Fratantoni JC, Martinez J. Fibrinogen Bethesda III: a hypodysfibrinogenemia. Blood 1979;53:28.
515. Carrell N, McDonagh J. Functional defects in abnormal fibrinogens. In: Henschen A, Hessel B, McDonagh J, Saldeen T, eds. Fibrinogen: structural variants and interaction. Berlin, Walter de Gruyter, 1985: 155.
516. Thorson LI, Stormoken H, Brosstad F, et al. A dysfibrinogenemia, Oslo I, acting as a more efficient cofactor in ADP stimulated platelet aggregation than normal fibrinogen. Thromb Haemost 1983;50:202.
517. Liu CY, Nossel HL, Kaplan KL. Defective thrombin binding by an abnormal fibrin associated with recurrent thrombosis. Thromb Haemost 1979;42:79.
518. Soria J, Soria C, Samama M, Caen JP. Study of 10 cases of congenital dysfibrinogenemia, clinical and molecular biological aspects. Thromb Haemost 1983;50:415.
519. Haverkate F, Mannucci P, d'Angelo A, et al. An abnormal fibrinogen (Milano II) with a defective thrombin binding and thrombin clotting time, but with normal reptilase and arvin times. Thromb Haemost 1983;50:337.
520. Caen JP, Soria J, Soria C. Structural anomaly of the fibrin clot with reduction of lys–plasminogen binding as a cause of familial thrombosis. C R Seances Acad Sci 1982;294:695.
521. Forman WB, Ratnoff OB, Boyer MH. An inherited qualitative abnormality in plasma fibrinogen: fibrinogen Cleveland. J Clin Med 1968;72: 455.
522. Brosstad F, Teige B, Olaisen B, et al. Two-dimensional electrophoretic characterization (iso-dalt) of fibrinogen and fibrin subunit chains from four different genetic dysfibrinogen variants. In: Haverkate F, Henschen A, Nieuwenhuizen W, Straub PW, eds. Fibrinogen: structure, functional aspects, metabolism. Berlin, Walter de Gruyter, 1983: 145.
523. Gralnick HR, Givelber HM, Shainoff JR, Finlayson JS. Fibrinogen Bethesda: a congenital dysfibrinogenemia with delayed fibrinopeptide release. J Clin Invest 1971;50:1819.
524. Latallo ZS, Fletcher AP, Alkjaersig N, Sherry S. Influence of pH, ionic strength, neutral ions, and thrombin on fibrin polymerization. Am J Physiol 1962;202:675.
525. Carr ME, Blatt PM, Roberts HR, et al. Detection of an abnormal plasma clot structure by a simple rigidity assay. Thromb Haemost 1979;42: 965.
526. Southan C. The elucidation of molecular defects in congenital dysfibrinogenemia. In: Francis JL, ed. Fibrinogen, fibrin stabilisation, and fibrinolysis: clinical, biochemical and laboratory aspects. Chichester, England, Ellis Horwood, 1988:100.
527. Bove JR. Fibrinogen: is the benefit worth the risk? Transfusion 1978;18: 129.
528. Gitlin D, Borges WH. Studies on the metabolism of fibrinogen in two patients with congenital afibrinogenemia. Blood 1953;8:697.
529. Mason DY, Ingram GIC. Management of the hereditary coagulation disorders. Semin Hematol 1971;8:158.
530. Tytgat GN, Collen D, Vermylen J. Metabolism and distribution of fibrinogen. II. Fibrinogen turnover in polycythemia, thrombocytosis, haemophilia A, congenital afibrinogenemia and during streptokinase therapy. Br J Haematol 1972;22:701.
531. Mammen EF. Congenital coagulation disorders: fibrinogen abnormalities. Semin Thromb Hemost 1983;9:1.
532. Bronnimann R. Kongenitale Afibrinogenamie. Acta Haematol 1954;11: 40.
533. de Vries A, Rosenberg T, Kochwa S, Boss JH. Precipitating antifibrinogen antibody appearing after fibrinogen infusions in a patient with congenital afibrinogenemia. Am J Med 1961;30:486.
534. Sasahara AA, Kakkar VV, Hull RD, Thomas DP. Treatment of venous thromboembolism. In: Bloom AL, Thomas DP, eds. Haemostasis and thrombosis, ed 2. Edinburgh, Churchill Livingstone, 1987:820.
535. Rijken DC, Collen D. Purification and characterization of the plasminogen activator secreted by human melanoma cells in culture. J Biol Chem 1981;256:7035.
536. Pennica D, Holmes WE, Kohr WJ, et al. Cloning and expression of human tissue-type plasminogen activator cDNA in *E. coli*. Nature 1983;301:214.
537. Collen D, Stassen JM, Marafino BJ, et al. Biological properties of human tissue-type plasminogen activator obtained by expression of recombinant DNA in mammalian cells. J Pharmacol Exp Ther 1984;231: 146.
538. Weimar W, Stibbe J, Van Seyen A, et al. Specific lysis of iliofemoral thrombus by administration of extrinsic (tissue-type) plasminogen activator. Lancet 1981;2:1081.
539. TIMI study group. Special report: the thrombolysis in myocardial infarction (TIMI) trial. N Engl J Med 1985;312:932.
540. Fretto LJ, Ferguson EW, Steinman HM, McKee PA. Localization of the α-chain crosslinking acceptor sites of human fibrin. J Biol Chem 1978;253:2184.
541. Mosher DF. Crosslinking of cold-insoluble globulin by fibrin-stabilizing factor. J Biol Chem 1975;250:6614.
542. Shainoff JR, Page LH. Deposition of modified fibrinogen within the aortic intima. Atherosclerosis 1972;16:287.
543. Shen L, Lorand L. Contribution of fibrin stabilization to clot strength. J Clin Invest 1983;71:1336.
544. Shen LL, McDonagh RP, McDonagh J, Hermans J. Early events in the plasmin digestion of fibrinogen and fibrin: effects of plasmin on fibrin polymerization. J Biol Chem 1977;252:6184.
545. Aoki N, Saito H, Kamiya T, et al. Congenital deficiency of α_2-plasmin inhibitor associated with severe hemorrhagic tendency. J Clin Invest 1979;63:877.
546. Sakata Y, Aoki N. Significance of crosslinking of α_2-plasmin inhibitor to fibrin in inhibition of fibrinolysis and in hemostasis. J Clin Invest 1982;69:536.
547. Sakata Y, Mimuro J, Aoki N. Differential binding of plasmin to crosslinked and noncrosslinked fibrins: its significance in hemostatic defect in factor XIII–deficiency. Blood 1984;63:1393.
548. Grinnell F. Fibronectin and wound healing. J Cell Biol 1984;26:107.
549. Ueyama M, Urayama T. The role of factor XIII in fibroblast proliferation. Jpn J Exp Med 1978;48:135.
550. Lanir N, Ciano PS, Van De Water L, et al. Macrophage migration in fibrin gel matrices: effects of clotting factor XIII, fibronectin and glycosaminoglycan content on cell migration. J Immunol 1988;140:2340.
551. Mishima Y, Nagao F, Ishibiki K, et al. Factor XIII in the treatment of postoperative refractory wound healing disorders: results of a controlled study. Chirurgie 1984;55:803.
552. Bruhn HD, Pohl J. Growth regulation of fibroblasts by thrombin, factor XIII and fibronectin. Klin Wochenschr 1981;59:145.
553. Duckert F. Documentation of the plasma factor XIII deficiency in man. Ann NY Acad Sci 1972;202:190.
554. McDonagh J, McDonagh RP Jr, Duckert F. Genetic aspects of factor XIII deficiency. Ann Hum Genet 1971;35:195.
555. Board PG. Genetic polymorphism of the A subunit of human coagulation factor XIII. Am J Hum Genet 1979;31:116.
556. Board PG. Genetic polymorphism of the B subunit of human coagulation factor XIII. Am J Hum Genet 1980;32:348.
557. Dykes DD, Polesky HF. The use of the serum protein factor XIIIB (FXIIIB) in parentage testing. Am J Clin Pathol 1987;88:627.
558. Skrzynia C, Reisner HM, McDonagh J. Characterization of the catalytic subunit of factor XIII by radioimmunoassay. Blood 1982;60:1089.
559. Ikematsu S, McDonagh RP, Reisner HM, et al. Immunochemical studies of human factor XIII: radioimmunoassay for the carrier subunit of the zymogen. J Lab Clin Med 1981;97:662.
560. Capellato MG, Lazzaro AR, Marafioti F, et al. A new family with congenital factor XIII deficiency showing a deficit of both subunit A and B: type I factor XIII deficiency. Haemotologia (Budap) 1987;20: 179.
561. Miloszewski KJA, Losowsky MS. Fibrin stabilisation and factor XIII–deficiency. In: Francis JL, ed. Fibrinogen, fibrin stabilisation and fibrinolysis. Chichester, England, Ellis Horwood, 1988:175.
562. Abbondanzo SL, Gootenberg JE, Lofts RS, McPherson RA. Intracranial hemorrhage in congenital deficiency of factor XIII. Am J Pediatr Hematol Oncol 1988;10:65.
563. Fisher S, Rikover M, Naor S. Factor 13 deficiency with severe hemorrhagic diathesis. Blood 1966;28:34.
564. Rodeghiero F, Castaman GC, Di Bona E, et al. Successful pregnancy in a woman with congenital factor XIII–deficiency treated with substitutive therapy: report of a second case. Blut 1987;55:45.
565. Beck E, Duckert F, Ernst M. The influence of fibrin-stabilizing factor on the growth of fibroblasts in vitro and wound healing. Thromb Diath Haemorrh 1961;6:485.
566. Claes L, Burri C, Gengross H, Mutschler W. Bone healing stimulated by plasma factor XIII: osteotomy experiments in sheep. Acta Orthop Scand 1985;56:57.
567. Karges HE, Clemens R. Factor XIII: enzymatic and clinical aspects. Behring Inst Mitt 1988;82:43.
568. McDonagh J. Structure and function of factor XIII. In: Colman RW, Hirsh J, Marden VJ, Salzman EW, eds. Hemostasis and thrombosis, ed 2. Philadelphia, JB Lippincott, 1987:289.
569. Winkelman L, Sims GE, Haddon ME, et al. A pasteurised concentrate of human plasma factor XIII for therapeutic use. Thromb Haemost 1986;55:402.
570. Daly HM, Haddon ME. Clinical experience with a pasteurised human plasma concentrate in factor XIII–deficiency. Thromb Haemost 1988;59:171.
571. Suzuki H, Kaneda T. Tooth extraction in two patients who had congenital deficiency of factor XIII. J Oral Maxillofac Surg 1985;43:221.
572. Francis JL. Detection and measurement of factor XIII. In: Francis JL, ed. Fibrinogen, fibrin stabilisation, and fibrinolysis. Chichester, England, Ellis Horwood, 1988:203.
573. Lorand L, Gotoh T. Fibrinoligase: the fibrin stabilizing factor system. Methods Enzymol 1970;19:770.
574. Nishida Y, Ikematsu S, Fukutake K, et al. A new, rapid and simple assay for factor XIII activity using dansylcadaverine incorporation and gel filtration. Thromb Res 1984;36:123.
575. Miraglia CC, Greenberg CS. Measurement of blood coagulation factor

XIIIa formation in plasma containing glycyl-L-prolyl-L-arginyl-L-proline. Anal Biochem 1985;144:165.
576. Stenberg P, Stenflo J. A rapid and specific fluorescent activity staining procedure for transamidating enzymes. Anal Biochem 1979;93:445.
577. Godal HC, Gravem K, Brosstad F, Nyvold N. Quantitation of factor XIII by SDS polyacrylamide gel electrophoresis. Thromb Res 1984;35: 577.
578. Muszbek L, Polgar J, Fesus L. Kinetic determination of blood coagulation factor XIII in plasma. Clin Chem 1985;31:35.
579. Ando Y, Imamura S, Yamagata Y, et al. High performance liquid chromatographic assay of transglutaminase and its application to the purification of human erythrocyte transglutaminase and platelet factor XIII. J Biochem (Tokyo) 1987;101:1331.
580. Lee KN, Birckbichler PJ, Patterson MK Jr. Colorimetric assay of blood coagulation factor XIII in plasma. Clin Chem 1988;34:906.
581. Laurell CB. Quantitative estimation of proteins by electrophoresis in agarose gel containing antibodies. Anal Biochem 1966;15:45.
582. Velasco PT, Karush F, Lorand L. Transamidating activities of factor XIIIa and of transglutaminases, measured by an ELISA procedure. Biochem Biophys Res Commun 1988;152:505.
583. Ballerini G, Guerra S, Rodeghiero F, Castaman G. A contribution to the pathology of acquired plasma factor XIII–deficiency. Semin Thromb Hemost 1985;11:357.
584. Adany R, Belkin A, Vasilevskaya T, Muszbek L. Identification of blood coagulation factor XIII in human peritoneal macrophages. Eur J Cell Biol 1985;38:171.
585. Duswald KH, Jochum M, Schramm W, Fritz H. Released granulocytic elastase: an indicator of pathobiochemical alterations in septicemia after abdominal surgery. Surgery 1985;98:892.
586. Galloway MJ, Mackie MJ, McVerry BA. Elastase-α 1 antitrypsin complexes in acute leukaemia. Thromb Res 1985;38:311.
587. Anders O, Gross EW, Ernst B, Konrad H. Detection of factor XIII–deficiency in acute leukemia with resonance thrombography. Folia Haematol (Leipz) 1987;114:670.
588. Rasche H, Haghou F, Gaus W, et al. Blutgerinnungs Faktor-XIII Substitution bei akunter Leu Kämie. Dtsch Med Wochenschr 1985;107: 1882.
589. Kloczko J, Wereszczynska U, Wojtukiewicz M, et al. Fibrin stabilization, factor XIII transamidase activity and subunits "A" and "B" concentration in plasma of patients with liver cirrhosis. Folia Haematol (Leipz) 1986;113:539.
590. Rus HG, Cucuianu M, Manasia M, et al. Plasma fibronectin and factor XIII in nephrotic syndrome. Med Interne 1987;25:105.
591. Kloczko J, Wojtukiewicz M, Bielawiec, Zuch A. Alterations of haemostasis parameters with special reference to fibrin stabilization, factor XIII and fibronectin in patients with obliterative atherosclerosis. Thromb Res 1988;51:575.
592. Kloczko J, Wojtukiewicz M, Bielawiec, et al. Plasma factor XIII and some other haemostasis parameters in patients with diabetic angiopathy. Acta Haematol 1986;76:81.
593. Kamitsuji H, Tani K, Yasui M, et al. Activity of blood coagulation factor XIII as a prognostic indicator in patients with Henoch-Schönlein purpura: efficacy of factor XIII substitution. Eur J Pediatr 1987;146: 519.
594. Henriksson P, Hender U, Nilsson IM. Factor XIII (fibrin stabilising factor) in Henoch-Schönlein's purpura. Acta Paediatr Scand 1977;66: 273.
595. Guillevin L, Chouvet B, Mery C, et al. Treatment of progressive systemic sclerosis using factor XIII. Pharmatherapeutica 1985;4:76.
596. Grivoux M, Pieron R. Brochiolo-alveolar carcinoma complicating systemic scleroderma under long-term treatment with factor XIII. Rev Pneumol Clin 1987;43:102.
597. Lorenz R, Heinmüller M, Classen M, et al. Substitution of factor XIII: a therapeutic approach to ulcerative colitis. Haemostasis 1991; 21:5.
598. Carrell M, McDonagh J. Fibrinogen Chapel Hill II: defective in reactions with thrombin, factor XIIIa, and plasmin. Br J Haematol 1982;52:35.
599. Lorand L, Losowsky MS, Miloszewski KJM. Human factor XIII: fibrin stabilizing factor. In: Spaet TH, ed. Progress in hemostasis and thrombosis, vol 5. New York, Grune & Stratton, 1980:245.
600. Lorand L, Velasco PT, Rinne JR, et al. Autoimmune antibody (IgG Kansas) against the fibrin stabilizing factor (factor XIII) system. Proc Natl Acad Sci USA 1988;85:232.
601. Fukue H, Anderson K, McPhedran P, Clyne, et al. A unique factor XIII inhibitor to a fibrin-binding site on factor XIIIA. Blood 1992;79: 65.
602. Lorand L, Urayama T, De Kiewiet JWC, Nossel HL. Diagnostic and genetic studies on fibrin-stabilizing factor with a new assay based on amine incorporation. J Clin Invest 1969;48:1054.
603. Henriksson P, McDonagh J, Villa M. Type I autoimmune inhibitor of factor XIII in a patient with congenital factor XIII deficiency. Thromb Haemost 1983;50:272.
604. Lorand L, Jacobsen A. Isonicotinic acid hydrazide as an inhibitor of transpeptidation: relevance for blood coagulation. Nature 1967;216: 508.

Blood: Principles and Practice of Hematology,
edited by Robert I. Handin, Samuel E. Lux, and Thomas P. Stossel.
J.B. Lippincott Company, Philadelphia © 1995.

42

Fibrinolytic System and Its Disorders

Désire Collen
H.R. Lijnen
Marc Verstraete

Mammalian blood contains an enzymatic system, called the fibrinolytic system, that is capable of dissolving blood clots. This system (Fig. 42-1) comprises an inactive proenzyme (plasminogen) that can be converted to the active enzyme (plasmin) that degrades fibrin into soluble fibrin-degradation products. Two immunologically distinct types of physiologic plasminogen activators have been identified: tissue plasminogen activator (tPA) and urokinase plasminogen activator (uPA). Inhibition of the fibrinolytic system may occur either at (1) the level of the plasminogen activators, by plasminogen activator inhibitor-1 (PAI-1) and plasminogen activator inhibitor-2 (PAI-2), or (2) the level of plasmin, by α_2-antiplasmin or α_2-macroglobulin. The physicochemical properties of these main components of the fibrinolytic system are summarized in Table 42-1. Plasminogen activation also may be induced by an intrinsic pathway involving several proteins, such as factor XII, high-molecular-weight (HMW) kininogen, and prekallikrein. Kallikrein, generated from prekallikrein by the action of factor XII and HMW kininogen, may convert single-chain uPA (scuPA) to two-chain uPA (tcuPA).

This chapter discusses tPA- and uPA-mediated fibrinolysis. Normal hemostasis requires precise regulation and control of the fibrinolytic system and depends on specific molecular interactions between its main components. Impaired fibrinolysis can cause thrombotic complications; excessive activation of the fibrinolytic system can cause a bleeding tendency. Some bleeding disorders may be treated with antifibrinolytic agents, while some thromboembolic complications may be treated with plasminogen activators, which can act as thrombolytic agents.

COMPONENTS OF THE FIBRINOLYTIC SYSTEM

Plasminogen Activators

Two types of physiologic plasminogen activator have been identified—one related to the activator found in tissues (tPA) and the other related to the activator found in urine (uPA). uPA may be obtained as a two-chain molecule (tcuPA) or as a single-chain form (scuPA or prourokinase).

Tissue Plasminogen Activator

Sources. Many reports on the purification and characterization of tPA are culled from various sources, including pig heart, hog ovaries, postmortem vascular perfusates, and postexercise blood. The first satisfactory purification of human tPA was from uterine tissue.[1] Using an antiserum raised against uterine plasminogen activator, it was shown that tPA, vascular plasminogen activator, and blood plasminogen activator are immunologically identical yet different from urokinase.[2] The major plasminogen activator found in blood is vascular plasminogen activator, which is synthesized and secreted by endothelial cells[3] and now called tPA.

tPA was purified from the culture fluid of a stable human melanoma cell line (Bowes, RPMI-7272) in sufficient amounts to study its biochemical and biologic properties.[4–6] tPA for clinical use is presently produced by recombinant DNA technology (Activase, Genentech Inc, or Actilyse, Boehringer Ingelheim GmbH).

The cDNA of human tPA was cloned and expressed in *Escherichia coli* and in mammalian cell systems.[7–12] Efficient expression of recombinant DNA encoding tPA was obtained in mammalian cells, yielding a properly processed and glycosylated molecule. This tPA is indistinguishable from the natural activator isolated from human melanoma cell cultures, with respect to biochemical properties, turnover in vivo, and specific thrombolytic activity.[13,14] The generation of Chinese hamster ovary (CHO) cells capable of producing human tPA has allowed the development of large-scale tissue culture fermentation and purification procedures.[15] The resulting product (Activase) consists primarily of a single-chain molecule.[16]

Structural Properties. tPA is a serine protease of about 70 kd and composed of a single polypeptide chain of 527 amino acids with Ser as NH_2-terminal amino acid.[7] Its primary structure—deduced from CDNA cloning—is illustrated in Figure 42-2. Native tPA contains an NH_2-terminal extension of three additional amino acids (Gly-Ala-Arg).[17] The molecule has 17 disulfide bonds and an additional free cysteine at position 83. tPA is converted by plasmin to a two-chain form by hydrolysis of the Arg 275–Ile 276 peptide bond (numbering based on a total of 527 residues). The NH_2-terminal region is composed of several domains with

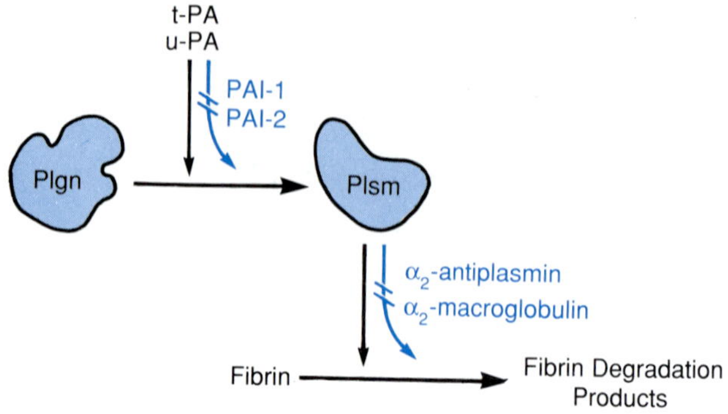

FIGURE 42-1. Schematic representation of the fibrinolytic system. Plgn, plasminogen; Plsm, plasmin.

homologies to other proteins: residues 1 to 43 are homologous to the finger domains (F) in fibronectin,[18] residues 44 to 91 are homologous to human epidermal growth factor (E), and residues 92 to 173 (K_1) and 180 to 261 (K_2) are homologous to the kringle regions of plasminogen. The region comprising residues 276 to 527 is homologous to that of other serine proteinases and contains the catalytic site, which is composed of His 322, Asp 371, and Ser 478.[7]

Melanoma tPA exists as two variants (types I and II) that differ in carbohydrate content. Type I tPA contains N-linked glycans at residues Asn 117, 184, and 448, whereas the type II tPA lacks the glycan at position 184.[19,20] The carbohydrate of melanoma-derived tPA contains sialic acid, fucose, mannose, galactose, N-acetylglucosamine and N-acetylgalactosamine.[21] Both forms of melanoma-derived tPA contain a high-mannose oligosaccharide at position 117.[20] Recombinant tPA (Activase) contains about 7% carbohydrate by weight, consisting of a high-mannose oligosaccharide at position 117 and complex fucosylated oligosaccharides at Asn 184 and Asn 448.[16]

The distinct domains in tPA appear to be involved in several enzyme functions including its binding to fibrin, rapid clearance in vivo, plasminogen-activating activity with fibrin specificity (enzymatic properties), and binding to endothelial cell receptors. As discussed below, construction, expression, and characterization of deletion mutants of tPA (those lacking one or more of these domains) allows a detailed study of structure–function relationships.

Binding to Fibrin. tPA has a specific affinity for fibrin. The dissociation constant of the tPA–fibrin complex is estimated to be 0.14 μmol/L in the presence of plasminogen.[22] Higgins and Vehar[23] found that significantly more (over 20%) one-chain tPA than two-chain tPA binds to fibrin, whereas Rijken and coworkers[24] found only a small difference. The stoichiometry of binding is about 1 mol of tPA per 1 mol of fibrin monomer.[23] Scatchard analysis of ^{125}I-tPA binding to fibrin in the absence of plasminogen suggests the existence of a single class of binding sites with K_a of 1.65×10^6 L/mol (which would correspond to a K_d of 0.6 μmol/L) and a maximum molar binding ratio of 0.88 mol tPA per 1 mol of fibrin.[25]

The structures involved in fibrin-binding of tPA are localized within the heavy chain (A chain), evidenced by the intact fibrin-affinity of the A chain that is isolated after mild reduction of two-chain tPA.[26,27] The finger domain of tPA (homologous to the finger-domains of fibronectin) was initially thought to be involved in the fibrin binding of the enzyme.[18] This was confirmed by demonstrating that a deletion mutant of tPA that encodes only the finger and serine protease domains binds to fibrin.[28] Kagitani and associates[29] report that tPA lacking the finger domain still has significant fibrin affinity, however. Evidence obtained with additional deletion mutants suggests that binding of tPA to fibrin is mediated via both the finger domain and the second kringle region (K_2).[30,31] A lysine-binding site is involved in the interaction of the (K_2) domain with fibrin (abolished by the lysine analogue, 6-aminohexanoic acid). A lysine-binding site is not involved, however, in the interaction of the finger domain with fibrin.[28] The presence of a weaker lysine-binding site in K_2[32] similar to the AH site observed in plasminogen[33] is also suggested. This AH site would interact with internal lysine residues in the fibrin matrix, whereas the lysine-binding site would interact with carboxyl-terminal lysine residues exposed on initial plasmic digestion of fibrin. However, a tPA variant lacking only the growth factor domain bound as poorly to fibrin as the finger domain deletion variant.[34] These results suggest that either both NH_2 terminal domains are required for high affinity to fibrin or the polypeptide region connecting the finger and growth factor domains is involved in binding to fibrin. A tPA variant lacking both the finger and growth factor domains, yet containing the kringle regions, had intact enzymatic activity but showed moderately[30] or markedly[34,35] reduced binding to fibrin.

Enzymatic Properties. The structures required for enzymatic activity of tPA are localized in the light chain (B chain) since the isolated B chain (separated chemically[26,27] or prepared by recombinant DNA technology[30,31]) retains full enzymatic activity. As expected, the plasminogen activating activity of the isolated B chain is not stimulated by the presence of fibrin.

The activation of plasminogen by tPA—in both the presence and the absence of fibrin—follows Michaelis-Menten kinetics. Hoylaerts and associates[22] found that the K_m was

TABLE 42-1. Physicochemical Properties of the Main Components of the Fibrinolytic System

	M_r (kd)	Carbohydrate Content (%)	No. Amino Acids	Plasma Concentration (mg/L)
Plasminogen	92	2	791	200
tPA	68	7	530	0.005
scuPA	54	7	411	0.008
α_2-Antiplasmin	70	13	452	70
α_2-Macroglobulin	725	8	4 × 1451	2500
PAI-1	52	—	379	0.05
PAI-2	47 (60)	—	393	<0.005

tPA, tissue plasminogen activator; scuPA, single-chain urokinase plasminogen activator; prourokinase, PAI-1, plasminogen activator inhibitor-1; PAI-2, plasminogen activator inhibitor-2.

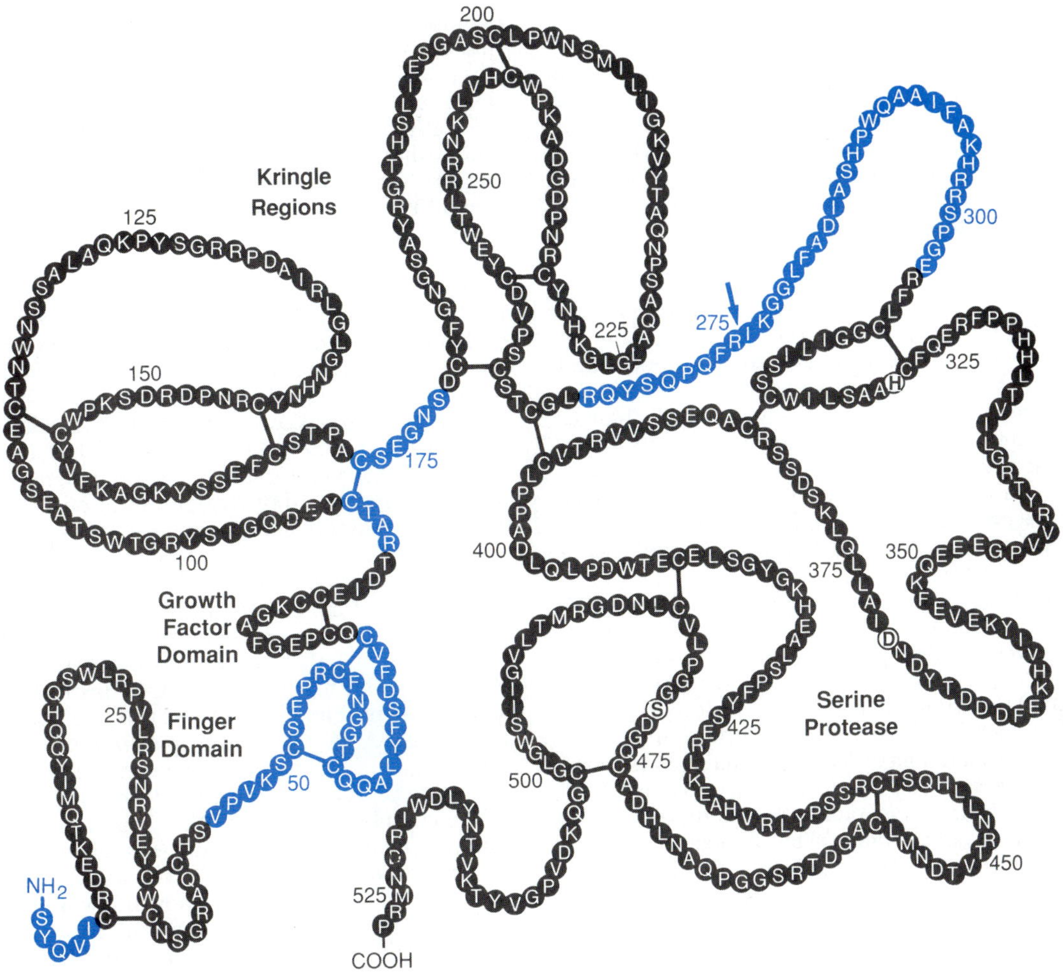

FIGURE 42-2. Schematic representation of the primary structure of tissue-type plasminogen activator. The arrow indicates the cleavage site for plasmin. The active site residues are indicated in white circles.

65 μmol/L, and the k_{cat} was 0.05 s^{-1} in the absence of fibrin; in the presence of fibrin, the K_m decreased to 0.16 μmol/L with only a minor change in k_{cat}. The catalytic efficiency (k_{cat}/K_m) of tPA for the activation of plasminogen thus increases about 1500 times in the presence of fibrin. A similar increase in catalytic efficiency was observed with CNBr-digested fibrinogen[14]; lysine residue 157 in the Aα-chain of fibrinogen was identified as the residue involved in fibrin-induced stimulation of plasminogen activation by tPA.[36] Rijken and coworkers,[24] using a system in which lysis of fibrin was prevented by an excess of aprotinin (a potent inhibitor of plasmin), found a K_m of 1.1 μmol/L. Ranby and colleagues[37] found that during the degradation of fibrin, the K_m decreased from 2 to 0.2 μmol/L. These changes and differences in K_m in the presence of fibrin are explained by the exposure of a strong plasminogen-binding site on initial fibrin degradation.[38] Nieuwenhuizen and coworkers,[39] however, report that fibrin affects both the K_m (with a 20-fold decrease) and the k_{cat} (with a 30-fold increase) of plasminogen activation by tPA. Although tPA in the single-chain form is less active with regard to low-molecular-weight (LMW) substrates and inhibitors,[40] it is now generally accepted that its activity with regard to plasminogen is comparable to that of the two-chain form.[24]

In addition to the interactions of tPA and plasminogen with fibrin, Miles and Plow[41] have shown that platelets bind plasminogen, and that platelet-bound plasminogen is more sensitive to activation by tPA. Stricker and associates[42] found that incubation of normal, washed human platelets with plasminogen at physiologic concentrations (180 mg/L) and tPA at concentrations achieved during thrombolytic therapy (40 to 800 μg/L) resulted in a 10- to 50-fold increase in plasmin activity relative to that obtained without platelets. These results suggest that platelets may also provide a surface for activation of plasminogen by pharmacologic concentrations of tPA.

The kinetics of plasminogen activation by tPA are also influenced by the presence of lipids: negatively charged lipids lower the K_m value 6- to 20-fold, whereas neutral lipids raise the K_m.[43] This finding suggests that plasminogen activation by cell-associated tPA may be influenced by the net charge of membrane lipids.

Both plasminogen[44] and tPA[45] bind specifically to cultured human umbilical vein endothelial cells. Binding of tPA results in a three- to four-fold increase of its apparent catalytic efficiency for plasminogen activation. Barnathan and coworkers[46] presented evidence for the existence of two distinct binding sites for tPA on cultured human umbilical vein endothelial cells. Binding to the higher-affinity site required an intact catalytic site of the molecule and resulted in inhibition of tPA by binding to PAI-1. Binding to the second site occurred with higher capacity but lower affinity with maintenance of tPA activity. Endothelial cells may thus serve as a focal point for plasmin generation in the blood vessel microenvironment by providing specific binding sites for the assembly of plasminogen and tPA.

Deletion mutants of tPA have been used to identify the domains in tPA that are involved in the stimulation of plasminogen activating potential by fibrin. Three groups[30,31,34] reported that tPA mutants lacking the finger domain are stimulated by fibrin to the same degree as intact tPA, whereas mutants lacking the K_2 structure, which retains the finger domain, show significantly reduced stimulation. This suggests that the interaction of the K_2 domain with fibrin may regulate fibrin stimulation.

Conversely, Kalyan and associates[35] reported that a deletion mutant of tPA lacking both the finger and growth factor domains (tPA-ΔFE) was less stimulated by fibrin than was wild-type tPA. This contrasts with the similar mutants described by Gething and colleagues[47] and by Larsen and associates[34] that showed no change in stimulation by fibrin. This difference may be due to conformational changes (caused by deletion) in the other domains of the heavy chain. The more extensive deletion (residues 2 to 89) was produced by Kalyan and colleagues[35]; the less extensive deletions were produced by Gething and associates[47] (residues 4 to 87) and Larsen and coworkers[34] (residues 6 to 86).

Several additional reports on the fibrin affinity of tPA deletion mutants add to the existing confusion. Ehrlich and others[48] constructed a tPA mutant that lacks the first kringle region (K_1) and K_2, and in which residue 86 at the COOH-terminal end of the E domain is linked to residue 262. This mutant had a specific activity and a fibrin affinity comparable to that of melanoma tPA. In plasma clot lysis systems in vitro, this mutant was an even more efficient thrombolytic agent than melanoma tPA, and systemic fibrinogenolysis was comparable. This indicates that the presence of the finger domain is sufficient for fibrin stimulation of tPA. These results apparently disagree with those of van Zonneveld and associates,[30] who found that tPA-ΔK_1K_2 (deletion of residues 89 to 254) has greatly reduced fibrin binding and reduced stimulation of plasminogen activating potential by fibrin.

In contrast, Gething and coworkers[47] reported that tPA mutants lacking both kringles are not stimulated by fibrin. Mutants containing only one kringle (either K_1 or K_2), however, are indistinguishable from one another and from wild-type tPA. This suggests that K_1 and K_2 are equivalent in their ability to mediate stimulation of the catalytic activity of tPA by fibrin. This conclusion is at variance with the results of van Zonneveld and colleagues[30] and those of Verheijen and associates,[31] which suggest that only K_2 and not K_1 is involved in fibrin binding and stimulation. Those conclusions are based on the properties of deletion mutants of tPA produced by excision of restriction fragments from tPA cDNA. One of the restriction sites used (the ScaI site at nucleotide 950) cleaves within the sequences coding for K_2—eight amino acids upstream of the exon–intron border that marks the end of this kringle.[49] These eight amino acids comprise two cysteine residues that normally form disulphide bonds with two other cysteines in the kringle.[50] None of the mutants created with this ScaI site bound efficiently to fibrin or were stimulated by fibrin. The defects exhibited by these mutants may result from incorrect folding of the protein, perhaps mediated by formation of improper disulfide bonds, rather than being a direct consequence of deletion of K_2.[47] In a review article, Pannekoek and coworkers[51] reported that they also constructed another set of deletion mutants that precisely obeyed the exon–intron positions in the tPA cDNA; however, they still could not demonstrate involvement of K_1 in fibrin binding and stimulation. These discrepancies indicate that loss of a function by deletion of a domain must be interpreted with care, because it may be due to conformational changes in the remaining part of the molecule rather than to the deletion itself. It seems more appropriate to look at the functions that are retained in particular deletion mutants; this provides unequivocal evidence that the retained function is not associated with the deleted domain.

Finally, a deletion mutant of tPA was constructed in which the last three COOH-terminal amino acids (Met-Arg-Pro) are lacking.[52] The activity of this mutant, relative to wild-type tPA, was lower in the absence but higher in the presence of fibrin, resulting in a more pronounced stimulation by fibrin. This suggests that the COOH terminal of tPA is involved in the active site of the enzyme and in its binding to fibrin. The observation remains unexplained.

Gene Structure. The gene coding for human tPA was localized to chromosome 8.[53–55] The tPA gene localization (chromosome 8, bands 8p12 → q11.2) coincides with a translocation breakpoint observed in myeloproliferative disorders.[55] The tPA gene was characterized in detail.[49,56,57] A total of 36,594 base pairs (bp) were sequenced (including 32,720 bp from the transciption initiation site to the polyadenylation site) in addition to 3530 bp of 5′ and 344 bp of 3′ flanking DNA. Thirteen intervening sequences (30,068 bp) divide the gene into 14 coding regions; the exons range from 43 to 914 bp, and the introns range in size from 111 bp to 14,257 bp. The transcription initiation site is an A residue with a TATA box nearby upstream (TATAAAAA at positions −22 to −29) and a CAAT box further upstream (CAATG at positions −112 to −116). The polyadenylation signal (AATAAA) is found at positions 32,688 to 32,693. The gene and 5′ flanking region contain 28 copies of Alu repetitive DNA and a single KpnI repeat.

The complete 2530-bp cDNA sequence of mature tPA[7] contains a single reading frame that begins with the ATG codon at nucleotides 85 to 87. This ATG probably serves as the site of translation initiation and is followed (562 codons later) by a TGA termination triplet at nucleotides 1771 to 1773. The serine residue originally[7] designated as the NH_2-terminal amino acid (disregarding the NH_2-terminal extension of 3 amino acids in native tPA[17]) is preceded by 35 amino acids, 20 to 23 of which (residues −35 to −13) probably constitute a hydrophobic signal peptide involved in the secretion of tPA. The remaining hydrophobic amino acids immediately preceding the start of mature tPA (residues −14 to −1) may constitute a *pro* sequence similar to that found for serum albumin. The 3′ untranslated region of 759 nucleotides contains the hexanucleotide AATAAA (positions 2496 to 2501), which precedes the site of polyadenylation in many eukaryotic mRNAs.

The assembly of the tPA gene is an example of the exon-shuffling principle. This is suggested by the findings that the different structural domains on the heavy chain (F, E, K_1, K_2) are encoded by a single exon or by two adjacent exons.[58] Because of the striking correlation between the exon–intron distribution of the gene and the putative domain structure of the protein, it is suggested that these domains are autonomous, structural, and functional entities (modules).[18,51] The validity of this exon-shuffling concept for tPA was directly investigated by constructing mutants with precise domain deletions, insertions, or substitutions (at the exon–intron junction of the gene), and evaluating their functional properties.

Assay. tPA antigen levels in human plasma at rest (measured by immunoradiometric assay[59] or by enzyme-linked immunosorbent assay [ELISA])[60,61] range between 3.4 ± 0.8 ng/mL and 6.6 ± 2.9 ng/mL. This level increases about three-fold by exhaustive physical exercise, venous occlusion, or infusion of 1-deamino-8-D-arginine vasopressin (DDAVP).[59] These immunologic methods detect active as well as inactive forms of antigen, however.

The classic method for measurement of fibrinolytic activity is the fibrin-plate method,[62] using euglobulin fractions. This assay is nonspecific, since both intrinsic and extrinsic plasminogen activators are measured. This method is used to express the activity of tPA in urokinase-like units through comparison of the fibrinolytic activity of tPA with that of a urokinase standard. The conversion of protein concentration to urokinase-like activity has, however, been a matter of dispute, since different values were reported for the specific activity (90,000 to 250,000 IU/mg), probably depending on the calibration system. An International Reference Preparation for tPA was established in 1985 in which 1 IU corresponds to 2 ng of protein.[63] This preparation was replaced by a second international standard for tPA, coded 86/670.[64]

Methods measuring the functionally active level of tPA were developed based on the stimulation of the activation of plasminogen by tPA in the presence of fibrin or fibrin fragments. Ranby and others[65] developed a sensitive parabolic rate assay (first described by Drapier[66]) in which plasminogen, tPA, fibrin monomer, and a plasmin-sensitive chromogenic substrate are incubated together. This method was adapted for euglobulin fractions, using CNBr-digested fibrinogen as stimulator.[67] Plasma in which proteinase inhibitors are neutralized by acidification was used in combination with fibrin monomer as stimulator.[68]

Alternatively, tPA in plasma was separated from inhibitors by adsorption on lysine-sepharose before to determination with the parabolic-rate assay using polylysine as stimulator.[69] In this way, the baseline activity at rest was determined to be 0.08 IU/mL (range, 0.01 to 0.26 IU/mL), corresponding to 0.32 ng/mL according to the calibration system used.

Using an ELISA based on a specific monoclonal antibody, detectable levels (4.5 ± 0.8 ng/mL) of free, single-chain tPA were found in plasma of 6 of 10 healthy subjects; this level increased to 7.6 ± 3.1 ng/mL after venous occlusion.[70]

Urokinase Plasminogen Activator

Sources. tcuPA, a trypsin-like serine proteinase composed of two polypeptide chains (20 and 34 kd), was isolated from human urine and from cultured human embryonic kidney cells.

Bernik and Oller[71] suggested in 1973 that urokinase might be secreted in an inactive form that can be activated by plasmin. Nolan and associates[72] reported that urokinase was secreted by human embryonic kidney cells in a precursor form. Several groups have isolated a single-chain form of urokinase (scuPA) from urine,[73,74] plasma,[75] or conditioned cell culture media.[76–83] It was also obtained by recombinant DNA technology and prepared from the translation product in *E coli* of an expression plasmid coding for human urokinase.[84,85] scuPA was efficiently purified from conditioned medium of the human lung adenocarcinoma cell line (CALU-3), with a yield of 65 to 100 μg/L of starting material, representing a 290-fold purification and a recovery of 30%.[83] Applying a similar procedure to human urine, highly purified scuPA was obtained with a yield of only 5 μg/L.[74] In addition to the 54-kd scuPA, we also obtained a previously unrecognized LMW form (32 kd) of scuPA (scuPA-32k) from the conditioned medium of CALU-3 cells.[86] This scuPA-32k was subsequently produced by recombinant DNA technology.[87]

Structural Properties. scuPA is a single-chain glycoprotein with of 54 kd containing 411 amino acids[84] (Fig. 42-3). On limited hydrolysis by plasmin or kallikrein of the Lys 158–Ile 159 peptide bond, the molecule is converted to a two-chain derivative. The light chain (A chain; NH_2 terminal) contains 158 amino acids and the heavy chain (B chain) contains 253[88–90]; both chains are connected by a Cys 148–Cys 279 interchain disulphide bond. Commercial, highly purified tcuPA, however, often has Phe instead of Lys as COOH-terminal amino acid of the light chain.[88] The

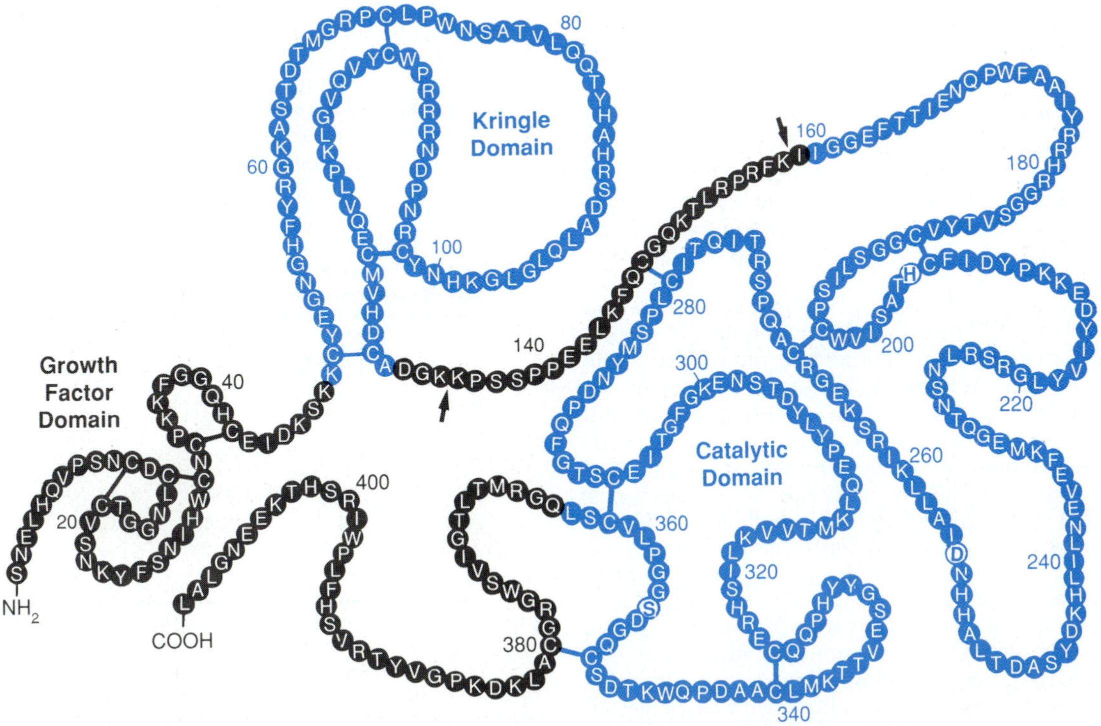

FIGURE 42-3. Schematic representation of the primary structure of single-chain urokinase-type plasminogen activator. The arrows indicate the cleavage sites for plasmin. The active site residues are indicated in white circles.

catalytic center is located in the carboxyl-terminal chain and is composed of Asp 255, His 204, and Ser 356. The amino-terminal chain contains regions homologous to human epidermal growth factor (residues 5 to 49) and one region homologous to the plasminogen kringles. A single carbohydrate moiety is attached to Asn 302. A LMW (33-kd) tcuPA can be generated with plasmin by hydrolysis of the Lys 135–Lys 136 peptide bond following previous cleavage of the Lys 158–Ile 159 bond.[88] scuPA-32k is generated by specific proteolytic cleavage of the Glu 143–Leu 144 peptide bond in scuPA.[86] Thrombin cleaves the Arg 156–Phe 157 peptide bond in scuPA, resulting in an inactive tcuPA molecule.[91]

A single-chain urokinase species was purified by chromatography on fibrin-cellite, suggesting a specific fibrin affinity.[73,78,79] In other studies, however, direct fibrin binding of scuPA,[83,92] or of scuPA-32k[86,87] has not been observed.

Gene Structure. The cDNA of uPA was isolated and the nucleotide sequence determined.[84,93,94] The cDNA sequence contains an open reading frame that starts with ATG at nucleotide positions 77 to 79 and extends for 1293 nucleotides until a TGA stop codon is reached at positions 1370 to 1372.[84] The open reading frame is preceded by at least 76 nucleotides of 5′ untranslated mRNA, which are extremely rich in G/C nucleotides (83%). Beyond the termination codon, the cDNA extends for another 932 nucleotides. The sequence includes 2 poly (A) adenylation signals (positions 2271 to 2276 and 2284 to 2289) preceding the polyadenylation site at position 2304.[84] The human uPA gene is 6.4 kb long and located on chromosome 10.[53] It contains 11 exons,[94] and the exon–intron organization of the gene closely resembles that of the tPA gene. Exons III, VIII, and IX of tPA are totally missing, however, and exon IV is partially missing in the uPA gene; this accounts for the absence of a finger domain and a K_2 in uPA. Exon II of the uPA gene codes for a signal peptide consisting of 20 amino acids; exons III and IV code for the growth factor domain, and exons V and VI code for the kringle region. The 5′ region of exon VII, which codes for the peptide connecting the light and the heavy chain, is 39 bp longer than the corresponding exon X of the tPA gene. The 3′ regions of exon VII and exons VIII to XI code for the heavy chain.

Enzymatic Properties

tcuPA. The activation of plasminogen by tcuPA obeys Michaelis-Menten kinetics. For the activation of native (Glu) plasminogen by urokinase in a purified system, kinetic parameters were reported ranging between 1.4 and 200 μmol/L for the Michaelis constant (K_m), and between 0.26 and 1.48 s^{-1} for the catalytic rate constant (k_{cat}). This yields second-order rate constants (k_{cat}/K_m) between 0.0074 and 0.5 $\mu mol^{-1} \cdot L \cdot s^{-1}$,[95,96] probably depending on the quality of the plasminogen preparation and on the experimental conditions used. Activation of Lys-plasminogen by tcuPA[97] appears to be 3 to 10 times faster than that of Glu-plasminogen. In the presence of certain ω-aminocarboxylic acids (eg, 6-aminohexanoic acid), the rate of activation of Glu-plasminogen by tcuPA increases 10 to 20 times, whereas that of Lys-plasminogen is unaffected.[98] This is probably because these amino acids induce a conformational change in the Glu-plasminogen moiety similar to that observed on conversion of Glu-plasminogen to Lys-plasminogen or to plasmin.[99] Activation of Glu-plasminogen by tcuPA is stimulated by the presence of fibrin,[100] and also by fibrinogen, fragment D, and fragment E[101]; activation of Lys-plasminogen is not affected. Addition of CNBr-digested fibrinogen also increases the activation rate of Glu-plasminogen by tcuPA about 10 times.[102]

scuPA. scuPA has a low reactivity toward LMW synthetic substrates or active-site titrants that are highly reactive toward tcuPA.[76,103] The synthetic urokinase inhibitor Glu-Gly-Arg-CH_2Cl irreversibly inhibits tcuPA, but it apparently acts as a reversible competitive inhibitor of scuPA.[104]

We investigated the activation of plasminogen by natural scuPA (nscuPA) purified from the human lung adenocarcinoma cell line CALU-3[83], by recombinant scuPA obtained by expression of cDNA in *E coli* (rscuPA-EC),[105] or CHO cells (rscuPA-CHO),[106] and by scuPA-32k, an LMW scuPA generated by specific cleavage of the Glu 143–Leu 144 peptide bond.[86,87]

In mixtures of scuPA and plasminogen, tcuPA and plasmin are quickly generated. Addition of plasmin inhibitors prohibits the conversion of scuPA to tcuPA but not the activation of plasminogen to plasmin, suggesting that scuPA activates plasminogen directly.[92] Kinetic analysis reveals that the conversion of scuPA and plasminogen to tcuPA and plasmin, respectively, can be described by a sequence of three reactions that each obey Michalis-Menten kinetics.[105,107] In a first reaction, scuPA directly activates plasminogen to plasmin; in the second reaction, plasmin then converts scuPA to tcuPA; plasminogen is activated by tcuPA in the third reaction. In the presence of an excess of a chromogenic plasmin substrate, the first reaction can be analyzed separately because generated plasmin is quantitatively bound, and conversion of scuPA to tcuPA or of Glu-plasminogen to Lys-plasminogen by plasmin is inhibited. The kinetic constants obtained are summarized in Table 42-2. rscuPA and nscuPA have a high affinity for plasminogen (K_m less than 1 μmol/L) but a low catalytic rate constant, suggesting that the high affinity of scuPA for plasminogen is a key property in the activation mechanism. The catalytic rate constant (K_{cat}) obtained with nscuPA is 15 to 20 times lower than that originally observed with rscuPA-EC but only 2 times lower than that obtained with rscuPA-CHO. Thus, the catalytic efficiency (k_{cat}/K_m) of nscuPA is significantly lower than that of rscuPA-EC[1], but it is comparable to that of rscuPA obtained from a mammalian cell system. The catalytic efficiency of rscuPA-EC[1] approaches that of tcuPA (K_m about 50 μmol/L; k_{cat} about 5 s^{-1}; k_{cat}/K_m 0.1 $\mu mol/L^{-1} \cdot s^{-1}$), whereas nscuPA and rscuPA-CHO are significantly less active (k_{cat}/K_m less than or equal to 1% of tcuPA). The molecular basis of the discrepancy between rscuPA-EC[1] and rscuPA-CHO is not clear. Furthermore, rscuPA-EC[2] had a lower catalytic efficiency for plasminogen activation[108] that more closely resembled that of nscuPA or rscuPA-CHO.

TABLE 42-2. Kinetic Constants for the Activation of Glu-Plasminogen by scuPA Moieties

	K_m (μmol)	k_{cat} (s^{-1})	k_{cat}/K_m (μmol/s)	Reference
nscuPA	0.83	0.0009	0.00112	83
nscuPA-32k	0.9	0.0028	0.00311	86
rscuPA-EC (1)	0.23	0.0170	0.07391	105
rscuPA-EC (2)	0.74	0.0020	0.00270	108
rscuPA-CHO	1	0.0020	0.00200	106
rscuPA-Glu^{158}	87	0.0100	0.00011	106
rscuPA-Gly^{158}	62	0.0110	0.00018	106

nscuPA, natural scuPA obtained from CALU-3 cells; nscuPA-32k, natural low-M_r scuPA obtained from CALU-3 cells; rscuPA-EC (1), recombinant scuPA obtained from *E coli* (supplied by Genentech Inc, San Francisco); rscuPA-EC (2), recombinant scuPA obtained from *E coli* (supplied by Grünenthal GmbH, Aachen); rscuPA-CHO, recombinant scuPA obtained from Chinese hamster ovary cells; rscuPA-Glu 158 and rscuPA-Gly 158, recombinant scuPA obtained by site-directed mutagenesis of Lys 158 to Glu or to Gly and expressed in Chinese hamster ovary cells.

Activation of Lys-plasminogen occurs with comparable affinity but with a higher catalytic rate constant, resulting in more efficient activation by scuPA (about 10-fold).[109] This high affinity is not mediated via the high-affinity lysine-binding site of plasminogen (located in kringles 1 to 3), nor via the low-affinity lysine-binding site comprised within kringle 4 (K_2), as evidenced by the comparable K_m of scuPA for native and LMW plasminogen (a derivative lacking these structures).[109] The similar kinetic constants obtained with scuPA-32k and scuPA (see Table 42-2) indicate that the plasminogen activating properties are independent of the NH_2-terminal 143 amino acids of scuPA.[86,87]

To further investigate the significance of the conversion of scuPA to tcuPA for the activation of plasminogen, we constructed mutants of rscuPA by site-specific mutagenesis of Lys 158 to Gly 158 or to Glu 158, thereby destroying the plasmic cleavage site for conversion to tcuPA.[106] At the plasminogen concentrations used to measure the kinetic parameters for activation by scuPA (around 1 μmol/L), no significant activation is observed with these mutants. When higher plasminogen concentrations are used (10 to 100 μmol/L), concentration-dependent activation of plasminogen is observed, following Michaelis-Menten kinetics. The kinetic constants (see Table 42-2) show that the mutants activate plasminogen with a catalytic rate constant (k_{cat}) that is about 5 times higher than that of rscuPA, but with a Michaelis constant (K_m) that is 60 to 80 times higher. The catalytic efficiency (k_{cat}/K_m) of both mutants is therefore 10 to 20 times lower than that of wild rscuPA. From these experiments, we conclude that scuPA has some intrinsic plasminogen activating potential. A low intrinsic plasminogen activating potential of scuPA is confirmed by others,[110] whereas some authors claim that scuPA has no enzymatic activity and is a genuine proenzyme.[111]

rtcuPA–Glu 158 (obtained by conversion of rscuPA–Glu 158 to a two-chain molecule by treatment with endoproteinase Glu-C) has a catalytic efficiency comparable to rtcuPA (obtained by conversion of rscuPA to a two-chain molecule by treatment with plasmin).[112]

Inactive thrombin-derived tcuPA (obtained by treatment of scuPA with thrombin) with Phe 157 as NH_2 terminal of the B chain can be converted to active tcuPA by hydrolysis of the Lys 158–Ile 159 peptide bond by plasmin, exposing Ile 159 as NH_2 terminal of the B chain of tcuPA.[113] These observations suggest that the structure of the NH_2-terminal region of the B chain of tcuPA is an important determinant for its enzymatic activity, whereas that of the COOH-terminal region of the A chain is not. Exposure of the Ile 159 residue apparently plays an important role converting low-activity scuPA to tcuPA with high enzymatic activity. The increased activity of tcuPA compared with scuPA may be related to a refolding of the Ile 159 residue into the binding pocket of the enzyme, as with other serine proteases.

Plasminogen

Physicochemical Properties

Human plasminogen is a single-chain glycoprotein of 92 kd, containing about 2% carbohydrate. The complete primary structure of the molecule was elucidated mainly by Sottrup-Jensen and coworkers[114,115] and by Wiman.[116] The plasminogen molecule consists of 790 amino acids; it contains 24 disulfide bridges and 5 homologous triple-loop structures or kringles.[115] The covalent structure of plasminogen is represented in Figure 42-4.

Plasminogen can be determined in plasma using immunologic methods, or by complex formation with streptokinase and measuring the plasminogen–streptokinase complex with a chromogenic substrate.[117] The normal plasma concentration is about 1.5 to 2 μmol/L. Native plasminogen has NH_2-terminal glutamic acid (Glu-plasminogen) but is easily converted by limited plasmic digestion to modified forms having NH_2-terminal lysine, valine, or methionine,[118,119] commonly designated Lys-plasminogen. This conversion occurs by hydrolysis of the Arg 67–Met 68, Lys 76–Lys 77, or Lys 77–Val 78 peptide bonds.

The method of choice for purifying human plasminogen is affinity chromatography on insolubilized lysine, a method introduced by Deutsch and Mertz.[120] Glu-plasminogen and Lys-plasminogen forms can be separated by chromatography on DEAE-Sephadex.[119] The hydrodynamic properties of both types have been reviewed elsewhere.[121]

The Glu-plasminogen occurring in human blood displays at least two types of microheterogeneity. Affinity chromatography on lysine-sepharose using gradient elution with 6-aminohexanoic acid separates plasminogen into two fractions (called type I and type II in the order of their elution from lysine-sepharose).[122] The first form appears more easily activatable than the second form and has a larger Stokes radius, as evidence by gel filtration.[123] Differences in carbohydrate and amino acid composition were invoked to explain this heterogeneity.[123,124] Each of these two fractions can be separated into about six forms having different isoelectric points using isoelectric focusing[118,125] or chromatography on DEAE-Sephadex.[123] These forms show differences in sialic acid content. All 12 molecular forms appear to be present in single-donor plasma.[123] Hayes and Castellino[126–128] have shown that type I plasminogen contains a glucosamine-based carbohydrate chain on Asn 288 and a galactosamine-based carbohydrate chain on Thr 345; type II plasminogen has only the latter. These differences in carbohydrate composition play a role in the interaction with α_2-antiplasmin and fibrin, with type II showing the strongest interaction with both.[129]

The turnover of both Glu-plasminogen and Lys-plasminogen labeled with radioiodine was studied in healthy subjects.[130,131] Glu-plasminogen had a plasma half-life of 2.2 ± 0.29 days and a fractional catabolic rate of 0.55 ± 0.1 of the plasma pool per day; Lys-plasminogen disappeared with a half-life of about 0.8 days. The two forms of Glu-plasminogen with different affinity for lysine-Sepharose have similar turnover characteristics in man.[130,131] The turnover of plasminogen increased during reptilase (Defibrase) treatment in patients with liver cirrhosis and in several clinical conditions associated with intravascular coagulation.[130,131]

Gene Structure

A 2.7-kb insert of a cDNA clone for human plasminogen containing the complete coding region was sequenced.[132] A 5′ noncoding region of 64 bp and a 3′ noncoding region of 253 bp are present in the full-length clone. A consensus AATAAA sequence is located at a position 46 nucleotides upstream of the polyadenylation site. The coding region contains an amino-terminal sequence of 19 amino acids having the characteristics of a signal sequence.[132] The amino acid sequence predicted from this cDNA is close to the published protein sequence[115] and differs only in four amide assignments (Glx, Asx) and in the presence of an extra isoleucine at position 85, giving a total of 791 amino acids for human plasminogen.

The plasminogen gene was mapped to the long arm of chromosome 6 at band q26 or q27.[133] A partial genomic organization of K_4 and kringle 5 (K_5) and part of the light chain in human plasminogen was presented.[134] Plasminogen K_4 and K_5 are encoded by two exons, as are K_1 of prothrombin and the two kringles of tPA. At least two introns are in the genomic region between exons and are

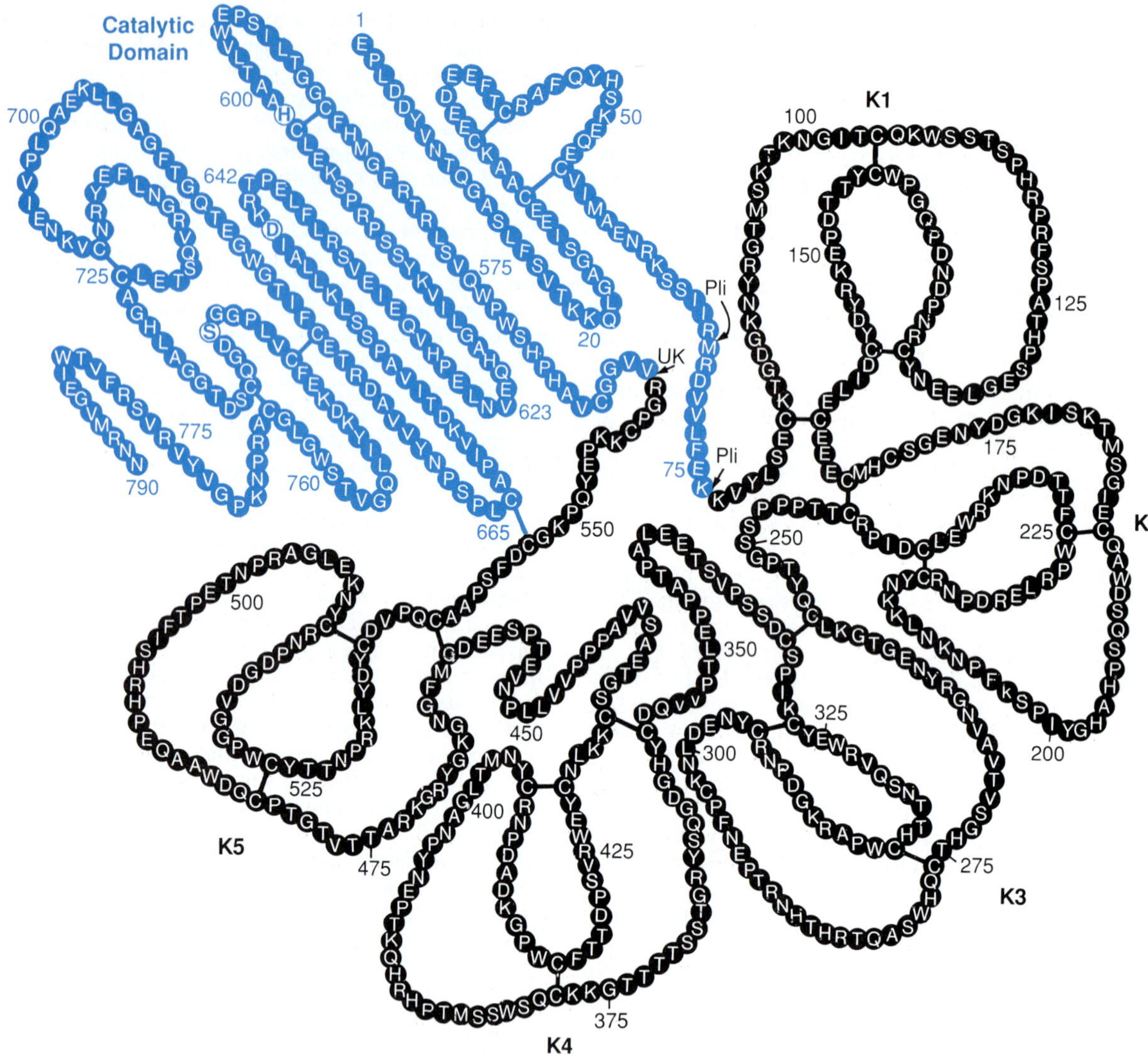

FIGURE 42-4. Schematic representation of the primary structure of plasminogen. Pli, plasma cleavage sties for conversion of Glu-plasminogen to Lys-plasminogen; UK, cleavage site for plasminogen activators, yielding plasmin.

encoding the active-site residues Asp and Ser in plasminogen (as in prothrombin). About 92% of the plasminogen gene appears to consist of noncoding regions, and the complete gene is probably larger than 30 kb.

Plasminogen Polymorphism

The heterogeneity of plasminogen observed in human plasma[122,125] appears to be genetically controlled. Structural polymorphism of human plasminogen was discovered in 1979 by Hobart[135] for the native protein, and by Raum and colleagues[136] for the desialylated protein. Plasminogen is coded by an autosomal gene with two common alleles and a number (about 11) of rare alleles.[135–137] A nomenclature for the designation of plasminogen variant alleles was proposed.[137] The technology of comparing plasminogen variants is based on isoelectric focusing of neuraminidase-treated sera and subsequent detection of plasminogen by caseinolytic overlay and Western blot analysis. Plasminogen variants are designated according to the relative direction of their isoelectric point (pI), by comparison with the two common types. The two common types found in all investigated races are designated PLG A (for more acidic pI) and PLG B (for more basic pI); the respective alleles are indicated PLG* A and PLG* B. Rare variants with a more acidic pI than common PLG A or a more basic pI than common PLG B receive a numerical suffix for the relative direction of their pI shift (suffix increases from basic to acidic direction of pI shift for PLG A variants and from acidic to basic direction for PLG B variants). The variants between common PLG A and PLG B are designated as PLG M1, PLG M2, PLG M3, and so forth (suffix increases from basic to acidic direction of pI shift).[137]

The allele frequencies differ substantially in various racial groups but are fairly constant within one race.[138–141] In the European populations, the distribution is roughly as follows: common PLG* A, 0.70; common PLG* B, 0.28; and rare PLG*, 0.020. The PLG B variant found in Japanese (allele frequency 0.022) had a normal antigen level but reduced activity to 40% of normal.[142,143] A direct correlation with thrombotic tendency was suggested but could not be established. The occurrence of a new silent allele (PLG^0) was reported in a Swiss family.[144]

Using plasminogen-specific probes, three common DNA polymorphisms were demonstrated by Southern blot analysis. These were observed with MspI, SacI, and RsaI digests of DNA. Significant linkage disequilibrium of the three common RFLPs and the protein polymorphism was seen.[133]

Linkage disequilibrium is the nonrandom association of an allele at one locus with an allele at another locus, and it provides evidence that the two markers describe variation at physically close loci. Very high association values were observed for PLG A and B with both SacI and MspI RFLPs. The lack of complete association of SacI and MspI alleles with PLG A and B suggests that neither of these RFLP sites represent exactly the nucleotide site of the DNA variation causing the protein polymorphism.

Mechanism of Activation to Plasmin

Lys-plasminogen is converted to plasmin by cleavage of a single Arg–Val peptide bond[145] corresponding to the Arg 560–Val 561 bond. The two-chain plasmin molecule is composed of a heavy chain (A chain) originating from the NH_2-terminal part of plasminogen, and of a light chain (B chain) constituting the COOH-terminal part.[146] The B chain contains (1) an active site similar to that of trypsin, composed of a histidine residue sensitive to tosyl-lysine chloromethyl ketone, and (2) a serine residue reactive toward diisopropyl-phosphofluoridate.[146] It appears that the active site of plasmin is composed of His 602, Asp 645, and Ser 740.[115]

Activation of Glu-plasminogen to plasmin by urokinase in purified systems occurs about 20 times slower than activation of Lys-plasminogen,[147–149] but Lys-plasmin is formed in either case. Rickli and Otavsky[150] demonstrated the release of an amino-terminal peptide from human plasminogen by urokinase. Wiman and Wallen[151] initially proposed that activation of Glu-plasminogen occurs in two steps: release of the NH_2-terminal preactivation peptide mainly by cleavage at Arg 67–Met 68 yielding Lys-plasminogen, followed by cleavage of the Arg 560–Val 561 bond to generate plasmin. When activation is carried out in excess plasmin inhibitor,[152,153] however, inhibited Glu-plasmin is obtained. In view of the great sensitivity of the Arg 67–Met 68 bond to plasmin, it was suggested that the major pathway for activation of plasminogen still is via Lys-plasminogen generated by plasmic cleavage of Glu-plasminogen.[148,153] Activation of Glu-plasminogen in the presence of the physiologic plasmin inhibitor α_2-antiplasmin generates inhibited Glu-plasmin, however.[154] Investigation of the activation pathways of plasminogen with the use of monoclonal antibodies specific for Lys-plasminogen reveals that activation of Glu-plasminogen in human plasma occurs by direct cleavage of the Arg 560–Val 561 peptide bond without generation of Lys-plasminogen intermediates.[155]

Lysine-Binding Sites

The plasminogen molecule contains lysine-binding site structures, which interact specifically with certain amino acids, such as lysine, 6-aminohexanoic acid, and *trans*-4-amino-methylcyclohexane-1-carboxylic acid (tranexamic acid).[122,156–160] Plasminogen contains one binding site with high affinity for 6-aminohexanoic acid (K_d of 9 μmol/L) and about four with low affinity (K_d of 5 mmol/L).[161] For tranexamic acid and Glu-plasminogen, these K_d values are 1.1 μmol/L for the high-affinity binding site and 750 μmol/L for the four or five sites with lower affinity.[162] Lys-plasminogen has one site that binds tranexamic acid with K_d of 2.2 μmol/L, one site with K_d of 36 μmol/L, and about two or three sites with K_d of 1000 μmol/L.[162] These lysine-binding sites are located in the plasmin A chain.[163] One site is located in the fourth triple-loop structure or K_4 (residues 354 to 439 based on a total of 790 amino acids), and at least one in the first three triple-loop structures (residues 79 to 337 to 353), shown by their affinities to lysine-sepharose. The LMW plasminogen (residues 442 to 790) has no affinity for lysine-sepharose.[114] The high-affinity lysine-binding site is comprised within the first three kringle structures of plasminogen[164] and is most probably located in K_1.[159,165] Binding of ω-aminocarboxylic acids to isolated K_4 is dependent on the presence of the Arg 70 and Asp 56 residues.[166] These essential residues are preserved in homologous positions in K_1 but are replaced by neutral amino acids in K_5, possibly explaining why K_5 has no ω-aminocarboxylic acid binding site. From nuclear magnetic resonance studies on K_4, it was also concluded that several aromatic residues (including Trp 71) may be lining the ω-aminocarboxylic acid binding site.[167] Using an antiserum raised with purified K_4 that blocks its lysine-binding site, it was shown that only K_4 containing derivatives of plasminogen interacts with this antibody, indicating that the lysine-binding sites are not identical.[168]

Plasminogen can specifically bind to fibrin through its lysine-binding sites. In both purified systems[169] and in plasma,[170] Lys-plasminogen has a higher affinity for fibrin than Glu-plasminogen. The differences in binding of Glu-plasminogen and Lys-plasminogen to fibrin might be due to an intramolecular interaction of one of the lysine-binding sites, with a specific site in the NH_2-terminal region of Glu-plasminogen[159,171] that is no longer present in Lys-plasminogen. The presence of 6-aminohexanoic acid prohibits the adsorption of plasminogen to fibrin in the purified system[169] and in the plasma system.[170] These findings indirectly indicate the importance of the lysine-binding sites in plasminogen for interaction with fibrin. More direct evidence was obtained by affinity chromatography of plasminogen and plasminogen derivatives on fibrin-sepharose.[172] Thus, one of the functions of the lysine-binding sites in plasminogen is to mediate its interaction with fibrin. In addition, Glu-plasminogen, Lys-plasminogen, and LMW plasminogen contain a weak lysine-binding site, termed the AH site; this site preferably interacts with ligands not carrying a free carboxylate function, and therefore may bind proteins via lysine side chains. It was suggested that the initial binding of plasminogen to fibrin is mainly determined by the AH site.[33]

The lysine-binding sites of plasmin(ogen) also mediate its interaction with α_2-antiplasmin, as discussed later. On the basis of these interactions, it is suggested that the lysine-binding sites play a crucial role in the regulation of fibrinolysis.[173,174]

Glu-plasminogen also binds in a specific and saturable manner to unstimulated human platelets, and this binding is enhanced 5-fold by thrombin stimulation.[42] Both phenomena occur through different pathways involving either glycoprotein IIb–IIIa or fibrin(ogen) for binding to unstimulated or stimulated platelets, respectively.[175] The region comprising the first three kringles (residues 79 to 337 or 353) appears to be the primary recognition site for plasminogen binding to both thrombin-stimulated and unstimulated platelets. Residues 354 to 439 (K_4) and 442 to 790 (LMW plasminogen) contribute differently to binding to stimulated and unstimulated platelets, confirming the occurrence of two distinct mechanisms.[176] Platelets apparently have the potential to enhance fibrinolysis by localizing plasminogen in a thrombus and enhancing its activation.

Inhibitors of the Fibrinolytic System

Inhibition of the fibrinolytic system may occur at the level of plasmin or at the level of plasminogen activators. For a long time, it was accepted that there were essentially two functionally important plasmin inhibitors in plasma: one immediately reacting inhibitor and one slower reacting inhibitor identical to α_2-macroglobulin and α_1-antitrypsin, respectively.[177] About 10 years ago, another plasmin inhibitor, α_2-antiplasmin, was identified in human plasma. On activation of plasminogen in plasma, plasmin is preferentially bound by this inhibitor. The complete activation of plasminogen (concentration, about 2 μmol/L), resulting in saturation of this plasmin inhibitor (concentration, about 1 μmol/L), must occur before the excess plasmin is neutralized by α_2-macroglobulin.

Inhibition of the physiologic plasminogen activators tPA and uPA in human plasma occurs mainly by PAI-1 and PAI-2.

α_2-Antiplasmin

Physicochemical Characterization. α_2-Antiplasmin was identified by several groups[178–181] and characterized by Moroi and Aoki[179] and by Wiman and Collen.[182] α_2-Antiplasmin is a single-chain glycoprotein of 70 kd containing about 13% carbohydrate. The molecule consists of 452 amino acids and contains two disulfide bridges[183–185] (Fig. 42-5). α_2-antiplasmin belongs to the serine protease inhibitor protein family (serpins).[183–185]

The concentration of the inhibitor in normal plasma is about 7 mg/dL (about 1 μmol/L).[179,182] The half-life of purified biologically intact iodine-labeled α_2-antiplasmin is 2.6 days, whereas the plasmin–α_2-antiplasmin complex disappears from plasma with a half-life of about half a day.[186]

The inhibitor in normal plasma is heterogeneous and consists of functionally active and inactive material. Complete activation of the plasminogen present in normal plasma converts only about 70% of the antigen material into a complex with plasmin; 30% of the inhibitor-related antigen appears to be functionally inactive.[180] Human plasma contains two forms of the inhibitor that differ in binding to plasminogen. The form that does not bind remains an active plasmin inhibitor[187–189] but reacts much slower with plasmin. This form lacks a 26-residue peptide from the carboxyl-terminal end of α_2-antiplasmin.[190] The peptide inhibits the interaction of α_2-antiplasmin with plasmin, which suggests that it contains the plasminogen-binding site.[190] Wiman and coworkers[191] measured the ratio of these forms in the plasma of pregnant women subjected to extensive plasmapheresis, and they concluded that the plasminogen-binding form of α_2-antiplasmin is primarily synthesized and it becomes partly converted to the non-plasminogen-binding form in the circulating blood.

Mechanism of Interaction With Plasmin. In purified systems[179,182] and in plasma,[178,180] α_2-antiplasmin forms a 1:1 stoichiometric complex with plasmin that is devoid of protease or esterase activity. α_2-Antiplasmin, like many other plasma proteinase inhibitors, has a broad in vitro inhibitory spectrum, but its physiologic role as an inhibitor of proteinases other than plasmin seems negligible.

Kinetics of Reaction. The kinetics of the inhibition of human plasmin by α_2-antiplasmin were studied in some detail.[192,193] The disappearance of plasmin activity after addition of excess α_2-antiplasmin does not follow first-order kinetics. Even though most of the plasmin is rapidly inactivated, the process slowly proceeds toward completion. This time of the reaction is compatible with a kinetic model composed of two successive reactions: a fast, reversible second-order reaction followed by a slower, irreversible first-order transition. The model can be represented by the following:

$$P + A \underset{k_{-1}}{\overset{k_1}{\rightleftharpoons}} PA \xrightarrow{k_2} PA'$$

where:
P = plasmin; A = α_2-antiplasmin
PA = reversible inactive complex
PA′ = an irreversible inactive complex

The second-order rate constant (k_1) is 2 to 4 × 10^7 $mol^{-1} \cdot L \cdot s^{-1}$. This is among the fastest protein–protein reactions described. Such rate constants approach the theoretical values for a diffusion-controlled process. The dissociation constant of the reversible complex is 2 × 10^{-10} mol/L. The half-time of the first-order transition, PA → PA′, is 166 seconds, corresponding to a k_2 value of 4.2 × $10^{-3} \cdot s^{-1}$.[193] Christensen and Clemmensen[192] report a value of 6.5 × $10^{-3} \cdot s^{-1}$ for k_2.

Plasmin molecules with a synthetic substrate bound to their active site or with 6-aminohexanoic acid bound to their lysine-binding sites[187,193] do not react or only react slowly with α_2-antiplasmin. The first step of the process thus clearly depends on the presence of a free lysine-binding site and active site in the plasmin molecule. This was further substantiated by studying the kinetics of the reaction between α_2-antiplasmin and a LMW form of plasmin (LMW plasmin) lacking lysine-binding sites.[194] The reaction scheme is identical to that observed with normal plasmin, but the rate constant of the first step is about 60 times smaller and is only slightly inhibited by 6-aminohexanoic acid.

These findings show that the first reversible step in the reaction between plasmin and α_2-antiplasmin can be divided into two parts: (1) a reaction between the lysine-binding sites in the plasmin A chain and the corresponding site in the α_2-antiplasmin molecule, and (2) a reaction between the active site of plasmin and a reactive site in α_2-antiplasmin. Because the reaction rate is strongly dependent on the availability of free lysine-binding sites, the main pathway is probably a consecutive reaction in this order. From competition experiments between plasminogen fragments containing lysine-binding sites and plasmin for binding of α_2-antiplasmin, it was concluded that the high-affinity lysine-binding sites situated in K_1 to K_3 of the plasmin A chain are mainly responsible for the interaction with α_2-antiplasmin.[164]

Mechanism of Irreversible Complex Formation. Plasmin and α_2-antiplasmin form a stoichiometric 1:1 complex of about 140 kd by interaction between the B chain of plasmin and the inhibitor. A nondisulfide-bonded pep-

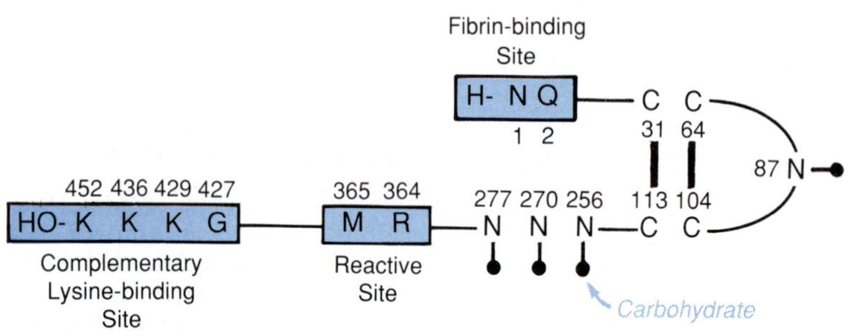

FIGURE 42-5. Schematic representation of the primary structure of α_2-antiplasmin.

tide (8 kd) is released concomitantly with complex formation. Upon disulfide bond reduction, the complex is dissociated in two parts: (1) an intact plasmin A chain (60 kd), and (2) a stable complex between the plasmin B chain and α_2-antiplasmin (80 kd), provided the complex formation is performed in excess α_2-antiplasmin.[154] The reactive-site peptide bond in α_2-antiplasmin cleaved by plasmin[195] consists of Arg 364–Met 365 (see Fig. 42-5). A bond is formed between the active-site seryl residue in plasmin and a specific arginyl residue in the inhibitor. Indirect evidence that an ester bond may play a role in stabilizing the plasmin–α_2-antiplasmin complex was reported.[196] The reaction rate between plasmin and α_2-antiplasmin in plasma may be reduced by the presence of plasma proteins, such as histidine-rich glycoprotein[197] or fibrinogen,[164] which interfere with the reaction. The half-life of plasmin molecules on the fibrin surface is estimated to be two to three orders of magnitude longer than that of free plasmin.[173]

α_2-Macroglobulin

α_2-Macroglobulin is a slower reacting inhibitor of plasmin than α_2-antiplasmin and acts as a second-line inhibitor. It is a glycoprotein of 725 kd containing 8% carbohydrate, which does not belong to the serpin superfamily. It is composed of two half-molecules held together by noncovalent bonds. Each half-molecule is composed of two chains of about 180 kd each that are held together by disulfide bonds. The complete amino acid sequence of α_2-macroglobulin was elucidated.[198] α_2-Macroglobulin forms complexes with serine proteases, thiol proteases, carboxyl proteases, and metal proteases.[199] The α_2-macroglobulin–bound enzymes have a low or negligible residual proteolytic activity on large natural substrates but a virtually normal hydrolytic activity on synthetic substrates.

Barrett and others[199,200] proposed the following mechanism for the interaction between α_2-macroglobulin and enzymes. Binding is initiated by a proteolytic attack on the α_2-macroglobulin molecule; this results in a conformational change, such that the enzyme is irreversibly trapped within α_2-macroglobulin. The inhibition of enzymatic activity results from the steric hindrance of the access of substrates to the enzyme in its enclosed environment. Binding of α_2-macroglobulin to proteinases is accompanied by cleavage of the α_2-macroglobulin subunits to 85-kd fragments.[201,202] The α_2-macroglobulin–proteinase complex contains a maximum of 2 mol proteinase per 1 mol α_2-macroglobulin.[201,203,204] α_2-Macroglobulin contains a "bait" region for proteinases that was identified as a 35-residue internal sequence containing two sites cleaved by elastase and one site cleaved by trypsin, plasmin, and thrombin.[205] In addition to limited proteolysis in the bait region, complex formation with proteinases also involves rapid cleavage of a thiol ester present in each of the four identical subunits of 180 kd.[206] Disruption of these internal thiol esters in α_2-macroglobulin is required for the conformational change involved in the formation of sterically inhibited α_2-macroglobulin–proteinase complexes but not for the receptor-mediated endocytosis of the complexes.[207] The receptor-recognition site of α_2-macroglobulin complexes is abolished by proteolysis with lysine-specific proteases, indicating that at least one lysine residue is located at or near the receptor-recognition site.[208] The detailed mechanism of action of α_2-macroglobulin is reviewed elsewhere.[209]

The concentration of α_2-macroglobulin in plasma is age dependent; it reaches a maximum of about 4.5 g/L at 1 to 3 years of age and declines slowly to the adult level of about 2 g/L at 25 years.[210] It is 10% to 20% higher in women than in men, and increased values are found in nephrosis and liver cirrhosis.[211] Decreased levels also have been found during thrombolytic therapy.[212,213] The restoration of a normal α_2-macroglobulin level following thrombolytic therapy requires several days.

Bergquist and Nilsson[214] described a suspected hereditary α_2-macroglobulin deficiency in a man with 25% of the normal level. The transmission was shown to be autosomal dominant. The gene for α_2-macroglobulin was localized to chromosome 12.[215]

Plasminogen Activator Inhibitor-1

Plasminogen activator inhibitor-1 was first identified in conditioned media of human endothelial cells[216,217] and rat hepatoma cells.[218,219] It has subsequently been identified in plasma,[220–225] platelets,[226–228] placenta,[228] and conditioned media of fibrosarcoma cells[229,230] and hepatocytes.[231] The inhibitor was purified from endothelial cells,[232,233] hepatoma cells,[234] fibrosarcoma cells,[229] and melanoma cells.[235] It is a single-chain glycoprotein of about 52 kd consisting of 379 amino acids. The PAI-1 gene is about 12.2 kb in length and consists of 9 exons and 8 introns. It was mapped to chromosome 7, bands q21.3-q22.[236] The cDNA was sequenced, revealing that PAI-1 is a member of the serine protease inhibitor (serpin) family. Its reactive site consists of Arg 346–Met 347.[233,237–242]

In healthy individuals, highly variable plasma levels of both PAI activity and PAI-1 antigen were observed. PAI activity ranges from 0.5 to 47 IU/mL with most values (80%) below 6 IU/mL. PAI-1 antigen in plasma ranges between 6 ng/mL to 85 ng/mL (geometric mean, 24 ng/mL).[243] PAI activity is rapidly cleared from the circulation via the liver; a half-life of 7 minutes in the rabbit was reported.[244]

PAI-1 is stabilized by binding to a plasminogen activator inhibitor–binding protein identified as S-protein or vitronectin.[245] PAI-1 is the primary inhibitor of tPA and uPA in human plasma.[221] It reacts with single-chain tPA, two-chain tPA, and tcuPA, but not with scuPA or streptokinase.[221,224,225,246] The second-order rate constant for the inhibition of single-chain tPA by PAI-1 is 10^7 $mol^{-1} \cdot L \cdot s^{-1}$,[221,222,234] whereas inhibition of two-chain tPA and tcuPA by PAI-1 is even more rapid. PAI-1 is released during platelet aggregation, resulting in a 10-fold level increase.[226,227,247]

PAI-1 is highly labile and is found in tissue-culture fluid in a latent form that can be partly reactivated by treatment with denaturing agents, such as urea, guanidine hydrochloride, SDS, and phospholipids.[248,249] Production and release of PAI-1 from various cells is regulated by several stimuli, including thrombin,[250,251] dexamethasone,[218,219] endotoxin,[244] interleukin-1,[252,253] transforming growth factor β,[254,255] and tumor necrosis factor.[256,257] PAI-1 levels are elevated in several disease states (see section below on pathophysiology).

Plasminogen Activator Inhibitor-2

PAI-2 was identified in human placenta[258] and in pregnancy plasma[259,260]; it is also secreted by leukoctyes[261–264] and by fibrosarcoma cells.[230] It was purified from placenta,[265,266] leukocytes,[261] and U-937 cells.[264] PAI-2 exists in two different forms having comparable inhibition properties: (1) an intracellular nonglycosylated form of 47 kd and with a pI of 5.0, and (2) a secreted glycosylated form with of 60 kd and with a pI of 4.4.[267,268] The cDNA was sequenced[269–271]; PAI-2 is a serpin, containing 393 amino acids with reactive site Arg 358–Thr 359.

PAI-2 inhibits tcuPA with a second-order rate constant (k_1) of 9×10^5 $mol^{-1} \cdot L \cdot s^{-1}$,[262,264] which is about 10 times slower than PAI-1. PAI-2 also efficiently inhibits two-chain tPA ($k_1 = 2 \times 10^5$ $mol^{-1} \cdot L \cdot s^{-1}$, inhibits single-chain tPA less efficiently ($k_1 = 9 \times 10^3$ $mol^{-1} \cdot L \cdot s^{-1}$), and does not inhibit scuPA.[264] PAI-2 does not occur as a latent form.[230] Secretion of PAI-2 is regulated by endotoxin[272] and by phorbol esters,[264,267] which act by stimulating the gene transcription of PAI-2 more than 50-fold.[269]

Although PAI-2 in plasma occurs most frequently in association with pregnancy, it has occasionally been identified in men and non-pregnant women.[273]

MECHANISM OF PHYSIOLOGIC FIBRINOLYSIS

Molecular Interactions Between Components of the Fibrinolytic System

Plasminogen interacts specifically but weakly with fibrin through lysine-binding site structures.[172] The presence of tPA increases binding of plasminogen to a fibrin clot.[274] tPA has a specific affinity for fibrin (Fig. 42-6); the dissociation constant of the activator-fibrin complex was estimated to be 0.14 μmol/L.[22] Neither tcuPA nor scuPA bind specifically to fibrin.[92]

α_2-Antiplasmin interacts weakly with Glu-plasminogen through the lysine-binding sites (K_d of 4 μmol/L).[164] It reacts rapidly with plasmin (second-order rate constant of 2 to 4 $\times 10^7$ $mol^{-1} \cdot L \cdot s^{-1}$); the rate of this inhibition is strongly dependent on the availability of free lysine-binding sites and on a free active site in the plasmin molecule.[193,194] α_2-Antiplasmin is cross-linked to the fibrin α-chain when blood is clotted in the presence of calcium ions and activated coagulation factor XIII,[275] thereby inhibiting endogenous fibrinolysis.

Mechanism of Action of Tissue Plasminogen Activator

Tissue plasminogen activator is a poor enzyme in the absence of fibrin, but the presence of fibrin strikingly enhances the activation rate of plasminogen.[22,100] The kinetic data support a mechanism where fibrin provides a surface

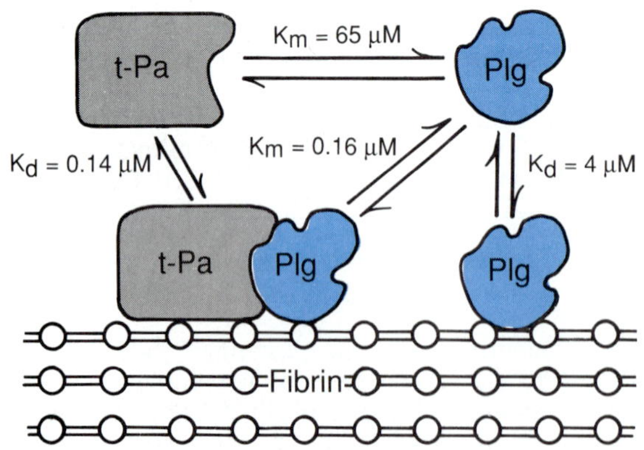

FIGURE 42-6. Schematic representation of the molecular interactions that regulate the fibrin-specific activation of the fibronolytic system by tissue-type plasminogen activator (tPA; t-Pa in figure). tPA in circulating plasma has a low affinity for its substrate plasminogen (Plg; K_m = 65 μmol/L), and no efficient plasminogen activation will occur. tPA binds specifically to fibrin (K_d = 0.14 μmol/L). The bimolecular tPA fibrin complex has high affinity for plasminogen (K_m = 0.16 μmol/L) compared with the low affinity of plasminogen for fibrin in the absence of tPA. Plasminogen binds to the binary tPA fibrin complex and is activated to plasmin at the fibrin surface. This in loco generated plasmin is protected from rapid inactivation by α_2-antiplasmin and degrades fibrin.

to which tPA and plasminogen adsorb in a sequential and ordered way, yielding a cyclic ternary complex. Fibrin essentially increases the local plasminogen concentration by creating an additional interaction between tPA and its substrate. The high affinity of tPA for plasminogen in the presence of fibrin thus allows efficient activation on the fibrin clot, whereas no efficient plasminogen activation by tPA occurs in plasma. Others, however, claim that fibrin influences both the K_m and k_{cat} of plasminogen activation by tPA.[39]

Plasmin formed on the fibrin surface has both its lysine-binding sites and active site occupied and is only slowly inactivated by α_2-antiplasmin (half-life of about 10 to 100 s); free plasmin, when formed, is rapidly inhibited by α_2-antiplasmin (half-life of about 0.1 second).[193] The fibrinolytic process thus seems to be triggered by and confined to fibrin.

It was proposed that initial binding of tPA to fibrin is governed by the finger domain, and following partial degradation of fibrin, newly exposed carboxyl-terminal lysine residues result in enhanced binding of tPA via K_2.[28] Higgins and Vehar[23] confirmed that when fibrin is degraded by plasmin, new tPA binding sites with markedly lower dissociation constants (two to four orders of magnitude) are formed. Thus, early fibrin digestion by plasmin could accelerate fibrinolysis by increasing binding of both tPA[28] and plasminogen.[39]

Mechanism of Action of Urokinase Plasminogen Activator

Two-chain urokinase plasminogen activator has no specific affinity for fibrin and activates fibrin-bound and circulating plasminogen relatively indiscriminately. Extensive plasminogen activation and depletion of α_2-antiplasmin may occur following treatment of thromboembolic diseases with tcuPA, leading to degradation of several plasma proteins including fibrinogen, factor V, and factor VIII.

scuPA, in contrast to tcuPA, has significant fibrin specificity. A hypothetical mechanism of action is proposed[92] on the basis of the following observations:

1. In purified systems, scuPA has some intrinsic plasminogen activating potential.
2. scuPA does not significantly activate plasminogen in plasma in the absence of fibrin. A component in plasma may interfere with plasminogen activation.
3. After preincubation of scuPA in plasma for up to 48 hours, efficient fibrinolysis without fibrinogenolysis is still observed on addition of a fibrin clot. Preliminary data suggest that the presence of fibrin reverses the inhibition exerted by plasma, although direct binding of scuPA to fibrin could not be demonstrated.

These findings suggest that the fibrin specificity of plasminogen activation by scuPA is due to neutralization by fibrin of components in plasma that impair plasminogen activation.

Alternatively, the presence of fibrin may enhance the activation rate of fibrin-bound plasminogen.[276] In clot lysis systems in human plasma in vitro, conversion of scuPA to tcuPA constitutes a major positive feedback mechanism for fibrinolysis.[277] Because 54-kd scuPA and scuPA-32k induce similar fibrin-specific clot lysis,[86,87] it appears that the structures responsible for the fibrin specificity of scuPA are independent of the NH_2-terminal portion of the protein. The molecular interactions that regulate the fibrin-specific activation of the fibrinolytic system by scuPA remain to be further detailed.

PATHOPHYSIOLOGY OF FIBRINOLYSIS

α_2-Antiplasmin Deficiency and Bleeding

Congenital α_2-Antiplasmin Deficiency

Patients with congenital α_2-antiplasmin deficiency may have a clinically severe bleeding tendency[278–286] (Table 42-3). Koie and associates[278] describe the first case of homozygous α_2-antiplasmin deficiency in a patient who presented with a hemorrhagic diathesis, characterized by prolonged bleeding and ecchymoses after minor trauma and by spontaneous joint hemorrhage.[278] Studies of family members indicate that this abnormality was inherited as an autosomal and recessive trait.[279] The bleeding tendency of the patient may be due to premature lysis of hemostatic plugs; in the absence of α_2-antiplasmin, plasmin molecules generated on the fibrin surface of the hemostatic plug would persist much longer than normal.

The first published families with α_2-antiplasmin deficiency were discovered through a homozygous propositus with severe bleeding. Several additional cases have now been reported where heterozygotes had no discernible bleeding symptoms.[279,282,284] In contrast, 6 of 16 heterozygotes in a group of Dutch families[281] and 2 of 5 heterozygotes in American families[286] presented with mild bleeding. Two additional heterozygotes having α_2-antiplasmin deficiencies and a mild[283] or severe[285] life-long bleeding history have been reported. The α_2-antiplasmin levels in all heterozygotes described thus far are similar—that is, 40% to 60% of normal (see Table 42-3).

Acquired α_2-Antiplasmin Deficiency

Increased fibrinolysis in liver disease, especially in cirrhosis, is a well-known phenomenon. The serum level of α_2-antiplasmin is significantly decreased in liver cirrhosis and in several other liver diseases. Teger-Nilsson and coworkers[287] report a mean value of 73% ± 15% for liver cirrhosis (controls, 100% ± 8%), and Aoki and Yamanaka found values of 4.24 ± 0.87 mg/dL and 2.56 ± 0.87 mg/dL for compensated and decompensated liver cirrhosis, respectively (controls, 6.2 ± 0.8 mg/dL).[288] Samama and colleagues [289] report a similar decrease in α_2-antiplasmin level in patients with liver cirrhosis having normal or elevated levels of fibrinogen degradation products. Thus, the decreased level of α_2-antiplasmin appears to be an important factor in the increased fibrinolytic activity observed in liver cirrhosis. Moreover, it is likely that the liver is the organ of synthesis or storage of α_2-antiplasmin.[290]

Decreased levels of α_2-antiplasmin also have been reported in patients having disseminated intravascular coagulation and some forms of renal disease.[291] α_2-Antiplasmin levels may be significantly reduced in patients undergoing thrombolytic therapy as a result of systemic activation of the fibrinolytic system. Following intravenous infusion of either recombinant tPA (rtPA) or streptokinase in patients with acute myocardial infarction, the observed decrease of α_2-antiplasmin was significantly greater in the streptokinase group.[292]

Dysfunctional α_2-Antiplasmin

An abnormal α_2-antiplasmin associated with a serious bleeding tendency was found in two siblings in a Dutch family; it is referred to as α_2-antiplasmin Enschede. These individuals have 3% of normal functional activity and 100% of normal antigen levels.[293] Their apparently heterozygous parents have 50% functional activity and 100% antigen levels. The ability of the protein to reversibly bind plasmin or plasminogen was not affected, but the abnormal α_2-antiplasmin is converted from an inhibitor of plasmin to a substrate. The molecular defect of α_2-antiplasmin Enschede was revealed by sequencing of cloned genomic DNA fragments.[294] It consists of the insertion of an extra alanine residue (GCG insertion) somewhere between amino acid residues 353 and 357 (4 Ala residues) 7 to 10 positions on the amino-terminal side of the P_1 residue (Arg 364) in the reactive site of α_2-antiplasmin. This 3-bp in-frame insertion within the gene of α_2-antiplasmin was identified in 2 true heterozygotes and in their 2 homozygous children.

Plasminogen Activator Inhibitor Activity and Thrombosis

Increased levels of PAI activity were reported in several thrombotic disease states. Increased levels of PAI were observed in coronary heart disease[295,296] and acute myocardial infarction.[297,298] In patients who had suffered a myocardial infarction, the depressed fibrinolytic activity was due to an increased PAI activity[299,300]; increased levels of PAI activity in these patients were associated with an increased risk of reinfarction.[301] Plasma PAI activity increased in patients with a recent episode of thrombosis.[302,303] In prospective studies, however, no difference was found in PAI activity in patients with or without deep-vein thrombosis (DVT).[304,305] In patients undergoing hip replacement, preoperative PAI activity was significantly elevated in those

TABLE 42-3. Congenital α_2-Antiplasmin Deficiency

Author	Propositus	α_2-Antiplasmin Level* (% Normal)	Bleeding
Koie et al[278,279]	Homozygote	0	Yes (severe)
	Heterozygotes, 9	±50	No
Kluft et al[280,281]	Homozygote	2	Yes (severe)
	Heterozygotes, 16	50–60	Yes, 6 (mild)
			No, 10
Yoshioka et al[282]	Homozygotes, 3	1–2	Yes (severe)
	Heterozygotes, 3	±50	Yes (mild)
Knot et al[283]	Heterozygote	±50	Yes (mild)
Stormorken et al[284]	Heterozygote	41–47	No
Kordich et al[285]	Heterozygote	±50	Yes (severe)
Miles et al[286]	Homozygotes, 2	<1	Yes
	Heterozygotes, 5	48 ± 12	Yes, 2 (mild)
			No, 3

* Functional and antigenic levels correspond well.

patients who would develop postoperative DVT.[306] Such a relation was not observed in patients undergoing major abdominal surgery, however.[305,307] These discrepancies suggest either that increased levels of PAI activity may constitute a risk factor for the development of DVT or that PAI actually increases as a result of DVT. In patients with recurrent DVT, a defective fibrinolytic response to venous occlusion is often observed as a result of either a decreased release of tPA or a high level of PAI.[308–310] Juhan-Vague and associates[310] investigated 120 patients with spontaneous or recurrent DVT and observed 3 groups based on their response to venous occlusion. A poor fibrinolytic response (less than 2-fold increase) to venous occlusion occurred in 35% of these patients; 25% of them (12 patients) had deficient tPA release and high risk for recurrent DVT; 75% (32 patients) had normal tPA release but increased level of PAI-1. Mellbring and coworkers[311] report that patients subjected to major abdominal surgery who have enhanced fibrinolytic activity preoperatively (as measured from the levels of plasmin–α_2-antiplasmin complex) have less tendency to develop postoperative DVT.

Plasminogen Deficiency and Thrombosis

Congenital Plasminogen Deficiency

The plasma concentration of plasminogen antigen in full-term newborns is about half that of adults,[312,313] whereas the functional activity is reported to be comparable[313] or lower[312] than expected on the basis of antigen concentration.

Plasminogen deficiency as a cause of thrombosis, characterized by a parallel decrease of functional and immunoreactive plasminogen, was reported in only a few cases.[314–318] Hasegawa and others[314] report three unrelated families with inherited low levels of plasminogen associated with recurrent pulmonary embolism and DVT. Ten Cate and associates[315] report an isolated plasminogen deficiency in a woman with recurrent thrombophlebitis and pulmonary embolism, characterized by a reduction of both plasminogen antigen and activity to 45%. Lottenberg and colleagues[316] identified a patient with pulmonary hypertension, a history of venous thrombosis, and severe plasminogen deficiency (30% of normal antigen and activity). All functional properties of the isolated plasminogen were normal, and no evidence for increased plasminogen activation or increased turnover was found. The authors concluded that this patient had a deficiency of normally functioning plasminogen, probably due to decreased synthesis. This abnormality was also found in two siblings and family members, but inheritance of the deficiency could not be established. Mannucci and others[317] reported a case of a young man having a history of venous thrombotic disease with a reduction of both antigenic and functional plasminogen to 50% of normal. This deficiency was inherited as an autosomal trait, and the propositus and his sister were heterozygotes. Administration of the anabolic steroid stanozolol transiently normalized the plasminogen level. A case of heterozygous plasminogen deficiency (50% of normal antigen and activity) was also observed in a mother (55 years) and daughter (10 years) and found to be inherited autosomally.[318] The mother showed a life-long thrombotic tendency.

In all these cases, other investigated hemostatic parameters were normal; thus, they apparently represent true isolated plasminogen deficiencies that are associated with severe thromboembolic complications.

Acquired Plasminogen Deficiency

Reduced levels of plasminogen have been observed in several clinical conditions, including liver disease[319] and sepsis (25% to 45% of normal activity).[320] Possible mechanisms for acquired plasminogen deficiency in severe liver disease are depression of synthesis and increased consumption.[321] Degradation of plasminogen into LMW plasminogen by leukocyte elastase is a possible explanation for the reduction observed in septic patients. In the plasma of some septic patients, a LMW plasminogen-like molecule has indeed been identified.[320] In severe Argentine hemorrhagic fever, plasminogen antigen levels were normal, but activity levels were significantly reduced. Proteolytic degradation of plasminogen by leukocyte enzymes (elastase) is a possible explanation.[322]

Human plasma contains at least two proteins—α_2-antiplasmin and hisitidine-rich glycoprotein (HRG)—that bind to the lysine-binding sites of plasminogen and thereby counteract plasminogen binding to fibrin. For the interaction of α_2-antiplasmin[164] or HRG[197] with plasminogen, dissociation constants of 4 or 1 μmol/L, respectively, were determined in purified systems. In the absence of other interactions in plasma, 50% of the plasminogen would be expected to circulate reversibly bound to HRG and 15% to circulate reversibly bound to α_2-antiplasmin. Jespersen and colleagues[323] found consistently higher concentrations of HRG in 34 patients with acute myocardial infarction associated with DVT. In a more extensive study, however, no significant change in the plasma level of HRG was found in a group of 40 patients with arterial thrombosis or in 152 patients with venous thrombosis.[324] Increased HRG levels, apparently associated with thrombosis, were observed only in a few families.

Dysplasminogenemia

Abnormalities in the plasminogen molecule resulting in defective activation to plasmin is described by several authors.

In 1978, Aoki and coworkers[325] identified a patient with recurrent thrombosis over a 15-year period who had an abnormally low plasminogen activity (about 50% of normal) but a normal level of plasminogen antigen. This antigen was a mixture of normal and abnormal molecules in about equal amounts. Studies of the patient's family members suggest that the molecular abnormality was inherited in an autosomal dominant pattern. One of the family members was a homozygote having virtually no plasminogen activity but normal antigen level. Functional analysis of this plasminogen (Tochigi)[326] revealed that (1) it forms a complex with streptokinase, but this complex does not incorporate the active-site titrant diisopropyl fluorophosphate; (2) it is converted to an inactive two-chain plasmin molecule by urokinase; and (3) the lysine-binding sites are functionally intact. An additional characteristic is the gel electrofocusing pattern of the purified plasminogen from the heterozygotes, which consists of 10 normal bands and 10 abnormal bands, each having a slightly higher isoelectric point than the respective corresponding normal component. The gel electrofocusing pattern of the homozygote plasminogen consists of abnormal bands only. Miyata and associates[327] demonstrated that the absence of proteolytic activity in plasminogen Tochigi is due to a single amino acid substitution (Ala 600 to Thr) near the His 602 residue of the active site. The genetic change responsible for this substitution is a G to A transition in the first nucleotide (5′ terminal) of the Ala 600 codon.[132,327] This Ala to Thr substitution in the plasmin light chain may affect the side chain of the Asp 645 or His 602 active-site residues and thereby disturb the active-site charge relay system, leading to loss of enzymatic activity. In trypsin, the methyl group of the corresponding Ala residue is spatially close to the imidazole ring of the active-site His and to the β-carboxyl group of the active-site Asp.[328]

Two additional abnormal plasminogens (plasminogen Tochigi II and plasminogen Nagoya) having the same molecular defect (ie, Ala 600 to Thr substitution) were identified in other members of the same family.[329] This heterozygote abnormal plasminogen phenotype was found in 3.6% of a Japanese population but could not be found in an American population.[330] A similar plasminogen polymorphism, characterized by normal antigen levels yet only half of normal activity, was also reported in Japanese by Nakamura and Abe.[331] They observed this type of polymorphism in 4.4% of a Japanese population with a gene frequency of 0.0233.

Besides these three dysplasminogenemias with an identical single amino acid mutation (Tochigi I, Tochigi II, and Nagoya), two identical cases (normal plasminogen antigen, 50% activity) with thrombotic complications were reported.[332,333] For both plasminogen Tokyo[332] and plasminogen Paris I,[333] the abnormality is presumably due to an active-site defect, which has not yet been identified. A similar case of heterozygous dysplasminogenemia combined with protein C deficiency was reported in a 21-year-old man with recurrent venous thrombosis.[334] In all these cases, the propositus suffered from thrombotic complications, whereas other family members with the same plasminogen abnormality usually had not presented with clinical symptoms of thrombosis.

Wohl and coworkers[335,336] characterized three human plasminogen variants (Chicago I, II, and III) identified in young males with a history of recurring DVT. No clear inheritance pattern was observed. Both homozygote plasminogens Chicago I and II have an activation defect characterized by a high Michaelis constant and impaired plasminogen activator binding, but normal cleavage of the Arg 560–Val 561 peptide bond.[335] The homozygote plasminogen Chicago III has both impaired affinity for plasminogen activators (evidenced by an increased Michaelis constant) and impaired cleavage of the Arg 560–Val 561 peptide bond.[336]

Another abnormal plasminogen, Frankfurt I, was identified in the plasma of a 42-year-old man with recurrent DVT.[337] A reduced antigen concentration—with only half the molecules having functional active sites—was found in the propositus and his mother. The molecular defect in this plasminogen has not been identified.

Characteristic of all these dysplasminogenemias is a low ratio of functional to immunoreactive plasminogen, ranging from 0.2 (plasminogen Tokyo) to 0.88 (plasminogen Chicago II). The main properties of the abnormal plasminogens are summarized in Table 42-4.

Plasminogen Activator Deficiency and Thrombosis

Release and Inhibition of Urokinase-Type Plasminogen Activator

Whereas tPA synthesis occurs mainly in endothelial cells,[3,338] immunocytochemical staining of tissues with antibodies directed against uPA reveals that cells of many different origins (including fibroblasts, epithelial cells, and pneumocytes) produce uPA.[339] The scuPA concentration in human plasma has not been clearly established, and mean values reported range between 2 and 20 ng/mL. With an ELISA based on murine monoclonal antibodies and using scuPA for the construction of a calibration curve, the level of uPA in normal resting plasma was about 2 ng/mL[340]; this is lower than values reported with other direct immunoassays calibrated with tcuPA.[75,341,342]

Many cells contain a receptor that is specific for scuPA and for HMW tcuPA, but it does not bind LMW tcuPA.[343–347] The amino acid sequence consisting of residues 18 to 30 in the growth factor domain of human uPA is probably involved in binding to this receptor.[348] The dissociation constant of the interaction of uPA with its receptor is 10^{-9} to 10^{-10} mol/L; about 50,000 binding sites are in the monocyte-like U-937 cell. The purified receptor is a glycoprotein of about 50 kd.[349] Membrane-bound uPA retains its plasminogen activating potential and is protected to some extent from extracellular inhibitors. The presence of uPA receptors on many normal and malignant cells may constitute a mechanism to remodel the extracellular matrix.[350] Phorbolmyristate acetate treatment of U-937 cells induces both an increase in synthesis and a decrease in affinity of the uPA receptor, which results in increased uPA binding.[347] This effect of phorbolmyristate acetate may be mediated by protein kinase C.[347]

tcuPA is slowly inhibited in human plasms by several protease inhibitors including α_2-macroglobulin,[351] α_1-antitrypsin,[352] antithrombin III,[353] α_2-antiplasmin,[354] and plasminogen activator inhibitor-3 (PAI-3),[355] which is identical to activated protein C inhibitor.[356] More specific and rapid inhibition occurs by PAI-1 and PAI-2. Urokinase inhibitor assays based on clot lysis depend strongly on the presence of plasmin inhibitors and therefore are not specific. Assayed with such clot lysis methods, the half-life of tcuPA was 9 to 16 minutes in vivo but 27 to 61 minutes in vitro[357]; this suggests that clearing the enzyme from the blood is important. In contrast to tcuPA, scuPA is not in-

TABLE 42-4. Characterization of Dysplasminogenemias

Designation	Molecular Defect	Antigen Level	Functional Level (% Normal)	Thrombosis	
				Propositus	Relatives
Tochigi I[325–327]	Active site Ala 600 → Thr substitution	Normal	40	Yes	No
Tochigi II[329]		Normal	50	No	No
Nagoya[329]		Normal	50	No	No
Tokyo[332]	Active site ?	Normal	20–30	Yes	No
Paris I[333]	Active site ?	Normal	45	Yes	No
Chicago I[335]	Lower affinity for activators	Normal	41	Yes	?
Chicago II[335]		Normal	88	Yes	?
Chicago III[336]	Lower affinity for activators + impaired cleavage of Arg 560–Val	Normal	80	Yes	?
Frankfurt I[337]	Active site ?	Low normal (78%)	37	Yes	?

hibited by plasma protease inhibitors and retains its activity after incubation in human plasma for up to 48 hours.[358,359]

Release and Inhibition of tPA

The mechanism of tPA secretion remains unknown. Cash[360] speculated that it may be under neurohumoral control and that a plasminogen activator–releasing hormone constitutes the major pathway for its release from endothelial cells. This hormone could not be identified in bovine pituitary or hypothalamic extracts, however.[361]

Comp and Esmon[362] infused activated protein C into dogs and found an increase in plasma fibrinolytic activity. This finding was not confirmed in squirrel monkeys using activated human protein C.[363] The profibrinolytic effect of activated protein C was later shown to result from a decrease in concentration of the fast-acting tPA inhibitor, PAI-1.[364] Agents that stimulate release of tPA from endothelial cells (such as thrombin) also stimulate secretion of PAI-1.[250,365] Dexamethasone increased tPA antigen levels in rat hepatoma cells moderately (1.5 times) but significantly increased PAI-1 antigen levels (4 to 5 times), resulting in inhibition of tPA activity.[366] Endotoxin stimulates the secretion of PAI-1 activity but not tPA antigen,[244,365] whereas histamine causes a secretion of tPA antigen but not PAI-1.[365]

Butyrate treatment of endothelial cells induces significant increases in tPA mRNA levels and in tPA production without influencing the level of PAI-1. A straight C_4 monocarboxylate structure with a methyl group at one end and a carboxyl moiety at the other is required for optimal induction of tPA in cultured endothelial cells.[367] Interleukin-1, derived from human placenta, stimulates preferentially the production of tPA by human articular chondrocytes.[368] Liu and associates[369] have shown that gonadotropin treatment increases tPA activity and antigen levels in ovarian cells to a maximum prior to ovulation. This gonadotropin regulation of tPA activity may play a role in follicle rupture. Quantitation of tPA mRNA levels in cell cultures by hybridization with a tPA cDNA probe[370] confirms that increased secretion of tPA induced by gonadotropins in rat granulosa cells is paralleled by increased steady-state levels of tPA mRNA.[371,372]

The mechanisms involved in removal of tPA from the blood are multiple. A main one is clearance by the liver, which results in a half-life of a few minutes both in animals and in humans.

tPA occurs in plasma in a free active form and in complexes with α_2-antiplasmin, α_1-antitrypsin,[373] and C_1-inhibitor.[374] A specific rapid-reacting inhibitor of tPA, PAI-1, having a molecular weight about 50,000 was more recently identified. PAI-1 is present in normal human plasma at a low concentration or at a higher concentration in many clinical conditions,[375] including venous thromboembolic disease.[310]

Pathophysiology of Impaired Fibrinolytic Activity

Impairment of fibrinolysis due to deficient synthesis, release of tPA from the vessel wall, or increased levels of PAI-1 is associated with a tendency to thrombosis.

Clayton and coworkers[376] determined several clinical and laboratory parameters preoperatively in women undergoing gynecologic surgery and measured the occurrence of postoperative DVT. Three clinical parameters (age, percentage overweight for height, and presence of varicose veins) and two laboratory tests (euglobulin clot lysis time and level of fibrinogen-related antigen in serum) were used to construct a preoperative index that clinically separated patients who subsequently developed DVT from those who did not. Of these parameters, a prolongation of the euglobulin clot lysis time was the most discriminating parameter. Rakoczi and coworkers[377] applied Clayton's index to a comparable group of gynecologic patients and confirmed that a low preoperative euglobulin fibrinolytic activity is associated with an increased risk of developing postoperative DVT.

Isacson and Nilsson[378] found a defective release of tPA from the vessel wall during venous occlusion or a decreased tPA content in walls of superficial veins in about 70% of patients with idiopathic recurrent venous thrombosis. This association of recurrent venous thrombosis with a defect in the fibrinolytic system is more frequent than with any other known disturbance of hemostasis. Phenformin combined with ethylestrenol stimulated release of fibrinolytic activity from the vessel wall and diminished the frequency of thrombotic episodes.[379] Korninger and associates[380] followed a group of 121 patients with a history of either venous thrombosis, pulmonary embolism, or both for 56 ± 19 months. They observed a significantly lower recurrence rate in patients with a postocclusion euglobulin lysis time shorter than 60 minutes (4.8% per year), compared with patients with a postocclusion euglobulin lysis time longer than 60 minutes (10.3% per year). In these two studies,[378,380] the potential cause of impaired fibrinolytic activity, defective release of tPA from the vessel wall, or increased rate of inactivation was not determined. Subsequent studies[310,381] show that both mechanisms may contribute to a deficient fibrinolytic response.

Excess tPA Levels and Bleeding

Excessive fibrinolysis due to increased tPA levels may cause bleeding complications. A life-long hemorrhagic disorder associated with enhanced fibrinolysis caused by increased levels of circulating plasminogen activator was described. No deficiency of any known inhibitor of fibrinolysis could be detected.[382] A similar case of an inherited increased fibrinolytic potential due to an excess of tPA was reported in a Spanish family.[383]

ANTIFIBRINOLYTIC AGENTS

Antifibrinolytic agents, which neutralize plasmin activity or reduce plasminogen activation in vivo include aprotinin, 6-aminohexanoic acid (epsilon aminocaproic acid), *p*-aminomethylbenzoic acid, and tranexamic acid.

Aprotinin

Aprotinin is a naturally occurring inhibitor of proteolytic enzymes. It was discovered independently by Kraut and colleagues[384] and by Kunitz and Northrop[385] as the trypsin-kallikrein inhibitor in bovine tissue.

Physiochemical and Pharmokinetic Properties

Aprotinin (a serine protease inhibitor) is 6512 daltons and consists of 58 amino acid residues in a single polypeptide chain cross-linked by 3 disulfide bridges. Aprotinin acts as an inhibitor of human trypsin, plasmin, plasma kallikrein, and tissue kallikreins by forming reversible stoichiometric enzyme-inhibitor complexes. The reactive site of this strongly basic protein consists of Lys 15–Ala 16.[386,387] The concentration and activity of commercial preparations of aprotinin are usually given in kallikrein inactivator units (KIU). One hundred thousand KIU are equivalent to 14 mg of the pure polypeptide.

After intravenous injection of aprotinin in humans, clearance is biphasic with an initial phase of rapid clearance from the circulation followed by a slower exponential decrease. The initial rapid decline in serum concentrations, with a half-life of about 9 minutes, represents equilibration with the extravascular compartment and rapid renal uptake. The half-life of the slow phases after intravenous administration are 2 hours and 7 hours, respectively, with the apparent explanation for the latter being accumulation of the drug in a "deep compartment."[388,389]

More of the infused aprotinin is excreted unchanged in the urine, even after a large dose (1 million KIU). Metabolic degradation into small peptides or amino acids apparently occurs by lysosomal activity in the kidney.[390]

Following administration of aprotinin to patients by constant intravenous infusion at a rate of 250,000 KIU/h over 24 hours, a steady-state plasma concentration of 40 to 50 KIU/mL was obtained, representing a concentration of about 1 μmol/L.[391]

Clinical Use

Several indications for the therapeutic and prophylactic use of aprotinin have been studied.

Acute Pancreatitis. A statistically significant reduction in mortality observed in one prospective controlled trial[392] could not be confirmed in two other controlled trials.[393,394] This leaves the issue unresolved whether aprotinin could possibly be effective in certain types of pancreatitis.

Prevention or Treatment of Abnormal Blood Loss. For this indication, the antifibrinolytic (antiplasmin) effect of aprotinin is important. Aprotinin is recommended for use mainly in acute acquired defects of the coagulation mechanism that arise secondary to a variety of clinical situations.

In a prospective, randomized, comparative study conducted on 40 patients with abruptio placenta complicated by fetal death, disseminated intravascular coagulation, and uterine inertia, aprotinin decreased the consumption of coagulation factors and reduced the overall complication rate.[395]

Women with intrauterine devices (IUDs) may have excessive blood loss. Intrauterine application of aprotinin or tranexamic acid was tried in 34 women with IUDs who complained of menorrhagia and the result compared with that of a placebo group. Both inhibitors reduced the length of the menstrual period by about 50%.[396]

Blood loss during and after surgery of the prostate was investigated by hemoglobin measurements in a comparative trial of different antifibrinolytic drugs. After administration of 200,000 KIU aprotinin in combination with either 5 g ϵ-aminocaproic acid or 1 g tranexamic acid, blood loss was significantly reduced compared with controls or with patients given either drug alone.[397] Another study revealed that a combination of a low dose (7 g/d) of ϵ-aminocaproic acid with 250,000 KIU aprotinin reduced blood loss after both transurethral and transvesical prostatectomy.[398]

A reduction in the frequency of recurrent hemorrhage in patients with subarachnoid bleeding was reported following combined treatment with a low dose of tranexamic acid (1 g three times a day) and aprotinin 500,000 KIU three times a day.[399,400]

Although excessive blood loss decreased with more refined cardiopulmonary bypass methodology and equipment, further reduction of postoperative bleeding in cardiac surgery is still needed.

Aprotinin given during open heart surgery diminished blood loss significantly.[401,402] But when aprotinin was administered at the end of bypass time (ie, immediately before neutralization of heparin by protamine), no distinct effect on coagulation parameters was found.[403] At a dose of 5,000,000 KIU/kg given before institution of cardiopulmonary bypass, myocardial protection from global ischemia resulted.[404] Aprotinin was used successfully to prevent fibrin-coated aortic allografts from leaking.[405,406]

Shock. One of the hallmarks of shock is early and profound derangement of microcirculation and of cell metabolism, the latter leading to lysosomal disruption and release of proteolytic enzymes, which contribute to the syndrome of "shock lung." Based on this pathogenetic rationale, the effect of protease inhibition in the therapy of various forms of shock was investigated; aprotinin favorably influenced several clinical parameters and improved survival.[407]

A large-scale therapeutic study of traumatic hemorrhagic shock (primarily from motor vehicle accidents) reveals a statistically significant difference in mortality between patients treated with aprotinin within 30 minutes of the accident as part of the emergency treatment compared with control patients.[408] In a randomized, controlled, double-blind study, posttraumatic respiratory insufficiency was selected as the relevant criterion of effectiveness of adjuvant aprotinin therapy in traumatic hemorrhagic shock. Both the frequency and severity of respiratory insufficiency were significantly diminished in 35 patients receiving aprotinin as soon as possible after hospital admission compared with a placebo control group.[409]

In another prospective clinical investigation in 81 polytrauma patients, no difference in the clinical outcome was found between a group given a standard intravenous heparin regimen (bolus of 1000 IU, followed 6 hours later by 200 IU/kg over 24 hours for 3 days) and the aprotinin group (bolus of 500,000 KIU, followed by 200,000 KIU every 4 hours for 5 days).[410]

Reduction of Infarct Size. Aprotinin may indirectly protect the myocardium from anoxic damage and maintain cell wall integrity by neutralizing kinin release in or from the damaged tissue. These intriguing observations stimulated a large-scale controlled trial. The results reveal that the survival curves of patients receiving aprotinin, heparin, or both were indistinguishable.[411]

The effect of aprotinin on the extent of myocardial necrosis and the development of Q-waves was studied in 25 patients admitted to hospital within 30 to 60 minutes after the onset of symptoms of acute myocardial ischemia. In comparison with a control group, there was a significantly smaller estimated infarct size (according to creatine phosphokinase measurements) in addition to improved electrocardiographic indicators of myocardial ischemic injury following treatment with aprotinin.[412]

Dosage and Side Effects. The initial loading dose for systemic administration of aprotinin is about 15,000 to 20,000 KIU/kg administered as a short intravenous infusion, followed by 200,000 KIU every 4 hours, preferably given as a continuous intravenous infusion (50,000 KIU/h).

Aprotinin has remarkably few side effects; the healthy individual apparently has a broad physiologic tolerance for protease inhibitors of similar specificity. This is in accordance with the available toxicity data for aprotinin and the good tolerance reported clinically.[413]

6-Aminohexanoic Acid

6-Aminohexanoic acid (ϵ-aminocaproic acid) was the first synthetic representative of a new class of drugs, the antifibrinolytic agents. The relation between its chemical structure and its antifibrinolytic action is well established, based on its action as a lysine substitute.[414] The five-carbon chain is important for its antifibrinolytic effect, which in principle is based on the same molecular interaction as for the other aminocarboxylic acids, tranexamic acid and *p*-aminomethylbenzoic acid. The antifibrinolytic potency of the aminocarboxylic acids depends on the presence of free amino and carboxylic groups, and on the distance between the carboxylic group and the carbon atom to which the amino group is attached.

Clinical Pharmacology

The clinical pharmacology of 6-aminohexanoic acid was investigated in detail.[415,416] Oral doses (100 mg/kg) are rapidly and nearly completely absorbed, giving peak plasma concentrations of 30 mg/L after about 2 hours, whereas the elimination half-life is between 1 and 2 hours. The drug is distributed throughout the extravascular space and readily crosses the erythrocyte membrane and diffuses into various tissues. Oral 6-aminohexanoic acid is concentrated and excreted in the urine in a chemically unchanged active form, 80% being excreted within 12 hours; only a small amount of the absorbed dose is believed to be metabolized. The rapid excretion means that parenteral administration for a systemic effect should be by continuous infusion; however, less frequent doses are adequate for its action in the renal tract where the drug is concentrated.

Intravenous administration of 100 mg/kg 6-aminohexanoic acid produces an initial serum concentration of about 1500 mg/L, which falls to 35 mg/L within 3 to 4 hours. About 90% of the administered dose is found in the urine within 4 to 6 hours. Thus, 6-aminohexanoic acid is concentrated many times during excretion, urinary levels being 50 to 100 times those found in plasma.

Dosage

Because of its short half-life, 6-aminohexanoic acid is administered in relatively large doses to reach and sustain an effective plasma concentration of 0.01 mol/L. An intravenous loading dose of 10 g followed by 1 g/h gives the desired blood level. The oral dose of 6-aminohexanoic acid is 0.1 g/kg every 6 hours.

Literature on the clinical use of 6-aminohexanoic acid in a variety of clinical conditions abounds, but its effectiveness was documented by controlled clinical trials in only a limited number of indications. As tranexamic acid is 7 to 10 times more potent than 6-aminohexanoic acid and has the same low toxicity, the latter drug is little used clinically and not discussed further.

p-Aminomethylbenzoic Acid

The study of the antifibrinolytic activity of a series of cyclic compounds with terminal amino or carboxylic groups led to the identification of *p*-aminomethylbenzoic acid.[417] Comparison of 6-aminohexanoic acid and *p*-aminomethylbenzoic acid showed that the latter is about three times more active than the former. The higher potency of this compound can likely be explained by the fixation of the distance between the amino and carboxylic groups because of its more rigid molecular structure.

p-Aminomethylbenzoic acid is readily absorbed after oral and intramuscular administration, with peak blood levels being reached after 2 to 3 hours and 30 to 60 minutes, respectively. The elimination half-life is about 1 hour. Excretion of *p*-aminomethylbenzoic acid is via the kidneys, and up to 70% is found in the urine in unchanged form within the first 24 hours; the remaining portion is thought to be excreted as an inert metabolic product.[418]

Clinical experience with *p*-aminomethylbenzoic acid is limited to case reports, and no controlled, randomized double-blind studies have been published. The initial intravenous dose is 50 to 100 mg followed by a continuous infusion of 100 mg/h. The recommended oral dose is 250 mg repeated at 4- to 8-hour intervals.[419] These doses are generally well tolerated.

Because no adequate clinical trials have been carried out, and more potent cyclic aminocarboxylic acids (such as tranexamic acid) have been developed, *p*-aminomethylbenzoic acid is not discussed further.

Tranexamic Acid

Chemical Definition

Tranexamic acid is the trans-stereoisomer of 4-aminomethylcyclohexane carboxylic acid, with a molecular weight of 157. Initial investigations with the drug were performed using a preparation containing a mixture of isomers, but it was subsequently found that only the trans-stereoisomer has antifibrinolytic activity.[420,421]

Mode of Action

The antifibrinolytic effect of the synthetic compounds 6-aminohexanoic acid, *p*-aminomethylbenzoic acid, and tranexamic acid is related mainly to a reversible complex formation with a modified plasminogen and the associated conformational changes of the proenzyme.[169] The binding of plasminogen to fibrin is mediated through the lysine-binding sites of plasminogen, and this interaction is virtually completely blocked by the synthetic antifibrinolytic amino acids. It is primarily the high-affinity lysine-binding site of plasminogen that is involved in its binding to fibrin; saturation of this binding site with tranexamic acid displaces plasminogen from the fibrin surface.[160] This results in retardation of fibrinolysis.

Defective fibrin formation or excessively rapid dissolution of fibrin results in excessive or recurrent bleeding. The untimely dissolution of hemostatic fibrin can be prevented by antifibrinolytic drugs, which stabilize the fibrin structures. Furthermore, antifibrinolytic treatment increases collagen synthesis and tensile strength within granulation tissue, presumably by preserving the fibrin matrix.[422]

Direct comparisons of the potencies of 6-aminohexanoic acid and tranexamic acid give results that vary substantially according to the test systems used, but values of 6 to 10 times higher potency of tranexamic acid have been reported; in fibrinolytic test systems, an overall figure of a 10-fold increment in potency seems to be the consensus. Tranexamic acid is a weak noncompetitive inhibitor of plasmin.

Pharmacokinetic Properties

At therapeutic concentrations (5 to 10 mg/L), about 3% of tranexamic acid is weakly bound to protein—primarily to plasminogen.[423] After oral doses of 10 to 15 mg/kg, the amounts recovered in the urine after 1, 3, and 24 hours were 1%, 13%, and 39%, respectively. Oral administration of 1 g as tablets to healthy adults produced peak plasma concentrations of 8 mg/L at 3 hours after dosing.[424]

Following intravenous administration of 10 mg/kg of tranexamic acid, plasma concentrations at 1, 3, and 5 hours after injection were 18, 10, and 5 mg/L, respectively. The elimination half-life is reported to be 80 minutes.[425] About 30% of the administered dose is recovered in the urine during the first hour after intravenous administration of 10 mg/kg, a total of about 45% during the first 3 hours, and about 90% after 24 hours. Tranexamic acid inhibits fibrinolytic activity in the urine.[416] After an oral dose of 10 mg/kg, there was substantial inhibition of urinary fibrinolytic activity for at least 24 hours.

Tranexamic acid displays a considerably higher and more sustained antifibrinolytic activity in tissues than does 6-aminohexanoic acid when measured in specimens from the large intestine, kidneys, and prostate.[416]

Clinical Use

Tranexamic acid is, on a molar basis, 6 to 10 times more potent than 6-aminohexanoic acid and twice as potent as p-aminomethylbenzoic acid, but it has the same low acute and chronic toxicity.[416,426] Since tranexamic acid also displays a considerably higher and more sustained antifibrinolytic activity in tissues than does 6-aminohexanoic acid and has a longer half-life, tranexamic acid is more commonly used in therapeutics.

Prevention of Bleeding After Surgery or Trauma

Tooth Extraction in Patients With Hemophilia. In a prospective, randomized double-blind study, Forbes and others[427] found that tranexamic acid 1 g three times per day for 5 days, given in conjunction with factor VIII or IX, significantly reduced blood loss and transfusion requirements after dental extraction in patients with hemophilia. Further worldwide experience confirms the favorable conclusion of the initial reports. Prior to dental extraction, 25 mg/kg tranexamic acid is given intravenously together with factor VIII or IX concentrate; after surgery, 25 mg/kg is administered orally three or four times daily for 8 days. Usually, no further substitution therapy with coagulation-factor concentrates is required after surgery. Tranexamic acid usage has reduced the need for factor VIII or IX concentrates by 80%, thereby avoiding potential hazards inherent to blood products.[428]

Cervical Conization. This operation has become more common for noninvasive cancer of the cervix. Postoperative bleeding requiring extra measures occurs in about 14% of cases when using the open technique. Because the uterine cervix contains a high concentration of plasminogen activator, it is logical to treat these patients with fibrinolytic inhibitors. Two double-blind trials (one using open surgical technique without suturing and one with suturing) revealed a significant reduction in blood loss (average of 70%) in patients who received 1.5 g tranexamic acid daily for at least 12 days postoperatively.[429,430]

Tonsillectomy and Adenoidectomy. The most common complication of tonsillectomy is rebleeding, with the frequency varying with the surgical technique used. The systemic administration of inhibitors of fibrinolysis after tonsillectomy, adenoidectomy, or both was evaluated in several trials. Two trials were with tranexamic acid, which showed a significant reduction in measured blood loss.[431,432]

Prostatic Surgery. Urine contains the plasminogen activator urokinase, which induces the breakdown of blood clots, thereby enhancing bleeding in the urinary tract. Moreover, prostatic tissue contains large amounts of plasminogen activator. Thus, there are two reasons for hemorrhage following prostatectomy.

In a randomized double-blind trial of patients undergoing prostatectomy, Hedlund[433] found that tranexamic acid in a dose of 10 g or 6 g during the 4 days immediately preceding and following prostatectomy significantly reduced urinary blood loss. These results confirmed the findings of a placebo-controlled trial in which the same doses of tranexamic acid were given.[434] Rö and associates,[435] in a randomized study of 22 patients undergoing reimplantation of ureters, found a significant reduction in bleeding in the tranexamic–acid-treated group (15 mg/kg orally on the day before operation; 10 mg/kg intravenously immediately before operation and again in the evening; for 7 days after operation, 15 mg/kg given two times per day). Six of the 10 patients treated with tranexamic acid had large clots in the urinary bladder, however.

The effect of tranexamic acid on the frequency of secondary hemorrhage during the 4-week postoperative period had been demonstrated in 2 controlled trials with 1 g tranexamic acid three times per day.[436,437] The incidence of secondary bleeding was reduced from 50% in the control group to 24% in the treatment group. For this indication, the recommended dose is 0.5 to 1 g (10 to 15 mg/kg) intravenously two or three times daily starting immediately after surgery during the first 3 postoperative days, and thereafter, 1 to 1.5 g orally three or four times daily until macroscopic hematuria is no longer present. One should be aware, however, that if bleeding is heavy, clot retention in the kidney (a high-bleeding site, for example, in nonoperated hemophiliacs) or in the ureter with subsequent urinary obstruction is a risk.

Ocular Trauma. The tissues in the body most richly endowed with endothelial plasminogen tissue activator are possibly the iris and choroid.[438] The anterior segment of the eye is filled with a fluid of low protein content, the aqueous humor, which has a diluent effect on blood in cases of intraocular bleeding. As a rule, intraocular blood coagulates, and dissolution of the clot is a necessary condition for adsorption of blood. But ophthalmic fibrinolysis also entails disadvantages, because dissolution of the fibrinous clot that seals the damaged blood vessel may result in secondary bleeding.

Accidental or surgical ocular trauma is often accompanied by hemorrhage in the anterior chamber of the eye. The most serious complication of traumatic hyphema is secondary bleeding, usually occurring in the second to seventh posttraumatic day in about 38% of patients. Impaired vision or blindness may be the consequence. The purpose of antifibrinolytic therapy is to prevent rebleeding in the anterior chamber and the vitrous body.

Two controlled trials show that tranexamic acid treatment (1 g tid) significantly reduces the frequency of secondary hemorrhage.[439,440] These findings support the favorable impression of other trials with historical controls.

Tranexamic acid appears to protect the hemostatic plug from premature dissolution, sealing the damaged vessel and preventing secondary hemorrhage after traumatic hyphema; the patient does not have to be confined to bed rest. Antifibrinolytic treatment delays dissolution of the primary clot, however, and therefore is contraindicated in massive (filling more than half the anterior chamber) intraocular hemorrhage.

Prevention of Subarachnoid Hemorrhage Rebleeding. Patients who survive the initial rupture of an intracranial aneurysm run a 20% risk of rebleeding and developing delayed ischemic cerebral deficits. In contrast to cerebral tissue, the meninges and the choroid plexus are rich in tPA. The goal of treatment with antifibrinolytic agents is to prolong the duration of the blood clot formed within and about the wall of the aneurysm so that the critical period of surgical delay can be reduced.

Numerous isolated case reports and 13 uncontrolled clinical trials provide data both for and against treatment with 6-aminohexanoic acid or tranexamic acid.[441] An American cooperative study and 7 randomized, controlled clinical trials using tranexamic acid in the management of ruptured cerebral aneurysm have been published. Four favor treatment in terms of rebleeding incidence, whereas four others were inconclusive.[442] These discrepancies may be because of multiple clinical and therapeutic variables and flaws in methodology.

Prevention of Spontaneous Bleeding in Hemophilia. Tranexamic acid in a dose of 2 g/d was used as prophylaxis against spontaneous bleeding episodes in hemophilia. One well-designed long-term (12 months) double-blind study failed to show benefit[443]; another trial using 3 g/d[444] in a double-blind crossover protocol found a reduction in spontaneous bleeding episodes, significant at the 5% level. Further studies are needed to elucidate the effect of tranexamic acid as long-term prophylactic therapy against spontaneous bleeding episodes in hemophilia.

Treatment of Primary or IUD-Induced Menorrhagia. Four clinical trials (three were randomized double-blind crossover studies with tranexamic acid,[445–447] one was a comparison between menstrual blood losses during a control period and a treatment period)[448] showed a dose-dependent reduction (35% to 51%) of menstrual blood loss in essential menorrhagia. The dose recommended for this indication is 1 to 1.5 g (12 to 25 mg/kg) of tranexamic acid orally three or four times daily for 3 to 4 days. The treatment is started when the bleeding has become profuse.

The use of inert or, to a lesser degree, copper intrauterine devices is frequently associated with excessive menstrual blood loss. In a well-designed controlled trial with random allocation, Weström and Bengtsson[449] demonstrated that 6 g of tranexamic acid daily reduced the incidence of heavy uterine blood loss after insertion of a copper-releasing IUD from 82.7% to 11.5%; this difference is highly significant.

Bleeding During or After Pregnancy. Bleeding during pregnancy is associated with a three- to four-fold increase in perinatal mortality. Tranexamic acid was used in a limited number of cases of threatened placental abruption with a low perinatal mortality (8%) and no maternal mortality.[450–452] Similarly, in the limited clinical experience with pregnant women, no harmful effects to the fetus have been reported.

Bleeding after parturition may be due to a variety of causes. The uterus is rich in plasminogen activators; when the placenta separates, fibrinolysis inhibitors (the placenta is well endowed with them) are lost. Therefore, a high fibrinolytic activity prevails at the ulcerated surface and adjuvant therapy with antifibrinolytic drugs may be of value. Extensive clinical experience is not available, however.

Treatment of Recurrent Epistaxis. Recurrent nose bleeds are rather common, and external trauma or a vascular change on the anterior septum is most frequently the cause. In other instances, the etiology is not clear; several factors—such as hypertension, upper respiratory tract infection, and aspirin ingestion—may play a role. In a randomized double-blind trial, tranexamic acid significantly reduced the severity of unexplained nose bleeds and the rebleeding frequency, also, when used at the usual dose of 1.5 g three times per day.[453]

Diffuse bleeding from the anterior portion of the nose can easily be treated with a cotton wool pledget impregnated with decongestant nose drops to decongest the mucous membrane. For persistent nose bleeds, the cotton wool or Spongostan can be impregnated with tranexamic acid solution and left in place until it falls out by itself after a few days. Patients treated by packing could be also given tranexamic acid orally.

Prevention of Spontaneous or Postoperative Corneal Edema. Endothelial dystrophy is a degenerative disease of the cornea (Fuchs' disease) that begins in the central portion of the corneal endothelium and causes pain and progressively impaired vision. Corneal edema is seen also in connection with cataract extraction and trabeculectomy.

Two double-blind trials were conducted with tranexamic acid in postoperative corneal edema after cataract operation[454] and trabeculectomy.[455] The antifibrinolytic drug appears to be effective in reducing corneal thickness, and this is followed by improved visual acuity. In a double-blind crossover study, central corneal thickness increased in response to aspirin and decreased in response to tranexamic acid. This finding provides further evidence that the fibrinolytic system is involved in the regulation of normal corneal thickness.

Treatment of Hereditary Angioneurotic Edema. Hereditary angioneurotic edema is characterized by recurrent, transient, nonitching edema of the skin, of the mucosa of the gastrointestinal tract (associated with acute attacks of abdominal pain), and of the mucosa of the upper respiratory tract (associated with risk of asphyxiation). It is an autosomal dominant disease and is due to a deficiency of C_1-esterase inhibitor. Deficiency of this inhibitor may lead to an uncontrolled activation of the complement system and overproduction of fragments, many having vasoactive properties. C_1-Esterase inhibitor also impedes the action of kallikrein on kininogen conversion and neutralizes plasmin.

Two randomized, double-blind crossover trials with tranexamic acid show a reduction in the number and severity of the attacks of edema.[456,457] Not all patients are helped, however, and the reason for this is not fully understood. The beneficial effect of tranexamic acid seems to be because of its antiplasmin effect and the inhibition of the conversion of C_1 into active C_1.

Scattered reports exist on the favorable effect of antifibrinolytic agents in urticaria and angioedema. But one double-blind crossover study with tranexamic acid in patients with chronic urticaria and low levels of C_1-esterase inhibitor does not favor this drug for management of patients with urticaria.[458]

Adjuvant Treatment of Ovarian Carcinoma. Malignant tumors possess coagulative properties that cause deposition of fibrin around them; they also possess tumor-plasminogen activator, which removes residual fibrin. Tranexamic acid is reported to interfere with ovarian tumor growth by maintaining the encapsulation of the tumor by fibrinoid substances.[460] Furthermore, tranexamic acid prevents the proliferation of vessels on which tumor growth also depends. Further studies of tranexamic acid in this area seem warranted.

Status of Tranexamic Acid in Therapeutics. The main indications for tranexamic acid are the prevention of excessive bleeding after tonsillectomy, in prostatic surgery, after cervical conisation, and in primary or IUD-induced menorrhagia. Gastric and intestinal bleeding might also be reduced, as might recurrent epistaxis. Tranexamic acid could prove useful after ocular trauma.

Dosage

The usual dose of tranexamic acid is 0.5 to 1 g (10 to 15 mg/kg) given intravenously 2 to 3 times daily starting immediately after surgery, and after a few days, 1 to 1.5 g orally 3 to 4 times daily. Treatment does not need to be started intravenously except in the first days after surgery.

A modified dosage in patients with decreased renal function further decreases the incidence of gastrointestinal side effects. In patients with serum creatinine concentrations of 120 to 150 μmol/L, 10 mg/kg tranexamic acid may be administered intravenously twice a day. Those having serum creatinine concentrations between 250 and 500 μmol/L may be given the same dose at 24-hour intervals; those having serum creatinine concentrations over 500 μmol/L may be given the same dose at 48-hour intervals.

Side Effects

Side effects of tranexamic acid are rare and mainly limited to nausea or diarrhea, or an occasional orthostatic reaction. The better tolerance of tranexamic acid compared with 6-aminohexanoic acid is probably because of the lower daily dose required with the former (3 to 6 g) than with the latter (18 to 30 g).

A few cases of acute renal failure and myopathy were described with 6-aminohexanoic acid, but this is most probably an idiosyncratic response. Theoretically, increased thrombotic tendency during treatment with fibrinolytic inhibitors is a risk. A few patients developed intracranial thrombosis during treatment with 6-aminohexanoic acid or tranexamic acid. This association may be fortuitous, so further observations are needed to assess the reality of this potential hazard.

No mutagenic activity of tranexamic acid could be demonstrated in several in vitro and in vivo test systems, and no fetal abnormalities were found in dysmorphology and reproductive studies.

REFERENCES

1. Rijken DC, Wijngaards G, Zaal-De Jong M, Welbergen J. Purification and partial characterization of plasminogen activator from human uterine tissue. Biochim Biophys Acta 1979;580:140.
2. Rijken DC, Wijngaards G, Welbergen J. Relationship between tissue plasminogen activator and the activators in blood and vascular wall. Thromb Res 1980;18:815.
3. Levin EG, Loskutoff DJ. Cultured bovine endothelial cells produce both urokinase and tissue-type plasminogen activators. J Cell Biol 1982;94:631.
4. Rijken DC, Collen D. Purification and characterization of the plasminogen activator secreted by human melanoma cells in culture. J Biol Chem 1981;256:7035.
5. Collen D, Rijken DC, Van Damme J, Billiau A. Purification of human tissue-type plasminogen activator in centigram quantities from human melanoma cell culture fluid and its conditioning for use in vivo. Thromb Haemost 1982;48:294.
6. Kruithof EKO, Schleuning WD, Bachmann F. Human tissue-type plasminogen activator. Production in continuous serum-free cell culture and rapid purification. Biochem J 1985;226:631.
7. Pennica D, Holmes WE, Kohr WJ, et al. Cloning and expression of human tissue-type plasminogen activator cDNA in E coli. Nature 1983;301:214.
8. Edlund T, Ny t, Ranby M, et al. Isolation of cDNA sequences coding for a part of human tissue plasminogen activator. Proc Natl Acad Sci USA 1983;80:349.
9. Fisher R, Waller EK, Grossi G, et al. Isolation and characterization of the human tissue-type plasminogen activator structural gene including its 5′ flanking region. J Biol Chem 1985;260:11223.
10. Kaufman R, Wasley LC, Spiliotes AJ, et al. Coamplification and coexpression of human tissue-type plasminogen activator and murine dihydrofolate reductase sequences in Chinese hamster ovary cells. Mol Cell Biol 1985;5:1750.
11. Harris TJR, Patel T, Marston FAO, et al. Cloning of cDNA coding for human tissue-type plasminogen activator and its expression in Escherichia coli. Mol Biol Med 1986;3:279.
12. Sambrook J, Hanahan D, Rodgers L, Gething MJ. Expression of human tissue-type plasminogen activator from lytic viral vectors and in established cell lines. Mol Biol Med 1986;3:459.
13. Collen D, Stassen JM, Marafino BJ, et al. Biological properties of human tissue-type plasminogen activator obtained by expression of recombinant DNA in mammalian cells. J Pharmacol Exp Ther 1984;231:146.
14. Zamarron C, Lijnen HR, Collen D. Kinetics of the activation of plasminogen by natural and recombinant tissue-type plasminogen activator. J Biol Chem 1984;259:2080.
15. Builder SE, Grossbard E. Laboratory and clinical experience with recombinant plasminogen activator. In: Murawski and Peetoom, eds. Transfusion medicine: recent technological advances. New York, AR Liss, 1986:303.
16. Vehar GA, Spellman MW, Keyt BA, et al. Characterization studies of human tissue-type plasminogen activator produced by recombinant DNA technology. In: Cold Spring Harbor Symposia on Quantitative Biology, vol LI. Cold Spring Harbor, NY, 1986:551.
17. Jörnvall H, Pohl G, Bergsdorf N, Wallen P. Differential proteolysis and evidence for a residue exchange in tissue plasminogen activator suggest possible association between two types of protein microheterogeneity. FEBS Lett 1983;156:47.
18. Banyai L, Varadi A, Patthy L. Common evolutionary origin of the fibrin-binding structures of fibronectin and tissue-type plasminogen activator. FEBS Lett 1983;163:37.
19. Bennett WF. Two forms of tissue-type plasminogen activator differ at a single specific glycosylation site. (Abstract) Thromb Haemost 1983;50:106.
20. Pohl G, Einarsson M, Nilsson B, Svensson S. The size heterogeneity in melanoma tissue plasminogen activator is caused by carbohydrate differences. Thromb Res 1985;50:163.
21. Rijken DC, Emeis JJ, Gerwig GJ. On the composition and function of the carbohydrate moiety of tissue-type plasminogen activator from human melanoma cells. Thromb Haemost 1985;54:788.
22. Hoylaerts M, Rijken DC, Lijnen HR, Collen D. Kinetics of the activation of plasminogen by human tissue plasminogen activator: role of fibrin. J Biol Chem 1982;257:2912.
23. Higgins DL, Vehar GA. Interaction of one-chain and two-chain tissue plasminogen activator with intact and plasmin-degraded fibrin. Biochemistry 1987;26:7786.
24. Rijken DC, Hoylaerts M, Collen D. Fibrinolytic properties of one-chain and two-chain human extrinsic (tissue-type) plasminogen activator. J Biol Chem 1982;257:2920.
25. Liu CY, Wallen P. The binding of tissue plasminogen activator by fibrin. Circulation 1984;70(Suppl II):365.
26. Rijken DC, Groeneveld E. Isolation and functional characterization of the heavy and light chains of human tissue-type plasminogen activator. J Biol Chem 1986;261:3098.
27. Holvoet P, Lijnen HR, Collen D. Characterization of functional domains in human tissue-type plasminogen activator with the use of monoclonal antibodies. Eur J Biochem 1986;158:173.
28. van Zonneveld AJ, Veerman H, Pannekoek H. On the interaction of the finger and kringle-2 domain of tissue-type plasminogen activator with fibrin. J Biol Chem 1986;261:14214.
29. Kagitani H, Tagawa M, Hatanaka K, et al. Expression in E coli of finger-domain lacking tissue-type plasminogen activator with high fibrin affinity. FEBS Lett 1985;189:145.
30. van Zonneveld AJ, Veerman H, Pannekoek H. Autonomous functions of structural domains on human tissue-type plasminogen activator. Proc Natl Acad Sci USA 1986;83:4670.
31. Verheijen JH, Caspers MPM, Chang GTG, et al. Involvement of finger domain and kringle 2 domain of tissue-type plasminogen activator in fibrin binding and stimulation of activity by fibrin. EMBO J 1986;5:3525.
32. Verheijen JH, Caspers MPM, de Munk GAW, et al. Sites in tissue-type plasminogen activator involved in the interaction with fibrin, plasminogen and low molecular weight ligands. (Abstract) Thromb Haemost 1987;58:491.
33. Christensen U. The AH-site of plasminogen and two C-terminal fragments: a weak lysine-binding site preferring ligands not carrying a free carboxylate function. Biochem J 1984;223:413.
34. Larsen GR, Henson K, Blue Y. Variants of human tissue-type plasminogen activator: fibrin binding, fibrinolytic, and fibrinogenolytic characterization of genetic variants lacking the fibronectin finger-like and/or the epidermal growth factor domains. J Biol Chem 1988;263:1023.
35. Kalyan NK, Lee SG, Wilhelm J, et al. Structure-function analysis with tissue-type plasminogen activator. Effect of deletion of NH_2-terminal domains on its biochemical and biological properties. J Biol Chem 1988;263:3971.
36. Voskuilen M, Vermond A, Veeneman GH, et al. Fibrinogen lysine residue Aα157 plays a crucial role in the fibrin-induced acceleration of plasminogen activation, catalyzed by tissue-type plasminogen activator. J Biol Chem 1987;262:5944.
37. Ranby M, Bergsdorf N, Norrman B, et al. Tissue plasminogen activator kinetics. In: Davidson JF, Bachman F, Bouvier CA, Kruithof EKO, eds. Progress in fibrinolysis, vol 6. Edinburgh, Churchill Livingstone, 1983:182.
38. Suenson E, Lützen O, Thorsen S. Initial plasmin-degradation of fibrin as the basis of a positive feed-back mechanism in fibrinolysis. Eur J Biochem 1984;140:513.
39. Nieuwenhuizen W, Voskuilen M, Vermond A, et al. The influence of fibrin(ogen) fragments on the kinetic parameters of the tissue-type plasminogen-activator–mediated activation of different forms of plasminogen. Eur J Biochem 1988;174:163.
40. Wallen P, Bergsdorf N, Ranby M. Purification and identification of two structural variants of porcine tissue plasminogen activator by affinity adsorption on fibrin. Biochim Biophys Acta 1982;719:318.
41. Miles LA, Plow EF. Binding and activation of plasminogen on the platelet surface. J Biol Chem 1985;260:4303.
42. Stricker RB, Wong D, Shiu DT, et al. Activation of plasminogen by tissue plasminogen activator on normal and thrombasthenic platelets: effects on surface proteins and platelet aggregation. Blood 1986;68:275.
43. Soeda S, Kakiki M, Shimeno H, Nagamatsu A. Some properties of tissue-type plasminogen activator reconstituted onto phospholipid and/or glycolipid vesicles. Biochem Biophys Res Comm 1987;146:94.
44. Hajjar KA, Harpel PC, Jaffe EA, Nachman RL. Binding of plasminogen to cultured human endothelial cells. J Biol Chem 1986;261:11656.
45. Hajjar KA, Hamel NM, Harpel PC, Nachman RL. Binding of tissue plasminogen activator to cultured human endothelial cells. J Clin Invest 1987;80:1712.
46. Barnathan ES, Kuo A, Van der Keyl H, et al. Tissue-type plasminogen activator binding to human endothelial cells: evidence for two distinct binding sites. J Biol Chem 1988;263:7792.
47. Gething MJ, Adler B, Boose JA, et al. Variants of human tissue-type plasminogen activator that lack specific structural domains of the heavy chain. EMBO J 1988;7:2731.
48. Ehrlich HJ, Bang NU, Little SP, et al. Biological properties of a kringleless tissue plasminogen activator (t-PA) mutant. Fibrinolysis 1987;1:75.

49. Ny T, Elgh F, Lund B. The structure of the human tissue-type plasminogen activator gene: correlation of intron and exon structures to functional and structural domains. Proc Natl Acad Sci USA 1984;81:5355.
50. Park CH, Tulinsky A. Three-dimensional structure of the kringle sequence: structure of prothrombin fragment 1. Biochemistry 1986;25:3977.
51. Pannekoek H, de Vries C, van Zonneveld AJ. Mutants of human tissue-type plasminogen activator (t-PA): structural aspects and functional properties. Fibrinolysis 1988;2:123.
52. Haigwood N, Pâques EP, Mullenbach G, et al. Improvement of t-PA properties by means of site directed mutagenesis. (Abstract) Thromb Haemost 1987;58:286.
53. Rajput B, Degen SF, Reich E, et al. Chromosomal locations of human tissue plasminogen activator and urokinase genes. Science 1985;230:672.
54. Verheijen JH, Visse R, Wijnen JT, et al. Assignment of the human tissue-type plasminogen activator gene (PLAT) to chromosome 8. Hum Genet 1986;72:153.
55. Yang-Feng TL, Opdenakker G, Volckaert G, Francke U. Human tissue-type plasminogen activator gene located near chromosomal breakpoint in myeloproliferative disorder. Am J Hum Genet 1986;39:79.
56. Browne MJ, Tyrrell AWR, Chapman CG, et al. Isolation of a human tissue-type plasminogen activator genomic DNA clone and its expression in mouse L cells. Gene 1985;33:279.
57. Degen SJF, Rajput B, Reich E. The human tissue plasminogen activator gene. J Biol Chem 1986;261:6972.
58. Patthy L. Evolution of the proteases of blood coagulation and fibrinolysis by assembly from modules. Cell 1985;41:657.
59. Rijken DC, Juhan-Vague I, De Cock F, Collen D. Measurement of human tissue-type plasminogen activator by a two-site immunoradiometric assay. J Lab Clin Med 1983;101:274.
60. Rijken DC, van Hinsbergh VWM, Sens EHC. Quantitation of tissue-type plasminogen activator in human endothelial cell cultures by use of an enzyme immunoassay. Thromb Res 1984;33:145.
61. Holvoet P, Cleemput H, Collen D. Assay of human tissue-type plasminogen activator (t-PA) with an enzyme-linked immunosorbent assay (ELISA) based on three murine monoclonal antibodies to t-PA. Thromb Haemost 1985;54:684.
62. Astrup T, Müllertz S. Fibrin plate method for estimating fibrinolytic activity. Arch Biochem Biophys 1952;40:346.
63. Gaffney PJ, Curtis AD. A collaborative study of a proposed international standard for tissue plasminogen activator (t-PA). Thromb Haemost 1985;53:134.
64. Gaffney PJ, Curtis AD. A collaborative study to establish the 2nd International Standard for Tissue Plasminogen Activator (t-PA). Thromb Haemost 1987;58:1085.
65. Ranby M, Norrman B, Wallen P. A sensitive assay for tissue plasminogen activator. Thromb Res 1982;27:743.
66. Drapier JC, Tenu JP, Lemaire G, Petit JF. Regulation of plasminogen activator secretion in mouse peritoneal macrophages. I. Role of serum studied by a new spectrophotometric assay for plasminogen activators. Biochimie 1979;61:463.
67. Verheijen JH, Mullaert E, Chang GTG, et al. A simple, sensitive spectrophotometric assay for extrinsic (tissue-type) plasminogen activator applicable to measurement in plasma. Thromb Haemost 1982;48:266.
68. Wiman B, Mellbring G, Ranby M. Plasminogen activator release during venous stasis and exercise as determined by a new specific assay. Clin Chim Acta 1983;127:279.
69. Gyzander E, Eriksson E, Teger-Nilsson AC. A sensitive assay for tissue plasminogen activator activity in plasma, using adsorption on lysine-sepharose. Thromb Res 1984;35:547.
70. Holvoet P, Boes J, Collen D. Measurement of free, one-chain tissue-type plasminogen activator in human plasma with an enzyme-linked immunosorbent assay based on an active site-specific murine monoclonal antibody. Blood 1987;69:284.
71. Bernik MB, Oller EP. Increased plasminogen activator (urokinase) in tissue culture after fibrin deposition. J Clin Invest 1973;52:823.
72. Nolan C, Hall L, Barlow GH, Tribby IIE. Plasminogen activator from human embryonic kidney cell cultures: evidence for a proactivator. Biochim Biophys Acta 1977;496:384.
73. Husain SS, Gurewich V, Lipinski B. Purification and partial characterization of a single-chain high-molecular-weight form of urokinase from human urine. Arch Biochem Biophys 1983;220:31.
74. Stump DC, Thienpont M, Collen D. Urokinase-related proteins in human urine: isolation and characterization of single chain urokinase (pro-urokinase) and urokinase-inhibitor complex. J Biol Chem 1986;261:1267.
75. Wun TC, Schleuning WD, Reich E. Isolation and characterization of urokinase from human plasma. J Biol Chem 1982;257:3276.
76. Wun TC, Ossowski L, Reich E. A proenzyme form of human urokinase. J Biol Chem 1982;257:7262.
77. Nielsen LS, Hansen JG, Skriver L, et al. Purification of zymogen to plasminogen activator from human glioblastoma cells by affinity chromatography with monoclonal antibody. Biochemistry 1982;21:6410.
78. Kohno T, Hopper P, Lillquist JS, et al. Kidney plasminogen activator: a precursor form of human urokinase with high fibrin affinity. Biotechnology 1984;2:628.
79. Sumi H, Maruyama M, Matsuo O, et al. Higher fibrin-binding and thrombolytic properties of single polypeptide chain-high molecular weight urokinase. Thromb Haemost 1982;47:297.
80. Sumi H, Kosugi T, Matsuo O, Mihara H. Physicochemical properties of highly purified kidney cultured plasminogen activator (single chain urokinase). Acta Haematol Jpn 1982;45:119.
81. Eaton DL, Scott RW, Baker JB. Purification of human fibroblast urokinase proenzyme and analysis of its regulation by proteases and protease nexin. J Biol Chem 1984;259:6241.
82. Kasai S, Arimura H, Nishida M, Suyama T. Proteolytic cleavage of single-chain pro-urokinase induces conformational change which follows activation of the zymogen and reduction of its high affinity for fibrin. J Biol Chem 1985;260:12377.
83. Stump DC, Lijnen HR, Collen D. Purification and characterization of single-chain urokinase-type plasminogen activator from human cell cultures. J Biol Chem 1986;261:1274.
84. Holmes WE, Pennica D, Blaber M, et al. Cloning and expression of the gene for pro-urokinase in Escherichia coli. Biotechnology 1985;3:923.
85. Winkler ME, Blaber M, Bennett GL, et al. Purification and characterization of recombinant urokinase from *Escherichia coli*. Biotechnology 1985;3:990.
86. Stump DC, Lijnen HR, Collen D. Purification and characterization of a novel low molecular weight form of single-chain urokinase-type plasminogen activator. J Biol Chem 1986;261:17120.
87. Lijnen HR, Nelles L, Holmes W, et al. Biochemical and thrombolytic properties of a low molecular weight form (comprising Leu^{144} through Leu^{411}) of recombinant single-chain urokinase-type plasminogen activator. J Biol Chem 1988;263:5594.
88. Steffens GJ, Günzler W, Ötting F, et al. The complete amino acid sequence of low molecular mass urokinase from human urine. Hoppe Seyler's Z Physiol Chem 1982;363:1043.
89. Günzler WA, Steffens GJ, Ötting F, et al. Structural relationship between human high and low molecular mass urokinase. Hoppe Seyler's Z Physiol Chem 1982;363:133.
90. Günzler WA, Steffens GJ, Ötting F, et al. The primary structure of high molecular mass urokinase from human urine. Hoppe Seyler's Z Physiol Chem 1982;363:1155.
91. Ichinose A, Fujikawa K, Suyama T. The activation of pro-urokinase by plasma kallikrein and its inactivation by thrombin. J Biol Chem 1986;261:3486.
92. Lijnen HR, Zamarron C, Blaber M, et al. Activation of plasminogen by pro-urokinase: I. mechanism. J Biol Chem 1986;261:1253.
93. Verde P, Stoppelli MP, Galeffi P, et al. Identification and primary sequence of an unspliced human urokinase poly$(A)^+$ RNA. Proc Natl Acad Sci USA 1984;81:4727.
94. Riccio A, Grimaldi G, Verde P, et al. The human urokinase-plasminogen activator gene and its promoter. Nucleic Acids Res 1985;13:2759.
95. Christensen U. Kinetic studies of the urokinase-catalysed conversion of NH_2-terminal glutamic acid plasminogen to plasmin. Biochim Biophys Acta 1977;481:638.
96. Wohl RC, Sinio L, Summaria L, et al. Comparative activation kinetics of mammalian plasminogen. Biochim Biophys Acta 1983;745:20.
97. Christensen U, Müllertz S. Kinetic studies on the urokinase catalysed conversion of NH_2-terminal lysine plasminogen to plasmin. Biochim Biophys Acta 1977;480:275.
98. Markus G, Evers JL, Hobika GH. Comparison of some properties of native (Glu) and modified (Lys) human plasminogen. J Biol Chem 1978;253:733.
99. Castellino FJ, Brockway WJ, Thomas JK, et al. Rotational diffusion analysis of the conformational alterations produced in plasminogen by certain antifibrinolytic amino acids. Biochemistry 1973;12:2787.
100. Camiolo SM, Thorsen S, Astrup T. Fibrinogenolysis and fibrinolysis with tissue plasminogen activator, urokinase, streptokinase-activated human globulin, and plasmin. Proc Soc Exp Biol Med 1971;138:277.
101. Lucas MA, Straight DL, Fretto LJ, et al. The effects of fibrinogen and its cleavage products on the kinetics of plasminogen activation by urokinase and subsequent plasmin activity. J Biol Chem 1983;258:12171.
102. Lijnen HR, Van Hoef B, Collen D. Influence of cyanogen-bromide-digested fibrinogen on the kinetics of plasminogen activation by urokinase. Eur J Biochem 1984;144:541.
103. Nielsen LS, Hansen JG, Skriver L, et al. Purification of zymogen to plasminogen activator from human glioblastoma cells by affinity chromatography with monoclonal antibody. Biochemistry 1982;21:6410.
104. Lijnen HR, Van Hoef B, Collen D. Differential reactivity of Glu-Gly-Arg-CH_2Cl, a synthetic urokinase inhibitor, with single-chain and two-chain forms of urokinase-type plasminogen activator. Eur J Biochem 1987;162:351.
105. Collen D, Zamarron C, Lijnen HR, et al. Activation of plasminogen by pro-urokinase. II. Kinetics. J Biol Chem 1986;261:1259.
106. Nelles L, Lijnen HR, Collen D, et al. Characterization of recombinant human single chain urokinase-type plasminogen activator mutants produced by site-specific mutagenesis of Lysine 158. J Biol Chem 1987;262:5682.
107. Lijnen HR, Van Hoef B, Collen D. Comparative kinetic analysis of the activation of human plasminogen by natural and recombinant single-

chain urokinase-type plasminogen activator. Biochim Biophys Acta 1986;884:402.
108. Dewerchin M, Lijnen HR, Van Hoef B, et al. Biochemical properties of conjugates of urokinase-type plasminogen activator with a monoclonal antibody specific for cross-linked fibrin. Eur J Biochem 1989;185: 141.
109. Lijnen HR, Zamarron C, Collen D. Characterization of the high-affinity interaction between human plasminogen and pro-urokinase. Eur J Biochem 1985;150:141.
110. Ellis V, Scully MF, Kakkar VV. Plasminogen activation by single-chain urokinase in functional isolation: a kinetic study. J Biol Chem 1987;262: 14998.
111. Petersen LC, Lund LR, Nielsen LS, et al. One-chain urokinase-type plasminogen activator from human sarcoma cells is a proenzyme with little or no intrinsic activity. J Biol Chem 1988;263:11189.
112. Lijnen HR, Van Hoef B, Nelles L, et al. Enzymatic properties of single-chain and two-chain forms of a $Lys^{158} \rightarrow Glu^{158}$ mutant of urokinase-type plasminogen activator. Eur J Biochem 1988;172:185.
113. Lijnen HR, Van Hoef B, Collen D. Activation with plasmin of two-chain urokinase-type plasminogen activator derived from single-chain urokinase-type plasminogen activator by treatment with thrombin. Eur J Biochem 1987;169:359.
114. Sottrup-Jensen L, Claeys H, Zajdel M, et al. The primary structure of human plasminogen: isolation of two lysine-binding fragments and one "mini"-plasminogen (MW 38,000) by elastase-catalyzed-specific limited proteolysis. In: Davidson JF, Rowan RM, Samama MM, Desnoyers PC, eds. Progress in chemical fibrinolysis and thrombolysis, vol 3. New York, Raven Press, 1978;191.
115. Sottrup-Jensen L, Petersen TE, Magnusson S. In: Dayhoff, ed. Atlas of protein sequence and structure, vol 5, suppl 3. Washington DC, National Biomedical Research Foundation, 1978:91.
116. Wiman B. Primary structure of the B-chain of human plasmin. Eur J Biochem 1977;76:129.
117. Friberger P, Knos M. Plasminogen determination in human plasma. In: Scully MF, Kakkar VV, eds. Chromogenic peptide substrates. Edinburgh, Churchill Livingstone, 1979:128.
118. Wallen P, Wiman B. Characterization of human plasminogen: I. on the relationship between different molecular forms of plasminogen demonstrated in plasma and found in purified preparations. Biochim Biophys Acta 1970;221:20.
119. Wallen P, Wiman B. Characterization of human plasminogen. II. Separation and partial characterization of different molecular forms of human plasminogen. Biochim Biophys Acta 1972;257:122.
120. Deutsch DG, Mertz ET. Plasminogen: purification from human plasma by affinity chromatography. Science 1970;170:1095.
121. Wiman B. Biochemistry of the plasminogen to plasmin conversion. In: Gaffney PJ, Balkuv-Ulutin S, eds. Fibrinolysis, current fundamental and clinical aspects. London, Academic Press, 1978:47.
122. Brockway WJ, Castellino FJ. Measurement of the binding of antifibrinolytic amino acids to various plasminogens. Arch Biochem Biophys 1972;151:194.
123. Collen D, De Maeyer L. Molecular biology of human plasminogen: I. physicochemical properties and microheterogeneity. Thromb Diath Haemorrh 1975;34:396.
124. Castellino FJ, Siefring GE Jr, Sodetz IM, et al. Amino terminal amino acid sequences and carbohydrate of the two major forms of rabbit plasminogen. Biochem Biophys Res Commun 1973;53:845.
125. Summaria L, Arzadon L, Bernabe P, Robbins KG. Studies on the isolation of the multiple molecular forms of human plasminogen and plasmin by isoelectric focusing methods. J Biol Chem 1972;247:4691.
126. Hayes ML, Castellino FJ. Carbohydrate of the human plasminogen variants. I. Carbohydrate composition, glycopeptide isolation and characterization. J Biol Chem 1979;254:8768.
127. Hayes ML, Castellino FJ. Carbohydrate of the human plasminogen variants. II. Structure of the asparagine-linked oligosaccharide unit. J Biol Chem 1979;254:8772.
128. Hayes ML, Castellino FJ. Carbohydrate of the human plasminogen variants. III. Structure of the O-glycosidically linked oligosaccharide unit. J Biol Chem 1979;254:8777.
129. Lijnen HR, Van Hoef B, Collen D. On the role of the carbohydrate side chains of human plasminogen in its interaction with α_2-antiplasmin and fibrin. Eur J Biochem 1981;120:149.
130. Collen D. Plasminogen and prothrombin metabolism in man. (Thesis) Louvain, Belgium, University of Louvain, 1974.
131. Collen D, Verstraete M. Molecular biology of human plasminogen: II. metabolism in physiological and some pathological conditions in man. Thromb Diath Haemorrh 1975;34:403.
132. Forsgren M, Raden B, Israelsson M. et al. Molecular cloning and characterization of a full-length cDNA clone for human plasminogen. FEBS Lett 1987;213:254.
133. Murray JC, Buetow KH, Donovan M, et al. Linkage disequilibrium of plasminogen polymorphisms and assignment of the gene to human chromosome 6q26-6q27. Am J Hum Genet 1987;40:338.
134. Malinowski DP, Sadler JE, Davie EW. Characterization of a complementary deoxyribonucleic acid coding for human and bovine plasminogen. Biochemistry 1984;23:4243.
135. Hobart MJ. Genetic polymorphism of human plasminogen. Ann Hum Genet 1979;42:419.
136. Raum D, Marcus D, Alper CA. Genetic polymorphism of human plasminogen. Am J Genet 1980;32:681.
137. Skoda U, Bertrams J, Dykes D, et al. Proposal for the nomenclature of human plasminogen (PLG) polymorphism. Vox Sang 1986;51:244.
138. Nishimukai H, Kera Y, Sakata K, Yamasawa K. Three new variants in the plasminogen system. Hum Hered 1982;32:130.
139. Nishimukai H, Shinmyozu K, Tamaki Y. Polymorphism of plasminogen in healthy individuals and patients with cerebral infarction. Hum Hered 1986;36:137.
140. Hitzeroth HW, Koda U, du Toit E, Mauff G. The plasminogen polymorphism in South African negro populations: genetics and anthropogenetics. Hum Genet 1986;74:341.
141. Dimo-Simonin N, Brandt-Casadevall C, Gujer HR. Gene frequencies of plasminogen in Switzerland. Hum Hered 1985;35:343.
142. Kera Y, Nishimukai H, Yamasawa K, Komura S. Comparative study of phenotypes on activity and plasma concentration in the genetic system of plasminogen. Hum Hered 1983;33:52.
143. Nishimukai H, Kera Y, Sakata K, Yamasawa K. Genetic polymorphism of plasminogen: a new basic variant (PLG B) and population study in Japanese. Vox Sang 1981;40:422.
144. Brandt-Casadevall C, Dimo-Simonin N, Gujer HR. A plasminogen silent allele detected in a Swiss family. Hum Hered 1987;37:389.
145. Robbins KC, Summaria L, Hsieh B, Shah RJ. The peptide chains of human plasmin:. mechanism of activation of human plasminogen to plasmin. J Biol Chem 1967;242:2333.
146. Groskopf WR, Summaria L, Robbins KC. Studies on the active center of human plasmin: partial amino acid sequence of a peptide containing the active center serine residue. J Biol Chem 1969;244:3590.
147. Claeys H, Vermylen J. Physico-chemical and proenzyme properties of NH_2-terminal glutamic acid and terminal lysine human plasminogen: influence of 6-aminohexanoic acid. Biochim Biophys Acta 1974;342: 351.
148. Wallen P, Wiman B. On the generation of intermediate plasminogen and its significance for activation. In: Reich E, Rifkin DB, Shaw E, eds. Proteases and biological control. Cold Spring Harbor NY, Cold Spring Harbor Laboratory, 1975:291.
149. Thorsen S, Kok P, Astrup T. Reversible and irreversible alterations of human plasminogen indicated by changes in susceptibility to plasminogen activators and in response to epsilon-aminocaproic acid. Thromb Diath Haemorrh 1974;32:325.
150. Rickli EE, Otavsky WI. Release of an N-terminal peptide from human plasminogen during activation with urokinase. Biochim Biophys Acta 1973;295:381.
151. Wiman B, Wallen P. Activation of human plasminogen by an insoluble derivative of urokinase: structural changes of plasminogen in the course of activation to plasmin and demonstration of a possible intermediate compound. Eur J Biochem 1973;36:25.
152. Summaria L, Arzadon L, Bernabe P, Robbins KC. The activation of plasminogen to plasmin by urokinase in the presence of the plasmin inhibitory trasylol: the preparation of plasmin with the same NH_2-terminal heavy (A) chain sequence as the parent zymogen. J Biol Chem 1975;250:3988.
153. Violand BN, Castellino FJ. Mechanism of the urokinase-catalyzed activation of human plasminogen. J Biol Chem 1976;251:3906.
154. Wiman B, Collen D. On the mechanism of the reaction between human α_2-antiplasmin and plasmin. J Biol Chem 1979;254:9291.
155. Holvoet P, Lijnen HR, Collen D. A monoclonal antibody specific for Lys-plasminogen: application to the study of the activation pathways of plasminogen in vivo. J Biol Chem 1985;260:12106.
156. Alkjaersig N. The purification and properties of human plasminogen. Biochem J 1964;93:171.
157. Abiko Y, Iwamoto M, Tomikawa M. Plasminogen-plasmin system: V. a stoichiometric equilibrium complex of plasminogen and a synthetic inhibitor. Biochim Biophys Acta 1969;185:424.
158. Winn ES, Hu SP, Hochschwender SM, Laursen RA. Studies on the lysine-binding sites of human plasminogen: the effect of ligand structure on the binding of lysine analogs to plasminogen. Eur J Biochem 1980;104:579.
159. Lerch PG, Rickli EE, Lergier W, Gillessen D. Localization of individual lysine-binding regions in human plasminogen and investigations in their complex-forming properties. Eur J Biochem 1980;107:7.
160. Hoylaerts M, Lijnen HR, Collen D. Studies on the mechanism of the antifibrinolytic action of tranexamic acid. Biochim Biophys Acta 1981;673:75.
161. Markus G, DePasquale JL, Wissler FC. Quantitative determination of the binding of ϵ-aminocaproic acid to native plasminogen. J Biol Chem 1978;253:727.
162. Markus G, Priore RL, Wissler FC. The binding of tranexamic acid to native (Glu) and modified (Lys) human plasminogen and its effect on conformation. J Biol Chem 1979;254:1211.
163. Rickli EE, Otavsky WI. A new method of isolation and some properties of heavy chain of human plasmin. Eur J Biochem 1975;9:441.
164. Wiman B, Lijnen HR, Collen D. On the specific interaction between the lysine-binding sites in plasmin and complementary sites in α_2-antiplasmin and in fibrinogen. Biochim Biophys Acta 1979;579:142.

165. Vali Z, Patthy L. Location of the intermediate and high affinity omega-aminocarboxylic acid–binding sites in human plasminogen. J Biol Chem 1982;257:2104.
166. Trexler M, Vali Z, Patthy L. Structure of the omega-aminocarboxylic acid-binding sites of human plasminogen: arginine 70 and aspartic acid 56 are essential for binding of ligand by kringle 4. J Biol Chem 1982;257:7401.
167. Trexler M, Banyai L, Patthy L, et al. The solution structure of kringle 4: NMR studies on native and several chemically modified kringle 4 species of human plasminogen. FEBS Lett 1983;154:311.
168. Plow EF, Collen D. Immunochemical characterization of a low affinity lysine binding site within plasminogen. J Biol Chem 1981;256:10864.
169. Thorsen S. Differences in the binding to fibrin of native plasminogen and plasminogen modified by proteolytic degradation: influence of omega-aminocarboxylic acids. Biochim Biophys Acta 1975;393:55.
170. Rakoczi I, Wiman B, Collen D. On the biological significance of the specific interaction between fibrin, plasminogen and antiplasmin. Biochim Biophys Acta 1978;540:295.
171. Wiman B, Wallen P. Structural relationship between "glutamic acid" and "lysine" forms of human plasminogen and their interaction with the NH_2-terminal activation peptide as studied by affinity chromatography. Eur J Biochem 1975;50:489.
172. Wiman B, Wallen P. The specific interaction between plasminogen and fibrin: a physiological role of the lysine binding site in plasminogen. Thromb Res 1977;10:213.
173. Wiman B, Collen D. Molecular mechanism of physiological fibrinolysis. Nature 1978;272:549.
174. Collen D. On the regulation and control of fibrinolysis. Thromb Haemost 1980;43:77.
175. Miles LA, Ginsberg MH, White JG, et al. Plasminogen interacts with human platelets through two distinct mechanisms. J Clin Invest 1986;77:2001.
176. Miles LA, Dahlberg CM, Plow EF. The cell-binding domains of plasminogen and their function in plasma. J Biol Chem 1988;263:11928.
177. Schwick HG, Heimburger N, Haupt H. Antiproteinasen des Humanserums. Z Inn Med 1966;7:1.
178. Collen D. Identification and some properties of a new fast-reacting plasmin inhibitor in human plasma. Eur J Biochem 1976;69:209.
179. Moroi M, Aoki N. Isolation and characterization of α_2-plasmin inhibitor from human plasma: a novel proteinase inhibitor which inhibits activator-induced clot lysis. J Biol Chem 1976;251:5956.
180. Müllertz S, Clemmensen I. The primary inhibitor of plasmin in human plasma. Biochem J 1976;159:545.
181. Bagge L, Bjork I, Saldeen T, Wallin R. Purification and characterization of an inhibitor of plasminogen activation from posttraumatic patients. Forensic Sci 1976;7:83.
182. Wiman B, Collen D. Purification and characterization of human antiplasmin, the fast-acting plasmin inhibitor in plasma. Eur J Biochem 1977;78:19.
183. Lijnen HR, Wiman B, Collen D. Partial primary structure of human α_2-antiplasmin: homology with other plasma protease inhibitors. Thromb Haemost 1982;48:311.
184. Holmes WE, Nelles L, Lijnen HR, Collen D. Primary structure of human α_2-antiplasmin, a serine protease inhibitor (serpin). J Biol Chem 1987;262:1659.
185. Lijnen HR, Holmes WE, Van Hoef B, et al. Amino-acid sequence of human α_2-antiplasmin. Eur J Biochem 1987;166:565.
186. Collen D, Wiman B. Turnover of antiplasmin, the fast-acting plasmin inhibitor of plasma. Blood 1979;53:313.
187. Christensen U, Clemmensen I. Purification and reaction mechanisms of the primary inhibitor of plasmin from human plasma. Biochem J 1978;175:635.
188. Wiman B. Affinity-chromatographic purification of human α_2-antiplasmin. Biochem J 1980;191:229.
189. Kluft C, Los N. Demonstration of two forms of α_2-antiplasmin in plasma by modified crossed immunoelectrophoresis. Thromb Res 1981;21:65.
190. Sasaki T, Morita T, Iwanaga S. Identification of the plasminogen-binding site of human α_2-plasmin inhibitor. (Abstract) Thromb Haemost 1983:50:170.
191. Wiman B, Nilsson T, Cedergren B. Studies on a form of α_2-antiplasmin in plasma which does not interact with the lysine-binding sites in plasminogen. Thromb Res 1982;28:193.
192. Christensen U, Clemmensen I. Kinetic properties of the primary inhibitor of plasmin from human plasma. Biochem J 1977;163:389.
193. Wiman B, Collen D. On the kinetics of the reaction between human antiplasmin and plasmin. Eur J Biochem 1978;84:573.
194. Wiman B, Boman L, Collen D. On the kinetics of the reaction betweeı. human antiplasmin and a low-molecular-weight form of plasmin. Eur J Biochem 1978;87:143.
195. Holmes WE, Nelles L, Lijnen HR, Collen D. Primary structure of human α_2-antiplasmin, a serine protease inhibitor (serpin). J Biol Chem 1987;262:1659.
196. Nilsson T, Wiman B. On the structure of the stable complex between plasmin and α_2-antiplasmin. FEBS Lett 1982;142:111.
197. Lijnen HR, Hoylaerts M, Collen D. Isolation and characterization of a human plasma protein with affinity for the lysine binding sites in plasminogen: role in the regulation of fibrinolysis and identification as histidine-rich glycoprotein. J Biol Chem 1980;255:10214.
198. Sottrup-Jensen L, Stepanik TM, Kristensen T, et al. Primary structure of human α_2-macroglobulin. V. The complete structure. J Biol Chem 1984;259:8318.
199. Barrett AJ, Starkey PM. The interaction of α_2-macroglobulin with proteinases: characteristics and specificity of the reaction, and a hypothesis concerning its molecular mechanism. Biochem J 1973;133:709.
200. Barrett AJ, Starkey PM, Munn EA. The unique nature of the interaction of α_2-macroglobulin with proteinases. In: Fritz H, Tschesche H, Green LJ, Truscheit E, eds. Proteinase inhibitors. Berlin, Springer-Verlag, 1974:72.
201. Harpel PC. Studies on human plasma α_2-macroglobulin-enzyme interactions: evidence for proteolytic modification of the subunit chain structure. J Exp Med 1973;138:508.
202. Werb Z, Burleigh MC, Barrett AJ, Starkey PM. The interaction of α_2-macroglobulin with proteinases. Biochem J 1974;139:359.
203. Hall PK, Roberts RC. Physical and chemical properties of human plasma α_2-macroglobulin. Biochem J 1978;171:27.
204. Swenson RP, Howard JB. Structural characterization of human α_2-macroglobulin subunits. J Biol Chem 1979;254:4452.
205. Sottrup-Jensen L, Lonblad PB, Stepanik TM, et al. Primary structure of the "bait" region for proteinases in α_2-macroglobulin. Nature of the complex. FEBS Lett 1981;127:167.
206. Sottrup-Jensen L, Hansen HF, Mortensen SB, et al. Sequence location of the reactive thiol ester in human α_2-macroglobulin. FEBS Lett 1981;123:145.
207. Van Leuven F, Marijnen P, Cassiman JJ, Van den Berghe H. Relation of internal thioesters to conformational change and receptor-recognition site in α_2-macroglobulin complexes. Biochem J 1982;203:405.
208. Marijnen P, Van Leuven F, Cassiman JJ, Van den Berghe H. Proteolysis at a lysine residue abolishes the receptor-recognition site of α_2-macroglobulin complexes. FEBS Lett 1982;137:241.
209. Travis J, Salvesen GS. Human plasma proteinase inhibitors. Ann Rev Biochem 1983;52:655.
210. Ganrot PO, Schersten B. Serum α_2-macroglobulin concentration and its variation with age and sex. Clin Chim Acta 1967;15:113.
211. Laurell CB. A screening test for α_1-antitrypsin deficiency. Scand J Clin Lab Invest 1972;29:247.
212. Nilehn JE, Ganrot PO. Plasmin, plasmin inhibitors and degradation products of fibrinogen in human serum during and after intravenous infusion of streptokinase. Scand J Clin Lab Invest 1967;20:113.
213. Arnesen H, Fagerhol MK. Alpha$_2$-macroglobulin, α_1-antitrypsin, and anti-thrombin III in plasma and serum during fibrinolytic therapy with urokinase. Scand J Clin Lab Invest 1972;29:259.
214. Bergqvist D, Nilsson IM. Hereditary α_2-macroglobulin deficiency. Scand J Haematol 1979;23:433.
215. Kan CC, Solomon E, Belt KT, et al. Nucleotide sequence of cDNA encoding human α_2-macroglobulin and assignment of the chromosomal locus. Proc Natl Acad Sci USA 1985;82:2282.
216. Loskutoff DJ, Edgington TS. Synthesis of a fibrinolytic activator and inhibitor by endothelial cells. Proc Natl Acad Sci USA 1977;74:3903.
217. Loskutoff DJ, van Mourik JA, Erickson LA, Lawrence D. Detection of an unusually stable fibrinolytic inhibitor produced by bovine endothelial cells. Proc Natl Acad Sci USA 1983;80:2956.
218. Seifert SC, Gelehrter TD. Mechanism of dexamethasone inhibition of plasminogen activator in rat hepatoma cells. Proc Natl Acad Sci USA 1978;75:6130.
219. Coleman PL, Barouski PA, Gelehrter TD. The dexamethasone-induced inhibitor of fibrinolytic activity in hepatoma cells. J Biol Chem 1982;257:4260.
220. Kruithof EKO, Ransijn A, Bachmann F. Inhibition of tissue plasminogen activator by human plasma. In: Davidson, Bachmann, Bouvier and Kruithof, eds. Progress in fibrinolysis, vol 6. Edinburgh, Churchill Livingstone, 1983:365.
221. Kruithof EKO, Tran-Thang C, Ransijn A, et al. Demonstration of a fast-acting inhibitor of plasminogen activators in human plasma. Blood 1984;64:907.
222. Chmielewska J, Rånby M, Wiman B. Evidence for a rapid inhibitor to tissue plasminogen activator in plasma. Thromb Res 1983;31:427.
223. Juhan-Vague I, Moerman B, De Cock F, et al. Plasma levels of a specific inhibitor of tissue-type plasminogen activator (and urokinase) in normal and pathological conditions. Thromb Res 1984;33:523.
224. Verheijen JH, Chang GTG, Kluft C. Evidence for the occurrence of a fast-acting inhibitor for tissue-type plasminogen activator in human plasma. Thromb Haemost 1984;51:392.
225. Thorsen S, Philips M. Isolation of tissue-type plasminogen activator-inhibitor complexes from human plasma: evidence for a rapid plasminogen activator inhibitor. Biochim Biophys Acta 1984;802:111.
226. Erickson LA, Hekman CM, Loskutoff DJ. The primary plasminogen activator inhibitors in endothelial cells, platelets, serum and plasma are immunologically related. Proc Natl Acad Sci USA 1985;82:8710.
227. Kruithof EKO, Tran-Thang C, Bachmann F. Studies on the release of a plasminogen activator inhibitor by human platelets. Thromb Haemost 1986;55:201.
228. Philips M, Juul AG, Thorsen S, et al. Immunological relationship between the fast-acting plasminogen activator inhibitors from plasma,

blood platelets and endothelial cells demonstrated with a monoclonal antibody against an inhibitor from placenta. Thromb Haemost 1986;55: 213.
229. Andreasen PA, Nielsen LS, Kristensen P, et al. Plasminogen activator inhibitor from human fibrosarcoma cells binds urokinase-type plasminogen activator, but not its proenzyme. J Biol Chem 1986;261:7644.
230. Cajot JF, Kruithof EKO, Schleuning WD, et al. Plasminogen activators, plasminogen activator inhibitors and procoagulant, analyzed in twenty human tumor cell lines. Int J Cancer 1986;38:719.
231. Sprengers ED, Princen HMG, Kooistra T, et al. Inhibition of plasminogen activators by conditioned medium of human hepatocytes and hepatoma cell line Hep G2. J Lab Clin Med 1985;105:751.
232. Van Mourik JA, Lawrence DA, Loskutoff DJ. Purification of an inhibitor of plasminogen activator (antiactivator) synthesized by endothelial cells. J Biol Chem 1984;259:14914.
233. Alessi MC, Declerck PJ, De Mol M, et al. Purification and characterization of natural and recombinant human plasminogen activator inhibitor-1 (PAI-1). Eur J Biochem 1988;175:531.
234. Coleman PL, Patel PD, Cwikel BJ, et al. Characterization of the dexamethasone induced inhibitor of plasminogen activator in HTC hepatoma cells. J Biol Chem 1986;261:4352.
235. Wagner O, Binder B. Purification of an active plasminogen activator inhibitor immunologically related to the endothelial type plasminogen activator inhibitor from the conditioned media of a human melanoma cell line. J Biol Chem 1986;261:14474.
236. Klinger KW, Winqvist R, Riccio A, et al. Plasminogen activator inhibitor type 1 gene is located at region q21.3-q22 of chromosome 7 and genetically linked with cystic fibrosis. Proc Natl Acad Sci USA 1987;84: 8548.
237. Ny T, Sawdey M, Lawrence D, et al. Cloning and sequence of a cDNA coding for the human β-migrating endothelial cell-type plasminogen activator inhibitor. Proc Natl Acad Sci USA 1986;83:6776.
238. Pannekoek H, Veerman H, Lambers H, et al. Endothelial plasminogen activator inhibitor (PAI): a new member of the serpin gene family. EMBO J 1986;5:2539.
239. Andreasen PA, Riccio A, Welinder KG, et al. Plasminogen activator inhibitory type-1: reactive center and amino-terminal heterogeneity determined by protein and cDNA sequencing. FEBS Lett 1986;209:213.
240. Ginsburg D, Zeheb R, Yang AY, et al. cDNA cloning of human plasminogen activator-inhibitor from endothelial cells. J Clin Invest 1986;78: 1673.
241. Wun TC, Kretzmer KK. cDNA cloning and expression in E coli of a plasminogen activator inhibitor (PAI) related to a PAI produced by Hep G2 hepatoma cell. FEBS Lett 1987;210:11.
242. Loskutoff DJ, Linders M, Keijer J, et al. Structure of the human plasminogen activator inhibitor 1 gene: nonrandom distribution of introns. Biochemistry 1987;26:3763.
243. Kruithof EKO, Gudinchet A, Bachmann F. Plasminogen activator inhibitor 1 and plasminogen activator inhibitor 2 in various disease states. Thromb Haemost 1988;59:7.
244. Colucci M, Paramo JA, Collen D. Generation in plasma of a fast-acting inhibitor of plasminogen activator in response to endotoxin stimulation. J Clin Invest 1985;75:818.
245. Declerck PJ, De Mol M, Alessi MC, et al. Purification and characterization of a plasminogen activator inhibitor-1 binding protein from human plasma: identification as a multimeric form of S protein (Vitronectin). J Biol Chem 1988;263:15454.
246. Wiman B, Chmielewska J, Ranby M. Inactivation of tissue plasminogen activator in plasma: demonstration of a complex with a new rapid inhibitor. J Biol Chem 1984;259:3644.
247. Kruithof EKO, Nicoloso G, Bachmann F. Plasminogen activator inhibitor 1: development of a radioimmunoassay and observations on its plasma concentration during venous occlusion and after platelet aggregation. Blood 1987;70:1645.
248. Hekman CM, Loskutoff D. Endothelial cells produce a latent inhibitor of plasminogen activators that can be activated by denaturants. J Biol Chem 1985;260:11581.
249. Levin EG. Quantitation and properties of the active and latent plasminogen activator inhibitors in cultures of human endothelial cells. Blood 1986;67:1309.
250. Gelehrter TD, Sznycer-Laszuk R. Thrombin induction of plasminogen activator-inhibitor in cultured human endothelial cells. J Clin Invest 1986 77:165.
251. Van Hinsbergh VWM, Sprengers ED, Kooistra T. Effect of thrombin on the production of plasminogen activators and PA-inhibitor-1 by human foreskin microvascular endothelial cells. Thromb Haemost 1987;57: 148.
252. Emeis JJ, Kooistra T. Interleukin-1 and lipopolysaccharide induce an inhibitor of tissue-type plasminogen activator in vivo and in cultured endothelial cells. J Exp Med 1986;163:1260.
253. Nachmann RL, Hajjar KA, Silverstein RL, et al. Interleukin-1 induces endothelial cell synthesis of plasminogen activator inhibitor. J Exp Med 1986;163:1595.
254. Laiho M, Saksela O, Andreasen PA, et al. Enhanced production and extracellular deposition of the endothelial-type plasminogen activator inhibitor in cultured human lung fibroblasts by transforming growth factor β. J Cell Biol 1986;103:2403.
255. Thalacker FW, Nilsen-Hamilton M. Specific induction of secreted proteins by transforming growth factor-β and 12-0-tetradecanoylphorbol-13-acetate. J Biol Chem 1987;262:2283.
256. Schleef RR, Bevilacqua MP, Sawdey M, et al. Cytokine activation of vascular endothelium: effects on tissue-type plasminogen activator and type 1 plasminogen activator inhibitor. J Biol Chem 1988;263:5797.
257. Van Hinsbergh VWM, Kooistra T, Fiers W, Emeis JJ. Tumor necrosis factor increases the production of plasminogen activator inhibitor in human endothelial cells in vitro and in rats in vivo. (Abstract) Thromb Haemost 1987;58:15.
258. Kawano T, Morimoto K, Uemura Y. Urokinase inhibitor in human placenta. Nature 1968;217:253.
259. Lecander I, Astedt B. Isolation of a new specific plasminogen activator inhibitor from pregnancy plasma. Br J Haematol 1986;62:221.
260. Kruithof EKO, Tran-Thang C, Gudinchet A, et al. Fibrinolysis in pregnancy: a study of plasminogen activator inhibitors. Blood 1987;69:460.
261. Kopitar M, Rozman B, Babnik J, et al. Human leucocyte urokinase inhibitor-purification, characterization and comparative studies against different plasminogen activators. Thromb Haemost 1985;54:750.
262. Chapman HA, Stone OL. Characterization of a macrophage-derived plasminogen activator inhibitor: similarities with placental urokinase inhibitor. Biochem J 1985;230:109.
263. Golder JP, Stephens RW. Minactivin: a human monocyte product which specifically inactivates urokinase-type plasminogen activators. Eur J Biochem 1983;136:517.
264. Kruithof EKO, Vassalli JD, Schleuning WD, et al. Purification and characterization of a plasminogen activator inhibitor from the histiocytic lymphoma cell-line U-937. J Biol Chem 1986;261:11207.
265. Astedt B, Lecander I, Brodin T, et al. Purification of a specific placental plasminogen activator inhibitor by monoclonal antibody and its complex formation with plasminogen activator. Thromb Haemost 1985;53: 122.
266. Wun TC, Reich E. An inhibitor of plasminogen activation from human placenta: purification and characterization. J Biol Chem 1987;262:3646.
267. Genton C, Kruithof EKO, Schleuning WD. Phorbol ester induces the biosynthesis of glycosylated and nonglycosylated plasminogen activator inhibitor 2 in high excess over urokinase-type plasminogen activator in human U-937 lymphoma cells. J Cell Biol 1987;104:705.
268. Wohlwend A, Belin D, Vassalli JD. Plasminogen activator-specific inhibitors produced by human monocytes/macrophages. J Exp Med 1987;165:320.
269. Schleuning WD, Medcalf RL, Hession C, et al. Plasminogen activator inhibitor 2: regulation of gene transcription during phorbol ester-mediated differentiation of U-937 human histiocytic lymphoma cells. Mol Cell Biol 1987;7:4564.
270. Ye RD, Wun TC, Sadler JE. cDNA cloning and expression in *Escherichia coli* of a plasminogen activator inhibitor from human placenta. J Biol Chem 1987;262:3718.
271. Webb AC, Collins KL, Snyder SE, et al. Human monocyte Arg-serpin cDNA: sequence, chromosomal assignment, and homology to plasminogen activator-inhibitor. J Exp Med 1987;166:77.
272. Chapman HA Jr, Stone OL. A fibrinolytic inhibitor of human alveolar macrophages: induction with endotoxin. Am Rev Respir Dis 1985;132: 569.
273. Lecander I, Astedt B. Occurrence of a specific plasminogen activator inhibitor of placental type, PAI-2, in men and non-pregnant women. Fibrinolysis 1989;3:27.
274. Tran-Thang C, Wyss P, Kruithof EKO, et al. Tissue-type plasminogen activator increases the binding of plasminogen to clots. (Abstract) Haemostasis 1984;14:17.
275. Ichinose A, Tamaki T, Aoki N. Factor XIII-mediated cross-linking of NH_2-terminal peptide of α_2-plasmin inhibitor to fibrin. FEBS Lett 1983;153:369.
276. Pannell R, Black J, Gurewich V. Complementary modes of action of tissue-type plasminogen activator and pro-urokinase by which their synergistic effect on clot lysis may be explained. J Clin Invest 1988;81: 853.
277. Lijnen HR, Van Hoef B, De Cock F, et al. The mechanism of plasminogen activation and fibrin dissolution by single chain urokinase-type plasminogen activator (scu-PA) in a plasma milieu in vitro. Blood 1989;73: 1864
278. Koie K, Ogata K, Kamiya T, et al. α_2-plasmin-inhibitor deficiency (Miyasato disease). Lancet 1978;2:1334.
279. Aoki N, Saito H, Kamiya T, et al. Congenital deficiency of α_2-plasmin inhibitor associated with severe hemorrhagic tendency. J Clin Invest 1979;63:877.
280. Kluft C, Vellenga E, Brommer EJP. Homozygous α_2-antiplasmin deficiency. Lancet 1979;2:206.
281. Kluft C, Vellenga E, Brommer EJP, Wijngaards G. A familial hemorrhagic diathesis in a Dutch family: an inherited deficiency of α_2-antiplasmin. Blood 1982;59:1169.
282. Yoshioka A, Kamitsuji H, Takase T, et al. Congenital deficiency of α_2-plasmin inhibitor in three sisters. Haemostasis 1982;11:176.
283. Knot EAR, ten Cate JW, Lamping RJ, Gie LK. α_2-Antiplasmin: functional characterization and metabolism in a heterozygote deficient patient. Thromb Haemost 1986;55:375.

284. Stormorken H, Gogstad GO, Brosstad F. Hereditary α_2-antiplasmin deficiency. Thromb Res 1983;31:647.
285. Kordich L, Feldman L, Porterie P, Lago O. Severe hemorrhagic tendency in heterozygous α_2-antiplasmin deficiency. Thromb Res 1985;40:645.
286. Miles LA, Plow EF, Donnelly KJ, et al. A bleeding disorder due to deficiency of α_2-antiplasmin. Blood 1982;59:1246.
287. Teger-Nilsson AC, Gyzander E, Myrwold H, et al. Determination of fast-acting plasmin inhibitor (α_2-antiplasmin) in plasma from patients with tendency to thrombosis and increased fibrinolysis. Haemostasis 1978;7:155.
288. Aoki N, Yamanaka T. The α_2-plasmin inhibitor levels in liver diseases. Clin Chim Acta 1978;84:99.
289. Samama MM, Schlegel N, Cazenave B, et al. α_2-Antiplasmin assay: amidolytic and immunological method. In: Lijnen HR, Collen D, Verstraete M, eds. Synthetic substrates in clinical blood coagulation assays. The Hague, Martinus Nijhoff, 1980:93.
290. Högstorp H, Jacobsson H, Saldeen T. Effect of hepatectomy on the post-traumatic fibrinolysis inhibition and the primary fibrinolysis inhibitor in the rat. Thromb Res 1980;18:361.
291. Collen D, Lijnen HR. The fibrinolytic system in man. CRC Crit Rev Oncool Hematol 1986;4:249.
292. Collen D, Bounameaux H, De Cock F, et al. Analysis of coagulation and fibrinolysis during intravenous infusion of recombinant human tissue-type plasminogen activator in patients with acute myocardial infarction. Circulation 1986;73:511.
293. Nieuwenhuis HK, Kluft C, Wijngaards G, et al. α_2-Antiplasmin Enschede: an autosomal recessive hemorrhagic disorder caused by a dysfunctional α_2-antiplasmin molecule. (Abstract) Thromb Haemost 1983;50:170.
294. Holmes WE, Lijnen HR, Nelles L, et al. α_2-Antiplasmin Enschede: alanine insertion and abolition of plasmin inhibitory activity. Science 1987;238:209.
295. Páramo JA, Colucci M, Collen D, et al. Plasminogen activator inhibitor in the blood of patients with coronary artery disease. Br Med J 1985;291:573.
296. Mehta J, Mehta P, Lawson D, et al. Plasma tissue plasminogen activator inhibitor levels in coronary artery disease: correlation with age and serum triglyceride concentrations. J Am Coll Cardiol 1987;9:263.
297. Almér LO, Öhlin H. Elevated levels of the rapid inhibitor of plasminogen activator in acute myocardial infarction. Thromb Res 1987;47:335.
298. Verheugt FWA, ten Cate JW, Sturk A, et al. Tissue plasminogen activator activity and inhibition in acute myocardial infarction and angiographically normal coronary arteries. Am J Cardiol 1987;59:1075.
299. Hamsten A, Wiman B, De Faire U, et al. Increased plasma levels of a rapid inhibitor of tissue plasminogen activator in young survivors of myocardial infarction. N Engl J Med 1985;213:1557.
300. Hamsten A, Blombäck M, Wiman B, et al. Haemostatic function in myocardial infarction. Br Heart J 1986;55:58.
301. Hamsten A, De Faire U, Walldius G, et al. Plasminogen activator inhibitor in plasma: risk factor for recurrent myocardial infarction. Lancet 1987;2:3.
302. Juhan-Vague I, Moerman B, De Cock F, et al. Plasma levels of a specific inhibitor of tissue-type plasminogen activator (and urokinase) in normal and pathological conditions. Thromb Res 1984;33:523.
303. Wiman B, Chmielewska J. A novel fast inhibitor to tissue plasminogen activator in plasma, which may be of great pathophysiological significance. Scand J Clin Lab Invest 1985;45(Suppl 177):43.
304. Mellbring G, Dahlgren S, Wiman B, et al. Relationship between preoperative status of the fibrinolytic system and occurrence of deep vein thrombosis after major abdominal surgery. Thromb Res 1985;39:157.
305. Kluft C, Jie AFH, Lowe GDO, et al. Association between postoperative hyper-response in t-PA inhibition and deep vein thrombosis. Thromb Haemost 1986;56:107.
306. Páramo JA, Alfaro MJ, Rocha E. Postoperative changes in the plasmatic levels of tissue-type plasminogen activator and its fast-acting inhibitor: relationship to deep vein thrombosis and influence of prophylaxis. Thromb Haemost 1985;54:713.
307. Mellbring G, Dahlgren S, Wiman B. Plasma fibrinolytic activity in patients undergoing major abdominal surgery. Acta Chir Scand 1985;151:109.
308. Stalder M, Hauert J, Kruithof EKO, Bachmann F. Release of vascular plasminogen activator (v-PA) after venous stasis: electrophoretic-zymographic analysis of free and complexed v-PA. Br J Haematol 1985;61:169.
309. Jorgensen M, Bonnevie-Nielsen V. Increased concentration of the fast-acting plasminogen activator inhibitor in plasma associated with familial venous thrombosis. Br J Haematol 1987;65:175.
310. Juhan-Vague I, Valadier J, Alessi MC, et al. Deficient t-PA release and elevated PA inhibitor levels in patients with spontaneous or recurrent deep venous thrombosis. Thromb Haemost 1987;57:67.
311. Mellbring G, Dahlgren S, Reiz S, Wiman B. Fibrinolytic activity in plasma and deep vein thrombosis after major abdominal surgery. Thromb Res 1983;32:575.
312. Benavent A, Estelles A, Aznar J, et al. Dysfunctional plasminogen in full term newborn: study of active site of plasmin. Thromb Haemost 1984;51:67.
313. Cederholm-Williams SA, Spender JAD, Wilkinson AR. Plasma levels of selected haemostatic factors in newborn babies. Thromb Res 1981;23:555.
314. Hasegawa DK, Tyler BJ, Edson JR. Thrombotic disease in three families with inherited plasminogen deficiency. Blood 1982;60(Suppl A):213a.
315. Ten Cate JW, Peters M, Büller H. Isolated plasminogen deficiency in a patient with recurrent thromboembolic complications. (Abstract) Thromb Haemost 1983;50:59.
316. Lottenberg R, Dolly FR, Kitchens CS. Recurring thromboembolic disease and pulmonary hypertension associated with severe hypoplasminogenemia. Am J Hematol 1985;19:181.
317. Mannucci PM, Kluft C, Traas DW, et al. Congenital plasminogen deficiency associated with venous thromboembolism: therapeutic trial with stanozolol. Br J Haematol 1986;63:753.
318. Girolami A, Marafioti F, Rubertelli M, Cappellato MG. Congenital heterozygous plasminogen deficiency associated with a severe thrombotic tendency. Acta Haematol 1986;75:54.
319. Davis RD, Picoff RC. Low plasminogen levels and liver disease. Am J Clin Pathol 1969;59:175.
320. Kordich LC, Porterie VP, Lago O, et al. Mini-plasminogen like molecule in septic patients. Thromb Res 1987;47:553.
321. Verstraete M, Vermylen J, Collen D. Intravascular coagulation in liver disease. Annu Rev Med 1974;25:447.
322. Molinas FC, Kordich L, Porterie P, et al. Plasminogen abnormalities in patients with Argentine hemorrhagic fever. Thromb Res 1987;48:713.
323. Jespersen J, Gram J, Bach E. A sequential study of plasma histidine-rich glycoprotein and plasminogen in patients with acute myocardial infarction and deep vein thrombosis. Thromb Haemost 1984;51:99.
324. Castel M, Horellou MH, Conard J, Samama M. Immunochemical determination of histidine-rich glycoprotein in healthy subjects and in a clinical population. In: Davidson JF, Bachman F, Bouvier CA, Kruithof EKO, eds. Progress in fibrinolysis, vol 6. Edinburgh, Churchill Livingstone, 1983:370.
325. Aoki N, Moroi M, Sakata Y, et al. Abnormal plasminogen: a hereditary molecular abnormality found in a patient with recurrent thrombosis. J Clin Invest 1978;61:1186.
326. Sakata Y, Aoki N. Molecular abnormality of plasminogen. J Biol Chem 1980;255:5442.
327. Miyata T, Iwanaga S, Sakata Y, Aoki N. Plasminogen Tochigi: inactive plasmin resulting from replacement of alanine-600 by threonine in the active site. Proc Natl Acad Sci USA 1982;79:6132.
328. Stroud RM, Kay LM, Dickerson RE. The structure of bovine trypsin: electron density maps of the inhibited enzyme at 5Å and at 2.7Å resolution. J Mol Biol 1974;83:185.
329. Miyata T, Iwanaga S, Sakata Y, et al. Plasminogens Tochigi II and Nagoya: two additional molecular defects with $Ala^{600} \rightarrow$ Thr replacement found in plasmin light chain variants. J Biochem 1984;96:277.
330. Aoki N, Tateno K, Sakata Y. Differences of frequency distributions of plasminogen phenotypes between Japanese and American populations: new methods for the detection of plasminogen variants. Biochem Genet 1984;22:871.
331. Nakamura S, Abe K. Genetic polymorphism of human plasminogen in the Japanese population: new plasminogen variants and relationship between plasminogen phenotypes and their biological activities. Hum Genet 1982;60:57.
332. Kazama M, Tahara C, Suzuki Z, et al. Abnormal plasminogen, a case of recurrent thrombosis. Thromb Res 1981;21:517.
333. Soria J, Soria C, Bertrand O, et al. Plasminogen Paris I: congenital abnormal plasminogen and its incidence in thrombosis. Thromb Res 1983;32:229.
334. Manabe SI, Matsueda M. Homozygous protein C deficiency combined with heterozygous dysplasminogenemia found in a 21-year-old thrombophilic male. Thromb Res 1985;39:333.
335. Wohl RC, Summaria L, Robbins KC. Physiological activation of the human fibrinolytic system: isolation and characterization of human plasminogen variants, Chicago I and Chicago II. J Biol Chem 1979;254:9063.
336. Wohl RC, Summaria L, Chediak J, et al. Human plasminogen variant Chicago III. Thromb Haemost 1982;48:146.
337. Scharrer IM, Wohl RC, Hach V, et al. Investigation of a congenital abnormal plasminogen, Frankfurt I, and its relationship to thrombosis. Thromb Haemost 1986;55:396.
338. Kristensen P, Larsson LI, Nielsen LS, et al. Human endothelial cells contain one type of plasminogen activator. FEBS Lett 1984;168:33.
339. Larsson LI, Skriver L, Nielsen LS, et al. Distribution of urokinase-type plasminogen activator immunoreactivity in the mouse. J Cell Biol 1984;98:894.
340. Darras V, Thienpont M, Stump DC, et al. Measurement of urokinase-type plasminogen activator (u-PA) with an enzyme-linked immunosorbent assay (ELISA) based on three murine monoclonal antibodies. Thromb Haemost 1986;56:411.
341. Huber K, Kirchheimer J, Binder BR. Characterization of a specific anti-human urokinase antibody: development of a sensitive competition radioimmunoassay for urokinase antigen. J Lab Clin Med 1984;103:684.
342. Kirchheimer J, Binder B. Urokinase antigen in plasma: age and sex dependent variations. Thromb Res 1984;36:643.

343. Vassalli JD, Baccino D, Belin D. A cellular binding site for the M_r 55,000 form of the human plasminogen activator, urokinase. J Cell Biol 1985;100:86.
344. Del Rosso M, Dini G, Fibbi G. Receptors for plasminogen activator, urokinase, in normal and rous sarcoma virus-transformed mouse fibroblasts. Cancer Res 1985;45:630.
345. Stoppelli MP, Corti A, Soffientini A, et al. Differentiation-enhanced binding of the amino-terminal fragment of human urokinase plasminogen activator to a specific receptor of U937 monocytes. Proc Natl Acad Sci USA 1985;82:4939.
346. Bajpai A, Baker JB. Urokinase binding sites on human foreskin cells: evidence for occupancy with endogenous urokinase. Biochem Biophys Res Commun 1985;133:994.
347. Blasi F. Surface receptors for urokinase plasminogen activator. Fibrinolysis 1988:2:73.
348. Blasi F, Stoppelli MP, Cubellis MV. The receptor for urokinase-plasminogen activator. J Cell Biochem 1986;32:179.
349. Nielsen LS, Kellerman GM, Behrendt N, et al. A 55,000–60,000 M_r receptor protein for urokinase-type plasminogen activator. Identification in human tumor cell lines and partial purification. J Biol Chem 1988;263:2358.
350. Bachmann F. Fibrinolysis. In: Verstraete M, Vermylen J, Lijnen R, Arnout J, eds. Thrombosis and haemostasis 1987. Leuven, Belgium, Leuven University Press, 1987:227.
351. Ogston D, Bennett B, Herbert RJ, Douglas AS. The inhibition of urokinase by α_2-macroglobulin. Clin Sci 1973;44:73.
352. Clemmensen I, Christensen F. Inhibition of urokinase by complex formation with human α_1-antitrypsin. Biochim Biophys Acta 1976;249: 591.
353. Clemmensen I. Inhibition of urokinase by complex formation with human antithrombin III in absence and presence of heparin. Thromb Haemost 1978;39:616.
354. Samama M, Castel M, Matsuo O, et al. Comparative study of the activity of high and low molecular weight urokinase in the presence of fibrin. Thromb Haemost 1982;47:36.
355. Stump DC, Thienpont M, Collen D. Purification and characterization of a novel inhibitor of urokinase from human urine. Quantitation and preliminary characterization in plasma. J Biol Chem 1986;261:12759.
356. Heeb MJ, España F, Geiger M, et al. Immunological identity of heparin-dependent plasma and urinary protein C inhibitor and plasminogen activator inhibitor-3. J Biol Chem 1987;262:15813.
357. Fletcher AP, Alkjaersig N, Sherry S, et al. The development of urokinase as a thrombolytic agent: maintenance of a sustained thrombolytic state in man by its intravenous infusion. J Lab Clin Med 1965;65:713.
358. Gurewich V, Pannell R, Louie S, et al. Effective and fibrin-specific clot lysis by a zymogen precursor form of urokinase (pro-urokinase): a study in vitro and in two animal species. J Clin Invest 1984;73:1731.
359. Zamarron C, Lijnen HR, Van Hoef B, Collen D. Biological and thrombolytic properties of proenzyme and active forms of urokinase: I. fibrinolytic and fibrinogenolytic properties in human plasma in vitro of urokinases obtained from human urine or by recombinant DNA technology. Thromb Haemost 1984;52:19.
360. Cash JD. Control mechanism of activator release. In: Davidson JF, Rowan RM, Samama MM, Desnoyers PC, eds. Chemical fibrinolysis and thrombolysis, vol 3. New York, Raven Press, 1978:65.
361. Colucci M, Stassen JM, Salwa J, Collen D. Identification of plasminogen activator releasing activity in the neurohypophysis. Br J Haematol 1984;58:337.
362. Comp PC, Esmon CT. Generation of fibrinolytic activity by infusion of activated protein C into dogs. J Clin Invest 1981;68:1221.
363. Colucci M, Stassen JM, Collen D. Influence of protein C activation on blood coagulation and fibrinolysis in squirrel monkeys. J Clin Invest 1984;74:200.
364. Bertina RM, van Hinsbergh VWM, Emeis SJ, et al. Inhibition of tissue-type plasminogen activator inhibitor activity by activated protein C. (Abstract) Circulation 1984;70(Suppl II):94.
365. Hanss M, Collen D. Secretion of tissue-type plasminogen activator and plasminogen activator inhibitor by cultured human endothelial cells: modulation by thrombin, endotoxin and histamine. J Lab Clin Med 1987;109:97.
366. Gelehrter TD, Sznycer-Laszuk R, Zeheb R, Cwikel BJ. Dexamethasone inhibition of tissue-type plasminogen activator (t-PA) activity: paradoxical induction of both t-PA antigen and plasminogen activator inhibitor. Mol Endocrinol 1987;1:97.
367. Kooistra T, Van den Berg J, Töns A, et al. Butyrate stimulates tissue-type plasminogen-activator synthesis in cultured human endothelial cells. Biochem J 1987;247:605.
368. Bunning RAD, Crawford A, Richardson HJ, et al. Interleukin 1 preferentially stimulates the production of tissue-type plasminogen activator by human articular chondrocytes. Biochim Biophys Acta 1987;924:473.
369. Liu YX, Cajander SB, Ny T, et al. Gonadotropin regulation of tissue-type and urokinase-type plasminogen activators in rat granulosa and theca-interstitial cells during the periovulatory period. Mol Cell Endocrinol 1987;54:221.
370. van Zonneveld AJ, Chang GTG, van den Berg J, et al. Quantification of tissue-type plasminogen activator (t-PA) mRNA in human endothelial cell cultures by hybridization with a t-PA cDNA probe. Biochem J 1986;235:385.
371. O'Connell ML, Canipari R, Strickland S. Hormonal regulation of tissue plasminogen activator secretion and mRNA levels in rat granulosa cells. J Biol Chem 1987;262:2339.
372. Ny T, Liu YX, Ohlsson M, et al. Regulation of tissue-type plasminogen activator activity and messenger RNA levels by gonadotropin-releasing hormone in cultured rat granulosa cells and cumulus-oocyte complexes. J Biol Chem 1987;262:11790.
373. Rijken DC, Juhan-Vague I, Collen D. Complexes between tissue-type plasminogen activator and proteinase inhibitors in human plasma, identified with an immunoradiometric assay. J Lab Clin Med 1983;101: 285.
374. Booth NA, Walker E, Maugham R, Bennett B. Plasminogen activator in normal subjects after exercise and venous occlusion: t-PA circulates as complexes with C_1-inhibitor and PAI-1. Blood 1987;69:1600.
375. Sprengers ED, Kluft C. Plasminogen activator inhibitors. Blood 1987;69: 381.
376. Clayton KJ, Anderson JA, McNicol GP. Preoperative prediction of postoperative deep vein thrombosis. Br Med J 1976;2:910.
377. Rakoczi I, Chamone D, Collen D, Verstraete M. Prediction of postoperative leg vein thrombosis in gynaecological patients. Lancet 1978;1: 509.
378. Isacson S, Nilsson IM. Defective fibrinolysis in blood and vein walls in recurrent "idiopathic" venous thrombosis. Acta Chir Scand 1972;138: 313.
379. Nilsson IM, Hedner U, Isacson S. Phenformin and ethyloestrenol in recurrent venous thrombosis. Acta Med Scand 1975;198:107.
380. Korninger C, Lechner K, Niessner H, et al. Impaired fibrinolytic capacity predisposes for recurrence of venous thrombosis. Thromb Haemost 1984;52:127.
381. Nilsson IM, Ljungner H, Tengborn L. Two different mechanisms in patients with venous thrombosis and defective fibrinolysis: low concentration of plasminogen activator or increased concentration of plasminogen activator inhibitor. Br Med J 1985;290:1453.
382. Booth NA, Bennett B, Wijngaards G, et al. A new life-long hemorrhagic disorder due to excess plasminogen activator. Blood 1983;61:267.
383. Aznar J, Estellés A, Villa V, et al. Inherited fibrinolytic disorder due to an enhanced plasminogen activator level. Thromb Haemost 1984;52: 196.
384. Kraut E, Frey EK, Werle E. Über die inaktivierung des kallikreins. Hoppe Seyler's Z Physiol Chem 1930;192:1.
385. Kunitz M, Northrop JH. Isolation from beef pancreas of crystalline trypsinogen, trypsin, a trypsin inhibitor, and an inhibitor trypsin compound. J Gen Physiol 1936;19:991.
386. Werle E. Contribution to the biochemistry of trasylol. In: Haberland, Matis, eds. New aspects of Trasylol therapy, vol 3. Stuttgart, FK Schattauer Verlag, 1970:51.
387. Werle E. Trasylol: a short survey on its history, biochemistry and activities. In: Brendel, Haberland, eds. New aspects of Trasylol therapy, vol 5. Stuttgart, FK Schattauer Verlag, 1972:9.
388. Kaller H, Patzschke K, Wegner LA, Horster FA. Pharmacokinetic observations following intravenous administration of radioactive labelled aprotinin in volunteers. Eur J Drug Metab Pharmacokinet 1978;3:79.
389. Naito SI, Hirano M, Yoshihara H, Ohta M. Pharmacokinetics on blood concentration of aprotinin (Trasylol) in humans. Basic Pharmacol Ther 1980;8:3613.
390. Fritz H, Oppitz KH, Meckl D, et al. Verteilung und Ausscheidung von natürlich vorkommenden und chemisch modifizierten Proteaseinhibitoren nach intravenöser Injektion bei Ratte, Hund (und Mensch). Hoppe Seyler's Z Physiol Chem 1969;350:1541.
391. Jochum M, Jonáková V, Dittmer H, Fritz H. An enzymatic assay convenient for the control of aprotinin levels during proteinase inhibitor therapy. Fresinius Z Anal Chem 1984;317:719.
392. Trapnell JE, Rigby CC, Talbot CH, Duncan EHL. A controlled trial of Trasylol in the treatment of acute pancreatitis. Br J Surg 1974;61:177.
393. Imrie CW, Benjamin SI, Ferguson JC, et al. A single-centre double-blind trial of Trasylol therapy in primary acute pancreatitis. Br J Surg 1978;65:337.
394. Medical Research Council Multicentre Trial. Morbidity of acute pancreatitis; the effect of aprotinin and glucagon. Gut 1980;21:334.
395. Sher G. Trasylol in the management of abruptio placentae with consumption coagulopathy and uterine inertia. J Reprod Med 1980;25: 113.
396. Tauber PF, Wolf AS, Herting W, Zaneveld LJD. Hemorrhage induced by intrauterine devices: control by local proteinase inhibition. Fertil Steril 1977;28:1375.
397. Kösters S, Wand H. Über die Beeinflussung des Blutverlustes nach Prostataoperationen durch prä-operative Applikation von Antifibrinolytika. Urologe [A] 1973;12:295.
398. Schmutzler R, Fürstenberg H. Fibrinolyse und Blutverlust nach Prostata-Operationen und deren Beeinflussbarkeit durch Antifibrinolytika. Dtsch Med Wochenschr 1966;91:297.
399. Beck OJ, Oeckler R. Frühdiagnose und Therapie der Aneurysmablutungen. Münch Med Wochenschr 1981;123:561.
400. Beck OJ, Oeckler R. Subarachnoid haemorrhage. Br Med J 1982;284: 1050.

401. Ambrus JL, Schimert G, Lajos TZ, et al. Effect of antifibrinolytic agents and estrogens on blood loss and blood coagulation factors during open heart surgery. J Med Exp Clin 1971;2:65.
402. Mammen EF. Natural proteinase inhibitors in extracorporeal circulation. Ann NY Acad Sci 1968;146:754.
403. Köstering H, Kirchhoff PG, Völker P, et al. Untersuchungen der Blutgerinnungsveränderungen während und nach Operationen mit Hilfe der Herz-Lungen-Maschine. Thoraxchir 1973;21:534.
404. Sunamori M, Amano J, Okamura T, Suzuki A. Cardioprotective effect of aprotinin in open heart surgery. Abstract presented at the 3rd International Symposium on Proteases: Antiproteases in Clinical Practice. Brussels, October 1982.
405. Borst HG, Haverich A, Walterbusch G, Maatz W. Fibrin adhesive: an important hemostatic ajunct in cardiovascular operations. J Thorac Cardiovasc Surg 1982;84:548.
406. Haverich A, Walterbusch G, Borst H-G. Abdichtung poröser Gefässprothesen under Teil-Heparinisierung und extrakorporaler Zirkulation. Angio 1983;5:215.
407. Haberland GL. The role of kininogenases, kinin formation and kininogenase inhibition in post traumatic shock and related conditions. Klin Wochenschr 1978;56:325.
408. Schneider B. Results of a field study on the therapeutic value of aprotinin in traumatatic shock. Arzneimittelforschung 1976;26:1606.
409. McMichan JC, Rosengarten DS, Philipp E. Prophylaxis of post-traumatic pulmonary insufficiency by protease-inhibitor therapy with aprotinin: a clinical study. Circ Shock 1982;9:107.
410. Hempelmann G, Trentz OA, Trentz O, et al. Behandlung des polytraumatischen Schocks. Unfallchirurgie 1981;7:116.
411. Horbach L, Just H. Trasylol in myocardial infarction. Intensivmed 1979;16:338.
412. Ceceña-Seldner FA, Villarreal F. Effect of the kallikrein inhibitor aprotinin on myocardial ischemia and necrosis in man. Angiology 1980;31:488.
413. Haberland GL, Matis P. Trasylol, ein Proteinaseninhibitor bei chirurgischen und internen Indikationen. Med Welt 1967;22:1367.
414. Okamoto S, Hijikata A. Rational approach to proteinase inhibitors. Drug Des 1975;6:143.
415. McNicol GP, Fletcher AP, Alkjaersig N, Sherry S. The absorption, distribution and excretion of epsilon-aminocaproic acid following oral or intravenous administration to man. J Lab Clin Med 1962;59:15.
416. Andersson L, Nilsson IM, Colleen S, et al. Role of urokinase and tissue activator in sustained bleeding and the management thereof with EACA and AMCA. Ann NY Acad Sci 1968;146:642.
417. Lohmann K, Markwardt F, Landmann H. Über neue Hemmstoffe der Fibrinolyse. Naturwissenschaften 1963;50:502.
418. Markwardt F, Klöcking HP. Über das Stoffwechselschicksal des Antifibrinolytikums p-Amino-methylbenzoesäure (PAMBA) beim Menschen. Acta Biol Med German 1965;14:519.
419. Markwardt F. Synthetic inhibitors of fibrinolysis. In: Markwardt F, ed. Fibrinolytics and antifibrinolytics. New York, Springer-Verlag, 1978: 511.
420. Okamoto S, Sato S, Takada Y, Okamoto U. An active stereo isomer (trans form) of AMCHA and its fibrinolytic (anti-plasminic) action in vitro and in vivo. Keio J Med 1964;13:177.
421. Melander B, Gliniecki G, Granstrand B, Hnashoff G. Biochemistry and toxicology of Amikapron: the antifibrinolytic active isomer of AMCHA. Acta Pharmacol Toxicol 1965;22:340.
422. Kwaan HC, Astrup T. Tissue repair in presence of locally applied inhibitors of fibrinolysis. Exp Mol Pathol 1969;11:82.
423. Widlund L, Strömberg S, Hellström H, et al. The disposition of tranexamic acid (AMCA) in various animal species and in man after oral dosage. (Data on file) Kabi AB, Stockholm, 1979.
424. Eriksson O, Kjellman H, Schannong M. The biological availability of Cyklokapron tablets compared with Cyklokapron solution administered orally. (Data on file) Kabi AB, Stockholm, 1971.
425. Kaller H. Enterale Resorption, Verteilung und Elimination von 4-Amino-Methylcyclohexancarbonsäure (AMCHA) und ϵ-Aminocapronsäure (EACS) beim Menschen. Naunyn Schmiedebergs Arch Pharmacol 1967;256:160.
426. Okamoto S, Oshiba S, Mihara H, Okamoto U. Synthetic inhibitors of fibrinolysis: in vitro and in vivo mode of action. Ann NY Acad Sci 1968;146:414.
427. Forbes CD, Barr RD, Reid G, et al. Tranexamic acid in control of haemorrhage after dental extraction in haemophilia and Christmas disease. Br Med J 1972;2:311.
428. Evans BE, Aledort LM. Hemophilia and dental treatment. J Am Dent Assoc 1976;96:827.
429. Landin LE, Weiner E. Late bleeding after conization: the effect of tranexamic acid (Cyclokapron). Opuscula Med 1975;20:280.
430. Rybo G, Westerberg H. The effect of tranexamic acid (AMCA) on postoperative bleeding after conization. Acta Obstet Gynecol Scand 1972;51: 347.
431. Verstraete M, Tyberghein J, de Greef Y, et al. Double-blind trials with ethamsylate, batroxobin or tranexamic acid on blood loss after adenotonsillectomy. Acta Clin Belg 1977;32:136.
432. Castelli G, Vogt E. Der Erfolg einer antifibrinolytischen Behandlung mit Tranexamsaure zur Reduktion der Blutverlustes während und nach Tonsillektomien. Schweiz Med Wochenschr 1977;107:780.
433. Hedlund PO. Antifibrinolytic therapy with Cyclokapron in connection with prostatectomy. Scand J Urol Nephrol 1969;3:177.
434. Kaufmann J, Siefker K. Medikamentöse Senkung postoperativer Blutungen nach Prostatiktomien. Urologe 1969;8:57.
435. Rö JS, Knutrud O, Stormorken H. Antifibrinolytic treatment with tranexamic acid (AMCHA) in pediatric urinary tract surgery. J Pediatr Surg 1970;5:315.
436. Gamba G, Fornasari PM, Grignani G, et al. Haemostasis during transvesical prostatic adenoctomy. Blut 1979;39:89.
437. Miller RA, May MW, Hendry WF, et al. The prevention of secondary haemorrhage after prostatectomy: the value of antifibrinolytic therapy. Br J Urol 1980;52:26.
438. Pandolifi M. Intraocular hemorrhages: a hemostatic therapeutic approach. Surv Ophthalmol 1978;22:322.
439. Jerndal T, Frisén M. Tranexamic acid (AMCA) and late hyphaema: a double-blind study in cataract surgery. Acta Ophthalmol 1976;54:417.
440. Varnek L, Dalsgaard C, Hansen A, Klie F. The effect of tranexamic acid on secondary haemorrhage after traumatic hyphaema. Acta Ophthalmol 1980;58:787.
441. Ramirez-Lassepas M. Antifibrinolytic therapy in subarachnoid hemorrhage caused by ruptured intracranial aneurysm. Neurology 1981;31: 316.
442. Verstraete M. Clinical application of inhibitors of fibrinolysis. Drugs 1985;29:236.
443. Bennett AE, Ingram GIC, Inglish PJ. Antifibrinolytic treatment in haemophilia: a controlled trial of prophylaxis with tranexamic acid. Br J Haematol 1973;24:83.
444. Rainsford SG, Jouhar AJ, Hall A. Tranexamic acid in the control of spontaneous bleeding in severe haemophilia. Thromb Diath Haemorrh 1973;30:272.
445. Callender ST, Warner GT, Cope E. Treatment of menorrhagia with tranexamic acid: a double blind trial. Br Med J 1970;4:214.
446. Nilsson L, Rybo G. Treatment of menorrhagia with an antifibrinolytic agent, tranexamic acid (AMCA): a double blind investigation. Acta Obstet Gynecol Scand 1967;46:572.
447. Vermylen J, Verhaegen-Declercq ML, Verstraete M, Fierens F. A double-blind study of the effect of tranexamic acid in essential menorrhagia. Thromb Diath Haemorrh 1968;20:583.
448. Nilsson L, Rybo G. Treatment of menorrhagia. Am J Obstet Gynecol 1971;110:713.
449. Weström L, Bengtsson LP. Effect of tranexamic acid (AMCA) in menorrhagia with intrauterine contraceptive devices. J Reprod Med 1970;5: 154.
450. Åstedt B, Nilsson IM. Recurrent abruptio placentae with the fibrinolytic inhibitor tranexamic acid. Br Med J 1978;1:756.
451. Svanberg L, Åstedt B, Nilsson IM. Abruptio placentae: treatment with the fibrinolytic inhibitor tranexamic acid. Acta Obstet Gynecol Scand 1980;59:127.
452. Walzman M, Bonnar J. Effects of tranexamic acid in the coagulation and fibrinolytic systems in pregnancy complicated by placental bleeding. Arch Toxicol 1982;5(Suppl):214.
453. Petruson B. A double-blind study to evaluate the effect of epistaxis with oral administration of the antifibrinolytic drug tranexamic acid (cyclokapron). Acta Otolaryngol 1974;317(Suppl):57.
454. Bramsen T, Ehlers N. Bullous keratopathy (Fuchs' endothelial dystrophy) treated systemically with 4-trans-amino-cyclohexano-carboxylic acid. Acta Ophthalmol Copenh 1977;55:665.
455. Bramsen T. A double-blind study on the influence of tranexamic acid on the intraocular pressure and the central corneal thickness after trabeculectomy for glaucoma simplex. Acta Ophthalmol 1978;56:998.
456. Blohmé G. Treatment of hereditary angioneurotic oedema with tranexamic acid: a random double-blind cross-over study. Acta Med Scand 1972;192:293.
457. Sheffer AL, Austen KF, Rosen FS. Tranexamic acid therapy in hereditary angioneurotic edema. N Engl J Med 1972;287:452.
458. Åstedt B, Glifberg I, Mattsson W, Trap C. Arrest of growth of ovarian tumor by tranexamic acid. JAMA 1977;238:154.
459. Laurberg G. Tranexamic acid (Cyclokapron) in chronic urticaria: a double-blind study. Acta Dermatovenereol 1977;57:369.

Blood: Principles and Practice of Hematology,
edited by Robert I. Handin, Samuel E. Lux, and Thomas P. Stossel.
J.B. Lippincott Company, Philadelphia © 1995.

43

Disseminated Intravascular Coagulation

Uri Seligsohn

The term disseminated intravascular coagulation (DIC) is most frequently used to describe a clinicopathologic syndrome in which widespread intravascular coagulation is induced by procoagulants that enter or are produced in the bloodstream and overcome its natural inhibitory mechanisms. DIC is by far the most complicated derangement of the coagulation system. It causes tissue ischemia from occlusive microthrombi and bleeding from the consumption of unregulated coagulation factors, and it results in anticoagulant effects of products of the ensuing compensatory or secondary fibrinolysis. DIC complicates a variety of disorders and has become the subject of an enormous literature. Entire books,[1–7] book chapters,[8–11] review articles,[12–25] and case studies[26–37] are devoted to the syndrome, its unresolved problems, and the controversies surrounding it. The goal of this chapter is to review new as well as previously neglected information on various aspects of DIC and to outline some approaches to its management. Two book chapters[10,11] and two issues of *Seminars in Thrombosis and Hemostasis* (1988, issue 4, and 1989, issue 1) can be consulted for additional information.

HISTORICAL ASPECTS

Some of the fundamental clinical and pathologic observations regarding DIC were made in the 19th century. On August 12, 1834, Dupuy[38] reported additional facts to the French Academy of Medicine on the fatal outcome of animals injected with brain material. Moreover, Dupuy stated that de Blainville had repeated his experiments and observed the death of two animals within 2 minutes of injection. "As expected," he said, "there were wide-spread clots in blood vessels and a fist-sized clot in the heart chambers." In the subsequent discussion, Emery commented that he had witnessed Gaspard and Magendie's experiments: they injected serosal fluids and milk intravenously and found hemorrhagic necrosis on the surface of the animals' lungs.[38] These were probably the first records of DIC induced through the extrinsic coagulation pathway.

Trousseau,[39] in 1865, described his and others' observations on the tendency of blood to clot and cause thrombosis, sometimes disseminated, in cachectic patients with malignancies. In 1873, Naunyn[40] showed that widespread thrombosis could be evoked by intravenous injection of dissolved red blood cells (RBCs). In 1886, Wooldridge[41] and later Barratt and York[42] demonstrated that the procoagulant was not hemoglobin but was contained in the stroma of the RBCs. Wooldridge added, "if only a moderate quantity be injected, the blood drawn off after injection clots slowly or not at all."[41] The active procoagulant of the RBC stroma appeared "similar if not identical to a proteid–lecithin compound," which Wooldridge had earlier extracted from other tissues.[41,43]

Many additional experimental and clinical observations were made during the ensuing years, but the way in which DIC can lead to bleeding was clarified only 33 years ago when Lasch and coworkers[44] introduced the concept of consumption coagulopathy. McKay[1] then established that DIC is an intermediary mechanism in many diseases and Hardaway[2] explored the relation between shock and DIC. Although extensive clinical experience was also gained during this period, studies of sizable series of cases were first carried out in the 1970s.[4] The introduction of assays for fibrinogen–fibrin degradation products and other tests that provide rigorously defined laboratory criteria for DIC enabled a more uniform diagnosis of DIC.[14] Despite the experience that has accrued during the past 20 years, DIC still constitutes a major clinicopathologic and therapeutic challenge.

PATHOLOGY

Manasse[45] was probably the first to observe and describe disseminated microthrombi in the cerebral blood vessels of patients who presumably had died from sepsis-related DIC. After these discoveries, extensive data have been accumulating on autopsy findings of patients with DIC.[1,28,34,37,46–61] These findings include diffuse multiorgan bleeding, hemorrhagic necrosis, microthrombi in small blood vessels, and thrombi in medium and large blood vessels. These pathologic findings were not evident in all patients who had had clearcut clinical and laboratory manifestations of DIC.[34,46,49,53] This apparent paradox was attributed to two possible causes: incomplete search for microthrombi and postmortem thrombolysis.[1,46,53] The latter explanation was challenged by Mori and Hizawa,[49] who did not find a correlation between the extent of microthrombi and the interval between the time of death and that of autopsy in a large series of patients with DIC. An additional problem arose when the results of many consecutive autopsies indicated that DIC also appeared to be a silent killer[50]; it was found in a significant number of patients whose clinical and laboratory manifestations had not been consistent with DIC.[34,47,49,50] Thus, the occasional lack of correlation between the clinical and the pathologic findings requires further investigation.

The distribution of microthrombi in various organs was determined in several pathologic studies of DIC.[28,34,37,46,47,49–54] Analysis of these data showed that in 510 patients in whom the diagnosis was established by clinical and laboratory criteria, and confirmed at autopsy, the organs most frequently involved by diffuse microthrombi were the lungs and kidneys, followed by the brain, heart, liver, spleen, adrenals, pancreas, and gut (Table 43-1). In studies using specific electron microscopic and staining techniques, microthrombi were found to consist mainly of fibrin monomers or fibrin polymers plus platelets.[48] Signs of thrombolysis and an inflammatory reaction were also noted.[55] If the DIC had lasted long enough, organization and endothelialization of the microthrombi occurred.[51,55] Of special interest were intraluminal globular hyaline thrombi unattached to the vessel walls that were found in some DIC cases[55] and in experimental DIC studies.[48] These thrombi were believed to consist of fibrin monomers.[48]

Detailed descriptions of the pathologic findings in the various organs can be found in several of the published series.[28,34,37,46,47,49–53] Certain features are worth mentioning:

Renal involvement: In rabbits, renal cortical necrosis is the hallmark of the generalized Shwartzman reaction mediated by DIC. In contrast, acute tubular necrosis was much more common than renal cortical necrosis in patients with DIC due to gram-negative septicemia as well as other causes.[34,46,49,55] Interestingly, kidney involvement was rarely observed in newborns with DIC.[56,57]

Nonbacterial thrombotic endocarditis: Nonbacterial thrombotic vegetations, predominantly on the mitral and aortic valves, have long been noted in autopsies of patients who had malignancies or chronic infectious diseases.[58,59] McKay was the first to suggest an association between these diseases and DIC.[1,60] This was later confirmed by the finding that in retrospect half of patients with nonbacterial thrombotic endocarditis had DIC.[59] Conversely, others found that a significant, but variable proportion of patients with DIC also had nonbacterial thrombotic endocarditis.[34,49,50,61,62] Nonbacterial thrombotic endocarditis in patients with DIC can be a significant source of arterial embolization leading to infarction of the brain, kidneys, and myocardium.[59]

TABLE 43-1. Organ Involvement by Microthrombi in Patients with Disseminated Intravascular Coagulation

Organ	Percentage of Patients With Microthrombi at Autopsy (Mean)
Kidney	70.4
Lung	70.0
Brain	41.1
Heart	40.4
Liver	39.6
Spleen	39.6
Adrenals	37.1
Pancreas	24.1
Gut	20.7

(Data compiled from 510 cases[28,34,46,47,49–54])

PATHOGENESIS

Simplified Mechanism of Disseminated Intravascular Coagulation

Disseminated intravascular coagulation is triggered when the inhibitory mechanisms fail to prevent formation of blood clots by procoagulants that have gained access to the circulation. The thrombin generated causes deposition of fibrin, which in turn obstructs blood vessels and results in tissue ischemia. When thrombosis is extensive, essential components of blood coagulation are consumed and bleeding ensues. Platelets, prothrombin, factors V and VIII, fibrinogen, antithrombin III (ATIII), and protein C are among the constituents most frequently depleted. Endothelial cells adjacent to intravascular thrombi secrete tissue plasminogen activator (tPA), which sets off compensatory thrombolysis. This reestablishes patency of the occluded vessels, but at the cost of formation of fibrin–fibrinogen degradation products which may impair platelet aggregation, act as an antithrombin, and interfere with fibrin polymerization, resulting in bleeding. Fibrin deposits in partially occluded vessels can damage traversing red cells and lead to microangiopathic hemolytic anemia, characterized by distorted erythrocytes (schistocytes), which are readily appreciated on examination of blood smears.

This simplified outline of the sequence of events in DIC seen in Figure 43-1 may be used to explain the initiation of DIC and its clinical manifestations, to facilitate diagnosis, and to establish guidelines for treatment.

Mechanisms of Initiation

The extrinsic and intrinsic pathways of blood coagulation are both initiated in the diseases and experimental conditions that trigger DIC. Thus, thrombin is generated either by exposure of tissue factor to blood or activation of factor XII by injured endothelial cells. Occasionally, DIC is triggered by introduction into the bloodstream of foreign or pathologic procoagulants such as snake venom or a cancer cell–derived factor X activator.

The major clinical conditions causing DIC and the presumptive initiating pathways are shown in Figure 43-2. (These conditions are discussed in detail later in this chapter.) The most complicated initiating pathways are those triggered by endotoxin. The first observations on disseminated thrombosis after injection of rabbits with heat-treated typhoid bacilli were made by Kusama[63] in 1913. His experiments preceded the classic descriptions of the generalized and localized Sanarelli-Shwartzman reactions and demonstrated numerous white blood cells incorporated in the thrombi as well as leukopenia in the endotoxin-treated rabbits.[64,65] He suggested that enzymes released from leukocytes, platelets, and endothelial cells participate in the formation of the disseminated microthrombi. Since then, extensive studies have been carried out to elucidate how endotoxin brings about DIC. These studies have been comprehensively reviewed.[66]

Although many questions are still open to discussion or exploration, it appears that a complex series of events are set off by endotoxin. Several points deserve special attention.

The intrinsic coagulation system is initiated either by endotoxin acting directly on factor XII[67] or by activation of factor XII by the injured vessel wall.[68] Both result in generation of kallikrein, which has two functions: it augments the deleterious effects of polymorphonuclear leukocytes (PMNs) on endothelial cells[66] and it cleaves bradykinin from high-molecular-weight kininogen. Bradykinin, in turn, causes vasodilation and hypotension.[68]

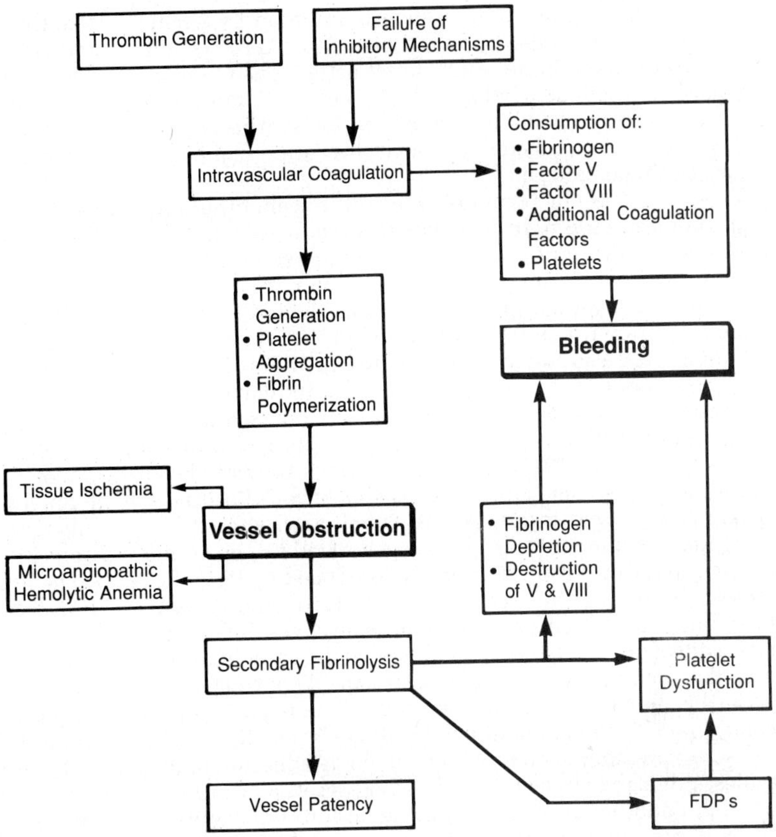

FIGURE 43-1. A simplified mechanism of disseminated intravascular coagulation. FDPs, fibrin degradation products.

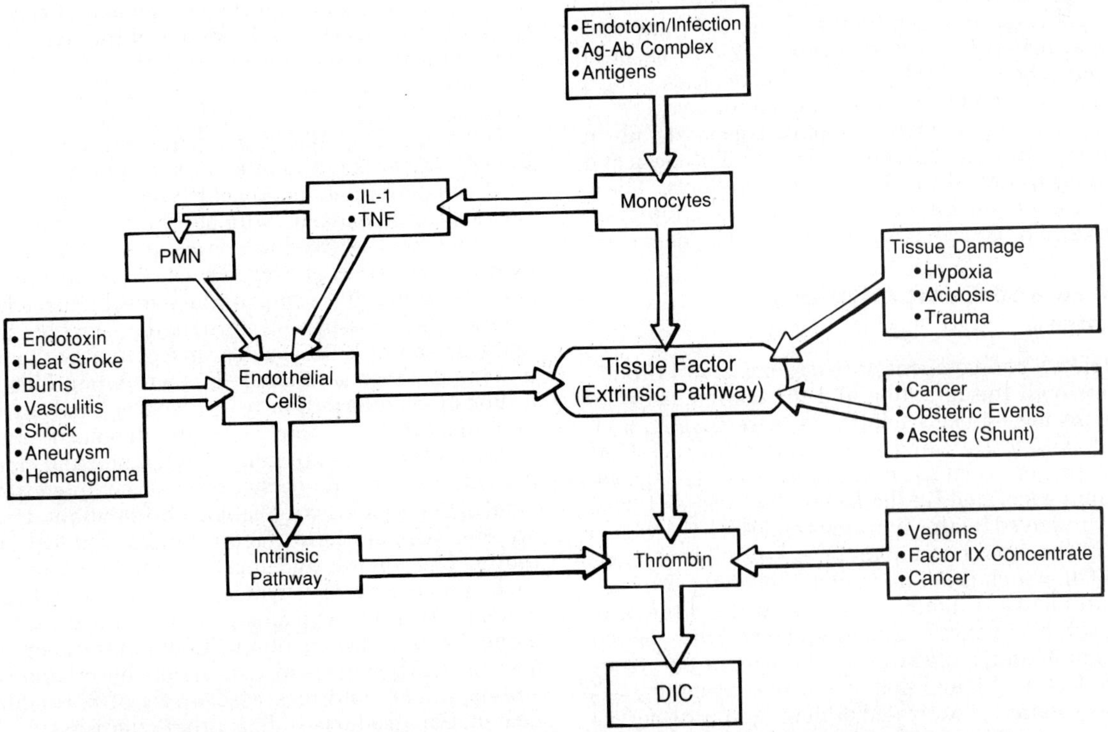

FIGURE 43-2. Main initiation pathways of disseminated intravascular coagulation (DIC) in a variety of underlying disorders. PMN, polymorphonuclear neutrophils; TNF, tumor necrosis factor; IL-1, interleukin-1; Ag-Ab, antigen–antibody.

The extrinsic coagulation system is initiated by tissue factor that is generated by monocytes and expressed on their surface membranes after direct activation by endotoxin.[69,70] This effect is enhanced by T cells.[71] Endothelial cells can also respond to endotoxin by synthesis and expression of tissue factor, although they are devoid of it under resting conditions.[72]

The profibrinolytic potential of the injured endothelium is curtailed as endotoxin decreases tPA production and release after a transient increase[73] and by increased release of plasminogen activator inhibitor-1.[74] The normal inhibitory effect of the endothelium on blood coagulation is also reduced by down-regulation of thrombomodulin.[75]

Platelets are also activated by endotoxin,[76] but this probably plays a minor role in DIC initiation.[77] Similarly, complement activation is not the crucial element in the development of DIC, but it may contribute to its evolution.[66]

The adhesion of PMNs to endothelium is promoted by the following agents: tumor necrosis factor (TNF); interleukin-1 (IL-1) and interleukin-8, which are secreted by macrophages (monocytes)[78–80]; C5a generated by the complement pathways[66]; leukotriene B4 produced by PMNs[81]; and finally platelet activation factor derived from PMNs, macrophages, and endothelial cells themselves.[66] The attachment of leukocytes inflicts damage on the endothelium, probably leading to release of factors capable of triggering both the extrinsic and intrinsic coagulation pathways. Adhesion of PMNs to endothelial cells is also mediated by surface expression of endothelial leukocyte adhesion molecules (although only several hours after triggers like TNF[82]), by the endothelial intercellular adhesion molecule-1, and by receptors on PMN membranes that consist of heterodimer complexes, CD11/CD18.[83] The endothelial adhesion molecules and the PMN receptor complexes interact strongly in the presence of endotoxin, TNF, or IL-1.[82] Damage by PMNs to the endothelium stems from production of oxygen metabolites such as hydrogen peroxide and HOCL; the latter also neutralizes plasma α_1-antitrypsin.[84] This neutralization paves the way for elastase, an enzyme secreted by PMNs, to attack both endothelial cells[85] and extracellular matrix.[84] All these events, which consist of cell–cell interactions and cell–substrate interactions, induce coagulation and simultaneously promote fibrinolysis.[86,87]

The reactions triggered by endotoxin generate fibrin monomers that form soluble complexes with fibrinogen and with fibrinogen and fibrin degradation products. These complexes can be precipitated throughout the circulation by endotoxin, a process that is not influenced by heparin.[88]

Defensive and Compensatory Mechanisms

Several defense and compensatory systems afford protection against both the initiation and the consequences of DIC. Defense mechanisms neutralize or remove components that initiate DIC, and compensatory mechanisms correct the pathophysiologic consequences of DIC (Fig. 43-3). Thrombin generated by the factors that trigger DIC is effectively removed by the enormous endothelial cell surface area of the microcirculation by means of two mechanisms: ATIII, which is bound to endothelial heparan sulfate, neutralizes thrombin by forming thrombin–antithrombin complexes[89] and thrombomodulin, which binds thrombin and abolishes its procoagulant effects on fibrinogen, factor XIII, and platelets, while promoting activation of protein C.[90] Activated protein C, in turn, serves as a physiologic anticoagulant by breaking down factors Va and VIIIa, and stimulates fibrinolysis by neutralizing plasminogen activator inhibitor-1.[90] It has also been found that thrombin, after binding to endothelial cells, stimulates release of tPA and prostacyclin.[91] The former augments compensatory fibrinolysis, and the latter inhibits platelet aggregation. Another physiologic anticoagulant is tissue factor pathway inhibitor. It inhibits factor Xa and inactivates tissue factor/factor VIIa in the presence of factor Xa but only when relatively small amounts of tissue factor gain access to circulating blood.[91a] Thus, as long as blood flow through the microcirculation is maintained, effective neutralization of procoagulant material exists unless overwhelming amounts have entered the circulation.

The reticuloendothelial system also plays a role in protection against DIC. It can remove tissue factor[92] and the soluble complexes of fibrin monomers.[93] Because tissue factor is a cell membrane component of tissues that are exposed to blood only under pathologic circumstances such as trauma and hematogenic metastasis or is expressed on monocytes and endothelial cells after stimuli like endotoxin, the reticuloendothelial system appears to be effective only for removal of circulating tissue factor bound to membrane microparticles.

The liver parenchymal cells also perform several defense as well as compensatory functions. These cells clear activated factors IX, X, XI,[94,95] and tPA[96] from the circulation and synthesize the depleted coagulation factors, components of the fibrinolytic system like plasminogen and α_2-antiplasmin and the inhibitor proteins, protein C, protein S, and ATIII.

The bone marrow, in addition to being a reticuloendothelial system organ, plays an important role in compensating for DIC by increasing the production of platelets. Bone marrow megakaryocytes need time to respond, so that it may take several days after an episode of DIC for the number of circulating platelets to rise.

In addition, it must be kept in mind that all defense and compensatory functions may be impeded by the underlying disease that caused the DIC, such as leukemia, which depletes or suppresses the megakaryocyte pool; hepatic disease, which impairs both the synthetic and clearance reticuloendothelial system functions of the liver; and septic shock in which blood flow through the microcirculation is decreased, thus diminishing its capacity to inhibit coagulation.

The outcome of DIC also depends on the magnitude of the DIC trigger and the rate of its introduction into or exposure to the circulation. What has been designated as *acute DIC*, such as in a patient with abruptio placentae, develops when blood is exposed to a large amount of tissue factor over a brief period of time. This overwhelms the defense systems before any compensatory mechanisms have had enough time to respond. Alternatively, what has been designated as *chronic DIC*, such as in a patient with metastatic mucinous adenocarcinoma, develops when blood is continuously or intermittently exposed to small amounts of tissue factor. In chronic cases, the defense and compensatory mechanisms are not overwhelmed and can control the DIC and provide partial or even complete replenishment of the depleted coagulation, fibrinolytic and inhibitory proteins. Under these circumstances, clinical signs are minimal or absent, and most coagulation tests are only slightly impaired. Nevertheless, an increased turnover of platelets and fibrinogen, a positive paracoagulation test (nonenzymatic aggregation of soluble intermediary products of fibrinogen–fibrin conversion by ethanol or protamine sulfate), and increased levels of fibrin–fibrinogen degradation products indicate that compensated DIC has taken place.[19] At times, overcompensation for a continuous DIC trigger results in thrombocytosis and elevated levels of fibrinogen and other clotting factors.[19]

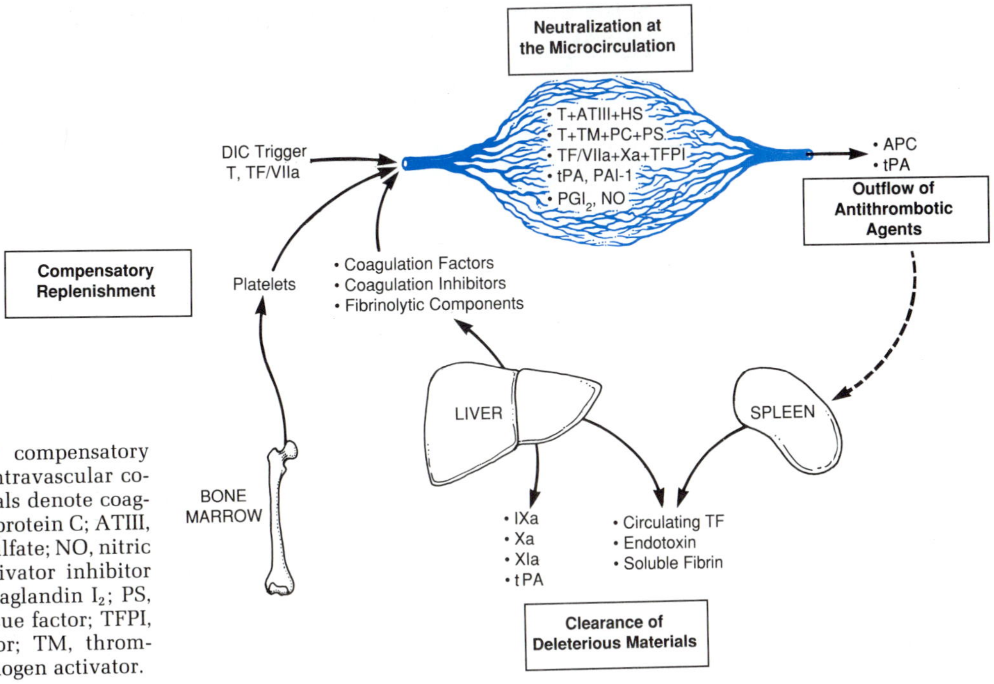

FIGURE 43-3. Defense and compensatory mechanisms in disseminated intravascular coagulation (DIC). Roman numerals denote coagulation factors. APC, activated protein C; ATIII, antithrombin III; HS, heparan sulfate; NO, nitric oxide; PAI-1, plasminogen activator inhibitor = 1; PC, protein C; PGI_2, prostaglandin I_2; PS, protein S; T, thrombin; TF, tissue factor; TFPI, tissue factor pathway inhibitor; TM, thrombomodulin; tPA, tissue plasminogen activator.

Self-Perpetuation of Disseminated Intravascular Coagulation

When the defense mechanisms fail, microthrombi are deposited throughout the vascular system with numerous pathophysiologic consequences. Many of these can amplify and perpetuate the DIC. Table 43-2 is a partial list of consequences of DIC and their immediate pathophysiologic effects. After DIC is initiated, the avalanche of its consequences and their deleterious effects can become extremely difficult to control and manage.

CLINICAL ASPECTS

Only a few retrospective clinical studies are available from which to draw conclusions about the clinical aspects of DIC.[26–37] Even these reports pose a problem for critical analysis because the studies were carried out in different types of medical centers with different inclusion criteria. In addition, the classification of the clinical manifestations and the underlying diagnoses were not uniform.

Incidence

Disseminated intravascular coagulopathy is relatively rare, although awareness on the part of clinicians and staff of coagulation laboratories undoubtedly increases the number of occasions on which the diagnosis is made. In five medical centers, which were alert to the possibility of DIC, the incidence ranged from 12 to 49 patients per year.[27,29–31,33] An Israeli study reported 1 case of DIC in 944 hospital admissions.[29] An exceptionally high rate of occurrence was documented in Japan, with 126 cases per year or 1 in 105 hospital admissions.[33]

Causes

Many diseases can provoke DIC (see Fig. 43-2). Only a limited number of the disorders listed are major causes of DIC. As shown in Table 43-3, infections and malignancies together account for 47% to 75% of DIC cases in the major series, except for one that included a disproportionately large number of obstetric cases.[37] In two series, trauma was a major cause of DIC, probably reflecting the specialized nature of the clinical material in the two centers.[29,31] It is interesting that in the two Japanese series, a relatively high proportion of malignant diseases and a relatively low proportion of obstetric cases were found.[33,34] One study included material from a large and active obstetric department.[29] Nevertheless, the relative rate of occurrence of DIC in obstetric cases in this center was low.

Manifestations

Patients with DIC display clinical manifestations that are attributable to DIC, to the underlying disease, or to both. Some of the manifestations common to severe forms of DIC are summarized in Table 43-4. The relative incidence of clinical symptoms varies according to the underlying disorders; this explains the considerable variations among the published series in the occurrence of shock and of dysfunction of liver, kidney, lungs, and central nervous system (Table 43-5). In contrast, the incidences of bleeding and thromboembolism were almost uniform in all the series and could be related to DIC. Bleeding was observed in 64% to 87% of the cases and was the most important symptom (and sign) of DIC.

Bleeding Sites

Acute DIC is frequently heralded by hemorrhage into the skin at multiple sites.[27,29] Petechiae, ecchymoses, and oozing from venipunctures, arterial lines, catheters, and injured tissues are common. Bleeding may also occur into mucosal surfaces throughout the body. Hemorrhage may be life threatening with massive bleeding into the gastrointestinal tract,[29] lungs,[27] central nervous system, and orbit.[37] Awareness of these fatal possibilities calls for a thorough physical examination supplemented by imaging procedures for the detection of occult hemorrhage.

Patients with chronic DIC have less dramatic hemorrhage but may have skin and mucosal bleeding.

TABLE 43-2. Consequences of Disseminated Intravascular Coagulation That Aggravate Its Manifestations

Consequences	Effects
General	
Shock	Compromised inhibitory functions of ATIII–heparan and thrombomodulin–protein C–protein S systems
	Release of tissue factor
Acidosis	Enhanced coagulation
Organ dysfunction	
Liver	Diminished synthesis of coagulation factors → bleeding
	Diminished synthesis of inhibitors → thrombosis
	Diminished removal of activated coagulation factors → thrombosis
	Diminished removal of tPA, and synthesis of α_2-antiplasmin → bleeding
Reticuloendothelial system	Decreased clearance of tissue factor, endotoxin, bacteria
Heart	Decreased output and tissue perfusion
	Embolization from nonbacterial thrombotic endocarditis
Lungs (ARDS)	Hypoxia, local consumption of hemostatic components
Consumption of platelet and coagulation factors	Bleeding
Consumption of ATIII, protein C, protein S	Thrombosis
Enhanced secondary fibrinolysis	
Fibrin degradation product	Bleeding
Excessive tPA release	Bleeding

ARDS, adult respiratory distress syndrome; ATIII, antithrombin III; tPA, tissue plasminogen activator.

Thromboembolism

Patients with acute and chronic DIC may have varied symptoms from thrombosis and embolism. Extensive organ dysfunction can accrue from multiple microvascular thrombi. For example, involvement of the skin can cause hemorrhagic bullae, acral necrosis, and gangrene.[27,37] Thrombosis of major veins and arteries and pulmonary embolism are rare but may appear during the course of acute or chronic DIC.[27,29] Cerebral–arterial embolism can occur as a consequence of nonbacterial thrombotic endocarditis in chronic DIC.[59]

Renal Dysfunction

Renal dysfunction in DIC stems from microthrombosis of afferent glomerular arterioles leading to cortical ischemia and hypotension from septicemia, hypovolemia, or DIC itself, leading to acute tubular necrosis. Thus, renal function is profoundly affected by both the underlying disease and by DIC. In one series,[27] the basic disorders were the predominant causes of renal dysfunction, whereas in another study group,[29] most cases of renal dysfunction were related to DIC. Notwithstanding these discrepancies, oliguria, anuria, azotemia, and hematuria were observed in 25% to 67% of patients in all series (see Table 43-5).

Liver Dysfunction

Hepatocellular jaundice has been reported in 24%[29] and 57%[37] of patients with DIC. Infectious diseases and prolonged hypotension contribute to hepatic dysfunction.

Central Nervous System Dysfunction

Microthrombi, macrothrombi, emboli, and hemorrhage all have been held responsible for the nonspecific symptoms and signs displayed by patients with DIC.[27,28] These include coma, delirium, stroke, and focal neurologic and meningeal lesions. Careful exclusion of causes other than DIC is essential because the detection of conditions such as bacterial meningitis, severe metabolic derangements, or metastatic involvement calls for different approaches in management.

Shock

Shock is a clinical syndrome brought about by tissue hypoperfusion and subsequent malfunction of organs vital to

TABLE 43-3. Percentage of Major Underlying Diseases in Disseminated Intravascular Coagulation*

Study	No. Cases	Infections	Malignant Diseases	Surgery and Trauma	Liver Diseases	Obstetric Complications	Miscellaneous Disorders
Minna et al[27]	60	41.7	30.0	1.7	5.0	1.7	19.9
Siegal et al[29]	118	39.8	6.8	23.7	4.2	4.2	21.3
Spero et al[31]	346	26.0	24.0	19.0	8.0	—	23.0
Matsuda et al[33]	503	15.3	60.8	2.4	5.6	3.8	12.1
Larcan et al[37]	361	15.0	6.1	13.6	3.3	38.8	12.1
Tanaka et al[34]	88	6.8	67.0	—	—	—	26.2
Kobayashi et al[35]	345	15.9	55.0	—	4.3	4.6	20.2

* Not included are two reports in which a major underlying disease was not given[30,32] and one study from a cancer center.[28]

TABLE 43-4. Clinical Manifestations of Severe Disseminated Intravascular Coagulation

System/Organ	Manifestations
Skin	Purpura, bleeding from injury sites, hemorrhagic bullae, focal necrosis, acral gangrene
Cardiovascular	Shock, acidosis, myocardial infarction, thromboembolism in large, medium, and small blood vessels and their consequences
Renal	Oliguria, azotemia, hematuria, acute tubular necrosis, renal cortical necrosis
Liver	Jaundice, parenchymal damage
Lungs	Adult respiratory distress syndrome, hypoxemia, edema, hemorrhage
Gastrointestinal	Bleeding, musocal necrosis and ulceration
Central nervous	Stupor, coma, convulsions, focal lesions, intracranial bleeding
Adrenals	Adrenal insufficiency (hemorrhagic necrosis)

survival. Both the diseases underlying DIC, and DIC itself, can cause shock. For example, septicemia or excessive blood loss due to trauma or obstetric complications can cause shock. In early studies, vehement claims were made that hemorrhagic shock per se could be a cause of DIC,[2] but more recent data from the same author indicate that additional triggers of DIC are important, for example, tissue factor release in trauma.[97] Whatever the cause of shock, its presence is of great concern and requires rapid intervention (see section on management).

Pulmonary Dysfunction

Symptoms resulting from respiratory dysfunction range from transient hypoxemia in mild cases to pulmonary hemorrhage and adult respiratory distress syndrome (ARDS) in severe cases. Although pulmonary hemorrhage is specific for DIC,[27] ARDS is not.[98–101] Pulmonary hemorrhage is heralded by hemoptysis, dyspnea, and chest pain, and physical examination reveals rales, wheezing, and occasionally a pleural friction rub. Chest radiographs show diffuse infiltration due to extensive intraalveolar hemorrhage.

ARDS is a clinicopathologic entity first described in 12 patients with multiple trauma on the basis of the following characteristics: tachypnea, no abnormalities on auscultation, hypoxemia, low lung compliance, a normal wedge pressure,[102] and coalescence into "white lungs" on chest radiographs.[103] The syndrome of ARDS stems from severe damage to the pulmonary vascular endothelium, whose increased permeability permits egress of blood components into the pulmonary interstitium and alveoli. This eventually leads to intraalveolar hyaline membrane formation and severe respiratory insufficiency.[100,101,104] ARDS can be caused by septic shock, severe trauma, fat embolism, amniotic fluid embolism,[103] and heat stroke,[105] all of which can also incite DIC. Initially, the trigger for ARDS was believed to be diffuse pulmonary microthrombosis associated with DIC.[97,103,104] Subsequent studies disclosed that only a small proportion of patients with ARDS exhibited signs of DIC.[99,101]

When DIC and ARDS are simultaneously triggered, it is likely that each will aggravate the other. Thus, in patients with ARDS the extensive endothelial injury associated mainly,[106–108] but not exclusively,[109] with activated neutrophils can set off the intrinsic coagulation pathway,[110] whereas DIC can augment the lung injury by vascular obstruction.[111,112] Regardless of the mechanism, ARDS is a common and serious complication in patients with severe DIC (see Table 43-5).

Mortality Rate

Disseminated intravascular coagulopathy per se, and its underlying disorders, contribute to the high rate of mortality reported in many series of patients with DIC. Mortality rate was independently correlated with the extent of organ (or system) involvement (Fig. 43-4), with the degree of hemostatic failure[29,36] and with increasing age.[29] The mortality rates given in several series of patients with DIC are shown in Table 43-6. Except for one series with a relatively low mortality rate,[32] a grave outcome was observed in all series, whether or not heparin had been administered.

LABORATORY FINDINGS

Acute and chronic DIC are encountered in relatively defined clinical circumstances. Knowledge of the potential underlying disorders can lead to early recognition and therefore rapid intervention. Laboratory tests have been invaluable for the following reasons:

1. They confirm or refute a presumptive diagnosis of DIC.
2. They help to differentiate acute from chronic DIC and to distinguish among DIC, primary fibrinogenolysis, and DIC associated with primary fibrino(geno)lysis.
3. They serve as guidelines for clinical decisions regarding treatment.
4. They provide a predictive value with regard to morbidity and mortality.
5. They are useful for monitoring therapy.
6. Assays of coagulation factors, inhibitors, and fibrinolytic parameters can shed light on the pathogenesis of DIC in different clinical settings and provide clues for the development of new approaches to therapy.

Evaluation of laboratory data must also take into account the possible effects of the underlying diseases. For example, substantial impairment of hemostasis, unrelated to DIC, can arise from hepatic disease, from bone marrow involvement by leukemia, during the neonatal period, and as a result of certain snake bites. Conversely, the above-normal levels of hemostatic components found during pregnancy may mask the presence of DIC. These limitations can be partially overcome by performing laboratory tests repeatedly (every 6 to 8 hours) so that if progressive abnormalities develop, the diagnosis of DIC can be established.

Acute Disseminated Intravascular Coagulation

Since patients with acute DIC are usually critically ill, rapid and relatively simple laboratory tests are required. If possible, these should include a platelet count, prothrombin time (PT), activated partial thromboplastin time (APTT), thrombin time (TT), levels of fibrinogen and fibrin degradation products (FDP), one of the paracoagulation tests, and a blood smear to check for fragmented RBCs. Several parameters represent the extent of consumption of hemostatic components and can be measured directly (platelets and fibrinogen) or indirectly by PT and PTT (factors V, VIII, and others). Other parameters represent the presence of by-products of in vivo thrombin generation, that is, fibrin monomers (paracoagulation tests) and secondary fibrinolysis (FDP and TT). The diagnostic value of the individual tests and the pitfalls in their interpretation are summarized in Table 43-7. In most instances, changes in three or more

TABLE 43-5. Percentage of Patients With Various Clinical Manifestations of Disseminated Intravascular Coagulation

Study	No. Patients	No Manifestations	Bleeding	Thromboembolism	Renal Dysfunction	Liver Dysfunction	Respiratory Dysfunction	Central Nervous System Manifestations	Shock	Acral Cyanosis
Minna et al[27]	60	8	87.0	22.0	67.0	*	78.0	65.0	*	14
Al-Mondhiry[28]	89	13.5	76.3	22.5	39.3	*	*	11.2	*	0
Siegal et al[29]	118	22.0	64.4	8.4	24.6	18.6	16.1	1.7	14.4	0
Mant & King[30]	47	—	87.2	46.8	40.4	†	38.3	†	*	†
Spero et al[31]	346	—	77.0	†	†	†	†	†	†	†
Larcan et al[37]	361	—	73.0	11.0	61.0	57.0	37.0	13.0	55.0	13‡

* Difficult to define relation to disseminated intravascular coagulation.
† Not mentioned.
‡ Including necrotizing purpura and acral gangrene.

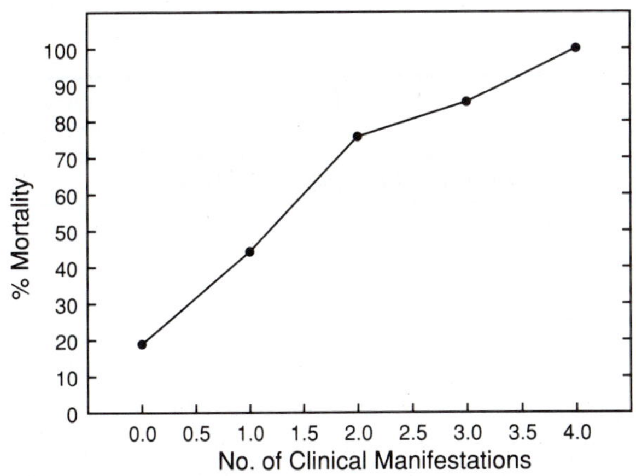

FIGURE 43-4. Correlation between mortality rate and number of defined clinical manifestations observed in 118 patients with disseminated intravascular coagulation. (After Siegal T, Seligsohn U, Aghai E, Modan M. Clinical and laboratory aspects of disseminated intravascular coagulation [DIC]: a study of 118 cases. Thromb Haemost 1978;39:122)

parameters in addition to a decreased platelet count are consistent with DIC, and no further tests are necessary.

Several scoring systems have been devised to determine the severity of DIC.[29,35,113] Some take into account only the laboratory data,[29,113] whereas others combine the data with clinical manifestations.[35] These scores are useful for prognostic evaluation, since a good correlation was found between the degree of abnormality of the laboratory results and the extent of organ involvement, as well as between the severity of hemostatic impairment and subsequent mortality.[29]

Analysis of the data given in six large series of a total of 932 patients (most with acute DIC) shows that the most common abnormality was a low platelet count (see Table 43-7). Thereafter, in decreasing order of incidence were found: elevated levels of FDP, prolonged PT, prolonged TT, prolonged APTT, and decreased fibrinogen levels. The value of paracoagulation tests was studied systematically in only two series, and the tests were positive in 66%[31] and in 100%[32] of the DIC cases, respectively.

Several investigators have used additional tests in the evaluation of patients with acute DIC. For instance, ATIII activity was decreased in 75%[31] and 97%[32] of DIC cases, respectively. Hepatic dysfunction may also be responsible for these results. A reduction in factor V was found to be helpful and was therefore included in one of the scoring systems.[113] Assay of D-dimer has also been introduced as a valuable test in DIC.[114–117] Its presence in plasma signifies that cross-linked fibrin has been degraded after thrombin and plasmin generation. Investigators in a study of 58 patients with DIC advocated the combination of assays of fibrin degradation products (highly sensitive but with low specificity) and of D-dimer (highly specific but less sensitive).[116]

Other hemostatic parameters investigated in patients with acute DIC did not provide further practical clinical information, but did afford important insights into its mechanism. The aberrations that were detected involve the following factors and steps in hemostasis: factor VIII coagulant activity was disproportionally decreased compared with von Willebrand factor because it is readily inactivated by thrombin, plasmin, and activated protein C[118] (hence, the ratio of factor VIII:von Willebrand factor was a good indicator of the severity of DIC[118]); diminished levels of factor XII and prekallikrein have been described by several authors,[68,113] indicating activation of the intrinsic coagulation pathway; an increased level of fibrinopeptide A, which specifically reflects thrombin generation, was found but may be observed in any type of thrombosis and is liable to in vitro artifacts.[119]

The presence of thrombin–ATIII complexes is characteristic in patients with acute DIC, and high levels were found in 25 of 41 patients with DIC.[120] A decline in activity of protein C and protein C antigen has been observed,[121–124] but this may be due at least partly to hepatic dysfunction. In this connection, a study has demonstrated diminished levels of protein C inhibitor,[123,124] as well as the presence of protein C–protein C inhibitor-2 complexes.[125] These findings suggest that during DIC, after protein C's activation by thrombin, it is complexed with one or both of its inhibitors and removed from the circulation. The amount of protein S is also decreased,[125,126] particularly that of the free protein S moiety.[126] Likewise, heparin cofactor II is low.[127] Reduced levels of the tissue factor pathway inhibitor have been reported[128] but not confirmed.[129]

A low level of plasminogen is specific but is not a sensitive indicator of acute DIC.[130] Increased values of tPA antigen (not activity) were frequently found and were associated with elevated levels of plasminogen activator inhibitor-1.[131] Complexes of plasmin–α_2-antiplasmin have been described specifically in patients with DIC related to acute promyelocytic leukemia.[132,133] The presence of these complexes and a low level of α_2-antiplasmin correlate well with serious bleeding.[132,133]

Chronic Disseminated Intravascular Coagulation

A state of chronic DIC develops when a moderate extent or slow rate of initiation of intravascular coagulation occurs. This complication can be observed in patients with distinct clinical entities, for example, metastatic carcinoma, the

TABLE 43-6. **Mortality Rate in Patients With Disseminated Intravascular Coagulation Treated With and Without Heparin**

			Mortality Rate (%)	
Study	**Patient Category**	**No. Patients**	Heparin Treatment	No Heparin Treatment
Colman et al[22]	Variable	60	62	67
Mant & King[30]	Variable	47	86	83
Siegal et al[29]	Variable	118	—	54
Spero et al[31]	Variable	346	42	32
Bick[32]	Variable	48	24	—
Corrigan[473]	Children, septic shock	222	79	76

TABLE 43-7. Value of Basic Laboratory Tests in Diagnosis of Acute Disseminated Intravascular Coagulation

Test	Abnormality*	Interpretations	DIC Patients With Abnormality† (%)	Causes Other Than DIC or Primary Fibrinolysis Contributing to Results of Tests
Platelet count	Decreased	Consumption by DIC	94.2	Leukemias, hypersplenism, sepsis
Fibrin degradation products	Increased	Secondary or primary fibrinolysis	83.8	Hematoma, transfusion of blood components, in vitro fibrinolysis when improperly processed
Paracoagulation tests	Positive	DIC with secondary fibrinolysis (sensitive to fibrin monomers and fibrin degradation products)	83.0‡	Thromboembolism, cirrhosis, improper drawing of blood, postoperative states
Prothrombin time	Prolonged	Consumption of fibrinogen and factors II, V, VII, X	82.0	Liver dysfunction, neonates
Partial thromboplastin time	Prolonged	Consumption of fibrinogen and factors II, V, VII, IX, X, XI, XII	60.0	Liver dysfunction, neonates (activated clotting factors produce normal results)
Thrombin time	Prolonged	Consumption of fibrinogen, elevated level of fibrin degradation products	72.4	Dysfibrinogenemia of liver disease and neonates
Fibrinogen level	Decreased	Consumption by DIC, breakdown by secondary or primary fibrinolysis	60.6	Pregnancy (states inducing acute phase reactants produce normal values)

* Beyond ±2 SD of mean values established in healthy controls.
† Based on data from six series encompassing 932 DIC cases.[27–29,31,32,35]
‡ Data from two series only.[31,32]

dead fetus syndrome, and giant hemangioma. In these conditions, the compensatory mechanisms counteract the consumption coagulopathy by augmenting the synthesis of the depleted components; consequently, variable values of these factors are obtained on testing. Thus, the platelet count may be mildly reduced, and fibrinogen levels may be normal or high, and the PT and APTT may be within normal limits. Usually an increase in fibrin degradation products and a positive paracoagulation test are seen. Fragmented RBCs in a blood smear can be confirmatory when other laboratory and clinical signs of DIC are present.

Primary Fibrino(geno)lysis

Primary fibrino(geno)lysis results from plasmin generation in the absence of DIC. It is a rare phenomenon occurring in hepatic disease, in certain malignancies, or without an apparent cause.[26] Primary fibrinogenolysis can be distinguished from DIC by finding: a normal platelet count; no D-dimers; a negative paracoagulation test (due to the absence of fibrin monomer); and tests reflecting increased fibrinolysis, that is, a rapid whole blood clot lysis, shortened euglobulin lysis time, and greatly elevated fibrinogen degradation products.

Primary fibrino(geno)lysis is more often found in association with DIC. In this situation, both the coagulation and the fibrinolytic systems are triggered simultaneously, that is, thrombin and plasmin are generated concomitantly. Consequently, typical laboratory signs of DIC are supplemented by whole blood lysis, shortened euglobulin lysis time, and a high concentration of fibrinogen degradation products. These crude parameters can also be abnormal when DIC and excessive secondary fibrinolysis are present; therefore, the distinction between DIC with secondary fibrinolysis from DIC with primary fibrino(geno)lysis is not at all clear. Notwithstanding these difficulties, accumulated evidence has shown that DIC is associated with primary fibrino(geno)lysis in acute promyelocytic leukemia, heat stroke, metastatic prostatic carcinoma, and amniotic fluid embolism (see specific sections).

MANAGEMENT

After the diagnosis of DIC is made, a hard decision-making process regarding management lies ahead. The various causes of DIC, its many clinical manifestations, and its different grades of severity have prevented execution of successful controlled studies; hence, widely divergent opinions remain concerning management. Nevertheless, some guidance can be obtained from consensus views, theoretical considerations, information gained from analysis of retrospective studies, and unequivocal evidence concerning specific causes of DIC. General guidelines for management are depicted in Figure 43-5.

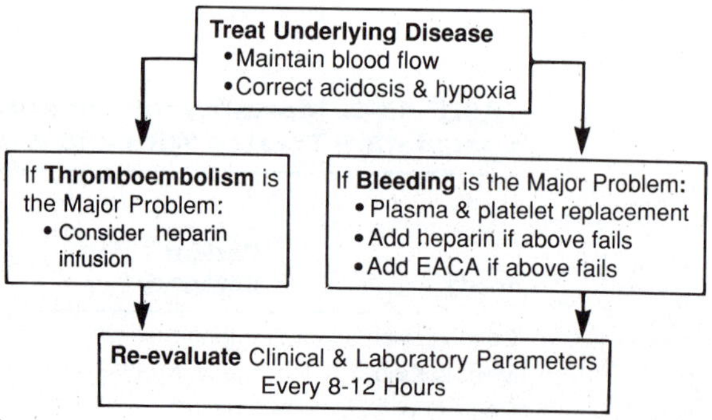

FIGURE 43-5. General guidelines for management of patients with disseminated intravascular coagulation. EACA, ε-aminocaproic acid.

Consensus Views

Vigorous Measures to Treat Underlying Disorders

The survival of patients with DIC requires successful management of the underlying disorders or curtailing the triggers of blood coagulation. Thus, specific therapy like hysterectomy in a patient with abruptio placentae, resection of an aortic aneurysm, débridement of crushed tissues, and intensive antibiotic treatment of gram-negative bacteremia are indispensable steps in management. Similarly, therapy in acute promyelocytic leukemia can completely eliminate associated DIC if the patient enters remission.

Support of Vital Functions

Vital functions are impaired both by the underlying disease and by DIC itself. Volume replacement and correction of hypotension and oxygenation improve blood flow through the microcirculation, thus restoring inhibitory functions of blood coagulation systems at the microcirculation (see Fig. 43-3). Although reperfusion may initially inflict further tissue injury, this is probably self-limited, and the influx of procoagulants soon stops. Careful monitoring of pulmonary, cardiac, and renal function enables prompt institution of supportive measures such as a respirator for better oxygenation, inotropic drugs for improvement of cardiac output, and maintenance of electrolyte balance.

Fibrinolytic Inhibitors

Patients with DIC should not be treated with antifibrinolytic agents like ϵ-aminocaproic acid and tranexamic acid. These drugs block the compensatory (secondary) fibrinolysis that accompanies DIC and partially preserves tissue perfusion. The use of these agents in patients with DIC was complicated by severe thrombosis.[134,135]

A different situation prevails in patients with DIC accompanied by primary fibrino(geno)lysis, as in acute promyelocytic leukemia, giant hemangioma, heat stroke, amniotic fluid embolism, and metastatic carcinoma of the prostate. In these conditions, the use of fibrinolytic inhibitors can be considered, provided that the patient is bleeding profusely and has not responded to replacement therapy and that extensive in vitro fibrinolysis can be demonstrated (rapid whole blood clot lysis or a short euglobulin lysis time). When these criteria have been met, it is advisable to precede the use of antifibrinolytic agents by continuous heparin infusion and replacement of depleted blood components.

Deliberate induction of thrombosis by inhibitors of fibrinolysis together with infusion of blood components has been performed in patients with giant hemangioma and DIC associated with primary fibrino(geno)lysis (see section on hemangioma).

Replacement Therapy

The readily available platelet concentrates, cryoprecipitate, and fresh frozen plasma contain the hemostatic factors commonly depleted in DIC. Replacement therapy should not be instituted in patients with only laboratory evidence of DIC. Eligible patients should have a well-established diagnosis of DIC, depleted hemostatic factors, and severe bleeding. Also eligible for replacement therapy are patients being prepared for emergency surgery. Gunshot-induced brain injury may be another indication for replacement therapy (see Fig. 43-5). The notion that replacement therapy in DIC fuels the fire has never been proved.

It is my practice to start replacement therapy by infusion of eight units of platelet concentrate, eight units of cryoprecipitate and one to two units of fresh frozen plasma. This triple component therapy is repeated every 8 hours with adjustment of doses according to the platelet count, PT, APTT, fibrinogen level, and volume load. Infusions are stopped as soon as normal or subnormal values of hemostatic factors are attained.

Fibrinogen concentrates are rarely used, and prothrombin complex concentrates are contraindicated in view of their potential prothrombotic effect.

Heparin

Theoretical Arguments Against Heparin

Clinicians were initially encouraged to use heparin after the demonstration of its efficacy in experimental models. Heparin was beneficial when given to animals before induction of DIC and not thereafter. In most clinical settings, physicians see patients when DIC is already well established, at which time heparin is expected to be less effective or ineffective.

Heparin administration can seriously aggravate bleeding in a patient with severe hemostatic failure due to consumption and to hepatic or renal dysfunction. Furthermore, when trauma is involved, it can induce bleeding from sites of injury.

Heparin may have a reduced anticoagulant effect because ATIII is depleted in patients with DIC. Fibrin monomers that are products of DIC also block the heparin-induced interaction between thrombin and ATIII.[136]

Finally, the interaction between heparin and elastase released from neutrophils impedes the interaction of heparin with ATIII,[137] which also diminishes its anticoagulant potential.

Clinical Arguments Against Heparin

None of the clinical reports has shown a reduction in mortality rate in patients treated with heparin (see Table 43-6). The use of heparin has at best improved the levels of hemostatic factors in the treated patients.[138]

The administration of heparin in DIC cases aggravated bleeding[30] or has even caused fatal hemorrhage.[28,30] In some cases, only a transient enhancement of bleeding occurred.[22]

Heparin can induce thrombocytopenia in about 5% of patients[139–141] and has been claimed to cause DIC on rare occasions.[142–145] The significance of the latter observations is not clear.

When to Consider the Use of Heparin

Administration of heparin may be of benefit in some of the rarer categories of acute or chronic DIC, including purpura fulminans, acute promyelocytic leukemia (not all authorities agree; see specific section on leukemias), before removal of a dead fetus from the uterus prior to resection of an aortic aneurysm; for thromboembolic complications in large vessels; and before surgery in patients with metastatic carcinoma (see Fig. 43-5 and specific sections). Other, less clearly established, indications include: skin necrosis and acral gangrene, septic abortion, mismatched transfusions, and amniotic fluid embolism.

When massive life-threatening bleeding occurs and intensive replacement fails to increase significantly the level of hemostatic factors so that DIC is uncontrolled and continuing, heparin administration combined with replacement therapy can be considered.[146]

Heparin should be used cautiously in all the previously mentioned conditions. The continuous intravenous technique is preferable. According to my experience, a continuous infusion of heparin, 500 to 750 IU/h, without a bolus injection is sufficient in chronic cases. If no response is obtained within 24 hours, the use of escalating dosages can be considered.

In hyperacute cases as in mismatched transfusions, amniotic fluid embolism, septic abortion, and purpura fulminans, an intravenous bolus injection of 10,000 IU heparin can be considered and followed by continuous infusion of 1000 IU/h with increasing dosage if necessary.

Other Treatment Modalities

Antithrombin III Concentrate

Antithrombin III infusion was first used in 1978 to treat three patients with DIC.[147] Since then, further studies have accumulated and have been reviewed.[148,149] ATIII concentrates were administered either alone[147,150–152] or in combination with heparin.[153–155] Unfortunately, most of these studies consisted either of small series of patients or were not well controlled. Nevertheless, they have demonstrated improved hemostatic function,[152,154] except in patients with LeVeen shunts,[153] but have not shown any improvement in mortality.[149,152] A study of sepsis-related DIC in baboons demonstrated that extremely high doses of an ATIII concentrate had to be given before injection of *Escherichia coli* to improve hemostasis and to prevent death.[156] The same dose given later was without benefit. Thus, no definitive recommendations regarding the clinical use of ATIII concentrate can be made.

Gabexate Mesilate

Gabexate mesilate (Foy), a synthetic serine protease inhibitor, was developed by Japanese investigators in 1972.[157] Both this drug[154,158] and nafamostat mesilate,[159,160] a newly developed derivative, have been used in the treatment of DIC. It was suggested that these preparations have an advantage over heparin because they do not depend on the patient's plasma ATIII level.[158] Conversely, their potential capacity to neutralize plasmin activity could constitute a disadvantage.[154] Thus, further experience with these drugs is desirable.

Prospective Treatment Modalities

Given the complexity of mechanisms that are set off by the common triggers of DIC, such as endotoxin, and the deleterious effects of the underlying disorders, it is unlikely that drugs that block only one pathway will improve the poor prognosis of most patients with DIC. Possibly, a better understanding of the complex mechanisms operating in DIC will promote development of a variety of means whose concerted effects yield better results. Several such preparations have already been tested in animals, for example, an activated protein C concentrate[161] and a genetically engineered mutant α_1-antitrypsin that exerts antithrombin and antikallikrein effects.[68] Other agents such as antitissue factor antibodies,[162] antiendotoxin antibodies, and peptides inhibitory for cytokines will probably follow.

DISSEMINATED INTRAVASCULAR COAGULATION IN SPECIFIC DISORDERS

Infectious Diseases

A large number of infectious agents initiate DIC, and infections constitute one of the most common causes of DIC[163] (see Table 43-3). The mechanism by which DIC is produced during infections is not fully understood. The complex effects of endotoxin have been discussed (see section on pathogenesis). Staphylococci produce an α toxin that can activate platelets and interact with macrophages to induce IL-1 secretion.[164] IL-1 induces expression of tissue factor by endothelial cells and down-regulates thrombomodulin, thereby favoring blood coagulation.[66] A different mechanism operates in viral infections: antigen–antibody complexes are formed that induce coagulation through the intrinsic pathway.[165] Viruses can also damage endothelial cells, which can activate the intrinsic coagulation pathway.[166,167] Thus, both the intrinsic and extrinsic coagulation systems may be activated by infectious agents.

Patients are particularly prone to infection-induced DIC in the presence of certain clinical conditions. For instance, in pregnancy with its diminished inhibitory and fibrinolytic capacities, the patient is susceptible to extremely severe infection-linked DIC complicated by renal cortical necrosis. Likewise, asplenic patients have a tendency to develop fulminant DIC, which is related to their inability to clear bacteria, particularly pneumococci.[168,169] Newborns (discussed in the section on DIC in neonates) have a similar vulnerability.

Infections are frequently superimposed on trauma and malignancies, which are themselves potential triggers of DIC. In addition, several consequences of infections can add fuel to the fire. For example, tissue ischemia and acidosis caused by septic shock enhance thrombosis; thrombocytopenia due to sepsis per se aggravates bleeding.[170]

Gram-Negative Infections

Meningococcemia is the most extreme example of a gram-negative infection associated with DIC. Its fulminant clinical course, characterized by extensive hemorrhagic necrosis and shock, was first described by Voelcker[171] in 1894, later by Waterhouse[172] in 1911 and Friderichsen[173] in 1918. A direct correlation was found between the patient's prognosis and the severity of the hemostatic derangements.[174] More recent work has revealed a good correlation between the coagulation abnormalities and the plasma levels of lipopolysaccharide, TNF, IL-1, and C3a, thus demonstrating the significance of these various mediators in this condition.[175] Heparin treatment is of questionable benefit in patients with meningococcemia.[138]

More common gram-negative infections associated with DIC are caused by *Pseudomonas aeruginosa*, *E coli*, and *Proteus vulgaris*. Patients affected by bacteremia with these agents may have only laboratory signs of DIC[29] or may present with severe DIC, especially when they have developed shock.[176] In extreme cases, the presentation may be reminiscent of the generalized Shwartzman reaction.[177] Mortality rate is high even when vigorous antibiotic therapy and supportive measures are promptly instituted.[178] A clear benefit of heparin administration has so far not been shown in controlled trials. Some investigations failed to demonstrate an effect on mortality, although a slight improvement in laboratory findings was shown.[138] Other studies did obtain an increased rate of survival in patients who had received heparin.[22] In view of these conflicting reports, definite guidelines for therapy with heparin cannot be given. Nevertheless, continuous heparin infusion should be considered only in pregnant women with hyperacute gram-negative septicemia (see sections on management and DIC during pregnancy) and in patients who develop skin necrosis.

Gram-Positive Infections

Staphylococcus aureus can cause fulminant DIC accompanied by renal cortical and dermal necrosis,[179,180] whereas streptococcal infections may underlie purpura fulminans.[181] *Streptococcus pneumoniae* infections have been associated with the Waterhouse-Friderichsen syndrome[182] and with acral gangrene,[183] particularly in asplenic patients.[168,169] The triggers of DIC in these circumstances were initially ascribed to the capsular antigen of the bacterium and to antigen–antibody complex formation.[184] Results of an experimental study did not support this view.[185] Instead, direct activation of factor XII by these bacteria or by their products was suggested as the trigger of DIC.[185]

Clostridia are also extremely virulent gram-positive bacteria, which were the pathogens described in septic abortions associated with severe DIC, renal failure, and microangiopathic hemolytic anemia.[163]

Insufficient data are available regarding the possible benefits of heparin therapy in patients with DIC-related gram-positive infections.

Viral Infections

Common viral infections such as influenza, chickenpox, rubella, and rubeola are sometimes complicated by DIC, but little information is available on treatment.[165] Of great interest are viral infections causing "hemorrhagic fevers," in which patients frequently exhibit fever, hypotension, bleeding, renal failure, and laboratory evidence of DIC.[165–167] Histopathologic examinations have revealed diffuse hemorrhagic necrosis and vasculitis but no fibrin microthrombi.[167] Consequently, the finding of hypofibrinogenemia and thrombocytopenia in the absence of elevated levels of FDP do not support the diagnosis of DIC in these disorders.

Other Infections

Fungal infections,[186,187] miliary tuberculosis,[188] and malaria[189] all have been associated at times with DIC. An early observation on the benefit of heparin administration in severe cases of falciparum malaria[189] was not confirmed.[190]

Purpura Fulminans

Purpura fulminans, first described by Henoch,[191] is a foudroyant disorder in which extensive areas of the skin become gangrenous within 2 to 4 weeks of a mild infection such as scarlet fever, chickenpox, or rubella. The disease predominantly affects children or infants,[192,193] but occasionally it also affects adults.[193,194] The onset of purpura fulminans is sudden, with sharply demarcated purple lesions on the skin. The lesions may be small (a few centimeters) or may extend over wide areas covering the extremities, buttocks, scrotum, and penis. Within a few days, necrosis sets in (Fig. 43-6), and sometimes bullae are formed. Biopsy of the involved skin reveals diffuse microthrombi in small blood vessels and also vasculitis, the picture being reminiscent of a local Shwartzman reaction.[192] The pathogenesis of the extensive damage to the dermal vasculature has not been determined. One predisposing state is recognized, namely homozygous protein C deficiency.[195–197] Neonates striken by this disorder present soon after birth with purpura fulminans[195,197] or massive intravascular thrombosis and abdominal wall gangrene.[196] Although the extremely deranged blood coagulation–inhibiting capacity is obvious in these patients, the procoagulant trigger operating so soon after birth remains to be elucidated.

Patients affected by purpura fulminans are acutely ill, with fever, hypotension, and hemorrhage from multiple sites. Laboratory examinations demonstrate typical signs of DIC.[192,193,198,199] The successful use of heparin in patients with purpura fulminans was reported in 1959[198] and confirmed by others.[192] Full heparinization should be supplemented by transfusion of the depleted hemostatic components. Excision of necrotic skin areas and grafting are usually necessary at a later stage.

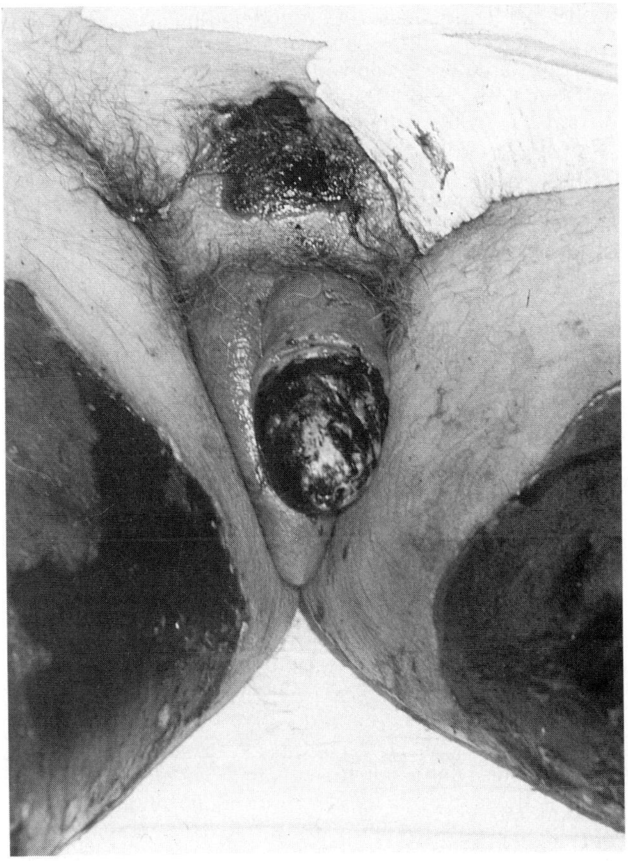

FIGURE 43-6. Extensive skin necrosis in a 63-year-old man with purpura fulminans. (After Tishler M, Abramov AL, Seligsohn U, Kahn Y. Purpura fulminans in an adult. Isr J Med Sci 1986;22:820)

Cancer

Neoplastic cells and tissues affect the hemostatic system by causing thromboembolism or bleeding. The hemostatic system influences the growth and spread of malignancies. This interrelation has long attracted the attention of clinicians and researchers, of whom Trousseau[39] was the first to describe the propensity to thrombosis of patients with cancerous cachexia. A comprehensive discussion of this subject is beyond the scope of this chapter; the reader is referred to several excellent reviews.[200–203]

Evidence for malignancy-related primary fibrino(geno)lysis and DIC, respectively, was provided more than 50 years ago by two studies. One study reported a fatal intracerebral hemorrhage in a 52-year-old man who had widespread metastases of prostatic carcinoma, a very low fibrinogen level, and a normal platelet count.[204] Another study documented the case of a young man with metastatic gastric carcinoma, who had focal tissue necrosis, thrombocytopenia, prolonged clotting time, whole blood fibrinolysis, and diffuse bleeding at time of death.[205]

In an extensive review, the incidence of excessive bleeding in patients with malignant disorders was high: 75 of 182 cases. The incidence of thromboembolism was even higher: venous thrombosis in 123 of 182, migratory thrombophlebitis in 96 of 182, arterial thrombosis in 45 of 182, and arterial embolism due to nonbacterial thrombotic endocarditis in 31 of 182 cases.[200] Also documented were multifocal hemorrhagic infarctions of the brain caused by fibrin microemboli.[206] These infarctions were manifested clinically as confusion and other disorders of consciousness. Patients with solid tumors and DIC are more prone to thrombosis, whereas patients with leukemia and DIC are more likely to exhibit hemorrhage. Varying rates of occurrence of DIC have been recorded for different solid tumors.[33] On the other hand, of the leukemias only acute promyelocytic leukemia is nearly always complicated by DIC (see section on leukemias).

Both bleeding and thromboembolism are apparently due to generation of procoagulants and seldom result from profibrinolytic materials that have gained access to circulating blood. Depending on the rate and quantity of influx, a decompensated, compensated, or overcompensated hemostatic state develops.[207] For instance, a patient may be asymptomatic when the tumor cells release procoagulants slowly or intermittently and the ensuing consumption of fibrinogen and platelet is compensated by overproduction of these components.[207] Conversely, massive thrombosis[208] or severe bleeding[28,30] may supervene in a patient whose circulation is deluged by powerful procoagulants.

The following procoagulants have been identified in or associated with malignant tissues:

- Tissue factor that was initially found in rabbit[209] and human[210] carcinomas as well as in leukemic cells[211]
- A protease that activates factor X[212]; a similar proteolytic activity has been identified in serosal fluids and in mucus, which helps to explain the predilection of DIC to patients with mucin-secreting adenocarcinomas[213]
- Tissue factor produced by circulating monocytes in response to an interaction with tumor antigens or complexes of tumor antigens with host antibodies[214]; a good correlation was found between the amount of tissue factor generated in vitro by monocytes and the circulating level of fibrinopeptide A, reflecting thrombin generation in patients with malignancies from whom these cells were obtained[214]
- Adhesion and aggregation of platelets[202] and extravascular fibrin deposition by malignant cells and tissues[215]; these accessory mechanisms promote intravascular clotting and consumption of hemostatic components

Primary fibrinogenolysis occurs mainly in patients with prostatic carcinomas[204,216] or acute promyelocytic leukemia (see next section). A fibrinogenolytic activity was identified in prostatic tissue in 1943.[217] Because this activity was not inhibited by the antifibrinolytic activity of normal plasma, it was considered to be different from fibrinolysin (plasmin).[216]

The intravascular coagulation or bleeding induced by the mechanisms just listed may be exacerbated because the neoplastic disorders predispose the patients to additional triggering factors. These factors are septicemia, immobilization, suppression of platelet production by chemotherapy, and involvement by metastases of organs responsible for the defense and compensatory mechanisms of hemostasis (see Fig. 43-3).

Generally, DIC may cause microangiopathic hemolytic anemia. This is particularly severe in patients with widespread intravascular metastases of mucin-secreting adenocarcinomas.[218–221]

The chronic DIC associated with malignancy has been treated successfully by administration of heparin.[200] Potential indications for therapy with heparin are arterial or venous thrombosis, significant bleeding, preparation for surgery, and before institution of intensive chemotherapy. Replacement of depleted blood components may be required during initial heparinization, but after appropriate anticoagulation has been achieved, DIC usually abates. Low-dose subcutaneous heparin can then effectively replace full heparinization; oral anticoagulants are useless.[203]

Impressive results with heparin administration have not been obtained in patients with neoplastic disorders who developed acute severe DIC.[28] Patients exhibiting primary fibrinogenolysis treatment with ϵ-aminocaproic acid or tranexamic acid can be considered, but the correctness of the diagnosis should be beyond any reasonable doubt in view of the hazards involved when these agents are used.[134,135]

Leukemias

In 1935, bleeding and a low fibrinogen level were noted in a patient with acute myelocytic leukemia.[222] Since then, numerous reports have been published on DIC and fibrinolysis complicating the course of leukemias.[223] Acute promyelocytic leukemia (APL) is the most common diagnosis made in these instances. In 1957, APL was the first disease entity characterized as being associated with severe hemorrhage, low levels of fibrinogen and other clotting factors, fibrinolysis, and thrombocytopenia.[224] These observations have since been confirmed,[225,226] but a controversy remains regarding the pathogenesis of the hemostatic disturbances and the implied therapeutic approach. One school of thought maintains that tissue factor expressed or released by malignant promyelocytes is responsible for the severe DIC and secondary fibrinolysis that are present before treatment and aggravated after chemotherapy.[225] In vitro studies have shown large amounts of tissue factor in leukemic cells,[227–230] and an immunologic study suggested that leukemic cell tissue factor and human brain thromboplastin are identical.[231]

Diffuse fibrin microthrombi in tissues of patients at autopsy constituted further support for the concept that DIC causes the hemostatic abnormalities in APL.[232–234] The proportion of patients with pathologically demonstrated DIC was relatively small[225]; this may be related to their intact inhibitory systems as manifested by the interesting finding of normal plasma levels of protein C and ATIII in these patients unlike in patients with other types of DIC.[235] Additional support for DIC in APL was provided by the demonstration of increased levels of prothrombin fragments 1 and 2 and thrombin–ATIII complexes.[236]

As a result of the preceding observations, heparinization was advocated in APL, especially at the time of induction chemotherapy, when augmentation of DIC with serious bleeding was anticipated.[225,237] In one study of 24 APL patients, bleeding was decreased and a higher rate of remission was obtained.[237] A retrospective analysis of APL cases has shown that fatal bleeding had occurred in 28% of 117 patients who received heparin compared with 19% of 179 patients who had not ($P > .05$).[226] Likewise, no significant improvement in the rate of remission induction was found between patients managed with or without heparin.[226]

Other authorities regard primary fibrinogenolysis as the predominant cause of the serious bleeding in patients with APL.[238] Low plasma levels of α_2-antiplasmin[239–242] and complexes of plasmin–antiplasmin have been detected in patients with APL.[241] These findings may be related to production of profibrinolytic proteases by leukemic cells.[240] Consequently, treatment by antifibrinolytic agents was recommended and in a small series of cases arrested bleeding.[238,243]

Patients with APL are not unlikely to have concomitant DIC and primary fibrino(geno)lysis, and both processes may be triggered by proteases released by leukemic cells. Introduction of sensitive tests recording the magnitude of thrombin and of plasmin generation (prothrombin fragments 1 and 2, thrombin–ATIII complex, α_2-antiplasmin,

plasmin–antiplasmin complex, and D-dimer) may provide guidelines as to when to administer heparin, when to use an antifibrinolytic agent, and when both agents may be indicated. In any case, treatment should be supplemented by blood components until balanced hemostasis is achieved.

Trauma

Trauma is a common cause of DIC (see Table 43-3), but this does not imply that trauma is frequently complicated by DIC. When it does occur, DIC usually manifests in severely injured patients by hemorrhage exceeding that commensurate with the trauma.

DIC as a consequence of trauma was first demonstrated in dogs whose femoral diaphyses were fractured.[244] Shortly thereafter, clinical and laboratory signs of DIC were extensively studied in series of patients.[2,245–250] Several mechanisms may be responsible for the development or aggravation of DIC in patients with traumatic injuries:

- Entry of tissue factor into the circulation, prominent in extensive trauma and injury of tissues rich in tissue factor such as the brain
- Trauma-induced hemorrhage and hemorrhagic shock leading to depletion of hemostatic factors, accelerated coagulation, and impaired clearance of procoagulants
- Superimposed infections and septicemia
- Multiple transfusions of stored blood that does not contain platelets, factor V, and factor VIII,[249] thus further diluting the concentration of these essential components
- Defense mechanisms that are impeded after direct injury to the liver or, if hepatic dysfunction follows hemorrhagic shock, from microthrombosis of hepatic vessels
- Respiratory distress syndrome, also termed *shock lung*, in which extensive damage to pulmonary vessels initiates the intrinsic coagulation system[251]
- Tissue damage inflicted by the complex mechanisms of postischemic reperfusion (generation of oxygen radicals, calcium overload as a consequence of severed blood vessels or application of tourniquets)

An additional complication is washout microembolization after release of arterial clamps.[252]

Fat embolism is another important factor to be considered. This syndrome, which was first described by Zenker[253] in the 19th century, can occur in patients within 48 hours of trauma.[254–256] Fat embolism is characterized by a triad of respiratory insufficiency, neurologic dysfunction, and bleeding[255,256]; in most cases, it stems from the entry into the circulation of marrow fat from injured bones. Occasionally, the syndrome follows trauma in which no involvement of bone is seen.[254] Three types of response to fat embolism were defined[256]:

- A hyperacute fatal type in which paradoxical systemic embolization is responsible for death soon after trauma
- The classic type of response characterized by respiratory distress due to obstruction of pulmonary capillaries and arterioles with fat droplets and by interstitial pulmonary edema and slight consumption of hemostatic factors; notable in this type of response is the absence of extensive alveolar hemorrhage or hyaline membrane formation
- A third type of response characterized by ARDS with diffuse fat embolization of pulmonary vessels, hemorrhagic necrosis, edema, hyaline membrane formation in alveoli, and prominent laboratory evidence of DIC; the initiation of fat embolism is probably caused by damage of the endothelium of pulmonary vessels, by release of tissue factor from ischemic pulmonary tissue or from other sites of fat embolization, and by inhibition of fibrinolysis[256]

The time interval between trauma and medical attention is also important. Experience with a large series of trauma cases managed during the Vietnamese war proved that fast evacuation and prompt medical care reduced the risk of complications by DIC.[249] This advantage probably stems from the shorter time of exposure of circulating blood to tissue factor.

After making a judgment as to what mechanisms contribute to DIC in a particular patient with trauma, the physician should institute appropriate management. Débridement of severely damaged tissues to arrest the influx of tissue factor into the circulation is of paramount importance. Vital functions such as blood flow through the microcirculation and respiratory, cardiac, and renal performance must be monitored and supported, and measures must be taken against potential infections. In the event of hemostatic derangement, transfusions should be given to replenish the consumed or lost clotting factors and platelets. Dextran is contraindicated because it can aggravate bleeding in thrombocytopenic patients.[246] I believe that heparin is not indicated.

Brain Injury

Brain tissue contains large amounts of tissue factor. The catastrophic effects of brain extracts, which were injected intravenously into animals, were first reported by Dupuy[38] in 1834. The earliest clinical observations on DIC and bleeding after brain injury were made in 1968[257] and thereafter were well established.[258–263] The course of DIC in brain-injured patients was self-limited,[258] probably because of the transient exposure of blood to tissue factor. The combination of severe injury and depleted hemostatic factors resulted in significant bleeding. Transfusion of platelets and plasma components effectively arrested the bleeding.[258] In fatal cases, DIC was confirmed by the presence of microthrombi in the brain, liver, lungs, kidneys, and pancreas.[264] Studies of adults and children with head injuries have shown a high rate of mortality when laboratory tests were indicative of DIC.[263,265,266] Moreover, a laboratory DIC score had a predictive value for prognosis of patients with head injuries, thereby supplementing the Glasgow Coma Scale.[266]

Therefore, although bleeding in patients with DIC related to brain injury can be managed by replacement therapy, it carries a grave prognosis.

Burns

Bleeding, laboratory tests indicative of DIC, and vascular microthrombi in biopsies of undamaged skin all have been described in patients with extensive burns.[267,268] Tissue factor released from burned areas, infection, and shock can be the triggers of DIC in these patients. The reduced levels of hemostatic factors in patients with burns cannot be solely related to DIC, since kinetic studies with labeled fibrinogen and platelets disclosed significant consumption of hemostatic factors by the burned areas themselves.[269]

Early experimental[270,271] and clinical[268,272,273] observations suggested that heparin administered locally and parenterally had some beneficial effects but had no influence on survival of the patients.[268] Subsequent investigations demonstrated that administration of heparin did not curtail the excessive consumption of hemostatic factors; therefore, its use was no longer advocated.[269,274]

These studies imply that replacement is the treatment of choice in patients with burns and bleeding due to low levels of hemostatic components.

Liver Diseases

As already pointed out, the liver plays a central role in hemostasis: it synthesizes most factors of the coagulation systems; it produces the proteins that control blood clotting (protein C, protein S, and ATIII), as well as the main components of the fibrinolytic system (plasminogen and α_2-antiplasmin). In addition, the liver clears the circulation of soluble fibrin monomer complexes and of the activated factors IX, X, and XI, and tPA.[96,275,276] Consequently, the abnormalities in hemostasis that occur in patients with severe liver disease predispose them to bleeding that is often aggravated by thrombocytopenia due to hypersplenism. The similarity between these hemostatic defects and those of patients with DIC has evoked an ongoing controversy on whether DIC is or is not involved in liver disease.[10,277,278] The opinions are reviewed below.

Several laboratory and clinical observations support the hypothesis that DIC accompanies hepatic disorders. These observations include a shortened half-life of radiolabeled fibrinogen and prolongation of its survival by administration of heparin[279,280]; failure of extensive replacement to increase significantly the levels of hemostatic factors, suggesting continuous consumption[281]; the beneficial effects of heparin in the management of some patients with acute hepatic failure[282]; and the increased blood levels of D-dimer[283] and fibrinopeptide A[284] indicative of thrombin generation.

Other investigators have maintained that DIC is not associated with liver disease. The observations and arguments in favor of this hypothesis include the presence of an extremely low incidence (2.2%) of microthrombosis in the tissues of patients who died of liver disease[285] and the fact that many of the hemostatic abnormalities of patients with hepatic disorders can stem from causes other than DIC or are not consistent with DIC. Examples are a prolonged thrombin time due to dysfibrinogenemia,[286] low levels of coagulation factors and inhibitors that may be related to reduced synthesis, increased FDP levels that may be a consequence of primary fibrinogenolysis, increased (rather than decreased) factor VIII clotting activity,[287] interpretation of excessive consumption of fibrinogen as loss of fibrinogen into extravascular spaces,[288] and data showing normal decay of endogenously labeled semethionine-75 fibrinogen and plasminogen.[289]

A third hypothesis maintains that patients with liver disease usually do not present with DIC but are extremely sensitive to the various triggers of DIC in view of their impeded capacity to clear procoagulants and synthesize essential components of coagulation inhibitory and fibrinolytic systems. An extreme sensitivity toward DIC has been demonstrated in patients who have primary or metastatic liver disease and who underwent a peritoneovenous shunt operation for severe ascites; this is in contrast to patients who underwent the same procedure for ascites due to other causes.[290]

Patients with liver disease and bleeding should be evaluated for possible underlying causes of DIC. Furthermore, their hemostatic profile should be examined repeatedly to detect any dynamic changes that may be helpful in recognizing DIC. Although stable abnormalities or slight decreases in hemostatic parameters can be related to the hepatic disease and bleeding, respectively, a dramatic reduction over short periods is indicative of DIC. An assay of factor VIII is time consuming but can be helpful because high and stable levels make the diagnosis of DIC unlikely. Sensitive assays that reflect thrombin generation have been devised, namely, levels of prothrombin fragments 1 and 2,[291] thrombin–ATIII complex[292] and D-dimer.[283] Routine application of these assays may help to establish the diagnosis of DIC in a patient with liver disease.

Given the present diagnostic limitations and the uncertainty as to whether a patient bleeds because of liver disease per se or because of superimposed DIC, the treatment should consist of replacement of hemostatic factors and, if a DIC trigger is identified, specific vigorous treatment. Concentrates containing activated clotting factors should be avoided in view of their potential thrombogenic effects.[293] Heparin administration has not been recommended by some authors,[280,294,295] but others were willing to consider its cautious use.[277,278] My opinion is that until evidence is provided that patients with well-established DIC and liver disease respond to heparin, this treatment modality should not be used.

Clinical and laboratory signs of DIC have been observed in some patients after a peritoneovenous shunt procedure (LeVeen shunt) for ascites associated with liver disease. The procoagulant effect of serosal fluids was already noted at the beginning of the 19th century.[38] Subsequently, ascites fluid was found to contain the following procoagulants: tissue factor,[296] a factor X activator,[297] collagen (which induces strong platelet aggregation),[298] and endotoxin in 6 of 11 cases.[299]

In one review of 278 patients with the LeVeen shunt, DIC was observed postoperatively in only 10 patients,[300] but other investigators have reported higher incidences[299,301–303] and even a fatal case.[304] As mentioned earlier, patients with primary liver disease or with hepatic metastases are more prone to DIC after shunt than are other patients after the same procedure.[290] Unsuccessful attempts have been made to control this shunt-related DIC with an ATIII concentrate,[305] whereas therapy with aspirin and dipyridamole has met with partial success.[306]

Heatstroke

The syndrome of heatstroke is caused by a rise in body temperature to over 42°C after collapse of the thermoregulatory mechanism. A high environmental temperature is the main cause of heatstroke, but several predisposing factors have been identified: strenuous physical activity, presence of infections, dehydration, and lack of acclimatization.[307] Multiple organ dysfunction occurs in patients with heatstroke,[308] and of these a bleeding tendency was already described in the 19th century. Thus, Wellstead, who wrote the book *Travels to the City of the Caliphs*, reported that in 1841, on an extremely hot day in the Persian Gulf, the decks of the ship Liverpool "resembled a slaughterhouse, so numerous were the bleeding patients."[309] Moreover, diffuse hemorrhage, unclottable blood, and venous engorgement were found in 1838 in postmortem examinations of patients who had died of heatstroke.[309] Since then, investigations on series of cases have confirmed that a severe hemorrhagic diathesis often accompanies heatstroke.[307,310–314]

Damage to the bone marrow and liver was at first thought to be responsible for the thrombocytopenia and the prolonged PT, but these developed so rapidly that additional reasons for bleeding appeared likely.[315,316] Primary fibrinolysis[317] and evidence of DIC were then revealed clinically[314,316,318] and experimentally.[319] Furthermore, diffuse fibrin deposition and hemorrhagic infarctions were found in fatal cases[311,320] and in dogs with experimental heatstroke.[319]

Triggers for initiation of primary fibrino(geno)lysis and DIC in patients with heatstroke include endothelial cell damage[321] and probably tissue factor released from heat-damaged tissues.

Both the severity of the syndrome and the stage of its development affect the type and magnitude of hemostatic alterations. Thus, one patient who was followed closely during the initial stages first manifested primary fibrinogenolysis, then thrombocytopenia and additional hemostatic derangements.[322] In a clinical study of 56 patients, three groups were distinguished: nonbleeders, bleeders without DIC but with slight consumption of hemostatic factors, and bleeders with typical signs of DIC.[314]

Prompt cooling and support of vital functions have substantially reduced the high mortality rate that was commonly observed in early studies.[307] Replacement of hemostatic components is the treatment of choice when bleeding occurs.[308] Several patients have been successfully treated by heparin,[323–326] but the hazards of this therapy were emphasized.[327] No controlled studies are available on this aspect of management. My opinion is that neither heparin nor antifibrinolytic agents should be administered because of their potential risks and because of the relatively good results obtainable by rapid intervention with general therapeutic measures.[307]

Snake Bites

Snakes belonging to the Viperidae family produce venoms containing a number of hemostatic poisons. Members of this family include the Viperidae (*Vipera*, *Echis* [*E carinatus* or *E coloratus*], and *Aspis* species) and the Crotalinae (*Crotalus, Bothrops*, and *Agkistrodon* species). Several excellent reviews are available on the biochemistry, pathophysiology, and clinical aspects of snake bites.[328–332]

The fact that blood remained fluid in animals bitten by vipers was reported during the 18th century,[333,334] and the procoagulant and anticoagulant effects of venoms were discovered in the late 19th century.[335,336] Detailed analysis of *Viperidae* venoms then disclosed that the active compounds are mainly enzymes or peptides with the following activities[331,332,337–339]:

- Thrombin-like activity—cleaving peptide A from the A–α chain of fibrinogen, thereby converting fibrinogen to fibrin; for example, the venom of *Agkistrodon rhodostoma*, the Malayan pit viper, has this activity
- Activation of prothrombin in the absence of calcium ions; the component possessing this activity is found in the venom of *E carinatus*
- Activation of factors X and V; such a substance is present in Russell viper venom
- Fibrinogenolytic activity (*Agkistrodon acutus* venom)[331]
- Induction of thrombocytopenia by platelet aggregation[331]
- Inhibition of platelet aggregation by the low-molecular-weight peptide, trigramin[340]
- Activation of protein C[341]; in addition, snakes belonging to the Viperidae family also produce compounds which damage endothelium and other vessel wall components leading to bleeding, tissue ischemia, and edema

Victims of snake bites rarely experience excessive bleeding or thromboembolism in spite of the powerful agents in venoms.[328,329,332,342] Nevertheless, serious derangements in laboratory tests are demonstrable. The major symptoms, which are related to other effects of envenomation, are vomiting, diarrhea, apprehension, hypotension, local swelling, ischemia, and necrosis. Unequivocal DIC was described after Viperidae snake bites,[342–345] but a controlled trial showed no advantage of administration of heparin and antivenom over administration of antivenom alone.[345] Consequently, victims of snake bites should be immobilized immediately and given reassurance. Local incisions, cooling, and application of tourniquet should be avoided.[329,332] Subsequently, administration of antivenom, fluids, and other general measures to preserve vital functions are recommended.[329,332] In the event of bleeding, replacement with platelet concentrates and plasma components is advisable. Heparin should be considered only when these measures fail.[343] I have treated two patients who were bitten by unidentified snakes and who presented with massive hematuria and laboratory indications of primary fibrinogenolysis. Both patients responded dramatically to brief administration of ϵ-aminocaproic acid.

Coagulation Factor Deficiencies: Infusion of Prothrombin Complex Concentrates

Concentrates of the vitamin K–dependent clotting factors (prothrombin complex) have been used for the past 30 years to treat patients with hemophilia B and other hereditary or acquired coagulation factor deficiencies. In 1972, intravascular coagulation was first described in rabbits injected with two such concentrates.[346] Soon after, thrombosis[293] and severe DIC[347,348] were reported in patients after administration of vitamin K–dependent clotting factors. Several procoagulants were identified in the prothrombin complex concentrates, including factor IXa, factor Xa,[349] and factor VIIa.[350] Factors IXa and Xa are neutralized by ATIII and removed by the parenchymal cells of the liver.[94,95] This explains why some of the severest episodes of DIC occurred in patients suffering from hepatic dysfunction.[347,348] Subsequent investigations have demonstrated that factor VIIa remains in the circulation for a relatively long time (half-life is 2.5 hours).[350] Therefore, patients with trauma in whom tissue factor is exposed to the blood may develop intravascular coagulation when factor VIIa is introduced by these concentrates. Newly prepared concentrates appear to be nonthrombogenic because they are almost completely free of activated clotting factors.[351]

Thus, prothrombin complex concentrates should not be given as replacement therapy to patients with DIC, and patients with hepatic dysfunction should receive prothrombin complex concentrates only after their nonthrombogenicity has been established.[352]

Hemangiomas

An association between giant hemangioma and a bleeding tendency was first described by Kasabach and Merritt[353] in 1940. Their 2-month-old patient had purpura, thrombocytopenia, and prolonged bleeding and clotting times, which normalized after regression of the hemangioma by irradiation. The bleeding tendency in this patient was initially attributed to consumption of fibrinogen and platelets because of coagulation and fibrinolysis within the hemangioma.[354,355] Studies using radiolabeled fibrinogen[356–358] and platelets[359–361] subsequently provided evidence for this hypothesis. The stimulus for the intravascular clotting and excessive fibrinolysis[362,363] is apparently related to local activation of the intrinsic coagulation pathway as well as release of large amounts of tPA by the abnormal endothelium lining the tumor vessels.

In addition to the hemostatic defects, patients with giant hemangioma[353–359] described in the early case reports frequently had unexplained anemia. Signs of microangiopathic hemolytic anemia in a patient with giant hemangioma were described in 1966 and attributed to the passage of blood through the abnormal vasculature of the tumor.[360] Soon thereafter, the concomitant occurrence of microangiopathic hemolytic anemia and laboratory signs of DIC was demonstrated in two additional patients with giant hemangiomas.[364,365] This raised the possibility that mechanical damage to the RBCs was inflicted not only by the microangiopathy but also by intravascular fibrin strands elsewhere. Figure 43-7 depicts the blood smear of one patient.[365]

Reviews have indicated that the Kasabach-Merritt syndrome occurs mainly in infants.[366] Accelerated growth of the tumor or its spontaneous involution is associated with augmented or diminished consumption of hemostatic factors. Spontaneous mild to moderate bleeding manifestations have been observed, but severe bleeding generally occurs only after surgery[354]; therefore, extreme caution should be exercised with every invasive procedure.

Signs of DIC have also been associated with other vascular lesions such as the Klippel-Trenaunay syndrome,[367,368] hemangiomas of the liver[369] and the spleen,[370] hemangioendotheliosarcoma,[371] and even Osler's disease.[372]

Effective management of patients with giant hemangiomas, particularly of the Kasabach-Merritt type, includes local irradiation and corticosteroids. Correction of hemostatic abnormalities by heparin has also been achieved by some investigators,[373] but others did not advocate heparin.[358,364]

The administration of ϵ-aminocaproic acid, another rather daring approach to management of giant hemangiomas, was used in an infant and resulted in regression of the giant hemangioma.[358] These authors had observed high levels of tPA and fibrinolytic activity beforehand in blood withdrawn from the tumor vessels. The use of antifibrinolytic agents was revived in the 1980s, and so far several studies have confirmed their beneficial effects. Tumor regression and improvement of hemostatic parameters have been attained by means of aminocaproic acid alone,[362] in combination with cryoprecipitate,[374,375] and with tranexamic acid, a more potent antifibrinolytic agent.[376,377] Recently, correction of hemostatic defects and some tumor regression were also achieved in a patient with Klippel-Trenaunay syndrome.[368]

Inhibition of fibrinolysis appears to permit coagulation of stagnant blood and thrombosis within the tumor, thereby preventing exposure to circulating blood of substantial areas of pathologic endothelium, thus curtailing the activation of clotting and fibrinolysis.

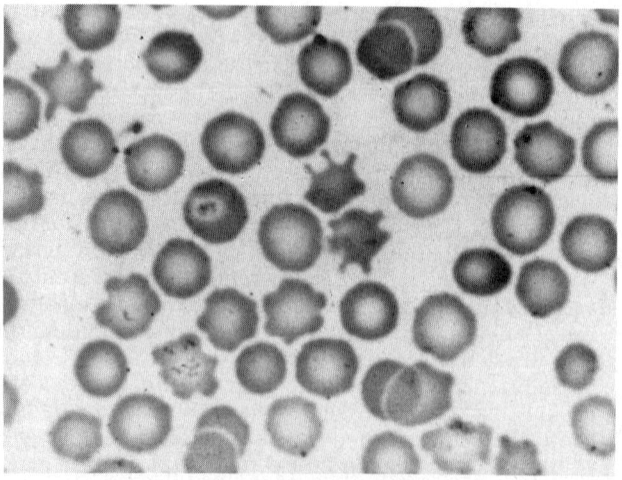

FIGURE 43-7. Appearance of RBCs in blood smear of a 42-year-old patient with giant hemangiomas of the left leg and the right hand, which are associated with chronic disseminated intravascular coagulation.

Aortic Aneurysm

A correlation between aortic aneurysm and DIC was first reported in 1967.[378] The patient experienced sudden extensive dissection of an aortic aneurysm and within several hours developed generalized bleeding; laboratory tests indicated DIC.[378] This association has been well documented since then,[379–385] but although 40% of patients with aortic aneurysm may have elevated levels of fibrin-split products, only 4% have significant bleeding and laboratory evidence of DIC.[383] Nevertheless, clinical and laboratory signs of DIC should be carefully sought in such patients, since bleeding may seriously complicate surgical repair of the aneurysm.[381–383]

Originally, the initiation of localized and generalized intravascular coagulation was ascribed to activation of the intrinsic coagulation pathway by exposure of the blood to collagen and elastin in the dissecting aneurysm.[378] Large amounts of tissue factor have been found in atherosclerotic plaques,[386] and it appears that the extrinsic coagulation pathway is also triggered by the wall of the aneurysm. Localized utilization of radiolabeled fibrinogen[379] and platelets[385] provided direct evidence that clotting takes place within the aneurysm.

Several factors predispose patients with an aortic aneurysm to the development of DIC: a large surface area,[383] dissection,[378] and expansion of the aneurysm.[379]

Heparin should not be given to patients with an aortic aneurysm who have laboratory indications of DIC but do not bleed. Spontaneous correction of the abnormal coagulation tests can take place and is attributed to packing of the aneurysm with blood clots.[379] When the patients present with significant bleeding or when surgery is planned, the hemostatic defects may be corrected by replacement therapy and continuous infusion of heparin.[384] A permanent solution to the problem of DIC associated with an aortic aneurysm can be attained by its surgical resection.

Hemolytic Anemias

Massive hemolysis can, under certain circumstances, be associated with DIC, and DIC can induce hemolysis. These reciprocal effects have been thoroughly investigated.[387] Early studies[40,41] described the strong in vitro and in vivo procoagulant effects of the stroma of RBCs, and a more recent report provided evidence showing that this activity bypasses the contact phase of the intrinsic coagulation system.[388] Conversely, fibrin deposition in the vasculature induced by injections of thrombin or thromboplastin caused intravascular hemolysis.[389,390] Hence, a vicious cycle of DIC causing hemolysis and hemolysis aggravating DIC is thought to develop in certain circumstances.[391] Whether this is operative in the clinical setting as well has not been clarified.[387]

Mismatched Transfusion

Severe bleeding was noted as one of the protean manifestations of incompatible blood transfusion, even in early case reports.[392,393] The bleeding was later related to initiation of DIC, as evidenced by typical laboratory findings[394] and disseminated thrombosis in fatal cases.[1] The trigger of DIC in these cases could not simply be ascribed to the release of RBC stroma, since patients with massive hemolysis due to favism (for example) did not develop DIC.[395] Furthermore, injection of autologous frozen thawed RBCs did not induce any hemostatic abnormalities.[396] Thus, it was suggested that additional triggers of DIC operate when mismatched blood is transfused. Candidates are antigen–antibody reactions and decreased reticuloendothelial system capacity.[395,397]

Microangiopathic Hemolytic Anemia

Hemolytic anemia associated with microangiopathy was first defined in patients with renal failure, disseminated malignancies, and thrombotic thrombocytopenic purpura.[398] The vasculopathy was initially held responsible for the RBC fragmentation and hemolysis, but later the "guillotine effect" of fibrin strands on RBCs was incriminated when intravascular coagulation was present.[399] Fibrin thrombi in the glomerular circulation, thrombocytopenia, and an elevated level of fibrin-split products were observed in infants with the hemolytic uremic syndrome.[400] The consumption of other coagulation factors in these cases is well compensated, since fibrinogen and levels of factors V and VIII are usually normal.[400,401]

RBC fragmentation probably does not promote intravascular coagulation, because a normal decay of radiolabeled fibrinogen was found in patients displaying this form of hemolytic anemia due to malfunctioning prosthetic heart valves.[391]

Consequently, microangiopathic hemolytic anemias and disseminated or localized intravascular coagulation may be initiated by the same disease processes (as in disseminated cancer), but only hemolytic anemia is aggravated by intravascular coagulation and not vice versa.

DISSEMINATED INTRAVASCULAR COAGULATION DURING PREGNANCY

Although the incidence of DIC during pregnancy is low (see Table 43-3), its dramatic occurrence during abruptio placentae and amniotic fluid embolism was responsible for some of the pioneering observations on DIC made by obstetricians. Substantial changes in hemostasis take place during normal pregnancy, and these have a direct bearing on the initiation, diagnosis, and treatment of DIC.

Pregnancy predisposes patients to DIC for two major reasons: (1) a hypercoagulable state manifested by evidence of low-grade thrombin generation, with elevated levels of fibrin monomer complexes and fibrinopeptide A (this is accompanied by increased levels of most coagulation factors[402]); and (2) a reduced fibrinolytic potential due to increased plasma plasminogen activator inhibitor levels and diminished tPA production.[402] The cause of these changes has not been elucidated.

When the diagnosis of DIC is considered in a pregnant patient, the results of the laboratory tests must be interpreted in the light of the foregoing physiologic changes in hemostasis. Thus, normal values of coagulation tests may actually indicate consumption of coagulation factors consistent with DIC. Helpful in this regard is a finding of thrombocytopenia, provided that other causes are excluded. Tests should be repeated several times to detect progressive alterations that confirm (or refute) the diagnosis of DIC.

Several reviews of DIC during pregnancy have been published.[402–404] Following is a discussion of the major entities in which DIC has been reported.

Abruptio Placentae

The dramatic clinical presentation of abruptio placentae was first reported by DeLee[405] in 1901. He described a 35-year-old woman who awoke at night in the seventh month of her fourth pregnancy with severe pain in the abdomen. On examination, she was found to have a hard uterus, profuse vaginal bleeding, and hematoma at injection sites. After extraction of a dead fetus, DeLee found a loose placenta in the uterine cavity and old, dark, firm clots. At that stage, the patient was restless, dyspneic, and pulseless; soon afterward, she died. DeLee noted that the patient had "a history of hemophilia: pains in joints, which were called rheumatic; prolonged hemorrhage when she pricked her finger or from any slight injury," and he wondered whether she was "a bleeder" or had "temporary hemophilia."[405] In retrospect, both conjectures were probably correct, namely, a bleeder (possible von Willebrand's disease) who developed abruptio placentae.

The immediate cause of sudden detachment of the placenta is unknown. Older multiparous women or patients with one of the hypertensive disorders of pregnancy are thought to be at risk.[406] The severe hemostatic failure accompanying abruptio placentae was initially attributed to three causes: excessive consumption of fibrinogen in a retroplacental clot, loss of fibrinogen during bleeding, and diminished synthesis of fibrinogen by the liver.[407] In 1947, it was shown that extracts of placenta possess thromboplastin activity,[408] which was later related to initiation of intravascular coagulation during abruptio placentae.[409] Since then, laboratory evidence of DIC and secondary fibrinolysis has repeatedly been obtained in patients with premature separation of the placenta.[406,410,411] Renal cortical necrosis, probably a consequence of DIC, was observed in 26 of 56 (46%) cases in an earlier series.[407] In a study of 141 patients in whom hypotension and hypovolemia were prevented, severe oliguria developed in only 5 patients.[406]

In two published series, the incidence of abruptio placentae among the total number of deliveries was 0.2%[407] and 0.37%,[406] and 38% of the patients had hypofibrinogenemia.[406] Thus, not all patients with abruptio placentae develop DIC; among those who do, different grades of severity are found with only the more severe forms resulting in shock and fetal death.[402]

Treatment for abruptio placentae consists of rapid volume replenishment and evacuation of the uterus and, when profuse bleeding occurs, transfusion of cryoprecipitate, fresh frozen plasma, and platelet concentrates. In the absence of severe bleeding, administration of blood components may not be necessary, since depleted coagulation factors increase rapidly after delivery.[410]

Therapy with heparin or an antifibrinolytic agent should not be used in patients with abruptio placentae. If the patient has had a cesarean section, administration of low-dose heparin, 5000 U twice daily subcutaneously should be considered to prevent venous thrombosis until she is completely mobile.[412]

Amniotic Fluid Embolism

The catastrophic disorder of amniotic fluid embolism, which may arise during parturition, was reported in 1926[413] but well defined by Steiner and Lushbaugh[414] in 1941. It happens in only 1 in 8000 to 80,000 deliveries but is regarded as a significant cause of maternal death.[415] Patients likely to have amniotic fluid embolism are multiparous women whose pregnancies are postmature with large fetuses and who undergo tumultuous labor after pharmacologic or surgical induction.[414–417] Apparently, amniotic fluid is introduced into the maternal circulation through tears in the chorioamniotic membranes, rupture of the uterus, and injury of uterine veins.[415] In fatal cases, extensive occlusion of the arterial pulmonary vessels by fetal debris, meconium, fat, and other elements of amniotic fluid occurred.[414]

The emboli provoke catastrophic clinical manifestations consisting of sudden dyspnea, cyanosis, acute cor pulmonale, shock, and convulsions followed by severe bleeding within minutes to several hours in 37% of the cases.[415] Hemorrhage is particularly severe from the atonic uterus and from puncture sites, but can also come from the gastrointestinal tract and other organs. Bleeding is caused by initiation of DIC by tissue factor[418–422] and by an activator of factor X,[423,424] both present in amniotic fluid. The mechanical obstruction of pulmonary blood vessels by the particulate matter in the amniotic fluid possibly enhances local fibrin platelet thrombi formation. Excessive fibrinogenolysis is also initiated, probably through direct activation of this system as well as indirectly by the DIC.[425,426]

An extremely high mortality rate (86%) in patients with amniotic fluid embolism was reported in a review of 272 cases.[415] Experience with specific treatment is entirely lacking. The best prospect for decreasing morbidity and mortality lies in early termination of parturition in predisposed patients and in prevention of hypertonic and tetanic uterine contractions during labor. When the syndrome has occurred, recognition in the early stages and immediate institution of vigorous pulmonary and cardiovascular support may save the patient. Insufficient data are available on the possible advantage of treatment by heparin or by antifibrinolytic agents. Platelet concentrates, fresh frozen plasma, and cryoprecipitate are given when bleeding and profound hemostatic impairment have supervened.

Preeclampsia and Eclampsia

Thrombocytopenia was noted in patients with eclampsia in 1922,[427] and widespread deposition of fibrin in blood vessels of the kidneys, liver, and brain was described in fatal cases.[428–431] These findings were interpreted as evidence of DIC,[1,432] triggered by placental thromboplastin, which entered the circulation.[433] More recent data imply that DIC is also related to activation of the intrinsic coagulation pathway.[434,435] Laboratory signs of DIC in preeclampsia and eclampsia were found in some series[432,436–441] but not in others.[442–444] In a large survey of eclamptic patients, 28 of 95 patients had thrombocytopenia, and only 2 of 65 patients had elevated levels of fibrin degradation products.[443] Similarly in another series, only 4 of 79 patients (2 eclamptic and 2 preeclamptic) had signs of DIC.[444] A critical analysis of the literature shows that the evidence for DIC appears relatively weak.[445] The increased consumption of platelets in these patients was suggested to be due to endothelial injury rather than DIC.[445,446]

In contrast, other investigators have provided evidence for significant DIC in preeclampsia and eclampsia. For example, in one study reduced fibrinolytic activity, elevated fibrin degradation products, and thrombocytopenia were reported.[436] In a large series of patients with uncomplicated hypertension, preeclampsia, or eclampsia, a good correlation was found between the severity of the clinical status and deviations in the platelet counts, fibrin degradation products, and reticulocyte counts.[438] Furthermore, results of assays of sensitive parameters of thrombin generation, such as ATIII activity, D-dimer, fibrinopeptide B-1-42, and factor VIII activity, compared with levels of von Willebrand factor, were consistent with findings seen in DIC.[439,441,447] Clearly, these conflicting data and opinions require further investigation and clarification.

Administration of heparin to patients with preeclampsia and eclampsia has not resulted in convincing benefits.[402] Therefore, no specific treatment for the hemostatic derangements can be recommended in these conditions.

HELLP Syndrome

The HELLP syndrome of hemolysis, elevated liver enzymes, low platelet count, and severe epigastric pain was described in 1982 as a complication of pregnancy-induced hypertension during the third trimester of pregnancy.[448] Two considerations led to the implication of DIC in the pathogenesis of this syndrome—liver biopsy findings of fibrin deposition in hepatic blood vessels and hemostatic impairment consistent with consumption coagulopathy.[449] What actually triggers the DIC in these cases is not known, because neither hypertension nor DIC are prerequisites for the HELLP syndrome. For example, the HELLP syndrome has been described in 6 women without hypertension or proteinuria[449]; in another report only 38% of 112 patients had laboratory signs of DIC.[450] In contrast, 18 patients with preeclampsia and HELLP syndrome had DIC and displayed progressive deterioration of hemostatic function, especially during labor.[451] Diffuse organ damage due to DIC may develop in patients with HELLP syndrome. The ensuing severe morbidity leads to a maternal mortality rate of 24% and a perinatal mortality rate of 60%.[450]

Management of patients with HELLP syndrome is controversial.[451] Some authors advocate immediate induction of labor, whereas others prefer to wait until signs of DIC develop to achieve greater fetal maturity.[451] Close clinical and laboratory evaluation of these patients is necessary.

Sepsis

Septicemia is a serious complication of pregnancy frequently accompanied by fulminant DIC. Initially described were the human equivalent of the generalized Shwartzman reaction during pregnancy complicated by endotoxemia[452] and severe DIC associated with septic abortion.[453] Gram-negative bacteria and *Clostridium perfringens* are the more common causes of sepsis encountered during pregnancy. These pathogens gain entry into the circulation during abortion, by the amnionitis that may follow invasive procedures, by the endomyometritis that develops during labor, and by the urinary tract. About 40% of bacteremic patients experience shock, which is fatal in 50% of cases.[402] In addition, a high rate of bleeding and dysfunctions of renal, pulmonary, and central nervous system occur.[402]

As in all cases of sepsis-related DIC, vigorous antibiotic treatment and measures to support impaired organ function should be instituted. If a local nidus of infection is present, surgical intervention such as abortion or even hysterectomy should be considered. Depleted hemostatic components should be replenished by cryoprecipitate, platelet concentrates, and fresh frozen plasma if bleeding is brisk or surgery is contemplated. Administration of heparin reportedly decreases the rate of DIC after septic abortion,[454,455] but controlled trials have not been conducted and definite recommendations cannot be made. It has been my practice and that of others[11] to advocate heparinization together with replacement therapy.

Dead Fetus Syndrome

Within several weeks of intrauterine fetal death, patients may display laboratory signs of DIC occasionally accompanied by bleeding.[456,457] In two clinical studies, the incidence of DIC in patients with the dead fetus syndrome was 18%[457] and 36%.[458] Presumably, thromboplastic materials from the retained dead fetus or placenta slowly enter the maternal circulation and initiate the extrinsic coagulation pathway, which sometimes also results in significant fibrinolysis.[459,460]

After the diagnosis of intrauterine fetal death is established, follow-up of blood coagulation tests is advisable. Fibrinogen level, PT, and a platelet count are the minimal criteria that should be taken into account. Progressive deterioration of these parameters is an indication for immediate evacuation of the uterus. Administration of heparin corrects the hemostatic defect and should be used to prepare patients for induction of labor.[461,462] A continuous heparin infusion at a rate of 1000 IU/h is recommended until normal fibrinogen levels and a normal platelet count are obtained. At this point, administration of heparin is discontinued, and 8 to 12 hours later the uterus is evacuated. When patients present with bleeding or when induction of labor becomes urgent, replacement therapy with cryoprecipitate is useful. Platelet transfusion is rarely needed.

Hypertonic Saline-Induced Abortion

Intraamniotic injection of hypertonic saline to induce abortion in the second trimester of pregnancy was shown to initiate DIC.[463] In most instances, only laboratory indications of DIC were present,[464,465] but significant bleeding did occur in a small percentage of patients.[466,467] Introduction of tissue factor into the maternal circulation, which coincided with the time of fetal death, possibly triggered the DIC.[468] An important factor in the initiation of the DIC was the hypertonicity of the solutions, whether saline, urea, or glucose.[469] After the introduction of prostaglandins E_2 and F_2 for induction of abortion during the second trimester of pregnancy,[469] this form of DIC is rarely seen.

DISSEMINATED INTRAVASCULAR COAGULATION IN NEONATES

Sick neonates frequently present with DIC.[470,471] This probably stems from the impaired capacity of newborns to cope with triggers of DIC; that is, their ability to clear soluble fibrin and activated factors is reduced; their fibrinolytic potential is diminished because of a low plasminogen level; their inhibitor function is decreased because of low levels of ATIII and protein C; and the capacity of their liver to synthesize coagulation factors is limited.[471]

In making the diagnosis of DIC in newborns, physiologic hemostatic deficiencies common at this age should be taken into account. These deficiencies include low levels of the vitamin K-dependent factors, reduced ATIII concentration, and prolonged TT. Therefore, laboratory evidence of DIC in the newborn is based on progressive decline of hemostatic parameters, thrombocytopenia, and reduced levels of fibrinogen, factor V, and factor VIII.[470–472]

The conditions associated with DIC in neonates have been outlined in several clinical series[472–474] and in a study of 201 consecutive autopsies.[56] The most common conditions are hyaline membrane disease (respiratory distress syndrome), asphyxia, sepsis, and necrotizing enterocolitis. More than one underlying cause can usually be identified in newborns with DIC.

The respiratory distress syndrome was originally thought to be due to DIC,[475] but this hypothesis was abandoned when a deficiency in pulmonary surfactant was discovered.[476] Nevertheless, for unknown reasons, DIC may accompany respiratory distress syndrome.[471] In severe cases, clinical and laboratory signs of DIC are common, and confirmatory histopathologic evidence is found.[477–479] A high rate of both intracranial and systemic bleeding occurs when DIC complicates the course of respiratory distress syndrome,[480] so that monitoring of hemostatic parameters is mandatory.

Regarding whether obstetric complications cause DIC in neonates, it has been assumed that placental tissue factor enters the circulation of the newborn during delivery.[471,475,479,481] No direct evidence corroborates this theory. Only a small proportion of obstetric complications (6 of 106) resulted in DIC in the neonate.[479]

Two series have reported a high mortality rate of newborns with DIC, namely, 76%[482] and 83%,[472] but in a later study of 33 intensely treated neonates, 68% survived.[474] Most authorities have not noted any benefit from administration of heparin,[470,472,473,483] although some observed slight improvements in bleeding[484] and in coagulation defects[485] but no influence on survival.[484,485] Likewise, exchange transfusion and infusion of platelet concentrates and plasma were of little help[474] although, in one study, protection against intracerebral bleeding was achieved by replacement therapy.[486] Consequently, vigorous therapeutic measures directed toward the underlying disorder and general support of vital functions are the best means at our disposal to treat neonates with DIC.

CONCLUDING REMARKS

The enormous literature on DIC that has accumulated during the past 30 years reflects the continuous striving of physicians and experimentalists to enlighten the "disseminated international confusion" that surrounds DIC and to improve its grim outlook that "death is coming." Many basic questions remain to be resolved and others are beginning to be clarified.

It is relatively easy to establish the diagnosis of DIC by combining knowledge of the underlying disorders with understanding of its mechanisms, by using simple serial diagnostic tests of blood coagulation, and by exercising good clinical judgment.

The use of advanced methodology, such as determination of D-dimers or ATIII–thrombin complex, has helped in the evaluation of the dynamic mechanisms operating in different forms of DIC; the methods have been useful in defining the state of DIC in individual patients at different points in time. More information is needed before these new methods can be applied routinely, especially in emergency cases.

Regarding the histopathology of DIC, a disturbing and unexplained lack of correlation remains in a substantial number of cases between the clinical and laboratory manifestations and the postmortem findings.

Understanding the pathogenesis of DIC is required for development of more effective means of cure. The main processes that operate in DIC such as initiation, amplification, self-perpetuation, defense, and compensation have been discussed in this chapter and are becoming the targets for development of new treatment modalities. For instance, initiation of DIC by the most common inciting agents—endotoxin and tissue factor—could be aborted by specific monoclonal antibodies; defense mechanisms could be reinforced by administration of recombinant activated protein C and ATIII concentrates; and endogenously produced amplifying agents such as TNF could be blocked either by monoclonal antibodies or by some other mechanisms. None of these sophisticated approaches can replace improved measures for treatment or cure of the basic disorders that cause DIC. A combination of better disease-oriented and better DIC-oriented means conceivably can reduce the present high mortality rate in patients with acute DIC.

Acknowledgments

The author is greatly indebted to Professor Bertha Frisch for her significant comments and suggestions, and to Mrs. Alice Nahum for outstanding secretarial help.

REFERENCES

1. McKay DG. Disseminated intravascular coagulation: an intermediary mechanism of disease. New York, Hoeber Medical Division of Harper & Row, 1965.
2. Hardaway RM. Syndromes of disseminated intravascular coagulation

with special reference to shock and hemorrhage. Springfield, IL, Charles C Thomas, 1966.
3. Mammen EF, Anderson GF, Barnhard MI, eds. Disseminated intravascular coagulation. Thromb Diath Haemorrh 1969;36(Suppl).
4. Minna JD, Robboy SJ, Colman RW. Disseminated intravascular coagulation in man. Springfield, IL, Charles C Thomas, 1974.
5. Bick RL. Disseminated intravascular coagulation and related syndromes. Boca Raton, FL, CRC Press, 1983.
6. Abe T, Yamanaka M, eds. Disseminated intravascular coagulation. Bibl Haematol 1983;49:9.
7. Larcan A, Lambert H, Gerard A. Consumption coagulopathies. New York, Masson Publishing USA, 1987.
8. Rapaport SI. Defibrination syndromes. In: Williams WJ, Beutler E, Erslev AJ, Rundles WR, eds. Hematology, ed 2. New York, McGraw-Hill, 1977: 1454.
9. Wintrobe MM, Lee GR, Boggs DR, et al. Clinical hematology, ed 8. Philadelphia, Lea & Febiger, 1981:1213.
10. Ratnoff OD. Disseminated intravascular coagulation. In: Ratnoff OD, Forbes CD, eds. Disorders of hemostasis. Orlando, Grune & Stratton, 1984:289.
11. Marder VJ, Martin SE, Francis CW, Colman RW. Consumptive thrombohemorrhagic disorders. In: Colman RW, Hirsh J, Marder VJ, Salzman EW, eds. Hemostasis and thrombosis: basic principles and clinical practice, ed 2. Philadelphia, JB Lippincott, 1987:975.
12. Rodriguez-Erdmann F. Bleeding due to increased intravascular blood coagulation: hemorrhagic syndromes caused by consumption of blood-clotting factors (consumption-coagulopathies). N Engl J Med 1965;273: 1370.
13. Verstraete M, Vermylen C, Vermylen J, et al. Excessive consumption of blood coagulation components as cause of hemorrhage diathesis. Am J Med 1965;35:899.
14. Merskey C, Johnson AJ, Kleiner GJ, et al. The defibrination syndrome: clinical features and laboratory diagnosis. Br J Haematol 1967;13:528.
15. Lasch HG, Heene DL, Huth K, Sandritter W. Pathophysiology, clinical manifestations and therapy of consumption-coagulopathy ("Verbrauchskoagulopathie"). Am J Cardiol 1967;20:381.
16. Deykin D. The clinical challenge of disseminated intravascular coagulation. N Engl J Med 1970;283:636.
17. Pitney WR. Disseminated intravascular coagulation. Semin Hematol 1971;8:65.
18. Straub PW. Chronic intravascular coagulation. Acta Med Scand 1971;526(Suppl):1.
19. Owen CA Jr, Bowie EJW. Chronic intravascular coagulation syndromes: a summary. Mayo Clin Proc 1974;49:673.
20. Sharp AA. Diagnosis and management of disseminated intravascular coagulation. Br Med Bull 1977;33:265.
21. Hamilton PJ, Stalker AL, Douglas AS. Disseminated intravascular coagulation: a review. J Clin Pathol 1978;31:609.
22. Colman RW, Robboy SJ, Minna JD. Disseminated intravascular coagulation: a reappraisal. Annu Rev Med 1979;30:359.
23. Bell WR. Disseminated intravascular coagulation. Johns Hopkins Med J 1980;146:289.
24. Feinstein DI. Treatment of disseminated intravascular coagulation. Semin Thromb Hemost 1988;14:351.
25. Muller-Berghaus G. Pathophysiologic and biochemical events in disseminated intravascular coagulation: dysregulation of procoagulant and anticoagulant pathways. Semin Thromb Hemost 1989;15:58.
26. Merskey C, Johnson AJ, Kleiner GJ, et al. The defibrination syndrome: clinical features and laboratory diagnosis. Br J Haematol 1967;13:528.
27. Minna JD, Robboy SJ, Colman RW. Disseminated intravascular coagulation in man. Springfield, IL, Charles C Thomas, 1974:1.
28. Al-Mondhiry H. Disseminated intravascular coagulation: experience in a major cancer center. Thromb Diath Haemorrh 1975;34:181.
29. Siegal T, Seligsohn U, Aghai E, Modan M. Clinical and laboratory aspects of disseminated intravascular coagulation (DIC): a study of 118 cases. Thromb Haemost 1978;39:122.
30. Mant MJ, King EG. Severe, acute disseminated intravascular coagulation: a reappraisal of its pathophysiology, clinical significance and therapy based on 47 patients. Am J Med 1979;67:557.
31. Spero JA, Lewis JH, Hasiba U. Disseminated intravascular coagulation: findings in 346 patients. Thromb Haemost 1980;43:28.
32. Bick RL. Disseminated intravascular coagulation: a clinical/laboratory study of 48 patients. Ann NY Acad Sci 1981;370:843.
33. Matsuda M, Aoki N. Statistics on underlying and causative diseases of DIC in Japan: a cooperative study. In: Abe T, Yamanaka M, eds. Disseminated intravascular coagulation. Basel, S Karger, 1983:15.
34. Tanaka K, Imamura T. Incidence and clinicopathological significance of DIC in autopsy cases. In: Abe T, Yamanaka M, eds. Disseminated intravascular coagulation. Basel, S Karger, 1983:79.
35. Kobayashi N, Maekawa T, Takada M, Tanaka H. Criteria for diagnosis of DIC based on the analysis of clinical and laboratory findings in 345 patients collected by the research committee on DIC in Japan. In: Abe T, Yamanaka M, eds. Disseminated intravascular coagulation. Basel, S Karger, 1983:265.
36. Sharp AA. Diagnosis of disseminated intravascular coagulation. In: Abe T, Yamanaka M, eds. Disseminated intravascular coagulation. Basel, S Karger, 1983:251.
37. Larcan A, Lambert H, Gerard A. Consumption coagulopathies. New York, Masson Publishing, 1987:59.
38. Dupuy M. Injections de matière cérébrale dans les veines. Gaz Med Paris 1834;2:524.
39. Trousseau A. Phlegmation alba dolens. Clin Med Hotel Dieu Paris 1865: 695.
40. Naunyn C. Untersuchungen uber Blutgerinnung im lebeden Tiere und ihre Folgen. Arch Exper Pathol Pharmacol Bd 1, 1873.
41. Wooldridge LC. Note on the relation of the red blood corpuscles to coagulation. Practitioner 1886;38:187.
42. Barratt JOW, York W. The production of general symptoms in haemoglobulinaemia. Br Med J 1914;1:235.
43. Wooldridge LC. Ueber intravasculare Gerinnungen. Arch Anat Physiol Physiol Abt (Leipzig) 1886;397.
44. Lasch HG, Krecke HJ, Rodriguez-Erdman F, Sessner HH, Schutterle G. Verbrauchskoagulopathien (Patogenese und Therapie). Folia Haematol 1961;6:325.
45. Manasse P. Ueber hyaline Ballen und Thromben in den Gehirngefassen bei acuten Infections: Krankheiten. Virchows Arch [A] 1882;130:217.
46. Robboy, SJ, Major MC, Colman RW, Minna JD. Pathology of disseminated intravascular coagulation (DIC): analysis of 26 cases. Hum Pathol 1972;3:327.
47. Kim HS, Suzuki M, Lie JT, Titus JL. Clinically unsuspected disseminated intravascular coagulation (DIC): an autopsy survey. Am J Clin Pathol 1976;66:31.
48. Bleyl U. Morphologic diagnosis of disseminated intravascular coagulation: histologic, histochemical and electronmicroscopic studies. Semin Thromb Hemost 1977;3:247.
49. Mori K, Hizawa K. Histopathological study of disseminated intravascular coagulation: an analysis of 114 autopsy cases. Tokushima J Exp Med 1982;29:47.
50. Watanabe T, Imamura T, Nakagaki K, Tanaka K. Disseminated intravascular coagulation in autopsy cases: its incidence and clinicopathologic significance. Pathol Res Pract 1979;165:311.
51. Shimamura K, Oka K, Nakazawa M, Kojima M. Distribution patterns of microthrombi in disseminated intravascular coagulation. Pathol Lab Med 1983;107:543.
52. Esaki Y, Hirokawa K, Fukazawa T, Matsuda T. Immunohistochemical study on the liver in autopsy cases with disseminated intravascular coagulation (DIC) with reference to clinicopathological analysis. Virchows Arch A 1984;404:229.
53. Wilde JT, Roberts KM, Greaves M, Preston FE. Association between necropsy evidence of disseminated intravascular coagulation and coagulation variables before death in patients in intensive care units. J Clin Pathol 1988;41:138.
54. Siegal A, Siegal T, Seligsohn U. Autopsy findings in 20 cases with disseminated intravascular coagulation. Unpublished data, 1978.
55. Kojima M, Shimamura K, Mori N, et al. A histological study on microthrombi in autopsy cases of DIC. Bibl Haematol 1983;49:95.
56. Dauraku M, Sueishi, Tanaka K. Disseminated intravascular coagulation in newborn infants: prevalence in autopsies and significance as a cause of death. Pathol Res Pract 1982;174:106.
57. Chessells JM, Hardisty RM. Bleeding problems in the newborn infant. Prog Hemost Thromb 1974;2:333.
58. Rohner RF, Prior JT, Sipple JH. Mucinous malignancies, venous thrombosis and terminal endocarditis with emboli: a syndrome. Cancer 1966;19:1805.
59. Kim HS, Suzuki M, Lie JT, Titus JL. Nonbacterial thrombotic endocarditis (NBTE) and disseminated intravascular coagulation (DIC). Arch Pathol Lab Med 1977;101:65.
60. McKay DG, Wahle GH. Disseminated thrombosis in colon cancer. Cancer 1955;8:970.
61. Sugiura M, Hiraoka K, Ohkawa S, et al. A clinico-pathological study on cardiac lesions in 64 cases of disseminated intravascular coagulation. Jpn Heart J 1977;18:57.
62. Kuramoto K, Matsushita S, Yamanouchi H. Nonbacterial thrombotic endocarditis as a cause of cerebral and myocardial infarction. Jpn Circ J 1984;48:1000.
63. Kusama S. Uber Aufbau und Entstehung der toxischen Thrombose und deren Bedeutung. Beitr Z Path Anat Allg Pathol 1913;55:459.
64. Sanarelli G. La pathogénie du choléra: reproduction expérimentale de la maladie. Presse Med 1916;24:505.
65. Shwartzman G. A new phenomenon of local skin reactivity to B. typhosus culture filtrate. Proc Soc Exp Biol Med 1928;25:560.
66. Muller-Berghaus G. Pathophysiologic and biochemical events in disseminated intravascular coagulation: dysregulation of procoagulant and anticoagulant pathways. Semin Thromb Hemost 1989;15:58.
67. Mason JW, Kleeberg U, Dolan P, Colman RW. Plasma kallikrein and Hageman factor in gram-negative bacteremia. Ann Intern Med 1970;73: 545.
68. Colman RW. Contact systems in infectious disease. Rev Infect Dis 1989;11(Suppl 4):S689.
69. Edwards RL, Rickles FR. Macrophage procoagulant. Prog Hemost Thromb 1984;7:183.
70. Nemerson Y. Tissue factor and hemostasis. Blood 1988;71:1.
71. Levy GA, Edgington TS. Lymphocyte cooperation is required for am-

plification of macrophage procoagulant activity. J Exp Med 1980;151:1232.
72. Stern D, Nawroth P, Handley D. An endothelial cell-dependent pathway of coagulation. Proc Natl Acad Sci USA 1985;82:2523.
73. Suffredini AF, Harpel PC, Parrillo JE. Promotion and subsequent inhibition of plasminogen activation after administration of intravenous endotoxin to normal subjects. N Engl J Med 1989;320:1165.
74. Colucci M, Paramo JA, Collen D. Generation in plasma of a fast-acting inhibitor of plasminogen activator in response to endotoxin stimulation. J Clin Invest 1985;75:818.
75. Moore KL, Andreoli SP, Esmon NL, et al. Endotoxin enhances tissue factor and suppresses thrombomodulin expression of human vascular endothelium in vitro. J Clin Invest 1987;79:124.
76. Hawiger J, Hawiger A, Steckley S, et al. Membrane changes in human platelets induced by lipopolysaccharide endotoxin. Br J Haematol 1977;35:285.
77. Bohn E, Muller-Berghaus G. The effect of leukocyte and platelet transfusion on the activation of intravascular coagulation by endotoxin in granulocytopenic and thrombocytopenic rabbits. Am J Pathol 1976;84:239.
78. Nawroth PP, Stern DM. Modulation of endothelial cell hemostatic properties by tumor necrosis factor. J Exp Med 1986;163:740.
79. Bevilacqua MP, Pober JS, Majeau GR, et al. Interleukin-1 (IL-1) induces biosynthesis and cell surface expression of procoagulant activity in human vascular endothelial cells. J Exp Med 1984;160:618.
80. Bagglioni M, Walz A, Kunkel SL. Neutrophil-activating peptide-1/interleukin 8, a novel cytokine that activates neutrophils. J Clin Invest 1989;84:1045.
81. Ford-Hutchinson AW. Leukotrienes: their formation and role as inflammatory mediators. Fed Proc 1985;44:25.
82. Bevilacqua MP, Stengelin S, Gimbrone MA, Seed B. Endothelial leukocyte adhesion molecule 1: an inducible receptor for neutrophils related to complement regulatory proteins and lectins. Science 1989;243:1160.
83. Luscinska FW, Brock AF, Arnaout MA, Gimbrone MA Jr. Endothelial-leukocyte adhesion molecule-1–dependent and leukocyte (CD11/CD18)–dependent mechanisms contribute to polymorphonuclear leukocyte adhesion to cytokine-activated human vascular endothelium. J Immunol 1989;142:2257.
84. Weiss SJ. Tissue destruction by neutrophils. N Engl J Med 1989;320:365.
85. Smedley LA, Tonnensen MG, Sandhaus RA, et al. Neutrophil-mediated injury to endothelial cells: enhancement by endotoxin and essential role of neutrophil elastase. J Clin Invest 1986;77:1233
86. Plow EF. Leucocyte elastase release during blood coagulation: a potential mechanism of the alternative fibrinolytic pathway. J Clin Invest 1981;69:564.
87. Machovich R, Owen WG. An elastase-dependent pathway of plasminogen activation. Biochemistry 1989;28:4517
88. Muller-Berghaus G, Hocke M. Effect of endotoxin on the formation of microthrombi from circulating fibrin monomer complexes in the absence of thrombin generation. Thromb Res 1972;1:541.
89. Rosenberg RD. Biochemistry of heparin antithrombin interactions and the physiologic role of this natural anticoagulant mechanism. Am J Med 1989;87(Suppl 3B):2S.
90. Esmon CT. Regulation of protein C activation by components of the endothelial cell surface. In: Gimbrone MA, ed. Vascular endothelium in hemostasis and thrombosis. Edinburgh, Churchill Livingstone, 1986:99.
91. Leroy-Viard K, Jandrot-Perrus G, Tobelem G, Guillin MC. Covalent binding of human thrombin to a human endothelial cell–associated protein. Exp Cell Res 1989;181:1.
91a. Rapaport SI. The extrinsic pathway inhibitor: a regulator of tissue factor–dependent blood coagulation. Thromb Haemost 1991;66:6.
92. Spaet TH, Horowitz HI, Zucker-Franklin D, et al. Reticuloendothelial clearance of blood thromboplastin by rats. Blood 1961;19:196.
93. Sherman LA, Lee J, Jacobson A. Quantitation of the reticuloendothelial system clearance of soluble fibrin. Br J Haematol 1977;37:231.
94. Deykin D. The role of the liver in serum-induced hypercoagulability. J Clin Invest 1966;45:256.
95. Deykin D, Cochios F, DeCamp G, Lopez A. Hepatic removal of activated factor X by the perfused rabbit liver. Am J Physiol 1968;214:414.
96. Korninger C, Stassen JM, Collen D. Turnover of human extrinsic (tissue-type) plasminogen activator in rabbits. Thromb Haemost 1981;46:658.
97. Hardaway RM. disseminated intravascular coagulation as a possible cause of acute respiratory failure. Surg Gynecol Obstet 1973;137:419.
98. Douglas ME, Downs JB, Dannemiller FJ, Hodges MR. Acute respiratory failure and intravascular coagulation. Surg Gynecol Obstet 1976;143:555.
99. Bone RC, Francis PB, Pierce AK. disseminated intravascular coagulation with the adult respiratory distress syndrome. Am J Med 1976;61:585.
100. Teplitz C. The core pathobiology and integrated medical science of adult acute respiratory insufficiency. Surg Clin North Am 1976;56:1091.
101. Rinaldo JE, Rogers RM. Adult respiratory-distress syndrome: changing concepts of lung injury and repair. N Engl J Med 1982;306:900.
102. Ashbaugh DG, Bigelow DB, Petty TL, Levine BE. Acute respiratory distress in adults. Lancet 1967;2:319.
103. Blaisdell FW, Schlobohm RM. The respiratory distress syndrome: a review. Surgery 1973;74:251.
104. Saldeen T. The microembolism syndrome. Stockholm, Alqvist & Wiksell International, 1979:7.
105. El-Kassimi FA, Al-Mashhadani S, Abdullah AK, Akhtar J. Adult respiratory distress syndrome and disseminated intravascular coagulation complicating heat stroke. Chest 1986;90:571.
106. Craddock PR, Fehr J, Dalmasso AP, et al. Hemodialysis leukopenia: pulmonary vascular leukostasis resulting from complement activation by dialyzer cellophane membrane. J Clin Invest 1977;59:879.
107. Craddock PR, Hammerschmidt DE, White JG, et al. Complement (C5a)-induced granulocyte aggregation in vitro: a possible mechanisms of complement-mediated leukostasis and leukopenia. J Clin Invest 1977;60:260.
108. Cochrane CG, Spragg R, Revak SD. Pathogenesis of the adult respiratory distress syndrome: evidence of oxidant activity in bronchoalveolar lavage fluid. J Clin Invest 1983;71:754.
109. Maunder RJ, Hackman RC, Riff E, et al. Occurrence of the adult respiratory distress syndrome in neutropenic patients. Am Rev Respir Dis 1986;133:313.
110. Carvhalo AC, DeMarinis S, Scott CF, et al. Activation of the contact system of plasma proteolysis in the adult respiratory distress syndrome. J Lab Clin Med 1988;112:270.
111. Barie PS, Malik AB. Role of intravascular coagulation and granulocytes in lung vascular injury after bone marrow embolism. Circ Res 1982;50:830.
112. Malik AB, Johnson A, Tahamont MV, et al. Role of blood components in mediating lung vascular injury after pulmonary vascular thrombosis. Chest 1983;83(Suppl): 21S.
113. Lammle B, Tran TH, Ritz R, Duckert F. Plasma prekallikrein, factor XII, antithrombin III, C_1-inhibitor and alpha-$_2$ macroglobulin in critically ill patients with suspected disseminated intravascular coagulation (DIC). Am J Clin Pathol 1984;82:396.
114. Lane DA, Preston FE, VanRoss ME, Kakkar VV. Characterization of serum fibrinogen and fibrin fragments produced during disseminated intravascular coagulation. Br J Haematol 1978;40:609.
115. Elms MJ, Bunce IH, Bundesen PG, et al. Measurement of cross linked fibrin degradation products: an immunoassay using monoclonal antibodies. Thromb Haemost 1983;50:591.
116. Carr JM, McKinney M, McDonagh J. Diagnosis of disseminated intravascular coagulation: role of D-dimer. Am J Clin Pathol 1989;91:280.
117. Wilde JT, Kitchen S, Kinsey S, et al. Plasma D-dimer levels and their relationship to serum fibrinogen/fibrin degradation products in hypercoagulable states. Br J Haematol 1989;71:65.
118. Tran TH, Lammle B, Duckert F. Factor VIII (procoagulant activity VIII:C, and antigen VIII:CAg, related antigen VIIIR:Ag and ristocetin cofactor: Cof) in intensive care patients with clinically suspected disseminated intravascular coagulation (DIC). Am J Clin Pathol 1984;82:565.
119. Nossel HL. Radioimmunoassay of fibrinopeptides in relation to intravascular coagulation and thrombosis. N Engl J Med 1976;295:428.
120. Hoek JA, Sturk A, ten Cate JW, et al. Laboratory and clinical evaluation of an assay of thrombin-antithrombin III complexes in plasma. Clin Chem 1988;34:2058.
121. Griffin JH, Mosher DF, Zimmerman TS, Kleiss AJ. Protein C, an antithrombotic protein, is reduced in hospitalized patients with intravascular coagulation. Blood 1982;60:261.
122. Mannucci PM, Vigano S. Definition of protein C, an inhibitor of blood coagulation. Lancet 1982;2:463.
123. Francis RB Jr, Thomas W. Behaviour of protein C inhibitor in intravascular coagulation and liver disease. Thromb Haemost 1984;52:71.
124. Marlar RA, Endres-Brooks J, Miller C. Serial studies of protein C and its plasma inhibitor in patients with disseminated intravascular coagulation. Blood 1985;66:59.
125. Heeb MJ, Mosher D, Griffin JH. Activation and complexation of protein C and cleavage and decrease of protein S in plasma of patients with intravascular coagulation. Blood 1989;73:455.
126. D'Angelo A, Vigano-D'Angelo S, Esmon CT, Comp PC. Acquired deficiencies of protein S. Protein S activity during oral anticoagulation, in liver disease, and in disseminated intravascular coagulation. J Clin Invest 1988;81:1445.
127. Tollefsen M, Pestka CA. Heparin cofactor II activity in patients with disseminated intravascular coagulation and hepatic failure. Blood 1985;66:769.
128. Bajaj MS, Rana SV, Wysolmerski RB, Bajaj SP. Inhibitor of the factor VIIa-tissue factor complex is reduced in patients with disseminated intravascular coagulation but not in patients with severe hepatocellular disease. J Clin Invest 1987;79:1874.
129. Warr TA, Rao LVM, Rapaport SI. Human plasma extrinsic pathway inhibitor activity. II. Plasma levels in disseminated intravascular coagulation and hepatocellular disease. Blood 1989;74:994.
130. Cembrowski GS, Griffin JH, Mosher DF. Diagnostic efficacy of six plasma proteins in evaluating consumptive coagulopathies: use of receiver operating characteristic curves to compare antithrombin III, plasminogen, α_2-plasmin inhibitor, fibronectin, prothrombin, and protein C. Arch Intern Med 1986;146:1997.

131. Francis RB Jr, Seyfert U. Tissue plasminogen activator antigen and activity in disseminated intravascular coagulation: clinicopathologic correlations. J Lab Clin Med 1987;110:541.
132. Takahashi H, Hanano M, Takizawa S, et al. Plasmin-alpha 2-plasmin inhibitor complex in plasma of patients with disseminated intravascular coagulation. Am J Hematol 1988;28:162.
133. Wolf PL. The importance of alpha$_2$-antiplasmin in the defibrination syndrome. Arch Intern Med 1989;149:1724.
134. Naeye RL. Thrombotic state after a hemorrhagic diathesis: a possible complication of therapy with epsilon-aminocaproic acid. Blood 1962;19: 694.
135. Gralnick HR, Greipp P. Thrombosis with epsilon aminocaproic acid therapy. Am J Clin Pathol 1971;56:151.
136. Hogg PJ, Jackson CM. Fibrin monomer protects thrombin from inactivation by heparin-antithrombin III: implications for heparin efficacy. Proc Natl Acad Sci USA 1989;86:3619.
137. Jordan RE, Nelson RM, Kilpatrick J, et al. Antithrombin inactivation by neutrophil elastase requires heparin. Am J Med 1989;87(Suppl 3B): 19S.
138. Corrigan JJ, Jordan CM. Heparin therapy in septicemia with disseminated intravascular coagulation. N Engl J Med 1970;283:778.
139. Bell WR, Royall RM. Heparin-associated thrombocytopenia: a comparison of three heparin preparations. N Engl J Med 1980;303:902.
140. King DJ, Kelton JG. Heparin-associated thrombocytopenia. Ann Intern Med 1984;100:535.
141. Kelton JG, Levine MN. Heparin-induced thrombocytopenia. Semin Thromb Hemost 1986;12:59.
142. Thodes GR, Dixon RH, Silver D. Heparin induced thrombocytopenia with thrombotic and hemorrhagic manifestations. Surg Gynecol Obstet 1973;136:409.
143. Klein HG, Bell WR. Disseminated intravascular coagulation during heparin therapy. Ann Intern Med 1974;80:477.
144. Zalckberg JR, Grotl KMc, Dauer R, Wiley JS. Heparin-induced thrombocytopenia with associated disseminated intravascular coagulation. Br J Haematol 1983;54:655.
145. Desmet G, Louwagie A, Criel A, et al. Heparin-induced thrombocytopenia with disseminated intravascular coagulation and white clot syndrome: a case report. Acta Clin Belg 1988;43:419.
146. Feinstein DI. Treatment of disseminated intravascular coagulation. Semin Thromb Hemost 1988;14:351.
147. Schipper HG, Kahle LH, Jenkins CSP, Ten Cate JW. Antithrombin-III transfusion in disseminated intravascular coagulation. Lancet 1978;1: 854.
148. Vinazzer H. Clinical use of antithrombin III concentrates. Vox Sang 1987;53:193.
149. Buller HR, Ten Cate JW. Acquired antithrombin III deficiency: laboratory diagnosis, incidence, clinical implications, and treatment with antithrombin III concentrate. Am J Med 1989;87(Suppl 3B):44S.
150. Blauhut B, Necek S, Vinazzer H, Bergman H. Substitution therapy with an antithrombin III concentrate in shock and DIC. Thromb Res 1982;27:271.
151. Hellgren M, Javelin L, Hagnevik K, et al. Antithrombin III concentrate as adjuvant in DIC treatment: a pilot study in 9 severely ill patients. Thromb Res 1984;35:459.
152. Blauhut B, Kramar H, Vinazzer H, Bergmann H. Substitution of antithrombin III in shock and DIC: a randomized study. Thromb Res 1985;39:81.
153. Buller HR, ten Cate JW. Antithrombin III infusion in patients undergoing peritoneovenous shunt operation: failure in the prevention of disseminated intravascular coagulation. Thromb Haemost 1983;49:128.
154. Maki M, Terao T, Ikenoue T, et al. Clinical evaluation of antithrombin III concentrate (BI 6.013) for disseminated intravascular coagulation in obstetrics: well-controlled multicenter trial. Gynecol Obstet Invest 1987;23:230.
155. Delshammar M, Lasson A, Nilsson IM, et al. Abnormal proteolysis (DIC): successful treatment with antithrombin III concentrate and a concentrate containing factor XIII and native von Willebrand factor. J Intern Med 1989;225:21.
156. Emerson TE Jr, Fournel MA, Redens TB, Taylor FB Jr. Efficacy of antithrombin III supplementation in animal models of fulminant Escherichia Coli endotoxemia or bacteremia. Am J Med 1989;87(Suppl 3B): 27S.
157. Muramatsu M, Fujii S. Inhibitory effects of ω-guanidino acid esters on trypsin, plasmin, plasma kallikrein and thrombin. Biochim Biophys Acta 1972;268:221.
158. Taenaka N, Shimada Y, Hirata T, et al. Gabexate mesilate (FOY) therapy of disseminated intravascular coagulation due to sepsis. Crit Care Med 1983;11:735.
159. Shibata A, Takahashi H, Aoki N, et al. Nafamostat mesilate as a therapy for disseminated intravascular coagulation (DIC): a well-controlled multicenter comparative study. Thromb Haemost 1989;62:371.
160. Takahashi H, Takizawa SI, Tatewaki W, et al. Nafamostat mesilate (FUT-175) in the treatment of patient with disseminated intravascular coagulation. Thromb Haemost 1989;62:372.
161. Taylor FB. Baboon model of E. coli septic shock: staging and observations on the role of the vascular endothelium. In: Fehraman BP, Shoemaker WC, eds. Critical care: state of the art, vol 10. Society of Critical Care Medicine, Fullerton, Fullerton California Publishers, 1989:251.
162. Warr TA, Rao LVM, Rapaport SI. DIC in rabbits induced by administration of endotoxin or tissue factor: effect of antitissue factor antibodies and measurement of plasma extrinsic pathway inhibitor activity. Blood 1990;75:1481.
163. Yoshikawa T, Tanaka KR, Guze LB. Infection and disseminated intravascular coagulation. Medicine 1971;50:237.
164. Bhakdi S, Muhly M, Mannhardt U, et al. Staphylococcal alpha-toxin promotes blood coagulation via attack on human platelets. J Exp Med 1988;168:527.
165. McKay DG, Margaretten W. Disseminated intravascular coagulation in virus diseases. Arch Intern Med 1967;120:129.
166. Viral haemorrhagic fevers. (Editorial) Lancet 1981;2:182.
167. Fisher-Hoch SP. The haemostatic defect in viral haemorrhagic fevers. Br J Haematol 1983;55:565.
168. Whitaker AN. Infection and the spleen: association between hypoplenism, pneumococcal sepsis and disseminated intravascular coagulation. Med J Aust 1969;1:1213.
169. Bisno AL, Freeman JC. The syndrome of asplenia, pneumococcal sepsis, and disseminated intravascular coagulation. Ann Intern Med 1970;72: 389.
170. Neame PB, Kelton JG, Walker IR, et al. Thrombocytopenia in septicemia: the role of disseminated intravascular coagulation. Blood 1980;56:88.
171. Voelcker AF. Report of the pathologist. In: Reports of the medical, surgical and pathological registers. London, The Middlesex Hospital 1894:244.
172. Waterhouse R. A case of suprarenal apoplexy. Lancet 1911;1:576.
173. Friderichsen C. Nebennierenappoplexie bei Kleinen Kindern. Jahrb Kinderh 1978;87:109.
174. Vik-Mo H, Lote K, Nordoy A. Disseminated intravascular coagulation in patients with meningococcal infection: laboratory diagnosis and prognostic factors. Scand J Infect Dis 1978;10:187.
175. Brandtzaeg P, Sandset PM, Joo GB, et al. The quantitative association of plasma endotoxin, antithrombin, protein C, extrinsic pathway inhibitor and fibrinopeptide A in a systemic meningococcal disease. Thromb Res 1989;55:459.
176. Corrigan JJ, Ray WL, May N. Changes in the blood coagulation system associated with septicemia. N Engl J Med 1968;279:851.
177. Rapaport SI, Tatter D, Coeur-Barron N, Hjort PF. Pseudomonas septicemia with intravascular clotting leading to the generalized Shwartzman reaction. N Engl J Med 1964;271:80.
178. Colman RW. Contact systems in infectious disease. Rev Infect Dis 1989;11(Suppl 4):S689.
179. Powell DEB. Non-suppurative lesions in staphylococcal septicaemia. J Pathol Bacteriol 1961;82:141.
180. Murray HW, Tuazon CU, Sheagren JN. Staphylococcal septicemia and disseminated intravascular coagulation. Arch Intern Med 1977;137: 844.
181. Dyggve H. A case of purpura fulminans with fibrinogenopenia in association with scarlatina. Acta Med Scand 1947;127:382.
182. Ratnoff OD, Nebehay WG. Multiple coagulative defects in a patient with Waterhouse-Friderichsen syndrome. Ann Intern Med 1962;56: 627.
183. Stossel TP, Levy R. Intravascular coagulation associated with pneumococcal bacteremia and symmetrical peripheral gangrene. Arch Intern Med 1970;125:876.
184. Rytel MW, Dee TH, Ferstenfeld JE, Hensley GT. Possible pathogenetic role of capsular antigens in fulminant pneumocóccal disease with disseminated intravascular coagulation (DIC). Am J Med 1974;57:889.
185. Hawley HB, Yamada T, Mosher DF, et al. Disseminated intravascular coagulopathy during experimental pneumococcal sepsis: studies in normal and asplenic monkeys. J Med Primatol 1977;6:203.
186. Philippidis P, Naiman JL, Sibinga MS, Valdes-Dapnea MA. disseminated intravascular coagulation in Candida albicans septicemia. J Pediatr 1971;78:683.
187. Falla A, Talavera-Terceco I, Rapkin RH. Candida sepsis in disseminated intravascular coagulation in a postoperative infant. Clin Pediatr 1975;14: 294.
188. Mavligit GM, Binder RA, Crosby WH. Disseminated intravascular in military tuberculosis. Arch Intern Med 1972;130:388.
189. Dennis LH, Eichenberger JW, Inman MM, Conrad ME. Depletion of coagulation factors in drug-resistant *Plasmodium falciparum* malaria. Blood 1967;29:713.
190. Vreeken J, Cremer-Goote TM. Haemostatic defect in non-immune patients with falciparum malaria: no evidence of diffuse intravascular coagulation. Br Med J 1978;2:533.
191. Henoch E. Ueber Purpura fulminans. Berl Klin Wochenschr 1887;24: 8.
192. Hjort PF, Rapaport SI, Jorgensen L. Purpura ulminans: report of a case successfully treated with heparin and hydrocortisone—review of 50 cases from the literature. Scand J Haematol 1964;1:169.
193. Spicer TE, Ran IM. Purpura fulminans. Am J Med 1976;61:566.
194. Tishler M, Abramov AL, Seligsohn U, Kahn Y. Purpura fulminans in an adult. Isr J Med Sci 1986;22:820.
195. Branson HE, Katz J, Marble R, Griffin JH. Inherited protein C deficiency

and a coumarin-responsive chronic relapsing purpura fulminans syndrome in a newborn infant. Lancet 1983;2:1156.
196. Seligsohn U, Berger A, Abend M, et al. Homozygous protein C deficiency manifested by massive venous thrombosis in the newborn. N Engl J Med 1984;310:559.
197. Marciniak E. Wilson D, Marlar RA. Neonatal purpura fulminans: a genetic disorder related to the absence of protein C in blood. Blood 1985;65:15.
198. Little JR. Purpura fulminans treated successfully with anticoagulation: report of a case. JAMA 1959;169:104.
199. Antley RM, McMillan CW. Sequential coagulation studies in purpura fulminans. N Engl J Med 1967;276:1287.
200. Sack GH Jr, Levin J, Bell WR. Trousseau's syndrome and other manifestations of chronic disseminated coagulopathy in patients with neoplasms: clinical, pathophysiologic, and therapeutic features. Medicine 1977;56:1.
201. Rickles FR, Edwards RL. Activation of blood coagulation in cancer: Trousseau's syndrome revisited. Blood 1983;62:14.
202. Donati MB, Davidson JF, Garattini S. Malignancy and the hemostatic system. New York, Raven Press, 1981.
203. Goldsmith GH. Hemostatic disorders associated with neoplasia. In: Ratnoff OD, Forbes CD, eds. Disorders of hemostasis. Orlando, Grune & Stratton, 1984:351.
204. Jurgens R, Trautwein H. Uber Fibrinopenie (Fibrinogenopenie) beim Erwaschsenen, nebst Bemerkungen uber die Herkunft des Fibrinogens. Deutsch Arch Klin Med 1930;169:28.
205. Jarcho S. Diffusely infiltrative carcinoma: a hitherto undescribed correlation of several varieties of tumor metastasis. Arch Pathol 1936;22: 674.
206. Collins RC, Al-Mondhiry H, Chernik NL, et al. Neurologic manifestations of intravascular coagulation in cancer: a clinicopathologic analysis of 12 cases. Neurology 1975;25:795.
207. Owen CA Jr, Bowie EJW. Chronic intravascular coagulation syndromes: a summary. Mayo Clin Proc 1974;49:673.
208. Bell WR, Starksen NF, Tong S, Porterfield JK. Trousseau's syndrome: devastating coagulopathy in the absence of heparin. Am J Med 1985;79: 423.
209. Lawrence EA, Bowman DE, Moore DB, Bernstein GI. A thromboplastic property of neoplasms. Surg Forum 1952;3:694.
210. O'Meara RAQ. Coagulative properties of cancers. Irish J Med Sci 1958;394:474.
211. Eiseman G, Stefanini M. Thromboplastic activity of leukemic white cells. Proc Soc Exp Biol Med 1954;86:763.
212. Gordon SG, Cross BA. A factor X–activating cysteine protease from malignant tissue. J Clin Invest 1981;67:1665.
213. Pineo GF, Regoeczi E, Hatton MWC, Brain MC. The activation of coagulation by extracts of mucus: a possible pathway of intravascular coagulation accompanying adenocarcinomas. J Lab Clin Med 1973;82: 255.
214. Edwards RL, Rickles FR, Cronlund M. Abnormalities of blood coagulation in patients with cancer: mononuclear cell tissue factor generation. J Lab Clin Med 1981;98:917.
215. Boneu A, Armand JP, Blasco A, et al. Demi-vie du fibrinogene marque à l'iode 131 chez les cancéreux: effets de l'heparine. Nouv Presse Med 1976;5:415.
216. Tagnon HJ, Whitmore WF, Shulman NR. Fibrinolysis in metastatic cancer of the prostate. Cancer 1952;5:9.
217. Huggins C, Vail VC. Plasma coagulation and fibrinogenolysis by prostatic fluid and trypsin. Am J Physiol 1943;139:129.
218. Joseph RR, Day HJ, Sherwin RM, Schwartz HG. Microangiopathic haemolytic anaemia associated with consumption coagulopathy in a patient with disseminated carcinoma. Scand J Haematol 1967;4:271.
219. Lynch EC, Bakken CL, Casey TH, Alfrey CP Jr. Microangiopathic hemolytic anaemia in carcinoma of the stomach. Gastroenterology 1967;52:88.
220. Seligsohn U, Weber H, Yoran C, et al. Microangiopathic hemolytic anemia and defibrination syndrome in metastatic carcinoma of the stomach. Isr J Med Sci 1968;4:69.
221. Brain MC, Azzopardi JG, Baker LRI, et al. Microangiopathic haemolytic anaemia and mucin-forming adenocarcinoma. Br J Haematol 1970;18: 183.
222. Risak E. Die Fibrinopenie. Zeitschr Klin Med 1935;128:606.
223. Bunjevacki PG, Sultan Y, Izrael V. Coagulation intravasculaire disséminée et fibrinolysée au cours des leucémies aigues. Nouv Rev Fr Hematol 1978;20:575.
224. Hillestad LK. Acute promyelocytic leukemia. Acta Med Scand 1957;159: 189.
225. Gralnick HR, Sultan C. Acute promyelocytic leukaemia: haemorrhagic manifestation and morphologic criteria. Br J Haematol 1975;29:373.
226. Goldberg MA, Ginsburg D, Mayer RJ, et al. Is heparin administration necessary during induction chemotherapy for patients with acute promyelocytic leukemia? Blood 1987;69:187.
227. Quigley HJ. Peripheral leukocyte thromboplastin in promyelocytic leukemia. (Abstract) Fed Proc 1967;26:648.
228. Heilmann-Gouault M, Varet B, Romano C, Josso F. Activité "thromboplastique" des leucocytes "in vitro" et coagulation intravasculaire au cours des leucémies. Pathol Biol 1972;20(Suppl 56).
229. Gralnick HR, Abrell E. Studies of the procoagulant and fibrinolytic activity of promyelocytes in acute promyelocytic leukaemia. Br J Haematol 1973;24:89.
230. Andoh K, Kubota T, Takada M, et al. Tissue factor activity in leukemia cells: special reference to disseminated intravascular coagulation. Cancer 1987;59:748.
231. Heilmann-Gouault M, Chardon E, Sultan C, Josso F. The procoagulant factor of leukaemic promyelocytes: demonstration of immunologic cross reactivity with human brain tissue factor. Br J Haematol 1975;30: 151.
232. Pittman GR, Senhauser DA, Lowney JF. Acute promyelocytic leukemia: a report of 3 autopsied cases. Am J Clin Pathol 1966;46:214.
233. Polliak A. Acute promyelocytic leukemia with disseminated intravascular coagulation. Am J Clin Pathol 1971;56:155.
234. Gralnick HR, Tan HK. Acute promyelocytic leukemia: a model for understanding the role of the malignant cell in hemostasis. Hum Pathol 1974;5:661.
235. Sandler RM, Liebman HA, Patch MJ, et al. Antithrombin III and antiactivated factor X activity in patients with acute promyelocytic leukemia and disseminated intravascular coagulation treated with heparin. Cancer 1982;50:2106.
236. Bauer KA, Rosenberg RD. Thrombin generation in acute promyelocytic leukemia. Blood 1984;64:791.
237. Drapkin RL, Gee TS, Dowling MD, et al. Prophylactic heparin therapy in acute promyelocytic leukemia. Cancer 1978;41:2484.
238. Avvisati G, Ten Cate JW, Buller HR, Mandelli F. Tranexamic acid for control of haemorrhage in acute promyelocytic leukemia. Lancet 1989;2:122.
239. Kahle LH, Avvisati G, Lamping RJ, et al. Turnover of alpha-2-antiplasmin in patients with acute promyelocytic leukemia. Scand J Clin Lab Invest 1985;178(Suppl 45):75.
240. Schwartz BS, Williams EC, Conlan MG, Mosher DF. Epsilon-aminocaproic acid in the treatment of patients with acute promyelocytic leukemia and acquired alpha-2-plasmin inhibitor deficiency. Ann Intern Med 1986;105:873.
241. Matsuda T, Asakura H, Ito K, et al. Changes in levels of t-PA and $alpha_2$ PI-plasmin complex in plasma in patients with DIC. Thromb Res 1988;8(Suppl):143.
242. Williams EC. Plasma $alpha_2$-antiplasmin activity: role in the evaluation and management of fibrinolytic states and other bleeding disorders. Arch Intern Med 1989;149:1769.
243. Keane TJ, Gorman AM, O'Connell LG, Fennelly JJ. Epsilon amino caproic acid in the management of acute promyelocytic leukemia. Acta Haematol 1976;56:202.
244. Bergentz SE, Nilsson IM. Effect of trauma on coagulation and fibrinolysis in dogs. Acta Chir Scand 1961;122:21.
245. Innes D, Sevitt S. Coagulation and fibrinolysis in injured patients. J Clin Pathol 1964;17:1.
246. McGehee WG, Rapaport SI. Systemic hemostatic failure in the severely injured patient. Surg Clin North Am 1968;48:1247.
247. McKay DG. Trauma and disseminated intravascular coagulation. J Trauma 1969;9:646.
248. Attar S, Boyd D, Layne E, et al. Alteration in coagulation and fibrinolytic mechanisms in acute trauma. J Trauma 1969;9:939.
249. Simmons RL, Collins JA, Heisterkamp CA, et al. Coagulation disorders in combat casualties. I. Acute changes after wounding. II. Effect of massive transfusion. III. Post-resuscitative changes. Ann Surg 1969;169: 455.
250. Ordog GJ, Wasserberger J, Balasubramanium S. Coagulation abnormalities in traumatic shock. Ann Emerg Med 1985;14:560.
251. Bone RC, Francis PB, Pierce AK. Intravascular coagulation associated with the adult respiratory syndrome. Am J Med 1976;61:585.
252. Blaisdell FW, Lim RC Jr, Amberg JR, et al. Pulmonary microembolism: a cause of morbidity and death after major vascular surgery. Arch Surg 1966;93:776.
253. Zenker FA. Beitrage zur normalen und pathologischen Anatomie der Lungen. Dresden, Braunsdorf, 1862.
254. Herndon JH, Riseborough EJ, Fischer JE. Fat embolism: a review of current concepts. J Trauma 1971;11:673.
255. Peltier LF. The diagnosis and treatment of fat embolism. J Trauma 1971;11:661.
256. McB Curtis A, Knowles GD, Putman CE, et al. The three syndromes of fat embolism: pulmonary manifestations. Yale J Biol Med 1979;52: 149.
257. McGehee WG, Rapaport SI. Systemic hemostatic failure in the severely injured patients. Surg Clin North Am 1968;48:1247.
258. Goodnight SH, Kenover G, Rapaport SI, et al. Defibrination after brain-tissue destruction: a serious complication of head injury. N Engl J Med 1974;290:1043.
259. Druskin MS, Drijansky R. Afibrinogenemia with severe head trauma. JAMA 1972;219:755.
260. Keimovitz RM, Annis BL. Disseminated intravascular coagulation associated with massive brain injury. J Neurosurg 1973;39:178.
261. Pondaag W. Disseminated intravascular coagulation related to outcome in head injury. Acta Neurochir 1979;28(Suppl):98.
262. Disseminated intravascular coagulation. Lancet Editorial 1982;2:531.
263. Miner ME, Kaufman HH, Graham SH, et al. Disseminated intravascular

coagulation fibrinolytic syndrome following head injury in children: frequency and prognostic implications. Pediatrics 1982;100:687.
264. Kaufman HH, Hui KS, Mattson JC, et al. Clinicopathological correlations of disseminated intravascular coagulation in patients with head injury. Neurosurgery 1984;15:34.
265. Kumura E, Sato M, Fukuda A, et al. Coagulation disorders following acute head injury. Acta Neurochir 1987;85:23.
266. Olson JD, Kaufman HH, Moake J, et al. The incidence and significance of hemostatic abnormalities in patients with head injuries. Neurosurgery 1989;24:825.
267. Gehrke CF, Penner JA, Niederhuber J, et al. Coagulation defects in burned patients. Surg Gynecol Obstet 1971;133:613.
268. McManus WF, Eurenius K, Pruitt BA. Disseminated intravascular coagulation in burned patients. J Trauma 1973;13:416.
269. Simon TL, Curreri PW, Harker LA. Kinetic characterization of hemostasis in thermal injury. J Lab Clin Med 1977;82:702.
270. Elrod PD, McCleery RS, Ball COT. An experimental study of the effect of heparin on survival time following lethal burns. Surg Gynecol Obstet 1951;92:35.
271. Johansson SA. Heparin and some coagulation factors in experimental burn injuries. Acta Chir Scand 1964;127:346.
272. Saliba MJ Jr. Heparin efficacy in burns. II. Human thermal burn treatment with large doses of topical and parenteral heparin. Aerospace Med 1970;41:1302.
273. Saliba MJ Jr, Dempsey WC, Kruggel JL. Large burns in humans: treatment with heparin. JAMA 1973;225:261.
274. Curreri PW, Wilterdink ME, Baxter CR. Coagulation dynamics following thermal injury: effect of heparin and protamine sulfate. Ann Surg 1975;181:161.
275. Deykin D, Chun R, Lopez A, Silversmith P. The role of the liver in serum-induced hypercoagulability. J Clin Invest 1966;45:256.
276. Fletcher AP, Biederman O, Moore D, et al. Abnormal plasminogen-plasmin system activity (fibrinolysis) in patients with hepatic cirrhosis: its cause and consequences. J Clin Invest 1964;43:681.
277. Bloom AL. Intravascular coagulation and the liver. Br J Haematol 1975;30:1.
278. Carr JM. Disseminated intravascular coagulation in cirrhosis. Hepatology 1989;10:103.
279. Tytgat GN, Collen D, Verstraete M. Metabolism of fibrinogen in cirrhosis of the liver. J Clin Invest 1971;50:1690.
280. Coleman M, Finlayson N, Bettigole RE, et al. Fibrinogen survival in cirrhosis: improvement by low dose heparin. Ann Intern Med 1975;83:79.
281. Tytgat GN, Piessens J, Collen D, De Groote J. Experience with exchange transfusion in the treatment of hepatic coma. Digestion 1968;1:257.
282. Rake MO, Pannell G, Flute PT, Williams R. Intravascular coagulation in acute hepatic necrosis. Lancet 1970;1:533.
283. Carr JM, McKinney M, McDonagh J. Diagnosis of DIC: role of D-dimer. Am J Clin Pathol 1989;91:280.
284. Coccheri S, Mannucci PM, Palaret G., et al. Significance of plasma fibrinopeptide A and high molecular weight fibrinogen in patients with liver cirrhosis. Br J Haematol 1982;52:503.
285. Oka K, Tanaka K. Intravascular coagulation in autopsy cases with liver diseases. Thromb Haemost 1979;42:564.
286. Palascak JE, Martinez J. Dysfibrinogenemia associated with liver disease. J Clin Invest 1977;60:89.
287. Corrigan JJ, Bennett BB, Bueffel B. The value of factor VIII levels in acquired hypofibrinogenemia. Am J Clin Pathol 1973;60:897.
288. Straub PW. Diffuse intravascular coagulation in liver disease? Semin Thrombos Hemost 1977;4:29.
289. Canoso RT, Hutton RA, Deykin D. The hemostatic defect of chronic liver disease: kinetic studies using ^{75}Se-seleno methionine. Gastroenterology 1979;76:540.
290. Tempero MA, Davis RB, Reed E, Edney J. Thrombocytopenia and laboratory evidence of disseminated intravascular coagulation after shunts for ascites in malignant disease. Cancer 1985;55:2718.
291. Bauer KA, Rosenberg RD. Thrombin generation in acute promyelocytic leukemia. Blood 1984;64:791.
292. Teitel JM, Bauer KA, Lau HK, et al. Studies of the prothrombin activation pathway utilizing radioimmunoassay for the F_2/F_{1+2} fragment and thrombin-antithrombin complex. Blood 1982;59:1086.
293. Kasper CK. Postoperative thromboses in hemophilia B. N Engl J Med 1973;289:160.
294. Hillenbrand P, Parbhoo SP, Jedrychowski A, Sherlock S. Significance of intravascular coagulation and fibrinolysis in acute hepatic failure. Scand J Gastroenterol 1973;19(Suppl 8):133.
295. Gazzard BG, Clark R, Borirakchanavat V, et al. A controlled trial of heparin therapy in the coagulation defect of paracetamol-induced hepatic necrosis. Gut 1974;15:89.
296. Lerner RG, Nelson JC, Corines P, et al. Intravascular coagulation complicating peritoneal-atrial shunts. Blood 1977;1(Suppl 50):274.
297. Phillips LL, Rodgers JB. Procoagulant activity of ascitic fluid in hepatic cirrhosis: in vivo and in vitro. Surgery 1979;86:714.
298. Salem HH, Koutts J, Handley C, et al. The aggregation of human platelets by ascitic fluid: a possible mechanism for disseminated intravascular coagulation complicating LeVeen shunts. Am J Hematol 1981;11:153.
299. Ragni MV, Lewis JH, Spero JA. Ascites-induced LeVeen shunt coagulopathy. Ann Surg 1983;198:91.
300. LeVeen HH, Wapnick S, Grosberg S, Kinney MU. Further experience with peritoneo-venous shunt for ascites. Ann Surg 1976;184:574.
301. Gibson PR, Dudley FJ, Jakobovits AW, et al. Disseminated intravascular coagulation following peritoneo-venous (LeVeen) shunt. Aust NZ J Med 1981;11:8.
302. Stein SF, Fulenwider JT, Ansley JD, et al. Accelerated fibrinogen and platelet destruction after peritoneovenous shunting. Arch Intern Med 1981;141:1149.
303. Rubinstein D, McInnes I, Dudley F. Morbidity and mortality after peritoneovenous shunt surgery for refractory ascites. Gut 1985;26:1070.
304. Matsehe JW, Beart RW, Bartholomew LG, Baldus WP. Fatal disseminated intravascular coagulation after peritoneovenous shunt for intractable ascites. Mayo Clin Proc 1978;53:526.
305. Buller HR, ten Cate JW. Antithrombin III infusion in patients undergoing peritoneovenous shunt operation: failure in the prevention of disseminated intravascular coagulation. Thromb Haemost 1983;49:128.
306. Salem HH, Dudley FJ, Merrett A, et al. Coagulopathy of peritoneovenous shunts: studies on the pathogenic role of ascitic fluid collagen and value of anti-platelet therapy. Gut 1983;24:412.
307. Shibolet S, Coll R, Gilat T, et al. Heatstroke: its clinical picture and mechanism in 36 cases. Quart J Med 1967;36:525.
308. Shibolet S, Lancaster MC, Danon Y. Heat stroke: a review. Aviat Space Environ Med 1976;47:280.
309. Wakefield EG, Hall WW. Heat injuries: a preparatory study for experimental heat stroke. JAMA 1927;89:92.
310. Gauss, Meyer KA. Heat stroke: report of one hundred and fifty-eight cases from Cook County Hospital, Chicago. Am J Med Sci 1917;154:554.
311. Malamud N, Haymaker W, Custer RP. Heat stroke: a clinicopathology study of 125 fatal cases. Milit Surg 1946;99:397.
312. Wright DO, Reppert LB, Cuttino JT. Purpuric manifestations of heatstroke: studies of prothrombin and platelets in twelve cases. Arch Intern Med 1946;77:27.
313. Hart GR, Anderson RJ, Crumpler CP, et al. Epidemic classical heat stroke: clinical characteristics and course of 28 patients. Medicine 1982;61:189.
314. Mustafa KY, Omer O, Khogali M, et al. Blood coagulation and fibrinolysis in heat stroke. Br J Haematol 1985;61:517.
315. Wilson SJ, Doan CA. The pathogenesis of hemorrhage in artificially induced fever. Ann Intern Med 1939;13:1214.
316. Meikle AW, Graybill JR. Fibrinolysis and hemorrhage in a fatal case of heat stroke. N Engl J Med 1967;276:911.
317. Shibolet S, Fisher S, Gilat T, Bank H, Heller H. Fibrinolysis and hemorrhages in fatal heatstroke. N Engl J Med 1962;266:169.
318. Gottschalk PG, Thomas JE. Heat stroke. Mayo Clin Proc 1966;41:470.
319. Rosenthal T, Shapiro Y, Seligsohn U, Ramot B. Disseminated intravascular coagulation in experimental heatstroke. Thromb Diath Haemorrh 1971;26:417.
320. Chao TC, Sinniah R, Pakiam JE. Acute heat stroke deaths. Pathology 1981;13:145.
321. Sohal RS, Sun SC, Colcolough HL, et al. Heat stroke: an electron microscopy study of endothelial cell damage and disseminated intravascular coagulation. Arch Intern Med 1968;122:43.
322. Beard MEJ, Hickton CM. Haemostasis in heat stroke. Br J Haematol 1982;52:269.
323. Weber MB, Blakely JA. The haemorrhagic diathesis of heatstroke: a consumption coagulopathy successfully treated with heparin. Lancet 1969;1:1190.
324. Cornell CJ, Fein SH, Reilly B, Cornwell GG. Heparin therapy for heat stroke. Ann Intern Med 1974;81:702.
325. Perschick JS, Winkelstein A, Shadduck RK. Disseminated intravascular coagulation in heat stroke. JAMA 1975;231:480.
326. Knochel JP. Disseminated intravascular coagulation in heat stroke: response to heparin therapy. JAMA 1975;231:496.
327. Shibolet S, Farfel Z. Heparin therapy for heatstroke. Ann Intern Med 1975;82:857.
328. De Vries A, Cohen I. Hemorrhagic and blood coagulation disturbing action of snake venoms. In: Poller L, ed. Recent advances in blood coagulation. London, JA Churchill, 1969:277.
329. Efrati P. Snake venoms and blood coagulation. In: Chen-Yuan Lee, ed. Snake venoms. Berlin, Springer-Verlag, 1979:956.
330. Russell FE. Snake venoms and blood coagulation. In: Chen-Yuan Lee, ed. Snake venoms. Berlin, Springer-Verlag,1979:978.
331. Seegers WH, Ouyang C. Snake venoms and blood coagulation. In: Chen-Yuan Lee, ed. Snake venoms. Berlin, Springer-Verlag, 1979:684.
332. Reid HA. Clinical hemostatic disorders caused by venoms. In: Ratnoff OD, Forbes CD, eds. Disorders of hemostasis. Orlando, Grune & Stratton, 1984.
333. Geoffroy EF, Hunauld I. Mémoire dans lequel on examine si l'huile d'olive est un specifique contre la morsure de vipères. Paris 1737, quoted by M. Phisalix in Les animaux venimeux et les venins. Paris, Masson Publishing, 1922.
334. Fontana F. Treatise on the venom of the viper. London, 1787.
335. Martin CJ. On some effects upon the blood produced by the injection of the venom of the Australian black snake. J Physiol 1893;15:380.

336. Phisalix C. Venin et coagulabilitéè du sang chez la vipère. CR Soc Biol (Paris) 1899;51:834.
337. Didisheim P, Lewis JH. Fibrinolytic and coagulant activities of certain snake venoms and proteases. Proc Soc Exp Biol Med 1956;93:10.
338. Nahas L, Denson KWE, MacFarlane RG. A study of the coagulant action of eight snake venoms. Thromb Diath Haemorrh 1964;12:355.
339. Markland FS, Kettner C, Schiffman S, et al. Kallikrein-like activity of crotalase: a snake venom enzyme that clots fibrinogen. Proc Natl Acad Sci USA 1982;79:1688.
340. Huang TF, Holt JC, Lukasiwicz H, Niewiarowski S. Trigramin: a low molecular weight peptide inhibiting fibrinogen interaction with platelet receptors expressed on glycoprotein IIb-IIIa complex. J Biol Chem 1987;262:16157.
341. Klein JD, Walker FJ. Purification of a protein C activator from the venom of the Southern copperhead snake (*Agkistrodon contortrix*). Biochemistry 1986;25:4175.
342. Schulchynska-Castel H, Dvilansky A, Keynan A. *Echis colorata* bites: clinical evaluation of 42 patients: a retrospective study. Isr J Med Sci 1986;22:880.
343. Weiss HJ, Phillips LL, Hopewell WS, et al. Heparin therapy in a patient bitten by a saw-scaled viper (*Echis carinatus*): a snake whose venom activates prothrombin. Am J Med 1973;54:653.
344. Fainaru M, Eisenberg S, Manny N, Hershko C. The natural course of defibrination syndrome caused by *Echis colorata* venom in man. Thromb Diath Haemorrh 1974;31:420.
345. Warrell DA, Pope HM, Prentice CRM. Disseminated intravascular coagulation caused by the carpet viper (*Echis carinatus*): trial of heparin. Br J Haematol 1976;33:335.
346. Triantaphyllopoulos DC. Intravascular coagulation following injection of prothrombin complex. Am J Clin Pathol 1972;57:603.
347. Blatt PM, Lundblad, RL, Kingdon HS, et al. Thrombogenic materials in prothrombin complex concentrates. Ann Intern Med 1974;81:766.
348. Cederbaum AI, Blatt PM, Roberts HR. Intravascular coagulation with use of human prothrombin complex concentrates. Ann Intern Med 1976;84:683.
349. Hultin MB. Activated clotting factors in factor IX concentrates. Blood 1979;54:1028.
350. Seligsohn U, Kasper CK, Osterud B, Rapaport SI. Activated factor VII: presence in factor IX concentrate and persistence in the circulation after infusion. Blood 1979;53:828.
351. Menache D, Behre HE, Orthner CL, et al. Coagulation factor IX concentrate: method of preparation and assessment of potential in vivo thrombogenicity in animal models. Blood 1984;64:1220.
352. Bick RL, Schmalhorst WR, Fekete L. Disseminated intravascular coagulation and blood component therapy. Transfusion 1976;16:361.
353. Kasabach HH, Merritt KK. Capillary hemangioma with extensive purpura. Am J Dis Child 1940;59:1063.
354. Gilon E, Ramot B, Sheba C. Multiple hemangiomata associated with thrombocytopenia: remarks on the pathogenesis of the thrombocytopenia in this syndrome. Blood 1958;14:74.
355. Beller FK, Rhurmann G. Zur Pathogenese des Kasabach-Meritt-Syndroms (Riesenhamangiom, Blutungen, Thrombopenie und Afibrinogenamie). Klin Wochenschr 1959;37:1078.
356. Blix S, Aas K. Giant hemangioma, thrombocytopenia, fibrinogenopenia, and fibrinolytic activity. Acta Med Scand 1961;169:63.
357. Straub PW, Kessler S, Schreiber A, Frick PG. Chronic intravascular coagulation in Kasabach-Merritt syndrome: preferential accumulation of fibrinogen ^{131}I in a giant hemangioma. Arch Intern Med 1972;129: 475.
358. Henriksson P, Nilsson IM, Bergentz SE, et al. Giant haemangioma with disorder of coagulation. Acta Paediat Scand 1971;60:227.
359. Brizel HE, Raccuglia G. Giant hemangioma with thrombocytopenia: radioisotopic demonstration of platelet sequestration. Blood 1965;26: 751.
360. Propp RP, Scharfman WB. Hemangioma-thrombocytopenia syndrome associated with microangiopathic hemolytic anemia. Blood 1966;28: 623.
361. Warrell RP, Kempin SJ, Benua RS, et al. Intra-tumoral consumption of Indium-111 labeled platelets in a patient with hemangiomatosis and intravascular coagulation (Kasabach-Merritt syndrome). Cancer 1983;52:2256.
362. Neidhart JA, Roach RW. Successful treatment of skeletal hemangioma and Kasabach-Merritt syndrome with aminocaproic acid: is fibrinolysis "defensive?" Am J Med 1982;73:434.
363. Henriksson RP, Nilsson IM, Bergentry SE, Ljungqvist U, Rosengren B. Giant hemangioma with a disorder of coagulation. Acta Paediatr Scand 1971;60:227.
364. Inceman S, Tangun Y. Chronic defibrination syndrome due to a giant hemangioma associated with microangiopathic hemolytic anemia. Am J Med 1969;46:997.
365. Seligsohn U, Ramot B. Angiopathic hemolytic anemias: report of 5 cases and review of the literature. J Isr Med Assoc 1968;74:39.
366. El Dessouky M, Azmy AF, Raine PA, Young DG. Kasabach-Merritt syndrome. J Pediatr Surg USA 1988;23:109.
367. D'Amico JA, Hoffman GC, Dyment PG. Klippel-Trenaunay syndrome associated with chronic disseminated intravascular coagulation and massive osteolysis. Clev Clin Q 1977;44:181.
368. Poon MC, Kloiber R, Birdsell DC. Epsilon-aminocaproic acid in the reversal of consumptive coagulopathy with platelet sequestration in a vascular malformation of Klippel-Trenaunay syndrome. Am J Med 1989;87:211.
369. Alpert LI, Benesch B. Hemangioendothelioma of the liver associated with microangiopathic hemolytic anemia. Am J Med 1970;48:624.
370. Shanberge JH, Tanaka K, Gruhl MC. Chronic consumption coagulopathy due to hemangiomatous transformation of the spleen. Am J Clin Pathol 1971;56:723.
371. Blix S, Jacobsen CD. The defibrination syndrome in a patient with hemangio-endothelio-sarcoma. Acta Med Scand 1963;173:377.
372. Bick RL. Hereditary hemorrhagic telangiectasia and disseminated intravascular coagulation: a new clinical syndrome. Ann NY Acad Sci 1981;370:851.
373. Hagerman LJ, Czapek EE, Donnellan WL, Schwartz AD. Giant hemangioma with consumption coagulopathy. J Pediatr 1975;87:766.
374. Warrell RP, Kempin SJ. Treatment of severe coagulopathy in the Kasabach-Merritt syndrome with aminocaproic acid and cryoprecipitate. N Engl J Med 1985;313:309.
375. Ortel TL, Onorato JJ, Bedrosian CL, Kaufman RE. Antifibrinolytic therapy in the management of the Kasabach-Merritt syndrome. Am J Hematol 1988;29:44.
376. Bell AJ, Chisholm M, Hickton M. Reversal of coagulopathy in Kasabach-Merritt syndrome with tranexamic acid. Scand J Haematol 1986;37: 249.
377. Hanna BD, Bernstein M. Tranexamic acid in the treatment of Kasabach-Merritt syndrome in infants. Am J Pediatr Hematol Oncol 1989;11:191.
378. Fine NL, Applebaum J, Elguezabal A, Castleman L. Multiple coagulation defects in association with dissecting aneurysm. Arch Intern Med 1967;119:522.
379. Straub PW, Kessler S. Umsatz und lokalisation von I^{131}-Fibrinogen bei chronischer intravasaler Gerinnung. Schweiz Med Wochenschr 1970;100:2001.
380. Bieger R, Vreeken J, Stibbe J, Loeliger EA. Arterial aneurysm as a cause of consumption coagulopathy. N Engl J Med 1971;285:152.
381. Ten Cate JW, Timmers H, Becker AE. Coagulopathy in ruptured or dissecting aortic aneurysm. Am J Med 1975;59:171.
382. Mulcare RJ, Royster TS, Phillips LL. Intravascular coagulation in surgical procedures on the abdominal aorta. Surg Gynecol Obstet 1976;143: 730.
383. Fisher DF, Yawn DH, Crawford S. Preoperative disseminated intravascular coagulation associated with aortic aneurysms. Arch Surg 1983;118:1252.
384. Goto H, Kimoto A, Kawaguchi H, et al. Surgical treatment of abdominal aortic aneurysm complicated with chronic disseminated intravascular coagulopathy. J Cardiovasc Surg 1985;26:280.
385. Mukaiyama H, Shionoya S, Ikezawa T, et al. Abdominal aortic aneurysm complicated with chronic disseminated intravascular coagulopathy: a case of surgical treatment. J Vasc Surg 1987;6:600.
386. Wilcox JN, Smith KM, Schwartz SM, Gordon D. Localization of tissue factor in the normal vessel wall and in the atherosclerotic plaque. Proc Natl Acad Sci USA 1989;86:2839.
387. Surgenor DM. Erythrocytes and blood coagulation. Thromb Diath Haemorrh 1974;32:247.
388. Quick AJ, Georgatsos JG, Hussey CV. The clotting activity of human erythrocytes: theoretical and clinical implications. Am J Med 1954;228: 207.
389. Brain MC, Esterly JR, Beck EA. Intravascular haemolysis with experimentally produced vascular thrombi. Br J Haematol 1967;13:868.
390. Rubenberg ML, Regoeczi E, Bull BS, et al. Microangiopathic haemolytic anaemia: the experimental production of haemolysis and red-cell fragmentation by defibrination in vivo. Br J Haematol 1968;14:627.
391. Baker LRI, Rubenberg ML, Dacie JV, Brain MC. Fibrinogen catabolism in microangiopathic haemolytic anaemia. Br J Haematol 1968;14:617.
392. Drinker CK, Brittingham HH. The cause of the reactions following transfusion of citrated blood. Arch Intern Med 1919;23:133.
393. Astrowe PS. Hemolysis following transfusion. JAMA 1923;79:1511.
394. Krevans JR, Jackson DP, Conley CL, Hartman RC. The nature of the hemorrhagic disorder accompanying hemolytic transfusion reactions in man. Blood 1957;12:834.
395. Mannucci PM, Lobina GF, Caocci L, Dioguardi N. Effect on blood coagulation of massive intravascular haemolysis. Blood 1969;33:207.
396. Spector JI, Crosby WH. Coagulation studies during experimental hemoglobinemia in humans. J Appl Physiol 1975;38:195.
397. Rabiner SF, Friedman LH. The role of intravascular haemolysis and the reticulo-endothelial system in the production of a hypercoagulable state. Br J Haematol 1968;14:105.
398. Brain MC, Dacie JV, Hourihane DO'B. Microangiopathic haemolytic anaemia: the possible role of vascular lesions in pathogenesis. Br J Haematol 1962;8:358.
399. Bull BS, Rubenberg ML, Dacie JV, Brain MC. Microangiopathic haemolytic anemia: mechanisms of red cell fragmentation: in vitro studies. Br J Haematol 1968;14.643.
400. Katz J, Lurie A, Kaplan BS, et al. Coagulation findings in the hemolytic-uremic syndrome of infancy: similarity to hyperacute renal allograft rejection. J Pediatr 1971;78:426.

401. Avalos JS, Vitacco M, Molinas F, et al. Coagulation studies in the hemolytic-uremic syndrome. J Pediatr 1970;76:538.
402. Von Hugo R, Graeff H. Thrombohemorrhagic complications in the obstetric patient. In: Colman RW, Hirsh J, Marder VJ, Salzman EW, eds. Hemostasis and thrombosis: basic principles and clinical practice. Philadelphia, JB Lippincott, 1987:926.
403. Graeff H, Kuhn W, eds. Coagulation disorders in obstetrics: pathobiochemistry, pathophysiology, diagnosis, treatment. Stuttgart, Georg Thieme Verlag, 1980.
404. Weiner CP. The obstetric patient and disseminated intravascular coagulation. Clin Perinatol 1986;13:705.
405. DeLee JB. A case of fatal hemorrhagic diathesis, with premature detachment of the placenta. Am J Obstet Gynecol 1901;44:785.
406. Pritchard JA, Brekken AL. Clinical and laboratory studies on severe abruptio placentae. Am J Obstet Gynecol 1967;97:681.
407. Dieckmann WJ. Blood chemistry and renal function in abruptio placentae. Am J Obstet Gynecol 1936;31:734.
408. Schneider CL. The active principle of placental toxin: thromboplastin: its inactivator in blood: antithromboplastin. Am J Physiol 1947;149:123.
409. Schneider CL. Fibrin embolism (disseminated intravascular coagulation) with defibrination as one of the end results during abruptio. Surg Gynecol Obstet 1951;92:27.
410. Kleiner GJ, Merskey C, Johnson AJ, Markus WB. Defibrination in normal and abnormal parturition. Br J Haematol 1970;19:159.
411. Basu HK. Fibrinolysis and abruptio placentae. J Obstet Gynecol Br Commonw 1969;76:481.
412. Beller FK, Uszynski M. Disseminated intravascular coagulation in pregnancy. Clin Obstet Gynecol 1974;17:250.
413. Meyer JR. Embolic pulmonar amnio-caseosa. Brazil Med 1926;2:301.
414. Steiner PE, Lushbaugh CC. Maternal pulmonary embolism by amniotic fluid as a cause of obstetric shock and unexpected deaths in obstetrics. JAMA 1941;117:1245, 1340.
415. Morgan M. Amniotic fluid embolism. Anaesthesia 1979;34:20.
416. Anderson DG. Amniotic fluid embolism: a re-evaluation. Am J Obstet Gynecol 1967;98:336.
417. Peterson EP, Taylor HB. Amniotic fluid embolism: an analysis of 40 cases. Obstet Gynecol 1970;35:787.
418. Weiner AE, Reid DE, Roby CC. The hemostatic activity of amniotic fluid. Science NY 1949;110:190.
419. Weiner AE, Reid DE. The pathogenesis of amniotic fluid embolism. III. Coagulant activity of amniotic fluid. N Engl J Med 1950;243:597.
420. Ratnoff OD, Vosburgh GJ. Observations on the clotting defect in amniotic fluid embolism. N Engl J Med 1952;247:970.
421. Attwood HD, Downing ES. Experimental amniotic fluid and meconium embolism. Surg Gynec Obstet 1965;120:255.
422. Yaffe H, Eldor A, Hornshtein E, Sadovsky E. Thromboplastic activity in amniotic fluid during pregnancy. Obstet Gynecol 1977;50:454.
423. Lang Phillips L, Davidson EC. Procoagulant properties of amniotic fluid. Am J Obstet Gynecol 1972;113:911.
424. Courtney LD, Allington M. Effect of amniotic fluid on blood coagulation. Br J Haematol 1972;22:353.
425. Alberchtsen OK, Storm O, Trolle D. Fibrinolytic activity in the circulating blood following amniotic fluid infusion. Acta Haematol 1955;14:309.
426. Beller FK, Douglas GW, Debrovner CH, Robinson R. The fibrinolytic system in amniotic fluid embolism. Am J Obstet Gynecol 1963;87:48.
427. Stahnke E. Uber das Verhalten der Blutplattchen bei Eklampsie. Zentralbl Gynak 1922;46:391.
428. McKay DG, Merrill SJ, Weiner AE, et al. The pathologic anatomy of eclampsia, bilateral renal cortical necrosis, pituitary necrosis, and other acute fatal complications of pregnancy, and its possible relationship to the generalized Schwartzman phenomenon. Am J Obstet Gynecol 1953;66:507.
429. Govan ADT. Renal changes in eclampsia. J Pathol 1954;67:311.
430. Vassali P, Morris RH, McClusky RT. The pathogenesis role of fibrin deposition in the glomerular lesions of toxemia of pregnancy. J Exp Med 1963;118:467.
431. Morris RH, Vassali P, Beller FK, et al. Immunofluorescent studies on renal biopsies in the diagnosis of toxemia of pregnancy. Obstet Gynecol 1964;24:32.
432. McKay DG. Chronic intravascular coagulation in normal pregnancy and pre-eclampsia. Contrib Nephrol 1981;25:108.
433. Page EW. On the pathogenesis of pre-eclampsia and eclampsia. J Obstet Gynecol Br Commonw 1972;79:883.
434. Vasiri ND, Toohey J, Powers D, et al. Activation of intrinsic coagulation pathway in pre-eclampsia. Am J Med 1986;8:103.
435. Hayakawa M, Maki M. Coagulation-fibrinolytic and Kinin-forming systems in toxemia of pregnancy. Gynecol Obstet Invest 1988;26:181.
436. Bonnar J, McNicol GP, Douglas AS. Coagulation and fibrinolytic systems in pre-eclampsia and eclampsia. Br Med J 1971;2:12.
437. McKay DG. Hematologic evidence of disseminated intravascular coagulation in eclampsia. Obstet Gynecol Surv 1972;27:399.
438. Giles C. Intravascular coagulation in gestational hypertension and pre-eclampsia: the value of haematological screening tests. Clin Lab Haematol 1982;4:351.
439. Borok Z, Weitz J, Owen J, et al. Fibrinogen proteolysis and platelet alpha granule release in pre-eclampsia/eclampsia. Blood 1984;63:525.
440. Friedman KD, Borok Z, Owen J. Heparin cofactor activity and antithrombin III antigen levels in pre-eclampsia. Thromb Res 1986;43:409.
441. Kobayashi T, Terao T. Preeclampsia as chronic disseminated intravascular coagulation: study of two parameters thrombin-antithrombin III complex and D-dimers. Gynecol Obstet Invest 1987;24:170.
442. Sher G, Davey DA, Ogilvie M, Jacobs P. Pregnancy, pre-eclampsia and disseminated intravascular coagulation. S Afr Med J 1975;49:1197.
443. Pritchard JA, Cunningham FG, Mason RA. Coagulation changes in eclampsia: their frequency and pathogenesis. Am J Obstet Gynecol 1976;124:855.
444. Roberts JM, May WJ. Consumptive coagulopathy in severe preeclampsia. Obstet Gynecol 1976;48:163.
445. Gibson B, Hunter D, Neame PB, Kelton JG. Thrombocytopenia in pre-eclampsia and eclampsia. Semin Thromb Hemost 1982;8:234.
446. Rakoczi I, Tallian F, Bagdani S, Gati I. Platelet life span in normal pregnancy and pre-eclampsia as determined by a non-radioisotopic technique. Thromb Res 1979;15:553.
447. Redman CWG, Denson KWE, Beilin LJ, et al. Factor VIII consumption in pre-eclampsia. Lancet 1977;2:1249.
448. Weinstein L. Syndrome of hemolysis, elevated liver enzymes, and low platelet count: a severe consequence of hypertension in pregnancy. Am J Obstet Gynecol 1982;142:159.
449. Aarnoudse JG, Houthoff HJ, Weits J, Vellenga E, Huisjes HJ. A syndrome of liver damage and intravascular coagulation in the last trimester of normotensive pregnancy: a clinical and histopathological study. Br J Obstet Gynaecol 1986;93:145.
450. Sibai BM, Taslimi MM, El-Naser A, et al. Maternal-perinatal outcome associated with the syndrome of hemolysis, elevated liver enzymes, and low platelets in severe pre-eclampsia-eclampsia. Am J Obstet Gynecol 1986;155:501.
451. Van Dam PA, Renier M, Baekelandt M, et al. Disseminated intravascular coagulation and the syndrome of hemolysis, elevated liver enzymes, and low platelets in severe pre-eclampsia. Obstet Gynecol 1989;73:97.
452. McKay DC, Jewett JF, Reid DE. Endotoxin shock and the generalized Shwartzman reaction in pregnancy. Am J Obstet Gyecol 1959;78:546.
453. Pfau von P, Lasch HG, Gunther O. Sanarelli-Shwartzman-Phaenomen bei febrilen Fehlgeburten und schweren Schock- und Blutungs-zustanden in der Geburtshilfe. Gynaecologia 1960;150:17.
454. Kuhn W, Graeff H. Infizierter Abort und disseminierte intravaskulare Gerinnung (DIG). Med Welt 1971;22:1199.
455. Koch HH, Keller O. Unsere Erfahrungen mit den prophylaktischen Massnahmen zur Verhinderung des Sanarelli-Shwartzman Phanomen (SSP) beim infizierten Abort. Geburtsh Frauenheilk 1973;33:460.
456. Weiner AE, Reid DE, Roby CC, Diamond LK. Coagulation defects with intrauterine death from Rh isosensitization. Am J Obstet Gynecol 1950;60:1015.
457. Pritchard JA, Ratnoff OD. Studies of fibrinogen and other hemostatic factors in women with intrauterine death and delayed delivery. Surg Gynecol Obstet 1955;101:467.
458. Pritchard JA. Fetal death in utero. Obstet Gynecol 1959;14:573.
459. Pritchard JA. Treatment of the defibrination syndromes of pregnancy. Mod Treat 1968;5:401.
460. Nossel HL, Niemetz J, Waxman SA, et al. Defibrination syndrome in a patient with chronic thrombocytopenic purpura. Am J Med 1969;46:591.
461. Lerner R, Margolin M, Slate WG, et al. Heparin in the treatment of hypofibrinogenemia complicating fetal death in utero. Am J Obstet Gynecol 1967;97:373.
462. Gallup DG, Lucas WE. Heparin treatment of consumption coagulopathy associated with intrauterine fetal death. Obstet Gynecol 1970;35:690.
463. Stander RW, Flessa HC, Glueck HI, et al. Changes in maternal coagulation factors after intra-amniotic injection of hypertonic saline. Obstet Gynecol 1971;37:660.
464. Spivak JL, Spangler DB, Bell WR. Defibrinogenation after intra-amniotic injection of hypertonic saline. N Engl J Med 1972;287:321.
465. Nossel HL, Wasser J, Kaplan KL, et al. Sequence of fibrinogen proteolysis and platelet release after intrauterine infusion of hypertonic saline. J Clin Invest 1979;64:1371.
466. Schwartz R, Greston W, Kleiner JG. Defibrination in saline abortion. Obstet Gynecol 1972;40:728.
467. Brown FD, Davidson EC, Phillips F, Phillips LL. Coagulation changes after hypertonic saline infusion for late abortions. Obstet Gynecol 1972;39:538.
468. Glueck H, Flessa H, Kisker CT, Stander R. Iatrogenic disseminated intravascular coagulation in patients, aborted with intraamniotic saline, correlated with time of fetal death. Abstracts Third Congress Thromb Haemost 1972;324.
469. McKenzie IZ, Sayers L, Bonnar J, Hillier K. Coagulation changes during second-trimester abortion induced by intra-amniotic prostaglandin E2 and hypertonic solutions. Lancet 1975;2:1066.
470. Hathaway WE, Mull MM, Peschet GS. Disseminated intravascular coagulation in the newborn. Pediatrics 1969;43:233.
471. Corrigan JJ Jr. Activation of coagulation and disseminated intravascular coagulation in the newborn. Am J Pediatr Hematol Oncol 1979;1:245.
472. Woods WG, Corman Luban NL, et al. Disseminated intravascular coagulation in the newborn. Am J Dis Child 1979;133:44.
473. Corrigan JJ. Disseminated intravascular coagulopathy. Pediatr Rev 1979;1:37.

474. Gross SJ, Filston HC, Anderson JC. Controlled study of treatment for disseminated intravascular coagulation in the neonate. J Pediatr 1982;100:445.
475. Stark CR, Abramson D, Erkan V. Intravascular coagulation and hyaline-membrane disease of the newborn. Lancet 1968;1:1180.
476. Hallman M, Gluck L. Respiratory distress syndrome: update 1982. Pediatr Clin North Am 1982;29:1057.
477. Alstatt LB, Dennis LH, Sundell H, et al. Disseminated intravascular coagulation and hyaline membrane disease. Biol Neonate 1971;19:227.
478. Markarian M, Githens JH, Rosenblut E, et al. Hypercoagulability in premature infants with special reference to the respiratory distress syndrome and hemorrhage. I. Coagulation studies. Biol Neonate 1971;17:84.
479. Hathaway WE, Mahasandana C, Makowski EL. Cord blood coagulation studies in infants of high-risk pregnant women. Am J Obstet Gynecol 1975;121:51.
480. McDonald MM, Johnson ML, Rumack CM, et al. Role of coagulopathy in newborn intracranial hemorrhage. Pediatrics 1984;74:26.
481. Boyd JF. Two possible cases of acquired hypofibrinogenemia in the newborns. Surg Gynecol Obstet 1958;106:176.
482. Whaun JM, Oski FA. Experience with disseminated intravascular coagulation in a children's hospital. Can Med Assoc J 1972;107:963.
483. Margolis CZ, Orzalesi MM, Schwartz AD. Disseminated intravascular coagulation in the respiratory distress syndrome. Am J Dis Child 1973;125:324.
484. Markarian M, Lubchenko LO, Rosenblut E, et al. Hypercoagulability in premature infants with special reference to the respiratory distress syndrome and hemorrhage. II. The effect of heparin. Biol Neonate 1971;17:98.
485. Gobel U, von Voss H, Jurgens H, et al. Efficiency of heparin in the treatment of newborn infants with respiratory distress syndrome and disseminated intravascular coagulation. Eur J Pediatr 1980;133:47.
486. Turner T, Prowse CV, Prescott RJ, et al. A clinical trial on the early detection and correction of haemostatic defects in selected high-risk neonates. Br J Haematol 1981;47:65.

Blood: Principles and Practice of Hematology,
edited by Robert I. Handin, Samuel E. Lux, and Thomas P. Stossel.
J.B. Lippincott Company, Philadelphia © 1995.

44

Natural Anticoagulants and the Prethrombotic State

Kenneth A. Bauer

The coagulation cascade is composed of a series of linked proteolytic reactions. In each reaction, a parent zymogen is converted to a corresponding serine protease that is responsible for a subsequent zymogen-serine protease transition. In most instances, protein cofactors are present that can be activated by serine proteases; they then possess the ability to bind the above reactants to specific cell surfaces. This process usually leads to a dramatic acceleration, as well as a partial localization, of the reactions. The result of these transformations is the generation of thrombin, which is able to act on fibrinogen and platelets to produce the hemostatic plug.

For coagulation-system enzymes to be generated at a significant rate, a zymogen, a cofactor, and a converting enzyme must form a multimolecular complex on a natural surface. These transformations are suppressed if the converting enzyme is inhibited, the protein cofactor is destroyed, or the surface receptors essential for the assembly of the macromolecular complex are sequestered. During the past two decades, considerable effort has been devoted to investigating several natural anticoagulant mechanisms that are able to exert damping effects on each step of the coagulation cascade via the mechanisms outlined above.[1,2] Two of these are the heparan sulfate–antithrombin III (ATIII) and protein C–thrombomodulin–protein S mechanisms (Fig. 44-1), which regulate the serine proteases and the activated cofactors, respectively. The biochemistry and physiology of these endogenous anticoagulant systems, in addition to an inhibitory mechanism for the factor VIIa–tissue factor complex, is described first. Then an approach to the diagnosis and management of the hypercoagulable patient is presented.

NATURAL ANTICOAGULANT MECHANISMS

Heparan Sulfate–Antithrombin III

Antithrombin III is a plasma glycoprotein of 58 kd. The complete primary structure of this protease inhibitor was first determined using protein chemical techniques; it is a single polypeptide chain composed of 432 amino acids.[3] Several investigators subsequently cloned cDNAs that code for ATIII.[4–6] ATIII neutralizes the activity of thrombin as well as other serine proteases of the coagulation cascade, including factors Xa, IXa, XIa, and XIIa, by forming a stoichiometric complex between enzyme and inhibitor via an arginine-active center on the inhibitor and the active-site serine on the enzyme.[7–13] Bjork and collaborators[14] provided evidence that the arginine reactive site of the protease inhibitor is located near the carboxy terminal end of this protein at Arg 393→Ser 394. Complex formation between hemostatic enzymes and ATIII occurs at a relatively slow rate in the absence of heparin. When heparin is present, however, it binds to lysyl residues on ATIII and dramatically accelerates the rate of complex formation.[9] The heparin-induced acceleration is due to an allosteric alteration in the position of the critical arginine residue that places it in a more favorable position to interact with thrombin.[14] Several groups of researchers[15,16] have shown that modification of Trp 49 prevents ATIII from binding to heparin-Sepharose. The altered protein is able to neutralize thrombin in a normal manner in the absence of heparin, but this interaction cannot be catalyzed by the addition of the mucopolysaccharide. Quantitative binding studies with ATIII that contains this Trp 49 modification suggest that this residue lies close to, but not within, the major binding region of the protease inhibitor.[17] It is likely to be involved in a conformational transition of the protein that is required for mucopolysaccharide-dependent acceleration of complex formation, however.

The heparin molecule possesses multiple functional domains that are responsible for accelerating interactions between coagulation serine proteases and ATIII.[18,19] The ATIII-binding site on this mucopolysaccharide consists of a unique sequence of sulfated and nonsulfated monosaccharide units.[20–22]

In 1973, Rosenberg and colleagues[11] suggested that the nonthrombogenic properties of blood vessels may be due, in part, to the presence of heparin-like species with anticoagulant activity on the vascular endothelium. The early studies of two groups of investigators[23,24] demonstrated that heparan sulfate, a heparin-like species with increased amounts of nonsulfated glucuronic acid and N-acetylated ester sulfated glucosamine residues, is found within the aorta and has trace amounts of anticoagulant activity. Subsequently, the manner by which this component expresses

Supported in part by National Institutes of Health Grant PO1 HL 33014 and the Medical Research Service of the Department of Veterans Affairs. Dr. Bauer is a recipient of an Established Investigatorship from the American Heart Association.

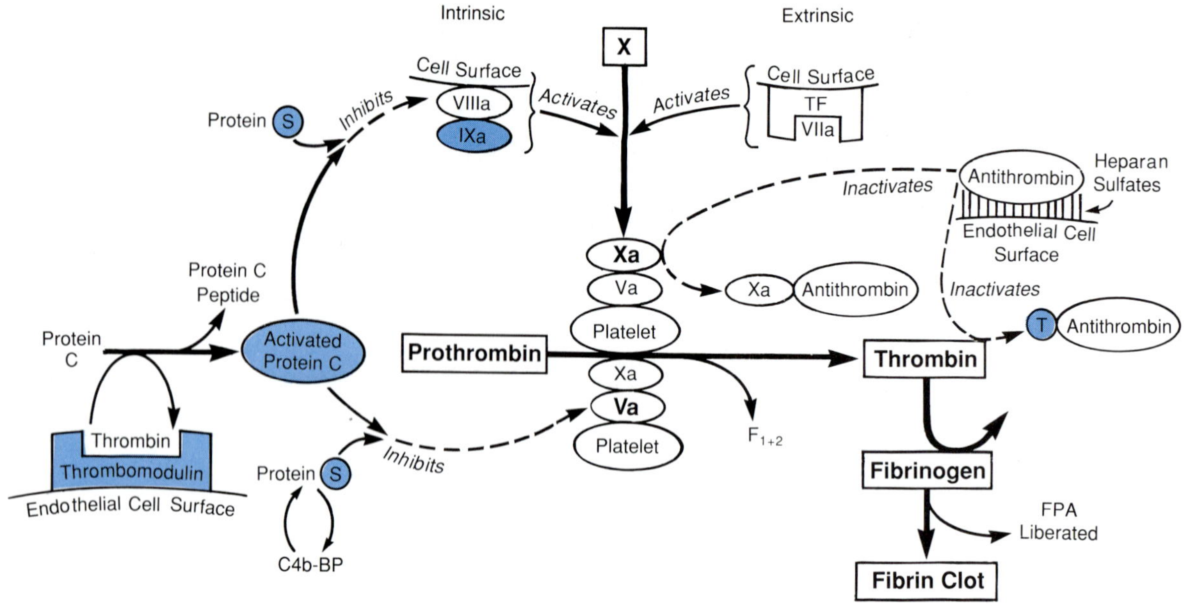

FIGURE 44-1. Schematic depiction of pathways that generate factor Xa and thrombin and of the natural anticoagulant mechanisms that regulate the activity of these enzymes.

Factor X can be activated by the extrinsic pathway (factor VIIa–tissue factor [TF]) or the intrinsic pathway (factor IXa/VIIIa–activated cell-surface complex). Factor Xa binds to factor Va on activated platelets and mediates the conversion of prothrombin to thrombin under physiologic conditions. During this process, the inactive F_{1+2} fragment is released from the amino terminus of prothrombin. Thrombin is then able to act on fibrinogen to form a fibrin clot; the initial step in this conversion results in the liberation of fibrinopeptide A (FPA).

Thrombin and factor Xa are inactivated by antithrombin III bound to heparan sulfate molecules associated with the vascular endothelium. This results in formation of factor Xa–antithrombin III and thrombin–antithrombin III complexes. Protein C is activated by thrombin bound to the endothelial cell receptor thrombomodulin, releasing a small peptide of about 1.4 kd. Quantification of protein C activation in humans has been accomplished by devising a radioimmunoassay for this protein C–activation peptide. Once evolved, activated protein C functions as a potent anticoagulant by inactivating factors VIIIa and Va. Protein S enhances the binding of activated protein C to phospholipid-containing membranes and accelerates the inactivation of factors VIIIa and Va. The complement component, C4b-binding protein (C4b-BP), forms complexes with protein S, which results in a reduction of its functional activity.

biologic activity and its location within vascular tissue was studied in detail.[25–31]

Heparin-like molecules were initially extracted from calf cerebral microvessels and aortae. Only a small portion of the heparan sulfate from the microvasculature (about 0.3%) accelerated the neutralization of hemostatic enzymes by ATIII. These moieties contained the critical monosaccharide sequences required for enhancing the activity of the protease inhibitor toward thrombin as well as factor Xa. But because mast cells beneath the endothelium are also able to synthesize anticoagulantly active mucopolysaccharides, mast cell free retinal microvessels were isolated. These preparations contained proteoglycans that function as an anticoagulant in a manner virtually identical to commercial heparin.[26] Next, to prove that endothelial cells are able to synthesize heparin-like molecules with anticoagulant activity, heparan sulfates were extracted from cloned endothelial cells.[27,28] The purified endothelial mucopolysaccharides contained the critical tetrasaccharide present in commercial heparin. Finally, the physiologic function of the endogenous heparan sulfate–ATIII mechanism was demonstrated using isolated rat hind-limb preparations that were free of mast cells.[30,31] Perfusion of thrombin and ATIII through the vascular tree accelerated enzyme-inhibitor complex formation 10- to 20-fold when compared with the calculated rate of reaction of thrombin with ATIII in solution.

The binding of ATIII to endothelial cell–associated heparan sulfates has been visualized by electron microscopy.[32] In addition, metabolic turnover studies with radiolabeled ATIII in humans suggest that a small portion of the total pool of ATIII is associated with heparin-like proteoglycans of the vessel wall.[33]

In summary, biochemical, cell biologic, and physiologic evidence indicate that heparan sulfate species with anticoagulant activity are associated with endothelial cells of the vascular tree. This permits a small fraction of plasma ATIII to be activated at blood–vessel wall interfaces where enzymes of the coagulation cascade are commonly generated and protects natural surfaces against thrombus formation. The catalytic nature of heparin-like species ensures the continual regeneration of these molecules, which are critical for maintaining the nonthrombogenicity of the endothelial cell layer.

Protein C–Thrombomodulin–Protein S Mechanism

Protein C is a vitamin K–dependent plasma glycoprotein of 62 kd. The amino acid sequences of the bovine and human glycoproteins were deduced from direct protein sequencing and the cloning of its cDNA.[34–37] Protein C consists of a heavy chain of 41 kd and a light chain of 21 kd, which are joined by a single disulfide bridge. In human plasma, a single-chain form of the zymogen has been identified that constitutes 5% to 15% of the total protein C in the circulation.[38] These observations suggest that the zymogen is initially synthesized as a single polypeptide chain and subsequently cleaved to generate a two-chain structure.

To perform its anticoagulant function, human protein C must be converted to a component with serine protease activity, which is designated activated protein C. This process involves the scission of a single Arg 12–Leu 13 bond at the amino-terminal end of the heavy chain of the zymogen with release of an activation peptide of about 1.4 kd.[39] The active-site serine residue is located on the heavy chain.[35] Both protein C and activated protein C possess γ-carboxyglutamic acid (Gla) residues in their light chains, which are required for the binding of protein to calcium ions and cell membranes.[34] β-Hydroxyaspartic acid, another posttranslational modification, was identified on the light chain of the protein.[40] Activated protein C is slowly neutralized by several protease inhibitors in human plasma—a 57-kd protease inhibitor designated protein C inhibitor,[41,42] α_1-antitrypsin,[43–45] and α_2-macroglobulin.[46,47] These three inhibitors neutralize activated protein C at a relatively slow rate, although the activity of the protein–C inhibitor is enhanced by high concentrations of heparin.[41]

Thrombin is the only physiologically relevant serine protease that can convert protein C to activated protein C.[39] The rate of this reaction is slow when blood is allowed to clot in vitro but is accelerated several thousand times by a cofactor on the surface of the vascular endothelium.[48,49] This receptor cofactor, thrombomodulin, was isolated from lung and placental tissue and endothelial cells of rabbits, cows, and humans.[50–54] The endothelial cell receptor has an apparent molecular weight of 74 kd and 105 kd, as determined by polyacrylamide sodium dodecyl sulfate-gel electrophoresis before and after the addition of reducing agents, respectively. The primary structure of thrombomodulin was deduced from the cloning of its cDNA by several groups of investigators.[54–58] This membrane receptor is structurally similar to coated-pit receptors and is organized into domains that resemble those of the low-density lipoprotein receptor.

Thrombin forms a 1:1 complex with thrombomodulin that rapidly activates protein C in the presence of calcium ions. Thrombin attached to thrombomodulin can be neutralized by antithrombin at a rate equivalent to that of the free enzyme. Data conflict, however, about the ability of the thrombin–thrombomodulin complex to clot fibrinogen, activate factor V, or trigger platelet activation. Experiments with the receptor isolated from rabbit lung indicate that the rabbit thrombin–thrombomodulin complex inhibits these procoagulant activities of thrombin,[59,60] whereas the human form of the receptor does not.[61]

Once evolved, activated protein C inactivates factors Va and VIIIa, which are cofactors of the coagulation cascade.[62–64] The procofactors—factors V and VIII—are relatively resistant to this proteolytic effect of activated protein C. Its first site of action is at the platelet surface where bound factor Va acts as a receptor for factor Xa. This multimolecular prothrombinase complex rapidly converts prothrombin to thrombin. Activated protein C functions in vivo as a naturally occurring anticoagulant by specifically cleaving peptide bonds of factor Va,[62] thereby preventing the assembly of the prothrombinase complex and suppressing the production of thrombin.[65] This inhibitory effect of activated protein C is modulated by factor Xa, which can bind to factor Va on phospholipid surfaces and can protect this cofactor from the proteolytic action of activated protein C.[66] The second site of action of activated protein C occurs at a locale where factor VIIIa regulates the interaction between factor IXa and factor X on phospholipid membranes. The predominant action of the enzyme is to destroy the biologic activity of factor VIIIa.[63,64,67–69] In this manner, it is able to prevent the conversion of factor X to factor Xa by factor IXa in the presence of calcium ions.

Another plasma protein, protein S, is involved in the activated protein C–dependent destruction of factors Va and VIIIa. Protein S enhances the binding of activated protein C to cell membranes and accelerates the cleavage of these cofactors by the enzyme.[70–74] Activated protein C and protein S form a stoichiometric complex in the presence of calcium ions and a phospholipid surface. The complement component, C4b-binding protein, can also complex with protein S and is involved in regulating the function of the latter protein,[75–78] since only the free form of protein S is active.

Human protein S is a vitamin K–dependent protein of about 69 kd.[79,80] Unlike the other vitamin K–dependent coagulation proteins, it is not a zymogen of a serine protease. The structure of protein S was deduced from the cloning of its cDNA.[81,82] It consists of a single polypeptide chain with an amine-terminal region that contains 10 Gla residues in addition to a number of β-hydroxyaspartic acid moieties.[80,83] This region is homologous to other vitamin K–dependent plasma proteins, while the carboxy-terminal end of the molecule is similar to that of androgen-binding proteins.[84]

The heparan sulfate–ATIII and protein C anticoagulant mechanisms undoubtedly act together to regulate the generation and neutralization of thrombin in the circulation. For example, ATIII inhibits many of the serine proteases generated by the coagulation cascade. But factor Xa, which is sequestered within the prothrombinase complex, is inaccessible to ATIII.[85,86] The factor Va in the prothrombinase complex is also relatively resistant to inactivation by activated protein C.[66,72] Protein S, however, is able to partially overcome this protection.[87] Hence, this portion of the protein C system is likely to play a particularly pivotal role in conjunction with the endogenous heparan sulfate–ATIII system.

Several independent lines of evidence, obtained from animal studies and clinical observations, indicate that the protein C–thrombomodulin mechanism functions in vivo to suppress thrombotic phenomena. Infusion of a small amount of thrombin into dogs induces protein–C activation before there are any observable changes in the levels of factor V, fibrinogen, or platelets.[88] Activated human protein C can prevent the accretion of radiolabeled fibrinogen onto preformed jugular–venous thrombi in dogs.[89] This enzyme can also inhibit platelet-dependent thrombus formation on prosthetic vascular grafts under arterial flow conditions in primates.[90] A monoclonal antibody directed against protein C induces thromboembolism in mice.[91] The administration of large amounts of activated human protein C into baboons just before the infusion of 100% lethal doses (LD_{100}) of *Escherichia coli* allowed the animals to survive and prevented the development of disseminated intravascular coagulation (DIC) and organ damage.[92] And prior blockade of endogenous protein C activation with a monoclonal antibody to protein C converted a sublethal dose of infused *E coli* organisms (10% of the LD_{100}) into a lethal dose. A radioimmunoassay for quantifying protein C–activation peptide concentrations in humans demonstrated elevated levels of this marker in DIC and deep-vein thrombosis.[93]

The potential role of the protein C–protein S system in the regulation of fibrinolysis remains controversial. Two groups of investigators demonstrated that activated protein C is able to increase the fibrinolytic activity of cultured endothelial cells, at least in part, by decreasing the level of plasminogen–activator inhibitor-1.[94,95] The influence of activated protein C on clot lysis in vitro is enhanced by protein S.[96] Studies also have been carried out in which activated protein C was infused into the bloodstream of animals, and the level of plasminogen activator and the extent of clot lysis were examined. The administration of activated protein C increased the activity of the fibrinolytic system in dogs,[97] but not in squirrel monkeys.[98] The importance of the link between the protein C–thrombomodulin–protein S and fibrinolytic mechanisms in humans is not yet established.

Inhibition of the Factor VIIa–Tissue Factor Mechanism

In studies done some years ago, it was suggested that serum contained a factor that neutralized the clotting activity of crude tissue factor preparations.[98] This phenomenon was reexamined, and it has been demonstrated that a serum component, tissue factor pathway inhibitor (TFPI; previously termed LACI for lipoprotein-associated coagulation inhibitor or EPI for extrinsic pathway inhibitor) forms a quaternary complex with factor Xa, factor VIIa, and tissue factor in the presence of calcium, and thereby suppresses the activity of the extrinsic cascade.[99–102] TFPI was purified to homogeneity from conditioned medium of human hepatoma cells.[104,105] It has a molecular weight of 38 kd and is functionally and antigenically similar to the plasma inhibitor.[106] There are multiple–molecular-weight forms in plasma and about half of the TFPI activity is found in the lipoprotein fraction of serum.[106,107] Human umbilical vein endothelial cells also secrete this inhibitor in culture,[108,109] and data indicate that vascular endothelium may be the major site of synthesis of this plasma protein. Platelets are able to secrete modest amounts of TFPI in response to agonists like thrombin and the calcium ionophore, A23187.[110] The presence of TFPI mRNA transcripts in platelet preparations suggests that megakaryocytes are also able to synthesize this inhibitor.

The sequence of TFPI was derived from cloning a full-length cDNA from a human endothelial cell cDNA library in λgt11.[111] It consists of a negatively charged NH_2 terminal end, three tandem Kunitz-type inhibitory domains, and a positively charged COOH terminal region. This information facilitated detailed structure-function analyses of TFPI. The second Kunitz domain binds to factor Xa and inhibits its enzymatic activity.[112] The factor Xa–TFPI complex can then bind to factor VIIa–tissue factor to inhibit its procoagulant activity. The first Kunitz domain presumably contains the binding site for factor VIIa, and both the first and second domains are required to inhibit factor VIIa–tissue factor. The function of the third domain is not known.

Several groups developed functional[109,113,114] or immunochemical[115] assays for measuring plasma concentrations of TFPI in humans. The mean antigenic level of the inhibitor in normal adults is 113 ng/mL with a range of 60 to 180 ng/mL. A hereditary deficiency associated with an increased risk of thrombotic disease has not been described. While Bajaj and colleagues[109] observed significant decrements in TFPI activity in patients with DIC, several other groups[115–117] reported normal levels in such individuals. The plasma measurements of this protein were also normal in subjects with severe chronic liver disease.[109,115–117] The infusion of intravenous heparin induces a marked rise in TFPI values,[115,118] however, suggesting that a large pool of TFPI is normally bound to the vascular endothelium.

Studies show that TFPI can inhibit tissue thromboplastin induced intravascular coagulation in rabbits.[119,120] It is speculated that, in humans, the in vivo activity of this inhibitor could help explain the bleeding diatheses associated with factor deficiencies of the intrinsic coagulation cascade.[121]

HYPERCOAGULABLE PATIENTS: CLINICAL FEATURES, LABORATORY EVALUATION, AND MANAGEMENT

From a clinical standpoint, patients suspected of having a hypercoagulable state can be divided into two broad categories.[122] The first group consists of the inherited thrombotic disorders or primary hypercoagulable states:

- Antithrombin III deficiency
- Protein C deficiency
- Protein S deficiency
- Dysfibrinogenemias
- Plasminogen deficiency
- Diminished plasminogen activator activity

In these instances, a specific defect in one of the three natural anticoagulant mechanisms (heparin–antithrombin III, protein C–thrombomodulin, or protein S mechanism; see Fig. 44-1), or in the plasminogen–plasminogen-activator mechanism (Fig. 44-2) has been identified. The second category consists of a heterogeneous array of clinical disorders in which there is an apparent increased risk of thromboembolism when compared with the general population; these disorders can be referred to as the acquired or secondary hypercoagulable states:

Diseases and Syndromes

- Lupus anticoagulant
- Malignancy
  - Disease related (includes migratory superficial thrombophlebitis [Trousseau's syndrome], nonbacterial thrombotic endocarditis, thrombosis associated with chronic DIC)
  - Treatment related (associated with the administration of various chemotherapeutic agents, including L-asparaginase, mitomycin, adjuvant programs for breast cancer)
- Estrogen administration (associated with oral contraceptive use, treatment of prostate cancer with diethylstilbestrol)
- Infusion of prothrombin complex concentrates
- Nephrotic syndrome
- Heparin-induced thrombocytopenia
- Thrombotic thrombocytopenic purpura
- Myeloproliferative disorders
- Paroxysmal nocturnal hemoglobinuria
- Hyperlipidemia
- Diabetes mellitus
- Homocystinuria
- Prosthetic vascular surfaces
- Hyperviscosity
- Congestive heart failure

Physiologic Factors

- Pregnancy, especially during the postpartum period
- Postoperative state
- Immobilization
- Advancing age
- Obesity

The pathophysiologic basis of increased coagulation system activity in most of these conditions is not known with any degree of certainty. Because of their complex pathophysiology, it seems unlikely that defects in a single component of the hemostatic mechanism accounts for the thrombotic tendency in most of these conditions. This section develops an approach to the diagnosis and treatment of the hypercoagulable patient and focuses on those disorders where laboratory studies (ie, deficiencies of one of the plasma components of the natural anticoagulant

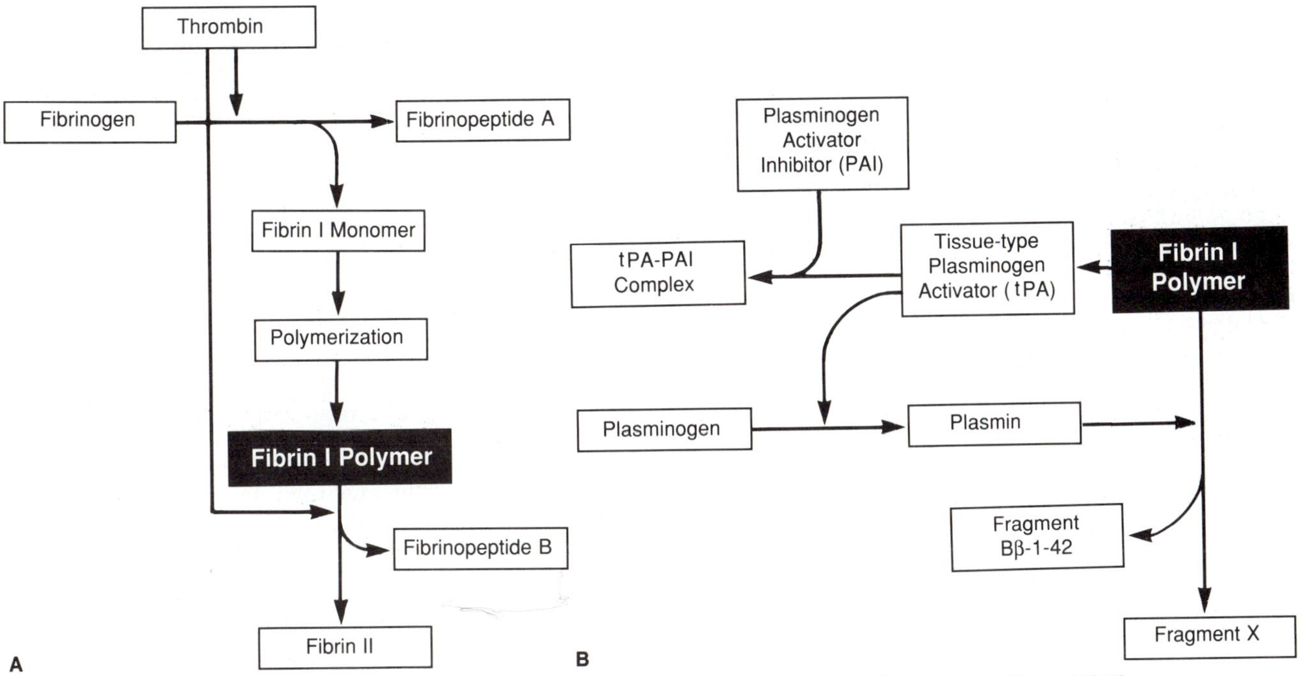

FIGURE 44-2. A model for the actions of thrombin on fibrinogen and of plasmin on fibrin. **(A)** The conversion of fibrinogen to fibrin by thrombin initially results in the formation of fibrin I monomer and the release of fibrinopeptide A. Fibrin I monomer is able to polymerize; thrombin can then cleave this polymer, resulting in the generation of fibrin II and the release of fibrinopeptide B. **(B)** The fibrinolytic activity of human plasma is determined primarily by the presence of tissue plasminogen activator (tPA) and its inhibitor (PAI), which are released from vascular endothelial cells. tPA is able to bind to fibrin I polymer, which allows plasminogen to be activated to plasmin at an increased rate. The action of the serine protease plasmin on fibrin I polymer results in the production of fragment X and other fragments, including Bβ-1-42. Plasmin subsequently can convert fragment X to soluble breakdown products.

mechanisms, dysfibrinogenemias, and the presence of lupus anticoagulants) can provide information that may be useful in the clinical management of such individuals.

INHERITED THROMBOTIC DISORDERS

The prevalence of inherited thrombotic disorders has been evaluated in several large studies of thrombotic patients with a positive family or personal history of spontaneous venous thrombosis. Deficiencies of protein C and protein S antigen of 4% and 5%, respectively, were present in 141 consecutive unrelated patients less than age 45 from Frankfurt.[123] This group also found deficiencies of ATIII as well as identifiable plasminogen and fibrinogen abnormalities in 3%, 2%, and 1% of the subjects, respectively. Similar results were obtained in such populations by investigators in the Netherlands,[124] Austria,[125] and Israel.[126] The prevalence of these genetic abnormalities has not been evaluated in a large group of unselected patients but is likely to be considerably lower if one includes a large number of older subjects.

Thus, with available tests, one can anticipate being able to make a diagnosis of a hereditary disorder in only 10% to 20% of young patients presenting with a documented episode of venous thromboembolism. The following clinical features, however, should suggest the presence of one of these diagnoses and prompt a screening laboratory evaluation (Table 44-1): (1) thrombosis occurring at an early age; (2) a family history of thrombotic disease; (3) thrombosis occurring at unusual sites (eg, mesenteric venous thrombosis, cerebral venous thrombosis); (4) recurrent thrombosis with or without apparent precipitating factors; and (5) recurrent thrombosis during anticoagulant therapy, or warfarin-induced skin necrosis. Individuals with congenital deficiencies of the proteins of the natural anticoagulant mechanisms (ie, ATIII, protein C, protein S) most often develop venous thromboembolic disease. The reasons for the absence of arterial thromboses in these disorders are unknown, though the traditional view is that arterial thrombosis may arise from defects in platelet or endothelial cell function.

TABLE 44-1. Screening Laboratory Evaluation for Patients Suspected of Having Inherited Thrombotic Disorders*

Functional assay of antithrombin III (heparin cofactor assay)
Immunologic and functional assays of protein C
Immunologic assays of total and free protein S
Screen for dysfibrinogenemias (immunologic and functional assays of fibrinogen, thrombin time)

* All assays are performed on platelet-poor plasmas obtained from blood samples drawn into a solution containing 3.8% (weight/volume) sodium citrate. The ratio of anticoagulant to blood is 0.1:0.9 (volume/volume). In the absence of an accompanying clinical history for the patient, the performance of a prothrombin time helps exclude the ingestion of warfarin, which affects the measurements of protein C and protein S. Performance of a thrombin time, as well as an activated partial thromboplastin time, helps exclude the administration of heparin.

Antithrombin III Deficiency

In 1965, Egeberg[127] reported a Norwegian family whose members had plasma ATIII concentrations that were 40% to 50% of normal and a history of repeated thrombotic events. Subsequently, other investigators described additional families with a similar constellation of clinical and laboratory abnormalities.[128–146] ATIII deficiency is inherited in an autosomal dominant fashion, and thus affects both sexes equally. The true prevalence of ATIII deficiency in the general population is unknown, but estimates reported in the literature range from about 1 in 2000 to 1 in 5000.[147,148] In a large review article published in 1981[149] that compiled the published cases of familial ATIII deficiency, about 55% of the biochemically affected patients had experienced at least one thrombotic event. Individuals rarely had thrombotic episodes before puberty, however, and increasing numbers of patients reported such events as they reached the age of 50. The initial clinical manifestations occurred spontaneously in about 42% of subjects but could be related to pregnancy, delivery, oral contraceptive ingestion, surgery, or trauma in the remaining 58% of patients. The most common sites of disease were the deep veins of the leg and the mesenteric veins. About 60% of individuals developed recurrent thrombotic episodes, and clinical signs of pulmonary embolism were evident in 40%.

Two major types of inherited ATIII deficiency have been delineated. The classic deficiency (type I) is a result of the reduced synthesis of biologically normal protease inhibitor molecules.[145,150] In these cases, the immunologic and biologic activity of ATIII in the blood is reduced to the same extent. The molecular basis of this disorder is either a deletion of a large segment of the gene or, more commonly, the occurrence of other alterations such as nonsense mutations, missense mutations, or base substitutions at splice sites.[151–154] The second type of ATIII deficiency is produced by a discrete molecular defect within the protease inhibitor (type II). Under these circumstances, the plasma levels of ATIII are greatly reduced as judged by biologic activity measurements, whereas the immunologic determinations of this inhibitor are essentially normal.

The first family with a functional deficiency of ATIII was reported by Sas and coworkers in 1974.[155] Many families with this type of deficiency have been reported, and they have been further subcategorized on the basis of two different functional assays of ATIII activity.[156] The first is the ATIII–heparin cofactor assay, which measures the ability of heparin to bind to lysyl residues on the inhibitor and catalyze the neutralization of coagulation enzymes such as thrombin and factor Xa. Another protein in human plasma exhibits heparin cofactor activity[157–159]; it has been termed *heparin cofactor* II. In contrast to ATIII, this inhibitor requires concentrations of heparin of at least 1 IU/mL to function as an effective inhibitor of thrombin. Therefore, it probably plays a minimal role when heparin is used clinically as an anticoagulant.[158] Heparin cofactor II does not interact with other serine proteases generated by the coagulation cascade and another mucopolysaccharide, dermatan sulfate, is able to accelerate the neutralization of thrombin by this inhibitor dramatically. Several patients were described with inherited deficiencies of heparin cofactor II and thrombotic phenomena,[160,161] but the causal relationship is uncertain.[162] The second test is the progressive ATIII activity assay, which quantifies the capacity of this inhibitor to neutralize the enzymatic activity of thrombin in the absence of heparin.

These two functional assays identify ATIII-deficient patients with reductions in heparin cofactor activity with or without concordant decrements in progressive ATIII activity. Using the techniques of classic protein chemistry or molecular biology, several abnormal ATIII molecules were identified with reductions in only heparin cofactor activity that have defects at a heparin-binding site. These variants generally have mutations at the amino-terminal end of the molecule[163–192] (Table 44-2). In one of these variants, the substitution of asparagine for isoleucine at residue 7 produces a new glycosylation site, and the resultant protein has a reduced affinity for heparin.[192] Variants with decreased activity in both ATIII activity assays generally have mutations near the thrombin-binding site at the carboxy-terminal end of the molecule[193–221] (see Table 44-2). All ATIII variants cannot be neatly characterized by this schema, however, since single amino acid substitutions can affect both functional domains of the molecule. This is perhaps best illustrated by a mutation in which arginine is replaced by histidine at residue 393.[205–213] This reactive-site mutation markedly decreases the ability of the protein to inhibit thrombin but also leads to a conformational alteration such that the abnormal molecule has increased heparin affinity.

Another type of mutation is described at the carboxy-terminal end of the ATIII molecule. In the plasma of ATIII-deficient patients derived from a large Utah family, trace amounts of an electrophoretically and functionally abnormal inhibitor molecule were identified.[222] It was determined by molecular cloning and sequencing techniques that leucine is substituted for proline at position 407 in the affected members of this kindred.[223,224] Small amounts of an electrophoretically abnormal inhibitor species were observed in the plasma of ATIII-deficient members of the Oslo kindred[225] first reported by Egeberg.[127] In this case, threonine replaces alanine at position 404 in the abnormal protein.[226] A variant from Kyoto is also described in which a methionine is substituted for arginine at position 406.[227] The ATIII-deficient subjects in the Utah, Oslo, and Kyoto pedigrees appear, however, to have a type I deficiency as determined by routine laboratory testing. The similar characteristics of these mutations suggest that the region of residues 404 to 407 is important for the maintenance of normal plasma levels of ATIII antigen.[228] It is possible that the mutant inhibitor molecules synthesized by the liver of these deficient individuals are susceptible to increased intracellular degradation, decreased extracellular export, or increased clearance on entry into the circulation. Finally, the mutation in the first reported ATIII variant, Budapest,[155] has been identified. The replacement of a proline by leucine at residue 429 leads to a molecular defect that can affect both the heparin- and thrombin-binding sites.[229,230]

The amino acid substitutions of a number of abnormal ATIII molecules from individuals with an inherited functional deficiency of the inhibitor have not yet been determined.[231–241]

A review of the literature suggests that the prevalence of thrombosis is different in patients with the two types of functional ATIII deficiency.[242] On one hand, heterozygous individuals with reductions in plasma ATIII–heparin cofactor activity to about 50% of normal with normal progressive ATIII activity have infrequent thrombotic episodes.[163,166,168,174,176,180] Several of these cases were brought to clinical attention when young children of these heterozygous subjects developed severe venous thrombosis, arterial thrombosis, or both,[163,168,174,238] accompanied by plasma ATIII–heparin cofactor levels below 10%. In each instance, there was a history of parental consanguinity, and these children were homozygous for an ATIII molecular defect. On the other hand, heterozygous type II patients with both progressive ATIII activity and ATIII–heparin cofactor activity diminished sustain venous thromboembolism as often as type I patients.

The mean concentration of ATIII in normal pooled

TABLE 44-2. Point Mutations in Antithrombin III

City or Region of Propositus	Substitution	Functional Domain of Antithrombin III
Rouen 3[187]	Ile 7→Asn	Heparin-binding domain
Rouen 4[189]	Arg 24→Cys	Heparin-binding domain
Basel,[185] Clichy[172]	Pro 41→Leu	Heparin-binding domain
Dublin II,[187] Franconville[188] Toyama,[165] Tours,[167] Alger[169] Paris 1,[172] Paris 2[172] Barcelona 2,[173] Kumamoto[175] Padua 2[191]	Arg 47→Cys	Heparin-binding domain
Rouen 1,[176] Padua 1[178] Bligny[179]	Arg 47→His	Heparin-binding domain
Rouen 2[180]	Arg 47→Ser	Heparin-binding domain
Geneva[182]	Arg 129→Gln	Heparin-binding domain
Hamilton[197]	Ala 382→Thr	Thrombin-binding domain
Charleville,[172] Cambridge 1[198] Vicenza[220]	Ala 384→Pro	Thrombin-binding domain
Cambridge 2[221]	Ala 384→Ser	Thrombin-binding domain
Glasgow,[205,207] Sheffield[209] Chicago,[211] Waikato[212] Avranches[172]	Arg 393→His	Thrombin-binding domain
Northwick Park,[205] Milano 1[204]	Arg 393→Cys	Thrombin-binding domain
Pescara[215]	Arg 393→Pro	Thrombin-binding domain
Denver,[194] Milano 2[196]	Arg 394→Ser	Thrombin-binding domain
Oslo[226]	Ala 404→Thr	These mutations result in the presence of trace amounts of abnormal antithrombin III in patient's plasma.
Kyoto[227]	Arg 406→Met	
Utah[224]	Pro 407→Leu	
Budapest[230]	Pro 429→Leu	Mutation produces altered conformation of antithrombin III resulting in abnormal heparin binding and reduced thrombin inhibitory activity.

plasma is about 140 μg/mL. In plasmas from normal individuals, the range of ATIII concentrations, determined by immunologic or functional tests, is narrow. Most laboratories report a normal range between 80% and 120% for ATIII–heparin cofactor determinations,[243] and a somewhat wider range for immunoassay results.[244] Given the various subtypes of the familial deficiency that might be encountered, the best single screening test for the disorder is the ATIII–heparin cofactor assay. Healthy newborns have about half the normal adult concentration[245,246] and gradually reach the adult level by 6 months of age.[247] The levels may be considerably lower in infants born between 30 to 36 weeks of gestation.[247]

A variety of pathophysiologic conditions can reduce the concentration of ATIII in the blood. While acute thrombosis does not lower ATIII levels substantially,[248] DIC usually reduces the level of this inhibitor.[249] Lowered ATIII concentrations are known to occur in patients with liver disease (mainly cirrhosis) due to decreased protein synthesis.[250] Decreased ATIII levels are also observed in individuals with the nephrotic syndrome as a consequence of urinary excretion.[251] Furthermore, modest reductions in plasma ATIII concentration are found in users of oral contraceptives,[252,253] as well as in individuals receiving estrogens for other purposes.[149] The levels of ATIII do not change substantially during normal pregnancies,[253,254] but may decrease significantly in women with pregnancy-induced hypertension, preeclampsia, or eclampsia.[254] Infusions of L-asparaginase, a chemotherapeutic agent employed in the treatment of acute lymphocytic leukemia, can substantially lower the plasma concentration of this inhibitor.[255] In addition, the administration of heparin decreases plasma ATIII levels,[256] presumably on the basis of accelerated in vivo clearance of the inhibitor. Evaluation of plasma samples from patients suspected of having congenital ATIII deficiency during a period of heparinization can therefore potentially lead to an erroneous diagnosis of the disorder.

Because of the number of clinical disorders that can be associated with reductions in the plasma concentration of ATIII, definitive diagnosis of the hereditary deficiency is often difficult. While an ATIII level in the normal range, drawn on clinical presentation, is usually sufficient to exclude the presence of the disorder, low levels should be confirmed by obtaining another sample at a subsequent time. This determination is ideally performed when the patient is no longer receiving oral anticoagulants, since these medications have occasionally been reported to raise plasma ATIII concentrations into the normal range in individuals with the hereditary deficiency.[130] In such situations, clinical assessment of the individual's risk of recurrent thrombosis determines whether this approach is feasible. In most ATIII-deficient subjects, however, this effect of oral anticoagulants is not of sufficient magnitude to obscure the diagnosis.[257] Confirmation of the hereditary nature of the disorder requires the investigation of other family members. Diagnosis of other biochemically affected family members also allows for appropriate counseling regarding the need for prophylaxis against venous thrombosis.

The indications for thrombolytic therapy in heterozygous ATIII-deficient patients are similar to those in other populations with acute venous thromboembolic episodes. These individuals can usually be treated successfully with intravenous heparin, however, though in some situations it may be found that unusually high doses of the drug are required to achieve adequate anticoagulation. Indeed, the diagnosis of ATIII deficiency is usually considered in the differential diagnosis of heparin resistance, and an occasional patient with this disorder is diagnosed in this manner. In ATIII-deficient patients receiving heparin for the treatment of acute thrombosis, the adjunctive role of ATIII concentrate purified from human plasma is not clearly defined, since controlled trials have not been performed. Based on the available data, however, administration of this product should be considered when difficulty is encountered in achieving adequate heparinization, or when recurrent thrombosis is observed despite adequate anticoagulation. It is also reasonable to treat ATIII-deficient subjects with concentrate before major surgery or in obstetric situations where the risks of bleeding from anticoagulation are unacceptable. The manufacturing processes used to prepare ATIII concentrate result in a product that is more than 95% pure and in which the hepatitis B virus and human immunodeficiency virus I have been inactivated.[258,259] Hence, it is preferable to administer ATIII concentrate rather than fresh frozen plasma in the above clinical settings.

The biologic half-life of ATIII is about 48 hours.[150] The infusion of 50 units of ATIII concentrate per kilogram of body weight (1 unit is defined as the amount of antithrombin in 1 mL of pooled normal human plasma) usually raises the plasma ATIII level to about 120% in a congenitally deficient individual with a baseline level of 50%.[259–263] Plasma levels should be monitored to ensure that they remain above 80%, and the administration of 60% of the initial dose at 24-hour intervals is recommended to maintain inhibitor levels in the normal range.[263]

Oral anticoagulants are highly effective in the management of patients with ATIII deficiency. Warfarin should be continued indefinitely in patients with recurrent venous thrombosis. Asymptomatic ATIII individuals from a thrombophilic kindred are not generally anticoagulated prophylactically unless they are exposed to situations that predispose them to developing thrombosis (eg, prolonged immobilization, surgery, pregnancy).

The management of pregnancies in women with congenital ATIII deficiency poses special problems.[264] A group of French investigators noted that the incidence of thrombotic complications during pregnancy and the postpartum period is greater in women with ATIII deficiency than in those with deficiencies of protein C or protein S.[265] Affected ATIII-deficient women who have not yet experienced thrombotic events should probably be given antithrombotic prophylaxis with heparin throughout pregnancy. Patients with a history of previous thrombotic episodes should definitely receive treatment. In women who chronically take oral anticoagulants, several approaches can be taken while planning pregnancy to minimize the risk of thrombotic complications as well as warfarin embryopathy. One approach is to stop warfarin and commence subcutaneous heparin therapy; this potentially exposes the patient to many months of heparin therapy while she is trying to conceive. Another approach is to use replacement therapy with ATIII concentrates until conception. This product needs to be administered intravenously at frequent intervals, however. Finally, warfarin therapy could be continued with the performance of pregnancy tests on a frequent basis. As soon as pregnancy is diagnosed and prior to the sixth week of gestation, oral anticoagulants must be discontinued and heparin therapy initiated. Though the risk of warfarin embryopathy appears to be small during the first 6 weeks of pregnancy,[266] even the small risk of this complication makes this the least preferable of the three approaches.

Anabolic steroids such as stanazolol and danazol raise plasma ATIII levels in individuals with normal[267,268] as well as reduced levels of this inhibitor.[269,270] Despite this effect, these drugs have not been shown to prevent thrombosis in patients with hereditary ATIII deficiency.[269] Stanazolol and danazol also have the potential for raising the levels of vitamin K–dependent procoagulant factors, which could lead to a lack of therapeutic benefit.

Protein C Deficiency

In 1981, Griffin and colleagues[271] described the first kindred in which several individuals had plasma levels of protein C antigen of about half of normal and a history of recurrent thrombotic events. Subsequently, other investigators[272–277] reported numerous other families with this disorder. This biochemical deficiency is inherited in an autosomal dominant fashion and has clinical features that are similar to those of hereditary ATIII deficiency. About 75% of these individuals experienced one or more thrombotic events. The initial episode occurred spontaneously in about 70% of the patients, with the remaining 30% having the usual associated risk factors at the time they developed acute thrombotic events (eg, pregnancy, delivery, oral contraceptive ingestion, surgery, or trauma). These patients are usually asymptomatic until their early twenties, with increasing numbers of individuals experiencing thrombotic events as they reach the age of 50. The most common sites of disease are the saphenous, the iliofemoral, and the mesenteric veins. Approximately 63% of the affected patients developed recurrent venous thrombosis with about 40% exhibiting signs of pulmonary embolism.[274] Investigators from the Netherlands noted a high frequency of superficial thrombophlebitis of the leg veins[273] as well as several cases of cerebral venous thrombosis in their protein C–deficient patients.[278]

Notably, other kindreds are reported in which individuals who are heterozygous for protein C deficiency have minimal symptoms. First, a number of case reports describe a homozygous or doubly heterozygous state in which newborns develop a syndrome described as purpura fulminans and exhibit laboratory evidence of DIC in association with protein C antigen levels less than 1% of normal.[279–288] The heterozygous parents of these infants have only infrequently had thromboses, however, in contrast to the patients with thrombotic histories and a hereditary partial deficiency of protein C. Second, Miletich and colleagues[289] observed that the frequency of heterozygous protein C deficiency is as high as 1 in 200 in a healthy adult population, and that many biochemically affected individuals had not yet developed thromboses. These data suggest that other undefined factors are likely to modulate the phenotypic expression of heterozygous protein C deficiency.

Coumarin-induced skin necrosis is associated with the presence of heterozygous protein C deficiency.[290–293] This syndrome typically occurs during the first several days of warfarin therapy, often in association with the administration of large loading doses of the medication. The skin lesions occur on the extremities, breasts, and trunk as well as the penis and marginate over a period of hours from an initial central erythematous macule. If vitamin K or a product containing protein C is not rapidly administered, the affected cutaneous areas become edematous, develop central purpuric zones, and ultimately become necrotic. Biopsies demonstrate fibrin thrombi within cutaneous vessels with interstitial hemorrhage. The dermal manifestations of coumarin-induced skin necrosis are clinically and pathologically similar to those seen in infants with purpura fulminans due to severe protein C deficiency.

The pathogenesis of warfarin-induced skin necrosis is attributable to the emergence of a transient hypercoagulable state. The initiation of the drug at standard doses leads to a decrease in protein C anticoagulant activity levels to about half of normal within a single day.[294] While factor VII activity measurements follow a pattern similar to that of protein C, the levels of the other vitamin K–dependent factors decline at slower rates consistent with their longer half-lives. Increased thrombin generation was documented in patients during this early phase of warfarin therapy utilizing a sensitive immunochemical assay for fragment F_{1+2}, an index of the in vivo activation of prothrombin mediated by factor Xa.[295] During this period, the drug's suppressive effect on protein C has a greater influence on the hemostatic mechanism than on factor VII. These effects are likely to be augmented when loading-dose schedules are used or the patient has an underlying hereditary deficiency of protein C. However, only a third of patients with warfarin-induced skin necrosis have an inherited deficiency of protein C,[296] and this complication is a rather infrequently reported event among individuals with the heterozygous deficiency. A case report also appeared in which this syndrome is described in association with an acquired functional deficiency of protein C.[297]

Two major subtypes of heterozygous protein C deficiency were delineated, using immunologic and functional assays. The classic, or type I, deficiency is the most common form and is characterized by a reduction in both the immunologic and biologic activity of the zymogen in the blood.[274] In one study of 14 protein C–deficient families, the use of genomic probes in conjunction with Southern blot analysis demonstrated that three kindreds had a deletion of the entire gene, and two had deletions or insertions of sequences that grossly altered restriction patterns of their DNA.[298] Most families with this disorder, however, have nonsense or missense point mutations.[299,300] The linkage between a rare polymorphism and a particular mutation in the protein C gene in several Dutch families with the deficiency suggests the presence of a founder effect (ie, the families are related).[301] In families with a type II deficiency, affected individuals have normal protein C levels on immunologic examination, yet possess lowered functional levels of the zymogen.[302–308]

As previously noted, a clinical disorder was reported in which newborns develop purpura fulminans in association with protein C antigen levels that are less than 1% of normal.[279–288] In some instances, there was a history of consanguinity in the family, making it highly likely that the affected infants were homozygous for the deficiency.[280,283,286] A number of case reports, however, document the existence of a form of severe protein C deficiency in which neonatal purpura fulminans is not present. These individuals generally have protein C levels of less than 20% of normal in the absence of oral anticoagulant therapy, and their clinical presentation is generally similar to that of severely affected subjects from thrombophilic kindreds with the heterozygous deficiency.[309–314] The parents of these subjects have a type I deficiency, as do those of babies with purpura fulminans. In addition, two reports describe patients who are doubly heterozygous for both type I and type II alleles that were inherited separately from each of the parents.[315,316] In one of these cases, a group of Japanese investigators determined that the type II defect resulted from the replacement of arginine by tryptophan at position 12 of the heavy chain. This residue is the site at which protein C is activated by the thrombin–thrombomodulin complex.[316]

A variety of immunologic and functional techniques were developed to measure protein C levels in plasma samples. The most commonly used procedures for antigen determinations are electroimmunoassay,[271,272] enzyme-linked immunosorbent assay,[309,317] or radioimmunoassay.[93,318] Functional assays utilize either thrombin[302,319] or the thrombin–thrombomodulin complex[303,320] to activate protein C after adsorbing the zymogen with aluminum hydroxide[302] or barium citrate.[319,320] With the exception of the method of Francis and Patch,[319] which measures the ability of activated protein C to prolong the activated partial thromboplastin time, the endpoint of these assays is the cleavage of a suitable synthetic substrate by the enzyme. Other methods use the thrombin–thrombomodulin complex to first activate protein C in plasma, followed by immunoadsorption of the enzyme with goat antihuman protein C IgG-agarose,[303] or alternatively, protein C is first adsorbed with a calcium-dependent monoclonal antibody and subsequently activated by the thrombin–thrombomodulin complex.[294] The activity of the enzyme is then assessed using a chromogenic substrate[302,303,320] or by measuring its anticoagulant activity in a factor Xa one-stage clotting assay.[294] The development of simpler functional assays has been facilitated by the observation that the venom from the Southern copperhead snake (*Agkistrodon contortrix*) is able to activate protein C in plasma.[321–323] This activation is followed by measuring the enzyme's amidolytic activity with a suitable chromogenic substrate or measuring its anticoagulant activity in a clotting assay.

Functional assays using amidolytic and clotting endpoints may give useful information regarding the nature of the molecular defect in patients with type II protein C–deficiency. Several individuals are described with normal protein C antigen measurements who have substantial reductions in protein C anticoagulant activity with normal or near normal amidolytic activity.[294,308] These defects may reflect a reduced ability of activated protein C to interact with protein S, membrane phospholipids, or its substrates such as factors V and VIII. Conversely, there are reports of abnormal protein C molecules that are normally activated by the thrombin–thrombomodulin complex but that fail to exhibit proteolytic activity as measured by amidolytic or anticoagulant assays.[305,307] This suggests that the mutations reside near the serine-reactive centers of the proteins.

Protein C normally circulates in human plasma at an average concentration of 4 μg/mL. The levels of protein C antigen in healthy adults are log-normal distributed with 95% of the values ranging from 70% to 140%.[289] There is no significant gender dependence, but mean protein C antigen concentrations increase by about 4% per decade. Similar results are seen with functional assays. The relatively wide normal range of protein C measurements in the general population frequently makes it difficult to identify a given individual as having heterozygous protein C deficiency. If medical and pharmacologic causes of low levels of protein C are excluded (see later discussion), patients with protein C values below 55% are likely to have the genetic abnormality, whereas levels of 55% to 65% are consistent with either a deficiency or the lower end of the normal distribution.[289] To document this disorder, it is useful to perform repeat determinations on the individual suspected of being protein C deficient in addition to performing family studies to document the presence of an autosomal dominant inheritance pattern.

Protein C levels in newborns are 20% to 40% of normal adult levels,[324,325] and preterm infants have even lower protein C levels.[326,327] Acquired protein C deficiency occurs in a number of clinical disorders, including liver disease,[294,324,328,329] DIC,[294,324,328,330,331] adult respiratory distress syndrome,[324] the postoperative state,[324] and in association with L-asparaginase therapy.[332] In contrast to ATIII, the antigenic concentrations of vitamin K–dependent plasma proteins, including protein C, are often elevated in patients with the nephrotic syndrome.[333,334]

Warfarin therapy reduces functional[294,302,320] and, to a lesser extent, immunologic measurements of protein C.[271,272] This makes it difficult to diagnose individuals with heterozygous protein C deficiency in this setting. Several research laboratories use a reduced ratio of protein C antigen to prothrombin antigen to identify patients with a type I deficiency.[271,272] This approach only can be used in subjects in a stable phase of oral anticoagulation, however, and the diagnostic criteria for the disorder vary with the intensity of warfarin therapy.[272] Therefore, in practice it is preferable to investigate patients suspected of having the deficiency after oral anticoagulation has been discontinued for at least 1 week; family studies should also be performed. If it is not possible to discontinue warfarin therapy because of the severity of the thrombotic diathesis, such individuals can be studied while receiving heparin therapy, which does not alter plasma protein C levels.

An acquired inhibitor of protein C was documented in an Australian patient who had a bleeding diathesis for several years and developed purpura fulminans before his death.[335] An autopsy showed arterial and venous thrombi in many organs. Laboratory evaluation demonstrated the presence of chronic DIC. The IgG fraction of the subject's plasma completely inhibited the functional anticoagulant activity of activated protein C.

Acute management of thromboembolic events in heterozygous protein C–deficient patients is similar to that of those without the disorder. It is advisable to keep the patient fully anticoagulated with heparin during the initiation of oral anticoagulation; large loading doses of the latter medication clearly should be avoided as has been recommended in other patient populations. Oral anticoagulants are effective in managing individuals with protein C deficiency, and the recommendations for its use in patients who have either sustained recurrent venous thrombosis or are asymptomatic are similar to those in patients with congenital ATIII deficiency. Many of the general guidelines for management of pregnancies in women with this latter disorder are also relevant to protein C–deficient women.

Stanazolol and danazol raise protein C levels substantially in heterozygous patients with type I protein C deficiency.[336–338] There is also a report of danazol treatment of a subject who is doubly heterozygous for both the type I and II deficiencies[315]; this resulted in a rise in protein C antigen concentration from 66% to 98% but no change in anticoagulant activity. As is the case for congenital ATIII deficiency, however, these drugs do not prevent thrombosis in patients with this disorder,[338] and an increase in fragment F_{1+2} levels (a measure of the in vivo activity of factor Xa on prothrombin) has been observed in conjunction with the rise in protein C levels in two French protein C–deficient patients who received stanazolol for 4 weeks.[337]

The infrequent occurrence of warfarin-induced skin necrosis and the diagnostic difficulty in making a rapid and definitive laboratory diagnosis of the deficiency are arguments against the routine measurement of plasma protein C levels in all individuals with venous thrombosis before the initiation of oral anticoagulants. If, however, one is starting oral anticoagulants in a patient who is already known or likely to be protein C deficient, it would be prudent to start the drug under the cover of full heparinization. It would also be wise to increase the dose of warfarin gradually, starting from a relatively low level (eg, 2 mg for the first 3 days, then increasing in increments of 2 to 3 mg until therapeutic anticoagulation is achieved). A case has been reported of successful oral anticoagulation of a subject with heterozygous protein C deficiency and a prior history of warfarin-induced skin necrosis.[293] Therapeutic doses of heparin in addition to protein C replacement in the form of fresh frozen plasma were used to prevent the development of this complication.

The management of neonatal purpura fulminans in association with severe protein C deficiency is more complicated, since heparin therapy and antiplatelet agents have not been effective.[279,281–285] The administration of a source of protein C appears to be critical in the initial treatment of these patients. Fresh frozen plasma has been used successfully in these infants. The half-life of protein C in the circulation is short (6 to 16 hours),[294,339] and the administration of plasma on a frequent basis is limited by the development of hyperproteinemia, hypertension, loss of venous access, and the potential for exposure to infectious viral agents. Protein C concentrate was successfully used in this disorder,[340] and highly purified concentrates of this protein are undergoing clinical trials for this indication. Warfarin was administered to these infants without the redevelopment of skin necrosis during the phased withdrawal of fresh frozen plasma infusions,[279,284,286,341,342] and this medication has been used chronically to control the thrombotic diathesis. Finally, there is a report of a 20-month-old child with liver failure and homozygous protein C deficiency undergoing successful liver transplantation.[343] The transplant normalized protein C levels and resolved the thrombotic diathesis.

Protein S Deficiency

In 1984, members from several kindreds who exhibited reduced levels of protein S were described who had a striking history of recurrent venous thrombotic disease.[344,345] Subsequently, many additional families with this disorder were reported.[78,346–360] The clinical presentation of patients with heterozygous protein S deficiency is similar to that outlined for ATIII or protein C deficiency. Among 71 protein S–deficient members from 12 Dutch pedigrees,[353] 74%, 72%, and 38% of the individuals have sustained deep venous thrombosis, superficial thrombophlebitis, or pulmonary emboli, respectively. The mean age of the first thrombotic event was 28 years, with a range between 15 and 68; 56% of the episodes were spontaneous, and the remainder were precipitated by an identifiable factor. Thrombosis was also reported in the axillary, mesenteric, and cerebral veins. Interestingly, a case report appeared describing warfarin-induced skin necrosis in a patient with heterozygous protein S deficiency.[361]

Under normal conditions, about 60% of the total protein S antigen in plasma is complexed to a complement component, C4b-binding protein. Only the free 40% is functionally active as a cofactor in mediating the anticoagulant effects of activated protein C.[78] This observation led to the development of methods for measuring total[345,362,363] and free protein S antigen.[350] The most reliable measurements of total protein S antigen are usually by radioimmunoassay[362–364] or enzyme-linked immunosorbent assay techniques that involve dilution of plasma samples and thereby favor dissociation of the protein S–C4b-binding protein complexes. After removing protein S–C4b-binding protein complexes from plasma by polyethylene glycol precipitation,[350,365] free protein S may be quantified by immunoassay of the supernatant fractions. Functional assay methods require immunodepleted protein S–deficient plasma or immobilized monoclonal antibodies to protein S.[344,366–370] They are based on the ability of protein S to serve as a cofactor for the anticoagulant effect of activated protein C.

The classic deficiency is associated with about 50% of the normal protein S antigen level,[345,347] and decrements in free protein S antigen and protein S–functional activity to less than about 40% of normal.[350] A molecular genetic analysis of this type of deficiency identified a partial protein S–gene deletion in one of six kindreds.[357] Thus, most families are likely to have point mutations as the basis for their disorders. Another type of hereditary deficiency has been described in which total protein S antigen measurements are in the normal range, but the levels of free protein S and protein S–functional activity are disproportionately reduced. The pathogenetic basis for this type of defect is not known, but possible explanations include a molecular abnormality in either protein S or C4b-binding protein that leads to a shift of the free protein S pool into the bound form.[344,350]

A family was reported that included two individuals with doubly heterozygous or homozygous protein S deficiency and recurrent venous thromboembolic disease.[78] The parents of these individuals were asymptomatic and had laboratory studies consistent with the classic protein S deficiency. In addition, a case report describes neonatal purpura fulminans in association with homozygous protein S deficiency.[371]

The average concentration of total protein S antigen in normal adults is 23 μg/mL.[362] The levels appear to increase significantly with advancing age and are significantly lower and more variable in females than males.[372,373] These factors confound the reliable estimation of the prevalence of heterozygous protein S deficiency in the normal population; also, they often make it difficult to make the diagnosis of heterozygous protein S deficiency by performing assays on a given individual at a single point in time. Therefore, resampling of patients, in addition to family studies, is usually required to firmly establish the diagnosis.

Acquired protein S deficiency occurs during pregnancy[364,365] and in association with the use of oral contraceptives.[373,374] Reduced protein S levels were noted in patients with DIC,[367,375] acute thromboembolic disease,[367] and in association with L-asparaginase therapy.[332] C4b-binding protein is an acute-phase protein, and the declines in protein S activity in the latter two conditions (as well as in other inflammatory disorders) is attributable to a shift of the protein to the complexed, inactive form.[367] Total protein S antigen measurements are generally increased in patients with the nephrotic syndrome,[333,334,376] though functional assays give reduced values. This is due in part to the loss of free protein S in the urine and elevations in C4b-binding protein levels. Total and free protein S antigen concentrations are moderately decreased in liver disease.[363,367] Total protein S antigen values in healthy newborns at term are 15% to 30% of normal, while C4b-binding protein is markedly reduced to less than 20%. Thus, the free form of the protein predominates in this setting and functional levels are only slightly reduced compared with those in normal adults.[370,377,378] Finally, interpretation of protein S measurements in individuals on oral anticoagulants is complicated, inasmuch as the antigenic and functional levels of the protein drop substantially in this setting. A few groups used reductions in the ratio of total protein S antigen to prothrombin antigen to infer a diagnosis of the classic type of protein S deficiency; this is accomplished by employing a strategy similar to that described for protein C–deficient subjects.[345,347]

Recommendations for the treatment of protein S–deficient patients with anticoagulants and thrombolytic agents are similar to those in individuals without this disorder. Heparin therapy is generally effective for the acute treatment of thrombotic episodes, and standard warfarin schedules appear to be effective in preventing recurrent venous thromboembolism. Anabolic steroids such as danazol or stanazolol have not been shown to have a role in the treatment of protein S–deficient patients.

Dysfibrinogenemias

Qualitative abnormalities of fibrinogen are usually inherited in an autosomal dominant manner. Because many different genetic mutations can result in the production of variant fibrinogen molecules by the liver, the dysfibrinogenemias are a heterogeneous group of clinical disorders that may present with either no clinical symptoms, a bleeding diathesis, or a history of recurrent venous or arterial thromboembolism.[379] Fewer than twenty cases of variant fibrinogens are reported to be associated with thrombotic complications. These defects can be discovered by screening patients with thrombin and reptilase times (often prolonged in these patients) and by performing fibrinogen assays. In one instance, the thrombin time was substantially shortened.[380,381] Functional fibrinogen measurements are generally substantially lower than antigenic measurements in the plasmas of these individuals. An occasional individual with a dysfibrinogenemia may have a prolonged prothrombin time or partial thromboplastin time, and the inability of some abnormal fibrinogens to clot completely in vitro can result in false-positive results in fibrin(ogen) degradation product tests.

The functional and biochemical defects of a number of abnormal fibrinogens associated with thromboembolic disease were characterized.[379] The conversion of fibrinogen to fibrin by thrombin results in the proteolytic cleavage of fibrinopeptides A and B from the molecule (see Fig. 44-2A). Defects in the release of these two peptides[382–386] or in thrombin binding[387–390] were also reported. This is not a surprising finding, since a prolonged thrombin time is often used to identify these variants. Other mutants were shown to cause abnormal fibrin polymerization.[389,391–393] Such functional defects do not, however, offer a ready explanation for the thrombotic diathesis seen in these subjects. Therefore, some of the abnormal fibrinogens were evaluated for their ability to resist or promote fibrinolysis on incorporation into a fibrin clot. The fibrin formed from fibrinogen Chapel Hill III is abnormally resistant to lysis by plasmin.[391] In contrast, plasminogen activation is decreased in the presence of the fibrin formed from fibrinogen Dusard despite normal tissue plasminogen activator binding to the substrate.[394,395] These abnormalities clearly have the potential for decreasing fibrinolytic activity in vivo, which could result in a familial thrombotic diathesis in biochemically affected persons.

Inherited Abnormalities of Fibrinolysis

Dysfunction of the fibrinolytic system certainly plays an important role in thrombus formation. While investigators have identified a few individuals with inherited abnormalities of the fibrinolytic mechanism and recurrent venous thromboembolism, the clinical association between these two conditions is considerably less striking than that observed in many kindreds with deficiencies of ATIII, protein C, or protein S. This relative lack of success in identifying fibrinolytic mechanism defects may be related to inadequacies in the laboratory methodologies available for the detection of clinically relevant abnormalities.

Dysplasminogenemia or hypoplasminogenemia is reported in about ten individuals with thromboembolic disease.[396–407] The first case of an abnormal plasminogen was identified in Japan by Aoki and colleagues.[396] The propositus had a history of recurrent thrombosis, and family studies demonstrated that the biochemical abnormality followed an autosomal dominant inheritance pattern. Despite the hereditary nature of the defect, none of the other biochemically affected members of the kindred had sustained thrombotic events. Other Japanese pedigrees have since been described with the same biochemical defect,[398,399] and the gene frequency of this abnormality in Japan is 0.018.[408] Population studies in the United States have not uncovered any cases of this particular dysplasminogenemia. The non-Japanese cases of dysplasminogenemia and hypoplasminogenemia are also remarkable for the lack of thrombotic episodes in biochemically affected family members other than the propositi.

A few reports document the existence of thrombophilic families with other inherited abnormalities of fibrinolysis.[409,410] Individuals from one of these kindreds were initially observed to have reduced fibrinolytic potential after venous occlusion[409] and they subsequently have been documented to have high levels of plasminogen activator inhibitor.[411] The pathogenetic basis for these abnormalities has yet to be determined, however.

Immunochemical methods for the measurement of tissue plasminogen activator and functional assays for the inhibitor are available and recently have been applied to the study of patients with documented venous thromboembolism. These studies suggest that defective synthesis or release of tissue-type plasminogen activator in addition to an increased concentration of the inhibitor of this serine protease may be important pathogenetic factors in as many as one third of these individuals.[412,413] The high incidence of such abnormalities, however, requires the execution of properly designed clinical studies to address issues regarding the clinical utility of these assay techniques in identifying individuals at high risk for subsequent thrombotic episodes. It is noteworthy that reduced fibrinolytic activity due to increased plasma levels of a rapid inhibitor of tissue plasminogen activator has been found in young survivors of myocardial infarction.[414] The measurements of this inhibitor correlated strongly with serum concentrations of triglycerides.

Management Decisions in Patients With Inherited Thrombotic Disorders

When a patient with one of the inherited thrombotic disorders is discovered, family studies should be conducted, since up to one half of the members of a given kindred may be affected. Affected individuals should receive counseling regarding the implications of the diagnosis and advice regarding the symptoms that require immediate medical attention. In women, oral contraceptives or estrogens are contraindicated in view of the increased thrombotic risk associated with the use of these medications. All biochemically affected individuals should be carefully evaluated prior to surgical, medical, or obstetric procedures that carry an increased thrombotic risk. These subjects should then receive appropriate prophylactic anticoagulation regimens. If specific concentrates are available for a patient with a particular deficiency, these can also be administered to raise the plasma levels of the protein to the normal range during the perioperative period. All women with previous thrombotic episodes should receive prophylactic anticoagulants throughout pregnancy, and asymptomatic women generally should also receive such treatment.

In patients with an inherited thrombotic disorder, the occurrence of two or more spontaneously occurring thromboembolic episodes should lead to the continuation of oral anticoagulants for life. Chronic warfarin therapy is generally not recommended until an individual has had at least one documented thrombotic episode.

Although it is clear that inherited deficiencies of ATIII, protein C, and protein S can be associated with thrombophilia, the rates of thrombosis cited for patients with these disorders in earlier sections of this chapter likely represent overestimates. This is the result of diagnostic bias on the part of physicians and of reporting bias in the literature for individuals from families with the most severe thrombotic diatheses. In addition, some of the reported episodes of venous thrombosis were not confirmed by objective tests, and it is known that the clinical diagnosis of such events is highly nonspecific. Thus, given that future events in an asymptomatic patient or an individual with only one prior thrombotic episode cannot be predicted with certainty, and given that there is a finite risk of bleeding associated with warfarin therapy, recommendations relating to long-term anticoagulation can be individualized. The clinical features that should be considered in making this decision include the following:

- The number, sites, and severity of thrombosis. For example, a patient who previously sustained a massive pulmonary embolus is more likely to receive long-term warfarin than a subject who developed deep venous thrombosis in a calf vein unless there were symptoms or signs of a significant postphlebitic syndrome.
- Whether the thrombotic episodes were spontaneous or the results of precipitating factors. For example, if a precipitant such as a major abdominal operation were present, it would be reasonable to manage the patient without long-term oral anticoagulation after the acute episode was adequately treated.
- The sex and life-style of the individual. Situations in which these factors may influence the decision-making process as to long-term anticoagulation include women of childbearing age planning to conceive (see section on ATIII deficiency), occupations that entail prolonged periods of immobilization and thereby might be associated with an increased risk of thromboembolism, and jobs or recreational activities with a higher than average chance of trauma that might lead to thrombotic or bleeding complications.
- A history of thromboembolism in other biochemically affected members of the family. While marked intrafamilial and interfamilial heterogeneity is observed in the phenotypic expression of the various inherited thrombotic disorders, it is reasonable to place asymptomatic, biochemically affected patients from severely affected kindreds on oral anticoagulants starting at puberty.

LUPUS ANTICOAGULANTS AND THE ANTICARDIOLIPIN SYNDROME

Lupus anticoagulants are antibodies (usually IgG, IgM, or both) that interfere with phospholipid-dependent coagulation tests in vitro, but not by directly inhibiting the activity of specific plasma coagulation factors. While activated partial thromboplastin time reagents sensitive to the presence of lupus anticoagulants are available for screening purposes,[415] more sensitive tests have been developed such as the dilute Russell's viper venom time,[416] the kaolin clotting time,[417] and the tissue thromboplastin inhibition test.[418] The increased sensitivity of these latter methods is attributable to the reduction of the phospholipid concentration in the assay system. Factor assays, the platelet neutralization procedure,[419] and the rabbit-brain neutralization procedure of Rosove and colleagues[420] are also useful in testing for the presence of lupus anticoagulants. In practice, these tests are best used to confirm the presence of such nonspecific inhibitors after the activated partial thromboplastin time has been found to be prolonged and the addition of an equal part of normal plasma does not normalize the result.

The term *lupus anticoagulant* is a misnomer, since this laboratory abnormality frequently occurs in patients without systemic lupus erythematosus. This phenomenon has been observed in other autoimmune diseases following exposure to drugs or various infectious agents, in malignancy, and in some individuals without any apparent underlying disease.[421,422] Furthermore, subjects with the lupus anticoagulant do not suffer from a bleeding diathesis unless other hemostatic defects are present (eg, thrombocytopenia, prothrombin deficiency). Paradoxically, the presence of lupus anticoagulants increases the apparent risk of both arterial and venous thromboembolism.[423,424] Compilation of published reports suggests that about one third of patients with such inhibitors have thrombotic events.[421] This is likely to be an overestimate since thrombophilic individuals with this abnormality are more likely to be detected than asymptomatic subjects. Prospective clinical studies have not been carried out to determine the risk of thrombosis in asymptomatic patients with lupus anticoagulants. Reports also appeared describing cutaneous lesions in association with lupus anticoagulants. These include livedo reticularis[425] and skin necrosis,[426] which likely represent manifestations of thrombosis in underlying vessels.

The presence of a lupus anticoagulant is also associated with the presence of biologic false-positive test for syphilis, since the VDRL assay is dependent on the presence of cardiolipin.[427] Some of these antibodies react with anionic phospholipids,[428,429] and the binding of antiphospholipid antibodies to cardiolipin requires the presence of a plasma cofactor, β_2-glycoprotein I (apolipoprotein H).[430,431] Sensitive radioimmunoassays[432] or enzyme-linked immunosorbent assays[433] were developed for the detection of antiphospholipid antibodies that are considerably more sensitive than the VDRL test. The relationship between the presence of lupus anticoagulants, antiphospholipid antibodies, and a thrombotic predisposition are complex. A study by Triplett and coworkers[434] demonstrates that antiphospholipid antibodies are not present in all patients with lupus anticoagulants, and that the presence of such immunoglobulins does not confer an increased thrombotic risk on these individuals.

From both the clinical and laboratory standpoint, patients with lupus anticoagulants constitute a heterogeneous population. It is therefore not surprising that numerous different mechanisms have been implicated in the pathogenesis of thrombosis in these subjects. Most studies attempted to demonstrate alterations in the function of one of the natural anticoagulant mechanisms of the endothelium, since phospholipids are essential components of vascular cell membranes. In one study, IgG from the plasma of a patient with arterial thrombosis and a lupus anticoagulant inhibited prostacyclin production by endothelial cells.[435] Other investigators report that immunoglobulins from such patients either increase prostacyclin production,[436,437] or have no effect.[438] In addition, there is evidence that immunoglobulins from some patients with lupus anticoagulants inhibit protein C activation mediated by the thrombin–thrombomodulin complex on the endothelial cell surface.[437,439,440] Abnormalities of the heparan sulfate–ATIII[441] or fibrinolytic mechanisms[442] are also suggested as explanations for the thrombotic tendency associated with lupus anticoagulants.

The management of acute venous thromboembolism in patients with lupus anticoagulants is similar to that of other individuals without this laboratory abnormality. The initial treatment of such subjects, however, is complicated by the fact that the activated partial thromboplastin time cannot reliably be used to monitor heparin dosage. The best way to monitor anticoagulant therapy in these individuals is to perform plasma heparin measurements using either factor Xa or thrombin, along with a chromogenic substrate.[443] To perform such amidolytic assay procedures, a plasma sample is first incubated with one of the enzymes. After an interval of time, the amount of p-nitroaniline released from a synthetic chromogenic substrate appropriate for the serine protease is quantified spectrophotometrically. A standard curve is constructed by assaying normal pooled plasma containing unfractionated heparin at several concentrations between 0.1 and 1 IU/mL. The range for therapeutic anticoagulation is 0.2 to 0.5 IU/mL, which generally corresponds to an activated partial thromboplastin time of 1.5 to 2.5 times the pretreatment value in patients without circulating inhibitors.[444] The presence of lupus anticoagulants can also interfere with heparin monitoring during cardiac surgery.[445]

The clinical heterogeneity of the patient populations that develop lupus anticoagulants makes it difficult to generalize regarding the long-term antithrombotic management of such individuals. For example, patients who develop transient lupus anticoagulants in association with infections do not usually sustain thromboembolic episodes. It is also unclear whether drug-associated lupus anticoagulants are associated with thrombosis. Thus, the presence of a persistent lupus anticoagulant, a high-titer antiphospholipid antibody, or both in an asymptomatic subject with no prior thrombotic history is not an indication for anticoagulant or antiplatelet medications. Given that it is not possible to reliably determine the risk of thrombosis in an asymptomatic patient with these laboratory abnormalities, all such individuals should receive appropriate prophylaxis in conjunction with major surgical procedures or a prolonged period of immobilization unless there is a strong contraindication to such treatment. Corticosteroids normalize clotting assay times or reduce antiphospholipid antibody titers in patients with lupus anticoagulants. These and other immunosuppressive medications do not prevent recurrent thrombosis, however.

The presence of lupus anticoagulants, anticardiolipin antibodies, or both has also been associated with obstetric complications such as habitual abortions, intrauterine death, and fetal growth retardation.[435,446–449] In some of these cases, pathologic examination demonstrates placental infarction due to decidual vessel thrombosis.[447] Data suggest that the administration of prednisone, 40 to 60 mg/d, and low-dose aspirin, 75 to 81 mg/d, or full-dose heparin may improve the outcome of pregnancies in women with lupus anticoagulants and poor obstetric histories.[449–451] A case report also appeared in which a woman with a lupus anticoagulant and recurrent fetal loss was successfully treated with intravenous γ-globulin.[452]

CONCLUSION

This chapter presented information regarding the natural anticoagulant mechanisms. Several inherited defects of the plasma proteins of these systems were described that predispose patients to venous thromboembolism. Laboratory tests have been developed to screen for these defects, though these assays are able to provide diagnoses in less than 20% of young patients with venous thromboembolism. This diagnostic armamentarium provides relatively little assistance in the evaluation of individuals with acquired risk factors for venous thrombosis or those with arterial vascular disease.

Advances in our understanding of the biochemistry of the hemostatic mechanism led to the development of sensitive immunochemical methods for measuring peptides or enzyme-inhibitor complexes that are liberated with the activation of the coagulation and fibrinolytic systems in vivo.[453–460] Studies using markers of coagulation-system activation indicate that a biochemical imbalance between procoagulant and anticoagulant mechanisms can be detected in the blood of humans prior to the appearance of thrombotic phenomena.[313,461,462] The continuing application of biochemical, molecular biologic, and clinical approaches to investigations of the hemostatic system leads to a greater appreciation of the molecular defects that lead to venous and arterial vascular disorders in humans. This new information should allow more precise identification of individuals who are entering a clinically relevant hypercoagulable state, and intervention with appropriate therapy before the onset of overt thrombotic disease.

REFERENCES

1. Rosenberg RD. Regulation of the hemostatic mechanism. In: Stamatoyannopoulos G, Nienhuis AW, Leder P, Majerus PW, eds. The molecular basis of blood diseases. Philadelphia, WB Saunders, 1987:534.
2. Esmon CT. Protein C: the regulation of natural anticoagulant pathways. Science 1987;235:1348.
3. Petersen EE, Dudek-Wojciechowska G, Sottrup-Jensen L, Magnusson S. The primary structure of antithrombin III (heparin-cofactor): partial homology between alpha$_1$-antitrypsin and antithrombin III. In: Collen D, Wiman B, Verstraete M, eds. The physiological inhibitors of coagulation and fibrinolysis. Amsterdam, Elsevier/North Holland, Biomedical Press, 1979:43.
4. Bock SC, Wion KL, Vehar GA, lawn RM. Cloning and expression of the endogenous anticoagulant protein, human antithrombin III. Nucleic Acids Res 1982;10:8113.
5. Prowchownik EV, Markham AF, Orkin SH. Isolation of a cDNA clone for human antithrombin III. J Biol Chem 1983;258:8389.
6. Chandra T, Stackhouse R, Kidd VJ, Woo SLC. Isolation and sequence characterization of a cDNA colone of human antithrombin III. Proc Natl Acad Sci USA 1983;80:1845.
7. Abildgaard U. Highly purified antithrombin III with heparin cofactor activity prepared by disc electrophoresis. Scand J Clin Lab Invest 1968;21:89.
8. Abildgaard U. Binding of thrombin to antithrombin III. Scand J Clin Lab Invest 1969;24:23.
9. Rosenberg RD, Damus PS. The purification and mechanism of action of human antithrombin-heparin cofactor. J Biol Chem 1973;248:6490.
10. Yin ET, Wessler S, Stoll PJ. Rabbit plasma inhibitor of the activated species of blood coagulation factor X: purification and some properties. J Biol Chem 1971;246:3694.
11. Damus PS, Hicks M, Rosenberg RD. Anticoagulant action of heparin. Nature 1973;246:355.
12. Rosenberg JS, McKenna P, Rosenberg RD. Inhibition of human factor IXa by human antithrombin-heparin cofactor. J Biol Chem 1975;250: 8883.
13. Stead N, Kaplan AP, Rosenberg RD. Inhibition of activated factor XII by antithrombin-heparin cofactor. J Biol Chem 1976;251:6481.
14. Bjork I, Jackson CM, Jornvall H, et al. The active site of antithrombin. J Biol Chem 1982;257:2406.
15. Blackburn MN, Sibley CC. The heparin binding site of antithrombin III. J Biol Chem 1980;255:824.
16. Villanueva GB, Perret V, Danishefsky I. Tryptophan residue at the heparin binding site in antithrombin III. Arch Biochem Biophys 1980;203:453.
17. Karp GI, Marcum JA, Rosenberg RD. The role of tryptophan residues in heparin-antithrombin interactions. Arch Biochem Biophys 1984;233: 712.
18. Oosta GM, Gardner WT, Beeler DL, Rosenberg RD. Multiple functional domains of the heparin molecule. Proc Natl Acad Sci USA 1981;78: 829.
19. Stone AL, Beeler D, Oosta G, Rosenberg RD. Circular dichroism spectroscopy of heparin-antithrombin interactions. Proc Natl Acad Sci USA 1982;79:7190.
20. Rosenberg RD, Armand G, Lam L. Structure-function relationship of heparin species. Proc Natl Acad Sci USA 1978;75:3065.
21. Rosenberg RD, Lam LH. Correlation between structure and function of heparin. Proc Natl Acad Sci USA 1979;76:1218.
22. Lindahl U, Backstrom G, Thunberg L, Leder IG. Evidence for a 3-O-sulfated D-glucosamine residue in the antithrombin-binding sequence of heparin. Proc Natl Acad Sci USA 1980;77:6551.
23. Teien AN, Abildgaard U, Hook M, Lindahl U. The anticoagulant effect of heparan sulfate and dermatan sulfate. Thromb Res 1977;11:107.
24. Thomas DP, Merton RE, Barrowcliffe TW, Mulloy B, Johnson EA. Anti-factor Xa activity of heparan sulfate. Thromb Res 1979;14:501.
25. Marcum JA, Rosenberg RD. Anticoagulantly active heparin-like molecules from vascular tissue. Biochemistry 1984;23:1730.
26. Marcum JA, Fritze L, Galli SJ, Karp G, Rosenberg RD. Microvascular heparinlike species with anticoagulant activity. Am J Physiol 1983;245: H725.
27. Marcum JA, Rosenberg RD. Heparinlike molecules with anticoagulant activity are synthesized by cultured endothelial cells. Biochem Biophys Res Commun 1985;126:365.
28. Marcum JA, Atha DH, Fritze LMS, et al. Cloned bovine aortic endothelial cells synthesize anticoagulantly active heparan sulfate proteoglycan. J Biol Chem 1986;261:7507.
29. Stern D, Nawroth P, Marcum JA, et al. Interaction of antithrombin III with bovine aortic segments: role of heparin in binding and enhanced anticoagulant activity. J Clin Invest 1985;75:272.
30. Marcum JA, McKenney JB, Rosenberg RD. The acceleration of thrombin-antithrombin complex formation in rat hindquarters via heparinlike molecules bound to the endothelium. J Clin Invest 1985;74:341.
31. Marcum JA, McKenney JB, Galli SJ, et al. Anticoagulantly active heparin-like molecules from mast cell-deficient mice. Am J Physiol 1986;19:H879.
32. de Agostini AI, Watkins SC, Slayter HS, et al. Localization of anticoagulantly active heparan sulfate proteoglycans in vascular endothelium: antithrombin binding on cultured endothelial cells and perfused rat aorta. J Cell Biol 1990;111:1293.
33. Carlson TH, Simon TL, Atencio AC. In vivo behavior of human radioiodinated antithrombin III: distribution among three physiologic pools. Blood 1986;66:13.
34. Fernlund P, Stenflo J. Amino acid sequence of the light chain of bovine protein C. J Biol Chem 1982;257:12170.
35. Stenflo J, Fernlund P. Amino acid sequence of the heavy chain of bovine protein C. J Biol Chem 1982;257:12180.
36. Foster D, Davie EW. Characterization of cDNA coding for human protein C. Proc Natl Acad Sci USA 1984;81:4766.
37. Beckmann RJ, Schmidt RJ, Santerre RF, et al. The structure and evolution of a 461 amino acid human protein C precursor and its messenger RNA, based upon the DNA sequence of cloned human liver cDNAs. Nucleic Acids Res 1985;13:5233.
38. Miletich JP, Leykam JF, Broze GJ. Detection of single chain protein C in human plasma. (Abstract) Blood 1983;62(Suppl 1):306a.
39. Kisiel W. Human plasma protein C: isolation, characterization, and mechanism of activation by α-thrombin. J Clin Invest 1979;64:761.
40. Drakenberg T, Fernlund P, Roepstorff P, Stenflo J. β-Hydroxyaspartic acid in vitamin K–dependent protein C. Proc Natl Acad Sci USA 1983;80:1802.
41. Suzuki K, Nishioka J, Hashimoto S. Protein C inhibitor: purification from human plasma and characterization. J Biol Chem 1983;258:163.
42. Suzuki K, Deyashiki Y, Nishioka J, et al. Characterization of a cDNA for human protein C inhibitor: a new member of the plasma serine protease inhibitor superfamily. J Biol Chem 1987;262:611.
43. Heeb MJ, Griffin JH. Physiologic inhibition of human activated protein C by α_1-antitrypsin. J Biol Chem 1988;263:11613.
44. Heeb MJ, Espana F, Griffin JH. Inhibition and complexation of activated protein C by two major inhibitors in plasma. Blood 1989;73:446.
45. Heeb MJ, Mosher D, Griffin JH. Activation and complexation of protein C and cleavage and decrease of protein S in plasma of patients with intravascular coagulation. Blood 1989;73::455.
46. Hoogendoorn H, Nesheim ME, Giles AR. A qualitative and quantitative analysis of the activation and inactivation of protein C in vivo in a primate model. Blood 1990;75:2164.
47. Hoogendoorn H, Toh CH, Nesheim ME, Giles AR. Identification of α2-macroglobulin as an APC-binding protein. Br J Haematol 1990;76 (Suppl 1):21.
48. Esmon CT, Owen WG. Identification of an endothelial cell cofactor for thrombin-catalyzed activation of protein C. Proc Natl Acad Sci USA 1981;78:2249.
49. Owen WG, Esmon CT. Functional properties of an endothelial cell cofactor for thrombin-catalyzed activation of protein C. J Biol Chem 1981;256:5532.
50. Esmon NL, Owen WG, Esmon CT. Isolation of a membrane bound cofactor for thrombin-catalyzed activation of protein C. J Biol Chem 1982;257:859.
51. Jakubowski HV, Kline MD, Owen WG. The effect of bovine thrombomodulin on the specificity of bovine thrombin. J Biol Chem 1986;261: 3876.
52. Salem HH, Maruyama I, Ishii H, Majerus PW. Isolation and characterization of thrombomodulin from human placenta. J Biol Chem 1984;259:12246.
53. Suzuki K, Kusomoto H, Hashimoto S. Isolation and characterization of thrombomodulin from bovine lung. Biochim Biophys Acta 1986;882: 343.
54. Jackman RW, Beeler DL, VanDeWater L, Rosenberg RD. Characterization of a thrombomodulin cDNA reveals structural similarity to the low density lipoprotein receptor. Proc Natl Acad Sci USA 1986;83: 8834.
55. Jackman RW, Beeler DL, Fritze L, Soff G, Rosenberg RD. Human thrombomodulin gene is intron depleted: nucleic acid sequences of the cDNA and gene predict protein structure and suggest sites of regulatory control. Proc Natl Acad Sci USA 1987;84:6425.
56. Suzuki K, Kusomoto H, Deyashiki Y, et al. Structure and expression of human thrombomodulin, a thrombin receptor on endothelium acting as a cofactor for protein C activation. EMBO J 1987;6:1891.
57. Wen DZ, Dittman WA, Ye RD, et al. Human thrombomodulin: complete

cDNA sequence and chromosome localization of the gene. Biochemistry 1987;26:4350.
58. Shirai T, Shiojiri S, Ito H, et al. Gene structure of human thrombomodulin, a cofactor for thrombin-catalyzed activation of protein C. J Biochem 1988;103:281.
59. Esmon CT, Esmon NL, Harris KW. Complex formation between thrombin and thrombomodulin inhibits both thrombin-catalyzed fibrin formation and factor V activation. J Biol Chem 1982;257:7944.
60. Esmon NL, Carroll RC, Esmon CT. Thrombomodulin blocks the ability of thrombin to activate platelets. J Biol Chem 1983;258:12238.
61. Maruyama I, Salem HH, Ishii H, Majerus PW. Human thrombomodulin is not an efficient inhibitor of the procoagulant activity of thrombin. J Clin Invest 1985;75:987.
62. Walker FJ, Sexton PW, Esmon CT. The inhibition of blood coagulation by activated protein C through the selective inactivation of activated factor V. Biochim Biophys Acta 1979;571:333.
63. Vehar GA, Davie EW. Preparation and properties of bovine factor VIII (antihemophilic factor). Biochemistry 1980;19:401.
64. Marlar RA, Kleiss AJ, Griffin JH. Mechanism of action of human activated protein C, a thrombin-dependent anticoagulant enzyme. Blood 1982;59:1067.
65. Dahlback B, Stenflo J. Inhibitory effect of activated protein C on activation of prothrombin by platelet-bound factor Xa. Eur J Biochem 1980;107:331.
66. Nesheim ME, Canfield WM, Kisiel W, Mann KG. Studies of the capacity of factor Xa to protect factor Va from inactivation by activated protein C. J Biol Chem 1982;257:1443.
67. Kisiel W, Canfield WM, Ericsson LH, Davie EW. Anticoagulant properties of bovine plasma protein C following activation by thrombin. Biochemistry 1977;16:5824.
68. Fulcher CA, Gardiner JE, Griffin JH, Zimmerman TS. Proteolytic inactivation of human factor VIII procoagulant protein by activated protein C and its analogy with factor V. Blood 1984;63:486.
69. Eaton D, Rodriguez H, Vehar GA. Proteolytic processing of human factor VIII: correlation of specific cleavages by thrombin, factor Xa, and activated protein C with activation and inactivation of factor VIII coagulant activity. Biochemistry 1986;25:505.
70. Walker FJ. The regulation of activated protein C by a new protein: the possible function for bovine protein S. J Biol Chem 1980;255:5521.
71. Walker FJ. Regulation of bovine activated protein C by protein S: the role of the cofactor protein in species specificity. Thromb Res 1981;22: 321.
72. Walker FJ. Regulation of protein C by protein S: the role of phospholipid in factor Va inactivation. J Biol Chem 1981;256:11128.
73. Gardiner JE, McGann MA, Berridge CW, et al. Protein S as a cofactor for activated protein C in plasma and in the inactivation of purified factor VIII:C. (Abstract) Circulation 1984;70(Suppl 2):205.
74. Walker FJ, Chavin SI, Fay PJ. Inactivation of factor VIII by activated protein C and protein S. Arch Biochem Biophys 1987;252:322.
75. Dahlback B, Stenflo J. High molecular weight complex in human plasma between vitamin K–dependent protein S and complement component C4b-binding protein. Proc Natl Acad Sci USA 1981;78:2512.
76. Dahlback B. Purification of human vitamin K–dependent protein S and its limited proteolysis by thrombin. Biochem J 1983;209:837.
77. Dahlback B. Purification of human C4b-binding protein and formation of its complex with vitamin K–dependent protein S. Biochem J 1983;209: 847.
78. Comp PC, Nixon RR, Cooper MR, Esmon CT. Familial protein S deficiency is associated with recurrent thrombosis. J Clin Invest 1984;74: 2082.
79. DiScipio RG, Hermodson MA, Yates SG, Davie EW. A comparison of human prothrombin, factor IX (Christmas factor), factor X (Stuart factor), and protein S. Biochemistry 1977;16:698.
80. DiScipio RG, Davie EW. Characterization of protein S, a γ-carboxyglutamic acid containing protein from bovine and human plasma. Biochemistry 1979;18:899.
81. Lundwall A, Dackowski W, Cohen E, et al. Isolation and sequence of the cDNA for human protein S, a regulator of blood coagulation. Proc Natl Acad Sci USA 1986;83:6716.
82. Hoskins J, Norman DK, Beckmann RJ, Long GL. Cloning and characterization of human liver cDNA encoding a protein S precursor. Proc Natl Acad Sci USA 1987;84:349.
83. Stenflo J, Fernlund P. β-Hydroxyaspartic acid in vitamin K–dependent proteins. J Biol Chem 1983;258:12509.
84. Baker ME, French FS, Joseph DR. Vitamin K–dependent protein S is similar to rat androgen-binding protein. Biochem J 1987;243:293.
85. Teitel JM, Rosenberg RD. The protection of factor Xa from neutralization by the heparin–antithrombin complex. J Clin Invest 1983;71:1383.
86. Dahlback B, Stenflo J. Binding of bovine coagulation factor Xa to human platelets. J Biol Chem 1978;255:1170.
87. Solymoss S, Tucker MM, Tracy PB. Kinetics of inactivation of membrane-bound Va by activated protein C. J Biol Chem 1988;263: 14884.
88. Comp PC, Jacocks RM, Ferrell GL, Esmon CT. Activation of protein C in vivo. J Clin Invest 1982;70:127.
89. Emerick SC, Bang NU, Yan SB, et al. Antithrombotic properties of activated human protein C. (Abstract) Blood 1985;66(Suppl 1):349a.
90. Gruber A, Griffin JH, Harker LA, Hanson SR. Inhibition of platelet-dependent thrombus formation by human activated protein C in a primate model. Blood 1989;73:639.
91. Kurosawa-Ohsawa K, Kimura M, Kume-Iwaki A, et al. Anti-protein C monoclonal antibody induces thrombus in mice. Blood 1990;75:2156.
92. Taylor FB Jr, Chang A, Esmon CT, et al. Protein C prevents the coagulopathic and lethal effects of Escherichia coli infusion in the baboon. J Clin Invest 1987;79:918.
93. Bauer KA, Kass BL, Beeler DL, Rosenberg RD. Detection of protein C activation in humans. J Clin Invest 1984;74:2033.
94. Sakata Y, Curriden S, Lawrence D, et al. Activated protein C stimulates the fibrinolytic activity of cultured endothelial cells and decreases antiactivator activity. Proc Natl Acad Sci USA 1985;82:1121.
95. van Hinsbergh VWM, Bertina RM, van Wijngaarden A, et al. Activated protein C decreases plasminogen activator-inhibitor activity in endothelial cell-conditioned medium. Blood 1985;65:444.
96. de Fouw NJ, Haverkate F, Bertina RM, et al. The cofactor role of protein S in the acceleration of whole blood clot lysis by activated protein C in vitro. Blood 1986;67:1189.
97. Comp PC, Esmon CT. Generation of fibrinolytic activity by infusion of activated protein C into dogs. J Clin Invest 1981;68:1221.
98. Colucci M, Stassen JM, Collen D. Influence of protein C activation on blood coagulation and fibrinolysis in squirrel monkeys. J Clin Invest 1984;74:200.
99. Hjort PF. Intermediate reactions in the coagulation of blood with tissue thromboplastin: chapter VI, anti-convertin. Scand J Clin Lab Invest 1957;9(Suppl 27):76.
100. Sanders NL, Bajaj SP, Zivelin A, Rapaport SI. Inhibition of tissue factor/factor VIIa activity in plasma requires factor X and an additional plasma component. Blood 1985;66:204.
101. Rao LV, Rapaport SI. Studies of a mechanism inhibiting the initiation of the extrinsic pathway of coagulation. Blood 1987;69:645.
102. Broze GJ Jr, Miletich JP. Characterization of the inhibition of tissue factor in serum. Blood 1987;69:150.
103. Broze GJ Jr, Warren LA, Novotny WF, et al. The lipoprotein-associated coagulation inhibitor that inhibits the factor VII–tissue factor complex also inhibits factor Xa: insight into its possible mechanism of action. Blood 1988;71:335.
104. Broze GJ Jr, Miletich JP. Isolation of the tissue factor inhibitor produced by Hep G2 hepatoma cells. Proc Natl Acad Sci USA 1987;84:1886.
105. Broze GJ Jr, Warren LA, Girard JJ, Miletich JP. Isolation of the lipoprotein associated coagulation inhibitor produced by HepG2 (human hepatoma) cells using bovine factor Xa affinity chromatography. Thromb Res 1987;48:253.
106. Novotny WF, Girard TJ, Miletich JP, Broze GJ Jr. Purification and characterization of the lipoprotein-associated coagulation inhibitor from human plasma. J Biol Chem 1989;264:18832.
107. Warn-Cramer BJ, Maki SL, Zivelin A, Rapaport SI. Partial purification and characterization of extrinsic pathway inhibitor (the factor Xa-dependent plasma inhibitor of factor VIIa/tissue factor). Thromb Res 1987;48:11.
108. Warn-Cramer BJ, Almus FE, Rapaport SI. Studies of the factor Xa-dependent inhibitor of factor VIIa/tissue factor (extrinsic pathway inhibitor) from cell supernates of cultured human umbilical vein endothelial cells. Thromb Haemost 1989;61:101.
109. Bajaj MS, Rana SV, Wysolmerski RB, Bajaj SP. Inhibitor of the factor VIIa–tissue factor complex is reduced in patients with disseminated intravascular coagulation but not in patients with severe hepatocellular disease. J Clin Invest 1987;79:1874.
110. Novotny WF, Girard TJ, Miletich JP, Broze GJ Jr. Platelets secrete a coagulation inhibitor functionally and antigenically similar to the lipoprotein associated coagulation inhibitor. Blood 1988;72:2020.
111. Wun T-C, Kretzmer KK, Girard TJ, et al. Cloning and characterization of a cDNA coding for the lipoprotein-associated coagulation inhibitor shows that it consists of three tandem Kunitz-type inhibitory domains. J Biol Chem 1988;263:6001.
112. Girard TJ, Warren LA, Novotny WF, et al. Functional significance of the Kunitz-type inhibitory domains of lipoprotein-associated coagulation inhibitor. Nature 1989;338:518.
113. Sandset PM, Abildgaard U, Pettersen M. A sensitive assay of extrinsic coagulation pathway inhibitor (EPI) in plasma and plasma fractions. Thromb Res 1987;47:389.
114. Warr TA, Warn-Cramer BJ, Rao LVM, Rapaport SI. Human plasma extrinsic pathway inhibitor activity. I. Standardization of assay and evaluation of physiologic variables. Blood 1989;74:201.
115. Novotny WF, Brown SG, Girard TJ, et al. Plasma LACI antigen in patient samples. (Abstract) Blood 1989;74(Suppl 1):209a.
116. Andersson TR, Bell H, Sandset PM, et al. "New" coagulation inhibitor levels in pneumonia, disseminated intravascular coagulation and liver diseases. (Abstract) Thromb Haemost 1987;58:1115.
117. Warr TA, Rao LVM, Rapaport SI. Human plasma extrinsic pathway inhibitor activity. II. Plasma levels in disseminated intravascular coagulation and hepatocellular disease. Blood 1989;74:994.
118. Sandset PM, Albildgaard U, Larsen ML. Heparin induces release of extrinsic coagulation pathway inhibitor (EPI). Thromb Res 1988;50: 803.
119. Day KC, Hoffman LC, Palmier MO, et al. Recombinant lipoprotein-

associated coagulation inhibitor inhibits tissue thromboplastin-induced intravascular coagulation in the rabbit. Blood 1990;76:1538.

120. Sandset PM, Warn-Cramer BJ, Rao VM, et al. The effect of tissue factor infusion in rabbits immunodepleted of extrinsic pathway inhibitor (EPI): evidence for a biologic role of EPI in blood coagulation. (Abstract) Circulation 1990;82(Suppl 2):133.
121. Rapaport SI. Inhibition of factor VIIa/tissue factor–induced blood coagulation: with particular emphasis upon a factor Xa–dependent inhibitory mechanism. Blood 1989;73:359.
122. Schafer AI. The hypercoagulable states. Ann Intern Med 1985;102:814.
123. Gladson CL, Scharrer I, Hach V, et al. The frequency of type I heterozygous protein S and protein C deficiency in 141 unrelated young patients with venous thrombosis. Thromb Haemost 1988;59:18.
124. Briet E, Engesser L, Brommer EJP, et al. Thrombophilia: its causes and a rough estimate of its prevalence. (Abstract) Thromb Haemost 1987;58:39.
125. Vikydal R, Korninger C, Kyrle PA, et al. The prevalence of hereditary antithrombin-III deficiency in patients with a history of venous thromboembolism. Thromb Haemost 1985;54:744.
126. Ben-Tal O, Zivelin A, Seligsohn U. The relative frequency of hereditary thrombotic disorders among 107 patients with thrombophilia in Israel. Thromb Haemost 1989;61:50.
127. Egeberg O. Inherited antithrombin deficiency causing thrombophilia. Thromb Diath Haemorrh 1965;13:516.
128. Van der Meer J, Stoepman-van Dalen EA, Jansen JMS. Antithrombin-III deficiency in a Dutch family. J Clin Pathol 1973;26:532.
129. Shapiro SS, Prager D, Martinez J. Inherited antithrombin III deficiency associated with multiple thromboembolic phenomena. (Abstract) Blood 1973;42:1001.
130. Marciniak E, Farley CH, DeSimone PA. Familial thrombosis due to antithrombin III deficiency. Blood 1974;43:219.
131. Gruenberg JC, Smallridge RC, Rosenberg RD. Inherited antithrombin-III deficiency causing mesenteric venous infarction: a new clinical entity. Ann Surg 1975;181:791.
132. Zucker ML, Metz J, Gomperts ED. Inherited antithrombin III deficiency as a cause of multiple venous thromboses. S Afr Med J 1975;49:1425.
133. Filip DJ, Eckstein JD, Veltkamp JJ. Hereditary antithrombin III deficiency and thromboembolic disease. Am J Hematol 1976;2:343.
134. Carvalho A, Ellman L. Hereditary antithrombin III deficiency: effect of antithrombin III deficiency on platelet function. Am J Med 1976;61:179.
135. Odegard OR, Abildgaard U. Antifactor Xa activity in thrombophilia: studies in a family with AT-III deficiency. Scand J Haematol 1977;18:86.
136. Stathakis NE, Papayannis AG, Antonopoulos M, Gardikas C. Familial thrombosis due to antithrombin III deficiency in a Greek family. Acta Haematol (Basel) 1977;57:47.
137. Mackie M, Bennett B, Ogston D, Douglas AS. Familial thrombosis: inherited deficiency of antithrombin III. Br Med J 1978;1:136.
138. Johansson L, Hedner U, Nilsson IM. Familial antithrombin III deficiency as pathogenesis of deep venous thrombosis. Acta Med Scand 1978;204:491.
139. Gyde OHB, Middleton MD, Vaughan GR, Fletcher DJ. Antithrombin III deficiency, hypertriglyceridaemia and venous thrombosis. Br Med J 1978;1:621.
140. Matsuo T, Ohki Y, Kondo S, Matsuo O. Familial antithrombin III deficiency in a Japanese family. Thromb Res 1979;16:815.
141. Pitney WR, Manoharan A, Dean S. Antithrombin III deficiency in an Australian family. Br J Haematol 1980;46:147.
142. Boyer C, Wolf M, Lavergne JM, Larrieu MH. Thrombin generation and formation of thrombin-antithrombin III complexes in congenital antithrombin deficiency. Thromb Res 1980;20:207.
143. Beukes CA, Heyns ADuP. A South African family with antithrombin III deficiency. S Afr Med J 1980;58:528.
144. Ambruso DR, Jacobson LJ, Hathaway WE. Inherited antithrombin III deficiency and cerebral thrombosis in a child. Pediatrics 1980;65:125.
145. Scully MF, De Haas H, Chan P, Kakkar VV. Hereditary antithrombin III deficiency in an English family. Br J Haematol 1981;47:235.
146. Winter JH, Fenech A, Ridley W, et al. Familial antithrombin III deficiency. Q J Med 1982;204:373.
147. Rosenberg RD. Actions and interactions of antithrombin and heparin. N Engl J Med 1975;292:146.
148. Odegard OR, Abildgaard U. Antithrombin III: critical review of assay methods: significance of variations in health and disease. Haemostasis 1978;7:127.
149. Thaler E, Lechner K. Antithrombin III deficiency and thromboembolism. Clin Haematol 1981;10:369.
150. Ambruso DR, Leonard BD, Bies RD, et al. Antithrombin III deficiency: decreased synthesis of a biochemically normal molecule. Blood 1982;60:78.
151. Winter JH, Bennett B, Watt JL, et al. Confirmation of linkage between antithrombin III and Duffy blood group and assignment of AT3 to 1q22–q25. Ann Hum Genet 1982;46:29.
152. Prochownik EV, Antonarkis S, Bauer KA, et al. Molecular heterogeneity of inherited antithrombin III deficiency. N Engl J Med 1983;308:149.
153. Bock SC, Prochownik EV. Molecular genetic survey of 16 kindreds with hereditary antithrombin III deficiency. Blood 1987;70:1273.
154. Olds RJ, Lane DA, Finazzi G, et al. A frameshift mutation leading to type I antithrombin deficiency and thrombosis. Blood 1990;76:2182.
155. Sas G, Blasko G, Banhegyi D, et al. Abnormal antithrombin III (antithrombin III "Budapest") as a cause of familial thrombophilia. Thromb Diathes Haemorrh 1974;32:105.
156. Bauer KA, Teitel JM, Rosenberg RD. Assays for the quantitation of antithrombin III thrombin-antithrombin complex and prothrombin activation fragments. In: Colman RW, ed. Disorders of thrombin formation. New York, Churchill Livingstone, 1983:142.
157. Tollefsen DM, Blank MK. Detection of a new heparin-dependent inhibitor of thrombin in human plasma. J Clin Invest 1981;68:589.
158. Tollefsen DM, Majerus DW, Blank MK. Heparin cofactor II: purification and properties of a heparin-dependent inhibitor of thrombin in human plasma. J Biol Chem 1982;257:2162.
159. Wunderwald P, Schrenk WJ, Port H. Antithrombin BM from human plasma: an antithrombin binding moderately to heparin. Thromb Res 1982;25:177.
160. Tran TH, Marbet GA, Duckert F. Association of hereditary heparin cofactor II deficiency with thrombosis. Lancet 1985;2:413.
161. Sie P, Dupouy D, Pichon J, Boneu B. Constitutional heparin cofactor II deficiency associated with recurrent thrombosis. Lancet 1985;2:414.
162. Bertina RM, van der Linden IK, Engesser L, et al. Hereditary heparin cofactor II deficiency and the risk of development of thrombosis. Thromb Haemost 1987;57:196.
163. Sakuragawa N, Takahashi K, Kondo S, Koide T. Antithrombin III Toyama: a hereditary abnormal antithrombin III of a patient with recurrent thrombophlebitis. Thromb Res 1983;31:305.
164. Koide T, Takahashi K, Odani S, et al. Isolation and characterization of a hereditary abnormal antithrombin III: "antithrombin III Toyama." Thromb Res 1983;31:319.
165. Koide T, Odani S, Takahashi K, et al. Antithrombin III Toyama: replacement of arginine-47 by cysteine in hereditary abnormal antithrombin III that lacks heparin-binding ability. Proc Natl Acad Sci USA 1984;81:289.
166. Chasse JF, Esnard F, Guitton JD, et al. An abnormal plasma antithrombin with no apparent affinity for heparin. Thromb Res 1984;34:297.
167. Duchange N, Chasse JF, Cohen GN, et al. Molecular characterization of the antithrombin III Tours deficiency. Thromb Res 1987;45:115.
168. Fischer AM, Cornu P, Sternberg C, et al. Antithrombin III Alger: a new homozygous AT III variant. Thromb Haemost 1986;55:218.
169. Brunel F, Duchange N, Fischer AM, et al. Antithrombin III Alger: a new case of Arg47-Cys mutation. Am J Hematol 1987;25:223.
170. Wolf M, Boyer C, Lavergne JM, Larrieu MJ. A new familial variant of antithrombin III: "antithrombin III Paris." Br J Haematol 1982;51:285.
171. Fischer AM, Beguin S, Sternberg C, Dautzenberg MD. Comparative effect of heparin and heparan sulphate on two abnormal antithrombin III type 3 variants. Br J Haematol 1987;66:213.
172. Molho-Sabatier P, Aiach M, Gaillard I, et al. Molecular characterization of antithrombin III (ATIII) variants using polymerase chain reaction: identification of the ATIII Charleville as an Ala 384 Pro mutation. J Clin Invest 1989;84:1236.
173. Owen MC, Shaw GJ, Grau E, et al. Molecular characterization of antithrombin Barcelona-2: 47 arginine to cysteine. Thromb Res 1989;55:451.
174. Okajima K, Ueyama H, Hashimoto Y, et al. Homozygous variant of antithrombin III that lacks affinity for heparin, AT III Kumamoto. Thromb Haemost 1989;61:20.
175. Ueyama H, Murakami T, Nishiguchi S, et al. Antithrombin III Kumamoto: identification of a point mutation and genotype analysis of the family. Thromb Haemost 1990;63:231.
176. Owen MC, Borg JY, Soria C, et al. Heparin binding defect in a new antithrombin III variant: Rouen, 47 Arg to His. Blood 1987;69:1275.
177. Girolami A, Pengo V, Patrassi GM, et al. Antithrombin III Padua: a "new" congenital antithrombin III abnormality with normal or near normal activity, normal antigen, abnormal migration and no thrombotic disease. Folia Haematol (Leipz) 1983;110:98.
178. Caso R, Lane DA, Thompson E, et al. Antithrombin Padua I: impaired heparin binding caused by an Arg47 to His (CGT to CAT) substitution. Thromb Res 1990;58:185.
179. Wolf M, Boyer-Neumann C, Molho-Sabatier P, et al. Familial variant of antithrombin III (AT III Bligny, 47Arg to His) associated with protein C deficiency. Thromb Haemost 1990;63:215.
180. Borg JY, Owen MC, Soria C, et al. Proposed heparin binding site in antithrombin based on arginine 47: a new variant Rouen-II, 47 Arg to ser. J Clin Invest 1988;81:1292.
181. de Moerloose PA, Reber G, Vernet Ph, et al. Antithrombin III Geneva: a hereditary abnormal antithrombin III with defective heparin cofactor activity. Thromb Haemost 1987;57:154.
182. Grandille S, Aiach M, Lane DA, et al. Important role of Arg 129 in heparin binding site of antithrombin III: identification of a novel mutation Arg 129 to Gln. J Biol Chem 1990;265:18997.
183. Tran TH, Bounameaux H, Bondeli C, et al. Purification and partial characterization of a hereditary abnormal antithrombin III fraction of a patient with recurrent thrombophlebitis. Thromb Haemost 1980;44:87.
184. Tran TH, Bondeli C, Marbet GA, Duckert F. Reactivity of a hereditary

abnormal antithrombin III fraction in the inhibition of thrombin and factor Xa. Thromb Haemost 1980;44:92.
185. Chang JY, Tran TH. Antithrombin III Basel: identification of a Pro-Leu substitution in a hereditary abnormal antithrombin with impaired heparin cofactor activity. J Biol Chem 1986;261:1174.
186. Aiach M, Francois D, Priollet P, et al. An abnormal antithrombin III (AT III) with low heparin affinity: AT III Clichy. Br J Haematol 1987;67: 515.
187. Daly M, Ball R, O'Meara A, Hallinan FM. Identification and characterization of an antithrombin III mutant (AT Dublin 2) with marginally decreased heparin activity. Thromb Res 1989;56:503.
188. de Roux N, Chadeuf G, Molho-Sabatier P, et al. Clinical and biochemical characterization of antithrombin III Franconville, a variant with Pro 41 Leu mutation. Br J Haematol 1990;75:222.
189. Borg JY, Brennan SO, Carrell RW, et al. Antithrombin Rouen-IV 24Arg Cys: the amino terminal contribution to heparin binding. FEBS Lett 1990;266:163.
190. Girolami A, Fabris F, Cappellato G, et al. Antithrombin III Padua 2: a new congenital abnormality with defective heparin co-factor activities but no thrombotic disease. Blut 1983;49:93.
191. Olds RJ, Lane DA, Caso R, et al. Antithrombin III Padua 2: a single base substitution in exon 2 detected with PCR and direct genomic sequencing. Nucleic Acids Res 1990;18:1926.
192. Brennan SO, Borg JY, George PM, et al. New carbohydrate site in mutant antithrombin (7 Ile–Asn) with decreased heparin affinity. FEBS Lett 1988;237:118.
193. Sambrano JE, Jacobson LJ, Reeve EB, et al. Abnormal antithrombin III with defective serine protease binding (antithrombin III "Denver"). J Clin Invest 1986;77:887.
194. Stephens AW, Thalley BS, Hirs CHW. Antithrombin III Denver, a reactive site variant. J Biol Chem 1987;262:1044.
195. Tripodi A, Krachmalnicoff A, Manucci PM. Characterization of an abnormal antithrombin (Milano 2) with defective thrombin binding. Thromb Haemost 1986;56:349.
196. Olds RJ, Lane D, Caso R, et al. Antithrombin III Milano 2: a single base substitution in the thrombin binding domain detected with PCR and direct genomic sequencing. Nucleic Acids Res 1989;17:10511.
197. Devraj-Kizuk R, Chui DHK, Prochownik EV, et al. Antithrombin-III–Hamilton: a gene with a point mutation (guanine to adeninine) in codon 382 causing impaired serine protease reactivity. Blood 1988;72:1518.
198. Perry DJ, Harper PL, Fairham S, et al. Antithrombin Cambridge, 384 Ala to Pro: a new variant identified using the polymerase chain reaction. FEBS Lett 1989;254:174.
199. Howarth DJ, Samson D, Stirling Y, Saghatchian MJ. Antithrombin III "Northwick Park": a variant antithrombin with normal affinity for heparin but reduced heparin cofactor activity. Thromb Haemost 1985;53:314.
200. Lane DA, Flynn A, Ireland H, et al. Antithrombin III Northwick Park: demonstration of an inactive high MW complex with increased affinity for heparin. Br J Haematol 1987;65:451.
201. Erdjument H, Lane DA, Ireland H, et al. Formation of a covalent disulfide-linked antithrombin-albumin complex by an antithrombin variant, antithrombin "Northwick Park." J Biol Chem 1987;262:13381.
202. Wolf M, Boyer C, Tripodi A, et al. Antithrombin Milano: a new variant with monomeric and dimeric inactive antithrombin III. Blood 1985;65: 496.
203. Wolf M, Boyer-Neumann C, Meyer D, et al. Purification and further characterization of antithrombin III Milano: lack of reactivity with thrombin. Thromb Haemost 1987;58:888.
204. Erdjument H, Lane DA, Ireland H, et al. Antithrombin Milano, single amino acid substitution at the reactive site, Arg 393 to Cys. Thromb Haemost 1988;60:471.
205. Erdjument H, Lane DA, Panico M, et al. Single amino acid substitutions in the reactive site of antithrombin leading to thrombosis: congenital substitution of arginine 393 to cysteine in antithrombin Northwick Park and to histidine in antithrombin Glasgow. J Biol Chem 1988;263: 5589.
206. Lane DA, Lowe GDO, Flynn A, et al. Antithrombin III Glasgow: a variant with increased heparin affinity and reduced ability to inactivate thrombin, associated with familial thrombosis. Br J Haematol 1987;66: 523.
207. Owen MC, Beresford CH, Carrell RW. Antithrombin Glasgow, 393 Arg to His: a P1 reactive site variant with increased heparin affinity but no thrombin inhibitory activity. FEBS Lett 1988;231:317.
208. Thein SL, Lane DA. Use of synthetic oligonucleotides in the characterization of antithrombin III Northwick Park (393 CGT—TGT) and antithrombin III Glasgow (393 CGT—CAT). Blood 1988;72:1817.
209. Lane DA, Erdjument H, Flynn A, et al. Antithrombin Sheffield: amino acid substitution at the reactive site (Arg 393 to His) causing thrombosis. Br J Haematol 1989;71:91.
210. Bauer KA, Ashenhurst JB, Chediak J, Rosenberg RD. Antithrombin "Chicago": a functionally abnormal molecule with increased heparin affinity causing familial thrombophilia. Blood 1983;62:1242.
211. Erdjument H, Lane DA, Panico M, et al. Antithrombin Chicago, amino acid substitution of arginine 393 to histidine. Thromb Res 1989;54: 613.
212. Owen M, Beresford CH. Antithrombin-III Waikato, 393 Arg to His: a P_1 reactive site variant with increased heparin affinity but no heparin cofactor activity. FEBS Lett 1988;231:317.
213. Aiach M, Roncato M, Chadeuf G, et al. Antithrombin III Avranches, a new variant with defective serine-protease inhibition: comparison with antithrombin III Charleville. Thromb Haemost 1988;60:94.
214. Leone G, De Stefano V, Di Donfrancesco A, et al. Antithrombin III Pescara: a defective AT III variant with no alterations of plasma crossed immunoelectrophoresis, but with an abnormal crossed immunoelectrofocusing pattern. Br J Haematol 1987;65:187.
215. Lane DA, Erdjument H, Thompson E, et al. A novel amino acid substitution in the reactive site of a congenital antithrombin: antithrombin Pescara, Arg393 to pro, caused by a CGT to CCT mutation. J Biol Chem 1989;264:10200.
216. Aiach M, Nora M, Fiessinger JN, et al. A functional abnormal antithrombin III (AT III) deficiency: AT III Charleville. Thromb Res 1985;39: 559.
217. Barbui T, Rodeghiero F. Hereditary dysfunctional antithrombin III (AT-III Vicenza). Thromb Haemost 1981;45:97.
218. Barbui T, Finazzi G, Rodeghiero F, Dini E. Immunoelectrophoretic evidence of a thrombin-induced abnormality in a new variant of hereditary dysfunctional antithrombin III (AT III 'Vicenza'). Br J Haematol 1983;54:561.
219. Finazzi G, Tran TH, Barbui T, Duckert F. Purification of antithrombin "Vicenza" a molecule with normal heparin affinity and impaired reactivity to thrombin. Br J Haematol 1985;59:259.
220. Caso R, Lane DA, Thompson EA, et al. Antithrombin Vicenza, Ala 384 to Pro (GCA to CCA) mutation, transforming the inhibitor into a substrate. Br J Haematol 1991;77:87.
221. Carrell RW, Evans DL, Stein P. Antithrombin: deduced structure of reactive centre, mutant dysfunction and heparin activation. (Abstract) Br J Haematol 1990;76(Suppl 1):2.
222. Cosgriff TM, Bishop DT, Hershgold EJ, et al. Familial antithrombin III deficiency: its natural history, genetics, diagnosis and treatment. Medicine 1983;62:209.
223. Bock SC, Harris JF, Schwartz CE, et al. Hereditary thrombosis in a Utah kindred is caused by a dysfunctional antithrombin III gene. Am J Hum Genet 1985;37:32.
224. Bock SC, Marrinan JA, Radziejewska E. Antithrombin III Utah: proline-407 to leucine mutation in a highly conserved region near the inhibitor reactive site. Biochemistry 1988;27:6171.
225. Hultin MB, McKay J, Abildgaard U. Antithrombin Oslo: type Ib classification of the first reported antithrombin-deficient family, with a review of hereditary antithrombin variants. Thromb Haemost 1988;59: 468.
226. Bock SC, Silbermann JA, Wikoff W, et al. Identification of a threonine for alanine substitution at residue 404 of antithrombin III Oslo suggests integrity of the 404–407 region is important for maintaining normal plasma inhibitor levels. (Abstract) Thromb Haemost 1989;62:494.
227. Nakagawa M. Antithrombin III deficiency and its molecular analysis. Presented at the XIIth Congress of ISTH, Kyoto Satellite Symposium, August 27–28, 1989.
228. Bock SC. Antithrombin III genetics. (Abstract) Thromb Haemost 1989;62: 468.
229. Sas G, Pepper DS, Cash JD. Further investigations on antithrombin III in the plasmas of patients with the abnormality of "antithrombin III Budapest." Thromb Diathes Haemorrh 1975;33:564.
230. Thein SL, Olds RJ, Caso R, et al. ATIII Budapest: A type IIa deficiency associated with a substitution (429 Pro to Leu) in a region highly conserved in the serpin superfamily. Br J Haematol 1990;76(Suppl 1):2.
231. Penner JA, Hassouna H, Hunter MJ, Chockley M. A clinically silent antithrombin III defect in an Ann Arbor family. (Abstract) Thromb Haemost 1979;42:186, 1979.
232. Sorensen PJ, Dyerberg J, Stoffersen E, Jensen MK. Familial functional antithrombin III deficiency. Scand J Haematol 1980;24:105.
233. Sorensen PJ, Sas G, Peto I, et al. Distinction of two pathologic antithrombin III molecules: antithrombin III "Aalborg" and antithrombin III "Budapest." Thromb Res 1982;26:211.
234. Sorensen PJ, Ezban M, Jessen TE, et al. Purification and characterization of the pathological antithrombin III "Aalborg." Thromb Res 1990;57: 807.
235. Girolami A, Marafioti F, Rubertelli M, et al. Antithrombin III Trento: a "new" congenital AT III abnormality with a peculiar crossed immunoelectrophoretic pattern in the absence of heparin. Acta Haematol (Basel) 1984;72:73.
236. Jorgensen M, Petersen LC, Thorsen S. Purification and characterization of hereditary abnormal antithrombin III with impaired thrombin binding. J Lab Clin Med 1984;104:245.
237. Tengborn L, Frohm B, Nilsson LE, Nilsson IM. A Swedish family with abnormal antithrombin III. Scand J Haematol 1985;34:412.
238. Boyer C, Wolf M, Vedrenne J, et al. Homozygous variant of antithrombin III: AT III Fountainebleau. Thromb Haemost 1986;56:18.
239. Leone G, Cotumaccio R, De Stefano V, et al. Different forms of AT-III congenital defect: a study by crossed immunoelectrofocusing. Scand J Haematol 1984;33:410.
240. Leone G, De Stefano V, Ferrelli R, et al. Antithrombin III molecular variants with defective binding to heparin or to serine proteases: ev-

idence of two different abnormal patterns identified by crossed immunoelectrofocusing. Thromb Haemost 1988;60:8.
241. De Stefano V, Leone G, Ferrelli R, et al. Further characterization of a pathological isoantithrombin with no affinity for heparin (antithrombin III Roma). Thromb Res 1987;48:23.
242. Finazzi G, Caccia R, Barbui T. Different prevalence of thromboembolism in the subtypes of congenital antithrombin deficiency: review of 404 cases. (Letter) Thromb Haemost 1987;58:1094.
243. Odegard OR, Lie M, Abildgaard U. Heparin cofactor activity measured with an amidolytic method. Thromb Res 1975;6:287.
244. Fagerhol MK, Abilgaard U. Immunological studies on human antithrombin III: influence of age, sex and use of oral contraceptives on serum concentration. Scand J Haematol 1970;1:10.
245. McDonald MM, Hathaway WE, Reeve EB, Leonard BD. Biochemical and functional study of antithrombin III in newborn infants. Thromb Haemost 1982;47:56.
246. Andrew M, Paes B, Milner R, et al. Development of the human coagulation system in the full-term infant. Blood 1987;70:165.
247. Andrew M, Paes B, Milner R, et al. Development of the human coagulation system in the healthy premature infant. Blood 1988;72:1651.
248. de Boer AC, van Riel LAM, den Ottolander GJH. Measurement of antithrombin III, α_2-macroglobulin and α_1-antitrypsin in patients with deep venous thrombosis and pulmonary embolism. Thromb Res 1979;15:17.
249. Damus PS, Wallace GA. Immunologic measurement of antithrombin III–heparin cofactor and α_2-macroglobulin in disseminated intravascular coagulation and hepatic failure coagulopathy. Thromb Res 1989;6:27.
250. von Kaulla E, von Kaulla KN. Antithrombin III and diseases. Am J Clin Pathol 1967;48:69.
251. Kauffman RH, Veltkamp JJ, Van Tilburg NH, Van Es LA. Acquired antithrombin III deficiency and thrombosis in the nephrotic syndrome. Am J Med 1978;65:607.
252. Panicucci F, Sagripanti A, Conte B, et al. Antithrombin III, heparin cofactor and antifactor Xa in relation to age, sex and pathological condition. Haemostasis 1980;9:297.
253. Weenink GH, Kahle LH, Lamping RJ, et al. Antithrombin III in oral contraceptive users and during normotensive pregnancy. Acta Obstet Gynecol Scand 1984;63:57.
254. Weenink GH, Treffers PE, Vijn P, et al. Antithrombin III levels in preeclampsia correlate with maternal and fetal morbidity. Am J Obstet Gynecol 1984;148:1092.
255. Buchanan GR, Holtkamp CA. Reduced antithrombin III levels during L-asparaginase therapy. Med Pediatr Oncol 1980;8:7.
256. Marciniak E, Gockemen JP. Heparin-induced decrease in circulating antithrombin III. Lancet 1978;2:581.
257. Kitchens CS. Amelioration of antithrombin III deficiency by coumarin administration. Am J Med Sci 1987;293:403.
258. Hoffman DL. Purification and large-scale preparation of antithrombin III. Am J Med 1989;87(Suppl 3B):23S–26S.
259. Menache D, O'Malley JP, Schorr JB, et al. Evaluation of the safety, recovery, half-life, and clinical efficacy of antithrombin III (human) in patients with hereditary antithrombin III deficiency. Blood 1990;75:33.
260. Mannucci PM, Boyer C, Wolf M, et al. Treatment of congenital antithrombin III deficiency with concentrates. Br J Haematol 1982;50:531.
261. Winter JH. Transfusion studies in patients with familial antithrombin III deficiency: half disappearance time of infused antithrombin III and influence of such infusion on platelet life span. Br J Haematol 1981;49:449.
262. Brandt P. Observations during the treatment of antithrombin III deficient women with heparin and antithrombin III during pregnancy, parturition, and abortion. Thromb Res 1981;22:15.
263. Schwartz RS, Bauer KA, Rosenberg RD, et al. Clinical experience with antithrombin III concentrate in treatment of congenital and acquired deficiency of antithrombin. Am J Med 1989;87(Suppl 3B):53S.
264. Hirsh J, Piovella F, Pini M. Congenital antithrombin III deficiency: incidence and clinical features. Am J Med 1989;87(Suppl 3B):34S.
265. Conard J, Horellou MH, Van Dreden P, et al. Thrombosis and pregnancy in congenital deficiencies in ATIII, protein C or protein S: study of 78 women. (Letter) Thromb Haemost 1990;63:319.
266. Iturbe-Alessio I, Fonseca MC, Mutchinik O, et al. Risks of anticoagulant therapy in pregnant women with artificial heart valves. N Engl J Med 1986;315:1390.
267. Walker ID, Davidson JF, Young P, Conkie JA. Effect of anabolic steroids on plasma antithrombin III α_2 macroglobulin and α_1 antitrypsin levels. Thromb Diath Haemorrh 1975;24:106.
268. Laurell C-B, Rannevik G. A comparison of plasma protein changes induced by danazol, pregnancy and estrogens. J Clin Endocrinol Metab 1979;49:719.
269. Winter JH, Fenech A, Bennett B, Douglas AS. Prophylactic antithrombotic therapy with stanazolol in patients with familial antithrombin III deficiency. Br J Haematol 1984;57:527.
270. Eyster ME, Parker ME. Treatment of familial antithrombin-III deficiency with danazol. Haemostasis 1985;15:119.
271. Griffin JH, Evatt B, Zimmerman TS, et al. Deficiency of protein C in congenital thrombotic disease. J Clin Invest 1981;68:1370.
272. Bertina RM, Broekmans AW, van der Linden IK, Mertens K. Protein C deficiency in a Dutch family with thrombotic disease. Thromb Haemost 1982;45:237.
273. Broekmans AW, Veltkamp JJ, Bertina RM. Congenital protein C deficiency and venous thromboembolism: a study of three Dutch families. N Engl J Med 1983;309:340.
274. Broekmans AW, Bertina RM Protein C. In: Poller L, ed. Recent advances in blood coagulation, no 4. New York, Churchill Livingstone, 1985: 117.
275. Horellou MH, Conard J, Bertina RM, Samama M. Congenital protein C deficiency and thrombotic disease in nine French families. British Medical J 1984;289:1285.
276. Pabinger-Fasching I, Bertina RM, Lechner K, et al. Protein C deficiency in two Austrian families. Thromb Haemost 1983;50:810.
277. Bovill EG, Bauer KA, Dickerman JD, et al. The clinical spectrum of heterozygous protein C deficiency in a large New England kindred. Blood 1989;73:712.
278. Wintzen AR, Broekmans AW, Bertina RM, et al. Cerebral hemorrhagic infarction in young patients with hereditary protein C deficiency: evidence for "spontaneous" cerebral venous thrombosis. Br Med J 1985;290:350.
279. Branson HE, Katz J, Marble R, Griffin JH. Inherited protein C deficiency and coumarin-responsive chronic relapsing purpura fulminans in a newborn infant. Lancet 1983;2:1165.
280. Seligsohn U, Berger A, Abend M, et al. Homozygous protein C deficiency manifested by massive venous thrombosis in the newborn. N Engl J Med 1984;310:559.
281. Sills RH, Marlar RA, Montgomery RR, et al. Severe homozygous protein C deficiency. J Pediatr 1984;105:409.
282. Estelles A, Garcia-Plaza I, Dasi A, et al. Severe inherited "homozygous" protein C deficiency in a newborn infant. Thromb Haemost 1984;52:53.
283. Marciniak E, Wilson HD, Marlar RA. Neonatal purpura fulminans: a genetic disorder related to the absence of protein C in blood. Blood 1985;65:15.
284. Yuen P, Cheung A, Lin HJ, et al. Purpura fulminans in a Chinese boy with congenital protein C deficiency. Pediatrics 1986;77:670.
285. Rappaport ES, Speights VO, Helbert B, et al. Protein C deficiency. South Med J 1987;80:240.
286. Peters C, Casella JF, Marlar RA, et al. Homozygous protein C deficiency: observations on the nature of the molecular abnormality and the effectiveness of warfarin therapy. Pediatrics 1988;81:272.
287. Tarras S, Gadia C, Meister L, Roldan E, Gregorios JB. Homozygous protein C deficiency in a newborn: clinicopathologic correlation. Arch Neurol 1988;45:214.
288. Auletta MJ, Headington JT. Purpura fulminans: a cutaneous manifestation of severe protein C deficiency. Arch Dermatol 1988;124:1387.
289. Miletich J, Sherman L, Broze G Jr. Absence of thrombosis in subjects with heterozygous protein C deficiency. N Engl J Med 1987;317:991.
290. Broekmans AW, Bertina RM, Loeliger EA, Hofmann V, Klingeman HG. Protein C and the development of skin necrosis during anticoagulant therapy. (Letter) Thromb Haemost 1983;49:244.
291. McGehee WG, Klotz TA, Epstein DJ, Rapaport SI. Coumarin necrosis associated with hereditary protein C deficiency. Ann Intern Med 1984;100:59.
292. Samama M, Horellou MH, Soria J, Conrad J, Nicolas G. Successful progressive anticoagulation in a severe protein C deficiency and previous skin necrosis at initiation of oral anticoagulant treatment. (Letter) Thromb Haemost 1984;51:132.
293. Zauber NP, Stark MW. Successful warfarin anticoagulation despite protein C deficiency and a history of warfarin necrosis. Ann Intern Med 1986;104:659.
294. D'Angelo SV, Comp PC, Esmon CT, D'Angelo A. Relationship between protein C antigen and anticoagulant activity during oral anticoagulation and in selected disease states. J Clin Invest 1986;77:416.
295. Conway EM, Bauer KA, Barzegar S, Rosenberg RD. Suppression of hemostatic system activation by oral anticoagulants in the blood of patients with thrombotic diatheses. J Clin Invest 1987;80:1535.
296. Broekmans AW, Teepe RGC, v d Meer FJM, et al. Protein C (PC) and coumarin-induced skin necrosis. (Abstract) Thromb Res 1986;6:137.
297. Teepe RGC, Broekmans AW, Vermeer BJ, et al. Recurrent coumarin-induced skin necrosis in a patient with an acquired functional protein C deficiency. Arch Dermatol 1986;122:1408.
298. Crabtree GR, Plutzky J, Marlar R, et al. The range of genotypes underlying human protein C deficiency. (Abstract) Thromb Haemost 1985;54:56.
299. Romeo G, Hassan HJ, Staempfli S, et al. Hereditary thrombophilia: identification of nonsense and missense mutations in the protein C gene. Proc Natl Acad Sci USA 1987;84:2829.
300. Reitsma PH. Molecular basis of hereditary thrombophilia. (Abstract) Br J Haematol 1990;76(Suppl 1):1.
301. Reitsma PH, te Lintel Hekkert W, Koenhen E, et al. Application of two neutral MspI DNA polymorphisms in the analysis of hereditary protein C deficiency. Thromb Haemost 1990;64:239.
302. Bertina RM, Broekmans AW, Krommenhoek-van Es C, et al. The use of a functional and immunologic assay for plasma protein C in the

study of the heterogeneity of congenital protein C deficiency. Thromb Haemost 1984;51:1.
303. Comp PC, Nixon RR, Esmon CT. Determination of functional levels of protein C, an antithrombotic protein, using thrombin–thrombomodulin complex. Blood 1984;63:15.
304. Barbui T, Finazzi G, Mussoni L, et al. Hereditary dysfunctional protein C (protein C Bergamo) and thrombosis. (Letter) Lancet 1984;2: 819.
305. Sala N, Borrell M, Bauer KA, et al. Dysfunctional activated protein C (PC Cadiz) in a patient with thrombotic disease. Thromb Haemost 1987;57:183.
306. Tirindelli MC, Franchi F, Tripodi A, et al. Familial dysfunctional protein C. Thromb Res 1986;44:893.
307. Faioni EM, Esmon CT, Esmon NL, Mannucci PM. Isolation of an abnormal protein C molecule from the plasma of a patient with thrombotic diathesis. Blood 1988;71:940.
308. Vasse M, Borg JY, Monconduit M. Protein C:Rouen, a new hereditary protein C abnormality with low anticoagulant but normal amidolytic activities. Thromb Res 1989;56:387.
309. Soria J, Soria C, Samama M, Nicolas G, Kissel W. Severe protein C deficiency in congenital thrombotic disease-description of an immunoenzymological assay for protein C determination. Thromb Haemost 1985;53:293.
310. Manabe S, Matsuda M. Homozygous protein C deficiency combined with heterozygous dysplasminogenemia found in a 21-year-old thrombophilic man. Thromb Res 1985;39:333.
311. Sharon C, Tirindelli MC, Mannucci PM, et al. Homozygous protein C deficiency with moderately severe clinical symptoms. Thromb Res 1986;41:483.
312. Kakkar S, Melissari E, VV Kakkar. Congenital severe protein C deficiency in adults. (Abstract) Thromb Haemost 1987;58:410.
313. Bauer KA, Broekmans AW, Bertina RM, et al. Hemostatic enzyme generation in the blood of patients with hereditary protein C deficiency. Blood 1988;71:1418.
314. Triplett DA, Sandquist DS, Musgrave KA. Clinical application of a functional assay for protein C. Hematol Pathol 1988;1:239.
315. Gruppo RA, Leimer P, Francis RB, et al. Protein C deficiency resulting from possible double heterozygosity and its response to danazol. Blood 1988;71:370.
316. Matsuda M, Sugo T, Sakata Y, et al. A thrombotic state due to an abnormal protein C. N Engl J Med 1988;319:1265.
317. Boyer C, Rothschild C, Wolf M, et al. A new method for the estimation of protein C by ELISA. Thromb Res 1984;36:579.
318. Epstein DJ, Begum PW, Bajaj SP, Rapaport SI. Radioimmunoassays for protein C and factor X: plasma antigen levels in abnormal hemostatic states. Am J Clin Pathol 1984;82:573.
319. Francis RB Jr, Patch MJ. A functional assay for protein C in human plasma. Thromb Res 1983;32:605.
320. Sala N, Owen WG, Collen D. Functional assay of protein C in human plasma. Blood 1984;63:671.
321. Martinoli JL, Stocker K. Fast functional protein C assay using Protac C, a novel protein C activator. Thromb Res 1986;43:253.
322. Francis RB Jr, Seyfert U. Rapid amidolytic assay of protein C in whole plasma using an activator from the venom of *Agkistrodon contortrix*. Am J Clin Pathol 1987;87:619.
323. Walker PA, Bauer KA, McDonagh J. A simple, automated functional assay for protein C. Am J Clin Pathol 1989;92:210.
324. Mannucci PM, Vigano S. Deficiencies of protein C, an inhibitor of blood coagulation. Lancet 1982;2:463.
325. Polack B, Pouzol P, Amiral J, Kolodie L. Protein C level at birth. Thromb Haemost 1984;52:188.
326. Karpatkin M, Mannucci P, Bhogal M, et al. Low protein C in the neonatal period. Br J Haematol 1986;62:137.
327. Manco-Johnson MJ, Marlar RA, Jacobson LJ, et al. Severe protein C deficiency in newborn infants. J Pediatr 1988;113:359.
328. Griffin JH, Mosher DF, Zimmerman TS, Kleiss AJ. Protein C, an antithrombotic protein, is reduced in hospitalized patients with intravascular coagulation. Blood 1982;60:261.
329. Rodeghiero F, Mannucci PM, Vigano S, et al. Liver dysfunction rather than intravascular coagulation as the main cause of low protein C and antithrombin III in acute leukemia. Blood 1984;63:965.
330. Marlar RA, Endres-Brooks J, Miller C. Serial studies of protein C and its plasma inhibitor in patients with disseminated intravascular coagulation. Blood 1985;66:59.
331. Mimuro J, Sakata Y, Wakabayashi K, Matsuda M. Level of protein C determined by combined assays during disseminated intravascular coagulation and oral anticoagulation. Blood 1987;69:1704.
332. Pui CH, Chesney CM, Bergum PW, et al. Lack of pathogenetic role of proteins C and S in thrombosis associated with asparaginase-prednisone-vincristine therapy for leukaemia. Br J Haematol 1986;64:283.
333. Cosio FG, Harker C, Batard MA, et al. Plasma concentrations of the natural anticoagulants protein C and protein S in patients with proteinuria. J Lab Clin Med 1985;106:218.
334. Vigano-D'Angelo S, D'Angelo A, Kaufman CE Jr, et al. Protein S deficiency occurs in the nephrotic syndrome. Ann Intern Med 1987;107: 42.
335. Mitchell CA, Rowell JA, Hau L, et al. A fatal thrombotic disorder associated with an acquired inhibitor of protein C. N Engl J Med 1987;317: 1638.
336. Gonzalez R, Alberca I, Sala N, Vicente V. Protein C deficiency-response to danazol and DDAVP. Thromb Haemost 1985;53:320.
337. Broekmans AW, Conard J, van Weyenberg RG, et al. Treatment of hereditary protein C deficiency with stanazolol. Thromb Haemost 1987;57:20.
338. De Stefano V, Leone G, Teofili L, et al. Transient ischemic attack in a patient with congenital protein-C during treatment with stanazolol. Am J Hematol 1988;29:120.
339. Vigano S, Mannucci PM, Solinas S, et al. Decrease in protein C antigen and formation of an abnormal protein soon after starting oral anticoagulant therapy. Br J Haematol 1984;57:213.
340. Vukovich T, Auberger K, Weil J, et al. Replacement therapy for a homozygous protein C deficiency-state using a concentrate of human protein C and S. Br J Haematol 1988;70:435.
341. Garcia-Plaza I, Jimenez-Astorga C, Borrego D, Marty ML. Coumarin prophylaxis for fulminant purpura syndrome due to homozygous protein C deficiency. (Letter) Lancet 1985;1:634.
342. Hartman KR, Manco-Johnson M, Rawlings JS, et al. Homozygous protein C deficiency: early treatment with warfarin. Am J Pediatr Hematol Oncol 1989;11:395.
343. Casella JF, Lewis JH, Bontempo FA, et al. Successful treatment of homozygous protein C deficiency by hepatic transplantation. Lancet 1988;1:435.
344. Comp PC, Esmon CT. Recurrent venous thromboembolism in patients with a partial deficiency of protein S. N Engl J Med 1984;311:1525.
345. Schwarz HP, Fischer M, Hopmeier P, et al. Plasma protein S deficiency in familial thrombotic disease. Blood 1984;64:1297.
346. Szatkowski NS, Miller CM, Endres-Brooks JL, et al. Clinical studies of human protein S and identification of a patient with protein S deficiency and thrombotic complications. (Abstract) Circulation 1984;70(Suppl 2):204.
347. Broekmans AW, Bertina RM, Reinalda-Poot J, et al. Hereditary protein S deficiency and venous thrombo-embolism: a study in three Dutch families. Thromb Haemost 1985;53:273.
348. Sas G, Blasko G, Petro I, Griffin J. A protein S deficient family with portal vein thrombosis. (Letter) Thromb Haemost 1985;54:724.
349. Kamiya T, Sugihara T, Ogata K, et al. Inherited deficiency of protein S in a Japanese family with recurrent venous thrombosis: a study of three generations. Blood 1986;67:406.
350. Comp PC, Doray D, Patton D, Esmon CT. An abnormal plasma distribution of protein S occurs in functional protein S deficiency. Blood 1986;67:504.
351. Mannucci PM, Tripodi A, Bertina RM. Protein S deficiency associated with "juvenile" arterial and venous thromboses. (Letter) Thromb Haemost 1986;55:440.
352. Pabinger I, Bertina RM, Lechner K, et al. Protein S deficiency in 7 Austrian families. (Abstract) Thromb Res 1986;42(Suppl 6):136.
353. Engesser L, Broekmans AW, Briet E, et al. Hereditary protein S deficiency: clinical manifestations. Ann Intern Med 1987;106:677.
354. Broekmans AW, van Rooyen W, Westerveld BD, et al. Mesenteric vein thrombosis as presenting manifestation of hereditary protein S deficiency. Gastroenterology 1987;92:240.
355. De Stefano V, Leone G, Ferrelli R, et al. Severe deep vein thrombosis in a 2-year-old child with protein S deficiency. (Letter) Thromb Haemost 1987;58:1089.
356. Boyer-Neumann C, Wolf M, Amiral J, et al. Familial type I protein S deficiency associated with severe venous thrombosis: a study of five cases. (Letter) Thromb Haemost 1988;60:128.
357. Ploos van Amstel HK, Huisman MV, Reitsma PH, et al. Partial protein S gene deletion in a family with hereditary thrombophilia. Blood 1989;73:479.
358. Schwarz HP, Heeb MJ, Lottenberg R, et al. Familial protein S deficiency with a variant protein S molecule in plasma and platelets. Blood 1989;74: 213.
360. Whitlock JA, Janco RL, Phillips JA III. Inherited hypercoagulable states in children. Am J Ped Hematol Oncol 1989;11:170.
361. Friedman KD, Marlar RA, Houston JG, Montgomery RR. Warfarin-induced skin necrosis in a patient with protein S deficiency. (Abstract) Blood 1986;68(Suppl 1):333a.
362. Fair DS, Revak DJ. Quantitation of human protein S in the plasma of normal and warfarin-treated individuals by radioimmunoassay. Thromb Res 1984;36:527.
363. Bertina RM, van Wijngaarden A, Reinalda-Poot J, et al. Determination of plasma protein S—the protein cofactor of activated protein C. Thromb Haemost 1985;53:268.
364. Comp PC, Thurnau GR, Welsh J, Esmon CT. Functional and immunologic protein S levels are decreased during pregnancy. Blood 1986;68: 881.
365. Malm J, Laurell M, Dahlback B. Changes in the plasma levels of vitamin K–dependent proteins C and S and of C4b-binding protein during pregnancy and oral contraception. Br J Haematol 1988;68:437.
366. Van de Waart P, Preissner KT, Bechtold JR, Muller-Berghaus G. A functional test for protein S activity in plasma. Thromb Res 1987;48: 427.
367. D'Angelo A, Vigano-D'Angelo S, Esmon CT, Comp PC. Acquired de-

ficiencies of protein S: protein S activity during oral anticoagulation, in liver disease, and in disseminated intravascular coagulation. J Clin Invest 1988;81:1445.
368. Suzuki K, Nishioka J. Plasma protein S activity measured using Protac, a snake venom derived activator of protein C. Thromb Res 1988;49: 241.
369. Kobayashi I, Amemiya N, Endo T, et al. Functional activity of protein S determined with use of protein C activated by venom activator. Clin Chem 1989;35:1644.
370. Schwarz HP, Muntean W, Watzke H, et al. Low total protein antigen but high protein S activity due to decreased C4b-binding protein in neonates. Blood 1988;71:562.
371. Mahasandana C, Suvatte V, Marlar R, et al. Neonatal purpura fulminans associated with homozygous protein S deficiency. (Abstract) Thromb Haemost 1989;62:301.
372. Miletich JP, Broze GJ Jr. Age and gender dependence of total protein S antigen in the normal adult population. (Abstract) Blood 1988;72(Suppl 1):371a.
373. Boerger LM, Morris PC, Thurnau GR, Esmon CT, Comp PC. Oral contraceptives and gender affect protein S status. Blood 1987;69:692.
374. Gilabert J, Fernandez JA, Espana F, Azner J, Estelles A. Physiological coagulation inhibitors (protein S, protein C and antithrombin III) in severe preeclamptic states and in users of oral contraceptives. Thromb Res 1988;49:319.
375. Heeb MJ, Mosher D, Griffin JH. Activation and complexation of protein C and cleavage and decrease of protein S in plasma of patients with disseminated intravascular coagulation. Blood 1989;73:455.
376. Gouault-Heilmann M, Gadelha-Parente T, Levent M, et al. Total and free protein S in nephrotic syndrome. Thromb Res 1988;49:37.
377. Malm J, Bennhagen R, Holmberg L, Dahlback B. Plasma concentrations of C4b-binding protein and vitamin K-dependent protein S in term and preterm infants: low levels of protein S-C4b-binding protein complexes. Br J Haematol 1988;68:445.
378. Melissari E, Nicolaides KH, Scully MF, Kakkar VV. Protein S and C4b-binding protein in fetal and neonatal blood. Br J Haematol 1988;70: 199.
379. McDonagh J, Carrell N. Disorders of fibrinogen structure and function. In: Colman RW, Hirsh J, Marder VJ, Salzman EW, eds. Hemostasis and thrombosis: basic principles and clinical practice, ed 2. Philadelphia, JB Lippincott, 1987:301.
380. Egeberg O. Inherited fibrinogen abnormality causing thrombophilia. Thromb Diath Haemorrh 1967;17:175.
381. Thorsen LI, Brosstad F, Solum NO, Stormorken H. Increased binding to ADP-stimulated platelets and aggregation effect of the dysfibrinogen Oslo I as compared with normal fibrinogen. Scand J Haematol 1986;36: 203.
382. Beck EA, Charache P, Jackson DP. A new inherited coagulation disorder caused by an abnormal fibrinogen (fibrinogen "Baltimore"). Nature 1965;208:143.
383. Beck EA, Shainoff JR, Vogel A, Jackson DP. Functional evaluation of an inherited abnormal fibrinogen: fibrinogen Baltimore. J Clin Invest 1971;50:1874.
384. Sandbjerg-Hansen M, Clemmensen I, Wither D. Fibrinogen Copenhagen: an abnormal fibrinogen with defective polymerization and release of fibrinopeptide A, but normal adsorption of plasminogen. Scand J Clin Lab Invest 1980;40:221.
385. Henschen A, Kehl M, Southan C, et al. Genetically abnormal fibrinogens-some current characterization strategies. In: Haverkate F, Henschen A, Nieuwenhuizen W, Straub PW, eds. Fibrinogen-structure functional aspects metabolism, vol 2. Berlin, Walter de Gruyter, 1983: 125.
386. Andes WA. Fibrinogen New Orleans II: a new dysfibrinogenemia with venous thrombosis. (Abstract) Thromb Haemost 1983;50:337.
387. Al-Mondhiry HAB, Bilezikian SB, Nossel HL. Fibrinogen "New York": an abnormal fibrinogen associated with thromboembolism: functional evaluation. Blood 1975;45:607.
388. Soria J, Soria C, Samama M, Caen JP. Study of 10 cases of congenital dysfibrinogenemia: clinical and molecular biological aspects. (Abstract) Thromb Haemost 1983;50:415.
389. Soria J, Soria C, Samama M, Caen JP. Study of 10 cases of congenital dysfibrinogenemia: clinical and molecular biological aspects. In: Henschen A, Hessel B, McDonagh J, Saldeen T, eds. Fibrinogen: structural variants and interactions, vol 3. Berlin, Walter de Gruyter, 1985: 165.
390. Haverkate F, Koopman J, Kluft C, et al. Fibrinogen Milano II: a congenital dysfibrinogenemia associated with juvenile arterial and venous thrombosis. Thromb Haemost 1986;55:131.
391. Carrell N, Gabriel DA, Blatt PM, et al. Hereditary dysfibrinogenemia in a patient with thrombotic disease. Blood 1983;62:439.
392. Carrell N, McDonagh J. Functional defects in abnormal fibrinogens. In: Henschen A, Hessel B, McDonagh J, Saldeen T, eds. Fibrinogen: structural variants and interactions, vol 3. Berlin, Walter de Gruyter, 1985:155.
393. Soria J, Soria C, Samama M, et al. Fibrinogen Haifa: fibrinogen variant with absence of protective effect of calcium on plasmin degradation of gamma chains. Thromb Haemost 1987;57:310.
394. Soria J, Soria C, Caen JP. A new type of congenital dysfibrinogenemia with defective fibrin lysis-Dusard syndrome: possible relation to thrombosis. Br J Haematol 1983;53:575.
395. Lijnen HR, Soria J, Soria C, et al. Dysfibrinogenemia (fibrinogen Dusard) associated with impaired fibrin-enhanced plasminogen activation. Thromb Haemost 1984;51:108.
396. Aoki N, Moroi M, Sakata Y, et al. Abnormal plasminogen: a hereditary abnormality found in a patient with recurrent thrombosis. J Clin Invest 1978;61:1186.
397. Sakata Y, Aoki N. Molecular abnormality of plasminogen. J Biol Chem 1980;255:5442.
398. Miyata T, Iwanaga S, Sakata Y, Aoki N. Plasminogen Tochigi: inactive plasmin resulting from replacement of alanine-600 by threonine in the active site. Proc Natl Acad Sci USA 1979;79:6132.
399. Miyata T, Iwanaga S, Sakata Y, et al. Plasminogens Tochigi II and Nagoya: two additional molecular defects with Ala-600—Thr replacement found in plasmin light chain variants. J Biochem 1984;96:277.
400. Wohl RC, Summaria L, Robbins KC. Physiological activation of the human fibrinolytic system: isolation and characterization of human plasminogen variants, Chicago I and Chicago II. J Biol Chem 1979;254: 9063.
401. Kazama M, Tahara C, Suzuki Z, et al. Abnormal plasminogen, a case of recurrent thrombosis. Thromb Res 1981;21:517.
402. Wohl RC, Summaria L, Chediak J, et al. Human plasminogen variant Chicago III. Thromb Haemost 1982;48:146.
403. Soria J, Soria C, Bertrand O, et al. Plasminogen Paris I: congenital abnormal plasminogen and its incidence in thrombosis. Thromb Res 1983;32:229.
404. Lottenberg R, Dolly FR, Kitchens CS. Recurring thromboembolic disease and pulmonary hypertension associated with severe hypoplasminogenemia. Am J Hematol 1985;19:181.
405. Mannucci PM, Kluft C, Traas DW, et al. Congenital plasminogen deficiency associated with venous thromboembolism: therapeutic trial with stanazolol. Br J Haematol 1986;63:753.
406. Scharrer IM, Wohl RC, Hach V, et al. Investigation of a congenital abnormal plasminogen, Frankfurt I, and its relationship to thrombosis. Thromb Haemost 1986;55:396.
407. Liu Y, Lyons RM, McDonagh J. Plasminogen San Antonio: an abnormal plasminogen with a more cathodic migration, decreased activation and associated thrombosis. Thromb Haemost 1988;59:49.
408. Aoki N, Tateno K, Sakata Y. Differences of frequency distributions of plasminogen phenotypes between Japanese and American populations: new methods for the detection of plasminogen variants. Biochem Genet 1984;22:871.
409. Johansson L, Hedner U, Nilsson IM. A family with thromboembolic disease associated with deficient fibrinolytic activity in vessel wall. Acta Med Scand 1978;203:477.
410. Jorgensen M, Mortensen JZ, Madsen AG, et al. A family with reduced plasminogen activator activity in blood associated with recurrent venous thrombosis. Scand J Haematol 1982;29:217.
411. Nilsson IM, Tengborn L. A family with thrombosis associated with high level of tissue plasminogen activator inhibitor. (Abstract) Haemostasis 1984;14:24.
412. Nilsson IM, Ljungner H, Tengborn L. Two different mechanisms in patients with venous thrombosis and defective fibrinolysis: low concentration of plasminogen activator or increased concentration of plasminogen activator inhibitor. Br Med J 1985;290:1453.
413. Wiman B, Ljungberg B, Chmielewska J, et al. The role of the fibrinolytic system in deep venous thrombosis. J Lab Clin Med 1985;105:265.
414. Hamsten A, Wiman B, de Faire U, Blomback M. Increased plasma levels of a rapid inhibitor of tissue plasminogen activator in young survivors of myocardial infarction. N Engl J Med 1985;313:1557.
415. Brandt JT, Triplett DA, Musgrave K, Orr C. The sensitivity of different coagulation reagents to the presence of lupus anticoagulants. Arch Pathol Lab Med 1987;11:120.
416. Thiagarajan P, Pengo V, Shapiro SS. The use of the dilute Russell viper venom time for the diagnosis of lupus anticoagulants. Blood 1986;68: 869.
417. Exner T, Rickard KA, Kronenberg H. A sensitive test demonstrating lupus anticoagulant and its behavioural patterns. Br J Haematol 1978;40: 143.
418. Schleider MA, Nachman RL, Jaffe EA, Coleman M. A clinical study of the lupus anticoagulant. Blood 1976;48:499.
419. Triplett DA, Brandt JT, Kaczor D, Schaeffer J. Laboratory diagnosis of lupus inhibitors: a comparison of the tissue thromboplastin inhibition procedure with a new platelet neutralization procedure. Am J Clin Pathol 1983;79:678.
420. Rosove MH, Ismail M, Koziol BJ, Runge E, Kasper CK. Lupus anticoagulants: improved diagnosis with a kaolin clotting time using rabbit brain phospholipid in standard and high concentrations. Blood 1986;68: 472.
421. Lechner K. Lupus anticoagulants and thrombosis. In: Verstraete J, Vermylen J, Lijnen R, Arnout J, eds. Thrombosis and haemostasis 1987. Leuven, Belgium, Leuven University Press, 1987:525.
422. Triplett DA, Brandt JT. Lupus anticoagulants: misnomer, paradox, riddle, epiphenomenon. Hematol Pathol 1988;2:121.
423. Mueh JR, Herbst KD, Rapaport SI. Thrombosis in patients with the lupus anticoagulant. Ann Intern Med 1980;92:156.

424. Gastineau DA, Kazmier FJ, Nichols WL, et al. Lupus anticoagulants: an analysis of the clinical and laboratory features of 219 cases. Am J Hematol 1985;19:265.
425. Weinstein C, Miller MH, Axtens R, et al. Livedo reticularis associated with increased titers of anticardiolipin antibodies in systemic lupus erythematosus. Arch Dermatol 1987;123:596.
426. Dodd HJ, Sarkany I, O'Shaughnessy D. Widespread cutaneous necrosis associated with lupus anticoagulant. Clin Exp Dermatol 1985;10:581.
427. Johansson EA, Lassus A. The occurrence of circulating anticoagulants in patients with syphilitic and biologically false positive antilipoidal antibodies. Ann Clin Res 1974;6:105.
428. Thiagarajan P, Shapiro S, DeMarco L. Monoclonal immunoglobulin M coagulation inhibitor with phospholipid specificity: mechanism of a lupus anticoagulant. J Clin Invest 1980;66:397.
429. Pengo V, Thiagarajan P, Shapiro SS, Heine MJ. Immunological specificity and mechanism of action of IgG lupus anticoagulants. Blood 1987;70:69.
430. McNeil HP, Simpson RJ, Chesterman CN, Krilis SA. Anti-phospholipid antibodies are directed against a complex antigen that includes a lipid-binding inhibitor of coagulation: β_2-glycoprotein I (apolipoprotein H). Proc Natl Acad Sci USA 1990;87:4120.
431. Galli M, Comfurius P, Maassen C, et al. Anticardiolipin antibodies (ACA) directed not to cardiolipin but to a plasma protein cofactor. Lancet 1990;335:1544.
432. Harris EN, Gharavi AE, Boey ML, et al. Anticardiolipin antibodies: detection by radioimmunoassay and association with thrombosis in systemic lupus erythematosus. Lancet 1983;2:1211.
433. Loizou S, McCrea JD, Rudge AC, et al. Measurement of anti-cardiolipin antibodies by an enzyme-linked immunosorbent assay (ELISA): standardization and quantitation of results. Clin Exp Immunol 1985;62:738.
434. Triplett DA, Brandt JT, Musgrave KA, Orr CA. The relationship between lupus anticoagulants and antibodies to phospholipid. JAMA 1988;259:550.
435. Carreras LO, Defreyn G, Machin SJ, et al. Arterial thrombosis, intrauterine death and "lupus" anticoagulant: detection of immunoglobulin interfering with prostacyclin production. Lancet 1981;1:244.
436. Petraiuolo W, Bovill E, Hoak J. The lupus anticoagulant stimulates the release of prostacyclin from human endothelial cells. Thromb Res 1988;50:847.
437. Cariou R, Tobelem G, Bellucci S, et al. Effect of lupus anticoagulant on antithrombogenic properties of endothelial cells-inhibition of thrombomodulin-dependent protein C activation. Thromb Haemost 1988;60:54.
438. Rustin MH, Bull HA, Machin SJ, et al. Effects of the lupus anticoagulant in patients with systemic lupus erythematosus on endothelial cell prostacyclin release and procoagulant activity. J Invest Dermatol 1988;90:744.
439. Freyssinet JM, Wiesel ML, Gauchy J, et al. An IgM lupus anticoagulant that neutralizes the enhancing effect of phospholipid on purified endothelial thrombomodulin activity: a mechanism for thrombosis. Thromb Haemost 1986;55:309.
440. Comp PC, DeBault LE, Esmon NL,Esmon CT. Human thrombomodulin is inhibited by IgG from two patients with non-specific anticoagulants. Blood 1983;62(Suppl 1):299a.
441. Faaber P, Rijke TP, Van de Putte LB, et al. Cross reactivity of human and murine anti-DNA antibodies with heparan sulfate. J Clin Invest 1986;77:1824.
442. Angles-Cano E, Sultan Y, Clauvel JP. Predisposing factors to thrombosis in systemic lupus erythematosus: possible relation to endothelial cell damage. J Lab Clin Med 1979;94:312.
443. Simon TL, Smith KJ. Heparin assays. In: Colman RW, ed. Disorders of thrombin formation. New York, Churchill Livingstone, 1983:119.
444. Kelton JG, Hirsh J. Bleeding associated with antithrombotic therapy. Semin Hematol 1980;17:259.
445. Wanger GP, Roberts W, Brandt JT. Misleading heparin monitoring leading to protamine sulphate overdose in a patient with a lupus anticoagulant (letter). Lancet 1981;2:1112.
446. Nilsson IM, Astedt B, Hedner U, Berezin D. Intrauterine death and circulating anticoagulant, "antithromboplastin." Acta Med Scand 1975;197:153.
447. de Wolf F, Carreras LO, Moerman P, et al. Decidual vasculopathy and extensive placental infarction in a patient with repeated thromboembolic events, recurrent fetal loss, and a lupus anticoagulant. Am J Obstet Gynecol 1982;142:829.
448. Lockshin MD, Druzin ML, Goei S, et al. Antibody to cardiolipin as a predictor of fetal distress or death in pregnant patients with systemic lupus erythematosus. N Engl J Med 1985;313:152.
449. Branch DW, Scott JR, Kochenour NK, Hershgold E. Obstetric complications associated with the lupus anticoagulant. N Engl J Med 1985;313:1322.
450. Lubbe WF, Butler WS, Palmer SJ, Liggins GC. Fetal survival after prednisone suppression of maternal lupus anticoagulant. Lancet 1983;1:1361.
451. Rosove MH, Tabsh K, Howard P, et al. Heparin therapy for prevention of fetal wastage in women with anticardiolipin antibodies and lupus anticoagulants. (Abstract) Blood 1987;70(Suppl 1):379a.
452. Carreras LO, Perez GN, Vega HR, Casavilla F. Lupus anticoagulant and recurrent fetal loss: successful treatment with gamma-globulin. (Letter) Lancet 1988;2:393.
453. Lau HK, Rosenberg JS, Beeler DL, Rosenberg RD. The isolation and characterization of a specific antibody population directed against the prothrombin activation fragments F_2 and F_{1+2}. J Biol Chem 1979;254:8751.
454. Teitel JM, Bauer KA, Lau HK, Rosenberg RD. Studies of the prothrombin activation pathway utilizing radioimmunoassays for the F_2/F_{1+2} fragment and thrombin-antithrombin complex. Blood 1982;59:1086.
455. Nossel HL, Younger LR, Wilner GD, et al. Radioimmunoassay of human fibrinopeptide A. Proc Natl Acad Sci USA 1971;68:2350.
456. Nossel HL, Yudelman I, Canfield RE, et al. Measurement of fibrinopeptide A in human blood. J Clin Invest 1974;54:43.
457. Nossel HL, Ti M, Kaplan KL, et al. The generation of fibrinopeptide A in clinical blood samples: evidence for thrombin activity. J Clin Invest 1976;58:1136.
458. Nossel HL, Wasser J, Kaplan KL, et al. Sequence of fibrinogen protolysis and platelet release after intrauterine infusion of hypertonic saline. J Clin Invest 1979;64:1371.
459. Weitz JI, Koehn JA, Canfield RE, et al. Development of a radioimmunoassay for the fibrinogen-derived peptide Bβ1-42. Blood 1986;67:1014.
460. Harpel PC. α_2-Plasmin inhibitor and α_2-macroglobulin-plasmin complexes in plasma: quantification by an enzyme-linked differential antibody immunosorbent assay. J Clin Invest 1981;68:46.
461. Nossel HL. Relative proteolysis of the fibrinogen B beta chain by thrombin and plasmin as a determinant of thrombosis. Nature 1981;291:165.
462. Owen J, Kvam D, Nossel HL, et al. Thrombin and plasmin activity and platelet activation in the development of venous thrombosis. Blood 1983;61:476.

Blood: Principles and Practice of Hematology,
edited by Robert I. Handin, Samuel E. Lux, and Thomas P. Stossel.
J.B. Lippincott Company, Philadelphia © 1995.

45

Antiplatelet and Anticoagulant Therapy

Laurence A. Harker

THROMBOGENESIS

Thrombosis is a leading cause of morbidity and mortality in the western world. Thrombus forms in vivo as a pathologic consequence of interactions between blood hemostatic mechanisms and components of the injured vessel wall under variable flow conditions. Arterial thrombotic occlusion complicates atherosclerosis causing acute myocardial or cerebral infarction; venous thromboembolic disease complicates a variety of clinical settings generally characterized by blood stasis, activated blood factors, and vascular dysfunction or damage. Typically, vascular injury with activation of platelet and coagulation mechanisms under high shear flow produces an arterial type of thrombus rich in platelets but poor in fibrin and red blood cells (RBCs; white thrombus). By contrast, the red thrombus seen in venous thromboembolic disease is rich in fibrin and RBCs and relatively poor in platelets.

The type and intensity of antithrombotic approaches differ for each of these two processes. Antiplatelet agents are effective in the treatment of arterial thrombosis by inhibiting platelet recruitment into forming thrombus. Anticoagulants are effective in venous thrombosis by inhibiting soluble thrombin or its production. Fibrinolytic agents remove already formed arterial and venous thrombus by degrading the fibrin network.

Intact endothelium maintains the fluidity of blood by multiple mechanisms. For example, the electronegative charge of the endothelial membrane prevents cell deposition on its surface.[1] Endothelial cells also rapidly degrade platelet proaggregatory adenosine diphosphate[2] and synthesize molecules that potently inhibit platelet reactivity, that is, prostacyclin (PGI_2),[3] and nitric oxide (endothelium-derived relaxing factor).[4] Moreover, endothelium interrupts fibrin deposition by thrombomodulin-dependent production of activated protein C (APC), which down-regulates thrombin generation and by heparan sulfate-dependent antithrombin III (ATIII) inhibition of thrombin activity.[5–10] Fibrinolytic mechanisms are also up-regulated by thrombin's direct action on endothelium to release tissue plasminogen activator.[11,12] Furthermore, coagulation may be controlled by the action of other plasma serine–protease inhibitors in addition to ATIII, including heparin cofactor II, α_2-macroglobulin, and α_1-antitrypsin.[13–15] Finally, activated prothrombotic molecules are diluted into flowing blood and rapidly removed from the circulation by the hepatic phagocytic systems.

Arterial thrombosis occurs typically after vascular damage produced by mechanical, chemical, immunologic, or thermal injury. Subendothelial structures are then exposed to circulating blood, and platelets, which normally circulate as single, disk-shaped cells, adhere to and spread over the subendothelium. Platelet adhesion, the first step in thrombosis is mediated by the interaction of platelet membrane glycoproteins with adhesive proteins bound to subendothelial connective tissue structures. These multiple redundant receptor–counterreceptor adhesion reactions are targets for potential therapeutic interventions. The platelet–von Willebrand factor (vWF) interaction is important for platelet adhesion, particularly at high shear rate (in small vessels).[16] vWF interacts with connective tissue collagen or as yet unidentified microfibrillar noncollagenous substances of the vessel wall to undergo conformational change permitting its interaction with platelet gpIb/IX.[17–20] vWF may also interact with platelet gpIIb/IIIa, the common receptor for several other adhesive proteins depending on the tripeptide sequence Arg-Gly-Asp,[21–23] including fibrinogen, fibronectin, vitronectin, thrombospondin, laminin, and nidogen.[24–29]

Adherent platelets change their shape to form irregular spheres that extend pseudopods along the thrombogenic vascular surface. These activated platelets also release their granule contents, contributing to both thrombogenesis (adenosine diphosphate, adenosine triphosphate, serotonin, Ca^{2+}, adhesive proteins, coagulation factors) and atherogenesis (platelet-derived and other growth factors).[30] Ambient platelets are thus recruited to form an enlarging thrombus. Adenosine diphosphate, thromboxane A_2, and thrombin are independent inducers of platelet recruitment. Thrombin is the most important physiologic agonist of platelet recruitment in vivo.

Platelets adhere at sites of mechanical vascular injury, undergo activation, and express functional gpIIb/IIIa receptors (also referred to as integrin $\alpha_{IIb}\beta_3$) for circulating adhesive ligand proteins (primarily fibrinogen). These functional gpIIb/IIIa receptors mediate the recruitment of ambient platelets by ligand interplatelet bridging, a process referred to as platelet cohesion.[21,22] Although functional gpIIb/IIIa receptors bind with other circulating adhesive molecules in plasma (including von Willebrand factor, fibronectin, vitronectin, and thrombospondin), fibrinogen is the predominant ligand because of its relative high concentration. The recognition peptide sequence ARG-GLY-ASP (RGD) present in these different adhesive molecules mediates binding with expressed gpIIb/IIIa receptors.[21–23] The expression of active receptors involves conformational reconfiguration of the membrane heterodimeric gpIIb/IIIa by realigning the cytoplasmic domains of this transmembrane complex. Monoclonal antibodies detect the conformational changes associated with receptor expression,[23] and are capable of inhibiting platelet recruitment by blocking interplatelet adhesive ligand binding.[31–33]

In vivo thrombin plays a central role in thrombus formation by cleaving the platelet thrombin receptor to create an agonist peptide neo–amino-terminus and by cleaving fibrinogen to form fibrin monomer.[34–37] Thrombin is formed by the intrinsic and extrinsic pathways of coagulation. Subendothelial tissues and disrupted endothelial cells activate the contact factors of the intrinsic pathway. Injured vascular wall cells and macrophage–monocytes express tissue factor.[38] Tissue factor complexes with factor VII/VIIa, which initiates activation of extrinsic coagulation. Tissue factor is a glycoprotein that is expressed by vascular wall cells, especially smooth muscle cells, and adventitial fibroblasts, as well as macrophage–monocytes. Although tissue factor does not circulate, vascular injury expresses surface-bound tissue factor. It complexes with factor VII/VIIa from plasma to convert factor X to Xa and factor IX to IXa. Factor Xa, and probably factor IXa, catalyze factor VII conversion to VIIa, resulting in greatly amplified coagulant activity.[38] Platelets may contribute to the activation of the contact factors,[39] perhaps by binding factor XIa by means of a specific receptor[40] and by providing the phospholipid surface for the formation of the "tenase" (factor IXa–VIIIa–Ca^{2+}–phospholipid) and prothrombinase (factor Xa–Va–Ca^{2+}–phospholipid) complexes.[37] By their rich membrane content of anionic phospholipid, platelets may also augment factor Xa–catalyzed factor VII activation.[41] Thus, platelets amplify the rate at which thrombin is formed, protect bound coagulation factors from inactivation by plasma inhibitors, and localize the subsequent coagulation reaction to the hemostatic plug. Thrombin greatly amplifies thrombotic processes by positive feedback mechanisms for both platelets and fibrin by activating membrane-bound coagulation factors V and VIII. Finally, the thrombotic mass is consolidated by the thrombin-dependent conversion of fibrinogen into fibrin and thrombin's activation of factor XIII, thereby providing a covalent structure to the fibrin clot.[42]

A number of products arising from the thrombotic process may serve as blood tests for ongoing thrombus formation (Fig. 45-1). Sensitive specific immunometric assays are able to detect activation products from platelets (PF4, β-TG, and thromboxane B_2 [TXB_2]), coagulation (fragments 1 + 2, FPA, FPB, fibrin, and T:AT) and fibrinolysis (D:D-dimer and P:PI).

Stasis contributes directly to the pathogenesis of venous thrombosis. In general, thrombi in veins are found at sites of maximum stasis, such as in valve pockets[43] where a captive annular vortex produces prolonged residence times

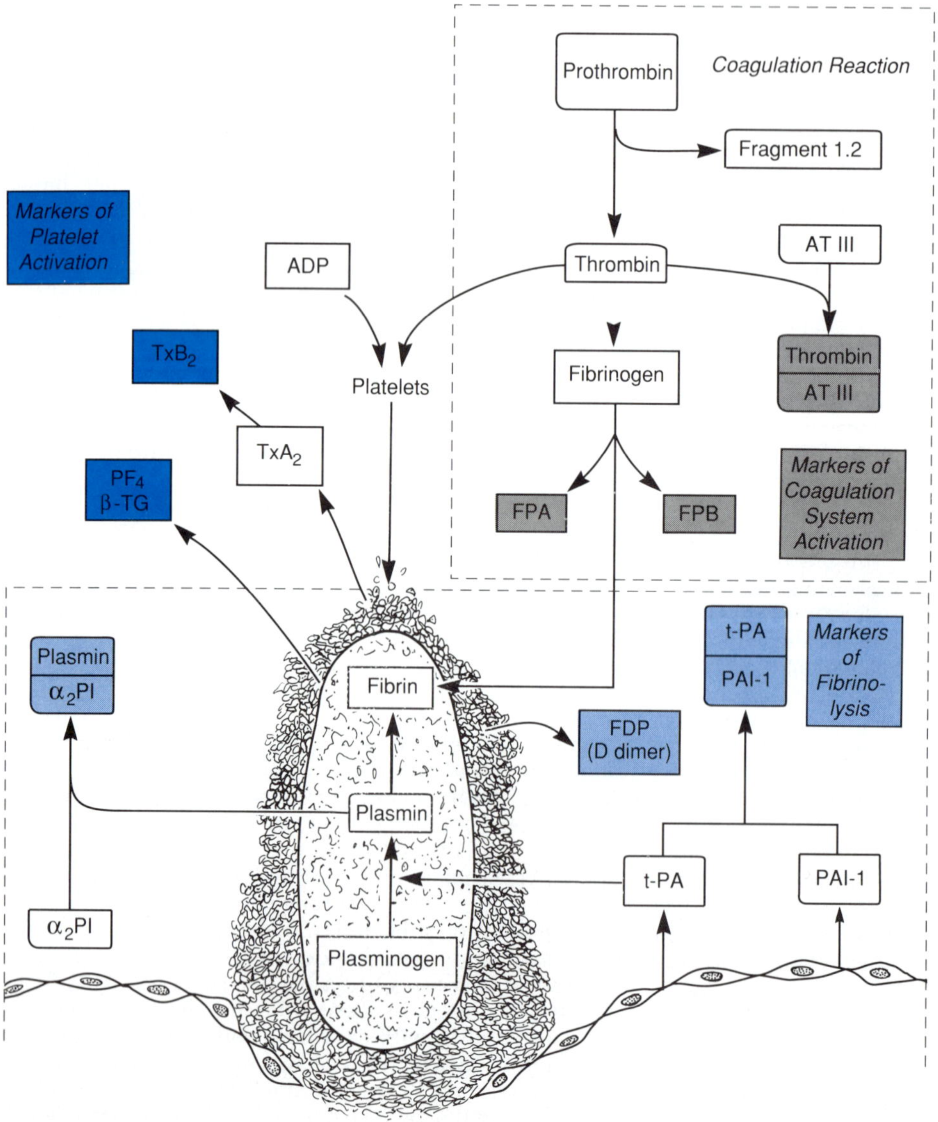

FIGURE 45-1. Biochemical blood markers of ongoing thrombus formation. Specific markers have been developed for detecting fibrin formation, fibrinolysis, platelet release, and for inhibitor complexes. Two platelet-specific proteins (platelet factor 4 [PF4] and β-thromboglobulin [βTG]) have been studied as markers of platelet activation. These proteins are localized in the α granules of resting platelets, and about 70% are released during the platelet release reaction. Care must be taken in drawing and preparing blood for assay to prevent artifactual release of these proteins during blood collection and processing. Increased levels of fibrinopeptide A (FPA) are sensitive to intravascular thrombin but are not entirely specific for intravascular thrombosis, since positive results are also found in patients with cellulitis and with generalized infections. Prothrombin activation fragment (fragment 1 + 2) circulates in humans under normal conditions and is detectably elevated in various thrombotic syndromes. Elevated levels of thrombin–antithrombin III (T-ATIII) complex are also found in patients with thrombosis. Assays for detection of plasmin–antiplasmin complex and D-dimer in plasma have been developed and show promise in clinical testing. These blood tests of ongoing thrombus formation are primarily useful for monitoring the effects of therapy with less certain usefulness in identifying patients at risk.

for blood cells and procoagulant species, thus increasing the likelihood that these elements will initiate the formation of thrombi.[44] Congenital or acquired hypercoagulability (deficiencies of plasma coagulation inhibitors, trauma, surgery, and others[45]) or hypofibrinolysis (decrease in tissue type plasminogen activator or increase in inhibitor of plasminogen activator[46]) predispose to the development of clinically evident venous thrombosis (Fig. 45-2). Platelets and endothelial cells are less important in venous thrombogenesis. Thrombosis after hip surgery because of local mechanical damage to the femoral vein produced during the surgical procedure is unusual. This may explain why thrombosis after hip surgery is less responsive to standard anticoagulant prophylaxis than other venous thrombotic events associated with surgery.[45]

A number of mechanisms limit the unwanted extension of thrombosis by modulating activation of platelets and coagulation. Since thrombin is the pivotal enzyme in the formation of thrombus, modifying thrombin production or its activity is a principal focus regulating thrombogenesis. Note that thrombin initiates antiaggregant,[3,4] anticoagulant,[6–10] and profibrinolytic properties[11,12] of endothelium. First, thrombin stimulates release of the antiaggregant molecules, PGI_2 and nitric oxide.[3,4] Second, ATIII complexes with heparin-like glycosaminoglycans at the surface of the endothelium and facilitates inactivation of thrombin by complex formation.[6,7] Third, the thrombin–thrombomodulin complex, with protein S as a cofactor, activates protein C. APC further destroys platelet-bound factors Va and VIIIa activity, thereby down-regulating the production of thrombin.[8–10] Fourth, thrombin activity is inhibited by several plasma serine–protease inhibitors, particularly antithrombin.[13–15]

Inhibition of the factor VIIa–tissue factor–induced blood coagulation by tissue factor pathway inhibitor limits thrombus extension associated with tissue injury or inflammation. This inhibitor initially forms a complex with factor Xa, which then inhibits further factor VIIa–tissue factor activation of factor X.[47]

Defective factors in these complex interactive protective mechanisms result in predisposition to thrombus formation (see Fig. 45-2).

The three classes of antithrombotic agents are antiplatelet, anticoagulant, and thrombolytic drugs. Their indi-

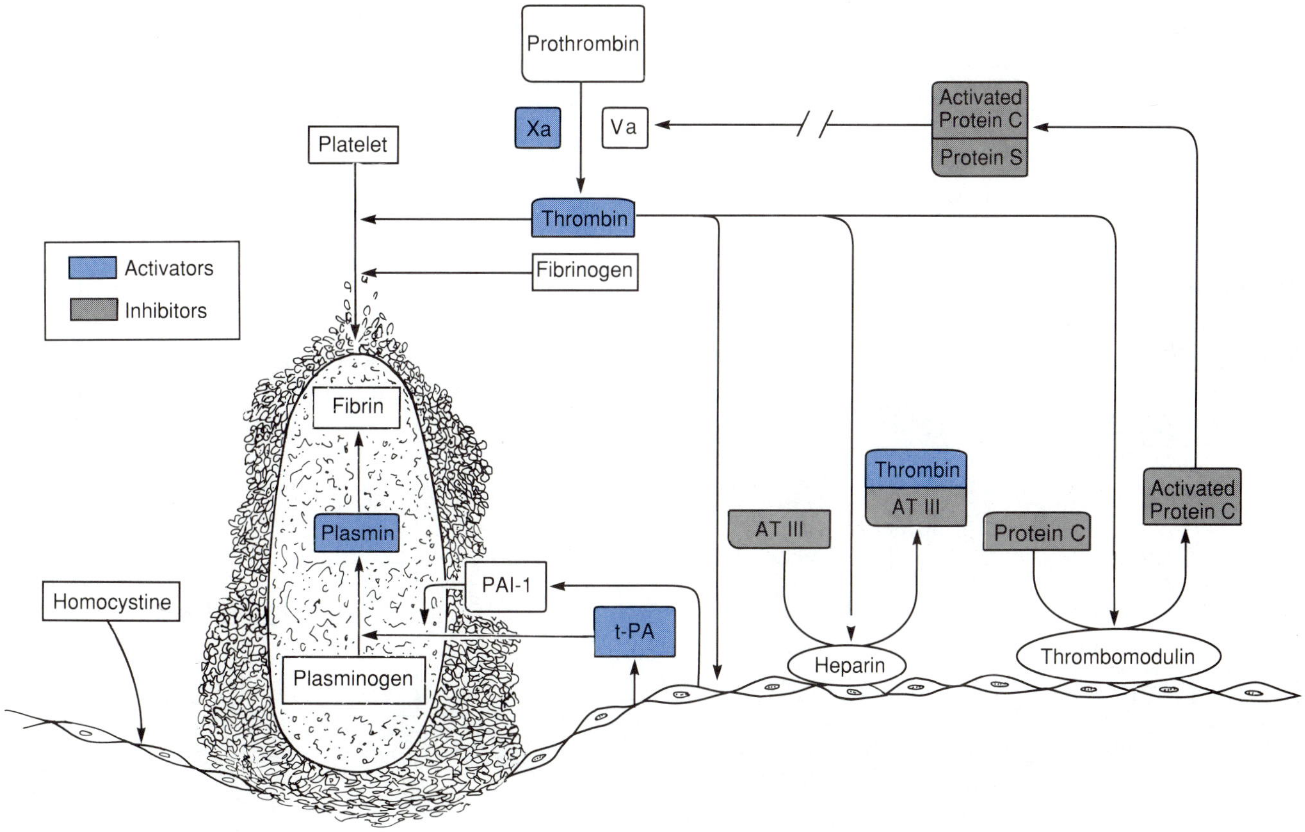

FIGURE 45-2. Genetic abnormalities predisposing to thrombotic disease. Kindred with various abnormalities affecting thrombus formation and its regulation have a predisposition to thrombosis (known disorders shown in the boldface boxes). Idiopathic and secondary venous thrombosis occurs in families with deficiency or dysfunction of antithrombin III (ATIII), protein C, and protein S. The traits are inherited in an autosomal dominant manner, and affected patients have ATIII levels of 40% to 60% of normal. Screening should be performed by functional assays. The inherited defects probably account for 8% to 10% of the venous thrombotic episodes occurring in patients aged 45 years or younger. Not all persons with these deficiencies develop thrombosis. By the age of 50, about 66% have symptoms. Inherited plasminogen defects or low plasma levels of tissue plasminogen activator are associated with about 2% to 3% of unexplained venous thromboembolism in younger patients, but only in a minority of family members is there a clear-cut association with thrombotic symptoms. Screening should be by functional assays. Occasionally, patients with congenital dysfibrinogenemia develop recurrent thrombosis. The inherited mechanisms for the occurrence of thrombosis in these patients are varied. The rare genetic recessive disorder of homocystinemia leads to focal endothelial denudation involving both arterial and venous endothelial surfaces so that thrombotic events in either or both systems may be observed.

cations differ according to the type of thrombotic process involved. The aim of antithrombotic therapy is to choose agents with an appropriate ratio of antithrombotic efficacy to hemostatic safety. These drugs may be administered separately or combined when broader or more potent antithrombotic effects are required.

ANTIPLATELET THERAPY

Antiplatelet drugs reduce platelet recruitment into forming thrombus (Fig. 45-3). Ideally, a clinically useful antiplatelet drug should be nontoxic and orally effective, should have sustained action, and should have good antithrombotic potency without excessive risk of abnormal bleeding. None of the clinically available agents satisfies all these requirements. Unequivocal evidence proves that aspirin[48–64] and ticlopidine[65–68] are effective antiplatelet agents in subgroups of patients with ischemic heart disease and cerebrovascular disease. The blockade of gpIIb/IIIa-dependent platelet recruitment is an appealing interventional strategy because gpIIb/IIIa is specific for platelets, platelet recruitment depends almost exclusively on the final phase of gpIIb/IIIa-dependent platelet cohesion, gpIIb/IIIa is the most abundant platelet membrane protein (ie, approximately 50,000 gpIIb/IIIa receptors per platelet), and high affinity monoclonal antibodies directed against gpIIb/IIIa have been engineered to be suitable for patient use.[21,32] The administration of these antibodies to patients undergoing high-risk angioplasty inhibits platelet recruitment and prevents acute coronary complications, albeit in association with significant abnormal bleeding.[33] Dipyridamole reduces thromboembolic complications of mitral valve prostheses when used in combination with oral anticoagulation.[69]

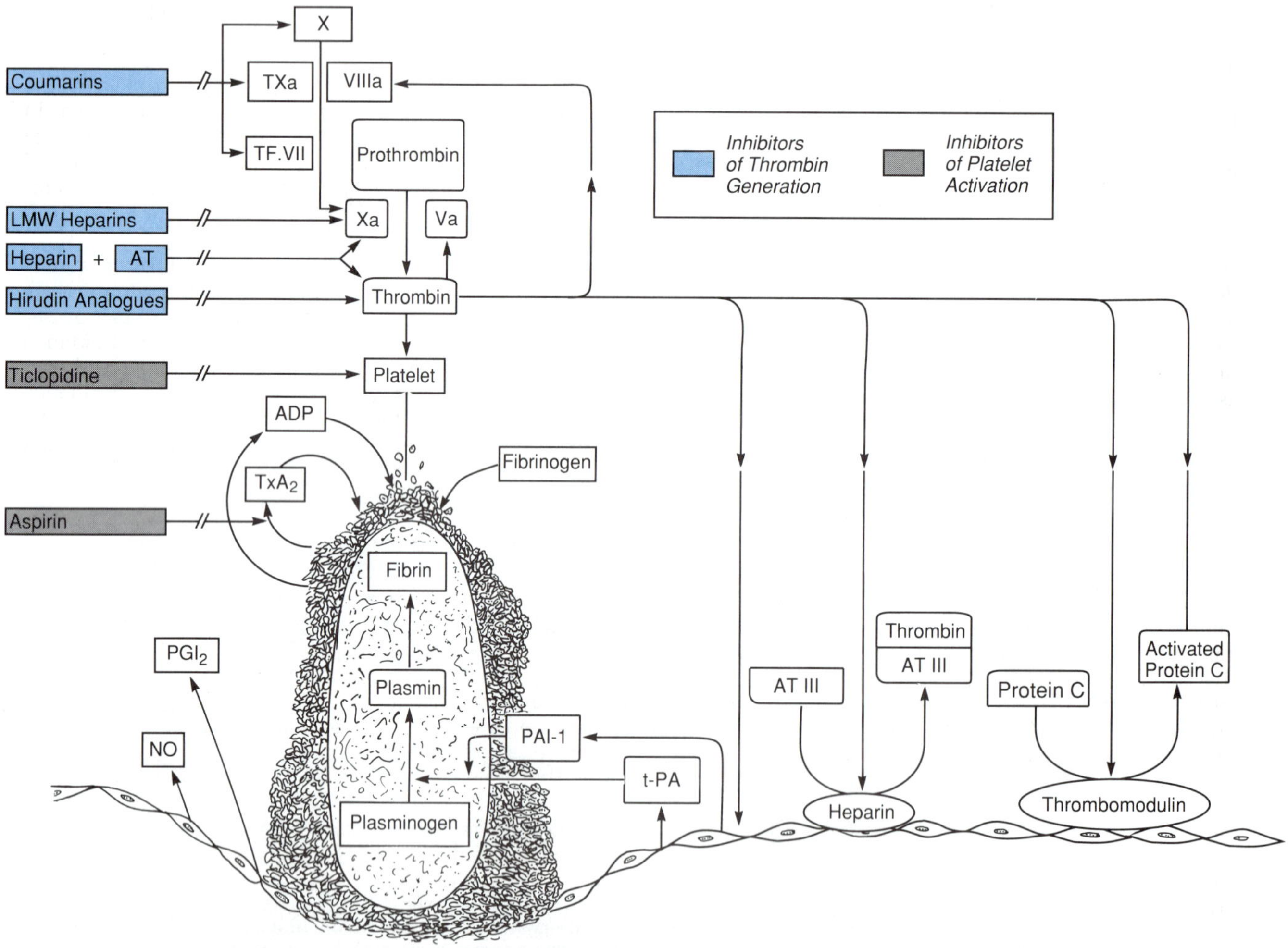

FIGURE 45-3. Antithrombotic therapies. Anticoagulation therapy, using heparin acutely and oral coumarin type anticoagulants chronically, interrupts and prevents venous thrombus formation. Heparin enhances antithrombin III (ATIII) activity through complex formation, acting primarily as an antithrombin, although anti–factor Xa activity is also detectable. The coumarins impair coagulation by producing dysfunctional Gla domains in factors II, VII, IX, and X. Low-molecular-weight (LMW) heparins exhibit anti–factor Xa activity in combination with varying lesser amounts of antithrombin activity. Aspirin inhibits the thromboxane A_2 (TxA_2) pathway of platelet recruitment by irreversibly inactivating cyclooxygenase. Ticlopidine blocks all pathways of platelet recruitment, perhaps by modifying membrane signal transduction. Dipyridamole appears to reduce platelet activation by increasing plasma adenosine, thereby elevating inhibitor cAMP. Other antithrombotic agents currently under development are antithrombins (synthetic or natural such as hirudin); activated protein C (reduces thrombin production); inhibitors of glycoprotein IIb/IIIa complex (dependent platelet recruitment); thrombus-directed thrombolytic agents (tissue plasminogen activator and single-chain urokinase); and agents that simulate or induce prostacyclin (PGI_2) and nitric oxide (NO) production.

Drugs That Inhibit the Arachidonate Pathway

Cyclooxygenase Inhibitors

Cyclooxygenase inhibitors consist of nonsteroid antiinflammatory drugs, such as aspirin, and indomethacin.

Although aspirin is not particularly potent in experimental animal models,[70] it has well-established beneficial effects in clinical trials and is the most widely used clinical antiplatelet agent. Aspirin irreversibly brings about acetylation of cyclooxygenase,[71] thereby abolishing both platelet production of thromboxane A_2 (TXA_2), the most potent natural vasocontrictor and platelet agonist, and endothelial synthesis of PGI_2, the potent vasodilator and antiplatelet agent. Aspirin's inhibitory effect on cyclooxygenase persists throughout the residual life-span of exposed platelets. Because endothelial cells resynthesize cyclooxygenase, aspirin's effect on endothelial production of PGI_2 reverses in 24 to 36 hours.

Antithrombotic effects of aspirin have been reported with doses that have varied between 100 mg/d to over 1.5 g/d.[48–61,64–68] Low doses of aspirin (100 mg/d) have been reported to be effective in preventing aortocoronary bypass shunt thrombosis[59] and thrombosis of arteriovenous shunts in patients undergoing long-term hemodialysis (160 mg/d).[61] Evidence also shows that aspirin is effective in cerebral ischemia at a dose of 300 mg/d.[50] No evidence exists that low doses of aspirin are either more effective or less effective than high doses. Evidence does show that low doses of aspirin produce fewer side effects.[63] The results of biochemical studies on the mechanism of action of aspirin, its dose-related side effects, and the results of clinical studies evaluating antithrombotic effects all support the use of low doses of aspirin in the treatment of thromboembolic disorders.[48,49]

Aspirin is rapidly absorbed in the stomach and upper intestine with peak plasma levels occurring at 15 to 20 minutes, and platelet function is inhibited within 1 hour.[71] Although the plasma concentration of aspirin decays with a half-life of 15 to 20 minutes, the platelet-inhibitory effect lasts for the life-span of the platelets (9 to 10 days) because of irreversible acetylation of platelet cyclooxygenase.[72] Aspirin also brings about acetylation of the enzyme in maturing megakaryocytes.

Since the side effects of aspirin are dose dependent,[73–75] and many of the clinical conditions in which aspirin is effective require that the drug be used long-term, the lowest effective dose should be administered. Aspirin administered in doses of about 1000 mg/d inhibits both platelet TXA_2 synthesis and vascular PGI_2 synthesis.[76] Daily administration of low doses of aspirin (about 40 mg/d) inhibits TXB_2 generation in vitro and urinary excretion of 2,3-dinor-TXB_2 without producing significant changes in the urinary excretion of metabolites of PGI_2 production (6-keto-PGF_{1a} and 2,3-dinor-6-keto-PGF_{1a}).[77,78] In contrast, similarly low doses of aspirin reduce PGI_2 synthesis by vascular tissue obtained from healthy volunteers,[79] and low doses (20 mg/d for 7 days) inhibit PGI_2 synthesis by 50% in both arterial and venous tissue in patients with atherosclerosis.[76] Additionally, low-dose aspirin (35 mg/d for 7 days) inhibits both TXA_2 and PGI_2 in blood emerging from a standardized skin bleeding time wounds by over than 80%.[62] Thus, a differential effect on inhibition of TXA_2 and PGI_2 biosynthesis has been reported with low- dose aspirin when these eicosanoids are measured as urinary metabolites; this differential effect is absent when the assays of TXA_2 and PGI_2 are performed on vascular wall biopsy tissue or when the assays are performed on blood sampled from standardized skin incisions. This apparent discrepancy may be caused by the short-lived effects of aspirin on PGI_2 formation, which is not reflected in the overall measurement of PGI_2 metabolites in the urine formed over 24 hours.

Moreover, increasing evidence suggests that the clinical relevance of inhibiting PGI_2 production has been exaggerated in the past and that it is, at most, of limited importance.[3] Epidemiologic studies of patients with rheumatoid arthritis treated with large doses of aspirin (about 2 to 3 g/d) do not show an increase in thrombosis or atherosclerosis, suggesting that these high doses of aspirin are not thrombogenic in man.[80,81] Furthermore, patients with congenital cyclooxygenase deficiency who lack both PGI_2 and TXA_2 do not suffer thrombotic episodes but have a mild bleeding tendency.[82] The antithrombotic effects of aspirin are similar when doses of 300 mg/d and 1.2 g/d are used.[50–61,64,83–90]

Good evidence shows that aspirin's side effects are reduced by using low doses of aspirin (325 mg/d).[50,56,57] In a case control study, a statistically significant association was found between heavy, regular aspirin use and major bleeding.[74] A similar association was found in patients with newly diagnosed, benign gastric ulcer (but not duodenal ulcer). Additionally, a number of trials using aspirin at a dose of 900 mg/d or more have reported an increase in incidence of stomach pain, heartburn, nausea, constipation, and occult gastrointestinal blood loss compared with that found in those taking the placebo.[84–90] In contrast, aspirin in doses of 324 mg or less does not increase gastrointestinal side effects when compared with side effects in a control group.[50,64,83] These side effects can be reduced by treatment with cimetidine, antacids, or enteric-coated or highly buffered aspirin.[91]

Aspirin does not cause a generalized bleeding abnormality unless it is given to patients with an underlying hemorrhagic defect (such as hemophilia or uremia) or unless it is combined with anticoagulants.[92–94] Good evidence shows that aspirin increases operative blood loss in heparinized patients undergoing open heart surgery.[60] Evidence also shows that, when combined with oral anticoagulants, aspirin produces a significant increase in gastrointestinal blood loss.[93,95]

Cerebrovascular Disease. Although the evaluation of antiplatelet therapy in cerebrovascular ischemia is difficult because of limited availability of suitable patients and because of the low incidence of the two clinically important outcome events, stroke and death, a number of large-scale multicenter trials with long-term follow-up testing of aspirin have been completed.[48–54] These multicenter trials studying aspirin in transient ischemic attacks (TIAs) are similar in that aspirin substantially reduces TIAs, stroke, and death, especially from vascular causes. The conclusions of these studies are convincing and consistent regarding mortality and stroke reduction with a range of 0.3- to 1.3-g daily aspirin treatment. In all studies, aspirin is well tolerated and the complications—mostly gastrointestinal—are dose dependent. No additional benefit has been shown by combining dipyridamole with aspirin,[51,96,97] and probably not with sulfinpyrazone.[52] In a Canadian study,[52] the benefit was seen predominantly in males. The French study[51] found benefit in both males and females. In the UK-TIA study,[50] 300- and 1200-mg dosages of aspirin were equally effective and were more effective than placebo.

Ischemic Heart Disease. Aspirin, 324 mg/d to 1.3 g/d, clearly reduces myocardial infarction and cardiac death in patients with unstable angina.[64,90] The efficacy of aspirin in patients with unstable angina over a wide dosage range parallels the results with aspirin in patients with transient cerebral ischemia and suggests the possibility of similar pathogenetic mechanisms for these two disorders.

Aspirin has been evaluated in a number of randomized trials in patients with acute myocardial infarction. Evidence from an overview analysis of these trials is convincing that aspirin is effective in preventing reinfarction and vascular death in patients who have suffered acute myocardial infarction.[48,56–58,83–89] The risk reduction is 31% plus or minus 5% for nonfatal reinfarction, 42% plus or minus 5% for nonfatal stroke, and 13% plus or minus 5% for vascular death.

The short-term effects of aspirin in patients presenting with acute myocardial infarction have also been evaluated in the ISIS-2 trial.[55] This trial, using a dose of aspirin of 300 mg/d and a factorial design, demonstrated a 5-week vascular mortality reduction of 17% with aspirin (odds reduction 21%), 22% with streptokinase (odds reduction 26%), and 39% with the combination (odds reduction 42%).

Two recent clinical trials of aspirin for primary prevention of myocardial infarction give conflicting results. At a dose of 325 mg every other day, aspirin reduced the incidence of fatal and nonfatal myocardial infarction significantly,[56] but in another study, it had no apparent effect at a dose of 500 mg daily.[57] Whether this discrepancy in results is a consequence of the difference in dose is not clear, particularly because the study reporting benefit with the smaller dose of aspirin included many more patients and therefore was more likely (because of increased power) to demonstrate a true benefit. Although this report of a study evaluating the effectiveness of aspirin, 325 mg every second day, in the primary prevention of vascular disease suggests a beneficial effect of aspirin, it would be prudent at this stage to recommend prophylactic aspirin only in persons who are at high risk for vascular disease.

Saphenous Vein Bypass Grafts. Patency of aortocoronary saphenous vein bypass grafts is improved by aspirin (325 mg/d).[60] The multicenter Veterans Administration study compared (1) aspirin, 325 mg/d; (2) aspirin, 325 mg three times daily; (3) aspirin plus dipyridamole, 325 and 75 mg, respectively, three times daily; (4) sulfinpyrazone, 267 mg three times daily; and (5) placebo three times daily. Therapy was started 48 hours before coronary artery bypass grafting except for aspirin, which was given as a single 325-mg dose 12 hours before surgery and maintained thereafter according to the assigned regimen. Patients in all aspirin-containing therapeutic regimens, but not sulfinpyrazone, showed equal improvement ($P < .05$) of graft patency compared with the placebo group. The addition of dipyridamole did not improve patency rates. This benefit persisted for at least 1 year.[98] Preoperative aspirin also increased chest tube drainage measured within the first 35 hours after coronary artery bypass grafting ($P < .02$), the requirements for whole blood and platelet transfusions ($P < .01$), and the reoperation rate ($P < .01$). In a subsequent study,[99] this group has shown that aspirin, 325 mg daily, started within 6 hours after bypass surgery gives the same patency benefit without the risks of increased blood loss, transfusion requirements, and reoperation rates. Thus, aspirin, 325 mg/d, is indicated for all bypass patients beginning within 6 hours of surgery and continuing for at least 1 year.

Aspirin may also reduce acute thrombotic complications associated with catheterization.[97] Acute coronary occlusion and restenosis after angioplasty are not prevented by aspirin or by the combination of aspirin and dipyridamole.[100]

Therefore, because doses of aspirin between 160 and 1500 mg/d in adults are probably equally antithrombotic and because low doses of 325 mg or less have minimal side effects, the general recommendation is that 325 mg of aspirin be given once daily for all documented indications.

Inhibitors of Thromboxane A_2 Production or Action

Blocking TXA_2 activation of platelets using TXA_2 synthetase inhibitor or TXA_2 receptor antagonists has the theoretical advantage over cyclooxygenase inhibitors of preserving endothelial PGI_2 production.[101] In vitro, such agents are weak platelet inhibitors, but no effects are established in vivo. The weak antithrombotic effects of TXA_2 synthetase inhibitors is ascribed to the continued production of PG endoperoxides, which may activate platelets.[102] Consequently, combining TXA_2 synthetase inhibition with antagonists to the shared TXA_2/prostaglandin endoperoxide receptor may produce more potent antithrombotic effects.[102] The in vivo effects of combined TXA_2 receptor antagonist with 5-HT_2 receptor antagonist are variable.[103–105]

Drugs That Increase Platelet Cyclic AMP Levels

Prostacyclin

Prostacyclin is a potent platelet inhibitor that acts by elevating platelet cyclic AMP (cAMP) through the stimulation of adenylate cyclase. Because of its instability and its potent vasodilator effects at doses that can produce useful antiplatelet effects, no significant clinical application of PGI_2 is known at present. A great number of related compounds have been developed with improved stability and somewhat reduced vascular effect. None of the available agents has improved the vasomotor:platelet inhibitor ratio.[106]

Although some studies have claimed that PGI_2 or related compounds reduce myocardial injury during acute myocardial infarction,[107,108] such results have not been confirmed in controlled trials.[109] These agents have also been administered in extracorporeal systems, including extracorporeal membrane oxygenation and hemodialysis, to preserve the platelet count, but the adequate antiplatelet doses produce unacceptable hypotensive consequences.[110,111] Similarly, these agents have been studied in the treatment of atherosclerotic peripheral vascular disease without benefit evident in controlled trials.[106]

Dipyridamole

Dipyridamole increases cAMP by inhibiting phosphodiesterase activity.[112] Experimentally, dipyridamole exhibits antiplatelet synergism when combined with aspirin.[113] Its clinical use is limited to the prevention of systemic embolism in patients with prosthetic heart valves when it is administered in combination with warfarin.[69,114] Dipyridamole is ineffective when given alone and provides no additional benefit when given in association with aspirin for the treatment of cerebrovascular or coronary thrombotic events or occlusion of saphenous vein bypass grafts.[97]

Ticlopidine

Ticlopidine is a global inhibitor of platelet function, but its mechanism of action remains undefined. It does not affect phosphodiesterase, adenylate cyclase, cyclooxygenase, or thromboxane synthetase activities. Perhaps it affects platelet receptor signal transduction after the binding of adenosine diphosphate, or it may block expression of the gpIIb/IIIa receptor site for fibrinogen.[65,66] Because ticlopidine is ineffective in vitro and requires several days of oral administration to manifest its maximum effect in vivo, its activity may be due to some membrane abnormality produced during megakaryocytopoiesis. In thrombosis models, ticlopidine is a more potent antithrombotic agent than aspirin.[70] The delay of several days before the drug is fully effective, and the persistent effect of ticlopidine for several days after discontinuing treatment complicates its clinical use. In addition, occasional idiosyncratic neutropenia and gastrointestinal side effects sometimes occur during its use.[66]

Clinically, ticlopidine, 250 mg twice a day, is effective in the secondary prevention of stroke. Recurrence of stroke and cardiovascular death are reduced by 30% compared with that seen in the placebo group.[67] At this dosage, ticlopidine is also more potent than aspirin, 650 mg twice daily, in preventing the occurrence of nonfatal stroke and death in patients with TIA. These events are reduced as much as 30% compared with that seen in patients treated with aspirin.[68] Other indications for ticlopidine include the treatment of peripheral vascular disease, in ischemic heart disease, in surgical bypass procedures (postendarterectomy), and in extracorporeal procedures.[68]

Newer Antiplatelet Strategies

Dietary n-3 Fatty Acids

A fish oil–rich diet produces changes in the lipid composition of cell membranes by incorporating n-3 polyunsaturated fatty acids instead of arachidonic acid.[115] Consequently, stimulated platelets produce TXA_3 rather than TXA_2. TXA_3 is a relatively weak platelet agonist. Concurrently, endothelial cells release PGI_3, a platelet inhibitor as potent as PGI_2.[116] Thus, inhibitory products are produced by the vessel wall without stimulator products being generated from platelets. Other antithrombotic effects of a fish oil–rich diet are reduction of macrophage–monocyte tissue factor expression, an augmentation of fibrinolytic activity,[117] and RBC membrane fluidity.[118]

Experimentally, dietary n-3 fatty acids reduce ex vivo platelet aggregation minimally and prolong bleeding time slightly.[119] In animal models of arterial thrombosis[120] and atherogenesis, substantial beneficial effects have been reported.[121–124] A recent experimental study demonstrated that dietary n-3 fatty acids are rapidly incorporated into blood and vascular tissues, modestly reduce the thrombotic responses of flowing blood to thrombogenic surfaces, and largely eliminate both the thrombotic and proliferative responses of endarterectomized carotid arteries, while producing trivial effects on platelet hemostatic function and no other notable adverse effects when administered in high doses to baboons. Dietary n-3 fatty acids are postulated to produce these striking biologic effects by disordering cellular membrane functions that are critical for both vascular thrombosis and vascular lesion formation at sites of arterial mechanical injury but largely inconsequential in hemostatic mechanisms.[125] Prospective controlled clinical trials report a decreased rate of restenosis after coronary angioplasty, but this effect has not been confirmed by other studies. Studies comparing the efficacy and toxicity (hemorrhagic, carcinogenic, or immunosuppressive effects) of such diet supplementation have not been reported.

Drugs That Interfere With Platelet–Adhesive Protein Interactions

A new group of oral agents have been recently designed to inhibit platelet recruitment by interrupting platelet binding with adhesive proteins, a process central to the formation of arterial thrombosis. This strategy is illustrated by the development of antibodies directed against gpIIb/IIIa that produce potent antihemostatic and antithrombotic effects in various animal models[124–129,132–135] and in patients undergoing high-risk angioplasty.[33] Monoclonal antibodies inhibiting the interaction of vWF with gpIb or against gpIb produces shear rate–dependent antithrombotic effects in pigs.[129–131] In vitro studies suggest that the interaction of vWF and gpIb may compensate in part for blockade of gpIIb/IIIa receptors or collagen receptor by antibodies.[22]

Antithrombin Therapy

Mechanical interventional approaches are commonly used in the management of symptomatic atherosclerotic vascular disease, such as balloon angioplasty, various types of endarterectomy, vascular grafting, endovascular stenting, and use of prosthetic cardiovascular devices. Such interventions of necessity produce direct vascular injury that promotes platelet-dependent thrombus formation and intimal smooth muscle cell proliferative lesion formation. For example, endarterectomy produces an arterial surface composed of disrupted vascular media (smooth muscle cells and collagen-containing connective tissue matrix). This surface initiates acute platelet thrombus formation and intimal proliferative lesions, resulting in a 35% rate of symptomatic arterial restenosis or occlusion. Available antithrombotic therapies consisting of aspirin and heparin do not prevent restenosis or occlusion. In the past, the resistance to heparin of platelet-mediated, high-shear arterial thrombosis has been interpreted to indicate that platelet-dependent processes are not thrombin mediated. Both the potent natural antithrombin hirudin[136,137] and the synthetic irreversible antithrombin 35,D-phenylalanyl-L-prolyl-L-arginyl-chloromethylketone[138] have been shown to prevent acute platelet-dependent thrombus formation on arterial endarterectomy sites or implanted prosthetic vascular grafts, indicating that thrombin is important in mediating platelet-dependent thrombosis.

Presumably, the mechanically injured vessel produces sufficient thrombin to induce platelet recruitment by means of ligands not dependent on gpIIb/IIIa such as thrombospondin, which binds to gpIV. Other synthetic antithrombins have been studied clinically.[139,140]

Because these findings establish the importance of thrombin in mediating platelet-dependent thrombotic responses, studies have also been made of the effect of inhibiting thrombin generation by infusing APC.[141,142] In these studies, human plasma-APC infused into baboons bearing prosthetic vascular grafts prolongs the partial thromboplastin time (PTT) and reduces vascular graft platelet deposition in a dose-dependent manner as determined by the real-time scintillation camera imaging of indium-111–labeled platelet deposition. APC infusion also preserves graft patency. Since platelet hemostatic plug formation remains normal (as measured by the template bleeding times), these results suggest that APC administration may produce immediate antithrombotic effects without a significantly increased risk of bleeding.

ANTICOAGULANTS

Anticoagulants act by inhibiting thrombin formation (see Fig. 45-3), thrombin activity, and coagulation serine proteases participating in the events preceding thrombin generation.[14,143] They are mainly used in the prevention and treatment of fibrin-dependent thrombotic events, including venous thrombosis, pulmonary embolism, and other venous thromboembolic complications. Because thrombin has a pivotal role in platelet-dependent thrombosis, some of these agents may also be useful at higher doses in the treatment of arterial thrombosis. For established deep-vein thrombosis (DVT) or pulmonary embolism, anticoagulation with heparin remains the mainstay of acute treatment, followed by warfarin therapy to reduce the risk of recurrence.

Oral anticoagulants are also effective in reducing thromboemboli and mural thrombi arising from the diseased heart in which interrupted and disturbed flow patterns produce venous type thrombus.

Drugs Accelerating Antithrombin III Action

Heparin

Standard unfractionated heparin is the most widely used antithrombotic agent in clinical practice.[143] Heparin is a heterodisperse mixture of polysaccharides of molecular weight ranging between 3 and 40 kd, and averaging about 15 kd. Heparin catalyzes bimolecular complex formation between plasma ATIII and serine proteases of the coagulation pathway; thrombin inhibition by heparin is primarily responsible for its anticoagulant action. In vitro at higher concentrations, heparin induces thrombin inhibition through heparin cofactor II, although this specific plasma antithrombin has uncertain clinical significance. A minor anticoagulant effect independent of both ATIII and heparin cofactor II has been also described.[143] Heparin is reported to activate, inhibit, or have no effect on platelets.[144]

Clinical studies have shown that both antithrombotic efficacy and bleeding complications are dose dependent. Heparin monitoring by coagulation tests is critical, since great variability exists in the anticoagulant response to heparin among different persons as well as in the same person at different times during the course of thromboembolic diseases.[145,146] Because the activated partial thromboplastin time (APTT), a global coagulation test, correlates relatively well with ex vivo plasma heparin levels, it is generally used to monitor therapy.[147] Laboratory monitoring of the platelet count is also important, since heparin-induced thrombocytopenia has been reported in about 5% of patients receiving therapeutic heparin.[148] The thrombin time is sensitive to the effects of heparin, whereas the prothrombin time is relatively insensitive to therapeutic levels of heparin.

Heparin may be administered by continuous intravenous injection or by intravenous or subcutaneous bolus injection. Subcutaneous administration is usually reserved for prophylaxis of venous thrombosis during surgery or for medical patients at bed rest. Continuous infusion is associated with fewer bleeding complications than intermittent bolus injection, and it provides equal protection against recurrent venous disease.[149] The half-life of heparin after bolus intravenous administration is around 90 minutes, depending on the dose and the patient.[145,150]

The variability in response to heparin that occurs may be explained by differences in heparin pharmacokinetics.[145,150] This variability also reflects varying levels of other basic proteins in plasma that bind heparin and thus compete with ATIII. Such proteins probably include acute phase reactants such as C-reactive protein, which is elevated several hundredfold during the first few days of an acute illness. These transient changes may explain the occasional phenomenon of an altered heparin requirement to achieve the same prolongation of the PTT a few days after the onset of therapy for thromboembolic disease. The 50% larger average dose needed in the patients with pulmonary embolism, compared with DVT without emboli, is explained by an increased rate of heparin clearance in patients with pulmonary embolism.[145,150]

When heparin is administered by intravenous bolus injection, the usual dose is 4000 to 8000 IU. Initially, this dose prolongs the PTT to infinity. By 30 minutes before the next dose, the PTT should be reduced to about twice that of baseline. The bolus regimen requires an average of 50% more heparin daily than does the continuous infusion regimen, and it is associated with more bleeding complications.[150]

When heparin is given by continuous infusion, an initial loading dose of 75 IU/kg is given as an intravenous bolus, and heparin is then infused at a rate of 10 to 25 IU/kg/h, depending on the patient and the clinical situation. When administered by continuous infusion, it is necessary to maintain the PTT at therapeutic levels of about 1.5 to 2 times baseline. Usually, the appropriate therapeutic PTT ranges from 50 to 80 seconds. Infusions require an accurate administration system and should be given in an intravenous line separate from other drugs or fluids. To adjust the PTT, it is usually sufficient to change the infusion rate without supplementing by additional bolus. After each adjustment, the PTT should be checked in another 4 hours to assess the effect of the change in administered dose. After the therapeutic level has been achieved, daily monitoring is sufficient.

Low-dose subcutaneous heparin, 5000 IU/12 h, is used for prophylaxis during surgery or for medical patients at bed rest.[151,152] Individual variations in heparin levels during administration of the low-dose regimen are seen. Some persons have no detectable heparin, whereas others occasionally have significantly prolonged PTTs from low-dose administration. Some increased risk of bleeding is encountered in these patients. Low-dose heparin is totally inadequate anticoagulation for established DVT or pulmonary embolism. Furthermore, it is clearly less effective than warfarin in preventing recurrence. A recent review of more than 70 randomized trials in 16,000 patients reports that the perioperative use of low-dose heparin (5000 IU twice daily) prevents about 50% of all pulmonary emboli and about two thirds of all DVT appearing after urologic, orthopedic, or general surgery.[153] Although this result may be achieved with a fixed low dose of heparin, the prevention of DVT in patients undergoing elective hip surgery requires subcutaneous heparin doses producing APTT values in the high normal range rather than fixed doses.[154]

Experimentally, heparin is also effective in the treatment of platelet-dependent thrombotic events, albeit at doses markedly higher than those required to block fibrin-dependent venous thrombosis.[155] Also, heparin reduces the development of acute platelet–thrombus deposition during angioplasty in pigs. In this model, other antiplatelet agents are either less effective or not effective.[156] Clinically, heparin has been reported to be more potent than aspirin in reducing the incidence of myocardial infarction in patients with unstable angina.[157,158]

Low-Molecular-Weight Heparins

Low-molecular-weight (LMW) heparins are effective and safe for the prevention and treatment of venous thrombosis.[159–161] They have recently been approved for clinical use for the prevention and treatment of venous thrombosis.

LMW heparins are fragments of standard commercial-grade heparin produced by either chemical or enzymatic depolymerization that are approximately one third of the size of heparin. Like standard heparin, they are heterogeneous in size with a molecular weight averaging 4 to 5 kd. Depolymerization of standard heparin changes its anticoagulant profile, bioavailability, and pharmacokinetics, and it affects platelet function and experimental bleeding. LMW heparins produce their major anticoagulant effect by binding to antithrombin III (ATIII) through a unique pentasaccharide sequence present on about one third of unfractionated heparin chains but present on a lower proportion of LMW heparin molecules. The binding of the pentasaccharide to ATIII produces a conformational change in the ATIII molecule, enhancing its ability to inactivate the coagulation enzymes thrombin and factor Xa. Standard and LMW heparins amplify the inactivation of thrombin by ATIII, acting as a template that binds both the plasma cofactor through the unique pentasaccharide sequence and thrombin to form a ternary complex. A minimum chain length of 18 saccharides (including the pentasaccharide sequence) is required for ternary complex formation. By contrast, inactivation of factor Xa by ATIII requires fewer bound heparin molecules. Accordingly, inhibition is achieved by LMW heparin fragments, provided that they contain the high-affinity pentasaccharide. The various commercial LMWHs have anti–factor Xa to antithrombin ratios of 4:1 to 2:1, compared with the ratio for standard heparin, which is 1:1.

Because LMW heparins bind much less avidly to heparin-binding plasma proteins and endothelium than does standard heparin, LMW heparins exhibit superior bioavailability, longer rates of elimination, and more predictable anticoagulant response.

When compared on a gravimetric basis in experimental models of venous thrombosis, LMW heparins are slightly less effective than heparin as antithrombotic agents, but they produce much less bleeding in models measuring blood loss from a standardized injury, perhaps related to their attenuated effects on platelet function and vascular permeability.

Clinically, LMW heparins also exhibit greater bioavailability, longer plasma half life, and a more predictable anticoagulant response than standard heparin, allowing them to be administered once daily and laboratory monitoring to be discontinued. Moreover, LMW heparins produce less bleeding than does standard heparin for an equivalent antithrombotic effect, thereby permitting patients to be treated with higher anticoagulant doses of LMW heparins without compromising patient safety. This latter potential advantage of LMW heparins has been demonstrated in one study evaluating prophylaxis in high-risk patients in which standard heparin produces a significant increase in bleeding when its dose was increased to match the anticoagulant effect ex vivo of a LMW heparin.[161] LMW heparins have been extensively evaluated for the prevention and treatment of venous thromboembolism and have been shown to be highly effective.[159]

Vitamin K Antagonists

Vitamin K is necessary for the glutamyl γ-carboxylation, an important posttranslation modification of clotting factors II, VII, IX, and X, as well as the anticoagulant proteins C and S. These same carboxylated residues are necessary for the binding of calcium ions, an essential step in the generation of the procoagulant and anticoagulant activities of these proteins. Vitamin K antagonists prevent γ-carboxylation, yielding biologically inactive proteins.[143,162–164] There are various types of vitamin K antagonists, and all are absorbed orally. Warfarin is the most widely used vitamin K antagonist in the United States because of its intermediate metabolism (half-life about 35 hours) and good bioavailability.[162–164] The anticoagulant effect of vitamin K antagonists is fully manifested 36 to 72 hours after drug administration and optimal when factors are reduced to about 10% of normal. Great individual variability exists in the response to vitamin K antagonists.[164]

The pharmacologic response of warfarin depends on the net effect on the levels of susceptible clotting factors in the circulation. The four clotting factors have different half-lives, and reduction in factor VII, which has the shortest half-life, can prolong the prothrombin time within 24 hours after large doses of warfarin before the other vitamin K–dependent factors have been significantly affected. Therefore, it is common practice to begin warfarin therapy with two daily doses of 10 mg each and to adjust the dose, usually downward, based on the results of the daily prothrombin time until it equilibrates in the therapeutic range. Prothrombin times, depending on the choice of thromboplastin reagent, vary considerably in their dose-response curves, so that they need to be carefully standardized. The range of response among different persons is particularly wide; from 1 to 20 mg/d may be required to maintain a patient in therapeutic range after equilibration has been achieved. The prothrombin time reflects the dose given 36 to 48 hours previously. To achieve antithrombotic effects without inordinant risks of bleeding, factors II, VII, IX, and X are reduced to about 10% of normal, that is, analogous to mild hemophilia.

A properly standardized prothrombin time should be used in monitoring warfarin therapy. The variability among commercial thromboplastins renders the prolongation in absolute times unsatisfactory for following changes in the prothrombin time. Moreover, because of the relatively greater sensitivity to lower levels of factor VII, the prothrombin time does not always reflect a patient's overall degree of anticoagulation, early or during unsteady periods. Newer tests, such as the use of chromogenic substrates or immunoassays for normal versus descarboxy prothrombin levels, may prove to be more useful in predicting patients at risk for hemorrhage or recurrent thrombosis.

The optimal therapeutic range for control of anticoagulant therapy has been a subject of considerable confusion, primarily because of varying responsiveness of different thromboplastin reagents to warfarin-induced decreases in vitamin K–dependent clotting factors.[151] Thromboplastins are prepared from brain, lung, or placental tissues and vary markedly in their responsiveness to the anticoagulant effects of warfarin, depending on their source and method of preparation.[165] For example, doubling of the PT over that of baseline requires a lower dose of warfarin using the more responsive thromboplastins used in Europe rather than the less responsive thromboplastins currently used in North America. This difference in thromboplastins appears to be responsible for clinically important differences in the dosage of anticoagulants used in different countries.[166] Consequently, an international reference preparation of thromboplastin has been designated and a calibration system has been developed based on the assumption that a linear relation exists between the logarithm of the PT ratios of the reference and test thromboplastins.[167]

Thus, to standardize the reporting of the PT, the observed PT ratio obtained with the local thromboplastin is converted into an International Normalized Ratio (INR), which is calculated as follows: INR = observed ratio^C, where C is the constant that represents the International Sensitivity Index (ISI). The INR, therefore, is the PT ratio that reflects the result that would have been obtained if the reference thromboplastin had been used to perform the test. For practical purposes, it is sufficient to know that the primary human brain reference thromboplastin, which is responsive to the anticoagulant effects of warfarin, has an ISI of 1.0 and that the ISI value of a thromboplastin increases as it becomes less responsive. The ISI values for the commercial rabbit brain thromboplastin used in North America vary between 2.2 and 2.6, whereas the thromboplastins generally used in Europe have ISI values of 1.1 to 1.2. Because the therapeutic PT ratio recommendations of 2 to 2.5 given 30 years ago were based on reactive thromboplastins, the more recent change in North America to less reactive thromboplastins requires that the therapeutic PT ratio be correspondingly reduced. The thrombotest reagent is a bovine thromboplastin that has not changed in for 30 years and has maintained a constant therapeutic recommendation, that is, a thrombotest value of 7% to 10%. That value is equivalent to a PT ratio using a less responsive rabbit brain thromboplastin of 1.5 to 1.7, compared with 2 to 2.5 for reactive thromboplastins.

Good evidence from well-designed controlled clinical trials suggests that a less intense oral anticoagulant regimen (by usual North American practice) with a targeted therapeutic ratio of 1.5 to 1.7 (INR range of 2 to 3) is effective in the prevention of venous thrombosis, the treatment of venous thrombosis after an initial course of heparin, and the prevention of systemic embolism in patients with acute myocardial infarction. Evidence also suggests that this less intense regimen prevents systemic embolism in patients with atrial fibrillation who undergo direct current cardioversion.[166,168–172]

Drug interactions play an important role in warfarin therapy.[173] Since warfarin contains an asymmetric carbon atom, there are two optically active isomers. In the presence of some drugs, the metabolic effects are different for the two isomers. Thus, the potentiating effect of phyenylbutazone, for example, is partly due to the increase in enzymes that metabolize the less active form in preference to the more active form.[174] This leads to no net change of plasma warfarin but a potentiation of the anticoagulant effect. Other drugs compete with the hydroxylase that initiates breakdown of either isomer of the active anticoagulant. Aspirin has a variable effect on synthesis, and occasionally some persons on large daily doses of aspirin may have reduced prothrombin complex proteins. Nearly any strongly acidic drug can displace albumin-bound warfarin in vitro, but interactions at other sites may predominate. Antagonism, leading to a shorter prothrombin time, may also occur. Barbiturates induce microsomal enzymes in the hepatocytes, which increase the metabolism of both forms of warfarin and thus antagonize the anticoagulant effect of the drug.

Disease states, blood lipid levels, alcohol ingestion, and dietary factors may also influence interactions, perhaps explaining effects observed occasionally in patients. Barbiturates and barbiturate-containing compounds account for 75% of the adverse drug interactions, and a strong correlation exists between total number of drugs prescribed to a patient and the likelihood that the patient will show effects of an interacting drug.[175]

Also, recognize that any drug independently impairing hemostasis potentiates the risk of bleeding in patients receiving warfarin, usually without further prolongation of the prothrombin time. This includes other antithrombotic agents and marrow suppressive drugs or drug-induced thrombocytopenias. Thus, additional hemostatic defects must be considered when bleeding occurs in patients who are receiving therapeutically appropriate doses of warfarin.

Newer Anticoagulants

A number of agents that inhibit thrombin activity or its formation are under study. Natural hirudin, a peptide found in medicinal leeches, is the most potent inhibitor of thrombin found in nature. It acts by forming a tight, stoichiometric complex with thrombin.[136,137,176] Although newly available recombinant forms of hirudin are less potent by order of magnitude, they have been shown to be effective in animal venous thrombosis models.[176] Recombinant hirudin is also potent in interrupting thrombus formation in arterial thrombosis models resistant to standard heparin.[136,137] A synthetic antithrombin, D-phenylalanyl-L-prolyl-L-arginylchloromethylketone, is equally potent.[138] It is interesting that a hirudin peptide, encompassing the minimal hirudin sequence with antithrombin activity, was found to be inactive with respect to platelets but effective in preventing fibrin-dependent thrombus formation. APC produces potent antithrombotic effects in the prevention of platelet-dependent thrombosis without significantly increasing the risk of bleeding, as determined by template bleeding time measurements.[141] Newly available recombinant APC is also effective.[142] These results are of particular interest because of the favorable ratio of antithrombotic efficacy to hemostatic safety.

Dermatan sulfate is a natural glycosaminoglycan recently proposed as an antithrombotic drug. In contrast to heparin, dermatan sulfate catalyzes specifically the HC II–thrombin interaction but has no action on ATIII–serine proteases interactions.[177] Experimentally, dermatan sulfate is an appealing antithrombotic agent as therapy for venous thrombotic events, since it is antithrombotic without evoking antihemostatic effects.[178] Also, the association of standard heparin and dermatan sulfate has been experimentally shown to be effective at doses that are not antithrombotic when the agents are used singly.[179] Clinical trials currently underway will determine the efficacy and safety hypothesis.

Approaches to Anticoagulant Therapy for Thrombotic Disorders

Venous Thrombosis and Thromboembolism

Immediate heparinization is the initial therapy for pulmonary embolism, and it markedly reduces mortality from recurrence.[180] Likewise, heparinization is used in DVT to prevent extension or embolization of thrombi, whereas endogenous fibrinolysis gradually removes thrombotic material. Treatment is associated with normalization of tests that reflect ongoing thrombosis, including circulating levels of fibrinopeptide A.[181] Incomplete normalization of this determination by therapy appears to predict a high risk of recurrence.

The standard approach to heparinization initially involves immediate anticoagulation with an intravenous bolus of heparin. This is followed by a continuous intravenous infusion. Platelet counts should be obtained before therapy on the fifth day or when any bleeding complication occurs. The infusion is maintained about 7 days. Oral anticoagulation with warfarin is begun at the time of admission concurrently with heparin; doses are adjusted according to the response of the prothrombin time which is itself relatively insensitive to heparin.

Recommendations for the length of time to maintain patients on oral anticoagulants are not precisely known. The risk of recurrence even in uncomplicated cases remains high for several weeks.[170] For straightforward, distal DVT, 6 weeks to 3 months usually suffice, whereas 3 to 6 months of treatment are generally recommended for proximal DVT or pulmonary embolism. Patients with recurrent venous thrombosis and a continuing risk factor such as ATIII deficiency, protein C deficiency, or malignancy should be treated with oral anticoagulants indefinitely.[151,182]

For the patient who continues to show new emboli despite adequate heparinization or who has an absolute contraindication to antithrombotic therapy, vena caval umbrella may protect the patient transiently from pulmonary emboli.[183] Recurrences of venous thrombosis or thromboemboli in patients on warfarin in anticoagulation range usually reflect a thrombotic tendency that exceeds the limited antithrombotic capacity of this drug. Monitored, full-dose heparinization by the subcutaneous route may be required.

Pregnant patients who develop DVT or pulmonary embolism or have prosthetic heart valves or atrial fibrillation with documented systemic embolization should be treated with adjusted-dose subcutaneous heparin (12 hourly subcutaneous heparin or continuous subcutaneous heparin administered by portable pumps, with a PTT 1.5 to 2 times that of control 6 hours after injection) from the time pregnancy is diagnosed until delivery.[151,184]

Surgical Prophylaxis

Moderate-risk patients should be treated prophylactically with low-dose heparin, 5000 IU/12 h subcutaneously, or intermittent pneumatic compression.[143,152,169] Because of the unacceptable consequences of any bleeding complication, patients undergoing neurosurgical procedures, major knee surgery, and urologic surgery should be treated with intermittent pneumatic compression only because the risks and consequences of excessive bleeding are considerable.[151,184]

Low-dose subcutaneous heparin (5000 IU/12 h), beginning before surgery and continuing until a patient is ambulatory, reduces the incidence of venous thrombosis by two thirds and pulmonary embolism by half.[152] These benefits also apply to medical patients at prolonged bed rest, such as patients with acute myocardial infarction or congestive failure.

Patients undergoing acute or elective hip surgery should be treated with LMW heparin beginning 24 hours after surgery or with adjusted-dose heparin or moderate-dose warfarin sodium (to prolong prothrombin time to an INR of 2 to 3, or 1.2 to 1.5 times that of control using rabbit brain thromboplastin).

Valvular Heart Disease and Atrial Fibrillation

Long-term warfarin therapy sufficient to prolong the prothrombin time to 1.5 to 2 times that of control using rabbit brain thromboplastin (standardized INR of 3 to 4.5) should be used in patients with rheumatic mitral valve disease who have documented systemic embolism.[151] Long-term antithrombotic therapy is not indicated in patients with aortic valve disease without associated mitral valve disease or atrial fibrillation. In addition, antithrombotic therapy is not indicated in patients with mitral valve prolapse who have not experienced systemic embolism, unexplained transient ischemic attacks, or atrial fibrillation.

Prosthetic Heart Valves

Patients with bioprosthetic valves in the mitral position should be treated for the first 3 months after valve insertion with warfarin (prothrombin time 1.2 to 1.5 using rabbit brain thromboplastin; INR of 2 to 3).[151] Patients with bioprosthetic valves who have a history of systemic embolism or evidence of a left atrial thrombus at surgery or atrial fibrillation should be treated with long-term warfarin therapy.

All patients with prosthetic heart valves should be treated with long-term warfarin, at a dose sufficient to prolong the prothrombin time to 1.5 to 2 times that of control using rabbit brain thromboplastin (standardized INR of 3 to 4.5). Dipyridamole, 400 mg/d, when combined with warfarin provides additional benefit.[69] Patients with prosthetic heart valves who suffer systemic embolism despite adequate therapy with warfarin should definitely be treated with dipyridamole, 400 g/d, in addition to warfarin. Antiplatelet agents alone, without warfarin, do not offer sufficient protection against systemic embolism.

Acute Myocardial Infarction

All patients with acute myocardial infarction should receive thrombolytic therapy (streptokinase, 1.5×10^6 IU intravenously, or tissue plasminogen activator, 100 mg) unless contraindicated, and they should receive 325 mg aspirin daily, beginning at the time of presentation and continuing for at least 1 year.[143] They should also receive low-dose heparin, 5000 IU/12 h subcutaneously, until fully ambulatory to prevent venous thromboembolism.[143,151] Patients with acute anterior transmural myocardial infarction are at increased risk of systemic embolism and should receive full-dose heparin therapy by continuous infusion followed by warfarin therapy to prolong prothrombin time to an INR of 2 to 3 (1.2 to 1.5 times that of control using rabbit brain thromboplastin) for 1 to 3 months. Patients with atrial fibrillation complicating acute myocardial infarction and a history of previous systemic embolism or pulmonary embolism, or congestive heart failure, should also receive heparin therapy followed by warfarin therapy to prolong prothrombin time to an INR of 2 to 3 (1.2 to 1.5 times that of control using rabbit brain thromboplastin) for at least 3 months.

Complications of Anticoagulant Therapy

The major risk of anticoagulant therapy is bleeding.[143,151,185–187] In several large studies, patients receiving standard doses of either heparin or warfarin exhibited a 2% to 4% per year incidence of major bleeding episodes (those requiring transfusion). The incidence of bleeding with heparin therapy is reduced when it is administered by continuous infusion and adjusted by monitoring, compared with that which occurs with the intermittent bolus regimen. The risk of a fatal hemorrhage is about 0.2% per year for patients on oral anticoagulants. The incidence of complications from warfarin is higher in patients monitored infrequently because the incidence of bleeding episodes increases with prolongation of the prothrombin time beyond the therapeutic range. In general, any new or painful symptom in an anticoagulated patient should be considered to be a manifestation of a potential bleeding complication until proved otherwise. Bleeding episodes in patients on warfarin occurring while the PT is within the therapeutic range are frequently due to focal pathologic lesions, such as an occult neoplasm that is unmasked by the therapy. The most common minor bleeding episodes involve urinary, gastrointestinal, and vaginal bleeding.

In patients who bleed because of heparin therapy, reversal of heparin is achieved by protamine sulfate, a basic nuclear histone that contains one third of its residues as arginine. Protamine binds heparin more tightly than any plasma protein, including ATIII. It is routinely given after heparinization during cardiopulmonary bypass surgery in about equal weight amounts to those of administered heparin. The protamine may dissociate or metabolize more rapidly than heparin, thereby accounting for the occasional open heart surgical patient who exhibits rebound heparinization, which is seen a few hours after surgery.

Management of bleeding in patients on warfarin depends on the seriousness of the bleeding episode. For immediate reversal, as for massive or life-threatening hemorrhage or emergency surgery, plasma (or whole blood) should be given. In adults, four to six bags of 250-mL fresh frozen plasma are usually required to raise the vitamin K–dependent factors to hemostatic levels, that is, above 30% to 40% of normal values. Vitamin K should also be given in this situation. Treatment with vitamin K alone corrects factor VII levels in several hours, and within 1 to 2 days hemostasis is sufficiently normalized to limit bleeding. If oral anticoagulants are truly indicated to prevent thrombosis and if the patient presents with only minor bleeding or if an abnormally prolonged prothrombin time alone is present, it is often more useful to reduce or withhold a warfarin dose, or that of a potentiating drug, and follow the prothrombin time until it returns to the therapeutic range.

Heparin-associated thrombocytopenia occurs in about 5% of treated patients.[188,189] Thus, it is prudent to check a platelet count before heparin administration on the fifth day or with any bleeding episode. Thrombocytopenia may occur with bovine or porcine heparin when it is given either intravenously or subcutaneously. The two main clinical types are a common, mild thrombocytopenia of early onset, possibly caused by the platelet proaggregating effect of some contaminating fraction of heparin itself,[190] and a severe delayed-onset thrombocytopenia caused by an immune mechanism.[189] Some patients with severe thrombocytopenia may have associated thromboembolic complications that may be attributed to an IgG heparin-dependent platelet antibody. The diagnosis of heparin-induced thrombocytopenia may be confirmed by the demonstration of the heparin-dependent antibody in vitro. In patients with severe thrombocytopenia, heparin should be stopped and warfarin commenced. Heparin may be continued in patients with asymptomatic mild thrombocytopenia provided that the patient's condition and the platelet counts are closely monitored. When recalcification times are used to monitor heparin effect, moderately severe thrombocytopenia will falsely prolong the test result, since it is dependent on platelets to provide phospholipids. Recombinant hirudin substitution for heparin may become useful in the management of heparin-induced thrombocytopenia when it becomes available for clinical use.[139]

Alopecia or osteoporosis also complicates heparin therapy after prolonged usage of full-dose heparin over several months. Rarely, "paradoxical thrombosis" occurs.

Warfarin therapy is associated with a fetal bony embryopathy when administered to women during their first trimester of pregnancy. Women receiving warfarin should be advised against pregnancy because of this risk. If pregnancy develops, full-dose subcutaneous heparin should be substituted for warfarin.[190] Poisoning with warfarin has occurred in children ingesting coumarin-type rat poisons and occasionally with factitious ingestion. Rarely, areas of skin necrosis are seen, particularly after large loading doses of warfarin. These lesions are associated with thrombi in vessels. In a percentage of these patients early depletion of proteins C and S by warfarin in the absence of heparin coverage may explain this thrombotic complication.[191]

Thrombosis is a complex process. In the future, combination of agents may be necessary to optimize efficacy and safety. Thus, effective treatment of acute myocardial infarction involves the combination of aspirin, streptokinase, and low-dose heparin. Also, combinations of warfarin and dipyridamole, heparin and aspirin, and heparin and PGI_2 have been successfully used in patients with prosthetic heart valves,[69] unstable angina,[157] and hemodialysis, respectively.[111] With new understanding of the complex systems for activation and inactivation of various pathways, together with development of the capability of molecular biology to produce many new specific and potent engineered therapeutic molecules, antithrombotic therapy is likely to undergo substantial innovation in the near future.

REFERENCES

1. Sawyer S, Srinivasan S. The role of electrochemical surface properties in thrombosis at vascular interfaces: cumulative experience of studies in animals and man. Bull NY Acad Med 1972;48:235.
2. Pearson JD, Carlton JS, Gordon JL. Metabolism of adenine nucleotides by ectoenzymes of vascular endothelial and smooth-muscle cells in culture. Biochem J 1980;190:421.
3. Moncada S, Vane JR. Arachidonic acid metabolites and their interactions between platelets and blood vessel wall. N Engl J Med 1979;300: 1142.
4. Moncada S, Palmer RMJ, Higgs EA. Prostacyclin and endothelium-derived relaxing factor: biological interactions and significance. In: Verstraete M, Vermylen J, Lijnen, Arnout J, eds. Thrombosis and haemostasis 1987. Leuven, Belgium, Leuven University Press, 1987:505.
5. Harker LA, Mann KG. Thrombosis and fibrinolysis. In: Fuster V, Verstraete M, eds. Thrombosis in cardiovascular disorders. Philadelphia, WB Saunders, 1992:1.
6. Marcum JA, McKenny JB, Rosenberg RD. Acceleration of thrombin antithrombin complex formation in rat hindquarters via heparin like molecules bound to the endothelium. J Clin Invest 1984;74:341.
7. Lollar P, Owen WG. Clearance of thrombin from the circulation in rabbits by high-affinity binding sites on the endothelium: possible role in the inactivation of thrombin by antithrombin III. J Clin Invest 1980;66: 1222.
8. Esmon CT, Owen GW. Identification of an endothelial cell cofactor for thrombin-catalyzed activation of protein C. Proc Natl Acad Sci USA 1981;78:2249.
9. Owen WG, Esmon CT. Functional properties of an endothelial cell cofactor for thrombin-catalyzed activation of protein C. J Biol Chem 1981;256:5532.
10. Esmon NL, Owen WG, Esmon CT. Isolation of a membrane-bound cofactor for thrombin-catalyzed activation of protein C. J Biol Chem 1982;257:859.
11. Levin EG, Loskutoff DJ. Cultured bovine endothelial cells produce urokinase and tissue-type plasminogen activators. J Cell Biol 1982;94: 631.
12. Levin EG, Marzec UM, Anderson J, Harker LA. Thrombin stimulates tissue plasminogen activator release from cultured human endothelial cells. J Clin Invest 1984;74:1988.
13. Harpel P. Blood proteolytic enzyme inhibitors: their role in modulating blood coagulation and fibrinolytic pathways. In: Colman RW, Hirsh J, Marder VJ, Salzman EW, eds. Hemostasis and thrombosis: basic principles and clinical practice, ed 2. Philadelphia, JB Lippincott, 1987: 219.
14. Rosenberg RD, Lam LH. Correlation between structure and function of heparin. Proc Natl Acad Sci USA 1979;76:1218.
15. Tollefsen DM, Blank MK. Detection of a new heparin-dependent inhibitor of thrombin in human plasma. J Clin Invest 1981;68:589.
16. Badimon L, Badimon JJ, Turitto VT, Fuster V: Role of von Willebrand factor in mediating platelet–vessel wall interaction at low shear rate: the importance of perfusion condition. Blood 1989;73:961.
17. de Groot PG, Sixma JJ. Role of von Willebrand factor in the vessel wall. Semin Thromb Hemost 1987;13:416.
18. Fressinaud E, Baruch D, Rothschild C, et al. Platelet von Willebrand factor: evidence for its involvment in platelet adhesion to collagen. Blood 1987;70:1214.
19. Sakariassen KS, Bolhuis PA, Sixma JJ. Human blood platelet adhesion to artery subendothelium is mediated by factor VIII–von Willebrand factor bound to the subendothelium. Nature 1979;279:636.
20. Kao KJ, Pizzo SV, McKee PA. Demonstration and characterization of specific binding sites for factor VIII/von Willebrand factor of human platelets. J Clin Invest 1979;63:656.
21. Coller BS, Peerschke EI, Scudder LE, Sullivan CA. A murine monoclonal antibody that completely blocks the binding of fibrinogen to platelets produces a thrombasthenic-like state in normal platelets and binds to glycoproteins IIb and/or IIIa. J Clin Invest 1983;72:325.
22. Phillips DR, Charo IF, Scarborough RM. GPIIb-IIIa: the responsive integrin. Cell 1991;65:359.
23. Frelinger AL III, Cohen I, Plow EF, et al. Selective inhibition of integrin function by antibodies specific for ligand-occupied receptor conformers. J Biol Chem 1990;265:6346.
24. Houdijk WPM, Sixma JJ. Fibronectin in artery subendothelium is important for platelet adhesion. Blood 1985;65:598.
25. Bastida E, Escolar G, Ordinas A, Sixma JJ. Fibronectin is required for platelet adhesion and thrombus formation on subendothelium and collagen surfaces. Blood 1987;70:1437.
26. Nievelstein PFEM, Sixma JJ. Glycoprotein IIb-IIIa and RGD(S) are not important for fibronectin-dependent platelet adhesion under flow conditions. Blood 1988;72:82.
27. Ill CR, Engvall E, Ruoslahti, E. Adhesion of platelets to laminin in the absence of activation. J Cell Biol 1984;99:2140.
28. Nieuwenhuis HK, Akkerman JWN, Houdijk WPM, Sixma JJ. Human blood platelets showing no response to collagen fail to express surface glycoprotein Ia. Nature 1985;318:470.
29. Nieuwenhuis HK, Sakariassen KS, Houdijk WPM, et al. Deficiency of platelet membrane glycoprotein Ia associated with a decreased platelet adhesion to subendothelium: a defect in platelet spreading. Blood 1986;68:692.
30. Holmsen H. Platelet secretion. In: Colman RW, Hirsh J, Marder VJ, Salzman EW, eds. Hemostasis and thrombosis: basic principles and clinical practice, ed 2. Philadelphia, JB Lippincott, 1987:606.

31. Coller BS. Platelets and thrombolytic therapy. N Engl J Med 1990;322:33.
32. Hanson SR, Pareti FI, Ruggeri ZM, et al. Effects of monoclonal antibodies against the platelet glycoprotein IIb/IIIa complex on thrombosis and hemostasis in the baboon. J Clin Invest 1988;81:149.
33. EPIC Investigators. Use of a monoclonal antibody directed against the platelet glycoprotein IIb/IIIa receptor in high-risk coronary angioplasty. N Engl J Med 1994;330:956.
34. Tollefsen DM, Majerus PW. Evidence for a single class of thrombin-binding sites on human platelets. Biochemistry 1976;15:2144.
35. Hanson SR, Harker LA. Interruption of acute platelet-dependent thrombosis by the synthetic antithrombin D-phenylalanyl-L-prolyl-L-arginyl chloromethyl ketone. Proc Natl Acad Sci USA 1988;85:1.
36. Lumsden AB, Kelly AB, Schneider PA, et al. Lasting safe interruption of endarterectomy thrombosis by transiently infused antithrombin peptide D-Phe-Pro-Arg CH_2Cl in baboons. Blood 1993;81:1762.
37. Vu T-KH, Hung DT, Wheaton VI, Coughlin SR. Molecular cloning of a functional thrombin receptor reveals a novel proteolytic mechanism of receptor activation. Cell 1991;64:1057.
38. Nemerson Y. Tissue factor and hemostasis. Blood 1988;71:1.
39. Walsh PN, Griffin JH. Contributions of human platelets to the proteolytic activation of blood coagulation factors XII and XI. Blood 1981;57:106.
40. Sinha D, Seaman FS, Koshy A, et al. Blood coagulation factors XIa binds specifically to a site on activated human platelets distinct from that for factor XI. J Clin Invest 1984;73:1550.
41. Rao LVM, Rapaport SI. The effect of platelets upon factor Xa-catalyzed activation of factor VII in vitro. Blood 1988;72:396.
42. Lorand L, Konishi K. Activation of the fibrin-stabilizing factor of plasma by thrombin. Arch Biochem Biophys 1964;105:58.
43. Sevitt S. The structure and growth of valve-pocket thrombi in femoral veins. J Clin Pathol 1974;27:517.
44. Kareno T, Motoniya M. Flow through a venous valve and its implication for thrombus formation. Thromb Res 1984;36:245.
45. Thomas DP. Overview of venous thrombogenesis. Semin Thromb Hemost 1988;14:1.
46. Nilsson IM, Ljunger H, Tengborn L. Two different mechanisms in patients with venous thrombosis and defective fibrinolysis: low concentration of plasminogen activator or increased concentration of plasminogen activator inhibitor. Br Med J 1985;290:1453.
47. Rapaport SI. Inhibition of factor VIIa/tissue factor-induced blood coagulation: with particular emphasis upon a factor Xa-dependent inhibitory mechanism. Blood 1989;73:359.
48. Antiplatelet Trialists' Collaboration. Collaborative overview of randomised trials of antiplatelet therapy. I. Prevention of death, myocardial infarction, and stroke by prolonged antiplatelet therapy in various categories of patients. Br Med J 1994;308:81.
49. Antiplatelet Trialists' Collaboration. Collaborative overview of randomised trials of antiplatelet therapy. II. Maintenance of vascular graft or arterial patency by antiplatelet therapy. Br Med J 1994;308:159.
50. UK-TIA Study Group. The UK-TIA Aspirin Trial: interim results. Br Med J 1987;296:316.
51. Bousser MG, Eschwege E, Haguenau M, et al. "AICLA" controlled trial of aspirin and dipyridamole in the secondary prevention of atherothrombotic cerebral ischemia. Stroke 1983;14:5.
52. The Canadian Cooperative Study Group. A randomized trial of aspirin and sulfinpyrazone in threatened stroke. N Engl J Med 1978;299:53.
53. Fields WS, Lemak NA, Frankowski RF, Hardy RJ. Controlled trial of aspirin in cerebral ischemia. Stroke 1977;8:301.
54. Antiplatelet Trialists' Collaboration. Secondary prevention of vascular disease by prolonged antiplatelet treatment. Br Med J 1988;296:320.
55. ISIS-2 Collaborative Group. Randomised trial of intravenous streptokinase, oral aspirin, both or neither among 17,187 cases of suspected acute myocardial infarction: ISIS-2. Lancet 1988;2:349.
56. The Steering Committee of The Physicians Health Study Research Group. Special report—preliminary report: findings from the aspirin components of the ongoing physicians' health study. N Engl J Med 1988;318:262.
57. Peto R, Gray R, Collins R, et al. Randomised trial of prophylactic daily aspirin in British male doctors. Br J Med 1988;296:313.
58. Hennekens CH, Peto R, Hutchison GB, Doll R. An overview of the British and American Aspirin Studies. N Engl J Med 1988;318:923.
59. Lorenz RL, Schacky CV, Weber M, et al. Improved aortocoronary bypass patency by low-dose aspirin (100 mg daily). Lancet 1984;1:1261.
60. Goldman S, Copeland J, Moritz T, et al. Improvement in early saphenous vein graft patency after coronary artery bypass surgery with antiplatelet therapy: results of a Veterans Administration cooperative study. Circulation 1988;77:1324.
61. Harter HR, Burch JW, Majerus PW, et al. Prevention of thrombosis in patients on hemodialysis by low-dose aspirin. N Engl J Med 1979;301:577.
62. Kyrle PA, Eichler HG, Jager U, Lechner K. Inhibition of prostaglandin and thromboxane A_2 generation by low-dose aspirin at the site of plug formation in man in vivo. Circulation 1987;75:1025.
63. Levy M. Aspirin use in patients with major upper gastrointestinal bleeding and peptic ulcer disease. N Engl J Med 1974;290:1158.
64. Lewis HD, Davis JW, Archibald DG, et al. Protective effects of aspirin against acute myocardial infarction and death in men with unstable angina. N Engl J Med 1983;309:396.
65. Maffrand JP, Defreyn G, Bernat A, et al. Reviewed pharmacology of ticlopidine. Angiologie 1988;77(Suppl):6.
66. Saltiel E, Ward A. Ticlopidine. A review of its pharmacodynamic and pharmacokinetic properties, and therapeutic efficacy in platelet-dependent disease states. Drugs 1987;34:222.
67. Gent M, Blakely JA, Easton JD, et al. The Canadian American Ticlopidine Study (CATS) in thromboembolic stroke. Lancet 1989;1:1215.
68. Hass WK, Easton JD, Adams HP, et al. A randomized trial comparing ticlopidine hydrochloride with aspirin for the prevention of stroke in high-risk patients. N Engl J Med 1989;321:501.
69. Sullivan JM, Harken DE, Gorlin R. Pharmacologic control of thromboembolic complications of cardiac-valve replacement. N Engl J Med 1971;284:1391.
70. Hanson SR, Harker LA. Baboon models of acute arterial thrombosis. Thromb Haemost 1987;58:801.
71. Pedersen AK, Fitzgerald GA. Dose-related kinetics of aspirin: presystemic acetylation of platelet cyclooxygenase. N Engl J Med 1984;311:1206.
72. Roth GJ, Majerus PW. The mechanism of the effect of aspirin on human platelets. I. Acetylation of a particulate fraction protein. J Clin Invest 1975;56:624.
73. Levy M. Aspirin use in patients with major upper gastrointestinal bleeding and peptic ulcer disease. N Engl J Med 1974;290:1158.
74. Silvoso GR, Ivey KJ, Butt JH, et al. Incidence of gastric lesions in patients with rheumatic disease on chronic aspirin therapy. Ann Intern Med 1979;91:517.
75. Graham DV, Smith LJ. Aspirin and the stomach. Ann Intern Med 1986;104:390.
76. Weksler BB, Pett SB, Richter RC, et al. Differential inhibition by aspirin of vascular and platelet prostaglandin synthesis in atherosclerotic patients. N Engl J Med 1983;308:800.
77. Patignani P, Filabozzi P, Patrono C. Selective cumulative inhibition of platelet thromboxane production by low-dose aspirin in healthy subjects. J Clin Invest 1982;69:1366.
78. Fitzgerald GA, Oates JA, Hawiger J, et al. Endogenous biosynthesis of prostacyclin and thromboxane and platelet function during chronic administration of aspirin in man. J Clin Invest 1983;71:678.
79. Preston FE, Whipps S, Jackson CA, et al. Inhibition of prostacyclin and platelet thromboxane A2 after low-dose aspirin. N Engl J Med 1981;304:69.
80. Davis RF, Engelman EG. Incidence of myocardial infarction in patients with rheumatoid arthritis. Arthritis Rheum 1974;17:527.
81. Linos A, Worthington JW, O'Fallon W, et al. Effect of aspirin on prevention of coronary and cerebrovascular disease in patients with rheumatoid arthritis: a long-term follow-up study. Mayo Clin Proc 1978;53:581.
82. Pareti FI, Mannucci PM, D'Angelo, et al. Congenital deficiency of thromboxane and prostacyclin. Lancet 1981;1:898.
83. Elwood PC, Cochrane AL, Burr ML. A randomized controlled trial of acetyl salicylic acid in the secondary prevention of mortality from myocardial infarction. Br Med J 1974;1:436.
84. Coronary Drug Project Group. Aspirin in coronary heart disease. J Chronic Dis 1976;29:625.
85. Breddin K, Loew D, Lechner K, et al. Secondary prevention of myocardial infarction: comparison of acetylsalicylic acid, phenprocoumon and placebo: a multicenter two-year prospective study. Thromb Haemost 1979;40:225.
86. Elwood PC, Sweetnam PM. Aspirin and secondary mortality after myocardial infarction. Lancet 1979;2:1313.
87. Aspirin Myocardial Infarction Study Research Group. A randomized controlled trial of aspirin in persons recovered from myocardial infarction. JAMA 1980;243:661.
88. Persantine-Aspirin Reinfarction Study Research Group. Persantine and aspirin in coronary heart disease. Circulation 1980;62:449.
89. Canner PL. Aspirin in coronary heart disease: comparison of six clinical trials. Isr J Med Sci 1983;19:413.
90. Cairns JA, Gent M, Singer J, et al. Aspirin, sulfinpyrazone, or both in unstable angina. N Engl J Med 1985;313:1369.
91. Mielants H, Veys EM, Verbruggen G, et al. Salicylate-induced gastrointestinal bleeding: comparison between soluble buffered, enteric-coated, and intravenous administration. J Rheumatol 1979;6:2.
92. Dale J, Myhre E, Storstein O, Stormorken H. Arterial thromboembolism and prosthetic heart valve: effects of acetylsalicylic acid. Thromb Diath Haemorrh 1975;34:587.
93. Chesebro JH, Fuster V, Elveback LR, et al. Trial of combined warfarin plus dipyridamole on aspirin therapy in prosthetic heart valve replacement: danger of aspirin compared with dipyridamole. Am J Cardiol 1983;51:1537.
94. Torosian M, Michelson EL, Morganroth J, et al. Aspirin-and-coumadin-related bleeding after coronary-artery bypass graft surgery. Ann Intern Med 1978;89:325.
95. Dale J, Myhre E, Storstein O, et al. Prevention of arterial thromboembolism with acetylsalicylic acid: a controlled clinical study in patients with aortic ball valves. Am Heart J 1977;94:101.

96. American-Canadian Cooperative Study Group. Persantine-aspirin trial in cerebral ischemia. Part II. Endpoint results. Stroke 1985;16:406.
97. Harker LA, Gent M. The use of agents that modify platelet function in the management of thrombotic disorders. In: Colman RW, Hirsh J, Marder VJ, Salzman EW, eds. Hemostasis and thrombosis: basic principles and clinical practice, ed 2. Philadelphia, JB Lippincott, 1987: 1438.
98. Veterans Administration Cooperative Study Group. Saphenous vein graft patency one year after coronary artery bypass surgery and effects of antiplatelet therapy: results of a Veterans Administration Cooperative Study. Circulation 1989;80:1190.
99. Veterans Administration Cooperative Study Group. Preoperative aspirin is not necessary to achieve improved vein graft patency after coronary artery bypass surgery. J Am Coll Cardiol 1989;13:165A.
100. Schwartz L, Bourassa MG, Lesperance J, et al. Aspirin and dipyridamole in the prevention of restenosis after percutaneous transluminal coronary angioplasty. N Engl J Med 1988;318:1714.
101. FitzGerald GA, Reilly IAG, Pedersen AK. The biochemical pharmacology of thromboxane synthase inhibition in man. Circulation 1985;72: 1194.
102. Fitzgerald DJ, Fragetta J, FitzGerald GA. Prostaglandin endoperoxydes modulate the response to thromboxane synthase inhibition during coronary thrombosis. J Clin Invest 1988;82:1708.
103. Golino P, Ashton JH, Glas-Greenwalt P, et al. Mediation of reocclusion by thromboxane A_2 and serotonin after thrombolysis with tissue-type plasminogen activator in a canine preparation of coronary thrombosis. Circulation 1988;77:678.
104. Golino P, Ashton JH, McNatt J, et al. Simultaneous administration of thromboxane A_2- and serotonin S_2-receptor antagonists markedly enhances thrombolysis and prevents or delays reocclusion after tissue-type plasminogen activator in a canine model of coronary thrombosis. Circulation 1989;79:911.
105. Lam JYT, Chesebro JH, Badimon L, et al. Serotonin and thromboxane A_2 receptor blockade decreases vasoconstriction but not platelet deposition after deep arterial injury. (Abstract) Circulation 1986;74(Suppl 2):97.
106. Moncada S, Higgs EA. Prostaglandins in the pathogenesis and prevention of vascular disease. Blood Rev 1987;1:141.
107. Henriksson P, Edajg O, Wennmaln A. Prostacyclin infusion in patients with acute myocardial infarction. Br Heart J 1985;53:173.
108. Chiariello M, Golino P, Cappelli-Bigazzi M, et al. Reduction in infarct size by the prostacyclin analogue iloprost (ZK 36374) after experimental coronary artery occlusion-reperfusion. Am Heart J 1988;115:499.
109. Armstrong PW, Langevin LM, Watts DG. Randomized trial of prostacyclin infusion in acute myocardial infarction. Am J Cardiol 1988;61: 455.
110. Malpass TW, Hanson SR, Savage B, et al. Prevention of acquired transient defect in platelet plug formation by infused prostacyclin. Blood 1981;57:736.
111. Turney JH, Williams LC, Fewell MR, et al. Platelet protection and heparin sparing with prostacyclin during regular dialysis therapy. Lancet 1980;2:219.
112. FitzGerald GA. Dipyridamole. N Engl J Med 1987;316:1247.
113. Hanson SR, Harker LA, Bjornsson TD. Effect of platelet-modifying drugs on arterial thromboembolism in baboons: aspirin potentiates the antithrombotic actions of dipyridamole and sulfinpyrazone by mechanism(s) independent of platelets cyclo-oxygenase inhibition. J Clin Invest 1985;75:1591.
114. Chesebro JH, Fuster V, Elveback LR, et al. Trial of combined warfarin plus dipyridamole or aspirin therapy in prosthetic heart valve replacement: danger of aspirin compared with dipyridamole. Am J Cardiol 1983;51:1537.
115. Goodnight SH Jr, Harris WS, Connor WE. The effects of dietary omega-3 fatty acids on platelet composition and function in man: a prospective, controlled study. Blood 1981;58:880.
116. Dyerberg J, Bang HO, Stoffersen E, et al. Eicosapentanoic acid and prevention of thrombosis and atherosclerosis? Lancet 1978;2:117.
117. Barcelli U, Glas-Greenwalt P, Pollack VE. Enhancing effect of dietary supplementation with omega-3 fatty acids on plasma fibrinolysis in normal subjects. Thromb Res 1985;39:307.
118. Popp-Snijders C, Schouten JA, van der Meer J, van der Veen EA. Fatty fish-induced changes in membrane lipid composition and viscosity of human erythrocyte suspensions. Scand J Clin Lab Invest 1986;46:253.
119. Goodnight SH Jr, Harris WS, Connor WE, Illingworth DR. Polyunsaturated fatty acids, hyperlipidemia, and thrombosis. Arteriosclerosis 1982;2:87.
120. Lam JYT, Chesebro JH, Badimon L, et al. Cod liver oil alters the platelet arterial wall response to injury by angioplasty. Circulation 1987;76(Suppl 4):601.
121. Weiner BH, Ockene IS, Levine PH, et al. Inhibition of atherosclerosis by cod-liver oil in a hyperlipidemic swine model. N Engl J Med 1986;315:841.
122. Davis HR, Bridenstine RT, Vesselinovitch D, Wissler RW. Fish oil inhibits development of atherosclerosis in rhesus monkeys. Arteriosclerosis 1987;7:441.
123. Hollander W, Hong S, Kirkpatrick BJ, et al. Differential effects of fish oil supplements on atherosclerosis. Circulation 1987;76(Suppl 4):1245.
124. Goodnight SH, Cairns JA, Fisher M, FitzGerald GA. Assessment of the therapeutic use of n-3 fatty acids in vascular disease and thrombosis. Chest 1992;102:374S.
125. Harker LA, Kelly AB, Hanson SR, et al. Interruption of vascular thrombus formation and vascular lesion formation by dietary n-3 fatty acids in fish oil in nonhuman primates. Circulation 1993;87:1017.
126. Gold HK, Coller BS, Yasuda T, et al. Rapid and sustained coronary artery recanalization with combined bolus injection of recombinant tissue-type plasminogen activator and monoclonal antiplatelet Gp IIb-IIIa antibody in a canine preparation. Circulation 1988;77:670.
127. Yasuda T, Gold HK, Fallon JT, et al. Monoclonal antibody against the platelet glycoprotein (Gp) IIb-IIIa receptor prevents coronary artery reocclusion after reperfusion with recombinant tissue-type plasminogen activator in dogs. J Clin Invest 1988;81:1284.
128. Torem S, Schneider PA, Hanson SR. Monoclonal antibody-induced inhibition of platelet function: effects on hemostasis and vascular graft thrombosis in baboons. J Vasc Surg 1988;7:172.
129. Cadroy Y, Kelly AB, Marzec UM, et al. Comparison of the antihemostatic and antithrombotic effects of monoclonal antibodies (MoA) against von Willebrand factor (vWF) and platelet (P) glycoprotein IIb/IIIa (GPIIb/IIIa). Circulation 1989;80(Suppl 2):24.
130. Bellinger DA, Nichols TC, Read MS, et al. Prevention of occlusive coronary artery thrombosis by a murine monoclonal antibody to porcine von Willebrand factor. Proc Natl Acad Sci USA 1987;84:8100.
131. Badimon L, Badimon JJ, Chesebro JH, Fuster V. Inhibition of thrombus formation: blockage of adhesive glycoprotein mechanisms versus blockage of the cyclooxygenase pathway. (Abstract) J Am Coll Cardiol 1988;11:30A.
132. Cadroy Y, Houghten RA, Hanson SR. RGDV peptide selectively inhibits platelet-dependent thrombus formation in vivo: studies using a baboon model. J Clin Invest 1989;84:939.
133. Huang TF, Holt JC, Lukasiewicz H, Niewiarowski. Trigramin: a low molecular weight peptide inhibiting fibrinogen interaction with platelet receptors expressed on glycoprotein IIb-IIIa complex. J Biol Chem 1987;262:16157.
134. Gan ZR, Gould RJ, Jacobs JW, et al. Echistatin: a potent platelet aggregation inhibitor from the venom of the viper, *Echis carinatus*. J Biol Chem 1988;263:19827.
135. Cook JJ, Huang TF, Rucinski B, et al. Inhibition of platelet hemostatic plug formation by Trigramin, a novel RGD containing peptide. (Abstract) Circulation 1978;78(Suppl II):313.
136. Kelly AB, Hanson SR, Marzec U, Harker LA. Recombinant hirudin (r-H) interruption of platelet-dependent thrombus formation. (Abstract) Circulation 1988;78(Suppl II):1242.
137. Heras M, Chesebro JH, Penny WJ, et al. Effects of thrombin inhibition on the development of acute platelet-thrombus deposition during angioplasty in pigs: heparin versus recombinant hirudin, a specific thrombin inhibitor. Circulation 1989;79:657.
138. Hanson SR, Harker LA. Interruption of acute platelet-dependent thrombosis by the synthetic antithrombin D-phenylalanyl-L-prolyl-L-arginyl chloromethylketone. Proc Natl Acad Sci USA 1988;85:3184.
139. Markwardt F, Fink E, Kaiser B, et al. Pharmacological survey of recombinant hirudin. Pharmazie 1988;43:202.
140. Markwardt F. Pharmacological approaches to thrombin regulation. Ann N Y Acad Sci 1986;485:204.
141. Gruber A, Griffin JH, Harker LA, Hanson SR. Inhibition of platelet-dependent thrombus formation by human activated protein C in a primate model. Blood 1989;73:639.
142. Gruber A, Hanson SR, Kelly AB, et al. Recombinant activated protein C (r-apC) inhibition of platelet-dependent thrombosis. Circulation 1988;78(Suppl II):1250.
143. Dalen JE, Hirsh J, eds. Third American College of Chest Physicians' Conference Report on Antithrombotic Therapy. Chest 1992;102:303S.
144. Moelker HCT. Heparins and platelet function. Prog Pharmacol 1982;44: 99.
145. Simon TL, Hyers TM, Gaston JP, Harker LA. Heparin pharmacokinetics: increased requirements in pulmonary embolism. Br J Haematol 1978;39: 111.
146. Hirsh J, van Aken WG, Gallus AS, et al. Heparin kinetics in venous thrombosis and pulmonary embolism. Circulation 1976;53:691.
147. Basu D, Gallus A, Hirsh J, Cade J. A prospective study of the value of monitoring heparin treatment with the activated partial thromboplastin time. N Engl J Med 1972;287:324.
148. King DJ, Kelton JG. Heparin-associated thrombocytopenia. Ann Intern Med 1984;100:536.
149. Salzman EW, Deykin D, Shapiro RM, Rosenberg R. Management of heparin therapy: controlled prospective trial. N Engl J Med 1975;292: 1046.
150. Hirsh J, van Aken WG, Gallus AS, et al. Heparin kinetics in venous thrombosis and pulmonary embolism. Circulation 1976;53:691.
151. ACCP-NHLBI National Conference on Antithrombotic Therapy. Chest 1986;89:1S.
152. Collins R, Scrimgeour A, Yusuf S, Peto R. Reduction in fatal pulmonary embolism and venous thrombosis by perioperative administration of subcutaneous heparin: overview of results of randomized trials in general, orthopedic, and urologic surgery. N Engl J Med 1988;318:1162.
153. Collins R, Scrimgeour A, Yusuf S, Peto R. Reduction in fatal pulmonary

embolism and venous thrombosis by perioperative administration of subcutaneous heparin. N Engl J Med 1988;318:1162.
154. Leyvraz PF, Richard J, Bachman F, et al. Adjusted versus fixed-dose subcutaneous heparin in the prevention of deep-vein thrombosis after total hip replacement. N Engl J Med 1983;309:954.
155. Cadroy Y, Harker LA, Hanson SR. Inhibition of platelet-dependent thrombosis by low molecular weight heparin (CY222): comparison with standard heparin. J Lab Clin Med 1989;114:349.
156. Heras M, Chesebro JH, Penny WJ, et al. The importance of adequate heparin dosage in arterial angioplasty in a porcine model. Circulation 1988;78:654.
157. Theroux P, Ouimet H, McCans J, et al. Aspirin, heparin, or both to treat acute unstable angina. N Engl J Med 1988;319:1105.
158. Castellot JJ JR, Cochran DL, Karnovsky MJ. Effect of heparin on vascular smooth muscle cells. I. Cell metabolism. J Physiol 1984;124:21.
159. Harker LA, Maraganore JM, Hirsh J. Novel antithrombotic agents. In: Colman RW, Hirsh J, Marder VJ, Salzman EW, eds. Hemostasis and thrombosis: basic principles and clinical practice. Philadelphia, JB Lippincott, 1994:1638.
160. Ofosu FA, Barrowcliffe TW. Mechanisms of action of low molecular weight heparins and heparinoids. In: Hirsh J, ed. Bailliere's clinical haematology, vol 3: antithrombotic therapy. London, Bailliere Tindall 1990:505.
161. Levine MN, Hirsh J, Gent M, et al. Prevention of deep vein thrombosis after elective hip surgery: a randomized trial comparing low molecular weight heparin with standard unfractionated heparin. Ann Intern Med 1991;114:545.
162. Deykin D. Warfarin therapy, part I. N Engl J Med 1970;283:691.
163. Deykin D. Warfarin therapy, part II. N Engl J Med 1970;283:801.
164. Kelly JG, O'Malley K. Clinical pharmacokinetics of oral anticoagulants. Clin Pharmacokinet 1979;4:1.
165. Kirkwood TBL. Calibration of reference thromboplastins and standardisation of the prothrombin time ratio. Thromb Haemost 1983;49: 238.
166. Hirsh J, Levine M. Confusion over the therapeutic range for monitoring oral anticoagulant therapy in North America. Thromb Haemost 1988;59: 129.
167. Loeliger EA. ICSH/ICTH recommendations for reporting prothrombin time in oral anticoagulant control. Thromb Haemost 54:155, 1985.
168. Hull R, Hirsh J, Jay R, et al. Different intensities of oral anticoagulant therapy in the treatment of proximal-vein thrombosis. N Engl J Med 1982;307:1676.
169. Hull R, Delmore T, Genton E, et al. Warfarin sodium versus low dose heparin in the long term treatment of venous thromboembolism. N Engl J Med 1979;301:855.
170. Hull R, Delmore T, Carter C, et al. Adjusted subcutaneous heparin versus warfarin sodium in the long term treatment of venous thrombosis. N Engl J Med 1982;306:189.
171. Tabener DA, Poller L, Burslem RW, Jones JB. Oral anticoagulants controlled by the British Comparative thromboplastin versus low dose heparin in prophylaxis of deep venous thrombosis. Br Med J 1978;1: 272.
172. Bjerkelund CJ, Orning OM. The efficacy of anticoagulant therapy in preventing embolism related to D.C. electrical conversion of atrial fibrillation. Am J Cardiol 1969;23:208.
173. O'Reilly RA. Vitamin K antagonists. In: Colman RW, Hirsh J, Marder VJ, Salzman EW, eds. Hemostasis and thrombosis: basic principles and clinical practice, ed 2. Philadelphia, JB Lippincott, 1987:1367.
174. O'Reilly RA, Trager WF, Motley CH, Howald W. Stereoselective interaction of phenylbutazone (with 12C/13C) warfarin pseudoracemates in man. J Clin Invest 1980;65:746.
175. Hull JH, Murray WJ, Brown S, et al. Potential anticoagulant drug interactions in ambulatory patients. Clin Pharmacol Ther 1978;24:644.
176. Markwardt F, Fink E, Kaiser B, et al. Pharmacological survey of recombinant hirudin. Pharmazie 1988;43:202.
177. Tollefsen DM, Pestka CA, Monafo WJ. Activation of heparin cofactor II by dermatan sulfate. J Biol Chem 1983;258:6713.
178. Fernandez F, van Ryn J, Ofosu F, et al. The haemorrhagic and antithrombotic effects of dermatan sulphate. Br J Haematol 1986;64:309.
179. Cadroy Y, Dol F, Caranobe C, et al. Standard heparin enhances the antithrombotic activity of dermatan sulfate in the rabbit but CY216 does not. Thromb Haemost 1988;59:295.
180. Barritt DW, Jordan SC. Anticoagulant drugs in the treatment of pulmonary embolism: a controlled trial. Lancet 1960;1:1309.
181. Yudelman IM, Greenberg J. Factors affecting fibrinopeptide A levels in patients with venous thromboembolism during anticoagulant therapy. Blood 1982;59:787.
182. Levin MN, Hirsh J. Hemorrhagic complications of anticoagulant therapy. Semin Thromb Hemost 1986;12:39.
183. Salzman EW. Surgical management of venous thromboembolism. In: Colman RW, Hirsh J, Marder VJ, Salzman EW, eds. Hemostasis and thrombosis: basic principles and clinical practice, ed 2. Philadelphia, JB Lippincott, 1987:1457.
184. Hirsh J. Venous thromboembolism: guide to management. Mississauga, Ontario, Du Pont Pharmaceuticals, 1988.
185. Colman RW, Hirsh J, Marder VJ, Salzman EW, eds. Hemostasis and thrombosis: basic principles and clinical practice, ed 2. Philadelphia, JB Lippincott, 1987.
186. Bloom AL, Thomas DP. Haemostasis and thrombosis, ed 2. New York, Churchill Livingstone, 1987.
187. Rodgers GM, Shuman MA. Congenital thrombotic disorders. Am J Hematol 1986;21:419.
188. King DJ, Kelton JG. Heparin-associated thrombocytopenia. Ann Intern Med 1984;100:535.
189. Chong BH. Heparin-induced thrombocytopenia. Blood Rev 1988;2:108.
190. Salzman EW, Rozenberg RD, Smith MH, et al. Effect of heparin and heparin fractions on platelet aggregation. J Clin Invest 1980;65:64.
191. Broekmans AW, Bertina RM, Loeliger EA, Kingeman HG. Protein C and the development of skin necrosis during anticoagulant therapy. Thromb Haemost 1983;49:244.

6

Blood Vessels and the Spleen

Blood: Principles and Practice of Hematology,
edited by Robert I. Handin, Samuel E. Lux, and Thomas P. Stossel.
J.B. Lippincott Company, Philadelphia © 1995.

46

Disorders of the Spleen

Susan Blakely Shurin

Hippocrates' and Aristotle's writings describe the gross anatomy of the spleen, which was regarded in ancient times as an "organ of mystery" (*misterii organum plenum*), as described by Galen. The earliest function ascribed to the spleen was the extraction of "melancholic humours," so large spleens resulted in more systemic humor. (Pliny the Elder, in AD 150, said, "great laughers have great spleens.") By the 17th century, localization of unhappiness in the spleen connoted spite, an attribute that persists. Anatomists of the 17th century described the microscopic structure of the spleen for the first time. In 1777, William Hewson assigned the spleen to the lymphatic system, recognizing a hematopoietic function as well. Virchow identified the malpighian follicles as being composed of lymphocytes.[1] The filtration function was described in 1885 by Ponfick, who recognized the role of the spleen in destruction of blood cells. The spleen was considered a nonessential organ because patients survived splenectomy without apparent ill effect. The association of asplenia with increased susceptibility to infection was not clear until 1952.[2]

EMBRYOLOGY, ANATOMY, PHYSIOLOGY

In mice, *Hox11*, one of the homeobox genes, controls the genesis of the spleen.[2a] Mice lacking Hox11, generated by a gene-knockout procedure, have no spleen but are otherwise normal. The spleen arises from the mesoderm, first evident at the fifth week of gestation in humans (0.8- to 1-cm embryo).[3] Layers of the left dorsal mesogastrium condense, and blood vessels appear in the eighth to ninth week of development.[3] Reticular cells and fibers form sheaths around arterioles as they develop. During the fourth month, lymphocytes appear; B cells (surface immunoglobulin bearing) and T cells (E-rosetting cells) are identifiable by the thirteenth week, with B cells predominating throughout gestation.[3] Red and white pulp can be identified by the sixth month, but germinal centers are not evident in fetal spleen.[3] Primitive inactive follicles are present at birth, with IgM and small amounts of IgG synthesized in the last trimester.[3] Macrophages in the cords of the spleen possess phagocytic activity by the end of the first trimester (12 weeks).[3]

Fetal studies on mammals other than humans demonstrate significant hematopoiesis (production of formed elements of blood) within the spleen. Human fetal spleen also has been regarded as a hematopoietic organ. The spleen certainly has the capacity to support hematopoiesis later in life in conditions of bone marrow dysfunction with extramedullary hematopoiesis (eg, myelofibrosis) and hemolytic anemias (eg, thalassemia). Hematopoietic precursors are seen in the spleen, peaking in the second trimester and tapering off during the last trimester.[4] Immature erythroid and myeloid precursors circulate in large numbers during fetal life, and their presence in the spleen may indicate little more than the filtering function of the spleen. The least mature blast forms and those in the mitotic pool are present in small numbers.[3] Since conditions of congenital asplenia are not associated with hematopoietic failure,[4] it appears that splenic hematopoiesis is not essential for normal maturation of blood cell production.

The anatomy of the spleen is shown schematically in Figure 46-1 and is covered in detail in Chapter 7. The spleen is covered with a fibrous capsule and coated by peritoneal mesothelium.[4] The capsule contains blood vessels, lymphatics, and nerves, but no muscular elements, and therefore has none of the contractile ability of the spleens of many animal species. The splenic artery exits from the celiac axis, enters the capsule at the hilum of the spleen, and branches into trabecular arteries. The central arteries branch from the trabecular arteries and enter the white pulp. The white pulp is grossly visible as white nodules 0.1 to 0.2 cm in diameter. The central arteries branching from the trabecular arteries are surrounded by a cuff of T lymphocytes, plasma cells, and macrophages; this is called the periarterial lymphoid sheath. As the arteries branch further, the sheath diminishes in size but continues down to the level of the penicilliary arterioles. At arterial branch points, follicles of B lymphocytes appear as clusters along the periarterial lymphoid sheath.[4] A reticulin network and supporting stromal cells with long cytoplasmic processes connect the parts of the white pulp. The appearance of the white pulp varies with age and with antigenic stimulation. At the time of birth, the white pulp is fully developed. The size of the nodules of the white pulp increases in childhood, especially with immunization and infection, peaks at puberty, and begins to involute in adulthood. Uninfected adults who are immunologically normal usually have no evident germinal centers, in contrast to children and adolescents.[4] The secondary germinal center, or follicle, is surrounded by a mantle zone of B lymphocytes, in turn engulfed by the marginal zone where the white and red pulps meet.[5] The marginal zone is part of the periarterial lymphoid sheath, so it consists mostly of T cells.[6] Around the marginal zone is an area of perifollicular venous sinuses. Some of the central arteries end within the periar-

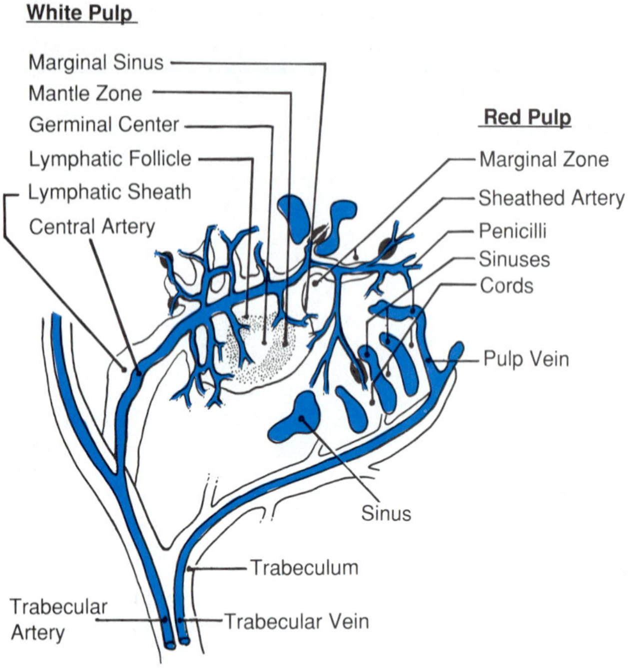

FIGURE 46-1. Schematic depiction of the spleen. (After Bellanti JA. In: Immunology: basic processes. Philadelphia, WB Saunders, 1979)

terial lymphoid sheaths, some enter the marginal zones, and some branches exit from the marginal zones into the red pulp as penicilliary arteries. The marginal zone of the white pulp is the site of initial antigen trapping and processing.[7]

The red pulp of the spleen consists of vascular sinuses, the cords of Billroth, and the terminal branches of the penicilliary arteries. Vascular sinuses are lined with endothelial cells with long cytoplasmic processes and a basement membrane beneath that has ring fibers at right angles to the endothelial cell processes. These ring fibers are attached to the macrophages' dendritic processes.[8] The cytoplasmic processes are close together without tight junctions or interdigitations. Intact blood cells can be seen squeezing through the potential spaces between these cells and between the ring fibers. Outside the sinus walls are processes of the reticular cells of the cords of Billroth, which also surround the periarterial lymphoid sheath and the marginal zones of the follicles. These macrophages attach to the ring fibers surrounding the sinuses.[8] The cords of Billroth are thus interspersed between the sinuses, and receive the terminations of the arterial capillaries. The cords are not lined with endothelium, unlike the sinuses and pulp veins. Circulation of blood through red pulp that is entirely lined with endothelial cells is relatively rapid and is referred to as *closed* circulation.[8,9] Circulation that goes directly into the cords is referred to as *open* circulation, is significantly slower, and encourages the cordal macrophages to remove cells that are damaged or aged in the hypoxic, hypoglycemic, and acidotic environment with stagnant flow.[10]

SPLENIC FUNCTIONS

Fetal and Extramedullary Hematopoiesis

Active hematopoiesis can be seen in the fetal spleen throughout the second trimester and, to a decreasing extent, in the third trimester.[11,12] Erythroid and megakaryocytic elements predominate, but myeloid elements are also present. After the fifth month in utero, bone marrow is the major hematopoietic organ, and the presence of immature hematopoietic elements may represent pooling of fetal blood in the spleen since hematopoietic elements circulate in considerable numbers in fetal blood.[13,14] Because the cells are represented in the approximate proportion that they are present in peripheral blood, it has been argued that the fetal spleen is not a hematopoietic organ.[15] Evidence that it can be comes from both mice and humans. In lethally irradiated mice given compatible bone marrow infusion, the spleen is the initial site of hematopoietic colonies.[16] Spleen cells reconstitute hematopoietic function in mice, but mononuclear cells from other lymphoid organs (nodes, thymus, thoracic duct) do not.[17]

Extramedullary hematopoiesis is a major cause of splenomegaly in human diseases affecting the bone marrow. It is most common in hemolytic anemias, either congenital (eg, thalassemia) or acquired, but production of myeloid and megakaryocytic elements is seen as well in myelofibrosis with myeloid metaplasia. It appears that the stromal cells of the spleen are capable of supporting hematopoiesis, which suggests that they resemble those of the bone marrow and produce the c-kit ligand needed for growth of stem cells.[18,19] Production of growth factors in the spleen is poorly defined, but the presence of appropriate cell types (lymphocytes, monocytes, fibroblasts, and stromal cells), and the occurrence of hematopoiesis in conditions of stress on the bone marrow make it clear that the spleen is capable of fulfilling this role. The normal bone marrow architecture seems to keep immature cells from circulating. The process of exiting from the marrow appears to require more active participation on the part of the cell than the spleen, and circulating nucleated erythroid elements and immature myeloid cells in addition to large platelets are characteristic of states in which splenic and other extramedullary sites of hematopoiesis are occurring. Reticulocytes mature in the spleen for 36 hours after leaving the bone marrow, and then reenter the circulation[8] (Table 46-1).

TABLE 46-1. Splenic Functions

CLEARANCE AND FILTRATION
Antibody-mediated clearance of blood cells, microorganisms, and other opsonized particles by macrophages
Culling and pitting of normal RBCs, trapping of abnormal RBCs by the reticular meshwork
IMMUNE FUNCTION
Marginal Zone
Promotes interaction of antigens with cells of monocytic and lymphocytic lines
Initiation of the immune response, processing of antigens
White Pulp
Periarteriolar lymphatic sheath (T cells): immune recognition
Lymphoid follicles (B cells): antibody production, immunoregulation
Red Pulp: Macrophages
Antigen processing, antigen preservation
Phagocytosis
HEMATOLOGIC FUNCTION
Hematopoiesis in utero, in severe hemolysis, in myeloid metaplasia, and transiently after bone marrow transplantation
Storage pool for erythrocytes, leukocytes, and platelets
HEMOSTATIC FUNCTION
Production of factor VIII and von Willebrand factor by endothelial cells

Culling and Pitting of Erythrocytes

The adult spleen receives about 2 L/min blood, or 5% of the cardiac output,[20] giving it an opportunity to view all circulating cells on a regular basis. The term *culling* is used to describe destruction of erythrocytes and may refer to either normal removal of aging erythrocytes or removal of damaged cells in pathologic conditions.[21] Other formed elements—leukocytes and platelets—are also culled from the blood by the spleen, especially when they are damaged. The spleen is probably not the normal site of destruction of most leukocytes and platelets, which adhere to vessel walls and migrate into tissues where they die and are removed.[22]

The removal of inclusions from within erythrocytes while releasing the cell back into the circulation is termed the *pitting* function. It is accomplished by passage of erythrocytes between or through the cordal macrophages, through the fenestrations of the basement membrane of the sinus, and then between the endothelial cells (Fig. 46-2). Cells that are poorly deformable are unable to enter the sinuses. The close apposition of the erythrocyte membrane with the macrophage membrane during this process enables the macrophage to identify aged or damaged membrane glycoproteins, or the presence of antibody or complement, and to phagocytize the cell. Cells that are poorly deformable (eg, spherocytes) may lyse in the process of passage into the sinus. Particulate matter within the erythrocyte is concentrated in the last part of the cell to pass through the sinusoidal wall, where it is removed by macrophages.[23] Among the particulate matter removed are Howell-Jolly bodies (remnants of nuclear material), Heinz bodies (denatured hemoglobin, usually adherent to the membrane), Pappenheimer bodies (iron-containing granules), and intraerythrocytic parasites, such as malarial organisms. Fragmentation of erythrocytes, with return of the rest of the red blood cell (RBC) to the circulating blood, is termed *erythroclasis*, and occurs in autoimmune hemolysis, the thalassemias, and RBC membrane disorders. These damaged fragments may be less deformable and may be removed on a subsequent passage through the spleen.

"Polishing" of the erythrocyte membrane also takes place in the spleen, with removal of excess membrane and "pocks" or "pits." These internal vesicles appear as if they are on the surface of the RBC using interference (Nomarski) optics[24,25] (Fig. 46-3). These pits are dramatically visible using scanning electron microscopy, but they are also visible when glutaraldehyde-fixed erythrocytes are examined under phase contrast microscopy. This simple examination is the easiest, cheapest, and least invasive approach to the identification of asplenia, and it is increasingly available in clinical laboratories. Less than 2% of the RBCs contain pits in individuals with normal splenic function.[26] Nearly half the erythrocytes of asplenic individuals may demonstrate pits. There is an inverse relationship between the pit count and the degree of splenic dysfunction or the amount of remaining splenic tissue.[27] Pits are removed with the protein-lipid components as the reticulocytes are polished by the spleen.[28] Other morphologic changes seen

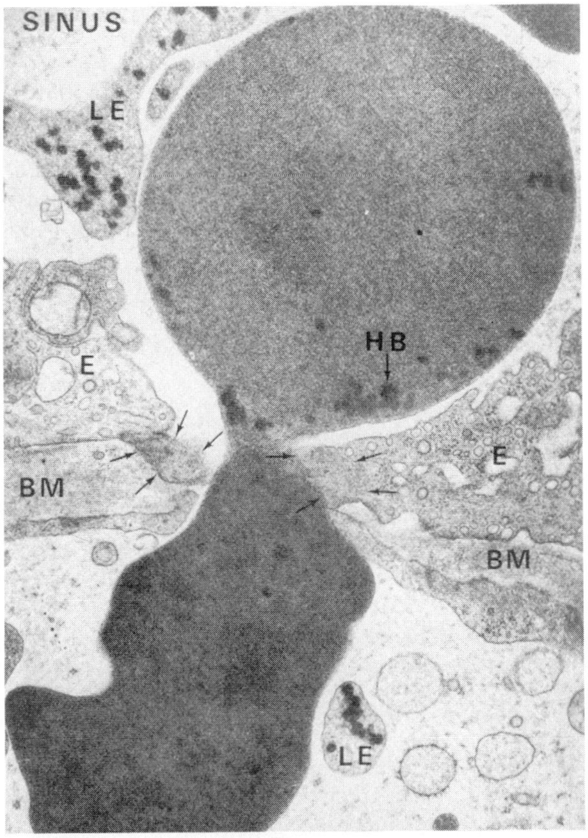

FIGURE 46-2. Heinz body (HB) being removed (culled) from an erythrocyte. BM, basement membrane; LE, hemolyzed erythrocyte fragments; E, sinus endothelial cell. (Chen LT, Weiss L. Role of the sinus wall in the passage of erythrocytes through the spleen. Blood 1973;41:529)

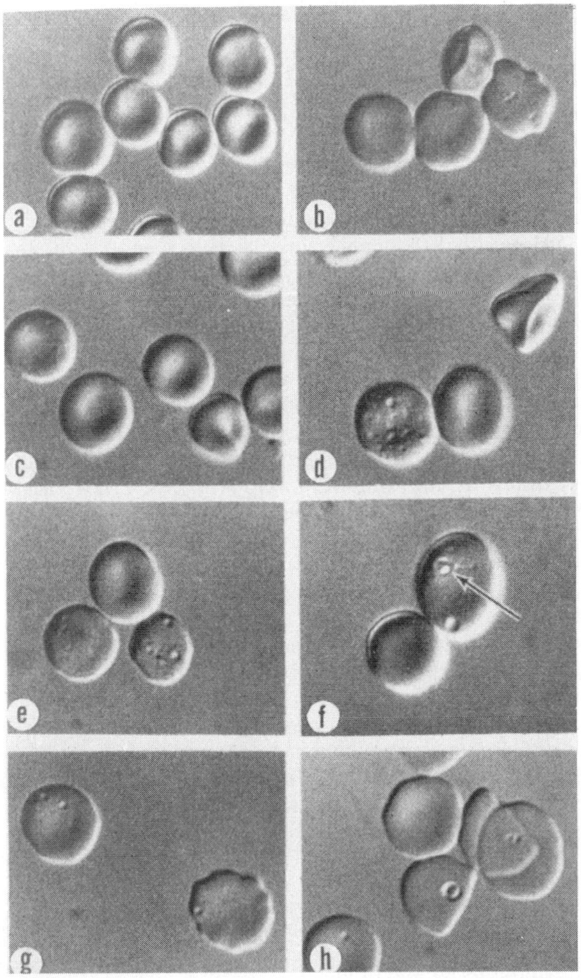

FIGURE 46-3. Pitted red blood cells. (Holroyde CP, Oski RA, Gardner FH. The "pocked" erythrocyte: red cell surface alterations in reticuloendothelial immaturity of the neonate. N Engl J Med 1969;281:516)

when the spleen is removed are increased numbers of target cells and acanthocytes.[29]

Senescence of Blood Cells

The blood in the pulp cords is concentrated and viscous, with a higher hematocrit than the blood in the splenic artery or vein. The environment is acidotic. Precise measurements within the red pulp are difficult to obtain without contamination by blood flowing more rapidly through the spleen. Best estimates indicate that pH within the red pulp ranges between 6.8 and 7.2. The oxygen tension appears to go as low as 54 mm Hg, and the glucose concentration is about 60% of that within the venous blood.[8,30] Normal erythrocytes tolerate such conditions, though glycolysis is probably impaired by acidosis and relative hypoglycemia. Normal reticulocytes are capable of oxidative phosphorylation and are imperiled by the hypoxic environment.[31] The importance of energy generation is demonstrated by pyruvate kinase deficiency, in which adenosine triphosphate generation from glucose is impaired. The spleen appears to be especially hostile to reticulocytes in protein kinase deficiency. Reticulocytes also have a less negative surface charge than mature erythrocytes and repel each other less.[28] They also are larger than mature erythrocytes and have excess membrane. Remodeling of erythrocytes and their removal from the circulation as they age are splenic contributions to erythrocyte maturation.

Host Defense

The white pulp of the spleen is the largest collection of lymphoid tissue in the body. The spleen is able to recognize and process antigens, produce lymphokines, activate T lymphocytes, and generate activated B cells to produce antibodies. Other lymphoid organs recognize and process antigens that enter locally; the spleen recognizes antigens in the blood stream and those administered systemically.[8,32–35]

The marginal zone, with abundant blood supply and large numbers of macrophages, appears to be most important in trapping and processing antigens.[36] After initial localization in the marginal zones, antigens penetrate the germinal center. T lymphocytes predominate in the periarterial lymphoid sheaths, while B lymphocytes predominate in the germinal centers and mantle zones.[37] The marginal-zone lymphocytes appear to be particularly adept at recognizing carbohydrate antigens, whose processing is markedly different from that of protein antigens.[38] Morphologic and metabolic (DNA synthesis) evidence of lymphocyte activation following administration of antigen occurs first in the periarterial lymphoid sheath and red pulp (T-cell areas), followed 3 to 4 days later by enlargement of the primary follicles and development of germinal centers (activation of B-lymphocyte areas).[39] These changes resolve over the month following removal of the antigenic stimulus. With reexposure to antigen (anamnestic response), the same sequence of events is repeated but greatly speeded up.

The key role of the spleen in defense against encapsulated organisms appears to derive from the marginal-zone lymphocytes (particularly important in recognizing the carbohydrate antigens found in bacterial capsules), and from the great sensitivity of splenic macrophages to small amounts of opsonin on the surface of particles. The spleen is particularly capable of recognizing and processing particulate antigens that the host has not previously encountered.[35,40] When an antigen is administered intravenously, an asplenic individual may fail to recognize it altogether.[40,41] Hepatic recognition of antigens is less efficient because of more-rapid transit of blood through the liver with less opportunity for macrophages to recognize and process the antigen.

The major impairment in antibody response following splenectomy is in IgM production.[42] Antigen-specific IgM antibody may not be made at all in an asplenic individual, even if IgG is produced.[41,42] The initial antibody response to an antigen is IgM, so the blunting of IgM production results in low levels of specific antibody early in an infectious process. Some splenectomized patients have low IgM levels,[43] but in immunologically normal adults, the total antibody levels are normal. Specific IgM production may still be impaired, however.[41]

Splenic macrophages phagocytize particles more effectively than hepatic macrophages when antibody is absent or present in low levels.[40,44–47] The receptors on the surface of splenic macrophages for the constant region of the immunoglobulin-G molecule (Fc receptors) appear to be able to bind to and recognize antibody more effectively than those in the liver.[48] This may be largely a function of longer exposure of opsonized particles to macrophages in the splenic sinusoids compared with the liver. When particles are well opsonized, with abundant surface IgG or C3b, they are removed with equal efficiency by the liver and spleen.[46,48]

Other Functions

Reservoir Function

The normal adult human spleen holds 20 to 40 mL of blood[49] and does not serve as a storage site for erythrocytes. Platelets and granulocytes are normally stored in the spleen, primarily in the red pulp. Up to one third of the total platelet mass is available for release into the systemic blood supply when factors that affect adhesiveness are released.[50] In some animals, the splenic capsule contains smooth muscle and is able to affect intravascular volume by relaxing and contracting, but this is not the case in humans.

In conditions associated with splenomegaly, the spleen does serve as a reservoir for all formed elements, including RBCs. Widening of the pulp cords creates an organ with greater volume, and secondary hypersplenism, or vascular pooling of cells within the cords and sinuses, occurs regardless of the underlying cause of the splenomegaly.[51] Thus, hypersplenism is a pathologic extension of the spleen's normal reservoir function. Because platelets and granulocytes are normally stored in the spleen, granulocytosis and thrombocytosis occur immediately after splenectomy. The increase in granulocyte and platelet counts partially resolves in the first 2 weeks after surgery, but the white blood cell and platelet counts are usually chronically elevated relative to normal values. In children, this is rarely a cause of difficulty. In children with polycythemia, however, and in adults with myeloproliferative disease, the thrombocytosis may lead to vascular complications, and antiplatelet agents may be needed.[29,52] Low-dose aspirin (80 mg/d) and dipyridamole are commonly used agents.

Response to Infection and Portal Hypertension

The increase in spleen size with pathologic conditions is associated with different microscopic findings, depending on the process used. With hemolysis or any destructive cytopenia, the major changes are in the red pulp and splenic sinusoids, with erythrophagocytosis or phagocytosis of leukocytes or platelets. The size of the spleen inversely correlates with the leukocyte and platelet counts[53] (Fig. 46-4). When the spleen is responding to infection, most of the increase in size is due to hyperplasia of the periarterial lymphoid tissue and germinal centers.[54] Regardless of the cause of splenomegaly, the increase in the blood flow to the spleen increases the portal venous pressure.[55,56] Portal hypertension may be mild, but it may increase with time and with the degree of splenomegaly. Both the incidence

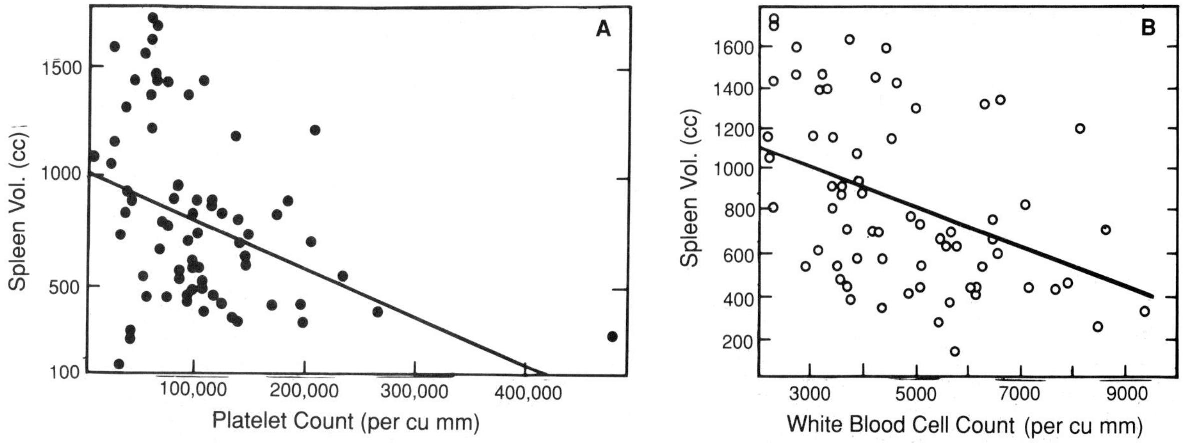

FIGURE 46-4. Correlation between spleen size and blood counts. (After El Khishen MA, Henderson JM, Millikan WJ, et al. Splenectomy is contraindicated for thrombocytopenia secondary to portal hypertension. Surg Gynecol Obstet 1985;160:233)

and the severity of hypersplenism in patients with portal hypertension depend on the underlying pathology. Portal hypertension may decrease intravascular volume, with secondary renin and aldosterone secretion followed by an increase in plasma volume.[57] These changes reverse following splenectomy when the portal hypertension is secondary to the splenomegaly.

Erythrokinetics

As the graveyard of normal and damaged erythrocytes, the spleen is the site of degradation of the contents of erythrocytes. Hemoglobin is broken down to bilirubin, which is released into the plasma, further metabolized in the liver, and excreted in bile and urine. The other major breakdown products that are handled by the spleen are membrane lipids and iron. Normally, the lipids in the membrane are also fully degraded and released into the plasma. In the lipid-storage diseases, absence of various degradative enzymes leads to accumulation of these membrane-lipid products, with engorgement of the macrophages and splenic enlargement.

Iron is also stored in the macrophages, as ferritin and hemosiderin.[58] In conditions of iron overload associated with hemolysis (eg, thalassemia major), splenic macrophages become engorged with iron. The bioavailability of iron stored in splenic macrophages is limited.[59] That transfused erythrocytes are the source of the iron in secondary hemochromatosis is demonstrated by the fact that the spleen, unlike the liver, does not store iron in primary hemochromatosis. As long as the spleen is in place, other organs that are affected by severe hemosiderosis (endocrine organs and the heart) appear to be somewhat protected.[60] In thalassemia, splenectomy for hypersplenism is usually performed late in the first decade or early in the second—about the time that iron overload is becoming clinically significant—and all subsequent iron absorption is directed to less expendable organs. In aplastic anemia and pure RBC aplasia in which iron is not reused, the presence of a normal spleen does not protect other organs from damage caused by iron.[61]

Developmental Changes in Splenic Function

Neonates have Howell-Jolly bodies in their erythrocytes and increased numbers of pocked erythrocytes, with a mean of 24% of erythrocytes pocked in the blood of term infants, and 47% in preterm infants[25] (Fig. 46-5). Some of the findings may be because of the high rate of erythrocyte production in the third trimester and because neonatal erythrocytes develop more membrane vesicles when incubated in vitro than do adult erythrocytes.[62] Nevertheless, the filtering function of the spleen is immature at birth.[63]

Both the Howell-Jolly bodies and the pocked erythrocytes disappear during the first few weeks of life (Fig. 46-6), and their persistence beyond a month in a term neonate should raise the suspicion of congenital hyposplenia or asplenia.[25] A consequence of normal maturation of splenic function is that neonates with isoimmune hemolytic disease who have a well-compensated hemolysis without anemia at

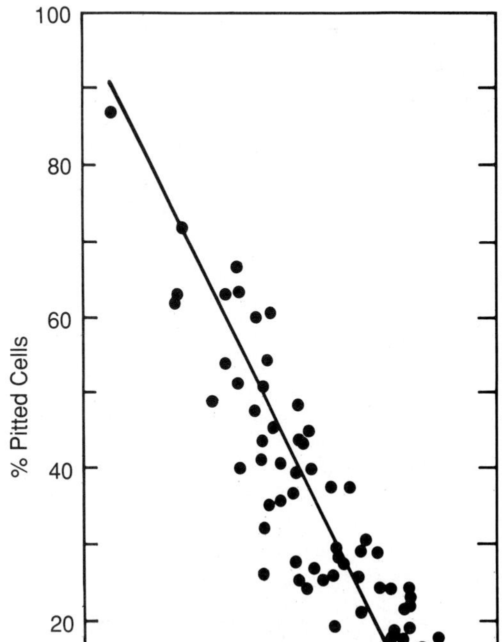

FIGURE 46-5. Graph of pit count versus birthweight. (After Holroyde CP, Oski RA, Gardner FH. The "pocked" erythrocyte: red cell surface alterations in reticuloendothelial immaturity of the neonate. N Engl J Med 1969;281:516)

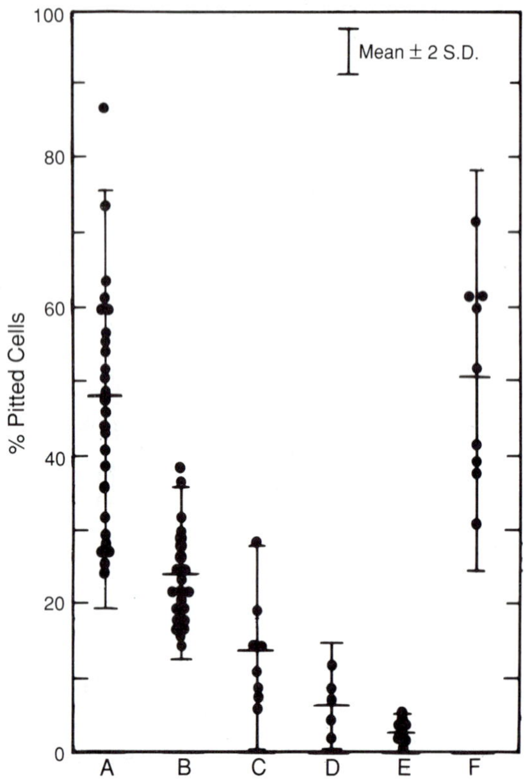

FIGURE 46-6. Disappearance of pitted cells relative to age. A, premature infants in first 24 hours; B, term infants in first 24 hours; C, term infants at 1 month; D, term infants at 2 months; E, adults; F, splenectomized adults. (After Holroyde CP, Oski RA, Gardner FH. The "pocked" erythrocyte: red cell surface alterations in reticuloendothelial immaturity of the neonate. N Engl J Med 1969;281:516)

birth may accelerate the rate of erythrocyte destruction as the spleen matures. Consequently, anemia may develop at a time when erythropoiesis has temporarily ceased.[64]

The relative impairment in the phagocytic function of the spleen of neonates may contribute to their immunoincompetence and susceptibility to infection, particularly with bacterial pathogens.[63] Macrophage dysfunction is also manifested by impaired processing of carbohydrate antigens,[65] a T-cell–independent function important in acquiring specific humoral immunity to many of the same particulate pathogens (encapsulated bacteria) phagocytosed by splenic macrophages.[67,68] Maturation of splenic phagocytic function is complete in term neonates by 2 months of age and slightly later in premature infants, as assessed by pit counts[25] (which may underestimate splenic function).[62] Development of the ability to process carbohydrate antigens occurs much later, progressing to adult norms by around 2 years.[69]

TESTS OF SPLENIC FUNCTION

Hematologic Changes in Asplenic Patients

Cell Numbers and Morphology

Absence of the spleen results in characteristic changes in the peripheral blood picture, some of which are used to diagnose asplenia, and the lack of which may indicate the existence of splenosis or accessory splenic tissue. Recognition of the hematologic impact of asplenia antedates the recognition of an infectious risk by two decades.[70,71] Changes are noted in erythrocyte morphology and in the numbers of leukocytes and platelets. Changes in erythrocytes are manifest by the presence of acanthocytes and target cells[72] on the Wright's stained smear, and of pocked erythrocytes when glutaraldehyde-fixed cells are examined in a microscope equipped with interference (Nomarski) optics.[25] Since the spleen removes senescent erythrocytes, the survival of erythrocytes is lengthened in asplenic conditions but only if the RBC survival was shorter than normal initially, as it is in many hemolytic anemias.[73] More dramatic than the changes in erythrocyte shape are the inclusions that are normally pitted from erythrocytes by the spleen. These include Howell-Jolly bodies, Heinz bodies, and Pappenheimer bodies.[74,75] Both leukocytes and platelets tend to pool in the spleen, and both are increased in number in asplenic patients compared with those with functional spleens.[76] The increase in leukocyte count is primarily of neutrophils without an increase in the numbers of immature cells.[29,77] The increase in platelet count may be dramatic immediately following splenectomy, especially if there was a shortened platelet survival that was compensated before splenectomy.[78–80]

Howell-Jolly Bodies

The most characteristic finding on the asplenic blood smear is the presence of Howell-Jolly bodies, which are dense, dark purple to black spheroidal inclusions (0.5 to 1.5 μm) that represent retained (incompletely extruded) nuclear material[29] (Fig. 46-7). Howell-Jolly bodies are visible and striking on routine peripheral blood smears with standard stains, and thus represent the simplest screening test for hyposplenism. Although Howell-Jolly bodies are fairly specific for hyposplenism, they are not seen unless splenic function is largely ablated[81] and may not be seen with lesser degrees of hyposplenism. Conversely, they may be seen with extensive hemolysis resulting in overload of splenic clearance of particles, indicating relative hyposplenia rather than anatomic or functional asplenia. The same is true for Pappenheimer bodies, which are siderotic granules that are normally removed by the spleen. Pappenheimer bodies tend to be particularly numerous in patients with hemolysis, particularly following splenectomy.[58]

Pitted Erythrocytes

Erythrocytes fixed in 0.5% to 1% buffered glutaraldehyde may be examined under interference optics for pocks or pits on their surface[24,25] (see Fig. 46-3). These pits are endocytic vesicles containing ferritin, hemoglobin, and remnants of mitochondria, which form spontaneously in erythrocytes.[21,23] They form in mature RBCs, and thus indicate ongoing membrane remodeling by the spleen.[82] Normally, less than 2% of erythrocytes have surface pits.[82] The number of cells that have pits is scored rather than the total number of pits. The number of pitted cells is inversely proportional to the degree of splenic function. The loss of splenic function with age in sickle cell disease has been examined using the pit count; this count reveals loss of splenic function earlier than radiologic methods.[83,84] In part, this may reflect the short RBC survival in sickle cell disease and the reticulocytosis that results in a higher proportion of the cells having pits to begin with; the total splenic burden is proportionately greater than when RBC survival is normal.[83]

Radionuclide Scans

In addition to assessing splenic size, a number of radionuclide scans provide information about splenic function. To assess the phagocytic function of the spleen, erythrocytes can be labeled with ^{51}Cr, ^{197}Hg, ^{81}Rb, or ^{99m}Tc and deliberately damaged with heat, antibody, or chemicals in vitro before reinfusion into the patient.[85] These manipu-

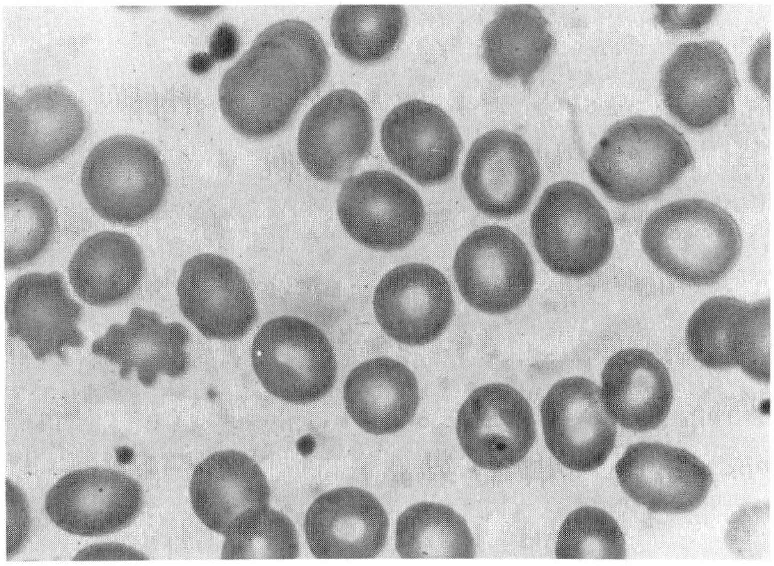

FIGURE 46-7. Postsplenectomy smear with acanthocytes and Howell-Jolly bodies.

lations ensure removal of the erythrocytes from the circulation by splenic macrophages, and the cytoplasmic radionuclide label permits external visualization.[86] These techniques have been supplanted by use of sulfur colloidal suspensions of radionuclides (eg, ^{99m}Tc) that are also sequestered in the spleen and are safer for patients. Other isotopes (eg, ^{198}Au and ^{113m}In) have also been used,[85] but they are not standard in most centers. A major use for these techniques is visualization of accessory or regenerated splenic tissue, particularly following splenectomy.[87]

To evaluate the extent to which particles or cells are sequestered in the spleen, reinfusion of the patient's own ^{111}In-labeled erythrocytes or platelets can be used to determine survival time.[88] Information is obtained about the in vivo survival of the cells and their relative extent of sequestration in liver and spleen. The half-life of platelet survival appears to predict response to splenectomy in immune thrombocytopenia (ITP).[89] The extent to which radioactivity accumulates in the spleen correlates poorly with the extent of prolongation of cell survival postsplenectomy in immunologically mediated processes. Because the liver is not a major site of cell destruction in many nonimmune cytopenias (eg, RBC membrane disorders), the spleen-to-liver accumulation is more meaningful in predicting response to splenectomy in these disorders.[89]

A third radionuclide imaging technique that may demonstrate splenic function is the use of ^{59}Fe to identify hematopoietic tissue. If the spleen is a site of extramedullary hematopoiesis, ^{59}Fe is concentrated in the spleen when ferrokinetic studies are performed. Often, these studies also demonstrate impaired hematopoiesis in the bone marrow.

Ultrasound

Ultrasonography is a noninvasive, readily available procedure for evaluation of splenic anatomy. Splenic size, shape, and several aspects of anatomy can be readily evaluated.[90] Cysts and abscesses are particularly readily identified. The technique is not sufficiently sensitive to exclude the presence of accessory spleens, which are frequently too small to be accurately identified.

Computed Tomographic Scanning

Computed tomography (CT) is the most useful imaging modality for evaluation of splenic pathology, since it elucidates both anatomy and certain aspects of function.[91] The visceral surface of the spleen is adjacent to the stomach, left kidney, tail of the pancreas, and splenic flexure of the colon. Thus, contrast media in the stomach, small bowel, and colon by oral administration may help identify splenic tissue when there is an external indentation on these organs. Intravenous administration of contrast is usually necessary to detect splenic lesions that are the same density as normal splenic parenchyma. The contrast is given as a bolus, but it is important not to scan during the arterial phase of the contrast administration. Inhomogeneous enhancement is often seen if scans are obtained in the first minute after the bolus is given, probably because of variable rates of blood flow in the red pulp.[92] Rapid scans may help distinguish accessory spleens from hilar lymph nodes (which do not enhance),[93] pancreatic tail masses, or vascular structures, however.[92] Without contrast medium, the spleen is slightly less dense than liver. With contrast enhancement, it fills just after the aorta. The liver has a delayed peak of contrast enhancement because of the later arrival of blood from the portal veins. Abscesses show rim enhancement and show up well on CT.[94]

The size of the spleen varies with the size of the patient and with age.[95] Children have relatively more splenic tissue than adults. Normal splenic volume in an adult is less than 175 mL.[96] With an electronic cursor, the volume of the spleen can be estimated by adding together areas of contiguous 1-cm slices on CT scans.[97] Accessory spleens have the same attenuation values and contrast enhancement as normal spleen, and are usually located in the gastrosplenic ligament near the hilum.[91,93]

Diffuse splenomegaly without evident abscess formation is seen with many viral infections (including Epstein-Barr virus, human immunodeficiency virus, and cytomegalovirus), parasitic infections (malaria, schistosomiasis), and some bacterial infections, including subacute bacterial endocarditis.[98] Most granulomatous diseases (including histoplasmosis tuberculosis) cause diffuse splenomegaly acutely, followed by calcified granulomata in a normal-size spleen, often noted incidentally.[99] Fungal infections also show focal lesions.[100] Leukemia, myeloproliferative disorders, histiocytosis X, and benign hematologic disorders (including hemolysis of any cause) produce diffuse splenomegaly.[101] The infarcted spleens of sickle cell disease are small and densely calcified.[102] Other inflammatory diseases (systemic lupus erythematosus, sarcoid, and rheumatoid arthritis) and storage diseases (Gaucher's, Niemann-Pick) also show diffuse splenomegaly.[103]

Congestive splenomegaly due to portal hypertension or splenic vein occlusion or thrombosis is associated with a nodular liver, ascites, gastroesophageal varices, and collateral veins. A dynamic scan, with rapid injection of contrast, may demonstrate an occluded splenic vein.[92]

Splenic trauma is extremely well visualized with CT.[104] Both subcapsular or intrasplenic hematomas and splenic laceration can be clearly identified. Subcapsular hematomas have a collection of low-density fluid in a crescent shape with a flattening of the surface.[104] Acutely (up to 4 hours), they are usually evident only with contrast enhancement, because the blood has the same density as the splenic tissue. As the hematoma organizes, it is evident without contrast administration and often keeps a crescent shape. This is then replaced with fluid of water density, which appears as a false cyst (ie, without epithelial lining) just below the capsule. Lacerations are more subtle. The splenic margins may be less clear, the parenchyma inhomogeneous, and lacerations may actually be evident. More commonly, a hematoma adjacent to the spleen or free blood or fluid in the left subphrenic space or in the peritoneal cavity is demonstrated on CT imaging. Contrast in the bowel is especially helpful to separate perisplenic blood or fluid from bowel.

Other focal abnormalities evident on CT scan include infarction, cysts, abscesses, and tumors. Infarction resulting from occlusion of a portion of the splenic artery is usually due to emboli (including tumor emboli) or to diseases of the arteries, such as atherosclerosis or polyarteritis.[102] It usually appears as a low-density, peripheral, wedge-shaped lesion without contrast enhancement. The rim of the infarcted region does enhance.[102]

Splenic cysts may be due to *Echinococcus granulosus*,[91] or they may be nonparasitic. Splenic hydatid cysts appear as well-defined, low-density masses with multiple septae and a thick, enhancing cyst wall. The CT findings are characteristic; with a suggestive history, serology, and eosinophilia, the diagnosis can be made before any invasive procedures are undertaken, since rupture poses the risk of hemorrhage and dissemination of infection. Nonparasitic cysts may be lined with epithelium (true cyst) or unlined (false cyst)—a differentiation that cannot be made on CT scan images. They are frequently not loculated, are thin-walled, and do not enhance with contrast. True cysts are developmental in origin. Unlined cysts represent previous splenic trauma with replacement of the hematoma by a cavity with serous fluid.[105] Cystic hemangiomas of the spleen may be multiple, and contain lymph.[106] Their attenuation is higher than other cystic lesions. Pancreatic pseudocysts may occur in or immediately adjacent or adherent to the spleen, usually in the context of pancreatitis. The fluid is high in amylase.[105]

Splenic abscesses produce focal cystic abnormalities on CT scan. Bacterial endocarditis, intravenous drug abuse, alcoholism, trauma, diabetes, sickle cell disease, and immunosuppression all predispose to splenic abscess formation. Systemic signs and symptoms suggestive of infection are usually present but may be absent, particularly in immunosuppressed or partially treated patients. Splenomegaly is more common than tenderness.[99,100] Blood cultures are frequently negative, necessitating percutaneous drainage or splenectomy.[93]

Malignancies involving the spleen may be focal on CT scan. Involvement with Hodgkin's disease may be evident on CT scan if the granulomas exceed 1 cm in diameter. For staging, CT does not exclude splenic involvement. Non-Hodgkin's lymphoma more often diffusely involves the spleen but may be nodular. Splenic enlargement and involvement with lymphoma may be more common in patients with acquired immunodeficiency syndrome. Metastatic disease is seen in the spleen, usually in the context of widespread metastasis to other organs, and rarely as the sole site of disease on CT scanning.[107,108]

CT-guided aspiration of cysts, drainage of hematomas and abscesses, and biopsies of lesions permit both diagnostic and therapeutic intervention in instances in which anatomic lesions are demonstrated. The availability of thin needles permits safe puncture of the splenic capsule as long as vascular structures have been excluded and portal hypertension is not present.

Magnetic Resonance Imaging

Magnetic resonance imaging (MRI) of the spleen may give better resolution than CT scanning but rarely displays abnormalities not evident on CT scanning. MRI is more expensive than CT scanning. It also is more difficult to image upper-abdominal contents, because there is motion artifact accompanying respiration and it takes longer to obtain the images with MRI. MRI complements CT scanning in imaging the spleen primarily for identification of vascular lesions that otherwise would require angiography.

STRUCTURAL DEFECTS

Accessory Spleens

Accessory spleens are noted in about one fourth of autopsies and may be single or multiple. They are identical to normal spleens anatomically and functionally but are usually small. They may be located at the splenic hilum, in the lienorenal and gastrosplenic ligaments, the jejeunal wall, the tail of the pancreas, mesentery and omentum. Their major importance is that they may hypertrophy following splenectomy for hematologic indications and may cause late (up to 25 years) relapse of a process for which splenectomy was performed.[109,110]

Splenic–Gonadal Fusion

During embryonic development, the spleen is close to the mesonephros. Occasionally, fusion of the spleen with the left gonad is noted.[111] Splenic–gonadal fusion occurs into the fifth to eighth week of intrauterine life, before the descent of the gonad and involution of the mesonephros. All cases have been described in males, since the condition may present with a nonpalpable testicle.[112] In the discontinuous variant of this anomaly, there is no physical connection between the spleen and the accessory splenic tissue associated with the gonad. In the continuous variant, fibrous connective tissue and ectopic splenic tissue link the spleen and gonad. Splenic tissue may be found in the scrotum, or the testicle may fail to descend into the scrotum. Associated hernias are found. All cases reported have been in males. If the process occurs in females, it appears to be clinically silent.

Asplenia–Polysplenia Syndrome

More serious congenital anomalies occur in association with major cardiovascular malformations. Asplenia is associated with severe cyanotic congenital heart disease and bilateral right-sidedness; polysplenia is associated with bilateral left-sidedness.[113] Asplenia is often accompanied by life-threatening cyanotic congenital heart lesions, including transposition of the great vessels, pulmonary artery atresia or stenosis, septal defects, anomalous venous drainage, and a single atrioventricular valve.[114] Typically, both lungs have 3 lobes, the liver is central, and the stomach is on the right side.[114] While the cardiovascular lesions are often fatal in early infancy, increased survival with better surgical management has resulted in survival of sufficient numbers of patients to permit clear identification of greatly increased risk of bacterial sepsis with a high mortality.[115] These patients have peripheral blood smears suggestive of asplenia. Imaging studies and autopsy demonstrate multiple small splenic nodules or no splenic tissue. In polysplenia, the splenic tissue is divided into two or more (up to nine described) masses.[116] Dextrocardia, bilateral superior venae cavae, septal defects, and anomalous pulmonary venous return are associated lesions. Both lungs tend to have two lobes, the liver is midline, and bowel malrotation is common.[117] These patients do not usually have evidence of hyposplenia on peripheral blood examination, and increased risk of infection has not been attributed to impaired splenic function.

Asplenia also may occur without heart disease, in which case it is less likely to be detected early in life than when it is associated with life-threatening lesions.[118] When it occurs with situs inversus, it represents a milder and later-occurring variant of the developmental processes of the syndromes described above. Less often, asplenia occurs without any other anatomic defect. In at least one case, isolated asplenia appears to have led to the death of an otherwise healthy adult from pneumococcal septicemia.[63] Some of these patients, like asplenic mice, may be found to have defects in the *Hox 11* gene.[2a]

Splenic Cysts

Splenic cysts are (1) parasitic (*Echinococcus granulosus*), (2) true cysts with epithelial lining, or (3) false cysts without such linings.[119]

Echinococcal (hydatid) cysts occur in patients with potential exposure, eosinophilia, and positive blood serology. The thick cyst wall is characteristic but not diagnostic, and there are usually multiple septate daughter cysts within the larger cyst, which are not seen with other types of cysts. *E granulosus* is endemic to the Mediterranean area, South America, Australia, and Alaska. Splenic involvement occurs in less than 4% of infected patients.[120] The fluid within the cyst is infected with organisms and is under pressure. The presence of daughter cysts and the serologic evidence of infection usually permit diagnosis of echinococcal cysts preoperatively. Total splenectomy is the treatment of choice and must be done with care to avoid spillage of the infectious contents within the abdomen, which may produce anaphylaxis. Surgery is easier if the cysts are drained and 1% formalin or 3% sodium chloride is used to kill the organisms. Mebendazole is used when spillage occurs or if cysts are present in other organs.

Nonparasitic true cysts (with an epithelial lining) develop as a consequence of several anomalies. The peritoneal mesothelium may infold after rupture of the splenic capsule, resulting in an intrasplenic cyst with mesothelial lining. Peritoneal mesothelial cells may be trapped in the sulci of the spleen, and these aggregates may form a cyst—again lined with mesothelium. Additionally, the lymphatics within the spleen may be dilated, creating lymphangiomata that are true cysts. Epidermoid and dermoid cysts are most common in young patients. Cystic lymphangiomas and true mesothelial cysts are often identified in older patients.[105,121,122] They tend to increase in size with time, and present with pressure, rupture, or secondary infection.[123] They are generally asymptomatic until enlarged. The treatment of choice is partial splenectomy, which can be performed by enucleating the cyst along a plane external to it, and achieving hemostasis in the residual splenic tissue.[124]

Non–epithelial-lined cysts, termed *false cysts* or *pseudocysts*, are generally posttraumatic in origin. Resolution of subcapsular or intraparenchymal hematomas results in a cavity with a thin, fibrous wall. The serous fluid replaces the earlier hematoma. The rim may be calcified. Pseudocysts do not tend to enlarge with time to the extent that true cysts do, since they lack an epithelial lining.[125] When they need surgery, splenic conservation or CT-guided aspiration usually can be performed. It is likely that these cysts will increase in frequency with the increasing use of splenic conservation for trauma and be more commonly diagnosed with more sensitive, noninvasive diagnostic techniques such as ultrasound and CT. With a previous history of trauma, their nature should be evident. Unless they pose a diagnostic dilemma or cause symptoms, no treatment is necessary.[124]

Splenic cysts may become large and may hemorrhage or lead to splenic rupture. When this is the case, splenectomy may be necessary to prevent rupture. Increasingly, as a consequence of spleen-preservation techniques developed for management of acute trauma, subtotal splenectomy with preservation of normal splenic tissue may be feasible, and is desirable when possible.[124]

Pancreatic pseudocysts may be adjacent to or actually extend into the spleen. These occasionally are loculated. Since pancreatic pseudocysts occur in the setting of acute or chronic pancreatitis, and the adjacent pancreas is inflamed, it is usually evident that this is the diagnosis. If questions remain, aspiration of the cyst yields fluid with a high amylase content,[126] which confirms the diagnosis. Specific treatment is not needed for the splenic cyst when it represents a pancreatic pseudocyst.

Splenic Tumors

Benign Tumors

Benign splenic hamartomas, cavernous hemangiomata, and adenomas are histologically similar to each other and to normal splenic tissue. These consist of large, thin-walled vascular spaces lined with endothelium, interspersed with normal pulp tissue.[127] Multiple benign tumors have been described at autopsy in the spleen.[128] These include dermoids, fibromata, leiomyomata, osteomata, chondromata, and lipomas. Because these rarely cause clinical problems, they appear not to require intervention.

Angiosarcoma

Splenic angiosarcoma is virtually the only primary malignant tumor seen in the spleen other than lymphoma. Angiosarcoma of the spleen has a high rate of metastasis to the liver (about 70%), and one third of patients experience spontaneous splenic rupture. Both hepatic and splenic angiosarcoma are associated with previous administration of the contrast medium, Thoratrast.[107]

Lymphomas

Lymphomas are the most common malignant tumors involving the spleen.[129] As detailed in the section on computed tomography of the spleen, imaging is unreliable in determining splenic involvement with lymphoma. Hodgkin's disease frequently involves the spleen with macroscopically visible nodules that are 1 cm or less in diameter, and thus tend not to be evident on CT scan. Additionally, granulomatous lesions that are not Hodgkin's disease (including tuberculosis, histoplasmosis, sarcoid and lymphatoid granulomatosis) may involve both the liver and spleen, so the presence of nodules in the spleen does not confirm Hodgkin's disease. The frequency of splenic involvement varies with the histologic subtype and is more common in mixed cellularity, nodular sclerosing, and lymphocyte depleted than in lymphocyte-predominant Hodgkin's disease. Staging laparotomy is commonly performed because there is about 25% discordance between clinical and pathologic staging, much of which is due to findings in the spleen at splenectomy. The spleen may be involved without being enlarged, and may be enlarged without being involved with Hodgkin's disease.

Non-Hodgkin's lymphomas may be primary in the spleen. They may have any histology or may be a manifestation of more widespread disease. In young patients, non-Hodgkin's lymphoma is virtually never truly a localized disease, and systemic therapy is needed regardless of histology or staging. In older patients, disease truly limited to the spleen, especially of low-grade histology, may be treated with splenectomy alone.[130,131] Non-Hodgkin's lymphomas are more commonly associated with diffuse splenomegaly, although this varies with histologic type. Splenic involvement is usually an indication of disseminated disease, although this is not always the case. Splenomegaly is common in all the leukemias, but the closest relation between disease activity and splenic function is seen in hairy cell leukemia.[132] Splenomegaly is a constant in hairy cell leukemia, and splenectomy remains frontline therapy for this disease. The pancytopenia accompanying hairy-cell leukemia usually improves if the marrow cellularity is less than 85%, and systemic therapy can often be delayed in these patients. Survival is unaffected, but clinical manifestations improve with splenectomy.[133]

Metastatic Tumors

Metastatic lesions involving the spleen develop as a consequence of the filtering function of the spleen for blood-borne contaminants. Unlike the lung (another filter organ), the spleen is rarely an isolated site of metastatic disease. Splenic metastasis occurs in the setting of widespread metastatic disease in other organs. Metastatic breast carcinoma may cause splenomegaly, which develops largely in response to splenic infarction from tumor clumps in the splenic arterial supply, with infarction and reactive splenomegaly.[134] Other metastatic tumors may also cause infarction. The tumors most likely to involve the spleen include melanoma, choriocarcinoma, seminoma, lung, pancreas, stomach, colon, breast, and neuroblastoma.[108,135–137]

FUNCTIONAL HYPOSPLENIA

Functional hyposplenia refers primarily to the phagocytic function of the spleen. It is defined by lack of uptake of heat-damaged labeled erythrocytes, sulfur colloid–^{99m}Tc, or other radionuclide imaging materials, and evidence of impaired remodeling of erythrocytes (increased numbers of pocked erythrocytes, Howell-Jolly bodies). In general, this appears to correlate well with macrophage processing of antigens, especially carbohydrate antigens and intravenously administered antigens such as sheep erythrocytes.[81,138] Actual atrophy of the spleen is less common than evidence of hypofunction without any change in the size of the spleen. Atrophy is seen in Fanconi's anemia,[139] after administration of Thoratrast[140] (also associated with development of angiosarcoma),[141] following irradiation therapy,[142,143] with infarction in sickle cell disease,[84] and accompanying a number of inflammatory disorders[144–147] (Table 46-2).

TABLE 46-2. Causes of Hyposplenism

HEMATOLOGIC
Sickle cell disease and variants
Lymphoma (Hodgkin's, non-Hodgkin's)
Fanconi's anemia
IMMUNOLOGIC
Systemic lupus erythematosus
Rheumatoid arthritis
Thyroiditis
Chronic active hepatitis
Sjögren's syndrome
Mixed connective tissue disease
Graft-versus-host disease
Ulcerative colitis
Crohn's disease
Celiac disease
Tropical sprue
Intestinal lymphangiectasia
ANATOMIC
Congenital absence or hypoplasia
Sarcoidosis
Amyloidosis
Occlusion of splenic artery or vein
Celiac artery thrombosis
Irradiation
Hemangiosarcoma

Sickle Cell Disease

Splenic Infarction

The spleen is a particularly hostile environment for sickle cells, which respond poorly to hypoxia, acidosis, and hypoglycemia. Sickle hemoglobin crystallizes when deoxygenated, and the poorly deformable cells then adhere to and block the small blood vessels in which they are circulating. Infarction of multiple organs is a major manifestation of the disease. Because the environment of the spleen predisposes to sickling, damage to the splenic vasculature is one of the earliest permanent consequences of sickle cell disease. The other major organ affected by these events in early childhood is the renal medulla, and both the concentrating ability of the kidney and the phagocytic function of the spleen can be restored by transfusion in young children with sickle cell disease (under about 2 years of age).[148] With time, however, the damage becomes permanent, and transfusion fails to restore the organs to health. By 6 to 8 years of age, the spleen is reduced to a fibrotic nubbin by repeated infarction, a process termed *autosplenectomy*.

The time course of splenic infarction and the development of hyposplenia in sickle cell disease are assessed with liver-spleen scans and by counting pocked erythrocytes.[49] Since a count of greater than 2% pocked erythrocytes correlates well with failure to visualize the spleen by ^{99m}Tc scanning,[84,148] this less-invasive and less-expensive test is used to screen for hyposplenia. In homozygous sickle cell disease and Sβ^0-thalassemia, hyposplenia is demonstrable in virtually all children by the time of their first birthdays[84] (Fig. 46-8). In patients with hemoglobin SC and Sβ^+-thalassemia, hyposplenia develops considerably later. The best predictor of hyposplenia is the level of fetal hemoglobin production.[149,150] With over 15% to 20% fetal hemoglobin, splenic function is preserved. This is predicted from observations of sickle cell patients in the eastern province of Saudi Arabia who retain fetal hemoglobin levels of above 20% and do not infarct their spleens.[151]

Patients with hemoglobin SC and sickle β^+-thalassemia often have persistent splenomegaly with evidence of impaired phagocytic function, despite the enlarged size.[152] It is important that those caring for such patients recognize that they are in fact hyposplenic[150] and therefore suscep-

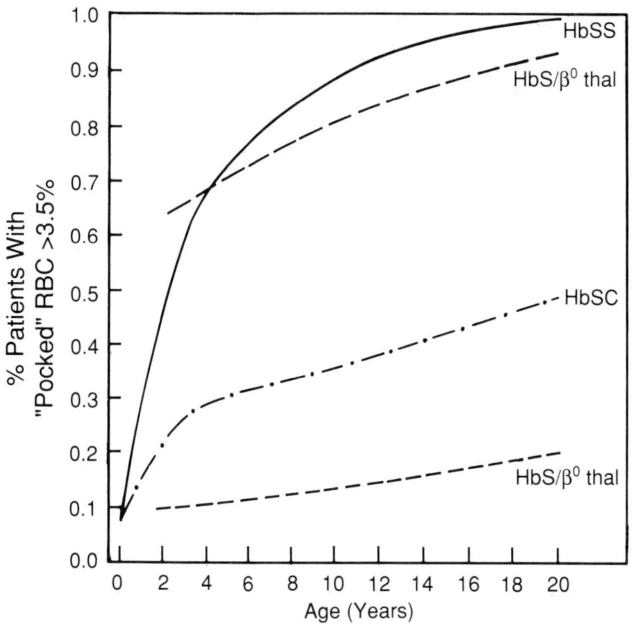

FIGURE 46-8. Development of asplenia in sickle syndrome. (After Pearson HA, Gallagher D, Chilcote R, et al. Developmental pattern of splenic dysfunction in sickle cell disorders. Pediatrics 1985;76:392)

tible to infection with encapsulated organisms, although the frequency of such events is less than for patients with SS or Sβ^0-thalassemia.[148]

The poor function of the spleen in sickle cell disease is reversible with transfusion in young children.[148] Neither the amount of blood needed to reverse the hypofunction nor the length of this reversibility is entirely clear. In general, sickling manifestations persist as long as hemoglobin S is the predominant hemoglobin; it is probable that transfusion to at least 50% hemoglobin A is needed to significantly affect sickling in the spleen as well. By 6 years of age, transfusion fails to restore splenic function.

The splenic infarction that leads to hyposplenia occurs primarily in the sinusoids. In sickling disorders, most of the infarction occurs in the capillaries and venules (where hemoglobin S is deoxygenated and sickled) rather than in the arterioles (where oxyhemoglobin S is in solution within the erythrocyte).

Splenic Sequestration Crisis

When sickling occurs in the venules and extends into the larger veins of the spleen, the immediate consequence is not infarction but obstruction of venous outflow. With unimpeded arterial blood supply and a distensible capsule, the spleen is capable of enlarging massively, and a significant portion of the systemic blood supply may pool within the spleen. This is termed a *splenic sequestration crisis*.[153,154] Similar events may occur within the liver but are rarely life-threatening, because the hepatic capsule is not as distensible. This is an event of early childhood, rarely occurring after 4 years of age, and may be fatal as a result of acute hypovolemia and severe anemia, with impaired perfusion, shock and acidosis.[155] Since acute splenic sequestration tends to recur and may be fatal, splenectomy is frequently recommended.[155]

Immunologic–Autoimmune Diseases

Hyposplenia occurs in a number of inflammatory and autoimmune disorders. In many instances, the function of the Fc receptors is impaired, with poor clearance of particles opsonized with IgG antibodies.[156] This common theme is demonstrated in systemic lupus erythematosus,[156] rheumatoid arthritis,[157] sarcoidosis,[147] systemic vasculitis,[157] ulcerative colitis,[81] amyloidosis,[158] and celiac disease, or sprue.[159,160]

Hyposplenia is an occasional feature of a variety of other diseases, including dermatitis herpetiformis,[161] sarcoidosis,[147] systemic mastocytosis,[144] thyrotoxicosis,[146] Fanconi's anemia,[139] splenic angiosarcoma[140] and graft-versus-host disease.[145] In the late stages of acquired immunodeficiency syndrome, atrophy of lymphoid follicles and severe depletion of all T-cell–dependent areas is seen.[162] Phagocytic function has not been specifically evaluated, but splenomegaly is common in acquired immunodeficiency syndrome and there is no suggestion of failure of macrophage function.[163] In many of the conditions mentioned, immunosuppressive therapy is administered, and patients are immunologically compromised for a variety of primary and secondary reasons. The fact that specific antibody production may be impaired adds to the risk of Fc receptor dysfunction. From the standpoint of patient management, rapid intervention to detect and treat infection with encapsulated organisms and gram-negative organisms that afflict hyposplenic patients may be life-saving. Immunization is rarely effective because of the underlying immunosuppression, but antibiotic administration with amoxicillin or equivalent coverage is recommended for febrile patients. The need for hospitalization and parenteral administration of antibiotics depends on the severity of the underlying process and concurrent immunosuppression.

Iatrogenic Splenic Dysfunction

Corticosteroids

Acquired splenic dysfunction accompanies several therapeutic maneuvers, especially treatment with systemic corticosteroids and irradiation therapy that affects the spleen. Corticosteroids decrease the affinity of the Fc receptors on splenic macrophages for the Fc fragment and may actually decrease the numbers of receptors on the macrophages themselves.[164] In addition, the phagocytic function of neutrophils and monocytes is diminished by corticosteroid treatment because of diminished surface adherence. This is also usually the cause of the acute effect of corticosteroid therapy on many processes mediated by humoral antibodies. The steroid-induced increase in the platelet count in ITP or the rise in hemoglobin in autoimmune hemolysis is due to diminished splenic clearance of opsonized particles.[165] The effect on hepatic macrophage function is much less marked than on splenic macrophages. Diminished antibody production is a later effect of steroid treatment but also affects the spleen, where antibody production takes place.[166]

Immunoglobulin-G

Blockade of Fc receptors in the liver and spleen is thought to be a major mechanism of action of high-dose intravenously administered immunoglobulin-G given for immune cytopenias, especially ITP.[167,168] This effect is transient and reversible within several weeks of administration, and therapy needs to be repeated to maintain Fc receptor blockade. The same mechanism is attributed to use of intravenous anti-D antibody in Rh-positive patients with ITP.[169,170]

Irradiation Therapy

Irradiation therapy to the spleen affects functions differently depending on the total dose administered. Lymphocytes are extremely sensitive to irradiation therapy, but the extent to which irradiation ablates lymphocyte function depends in part on the cell type and the extent to which the cell is activated. Less than 500 cGy ablates much B-cell function.[171] Exposure to 3000 cGy eliminates over 95% of T-lymphocyte thymidine incorporation.[171] Because blastogenesis and proliferation are an integral part of specific lymphocyte responses, low doses to areas that include the spleen impair lymphocyte function. These changes are transient, since circulating blood lymphocytes originating in the bone marrow, thymus, and lymph nodes repopulate the spleen within a matter of weeks, and no pathologic changes are noted years after 600 to 800 cGy of irradiation exposure.[172] In contrast, macrophages are much more tolerant of irradiation exposure than lymphocytes, and the phagocytic function of the spleen is rarely affected by doses below 2000 cGy. It is, however, ablated at high doses, and functional hyposplenia (ie, phagocytic dysfunction) can be expected with the doses of irradiation (4000 cGy) given for Hodgkin's disease.[142,143] Thus, a child receiving 1080 cGy to the left renal bed for Wilms' tumor may lose some lymphocyte function but is not likely to have increased susceptibility to bacterial infection on the basis of poor clearance of particles by the spleen. The anatomic changes with higher-dose irradiation are similar to those seen with infarction of the spleen for any reason, and susceptibility to bacterial infection is well known.[173]

SPLENECTOMY AND RELATED PROCEDURES

Indications

Some indications for splenectomy are listed in Table 46-3. None of these indications is absolute. In each instance, the relative risks and benefits must be weighed to make a rational decision.

In hemolytic disorders, splenectomy is indicated if the patient has significant compromise related to anemia (poor physical growth, inadequate stamina), requires repeated

TABLE 46-3. Indications for Splenectomy

CHRONIC HEMOLYTIC ANEMIAS
Diseases that respond reliably to splenectomy
Hereditary spherocytosis
Hereditary elliptocytosis or pyropoikilocytosis
Hereditary stomatocytosis
Diseases that respond variably to splenectomy when a partial response would be clinically significant
Autoimmune hemolytic anemia
Glycolytic defects
Unstable hemoglobinopathies
Congenital erythropoietic porphyria
Thalassemia intermedia
Thalassemia with increasing transfusion requirement due to hypersplenism
Hb S syndromes with recurrent splenic sequestration crises
CHRONIC THROMBOCYTOPENIAS
Idiopathic thrombocytopenic purpura
Human immunodeficiency virus infection with refractory thrombocytopenia
Thrombotic thrombocytopenic purpura refractory to plasma therapy
Wiskott-Aldrich syndrome (occasionally)
CHRONIC NEUTROPENIAS
Rheumatoid arthritis (Felty's syndrome) and recurrent infections (occasionally)
PRIMARY SPLENIC MALIGNANCIES
Splenic lymphoma
Angiosarcoma
SEVERE HYPERSPLENISM (SEVERE CYTOPENIAS) OR OTHER SYMPTOMS OF MARKED SPLENOMEGALY (PRESSURE SYMPTOMS, SPLENIC INFARCTION)
Lymphoproliferative diseases
Hairy cell leukemia (leukemic reticuloendotheliosis)
Chronic lymphocytic leukemia
Myeloproliferative diseases (without significant splenic hematopoiesis)
Myeloid metaplasia
Spent polycythemia vera (occasionally)
Congestive splenomegaly
Cirrhosis
Portal, splenic, or hepatic vein thrombosis
Storage diseases (especially Gaucher's disease)
Renal disease on chronic hemodialysis (occasionally)
SURGICAL INDICATIONS
Staging for Hodgkin's disease
Splenic cysts, including echinococcal cysts
Ruptured spleen that cannot be repaired
En bloc resection for certain carcinomas
Splenorenal shunt
DIAGNOSTIC SPLENECTOMY

exposure to blood products, demonstrates impaired function and energy sufficient to interfere with normal activities, or requires medications that have significant side effects. These indications apply only if the disorder can be expected to improve, or if the medication (such as corticosteroids) can be discontinued or decreased to significantly less toxic doses following splenectomy. Newer approaches to gallstones and better recognition that such stones are frequently silent and cause no symptoms make prevention of gallstones a poor sole indicator for splenectomy in hemolytic anemia. When splenectomy is needed, it is worthwhile to delay it until the patient has reached at least the age of 2 years. Doing so allows maturation of lymphoid immunity to a degree sufficient to minimize the risks of postsplenectomy septicemia and increases the probability of a good response to active immunization measures.

Young children with sickle cell disease are susceptible to acute splenic sequestration crises in which the venous drainage of the spleen is occluded by sickled cells, and the arterial supply is patent. The result is rapid distention of the spleen with pooling of a substantial portion of the total blood volume. This complication is accompanied by a high mortality rate unless rapid intervention with either transfusion, splenectomy, or both occurs.[153,154] Exchange transfusion is usually successful in reversing the venous occlusion, but the relapse rate is high, and acute splenic sequestration is usually considered an indication for splenectomy.[154] Since this is a process primarily seen in very young children, chronic transfusion to delay splenectomy until the child is 2 years of age is commonly undertaken. This permits the lymphoid function of the spleen to mature, and may lessen the risk of postsplenectomy sepsis. Prophylactic antibiotics are imperative in these children.

In ITP, splenectomy depends heavily on the age of the patient and whether the thrombocytopenia is acute or chronic. In children, most acute ITP resolves without requiring splenectomy or long-term steroid therapy. In adults and older children with chronic ITP, spontaneous resolution is uncommon, and splenectomy may be indicated early in the course of the illness. In both instances, it is important to use clinical rather than laboratory indications for splenectomy to prevent potentially hazardous surgery that improves the patient on paper but does not result in better function.

Splenectomy should be undertaken with extreme caution in patients with underlying immunologic impairment (eg, Wiskott-Aldrich syndrome and acquired immunodeficiency syndrome), since the loss of lymphocyte and macrophage mass may further compromise an already tenuous balance between host and pathogens.[174,175] With antibiotic prophylaxis, this may be manageable if the indications are strong. Autoantibodies may cause splenic destruction of platelets and worsen the primary thrombocytopenia in Wiskott-Aldrich syndrome. In these instances, the platelet count may improve with splenectomy.

Thrombotic thrombocytopenic purpura that is relapsing and recurrent has been successfully treated with splenectomy. The mechanism of benefit is unclear but appears to relate to abnormal platelet aggregation and von Willebrand multimers.[176] It is difficult to predict those patients who are likely to improve.

Splenectomy is indicated in hypersplenism when hypersplenism is the principal cause of thrombocytopenia, neutropenia, anemia, or increased transfusions. Splenomegaly may cause substantial local symptoms (especially in portal hypertension and cirrhosis where the spleen presses on the stomach), including impaired growth and nutrition. Clinical problems, such as infection or bleeding, rather than laboratory abnormalities should be used in determining whether splenectomy is needed in portal hypertension.

In Gaucher's disease, the spleen protects the bones against accumulation of material that causes thinning of the cortex, and splenectomy may be followed by increased orthopedic problems and hepatomegaly.[177] Timing of splenectomy should be carefully balanced so that the consequences of hypersplenism are sufficiently great to justify this additional risk. Specific benefits (improved blood counts or nutrition) should be anticipated from splenectomy, which should be done after the teen years if possible.

In thalassemia and other disorders in which patients are transfusion dependent, the spleen may absorb a considerable amount of iron that will be stored in other, less expendable organs such as the liver and heart. Again, documentation that the transfusion requirement is increased sufficiently to warrant this possible risk is imperative before splenectomy is performed.

Splenectomy is performed to ameliorate the pancytopenia of hairy cell leukemia. Some patients with enlarged spleens are not cytopenic, and some fail to respond to splenectomy, which should be done for clinical rather than laboratory indications.[133] This remains a useful modality despite availability of systemic therapies for this disease.

In addition to staging of Hodgkin's disease, splenectomy may be useful for treatment if the spleen is massively enlarged. Irradiating a large spleen subjects the stomach and the left kidney to doses of irradiation that are poorly tolerated by those organs, both acutely and in the long term. Thus, splenectomy with irradiation only to the splenic pedicle may be a less damaging approach to massive involvement of the spleen in Hodgkin's disease. The indications for staging laparotomy with splenectomy have changed during the past 20 years as therapies changed. The late effects of 4000 cGy of total nodal irradiation are significant, and systemic chemotherapy is being used in a greater number of patients with lower-stage disease, particularly children.

Occasionally, it is necessary to do a splenectomy to make a diagnosis.[178] Under no circumstances should a splenectomy be undertaken for diagnostic purposes without confirmation that the bone marrow is not fibrotic. Conditions associated with myelofibrosis may result in myeloid metaplasia, with hematopoiesis occurring in the spleen. This is perhaps the single true contraindication to splenectomy,[179,180] since splenectomy performed under these circumstances leaves a patient without adequate resources for hematopoiesis, and may be followed by aplasia. The risks of the splenectomy itself must be acceptable if the procedure is to be performed.

Techniques of Splenectomy

Partial Splenectomy

Surgical procedures have become more sophisticated in recent years because of improvements in surgical techniques motivated by an appreciation that splenectomy leaves patients at risk for serious medical complications in later years. The intrasplenic surgical arterial anatomy is well enough defined[181,182] to permit subtotal splenectomy in instances where total splenectomy is not desirable. Hemostatic techniques have been developed for partial excision, including mattress sutures, wedge resection with sutures, cyanoacrylate adhesives, and microfibrillar collagen omental packs.[183] Hilar artery ligation minimizes blood loss. By approaching the spleen through the intersegmental planes, partial excision with lesser degrees of blood loss can be planned. These techniques are appropriate for elective partial resection (eg, for removal of cysts[184] or tumors), for Gaucher's disease,[185,186] for some studies on patients with Hodgkin's disease, and for splenic preservation following traumatic rupture.[183,187–189]

Partial splenectomy leaves an obvious risk of regeneration of splenic tissue and is not generally indicated when the spleen is causing cell destruction. It is potentially desirable for removal of cysts or other localized anatomic structures, and for staging for Hodgkin's disease. The lack of homogeneous involvement of the spleen in Hodgkin's disease has relegated this procedure to a minor or investigational role, as failure to identify disease of clinical significance is clearly possible with partial splenectomy. Partial splenectomy, splenic repair, and nonoperative management have become prominent in the management of splenic trauma, and permit the salvage of more than half of ruptured spleens.[183] Improvements in nonoperative diagnosis (CT scan and ultrasound) and a greater appreciation of the risks of postsplenectomy sepsis contribute substantially to the development of conservative management plans.[189]

Total Splenectomy

Massive splenomegaly presents some challenges to the surgeon, since the risk of intraoperative splenic rupture is significantly greater than when the spleen is moderately enlarged.[190,191] A sufficiently large incision to permit full visualization and mobilization is imperative.[192–194] A flank incision may permit identification of the vessels at the splenic hilum, through which the splenic artery may be ligated, but removal of a massively enlarged spleen is rarely possible through such an approach.

When splenectomy is performed for hematologic indications to reduce the rate of destruction of formed elements of the blood, a thorough search for accessory spleens must be performed. Since most accessory spleens are located at the splenic hilum, gastrosplenic ligament, and tail of the pancreas,[110] most are readily identified at the time of splenectomy. They may be found at any place in the peritoneal cavity,[195] however, and may later hypertrophy to resume destruction of formed elements, even years later. Thus, late relapse after splenectomy for ITP, autoimmune hemolytic anemia, hereditary spherocytosis, or pyruvate kinase deficiency should raise the question of whether an accessory spleen has hypertrophied and is causing destruction of cells.

Preliminary ligation of the splenic artery should be performed in the lesser sac before the spleen is mobilized to permit control of the major blood supply to the spleen. Accessory spleens should be sought at the beginning of the dissection and again after the spleen is mobilized. The lateral peritoneal attachments must be incised, followed by the gastrosplenic and splenocolic ligaments. The lower pole of the spleen is raised by division of the gastroepiploic vessels, and the upper by division of the short gastric vessels. This leaves the spleen attached at the hilum and the tail of the pancreas. Dissection of the splenic artery and vein must be done with special attention to protection of the tail of the pancreas, which may extend into the splenic hilum. The artery should be ligated before the vein so that blood is not sequestered in the spleen. An inflamed or massively enlarged spleen may be particularly difficult to free because of dense adhesions to the pancreas or diaphragm.

Surgical complications of splenectomy include splenic rupture with bleeding, postoperative atelectasis (especially in the lower lobes), and subphrenic abscess.[194,196] When splenectomy is performed for causes associated with serious systemic disease (especially portal hypertension), operative and postoperative complications, including bleeding, are more likely to develop. Postoperative splenic vein thrombosis with bleeding varices is an occasional complication.[197] In patients without underlying disease, splenectomy is extremely well tolerated and has been performed without significant bleeding in many patients with thrombocytopenia.[196]

Splenic Embolization

Splenic embolization is used to diminish splenic blood flow in patients with portal hypertension.[198–201] This can be done in patients whose condition makes surgery risky. The procedure may raise the platelet count for a period of months.[202,203] Because collateral blood vessels tend to develop readily, responses may not be sustained.[204] Embolization appears to be of greatest use in patients whose surgical risks and anticipated survival times make a less-invasive approach desirable.[205–207]

Splenic Autotransplantation

Autotransplantation, or deliberate introduction of splenic tissue into the peritoneal cavity with the intention of inducing splenosis is performed in an attempt to minimize the risk of postsplenectomy septicemia in patients for whom residual splenic tissue is not a problem. This is done primarily during splenectomy for trauma or removal of cysts.[208] Animal studies show improved clearance of bacterial inocula following autotransplantation.[209,210] It is unclear if this benefit translates to improvement in host defenses in humans. An apparent difficulty with autotransplantation is the restoration of the arterial blood supply to the splenic remnant.[211] Random regeneration in the peritoneum appears not to restore the blood supply to the autotransplanted splenic tissue as does growth of splenic tissue in the gastrosplenic ligament.

SPLENOSIS

Splenosis is the regrowth of splenic tissue following splenic rupture.[212] This may occur during the traumatic rupture that occasioned splenectomy,[213] or when intraoperative rupture of the spleen occurs. Splenosis may occur throughout the peritoneal cavity, on the pleural and pericardial surfaces, and in skin scars.[212] Usually, they range from 1 to 7 cm in diameter.[208] The splenic function of these regenerated remnants is sufficient to be visualized on radionuclide scans, and they remodel erythrocyte membranes sufficiently to normalize the pit count in some patients.[214] Because the risk of postsplenectomy septicemia is already low in patients who undergo splenectomy for trauma, it is difficult to assess whether patients with splenosis actually have a lower risk of such infections. The functional capacity of these splenotic nodules is real, however, and splenosis appears to be potentially beneficial for patients whose spleens were removed for nonhematologic indications. Animal studies of splenosis suggest that preservation of the arterial supply and of the architecture of splenic tissue is important for the splenic nodules to retain their protective filter function.[6,211,215–217] Splenic implants without adequate blood supply may not be protective against pneumoccal septicemia even if the volume of tissue is considerable.[208,218–221] The volume of splenic tissue appears to be regulated by humoral factors that are poorly defined.[222] After splenectomy, the accessory spleens or implants hypertrophy in response to these factors.

POSTSPLENECTOMY SEPSIS

Bacterial infection with septicemia rapidly progressing to circulatory collapse and death is a recognized syndrome following splenectomy.[223–225] Abrupt onset, rapid development of shock, and frequent accompaniment of meningitis are characteristic of overwhelming postsplenectomy sepsis.[226] Its occurrence is more frequent in younger patients[227] and during the first few years after splenectomy, but it may occur in older patients and years after splenectomy.[228–230] Patients generally run high fevers and may appear well at the time of initial evaluation.[223] Once cardiovascular decompensation occurs, the process is frequently fatal regardless of therapy. Adrenal hemorrhage (Waterhouse-Friderichsen syndrome) accompanies cardiovascular collapse with the septicemia.[231] Encapsulated organisms that evade normal clearance mechanisms and intraerythrocyte parasites are the greatest threats to these patients.

Streptococcus pneumoniae is the most common cause of septicemia in asplenic children and adults, accounting for 60% of cases[232,233] (Table 46-4). *Neisseria meningitidis* and *Haemophilus influenzae* type b account for another 25%, with the remainder caused by *Escherichia coli*, *Streptococcus* sp, *Staphylococcus aureus*, *Klebsiella* sp, *Salmonella* sp, anaerobic oral organisms such as the DF-2 group, and *Pseudomonas aeruginosa*.[234–241] Severe infections with *Brucella* sp and *Pasteurella tularensis* are also described after splenectomy. Fatal malaria[242] and severe babesiosis[243] are other potential complications of asplenia.

Bacteria proliferate in the blood stream when they are not cleared by the splenic macrophages. Studies in animals demonstrate the intravascular growth of bacteria in the absence of the spleen.[22] The ability of hepatic, pulmonary, and bone marrow macrophages to compensate for the absence of the spleen is especially compromised in the absence of specific antibody to the encapsulated organisms.[48] Splenic macrophages ingest particles with far fewer antibody and complement molecules on their surfaces than do hepatic macrophages, and the contact between particles and the phagocytes is much closer in the spleen than the liver.[244] Deposition of complement via the alternative pathway is insufficient in the absence of type-specific antibody to opsonize bacteria for the liver.[48,244] In the presence of type-specific antibody, the liver is able to recognize encapsulated organisms, and complement is activated by means of the classic pathway.[245] The role of antibody is important in the prevention of postsplenectomy sepsis, and contributes to the greater susceptibility of younger (preimmune) children to the development of this complication (Fig. 46-9). Because young children fail to respond well to carbohydrate antigens,[246,247] immunization frequently is not protective for the group at highest risk.[248,249]

TABLE 46-4. Organisms Causing Severe Infections in Asplenic Patients

BACTERIA
Streptococcus pneumoniae
Haemophilus influenzae types b and f
Neisseria meningitidis
Pseudomonas aeruginosa
Escherichia coli
Dysgonid fermenter 2
Other encapsulated organisms
PROTOZOA
Babesia species
Plasmodium species

The incidence of overwhelming postsplenectomy septicemia is affected not only by the age and immune status of the patient but also by the underlying disease (Fig. 46-10). Whereas children who undergo splenectomy as a result of trauma have a 58 times greater risk of death from sepsis than healthy children, those who undergo splenectomy for thalassemia have a 1000 times greater risk.[226] The patients at lowest risk have no associated underlying immunologic deficits (eg, ITP and congenital hemolytic anemias). Those at highest risk have associated reticuloendothelial blockade, especially associated with iron overload (thalassemia), or lymphoid immunodeficiency (including Hodgkin's disease, other lymphomas, and congenital or acquired immunodeficiency [eg, Wiskott-Aldrich syndrome]).[175,250] Additionally, patients with nonsurgical asplenia induced by irradiation or splenic infarction,[173] as in sickle cell disease,[27] share the high risk of sepsis accompanying asplenia. Complicating factors may be genetic differences in antibody production in response to carbohydrate antigens, which appear to develop later or to a lesser extent in African Americans and native Americans.[246,247]

Gorse[251] combined several series of reports, and estimated the incidence of postsplenectomy septicemia in various conditions (Table 46-5). The number of fatalities ranged from 33% to 71% of those who developed septicemia.[251] These data are imperfect, since the studies were all retrospective. Because most patients are immunized against

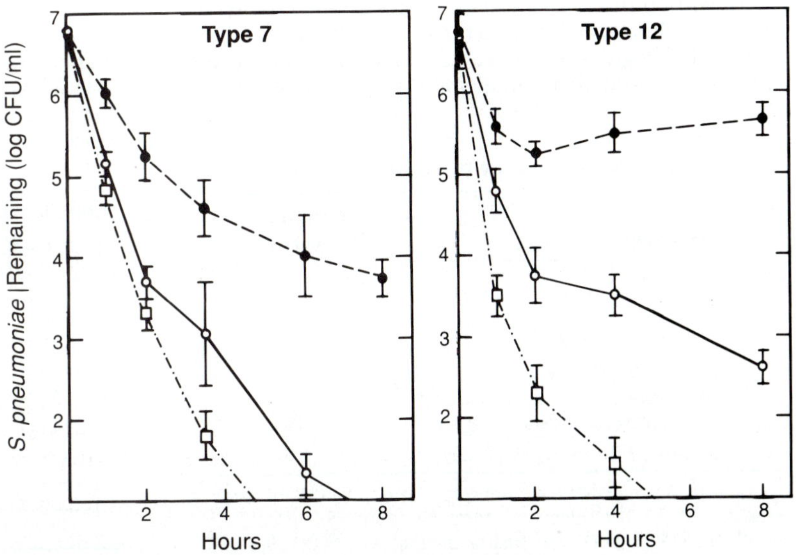

FIGURE 46-9. Clearance of pneumococci from the blood of guinea pigs. Immunization corrects the clearance defect for both types of pneumococci. Squares, splenectomized guinea pig immunized to the specific pneumococcal serotype indicated; open circles, intact, unimmunized guinea pig; filled circles, splenectomized, unimmunized guinea pig. (After Brown EJ, Hosea SW, Frank MM. The role of the spleen in experimental pneumococcal bacteremia. J Clin Invest 1981;67: 975)

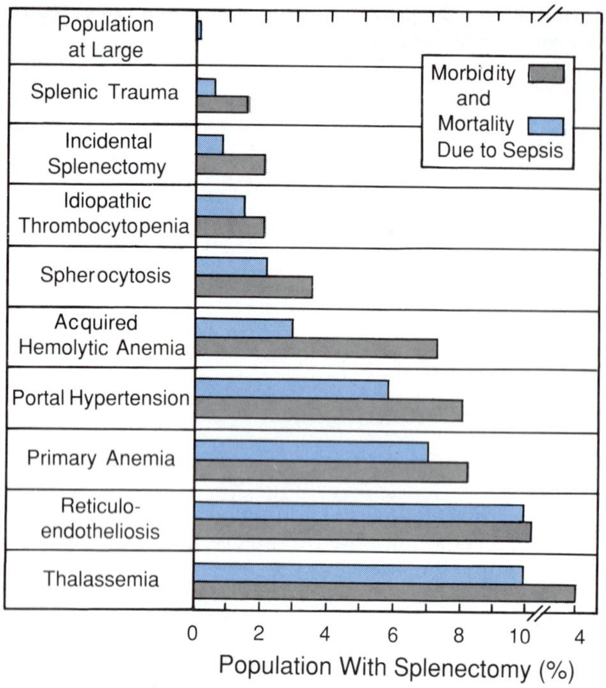

FIGURE 46-10. Postsplenectomy sepsis. (After Singer DB. Postsplenectomy sepsis. In: Rosenberg HS, Bolande RP, eds. Perspectives in pediatric pathology, vol 1. Chicago, Year Book, 1973:285)

the most common organisms before splenectomy, and high-risk patients are often maintained on prophylactic antibiotics or treated early for potential septicemia because they and their caregivers are aware of the risks, it may be difficult to obtain better estimates of these risks in the future.

The risk of infection appears to be greatest in the first 2 years after splenectomy[238] but may occur years later.[228,239,240] Infants and children appear to be at greater risk.[224–227] In Singer's review,[226] serious bacterial infection occurred in 21% of children who underwent splenectomy for hereditary spherocytosis before 1 year of age but in only 3.5% of children who underwent splenectomy later in life (see Fig. 46-9). Chaikof,[229] in a retrospective review done 10 to 20 years after surgery, found an incidence of overwhelming postsplenectomy septicemia of 3.77% in children who underwent splenectomy before 16 years of age, and 0.34% in patients who underwent splenectomy as adults.

Prevention of this devastating consequence of asplenia depends primarily on having the patient, family, and medical staff recognize the risk, undertake preventive measures, and treat with antibiotics at the first sign of a possible

TABLE 46-5. Incidence of Postsplenectomy Sepsis

Disorder	Incidence of Sepsis (%)
Thalassemia	25
Sickle cell disease	15
Hodgkin's disease	10
Portal hypertension	8.2
Miscellaneous hematologic diseases	3.5
Trauma	1.5

(Data from Gorse GJ. The relationship of the spleen to infection. In: Bowlder AJ, ed. The spleen: structure, function, and clinical significance. New York, van Nostrand Reinhold, 1990:269)

TABLE 46-6. Prevention of Postsplenectomy Septicemia

- Avoid splenectomy when possible
- Delay splenectomy until patient is over 5 years of age
- Immunize before splenectomy with polyvalent pneumococcal and meningococcal vaccines, and conjugated hemophilus vaccine
- Prophylactic antibiotic administration (250 mg penicillin or amoxacillin by mouth, twice daily, or erythromycin for penicillin-allergic patients), for all patients at high risk of development of sepsis (younger patients, underlying disease)
- Aggressive education of patient and family to ensure rapid medical attention
- Obtain MedicAlert or equilavent warning system

infection. All patients who are at risk of having or developing splenic hypofunction because of an underlying disease should have their splenic function assessed and should be immunized and receive prophylactic antibiotics.[252] Early recognition is most important in children with sickle cell syndromes and cardiac lesions associated with asplenia or polysplenia. The polyvalent pneumococcal vaccine induces a poor response in children under the age of 2 years[253] and should not be given before that time. It remains unclear if the vaccine should be repeated, but it is probably wise to do so 5 to 10 years after initial immunization. Vaccines against other encapsulated organisms should also be given. The trivalent meningococcal vaccine should also be given after the age of 2 years. The conjugated Hib vaccines can be given in the first few months of life. New vaccines are being developed that are immunogenic in populations previously poorly responsive to these vaccines and should be used as soon as efficacy is established.[253]

Patients scheduled for elective splenectomy should receive the polyvalent pneumococcal vaccine, trivalent meningococcal vaccine, and (if not previously given) the Hib vaccine at least 72 hours before splenectomy for greatest efficacy. This permits antigen processing and maximizes the immune response to the vaccine before splenectomy.[252] Ideally, splenectomy should be delayed until a child is 5 years old to permit lymphoid maturation and minimize the risks of postsplenectomy sepsis.

TABLE 46-7. Emergency Management of Febrile Asplenic Patient

TEMPERATURE BELOW 38.5°C

- Examine patient (vital signs, localizing findings)
- Obtain blood cultures, other cultures as indicated
- Administer intravenous or intramuscular antibiotics (ceftriaxone, ampicillin, or equivalent coverage)
- Begin oral antibiotics to cover encapsulated organisms (choice depends upon local epidemiology and whether the patient is receiving prophylactic antibiotics)

TEMPERATURE ABOVE 38.5°C

- Examine patient (vital signs, localizing findings, especially any indication of meningitis)
- Obtain blood cultures, complete blood count, other cultures as indicated
- Administer intravenous antibiotics (ceftriaxone, ampicillin, or equivalent coverage)
- Maintain intravenous hydration and observe patient for at least 6 to 12 hours in medical facility
- Consider admission, depending upon local circumstances, ability to monitor patient, proximity to medical facility; discharge requires a responsible adult immediately available to bring patient back in event of change in clinical status

Prophylactic antibiotics are of demonstrated benefit in prevention of bacterial infections in patients with sickle cell syndromes.[249] All children in the highest-risk groups (underlying disorders and young age) should receive prophylactic antibiotics following splenectomy or when at risk for splenic infarction. Benefits of prophylactic antibiotics in patients of lower risk (patients over 5 years of age who have undergone splenectomy for trauma and hematologic indications) are unproven. If compliance is poor, it may not be worth the risk of selecting resistant organisms, which accompanies use of prophylactic antibiotics. Since pneumococcal infection is the greatest risk, and it is possible to immunize against *Haemophilus*, penicillin or amoxicillin, 125 to 250 mg (depending on the size of the patient) twice daily, is the most frequently used antibiotic regimen (Table 46-6).

The single best protection against overwhelming postsplenectomy septicemia is a high index of suspicion and a rapid response to fever on the part of the patient, family, and medical staff. Antibiotics should be readily available,

TABLE 46-8. Diseases Associated With Splenomegaly

ANATOMIC

Cysts
Hamartomas
Pseudocysts
Peliosis
Systemic cystic angiomatosis
Hemangiomas

HYPERPLASIA DUE TO HEMATOLOGIC DISORDERS

Acute and chronic hemolysis
- HS, HE, SS, SC, S-thal, thalassemias, unstable hemoglobins, PK deficiency, autoimmune hemolytic anemia, isoimmune hemolysis, etc

Extramedullary hematopoiesis
- Severe hemolytic anemias, especially in fetus and neonates
- Myeloproliferative diseases: polycythemia vera, chronic myelogenous leukemia, thrombocythemia, myelofibrosis with myeloid metaplasia
- Osteopetrosis

INFECTIONS

Bacterial

Acute sepsis: *Salmonella* (typhoid fever), *Streptococcus pneumoniae, Haemophilus influenzae, Staphylococcus aureus,* etc
Chronic infections: subacute bacterial endocarditis, chronic meningococcemia, brucellosis, tularemia, etc
Local infections: splenic abscess, pyogenic liver abscess, cholangitis

Viral

Acute viral infections, especially in children
Congenital: cytomegalovirus, herpes simplex, rubella
Hepatitis A, B, C, cytomegalovirus
Epstein-Barr virus
Psittacosis
Viral hemophagocytic syndromes
Human immunodeficiency virus

Spirochetal

Syphilis (especially congenital)
Lyme disease
Leptospirosis

Rickettsial

Rocky Mountain spotted fever
Q fever
Typhus

Fungal or Mycobacterial

Disseminated tuberculosis
Disseminated histoplasmosis
South American blastomycosis

Parasitic

Malaria
Babesiosis
Toxoplasmosis, especially congenital
Visceral larval migrans (*Toxocara canis, Toxocara catis*)
Leishmaniasis (Kala-azar)
Schistosomiasis
Trypanosomiasis
Fascioliasis

IMMUNOLOGIC, INFLAMMATORY

Collagen vascular

Systemic lupus erythematosus
Rheumatoid arthritis (Felty's syndrome)
Mixed connective tissue disease
Systemic vasculitis

Other

Serum sickness
Drug hypersensitivity, especially phenytoin
Graft-versus-host disease
Sjögren's syndrome
Cryoglobulinemia
Amyloidosis
Inflammatory bowel disease
Myasthenia gravis
Sarcoidosis
Large granular lymphocytosis and neutropenia
Hyperimmune B-lymphocyte disorder
Weber-Christian disease
Familial Mediterranean fever
Histiocytosis syndromes
Systemic mastocytosis

MALIGNANCIES

Primary: leukemia, lymphoma, angiosarcoma, etc
Metastatic

STORAGE DISEASES

Gaucher's disease, Niemann-Pick disease, GM-1 gangliosidosis, etc
Glycogen storage disease type IV
Tangier disease
Wolman's disease
Hyperchylomicronemia types I and V
Mucopolysaccharidoses

CONGESTIVE DISORDERS

Congestive heart failure
Intrahepatic cirrhosis
Extrahepatic portal, splenic, hepatic vein obstruction (Budd-Chiari syndrome)

IDIOPATHIC DISORDERS

and patients with documented fever exceeding 38.5°C should be treated. Controversy exists regarding whether all therapy needs to be administered in the hospital or parenterally. It is possible to treat selected outpatients with oral or parenteral agents.[254] It is important to keep in mind that patients may appear well minutes before developing circulatory collapse, and these patients must be considered at high risk regardless of how well they appear. In addition, the risk of organisms other than those sensitive to penicillin (including gram-negative organisms) must be kept in mind.[255] Choice of empiric antibiotics depends on local epidemiology. In areas where penicillin-resistant pneumococcus and ampicillin-resistant *Haemophilus* are uncommon, ampicillin may be sufficient, but a second- or third-generation cephalosporin is more commonly chosen. While it is important not to alarm families unnecessarily, a well-educated patient and family is the best first-line defense and prevents most fatal outcomes[256] (Table 46-7).

OTHER COMPLICATIONS OF SPLENECTOMY

The increase in platelet count following splenectomy may be associated with a tendency to develop thrombosis in adults. Antiplatelet agents (aspirin and dipyridamole) may be used to reduce the risk of thrombosis.[257] Even marked thrombocytosis rarely causes clinical problems in children, but thrombosis may occur in older patients with myeloproliferative disorders or preexisting arteriosclerosis.

Removal of the spleen also removes a major site of antibody production, and the serum IgM and properdin levels are lower following splenectomy than before.[245,258]

The risk of ischemic heart disease may also increase after splenectomy. In one study,[258a] death from ischemic heart disease was 1.86 times more frequent in splenectomized men than in men who had their spleens during a 28-year follow-up, a significant difference. Chronically elevated platelet counts may contribute to this risk, although the precise etiology is unclear.

SPLENOMEGALY

Spleens that are palpable more than 2 cm below the left costal margin are usually abnormal.[222] Many enlarged spleens are not palpable on physical examination, however, because of their relationship to other organs and the thoracic cage. And some spleens that are repeatedly palpable are not affected with clear-cut pathology. Patients with low diaphragms often have palpable spleens. About 3% of college freshmen[259] and 5% to 15% of younger children[260] have palpable spleens. A relaxed patient must be examined supine and in the right lateral decubitus position with the knees up to maximize the probability that a palpable spleen will be appreciated by the examiner. In adults, the spleen ranges from 100 to 250 g, with an upper limit of 15 cm in length on ultrasound examination. The spleen is proportionally larger in normal children and adolescents, and involutes with age so that a barely palpable spleen in an older person is far more likely to represent pathology than in a younger patient.

A wide variety of conditions can cause splenomegaly (Table 46-8). Chronic splenomegaly may be due to several types of processes, such as the "work hypertrophy" seen with acute and chronic infections and in hemolytic anemias; congestive enlargement due to heart failure, cirrhosis, or portal hypertension; infiltration with sarcoidosis, amyloidosis, or storage diseases such as Gaucher's; myeloproliferative as in chronic myelogenous leukemia and myeloid metaplasia; and neoplastic causes, as in lymphomas, hemangiomas, and cysts. Acute enlargement of the spleen is usually due to trauma or to sequestration crises in sickle syndromes.

REFERENCES

1. Virchow, R. Weisses Lut und Ilztumoren. Med Zeit 1846;15:157.
2. King H, Shumacher HB. Splenic studies. 1. Susceptibility to infection after splenectomy performed in infancy. Ann Surg 1952;136:239.

2a. Roberts CWM, Shutter JR, Korsmeyer SJ. *Hox 11* controls the genesis of the spleen. Nature 1994;368:747.

3. Tischendorf F. On the evolution of the spleen. Experientia 1985;41:145.
4. Weiss L. The spleen. In: Weiss L, ed. Histology, cell, and tissue biology, ed 5. New York, Elsevier, 1983:236.
5. Eikelenboom P, et al. Characterization of lymphoid and nonlymphoid cells in the white pulp of the spleen using immunohistoperoxidase techniques and enzyme histochemistry. Experientia 1985;41:209.
6. van Wyck DB, Witte MH, Witte CL. Compensatory spleen growth and protective function in rats. Clin Sci 1986;71:573.
7. Kashimura M, Fujita T. A scanning electron microscope study of human spleen: relationship between the microcirculation and function. Scanning Microsc 1987;1:841.
8. Groom AC. Microcirculation of the spleen: new concepts, new challenges. Microvasc Res 1987;34:269.
9. Weiss L. A scanning electron microscopic study of the spleen. Blood 1974;43:665.
10. Weiss L. The red pulp of the spleen: structural basis of blood flow. Clin Haematol 1983;12:375.
11. Theil GA, Downey H. The development of the mammalian spleen with special reference to its hematopoietic activity. Am J Anat 1921;28:279.
12. Freeman MH, Saunders EF. Hematopoiesis in the human spleen. Am J Hematol 1981;11:271.
13. Playfair JHL, Wolfendale MR, Kay HEM. The leukocytes of the peripheral blood in the human foetus. Br J Haematol 1963;9:336.
14. Linch DC, Knott RJ, Rodeck CH, et al. Studies of circulating hematopoietic progenitor cells in human fetal blood. Blood 1982;59:976.
15. Wolf BC, Luevano E, Neiman RS. Evidence to suggest that the human fetal spleen is not a hematopoietic organ. Am J Clin Pathol 1983;80:140.
16. McCulloch AE, Till JE. The sensitivity of cells from normal mouse bone marrow to gamma radiation in vitro and in vivo. Radiat Res 1962;16:882.
17. Ford CE, Micklem HS. The thymus and lymph nodes in radiation chimaeras. Lancet 1963;1:359.
18. Copeland NG, Gilbert DJ, Cho BC. Mast cell growth factor maps near the steel locus on mouse chromosome 10 and is deleted in a number of steel alleles. Cell 1990;63:175.
19. Flanagan JG, Leder P. The kit ligand: a cell surface molecule altered in steel mutant fibroblasts. Cell 1990;63:185.
20. Bowdler AJ. Regional variations in the proportion of red cells in the blood in man. Br J Haematol 1969;16:557.
21. Weiss L, Javassoli M. Anatomical hazards to the passage of erythrocytes through the spleen. Semin Hematol 1970;7:372.
22. McBride JA, Dacie JV, Shapley R. The effect of splenectomy on the leucocyte count. Br J Haematol 1968;14:225.
23. Nathan DG. Rubbish in the red cell. N Engl J Med 1969;281:558.
24. Crosby WH. Splenic remodeling of red cell surfaces. Blood 1977;50:643.
25. Holroyde CP, Oski RA, Gardner FH. The "pocked" erythrocyte: red cell surface alterations in reticuloendothelial immaturity of the neonate. N Engl J Med 1969;281:516.
26. Corrigan JJ Jr, VanWyck DB, Crosby WH. Clinical disorders of splenic function: the spectrum from asplenism to hypersplenism. Lymphology 1983;16:101.
27. Buchanan GR, Holtkamp CA, Horton JA. Formation and disappearance of pocked erythrocytes: studies in human subjects and laboratory animals. Am J Hematol 1987;25:243.
28. Lux SE, John KM. Isolation and partial characterization of a high molecular weight red cell membrane protein complex which is normally removed by the spleen. Blood 1977;50:625.
29. Lipson RL, Bayrd ED, Watkins CH. The post-splenectomy blood picture. Am J Clin Pathol 1959;32:526.
30. Groom AC, Levesque MJ, Bruckschweiger D. Flow stasis, blood gases and glucose levels in the red pulp of the spleen. Adv Exp Med Biol 1977;94:567.
31. Song SH, Groom AC. Sequestration and possible maturation of reticulocytes in the normal spleen. Can J Physiol Pharmacol 1972;50:400.
32. Aguado MT, Mannik M. Clearance kinetics and organ uptake of complement-solubilized immune complexes in mice. Immunology 1987;60:255.
33. Amlot PL, Hayes AE. Impaired human antibody response to the thymus-independent antigen, DNP-Ficoll, after splenectomy: implications for post-splenectomy infections. Lancet 1985;1:1008.

34. Mitchell J, Abbot A. Antigens in immunity. XVI. A light and electron microscope study of antigen localization in the rat spleen. Immunology 1971;21:207.
35. Nossal GJV, Austin CM, et al. Antigens in immunity. XII. Antigen trapping in the spleen. Int Arch Allergy 1966;29:368.
36. Humphrey JH, Grennan D. Different macrophage populations distinguished by means of fluorescent polysaccharides: recognition and properties of marginal-zone macrophages. Eur J Immunol 1981;11:221.
37. Kumararatne DS, Bazin H, MacLennan ICM. Marginal zones: the major B cell compartment of rat spleens. Eur J Immunol 1981;11:858.
38. Hammarstrom L, Smith CIE. Development of anti-polysaccharide antibodies in asplenic children. Clin Exp Immunol 1986;66:457.
39. MacLennan ICM, et al. The lymphocytes of splenic marginal zones: A distinct B cell lineage. Immunol Today 1981;3:305.
40. Brown JC, et al. Lymphocyte-mediated transport of aggregated gammaglobulin into germinal centre areas of normal mouse spleen. Nature 1973;228:367.
41. Sullivan JL, Schiffman G, Miser J, et al. Immune response after splenectomy. Lancet 1978;1:178.
42. Claret I, Morales L, Montaner A. Immunological studies in the postsplenectomy syndrome. J Pediatr Surg 1975;10:59.
43. Schumacker MJ. Serum immunoglobulin and transferrin levels after childhood splenectomy. Arch Dis Child 1970;45:114.
44. Jandl J, Greenberg MS, et al. Clinical determination of the sites of red cell destruction in the hemolytic anemias. J Clin Invest 1956;35:842.
45. Brown EJ, Hosea SW, et al. A quantitative analysis of the interactions of anti-pneumoccal antibody and complement in experimental pneumococcal antibody and comlement in experimental pneumococcal bacteremia. J Clin Invest 1982;69:85.
46. Brown EJ, Hosea SW, Frank MM. The role of antibody and complement in the reticuloendothelial clearance of pneumococci from the bloodstream. Rev Infect Dis 1983;5(Suppl):8797.
47. Brown EJ, Hosea SW, Frank MM. The role of the spleen in experimental pneumococcal bacteremia. J Clin Invest 1981;67:975.
48. Hosea SW, et al. Opsonic requirements for intravascular clearance after splenectomy. N Engl J Med 1981;304:245.
49. Davies BN, Withrington PG. The action of drugs on smooth muscle of the capsule and blood vessels of the spleen. Pharmacol Rev 1973;25:373.
50. Aster RH. Pooling of platelets in the spleen: role in the pathogenesis of "hypersplenic" thrombocytopenia. J Clin Invest 1966;45:645.
51. Jandl JH, Aster RH. Increased splenic pooling and the pathogenesis of hypersplenism. Am J Med Sci 1967;253:383.
52. Dawson AA, et al. Thrombotic risks of staging laparotomy with splenectomy in Hodgkin's disease. Br J Surg 1981;68:842.
53. el Kishen MA, et al. Splenectomy is contraindicated for thrombocytopenia secondary to portal hypertension. Surg Gynecol Obstet 1985;160:233.
54. Jandl JH, Files NM, et al. Proliferative response of the spleen and liver to hemolysis. J Exp Med 1965;122:299.
55. Blendis LM, et al. Spleen blood flow and splanchic haemodynamics in blood dyscrasias and other splenomegalies. Clin Sci 1970;38:73.
56. Stathers GM, Ma MH, Blackburn CRB. Extra-hepatic portal hypertension: the clinical evaluation, investigation and results of treatment of 28 patients. Aust Ann Med 1968;17:12.
57. Hess CE, Ayers CR, Sandusky WR, et al. Mechanism of dilutional anemia in massive splenomegaly. Blood 1976;47:629.
58. Crosby WH. Siderocytes and the spleen. Blood 1956;12:165.
59. Barzanju J, Every JL. Changes in the spleen related to birth. J Anat 1979;129:819.
60. Blendis LM, Modell CB, et al. Some effects of splenectomy in thalassemia major. Br J Haematol 1974;28:77.
61. Heaton LD, Crosby WH, et al. Splenectomy in the treatment of hypoplasia of the bone marrow: with a report of 12 cases. Ann Surg 1957;146:634.
62. Sills RH, Tamburlin JH, Barrios NJ, et al. Formation of intracellular vesicles in neonatal and adult erythrocytes: evidence against the concept of neonatal hyposplenism. Pediatr Res 1988;24:703.
63. Freeman RM, Johnston D, Mahoney MJ, et al. Development of splenic reticuloendothelial function in neonates. J Pediatr 1980;96:466.
64. Diamond LK. The concept of functional asplenia. N Engl J Med 1969;281:958.
65. Sullivan JL, Ochs HD, Schiffman G, et al. Immune response after splenectomy. Lancet 1978;1:178.
66. Auerbach R. Ontogeny of immune responsiveness in the absence of the spleen: a review. Dev Comp Immunol 1978;2:219.
67. Llende M, Santiago-Delpin EA, Lavergne J. Immunobiological consequences of splenectomy: a review. J Surg Res 1986;40:85.
68. Timens W, Poppema A. Impaired immune response to polysaccharides. N Engl J Med 1987;317:837.
69. Ozsoylu S, Hosain F, et al. Functional development of phagocytic activity of the spleen. J Pediatr 1977;90:560.
70. Polhemus DW, Schaefer WB. Absent spleen syndrome: hematologic findings as an aid to diagnosis. Pediatrics 1959;24:254.
71. Krumbhaar EB. The changes produced in the blood by removal of the normal mammalian spleen. Am J Med Sci 1932;184:215.
72. Dean HW. Acanthocytes after splenectomy. N Engl J Med 1968;279:947.
73. Weiss L. The role of the spleen in the removal of normal aged red cells. Am J Anat 1962;111:175.
74. Douglas AS, Dacie JV. Incidence and significance of iron-containing granules in human erythrocytes and their precursers. J Clin Pathol 1953;6:307.
75. Acevedo G, Mauer AM. The capacity for removal of erythrocytes containing Heinz bodies in premature infants and patients following splenectomy. J Pediatr 1963;63:61.
76. Peters AM. Splenic blood flow and blood cell kinetics. Clin Haematol 1983;12:421.
77. McBride JA. The effect of splenectomy on the leukocyte count Br J Haematol 1968;14:225.
78. Aster RH. Pooling of platelets in the spleen: role in the pathogenesis of "hypersplenic" thrombocytopenia. J Clin Invest 1966;45:645.
79. Penny R, Rozenberg MC, et al. The splenic platelet pool. Blood 1966;27:1.
80. Libre EB, Cowan DH, et al. Relationship between spleen, platelets, and factor VIII levels. Blood 1968;31:358.
81. Robertson DAF, et al. Blood film appearances in the hyposplenism of coeliac disease. Br J Clin Pract 1983;37:19.
82. Holyroyde CP, Gardner FH. Acquisition of autophagic vacuoles by human erythrocytes: physiological role of the spleen. Blood 1970;36:566.
83. Pearson HA, Gallagher D, et al. Developmental patterns of splenic dysfunction in sickle cell disorders. Pediatrics 1985;76:392.
84. Pearson HA. Developmental aspects of splenic function in sickle cell disease. Blood 1979;53:358.
85. Mettler FA. Essentials of nuclear medicine imaging. Orlando, Grune & Stratton, 1986:223.
86. Armas RR, Thakur ML, Gottschalk A. A simplified method of selective spleen scintigraphy with Tc-99m–labeled erythrocytes: clinical applications. J Nucl Med 1980;21:413.
87. Nielsen JL, Ellegaard J, Marqversen J, et al. Detection of splenosis and ectopic spleens with 99mTc-labelled heat damaged autologous erythrocytes in 90 splenectomized patients. Scand J Haematol 1981;27:51.
88. Peters AM, et al. Methods of measuring splenic blood flow and platelet transit time with "In-labelled" platelets. J Nucl Med 1984;25:86.
89. Siegel RS, Rae JL, Barth S, et al. Platelet survival and turnover: important factors in predicting response to splenectomy in immune thrombocytopenic purpura. Am J Hematol 1989;30:206.
90. Cooperberg PL. Ultrasonography of the spleen. In: Sarti DA, ed. Diagnostic ultrasound: text and cases. Chicago, Year Book, 1987:312.
91. Federle M, Moss AA. Computer tomography of the spleen. Crit Rev Diagn Imaging 1983;19:1.
92. Glazer GM, et al. Dynamic CT of the normal spleen. Am J Radiol 1981;137:343.
93. Beahrs JR, Stephens DH. Enlarged accessory spleens: CT appearance in postsplenectomy patients. Am J Radiol 1980;135:483.
94. Johnson FD, et al. Radiology in the diagnosis of splenic abscess. Rev Infect Dis 1985;7:10.
95. Heymsfield SB, et al. Accurate measurement of liver, kidney and spleen volume and mass by CT. Ann Intern Med 1979;90:185.
96. Henderson JM, et al. Measurements of liver and spleen volume by CT. Radiology 1981;141:525.
97. Moss AA, Friedman MA, Brito AC. Determination of liver, kidney and spleen volumes by computed tomography: an experimental study in dogs. J Comput Assist Tomogr 1981;5:12.
98. Pierkarski J, et al. Difference between liver and spleen CT numbers in the normal adult: its usefulness in predicting the presence of diffuse liver disease. Radiology 1980;137:727.
99. Miller JH, Greenfield LD, Wald BR. Candidiasis of the liver and spleen in childhood. Radiology 1982;142:375.
100. Bartley DL, Hughes WT, Parvey LS, et al. Computed tomography of hepatic and splenic fungal abscesses in leukemic children. Pediatr Infect Dis 1982;1:317.
101. Ellert J, Kneel L. The role of computed tomography in the initial staging and subsequent management of the lymphomas. J Comput Assist Tomogr 1980;4:368.
102. Balcar I, et al. CT patterns of splenic infarction: a clinical and experimental study. Radiology 1984;151:723.
103. Pierkarski J, et al. Computed tomography of the spleen. Radiology 1980;135:683.
104. Federle MP, et al. Evaluation of abdominal trauma by computed tomography. Radiology 1981;138:637.
105. Dachman AH, et al. Nonparasitic splenic cysts: a report of 52 cases with radiologic-pathologic correlation. Am J Roentgenol 1986;147:537.
106. Ros PR, et al. Hemangioma of the spleen: radiologic pathologic correlation in ten cases. Radiology 1987;162:73.
107. Levy DW, et al. Thoratrast-induced hepatosplenic neoplasia: CT identification. Am J Radiol 1986;146:997.
108. Berge T. Splenic metastases: frequencies and patterns. Acta Pathol Microbiol Scand (A) 1974;82:499.
109. Bart JB, Appel MF. Recurrent hemolytic anemia secondary to accessory spleens. South Med J 1978;71:608.

110. Wallace D, Fromm D, Thomas D. Accessory splenectomy for idiopathic thrombocytopenic purpura. Surgery 1982;91:134.
111. Putschar WGJ, Manion WC. Splenic–gonadal fusion. Am J Pathol 1986;32:15.
112. Wick MR, Rife CC. Paratesticular accessory spleen. Mayo Clin Proc 1981;56:455.
113. Moller JH, Nakib A, Anderson RC, et al. Congenital cardiac disease associated with polysplenia: a development complex of bilateral "leftsidedness." Circulation 1967;36:789.
114. Ivemark BI. Implications of agenesis of the spleen on the pathogenesis of cono-truncus anomalies in childhood: analysis of the heart malformations of the splenic agenesis syndrome with fourteen new cases. Acta Paediatr 1955;44(Suppl 104):1.
115. Waldman JD, Rosenthal A, Smith AL, et al. Sepsis and congenital asplenia. J Pediatr 1977;90:555.
116. van Mierop LHS, Gessner IHS, Schiebler GL. Asplenia and polysplenia syndromes. Birth Defects 1972;8:36.
117. Freedom RM. The asplenia syndrome: a review of significant extracardiac structural abnormalities in twenty-nine necropsied patients. J Pediatr 1972;81:1130.
118. Pearson HA, Schiebler GL, Spencer RP. Functional hyposplenia in cyanotic congenital heart disease. Pediatrics 1971;48:277.
119. Burrig K-F. Epithelial (true) splenic cysts: pathogenesis of the mesothelial and so-called epidermoid cyst of the spleen. Am J Surg Pathol 1988;12:275.
120. Al Mohaya S, et al. Hydatid cyst of the spleen. Am J Trop Med Hyg 1986;35:995.
121. Browne MK. Epidermoid cyst of the spleen. Br J Surg 1963;50:838.
122. Sirinek KR, Evans WE. Nonparasitic splenic cysts: case report of epidermoid cyst with review of the literature. Am J Surg 1973;126:8.
123. Didlake RH, Miller RC. Epidermoid cyst of the spleen manifested as an abdominal abscess. South Med J 1986;79:635.
124. Morgenstern L, Shapiro SJ. Partial splenectomy for nonparasitic splenic cysts. Am J Surg 1980;139:278.
125. Martin JW. Congenital splenic cysts. Am J Surg 1958;96:302.
126. Ugochukwu AI, Irving M. Intraperitoneal low-pressure suction drainage following splenectomy. Br J Surg 1985;72:247.
127. Rappaport H. Tumors of the hematopoietic system. In: Atlas of tumor pathology. Armed Forces Institute of Pathology, fascicle 8, section 3, 1966:357.
128. Garvin DF, King FM. Cysts and nonlymphomatous tumors of the spleen. Pathol Ann 1981:16:61.
129. Mauch P, Larson D, Osteen R, et al. Prognostic factors for positive surgical staging in patients with Hodgkin's disease. J Clin Oncol 1989;8: 257.
130. Falk S, Stutte JH. Primary malignant lymphomas of the spleen. Cancer 1990;64:2612.
131. Strauss KJ. Primary lymphomas of the spleen: clinical features and outcome after splenectomy. Cancer 1988:62:433.
132. Ratain MJ, Vardiman JW, Barker CM, et al. Prognostic variables in hairy cell leukemia after splenectomy as initial therapy. Cancer 1988;62:2420.
133. Golomb HM. The treatment of hairy cell leukemia. Blood 1987;69: 979.
134. Klein B, et al. Splenomegaly and solitary spleen metastasis in solid tumors. Cancer 1987;60:100.
135. Zamora JU, Halpern NB. Splenectomy for metastatic neoplasms. South Med J 1987;80:805.
136. Willey RF, Ridger A, Webb JN. Seminoma presenting as gross splenomegaly. Scott Med J 1982;27:254.
137. Carr AJ, et al. Male choriocarcinoma of the spleen: a case report. Eur J Surg Oncol 1987;13:75.
138. Spencer RP, et al. "Reversible" functional asplenia in combined immunodeficiency. Int J Nucl Med Biol 1978;5:125.
139. Garriga S, Crosby WH. The incidence of leukemia in families with hypoplasia of the marrow. Blood 1959;14:1008.
140. Bensinger TA, et al. Thorotrast-induced reticuloendothelial blockade in man. Am J Med 1970;51:663.
141. Levy DW, et al. Thoratrast-induced hepatosplenic neoplasia: CT identification. Am J Roentgenol 1986;146:997.
142. Dailey MO, Coleman CN, Kaplan HS. Radiation-induced splenic atrophy in patients with Hodgkin's disease and non-Hodgkin's lymphoma. N Engl J Med 1980;302:215.
143. Coleman CN, et al. Functional hyposplenia after splenic irradiation for Hodgkin's disease. Ann Intern Med 1982;96:44.
144. Roth J, Brudler O, Henze E. Functional asplenia in malignant mastocytosis. J Nucl Med 1985;26:1149.
145. Al-Eid MA, et al. Functional asplenia in patients with graft-versus-host disease. J Nucl Med 1983;24:1123.
146. Jellinek EH, Ball K. Hashimoto's disease, encephalopathy and splenic atrophy. Lancet 1976;1:1248.
147. Stone RW, et al. Acquired functional asplenia in sarcoidosis. J Natl Med Assoc NY 1985;77:930.
148. Pearson HA, Cornelius EA, et al. Transfusion reversible functional asplenia in young children with sickle cell anemia. N Engl J Med 1970;283:334.
149. Stevens MCG, Vaidya S, Serjeant GR. Fetal hemoglobin and clinical severity of homozygous sickle cell disease in early childhood. J Pediatr 1981;98:37.
150. Rogers DW, Serjeant BE, Serjeant GR. Early rise in 'pitted' red cell count as a guide to susceptibility to infection in childhood sickle cell anaemia. Arch Dis Child 1982;57:338.
151. Al-Alwamy B, Wilson W, et al. Splenic function in sickle cell disease in the eastern province of Saudi Arabia. J Pediatr 1984;104:714.
152. Rogers DW, Vaidya S, Serjeant GR. Early splenomegaly in homozygous sickle cell disease: an indicator of susceptibility to infection. Lancet 1978;2:963.
153. Seeler RA, Shwaiki MZ. Acute splenic sequestration crises (ASSC) in young children with sickle cell anemia. Clin Pediatr 1972;11:701.
154. Edmond AM, et al. Acute splenic sequestration in homozygous sickle cell disease; natural history and management. J Pediatr 1985;107:201.
155. Topley DW, Rogers MC, Stevens C, et al. Acute splenic sequestration and hypersplenism in the first five years in homozygous sickle cell disease. Arch Dis Child 1981;56:765.
156. Frank MM, Hamburger MI, Lawley TJ, et al. Defective reticuloendothelial system Fc-receptor function in systemic lupus erythematosus. N Engl J Med 1979;300:518.
157. Frank MM, et al. Immunoglobulin G Fc-receptor–mediated clearance in autoimmune diseases. Ann Intern Med 1983;98:206.
158. Gertz MA, Kyle RA, Griepp RP. Hyposplenism in primary systemic amyloidosis. Ann Intern Med 1983;98:475.
159. Corazza GR, et al. Splenic function in childhood coeliac disease. Gut 1982;23:415.
160. Corazza GR, et al. Effect of gluten-free diet on splenic hypofunction of adult coeliac disease. Gut 1983;24:228.
161. Corazza GR, et al. Simple method of assessing splenic function in coeliac disease. Clin Sci 1981;60:109.
162. Bender BS, Quinn TC, Lawley TJ. Acquired immune deficiency syndrome (AIDS): a defect in Fc-receptor–specific clearance. Clin Res 1984;32:511A.
163. Falk S, Muller H, Stutte J-J. The spleen in acquired immunodeficiency syndrome (AIDS). Pathol Res Pract 1988;183:425.
164. Schreiber AD, Parsons J, McDermott P, et al. The effects of corticosteroids on the human monocyte IgG and complement receptors. J Clin Invest 1975;56:1189.
165. Schreiber AD, et al. Effect of corticosteroids on the human monocyte IgG and complement receptors. J Clin Invest 1975;56:1189.
166. Rosse WF. Quantitative immunology of immune hemolytic anemia: II. the relationship of cell-bound antibody to hemolysis and the effect of treatment. J Clin Invest 1971;50;734.
167. Kelton JG. Platelet and red cell clearance is determined by the interaction of the IgG and complement on the surface of the cells and activity of the reticuloendothelial system. Transfus Med Rev 1987;1: 75.
168. Kawada K, Terasaki PI. Evidence for immunosuppression by high-dose gammaglobulin. Exp Hematol 1987;15:133.
169. Petri IB, Lorincz A, Berek I. Detection of Fc-receptor blocking antibodies in anti-Rh (D) hyperimmune gammaglobulin. Lancet 1984;2: 1478.
170. Bussel JB, Graziano JN, Kimberley RP, et al. Intravenous anti-D treatment of immune thrombocytopenic purpura: analysis of efficacy, toxicity and mechanism of effect. Blood 1991;77:1884.
171. Paule B, Cosset HN, LeBourgeois JP. The possible role of radiotherapy in chronic lymphocytic leukemia: a critical review. Radiother Oncol 1985;4:45.
172. Singh AK, Bates T, Wetherley-Mein G. A preliminary study of low-dose splenic irradiation for the treatment of chronic lymphocytic and prolymphocytic leukemias. Scand J Haematol 1986;37:50.
173. Coleman CN, McDougall IR, Dailey MO, et al. Functional hyposplenia after splenic irradiation for Hodgkin's disease. Ann Intern Med 1982;96: 44.
174. Barbui T, et al. Does splenectomy enhance risk of AIDS in HIV-positive patients with chronic thrombocytopenia? Lancet 1987;2:342.
175. Lum LG et al. Splenectomy in the management of the thrombocytopenia of the Wiskott-Aldrich syndrome. N Engl J Med 1980;302: 892.
176. Rowe JM, Francis CW, Cyran EM, et al. Thrombotic thrombocytopenic purpura: recovery after splenectomy associated with persistence of unusually large von Willebrand's factor multimers. Am J Hematol 1985;20:161.
177. Ashkenazi A, Zizov R, Mathoth Y. Effect of splenectomy on destructive bone changes in children with chronic (type I) Gaucher disease. Eur J Pediatr 1986;145:138.
178. Goonewardene A, et al. Splenectomy for undiagnosed splenomegaly. Br J Surg 1979;66:62.
179. Coon WW, Liepman MK. Splenectomy for agnogenic myeloid metaplasia. Surg Gynecol Obstet 1982;154:561.
180. Towell BL, Levine SP. Massive hepatomegaly following splenectomy for myeloid metaplasia. Am J Med 1987;82:371.
181. Cooney DR, et al. Relative merits of partial splenectomy, splenic reimplantation, and immunization in preventing postsplenectomy infection. Surgery 1979;86:561.

182. Dawson DL, Molina ME, Scott-Conner CEH. Venous segmentation of the human spleen: a corrosion cast study. Am Surg 1986;52:253.
183. Sherman R. Management of trauma to the spleen. In: Shires GT, ed. Advances in surgery, vol 17. Chicage, Year Book, 1984.
184. Kamel R, Dunn MA. Segmental splenectomy in schistosomiasis. Br J Surg 1982;69:311.
185. Guzzetta PE, et al. Operative technique and results of subtotal splenectomy for Gaucher disease. Surg Gynecol Obstet 1987;164:359.
186. Rodgers BM, Tribble C, Joob A. Partial splenectomy for Gaucher's disease. Ann Surg 1987;205:693.
187. Dixon JA, Miller F, McCloskey D, et al. Anatomy and techniques in segmental splenectomy. Surg Gynecol Obstet 1980;150:520.
188. Scher KS, Scott-Conner C, Jones CW, et al. Methods of splenic preservation and their effect on clearance of pneumococcal bacteremia. Ann Surg 1985;202:595.
189. Luna GK, Dellinger EP. Nonoperative observation treatment for splenic injuries: a safe therapeutic option? Am J Surg 1987;153:462.
190. Wobbes T, Van der Sluis RF, Lubbers E-JC. Removal of the massive spleen: a surgical risk? Am J Surg 1984;147:800.
191. Goldstone J. Splenectomy for massive splenomegaly. Am J Surg 1978;135:385.
192. Taylor MA, Kaplan HS, Nelson TS. Staging laparotomy with splenectomy for Hodgkin's disease: the Stanford experience. World J Surg 1985;9:449.
193. Williams SF, Golomb HM. Perspective on staging approaches in the malignant lymphomas. Surg Gynecol Obstet 1986;163:193.
194. Kieswetter WB. Pediatric splenectomy: indications, technique, complications, and mortality. Surg Clin North Am 1975;55:449.
195. Appel MF, Bart JB. The surgical and hematologic significance of accessory spleens. Surg Gynecol Obstet 1976;143:191.
196. Ellison EC, Fabri PJ. Complications of splenectomy: etiology, prevention and management. Surg Clin North Am 1983;63:1313.
197. Roder OC. Splenic vein thrombosis with bleeding gastro-oesophageal varices: reports of two splenectomised cases and review of the literature. Acta Chir Scand 1984;150:265.
198. Jonasson O, Spigos DG, Mozes MF. Partial splenic embolisation: experience in 136 patients. World J Surg 1985;9:461.
199. Levy JM, Wasserman P, Pitha N. Presplenectomy transcatheter occlusion of the splenic artery. Arch Surg 1979;114:198.
200. Back LM, et al. Hazards of splenic embolization. Clin Pediatr 1987;26: 292.
201. Yoshioka H, et al. Splenic embolization for hypersplenism using steel coils. Am J Radiol 1985;144:1269.
202. Maddison FE. Embolic therapy of hypersplenism. Invest Radiol 1973;8: 280.
203. Chuang VP, Reuter SR. Experimental diminution of splenic function by selective embolization of the splenic artery. Surg Gynecol Obstet 1975;140:715.
204. Politis E, et al. Partial splenic embolisation for hypersplenism of thalassaemia major: five year follow up. Br Med J 1987;294:665.
205. Owman T, Lunderquist A, Alwmark A, et al. Embolization of the spleen for treatment of splenomegaly and hypersplenism in patients with portal hypertension. Invest Radiol 1979;14:457.
206. Mozes MF, et al. Partial splenic embolization: an alternative to splenectomy—results of a prospective, randomized study. Surgery 1984;96: 694.
207. Thanopoulos BD, Frimas CA. Partial splenic embolisation in the management of hypersplenism secondary to Gaucher disease. J Pediatr 1982;101:740.
208. Pabst R, Kamran D. Autotransplantation of splenic tissue. J Pediatr Surg 1986;21:120.
209. Dickerman JD, Horner SR, Coil JA, et al. The protective effect of intraperitoneal splenic autotransplants in mice exposed to an aerosolized suspension of type III *Streptococcus pneumoniae*. Blood 1979;54:354.
210. Patel J, Williams JS, Shmigel B, et al. Preservation of splenic funcion by autotransplantation of traumatized spleen in man. Surgery 1981;90: 683.
211. Horton J, et al. The importance of splenic blood flow in clearing pneumococcal organisms. Ann Surg 1982;195:172.
212. Fleming CR, Dickson ER, Harrison EG. Splenosis: autotransplantation of splenic tissue. Am J Med 1976;61:414.
213. Willis BK, Deitch EA, McDonald JC. The influence of trauma to the spleen on postoperative complications and mortality. J Trauma 1986;26:1073.
214. Pearson HA, Johnston D, et al. The born-again spleen: return of splenic function after splenectomy for trauma. N Engl J Med 1978;298:1389.
215. Traub A, et al. Splenic reticuloendothelial function after splenectomy, spleen repair and spleen autotransplantation. N Engl J Med 1987;317: 559.
216. Steely WM, et al. Comparison of omental splenic autotransplant to partial splenectomy: protective effect against septic death. Am Surg 1987;53:702.
217. Livingston CD, Levine BA, Sirinek KR. Improved survival rate for intraperitoneal autotransplantation of the spleen after pneumococcal pneumonia. Surg Gynecol Obstet 1983;156:761.
218. Moore GE, et al. Failure of splenic implants to protect against fatal postsplenectomy infection. Am J Surg 1983;146:413.
219. Scher KS, Wroczynski AF, Scott-Conner CEH. Intraperitoneal splenic implants do not alter clearance of pneumococcal bacteremia. Am Surg 1985;51:269.
220. Sass W, et al. Overwhelming infection after splenectomy in spite of some spleen remaining and splenosis: a case report. Klin Wochenschr 1983;61:1075.
221. Rice HM, James PD. Ectopic splenic tissue failed to prevent fatal pneumococcal septicemia after splenectomy for trauma. Lancet 1980;1: 565.
222. Jacob HS, McDonald RA, Jandl JH. Regulation of spleen growth and sequestering function. J Clin Invest 1963;42:1476.
223. Bisno AL, Freeman JC. The syndrome of asplenia, pneumococcal sepsis, and disseminated intravascular coagulation. Ann Intern Med 1970;72:389.
224. Heier HE. Splenectomy and serious infections. Scand J Haematol 1980;24:5.
225. Horan M, Colebatch FH. Relation between splenectomy and subsequent infection: a clinical study. Arch Dis Child 1962;37:398.
226. Singer DB. Postsplenectomy sepsis. Perspect Pediatr Pathol 1973;1: 285.
227. Eraklis AJ, et al. Hazards of overwhelming infection after splenectomy in childhood. N Engl J Med 1967;276:1225.
228. Rosner F, Zarrabi MH. Late infections following splenectomy in Hodgkin's disease. Cancer Invest 1983;1:57.
229. Chaikof EL, McCabe CJ. Fatal overwhelming postsplenectomy infection. Am J Surg 1985;149:534.
230. O'Neal BJ, McDonald JC. The risk of sepsis in the asplenic adult. Ann Surg 1981;194:775.
231. Kingston ME, MacKenzie CR. The syndrome of pneumococcaemia, disseminated intraveascular coagulation and asplenia. Can Med Assoc J 1979;121:57.
232. Wara DW. Host defense against Streptococcus pneumoniae: the role of the spleen. Rev Infect Dis 1981;3:299.
233. Barrett-Connor E. Bacterial infection and sickle cell anemia. an analysis of 250 infections in 166 patients and a review of the literature. Medicine 1971;50:97.
234. Mower WR, Hawkins JA, Nelson EW. Postsplenectomy infection in patients with chronic leukemia. Am J Surg 1986;152:583.
235. Askergren J, Bjorkholm M. Postsplenectomy septicaemia in Hodgkin's disease and other disorders. Acta Chir Scand 1980;146:569.
236. Buchanan GR, et al. Bacterial infection and splenic reticuloendothelial function in children with hemoglobin SC disease. Pediatrics 1983; 72:93.
237. Loggie BW, Hinchey J. Does splenectomy predispose to meningococcal sepsis? An experimental study and clinical review. J Pediatr Surg 1986;21:326.
238. Hitzig WH. Immunological and hematological consequences of deficient function of the spleen. Prog Pediatr Surg 1985;18:132.
239. Wahlby L, Domellof L. Splenectomy after blunt abdominal trauma: a retrospective study of 413 children. Acta Chir Scand 1981;147:131.
240. Zarrabi MH, Rosner F. Serious infections in adults following splenectomy for trauma. Arch Intern Med 1984;144:1421.
241. Hicklin H, Verghese A, Alvarez S. Dysgonic fermenter 2 septicemia. Rev Infect Dis 1987;9:884.
242. Israeli A, Shapiro M, Ephros MA. Plasmodium falciparum malaria in an asplenic man. Trans R Soc Trop Med Hyg 1987;81:233.
243. Rosner F, et al. Babesiosis in splenectomized adults: review of 22 reported cases. Am J Med 1984;76:696.
244. Jandl JH, Jones AR, et al. The destruction of red cells by antibodies in man: I. observations on the sequestration and lysis of red cells altered by immune mechanisms. J Clin Invest 1957;36:1428.
245. Carlisle HN, Saslaw S. Properdin levels in splenectomized persons. Proc Soc Exp Biol Med 1959;102:150.
246. Petersen GM, Silimperi DR, Rotter JI, et al. Genetic factors in Haemophilus influenzae type b disease susceptibility and antibody acquisition. J Pediatr 1987;110:228.
247. Siber GR, Santosham M, Reid GR, et al. Impaired antibody response to Haemophilus influenzae type b polysaccharide and low IgG2 and IgG4 concentrations in Apache children. N Engl J Med 1990;323:1387.
248. Hosea SW, Burch CG, Brown EF, et al. Impaired immune response of splenectomized patients to polyvalent pneumococcal vaccine. Lancet 1981;1:804.
249. Gaston MH, Verter JI, Woods G et al. Prophylaxis with oral penicillin in children with sickle cell anemia: a randomized trial. N Engl J Med 1986;314:1593.
250. Chilcote RR, Baehner RL, Hammond D, et al. Septicemia and meningitis in children splenectomized for Hodgkin's disease. N Engl J Med 1980;302:892.
251. Gorse GJ. The relationship of the spleen to infection. In: Bowlder AJ, ed. The spleen: structure, function, and clinical significance. New York, van Nostrand Reinhold, 1990:269.
252. Goodman RA, Ahtone JL, Finton RJ. Prevention of fatal bacterial in-

fection in patients with anatomic or functional asplenia. Ann Intern Med 1982;96:117.
253. Committee on Infectious Diseases. In: Peter G, ed. Immunization in special clinical circumstances: asplenic children. 1994 Red Book. Elk Grove, IL, American Academy of Pediatrics, 1994:57.
254. Rogers ZR, Morrison RA, Vedro DA, et al. Outpatient management of febrile illness in infants and young children with sickle cell anemia. J Pediatr 1990;117:736.
255. Istre GR, et al. Invasive disease due to *Streptococcus pneumoniae* in an area with a high rate of relative penicillin resistance. J Infect Dis 1987;156:732.
256. Zarrabi MH, Rosner F. Rarity of failure of penicillin prophylaxis to prevent postsplenectomy sepsis. Arch Intern Med 1986;146:1207.
257. Pedersen AK, FitzGerald. Dose-related kinetics of aspirin: presystemic acetylation of platelet cyclooxygenase. N Engl J Med 1984;311:1206.
258. Schumacher MJ. Serum immunoglobulin and transferrin levels after childhood splenectomy. Arch Dis Child 1970;45:114.
258a. Robinette CD, Fraumeni JF Jr. Splenectomy and subsequent mortality in veterans of the 1939–45 war. Lancet 1977;2:127.
259. McIntyre OR, Ebaugh FG. Palpable spleens in college freshmen. Arch Int Med 1967;66:301.
260. DeLand FH. Normal spleen size. Radiology 1970;97:589.

7

Red Blood Cells

Blood: Principles and Practice of Hematology,
edited by Robert I. Handin, Samuel E. Lux, and Thomas P. Stossel.
J.B. Lippincott Company, Philadelphia © 1995.

47

Introduction to Anemias

Samuel E. Lux

The chapters that follow, and some earlier chapters (Chaps. 9 to 11), are devoted to specific anemias. This chapter focuses on the classification of anemias and an approach to their diagnosis.

DEFINITION OF ANEMIA

Theoretically, anemia refers to a reduction in red blood cell mass, but practically it refers to a decrease in the hemoglobin (Hb) concentration or the hematocrit (packed red cell volume). The hemoglobin value is more accurate since automated cell counters measure it directly. The hematocrit used to be directly measured and now is usually calculated from the red cell count and the mean corpuscular volume (MCV; see Chap. 2). The hemoglobin concentration also relates more directly to physiologically important measures, like oxygen carrying capacity. Nevertheless, old habits die hard and for many the hematocrit is easier to use.

The normal values of hemoglobin, hematocrit, and MCV for persons at different ages are presented in Table 47-1. The values shown in the neonatal period are for term infants. Premature babies have less time in utero to synthesize red cells and are born with lower hemoglobins and hematocrits (see Chap. 64). The lower limits of normal in the table—2 SD below the mean for each age group—mathematically define 2.5% of the population as anemic. Other findings, such as symptoms or signs of anemia, abnormal red cell indices or morphology, and coexisting leukopenia or thrombocytopenia, help to determine the significance of the hemoglobin and hematocrit.

Conversely, persons who are in the upper normal range when they are well may still be within the "normal" range when anemic. Also, patients with cardiorespiratory diseases or vascular compromise to a vital organ like the heart or brain may sometimes be functionally anemic at hemoglobin values that are technically normal. In both these situations, "anemia" may be recognized only after treatment.

Finally, remember that patients with hemolytic diseases can compensate for red cell destruction to a considerable degree and may have little or no anemia in their usual, steady-state condition. This occurs surprisingly often: about half of children and adults with hereditary spherocytosis have compensated or nearly compensated hemolysis (hemoglobin 12 g/dL or higher in adults[1,2]; see Chap. 54). Such patients may be recognized only when a reticulocyte count is obtained or when other signs or symptoms (such as splenomegaly, jaundice, or cholecystitis) reveal the hemolytic process.

CLASSIFICATION OF ANEMIAS

Anemias are usually classified according to pathophysiology (Table 47-2) or red cell size (Table 47-3). In practice, elements from both classification schemes are often used in differential diagnosis, along with information about red cell morphology (Table 47-4). The pathophysiologic classification divides anemias into four categories: (1) decreased production due to inadequate erythropoietin (such as renal disease) or bone marrow failure (such as aplasias, marrow invasion); (2) disorders of red cell nuclear or cytoplasmic maturation (such as cobalamin, folate, and iron deficiencies; thalassemias); (3) hemolytic anemias; and (4) bleeding. Morphologic classification divides anemias into microcytic, normocytic, and macrocytic groups, based on the MCV, and subdivides them into hemolytic and marrow failure or dysplasia categories. Conflicts arise in each of the schemes, as might be expected.

Thalassemias are disorders of cytoplasmic maturation caused by poor synthesis of one globin chain, but they are also hemolytic anemias caused by membrane damage from the unpaired complementary globin chain. Red cells are macrocytic in patients with many hemolytic anemias because of the presence of reticulocytes, which have a high MCV (about 140 to 150 fL), and young red cells, which are also larger than average. Patients with mild variants of the same hemolytic anemias have lower reticulocyte counts and slightly older cells and may be classified as normocytic. Similarly, patients with severe hemolytic anemias and marked reticulocytosis have normocytic red cells if the underlying disease process causes cellular dehydration, as in hereditary spherocytosis and sickle cell disease. Many other examples are possible. The point is that the classification schemes are not perfect; nevertheless, they are diagnostically useful.

EVALUATION OF ANEMIA

History, Physical Examination, and Initial Laboratory Studies

The initial diagnostic encounter includes a detailed history and physical examination and a minimum of laboratory tests. The features of the history and physical examination

(text continues on page 1388)

TABLE 47-1. Normal Values (Mean and Lower Limit of Normal [−2 SD]) for Hemoglobin, Hematocrit, and Mean Corpuscular Volume at Various Ages

Age	Hemoglobin (g/dL)		Hematocrit (%)		MCV (fL)	
	Mean	−2 SD	Mean	−2 SD	Mean	−2 SD
Cord blood	16.5	13.5	51	42	108	98
1 wk	17.5	13.5	54	42	107	88
2 wk	16.5	12.5	51	39	107	86
1 mo	14.0	10.0	43	31	104	85
2 mo	11.5	9.0	35	28	96	77
3–6 mo	11.5	9.5	35	29	91	74
0.5–2 yr	12.0	10.5	36	33	78	70
2–6 yr	12.5	11.5	37	34	81	75
6–12 yr	13.5	11.5	40	35	86	77
12–18 yr						
Female	14.0	12.0	41	36	90	78
Male	14.5	13.0	43	37	88	78
18–49 yr						
Female	14.0	12.0	41	36	90	80
Male	15.5	13.5	47	41	90	80

MCV, mean corpuscular volume.
(Dallman PR. In: *Pediatrics*, Rudolph A, ed. ed 16, New York, Appleton-Century-Crofts, 1977:1111. Data were compiled from several sources, with emphasis on data obtained with electronic counters, and excluding persons likely to have iron deficiency.)

TABLE 47-2. Pathophysiologic Classification of Anemias

DECREASED PRODUCTION OF RED CELLS RELATIVE TO DEGREE OF ANEMIA

Decreased Erythropoietin Production

Renal disease
Protein malnutrition
Low-affinity hemoglobins
Hypothyroidism
Hypopituitarism

Bone Marrow Failure

Aplastic anemia
- Congenital
  - Fanconi's anemia
  - Shwachman-Diamond syndrome
  - Dyskeratosis congenita
- Acquired
  - Radiation
  - Drugs, chemicals (including alcohol)
  - Viruses: Epstein-Barr virus (EBV), hepatitis
  - Autoimmune disease
  - Pregnancy
  - Preleukemia
  - Paroxysmal nocturnal hemoglobinuria (PNH)
  - Protein malnutrition, anorexia nervosa

Pure red cell aplasia
- Congenital: Diamond-Blackfan anemia
- Acquired
  - Transient erythroblastopenia of childhood
  - Thymoma
  - Lymphoma, chronic lymphocytic leukemia, myeloma
  - Other malignancies
  - Autoimmune diseases
  - Viruses, especially parvovirus B19
  - Drugs

Bone Marrow Invasion (Myelophthisis)

Leukemias, lymphomas
Myeloma, macroglobulinemia
Histiocytosis syndromes
Metastatic tumors (especially breast, prostate, small cell lung, neuroblastoma, melanoma, hypernephroma, seminoma, thyroid, stomach)
Granulomas
Storage diseases (advanced)
Myelofibrosis
Osteopetrosis

DISORDERS OF ERYTHROPOIETIC MATURATION

Defects Involving Nuclear Maturation (Megalobastic Anemias)

Cobalamin (vitamin B_{12}) deficiency
- Inherited disorders in absorption, transport, or cellular metabolism
- Acquired disorders
  - Inadequate intrinsic factor
  - Small bowel disease
  - Dietary deficiencies
  - Drugs (especially N_2O)

Folic acid deficiency
- Inherited defects in absorption or metabolism
- Acquired disorders
  - Dietary deficiency
  - Small bowel disease
  - Increased requirements (pregnancy, hemolysis)
  - Drugs (methotrexate, trimethoprim, pyrimethamine)

Other causes
- Orotic aciduria
- Myelodysplasia
- Erythroleukemia
- Thiamine-responsive anemia
- Pyridoxine-responsive anemia
- Congenital dyserythropoietic anemias (CDA) I and III

Defects Involving Cytoplasmic Maturation

Iron deficiency
- Nutritional deficiency
- Increased requirements (e.g., growth, pregnancy)
- Chronic blood loss (GI, GU, lungs)
- Decreased iron reutilization: anemia of chronic disease
  - Chronic infections (including HIV)

(continued)

- Connective tissue diseases
- Malignancies

Globin deficiency
- α-Thalassemias
- β-Thalassemias
- γ-Thalassemias
- Very unstable hemoglobins

Sideroblastic anemias
- Inherited
- Acquired
  - Alcohol
  - Myelodysplasia, preleukemia
  - Drugs

CDA II or HEMPAS (hereditary erythroblastic multinuclearity with positive acid serum test)

Lead poisoning

HEMOLYTIC ANEMIAS

Extrinsic Defects

Antibody mediated
- Warm antibody, autoimmune
  - Idiopathic
  - Lymphoproliferative diseases
  - Connective tissue diseases
  - Drugs
- Cold antibody, autoimmune
  - Idiopathic
  - Infections: *Mycoplasma*, EBV
  - Lymphoproliferative
- Paroxysmal cold hemoglobinuria
- Neonatal isoimmune
  - Rh(D) hemolytic disease
  - ABO hemolytic disease
  - Other blood group incompatibilities
- Transfusion reactions

Thermal injury: severe burns

Vascular injury (fragmentation syndromes)
- Large blood vessels
  - Replaced valve, prosthesis, grafts
  - Aortic stenosis (severe), regurgitant jets
- Small blood vessels
  - Disseminated intravascular coagulation
  - Thrombotic thrombocytopenic purpura
  - Hemolytic uremic syndrome
  - Preeclampsia/eclampsia
  - Polyarteritis
  - Acute glomerulonephritis, malignant hypertension, allograft rejection
  - Disseminated carcinoma
  - Rickettsial diseases
- Arteriovenous malformations
  - Kasabach-Merritt syndrome
  - Hemangioendotheliomas
- Drugs: mitomycin C, cyclosporine

Mechanical trauma
- March hemoglobinuria
- Cardiopulmonary bypass

Osmotic hemolysis: freshwater drowning

Infections
- Erythrocyte parasites
  - Malaria
  - *Babesia microti*
  - *Bartonella bacilliformis*
- Red cell damage from bacterial products: clostridial sepsis

Venoms, toxins: snakes, spiders

Extrinsic oxidant hemolysis
- Drugs, chemicals
- Copper: acute poisoning, Wilson's disease

Intrinsic Defects

Red cell membrane
- Membrane skeleton
  - Hereditary spherocytosis
  - Hereditary elliptocytosis
  - Hereditary pyropoikilocytosis
- Defective phosphoinositide-based membrane protein anchors: PNH
- Blood group antigen deficiencies: Rh_{null}, McLeod's syndrome, In(Lu)
- Cation permeability disorders
  - Hereditary stomatocytosis
  - Hereditary xerocytosis
- Photooxidation: erythropoietic and hepatoerythropoietic porphyrias
- Membrane lipids
  - Hepatocellular disease: spur cell anemia
  - Lecithin:cholesterol acyltransferase deficiency
  - High phosphatidylcholine hemolytic anemia
  - Vitamin E deficiency
  - Abetalipoproteinemia
  - Tangier disease
- Other presumed membrane disorders
  - Acanthocytosis with neurologic disease and normal lipoproteins
  - Infantile pyknocytosis

Hemoglobin
- Structural defects
  - Unstable hemoglobins (including Hb E)
  - Hemoglobin S
  - Hemoglobins C, D
- Synthesis defects: thalassemia syndromes

Red cell metabolism
- Inherited glycolytic defects
  - Hexokinase
  - Glucose phosphate isomerase
  - Phosphofructokinase
  - Triose phosphate isomerase
  - Phosphoglycerate kinase
  - Pyruvate kinase
- Acquired glycolytic defects
  - Malignancies, myelodysplasia
  - Hypophosphatemia (severe)
- Hexose monophosphate shunt defects: glucose-6-phosphate dehydrogenase deficiency
- Glutathione metabolism defects
- Nucleotide metabolism defects
  - Pyrimidine 5′-nucleotidase
  - Adenylate kinase
  - Adenosine deaminase overproduction

Hypersplenism

Hemophagocytic Syndromes

BLEEDING

Internal

Intracranial: especially premature infants

Cephalohematoma

Pulmonary cavity

Peritoneal, retroperitoneal

External (including GI)

GI, gastrointestinal; GU, genitourinary.

TABLE 47-3. Classification of Anemias by Red Blood Cell Size

MICROCYTIC ANEMIAS

Microcytic–Hypochromic

- Iron deficiency
- Thalassemias
- Anemia of chronic disease*
- Lead poisoning*
- Sideroblastic anemias†
- Very unstable hemoglobins*

Microcytic–Normochromic (Red Cell Fragments)

- Hereditary pyropoikilocytosis
- Homozygous hereditary elliptocytosis

NORMOCYTIC ANEMIAS

Hypoplastic/Dysplastic Bone Marrow

- Aplastic anemias†
  - Radiation, drugs, alcohol
  - Viruses (Epstein-Barr, hepatisis)
  - Autoimmune
  - Pregnancy
  - Preleukemia
  - Paroxysmal nocturnal hemoglobinuria†
  - Anorexia nervosa, starvation
- Myelophthisis (bone marrow invasion) syndromes
  - Leukemias, lymphomas
  - Myelomas, macroglobulinemia
  - Metastatic tumors
  - Granulomas
  - Storage diseases (advanced)
  - Myelofibrosis
  - Osteopetrosis
- Myelodysplastic syndromes

Erythroid Aplasia/Hypoplasia

- Pure red cell aplasia
  - Parvovirus B19
  - Transient erythroblastopenia of childhood
  - Thymoma, lymphoma, CLL
  - Autoimmune
  - Diamond-Blackfan anemia†
- Renal disease
- Liver disease
- Endocrine disease
  - Hypothyroid
  - Hypopituitary
  - Hyperparathyroid
- Anemia of chronic disease
- Early iron deficiency
- Low-affinity hemoglobins

Hemolysis With Ineffective Erythropoiesis: Congenital Dyserythropoietic Anemia, Type II (HEMPAS)

Hemolytic Anemias

- Hemolysis with red cell dehydration
  - Hereditary spherocytosis
  - Sickle cell disease
  - Sickle syndromes
  - Hb C disease
  - Hereditary xerocytosis†
- Hemolysis with mild red cell fragmentation
  - Microangiopathic and macroangiopathic hemolytic anemias
  - Hereditary elliptocytosis
- Mild variants of other hemolytic disorders
- Hypersplenism
- Hemophagocytic syndromes

Bleeding (Recent)

MACROCYTIC ANEMIAS

Hypoplastic Bone Marrow With Stress Erythropoiesis

- Hypoplastic anemias
  - Inherited
    - Fanconi's anemia
    - Dyskeratosis congenita
    - Shwachman-Diamond syndrome
  - Acquired*
- Pure red cell aplasia, especially Diamond-Blackfan anemia

Dysplastic Bone Marrow

- Myelodysplastic syndromes
- Erythroleukemia
- Alcohol toxicity
- Congenital dyserythropoietic anemias I and III

Megaloblastic Bone Marrow

- Cobalamin (vitamin B_{12}) deficiency
- Folic acid deficiency
- Other defects of DNA synthesis
  - Inherited
  - Chemotherapy

With Reticulocytosis

- Hemolysis without red cell dehydration or fragmentation
  - Enzyme disorders
  - Immunohemolysis: warm antibody, cold agglutinin, paroxysmal cold hemoglobinuria
  - Unstable hemoglobins
  - PNH‡
  - Hereditary stomatocytosis
- Hemolysis and macrocytosis despite red cell dehydration: hereditary xerocytosis
- Bleeding (with reticulocytosis)
- Treated cobalamin (vitamin B_{12}) or folate deficiency

* Often normocytic, normochromic.
† Sometimes macrocytic.
‡ Often normocytic due to accompanying aplasia.

TABLE 47-4. Classification of Anemias by Predominant Morphology

SPHEROCYTES

Hereditary spherocytosis*
Immunohemolysis with IgG- or C3-coated red cells*†
Acute oxidant injury (HMP shunt defects during hemolytic crisis, oxidant drugs and chemicals)*
ABO incompatibility in neonates*
Hemolytic transfusion reactions*†
Clostridial sepsis*
Severe burns, other red cell thermal injuries*
Snake venoms*
Severe hypophosphatemia*
Hypersplenism*‡

ELLIPTOCYTES

Hereditary elliptocytosis§
Thalassemias*
Iron deficiency, severe
Sideroblastic anemias
Megaloblastic anemias

BIZARRE POIKILOCYTES

Red cell fragmentation syndromes: microangiopathic and macroangiopathic hemolytic anemias*
Acute oxidant injury*‡
Hereditary elliptocytosis in neonates*‡
Hereditary pyropoikilocytosis*
Homozygous hereditary elliptocytosis*

STOMATOCYTES

Hereditary stomatocytosis*
Hereditary cryohydrocytosis*
Liver disease, especially acute alcoholism
Rh_{null} or Rh_{mod} blood groups*
Adenosine deaminase hyperactivity*‡
Tangier disease‡
Mediterranean stomatocytosis§
Duchenne's muscular dystrophy‡§
Marathon runners‡§

PROMINENT BASOPHILIC STIPPLING

Thalassemias*
Unstable hemoglobinopathies*
Pyridine 5′-nucleotidase deficiency*
Lead poisoning
Sideroblastic anemias

IRREVERSIBLY SICKLED CELLS

Sickle cell anemia*
Symptomatic sickle syndromes*

INTRAERYTHROCYTIC PARASITES

Malaria*
Babesiosis*
Bartonellosis*

SPICULATED OR CRENATED RBCs

Acute hepatic necrosis (spur cell anemia)*
Embden-Meyerhof pathway (glycolytic) defects*‡
Red cell fragmentation syndromes*‡
Uremia‡
McLeod blood group*
In(Lu) blood group§
Abetalipoproteinemia*
Acanthocytosis with neurologic disease and normal lipoproteins§
Postsplenectomy§
Anorexia nervosa
Vitamin E deficiency*‡
Infantile pyknocytosis*
Heat stroke*‡
Transiently after massive transfusion of stored blood
Hypothyroidism

TARGET CELLS

Hemoglobins S, C, D, E*
Obstructive liver disease§
Hereditary xerocytosis*
Thalassemias*
Iron deficiency
Sideroblastic anemias
Postsplenectomy§
Lecithin:cholesterol acyltransferase deficiency

TEARDROP ERYTHROCYTES

Extramedullary hematopoiesis
Myelofibrosis
Neoplastic invasion of the bone marrow‡
Granulomatous diseases involving the bone marrow‡
Osteopetrosis

NONSPECIFIC OR NORMAL MORPHOLOGY

Anemia of chronic diseases
Aplastic anemias
Pure red cell aplasias
Embden-Meyerhof pathway (glycolytic) defects*
HMP shunt defects*
Other red cell enzyme deficiencies*
Unstable hemoglobinopathies*
α-Thalassemia (heterozygous)§
Warm antibody immunohemolytic anemias*†‡
Cold agglutinin disease*†
Rh hemolytic disease in neonates*†
Paroxysmal cold hemoglobinuria*†‡
Paroxysmal nocturnal hemoglobinuria*
Congenital dyserythropoietic anemias*
Hypothyroidism
Hemolysis with infections*‡
Erythrophagocytic disorders*
Wilson's disease*
Hereditary xerocytosis*‡
Erythropoietic or hepatoerythropoietic porphyria*
Vitamin E deficiency*
Hypersplenism*
Leukemias, lymphomas
Refractory anemia, preleukemia‡
Myelomas, macroglobulinemia
Metastatic tumors‡
Storage diseases (advanced)
Granulomatous diseases involving the bone marrow‡
Bleeding

HMP, hexose monophosphate.
* Usually associated with increased red cell destruction.
† Usually associated with a positive Coombs' test.
‡ Disorder sometimes associated with this morphology.
§ Usually no anemia.

relevant to the differential diagnosis of anemias are covered in detail in Chapter 1. The initial laboratory tests should include determinations of the hemoglobin, hematocrit, red cell indices, reticulocyte count, platelet count, white blood cell count and differential, an examination of the peripheral blood smear, and additional studies of the patient or family members that derive from the history and physical examination.

The Blood Smear

In evaluation of anemias, the physician should always examine the blood smear personally and not simply take the word of others regarding the red cell morphology. It is impossible to encompass the subtleties of the smear with terms like *anisocytosis* and *poikilocytosis*. Great care must be taken to ensure that good peripheral blood smears are obtained and that artifact-free areas of the smear are examined. This is a particular problem in very anemic or polycythemic patients (hematocrit less than 15 or more than 65). In these patients, it is sometimes useful to concentrate the red cells by gentle centrifugation and removal of some plasma before preparing the smear. Conversely, in polycythemic patients (or neonates), it is sometimes necessary to dilute a drop of the patient's blood with a drop of plasma (obtained from a hematocrit tube) to prepare a smear with optimal morphology.

The blood film should first be examined under low power to assess the adequacy of staining and to find an optimal site for morphologic study. The best site is usually a few millimeters inside the feather edge of a slide smear and toward the middle of a coverslip smear. Coverslip smears, prepared by an experienced technician, generally provide the best morphology. Unfortunately, such experience is disappearing in our increasingly automated hematology laboratories.

In a satisfactory area, the red cells are separated from each other and central pallor is evident in most of the red cells. This is true even in blood of patients with diseases like hereditary spherocytosis where central pallor is diminished. The red cells should not overlap significantly, or line up in "rouleaux," and they should not deform each other into polygonal shapes, as they often do at the edges of the smear. The red cells also must not be artifactually deformed by excessive water in the stain (the so-called humidity artifact) or peppered by precipitated stain. It cannot be overemphasized that it is risky and often useless to assess red cell morphology on a poorly spread or poorly stained blood smear. Another smear must be prepared.

Target cells, crenated cells, stomatocytes, and spherocytes may be produced by artifact as well as disease. Real findings should be evident in multiple areas of the smear and on multiple smears. Artifactual spherocytes are particularly common and are recognized by their complete loss of central pallor and by the fact that they are larger, not smaller, than normal red cells. It is sometimes useful, particularly with spiculated cells and stomatocytes, to dilute freshly drawn blood into phosphate-buffered saline containing 0.5% glutaraldehyde, place a drop under a coverslip, blot to remove excess liquid, and examine the wet preparation by phase microscopy (or, if necessary, under brightfield conditions with the condenser lowered). Under these conditions, the artifacts and morphologic distortions induced by drying are eliminated.

Semipermanent mounts can be prepared by sealing the coverslips with nail polish. Unfixed wet preps can also be examined, prepared by diluting the patient's blood with his or her own plasma, but the cells must be examined immediately. They gradually change shape because of local pH changes and the so-called glass effect.[3,4]

DIAGNOSTIC APPROACH TO ANEMIA

One useful diagnostic approach is illustrated in Figure 47-1. Anemias are first divided into microcytic, normocytic, and macrocytic categories, according to the MCV.* Each of these categories is subdivided into various pathophysiologic categories, depending on the white cell, platelet, and reticulocyte counts and on whether the bone marrow is hypoplastic, dysplastic, or megaloblastic.

Microcytic Anemias

Microcytic anemias usually result from inadequate hemoglobin synthesis and are characterized by the presence of hypochromic red cells (enlarged central pallor), target cells, and in more severe cases by elliptocytes and other poikilocytes.

Laboratory studies typically include examination of the peripheral blood smear; measurements of serum iron, total iron-binding capacity (TIBC) a measure of the serum transferrin concentration, and serum ferritin; and a hemoglobin electrophoresis. In young children, a blood lead or free erythrocyte protoporphyrin concentration should also be obtained. In some cases, a bone marrow aspirate may also be necessary to assess iron stores and the presence or absence of ringed sideroblasts.

Iron deficiency anemia (see Chap. 49) is by far the most common cause of microcytic anemias. The diagnosis is particularly common in infants from 6 months to 2 years of age and in women of reproductive age. At other ages, iron deficiency is much less common and the physician must carefully confirm the diagnosis and establish its cause. Iron deficiency is only rarely caused by a poor diet in older children and adults who are not obviously malnourished. Chronic gastrointestinal blood loss must always be excluded in adult men and postmenopausal women, and it also must be considered in older children. Infants younger than 6 months of age should have adequate iron stores left over from intrauterine life and should not be iron deficient unless considerable bleeding or blood drawing has occurred.

Typically, the serum iron concentration is low, the TIBC is high, and the iron saturation is less than 10% in persons with iron deficiency anemia[6]; these measurements are unreliable in patients who have recently taken iron supplements. Fortunately, the serum ferritin concentration is almost always low, regardless of the history of iron therapy.[7]

Although *lead poisoning* (see Chap. 50) is always included in the differential diagnosis of hypochromic–microcytic anemias, anemia is a late complication of lead intoxication and may be normocytic as well as microcytic. In many patients, the anemia of lead poisoning is actually due to concomitant iron deficiency. Both diseases occur in the same age children, and some evidence exists that iron deficiency may exacerbate the pathophysiology of lead.[8] For these reasons, all children with either disease should be tested for the other disease.

β-Thalassemia major and *β-thalassemia intermedia* (see Chap. 51) are severe conditions that usually become evident between 6 and 18 months of life. The marked microcytic anemia, splenomegaly, and bony changes of β-

* It is important to remember that children have lower MCVs than adults do (see Table 47-1). From 1 to 6 years of age, the lower limit of normal is approximated by $MCV_{lower\ limit}$ = 69 fL + (age in years); after that, the limit rises about 1 fL every other year until the lower adult limit (80 fL) is reached.[5] The upper limit for the MCV rises linearly (0.6 fL/y) from 84 fL at 1 year to the upper limit of normal for adults (96 fL).[5]

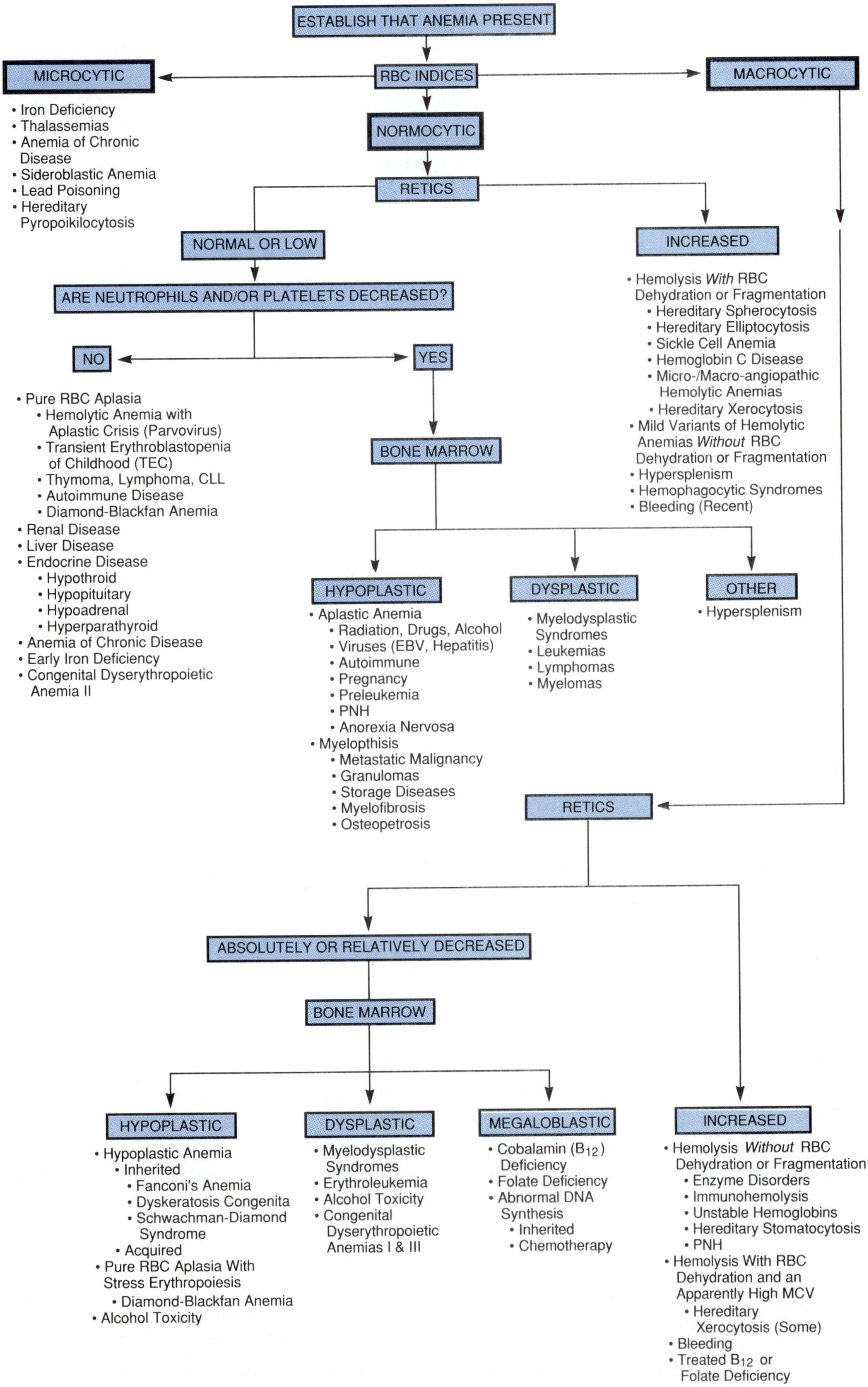

FIGURE 47-1. Diagnostic approach to anemias.

thalassemia major or intermedia and the presence of thalassemia trait in both parents make the diagnosis relatively easy, although subsequent complications can pose many diagnostic dilemmas.

β-Thalassemia trait (see Chap. 51) is a common condition and must often be distinguished from other mild hypochromic–microcytic anemias, especially iron deficiency and the anemia of chronic disease. Plasma color (observed in a spun hematocrit tube) is frequently clear in iron deficiency, but is a normal (straw) color or even abnormally yellow (due to increased bilirubin) in thalassemia trait. The blood smear also provides clues. Poikilocytosis ("animal cracker" cells) and basophilic stippling are more pronounced in thalassemia trait than iron deficiency when patients with the same degree of anemia are compared. The red cell count is increased in patients with thalassemia trait compared with that of those with iron deficiency, which is the basis of the Mentzer index (MCV/red cell count; less than 13 in thalassemia trait, more than 13 in iron deficiency)[9] and the England and Fraser index (MCV − red cell count − [5 × Hb] − 8.4; negative in thalassemia trait, positive in iron deficiency),[10] which attempt to differentiate the two diseases. Most patients with thalassemia trait also have an increased Hb A2 (and less reliably an increased Hb F [fetal Hb]), have a parent with microcytosis, and have normal or increased serum iron and ferritin values.[11] It is important to remember that the elevation in Hb A2 is muted by iron deficiency and is not observed in forms of thalassemia that involve the δ chain (such as δβ-thalassemia).

Patients with *α-thalassemia trait* (see Chap. 51) also have microcytosis, usually without anemia, and a normal hemoglobin electrophoresis. A definitive diagnosis of αDthalassemia requires DNA analysis of the α-globin loci. This is not routinely available and is rarely needed.

The *anemia of chronic disease* (see Chap. 59) is often the most difficult disease to diagnose in this category. In most patients, diagnosis can be made only by exclusion. Classically, the disorder is characterized by mild to moderate anemia, a low or low-normal serum iron concentration, a low TIed cell, an iron saturation higher than 10%, and an elevated serum ferritin[12]; some of these features are often missing. The bone marrow exam demonstrates adequate iron stores. The MCV is only mildly decreased in patients with anemia of chronic disease, less so than in those with iron deficiency or thalassemia trait, and it is often normocytic.

Sideroblastic anemias (see Chaps. 12 and 49) are characterized by failure to incorporate iron into heme. The serum iron and ferritin concentrations are normal to high, and the iron binding capacity is normal or mildly decreased.[13] Usually X-linked, the inherited sideroblastic anemias present in childhood are rare. Acquired forms, caused by alcohol, isoniazid, and other drugs and especially myelodysplasia, occur in adults. Some patients have the classic dimorphic blood smear (hypochromic–microcytic erythrocytes coexisting with normally hemoglobinized cells or even macrocytes), but many do not. The diagnosis of sideroblastic anemia is confirmed by demonstrating ringed sideroblasts on a Prussian blue (iron) stain of the bone marrow aspirate.

Finally, patients with extreme red cell fragmentation may also present with microcytosis. The best examples are hereditary pyropoikilocytosis and homozygous hereditary elliptocytosis (see Chap. 54), in which MCV counts in the 50s are reported, despite reticulocytosis.[14] It is surprising that the microangiopathic hemolytic anemias that occur in disseminated intravascular coagulation, thrombotic thrombocytopenic purpura, hemolytic–uremic syndrome, and a variety of other diseases are usually not microcytic. The percentages of fragmented cells (typically 5% to 20%) are too small to affect the MCV. Anemias characterized by severe red cell dehydration, such as homozygous Hb C disease, may also have a slightly low MCV, although generally they are classified as normocytic anemias.

Macrocytic Anemias With Normal or Low Reticulocyte Count

Macrocytic anemias are first subdivided according to the reticulocyte count. Patients with reticulocytosis and macrocytosis usually have bleeding or hemolysis and are considered in the section on hemolytic anemias. Macrocytosis results from the large size of reticulocytes (MCV of about 140 to 150 fL). Patients with macrocytosis and a normal to low reticulocyte count (relative to the degree of anemia) have disorders characterized by inadequate red cell production, which can be further subdivided into bone marrow failure syndromes and megaloblastic anemias. Macrocytosis in bone marrow failure syndromes is caused by stress erythropoiesis, that is, the production of red cells with characteristics of fetal erythrocytes (large size, increased Hb F and i antigen).[15] Many classification schemes also group hypothyroidism and liver disease among the macrocytic anemias, but both diseases are more commonly associated with normocytic morphology.[16–18]

Initial blood studies should include serum (and possibly red cell) folate measurements, a serum cobalamin assay, and a bone marrow aspirate and biopsy. Patients who have macrocytosis and evidence of marrow failure should always have a bone marrow examination unless the diagnosis is clear from history (such as chemotherapeutic agents, AZT) or laboratory studies (such as folate deficiency). Additional studies will be dictated by the history, physical examination, and age of the patient and may include bone marrow chromosomes; diepoxybutane test[19] and radiographic studies for Fanconi's anemia; tests for evidence of stress erythropoiesis (Hb F, red cell i antigen); red cell adenosine deaminase activity (increased in Diamond-Blackfan anemia [DBA])[20]; bone marrow special stains (iron, periodic acid-Schiff, and others) for evidence of sideroblastic, erythroleukemic, or other myelodysplastic features; blood alcohol concentration; liver function tests; Schilling test; serum anti-IF and other autoantibodies; gastric hydrochloric acid secretion test; or a therapeutic trial of cobalamin or folic acid.

Megaloblastic disorders, such as cobalamin (vitamin B_{12}) deficiency, folic acid deficiency, and inherited disorders of DNA metabolism, often leave diagnostic clues in the peripheral blood smear, particularly hypersegmented polymorphonuclear leukocytes and macroovalocytes. They damage all rapidly proliferating cells—neutrophils and megakaryocytes as well as erythrocytes—and may cause pancytopenia. Uncomplicated megaloblastic anemias are relatively easy to recognize, especially if the bone marrow is examined; however, some conditions that lead to megaloblastic hematopoiesis also cause gastrointestinal bleeding and iron deficiency (such as cirrhosis, alcoholism), which can mask macrocytosis and some of the megaloblastic morphology. Fortunately, the leukocyte changes (giant metamyelocytes and hypersegmented neutrophils) are not altered and serve as a marker to the underlying condition.[21]

In addition to its effects on gastric mucosa and the liver, *alcohol* (see Chap. 59) can also cause anemia through a direct toxic effect on the bone marrow. This is manifested by vacuolization of erythroid precursors[22] and a mild macrocytosis[23] that persists for several weeks after withdrawal of alcohol,[24] or by dysplastic features (megaloblastic changes and ringed sideroblasts).[25]

In adults with macrocytic anemia, the most difficult diagnostic challenge is identification of *myelodysplastic syndromes* (see Chap. 12). The typical picture is an elderly patient with macrocytosis and bi- or pancytopenia combined with a normocellular or hypercellular bone marrow, dysplastic features in one or more cell lines and, in some patients, excess myeloblasts. The dysplastic features in the erythroid series include the megaloblastic attributes, multinuclearity, nuclear budding, and internuclear bridging, and ringed sideroblasts. Disordered myelopoiesis (such as left-shifted maturation, hypogranulation, pseudo–Pelger-Huët cells, Auer rods) and megakaryocytopoiesis (such as micromegakaryocytes, nuclear–cytoplasmic asynchrony) are also common.[26] Clonal cytogenetic abnormalities are found in 40% to 70% of patients.[27]

In children, macrocytic anemias are more often due to bone marrow failure. Megaloblastic anemias and myelodysplastic syndromes occur but are uncommon. Hypoplastic anemias may be either macrocytic or normocytic (see Chaps. 9 and 10). In general, they are macrocytic when the marrow insult is chronic and mild enough so that a patient can produce some red cells, but less than normal. Under these conditions of stress erythropoiesis, the red cells have fetal characteristics, including macrocytosis and the presence of increased Hb F and i antigen.[15] In patients with severe aplastic anemia, virtually no erythropoiesis occurs and the anemia is normocytic and normochromic.

Acquired aplastic anemias are often severe and normocytic, whereas congenital marrow failure syndromes are typically macrocytic. *Fanconi's anemia* (see Chap. 9), the most common syndrome, is characterized by pancytopenia, recessive inheritance, physical anomalies (especially hyperpigmentation, café-au-lait spots, microsomy, microcephaly, thumb and radial anomalies, hypogenitalia, and renal malformations), and increased chromosomal breaks (see Chap. 9). The latter occur spontaneously, but are especially common after clastogenic agents, such as diepoxybutane.[19] This forms the basis for a sensitive diagnostic test. The clinician must remember that Fanconi's anemia can present in young adults as well as children (up to 35 years) and occurs fairly often without physical defects (about 25%)[28] or with subtle defects that can be detected only by an astute observer (such as loss of radial pulses or hypoplasia of the first metacarpal or of the thenar eminence).

Shwachman-Diamond syndrome (see Chap. 9) begins in infancy as bicytopenia or pancytopenia, combined with pancreatic insufficiency (fat malabsorption, failure to thrive), short stature, and, in some patients, metaphyseal dysostosis[29,30] (see Chap. 9).

Dyskeratosis congenita (see Chap. 9) is an X-linked form of ectodermal dysplasia and pancytopenia that presents from infancy to about 30 years. The characteristic dermatologic features are reticulated hyperpigmentation of skin, dystrophic nails, and leukoplakia.

Syndromes of pure red cell aplasia, like the aplastic anemias, are usually normocytic when acquired and macrocytic when congenital. Diamond-Blackfan anemia, an uncommon but not rare congenital disorder, classically presents in infancy (1 year or earlier) with macrocytic anemia, reticulocytopenia, selective absence of erythroid precursors beyond proerythroblasts, and sometimes (about 25%) physical anomalies of various types.[31] Only about 30% of patients have an increased MCV at presentation, presumably because red cell production is so suppressed that even stress erythropoiesis cannot occur. As expected, almost all patients are macrocytic during recovery. For unknown reasons, adenosine deaminase activity is increased in DBA erythrocytes.[20] This can be a useful differentiating point in distinguishing DBA from transient *erythroblastopenia of childhood* (TEC; see Chap. 9), a more common cause of childhood red cell aplasia. TEC typically occurs in toddlers and children (1 year or older) who previously had normal hemoglobin levels. It is a normocytic anemia with reticulocytopenia and marrow erythroblastopenia at presentation, although macrocytosis is observed during recovery, which occurs usually within 1 to 2 months.

Normocytic Anemias With Normal or Low Reticulocyte Count

Normocytic anemias with an increased reticulocyte count are due to red cell destruction (hemolysis) or bleeding and are discussed in the following section. Anemias with normal or low reticulocyte counts are due to bone marrow failure (see Fig. 47-1 and Table 47-3). The differential diagnosis includes many of the disorders described in the previous sections. Under certain circumstances, particularly early in the disease, patients with iron deficiency, anemia of chronic disease, lead poisoning, acquired sideroblastic anemias, DBA, and myelodysplastic syndromes may have a normocytic anemia. Patients with combinations of disease that balance and camouflage each other, such as iron deficiency and cobalamin or folate deficiency, may also be normocytic, as may mild variants of hemolytic anemias that are macrocytic when reticulocyte counts are high. Thus, knowing that red cell size is normal is not as useful diagnostically as knowing that red cells are large or small. Some conditions are typically normocytic and deserve special consideration in the workup of anemias in this category.

Patients with normocytic anemia and low reticulocyte counts should be further categorized depending on whether the granulocyte and platelet counts are normal or low. Those with bi- or pancytopenia often have serious diseases and require a thorough workup, including a bone marrow aspirate and biopsy, and often chromosome studies. Patients with isolated anemia and reticulocytopenia should also have a bone marrow examination if the condition is severe.

By definition, an empty or markedly hypoplastic bone marrow represents *aplastic anemia* (see Chap. 10). Aplastic anemia has many causes (see Table 47-2). In addition to drugs, radiation, toxins, and relatively obvious conditions like anorexia nervosa and postpregnancy aplasia, the physician must consider viruses (especially hepatitis viruses and Epstein-Barr virus), autoimmune pancytopenia, hypoplastic preleukemia (often clonal), and paroxysmal nocturnal hemoglobinuria (positive sugar water and Ham tests; see Chap. 11). In addition, in children and young adults, congenital bone marrow failure syndromes must be considered, although most patients with these syndromes have macrocytosis.

Myelophthisis is a term used to classify disorders that interfere with normal hematopoiesis due to the accumulation of malignant or reactive cells or cell products. These include malignancies of cells that are intrinsic to the marrow, such as leukemias (see Chaps. 18, 27, and 28), lymphomas (see Chaps. 29 and 30), myelomas (see Chap. 31), macroglobulinemias (see Chap. 31), and histiocytoses (see Chap. 32) and metastatic tumors. In the latter category, neuroblastomas, melanomas, seminomas, and a variety of carcinomas (breast, prostate, thyroid, stomach, renal, and small cell lung) are especially likely to involve the marrow. Myelophthisis can also be produced by granulomatous diseases, such as disseminated tuberculosis, histoplasmosis, or sarcoid; myelofibrosis (agnogenic myelofibrosis with myeloid metaplasia; see Chap. 13); disseminated vasculitis; storage diseases in advanced stages; and osteopetrosis (see Chap. 9), a rare defect of osteoclasts in which bone overgrowth occludes the marrow cavity. In addition to cytopenias, myelophthisic processes are usually accompanied by a characteristic blood smear featuring various combinations of teardrop erythrocytes, poikilocytes, nucleated erythrocytes, immature myeloid cells, and giant platelets or megakaryocyte fragments—the so-called leukoerythroblastic blood smear.[32,33] Leukoerythroblastosis is also observed in patients with severe hypoxia or acidosis, especially infants; in diseases in which extramedullary hematopoiesis occurs without myelophthisis (such as thalassemia major (see Chap. 51) and erythroblastosis fetalis (see Chap. 64); with intrauterine infections (syphilis, cytomegalovirus, herpes simplex virus, rubella, and toxoplasmosis); with bacterial or fungal osteomyelitis (rarely); and with the transient myeloproliferative disease associated with Down's syndrome in infancy (see Chap. 18).

Isolated cytopenias or pancytopenia in a patient with splenomegaly may also be due to *hypersplenism*. Usually, the spleen is large enough to be detected on physical examination; often it is massive, but ultrasound detection occasionally is required. The thrombocytopenia and neutropenia are caused by splenic pooling and are generally not severe unless underlying disease also contributes to the splenomegaly. Bone marrow examination shows normocellularity or hypercellularity of all lines, without dysplasia, unless the marrow is also affected by the underlying disease. Indium-111 platelet survival studies can aid in the diagnosis by showing reduced platelet recovery and a normal platelet survival, the characteristics of platelet pooling.

Patients with normocytic anemia and reticulocytopenia with *normal* neutrophil and platelet counts may have pure red cell aplasia or anemias secondary to certain systemic diseases (renal disease, liver disease, endocrine disease, or anemia of chronic disease). *Acquired pure red cell aplasia* (see Chap. 10) may develop as a primary autoimmune disease, with antibody-mediated or T-cell–mediated marrow inhibition, and as a secondary condition, in association with thymomas (5% to 10% of thymomas), lymphomas, leukemias (especially chronic lymphocytic leukemia), myelofibrosis, systemic lupus erythematosus, rheumatoid arthritis, and a variety of other conditions.[34] Erythroblasts are almost completely lacking from the bone marrow. Other cell lines are normal.

Transient erythroblastosis of childhood (TEC) probably represents a temporary immune reaction to erythroid precursors, perhaps stimulated by childhood viral infections, although this has been difficult to prove. A transient form of red cell aplasia also occurs in older children and adults from drugs[34] or viruses, especially B19 parvovirus.[35] Parvovirus infections rarely produce significant anemia in normal individuals, but they can cause life threatening aplastic crises in persons with chronic hemolytic anemias (see Chap. 10).

The anemia of *renal disease* (see Chap. 59) is complex. It is primarily an erythropoietin deficiency state, but bleeding, microangiopathic hemolysis, and hyperparathyroidism may also be contributors.[36]

Liver disease (see Chap. 59) also produces a normocytic anemia, partly caused by hemodilution and hypersplenism; its complications may lead to either macrocytosis (such as folate deficiency, alcoholism, spur cell hemolysis) or microcytosis (such as chronic gastrointestinal blood loss). Hyperbilirubinemia, increased lactate dehydrogenase (LDH), and decreased haptoglobin all may result from liver disease and not be caused by hemolysis.

Hypopituitarism, hypothyroidism, and *hyperparathyroidism* are associated with anemia (see Chap. 59), which is usually normocytic, although patients with hypothyroidism may have macrocytic red cells. Whether this is due to accompanying pernicious anemia or is a direct effect of the lack of hormone is unclear.

HEMOLYTIC ANEMIAS

Presentation, History, and Physical Examination

Most of the signs and symptoms of anemia and hemolysis are well known to physicians and do not require detailed discussion. It is important to remember that patients with chronic hemolysis often have little or no anemia as a result of bone marrow compensation and that those who are anemic often are asymptomatic until hemoglobin levels fall to 8 g/dL or lower because of adjustments in the cardiovascular system and in hemoglobin–oxygen dissociation[37] (see Chap. 52). This is particularly true in children.[38] It is also important to remember that patients with acute hemolysis may present with unusual symptoms such as isolated dizziness or fainting or with symptoms resembling an acute febrile illness, including headache, fever, shaking chills, vomiting, diarrhea, and abdominal or back pain. The latter symptoms are particularly likely with disorders producing acute intravascular hemolysis (Table 47-5), but may be seen as part of the picture of a hemolytic crisis in any chronic hemolytic anemia.

In patients with suspected hemolysis, special attention should be directed toward the family history and toward defining whether the process is acute or chronic, congenital or acquired. A history of consanguinity, anemia, jaundice, splenomegaly, splenectomy, and gallbladder disease should

TABLE 47-5. Hemolytic Anemias With Predominantly Intravascular Destruction and Hemoglobinuria

IMMUNOHEMOLYTIC ANEMIAS
Hemolytic transfusion reactions*
Paroxysmal cold hemoglobinuria
Acute onset autoimmune hemolytic anemia*
ACUTE OXIDANT HEMOLYSIS
Glucose-6-phosphate dehydrogenase deficiency (after infections, drugs, favism)*
Oxidant drugs, chemicals
PAROXYSMAL NOCTURNAL HEMOGLOBINURIA
RED CELL FRAGMENTATION SYNDROMES
Cardiac hemolytic anemia
Disseminated intravascular coagulation
March hemoglobinuria
CERTAIN INFECTIONS
Clostridial sepsis
Blackwater fever in falciparum malaria
SEVERE BURNS AND OTHER RED CELL THERMAL INJURIES
CHEMICALS AND TOXINS
Copper toxicity*
Snake venoms
Arsine poisoning
Water: osmotic hemolysis (freshwater drowning, infusion of hypotonic solutions)

* Sometimes associated with intravascular hemolysis.

be sought through several generations. Unstable hemoglobins, hemolytic anemia with elevated red cell adenosine deaminase,[39] and certain membrane diseases (hereditary spherocytosis, hereditary elliptocytosis, hereditary stomatocytosis, hereditary xerocytosis) are dominantly inherited and may be discovered in abundance when family studies are pursued (Table 47-6). Neonatal jaundice is common in patients with congenital hemolytic anemias (as is present by history in half the patients with hereditary spherocytosis) but may be dismissed as "physiologic."[40] Subsequent jaundice is often mild or transiently present in association with viral illnesses and may be ignored unless it is brought out by careful questioning.

Diagnosis of Hemolysis

Hemolysis, in the steady state, is characterized by evidence of both increased red cell production and destruction. Many tests are available for assessing each of these processes, but only a few are really useful.

Tests for Increased Red Cell Destruction

The most widely used test for detecting hemolysis is the test for unconjugated (indirect) serum *bilirubin* level. In general, a level over 1 mg/dL is considered abnormal. Nonhemolytic causes of unconjugated hyperbilirubinemia are discussed in Chapter 50. With the exception of the neonatal period, *unconjugated bilirubin concentrations in patients with hemolytic anemia do not exceed 4 mg/dL unless hepatic disease coexists.*[41] Unfortunately, the test is only moderately sensitive because the normal range for unconjugated bilirubin is so great.[41] For example, 25% of patients with hereditary spherocytosis[42] and almost 50% of patients with immunohemolytic anemia[43] have normal bilirubin levels.

TABLE 47-6. Anemias With a Dominant or X-Linked Pattern of Inheritance

AUTOSOMAL DOMINANT
Membrane Disorders
Hereditary spherocytosis
Hereditary elliptocytosis
Hereditary stomatocytosis and cryohydrocytosis
Hereditary xerocytosis
Hemoglobin Disorders
Unstable hemoglobinopathies
Heterozygous thalassemias
Hemoglobins with diminished oxygen affinity
Metabolic Disorders
Adenosine deaminase overproduction
Disorders of Red Cell Production or Maturation
Diamond-Blackfan syndrome*
Congenital dyserythropoietic anemia, type III
Osteopetrosis, benign form
X-LINKED RECESSIVE
Metabolic Disorders
Glucose-6-phosphate dehydrogenase deficiency
Phosphoglycerate kinase deficiency
Disorders of Red Cell Production or Maturation
Congenital sideroblastic anemia*
Dyskeratosis congenita
Other Diseases
X-linked lymphoproliferative syndrome

* Sometimes associated with this pattern of inheritance.

The most sensitive test for red cell destruction is the serum *haptoglobin* concentration (see Chap. 50). In most patients, haptoglobin is absent from the plasma when the rate of red cell destruction exceeds twice normal, regardless of diagnosis.[44] The haptoglobin test is very sensitive. In one large family with mild hereditary elliptocytosis and no detectable hyperbilirubinemia, 92% had low haptoglobin levels.[45] The usefulness of haptoglobin determinations is complicated by the fact that the haptoglobin is an acute-phase reactant and its *concentration may be normal, despite hemolysis,* in patients with coexisting acute inflammation or malignancy or in patients taking androgens.[44] This problem may be remedied if haptoglobin levels are compared with those of other acute-phase reactants (such as α_1-antitrypsin or orosomucoid), but these controls are not always available. In addition, haptoglobin is not a useful measure of hemolysis in the neonatal period, since it is usually absent or diminished during the first few months of life.[46] Normal adult haptoglobin concentrations are not reached until the infant is about 4 months of age.[47] Hereditary absence of haptoglobin is uncommon in white subjects but is found in about 4% of American blacks for unknown reasons.[48]

Hemoglobinemia, hemoglobinuria, and hemosiderinuria are useful measures of hemolysis when red cell destruction is intravascular (see Table 47-5). *Plasma hemoglobin* is readily detectable by visual observation when the concentration exceeds about 50 mg/dL (normal is less than 5 mg/dL). The color may range from pink to brown, depending on the relative concentration of hemoglobin (red), bilirubin (yellow–green), methemoglobin (brown), and methemalbumin (brown). Hemoglobin that passes through the glomerulus is reabsorbed by proximal tubular cells (threshold is about 100 to 150 mg/dL), where it is metabolized and the iron stored as ferritin and hemosiderin. Hemoglobinuria occurs if this reabsorption capacity is exceeded; it is characterized by heme-positive urine in the presence of red cells. Care must be taken to examine freshly voided specimens, since hemolysis may occur in dilute urine on standing. The color varies from pink to red to brown to almost black ("coca-cola urine").

Myoglobinuria gives a similar color but it can be differentiated from hemoglobinuria by electrophoresis, gel filtration chromatography, or spectrophotometry or by the fact that myoglobin remains in solution in fresh urine that is 80% saturated with ammonium sulfate.[49] Inspection of the plasma (such as in a hematocrit tube) is also useful since myoglobin, because of its low molecular weight (17 kd, compared with 68 kd for hemoglobin) is rapidly filtered by the kidneys and does not accumulate to visibly detectable levels. In addition, myoglobin does not bind to haptoglobin, so haptoglobin levels remain normal.[50]

Even after intravascular hemolysis abates, iron-laden renal tubular cells continue to be sloughed, sometimes for months, and may be detected as *urine hemosiderin.*[51] This is a useful test because it is simple, reliable, and sensitive and because it permits detection of intermittent intravascular hemolysis (such as in paroxysmal nocturnal hemoglobinuria), but it may be negative in the first few days after a hemolytic episode.[52] In the usual qualitative test, a smear of cells, prepared from the urine sediment, is stained with Prussian blue (as for bone marrow iron). Hemosiderinuria also occurs in patients with hemosiderosis or hemochromatosis.

The serum *LDH* level is elevated in many hemolytic anemias, especially with intravascular hemolysis or ineffective erythropoiesis, because of the release of the red cell isoenzyme (LDH-2).[53] Comparisons of the sensitivity of this

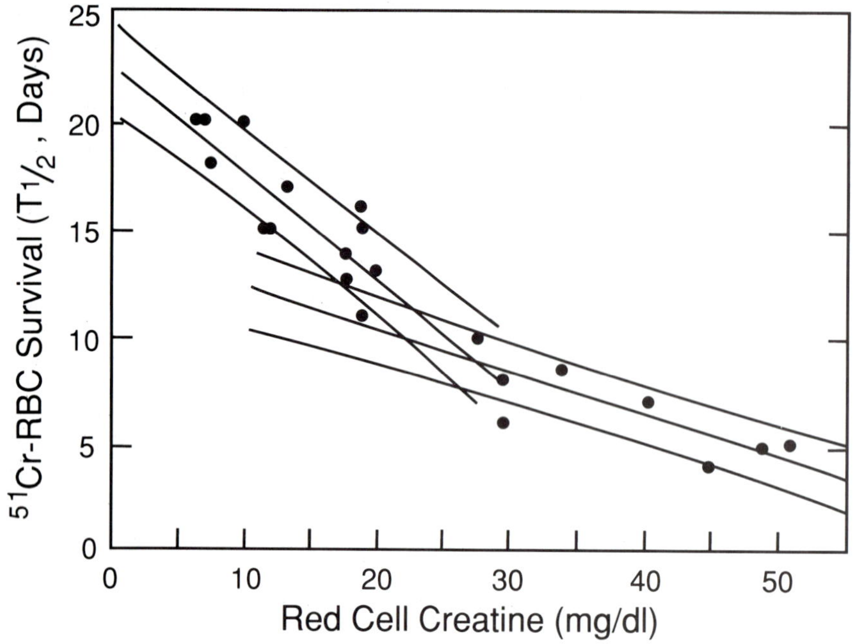

FIGURE 47-2. Relation of mean red cell creatine concentration and red cell survival, measured as the half-life of ^{51}Cr-labeled erythrocytes (normal, 25 to 31 days; regression lines ± 1 SD). (After Fehr J, Knob M. Comparison of red cell creatine level and reticulocyte count in appraising the severity of hemolytic processes. Blood 1979;53:966)

readily available test relative to other tests of hemolysis have been made in patients with selected hemolytic anemias such as cardiac hemolysis, but its usefulness in many hemolytic anemias is unknown. One extensive study compared haptoglobin, red cell hemoglobin, plasma hemoglobin, LDH, schistocyte counts, transferrin levels, and urine hemosiderin in 1091 patients and concluded that the haptoglobin level is the most sensitive test, but the serum LDH concentration value is best for quantitating intravascular hemolysis.[54] Another study found haptoglobin and LDH levels to be similarly sensitive, but each was less sensitive than the chromium-51 (^{51}Cr)–red cell life-span.[55]

Another useful test is that for red cell *creatine* concentration.[56] Its concentration correlates closely with red cell life-span, even in patients with mild hemolysis (Fig. 47-2). It is easily measured, the measurement requires little blood (0.1 to 0.2 mL), and the blood may be stored at 4°C for up to 1 week.

Other tests are available for assessing red cell destruction but are rarely needed. Tests for methemalbumin and hemopexin concentrations are insufficiently sensitive, and fecal urobilinogen levels are insufficiently practical to be useful.[57,58] Carbon monoxide production tests can be precise and sensitive, but they are difficult to perform and require special apparatus.[59] Carboxyhemoglobin tests are an indirect measure of carbon monoxide production, but are less sensitive. ^{51}Cr-labeled red cell life-span measurements are the gold standard. They are sensitive and can be valuable, but they are time-consuming and expensive and are only rarely required.

Tests for Increased Red Cell Production

The most useful test for assessing red cell production and generally for detecting hemolysis is the *reticulocyte count*. Expressed as a percentage of the red cell count, the normal range is about 0.5% to 1.5%. It is difficult to use the percentage of reticulocytes to make accurate estimates of red cell production in anemic patients because the value is increased by the fall in red cell count (the denominator) and the premature, erythropoietin-induced release of bone marrow reticulocytes (identifiable on smears by their polychromatophilia), which take longer to mature in the circulation. The reticulocyte production index (RPI) takes these factors into account and has been shown to correlate closely with ferrokinetic studies of red cell turnover.[60] The usual formula for RPI corrects the hematocrit to a normal of 45%:

$$\text{RPI} = \frac{\text{\% reticulocytes}}{\text{reticulocyte maturation time (days)}} \times \frac{\text{hematocrit}}{45}$$

The maturation time of the reticulocyte in the circulation is taken to be 1 day at a hematocrit value of 45%, 1.5 days at 35%, 2 days at 25%, and 2.5 days at 15%. Unfortunately, this formula is not standardized for women or children,

TABLE 47-7. Conditions Mistaken for Hemolytic Anemia

ANEMIA AND UNCONJUGATED HYPERBILIRUBINEMIA WITHOUT RETICULOCYTOSIS
Internal bleeding
Ineffective erythropoiesis
UNCONJUGATED HYPERBILIRUBINEMIA WITHOUT ANEMIA OR RETICULOCYTOSIS
Defective bilirubin conjugation: neonates, Crigler-Najjar and Arias syndromes
Breast milk jaundice
Gilbert's syndrome
ANEMIA AND RETICULOCYTOSIS WITHOUT HYPERBILIRUBINEMIA
Bleeding
Recovery from aplastic or nutritional (iron, vitamin B_{12}, folate) anemia
LEUKOERYTHROBLASTOSIS
Marrow invasion (myelophthisis): neoplastic disease, granulomas, myelofibrosis, osteopetrosis
Severe hypoxia or acidosis (especially in infants)
MYOGLOBINURIA
DECREASED HAPTOGLOBIN WITHOUT HEMOLYSIS
Normal neonate
Congenital haptoglobin deficiency

whose normal hematocrit levels are less than 45%.[5] The error is not serious, considering the limited accuracy of the method. Thus, in a 40-year-old man with a hematocrit level of 25% and reticulocytes of 15%, the RPI = 15/2 × 25/45 = 4.2, indicating that the red cell production rate is about four times normal. In general, anemias are due to hemolysis if the RPI exceeds about 2.5. In practice; the RPI is a very sensitive indicator of relative hypoproduction, and it is particularly useful in detecting an early aplastic crisis. The RPI may be misleading in the initial assessment of hemolysis, presumably because patients are often evaluated during illnesses. For example, if the RPI is calculated for patients with hereditary spherocytosis, using the extensive data of Emerson and associates,[61] only 67% had an RPI greater than 2.5 on their initial evaluation.

In patients with severe hemolysis, nucleated red cells may appear in the peripheral blood and granulocytosis and thrombocytosis may develop; in such patients, the reticulocyte count is almost always elevated. More sophisticated measures for assessing red cell production such as the bone marrow examination or ferrokinetic studies are rarely needed.

Diagnostic Problems

Patients with evidence of either increased red cell destruction or increased erythropoiesis (not both) may cause diagnostic difficulties. Conditions to consider are listed in Table 47-7.

Hemolysis in the Neonate

Hemolysis may be difficult to document in the first few days of life because indirect hyperbilirubinemia is common and multifaceted during this period and serum haptoglobin levels are depressed.[46] Generally, the reticulocyte count is

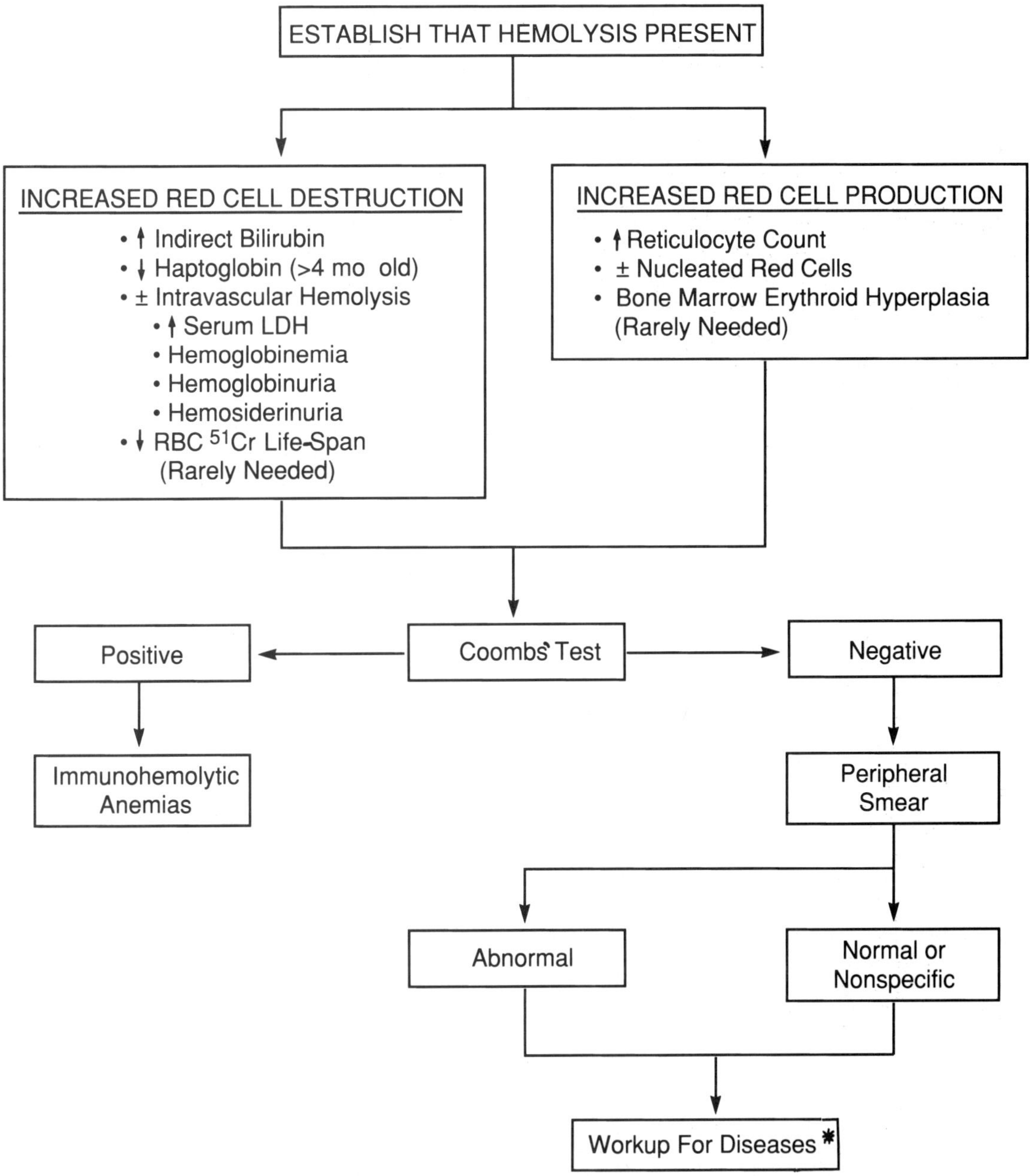

FIGURE 47-3. Diagnostic approach to hemolytic anemias. *See Table 47-4 for diseases included in workup.

the most useful parameter. The reticulocytosis evident in cord blood and during the first day of life (3% to 7%) normally falls to less than 3% by day 3 and to less than 1% by day 7 as a result of the termination of erythropoiesis.[62] Reticulocytosis usually persists in the presence of severe hemolysis (often with nucleated red cells) but may be unimpressive in neonates with only mild to moderate hemolysis.[63] Unfortunately, anoxia, infection, and acidosis also stimulate reticulocytes and nucleated red cells in neonates, and blood drawing may produce enough anemia to induce reticulocytosis and simulate hemolysis. To make matters worse, poikilocytes are common in normal neonatal blood smears (see Chap. 64), particularly in premature infants, and subtle morphologic defects can easily be missed. Fortunately, time is on the side of the diagnostician. Within a few months, fetal red cells disappear, the blood smear becomes simpler to interpret, and hemoglobin, bilirubin, haptoglobin, and reticulocyte levels come to equilibrium.

Initial Evaluation of the Hemolytic Process

Patients with documented hemolysis are separated into a Coombs' test–positive group (immunohemolytic anemias) and a Coombs' test–negative group. The latter group is then further divided, depending on whether the blood smear is characterized by a predominant red cell morphology (smear "abnormal" in Fig. 47-3) or by a normal or nonspecific red cell morphology. The anemias are classified according to their morphologic characteristics in Table 47-4. This classification is extensive but not inclusive. Occasional patients have inexplicable morphologic findings or combinations of diseases (such as hereditary spherocytosis and obstructive jaundice) that conspire to cause morphologic and diagnostic confusion.

REFERENCES

1. MacKinney AA Jr. Hereditary spherocytosis: clinical family studies. Arch Intern Med 1965;116:257.
2. Krueger HC, Burgert EO Jr. Hereditary spherocytosis in 100 children. Mayo Clin Proc 1966;41:821.
3. Furchgott RF. Disk–sphere transformation in mammalian red cells. J Exp Biol 1940;17:30.
4. Brecher G, Bessis M. Present status of spiculated red cells and their relationship to the discocyte–echinocyte transformation: a critical review. Blood 1972;40:333.
5. Dallman PR, Siimes MA. Percentile curves for hemoglobin and red cell volume in infancy and childhood. J Pediatr 1979;94:26.
6. Beutler E. Clinical evaluation of iron stores. N Engl J Med 1957;256: 692.
7. Lipschitz DA, Cook JD, Finch CA. A clinical evaluation of serum ferritin as an index of iron stores. N Engl J Med 1974;290:1213.
8. Piomelli S. Lead poisoning. In: Nathan DG, Oski FA, eds. Hematology of infancy and childhood, ed 3. Philadelphia, WB Saunders, 1987:389.
9. Mentzer WC. Differentiation of iron deficiency from thalassemia trait. Lancet 1973;1:882.
10. England JM, Fraser PM. Differentiation of iron deficiency from thalassemia trait by routine blood count. Lancet 1973;1:449.
11. Johnson CS, Tegos C, Beutler E. Thalassemia minor: routine erythrocyte measurements and differentiation from iron deficiency. Am J Clin Pathol 1983;80:31.
12. Lee GR. The anemia of chronic disease. Semin Hematol 1983;20:61.
13. Hines JD, Grasso JA. The sideroblastic anemias. Semin Hematol 1970;7: 86.
14. Palek J. Hereditary elliptocytosis and related disorders. Clin Haematol 1985;14:45.
15. Alter BP. Fetal erythropoiesis in stress hematopoiesis. Exp Hematol 1979;7:200.
16. Daughday WH, Williams RH, Daland GA. The effect of endocrinopathies on the blood. Blood 1948;3:1342.
17. Horton L, Coburn R, England J, et al. The haematology of hypothyroidism. Q J Med 1985;45:101.
18. Mazzaferri EL. Adult hypothyroidism: manifestations and clinical presentation. Postgrad Med 1986;29:64.
19. Auerbach AD, Wolman SR. Susceptibility of Fanconi's anemia fibroblasts to chromosome damage by carcinogens. Nature 1976;261:494.
20. Glader BE, Backer K, et al. Elevated erythrocyte adenosine deaminase activity in congenital hypoplastic anemia. N Engl J Med 1983;309:1486.
21. Spivak JL. Masked megaloblastic anemia. Arch Intern Med 1982;142: 2111.
22. McCurdy P, Rath CE. Vacuolated nucleated bone marrow cells in alcoholism. Semin Hematol 1980;17:100.
23. Unger KW, Johnson D. Red blood cell mean corpuscular volume: a potential indicator of alcohol usage in a working population. Am J Med Sci 1974;267:281.
24. Wu A, Chanarin I, Levi AJ. Macrocytosis of chronic alcoholism. Lancet 1974;1:829.
25. Eichener ER, Hillman RS. The evolution of anemia in alcoholic patients. Am J Med 1971;50:218.
26. Bennett JM. Classification of the myelodysplastic syndromes. Clin Haematol 1986;15:909.
27. Yunis JJ, Lobell M, Arnesen MA, et al. Refined chromosome study helps define prognostic subgroups in most patients with primary myelodysplastic syndrome and acute myelogenous leukaemia. Br J Haematol 1988;68:189.
28. Glanz A, Fraser FC. Spectrum of anomalies in Fanconi's anemia. J Med Genet 1982;19:412.
29. Shwachman H, Diamond LK, et al. The syndrome of pancreatic insufficiency and bone marrow dysfunction. J Pediatr 1964;65:645.
30. Aggett PJ, Cavanagh NPC, et al. Shwachman's syndrome: a review of 21 cases. Arch Dis Child 1980;55:331.
31. Alter BP. Childhood red cell aplasia. Am J Pediatr Hematol Oncol 1980;2: 121.
32. Weick J, Hagedorn A, Linman J. Leukoerythroblastosis: diagnostic and prognostic significance. Mayo Clin Proc 1974;49:110.
33. Sills RH, Hadley RAR. The significance of nucleated red blood cells in the peripheral blood of children. Am J Pediatr Hematol Oncol 1983;5: 173.
34. Dessypris EN. Pure red cell aplasia. Baltimore, Johns Hopkins University Press, 1988.
35. Young NS, Mortimer PP. Viruses and bone marrow failure. Blood 1984;63: 729.
36. Klahr S, Slatopolsky E. Toxicity of parathyroid hormone in uremia. Annu Rev Med 1986;37:71.
37. Dawson AA, Ogston D, et al. Evaluation of diagnostic significance of certain symptoms and physical signs in anaemic patients. Br Med J 1969;3:436.
38. Cropp GJA. Cardiovascular function in children with severe anemia. Circulation 1969;39:775.
39. Valentine WM, Paglia DE, Tartaglia AP, Gilsanz F. Hereditary hemolytic anemia with increased red cell adenosine deaminase (45- to 70-fold) and decreased adenosine triphosphate. Science 1977;195:783.
40. Stamey CC, Diamond LK. Congenital hemolytic anemia in the newborn. Am J Dis Child 1957;94:616.
41. Berk PD, Martin JF, et al. Unconjugated hyperbilirubinemia: physiologic evaluation and experimental approach to therapy. Ann Intern Med 1975;82:552.
42. MacKinney AA Jr, Morton NE, et al. Ascertaining genetic carriers of hereditary spherocytosis by statistical analysis of multiple laboratory tests. J Clin Invest 1962;41:554.
43. Pirofsky B. Autoimmunization and the autoimmune hemolytic anemias. Baltimore, Williams & Wilkins, 1969.
44. Brus I, Lewis SM. The haptoglobin content of serum in haemolytic anaemia. Br J Haematol 1959;5:348.
45. Geerdink RA, Hellman PW, Verloop MC. Hereditary elliptocytosis and hyperhaemolysis: a comparative study of six families with 145 patients. Acta Med Scand 1966;179:715.
46. Bergstrand CG, Czar B, Tarukoski PH. Serum haptoglobin in infancy. Scand J Clin Lab Invest 1961;13:576.
47. Landaas S, Skrede S. The levels of serum enzymes, small proteins and lipids in normal infants and small children. J Clin Chem Clin Biochem 1981;19:1075.
48. Giblett ER. Haptoglobin types in American negroes. Nature 1959;183: 192.
49. Blondheim SH, Margoliash E, et al. A simple test for myohemoglobinuria (myoglobinuria). JAMA 1958;167:453.
50. Javid J, Horowitz JI, et al. Idiopathic paroxysmal myoglobinuria: report of a case with studies on serum haptoglobin levels. Arch Intern Med 1959;104:628.
51. Roesser HP, Powell LW. Urinary iron excretion in valvular heart disease and after heart valve replacement. Blood 1970;36:785.
52. Crosby WH, Dameshek W. The significance of hemoglobinemia and associated hemosiderinuria, with particular references to various types of hemolytic anemia. J Lab Clin Med 1951;38:829.
53. Emerson PM, Wilkerson JH. Lactate dehydrogenase in the diagnosis and assessment of response to treatment of megaloblastic anemia. Br J Haematol 1966;12:678.
54. Horstkotte D, Aul C, Seipl L, et al. Einfluss von Klappentyp und Klappenfunktion auf die chronische intravasale Hämolyse nach allopro-thetischem Mitral- und Aortenklappenersatz. Z Kardiol 1983;72:119.
55. Madhu Sudana Rao K, Learoyd PA, Suba Rao R, et al. Chronic haemolysis after Lillehei-Kaster valve replacement: comparison with the findings

after Björk-Shiley and Starr-Edwards mitral valve replacement. Thorax 1980;35:290.

56. Fehr J, Knob M. Comparison of red cell creatine level and reticulocyte count in appraising the severity of hemolytic processes. Blood 1979;53: 966.
57. Muller-Eberhard U, Javid J, Liern HH, et al. Plasma concentrations of hemopexin, haptoglobin and heme in patients with various hemolytic diseases. Blood 1968;32:811.
58. Lundh B, Oski FA, Gardner FH. Plasma hemopexin and haptoglobin in hemolytic diseases of the newborn. Acta Paediatr Scand 1970;59:121.
59. Maisels MJ, Pathak A, Nelson NM, Nathan DG. Endogenous production of carbon monoxide in normal and erythroblastic newborn infants. J Clin Invest 1971;50:1.
60. Rhyner K, Ganzoni A. Erythrokinetics: evaluation of red cell production by ferrokinetics and reticulocyte counts. Eur J Clin Invest 1972;2:96.
61. Emerson CP Jr, Shen SC, et al. Studies on the destruction of red blood cells. IX. Quantitative methods for determining the osmotic and mechanical fragility of red cells in the peripheral blood and splenic pulp: the mechanism of increased hemolysis in hereditary spherocytosis (congenital hemolytic jaundice) as related to the function of the spleen. Arch Intern Med 1956;97:1.
62. Oski FA, Naiman JL. Normal blood values in the newborn period. In: Hematologic problems in the newborn. Philadelphia, WB Saunders, 1972:1.
63. Trucco JI, Brown AK. Neonatal manifestations of hereditary spherocytosis. Am J Dis Child 1967;113:263.

Blood: Principles and Practice of Hematology,
edited by Robert I. Handin, Samuel E. Lux, and Thomas P. Stossel.
J.B. Lippincott Company, Philadelphia © 1995.

48

Disorders of Cobalamin and Folic Acid Metabolism

Bernard A. Cooper
David S. Rosenblatt

Cobalamin (Cbl; vitamin B_{12}) and folate are vitamins that are necessary coenzymes of intracellular reactions required for the endogenous synthesis of purines, thymidylate, and methionine, and they remove metabolic intermediates that may accumulate without such reactions. These metabolic intermediates include methylmalonic acid (MMA), homocysteine, formiminoglutamate, and formate, some of which are toxic.

Deficiency of folate or Cbl, or disturbance of their metabolism, causes megaloblastic anemia in addition to other metabolic and clinical effects. The function of these vitamins in human metabolism was discovered as a result of investigation of the cause of megaloblastic anemia.

MEGALOBLASTIC ANEMIA

Megaloblastic anemia is a syndrome of characteristic bone marrow morphology affecting erythroid, myeloid, and platelet precursors and usually producing one or more cytopenias in the peripheral blood. The term is sometimes used even in the absence of true anemia. Megaloblastic anemia is caused by deficiency of folate or Cbl. Similar morphology occurs with some myelotoxic agents, certain retroviruses, or myelodysplasia and acute leukemia. The syndrome appears to occur when methionine synthesis in bone marrow cells is impaired by deficiency of folate or Cbl. How this causes the apparent DNA defect of the megaloblastic anemia of deficiency of Cbl or folate is unknown.

History

The Blood

Anemia associated with erythrocytes of abnormal morphology was observed in patients with pernicious anemia in 1876 to 1877; by 1883, macrocytosis had been noted.[1–3] Megaloblastic erythroid precursors were stained and defined by Ehrlich[4] in 1891. Increased numbers of nuclear segments in neutrophils in stained blood smears from these patients were described in 1923 to 1927, the giant myeloid band forms in megaloblastic bone marrow having been reported in 1920.

Megaloblastic changes in the bone marrow during relapse with return of normal morphology during remission were described in 1921 to 1922, 5 to 6 years before therapy for the disease was discovered.

Conversion of megaloblastic to normoblastic bone marrow with reticulocytosis and correction of the anemia by treatment with liver was described by Minot and Murphy[5] in 1926. The sequence of these events is summarized in several reviews.[1,2]

Other Observations

Many important observations followed:

1. Folate was found to produce a similar clinical syndrome (Wills' syndrome).[6]
2. In pernicious anemia patients, the stomach was found to lack intrinsic factor[7] (IF) because of atrophy (destruction) of the gastric mucosa.[8] The disease is caused by failure to absorb adequate quantities of Cbl.[1,9]
3. Cbl injections corrected pernicious anemia, and folate corrected the anemia described by Wills.[10] Each vitamin in large doses could produce some effect on the hematologic abnormalities caused by the other.[11,12]
4. Transcobalamin II (TCII) was shown to function as an IF within the body, permitting endocytosis-mediated utilization of Cbl by cells.[13,14]
5. Assays of Cbl and folate in serum and tissues of patients with megaloblastic anemia made chemical definition of the deficiency possible.[15–17]
6. A neurologic syndrome was described in classic pernicious anemia, but usually not in the syndrome caused by folate deficiency.[1,18]
7. Pernicious anemia was shown to be an autoimmune disease,[19] probably caused by lymphocyte-mediated destruction of gastric parietal cells.[20–22]
8. Inherited defects of the Cbl and folate metabolism were found to cause abnormal development in addition to megaloblastic anemia.[23,24]
9. The purification and cloning of some of the binding proteins and receptors have helped to define their function.[25–31]

Physiology

The megaloblastic bone marrow is hyperactive, stimulated by erythropoietin acting on erythroid stem cells (erythroid colony-forming units [CFU-E]). These CFU-E are increased in number[32] but probably are abnormal, since the descendants they generate are megaloblastic. Maturing megaloblastic erythroid cells are more likely than normoblastic cells to be destroyed or to die during maturation,[33,34] so that the proportion of young erythroid cells in the bone marrow is greater than normal. This ineffective erythropoiesis is the cause of elevated levels of lactate dehydrogenase and iron in plasma (derived from dying erythroid precursors). Typically, mature erythrocytes have abnormal shapes and variable sizes, mean cell volume is greater than normal, and erythrocytes have membrane defects including decreased membrane-associated cholinesterase. Mature megaloblastic erythrocytes entering the blood often have a short life-span due to random destruction.

Myeloid precursors in the bone marrow are slightly larger than normal, but the most striking abnormality in megaloblastic bone marrow is the accumulation of giant metamyelocytes and bands affecting a minority of late myeloid cells. These metamyelocytes and bands have a DNA content of 4n, and many label with tritiated thymidine, unlike normal myeloid cells of comparable maturity. Giant bands and metamyelocytes may persist for 10 to 14 days in bone marrow after treatment of megaloblastic anemia.[35] Giant band neutrophils and late metamyelocytes usually are not seen in the megaloblastoid bone marrows of patients with leukemia and myelodysplasia. Similar abnormalities probably affect the precursors of the megakaryocytic series, but these are less well defined.

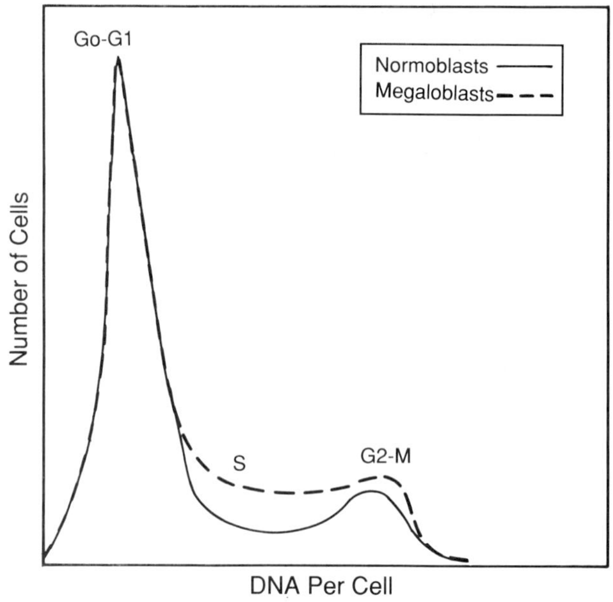

FIGURE 48-1. The cell cycle in the bone marrow, measured by flow cytometry using a dye that binds to DNA. The idealized drawing represents cells in G0 or G1 as having DNA corresponding to 2n (46 chromosomes) and those in G2-M as having DNA corresponding to 4n (92 chromosomes). Cells with intermediate quantities of DNA in normal bone marrow are synthesizing DNA (S phase), but some of these in megaloblastic bone marrow are not. (After Yoshida Y, Todo A, Shirakawa S, Wakisaka G, Uchino H. Proliferation of megaloblasts in pernicious anemia as observed from nucleic acid metabolism. Blood 1968;31:292)

DNA Synthesis in Normal and Megaloblastic Cells

When human bone marrow is incubated with tritiated thymidine and radioautographed, cells synthesizing DNA (S phase) are labeled. In normal bone marrow, 20% to 25% of erythroid cells are in S phase. The remainder of the cells are distributed in the other phases of the cell cycle: G1, which describes cells with a 2n complement of DNA and which are not making DNA; and G2-M, which describes cells with a 4n complement of DNA after completion of S phase. All cells with DNA content between 2n and 4n are in S phase (Fig. 48-1). In megaloblastic anemia, 40% to 50% of erythroid cells are in S phase. In addition, some cells that are not labeled with thymidine have DNA contents that are between 2n and 4n. These cells appear to have entered S phase, but have stopped DNA synthesis before the 4n complement was achieved. They have been called U cells and have been found not to be engaged in active protein synthesis, as are all other maturing erythroid precursors. It is presumed that these U cells will die and have stopped cycling because of deficiency of intracellular nutrients.[36–39]

As already noted, how deficiency of Cbl or folate causes megaloblastic anemia remains unclear. The synthesis of DNA in mammalian cells requires a supply of deoxynucleotides (phosphates of deoxyadenosine, deoxythymidine, deoxycytidine, and deoxyguanosine). These are synthesized from small molecules (endogenous synthesis) and can also be supplied from preformed bases that are phosphorylated by various kinase enzymes (salvage pathway).

DNA synthesis requires unwinding of coiled DNA strand pairs to uncover the DNA from its protein coating. The paired DNA strands then separate at specific areas (initiation sites) to permit pairing of nucleotides with those exposed in the open loop between strands (each such loop is a *replicon*). The newly attached nucleotides are linked to form a strand by the enzyme DNA polymerase A, which elongates short strands provided by RNA primers. New DNA strands, which are synthesized, extend from these primers. The strand extending 5′ toward 3′ is generated as a single strand and extends to the edge of the adjacent initiation site. The strand being generated in the 3′ to 5′ direction is generated as short, about 200–base fragments (Okazaki fragments). Spaces between these, and that taken by the RNA primer, are then filled by the action of the same DNA polymerase and several other enzymes. Although in most studies of DNA synthesis, nucleotide triphosphates are used, since the final form in DNA is the triphosphate, it remains unclear when DNA synthesis by enzyme complexes in vivo requires nucleotide triphosphates, diphosphates,[40] or even nucleotide monophosphates.[41]

Polyglutamyl 5,10-methylene tetrahydrofolate (THF) is the methyl source for conversion of deoxyuridylate to thymidylate. If this folate were deficient, thymidylate supply and synthesis might be inadequate to complete DNA synthesis during the normal S phase of the cell cycle (8 to 12 hours). Published data[41] indicate that in lymphocytes from patients with megaloblastic anemia, ligation of Okazaki fragments may be slower than in normal cells, and mean replicon size may be smaller. In the deoxyuridine suppression test (described later), utilization of labeled deoxyuridine for DNA synthesis is impaired in megaloblastic bone marrow caused by deficiency of either Cbl or folate. The biochemical defect is corrected in vitro within 1 to 2 hours when 5-formyl-THF is added to the cells. This suggests that the critical lesion in these cells is in thymidylate synthesis and that it can be corrected with excess folate.

Deficient thymidylate for the process just described would be a compelling explanation of megaloblastic anemia, producing slower DNA replication and less condensation of DNA into tight, protein-associated coils (nucleosomes). Nucleotide pools in megaloblastic cells are normal or increased. If thymidylate deficiency is the cause of megaloblastic anemia, the thymidylate deficiency must be compartmentalized, affecting only selected portions of the nucleotide pool, such as those mentioned above. It has also been suggested that megaloblastic morphology may be caused by incorporation of excess deoxyuridylate into DNA instead of thymidylate because of accumulation of the former in the thymidylate-deficient cells. Such incorporation of deoxyuridylate would be followed by rapid removal of the incorporated deoxyuridine by deoxyuridine triphosphatase, leaving strand breaks requiring repair that would be slow because of inadequate thymidylate.

In addition to the nucleic acid abnormalities previously described, the nuclei of megaloblasts have been shown to contain more homocysteine than the nuclei of normal cells.[42] Whether this is critical for the formation of megaloblasts is unknown. Further studies are required to determine the cause of megaloblastic anemia.

Megaloblastic Erythroid Precursors

The maturing erythroid precursors in megaloblastic anemia contain less DNA per RNA unit and are larger than normal cells of the same level of maturation[38,43]; thus, they have about a normal DNA content per cell and an elevated RNA content. Their nuclear morphology appears looser than normal on stained smears, giving the characteristic appearance of the megaloblast (Fig. 48-2). In addition, the stage of maturation of the nucleus often appears less mature than does that of the cytoplasm. Therefore, erythroblasts with considerable accumulation of hemoglobin in the cytoplasm (polychromatophilic erythroblasts) may have vesicular, open, or immature nuclei, and orthochromic erythroblasts (red-staining cytoplasm) may contain nuclei that are not the dense, small, purple-staining nuclei of normal orthochromic erythroid cells. Experienced observers usually recognize megaloblastic erythropoiesis by noting vesicular and open nuclei in the earliest erythroblasts (proerythroblasts and basophilic erythroblasts).

Leukocyte Abnormalities

Some of the maturing myeloid cells are abnormal. Continued DNA synthesis beyond the stage of maturation at which cell division occurs (delayed nuclear maturation of neutrophils) produces large metamyelocytes and band neutrophils. Mature neutrophils may be larger than normal or of normal size, and some contain more nuclear lobes than normal. The cause of nuclear hyperlobation is unknown. Although it is tempting to assume that multilobed neutrophils are derived from giant bands and metamyelocytes, the DNA content of giant bands has been reported to be 2n, rather than 4n as observed in metamyelocytes.[44–47] Giant band neutrophils are readily recognized in smears of bone marrow, contain more DNA per cell than do normal cells, synthesize DNA, and are diagnostic of megaloblastic anemia. Multilobed neutrophils, when observed in smears of peripheral blood, also are diagnostic of megaloblastic anemia (see Fig. 48-2). Neutropenia may be noted in patients with megaloblastic anemia. In those with a nutritional cause, neutropenia is more common in patients with severe anemia, and uncommon in patients without significant anemia (Fig. 48-3*A*). In megaloblastic anemia provoked by some mild antifolates (such as trimethoprim), neutropenia usually precedes abnormalities of erythrocytes. The clinical application of these are discussed in the section on clinical manifestations of deficiency.

Platelet Abnormalities

Thrombocytopenia is observed in patients with megaloblastic anemia. Like neutropenia, it is more common in patients with severe anemia (see Fig. 48-3*B*) than in those without anemia, except in the presence of drug-induced megaloblastic change. In the bone marrow, megakaryocytes may be abundant or decreased. Diminished lobation of megakaryocyte nuclei has been described in megaloblastic anemia, but this is difficult to observe and is an unreliable sign. The physiologic abnormality in megakaryocyte maturation, or the stage of maturity in which maturation and proliferation are delayed, has not been defined.

Other Tissues

Macrocytosis of buccal cells, obtained by scraping the buccal mucosa, has been reported in patients with megaloblastic anemia. Similar abnormalities have been described in cells of the tongue, vaginal epithelium, urinary tract, nasal epithelium, and other lining tissues. Decreased height of gastric cells and enterocytes has also been described. These changes reverse after treatment of the megaloblastic anemia and are not found in all patients.[1,48]

Causes of Megaloblastic Anemia

Megaloblastic anemia occurs under the following conditions:

Cobalamin Deficiency

- Inadequate Cbl intake
- Malabsorption from the gut
  - Intestinal disease
  - Lack of IF or its receptor
  - Competition for Cbl by large quantities of the fish tapeworm, *Diphyllobothrium latum*, or bacteria in areas of stasis (blind loop syndrome)
  - Combinations of these
- TCII deficiency
- Defective intracellular metabolism

Folate Deficiency

- Inadequate folate intake
- Increased folate loss or need
- Malabsorption from the gut
- Defective intracellular metabolism
  - Inherited defects
  - Antimetabolites

Other Metabolic Abnormalities

- Neoplastic or viral effects on stem cells

COBALAMIN

Cobalamin in nature is synthesized by bacteria and fungi and is required as a vitamin by animals but not by higher plants. Plants consequently do not accumulate Cbl and do not contribute it to the diet.

Chemistry

Cobalamins have the chemical structure shown in Figure 48-4.[49–51] They represent a subgroup of substances called *corrins*, which have structural similarity to porphyrins. In the Cbl, the tetrapyrrole corrin ring contains a cobalt atom in the center, and a nucleotide (5,6-dimethylbenzimidazole) bound to one side of the corrin ring through α-ribofuranose-5-phosphate, which in turn binds through 1-amino-2-propanol to propionamide on one of the pyrrole rings of the corrin plate. This produces the structure of a flat horizontal plate (corrin), with nucleotide-phosphate-aminopropanol hanging from one face of the plate and a methyl or 5′-deoxyadenosyl group protruding up from the other face. The methyl or 5′-deoxyadenosyl groups are split from the corrin by light and are readily replaced by water, cyanide, sulfite, or other ligands. One end of the nucleotide chain attaches to one of the pyrrole rings of the corrin, while the other end either binds to the cobalt (base-on con-

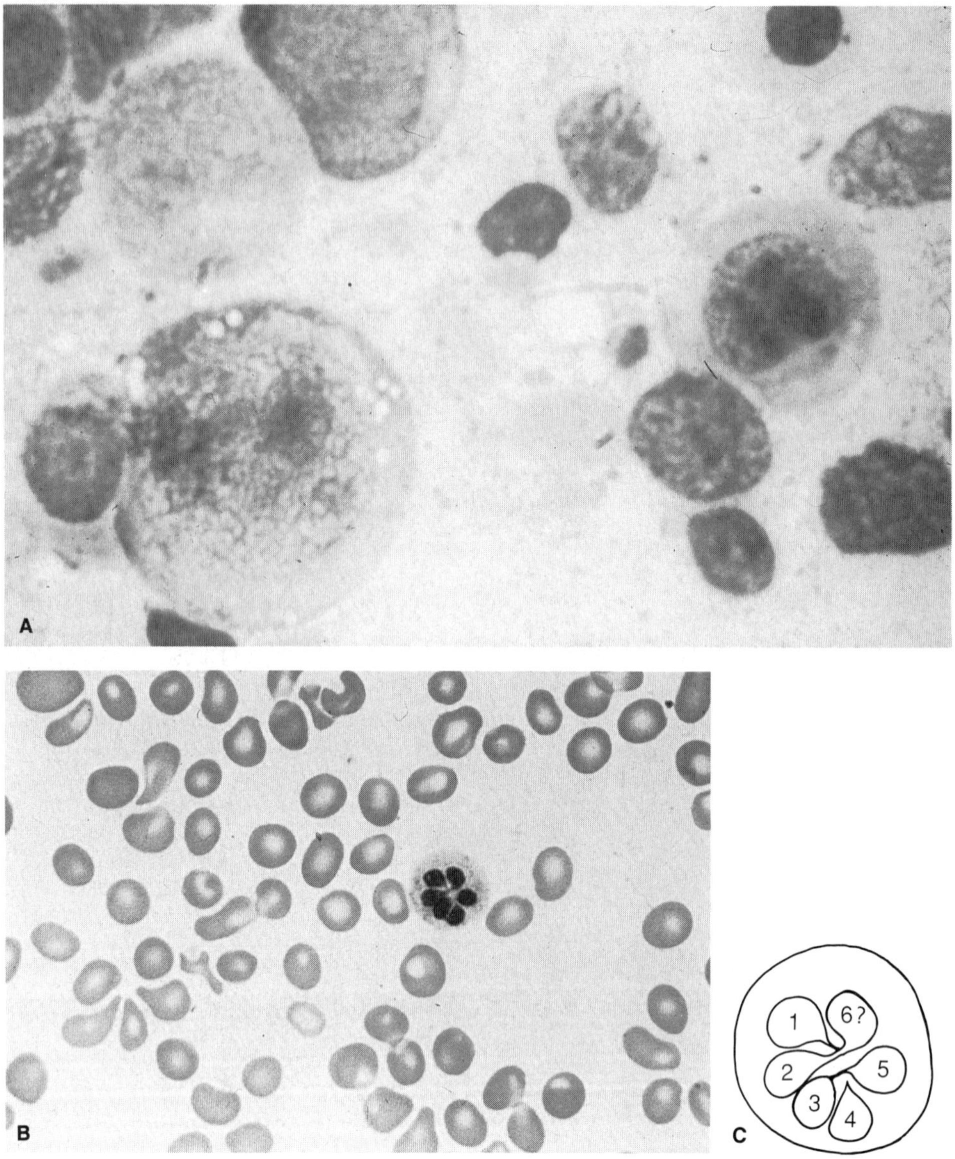

FIGURE 48-2. Megaloblasts in bone marrow (**A**), a multilobed neutrophil in blood (**B**), and a lobe count of the neutrophil (**C**). The chromatin linking lobes 2 and 6 is thicker than should be accepted for separate lobes, so we count this as having five lobes. Others may define this as six lobed but must then apply this definition to all cells counted. (Courtesy of Irma Pereira, Hematology Laboratory of Stanford University Medical Center)

figuration) or dangles free of the cobalt (base-off configuration).

In this review, vitamin B_{12} refers to Cbls that either have coenzyme activity in cells or can be converted to such substances when presented to mammalian cells. These include both base-on and base-off configurations of Cbl with CN, OH, H_2O, SH, SO_3, glutathione, methyl, 5′-deoxyadenosyl bound to the cobalt, or Cbl with the cobalt atom reduced to the divalent (cob[II]alamin, B_{12R}), or monovalent (cob[I]alamin, B_{12S}) states. When the cobalt atom is in its natural, oxidized, trivalent state, the compounds are called cob(III)alamin or are named for the group binding to the cobalt (cyanocobalamin [CN-Cbl], hydroxocobalamin [OH-Cbl], aquocobalamin, and so on).

Biochemistry

Vitamin B_{12} functions in mammalian cells as a coenzyme in two reactions: synthesis of methionine from homocysteine and 5-methyl-THF[52] and conversion of methylmalonyl-CoA to succinyl-CoA.[1,53] Both reactions serve to detoxify potentially toxic materials (homocysteine and methylmalonate). In addition, conversion reaction is the major pathway for resynthesis of methionine in humans, and low plasma levels of methionine develop when it is inactive.[54]

Cobalamin-Dependent Enzymes

The only enzymes that require Cbl in human cells are the mitochondrial methylmalonyl CoA-mutase (EC 5.4.99.2)[55–63] and the cytoplasmic methionine synthase (5-methyl-THF: homocysteine methyltransferase ECC 2.1.1.13). In prokaryotes, a variety of other enzymes utilize Cbl for reactions that appear not to occur in mammalian cells.

Cbl entering the cytoplasm of a cell appears to leave the cell if it does not bind either to methionine synthase in the cytoplasm[64] or enter the mitochondria to react with the mitochondrial enzyme, adenosine triphosphate (ATP): cob(II)alamin transferase to form 5′-deoxyadenosylcobalamin (AdoCbl) and bind to MMA mutase.[65–70] In mitochondria from rat liver, most of the Cbl appears to be AdoCbl.[69] Before binding to methionine synthase, the Cbl is probably reduced to cob(II)alamin. Cob(III)alamin appears

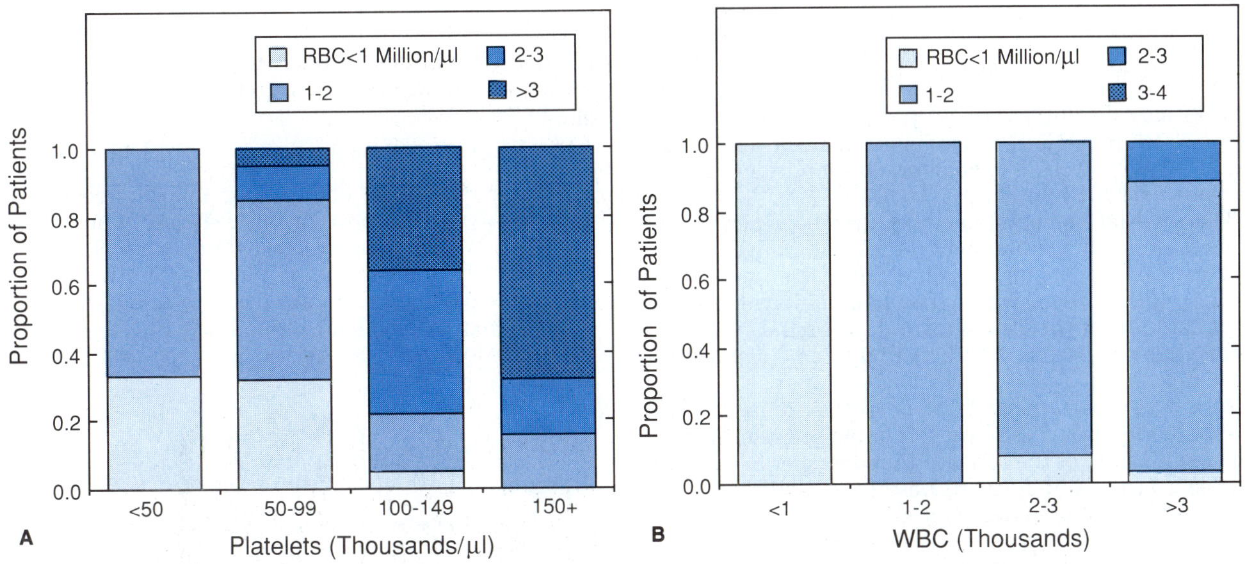

FIGURE 48-3. The proportion of patients with platelet counts (**A**) or leukocytes (**B**) in the range indicated on the horizontal axis is compared with their degree of anemia. Neutropenia and thrombocytopenia were more common in but not restricted to patients with severe anemia. (After Cooper BA, Rosenblatt DS, Whitehead V. Megaloblastic anemia. In: Nathan DG, Oski FA, eds. Hematology of infancy and childhood. Philadelphia, WB Saunders, 1993:358)

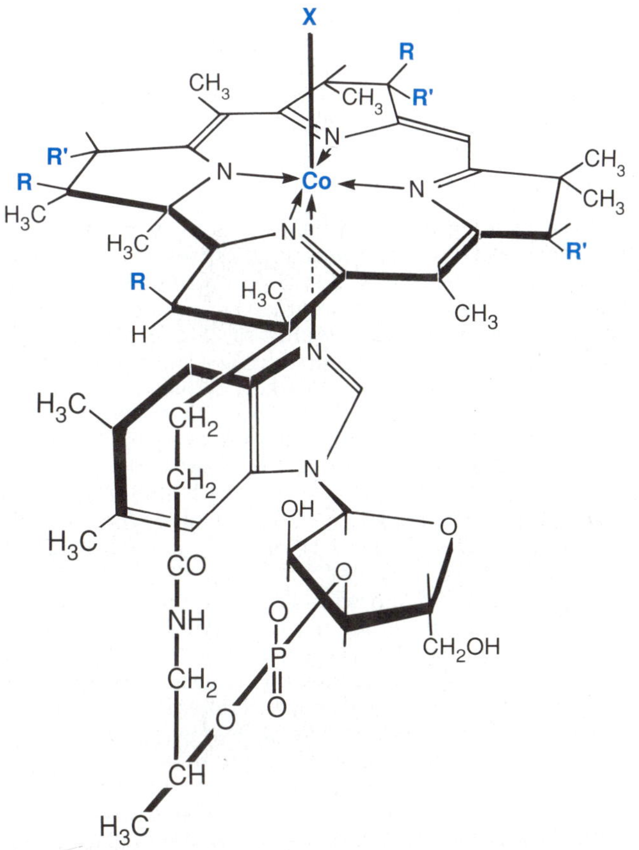

FIGURE 48-4. Cobalamin. When X is methyl, the compound is methylcobalamin (MeCbl), when X is adenosyl, it is 5′-deoxyadenosylcobalamin (AdoCbl), when CN, cyanocobalamin, and so on. (After Cooper BA, Rosenblatt DS, Whitehead V. Megaloblastic anemia. In: Nathan DG, Oski FA, eds. Hematology of infancy and childhood. Philadelphia, WB Saunders, 1993:359)

incapable of binding to methionine synthase.[64] It is possible that entry into mitochondria also requires reduction or chemical modification of cob(III)alamin. Intact (unswollen) mitochondria from rat liver appear to be impermeable to cobalamins.[71] Cbl bound to TCII associates with mitochondria. The physiologic relevance of this observation is unclear.

Biochemistry of Cobalamin-Mediated Reactions

Reactions proved to require Cbl in human cells are limited to the following:

Reaction 1: homocysteine + 5-methyl-THF → methionine + THF

Reaction 2: methylmalonyl-CoA → succinyl-CoA

In reaction 1, methyl-Cbl (MeCbl) is converted to cob(I)alamin and accepts a methyl group from 5-methyl-THF to regenerate MeCbl. In reaction 2, an intramolecular rearrangement converts potentially toxic methylmalonyl-CoA to succinyl-CoA, which is readily metabolized.

Methionine Synthesis

Methionine is consumed in the diet and is absorbed from the intestine by a transport system, which it shares with other neutral amino acids or dipeptides.[54,72–75] Plasma methionine enters cells and the cerebrospinal fluid (CSF) by similar membrane transport systems. Methionine is an essential amino acid, but the mammalian requirement for methionine is decreased by two thirds when cysteine is abundant in the diet.

The methionine in the cytoplasm of the cell may take several pathways:

1. It may remain as the amino acid.
2. It may be converted to S-adenosylmethionine (SAM)

by the enzyme ATP: L-methionine-S-adenosyltransferase (EC 2.5.1.6).
3. It may be incorporated into protein.

SAM may donate its methyl group leaving S-adenosylhomocysteine (SAH). SAH is toxic in the cells and is metabolized by hydrolysis to homocysteine and adenosine by the enzyme SAH-hydrolase (EC 3.3.1.1).

The residual homocysteine may then be remethylated to methionine by methionine synthase, or, in liver, by the enzyme betaine: L-homocysteine methyltransferase (EC 2.1.1.5). It may react with cystathionine-β synthase (EC 4.2.1.22) to form cystathionine and, in tissues, with cystathionine γ-lyase (EC 4.4.1.1) activity, to be degraded to cysteine.

At low concentrations of homocysteine, remethylation to methionine is favored over formation of cystathionine. The equilibrium of the reaction that degrades SAH favors SAH synthesis, so that hydrolysis of this toxic substance requires removal of homocysteine and adenosine.[76]

Cystathionine γ-lyase activity is absent from many tissues (including spleen and brain). When excess methionine is administered, cystathionine accumulates in these tissues. In liver, homocysteine may react with betaine to form dimethylglycine and sarcosine.

In remethylation of homocysteine by methionine synthase, it is required that Cbl be bound to the enzyme as a prosthetic group or coenzyme. If cob(I)alamin is bound to the enzyme, cob(I)alamin is readily methylated by 5-methyl-THF to form MeCbl bound to the enzyme. The methionine synthase then mediates transfer of this methyl from methyl-Cbl to homocysteine to form methionine.

Cob(I)alamin is readily oxidized, and appears to spontaneously undergo oxidation to cob(II)alamin. The latter will not accept a methyl from 5-methyl-THF. Cob(II)alamin bound to enzyme appears to be converted to MeCbl by donation of a methyl from SAM, which then permits continued acceptance of a methyl group from 5-methyl-THF. The number of 5-methyl-THF transfers permitted before transfer is again required from SAM in vivo is unknown, but in vitro, SAM appears to methylate the reaction every 300 to 500 methylation cycles.[52,77]

In *Escherichia coli*, two flavoproteins have been described which maintain cob(I)alamin or provide other necessary reduction in the reaction.[78] In mammalian cells, this function may be provided by an iron atom that is a part of the methionine synthase enzyme,[64] whereas a copper atom appears to serve this function in the *E coli* enzyme. Evidence for the importance of some type of reduction reaction associated with methionine synthesis is provided by cblE mutants (described in the section on methyl-Cbl deficiency), in whom this activity appears to be abnormal.[79] In one patient with cblG mutation, the SAM-dependent methylation of cob(II)alamin appears to be abnormal.

Methylfolate Trap

In the early 1960s, the role of Cbl in folate-dependent methionine metabolism was discovered. A concept was presented that deficiency of Cbl induced megaloblastic anemia by trapping folate as 5-methyl-THF, thus creating intracellular deficiency of other folates with consequent megaloblastic anemia indistinguishable from that caused by deficiency of folate. Many of the predictions of this hypothesis have been challenged in subsequent studies, but the interference with folate metabolism by means of slowing of the methionine synthase reaction by Cbl deficiency is clearly correct and is the cause of megaloblastic anemia and homocyst(e)inemia in Cbl deficiency.

Methylmalonic Acid Mutase

For this intramitochondrial reaction (reaction 3), Cbl must enter the mitochondria and receive a 5′-deoxyadenosyl group from ATP:

Reaction 3: ATP + cob(I)alamin → AdoCbl + phosphate

It appears that Cbl entering the mitochondria must be reduced to cob(I)alamin for this reaction to proceed. The resulting AdoCbl then appears to bind to the MMA mutase enzyme to produce the active enzyme. This pathway thus appears to require penetration of mitochondria by Cbl (by an unknown mechanism), reduction of Cbl to cob(I)alamin (either before entry or in the mitochondria), and reaction 3.

Utilization

Transport

Cobalamin crosses cell membranes poorly, and effective transmembrane transport by mammalian cells at the low Cbl levels found in nature (nmol/L) always requires mediation of a Cbl-binding protein reacting with a receptor on the cell surface. In some unicellular organisms, Cbl accumulation is by a surface receptor that binds free Cbl. The latter transport system, which is almost completely defined in *E coli* mutants, involves a Cbl binder on the outer membrane, a gene product required to release membrane-bound Cbl from the outer membrane into the periplasmic space, a possible Cbl binder in the periplasmic space, and two different gene products on the inner cell membrane—either of which can translocate periplasmic Cbl into the cytoplasm.[81–83] This mechanism is not identical to the transport system of eukaryotic cells. These cells permit entry of a small proportion of Cbl when extracellular concentrations are very high.

Cobalamin-Binding Proteins

Transcobalamin II. TCII mediates entry of plasma Cbl into cells. It is found in plasma, CSF, seminal fluid, and transudates; is synthesized in a variety of cells (including fibroblasts, macrophages, enterocytes, renal cells, hepatocytes, spleen, heart, gastric mucosa, and endothelium)[84]; and is a nonglycosylated protein with a short plasma half-life and a molecular size of 43 kd.[85] It readily penetrates extracellular fluids and polymerizes with itself or with another protein when it binds Cbl. In the rat, but not in the dog, TCII–Cbl filters through the renal glomerulus.[86–88] Plasma turnover of TCII is rapid.[89,90] TCII binds Cbl tightly (dissociation constant $[K_d]$ = 5 to 18 pmol/L) and has little affinity for corrins without vitamin B_{12} activity. A cDNA for TCII has been described.[25,26,91]

Haptocorrin. Haptocorrin (TCO, I, III, R binder, cobalophyllin) is a family of proteins with similar structures but variably glycosylated. These proteins are present in many tissues and are synthesized by myeloid cells and probably by many other cells. Haptocorrin is present in many secretions including plasma, bile, saliva, tears, breast milk, amniotic fluid, and seminal fluid, and in extracts of granulocytes, salivary gland, platelets, hepatoma cells, and breast tumors.[84,92,93] The fully glycosylated haptocorrin, with a low isoelectric point, which is found in plasma, has a half-life of 9 days; those with higher isoelectric points are cleared rapidly from the plasma by hepatocytes into the bile. Seventy to ninety percent of the Cbl in plasma is bound to haptocorrin. The remainder is attached to TCII. Most of the Cbl bound to human haptocorrin is methyl-Cbl, unlike the mixture of cobalamins described as bound to TCII.[94] Haptocorrin has the greatest affinity for corrins of all of the vitamin B_{12}–binding proteins. Its K_d for Cbl is 3 to 7 pmol/L, but it has considerable binding affinity for cobalamins and other corrins without vitamin B_{12} activity. The function of haptocorrin in vivo is not clear. Because of its strong affinity for cobalamins as well as corrins without vitamin B_{12} activity, it has been suggested that haptocorrin functions to bind and excrete such vitamin B_{12} analogues into the bile by binding to the galactose receptor on the surface of hepatocytes.[95] Cbl binders in gastric juice include haptocorrin, which probably is derived from saliva and perhaps from gastric parietal cells[93] and IF. A cDNA has been isolated.[96]

Intrinsic Factor. IF is a glycoprotein that is synthesized in gastric parietal cells in humans and guinea pigs and in chief (pepsinogen) cells in rat stomach. It may also be secreted by pancreatic cells in dogs.[97] It is readily digested by pepsin but not by trypsin.[98] Cbl bound to IF in the gut lumen is available for absorption. IF is not absorbed from the gut and is thus not reutilized. IF binds cobalamins less tightly than do the transcobalamins (K_d of 0.1 to 1 nmol/L),[99] but binds only those cobalamins with vitamin B_{12} activity.

Within the cells, Cbl appears to be bound to its enzymes. No significant free Cbl is found within cells.

Physiology

Absorption From the Gut

Cobalamin bound to intracellular enzymes in food is readily released by chewing or cooking and binds to haptocorrin from the saliva or from the animal tissues from which it is derived. This mixture of corrins enters the intestine, where haptocorrin is digested by trypsin, permitting binding of Cbl to IF. The IF–Cbl complex binds to receptors on the ileal brush border from which the Cbl slowly enters the portal vein bound to TCII. Whereas the maximum velocity of appearance into the portal vein of Cbl fed in large quantities without IF is 1 hour after feeding, that of Cbl bound to IF is about 12 hours after feeding, and 8 to 12 hours after reaching the ileal lumen.[100] Synthesis of TCII by ileal cells may be required for transport.[101,102]

The receptor for the IF–Cbl complex is on the brush border of the ileal enterocyte. The distribution of these receptors varies in different subjects. In some subjects, removal of a small segment of ileum removes most of the absorptive surface and causes malabsorption of Cbl; in other subjects, the absorptive mechanism extends through a considerable portion of the ileum. The receptor appears to disappear from the surface of the enterocyte during absorption of IF-bound Cbl. The maximum IF–Cbl complex that can be bound to receptor is about 1.5 μg.[1] Larger doses of Cbl, even when bound to IF, probably are not absorbed by this mechanism. Receptor activity reappears rapidly after absorption of Cbl, so that a second bolus can be absorbed soon after. When massive quantities of Cbl (100 to 1000 μg) are fed to patients without IF in the gut, a small proportion (0.1% to 1%) is absorbed from the jejunum. The receptor for IF–Cbl complex has been purified[103,104] and seems to be expressed in several other tissues.[105] Failure to express the receptor results in malabsorption of vitamin B_{12} in dogs.[106]

Malabsorption of Cbl caused by competition for the Cbl in the intestinal lumen has generated some of the most exotic studies in this field. After it was demonstrated that, in some patients in Finland, megaloblastic anemia could be corrected by removal of massive quantities of infecting fish tapeworm (*Diphyllobothrium latum*), it was observed that the worm had the capacity to release Cbl from IF and to accumulate the released Cbl.[107,108] Although this competition by 100 m of worm length was well documented, the Cbl deficiency caused by the worm clearly occurred only in patients with marginal secretion of IF and not in persons with normal gastric secretion. The increase in ingestion of raw fish among some social groups probably will generate new cases of this previously extinct illness.

In some patients with intestinal blind loops, or stenotic areas of the small bowel, Cbl malabsorption has been observed. Absorption has improved after treatment with some antibiotics (tetracycline). This malabsorption of Cbl appears to be due to accumulation of Cbl by bacteria in the stagnant intestinal areas, but the physiology remains unclear. In many patients, serum folate levels are above normal, apparently because of generation of folate by the intestinal bacteria. The means by which Cbl is transported across the ileal cell is unknown. Indirect evidence suggests that the process may be by endocytosis with digestion of the Cbl free of IF in lysosomes.[109–113] The subsequent transport of the vitamin appears to require the correct chemical configuration of the Cbl[114] and probably involves specific binding of the Cbl to a transporter, which might be TCII. Chemical modification of absorbed Cbl is not required for absorption, although when the Cbl enters ileal cells, it may be metabolized to coenzymes as described in the following section.

Entry of Cobalamin Into Cells

Cbl bound to TCII enters cells by endocytosis after the complex associates with receptors on the cell surface.[13,14,99,115] The receptor has been purified.[116] The Cbl enters the cytoplasm with no chemical modification required for transport. Entry into the cytoplasm is probably from lysosomes, and requires lysosome-mediated digestion of the transcobalamin before the free Cbl penetrates into the cell.[13] Entry into the cytoplasm is prevented by treatment of cells with agents, such as chloroquine and ammonium chloride, that prevent generation of low pH in endosomes and probably prevent formation of lysosomes.[13,117] In these situations, TCII–Cbl complex accumulates. Penetration of free Cbl from lysosomes into cytoplasm appears to require a transport system. This transport system was defective in two children with cblF disease.[122]

Biochemical Effects of Cobalamin Deficiency

Direct biochemical effects of Cbl deficiency expected (and observed) are the following:

- Methylmalonic acidemia and aciduria of magnitude determined by the flow of odd chained fatty acids, valine and threonine, through the pathway. The secondary effects of MMA accumulation include acidosis, hyperglycinemia, and possibly inhibition of other enzymes and of bone marrow stem cells by accumulated MMA[118–121]
- Homocyst(e)inemia and homocyst(e)inuria
- Inadequate levels of THF in cells, producing defective rates of polyglutamyl folate synthesis and deficiency of folates required for some intracellular reactions
- Defective thymidylate synthesis
- Defective synthesis of endogenous purines
- Defective detoxification of formate
- Accumulation of formiminoglutamate, 5(4)-amidoimidazole-4(5) carboxyribonucleotide, and other intermediates of folate-dependent reactions

- Biochemical central nervous system (CNS) changes, which might relate to defective methylation of myelin basic protein, although data are conflicting[122–124]
- Lower intracellular folate levels than expected for the concentration folate in plasma

Nutritional Needs

Because all of Cbl and folate utilized by the body is ultimately absorbed from the diet, inadequate intake may cause deficiency. Neither dietary needs nor the prevalence of dietary deficiency in different populations is well defined, but some conclusions are possible based on published data.[125,126]

In India, where vegetarianism is common, and elsewhere, also among strict vegetarians (vegans), the concentration of Cbl in serum and tissues is low[127–131] and megaloblastic anemia due to inadequate intake occurs. In vegans, neurologic disease (subacute combined degeneration of the spinal cord) has been described, but its prevalence among strict vegetarians who take no animal products or vitamin supplements appears to be very low.[132,133] It is not clear whether the low incidence of neurologic disease in patients with very low levels of Cbl in plasma is due to secret noncompliance with their avowed vegetarianism. Studies of homocysteine and MMA levels in vegan communities are required to determine the incidence of biologic deficiency and to compare this with the incidence of neurologic disease. The World Health Organization (WHO) calculated that mean Cbl intake per day was less than 1 μg in many countries.[134] Despite inadequate information about the incidence of significant deficiency of Cbl, the WHO recommended a daily intake of 0.1 μg/d for infants, 1 μg/d for normal adults, and 0.3 to 0.4 μg more for lactating and pregnant women, respectively, based on known physiology and turnover of Cbl, the quantity required to treat deficiency, and a variety of other factors.

Inborn Errors of Cobalamin Metabolism and Transport

Intrinsic Factor Deficiency

Absence of effective IF has been recognized as a cause of megaloblastic anemia and developmental delay in a number of children. In these children, evidence of Cbl deficiency usually appears after the first year but before age 5, although in cases of partially defective IF, clinical deficiency has appeared as late as age 12 years.[135] Patients with IF deficiency have normal gastric acid excretion and normal gastric cytology. In some patients, immunologically active but nonfunctional IF is produced, whereas in others no immunologically active IF is present. An unstable IF, labile to destruction by acid and pepsin and with a low affinity for vitamin B_{12}, has also been reported.[136] In children with IF deficiency, absorption of Cbl is abnormal but is normalized when the vitamin is mixed with a source of normal IF, such as human gastric juice from an unaffected person. As with the other disorders of Cbl transport, inheritance appears to be autosomal recessive.

Defective Transport of Cobalamin by Enterocytes

Defective Cbl transport by enterocytes, also known as Imerslund-Graesbeck syndrome, usually presents with clinical manifestations of Cbl deficiency between the ages of 1 and 15 years, although the disease has appeared later.[137–142] Patients with this disease have normal IF, no evidence of antibodies to IF, and normal intestinal morphology. A selective defect in Cbl absorption was found that was not corrected by treatment with IF. In some patients, proteinuria was found, and in a few cases, this was of the tubular type, with all species of protein represented rather than albumin alone. Patients who excreted protein during childhood continued to excrete protein in adulthood, but the renal lesions were not progressive.[138] The literature on the renal pathology has been reviewed recently.[143] Neurologic abnormalities such as spasticity, truncal ataxia, and cerebral atrophy may be present as a result of Cbl deficiency.

In one sibship, homogenates of ileal biopsy specimens bound IF-Cbl normally, suggesting that the defect does not lie in the absence of receptors.[144] In other patients, an apparent absence of the ileal receptor has been described.[145] Recent observations indicate that in a canine model of Imerslund-Graesbeck syndrome, Cbl malabsorption may be due to a mutation in the IF-Cbl receptor that results in retention of an early biosynthetic compartment and inefficient expression in the brush border membrane of the intestine and kidney.[146,147]

Imerslund-Graesbeck syndrome is inherited as an autosomal recessive disorder and is most commonly found in Finland and among North African Jews. It is not restricted to those ethnic groups, however, and some 150 cases have been reported.[141–143] Treatment with systemic Cbl corrects the anemia and neurologic findings but not the proteinuria.

R-Binder (Haptocorrin) Deficiency

Deficient or absent R binder has been described in the plasma, saliva, and leukocytes of six persons in five families.[79,148–152] No clear evidence proves that the R-binder deficiency is the cause of disease in any of these patients. Although serum Cbl levels are low, TCII–Cbl levels are normal and the patients are not clinically deficient in Cbl. Two of the six patients in the literature had neurologic disease of unknown cause. It has been postulated that because of the possible role of R binder in scavenging Cbl analogues, the deficiency of R binder may be playing a role in protecting the brain from the effects of these analogues.

Transcobalamin II Deficiency

Clinical Findings. TCII deficiency has been reported in 18 patients, and data on an additional 10 have been reviewed.[79] Patients are not clinically deficient in Cbl at birth even though the only TCII found in cord blood was of fetal origin. There has not been a description of a fetal TCII, and maternal TCII does not cross the placenta. Perhaps in the presence of adequate folate and removal of intermediate proteins, Cbl is not required. TCII-deficient patients develop severe anemia much earlier than patients with other causes of Cbl malabsorption, usually developing symptoms in the first few months of life. These symptoms include failure to thrive, weakness, and diarrhea in addition to pallor. The anemia is usually clearly megaloblastic, but some patients present with pancytopenia or even isolated erythroid hypoplasia.[153] The presence of immature white cell precursors in a marrow that is otherwise hypocellular can lead to the misdiagnosis of leukemia. Neurologic disease has appeared in patients from 6 months to 30 months after the onset of symptoms.[154–157] Severe immunologic deficiency with defective cellular and humoral immunity has been seen, as well as defective granulocyte function.

Homocyst(e)inuria has been looked for in only two patients prior to Cbl therapy. In one of these patients, homocyst(e)inuria was found. In 60% of patients who were tested before therapy was initiated, methylmalonic aciduria was found. After discontinuation of therapy, MMA may return.[79,148]

In all but one patient, functional TCII as determined by an ability to bind Cbl was absent. Immunologically reactive TCII was found in three patients. In one patient, TCII was able to bind Cbl but the complex did not mediate Cbl uptake into cells. An abnormal Schilling test is usually found in patients with TCII deficiency (five of seven); in the two patients in whom the absorption of Cbl was normal, immunoreactive TCII was present. This suggests that the TCII molecule may play a role in the IF–Cbl mediated transport across the ileal cell, even if it is not functional in transporting the vitamin in the circulation.

Inheritance. Using the inherited polymorphisms of TCII in human plasma, the gene for TCII was found by genetic linkage analysis to lie close to the P blood group system on chromosome 22q.[159,160] The cDNA and the amino acid sequence of TCII have recently been described,[161] as has sequence analysis of variants.[162] Mutation analysis of TCII-deficient patients is in progress. TCII deficiency is inherited as an autosomal recessive disease. TCII is synthesized by cultures cells, and prenatal diagnosis is possible.

Management. It is necessary to keep serum Cbl levels very high to treat TCII-deficient patients successfully. Levels ranging from 1000 to 10,000 pg/mL have been required, achieved with doses of oral OH-Cbl or CN-Cbl, 500 to 1000 μg twice weekly, or systemic OH-Cbl, 1000 μg weekly or more often. Folate in the form of folic acid or folinic acid in milligram doses has been successful in reversing the hematologic findings in most patients. Folate should not be given as the only therapy because of the danger of hematologic relapse and of neurologic damage if Cbl is not also given.

Methylmalonic Acidurias

The disorders causing methylmalonic aciduria are characterized by severe metabolic acidosis and by the accumulation of large amounts of MMA in the blood, urine, and CSF.[163] Patients with methylmalonic aciduria have a defect in the mitochondrial matrix enzyme methylmalonyl-CoA mutase, which requires AdoCbl as a cofactor, and catalyzes the conversion of L-methylmalonyl-CoA to succinyl-CoA (Fig. 48-5). Classification of the methylmalonic acidurias has been based largely on the studies in cultured fibroblasts in which complementation groups have been established according to whether two lines partially correct a defect in propionate incorporation after cell fusion.

MMA Mutase Deficiency (Deficiency of Methylmalonyl-CoA Mutase)

Background. Disorders of the mutase apoenzyme result in MMA mutase deficiency and methylmalonic aciduria unresponsive to Cbl therapy. Mature mutase purified from human liver is a homodimer of 77-kd subunits, which is coded by a nuclear gene found in the cytoplasm as a precursor with a leader sequence and processed to a mature protein in the mitochondria.[61] At least two separate alleles are found at the MUT locus. The mut° cell lines have no residual mutase activity, whereas the mut⁻ cell lines show some residual mutase activity in the presence of AdoCbl. The mutase in mut⁻ cell lines show decreased affinity for AdoCbl. Several of the mut° cell lines synthesize no detectable protein, whereas some synthesize unstable proteins and at least one has a mutation that interferes with transfer of the mutase to the mitochondria.[59] Similarly variable levels of mRNA have been demonstrated in different mut° lines. Usually, no complementation between mut° and mut⁻ cell lines is seen, but recently cell lines have been shown to complement with most mut⁻ and some mut° cell lines.[164]

Clinical Findings. Patients with mutase deficiency are clinically well at birth but rapidly become symptomatic with protein feeding. They usually come to medical attention because of lethargy, vomiting, failure to thrive, muscular hypotonia, respiratory distress, and recurrent vomiting and dehydration. In normal children, MMA in urine is usually less than 15 to 20 μg/g creatinine, whereas in MMA mutase deficiency, excretion is usually more than 100 mg, and up to several g/d. In addition to MMA deficiency, these patients may have ketones and glycine in both blood and urine and metabolic acidosis with elevated levels of ammonia. Many also have hypoglycemia, leukopenia, and thrombocytopenia. One study has demonstrated that MMA mutase deficiency inhibits bone marrow stem cells in a concentration-dependent manner.[165] Follow-up of children identified by newborn screening has shown a

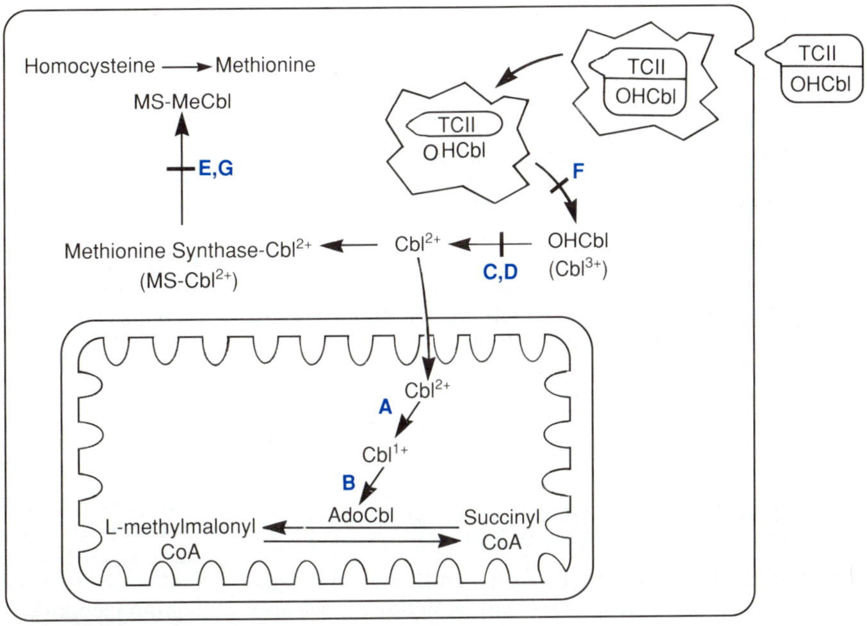

FIGURE 48-5. Scheme of cobalamin (Cbl) metabolism. Letters A through G represent the sites of known inherited defects (CblA–CblG). $Cbl^{1+,2+,3+}$, Cbl with 1+, 2+, or 3+ oxidation states of the central cobalt; AdoCbl, 5′-adenosylcobalamin; OHCbl, hydroxocobalamin; MS, methionine synthase; TCII, transcobalamin II.

number of persons who excrete MMA, have mutase deficiency by complementation analysis, and are clinically well and have never developed acidosis.[166] It is unclear whether these children are at risk for catastrophic acidosis later in life. The incidence of all forms of methylmalonic acidurias in Massachusetts is 1 in 48,000. About half of affected children respond to Cbl therapy. Patients with mut^- seek medical attention later than do mut^o patients, and they tend to have better prognoses. Neurologic sequelae may occur in mut patients, even in the absence of a documented acidotic episode.[167]

Inheritance. The gene for the mutase has been cloned and the primary amino acid sequence determined. The gene is located on the short arm of chromosome 6 (6p12-21.1).[56,60,168,169] All of the methylmalonic acidurias appear to be inherited in an autosomal recessive manner, and a number of the responsible mutations have been identified.[164,170,171]

Management. Therapy consists of protein restriction with an aim to limiting the amino acids that use the propionate pathway. Formula deficient in valine, isoleucine, methionine, and threonine is used. Mutase-deficient patients are nonresponsive to Cbl; therefore, their dietary control is essential. Maintenance of acid–base balance and therapy with carnitine in patients who are deficient has been advocated.[172,173] Even with therapy, prognosis is guarded with reports of brain infarcts and renal dysfunction as late complications.[163]

5′-Deoxyadenosylcobalamin Deficiency: cblA and cblB

Background. Two disorders result in Cbl-responsive MMA and an intracellular deficiency in AdoCbl. They are distinguished by complementation analysis and by the fact that cblA is capable of AdoCbl synthesis in cell extracts but not in intact cells, and that cblB is deficient in both systems. The defect in cblA is in a reducing system, presumably in mitochondria, which results in the conversion of cob(III)alamin to cob(I)alamin. The defect in cblB lies in the adenosyltransferase, which is the final step in the synthesis of AdoCbl (see Fig. 48-5).

Clinical Findings. In 5 of 12 patients with cblA, illness began in the first week of life; in 6 patients, it began before the end of the first year of life. Of 8 patients with cblB disease, 4 presented before the age of 1 month and 1 patient presented after the age of 1 year. Symptoms were similar to those reported for mutase deficiency, although usually they are less severe and are dependent on the clinical response to Cbl therapy.[174] Most (90%) of cblA patients responded to Cbl, and almost 70% were well at up to 14 years of age. Forty percent of cblB patients responded to therapy, and only 30% had a long-term survival. Therapy has been with either OH-Cbl or CN-Cbl by injection. It is not clear whether AdoCbl offers any therapeutic advantage.

Inheritance. Both cblA and cblB are presumed to be inherited in an autosomal recessive manner. Roughly equal numbers of patients of both sexes have been reported, and obligate heterozygotes of cblB patients show decreased adenosyltransferase activity.[158] The mutations behave as recessives in complementation analyses.

Management. One report has been made of prenatal Cbl therapy with good therapeutic results.[175] It is not certain whether therapy at birth would have been equally effective.

Combined Deficiencies of 5′-Deoxyadenosylcobalamin and Methylcobalamin: cblC, cblD, and cblF

Background. Patients with cblC, cblD, and cblF disorders have a functional deficiency in both the mutase and methionine synthase. The precise defect in these three disorders is not known but all result in a failure of the cell to synthesize both Cbl cofactors, methyl-Cbl and AdoCbl. Clinically, this can lead to combined homocyst(e)inuria and hypomethioninemia along with methylmalonic aciduria. The defect in all three disorders occurs subsequent to the endocytosis of TCII–Cbl and to hydrolysis of the TCII–Cbl complex. In cblF, the defect appears to be in the transfer of free Cbl from the lysosome to the cytoplasm, whereas in cblC and cblD the defect is presumed to be in a cytosolic cob(III)alamin reductase, which is needed to reduce the trivalent cobalt of Cbl subsequent to further Cbl metabolism (see Fig. 48-5). When incubated with labeled CN-Cbl, fibroblasts from cblC and cblD accumulate little intracellular Cbl and virtually no AdoCbl or MeCbl. In contrast, cblF fibroblasts accumulate excess Cbl but it is all free, unmetabolized, and localized to lysosomes.

Clinical Findings. We are aware of more than 80 cases of cblC: 2 patients in 1 sibship with cblD and 5 unrelated patients with cblF.

Most patients with cblC are symptomatic in the first 2 months of life with poor feeding, failure to thrive, and lethargy. Most have megaloblastic macrocytic anemia, and some have hypersegmented neutrophils and thrombocytopenia. Others have a later onset; reports were made of a 4-year-old boy presenting with fatigue, delirium, and spasticity[176] and of a 15-year-old girl presenting with mental deterioration and myelopathy.[177] In three patients, a retinal abnormality associated with perimacular degeneration was described.[79,176,178] In at least two patients, neonatal screening for methylmalonic aciduria was the method by which diagnosis was made. The methylmalonic aciduria in these patients is less severe than that seen in children with mutase deficiency but higher than that reported for those with defects in Cbl transport. Elevated serum Cbl and folate levels have been reported in several patients, but levels were never low.

The cblD patients were more mildly affected and came to attention because of mild mental retardation and behavioral problems.

The findings common to both reported patients with cblF include their being small for gestational age, poor feeding, growth retardation, and persistent stomatitis.[179,180] The first patient had glossitis, and the other had a persistent skin rash. Both patients had minor facial abnormalities, and the first had dextrocardia. Only the second patient had macrocytosis and homocyst(e)inemia as reflected by elevated total blood homocysteine.[179] Both patients were female. The second patient died suddenly, despite apparent clinical response to therapy with Cbl.

Inheritance. Males and females are affected with cblC about equally, and level of severity is equal in both sexes. The disorder is probably inherited as an autosomal recessive. The two siblings with cblD are both males, so that the possibility of sex linkage cannot be excluded.

All these defects are reflected in cultured fibroblasts. Uptake of labeled CN-Cbl can distinguish cblC and cblD from all other Cbl mutations because it is reduced in these two disorders. The incorporation of the substrates, propionate and methyl-THF, is reduced in all three disorders, as is synthesis of the two Cbl cofactors, AdoCbl and MeCbl. Direct measurements of total mutase and methionine synthase activity in cell extracts should be low (not measured in cblF). Complementation analysis between an unknown cell line and previously defined groups provides the specific diagnosis. Prenatal diagnosis has been successfully accomplished in cblC disease using amniocytes, and the diagnosis has been ruled out using chorionic villous biopsy material and cells (from unpublished data).

Management. Therapy in cblC disease can be difficult,

particularly in infants with early onset. Four of the six patients with the earliest onset have died.[158] Most patients have improved with OH-Cbl therapy (1 mg/d) by injection by reducing MMA and homocyst(e)ine excretion. Both because of studies in cultured cells[158] and because of clinical confirmation,[181] OH-Cbl rather than CN-Cbl should be used. Therapy with MeCbl and AdoCbl has been used, but it is not clear whether this offers a therapeutic advantage. In the thorough report of therapy, the effectiveness of oral as opposed to systemic OH-Cbl was compared along with the effect of carnitine, folinic acid, and betaine (250 mg/kg/d). Systemic OH-Cbl was much better than oral therapy; betaine appeared to be helpful in combination with OH-Cbl. Neither folinic acid nor carnitine had any effect. The result of therapy with daily oral betaine and biweekly injections of OH-Cbl was reduced MMA excretion, normal serum methionine and homocyst(e)ine concentration, and resolution of lethargy, irritability, and failure to thrive. All the neurologic and retinal findings were not reversed, making it apparent that early diagnosis and treatment are essential.

Patients with cblF appeared to respond to therapy with OH-Cbl in one case only by injection[179] and in the other first by injection and then by mouth.[180] Experience is too limited to know whether systemic therapy is essential. Schilling tests in one cblF patient showed an inability to absorb physiologic levels of Cbl with or without IF (from unpublished data). The theoretical consideration is that cblF patients might store Cbl in lysosomes to an extent that in itself causes symptoms after prolonged therapy. The disease has been excluded in twins and in a single pregnancy by studies on amniocytes.

Methylcobalamin Deficiency: cblE and cblG

Background. Functional methionine synthase deficiency is characterized by homocystinuria and hypomethioninemia without methylmalonic aciduria. On the basis of complementation analysis, two distinct groups have been identified, cblE and cblG (see Fig. 48-5).

Clinical and Laboratory Findings. Methyl-Cbl–deficient patients usually come to medical attention in the first 2 years of life, but one patient presented at age 21 with symptoms that caused her to be diagnosed with multiple sclerosis. There have been 23 patients with these diseases, 9 with cblE and 14 with cblG. Seven of the cblE patients were boys, and there were 9 boys with cblG.

The most common findings in both disorders include megaloblastic anemia and various neurologic problems, of which developmental delay and cerebral atrophy were the most common.[182] Other findings included electroencephalographic (EEG) abnormalities, nystagmus, hypotonia, hypertonia, seizures, blindness, and ataxia. Fibroblasts from both cblE and cblG patients show decreased intracellular levels of MeCbl in the presence of normal levels of AdoCbl. In cultured fibroblasts, normal total CN-Cbl uptake and binding to the intracellular enzymes in cblE were found; in most (7 of 10) cblG cells studied, there was normal binding to Cbl to methionine synthase, but in three lines no binding was seen.[183] Decreased incorporation of methyl-THF reflects the functional methionine synthase deficiency. The standard assay for methionine synthase in cell extracts fell within the range of controls in cblE patients, but most cblG patients have low methionine synthase activity in cell extracts. In cblE cells, a relative deficiency in methionine synthase activity can be seen when the assay is performed under suboptimal reducing conditions, suggesting that the defect lies in a reducing system associated with methionine synthase.[184,185] It has been suggested that the defect in cblG may lie in the interaction of methionine synthase with S-adenosylmethionine.[186]

One patient with cblE disease had transient methylmalonic aciduria.[187] The clinical heterogeneity is evidenced by the patient who did not present until adulthood. Her presentation was mainly neurologic, and the anemia was recognized only later.

Inheritance. Both cblE and cblG are presumed to be inherited in an autosomal recessive pattern. Decreased MeCbl levels have been seen in fibroblasts from obligate heterozygotes in cblE.[188]

Management. Therapy with OH-Cbl systemically first daily, then once or twice weekly, has been used. Usually, Cbl therapy results in correction of the anemia and metabolic abnormalities. The neurologic findings have been difficult to reverse, particularly in those affected with cblG. This stresses the importance of early diagnosis and therapy.

Prenatal diagnosis of cblE in amniocytes has been successful, and the mother carrying an affected fetus was treated from the second trimester with systemic Cbl. The baby was treated from birth and has subsequently done well. It is uncertain whether prenatal therapy is needed.

FOLATE

Folate is widespread in the diet.[1,189–192] Foods with high folate content include liver, kidney, orange juice, and spinach.[193–196] In studies of replete populations, about one third of the daily folate intake is provided by each of the following food groups: cereals and bread, fruits and vegetables, meats and fish.[197]

Chemistry

Pteroylglutamates or folates are conjugates of pterin, para-aminobenzoate, and glutamate.[198] Pterins contain two rings: one 6-membered unsaturated pyrimidine ring containing nitrogen at positions 1 and 3, and one pyrazole ring containing nitrogen at positions 5 and 8 of the pterin, which may be saturated or unsaturated. The pterin is in the form of pteridine, that is, 2-amino-4-hydroxypteridine in (Fig. 48-6). In folates, PABGlu binds to the pteridine through an aminomethyl group attached to position 6 of the pteridine. The C9–N10 bond is labile in many of the reduced folates, and cleavage of the molecule occurs readily at this point.

Folic acid, the stable yellow powder sold commercially, is synthesized chemically and sold 95% or more pure. It has both rings unsaturated and without reduction of the pyrazole ring. Folic acid is not a coenzyme for any known reaction. Folic acid is not particularly soluble in aqueous solutions or at acid pH and may thus precipitate when present at high concentrations (such as in the kidney). Folates, especially reduced folates, are photolabile and susceptible to destruction by oxidation. THF, in which the pyrazole ring is completely reduced, is labile and readily breaks at the C9–N10 bond, producing inactive catabolites.

Biochemistry

Folates bind to enzymes for which they act as cofactors or coenzymes.[1,198] They function to receive single-carbon fragments from selected reactions and to transfer these to other molecules with the aid of their enzymes. The transferred fragments are at different states of oxidation, such as those of formaldehyde, formate, or methyl; different enzymes transfer these different fragments. Folate-dependent enzymes are therefore completely inactive without their folate cofactors.[199] A scheme of folate metabolism is illustrated in (Fig. 48-7).

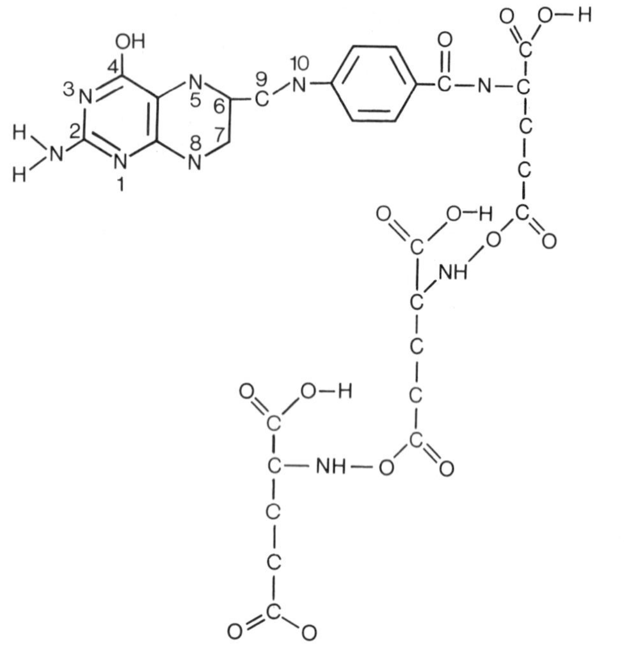

FIGURE 48-6. Tetrahydrofolyltriglutamate. Glutamates are attached by ester linkage from the α amino group of the new glutamate to the γ-carboxyl of the previously added one. This produces a chain of OH-binding carbons with carboxyl groups protruding at regular intervals—that is, a cation exchanger. The pterin (*left corner*) may be in the form of any of the folates. (Only the skeleton of the pterin is shown, many of the protons have been omitted for clarity.)

The concentrations of folates found within cells is much less than the affinity constants of most of the folate-dependent enzymes for them.[200–202] Intracellular metabolism would thus not occur if these affinities were not increased. This appears to depend on folyl polyglutamate synthetase (FPGS), an enzyme within both cytosol and mitochondria, which utilizes ATP to phosphorylate the γ-carboxyl of the folate molecule[203] and then to replace this phosphate with another glutamate.[204] Almost all intracellular folate is in the form of polyglutamyl folate, with the predominant form in most cells containing a total of five or six glutamates.[202] The affinity of polyglutamyl folates for most of these enzymes is much greater than that of monoglutamyl folates, so that most intracellular folate-dependent reactions utilize polyglutamyl folates and would not function without these forms of the folates. Cells without FPGS are auxotrophic for the products of the folate-dependent reactions, that is, they grow only in media from which they can obtain the products of folate-dependent reactions,[205] and a fluorinated folate that cannot add glutamyl residues to its γ-carboxyl sustains growth of cultured cells only at very high concentrations.[206]

Folate-dependent reactions include the following (see Fig. 48-7):

Reaction 1: Folic acid, or dihydrofolate (DHF) → THF
Reaction 2: THF + serine ↔ 5,10-methylene-THF + glycine
Reaction 3: 5,10-methylene-THF + deoxyuridylate → thymidylate + DHF
Reaction 4: 5,10-methylene-THF → N-5-methyl-THF
Reaction 5: 5,10-methylene-THF ↔ 5,10-methenyl-THF ↔ 10-formyl-THF
Reaction 6: THF + formate ↔ 10 formyl-THF
Reaction 7: 10-formyl-THF + glycinamide ribonucleotide (GAR) → N-formylglycinamide ribotide
Reaction 8: 10-formyl-THF + AICAR → formyl-AICAR
Reaction 9: N-5-methyl-THF + homocysteine → methionine
Reaction 10: 5,10-methylene THF + glycine → methylglycine
Reaction 11: THF + formiminoglutamate → N-5-formimino-THF → 5,10-methenyl-THF
Reaction 12: 5-formyl-THF → 5,10-methenyl-THF

Reaction 5 occurs on a single peptide, called C1 synthase, which contains three different enzyme sites; both enzyme sites listed as 11 are on a single protein. Reaction 11 appears restricted to hepatocytes.

DNA synthesis requires reactions 3 and 1, which are combined in the formation of thymidylate and subsequent DNA synthesis. Failure to reduce the DHF to THF causes accumulation of polyglutamyl DHF and inhibition of several reactions. Endogenous synthesis of purines (inosinic acid [IMP]) requires reactions 7 and 8.

Methionine resynthesis from homocysteine requires reaction 9. Reaction 9, methionine synthase, runs effectively with monoglutamyl N-5-methyl-THF and is the pathway for entry of plasma folate into cellular folate metabolism.

Cells in culture with defects in reaction 3, thymidylate synthase, require exogenous thymidine for growth. Those with defects in reactions 7, GAR transformylase, or 8, AICAR transformylase, cannot grow without exogenous purines. Those with defects of reaction 9 cannot grow without exogenous methionine even if homocysteine and methyl-THF are provided.

A group of enzymes, found mostly but not exclusively in lysosomes, can hydrolyze polyglutamyl folate chains to release monoglutamyl folate. These are called *folyl polyglutamate hydrolases*, or conjugases.[207] Monoglutamyl folates cross cell membranes much better than do polyglutamyl folates, and adequate cellular nutrition is impossible without this hydrolysis. Trypsin, pepsin, and other esterases do not hydrolyze folyl polyglutamates to monoglutamates. Lysosomal conjugases have a low pH optimum and seem to function almost solely in lysosomes. Conjugases that function at neutral pH are present in chick pancreas and associated with the brush border of intestinal cells. Under physiologic conditions, the relative contribution of lysosomal and neutral conjugases is unclear, but most conjugase action in vivo probably occurs within lysosomes.

Utilization

Dietary folate is mostly polyglutamyl folate. It must be hydrolyzed within the gut lumen or brush border or in the lysosomes of enterocytes to monoglutamyl folate. Polyglutamyl folates are progressively converted to monoglutamyl forms within the lumen of the small intestine.[208,209]

Physiology

Absorption From the Gut

Monoglutamyl folate is transported by a carrier-mediated transport system from the intestine into portal venous plasma. In addition to this transport system, it also can diffuse across the intestine by unidentified pathways that are not saturated by large quantities of folate. The saturable system utilizes a folate binder on the enterocyte surface, which has little selectivity for the chemical form of monoglutamyl folate. This transport is pH-dependent,[210–214] and dependent on Na^+ transport. Folate presented to the intestinal lumen does not require metabolism to other folate forms for transport,[215] appears in the portal venous blood within 15 minutes of entering the stomach, and reaches a maximal level in portal venous plasma about 1 hour later.

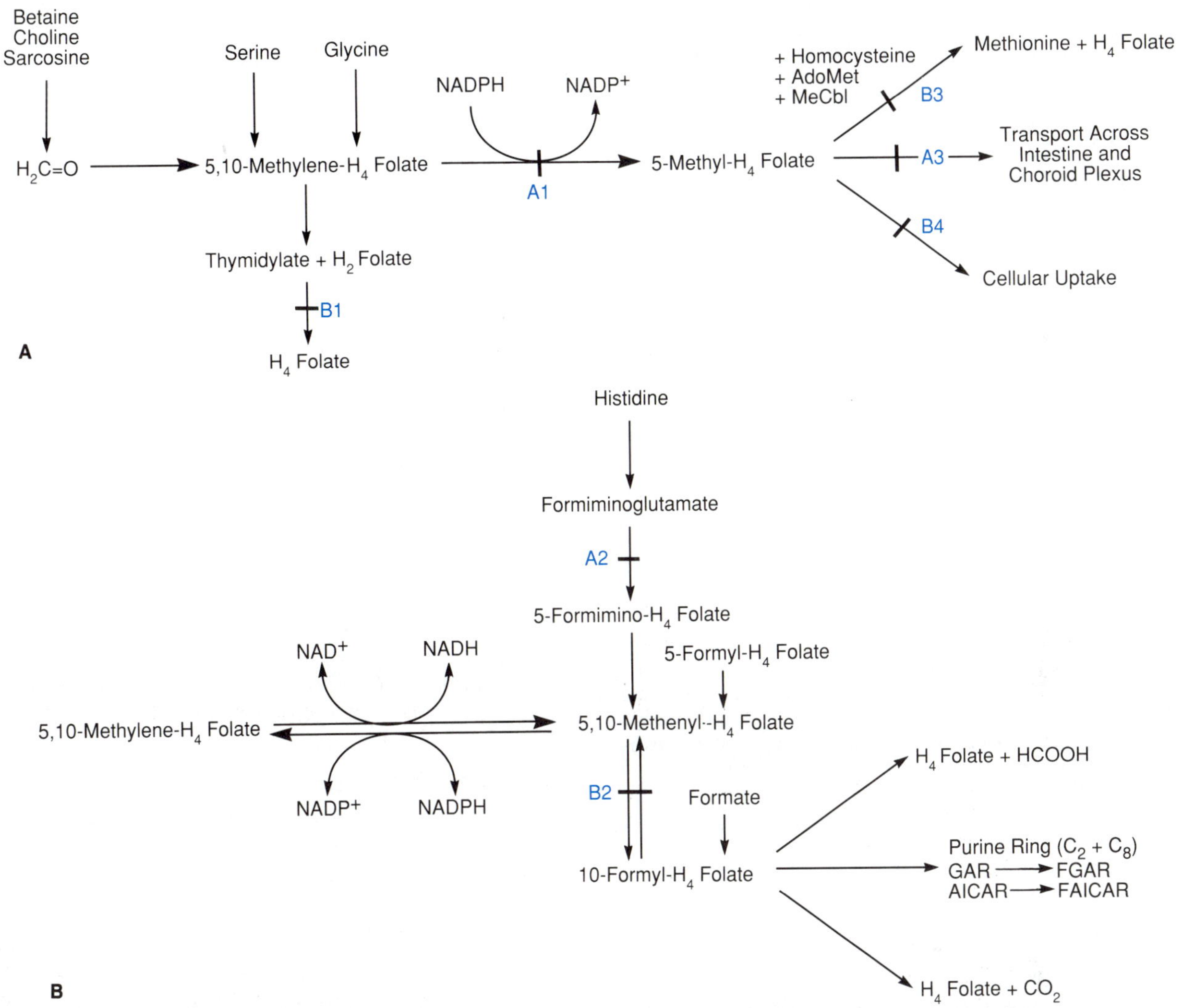

FIGURE 48-7. Folate metabolism. (**A**) The generation of 5-methyltetrahydrofolate (5-methyl-H_4-folate) and its disposition. (**B**) The remainder of the folate pathway. The sites of the confirmed (A series) and suspected (B series) inborn errors of folate metabolism and transport are indicated. GAR, glycinamide ribonucleotide; FGAR, formyl-GAR; AICAR, 5(4)-aminoimidazole-4(5) carboxamide ribonucleotide; FAICAR, formyl-AICAR. (After Cooper BA, Rosenblatt DS, Whitehead V. Megaloblastic anemia. In: Nathan DG, Oski FA, eds. Hematology of infancy and childhood. Philadelphia, WB Saunders, 1993:378)

Plasma folate then declines slowly over several hours. Reduced folates, such as 5-formyl-THF, are rapidly converted to 5-methyl-THF by the enterocyte during absorption.[216] This conversion is not required for transport and may reflect the apparent absence of methionine synthase in enterocytes.[54]

Some folate that is presented to the liver and some hepatic folate are excreted into the bile and reabsorbed.[1,217,218] This enterohepatic circulation of folate provides a slow and more even absorption than would occur without it. Some evidence shows that this enterohepatic circulation is disturbed by alcohol ingestion,[218,219] so that folate deficiency occurs more rapidly during alcohol ingestion.[220–222]

The efficiency of utilization of folic acid, polyglutamyl folate, and food folate is variable in different subjects. In general, polyglutamyl folate is absorbed about 80% as effectively as is monoglutamyl,[223] but food folate availability varies depending on the diet. Folate absorption from a mixed diet is, on average, about 50% as efficient as absorption of folic acid; that is, about twice as much folate in food is required as is folic acid.[134,193]

Transport in Plasma

Plasma folate is almost all monoglutamyl N-5-methyl-THF.[224] Most probably is unbound, although some may be bound to albumen. Treatment of volunteers with aspirin reduces their plasma folate, which suggests that albumen binding may be important.[225] Folate clearance through the kidney is about 10% of the administered folate. Proximal convoluted tubular renal cells contain folate-binding protein (FBP) on their brush borders and appear to reabsorb much of the folate that filters through the glomerulus. Renal clearance increases during pregnancy, but urinary folate remains a minority of circulating folate.[214,226–230] Because folate leaves the plasma to enter extracellular fluid compartments, cells, and the kidney, plasma folate reflects folate absorption. When absorption of folate is stopped, plasma folate decreases rapidly over days and becomes very low within 1 to 2 weeks.[231]

A minority of plasma folate is bound to an FBP,[232–235] which is homologous to or identical with the protein on the surfaces of some cells,[235–237] and is secreted by some cells. Such proteins are found on many cells types, and plasma FBP increases in pregnancy, during folate deficiency, in renal failure and cancer, and during some types of inflammation. Its function is unclear.[226,238–240] In milk, FBP may function to improve the utilization of milk folate by the newborn animal.[239,241,242]

Entry Into Cells

Folate transport into cells appears to be through a major transport system, which has much greater affinity for reduced (tetrahydro-) folates than for folic acid.[243–245] Transport is mediated by a carrier of about 35 kd that has greater affinity for 5-methyl-THF and other reduced folates than for folic acid and that appears to function by exchanging folate for intracellular anions. Divalent anions are more effective than monovalent ions, and the transport system may also serve to remove organic anions such as adenosine monophosphate and phosphate from the cell.

As already indicated, proteins homologous with the FBP of plasma are found on most body cells. Some evidence exists that on cells, FBP represents an auxiliary folate transport protein, which preferentially transports folic acid over reduced folates and is responsible for a minority of folate-entering cells. Mutant cells in culture that have lost the reduced folate binder and transport system can survive using this folate transport pathway.[246]

Monoglutamyl folate also is transported from cells, the sum of influx and efflux being the net intake by the cells. The reduced folate binder can function to exchange intracellular folyl monoglutamate with extracellular anions. Two other efflux pathways have been found, one of which is inhibited by verapamil and sulfobromophthalein and which uses vincristine as a substrate. It may be related to the multidrug resistance gene product.

Nutrition

Folate Requirements

Inadequate folate intake causes megaloblastic anemia. Most reduced folates are labile to light and oxidation and are readily destroyed by cooking. The dietary folate requirement is a matter of dispute, but the daily intake recommended by the WHO is listed in Table 48-1. The assay of folate in diets is not standardized, and different results are obtained using different techniques for hydrolysis of polyglutamyl folates, homogenization of diets, and assay of folate content. Folate is readily destroyed by cooking, so that food preparation techniques using prolonged cooking and dilution in water deplete folate (and some other water-soluble vitamins) from food. Within these limits, in populations in which folate deficiency is unusual, mean dietary folate intake has been about 3 μg of total folate per kilogram of body weight: about 150 μg/d for women and 200 μg/d for men. In this population, 500 liver specimens—most obtained from victims of trauma—showed adequate concentrations of hepatic folate.[247] In volunteers ingesting diets of known folate content,[248,249] plasma and erythrocyte folate levels remained within the normal range on such intakes. Intakes of this magnitude were calculated for normal subjects by measurements of a catabolite of folate (para-acetamido *para*-aminobenzyl glutamate), which is excreted in the urine.[250,251]

TABLE 48-1. Recommended Daily Intake of Folate and Cobalamin

Age	Folate (μg/kg/d)	Cobalamin (μg/d)
Infants	3.6	0.1
Age 1–16 y	3.3	—
Adults*	3.1	1.0

* For pregnant or lactating women: folate supplement with 300 to 1000 μg/d; cobalamin 0.3 to 0.4 μg/d.

(Adapted from Beaton G. Requirements of vitamin A, iron folate and vitamin B_{12}: report of a Joint FAO/WHO Expert Consultation Food and Agriculture Organization of the United States, Rome, 1988)

Persons With Greater Folate Requirements

Folate requirements appear greater per kilogram in the newborn infant and young child[134] (see Table 48-1), in pregnant women in whom folate is shunted to the developing fetus and urinary folate loss is increased, and in lactating women who secrete 50 μg or more into each liter of milk. The folate content of milk does not correlate with the mother's plasma folate,[252] since folate is concentrated in milk above the level of plasma folate. Some milk folate is bound to the FBP as indicated above.

Other groups with higher than normal folate requirements appear to include the following:

- Persons with sprue and other diseases of the small intestine
- Persons taking antiepileptic medication
- Women taking birth control pills
- Persons with hemolytic anemia, including those with sickle cell anemia and thalassemia

Folate Antimetabolites

Recognition of the importance of folates for cell growth prompted attempts to employ analogues for treatment of neoplastic disease. Aminopterin (4-aminopteroylglutamate) differs from folic acid in having the OH- at C4 replaced by an amino group. This material was found to be cytotoxic and was replaced for cytotoxic therapy by methotrexate, or amethopterin, which differs from aminopterin by the addition of a methyl group at C10. These materials rapidly produce neutropenia and thrombocytopenia and were found to be useful in treatment of patients with leukemia, choriocarcinoma, and subsequently a variety of other neoplastic diseases. Their effects on cell proliferation may explain their effectiveness as therapy for psoriasis, and their effect on lymphocyte metabolism and the immune system may explain their effectiveness as agents for treatment of graft-versus-host disease, rheumatoid arthritis,[253] and a variety of other diseases. Methotrexate with nicotinamide adenine dinucleotide phosphate binds tightly to dihydrofolate reductase (DHFR) and prevents binding of folate and DHF to DHFR.

Studies of the three-dimensional structure of DHFR[254,255] and the mechanism of folate and methotrexate binding have revealed that methotrexate is not a true analogue of folate because it binds to this enzyme in a different orientation than does folate, with its four-amino group in the site normally occupied by the two-amino group of folate. The three-dimensional structure that causes inhibition of this important folate enzyme could not have been predicted by examination of its two-dimensional formula.

Other Effects of Methotrexate

Methotrexate is a substrate for human FPGS and can form polyglutamates, which have a greater affinity for folate enzymes than does the monoglutamyl form and are selectively retained in cells over monoglutamyl methotrexate.[204,256] Methotrexate has a much higher K_m for FPGS than does THF (smaller affinity), so that its access to this enzyme may be blocked in the presence of large concentrations of reduced monoglutamyl folates; conversely, more methotrexate polyglutamates will be formed in folate-deficient cells. Polyglutamyl methotrexate inhibits thymidylate synthase and GAR transformylase at concentrations of methotrexate achieved in mammalian cells.[257–260] It thus inhibits endogenous thymidylate synthesis and purine synthesis. Polyglutamyl methotrexate also has a greater affinity for DHFR than does monoglutamyl methotrexate. The inhibition of DHFR by monoglutamyl and polyglutamyl methotrexate also induces accumulation of polyglutamyl DHF, which inhibits GAR transformylase and thymidylate synthase.[257,258]

Methotrexate is lost through the kidney by filtration and tubular secretion. The latter may represent a small component of methotrexate clearance.[229] Renal failure, or competition for reabsorption (or secretion) by a number of other drugs, may delay its clearance, as will accumulation of methotrexate in pleural or peritoneal effusions.[261] Methotrexate is not easily cleared from the plasma by renal dialysis. Methotrexate penetrates poorly into the CNS, but at high doses, significant concentrations are achieved in CSF. Methotrexate is lost from the CNS more slowly than from plasma.[262,263]

Normal hematopoietic cells appear to tolerate exposure to high concentrations of methotrexate for up to 24 hours under conditions that appear to kill many neoplastic cells and lymphocytes. High-dose methotrexate, with leucovorin rescue is thus efficacious in treatment of some neoplastic conditions. The means by which leucovorin (racemic mixture of R and S5-formyl-THF) rescue works is unclear. The latter enters cells readily, competing for entry with methotrexate and reducing methotrexate entry. The biologically active S5-formyl-THF is converted to 5,10-methenyl-THF by the enzyme 5,10-methenyl-THF cyclohydrase and ATP, and enters intracellular pool of reduced folate.[264–266]

Resistance to Methotrexate

Resistance to methotrexate is developed by cells in a variety of ways[267]:

- Duplication of DHFR gene with overproduction of DHFR
- Diminished transport of methotrexate (and of reduced folates) into the cells
- Decreased FPGS activity with consequent diminished polyglutamylation of methotrexate

Antifolates Other Than Methotrexate

A variety of folate inhibitors have been synthesized. Some have much greater affinity for prokaryotic than for mammalian DHFR and are used as antimalarials, antihelminthics (pyrimethamine), and antibacterials (trimethoprim). These bacterial antifolates have some affinity for mammalian DHFR, and when intracellular folate concentrations are low (as in folate deficiency), they may inhibit human DHFR and produce acute deficiency of folate. Lipid-soluble folate antagonists (such as trimetrexate) can penetrate cells in which the folate transport system will not transport methotrexate.

Inborn Errors of Folate Metabolism and Transport

Methylenetetrahydrofolate Reductase Deficiency (A_1)

Although it is the most common of the inborn errors of folate metabolism[268,269] with more than 25 cases known, methylene-THF reductase deficiency (MRD) is not associated with megaloblastic anemia. This is because the block is in the conversion of 5,10-methylene-THF to methyl-THF and therefore prevents the trapping of folates as methyl-THF. Reduced folates are available for purine and pyrimidine metabolism. Because methyl-THF serves as a methyl donor for the conversion of homocysteine to methionine (see Fig. 48-7), MRD results in elevated homocyst(e)ine levels and decreased levels of methionine.

Clinical Findings. Patients may become symptomatic at any time from infancy to adulthood. In general, the clinical severity of MRD is inversely related to the proportion of methyl-THF in cells. Most frequently, the disease appears in infancy with the most common clinical manifestation being developmental delay. More than half of patients have been diagnosed in the first year of life. Breathing disorders and seizures are often present, as is microcephaly. Motor and gait abnormalities and psychiatric manifestations have been reported. The report of a black girl with schizophrenia and MRD led to intense interest in the role of MRD in psychiatric disease. Most patients with MRD have developmental delay in contrast to psychiatric disease.

Laboratory Investigation. Homocystinuria is seen in all patients with a range of 15 to 667 μmol/24 h and a mean of 130 μmol/24 h.[268] These values are much lower than those found in patients with classic homocystinuria due to cystathionine synthase deficiency. If MRD is suspected, more than one determination of homocyst(e)ine excretion should be performed to eliminate the possibility of a false-negative value. These values are those for free homocyst(e)ine, which is normally not found in plasma or urine. Interest has developed in the measurements of both protein-bound and total homocyst(e)ine. These measurements are performed by treating plasma or serum with reducing agents to free the homocyst(e)ine from proteins to which it is bound. These measurements have defined several patients with elevated levels of homocyst(e)ine and clinical findings not typical of MRD.[270] Measurement of methylene-THF reductase in cell extracts has revealed unusual thermolability, and the term *intermediate homocystinuria* was coined. Patients with this condition were adults without the usual manifestations of MRD, particularly no neurologic manifestations. Some of these patients may be at increased risk for early coronary disease.[271,272]

Methionine levels in plasma have been low, with values from 0 to 18 μmol/L (mean, 12 μmol/L)[268]; normal fasting plasma methionine levels vary among laboratories but are usually in the range of 23 to 35 μmol/L. Although neurotransmitter levels have been measured in the CSF of only a few patients, these levels have usually been low.[268]

The diagnosis of MRD has been confirmed by direct measurement of enzyme activity in liver, leukocytes, and cultured fibroblasts and lymphocytes. In cultured fibroblasts, the specific activity of methylene-THF reductase depends on the stage of the culture cycle being several-fold higher at confluency than during logarithmic growth. Thus, it is important to compare activities of unknown samples and control cell lines at confluency. A rough correlation exists between residual enzyme activity and clinical severity.[273]

In cultured fibroblasts, the proportion of total folate that is methyl-THF and the extent of labeled formate incorporated into methionine provide better correlations with clinical severity.[273,274] Cultured fibroblasts from patients with MRD do not grow on tissue culture medium in which homocysteine replaces methionine.[275,276] This absolute growth requirement for methionine is shared by the inborn errors of Cbl metabolism that affect methionine synthase activity (cblC, cblD, cblE, cblF, and cblG).

The clinical heterogeneity in MRD is reflected at the biochemical level. Enzyme from fibroblasts of the first reported case of MRD had increased thermolability compared with control enzyme, especially when the assay was performed in the presence of the cofactor, flavin-adenine dinucleotide.[276] Recent studies have demonstrated increased thermolability in enzyme from adults who have been detected on the basis of increased plasma protein-bound homocysteine. These patients were detected as a result of screening either patients with coronary heart disease or those with low folate and Cbl levels; they had none of the other manifestations of MRD.

Autopsy Findings. Findings at autopsy in MRD patients include dilated cerebral vessels, internal hydrocephalus, microgyria, and low birth weight.[277–284] Perivascular changes, demyelination, macrophage infiltration, gliosis, and astrocytosis have been reported. The major factor in the death of some patients was thrombosis of both arteries and cerebral veins.[277] The neurovascular findings in methylene-THF reductase are not unlike those seen in classic homocystinuria due to cystathionine synthase deficiency. Two reports have been made of patients with classic findings of subacute combined degeneration of the cord similar to that described for Cbl deficiency.[283,284] Methionine deficiency may cause demyelination by interfering with methylation. Since methylene-THF reductase is present in the mammalian brain and since only methyl-THF can cross the blood–brain barrier, MRD may result in functionally low levels of folate in the brain. Because neurologic findings in MRD may be present in the absence of low methionine levels, it is possible that they are due to impaired purine and pyrimidine synthesis as opposed to methionine depletion. Also, since methylene-THF reductase has dihydropteridine reductase activity, it may have a direct role in neurotransmitter synthesis.[285] It is not resolved whether the major contribution to the neuropathology is from elevated homocysteine, decreased methionine, or other effects of low folate removed from the methylation of homocysteine to methionine. It is important that except for the absence of megaloblastic anemia, the findings in methylene-THF reductase are similar to those found in cblE and cblG disease and to a lesser extent in cblC disease in which there is also methylmalonic aciduria.

Inheritance and Prenatal Recognition. Because of the occurrence of more than one case in several families and because of the presence of both affected males and females with unaffected parents, including reports of consanguineous parents, autosomal recessive inheritance of MRD is presumed. Decreased methylene-THF reductase activity has been found in the cells of obligate heterozygotes. Prenatal diagnosis has been reported using amniocytes,[286] and the enzyme is present in chorionic villi. A cDNA for methylene-THF reductase has recently been isolated, and two mutations have been identified: a missense (ARG→GLN) in a residue conserved in bacterial enzymes, or a nonsense mutation (ARG→TER). The human gene has been localized to the p 36.3 region of chromosome 1.[286a]

Management. Early diagnosis of MRD is important because the prognosis is poor after neurologic involvement is evident. Patients with MRD are difficult to treat. Therapeutic agents that have been used include (1) folates to maximize any residual activity; (2) methyl-THF to specifically replace the missing product of methylene-THF reductase; (3) methionine to correct the deficiency of this amino acid, which requires methyl-THF for synthesis; (4) pyridoxine because it is a cofactor for cystathionine synthase and therefore may lower homocyst(e)ine levels; (5) Cbl because methyl-Cbl is a cofactor for methionine synthase; (6) carnitine because of its requirement for adenosylmethionine; (7) betaine because along with homocysteine it is a substrate for betaine methyltransferase, an enzyme that also converts homocysteine to methionine but is primarily active in the liver. Betaine has the advantage of both raising methionine levels and decreasing homocysteine levels. Because betaine methyltransferase is a liver enzyme, effects of betaine on the brain are thought to be mediated through changes in circulating levels of metabolites.

A summary of the treatment protocols for individual patients with MRD has been published.[268] These protocols have been highly variable and for the most part unsuccessful until the introduction of betaine. Therapy with either methionine alone or with methyl-THF has not been effective. We have suggested a regimen consisting of oral betaine, folinic acid, and Cbl and vitamin B_6.[287] Early therapy with betaine after prenatal diagnosis has resulted in the best outcome to date.[288]

Glutamate Formiminotransferase Deficiency (A_2)

Clinical Findings. The clinical manifestations of glutamate formiminotransferase deficiency (GFD) remain unclear. More than 12 patients have been described. The catabolism of histidine is associated with the transfer of a formimino group to THF followed by the release of ammonia and the formation of 5,10-methenyl-THF. Two activities that share a single octameric enzyme are involved in these reactions, glutamate formiminotransferase and formimino-THF cyclodeaminase. These activities are found only in the liver and kidney, and defects in these activities result in the excretion of formiminoglutamate (FIGLU). FIGLU excretion is the one constant feature of GFD.

Two distinct phenotypes have been described, one mild and one severe. In the severe form of GFD, mental and physical retardation, abnormal EEG, and dilation of the cerebral ventricles with cortical atrophy are seen. In the mild form, no mental retardation is found but excretion of FIGLU is higher. It has been proposed that, without direct enzyme measurements, the mild form of GFD is caused by a defect in the formiminotransferase enzyme, whereas the severe form is caused by a block in the cyclodeaminase enzyme.[289]

Laboratory Investigation. In most cases in which it has been examined, enzyme activity in liver has been higher than would be expected for an enzymatic block causing disease. The activity measured in the livers of five patients ranged from 14% to 54% of control values. Because the enzyme activity is expressed only in liver, it has not been possible to confirm the diagnosis of GFD using cultured cells. Also, considerable debate concerns whether the enzyme is expressed in erythrocytes.[268,290] Patients with GFD range in age from 3 months to 42 years at diagnosis. Several of the patients had macrocytosis and hypersegmentation of neutrophils. Three had delayed speech, two had seizures, and two had mental retardation as their presenting findings. Two patients were studied because they were siblings of known patients. Mental retardation was described in most of the original patients from Japan[291] but of the remaining eight patients, only three showed mental retardation.

Elevated FIGLU excretion, as well as increased FIGLU in the blood after histidine load, and high to normal serum folate levels have been reported in patients with GFD. Amino acid levels, including histidine levels, were usually normal in plasma, although occasionally hyperhistidinemia and hyperhistidinuria have been found as well as low plasma methionine levels. The excretion of two other metabolites has also been reported: hydantoin-5-propionate, the stable oxidation product of the FIGLU precursor, 4-imidazolone-5-propionate, and 4-amino-5-imidazolecarboxamide, an intermediate in purine synthesis.

Inheritance. GFD has been found in offspring of both sexes with unaffected parents. No enzyme levels in the livers of the parents and instances of consanguinity have been reported. Autosomal recessive inheritance is the probable means of transmission. Because of the lack of expression of glutamate formiminotransferase cyclodeaminase in cultured cells, definitive understanding of the inheritance of this disorder awaits the cloning of the gene and localization of the molecular defect.

Management. Two patients in one family with GFD responded with decreased FIGLU excretion to therapy with folates.[292] Six other patients did not.[268] One of two patients responded to methionine supplementation.[293,294] Since the relation between clinical expression and FIGLU excretion has not been easy to define, it is uncertain whether reducing FIGLU excretion is of any value.

Hereditary Folate Malabsorption (A_3)

Clinical and Laboratory Studies. Hereditary folate malabsorption (HFM) is characterized by severe megaloblastic anemia, diarrhea, mouth ulcers, failure to thrive, and usually progressive neurologic deterioration. Megaloblastic anemia in the first few months of life and low serum folate levels are the most important diagnostic features.

Excretion of FIGLU and orotic acid may be found in patients with hereditary folate malabsorption. All patients have a severe abnormality in the absorption of oral folic acid or of reduced folates such as folinic acid or methyl-THF. Patients with hereditary folate malabsorption provide the best evidence for a specific transport system for folates across both the intestine and the choroid plexus. Except in the case of the one affected male,[295] even when blood folate levels were raised sufficiently to correct the anemia, levels in the CSF remained low. This provides evidence that the carrier system in both intestine and brain is coded by a single gene product. The uptake of folate into other cells is probably not defective in hereditary folate malabsorption, because the hematologic findings are reversed by relatively low levels of folate and uptake of folate into cultured cells is not abnormal.

Management. Oral folate in pharmacologic doses caused a therapeutic response in some patients through correction of the hematologic abnormality. Parenteral folates have been effective in reversing the anemia but less effective in correcting the low level of folate in the CSF. 5-Formyl-THF or methyl-THF may be more effective in getting into the CSF in hereditary folate metabolism. The clinical response to therapy with folates has varied among patients. In some patients, seizures improved, and in others seizures worsened with folate therapy.[269,296]

In treating HFM patients, levels of folate must be maintained in the blood and the CSF in the range that is associated with folate sufficiency. Oral doses of folates may be increased to 100 mg or more daily if necessary, and if oral therapy is not effective, systemic therapy must be instituted. It may be necessary to give intrathecal folate if CSF levels cannot be normalized. As mentioned previously, it is thought that reduced folates such as folinic acid or methyl-THF may be more effective than folic acid in treating hereditary folate metabolism.

Inheritance. Hereditary folate metabolism has been described in only 12 patients.[295] All but one have been female, and the one male had atypical clinical findings including a lack of mental retardation and lack of correction of CSF folate levels in conjunction with correction of serum folate levels. There may be unrecognized cases of HFM, since several of the patients with hereditary folate malabsorption had siblings who died. Consanguinity has been reported in four families, and the father of one patient has intermediate levels of folate absorption. This makes autosomal recessive inheritance likely, but an explanation for the preponderance of female patients is not yet available.

The following disorders have been postulated as being due to inborn errors of folate transport or metabolism, but it is not clear whether they represent primary genetic defects.

Dihydrofolate Reductase Deficiency (B_1)

Three patients in two published reports have been postulated to have DHFR deficiency, but the existence of DHFR deficiency as a true disorder remains in doubt. The clinical manifestations are megaloblastic anemia developing shortly after birth with a better response to reduced folates such as folinic acid (citrovorum; 5-formyltetrahydrofolate) than to folic acid. DHFR converts DHF, which is generated as a by-product of the thymidylate synthase reaction to THF.

The original patient described with DHFR deficiency presented at age 6 weeks with anemia. Residual activity of DHFR in the liver was 35% of control levels. Treatment with physiologic doses of folic acid did not give a therapeutic response, but pharmacologic doses (5 mg/d orally) produced a sustained remission. After 3 years, the patient had a relapse when the folic acid was withdrawn. He did respond to small doses of folinic acid. He was restudied at age 19 years and found to be still folate-dependent.[297] Studies on fibroblasts from this patient did not show any abnormalities in DHFR activity, kinetics, or thermolability. Two other infants have been reported with megaloblastic anemia of infancy and reduced DHFR activity in liver biopsies.[298] One of these was subsequently shown to have TCII deficiency[299] and the other an inborn error of Cbl metabolism (from unpublished data).

No further reports have been made of DHFR deficiency. It is difficult to determine whether the reduced enzyme activities in liver reflect a primary deficiency of DHFR. Since the gene for DHFR has been cloned, molecular studies could clarify whether there is a a defect in a patient postulated to have this disorder.[300,301] Because it is essential not to miss a diagnosis of TCII deficiency, HFM, or an inborn error of Cbl metabolism, the diagnosis of DHFR deficiency should be considered only after ruling out other disorders.

Methylenetetrahydrofolate Cyclohydrolase Deficiency (B_2)

Three patients were reported with microcephaly, mental retardation, abnormal EEG findings, and reduced activity of methylene-THF cyclohydrolase in liver biopsy and in erythrocytes.[291] The original diagnosis was subsequently retracted, and no further cases have been reported.

Methionine Synthase Deficiency (B_3)

Functional deficiency in methionine synthase (methyl-THF: homocysteine methyltransferase) have been discussed in conjunction with cblE and cblG diseases. A single report has been made of a 6-month-old girl with megaloblastic anemia, seizures, dilated cerebral ventricles, elevated serum folate levels, and no homocystinuria.[302] Specific activity of methionine synthase was reduced to 36% of control values. Subsequent study of fibroblasts from this patient showed normal methionine synthase activity. Because the patient did not have homocystinuria, the confirmation of this disorder awaits more reports. Patients with a functional deficiency of methionine synthase due to defects in the generation of MeCbl (cblE, cblG) have both megaloblastic anemia and homocystinuria. A subset of cblG patients have decreased binding of Cbl to methionine synthase. The primary defect in cblG may indeed be in methionine synthase.

Cellular Uptake Defects (B_4)

A series of patients has been described with well-characterized abnormalities of folate uptake into cells, but it remains unclear as to whether any of these abnormalities represents primary defects.

In one large kindred, a high incidence of severe hematologic disease was seen including anemia, pancytopenia, and leukemia in 34 persons, resulting in the death of 18.[303] The proband had severe aplastic anemia that responded to folate therapy. In stimulated lymphocytes from the proband and from four family members, a marked reduction occurred in the uptake of methyl-THF despite normal uptake of folic acid. Both the proband and his son also had a lesser reduction of methyl-THF uptake in bone marrow cells. One son developed only the transport defect after becoming neutropenic, suggesting that the abnormality may not be the primary defect.[296]

In another family in which the proband and three daughters had dyserythropoiesis without anemia, an abnormality of methyl-THF uptake was seen in red blood cells and bone marrow cells but not in lymphocytes.[304] No clear correlation was found in the family between the clinical findings and the putative disorder of cellular uptake.

Orotic Aciduria

Background. Uridine-5′-monophosphate synthase (UMPS) is a bifunctional protein that contains activities for orotate phosphoribosyltransferase and orotidine-5′-monophosphate decarboxylase (ODC), resulting in the de novo synthesis of uridine-5′-monophosphate. The protein is coded by a gene located on the long arm of chromosome 3.

Clinical Symptoms. Thirteen documented patients with UMPS deficiency have been summarized.[305] More than half came to medical attention in the first few months of life, but two did not present until the age of 7 years. The most common findings in hereditary orotic aciduria are megaloblastic anemia, orotic aciduria with crystalluria, and developmental delay. If treated with pyrimidine replacement therapy, clinical response appears to be good, although even with therapy, death resulted in two patients who had been treated with uridine. Numbers of affected male and female patients have been roughly equal. Clinical heterogeneity is seen in orotic aciduria patients, and some patients have other clinical findings including immune deficiencies and congenital malformations. Four patients had evidence of cardiac malformations, and altered immune function has been suggested in a few patients.

Laboratory Diagnosis. Orotic aciduria can be differentiated from other hereditary causes of megaloblastic anemia by the excretion of orotic acid. Although excretion of orotic acid has been described in a patient with GFD,[290] the levels were lower than those seen in orotic aciduria. Whereas the excretion of orotic acid is usually less than 10 μmol/mmol creatinine in children, in orotic aciduria patients the excretion is between 1 and 10 mmol/mmol creatinine. Crystalluria may be sufficient to cause an obstructive uropathy.

Orotic aciduria is almost always associated with a deficiency of both orotate phosphoribosyltransferase and ODC. The deficiency has been seen in both erythrocytes and cultured cells. In one patient, only ODC was decreased. In patients who have been examined, mRNA of appropriate size is produced, as is immunoreacting protein. Some patients have residual enzyme activity that is more thermolabile and of different electrophoretic mobility than control enzyme.[306,307] The activities are expressed in both amniocytes and chorionic villi.[305] Orotic aciduria is inherited as an autosomal recessive disorder, and heterozygotes can be detected within families by the combined study of orotic acid excretion and enzyme activity of UMPS in erythrocytes or fibroblasts.

Management. Treatment with pyrimidine replacement has been successful in most patients with orotic aciduria resulting in disappearance of megaloblastic anemia and general improvement. Oral uridine in doses ranging from 100 to 200 mg/kg/d has been used. In two patients, therapy with cortisone and prednisone had some beneficial effect.

Dihydropteridine Reductase Deficiency

Background. Disorders of tetrahydrobiopterin metabolism affect the hydroxylation of not only phenylalanine but also of tyrosine and tryptophan.[308] The major manifestations of dihydropteridine reductase (DHPR) deficiency are related to neurologic deterioration in patients who are otherwise controlled by diet for hyperphenylalaninemia. More than 30 patients have been reported with this deficiency. Related disorders of biopterin synthesis include biopterin synthase deficiency and guanosine triphosphate cyclohydrolase deficiency. Patients with these disorders are deficient in neurotransmitters because the tetrahydrobiopterin is required for the proper function of tyrosine and tryptophan hydroxylases.[309–311] DHPR may also be required to keep folates fully reduced,[312] and folate deficiency has been reported in some cases. Megaloblastic anemia is not a primary feature of DHPR deficiency.

Diagnosis. The diagnosis of DHPR deficiency can be considered on the basis of the measurement of related metabolites in the urine, blood, and CSF. The enzyme can be measured in both cultured cells and in erythrocytes and leukocytes. DHPR is present in amniocytes, and diagnosis can been achieved prenatally.[313]

Inheritance. DHPR deficiency is an autosomal recessive disorder. Decreased enzyme activity has been demonstrated in obligate heterozygotes. Significant biochemical heterogeneity is found among patients.

Management. Therapy of DHPR deficiency involves controlling elevated phenylalanine levels by dietary restriction and by elevating neurotransmitter levels by the oral administration of L-dopa, 12 mg/kg/d, and 5-hydroxytryptophan, 10 mg/kg/d. Because of the finding of low serum and brain folate in patients with DHPR deficiency, reduced folates in the form of folinic acid in milligram doses has been added to the therapeutic regimen. DHPR deficiency is difficult to treat, and neurologic damage is possibly already present at birth.

Methionine Adenosyltransferase Deficiency

Clinical and Laboratory Findings. Patients with methionine adenosyltransferase (MAT) deficiency usually have elevated plasma methionine levels and deficient liver activity of MAT.[73,314–318] In five of six of patients, the elevated methionine levels were detected on newborn screening with levels ranging from 250 to 1270 μmol/L (control less than 30 μmol/L). The plasma and urine also contain high levels of methionine sulfoxide. No elevation of either homocyst(e)ine or tyrosine is found in plasma or urine. One patient, diagnosed at age 31, had an unusual breath odor due to the presence of high levels of dimethylsulfide. MAT activity in erythrocytes, fibroblasts, and lymphoblasts was in the range of control values in those patients studied. Findings on liver studies suggested an abnormality in the hepatic high-K_m form of MAT with sparing of the low-K_m form. Despite the fact that SAM inhibits methylene-THF reductase, no clinical manifestations related to folate deficiency or to anything else has been reported. Significant methylation of homocysteine to methionine is present presumably because methylene-THF reductase is not inhibited. The inheritance of MAT remains undefined, although one father had decreased enzyme activity. Equal numbers of affected males and females have been reported. No treatment is necessary.

CLINICAL MANIFESTATIONS OF DEFICIENCY

Cobalamin Deficiency

In well-nourished subjects, deficiency of Cbl (vitamin B_{12}) takes many months to develop because of the long half-life of Cbl within the body (about 0.05% to 0.2% is lost per day)[319] and the large hepatic stores of the vitamin. The earliest evidence of impending deficiency in such subjects with pernicious anemia is reduced capacity to absorb Cbl because of loss of gastric IF. Some evidence suggests that at this stage, the proportion of Cbl in plasma that is associated with TCII is below normal.[320]

During development of deficiency, the quantity of Cbl in the liver and the plasma decreases progressively. In most persons, the concentration of Cbl in plasma seems to decrease to below the normal range before other manifestations of deficiency can be measured. In some patients, although plasma Cbl has decreased to below its previous level, other manifestations of deficiency may appear before the concentration of Cbl in plasma reaches levels that are usually associated with deficiency.[321,322]

The appearance of hypersegmented neutrophils in the peripheral blood smear, and the accumulation of MMA and homocysteine in plasma precede the development of classic megaloblastic anemia, although bone marrow morphology probably will be noted to be abnormal if examined, and oval macrocytes may be observed on blood smears. Neurologic and mental disease may develop at this stage and may not be recognized to be caused by Cbl deficiency in the absence of anemia, elevated MCV, or abnormal concentration of Cbl in plasma.[168]

More prolonged deficiency results in anemia with megaloblastic bone marrow, sometimes with neutropenia and thrombocytopenia. The latter are more common in patients with the most severe anemia, but may sometimes be observed without severe anemia[1,323] (see Fig. 48-3).

From the foregoing, it is apparent that patients with deficiency of Cbl without symptoms may be identified by laboratory testing, may appear with unexplained neurologic signs or dementia, or may develop the full picture of megaloblastic anemia. The progression is more rapid in patients with small stores and in those with an added metabolic insult (exposure to nitrous oxide,[324] simultaneous deficiency of folate, or exposure to antifolates).

General Clinical Findings

No clinical manifestations of deficiency of Cbl may be detectable, but many deficient patients volunteer that they feel better when treated. Complaints relating to Cbl deficiency may include the following:

- Weakness and shortness of breath secondary to anemia
- Gastrointestinal symptoms
  - Loss of appetite, with small weight loss (5% to 10% of body weight)
  - Nausea, usually without vomiting
  - Constipation, but diarrhea occasionally
  - Sore tongue or cankers of the tongue, aggravated by eating spicy or acid foods
- Sterility[325]

Neurologic Findings

Neurologic problems seen in patients with Cbl deficiency are the following:

- Loss of memory rarely producing the syndrome of senile dementia or Alzheimer's disease
- Numbness and tingling of the toes or fingers or both (usually symmetric)
- Loss of balance when losing a visual horizon (as in closing the eyes)
- Difficulty in walking due to pyramidal tract or peripheral nerve involvement, which may progress to paralysis, and loss of bowel and bladder[326] control
- Blindness due to optic atrophy (rare)
- Depression[327,328]

The frequency of occurrence of the above symptoms in patients with pernicious anemia appears to have changed over the past 30 years. In a study published in 1961, weakness and dyspnea were among the complaints of almost 60% of patients with this diagnosis, 10% to 30% of patients complained of gastrointestinal symptoms, and 10% to 15% complained of neurologic symptoms.[1] Hall[329] reported that neurologic symptoms were found in 35% of patients with Cbl deficiency. In a study of such patients in 1986 in California, neurologic or mental disorders were present in 50% of patients.[330] Because no data on possible change of incidence have been published, it is unclear whether the spectrum of the disease has changed or whether patients without anemia are now being recognized because of the availability of measurements of MCV and serum Cbl. Probably the latter is the case.

Laboratory Findings

The following are findings secondary to megaloblastic anemia:

- Macrocytic anemia with or without neutropenia and thrombocytopenia; blood smear showing oval macrocytes and multilobated neutrophils
- Increased lactate dehydrogenase and sometimes bilirubin in the plasma
- Bone marrow showing megaloblastic morphology
- Increased plasma iron content and saturation of transferrin
- Decreased serum cholesterol and lipids[1]
- Decreased ratio of erythrocyte folate to serum folate
- Decreased immunoglobulins in plasma with correction after therapy[331,332]

Direct evidence of folate deficiency includes the following:

- Decreased serum Cbl
- Excess methylmalonic acid in the urine or serum
- Homocyst(e)inemia and sometimes homocyst(e)inuria
- Abnormal deoxyuridine suppression test in bone marrow, corrected in vitro by addition of MeCbl or 5-formyl-THF but not by methyl-THF

Explanation of Clinical and Laboratory Abnormalities. Anemia reduces exercise tolerance. In patients whose cardiac function cannot tolerate the increased cardiac output in response to the anemia, cardiac failure will appear. This probably is the cause of the weakness and shortness of breath secondary to anemia in these patients. Anemia induces increased cardiac output, which, with decreased oxygen transport to the myocardium, probably produces failure secondary to ischemia. Sodium retention by the kidney occurs with anemia. Megaloblastic anemia usually is macrocytic, with MCV of 120 fL or more, unless reduced by coexisting iron deficiency or other associated illness.[333–336] Not all patients with macrocytosis have megaloblastic anemia. In one study, the probability of such a patient having megaloblastic bone marrow increased with an increase of MCV; most of those with MCV greater than 106 had megaloblastic bone marrow. The incidence of anemia and the MCV values for some patients with Cbl deficiency are illustrated in (see Table 48-2).

Gastrointestinal symptoms may be secondary to megaloblastic changes in gut cells, but although morphologic changes are noted in buccal, esophageal, and enteric cells,[48] the relation of these to anorexia and to occasional diarrhea is unknown.

Neurologic degeneration (subacute combined degeneration of the spinal cord) consists of degeneration of posterior and lateral columns of the cord and a peripheral nerve lesion,[337,338] more severe in the lower extremities and characterized by demyelination that may be secondary to axonal degeneration. Decreased vibration and position sense usually are the first objective manifestations of this, with pyramidal signs observed later. The latter may be masked by decreased tendon reflexes secondary to the peripheral nerve lesion.[339–341] Cerebral symptoms and optic nerve degeneration also may occur.

Pathogenesis. The pathogenesis of the neurologic disease caused by deficiency of Cbl is not clear. It is produced in primates (including humans) and pigs by chronic exposure to nitrous oxide,[342] which also produces megaloblastic anemia in humans. Nitrous oxide penetrates cells readily and oxidizes Cbl bound to methionine synthase when the MeCbl transfers its methyl group to homocysteine. The cob(I)alamin remaining after methyl transfer is oxidized irreversibly by nitrous oxide to Cbl catabolites, which remain bound to the enzyme. This irreversibly inactivates methionine synthase. The neurologic lesion can be prevented in monkeys and pigs with methionine supplements. How this inactivation of methionine synthase causes neurologic disease and how it is prevented by methionine are unknown, but subacute combined degeneration of the spinal cord probably is caused by the same mechanism. The concentration of MMA in spinal fluid exceeds that in plasma.[343]

Plasma or Serum Levels of Vitamin B_{12}. Cbl circulates in plasma but usually is assayed in serum. Quantitation of Cbl in serum permitted unambiguous recognition of patients deficient in Cbl with megaloblastic bone marrow.[323] This analysis requires release of plasma Cbl from haptocorrin and either microbiologic analysis of the released Cbl or saturation of a high-affinity binder by a mixture of released endogenous Cbl and added labeled Cbl.

Early evaluations of measurement of Cbl in serum as a diagnostic test of deficiency revealed that serum Cbl was less than 100 pg/mL (78 pmol/L) in most patients with megaloblastic anemia due to Cbl deficiency but that in occasional patients, serum Cbl was greater than this.[323] In only 20% to 30% of patients with such low levels of serum Cbl was the bone marrow megaloblastic.[335,344] The wide availability of radiodilution assays for Cbl was followed by use of serum Cbl alone as a screening test for deficiency without proof that normal levels excluded deficiency. Serum Cbl has been shown to reflect hepatic Cbl in a small number of subjects.[1] Serum Cbl was not invariably very low in all patients with little Cbl in the liver. The clinical significance of isolated low levels of Cbl in serum without other evidence of Cbl deficiency has never been evaluated. The fact that in some patients with true deficiency of Cbl, serum Cbl was in the normal range,[345] was presumed by an investigating committee to reflect defects in the assay procedure; therefore, modified assays were introduced.

In many patients in whom serum Cbl is higher than the usual deficient range (over 100 pg/mL), neuropsychiatric symptoms and signs may be associated with methylmalonic acidemia, all of which may disappear after treatment with large doses of Cbl. This confirms previous evidence that in some patients with low serum concentrations of Cbl, hepatic Cbl was normal, and conversely, in a minority of patients with hepatic deficiency of Cbl, serum Cbl was not in the deficient range.[346] Methylmalonic acidemia may be abnormal in 10% to 15% of persons with serum Cbl levels between 100 and 300 pg/mL[346–352] (Table 48-2). It is abnormal in most patients with serum Cbl concentrations below 100 pg/mL. This indicates that although megaloblastic anemia due to deficiency of Cbl is unusual among patients with serum Cbl levels above 100 to 140 pg/mL (74 to 100 pmol/L), other manifestations of deficiency cannot be excluded without measurement of MMA or a therapeutic trial with Cbl.

Another cause of low levels of serum Cbl is folate deficiency. In a proportion of patients with folate deficiency, serum Cbl is decreased and may be in the range of deficiency. This Cbl level increases over 7 days when folate is administered, whereas the level does not increase in patients deficient in Cbl.[354] The cause of this is unknown and probably represents redistribution of Cbl between cells and plasma. It may be speculated that in intracellular deficiency of methyl-THF, MeCbl synthesis may be impaired, with decreased release of MeCbl (the predominant form) into plasma. The practical implication is that low serum Cbl levels may be observed in patients deficient only in folate.

As previously indicated, only 20% to 30% of patients with concentrations of Cbl in serum within the deficient range can be proved to be deficient in Cbl. A minority of the remainder are deficient in folate. The others are not known to be deficient and do not demonstrate abnormal metabolism of methylmalonate or homocysteine. Deoxyuridine suppression tests when performed on such patients are often slightly abnormal, but not clearly deficient. Often these patients are treated with Cbl, but no clinical benefit can be recognized.

Although a normal concentration of Cbl in serum does not completely exclude Cbl deficiency and most patients with low concentration in serum cannot be proved to be deficient, the analysis is clinically useful. It appears that the probability of Cbl deficiency decreases with increasing serum Cbl, but there is no level above which deficiency can be excluded or below which deficiency is always present. Cbl levels must be interpreted with other clinical and laboratory data, and if other evidence of Cbl deficiency is found, they may aid in confirmation. Their use as a single screening test to exclude Cbl deficiency despite the clinical picture can only be condemned.

TABLE 48-2. Frequency of Abnormal Metabolites in Patients With Ranges of Serum Cobalamin

Population	Serum Cobalamin (pg/mL)			Reference
	<100	<200	<300	
Elderly outpatients	—	80%	—	346
Referred patients	—	74%*	—	347
	—	40%	—	348
Patients referred by neurologists	53%	39%	27%	349
Macrobiotic subjects	50%	33%	—	350
Lactating vegetarians	—	70%	—	351
Outpatients	—	74%	62%	352

* Serum cobalamin level below 135 pg/mL.

Folates in Cbl Deficiency. Because intracellular folate is derived from the 5-methyl-THF of plasma, intracellular folate concentration should be proportional to that of plasma folate. This appears to be true of maturing erythroid precursors, and much of the polyglutamyl (pentaglutamyl) methyl-THF of the maturing cells is retained within the mature erythrocyte, bound to deoxyhemoglobin. Intracellular accumulation and retention of folate require the formation of polyglutamyl folate from the monoglutamyl form that enters the cell. The inactivity of methyl-THF as substrate for FPGS requires that this folate be converted to THF by methionine synthase, which has decreased activity when the cell is deficient in Cbl. Such decreased synthesis of polyglutamyl folate by maturing erythroblasts is reflected in less intracellular folate in mature erythrocytes, with consequent decreased ratio of erythrocyte folate to serum folate.[355] The decreased activity of methionine synthase in liver caused by deficiency either of Cbl or of folate may be reflected in homocyst(e)inemia and by decreased methionine levels in plasma and urine.

Deoxyuridine Suppression Test. Cells that are deficient in folate or Cbl have an expanded intracellular pool of deoxyuridylate. Incubation of such cells with deoxyuridine further expands this pool if thymidylate synthase cannot rapidly convert this to thymidylate. Based on the assumption that in cells deficient in Cbl or folate, the activity of thymidylate synthase would be decreased because of intracellular deficiency of the required folate, polyglutamyl 5,10-methylene-THF, the deoxyuridine suppression test was developed.[356,357] In this test, washed bone marrow cells are incubated with 0.1 mmol/L of deoxyuridine for 1 hour, followed by incubation with labeled thymidine for 1 hour. In normal cells, this preincubation reduces the amount of label from thymidylate incorporated into a trichloracetic acid precipitate to less than 10% of that observed without preincubation with deoxyuridylate. In cells deficient in Cbl or folate, the preincubation with deoxyuridylate reduces incorporation of label from thymidine to only 30% to 40% of that observed without preincubation with deoxyuridylate. Addition of methyl-THF to the preincubation with deoxyuridylate corrects the defect in cells deficient in folate but not in those deficient in Cbl. The defect in Cbl-deficient cells is corrected by incubation with deoxyuridylate and either methyl-Cbl or 5-formyl-THF (folinic acid). The precise biochemical basis of this phenomenon is not completely clear, but the deoxyuridine suppression test is a reliable determinant of deficiency of Cbl or folate, except in the presence of iron deficiency, which corrects the abnormal result in cells also deficient in folate or Cbl.

MMA and Homocysteine Accumulation in Plasma and Urine. As would be predicted by the biochemical reactions just described, tissues deficient in Cbl may not efficiently metabolize substrates of Cbl-dependent enzymes. The presence of MMA in the urine of some patients with pernicious anemia was described 30 years ago, as was the slow correction of this abnormal excretion after treatment with Cbl in doses adequate to correct the anemia. Most persons (over 90%) who are deficient in Cbl accumulate MMA in the plasma when the test is standardized using an internal standard.[358–362] Abnormal levels of MMA are found in plasma in some patients whose deficiency has not produced macrocytosis or anemia, but these return to the normal range after several days or weeks of Cbl treatment.

Homocysteine also accumulates in plasma in patients deficient in Cbl or folate.[321,322,363–365] The homocysteine reacts with free SH groups on proteins and is not measurable when present in low concentration if it is not released from proteins by reducing agents. Abnormal concentrations of total homocysteine are found in the plasma of over 80% of patients who are deficient in Cbl or folate. As with MMA, the homocysteine concentration returns to normal after several days or weeks of therapy with the vitamin that was deficient (Cbl or folate) but does not decrease when the other vitamin is given.

Folate Deficiency

Clinical Evidence

Hematologic. Clinically significant folate deficiency probably always has some megaloblastic component in the bone marrow, which may be reflected by anemia, as described for Cbl deficiency. In these manifestations, folate deficiency is identical with Cbl deficiency. A model of folate deficiency in mice permits study of the hematologic aspects of folate deficiency.[366]

Gastroenterologic. Patients with deficiency of folate may have gastrointestinal symptoms as described for patients deficient in Cbl. In patients with tropical sprue, diarrhea often improves after treatment with both antibacterial agents and folic acid, strongly supporting the contribution of folate deficiency in gut malfunction. Patients deficient in folate may have glossitis, anorexia, a sense of gastrointestinal discomfort, or occasionally diarrhea.

Immunologic. Evidence for immunologic deficiency affecting both humoral and cell-mediated immunity has been published for folate deficiency as for Cbl deficiency.[367,368]

Neurologic. Depression, poor judgment, and some affective disorders have been reported in patients with folate deficiency, and evidence for improvement of these with folate therapy has been presented.[369] The evidence that folate deficiency causes neurologic or affective disorders is much weaker than for the well-established defects associated with Cbl deficiency; therefore, a folate-deficient cause of these defects remains to be proved. A small number of cases have been reported of classic subacute combined degeneration of the spinal cord in patients who appeared not to be Cbl deficient and who appeared to respond to therapy with folate.[370] Other small series have reported improvement of bedridden patients hospitalized for organic brain disorders and senility after treatment with large quantities of folic or folinic acid.[371] The significance of these responses has been difficult to assess, and possible placebo effects of therapy have been difficult to determine.

Other Evidence. Increased birthweight of infants born after a longer gestation period has been reported in apparently folate-replete women treated during pregnancy with large doses of folic acid compared with similar women not so treated.[372]

Data recently published[373] have confirmed the preliminary reports that suggested an association between folate and the risk of neural tube defect.[374–378] The following have become clear:

1. The risk of such birth defects is 1 to 5 per 1000 live births in the population and about 10 times this among women who have borne a previous child with a defect in the neural tube.
2. The risk among populations with poor nutrition and consequent high frequency of folate deficiency is greater than among well-nourished populations.
3. When susceptible women received supplements of folic acid *before they became pregnant*, the incidence of neural tube defect decreased by 72%. In a general population without particular risk, no neural tube defect cases were observed among 2052 women who received folate supplements compared with 6 cases among 2104 women who received multivitamins without folate.[378a,378b]

Whether large doses of folic acid (4 mg/d) were more effective than smaller doses (0.36 to 0.8 mg/d) is unknown.

Not all cases of neural tube defect were prevented by folate supplementation. It is probable that the genetic effect that causes the abnormality can be partially masked by preventing slowing of cell proliferation caused by deficiency of folate. The effectiveness with which the fetus accumulates folate at the expense of the mother attests to the need to prevent a fetal deficiency of folate. It may be that mild defects are of such severity as to require supernormal concentrations of intracellular folate to mediate an undefined critical reaction.

The published data support routine supplementation before pregnancy of all women who might become pregnant. The dose recommended is about 0.4 mg/d folic acid, the largest dose that seems not to have masked Cbl deficiency. Whether routine supplementation of such women with Cbl would also be useful remains speculative.[378c]

Some evidence has been published that women with lower levels of folate in plasma and erythrocytes have more abortions and premature terminations of pregnancy than do women with normal folate levels.[379,379a]

Laboratory Findings

The following are laboratory findings secondary to megaloblastic anemia:

- Macrocytic anemia with or without neutropenia and thrombocytopenia, blood smear showing oval macrocytes and multilobated neutrophils
- Increased lactate dehydrogenase and sometimes bilirubin in plasma
- Bone marrow showing megaloblastic morphology
- Increased plasma iron content and saturation of transferrin
- Decreased serum cholesterol and lipids

Direct evidence of deficiency of folate is indicated by the following:

- Decreased serum folate
- Decreased erythrocyte folate
- Homocyst(e)inemia and sometimes homocystinuria
- Abnormal deoxyuridine suppression test in bone marrow, corrected in vitro by addition of N-5-methyl-THF or other folates
- Excretion of formiminoglutamate in the urine

Most of the laboratory manifestations are similar to those observed in Cbl deficiency except that methylmalonic acidemia is not observed. The sensitivity of elevated concentrations of homocyst(e)ine in plasma in detecting folate deficiency is unknown. When present and responsive to treatment with folate, it proves deficiency, but we remain ignorant of the proportion of folate deficient subjects in whom these values are elevated and whether significant deficiency of folate can be associated with normal values.

Measurements of Folate in Serum or Plasma and Erythrocytes

Folate in plasma (measured in serum) reflects recent folate absorption from the gut, so that short periods (such as 2 weeks) of diminished folate intake cause low levels of folate in plasma.[231] For this reason, the incidence of low levels of serum folate is extremely high in patients admitted to the hospital because of illness.[193] In Western countries, serum folate concentrations in the range within which deficiency is observed are found in about 40% of hospitalized patients, but in only 5% to 10% of nonhospitalized, apparently normal subjects. In subjects other than those ingesting alcohol, megaloblastic anemia and other objective evidence of folate deficiency appear to require 3 to 4 months of poor folate intake.[231,249] The problem of published normal and abnormal ranges of values complicate the interpretation of data generated by these assays. The range of normal was originally based on values obtained from a selected group of persons working in a hospital, and the range of deficient on values obtained from the range of folate values measured in groups of subjects with megaloblastic anemia that responded to folate. The lower limit of the range of normal (between 5 and 6 ng/mL in different studies) did not overlap the upper limit of the range of folate-deficient patients (3.5 or 4 ng/mL), whereas studies of folate levels in populations showed only a single population. A similar observation was made with measurements of erythrocyte folate. Since folate stores are exhausted after 3 to 4 months of folate starvation, the values would not give useful information about folate stores.

Folate in circulating erythrocytes reflects the mean folate in plasma during maturation of the precursors of the erythrocytes. In normal subjects, erythrocyte folate indicates folic acid available over the previous 3 months, and thus would be expected to correlate better than serum folate with folate status. In most patients with megaloblastic anemia due to folate deficiency, erythrocyte folate is low. Erythrocyte folate levels are in the same low range in up to 10% of apparently normal subjects, yet megaloblastic anemia occurs only in a minority. In women with megaloblastic anemia of pregnancy,[1] in patients with acute symptomatic folate deficiency (sometimes observed in intensive care units),[380–382] and in patients with combined deficiency of folate and iron, erythrocyte folate is not always in this low range. These data indicate that although erythrocyte folate levels in the deficient range may reflect low folate intake over a long period, the level of folate measured in erythrocytes does not measure whether enough folate is available to the body to prevent megaloblastic anemia but correlates with the duration of deficiency. In a study of students in Germany, multilobed neutrophils were observed in 70% of students with erythrocyte folate levels in the deficient range[383] and in a minority of those with higher levels but not in subjects with erythrocyte folate levels within the normal range.

PERNICIOUS ANEMIA

Pernicious anemia is a disease in which Cbl is not absorbed because of a lack of functioning IF. Patients in whom gastric resections have produced the IF insufficiency usually are not considered to have pernicious anemia. A small number of cases are caused by genetically determined production of no or defective IF; the remainder are caused by destruction of gastric parietal cells by lymphocyte-mediated immune destruction.

Age and Sex

The incidence of pernicious anemia increases with age, with most new cases detected in the fifth to seventh decades. In most surveys, men and women have been equally affected, but in 1968 in Sweden, the disease was twice as frequent in women over the age of 50 as in men. The incidence of the disease is reported to be 100 to 130 per 100,000 population (studies in Sweden, Denmark, and the United Kingdom between 1942 and 1968). The incidence increases with age so that with progressive aging of Western populations, the incidence is probably greater than reported above. In the seventh decade, the incidence is calculated to be 0.25 to 0.5 cases per 1000 population.

Race

Pernicious anemia is predominantly a disease of whites, being less common in blacks (in whom it may appear at a younger age than in whites) and East Indians and rare in Asians. Among whites, the disease is more common among those of northern European origin than among those originating in the Mediterranean area. Such a North–South gradient of cases has even been reported within the United Kingdom and Holland.

Genetics

Several attempts to link pernicious anemia with HLA phenotypes have not shown reliable relations. An increased risk of pernicious anemia is seen in identical twins.

Clinical Manifestations

Megaloblastic Anemia

The manifestations of megaloblastic anemia as already described are anemia, gastrointestinal symptoms, and neurologic symptoms.

Neurologic Disease

Decreased sense of vibration in the legs and some paresthesias probably affect many patients with symptomatic pernicious anemia, but subacute combined degeneration of the spinal cord affects no more than 30%. In one series,[1] paresthesias were noted in 30%, and subacute combined degeneration appeared to affect 6% to 9% of patients.

The neurologic syndrome of subacute combined degeneration of the spinal cord includes the following:

- Degeneration of posterior spinal columns causing decreased vibration sense below the iliac crests (48% of one series)[1] and less frequently causing loss of position sense in the feet (42%) and ataxia (64%)
- Degeneration of pyramidal tracts, causing spasticity and upgoing toes (Babinski's response; 56%)
- Peripheral neuropathy with distal symptomatology, causing paresthesia, anesthesia, and muscular weakness (90%)
- Dementia, mimicking Alzheimer's disease
- Optic atrophy (very rare in pernicious anemia)
- Depression, with some dementia and depression affecting virtually all symptomatic patients (90%)

Abnormalities are secondary to deficiency of Cbl, and may include all of those listed here.

Clinical Presentations

Four clinical syndromes predominate:

- Severe anemia, associated with cardiac failure, and usually associated with neutropenia, thrombocytopenia, some neurologic symptoms, glossitis, and sometimes decreased immunoglobulins
- Gastrointestinal presentation, in which gastrointestinal symptoms predominate. Glossitis usually is present. Mild anemia, which is macrocytic with a megaloblastic bone marrow, and neurologic symptoms may be present. Neutropenia, thrombocytopenia, and abnormal immunoglobulins usually are absent.
- Primarily neurologic disease with little evidence of anemia. In most patients, the MCV is elevated, but in patients with little anemia and primarily neurologic disease, serum Cbl levels are frequently found to be above the range of deficiency. The diagnosis of Cbl deficiency should not be excluded based only on serum Cbl level.
- Macrocytosis of erythrocytes determined during routine blood analysis in many patients with pernicious anemia

INVESTIGATION OF SUSPECTED DEFICIENCY OF COBALAMIN OR FOLATE

Deficiency of folate or Cbl is suspected in patients with macrocytic erythrocytes or multilobed neutrophils, a history of inadequate dietary intake, or dysfunction of the small bowel. Pernicious anemia as a cause of deficiency of Cbl is suspected in patients with unexplained neurologic disease or organic types of brain disease and in those with other autoimmune diseases. Folate deficiency is suspected in patients treated with antibiotics for several weeks and in those with poor nutrition and exposure to trimethoprim.

Screening

Measurement of serum concentrations of Cbl and folate and of erythrocyte folate determine or exclude deficiency in most patients. In patients deficient in Cbl, serum Cbl levels are usually less than 30 pg/mL; in many, erythrocyte folate is less than 15 times the serum folate level. In most patients who are deficient in folate, both serum folate and erythrocyte folate are below the normal range (less than 3 and 150 ng/mL, respectively). If multilobed neutrophils are found in the smear and the vitamin levels are in the ranges indicated, deficiency is almost certain.

If the clinical situation suggests deficiency, but screening does not confirm it, the clinical situation must be reassessed. If abnormalities of neurologic or mentation function or severe anemia, neutropenia, or thrombocytopenia are present, recognition and treatment of deficiency must not be delayed. In such patients, the tests described in the following section on confirmation of deficiency should be performed.

If neurologic abnormalities or severe cytopenias are not present and the patient understands the problem and is reliable, further investigation may be delayed pending repetition of the above tests after 1 to 2 months. Such delay cannot be justified in patients in whom subsequent study is not certain.

Confirmation of Deficiency

Confirmation of deficiency requires bone marrow aspiration for examination for megaloblastic morphology or measurement of concentrations of MMA or homocysteine in plasma, followed by a therapeutic trial (see section on therapeutic test). Methylmalonic acidemia or homocyst(e)inemia without examination of bone marrow morphology is not adequate to confirm deficiency unless that abnormality disappears after treatment. MMA may accumulate in patients with defective renal function and in those with bacterial overgrowth of the small bowel. In the latter, it decreases after administration of antibiotics.

Deficiency can also be confirmed by abnormal deoxyuridine suppression tests on freshly collected bone marrow cells, but not by this test performed on lymphocytes or other cells.

Determination of Cause of Deficiency

Cobalamin deficiency can be proved to be caused by pernicious anemia if malabsorption of free Cbl is demonstrated and is corrected by administration of a source of IF (porcine or human). This can usually be done with the *Schilling test*. The authors recommend that absorption of free Cbl be tested separately from that of Cbl bound to IF and that the commercial kits designed to evaluate both simultaneously not be used.

Pernicious anemia can almost definitively be proved in a patient with antibody to IF in serum (sensitivity around 55%, specificity almost 100%). Pernicious anemia can be definitively diagnosed in patients in whom IF is absent from the gastric juice after stimulation with histamine or another gastric stimulant.

Tests of folate absorption are unreliable. Folate malabsorption may be presumed to be present in patients ingesting a reasonable diet in whom folate deficiency is proved.

Therapeutic Test for Deficiency of Cobalamin

After treatment with one or more injections of 100 μg of CN-Cbl or OH-Cbl, a positive therapeutic test can be shown by disappearance of megaloblastic changes in the erythroid series in the bone marrow after 48 hours or by any *two* of the following:

- Decrease in MCV by 5 fL or more over 2 weeks[384,385]
- Decrease in polymorphonuclear leukocyte lobe count from the abnormal into the normal range over 4 weeks
- Decrease in serum iron by 50% over 24 hours
- Correction of anemia over 2 to 4 weeks
- Correction of thrombocytopenia over 2 weeks
- Correction of neutropenia over 2 weeks

Early Evidence of Deficiency

Some evidence shows that in patients who cannot absorb Cbl, the Cbl bound to TCII decreases before the decrease of total serum Cbl (mostly bound to haptocorrin). In such patients, poly lobe count may increase within 6 to 8 weeks after Cbl injections are discontinued and decreases again after injection of CN-Cbl. Plasma homocysteine and MMA sometimes increase into the abnormal range in less than 6 months.[385] The test that measures Cbl associated with TCII (holoTCII) might then be an early indicator of impending deficiency of Cbl. Further studies are required to evaluate the reproducibility of this test in the field, and its reliability as an early indicator of deficiency of Cbl.

Gastrin Levels and Antibodies Against Gastric Parietal Cells

In patients with atrophic gastritis and pernicious anemia, gastrin levels and antibodies against gastric parietal cells are usually abnormal, apparently reflecting the destruction of gastric parietal cells. The values do not show a differentiation between atrophic gastritis with adequate residual IF secretion and pernicious anemia.

Food Schilling Test

In patients with atrophic gastritis and inadequate gastric peptic activity, Cbl may be absorbed when fed in water, but food Cbl may not be adequately absorbed. Cbl in a variety of cooked foods has been demonstrated to be poorly absorbed by such patients, and this may produce decreased body stores of Cbl, sometimes even true deficiency.[125,126] In such patients, the usual Schilling test is normal.

Tests for Cbl absorption are not well standardized. Measurement of absorption of Cbl naturally incorporated into eggs, meat, or liver may require fecal excretion rather than urinary excretion tests. Most naturally occurring Cbl in food is as AdoCbl. This decomposes to OH-Cbl during food preparation and cooking, which binds to proteins and may not be excreted into the urine during routine Schilling tests. Absorption of 1 μg of labeled CN-Cbl added to eggs and fed, cooked or uncooked or mixed with 3 mL of chicken serum can be tested by the standard protocol for the Schilling test. Clinical studies are inadequate so far to define normal ranges, reliability, and precise procedures.[386–388] At this time, such tests must be standardized within the institution using them, with development of normal ranges for each batch of food Cbl produced. If possible, the total Cbl fed in the test (including the Cbl naturally in the food) should not exceed 2 μg.

Single-Sample Fecal Excretion Test

The single-sample fecal test of Cbl absorption is convenient and simple and probably avoids pitfalls of tests using urinary excretion. The basis of this test is the simultaneous feeding of labeled Cbl (free or bound to food) with 2 g of a nonabsorbable dye (carmine) and 10 μCi (1 mg) of chromium-51 (^{51}Cr) chromic chloride. The ^{51}Cr is not absorbed. A 2- to 3-g sample of the first or second carmine (red) stained stool is added to a counting vial, shaken with 1 to 3 mL of water, and counted for ^{51}Cr and cobalt-57 (^{57}Co). The ratio of counts is compared with the ratio in the sample fed. In normal subjects, 36% to 88% of a 1- to 2-μg dose of ^{57}Co-labeled Cbl is absorbed.[389]

TREATMENT OF DEFICIENCY

General Therapy

Patients admitted to the hospital because of severe anemia usually are symptomatic because of heart failure caused by inadequate oxygenation of tissues, induction of tachycardia and increased cardiac output, and sodium retention due to the anemia. The danger in such patients is from cardiac failure. Treatment using diuretics, limited transfusion, and oxygen should prevent death and permit investigation and treatment. Emergency administration of Cbl or folate is never required. Massive transfusion may induce cardiac failure and generally is not required because the anemia usually develops gradually. When the patient is clinically stable, investigation and appropriate therapy can be administered.

Clinical disasters sometimes occur during therapy. Treatment of severely anemic patients with pernicious anemia has been reported to be associated with a mortality rate of 14%,[390] but studies do not appear to confirm this.[391] Disasters include thrombotic events (usually strokes due to cerebral thrombosis or embolism) and hypokalemia. The latter occurs only during therapy with large doses of Cbl in patients with severe anemia and appears to be due to delay in conserving potassium, since cellular potassium loss is rapidly stopped by therapy. Although hypokalemia appears not to explain the deaths described previously, it can be prevented with potassium supplements (sometimes requiring massive supplementation), by less abrupt therapy or by transfusion to partially correct the anemia. Thrombotic disorders also might be prevented by these maneuvers, but this has not been proved. The role of potentially thrombogenic homocyst(e)inemia in causing these thrombotic episodes has not been explored.

Specific Therapy

Establish the presence of megaloblastic anemia and the cause of the deficiency by taking of serum for measurement of Cbl and folate and whole blood (citrated or in EDTA before transfusion) for erythrocyte folate determination. Serum values are not significantly altered by transfusion, but specimens should be taken before Cbl is administered. The same serum specimens can be used for measurement of MMA and homocysteine if desired.

If Cbl deficiency is suspected, treat with CN-Cbl, 10 μg/d subcutaneously for 2 days, then 100 to 1000 μg/d for 2 to 7 days. In some patients, complete conversion of megaloblastic erythropoiesis occurs with as little as 15 μg; in others, as much as 150 μg of Cbl is required. Weekly and then monthly injections are required to replete body stores.

If folate deficiency is suspected, treat with folic acid, 0.5 mg/d orally for 2 to 3 days, then with tablets of convenient size (2 to 5 mg). Unlike Cbl, folate is not stored in significant amounts. In both cases, monitor response as described earlier:

- Reticulocyte count: 2 to 5 mg of folic acid induces reticulocytosis in almost all cases of Cbl deficiency, and 100 to 1000 μg of Cbl induces reticulocytosis in some patients with folate deficiency.
- Decrease of serum iron over 24 to 48 hours. Iron deficiency may appear, which may have been masked by the megaloblastic anemia.
- Conversion of bone marrow from megaloblastic to normoblastic. The morphology of early erythroid cells is normoblastic 48 hours after enough Cbl or folate has been given.
- Decrease of MCV by 5 fL over 2 weeks
- Decrease to normal of elevated plasma homocysteine or MMA
- A sense of clinical improvement noted by the patient. Neurologic abnormalities caused by Cbl deficiency, except for dementia and depression, usually improve slowly over 1 to 6 months and the patient may not return to normal. The authors have seen one case of complete recovery from subacute combined degeneration of the spinal cord in a patient who was bedridden and had Babinski's responses over 1 to 2 weeks after institution of Cbl treatment. Dementia may sometimes improve slowly.[392]

Maintenance Therapy

Patients proved to be deficient in Cbl and who cannot absorb it require monthly injections of CN-Cbl. A prudent dose is 100 μg/mo injected subcutaneously. Failure of this regimen to maintain normal body stores is extremely rare. Similar maintenance of stores and repletion appears to follow injections of 1000 μg (1 mg) of OH-Cbl every 3 months,[393] or of 1 mg of OH-Cbl daily for 1 to 2 weeks every 6 to 12 months. The binding of OH-Cbl to tissues permits such infrequent injections, but a small proportion of such patients develop antibodies to the TCII–Cbl complex.[394] These antibodies have not been found to affect health, but they cause the accumulation of large concentrations of the TCII in plasma. It is unclear whether the rare allergy to Cbl is more common after injections of OH-Cbl than CN-Cbl.

In some patients with pernicious anemia, Cbl levels in serum or plasma can be maintained in the normal range with daily ingestion of 200 to 600 μg of CN-Cbl, taken well after meals, and perhaps by daily nasal instillation of CN-Cbl as snuff or even as a fine aerosol that is deeply inhaled. All routes except injections remain experimental.

In patients with apparent deficiency of Cbl secondary to defective peptic digestion (normal Schilling test but abnormal absorption of Cbl bound to food), normal Cbl levels and stores should be maintained by feeding 10 to 25 μg/d of CN-Cbl, but this should be verified periodically using the previously mentioned tests.

In patients with deficiency in folate, the diet should be corrected. In those with intestinal disease, 5 mg of folic acid daily by mouth is always enough therapy.

LATE COMPLICATIONS

Cancer of the stomach is associated with pernicious anemia.[395–397] Its incidence and the increased risk in such patients are not clear. Estimates have ranged from 10 times that of control subjects to minimally increased risk. Survival data of patients with pernicious anemia reported from Denmark did not demonstrate a statistically greater risk of death among patients receiving treatment for pernicious anemia than for the general population. The survival curve for men was steeper than for control subjects, but this was not statistically significant. Some evidence shows that argentaffin tumors and gastric carcinoids are more common in patients with pernicious anemia than in other subjects, and some gastroenterologists recommend periodic gastroscopy to find and remove these.[398–404] The frequency of occurrence of other tumors of the gastrointestinal tract (esophagea carcinoma, carninoid) has also been reported to be increased in patients with pernicious anemia.[405,406]

MISCELLANEOUS CLINICAL SITUATIONS

Effect of Exposure to Nitrous Oxide

Background

Nitrous oxide (laughing gas) is lipid soluble and distributes within both intracellular and extracellular spaces. Patients treated for many consecutive hours with this anesthetic have developed megaloblastic anemia despite normal plasma concentrations of folate and Cbl. Other subjects, exposed intermittently, have developed neurologic disease (subacute combined degeneration of the spinal cord) typical of deficiency of Cbl. In experimental animals (monkeys, pigs, bats), the neurologic disease caused by intermittent or chronic exposure to nitrous oxide is prevented by supplements of methionine.[404–410] The Cbl lesion is caused by oxidative destruction of intracellular Cbl by nitrous oxide.[411] Under usual conditions, only Cbl on methionine synthase is destroyed and only during turnover of the enzyme after transfer of a methyl group to homocysteine to form methionine and before the remaining Cbl is remethylated. Short exposure to nitrous oxide has no effect on cells in which methionine synthase is not turning over; during prolonged exposure, other effects may occur.[412]

The molecules of methionine synthase binding the altered Cbl are permanently inactivated. Under normal conditions, only a portion of methionine synthase binds Cbl. After inactivation by nitrous oxide, enzyme activity can consequently be restored by administration of Cbl, which binds to the residual apoenzyme of methionine synthase.

Clinical Implications

Patients exposed to nitrous oxide for more than 6 hours develop megaloblastic changes in the bone marrow, detected by abnormal deoxyuridine suppression test, and subsequently by a morphologically typical megaloblastic marrow. The acute development of megaloblastic anemia causes neutropenia and thrombocytopenia before anemia or macrocytosis. The megaloblastic anemia responds to injections of Cbl (such as CN-Cbl) if all intracellular enzyme has not previously been saturated by treatment with large doses of Cbl.

The anti-Cbl activity of nitrous oxide may cause increased sensitivity to methotrexate and to other antifolates.[413,414]

Variations in Transcobalamin Concentration

Measurement

The binding capacity of plasma or serum for Cbl is readily measured. The components binding the Cbl include TCII and haptocorrin from circulating plasma and other haptocorrins released from granulocytes during collection and separation of the blood components. Release in vitro of myeloid-associated haptocorrin also occurs in blood samples that contain EDTA. Addition of fluoride to blood during collection reduces in vitro release by preventing myeloid degranulation.

Most measures of binding capacity use serum. For empiric comparison of Cbl binding capacity with values in the literature, no special precautions need to be taken. For detailed studies of circulating haptocorrins, precautions must be taken to prevent degranulation of myeloid cells during blood collection and preparation.

Binding capacity is readily measured by mixing an excess of labeled Cbl with serum, incubating for 30 minutes and removing unbound Cbl with charcoal or another agent. Cbl remains bound to haptocorrin at pH 2.0, whereas that bound to TCII is released.[415] Binding capacity for Cbl, measured at pH2 and neutral pH thus quantitates binding to the two types of binders.

Leukemia

Elevated levels of haptocorrin were noted in patients with chronic myelocytic leukemia and found to correspond to the elevation of leukocyte count. Elevations of haptocorrin levels in patients with other myeloid diseases were expected and noted. Binding capacity of serum for Cbl is used as a measure of activity of disease in polycythemia vera and chronic myelocytic leukemia. Elevated levels of haptocorrin have also been described in some cases of eosinophilic leukemia.

Haptocorrin levels have been used to measure myeloid mass in patients with aplastic anemia, but this method has not been widely used and may not be of significant clinical usefulness.

Cancer

Elevated plasma content of haptocorrin has been noted in a few patients with carcinoma, especially adenocarcinoma of the breast and cancers in the liver, either primary or metastatic.[416,417] Haptocorrin has been detected in these cancer cells. This has not been explored clinically.

Other

Transcobalamin II in plasma decreases in patients with bone marrow aplasia and increases early during bone marrow regeneration after bone marrow transplantation. TCII levels are strikingly elevated in patients with Gaucher's disease,[418] apparently reflecting its synthesis by macrophages.[419]

Management of Asymptomatic Patients With Low Levels of Plasma Cobalamin

Normal ranges of plasma Cbl established in clinical laboratories usually include values of a normal population extending 2 standard deviations above and below the mean, thus including 95% of normal subjects. For this reason, 2.5% of all normal subjects will have values below the normal range. By these calculations, in Western populations, more normal subjects than deficient patients in a group of subjects would be expected to have values of serum Cbl below the range of normal. Because serum Cbl in some patients with true deficiency may not be very low, patients with abnormal levels of serum Cbl require detailed clinical and laboratory investigation to separate normals from patients with true deficiency. No recent and detailed studies have been done of apparently normal subjects with low levels of Cbl but no other evidence of deficiency to determine what proportion of such subjects have clinically significant deficiency. These studies are made difficult because in many of these patients, absorption of Cbl from the gut is assessed using the Schilling test; therefore, the patients have received injections of Cbl.

In asymptomatic subjects with low concentrations of Cbl in serum, without evidence of folate deficiency, and in whom absorption of CN-Cbl is shown subsequently to be normal, the presence of multilobed neutrophils in the blood smear, megaloblastic bone marrow, or elevated levels of homocysteine or MMA in plasma suggests physiologically significant deficiency and demands treatment. In such patients, treatment with oral Cbl (2 μg/d) should be effective, but response to therapy and proof of maintenance of normal levels of serum Cbl and other parameters must be documented 2 to 4 times per year. If these are not maintained in the normal range, monthly injections of Cbl are required. In such patients, one may presume that the absorption is less effective than is absorption of the free Cbl that is evaluated by the Schilling test. The investigation may also be supplemented by measuring absorption of CN-Cbl mixed with eggs or chicken serum.

In patients with low levels of folate in plasma or erythrocytes, nutritional counseling is recommended to teach them to increase folate intake in the diet. In patients whose plasma or erythrocyte folate concentrations chronically return to deficient levels, supplementation with folate (2 to 5 mg of folate twice weekly) or daily orange juice may be used.

Megaloblastic Anemia Patients Who Do Not Respond to Cobalamin or Folate Treatment

Nutritional anemia always responds to correction of the deficiency when the nutrient enters the body. If megaloblastic anemia persists after treatment and correction of plasma levels of the vitamin, either a metabolic abnormality is present, requiring larger doses of Cbl (such as in cblC, TCII deficiency), or the defect is not caused by the deficiency. Such patients often have myelodysplasia or other clonal neoplastic disease, but they may have viral infection (such as HIV) that produces megaloblastic morphology of erythroid precursors, or they may be taking antimetabolic drugs. Antimetabolic drugs (6-mercaptopurine, cytosine arabinoside) produce megaloblastic changes that usually are restricted to erythroid cells, whereas both megaloblastic erythroid cells and macrogranulocytes are observed in patients treated with hydroxyurea. Methotrexate and other antifolates produce morphologic abnormalities in bone marrow that are megaloblastic but less striking than would be expected for the degree of cytopenia.

Pregnant Women

It is apparent that folate intake should be increased during pregnancy and that some risk to the fetus of a folate-deficient pregnant woman does exist. Good nutrition, including foods rich in folate (orange juice, liver, kidney, spinach), is recommended for women in whom pregnancy is likely. Folate supplementation of grain for the entire population may take place in an attempt to reduce neural tube defects.[378c]

After pregnancy has begun and reaches the second trimester, the major benefit of folate sufficiency probably is to the mother. In women who do not take in the quantities of folate and iron recommended by the WHO, supplementation with iron, folate, and Cbl prevent megaloblastic anemia of pregnancy and may reduce maternal morbidity. Oral folic acid probably must be taken daily, since weekly administration does not prevent megaloblastic anemia of pregnancy. Tablets containing multiple nutrients may cause destruction of Cbl in the tablets, so that Cbl probably should be taken alone and not as part of a vitamin–mineral mixture.

Young Patients With Pernicious Anemia

The age at which inherited defects of Cbl cause disease varies in patients with different defects and according to the degree of abnormality of the defect. Thus, the first patient described with structurally abnormal IF remained well until age 11, apparently because his IF retained 1% to 2% of the activity of normal IF. Megaloblastic anemia was noted in the patient with structurally abnormal TCII in the second decade. Disease first appears in early infancy in most patients with cblC disease or TCII deficiency.

Classic pernicious anemia occurs in young persons, perhaps in a higher proportion of blacks than whites.[420] In these young patients with autoimmune destruction of gastric mucosa and consequent lack of IF (pernicious anemia), antibody to IF is almost always detectable in serum.

As the age of the patient deficient in Cbl increases, the likelihood that Cbl deficiency is due to pernicious anemia and not to an inherited defect of Cbl metabolism increases. However, rare cases of inherited disorders (cblC, cblG) do occur in adults.

Mutilobed Neutrophils

From the foregoing text, it is apparent that recognition of the biologic effects of deficiency of Cbl and folate are vital to the adequate management of patients. Although megaloblastic hematopoiesis in bone marrow and its replacement with normoblastic hematopoiesis after therapy are definitive of deficiency and its cause, frequent bone marrow aspirations are difficult to obtain and uncomfortable for patients. In most clinical settings, practical considerations require a less invasive technology. Measurement of changes in plasma levels of MMA and homocysteine may become available and less expensive in the future, and new data generated probably will validate these as objective measures of deficiency and its correction. Recognition of multilobation of neutrophils in smears of peripheral blood remains the single least expensive and reproducible measure of significant deficiency of folate or Cbl.[35,322,383,419,421] Disappearance of multilobation 10 to 15 days after therapy can be used to evaluate response.

Lobe Counts

Lobe counts differ in different studies, according to the criteria used for lobation and the quality of the smears. It remains unclear whether hyperlobation reflects the entry into the blood of a population of abnormal cells or whether physiologic lobe formation becomes exaggerated in megaloblastic anemia. Also unclear is whether the multilobed neutrophils contain more DNA and are larger than normal.

Measures of Hyperlobation

Counting Six-Lobed Neutrophils. Even a single six-lobed neutrophil among 100 neutrophils appears to be diagnostic of hyperlobation. It remains unclear whether six-lobed neutrophils are more significant than increased numbers of five-lobed neutrophils.

Counting Five-Lobed Neutrophils. In normal blood, five-lobed neutrophils represent about 2% of all lobated neutrophils (excluding band forms).The presence of more than five cells containing five lobes among 100 segmented neutrophils counted has been considered abnormal. Mathematically, if 5% of all segmented neutrophils contain five lobes, by repeatedly counting 100 cells, one would count between 0.5 and 9.5, five-lobed polys 95% of the time, and 0 to 7.2 five-lobed polys will be counted among 100 cells 68% of the time. This indicates that although counting 5 five-lobed polys per 100 cells may indicate hyperlobation, finding fewer five-lobed polys does not exclude hyperlobation.

Poly Lobe Count. This technique counts the total number of lobes found when 100 segmented neutrophils are counted. In normal smears in most laboratories, poly lobe count is usually less then 3.4. One standard deviation equals the square root of the number of lobes counted, so that if 340 lobes are found among 100 polys, 95% of the time another count will be greater than 303 lobes in 100 polys.

Comments

The technique used is immaterial, but it must be validated by determining normal ranges and reproducibility of counts on single samples; then it must be applied with confidence to smears from patients. In patients with inflammation and left shift of neutrophils, all values decrease. The error caused by this left shift may be reduced by omitting band neutrophils from counts. The definition of a lobe rests with the observer; it requires only that the definition be consistent. We find that to obtain consistent poly lobe counts (the number of neutrophils with five or more lobes or the mean lobe count per 100 segmented cells), it is necessary to limit lobes counted to those separated from the next area of chromatin by a thin thread (see Fig. 48-2). Others believe that "if it's separate, then it's separate."

Are multilobed neutrophils ever seen in patients without megaloblastic myelopoiesis? Multilobed neutrophils have been described in patients with iron deficiency, uremia, chronic myelocytic leukemia; in patients receiving hydroxyurea; and in several other conditions. Hyperlobation that disappears 10 to 14 days after therapy with Cbl or folate indicates megaloblastic myelopoiesis.[35]

REFERENCES

1. Cooper BA, Rosenblatt DS, Whitehead V. Megaloblastic anemia. In: Nathan DG, Oski FA, eds. Hematology of infancy and childhood. Philadelphia, WB Saunders, 1993:354.

1a. Chanarin I. The megaloblastic anaemias. London, Blackwell Scientific Publications, 1979.

2. Wintrobe MM. Hematology, the blossoming of a science: a story of inspiration and effort. Philadelphia, Lea & Febiger, 1985.

3. Castle WB. The conquest of pernicious anemia. In: Wintrobe MM, ed. Blood: pure and eloquent. New York, McGraw-Hill, 1979:283.

4. Ehrlich P. Untersuchungen zur Histologie und Klinik des Blutes. Berlin, Hirschwald, 1891.

5. Minot GR, Murphy RP. Treatment of pernicious anemia by a special diet. JAMA 1926;87:470.

6. Wills L. Treatment of "pernicious anaemia of pregnancy" and "tropical anaemia" with special reference to yeast extract as curative agent. Br Med J 1931;1:1059.

7. Castle WB. Observations on the etiologic relationship of achylia gastrica to pernicious anemia. I. The effect of administration to patients with pernicious anemia of the contents of the normal human stomach recovered after ingestion of beef muscle. Am J Med Sci 1929;178:748.

8. Fenwick S. On atrophy of the stomach. Lancet 1870;2:78.
9. Cooper BA, Castle W. Sequential mechanisms in the enhanced absorption of vitamin B_{12} by intrinsic factor in the rat. J Clin Invest 1960;39:199.
10. Ungley CC. Vitamin B_{12} in pernicious anaemia: parenteral administration. Br Med J 1949;2:1370.
11. Zalusky R, Herbert V, Castle WB. Cyanocobalamin therapy effect in folic acid deficiency. Arch Intern Med 1962;109:545.
12. Hall BE, Watkins CH. Experience with pteroylglutamate synthetic folic acid in treatment of pernicious anemia. J Lab Clin Med 1947;32:622.
13. Youngdahl-Turner P, Rosenberg LE. Binding and uptake of TC II by human fibroblasts. J Clin Invest 1978;61:1331.
14. Cooper BA, Paranchych W. Selective uptake of specifically-bound cobalt-58 vitamin B_{12} by human and mouse tumour cells. Nature 1961;191:393.
15. Gottlieb CW, Lau K-S, Wasserman LR, Herbert V. Rapid charcoal assay for intrinsic factor (IF), gastric juice unsaturated binding capacity, antibody to IF, and serum unsaturated binding capacity. Blood 1965;25:875.
16. Mollin DL, Ross GIM. The vitamin B_{12} concentrations of serum and urine of normals and of patients with megaloblastic anaemias and other diseases. J Clin Pathol 1952;5:129.
17. Adams JF, Tankel HI, MacEwan F. Estimation of the total body vitamin B_{12} in the live subject. Clin Sci 1970;39:1.
18. Russell JSR, Batten FE, Collier J. Subacute combined degeneration of the spinal cord. Brain 1900;23:39.
19. Jeffries GH, Hoskins DW, Sleisinger MH. Antibody to intrinsic factor in serum of patients with pernicious anemia. J Clin Invest 1962;41:1106.
20. Dow CA, Aizpura HJ, Pedersen JS, Ungar B, Toh BH. 65- to 70-kd protein identified by immunoblotting as the presumptive gastric microsomal autoantigen in pernicious anaemia. Clin Exp Immunol 1985;62:732.
21. Aizpura HJ, Ungar B, Toh B-H. Autoantibody to the gastric receptor in pernicious anemia. N Engl J Med 1985;313:479.
22. Burman P, Mårdh S, Norberg L, Karlsson FA. Parietal cell antibodies in pernicious anemia inhibit H^+,K^+-adenosine triphosphatase, the proton pump of the stomach. Gastroenterology 1989;96:1434.
23. Hakami N, Nieman PE, Canellos GP, Lazerson J. Neonatal megaloblastic anemia due to inherited TCII deficiency in two siblings. N Engl J Med 1971;285:1163.
24. Levy HL, Mudd SH, Schulman JD, Dreyfus PM, Abeles RH. A derangement in B_{12} metabolism associated with homocystinemia, cystathioninemia, hypomethioninemia and methylmalonic aciduria. Am J Med 1970;48:390.
25. Platica O, Janeczko R, Regec A, Quadros EV, Rothenberg SP. Isolation of the complementary DNA for human TCII. Proc Soc Exp Biol Med 1989;192:95.
26. Platica O, Janeczko R, Quadros EV, Regec A, Romain A, Rothenberg SP. The cDNA sequence and the deduced amino acid sequence of human TCII show homology with rat intrinsic factor and human TCI. J Biol Chem 1991;266:7863.
27. Johnston J, Bollekens J, Allen RH, Berliner N. Structure of the cDNA encoding TC I: a neutrophil granule protein. J Biol Chem 1989;264:15754.
28. Hansen MR, Nexo E, Svendsen I, Bucher D, Olesen H. Human intrinsic factor: its primary structure compared to the primary structure of rat intrinsic factor. Scand J Clin Lab Invest 1989;49(Suppl 194):19.
29. Gueant JL, Jokinen O, Schohn H, Monin B, Nicolas JP, Gräsbeck R. Purification of intrinsic factor receptor from pig ileum using as affinity medium human intrinsic factor covalently bound to Sepharose. Biochim Biophys Acta 1989;992:281.
30. Dieckgraefe BK, Seetharam B, Banaszak L, Leykam JF, Alpers DH. Isolation and structural characterization of a cDNA clone encoding rat gastric intrinsic factor. Proc Natl Acad Sci USA 1988;85:46.
31. Grasbeck R, Simons K, Sinkkonen I. Isolation of intrinsic factor and its probable degradation product as their vitamin B_{12} complexes, from human gastric juice. Biochim Biophys Acta 1968;158:292.
32. Rickard KA, Brown RD, Dunleavy L, Robin H, Kronenberg H. The bone marrow colony forming cell in megaloblastic anaemia and iron deficiency anaemia. Aust NZ J Med 1975;5:424.
33. Finch CA, Coleman DH, Motulsky AG, Donohue DH, Reiff RH. Erythrokinetics in pernicious anemia. Blood 1956;11:807.
34. London IM, West R. The formation of bile pigments in pernicious anemia. J Biol Chem 1950;184:359.
35. Nath BJ, Lindenbaum J. Persistence of neutrophil hypersegmentation during recovery from megaloblastic granulopoiesis. Ann Intern Med 1979;90:757.
36. Wickramasinghe SN, Cooper EH, Chalmers DG. A study of erythropoiesis by combined morphologic qualitative cytochemical and autoradiographic methods: normal bone marrow, vitamin B_{12} deficiency and iron deficiency anemia. Blood 1968;31:304.
37. Schmid JR, Moeschlin S, Haegi V. Pernicious anaemia: an erythrokinetic and autoradiographic study, using ^{3}H-thymidine, ^{3}H-uridine, and ^{3}H-cytidine. Acta Hematol 1964;32:65.
38. Reisner EH Jr, Korson R. Microspectrophotometric determination of desoxyribosenucleic acid in megaloblasts of pernicious anemia. Blood 1951;6:344.
39. Yoshida Y, Todo A, Shirakawa S, Wakisaka G, Uchino H. Proliferation of megaloblasts in pernicious anemia as observed from nucleic acid metabolism. Blood 1968;31:292.
40. Castellot JJ Jr, Miller MR, Lehtomaki DM, Pardee AB. Comparison of DNA replication and repair enzymology using permeabilized baby hamster kidney cells. J Biol Chem 1979;254:6904.
41. Hoffbrand AV, Wickramasinghe RG. Biochemical basis of megaloblastosis. In: Zittoun J, Cooper BA, eds. Folates and cobalamins. Berlin, Springer-Verlag, 1989:1.
42. Kass L. Cytochemical detection of homocysteine in pernicious anemia and in chronic erythremic myelosis. Am J Clin Pathol 1977;67:53.
43. Glazer HS, Mueller JF, Jarrold T, Sakurai K, Vilter .W. Effect of vitamin B_{12} and folic acid on nucleic acid composition of bone marrow of patients with megaloblastic anemia. J Lab Clin Med 1954;43:905.
44. Wickramasinghe SN, Longman JE. Rate of incorporation of tritiated thymidine into DNA of normoblastic and megaloblastic bone marrow cells in vitro. Acta Hematol 1974;52:14.
45. Hawkins CF. Value of serum iron levels in assessing effect of haematinics in macrocytic anaemias. Br Med J 1955;1:383.
46. Heinivaara O, Kaipainen WJ. Occurrence of large cells in myelopoiesis of megaloblastic anaemias. Ann Med Intern Fenn 1959;48:177.
47. Fliedner TM, Cronkite EP, Killmann SA, Bond VP. Granulopoiesis. II. Emergence and pattern of labeling of neutrophilic granulocytes in humans. Blood 1964;24:683.
48. Mitchell K, Ferguson MM, Lucie NP, Macdonald DG. Epithelial dysplasia in the oral mucosa associated with pernicious anaemia. Br Dent J 1986;161:259.
49. Dolphin D. B_{12}. In: Chemistry, vol 1. New York, John Wiley & Sons, 1982.
50. Pratt JM. Inorganic chemistry of vitamin B_{12}. New York, Academic Press, 1972.
51. Hogenkamp HPC. Chemistry of vitamin B_{12}. In: Babior BM, ed. Cobalamin: biochemistry and pathophysiology. New York, Wiley Interscience, 1975:21.
52. Taylor RT. B_{12}-dependent methionine biosynthesis. In: Dolphin D, ed. B_{12}. Biochemistry and medicine, vol 2. New York, John Wiley & Sons, 1982:307.
53. Retey J. Methylmalonyl-CoA mutase. In: Dolphin D, ed. Biochemistry and medicine, vol 2. New York, John Wiley & Sons, 1982:357.
54. Finkelstein JD. Regulation of methionine metabolism in mammals. In: Usdin E, Borchardt RT, Creveling CR, eds. Transmethylation. New York, Elsevier/North Holland, 1978:49.
55. Kolhouse JF, Utley C, Fenton WA, Rosenberg LE. Immunochemical studies on cultured fibroblasts from patients with inherited methylmalonic acidemia. Proc Natl Acad Sci USA 1981;78:7737.
56. Ledley FD, Lumetta M, Nguyen PN, Kolhouse JF, Allen RH. Molecular cloning of L-methylmalonyl-CoA mutase: gene transfer and analysis of mut cell lines. Proc Natl Acad Sci USA 1988;85:3518.
57. Marsh EN, McKie N, Davis NK, Leadlay PF. Cloning and structural characterization of the genes coding for adenosylcobalamin-dependent methylmalonyl-CoA mutase from *Propionibacterium shermanii*. Biochem J 1989;260:345.
58. Cameron B, Briggs K, Pridmore S, Refort G, Crouzet J. Cloning and analysis of genes involved in coenzyme-B_{12} biosynthesis in pseudomonas denitrificans. J Bacteriol 1989;171:547.
59. Fenton WA, Hack AM, Kraus JP, Rosenberg LE. Immunochemical studies of fibroblasts from patients with methylmalonyl-CoA mutase apoenzyme deficiency: detection of a mutation interfering with mitochondrial import. Proc Natl Acad Sci USA 1987;84:1421.
60. Ledley FD, Lumetta MR, Zoghbi HY, VanTuinen P, Ledbetter D.H. Mapping of human methylmalonyl CoA mutase (MUT) locus on chromosome 6. Am J Human Genet 1988;42:839.
61. Fenton WA, Hack AM, Helfgott D, Rosenberg LE. Biogenesis of the mitochondrial enzyme methylmalonyl-CoA mutase: synthesis and processing of a precursor in a cell-free system and in cultured cells. J Biol Chem 1984;259:6616.
62. Barness LA, Morrow G III. Methylmalonic aciduria: a newly discovered inborn error. Ann Intern Med 1968;69:633.
63. Morrow G III, Revsin B, Clark R, Lebowitz J, Whelen DT. A new variant of methylmalonic acidemia–defective coenzyme-apoenzyme binding in cultured fibroblasts. Clin Chem Acta 1978;85:67.
64. Utley CS, Marcell PD, Allen RH, Asok CA, Kolhouse JF. Isolation and characterization of methionine synthase from human placenta. J Biol Chem 1985;260:13656.
65. Fenton WA, Ambani LM, Rosenberg LE. Uptake of hydroxocobalamin by rat liver mitochondria: binding to a mitochondrial protein. J Biol Chem 1976;251:6616.
66. Fenton WA, Rosenberg LE. Genetic and biochemical analysis of human cobalamin mutants in cell culture. Annu Rev Genet 1978;12:223.
67. Fenton WA, Rosenberg LE. The defect in the cbl B class of human methylmalonic acidemia: deficiency of cob(I)alamin adenosyltransferase activity in extracts of cultured fibroblasts. Biochem Biophys Res Commun 1981;98:283.
68. Abe T, Gibbs B, Cooper BA. Forms of vitamin B_{12} in blood and bone marrow in patients with pernicious anaemia. Br J Hematol 1975;31:493.
69. Beck WS, Cohen R, Jorgensen J. Mitochondrial cobalamins: evidence

of their noninvolvement in mitochondrial DNA synthesis. In: Zagalak B, Friedrich W, eds. Vitamin B_{12}. Berlin, Walter de Gruyter, 1979:975.
70. Quadros EV, Jackson B, Linnell JC. Interconversion of cobalamins in human lymphocytes in in vitro and the influence of nitrous oxide on synthesis of cobalamin coenzymes. In: Zagalak B, Friedrich W, eds. Vitamin B_{12}. Berlin, Walter de Gruyter, 1979:1045.
71. Fenton N, Rosenberg LE. Mitochondrial metabolism of hydoxocobalamin: synthesis of adenosylcobalamin by intact rat mitochondria. Arch Biochem Biophys 1978;189:441.
72. Storch KJ, Wagner DA, Burke JF, Young VR. Quantitative study in vivo of methionine cycle in humans using [methyl-2H3]- and [1-13C]methionine. Am J Physiol 1988;255:E322.
73. Gahl WA, Finkelstein JD, Mullen KD, et al. Hepatic methionine adenosyltransferase deficiency in a 31-year-old man. Am J Hum Genet 1987;40:39.
74. Gahl WA, Bernardini I, Finkelstein JD, et al. Transsulfuration in an adult with hepatic methionine adenosyltransferase deficiency. J Clin Invest 1988;81:390.
75. Blom HJ, Boers GHJ, Trijbels JMF, Van Roessel JJM, Tangerman A. Cystathionine-synthase-deficient patients do not use the transamination pathway of methionine to reduce hypermethioninemia and homocystinemia. Metabolism 1989;38:577.
76. Finkelstein JD. Regulation of methionine metabolism in mammals. In: Usdin E, Borchardt RT, Creveling CR, eds. Transmethylation. New York, Elsevier/North Holland, 1978:49.
77. Matthews RG, Jencks DA, Frasca V, Matthews KD. Methionine biosynthesis in chemistry and biology of pteridines. In: Cooper BA, Whitehead VM, eds. Pteridines and folic acid derivatives. New York, Walter de Gruyter, 1986:698.
78. Fujii K, Galivan JH, Huennekens FM. Activation of methionine synthase: further characterization of the flavoprotein system. Arch Biochem Biophys 1979;178:662.
79. Cooper BA, Rosenblatt DS. Inherited defects of vitmain B_{12} metabolism. Annu Rev Nutr 1987;7:291.
80. Frasca V, Dunham WR, Sands RH, Riazzi BS, Matthews RG. Studies of cobalamin-dependent methionine synthase from Escherichia coli. In: Cooper BA, Whitehead VM, eds. Chemistry and biology of pteridines 1986: pteridines and folic acid derivatives. Berlin, Walter de Gruyter, 1986:917.
81. Rioux CR, Kadner RJ. Two outer membrane transport systems for vitamin B_{12} in Salmonella typhimurium. J Bacteriol 1989;171:2986.
82. Lundrigan MD, Kadner RJ. Altered cobalamin metabolism in *Escherichia coli* btuR mutants affects btuB gene regulation. J Bacteriol 1989;171:154.
83. Friedrich MJ, Deveaux LC, Kadner RJ. Nucleotide sequence of the BtuCED genes involved in vitamin B_{12} transport in *Escherichia coli* and homology with components of periplasmic-binding-protein–dependent transport systems. J Bacteriol 1986;167:928.
84. Fernandez-Costa F, Metz J. Vitamin B_{12} binders (transcobalamins) in serum. CRC Crit Rev Clin Lab Sci 1982;18:1.
85. Quadros EV, Rothenberg SP, Pan YC, Stein S. Purification and molecular characterization of human TC II. J Biol Chem 1986;261:15455.
86. Newmark P, Newman GE, OBrien JR. Vitamin B_{12} in the rat kidney: evidence for an association with lysosomes. Arch Biochem Biophys 1970;141:121.
87. Newmark PA. The mechanism of vitamin B_{12} by the kidney of the rat in vivo. Biochim Biophys Acta 1972;261:85.
88. Cooper BA, Dirks J. Evidence for complexing of TC II in canine and human plasma and serum. Am J Physiol 1973;224:758.
89. Pletch QA, Coffey JW. Properties of the proteins that bind vitamin B_{12} in rat liver. Arch Biochem Biophys 1972;15(1):157.
90. Tan CH, Hansen HJ. Studies on the site of synthesis of TCII. Proc Soc Biol Med 1968;127:740.
91. Li N, Seetharam S, Lindemans J, Alpers DH, Arwert F, Seetharam B. Isolation and sequence analysis of variant forms of human transcobalamin II. Biochim Biophys Acta 1993;1172:21.
92. Ogawa K, Kudo H, Kim YC, Nakashima Y, Ohshio G, Yamabe H. Expression of vitamin B_{12} R-binder in breast tumors: an immunohistochemical study. Arch Pathol 1988;112:1117.
93. Lee EY, Seetharam B, Alpers DH, DeSchryver-Kecskemeti K. Immunohistochemical survey of cobalamin-binding proteins. Gastroenterology 1989;97:1171.
94. Nexo E. Characterization of cobalamins attached to TC I and TC II in human plasma. Scand J Haematol 1977;18:358.
95. Kolhouse JF, Kondo H, Allen NC, Podell E, Allen RH. Cobalamin analogues are present in human plasma and can mask cobalamin deficiency because current radioisotope dilution assays are not specific for true cobalamin. N Engl J Med 1978;299:785.
96. Hewitt JE, Seetharam B, Leykam J, Alpers DH. Isolation and characterization of a cDNA encoding porcine gastric haptocorrin. Eur J biochem 1990;189:125.
97. Batt RM, Horadagoda NU. Gastric and pancreatic intrinsic factor–mediated absorption of cobalamin in the dog. Am J Physiol 1989;257: G344.
98. Allen RH, Seetharam B, Podell E, Alpers DH. Effect of proteolytic enzymes on the binding of cobalamin to R protein and intrinsic factor. J Clin Invest 1978;61:47.
99. Sennett C, Rosenberg LE, Mellman IS. Transmembrane transport of cobalamin in prokaryocytic and eukaryocytic cells. Annu Rev Biochem 1981;50:1053.
100. Doscherholmen A, Hagen PS. Delay of absorption of radiolabeled cyanocobalamin in the intestinal wall in the presence of intrinsic factor. J Lab Clin Med 1959;54:434.
101. Rothenberg SP, Weiss JP, Cotter R. Formation of TC II–vitamin B_{12} complex by guinea-pig ileal mucosa in organ culture after in vivo incubation with intrinsic factor–vitamin B_{12}. Br J Haematol 1978;40:401.
102. Chanarin I, Muir M, Hoffbrand AV, Hughes A. Evidence for an intestinal origin of TC II during vitamin B_{12} absorption. Br Med J 1978;11:1453.
103. Katz M, Cooper BA. Solubilization of the receptor for intrinsic factor—B_{12} complex from guinea pig intestinal mucosa. Methods Enzymol 1980;67:67.
104. Radford DM, Eddy R, Haley L, et al. Gene sequences coding for S-adenosylmethionine decarboxylase are present on human chromosome 6 and the X and are not amplified in colon neoplasia. Cytogenet Cell Genet 1988;49:285.
105. Seetharam S, Ramaujam KS, Seetharam B. Intrinsic factor receptor activity and cobalamin transport in bile duct–ligated rats. Am J Physiol 1992;262:G210.
106. Fyfe JC, Ramanujam KS, Ramaswamy K, Patterson DF, Seetharam B. Defective brush border expression of intrinsic factor–cobalamin receptor in canine inherited intestinal cobalamin malabsorption. J Biol Chem 1991;266:4489.
107. Von Bonsdorf B. On the remission after removal of the worm in pernicious anemia in presence and absence of extrinsic factor in the food. Acta Med Scand 1943;116:77.
108. Nyberg W, Grasbeck R, Saarni M, Von Bonsdorf B. Serum vitamin B_{12} levels and incidence of tape worm anemia in a population heavily infected with Diphyllobothrium latum. Am J Clin Nutr 1961;9:606.
109. Robertson JA, Gallagher ND. Intrinsic factor-cobalamin accumulates in the ilea of mice treated with chloroquine. Gastroenterology 1985;89: 1353.
110. Robertson JA, Gallagher ND. In vivo evidence that cobalamin is absorbed by receptor-mediated endocytosis in the mouse. Gastroenterology 1985;88:908.
111. Kapadia CR, Serfilippi D, Voloshin K, Donaldson RM Jr. Intrinsic factor–mediated absorption of cobalamin by guinea pig ileal cells. J Clin Invest 1983;71:440.
112. Gueant JL, Monin GB, Champigneulle B, Gerard H, Nicolas JP. Radioautographic localization of iodinated human intrinsic factor in the guinea pig ileum using electron microscopy. Gut 1988;29:1370.
113. Cooper BA. Complex of intrinsic factor and B_{12} in human ileum during vitamin B_{12} absorption. Am J Physiol 1968;214:832.
114. Kolhouse JF, Allen RH. Absorption, plasma transport, and cellular retention of cobalamin analogues. J Clin Invest 1977;60:1381.
115. Kishimoto T, Tavassoli M, Green R, Jacobsen DW. Receptors for transferrin and TCII display segregated distribution on microvilli of leukemia L1210 cells. Biochem Biophys Res Commun 1987;146:1102.
116. Seligman PA, Allen RH. Characterization of the receptor for TCII isolated from human placenta. J Biol Chem 1978;253:1766.
117. Rosenblatt DS, Hosack A, Matiaszuk N. Expression of TCII by amniocytes. Prenat Diagn 1987;7:35.
118. Rosenberg LE. The inherited methylmalonic acidemias. Prog Clin Biol Res 1982;103:187.
119. Coulombe JT, Shih VE, Levy HL. Massachusetts metabolic disorders screening program. II. Methylmalonic aciduria. Pediatrics 1981;67:26.
120. Halperin ML, Schiller CM, Fritz IB. The inhibition by methylmalonic acid of malate transport by the dicarboxylate carrier in rat liver mitochondria: a possible explanation for hypoglycemia in methylmalonic aciduria. J Clin Invest 1971;50:2276.
121. Montgomery JA, Mamer OA, Scriver CR. Metabolism of methylmalonic acid in rats. J Clin Invest 1983;72:1937.
122. Young PR, Waickus CM. Time dependence of the methylation of myelin basic protein from bovine brain: evidence for protein-methylarginine demethylation. Biochem Biophy Res Comm 1987;142:200.
123. Deacon R, Purkiss P, Green R, Lumb M, Perry J, Chanarin I. Vitamin-B_{12} neuropathy is not due to failure to methylate myelin basic protein. J Neurol Sci 1986;72:113.
124. Van Tonder SV, Ruck A, Van der Westhuyzen J, Fernandez-costa F, Metz J. Dissociation of methionine synthetase (ec 2.1.1.13) activity and impairment of DNA synthesis in fruit bats (*Rousettus augyptiacus*) with nitrous oxide–induced vitamin B_{12} deficiency. Br J Nutr 1986;55:187.
125. Levine AS, Doscherholmen A. Vitamin B_{12} bioavailability from egg yolk and egg white: relationship to binding proteins. Am J Clin Nutr 1983;38:436.
126. Doscherholmen A, McMahon J, Economon P. Vitamin B_{12} absorption from fish. Proc Soc Exp Biol Med 1981;167:480.
127. Bakker HD, van Gennip AH, Duran M, Wadman SK. Methylmalonate excretion in a pregnancy at risk for methylmalonic acidaemia. Clin Chim Acta 1978;86:349.
128. Baker SJ, Mathan VI. Evidence regarding the minimal daily requirement of dietary vitamin B_{12}. Am J Clin Nutr 1981;34:2423.
129. Roberts RD, Webb JKG, Vaishnava S, Baker SJ. Vitamin B_{12} deficiency in Indian infants. Br Med J 1973;3:67.
130. Banerjee DK, Chatterjea JB. Vitamin B_{12} content of some articles of Indian diets and effect of cooking on it. Br J Nutr 1963;17:385.

131. Chanarin I, Stephenson E. Vegetarian diet and cobalamin deficiency: their association with tuberculosis. J Clin Pathol 1988;41:759.
132. Armstrong BK, Davis RE, Nicol DJ, van Merwyk AJ, Larwood CJ. Hematological vitamin B_{12} and folate studies on Seventh Day Adventist vegetarians. Am J Clin Nutr 1974;27:712.
133. Abdulla M, Anderson I, Asp N-G, et al. Nutrient uptake and health status of vegans: chemical analyses of diets using the duplicate portion sampling technique. Am J Clin Nutr 1981;34:2464.
134. Beaton G. Requirements of vitamin A, iron, folate and vitamin B_{12}: report of a Joint FAO/WHO Expert Consultation Food and Agriculture Organization of the United Nations, Rome, 1988.
135. Katz M, Lee SK, Cooper BA. Vitamin B_{12} malabsorption due to a biologically inert intrinsic factor. N Engl J Med 1972;287:425.
136. Yang Y-M, Ducos R, Rosenberg AJ, et al. Cobalamin malabsorption in three siblings due to abnormal intrinsic factor that is markedly susceptible to acid and proteolysis. J Clin Invest 1985;76:2057.
137. Gräsbeck R. Familial selective citamin B_{12} malabsorption. (Letter) N Engl J Med 1972;287:358.
138. Brocj H, Imerslund O, Monn E, Seip M. Imerslund-Grasbeck anemia: a long-term follow-up study. Acta Pediatr Scand 1984;73:248.
139. el Mauhoub M, Sudarshan G, Aggarwal V, Banerjee G. Imerslund-Grasbeck syndrome in a Libyan boy. Ann Trop Paediatr 1989;9:180.
140. el Bez M, Souid M, Mebazaa R, Ben dridi MF. L'anemie d'Imerslund-Grasbec: a propos d'un cas. Ann Pediatr (Paris) 1992;39:305.
141. Salameh MM, Banda RW, Mohdi AA. Reversal of severe neurological abnormalities after vitamin B_{12} replacement in Imerslund-Grasbeck syndrome. J Neurol 1991;238:349.
142. Kulkey O, Reusz G, Sallay P, Mitenyi M. Szeletiv B12-vitamin felszivasi zavar (Imerslund-Grabeck syndroma). Orv Hetil 1992;133:3311.
143. Liang DC, Hsu HC, Huang FY, Wei KN. Imerslund-Grasbeck syndrome in two brothers: renal biopsy and ultrastructural findings. Pediatr Hematol Oncol 1991;8:361.
144. Mackenzie IL, Donaldson RM Jr, Trier JS, Mathan VI. Ileal mucosa in familial selective vitamin B_{12} malabsorption. N Engl J Med 1972;286: 1021.
145. Burman JF, Walker WJ, Smith JA, et al. Absent ileal uptake of IF-bound vitamin B_{12} in the Imerslund-Grasbeck syndrome (familial vitamin B_{12} malabsorption with proteinuria). Gut 1985;26:311.
146. Fyfe JC, Giger U, Hall CA, Jezyk PF, Klumpp SA, Levine J, Patterson DF. Inherited selective intestinal cobalamin malabsorption and cobalamin deficiency in dogs. Pediatr Res 1991;29:24.
147. Fyfe JC, Ramanujam KS, Patterson DF, Seetharam B. Defective brush-border expression of intrinsic factor–cobalamin receptor (IFCR) in canine inherited intestinal cobalamin malabsorption. J Biol Chem 1991;266:4489.
148. Barshop BA, Wolff J, Nyhan WL, et al. TCII deficiency presenting with methylmalonic aciduria and homocystinuria and abnormal absorption of cobalamin. Am J Med Genet 1990;35:222.
149. Carmel R. A new case of deficiency of the R binder for cobalamin, with observations on minor cobalamin binding proteins in serum and saliva. Blood 1982;59:152.
150. Carmel R. R-binder deficiency. A clinically benign cause of cobalamin pseudodeficiency. JAMA 1983;250:1886.
151. Deficiency of vitamin B_{12} alpha globulin in two brothers. Blood 1969;33: 1.
152. Jenks J, Begley J, Howard L. Cobalamin-R binder deficiency in a woman with thalassemia. Nutr Rev 1983;41:277.
153. Nierbrugge DJ, Benjamin DR, Christie D, Scott CR. Hereditary TC II deficiency presenting as red cell hypoplasia. J Pediatr 1982;101:732.
154. Burman JF, Mollin DL, Sourial NA, Sladden RA. Inherited lack of TC II in serum and megaloblastic anemia: a further patient. Br J Hematol 1979;43:27.
155. Meyers PA, Carmel R. Hereditary TC II deficiency with subnormal serum cobalamin levels. Pediatrics 1984;74:866.
156. Thomas PK, Hoffbrand AV, Smith IS. Neurological involvement in hereditary TC II deficiency. J Neurol Neurosurg Psychiatry 1982;45: 74.
157. Zeitlin HC, Sheppard K, Bolton FG, Hall CA. Homozygous TCII deficiency maintained on oral hydroxocobalamin. Blood 1985;66:1022.
158. Fenton W, Rosenberg LE. Inherited disorders of cobalamin transport and metabolism. In: Scriver CR, Beaudet AL, Sly WS, Valle D, eds. The metabolic basis of inherited disease. New York, McGraw-Hill, 1989: 2065.
159. Daiger SP, Labowe ML, Parsons M, Wang L, Cavalli-Sforza LL. Detection of genetic variation with radioactive ligands. III. Genetic polymorphism of TC II in human plasma. Am J Hum Genet 1978;30:202.
160. Eiberg H, Moller N, Mohr J, Nielsen LS. Linkage of TC II to the P blood group system and assignment to chromosome 22. Clin Genet 1986;29: 354.
161. Platica O, Janeczko R, Quadros EV, Regee A, Romain R, Rothenberg SP. The cDNA sequence and the deduced amino acid sequence of human transcobalamin II show homology with rat intrinsic factor and human transcobalamin I. J Biol Chem 1991;266:7860.
162. Li N, Seetaran S, Lindemans J, Alpers DH, Arwert F, Seetharan B. Isolation and sequence analysis of variant forms of human transcobalamin II. Biochem Biophys Acta 1993:1172;21.
163. Mahoney MJ, Bick D. Recent advances in the inherited methylmalonic acidemias. Acta Paediatr Scand 1987;76:689.
164. Raff ML, Crane AM, Jansen R, Ledley FD, Rosenblatt DS. Genetic characterization of a mut locus mutation discriminating heterogeneity in *mut°* and *mut⁻* methylmalonic aciduria by interallelic complementation. J Clin Invest 1991;87:203.
165. Inque S, Kreiger I, Sarnaik A, Ravindranath Y, Fracassa M, Ottenbreit MJ. Inhibition of bone marrow stem cell growth in vitro by methylmalonic acid: a mechanism for pancytopenia in a patient with methylmalonic acidemia. Pediatr Res 1981;15:95.
166. Ledley FD, Levy HL, Shih VE, Benjamin R, Mahoney MJ. Benign methylmalonic aciduria. N Engl J Med 1984;311:1015.
167. Shevell MI, Matiaszuk N, Ledley FD, Rosenblatt DS. Varying neurologic phenotypes among mut° and mut⁻ patients with methylmalonyl CoA mutase deficiency. Am J Med Genet 1993;45:619.
168. Zoghbi HY, O'Brien WE, Ledley FD. Linkage relationships of the human methylmalonyl-CoA mutase to the HLA and D6S4 loci on chromosome 6. Genomics 1988;3:396.
169. Jansen R, Kalousek F, Fenton WA, Rosenberg LE, Ledley FD. Cloning of full-length methylmalonyl-CoA mutase from a CDNA library using the polymerase chain reaction. Genomics 1989;4:198.
170. Crane AM, Martin LS, Valle D, Ledley FD. Phenotype of disease in three patients with identical mutations in methylmalonyl CoA mutase. Hum Genet 1992;89:259.
171. Crane AM, Jansen R, Andrews R, Ledley FD. Cloning and expression of a mutant methymalonyl coenzyme A mutase with altered cobalamin affinity that causes mut⁻ methylmalonic aciduria. J Cl∞ Invest 1992;89: 385.
172. Chalmers RA, Stacey TE, Tracey BM, et al. L-Carnitine insufficiency in disorders of organic acid metabolism: response to L-carnitine by patients with methylmalonic aciduria and 3-hydroxy-3-methylglutaric aciduria. J Inherit Metab Dis 1984;7:109.
173. Wolff JA, Carroll JE, Le Phuc Thuy, Prodanos C, Haas R, Nyhan WL. Carnitine reduces fasting ketogenesis in patients with disorders of propionate metabolism. Lancet 1986;1:289.
174. Matsui SM, Mahoney MJ, Rosenberg LE. The natural history of the inherited methylmalonic acidemias. N Engl J Med 1983;308:857.
175. Ampola MG, Mahoney MJ, Nakamura E, Tanaka K. Prenatal therapy of a patient with vitamin B_{12} responsive methylmalonic acidemia. N Engl J Med 1975;293:313.
176. Mitchell GA, Watkins D, Melancon SB, et al. Clinical heterogeneity in cobalamin C variant of combined homocystinuria and methylmalonic aciduria. J Pediatr 1986;108:410.
177. Shinnar S, Singer HS. Cobalamin C mutation (methylmalonic aciduria and homocystinuria) in adolescence: a treatable cause of dementia and myelopathy. N Engl J Med 1984;311:451.
178. Robb RM, Dowton SB, Fulton AB, Levy HL. Retinal degeneration in vitamin B_{12} disorder associated with methylmalonic aciduria and sulfur amino acid abnormalities. Am J Ophthalmol 1984;97:691.
179. Shih VE, Axel SM, Tewksbury JC, Watkins D, Cooper BA, Rosenblatt DS. Defective lysosomal release of vitamin B_{12} (cblF): a hereditary metabolic disorder associated with sudden death. Am J Hum Genet 1989;33: 555.
180. Rosenblatt DS, Laframboise R, Pichette J, Langevin P, Cooper BA, Costa T. New disorder of vitamin B_{12} metabolism (cobalamin F) presenting as methylmalonic aciduria. Pediatrics 1986;78:51.
181. Bartholomew DW, Batshaw ML, Allen RH, et al. Therapeutic approaches to cobalamin-C methylmalonic acidemia and homocystinuria. J Pediatr 1988;112:32.
182. Watkins D, Rosenblatt DS. Functional methionine synthase deficiency (cblE and cblG): clinical and biochemical heterogeneity. Am J Med Genet 1989;34:427.
183. Sillaots SL, Hall CA, Rosenblatt DS. Heterogeneity in cblG: differential binding of vitamin B_{12} to methionine synthase. Am Soc Hum Genet 1990;47:A167.
184. Rosenblatt DS, Cooper BA, Pottier A, Lue-Shing H, Matiaszuk N, Grauer K. Altered vitamin B_{12} metabolism in fibroblasts from a patient with megaloblastic anemia and homocystinuria due to a new defect in methionine biosynthesis. J Clin Invest 1984;74:2149.
185. Rosenblatt DS, Cooper BA. Selective deficiencies of methyl B_{12} (cblE and cblG). Clin Invest Med 1989;12:270.
186. Hall CA, Lindenbaum RH, Arenson E, Begley JA, Chu RC. The nature of the defect in cobalamin G mutation. Clin Invest Med 1989;12:262.
187. Tuchman M, Kelly P, Watkins D, Rosenblatt DS. Vitamin B_{12}-responsive megaloblastic anemia, homocystinuria, and transient methylmalonic aciduria in cb1E disease. J Pediatr 1988;113:1052.
188. Rosenblatt DS, Cooper BA, Schmutz SM, Zaleski SM, Casey RE. Prenatal vitamin B_{12} therapy of a fetus with methylcobalamin deficiency (cobalamin E disease). Lancet 1985;1:1127.
189. Chung ASM, Pearson MN, Darby WI, Miller ON, Goldsmith GA. Folic acid, vitamin B6, pantothenic acid and vitamin B_{12} in human dietaries. Am J Clin Nutr 1961;9:573.
190. Collins RA, Harper AE, Schreiber M, Elvehjem CA. The folic acid and vitamin B_{12} content of the milk of various species. J Nutr 1951;43:313.
191. Moscovitch LF, Cooper BA. Folate content of diets in pregnancy: comparison of diets collected at home and diets prepared from dietary records. Am J Clin Nutr 1973;26:707.
192. Clifford AJ, Wilson DS, Casey SM, Stedman LJ, Bills ND. A rat bioassay of the comparative availability of food folates. (Abstract) FASEB J 1989;3: 667.

193. Cooper BA. Reassessment of folic acid requirements. In: White PL, Selvey N, eds. Nutrition in transition: Proceedings of the Western Hemisphere Nutrition Congress V. Monroe, WI, American Medical Association, 1978:281.
194. Zittoun J. Folate and nutrition. Chemioterapia 1985;4:388.
195. Senti FR, Pilch SM. Analysis of folate data from the second National Health and Nutrition Examination Survey (NHANES II). J Nutr 1985;115:1398.
196. Herbert V. Making sense of laboratory tests of folate status: folate requirements to sustain normality. In: Zittoun J, Cooper BA, eds. Folates and cobalamins. Berlin, Springer-Verlag, 1989:119.
197. Canada Department of National Health and Welfare. Food Consumption Patterns Report: a report from Nutrition Canada by the Bureau of Nutritional Sciences, Health Protection Branch, Ottawa, Department of Health and Welfare Health and Welfare Canada, 1976.
198. Blakley RL, Benkovic SJ. Folates and pterins, vol 1. Chemistry and biochemistry of folates. New York, John Wiley & Sons, 1984.
199. Mackenzie RE. Biogenesis and interconversion of substituted tetrahydrofolates. In: Blakley RL, Benkovic SJ, eds. Folates and pterins: chemistry and biochemistry of folates. New York, John Wiley & Sons, 1984:255.
200. Matthews RG, Lu Y-Z, Green JM, Mackenzie RE. The polyglutamate specificities of four folate-dependent enzymes from pig liver. In: Goldman ID, ed. Proceedings of the Second Workshop on Folyl and Antifolyl Polyglutamates. New York, Praeger, 1985:65.
201. Hilton JG, Cooper BA, Rosenblatt DS. Folate polyglutamate synthesis and turnover in cultured human fibroblasts. J Biol Chem 1979;254: 8398.
202. Foo SK, Shane B. Regulation of folylpoly-gamma-glutamate synthesis in mammalian cells In vivo and in vitro synthesis of pteroylpoly-gamma-glutamates by Chinese hamster ovary cells. J Biol Chem 1982;257:13587.
203. Mejillano MR, Jahansouz H, Matsunaga TO, Kenyon GL, Himes RH. Formation and utilization of formyl phosphate by N10-formyltetrahydrofolate synthetase: evidence for formyl phosphate as an intermediate in the reaction. Biochemistry 1989;28:5136.
204. Cichowitz DJ, Hynes JB, Shane B. Substrate specificity of mammalian folylpolygamma-glutamate synthetase for 5,8-dideazafolates and 5,8-dideaza analogues of aminopterin. Biochim Biophys Acta 1988;957: 363.
205. McBurney MW, Whitmore GF. Characterization of a Chinese hamster cell with a temperature-sensitive mutation in folate metabolism. Cell 1974;2:183.
206. Coward JK, McGuire JJ, Galivan J. Fluoroglutamate-containing folates and antifols: probing the role of polyglutamylation in vitro. In: Curtius HC, Ghisla S, Blau N, eds. Chemistry and biology of pteridines 1989: pteridines and folate derivatives. Berlin, Walter de Gruyter, 1990:1198.
207. McGuire JJ, Coward JK. Pteroylpolyglutamates: biosynthesis, degradation, and function. In: Blakley RL, Benkovic SJ, eds. Folates and pterins: chemistry and biochemistry of folates. New York, John Wiley & Sons, 1984:135.
208. Halsted CH, Baugh CM, Butterworth CE. Jejunal perfusion of simple and conjugated folates in man. Gastroenterology 1975;68:261.
209. Chandler CJ, Wang TT, Halsted CH. Pteroylpolyglutamate hydrolase from human jejunal brush borders: purification and characterization. J Biol Chem 1986;261:928.
210. Rosenberg IH, Zimmerman J, Selhub J. Folate transport. Chemioterapia 1985;4:354.
211. Selhub J, Rosenberg IH. Folate transport in isolated brush border membrane vesicles from rat intestine. J Biol Chem 1981;256:4489.
212. Schron CM, Washington C Jr, Blitzer BL. Anion specificity of the jejunal folate carrier: effects of reduced folate analogues on folate uptake and efflux. J Membr Biol 1988;102:175.
213. Blakeborough P, Salter DN. Folate transport in enterocytes and brush-border membrane vesicles isolated from the small intestine of the neonatal goat. Br J Nutr 1988;59:485.
214. Browman BB, McCormick DB, Rosenberg IH. Epithelial transport of water-soluble vitamins. Annu Rev Nutr 1989;9:187.
215. Whitehead VM, Cooper BA. Absorption of unaltered folic acid from the gastrointestinal tract in man. Br J Hematol 1967;13:679.
216. Whitehead VM, Pratt R, Viallet A, Cooper BA. Intestinal conversion of folinic acid to 5-methyltetrahydrofolate in man. Br J Hematol 1972;22: 63.
217. Herbert V. Excretion of folic acid in the bile. Lancet 1965;1:913.
218. Hillman RS, McGuffin R, Campbell C. Alcohol interference with the folate enterohepatic cycle. Trans Assoc Am Physicians 1978;91:145.
219. Eisenga BH, Collins TD, McMartin KE. Differential effects of acute ethanol on urinary excretion of folate derivatives in the rat. J Pharmacol Exp Ther 1989;248:916.
220. Blocker EB, Thenen SW. Intestinal absorption, liver uptake, and excretion of 3H-folic acid in folic acid–deficient, alcohol-consuming nonhuman primates. Am J Clin Nutr 1987;46:503.
221. Eichner ER, Pierce HI, Hillman RS. Folate balance in dietary-induced megaloblastic anemia. N Engl J Med 1971;284:933.
222. Lane F, Goff P, McGuffin R, Eichner ER, Hillman RS. Folic acid metabolism in normal, folate deficient and alcoholic man. Br J Hematol 1976;34:489.
223. Halsted CH. The intestinal absorption of folates. Am J Clin Nutr 1979;32: 846.
224. Herbert V, Larrabee AR, Buchanan JM. Studies on the identification of a folate compound of human serum. J Clin Invest 1962;41:1134.
225. Lawrence VA, Loewenstein JE, Eichner ER. Aspirin and folate binding: in vivo and in vitro studies of serum binding and urinary excretion of endogenous folate. J Lab Clin Med 1984;103:944.
226. Hansen SI, Holm J, Hoier-Madsen M. A high-affinity folate binding protein in human urine. Radioligand binding characteristics, immunological properties and molecular size. Biosci Rep 1989;9:93.
227. Bhandari SD, Joshiu SK, McMartin KE. Folate binding and transport by rat kidney brush-border membrane vesicles. Biochim Biophys Acta 1988;9370:211.
228. Deutsch JC, Kolhouse JF. Folate and methotrexate interactions in the rat kidney. Cancer Res 1989;49:5858.
229. Besseghir K, Mosig D, Roch-Ramel F. Transport of methotrexate by the in vitro isolated rabbit proximal tubule. J Pharmacol Exp Ther 1989;250:688.
230. Fink M, Henry M, Tange JD. Experimental folic acid nephropathy. Pathology 1987;19:143.
231. Herbert V. Experimental nutritional folate deficiency in man. Trans Assoc Am Physicians 1962;75:307.
232. Waxman S, Schreiber C. Characteristics of folic acid–binding protein in folate deficient serum. Blood 1973;42:291.
233. Wagner C. Folate-binding proteins. Nutr Rev 1985;43:293.
234. Eichner ER, McDonald CR, Dickson VL. Elevated serum levels of unsaturated folate binding protein: clinical correlates in a general hospital population. Am J Clin Nutr 1978;31:1988.
235. Sadasivan E, Rothenberg SP. The complete amino acid sequence of a human folate binding protein from KB cells determined from the cDNA. J Biol Chem 1989;264:5806.
236. Sadasivan E, Rothenberg SP. Molecular cloning of the complementary DNA for a human folate binding protein. Proc Soc Exp Biol Med 1988;189:240.
237. Djurhuus R, Svardal AM, Ueland PM. Differential effects on growth, homocysteine, and related compounds of two inhibitors of S-adenosylhomocysteine catabolism, 3-deazaadenosine, and 3-deazaaristeromycin, in C3H/10T1/2 cells. Cancer Res 1989;49:324.
238. Deutsch JC, Elwood PC, Portillo RM, Macey MG, Kolhouse JF. Role of the membrane-associated folate binding protein (folate receptor) in methotrexate transport by human KB cells. Arch Biochem Biophys 1989;274:327.
239. Transport properties of folate bound to human milk folate-binding protein. (Editorial) Nutr Rev 1988;46:230.
240. Ratnam M, Marquardt H, Duhring JL, Freisheim JH. Homologous membrane folate binding proteins in human placenta: cloning and sequence of a cDNA. Biochemistry 1989;28:8249.
241. Lonnerdal B. Biochemistry and physiological function of human milk proteins. Am J Clin Nutr 1985;42:1299.
242. Said HM, Horne DW, Wagner C. Effect of human milk folate binding protein on folate intestinal transport. Arch Biochem Biophys 1986;251: 114.
243. Henderson GB, Tsuji JM, Kumar HP. Mediated uptake of folate by a high-affinity binding protein in sublines of L1210 cells adapted to nanomolar concentrations of folate. J Membr Biol 1988;101:247.
244. Freisheim JH, Ratnam M, Smith PL, Delcamp TJ, Price EM. Photoaffinity analogues of methotrexate as folate antagonist binding probes. Adv Enzyme Regul 1988;27:15.
245. Price EM, Freisheim JH. Photoaffinity analogues of methotrexate as folate antagonist binding probes. 2. Transport studies, photoaffinity labeling, and identification of the membrane carrier protein for methotrexate from murine L1210 cells. Biochemistry 1987;26:4757.
246. Jansen G, Westerhof GR, Kathmann I, Rademaker BC, Rijksen G, Schornagel JH. Identification of a membrane-associated folate-binding protein in human leukemic CCRF-CEM cells with transport-related methotrexate resistance. Cancer Res 1989;49:2455.
247. Hoppner K, Lampi B. Folate levels in human liver from autopsies in Canada. Am J Clin Nutr 1980;33:862.
248. Milne DB, Johnson L, Mahalko JR, Sandstead HH. Folate status of adult males living in a metabolic unit: possible relationships with iron nutrition. Am J Clin Nutr 1983;37:768.
249. Banerjee DK, Maitra A, Basu AK, Chatterjea JB. Minimal daily requirement of folic acid in normal Indian subjects. Indian J Med Sci 1975;63:45.
250. McNulty H, McPartlin JM, Weir DG, Scott JM. Folate catabolism in normal subjects. Hum Nutr 1987;41A:338.
251. Scott JM. Catabolism of folates. In: Blakley RL, Benkovic SJ, eds. Folates and pterins, vol 1. Chemistry and biochemistry of folates. New York, John Wiley & Sons, 1984:307.
252. Ek J. Plasma, red cell, and breast milk folacin concentration in lactating women. Am J Clin Nutr 1983;38:929.
253. Boerbooms AMT, Jeurissen MEC, Van de Putte LBA. Pulse methotrexate therapy in rheumatoid arthritis. Ann Intern Med 1988;108:905.
254. Benkovic SJ, Adams JA, Fierke CA, Naylor AM. Insights into enzymatic catalysis from studies on dihydrofolate reductase. Pteridines 1989;1: 37.
255. Barclay BJ, Huang T, Nagel MG, Misener VL, Game JC, Wahl GM. Mapping and sequencing of the dihydrofolate reductase gene (DFR1) of Saccharomyces cerevisiae. Gene 1988;63:175.

256. Whitehead VM. Synthesis of methotrexate polyglutamates in 11210 murine leukemia cells. Cancer Res 1977;37:408.
257. Allegra CJ, Chabner BA, Drake JC, Lutz R, Rodbard D, Jolivet J. Enhanced inhibition of thymidylate synthase by methotrexate polyglutamates. J Biol Chem 1985;260:9720.
258. Kumar P, Kisliuk RL, Gaumont Y, Fresheim JH, Nair MG. Inhibition of human dihydrofolate reductase by antifolyl polyglutamates. Biochem Pharmacol 1989;38:541.
259. Rosenblatt DS, Whitehead VM, Vera N, Pottier A, Dupont M, Vuchich MJ. Prolonged inhibition of DNA synthesis associated with the accumulation of methotrexate polyglutamates by cultured human cells. Mol Pharmacol 1978;14:1143.
260. Chabner BA, Allegra CJ, Curt GA, et al. Polyglutamation of methotrexate: is methotrexate a prodrug? J Clin Invest 1985;76:907.
261. Christophides N, Louis WJ, Lucas I, Moon W, Vajda FJE. Renal clearance of methotrexate in man during high-dose oral and intravenous infusion therapy. Cancer Chemother Pharmacol 1981;6:59.
262. Shapiro WR, Young DF, Mehta BM. Methotrexate distribution in cerebrospinal fluid after intravenous, intraventricular and lumbar injections. N Engl J Med 1975;293:161.
263. Balis FM, Mirro J Jr, Reaman GH, et al. Pharmacokinetics of subcutaneous methotrexate. J Clin Oncol 1988;6:1882.
264. Bertrand R, Mackenzie RE, Jolivet J. Human liver methenyltetrahydrofolate synthetase: improved purification and increased affinity for folate polyglutamate substrates. Biochim Biophys Acta 1987;911:154.
265. Bertrand R, Jolivet J. Methenyltetrahydrofolate synthetase prevents the inhibition of phosphoribosyl 5-aminoimidazole 4-carboxamide ribonucleotide formyltransferase by 5-formyltetrahydrofolate polyglutamates. J Biol Chem 1989;264:8843.
266. Seither RL, Trent DF, Mikulecky DC, Rape TJ, Goldman ID. Folate-pool interconversions and inhibition of biosynthetic processes after exposure of L1210 leukemia cells to antifolates: experimental and network thermodynamic analyses of the role of dihydrofolate polyglutamylates in antifolate action in cells. J Biol Chem 1989;264:17016.
267. Jolivet J. Methotrexate and 5-fluorouracil: cellular interactions with folates. In: Zittoun J, Cooper BA, eds. Folates and cobalamins. Berlin, Springer-Verlag, 1989:247.
268. Erbe RW. Inborn errors of folate metabolism. In: Blakley RL, Whitehead VM, eds. Folates and pterins: nutritional, pharmacological and physiological aspects, vol 3. New York, John Wiley & Sons, 1986:413.
269. Rosenblatt DS. Inherited disorders of folate transport and metabolism. In: Scriver CR, Beaudet AL, Sly WS, Valle D, eds. The metabolic basis of inherited disease. New York, McGraw-Hill, 1989:2049.
270. Kang SS, Zhou J, Wong PWK, Kowalisyn J, Strokosch G. Intermediate homocysteinemia: a thermolabile variant of methylenetetrahydrofolate reductase. Am J Hum Genet 1988;43:414.
271. Kang S-S, Wong WK, Bock H-GO, Horwitz A, Grix A. Intermediate hyperhomocysteinemia resulting from compound heterozygosity of methylenetetrahydrofolate reductase muatation. Am J Hum Genet 1991;48:546.
272. Kang S-S, Wong PWK, Susmano A, Sora J, Norusis M, Ruggie N. Thermolabile methylenetetrahydrofolate reductase: an inherited risk factor for coronary artery disease. Am J Hum Genet 1991;48:536.
273. Rosenblatt DS, Cooper BA, Lue-Shing S, et al. Folate Distribution in cultured human cells: studies on 5,10-CH2-H4PteGlu reductase deficiency. J Clin Invest 1979;63:1019.
274. Boss GR, Erbe RW. Decreased rates of methionine synthesis by methylenetetrahydrofolate reductase-deficient fibroblasts and lymphoblasts. J Clin Invest 1981;67:1659.
275. Mudd SH, Uhlendorf BW, Freeman JM, Finkelstein JD, Shih VE. Homocysteinuria associated with decreased methylenetetrahydrofolate reductase activity. Biochem Biophys Res Commun 1972;46:905.
276. Rosenblatt DS, Erbe RW. Methylenetetrahydrofolate reductase in cultured human cells. II. Studies of methylenetetrahydrofolate reductase deficiency. Pediatr Res 1977;11:1141.
277. Kanwar YS, Manaligod JR, Wong PWK. Morphologic studies in a patient with homocystinuria due to 5,10-methylenetetrahydrofolate reductase deficiency. Pediatr Res 1976;10:598.
278. Wong PWK, Justice P, Hruby M, Weiss EB, Diamond E. Folic acid nonresponsive homocystinuria due to methylenetetrahydrofolate reductase deficiency. Pediatrics 1977;59:749.
279. Baumgartner ER, Schweizer K, Wick H. Different congenital forms of defective remethylation in homocystinuria: clinical, biochemical, and morphological studies. Pediatr Res 1977;11:1015.
280. Haan EA, Rogers JG, Lewis GP, Rowe PB. 5,10-methylenetetrahydrofolate reductase deficiency: clinical and biochemical features of a further case. J Inherit Metab Dis 1985;8:53.
281. Hyland K, Smith I, Howell DW, Clayton PT, Leonard JV. The determination of pterins, biogenic amino metabolites, and aromatic amino acids in cerebrospinal fluid using isocratic reverse phase liquid chromatography within series dual cell coulometric electrochemical and fluorescence determinations: use in the study of inborn errors of dihydropteridine reductase and 5,10-methylenetetrahydrofolate reductase. In: Wachter H, Curtius H, Pfleiderer W, eds. Biochemical and clinical aspects of pteridines, vol 4. Berlin, Walter de Gruyter, 1985:85.
282. Baumgartner ER, Stokstad ELR, Wick H, Watson JE, Kusano G. Comparison of folic acid coenzyme distribution patterns in patients with methylenetetrahydrofolate reductase and methionine synthetase deficiencies. Pediatr Res 1985;19:1288.
283. Clayton PT, Smith I, Harding B, Hyland K, Leonard JV, Leeming RJ. Subacute combined degeneration of the cord, dementia, and parkinsonism due to an inborn error of folate metabolism. J Neurol Neurosurg Psychiatry 1986;49:920.
284. Beckman DR, Hoganson G, Berlow S, Gilbert EF. Pathological findings in 5,10-methylenetetrahydrofolate reductase deficiency. Birth Defects 1987;23:47.
285. Matthews RG, Kaufman S. Characterization of dihydropteridine reductase activity of pig liver methylenetetrahydrofolate reductase. J Biol Chem 1980;255:6014.
286. Christensen E, Brandt NJ. Prenatal diagnosis of 5,10-methylenetetrahydrofolate reductase deficiency. N Engl J Med 1985;313:50.
286a. Goyette R, Sumner JS, Milos R, et al. Human methylenetetrahydrofolate reductase: isolation of cDNA, mapping and mutation identification. Nature Genet 1994 (in press).
287. Cooper BA. Anomalies congenitales du metabolisme des folates. In: Zittoun J, Cooper BA, eds. Folates et cobalamines. Paris, Doin, 1987: 193.
288. Brandt NJ, Christensen E, Skovby F, Djernes B. Treatment of methylenetetrahydrofolate reductase deficiency from the neonatal period. (Abstract) Amersfoort, The Netherlands, The Society for the Study of Inborn Errors of Metabolism, 1986.
289. Rowe PB. Inherited disorders of folate metabolism. In: Stanbury JB, Wyngaarden JB, Frederickson DS, Goldstein JL, Brown MS, eds. The metabolic basis of inherited diseases, New York, McGraw-Hill, 1983: 498.
290. Shin YS, Reiter S, Zelger O, Brunstler I, Vrucker A. Orotic aciduria, homocystinuria, formiminoglutamic aciduria and megalobastosis associated with the formiminotransferase/cyclodeaminase deficiency. In: Nyhan WL, Thompson LF, Watts RWE, eds. Purine and pyrimidine metabolism in man. New York, Plenum Press, 1986:71.
291. Arakawa T. Congenital defects in folate utilization. Am J Med 1970;48: 594.
292. Perry TL, Applegarth DA, Evans ME, Hansen S. Metabolic studies of a family with massive formiminoglutamic aciduria. Pediatr Res 1975;9: 117.
293. Russel A, Statter M, Abzug S. Methionine-dependent formiminoglutamic acid transferase deficiency: human and experimental studies in its therapy. Hum Hered 1977;27:205.
294. Duran M, Ketting D, deBree PK, et al. A case of formiminoglutamic aciduria. Eur J Pediatr 1981;136:319.
295. Urbach J, Abramov A, Grossowicz N. Congenital isolate folate acid malabsorption. Arch Dis Child 1987;62:78.
296. Buchanan JA. Fibroblast plasma membrane vesicles to study inborn errors of transport. (Doctoral thesis) Montreal, McGill University, 1984.
297. Erbe RW. Genetic aspects of folate metabolism. Adv Hum Genet 1979;9: 293.
298. Tauro GP, Danks DM, Rowe PB, et al. Dihydrofolate reductase deficiency causing megaloblastic anemia in two families. N Engl J Med 1976;294:466.
299. Hoffbrand AV, Tripp E, Jackson BFA, Luck WE, Frater-Schroder M. Hereditary abnormal TCII previously diagnosed as congenital dihydrofolate reductase deficiency. N Engl J Med 1984;310:789.
300. Anagnou NP, O'Brien SJ, Shimada T, Nash WG, Chen M-J, Nienhouse AW. Chromosomal organization of the human dihydrofolate reductase genes: dispersion, selective amplification, and a novel form of polymorphism. Proc Natl Acad Sci USA 1984;81:5170.
301. Funanage VL, Myoda TT, Moses PA, Cowell HR. Assignment of the human dihydrofolate reductase gene to the q11-q22 region of chromosome 5. Mol Cell Biol 4:2010 1984.
302. Arakawa T, Narisawa K, Tanno K, et al. Megaloblastic anemia and mental retardation with hyperfolic acidemia: probably due to N5-methyltetrahydrofolate transferase deficiency. Tohoku J Exp Med 1967;93:1.
303. Branda RF, Moldow CF, MacArthur JR, Wintrobe MM, Anthony BK, Jacob HS. Folate-induced remission in aplastic anemia with familial defect of cellular folate uptake. N Engl J Med 1978;298:469.
304. Howe RB, Branda RF, Douglas SD, Brunning RD. Hereditary dyserythropoiesis with abnormal membrane folate transport. Blood 1979;54: 1080.
305. Suttle DP, Becroft DMO, Webster DR. Hereditary orotic aciduria and other disorders of pyrimidine metabolism. In: Scriver CR, Beaudet AL, Sly WS, Valle D, eds. The metabolic basis of inherited disease. New York, McGraw-Hill, 1989:1095.
306. Howell RR, Klineberg JR, Krooth RS. Enzyme studies on diploid cell strains developed from patients with hereditary orotic aciduria. Johns Hopkins Med J 1967;120:81.
307. Worthy TE, Grobner W, Kelley WN. Hereditary orotic aciduria: evidence for a structural gene mutation. Proc Natl Acad Sci USA 1974;71: 3031.
308. Scriver CR, Kaufman S, Woo SLC. The hyperphenylalaninemias. In: Scriver CR, Beaudet AL, Sly WS, Valle D, eds. The metabolic basis of inherited disease. New York, McGraw-Hill, 1989:495.
309. Brenneman AR, Kaufman S. The role of tetrahydropteridine in the enzymatic conversion of tyrosine to 3,4-dihydroxyphenylalanine. Biochem Biophys Res Commun 1964;17:177.

310. Shiman R, Akino M, Kaufman S. Solubilization and partial purification of tyrosine hydroxylase from bovine adrenal medulla. J Biol Chem 1971;246:1330.
311. Friedman PA, Kappelman AH, Kaufman S. Partial purification and characterization of tyrosine hydroxylase from rabbit hindbrain. J Biol Chem 1972;247:4167.
312. Pollock RJ, Kaufman S. Dihydropteridine reductase may function in tetrahydrofolate metabolism. J Neurochem 1978;31:115.
313. Firgaira FA, Cotton RGH, Danks DM, Fowler K, Lipson A, Yu JS. Prenatal determination of dihydropteridine reductase in a normal fetus at risk for malignant hyperphenylalaninemia. Prenat Diagn 1983;3:7.
314. Mudd SH, Levy HL, Skovby F. Disorders of transsulfuration. In: Scriver CR, Beaudet AL, Sly WS, Valle D, eds. The metabolic basis of inherited disease, New York, McGraw-Hill, 1989:693.
315. Gaull GE, Tallan HH. Methionine adenosyltransferase deficiency: new enzymatic defect associated with hypermethioninemia. Science 1974;186:59.
316. Gout J-P, Serre J-C, Dieterlen M, et al. Une nouvelle cause d'hypermethionin de l'enfant: le deficit en S-adenosyl-methionine-synthetase. Arch Fr Pediatr 1977;34:416.
317. Finkelstein JD, Kyle WE, Martin JJ. Abnormal methionine adenosyltransferase in hypermethioninemia. Biochem Biophys Res Commun 1975;66:1491.
318. Gaull GE, Tallan HH, Lonsdale D, Przyrembel H, Schaffner F, von Bassewitz DB. Hypermethioninemia associated with methionine adenosyltransferase deficiency: clinical, morphological and biochemical observations on four patients. J Pediatr 1981;98:734.
319. Reizenstein PG, Matthews CME. Vitamin B_{12} kinetics in man: implications on total-body B_{12} determinations, human requirements, and normal and pathological cellular B_{12} uptake. Physics Med Biol 1966;11: 295.
320. Herzlich B, Herbert V, Drivas G. Depletion of serum holotranscobalamin-II: an early sign of negative vitamin-B_{12} balance. Lab Invest 1988;58:332.
321. Lindenbaum J, Healton EB, Savage DG, et al. Neuropsychiatric disorders caused by cobalamin deficiency in the absence of anemia or macrocytosis. N Engl J Med 1988;318:1720.
322. Lindenbaum J, Savage DG, Stabler SP, Allen RH. Diagnosis of cobalamin deficiency. II. Relative sensitivities of serum cobalamin, methylmalonic acid and total homocysteine concentrations. Am J Hematol 199034: 99.
323. Mollin DL, Anderson BB, Burman JF. The serum vitamin B_{12} level: its assay and significance. Clin Haematol 1976;5:521.
324. Landon MJ, Creagh-Barry P, McArthur S, Charlett A. Influence of vitamin B_{12} status on the inactivation of methionine synthase by nitrous oxide. Br J Anaesth 1993;69:81.
325. Girdwood RH, Eastwood MA, Finlayson NDC, Graham GS. Pernicious anaemia as a cause of infertility in twins. Lancet 1971;1:528.
326. Hogan DB, Cadogan M, Auld RB, Fox RA. Micturition difficulties in the setting of pernicious anemia. J Am Geriatr Soc 35:823.
327. Shulman R. The present status of vitamin B 12 and folic acid deficiency in psychiatric illness. Can Psychiatr Assoc J 1972;17:205.
328. Shulman R. Psychiatric aspects of pernicious anaemia: a prospective controlled investigation. Br Med J 1967;3:266.
329. Hall CA. The nondiagnosis of pernicious anemia. Ann Intern Med 1965;63:951.
330. Carmel R, Karnaze DS, Weiner JM. Neurologic abnormalities in cobalamin deficiency are associated with higher cobalamin "analogue" values than are hematologic abnormalities. J Lab Clin Med 1988;111: 57.
331. Kafetz K. Immunoglobulin deficiency responding to vitamin B_{12} in two elderly patients with megaloblastic anaemia. Postgrad Med J 1985;61: 1065.
332. Wright PE, Sears DA. Hypogammaglobulinemia and pernicious anemia. South Med J 1987;80:243.
333. Saxena S, Weiner JM, Carmel R. Red blood cell distribution width in untreated pernicious anemia. Am J Clin Pathol 1988;89:660.
334. Thong KL, Hanley SA, McBride JA. Clinical significance of a high mean corpuscular volume in nonanemic patients. Can Med Assoc J 1977;117: 908.
335. Pierce HI, Hillman RS. The value of serum vitamin B_{12} level in diagnosing B_{12} deficiency. Blood 1974;43:915.
336. Carmel R, Karnaze DS. Physician response to low serum cobalamin levels. Arch Intern Med 1986;146:1161.
337. Botez MI. Neuropsychiatric illness and deficiency of vitamin B_{12} and folate. In: Zittoun JA, Cooper BA, eds. Folates and cobalamins. Berlin, Springer-Verlag, 1989:145.
338. Ditrapani G, Barone C, La Cara A, Laurienzo P. Dementia-peripheral neuropathy during combined deficiency of vitamin B_{12} and folate: light microscopy and ultrastructural study of sural nerve. Ital J Neurol Sci 1986;7:545.
339. Steiner I, Kidron D, Soffer D, Wirguin I, Abramsky O. Sensory peripheral neuropathy of vitamin B_{12} deficiency: a primary demyelinating disease? J Neurol 1988;235:163.
340. Zegers de Beyl D, Delecluse F, Borenstein S, Capel P, Brunko E. Somatosensory conduction in vitamin B_{12} deficiency. Electrophysiol Clin Neurophysiol 1988;69:313.
341. Perkin GD, Roche SW, Abraham R, Roche S. Delayed somatosensory evoked potentials in pernicious anaemia with intact peripheral nerves. J Neurol Neurosurg Psychiatry 1989;52:1017.
342. Weir DG, Keating S, Molloy A, et al. Methylation deficiency causes vitamin B_{12}–associated neuropathy in the pig. J Neurochem 1988;51: 1949.
343. Stabler SP, Allen RH, Barrett RE, Savage DG, Lindenbaum, J. Cerebrospinal fluid methylmalonic acid levels in normal subjects and patients with Cbl deficiency. Neurology 1991;41:1627.
344. Cooper BA, Fehedy V, Blanshay P. Recognition of deficiency of vitamin B_{12} using measurement of serum concentration. J Lab Clin Med 1986;107:447.
345. Cooper BA, Whitehead VM. Evidence that some patients with pernicious anemia are not recognized by radiodilution assay for cobalamin in serum. N Engl J Med 1978;299:816.
346. Yao Y, Slau Y, Ssau Y, Gau Y, Lou W. Prevalence of vitamin B_{12} deficiency among geriatric populations. J Fam Pract 1992;35:524.
347. Moelby L, Rasmussen K, Jensen MK, Pedersen KO. The relationship between clinically confirmed cobalamin deficiency and serum methylmalonic acid. J Intern Med 1990;228:373.
348. Stabler SP, Allen RH, Savage DG, Lindenbaum J. Clinical spectrum and diagnosis of cobalamin deficiency. Blood 1990;76:871.
349. Chadefaux B, Cooper BA, Gilfix BM, et al. Homocysteinemia: relationship to serum cobalamin and folate, erythrocyte folate and lobation neutrophils. Clin Invest Med 1994 (in press).
350. Miller DR, Specker BL, Ho ML, Normal EJ. Vitamin B_{12} status in a macrobiotic community. Am J Clin Nutr 1991;53:524.
351. Specker BL, Black A, Allen L, Morrow R. Vitamin B_{12}: low milk concentrations are related to low serum concentrations in vegetarian women and to methylmalonic aciduria in their infants. Am J Clin Nutr 1990;52:1073.
352. Pennypacker LC, Allen RH, Kelly JP, et al. High prevalence of cobalamin deficiency in elderly outpatients. J Am Geriatr Soc 1992;40:1197.
353. Cox EV, White M. Methylmalonic acid excretion: an index of vitamin-B_{12} deficiency. Lancet 1962;2:853.
354. Cooper BA, Lowenstein L. Vitamin B-12–folate interrelationships in megaloblastic anaemia. Br J Haematol 1966;12:283.
355. Cooper BA, Lowenstein L. Relative folate deficiency of erythrocytes in pernicious anemia. Blood 1964;24:502.
356. Waxman S, Metz J, Herbert V. Defective DNA synthesis in human megaloblastic bone marrow: effects of homocysteine and methionine. J Clin Invest 1969;48:284.
357. Wickramasinghe SN. The deoxeuridine suppression test. In: Hall CA, ed. The cobalamins. Edinburgh, Churchill Livingstone, 1983:196.
358. Norman EJ. New urinary methylmalonic acid test is a sensitive indicator of cobalamin (vitamin B_{12}) deficiency: a solution for a major unrecognized medical problem. J Lab Clin Med 1987;110:369.
359. Stabler SP, Marcell PD, Podell ER, Allen RH, Lindenbaum J. Assay of methylmalonic acid in the serum of patients with cobalamin deficiency using capillary gas chromatography-mass spectrometry. J Clin Invest 1986;77:1606.
360. Hawkins CF. Value of serum iron levels in assessing effect of haematinics in macrocytic anaemias. Br Med J 1955;1:383.
361. Ho C-H, Chang H-C, Yeh S-F. Quantitation of urinary methylmalonic acid by gas chromatography mass spectrometry and its clinical applications. Eur J Haematol 1987;38:80.
362. Matchar DB, Feusser JR, Millington DS, Wilkinson RH, Watson DJ, Gale D. Isotope-dilution assay for urinary methylmalonic acid in the diagnosis of vitamin B_{12} deficiency. Ann Intern Med 1987;106:707.
363. Stabler SP, Marcell PD, Podell ER, Allen RH. Elevation of total homocysteine in the serum of patients with cobalamin and folate deficiency detected by capillary gas chromatography-mass spectrometry. J Clin Invest 1988;810:4660.
364. Kang S-S, Wong PWK, Norusis M. Homocystinemia due to folate deficiency. Metabolism 1987;36:458.
365. Refsum H, Ueland PM, Svardal AM. Fully automated fluorescence assay for determining total homocysteine in plasma. Clin Chem 1989;35: 1921.
366. Bills ND, Koury MJ, Clifford AJ, Dessypris EN. Ineffective hematopoiesis in folate-deficient mice. Blood 1992;79:2273.
367. Gross RL, Reid JVO, Newberne PM, Burgess B, Marston R, Hift W. Depressed cell-mediated immunity in megaloblastic anemia due to folic acid deficiency. Am J Clin Nutr 1975;28:225.
368. Hitzig WH, Kenny AB. The role of vitamin B_{12} and its transport in globins in the production of antibodies. Clin Exp Immunol 1975;20: 105.
369. Reynolds EH. Interrelationships between the neurology of folate and vitamin B_{12} deficiency. In: Botez MI, Reynolds EH, eds. Folic acid and neurology, psychiatry, and internal medicine. New York, Raven Press, 1978:501.
370. Lever EG, Elwes RDC, Williams A, Reynolds EH. Subacute combined degeneration of the cord due to folate deficiency: response to methyl folate treatment. J Neurol Neurosurg Psychiatry 1986;49:1203.
371. Brocker P, Lebel C, Maurin H, Lods JC. Carences en folates chez les sujets âgés: intérêt de leur correction dans le traitement des troubles due comportment. Semin Hop Paris 1986;62:2135.
372. Ek J. Plasma and red cell folate in mothers and infants in normal pregnancies: relation to birth weight. Acta Obstet Gynecol Scand 1982;61: 17.

373. MRC Vitamin Research Group. Prevention of neural tube defects: results of the Medical Research Council Vitamin Study. Lancet 1991;338: 131.
374. Mulinsky A, Jick H, Jick SS, et al. Multivitamin/folic acid supplementation in early pregnancy reduces the prevalence of neural tube defects. JAMA 1989;262:2847.
375. Yates JRW, Ferguson-Smith MA, Shenkin A, Guzman-Rodriguez R, White M, Clark BJ. Is disordered folate metabolism the basis for the genetic predisposition to neural tube defects? Clin Genet 1987;31:279.
376. Rhoads GG, Mills JL. Can vitamin supplements prevent neural tube defects? Current evidence and ongoing investigations. Clin Obstet Gynecol 1986;29:569.
377. Griffin JP. Vitamins and neural tube defects. Br Med J 1988;296:430.
378. Molloy AM, Kirke I, Hillary I, Weir DG, Scott JM. Maternal serum folate and vitamin B_{12} concentrations in pregnancies associated with neural tube defects. Arch Dis Child 1985;60:660.
378a. Czeisel AE, Dudas I. Prevention of the first occurrence of neural-tube defects by periconceptual vitamin supplementation. N Engl J Med 1992;327:1832.
378b. Werler MM, Shapiro S, Mitchell AA. Periconceptual folic acid exposure and risk of occurrent neural tube defects. JAMA 1993;269:1257.
378c. Centers for Disease Control and Prevention. Recommendations for the use of folic acid to reduce the number of cases of spina bifida and other neural tube defects. MMWR 1992;41:1233.
379. Dansky LV, Andermann E, Rosenblatt DS, Sherwin AL, Andermann F. Anticonvulsants, folate levels, and pregnancy outcome: a prospective study. Ann Neurol 1987;21:176.
379a. Dansky LV, Rosenblatt DS, Andermann E. Mechanism of teratogenesis: folic acid and antiepileptic therapy. Neurology 1992;42:32.
380. Campillo B, Zittoun J, de Gialluly E. Prophylaxis of folate deficiency in acutely ill patients: results of a randomized clinical trial. Intens Care Med 1988;14:640.
381. Boeschoten EW, Schrijver J, Krediet RT, Schreurs WH, Arisz L. Deficiencies of vitamins in CAPD patients: the effect of supplementation. Nephrol Dial Transplant 1988;3:187.
382. Campillo B, de Gialluly E, Marquet J, Jouault H, Zittoun J. Folate deficiency in medical intensive care: incidence, predictive factors and consequences—results of a prospective study with 105 patients [in French]. Presse Med 1988;17:1071.
383. Hages M, Pietrzik K. Evaluation of the folacin status in children with regard to the cobalamin and iron status. 2. Incidence and severity of folate deficiency. Int J Vitam Nutr Res 1985;55:69.
384. Allen RH, Stabler SP, Savage DG, Lindenbaum J. Diagnosis of cobalamin deficiency. I. Usefulness of serum methylmalonic acid and total homocysteine concentrations. Am J Hematol 1990;34:90.
385. Lindenbaum J, Savage DG, Stabler SP, Allen RH. Diagnosis of cobalamin deficiency. II. Relative sensitivities of serum cobalamin, methylmalonic acid, and total homocysteine concentrations. Am J Hematol 1990;34: 99.
386. Carmel R, Sinow RM, Siegel ME, Samloff IM. Food cobalamin malabsorption occurs frequently in patients with unexplained low serum cobalamin levels. Arch Intern Med 1988;148:1715.
387. Gozzard DI, Dawson DW, Lewis MJ. Experiences with dual protein bound aqueous vitamin B_{12} absorption test in subjects with low serum vitamin B_{12} concentrations. J Clin Pathol 1987;40:633.
388. Jones BP, Broomhead AF, Kwan YL, Grace CS. Incidence and clinical significance of protein-bound vitamin B_{12} malabsorption. Eur J Haematol 1987;38:131.
389. Hippe E, Gimsing P, Hollander NH. A simplified method for quantitative determination of vitamin B_{12} absorption. In: Zagalak B, Friedrich W, eds. Vitamin B_{12}. Berlin, Walter de Gruyter, 1979;939.
390. Lawson DH, Parker JWL. Deaths from severe megaloblastic anaemia in hospitalized patients. Scand J Haematol 1976;17:347.
391. Carmel R. Treatment of severe pernicious anemia: no association with sudden death. Am J Clin Nutr 1988;48:1443.
392. Martin DC, Francis J, Protetch J, Huff FJ. Time dependency of cognitive recovery with cobalamin replacement: report of a pilot study. J Am Geriatr Soc 1992;40:168.
393. Skouby AP. Hydroxocobalamin for initial and long-term therapy for vitamin B_{12} deficiency. Acta Med Scand 1987;221:399.
394. Olesen H, Hom B, Schwartz M. Antibody to TCII in patients treated with long-acting vitamin B_{12} preparations. Scand J Haematol 1968;5: 5.
395. Brinton LA, Gridley G, Hrubec Z, Hoover R, Fraumeni JF Jr. Cancer risk following pernicious anaemia. Br J Cancer 1989;59:810.
396. Talley NJ, Chute CG, Larson DE, Epstein R, Lydick EG, Melton LJ III. Risk for colorectal adenocarcinoma in pernicious anemia: a population-based cohort study. Ann Intern Med 1989;111:738.
397. Berendt RC, Jewell LD, Shnitka TK, Manickavel V, Danyluk J. Multicentric gastric carcinoids complicating pernicious anemia: origin from the metaplastic endocrine cell population. Arch Pathol Lab Med 1989;113:399.
398. Mendelsohn G, De La Monte S, Dunn JL, Yardley JH. Gastric carcinoid tumors, endocrine cell hyperplasia, and associated intestinal metaplasia: histologic, histochemical and immunohistochemical findings. Cancer 1987;60:1022.
399. Ranaldi R, Lorenzini I, Montesi A, Bearzi I. Multiple gastic carcinoids and pernicious anemia: report of a case. Tumori 1986;72:439.
400. Magnusson I, Uvnas-MoberG K, Ost A. Gastric carcinoid tumors: endoscopic removal or gastric resection? Acta Chir Scand 1986;152:707.
401. Stalnikowicz R, Eliakim R, Steiner D, Gross D, Okon E. Should gastric carcinoid tumors associated with pernicious anemia be treated aggressively? J Clin Gastroenterol 1987;9:521.
402. Sjoblom S-M, Sipponen P, Karonen S-L, Järvinen HJ. Mucosal argyrophil endocrine cells in pernicious anaemia and upper gastrointestinal carcinoid tumours. J Clin Pathol 1989;42:371.
403. Borch K. Atrophic gastritis and gastric carcinoid tumours. Ann Med 1989;21:291.
404. Duffield MS, Phillips JI, Vieira-Makings E, van der Westhuyzen J, Metz J. Demyelinisation in the spinal cord of vitamin B_{12} deficient fruit bats. Comp Biochem Physiol [C] 1990;96C:291.
405. Hsing AW, Hansson LE, McLaughlin JK, et al. Pernicious anemia and subsequent cancer: a population-based cohort study. Cancer 1993;71: 745.
406. Sjoblom SM, Sipponen P, Juruinen H. Gastroscopic follow-up of pernicious anaemia patients. Gut 1993;34:28.
407. Colman M, Drivas G, Herbert V, Van Der Westhuyzen J, Metz J. Appearance of cobalamin analogs in brain and increased ratio in liver during development of nitrous oxide induced vitamin B_{12} deficiency in fruit bats. Clin Res 1984;32:696A.
408. Bakker HD, van Gennip AH, Duran M, Wadman SK. Methylmalonate excretion in a pregnancy at risk for methylmalonic acidaemia. Clin Chim Acta 1978;86:349.
409. Long M, Weir D, Scott J. Source of methyl groups in brain and nerve tissue in the rat. J Neurochem 1989;52:377.
410. Weir DG, Keating S, Molloy A, McPartlin J, Kennedy S, Blanchflower J, Kennedy DG, Rice D, Scott JM. Methylation deficiency causes vitamin B_{12} associated neuropathy in the pig. J Neurochem 51:1949.
411. Koppenol WH. Thermodynamic considerations on the generation of hydroxyl radicals from nitrous oxide: no laughing matter. Free Radic Biol Med 1991;10:85.
412. Kondo H, Osborne ML, Kolhouse JF, et al. Nitrous oxide has multiple deleterious effects on cobalamin metabolism and causes decreases in activities of both mammalian cobalamin-dependent enzymes. J Clin Invest 1981;67:1270.
413. Ueland PM, Refsum H, Wesenberg F, Kvinnsland S. Methotrexate therapy and nitrous oxide anesthesia. N Engl J Med 1986;314:1514.
414. Ermens AAM, Schoester M, Lindemans J, Abels J. Effect of nitrous oxide and methotrexate on folate coenzyme pools of blast cells from leukemia patients. Leuk Res 1991;15:165.
415. Gilbert HS. Inhibition of vitamin B_{12} binding to TC II at low pH: basis of a procedure for quantitation of circulating TC II and R binders. J Lab Clin Med 1977;89:13.
416. Pajunen A, Crozat A, Jänne OA, et al. Structure and regulation of mammalian S-adenosylmethionine decarboxylase. J Biol Chem 1988;263:17040.
417. Kudo H, Ohshio G, Ogawa K, et al. Distribution of vitamin B_{12} R-binder in carcinomas of the digestive tract. J Clin Pathol 1988;41:320.
418. Gilbert HS, Weinreb N. Increased circulating levels of TC II in Gaucher's disease. N Engl J Med 1976;295:1096.
419. Mukiibi JM, Kyobe J. Detection of incipient megaloblastic anaemia in peripheral blood. East Afr Med J 1979;56:375.
420. Burman P, Kampe O, Kraaz, et al. A study of autoimmune gastritis in the postpartum period and at a 5-year follow-up. Gastroenterology 1992;103:934.
421. Pietrzik K, Urban G, Hotzel D. Biochemical and hematological parameters for the estimation of folate status in man. 3. Importance of formiminoglutamic acid excretion in the urine in comparison to other measurements. Int J Vitam Nutr Res 1980;50:261.

Blood: Principles and Practice of Hematology,
edited by Robert I. Handin, Samuel E. Lux, and Thomas P. Stossel.
J.B. Lippincott Company, Philadelphia © 1995.

49

Disorders of Iron Metabolism

Kenneth R. Bridges
Paul A. Seligman

Although Aristotle was one of the greatest thinkers in human history, his belief that the world consisted of air, earth, water, fire, and ether was incorrect. An analysis of this planet's composition shows, in fact, that the fourth most common element is iron.[1] Iron participated in important biochemical reactions during the evolution of the earliest life forms and is recognized as an essential nutrient for all living organisms.[1–3] Iron catalyzes a number of enzymatic reactions involving electron transfer.[2,3] These enzymes use iron found either in heme or in nonheme forms (such as iron–sulfur complexes).[3] Heme (iron protoporphyrin IX) is the prosthetic group found in respiratory enzymes involved in oxidative phosphorylation, enzymes involved in splitting hydrogen peroxide, and other enzymes associated with detoxification of various chemical agents or drugs. Heme also is the functional group for oxygen transport by hemoglobin in red cells and oxygen storage by myoglobin in the muscle of higher organisms.[2–5]

All organisms require a mechanism for assimilating iron to avoid the ill effects of iron deficiency.[1–3] Despite its abundance, two factors associated with iron's unique chemistry required that organisms with intact circulatory systems evolve complex systems of iron delivery.[2,6] First, the predominant form of ionic iron, Fe(III), is relatively insoluble at physiologic pH in aqueous solutions.[2] Therefore, vertebrate plasma contains the iron transport protein, transferrin, which maintains iron in a soluble state for cellular assimilation at neutral pH.[6–8] Specific cell surface receptors for transferrin permit efficient iron uptake.[7,9,10] In addition, these receptors regulate the amount of iron taken up by cells.

Iron must be appropriately compartmentalized within cells because the element can be extremely toxic. Relatively low concentrations of excess free intracellular iron can severely damage a number of cellular components, including membranes and DNA.[2,3,6,11] Enough free iron must be present intracellularly for the enzymatic reactions just described, but detoxification mechanisms must be available to keep the free iron below a toxic level. The precise mechanisms that regulate this free intracellular iron pool have not been defined. Ferritin, a specialized protein that exists in many forms (called isoferritins) clearly plays an important role in the compartmentalization and detoxification of intracellular iron.[6,12]

Molecular mechanisms level have evolved that regulate the synthesis of various proteins involved in iron transport and intracellular compartmentalization. We are only beginning to understand the impact of these processes on the clinical spectrum of abnormal iron metabolism. Some disorders, such as simple iron deficiency, are easily explained, whereas others, such as hereditary hemochromatosis, remain mysterious despite intense investigation. The pathways of cellular iron use provide a context in which to understand the mechanisms of many disorders and a starting point to explore the etiology of others.

IRON BALANCE

By birth, infants have acquired about 350 mg of iron from their mothers.[3] This iron is distributed in four main body compartments (discussed in the follow sections). After birth, iron balance is maintained by gastrointestinal absorption of iron from the diet.[12,13] No physiologic mechanism of iron excretion exists. Obligatory losses result from shedding of epithelial cells from the intestinal and urinary tracts, from desquamation of the skin, and from menstruation by women in their childbearing years. The magnitude of these losses varies but usually totals only 1 to 2 mg/d and seldom exceeds 3 mg.[13,14] Small increases in iron loss can be compensated by increased iron absorption. Three factors help to maintain the balance and availability of iron for specific reactions: reuse of erythrocyte iron, minimization of blood loss, and uptake of adequate quantities of iron from the diet.

IRON COMPARTMENTALIZATION

The major iron compartments in humans are detailed in Table 49-1 and Figure 49-1 and can be distinguished according to function.[15]

Operational Iron

This largest compartment is composed of iron necessary for specific reactions. In humans, most operational iron consists of a heme moiety attached to hemoglobin or myoglobin. Heme is formed by the insertion of a ferrous iron atom (Fe^{2+}) into protoporphyrin IX. The reaction is catalyzed by the enzyme ferrochelatase.[16–18] When oriented appropriately in hemoglobin, the iron component of heme mediates oxygen uptake by erythrocytes in the pulmonary vessels and, later, release of oxygen to the tissues.[13] As

TABLE 49-1. Composition of Iron Compartments

Operational Compartment	Optimal Amount of Iron (g)	Percentage of Total Body Iron
Hemoglobin	2.67	65.6
Myoglobin	0.20	3.3
Other heme enzymes: cytochromes, peroxidases	0.008	0.1
Nonheme enzymes	<0.0001	
Intracellular storage compartment (ferritin iron)	1.0	30.0
Intracellular labile compartment	0.07	1.0
Intracellular transport compartment	0.003	0.07

noted in Table 49-1, hemoglobin contains most of the iron present in the body. Each hemoglobin molecule consists of about 0.35% iron,[15] which means that 1 mL of packed red cells contains about 1 mg of elemental iron. In addition to myoglobin, other important heme-containing enzymes include most cytochromes, various peroxidases, and catalase.[15] Nonheme iron is found in many important enzymes, including those involved in the metabolism of the amine neurotransmitters,[19,20] reduction of ribonucleotides,[21] and methionine synthetase.[22] Abnormalities in these and other metabolic processes may account for some of the ill-defined effects of iron deficiency.

Storage Iron

Storage iron accounts for the second largest iron compartment in the body[15] (see Fig. 49-1 and Table 49-1). Most storage iron is found in hepatocytes. Macrophages, particularly those in the bone marrow, liver, and spleen are another prominent site. Macrophages acquire a large part of their iron by engulfing senescent erythrocytes. As these cells catabolize hemoglobin, the iron is oxidized to the trivalent state, forming methemoglobin.[23] Methemoglobin has a much lower affinity for heme. The molecule dissociates from globin, and iron is liberated from heme by the enzyme heme oxygenase. The iron is then deposited in ferritin, which sequesters iron from the rest of the cell, thereby preventing damage from uncontrolled oxidation.[24]

Ferritin Structure

Each ferritin molecule is composed of 24 subunits. In the absence of stored iron, ferritin is termed *apoferritin*. Two distinct subunits have been identified, a light and a heavy chain.[25,26] The human light chain contains 174 residues with a molecular weight of 19.7 kd, whereas the heavy chain has 182 residues with a molecular weight of 21.1 kd. Ferritins from different tissues can differ substantially in composition (hence, the term *isoferritins*), reflecting differences in the proportion of heavy chains and light chains that make up the individual ferritin molecules.[24–26] Liver ferritin, for example, is composed mainly of light chains. In contrast, ferritin obtained from many neoplastic tissues, including lymphoma cells, is composed mainly of heavy chains. How variations in ferritin composition affect iron uptake and iron release from the molecule is not well understood.

The 24 subunits that form the ferritin shell are arranged in 4-3-2 symmetry, creating a cavity in which crystalline iron is stored.[27] Eight channels lined by hydrophilic amino acid residues lie along the axes of three-fold symmetry, whereas six hydrophobic channels are aligned along the four-fold axes of symmetry. Although the heavy and light chains of ferritin demonstrate only 50% homology in amino acid sequence, the residues that form the hydrophilic channels are strongly conserved.[28,29] In contrast, marked differences exist in the amino acids that form the hydrophobic channels. Such data suggest that the hydrophilic channels play some central role in the function of the ferritin molecule.

Ferritin Function

Ferritin channels may provide a route for iron entry into and exit from ferritin. One hypothesis is that iron enters and leaves ferritin by way of the hydrophilic three-fold channels, whereas phosphate and dioxygen, other important components of the iron crystals in the central cavity, gain access to the interior of the shell by the hydrophobic four-fold channels.[30] Examination of metal binding to apoferritin in solution indicates that one and perhaps two metal ions bind within the hydrophilic channels of the protein, after which the Fe^{2+} is oxidized to Fe^{3+}.[31] Subsequently, Fe^{3+} migrates to sites of polymer nucleation. The iron precipitates, producing a thermodynamic drive toward iron flow into the shell.

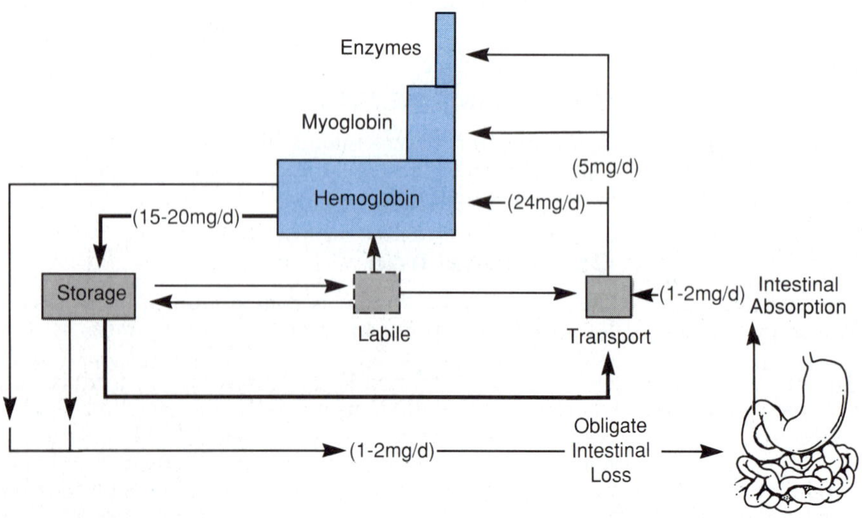

FIGURE 49-1. A kinetic scheme of iron exchange among different body compartments under optimal conditions in a 70-kg subject. About 1 to 2 mg of iron absorbed daily through the gastrointestinal tract is found on transferrin. The transport compartment, containing transferrin-bound iron, delivers about 24 mg/d of iron to the erythroid compartment for hemoglobin production and an additional 5 mg/d to parenchymal tissues, including muscles for myoglobin formation, and to other tissues, including liver for incorporation into iron-requiring enzymes. Most of the 15 to 20 mg/d of iron incorporated into the storage compartment that contains mainly ferritin-bound iron is derived from senescent red cells. A small amount of iron is found in the labile intracellular pool for incorporation into various operational iron components. About 1 to 2 mg/d of iron is lost (see text for further details).

The role of the ferritin channels in the function of the protein has been tested by the construction of homopolymers of heavy-chain ferritin and of heavy-chain ferritin mutants, using an *Escherichia coli* expression system.[32] A mutant heavy-chain ferritin lacking the first 13 amino acids of the N terminal forms a stable protein shell and also accumulates an iron core when incubated with ferrous ammonium sulfate. In contrast, another mutant in which the last 22 amino acids are deleted assembles into an unstable homopolymer that denatures when heating to 75°C. This structurally defective shell also fails to store iron properly. The missing 22 amino acids form a portion of the hydrophobic channel of the heavy chain. The hydrophilic channels are unchanged in the mutant protein. These data support the hypothesis that the hydrophobic channels are also required for ferritin to form its iron core.

Despite in vitro information concerning the redox characteristics of ferritin iron, the mechanism by which iron is released from ferritin in vivo remains a mystery. At one time, xanthine oxidase, an enzyme that mobilizes iron from ferritin effectively in vitro, was a strong candidate,[33] but its role has been disproved in vivo.[34]

Reduced flavin mononucleotides (FMN) effectively reduce ferritin iron in vitro and have also been evaluated as possible in vivo mediators of iron release from the protein.[35] The fact that the concentration of reduced flavins is very low argues against a physiologic role in iron mobilization from ferritin. Further, net production of $FMNH_2$ occurs most efficiently at unphysiologically low oxygen tensions, generally less than 5 nmol/L.[36]

Other small molecules can mobilize iron from ferritin in vitro. Both cysteine and glutathione reduce and mobilize iron from horse spleen ferritin.[37] The rate of iron reduction in either case is low, suggesting that neither agent plays an important role in iron mobilization from ferritin in vivo. Citrate, another small molecule that can mobilize ferritin iron, is largely confined to the mitochondria, whereas ferritin is found in the cytosol.

Certain bacterial proteins, such as flavoproteins or ferrodoxins, can mediate iron mobilization from ferritin. In some cases, these proteins are too large to enter the shell through the pores, suggesting that iron oxidation and reduction can be mediated by electrons transported across the ferritin shell.[38] The mechanism of such a possible transfer is unknown. Electron tunneling through the ferritin shell could be responsible, but would require movement across large distances (20 to 25 Å). An alternative explanation is that ferritin is sufficiently elastic in solution to allow molecules that exceed the crystallographically determined pore sizes to enter the shell. The one definite statement on this process is that iron mobilization from ferritin in vivo is complex.

Ferritin Catabolism and Hemosiderin

Iron is electron dense. The lysosomal degradation of ferritin was demonstrated by ultrastructural studies that capitalized on the opacity of the molecule's iron core.[39,40] Ferritin is slowly proteolyzed within lysosomes to a nonspecific complex containing iron, partially degraded protein, and lipid. This material, called hemosiderin, lacks a constant stoichiometric relation between its components[41,42] and is prominent in cells heavily loaded with iron. The iron-engorged lysosomes eventually form dense structures termed residual bodies. Hemosiderin appears to be a dead end in the metabolism of iron and ferritin. Iron can be leached out of this complex only under certain unusual conditions, such as high concentrations of chelators.

Ferritin particles in the cytoplasm are prominent in hemochromatosis and often form visible aggregates in the cytosol that appear almost crystalline. The structures are found in many organs including the liver[43] and heart[44] of people with iron overload. The mechanism of aggregate formation is unknown. Purified ferritin aggregates in vitro,[45] but the relation of this property to structures seen in vivo is unclear.

Biochemical data support the concept that ferritin forms aggregates in cells as a preliminary to lysosomal uptake and degradation. Fractionation of the cytoplasm from cells labeled with radioactive iron (^{59}Fe) by gel filtration reveals the existence of ferritin with low and high molecular weights.[46] Pulse chase analysis using an ^{59}Fe label indicates that iron taken into the cell is initially deposited in either monomeric or aggregated ferritin in the cytoplasm. After 24 hours, the label shifts from cytoplasmic ferritin to lysosomes, indicating that over time the ferritin clusters in the cytoplasm are taken into lysosomes.

In total, these data present a consistent picture of ferritin turnover in cells (Fig. 49-2). Individual ferritin shells are formed from subunits synthesized on free polyribosomes. The shells accumulate iron, and over time form aggregates that are taken into autophagic vacuoles. These structures fuse with secondary lysosomes, and the ferritin is degraded to hemosiderin. Although the factors that control ferritin aggregation and the recognition signals that lead to its entry into lysosomes are unknown, the process appears not to be random. The implication is that more mature ferritin shells encasing abundant iron are engulfed more efficiently by lysosomes than newly formed shells that contain little or none of the mineral.[47]

Ferritin degradation undoubtedly plays an important role in iron accessibility in cells because a change occurs in both the subcellular location and structure of the protein. Cytoplasmic ferritin is structurally intact, favoring the possibility of controlled interactions with enzyme-generated reducing agents that could mobilize iron. The iron released from cytoplasmic ferritin would move directly into the cytosol and the metabolic mainstream of the cell. Cellular access to ferritin iron could be closely controlled by the redox state of the cell, whereas other proteins and lipids are protected by ferritin from the potentially deleterious effects of iron-catalyzed oxidation.

In contrast, ferritin within lysosomes is under proteolytic attack, with its protein structure deteriorating during its existence in the organelle. Iron released from lysosomal ferritin would be separated from the "active pool" in the cell by the lysosomal membrane. A membrane pump or some similar mechanism would be needed to shuttle the iron out into the cytosol. No evidence supports the existence of such a pump. The cytosol, therefore, appears to be the most common site for iron release from ferritin. As such, any factor that shifts the relative distribution of storage iron between the two compartments alters iron availability.

Labile Iron

The labile iron compartment contains a poorly defined quantity of iron that was first identified in early studies of iron kinetics.[48] This compartment includes iron that is bound to cell membranes or to intracellular carriers for relatively brief periods before incorporation into heme, ferritin, or nonheme iron-containing enzymes. Based on these kinetic studies, the labile pool has been estimated to contain about 70 mg of iron[48] (see Table 49-1; Fig. 49-1). Loosely bound iron found on certain enzymes that require iron as a coenzyme may account for a portion of this pool, some of which may be iron in the process of incorporation into ferritin.

Techniques using cells in tissue culture have further de-

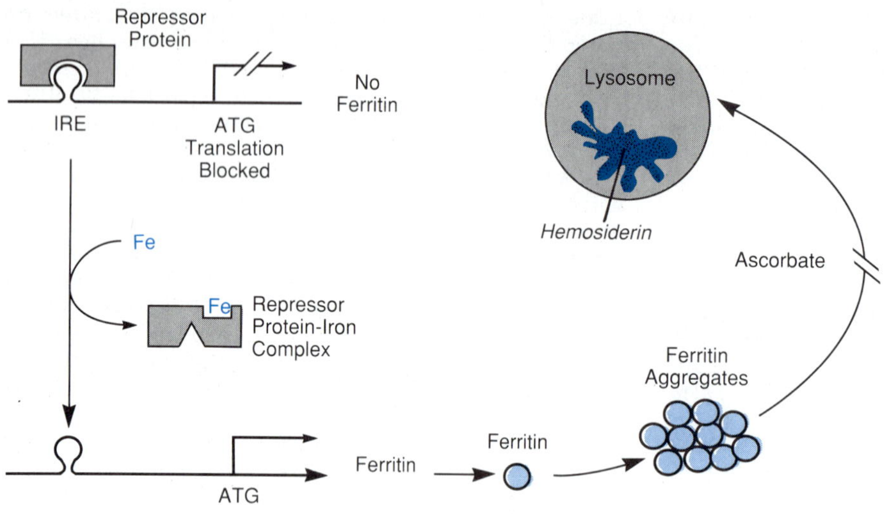

FIGURE 49-2. Ferritin biosynthesis and turnover. Ferritin mRNA exists as a stable complex in the cytoplasm of the cell. A protein binds to a consensus sequence in the 5′ untranslated region of the message, inhibiting translation. Iron frees the message from the suppressor protein, allowing translation of ferritin subunits. Twenty-four subunits assemble to form the mature ferritin shell. As they age and accumulate iron, the shells aggregate, are taken up by lysosomes, and are degraded to hemosiderin.

fined a subset of iron that appears to make up the major part of the labile iron pool identified in kinetic studies.[49,50] This chelatable iron appears to be intracellular iron released from transferrin that is used for various functional cellular processes just described and is in the process of being incorporated into various iron-requiring proteins. Some of this chelatable iron binds to a specific cytosolic protein that regulates the synthesis of ferritin and of the transferrin receptor in response to changing cellular iron requirements.

Transport Iron

The transport iron compartment is composed almost exclusively of transferrin-bound iron, which is either in the plasma or bound to cell membrane receptors. Human transferrin is a member of a family of proteins that contain two iron-binding sites.[7] A well-known member of this category of proteins is *lactoferrin*, a constituent of mammalian milk and other body fluids.[7] Serum transferrin contains 679 amino acids that, together with two oligosaccharide chains, give a calculated molecular weight of about 79.5 kd.[51–53] The molecule consists of two homologous domains of about 330 amino acids each. Designated the N (for N terminal) and C (for C terminal) domains, each domain has a single iron-binding site.[7,51–53] A statistical comparison of cDNA sequences of the two domains identified three regions in each that have extensive internal nucleotide sequence homology with corresponding regions in the homologous domain. Nucleotide sequence identity in each of the three pairs of regions is greater than 60%.[54–56] Whether any or all of these homologous "blocks" are associated with the primary function of transferrins (iron transport or transferrin receptor binding) is unknown.

The metal-binding sites of transferrin each bind Fe^{3+} with high affinity (K_a, 10^{26}) and have little or no affinity for Fe^{2+}.[7] Metal binding is a complex process in which each metal ion interacts with a sterochemically suitable anion to achieve a high-binding affinity. The bicarbonate ion serves this role under physiologic conditions.[7,57,58] Histidine residues in close proximity to each of the metal-binding sites also participate in the binding complex.[51,57,58]

Transferrin binds a number of multivalent cations, including transition metals (Cr^{3+}, Mn^{3+}, Cu^{2+}), Zn^{2+}, the class 3A metals (Al, Ga, In), and a number of rare earth ions.[7,59,60] Although the binding of other metals may be manipulated for diagnostic or therapeutic purposes, overwhelming volumes of data indicate that, under physiologic conditions, transferrin functions exclusively as the plasma iron transport protein.

Plasma transferrin is normally about one third saturated with iron, with the element randomly distributed between the two metal-binding sites.[7,53] Based on a transferrin concentration of about 3 mg/mL of plasma, the total transferrin-bound iron in the body is about 3 mg (see Table 49-1). Kinetic studies substantiate that, under normal conditions, about 10 times this amount of iron is delivered by transferrin to cells daily[48,53] (see Fig. 49-1). Therefore, small fluctuations in iron saturation of transferrin may profoundly change the rate of iron delivery to cells as well as the distribution of iron in tissues. This may explain why the extremely low transferrin saturation seen in iron deficiency is associated with an increased percentage of available iron delivered to erythroid cells, whereas the high transferrin saturation seen in iron overload states is associated with relatively more iron delivered to parenchymal cells found in the liver, pancreas, pituitary gland, and other selected organs. Even under normal conditions, the rate of iron delivery may vary with the diurnal change in transferrin saturation, with the level increasing slowly during the early part of the day (even under fasting conditions), followed by a steady decrease to the the evening trough.[7,61] The increase in saturation reflects an increase in serum iron that averages 15 to 20 $\mu g/dL$.[61]

In addition to changes in iron–transferrin saturation, iron transport is also regulated by changes in transferrin synthesis. Plasma transferrin appears to be exclusively derived from transferrin that is synthesized by the liver.[62,63] Hepatocyte transferrin synthesis increases with iron deficiency or under conditions of increased tissue iron requirements (eg, the latter part of pregnancy).[64,65] The plasma transferrin concentration depends primarily on the rate of protein synthesis because its half-life ($T_{1/2}$) remains relatively constant at about 7 days.[7,62] Infection and inflammation decrease transferrin synthesis, which probably accounts for the decreased transferrin concentration seen with the anemia of chronic disease.[7,62] Rarely, clinically significant transferrin degradation or loss occurs because of increased protein catabolism or urinary loss such as occurs in some patients with severe proteinuria.[66]

Plasma delivery of iron to cells is mediated by the binding of the iron–transferrin complex to specific cell surface receptors.[54,55,67,68] As discussed in detail in the section that follows on cellular iron metabolism, cellular iron uptake is regulated primarily by the number of transferrin receptors on the cell surface. In most instances, the transferrin receptor binds iron–transferrin with high affinity at physiologic pH. The receptor binds apotransferrin with a 1500-fold lower affinity.[69,70] The binding of monoferric transferrin to the transferrin receptor appears to be only slightly lower than diferric transferrin.[71,72]

Some physical–chemical data indicate that the two binding sites of transferrin are not identical. This view is most strongly supported by the fact that one transferrin-binding site releases iron at a relatively higher pH (5.5) compared with that of the other more acid-stable binding site (5.0).[7,73] In vivo as well as in vitro evidence attained to date indicates that the binding sites do not differentially donate iron to cells.[71,72] These studies, mainly using erythroid cells, have shown that under normal conditions, transferrin-mediated iron uptake is equivalent irrespective of the metal-binding site that contains the element.

Although most cellular iron is acquired from transferrin-bound iron in plasma, certain tissues may have limited access to transferrin-bound plasma iron because of poor penetration or other considerations (eg, blood–testes barrier). Good evidence shows that under certain conditions tissues, including the testes, lymph nodes, and certain tumors, synthesize transferrin,[74–76] permitting local regulation of the iron supply.[77,78] In these instances, the cells synthesize apotransferrin that is secreted and appears to bind small amounts of iron present in the interstitial fluid.[78] The iron-saturated transferrin then binds to cell surface transferrin receptors and is internalized in much the same way as plasma iron transferrin. The Sertoli's cells of the testes synthesize transferrin to provide iron to proliferating spermatocytes.[76] Transferrin synthesis by lymphocytes, specifically the T4-inducer subset of T lymphocytes, may permit T-lymphocyte proliferation in certain poorly vascularized areas of the lymph node.[77] Transferrin synthesis in these instances may constitute an important component of a paracrine (Sertoli's cells) or autocrine pathway (lymphocytes) that regulates cellular proliferation.

Extensive investigation has not revealed how transferrin acquires iron for plasma transport. At least one mechanism involves transferrin uptake of iron from storage sites. This storage iron appears to be mainly the iron incorporated into ferritin found in macrophages. The process can be facilitated by specialized transferrin receptors found on tissue macrophages that have a relatively high affinity for apotransferrin.[79] This form of transferrin uptake differs from the model for receptor-mediated uptake described in the text that follows. Thus, only in this specialized uptake system does the cell internalize unsaturated transferrin to acquire storage iron (by poorly defined mechanisms). The second important source of iron for transferrin is that absorbed from the diet. Whether transferrin acquires iron from duodenal cells in a manner similar to acquisition of iron from macrophages or whether transferrin directly participates in absorption of iron at the mucosal surface is not completely understood (see following section).

REGULATION OF GASTROINTESTINAL IRON ABSORPTION

Adequate gastrointestinal iron absorption is necessary to maintain optimal iron balance. Men require only about 1 mg of absorbed iron daily to make up for the obligatory losses (previously described).[80] This baseline iron requirement increases under certain normal circumstances such as periods of rapid growth (adolescence). Women require additional iron to balance losses during menstruation or pregnancy. Increased iron requirements are coupled with increased iron absorption by an undefined process.[81] Also, poorly understood is the increase in absorption often seen in patients with ineffective erythropoiesis owing to such diverse conditions as thalassemia and myelodysplastic syndromes.[62] Further, the primary defect leading to inappropriately high iron absorption in patients with homozygous hemochromatosis is unexplained.

Explanations of defective iron absorption are impossible without a better understanding of the normal mechanics of the process. Human trials have clearly shown that increased erythropoiesis is associated with increases in iron absorption, particularly with severe ineffective erythropoiesis.[62] An extremely rapid increase in iron absorption occurs in animals subjected to exchange transfusion with reticulocyte-rich blood.[82] These studies demonstrate that increased iron requirements associated with very high rates of erythropoiesis somehow convey a signal to the iron absorption machinery of the intestinal mucosa, triggering an increase in iron uptake. Depletion of body iron stores (through blood loss) likewise induces increased iron absorption. Increased iron stores are associated with a reduction of absorption, sometimes without any demonstrable change in plasma iron concentration or transferrin saturation.[82,83] Body iron stores may affect iron absorption by changes in gastrointestinal mucosal ferritin content (the mucosal block theory)[84] and possibly by elevations in ferritin composition. According to this hypothesis, depleted iron stores would lower the content of mucosal ferritin, permitting a more rapid transfer of iron to the portal circulation. Also, when intracellular ferritin is lower, less iron loss occurs when the cell is shed into the gastrointestinal tract.

External factors can significantly affect the amount of iron absorbed by the gastrointestinal tract. For example, different forms of iron found in the diet differ in bioavailability primarily because of differences in gastrointestinal absorption.[12,85–88] Dietary heme iron derived from the blood or meat of animals is absorbed with great facility. Heme iron uptake by mucosal cells is accomplished by specialized receptors on the mucosal cell membrane.[87,88] Heme oxygenase releases the iron within the mucosal cell.[87,88]

Nonheme iron or iron salts found in foods derived from plants, must be taken up as free iron or in protein-bound form. Most iron salts contain Fe^{3+}. The solubility of these salts is low. Conversion to Fe^{2+}, which is more soluble, is facilitated by gastric acid.[89] Absorption of these iron salts can be affected by other components of the diet.[90,91] Ascorbic acid facilitates elemental iron absorption probably by increasing solubility, although the exact physical–chemical change is unknown.[92,93] Iron absorption from iron salts may be blocked by tannin (a component of tea),[94] antacids such as calcium carbonate or magnesium oxide,[95] or the phytates found in wheat. These compounds are important mainly when simultaneously taken with iron salts, such as when calcium carbonate is incorporated into a multivitamin mineral preparation.[92–95] In addition to maintaining iron in a soluble state, gastric acidity also creates a lower pH in the upper duodenum, which appears to facilitate iron absorption.[96]

IRON PASSAGE THROUGH THE ENTEROCYTE

The uptake of iron salts is best accomplished in the duodenum, particularly in the epithelial cells at the tip of the crypts.[97] Although some ionized iron may diffuse between mucosal cells, most of the iron initially interacts with the intestinal brush border and is taken up by the cells.[98–101] Whether this is an active process or passive diffusion has not been completely defined. A newly discovered protein called *mobilferrin* in the mucosa of the duodenum may facilitate iron absorption.[102] When inside the cell, the liberated iron is either incorporated into ferritin or is transferred to iron-binding components that may be important for the "shuttling" of the iron to the portal circulation.[100,101] Some investigations have suggested that intraluminal transferrin provides a second pathway by which nonheme iron enters the mucosal cell.[103,104] Other studies, however, do not support the concept of transferrin-mediated gastrointestinal iron uptake.[105]

The pool of intracellular iron not incorporated into ferritin is quickly shuttled onto transferrin in the portal circulation. How mucosal cell iron-binding proteins[106,107] actively participate in the transfer of iron to the portal circulation has not been determined.

CELLULAR IRON METABOLISM

The handling of iron by an individual cell is directly related to its iron needs. This process is regulated by two main factors: the amount of transferrin-bound iron available and the number of functional transferrin receptors on the cell surface. Because individual cells cannot control the availability of transport iron, the main regulatory process at their disposal is the synthesis and expression of functional transferrin receptors. In conjunction with modulation of transferrin receptor expression, the cell regulates the appropriate compartmentalization of the internalized iron by changes in ferritin synthesis, a process that has been found to be coordinated with transferrin receptor synthesis.

Receptor-Mediated Uptake

Kinetic studies performed several decades ago first demonstrated that ^{59}Fe bound to transferrin was distributed to specific tissues. Under optimal conditions, over 90% of the radioactivity is incorporated into erythroid progenitors, as evidenced by increased radioactive uptake over sites of active bone marrow.[8,48] Because these cells require most of the body iron for hemoglobin synthesis, the first studies describing a specific receptor for transferrin not surprisingly were performed on normoblasts and reticulocytes.[49,108] In fact, the studies performed by Jandl and associates[108] on reticulocytes help to provide the first evidence that specific cell surface receptors existed for plasma transport proteins. In vivo studies have quantitated total body transferrin receptors and document that under normal conditions, transferrin-mediated iron uptake is dominated by hemoglobin synthesizing cells and hepatocytes.[53,71]

Transferrin Receptor Structure

The transferrin receptor is composed of two identical polypeptides, each containing 760 amino acids with a molecular weight of about 90 kd.[9,10,109] Carbohydrate contributes 5% of the molecular weight and consists of 3 N–linked oligosaccharide chains.[9,110,111] The two polypeptides are linked by a single disulfide bridge to form a 180-kd molecule[9,10] (Fig. 49-3). The transferrin receptor is oriented in the cell membrane with the C terminal exposed to the exterior of the cell.[112–114] This extracellular segment contains 671 amino acid residues, while the N-terminal cytoplasmic domain contains 61 amino acids. The amino acids between residues 62 and 89 are mainly hydrophobic and form a transmembrane segment.[112–114] The functional receptor also contains covalently bound fatty acid, which may play a role in proper orientation of the receptor in the membrane.[115] In addition, phosphorylation of serine residues found near the N terminal may affect membrane orientation, particularly during endocytosis.[109]

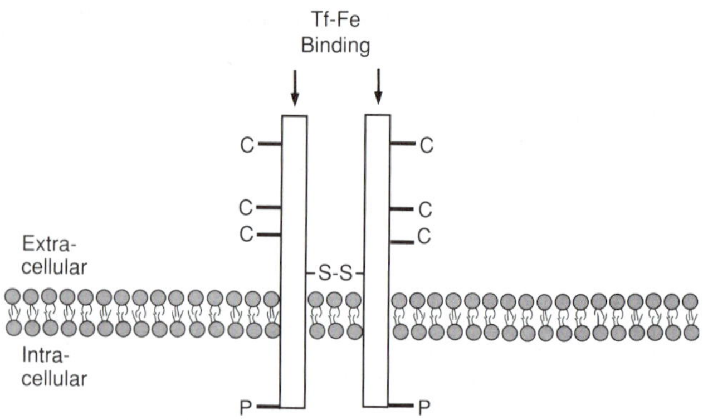

FIGURE 49-3. Schematic representation of the transferrin receptor molecule. The carboxy terminals of the two subunits of the transferrin receptor are joined by a disulfide bridge (S-S). The carboxy terminal extends into the extracellular space, and each subunit binds a transferrin–iron molecule. The short intracellular segment contains the amino termini. The P represents the phosphorylation site of a serine amino acid. The Cs indicate the likely positions of carbohydrate chains.

Transferrin Receptor Function: Receptor-Mediated Endocytosis

The transferrin receptor, like many other receptors,[116–118] is internalized with its ligand during the process of iron–transferrin uptake.[119–122] In general, receptor-mediated endocytosis regulates the action of hormones, neurotransmitters, growth factors, differentiation factors, and other important cell effector molecules. Studies performed more than 30 years ago first documented endocytosis of proteins by membrane structures described as coated pits.[123,124] The prototype pathway of receptor-mediated endocytosis is that of the low-density lipoprotein receptor system. Studies showed that ligand bound to the receptor enters the cell through an endosome, and, after a complex journey through various membrane-bound compartments, the ligand is delivered to lysosome where it is degraded and cholesterol is released.

Transferrin receptor-mediated endocytosis begins with the binding of monoferric or diferric transferrin to receptors on the cell surface that then cluster in coated pits[125] (Fig. 49-4). Investigations using truncated transferrin receptor mutants demonstrated that a small segment of the cytoplasmic domain is essential for endocytosis.[126] The "coat" in these coated pits is composed of a polygonal structure formed by a protein called *clathrin*.[127] The coated pit region invaginates and closes into a completed cytoplasmic vesicle referred to as a *coated vesicle*. The coat is usually lost, and the smooth-walled vesicle formed that contains newly internalized material is referred to as an *endosome*.[128] The endosome is acidic with a pH of 5.5 or slightly higher. The acidity of this environment facilitates the release of iron from transferrin and leaves apotransferrin bound to its receptor. The acidity of this compartment may be maintained by a specific H^+-ATPase; these specific enzymes may differ from compartment to compartment as evidenced by differing characteristics of a purified H^+-ATPase from Golgi apparatus.[129] The affinity of apotransferrin for the receptor at pH 5.5 is much higher than at neutral pH; therefore, apotransferrin remains bound to the receptor in the acidic endosome, and the receptor apotransferrin complex is carried back to the cell surface.[69,70,130,131] On reaching the neutral pH of the extracellular environment, the apotransferrin dissociates from the receptor and is available for binding and transport of more iron molecules. This recycling of transferrin is different from most receptor ligand interac-

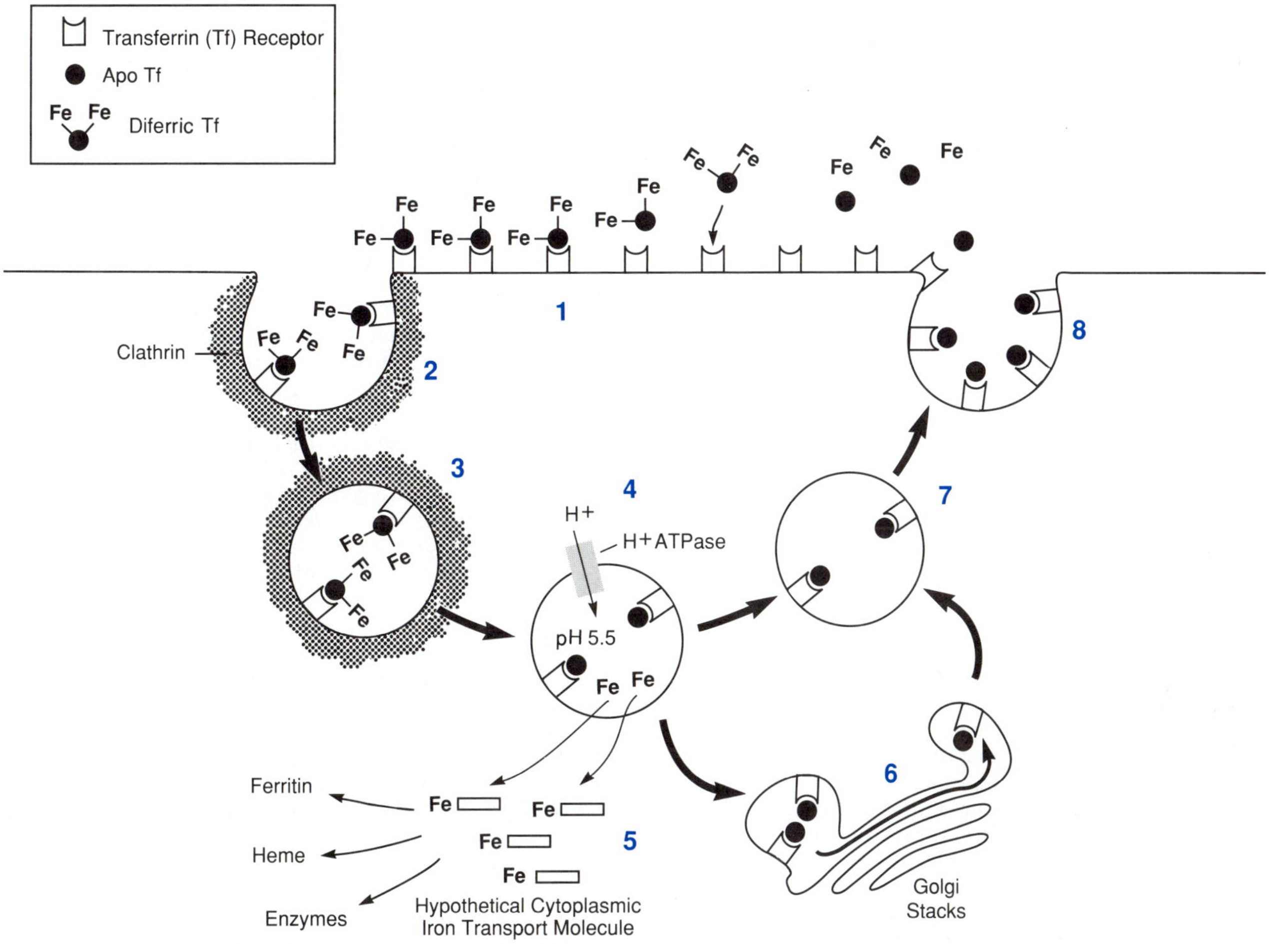

FIGURE 49-4. Schematic representation of receptor-mediated transferrin endocytosis. Iron–transferrin complex binds to specific transferrin receptors found on the cell surface (*1*). The receptor molecules with their bound transferrin cluster in specific areas of the membrane called *coated pits* (*2*). The coated pit region invaginates, creating a cytoplasmic vesicle referred to as a *coated vesicle* (*3*). The coat is then lost, and the smooth-walled vesicle formed is referred to as an *endosome* (*4*). This structure has an acidic milieu with a pH of 5.5 or slightly higher. The acidity of the environment promotes iron release from transferrin (*5*). The iron is then shuttled into the cytoplasm. Apotransferrin remains bound to the receptor and is either carried back to the cell surface (*8*) by the same endosome (*7*) or is cycled through portions of the Golgi apparatus (*6*). Apotransferrin dissociates, is released to the plasma, and is again available for binding and transport of more iron molecules.

tions in which the ligand is degraded during the process of internalization (previously described). The absence of significant degradation of transferrin during uptake may explain, in part, why early studies that suggested transferrin is internalized[132,133] were initially met with skepticism. In a single cycle through the cell, over 95% of the iron–transferrin is released as apotransferrin after about 10 minutes.[130,131]

Regulation of Transferrin Receptor Expression

Transferrin receptor density appears to be the most important determinant of cellular iron uptake. Therefore, it is not surprising that studies of erythroid progenitors including reticulocytes have shown that the number of cell surface receptors is directly related to the rate of hemoglobin production.[134] Hepatocytes also express large numbers of transferrin receptors, probably reflecting the synthesis of large quantities of heme for incorporation into enzymes.[49]

Rapidly proliferating cells also display a high density of transferrin receptors.[135–139] Transferrin is necessary for cell growth. When cells are cultured in serum-free (defined) medium, growth arrest occurs when transferrin is omitted.[140] Most studies support the concept that transferrin maintains cellular proliferation by providing iron and triggers no independent cellular signaling process.[141–143] At least part of this iron requirement can be explained by the iron-requiring enzyme, ribonucleotide reductase—an enzyme necessary for DNA synthesis.[90]

Receptor density on proliferating cells is directly related to intracellular iron availability because iron deprivation caused by the addition of chelators such as desferrioxamine to the growth medium of cultured cells rapidly induces transferrin receptor synthesis.[144,145] Other studies indicate that receptor density is five times greater in rapidly proliferating cells than in cells that are quiescent and have a lower iron requirement.[146] The increase in transferrin receptor seen during cellular proliferation and at least part of the increase seen with iron deprivation is due to increased transcription of the transferrin receptor gene.[147] Other studies show that transferrin receptor messenger ribonucleic acid (mRNA) has a relatively short $T_{1/2}$, which allows its level within cells to change quickly in response to MRNA stability.[148] The 3′ untranslated end of the message contains a series of conserved stem loops, called *iron-responsive elements* (IRE), that modulate message stability. Thus, posttranslational mechanisms profoundly influence transferrin receptor synthesis. The IRE closely links transferrin receptor synthesis to the synthesis of ferritin, whose mRNA also has an IRE (discussed later).

About two thirds of the transferrin receptors in a cell are sequestered in cytoplasmic vesicles, with only about one third displayed on the surface. Receptors can shift between internal and surface compartments, however. For example, cells in S phase of the cell cycle express more functional surface transferrin receptors than cells in G1 phase.[146,149,150] Also, certain agents such as phorbol esters increase receptor phosphorylation with an associated increase in the fraction of internal receptors.[151] Other evidence suggests that cells may exhibit different patterns of cellular processing of transferrin receptor during internalization[152] or with minor alterations in receptor structure (see Fig. 49-4), indicating that the rate of receptor degradation may vary.

INTRACELLULAR IRON METABOLISM

After iron is released from transferrin in the acidic milieu of the endosome, it is shuttled across the endosomal membrane and into the cytoplasm. At some point in this process, the iron atom is coupled to a molecule that transports the element within the cytoplasm to areas of use, such as cytoplasmic enzymes, the mitochondria, the nucleus, and the protein that binds to mRNA iron-responsive elements, or directly to intact ferritin molecules for storage.[153] Only sketchy data are available on the nature of this low-molecular-weight transport molecule because attempts at characterization have been only partially successful. One major problem is that iron forms complexes with a variety of intracellular molecules such as adenosine diphosphate (ADP) and amino acids. When cells are disrupted for biochemical evaluation, the true intracellular carrier is difficult to distinguish from artifactual complexes between iron and anionic molecules in the cytoplasm. This technical problem best explains why investigations into the nature of the transport molecule have been contradictory.

Examination of a low-molecular-weight iron-binding fraction from reticulocytes in one instance revealed an average molecular weight of 550 daltons.[154] Analysis of the fraction demonstrated several amino acids including glycine, cysteine, and aspartic acid. In addition, citric acid was present in the fractions. In contrast, other studies have identified low-molecular-weight iron-binding fractions that contain no amino acids, nucleotides, or sugars.[155] In the latter instance, iron recovery was greater under anaerobic isolation conditions, suggesting that the iron was in the Fe^{2+} oxidation state. The lack of agreement on the nature of the iron binding may persist until new characterization techniques are available.

Role of Iron in Coordinating Ferritin and Transferrin Receptor Synthesis

The expression of a number of proteins is modulated by the intracellular iron concentration. Of the systems examined to date, the role of iron in coordinating the synthesis of ferritin and of the transferrin receptor is best understood. Through its influence on the expression of these proteins, iron exerts feedback control on its bioavailability in cells.

Ferritin synthesis increases dramatically in animals treated with large amounts of iron.[156,157] The lack of effect of actinomycin D on the iron-dependent induction of ferritin synthesis indicates that the increase is due to control of ferritin mRNA expression at a posttranscriptional level.[158] Intensive evaluation revealed the control to be translational in nature.

In rats loaded with iron, the distribution of ferritin mRNA in liver extracts shifts to the polyribosomes from a free cytosolic pool.[159] This change in ferritin mRNA distribution increases its translation and consequently the level of ferritin protein in the tissue (see Fig. 49-2). Similar results are obtained with hepatoma cells in culture.[160] Here, the iron chelator desferrioxamine (which penetrates into the cell) decreases the ferritin mRNA shift onto polyribosomes and reduces the synthesis of ferritin protein. The chelator, diethylenetriaminepentaacetic acid (DTPA), which is confined to the extracellular space, does not interfere with translation of the ferritin message. These data indicate that a chelatable pool of intracellular iron is responsible for this regulation.

Ferritin mRNA from mouse fibroblasts can be translated in vitro using a reticulocyte lysate translation system. When the mRNA is derived from fibroblasts grown in iron-deficient medium, the translation of the message is inefficient.[161] Phenol extraction of the mRNA to remove associated protein increases the efficiency of ferritin translation. In contrast, cells grown in medium supplemented with iron display efficient translation of ferritin mRNA without manipulation. This indicates that in the absence of iron, a protein inhibitor blocks the translation of the ferritin message.

Gel retardation experiments confirm that a protein that binds to the ferritin message in an iron-dependent fashion is responsible for regulating the translation of the mRNA.[162,163] The partially purified protein has a molecular weight of about 180 kd[164] and interacts with the 5′ noncoding region of ferritin mRNA, blocking ferritin synthesis. These results were confirmed by the cloning of the IRE-binding protein (IRE-BP).[165]

Figure 49-5 illustrates how transferrin receptor synthesis is coordinated with ferritin synthesis. The overall control of ferritin expression is undoubtedly more complicated than the picture derived from merely examining the 5′ noncoding region. With prolonged exposure to iron, for instance, the level of ferritin message in some cells increases because of enhanced stability.[166] Also, the role of other factors that may modify ferritin expression, including growth factors, remains to be explored in detail.

As previously noted, the influence of iron on the expression of transferrin receptors is indicated by the increase in receptor number that occurs in cells grown in culture me-

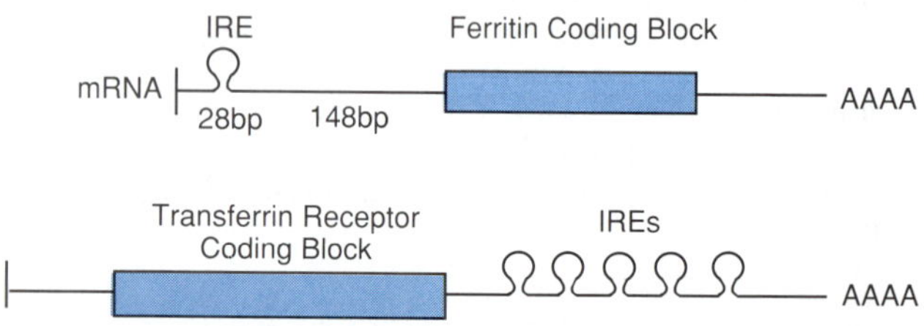

FIGURE 49-5. Coordination of ferritin and transferrin receptor synthesis. Ferritin mRNA has a conserved sequence called the *iron-responsive element* (IRE) in its 5′ untranslated region. A specific cytoplasmic protein, the *iron regulatory protein* (IRP), attaches to the IRE and blocks translation of the ferritin message into protein. When iron enters the cell, the IRP detaches from the message, permitting ferritin synthesis. The transferrin receptor message has five IREs in the 3′ untranslated region. When the IRP binds to the transferrin receptor message, the mRNA is stabilized. In the presence of iron, the IRP detaches, and transferrin receptor message stability and mRNA levels decrease. Thus, iron stimulates ferritin synthesis (providing cellular storage sites) while decreasing transferrin receptor production (and secondarily, iron influx into the cell).

dium supplemented with chelators that have access to the interior of the cell.[144,167,168] This increase results from elevated transferrin receptor mRNA levels.[147]

Experiments in mouse cells transfected with human transferrin receptor mRNA subcloned into expression vectors demonstrate that the iron-responsive translational regulation of receptor expression depends critically on segments of the 3′ noncoding region.[169] The transferrin receptor promoter is not required for this effect. Growth arrest in cells decreases the level of transferrin receptor expression by a transcriptional mechanism. This phenomenon is unaffected by deletions in the 3′ noncoding region, suggesting that growth-dependent regulation of transferrin receptor expression may not be controlled by message stability.

The stability of the transferrin receptor message is mediated through its 3′ untranslated region.[170] Computer analysis of the secondary structure of the 3′ noncoding region of transferrin receptor mRNA suggests that five IRE stem loops are involved in the regulatory process. When the IRE-BP binds to the IRE, the transferrin receptor message is stabilized (see Fig. 49-5). These loops are homologous to those in the 5′ noncoding segment of ferritin mRNA. As illustrated in Figure 49-5, the IRE loops modulate message translation when they occur 5′ to the coding block, as in ferritin mRNA. When located in the 3′ noncoding region, as in transferrin receptor mRNA, they alter message availability by altering mRNA stability. With iron excess, the IRE-BP detaches from the 3′ region of receptor mRNA, decreasing its stability and consequently receptor synthesis. At the same time, detachment of the IRE-BP from the 5′ IRE of ferritin mRNA releases the block to ferritin synthesis.[148] Counterbalancing synthesis of the transferrin receptor and of ferritin ensures an adequate, but subtoxic, supply of iron for the cell.

Control of gene expression by the IRE is not limited to ferritin and the transferrin receptor. δ-Aminolevulinic acid synthetase, the first enzyme in the biosynthetic pathway for heme, has two isoforms: a "housekeeping" form that is expressed in all tissues and an erythroid-specific form.[171] The erythroid-specific form has an IRE in the 3′ untranslated region of the message, suggesting that translation of the message may be regulated by iron (analogous to the situation with ferritin).[172,173]

IRON DEFICIENCY

The correct definition of iron deficiency implies that there is a decrease in normal body iron stores.[174] The main difficulty with this definition in assessing an iron-deficient state is defining the word "normal." Under optimal conditions, a person who experiences only the obligatory 1-mg/d loss of iron can easily obtain this amount from a normal diet. Certain normal conditions such as growth (in young children or adolescents), menstruation, and pregnancy result in iron losses that cannot always be counterbalanced by dietary iron, even with maximal increases in gastrointestinal iron absorption.[174,175] As noted in Table 49-2, a significant number of these people may suffer from iron deficiency.

Iron deficiency is represented by a continuum comprising the following stages[174,176]:

Stage 1—a depletion of body iron stores with normal laboratory values including hemoglobin levels

Stage 2—iron deficiency without anemia with laboratory evidence suggestive of decreased body iron, absent iron stores, and a normal hemoglobin level

Stage 3—iron deficiency with anemia with diagnostic laboratory abnormalities including a mild anemia generally associated with a normal mean corpuscular volume (MCV)

Stage 4—severe iron deficiency with obvious hypochromic microcytic anemia and clear evidence of some of the nonhematologic effects of iron deficiency (discussed later in text)

Iron deficiency must be recognized as early as possible so that its cause can be determined and appropriate treatment instituted.

TABLE 49-2. Specific Groups That May Develop Iron Deficiency

Group	Prevalence (%)	Contributing Factors
Infants	20–50	Low birthweight and breastfeeding beyond 6 mo
Children (2–5 y)	≈5*	Uncorrected iron deficiency in infancy and poor diet
Adolescents	≈5*	Poor diet and rapid growth
Menstruating females	20	Heavy menses
Pregnancy	50*	Multiple previous pregnancies

* The prevalence of deficiency in these groups may be affected by previous iron supplementation when younger.

Causes of Iron Deficiency

In evaluating the cause of iron deficiency, an analogy can be made with basic accounting principles. A negative balance sheet (iron deficiency) results when credits (iron absorbed from the gastrointestinal tract) fall short of debits (iron loss). For example, a menstruating woman with relatively heavy menses may be able to balance the increased iron loss with a diet high in heme iron or one containing a large quantity of iron salts. However, the deficit cannot be corrected on a low caloric diet without red meat. In another common example, people in Third-World countries, particularly children who suffer iron loss associated with hookworm infestation, are more likely to develop iron deficiency when the infection is combined with poor nutrition.[49]

In Adults

In most adult cases, iron deficiency results from blood loss.[174,177] Although absorption of dietary iron may increase significantly in response to increased iron loss, the maximal amount of iron that can be obtained from the diet is limited. About 6 mg of iron is present per 1000 calories in the average American diet. An adult male in normal balance requires about 1 mg of iron to compensate for obligatory iron loss.[174] Therefore, with an optimal diet containing about 3000 calories, he needs to absorb only about 6% of dietary iron. On the other hand, a person with a normal gastrointestinal tract eating the same diet who is significantly iron deficient can, at best, absorb about 40% of this dietary iron, or slightly less than 6.5 mg. Assuming a normal hematocrit of 50 mL/dL and an average blood loss exceeding as little as 11 mL/d (5.5 mg iron) combined with obligatory losses (1 mg), the result would be a negative iron balance.

Blood loss can be described as either occult (meaning the source of the blood loss must be investigated) or obvious. As noted in Table 49-3, a common site of occult bleeding is the gastrointestinal tract. Occult gastrointestinal bleeding

TABLE 49-3. Causes of Blood Loss Leading to Iron Deficiency

GASTROINTESTINAL	
Upper	
	Nosebleeds (including telangiectasia)
	Varices
	Gastritis
	Ulcer
	Tumor
Lower	
	Meckel's diverticulum (children)
	Milk-induced enteropathy (children)
	Helminthiasis
	Tumor or polyps
	Ulcerative colitis
	Arteriovenous malformation
	Diverticuli
	Hemorrhoids
VAGINAL	
	Increased menstrual flow
	Tumor
URINARY	
	Tumor
	Chronic infection
PULMONARY	
	Pulmonary hemosiderosis
	Tuberculosis
	Bronchiectasis

may originate from a wide variety of anatomic lesions, including the small but significant amount of bleeding that can result from gastric irritation caused by common medications, such as aspirin[178] or nonsteroidal antiinflammatory drugs (NSAIDs).[179] In some cases, such as excessive menstrual bleeding, a careful history may be required to unveil the source of blood loss.[180,181]

Rarely, occult bleeding occurs in the urinary tract manifesting as tumors, chronic infections, congenital malformations, and glomerular disease.[174] Although hematuria is usually easily recognizable, urine with a packed red cell volume of 0.5% may appear normal to the patient, but may result in more than 10 mL of lost red cells per day. Bleeding into the lungs in the rare entity called *idiopathic pulmonary hemosiderosis* is associated with profound iron loss, hemosiderin-laden pulmonary macrophages, and iron deficiency.[182]

Occasionally, hemolytic anemia causes significant loss of iron. This is particularly true in intravascular hemolysis, in which liberated hemoglobin saturates hepatoglobin-binding sites and is excreted in the urine. When the hemolysis is brisk, as often occurs with paroxysmal nocturnal hemoglobinuria, iron loss in the form of hemoglobinuria becomes obvious.[183] Mild intravascular hemolysis, as occurs with defective heart valves, may not produce dark urine and often is recognized only when the sediment from a spun urine specimen is stained for iron using a Prussian blue reagent.[184,185] In such cases, large quantities of hemosiderin are identified in desquamated renal tubular epithelial cells, indicating the uptake of small but significant amounts of urinary hemoglobin. Iron is released from the catabolized protein and is deposited in ferritin.

Finally, there is a single report of a previously healthy woman with a severe microcytic anemia and high serum iron who was discovered to have autoantibodies to the transferrin receptor.[185a] A complete remission occurred with prednisone and azathioprine treatment.

Hereditary Causes in Infants and Young Children

A small number of hereditary diseases that produce iron deficiency have been described. These physiologically instructive disorders generally present early in life.

Atransferrinemia. Atransferrinemia is a rare recessive genetic disorder that produces severe hypochromic microcytic anemia that is resistant to iron therapy.[186–188] In some cases, inappropriately large amounts of iron are deposited in the reticuloendothelial cells. The deficiency of transferrin substantially impairs iron delivery to normoblasts. Although only a few kindred of atransferrinemic patients have been described, in all instances in which either iron-binding ability or immunoreactive transferrin was measured, detectable amounts of iron–transferrin were present in plasma.[186–188] This suggests, not surprisingly, that the total absence of transferrin would be incompatible with fetal development. Molecular biology techniques to assess the transferrin gene in these people have not been performed. The advent of a mouse model of atransferrinemia may shed light on this rare cause of iron deficiency.[189]

Abnormal Iron Metabolism. A few reports have surfaced of children with abnormal iron metabolism associated with decreased or absent stainable bone marrow iron, hypochromic microcytic anemia, and increased parenchymal cell iron, particularly in the liver. An ill-defined biochemical defect resulting in inappropriate iron use appears to be the culprit.[190,191]

Another report describes three children with functional iron deficiency (low serum iron, low transferrin saturation, and hypochromic-microcytic anemia); hyperglobulinemia; benign lymphoid hamartomas in the thorax and abdomen; and marked hemosiderosis of the liver and tumors.[191a] The cause of this unusual syndrome is unknown.

Arteriovenous Malformation. Some congenital diseases are associated with a bleeding tendency and resultant iron deficiency. Any of the hereditary disorders of hemostasis that cause increased blood loss lead to iron deficiency. For these relatively common conditions, prior acute bleeding usually is obvious. Disorders of blood vessels, particularly arteriovenous (AV) malformations involving the gastrointestinal or urinary tract, may lead to chronic iron deficiency. An interesting but poorly understood syndrome associated with multiple small AV malformations in the colon and aortic stenosis[192,192a] has been described in patients over the age of 50 years. Some of these patients present with iron-deficiency anemia caused by gastrointestinal blood loss.

Hereditary hemorrhagic telangiectasia is a rare syndrome that can be manifested by iron deficiency and a history of intermittent blood loss, usually originating from the nose and gastrointestinal tract.[193] The diagnosis may first be evident in early adulthood or as late as middle age.

Nonhereditary Causes in Infants and Young Children

Iron Supplementation in Infancy and Early Childhood. Iron deficiency in infancy is a serious problem because of the rapid growth that occurs during this phase of life. As a result, the issue of iron availability in milk and formula is important. Both human breast milk and cow's milk contain iron at an average concentration of about 0.75 mg/L.[194] The daily volume consumed by infants is about 0.5 L, so that about 0.4 mg of iron enters the gastrointestinal tract from either source. When the daily loss of iron by infants is factored together with the amount of iron required for growth, the quantity of the mineral needed is about 1 mg/d.

Despite the roughly equal concentrations of iron in breast milk and cow's milk, the former provides a significantly greater amount of iron to the infant. Administration of labeled iron to 6-month-old infants either nursing on breast milk or receiving unfortified cow's milk shows an uptake of 50% of the label by infants in the former group compared with a 10% uptake by the latter cohort.[195] Serum ferritin levels, transferrin saturation, hemoglobin concentrations, and MCV are higher in infants on breast milk. These data indicate that breast milk provides more bioavailable iron than does cow's milk and that breastfed infants have higher body iron stores.

Coffee may pose a problem in iron acquisition for infants, particularly those that nurse. Women of 8 months' gestation who drink coffee have slightly but significantly lower hematocrit and hemoglobin values than those who abstain.[296] At birth, the cord hematocrit and hemoglobin are lower in infants born to coffee-drinking mothers than those born to mothers who avoid the beverage. After 1 month of lactation, the coffee-drinking mothers also have a lower iron content in their breast milk than do controls. These associations occur independently of maternal iron status. When iron-supplemented formula is used as a source of nutrition; maternal coffee consumption is of no concern. Among the large number of infants who depend on breast milk, coffee drinking by the mother must be taken into account in the evaluation of potential health risks.

Evaluation of the relation between the iron status of mothers and that of their children reveals that infants fed entirely on breast milk have normal iron stores at 6 months of age regardless of maternal iron status.[297] The fact that no relation exists between the iron content of breast milk and the body iron status of the mother probably accounts for this finding. Mothers who are iron deficient and breastfeed their infants are no more likely to induce a secondary iron deficiency in their infants than are mothers with normal iron stores.[297]

One of the most common means of iron supplementation is iron-fortified formulas. Soy formulas are commonly used because the incidence of allergic reactions to the proteins in these mixtures is lower than in formulas that contain wheat agglutinins. In adult volunteers, only about 2% of the iron in soy formula supplemented with iron and ascorbate is absorbed.[198] Comparison at 9 months of age of infants fed with iron-supplemented soy formula, iron-supplemented cow's milk, and breast milk shows essentially identical values in the first two cohorts for hemoglobin, MCV, transferrin saturation, serum ferritin, and free erythrocyte protoporphyrin. In contrast, the breastfed infants at 9 months have substantially lower values, suggesting iron deficiency. The presence of frank anemia in 27% of these children (compared with 4% and 2% of those on iron-supplemented soy formula or iron-supplemented cow's milk, respectively) confirms this suspicion.

One of the reasons that older nursing infants become iron deficient is that the iron content of breast milk is not constant over time. In a group of women evaluated serially during lactation for periods of up to 9 months, the iron content of the breast milk declined from roughly 0.6 to 0.3 mg/L.[199] A wide scatter in values existed, and a decline did not occur in every mother. Nonetheless, these data raise the question of whether iron supplementation is needed in infants who are breastfed for prolonged periods of time. Based on these findings, pediatricians generally recommend vitamin supplements containing about 10 mg of elemental iron for all infants ages 6 months to 2 years. Recommendations for older children are less uniform, particularly since the exact incidence of iron deficiency is unknown and a major cause of iron deficiency in this age group is uncorrected iron deficiency during infancy (see Table 49-2). The recommendations stated above are based on the finding that 20% or more of children at age 12 months show evidence of iron-deficiency anemia.[200] This percentage is even higher in black intercity children,[201] although in most instances, particularly in infants, iron deficiency is due to dietary factors. Along with increased requirements, there is some evidence that blood loss, possibly due to intestinal mucosal changes, is associated with iron-deficiency anemia in about 50% of children.[202] In unusual circumstances, excessive intake of cow's milk can result in a milk-induced enteropathy associated with blood loss and iron-deficiency anemia.[203]

Infants born prematurely are often deficient in vitamin E. Iron supplementation exacerbates the vitamin E deficiency and may contribute to the anemia suffered by many of these patients.[204] The level of total tocopherol required for effective antioxidant activity in these children is 0.64 mg/dL and that of α-tocopherol is greater than 0.50 mg/dL.[205] Correction of the iron deficiency in premature infants should be accompanied by vitamin E supplementation.[206] The supplementation should be continued for at least 3 months.

Gastrointestinal Malabsorption of Iron. Isolated malabsorption of iron is uncommon. When it occurs, the result often is severe iron deficiency. A number of gastric surgical procedures can produce malabsorption of iron. These operations include total gastrectomy,[207] partial gastrectomy (particularly when the duodenum is bypassed),[208] and other bypass procedures associated with vagotomy. The slow depletion of iron associated with inadequate absorption means that iron deficiency may not become evident until more than 10 years after the operation.[209] The cause of postsurgical iron malabsorption is multifactorial. One major contributor is *achlorhydria*, which inhibits absorption of iron salts.[209] Also, the rapid gastric emptying seen with some surgical procedures may allow insufficient time for dietary iron to be absorbed in the duodenum. Achlorhydria alone, whether it is a natural occurrence (particularly in the elderly)[209,210] or is associated with histamine H_2 blocker therapy, may result in malabsorption of iron. These circumstances can also contribute to iron deficiency by rendering treatment with oral iron ineffective after iron deficiency is diagnosed.

Diseases of the small intestine, including various forms of sprue and extensive Crohn's disease, may cause iron malabsorption and deficiency. Patients with these diseases rarely present with iron deficiency alone. Other clinical manifestations make the diagnosis relatively straightforward. These disorders frequently are accompanied by the anemia of chronic inflammation, a condition that can be confused with iron deficiency.

Clinical Manifestations of Iron Deficiency

The variable and sometimes subtle signs and symptoms of iron deficiency and its association with other diseases have sometimes led to confusion in arriving at a proper diagnosis (Table 49-4). The best example of this confusion is chlorosis, a syndrome first described in the 1600s that persisted until the turn of the 20th century. The word *chlorosis* was coined because of what observers described as a "green sickness" that occurred in young women beginning in the early teenaged years and ending in their early 20s.[211] Although anemia was thought to be a major component of the disease, many medical observers suggested that the malaise, alternating with irritability that the young ladies manifested, was the effect primarily of "love sickness."[211,212] Although

TABLE 49-4. Stages of Iron Deficiency

	Optimal Iron Balance	Iron Depletion	Iron Deficiency Without Anemia	Iron-Deficient Erythropoiesis	Iron-Deficiency Anemia	Severe Iron Deficiency
Bone marrow iron	N	N or ↓	Absent	Absent	Absent	Absent
Hemoglobin	N	N	N	N or ↓N	↓N or ↓	↓
MCV	N	N	N	N or ↓N	↓N or ↓	↓
RDW	N	N	N	N or ↑N	↑	↑
ZPP	N	N	N	N or ↑N	↑	↑
% Iron saturation	N	N	N	↓N or ↓	↓	↓
Ferritin	N	N	N or ↓N	↓N or ↓	↓	↓
Symptoms	None	None	?Decreased exercise tolerance	Pica; decreased exercise tolerance	Pica; decreased exercise tolerance; ?weakness	Weakness; sore mouth
Signs	None	None	None	None	Anemia	Anemia, pallor; abnormalities of epithelial cells including fingernails and mucosa

N, normal (95% confidence limits); ↑, increased; ↓, decreased; ↓N, lower than mean value but in normal range; ↑N, higher than mean value but in normal range; MCV, mean corpuscular volume; RDW, RBC distribution width; ZPP, zinc protoporphyrin.

the early literature abounds with treatments of the condition with oral iron or heme-containing food products, the use of iron therapy for any form of anemia was controversial until the 1930s. At that time, it became clear that both parenteral and oral iron were effective in the treatment of a large number of patients with anemia. Few reports of chlorosis were made after 1910, and certain medical historians believed that iron deficiency may have been only one component of the disease,[213] particularly because the syndrome disappeared at about the same time that extremely tight corsets were abandoned.[213] Tight corsets may have complicated iron deficiency by decreasing food intake and causing esophageal reflux and gastrointestinal blood loss. On the other hand because no satisfactory explanation exists for the appearance of the green skin color and organ dysfunction, hepatocellular disease caused by tight corsets may offer a better explanation for these signs.

Although iron therapy was not accepted as beneficial until this century,[214] examples of bioavailable iron given as a remedy for certain signs and symptoms of iron deficiency are abundant in folklore. This includes therapy given in Eastern Europe before 1900, in which pregnant women were fed apples pierced by iron nails with the nails removed 24 hours later. This therapy was given for pica and apparently reversed that condition.

Patients with iron-deficiency anemia may experience generalized weakness, malaise, and lassitude and may require more sleep. The question of whether vague neurologic complaints, including irritability and lack of energy, are due to the nonhematologic effects of iron deficiency is controversial.

Severe Iron Deficiency

Severe iron deficiency is associated with significant hypochromic microcytic anemia with hemoglobin levels often below 10 g/dL[215] (see Table 49-4). In most instances, weakness progresses gradually (over weeks or months) and sometimes leaves the patient bed ridden. Sometimes, particularly with children, the symptoms can develop rapidly despite slow progression of the anemia. These patients often are strikingly pale. When generalized pallor is difficult to evaluate, such as with black patients, examination of the nail beds, conjunctiva, and creases of the palm is sometimes helpful in evaluating the severity of the anemia.

Symptoms such as a sore tongue or mouth are related to the abnormal regeneration of rapidly proliferating cells, particularly those of the alimentary tract.[215] The physical findings associated with this abnormality are glossitis (smooth red tongue that may be indistinguishable from the findings encountered in folate or cobalamin deficiency), stomatitis, and angular chelosis (inflammation and fissuring occurring at the angles of the mouth).[215] Esophageal webs that impair swallowing (Plummer-Vinson syndrome) have been reported in patients with severe, long-standing iron deficiency but are rare.[216] Atrophic gastritis[217] and abnormalities of the small intestinal mucosa that often result from severe iron deficiency may actually make the patient resistant to oral iron therapy due to malabsorption.

Koilonychia, or "spooning" of the fingernails, is another condition seen occasionally with severe, long-standing iron deficiency.[218] The cells of the nail bed normally proliferate rapidly. Their growth is impaired with iron deficiency, producing thin nails that are soft and friable. The spooning, or concavity, of the surface of the nail is most evident when the finger is viewed edgewise.

The aforementioned abnormalities were found in 10% to 60% of patients with iron deficiency studied before 1960.[215,219] These abnormalities are now rare, particularly in children with iron deficiency. Nonetheless, they are obvious clinical signs that are diagnostically important when present.

Mild Iron Deficiency

Most patients newly diagnosed with iron deficiency have few, if any, symptoms. Certain subtle signs and symptoms may exist that can be elicited only by a carefully directed history and physical examination.

Hematologic Effects. Mild anemia can produce subtle findings such as the inability to perform strenuous exercise that was easily performed previously. In a significant number of patients, symptoms of weakness and poor exercise tolerance may actually occur with normal hemoglobin values.[220] Although these nonspecific complaints can be caused by the nonhematologic effects of iron deficiency, a normal hemoglobin level may not be optimal for a particular person. Two case histories help to illustrate this point. A young woman who was an avid mountain climber noted that she was more fatigued than usual with weekend climbing trips. Although her hemoglobin was 13.8 g/dL, serum values were diagnostic of iron deficiency. With oral iron therapy, her hemoglobin value after 3 months had risen to 15 g/dL, and her climbing tolerance improved considerably.

In the other example, a marathon runner was seen because of deteriorating clock times in recent events. Again, serum values substantiated iron deficiency despite a hemoglobin level of 13.6 g/dL. Long-distance runners of both sexes appear to be at risk for iron deficiency based on several factors, including hemoglobin loss in the urine from march hemoglobinuria,[220] and occult gastrointestinal blood loss[221] from stress as well as frequent use of aspirin and NSAIDs. After 2 months of iron therapy, the patient's hemoglobin reached 14.8 g/dL, and she noted a significant improvement in her running performance.

Nonhematologic Signs and Symptoms of Iron Deficiency

Pica. Pica is a striking condition that develops in some patients with iron deficiency. It is characterized by the compulsive consumption of various materials, most of which are not foods.[213] Food pica, which is the compulsive eating of a single entity such as celery or potato chips, has no particular association with iron deficiency.[222] Although obvious changes in epithelial or mucosal surfaces are seen with severe iron deficiency, pica is thought to be a manifestation of subclinical stomatitis or glossitis. Pica can exacerbate, or at least complicate, iron deficiency because many people eat dirt, clay, or corn starch, materials that impede iron absorption.[222] The form of pica most frequently seen is termed *pagophagia*—compulsive eating of ice. The condition is characterized as the consumption of at least one tray of ice per day for 2 months, and it occurs in 20% or more of patients with iron-deficiency anemia.[223] Although people commonly chew leftover ice after consuming a soft drink, true pagophagia involves strikingly higher levels of ice consumption, sometimes to the point where additional ice trays must be purchased. In these patients, pagophagia is almost certainly due to iron deficiency, and the patient always responds to appropriate iron supplementation within the first month of therapy.[224]

Exercise Intolerance. Weakness and poor exercise tolerance occur with anemia irrespective of its cause. Severe iron deficiency could exacerbate these symptoms by reducing the quantity of myoglobin in muscles and by lowering the activity of enzymes responsible for oxidative phosphorylation. Such changes are difficult to measure in patients with severe iron deficiency. On the other hand, studies of severely iron-deficient rats that were transfused to correct their hemoglobin levels clearly demonstrated a marked decrease in exercise tolerance.[225] Whether these changes seen in severely iron-deficient animals can be extrapolated to humans with early iron deficiency associated with mild or no anemia is unknown. Some patients with mild iron deficiency have impaired exercise endurance, particularly when the endpoint activity level is extremely high. A study of adolescent females demonstrated that mildly iron-deficient people with no anemia can improve their exercise performance with iron supplementation compared with what occurs in a group given placebo.

Central Nervous System Effects. The central nervous system effects of iron deficiency have generated considerable interest. An abnormality of dopaminergic neurotransmission may cause some of the subtle and slightly elusive central nervous system symptoms.[20,226] This hypothesis is supported most strongly by data that show that behavioral responses to presynaptic (amphetamine) and postsynaptic (apomorphine) dopaminergic-acting drugs are significantly diminished in rats made iron deficient by dietary manipulation.[227] In other studies, iron deficiency in rats has been shown to significantly diminish dopamine D_2 receptor–binding sites.[228] Indirect support for the hypothesis arises from the fact that iron is highly localized in areas of the brain (such as the caudate nucleus) that contain large amounts of dopamine and neuropeptides.[229]

A number of investigations of people have indicated that iron deficiency adversely affects behavior by impairing cognitive function, producing noncognitive disturbance, and limiting activity and work capacity.[226,230–232] Studies of cognitive function in older children and adults with iron deficiency have mainly demonstrated attention-deficit defects. Iron deficiency in young children appears to impair cognitive function significantly. Some of the subtle central nervous system symptoms seen in infants and young children with iron deficiency can occur with mild iron deficiency, even without anemia.[232] When rigorous tests are applied, such as the mental development index, mild iron deficiency is associated with some abnormalities, but significant differences in test scores occur only in iron-deficient infants or children who are also anemic.[231] In this anemic group, central nervous system disturbances are not a direct result of anemia because infants treated for iron deficiency for more than 3 months experienced correction of the anemia but had significantly lower test scores two thirds of the time.[231] These persistently lower scores suggest that iron therapy adequate to correct the anemia is not sufficient to reverse behavioral and developmental disturbances in many infants. Substantial iron supplementation may eventually reverse some of these abnormalities.

These human data concur with animal studies in which rats that were made iron deficient at birth exhibited behavior abnormalities after adequate iron supplementation. In contrast, the behavior of older iron-deficient rats normalized when they were given adequate iron supplementation.[227,233,234] These data taken together support the need for maternal and infant iron supplementation in which the main goal is prevention of iron deficiency in infancy and childhood.

Whether mild iron deficiency without anemia impairs long-term behavioral or learning development is unresolved. At an international conference on iron deficiency and behavioral development, a number of studies clearly showed an association between iron-deficiency anemia in infants and children and suboptimal test scores in development, learning, and school achievement.[235,236] The conference participants concluded that aggressive measures be taken to prevent or to treat iron-deficiency anemia in childhood. Further, they recommended investigations into the specific mechanism and functional significance of behavioral changes in iron-deficiency anemia and an assessment of their reversibility. Finally, the importance of lesser degrees of iron deficiency in children must be determined.

Delayed Growth. Given the central role of iron in cell metabolism, the association of childhood iron deficiency and delayed growth is not surprising.[174,237] The frequent association of iron deficiency and nutritional deficiency complicates the clinical picture in many instances. Correction of childhood iron deficiency usually produces an acceleration in the rate of growth.[237]

Laboratory Features of Iron Deficiency

Iron deficiency is not a single entity but rather a spectrum of disorders, as shown in Table 49-4. The clinical picture and laboratory data of a particular patient depend on where the patient falls in the continuum. Consequently, laboratory findings may vary from subtle changes to profound abnormalities.

Analysis of Peripheral Blood

Dwindling iron stores in patients with iron deficiency (see Table 49-4) means that less of the element is available to erythroid precursors. The result is iron-deficient erythropoiesis. Initially, the red cells formed under this condition show only a slight decrease in hemoglobin concentration. Given the broad range of hemoglobin concentrations in the population as a whole, a particular patient can have a substantial fall in hemoglobin with the value still in the normal range. Examination of the blood smear often reveals no discernible change. As the iron depletion continues, the patient can become frankly anemic without clearcut abnormalities on the peripheral blood smear.[238] One study, in which nine experienced hematologists examined coded blood films, demonstrated that most of a panel of expert morphologists could not identify iron deficiency by blood smear in a woman with confirmed iron-deficiency anemia and a hemoglobin of 10.1 g/dL.[239]

Automated analysis of the peripheral red cells in early iron deficiency may be more helpful but is not diagnostic. A patient with isolated iron deficiency from bleeding and a hemoglobin of 11 g/dL almost always exhibits a normal MCV (directly measured by the automated apparatus), a normal mean corpuscular hemoglobin (MCH), and a normal mean corpuscular hemoglobin concentrations (MCHC). Because mild iron-deficiency anemia often displays variation in cell size, the RDW (red cell width distribution) may be of more value in the diagnosis of early iron deficiency.[240] Because most automated blood analyses now report the RDW, a number of recently published studies have evaluated the RDW value alone or in conjunction with other tests for the correct diagnosis of iron deficiency.

In these studies, performed on adults in an outpatient setting, a high RDW (over 15%) proved to be highly sensitive (71% to 100%) in diagnosing iron deficiency,[240,241] but as might be expected, specificity is low (about 50%). Specificity improved greatly if a high RDW was associated with a low MCV, but sensitivity was compromised.[240] Based on these findings, the conclusion is that a patient with a high RDW value who gives a history suggestive of iron deficiency should have further tests performed to confirm the diagnosis. Using the RDW alone as a screening test for the diagnosis of early iron deficiency is not appropriate given the low specificity. When assessing changes in children, laboratory finding must be compared with age-matched normal values (see Appendix). For example, the MCV is high at birth, falls to a minimum at about 1 year of age, and then gradually increases until about age 16 years, when values are similar to those of normal adults.

As with all disease states, the diagnosis of iron-deficiency anemia becomes more obvious as the severity of the condition increases. Thus, as the hemoglobin level falls to below 9 g/dL because of iron deficiency, the peripheral blood smear shows frank hypochromia, microcytosis, some occasional target cells, and anisocytosis.[238] The MCV falls to well below the normal range, as do the MCH and MCHC (the last value to significantly decrease). The RDW can reach extremely high levels (greater than 20%), reflecting the obvious differences in size among the red cells seen on the blood smear.

With uncomplicated iron deficiency, the relative level of erythropoiesis is low.[177] Erythropoiesis can be assessed by the absolute reticulocyte count or the reticulocyte index.[177] The absolute reticulocyte count is determined by the percentage of the red cells that are reticulocytes. Most models of automated blood analyzers provide the red cell number, and some can even determine the percentage of red cells that are reticulocytes. The absolute reticulocyte count normally ranges between 40,000 and 60,000 cells/μL.

The absolute reticulocyte count often rises four- or fivefold with an acute bleeding episode. Prolonged, low-grade bleeding eventually produces iron deficiency with a consequent blunted reticulocyte response to anemia.[242]

In certain complicated clinical conditions, the reticulocyte count can rise despite chronic iron deficiency. This can occur, for example, with a patient who is iron deficient owing to excessive menstrual blood loss and who only intermittently takes iron tablets (eg, only during menses). In this case, the patient may be able to mount an increased reticulocyte response transiently during the time of iron supplementation.

Pure iron deficiency rarely, if ever, lowers the white blood cell (WBC) count. Some animal studies have indicated that dietary iron deficiency produces susceptibility to certain infections requiring cell-mediated immunity.[243] In vitro studies of human cells suggest that neutrophil function and T-cell proliferation can both be defective in patients with iron-deficiency anemia.[243,244]

Iron deficiency often produces thrombocytosis. Particularly high platelet counts, sometimes in excess of 1,000,000 cells/μL, can be seen when the patient is actively bleeding.[245,246] Rarely, severe iron-deficiency anemia is associated with thrombocytopenia.[247] This scenario is more common in children than in adults.

Because the diagnosis of early iron deficiency is difficult to make based on changes in the complete blood count, specialized tests have been developed that help to confirm the diagnosis. The gold standard for the diagnosis of early iron deficiency is a bone marrow examination with iron stains. Because bone marrow aspirates generally are performed only by hematologists and oncologists, the measurements detailed in the following section are particularly valuable in a general medical evaluation. In patients in whom these tests are equivocal but in whom iron deficiency is still suspected, a bone marrow examination is indicated.

Serum Iron and Total Iron-Binding Capacity

The methods of performing these tests are similar, and they should always be performed in tandem to differentiate iron deficiency from other diseases.[176,248] The serum iron is measured using *ferrizone*, a sulfonate derivative of a diphenyltrizine, which forms a water-soluble blue complex when it binds iron.[248] The reaction is conducted at acid pH to dissociate the iron in serum from transferrin, and with a reducing agent that forms soluble Fe^{2+} ions. The serum iron does not fall substantially in iron deficiency until the iron stores have been completely depleted. At this time, transferrin synthesis by the liver increases markedly.

The increase in transferrin concentration increases the total iron-binding capacity of the serum. An excess of iron is added to the serum in a separate tube, where it is bound by transferrin. From this, the total quantity of unsaturated transferrin-binding sites present in plasma (UIBC) can be calculated. The values obtained for the serum iron and the UIBC are then added to determine the total iron-binding capacity. The percentage of transferrin saturation is then determined by dividing the serum iron by the total iron-binding capacity. A value of 10% or less is diagnostic of iron deficiency. A value lower than 16% is highly suggestive of iron deficiency, and the clinical situation would dictate whether further studies should be performed.[176]

Patients with chronic inflammatory diseases without iron deficiency can have transferrin saturations less than 16%

and, rarely, less than 10%. In these cases, a markedly low serum iron is associated with a lower than normal total iron-binding capacity (less than 200 mg/dL). A bone marrow study is required to document iron deficiency in a patient with chronic inflammatory disease. Iron therapy does not benefit the anemia of chronic disease.

Serum iron and total iron-binding capacity should be obtained early in the morning after the patient has fasted for more than 8 hours because serum iron values can be affected by a meal. Also, a well-documented diurnal fluctuation in serum iron occurs.[249] Iron-deficient patients sometimes take multivitamin mineral preparations that contain subtherapeutic quantities of iron (eg, 20 mg). These preparations can transiently increase the serum iron without correcting the body iron deficit.[250]

Serum Ferritin

The serum ferritin assay was introduced in the mid-1970s as a test that correlated with total body iron stores.[251,252] A number of reliable commercial kits using various immunoassay techniques for the measurement of serum ferritin are available. The precise origin of the ferritin found in serum is unknown.[253] Data indicate that ferritin is synthesized by reticuloendothelial cells in response to cellular iron uptake.[253] This ferritin, which is secreted by the cell, appears to contain little or no iron (apoferritin).

Concentrations of ferritin are measured as nanograms per milliliter of blood, whereas tissue ferritin can be found in milligram concentrations per gram of tissue. Therefore, any disease that destroys tissues with a high ferritin content, such as hepatitis, leads to erroneously high serum ferritin values that may obscure the diagnosis of iron deficiency.[252] Chronic inflammatory diseases, such as rheumatoid arthritis, are also associated with spuriously high serum ferritin levels.

Because few conditions artifactually depress the serum ferritin value, the test is most valuable when it is low. Serum ferritin concentrations of less than 10 μg/L are generally considered to be diagnostic of iron deficiency, and values of less than 20 μg/L are suggestive of a deficient state.[252] These relative values may be even more specific when screening anemic people. In a study of anemic patients older than 65 years, 95% of patients with ferritin values less than or equal to 18 μg/L had absent bone marrow iron stores.[254] Extremely high serum ferritin concentrations can be helpful in evaluating patients with iron overload. Even with iron overload, the serum ferritin value is not linearly related to total body iron stores.[255] In individual patients, serial values obtained during iron supplementation may be helpful in determining whether the body iron stores have been replenished.

Erythrocyte Protoporphyrin Levels

Assay of free erythrocyte protoporphyrin levels is performed most commonly in children to distinguish various disorders that may be confused with iron deficiency.[256–258] Thus, measurements of free erythrocyte protoporphyrin can help distinguish between iron-deficiency anemia, in which the level is high (less iron available for conversion of protoporphyrin to heme), and thalassemia, in which the level is low.[257,258] (Decreased globin chain synthesis produces a commensurate decrease in protoporphyrin synthesis.) The free erythrocyte protoporphyrin levels are particularly high in children with lead intoxication because lead directly inhibits the enzyme ferrochelatase.[257]

Based on a need to screen large populations potentially at risk for lead intoxication, another test has been developed, the erythrocyte zinc protoporphyrin level.[259] Under conditions in which iron is not made available for incorporation into protoporphyrin, the zinc chelate of protoporphyrin forms readily.[259] Zinc protoporphyrin measurements are simple. The substance is measured using a direct fluorometric assay of whole blood without the extraction procedures necessary for measurements of erythrocyte protoporphyrin. The zinc protoporphyrin determination requires only a drop of blood placed on a long coverslip with low background fluorescence; a hematofluorometer measures the absorbance of zinc protoporphyrin at 420 nm.[259] The determination must be made on oxygenated blood, but the results are not influenced by the hematocrit. The values obtained so far have shown that this rapid technique, requiring minimal amounts of blood, is useful in diagnosing lead poisoning. Recently, the method has been used to assess iron deficiency in selected adult patients. A more sensitive measure of iron-deficient erythropoiesis uses the free erythrocyte or zinc protoporphyrin/heme ratio.[260] Unfortunately, even this very sensitive test is not useful in differentiating iron deficiency from many other common causes of anemia. The zinc protoporphyrin/heme ratio is also elevated in patients with anemia of chronic inflammation, for instance.

Despite their sophistication, the available laboratory tests, taken individually, are suboptimal for the diagnosis of iron deficiency. Data compiled from several tests are more likely to be informative than the separate values.[261] Sensitivity and specificity are greatest when a high clinical suspicion of iron deficiency is combined with appropriate testing.

Bone Marrow Examination

The bone marrow examination is the gold standard in the evaluation of iron deficiency. If the blood and serum studies are equivocal or suggest multiple disorders (eg, iron deficiency in the face of anemia of chronic inflammation), a bone marrow aspirate to assess iron stores may be the only way to diagnose iron deficiency.

With routine marrow staining techniques, the changes seen in iron deficiency are nonspecific. Some normoblasts have irregular cytoplasmic borders, reflecting poor hemoglobin production. Quantitation of erythropoiesis varies considerably because, with mild iron deficiency, an increase in erythropoiesis can be observed, while longstanding chronic or severe iron deficiency decreases erythropoiesis. Generally, the WBC and megakaryocytic series appear to be normal.[176]

Given the unimpressive morphologic changes associated with iron deficiency, the diagnostic test performed on bone marrow specimens is specific staining for iron. The technique used almost exclusively by histology laboratories is the Prussian blue reaction.[262] This method is reliable and easily distinguishes iron, which is bluish green against a light background. Because extracellular precipitates can stain with Prussian blue, it is important to look specifically for intracellular iron, particularly by examining macrophages. Macrophage iron is generally seen as round granules that often are clumped. These granules appear to represent hemosiderin iron in lysosomes and are particularly pronounced with iron overload.[263] Small round specks of iron are seen under normal conditions in about 20% of normoblasts and probably represent cytosolic ferritin aggregates.[264]

Chronic inflammatory diseases impair the release of iron from the macrophage storage pools, thereby the proper formation of hemoglobin by red cells. In sideroblastic anemias, the normoblasts show a ring of iron granules that partially, if not completely, surrounds the nucleus.[265] The iron is localized in the mitochondria because it cannot be incorporated into protoporphyrin to form heme.

Reduced stainable iron in the bone marrow is suggestive of iron-deficiency anemia.[263] To ascertain whether the iron content is reduced, at least one other bone marrow specimen stained for iron at the same time should be examined. In general, even mild anemia caused by iron deficiency is associated with completely absent bone marrow iron stores[266]; in mildly anemic patients in whom the iron is present but reduced, a therapeutic trial of iron may clinch the diagnosis of iron-deficiency anemia.

Sometimes, the absence of stainable iron is artifactual. Thus, even with an appropriate control specimen, analysis of bone marrow sections may show less than the expected amount of iron because of the processing technique.[267] Bone marrow core specimens subjected to decalcification with acidic fixatives (or even nonbuffered formalin) increases the solubility of iron and releases the element from the specimen if left in the solution for extended periods of time (eg, overnight). Because of this problem, some laboratories have used bone marrow clot sections to assess iron stores because this preparation does not have to be decalcified or exposed to fixatives. If the bone marrow core is fixed in buffered formalin or neutral pH fixative, appropriate assessment of iron stores and identification of sideroblasts should be possible.

Other Laboratory Tests That May Be Used in the Evaluation of Iron Deficiency

In the past, studies of *iron kinetics* were performed by injecting intravenous ^{59}Fe. Clearance measurements, distribution in various body organs by using external counting techniques, and the appearance of the radioactive label in the hemoglobin of circulating erythrocytes all were used for the assessment of abnormalities in iron metabolism.[48] These studies were extremely helpful in the identification of the various iron compartments in the body. Few laboratories presently perform iron kinetic studies, and results are difficult to interpret because they are performed so infrequently. If the test is performed on iron-deficient people, the already high rate of incorporation of the ^{59}Fe label into hemoglobin rises, and the plasma iron clearance is relatively rapid.[48] Because ferrokinetic studies rely on plasma iron turnover, the turnover of an injected dose of ^{59}Fe is affected profoundly by the quantity of nonradioactive iron in the plasma as well as transferrin saturation.[268] At high transferrin saturation, the proportion of radioiron that is incorporated into transferrin and that becomes diferric with the binding is high. Diferric transferrin binds to transferrin receptors more avidly than does monoferric transferrin. Therefore, for a given rate of erythropoiesis, radiolabeled iron uptake is greater at higher transferrin saturations.

With this information, it is possible to first calculate the plasma iron turnover and then, by accounting for transferrin saturation, to calculate the erythron transferrin uptake.[269–271] This value can then be used to differentiate among various forms of anemia. Specifically, hyperproliferative anemias associated with increased red cell destruction or ineffective erythropoiesis have profoundly increased erythron transferrin uptake compared with that which occurs with hypoproliferative anemias.[272]

Based on the fact that the erythron transferrin turnover is an indirect measurement of erythroid transferrin receptors, studies suggest that direct measurements of transferrin receptors in plasma could become a diagnostic tool.[273,274] *Plasma transferrin receptors* appear to be molecules that have been shed from erythroid and other normal cells.[275,276] In some instances, rapidly proliferating tumor cells appear to account for a portion of plasma transferrin receptors.[275] Plasma transferrin receptor levels rise both with iron deficiency and with elevated erythroid turnover, as occurs, for instance, with hemolytic anemia.[277] Investigations continue in an effort to determine the operational limits of the plasma transferrin receptor assay in clinical medicine.

Another clinical test that has fallen from favor is the measurement of absorption of trace doses of ^{59}Fe or radioactive cobalt (^{27}Co).[278] Absorption of the radioactive label increases markedly in iron-deficient subjects. Interest in measurement of *gastrointestinal iron absorption* has been rekindled by reports that absorption of small amounts of nonradioactive iron (eg, 20 mg of elemental iron) can be measured accurately by serial assays of the plasma iron concentration.[250] In even mildly iron-deficient people, plasma iron levels increase substantially 2 to 4 hours after ingestion of the iron test dose relative to iron-replete subjects. This test may be used to identify certain patients with mild iron deficiency. A variation of the test using high doses of iron (described in the text that follows) can be employed to assess a person's ability to absorb oral iron.

A test not available commercially is the assay for red cell ferritin. This assay measures the total amount of *ferritin* in a given number of red cells and may be useful in people who are iron deficient but have spuriously high serum ferritin levels (eg, caused by hepatic disease).[279] Another test that may soon be available is the assay of the erythrocyte *zinc protoporphyrin/heme ratio*. As previously noted, this ratio could be even more sensitive in defining iron deficiency and impaired heme synthesis. The test does not distinguish iron deficiency from the anemia of chronic disease or defects of porphyrin metabolism such as lead poisoning.

Despite a plethora of diagnostic tests, an accurate determination of iron deficiency by laboratory means can be elusive at times. Even definitive tests such as bone marrow examination are equivocal on occasion. The diagnosis can then be made by assessing the response to iron therapy. This therapeutic trial is most often performed when iron deficiency complicates another condition that causes anemia.

Diseases That Complicate the Diagnosis of Iron Deficiency

Table 49-5 lists several common diseases and a number of uncommon entities that can be confused with iron deficiency.

Anemia of Chronic Disease

Anemia of chronic disease includes the anemia associated with chronic infections and inflammation as well as the anemia associated with malignancy. The defect involves

TABLE 49-5. Diseases That Can Complicate or Be Confused With Iron Deficiency

Disease	Manifestation*
Anemia of chronic disease	Not responsive to iron therapy; associated diseases may also cause blood loss and coexistent iron deficiency
β-Thalassemia	May have normalization of hemoglobin A_2 levels if iron deficiency coexists
α-Thalassemia	Low MCV, even with normal hemoglobin level
Sideroblastic anemia	Hypochromic blood picture, but bone marrow confirms diagnosis
Folate or cobalamin deficiency	Tends to normalize peripheral blood values (MCV) when coexistent with iron deficiency

* See text for further details.

an inhibition of iron use despite adequate, if not increased, iron stores.[280] The serum ferritin level is normal or slightly increased. The serum iron is low, but the serum transferrin concentration is normal or decreased.[280,281] The diagnosis should be suspected if a chronic inflammatory disease or malignancy exists and the hemoglobin level is low but has not changed abruptly.

On bone marrow examination, normal or increased iron is seen in reticuloendothelial cells.[280] The blockade in red cell iron uptake produces iron-deficient erythropoiesis and markedly decreases the number of sideroblasts. The resulting anemia is usually normocytic, although at hemoglobin levels below 10 g/dL, a low MCV can occur.[280] The degree of anemia is related to the duration of the underlying disease. Hemoglobin levels in uncomplicated anemia of chronic disease seldom fall below 8 g/dL. Lower hemoglobin values or an abrupt fall in hemoglobin raises the prospect that a second process is contributing to the anemia. Iron deficiency commonly complicates a number of diseases associated with the anemia of chronic inflammation. An important example is that of gastrointestinal blood loss that occurs in patients with chronic arthritis who are taking aspirin or NSAIDs. People on NSAID therapy for more than a few months develop peptic ulcer disease associated with bleeding or perforation in about 2% of instances.[179] Certainly, the incidence of bleeding from chronic gastric irritation due to NSAID therapy is much higher.

β-Thalassemia Trait

Thalassemia is another common disease that frequently is confused with iron deficiency. All the β-thalassemias, including hereditary persistence of fetal hemoglobin and δβ-thalassemia, can be diagnosed by various abnormalities seen on a hemoglobin electrophoresis. A diagnosis of β-thalassemia should be suspected when the patient has a family history of microcytic anemia, has been known to have anemia since infancy, or has been known to be anemic and has received an adequate trial of iron supplementation with no improvement. Patients with β-thalassemia can also have iron-deficiency anemia. This complication occurs commonly in women of childbearing age. When iron deficient, normalization of hemoglobin A_2 levels occurs in some patients with β-thalassemia, frequently producing diagnostic confusion.[282] These patients may have laboratory evidence of iron deficiency. Despite adequate iron supplementation and measures to correct blood loss, they never reach a normal hemoglobin level. After the iron stores have been replenished, a hemoglobin electrophoresis shows a pattern consistent with a diagnosis of β-thalassemia (including elevated levels of hemoglobin A_2).[282]

α-Thalassemia

The form of thalassemia most frequently confused with iron-deficiency anemia, particularly in blacks, is α-thalassemia. Population studies indicate that the incidence of α-thalassemia trait (two of the four α chains deleted) is close to 3% in the African American population.[283] A routine hemoglobin electrophoresis is usually normal. Bart's hemoglobin (the γ-chain tetramer) is detectable in neonates with α-thalassemia trait but is absent in older children and adults.[283] The hemoglobin of patients with α-thalassemia ranges from normal to slightly lower than normal. Even with normal hemoglobin levels, the MCV is low.

Analysis of the peripheral blood can help to differentiate α-thalassemia and iron deficiency. People with α-thalassemia trait tend to have a lower MCV for the level of hemoglobin than patients with iron deficiency. The MCV of the latter group usually is normal until the hemoglobin falls below 10 g/dL. Further, the RDW is minimally elevated in α-thalassemia patients, despite a very low MCV. Patients with iron deficiency usually have a high RDW, particularly when their cells are microcytic. Given the high frequency of α-thalassemia in many segments of the population, all patients in whom iron deficiency is suspected clinically must have the diagnosis substantiated by appropriate laboratory studies.

Other Diseases

A number of less common diseases can also be confused with iron deficiency. Both hereditary and acquired sideroblastic anemias can have a hypochromic, microcytic blood picture. This heterogenous group of diseases is associated with defective heme synthesis. Many patients have excessive amounts of bone marrow storage iron. The diagnosis is confirmed by the presence of ringed sideroblasts seen on the Prussian blue iron stain of the bone marrow. The frequent association of defects in other peripheral blood cells, often manifested as thrombocytopenia or neutropenia, further distinguishes sideroblastic anemia from iron deficiency.

Lead intoxication, which occurs in children who eat lead-based paint, can produce a hypochromic microcytic anemia due to inhibition of ferrochelatase. Although lead has been removed from present-day paints, children who reside in older buildings are at risk for developing the disease. Also, cases of lead poisoning have been described in certain areas where lead has seeped into the ground water and contaminated the water supply. Lead and some other heavy metals can be taken up in the gut by the iron-absorption machinery. As a result, increased iron absorption due to iron deficiency also leads to increased absorption of other metals, including lead.[284] Children who are iron deficient should also have lead levels checked.

Occasionally, other types of anemia mask iron deficiency.[285] For example, the ineffective erythropoiesis seen in patients with severe folate or cobalamin deficiency is often associated with high serum iron and ferritin values. When patients with this deficiency are treated with cobalamin or folic acid, the serum iron level falls, reflecting the rapid generation of new cells. Mild iron deficiency in these patients may become obvious only when the megaloblastic anemia is adequately treated with folate or cobalamin.

Although most patients with hemolytic anemia have replete or even increased iron stores, iron deficiency can complicate a few hemolytic disorders. Some patients with intravascular hemolysis, for instance, lose substantial amounts of hemoglobin and iron in their urine. These patients often have transferrin saturation and ferritin values that are in the low-normal range. Bone marrow iron stores may be decreased or even absent. Red cell free erythrocyte protoporphyrin or zinc protoporphyrin levels are often high, indicating relative tissue iron deficiency. In some instances, iron and folate supplementation significantly increase the rate of erythropoiesis. A therapeutic iron trial should be monitored carefully because some patients fail to respond and can actually develop iron overload.

IMPLICATIONS OF A DIAGNOSIS OF IRON DEFICIENCY

A diagnosis of iron deficiency has two major implications: the patient will respond beneficially if treated with appropriate iron supplementation, and an underlying problem has caused the iron deficiency. In most cases, iron deficiency is caused by a physiologic condition such as menstruation or pregnancy. Even in patients with high-risk factors, however, iron deficiency cannot be a priori attributed to the risk condition. The cardinal rule in adults and children over 2 or 3 years of age is that pathological blood loss is the cause of iron deficiency until proved otherwise. In infants and young children, poor nutrition in utero or after birth may account for a higher number of cases of iron deficiency. Even in infants, blood loss must be assessed, and a careful history and physical examination must be performed to assess for possible bleeding.

Evaluation for Blood Loss

In iron-deficient adults without gastrointestinal disease or intravascular hemolysis, blood loss almost invariably is the culprit. As noted in Table 49-3, the blood loss can originate from a number of sources. In women of childbearing age, menstrual loss is a primary consideration; in males or females of other ages, gastrointestinal blood loss must be considered first.

A careful history and physical examination are the keys to evaluation of menstrual blood loss. Often, many women initially comment that their menstrual blood loss is normal, not realizing that individual variability is substantial and that they have much higher than normal menstrual flow. A number of questions may help to define the extent of menstrual blood loss:

1. If blood flow is experienced for more than 5 days, the blood loss can be excessive; blood flow does not include spotting, in which small amounts of brown discharge are seen for several days after the usual menstrual flow.
2. Counting the number of tampons or pads used is not a useful measure unless it can be definitely determined that more than six saturated tampons or pads are used daily for more than 3 days.
3. Perhaps the best measure of increased menstrual flow is the presence of clots found daily that measure more than 1 inch in length. The presence of clots demonstrates that the menstrual blood loss has exceeded the normal fibrolytic activity present in the urogenital tract.

Heavier than normal menstrual flow may not be associated with iron deficiency until the patient has other reasons for increased iron loss, such as a previous pregnancy. Superimposed evaluation of excessive menstrual flow include a gynecologic examination. A pathological source of bleeding may be superimposed on menstrual blood losses. Vaginal bleeding that occurs between menstrual periods or after menopause reflects dysfunctional bleeding and requires immediate gynecologic evaluation.

The diagnosis of gastrointestinal blood loss is often obvious, particularly if the patient has a history of prior peptic ulcer disease or explicitly states that hematemesis, hematochezia, or melena are recurring symptoms. Usually, gastrointestinal bleeding that produces iron deficiency is occult, and the diagnosis requires fecal occult blood testing. The Hemoccult test is the most common approach to evaluating occult blood loss[286]; a small amount of stool is placed by the patient on paper impregnated with the indicator substance, guaiac. The patient returns the test paper to the physician's office where hydrogen peroxide is added. In the presence of hemoglobin and hydrogen peroxide, the guaiac is oxidized, producing a blue color on the test paper. The test is inexpensive and relatively easy to perform but has numerous confounding problems that affect accurate interpretation. Peroxidases found in red meats may give false-positive reactions. Certain drugs, including high-dose aspirin, can cause a peroxidase reaction. Because of these type of errors, the false-positive rate is about 2%.[286,287] The hemoglobin or myoglobin present in red meat does not give false-positive reactions unless exceptionally large quantities of meat containing substantial amounts of blood are ingested.

The Hemoccult reaction can detect 7 mg or more of hemoglobin per g of stool. Consequently, lower gastrointestinal blood losses of 10 mL/d or more should give a positive Hemoccult test.[287] Since blood loss can be intermittent with some lesions (eg, colon carcinoma), at least six Hemoccult specimens should be examined to obtain adequate sensitivity. This test is much less sensitive if the specimen is dried. Wetting the sample with normal saline before application of the hydrogen peroxide restores sensitivity.[286,287]

The Hemoccult test is also less sensitive to upper gastrointestinal bleeding because the hemoglobin in the specimen tends to be more dilute. Further, hemoglobin released in the upper gastrointestinal tract tends to lose its heme, and free heme is less reactive.[287-289] Also, the reaction does not measure porphyrin degradation products that are frequently produced with bleeding in the stomach or upper part of the duodenum.[287] The HemoQuant, a quantitative fecal assay based on conversion of heme to a fluorescent porphyrin, is not affected by many of these factors, making it more sensitive to upper gastrointestinal bleeding. Unfortunately, the HemoQuant assay requires larger stool samples. Also, greater technical expertise is needed for the HemoQuant test because analytic measurement of porphyrin is required.[286,287]

Other tests of gastrointestinal bleeding, including immunochemical methods, are still not available for widespread use. An algorithm for the evaluation of gastrointestinal bleeding in children over age 13 years and in adults is shown in Figure 49-6. A negative test for occult blood in the stool warrants a gastrointestinal work-up in males over the age of 40 years and in women who are postmenopausal without a history of previous iron deficiency because of heavy menses or numerous pregnancies. Even with a negative work-up, medications associated with gastric irritation such as NSAIDs should be discontinued. A careful menstrual history should be performed in younger women to evaluate possible excessive blood loss. In some cases, a meticulous diary should be kept to document the length of the menstrual period, the number of tampons or pads used, and whether clots were identified. A careful history for recurrent nosebleeds should be obtained both in young men and young women. Young patients with iron deficiency who lack good evidence for blood loss from other sites should have at least an upper gastrointestinal evaluation (see Fig. 49-6). If the physician still suspects gastrointestinal blood loss despite a negative work-up, stools specimens should again be assessed for occult blood, even if the patient is being treated appropriately with iron. Iron darkens the stool but does not give a false-positive reaction to the guaiac test.[286]

IRON REPLACEMENT THERAPY

After the diagnosis of iron deficiency is documented, iron replacement therapy should begin, even while the evaluation for blood loss is conducted. For infants and young children, the treatment of choice is a liquid iron preparation that provides 2 mg/kg of elemental iron given three times per day.[290] Iron replacement therapy for older children and adults consist of tablets containing various iron salts that provide about 60 mg of elemental iron each.[289] The most common iron salt used, ferrous sulfate, usually is prescribed as a 330-mg tablet containing 60 mg of elemental iron. Other oral iron preparations are listed in Table 49-6. The tablets are coated to decrease the rate of oxidation of the Fe^{2+} to the less soluble Fe^{3+}. Ferrous fumarate is more resistant to

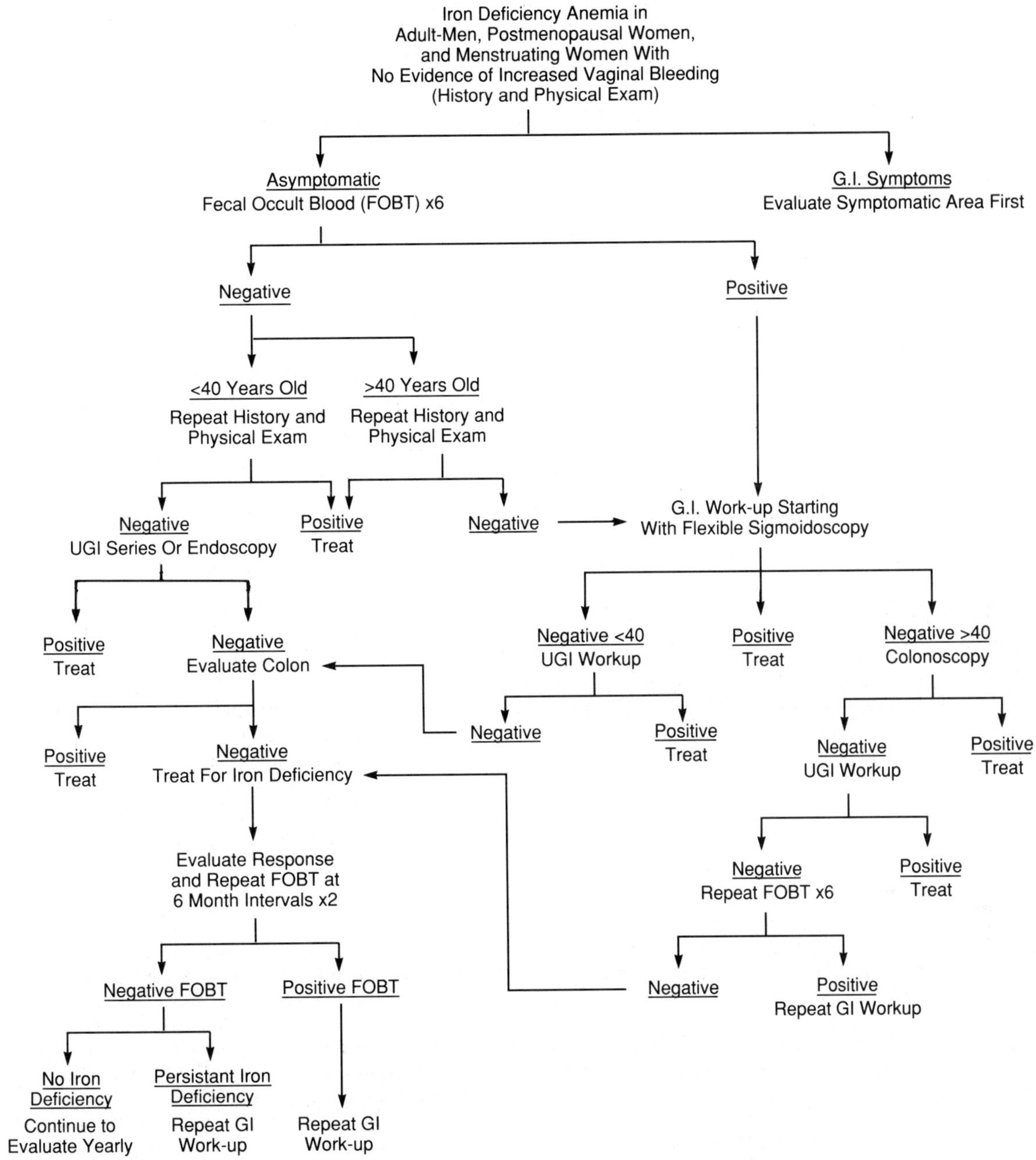

FIGURE 49-6. A suggested scheme for evaluation of the gastrointestinal tract in the presence of iron-deficiency anemia.

oxidation than other iron salts and need not be coated. Apparently, the unappealing grayish color of ferrous fumarate prompted most pharmaceutical companies to apply a waxy enteric coating with more pleasing pastel shades. Unfortunately, some people have difficulty absorbing the iron because of poor dissolution of the coating.[95] For these patients, a liquid iron preparation may provide more bioavailable elemental iron. Polysaccharide iron complex is not a salt. The capsules contain iron that is held in soluble form through charge–charge interactions with the side chains of complex sugars. Each capsule contains about three times the amount of elemental iron as other iron preparations (see Table 49-6).

Although ferrous sulfate tablets are the least expensive preparation, oral iron therapy—whatever the preparation—costs $5 or less per month. Preparations that contain only iron salts can be purchased over the counter. When iron is provided in combination with other nutrients in a multivitamin and mineral tablet, the cost is much higher, and the preparation may come only in prescription form (if 1 mg or more of folic acid is included). Some of these additives may actually inhibit iron absorption, particularly certain mineral salts that act as antacids, such as calcium carbonate and magnesium oxide.[95] Even with bioavailable iron present, combination hematinic agents containing other minerals and vitamins should be avoided. Some preparations containing iron are designated as sustained release and purport to cause fewer side effects. Most of these preparations are more expensive than routine supplements and are not of proven greater benefit,[291] although some patients may prefer them. Polysaccharide iron complex is well tolerated by some patients who are unable to take iron salts.

For the treatment of iron deficiency in adults, three iron salt tablets containing about 60 mg of elemental iron should be taken per day.[289,292] Some clinicians recommend that

TABLE 49-6. Oral Iron Preparations Commonly Used for Iron Replacement Therapy

Preparation	Elemental Iron Content	Recommended Dose
IRON SALT TABLETS		
Ferrous sulfate, 330 mg	60 mg	3/d
Ferrous gluconate, 325 mg	37 mg	5/d
Ferrous fumerate, 200 mg	66 mg	3/d
LIQUID		
Ferrous gluconate ([Fergon] elixir = 300 mg/tsp)	35 mg/tsp	2 tsp 3×/d (adults) 1 mg elemental iron/kg 2–3×/d (pediatric dose)
Ferrous sulfate (elixir = 220 mg/tsp)	44 mg/tsp	2 tsp 2–3×/d (adults) 1 mg elemental iron/kg 2–3×/d (pediatric dose)
IRON SACCHARIDES		
Polysaccharide iron complex	150 mg	2/d

only two tablets are necessary because little benefit is derived from the third dose. This recommendation is supported by the fact that ingestion of 60 mg of elemental iron produces serum iron levels sufficiently high to saturate substantially transferrin for 6 hours or longer. The implication is that another tablet taken during this period would be absorbed poorly.[95] Because poor compliance is often a problem with oral iron supplementation, the recommendation of three tablets per day is reasonable because patients may then take at least two tablets.

Various elements found in food may inhibit absorption of iron salts. Therefore, whenever possible, iron should be taken on an empty stomach. The side effects associated with oral iron therapy, such as upper gastrointestinal irritation (including nausea) and constipation, can adversely affect patient compliance. The contention that upper gastrointestinal symptoms are associated with increased iron absorption has no experimental support.[293] Iron taken with food has fewer side effects than when taken on an empty stomach, but the improvement in compliance produced by this approach must be weighed against inferior absorption. The constipating effect of iron therapy varies and sometimes is alleviated by bulk laxatives or stool softeners. Polysaccharide iron complex is generally tolerated much better than iron salts despite its higher iron content. All iron preparations cause dark green or black stools. This discoloration is not harmful.

Response to Oral Iron Therapy

The response to oral iron therapy varies according to factors such as patient compliance, individual variation in absorption of iron, and the rate of continued iron loss. The severity of iron deficiency does not affect the rate of response because patients with lower iron levels show a more rapid increase.[294] The reticulocyte count should increase within 7 to 10 days of initiation of therapy in an iron-deficient patient[295]; a significant increase in the hemoglobin level should occur after 2 to 3 weeks[294]; and after 2 months, the hemoglobin level should reach the normal range.[294] The iron should be continued until iron body stores have been replenished. This usually requires an additional 2 to 4 months of therapy after the hemoglobin level has been corrected.[288,289] The total duration of therapy needed to correct the iron status of a deficient patient ranges from 6 to 10 months. Failure to replenish iron stores makes the patient extremely vulnerable to the rapid recurrence of iron-deficiency anemia, particularly if bleeding continues or the diet is inadequate. It is often difficult to convince patients who are not anemic to continue taking iron supplementation. Vigilance always and reinforcement frequently are necessary.

Failure to Respond to Oral Iron Therapy

Some reasons that patients fail to respond at all or respond partially to oral iron therapy are listed here:

- Blood loss greater than hemoglobin regeneration
- Incorrect diagnosis (eg, thalassemia trait)
- Superimposed infection, inflammation, malignancy, or uremia
- Noncompliance with medication regimen
- Lead poisoning
- Defective gastrointestinal iron absorption
- Concomitant folate or cobalamin deficiency
- Copper deficiency
- Renal failure and erythropoietin deficiency

The most serious problem is continued blood loss, which often results from a failure to identify the source. Sometimes, a repeat work-up for gastrointestinal bleeding is fruitful because small lesions in the colon that initially were missed can become detectable with time. Transient responses to iron replacement are often the result of continued occult gastrointestinal bleeding (see Fig. 49-6).

Patients with other reasons for anemia such as mild thalassemia or anemia of chronic disease who are also iron deficient respond only partially to iron supplementation. In many of these patients, the diagnosis of iron deficiency is not clearcut from laboratory data, and a bone marrow examination is required. If a bone marrow examination is not feasible, the patient should be given a trial of iron therapy for 2 months. If the hemoglobin initially improves but stabilizes at a level lower than normal in the absence of continued blood loss, then a second anemia probably coexists with the iron deficiency. Despite the subnormal response, iron supplementation should be continued for an additional 4 months to replenish iron stores.

The most common reason for a failure of oral iron therapy is poor compliance.[296] In many instances, the side effects of iron therapy, particularly upper gastrointestinal symptoms, make compliance with the recommended oral supplementation program impossible. In most cases, the long duration of iron therapy, particularly after the hemoglobin has reached normal levels, leads to patients or parents of patients simply forgetting the medication. Compliance must be documented to rule out other causes of response failures.

If gastrointestinal side effects are a problem, the therapy can be changed appropriately. Pillboxes, marked calendars, and other mnemonic strategies can supplement the memory. Serum iron measurements are useless in determining compliance because taking medication only before office visits would give a high serum iron value on that particular day. One study of iron-deficient adolescents showed that serum ferritin and zinc protoporphyrin levels are helpful in determining compliance, but the simple approach of seeing patients frequently (every 2 weeks to 1 month) and counting tablets was equally as effective.[297]

Occasionally, malabsorption produces a poor response to iron replacement therapy. Sometimes, as in patients with nontropical sprue, the cause of the malabsorption is obvious. More often, however, poor iron absorption is associated with no obvious gastrointestinal disease. Gastric achlorhydria, a common condition found in the elderly, is the culprit at times. Increased gastric emptying or rapid duodenal transit time can impair iron absorption by reducing exposure to the absorption machinery in the duodenum. In other instances, a particular iron preparation is poorly absorbed. For instance, the coating on the tablet can be too thick to allow complete dissolution, or the preparation may include various supplements that inhibit absorption.[95] Drugs that inhibit the secretion of gastric acid are among the most commonly prescribed medications and can inhibit iron absorption. Iron absorption is inhibited significantly but not completely by cimetidine.[298,299] Some of the newer preparations that neutralize gastric acidity even more profoundly can render oral iron therapy useless.

Gastrointestinal absorption of a particular iron preparation can be measured by examining serial changes in serum iron. A preparation containing 60 mg of elemental iron should produce a rapid change in serum iron level even in iron-replete subjects[95] (Fig. 49-7). Even more profound increases in serum iron occur in patients with iron deficiency who can attain serum iron levels that completely saturate transferrin transiently.

Although several serial values make the test more sensitive, only two serum iron determinations are required. After a 12-hour fast, the serum iron level is drawn, and the patient takes one of the iron supplement tablets. Three hours later (still fasting), another iron value is obtained. Milligrams of iron absorbed from the preparation can be estimated by the following formula: milligrams of iron absorbed = .062 × the change in serum iron (3-hour value minus 0-hour value) + 0.45.[95] Although there is great variation among individual patients, iron-deficient subjects should absorb at least 7 mg of iron, the value seen with iron-replete subjects (see Fig. 49-7). A presumptive diagnosis of gastrointestinal malabsorption is made if less than 3 mg of iron are taken up.

Liquid iron preparations similarly can be tested. The patient is given a small dose of iron (eg, 20 mg), and the plasma iron concentration is measured 2 to 4 hours after ingestion.[250] People with normal iron stores show little change in serum iron levels with this dose. In contrast, relatively large increases occur in iron-deficient people.[250] If a sufficiently high increase occurs with this test (greater than 75 μg/dL change), the oral iron therapy could be changed to a liquid preparation. If the increase is below 75 μg/dL, parenteral iron therapy should be considered. A patient who malabsorbs iron may exhibit other evidence of gastrointestinal malabsorption, but more often malabsorption of other nutrients is not a problem and a work-up for malabsorption is not necessary. The rapid uptake of iron salts from the duodenum makes the rapid serum iron test possible. The kinetics could be different with polysaccharide iron complex because this material has to be processed by the cell before iron is released into the circulation.

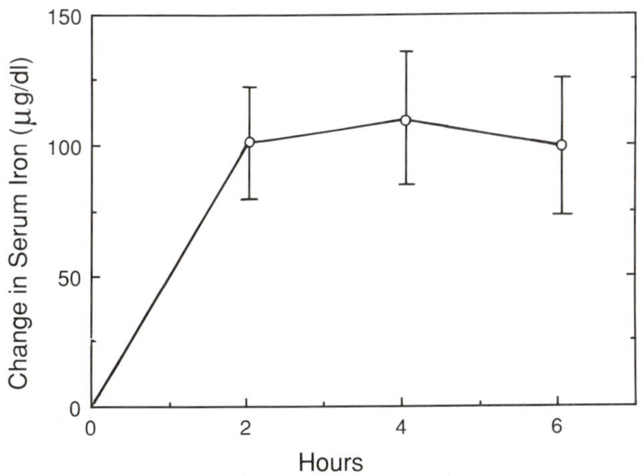

FIGURE 49-7. Change in serum iron after ingestion of a single iron salt tablet by 16 women of childbearing age with normal hematologic indices and ferritin values of 20 mg/L or more. After an overnight fast, the subjects ingested a single ferrous fumarate table containing 65 mg of elemental iron. The values represent the mean (±SEM) for the change in serum iron from time zero at 2, 4, and 6 hours after the preparation was taken (with subjects still fasting).

TABLE 49-7. Reactions to Intravenous Iron Dextran*

Reaction	Estimated Incidence (%)
Life-threatening anaphylaxis	<1
Hypotension or flushing or both	2
Delayed reactions including rash and arthritis	
Severe	5
Mild to moderate	20
Phlebitis at site of injection (more frequent with too-rapid injection)	10

* Data reported are for adult patients.

Indications for Intravenous Iron Therapy

Indications for the use of intravenous iron dextran are as follows[300,301]:

- Chronic, uncorrectable bleeding
- Gastrointestinal malabsorption of iron
- Gastrointestinal inflammatory disease
- Oral iron intolerance
- Uncooperative or persistently noncompliant patient
- Extremely low Hg (less than 6 g/dL) with signs of poor perfusion and transfusion is contraindicated (eg, religious objection)

The main advantage of parenteral iron therapy is that the clinician is assured that the patient has received a known amount of iron replacement. Although iron dextran therapy can be given intramuscularly, the drug is routinely given intravenously. Intramuscular injections are painful, can produce sterile abscess formation, and can induce hyperpigmentation of the skin in the area of the injection.[301] The main side effects of intravenous iron dextran therapy are illustrated in Table 49-7. Although iron dextran is more expensive than oral iron, the cost is more than offset by fewer office visits.

Because the most dangerous side effect of iron dextran is an acute anaphylactic reaction, the patient should receive a test dose before the therapeutic dose is given. A total of 10 mg of intravenous iron dextran is infused over 30 minutes as a test. A physician must be present with resuscitation equipment. The intravenous form of iron dextran is then diluted in an equal amount of normal saline, and as much as 3 g of iron dextran are infused over a 6-hour period.[301] The day after the infusion, up to 20% of patients experience mild to moderate myalgia and arthralgia. The symptoms are usually relieved with NSAIDs. Lasting sequelae do not occur. Intravenous iron dextran should be used cautiously in patients with rheumatoid arthritis because it may cause flares in their disease.

A patient's iron requirements can be easily calculated to allow replacement with iron dextran. For example, if a patient has a hematocrit of 30 mL/dL and the desired level should be 45 mL/dL, then a 15% increase in packed red cell volume is necessary, and the appropriate dose of iron dextran is 750 mg (blood volume is 5000 mL × 0.15, or 750 mL of packed red cells at 1 mg/mL). Replenishment of the iron stores requires another 1000 mg. Two grams of intravenous iron dextran would then provide for the total iron needs.

ROUTINE IRON SUPPLEMENTATION

The routine use of oral iron supplements has dramatically increased over the past decade. In some instances, supplementation is aimed at high-risk groups, including low-birthweight infants, growing children, and pregnant women. In other cases, iron supplementation is based on the belief that the probability is high that iron deficiency will develop in the long run. Such diverse groups as normal menstruating women and long-distance runners fall under this heading. A large number of multivitamin supplements and other iron-containing products have saturated the market. These products are frequently used not only by high-risk groups but also by members of the general population who have been convinced by mass advertising campaigns and other vehicles that they need nutritional supplements.

Table 49-8 lists some of these iron-containing supplements. The supplements are grouped according to the perceived indications, but they frequently are taken by other family members or, in the case of prenatal tablets, continued for years after the pregnancy. In general, these compounds are not harmful, and when the supplement contains a relatively small amount of iron (eg, less than 20 mg), the additional dietary iron is minimal. Routine use of these preparations by all members of the population is unwise, however, because they may be harmful in certain instances. For example, iron deficiency caused by a colonic tumor can be masked so that a diagnosis is delayed until the tumor is less amenable to local therapy. In addition, routine unmonitored iron supplementation always poses a risk to the small but significant number of people who are prone to iron overload, including patients with hereditary hemochromatosis. Certain groups, however, such as infants, young children, and pregnant women, are at sufficiently high risk of iron deficiency to warrant supplementation.

TABLE 49-8. Recommended Over-the-Counter Multivitamin and Mineral Preparations

Routine Use	Amount of Iron/Tablet (mg)	Cost* (Per Daily Dose)
FOR ADULTS		
Geritol Complete	50	10¢
Myadec Professional	30	8¢
Theragran M	27	5¢
Centrum	18	6¢
One-A-Day "Stress Guard"	18	10¢
Nature Made Stress Pak†	8.3	25¢
FOR CHILDREN		
Flintstones Complete	18	8¢
Flintstones Plus Iron	18	7¢
FOR WOMEN		
One-A-Day (Within)	27	5¢
Nature Made Women's Pak†	8.3	20¢
HEMATINICS‡		
Stuartinic	100	26¢
FOR PREGNANT WOMEN‡		
Mission F.A.	30	13¢
Stuart Prenatal	60	15¢

* Approximate retail cost is based on a single survey.
† Daily packet contains a number of tablets.
‡ Contain less than 1 mg of folic acid. Preparations that contain 1 mg or more of folic acid require a prescription. Based on their folic acid content, most hematinics and prenatal vitamins require a prescription and are not included in this table.

IRON SUPPLEMENTATION DURING PREGNANCY

In the United States, most obstetricians recommend routine iron supplementation during pregnancy. Generally, the supplementation is the 60 mg of elemental iron found in average multivitamin mineral prenatal preparations[302,303] (see Table 49-8). Studies of iron absorption from these supplements indicate that some provide less than the desired amount of bioavailable iron.[95]

Studies performed in the 1960s indicated that 50% to 80% of pregnant women were iron deficient.[304] The risk of iron deficiency during pregnancy is higher in women with a history of previous pregnancies, heavy menses, or poor diet. The average iron loss during pregnancy, including iron used by the fetus for growth and erythropoiesis, blood loss at delivery, and iron loss in breast milk for 6 months postpartum, is about 900 mg, nearly equivalent to the quantity of iron found in four units of blood.[305] The average daily iron requirement during pregnancy is greatest in the third trimester of pregnancy, when 6.5 mg/d of iron are required for the fetus, placenta, and mother. These data are a solid basis on which to recommend iron supplementation during pregnancy.

Controversy continues in Great Britain over routine iron supplementation practices.[302,303] Even in the medicinally conservative United States, however, the case for routine iron supplementation is strong. This is particularly true because the elimination of routine iron supplementation would require that iron-deficient people in high-risk groups be identified by serial ferritin determinations, a more expensive proposition than routine supplementation.[303]

The increase in plasma volume that occurs during pregnancy and peaks at the 24th week lowers hemoglobin values even in women on optimal supplementation. Pregnant women who daily take one multivitamin–multimineral tablet containing 60 mg of iron still frequently develop iron deficiency, particularly during the last trimester.[95] Iron deficiency in these women can result from poor absorption of iron from the multivitamin–multimineral preparation and from preexisting iron deficiency. Therefore, routine blood counts should be obtained from pregnant women during the last trimester. Failure of the hemoglobin to rise from the level seen at 24 weeks' gestation suggests iron deficiency.

Plasma iron profiles are difficult to interpret in pregnancy when the deviations are small. Pregnancy per se lowers plasma iron and raises the total iron-binding capacity. Ferritin values tend to fall during pregnancy. These changes reflect physiologic iron deficiency to some extent. The trend is the same, however, even in well-supplemented women. Iron supplementation certainly should be increased in women whose transferrin saturation and serum ferritin levels fall into the range known to reflect iron deficiency. Iron supplementation should be continued for at least 6 months postpartum in women who breastfeed their infants.[302]

ROUTINE IRON SUPPLEMENTATION FOR MENSTRUATING WOMEN

Menstruating women generally require 1 mg of iron in addition to the 1 mg required for obligatory losses. Because blood lost during menstruation varies markedly and dietary iron uptake may be suboptimal (particularly for young menstruating women who are dieting), probably 20% or more or these women are iron deficient.[306] For these reasons, menstruating women on average have about one third the storage iron found in men.[306] Since the prevalence of iron depletion is extremely high in this population, most laboratories have a separate normal range for serum ferritin determinations in women of childbearing age. The lower end of this range may fall below a value indicative of iron deficiency, that is, below 18 ng/mL. Ferritin values of less than 18 ng/mL still strongly suggest iron deficiency, even if the value is in the normal range for women in this group. A history of excessive blood loss (particularly menstrual blood loss) should be sought in these patients. Therapeutic iron supplementation is indicated.

Although menstruating women have a high incidence of iron deficiency, and most have less than optimal iron stores, clinical or laboratory evidence of iron depletion should be sought to justify supplementation. The relatively small quantity of elemental iron (10 to 18 mg) in multivitamin–multimineral supplements rarely, if ever, would be harmful to anyone. However, the routine use of preparations that contain higher amounts of elemental iron (30 mg or more) should definitely be discouraged without an indication because a small but significant number of people have a condition associated with iron overload.

Menstruating women are not routinely screened for iron deficiency, although most clinicians anticipate that this group of patients can become iron deficient, and the diagnosis is seldom delayed to the point at which significant anemia develops. One study analyzed a number of different tests for iron deficiency and concluded that the serum ferritin is the most sensitive test in defining iron deficiency in nonanemic people.[307] Because of problems with specificity, the serum ferritin is a good screening test only if 20% or more of a population is at risk for iron deficiency. Unfortunately, no large-scale trial has been performed on menstruating women to clearly define how best to assess and treat iron deficiency in this large population.

CLINICAL DISORDERS OF IRON OVERLOAD

Excessive body iron stores always reflect iron intake that exceeds the daily requirement. The obligatory daily loss of iron is about 1 mg. This reflects mainly iron lost from desquamated epithelial cells. Although people with iron overload may increase the obligatory loss to a maximum of 2 mg/d because of nonspecific increases in intracellular ferritin iron, no mechanism regulates iron excretion. Conversely, excessive buildup of the element does not occur because of impaired elimination, as with phosphate overload in renal failure. Consequently, iron overload can develop only from inordinately increased iron absorption or from parenteral administration of iron (Table 49-9). Gastrointestinal iron absorption is enhanced in idiopathic hemochromatosis, certain iron-loading anemias characterized by ineffective erythropoiesis (eg, thalassemia intermedia), or, rarely, intemperate ingestion. Parenteral iron loading is usually due to transfusions for refractory forms of anemia. Only rarely does iatrogenic iron overload result from overzealous administration of iron dextran supplements.

TABLE 49-9. Conditions That Cause Clinical Disorders of Iron Overload

Homozygous hereditary hemochromatosis
Anemia associated with ineffective erythropoiesis (with or without transfusions)
Thalassemia (intermedia and major)
Hereditary and acquired sideroblastic
Dysmyelopoietic refractory anemias
Congenital dyserythropoietic anemias (HEMPAS and others)
Hereditary hemolytic anemias without transfusion (associated heterozygosity for idiopathic hemochromatosis described)
Hereditary spherocytosis
Thalassemia minor
Intemperate ingestion (rare)
Chronic iron tablet ingestion
Transfusional iron overload
Severe hemolytic anemias (especially thalassemia major, sickle cell anemia)
African iron overload

Hereditary Hemochromatosis

Hereditary hemochromatosis (HHC) is an inborn error of metabolism in which systemic iron loading results from increased gastrointestinal absorption of the element. Daily iron absorption increases from about 1 mg to 2 or 3 mg with the disorder.[308] The result over the course of 40 to 60 years is a rise in body iron stores from the normal of about 1 g in the adult male to anywhere between 15 and 50 g. According to most estimates, about 20 g of excess iron is required to cause enough tissue damage to result in clinical disease.[308] The increased iron loss by women during menstruation and pregnancy prolongs significantly the time required to raise body iron stores compared with men. Thus, women who have HHC typically exhibit a lower incidence of clinically significant disease and present with phenotypic disease later in life. This conclusion is best illustrated by the following example: a 55-year-old man with excessive iron absorption of 1 mg/d will have accumulated 20.1 g of excess iron; a woman with excessive iron absorption of 1 mg/d except for years 12 through 50 would require 93 years to accumulate the same amount of excess iron.

The basis for the defect in HC is unknown. With so little known about the mechanism of iron absorption, the foundation on which to develop hypotheses concerning the biochemical basis of HHC is weak. Studies of patients with HHC have to date demonstrated no defect in other aspects of iron metabolism, including the serum levels and sialic acid content of transferrin[309] and the expression of transferrin receptors.

A genetic basis for HHC is suggested by its association with the human leukocyte antigen (HLA) system on chromosome 6. The gene that encodes the defect is closely linked to the HLA-A allele.[310] Thus, whereas 29% of controls express the HLA-A3 allele, HLA-A3 is found in 74% of patients with HHC.[310] The association between HHC and the HLA-B14 and HLA-B7 alleles is due to their linkage to HLA-A3. The disorder displays a recessive mode of inheritance. Within a given family, the HLA linkage often varies from the classic A3, B14, B7 pattern, but the defective gene will breed true in a particular kindred because it is linked to a particular HLA haplotype. Therefore, a patient with clinically evident homozygous hemochromatosis with a certain HLA haplotype (eg, A10, B17, A5, B12) presumably acquired the defective genes linked to an abnormal haplotype from each parent. Therefore, siblings with identical

HLA haplotypes almost certainly have homozygous hemochromatosis, whereas a sibling with only one of these haplotypes (only the A10, B17 haplotype) is heterozygous for the disease (unless one of the parents is homozygous).

HHC is a more common disorder than has generally been appreciated. One investigation found a gene frequency of 0.056, which places the frequency of heterozygotes at 0.104 and that of homozygotes at 0.003.[311] A population in central Sweden displays the very high gene frequency of 0.08, placing the frequency of heterozygotes at 0.160 in this group.[312] Such data indicate that HHC is one of the most common inborn errors of metabolism. People who are homozygous for the HHC gene can develop the complete picture of iron overload with all its potential complications. Heterozygotes generally are asymptomatic, although body iron stores may be elevated.[313]

Iron overload occurs frequently in sub-Saharan Africans.[314] Reports from the 1950s and 1960s suggested that iron loading was due to the consumption of excessive amounts of the element that occurred in homemade beer produced in iron kettles.[315] The condition was called *Bantu siderosis* after the South African population on which many of the early reports were based. More recent reports have debunked this hypothesis.[314,316]

Iron overload occurs frequently in many African populations and is unrelated to alcohol or excessive iron ingestion. The disorder is differentiated from the European hereditary hemochromatosis by its lack of linkage to the HLA locus. Another distinguishing feature is the fact that liver biopsy shows excessive iron in both hepatocytes and Kupffer cells. In HLA-linked hereditary hemochromatosis, excessive iron is seen only in hepatocytes. Sufficiently extensive and controlled studies to determine whether non-HLA–linked iron loading occurs with any frequency in African Americans are lacking.

Laboratory Diagnosis

In view of the fact that more is known regarding the genetics of HHC and the routine use of screening laboratory tests such as the serum iron, the diagnosis of HHC is made at a much earlier clinical stage. The classic triad of bronze skin, diabetes, and cirrhosis that was frequently seen in patients who presented with HHC 20 years ago is now encountered less than 10% of the time.[311] A large percentage of patients are identified who have subclinical homozygous hemochromatosis with no discernible clinical or laboratory abnormality indicative of organ dysfunction.[311]

The initial laboratory tests that should be performed on people who have a family member diagnosed with homozygous hemochromatosis or who exhibit a markedly increased serum iron on screening chemistry panels include the transferrin saturation and serum ferritin. A number of extensive studies performed on kindreds with HHC have helped to define values that indicate homozygosity, even in the early or subclinical state[310–313] (Table 49-10). Heterozygotes tend to have test results that are intermediate between normal subjects and those with homozygous disease.

The most useful screening test is the transferrin saturation test. A saturation of over 61% on two occasions strongly suggests the diagnosis of HHC. Some people with subclinical disease, particularly women and children, may not always exhibit high saturations, and the diagnosis is substantiated using analysis of HLA haplotypes. The serum ferritin correlates with the degree of iron overload. Higher than normal values suggest the presence of excess tissue iron deposition, even in asymptomatic patients. The serum ferritin value does not form a perfectly linear relation with total body iron stores. Thus, the absolute degree of iron

TABLE 49-10. Diagnosis of Subclinical or Early Hemochromatosis

Screening Test	Normal*	Homozygous Hemochromatosis
Serum iron (μg/dL)	<160	160–307
Transferrin saturation (%)	<50	61–100
Ferritin (ng/mL)		
Males	<325	45–688
Females	<125	25–549

* 95% confidence levels.

overload can be estimated only from the serum ferritin values in individual patients. Therefore, a high transferrin saturation and a high serum ferritin value indicative of homozygous hemochromatosis warrant a liver biopsy.

The liver biopsy is necessary to confirm the diagnosis of HHC because specific biochemical markers are not available. A quantitative estimate of iron overload on examination of a Prussian blue stain of the liver biopsy sections can be determined (Table 49-11). The diagnosis is confirmed by identifying iron in liver parenchymal cells.[311,312] A sample of liver should also be sent for quantitative iron analysis using atomic absorption spectroscopy. A number of commercial laboratories perform this test. Quantitative iron determination in liver may help define the extent of iron overload after the diagnosis has been made by histologic means.

A number of other tests are available for estimating the degree of iron overload. Measurement of the 24-hour urinary iron excretion after a desferrioxamine infusion is rarely performed and may therefore be difficult to interpret.[311,312]

Alcohol and Iron Overload. Alcoholics may occasionally have a clinical presentation that mimics HHC with increases in serum iron and ferritin levels as well as stainable iron in the liver.[317] Although this clinical picture is not common in the total population of alcoholics, the incidence of excessive alcohol ingestion is sufficiently high that the absolute number of people who fall into this category is large. This form of iron loading may in part be secondary to anemias associated with ineffective erythropoiesis, including alcohol-related sideroblastic anemia and folate deficiency. The massive iron loading seen in some patients was at one time also attributed to an acquired defect in iron absorption caused by excessive alcohol ingestion.[318] Alcohol alone (without the presence of ineffective erythropoiesis) has a small effect, at best, on iron absorption.

In other studies assessing the effects of alcohol, HLA typing of families affected by the HHC gene permits the identification of people who are heterozygous for the defect.[319] Comparison of HHC heterozygotes who consume alcohol with those who do not reveals similar iron stores in the two groups.[320] In patients who are alcoholic with evidence of mild iron overload, the incidence of HLA-A3 is similar to that in the population as a whole and is much lower than that found in HHC heterozygotes.[321] When iron-loaded people are divided into those with excessive alcohol ingestion and those who consume little or none, no difference is found in clinical manifestations (increased skin pigmentation, diabetes mellitus, hypogonadism, arthropathy, cardiomyopathy).[322] In addition, body iron stores as determined by phlebotomy are identical in the two groups. Finally, the incidence of the HLA-A3 allele is much greater in the iron-loaded group as a whole than in the general population. The gene frequency is elevated equally in the alcoholic and nonalcoholic subgroups with iron overload,

TABLE 49-11. Liver Biopsy Results in Subclinical or Early Homozygous Hemochromatosis

	Normal	Hemochromatosis
Hepatic parenchymal cell iron (grade 0 = none; grade 4 = most)	≤1	1–4
Hepatic iron concentration (μg iron/100 mg tissue dry weight)	<140	240–1682

indicating that alcohol by itself is not a significant contributor to the development of clinical HHC. At the same time, alcohol intake in patients with iron overload must be discouraged because both conditions can damage the same organs, particularly the liver.

Impact of Hereditary Hemochromatosis on Iron Loading in Other Disorders

A number of clinical conditions that once were believed to induce iron overload appear to do so only in association with the allele encoding the HHC defect. People with hereditary spherocytosis[323] and β-thalassemia trait,[324] for example, who are also heterozygous for HHC may manifest iron overload that results in clinical disease. In contrast to the situation with β-thalassemia trait, thalassemia intermedia clearly produces iron overload independent of the HHC gene.[325] The ineffective erythropoiesis associated with this disorder is thought to be the basis of the iron loading.

One disorder that has been problematic in its relation to iron loading and the HHC gene is idiopathic acquired sideroblastic anemia. Although many patients receive transfusions frequently to maintain an acceptable hematocrit, some with this disorder develop iron loading in the absence of transfusion. One study of seven patients with sideroblastic anemia and iron loading in the absence of transfusion found that five carried the HLA-A3 allele.[326] This finding prompted the proposal that iron overload in sideroblastic anemia results from an association with the gene for HHC. Subsequently, evaluations that included larger numbers of patients failed to show any association between the HLA-A3 allele and sideroblastic anemia.[327] In those cases, the iron loading most likely results from ineffective erythropoiesis.

Hereditary Hemochromatosis and Hepatocellular Carcinoma

A lethal complication of HHC is hepatocellular carcinoma. The risk of patients with idiopathic hemochromatosis developing this malignancy is significantly greater than that of the general population.[328] The index case in most kindreds of patients with HHC displays massive hepatic iron overload at presentation. The incidence of cirrhosis under these circumstances may be as high as 85%.[329] Only about two thirds of such patients survive for 4 years owing to complications of cirrhosis and the development of hepatocellular carcinoma. When these patients survive from 4 to 10 years after the diagnosis of HHC, their survival curve follows the trend of the general population.[329]

One of the important questions in the management of patients with HHC is the relation of cirrhosis to the development of hepatocellular carcinoma and the impact of therapy on these complications.

Phlebotomy reduces the incidence of cirrhosis in HHC. When followed by repeated liver biopsies during venesection therapy for a mean of 7 years, 60% of patients demonstrate no change in hepatic histology, and progression occurs in 30%.[330] Although an actual improvement in histology occurs in only 5% of patients, progression to more severe liver damage is prevented in most. Hepatocellular carcinoma occurs in 20% of these patients despite long-term phlebotomy. Therefore, hepatocellular carcinoma clearly can occur with HHC independent of cirrhosis.[331] The mechanism of this effect is unknown.

In areas where the hepatitis B virus is endemic, the incidence of cirrhosis and hepatocellular carcinoma is probably increased in patients with HHC by a synergistic impact of the virus and iron loading on the liver.[332] Hepatocellular carcinoma is resistant to chemotherapy, and even surgical intervention is usually futile.

Transfusional Iron Overload

At one time, transfusional iron overload was termed *hemosiderosis* to distinguish it from HHC (see section on pathologic differences in iron loading). Except for iron deposition in the reticuloendothelial cells of transfused patients, the pattern of parenchymal iron deposits is identical in the two conditions. *Hemochromatosis*, which is a descriptive term describing parenchymal iron deposit, sufficiently encompasses both conditions.

At least two criteria must be met to permit the development of clinically significant transfusional iron overload in the setting of chronic intractable anemias. First, chronic blood loss, for example, menorrhagia, cannot be the cause of the anemia because iron is lost in the process. Second, the anemia must be associated with a relatively long life expectancy. For example, patients with acute myelogenous leukemia in relapse may require frequent transfusions, but their life expectancies are insufficient to allow important sequelae of iron overload to develop. A number of common conditions fulfill both criteria: (1) thalassemia major and intermedia, (2) myelodysplastic anemia and congenital dyserythropoietic anemias, (3) mild aplastic anemia and related syndromes including red cell dysplasia, and (4) anemia of renal failure.

The introduction of recombinant erythropoietin for general use in anemic patients with renal failure is rapidly eliminating the last category from the list. Less common conditions that fall under this rubric include Diamond-Blackfan syndrome, pure red cell aplasia, and Fanconi's anemia. Significant iron overload generally occurs in patients who have received about 30 units of blood. With ineffective erythropoiesis, clinically important iron loading can be reached even more rapidly.

Mechanisms for Cellular Injury Caused by Iron Loading

The high transferrin saturation that occurs in hemochromatosis increases iron deposition in almost all parenchymal cells. When transferrin is 100% saturated with iron, a small but significant amount of free or loosely protein-bound iron in the serum may also be taken up by cells in a nonspecific fashion. The resulting increase in cellular iron probably leads to free radical damage to membranes and proteins. Rats fed diets supplemented with carbonyl iron absorb large quantities of the mineral and develop a pattern of iron deposition in the tissues that mimics that seen with HHC.[333] The livers and other organs of these animals demonstrate considerable membrane oxidative damage as manifested by the production of malonyl dialdehyde, a product of lipid oxidation. Iron overload in humans produces similar patterns of tissue injury.

The other factor that probably contributes to cellular damage with iron overload is lysosomal fragility. When the medium of cells in continuous culture is supplemented with iron salts, the iron taken into the cell induces the synthesis of ferritin and the formation of hemosiderin-laden lysosomes.[334,335] The lysosomes isolated from such cell preparations are mechanically fragile.[336] These organelles tend to fracture and release hydrolases during the isolation process. A similar fragility within the cell potentially allows the escape of hazardous hydrolases into the cytosol, where they may wreak havoc. An analogous lysosomal fragility is seen when the organelles are isolated from the livers of iron-loaded rats.[337,338]

Pathologic Differences in Iron Loading (Hemosiderosis and Hemochromatosis)

Iron is deposited in large quantities throughout the tissues of patients with iron overload. With increased intestinal absorption, as occurs in HHC or ineffective erythropoiesis, iron is most prominent in parenchymal cells. Transfusional iron loading begins in the reticuloendothelial cells, which degrade the allogeneic red cells as they become senescent. Iron in the reticuloendothelial cells is cycled to transferrin and redistributed to the parenchymal cells (Fig. 49-8). After iron is deposited in parenchymal cells, tissue damage is similar to that seen in HHC. Clinically, when parenchymal cell iron loading is excessive, the two conditions are identical in their effect on organs.

ORGANS DAMAGED BY IRON OVERLOAD

Liver

Dramatic hepatic iron deposition can occur in patients with HHC. The brownish granules seen in the hepatocytes with hematoxylin and eosin staining prove to be iron deposits by Prussian blue staining. Electron microscopy shows iron deposition both in ferritin and in hemosiderin inclusions.[339] Along with a quantitative increase in ferritin, the electron density of many of the ferritin particles is significantly greater than normal.[340] Ferritin aggregates form, which at times appear to be paracrystalline in structure.

As with many other types of hepatic injury, liver fibrosis is a secondary consequence of excessive iron deposition.[341] Coincident insults to the liver by other toxins such as alcohol may further exacerbate the injury. Hepatic damage is manifested by increases in the levels of serum transaminases and lactate dehydrogenase, although these elevations usually are modest because iron overload produces little hepatic inflammation. Therefore, the amount of the iron-induced injury can be misleading in the clinical evaluation of patients with HHC. Liver injury can progress to irreversible fibrosis and cirrhosis, whereas the serum transaminase levels give little indication that anything is awry.[342] As a result, reliance on these values to monitor the severity or progression of the disorder can be disastrous. The first alarming sign may be compromised hepatic biosynthetic capacity, manifested by a falling serum albumin level and a rising prothrombin time. These developments indicate life-threatening hepatocellular dysfunction. As previously noted, the development of hepatoma is a common and deadly complication of hepatic iron damage, particularly in patients with HHC.

Besides confirming the diagnosis by the presence of parenchymal cell iron deposition, liver biopsy remains the benchmark for the evaluation of body iron stores in HHC patients. The biopsy sample not only gives accurate data on iron content, but also the degree to which iron deposition has resulted in tissue damage can be assessed by histologic examination. Liver biopsy does carry a risk of internal bleeding, but death rarely results from complications of the procedure. Consequently, under certain conditions, when HHC has been diagnosed using HLA markers, for example, noninvasive approaches may be important in the evaluation of the liver in HHC patients.

Noninvasive diagnostic methods are becoming more accurate. Liver density as determined by dual-energy computed tomography (CT) correlates well with biopsy determinations of liver iron content.[343] Iron has a high atomic number, producing a characteristic difference in attenuation when the liver is probed by x-rays of differing energies. The iron content of the tissue can be estimated from these data. Rather than a complete abdominal CT evaluation, only a single CT "slice" through the liver is necessary because iron in the liver is relatively uniform in distribution. Because the determinations can be performed repeatedly without injury, the usefulness of long-term follow-up is obviously great. CT scans performed without the dual-energy technique can also provide useful information about liver density, particularly when the liver density is compared with other tissues such as muscle, which show a much smaller degree of iron deposition. Liver CT scans can be misleading with conditions that influence the CT density of the organ. For example, patients with significant alcohol intake may have increased fat deposition in the liver, which reduces its overall density.

The paramagnetic properties of storage iron have been exploited in the development of two other useful methods of determining body iron stores. Magnetic resonance imaging (MRI) is a powerful technique for the assessment of the iron content of tissues, particularly the liver.[344] The relatively homogenous structure of the liver lessens some of the technical difficulties that occur with imaging of some other organs. Striking images are obtained in patients with HHC, and the technique promises ultimately to be more useful than CT imaging.[345] The other method of iron determination involves the measurement of magnetic susceptibility in tissues, which directly reflects the levels of the element.[346] Magnetic susceptibility measurement is by far the most accurate noninvasive test of storage iron. Unfortunately, the availability of this technique is limited.

Heart

Cardiac abnormalities in HHC patients may present a variety of serious and life-threatening complications, particularly in those in whom anemia constitutes a further cardiac stress. Clinically, the most common cardiac abnormality is congestive cardiomyopathy, but others have been described, including pericarditis, restrictive cardiomyopathy, and angina without coronary artery disease.[347–351] A strong correlation exists between the cumulative number of blood transfusions and functional cardiac derangements in patients with transfusional iron overload[352] (Fig. 49-9). A direct comparison of cardiac iron content and cardiac function has not been made. Of 41 patients with severe thalassemia or aregenerative anemia and secondary hemochromatosis reported in one series, 26 succumbed to congestive heart failure.[353] With the exception of 8 patients, all patients over the age of 8 years showed cardiac abnormalities—atrial arrhythmias and conduction defects in most cases and pericarditis in others. When these clinical findings were correlated with postmortem studies, extensive cardiac iron deposition was found in each instance. The heaviest involvement occurred in the ventricular myocardium. In addition, many of the necropsy specimens showed extensive fibrosis.

In another study including patients with HHC, Buja and Roberts[354] reported postmortem studies from 19 people with cardiac iron deposits. In patients with anemia, extensive

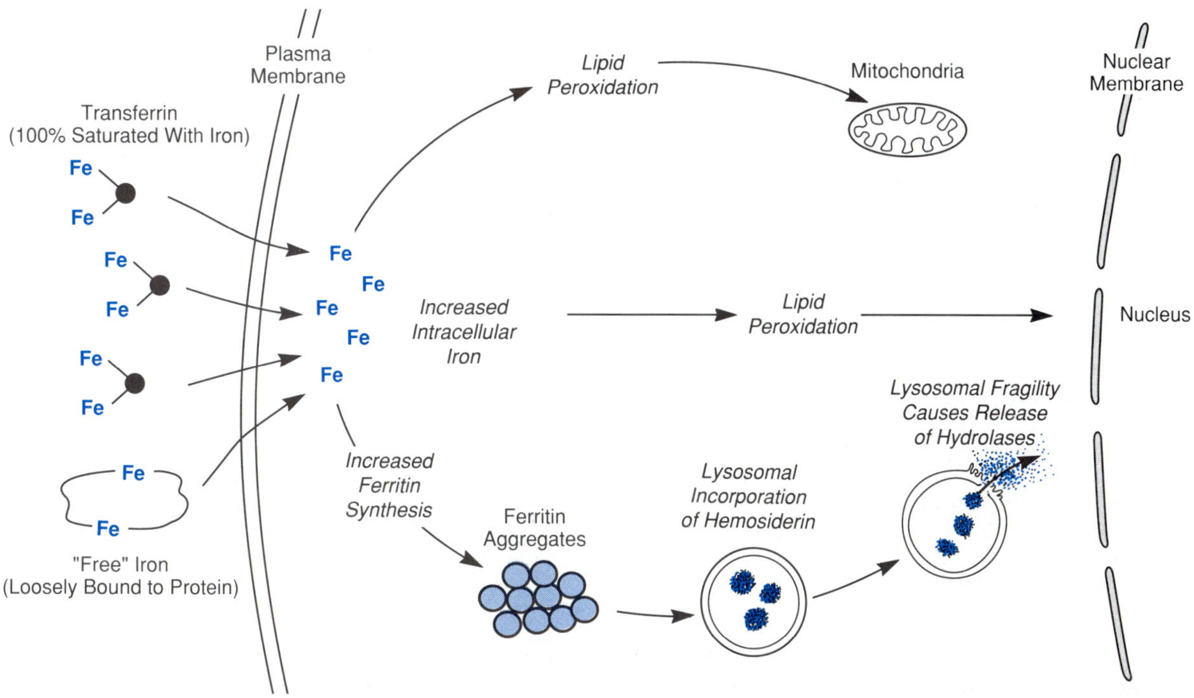

FIGURE 49-8. Damage to tissues in iron overload results from increased iron uptake by parenchymal cells when serum transferrin is highly saturated with iron. Cellular damage results from lipid peroxidation of membranes and the cytosolic release of lysosomal hydrolases.

iron deposition was believed to occur only in those who received more than 100 units of blood. We now know that substantial iron loading can occur with fewer than 20 transfused units. Iron deposits initially occur in ventricular myocardium and are usually more pronounced in ventricular than in atrial muscle. No difference exists in the degree of iron deposition in the left and right ventricles. Conducting myocardium is relatively spared. Within the ventricular myocardium, iron deposition is not uniform; iron deposition is heaviest in the subepicardial myocardium, less pronounced in the subendocardium, and lightest in the region between. Consequently, endomyocardial biopsy can underestimate the extent of cardiac iron deposition. Iron deposition occurs both within myocytes and in the interstitial tissue. How these findings correlate with clinical consequences is unknown. Myocardial iron deposits are associated with prominent iron deposition in other organs, although the reverse is not always true. As might be expected, as far as cardiac histology is concerned, there is no significant difference between primary and transfusion-associated hemochromatosis. A postmortem evaluation of 14 patients from the Mayo Clinic with hemochromatosis confirmed most of the conclusions of Buja and Roberts.[355] This study also found that iron deposition was exclusively sarcoplasmic.

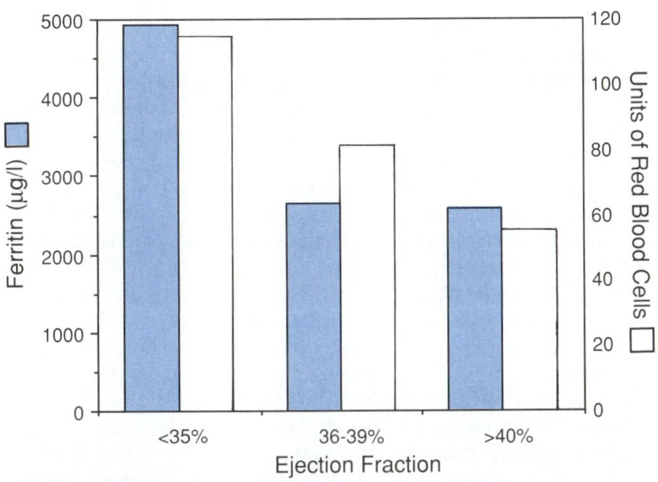

FIGURE 49-9. Correlation of cardiac ejection fraction with serum ferritin and number of transfusions in patients with iron overload.

Antemortem investigations of cardiac pathology in patients with anemia and iron overload have been reported in only two instances. In one, evaluation of four such patients using either left or right ventricular endomyocardial biopsy, evidence of excessive iron deposition was found in only one person.[356] In another investigation, right ventricular endomyocardial biopsy was used to study a patient with severe cardiac failure from iron overload secondary to the excessive iron absorption associated with ineffective erythropoiesis.[357] The initial biopsy showed extensive intracellular iron deposition without inflammation or fibrosis. The biopsy specimen obtained after chelation therapy demonstrated a marked reduction in iron content associated with significant improvement in cardiac function.

Myocardial cell dysfunction appears to develop only after the intracellular concentration of iron reaches a critical threshold. Indirect evidence to support this hypothesis comes from clinical studies showing that extensive cardiac iron deposits need not be associated with myocardial dysfunction.[354] After the first symptoms of cardiac failure appear, a rapid deterioration in cardiac function ensues, which is often unresponsive to medical therapy.

Evaluation of Cardiac Function in Hemochromatosis

Accurate evaluation of cardiac function in patients with HHC is extremely important because potentially lethal cardiac injuries can be reversible if diagnosed early. The ideal test of cardiac performance in such people would be noninvasive and sensitive and would demonstrate perturbations prior to significant deterioration in cardiac status. None of the available modalities meets these criteria. The physical examination in most patients is relatively unremarkable until heart failure produces a third heart sound. With advanced disease, dilated cardiomyopathy may occur with cardiomegaly on the chest radiograph. Earlier in the course, routine chest radiograph is unrevealing. Electrocardiographic abnormalities may include atrial arrhythmias. Since the atria and conducting tissue are relatively spared from iron deposition, these disturbances usually indicate substantial cardiac iron deposition.

The most useful noninvasive techniques are echocardiography and radionuclide ventriculography. Echocardiographic abnormalities are more prominent in patients who have received a greater number of transfusions.[358] This correlation exists, as shown in Figure 49-9, but is not absolute. In some instances, radionuclide ventriculograms have been more useful in the detection of early cardiac dysfunction, particularly when combined with exercise. In no case has a systematic correlation been found between these noninvasive tests and pathologically determined deposition of iron in the heart. Usually, a relation is sought between the test and parameters such as the number of transfusions or patient compliance with chelation therapy. Given the approximate nature of the association between these values and the actual iron deposition in the heart, the conclusions must be viewed with some caution.

The limitations of the noninvasive techniques of cardiac evaluation combined with the relative inaccessibility of the organ to biopsy evaluation leave a number of important questions unanswered concerning the heart in HHC patients. One issue is the exact prevalence of myocardial iron deposition. As previously noted, the most thorough studies of cardiac involvement have been postmortem evaluations. These investigations are by their nature skewed toward those with more severe degrees of iron deposition. Therefore, the condition of the heart of patients early in the course of their disease is unknown.

Likewise, the relation between the quantity of iron in the heart and the degree of cardiac dysfunction is unknown. Noninvasive tests, such as the radionuclide ventriculogram and exercise tolerance test, are more readily available to the general medical community than endomyocardial biopsy. The degree to which individual tests or combinations of tests reflect myocardial iron loading in patients at risk has not been clarified. Data on this subject would provide valuable decision-making information for physicians with the responsibility of caring for these at-risk people. Rational decisions then can be made regarding the need for therapeutic intervention or the efficacy of individual treatment regimens.

Endocrine Dysfunction

Dysfunction of the endocrine pancreas is common in patients with iron overload.[359] In some instances, overt diabetes mellitus requiring insulin treatment develops. Most often, the perturbations in carbohydrate metabolism are more subtle, and an oral glucose tolerance test may be necessary to demonstrate abnormalities in insulin production. With vigorous treatment of the iron overload, islet cell dysfunction can be reversed in some people, including patients requiring insulin treatment.[360] Exocrine function is usually well preserved in HHC, indicating that the cells in the islets of Langerhans are more susceptible to iron-induced injury than those of the exocrine pancreas.

Pituitary dysfunction may be manifested in a variety of ways. Reduced gonadotropin levels are common and may be the best screening test for subclinical endocrine dysfunction.[361] When this phenomenon is combined with primary reductions in gonadal sex corticosteroid production, delayed sexual maturation may occur in children and libido is frequently lost in adults. Many people are reluctant to mention the subject of their declining sexual drive and must be questioned specifically about the issue. Although overt adrenal failure leading to Addison's disease is uncommon, deficient production of adrenocorticotropic hormone (ACTH) is seen occasionally.[362] A metyrapone stimulation test may show either delayed or diminished pituitary ACTH secretion in patients with significant iron overload. Rarely, iron deposition in the adrenal gland itself may result in a primary reduction in adrenocorticoid production. Aldosterone production is usually well preserved.

Less common endocrine problems include thyroid and parathyroid dysfunction. Occasionally, iron deposition in these glands may be heavy. Subclinical parathyroid dysfunction can be detected in most patients when challenged with the chelator EDTA.[363] This sensitive method of detecting endocrine dysfunction involves the infusion of chelator with simultaneous serial assessments of the levels of parathyroid hormone. If the elevation of parathyroid hormone in response to EDTA infusion is blunted, significant subclinical damage to the parathyroid glands has occurred. Therapeutic iron removal should be strongly considered in this instance. Thyroid-stimulating hormone (TSH) production in response to thyroid-releasing hormone is impaired in some patients.[362] Elevated baseline TSH levels suggestive of subclinical thyroid dysfunction may be seen. Frank thyroid deficiency is uncommon.

Other Organs Involved in Hemochromatosis

Hyperpigmentation is a nonspecific response by the skin to injury. In much the fashion that cirrhosis is a common endpoint in injury to the liver, hyperpigmentation is a stereotypic response by the skin to a variety of insults including excessive ultraviolet light exposure (tanning), thermal injury, and drug reactions. In hemochromatosis, the degree of hyperpigmentation correlates poorly with the level of iron overload. The classic triad of bronze diabetes consisting of hyperpigmentation, diabetes, and cirrhosis is rarely seen, and some massively overloaded patients show no increase in skin pigmentation. The injury from iron and light exposure often are synergistic in the pigmentation process, and rather than having baseline hyperpigmentation, some patients tan easily.

The hyperpigmentation in HHC is due to increased melanin production by melanocytes.[310,311] Iron deposition in these cells is the apparent culprit.[364] Some people with particularly heavy iron overload have visible iron in the skin, which manifests as a grayish discoloration. Treatment for HHC reverses this defect, although the hyperpigmentation often disappears more quickly than the grayish color.

In patients with clinical HHC, arthropathy involving the distal phalangeal joints of the hands is common,[310,311] although large joints including the knees can be affected as well. Severe pain and swelling of the joints can occur, but the signs and symptoms are indistinguishable from those of osteoarthritis. The pathologic defect seen on radiograph is usually identified as chondrocalcinosis, although in some cases actual iron deposition in the synovium occurs.[365] Synovial biopsy may be necessary to clarify the situation. Biopsy may show iron deposition in the myocytes, but the precise mechanism leading to the pain and muscle cramps seen in hemochromatosis is unknown. Arthritis frequently does not respond to iron removal therapy because synovial tissues are irreversibly damaged.

Opportunistic Infections in Hemochromatosis

The fact that iron is indispensable to the growth and survival of all organisms means that withholding the element from potential pathogens provides a degree of protection from infection.[11,366] Transferrin, in fact, was discovered as a result of its ability to retard the growth of bacteria in culture. The extremely high affinity of the protein for iron, together with the fact that two thirds of transferrin-binding sites are normally unoccupied, makes free iron essentially nonexistent in plasma. Other iron-binding proteins also have a bacteriostatic effect. Lactoferrin is structurally similar to transferrin and likewise binds iron very tightly.[367] The protein is found in many secretions as well as the granules of polymorphonuclear leukocytes from which it is released at the site of infection. Egg white contains the protein ovotransferrin, which is bacteriostatic and provides some protection to the developing embryo inside the semiporous egg shell.

Patients with iron overload often have transferrin saturations that approach and sometimes exceed 100%.[368] As a result, the bacteriostatic ability of the protein is compromised. Because iron withholding by transferrin is not part of the front line in the body's defensive network, susceptibility to infection is not markedly increased. Nonetheless, a number of infections, often with unusual organisms, have been described in iron overload patients. When considering risk of infections, evaluation of people with myelodysplastic syndromes and iron overload secondary to transfusion may be misleading since granulocyte dysfunction is common. Even patients with iron overload, in whom no known defect in the immune or phagocytic systems exists, occasionally develop opportunistic infections.

Mucormycosis due to *Rhizopus oryzae* has been reported in a number of people with iron overload.[369,370] Mucomycosis is often seen in diabetic patients with poor control of blood glucose levels. The roll call of other rare organisms reported in patients with iron overload is extensive and includes *Cunninghamella bertholletiae*, *Listeria monocytogenes*, and *Salmonella typhimurium*, as well as more common organisms such as *Escherichia coli*.[371–373] Often, these infections occur suddenly and without any apparent previous predisposition. Nearly all the information on such infectious complications comes from case reports so that the actual disease incidence is unknown. The extreme rarity of infections with organisms such as *R oryzae* in the general population suggests that the cases reported in iron overload are significant. Evidence that some bacteria including certain strains of *Neisseria* have transferrin receptors that permit transferrin-mediated iron uptake suggests that these organisms may be more virulent in patients with iron overload.[374,375] Clinical support for this suggestion requires prospective studies.

In a few patients with transfusional hemochromatosis, infections have been linked to the use of desferrioxamine. Some bacteria, such as *Yersinia enterocolitica*, display a decreased LD_{50} level when inoculated into mice in the presence of the siderophore because of the ability of the microbes to extract iron from the compound.[376] One report was made of several patients with renal failure on peritoneal dialysis who developed peritonitis with *Rhizopus* while receiving desferrioxamine for transfusional iron overload.[377] Desferrioxamine was shown to support the growth of the organism in iron-deficient culture medium. The presumption is that these infections were fueled by the delivery of iron to the organisms by the chelator.

Pregnancy and Hemochromatosis

In contrast to iron deficiency, iron overload is an infrequent problem during pregnancy. Although the genetic defect in iron overload is present from birth, affected females do not develop significant iron overload until after the reproductive years because of the blood loss that occurs with menstruation. Obviously, iron overload is more likely to complicate pregnancy in disorders that necessitate repeated transfusions.

The condition that most often produces iron overload during the reproductive years is thalassemia. In thalassemia major and intermedia, normal reproduction is often thwarted by endocrine dysfunction secondary to the iron loading. With impaired gonadotropin production and secondary ovarian failure, ovulation and fertility are compromised. Consequently, iron overload and pregnancy do not often overlap, even in this population. When the conditions do occur simultaneously, the placenta shields the fetus from the possibly deleterious consequences of iron overload by regulating iron delivery from the mother.

Neonatal Hemochromatosis

The great efficiency with which the placenta extracts iron for fetal use in the face of a maternal dearth of the mineral appears to be matched or exceeded by the protective wall formed by this organ when there is maternal overload. In rats, dams loaded with iron by repeated injection show widespread tissue deposition, but no increase in the amount of iron in the fetuses relative to the control animals.[378] Iron deposition in the placenta is elevated, indicating that a barrier to the transfer of excess iron to the fetus exists in the placenta. Thus, placenta shuttles to the fetus only that amount of iron that is needed for growth.

The placental barrier to excessive iron deposition in the fetus makes fetal iron overload exceedingly rare. The barricade is not impregnable, as shown by the rare disorder, idiopathic neonatal iron overload.[379,380] This apparently autosomal recessive disorder is manifested by massive iron overload present from birth. The pattern of tissue deposition and injury is similar to that seen with idiopathic hemochromatosis. The liver is the most heavily affected organ, showing prominent iron granules, diffuse fibrosis, and cirrhosis. Relatively little iron deposition is found in Kupffer cells. Pancreatic acinar cells are diffusely infiltrated with iron, whereas cardiac cells have fine, particulate, intracytoplasmic iron deposits. Because the probands are iron overloaded at birth, the defect is a consequence of transplacental iron loading. Death usually occurs within days to weeks of birth. Healthy siblings to the affected people exist in several families. The nature of the metabolic defect that thwarts the placental iron barrier is a mystery.[381]

TREATMENT OF IRON OVERLOAD

Phlebotomy

Phlebotomy is the most effective way to remove iron from the body and is the treatment of choice for patients with HHC. One to two units can be removed safely each week. When a phlebotomy is performed each week, iron is removed at the rate of about 1000 mg per month. Patients with HHC often have body iron stores of 20 g or more so that this initial phase of treatment may last for more than a year. The therapy is continued until early signs of iron deficiency develop as manifested by mild hypochromic anemia. The serum ferritin value declines during phlebotomy, followed by transferrin saturation. Patients with low serum ferritin values and normal levels of transferrin saturation can still have significant iron stores. The onset of mild iron-deficiency anemia, however, is clear evidence that iron stores have been depleted. The hematocrit begins to fall with phlebotomy but quickly returns to normal. The rate of phlebotomy should be decreased to one or two units per month if these troughs produce symptoms. The process should be continued until microcytic, hypochromic red cells appear. Changes in the various parameters of iron metabolism during phlebotomy therapy are illustrated in Figure 49-10. Of all the indirect measures of iron stores, transferrin saturation is the last value to decline.[382]

A program of maintenance phlebotomy is initiated after the initial phase of treatment. In most instances, patients can be maintained in proper iron balance with the removal of 4 to 5 units per year. In patients with subclinical hemochromatosis who have normal or slightly increased ferritin values, the maintenance program is the initial form of treatment.

One problem that sometimes develops during the initial treatment phase with its frequent phlebotomies is a loss of venous access caused by collapse and scarring of veins. Rotation of the venipuncture sites and care in prevention of hematomas and other unnecessary trauma to the veins greatly increase their useful life-span. Occasionally, a patient loses all readily accessible peripheral veins despite the best of care. In such circumstances, the temporary placement of a central access line, such as a Port-A-Cath catheter, allows the phlebotomy program to be completed. The significantly fewer venipunctures of the second phase of the treatment allow adequate healing of veins so that access is usually not a problem during this time. Although chelation therapy removes iron from patients with HHC,[383] the expense and inefficiency of this treatment relative to phlebotomy makes it contraindicated in these patients.

Iron Chelation Therapy

In patients with transfusion-dependent anemia, chelation is the only route for effective iron removal. Compounds that bind iron vary widely in their structure and origin (Fig. 49-11). Some, such as rhodotorulic acid, are hydrophilic in nature and water soluble. Others, such as α,α'-bipyridyl, are lipophilic in character and readily partition into biologic membranes. Many iron chelators are microbial siderophores. These molecules, such as aerobactin from *Aerobacter aerogenes*, are produced by a variety of bacteria and other microorganisms. They are released into the environment, where they bind available iron and then are taken back into the cells by specific receptors. Other chelators, as exemplified by ethylenediamine-*N,N'*-bi(o)-hydroxyphenylglycine (EHPG), are synthetically derived.

Clinically useful chelators must fulfill certain criteria. First, they must have a high specificity for iron. Ethylenediaminetetraacetic acid (EDTA) binds iron, but also has a high affinity for a number of biologically important cations such as Ca^{2+}. As such, this agent is of no use in the treatment of iron overload. Second, a perspective chelator must have few nonspecific side effects. Diethylenetriaminepentaacetic acid (DTPA) binds iron effectively but produces significant toxicity.[384] Finally, the chelator should have access to the intracellular sites where the excess iron is deposited.

Iron chelators fall into two clinically important groups. Hydrophilic chelators, and desferrioxamine in particular, dominated the treatment of transfusional iron overload for the past 20 years. Promising new lipophilic chelators have undergone testing in animals and in human subjects.

Desferrioxamine

Of the large number of hydrophilic iron chelators, only desferrioxamine is useful in the treatment of patients with iron overload. Agents such a EDTA, DTPA, and rhodotorulic acid have proved to be either excessively toxic or ineffective in clinical trials.[385,386] A product of *Streptomyces pilosis*, desferrioxamine is small (molecular weight, 560 daltons) and contains a number of hydroxamic acid groups that interact with iron, forming a tight association.[387] The stability constant of ferrioxamine (iron bound to desferrioxamine) is 10^{31} and exceeds that of the iron–transferrin complex. Desferrioxamine removes iron from transferrin only with the aid of small chelating compounds such as citrate.[388] These agents dislodge the iron atom from the binding pocket of the transferrin molecule, thereby making it available to desferrioxamine. Desferrioxamine does not remove iron from heme.[387]

Desferrioxamine is poorly absorbed from the gastrointestinal tract, and when it reaches the bloodstream, renal filtration of the drug is rapid. When administered as an intravenous bolus, the half-life of desferrioxamine is only

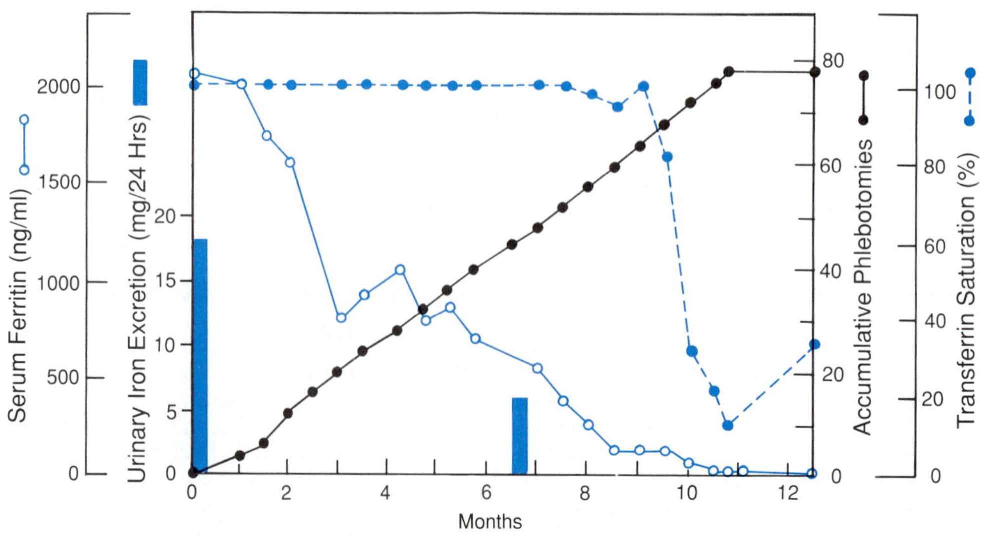

FIGURE 49-10. Changes in the parameters of iron metabolism during phlebotomy therapy.

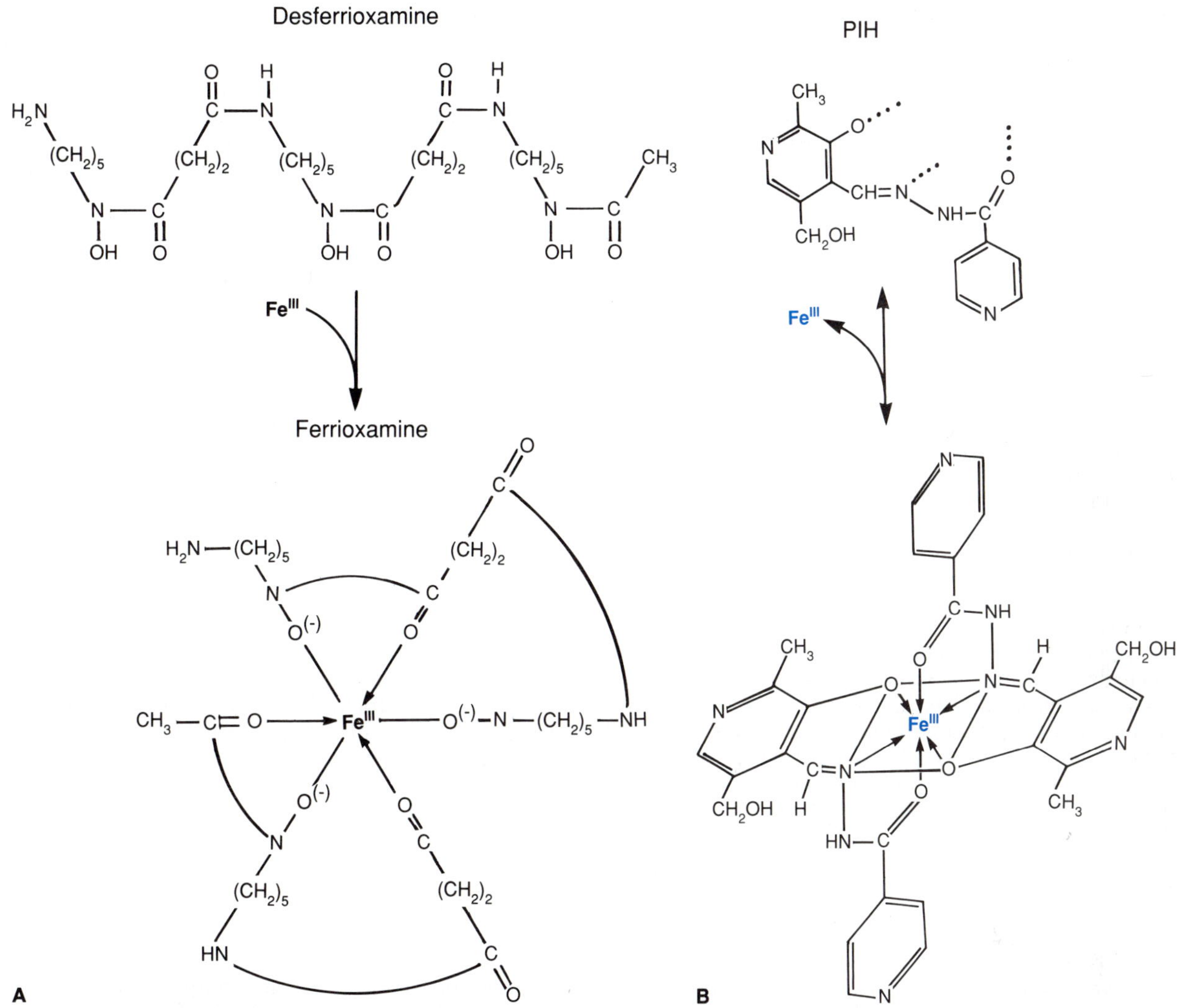

FIGURE 49-11. Structures of representative hydrophilic and lipophilic iron chelators. (**A**) Desferrioxamine is a water-soluble iron-chelating agent that binds iron in a 1:1 molecular ratio. Desferrioxamine forms ferrioxamine as illustrated in the figure. (**B**) Pyridoxal isonicotinoyl hydrazone (PIH) is a lipophilic chelator. Three of these molecules form a coordination complex with a single iron atom.

10 to 15 minutes.[387] The chelator binds little iron during such a short period of time so that most of the desferrioxamine passes into the urine devoid of iron. This property of the drug places severe constraints on its clinical use.

Desferrioxamine binds iron in a chelatable pool within the cell. As noted, the physical nature of the iron in the chelatable pool is unknown but may consist of that fraction complexed to the intracellular carrier molecule. Chang cells incubated with ^{59}Fe transferrin in culture incorporate the label both into ferritin and a low-molecular-weight fraction.[389] Desferrioxamine preferentially removes the iron from the nonferritin low-molecular-weight component.[390] After 6 hours of incubation with desferrioxamine, 61% of the ferritin iron in these cells is removed by the chelator, indicating that the iron in the ferritin shell is ultimately available to desferrioxamine.

Thus, although iron removal from purified ferritin in solution with desferrioxamine is inefficient,[391] the chelator is able to remove labeled iron from ferritin in cultures both of Chang cells and K562 cells.[389,392] Data are lacking on whether iron is removed from ferritin owing to the molecule directly entering the shell and binding the element or to a shift in the kinetics of iron dispersal and more rapid release from the protein. The preferential chelation of the nonferritin, low-molecular-weight iron in Chang cells supports the latter mechanism. In such an instance, iron removal from ferritin by desferrioxamine would be indirect, reflecting a siphoning off of the element as it leaves the ferritin shell coupled to the intracellular transport molecule.

After forming a complex with iron, ferrioxamine exits from the cell and is excreted. The pattern of excretion differs in various species. In rats, for example, the bulk of the ferrioxamine formed is released into bile and from there into the feces.[393] Humans, in contrast, excrete about 80% of the ferrioxamine in the urine, with the remaining 20% leaving by the biliary route.

Clinical Use. Desferrioxamine was enthusiastically introduced into the clinical armamentarium, but interest in it soon flagged for a number of reasons. Most important was the fact that despite the striking avidity of desferrioxamine for iron, results in patients were poor. When given as an intravenous bolus, most of the drug was excreted in the urine without iron. Intramuscular injections were more effective, but significant inflammation often developed at the deposition site. Another approach was to add desferrioxamine to the blood transfusions that patients received, but this was of no benefit. The desferrioxamine added to a unit of blood removes no iron from the heme embedded in hemoglobin. After transfusion, the compound is rapidly excreted in the urine without chelating a significant amount of iron from body stores. Because of these problems, use of the drug declined significantly.

A major advance occurred when in 1974 Barry and colleagues[394] showed that long-term chelation therapy in children with transfusion-dependent thalassemia had significant benefits. Many of the children were initially treated with daily intramuscular injections of DTPA. Because of the toxicity of this agent, all the patients were eventually switched to intramuscular desferrioxamine. After several years of treatment, less hepatic fibrosis and iron deposition were found in the treated children compared with what was found in an untreated control group. Sustained treatment was clearly beneficial, but years of therapy were required to show a difference. Later, continuous intravenous infusion of desferrioxamine was found to be much more effective in mobilizing iron. This approach was clearly not practical for long-term clinical treatment. The demonstration that continuous subcutaneous infusion of desferrioxamine was nearly as efficacious as when it was given intravenously meant that there was a practical means of large-scale iron mobilization in these patients.[395,396]

Desferrioxamine is readily solubilized in sterile water for subcutaneous administration. In adults, the maximum quantity of the drug that is tolerated with subcutaneous infusion is about 2.5 to 3 g/d. In children, desferrioxamine can be given at a rate of 25 to 50 mg/kg/d. The infusion pump is set to deliver the drug over about 12 to 16 hours because the amount of iron excreted may be reduced with shorter times. The site of infusion is rotated daily to minimize local subcutaneous irritation. The pump is easily portable and usually attached to a belt. Since desferrioxamine is stable in solution at room temperature for several days, a 3- or 4-day supply can be mixed at a single sitting.

The risk of cellular injury due to iron overload increases when the iron is in a free state, that is, not stored in ferritin or hemosiderin. Desferrioxamine binds free iron, thereby preventing the generation of free radicals by the element and secondary cellular damage. When desferrioxamine is used in a fashion that increases its time of exposure to iron stores, the risk of injury is decreased. The drug should be used daily for periods of greater than 12 hours if tolerated by the patient. The optimal dose of desferrioxamine varies for each patent. The initial infusion of desferrioxamine should be given in the presence of a physician with appropriate resuscitation equipment. Anaphylaxis or explosive urticaria occur rarely, but the consequences can be devastating. The excretion of the iron–desferrioxamine complex in the urine should be monitored to determine the maximum effective drug dose. Later, periodic urine tests for iron should be performed to ensure continued drug efficacy.

Ascorbic acid increases the iron excretion by desferrioxamine, but is toxic to some patients when administered at high levels.[396] Thus, cardiac arrhythmias and sudden death have been reported in patients receiving more than 1 g/d. By reducing the ascorbate intake to between 200 and 500 mg/d and by beginning vitamin treatment only after desferrioxamine therapy is well established, enhancement of iron excretion without the potential of excessive mobilization is possible.

Efficacy. The benefits of desferrioxamine treatment in patients with transfusional hemochromatosis are well established. Children treated with the drug have a lower incidence of diabetes and show improvements in liver function tests.[397] In addition, there is a reduced incidence of cardiac dysfunction in compliant children treated with the drug when compared with noncompliers.[398] Adults show improvement in liver function tests as well as a reversal of endocrine dysfunction in some cases.[189] Since the rate of iron removal is low, 1 to 2 years of treatment is often necessary to show any improvement. Whether desferrioxamine therapy improves patient survival is unknown. Because cardiac injury, the leading cause of death, is reduced by the treatment, there is a reason for optimism about the long-term efficacy of the drug. Even patients with improved end-organ function often continue to have evidence of iron overload as measured by the indirect tests such as serum iron, iron-binding capacity, and ferritin. Follow-up of cardiac, hepatic, and endocrine function is therefore important in assessing treatment efficacy.

Compliance is a major problem in the transfusional treatment of children. The elaborate paraphernalia is often perplexing and sometimes frightening to young children. Adolescents sometimes rebel against a mode of therapy that makes them stand out from their peers. By timing the infusions so that the bulk of the drug is given overnight, this anger and intransigence can at times be defused. Although the pump is relatively compact, children may feel constrained in their activities. Counseling with child psychologists and a close doctor–parent relationship may aid in reducing some of these problems.

Compliance is a lesser problem in adults, but many patients fear giving themselves parenteral medication or despair at the apparent complexity of the process. Pumps, needles, vials, and syringes all can incite anxiety in people who are unfamiliar with medical technology. Through repetitive teaching, even inexperienced patients can learn to use the infusion pump and to administer the desferrioxamine. Other family members should also learn the procedures and can aid in the treatment process. An increasing number of home-infusion pharmaceutical companies supply desferrioxamine. This relieves much of the burden from patient and family. Effective iron mobilization occurs in patients who generally use the pump 5 to 6 days per week. This flexibility allows patients the freedom to be unencumbered for special events such as a wedding or a day at the beach. The pump can be worn even during some athletic activities such as golf or bicycling and over time may become second nature.

Some patients on hemodialysis who are overloaded with iron because of repeated transfusions are treated with desferrioxamine.[399] With the continued improvements in survival of dialysis patients, some people receive more than 100 transfusions and have manifestations of significant iron overload. Desferrioxamine is given as an intravenous bolus at the end of a dialysis session since the rapid urinary excretion of the drug seen in patients with normal renal function obviously does not occur. The chelator penetrates the tissues and removes storage iron. The ferrioxamine is removed both in the bile and with subsequent dialysis. The initial studies have been encouraging, but information about long-term efficacy is not available.[400] Anemia in these cases is due largely to a deficiency of erythropoietin seen with end-stage renal failure. The release of recombinant erythropoietin may eliminate this problem because the hormone corrects completely the anemia of renal failure.[401,402]

Complications. A large number of side effects have been reported with desferrioxamine, but most occur infrequently.[403] Rare allergic reactions with anaphylaxis are the most serious. The occurrence of an immediate hypersensitivity reaction presumably is the result of desferrioxamine cross-reactivity to antibodies produced against other siderophores released by bacteria in the gastrointestinal tract. Desensitization has been accomplished in a few patients who have had significant allergic reactions including anaphylaxis and local urticaria. Such a procedure should be performed in a setting where life support systems, including an anesthesiologist, are available.

Other side effects of desferrioxamine are less threatening, but troublesome nonetheless. The most common of these is inflammation at the site of the infusion. This is a chemical irritation and not an allergic phenomenon and is much more common in adults than in children. Erythema, swelling, tenderness, and occasionally blistering and ulceration can occur. Hydrocortisone greatly reduces this local reaction. Two or three mg of hydrocortisone in solution are mixed with the desferrioxamine and included in the infusion, or 1% hydrocortisone ointment is applied to the site of the infusion.

Cataracts have developed in some experimental animals treated with desferrioxamine and have been reported on rare occasions in patients receiving the drug.[404] This appears to be a dose-dependent phenomenon. Before beginning treatment, patients should be checked for cataracts by an ophthalmologist. Thereafter, they should have yearly ophthalmologic examinations. Cessation of desferrioxamine therapy halts and may even reverse the progression of cataracts. One group of children treated with doses of desferrioxamine ranging from 34 to 150 mg/kg over 12 hours developed optic and vestibular neurotoxicity, resulting in impaired vision and balance.[405] These toxic effects were also reversed with the cessation of treatment.

A major factor limiting the usefulness of desferrioxamine therapy is its expense. The infusion pump alone costs about $1000. The drug is expensive, and with the associated needles, infusion tubing, and other supplies, the annual total may exceed $12,000 to $15,000. Third-party payers generally cover only 80% of this cost at most, leaving a very large bill for the patient and family. In addition, the socioeconomic profiles of the patients tend to magnify the problem. Because thalassemia is a hereditary disorder, more than one child may be affected in a given family, creating a tremendous financial burden. Moreover, some of the countries in which thalassemia is prevalent lack the financial resources to provide such an expensive form of treatment. The myelodysplastic anemias of adulthood, on the other hand, present in older patients who often are near the age of retirement. The expense of desferrioxamine treatment can be devastating to families on fixed incomes.

Compliance with desferrioxamine therapy is often poor. Consequently, a search is continuing for orally active iron chelators that are less expensive to administer than desferrioxamine. Some of the newer lipophilic chelators appear poised to fill this role.

Lipophilic Iron Chelators

The mechanism by which lipophilic chelators mobilize iron from cells is complex. The relative lipid solubility of the free and iron-complexed forms of the chelators greatly influences iron mobilization, as do the iron-binding constants of the molecules.[406] With the hydroxypyridin-4-one class of chelators, iron mobilization from primary hepatocyte cultures is most effective when the components are about equally soluble in lipid or aqueous phases. Highly hydrophilic compounds may fail to mobilize enough iron, whereas the highly lipophilic compounds tend to be toxic. Comparison of chelators with similar lipid partition coefficients and different iron-binding constants reveals that the affinity of the chelator for Fe^{3+} is especially important at concentrations of less than 10 μmol/L. At concentrations exceeding 500 μmol/L, the size of the chelatable iron pool in the cells determines the degree of iron mobilization. The ability of iron chelators to cross the barrier presented by the cell membrane greatly influences their ability to mobilize iron. The fact that the most active hydroxypyridin-4-one type chelators release more iron than equimolar concentrations of desferrioxamine reflects this point.

Pyridoxal isonicotinylhydrase (PIH) is a potent and clinically promising lipophilic chelator. In reticulocytes, the primary site from which the drug mobilizes iron appears to be the mitochondria.[407] The agent mobilizes little iron in reticulocytes in which heme biosynthesis is not blocked either by isoniazid or by succinylacetone, an inhibitor of δ-aminolevulinic acid dehydrase, which is the second enzyme in the heme biosynthetic pathway. The uptake of PIH into reticulocytes is rapid, attaining a plateau after 10 to 15 minutes.[407] The compound crosses the membrane by passive diffusion, reflecting its lipophilic character. One characteristic of PIH that makes it particularly effective in iron mobilization from cells is that the agent retains a relatively high lipid partition coefficient even after it binds iron. Some lipophilic chelators, such as α,α'-bipyridyl, assume a much lower lipid partition coefficient after binding iron. As a result, the agents may enter cells readily, but become entrapped after iron chelation.[408]

When tested for their ability to inhibit the uptake of labeled iron into primary cultures of rat hepatocytes, PIH and the related chelator, pyridoxal benzoylhydrazone, are at least as efficient as desferrioxamine in this regard.[409] The chelators reduce both the net uptake of ^{59}Fe into the cells and the incorporation of the iron into ferritin. Pyridoxal benzoylhydrazone, a more lipophilic compound, in fact exceeds both PIH and desferrioxamine in this capacity, bolstering the conclusion that lipophilicity plays an important role in iron mobilization by these chelators.

Oral Iron Chelation

Despite its impressive clinical record of safety and efficacy in the treatment of transfusional iron overload, the requirement for parenteral administration has been a severe stumbling block in the use of desferrioxamine. The drug is not completely inactive when given orally and when administered in this fashion in doses ranging from 3 to 9 g/d, desferrioxamine mesylate substantially increases iron excretion in patients with transfusional hemochromatosis.[410] In no instance does the level of iron excretion in response to orally administered desferrioxamine approach that achieved when the drug is given parenterally.

The search for alternative, orally active chelating agents had a number of false starts and disappointing leads.[411] Some promising leads have developed, but no agent has received endorsement for general clinical use.[412] The prospect has improved for an effective and safe orally active chelator to be available in the near future.

ACUTE IRON TOXICITY

Iron poisoning is rare except in children who have accidentally ingested iron preparations. The clinical sequelae to the ingestion of 2 g of ferrous sulfate occurs in two stages, with the first developing in about 30 minutes.[413–415] The iron salt produces irritation of the stomach and duodenum manifested by nausea, vomiting, and abdominal pain. Necrosis of the epithelial cells of the gastrointestinal tract leads to hemorrhage and hematemesis, which may be followed by shock. Diarrhea, drowsiness, and coma can develop, and death can occur in 5 to 6 hours after ingestion of the iron.

Often, the patient with acute iron toxicity survives the initial phase and appears to enter a period of recovery. Rapid influx of iron into the plasma overwhelms the binding capacity of transferrin, leaving much of the mineral in loose association with other proteins such as albumin.[414,415] This excess free iron can cause cardiovascular collapse and death. In other cases, the excess iron is deposited in the liver, producing hepatic necrosis and fibrosis. Other long-term complications in survivors of iron overdose include pyloric stenosis and severe gastric scarring from the initial necrotizing mucosal injury.

Treatment of acute iron overdose includes gastric lavage to remove as much iron as possible, followed by administration of desferrioxamine, both orally and intravenously. The orally administered chelator binds the free iron that remains in the gastrointestinal tract. The chelator given parenterally binds and inactivates excess iron in the plasma and tissues.[414,415] Intravenous desferrioxamine should be continued until the transferrin saturation is consistently maintained below about 80%. The patient should be supported with fluid and electrolytes as needed to correct any imbalances that could occur. Iron overdose, particularly in children, requires consultation with an experienced clinical toxicologist, who should individualize the therapeutic plan.

REFERENCES

1. Bothwell TH, Charlton RW, Cook JD, Finch CA. Iron metabolism in man. Oxford, Blackwell Scientific Publications, 1979.
2. Emery T. Iron metabolism in humans and plants. Am Sci 1982;70: 626.
3. London I. Iron and heme: Crucial carriers and catalysts. In: Wintrobe MM, ed. Blood, pure and eloquent. New York; McGraw-Hill, 1980.
4. Finch CA, Huebers HA. Iron metabolism. Clin Physiol Biochem 1986; 4:5.
5. Lewin R. How micro-organisms transport iron. Science 1985;225:401.
6. Spik G, Montreuil J, Crichton RR, Mazurier J. Proteins of iron storage and transport. New York, Elsevier, 1985.
7. Aisen P, Brown EB. Structure and function of transferrin. In: Brown EB, ed. Progress in hematology. New York, Grune & Stratton, 1975: 25.
8. Morgan EH. Transferrin: biochemistry, physiology and clinical significance. In: Molecular aspects of medicine. Oxford, Pergamon Press, 1981.
9. Seligman PA, Schleicher RB, Allen RH. Isolation and characterization of the transferrin receptor from human placenta. J Biol Chem 1979;254: 9943.
10. Enns CA, Sussman HH. Physical characterization of the transferrin receptor in human placentae. J Biol Chem 1981;256:9820.
11. Weinberg ED. Roles of iron in infection and neoplasia. J Pharmacol 1985;16:358.
12. Finch CA, Huebers H. Perspectives in iron metabolism. N Engl J Med 1982;306:1520.
13. Finch CA, Huebers HA. Iron metabolism. Clin Physiol Biochem 1986; 4:5.
14. Green R, et al. Body iron excretion in man. Am J Nutr 1968;45:336.
15. Granick S. Iron metabolism. In: Trace elements. New York, Academic Press, 1954:122.
16. Goldberg A, Ashenbrucker H, Cartwright GE, Wintrobe MM. Studies on the biosynthesis of heme in vitro by avian erythrocytes. Blood 1956;11:821.
17. Jones MS, Jones OTG. Evidence for the location of ferrochelatase on the inner membrane of rat liver mitochondria. Biochem Biophys Res Commun 1968;31:977.
18. Yoshikawa H, Yoneyama Y. Incorporation of iron in the haem moiety of chromoproteins. In: Gross F, ed. Iron metabolism. Berlin, Springer-Verlag, 1964:24.
19. Hill JM, Ruff MR, Weber RJ, Pert CB. Transferrin receptors in rat brain: neuropeptide-like pattern and relationship to iron distribution. Proc Natl Acad Sci USA 1985;82:4553.
20. Youdim MBH, Yehuda S, Ben-Shachar D, Askenazi R. Behavioral and brain biochemical changes in iron-deficient rats: the involvement of iron in dopamine receptor function. In: Pollitt E, Leibel RL, eds. Iron deficiency: brain biochemistry and behavior. New York, Raven Press, 1982:39.
21. Graslund A, Ehrenberg A, Thelander L. Characterization of the free radical mammalian ribonucleotide reductase. J Biol Chem 1982;257: 5711.
22. Utley CS, Marcell PD, Allen RH, Antony AC, Kolhouse JF. Isolation and characterization of methionine synthetase from human placenta. J Biol Chem 1985;260:13656.
23. Noyes WD, Bothwell TH, Finch CA. The role of the reticulo-endothelial cell in iron metabolism. Br J Haematol 1960;6:43.
24. Aisen P, Listowski I. Iron transport and storage proteins. Annu Rev Biochem 1980;49:357.
25. Drysdale J, Jain SK, Boyd D, et al. Human ferritins: genes and proteins. In: Spik G, Montreuil J, Crichton RR, Mazurier J, eds. Proteins of iron storage and transport. New York, Elsevier, 1985:343.
26. Munro HN, Leibold EA, Vass JK, et al. Ferritin gene structure and expression. In: Spik G, Montreuil J, Crichton RR, Mazurier J, eds. Proteins of iron storage and transport. New York, Elsevier, 1985:331.
27. Harrison PM, Treffry A, Lilley TH. Ferritin as an iron storage protein: mechanisms of iron uptake. J Inorgan Biochem 1986;27:287.
28. Boyd D, Vecoli C, Belcher DM, Jain SK, Drysdale JW. Structural and functional relationships of human ferritin h and l chains deduced from cDNA clones. J Biol Chem 1986;260:11755.
29. Wilkins Stevens P, Dodgson JB, Engel JD. Structure and expression of the chicken ferritin H-subunit gene. Mol Cell Biol 1987;7:1751.
30. Treffry A, Harrison PM, Cleton MI, deBruijn WC, Mann S. A note on the composition and properties of ferritin iron cores. J Inorgan Biochem 1987;31:1.
31. Wardeska JG, Viglione B, Chasteen ND. Metal iron complexes of apoferritin: evidence for initial binding in the hydrophilic channels. J Biol Chem 1986;261:6677.
32. Levi S, Luzzago A, Cesareni G, et al. Mechanism of ferritin iron uptake: activity of the H-chain and deletion mapping of the ferro-oxidase site—a study of iron uptake and ferro-oxidase activity of human liver, recombinant H-chain ferritins, and of two H-chain deletion mutants. J Biol Chem 1988;263:18086.
33. Mazur A, Green S, Salia A, Carleton A. Mechanism of release of ferritin iron in vitro by xanthine oxidase. J Clin Invest 1958;37:1809.
34. Grace ND, Greenwald MA, Greenberg MS. Effect of allopurinol on iron mobilization. Gastroenterology 1970;59:103.
35. Sirivech S, Freiden E, Osaki S. The release of iron from horse spleen ferritin by reduced flavins. Biochem J 1974;143:311.
36. Ulvik RJ, Romslo I. Reduction of exogenous FMN by isolated rat liver mitochondria: significance to the mobilization of iron from ferritin. Biochem Biophys Acta 1981;635:457.
37. Dognin J, Crichton RR. Mobilization of iron from ferritin fractions of defined iron content by biological reductants. FEBS Lett 1975;54:234.
38. Watt GD, Jacobs D, Frankel RB. Redox reactivity of bacterial and mammalian ferritin: is reductant entry into the ferritin interior a necessary step for iron release? Proc Natl Acad Sci USA 1988;85: 7457.
39. Richter GW. Studies of iron overload: rat liver sidersome ferritin. Lab Invest 1984;50:26.
40. Hultcrantz R, Glaumann H. Studies on the rat liver following iron overload: biochemical studies after iron mobilization. Lab Invest 1982;46:383.
41. Weir MP, Sharp GA, Peters TJ. Electron microscopic studies of human haemosiderin and ferritin. J Clin Pathol 1985;38:915.
42. Wixom RL, Prutkin L, Munro HN. Hemosiderin: nature, formation and significance. Int Rev Exp Pathol 1980;22:193.
43. Iancu TC, Neustein HB, Landing BH. The liver in thalassemia major: ultrastructural observations. In: Iron metabolism: Ciba Foundation Symposium 51. New York, Elsevier, 1977:293.
44. Schellhammer PF, Engle MA, Hagstrom JW. Histochemical studies of the myocardium and conduction system in acquired iron-storage disease. Circulation 1967;35:631.
45. Lee SSC, Richter GW. The monomers and oligomers of ferritin and apoferritin: association and dissociation. Biochemistry 1976;15:65.
46. Bridges KR. Ascorbic acid inhibits lysosomal autophagy of ferritin. J Biol Chem 1987;262:14773.
47. Richter GW. Studies of iron overload: lysosomal proteolysis of rat liver ferritin. Pathol Res Pract 1986;181:159.
48. Pollycove M, Mortimer R. The quantitative determination of iron kinetics and hemoglobin synthesis in human subjects. J Clin Invest 1961;40:753.
49. Seligman PA, Klausner RD, Huebers HA. Molecular mechanisms of iron metabolism. In: Leder P, Majerus P, Neinhuis A, Stamatoyauopolous G, eds. Molecular basis of blood disease. 1988:219.
50. Mattia E, Josic D, Ashwell G, Klausner R, van Renswoude J. Regulation of intracellular iron distribution in K562 human erythroleukemia cells. J Biol Chem 1986;261:4587.
51. MacGillivroy RTA, Mendez E, Shewale JG, Sinha S, Lineback-Zins J, Brew K. The primary structure of human serum transferrin: the structures of seven cyanogen bromide fragments and the assembly of the complete structure. J Biol Chem 1983;258:3543.
52. Williams J. The structure of transferrins. In: Spik G, Montreuil J, Crichtion RR, Mazurier J, eds. Proteins of iron storage and transport. New York, Elsevier, 1985:13.
53. Huebers HA, Finch CA. Transferrin: physiologic behavior and clinical implications. Blood 1984;64:763.
54. Uzan G, Frain M, Park I, et al. Molecular cloning and sequence analysis of cDNA for human transferrin. Biochem Biophys Res Commun 1984;119:273.
55. Yang F, Lum JB, McGill JR, et al. Human transferrin: cDNA characterization and chromosomal localization. Proc Natl Acad Sci USA 1984;81:2752.
56. Park I, Schaeffer E, Sidoli A, Baralle FE, Cohen GN, Zakin MM. Organization of the human transferrin gene: direct evidence that it originated by gene duplication. Proc Natl Acad Sci USA 1985;82:3149.

57. Chasteen ND. The identification of the probable locus of iron and anion binding in the transferrins. Trends Biol Sci 1983;2:272.
58. Aisen P, Leibman A, Zweier J. Stoichiometric and site characteristics of the binding of iron to human transferrin. J Biol Chem 1978;253: 1930.
59. Chitambar CR, Massey EJ, Seligman PA. Regulation of transferrin receptor expression on human leukemic cells during proliferation and induction of differentiation: effects of gallium and dimethylsulfoxide. J Clin Invest 1983;72:1314.
60. Harris WR. Thermodynamic binding constants of the zinc–human transferrin complex. Biochemistry 1983;22:3920.
61. Kuhn E, Brodan V. Changes in the circadian rhythm of serum iron induced by a 5-day sleep deprivation. Eur J Appl Physiol 1983;49: 215.
62. Katz JH. Iron and protein kinetics studied by means of doubly labeled human crystallin transferrin. J Clin Invest 1961;409:2143.
63. Morgan EH, Peters T Jr. The biosynthesis of rat transferrin: evidence for rapid glycosylation, disulfide bond formation, and tertiary folding. J Biol Chem 1985;260:14793.
64. McKnight GS, Lee DC, Hemmaplardh D, Finch CA, Palmiter RD. Transferrin gene expression: effects of nutritional iron deficiency. J Biol Chem 1980;255:144.
65. Idzerda RL, Huebers H, Finch CA, McKnight GS. Rat transferrin gene expression: tissue-specific regulation by iron deficiency. Proc Natl Acad Sci USA 1986;83:3723.
66. Rifkind D, Krauetz HM, Knight V, Schade AL. Urinary excretion of iron-binding protein in nephrotic syndrome. N Engl J Med 1961;265: 115.
67. Finch CA, Deubelbeiss K, Cook JD, et al. Ferrokinetics in man. Medicine 1970;49:17.
68. Jandl JH, et al. Transfer of iron from serum iron-binding protein to human reticulocytes. J Clin Invest 1959;38:161.
69. Klausner RD, van Renswounde J, Ashwell G, et al. Receptor-mediated endocytosis of transferrin in K562 cells. J Biol Chem 1983;258:4715.
70. Ciechanover A, Schwartz AL, Dautry-Varsat A, Lodish HF. Kinetics of internalization and recycling of transferrin and the transferrin receptor in a human hepatoma cell line. J Biol Chem 1983;258:9681.
71. Huebers HA, Huebers E, Csiba E, Finch CA. Heterogeneity of the plasma iron pool: explanation of the Fletcher-Huehns phenomenon. Am J Physiol 1984;247:R280.
72. Huebers H, Csiba E, Huebers E, Finch CA. Molecular advantage of diferic transferrin in delivering iron to reticulocytes: a comparative study. Proc Soc Exp Biol Med 1985;179:222.
73. Lestas AN. The effect of pH upon human transferrin: selective labelling of the two iron-binding sites. Br J Haematol 1976;32:341.
74. Bloch B, Popovici T, Levin MH, Tuil D, Kahn A. Transferrin gene expression visualized in oligodendrocytes of the rat brain by using in situ hybridization and immunohistochemistry. Proc Natl Acad Sci USA 1985;82:6706.
75. Levin MJ, Tuil D, Uzan G, Dreyfus JC, Kahn A. Expression of the transferrin gene during development of non-hepatic tissues: high level of transferrin mRNA in fetal muscle and adult brain. Biochem Biophys Res Commun 1984;122:212.
76. Skinner MK, Cosand WL, Griswold MD. Purification and characterization of testicular transferrin secreted by rat Sertoli cells. Biochem J 1984;218:313.
77. Lum JB, Infante A, Makker DM, Yang F, Bowman BA. Transferrin synthesis by inducer T lymphocytes. J Clin Invest 1986;77:841.
78. Vostrejs M, Moran PL, Seligman PA. Transferrin synthesis by small cell lung cancer cells acts as an autocrine regulator of cellular proliferation. J Clin Invest 1988;82:331.
79. Saito KT, Nishisato A, Grasso A, Aisen P. Interaction of transferrin with iron-loaded peritoneal macrophages. Br J Haematol 1986;62:275.
80. Hallberg L. Bioavailability of dietary iron in man. Annu Rev Nutr 1981;1:123.
81. Savin MA, Cook JD. Mucosal iron transport by rat intestine. Blood 1980;56:1029.
82. Finch CA, Huebers H, Eng M, Miller L. Effect of transfused reticulocytes on iron exchange. Blood 1982;59:364.
83. Cook JD, Monsen ER. Food iron absorption. I. Use of a semisynthetic diet to study absorption of non-heme iron. Am J Clin Nutr 1975;28: 1289.
84. Klausner RD, Harford JB, Rao K, et al. Molecular aspects of the regulation of cellular iron metabolism. In: Spik G, Montreuil J, Crichton RR, Mazurier J, eds. Proteins of iron storage and transport. New York, Elsevier, 1985:111.
85. Finch CA, Cook JD. Iron deficiency. Am J Clin Nutr 1985;39:471.
86. Huebers H, Rummel W. Protein mediated epithelial iron transfer. In: Csaky TZ, ed. Pharmacology of intestinal permeation. Berlin, Springer Verlag, 1984:513.
87. Callender ST, Mallett BJ, Smith MD. Absorption of hemoglobin iron. Br J Haematol 1957;3:186.
88. Wheby MS, Spyker DA. Hemoglobin iron absorption kinetics in the iron-deficient dog. Am J Clin Nutr 1981;34:1686.
89. Charlton RW, Bothwell TH. Iron absorption. Annu Rev Med 1983;34: 55.
90. Hallberg L, Rossander L. Bioavailability of iron from Western-type whole meals. Scand J Gastroenterol 1982;17:151.
91. Hallberg L. Iron nutrition and food iron fortification. Semin Hematol 1982;19:31.
92. Sorensen EW. Studies on iron absorption. V. The effect of ascorbic acid and ethyl alcohol on the absorption of iron in iron-deficient subjects. Acta Med Scand 1966;180:241.
93. Hunt JR, Mullen LM, Lykken GI, Gallagher SK, Nielsen FH. Ascorbic acid: effect on ongoing iron absorption and status in iron-depleted young women. Am J Clin Nutr 1990;51:649.
94. Morck TA, Lynch SR, Cook JD. Inhibition of food iron absorption by coffee. Am J Clin Nutr 1983;37:416.
95. Seligman PA, Caskey JH, Frazier JL, Zucker RM, Podell ER, Allen RH. Measurements of iron absorption from prenatal multivitamin–mineral supplements. Obstet Gynecol 1983;61:356.
96. Jacobs A, Rhodes J, Peters DK, Campbell H, Eakins JD. Gastric acidity and iron absorption. Br J Haematol 1966;12:728.
97. Crosby WH. Iron absorption. In: Handbook of physiology. Washington, DC, American Physiology Society, 1968:1553.
98. Bedard YC, Pinkerton PH, Simon GT. Radioautographic observations on iron absorption by the duodenum of mice with iron overload, iron deficiency, and X-linked anemia. Blood 1973;42:131.
99. Conrad ME, Crosby WH. Intestinal mucosal mechanisms controlling iron absorption. Blood 1963;22:406.
100. Parmley RT, Barton JC, Conrad ME. Ultrastructural cytochemical identification of the siderophilic enterocyte. J Histochem Cytochem 1984;2:724.
101. Humphrys J, Walpole B, Worwood M. Intracellular iron transport in rat intestinal epithelium: biochemical and ultrastructural observations. Br J Haematol 1977;36:209.
102. Conrad ME, Umbreit JN, Moore EG, Peterson RDA, Jones MB. A newly identified iron binding protein in duodenal mucosa of rats: purification and characterization of Mobilferrin. J Biol Chem 1990;265:5273.
103. Huebers H, Huebers E, Rummel W, Crichton R. Isolation and characterization of iron-binding proteins from rat intestinal mucosa. Eur J Biochem 1976;66:447.
104. Huebers HA, Huebers E, Csiba E, Rummel W, Finch CA. The significance of transferrin for intestinal iron absorption. Blood 1983;61:283.
105. Whittaker P, Skikne BS, Covell AM. Duodenal iron proteins in idiopathic hemachromatosis. J Clin Invest 1989;83:261.
106. Johnson G, Jacobs P, Purves LR. Iron binding proteins of iron-absorbing rat intestinal mucosa. J Clin Invest 1983;71:1467.
107. Conrad ME, Umbreit JN, Moore EG, Rodning CR. Newly identified iron-binding protein in human duodenal mucosa. Blood 1992;79:244.
108. Jandl JH, Katz JH. The plasma-to-cell cycle of transferrin. J Clin Invest 1963;42:314.
109. Schneider C, Sutherland R, Newman R, Greaves M. Structural features of the cell surface receptor for transferrin that is recognized by the monoclonal antibody OKT9. J Biol Chem 1982;257:8516.
110. Omary MB, Trowbridge IS. Biosynthesis of the human transferrin receptor in cultured cells. J Biol Chem 1981;256:12888.
111. Seligman P, Chitambar C, Massay EJ. Structure and regulation of the transferrin receptor. In: Schecter A, ed. Biochemical and biophysical properties of membranes and proteins. Amsterdam, Elsevier, 1983.
112. Schneider C, Owen MJ, Banville D, Williams JG. Primary structure of human transferrin receptor deduced from the mRNA sequence. Nature 1984;311:675.
113. Kuhn LC, McClelland A, Ruddle FH. Gene transfer, expression and molecular cloning of the human transferrin receptor gene. Cell 1984;37:95.
114. McClelland A, Kuhn LC, Ruddle RH. The human transferrin receptor gene: genomic organization, and the complete primary structure of the receptor deduced from a cDNA sequence. Cell 1984;39:267.
115. Omary MB, Trowbridge IS. Covalent binding of fatty acid to the transferrin receptor in cultured human cells. J Biol Chem 1981;256: 4715.
116. Goldstein JL, Anderson RG, Brown MS. Coated pits, coated vesicles and receptor-mediated encocytosis. Nature 1979;279:679.
117. Pastan IH, Willingham MC. Receptor-mediated endocytosis: coated pits, receptosomes and the Golgi. Trends Biochem Sci 1983;8:250.
118. Steinman RM, Mellman IS, Muller WA, Cohn ZA. Endocytosis and the recycling of plasma membrane. J Cell Biol 1983;96:1.
119. Morgan EH, Appleton TC. Autoradiographic location of ^{125}I-labeled transferrin in rabbit reticulocytes. Nature 1969;223:1371.
120. Sullivan AL, Grasso JA, Weintraub LR. Micropinocytosis of transferrin by developing red cells: an electron microscopic study utilizing ferritin-conjugates antibodies to transferin. Blood 1976;47:133.
121. Karin M, Minz B. Receptor-mediated endocytosis of transferrin in developmentally totipotent mouse teratocarcinoma cells. J Biol Chem 1981;256:3245.
122. Bleil JD, Bretscher MS. Transferrin receptor and its recycling in HeLA cells. EMBO J 1982;1:351.
123. Cambell CH, Fine RE, Squicciarini J, Rome LH. Coated vesicles from rat livers and calf brain contain cryptic mannose-6-phosphate receptors. J Biol Chem 1983;258:2628.
124. Limet JN, Quintart, Schneider Y-J, Courtoy PJ. Receptor-mediated endocytosis of polymeric IgA and galactosylated serum albumin in rat liver. Eur J Biochem 1985;146:539.
125. Pastan I, Willingham MC. The pathway of endocytosis. In: Pastan I, Willingham MC, eds. Endocytosis. New York, Plenum Press, 1985:1.

126. Girones N, Alverez E, Seth A, Lin IM, Latour DA, Davis RJ. Mutational analysis of the cytoplasmic tail of the human transferrin receptor: identification of a sub-domain that is required for rapid endocytosis. J Biol Chem 1991;266:19006.
127. Pearse BMF. On the structural and functional components of coated vesicles. J Mol Biol 1978;126:803.
128. Helenius A, Mellman I, Wall D, Hubbard A. Endosomes. Trends Biochem Sci 1983;8:245.
129. Yilla M, Tan A, Ito K, Miwa K, Ploegh HL. Involvement of the vacuolar H(+)-ATPases in the secretory pathway of HepG2 cells. J Biol Chem 1993;268:19092.
130. van Renswoude JK, Bridges KR, Harford JB, Klausner RD. Receptor-mediated endocytosis of transferrin and the uptake of Fe in K562 cells: identification of a non-lysosomal acidic compartment. 1982;79: 6186.
131. Klausner RD, Ashwell G, van Renswoude J, Harford JB, Bridges KR. Binding of the apotransferrin to K562 cells: explanation of the transferrin cycle. Proc Natl Acad Sci USA 1983;80:2263.
132. Morgan EH. Exchange of iron and transferrin across endothelial surfaces in the rat and rabbit. J Physiol 1963;169:339.
133. Morgan EH. Inhibition of reticulocyte iron uptake by NH_4Cl and methylamine. Biochim Biophys Acta 1981;642:119.
134. Frazier JL, Caskey JH, Yoffe M, Seligman PA. Studies of the transferrin receptor on both human reticulocytes and nucleated human cells in culture. J Clin Invest 1982;69:853.
135. Larrick JW, Creswell P. Modulation of cell surface iron transferrin receptors by cellular density and state of activation. J Supramol 1979;11:579.
136. Trowbridge IS, Omary MB. Human cell surface glycoprotein related to cell proliferation is the receptor for transferrin. Proc Natl Acad Sci USA 1981;78:3039.
137. Galbraith RM, Galbraith GM. Expression of transferrin receptors on mitogen-stimulated human peripheral blood lymphocytes: relation to cellular activation and related metabolic events. Immunology 1981;44:703.
138. Hamilton TA. Regulation of transferrin receptor expression in concanavalin A stimulated and gross virus transformed rat lymphoblasts. J Cell Physiol 1982;113:40.
139. Ward JH, Kushner JP, Kaplan J. Regulation of HeLa cell transferrin receptors. J Biol Chem 1982;257:10317.
140. Hayashi I, Sato GH. Replacement of serum by hormones permits growth of cells in defined media. Nature 1976;259:132.
141. Stragand JJ, Hagemann RF. An iron requirement for the synchronous progression of colonic cells following fasting and refeeding. Cell Tissue Kinet 1978;11:513.
142. Soyano A, Chinea M, Romano EL. The effect of desferrioxamine on the proliferative response of rat lymphocytes stimulated with various mitogens in vitro. Immunopharmacology 1984;8:163.
143. Lederman HM, Cohen A, Lee JW, Freedman MHJ, Gelfand EW. Deferoxamine: a reversible S-phase inhibitor of human lymphocyte proliferation. Blood 1984;64:748.
144. Mattia E, Rao K, Shapiro DS, Sussman HH, Klausner RD. Biosynthetic regulation of the human transferrin receptor by desferrioxamine in K562 cells. J Biol Chem 1984;529:2689.
145. Louache F, Pelosi E, Titieux M, Peschle C, Testa U. Molecular mechanisms regulating the synthesis of transferrin receptors and ferritin in human erythroleukemic cell lines. FEBS Lett 1985;183:223.
146. Chitambar CR, Massey EJ, Seligman PA. Regulation of transferrin receptor expression on human leukemic cells during proliferation and induction of differentiation: effects of gallium and dimethylsufoxide. J Clin Invest 1983;72:1314.
147. Rao D, Harford JB, Rouautl T, McClelland A, Ruddle FH, Klausner RD. Transcriptional regulation by iron of the gene for the transferrin receptor. Mol Cell Biol 1986;6:236.
148. Mullner EW, Kuhn LC. A stem-loop in the 3 untranslated region mediates iron-dependent regulation of transferrin receptor mRNA stability in the cytoplasm. Cell 1988;53:815.
149. Musgrove E, Rugg C, Taylor I, Hedley D. Transferrin receptor expression during exponential and plateau phase growth of human tumour cells in culture. J Cell Physiol 1984;118:6.
150. Sager PR, Brown PA, Berlin RD. Analysis of transferrin recycling in mitotic and interphase HeLa cells by quantitative fluorescence microscopy. J Cell Physiol 1984;39:275.
151. May WS, Jacobs S, Cuatrecasas P. Association of phorbol ester-induced hyperphosphorylation and reversible regulation of transferrin membrane receptors in HL60 cells. Proc Natl Acad Sci USA 1984;81:2016.
152. Stein BS, Sussman HH. Demonstration of two distinct transferrin receptor recycling pathways and transferrin-independent receptor internalization in K562 cells. J Biol Chem 1986;261:10319.
153. Jacobs A. Low molecular weight intracellular iron transport compounds. Blood 1977;50:433.
154. Bakkeren DL, de Jeu-Jaspars CMH, Van der Heul C, Van Eijk HG. Analysis of iron-binding components in the low molecular weight fraction of rat reticulocyte cytosol. Int J Biochem 1985;17:925.
155. Pollack S, Campaua T, Weaver J. Low molecular weight iron in guinea pig reticulocytes. Am J Hematol 1985;19:75.
156. Yoshino Y, Manis J, Schachter D. Actinomycin D and the regulation of apoferritin synthesis in rat liver. Nature 1966;210:53.
157. Millar JA, Cumming JL, Smith JA, Goldberg A. Effect of actinomycin D, cycloheximide, and acute blood loss on ferritin synthesis in rat liver. Biochem J 1970;119:643.
158. Zahringer J, Baliga BS, Munro HN. Novel mechanism for translation control in regulation of ferritin synthesis by iron. Proc Natl Acad Sci 1976;73:857.
159. Aziz N, Munro HN. Both subunits of rat liver feritin are regulated at a translational level by iron induction. Nucleic Acids Res 1986;14: 915.
160. Rogers J, Munro H. Translation of ferritin light and heavy subunit mRNA's is regulated by intracellular chelatable iron levels in rat hepatoma cells. Proc Natl Acad Sci USA 1987;84:2277.
161. Walden WE, Thach RE. Translational controls of gene expression in a normal fibroblast: characterization of a subclass of mRNA's with unusual kinetic properties. Biochemistry 1986;25:2033.
162. Liebold EA, Munro HN. Cytoplasmic protein binds in vitro to a highly conserved sequence in the 5′ untranslated region of ferritin heavy- and light-subunit mRNA. Proc Natl Acad Sci USA 1988;85:2171.
163. Rouault TA, Hentze MW, Caughman SW, Harford JB, Klausner RD. Binding of a cytosolic protein to the iron responsive element of human ferritin messenger RNA. Science 1988;241:1207.
164. Walden WE, Daniels-McQueen S, Brown PH, et al. Translational repression in eukaryotes: partial purification and characterization of a repressor of ferritin mRNA translation. Proc Natl Acad Sci USA 1988;85:9503.
165. Klausner RD, Harford JB. *Cis-trans* models for post-transcriptional gene regulation. Science 1989;246:870.
166. Mattia E, den Blaauwen J, Ashwell G, van Renswoude J. Multiple post-translational regulatory mechanisms in ferritin gene expression. Proc Natl Acad Sci USA 1989;86:1801.
167. Bridges KR, Cudkowicz A. Effect of iron chelators on the transferrin receptor in K562 cells. J Biol Chem 1984;259:12970.
168. Louache F, Testa U, Pelicci P, Thompoulous P, Titeuz M, Rochant H. Regulation of transferrin receptors in human hematopoietic cell lines. J Biol Chem 1984;259:11576.
169. Casey JL, Hentze MW, Koeller DM, et al. Iron-responsive elements: regulatory RNA sequences that control mRNA levels and translation. Science 1988;240:924.
170. Koeller DM, Casey JL, Hentze MW, et al. A cytosolic protein binds to structural elements within the iron-responsive regulatory region of the transferrin receptor mRNA. Proc Natl Acad Sci USA 1989;86: 3574.
171. Elferink CJ, Sassa S, May BK. Regulation of 5-aminolevulinate synthase in mouse erythroleukemic cells is different from that in liver. J Biol Chem 1988;263:13012.
172. Goessling LS, Daniels-McQueen S, Bhattacharyya-Pakrasi M, Lin JJ, Thach RE. Enhanced degradation of the ferritin repressor protein during induction of ferritin messenger RNA translation. Science 1992;256:670.
173. Melefors O, Hentze MW. Translational regulation by mRNA/protein interactions in eukaryotic cells: ferritin and beyond. Bioessays 1993;15: 85.
174. Committee on Iron Deficiency, AMA Council on Foods and Nutrition. Iron deficiency in the United States. JAMA 1968;203:497.
175. Fairbanks VF, Fahey JL, Beutler E. Clinical disorders of iron metabolism, ed 2. New York, Grune & Stratton, 1971.
176. Bainton DF, Finch CA. The diagnosis of iron deficiency anemia. Am J Med 1964;37:62.
177. Charlton RW, Bothwell TH. Definition, prevalence and prevention of iron deficiency. Clin Haematol 1982;11:309.
178. Roth WA, Waldes-Dapnea A, Pieses P, Buchman E. Topical action of salicylates in gastrointestinal erosion and hemorrhage. Gastroenterology 1963;44:146.
179. Fries JF, Miller SR, Spitz PW, Williams CA, Hubert H, Bloch DA. Toward an epidemiology of gastropathy associated with nonsteroidal antiinflammatory drug use. Gastroenterology 1989;96:647.
180. Galberg L, Hogdahl AM, Nilsson L, Rybo G. Menstrual blood loss: a population study. Acta Obstet Gynecol Scand 1966;45:320.
181. Jacobs A, Butler EB. Menstrual blood loss in iron deficiency anemia. Lancet 1965;2:407.
182. Soergel KH, Sommers SC. Idiopathic pulmonary hemosiderosis and related syndromes. Am J Med 1962;32:499.
183. Hartmann RC, et al. Paroxysmal nocturnal hemoglobinuria: clinical and laboratory studies relating to iron metabolism and therapy with endrogen and iron. Medicine 1966;45:331.
184. Hunter CA. Iron deficiency anemia in pregnancy. Surg Gynecol Obstet 1960;110:210.
185. Harvey GW, et al. Low hemoglobin levels in women as revealed by blood donor records. JAMA 1952;149:1127.
185a. Larrick JW, Hyman ES. Acquired iron-deficiency anemia caused by an antibody against the transferrin receptor. N Engl J Med 1984;311: 214.
186. Metz-Boutique MH, Jolies J, Mazurier J, et al. Human lactotransferrin: amino acid sequence and structural comparison with other transferrins. Eur J Biochem 1984;145:659.
187. Heilmeyer L, Keller W, Vivell O. Congenital transferrin deficiency in a seven-year old girl. German Med Meth 1961;6:385.

188. Sakata T. Atransferrinemia. J Pediatr Pract 1969;32:1523.
189. Kaplan J, Craven C, Alexander J, Kushner J, Lamb J, Bernstein S. Regulation of the distribution of tissue iron. Ann NY Acad Sci 1988;526:124.
190. Shahidi NT, Nathan DG, Diamond LK. Iron deficiency anemia associated with an error of iron metabolism in two siblings. J Clin Invest 1964;43:510.
191. Stavem P, Saltvedt E, Elgjo K, Rootwelt K. Congenital hypochromic microcytic anaemia with iron overload of the liver and hyperferraemia. Scand J Haematol 1973;10:153.
191a. Neerhout RC, Larson W, et al. Mesenteric lymphoid harmartoma associated with chronic hypoferremia, anemia, growth failure and hyperglobulinemia. N Engl J Med 1969;280:922.
192. Meyer CT, Troncale FJ, Galloway S, Sheahan DG. Arteriovenous malformations of the bowel: an analysis of 22 cases and a review of the literature. Medicine 1981;60:36.
192a. Shbeeb I, Prager E, Love J. The aortic valve-colonic axis. Dis Colon Rectum 1984;27:38.
193. Osler W. On a family form of recurring epistaxis associated with multiple telangiectases of the skin and mucous membrane. Bull Johns Hopkins Hosp 1901;12:333.
194. Burman D. Iron deficiency in infants and children. Clin Haematol 1973;2:257.
195. Sarrinen UM, Siimes MA, Dallman PR. Iron absorption in infants: high bioavailability of breast milk iron as indicated by the extrinsic tag method of iron absorption and by the concentration of serum ferritin. J Pediatr 1977;91:36.
196. Munoz LM, Lonnerdal B, Keen CL, Dewey KG. Coffee consumption as a factor in iron deficiency anemia among pregnant women and their infants in Costa Rico. Am J Clin Nutr 1988;48:645.
197. Murray MJ, Murray AB, Murray NJ, Murray MB. The effect of iron status of Nigerian mothers on that of their infants at birth and 6 months, and on the concentration of Fe in breast milk. Br J Nutr 1978;39:627.
198. Hertrampf E, Cayazzo M, Pizarro F, Stekel A. Bioavailability of iron in soy-based formula and its effect on iron nutriture in infancy. Pediatrics 1986;78:640.
199. Siimes MA, Kuitunen VE. Breast milk iron: a declining concentration during the course of lactation. Acta Paediatr Scand 1979;68:29.
200. Cook JD, Skikne BS, Lynche SR, Reusser ME. Estimates of iron sufficiency in the US population. Blood 1986;68:726.
201. James J, Lawson P, Male P, Oakhill A. Preventing iron deficiency in preschool children by implementing an educational and screening programme in an inner city practice. Br Med J 1989;299:838.
202. Ziegler EE, Fomon SJ, Nelson SE, et al. Cow milk feeding in infancy: further observations on blood loss from the gastrointestinal tract. J Pediatr 1990;116:11.
203. American Academy of Pediatrics Committee on Nutrition. The use of whole cow's milk in infancy. Pediatrics 1992;89:1105.
204. Williams ML, Shoot RJ, O'Neal PI, Oski FA. Role of dietary iron and vitamin E deficiency in anemia of infancy. N Engl J Med 1975;292: 887.
205. Gutcher GR, Raynor WJH, Farrell PM. An evaluation of vitamin E status in premature infants. Am J Clin Nutr 1984;40:1078.
206. Ronnholm KA, Dostalova L, Siimes MA. Vitamin E supplementation in very-low-birth-weight infants: long-term follow-up at two different levels of vitamin E supplementation. Am J Clin Nutr 1987;49:121.
207. Adams JF. The clinical and metabolic consequences of total gastrectomy. Scand J Gastroenterol 1968;3:145.
208. Hobbs JR. Iron deficiency after partial gastrectomy. Gut 1961;2:141.
209. Sutton DR. "Free" iron loss in atrophic gastritis, post-gastrectomy states and adult celiac disease. Lancet 1970;2:387.
210. Murray MJ, Stein N. Experimental achylia gastrica and iron absorption. Br J Haematol 1971;21:113.
211. Lange J. Medicinalium epistolarum miscelanea varia et rara, 1554. Am J Dis Child 1932;48:393.
212. Cabot RC. Diseases of the blood. In: Modern medicine, ed 4. Philadelphia, Lea & Febiger, 1915:650.
213. Schwartz E. Chlorosis. Acta Med Belg (Suppl) 1951.
214. Haden RL. Historical aspects of iron therapy in anemia. JAMA 1938;111:1059.
215. Beveridge BR, et al. Hypochromic anemia. Q J Med 1965;34:135.
216. Vinson PP. Hysterical dysphagia. Minn Med 1922;5:107.
217. Davidson WMB, Markson JL. The gastric mucosa in iron deficiency anaemia. Lancet 1955;2:639.
218. Hogan GR, Jones B. The relationship of koilonychia and iron deficiency in infants. J Pediatr 1970;77:1054.
219. Jacobs A, Cavill I. The oral lesions of iron deficiency anaemia: pyridoxine and riboflavin status. Br J Haematol 1968;14:291.
220. Beutler E, et al. Iron therapy in chronically fatigued non-anemic women. Ann Intern Med 1960;52:378.
221. McMahon LF, Ryan MJ, Larson D, Fisher R. Occult gastrointestinal blood loss in marathon runners. Ann Intern Med 1984;100:846.
222. Crosby WH. Pica. JAMA 1976;235:2765.
223. Coltman CA Jr. Pagophagia and iron lack. JAMA 1969;207:513.
224. Reynolds RD, et al. Pagophagia and iron deficiency anemia. Ann Intern Med 1968;69:435.
225. Finch CA, Miller LR, Inamdar AR, Person R, Seiler K, Mackler B. Iron deficiency in the rat: physiological and biochemical studies of muscle dysfunction. J Clin Invest 1976;58:447.
226. Beard J, Finch CA, Mackler B. Deleterious effects of iron deficiency. In: Nutrition in health and diseases and international development. New York, Alan R Liss, 1981:305.
227. Ben-Schachar D, Ashkenazi R, Youdim MBH. Long-term consequence of early iron deficiency on dopaminergic neurotransmission in rats. Int J Dev Neurosci 1986;4:81.
228. Ashkenzzi R, Ben-Schachar D, Youdim MBH. Nutritional iron and dopamine binding sites in the rat brain. Pharmacol Biochem Behav 1982;17:43.
229. Hill JM, Ruff MR, Weber RJ, Pert CB. Transferrin receptors in rat brain: neuropeptide-like pattern and relationship to iron distribution. Proc Natl Acad Sci USA 1985;82:4553.
230. Lozoff B, Brittenham GM. Behavioral alterations in iron deficiency. Pediatr Hematol 1987;1:449.
231. Lozoff B, Brittenham GM, Wolf AW, et al. Iron deficiency anemia and iron therapy effects on infant developmental test performance. Pediatrics 1987;79:981.
232. Walter T, Kovalskys J, Stekel A. Effect of mild iron deficiency on infant mental development scores. J Pediatr 1983;102:519.
233. Findlay E, Ng KT, Reid RL, Armstrong SM. The effect of iron deficiency during development on passive avoidance learning in the adult rat. Physiol Behav 1981;27:1084.
234. Weinberg J, Dallman PR, Levine S. Iron deficiency during early development in the rat: behavorial and physiological consequences. Pharmacol Biochem Behav 1980;12:493.
235. Burman D. Iron deficiency in infants and children. Clin Haematol 1973;2:257.
236. Palti H, Pevsner B, Adler B. Does anemia in infancy affect acheivement on developmental and intelligence tests? Hum Biol 1983;55:189.
237. Bomford A, Conlon-Hollingshead C, Munro HM. Adaptive responses of rat tissue isoferritins to iron administration: changes in subunit synthesis, isoferritin abundance, and capacity for iron storage. J Biol Chem 1981;256:948.
238. Conrad ME, Crosby WH. The natural history of iron deficiency induced by phlebotomy. Blood 1962;20:173.
239. Fairbanks VF. Is the peripheral blood film reliable for the diagnosis of iron deficiency anemia. Am J Clin Pathol 1971;55:447.
240. Thompson WG, Meola T, Lipkin M, Freedman ML. Red cell distribution width, mean corpuscular volume, and transferrin saturation in the diagnosis of iron deficiency. Arch Intern Med 1988;148:2128.
241. McClure S, Custer E, Bessman JD. Improved detection of early iron deficiency in nonanemic subjects. JAMA 1985;253:1021.
242. Oski FA. Iron deficiency in infancy and childhood. N Engl J Med 1993;329:190.
243. Good MF, Powell LW, Holliday JW. Iron status and cellular immune competence. Blood Rev 1988;2:43.
244. Beard J, Finch CA, Mackler B. Deleterious effects of iron deficiency. In: Nutrition in health and disease and international development. New York, Alen R Liss, 1981:305.
245. Choi SI, Simone JV. Platelet production in experimental iron deficiency anemia. Blood 1973;42:219.
246. Dinol K, Aksoy M. On the platelet level in chronic iron deficiency anemia. Acta Haematol 1969;41:135.
247. Gross S, Keefer V, Newman AJ. The platelet in iron deficiency anemia: the response to oral and parenteral iron. Pediatrics 1964;34:315.
248. Burrows S. Comparison of methods designed to measure transferrin and iron binding capacity of serum. Am J Clin Pathol 1967;47:326.
249. Casale G, Migliavacca A, Bonora C, Zurita I, deNichola P. Circadian rhythm of plasma iron, total iron binding capacity and serum ferritin arteriosclerotic aged patients. Age Ageing 1981;10:115.
250. Crosby WH, O'Neil-Cutting MA. A small-dose iron tolerance test as an indicator of mild iron deficiency. Clin Invest 1984;251:1986.
251. Jones BM, Worwood M. Ferritin in serum. N Engl J Med 1975;292: 951.
252. Lipschitz DA, Cook JD, Finch CA. A clinical evaluation of serum ferritin as an index of iron stores. N Engl J Med 1974;290:1213.
253. Holliday JW, Powell LW. Ferritin and cellular iron metabolism. Ann NY Acad Sci 1988;526:101.
254. Guyatt GH, Patterson C, Ali M, et al. Diagnosis of iron-deficiency in the elderly. Am J Med 1990;88:205.
255. Jacobs A, Worwood J. Ferritin in serum. N Engl J Med 1975;292:951.
256. Wranne L. Free erythrocyte copro- and protoporphyrin. Acta Paediatr Scand 1960;49:1.
257. Piomelli S. A micromethod for free erythrocyte porphyrins: the FEP test. J Lab Clin Med 1973;81:932.
258. Stockman JA, Weiner LS, Simon GE, Stuart MJ, Oski FA. The measurement of free erythrocyte porphyrin (FEP) as a simple means of distinguishing iron deficiency from beta-thalassemia trait in subjects with microcytosis. J Lab Clin Med 1975;85:113.
259. Trundle DS. Erythrocyte zinc protoporphyrin. Clin Chem News 1984;10:19.
260. Rajkumar S, Geibel V, Devanagondi B, Kaul B, Brown AK. The diagnostic significance of free erythrocyte protoporphyrin and the FEP/hemoglobin ratio in plumbism. NY State J Med 1987;87:542.
261. Saarinen UM, Siimes MA. Developmental changes in serum iron,

total iron-binding capacity, and transferrin saturation in infancy. J Pediatr 1977;91:875.
262. Rath CE, Finch CA. Sternal marrow hemosiderin. A method for determination of available iron stores in man. J Lab Clin Med 1948;3:81.
263. Ellis LD, Jensen WN, Westerman MP. Marrow iron: an evaluation of depleted stores in a series of 1,322 needle biopsies. Ann Intern Med 1964;61:44.
264. Baumgartner-Staubli R, Beck EA. Sideroblast score: a sensitive indicator of iron deficiency and hypoproliferative anemia. Acta Haematol 1977;57:24.
265. Bessis MC, Jensen WN. Sideroblastic anaemia, mitochondria and erythroblast iron. Br J Haematol 1965;11:49.
266. Fairbanks VR, Beutler E. Iron deficiency. In: Williams WW, ed. Erythrocyte disorders: anemias related to disturbances of hemoglobin synthesis. New York, McGraw-Hill, 1982:466.
267. Fong TP, et al. Stainable iron in aspirated and needle-biopsy specimens of marrow: a source of error. Am J Hematol 1977;2:47.
268. Beguin Y, Stray SM, Cazzola M, Huebers H, Finch CA. Ferrokinetic measurements of erythropoiesis. Acta Haematol 1988;79:121.
269. Cook JD, Marsaglia G, Eshbach JW, Funk DD, Finch CA. Ferrokinetics: a biologic model for iron exchange in man. J Clin Invest 1970;49:197.
270. Ricketts C, Cavill I, Napier JA, Jacoby AF. Ferrokinetics and erythropoiesis in man: an evaluation of ferrokinetic measurements. Br J Haematol 1977;35:41.
271. Cazzola M, Huebers HA, Sayers MH, et al. Transferrin saturation, plasma iron turnover, and transferrin uptake in normal humans. Blood 1985;66:935.
272. Cazzola M, Pootrakul P, Huebers HA, Eng M, Esbach J, Finch CA. Erythroid marrow function in anemic patients. Blood 1987;69:296.
273. Kohgo Y, Nishisato T, Kondo H, Tsushima N, Niitsu Y, Urushizaki I. Circulating transferrin receptor in human serum. Br J Haematol 1986;64:277.
274. Flowers CH, Skikne BS, Covell AM, Cook JD. The clinical measurement of serum transferrin receptors. J Lab Clin Med 1989;114:368.
275. Shih YJ, Baynes RD, Hudson BG, Flowers CH, Skikne BS, Cook JD. Serum transferrin receptor is a truncated form of tissue receptor. J Biol Chem 1990;265:19077.
276. Shih YJ, Baynes RD, Hudson BG, Cook JD. Characterization and quantitation of the circulating forms of serum transferrin receptor using domain-specific antibodies. Blood 1993;81:234.
277. Huebers HA, Beguin Y, Pootrakul P, Einspahr D, Finch CA. Intact transferrin receptors in human plasma and their relation to erythropoiesis. Blood 1990;75:102.
278. Valgerg LS, et al. Cobalt test for the detection of iron deficiency anemia. Ann Intern Med 1972;77:186.
279. Isa L, Jean G, Silvani A, et al. Evaluation of iron stores in patients with alcoholic liver disease: role of red cell ferritin. Acta Haematol Base 1988;80:85.
280. Cartwright GE. The anemia of chronic disorders. Semin Hematol 1966;3:351.
281. Banerjee RN, Narang RM. Haematological changes in malignancy. Br J Haematol 1967;13:829.
282. Wasi P, et al. The effect of iron deficiency on the levels of hemoglobin A_2 and E. J Lab Clin Med 1968;71:85.
283. Dozy AM, et al. Alpha globin gene organization in blacks precludes the severe form of α-thalassemia. Nature 1979;280:605.
284. Forth W, Rummel W. Gastrointestinal absorption of heavy metals. In: IEPT. Pharmacology of intestinal absorption: gastrointestinal absorption of drugs. Oxford, Pergamon Press, 1975:599.
285. Herbert V. Polymorphonuclear hypersegmentation. Br J Haematol 1979;39:357.
286. Levine JS. Occult blood in stool (iron deficiency) In: Decision making in gastroenterology. Burlington, Ont, BC Decker, 1985:102.
287. Schwartz S, Ellefson M. Quantitative fecal recovery of ingested hemoglobin-heme in blood: comparisons by HemoQuant assay with ingested meat and fish. Gastroenterology 1985;89:19.
288. Barry MJ, Mulley AG, Richter JM. Effect of workup strategy on the cost-effectiveness of fecal occult blood screening for colorectal cancer. Gastroenterology 1987;93:301.
289. O'Sullivan DJ, Higgins PG, Wilkinson JF. Oral iron compounds: a therapeutic comparison. Lancet 1955;2:482.
290. Reeves JD, Yip R. Lack of adverse side effects of oral ferrous sulfate therapy in 1-year-old infants. Pediatrics 1985;75:352.
291. Beutler E, Meerkreebs G. Doses and dosing. N Engl J Med 1966;274: 1152.
292. Mitchell ABS, Gill AM. Choice of iron therapy. Practitioner 1974;213: 370.
293. Hallberg L, Ryttinger L, Solvell L. Side-effects of oral iron therapy: a double-bind study of different iron compounds in tablet form. Acta Med Scand 1966;459:3.
294. Swan HT, Jowett GH. Treatment of iron deficiency with ferrous fumarate. Br Med J 1959;2:782.
295. Swan HT, Jowett GH. Treatment of iron deficiency with ferrous fumarate: assessment by a statistically accurate method. Br Med J 1959;2: 782.
296. Maddock RK. Patient cooperation in taking medicines. JAMA 1967;199: 137.
297. Cromer BA, Steinberg K, Gardner L, et al. Psychosocial determinants of compliance in adolescents with iron deficiency. Am J Dis Child 1989;143:55.
298. Bianchi FM, Cavassini GB, Leo P. Iron protein succynilate in the treatment of iron deficiency: potential interaction with H_2-receptor antagonists. Int J Clin Pharmacol Ther Toxicol 1993;31:209.
299. Skikne BS, Lynch SR, Cook JD. Role of gastric acid in food iron absorption. Gastroenterology 1981;81:1068.
300. Wallerstein RO. Intravenous iron–dextran complex. Blood 1968;32: 690.
301. Hamstra RD, Block MH, Schocket AL. Intravenous iron dextran in clinical medicine. JAMA 1980;243:1726.
302. Horn E. Iron and folate supplements during pregnancy: supplementing everyone treats those at risk and is cost effective. Br Med J 1988;297: 1325.
303. Hibbard BM. Iron and folate supplements during pregnancy: supplementation is valuable only in selected patients. Br Med J 1988;297: 1324.
304. Allaire BI, Campagna A. Iron deficiency anemia in pregnancy. Obstet Gynecol 1961;17:605.
305. Hunter CA. Iron deficiency anemia in pregnancy. Surg Gynecol Obstet 1960;110:210.
306. Valberg LS, et al. Serum ferritin and the iron status of Canadians. Can Med Assoc J 1976;114:417.
307. Zanella A, Gridelli L, Berzuini A, et al. Sensitivity and predictive value of serum ferritin and free erythrocyte protoporphyrin for iron deficiency. J Lab Clin Med 1989;113:73.
308. Cox TM, Peters TJ. Uptake of iron by duodenal biopsy specimens from patients with iron-deficiency anaemia and primary haemochromatosis. Lancet 1978;1:123.
309. Tsan MF, Scheffel U. Transferrin sialic acid contents of patients with hereditary hemochromatosis. Am J Hematol 1985;20:359.
310. Worwood M. Iron and haemochromatosis. J Inherit Metab Dis 1983;6: 63.
311. Cartwright GE, Edwards CQ, Kravitz K, et al. Hereditary hemochromatosis: phenotypic expression of the disease. N Engl J Med 1979;301: 175.
312. Olsson KS, Ritter B, Rosen U, Heedman PA, Staugard F. Prevalence of iron overload in central Sweden. Acta Med Scand 1983;213:145.
313. Beaumont C, Simon M, Fauchet R, et al. Serum ferritin as a possible marker of the hemochromatosis allele. N Engl J Med 1979;301:79.
314. Gordeuk VR, Mukiibi J, Hasstedt SJ, et al. Iron overload in Africa: interaction between a gene and dietary iron content. N Engl J Med 1992;326:95.
315. Bothwell TH, Seftel H, Jacobs P, Torrance JD, Baumslag N. Iron overload in Bantu subjects: studies on the availability of iron in Bantu beer. Am J Clin Nutr 1964;14:47.
316. MacPhail AP, Simon MO, Torrance JD, Charlton RW, Bothwell TH, Issacson C. Changing patterns of dietary iron overload in black South Africans. Am J Clin Nutr 1979;32:1272.
317. Chejfec G. Liver biopsy: conventional histologic techniques. Lab Res Method Biol Med 1983;7:491.
318. MacDonald RA. Idiopathic hemochromatosis: genetic or acquired? Arch Intern Med 1963;112:184.
319. Powell LW. The role of alcoholism in hepatic iron storage disease. NY Acad Sci 1975;252:124.
320. Bassett ML, Halliday JW, Powell LW. HLA typiong in idiopathic hemochromatosis: distinction between hemozygotes and heterozygotes with biochemical expression. Hepatology 1981;1:120.
321. Simon M, Bourel M, Genete B, Fauchet R, Edan G, Brissot P. Idiopathic hemochromatosis and iron overload in alcoholic liver disease: differentiation by HLA phenotype. Gastroenterology 1977;73:655.
322. Lesage GD, Baldus WP, Fairbanks WF, et al. Hemochromatosis: genetic or alcohol-induced? Gastroenterology 1983;84:1471.
323. Edwards CQ, Skolnick MH, Padone MM, Kushner JP. Iron overload in hereditary spherocytosis: association with HLA-linked hemochromatosis. Am J Hematol 1982;14:101.
324. Edwards CQ, Skolnick MH, Kushner JP. Coincidential nontransfusional iron overload and thalassemia minor: association with HLA-lined hemochromatosis. Blood 1981;58:844.
325. Pippard MJ, Callender ST, Warner GT, Weatherall DJ. Iron absorption and loading in beta-thalassaemia intermedia. Lancet 1979;2:819.
326. Cartwright GE, Edwards CQ, Skolnick MH, Amos DB. Association of HLA-linked hemochromatosis with idiopathic refractory sideroblastic anemia. J Clin Invest 1980;65:989.
327. Simon M, Beaumont C, Briere J, et al. Is the HLA-linked haemochromatosis allele implicated in idiopathic refractory sideroblastic anaemia? Br J Haematol 1985;60:75.
328. Bradbear RA, Bain C, Siskind V, et al. Cohort study of internal malignancy in genetic hemochromatosis and other nonalcoholic liver diseases. J Natl Cancer Inst 1985;75:81.
329. Conte D, Piperno A, Mandelli C, et al. Clinical, biochemical and histologic features of primary haemochromatosis: a report of 67 cases. Liver 1986;6:310.
330. Tiniakos G, Williams R. Cirrhotic process, liver cell carcinoma and

extrahepatic malignant tumors in idiopathic haemochromatosis: study of 71 patients treated with venesection therapy. Appl Pathol 1988;6: 128.
331. Fellows IW, Stewart M, Jeffcoate WJ, Smith PG, Toghill PG. Hepatocellular carcinoma in primary haemochromatosis in the absence of cirrhosis. Gut 1988;29:1603.
332. Blumberg RS, Chopra S, Ibrahim R, et al. Primary hepatocellular carcinoma in idiopathic hemochromatosis after reversal of cirrhosis. Gastroenterology 1988;95:1399.
333. Park CH, Bacon BR, Brittenham GM, Tavill AS. Pathology of dietary iron overload in rats. Lab Invest 1987;57:555.
334. Iancu TC, Shiloh H, Link G, Bauminger ER, Pinson A, Hershko C. Ultrastructural pathology of iron-loaded rat myocardial cells in culture. Br J Exp Pathol 1987;68:53.
335. Link G, Pinson A, Hershko C. Heart cells in culture: a model of myocardial iron overload and chelation. J Lab Clin Med 1985;106:147.
336. Abok K, Hirt T, Ericsson JLE, Brunk U. Effect of iron on the stability of macrophage lysosomes. Virchow Arch (Cell Pathol) 1983;43:85.
337. Hultcrantz R, Ahlberg J, Glaumann H. Isolation of two lysosomal populations from iron-overloaded rat liver with different iron concentrations and proteolytic activity. Virchow Arch (Cell Pathol) 1984;47: 55.
338. Ahlberg J, Glaumann H. Uptake, microautophagy and degradation of exogenous proteins by isolated rat liver lysosomes: effects of pH ATP inhibitors of proteolysis. Exp Mol Pathol 1985;42:78.
339. Cappell DF, Hutchison HE, Jowell M. Transfusional siderosis: the effects of excessive iron deposits on the tissues. J Pathol Baceriol 1957;74: 245.
340. Iancu TC. Iron overload. Mol Aspect Med 1983;6:1.
341. Peters TJ, Seymour CA. Acid hydrolase activities and lysosomal integrity in liver biopsies from patients with iron overload. Clin Sci Mol Med 1976;50:75.
342. Milder MS, Cook JD, Stray S, Finch CA. Idiopathic hemochromatosis: an interim report. Medicine 1980;59:34.
343. Howard JM, Ghent CN, Carey LS, Flanagan PR, Valberg LS. Diagnostic efficacy of hepatic computed tomography in the detection of body iron overload. Gastroenterology 1983;8:209.
344. Leung AW, Steiner RE, Young IR. NMR imaging of the liver in two cases of iron overload. J Comput Assist Tomogr 1984;8:446.
345. Kaltwasser JP, Gottschalk R, Schalk KP, Harti W. Non-invasive quantitation of liver iron-overload by magnetic resonance imaging. Br J Haematol 1990;74:360.
346. Brittenham GM, Farrell DE, Harris JW, et al. Magnetic susceptibility measurement of human iron stores. N Engl J Med 1982;307:1671.
347. Wasserman AJ, Richardson DW, Baird CL, Wyso EM. Cardiac hemochromatosis simulating constrictive pericarditis. Am J Med 1962;32: 316.
348. Jacobs A. Iron overload: clinical and pathological aspects. Semin Haematol 1977;14:89.
349. Cutler DJ, Isner JM, Bracey AW. Hemochromatosis heart disease: an unemphasized cause of potentially reversible restrictive cardiomyopathy. Am J Med 1980;69:923.
350. Feely J, Counihan TB. Hemochromatosis presenting as angina and responding to venesection. Br Med J 1977;2:681.
351. Sanyal SK, Johnson W, Jayalakshamma B, Green AA. Fatal "iron heart" in an adolescent: biochemical and ultrastructural aspects of the heart. Pediatrics 1975;55:336.
352. Leon MB, Borer JS, Bacharach SL, et al. Detection of early cardiac dysfunction in patients with severe beta-thalassemia and chronic iron overload. N Engl J Med 1979;301:1143.
353. Engle MA, Erlandson M, Smith CH. Late cardiac complications of chronic severe refractory anemia with hemochromatosis. Circulation 1974;300:698.
354. Buja LM, Roberts WC. Iron in the heart. Am J Med 1971;51:209.
355. Olson LJ, Edwards WD, McCall JT, Ilstup DM, Gersh BJ. Cardiac iron deposition in idiopathic hemochromatosis: histologic and analytic assessment of 14 hearts from autopsy. J Am Coll Cardiol 1987;10:1239.
356. Fitchett DH, Coltart DJ, Littler WA, et al. Cardiac involvement in secondary hemochromatosis. Cardiovasc Res 1980;14:7199.
357. Rahko PS, Salerni R, Uretsky BF. Successful reversal by chelation therapy of congestive cardiomyopathy due to iron overload. J Am Coll Cardiol 1986;8:436.
358. Henry WL, Neinhuis AW, Wiener M, Miller DR, Canale VC, Piomelli S. Echocardiographic abnormalities in patients with transfusion-dependent anemia and secondary myocardial iron deposition. Am J Med 1978;64:547.
359. Walton C, Kelly WF, Laing I, Bulock E. Endocrine abnormalities in idiopathic haemochromatosis. Q J Med 1983;205:99.
360. Schafer AI, Cheron RG, Dluhy R, et al. Clinical consequences of acquired transfusion overload in adults. N Engl J Med 1981;304:319.
361. Bezwoda WR, Bothwell TH, Van der Walt LA, Srohnheim S, Pimstone BL. An investigation into gonadal dysfunction in patients with idiopathic haemochromatosis. Clin Endocrinol 1976;6:377.
362. Schafer AI, Cheron RG, Dluhy R, et al. Clinical consequences of acquired transfusional iron overload in adults. N Engl J Med 1981;304: 319.
363. Gertner JM, Broadus AE, Anast CS, Grey M, Pearson H, Genel M. Impaired parathroid response to induced hypocalcemia in thalassemia major. J Pediatr 1979;95:210.
364. Tsuji T. Experimental hemosiderosis: relationship between skin pigmentation and hemosiderosis. Acta Dermatol Venereol (Stockh) 1980;60:109.
365. Isaacson C, Bothwell TH. Synovial iron deposits in black subjects with iron overload. Arch Pathol Lab Med 1981;105:487.
366. Weinberg ED. Iron and infection. Microb Rev 1978;2:46.
367. Weinberg ED. Iron, infection and neoplasia. Clin Physiol Biochem 1985;4:50.
368. Bridges KR. Transfusion medicine. Cambridge, MA, Blackwell Scientific Publications, 1988:129.
369. Rex JH, Ginsberg AM, Fries LF, Pass HI, Kwon-Chung KJ. *Cunninghamella bertholletiae* infection associated with deferoxamine therapy. Rev Infect Dis 1988;10:1187.
370. Segaert MF. The role of desferioxamine in dialysis-associated mucormycosis: report of three cases and review of the literature. Clin Nephrol 1988;29:261.
371. Abbott M, Galloway A, Cunningham JL. Haemochromatosis presenting with a double *Yersinia* infection. J Infect 1986;13:143.
372. Christopher GW. *Escherichia coli* bacteremia, meningitis, and hemochromatosis. Arch Intern Med 1985;145:1908.
373. Brennan RO, Brain BJ, Proctor AM, Burack DT. *Cunninghamella*: a newly recognized cause of rhinocerebral mucomycosis. Am J Clin Pathol 1983;80:98.
374. Tsai J, Dyer DW, Sparling PF. Loss of transferrin receptor activity in *Neisseria meningitidis* correlates with inability to use transferrin as an iron source. Infect Immun 1988;56:3132.
375. Schryvers AB. Identification of the transferrin- and lactoferrin-binding proteins in *Haemophilus influenzae*. J Med Microbiol 1987;29:121.
376. Robins-Browne RM, Prpic JK. Effects of iron and desferrioxamine on infections with *Yersinia enterocolitica*. Infect Immun 1985;47:774.
377. Windus DW, Stokes TJ, Julian BA, Fenves AZ. Fatal *Rhizopus* infections in hemodialysis patients receiving deferoxamine. Ann Intern Med 1987;107:678.
378. McArdle HJ, Morgan EH. Transferrin and iron movements in the rat conceptus during gestation. J Reprod Fertil 1982;66:529.
379. Goldfischer S, Grotsky HW, Chang CH, et al. Idiopathic neonatal iron storage involving the liver, pancreas, heart, and endocrine and exocrine glands. Hepatology 1981;1:58.
380. Silver MM, Beverley DW, Valberg LS, Cutz E, Phillips MJ, Shaheed WA. Perinatal hemochromatosis: clinical, morphologic, and quantitative iron studies. Am J Pathol 1987;128:538.
381. Knisely AS, Harford JB, Klausner RD, Taylor SR. Neonatal hemochromatosis: the regulation of transferrin-receptor and ferritin synthesis by iron in cultured fibroblastic-line cells. Am J Pathol 1989;134: 439.
382. Dadone MM, Kushner JP, Edwards CQ, Bishop DT, Skolnick MH. Hereditary hemochromatosis: analysis of laboratory expression of the disease by genotype in 19 pedigrees. Am J Clin Pathol 1982;78:196.
383. Conte D, Brunelli L, Ferrario L, et al. Effect of ascorbic acid on desferrioxamine-induced urinary iron excretion in idiopathic hemochromatosis. Acta Haematol 1984;72:117.
384. Fairbanks VF, Warson MD, Beutler E. Drugs for iron overload. Br Med J 1963;1:1577.
385. Brown EB. Development of iron chelators for clinical use. New York, Elsevier/North-Holland, 1981:47.
386. Grady RW, Peterson CM, Jones RL, et al. Rhodotorulic acid: investigation of its potential as an iron-chelating drug. J Pharmacol Exp Ther 1979;209:342.
387. Keberle H. The biochemistry of desferrioxamine and its relation to iron metabolism. Ann NY Acad Sci 1964;119:758.
388. Pollack S, Aisen P, Lasky FD, Vanderhoff G. Celate-mediated transfer of iron from transferrin to desferrioxamine. Br J Haematol 1976;34: 21.
389. White GP, Jacobs A, Grady RW, Cerami A. The use of Chang cells cultured in vitro to evaluate potential iron chelating drugs. Br J Haematol 1976;33:487.
390. White GP, Bailey-Wood R, Jacobs A. The effect of chelating agents on cellular iron metabolism. Clin Sci Mol Med 1976;50:145.
391. Harris DC. Iron exchange between ferritin and transferrin in vitro. Biochemistry 1978;17:3071.
392. Bottomley SS, Wolfe LC, Bridges KR. Iron metabolism in K562 erythroleukemia cells. J Biol Chem 1985;260:6811.
393. Hershko C, Cook JD, Finch CA. Storage iron kinetics. III. Study of desferrioxamine action by selective radioiron labels of RE and parenchymal cells. J Lab Clin Med 1973;81:876.
394. Barry M, Flynn DM, Letsky EA, and Risdon RA. Long-term chelation therapy in thalassaemia major: effect on liver iron concentration, liver histology and clinical progress. Br Med J 1974;2:16.
395. Hussain MAM, Green N, Flynn DM, Hussein S, Hoffbrand AV. Subcutaneous infusion and intramuscular injection of desferrioxamine in patients with transfusional iron overload. Lancet 1976;2:1278.
396. Propper RD, Cooper B, Rufo RR, et al. Continuous subcutaneous administration of deferoxamine in patients with iron overload. N Engl J Med 1977;297:418.
397. Flynn DM, Hoffbrand AV, Politis D. Subcutaneous desferrioxamine:

the effect of three years' treatment on liver, iron, serum ferritin, and comments on echocardiography. Birth Defects 1982;18:347.
398. Wolfe L, Oliver N, Sallan D, et al. Prevention of cardiac disease by subcutaneous deferoxamine in patients with thalassemia major. N Engl J Med 1985;312:1600.
399. Falk RJ, Mattern WD, Lammanna RW, et al. Iron removal during continuous ambulatory peritoneal dialysis using deferoxamine. Kidney Int 1983;24:110.
400. Gomez RA, Campbell F, Savory J, Chevalier RL. Deferoxamine for the treatment of hemosiderosis during CAPD. Int J Pediatr Nephrol 1987;8:21.
401. Winearls CG, Oliver DO, Pippard MJ, Reid C, Downing MR, Cotes PM. Effect of human erythropoietin derived from recombinant DNA on the anaemia of patients maintained by chronic haemodialysis. Lancet 1986;2:1175.
402. Esbach JW, Egrie JC, Downing MR, Browne JK, Adamson JW. Correction of the anemia of end-stage renal disease with recombinant human erythropoietin. N Engl J Med 1987;316:73.
403. Deferoxamine. Drug Information for the Health Care Professional, U.C. Pharmacopeial Convention. Rockville, MD, 1988.
404. Davies SC, Marcus RE, Hungerfod JL, Miller MH, Arden GB, Huehns ER. Ocular toxicity of high dose intravenous desferrioxamine. Lancet 1983;2:181.
405. Olivieri NF, Buncic Jr, Chew E, et al. Visual and auditory neurotoxicity in patients receiving subcutaneous deferoxamine infusions. N Engl J Med 1986;314:869.
406. Porter JB, Gyparaki M, Burke LC, et al. Iron mobilization from hepatocyte monolayer cultures by chelators: the importance of membrane permeability and the iron-binding constant. Blood 1988;72:1497.
407. Huang AR, Ponka P. A study of the mechanism of action of pyridoxal isonicotinoyl hydrazone at the cellular level using reticulocytes loaded with non-heme ^{59}Fe. Biochem Biophys Acta 1983;757:306.
408. Ponka P, Grady RW, Wilcznska A, Schulman HM. The effect of various chelating agents on the mobilization of iron from reticulocytes in the presence and absence of pyridoxal isonicotinoyl hydrazone. Biochem Biophys Acta 1984;802:477.
409. Baker E, Vitolo ML, Webb J. Iron chelation by pyridoxal isonicotinoyl hydrazone and analogues in hepatocytes in culture. Biochem Pharmacol 1985;34:3011.
410. Callender ST, Weatherall DJ. Iron chelation with oral desferrioxamine. Lancet 1980;2:689.
411. Hershko C, Grady RW, Link G. Phenolic ethylenediamine derivatives: a study of orally effective iron chelators. J Lab Clin Med 1984;10:337.
412. Kontoghiorghes GJ. The study of iron mobilization from transferrin using alpha-ketohydroxy-heteroaromatic chelators. Biochim Biophys Acta 1986;869:141.
413. Westlin WF. Deferoxamine in the treatment of acute iron poisoning: clinical experiences with 172 children. Clin Pediatr 1966;5:531.
414. Greengard J, McEnery JT. Iron poisoning in children. Gen Pract 1968;37:88.
415. Whitten CF, Brough AJ. The pathophysiology of acute iron poisoning. Clin Toxicol 1971;4:585.

Blood: Principles and Practice of Hematology,
edited by Robert I. Handin, Samuel E. Lux, and Thomas P. Stossel.
J.B. Lippincott Company, Philadelphia © 1995.

50

Disorders of Heme Production and Catabolism

Shigeru Sassa and Attallah Kappas

HEME SYNTHESIS

Structure of Heme

Heme is a complex of an iron atom and a cyclic tetrapyrrole, protoporphyrin IX (Fig. 50-1). The iron atom is coordinated to the pyrrole rings of the porphyrin through the nitrogen atom in each ring. Pyrrolic rings are linked to each other through their α-carbon atoms by methene bridges. The rings are conventionally designated as A, B, C, and D, and the bridge carbons are labeled α, β, γ, and δ.[1] A revised nomenclature has also been recommended by the International Union of Applied Chemistry and the International Union of Biochemistry,[2] but it has rarely been used in medical literature.

Porphyrins are molecules of ancient derivation. For example, corrin, a porphyrin derivative that makes up the backbone of vitamin B_{12}, probably existed in early bacteria 3.8×10^9 years ago.[3] Structures of some porphyrins of biologic interest are shown in Figure 50-2. Uroporphyrin has acetic acid and propionic acid side chains on each ring; coproporphyrin has a methyl group and a propionic acid side chain on each ring. There are four possible isomers of these compounds. In isomer I, side chains are arranged symmetrically around the rings; in isomer III, the substituents on ring D are reversed. Only type I and III isomers of uroporphyrin and coproporphyrin occur in nature, and hemes, chlorophylls, and the corrin ring of vitamin B_{12} all have the type III structure. Protoporphyrin IX is derived from the type III coproporphyrinogen; it has both methyl and vinyl groups on rings A and B and both methyl and propionyl groups on rings C and D. Protoporphyrin IX is the only naturally occurring protoporphyrin of the 15 possible isomers. Substitutions or deletions at methene bridge carbons occur in vitamin B_{12} and in chlorophylls, but not in porphyrins or heme.[1]

Porphyrins are readily excited by light at around 400 nm (the region of the Soret band) and emit intense red fluorescence. In acidic solution, porphyrins display two strong emission bands, one at 590 to 610 nm and the other at 640 to 660 nm. Porphyrins are reduced in vitro by agents such as sodium amalgam and sodium borohydride to colorless, nonfluorescent hexahydroporphyrins (porphyrinogens). Porphyrinogens also occur in nature as the actual intermediates in the biosynthesis of heme. Free porphyrins occur only in small amounts in nature and have no known useful biologic functions.

The iron atom of heme (ferrous protoporphyrin IX) is readily autooxidized to form ferric protoporphyrin IX. The ferric complex has one residual positive charge and is generally isolated as a halide, usually as the chloride. Thus, heme in isolated form is usually hemin(chloride); in alkaline solution, it becomes hematin, in which the halide is replaced by a hydroxyl ion (Fig. 50-3). Ferrous protoporphyrin can form hexacoordinated complexes with nitrogenous bases, which are called *hemochromes* or *hemochromogens*. Hemochromogens, such as pyridine hemochromogen, have intense absorption in the region of 520 to 560 nm, arising from the ferroprotoporphyrin–pyridine complexes, and are useful for identifying and quantifying heme in biologic samples.

Ferrous ions have six electron pairs per atom. Thus, the ferrous atom in heme, bound to the pyrrolic nitrogens by four electron pairs, has two unoccupied electron pairs, one above and one below the plane of the porphyrin ring. In hemoglobin, one of these pairs is coordinated with a histidyl residue of the globin chain. This histidine is an essential residue found in all functionally active globins; when substituted with other amino acids, the resulting abnormal hemoglobins, termed *hemoglobin M*, have decreased oxygen affinity. The other coordination site of iron, the sixth coordination site, is open in deoxyhemoglobin and protected from oxidation by the nonpolar environment provided by the amino acid residues surrounding the heme moiety. This coordination position of the iron atom in hemoglobin is the site of oxygen binding. Iron in hemoglobin must be in the ferrous form for this binding to occur. Erythrocytes contain NADH-cytochrome b_5 reductase, which reduces methemoglobin (Fe^{3+}) to hemoglobin (Fe^{2+}).

Heme Biosynthetic Pathway

Outline of the Pathway

The heme biosynthetic pathway is illustrated in Figure 50-4. In higher organisms, the first step, which is the formation of δ-aminolevulinic acid (ALA), and the last three steps—the conversion of coproporphyrinogen to heme—take place in mitochondria; the intermediate steps take place in the cytosol. Thus, hemoglobin is made entirely in the precur-

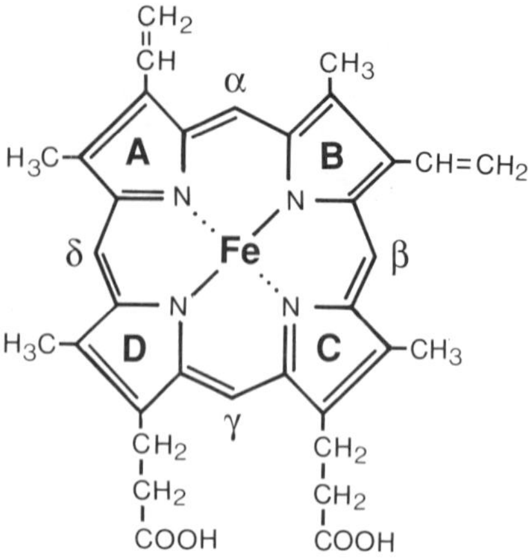

FIGURE 50-1. Structure of heme.

sors of erythrocytes, such as erythroblasts or reticulocytes, which still contain mitochondria. More detailed information on the biosynthesis of heme can be found in recent reviews.[4,5]

Formation of ALA From Glycine and Succinyl-CoA by ALA Synthase

ALA synthase (succinyl-CoA:glycine C succinyltransferase[decarboxylating]), the first enzyme of the pathway, catalyzes the condensation of glycine and succinyl-CoA (see Fig. 50-4, *step 1*) to form ALA; α-amino-β-ketoadipic acid is the presumed intermediate. Pyridoxal 5′-phosphate is a cofactor for the enzyme. In liver, ALA synthase activity is very low, and rate limiting for heme formation.[6–8] The turnover time of hepatic ALA synthase is rapid; for example, the half-life is 68 minutes for the rat liver enzyme, which is consistent with its rate-limiting nature.[9] In mam-

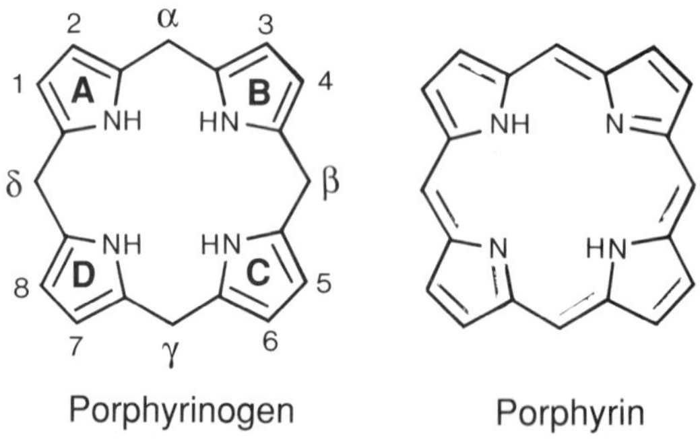

	1	2	3	4	5	6	7	8
Uroporphyrinogen I	A	P	A	P	A	P	A	P
Uroporphyrinogen III	A	P	A	P	A	P	P	A
Heptacarboxylate porphyrinogen	A	P	A	P	A	P	P	M
Hexacarboxylate porphyrinogen	M	P	A	P	A	P	P	M
Pentacarboxylate porphyrinogen	M	P	M	P	A	P	P	M
Isocoproporphyrinogen	M	E	M	P	A	P	P	M
Coproporphyrinogen I	M	P	M	P	M	P	M	P
Coproporphyrinogen III	M	P	M	P	M	P	P	M
Harderoporphyrinogen	M	V	M	P	M	P	P	M
Isoharderoporphyrinogen	M	P	M	V	M	P	P	M
Portoporphyrin(ogen)	M	V	M	V	M	P	P	M

M: $-CH_3$ V: $-CH{=}CH_2$ A: $-CH_2COOH$ P: $-CH_2CH_2OOH$ E: $-CH_2CH_3$

FIGURE 50-2. Structures of biologically important porphyrinogens and porphyrins.

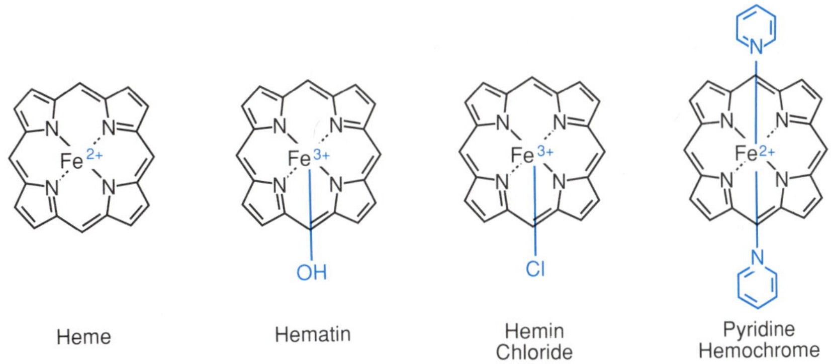

FIGURE 50-3. Heme and its derivatives.

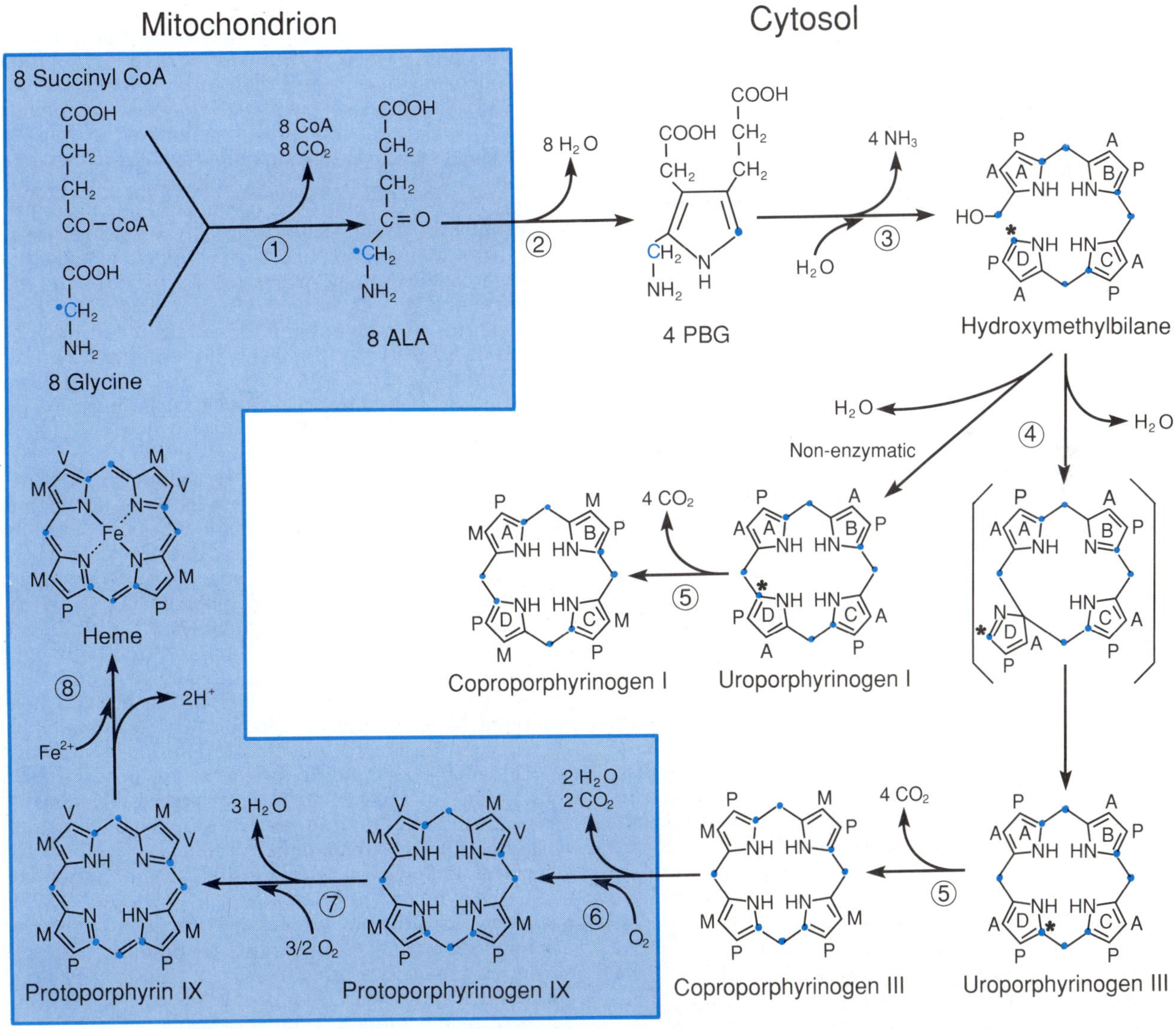

FIGURE 50-4. Enzymes and intermediates of the heme biosynthetic pathway. (*Step 1*) δ-Aminolevulinic acid synthase. (*Step 2*) ALA dehydratase. (*Step 3*) Porphobilinogen deaminase. (*Step 4*) Uroporphyrinogen III cosynthase. (*Step 5*) Uroporphyrinogen decarboxylase. (*Step 6*) Coproporphyrinogen oxidase. (*Step 7*) Protoporphyrinogen oxidase. (*Step 8*) Ferrochelatase. A, $-CH_2-COOH$; M, $-CH_3$; P, $-CH_2-CH_2-COOH$; V, $-CH{=}CH_2$. The carbon atom derived from the α carbon of glycine is shown in color. The structure denoted by the brackets after step 4 is the presumed intermediate whose pyrrole ring D becomes rearranged to yield uroporphyrinogen III. At step 7, 1 mol of oxygen is consumed per 1 mol of water produced.

malian liver, the enzyme is loosely bound to the inner membrane or is present in the matrix of mitochondria. The enzyme activity has been identified in many organisms and tissues.[4] Regulation of ALA synthase differs depending on tissue site, and the enzyme may not always be rate-limiting for heme formation in nonhepatic tissues.

ALA formation that does not involve glycine and succinyl-CoA has been described in plants and algae and also in mammalian livers.[10–12] In this reaction, the intact carbon skeleton of glutamate is used for the synthesis of ALA, and C_1 of glutamate becomes C_5 of ALA. This is the major route of synthesis of ALA in plants and algae, but its significance in mammalian cells is not clear.

Properties. Hepatic ALA synthase purified from several sources has K_m values for glycine, succinyl-CoA, and pyridoxal 5′-phosphate in the range of 5 to 19 mmol/L, 60 to 200 μmol/L, and 1 to 10 μmol/L, respectively.[4] The relatively high K_m (low affinity) for glycine suggests that alterations in glycine concentrations in the physiologic range could regulate the enzyme.[13] The V_{max} of liver ALA synthase purified from various sources is in the range of 2000 to 20,000 nmol/h/mg protein.[14,15]

ALA synthase represents less than 0.005% by weight of total liver protein.[14] The mature enzymes from chick embryo liver and rat liver mitochondria have similar molecular weights.[16,17] The enzyme synthesized in vitro using rat liver polysomes has a molecular weight of 73 kd, which is considerably larger than that of the mitochondrial enzyme.[18]

Hepatic ALA synthase is encoded by a nuclear gene and is synthesized on free cytoplasmic polyribosomes as a cytosolic precursor. The exact molecular weights of the precursor and the mature mitochondrial enzyme in the chick embryo liver have been deduced from their cDNAs to be 70,029 and 63,903 daltons, respectively.[19] The enzyme apparently exists as a dimer of molecular weight 140 kd.[16] Electron micrographic studies of the purified enzyme protein suggest that it consists of two curved and identical subunits associated in opposite polarities[20] (Fig. 50-5). The precursor contains an N-terminal extension of 56 amino acids. The presequence of ALA synthase is processed during transfer into mitochondria to yield the mature enzyme,[19] presumably by matrix-localized proteases.[21] Incorporation of the precursor into mitochondria with processing to the mature enzyme and inhibition of the translocation by hemin can be demonstrated in vitro.[22]

From DNA sequence comparison, mRNA distribution, relative abundance of mRNA, and genetic mapping of genomic loci encoding the mRNAs, it has been shown that at least two separate genes encode ALA synthase mRNAs in avian cells[23]; that is, the genes for the ALA synthase isozymes in erythroid and liver tissues are different. The product of the erythroid gene is expressed solely in erythroid cells; the hepatic gene is expressed ubiquitously.[23]

Reaction Mechanism. Using ALA synthase purified from *Rhodopseudomonas spheroides*, the following reaction mechanism has been proposed[24–26]:

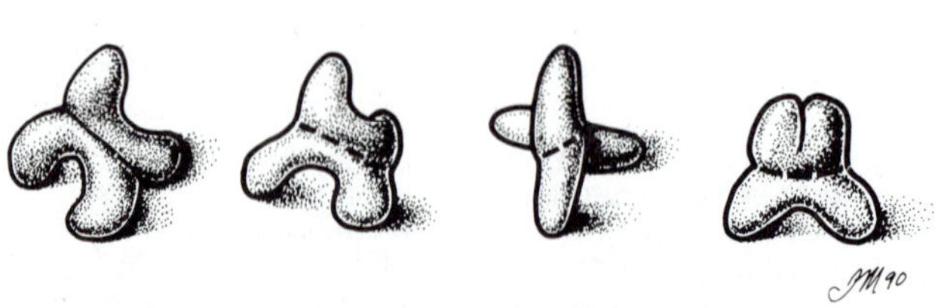

FIGURE 50-5. A proposed structure model of ALA synthase. The model consists of two curved subunits of identical size, attached to each other in opposite polarities. (After Pirola BA, Mayer F, Borthwick IA, et al. Electron microscopic studies on liver δ-aminolevulinate synthase. Eur J Biochem 1984;144:577)

- Glycine forms a Schiff base with pyridoxal 5′-phosphate, which is bound to the enzyme yielding a stable carbanion
- A proton (R configuration) is removed from the methylene carbon atom of glycine
- Succinyl-CoA condenses to the carbon ion to form α-amino-β-ketoadipic acid, with loss of CoA
- α-Amino-β-ketoadipic acid is decarboxylated to yield ALA

Decarboxylation occurs on the enzyme, and ALA is then released from the pyridoxal–enzyme complex.[2]

Formation of Porphobilinogen From ALA by ALA Dehydratase

Two molecules of ALA are converted by a cytosolic enzyme, ALA dehydratase (δ-aminolevulinate hydrolase; porphobilinogen [PBG] synthase) to a monopyrrole, PBG, with the removal of two molecules of water (see Fig. 50-4, *step 2*). ALA dehydratase has been isolated from animals,[27] plants,[28] and bacteria.[29] The bovine liver and human erythrocyte enzymes have a molecular weight of 285 kd[30] and 252 kd,[31] respectively, with each having eight identical subunits.[31,32] The enzyme in mammalian erythrocytes and liver requires sulfhydryl compounds such as reduced glutathione or dithiothreitol,[31–33] as well as Zn^{2+}, for maximal activity.[31,34] ALA dehydratase contains 1 atom of Zn per 1 mol of subunit.[35,36] Its activity is quickly lost when the sulfhydryl groups of the enzyme are inactivated by oxidation, or by mercaptide formation, or when Zn^{2+} is displaced from the enzyme.[35]

ALA forms a covalent bond to the enzyme through formation of a Schiff base between the ε-amino group of a lysine residue and the keto group of ALA.[37] The ALA molecule initially bound to the enzyme contributes to the propionic acid side chain of PBG.[38]

ALA dehydratases purified from different mammalian tissues are remarkably similar[39]; K_m values for ALA are 1 to 4×10^{-4} mol/L; V_{max} values are 20 to 24 μmol/h/mg protein, 37°C. No tissue-specific isozymes of ALA dehydratase or strain-specific differences are found in mice and rats.[40,41] There is a clear species specificity of the enzyme consistent with phylogenetic development.[40]

ALA dehydratase activity is subject to inhibition by lead,[42] levulinic acid,[43] hemin,[44,45] and succinylacetone (4,6-dioxoheptanoic acid).[46,47] Among other agents lead inhibits the enzyme by displacing Zn^{2+} from the protein. Lead-inhibited ALA dehydratase can be completely reactivated by the addition of Zn^{2+} or dithiothreitol or both, both of which reduce the binding of lead to the enzyme.[42] The most potent inhibitor of the enzyme is probably succinylacetone, which is found in the urine and blood of patients with hereditary tyrosinemia.[46–48] Succinylacetone is a structural analogue of ALA (Fig. 50-6); its inhibition constant for the bovine enzyme is 5×10^{-8} M, which is about $1/_{10,000}$ the K_m of the enzyme for ALA.[49]

Erythrocyte ALA dehydratase in humans and mice shows a three- to four-fold range of enzyme activity among individuals. In contrast, identical twins, or mice from the same strain, have similar values of enzyme activity.[50] These findings strongly suggest genetic control of the enzyme synthesis in humans as well as in experimental animals.

The enzyme activity in erythroid cells changes during erythroid cell maturation. The activity increases early and sharply during erythroid differentiation and precedes the appearance of hemoglobin.[51–53] It falls with the maturation of reticulocytes into erythrocytes.[54] For example, ALA dehydratase activity in mouse reticulocytes is about 15 times higher than in erythrocytes. A similar decline of the en-

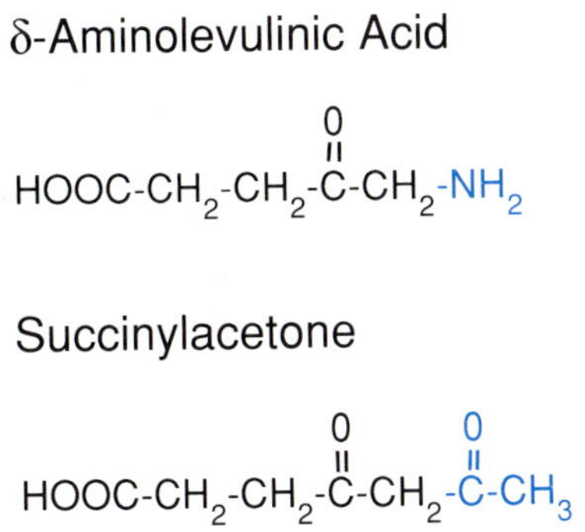

FIGURE 50-6. Structural formulae of ALA and succinylacetone. Succinylacetone (4,6-dioxoheptanoic acid) is a structural analogue of ALA and a potent inhibitor of ALA dehydratase. (After Kappas A, Sassa S, Galbraith RA, Nordmann Y. The porphyrias. In: Scriver CR, Beaudet AL, Sly WS, Valle D, eds. The metabolic basis of inherited disease. New York, McGraw-Hill, 1989;1305)

zyme activity with red blood cell (RBC) age is observed in human RBCs.[55]

Sequence determination of cDNA clones encoding human ALA dehydratase revealed an open reading frame of 990–base pair (bp) coding for a protein of molecular weight of 36,274. Extensive homologies exist between sequences of human and bovine ALA dehydratase peptides[56] and between human and rat liver nucleotide sequences of the cDNA coding for ALA dehydratase.[57,58] The sequences corresponding to the active lysine residue at the catalytic site and the cysteine- and histidine-rich Zn^{2+} binding site of the protein were identified.[59]

Formation of Hydroxymethylbilane From PBG by PBG Deaminase

PBG deaminase (porphobilinogen ammonia-lyase [polymerizing]; hydroxymethylbilane synthase) catalyzes the condensation of four PBG molecules to yield a linear tetrapyrrole, hydroxymethylbilane.[60,61] In this reaction, 4 units of PBG are assembled head to tail, starting with ring A followed by rings B, C, and D (see Fig. 50-4, *step 3*). In the absence of the subsequent enzyme, uroporphyrinogen III cosynthase, the bilane is released into the medium as hydroxymethylbilane,[61] which then spontaneously cyclizes into the first tetrapyrrole, uroporphyrinogen I. This enzyme is frequently referred to as *uroporphyrinogen I synthase*. This term should not be used, since the enzyme furnishes a straight-chain tetrapyrrole, not a cyclic tetrapyrrole.[62]

PBG deaminase purified from human erythrocytes forms stable covalent complexes bearing up to four PBG molecules.[63] It was also shown that erythrocyte-specific and tissue-specific enzymes show different migration in isoelectric focusing[64] and in sodium dodecyl sulfate-polyacrylamide gel electrophoresis.[65] These findings suggest that there are erythroid- and tissue-specific isozymes of PBG deaminase.

Properties. PBG deaminase purified from human erythrocytes has a specific activity of about 2300 nmol uroporphyrinogen per hour per milligram of protein.[63] The pH optimum of the enzyme is 8.2, and the K_m is 6 μmol/L. Molecular weights of deaminases from human and other sources are in the range of 36 to 40 kd.[63,66,67] PBG deaminase appears more stable when bound to its substrate than when free.[68] The gene locus encoding the human enzyme has been assigned to chromosome 11q23 → 11qter.[69,70]

Molecular cloning and the complete primary sequence of cDNA complementary to human PBG deaminase have been reported.[71,72] Human PBG deaminase cDNA encodes 344 amino acids and accounts for a protein of molecular weight 37,627.[73] Southern blot analysis of human genomic restriction fragments is compatible with the existence of only one gene coding for the enzyme.

Two distinct molecular forms of PBG deaminase were identified in mouse erythroleukemia cells by gel electrophoresis.[74] The heavier (44 kd) corresponds to a nonerythroid enzyme, whereas the lighter (42 kd) represents an erythroid-specific form. Similar findings were obtained in human cells.[65] Analysis of cell-free translation products directed by mRNAs from human erythropoietic spleen and human liver showed that the two isoforms of PBG deaminase were encoded by distinct mRNAs. Comparison of the sequences from human erythroid mRNA[71] with those of nonerythroid (lymphoblastoid cells) mRNA[65] revealed a 1320-bp stretch of near-identity; the two mRNA species differed at their 5′ extremities; and an additional in-frame AUG codon was found 51 bp upstream from the initiating codon of the nonerythroid cDNA. It could be deduced that a peptide of 17 amino acid residues at the NH_2 terminal of the nonerythroid isoform accounts for its higher molecular mass. From human cell type studies, it is clear that the presence of the erythroid type of mRNA is exclusively restricted to cells of erythroid lineage. The generation of alternative mRNAs from a single gene arises from two overlapping transcription units.[75] The first (upstream) is active in all tissues and its promoter has some structural features of a housekeeping promoter, whereas the second (3 kb downstream) is active only in erythroid cells and its promoter has structural homology to β-globin gene promoters.

PBG deaminase activity is decreased in the tissues of patients with acute intermittent porphyria (AIP). The enzyme deficiency is usually about 50% of the normal level, and the deficiency has been identified in erythrocytes,[50,76–78] skin fibroblasts,[79–81] liver,[82,83] lymphocytes,[84] and amniotic cells.[79] In some AIP families, the PBG deaminase deficiency seems restricted to nonerythroid tissues.[85] The defect in the PBG deaminase gene in this type of AIP is due to a single-base substitution (G → A) in the canonical 5′ splice donor site of intron 1.[86] This mutation results in abnormal splicing, leading to a detrimental effect on the gene product in nonerythroid cells; it does not affect the transcription of the erythroid PBG deaminase mRNA, since transcription of the erythroid mRNA starts about 3 kb downstream from the mutated site.[86]

Formation of Uroporphyrinogen III From Hydroxymethylbilane by Uroporphyrinogen III Cosynthase

Uroporphyrinogen III cosynthase catalyzes the formation of uroporphyrinogen III from hydroxymethylbilane (see Fig. 50-4, *step 4*). This involves an intramolecular reversal of ring D. Evidence suggests an association of the deaminase and cosynthase molecules, which would account for the rapid formation of uroporphyrinogen III.[87–89] Normal human erythrocytes[90] and mouse spleen[91] contain an excess of the cosynthase relative to the deaminase activity, which favors predominant synthesis of type III uroporphyrinogen. In erythrocytes from patients with congenital erythropoietic porphyria (CEP), or from cattle with CEP, cosynthase activity is greatly reduced (about 40% of normal),[91,92] and the disease is accompanied by overproduction of uroporphyrinogen I.

Properties. Uroporphyrinogen cosynthase purified to homogeneity from human erythrocytes has a specific activity of more than 300,000 nmol of uroporphyrinogen III formed per hour per milligram of protein and is thermolabile (half-life at 60°C at about 1 minute).[93] Gel filtration and analytical gel electrophoresis studies indicate that the enzyme is a monomer (molecular weight of 30 kd). The K_m for hydroxymethylbilane is 5 to 20 μmol/L.

Formation of Coproporphyrinogen From Uroporphyrinogen by Uroporphyrinogen Decarboxylase

Uroporphyrinogen decarboxylase catalyzes sequential removal of the carboxylic groups of the four acetic acid side chains in uroporphyrinogen to yield coproporphyrinogen (see Fig. 50-4, *step* 5). The enzyme decarboxylates all four isomers of uroporphyrinogen, but the naturally abundant type III isomer is decarboxylated most rapidly, followed by the type IV, II, and I isomers in decreasing order.[94,95] Only one enzyme catalyzes the four successive decarboxylation steps from the eight carboxylic uroporphyrinogens to the four carboxylic coproporphyrinogens.[96] The reaction catalyzed by purified uroporphyrinogen decarboxylase yields all of the intermediates from uroporphyrinogen (heptacarboxylate, hexacarboxylate, pentacarboxylate and tetracarboxylate porphyrinogens).[97,98]

Properties. Uroporphyrinogen decarboxylase is active only on porphyrinogen substrates and does not require a cofactor.[99] With uroporphyrinogen III as substrate, the decarboxylations on each pyrrolic ring proceed in a clockwise fashion starting from ring D (see Fig. 50-4, *step* 5). All series III isomers have a higher affinity for the enzyme than the corresponding series I isomers. The affinity of the enzyme for the substrate decreases with each decline in the number of carboxylic groups in the substrate.[97] Type I and type III porphyrinogens with the same number of carboxylic groups are decarboxylated at the same active center, whereas decarboxylation of porphyrinogen substrates with different numbers of carboxylic groups appears to occur at different active centers.[97] Uroporphyrinogen decarboxylase purified from human erythrocytes has a molecular weight of 46 kd and a specific activity of 9970 nmol coproporphyrinogen formed/h/mg protein using uroporphyrinogen III as substrate.[96] Enzyme activity is sensitive to sulfhydryl modification. The direct effect of iron on the enzyme remains controversial. Using a purified enzyme preparation, it has been reported that the enzyme activity is uninhibited by Fe^{2+} and Fe^{3+},[96,100] inhibited by Fe^{2+},[101] or stimulated by Fe^{2+}.[102] Clear evidence is seen that in vivo iron potentiates inhibition of uroporphyrinogen decarboxylase by 2,3,7,8-tetrachloro-dibenzo-*p*-dioxin (TCDD)[103] and hexachlorobenzene.[104] This synergism may depend on the ability of divalent iron to catalyze peroxidative and free radical reactions.[105]

The enzyme activity is decreased in the liver of patients with porphyria cutanea tarda (PCT)[98,106] as well as in erythrocytes in most patients with familial PCT[107,108] and is also reduced in the liver of rats fed hexachlorobenzene.[109–111] Uroporphyrinogen decarboxylase in rat liver has a long half-life and does not show decay for at least 10 hours after treatment with cycloheximide.[112] Iron removal by venesection is known to be highly beneficial in the treatment of patients with PCT,[113–115] presumably decreasing free radical reactions. An experimental porphyria inducible with TCDD in mice does not occur in animals made iron deficient by phlebotomy.[103] Rats with genetic[104] or acquired[116,117] siderosis are more susceptible to hexachlorobenzene-induced porphyria than nonsiderotic rats. A gene locus encoding human uroporphyrinogen decarboxylase has been assigned to chromosome 1 pter→p21.[118]

cDNA sequences complementary to uroporphyrinogen decarboxylase mRNA from rats and humans have been cloned.[71,119] The deduced molecular weight of the human enzyme was 40,831, in good agreement with the value of 42 kd estimated by sodium dodecyl sulfate-polyacrylamide gel electrophoresis. Southern blot analysis of human genomic DNA suggests that the uroporphyrinogen decarboxylase gene is present as a single copy in the human genome. Northern blot analysis shows the presence of a single-size species of mRNA in erythroid and nonerythroid tissues; the level of uroporphyrinogen decarboxylase mRNA is higher in erythroid than in nonerythroid tissues, suggesting that the enzyme expression is differentially regulated at a pretranslational level in a tissue-specific manner.

Formation of Protoporphyrinogen From Coproporphyrinogen by Coproporphyrinogen Oxidase

Coproporphyrinogen oxidase (coproporphyrinogen: oxygen oxidoreductase [decarboxylating]) in mammalian cells is a mitochondrial enzyme that catalyzes removal of the carboxyl group and two hydrogens from the propionic groups of pyrrole rings A and B of coproporphyrinogen to form vinyl groups at these positions (see Fig. 50-4, *step* 6). The reaction thus yields a divinyl compound, protoporphyrinogen.[120]

This mitochondrial enzyme is easily solubilized without use of detergent[121–123] and evidently is not membrane-bound. Using a technique for preferentially rupturing the outer mitochondrial membrane,[124] coproporphyrinogen oxidase was shown to be localized to the intermembrane space of rat liver mitochondria.[125,126] The intermembrane localization of coproporphyrinogen oxidase implies that either protoporphyrinogen or protoporphyrin must cross the inner membrane where heme is formed.

Purified coproporphyrinogen oxidase from bovine liver has a molecular weight of 71 to 74 kd[127]; the enzyme has a specific activity of 6920 nmol protoporphyrinogen formed per hour per milligram of protein and a K_m of 48 μmol/L for coproporphyrinogen III. Oxygen is an absolute requirement for the enzymatic function. This oxidase is unusual in that it does not contain any metal atom.[127]

The decarboxylation of coproporphyrinogen by the enzyme proceeds only at the β-carbon atom at the propionate side chains, with a stereospecific loss of one of the hydrogen atoms.[128,129] An intermediate 3-carboxylate porphyrinogen, termed *harderoporphyrinogen*, in the decarboxylation of hydroxypropionic porphyrin to protoporphyrin has also been isolated. The corresponding porphyrin was originally isolated from the harderian gland of rodents, which is an orbital structure associated with the nictitating membrane.[130]

Formation of Protoporphyrin From Protoporphyrinogen by Protoporphyrinogen Oxidase

The oxidation of protoporphyrinogen to protoporphyrin is mediated by protoporphyrinogen oxidase, which catalyzes removal of six hydrogen atoms from the porphyrinogen nucleus (see Fig. 50-4, *step* 7).

Properties. The enzyme that catalyzes this oxidation step has been identified in many cells and tissues.[131] Protoporphyrinogen oxidase has been purified from rat liver mitochondria and has a molecular weight of 35 kd, a K_m of 11 μmol/L, a V_{max} of 8.7 nmol/min/mg protein, and an absolute requirement for oxygen. The enzyme acts specifically on protoporphyrinogen and does not catalyze the oxidation of coproporphyrinogen I or III or uroporphyrinogen I. Hemin (50 μmol/L) inhibits the enzyme activity by about 50%; the inhibition is apparently noncompetitive and irreversible.[132] Fibroblasts from patients with variegate porphyria, but not from patients with erythropoietic protoporphyria (EPP), have decreased levels of protoporphyrinogen oxidase activity.[133]

Formation of Heme From Protoporphyrinogen by Ferrochelatase

The final step of heme biosynthesis involves the insertion of iron into protoporphyrin (see Fig. 50-4, *step 8*). This reaction is catalyzed by the enzyme ferrochelatase (heme synthase, heme synthetase or protoheme-ferrolyase).

Properties. Ferrochelatase in mammalian cells is localized to the inner membrane of mitochondria. The enzyme activity is also found in plant chloroplasts and chromatophores of photosynthetic bacteria. Unlike other enzymatic steps in the heme biosynthetic pathway that utilize porphyrinogens, ferrochelatase utilizes protoporphyrin as substrate. In addition to protoporphyrin, other 2-carboxylate porphyrins such as deuteroporphyrin and mesoporphyrin serve as good substrates for the enzyme in vitro.[134–136] Only the reduced form of iron (Fe^{2+}) is incorporated into protoporphyrin by the enzyme.[136] Co^{2+} and Zn^{2+} are more efficient enzyme substrates than Fe^{2+}.[135] Therefore, various rates of ferrochelatase activity are obtained, depending on which metal and porphyrin substrates are used.[135]

Ferrochelatase has been purified to apparent homogeneity from rat liver mitochondria.[137,138] The molecular weight of the enzyme was reported to be either 63[137] or 42 kd,[138] as determined by sodium dodecyl sulfate-polyacrylamide gel electrophoresis. The purified rat liver has a specific activity of 3500 nmol heme formed per 30 minutes per milligram of protein and a K_m of 28.5 μmol/L. These properties were determined using iron and protoporphyrin as substrates.[138] The enzyme activity (using iron as the metal substrate) is markedly stimulated by fatty acids, whereas it is inhibited by metals such as Co, Zn, Pb, Cu, or Mn.[138] Human liver mitochondrial membranes contain large amounts of endogenous metals, especially Zn^{2+}, which act as substrates for ferrochelatase, thus competing with iron and leading to a lack of linearity of the activity as a function of protein concentration.[139]

Biochemical Findings. Ferrochelatase deficiency has been reported in tissues from patients with EPP (about 20% of normal levels)[140,141] and from cattle with the same disorder (5% to 10% of normal).[142] The cattle disease is inherited as an autosomal recessive trait, whereas the human disease is inherited as an autosomal dominant trait. Ferrochelatase deficiency in EPP can be functionally demonstrated in cultured lymphocytes from human patients[143] or in skin fibroblasts from affected cattle.[144] In the cattle disease, gene dosage-dependent protoporphyrin accumulation was demonstrated when cells were incubated with ALA.[144]

Control of Heme Synthesis

Regulation of Hepatic ALA Synthase

Biosynthesis of heme in the liver is controlled largely by the rate of formation of ALA synthase.[7,8] The enzyme activity in normal liver is very low, whereas it increases dramatically when the liver needs to make more heme in response to various chemical treatments.[145] Hepatic ALA synthase turnover is rapid; for example, half-life is 68 min in rat liver,[146] which is considerably shorter than the half-life of other mitochondrial proteins. Synthesis of the enzyme is regulated in a feedback fashion by heme.[147] At higher heme concentrations than those that repress the synthesis of ALA synthase, heme induces microsomal heme oxygenase, resulting in an enhancement of its own catabolism.[148] Thus, it can be visualized that the hepatic heme concentration is maintained by a balance between the syntheses of ALA synthase and heme oxygenase, both of which are under the regulatory influence of heme. The regulatory effect of heme is thought to be exerted by a small pool of free heme, for example, 10 to 100 nmol/L, rather than by general heme or hemeprotein content in hepatocytes.[149]

Control by Free Heme. Evidence for the regulation of ALA synthase by heme was first deduced by studies with chemicals known to deplete the cellular heme pool either by destroying the heme moiety of cytochrome P-450 or by inhibiting the biosynthesis of heme. Thus, in experiments with animals treated with 3,5-diethoxycarbonyl-1,4-dihydrocollidine (DDC), hepatic ALA synthase activity was markedly increased; similar induction of ALA synthase was demonstrated in animals treated with 2-allyl-2-isopropylacetamide (AIA),[150] allyl-containing barbiturates,[151] and griseofulvin.[152] Using cultured chick embryo hepatocytes, it was shown that ALA synthase levels in the cells were markedly increased when cells were treated with a number of drugs, chemicals, or steroids, and that the increase of the enzyme was prevented by hemin.[7,153,154] More recently, alterations in the level of hepatic ALA synthase activity after drug or hemin treatment of chick embryos have been shown to be accompanied by similar changes in immunoprecipitable ALA synthase protein.[155] Experimental evidence suggests that regulation of hepatic ALA synthase activity by heme occurs at four different levels: enzyme activity, transport of the precursor, translation, and transcription.[4]

The regulatory role of heme in the synthesis of ALA synthase and in the induction of heme oxygenase can be best explained by assuming one or more free heme pools (Fig. 50-7). Free heme can be defined as heme that is newly synthesized and has not been incorporated into hemeproteins, or heme that has recently been released from hemeproteins and not immediately reutilized or catabolized. Conceptionally, free heme pools should exist at least in mitochondria, cytosol, and endoplasmic reticulum. All free heme pools are presumed to be small and to turn over rapidly. With respect to their rapid turnover, a certain proportion of hepatic heme is known to be rapidly labeled (1 to 2 hour) after pulse labeling with [^{14}C]glycine in the rat.[156] The appearance of the radiolabeled heme is so rapid that it probably cannot be derived from the turnover of hemeproteins.[8] In cultured rat hepatocytes, as much as 20% of newly synthesized heme appears to be directly converted to bilirubin without being incorporated into hemeproteins.[157]

Regulatory heme can be considered as that specific fraction of free heme that represses the synthesis of ALA synthase or induces heme oxygenase. Because both enzymes are encoded by nuclear genes, it is possible that free heme may also be in the nucleus. The presence of heme in the nucleus and its potential influence on gene expression have been demonstrated in mouse erythroleukemia (MEL) cells.[158]

It has been proposed that cytosolic free heme is closely associated with tryptophan pyrrolase, but not with microsomal cytochrome P-450.[159] Tryptophan pyrrolase in rat liver exists in two forms—heme-free apoenzyme and heme-saturated holoenzyme—and the holoenzyme catalyzes the oxidative cleavage of the pyrrole ring of L-tryptophan to yield N^1-formylkynurenine. Inhibition of heme synthesis, increased destruction of heme, and increased utilization of heme all decrease the saturation of tryptophan pyrrolase and thus the activity of the enzyme.

Regulation of ALA Synthase in Erythroid Cells

Studies using a variety of model systems suggest that distinct regulatory features of heme synthesis are in erythroid cells, compared with that found in hepatic cells, particu-

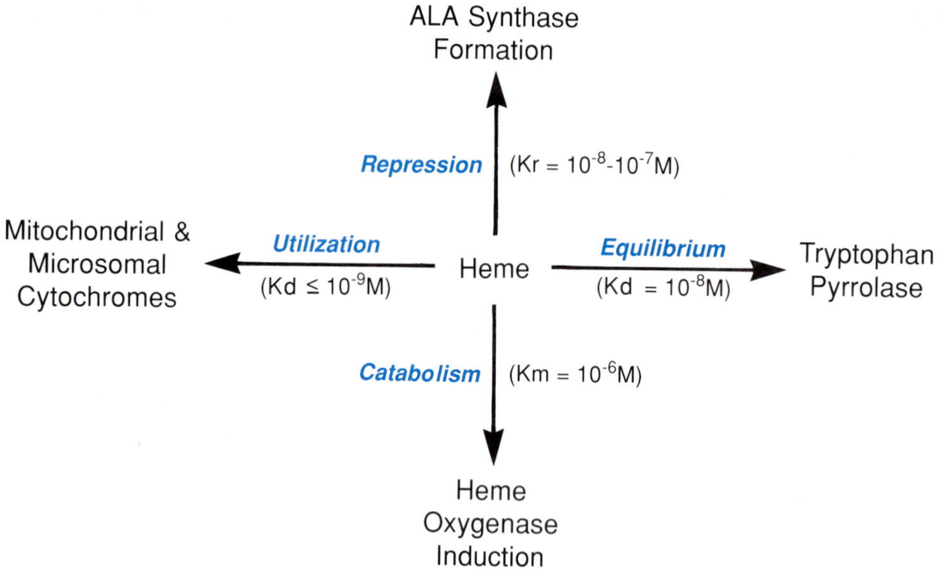

FIGURE 50-7. Regulation of hepatic ALA synthase by free heme. Regulatory free heme in the cytosol is considered to be in equilibrium with the heme moiety of tryptophan pyrrolase. Its concentration, which can be determined only by indirect methods, has been reported to be 10^{-8} to 10^{-7} mol/L. Regulatory heme may inhibit (1) the activity of ALA synthase, (2) the transport of the precursor into mitochondria, (3) translation, and (4) transcription of the mRNA for ALA synthase in the liver. Repression of transcription appears to be most important. Increased utilization of heme for hemoprotein synthesis, increased catabolism of heme by heme oxygenase, and enzyme defects in the porphyrias all contribute to increased production of hepatic ALA synthase.

larly at the level of ALA synthase,[51,53,160–162] and that this pathway is controlled in a different manner than that in the liver.

The kinetic and ligand-binding properties of guinea pig hepatic and erythroid ALA synthase are different.[41] Chicken erythroid ALA synthase is synthesized as a 55 kd precursor, which is then processed to a 53 kd form during transport into mitochondria.[18] These molecular weights are different from their liver enzyme counterparts. Immunologic studies on chicken[18] and rat[163] ALA synthase in liver and erythroid cells provide the most compelling evidence for the isozymic nature of the enzyme in these tissues, since there is a complete lack of antibody cross-reactivity between ALA synthase in erythroid and hepatic tissues.[18]

cDNA clones encoding ALA synthase have been isolated from a chicken erythroid cDNA library.[163] The mRNA encoding this enzyme species was about 2000 bp in length and was expressed in liver, brain, and especially erythroid cells. Based on these findings, it was suggested that ALA synthase isozymes are encoded by a multigene family that is subject to different developmental stimuli and regulation.[164]

In contrast to the regulation of hepatic ALA synthase, which is principally transcriptional, the level of ALA synthase protein in MEL cells during erythroid differentiation appears to be regulated by a major posttranscriptional mechanism.[165] Transcription of the ALA synthase gene and mRNA levels were both significantly increased during erythroid differentiation of cells induced by dimethyl sulfoxide, but were not markedly altered by succinylacetone or hemin treatment. These findings indicate that levels of ALA synthase in MEL cells are regulated by a significant posttranscriptional mechanism, possibly at the translational level. Thus, the regulation of ALA synthase in differentiating erythroblasts is complex, but clearly differs from that in liver cells.

Recently, it has been demonstrated that there are two separate genes encoding ALA synthases—erythroid-specific (ALAS-E) and nonspecific (ALAS-N) isoforms[23]; each is under separate control. The human ALAS-E gene encodes a precursor of 587 amino acids, with a molecular weight of 64.6 kd. Nucleotide sequences for the ALAS-E and ALAS-N isoforms are about 60% similar; there is no homology in the amino-terminal region, whereas there is a high homology (about 73%) after the hepatic residue 197.[165a] The gene locus for the human ALAS-N is at 3p.21; that for the erythroid ALA synthase is at Xp11.21.[165b]

The promoter in the human ALAS-E gene contains several putative erythroid-specific *cis*-acting elements, including both a GATA-1 and an NF-E2 binding site.[165c] Both GATA-1 and NF-E2 are erythroid-specific transcription factors that bind to multiple DNA sites such as the promoter of the human β-globin gene and the erythroid porphobilinogen deaminase gene.[165d] Additionally, ALAS-E mRNA contains an iron-responsive element (IRE) in its 5′ untranslated region,[165c,165e] similar to mRNAs encoding ferritin[165f] and transferrin receptor,[165g] suggesting that translation of ALAS-E mRNA can be upregulated by the availability of iron, or heme, in erythroid cells.[165h] In contrast to ALAS-N, which is regulated in a feedback manner by heme,[22,149] ALAS-E in erythroid cells has in fact been shown to be upregulated by hemin treatment.[165e,165i] Thus, the regulation of heme synthesis in erythroid cells is distinct from that in the liver.[165j]

Hemin was also reported to increase the formation of hemoglobin in normal mouse bone marrow cultures.[166] Increases in ALA synthase and heme synthesis in response to hemin treatment in normal and virus-transformed erythroid cells are in striking contrast to the inhibitory effect of hemin on these indices in the liver.

Several studies suggest the importance of ferrochelatase, the terminal enzyme in the heme biosynthetic pathway, in hemoglobin formation in erythroid cells. For example:

1. Hemoglobin formation does not occur until ^{59}Fe incorporation into heme is increased in MEL cells.[51]
2. Hemin, but not ALA, PBG, or protoporphyrin, can increase hemoglobin in MEL cells.[167–169]
3. In the mutant clone of MEL cells, which displays normal induction of ALA synthase, ALA dehydratase, and PBG deaminase but which is unable to make hemoglobin after treatment with dimethyl sulfoxide, simultaneous treatment of cells with dimethyl sulfoxide and hemin can correct for the defect of hemoglobin formation.[160,161]
4. The ferrochelatase deficiency in patients with EPP is clinically expressed mainly in erythroid cells as a marked elevation of protoporphyrin, despite the fact that this enzymatic deficiency can be demonstrated in all tissues so far examined.

These findings suggest that ferrochelatase may become rate limiting for heme synthesis in erythroid cells when its activity is decreased, as in patients with EPP, or when an increased synthesis of earlier enzymes of the heme biosynthetic pathway occurs as in erythroid differentiation.

Regulation of ALA Synthase in Other Tissues

Control of ALA synthase in tissues other than hepatocytes and erythroid cells is poorly understood. Available evidence suggests that the regulation of heme synthesis in such nonhepatic cell types may be different from that in liver. For example, ALA synthase activity in nonhepatic cells is generally not inducible by chemicals that induce hepatic ALA synthase[170–172]; the enzyme is usually refractory to inhibition or repression by hemin[170,171]; and ALA synthase is hardly derepressed by heme deficiency.[80,81,84]

Assembly of Heme and Globin

The orderly assembly of heme and globin is essential for the formation of a functional hemeprotein. For example, in the anucleate reticulocyte, the proportions of α subunits, non–α subunits, and heme are nearly always equal, indicating that a tight regulatory mechanism exists in cytoplasm for these components and that this process is independent of genetic control. The assembly of heme and apoprotein occurs in a highly specific manner. For example, cytochrome c oxidase subunit I–III in mitochondria requires a specific heme for its component subunits, heme a, and the assembly does not take place when mitochondria are incubated with protoheme, or heme b, the heme moiety of hemoglobin.[173] Heme a differs from protoheme in that the substituent at position 8 of the macrocycle is formyl, instead of methyl, and the vinyl group at position 2 is replaced by a 1-hydroxy-2-(E, E-farnesyl) ethyl group.

The reaction of heme and globin in vitro is rapid (about 5×10^4 mol/L/s).[174] The formation of hemoglobin from free carbon monoxide (CO) heme (to prevent aggregation of hemin) and globin proceeds by a two-step mechanism. The first step is a rapid equilibration of the heme groups with hydrophobic regions of the globin molecule. The second step is a unimolecular process, which involves a large conformational transition, resulting in iron–histidine bond formation.[175] Affinity of the α-chains of globin for heme has been reported to be either similar to[175] or higher than[176] that of the β-chains.

Despite evidence in vitro that suggests rapid binding of heme with globin, no evidence indicates that heme is bound to nascent globin chains during translation.[177,178] In contrast, experiments using dual labeling for both the heme and the globin moieties indicated that the interaction of heme and globin occurs after completion of the primary structure of the globin chains.[179] Hemin also does not appear to influence the release of nascent globin chains from polyribosomes.[178] The function of hemin in globin synthesis is not solely limited to binding with completed globin chains; rather, the heme moiety is also involved in an initiation process that results in continued synthesis of new nascent globin chains.[180]

After the association of heme with globin chains, a heme-intact α subunit and a heme-intact β subunit interact to form an $\alpha\beta$-dimer. Under normal circumstances, the balance between α- and non–α-subunit synthesis is coordinately maintained, and no excess subunits are found. After $\alpha\beta$-dimer formation, two of the dimers bind with each other to form an $\alpha_2\beta_2$ tetramer, Hb A. The rate-limiting step in this series of reactions is the formation of the $\alpha\beta$-dimer, which is largely irreversible, whereas the formation of the tetramer from the dimer is readily reversible. Formation of the tetramer, consisting of α and non–β subunits, also occurs in a similar manner; rate constants governing each association–dissociation step are different from those of Hb A. A detailed account of this topic is available in a comprehensive review.[181]

DISORDERS OF HEME SYNTHESIS

Normal and Abnormal Levels of Porphyrins and Porphyrin Precursors in Various Tissues and Excreta

Normal values for activities of enzymes in the heme biosynthetic pathway in human tissues and excreta are summarized in Table 50-1; abnormal values observed in patients with the porphyrias are summarized in Table 50-2. The porphyrias are inherited and acquired disorders in which the activities of the enzymes of the heme biosynthetic pathway are partially deficient. As a result, abnormally elevated levels of porphyrins and their precursors, such as ALA and PBG, are produced, accumulate in tissues, or are excreted in urine and stool.

Classification of Porphyrias

Porphyrias are classified as either hepatic or erythropoietic, depending on the principal site of expression of the specific enzymatic defect in each disorder. Eight enzymes are involved in the synthesis of heme and, with the exception of the first enzyme, ALA synthase, an enzymatic defect at each step of heme synthesis is associated with each form of porphyria (Fig. 50-8). There are also recent reviews on these disorders.[4,182]

Pathophysiology of Porphyrins and Porphyrin Precursors

Photosensitivity

Free porphyrins occur only in small amounts in nature. Upon illumination at wavelengths of around 400 nm and in the presence of oxygen, metal-free and diamagnetic metalloporphyrins cause photodynamic effects on tissues, cells, subcellular elements, and biomolecules by the formation of singlet oxygen.[183] Patients with cutaneous porphyrias have elevated plasma porphyrin contents and suffer from skin damage caused by the photoexcitation of porphyrins in the skin. The action spectrum for the induction of cutaneous lesions in porphyrias is the same as the maximal absorption peak of porphyrins (about 400 nm).[184] Erythrocytes that contain high concentrations of porphyrins also undergo photochemical hemolysis.[185]

Neurologic Disturbances

Acute hepatic porphyrias, such as ALA dehydratase porphyria, AIP, hereditary coproporphyria, and variegate porphyria, are characterized by neurologic disturbances that manifest as abdominal pain, disordered intestinal motility (diarrhea and constipation), dysesthesia, muscular paralysis, and potentially fatal respiratory failure. Several hypotheses have been proposed to explain the neurologic disturbances in these acute hepatic porphyrias.

The first hypothesis deals with a putative heme deficiency in the CNS. Heme pathway enzymes,[186,187] microsomal and mitochondrial cytochromes P-450, and their associated functions are also present in brain.[188,189] PBG deaminase deficiency, which is thought to be expressed in all tissues in persons with AIP, could therefore limit the formation of heme, resulting in decreased amounts of cytochromes in nervous tissue. A problem with this hypothesis is that ALA synthase in the brain of animals is refractory to treatment with porphyrogenic chemicals that act to induce the enzyme in the liver.[186,187,190–192]

TABLE 50-1. Normal Values of Heme Pathway Enzymes in Human Tissues

Enzyme	Liver	Erythroid Cells	Fibroblasts	Lymphocytes
ALA synthase, nmol/h of ALA per gram	24	49[a,b]	5.3[c]	120[c,d]
ALA dehydratase, nmol/h of PBG per gram	1100, 1300	2500[e]	120[c,f]	290[c,d]
PBG deaminase, nmol/h of uroporphyrinogen I per gram	2.8	36[e]	6.1[c,g]	6.1[c,d] 10[c,j]
Uroporphyrinogen III cosynthase, nmol/h of uroporphyrinogen III per gram	—	6600[e,h,i]	8800[c,i]	—
Uroporphyrinogen decarboxylase, nmol/h of coproporphyrinogen per gram	170[c]	720[k]	310[c]	480[c,l]
Coproporphyrinogen oxidase, nmol/h of protoporphyrinogen per gram	220[c]	—	87[c]	73[c,l]
Protoporphyrinogen oxidase, nmol/h of protoporphyrin per gram	—	—	300[c]	658[c,l]
Ferrochelatase, nmol/h of heme per gram	350	18[a,b]	3.7[c,m] 6.2[m]	310[c,l] 1900[n]

Note: Only mean values are cited in this table. To make comparisons of enzymatic activities, certain assumptions were made to recalculate reported data so that they can be expressed per gram of tissue per hour of incubation.

[a] Assuming 2 × 10^8 erythroblasts per gram of bone marrow.
[b] Bone marrow.
[c] Assuming 150 mg of protein per gram of tissue.
[d] Mitogen-stimulated lymphocytes.
[e] Erythrocytes.
[f] Sassa et al, unpublished data, 1993.
[g] At 60°C.
[h] Assuming 300 g hemoglobin per gram of erythrocytes.
[i] At 31°C.
[j] EBV-transformed lymphocytes.
[k] Assuming that uroporphyrinogen III is used as substrate (about 5 times faster than 5-carboxylate porphyrinogen I).
[l] Nonstimulated lymphocytes.
[m] Protoporphyrin as substrate.
[n] Mesoporphyrin as substrate.

The second hypothesis relates to the toxic consequence of elevated concentrations of heme pathway intermediates. The effects of ALA in vitro include, among others, changes in motor nerve conduction velocity,[193] acetylcholine release,[194] stretch receptors,[195] muscle-resting membrane potential,[196] porphyrin synthesis,[197] duodenal contraction,[198] and [Na^+,K^+]ATPase activity.[199] ALA has also been shown to compete for the binding of γ-aminobutyric acid (GABA) associated with synaptic GABA receptors,[200] and to facilitate GABA release. Although plasma levels of ALA as high as 10^{-4} mol/L have been reported in AIP patients, spinal fluid taken simultaneously from such patients contained signif-

TABLE 50-2. Activities of Heme Pathway Enzymes in Human Porphyrias

Enzyme	Disease Displaying Abnormal Enzyme Activity	Enzyme Activity (Percentage of Normal Controls)				
		Liver	Bone Marrow	Erythrocytes	Fibroblasts	Lymphocytes
ALA synthase	ADP AIP HCP VP	1000–2000			Normal	Normal
ALA dehydratase	ADP	<2		<2		<2
PBG deaminase	AIP	~50		~50	~50	~50
Uroporphyrinogen III cosynthase	CEP			10–20	10–20	
Uroporphyrinogen decarboxylase	PCT (type I)	<50		Normal	Normal	Normal
	PCT (type II)	~50		~50	~50	~50
	PCT (type III)	~50		Normal		
	HEP	<2		<10		<10
Coproporphyrinogen oxidase	HCP				~50	~50
Protoporphyrinogen oxidase	VP				~50	~50
Ferrochelatase	EPP		~50		~20	~50

ADP, ALA dehydratase porphyria; AIP, acute intermittent porphyria; HCB, hereditary coproporphyria; VP, variegate porphyria; CEP, congenital erythropoietic porphyria; PCT, porphyria cutanea tarda; HEP, hepatoerythropoietic porphyria; EPP, erythropoietic protoporphyria.

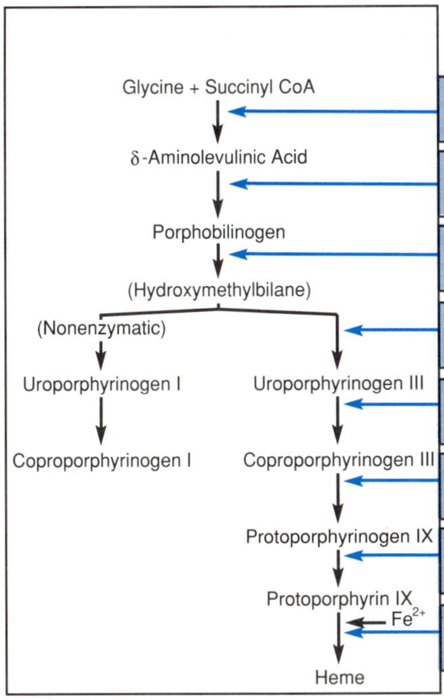

Enzyme	Disease	Major Symptoms	Accumulation Products
δ-Aminolevulinic Acid Synthase			
δ-Aminolevulinic Acid Dehydratase	ALAD Deficiency Porphyria	Neurovisceral	Urinary ALA
Porphobilinogen Deaminase	Acute Intermittent Porphyria	Neurovisceral	Urinary ALA and PGB
Uroporphyrinogen III Cosynthase	Congenital Erythropoietic Porphyria	Photosensitivity	Erythrocyte and Urinary Uro I and Copro I
Uroporphyrinogen Decarboxylase	Porphyria Cutanea Tarda; Hepatoerythropoietic Porphyria	Photosensitivity	Urinary Uro, 7-c Porphyrin; Fecal Isocopro
Coproporphyrinogen Oxidase	Hereditary Coproporphyria	Neurovisceral; Photosensitivity	Urinary ALA, PGB, Copro; Fecal Copro
Protoporphyrinogen Oxidase	Variegate Porphyria	Neurovisceral; Photosensitivity	Urinary ALA, PGB, Copro; Fecal Proto
Ferrochelatase	Erythropoietic Protoporphyria	Photosensitivity	Erythrocyte Proto; Fecal Proto

FIGURE 50-8. Classification and major symptoms of the porphyrias. PGB, porphobilinogen. With the exception of δ-aminolevulinate synthase, each enzymatic defect in the heme biosynthetic pathway leads to the development of porphyrias.

icantly lower levels of the compound (about 15% of the plasma concentration).[201] Thus, it has not been clearly established that ALA concentrations in the spinal fluid can reach the level that elicits the various neurologic effects observed in vitro.

Administration of ALA to rats has been reported to induce behavioral changes,[202] and direct instillation of ALA into the brain causes both behavioral effects[203] and convulsions[203,204]; convulsions are also seen after PBG administration into the brain.[204] Most of these in vitro studies have used pharmacologic concentrations of ALA (10^{-3} to 10^{-4} mol/L). Although plasma concentrations of ALA may occasionally reach such levels, patients with AIP rarely demonstrate CSF concentrations in this range.[205,206] Furthermore, some investigators have concluded that their results are inconsistent with a neuropharmacologic role for ALA in causing neurologic dysfunction.[206,207]

A more recent hypothesis proposes an indirect metabolic consequence of a relative hepatic heme deficiency. Brain levels of tryptophan and the subsequent synthesis of brain 5-hydroxytryptamine are largely determined by plasma concentrations of the amino acid.[208] In turn, plasma tryptophan concentrations are largely determined by the activity of hepatic tryptophan pyrrolase, a heme-dependent enzyme that converts tryptophan to kynurenine.[209] In acute attacks of AIP, deficiency of heme may lead to decreased activity of hepatic tryptophan pyrrolase, enhanced plasma levels and brain uptake of tryptophan, and ultimately increased 5-hydroxytryptamine synthesis. Experimental evidence for this sequence of events has been reported in a rodent model of porphyria (DDC-treated, phenobarbital-primed rat).[210,211] In another chemically induced model of porphyria (ALA-treated rat), tryptophan pyrrolase activity was increased,[212] which would predict a decrease in brain 5-hydroxytryptamine synthesis.

Thus, none of the above theories can sufficiently explain the neurologic disturbances observed in the acute hepatic porphyrias in humans, and this issue remains unsettled.

The Porphyrias

In this chapter, each porphyric disorder is described according to the order of the enzymes in the heme biosynthetic sequence.

ALA Dehydratase Porphyria

Definition. ALA dehydratase porphyria (ADP) is an autosomal recessive disorder resulting from a homozygous deficiency in ALA dehydratase activity.[213,214] The symptomatology is similar to that seen in patients with AIP. Four cases in males have been reported to date: two with postpubertal onset, one with onset immediately after birth, and another with late onset in the 60s.

Clinical Findings. The two German male postpubertal patients with ADP both presented at 16 years of age with vomiting, pain in the arms and legs, and neuropathy.[213,214] Both patients displayed clinical exacerbations after stress, alcohol use, or decreased food intake; one patient responded favorably to intravenous glucose infusions.[213–215] The third patient was a Swedish child, diagnosed at age 2 years but with a stormy clinical course from birth onward.[216] General muscle hypotonia and respiratory insufficiency necessitated assisted ventilation for several weeks during the slow recovery of muscle tone and tendon reflexes; electromyography changes had normalized by the time the patient reached 10 months of age although he still vomited frequently. Thirteen months later, decreased food intake heralded the onset of bilateral paralysis of the legs and abnormal porphyrin metabolism. Subsequently, his clinical course consisted of a series of exacerbations and remissions leading to ankle contractions, atrophy of the calf muscles, and impaired hand movements.[216] The fourth patient was a late-onset Belgian male who developed acute hepatic porphyria for the first time at the age of 63. His symptoms were subacute polyneuropathy, predominantly of the motor type, in the upper limbs.[217]

Biochemical Findings. Urinary ALA excretion has been markedly elevated in patients with ADP, but urinary PBG excretion has been little affected. Urinary and erythrocyte porphyrins have also been about 100-fold elevated; no satisfactory explanation has been advanced to account for this observation. Fecal porphyrin excretion has been normal or marginally elevated.

All patients have displayed decreased activities of ALA dehydratase in erythrocytes and, in two patients, in bone marrow cells (2% or less of normal) with about 50% decreases in activity of the parents' RBC enzyme and normal activities in siblings. In all four patients, a defective enzyme has been detected immunologically.[218,219] The 2-year-old patient had hemolytic anemia that required transfusion.

The molecular defect of ALA dehydratase in one of the two German patients has been determined.[219a] The proband had compound heterozygosity for two distinct point mutations of the ALA dehydratase gene, A820 → G and C718 → T, at each allele, resulting in amino acid changes Ala274 → Thr and Arg240 → Trp, respectively.[219b,219c] The A820 → G mutation was present within the substrate-binding site, and the C718 → T mutation was present downstream of this site. The mother, the brother, and the sister were shown to have the A820 → G mutation. Expression of the A820 → G cDNA in Chinese hamster ovary cells produced ALA dehydratase protein with little activity; the C718 → T cDNA produced the enzyme with about 50% normal enzyme activity. Pulse-labeling studies demonstrated that the A820 → G enzyme had a normal half-life, whereas the C718 → T enzyme had a markedly decreased half-life. These findings demonstrated that the proband was a compound heterozygote for two separate point mutations of the ALA dehydratase gene, and it also accounted for the almost complete lack of enzymatic activity in the proband's cells and the half-normal activity in cells from the family members.

The molecular defect in the Swedish infant with ADP was also reported.[219c] A maternal G397 → A transition predicted a Gly133 → Arg change, which occurred at the carboxyl end of the zinc-binding site in the enzyme. The paternal mutation was G823 → A, resulting in an amino acid change, Val275 → Met. These mutations were thought to be responsible for the altered function of the enzyme, though no direct demonstration by expression studies of the mutant cDNAs was made. The four distinct point mutations in two pedigrees suggest a marked heterogeneity in this disorder.

Diagnosis. Definitive diagnosis of ADP depends on the demonstration of impaired ALA dehydratase activity and deficiency of enzyme protein in erythrocytes. Supporting evidence for the diagnosis includes massive elevations in urinary ALA, substantial elevations of porphyrins in urine and erythrocytes, and possibly modest elevations in fecal porphyrins. Clinical symptoms of ADP occur only in homozygous patients, whereas heterozygous subjects (parents and certain siblings of the probands) remain clinically unaffected.

Treatment. The similarities between ADP and AIP suggest that prudent management of ALA dehydratase porphyria should probably be directed along the same lines as the management of AIP (discussion follows).

Acute Intermittent Porphyria

Definition. AIP (synonyms: Swedish porphyria, pyrroloporphyria, intermittent acute porphyria) is an autosomal dominant disorder resulting from a deficiency in PBG deaminase activity. The deficient enzyme activity is almost always about 50% of normal, consistent with the heterozygous state of affected persons. Most (about 90%) persons with this genetic enzyme deficiency remain otherwise biochemically and clinically normal, that is, latent, throughout life. Clinical expression of the disease is usually linked to environmental or acquired factors such as nutritional status, drugs, and other chemicals of endogenous origin such as steroids, or those of exogenous origin, and others. The cardinal pathobiology of the disease is a neurologic dysfunction that may affect the peripheral, autonomic system or the CNS; the resulting neuropathic clinical presentation may be highly diverse.

Prevalence. The highest incidence of AIP occurs in Lapland, Scandinavia, and in the United Kingdom, although it has been reported in many population groups.[4] The incidence of the defective gene in the United States has been estimated at between 5 and 10 per 100,000.[220] The incidence of AIP in psychiatric populations is higher than that in the normal population (0.21% of 3867 patients).[221] The disorder is expressed clinically almost invariably after puberty and more frequently in women than in men. AIP is probably the most common of all the genetic porphyrias.

Clinical Findings. Abdominal pain is nearly always present and is often the initial symptom of an acute attack of AIP. It may be generalized or localized, and in severe cases may mimic an acute surgical abdomen. Surgical explorations combined with barbiturate induction of anesthesia may occasionally lead to disastrous exacerbations of an already initiated porphyria attack. Other gastroenterologic features are nausea, vomiting, constipation or diarrhea, abdominal distention, and ileus. Urinary incontinence, dysuria, and urinary frequency may occur, although urinary retention is probably more common. In severe cases of AIP, the urine may develop a port-wine color due to a high content of porphobilin, an autooxidized product of PBG, and some porphyrins that are formed by nonenzymatic cyclization of PBG.

Tachycardia and hypertension, and, less frequently, fever, sweating, restlessness, and tremor are also observed in patients with AIP. Catecholamine hypersecretion, when severe, has been implicated in sudden death, possibly secondary to cardiac arrhythmias.[222,223] In up to 40% of AIP patients, hypertension may become sustained between acute attacks.

Neuropathy is a common feature of AIP. Muscle weakness often begins proximally in the legs but may involve the arms or the distal extremities; involvement may be symmetric, asymmetric, or focal[224] and in some patients may be associated with a decrease or loss of tendon reflexes.[223] Motor neuropathy may also involve the cranial nerves (most frequently the 7th and 10th) or may lead to bulbar paralysis, respiratory deficiency, and death; AIP rarely presents as respiratory failure.[225] Sensory patchy neuropathy also occurs when motor neuropathy is severe and may be manifested by acute or chronic paresthesia, numbness, or dysesthesia.[226]

Acute attacks of AIP may be accompanied by seizures, especially in patients with hyponatremia due to vomiting, to inappropriate fluid therapy, or to the syndrome of inappropriate antidiuretic hormone release. The course of an acute attack of AIP is highly variable among patients and within individuals, with attacks lasting from a few days to several months.

Precipitating Factors. Asymptomatic heterozygotes (about 90% of subjects with documented PBG deaminase deficiency) may display neither abnormal levels of heme pathway intermediates nor clinical symptoms. Persons with both latent or previously clinically expressed AIP may be precipitated into an acute attack by endogenous or exogenous environmental factors. It is not certain whether all latent gene carriers of AIP can be precipitated into clinical expression of the disorder; the distinction between those

PBG deaminase-deficient persons who ultimately show clinical expression of AIP and those who never display the overt disease is an important unanswered aspect of the pathogenesis of this genetic disorder. Most, if not all, precipitating factors in AIP can be related to an associated increase in the activity of ALA synthase in liver.[227,228] The clinical disease is more common in women, especially at the time of menses[229]; a subset of female patients experiences regular cyclical premenstrual exacerbations of their disease.

In vitro studies using primary cultures of chick embryo hepatocytes as well as whole avian liver have established that hepatic ALA synthase is induced by sex steroid metabolites. AIP patients with the clinically expressed disorder excrete increased amounts into the urine[230–232] of steroids with a predominantly 5β configuration due to impaired hepatic 5α-reductase activity[233–235]; AIP gene carriers who have remained entirely latent display no such abnormality in steroid metabolism.[236]

Reduced calorie intake often leads to exacerbations of AIP.[237] Urinary ALA and PBG excretion may increase in AIP patients after only a 20% decrease in caloric intake[238]; conversely, additional carbohydrate-derived calories added to a preexisting adequate diet decreases PBG excretion.[238,239] The ratio of 5β to 5α steroid metabolism is also considerably decreased by increasing the amount of carbohydrate in the diet.[240] This effect of the protein:carbohydrate ratio mimics that produced by the porphyria-inducing drug, phenobarbital, in humans[241] and in experimental animals.[240] An attenuated ALA synthase induction response to allyl isopropylacetamide in rat liver occurs after glucose administration both in vivo[150] and in vitro.[242] Despite considerable study, the mechanism of this glucose effect remains unclear.

Drugs and other foreign chemicals constitute a major category of inducers of acute attacks of AIP. Barbiturates are the most widely recognized and potentially the most injurious group of such agents. Many chemicals that exacerbate porphyria have the potential to induce cytochrome P-450, and the resultant enhanced demand for de novo heme synthesis is presumed to lead to hepatic ALA synthase induction. These chemicals include sex steroids, as studies in avian liver have shown,[243,244] as well as barbiturates and other foreign chemicals.

Stress is also considered to exacerbate AIP. Similarly, intercurrent illnesses, infections,[245] alcoholic excess, and surgery may contribute to the genesis of an acute attack of this disorder. Most of these conditions elicit an acute-phase reaction, probably by a mechanism involving the production of certain cytokines. Recent studies indicate that ALA synthase activity can also be induced in a human hepatoma-derived cell line in culture by treatment with acute-phase inducers.[246]

Biochemical Findings. Patients with clinically expressed AIP, as well as a few persons with latent AIP, excrete increased amounts of ALA and PBG in the urine between attacks. In most patients, the onset of an acute attack is accompanied by further marked-to-massive increases in excretion of these precursors (ALA, 25 to 100 mg/d; PBG, 50 to 200 mg/d[247]). Acute attacks may also be associated with elevations in the plasma concentrations of ALA, PBG, and porphyrins, which are normally undetectable. Stool porphyrins are usually normal or slightly elevated.[248]

The Watson-Schwartz test is widely used to screen for urinary PBG.[249,250] PBG chromogens are generated with Ehrlich's reagent, and contaminating chromogens (such as indoles, urobilinogen) can be extracted with chloroform and butanol. PBG chromogens are quantitated colorimetrically in the aqueous fraction. The Watson-Schwartz test is neither as sensitive nor as specific as the quantitative column method of Mauzerall and Granick,[251] which should be used to verify positive results from either screening test. Hematologic profiles are usually normal unless aberrations of salt or water balance supervene.[252] Hemoglobin synthesis and bilirubin production are normal in patients with AIP.[252,253]

Diagnosis. Diagnosis of AIP can be made by demonstrating decreased PBG deaminase activity in erythrocytes, whereas the distinction between carrier or latent status and clinically expressed AIP depends on the demonstration of elevated excretion of PBG and ALA and on the natural history of the person. Elevated levels of ALA and PBG may also be seen in patients with hereditary coproporphyria and variegate porphyria; measurement of urinary and stool porphyrins usually differentiates these conditions from AIP. The diagnosis of the subset of AIP expressing the PBG deaminase gene defect only in nonerythroid tissues requires either the demonstration of PBG deaminase deficiency in nonerythroid cells[79,84] or DNA hybridization using allele-specific oligonucleotides.[86]

Treatment. The treatment of patients with AIP as well as those with ALA dehydratase porphyria, hereditary coproporphyria, and variegate porphyria is essentially identical. The following discussion applies to patients with all four forms of these acute hepatic porphyrias. All such patients should be provided with Medi-Alert bracelets. Treatment between attacks consists of adequate nutritional intake, avoidance of drugs known to exacerbate porphyria, and prompt treatment of intercurrent diseases or infections. Unresponsive patients with severe disease should be admitted to the hospital and intravenous administration of carbohydrate initiated with dextrose to provide a minimum of 300 g/d carbohydrate.

The use of intravenous hematin is generally effective in reducing ALA and PBG excretion, in curtailing acute attacks, and perhaps in reducing the severity of neuropathies.[254–256] Hematin (Panhematin, Abbott Laboratories, Chicago), up to 4 mg/kg, is given intravenously, preferably over 30 minutes every 12 hours. Hematin therapy is frequently associated with phlebitis or thrombophlebitis,[257] which in normal subjects, was found to occur in 50% of patients after infusion with doses of 4 mg/kg.[258] Coagulopathy[258–260] and hemolysis[261] have also been reported after hematin infusion but not in association with frank hemorrhage. Heme arginate (Normosang, Huhtamaki Oy Pharmaceuticals, Finland) is a highly water-soluble compound and causes local phlebitis less frequently when injected into the ear vein of rabbits than does hematin.[262] It is being widely used to treat active AIP in replacement of hematin for this purpose.[263] Four daily infusions of heme arginate at doses of 2 to 3 mg/kg to AIP patients in relapse were reported to result in virtual normalization of ALA and PBG excretion.[264]

Nasal or subcutaneous administration of long-acting agonistic analogues of luteinizing hormone-releasing hormone (Hoechst or Salk Institute) in doses of 400 to 1200 μg/d has been shown to inhibit ovulation and greatly reduce the incidence of perimenstrual attacks of AIP in some women with cyclic exacerbations of the disease.[265–267] Synthetic heme analogues (Porphyrin Products, Logan, UT), such as Sn-protoporphyrin, 1 μmol/kg, and Sn-mesoporphyrin, 0.5 μmol/kg/d for 4 days, have also been shown to diminish the output of ALA, PBG, and porphyrins in stable hyperexcretors with acute hepatic porphyria.[268] The advantages of the latter compounds are that they may be administered intramuscularly; they are not degraded to bile pigments by heme oxygenase; and they simultaneously suppress induction of ALA synthase and potently inhibit the rate of heme catabolism, thus preserving cellular heme concentrations in liver.[268]

Congenital Erythropoietic Porphyria

Definition. CEP (synonyms: Günther's disease, erythropoietic porphyria, congenital porphyria, congenital hematoporphyria, erythropoietic uroporphyria) is inherited in an autosomal recessive fashion. The primary abnormality in the affected homozygote is a decreased activity of uroporphyrinogen III cosynthase activity that results in accumulation and hyperexcretion of predominantly type I porphyrins. Clinically, this enzymatic defect is expressed in infancy and results in cutaneous photosensitivity, hemolysis, and a decreased life expectancy.

Prevalence. CEP is rare, with fewer than 200 cases reported by 1992, and some of these patients may really have had PCT[269,270] or hepatoerythropoietic porphyria (HEP). No clear racial or sexual predominances have been found.

Clinical Findings. Pink to dark brown staining of the diapers in infants is often the first clue to a diagnosis of CEP; this discoloration is caused by large amounts of porphyrins in urine. Early onset of cutaneous photosensitivity is characteristic and is exacerbated by exposure to sunlight. Subepidermal bullous lesions progress to crusted erosions that heal, with scarring and either hyperpigmentation or, less frequently, hypopigmentation. Hypertrichosis and alopecia are common, and erythrodontia (with red fluorescence under ultraviolet light) is virtually pathognomonic of CEP[271–273] (Fig. 50-9).

Patients may display symptoms and signs of anemia (usually hemolytic) with splenomegaly and porphyrin-rich gallstones.[274] Compensatory expansion of hyperactive bone marrow may result in pathologic fractures or vertebral compression–collapse and shortness of stature. Although onset of symptoms of CEP is most often observed in early infancy, a few patients may first present with the syndrome as adults.[272,275–278]

Pathogenesis of Clinical Findings. Autopsy findings in patients with CEP reveal an orange-red fluorescence of all viscera, skin, and bones under ultraviolet light.[279] Microscopy shows fluorescence of erythrocytes, skin, bile duct, and nephrons but not of hepatocytes. Atrophic epidermis with thickened dermis containing periodic acid-Schiff–positive staining vessels is found.

The primary site of expression of the enzymatic defect is the bone marrow wherein fluorescence secondary to porphyrin accumulation is variably distributed but invariably present. Most marrow normoblasts display fluorescence, principally localized in the nuclei of the cells.[270,280–283] Such fluorescent cells are morphologically abnormal and also display heme deposition in nuclear vacuoles, whereas nonfluorescent cells are morphologically normal.[270] Massive elevations of systemic porphyrins in CEP are derived from porphyrin-laden erythrocytes and largely account for the multiple pathologies of the integument.

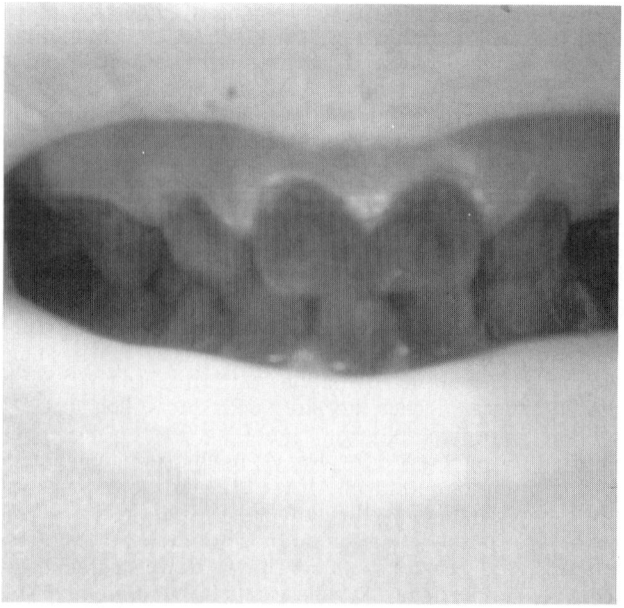

FIGURE 50-9. Erythrodontia of a patient with congenital erythropoietic porphyria. (See Color Fig. 50-9.) (Courtesy of Dr. H.L. Nitowsky)

Although hemolysis is usually present, it is not always accompanied by anemia, since the hypertrophied and hyperactive marrow may compensate for the increased rate of erythrocyte destruction. Often, the degree of compensation varies over time leading to exacerbations and remissions of hemolysis and anemia.[270,284] All CEP patients show increased plasma iron turnover.[272,285,286]

Hemolysis of erythrocytes may result from photolysis of porphyrin-laden cells that are exposed to light in the dermal capillaries. Wavelengths of light suitable for porphyrin photoactivation are known to penetrate the skin to a depth sufficient to produce this phenomenon.[285] When porphyric cattle were exposed to sunlight, their RBCs showed marked shortening of survival.[287] Light shielding was also reported to be effective in ameliorating anemia in a human with CEP.[288] In contrast to these findings, it is known that no seasonal differences appear in anemia and hemolysis of patients with CEP.

Biochemical Findings. Urinary porphyrins are always elevated (20- to 60-fold) above normal levels in patients with CEP. Uroporphyrin levels are higher than coproporphyrin levels and, although type I isomers predominate, type III isomers are also elevated. Smaller amounts of 7-, 6-, and 5-carboxylic porphyrins are also excreted.[284,286,289] Urinary ALA and PBG excretion is generally within normal limits. Fecal porphyrin excretion is usually increased and is predominantly type I coproporphyrin with lesser and variable elevations of uroporphyrin, or rarely protoporphyrin. Elevated type I uroporphyrin and sometimes coproporphyrin concentrations are found in plasma and erythrocytes. Erythrocyte protoporphyrin level is usually normal or mildly elevated, although it is the dominantly elevated porphyrin in erythrocytes in some patients.[272,276,286] Also, some patients with HEP who show marked elevation of erythrocyte protoporphyrin could have mistakenly been diagnosed as having CEP.

Fluctuating degrees of anemia may be present and erythrocytes may exhibit polychromasia, poikilocytosis, anisocytosis, and basophilic stippling. Increased reticulocytes and normoblasts may be detected in the peripheral circulation. Occasionally, anemia may be severe and may require transfusion.[281,290] Rarely, thrombocytopenia or leukopenia occurs in association with hypersplenism; thrombocytopenia may predispose to bleeding diatheses.[272,277,278,280,289] Although protoporphyrin and hemin are known to activate factor XII–dependent pathways with the generation of kallikrein activity,[291] no such studies on the effects of uroporphyrin or coproporphyrin on platelet functions or coagulation pathway have been reported.

Diagnosis. Pink urine or the onset of severe cutaneous photosensitivity in infancy (or rarely in adults) should suggest the diagnosis of CEP. Demonstration of elevated urinary, fecal, and erythrocyte porphyrins with elevated type I isomers of uroproporphyrin and coproporphyrin establishes the diagnosis of CEP. Demonstration of a deficiency of uroporphyrinogen III cosynthase activity constitutes the definitive diagnosis, but the enzyme assay is usually a research procedure. Patients with HEP may also present with

TABLE 50-3. Subsets of Porphyria Cutanea Tarda

Type	Familial Occurrence	Uroporphyrinogen Decarboxylase	
		Liver	Erythrocytes
I	(−)	Decreased	Normal
II	(+)	Decreased	Decreased
III	(+)	Decreased	Normal

photosensitivity, excessive porphyrin excretion, and elevated erythrocyte protoporphyrin in children, but such patients (in contrast to CEP) have elevated fecal levels of isocoproporphyrin and 5-carboxylic porphyrins and often excrete Zn-protoporphyrin into the urine.[292,293]

Treatment. The avoidance of sunlight, trauma to the skin, and infections is the most important preventive measure for patients with CEP. Topical sunscreens may be of help as may oral treatment with β-carotene.[294] Transfusions with packed erythrocytes transiently decrease hemolysis and its attendant drive to increased erythropoiesis and also decrease porphyrin excretion.[295,296] Splenectomy has been used fairly frequently and has produced short-term reductions in hemolysis, porphyrin excretion, and skin manifestations,[280,297] but not all patients respond.[273,281,298] Hematin has been administered to a woman with CEP and were reported to reduce porphyrin output with about the same efficacy as packed erythrocyte transfusions, but over a shorter duration.[275] In a patient with CEP, treatment with oral charcoal, 60 g three times daily for 9 months, was found to suppress porphyrin levels in plasma and skin and resulted in a complete clinical remission in which the effect lasted only during therapy.[299]

Porphyria Cutanea Tarda and Hepatoerythropoietic Porphyria

Porphyria cutanea tarda is due to a heterozygous deficiency, and HEP is due to a homozygous deficiency of uroporphyrinogen decarboxylase.

Porphyria Cutanea Tarda

Definition. PCT (synonyms: symptomatic porphyria, porphyria cutanea symptomatica, idiosyncratic porphyria) refers to a heterogeneous group of porphyric diseases that may be inherited (familial or type II) or, more commonly, acquired (sporadic or type I; Table 50-3). Both forms display reductions in the activity of uroporphyrinogen decarboxylase; in the autosomal dominant inherited form the enzyme is deficient in all tissues, whereas in the acquired form the defect is confined to the liver. Acquired PCT typically presents in adults, either spontaneously or more commonly in conjunction with precipitating environmental factors such as alcohol, estrogen, or polyhalogenated aromatic hydrocarbons, or in association with other disorders. Another form, termed *type III PCT*, has been reported in which normal erythrocyte uroporphyrinogen decarboxylase activity and concentrations were found in more than one member in a single family, but with decreased hepatic uroporphyrinogen decarboxylase activity[300,301] (see Table 50-3). The hallmark of all forms of PCT is cutaneous photosensitivity due to increased production of uroporphyrin and 7-carboxylic porphyrin.

Cutaneous lesions in the light-exposed areas such as the face, tip of the nose, and dorsa of hands include skin fragility, vesicles and bullae formation (Fig. 50-10), atrophic changes, and scar formation. The lesions are often followed by hypopigmentation and hyperpigmentation, hypertrichosis, and pseudosclerodermoid changes. Dystrophic calcifications may occur in severely scarred tissues, forming protrusion of calcium spicules through the epidermis, while leading to chronic nonhealing ulcerations as well.

Prevalence. PCT is probably the most common of all the porphyrias, but its exact incidence is not clear. The disease is recognized worldwide and no racial predilection exists except among the Bantus in South Africa,[302,303] probably because of their high incidence of hemosiderosis. Sporadic PCT is generally more common than familial PCT in Europe, South Africa, and South America,[304] although the trend may be less obvious or even reversed in North America.[305] Previously, PCT was held to be more common, perhaps secondary to higher alcohol intake, in men than in women, but the incidence in females has increased of late to the level seen in males, perhaps due to increased use of contraceptive steroids, postmenopausal estrogens, and alcohol.[306,307]

Pathogenesis of Clinical Findings. Phototoxic porphyrins in the skin may be largely derived from the liver and, to some extent, formed locally in the skin.[308] Activation of the complement system after irradiation has been demonstrated in PCT patients both in vivo[309,310] and in vitro in sera[311,312] and is presumed to result from the generation of reactive oxygen species, most likely singlet oxygen.[313] Bul-

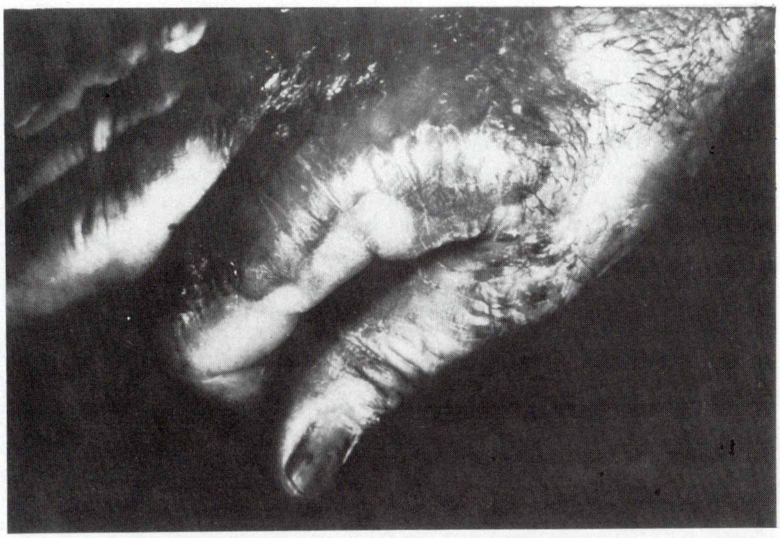

FIGURE 50-10. Bullous eruption of a hand of a patient with porphyria cutanea tarda. (Poh-Fitzpatrick MB. Porphyrin-sensitized cutaneous photosensitivity. Clin Dermatol 1985;3:41)

lous fluid is known to contain prostaglandin E_2[314] and photoactivation of uroporphyrin damages lysosomes[315]; inflammation and autolysis may be partly attributable to these factors.

Liver biopsy specimens from patients with PCT almost invariably display siderosis but of widely varying degrees, with fatty changes, necrosis, chronic inflammatory changes, and granuloma formation.[316] Red autofluorescence and needle-like cytoplasmic inclusion bodies, which most likely represent porphyrin crystals, have also frequently been reported.[316,317] Iron, estrogens, alcohol, and chlorinated hydrocarbons, all of which are potential hepatotoxins, may aggravate PCT. The incidence of hepatitis B infection may be higher than normal in PCT patients.[318,319] Any or all of these factors, or perhaps porphyrins themselves, may predispose the liver of PCT patients to neoplastic change, and the incidence of hepatocellular carcinoma in PCT is known to be greater than in the general population.[316,320–322] Rarely, primary hepatomas may secrete porphyrins and simulate PCT.[323]

Biochemical Findings. Increased concentrations of uroporphyrin (mainly isomer I) and 7-carboxylic porphyrins (mainly isomer III) are found in the urine in PCT patients, with lesser increases of coproporphyrin and 5- and 6-carboxylic porphyrins.[324,325] Porphyrins can be separated by thin-layer chromatography or high-performance liquid chromatography.[326] Small quantities of isocoproporphyrin may be detected in plasma or urine, but in feces isocoproporphyrin is often the dominant porphyrin excreted[327,328] and represents the most important diagnostic criterion for PCT. Coproporphyrin, 7-carboxylic porphyrin, uroporphyrin, and X-porphyrin (ether-acetic acid–insoluble, extractable with urea-triton) content of stool all may be increased in patients with PCT.[329] Total daily fecal porphyrin excretion exceeds total urinary porphyrin excretion. Skin porphyrins are especially increased in areas that are protected from photoactivation.[330]

Biochemical indices of liver dysfunction may also be present. Elevated levels of serum transaminases and γ-glutamyltranspeptidase, especially in alcoholics, are often seen. Serum iron and ferritin concentrations are frequently elevated.

Diagnosis. The clinical picture in patients with PCT is fairly specific but can be confused with that of other porphyric (variegate porphyria) and nonporphyric (systemic lupus erythematosus) diseases. Urinary fluorescence under ultraviolet light illumination and quantitation of porphyrins and separation and identification of porphyrins by thin-layer chromatography and high-performance liquid chromatography assist the diagnosis. Plasma porphyrins are elevated in patients with PCT and other photosensitizing porphyrias. Fecal porphyrins are often elevated; isocoproporphyrin (or an isocoproporphyrin/coproporphyrin ratio of 0.1 or more) is virtually diagnostic of PCT.[331] The catalytic activity and the concentration of immunoreactive uroporphyrinogen decarboxylase are about 50% of normal in patients with type II PCT, and decreased uroporphyrinogen decarboxylase in type II PCT segregates as an autosomal dominant trait in patients' families. In contrast, patients with type I PCT show normal erythrocyte uroporphyrinogen decarboxylase activity and concentrations and familial occurrence of the disorder. Patients with type III PCT show familial occurrence with normal erythrocyte uroporphyrinogen decarboxylase activity.

Treatment. In patients with type I PCT, the identification and avoidance of precipitating factors are essential to treatment.[332] The clinical response to cessation of alcohol ingestion is highly variable[333,334]; nonetheless, abstinence should be recommended.

Phlebotomy is usually effective in reducing urinary porphyrin concentrations and inducing clinical remissions. Strong evidence shows that the beneficial effects of phlebotomy result from a diminution in body iron stores.[113,335,336] Replenishment of iron after remission of PCT may accelerate the onset of subsequent relapse,[337] which, in the absence of supplemental iron administration, may occur from 1 to 8 years later. Reduction of porphyrin excretion usually precedes clinical improvement, which starts with an abatement of new skin lesions and may eventually progress to healing of scars and loss of skin fragility.

If phlebotomy is ineffective or contraindicated because of the presence of other diseases such as anemia, low-dose chloroquine therapy may be effective. Efficacy of chloroquine therapy and phlebotomy is probably similar,[338,339] and some reports suggest that a combined approach is useful and may diminish the incidence of side effects.[340,341] The mechanism of action of chloroquine therapy is thought to be related to its ability to chelate porphyrins in a water-soluble and hence more easily excretable form.[342]

Hepatoerythropoietic Porphyria

Definition. HEP is a rare form of porphyria, probably resulting from a homozygous defect in uroporphyrinogen decarboxylase activity. Clinically, HEP is indistinguishable from CEP and characterized by the childhood onset of severe photosensitivity and skin fragility. The term *hepatoerythropoietic porphyria* was coined to reflect the fact that excess porphyrins are synthesized in both the liver and the bone marrow.

Incidence. HEP is extremely rare; some 20 cases have been reported worldwide to date.[343]

Clinical Findings. Clinical findings in patients with HEP are similar to those seen in CEP. Pink urine, severe photosensitivity leading to scarring and mutilation of sun-exposed areas of skin, sclerodermoid changes, hypertrichosis, erythrodontia, anemia (often hemolytic), and hepatosplenomegaly characterize HEP. Onset is usually in early infancy or childhood,[344] but adult onset has also been described.[345,346] In contrast to those found in PCT patients, serum iron concentrations have usually been normal in HEP patients. Likewise, the incidence of bone marrow and liver fluorescence (Fig. 50-11), anemia, and evidence of abnormal liver function and histology have been highly variable. Skin biopsies have shown subepidermal bullae and other findings similar to the lesions of PCT.[293]

Recent availability of a human uroporphyrinogen decarboxylase cDNA clone[71] allowed de Verneuil and colleagues[347,348] to investigate the mutant gene and its expression in lymphoblastoid cell lines from a family with

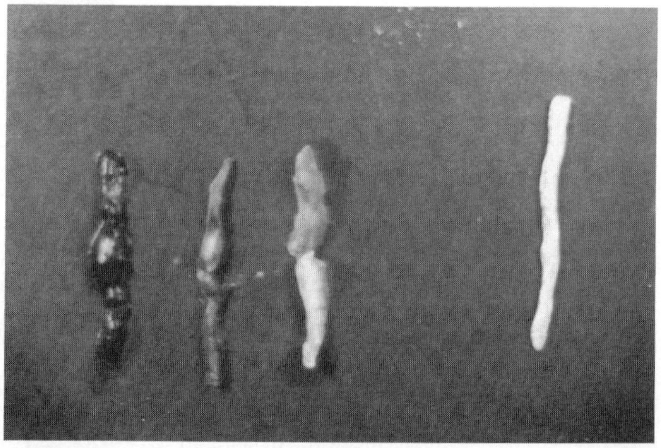

FIGURE 50-11. Liver biopsy sample from a patient with hepatoerythropoietic porphyria shows autofluorescence (*far right*), whereas samples from nonporphyric patients do not. (See Color Fig. 50-11.)

two cases of HEP. Southern blot analysis after digestion of genomic DNA showed the same restriction fragments in DNA isolated from a normal cell line and from both patients, thus excluding large deletions or rearrangements in the mutant gene. Northern and dot blot analyses demonstrated that the concentration of mRNA was similar in cell lines from controls, heterozygous parents, or homozygous patients. Synthesis, processing, and cell-free translation of the specific transcripts appeared to be normal.[347] Size and molecular weight of the protein were identical with those of the marker enzyme. The only explanation for the very low level of uroporphyrinogen decarboxylase protein in cells (5% of control value) was provided by a study of the half-life of the enzyme[347]; half-life was 82 hours in control cells and only 7 hours in the patients' cells. Thus, the enzyme defect appears to result from rapid degradation in vivo of an unstable protein.

Cloning and sequencing of a cDNA of the mutated gene in one patient from the family revealed the nature of the mutation that consists of a G to A change at nucleotide 860 in the cDNA sequence leading to a Gly (GGG) to Glu (GAG) change in the amino acid sequence at position 281.[347] In vitro experiments revealed that the cDNA with this mutation encoded a polypeptide product that was very rapidly degraded when compared with the polypeptide encoded by the normal cDNA in the presence of cell lysate. This observation is consistent with decreased stability of the mutant protein in vivo. Subsequent studies showed that there are different types of mutations in this disorder, such as another homozygous mutation involving a single base substitution within the coding region leading to the replacement of a glutanic acid by a lysine at codon 167,[348a] compound heterozygosity involving two separate point mutations,[348b] or a missense mutation combined with a large deletion.[348c]

Biochemical Findings. Most HEP patients have displayed elevations in urinary porphyrins, predominantly uroporphyrin I with lesser quantities of 7-carboxylic porphyrins, mainly type III. Isocoproporphyrin concentrations equal to or greater than coproporphyrin have also been detected in urine and feces. Elevated erythrocyte protoporphyrin (usually zinc protoporphyrin) has also been observed in HEP. Anemia and biochemical evidence of impaired hepatic function are highly variable. Serum iron is usually normal.

Diagnosis. The diagnosis must be suspected in patients with severe photosensitivity and especially considered in the differential diagnosis of CEP. Diagnostic criteria include elevated levels of fecal or urinary isocoproporphyrin and erythrocyte Zn-protoporphyrin. Included in the differential diagnosis is EPP in which erythrocyte protoporphyrin is also elevated but in which, in contrast to HEP, urinary porphyrins are normal. EPP is also clinically milder than HEP. Measurement of erythrocyte or fibroblast uroporphyrinogen decarboxylase activities typically shows reductions to 2% to 10% of normal control values with intermediate reductions of uroporphyrinogen decarboxylase activities in family members.[344]

Treatment. Avoidance of sun exposure and use of topical sun screens are essentially all that can be offered to HEP patients. Responses to phlebotomy have not been observed, although this is perhaps not surprising since serum iron levels, in contrast to those in PCT patients, are invariably normal.[344]

Hereditary Coproporphyria

Hereditary coproporphyria (HCP) is a heterozygous deficiency of coproporphyrinogen oxidase activity, which is inherited in an autosomal dominant manner. Clinically, HCP is similar to ALA dehydratase porphyria, or AIP, although it is often milder; in addition, HCP may be associated with photosensitivity. Expression of HCP is variable and influenced by the same factors responsible for exacerbating AIP. Rarely, homozygous deficiency of this enzyme may occur and is associated with a more severe form of the disease.

Prevalence. Clinically expressed HCP is much less common than clinically expressed AIP, but as with the latter disease, latent HCP or HCP gene carriers are being recognized more frequently since the advent of improved laboratory techniques for their detection. As of 1977, 111 cases had been reported.[349]

Clinical Findings. Neurovisceral symptomatology predominates and is essentially indistinguishable from that of ALA dehydratase porphyria or AIP. Thus, abdominal pain, vomiting, constipation, neuropathies, and psychiatric manifestations were reported to be most common in a review of 111 cases.[349] Cutaneous photosensitivity was a feature in about 30% of cases.[349] Attacks have been precipitated by pregnancy, menses, and contraceptive steroids,[232,350,351] but the most common precipitating factor has been drug administration, notably barbiturates.[352,353]

Biochemical Findings. The biochemical hallmark of HCP is hyperexcretion of coproporphyrin (predominantly type III) into the urine and feces. Fecal coproporphyrin may be chelated with copper,[354] and fecal protoporphyrin may be modestly elevated. Hyperexcretion of ALA, PBG, and uroporphyrin into the urine may accompany exacerbations of the disease, but in contrast to that seen in AIP, these findings generally normalize between attacks. Coproporphyrinogen oxidase activity is typically reduced by about 50% in heterozygotes and by about 90% to 98% in homozygotes. Homozygotes also show elevations in urinary ALA, PBG, and uroporphyrins; in addition, patients with harderoporphyria have elevated erythrocyte protoporphyrin levels and higher total fecal porphyrins, of which about 60% is harderoporphyrin.

Diagnosis. HCP should be suspected in patients with the symptoms and clinical course characteristic of the acute hepatic porphyrias (ALA dehydratase porphyria, AIP, HCP, and variegate porphyria), but in whom PBG deaminase activity is normal. Urinary excretion of heme precursors is similar in patients with HCP and variegate porphyria, but the predominant or exclusive presence of fecal coproporphyrin is more suggestive of HCP than variegate porphyria, in which fecal coproporphyrin and protoporphyrin concentrations are usually about equal. Fecal or urinary predominance of harderoporphyrin, with greatly reduced coproporphyrinogen oxidase activity, indicates harderoporphyria.

Harderoporphyria

Harderoporphyria is a variant of HCP described in a white family.[355] Coproporphyrinogen oxidase catalyzes the oxidative decarboxylation of the two propionyl groups at positions 2 and 4 of coproporphyrinogen to yield the two vinyl groups of protoporphyrinogen. Harderoporphyrin, a tricarboxylate porphyrinogen, is an intermediate in this reaction. Coproporphyrinogen oxidase activity determined in lymphocytes from three patients with harderoporphyria was only 10% of that of normal controls, suggesting that harderoporphyria patients were homozygous for the enzymatic defect. Enzyme kinetic studies showed that coproporphyrinogen oxidase in patients had an unusually high K_m (15- to 20-fold higher than the normal enzyme), and a half-maximal velocity. The enzyme activity in these patients was also abnormally sensitive to heat. The unique porphyrin excretion profile (harderoporphyrin predominating) and the properties of coproporphyrinogen oxidase in these patients are different from those of the homozygous case of HCP. It has been suggested that harderoporphyria is caused by a homozygous deficiency of a structurally altered enzyme, whereas a homozygous HCP is caused by a homozygous deficiency of the normal coproporphyrinogen oxidase.

Treatment. The identification and avoidance of precipitating factors are essential. Treatment of patients with acute attacks of HCP and harderoporphyria is similar to treatment of those with AIP.

Variegate Porphyria

Definition. Variegate porphyria (synonyms: porphyria variegata, protocoproporphyria, South African genetic porphyria, Royal malady) is caused by a heterozygous deficiency in protoporphyrinogen oxidase activity and is inherited in an autosomal dominant manner. Patients with this disorder may show neurovisceral symptoms, photosensitivity, or both. Very rare forms of variegate porphyria are seen with homozygous deficiencies in protoporphyrinogen oxidase activity.

Prevalence. The incidence of variegate porphyria of 3 per 1000 in South Africa is substantially higher than that found elsewhere. In 1980, an estimated 10,000 persons were affected in South Africa,[356] and good evidence indicates that all are descendants of a single union between two Dutch settlers in 1680.[303] Nevertheless, the disease has now been reported worldwide, and, with the exception of South Africa, probably no racial or geographic predilection exists. The incidence in Finland is reported at 1.3 per 100,000.[357] Outside South Africa, variegate porphyria is probably less common than AIP.

Clinical Findings. The neurovisceral symptomatology seen in patients with variegate porphyria is indistinguishable from that observed in ADP, AIP, and HCP (just described). Photosensitivity is more common, and the resulting lesions tend to be more chronic in patients with variegate porphyria than in patients with HCP. Cutaneous manifestations consist of vesicles, bullae, hyperpigmentation, milia, hypertrichosis, and increased skin fragility. Lesions are clinically and histologically indistinguishable from those affected with PCT, and in the absence of neurovisceral symptoms the diagnosis of variegate porphyria is easily overlooked.[358] Skin manifestations are less frequently observed in cold climates (45% in a series from Finland[357]) than in hot climates (85% in a series from South Africa[356]).

The same spectrum of factors that leads to activation of ALA dehydratase porphyria, AIP, and HCP also appears to exacerbate variegate porphyria. Thus, barbiturates,[359] dapsone,[360] lead from moonshine whiskey,[361] contraceptive steroids,[362] pregnancy,[349,363] and decreased carbohydrate intake[364,365] all have been reported to exacerbate variegate porphyria.

Pathogenesis of Clinical Findings. Protoporphyrinogen oxidase activity appears to be decreased in patients with variegate porphyria.[133,366,367] Homozygous variegate porphyria has been documented by virtual absence of this enzyme activity in three patients and suspected in another.[368,369] Symptoms were severe photosensitivity, growth and mental retardation, and marked neurologic abnormalities (in two patients); onset was in childhood in all cases.

Biochemical Findings. The biochemical hallmark of variegate porphyria is elevated fecal porphyrin excretion, usually with protoporphyrin exceeding coproporphyrin (mostly isomer III). Fecal mesoporphyrins and deuteroporphyrins may also be elevated. Fecal "X-porphyrins", a heterogeneous group of porphyrin–peptide conjugates, are elevated in patients with variegate porphyria more than with any other type of porphyria. Urinary coproporphyrin III, ALA, and PBG are often normal between attacks but may become markedly elevated during acute attacks. Plasma invariably contains a porphyrin with a fluorescence emission that is maximal at 626 nm and appears specific for variegate porphyria[370] and a porphyrin–peptide conjugate.[371]

Diagnosis. Variegate porphyria should be considered in the differential diagnosis of acute porphyria, especially if PBG deaminase activity is normal. Characteristic plasma porphyrin fluorescence, having a different fluorescence emission maximum from that of PCT, is seen in variegate porphyria.[370] The differentiation of variegate porphyria from HCP is usually possible after fecal porphyrin analysis in patients with only cutaneous manifestations. The demonstration of urinary 8- and 7-carboxylic porphyrins and isocoproporphyrin in PCT is usually sufficient for differentiation from variegate porphyria. Protoporphyrinogen oxidase activity can be measured in fibroblasts or lymphocytes.

Treatment. Identification and avoidance of precipitating factors are essential. Photosensitivity can be minimized by protective clothing and canthaxanthrin (a β-carotene analogue) may be of some help.[372] The treatment of patients with neurovisceral symptoms is identical with that described for AIP patients.

Erythropoietic Protoporphyria

Definition. EPP (synonyms: protoporphyria, erythrohepatic protoporphyria) is inherited in an autosomal dominant fashion and is associated with decreased activity of ferrochelatase. Biochemically, this defect results in massive accumulations of protoporphyrin in erythrocytes, plasma, and feces. Clinically, the disease is characterized by the childhood onset of cutaneous photosensitivity in light-exposed areas, but skin lesions are milder and less disfiguring than those seen in CEP.

Prevalence. EPP is the most common form of erythropoietic porphyria. Three hundred case reports were published as of 1976.[373] No racial or sexual predilection is found, and onset is typically in childhood.

Clinical Findings. Symptoms of EPP are usually worse during spring and summer and occur in light-exposed areas, especially on the face and hands. Within 1 hour of exposure to the sun, stinging or painful burning sensations in the skin occur and are followed several hours later by erythema and edema. Petechiae or, more rarely, purpura, vesicles, and crusting may develop and persist for several days after sun exposure. Some patients experience burning sensations in the absence of such objective signs of cutaneous phototoxicity. Artificial lights may also cause photosensitivity, especially theater lights.[374] Intense and repeated exposure to the sun may result in oncolysis, leathery hyperkeratotic skin over the dorsa of the hands, and mild scarring (Fig. 50-12). Gallstones, sometimes presenting at an unusually early age, are fairly common. Hepatic disease, although unusual, may be severe and associated with significant morbidity. Anemia is not common. No precipitating factors and no neurovisceral manifestations are known.

Pathogenesis of Clinical Findings. The peak light absorption range for porphyrins, that is, in the region of the Soret band, corresponds well to the wavelength of light (about 400 nm) known to trigger photosensitivity reactions in the skin of EPP patients.[375] Protoporphyrin, but not zinc protoporphyrin, is released from erythrocytes after light exposure, which may explain why lead intoxication and iron deficiency are not associated with photosensitivity.[376] Forearm irradiation in EPP patients leads to complement activation and polymorphonuclear chemotaxis.[309] Similar

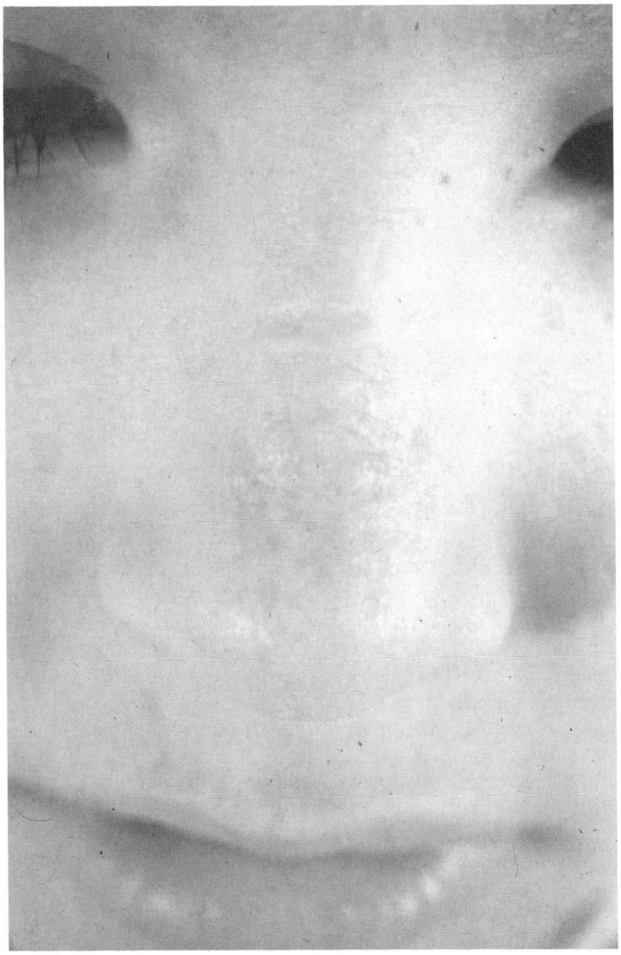

FIGURE 50-12. Typical shallow, elliptical scars over the nose in a child with erythropoietic protoporphyria. (See Color Fig. 50-12.) (Poh-Fitzpatrick MB. Porphyrin-sensitized cutaneous photosensitivity. Clin Dermatol 1985;3:41)

results have been obtained in vitro,[377,378] and these events may also contribute to the pathogenesis of skin lesions in EPP.

Biochemical Findings. The biochemical hallmark of EPP is excessive concentrations of protoporphyrin in erythrocytes, plasma, bile, and feces, but not in urine. Available evidence tends to favor the bone marrow and the newly released reticulocyte–erythrocyte as the major source of elevated protoporphyrin concentrations[140,379,380] (Fig. 50-13), although the liver may contribute in certain cases.[381,382] Mild anemia with hypochromia and microcytosis may occasionally be seen (in about 20% of patients).[140,373] One patient with EPP also had a hematologic feature compatible with sideroblastic anemia.[383] In general, heme synthesis in EPP appears normal, despite a large overproduction of protoporphyrin.[375] A single case of homozygous ferrochelatase deficiency has been described in an 18-year-old man who had normal growth and normal hematologic picture.[384] Bovine protoporphyria, which is due to a homozygous deficiency of ferrochelatase, is also not associated with anemia.[142] Although erythrocyte protoporphyrin concentration is markedly increased in EPP, it is still a small fraction compared with the overall rate of protoporphyrin production for heme synthesis; an increase of protoporphyrin in EPP can be explained by an increase in overall synthesis of protoporphyrin of only 5% to 8%.[385] Increased hepatic ALA synthase activity has also been implicated in the elevation of erythrocyte protoporphyrin in EPP patients,[386,387] which may contribute to the maintenance of heme concentrations in erythroid cells in this disease. In support of this hypothesis, hematin administration, which presumably suppresses ALA synthase activity, was also shown to reduce the rate of protoporphyrin formation in patients with EPP.[388] Mild hypertriglyceridemia also occurs with increased incidence in patients with EPP.[389]

The molecular basis of the defect of ferrochelatase in two patients has recently been described. The first case was a patient with heterozygous ferrochelatase deficiency.[389a] The enzyme activity, the immunoquantifiable

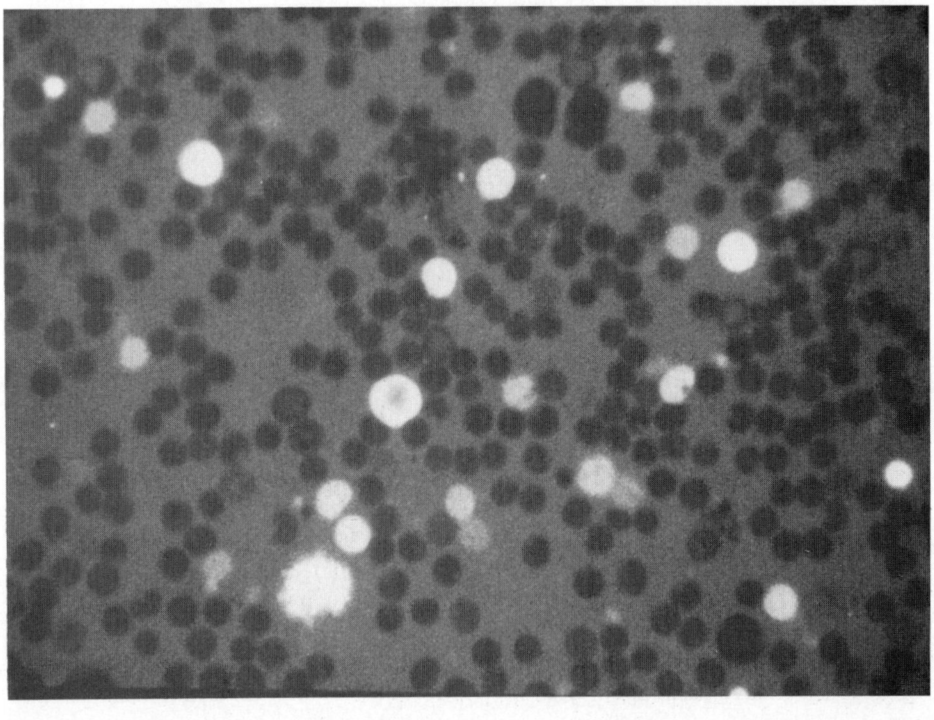

FIGURE 50-13. Fluorescent erythroblasts in a bone marrow smear from a patient with erythropoietic protoporphyria. (See Color Fig. 50-13.) (Poh-Fitzpatrick MB. Porphyrin-sensitized cutaneous photosensitivity. Clin Dermatol 1985;3:41)

protein, and the mRNA content of ferrochelatase were about half the normal level. However, the rate of transcription of ferrochelatase mRNA was normal, suggesting that the decrease in ferrochelatase mRNA was due to an unstable transcript. cDNA clones encoding ferrochelatase in the proband were found to be classified either into those encoding the normal protein, or into those encoding an abnormal protein with a deletion of 127 bp corresponding to nucleotides 67 to 194 of the normal ferrochelatase cDNA. Comparison of this sequence with that of normal genomic DNA showed that the missing fragment corresponded to the entire region of exon 2. Genomic DNA analysis revealed that the abnormal allele had a point mutation, C → T, near the acceptor site of intron 1.

The other patient was a homozygous case with ferrochelatase activity at 10% of the normal level.[384] Two mutations were identified[389b]: one was the replacement of glycine with cysteine at position 55, and the other was the replacement of methionine with isoleucine at position 267. This patient was therefore doubly heterozygous for the gene defect, and as expected, each of his parents carried one of these mutations. These findings suggest that EPP is a heterogeneous disease. Its mode of inheritance seems to be generally dominant but can sometimes be recessive[389c]; the difference may depend on the types of mutations.[389d] Recessive inheritance may occur if a mutation in the ferrochelatase gene is not entirely lethal so that it permits some degree of heme synthesis. In contrast, the dominant inheritance may occur as a result of a lethal mutation of the ferrochelatase gene, which is then unable to synthesize heme. Thus, a homozygous case with the dominant type of mutation would be incompatible with life, whereas a heterozygote may be expressed as EPP. Furthermore, not all gene carriers of ferrochelatase deficiency express themselves as EPP; there is a variable degree of clinical expression in this disorder, suggesting that other factors may be involved in the clinical expression of this enzyme defect, as is the case with other dominantly inherited porphyrias.

Diagnosis. Photosensitivity should suggest the diagnosis of EPP, which can be confirmed by elevated concentrations of free protoporphyrin in erythrocytes, plasma, and stools with normal urinary porphyrins. The presence of protoporphyrin (as evidenced by its characteristic spectrum) in both plasma and erythrocytes is a finding specific for EPP. Fluorescent reticulocytes on examination of peripheral blood smear may also suggest the diagnosis.

Treatment. Avoidance of sun exposure and use of topical sunscreen agents may be helpful. Oral administration of β-carotene may afford systemic photoprotection resulting in improved, although highly variable, tolerance to the sun.[390,391] The recommended serum β-carotene level of 600 to 800 μg/dL is usually achieved with oral doses of 120 to 180 mg/d, and beneficial effects are typically seen 1 to 3 months after the onset of therapy.[373] The mechanism of protection probably involves quenching of activated oxygen radicals.[294]

Prenatal Diagnosis of Porphyria

Note that in the heterozygous porphyrias, even though prenatal diagnosis is possible, clinical expression of inherited defective enzyme activity is far from inevitable (only 1 in 10 cases of AIP). Consequently, the demonstration of decreased enzyme activities compatible with a heterozygous form of an autosomal dominant porphyria is not considered an indication for termination of pregnancy. In contrast, decreased enzyme activities consistent with homozygous porphyrias, because of their more severe clinical course, may be considered indications for termination of pregnancy. Such cases are exceedingly rare.

LEAD POISONING

Adverse Effects of Lead

Lead poisoning has been recognized as a health hazard for more than 2000 years. This potentially preventable disorder is still a public health problem despite extensive efforts to eliminate the sources of exposure. In humans, three major tissues are principally affected by lead: kidney, hematopoietic tissues, and CNS. If proper measures are taken, the renal and hematopoietic effects of lead are reversible, whereas the CNS effects are almost always irreversible, leaving clinically serious sequelae in afflicted persons. The major biochemical interactions of lead in the organism can be grouped into three categories: its high affinity for sulfhydryl groups; its competition with other biologically important divalent metals; and its effects on nucleic acid metabolism.[392]

Adults and developing children show distinct clinical presentations of lead poisoning. Specifically, adults acquire lead poisoning mainly by occupational exposure and almost always show signs of chronic lead poisoning. This presentation is characterized by abdominal pain and peripheral motor neuropathy, such as radial palsy and house painter's wristdrop.[393–395] In contrast, infants and children acquire lead poisoning mostly from ingestion of the metal and generally develop acute CNS symptoms.

The three basic stages in childhood lead poisoning are asymptomatic lead poisoning, in which measurable metabolic changes but no clinical symptoms occur; symptomatic lead poisoning, which manifests clinically as anorexia, vomiting, apathy, ataxia, drowsiness, or irritability; and lead encephalopathy with cerebral edema that may progress to convulsions or coma.[396,397] The sequelae of lead encephalopathy include chronic seizures, severe mental retardation, or death. Even with a less severe form of lead poisoning, minimal brain dysfunctions are common and various behavioral and functional abnormalities such as hyperactivity, compulsive behavior, prolonged reaction time, perceptual disorders, and learning disability may develop.

The term *critical effect* is used in lead poisoning to indicate the first definable effect of the toxic metal. The critical effect denotes the most sensitive and specific biologic change, which is beyond acceptable physiologic variation, rather than the most serious effect caused by metal. The critical effect occurs in the hematopoietic system, and environmental limits to prevent irreversible effects of lead on the CNS are determined using reversible effects in the hematopoietic system. The first metabolic effects in children become evident when the blood lead concentration exceeds 15 to 20 μg/dL. Potent inhibition of erythrocyte ALA dehydratase activity and moderate increases in erythrocyte protoporphyrin are observed at these blood lead levels.[42,398] More detailed information can be found in comprehensive accounts.[399–401]

Sources of Lead in the Environment

Lead occurs in nature mainly as a sulfide. Natural sources contribute little to the present daily concentrations of lead in our environment. The most useful records of the natural concentrations of lead are found in chronologic layers of snow strata, which are present in quiescent ice sheets in perpetually frozen polar regions.[402] Annual ice layers from the interior of northern Greenland show that lead concentrations in 800 BC were less than 0.0005 μg/kg, whereas they were greater than 0.2 μg/kg in AD 1965, which is more than a 400-fold increase in 2000 years and more than a 16-fold increase after the start of the Industrial Revolution.

Antarctic continental ice sheets fail to show similar changes, perhaps due to barriers to north–south tropospheric mixing, which prevent the migration of the aerosol pollutants, mainly emitted in the northern hemisphere, to the Antarctic.

The relative inertness and malleability of the metal are useful features for many purposes. Lead is used widely in the electric storage battery, petroleum, and paint industries. Until the ban on the use of lead in gasoline recently, 98% of airborne lead could be traced to this source—the combustion of gasoline containing lead additives. The levels of atmospheric lead in large cities are significantly higher than in small rural towns because of emissions from automobiles. The number of children with blood lead levels of 60 μg/dL doubled in areas of vehicular densities greater than 24,000 as a weekday average, compared with a city-wide basis of vehicular densities less than 24,000.[403]

Occupational lead exposure results largely from inhalation of lead dust. In contrast, gastrointestinal absorption represents the most important route of lead absorption in children. In addition, a small amount of lead can be absorbed through the skin; this is usually of minor significance. About 300 μg/d lead is ingested naturally.[404] Adults may absorb less than 10% of the daily intake of lead,[399,405] whereas young children may absorb as much as 50% through the gut.[406] A daily intake up to 40 μg/d may be tolerated for a lifetime with no apparent detrimental effects.[407]

Lead in paint films is less well absorbed than dietary lead. About 17% of lead in paint would be absorbed by a young child, compared with 50% absorption of dietary lead. Pica, the repetitive ingestion of nonfood substances, occurs in about 50% of children between 1 and 3 years of age. It is considered normal behavior until a child is 3 years of age; persistence of the habit beyond this age is associated with psychosocial complications or organic brain damage. Children with pica may ingest 1 to 3 g of paint chips per week.[408] Children with normal blood lead levels of 20 μg/dL on a normal diet absorb lead at a rate of about 4.5 μg/kg/d.[408] A child with pica for paint (containing the legal limit of 0.5% [weight to volume], or 5000 μg lead per gram of paint) may absorb three to seven times more lead than a child with a normal diet. Thus, for a child with pica, 0.5% lead in paint clearly represents a hazard.[408] Lipids or milk in the diet may facilitate the retention of ingested lead. In addition, dietary deficiencies of calcium, copper, and iron increase the absorption of lead in experimental animals.

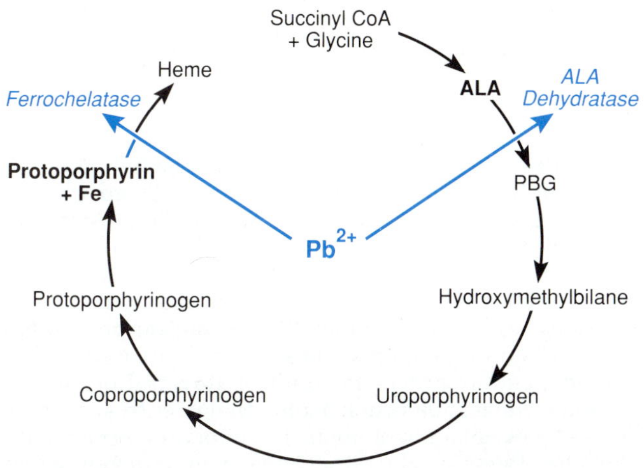

FIGURE 50-14. Effects of lead on heme biosynthesis.

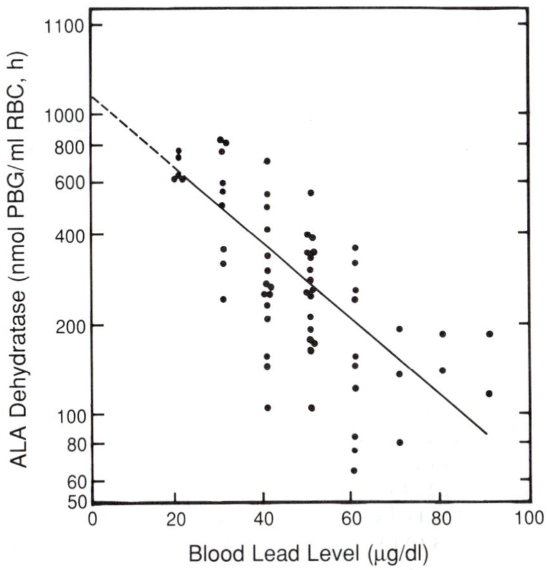

FIGURE 50-15. The log of erythrocyte ALA dehydratase activity is inversely related to blood lead concentrations (r = .72). (After Granick JL, Sassa S, Granick S, Levere RD, Kappas A. Studies in lead poisoning. II. Correlation between the ratio of activated to inactivated δ-aminolevulinic acid dehydrogenase of whole blood and the blood lead level. Biochem Med 1973;8:149)

Hematologic Effects of Lead

One of the most evident sites of the toxic effects of lead is the hematopoietic system. Both anemia and disturbances in heme biosynthesis occur in lead poisoning. Two principal enzymic sites in the heme biosynthetic pathway are subject to inhibition by lead, ALA dehydratase, and ferrochelatase (Fig. 50-14). Both enzymes are sulfhydryl dependent, and lead interferes with their activities by binding to critical sulfhydryl groups.

ALA Dehydratase

Lead displaces the zinc atom in ALA dehydratase by mercaptide formation, resulting in inactivation of the enzyme. Zinc supplementation can restore the lead-inhibited enzyme activity in vitro.[34] Lead does not interfere with the synthesis of ALA dehydratase. On the contrary, evidence both in experimental animals and in humans suggests that the synthesis of ALA dehydratase is stimulated in reticulocytes in lead poisoning.[409–411]

The inhibition of ALA dehydratase by lead in vivo results in accumulation of the substrate, ALA, which is then excreted in the urine. Lead inhibition of ALA dehydratase activity in erythrocytes represents one of the most sensitive indices of the biologic effects of the metal. The log of enzyme activity is inversely related to lead concentration in blood[42] (Fig. 50-15). The enzyme activity is decreased about 50% with an increase in blood lead concentration of 20 μg/dL. Lead-inhibited ALA dehydratase activity can be completely reactivated, over a wide range of blood lead concentrations, by incubating blood samples in the presence of sulfhydryl-donating reagents such as dithiothreitol or reduced glutathione. Erythrocyte ALA dehydratase in normal blood is also activated two-fold by dithiothreitol, suggesting that the enzyme in normal blood is present in a partially inactivated form.[42]

The broad distribution of enzyme activities compared with blood lead concentrations (r = .72; see Fig. 50-15) is partly due to genetic variation of enzyme activity.[42] On the other hand, the ratio of dithiothreitol-activated enzyme to nonactivated enzyme activity is not influenced by genetic variation of the enzyme activity and shows a linear regression compared with blood lead levels with a higher correlation coefficient (r = .8; Fig. 50-16).[42] The minimum blood lead level that displays any evident effect on erythrocyte ALA dehydratase activity is about 15 μg/dL[42]; this level can thus be considered the critical effect concentration of lead in humans.

Ferrochelatase

Ferrochelatase, the terminal enzyme of the heme biosynthetic pathway, is also subject to marked inhibition by lead. Abnormal accumulations of iron have been reported in the mitochondria of erythroblasts from animals with experimental lead poisoning,[412] presumably due to a block at the ferrochelatase step. Ferrochelatase activity in erythropoietic tissues appears to be more vulnerable to inhibition by lead than the enzyme in nonerythropoietic tissues, since the hepatic enzyme is not influenced in animals treated with the metal.[413] Inhibition of ferrochelatase in erythropoietic tissues in vivo results in the accumulation of erythrocyte protoporphyrin. Since circulating erythrocytes in mammals do not contain mitochondria, the elevated erythrocyte protoporphyrin in lead-poisoned subjects must reflect the inhibition of ferrochelatase in bone marrow erythroblasts and reticulocytes.

The levels of erythrocyte protoporphyrin represent an average of the effects of bone marrow lead on erythroid ferrochelatase during the 3-month (approximate) life-span of circulating erythrocytes.[398] Erythrocyte protoporphyrin is therefore a good indicator of chronic lead exposure (see also a review[414]). The log of erythrocyte protoporphyrin is linearly correlated with blood lead levels (Fig. 50-17).

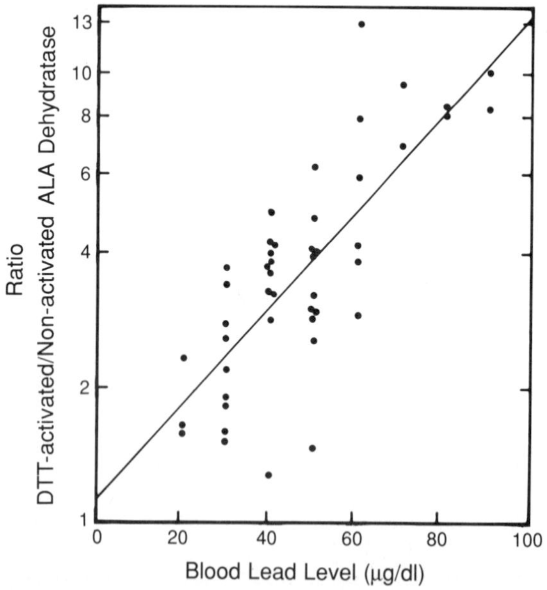

FIGURE 50-16. Ratio of activated ALA dehydratase to nonactivated ALA dehydratase and blood lead concentrations. Dithiothreitol (DTT) activates lead-inhibited ALA dehydratase activity and completely restores enzyme activity. Thus, the ratio between DTT-activated and nonactivated ALA dehydratase activity is independent of genetic variation, and is linearly correlated with blood lead concentrations. A higher correlation coefficient (r = .80) than that in Figure 50-15 is considered to reflect the normalization of genetic variation in enzyme activity in this figure. (After Granick JL, Sassa S, Granick S, Levere RD, Kappas A. Studies in lead poisoning. II. Correlation between the ratio of activated to inactivated δ-aminolevulinic acid dehydrogenase of whole blood and the blood lead level. Biochem Med 1973;8:149)

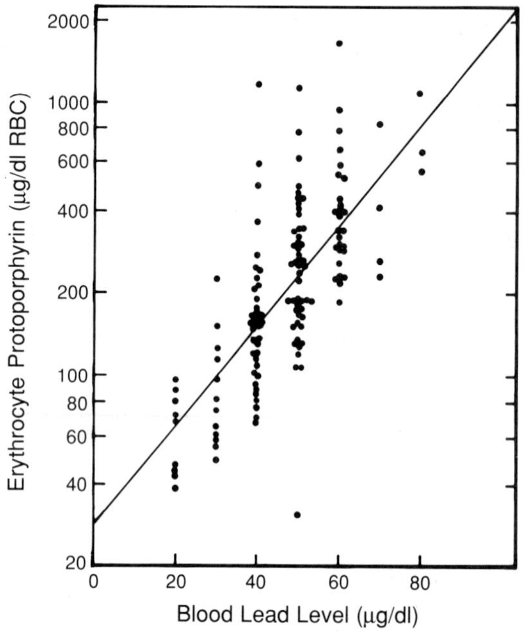

FIGURE 50-17. The log of erythrocyte protoporphyrin concentrations is correlated with blood lead levels (r = .72). (After Sassa S, Granick JL, Granick S, Kappas A, Levere RD. Studies in lead poisoning. I. Microanalysis of erythrocyte protoporphyrin levels by spectrophotometry in the detection of chronic lead intoxication in the subclinical range. Biochem Med 1973;8:135)

Erythrocyte protoporphyrin has been frequently referred to as *free erythrocyte protoporphyrin*; the porphyrin is largely chelated with zinc in humans.[415] Zinc cytochrome c has also been found in lead-poisoned animals.[416] These findings suggest that zinc may be incorporated into protoporphyrin in place of iron when iron incorporation into heme is inhibited by lead.

Effects of lead on other steps in the heme biosynthetic pathway are of lesser significance in vivo. Lead intoxication is known to cause coproporphyrin excretion into the urine. Studies in rabbits experimentally poisoned with lead indicate that decarboxylations of porphyrins leading to diminished production of coproporphyrin are only minimally affected by the metal.[417] The source of coproporphyrin may not be erythroid but rather other tissues such as kidney. Although lead-mediated inhibition of ALA dehydratase and ferrochelatase represents one of the most sensitive measures of the biologic effects of lead, this enzyme inhibition is rarely accompanied by severe heme deficiency in the erythropoietic system. For example, anemia of lead poisoning is almost always normochromic and normocytic in nature and is distinct from the anemia caused by iron deficiency that is hypochromic and microcytic.

Lead-Induced Inclusion Bodies

Lead forms several inclusion bodies in the cell. Nuclear inclusion bodies in renal tubular lining cells are characteristic signs of lead poisoning (Fig. 50-18). They occur most frequently in the proximal tubule and appear as dense bodies under light microscopy. The inclusion body is a lead–protein complex, and most of the lead in the kidney is sequestered in the complex.[418] The nuclear protein has been found to be a nonhistone acidic protein, enriched in glutamic and aspartic acid residues. Reversal of the formation of nuclear inclusion bodies, that is, extrusion of the bodies by evagination of nuclear membranes, occurs after chelation therapy. Thus, the nuclear protein complexes represent a labile and removable pool of the toxic metal.[419]

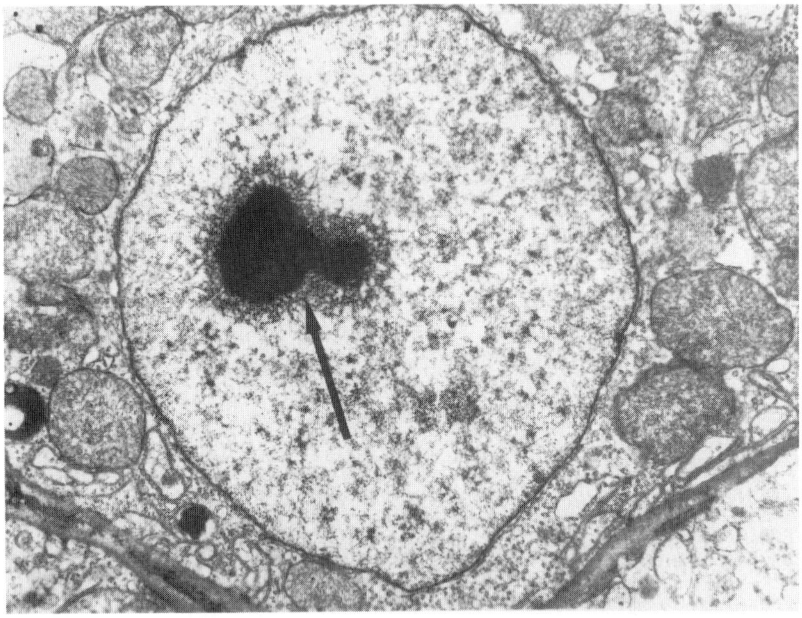

FIGURE 50-18. A nuclear inclusion body of the proximal renal tubular lining cell of lead-poisoned rat. (Goyer RA, May P, Cates M, et al. Lead and protein content of isolated intranuclear inclusion bodies from kidneys of lead-poisoned rats. Lab Invest 1970;22:245)

A partial impairment of the respiratory and oxidative activities of kidney mitochondria has been reported in lead-poisoned rats. The adenosine diphosphate-stimulated respiration of mitochondria isolated from kidneys of normal rats can be inhibited by lead in vitro as low as 0.15 to 0.2 μg/mg of mitochondrial protein. The maturing brain may be most vulnerable to the toxicity of lead at the critical period when rapid synthesis and increasing activity of respiratory enzymes take place. Lead feeding to suckling rats produces an encephalopathy similar to that seen in infants, and mitochondria isolated from brain, particularly from cerebellum, show decreased NAD-linked respiration and cytochrome oxidase activity.[420]

Pyrimidine 5′-Nucleotidase

Pyrimidine nucleotides, which result from degradation of ribosomal RNA by ribonucleases in reticulocytes, are usually present in only minute amounts in normal erythrocytes.[421] Erythrocytes that are deficient in or have inhibited pyrimidine 5′-nucleotidase activity are unable to dephosphorylate; thus, they render diffusible, pyrimidine 5′-nucleotide monophosphates.[422] The accumulated pyrimidine nucleotides are believed to retard RNA breakdown and result in the aggregation of undegraded and partially degraded ribosomes that are observed as basophilic stippling[422] (Fig. 50-19). Pyrimidine 5′-nucleotidase activity in normal erythrocytes can be markedly inhibited by lead or certain other heavy metals, and lead poisoning in vivo is associated with marked decreases in erythrocyte pyrimidine 5′-nucleotidase activity[423] (Fig. 50-20). Also, a significant correlation exists between pyrimidine 5′-nucleotidase activity and the levels of cytidine 5′-nucleotidase (CTP; Fig. 50-21) as well as between erythrocyte protoporphyrin concentration and CTP levels[424] (Fig. 50-22). The increase in CTP and uridine triphosphate antedates basophilic stippling in lead-treated animals.[424] Clinically, erythrocyte pyrimidine 5′-nucleotidase activity has been shown to be a reliable and sensitive index of lead exposure.[425] Decreased pyrimidine 5′-nucleotidase activity in erythrocytes reflects chronic effects of lead on reticulocytes rather than acute effects.[426] In this respect, pyrimidine 5′-nucleotidase activity

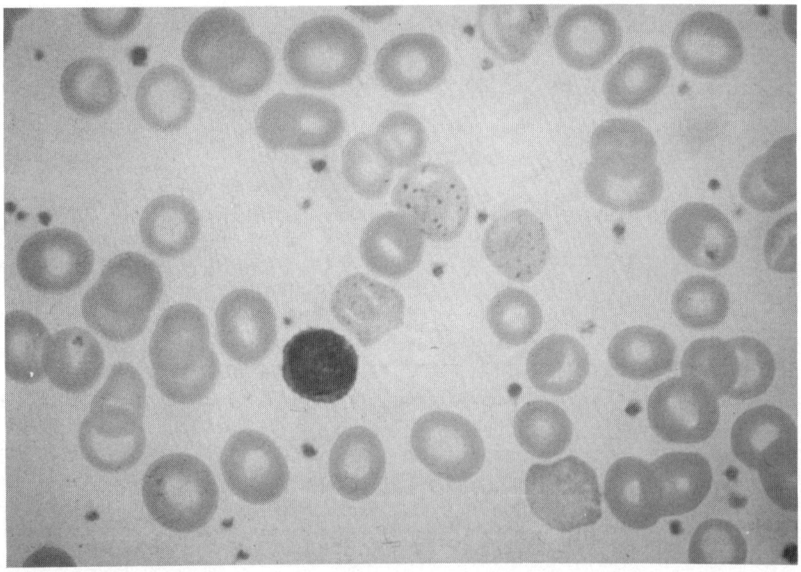

FIGURE 50-19. Basophilic stippling of erythrocytes. (See Color Fig. 50-19.) (Courtesy of Dr. F.H. Bunn)

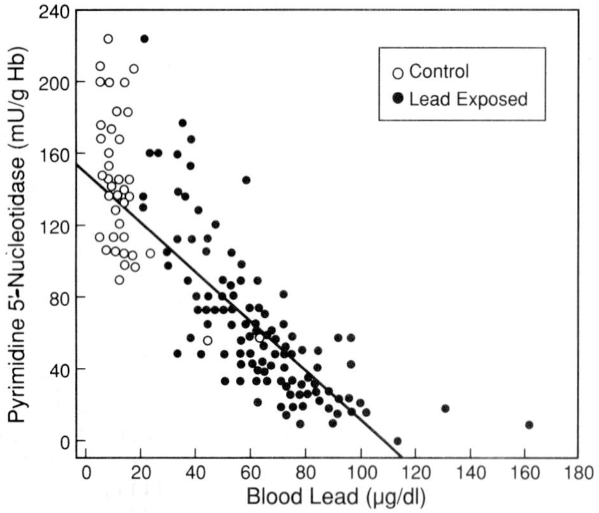

FIGURE 50-20. Inverse relation between blood lead and erythrocyte pyrimidine 5'-nucleotidase activity (mU/g hemoglobin; 1 U = 1 nmol CMP hydrolyzed/min). (After Angle CR, Stohs SJ, McIntire MS, et al. Lead-induced accumulation of erythrocyte pyrimidine nucleotides in the rabbit. Toxicol Appl Pharmacol 1980;54:161)

provides information similar to that provided by erythrocyte protoporphyrin levels. Both the genetic deficiency of pyrimidine 5'-nucleotidase and certain cases of lead poisoning are characterized by hemolytic anemia and basophilic stippling, and these features can be explained in part by the decreased pyrimidine 5'-nucleotidase activity observed in both disorders. A general discussion on hemolytic anemia and erythrocyte enzymopathies including pyrimidine 5'-nucleotidase deficiency can be found in a comprehensive review.[427]

Anemia

Anemia in lead poisoning is usually normochromic and normocytic and not associated with hypochromia. This finding suggests that sufficient heme is made to completely supplement the need for heme for hemoglobin formation, even in the presence of inhibition of certain enzymes in the heme biosynthetic pathway. In patients with lead poisoning, osmotic fragility of RBCs is decreased, whereas mechanical fragility is increased.[428,429] Although lead is known

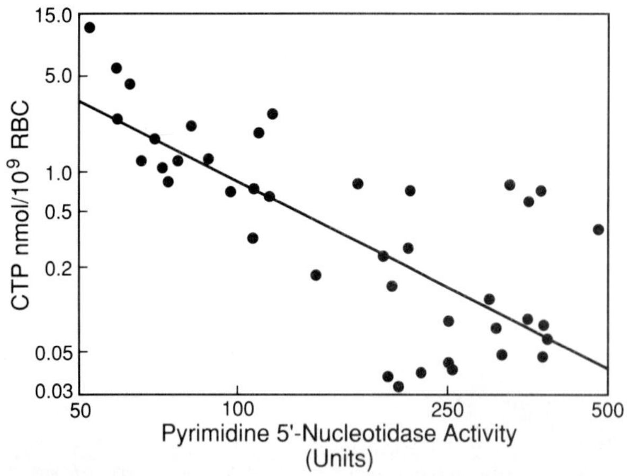

FIGURE 50-21. Inverse relation between erythrocyte cytidine 5'-triphosphate (CTP) and pyrimidine 5'-nucleotidase activity. (After Torrance JD, Mills W, Kilroe-Smith TA, et al. Erythrocyte pyrimidine 5'-nucleotidase activity as a sensitive indicator of lead exposure. S Afr Med J 1985;67:850)

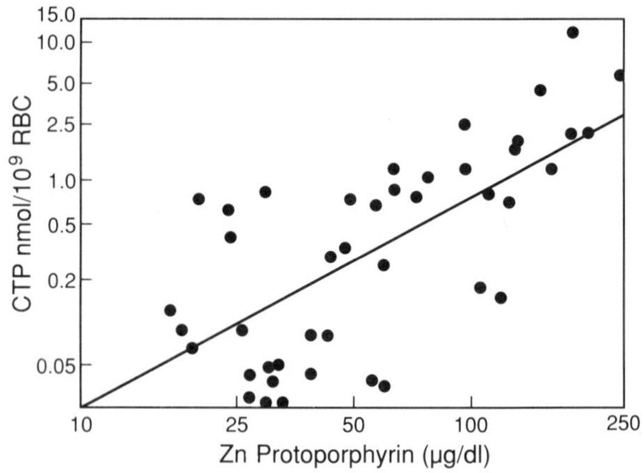

FIGURE 50-22. Relation between erythrocyte cytidine 5'-triphosphate (CTP) and zinc protoporphyrin. (After Angle CR, Stohs SJ, McIntire MS, et al. Lead-induced accumulation of erythrocyte pyrimidine nucleotides in the rabbit. Toxicol Appl Pharmacol 1980;54:161)

to bind firmly to phosphatidylcholine in membranes in vitro,[430] it is not known whether such a mechanism is responsible for the abnormal fragility of lead-poisoned RBCs. Incubation of human erythrocytes with lead in vitro results in marked loss of K^+.[431,432] Membrane Na^+-K^+-ATPase activity is decreased by incubation of erythrocytes with lead,[433] but this may not account for the leakage of K^+ from cells, since the passive influx of Na^+ is greater than the efflux of K^+. Renal tubular Na^+-K^+-ATPase activity is also markedly inhibited by incubation with lead.[434]

Some studies using lead tracers showed that the metal apparently accumulates in cell membranes,[435] whereas others showed that the metal is preferentially bound to hemoglobin and some low molecular weight material in the cytosol.[436] At any rate, these findings suggest that anemia in lead poisoning is more likely due to a shortened life-span of erythrocytes than to impaired heme synthesis. The extent to which the RBC life-span is diminished also correlates most closely with the reticulocyte count.[437] It should also be noted that the anemia in acute severe lead exposure is characterized by hemolysis, whereas prolonged and increased exposure leads ultimately to erythroid hypoplasia and marked morphologic changes in the bone marrow.[408]

When normal erythrocytes are incubated with lead in vitro, suppression of pentose phosphate shunt activity is observed, together with decreased glutathione and Heinz body formation.[438] This suggests that lead-poisoned erythrocytes are more sensitive to oxidant stress than normal cells, and that the suppression of the pentose phosphate shunt may, in part, account for the shortened life-span of erythrocytes in lead poisoning.

Treatment

Chelation therapy should be instituted when evidence of increased absorption or accumulation of lead in tissues is found. In addition, patients should be removed from the source of lead exposure. In the case of occupational exposure, this can be achieved by permanent isolation, or sometimes even by rotation of workers. Physicians need to identify unusual sources of lead exposure, such as the burning of battery casings,[439,440] improperly lead-glazed culinary ware,[441,442] old tapestry containing high amounts of lead,[443] glass-making materials,[444] artists' paint pigments,[443] lead dust in shooting galleries,[445] and other sources. Patients with blood lead levels lower than 80 μg/dL blood can be treated with chelating agents on an ambulatory basis, whereas those with higher blood lead levels should probably be treated in hospitals.

Three chelating agents are commonly used to treat lead poisoning. British antilewisite (BAL; 2,3-mercaptopropanol) is given as a single injection of up to 4 mg/kg to promote excretion of lead. In adults, 3 mg/kg appears to be better tolerated.[446] Although some authorities consider that BAL has a place either singly or in combination therapy, this agent has been largely superseded by calcium disodium ethylene diamine tetraacetic acid (Ca-Na_2EDTA, edathamil calcium disodium, or calcium versenate) and penicillamine.[446] Ca-Na_2EDTA, 12.5 mg/kg, is administered intramuscularly and increases the urinary excretion of lead by 30- to 50-fold.[446] D-Penicillamine can be administered orally in doses of 150 mg twice daily for 4 to 6 weeks in children; 250 to 500 mg twice daily for adults increases renal lead excretion three to eight times,[447] although it produces a marked zincuresis as well.[448] In addition to chelation therapy, subsequent exposure to lead should be carefully monitored, since this will ensure the most effective means of preventing the accumulation of an increased body burden of lead. During treatment, patients should be monitored by daily total urinary lead excretion and blood lead concentrations.

HEME DEGRADATION AND BILIRUBIN FORMATION

Heme Transport

Senescent erythrocytes are removed and catabolized by macrophages. Heme in the circulation is essentially all bound to albumin and hemopexin; thus, free heme is not usually found in plasma. Free hemoglobin is also bound with haptoglobin and rapidly cleared from plasma by hepatic uptake (Fig. 50-23).

Haptoglobin

Structure. Haptoglobin is a plasma protein that belongs to the class of α_2-glycoproteins. It is synthesized in the liver, and its function appears to be to sequester free hemoglobin that may be released from erythrocytes as a result of hemolysis injury or inflammation. Haptoglobin has been identified in all mammals and vertebrates so far studied.[449] The protein forms a stable, effectively irreversible complex with free hemoglobin. The stable hemoglobin–haptoglobin complex is then removed from the bloodstream by incorporation exclusively into liver parenchymal cells through a receptor-mediated mechanism. It is degraded there, and the iron atom of heme recycled.[450] In this manner, cellular injury in the kidney glomerulus by free hemoglobin is circumvented.[451] The complex is also taken up by reticuloendothelial cells in the liver and spleen.[449] The role of haptoglobin is thought to be related to the recycling of hemoglobin iron, but it has also been suggested that one of its functions is to deny heme iron to pathogenic organisms.[452]

Native rat haptoglobin is a heterotetramer consisting of two α subunits (about 9.5 kd) and two glycosylated β subunits (about 38 kd), which are covalently attached by interchain disulfide bonds. The α and β subunits are also called light (L) and heavy (H) chains, respectively. A single disulfide bond exists between the α subunits, each of which is linked to a glycosylated β subunit by a single disulfide linkage.[453] About 35% homology exists between the hap-

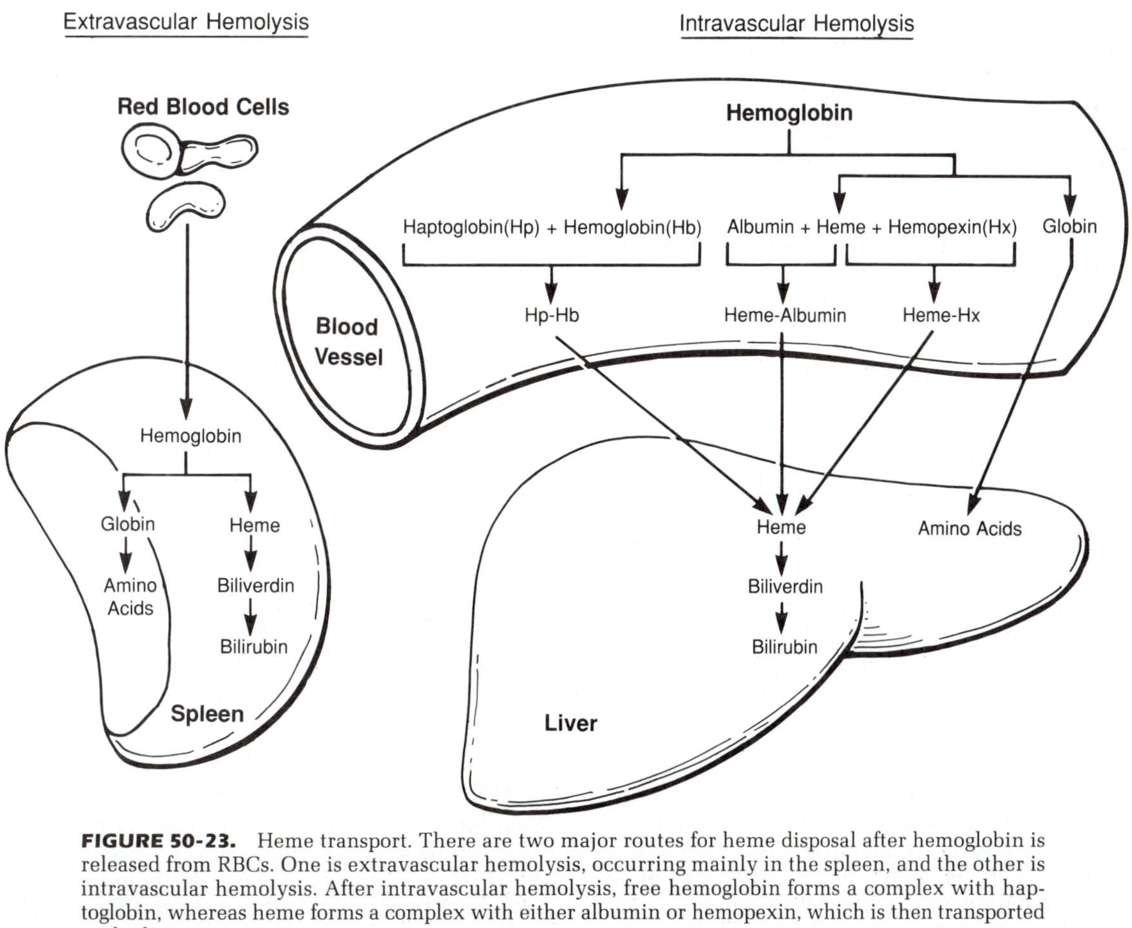

FIGURE 50-23. Heme transport. There are two major routes for heme disposal after hemoglobin is released from RBCs. One is extravascular hemolysis, occurring mainly in the spleen, and the other is intravascular hemolysis. After intravascular hemolysis, free hemoglobin forms a complex with haptoglobin, whereas heme forms a complex with either albumin or hemopexin, which is then transported to the liver.

toglobin structure and the structure of several serine proteases. Haptoglobin does not exhibit serine protease activity, since two of the three active site amino acids of serine proteases have been substituted in haptoglobin.[454] The amino acid sequence of the β subunit of haptoglobin from several species has been partially analyzed.[455] The synthesis of haptoglobin is encoded by a single mRNA, and the primary in vitro translation product is a single polypeptide, preprohaptoglobin (about 40 kd), which contains both an NH_2-terminal signal sequence, an α-subunit region, and a β-subunit region.[456]

Preprohaptoglobin is processed to prohaptoglobin cotranslationally, whereas prohaptoglobin undergoes dimerization in the endoplasmic reticulum, followed by processing into the individual α and β subunits.[454] Some prohaptoglobin is secreted from hepatocytes as a dimer, which then undergoes conversion to α and β subunits after secretion.[454] The molecular weight of the complete protein is about 85 kd in rats, and the protein can be symbolized as H-L-L-H, or $(\alpha\beta)_2$.[457] This form of the complex in humans is referred to as Hp1-1.

Clearance of the hemoglobin–haptoglobin complex in humans occurs at a rate of about 15 mg hemoglobin per 100 mL of plasma per hour.[458,459] When the hemoglobin tetramer splits into two dimers, the $\alpha_1\beta_2$ interface is exposed, whereas the $\alpha_1\beta_1$ interface is preserved. These dimers, termed *$\alpha_1\beta_1$-dimers*, form a complex with Hp1-1 (the haptoglobin–hemoglobin complex).[460–465] Each $\alpha_1\beta_1$-dimer binds to an H chain of haptoglobin; the L chain does not interact with hemoglobin.[466,467] Since the $\alpha\beta$ dimers, not the tetramers, bind to haptoglobin and many different species of hemoglobin bind to human haptoglobin, the sequence-invariant $\alpha_1\beta_2$-interdimer interface is probably the region of hemoglobin that binds to the H chain.[462] Residues around 130 to 137 in the H chain have been suggested to be the most likely sites of hemoglobin binding.

Polymorphism. Haptoglobin has been extensively studied from a genetic point of view, since it consists of several different phenotypes in animals and humans. For example, when plasma from different persons is examined by starch gel electrophoresis, several distinct and characteristic haptoglobin types can be recognized. The most commonly observed types are called Hp1-1, Hp2-1, and Hp2-2.[468] The types are genetically determined, and a pair of alleles at an autosomal locus is involved.[469,470] These are termed Hp^1 and Hp^2. It is supposed that Hp1-1 persons are homozygous for Hp^1; Hp2-2 persons are homozygous for Hp^2; and Hp2-1 persons are heterozygous for Hp^1/Hp^2. In European populations, about 16% of persons are type 1-1, about 48% are type 2-1, and about 36% are type 2-2,[471] whereas the percentages are 7%, 35%, and 58%, respectively, in Japanese populations.[472]

The multiple components in Hp2-1 and Hp2-2 represent a series of polymers of increasing molecular weight.[473] Electrophoretic studies of the separated α chains from different types indicate further genetic heterogeneity.[474–476] Two kinds of electrophoretically distinct α chains come from Hp1-1; these are termed *hp1Fα* and *hp1Sα*, with hp1Fα having a slightly faster electrophoretic mobility than hp1Sα. These concealed differences within the Hp1-1 type are also genetically determined and family studies indicate that there are two types of Hp^1 alleles, Hp^{1F} and Hp^{1S}. HpF and HpS differ from each other in the amino acid at position 53 of the α chain, whereas Hp^2 shows a partial duplication of the α chain.[477] Studies of families have suggested the presence of only one expressed gene in each individual, whereas there are clearly two haptoglobin genes per haploid genome.[478] Thus, the additional Hp gene may either be an unexpressed pseudogene or a second functional gene that is expressed at particular stages of development or in a particular tissue. All haptoglobins are able to bind with free hemoglobin, that is, circulating methemoglobin, at a constant ratio. Haptoglobin does not bind with free heme. More detailed discussion on the properties and genetics of haptoglobin can be found in comprehensive reviews.[479,480]

Normal Values in Children and Adults. Normal levels of haptoglobin in cord blood are undetectable. Ahaptoglobinemia is also common in newborns (80% to 90%) or infants, and it is difficult to demonstrate haptoglobin by electrophoretic means up to 3 months.[481] The absence of haptoglobin in the neonate is attributed to the intravascular hemolysis of fetal RBCs as well as to the immaturity of the liver to synthesize the protein.

Normal values of haptoglobin in adults vary from 40 to 180 mg/dL plasma.[482,483] Several quantitative variants of haptoglobin particularly affect the $Hp\alpha^2$ gene. The fast-moving band (monomeric $Hp\alpha^1$) becomes intense and slower migrating bands may disappear. The mean levels of plasma haptoglobin in subjects with Hp1-1 are generally higher than those for Hp2-2.[484] Persons with the Hp1-1 phenotype are seldom associated with ahaptoglobinemia, whereas persons with Hp2-1 phenotype are often associated with this condition. Thus, there is rather a high incidence of ahaptoglobinemia among healthy Africans (about 30%).[485] The area of high prevalence of ahaptoglobinemia in Africa is also closely related to the belt of malaria endemicity, and the high incidence of this condition has been suggested to be partly due to malaria infection. Ahaptoglobinemia also exists in 4% to 10% of US blacks, 2% of Micronesians, 1% or less of Europeans, and in other populations.[486] In addition, normal persons may show intermittent ahaptoglobinemia without any apparent cause.[487] Sickle cell trait was implicated in increased ahaptoglobinemia among blacks due to possible modification of expression of Hp determinants by the genetic abnormality associated with sickle cell trait[488]; the tendency for ahaptoglobinemia among Greek children with HbSA was also found to be higher than in those with HbA.[489]

Haptoglobin levels are decreased in females,[490] during pregnancy,[491] and during severe malnutrition.[381] Several hemolytic diseases also accompany very low to undetectable levels of plasma haptoglobin, a fact that has been confirmed by numerous reports.[492] For example, low haptoglobin levels were found in paroxysmal nocturnal hemoglobinuria, hereditary spherocytosis, sickle cell disease, thalassemia major, and untreated pernicious anemia.[493] On the other hand, increased levels of haptoglobin are found as a result of aging, smoking, and the occurrence of malignant lymphomas, chronic and acute leukemias, alcoholic and viral hepatitis, tuberculosis, and acute pneumonia.[494] Haptoglobin is one of the acute phase proteins that increase during acute inflammation or after exposure to toxic stimuli.[495] Thus, even in some patients with hemolysis, haptoglobin levels may not be decreased during an acute phase reaction.

Haptoglobin concentrations can be determined by its capacity for binding hemoglobin[388] or by electrophoresis of the haptoglobin–hemoglobin complex.[496] In both cases, the haptoglobin–hemoglobin complex can be visualized by peroxidase activity using benzidine. A double-decker rocket immunoelectrophoresis has also been used to determine both free haptoglobin and its complex with hemoglobin.[497]

Hemopexin

Free heme found in the circulation is largely bound to plasma proteins such as albumin, α_1-fetoprotein, and hemopexin; free heme is normally not found in plasma. Free heme can be toxic to cells by promoting peroxidation of lipids and proteins.[498] The role of plasma proteins in heme binding includes prevention of potential oxidative damage of cellular constituents by heme and transport of heme to its site of metabolism. Human plasma albumin has a specific heme binding site, with a dissociation constant of about 1 $\times 10^{-8}$ mol/L, which is distinct from the principal bilirubin binding site.[499] α_1-Fetoprotein, the fetal counterpart of albumin, also binds heme, but with lesser affinity than albumin (dissociation constant about 1.5×10^{-7} mol/L).[500] Hemopexin is a glycoprotein that is synthesized by the liver. Its concentration in plasma ranges from 0.5 to 2 mg/dL,[501] and it has an extremely high affinity for heme (dissociation constant less than 10^{-13} mol/L).[502] Hemopexin binds heme in a 1:1 molar ratio by histidine–iron coordination. A review article discusses these aspects in more details.[501]

Albumin appears to be the most important protein with respect to the delivery of heme to the liver.[503] Although hemopexin is removed from the circulation after intravenous administration of large amounts of heme, its role in heme transport remains unclear.[504,505] The protein may possibly serve to tightly bind heme so that it can prevent heme-coupled peroxidation of other cellular constituents. Heme may also be taken up by the liver directly by a membrane heme receptor.[506]

Heme Catabolism

Human erythrocytes have an average life-span of about 120 days in the circulation; they are then phagocytosed by macrophages in the reticuloendothelial system. Hemoglobin is broken down intracellularly with the following results: (1) the protoporphyrin macrocycle is cleaved at the α-methene bridge; (2) one atom of iron is released; (3) one molecule of CO is produced; and (4) the globin moiety is ultimately hydrolyzed into its component amino acids (Fig. 50-24). The porphyrin moiety is converted into biliverdin IXα, a straight chain tetrapyrrole, which is then rapidly reduced to bilirubin IXα by cytosolic biliverdin reductase. Iron is transported to the bone marrow and reutilized in the formation of heme. CO is bound to hemoglobin to form carboxyhemoglobin, which is transported to the lungs, where it is excreted in expired air. Amino acids resulting from the hydrolysis of globin peptides are reutilized for protein synthesis.

In humans, 250 to 400 mg of bilirubin are formed daily, about 75% of which is accounted for by the degradation of hemoglobin heme.[507,508] If one assumes that heme catabolism is the sole source of CO in the body, the rate of bilirubin production in humans would be 4.4 ± 0.7 (mean $\pm$ SE) mg/kg/d.[509,510] The estimated hepatic contribution to total bilirubin production ranges from 23% to 37%.[511–513] The turnover of hepatic heme is reflected in the so-called early labeled bilirubin (ELB),[514] of which heme from microsomal cytochrome P-450 is the most significant.[284] A significant percentage of ELB is also derived from an erythroid source, that is, ineffective erythropoiesis, and from hepatic free heme, which serves both as a precursor for hepatic hemeprotein synthesis and as a regulator of the synthesis of ALA synthase and of heme oxygenase.[149,157,515,516] Exogenously administered hemin is quickly incorporated into the hepatic free heme pool,[517] as determined by the fact that (1) a small proportion can be incorporated into microsomal[518] or cytosolic hemeproteins[519]; (2) it suppresses the synthesis of ALA synthase[520]; and (3) it induces heme oxygenase and is itself converted to bilirubin.[521]

Heme Oxygenase

The microsomal heme oxidation system consists of NADPH–cytochrome P-450 reductase (also known as NADPH–cytochrome c reductase) and microsomal heme oxygenase, which is the rate-limiting enzyme in the oxidative catabolism of heme to bile pigments. Heme oxygen-

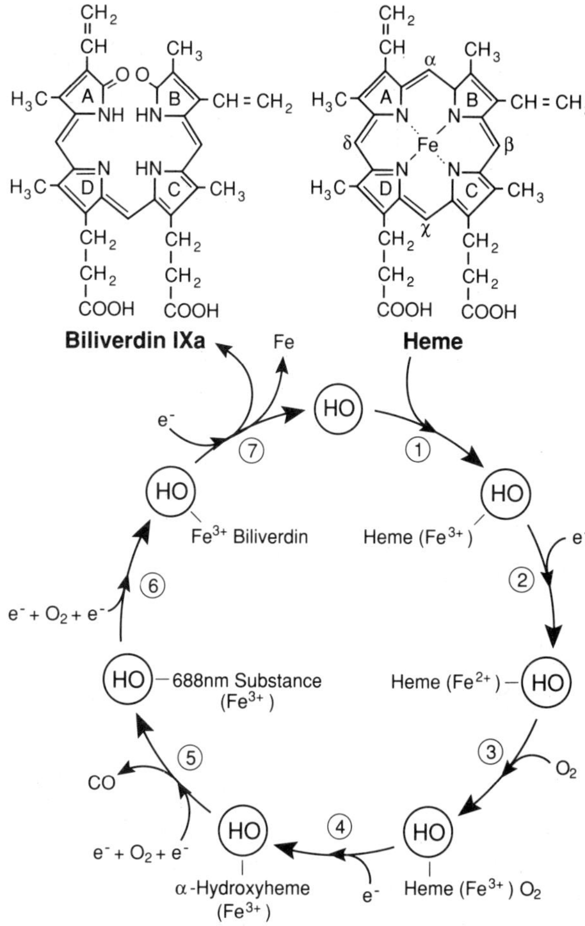

FIGURE 50-24. Oxidative catabolism of heme. A possible scheme for oxidative heme degradation is shown. (1) Heme is first bound to heme oxygenase (HO), yielding a ferric heme–HO complex. (2) Ferric heme is reduced on the complex by an electron provided by the NADPH–cytochrome c reductase system. (3) One oxygen atom binds with the ferrous heme–HO complex to form the oxygenated heme–HO complex. (4) Another reducing equivalent, provided by NADPH–cytochrome c reductase, binds with the complex and oxidative degradation of heme is initiated; the first oxidation product is α-hydroxyheme. (5) Consuming another reducing equivalent, α-hydroxyheme is oxidized to a 688-nm substance, which occurs on the complex. α-Methene bridge carbon is released as CO at this oxidation step. (6) Conversion of the 688-nm substance to the biliverdin–Fe^{3+} complex requires molecular oxygen and reducing equivalents, presumably involving another hydroxylation reaction. (7) Finally Fe^{3+} and biliverdin are released from the complex, consuming another reducing equivalent. In this series of reactions, all electrons are provided by NADPH–cytochrome c reductase.

ases purified from various sources have a minimum molecular weight of 31 to 32 kd. Recently, two forms of heme oxygenase, termed *HO-1* and *HO-2*, have been reported in rat liver and testis microsomes.[522] HO-1 and HO-2 have been suggested to be isozymes, representing two gene products.[523] HO-2 has a molecular weight of about 36 kd and appears not to be inducible by chemical treatment.[525]

Heme oxygenase binds heme at an equimolar ratio and exhibits properties similar to those of hemoglobin and myoglobin.[526] NADPH-cytochrome P-450 reductase, heme oxygenase, and biliverdin reductase, which reduces biliverdin IXα to bilirubin IXα, have been shown to form a ternary complex in vitro in an equimolar ratio.[527] This finding suggests that not only an enzyme–enzyme interaction within the endoplasmic reticulum between the membrane-bound NADPH-cytochrome P-450 reductase and heme oxygenase may occur, but also a further interaction between the binary complex with the cytoplasmic biliverdin reductase. Thus, biliverdin IXα produced by the membrane-bound NADPH-cytochrome P-450 reductase–heme oxygenase complex may be converted to bilirubin IXα by biliverdin reductase without leaving the enzyme complex in the membrane.

Heme catabolism by the heme oxidation system proceeds essentially in an autocatalytic fashion on heme bound to heme oxygenase.[526] The initial step of the heme oxygenase-dependent heme catabolic process is the formation of a heme–heme oxygenase complex. This complex is then oxidized by a reducing equivalent provided by NADPH-cytochrome P-450 reductase in the presence of NADPH,[528] yielding the first product, α-hydroxyheme.[529] α-Hydroxyheme is further oxidized to a 688-nm absorbing substance,[530] consuming another reducing equivalent. The α-methene carbon is released as CO at this step of the oxidation process.[531,532] In the heme oxygenase reaction, the molecular oxygen that is bound to heme on heme oxygenase is probably reduced to a peroxo form of dioxygen,[533] and this activated form of oxygen attacks the α-methene bridge of heme, yielding one molecule each of biliverdin IXα, iron, and CO[534,535] (Fig. 50-24).

Induction of Heme Oxygenase

HO-1 is an inducible enzyme in various tissues of many animal species by treatment with the natural substitute of the enzyme, hemin. Induction of the enzyme has also been demonstrated in isolated macrophages,[536,537] and in cultured hepatocytes[538] after treatment with hemin. The enzyme can also be induced by treatment of animals or cultured cells with a number of nonheme substrates, such as insulin, epinephrine, endotoxin, carbon disulfide, certain trace elements and heavy metals, diethylmaleate, bromobenzene, chlorinated benzenes, and interferon-inducing agents. Some of these agents such as heavy metals induce the enzyme directly, that is, by a heme-independent mechanism. Studies using isolated macrophages suggest that inductions of HO-1 by carbon disulfide, endotoxin, insulin, and epinephrine are probably due to a heme-dependent mechanism, whereas inductions by metal ions, diethylmaleate, and bromobenzene appear to be produced by mechanisms that do not involve the intermediation of heme.[526,539]

The HO-1 gene has been isolated from a rat genomic DNA library, and its complete nucleotide sequence has been determined.[540] The gene is composed of 6830 nucleotides and is organized into four introns and five exons. In the 5′-flanking region of the gene, several potential binding sites for different transcription factors were identified: a transcription factor (Sp1), a positive regulator for the control of amino acid synthesis (GCN4), a heat-shock transcription factor, and a metal-dependent transcription factor.[540] The human HO-1 cDNA has also been isolated using rat cDNA.[541] The deduced human HO-1 is composed of 288 amino acids with a molecular weight of 32 kd. The homology in amino acid sequences between rat and human HO-1 is about 80%. Both the rat and the human enzymes contain a putative membrane segment at the carboxy terminal, which is probably essential for the insertion of heme oxygenase into the endoplasmic reticulum. Both heat shock and hemin treatment in rat cells induce HO-1 at the transcriptional level.[542] The 5′-flanking region of the rat HO-1 gene bearing the heat shock element can also confer.[542] Human HO-1 and its mRNA have been reported to be either noninducible[541] or inducible with heat treatment.[544] Induction of HO-1 mRNA has also been demonstrated in human skin fibroblasts when cells were treated with arsenite, cadmium, hydrogen peroxide, ultraviolet light, or sulfhydryl reagents.[543] It appears that the induction of HO-1 may be a general response to oxidant stress to the cell. More detailed accounts of the gene expression of HO-1 can be found in a review article.[524]

Competitive Inhibition of Heme Oxygenase

Heme oxygenase can be regulated not only by induction of new enzyme protein, but also by inhibition of its activity. A number of synthetic heme analogues, in which the central iron atom of heme has been replaced by another element, bind more tightly to the catalytic site of the enzyme than does heme; this results in various degrees of competitive inhibition of heme degradation to bile pigments.[521,545] Such inhibitors include, among others, Sn-, Zn-, Cr-, and Mn-protoporphyrin and mesoporphyrin derivatives. Sn-protoporphyrin and Sn-mesoporphyrin have been the most well studied of this class of compounds and have the capacity to inhibit heme oxidation to such an extent that they can in small doses significantly lower the levels of plasma bilirubin in experimental animals, in normal and jaundiced adult humans, and in infants with hemolytic disease of the newborn.[268,546,547]

Extensive toxicologic examination of these compounds has shown them to be essentially innocuous; the only side effect noted in humans has been the occurrence of transient photosensitivity when they have been administered in doses of 1 μmol/kg (or more) and when the treated subject is then exposed to sunlight or when newborns receive concurrent phototherapy with broad-spectrum white-light lamps. The use of high-intensity blue lamps, whose emission spectrum does not extend into the region of peak porphyrin absorbance (400 to 410 nm), has for practical purposes eliminated this side effect in infants.

Sn-protoporphyrin and Sn-mesoporphyrin inhibit heme oxygenase potently and rapidly (in less than 1 hour) after subcutaneous, intramuscular, and intravenous administration; their effect is manifested by a prompt lowering of biliary bilirubin output; a decrease in respiratory CO production[548,549]; a transient (about 6 hours) complete saturation of hepatic tryptophan pyrrolase, reflecting a temporary cellular accumulation of heme; and the rapid excretion of unmetabolized heme into bile to an extent that quantitatively accounts for the diminution of bilirubin production produced by the inhibitors.[521,548–551] The incorporation of heme oxygenase inhibitors into liposomes markedly enhances inhibition of splenic heme oxygenase. Targeting this major tissue site of heme oxygenase activity in this manner produces a profound decrease in biliary bilirubin output and a near-total inhibition of splenic heme catabolism, lasting many days after a single dose of the inhibitor–liposome preparation.[552] These findings raise the possibility that a single-dose treatment for suppressing hyperbilirubinemia in newborns or in patients with the lethal disorder Crigler-Najjar syndrome type I can be developed.

The discovery of competitive inhibitors of heme oxygenase activity, combined with the known inducibility of the enzyme by many foreign chemicals, offers an important new means for experimental examination of the rate of heme catabolism and its relation to the overall regulation of heme and hemeprotein metabolism. The clinical potential for use of these compounds in the amelioration of severe hyperbilirubinemic conditions is also considerable. Reports summarize the status of this work in detail.[553–557]

Carbon Monoxide Production as a Measure of Heme Catabolism

Plasma bilirubin concentrations may be influenced by a number of factors and may not necessarily reflect the rate of heme degradation. In contrast, under steady-state conditions, the pulmonary CO excretion rate can be considered to largely reflect the rate of heme catabolism.[558] Like bilirubin, CO excretion rates also have an early labeled peak (ELP), which mostly reflects the catabolism of hepatic free heme.[559] Both ELP and ELB are increased by treatment with phenobarbital or allylisopropylacetamide, agents known to increase hepatic heme turnover.[558] The magnitude of the ELP can also be increased after phlebotomy, phenylhydrazine, iron-deficiency anemia, and hemolysis,[558] presumably reflecting a pool of the erythropoietic component of CO in the ELP fraction. More detailed information is available in a review article on this topic.[556] More detailed discussion on the chemistry, transport, conjugation and excretion of bilirubin can be found in another article.[560]

Biliverdin Reductase

Biliverdin reductase is a cytosolic enzyme that reduces biliverdin to bilirubin. This enzyme is present in excess in the liver, and all biliverdin IXα formed is promptly converted to bilirubin IXα. The molecular weight of the purified enzyme from pig spleen and rat liver is in the range of 34 to 36 kd,[561,562] and the enzyme requires NADPH as a cofactor. In normal rat liver, the enzyme is known to exist in two major molecular forms, form *1* and *2*, which can be separated by anion exchange chromatography.[563] The major molecular form, *1*, is converted to a new form, *3*, after treatment of animals with $CoCl_2$, or treatment of the enzyme with thioredoxin in vitro.[564] Form *1* preferentially reduces biliverdin IXα, whereas form *2* (a minor form) reduces biliverdin IXα and IXβ. Form *3* can reduce both biliverdin IXα and IXβ at comparable rates. The physiologic significance of these different molecular forms is not clear, but the form *2* enzyme may explain the existence of the small amount of bilirubin IXβ in the bile of adults, newborn babies, rhesus monkeys, and dogs.[565,566]

Chemistry of Bilirubin

Bilirubin is lipophilic in solution in vitro, whereas it behaves as a relatively polar compound in circulation by binding to albumin.[567] Its solubility at physiologic pH is difficult to estimate because of its colloid formation in aqueous solutions. Binding of bilirubin with polar lipids may be an important factor in directing its transit through cellular membranes. Although both biliverdin IXα and bilirubin IXα have two propionic acid side chains, the latter is far less soluble in aqueous solutions than the former, probably because it takes a "ridge tile" conformation by intramolecular hydrogen bonding involving the two propionic acid side chains.[568–570] As a result, rings A and B of bilirubin IXα lie in one plane, and rings C and D lie in another.

Bilirubin IXα in organic solvents has a strong absorption band at about 460 nm with a molar extinction coefficient of about 60,000.[571] Pure bilirubin does not fluoresce; it emits an intense fluorescence (maxima occurring at 510 to 530 nm) when dissolved in detergent, alkaline methanol, or albumin solution.[572,573] When bilirubin in solution is exposed to light under air, it undergoes photooxidation resulting in colorless products.[573] These products are a mixture of maleimides and propentdyopents and reflect random fission of the tetrapyrrole structure by singlet oxygen. Bilirubin also undergoes geometric isomerization by light to yield more polar isomers, termed *photobilirubin*, or *lumirubin*. Both propentdyopents and photobilirubin are more polar than bilirubin, which probably explains the efficacy of phototherapy in lowering plasma bilirubin levels.[574–576]

Bilirubin is toxic to a wide variety of biochemical functions in many cell types.[577] For example, oxidative phosphorylation and ATPase activity of brain mitochondria are inhibited by bilirubin, and mitochondria swelling can be demonstrated after bilirubin treatment.[578–580] Rapidly developing and irreversible actions of bilirubin on CNS cells have also been recently described.[581,582] Toxic effects of bilirubin may be decreased by albumin in vitro and in vivo.[578,583]

Bilirubin has generally been considered to be a functionless metabolite of heme catabolism. Both bilirubin and bilirubin glucuronides exhibit significant antioxidant activities in vitro.[584,585] Unconjugated bilirubin scavenges singlet oxygen,[586] reacts with superoxide anion[587] and peroxyl radicals,[584] and serves as a reducing substrate in the presence of hydrogen peroxide or organic hydroperoxides.[588,589] The antioxidant activity of bilirubin appears to be due to its hydrogen-donating activity.[584,590] It is not known whether the antioxidant activity is physiologically important or at what blood level the deleterious effects of the pigment exceed its potentially useful actions.

Transport and Uptake of Bilirubin

Bilirubin in the plasma is essentially all bound, but in a reversible manner, with albumin. Binding of the pigment occurs at a primary site and one or more secondary sites on the protein, and the affinity of the protein for the bile pigment can be altered by other ligands such as certain drugs and fatty acids.[560] Thus, the administration of drugs such as sulfonamides to the newborn increases the likelihood of bilirubin toxicity, presumably by displacing bilirubin from its binding to albumin.[591,592] Bilirubin is rapidly removed from the circulation by the liver (Fig. 50-25). In this process, the pigment is extracted from albumin, and albumin does not enter the liver.[593] Although a receptor-like mechanism has been proposed for the uptake of the bilirubin–albumin complex by the liver,[594] its physiologic role has not been established. Conjugated bilirubin can also covalently bind to albumin.[595,596]

In healthy subjects, essentially all bilirubin is unconjugated. In contrast, when bile ducts are obstructed or liver cells are diseased, conjugated bilirubin refluxes into plasma and a portion of such conjugated bilirubin is found as a covalent complex with albumin.[492] The formation of the albumin–bilirubin complex in vivo is apparently nonenzymatic and appears to occur by acyl migration of bilirubin from a bilirubin–glucuronide acid ester to a nucleophilic site on albumin.[597] The protein-bound bilirubin cannot be taken up by the liver and is eliminated only when its albumin is degraded. Thus, its half-life approximates the decay of albumin (12 to 14 days).[492] Because this complex is not eliminated as readily as the pigment itself and is only slightly filtered through the glomerulus in the kidney,[598] the resolution of jaundice generally lags behind the recovery of the hepatobiliary disease and the plasma usually remains jaundiced longer than the urine.

Bilirubin in the hepatocyte is bound to a cytosolic protein, ligandin (glutathione S-transferase B)[599,600] and Z protein.[601] Ligandin is a basic protein with a molecular weight of 47 kd and accounts for about 5% of the soluble protein in rat and human liver. Structural and immunologic studies have shown that ligandin is also identical with the protein that has been demonstrated to be an azo-dye carcinogen-binding protein,[602] a cortisol-metabolite–binding protein,[603] or glutathione S-transferase B.[604] Rat liver ligandin consists of one each of subunits A and B, with molecular weights of 22 and 25 kd, respectively.[605] For glutathione S-transferase activity, both subunits are necessary, whereas bilirubin binding occurs exclusively on subunit A. Immunochemical studies indicate that ligandin is localized in the cytosol

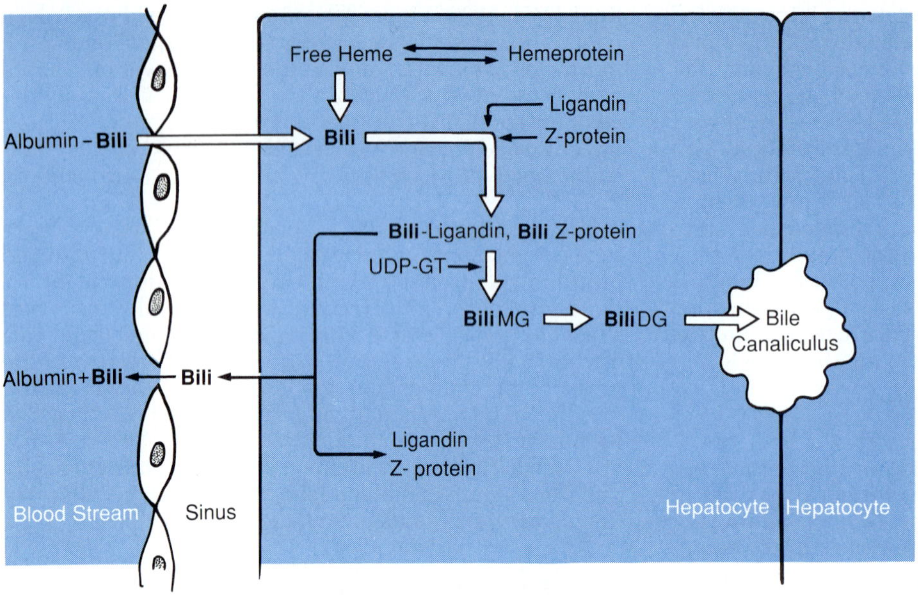

FIGURE 50-25. Transport and uptake of bilirubin (Bili) by the liver. Bilirubin in circulation is largely bound with albumin, which is taken up by the liver. In hepatocytes, bilirubin is bound with bilirubin binding proteins, such as ligandin or Z-protein, the major one being ligandin. Bilirubin is conjugated by UDP-glucuronyl transferase before excretion into bile canaliculi.

with highest concentration in close vicinity to the endoplasmic reticulum. Whether this finding reflects the directional movement of ligandin in the cell is not clear, and the exact role of ligandin in intracellular bilirubin transport remains conjectural.[606] Intracellular movement of bilirubin may also occur by membrane–membrane transfer.[607]

Much less is known about Z protein, which is a fatty acid–binding protein but which also binds bilirubin. Z protein purified from human liver has a molecular weight of 11 kd.[608] It has a lower binding affinity for bilirubin and has a higher binding capacity than ligandin.[608] Plasma concentrations of Z protein in patients with Gilbert's syndrome are decreased,[608] whereas those of ligandin are not.[609]

When bilirubin metabolism was studied using radiolabeled precursors such as ALA,[511,512,610,611] heme,[612] or biliverdin,[613] a large proportion of bilirubin that initially was taken up by the liver refluxed into plasma.[508,614] Bidirectional flux of unconjugated bilirubin was also predicted from kinetic analysis and mathematical modeling of plasma disappearance and bile excretion curves of radiolabeled bilirubin.[615]

Bilirubin Conjugation

Under physiologic conditions, bilirubin is conjugated before excretion into bile. One or both of the two propionic acid side chains are esterified with a glucuronide moiety yielding bilirubin monoglucuronide or bilirubin diglucuronide, respectively. Glucuronic acid is the major conjugating group, although xylosyl and glucosyl conjugates are also found to a minor degree in normal mammalian bile.[616,617] Bilirubin diglucuronide constitutes a large proportion of the total bilirubin conjugates in bile in humans, dogs, rats, and cats, whereas bilirubin monoglucuronide is the major form in bile of guinea pigs, sheep, mice, and rabbits.[618]

Conjugation of bilirubin with glucuronic acid is carried out by one or more microsomal enzymes, uridine diphosphate (UDP)-glucuronyl transferase, which transfers the glucuronyl moiety of UDP-glucuronate to a variety of aglycones, yielding ethers, esters, thiols, and N-glucuronides.[619,620] Bilirubin appears to be freed from ligandin and taken into the endoplasmic reticulum before it is glucuronidated by the membrane-bound glucuronyl transferase.[621] In addition to bilirubin, UDP-glucuronyl transferase plays an important role in conjugating a variety of other substrates including thyroxine, steroids, and various exogenous chemicals. UDP-glucuronyl transferase appears to consist of a group of related enzymes. Many xenobiotics metabolized by the cytochrome P-450–dependent mixed function oxidase system in the liver undergo glucuronidation in the endoplasmic reticulum by UDP-glucuronyl transferase prior to their excretion into bile. The enzyme catalyzing the conjugation of *p*-nitrophenol, 1-naphthol, and 3-hydroxybenzo(a)pyrene appears to be different from the enzyme involved in the conjugation of bilirubin and steroids.[622,623] For example, the UDP-glucuronyltransferase catalyzing the conjugation of *p*-nitrophenol, 1-naphthol, and 3-hydroxybenzo(a)pyrene is inducible by treatment of animals with 3-methylcholanthrene, whereas the enzyme responsible for the conjugation of bilirubin and steroids is inducible by phenobarbital.[624,625]

Certain structural similarities among different UDP-glucuronyl transferases exist, since an antibody against purified rat *p*-nitrophenol UDP-glucuronyl transferase also precipitates bilirubin UDP-glucuronyl transferase activity.[626] Gunn rats that are genetically deficient in bilirubin UDP-glucuronyl transferase activity also have decreased activities of UDP-glucuronyl transferase activity for *p*-nitrophenol, *o*-aminophenol, 1-naphthol, and methylumbelliferone.[626]

Unconjugated and conjugated bilirubin can be distinguished by the diazo reaction.[627,628] Conjugated bilirubin reacts with the sulfanilic acid diazo reagent within minutes, whereas unconjugated bilirubin reacts only when an accelerator, such as methanol or caffeine, is added.[627] More recently, diazotized ethylanthranilate and *p*-iodoaniline have been used in place of sulfanilic acid, since they offer better sensitivity and greater specificity.[629] The most accurate, sensitive, and quantitative determination of bile pigments is accomplished by high-performance liquid chromatography.[630–632] The irreversibly albumin-bound bilirubin can be determined by reverse-phase, high-performance liquid chromatography.[633] A rapid fluorometric method for determining both unconjugated and conjugated bilirubin and bilirubin-binding capacity using Ektachem slides has also been reported. The results obtained by the slide test were consistent with those verified by high-performance liquid chromatography.[634,635]

cDNA clones for multiple rat UDP-glucuronyl transferases have been isolated. They include the transferase isoform for the steroid, androsterone,[636] and isoforms that are inducible by treatment with 3-methylcholanthrene[637] and phenobarbital.[638] Nucleotide sequences of these isoforms indicate that UDP-glucuronyl transferases differ in their primary structure.[636–638]

Biliary Excretion of Bilirubin

In mammals, conjugation of bilirubin is, for practical purposes, a prerequisite for excretion of the compound into bile canaliculi. In normal humans and in animals, the rate-limiting step for bilirubin excretion appears to be related to canalicular transport rather than the conjugation rate.[639,640] In contrast, in Gunn rats and in patients with type I Crigler-Najjar syndrome, that is, homozygous deficiencies of UDP-glucuronyl transferase activity, the conjugation step may become rate limiting in the excretion process.

Biliary excretion of bilirubin appears to be an energy-dependent concentration process in that bile bilirubin concentrations are about 100-fold greater than those in the hepatic cytosol.[641] Bilirubin excretory capacity is affected by various factors. The maximal bilirubin excretory capacity is influenced by bile flow that can be increased by infusion of micelle-forming bile acids such as taurocholate[642] or by phenobarbital treatment.[643] The latter increases bile flow by a different mechanism than that mediated by bile acids. Even at very high concentrations, bilirubin in bile has little effect on osmolarity,[641] suggesting that it is largely incorporated into bile salt micelles, as is the case with biliary cholesterol and lecithin.

The plasma concentration of unconjugated bilirubin is known to increase linearly with increased rates of bilirubin production, if hepatic bilirubin clearance is within the relatively normal range.[644] The highest value for plasma unconjugated bilirubin that can occur as the result of sustained hemolysis in a person with normal hepatic bilirubin clearance has been estimated to be 4 mg/dL.[496] When hepatic bilirubin clearance is impaired as in hepatitis, in obstructive disorders of bile flow, and in certain metabolic disorders, bilirubin and bile salts are largely retained in the liver (cholestasis)[641] and some of these biliary components are refluxed into plasma.

Enteric Bilirubin Absorption and Processing

In contrast to that which occurs for conjugated bilirubin, unconjugated bilirubin can be reabsorbed from the intestine and the reabsorbed unconjugated bilirubin may therefore contribute to hyperbilirubinemia in the neonate.[645] A small amount of conjugated bilirubin may also undergo some nonenzymatic (alkaline hydrolysis in the duodenum or jejunum) or enzymatic deconjugation (by bacterial or intestinal mucosal β-glucuronidase) to yield unconjugated bilirubin.[645]

Bilirubin in the intestinal tract is degraded by various bacteria, primarily by *Clostridium perfringens* and *E coli*, resulting in the formation of a series of products, termed *urobilinoids*.[646] Urobilinoids include urobilin, urobilinogens, stercobilinogens, and stercobilins, in the order of their reduction steps.[647,648] Complete lack of bile flow such as obstruction by tumor is consequently associated with the absence of urobilinoids in intestinal contents. In contrast, urobilinoids such as urinary urobilinogen are increased in liver disease and in conditions associated with increased bilirubin production as in hemolysis. Urobilinogen in the circulation is largely bound to plasma proteins (80% or more), and only a small percentage is filtered through the glomerulus. Urobilinogen excretion is influenced by a number of factors, including urinary pH[649] and diurnal rhythm[650]; thus, it usually carries little clinical significance in the estimation of hepatic dysfunction.

DISORDERS OF BILIRUBIN METABOLISM IN THE NEONATE: NEONATAL JAUNDICE

Normal Bilirubin Metabolism and Physiologic Jaundice

Definition. In normal, healthy, full-term neonates, the plasma bilirubin concentration generally rises during the first few days of life, reaching a maximum at about 3 days, then reverts to the normal range by the end of the second week of life[651] (Fig. 50-26). Occasionally, some infants show marked increases in plasma bilirubin during the immediate postnatal period. In a study of 4000 newborns, 16% were found to reach peak bilirubin levels higher than 10 mg/dL and 5% had levels greater than 15 mg/dL.[652] Generally, an inverse correlation exists between bilirubin levels and body weights in newborns[652,653]; more specifically, this correlation is with gestational age. This pattern of hyperbilirubinemia, usually observed in the absence of documentable abnormalities, is called *physiologic jaundice* and generally is not accompanied by serious clinical consequences. Two functionally distinct periods of physiologic jaundice are seen in human newborns.[654] During the first period, *phase I*, bilirubin concentrations rise to an average peak level of 6 mg/dL by the third day of life as already noted, whereas both the peak period and the bilirubin concentrations are exaggerated in premature babies. In full-term infants, plasma bilirubin concentrations rapidly decline from the third day until the fifth day, when another increase in bilirubin concentration takes place. The latter increase is called *phase II*, and plasma bilirubin levels in phase II average about 2 mg/dL, a level that may persist until the 14th day of life. At that time, usually a return to normal concentrations of 1 mg/dL or less occurs. In the premature infant, both the time and the magnitude of the initial peak bilirubin concentration and the duration of phase II are exaggerated.

Mechanism. Physiologic jaundice reflects several factors including overproduction of bilirubin from the catabolism of fetal hemoglobin heme during the postnatal period; insufficient activity of UDP-glucuronyl transferase in newborns, which is essential for the hepatic excretion of bilirubin; and reabsorption in newborns of unconjugated bilirubin through the gastrointestinal tract. The erythrocyte life-span in neonates is 70 to 90 days,[655,656] which is significantly shorter than that in the adult (120 days); this results

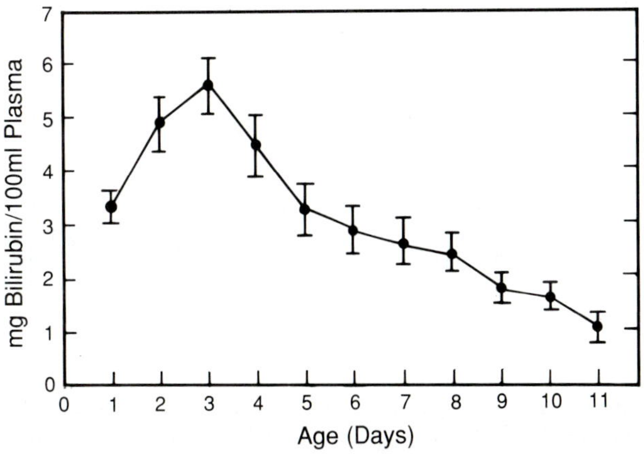

FIGURE 50-26. Mean total daily bilirubin concentrations in sera from 29 full-term human infants. Vertical bars are 1 standard error of the mean. (After Gartner LM, Lee KS, Vaisman S, et al. Development of bilirubin transport and metabolism in the newborn rhesus monkey. J Pediatr 1977;90:513)

in an overload of heme with respect to the heme degrading system in the infant. This heme overload would be expected to induce heme oxygenase in human newborns and may account for developmental changes in the enzyme in fetal and newborn experimental animals[657,658]; heme oxygenase induction would result in a greater rate of formation of bilirubin in the presence of excess heme substrate. Premature infants may also have an even shorter erythrocyte life-span than full-term infants. Estimates of CO or carboxyhemoglobin production indicate that newborn infants have a several-fold higher heme turnover rate than do normal adults.[659,660]

UDP-glucuronyl transferase activity in the newborn is very low and is insufficient to cope with the enhanced load of bilirubin produced during the postnatal period.[654,661,662] For example, the enzyme activity in human full-term and premature infants during the first 10 days of life is usually less than 0.1% of that of the normal adult value[554]; this increases rapidly during the subsequent several days, ultimately reaching adult values by 6 to 14 weeks of age[663] (Fig. 50-27). With the rise in UDP-glucuronyl transferase activity, the plasma bilirubin concentration rapidly drops, an effect observed by 24 hours in the newborn monkey, and at or after 72 hours in the human infant.[654] Studies in newborn monkeys suggest that a large proportion of the bilirubin present in the liver cytosol is derived from intestinal reabsorption of the pigment and not from its de novo synthesis.[664] Thus, a significant percentage of plasma bilirubin in human infants possibly originates from the enterohepatic circulation.

Ethnic Factors. In full-term, healthy newborns, levels of unconjugated hyperbilirubinemia are known to be higher in infants of Asian parentage than in those of whites and blacks.[665–669] In Asian infants, hyperbilirubinemia occurs in the absence of hemolysis and appears to be due to delayed maturation of the bilirubin conjugating system, a process for which there are presumably genetic determinants. Also, reports have been made of unexplained hyperbilirubinemia in geographically localized areas.[670] Several review articles deal with these aspects of bilirubin metabolism in more detail.[554,671]

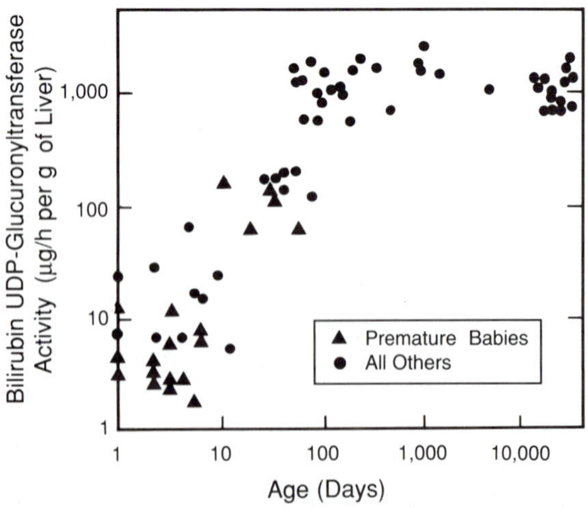

FIGURE 50-27. Developmental changes of human hepatic UDP-glucuronyl transferase activity toward bilirubin. (After Onishi S, Itho S, Kawade N, et al. An accurate and sensitive analysis by high pressure liquid chromatography of conjugated and unconjugated bilirubin IX and in various biological fluids. Biochem J 1980;185: 281)

TABLE 50-4. Disorders of the Newborn Predominantly Associated With Unconjugated Hyperbilirubinemia

TRANSIENT NEONATAL HYPERBILIRUBINEMIA
Delayed development of hepatic uptake and conjugation system: physiologic jaundice
Inhibitors of conjugation
Novobiocin
? Certain breastmilks
Unknown mechanisms
Pyloric stenosis
Upper intestinal obstruction
Transient familial neonatal bilirubinemia
Infants of diabetic mothers
OVERPRODUCTION OF BILIRUBIN
Isoimmune hemolysis
Rh(D) hemolytic disease
ABO hemolytic disease
Other blood groups incompatibilities
Hereditary hemolytic anemias
Hereditary spherocytosis
Hereditary elliptocytosis with neonatal polkilocytosis
Hereditary stomatocytosis or xerocytosis
G-6-PD deficiency
Pyruvate kinase deficiency and other glycolytic defects
Nucleotide metabolism defects
α or γ-thalassemias or unstable hemoglobinopathies
Acquired hemolytic anemia
Oxidant (Heinz body) hemolytic anemias
Vitamin E deficiency
Infantile pyknocytosis
Extravascular blood
Cephalohematoma
Occult hemorrhage
MIXED OR UNKNOWN MECHANISM
Sepsis
Hypothyroidism
INHERITED DEFECTS IN BILIRUBIN CONJUGATION
Crigler-Najjar syndrome types I and II
Gilbert's syndrome

Neonatal Jaundice Due to Unconjugated Hyperbilirubinemia

If abnormalities of hepatic uptake, intracellular binding, or conjugation of bilirubin are present, unconjugated bilirubin accumulates in the plasma. In contrast, an obstruction to the flow of conjugated bilirubin through the biliary system into the gastrointestinal tract at any level in the canalicular-ductal system results in an increase in conjugated bilirubin in the plasma. In the case of diffuse hepatic injuries such as viral hepatitis and cirrhosis, a combined abnormality of one or more hepatic bilirubin-metabolizing systems results in a mixed type of hyperbilirubinemia. The disorders predominantly associated with unconjugated hyperbilirubinemia are listed in Table 50-4. Those related to erythroblastosis fetalis and other hemolytic diseases are discussed in Chapter 64. Also, certain articles discuss these topics.[554,672] The following disorders are attributable to UDP-glucuronyl transferase deficiencies.

Crigler-Najjar Syndrome Type I

The Crigler-Najjar type I syndrome (congenital nonhemolytic jaundice) is an extremely rare condition that is characterized by early onset of unconjugated hyperbilirubinemia and kernicterus.[673] About 100 cases have been reported. Affected infants usually die within 18 months of birth because of severe brain damage. Plasma bilirubin concentrations in Crigler-Najjar patients may range from 25 to 45 mg/dL, and the bile of the affected children is colorless and contains no glucuronides. A few Crigler-Najjar patients survive until or past puberty[674]; they may thereafter develop bilirubin encephalopathy.[675,676] Hepatic UDP-glucuronyl transferase activity in this homozygous genetic disorder is virtually absent, and the enzyme activity in the patient's parents who are clinically unaffected is about 50% of the normal control.[677,678] In normal liver, there are at least three immunodetectable bands of UDP-glucuronyl transferase (53 to 56 kd), whereas a protein of 53 kd is completely lacking in the liver of Crigler-Najjar children.[679]

Treatment of patients with Crigler-Najjar type I syndrome has been attempted by phlebotomy,[680] plasmapheresis,[675] and phototherapy[676,681]; some reductions in plasma bilirubin levels have been attained but these responses are only temporary. Bilirubin production in patients with Crigler-Najjar syndrome is essentially normal, whereas hepatic clearance of bilirubin and fecal urobilinoids is greatly reduced (1% or less of the normal level).[676,680,682] This reflects the complete absence of conjugation. Administration of phenobarbital or glutethimide, which induces UDP-glucuronyl transferase activity in patients with the type II form of the Crigler-Najjar syndrome or Gilbert's syndrome, does not have a similar effect on bilirubin metabolism in Crigler-Najjar type I patients.[676] As patients with this form of icterus live beyond 4 to 5 years, phototherapy becomes increasingly ineffective in lowering plasma bilirubin levels. No effective long-term therapy is available for patients with this condition. Liver transplantation in the type I Crigler-Najjar syndrome has been reported to be successful.[683] In one patient, plasma bilirubin levels fell from the preoperative value of 31 mg/dL to the normal range postoperatively. In another case, administration of the heme oxygenase inhibitor Sn-protoporphyrin in doses of 1 μmol/kg parenterally over the first 4 months of postnatal life considerably decreased, although not entirely, the requirement for phototherapy in an infant with this syndrome.[684] In two adolescent patients with type I Crigler-Najjar syndrome, Sn-mesoporphyrin was successfully used to lower bilirubin levels for an extended period.[684a]

Crigler-Najjar Syndrome Type II

Type II Crigler-Najjar syndrome, which was described by Arias,[685] is a relatively common disorder characterized by substantial unconjugated hyperbilirubinemia in the newborn (8 to 20 mg/dL) and reduced hepatic UDP-glucuronyl transferase activity. In contrast to that seen in patients with Crigler-Najjar type I syndrome, the clinical course of type II patients is always benign.[685,686] The Crigler-Najjar type II syndrome can be differentiated from the type I syndrome by a reduction in plasma bilirubin concentrations after treatment with phenobarbital[677,687] or other agents that induce hepatic UDP-glucuronyl transferase activity such as glutethimide[688] and by the presence of monoglucuronidated bilirubin in bile (90% or more).[689,690] The Crigler-Najjar type II syndrome commonly occurs in families, but its mode of inheritance has not been established. Some family members of Crigler-Najjar type II patients have a condition that matches the description of Gilbert's syndrome. This suggests that the Crigler-Najjar syndrome and Gilbert's syndrome may have a similar pathogenesis, although it has not been established whether patients with Gilbert's syndrome represent heterozygotes for the UDP-glucuronyl transferase deficiency, which characterizes Crigler-Najjar type I disorder in patients in the homozygous state.

Administration of phenobarbital reduces plasma bilirubin levels to within the normal range after about 3 days of treatment. A low plasma bilirubin level can be maintained so long as the drug is continuously administered; plasma bilirubins are known to return to pretreatment levels if the drug is discontinued. After the immediate neonatal period, little risk of developing kernicterus is seen in patients with the type II syndrome.

Gilbert's Syndrome

Gilbert's syndrome (familial nonhemolytic jaundice, constitutional hepatic dysfunction), described by Gilbert and Lereboullet[691] in 1901, is a common disorder characterized by mild fluctuating hyperbilirubinemia, usually less than 3 mg/dL (Table 50-5). This disorder has been reviewed in a comprehensive manner.[692] Familial occurrence is common; it has been proposed that the disorder is transmitted in an autosomal dominant mode of inheritance,[693,694] but

TABLE 50-5. Characteristic Symptoms of Hereditary Unconjugated Hyperbilirubinemia

	Crigler-Najjar Syndrome		
Symptoms	**Type I**	**Type II**	**Gilbert's Syndrome**
Liver histology	Normal	Normal	Normal
Serum bilirubin	20–45 mg/dL	<20 mg/dL	<3 mg/dL
Liver function	Normal	Normal	Normal
Bromsulphalein clearance	Normal	Normal	Usually normal; occasionally enhanced
Hepatic UDP-glucuronyl transferase activity	Absent	Decreased	Decreased
Phenobarbital	No effect	Decreased serum bilirubin	Decreased serum bilirubin
Inheritance	Autosomal recessive	Autosomal recessive (?)	Autosomal dominant (?)
Prognosis	Kernicterus	Benign	Benign

this has not been established with certainty. A male preponderance has been reported, but does not reflect sex-linked inheritance and probably relates to the known lower plasma bilirubin concentrations in females.[695,696] Plasma unconjugated bilirubin concentrations in Gilbert's syndrome patients increase during fasting, stress, intercurrent illness, hyperthyroidism, and menses.[697] No indication of increased hemolysis or increased bilirubin production is found in patients with the syndrome, and hyperbilirubinemia appears to be exclusively due to decreased hepatic clearance of bilirubin. Decreased hepatic UDP-glucuronyl transferase activity has been consistently shown in Gilbert's syndrome.[698,699] In addition, a hepatic uptake defect of bilirubin has been suggested.[700,701] Biliary bilirubin in Gilbert's syndrome or in type II Crigler-Najjar syndrome contains an increased percentage of monoglucuronidated bile pigment (20% to 60%).[497] Other than mild jaundice, no clinical abnormalities are seen in these subjects. Despite the fact that Gilbert's syndrome persists for life, patients do not develop any deleterious consequences of their hyperbilirubinemia and thus do not require treatment.

Elevated fasting levels of plasma cholyl-conjugated bile acids have been found to be a useful aid in the diagnosis of Gilbert's syndrome.[702] Two provocative tests, the 48-hour caloric restriction test and the nicotinic acid test, have been publicized, but neither test seems specific enough to be clinically useful.[703,704] Hepatic cytochrome P-450 inducers, such as phenobarbital and glutethimide, decrease plasma bilirubin concentrations in patients with Gilbert's syndrome to the normal level.[705] The normalization of plasma bilirubin levels is not due to decreased bilirubin production but to increased hepatic clearance of bilirubin.[596] Unequivocal diagnosis of the syndrome depends on the determination of radiobilirubin clearance and glucuronyl transferase activity in liver biopsy, but they are available only at a few research centers. This syndrome should not be considered a disease, but rather a slow bilirubin glucuronidation phenotype, which occurs in about 8% of the population.[679]

Breast Milk Jaundice

Plasma bilirubin concentrations are also known to be increased in newborn infants who are breastfed, compared with those who are fed formula.[706] Increments in bilirubin concentrations are usually small and are not associated with any clinical problems. The initial suspected causative agent, pregnan-3α,20β-ol, a steroid reported to have been found in maternal milk, which inhibits hepatic UDP-glucuronyl transferase activity in the rat and the rabbit,[707,708] was not shown to have such activity.[709] Plasma bilirubin levels in breastfeeding infants may remain elevated for 3 to 16 weeks and have occasionally been reported to reach concentrations of 15 to 24 mg/dL; they slowly and steadily decline after this period. No infants with breast milk jaundice have been reported to develop kernicterus.[707] Temporary interruption of nursing may help to establish the diagnosis by the resultant decrease in plasma bilirubin concentration followed by a rise when nursing is resumed, but interruption of nursing is not needed in most cases[710] and should not be indicated unless the plasma bilirubin concentration is near the risk level for bilirubin toxicity.

Transient Familial Neonatal Hyperbilirubinemia

Transient familial neonatal hyperbilirubinemia is a condition characterized by marked hyperbilirubinemia, which develops by 4 days of life but which is neither associated with breastfeeding nor with overt, excess hemolysis. Peak bilirubin concentrations have been reported in the range of about 9 to 65 mg/dL, and the condition was said to be due to an unidentified circulating inhibitor of UDP-glucuronyl transferase, which was found in the sera of both mother and infant.[711] Since kernicterus was observed in some infants, exchange transfusion may be required in some newborns with this disorder to prevent the development of bilirubin toxicity. The circulating inhibitor, whose nature has not been defined, disappears by the end of the second week of life, and plasma bilirubin concentrations in the affected infant return to normal. Transient familial neonatal hyperbilirubinemia was first described by Arias and colleagues[711] in 24 infants born to 8 mothers, but there have been no further reports on this condition.

Other Disorders Associated With Unconjugated Hyperbilirubinemia

Infants with pyloric stenosis and proximal small intestinal obstruction may display unconjugated hyperbilirubinemia in the absence of hemolysis. Affected infants have decreased hepatic UDP-glucuronyl transferase activity,[12] which may account for the development of this form of jaundice; pathogenesis of the decreased bilirubin UDP-glucuronyl transferase activity is not clear. Novobiocin, an antibiotic no longer used in the United States, has been reported to cause unconjugated hyperbilirubinemia in treated infants; this drug has also been shown to inhibit hepatic UDP-glucuronyl transferase activity.[713] Infants with congenital hypothyroidism occasionally develop neonatal unconjugated hyperbilirubinemia.[714] Infants born from mothers who have diabetes mellitus are also at high risk for the development of unconjugated hyperbilirubinemia.[715]

Bilirubin Toxicity

Signs and Symptoms

Clinical findings of bilirubin toxicity range from little or no overt signs or symptoms in some affected infants to the severe expression of this toxicity, termed *kernicterus*, and characterized by progressive lethargy, hypotonia, muscular rigidity, opisthotonus, spasticity, high-pitched cry, fever, convulsions, and ultimately death.[716] Hearing defects are probably the mildest overt neurologic expression of bilirubin toxicity.[717] Aberrations of auditory brain stem responses have also been reported in the Gunn rat, which represents an animal equivalent of the human disorder, Crigler-Najjar type I syndrome.[718] Infants who have survived severe bilirubin toxicity may show high-frequency deafness, sustained choreoathetosis, mental retardation, and cerebral palsy.[719] Seemingly unaffected infants with unconjugated hyperbilirubinemia may also display subtle neurologic abnormalities such as impaired motor functions, hearing loss, an aberrant cry, and psychologic dysfunction.[720–723] A national collaborative survey of the relation of hyperbilirubinemia to neurodevelopmental outcome in preterm infants carried out in Holland has indicated that the risk of an adverse neurodevelopmental outcome at the age of 2 years increased by 30% for each increment of 2.9 mg/dL in maximal plasma bilirubin concentrations in the neonatal period.[724]

Pathophysiology

Brains of infants with kernicterus examined at autopsy show characteristic yellowish staining of basal ganglia, hippocampal cortex, cerebellum, and subthalamic regions due to deposits of bilirubin.[725] Conditions such as prematurity, hypoalbuminemia, hypoxia, acidosis, and hemolysis in the infant greatly enhance the risk of kernicterus. Conjugated bilirubin does not enter the CNS, whereas free bilirubin can diffuse into the brain and exert toxic effects. Unconjugated bilirubin in plasma is bound to albumin.[726] Similarly, bilirubin in interstitial fluid, which represents about 20% of the circulating concentration, is also bound to albumin.[727] Albumin-bound bilirubin is also in equilibrium with a small amount of unbound bilirubin (0.5 mg/dL or less).[727] This equilibrium can be greatly influenced by factors that compete for bilirubin binding in favor of the release of free bilirubin. These factors are hypoalbuminemia, acidosis, and the presence of organic anions that bind to albumin such as sulfonamides, salicylates, caffeine, heparin and sodium benzoate, and certain nonesterified fatty acids.[727,728]

Free bilirubin has been shown to exert a variety of other toxic effects on cells, as already described. Bilirubin toxicity may also be exaggerated in the presence of hypoxia, and resultant tissue acidosis may enhance this toxicity.[729] Also, evidence shows that bilirubin may gain access to the CNS if the blood–brain barrier is disrupted.[730,731] The blood–brain barrier appears to be also selective to bilirubin. A recent study using iodine-125–albumin-bound bilirubin in newborn piglets showed that the blood–brain barrier is more permeable to bilirubin than to albumin, whereas the permeability of the blood–brain barrier to bilirubin decreases with age, without alterations in the permeability to albumin.[732]

Prevention of Bilirubin Toxicity

The two principal modes of treatment in current use to lower dangerously high plasma bilirubin levels are phototherapy and exchange transfusion. Experimental therapies include the use of phenobarbital to induce hepatic UDP-glucuronyl transferase for bilirubin and the use of heme oxygenase inhibitors to diminish heme degradation to bile pigment and thus to moderate hyperbilirubinemia in newborns.

Phototherapy. Products of photocatalyzed isomerization of bilirubin are more polar than the parent compound and are readily excreted in bile and urine. Phototherapy has been shown to be highly effective in lowering plasma bilirubin concentrations in infants with unconjugated hyperbilirubinemia[733–735] and Gunn rats.[736–738] When shaved Gunn rats were irradiated with blue light, bile pigment was immediately excreted into bile. The pigment concentration reached a steady state by 60 to 90 minutes and decreased abruptly when light was shut off.[736–738] Exposure of bilirubin to light in the range of 400 to 500 nm in vitro induces three major changes: configurational isomerization, structural isomerization, and photooxidation.[739] The efficiencies of these processes are defined by the relative values of their quantum yields, that is, the number of product molecules divided by the number of photons absorbed by bilirubin.

Configurational isomerization of bilirubin bound to human plasma albumin has a high quantum yield, is reversible, and is completely regioselective for the 4Z, 15E isomers[740] (Fig. 50-28). This isomer appears to be excreted only slowly into bile, so that it may reach a photostationary state during phototherapy with sufficiently bright light. Structural isomerization of bilirubin has a much lower quantum yield, but the reaction is irreversible and the primary product, lumirubin, is excreted much faster into bile and urine than in the configurational isomer. Photooxidation of bilirubin has the lowest quantum yield among the three photoprocesses and yields colorless water-soluble products, that is, oxidized monopyrroles and dipyrroles, which are excreted rapidly into urine. Photoisomerization is a more important process than photooxidation, and lumirubin is a major contributor to the effectiveness of phototherapy.[741] Lumirubin results from a "flipping-over" of one or both of the outer pyrrole rings of bilirubin IXα (Z,Z geometric isomer), which yields a mixture of geometric isomers (Z,E; E,Z; E,E).[576,742–745] Unlike the stable ground state Z,Z isomer, lumirubin cannot form intramolecular hydrogen bonds. Thus, they are more polar than the Z,Z isomer and can be excreted without glucuronidation. After excretion, they rapidly undergo reverse isomerization to form the more stable Z,Z form. This is probably the reason why unconjugated bilirubin can be found in bile and intestine after phototherapy.

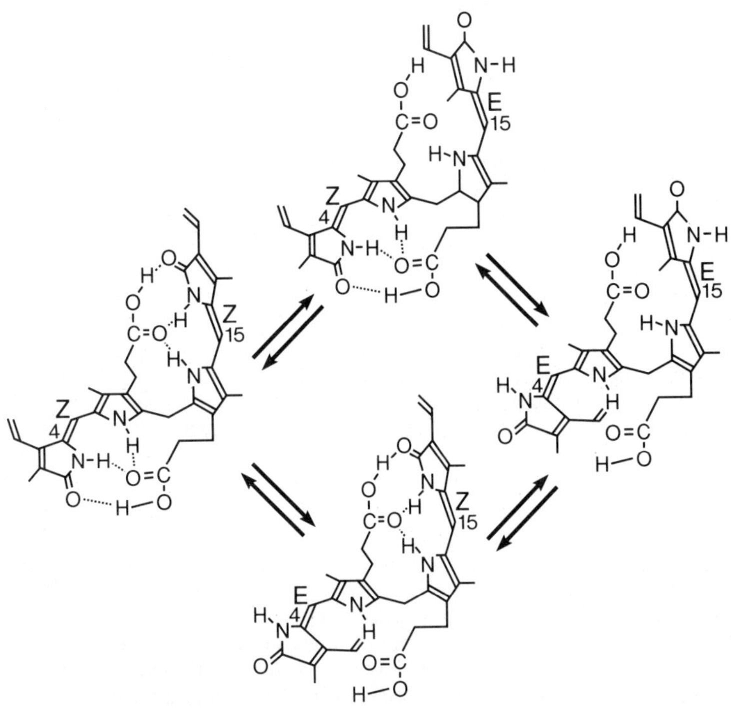

FIGURE 50-28. The four bilirubin configurational isomers. (*From left, clockwise*) ZZ, ZE, EE and EZ isomers. ZZ is the stable ground state isomer, while ZE, EE and EZ are lumirubins. Lumirubin, like a bilirubin monoglucuronide, has a polar end and a nonpolar end. Like a monoglucuronide, it undergoes monoglucuronidation if the glucuronidating enzyme system in the liver is functional, and it can be excreted into bile if the glucuronidating enzyme is insufficient or inactive, as in newborns or jaundiced Gunn rats. (After Lightner DA, McDonagh AF. Molecular mechanisms of phototherapy for neonatal jaundice. Acc Chem Res 1984;17:417)

Phototherapy, first used by Cremer and colleagues[741] to treat infants with hyperbilirubinemia and developed as a preventive form of therapy for newborn jaundice by Lucey and associates,[733] is an effective treatment modality for this common clinical problem. It is important to monitor plasma bilirubin concentrations before and during light treatment and to be aware of certain clinical concerns associated with its use, such as thermoregulatory and hydration problems.[746] Otherwise, no significant long-term deleterious effects of phototherapy in newborns have been described,[747] and the procedure has represented a remarkable advance in therapeutics.

Green light has been shown to be as effective as blue light in reducing plasma bilirubin concentrations in infants with hyperbilirubinemia.[748] The reason for green light's effectiveness in the photodestruction of bilirubin is not clear, but an effective spectral range and light intensity in tissues may possibly be attained by such light, since the depth of penetration of visible light increases with increasing wavelengths.[749] The use of green light may also be beneficial in reducing potential side effects of blue light.[750] Phototherapy was demonstrated to be more effective than exchange transfusion in achieving prolonged reduction of bilirubin levels for nonhemolytic hyperbilirubinemia.[751] An excellent account of this topic can be found in recent articles.[576,752]

Exchange Transfusion. Exchange transfusion was initially used to treat infants with Rh erythroblastosis but is also used in the treatment of infants with other types of unconjugated hyperbilirubinemia who are at risk for developing kernicterus.[753–756] Small volumes of the infant's blood are replaced with 10 to 20 mL of donor blood.[757] This is usually repeated until the volume of donor blood is about 180 mL/kg, or twice the blood volume of the infant. About 90% of the RBCs can be replaced with donor RBCs by this procedure.[758] A contemporary list of conditions warranting consideration for exchange transfusion, with a summary of the various techniques for performing exchange transfusions is available.[759] Exchange transfusion physically removes bilirubin and other organic substances that may compete for binding with bilirubin to carrier proteins. The procedure also supplies albumin to help correct hypoalbuminemia, which is commonly seen in infants with Rh erythroblastosis. For example, in a study with a typical exchange of blood, it was found that plasma bilirubin concentrations decreased by 50%, and plasma bilirubin binding capacity increased by 20% for each blood replacement.[760]

A two-volume exchange transfusion is also known to replace about 150% of the bilirubin calculated to be in the intravascular pool suggesting that a significant amount of albumin is located extravascularly and is in a readily exchangeable state with the intravascularly located albumin.[758] Exchange transfusion can be carried out in conjunction with albumin administration to augment bilirubin binding capacity.[728,761,762] In addition to complications that are common to any transfusion, complications of exchange transfusion include acidosis due to citrated blood, hyperkalemia resulting from aged blood, hypocalcemia due to calcium binding by citrate, pulmonary as well as intravascular hemorrhage, and thrombosis of the portal vein with hemorrhagic infarction of the bowel.[763] Mortality rate from the procedure ranges from about 1%[764] to 4.2%.[760]

A cut-off level of 20 mg of bilirubin per 100 mL plasma for administering exchange transfusion has been widely used.[756] In fact, it is unlikely that an otherwise well full-term infant with a plasma bilirubin concentration of less than 25 mg/dL would develop classic kernicterus.[721,765,766] On the other hand, the occurrence of kernicterus at plasma bilirubin levels lower than 20 mg/dL is also well documented in association with drug administration, hypoalbuminemia, hypoxia, and acidosis, particularly in the premature infant.[767–770] The cut-off value of 20 mg/dL was determined on the basis of studies performed 30 to 40 years ago,[756,771] which did not include sufficiently long follow-up studies (1 year or more). Thus, the value, 20, particularly in low-birthweight infants, cannot be considered an absolute limit, and other factors or conditions that may complicate hepatic bilirubin metabolism must also be taken into consideration in deciding if and when to initiate exchange transfusion or phototherapy.[772,773] A rate of rise in the plasma bilirubin levels greater than 1 mg/dL/h is considered to be a dangerously rapid rise that warrants early exchange.[774] Graphs are also available from which the risk level of bilirubin can be predicted to determine the need for exchange[671,754] (see Chap. 64).

Severely affected infants with Rh erythroblastosis of less than 32 weeks' gestational age are candidates for intrauterine RBC transfusions.[775] RBCs are transfused directly into the peritoneal cavity, are taken up by the lymphatic system, and enter the systemic circulation. The injected Rh-negative cells replace fetal cells, resulting in a negative Coombs' test and no fetal hemoglobin in the infant at birth. Babies may continue to synthesize RBCs; thus, significant and delayed postnatal hyperbilirubinemia may be present.

Phenobarbital Treatment. Administration of drugs and other compounds that are metabolized by the liver often results in significant induction of the cytochrome P-450–dependent, mixed-function drug system, as well as such enzymes in the endoplasmic reticulum as the UDP-glucuronyl transferases. With respect to bilirubin, phenobarbital treatment leads to enhanced hepatic uptake, conjugation,[727,776,777] UDP-glucuronyl transferase activity,[670,677,776,778–782] and secretion into bile of this pigment.[657,776,783] Phenobarbital also increases ligandin concentrations that contribute to the higher intracellular bilirubin binding capacity, resulting in reduced hepatic efflux of bilirubin.[784] Infants are treated with 5 to 6 mg/kg/d,[785] whereas mothers are treated with 30 to 100 mg/d for 2 to 4 weeks before delivery.[786,787]

Glutethimide produces effects similar to those of phenobarbital in normal volunteers and in patients with Gilbert's syndrome.[788] Potential side effects of phenobarbital have been indicated in studies using rats, which include enhanced metabolism of drugs, vitamin D,[789–791] and corticosteroids.[792] These effects may result in growth retardation, including brain growth.[793] Because of the potential side effects, phenobarbital treatment has not found clinical favor and has essentially been replaced by phototherapy and exchange transfusion in the United States.

Inhibition of Bilirubin Formation. Two heme oxygenase inhibitors, Sn-protoporphyrin and Sn-mesoporphyrin, have been studied extensively at the clinical level during the past several years with respect to their ability to ameliorate hyperbilirubinemia or lower normal levels of plasma bilirubin in humans.[268,545–547,557,794] Subjects of study have included normal volunteers, patients with various forms of jaundice, a newborn infant with Crigler-Najjar type I syndrome,[684] and a group of full-term newborns with jaundice associated with direct Coombs'-positive ABO incompatibility.[546] In the latter studies, incremental changes in plasma bilirubin levels were determined in control babies and inhibitor-treated infants (0.5 μmol/kg $\times$ 1, or 0.75 μmol/kg $\times$ 2 or 3) in the 96-hour period after birth; some infants were followed up for up to 176 hours postnatally.

The results indicated that inhibitor treatment diminished the incremental changes in plasma bilirubin levels at all time points studied after birth, with the effects being statistically significant at 48 hours and thereafter in infants receiving a total of either 1.5 μmol/kg (15 infants) or 2.25 μmol/kg (9 infants). The only clinical side effect noted was transient erythema during concurrent phototherapy with broad-spectrum lights in two infants. No sequelae were seen in children who developed erythema.

The overall requirement for phototherapy was diminished by about 40% in the combined treatment groups compared with that in the control group. Inhibitor alone was sufficient to moderate the severity of jaundice in treated infants, since plasma bilirubin levels in newborns receiving Sn-protoporphyrin alone were consistently lower than those in control babies.[546] In this comparison, 15 of 55 control infants required phototherapy, whereas only 1 of 35 inhibitor-treated babies required such treatment.[546] These preliminary studies suggest that heme oxygenase inhibitors may prove to be useful in the clinical management of jaundice in certain newborns.

Neonatal Jaundice Due to Conjugated Hyperbilirubinemia

Marked elevations of conjugated bilirubin in the newborn are not physiologic and are almost always associated with hepatocellular injuries or with obstructive lesions in the bile flow system (Table 50-6). Hepatocellular injuries result in the impaired excretion of conjugated bilirubin into the bile, whereas an obstruction in the bile flow (cholestasis) results in the accumulation of conjugated bilirubin in the circulation. Obstruction to bile flow can be either intrahepatic (from the level of the bile canaliculi to an intrahepatic duct) or extrahepatic (the common hepatic duct). In addition, certain disorders such as Dubin-Johnson syndrome or Rotor's syndrome are associated with specific excretory defects for bilirubin.

TABLE 50-6. Disorders of the Newborn Predominantly Associated With Conjugated Hyperbilirubinemia

OBSTRUCTION TO BILE FLOW
Extrahepatic
Extrahepatic biliary atresia
Extrahepatic stenosis/choledochal cyst
Extrahepatic mass (tumor, stone)
Bile plug syndrome/inspissated bile syndrome
Intrahepatic
Paucity of the intrahepatic ducts
Congenital hepatic cirrhosis
Intrahepatic biliary atresia
HEPATOCELLULAR INJURIES
Infection
Bacterial
Syphilis
Listeria
Tuberculosis
Viral
Hepatitis B (HB_sAg+), hepatitis A (?)
Hepatitis non-A, non-B (?)
Rubella
Cytomegalovirus
Coxsackie virus B
Protozoal: toxoplasmosis
Toxic
Bacterial sepsis
Intestinal obstruction
Diarrhea
Intravenous alimentation
Drugs
METABOLIC DISORDERS
Disorders of amino acid metabolism: tyrosinemia
Disorders of carbohydrate metabolism
Galactosemia
Fructosemia
Glycogenosis IV
Miscellaneous
α_1-Antitrypsin deficiency
Zellweger's syndrome
OVERPRODUCTION OF BILE PIGMENTS
Erythroblastosis fetalis
Hemolytic anemia due to erythrocyte enzyme deficiencies (glucose-6-phosphate dehydrogenase deficiency and others)
Hemolytic anemia due to erythrocyte membrane structural defects (spherocytosis, elliptocytosis, pyknocytosis, and others)
Congenital erythropoietic porphyria

DISORDERS OF BILIRUBIN METABOLISM IN OLDER CHILDREN, ADOLESCENTS, AND ADULTS

Disorders Associated With Unconjugated Hyperbilirubinemia

Unconjugated hyperbilirubinemia in older children and in adults is associated either with hemolysis or Gilbert's syndrome. Prolonged, mild, unconjugated hyperbilirubinemia in the absence of signs of hemolysis suggests Gilbert's syndrome. A 48-hour fasting period aggravates plasma bilirubin levels in those with Gilbert's syndrome, and intravenous administration of nicotinic acid provokes jaundice in affected persons.[795,796] Distinction from normals may be difficult, since similar changes are also observed to a certain extent in normal controls. No treatment is necessary for this condition.

Disorders Associated With Conjugated Hyperbilirubinemia

Dubin-Johnson Syndrome

Dubin-Johnson syndrome is an autosomal recessive benign disorder characterized by chronic conjugated hyperbilirubinemia. Plasma bilirubin concentrations in patients with this syndrome are usually 2 to 5 mg/dL, but may occasionally be elevated to as high as 17 mg/dL. The liver tissue has a dark color that is characteristic of this disorder; this is due to a lysosomal pigment.[797] Plasma bilirubin is predominantly direct reacting with the sulfanilic acid diazo reagent (50% or more).[798,799] A major portion of plasma bilirubin in patients with Dubin-Johnson syndrome is covalently bound with albumin, a finding commonly observed in patients with chronic conjugated hyperbilirubinemia.[596,800] In addition to conjugated hyperbilirubinemia, hepatic transport (but not uptake) of organic anions such as sulfobromophthalein, indocyanine green, metanephrine glucuronide, and iopanoic acid is decreased in this disorder.[801] The total amount of urinary coproporphyrin in patients with Dubin-Johnson syndrome is normal, but the type I isomer of coproporphyrin is greatly increased (over 80%), compared with that in normal subjects[802] (20% to 25%; Table 50-7).

A mutant strain of Corriedale sheep has an inherited disorder similar to the human Dubin-Johnson syndrome.[803–805] The animals have chronic conjugated hyperbilirubinemia

TABLE 50-7. Characteristic Symptoms of Inherited Conjugated Hyperbilirubinemia Syndromes

Symptoms	Dubin-Johnson Syndrome	Rotor's Syndrome
Liver	Dark-stained	Normal
Serum bilirubin	2–5 mg/dL; occasionally as high as 25 mg/dL; mostly direct reacting	2–5 mg/dL; usually ≤15 mg/dL; mostly direct reacting
Liver function	Normal except for bilirubin and certain organic anions	Normal except for bilirubin and certain organic anions
Bromsulphalein clearance	Normal or elevated; secondary rise	Elevated; no secondary rise
Urinary coproporphyrin	Normal; predominantly type I (>80%)	Elevated; type I less than 80%
Inheritance	Autosomal recessive	Autosomal recessive

and the characteristic lysosomal pigment of Dubin-Johnson syndrome.

Rotor's Syndrome

Rotor's syndrome is a rare benign disorder characterized by conjugated hyperbilirubinemia. It is inherited in an autosomal recessive fashion.[806] Plasma bilirubin concentrations rarely exceed 10 mg/dL. In contrast to that found in patients with Dubin-Johnson syndrome, no hepatocyte lysosomal pigmentation is present, and the hepatic uptake of bilirubin is diminished. Plasma disappearance curves for both sulfobromosulphthalein and indocyanine green are also different from those with Dubin-Johnson syndrome. Specifically, the first slope of plasma disappearance is impaired (suggesting impaired hepatic uptake), whereas no secondary rise in plasma bilirubin occurs in those with Rotor's syndrome[807] (Table 50-7). Unlike in patients with Dubin-Johnson syndrome, in whom total urinary coproporphyrin concentration is normal with the predominance of coproporphyrin I, a significant increase in total urinary coproporphyrin is found in those with Rotor's syndrome (2.5 to 5-fold) with a more balanced coproporphyrin I and III excretion.[808] Kinetic analyses of plasma sulfobromosulphthalein clearance suggested that this syndrome is due to a defect of hepatic storage and, to a lesser extent, of hepatic uptake.[679] The unconjugated hyperbilirubinemia of Rotor's syndrome appears to have no pathologic consequences of note.

REFERENCES

1. Falk JE. Porphyrins and metalloporphyrins: their general, physical and coordination chemistry, and laboratory methods. Amsterdam, Elsevier, 1964:1.
2. IUPAC-IUB Joint Commission on Biochemical Nomenclature (JCBN). Nomenclature of tetrapyrroles: recommendations 1978. Eur J Biochem 1978;108:1.
3. Gilbert DL. Significance of oxygen on earth. In: Gilbert DL, ed. Oxygen and living processes: an interdisciplinary approach. New York, Springer-Verlag, 1981:73.
4. Kappas A, Sassa S, Galbraith RA, Nordmann Y. The porphyrias. In: Scriver CR, Beaudet AL, Sly WS, Valle D, eds. The metabolic basis of inherited disease. New York, McGraw-Hill, 1989:1305.
5. Dailey HA. Biosynthesis of heme and chlorophylls. New York, McGraw-Hill, 1990.
6. Granick S, Urata G. Increase in activity of δ-aminolevulinic acid synthetase in liver mitochondria induced by feeding of 3,5-dicarbethoxy-1,4-dihydrocollidine. J Biol Chem 1963;238:821.
7. Granick S. The induction in vitro of the synthesis of δ-aminolevulinic acid synthetase in chemical porphyria: a response to certain drugs, sex hormones, and foreign chemicals. J Biol Chem 1963;241:1359.
8. Granick S, Sassa S. δ-Aminolevulinic acid synthetase and the control of heme and chlorophyll synthesis. In: Vogel HJ, ed. Metabolic pathway, vol 5: metabolic regulation. New York, Academic Press, 1971: 77.
9. Hayashi N, Yoda B, Kikuchi G. Mechanism of allylisopropylacetamide-induced increase of δ-aminolevulinate synthetase in liver mitochondria. IV. Accumulation of the enzyme in the soluble fraction of rat liver. Arch Biochem Biophys 1979;131:83.
10. Beale SI. δ-Aminolevulinic acid in plants: its biosynthesis, regulation and role in plastid development. Annu Rev Plant Physiol 1978;29: 95.
11. Huang D-D, Wang W-Y, Gough S, Kannangara CG. δ-Aminolevulinic acid–synthesizing enzymes need an RNA moiety for activity. Science 1984;225:1482.
12. Varticovski L, Kushner JP, Burnham BF. Biosynthesis of porphyrin precursors: purification and characterization of mammalian L-alanine gamma, δ-dioxovaleric acid aminotransferase. J Biol Chem 1980;355: 3742.
13. Sinclair P, Granick S. Two methods for determining the activity of δ-aminolevulinic acid synthetase within inteact liver cells in culture. Anal Biochem 1977;79:380.
14. Whiting MJ, Granick S. δ-Aminolevulinic acid synthase from chick embryo liver mitochondria. I. Purification and some properties. J Biol Chem 1976;251:1340.
15. Paterniti JR, Beattie DS. δ-Aminolevulinic acid synthetase from rat liver mitochondria: purification and properties. J Biol Chem 1979;254: 6112.
16. Borthwick IA, Srivastava G, Brooker JD, et al. Purification of δ-aminolevulinate synthase from liver mitochondria of chick embryo. Eur J Biochem 1982;129:615.
17. Srivastava G, Borthwick IA, Brooker JD, et al. Purification of rat liver mitochondrial δ-aminolevulinate synthase. Biochem Biophys Res Commun 1982;109:305.
18. Watanabe N, Hayashi N, Kikuchi G. δ-Aminolevulinate synthase isozymes in the liver and erythroid cells of chicken. Biochem Biophys Res Commun 1983;113:377.
19. Borthwick IA, Srivastava G, Hobbs AA, et al. Molecular cloning of hepatic δ-aminolevulinate synthase. Eur J Biochem 1984;144:95.
20. Pirola BA, Mayer F, Borthwick IA, et al. Electron microscopic studies on liver δ-aminolevulinate synthase. Eur J Biochem 1984;144:577.
21. Horwich AL, Fenton WA, Williams KR, et al. Structure and expression of a completmentary DNA for the nuclear coded precursor of human mitochondrial ornithine transcarbamylase. Science 1984;224:1068.
22. Hayashi N, Watanabe N, Kikuchi G. Inhibition by hemin of in vitro translocation of chicken liver δ-aminolevulinate synthase into mitochondria. Biochem Biophys Res Commun 1983;115:700.
23. Riddle RD, Yamamoto M, Engel JD. Expression of δ-aminolevulinic synthase in avian cells: separate genes encode erythroid-specific and nonspecific isozymes. Proc Natl Acad Sci USA 1989;86:792.
24. Zaman Z, Jordan PM, Akhtar M. Mechanism and stereochemistry of the δ-aminolevulinate synthetase reaction. Biochem J 1973;135:257.
25. Akhtar M, Abboud MM, Barnard G, et al. Mechanism and stereochemistry of enzymic reactions involved in porphyrin biosynthesis. Philos Trans R Soc Lond [Biol] 1976;273:117.
26. Abboud MM, Jordan PM, Akhtar M. Biosynthesis of δ-Aminolevulinic acid: involvement of a retention-inversion mechanism. J Chem Soc Chem Commun 1974;643.
27. Gibson KD, Neuberger A, Scott JJ. The purification and properties of δ-aminolevulinic acid dehydrase. Biochem J 1955;61:618.
28. Granick S. Enzymatic conversion of δ-aminolevulinic acid to porphobilinogen. Science 1954;120:1105.
29. Burnham BF, Lascelles J. Control of porphyrin biosynthesis through a negative-feedback mechanism: studies with preparation of δ-aminolevulinate synthase and δ-aminolevulinate dehydratase from *Rhodopseudomonas spheroides*. Biochem J 1963;87:462.
30. Wu WH, Shemin D, Richards KE, et al. The quarternary structure of δ-aminolevulinate dehydratase from bovine liver. Proc Natl Acad Sci USA 1974;71:1767.
31. Anderson PM, Desnick RJ. Purification and properties of δ-aminolevulinate dehydratase from human erythrocytes. J Biol Chem 1979;254: 6924.
32. Bevan DR, Bodlaender P, Shemin D. Mechanism of porphobilinogen

synthase: requirement of Zn2+ for enzyme activity. J Biol Chem 1979;254:6924.
33. Barnard GF, Itoh R, Hohberger LH, et al. Mechanism of porphobilinogen synthase: possible role of essential thiol groups. J Biol Chem 1977;252:8965.
34. Tsukamoto I, Yoshinaga T, Sano S. Zinc and cysteine residues in the active site of bovine liver δ-aminolevulinic acid dehydratase. Int J Biochem 1980;12:751.
35. Tsukamoto I, Yoshinaga T, Sano S. The role of zinc with special reference to the essential thiol groups in δ-aminolevulinic acid dehydratase of bovine liver. Biochim Biophys Acta 1979;570:167.
36. Sommer R, Beyersmann D. Zinc and cadmium in 5-aminolevulinic acid dehydratase: equilibrium, kinetic and ^{113}Cd-nmr-studies. J Inorg Biochem 1984;20:131.
37. Nandi DL, Shemin D. δ-Aminolevulinic acid dehydratase of *Rhodopseudomonas spheroides*: III. Mechanism of porphobilinogen synthesis. J Biol Chem 1968;234:1236.
38. Jordan PM, Seehra JS. Mechanism of action of δ-aminolevulinic acid dehydratase: stepwise order of addition of the two molecules of δ-aminolevulinic acid in the enzyme synthesis of porphobilinogen. J Chem Soc Chem Commun 1980;240.
39. Shemin D. δ-Aminolevulinic acid dehydratase. In: Boyer PD, ed. The enzymes, vol 7. New York, Academic Press, 1972:323.
40. Chang CS, Sassa S, Doyle D. An immunological study of δ-aminolevulinic acid dehydratase specificity consistent with the phylogeny of species. Biochim Biophys Acta 1984;797:297.
41. Yamamoto M, Fujita H, et al. An immunochemical study of δ-aminolevulinate synthase and δ-aminolevulinate dehydratase in liver and erythroid cells of rat. Arch Biochem Biophys 1986;245:76.
42. Granick JL, Sassa S, Granick S, Levere RD, Kappas A. Studies in lead poisoning. II. Correlation between the ratio of activated to inactivated δ-aminolevulinic acid dehydratase of whole blood and the blood lead level. Biochem Med 1973;8:149.
43. Beale SI. The biosynthesis of δ-aminolevulinic acid in *Chlorella*. Plant Physiol 1970;45:505.
44. Doyle D, Schimke RT. The genetic and developmental regulation of hepatic δ-aminolevulinate dehydratase in mice. J Biol Chem 1969;244: 5440.
45. Weissberg JB, Lipschutz F, Oski FA. δ-Aminolevulinic acid dehydratase activity in circulating blood cells: a sensitive laboratory test for the detection of childhood lead poisoning. N Engl J Med 1971;284: 565.
46. Lindblad B, Lindstedt S, Steen G. On the genetic defects in hereditary tyrosinemia. Proc Natl Acad Sci USA 1977;74:4641.
47. Tschudy DP, Hess RA, Frykholm BD. Inhibition of δ-aminolevulinic acid dehydratase by 4,6-dioxoheptanoic acid. J Biol Chem 1981;256: 9915.
48. Stoner E, Starkman H, Wellner D, et al. Biochemical studies of a patient with hereditary hepatorenal tyrosinemia: evidence of glutathione deficiency. Pediatr Res 1984;18:1332.
49. Sassa S, Kappas A. Hereditary tyrosinemia and the heme biosynthetic pathway: profound inhibition of δ-aminolevulinic acid dehydratase activity by succinylacetone. J Clin Invest 1983;71:625.
50. Sassa S, Granick S, Bickers DR, Levere RD, Kappas A. Studies on the inheritance of human erythrocyte δ-aminolevulinate dehydratase and uroporphyrinogen synthetase. Enzyme 1973;16:326.
51. Sassa S. Sequential induction of heme pathway enzymes during erythroid differentiation of mouse Friend leukemia virus–infected cells. J Exp Med 1975;143:305.
52. Sassa S. Control of heme biosynthesis in erythroid cells. In: Rossi GB, ed. In vitro and in vivo erythropoiesis: the Friend system. Amsterdam, Elsevier/North-Holland Biochemical Press, 1980:219.
53. Hoffman R, Ibrahim N, Murnane MJ, et al. Hemin control of heme biosynthesis and catabolism in a human leukemia cell line. Blood 1980;56:567.
54. Sassa S, Bernstein SE. Levels of δ-aminolevulinate dehydratase, uroporphyrinogen-I synthase, and protoporphyrin IX in erythrocytes from anemic mutant mice. Proc Natl Acad Sci USA 1977;74:1181.
55. Anderson KE, Sassa S, Peterson CM, Kappas A. Increased erythrocyte uroporphyrinogen-1-synthetase, δ-aminolevulinic acid dehydratase and protoporphyrin in hemolytic anemias. Am J Med 1977;63:359.
56. Lingner B, Kleinschmidt T. N-terminale Sequenz einer Porphobilinogen-Synthase. Z Naturforsch 1983;38:1059.
57. Bishop TR, Cohen RJ, Boyer SH, et al. Isolation of a rat liver δ-aminolevulinate dehydratase (ALAD) cDNA clone: evidence for unequal ALA gene dosage among inbred mouse strains. Proc Natl Acad Sci USA 1986;83:5568.
58. Bishop TR, Frelin LP, Boyer SH. Nucleotide sequence of rat liver δ-aminolevulinic acid dehydratase cDNA. Nucleic Acids Res 1986;14: 10115.
59. Gibbs PN, Jordan PM. Identification of lysine at the active site of human 5-aminolaevulinate dehydratase. Biochem J 1986;236:447.
60. Battersby AR, Fookes CJR, Matcham GWJ, et al. Order of assembly of the four pyrrole rings during biosynthesis of the natural porphyrins. J Chem Soc Chem Commun 1979;539.
61. Battersby AR, Fookes CJR, Matcham GWJ, et al. Biosynthesis of the natural porphyrins: experiments on the ring closure steps and with the hydroxy-analogue of porphobilinogen. J Chem Soc Chem Commun 1979;316.
62. Battersby AR, Fookes CJR, Matcham GWJ, et al. Biosynthesis of the pigments of life: formation of the macrocycle. Nature 1980;285:17.
63. Anderson PM, Desnick RJ. Purification and properties of uroporphyrinogen. I. Synthase from human erythrocytes: identification of stable enzyme-substrate intermediates. J Biol Chem 1980;255:1993.
64. Meisler MH, Carter MLC. Rare structural variants of human and murine uroporphyrinogen I synthase. Proc Natl Acad Sci USA 1980;77: 2848.
65. Grandchamp B, de Verneuil H, et al. Tissue-specific expression of porphobilinogen deaminase: two isozymes from a single gene. Eur J Biochem 1987;162:105.
66. Jordan PM, Shemin D. Purification and properties of uroporphyrinogen. I. Synthase from *Rhodopseudomonas spheroides*. J Biol Chem 1973;248:1019.
67. Miyagi K, Kaneshima M, Kawakami J, et al. Uroporphyrinogen I synthase from human erythrocytes: separation, purification, and properties of isoenzymes. Proc Natl Acad Sci USA 1979;76:6172.
68. Beaumont C, Grandchamp B, Bogard M, et al. Porphobilinogen deaminase is unstable in the absence of its substrate. Biochim Biophys Acta 1986;882:384.
69. Wang A-L, Arredondo-Vega FX, Giampietro PF, et al. Regional gene assignment of human porphobilinogen deaminase and esterase A_4 to chromosome 11 23 11qter. Proc Natl Acad Sci USA 1981;78:5734.
70. de Verneuil H, Phung N, Nordmann Y, et al. Assignment of human uroporphyrinogen-I synthase locus to region 11qter by gene dosage effect. Hum Genet 1982;60:212.
71. Romeo P-H, Raich N, et al. Molecular cloning and nucleotide sequence of a complete human uroporphyrinogen decarboxylase cDNA. J Biol Chem 1986;261:9825.
72. Raich N, Romeo P-H, et al. Molecular cloning and complete primary sequence of human erythrocyte porphobilinogen deaminase. Nucl Acids Res 1986;14:5955.
73. Grandchamp B, Romeo P-H, Dubart A, et al. Molecular cloning of a cDNA sequence complementary to porphobilinogen deaminase mRNA from rat. Proc Natl Acad Sci USA 1984;81:5036.
74. Grandchamp B, Beaumont C, de Verneuil H, et al. Genetic expression of porphobilinogen deaminase and uroporphyrinogen decarboxylase during the erythroid differentiation of mouse erythroleukemic cells. In: Nordmann Y, ed. Porphyrins and porphyrias. Colloque INSERM, vol 134. London, John Libbey Eurotext, 1986:35.
75. Chretien S, Dubart A, Beaupain D, et al. Alternative transcription and splicing of the human porphobilinogen deaminase gene results either in tissue-specific or in housekeeping expression. Proc Natl Acad Sci USA 1988;85:6.
76. Meyer UA, Strand LJ, Doss M, et al. Intermittent acute porphyria: Demonstration of a genetic defect in porphobilinogen metabolism. N Engl J Med 1972;286:1277.
77. Strand LJ, Meyer UA, Felsher BF, et al. Decreased red cell uroporphyrinogen I synthetase activity in intermittent acute porphyria. J Clin Invest 1972;51:2530.
78. Sassa S, Granick S, Bickers DR, Bradlow HL, Kappas A. A microassay for uroporphyrinogen I synthase, one of three abnormal enzyme activities in acute intermittent porphyria, and its application to the study of the genetics of this disease. Proc Natl Acad Sci USA 1974;71: 732.
79. Sassa S, Solish G, Levere RD, Kappas A. Studies in porphyria. IV. Expression of the gene defect of acute intermittent porphyria in cultured human skin fibroblasts and amniotic cells: prenatal diagnosis of the porphyric trait. J Exp Med 1975;142:722.
80. Bonkowsky HL, Tschudy DP, Weinbach EC, et al. Porphyrin synthesis and mitochondrial respiration in acute intermittent porphyria: studies using cultured human fibroblasts. J Lab Clin Med 1975;85:93.
81. Meyer UA. Intermittent acute porphyria: clinical and biochemical studies of disordered heme biosynthesis. Enzyme 1973;16:334.
82. Strand LJ, Felsher BF, et al. Heme biosynthesis in intermittent acute porphyria: decreased hepatic conversion of porphobilinogen to porphyrins and increased δ-aminolevulinic acid synthetase activity. Proc Natl Acad Sci USA 1970;67:1315.
83. Miyagi K, Cardinal R, Bossermaier I, et al. The serum porphobilinogen and hepatic porphobilinogen deaminase in normal and porphyric individuals. J Lab Clin Med 1971;78:683.
84. Sassa S, Zalar GL, Kappas A. Studies in porphyria. VII. Induction of uroporphyrinogen-I synthase and expression of the gene defect of acute intermittent porphyria in mitogen-stimulated human lymphocytes. J Clin Invest 1978;61:499.
85. Mustajoki P. Normal erythrocyte uroporphyrinogen I synthetase in a kindred with acute intermittent porphyria. Ann Intern Med 1981;95: 162.
86. Grandchamp B, Picat C, Mignotte V, et al. Tissue-specific splicing mutation in acute intermittent porphyria. Proc Natl Acad Sci USA 1989;86:661.
87. Frydman RB, Feinstein G. Studies on porphobilinogen deaminase and uroporphyrinogen III cosynthase from human erythrocytes. Biochim Biophys Acta 1974;350:358.
88. Higuchi M, Bogorad L. The purification and properties of uropor-

phyrinogen I synthase and uroporphyrinogen III cosynthase: interactions between the enzymes. Ann NY Acad Sci 1975;244:401.
89. Rossetti MV, de Geralnick AAJ, Kotler M, et al. Occurrence of multiple molecular forms of porphobilinogenase in diverse organisms: the minimum quarternary structure of porphobilinogenase is a promoter of one deaminase and one isomerase domain. Int J Biochem 1980;12: 761.
90. Stevens E, Frydman RB, Frydman B. Separation of porphobilinogen deaminase and uroporphyrinogen III cosynthase from human erythrocytes. Biochim Biophys Acta 1968;158:496.
91. Levin EY. Uroporphyrinogen III cosynthase from mouse spleen. Biochemistry 1968;7:3781.
92. Romeo G, Levin EY. Uroporphyrinogen III cosynthetase in human congenital erythropoietic porphyria. Proc Natl Acad Sci USA 1969;63: 856.
93. Tsai S-F, Bishop DF, Desnick RJ. Purification and properties of uroporphyrinogen III synthase from human erythrocytes. J Biol Chem 1987;262:1268.
94. Cornford P. Transformation of porphobilinogen into porphyrins by preparations from human erythrocytes. Biochem J 1964;91:64.
95. Smith AG, Francis JE. Decarboxylation of porphyrinogens by rat liver uroporphyrinogen decarboxylase. Biochem J 1979;183:455.
96. de Verneuil H, Sassa S, Kappas A. Purification and properties of uroporphyrinogen decarboxylase from human erythrocytes: a single enzyme catalyzing the four sequential decarboxylations of uroporphyrinogens I and III. J Biol Chem 1983;258:2454.
97. de Verneuil H, Grandchamp B, Nordmann Y. Some kinetic properties of human red cell uroporphyrinogen decarboxylase. Biochim Biophys Acta 1980;611:174.
98. Elder GH, Tovey JA. Uroporphyrinogen decarboxylase activity of human tissues. Biochem Soc Trans 1977;5:1470.
99. Jackson AH, Sancovich HA, Ferramola AM, et al. Macrocyclic intermediates in the biosynthesis of porphyrins. Philos Trans R Soc Lond [Biol] 1975;273:119.
100. Zuyderhoudt FMJ, Sindram JW, Marx JJM, et al. The amount of ferritin and hemosiderin in the liver of patients with iron-loading diseases. Hepatology 1983;3:232.
101. Straka JG, Kushner JP. Purification and characterization of bovine hepatic uroporphyrinogen decarboxylase. Biochemistry 1983;22:4664.
102. Blekkenhorst GH, Eales L, Pimstone NR. Activation of uroporphyrinogen decarboxylase by ferrous iron in porphyria cutanea tarda. S Afr Med J 1979;56:918.
103. Sweeney GD, Jones KG, Cole FM, et al. Iron deficiency prevents liver toxicity of 2,3,7,8-tetrachlorodibenzo-p-dioxin. Science 1979;204:332.
104. Smith AG, Cabral JRP, De Matteis F. A difference between two strains of rats in their liver non-haem iron content and in their response to the porphyrogenic effect of hexochlorobenzene. Chem Biol Interact 1979;27:353.
105. Winterbourn CC, Sutton HC. Iron and xanthine oxidase catalyze formation of an oxidant species distinguishable from OH: comparison with the Harber-Weiss reaction. Arch Biochem Biophys 1986;244:27.
106. Elder GH, Lee GB, Tovey JA. Decreased activity of hepatic uroporphyrinogen decarboxylase in sporadic porphyria cutanea tarda. N Engl J Med 1978;299:274.
107. Kushner JP, Barbuto AJ, Lee GR. An inherited enzymatic defect in porphyria cutanea tarda. J Clin Invest 1976;58:1089.
108. Felsher BF, Norris ME, Shih JC. Red-cell uroporphyrinogen decarboxylase activity in porphyria cutanea tarda and in other forms of porphyria. N Engl J Med 1978;299:1095.
109. Taljaard JJF, Shanley BC, Joubert SM. Decreased uroporphyrinogen decarboxylase activity in experimental symptomatic porphyria. Life Sci 1971;10:887.
110. Taljaard JJF, Shanley BC, Deppe WM, et al. Porphyrin metabolism in experimental hepatic siderosis. II. Combined effect of iron overload and hexachlorobenzene. Br J Haematol 1972;23:513.
111. Taljaard JJF, Shanley BC, Deppe WM, et al. Porphyrin metabolism in experimental hepatic siderosis. III. Effect of iron overload and hexachlorobenzene on liver haem biosynthesis. Br J Haematol 1972;23: 587.
112. Smith AG, Francis JE. Investigations of rat liver uroporphyrinogen decarboxylase. Biochem J 1981;195:241.
113. Ippen H. Treatment of porphyria cutanea tarda by phlebotomy. Semin Hematol 1977;14:253.
114. Danby CWE, Koval A, Wyllie J. Acquired porphyria cutanea tarda: two cases treated by repeated phlebotomies. Can Med Assoc J 1966;94: 1358.
115. Epstein JH, Redeker AG. Porphyria cutanea tarda symptomatica (PCT-S): a study of the effect of phlebotomy therapy. Arch Dermatol 1965;92: 286.
116. Blekkenhorst GH, Day RS, Eales L. The effect of bleeding and iron administration on the development of hexachlorobenzene-induced rat porphyria. Int J Biochem 1980;12:1013.
117. Louw M, Neethling AC, Percy VA, et al. Effects of hexachlorobenzene feeding and iron overload on enzymes of haem biosynthesis and cytochrome P-450 in rat liver. Clin Sci Mol Med 1977;53:111.
118. McLellan T, Pryor MA, Kushner JP, et al. Assignment of uroporphyrinogen decarboxylase (UROD) to the pter→p21 region of human chromosome 1. Cytogenet Cell Genet 1985;39:224.
119. Romeo P-H, Dubart A, et al. Isolation and identification of cDNA clone coding for rat uroporphyringen decarboxylase. Proc Natl Acad Sci USA 1984;81:3346.
120. Granick S, Mauzerall D. Enzymes of porphyrin synthesis in red blood cells. Ann NY Acad Sci 1958;75:115.
121. Sano S, Granick S. Mitochondrial coproporphyrinogen oxidase and protoporphyrinogen formation. J Biol Chem 1961;236:1173.
122. Battle AM del C, Benson A, Rimington C. Purification and properties of coproporphyrinogenase. Biochem J 1965;97:731.
123. Poulson R, Polgase WJ. Aerobic and anaerobic coproporphyrinogenase activities in extracts from *Saccharomyces cerevisiae*: purification and characterization. J Biol Chem 1974;249:6367.
124. Greenawalt JW. The isolation of outer and inner mitochondrial membranes. Methods Enzymol 1974;31:310.
125. Elder GH, Evans JO. Evidence that the coproporphyrinogen oxidase activity of rat liver is situated in the intermembrane space of mitochondria. Biochem J 1978;172:345.
126. Grandchamp B, Phung N, Nordmann Y. The mitochondrial localization of coproporphyrinogen III oxidase. Biochem J 1978;176:97.
127. Yoshinaga T, Sano S. Coproporphyrinogen oxidase. 1. Purification, properties and activation by phospholipids. J Biol Chem 1980;255: 4722.
128. Zaman Z, Abboud MM, Akhtar M. Mechanism and stereochemistry of vinyl group formation in heme biosynthesis. J Chem Soc Chem Commun 1972;1263.
129. Battersby AR, Baldas J, Collins J, et al. Mechanism of biosynthesis of the vinyl groups of protoporphyrin IX. J Chem Soc Chem Commun 1972;1265.
130. Jackson AH, Jones DM, Philip G, et al. Synthetic and biosynthetic studies of porphyrins. IV. Further studies of the conversion of coproporphyrinogen III to protoporphyrin IX: mass spectrometric investigation of the incubation of specifically deuterized coproporphyrinogen III with chicken red cell haemolysates. Int J Biochem 1980;12:681.
131. Poulson R. The enzymic conversion of protoporphyrinogen IX to protoporphyrin IX in mammalian mitochondria. J Biol Chem 1976;251: 3730.
132. Poulson R, Polgase WJ. The enzymic conversion of protoporphyrinogen IX to protoporphyrin IX: protoporphyrinogen oxidase activity in mitochondrial extracts of *Saccharomyces cerevisiae*. J Biol Chem 1975;250:1269.
133. Brenner DA, Bloomer JR. The enzymatic defect in variegate porphyria: studies with human cultured skin fibroblasts. N Engl J Med 1980;302: 769.
134. Jones MS, Jones OTG. The structural organization of haem synthesis in rat liver mitochondria. Biochem J 1969;113:507.
135. Johnson A, Jones OTG. Enzymic formation of hemes and other metalloporphyrins. Biochim Biophys Acta 1964;93:171.
136. Porra RJ, Jones OTG. Studies on ferrochelatase. I. Assay and properties of ferrochelatase from a pig liver mitochondrial extract. Biochem J 1963;87:186.
137. Mailer K, Poulson R, Dolphin D, et al. Ferrochelatase: isolation and purification via affinity chromatography. Biochem Biophys Res Commun 1980;96:777.
138. Taketani S, Tokunaga R. Rat liver ferrochelatase: purification, properties and stimulation by fatty acids. J Biol Chem 1981;256:12738.
139. Camadro JM, Ibrahim NG, Levere RD. Kinetics of studies of human liver ferrochelatase: role of endogenous metals. J Biol Chem 1984;259: 5678.
140. Bottomley SS, Tanaka M, Everett MA. Diminished erythroid ferrochelatase activity in protoporphyria. J Lab Clin Med 1975;86:126.
141. Bloomer JR, Brenner DA, Mahoney MJ. Study of factors causing excess protoporphyrin accumulation in cultured skin fibroblasts from patients with protoporphyria. J Clin Invest 1977;60:1354.
142. Ruth GR, Schwartz S, Stephenson B. Bovine protoporphyria: the first nonhuman model of this hereditary photosensitizing disease. Science 1977;198:199.
143. Sassa S, Zalar GL, Poh Fitzpatrick MB, Anderson KE, Kappas A. Studies in porphyria: functional evidence for a partial deficiency of ferrochelatase activity in mitogen-stimulated lymphocytes from patients with erythropoietic protoporphyria. J Clin Invest 1982;69:809.
144. Sassa S, Schwartz S, Ruth G. Accumulation of protoporphyrin IX from δ-aminolevulinic acid in bovine skin fibroblasts with hereditary erythropoietic protoporphyria: a gene-dosage effect. J Exp Med 1981;153:1094.
145. Sassa S, Kappas A. Genetic, metabolic, and biochemical aspects of the porphyrias. In: Harris H, Hirschhorn K, eds. Advances in human genetics. New York, Plenum, 1981:121.
146. Tschudy DP, Marver HS, Collins A. A model for calculating messenger RNA half-life: short-lived messenger RNA in the induction of mammalian δ-aminolevulinic acid synthetase. Biochem Biophys Res Commun 1965;21:480.
147. Sassa S, Granick S. Induction of δ-aminolevulinic acid synthetase in chick embryo liver cells in culture. Proc Natl Acad Sci USA 1970;67: 517.
148. Tenhunen R, Marver HS, Schmid R. The enzymatic catabolism of hemoglobin: stimulation of microsomal heme oxygenase by hemin. J Lab Clin Med 1970;75:410.
149. Granick S, Sinclair P, Sassa S, Grieninger G. Effects by heme, insulin,

and serum albumin on heme and protein synthesis in chick embryo liver cells cultured in a chemically defined medium, and a spectrofluorometric assay for porphyrin composition. J Biol Chem 1975;250:9215.
150. Marver HS, Collins A, et al. δ-Aminolevulinic acid synthetase. J Biol Chem 1966;241:4323.
151. Abbritti G, De Matteis F. Decreased levels of cytochrome P-450 and catalase in hepatic porphyria caused by substituted acetamides and barbiturates: importance of the allyl group in the molecule of the active drugs. Chem Biol Interact 1971;4:281.
152. Nakao K, Wada O, Takaku F, Sassa S, Yano Y, Urata G. The origin of the increased protoporphyrin in erythrocytes of mice with experimentally induced porphyria. J Lab Clin Med 1967;70:923.
153. Granick S, Kappas A. Steroid induction of porphyrin synthesis in liver cell culture. I. Structural basis and possible physiological role in the control of heme formation. J Biol Chem 1967;242:4587.
154. Kappas A, Granick S. Steroid induction of porphyrin synthesis in liver cell culture. II. The effects of heme, uridine diphosphate glucuronic acid, and inhibitors of nucleic acid and protein synthesis on the induction process. J Biol Chem 1968;243:346.
155. Whiting MJ, Granick S. δ-Aminolevulinic acid synthetase from chick embryo liver mitochondria. II. Immunochemical correlation between synthesis and activity in induction and repression. J Biol Chem 1976;251:1347.
156. Yannoni CZ, Robinson SH. Early-labeled heam in erythroid and hepatic cells. Nature 1975;258:330.
157. Grandchamp B, Bissell DM, Licko V, Schmid R. Formation and disposition of newly synthesized heme in adult rat hepatocytes in primary culture. J Biol Chem 1981;256:11677.
158. Lo SC, Aft R, Mueller GC. Role of nonhemoglobin heme accumulation in the terminal differentiation of Friend erythroleukemia cells. Cancer Res 1981;41:864.
159. Ades IZ. Biogenesis of mitochondrial proteins: regulation of maturation of δ-aminolevulinate synthase by hemin. Biochem Biophys Res Commun 1983;110:42.
160. Sassa S, Granick JL, Eisen H, et al. Regulation of heme synthesis in mouse Friend virus-transformed cells in culture. In: Murphy MJ Jr, ed. In vitro aspects of erythropoiesis. New York, Springer-Verlag, 1978:135.
161. Eisen H, Keppel-Ballivet F, Georgopoulos CP, et al. Biochemical and genetic analysis of erythroid differentiation in Friend-virus transformed murine erythroleukemia cells. In: Clarkson B, Marks PA, Till JE, eds. Differentiation of normal and neoplastic hematopoietic cells, vol 5. Cold Spring Harbor, NY, Cold Spring Harbor Laboratory, 1978:277.
162. Rutherford T, Thompson GG, Moore MR. Heme biosynthesis in Friend erythroleukemia cells: Control by ferrochelatase. Proc Natl Acad Sci USA 1979;76:833.
163. Yamamoto M, Yew NS, Federspiel M, et al. Isolation of recombinant cDNAs encoding chicken erythroid δ-aminolevulinic acid synthase. Proc Natl Acad Sci USA 1985;82:3701.
164. Schoenhaut DS, Curtis PJ. Nucleotide sequence of mouse δ-aminolevulinic acid synthase cDNA and expression of its gene in hepatic and erythroid tissues. Gene 1986;48:55.
165. Elferink CJ, Sassa S, May BK. Regulation of 5-aminolevulinate synthase in mouse erythroleukemic cells is different from that in liver. J Biol Chem 1988;263:13012.
165a. Bishop DF. Nucl Acids Res 1990;18:7187.
165b. Bishop DF, Astrin KH, Ioannou YA. Am J Hum Genet 1989;45:A176.
165c. Cox TC, Bawden MJ, Martin A, May BK. EMBO J 1991;10:1891.
165d. Mignotte V, Eleouet JF, Raich N, Romero P-H. Proc Natl Acad Sci USA 1989;86:6548.
165e. Dandekar T, Stripecke R, Gray NK, et al. EMBO J 1991;10:1903.
165f. Aziz N, Munro HN. Proc Natl Acad Sci USA 1987;84:8478.
165g. Casey JL, DiJeso B, Rao K, Rouaolt TA, Klausner RD, Harford JB. Ann NY Acad Sci 1988;526:54.
165h. Melefors O, Goossen B, Johansson HE, Stripecke R, Gray NK, Hentze MW. J Biol Chem 1993;268:5974.
165i. Fujita H, Yamamoto M, Yamagami T, Hayashi N, Sassa S. J Biol Chem 1991;266:17494.
165j. Sassa S. Int J Cell Cloning 1990;8:10.
166. Porter PN, Meints RH, Mesner K. Enhancement of erythroid colony growth in culture by hemin. Exp Hematol 1979;7:11.
167. Ross J, Sautner D. Induction of globin mRNA accumulation by hemin in cultured erythroleukemia cells. Cell 1976;8:513.
168. Dabney BJ, Beaudet AL. Increase in globin chains and globin mRNA in erythroleukemia cells in response to hemin. Arch Biochem Biophys 1977;179:106.
169. Granick JL, Sassa S. Hemin control of heme biosynthesis in mouse Friend virus–transformed erythroleukemia cells in culture. J Biol Chem 1978;253:5402.
170. Briggs DW, Condie LW, Sedman RM, Tephly TR. δ-Aminolevulinic acid synthetase in the heart. J Biol Chem 1976;251:4996.
171. Condie LW, Baron J, Tephly TR. δ-Aminolevulinic acid synthetase. Arch Biochem Biophys 1976;172:123.
172. Held H, Przerwa M. Effect of the female sexual cycle on the activity of δ-aminolevulinate synthase in rat liver. Eur J Clin Invest 1976;6:411.
173. Wielburski A, Nelson BRD. Heme *a* induces assembly of rat liver cytochrome c oxidase subunits I-III in isolated mitochondria. FEBS Lett 1984;177:291.
174. Gibson QH, Antonini E. Kinetic studies on the reaction between native globin and haem derivatives. Biochem J 1960;77:328.
175. Rose MY, Olson JS. The kinetic mechanism of heme binding to human apohemoglobin. J Biol Chem 1983;258:4298.
176. Cassoly R, Banerjee R. Structure and function of human semihemoglobins α and β. Eur J Biochem 1971;19:514.
177. Waxman HS, Freedman ML, Rabinovitz M. Studies with ^{59}Fe-labeled hemin on the control of polyribosome formation in rabbit reticulocytes. Biochim Biophys Acta 1967;145:353.
178. Rabinovitz M, Freedman ML, Fisher JM, et al. Translational control in hemoglobin synthesis. Cold Spring Harbor Symp Quant Biol 1969;34:567.
179. Morris AJ, Liang K. Interaction of globin and heme during hemoglobin biosynthesis. Arch Biochem Biophys 1968;125:468.
180. Hunt T, Vanderhoff G, London IM. Control of globin synthesis: the role of hemin. J Mol Biol 1972;66:471.
181. Bunn HF. Subunit assembly of hemoglobin: an important determinant of hematologic phenotype. Blood 1987;69:1.
182. Moore MR, McColl KEL, Rimington C, Goldberg A. Disorders of porphyrin metabolism. New York, Plenum, 1987:1.
183. Spikes JD. Porphyrins and related compounds as photodynamic sensitizers. Ann NY Acad Sci 1975;244:496.
184. Lim HW. Pathophysiology of cutaneous lesions in porphyrias. Semin Hematol 1989;26:114.
185. Goldstein BD, Harber LC. Erythropoietic protoporphyria: lipid peroxidation and red cell membrane damage associated with photohemolysis. J Clin Invest 1972;51:892.
186. Gibson SIM, Goldeberg A. Defects in haem synthesis in mammalian tissues in experimental lead poisoning and experimental porphyria. Clin Sci 1970;38:63.
187. Percy VA, Shanley BC. Studies on haem biosynthesis in rat brain. J Neurochem 1979;33:1267.
188. Cohn J, Alvares AP, Kappas A. On the occurrence of cytochrome P-450 and aryl hydrocarbon hydroxylase activity in rat brain. J Exp Med 1977;145:1607.
189. Das M, Seth PK, Mukhtar H. NADH-dependent inducible aryl hydrocarbon hydroxylase activity in rat brain mitochondria. Drug Metab Dispos 1981;9:69.
190. Paterniti JR Jr, Simone JJ, Beattie DS. Detection and regulation of δ-aminolevulinic acid synthetase activity in the rat brain. Arch Biochem Biophys 1978;189:186.
191. Feuer G, Sosa-Lucero JC, Lund G, et al. Failure of various drugs to induce drug-metabolizing enzymes in extrahepatic tissues of the rat. Toxicol Appl Pharmacol 1971;19:579.
192. Nabeshima T, Fontenot J, Ho JK. Effects of chronic administration of phoenobarbital or morphine on the brain microsomal cytochrome P-450 system. Biochem Pharmacol 1981;30:1142.
193. Sima AAF, Kennedy JC, Blakeslee D, et al. Experimental porphyric neuropathy. J Can Sci Neurol 1981;8:105.
194. Bornstein JC, Pickett JB, Diamond I. Inhibition of the evoked release of acetylcholine by the porphyrin precursor δ-aminolevulinic acid. Neurology 1979;5:94.
195. Dichter HN, Taddeini L, Lin S, et al. δ-Aminolevulinic acid: effect of a porphyrin precursor on an isolated neuronal preparation. Brain Res 1977;126:189.
196. Becker DM, Goldstuck N, Kramer S. Effect of δ-aminolevulinic acid on the resting membrane potential of frog sartorius muscle. S Afr Med J 1975;49:1790.
197. Durko I, Juhasz A. Porphyrin synthesis in primary nervous tissue cultures from 10^{-3} M δ-aminolevulinic acid in the presence of metatonin and neuropeptides. Neurochem Res 1986;11:607.
198. Culter MG, Moore MR, Dick JM. Effects of δ-aminolevulinic acid on contractile activity of rabbit duodenum. Eur J Pharmacol 1980;64:221.
199. Becker DM, Viljoen D, Kramer S. The inhibition of red cell and brain ATPase by δ-aminolevulinic acid. Biochim Biophys Acta 1971;225:26.
200. Mueller WE, Snyder SH. δ-Aminolevulinic acid: influences on synergistic GABA receptor binding may explain CNS symptoms of porphyria. Ann Neurol 1977;2:340.
201. Sweeney VP, Pathak MA, Asbury AK. Acute intermittent porphyria: increased ALA synthetase activity during an acute attack. Brain 1970;93:369.
202. McGillon FB, Moore MR, Goldberg A. The effect of δ-aminolevulinic acid on the spontaneous activity of mice. Scott Med J 1973;18:133.
203. Shanley BC, Neathling AC, Percy VA, Carstens M. Neurochemical aspects of porphyria: studies on the possible neurotoxicity of δ-aminolevulinic acid. S Afr J Lab Clin Med 1975;49:576.
204. Pierach CA, Edwards PS. Neurotoxicity of δ-aminolevulinic acid and porphobilinogen. Exp Neurol 1978;62:810.
205. Percy VA, Shanley BC. Porphyrin precursors in blood, urine and cerebrospinal fluid in acute porphyria. S Afr Med J 1977;52:219.
206. Gorchein A, Webber R. δ-aminolevulinic acid in plasma, cerebrospinal fluid, saliva and erythrocytes: studies in normal, uremic and porphyric subjects. Clin Sci 1987;72:103.

207. Edwards SR, Shanley BC, Reynoldson JA. Neuropharmacology of δ-aminolevulinic acid. Neuropharmacology 1984;23:477.
208. Green H, Greenburg SM, Erickson RW, et al. Effect of dietary phenylanine and typtophan upon rat brain anine levels. J Pharmacol Exp Ther 1962;136:174.
209. Knox WE. The regulation of tryptophan pyrrolase activity by tryptophan. Adv Enzyme Regul 1966;4:287.
210. Litman DA, Correia MA. L-Tryptophan: a common denominator of biochemical and neurological events of acute hepatic porphyria. Science 1983;222:1031.
211. Litman DA, Correia MA. Elevated brain tryptophan and enhanced 5-hydroxytryptamine turnover in acute heme deficiency: clinical implications. J Pharmacol Exp Ther 1985;232:337.
212. Yuwiler A, Wetterberg L, Geller E. Tryptophan pyrrolase, tryptophan and tyrosine transaminase changes during allisopropylacetamide-induced porphyria in the rat. Biochem Pharmacol 1970;19:189.
213. Doss M, von Tiepermann R, Schneider J, Schmid H. New types of hepatic porphyria with porphobilinogen synthase defect and intermittent acute clinical manifestation. Klin Wochenschr 1979;57:1123.
214. Doss M, von Tiepermann R, Schneider J. Acute hepatic porphyria syndrome with porphobilinogen synthase defect. Int J Biochem 1980;12:823.
215. Doss M, Schneider J, von Tiepermann R, Brandt A. New type of acute porphyria with porphobilinogen synthase (δ-aminolevulinic acid dehydratase) defect in the homozygous state. Clin Biochem 1982;15:52.
216. Thunell S, Holmberg L, Lundgreen J. Aminolevulinate dehydratase porphyria in infancy: a clinical and biochemical study. J Clin Chem Clin Biochem 1987;25:5.
217. Hassoun A, Verstraeten L, Mercelis R, Martin J-J. Biochemical diagnosis of an hereditary aminolaevulinate dehydratase deficiency in a 63 year-old man. J Clin Chem Clin Biochem 1989;27:781.
218. de Verneuil H, Doss M, Brusco N, et al. Hereditary hepatic porphyria with δ-aminolevulinate dehydratase deficiency: immunological characterization of the non-catalytic enzyme. Hum Genet 1985;69: 174.
219. Fujita H, Sassa S, Lundgren J, Holmberg L, Thunell S, Kappas A. Enzymatic defect in a child with hereditary hepatic porphyria due to homozygous δ-aminolevulinic acid dehydratase deficiency: immunochemical studies. Pediatrics 1987;80:880.
219a. Ishida N, Fujita H, Noguchi T, Doss M, Happas A, Sassa S. Biochem Biophys Res Commun 1990;172:237.
219b. Ishida N, Fujita H, Fukada Y, et al. J Clin Invest 1992;89:1431.
219c. Plewinska M, Thunell S, Holmberg L, Wetmur JG, Desnick RJ. Am J Hum Genet 1991;49:167.
220. Bonkowsky HL. Porphyrin and heme metabolism and the porphyrias. In: Zakim D, Boyer TD, eds. A textbook of liver disease. Philadelphia, WB Saunders, 1982:351.
221. Tishler PV, Woodward B, O'Connor J, et al. High prevalence of intermittent acute porphyria in a psychiatric patient population. Am J Psychiatry 1985;142:1430.
222. Stein JA, Curl FD, Valsamis M, Tschudy DP. Abnormal iron and water metabolism in acute intermittent porphyria with new morphologic findings. Am J Med 1972;53:784.
223. Ridley A. Porphyric neuropathy. In: Dyck PJ, Thomas PK, Lambert EH, eds. Peripheral neuropathy, vol 2. Philadelphia, WB Saunders, 1975:942.
224. Poser CM, Edwards K. Transient monoparesis in acute intermittent porphyria. Arch Neurol 1978;35:550.
225. Greenspan GH, Block AJ. Respiratory insufficiency associated with acute intermittent porphyria. South Med J 1981;74:954.
226. Sorensen HWS, With TK. Persistent pareses after porphyric attacks. Acta Med Scand 1971;190:219.
227. Tschudy DP, Perlroth MG, Marver HS, Collins A, Hunter G Jr, Rechcigl M Jr. Acute intermittent porphyria: the first "overproduction disease" localized to a specific enzyme. Proc Natl Acad Sci USA 1965;53:841.
228. Nakao K, Wada O, Kitamura T, Uono K. Activity of aminolevulinic acid synthetase in normal and porphyric human livers. Nature 1966;210:838.
229. McColl KEL, Wallace AM, et al. Alterations in haem biosynthesis during the human menstrual cycle: studies in normal subjects and patients with latent and active acute intermittent porphyria. Clin Sci 1982;62:183.
230. Goldberg A, Moore MR, Beattie AD, et al. Excessive urinary excretion of certain porphyrinogenic steroids in human acute intermittent porphyria. Lancet 1969;1:115.
231. Paxton JR, Moore MR, Beattie AD, Goldberg A. 17-Oxosteroid conjugates in plasma and urine of patients with acute intermittent porphyria. Clin Sci Mol Med 1974;46:207.
232. Paxton JR, Moore MR, Beattie AD, Goldberg A. Urinary excretion of 17-oxosteroids in hereditary coproporphyria. Clin Sci Mol Med 1975;49:441.
233. Kappas A, Bradlow HL, Gillette PN, Gallagher TF. Abnormal steroid hormone metabolism in the genetic liver disease acute intermittent porphyria. Ann NY Acad Sci 1971;179:611.
234. Kappas A, Bradlow HL, Gillette PN, Levere RD, Gallagher TF. A defect of steroid hormone metabolism in acute intermittent porphyria. Fed Proc 1972;31:1293.
235. Bradlow HL, Gillette PN, Gallagher TF, Kappas A. Studies in porphyria. II. Evidence for a deficiency of steroid Δ^4-5-α-reductase activity in acute intermittent porphyria. J Exp Med 1973;138:754.
236. Anderson KE, Bradlow HL, Sassa S, Kappas A. Studies in porphyria. VIII. Relationship of the 5α-reductive metabolism of steroid hormones to clinical expression of the genetic defect in acute intermittent porphyria. Am J Med 1979;66:644.
237. Felsher BF, Redeker AG. Acute intermittent porphyria: effect of diet and griseofulvin. Medicine 1967;46:217.
238. Welland FH, Hellman ES, Gaddis EM, et al. Factors affecting the excretion of porphyrin precursors by patients with acute intermittent porphyria. I. The effects of diet. Metabolism 1964;13:251.
239. Bonkowsky HL, Magnussen CR, Collins AR, et al. Comparative effects of glycerol and dextrose on porphyrin precursor excretion in acute intermittent porphyria. Metabolism 1976;25:405.
240. Kappas A, Anderson KE, Conney AH, Pantuck EJ, Fishman J, Bradlow HL. Nutrition-endocrine interactions: induction of reciprocal changes in the Δ^4-5α-reduction of testosterone and the cytochrome P-450–dependent oxidation of estradiol by dietary macronutrients in man. Proc Natl Acad Sci USA 1983;80:7646.
241. Kappas A, Bradlow HL, Bickers DR, Alvares AP. Induction of a deficiency of steroid Δ^4-5α-reductase activity in liver by a porphyrinogenic drug. J Clin Invest 1977;59:159.
242. Canepa ET, Llambias EBC, Grinstein M. The effect of glucose on the induction of δ-aminolevulinic acid synthase and ferrochelatase in isolated rat hepatocytes by ALA. Biochem Biophys Acta 1984;804:8.
243. Stephens JK, Fisher PWF, Marks GS. Porphyrin induction: equivalent effect of 5αH and 5βH steroids in chick embryo liver cells. Science 1977;197:659.
244. Sassa S, Bradlow HL, Kappas A. Steroid induction of δ-aminolevulinic acid synthase and porphyrins in liver: structure-activity studies and the permissive effects of hormones on the induction process. J Biol Chem 1979;254:10011.
245. Dudzinski B, Weinstein AJ. Infectious mononucleosis presenting as acute intermittent porphyria. South Med J 1984;77:523.
246. Iwasa F, Sassa S, Kappas A. The effects of acute-phase inducers and dimethyl sulphoxide on δ-aminolaevulinate synthase activity in human HepG2 hepatoma cells. Biochem J 1989;259:605.
247. Granick S, van den Schreieck HG. Porphobilinogen and δ-aminolevulinic acid in acute porphyria. Proc Soc Exp Biol Med 1955;88:270.
248. Wetterberg L, Haeger-Aronsen B, Stathers G. Faecal porphyrins as a diagnostic index between acute intermittent porphyria and porphyria variegata. Scand J Clin Lab Invest 1968;22:131.
249. Watson CJ, Schwartz S. A simple test for urinary porphobilinogen. Proc Soc Exp Biol Med 1941;47:393.
250. Watson CJ, Taddeini L, Bossermaier I. Present status of the Ehrlich aldehyde reaction for urinary porphobilinogen. JAMA 1964;190:501.
251. Mauzerall D, Granick S. The occurrence and determination of δ-aminolevulinic acid and porphobilinogen in urine. J Biol Chem 1956;219: 435.
252. Bloomer JR, Berk PD, et al. Blood volume and bilirubin production in acute intermittent porphyria. N Engl J Med 1971;284:17.
253. Jones EA, Bloomer JR, Berlin NI. The measurement of the synthetic rate of bilirubin from hepatic hemes in patients with acute intermittent porphyria. J Clin Invest 1971;50:2259.
254. Bonkowsky HL, Tschudy DP, Collins A, et al. Repression of the overproduction of porphyria precursors in acute intermittent porphyria by intravenous infusions of hematin. Proc Natl Acad Sci USA 1971;68: 2725.
255. Pierach CA. Hematin therapy for the porphyria attack. Semin Liver Dis 1982;2:125.
256. Watson CJ, Pierach CA, Bossenmaier I, Cardinal R. Postulated deficiency of hepatic heme and repair by hematin infusions in the "inducible" hepatic porphyrias. Proc Natl Acad Sci USA 1977;74:2118.
257. Lamon JM, Frykholm BC, Tschudy DP. Hematin administration to an adult with lead intoxication. Blood 1979;53:1007.
258. Simionatto CS, Galbraith RA, Jones R, et al. Hematin infusions impair hemostasis in normal subjects. Clin Res 1986;34:651A.
259. Morris DL, Dudley MD, Pearson RD. Coagulopathy associated with hematin treatment for acute intermittent porphyria. Ann Intern Med 1981;95:700.
260. Glueck R, Green D, Cohen I, Ts'ao CH. Hematin: unique effects on hemostasis. Blood 1983;61:243.
261. Petersen JM, Pierach CA. Hematin-induced hemolysis in acute porphyria. Ann Intern Med 1984;101:877.
262. Tenhunen R, Tokola O, Linden I-B. Haem arginate: a new stable haem compound. J Pharm Pharmacol 1987;39:780.
263. Mustajoki P, Tenhunen R, Pierach C, Volin L. Heme in the treatment of porphyrias and hematological disorders. Semin Hematol 1987;26: 1.
264. Mustajoki P, Tenhunen R, Tokola O, Gothoni G. Haem arginate in the treatment of acute hepatic porphyrias. Br Med J 1986;293:538.
265. Anderson KE, Spitz IM, Sassa S, Bardin CW, Kappas A. Prevention of cyclical attacks of acute intermittent porphyria with a long-acting agonist of luteinizing hormone-releasing hormone. N Engl J Med 1984;311:643.
266. Semon C, Dupond JL, Mallet H, et al. Traitment d'une porphyrie

aigue intermittente avec attaques cycliques par un agoniste Lh-RH administre par voie nasale. Ann Endocrinol (Paris) 1986;47:399.
267. Anderson KE. LHRH analogues for hormonal manipulation in acute intermittent porphyria. Semin Hematol 1989;26:10.
268. Galbraith RA, Kappas A. Pharmacokinetics of tin-mesoporphyrin in man and the effects of tin-chelated porphyrins on hyperexcretion of heme pathway precursors in patients with acute inducible porphyria. Hepatology 1989;9:882.
269. Schmid R, Schwartz S, Watson CJ. Porphyrin content in bone marrow and liver in the various forms of porphyria. Arch Intern Med 1954;93:416.
270. Schmid R, Schwartz S, et al. Erythropoietic (congenital) porphyria: a rare abnormality of the normoblasts. Blood 1955;10:416.
271. Poh-Fitzpatrick MB. The erythropoietic porphyrias. Dermatol Clin 1986;4:291.
272. Kramer S, Viljoen E, Meyer AM, Metz J. The anemia of erythropoietic porphyria with the first description of the disease in an elderly patient. Br J Haematol 1965;11:666.
273. Kaufman BM, Vickers HR, Rayne J, Ryan TJ. Congenital erythropoietic porphyria: report of a case. Br J Dermatol 1967;79:210.
274. Feurle GE, Ho AD, Wosiewitz U, Encke A. Cholelithiasis bei einem bisher nicht beschriebenen: Fall von Porphyria erythropoietica congenita. Dtsch Med Wochenschr 1980;105:1153.
275. Watson CJ, Bossenmaier I, et al. Repression by hematin of porphyrin biosynthesis in erythrocyte precursors in congenital erythropoietic porphyria. Proc Natl Acad Sci USA 1974;71:278.
276. Deybach J-C, de Verneuil H, et al. Congenital erythropoietic porphyria (Gunther's disease): enzymatic studies on two cases of late onset. J Lab Clin Med 1981;97:551.
277. Pain RW, Welch FW, et al. Erythropoietic uroporphyria of Gunther first presenting at 59 years with positive family studies. Br Med J 1975;3:621.
278. Weston MJ, Nicholson DC, et al. Congenital erythropoietic uroporphyria (Gunther's disease) presenting in a middle-aged man. Int J Biochem 1978;9:921.
279. Bhutani LK, Sood SK, Das PK, et al. Congenital erythropoietic porphyria: an autopsy report. Arch Dermatol 1974;110:427.
280. Varadi S. Haemotological aspects in a case of erythropoietic porphyria. Br J Haematol 1958;4:270.
281. Gross S. Hematologic studies on erythropoietic porphyria: a new case with severe hemolysis, chronic thrombocytopenia and folic acid deficiency. Blood 1964;23:762.
282. Watson CJ, Perman V, Spurrel FA, et al. Some studies of the comparative biology of human and bovine porphyria erythropoietica. Trans Assoc Am Physicians 1958;71:196.
283. Heilmeyer VL, Clotten R, Kerp L, et al. Porphyria erythropoietica congenita Gunther Dtsch Med Wochenschr 1963;51:2449.
284. Marver HS, Schmid R. The porphyrias. In: Stanbury JB, Wyngaarden JB, Fredrickson DS, eds. The metabolic basis of inherited disease. New York, McGraw-Hill, 1972:1087.
285. Nordmann Y, Deybach J-C. Congenital erythropoietic porphyria. Semin Liver Dis 1982;2:154.
286. Haining RG, Cowger ML, Shurtleff DB, Labbe RF. Congenital erythropoietic porphyria. I. Case report, special studies and therapy. Am J Med 1968;45:624.
287. Johnson LW, Schwartz S. Isotopic studies of erythrocyte survival in normal and porphyric cattle: influence of light exposure, blood withdrawal and splenectomy. Am J Vet Res 1970;31:2167.
288. Eriksen L, Hofstad F, Seip M. Congenital erythropoietic porphyria: the effect of light shielding. Acta Paediatr Scand 1973;62:385.
289. Aldrich RA, Hawkinson V, Grinstein M, Watson CJ. Photosensitive or congenital porphyria with hemolytic anemia. I. Blood 1951;6:685.
290. Sato A, Takahashi N. A new form of congenital hematoporphyria: oligochromia, porphyrinuria (megalosplenica congentia). Am J Dis Child 1926;32:325.
291. Becker CG, Wagner M, Kaplan AP, et al. Activation of factor XII–dependent pathways in human plasma by hemin and protoporphyrin. J Clin Invest 1985;76:413.
292. Elder GH, Smith SG, Herrero C, et al. Hepatoerythropoietic porphyria: a new uroporphyrinogen decarboxylase defect on homozygous porphyria cutanea tarda? Lancet 1981;1:916.
293. Lim HW, Poh-Fitzpatrick MB. Hepatoerythropoietic porphyria: a variant of childhood-onset porphyria cutanea tarda. J Am Acad Dermatol 1984;11:1103.
294. Mathews-Roth MM. β-Carotene in congenital porphyria. Arch Dermatol 1979;114:641.
295. Eriksen L, Seip M. The effect of various therapeutic trials on the porphyrin excretion in a case of congenital erythropoietic porphyria. Acta Paediatr Scand 1975;64:287.
296. Piomelli S, Poh-Fitzpatrick MB, et al. Complete suppression of the symptoms of congenital erythropoietic porphyria by long-term treatment with high-level transfusions. N Engl J Med 1986;314:1029.
297. Rosenthall IM, Lipton EL, Asrow G. Effect of splenectomy on porphyria erythropoietica. Pediatrics 1955;15:663.
298. Gray CH, Neuberger A. Effect of splenectomy in a case of congenital porphyria. Lancet 1952;1:851.
299. Pimstone NR, Gandhi SN, Mukerji SK. Medical intelligence: therapeutic efficacy of oral charcoal in congenital erythropoietic porphyria. N Engl J Med 1987;316:390.
300. Elder GH. Human uroporhyrinogen decarboxylase defects. In: Orfanos CE et al, eds. Dermatology in five continents. Berlin, Springer-Verlag, 1988:857.
301. Held J, Sassa S, et al. Erythrocyte uroporphyrinogen decarboxylase activity in porphyria cutanea tarda: a study of 40 consecutive patients. J Invest Dermatol 1989;93:332.
302. Banes HD. Porphyrias in the Bantu races on the Witwatersrand. S Afr Med J 1955;29:781.
303. Dean G. The porphyrias: a study of inheritance and environment. London, Pitman Medical, 1971.
304. Elder GH. Recent advances in the identification of enzyme deficiences in the porphyrias. Br J Dermatol 1983;108:729.
305. Kushner JP. The enzymatic defect in porphyria cutanea tarda. N Engl J Med 1982;306:799.
306. Behm AR, Unger WP. Oral contraceptives and porphyria cutanea tarda. Can Med Assoc J 1974;110:1052.
307. Grossman ME, Bickers DR, et al. Porphyria cutanea tarda: clinical features and laboratory findings in forty patients. Am J Med 1979;67:277.
308. Bickers DR, Keogh L, Rifkind AB, Harber LC, Kappas A. Studies in porphyria. VI. Biosynthesis of porphyrins in mammalian skin and in the skin of porphyric patients. J Invest Dermatol 1977;68:5.
309. Lim HW, Poh-Fitzpatrick MB, Gigli I. Activation of the complement system in patients with Porphyrias after irradiation in vivo. J Clin Invest 1984;74:1961.
310. Meurer M, Schulte C, Weiler A, Goerz G. Photodynamic action of uroporphyrin on the complement system in porphyria cutanea tarda. Arch Dermatol Res 1985;277:293.
311. Torinuki W, Miura T, Tagami H. Activation of complement by 405-nm light in serum from porphyria cutanea tarda. Arch Dermatol Res 1985;277:174.
312. Pigatto PD, Polenghi MM, Altomare GF, et al. Complement cleavage products in the phototoxic reaction of porphyria cutanea tarda. Br J Dermatol 1986;114:567.
313. Sandberg S, Romslo I. Protoporphyrin-induced photodamage at the cellular and the subcellular level as related to the solubility of the porphyrin. Clin Chim Acta 1981;109:193.
314. Strandberg K, Hagermark O. Prostaglandin E_2 in blister fluid of bullous diseases and experimental suction blisters. Acta Derm Venereol (Stockh) 1977;57:487.
315. Sandberg S, Romslo I, Hovding G, Bjorndal T. Porphyrin-induced photodamage as related to the subcellular localization of the porphyrins. Acta Derm Venereol 1982;100(Suppl):75.
316. Cortes JM, Oliva H, Paradinas FJ, Hernandez-Guio C. The pathology of the liver in porphyria cutanea tarda. Histopathology 1980;4:471.
317. James KR, Cortes JM, Paradinas FJ. Demonstration of intracytoplasmic needle-like inclusions in hepatocytes of patients with porphyria cutanea tarda. J Clin Pathol 1980;33:899.
318. Uthemann H, Kottschke R, Lissner R, Goergz G. Serologische hepatitis-B–marker bei Porphyria Cutanea Tarda. Dtsch Med Wochenschr 1980;105:1718.
319. Bel A, Girard D. Porphyrie cutanee tardive avec antigene HBs of hepatite chronique agressive. Nouv Presse Med 1980;9:2027.
320. Pierach CA. Porphyria and hepatocellular carcinoma. Br J Cancer 1987;55:111.
321. Packe GE, Clarke CWF. Is porphyria cutanea tarda a risk factor in the development of hepatocellular carcinoma? Oncology 1985;42:44.
322. Kordac V. Frequency of occurrence of hepatocellular carcinoma in patients with porphyria cutanea tarda in long-term follow-up. Neoplasma 1972;19:135.
323. Tio TH, Leijnse B, Jarrett A, Rimington C. Acquired porphyria from a liver tumor. Clin Sci Mol Med 1959;16:517.
324. Nacht S, San Martin de Viale LC, Grinstein M. Human porphyria cutanea tarda: isolation and properties of the urinary porphyrins. Clin Chim Acta 1970;27:445.
325. Smith SG, Rao KR, Jackson AH. The porphyrins of normal human urine, with a comparison of the excretion pattern in porphyria cutanea tarda. J Biochem (Tokyo) 1980;12:873.
326. Johansson IM, Niklasson FA. Determination of porphyrins in urine by direct injection on a liquid chromatographic column coated with tributylphosphate. J Chromatogr 1983;275:51.
327. Elder GH. The metabolism of porphyrins of the isocoproporphyrin series. Enzyme 1974;17:61.
328. Smith SG. Porphyrins found in urine of patients with symptomatic porphyria. Biochem Soc Trans 1977;5:1472.
329. Elder GH, Magnus IA, et al. Faecal "X-porphyrin" in the hepatic porphyrias. Enzyme 1973;17:29.
330. Malina L, Miller VI, Magnus IA. Skin porphyrin assay in porphyria. Clin Chim Acta 1978;83:55.
331. Elder GH. The differentiation of porphyria cutanea tarda symptomatica from other types of porphyria by the measurement of isocoproporphyrin in faeces. J Clin Pathol 1975;28:601.
332. Topi GC, Amantea A, Griso D. Recovery from porphyria cutanea tarda with no specific therapy other than avoidance of hepatic toxins. Br J Dermatol 1984;111:75.

333. Addy JH. Pathogenesis and natural history of porphyria cutanea tarda. Lancet 1974;2:213.
334. Ramsay CA, Magnus IA, Turnbull A, Baker H. The treatment of porphyria cutanea tarda by venesection. Q J Med 1974;169:1.
335. Epstein JH, Redeker AG. Porphyria cutanea tarda: a study of the effect of phlebotomy. N Engl J Med 1968;279:1301.
336. Sweeney GD. Porphyria cutanea tarda, or the uroporphyrinogen decaroxylase deficiency diseases. Clin Biochem 1986;19:3.
337. Lundvall O. Phlebotomy treatment of porphyria cutanea tarda. Acta Derm Venereol 1982;100(Suppl):107.
338. Malina L, Chlumsky J. A comparative study of the results of phlebotomy therapy and low-dose chloroquine treatment in porphyria cutanea tarda. Acta Derm Venereol (Stockh) 1981;61:346.
339. Cainelli T, Di Padova C, et al. Hydroxychloroquine versus phlebotomy in the treatment of porphyria cutanea tarda. Br J Dermatol 1983;108: 593.
340. Swanbeck G, Wennersten G. Treatment of porphyria cutanea tarda with chloroquine and phlebotomy. Br J Dermatol 1977;97:77.
341. Wennersten G, Ros AM. Chloroquine in treatment of porphyria cutanea tarda. Acta Derm Venereol 1982;100(Suppl):119.
342. Scholnick PL, Epstein J, Marver HS. The molecular basis of the action of chloroquine in porphyria cutanea tarda. J Invest Dermatol 1973;61: 226.
343. Fujita H, Sassa S, Toback AC, Kappas A. Immunochemical study of uroporphyrinogen decarboxylase in a patient with mild hepatoerythropoietic porphyria. J Clin Invest 1987;79:1533.
344. Toback AC, Sassa S, Poh Fitzpatrick MB, et al. Hepatoerythropoietic porphyria: clinical, biochemical, and enzymatic studies in a three-generation family lineage. N Engl J Med 1987;316:645.
345. Simon N, Berko GY, Schneider I. Hepatoerythropoietic porphyria presenting as scleroderma and acrosclerosis in a sibling pair. Br J Dermatol 1977;96:663.
346. Pinol-Aguade J, Castells A, Indacochea A, Rodes J. A case of biochemically unclassifiable hepatic porphyria. Br J Dermatol 1969;81: 270.
347. de Verneuil H, Grandchamp B, Romeo P-H, et al. Molecular analysis of uroporhyrinogen decarboxylase deficiency in a family with two cases of hepatoerythropoietic porphyria. J Clin Invest 1986;77:431.
348. de Verneuil H, Grandchamp B, Romeo P-H, et al. Molecular heterogeneity of uroporphyrinogen decarboxylase deficiency in hepatoerythropoietic porphyria. In: Nordmann Y, ed. Porphyrins and porphyrias. Paris, John Libbey, 1986:201.
348a. Romana M, Grandchamp B, Dubart A, et al. Identification of a new mutation responsible for hepatoerythropoietic porphyria. Eur J Clin Invest 1991;21:225.
348b. Meguro K, Fujita H, Ishida N, et al. Molecular defects of uroporphyrinogen decarboxylase in a patient with mild hepatoerythropoietic porphyria. J Invest Dermatol 1994;102:681.
348c. de Verneuil H, Bourgeois F, de Rooij F, et al. Characterization of a new mutation (R292G) and a detection at the human uroporphyrinogen decarboxylase locus in two patients with hepatoerythropoietic porphyria. Hum Genet 1992;89:548.
349. Brodie MJ, Thompson GG, Moore MR, Beattie AD, Goldberg A. Hereditary coproporphyria: demonstration of the abnormalities in haem biosynthesis in peripheral blood. Q J Med 1977;46:229.
350. Roberts DT, Brodie MJ, Moore MR, et al. Hereditary coproporphyria presenting with photosensitivity induced by the contraceptive pill. Br J Dermatol 1977;96:549.
351. Hunter JAA, Khan SA, Hope E, et al. Hereditary coproporphyria: photosensitivity, jaundice and neuropsychiatric manifestations associated with pregnancy. Br J Dermatol 1971;84:301.
352. Andrews J, Erdjument H, Nicholson DC. Hereditary coproporphyria: incidence in a large English family. J Med Genet 1984;21:341.
353. Houston AB, Brodie MJ, et al. Hereditary coproporphyria and epilepsy. Arch Dis Child 1977;52:646.
354. Carlson RE, Dolphin D, Bernstein M. Copper coproporphyrin: excretion in familial coproporphyria. Clin Chem 1978;24:2009.
355. Nordmann Y, Grandchamp B, et al. Harderoporphyria: a variant hereditary coproporphyria. J Clin Invest 1983;72:1139.
356. Eales L, Day RS, et al. The clinical and biochemical features of variegate porphyria: an analysis of 300 cases studied at Groote Schuur Hospital, Cape Town. Int J Biochem 1980;12:837.
357. Mustajoki P. Variegate porphyria: twelve years' experience in Finland. Q J Med 1980;194:191.
358. Poh-Fitzpatrick MB. A plasma porphyrin fluorescence marker for variegate porphyria. J Am Acad Dermatol 1983;8:115.
359. Mustajoki P, Heinonen J. General anesthesia in "inducible" porphyria. Anesthesiology 1980;53:15.
360. Mustajoki P, Vuoristo M, Reunala T. Celiac disease or dermatitis herpetiformis in three patients with porphyria. Dig Dis Sci 1981;26: 618.
361. Hughes GS, Davis L. Variegate porphyria and heavy metal poisoning from ingestion of "moonshine." South Med J 1983;76:1027.
362. Folwer CJ, Ward JM. Porphyria variegata provoked by contraceptive pill. Br Med J 1975.663.
363. Handa F, Kumar K, Kumar R. A case of variegate porphyria in an Indian. Br J Dermatol 1975;92:347.
364. Quiroz-Kendall E, Wilson FA, King LE. Acute variegate porphyria following a Scarsdale gourmet diet. J Am Acad Dermatol 1983;8:46.
365. Perloth MG, Tschudy DP, et al. The effect of diet in variegate porphyria. Metabolism 1968;17:571.
366. Meissner PN, Day RS, Moore MR, et al. Protoporphyrinogen oxidase and porphobilinogen deaminase in variegate porphyria. Eur J Clin Invest 1986;16:257.
367. Siepker L, Kramer S. Protoporphyrin accumulation by mitogen stimulated lymphocytes and protoporphyrinogen oxidase activity in patients with porphyria variegata and erythropoietic porphyria: evidence for a deficiency of protoporphyrinogen oxidase and ferrochelatase in both diseases. Br J Haematol 1985;60:65.
368. Kordac V, Deybach JC, Martasek P, et al. Homozygous variegate porphyria. Lancet 1984.851.
369. Murphy GM, Hawk JLM, Magnus IA, et al. Homozygous variegate porphyria: two similar cases in unrelated families. J R Soc Med 1986;79: 361.
370. Poh-Fitzpatrick MB. A plasma porphyrin fluorescence marker for variegate porphyria. Arch Dermatol 1980;116:543.
371. Rimington C, Lockwood WH, Belcher RV. The excretion of porphyrin-peptide conjugates in porphyria variegata. Clin Sci 1968;35:211.
372. Eales L. The effects of canthaxanthrin on the photocutaneous manifestations of porphyrias. S Afr Med J 1978;54:1050.
373. DeLeo VA, Poh-Fitzpatrick MB, Mathews-Roth MM, Harber LC. Erythropoietic protoporphyria: 10 years experience. Am J Med 1976;60:8.
374. Mooney B, Tennant F. Operating theatre lights as hazard in photosensitive patients. Br Med J 1983;287:1028.
375. Magnus IA, Jarrett A, Prankert TAJ, Rimington C. Erythropoietic protoporphyria: a new porphyria syndrome with solar urticaria due to protoporphyrinaemia. Lancet 1961;2:448.
376. Sandberg S, Talstad I, Hovding G, Bejelland N. Light-induced release of protoporphyrin, but not of zinc protoporphyrin, from erythrocytes in a patient with greatly elevated erythropoietic protoporphyria. Blood 1983;62:846.
377. Gigli I, Schothorst AA, Soter NA, Pathak MA. Erythropoietic protoporphyria: photoactivation of the complement system. J Clin Invest 1980;66:517.
378. Lim HW, Perex HD, Goldstein IM, Gigli I. Complement-derived chemotactic activity is generated in human serum containing uroporphyrin after irradiation with 405 nm light. J Clin Invest 1981;67:1072.
379. Clark KGA, Nicholson DC. Erythrocyte protoporphyrin and iron uptake in erythropoietic protoporphyria. Clin Sci 1971;41:363.
380. Porter S. Congenital erythropoietic protoporphyria II. Blood 1963;22: 532.
381. Scholnick P, Marver HS, Schmid R. Erythropoietic protoporphyria: evidence for multiple sites of excess protoporphyrin formation. J Clin Invest 1971;50:203.
382. Nicholson DC, Cowger ML, Kalivas J, et al. Isotopic studies of the erythropoietic and hepatic components of congenital Porphyria and "Erythropoietic" Protoporphyria. Clin Sci 1973;44:135.
383. Scott AJ, Ansford AJ, Webster BH, Stringer HCW. Erythropoietic protoporphyria with features of a sideroblastic anaemia terminating in liver failure. Am J Med 1973;54:251.
384. Deybach JC, Da Silva V, Paquier Y, Nordmann Y. Ferrochelatase in human erythropoietic protoporphyria: the first case of a homozygous form of the enzyme deficiency. In: Nordmann Y, ed. Porphyrins and porphyrias. Colloque INSERM. London, John Libbey Eurotext, 1986: 163.
385. Piomelli S, Lamola AA, Poh-Fitzpatrick MB, Seaman C, Harber LC. Erythropoietic protoporphyria and lead intoxication: the molecular basis for difference in cutaneous photosensitivity. I. Different rates of disappearance of protoporphyrin from the erythrocytes, both in vivo and in vitro. J Clin Invest 1975;56:1519.
386. Pimstone NR, Webber BL, Blekkenhorst GH, Eales L. The hepatic lesion in protoporphyria (PP): preliminary studies on haem metabolism, liver structure and ultrastructure. Ann Clin Res 1976;8:122.
387. Cripps DJ, MacEachern WN. Hepatic and erythropoietic protoporphyria. Arch Pathol 1971;91:497.
388. Bloomer JR, Pierach CA. Effect of hematin administration to patients with protoporphyria and liver disease. Hepatology 1982;2:817.
389. Poh-Fitzpatrick MB, Palmer RH. Elevated plasma triglyceride levels are associated with human protoporphyria. J Lab Clin Med 1984;104: 257.
389a. Nakahashi Y, Fujita H, Taketani S, Ishida N, Kappas A, Sassa S. Proc Natl Acad Sci USA 1992;89:281.
389b. Lamoril J, Boulechfar S, de Verneuil H, Grandchamp B, Nordmann Y, Deybach JC. Biochem Biophys Res Commun 1991;181:594.
389c. Went LN, Klasen EC. Ann Hum Genet 1984;48:105.
389d. Norris PG, Nunn AV, Hawk JL, Cox TM. J Invest Dermatol 1990;95: 260.
390. Mathews-Roth MM, Pathak MA, Fitzpatrick TB, et al. B-carotene as an oral photoprotective agent in erythropoietic protoporphyria. JAMA 1974;228:1004.
391. Krook G, Haeger-Aronsen B. B-carotene in the treatment of Erythropoietic protoporphyria. Acta Derm Venereol 1982;100(Suppl):125.
392. Granick JL, Sassa S, Kappas A. Some biochemical and clinical aspects

of lead intoxication. In: Bodansky O, Latner AL, eds. Advances in clinical chemistry. New York, Academic Press, 1978:287.
393. Campbell AM, Williams ER. Chronic lead intoxication mimicking motor neuron disease. Br Med J 1968;4:582.
394. Lampert PW, Schochet SS Jr. Demyelination and remyelination in lead neuropathy: electromicrographic studies. J Neuropathol Exp Neurol 1968;27:527.
395. Livesley B, Sissons CE. Chronic lead intoxication mimicking motor neuron disease. Br Med J 1968;4:387.
396. Benson P. Lead poisoning in children. Dev Med Child Neurol 1965;7:569.
397. Perlstein MA, Attala R. Neurologic sequelae of plumbism in children. Clin Pediatr 1966;5:292.
398. Sassa S, Granick JL, Granick S, Kappas A, Levere RD. Studies in lead poisoning. I. Microanalysis of erythrocyte protoporphyrin levels by spectrophotometry in the detection of chronic lead intoxication in the subclinical range. Biochem Med 1973;8:135.
399. Committee on Biologic Effects of Atmospheric Pollutants. Lead, airborne lead in perspective. Washington, DC, National Academy of Sciences, 1972:5.
400. Grandjean P. Widening perspectives of lead toxicity: a review of health effects of lead exposure in adults. Environ Res 1978;17:303.
401. Moore MR. Hematological effects of lead. Sci Total Environ 1988;71:419.
402. Murozumi M, Chow TJ, Patterson C. Chemical concentrations of pollutant lead aerosols, terrestrial dusts, and sea salts in Greenland and Antarctic snow strata. Geochim Cosmochim Acta 1969;33:1247.
403. Caprio RJ, Margulis HL, Joselow MM. Lead absorption in children and its relationship to urban traffic densities. Arch Environ Health 1974;28:195.
404. Kehoe RA. Normal metabolism of lead. Arch Environ Health 1964;8:232.
405. Thompson JA. Balance between intake and output lead in normal individuals. Br J Ind Med 1971;28:189.
406. Alexander FW, Delves HT, Clayton BE. The uptake and excretion by children on lead and other contaminants. In: Proceedings of an International Symposium on the Environmental Health Aspects of Lead, Luxembourg, May 1973:319.
407. Kehoe RA. Metabolism of lead under abnormal conditions. Arch Environ Health 1964;8:235.
408. Committee on Toxicology of the National Research Council. Recommendations for the prevention of lead poisoning in children. Washington, DC, National Academy of Sciences, 1976:37.
409. Maes J, Gerber GB. Increased ALA dehydratase activity and spleen weight in lead-intoxicated rats: a consequence of increased blood cell destruction. Experientia 1978;34:381.
410. Fujita H, Orii Y, Sano S. Evidence of increased synthesis of δ-aminolevulinic acid dehydratase in experimental lead-poisoned rats. Biochim Biophys Acta 1981;678:39.
411. Fujita H, Sato K, Sano S. Increase in the amount of erythrocyte δ-aminolevulinic acid dehydratase in workers with moderate lead exposure. Int Arch Occup Environ Health 1982;50:287.
412. Jensen WN, Moreno G. Les ribosomes et les ponctuations basophiles des erythrocytes dans l'intoxication par le plomb. C R Acad Sci 1964;258:3596.
413. Wada O, Takeo K, Yano Y, et al. δ-Aminolevulinic acid dehydratase in low level lead exposure. Arch Environ Health 1976;31:211.
414. Piomelli S, Seaman C, Kapoor S. Lead-induced abnormalities of porphyrin metabolism: the relationship with iron deficiency. Ann NY Acad Sci 1987;514:278.
415. Lamola AA, Yamane T. Zinc protoporphyrin in the erythrocytes of patients with lead intoxication and iron deficiency anemia. Science 1974;186:936.
416. Vanderkooi JM, Landsberg R. In vivo synthesis of iron-free cytochrome c during lead intoxication. FEBS Lett 1977;73:254.
417. San Martin de Viale LC, De Calmanovici RW, et al. Studies on porphyrin biosynthesis in lead-intoxicated rabbits. Clin Chim Acta 1976;69:375.
418. Goyer RA, Leonard DL, Moore JF, et al. Lead dosage and the role of the intranuclear inclusion body: an experimental study. Arch Environ Health 1970;20:705.
419. Goyer RA. Intracellular sites of toxic metals. Neurotoxicology 1983;4:147.
420. Holtzman D, Hsu JS. Early effects of inorganic lead on immature rat brain mitochondrial respiration. Pediatr Res 1976;10:70.
421. Minakami S, Suzuki C, Saito T, et al. Studies on erythrocyte glycolysis. I. Determination of the glycolytic intermediates in human erythrocytes. J Biochem (Tokyo) 1965;58:543.
422. Valentine WN, Fink K, Paglia DE, et al. Hereditary hemolytic anemia with human erythrocyte pyrimidine 5′-nucleotidase deficiency. J Clin Invest 1974;54:866.
423. Paglia DE, Valentine WN, Dahlgren JG. Effects of low-level lead exposure on pyrimidine 5′-nucleotidase and other erythrocyte enzymes: possible role of pyrimidine 5′-nucleotidase in the pathogenesis of lead-induced anemia. J Clin Invest 1975;56:1164.
424. Angle CR, Stohs SJ, McIntire MS, et al. Lead-induced accumulation of erythrocyte pyrimidine nucleotides in the rabbit. Toxicol Appl Pharmacol 1980;54:161.
425. Torrance JD, Mills W, Kilroe-Smith TA, et al. Erythrocyte pyrimidine 5′-nucleotidase activity as a sensitive indicator of lead exposure. S Afr Med J 1985;67:850.
426. Swanson MS, Angle CR, Stohs SJ. Effect of lead chelation therapy with EDTA in children on erythrocyte pyrimidine 5′-nucleotidase and with cytidine triphosphate levels. Int J Clin Pharmacol Toxicol 1982;20:497.
427. Valentine WN, Tanaka KR, Paglia DE. Hemolytic anemia and erythrocyte enzymopathies. Ann Intern Med 1985;103:245.
428. Aub JC, Minot AS, Fairhall LT, Reznikoff P. Recent investigations of absorption and excretion of lead in organism. JAMA 1924;83:588.
429. Aub JC, Fairhall LT, Minot AS, Reznikoff P. Lead poisoning. Medicine 1925;4:1.
430. Hoogeveen JY. In: Maniloff J, Coleman JR, Miller MW, eds. Effects of metals on cells, subcellular elements, and macromolecules. Springfield, IL, Charles C Thomas, 1990:207.
431. Joyce CRB, Moore H, Weatherall M. Effects of lead, mercury and gold on potassium turnover of rabbit blood cells. Br J Pharmacol 1954;9:463.
432. Hasan J, Hernberg S, Metsala P, Vihko V. Enhanced potassium loss in blood cells from men exposed to lead. Arch Environ Health 1967;14:309.
433. Galzigna L, Corsi GC, Saia B, Rizzoli AA. Inhibitory effect of triethyl lead on serum cholinesterase in vitro. Clin Chim Acta 1969;26:391.
434. Stankovic M, Mokranjac M. International Congress on Occupational Health, 14th Madrid International Congress Series 62. Amsterdam, Excerpta Medica Foundation II, 1963:831.
435. Castellino N, Aloj S. Intracellular distribution of lead in the liver and kidney of the rat. Br J Ind Med 1969;26:139.
436. Barltrop D, Smith A. Lead binding to human haemoglobin. Experientia 1971;27:92.
437. Hernberg S, Nurminen M, Hasan J. Nonrandom shortening of red cell survival times in men exposed to lead. Environ Res 1967;1:247.
438. Lachant NA, Tomoda A, Tanaka KR. Inhibition of the pentose phosphate shunt by 2,3,-diphosphoglycerate in erythrocyte pyruvate kinase deficiency. Blood 1984;63:518.
439. Williams H, Schulze WH, Rothchild HB, et al. Lead poisoning from the burning of battery casings. JAMA 1933;100:1485.
440. Gillet JA. An outbreak of lead poisoning in the Canklow district of Rotherham. Lancet 1955;1:1118.
441. Harris RW, Elsea WR. Ceramic glaze as a source of lead poisoning. JAMA 1967;202:344.
442. Klein M, Namer R, Harpur E, et al. Earthenware containers as a source of fatal lead poisoning: case study and public-health considerations. N Engl J Med 1970;283:669.
443. Fischbein A, Wallace J, Anderson KE, et al. Lead poisoning in an art conservator. JAMA 1982;247:2007.
444. Landrigan PJ, Tanblyn PB, Nelson M, et al. Lead exposure in stained glass workers. Am J Ind Med 1981;1:177.
445. Anderson KE, Fischbein A, Kestenbaum D, Sassa S, Alvares AP, Kappas A. Plumbism from airborne lead in a firing range: an unusual exposure to a toxic heavy metal. Am J Med 1977;63:306.
446. Chisolm JJ. The use of chelating agents in the treatment of acute and chronic lead intoxication in childhood. J Pediatr 1968;73:1.
447. Selander S, Cramer K, Hallberg L. Studies in lead poisoning: oral therapy with penicillamine: relationship between lead in blood and other laboratory tests. Br J Ind Med 1966;23:282.
448. Rosenberg DW, Kappas A. Comparative ability of exogenously administered metals to alter tissue levels and urinary output of copper and zinc. Pharmacology 1989;38:159.
449. Putnam FW. The plasma proteins: structure, function, and genetic control, vol 2. New York, Academic Press, 1975:1.
450. Kino K, Tsunoo H, Higa Y. Hemoglobin-haptoglobin receptor in rat liver plasma membrane. J Biol Chem 1980;255:9616.
451. Hinton RH, Dobrota M, Mullock BM. Haptoglobin-mediated transfer of hemoglobin from serum into bile. FEBS Lett 1980;112:247.
452. Eaton JW, Brandt P, Mahoney JR, et al. Haptoglobin: a natural bacteriostat. Science 1982;215:691.
453. Kurosky A, Barnett DR, Lee T, et al. Covalent structure of human haptoglobin: a serine protease homolog. Proc Natl Acad Sci USA 1980;77:3388.
454. Hanley JM, Haugen TH, Heath EC. Biosynthesis and processing of rat haptoglobin. J Biol Chem 1983;258:7858.
455. Kurosky A, Kim H-H, Touchstone B. Comparative sequence analysis of the N-terminal region of rat, rabbit and dog haptoglobin β-chains. Comp Biochem Physiol [B] 1976;55:453.
456. Haugen TH, Hanley JM, Heath EC. Haptoglobin: a novel mode of biosynthesis of a liver secretory glycoprotein. J Biol Chem 1981;256:1055.
457. Black JA, Dixon GH. Amino acid sequence of chains of human haptoglobins. Nature 1968;218:736.
458. Faulstick DA, Lowenstein J, Yiengst MJ. Clearance kinetics of haptoglobin-hemoglobin complex in the human. Blood 1962;20:65.
459. Gabrieli ER, Pyzikiewicz T. Plasma hemoglobin clearance: a clinical study. J Reticuloendothel Soc 1966;3:163.

460. Laurell CB. Purification and properties of different haptoglobins. Clin Chim Acta 1959;4:79.
461. Nagel RL, Gibson QH. Kinetics and mechanism of complex formation between hemoglobin and haptoglobin. J Biol Chem 1967;242:3428.
462. Nagel RL, Gibson QH. The binding of hemoglobin to haptoglobin and its relation to subunit dissociation of hemoglobin. J Biol Chem 1971;246:69.
463. Peacock AC, Pastewka JV, Reed RA, et al. Haptoglobin–hemoglobin interaction: stoichiometry. Biochemistry 1970;9:2275.
464. Hwang PK, Greer J. Identification of residues involved in the binding of hemoglobin α chains to haptoglobin. J Biol Chem 1979;254:2265.
465. Hwang PK, Greer J. Interaction between hemoglobin subunits in the hemoglobin. J Biol Chem 1980;255:3038.
466. Valette I, Waks M, Wejamn JC, et al. Haptoglobin heavy and light chains: structural properties, reassembly, and formation of mini complex with hemoglobin. J Biol Chem 1981;256:672.
467. Bernini LF, Borri-Voltattorni C. Studies on the structure of human haptoglobins. I. Spontaneous refolding after extensive reduction and dissociation. Biochim Biophys Acta 1970;200:203.
468. Smithies O. Zone electrophoresis in starch gels: group variations in the serum proteins of normal human adults. Biochem J 1955;61:629.
469. Smithies O, Walker NF. Genetic control of some serum proteins in normal humans. Nature 1955;176:1265.
470. Smithies O, Walker NF. Notation for serum protein groups and the genes controlling their inheritance. Nature 1956;178:694.
471. Harris H. The principles of human biochemical genetics. New York, Elsevier, 1971:67.
472. Terano Y. Haptoglobin. Nihon Rinsho 1985;43:116.
473. Smithies O, Connell GE. Biochemical aspects of the inherited variations in human serum haptoglobins and transferrins. In: Wolstenholme GE, O'Connor CM, eds. Ciba Foundation Symposium on Biochemistry of Human Genetics. London, Churchill, Livingstone, 1959.
474. Connell GE, Dixon GH, Smithies O. Subdivision of the three common haptoglobin types based on hidden differences. Nature 1962;193:505.
475. Smithies O, Connell GE, Dixon GH. Inheritance of haptoglobin subtypes. Am J Hum Genet 1962;14:14.
476. Smithies O, Connell GE, Dixon GH. Gene action in the human haptoglobins. I. Dissociation into constituent polypeptide chains. J Mol Biol 1966;21:213.
477. Bowman BH, Kurosky A. Haptoglobin: the evolutionary product of duplication, unequal crossing over, and point mutation. In: Harris H, Hirschhorn K, eds. Advances in human genetics, vol 12. New York, Plenum, 1982:189.
478. Raugei G, Bensi G, Colantuori V, et al. Sequence of human haptoglobin cDNA: Evidence that the α and β subunits are coded by the same mRNA. Nucleic Acids Res 1983;11:5811.
479. Maeda N, Smithies O. The evolution of multigene families: human haptoglobin genes. Annu Rev Genet 1986;20:81.
480. Bowman BH, Kurosky A. Haptoglobin: The evolutionary product of duplication, unequal crossing over, and point mutation. Adv Hum Genet 1982;12:189.
481. Gitlin D, Biasucci A. Development of γG, γA, γM, βIC/βIA C1 esterase, hemopexin, haptoglobin, fibrinogen, plasminogen, α1-antitrypsin, orosomucoid, β-lipoprotein, α2-macroglobulin and prealbumin in human conceptus. J Clin Invest 1969;48:1433.
482. Ferris TC, Easterling RE, Nelson KJ, Budd RE. Determination of serum-hemoglobin binding capacity and haptoglobin type by acrylamide gel electrophoresis. Am J Clin Pathol 1966;46:385.
483. Shinton NK, Richardson RW, Williams JDF. Diagnostic value of serum haptoglobins. J Clin Pathol 1965;18:114.
484. Nyman M. Serum haptoglobin: Methodological and clinical studies. Scand J Clin Lab Invest 1959;39(Suppl):11.
485. Allison AC, Blumberg BS, Rees W. Haptoglobin types in British, Spanish Basque and Nigerian African populations. Nature 1958;181: 824.
486. Blumberg BS. Clinical significance of serum haptoglobins. In: Sunderman FW, Sunderman FW Jr, eds. Hemoglobin: its precursors and metabolites. Philadelphia, JB Lippincott, 1964:318.
487. Blumberg BS, Gentile Z. Haptoglobins and transferrins in two tropical populations. Nature 1961;189:897.
488. Mehta SR, Jensen WR. Haptoglobins in haemoglobinopathy: a genetic and clinical study. Br J Haematol 1960;6:250.
489. Blumberg BS, Murray RF, Allison AC, Barnicot NA. Serum protein polymorphisms in Greek populations. Ann Hum Genet 1964;28:189.
490. Barnicot NA, Garlick JP, Roberts DF. Haptoglobin and transferrin inheritance in northern Nigerians. Ann Hum Genet 1960;24:171.
491. Coryell MN, Beach EF, Robinson AR, Macy IG, Mack HC. Metabolism of women during the reproductive cycle. XVII. Changes in electrophoretic pattern of plasma proteins throughout the cycle and following delivery. J Clin Invest 1950;29:1559.
492. Pintera J. The biological and clinicopathological aspects of haptoglobin. Semin Hematol 1971;4:12.
493. Allison AC. The genetical and clinical significance of the haptoglobins. Proc R Soc Med 1958;51:641.
494. Swain BK, Talukder G, Sharma A. Genetic variations in serum proteins in relation to diseases. Med Biol 1980;58:246.
495. Baumann H, Held WA, Berger FG. The acute phase response of mouse liver: genetic analysis of the major acute phase reactants. J Biol Chem 1984;259:566.
496. Javid J, Horowitz H. An improved technique for the quantitation of serum haptoglobin. Am J Clin Pathol 1960;34:35.
497. Brandslund I, Svehag SE. RES-saturation with accumulation of hemoglobin-haptoglobin complexes in plasma: a method for simultaneous quantitation of free haptoglobin and hemoglobin-haptoglobin complexes. Adv Exp Med Biol 1982;155:629.
498. Vincent SH, Grady RW, Shaklai N, et al. The influence of heme-binding proteins in heme-catalyzed oxidations. Arch Biochem Biophys 1988;265:539.
499. Beaven GH, Chen SH, d'Albis A, et al. A spectroscopic study of the haemin-human-serum-albumin system. Eur J Biochem 1974;41:539.
500. Zizkovsky V, Havranova M, Storp P, et al. Spectroscopic study of the hemin–human-α-fetoprotein system. Ann NY Acad Sci 1983;417:57.
501. Muller-Eberhard U. Hemopexin. Methods Enzymol 1988;163:536.
502. Hrkal Z, Vodrazka Z, Kalousek I. Transfer of heme from ferrihemoglobin and ferrihemoglobin isolated chains to hemopexin. Eur J Biochem 1974;43:73.
503. Muller-Eberhard U, Nikkila H. Transport of tetrapyrroles by proteins. Semin Hematol 1989;26:86.
504. Lane RS, Rangley DM, Liem HH, et al. Plasma clearance of 125I-labelled haemopexin in normal and haem-loaded rabbits. Br J Haematol 1973;25:533.
505. Wochner RD, Spilberg I, Iio A, et al. Hemopexin metabolism in sickle-cell disease, porphyrias and control subjects: effects of heme injection. N Engl J Med 1974;290:820.
506. Galbraith RA, Sassa S, Kappas A. Heme binding to murine erythroleukemia cells: evidence for a heme receptor. J Biol Chem 1985;260: 12198.
507. London IM, West R, Shemin D, Rittenberg D. On the origin of bile pigment in normal man. J Biol Chem 1950;184:351.
508. Berk PD, Howe RB, Bloomer JR, et al. Studies of bilirubin kinetics in normal adults. J Clin Invest 1969;48:2176.
509. Berk PD, Rodkey FL, Blaschke TF, et al. Comparison of plasma bilirubin turnover and carbon monxide production in man. J Lab Clin Med 1974;83:29.
510. Landaw SA. Carbon monoxide production as a measurement of heme catabolism. In: Goresky CA, Fischer MM, eds. Jaundice. New York, Plenum, 1975:103.
511. Jones EA, Shrager R, Bloomer JR, et al. Quantitative studies of the delivery of hepatic synthesized bilirubin to plasma utilizing δ-aminolevulinic acid 4-^{14}C and bilirubin-^{3}H in man. J Clin Invest 1972;51: 2450.
512. Kirshenbaum G, Shames DM, Schmid R. An expanded model of bilirubin kinetics: effect of feeding, fasting and phenobarbital in Gilbert's syndrome. J Pharmacokinet Biopharm 1976;4:115.
513. Berk PD, Scharschmidt BF, Waggoner JG, et al. The effect of repeated phlebotomy on bilirubin turnover, bilirubin clearance and unconjugated hyperbilirubinemia in the Crigler-Najjar syndrome and the jaundiced Gunn rat: application of computers to experimental design. Clin Sci Mol Med 1976;50:333.
514. Wolkoff AW, Chowdhury JR, Arias IM. Hereditary jaundice and disorders of bilirubin metabolism. In: Stanbury JB, Wyngaarden JB, Fredrickson DS, Goldstein JL, Brown MS, eds. The metabolic basis of inherited disease. New York, McGraw-Hill, 1983:1385.
515. Bissell DM, Hammaker LE. Cytochrome P-450 and the regulation of δ-aminolevulinic acid synthetase in the liver. Arch Biochem Biophys 1976;176:91.
516. Bissell DM, Hammaker LE. Effect of endotoxin on tryptophan pyrrolase and δ-aminolevulinate synthetase: evidence for an endogenous regulatory haem fraction in rat liver. Biochem J 1977;166:301.
517. Farrell GC, Correia MA. Structural and functional reconstitution of hepatic cytochrome P-450 in vivo. Reversal of allylisopropylacetamide-mediated destruction of the hemoprotein by exogenous heme. J Biol Chem 1980;255:10128.
518. Correia MA, Farrell GC, Schmid R, et al. Incorporation of exogenous heme into hepatic cytochrome P-450 in vivo. J Biol Chem 1979;254: 15.
519. Feigelson P, Greengaard O. A microsomal iron-porphyrin activator of rat liver tryptophan pyrrolase. J Biol Chem 1961;236:153.
520. Hayashi N, Kurashima Y, et al. Mechanism of allylisopropylacetamide-induced increase of δ-aminolevulinate synthetase in liver mitochondria. V. Mechanism of regulation by hemin of the level of δ-aminolevulinate synthetase in rat liver mitochondria. Arch Biochem Biophys 1972;148:10.
521. Kappas A, Simionatto CS, Drummond GS, Sassa S, Anderson KE. The liver excretes large amounts of heme into bile when heme oxygenase is inhibited competitively by Sn-protoporphyrin. Proc Natl Acad Sci USA 1985;82:896.
522. Maines MD, Trakshell GM, Kutty RK. Characterization of two constitutive forms of rat liver microsomal heme oxygenase: only one molecular species of the enzyme is inducible. J Biol Chem 1986;261: 411.
523. Cruse I, Maines MD. Evidence suggesting that the two forms of heme oxygenase are products of different genes. J Biol Chem 1988;263:3348.

524. Shibahara S. Regulation of heme oxygenase gene expression. Semin Hematol 1988;25:370.
525. Maines MD. Heme oxygenase: function, multiplicity, regulatory mechanisms, and clinical applications. FASEB J 1988;2:2557.
526. Kikuchi G, Yoshida T. Function and induction of the microsomal heme oxygenase. Mol Cell Biochem 1983;53/54:163.
527. Yoshinaga T, Sassa S, Kappas A. The occurrence of molecular interactions among NADPH-cytochrome c reductase, heme oxygenase, and biliverdin reductase in heme degradation. J Biol Chem 1982;257:7786.
528. Yoshida T, Noguchi M, Kikuchi GJ. Oxygenated from of heme: heme oxygenase complex and requirement for second electron to initiate heme degradation from the oxygenated complex. Biol Chem Hoppe Seyler 1980;255:4418.
529. Yoshida T, Noguchi M, Kikuchi G, et al. Degradation of mesoheme and hydroxymesoheme catalyzed by the heme oxygenase system: involvement of hydroxyheme in the sequence of heme catabolism. J Biochem (Tokyo) 1981;90:125.
530. Yoshida T, Noguchi M, Kikuchi GJ. A new intermediate of heme degradation catalyzed by the heme oxygenase system. Biochem J 1980;88:557.
531. Sjostrand T. The formation of carbon monoxide by in vitro decomposition of haemoglobin in bile pigments. Acta Physiol Scand 1952;26:328.
532. Yoshida T, Noguchi M, Kikuchi GJ. The step of carbon monoxide liberation in the sequence of heme degradation catalyzed by the reconstituted microsomal heme oxygenase system. Seikagaku 1982;257:9345.
533. Noguchi M, Yoshida T, Kikuchi G. Identification of the products of heme degradation catalyzed by the heme oxygenase system as biliverdin IX-α by reversed-phase high-performance liquid chromatography. J Biochem (Tokyo) 1982;91:1479.
534. Frydman RB, Awruch J, Tomaro ML, et al. Concerning the specificity of heme oxygenase: the enzymatic oxidation of synthetic hemins. Biochem Biophys Res Commun 1979;87:928.
535. Docherty JC, Masters BSS, Firneisz GD, et al. Heme oxygenase provides α-specificity to physiological heme degradation. Biochem Biophys Res Commun 1982;105:1005.
536. Gemsa D, Woo CH, Fudenberg HH, Schmid R. Erythrophagocytosis by macrophages: suppression of heme oxygenase by cyclic AMP. J Clin Invest 1973;52:812.
537. Shibahara S, Yoshida T, Kikuchi G. Mechanism of increase of heme oxygenase activity induced by hemin in cultured pig alveolar macrophages. Arch Biochem Biophys 1979;197:607.
538. Sardana MK, Sassa S, Kappas A. Hormonal regulation of heme oxygenase induction in avian hepatocyte culture. Biochem Pharmacol 1985;34:2937.
539. Maines MD, Kappas A. Studies on the mechanism of induction of haem oxygenase by cobalt and other metal ions. Biochem J 1976;154:125.
540. Muller RM, Taguchi H, Shibahara S, et al. Nucleotide sequence and organization of the rat heme oxygenase gene. J Biol Chem 1987;262:6795.
541. Yoshida T, Biro P, Cohen T, et al. Human heme oxygenase cDNA and induction of its mRNA by hemin. Eur J Biochem 1988;171:457.
542. Shibahara S, Muller RM, Taguchi H. Transcriptional control of rat heme oxygenase by heat shock. J Biol Chem 1987;262:12889.
543. Keyse SM, Tyrrell RM. Heme oxygenase is the major 32-kDa stress protein induced in human skin fibroblasts by UVA radiation, hydrogen peroxide, and sodium arsenite. Proc Natl Acad Sci USA 1989;86:99.
544. Mitani K, Fujita H, Sassa S, Kappas A. Heat shock induction of heme oxygenase mRNA in human Hep 3B hepatoma cells. Biochem Biophys Res Commun 1989;165:437.
545. Kappas A, Drummond GS, Simionatto CS, Anderson KE. Control of heme oxygenase and plasma levels of bilirubin by a synthetic heme analogue, tin-protoporphyrin. Hepatology 1984;4:336.
546. Kappas A, Drummond GS, Manola T, Petmezaki S, Valaes T. Sn-protoporphyrin use in the management of hyperbilirubinemia in term newborns with direct Coombs-positive ABO incompatibility. Pediatrics 1988;81:485.
547. Berglund L, Angelin B, Blomstrand R, et al. Sn-protoporphyrin lowers serum bilirubin levels, decreases biliary bilirubin output, enhances biliary heme excretion and potently inhibits hepatic heme oxygenase activity in normal human subjects. Hepatology 1988;8:625.
548. Milleville GS, Levitt MD, Engel RR. Tin protoporphyrin inhibits carbon monoxide production in adult mice. Pediatr Res 1985;19:94.
549. Landaw SA, Sassa S, Drummond GS, Kappas A. Proof that Sn-protoporphyrin inhibits the enzymatic catabolism of heme in vivo. Suppression of ^{14}CO generation from radiolabeled endogenous and exogenous heme sources. J Exp Med 1987;165:1195.
550. Simionatto CS, Anderson KE, Drummond GS, Kappas A. Studies on the mechanism of Sn-protoporphyrin suppression of hyperbilirubinemia: inhibition of heme oxidation and bilirubin production. J Clin Invest 1985;75:513.
551. Kappas A, Drummond GS, Sardana MK. Sn-protoporphyrin rapidly and markedly enhances the heme saturation of hepatic tryptophan pyrrolase: evidence that this synthetic metalloporphyrin increases the functional content of heme in the liver. J Clin Invest 1985;75:302.
552. Landaw SA, Drummond GS, Kappas A. Targeting of heme oxygenase inhibitors to the spleen markedly increases their ability to diminish bilirubin production. Pediatrics 1989;84:1091.
553. Whiting PF, Moscioni AD, Gartner LM. The effect of Tin(IV)-protoporphyrin-IX on bilirubin production and excretion in the rat. Pediatr Res 1987;21:487.
554. Maisels MJ. Neonatal jaundice. Semin Liver Dis 1988;8:148.
555. Ostrow JD. Therapeutic amelioration of jaundice: old and new strategies. Hepatology 1988;8:683.
556. Sassa S. Inhibition of carbon monoxide production by tin-protoporphyrin. J Pediatr Gastroenterol Nutr 1987;6:167.
557. Kappas A, Drummond GS. Control of heme metabolism with synthetic metalloporphyrins. J Clin Invest 1986;77:335.
558. Landaw SA. Kinetic aspects of endogenous carbon monoxide production in experimental animals. Ann NY Acad Sci 1970;174:32.
559. White P. Carbon monoxide production and heme catabolism. Ann NY Acad Sci 1970;174:23.
560. Roy Chowdhury J, Wolkoff AW, Arias IM. Hereditary jaundice and disorders of bilirubin metabolism. In: Scriver CR, Beaudet AL, Sly WS, Valle D, eds. The metabolic basis of inherited disease. New York, McGraw-Hill, 1989.
561. Noguchi M, Yoshida T, Kikuchi G. Purification and properties of biliverdin reductase from pig spleen and rat liver. Seikagaku 1979;86:833.
562. Kutty RK, Maines MD. Purification and characterization of biliverdin reductase from rat liver. J Biol Chem 1981;256:3956.
563. Frydman RB, Tomaro ML, Awruck J, Frydman B. Molecular forms of biliverdin reductase from rat liver with different reduction rates for biliverdin-IX. Biochem Biophys Res Commun 1982;105:752.
564. Frydman RB, Tomaro ML, Awruch J, Frydman B. Interconversion of the molecular forms of biliverdin reductase from rat liver. Biochim Biophys Acta 1983;759:257.
565. Blumenthal SG, Taggart DB, Ikeda RM, et al. Conjugated and unconjugated bilirubins in bile of humans and rhesus monkeys: structural identity of adult human and rhesus monkey bilirubins. Biochem J 1977;167:535.
566. Blumenthal SG, Taggart DB, Rasmussen RD, et al. Conjugated and unconjugated bilirubins in humans and rhesus monkeys: structural identity of bilirubins from biles and meconium of newborn humans and rhesus monkeys. Biochem J 1979;179:537.
567. McDonagh AF. Bile pigments, bilatrienes and 5,15-biladienes. In: The porphyrins, vol 26. New York, Academic Press, 1979.
568. Fog J, Jellum E. Structure of bilirubin. Nature 1963;198:88.
569. Kuenzle CC, Weibel MH, Pelloni RR. A proposed novel structure for the metal chelates of bilirubin. Biochem J 1973;130:1147.
570. Kuenzle CC, Weibel MH, Pelloni RR. The reaction of bilirubin with diazomethane. Biochem J 1973;133:357.
571. Kuenzle CC. Bilirubin conjugates of human bile: nuclear magnetic resonance, infrared and optical spectra of model compounds. Biochem J 1970;119:395.
572. Cu A, Bellah GG, Lightner DA. On the fluorescence of bilirubin. J Am Chem Soc 1975;97:2579.
573. McDonagh AF, Palma LA. Mechanism of bilirubin photodegradation: role of singlet oxygen. In: Berk PD, Berlin NI, eds. Chemistry and physiology of bile pigments (DHEW publication no. [NIH] 77-1100). Washington, DC, US Government Printing Office, 1977:81.
574. McDonagh AF. Phototherapy of neonatal jaundice. Biochem Soc Trans 1976;4:219.
575. McDonagh AF. Light effects on transport and excretion of bilirubin in newborns. Ann NY Acad Sci 1985;453:65.
576. Ennever JF. Phototherapy for neonatal jaundice. Photochem Photobiol 1988;47:871.
577. Schneider J, Sassa S, Kappas A. Metabolism of estradiol in liver cell culture: Differential responses of C-2 and C-16 oxidations to drugs and other chemicals that induce selective species of cytochrome P-450. J Clin Invest 1983;72:1420.
578. Mustafa MG, Cowger ML, King TW. Effects of bilirubin on mitochondrial reaction. J Biol Chem 1969;244:6403.
579. Diamond I, Schmid R. Oxidative phosphorylation in experimental bilirubin encephalopathy. Science 1967;155:1288.
580. Menken M, Waggoner JG, Berlin NI. The influence of bilirubin on oxidative phosphorylation and related reactions in brain and liver mitochondria: effects of protein binding. J Neurochem 1966;13:1241.
581. Amit Y, Chan G, Fedunec S, et al. Bilirubin toxicity in a neuroblastoma cell line N-115. I. Effects on Na^+K^+ ATPase, [^{3}H]-thymidine uptake, L-[^{35}S]-methionine incorporation, and mitochondrial function. Pediatr Res 1989;25:364.
582. Amit Y, Posnansky MJ, Schiff D. Bilirubin toxicity in a neuroblastoma cell line N-115. II. Delayed effects and recovery. Pediatr Res 1989;25:369.
583. Odell GB. Influence of binding on the toxicity of bilirubin. Ann NY Acad Sci 1973;226:225.
584. Stocker R, Yamamoto Y, McDonagh AF, et al. Bilirubin is an antioxidant of possible physiological significance. Science 1987;235:1043.
585. Stocker R, Ames BN. Potential role of conjugated bilirubin and copper

in the metabolism of lipid peroxides in bile. Proc Natl Acad Sci USA 1987;84:8130.
586. Stevens B, Small RD Jr. The photoperoxidation of unsaturated organic molecules-XV: O21 δ g quenching by bilirubin and biliverdin. Photochem Photobiol 1976;23:33.
587. Kaul R, Kaul HK, Murti CRK. An alternatate pathway for bilirubin catabolism. FEBS Lett 1980;111:240.
588. Brodersen R, Bartels P. Enzymatic oxidation of bilirubin. Eur J Biochem 1969;10:468.
589. Jacobsen J, Fedders O. Determination of non–albumin-bound bilirubin in human serum. Scand J Clin Lab Invest 1970;26:237.
590. Stocker R, Glazer AN, Ames BN. Antioxidant activity of albumin-bound bilirubin. Proc Natl Acad Sci USA 1987;84:5918.
591. Silverman WA, Anderson DH, Bland DA, Crozier DN. A difference in mortality rate and incidence of kernicterus among premature infants allotted to prophylactic antibacterial regimens. Pediatrics 1956;18:614.
592. Odell GB. The dissociation of bilirubin from albumin and its clinical implications. J Pediatr 1959;55:268.
593. Bloomer JR, Berk PD, Bergalla J, Berlin NI. Influence of albumin on the hepatic uptake of unconjugated bilirubin. Clin Sci Mol Med 1973;45:505.
594. Weisiger RA. Dissociation from albumin: a potential rate-limiting step in the clearance of substances by the liver. Proc Natl Acad Sci USA 1985;82:1563.
595. Blankaert N, D'Argenio G. Presence of bilirubins linked covalently to albumin in serum of patients with cholestasis. Gastroenterology 1982;82:1222.
596. Weiss JS, Gautam A, Lauff JJ, et al. The clinical importance of a protein-bound fraction of serum bilirubin in patients with hyperbilirubinemia. N Engl J Med 1983;309:147.
597. McDonagh AF, Palma LA, Lauff JJ, Wu T-W. Origin of mammalian biliprotein and rearrangement of bilirubin glucuronides in vivo in the rat. J Clin Invest 1984;74:763.
598. Gollan JL, Dallinger KJC, Billing BH. Excretion of conjugated bilirubin in the isolated perfused rat kidney. Clin Sci Mol Med 1978;54:381.
599. Kaplowitz N. Physiological significance of glutathione S-transferases. Am J Physiol 1980;239:G439.
600. Bhargava MM, Arias IM. Ligandin. Trends Biochem Sci 1981;6:131.
601. Levi AJ, Gatmaitan Z, Arias IM. Two hepatic cytosolic protein fractions, Y and Z, and their possible role in the hepatic uptake of bilirubin, sulfbromophthlein and other anions. J Clin Invest 1969;48:2156.
602. Ketterer B, Ross-Mansell P, Whitehead JK. The isolation of carcinogen-binding protein from livers of rats given 4-dimethylaminoazobenzene. Biochem J 1967;103:316.
603. Morley KS, Litwack G. Isolation and properties of cortisol metabolite binding proteins of rat liver cytosol. Biochemistry 1969;8:4813.
604. Habig WH, Pabst MJ, Fleischner G, et al. The identity of glutathione S-transferase B with ligandin, a major binding protein of liver. Proc Natl Acad Sci USA 1974;10:3879.
605. Bhargava MM, Listowsky J, Arias IM. Studies on subunit structure and evidence that ligandin is a heterodimer. J Biol Chem 1978;253:4116.
606. Wolkoff AW, Goresky CA, Sellin J, et al. Role of ligandin in transfer of bilirubin from plasma into liver. Am J Physiol 1978;236:E638.
607. Gollan JL, Schmid R. Bilirubin update: formation, transport, and metabolism. Prog Liver Dis 1982;7:261.
608. Kamisaka K, Maezawa H, Inagaki T, Okano K. A low molecular weight binding protein for organic anions (Z protein) from human hepatic cytosol: purification and quantitation. Hepatology 1981;1:221.
609. Fleischner G, Kamisaka K, Habig W, et al. Human ligandin: characterization and quantitation. (Abstract) Gastroenterology 1975;69:821.
610. Jones EA, Bloomer JR, Berk PD, et al. Quantitation of hepatic bilirubin synthesis in man. In: Berk PD, Berlin NI, eds. The chemistry and physiology of bile pigments, (DHEW publication no. [NIH] 77-1100). Washington, DC, US Government Printing Office, 1977:189.
611. Anwer MS, Gronwall R. A compartmental model for bilirubin kinetics in isolated perfused rat liver. Can J Physiol Pharmacol 1976;54:277.
612. Farrell GC, Gollan JL, Schmid R. Efflux of bilirubin into plasma following hepatic degradation of exogenous heme. Proc Soc Exp Biol Med 1980;163:504.
613. Gollan JL, McDonagh AF, Schmid R. Biliverdin IX: a new probe of hepatic bilirubin metabolism. (Abstract) Gastroenterology 1977;72:1186.
614. Gollan JL, Hammaker L, Licko V, Schmid R. Bilirubin kinetics in intact rats and isolated perfused liver: evidence for hepatic deconjugation of bilirubin glucuronides. J Clin Invest 1981;67:1016.
615. Carson ER, Jones EA. Use of kinetic analysis and mathematical modeling in the study of metabolic pathways in vivo: applications to hepatic organic anion metabolism. N Engl J Med 1979;300:1016.
616. Heirwegh KPM, van Hees GP, Leroy P, et al. Heterogeneity of bile pigment conjugates as revealed by chromatography of their ethyl anthranilate azopigments. Biochem J 1970;120:877.
617. Fevery J, van Damme B, Michiels R, et al. Bilirubin conjugates in bile of man and rat in the normal state and in liver disease. J Clin Invest 1972;51:2482.
618. Fevery J, van de Vijver M, Michiels R, Heirwegh KP. Comparison in different species of biliary bilirubin-IXα conjugates with the activities of hepatic and renal bilirubin-IXα-uridine diphosphate glycosyltransferases. Biochem J 1977;164:737.
619. Dutton GJ, Burchell B. Newer aspects of glucuronidation. Prog Drug Metab 1977;2:1.
620. Tephly T, Green M, Puig J, Irshaid Y. Endogenous substrates for UDP-glucuronosyltransferases. Xenobiotica 1988;26:975.
621. Whitmer DL, Russell PE, Ziurys JC, et al. Hepatic microsomal glucuronidation of bilirubin is modulated by the lipid microenvironment of membrane-bound substrate. J Biol Chem 1986;261:7170.
622. Tomlison GA, Yaffe SJ. The formation of bilirubin and p-nitrophenol glucuronides by rabbit liver. Biochem J 1964;99:507.
623. Halac E, Reff A. Studies on bilirubin UDP-glucuronyl transferase. Biochim Biophys Acta 1967;139:328.
624. Bock KW, Josling D, Lilenblum WM, et al. Purification of rat liver glucuronyl transferase: separation of two enzymic forms inducible with 3-methylcholanthrene or phenobarbital. Eur J Biochem 1977;98:19.
625. Bock KW, Kittel J, Josting D. Purification of rat liver UDP glucuronyl transferase: separation of two enzyme forms with different substrate specificity and differential inducibility. In: Aitio A, ed. Conjugation reactions in drug biotransformation. Amsterdam, Elsevier/North-Holland, 1978:357.
626. Nakata D, Zakim D, Vassey DA. Defective function of a microsomal UDP-glucuronyl transferase in Gunn rats. Proc Natl Acad Sci USA 1976;73:289.
627. Van den Bergh AAH, Muller P. Uber eine direkte und eine indirekte Diazoreaktion aus Bilirubin. Biochem Z 1916;77:90.
628. Hutchinson DW, Johnson B, Knell AJ. The reaction between bilirubin and aromatic diazo compounds. Biochem J 1972;127:907.
629. Heirwegh KPM, Fevery JB, Meuwissen JATP, et al. Recent advances in the separation and analysis of diazo-positive bile pigments. Methods Biochem Anal 1974;22:205.
630. Blankaert N, Kabra PM, Farina FA, et al. Measurement of bilirubin and its mono- and di-conjugates in human serum by alkaline methanalysis and high performance liquid chromatography. J Lab Clin Med 1980;96:198.
631. Onishi S, Itho S, Kawade N, et al. An accurate and sensitive analysis by high pressure liquid chromatography of conjugated and unconjugated bilirubin IX and in various biological fluids. Biochem J 1980;185:281.
632. Roy Chowdhury J, Arias IM. Dismutation of bilirubin. Methods Enzymol 1981;77:192.
633. Lauff JJ, Kasper ME, Ambros RT. Quantitative liquid chromatography estimation of bilirubin species in pathological serum. Clin Chem 1983;29:800.
634. Dappen GM, Smedberg MW, Wu TW, et al. A diazo-based dry film for determination of total bilirubin in serum. Clin Chem 1983;29:37.
635. Brown AK, Eisinger J, Blumberg WE, et al. A rapid fluorometric method for determining bilirubin levels and binding in the blood of neonates: comparison with other methods. Pediatrics 1980;65:762.
636. Jackson MR, Burchell B. The full length coding sequence of rat liver androsterone UDP-glucuronyl transferase cDNA and comparisons with other members of the gene family. Nucleic Acids Res 1986;14:779.
637. Iyanagi T, Haniu M, Sogawa K, et al. Cloning and characterization of cDNA encoding 3-methylcholanthrene-inducible rat mRNA for UDP-glucuronyl transferase. J Biol Chem 1986;261:15607.
638. MacKenzie PI. Rat liver UDP-glucuronyl transferase: sequence and expression of a cDNA encoding a phenobarbital-inducible form. J Biol Chem 1986;261:6119.
639. Jansen PLM, Roy Chowdhury J, Fischberg EB, Arias IM. Enzymatic conversion of bilirubin monoglucuronide to diglucuronide by rat liver plasma membranes. J Biol Chem 1977;252:2710.
640. Roy Chowdhury J, Fischberg EB, Daniller A, et al. Hepatic conversion of bilirubin monoglucuronide to bilirubin diglucuronide in uridine diphosphate glucuronyltransferase deficient in man and rat by bilirubin glucuronyl transferase. J Clin Invest 1978;62:191.
641. Gartner LM, Lane DL, Cornelius CE. Bilirubin transport by liver in adult Macaca Mulatta. Am J Physiol 1971;220:1528.
642. Upson DW, Gronwall RR, Cornelius CE. Maximal hepatic excretion of bilirubin in sheep. Proc Soc Exp Biol Med 1970;134:9.
643. Klaassen CD, Plaa GL. Studies on the mechanism of phenobarbital-enhanced sulfobromophthalein disappearance. J Pharmacol Exp Ther 1968;161:361.
644. Berk PD, Martin JF, Blaschke TF, Scharschmidt BF, Plotz PH. NIH conference: unconjugated hyperbilirubinemia: physiologic evaluation and experimental approaches to therapy. Ann Intern Med 1975;82:552.
645. Brodersen R, Herman LS. Intestinal reabsorption of unconjugated bilirubin: a possible contributing factor in neonatal jaundice. Lancet 1963;1:1242.
646. Schmid R, McDonagh AF. The enzymatic formation of bilirubin. Ann NY Acad Sci 1975;244:533.
647. Watson CJ. The urobilinoids: Milestones in their history and some recent developments. In: Berk PD, Berlin NI, eds. The chemistry and physiology of bile pigments (USDHEW publication no. [NIH] 77-1100). Washington, DC, US Government Printing Office, 1977:469.
648. Stoll MS, Lim CK, Gray CH. Chemical variants of the urobilins. In:

Berk PD, Berlin NI, eds. The chemistry and physiology of bile pigments (USDEW publication [NIH]). Washington, DC, US Government Printing Office, 1977:483.
649. Levy M, Lester R, Levinsky NG. Renal excretion of urobilinogen in the dog. J Clin Invest 1968;47:2117.
650. Watson CJ. Recent studies of the urobilin problem. J Clin Pathol 1963;16:1.
651. Davidson LT, Merritt KK, Weech AA. Hyperbilirubinemia in the newborn. Am J Dis Child 1941;61:958.
652. Hardy JB, Peeples MO. Serum bilirubin levels in newborn infants: distributions and associations with neurological abnormalities during the first year of life. Johns Hopkins Med J 1971;128:265.
653. Lang FC, Stroder J, Alao M. Die Korrelation zwischen Hyperbilirubinaemie und Korpergewicht bei reifen Neugeborenen. Z Kinderh 1968;104:161.
654. Gartner LM, Lee KS, Vaisman S, et al. Development of bilirubin transport and metabolism in the newborn rhesus monkey. J Pediatr 1977;90:513.
655. Pearson H. Life-span of the fetal red blood cell. J Pediatr 1967;70:166.
656. Vest MF, Grieder AR. Erythrocyte survival in newborn infants as measured by chromium 51 and its relation to postnatal serum bilirubin level. J Pediatr 1961;54:194.
657. Thaler MM. Effect of phenobarbital on hepatic transport and excretion of ^{131}I-rose bengal in children with cholestasis. Pediatr Res 1972;6:100.
658. Maines MD, Kappas A. Study of the developmental pattern of heme catabolism in liver and the effects of cobalt on cytochrome P-450 and the rate of heme oxidation during the neonatal period. J Exp Med 1975;141:1400.
659. Maisels MJ, Pathak A, Nelson NM, et al. Endogenous production of carbon monoxide in normal and erythroblastotic newborn infants. J Clin Invest 1971;50:1.
660. Bartoletti AL, Stevenson DK, Ostrander CR, Johnson JD. Pulmonary excretion of carbon monoxide in the human infant as an index of bilirubin production. I. Effects of gestational and postnatal age and some common neonatal abnormalities. J Pediatr 1979;94:952.
661. Brown AK, Zuelzer WW. Studies on the neonatal development of the glucuronide conjugating system. J Clin Invest 1958;37:332.
662. Lathe GH, Walker MJ. The synthesis of bilirubin glucuronide in animal and human liver. Biochem J 1958;70:705.
663. Onishi S, Kawade N, Itoh S, Isobe K, Sugiyama S. Postnatal development of uridine diphosphate glucuronyl transferase activity towards bilirubin and 2-aminophenol in human liver. Biochem J 1979;184:705.
664. Gartner LM. Disorders of bilrubin metabolism. In: Nathan DG, Oski FA, eds. Hematologic disorders of the fetus and newborn. Philadelphia, WB Saunders, 1981:86.
665. Brown WR, Boon WH. Ethnic group differences in plasma bilirubin levels of full-term healthy Singapore newborns. Pediatrics 1965;36:745.
666. Horiguchi T, Bauer C. Ethnic differences in neonatal jaundice: comparison of Japanese and caucasian newborn infants. Am J Obstet Gynecol 1975;121:71.
667. Lu T-C, Wei H, Blackwell RQ. Increased incidence of severe hyperbilirubinemia among newborn Chinese infants with G-6-PD deficiency. Pediatrics 1966;37:994.
668. Ose T, Tsuruhara T. Follow-up study of exchanges transfusion for hyperbilirubinemia in infants in Japan. Pediatrics 1976;40:196.
669. Sutow WW, Moloney WC, Margoles C. Kernicterus in Japanese infants. I. Clinical and serological data from 25 patients. Pediatrics 1956;17:349.
670. Valaes T, Petmezaki S, Doxiadis SA. Effect on neonatal hyperbilirubinemia of phenobarbital during pregnancy or after birth: practical value of the treatment in a population with high risk of unexplained severe neonatal jaundice. Birth Defects 1970;6:46.
671. Lee K-S, Gartner LM. Management of unconjugated hyperbilirubinemia in the newborn. Semin Liver Dis 1983;3:52.
672. Levine RL. Neonatal jaundice. Acta Paediatr Scand 1988;77:177.
673. Crigler JF, Najjar VA. Congenital familial nonhemolytic jaundice with kernicterus. Pediatrics 1952;10:169.
674. Blumenschein SD, Kallen RJ, Storey B, et al. Familial nonhemolytic jaundice with late onset of neurological damage. Pediatrics 1968;42:786.
675. Berk PD, Martin JF, Blaschke TF, et al. Unconjugated hyperbilirubinemia. Physiologic evaluation and experimental approaches to therapy. Ann Intern Med 1975;82:552.
676. Blaschke TF, Berk PD, Scharschmidt BF, et al. Crigler-Najjar syndrome: an unusual course with development of neurologic damage at age eighteen. Pediatr Res 1974;8:573.
677. Arias IM, Gartner LM, Cohen M, et al. Chronic non-hemolytic unconjugated hyperbilirubinemia with glucuronyl transferase deficiency: clinical, biochemical, pharmacologic, and genetic evidence for heterogeneity. Am J Med 1969;47:395.
678. Axelrod J, Schmid R, Hammaker L. A biochemical lesion in congenital, non-obstructive, non-hemolytic jaundice. Nature 1957;180:1426.
679. Jansen PLM, Elferink RPJO. Hereditary hyperbilirubinemias: a molecular and mechanistic approach. Semin Liver Dis 1988;8:168.
680. Berk PD, Blaschke TF, Scharschmidt BF, et al. A new approach to quantitation of the various sources of bilirubin in man. J Lab Clin Med 1976;87:767.
681. Odievre M. Case of congenital nonobstructive nonhaemolytic jaundice: successful long-term therapy at home. Arch Dis Child 1978;53:81.
682. Schmid R, Hammaker L. Metabolism and disposition of C^{14} bilirubin in congenital nonhemolytic jaundice. J Clin Invest 1963;42:1720.
683. Kaufman SS, Wood RP, Shaw BW, et al. Orthotopic liver transplantation for type I Crigler-Najjar syndrome. Hepatology 1986;6:1259.
684. Rubaltelli FF, Guerrini P, Reddi E, Jori G. Tin-protoporphyrin in the management of Crigler-Najjar Disease. Pediatrics 1989;84:728.
684a. Galbraith RA, Drummond GS, Kappas A. Suppression of bilirubin production in the Crigler-Najjar Type I syndrome: studies with the heme oxygenase inhibitor, Sn-mesoporphyrin. Pediatrics 1992;89:175.
685. Arias IM. Chronic unconjugated hyperbilirubinemia without overt signs of hemolysis in adolescents and adults. J Clin Invest 1962;41:2233.
686. Berk PD, Wolkoff AW, Berlin NI. Inborn errors of bilirubin metabolism. Med Clin North Am 1975;59:803.
687. Arias IM, Gartner LM, Furman M, Wolfson S. Studies of the effect of several drugs on hepatic glucuronide formation in newborn rats and humans. Ann NY Acad Sci 1963;111:274.
688. Black M, Fevery J, Parker D, et al. Effect of phenobarbitone on plasma ^{14}C bilirubin clearance in patients with unconjugated hyperbilirubinemia. Clin Sci Mol Med 1974;46:1.
689. Gordon EF, Shaffer EA, Sass-Kortsaka A. Bilirubin secretion and conjugation in the Crigler-Najjar syndrome type II. Gastroenterology 1976;70:761.
690. Fevery J, Blankaert N, Heirwegh KPM, Preaux A-M, Berthelot P. Unconjugated bilirubin and an increased proportion of bilirubin monoconjugates in the bile of patients with Gilbert's syndrome and Crigler-Najjar syndrome. J Clin Invest 1977;60:970.
691. Gilbert A, Lereboullet P. La cholemie simple familiale. Sem Med 1901;21:241.
692. Watson KJ, Gollan JL. Gilbert's syndrome. Baillieres Clin Gastroenterol 1989;3:337.
693. Powell LW, Hemingway E, Billing BH, et al. Idiopathic unconjugated hyperbilirubinemia (Gilbert's syndrome): a study of 42 families. N Engl J Med 1967;277:1108.
694. Thompson RPH. Genetic transmission of Gilbert's syndrome. In: Okolicsanyi L, ed. Familial hyperbilirubinemia. New York, John Wiley & Sons, 1981:91.
695. Powell LW, Hemingway EH, Billing BH, Sherlock S. Idiopathic unconjugated hyperbilirubinemia (Gilbert's syndrome): a study of 42 families. N Engl J Med 1967;217:1108.
696. Owens D, Evans J. Population studies on Gilbert's syndrome. J Med Genet 1975;12:152.
697. Foulk WT, Butt HR, Owen CA, Whitcomb FF. Constitutional hepatic dysfunction (Gilbert's disease): its natural history and related syndrome. Medicine 1959;38:25.
698. Black M, Billing BH. Hepatic bilirubin UDP-glucuronyltransferase activity in liver disease and Gilbert's syndrome. N Engl J Med 1969;280:1266.
699. Felsher BF, Craig JR, Carpio N. Hepatic bilirubin glucuronidation in Gilbert's syndrome. J Lab Clin Med 1973;81:829.
700. Berk PD, Bloomer JR, Howe RB, et al. Constitutional hepatic dysfunction (Gilbert's syndrome): a new definition based on kinetic studies with unconjugated radiobilirubin. Am J Med 1970;49:296.
701. Okolicsanyi L, Ghidini O, Orlando R, Naccarato R, Manitto P. An evaluation of bilirubin kinetics with respect to the diagnosis of Gilbert's syndrome. Clin Sci Mol Med 1978;54:539.
702. Vierling JM, Berk PD, Hofmann AF, Martin JF, Wolkoff AW, Scharschmidt BF. Normal fasting-state levels of serum cholyl-conjugated bile acids in Gilbert's syndrome: an aid to the diagnosis. Hepatology 1982;2:340.
703. Okolicsanyi L, Orlando R, Venuti M, et al. A modeling study of the effect of fasting on bilirubin kinetics in Gilbert's syndrome. Am J Physiol 1981;240:266.
704. Fromke VL, Miller D. Constitutional hepatic dysfunction (CHD: Gilbert's disease): a review with special reference to a characteristic increase and prolongation of the hyperbilirubinemic response to nicotinic acid. Medicine 1972;51:451.
705. Blaschke TF, Berk PD, Rodkey FL, Scharschmidt BF, Collision HA, Waggoner JG. Drugs and the liver. I. Effects of glutethimide and phenobarbitone on hepatic bilirubin clearance, plasma bilirubin turnover and carbon monoxide production in man. Biochem Pharmacol 1974;23:2795.
706. Arthur LJH, Beva BR, Holton JB. Neonatal hyperbilirubinemia and breast feeding. Dev Med Child Neurol 1966;8:279.
707. Arias IM, Gartner LM, Seifter S, Furman M. Prolonged neonatal unconjugated hyperbilirubinemia associated with breast feeding and a steroid, pregnane-3-α, 20-β-diol, in maternal milk that inhibits glucuronide formation in vitro. J Clin Invest 1964;43:2037.
708. Holton JB, Lathe HGH. Inhibitors of bilirubin conjugation in newborn infant serum and male urine. Clin Sci 1963;25:499.
709. Adlard BP, Lathe GH. Breast milk jaundice: effect of 3-α, 20-β-pregnanediol on bilirubin conjugation by human liver. Arch Dis Child 1970;45:186.

710. Maisels MJ, Gifford K. Normal serum bilirubin levels in the newborn and the effect of breast-feeding. Pediatrics 1986;78:839.
711. Arias IM, Wolfson S, Lucey JF, McKay RJ Jr. Transient familial neonatal hyperbilirubinemia. J Clin Invest 1965;44:1442.
712. Woolley MM, Felsher BF, Asch J, et al. Jaundice, hypertrophic pyrolic stenosis and hepatic glucuronyl transferase. J Pediatr Surg 1974;9:359.
713. Lokietz H, Dowben RM, Hsia DY-H. Studies on the effect of novobiocin on glucuronyl transferase. Pediatrics 1963;32:47.
714. Akerren Y. Prolonged jaundice in the newborn associated with congenital myxedema. Acta Paediatr 1954;43:411.
715. Taylor PM, Wolfson JH, Bright NH, et al. Hyperbilirubinemia in infants of diabetic mothers. Biol Neonate 1963;5:289.
716. Van Praagh R. Diagnosis of kernicterus in the neonatal period. Pediatrics 1961;28:870.
717. Perlstein MA. The late clinical syndrome of post-icteric encephalopathy. Pediatr Clin North Am 1960;7:665.
718. Shapiro SM, Hecox KE. Brain stem auditory evoked potentials in jaundiced Gunn rats. Ann Otol Rhinol Laryngol 1989;98:308.
719. Hyman CB, Keaster J, Hanson V, et al. CNS abnormalities after neonatal hemolytic disease or hyperbilirubinemia. Arch Dis Child 1969;117:395.
720. Johnson L, Boggs TR. Bilirubin-dependent brain damage. Incidence and indications for treatment. In: Odell GB et al, eds. Phototherapy in the newborn: an overview. Washington, DC, National Academy of Science, 1974:122.
721. Johnston WH, Angara V, Baumal R, et al. Erythroblastosis fetalis and hyperbilirubinemia: a five-year follow-up with neurological, psychological and audiological evaluation. Pediatrics 1967;39:88.
722. Scheidt PC, Mellits ED, Hardy JB, et al. Toxicity to bilirubin in neonates: infant development during first year in relation to maximal neonatal serum bilirubin concentration. J Pediatr 1977;91:292.
723. Corwin MJ, Golub HL. Spectral analysis of a cry is abnormal in infants who have moderate hyperbilirubinemia. Pediatr Res 1984;18:102A.
724. van de Bor M, van Aeben-van der Aa TM, Verloove-Vanhorick SP, et al. Hyperbilirubinemia in preterm infants and neurodevelopmental outcome at 2 years of age: results of a national collaborative survey. Pediatrics 1989;83:915.
725. Rose AL, Johnson A. Bilirubin encephalopathy: neurological and histochemical studies in the Gunn rat model. Neurology 1972;22:420.
726. Odell GB. Studies in kernicterus: the protein binding of albumin. J Clin Invest 1959;38:823.
727. Odell GB. The distribution and toxicity of bilirubin. Pediatrics 1970;46:16.
728. Odell GB. Neonatal jaundice. In: Popper H, Schaffner F, eds. Progress in liver disease, vol 5. New York, Grune & Stratton, 1977:457.
729. Brodersen R. Prevention of kernicterus, based on recent progress in bilirubin chemistry. Acta Paediatr Scand 1977;66:625.
730. Levine RL, Fredericks WR, Rapoport SI. Entry of bilirubin into the brain due to opening of the blood-brain barrier. Pediatrics 1982;69:255.
731. Hansen TW, Bratlid D. Bilirubin and brain toxicity. Acta Paediatr Scand 1986;75:513.
732. Lee C, Oh W, Stonestreet BS, Cashore WJ. Permeability of the blood brain barrier of 125I-albumin–bound bilirubin in newborn piglets. Pediatr Res 1989;25:452.
733. Lucey JF, Ferreiro M, Hewitt J. Prevention of hyperbilirubinemia of prematurity by phototherapy. Pediatrics 1968;41:1047.
734. Hodgman JE, Schwartz A. Phototherapy and hyperbilirubinemia of the premature. Am J Dis Child 1973;119:473.
735. Lucey JF. Phototherapy of jaundice. In: Bergsma D et al, eds. Bilirubin metabolism of the newborn. New York, National Foundation for Birth Defects, Original Article Series, 1970:63.
736. Ostrow JD. Bilirubin and jaundice. In: Becker FF, ed. The liver, part A. New York, Marcel Dekker, 1975:303.
737. Ostrow JD, Berry CS, Knodell RG, et al. Effect of phototherapy on bilirubin excretion in man and the rat. Birth Defects 1976;12:81.
738. Ostrow JD, Berry CS. Effect of phototherapy on hepatic excretory function in normal and Gunn rats. Gastroenterology 1971;62:168.
739. McDonagh AF, Agati G, Fusi F, Pratesi R. First observation of the wavelength-dependent photoproduction of the 4E, 15Z configurational isomer of bilirubin bound to human serum albumin. Soc Photo-Opt Instr Engin 1987;701(ECOOSA '86):367.
740. Lightner DA, McDonagh AF. Molecular mechanisms of phototherapy for neonatal jaundice. Acc Chem Res 1984;17:417.
741. Cremer RJ, Perryman PW, Richards DW. Influences of light on the hyperbilirubinemia of infants. Lancet 1958;1:1094.
742. Lightner DA, Wooldridge TA, McDonagh AF. Photobilirubin: an early bilirubin photoproduct detected by absorbance difference spectroscopy. Proc Natl Acad Sci USA 1979;76:29.
743. Lightner DA, Wooldridge TA, McDonagh AF. Configuration isomerization of bilirubin and mechanism of jaundice phototherapy. Biochem Biophys Res Commun 1979;86:235.
744. Stoll MS, Zenone FA, Ostrow JD, et al. Preparation and properties of bilirubin photoisomers. Biochem J 1979;183:139.
745. Cohen AN, Ostrow JD. New concepts in phototherapy: photoisomerization of bilirubin IXα and potential toxic effects of light. Pediatrics 1980;65:740.
746. Sisson TRC, Voge TP. Phototherapy of hyperbilirubinemia. In: Regan JD, Parrish JA, eds. The science of photomedicine. New York, Plenum, 1982:477.
747. National Institutes of Child Health and Human Development. Randomized controlled trial of phototherapy for neonatal hyperbilirubinemia. Pediatrics 1985;75(Suppl):385.
748. Vecchi C, Donzelli GP, Migliorini MG, Sbrana G. Green light in phototherapy. Pediatr Res 1983;17:461.
749. Anderson RR, Parrish JA. The optics of human skin. J Invest Dermatol 1981;77:13.
750. Donzelli GP. Green light phototherapy: towards new trends. Photochem Photobiol 1989;126.
751. Tan KL. Comparison of the effectiveness of phototherapy and exchange transfusion in the management of nonhemolytic neonatal hyperbilirubinemia. J Pediatr 1975;87:609.
752. McDonagh AF, Lightner DA. Phototherapy and the photobiology of bilirubin. Semin Liver Dis 1988;8:272.
753. Allen FH Jr, Diamond LK. Erythroblastosis fetalis including exchange transfusion technique. Boston, Little, Brown, 1958.
754. Allen FH Jr, Diamond LK, Vaughan VC III. Erythroblastosis fetalis. VI. Prevention of kernicterus. Am J Dis Child 1950;80:779.
755. Diamond LK. Replacement transfusion as a treatment for erythroblastosis. Pediatrics 1948;2:520.
756. Hsia DY-Y, Allen FH, Gellis SS, et al. Erythroblastosis fetalis: studies of serum bilirubin in relation to kernicterus. N Engl J Med 1952;247:668.
757. Allen FH Jr, Diamond LK. Erythroblastosis fetalis including exchange transfusion technique. N Engl J Med 1957;257:659.
758. Valaes T. Bilirubin distribution and dynamics of bilirubin removal by exchange transfusion. Acta Paediatr 1963;149(Suppl):1.
759. Baumgart S, Kim HC. Exchange transfusion in the neonate. In: Stockman JA III, Pochedly C, eds. Developmental neonatal hematology. New York, Raven Press, 1988:199.
760. Keenan WJ, Novak KK, Sutherland JM, Bryla DA, Fetterly KL. Morbidity and mortality associated with exchange transfusion. Pediatrics 1985;75:417.
761. Odell GB. Administration of albumin in the management of hyperbilirubinemia by exchange transfusion. Pediatrics 1962;30:613.
762. Waters WJ, Porter E. Indications for exchange transfusion based upon the role of albumin in the treatment of hemolytic disease of the newborn. Pediatrics 1964;33:749.
763. Oski FA, Naiman JL. Hematologic problems in the newborn. Philadelphia, WB Saunders, 1972.
764. Boggs TR Jr, Westphal MD Jr. Mortality of exchange transfusion. Pediatrics 1960;26:745.
765. Culley P, Powell J, Waterhouse J, et al. Sequelae of jaundice. Br Med J 1970;3:383.
766. Rubin RA, Balow B, Fisch RO. Neonatal serum bilirubin levels related to cognitive development at ages 4 through 7 years. J Pediatr 1979;94:601.
767. Gartner IM, Snyder RN, Chabon RS, et al. High incidence in premature infants with low serum bilirubin concentrations. Pediatrics 1970;45:906.
768. Keenan WJ, Perlstein PH, Light IJ, et al. Kernicterus in small sick premature infants receiving phototherapy. Pediatrics 1972;49:652.
769. Odell GB, Storey GN, Rosenberg LA, et al. Studies in kernicterus. III. The saturation of serum proteins with bilirubin during neonatal life and its relationship to brain damage at five years. J Pediatr 1970;76:12.
770. Stern L, Denton RL. Kernicterus in small premature infants. Pediatrics 1965;35:483.
771. Mollison PL, Cutbush M. Haemolytic disease of the newborn. In: Gardiner D, ed. Recent advances in pediatrics. New York, P Blakiston & Sons, 1954:110.
772. Lucey JF. Bilirubin and brain damage: a real mess. Pediatrics 1982;69:381.
773. Watchko JF, Oski FA. Bilirubin 20 mg/dl = vigintiphobia. Pediatrics 1983;71:660.
774. Phipps RH. Hemolytic anemias: hemolytic diseases of the newborn (erythroblastosis fetalis). In: Rudolph AM, Hoffman JIE, eds. Pediatrics. Norwalk, CT, Appleton-Century-Crofts, 1982:1057.
775. Liley AW. Intrauterine transfusion of fetus in hemolytic disease. Br Med J 1963;2:1107.
776. Catz C, Yaffe SJ. Barbiturate enhancement of bilirubin conjugation and excretion in young and adult animals. Pediatr Res 1968;2:361.
777. Flodgaard H, Brodersen R. Bilirubin glucuronide formation in developing guinea pig liver. Scand J Clin Lab Invest 1967;19:149.
778. Catz C, Yaffe SJ. Pharmacological modification of bilirubin modification in the newborn. Am J Dis Child 1962;104:516.
779. Halac E Jr, Sicignano C. Re-evaluation of influence of sex, age, pregnancy, and phenobarbital on the activity of UDP-glucuronyl transferase in rat liver. J Lab Clin Med 1969;73:677.
780. Yaffe SJ, Levy G, Matsuzawa T, et al. Enhancement of glucuronide-conjugating capacity in a hyperbilirubinemic infant due to apparent enzyme induction by phenobarbital. N Engl J Med 1966;275:1461.
781. Zaidenberg P, Orrenius S, Ernster L. Increase in levels of glucuronylating enzymes and associated rise in activities of microsomal oxi-

dative enzymes upon phenobarbital administration the rat. J Cell Biol 1967;32:528.
782. Valaes T. Bilirubin metabolism: review and discussion of inborn errors. Clin Perinatol 1976;3:177.
783. Robinson SH, Yannoni C, Nagasawa S. Bilirubin excretion in rats with normal and impaired bilirubin conjugation. J Clin Invest 1971;50: 2606.
784. Wolkoff AW, Ketley GN, Waggoner JG, et al. Hepatic accumulation and intracellular binding of conjugated bilirubin. J Clin Invest 1978;61: 142.
785. Yeung CY, Field CE. Phenobarbitone therapy in neonatal hyperbilirubinemia. Lancet 1969;2:135.
786. Trolle D. Decrease of total serum-bilirubin concentration in newborn infants after phenobarbitone treatment. Lancet 1968;2:705.
787. Maurer HM, Wolff JA, Finster M, et al. Reduction in concentration of total serum-bilirubin in offspring of women treated with phenobarbitone during pregnancy. Lancet 1968;2:122.
788. Berk PD, Blaschke TF. Effect of glutethimide on the plasma concentration of unconjugated bilirubin. Clin Res 1971;19:347.
789. Burns JJ, Conney AH, Koster R. Stimulatory effect of chronic drug administration on drug-metabolizing enzymes in liver microsomes. Ann NY Acad Sci 1963;104:881.
790. Conney AH. Pharmacological implications of microsomal enzyme induction. Pharmacol Rev 1967;19:317.
791. Conney AH, Schneidman K, Jacobson M, et al. Drug-induced changes in steroid metabolism. Ann NY Acad Sci 1965;123:98.
792. Wilson JT. Phenobarbital in the neonatal period. Pediatrics 1969;43: 324.
793. Diaz J, Schain RJ. Phenobarbital: effects of long-term administration on behavior and brain of artificially reared rats. Science 1978;199:90.
794. Anderson KE, Simionatto CS, Drummond GS, Kappas A. Disposition of tin-protoporphyrin and suppression of hyperbilirubinemia in humans. Clin Pharmacol Ther 1986;39:510.
795. Okolicsanyi L, Orlando R, Venuti M, et al. A modeling study of the effect of fasting on bilirubin kinetics in Gilbert's syndrome. Am J Physiol 1981;240:266.
796. Ohkubo H, Musha H, Okuda K. Studies on nicotinic acid interaction with bilirubin metabolism. Digest Dis Sci 1979;24:700.
797. Seymour CA, Neale G, Peters TJ. Lysosomal changes in liver tissue from patients with Dubin-Johnson-Sprinz syndrome. Clin Sci Mol Med 1977;52:241.
798. Cohen L, Lewis C, Arias IM. Pregnancy, oral contraceptives, and chronic hyperbilirubinemia (Dubin-Johnson syndrome). Gastroenterology 1972;62:1182.
799. Kondo T, Kuchiba K, Ohtsuka Y, et al. Clinical and genetic studies on Dubin-Johnson syndrome in a clustered area in Japan. Jinrui Idengaku Zasshi 1974;18:378.
800. Jansen PLM, Peters WHM, Janssens AR. Clinical value of serum bilirubin subfractionation by high-performance liquid chromatography and conventional methods in patients with primary biliary cirrhosis. J Hepatol 1986;2:485.
801. Schoenfield LJ, McGill DB, Hutton DB, et al. Studies of chronic idiopathic jaundice (Dubin-Johnson syndrome). I. Demonstration of hepatic excretory defect. Gastroenterology 1963;44:101.
802. Kaplowitz N, Javitt N, Kappas A. Coproporphyrin I and 3 excretion in bile and urine. J Clin Invest 1972;51:2895.
803. Cornelius CE, Arias IM, Osburn BI. Hepatic pigmentation with photosensitivity: a syndrome in Corriedale sheep resembling Dubin-Johnson syndrome in man. J Am Vet Med Assoc 1965;146:709.
804. Cornelius CE, Osburn BI, Gronwall RR, Cardinet GH. Dubin-Johnson syndrome in immature sheep. Am J Dig Dis 1968;13:1072.
805. Mia AS, Gronwall RR, Cornelius CE. Unconjugated bilirubin transport in normal and mutant Corriedale sheep with Dubin-Johnson syndrome. Proc Soc Exp Biol Med 1970;135:33.
806. Rotor AB, Manahan L, Florentin A. Familial non-hemolytic jaundice with direct Van den Bergh reaction. Acta Med Philipp 1948;5:37.
807. Wolpert E, Pascasio FM, Wolkoff AW, et al. Abnormal sulfobromophthalein metabolism in Rotor's syndrome and obligate heterozygotes. N Engl J Med 1977;296:1091.
808. Wolkoff AW, Wolpert E, Pascasio FN, et al. Rotor's syndrome, a distinct inheritable pathophysiologic entity. Am J Med 1976;60:173.

Blood: Principles and Practice of Hematology,
edited by Robert I. Handin, Samuel E. Lux, and Thomas P. Stossel.
J.B. Lippincott Company, Philadelphia © 1995.

51

Hemoglobin Synthesis and the Thalassemias

Bernard G. Forget
Howard A. Pearson

HEMOGLOBIN SYNTHESIS

Normal Human Hemoglobins and Their Genes

Many different normal human hemoglobins exist, as well as numerous abnormal hemoglobins. Before precise knowledge of globin gene organization by gene mapping and gene cloning procedures was gained, a general picture of the number and arrangement of the normal human globin genes emerged from the genetic analysis of normal and abnormal hemoglobins and their pattern of inheritance. The number and subunit composition of different normal human hemoglobins (Fig. 51-1) indicated that there must be at least one different globin gene for each of the different globin chains: α, β, γ, δ, ε, and ζ. Evidence then accumulated from the study of hemoglobin variants and the analysis of the biochemical heterogeneity of the chains in fetal hemoglobin (Hb F) that the α- and γ-globin genes were duplicated. Persons were identified whose red blood cells (RBCs) contained more than two structurally different α-globin chains that could be best explained by duplication of the α-globin gene locus, and the characterization of the structurally different $^{G}\gamma$- and $^{A}\gamma$-globin chains of Hb F imposed a requirement for duplication of the γ-globin gene locus.

From the study of the pattern of inheritance of hemoglobin variants from persons carrying both an α-chain and a β-chain variant, it became clear that the α- and β-globin genes must be on different chromosomes or at least widely separated if on the same chromosome; α- and β-chain hemoglobin variants were always observed to segregate independently in offspring of doubly affected parents.[1] Linkage of the various β-like globin genes to one another was established from the study of interesting hemoglobin variants, which contained fused globin chains presumably resulting from nonhomologous crossover among different β-like globin gene loci. The characterization of Hb Lepore,[2] with its $\delta\beta$ fusion chain, established that the δ-globin gene was linked to and located on the 5′ (or N-terminal) side of the β-globin gene, whereas the analysis of Hb Kenya,[3] with its $^{A}\gamma\beta$-fusion chain, provided evidence for linkage of the $^{A}\gamma$ gene, and presumably the $^{G}\gamma$ gene as well, to the 5′ side of the δ- and β-globin genes.

Thus, the general concept of the arrangement of the globin genes that emerged from these various genetic analyses can be represented as illustrated in Figure 51-1. It was also assumed, but unsupported by genetic evidence, that the embryonic α-like (ζ) and β-like (ε) globin genes were likely to be linked to the loci for their adult counterparts.

Chromosomal Localization of Globin Genes

By the use of rodent–human somatic hybrid cells containing only one or a limited number of human chromosomes, Deisseroth and colleagues[4,5] clearly established that the human α- and β-globin genes resided on different chromosomes and that the α genes were located on chromosome 16, whereas the β-like genes were located on chromosome 11. The latter results were obtained by solution hybridization assays of total cellular DNA from the various somatic hybrid cells hybridized to radioactive cDNAs synthesized from α- and β-globin mRNAs by use of the enzyme reverse transcriptase. These results were later confirmed and extended by various groups using the gene mapping procedure of Southern blot analysis with DNA from various hybrid cell lines containing different translocations or deletions of the involved chromosomes.

These studies led to the regional localization of the globin gene loci on their respective chromosomes: the β-globin gene cluster to the short arm of chromosome 11 and the α-globin gene cluster to the short arm of chromosome 16. These chromosomal assignments were further confirmed and refined by in situ hybridization of radioactive cloned globin gene probes to metaphase chromosomes. Thus, the β-globin gene cluster was assigned to 11p15.5 and the α-globin gene cluster to 16p13.3.

Detailed Chromosomal Organization of Human Globin Genes

A precise picture of the chromosomal organization of the α-like and β-like human globin gene clusters, with respect to the number of structural loci and intergene distances, was obtained by the technique of restriction endonuclease mapping using the gel blotting procedure of Southern as well as actual isolation, gene cloning technology, and characterization of large fragments of human DNA containing the various globin genes.[6–8] Sets of overlapping genomic DNA fragments spanning the entire α- and β-globin gene clusters have been obtained by gene cloning, initially in

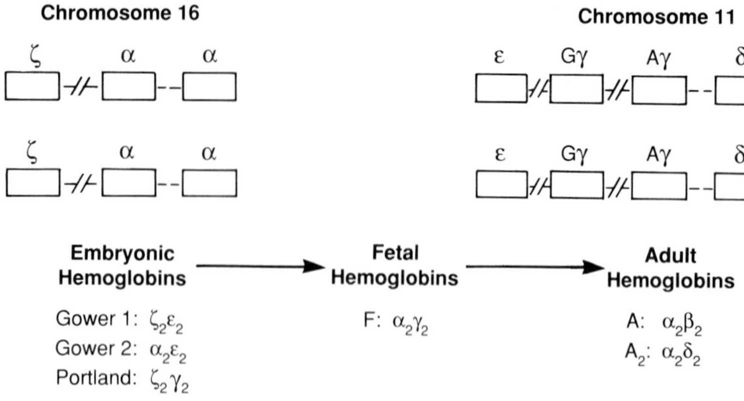

FIGURE 51-1. Model of the human globin gene system based on genetic information available before the actual cloning of the genes. The various hemoglobins expressed at different stages of development are indicated below the model.

bacteriophage λ as well as larger fragments in cosmid vectors. Detailed analysis of these recombinant DNA clones has led to the determination of the gene organization illustrated in Figure 51-2. Some of the results were expected, such as the finding of single δ- and β-globin gene loci and duplication of the α- and γ-globin gene loci. In addition, single loci for the embryonic ζ- and ε-globin chains were found to be linked to the α- and β-globin gene clusters, respectively.

An unexpected finding was the presence in the globin gene clusters of additional gene-like structures with structural homology to the authentic globin genes: one in the β-gene cluster between the γ- and δ-globin genes and three in the α-gene cluster, between the ζ- and authentic α-globin genes. These structures have been called pseudogenes. They are characterized by the presence of one or more mutations that render them incapable of encoding a functional globin chain. These pseudogenes appear to have arisen by gene duplication events within the globin gene clusters followed by mutation and inactivation of the duplicated gene and subsequent accumulation of additional mutations through loss of selective pressure.

Another α-like globin gene has been identified and characterized in the α-globin gene cluster: the θ gene located toward the 3′ or C-terminal side of the duplicated α-globin genes.[9] This gene is evolutionally related to and coexpressed with the α-globin genes.[10,11] mRNA transcripts are only at very low levels (less than 1% of α), and no hemoglobin containing the θ-globin chains has been identified. Furthermore, the predicted structure (translated amino acid sequence) of the θ-globin chain suggests that it is unlikely to function normally as a hemoglobin subunit.[12]

Globin Gene Structure

Intervening Sequences or Introns

The coding region of the globin genes of humans and other animals is interrupted at two positions by considerable stretches of noncoding DNA called intervening sequences or introns.[6–8] In the β-like globin genes, the intervening sequences interrupt the sequence between codons 30 and 31 and between codons 104 and 105; in the α-globin gene family, the intervening sequences interrupt the coding sequence between codons 31 and 32 and between codons 99 and 100 (Fig. 51-3). Although the precise codon position numbers at which the interruption occurs differ between the α- and β-like globin genes, the introns occur at precisely the same position with regard to the regions of the primary structure of the α- and β-globin chains that are homologous and can be aligned if one assumes that the α- and β-globin gene families originally evolved from a single ancestral globin gene. The first intervening sequence (IVS-1) is shorter than the second intervening sequence (IVS-2) in both α- and β-globin genes, but IVS-2 of the human β-globin gene is considerably larger than that of the α-globin gene.

As illustrated in Figure 51-2, the pattern of intron sizes of the ζ-like globin genes is different from that of the other α-like globin genes, whereas the introns in the α and ψα genes are small (fewer than 150 base pairs [bp]), those of the ζ and ψζ gene are considerably larger and, furthermore, IVS-1 is much larger than IVS-2, being 8 to 10 times larger than the IVS-1 of any other globin gene.

The presence of intervening sequences that interrupt the coding sequences of structural genes imposes a requirement for some cellular process to prevent the occurrence of these

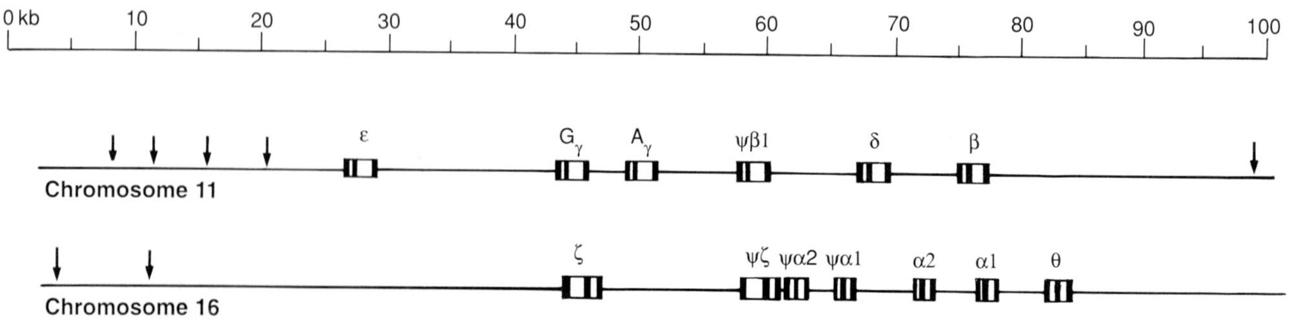

FIGURE 51-2. Structure of the human α- and β-globin gene loci based on information obtained by gene cloning and DNA sequence analysis. The vertical arrows indicate the positions of developmentally stable, erythroid-specific DNase I–hypersensitive sites located in the locus control region (LCR) of the two gene clusters. The fine structure of the genes (exon–intron organization) is shown in Figure 51-3. (After Bunn HF, Forget BG. Hemoglobin: molecular, genetic and clinical aspects. Philadelphia, WB Saunders, 1986)

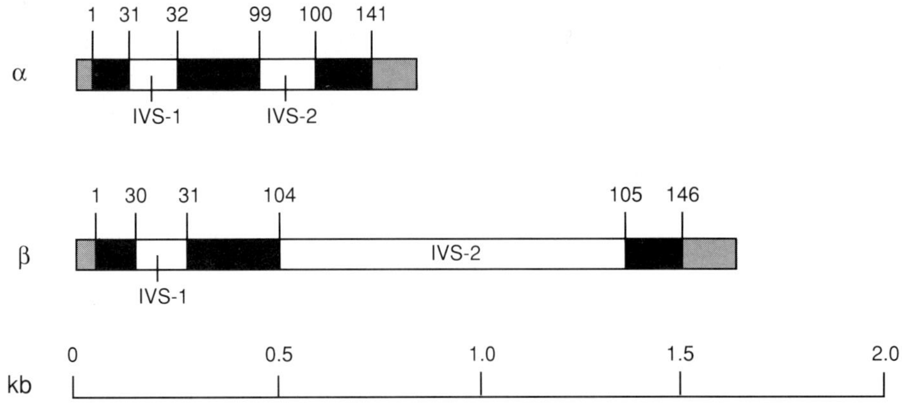

FIGURE 51-3. Fine structure of the human α- and β-globin genes. The black blocks represent the coding regions of the gene; the gray blocks at either end represent the 5′ and 3′ untranslated sequences; IVS-1 and IVS-2 are the intervening sequences (introns) that interrupt the coding sequences of the genes. The numbers above the diagram indicate the amino acid codon positions of the coding sequence. (After Bunn HF, Forget BG. Hemoglobin: molecular, genetic and clinical aspects. Philadelphia, WB Saunders, 1986)

sequences in the mature mRNA. Intervening sequences have been found to be transcribed into globin (and other) precursor mRNA molecules but subsequently excised and the proper ends of the coding sequences religated to yield the mature mRNA. This posttranscriptional processing of mRNA precursors has been termed *splicing* and is illustrated schematically in Figure 51-4.

A crucial prerequisite for the proper splicing of globin (and other) precursor mRNA molecules is the presence of specific nucleotide sequences at the junctions between coding sequences (exons) and intervening sequences (introns). Comparison of these sequences in many different genes has permitted the derivation of two different "consensus" sequences, which are universally found at the 5′ and 3′ ends, respectively, of introns.[13,14] The consensus sequences thus derived are the following:

donor splice site — acceptor splice site

(5′)(C/A) AG <u>GT</u> (A/G) AGT . . . $(T/C)_n$N(C/T)<u>AG</u> G(3′)

▲ ▲

where:

N = any nucleotide

n = a variable number of pyrimidine nucleotides, equal to or greater than 11

The 5′ sequence is sometimes called the donor splice site and the 3′ sequence, the acceptor splice site. The underlined dinucleotides GT and AG, located at the 5′ and 3′ ends, respectively, of the intron, are essentially invariant and are thought to be required for proper splicing: the so-called GT-AG rule. Rare examples have been described where GC instead of GT is found at the donor splice site junction. The importance or significance of these consensus sequences is underscored by the fact that mutations that alter these normal consensus sequences, or mutations that create consensus sequences at new sites in a globin gene, lead to abnormal processing of globin mRNA precursors and constitute the molecular basis for many types of thalassemia.

Conserved Functional Sequences of Mature Globin mRNA

The transcript of the human globin genes that is represented in mature globin mRNA contains additional sequences at both extremities of the mRNA in addition to the information required to encode the globin polypeptide chains. These additional untranslated nucleotides account for about 30% of the total length of globin mRNA. The 3′ (C-terminal) untranslated sequences are two to three times the length of the 5′ (N-terminal) untranslated sequences. The lengths of these sequences in the major human globin mRNAs are illustrated in Figure 51-5. In addition to the nucleotides that are transcribed from the globin gene, the globin mRNA contains additional nucleotides that are added to it within the cell nucleus after transcription: a

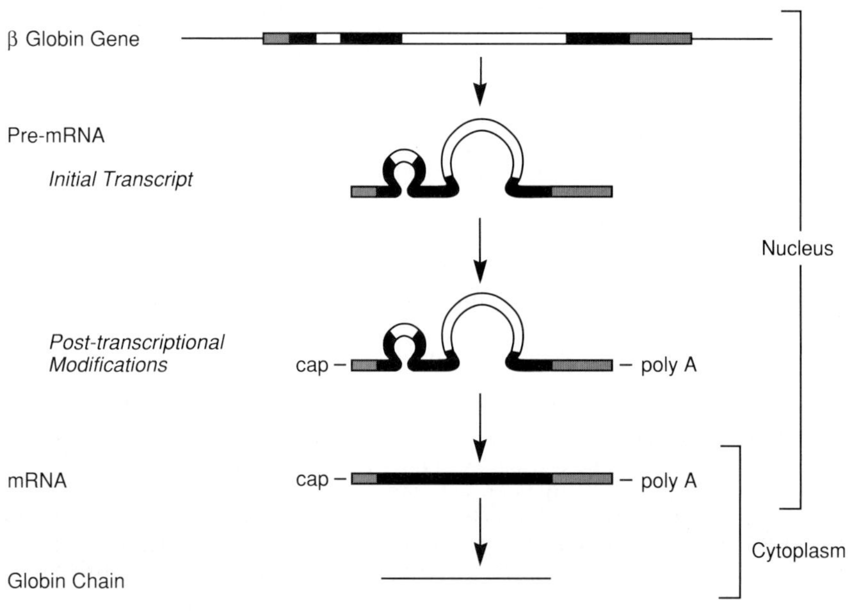

FIGURE 51-4. Schematic representation of the process of β-globin gene expression, including gene transcription, posttranscriptional processing of the mRNA, transport of mRNA from nucleus to cytoplasm, and mRNA translation. (After Bunn HF, Forget BG. Hemoglobin: molecular, genetic and clinical aspects. Philadelphia, WB Saunders, 1986)

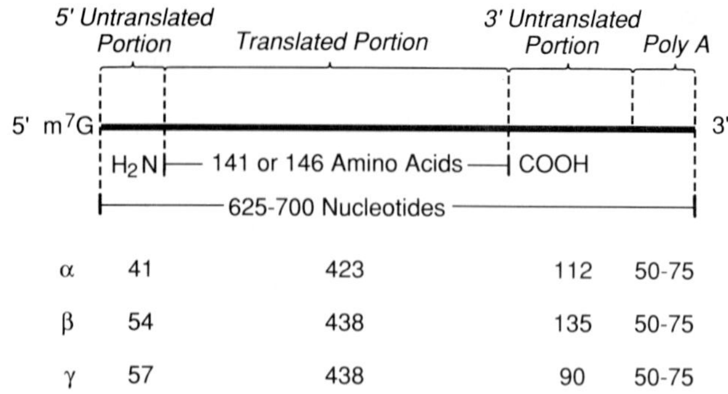

FIGURE 51-5. Diagram of the relative sizes of translated and untranslated regions of the major human globin messenger RNAs. (After Forget BG. Molecular genetics of human hemoglobin synthesis. Ann Intern Med 1979;91:605)

methylated guanylic acid (m^7G) cap structure at the 5′ end of the mRNA and a number of adenylic acid residues forming a poly(A) tail at the 3′ end of the mRNA. The precise functions of these untranslated sequences in globin and other mRNAs are not completely known. The 5′-methylated cap structure appears to be important for the initiation of polypeptide chain synthesis through its interaction with specific initiation factors. The poly(A) tail of mRNAs appears to contribute to the stability of the mRNA.[6–8]

Two general consensus sequences are at or near the extremities of these untranslated sequences and are important for the efficient processing of mRNA transcripts. The cap site in globin (and most eukaryotic) mRNAs is usually located at an A residue that is preceded in genomic DNA by a C. The DNA sequence to either side of the CA is generally rich in pyrimidines. The cap site consensus sequence appears to be important not only for accurate initiation of transcription and 5′ processing of the mRNA but also for serving as a promoter element called the initiator or Inr element,[15] which is capable of influencing both the efficiency and the accuracy of transcription initiation. This is especially true in the case of certain genes that lack a TATA box in their promoters (see the following section). At least one β-thalassemia mutation involves a base substitution in the cap site consensus sequence.

The one common feature of the 3′ noncoding sequence of globin and other mRNAs is the presence of the hexanucleotide AAUAAA (AATAAA in the DNA) about 20 nucleotides from the poly(A) tail.[16,17] It was initially assumed and subsequently demonstrated experimentally that this consensus sequence constitutes a necessary signal for the proper processing and polyadenylation of the 3′ end of mRNA transcripts. Base substitutions in this consensus sequence have also been shown to be responsible for certain types of thalassemia as a result of faulty processing and polyadenylation of globin mRNA transcripts. It appears that the AAUAAA is a signal not only for poly(A) addition but also (perhaps more important) for the proper cleavage, before polyadenylation, of the primary RNA transcripts of globin (and other) genes that normally extend well beyond the site of polyadenylation.[16,17] The nucleotide immediately preceding the site of poly(A) addition in globin and other mRNAs is almost always C, and GC is the most common, although not invariant, dinucleotide at this site.

Translation of globin (and other eukaryotic) mRNAs starts at the initiator codon ATG, which is generally the first ATG encountered in any reading frame of the mature mRNA. The initiator ATG, like ATG codons elsewhere in the mRNA, encodes the amino acid methionine, which is present at the N terminal of all nascent polypeptide chains. During the process of peptide chain elongation, the N-terminal methionine is cleaved from nascent globin chains and is thus absent from the full-length chains. The nature of the first two amino acids encoded immediately after the initiator methionine is important in determining whether the N-terminal methionine is cleaved from a nascent peptide chain. Generally, if the second amino acid is also a methionine or is a charged residue or if the third amino acid is a proline, the N-terminal methionine is retained.[18] A number of human β-globin chain variants in which such amino acid replacements have occurred at codon positions 2 or 3 have retained the initiator methionine at the N terminal of the full-length mutant globin chain.

The sequence surrounding the initiator ATG is important for the efficiency of peptide chain initiation. Comparison of the nucleotide sequence of a large number of eukaryotic mRNAs has revealed the presence of a conserved consensus sequence flanking the initiator ATG, the so-called Kosak consensus sequence: CC(**A/G**)CCATG**G**.[19] The most important features of this consensus sequence are the presence of a purine (A or G) at position −3 and the presence of a G at position +4 (where position +1 is the A of the initiator ATG). These positions are indicated in boldface type. The consensus sequence presumably facilitates efficient binding of the mRNA to ribosomes. One form of α-thalassemia is caused by a base substitution changing the purine to a pyrimidine at position −3 of the consensus sequence. Other α- and β-thalassemia mutations are due to base substitutions in the ATG itself, resulting in a complete block to normal globin chain initiation (see sections on molecular basis of α- and β-thalassemia).

Termination of globin chain synthesis occurs when one of the three possible chain termination codons (UAA, UAG, or UGA) is encountered in the mRNA sequence. Point mutations in the termination codon result in the insertion of a novel amino acid residue at that position and translation of the normally untranslated 3′ portion of the mRNA into an abnormally elongated peptide chain until a new in-phase termination codon is encountered. A number of different termination codon mutations are the cause of hemoglobin variants associated with α-thalassemia (see section on Hb Constant Spring and related variants).

The synthesis of normal globin chains requires that the triplet codons of the mRNA encoding each amino acid of the peptide chain be arrayed in the proper uninterrupted alignment. Nucleotide insertions or deletions other than those in multiples of 3 will lead to a shift in the reading frame (frameshift) of mRNA translation and the synthesis of a novel peptide sequence until a new in-phase termination codon is encountered, which usually occurs within a relatively short distance. The mutant globin chain thus encoded usually accumulates in markedly reduced amounts because either the mutant globin chain itself or its mRNA is unstable, resulting in a thalassemia phenotype. A large number of different forms of α- and β-thalassemia are the result of such frameshift mutations. Point mutations (nonsense mutations) can also change a normal amino acid codon to a chain termination codon, resulting in the synthesis of a truncated, unstable globin chain and a thalassemia phenotype. A number of such nonsense mutations have also been documented as causes of α- and β-thalassemia (see sections on molecular basis of α-and β-thalassemia).

Conserved Sequences in 5′ Flanking DNA of Globin Genes

The DNA flanking the 5′ extremity of the globin genes contains a number of sequences (Fig. 51-6) that are common to all of these genes and are situated at relatively similar

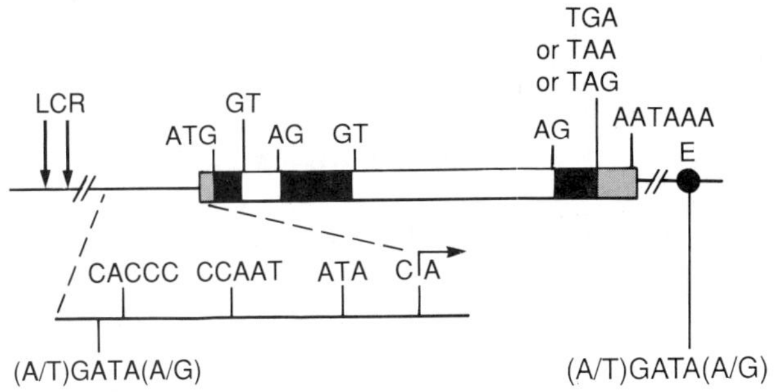

FIGURE 51-6. Model of the structure of a typical globin gene showing specific sequences and *cis*-acting elements that are important for the regulation of gene expression. The same conventions are used as in Figure 51-3. The following elements and consensus sequences are shown: LCR, locus control region; consensus sequences of the promoter, CACCC, CCAAT, ATA; cap site, CA; initiator codon, ATG; consensus dinucleotides at exon–intron junctions, 5′ GT . . . AG 3′; termination codons, TGA, TAA, or TAG; polyadenylation signal, AATAAA; and enhancer element, E. The bottom line shows the consensus binding sequences, for the erythroid-specific factor GATA-1, found within the LCR, promoter, and enhancer.

distances from the site of initiation of transcription of the genes (cap site).[6–8] The first preserved sequence is ATA situated about 30 nucleotides from the cap site. A second preserved sequence is CCAAT situated about 70 to 80 nucleotides from the cap site. In the case of the human δ-globin gene, there are three CCAAT-like sequences, but neither has the perfect canonical sequence; the closest is CCAAC. In the case of both γ-globin genes, the CCAAT sequence is duplicated. A third preserved 5′ flanking sequence is slightly more variable in location and is found 80 to 140 nucleotides from the cap site. It has the general structure CACCC or the inverted form GGGTG and is duplicated in the 5′ flanking DNA of the β gene.

Site-directed mutagenesis or deletion of these preserved sequences, followed by testing of the modified genes in various cell-free and tissue culture cell systems capable of transcribing cloned genes, have demonstrated the importance of these sequences for the efficiency and accuracy of gene transcription. Their importance for normal globin gene expression is also underscored by the fact that decreased expression of the β-globin genes in certain forms of β-thalassemia has been found to be due to base substitutions in these sequences, specifically in and around the ATA box and the proximal as well as distal CACCC box of the β-globin gene (see section on molecular basis of β-thalassemia).

The promoter sequences previously described are common to a large number of other nonglobin eukaryotic genes and constitute binding sites for the general transcription apparatus of the cell: RNA polymerase II and its associated accessory transcription factors.[20] In addition, the 5′ flanking DNA of the globin genes contains one or more copies of a consensus sequence having the motif (A/T)GATA(A/G), which has been shown to be the binding site of an erythroid-specific transcription factor originally called GF-1,[21,22] NF-E1, or Eryf-1, but subsequently renamed GATA-1.[23–25] The importance of GATA-1 for gene expression in erythroid cells is underscored by the fact that chimeric mice that developed from embryonal stem (ES) cells with a disrupted GATA-1 gene failed to produce erythroid cells of the ES cell lineage.[26] Furthermore, the ability of the mutant ES cell line to give rise to erythroid cells was restored following transfer of a functional GATA-1 gene.[27] In the γ-globin gene promoters, two GATA-1 binding sites flank the octameric consensus sequence ATTTGCAT for a ubiquitous octamer-binding transcription factor (OTF-1 or OCT-1), which is related to the lymphoid-specific octamer-binding transcription factor (OTF-2 or OCT-2) involved in immunoglobulin gene regulation.[20] A base substitution involving the one nucleotide overlapping one of the GATA-1 consensus sequences and the OCT-1 consensus sequence is associated with one form of nondeletion hereditary persistence of fetal hemoglobin (HPFH). See section on nondeletion HPFH. More recently, Orkin and coworkers have characterized a second erythroid-specific *trans*-acting factor, called NF-E2, that binds to the locus control region (LCR) of the β gene cluster (see following section).[28]

Enhancers and Other *cis*-Acting Sequences That Influence Globin Gene Expression

Enhancer elements are *cis*-acting DNA sequences in the vicinity of a gene, which confer to the gene a high level of expression, frequently in a tissue-specific or developmentally specific manner. Originally described in viral genomes, enhancer elements were subsequently discovered in many chromosomal genes, either in 5′ or 3′ flanking DNA or in introns.[29] Typically, enhancers are functional in a position- and orientation-independent fashion, when tested in various gene transfer–expression systems. The mechanisms of action of enhancers are not completely understood. Enhancers are known to bind various ubiquitous as well as tissue-specific *trans*-acting protein factors with resulting alterations in the configuration of the local chromatin such as the creation of sites that are hypersensitive to various nucleases such as DNase I.[30] Such perturbations in the structure or configuration of chromatin are probably associated with activation of transcription of the adjacent gene through various protein–protein interactions.[31,32]

A well-defined tissue-specific and developmental stage-specific enhancer element has been identified and characterized in the 3′ flanking DNA of the β-globin gene in humans[33–37] as well as other animal species, particularly the chicken. This element confers a high level of gene expression specifically in adult erythroid cells and contains multiple binding sites for the erythroid-specific transcription factor GATA-1.[38] A less well-defined enhancer element has also been identified in the 3′ flanking DNA of the human $^{A}\gamma$-globin gene.[39] Thus far, no analogous enhancer elements have been identified in proximity to the human α-globin genes, although an enhancer has been found in the 3′ flanking DNA of the chicken α-globin gene.[40] In contrast to such positive regulatory sequences, which are found adjacent to adult and fetal globin genes, negative regulatory sequences in 5′ flanking DNA have been shown to influence the function of the human embryonic ε- and ζ-globin gene promoters.[41,42]

Another important group of cis-acting DNA elements are present at some distance from the globin genes that they influence, within regions of chromatin that are particularly hypersensitive to digestion by DNase I in erythroid cell nuclei. Four major hypersensitive sites were identified by Tuan and coworkers[43] and Forrester and colleagues[44] in the DNA located 6 to 18 kb 5′ to the ε-globin gene and an additional site was found in the DNA about 20 kb 3′ to the β-globin gene. In contrast to hypersensitive sites located in promoter regions of the individual globin genes that are usually present only at developmental stages when the particular globin gene is expressed, these remote hypersensitive sites were found to be present in erythroid cells at all developmental stages. The functional significance of the DNA encompassing these DNase I hypersensitive sites was initially demonstrated by Grosveld and colleagues[45] and subsequently by other investigators in experiments involving transfer of human globin genes into transgenic mice and mouse erythroleukemia (MEL) cells.[46]

When DNA containing the DNase I hypersensitive sequences normally located 5′ to the ε gene is linked to a human β-globin gene that is used to produce transgenic mice, the level of expression of the transferred β-globin gene is virtually equivalent, on a per-copy basis, to that of the endogenous murine β-globin gene and does not vary significantly with the site of integration of the transgene (i.e., there is position-independent high level of gene expression).[45] Similar results were also obtained in MEL cells. Previous gene transfer–expression studies in transgenic mice and MEL cells using human β-globin genes without these sequences resulted in low levels of expression of the transferred gene. The expression level on the average was less than 10% of that of the endogenous murine β-globin gene and frequently varied depending on the site of integration of the transferred gene. Because of its functional properties, this region of DNA was initially called the locus activating region[47] or the dominant control region,[48] but subsequently renamed the LCR.[23] The LCR of the β cluster appears not only to be crucial for high levels of globin gene expression in erythroid cells but also to play a role in the fetal to adult globin gene switch (see the following section). An analogous LCR has been identified in the α-globin gene cluster in the DNA located between 28 and 65 kb 5′ to the ζ-globin gene.[49] The importance of the LCRs in the control of normal human globin gene expression is underscored by the finding that certain forms of thalassemia are due to deletions of LCR sequences that leave the globin genes themselves structurally intact but nevertheless inactive in erythroid cells (see sections on α-thalassemia and γδβ-thalassemia).

The mechanisms by which the LCR exerts its influence on globin gene expression from its remote location are poorly understood. The LCR is known to be the binding site for a number of ubiquitous as well as erythroid-specific transcription factors. These include GATA-1, AP-1, and NF-E2.[50–54] The ubiquitous factor AP-1 and the erythroid-specific factor NF-E2 show a similar DNA binding consensus sequence; evidence shows that competitive binding of these two factors occurs at a duplicated consensus sequence in hypersensitive site 2 of the LCR, which is critical for the activity of the LCR.[55–57] A looping model has been proposed[23,46,58–60] for the interaction of the LCR with the promoters or enhancers of the β-like globin genes, perhaps through protein–protein interactions, during the fetal to adult hemoglobin switch (see following section).

Ontogeny of Globin Gene Expression

The pattern of human globin gene expression during development is illustrated in Figure 51-7. Two switches in globin gene expression are observed during development[1,6,23,61,62]: an embryonic to fetal switch, which occurs in the early weeks of gestation and during which α- and γ-chain synthesis replaces ζ- and ε-chain synthesis, and a perinatal fetal to adult switch during which β-chain synthesis replaces γ synthesis. The α-like globin genes switch only once at the time of the ζ→ α switch, whereas the β-like globin genes switch twice: ε→γ→β. The embryonic to fetal switch coincides with the shift of erythropoiesis from yolk sac to fetal liver and is associated with a dramatic change in the morphology of circulating erythroid cells from nucleated megaloblastic cells to anucleated macrocytic cells. It was long assumed that this embryonic to fetal switch represented the replacement of one population or lineage of erythropoietic stem cells by another. Evidence suggests that a population of yolk sac–derived erythroid cells synthesize α and γ chains.[63] Therefore, the embryonic to fetal globin gene switch may not be strictly regulated at the level of cell lineage; it is feasible that the definitive lineage of erythroid cells may derive from seeding of the liver by yolk sac–derived hematopoietic stem cells. In the absence of separate stem cell lineages, the basis for the dramatic change in gene expression program and phenotype in fetal versus embryonic erythroid cells remains essentially unexplained.

The mechanism by which erythroid cells switch from the synthesis of Hb F ($\alpha_2\gamma_2$) to that of Hb A ($\alpha_2\beta_2$) during the perinatal period has been the subject of much study and speculation. The issue has generated a great deal of interest because it constitutes an excellent model system for study of the developmental regulation of gene expression and also because of the practical consideration that reactivation, or prevention of suppression, of γ-globin gene expression could potentially constitute a form of gene therapy for serious β-chain hemoglobinopathies such as sickle cell anemia and β-thalassemia. Despite a large body of work on this topic, the precise mechanisms that regulate the normal switch from γ- to β-globin gene expression remain essentially unknown.

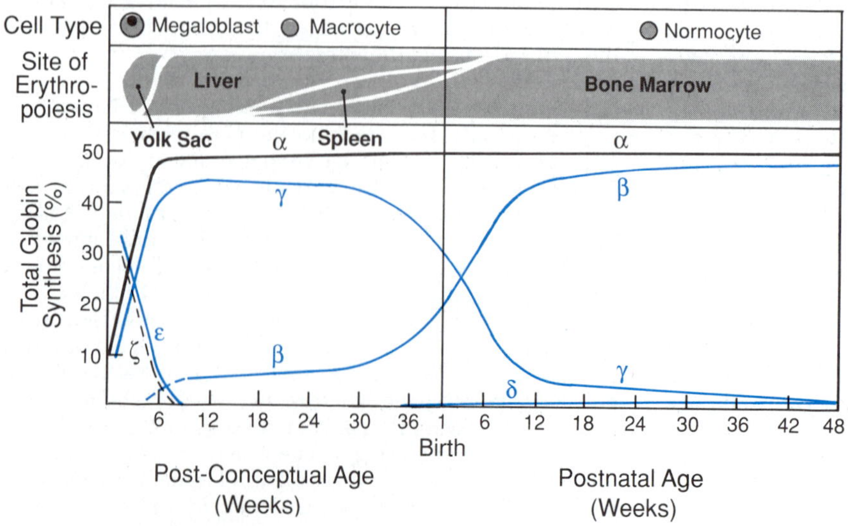

FIGURE 51-7. Schematic representation of the pattern of synthesis of the different globin chains at various stages of development, showing the sites of erythropoiesis as well as the morphologic features of the red cells at the different developmental stages. (After Weatherall DJ, Clegg JB. The thalassemia syndromes, ed 3. Oxford, Blackwell Scientific Publications, 1981)

The Developmental Clock

The switch seems to be regulated more by a developmental "clock" and by gestational age than by intra- or extrauterine environmental factors, as evidenced by the fact that prematurity has little effect on the process.[64,65] The apparent developmental programming of fetal versus adult globin gene expression, independent of environmental factors, is also illustrated by a number of transplantation experiments between fetal and adult donor–recipient pairs in sheep as well as in humans. When fetal liver cells were transplanted into lethally irradiated adult sheep, the pattern of hemoglobin synthesis in reconstituted animals was essentially the same as that observed with fetal liver erythroid cells of a fetal lamb of the same gestational age as the donor; substantial synthesis of Hb F was found and only slightly more than expected Hb A synthesis for the age of the donor cells.[66,67] Analogous results were obtained when human fetal liver (instead of adult bone marrow) was transplanted into children after marrow ablation for therapy of acute leukemia; the pattern of hemoglobin synthesis after engraftment was similar to that expected for the donor cells.[68,69]

The reverse experiment was also performed in which adult bone marrow cells were transplanted into fetal lambs in utero at a time when they synthesized only Hb F. The transplanted cells were derived from animals who were homozygous for the adult variant Hb B, whereas the recipient animals were homozygous for adult Hb A. Repeated sampling of the blood of the transplanted fetuses revealed the appearance of substantial amounts of β^B-globin chains at a time preceding the appearance of β^A-globin chains resulting from the fetal to adult switch in the recipient's endogenous erythroid cells.[70] The results were consistent with the lack of influence of the fetal environment on the pattern of globin gene expression by the transplanted adult erythroid cells.

Taken together, these various transplantation experiments provide convincing evidence for a predetermined program of γ- and β-globin gene expression that is intrinsic to erythroid precursor cells derived from different developmental stages or ages and that cannot be significantly altered by transferring the cells into a different developmental environment.

The intrinsic programming of the β-globin gene cluster during the period of the fetal to adult switch is also illustrated by experiments using hybrid tissue culture cell lines, established by fusion between human fetal erythroid cells and MEL cells, which were selected for retention of human chromosome 11 bearing the human β-globin gene cluster.[71] MEL cells express adult mouse globin genes after induction of erythroid differentiation by various chemical agents and are considered to provide an adult erythroid environment for globin gene expression. After induction, the hybrid cell lines initially produced both human γ- and β-globin chains but with a marked predominance of cells expressing γ-globin. While the cell lines were maintained in culture for longer periods of time before induction, the proportion of cells expressing human β-globin progressively increased in a manner similar to the pattern of hemoglobin switching in vivo during the same period of time.

The Clonal Model

Another issue related to the mechanisms of hemoglobin switching is whether fetal and adult erythroid cells derive from the same family or lineage of erythroid progenitor or stem cells. This issue is the subject of controversy and is not totally resolved. One hypothetic model (clonal model) for the mechanism of the fetal switch would be the progressive replacement of cells derived from a fetal stem cell or progenitor cell lineage by cells derived from an adult cell lineage. The apparent correlation between the switch in the site of erythropoiesis from liver to bone marrow and the switch in type of hemoglobin synthesized from Hb F to Hb A initially suggested the possibility of different, organ-specific, erythroid cell populations with different programs of hemoglobin synthesis. The available data suggest no clearcut difference in the lineage of marrow-derived and liver- or spleen-derived erythroid cells.

Throughout fetal development, the ratio of γ- to β-globin chain synthesis is the same in erythroid cells isolated from different sites of erythropoiesis, indicating the presence of a common progenitor cell population in the fetal liver, spleen, and bone marrow.[72,73] Furthermore, during the perinatal switching period, virtually all of the RBCs contain both Hb F and Hb A in variable amounts, consistent with a gradual and progressive change in the program of globin gene expression in cells derived from a single lineage of progenitor cells. If the switch were due to the differential proliferation or output of two totally distinct progenitor cell pools (one strictly fetal and the other strictly adult), one would expect to find variable admixtures of two different RBC populations during the perinatal switch: one containing exclusively (or predominantly) Hb F and the other containing Hb A. Such a phenomenon is not observed, and the postnatal decline in Hb F synthesis is generally smooth and gradual.[64,65] In addition, studies of globin chain synthesis in individual erythroid colonies derived from neonatal progenitor cells revealed a continuous distribution of γ/β synthesis ratios consistent with a range of globin gene expression programs in different progenitors, rather than a biphasic distribution, as would be expected with two different progenitor cell populations.[61]

Nevertheless, some evidence exists of a change in the characteristics of the erythroid progenitor cell population at the time of the neonatal hemoglobin switch in humans. Analysis of the time course of the transition from Hb F to Hb A production in the postnatal period has revealed two distinct phases: the first phase (from birth to 6 weeks), in which erythropoiesis is markedly suppressed but during which the proportion of Hb F remains relatively constant, and the second phase, which occurs after the reactivation of erythropoiesis, in which the proportion of Hb A rapidly increases.[74,75] Earlier histochemical studies of the distribution of Hb F in neonatal RBCs also revealed the relatively sudden appearance of cells containing predominantly Hb A at about 2 months of age after after recovery from the neonatal period of suppression of erythropoiesis.[76]

The most convincing evidence for a change in progenitor cell population during the neonatal period has been obtained from the study of hemoglobin synthesis in erythroid colonies derived from the blood of newborn infants.[77] By analyzing the characteristics of globin chain synthesis in individual colonies that developed at different times in culture, two different populations of colonies were identified: colonies unique to cord blood (fetal colonies), in which a strong negative correlation was found between the levels of $^G\gamma$- and β-globin chain synthesis, and colonies analogous to those found in adults (adult colonies), in which the proportion of $^G\gamma$ synthesis did not correlate with the proportion of total γ (or β) synthesis.[77] The ratio of $^G\gamma$ to $^A\gamma$ chain synthesis normally differs in fetal and adult erythroid cells, with $^G\gamma$ predominating in fetal cells but being about equal to $^A\gamma$ in adult cells.[1]

Qualitatively different progenitor cell populations were also identified in studies of the Hb F switch in rhesus monkeys.[78] The results of these various studies were interpreted as being consistent with a clonal model for hemoglobin switching in which fetal progenitors are gradually replaced during ontogeny by adult progenitors. It is not clear whether these progenitors with different globin synthesis programs derive from distinct populations of pluripotential stem cells or whether they result from qualitative differences in the pattern of maturation or differentiation among the progeny of a single population of pluripotential stem cells.

Humoral Influences

Considerable speculation has focused on the possibility that some hormonal or humoral factor or factors may normally regulate hemoglobin switching, but little evidence supports this contention. A number of ablation experiments of endocrine organs in fetal sheep have been performed to study this question. In one study, hypophysectomy in utero did not affect the time of onset of the fetal to adult hemoglobin switch, but it did result in a moderate slowing of the rate at which switching occurred, concomitant with an overall delay in the development of the animals.[73,79] In another study, adrenalectomy in utero did not affect the initiation of the switch but was associated with a significant delay in its completion, which could be reversed by replacement therapy with cortisol.[80] In humans, a number of observations have suggested the possible influence of humoral or hormonal factors on hemoglobin switching.[1,6] These include increased maternal synthesis of Hb F during pregnancy shortly after the time of peak secretion of human chorionic gonadotropin (hCG) by the placenta; increased Hb F production in patients with hCG-producing tumors or with thyrotoxicosis; and an apparent delay in the switch in infants of insulin-dependent diabetic mothers.[81,82] It has been suggested that butyrate, a metabolite that is elevated in diabetic mothers and their infants, may mediate this effect. In fact, butyrate has been shown to be capable of increasing the level of expression of embryonic or fetal globin genes in a number of animal and cell culture model systems,[83–88] as well as in humans[89,90] (see section on manipulation of endogenous globin gene expression).

In most circumstances in which there is increased synthesis of Hb F in adults, usually some accelerated production of erythroid cells (erythropoietic stress) is found in association with the presence of substantial amounts of Hb F in some of the circulating erythrocytes. This subpopulation of Hb F-containing cells is referred to as F cells (see following section). The increased production of F cells in the face of erythropoietic stress is usually associated with increased erythropoietin levels, but no evidence exists that the physiologic neonatal fetal to adult switch is induced by changes in the amount or type of erythropoietin produced.

Stress Erythropoiesis and Increased F-Cell Production

The normal level of Hb F in adults is rarely above 1%, and it is distributed within a subset of only 1% to 7% of the total RBCs called F cells.[91,92] F cells contain both Hb A and Hb F (in a ratio of about 2:1) and have membrane antigens as well as other characteristics of adult rather than fetal erythrocytes. A model for the origin of normal F cells and their increase in conditions of erythropoietic stress has been proposed by Stamatoyannopoulos and coworkers[61] and is illustrated in Figure 51-8. Erythroid progenitor cells at the early or BFU-E (burst-forming unit—erythroid) stage of committed erythroid progenitor cell maturation are thought to have the potential to express both Hb F and Hb A. Nevertheless, during the progressive maturation of these progenitor cells from BFU-Es to CFU-Es (colony-forming units—erythroid), most of the progenitors lose their potential for γ-globin gene expression and their progeny become predominantly A cells with relatively few progenitors giving rise to F cells (which should be more accurately designated as A+F cells).

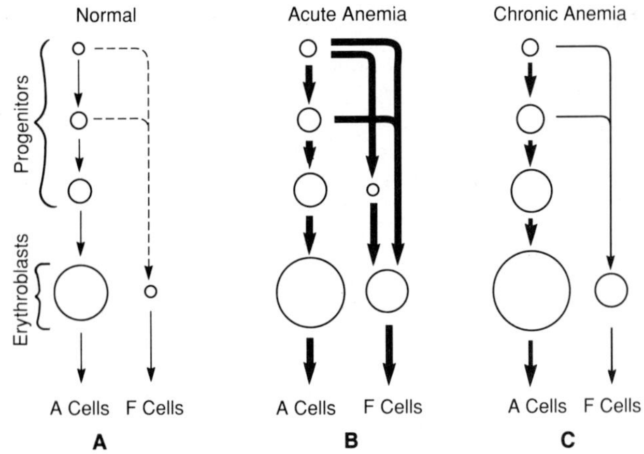

FIGURE 51-8. Model of F cell formation in a normal situation (**A**), in acute anemia or sudden erythroid regeneration (**B**), and in chronic anemia with expanded erythropoiesis (**C**). (After Stamatoyannopoulos G, Veith R, Al-Khatti A, Papayannopoulou T. Induction of fetal hemoglobin by cell-cycle–specific drugs and recombinant erythropoietin. Am J Pediatr Hematol Oncol 1990; 12:21)

A hypothetic corollary of the model shown in Figure 51-8 is that normal F cells may derive directly from BFU-E progenitor cells that short-circuit the normal pathway of maturation through the CFU-E stage and give rise slightly prematurely to differentiated erythroid cell progeny that manifest the early potential of their immediate progenitors and contain both Hb F and Hb A (see Fig. 51-8*A*). This model is attractive because it reconciles both the results of in vitro culture experiments and the in vivo observations of increased F-cell production in conditions associated with erythropoietic stress. The model proposes that under conditions of erythropoietic stress, the short circuit pathway of progenitor cell maturation becomes favored and quantitatively more significant, thereby resulting in the production of increased numbers of erythroid cells containing Hb F (see Fig. 51-8*B* and *C*). This model also potentially explains, at least partially, how the administration of some chemotherapeutic agents such as 5-azacytidine, cytosine arabinoside, and hydroxyurea can result in increased Hb F and F-cell production[61,62] (see section on manipulation of endogenous globin gene expression).

Molecular Mechanisms and Models

Studies of DNA methylation and chromatin structure by nuclease sensitivity have demonstrated that hypomethylation and DNase I hypersensitivity of the 5′ flanking DNA of the γ-globin genes are associated with activity of these genes and that hypermethylation and loss of DNase I hypersensitivity are associated with lack of gene activity.[61] These phenomena are probably secondary to other regulatory events that are not well understood.

Further insights into the mechanisms of the hemoglobin switch were hoped to be provided by elucidation of the molecular basis of the HPFH syndromes in which Hb F expression persists at a high level and in a pancellular fashion in adult erythroid cells. In the deletion types of HPFH, it was once thought that the basis of the marked increase in γ-globin gene expression might be the loss of regulatory sequences located in the intergene DNA between the $^{A}\gamma$- and δ-globin genes, which would be preserved in other deletion syndromes such as $\delta\beta$-thalassemia, in which Hb F is produced at a lower level and in a heterocellular fashion.[93] Comparison of the 5′ deletion endpoints in HPFH with those in a large number of $\delta\beta$-thalassemia syndromes does not allow construction of a comprehensive model for the regulation of γ-globin gene expression by putative control sequences in the intergene DNA between the $^A\gamma$- and δ-globin genes (see sections on deletions associated with $\delta\beta$-thalassemia Hb Kenya and hereditary persistence of fetal hemoglobin).

In nondeletion forms of HPFH, a number of point mutations have been identified in the promoter region of the affected γ-globin genes (see section on nondeletion forms of $\delta\beta$-thalassemia and hereditary persistence of fetal hemoglobin). These mutations are thought to interfere with the normal pattern of binding of various transcriptional regulatory protein factors to the affected γ-gene promoter and thereby prevent the normal postnatal suppression of γ-gene expression. Even though a number of human erythroid-specific *trans*-acting factors have been described, their role in the regulation of hemoglobin switching remains to be determined. In particular, the mRNA for the erythroid-specific factor GATA-1 is present in erythroid cells of all developmental stages.[22,94–96] Therefore, if GATA-1 plays a role in hemoglobin switching, it is not by its de novo appearance or disappearance during development. Nonetheless, subtle quantitative differences in the level of GATA-1 or its posttranslational modification (resulting in activation or inactivation) could play roles in the human hemoglobin switching process. Furthermore, in the mouse, the levels of GATA-1 mRNA in fetal liver erythroid cells are markedly higher than those of yolk-sac derived cells; this suggests a role for GATA-1 in the embryonic to definitive hemoglobin switch.[97] Differences in levels of various transcription factors, including GATA-1, have also been observed during the embryonic to definitive hemoglobin switch in the chicken.[98]

In addition, GATA-1 binding to the γ promoter is essential for the increased promoter activity of one type of nondeletion HPFH with a point mutation at position −175 of the promoter because mutations that abolish GATA-1 binding to this promoter also abolish its overexpression.[21,99]

The most convincing evidence for the role of a *trans*-acting factor in hemoglobin switching is found in the embryonic to adult hemoglobin switch in the chicken, in which the onset of adult β-globin chain synthesis coincides with the appearance of an erythroid-specific *trans*-acting factor (NF-E4).[100] This factor appears to promote, in a looping model, the competitive interaction between the 3′ β enhancer and β promoter at the expense of the interaction between the 3′ β enhancer and the downstream chicken embryonic ε-globin gene promoter.[100,101] Developmental stage-specific factors that are capable of binding to the γ-gene promoters and the $^A\gamma$-gene enhancer element have been identified in fetal erythroid cells of humans and nonhuman primates.[102–105]

As discussed previously in the section on enhancers and other *cis*-acting sequences, a major advance in the field has been the demonstration of the functional importance of the region of DNA, located 6 to 20 kb 5′ to the ε-globin gene, which contains a number of erythroid-specific but developmentally stable DNase I hypersensitive sites and has been called the *locus control region*. It has been proposed that the LCR plays a role in hemoglobin switching.[23,46,58–60,62] When linked to an isolated human ε-globin gene, the LCR allows proper developmental control of the gene, which is expressed in yolk sac erythroid cells of transgenic mice but not at later stages.[106] On the other hand, when linked to isolated γ- or β-globin genes, the LCR appears to disrupt the normal developmental pattern of globin gene expression by conferring activity to the γ genes in adult erythroid cells and to β genes in embryonic erythroid cells of transgenic mice.[107–109] However, in another study[110] the LCR-γ gene was expressed in a developmentally appropriate manner; this suggests that the expression of the γ gene, like that of the ε gene, can be appropriately regulated in the absence of a linked β gene, most likely due to the binding of *trans*-acting factors to silencer elements near the genes.[41,105,106,110] When the LCR is linked to larger DNA fragments containing both γ- and β-globin genes, or when the entire β-gene cluster is used as a transgene, proper developmental regulation is observed.[108–112] A looping model has been proposed in which the fetal to adult switch may be associated with differential competition between the β- and γ-globin gene promoter or enhancer elements for the influence of the LCR,[23,46,58–60,108,109] as illustrated schematically in Figure 51-9. This is possibly mediated by the presence or absence of developmentally specific *trans*-acting factors.

INTRODUCTION TO THE THALASSEMIAS

Definition

The thalassemia syndromes are a group of hereditary disorders in which a defect in the synthesis of one or more of the globin polypeptide chains of hemoglobin is present.[1] This defect causes absent or decreased synthesis of the affected globin chain. As a result, the erythrocytes are characterized by decreased intracellular hemoglobin content (hypochromia) and small size (microcytosis). In addition, the continued normal synthesis of the unaffected globin chain leads to the accumulation of unstable aggregates of these unmatched globin chains. These unstable aggregates precipitate within the erythroid cell, leading to oxidative membrane damage and premature destruction of erythroid cells in the peripheral circulation as well as at earlier stages of maturation in the bone marrow. In α-thalassemia, syn-

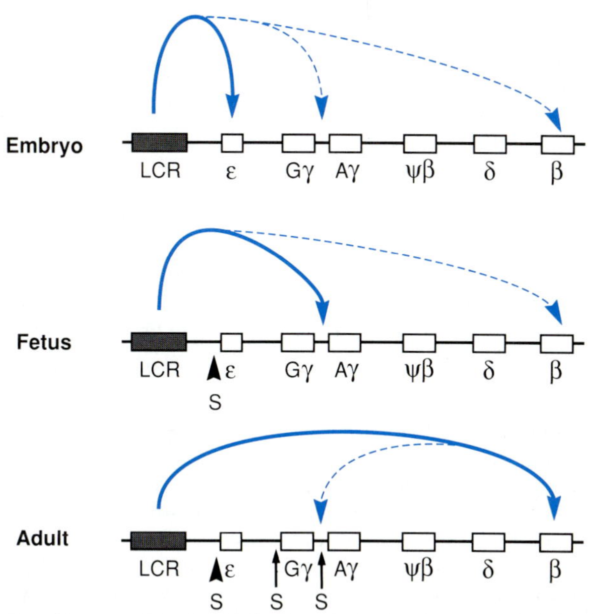

FIGURE 51-9. Model of the regulation of human globin gene switching. Arrows illustrate the competition between genes for interaction with the locus control region. S denotes silencing sequences; the arrowhead indicates a proven silencer, and the thin arrows indicate postulated silencing sequences. (After Stamatoyannopoulos G. Human hemoglobin switching. Science 1991;252:383)

thesis of the α chain of Hb A ($\alpha_2\beta_2$) is impaired, whereas in β-thalassemia, the synthesis of β-chains is reduced or absent.

Prevalence, Geographic Distribution, and Influence of Malaria

Thalassemia affects primarily people of Mediterranean, African, and Asian ancestry. Sporadic cases have been reported in many varied ethnic groups. Malaria is believed to have exerted selective pressure for the increased prevalence of the thalassemia genes in certain populations, although the precise scientific basis for the probable protection of the thalassemia heterozygote against malaria is unknown.[2] It has been proposed that in β-thalassemia heterozygotes, the main protection may be against cerebral malaria in the first 1 to $1\frac{1}{2}$ years of life because of a slower than normal decline of neonatal Hb F levels and growth retardation of malarial parasites in RBCs containing Hb F.[1,114] An alternative explanation proposes that the RBC membrane in heterozygous thalassemia is particularly susceptible to damage by oxidation and that infection with the malaria parasite gives rise to sufficient oxidative stress to perturb intracellular metabolism in a manner that leads to premature death of the parasite.[115,116] This latter hypothesis provides a unifying theory for the selective survival of heterozygotes for α-thalassemia as well as β-thalassemia, glucose-6-phosphate dehydrogenase deficiency, and sickle hemoglobin (Hb S).

The prevalence of thalassemia in various populations has been estimated in a number of surveys.[1] In Southern Italian, Sicilian, and Greek populations, about 10% are heterozygotes for β-thalassemia. In certain Greek islands and some villages of Sardinia, the incidence reaches 20% to 30%. In Southeast Asian populations, the incidence of heterozygous β-thalassemia is about 5%, although a higher incidence is encountered in certain regions. In African and American blacks, the percentage of heterozygous β-thalassemia is about 1.5%.

The highest incidence of heterozygous α-thalassemia occurs in blacks and Southeast Asians. As will be discussed in detail in the section on the molecular basis of α-thalassemia, phenotypically apparent α-thalassemia trait with hypochromic and microcytic RBCs is almost always associated with the deletion or malfunction of two of the four α-globin genes. This is referred to as α-thalassemia-1. When only one of the four α genes is deleted or dysfunctional, the RBCs are usually phenotypically normal (without apparent hypochromia and microcytosis), and the condition is referred to as α-thalassemia-2 or the silent carrier state. About 3% of blacks have phenotypically apparent α-thalassemia trait (α-thalassemia-1 phenotype); this phenotype results from homozygosity for the α-thalassemia-2 genotype, with the deletion of a single α-globin gene on each chromosome that is, there is the deletion of two α-globin genes in *trans*.

Thus, to account for the 3% incidence of the α-thalassemia-1 phenotype due to homozygosity for α-thalassemia-2, about 25% to 30% of blacks must be heterozygous for the α-thalassemia-2 gene deletion; this fact has been confirmed experimentally.[117] The cause of this extraordinarily high gene frequency is poorly understood. It is difficult to explain a selective advantage against malaria when the RBCs in heterozygous α-thalassemia-2 are difficult to distinguish hematologically from normal RBCs.

In Thailand, where the α-thalassemia-1 phenotype is due to the deletion of two α-globin genes on the same chromosome (in *cis*), the prevalence of this form of heterozygous α-thalassemia is about 10%. An additional 10% or so of Thais are heterozygous for α-thalassemia-2. Thus, the combined prevalence of heterozygous α-thalassemia in Thailand is about 20%, although in northern Thailand it is higher and approaches 30%. In certain regions of New Guinea, the combined prevalence of heterozygous and homozygous α-thalassemia-2 is greater than 80%.[118] In other Southeast Asian populations, the evidence of heterozygous α-thalassemia is about 5%. In Mediterranean populations, α-thalassemia is less common than β-thalassemia, with an incidence of about 5% in Sardinia and Greece and a slightly higher incidence of about 10% in Cyprus.

Pathophysiology of the Anemia

As previously stated, the primary biochemical abnormality in thalassemia is a quantitative defect in the synthesis or accumulation of one or more of the polypeptide chains of hemoglobin. As a result of the deficient production of the affected globin chain, an overall deficit of Hb A occurs in thalassemic erythrocytes. As a consequence, these cells are microcytic and hypochromic in both the heterozygous and homozygous states.

The imbalance of globin chain synthesis that is characteristic of thalassemia can be directly demonstrated by a technique that consists of incubating peripheral blood reticulocytes for 1 to 2 hours in the presence of a radioactive amino acid precursor, usually leucine, followed by separation of the individual globin chains by column chromatography and quantitation of incorporated radioactivity into the different peaks.[1,6] The results are usually expressed as the ratio of β- to α-globin chain radioactivity (β/α synthetic ratio), which in normal cells is equal to 1.

When applied to the study of thalassemic reticulocytes, a decrease in β-chain synthesis relative to α-chain synthesis can be demonstrated in β-thalassemia, and a decrease in α-chain synthesis relative to β-chain synthesis can be demonstrated in α-thalassemia. In the usual heterozygotes for β-thalassemia, about half as much radioactivity is incorporated into β chains as into α chains. In homozygotes for β-thalassemia, either a total absence of β-chain radioactivity (β-thalassemia) or a marked decrease in β-chain radioactivity (β^+-thalassemia) with β/α ratios of 0.1:0.3 is observed.

When globin chain synthesis is studied in reticulocytes of α-thalassemia heterozygotes, the observed imbalance in globin chain synthesis is less striking than in β-thalassemia heterozygotes. In the phenotypically apparent form of heterozygous α-thalassemia (α-thalassemia-1), the α/β ratio is 0.7 to 0.8, whereas in the mild form of heterozygous α-thalassemia (silent carrier state or α-thalassemia-2 trait), it is 0.8 to 0.95. In homozygous α-thalassemia-1 (hydrops fetalis with Hb Bart's), there is a total absence of α-chain synthesis. In Hb H disease, which is a less severe α-thalassemia syndrome usually due to double heterozygosity for α-thalassemia-1 and α-thalassemia-2, the globin synthesis profile reveals decreased incorporation of radioactivity into α chains compared with that into β chains, with an α/β ratio of 0.3 to 0.6.

It is easy to understand how reduced synthesis of one or another of the globin chains of Hb A can result in an overall deficit of Hb A accumulation in RBCs and cause a hypochromic, microcytic anemia. In the homozygous state, another pathophysiologic process worsens the anemia and is responsible for the major clinical and hematologic manifestations of thalassemia. The continued synthesis in normal amounts of the nonaffected globin chain results in the accumulation within the thalassemic erythroid cells of excessive amounts of these normal chains.[1,6] Not finding complementary globin chains with which to bind, these chains form unstable aggregates that become oxidized and precipitate within the cell. These precipitates lead to physical and oxidative damage of the cell membrane, resulting in premature destruction of erythroid cells.

In β-thalassemia, the resulting α-chain aggregates are called inclusion bodies or, perhaps improperly, Heinz bodies. In contrast to true Heinz bodies, which are made up of total precipitated hemoglobin ($\alpha_2\beta_2$), the β-thalassemic inclusions consist of only α-globin chains, which have some attached heme in the form of hemichromes. The process of inclusion body formation occurs extensively in the erythroid precursor cells of the marrow and is responsible for the marked ineffective erythropoiesis that characterizes homozygous β-thalassemia.

In α-thalassemia, the resulting β_4 tetramers constitute Hb H, which is less insoluble than α-chain aggregates. In the neonatal and fetal periods, γ_4-tetramers are formed and constitute Hb Bart's.

In β-thalassemia, the role of thalassemic inclusions in the pathophysiology of the hemolytic anemia provides an explanation for the genesis of the heterogeneous RBC population found in this disorder. The peripheral blood of patients with homozygous β-thalassemia usually contains increased amounts of Hb F. The Hb F is heterogeneously distributed among such β-thalassemic RBCs, consistent with a relative increase in the normal number of circulating F cells (see section on ontogeny of globin gene expression). The cells with the most Hb F are those that have the least relative excess of α chains, since the γ chains can combine with α chains to form Hb F. It has been demonstrated in β-thalassemia that Hb A has a more rapid turnover (shorter half-life) than Hb F. This finding is consistent with the presence of at least two different populations of RBCs; those containing mainly Hb A are short-lived and those containing much more Hb F (F cells) have a longer survival.

Differential centrifugation of RBCs in β-thalassemia reveals that the older, more rapidly sedimenting RBCs contain much Hb F and have relatively few α-chain inclusions, whereas the younger, more slowly sedimenting cells are relatively deficient in Hb F and contain many α-chain inclusions. These results are consistent with selective survival of F cells in homozygous β-thalassemia and this selective survival of F cells, combined with some increase in F-cell production due to stress erythropoiesis, are the major causes of the increased Hb F levels observed in this condition. The severity of the disease in homozygous β-thalassemia correlates well with the size of the free α-chain pool and the degree of α-chain to non–α-chain imbalance. Furthermore, coinheritance of α-thalassemia, together with homozygous β-thalassemia reduces the degree of α-globin to non–α-globin chain imbalance and leads to a milder clinical course.

Finally, persons with high Hb F levels and therefore less α-chain/non–α-chain imbalance due to higher $\alpha-/(\beta+\gamma)$-globin chain synthetic ratios also generally have a milder clinical course. These findings indicate that a relation exists between α-chain inclusion body formation and processes of peripheral hemolysis and intramedullary ineffective erythropoiesis. They also illustrate the beneficial role of γ-chain synthesis in decreasing the imbalance of globin chain synthesis, decreasing the formation of α-chain inclusions, and thus increasing the effective production of RBCs and prolonging their survival in the circulation.

In homozygous β-thalassemia, the α-chain inclusions are found in large quantities in the maturing bone marrow erythroid precursor cells, a phenomenon that is thought to be the cause of the marked ineffective erythropoiesis or intramedullary destruction of erythroid cells observed in this condition. Before splenectomy, these inclusion bodies are practically never seen in peripheral RBCs, but after splenectomy they appear in large numbers. This observation correlates well with the demonstrated role of the spleen (and reticuloendothelial system) in removing inclusion bodies of the Heinz body type from RBCs, thereby damaging or destroying these cells.

One cause of RBC injury and destruction in homozygous β-thalassemia may be direct physical trauma due to the presence of the rigid α-chain inclusions and the mechanical injury resulting from the interactions between the abnormal erythroid cells and the reticuloendothelial cells. In addition, other abnormalities of RBC metabolism occur that further damage the erythroid cell membrane and contribute to the premature destruction of the cell.[1,119,120] These abnormalities include oxidant damage to the membrane (lipid peroxidation and protein oxidation or cross-linking) resulting from increased superoxide generation and hemichrome formation due to excessive oxidation of the unstable globin chain aggregates. Such oxidant effects may be further enhanced by vitamin E deficiency and iron overload resulting from transfusions. β-Thalassemic RBCs exhibit markedly reduced cellular deformability. Their membranes, to which are associated large amounts of α-globin chains, are characterized by increased rigidity as well as decreased mechanical stability.[121] These changes are consistent with damage to the RBC membrane skeleton. In fact, a number of abnormalities of the membrane and membrane skeleton proteins has been identified in β-thalassemic RBCs,[121–128] including a specific acquired abnormality in the ability of protein 4.1 molecules to bind normal spectrin.[122]

In addition, cross-linking of protein 3 molecules by hemichromes may occur and result in the formation of an external antigenic site for the binding of a specific antibody, which leads to premature destruction of the RBCs in the reticuloendothelial system.[120,128]

In the α-thalassemia syndrome of Hb H disease, the resulting β_4-tetramers (Hb H) are more stable than α-chain aggregates and precipitate more slowly. Therefore, one does not observe the marked ineffective erythropoiesis and intramedullary destruction of erythroid precursor cells that is characteristic of homozygous β-thalassemia, although some Hb H inclusions are occasionally seen in marrow normoblasts. The precipitation of β_4-tetramers (Hb H) to form inclusion bodies proceeds more gradually and occurs mainly in mature RBCs rather than in nucleated erythroid precursor cells. The spleen removes these inclusion bodies and thus damages the RBCs, resulting in their premature destruction. Before splenectomy, no preformed Hb H inclusion bodies are seen in the peripheral RBCs, although soluble Hb H is present and can be induced to precipitate in the form of small, stippled inclusions after in vitro incubation of the blood with the oxidant compound brilliant cresyl blue. After splenectomy, large, usually single, round preformed inclusion bodies are seen in the RBCs after staining with supravital stains, by phase and electron microscopy, and occasionally on routine blood smears. The membrane lesion that develops in Hb H disease erythrocytes is different from that observed in homozygous β-thalassemia. The RBCs in both disorders display increased membrane rigidity and viscosity.[123] The mechanical stability of the RBC membrane is normal or slightly increased in Hb H disease, whereas it is markedly decreased in homozygous β-thalassemia.[123]

Analysis of membrane skeleton protein interactions has also revealed a different defect in Hb H disease compared with that in homozygous β-thalassemia: a qualitative defect in the binding of normal spectrin to inside-out vesicles, suggesting either oxidative damage to the protein ankyrin or interference of spectrin binding to ankyrin due to steric hindrance by Hb H that is bound to the membrane.[122]

In addition to the primary pathophysiologic processes operative in thalassemia, a number of secondary abnormalities occur that can worsen the anemia or its consequences on the affected patient. In patients with β-thalassemia intermedia with no transfusion or in patients on low transfusion programs, the anemia may be aggravated by folic acid deficiency. This can easily develop because of the high folic acid requirement resulting from the massive marrow erythroid hyperplasia and cellular turnover. Such patients may also experience sudden worsening of their anemia during aplastic crises induced by various bacterial or viral infections including that caused by parvovirus B19, as also occurs in patients with sickle cell anemia and other chronic hemolytic anemias. The splenomegaly invariably associated with homozygous β-thalassemia also contributes to the anemia either by simply acting as a third space, increasing intravascular volume and causing hemodilution, or by causing true hypersplenic destruction of RBCs. After splenectomy, the liver may act in a similar fashion but less effectively. Finally, since RBCs containing Hb F have a high oxygen affinity, actual tissue hypoxia may exist at hemoglobin levels that would otherwise be adequate to provide proper tissue oxygenation if the hemoglobin were all normal adult Hb A. In fact, thalassemic RBCs appear to adapt poorly to anemia, as reflected by inappropriately low levels of RBC 2,3-diphosphoglycerate (DPG) and relatively increased oxygen affinity.[1]

A schematic outline of the interactions between the various pathophysiologic processes in severe β-thalassemia is illustrated in Figure 51-10.

Classification of the Thalassemia Syndromes

The thalassemia syndromes are usually classified according to the type of globin chain that is absent or present in decreased amounts. The clinical types of thalassemia syndromes are listed in Table 51-1. The two major categories consist of the α- and β-thalassemias, each of which can be subdivided into a number of different subtypes that may be inherited in the heterozygous state, in the homozygous state, or in various doubly heterozygous states to generate

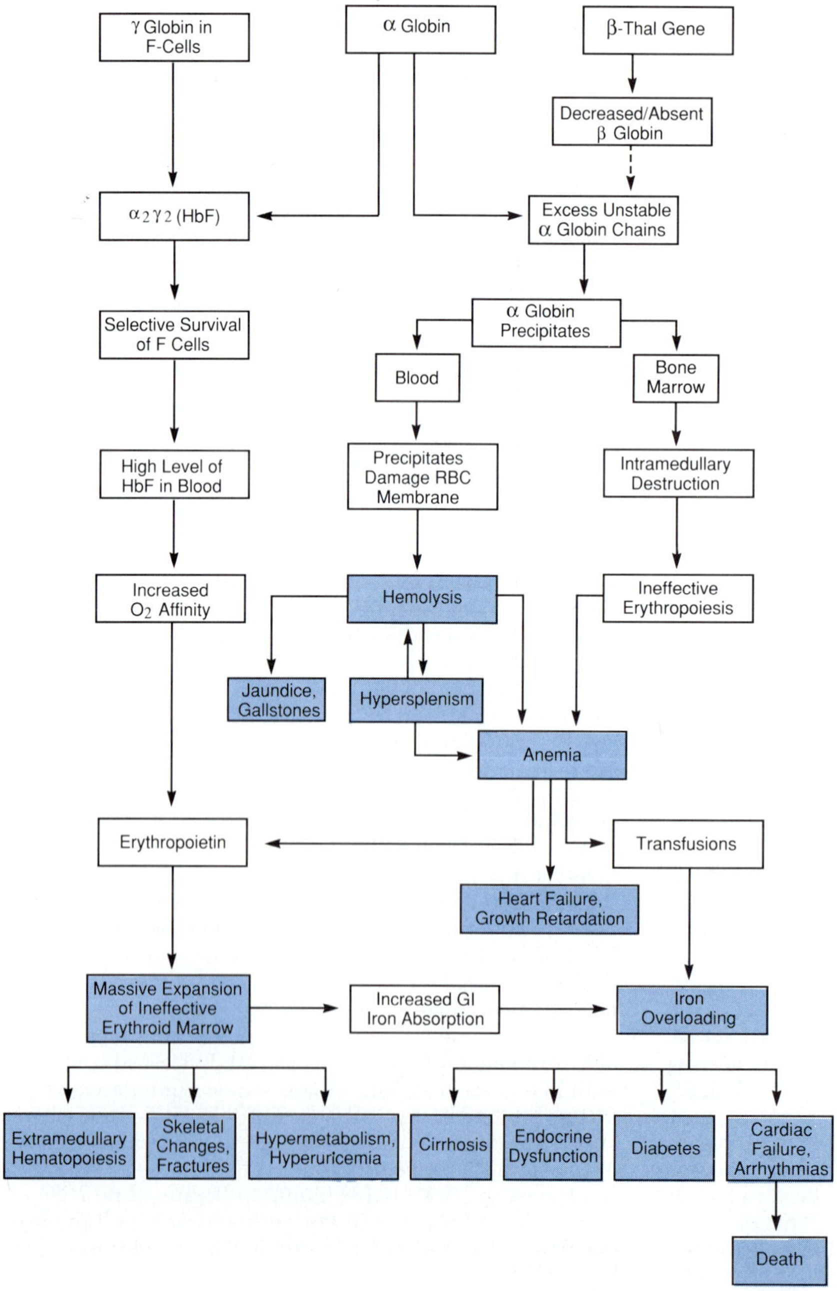

FIGURE 51-10. Pathophysiology of severe β-thalassemia. The colored boxes indicate clinical consequences. (After Weatherall DJ, Clegg JB. The thalassemia syndromes, ed 3. Oxford, Blackwell Scientific Publications, 1981)

TABLE 51-1. Clinical and Hematologic Classification of the Thalassemias and Thalassemia-Like Syndromes

α-THALASSEMIA SYNDROMES

- Heterozygous α-thalassemia-2 or silent-carrier state
- Heterozygous α-thalassemia-1 or α-thalassemia trait
- Hb H disease: double heterozygosity for α-thalassemia-1 and α-thalassemia-2
- Hydrops fetalis with Hb Bart's: homozygous α-thalassemia-1
- Hb Constant Spring syndromes
- α + β-Thalassemia
- Hb S or Hb SS/α-thalassemia

β-THALASSEMIA SYNDROMES

- Heterozygous β-thalassemia, β-thalessemia trait, or β-thalassemia minor
  - With elevated Hb A_2, with or without elevated Hb F
  - With normal Hb A_2 and elevated Hb F: $\delta\beta$-thalassemia, or F-thalassemia
    - $^G\gamma^A\gamma(\delta\beta)^0$-Thalassemia
    - $^G\gamma(^A\gamma\delta\beta)^0$-Thalassemia
  - With normal Hb A_2 and Hb F
    - Silent carrier, including Hb Knossos
    - Concomitant δ- + β-thalassemia, in *cis* or in *trans*
    - $\gamma\delta\beta$-Thalassemia
    - Other: atypical $\delta\beta$-thalassemia, concomitant iron deficiency
  - Hb Lepore trait
- Homozygous β-thalassemia, Cooley's anemia, or β-thalassemia major
  - True homozygosity for one β-thalassemia gene
  - Double heterozygosity for any two different β-thalassemia genes
  - β-Thalassemia intermedia

RARE FORMS OF THALASSEMIA

- γ-Thalassemia
- δ-Thalassemia
- $\gamma\delta\beta$-Thalassemia

INTERACTING THALASSEMIA

- α-Thalassemia + α-chain variant
  - Hb Q/α-thalassemia
  - Hb G/α-thalassemia
- β-Thalassemia + β-chain variant
  - Sickle/β-thalassemia
  - Hb C/β-thalassemia
  - Hb E/β-thalassemia

HEREDITARY PERSISTENCE OF FETAL HEMOGLOBIN (HPFH)

- Pancellular
  - $^G\gamma^A\gamma(\delta\beta)^0$ HPFH
  - Hb Kenya ($^G\gamma$ HPFH)
  - Black $^G\gamma\beta^+$ HPFH with high Hb F
  - Greek $^A\gamma$ HPFH
  - Chinese $^A\gamma$ HPFH
- Heterocellular
  - Swiss type $^G\gamma^A\gamma$ HPFH
  - British type $^A\gamma$ HPFH
  - Other: Seattle-type $^G\gamma^A\gamma$ HPFH; Atlanta-type—black $^G\gamma\beta^+$ HPFH with low Hb F; Saudi high Hb F determinant

a large number of diverse clinical and hematologic syndromes.

In the α-thalassemia syndromes, heterozygous α-thalassemia can occur in two forms: a phenotypically apparent form, referred to as α-thalassemia-1, and a mild defect, with minimal or no hematologic abnormalities, called α-thalassemia-2 or the silent carrier state. The α-thalassemia-1 phenotype can also result from homozygosity for α-thalassemia-2. The heterozygous state for the structurally abnormal hemoglobin Hb Constant Spring is phenotypically similar to α-thalassemia-2, except that small amounts (1% to 2%) of the abnormal hemoglobin are detectable. The homozygous state for α-thalassemia-1 is the syndrome of hydrops fetalis with Hb Bart's. The doubly heterozygous state for α-thalassemia-1 and α-thalassemia-2 (or Hb Constant Spring) results in the less severe syndrome of Hb H disease.

In the β-thalassemia syndromes, the heterozygous state for β-thalassemia (β-thalassemia minor or β-thalassemia trait) is heterogeneous, as indicated by the variations in the amounts of the minor components of hemoglobin present in RBCs of affected persons. The various heterozygous states include (1) β-thalassemia with elevated Hb A_2; (2) $\delta\beta$-thalassemia or F-thalassemia, characterized by normal Hb A_2 but elevated Hb F; (3) β-thalassemia trait with normal levels of Hb F and Hb A_2; and (4) Hb Lepore trait, a condition that is phenotypically similar to heterozygous β-thalassemia but characterized by normal levels of Hb A_2, the presence of small amounts (10% to 15%) of the structurally abnormal hemoglobin (Hb Lepore), and usually some elevation of Hb F. β-Thalassemia major or Cooley's anemia may result from the combination of any two of these genes.

Occasionally, a person inherits a combination of thalassemic genes that result in a syndrome that is clinically less severe than the typical cases of homozygous β-thalassemia. Typically, such a condition is not associated with a chronic transfusion requirement and is referred to as β-thalassemia intermedia. A number of different genotypes can be associated with β-thalassemia intermedia, including a form of unusually severe heterozygous β-thalassemia associated with inclusion body formation (see section on molecular basis of β-thalassemia).

Thalassemia can also be classified according to the nature of the molecular defect. In the sections that follow, the various molecular lesions associated with α- and β-thalassemia and their related syndromes are discussed.

MOLECULAR PATHOPHYSIOLOGY

Despite having a relatively homogeneous clinical, hematologic, and biochemical phenotype, the thalassemias have been shown to be due to a surprisingly large number of different genetic defects. The review of normal gene structure and function presented at the beginning of this chapter (and also in Chap. 4) illustrates the many steps of gene expression at which a mutation can result in the absent or markedly decreased production or accumulation of a normal gene product such as α- or β-globin. The α-thalassemias are generally due to deletions in the α-globin gene cluster, whereas the β-thalassemias are generally due to point mutations in the β-globin gene. Nondeletion forms of α-thalassemia and deletion forms of β-thalassemia have also been identified. In the following sections, we describe the different genetic lesions that result in α- and β-thalassemia.

Molecular Basis of β-Thalassemia

Most mutations that cause β-thalassemia are due to point mutations in functionally important regions of the β-globin gene. More than 125 different point mutations have thus far been identified as causes of β-thalassemia, although a relatively small number of mutations account for the majority of cases in a given racial group (see section on prenatal diagnosis). These point mutations can be classified according to the type or category of defect in gene expression that they cause (Table 51-2).

TABLE 51-2. Mutations Causing β-Thalassemia (Reported Through May 1993)

Mutation	Phenotype β^0 or β^+	Racial Group	References
PROMOTER MUTATIONS			
ATA Box			
−28 (A → G)	+	Chinese	129
−28 (A → C)	+	Kurdish	130
−29 (A → G)	+	American black, Chinese	131, 132
−30 (T → C)	+	Chinese	133
−30 (T → A)	+	Eastern Mediterranean	134
−31 (A → G)	+	Japanese	135
−32 (C → A)	+	Taiwanese	136
CACCC Box			
−86 (C → G)	+	Lebanese	137, 138
−86 (C → A)	+	Italian	139
−87 (C → G)	+	Mediterranean	140
−87 (C → T)	+	German, Italian	141
−87 (C → A)	+	Yugoslavian	142
		American black	143
−88 (C → A)	+	Kurdish	144
−88 (C → T)	+	American black, Asian Indian	145
−90 (C → T)	+	Portuguese	146
		Ashkenazi Jewish	147
−92 (C → T)	+	Mediterranean	137, 138
−101 (C → T)	+	Italian, Eastern Mediterranean	148
Cap Site			
+1 (A → C)	+	Asian Indian	149
CLEAVAGE AND POLYADENYLATION MUTATIONS			
AATAAA → AACAAA	+	American black	151
AATAAA → AATAAG	+	Kurdish	144
AATAAA → AATAGA	+	Malaysian	152
AATAAA → AATGAA	+	Mediterranean	152
AATAAA → A(−AATAA)	+	Arab	153
AATAAA → AAAA(−AT)	+	French	154
SPLICING MUTATIONS			
Splice Site Junction Mutations			
IVS-1 position 1 (G → A)	0	Mediterranean	140
IVS-1 position 1 (G → T)	0	Asian Indian, Chinese	155
IVS-1 position 2 (T → G)	0	Tunisian	156
IVS-1 position 2 (T → C)	0	American black	157
		Algerian	158
IVS-1 position 2 (T → A)	0	Algerian	159
IVS-1 5′-end (−44 bp)	0	Mediterranean	160
IVS-1 position 130 (G → A)	0	Egyptian	161
IVS-1 position 130 (G → C)	0	Italian	137, 138
		Turkish	162
		Japanese	163
IVS-1 3′-end (−17 bp)	0	Kuwaiti	160
IVS-1 3′-end (−25 bp)	0	Asian Indian	164
IVS-2 position 1 (G → A)	0	Mediterranean	165
		Tunisian	156
		American black	166
		Japanese	167
IVS-2 position 1 (G → C)	0	Iranian	168
IVS-2 position 849 (A → G)	0	American black	131, 169
IVS-2 position 849 (A → C)	0	American black	170
IVS-2 position 850 (G → C)	0	Yugoslavian	171
IVS-2 position 850 (−G)	0	Italian	172

(continued)

TABLE 51-2. *(Continued)*

Mutation	Phenotype β^0 or β^+	Racial Group	References
Consensus Sequence Mutations			
IVS-1 position −3 (C → T) (codon 29)	?	Lebanese	173
IVS-1 position −1 (G → C) (codon 30) (Hb Kairoran or Monroe)	+	Tunisian, American black	156, 174, 175
IVS-1 position −1 (G → A) (codon 30)	?	Bulgarian	176
IVS-1 position 5 (G → C)	+	Asian Indian	155
		Chinese	177
		Melanesian	178
IVS-1 position 5 (G → T)	+	Mediterranean	179
		American black	180
IVS-1 position 5 (G → A)	+	Greek*	181, 182
		Algerian	183
IVS-1 position 6 (T → C)	+	Mediterranean	140
IVS-1 position 128 (T → G)	+	Saudi Arabian	184
		Chinese	185
IVS-2 positions 4–5 (−AG)	0	Portuguese	146
IVS-2 position 848 (C → A)	+	Mediterranean, Iranian, Egyptian, American black	182, 184, 186
IVS-2 position 848 (C → G)	+	Japanese	167
IVS-2 position 844 (C → G)	+	Italian	187
IVS-2 position 843 (T → G)	+	Algerian	188
IVS-2 position 837 (T → G)	?	Asian Indian	189
Mutations Creating Alternative Splice Sites			
In introns			
IVS-1 position 110 (G → A)	+	Mediterranean	190, 191
IVS-1 position 116 (T → G)	0	Mediterranean	192
IVS-2 position 654 (C → T)	0	Chinese	177
IVS-2 position 705 (T → G)	0	Mediterranean	193
IVS-2 position 745 (C → G)	+	Mediterranean	140
In exons			
Codon 19 (A → G) Hb Malay	+	Malaysian	194
Codon 24 (T → A)	+	American black	195
		Japanese	196
Codon 26 (G → A) Hb E	+	SE Asian	197
Codon 27 (G → T) Hb Knossos	+	Mediterranean	198
MUTATIONS PRODUCING NONFUNCTIONAL mRNAs			
Nonsense Mutations			
Codon 15 (TGG → TAG)	0	Asian Indian	155
Codon 15 (TGG → TGA)	0	Portuguese	199
Codon 17 (A → T)	0	Chinese	200
Codon 22 (G → T)	0	Reunion Islander	138, 154
Codon 26 (G → T)	0	Thai	201
Codon 35 (C → A)	0	Thai	202
Codon 37 (G → A)	0	Saudi Arabian	203
Codon 39 (C → T)	0	Mediterranean, European	204–210
Codon 43 (G → T)	0	Chinese	211
Codon 61 (A → T)	0	American black	186
Codon 90 (G → T)	0	Japanese	167, 212
Codon 112 (T → A)	0	Czechoslovakian	213
Codon 121 (G → T) truncated β-chain variant	(+)	Polish, Swiss, British, Japanese	163, 214–216
Codon 127 (C → T)	0	English	217
Frameshift Mutations			
Codon 1 (−G)	0	Mediterranean	218
Codon 5 (−CT)	0	Mediterranean	219
Codon 6 (−A)	0	Mediterranean, American black	186, 220, 221
Codon 8 (−AA)	0	Turkish	222

(continued)

TABLE 51-2. *(Continued)*

Mutation	Phenotype β^0 or β^+	Racial Group	References
Codons 8/9 (+G)	0	Asian Indian	155
		Mediterranean	182
Codon 11 (−T)	0	Mexican	223
Codons 14/15 (+G)	0	Chinese	224
Codon 15 (−T)	0	Asian Indian, Thai	154
Codon 16 (−C)	0	Asian Indian	155
Codons 20/21 (+G)	0	Ashkenazi Jewish	147
Codon 24 (−G, +CAC)	0	Egyptian	225
Codons 25/26 (+T)	0	Tunisian	226
Codons 27/28 (+C)	0	Chinese	227
Codon 35 (−C)	0	Malaysian	194
Codons 36/37 (−T)	0	Kurdish (Iranian)	144
Codons 37–39 (−GACCCAG)	0	Turkish	228
Codons 38/39 (−C)	0	Czechoslovakian	229
Codon 41 (−C)	0	Thai	230
Codons 41/42 (−TTCT)	0	Asian Indian	155
		Chinese	231
Codon 44 (−C)	0	Kurdish	232
Codon 47 (+A)	0	Surinamese black	233
Codon 54 (+G)	0	Japanese	234
Codon 64 (−G)	0	Swiss	235
Codon 71 (+T)	0	Chinese	236
Codons 71/72 (+A)	0	Chinese	177
Codons 74/75 (−C)	0	Turkish	237
Codon 76 (−C)	0	Italian	238
Codons 82/83 (−G)	0	Azerbaijani	239
		Czechoslovakian	240
Codon 88 (+T)	0	Asian Indian	189
Codon 94 (+ TG) β Agnana	(+)	Italian	241
Codon 95 (+A)	0	Thai	154
Codons 106/107 (+G)	0	American black	149
Codons 109/110 (−G) β Manhattan	(+)	Lithuanian	242
+1 codon 114 (−CT, +G) β Geneva	(+)	French	243
Codon 123 (−A) β Makabe	(+)	Japanese	244
Codons 123–125 (−ACCCCACC) β Khon Kaen	0	Thai	245
Codon 126 (−T) β Vercelli	(+)	Italian	187
Codons 127/128 (−AGG) β Gunma	(+)	Japanese	196, 246
Codons 128/129 (−4, +5) (−GCTG, +CCACA) and codons 132–135 (−11) (−AAAGTGGTGGC)	(+)	Irish	216
Codons 134–137 (−10, +4) (−TGGCTGGTGT, +GCAC)	0	Portuguese	247
Initiation Codon Mutations			
ATG → AGG	0	Korean	154
		Chinese	248
		Japanese	249
ATG → ACG	0	Yugoslavian	250
		Swiss	251
ATG → GTG	0	Japanese	252
ATG → ATT	0	White	253
OTHER			
5′ Untranslated Sequence			
+22 G → A	+	Eastern Mediterranean	254
		Italian	255
+43 → +40 (−AAAC)	+	Chinese	256
3′ Untranslated Sequence			
Cap site + 1570 (T → C)†	+	Irish	255, 257
Termination codon +6 (C → G)	+	Greek	258

(continued)

TABLE 51-2. *(Continued)*

Mutation	Phenotype β^0 or β^+	Racial Group	References
UNSTABLE GLOBIN CHAINS WITH THALASSEMIC PHENOTYPE DUE TO MISSENSE MUTATIONS‡			
Codon 28 (Leu → Arg) β Chesterfield	+	English	259
Codon 60 (Val → Glu)	+	Italian	260
Codon 106 (Leu → Arg) β Terre Haute, formerly β Indianapolis	+	European	261
Codon 110 (Leu → Pro) β Showa-Yakushiji	+	Japanese	262
Codon 114 (Leu → Pro) β Durham N.C.	+	Irish	263
Codon 127 (Gln → Pro) β Houston	+	British	242
Codon 127 (CAG → CGG)	+	French	154

* Combined with 7.2-kb deletion of δ-globin gene (Corfu δβ-thalassemia).[181]
† This base change has subsequently been determined to be a polymorphism linked to the IVS-2 position 654 mutation.[256]
‡ See also frameshift mutations for additional unstable β chains or variants associated with inclusion bodies, indicated by (+). A number of additional, usually unstable, β-chain variants are also associated with a mild β-thalassemia phenotype.[154,279]

Promoter Mutations

As discussed at the beginning of this chapter, a number of conserved sequence motifs in the 5′ flanking DNA of globin (and other) genes constitute important functional elements of the gene promoter and are therefore important for efficient transcription of the gene. Three of these consensus sequences are found in the promoter regions of all globin genes: the CACCC box, the CCAAT box, and the ATAA (or TATA) box. Mutations in two of these three conserved sequence motifs have been identified in different patients with β-thalassemia, that is, in the CACCC and ATAA boxes. No mutations of the CCAAT box have been identified as causes of β-thalassemia, although mutations in this motif are associated with certain cases of HPFH (see section on nondeletion forms of δβ-thalassemia and hereditary persistence of fetal hemoglobin).

In general, the degree of diminished β-chain synthesis associated with mutations of the β-globin gene promoter is relatively minor. Patients have β^+-thalassemias which, in the homozygous or doubly heterozygous form, is relatively mild and frequently associated with the clinical phenotype of β-thalassemia intermedia. This finding is consistent with studies of transcription of the mutant genes in gene transfer–expression studies in tissue culture cells, which reveal only a mild to moderate decrease in transcriptional activity of these genes.[129,131,135,145]

As listed in Table 51-2, there are seven mutations at five different positions of the ATAA box (nucleotides −28 to −32 from the cap site) and nine mutations at five different positions of the proximal CACCC box (nucleotides −86, −87, −88, and −92 from the cap site). One mutation has been identified at position −101 within a second (distal) CACCC element of the β-globin gene promoter. This mutation is extremely mild and is associated in heterozygotes with the silent carrier phenotype characterized by little or no hypochromia and microcytosis of the RBCs. The ATAA box mutations at position −28 (A→G) and −29 (A→G) are relatively common causes of β-thalassemia in Chinese and black populations, respectively. Although the −29 mutation results in a relatively mild disorder in blacks,[131] the same mutation is associated with severe transfusion-dependent thalassemia in a homozygous Chinese patient.[132] The cause of this striking difference in phenotype is not known but may be related to different levels of γ-gene expression associated with the different chromosomal backgrounds on which these apparently identical mutations occurred in the two different racial groups.[132,137,149]

As previously discussed, the cap site or transcription initiation site is part of a conserved sequence motif which, in the case of genes lacking a TATA box, serves as a promoter element (Inr element).[15] It is not known if the Inr element plays a significant role in transcription of the globin genes that do contain a TATA box. Nevertheless, one mutation of the cap site (+1 A→C) has been found to be associated with a mild form of β-thalassemia similar to the silent carrier state.[150] It is not known whether this mutation causes β-thalassemia by decreasing β-globin gene transcription or by decreasing the efficiency of capping (posttranscriptional addition of m^7G) and mRNA translation.

Mutations Causing Abnormal Posttranscriptional Modification

As discussed earlier in this chapter, the nascent precursor globin mRNA molecule is modified at both of its ends: a methylated (m^7G) cap structure is added at the 5′ end, and a poly(A) tail is added at the 3′ end of the mRNA. One mutation of the cap site has been described, although it is not known whether the principal effect of the mutation is on transcription or on the capping modification. On the other hand, a number of different β-thalassemias have been associated with defective polyadenylation due to mutations involving the consensus sequence AATAAA required for the cleavage–polyadenylation reaction: four base substitutions at different positions of the consensus sequence and two short deletions (2 and 5 bp; see Table 51-2). These mutations markedly decrease the efficiency of the cleavage–polyadenylation process but do not abolish it completely. Therefore, the associated phenotype is that of β^+-thalassemia of typical severity because only about 10% of the β mRNA is properly modified. The remainder of the transcripts extend far beyond the normal polyadenylation site and are probably cleaved and polyadenylated after the next AATAAA consensus sequences, which occur about 0.9 to 3 kb downstream.[151] These elongated transcripts are presumably unstable because they constitute only a minor portion of the β mRNA in affected erythroid cells.

Mutations Causing Abnormal Precursor mRNA Splicing

The precursor globin mRNA must be processed posttranscriptionally to remove sequences corresponding to the introns of the gene. The complex, multistep process is referred to as splicing, and the consensus sequences required for efficient and accurate splicing were discussed at the beginning of this chapter. Defects in splicing can be either complete or partial, resulting in β^0 or β^+-thalassemia, respectively. These are described individually in the sections that follow.

Mutations of the Splice Site Junction That Totally Abolish Normal Splicing. The dinucleotides GT and AG are nearly always present at the 5′ (donor) and 3′ (acceptor) splice junctions, respectively, forming the boundaries of the intronic sequence. Base substitutions that change one or the other of these invariant dinucleotides, or short deletions that remove them, are associated with total absence of normal pre-mRNA splicing. Therefore, the phenotype is that of β^0-thalassemia. A total of sixteen base substitutions or short deletions involving the invariant dinucleotides of the β-globin gene introns have been identified (see Table 51-2): six involving the 5′ GT of IVS-1; two involving the 5′ GT of IVS-2; four involving the 3′ AG of IVS-1; and four involving the 3′ AG of IVS-2. In some cases, the mutated intron is totally retained within the mutant mRNA. In other cases, the mutation appears to activate (or facilitate the use of) cryptic splice sites present elsewhere in the intron or, in the case of mutations of the IVS-1 5′ splice junctions, in the adjacent exon, thus resulting in partial splicing of the mutant intron or removal of the intron together with a portion of the 5′ flanking exon.[131,165,169,177,264] The partially or abnormally spliced mRNA species can sometimes be detected in small amounts in affected erythroid cells. They are presumably unstable or poorly transported from nucleus to cytoplasm to account for their low abundance, and they are nonfunctional because translation of the abnormally spliced or frameshifted mRNAs would usually stop prematurely because of the presence of chain termination (nonsense) codons (see section on mutations that produce nonfunctional β-globin mRNAs).

Mutations of Splice Site Consensus Sequence That Partially Block Normal Splicing. The invariant dinucleotides GT at AG, which are present at the 5′ and 3′ splice junctions, respectively, are necessary but not sufficient to ensure efficient and accurate splicing. They are normally part of a larger consensus sequence that contains a number of other conserved sequence features, as previously discussed in this chapter. Mutations of certain residues in this consensus sequence result in a partial block of normal mRNA splicing, the severity of which varies with the site of the mutation within the consensus sequence. As a group, these mutations

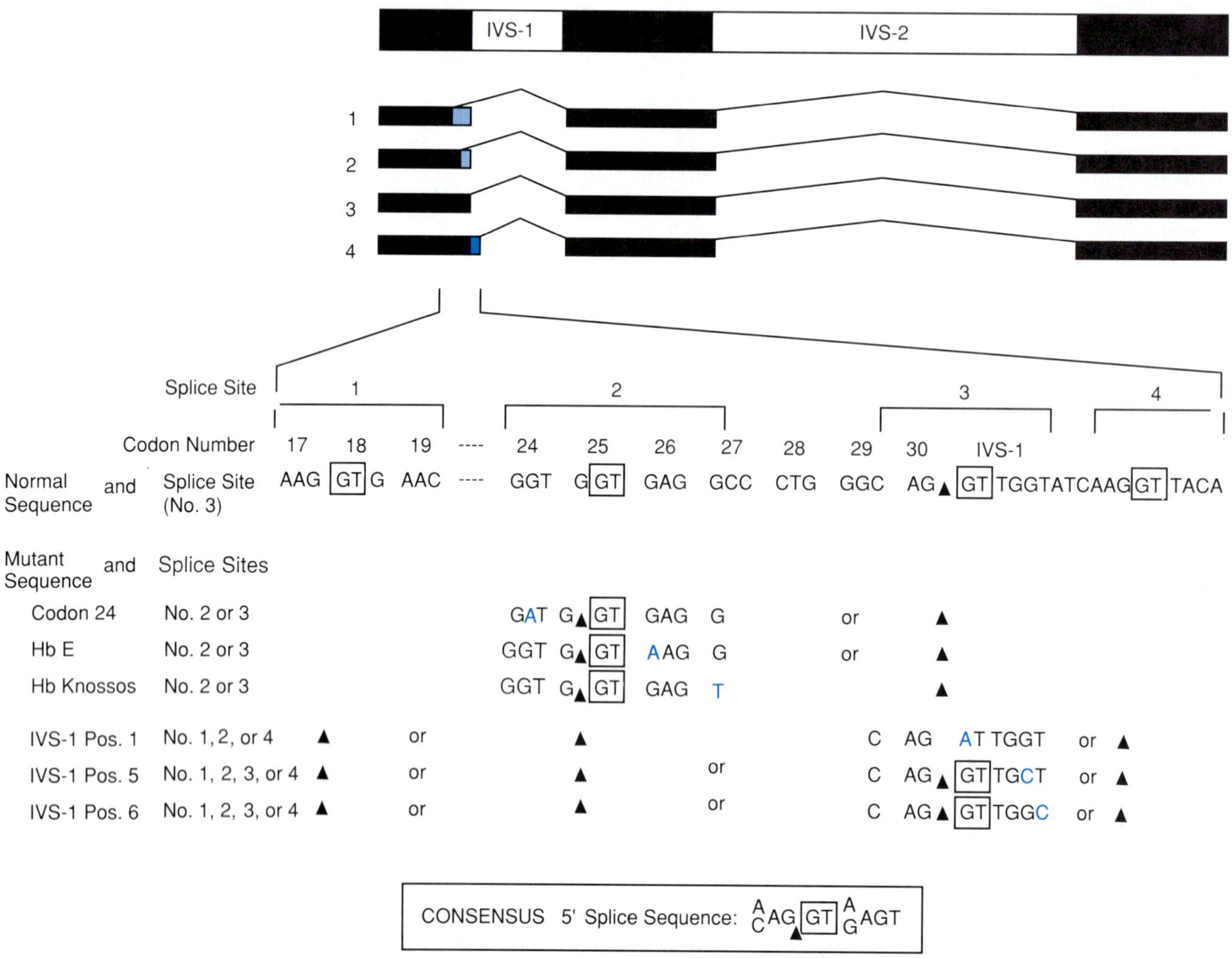

FIGURE 51-11. Splicing patterns associated with different thalassemic mutations in exon 1 and IVS-1 of the β-globin gene. The normal and abnormal 5′ (donor) splice sites are indicated by arrowheads. The GT dinucleotide sequences required for the splicing events are indicated by the boxes. The nucleotide base substitutions resulting from the mutations are indicated in color. The lightly colored boxes indicate the portions of exon 1 that are removed from the processed mRNA by alternative splicing; the open box represents the portion of IVS-1 retained in the processed mRNA. (After Bunn HF, Forget BG. Hemoglobin: molecular, genetic and clinical aspects. Philadelphia, WB Saunders, 1986)

are generally associated with a phenotype of β^{+}-thalassemia. The mutation at position +6 of the IVS-1 5′ (donor) consensus sequence is particularly mild and is usually associated with β-thalassemia intermedia because of a relatively high level of normal mRNA splicing. In contrast, three different mutations at position +5 of the same consensus sequence result in a severe form of β-thalassemia with a markedly reduced amount of normally spliced β-globin mRNA.

Other positions of the donor consensus sequences affected by mutations include positions −1 and −3 from the GT. A total of 14 mutations of the β-globin gene have been described in this category, seven of which involve the 5′ consensus sequence of IVS-1; one involves the 3′ consensus sequence of IVS-1; one involves the 5′ consensus sequence of IVS-2; and five involve the 3′ consensus sequence of IVS-2 (see Table 51-2). The 3′ consensus mutations affect nucleotides at four different positions of the polypyrimidine tract upstream from the acceptor AG.

The pattern of splicing that occurs with mutations of the 5′ consensus sequence of IVS-1 is complex. Mutations at this site result in the activation or use of three neighboring alternative or cryptic splice sites, two of which are present in adjacent exon 1 and one of which is located downstream in IVS-1[179,264] (Fig. 51-11). The alternative splice site that is preferentially used over all others is located within exon 1 at codon positions 24 to 27. This cryptic splice site, GTGGTGAGG, consists of a good, although imperfect, match with the generic or canonical consensus sequence (A/C)AGGT(A/G)AGT Preferential use of this same alternative or cryptic splice site also occurs in the case of Hb E,[197] as well as two other Hb variants with base substitutions in the same region of the β mRNA[195,198] and is presumably responsible for the β-thalassemia phenotype associated with these disorders (see section on mutations that create new alternative splice sites in exons). The resulting abnormally spliced mRNA species have been characterized after gene transfer and expression in tissue culture cells. They are presumably highly unstable in vivo because they are not present in easily detectable amounts in erythroid cells of affected patients. Even if these abnormally spliced β-globin mRNAs did accumulate within the cell, the two main species would be nonfunctional because of premature termination due to frameshift (see section on mutations that produce nonfunctional β-globin mRNAs).

Mutations That Create New Alternative Splice Sites in Introns. A third category of splicing mutation is due to base substitutions in introns that generate new splicing signals preferentially used instead of the normal splice sites. Five such mutations have been identified in the β-globin gene: two in IVS-1 and three in IVS-2 (see Table 51-2). The associated phenotype may be either β^{+} or β^{0}-thalassemia, depending on the site and nature of the mutation.

The first base substitution identified in a β-thalassemia gene was at position 110 of IVS-1. This mutation has subsequently been shown to be the most common form of β-thalassemia in the Mediterranean population. The mutation is a substitution of G to A that creates an acceptor AG in a favorable consensus sequence environment, 19 bp 5′ to the normal acceptor AG of IVS-1 (Fig. 51-12*A*). Gene transfer and expression studies in tissue culture cells have demonstrated that this newly created alternative splice site is preferentially used in 80% to 90% of the transcripts, whereas the normal splice site is used in only 10% to 20% of the transcripts,[265,266] thus giving the phenotype of β^{+}-thalassemia (see Fig. 51-12*B*). The mutant mRNA is presumably unstable or poorly transported from nucleus to cytoplasm because it is not detected in significant quantity in affected erythroid cells. Even if it were to accumulate, it would be nonfunctional because the 19-bp segment of

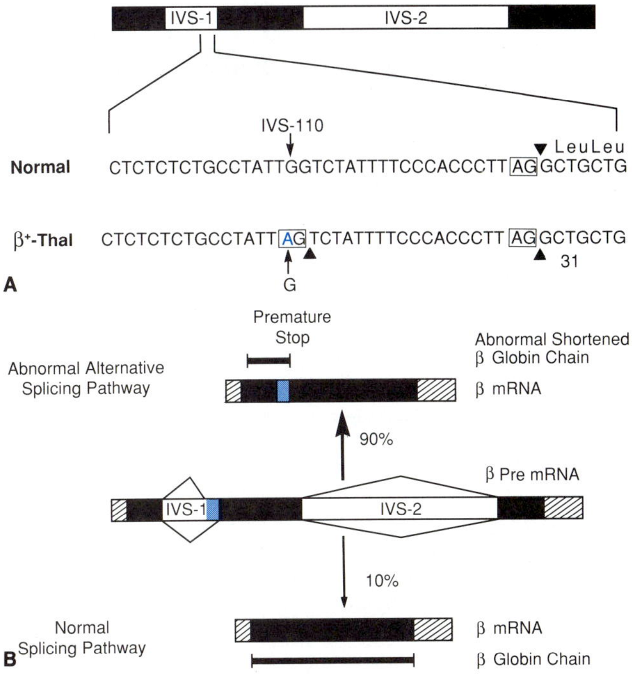

FIGURE 51-12. Alternative splicing of precursor β-globin mRNA resulting in β^{+}-thalassemia associated with the mutation at IVS-1 position 110. (**A**) Diagram of the β-globin gene showing the DNA sequence at the 3′ end of IVS-1 and the G → A base substitution at position 110, creating an AG dinucleotide within a potential consensus 3′ (acceptor) splice site in the β^{+} thalassemic gene. The arrowheads indicate potential splice sites. (**B**) Schematic representation of alternative splicing pathways caused by the mutation. The colored area in IVS-1 indicates the portion of IVS-1 that is abnormally spliced into the β mRNA. (After Bunn HF, Forget BG. Hemoglobin: molecular, genetic and clinical aspects. Philadelphia, WB Saunders, 1986)

retained intronic sequence contains an in-phase termination codon; thus, a truncated β-globin peptide would be synthesized.

Another mutation was later identified in a different Mediterranean family, 6 bp farther 3′ in IVS-1 at position 116.[192] This mutation (T→G) also creates a new acceptor AG in a good consensus sequence, but in this case the phenotype is that of β^{0}-thalassemia. The normal acceptor sequence, although intact, is not used presumably because the new AG occurs at a position that is too proximal to the normal AG and thus totally interferes with its recognition and use as a splice site.[192] In a survey of normal acceptor sites, a second AG was virtually never found at positions −5 to −15 from the normal acceptor AG[14]; the new AG in the IVS-1 position 116 mutation occurs at positions −13 and −14.

In IVS-2, a mutation at position 654 (C→T) has been identified as a relatively common cause of β^{0}-thalassemia in Chinese persons.[177] The mutation creates a new donor GT splice site within IVS-2. Gene transfer and expression studies revealed that IVS-2 sequences of the mutant precursor β mRNA are partially spliced out in two steps: from the normal 5′ donor GT to a cryptic acceptor at position 579, then from the mutant donor site at position 654 to the normal 3′ acceptor.[177] As a result, a 75-bp segment of IVS-2 sequence is retained in the abnormally processed mRNA (Fig. 51-13). It is surprising that although the normal splice sites of IVS-2 are intact and located at a considerable distance from the mutation, no normal splicing is observed. A similar phenomenon occurs in the case of the mutation of IVS-2 at position 705 (T→G). There is an apparent absence of normal splicing, and two-step partial excision of

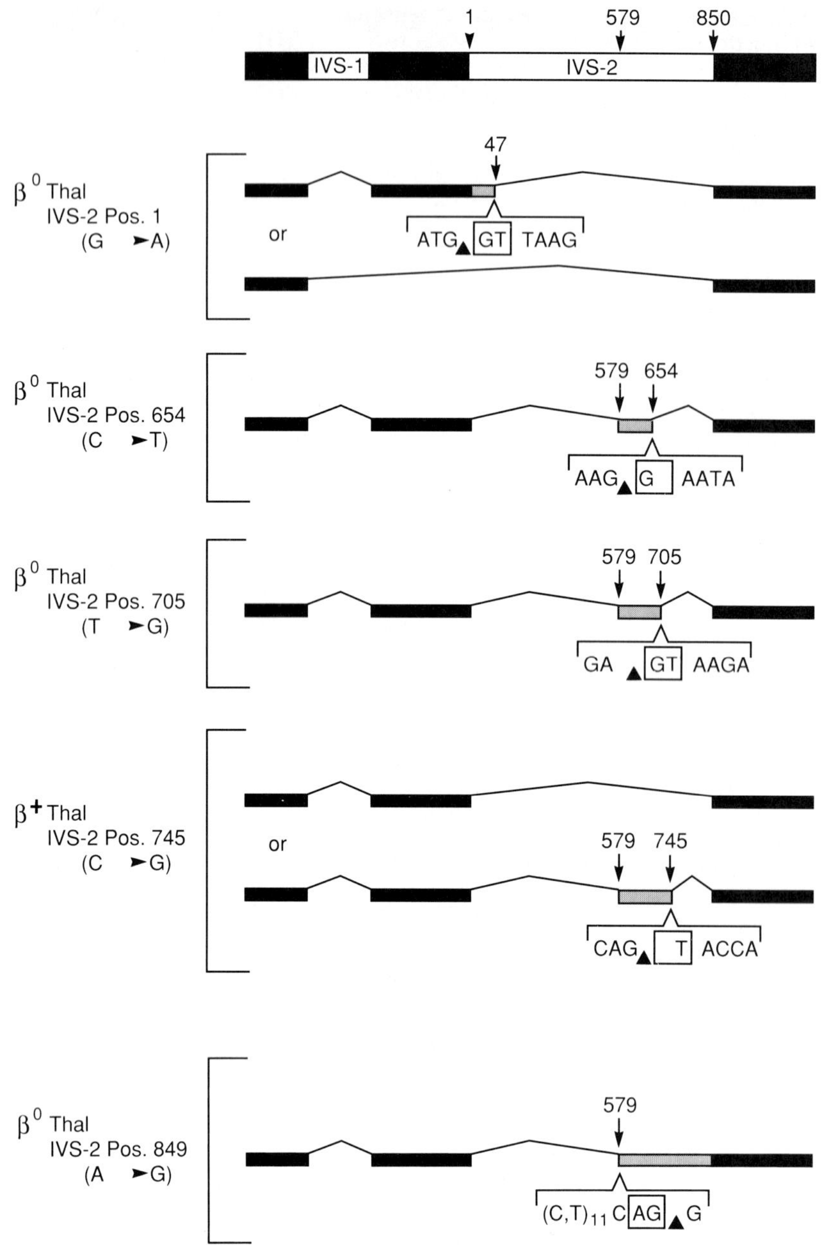

FIGURE 51-13. Splicing patterns associated with different thalassemic mutations in IVS-2 of the β-globin gene. The nucleotide sequences at the cryptic or alternative splicing sites are indicated, with the same conventions as in Figure 51-11. The same cryptic acceptor site at IVS-2 position 579 is used in many of the mutations. The portions of IVS-2 retained in the processed mRNAs are indicated by the gray boxes. (After Bunn HF, Forget BG. Hemoglobin: molecular, genetic and clinical aspects. Philadelphia, WB Saunders, 1986)

IVS-2 occurs (1) from the normal 5′ GT to the naturally occurring cryptic acceptor at position 579 and (2) from the cryptic donor site created by the mutation at position 705 to the normal 3′ acceptor AG.[193,267]

In contrast, another mutation of IVS-2 at position 745 also creates a new alternative donor splice site and is associated with a similar two-step excision of IVS-2 with use of the cryptic acceptor at position 654.[264] Some normal splicing of IVS-2 does occur[264]; therefore, this mutation results in β^+- rather than β^0-thalassemia.[264] The β^0 versus β^+ phenotype associated with these different mutations must be related to different affinities of the enzymatic splicing complex for a given mutant splice site versus the normal splice sites.

Mutations That Create New Alternative Splice Sites in Exons. Four mutations have been identified in exon 1 that are associated with activation of cryptic or alternative splice sites within exon 1 in a manner analogous to the mutations of the normal IVS-1 5′ consensus sequence (see previous section on mutations of the splice site consensus sequence that partially block normal splicing). In contrast to the latter group of mutations that activate three cryptic splice sites, the exon mutations activate only the one cryptic splice site that they modify. Three of these mutations are located in codons 24 to 27 (see Table 51-2) and activate the previously mentioned cryptic donor site that has a preexisting GT derived from codon 25. The mutations involve the nucleotides at positions −2, +3, and +6 of the consensus sequence. These mutations presumably increase the affinity of the preexisting cryptic splice site for the enzymatic splicing complex so that it is more readily recognized and used. The mutation at codon 24 is silent and does not change the encoded amino acid in the normally spliced β mRNA.[195]

The mutations at codon positions 26 and 27 do result in the encoding of amino acid replacements by the normally spliced β mRNA and the synthesis of structurally abnormal variant hemoglobins: *Hb E*[197] and *Hb Knossos*,[198] respectively. The phenotype associated with these mutations is that of β^+-thalassemia, because the normal 5′ splice site of IVS-1 is intact and variably used instead of the cryptic site at codon positions 24 to 27. The mutation at codon 24 is associated with a β^+-thalassemia phenotype of typical severity.[195] In contrast, Hb E and Hb Knossos are associated with relatively mild forms of β^+-thalassemia. In fact, Hb Knossos is usually associated with the silent carrier state for β-thalassemia.[268,269] Hb E, which is a common hemoglobin variant in Southeast Asia, was long known to be associated with the phenotype of mild β-thalassemia with hypochromia, microcytosis, and interaction with typical β-thalassemia resulting in a more severe clinical syndrome. The basis for the thalassemic phenotype did not become clear until gene cloning and expression studies.[197]

A mutation at codon 19 also results in a hemoglobin variant, *Hb Malay*, which is associated with a mild β^+-thalassemia phenotype.[194] The mutation involves the nucleotide at position +5 of the consensus sequence of a preexisting cryptic donor site at codon positions 17 to 19 of exon 1. This same cryptic site is also used in the case of mutations of the normal IVS-1 donor consensus sequence (see previous section on mutations of splice consensus sequence that partially block normal splicing). Gene expression studies have demonstrated that about 25% of the mRNA from the β Malay gene is abnormally spliced at the alternative splice site.[270]

Mutations That Produce Nonfunctional β-Globin mRNAs

Nonsense Mutations. Nonsense mutations result from single base substitutions that change a codon for a given amino acid to a chain termination codon and cause premature cessation of mRNA translation. Three mRNA chain termination codons are possible: UAA, UAG, and UGA or their DNA codons TAA, TAG, and TGA.

Truncated globin chains should be produced as a result of such mutations, but they are not usually detected, presumably because they are unstable and rapidly degraded. The phenotype is that of β^0-thalassemia with total absence of normal β-chain synthesis from the affected gene. In the nonsense mutation at codon 121 in exon 3, the phenotype in heterozygous persons is unusually severe and is associated with inclusion bodies and hemolytic anemia, as is also observed in frameshift mutations in exon 3 (see sections on frameshift mutations and on mutations resulting in unstable globin chains).

One of the first nonsense mutations to be characterized and extensively studied is the mutation at codon 39 (CAG to TAG), which is the second most common cause of β-thalassemia in the Mediterranean population. An interesting and poorly understood feature of this and other nonsense mutations is the finding of very low levels of the mutant β-globin mRNA in affected erythroid cells. Although the gene is transcribed normally, there appears to be defective mRNA stability in the nucleus or defective processing or transport of the mRNA from nucleus to cytoplasm. mRNA stability in the cytoplasm appears to be normal.[271–274] Thus, the basis for mRNA deficiency does not appear to be increased degradation due to lack of protection of the mRNA by ribosomes engaged in its full-length translation. In some as-yet-undetermined way, the inability of the mRNA to be normally translated interferes with the normal process of β-globin mRNA accumulation in affected erythroid cells.

Frameshift Mutations. Frameshift mutations result from the deletion or insertion of one or more nucleotides (other than multiples of three) in the protein encoding region of the gene. This causes a change in the normal reading frame of the encoded mRNA at the site of the mutation. Such mutations usually allow the continued translation of the mRNA for some distance, yielding a novel abnormal amino acid sequence until a chain termination codon is encountered in the new reading frame. Chain termination usually occurs at a position well before the normal termination codon and results in the synthesis of a truncated unstable mutant globin chain that is presumably rapidly degraded. The frameshift due to a 4-bp deletion at codon positions 41 and 42 is a particularly common mutation in persons of Chinese and Asian Indian ancestry.[155,231] The frameshift due to a single base deletion at codon 44 in Kurdish Jewish persons is associated with an unusually short β-globin mRNA half-life of 30 minutes.[275] The basis for this marked mRNA instability is unknown but appears to be restricted to erythroid cells, because the abnormal β-globin mRNA is stable after gene transfer and expression in HeLa cells.[276]

Although most frameshift mutations are associated with β^0-thalassemia, those that occur relatively far into the coding sequence (in exon 3) can result in the synthesis of detectable amounts of mutant β-globin chains and are therefore classified as $\beta^{(+)}$-thalassemia (see Table 51-2). In such cases, heterozygotes are more severely affected than persons with typical forms of heterozygous β^+- or β^0-thalassemia and manifest moderately severe anemia, splenomegaly, and inclusion body formation. The nonsense mutation at codon 121 of exon 3 is also associated with such a phenotype. The striking difference in phenotype between these cases and the more common forms of heterozygous β-thalassemia is probably due to the length and stability of the mutant β-globin chain, together with its ability to bind heme and produce aggregates that are relatively resistant to proteolytic degradation.[216,277] Other mechanisms may also be responsible for the dominant β-thalassemia phenotype associated with mutations in exon 3.[242]

Initiation Codon Mutations. As discussed earlier in this chapter, translation of globin mRNAs begins at the initiation codon AUG (or ATG in DNA), which encodes methionine. The initiator ATG is usually located within a consensus sequence (Kozak consensus) that probably constitutes part of the ribosome binding site of the mRNA.[19] Four different point mutations of the initiator ATG have been identified as causes of β^0-thalassemia (see Table 51-2). It is theoretically possible for the mutant mRNAs to be initiated at the next downstream ATG. In β-globin mRNA, the next ATG occurs in a different reading frame at codon positions 21 and 22 and the abnormal translation product would terminate about 40 codons further downstream, giving a short missense peptide unrelated to β-globin. In addition, this ATG is not located within a good Kozak consensus sequence. The only other inframe ATG in β-globin mRNA is at codon 55, and it is part of a better Kozak consensus sequence. Even if it were used, a nonfunctional and possibly unstable N-terminal truncated globin chain would be produced.

Mutations Resulting in Unstable Globin Chains

Many base substitutions result in amino replacements at residues that are crucial for globin chain stability. The globin chain that is synthesized is so unstable that little or no soluble mutant hemoglobin is detectable. In certain cases, such as in *Hb Terre Haute* (formerly called Hb Indianapolis),[261] the phenotype may be similar to that previously described for nonsense and frameshift mutations involving exon 3: hypochromia, microcytosis, and hemolytic anemia in heterozygotes, presumably due to membrane damage caused by precipitation and association of the mutant globin chain aggregates with the erythrocyte membrane.[278] In other cases, simply hypochromia and microcytosis without inclusion body formation or hemolysis are present, presumably because of more rapid and efficient proteolysis of the mutant globin chain. A number of such mutations have been identified in the β-globin gene (see Table 51-2; see also Chap. 52). A mild degree of hypochromia can also be associated with a number of additional unstable hemoglobins caused by the progressive loss of intracellular hemoglobin from precipitation and degradation.[279] In these cases, the β-globin chain that is initially synthesized is stable and assembled into hemoglobin tetramers that become progressively unstable. Variants of this type are not included in Table 51-2.

Deletions of the β-Globin Gene Resulting in β⁰-Thalassemia

Although most cases of β-thalassemia are due to point mutations, a few cases occur in which the cause is a partial or total deletion of the β-globin gene (Fig. 51-14). These deletions involve only the β-globin gene and its flanking DNA without affecting any of the other neighboring β-like globin genes.[160,280–293] In contrast, δβ-thalassemia and HPFH are associated with deletions, which encompass multiple genes in the cluster (see sections on deletions associated with δβ-thalassemia, γδβ-thalassemia, and hereditary persistence of fetal hemoglobin). The β-thalassemic deletions vary in size between 290 bp and 12.6 kb, excluding the smaller intragenic deletions of 17, 25, and 44 bp listed in Table 51-2 under splice site junction mutations. The phenotype associated with these deletions is that of β⁰-thalassemia.

The 0.6-kb deletion involving the 3′ of the β-globin gene is a relatively common cause of β⁰-thalassemia in Asian Indians and accounts for about one third of cases of β-thalassemia in this population.[155,290] The other β-gene deletions are relatively rare but have an interesting phenotype with *unusually high levels of HbA2 in heterozygotes.*[281–283,286,291,292] A common feature of these mutations is the deletion of the promoter region of the β-globin gene. It has been proposed that the unusually high level of HbA_2 may be due to the lack of competition between δ- and β-globin gene promoters for transcription factors, thus allowing more efficient expression of the δ-globin gene.[286] In this regard, the β-gene promoter mutation at position −88, and possibly that at position −29, are also associated with unexpectedly high levels of Hb A_2.[294]

Unknown, Possibly Distant, Mutations Causing β-Thalassemia

A small number of β-thalassemic patients carry β-globin genes that are entirely normal in structure. The cause of β-thalassemia in these cases is presumably a more remote mutation either within the β-globin gene cluster (perhaps in the LCR) or in another gene such as one for a specific transcription factor. The first family of this type to be studied was an Albanian family in which two children had β-thalassemia of intermediate severity (β-thalassemia intermedia). The mother had typical β-thalassemia trait, whereas the father apparently had the silent carrier trait.[295] One of the cloned β-globin genes from one of the affected children had a normal DNA sequence except for some sequence variation (−T, +ATA) at position −530 from the cap site.[296] This region of DNA is characterized by the presence of variable numbers of repeated AT and T residues, in different persons, that is suggestive of a polymorphism[297–299] (see the following section). Analysis of other β-globin cluster polymorphisms in this family initially indicated that the two affected children had inherited different β-globin gene clusters from their father. This suggests that the β-thalassemia determinant in the father did not reside nearby on chromosome 11 and could even be located on a different chromosome.[296]

Subsequent analysis revealed that both of the affected children had inherited the same sequence variation at −530, and the difference in the polymorphisms was attributed to a first-generation crossover between the two paternal alleles.[300] It has been proposed that the base changes found in the −530 region of the β gene in this family may be responsible for the β-thalassemia phenotype because of the increased binding of a putative negative regulatory *trans*-acting factor.[301] The same changes were also found in three siblings (of a Southern Italian family) who had β-thalassemia intermedia and an otherwise normal β gene,[302] further suggesting that the sequence variation point −530 might be functionally significant.

In another Italian family, two brothers with β-thalassemia intermedia also had the complex rearrangement at −530 (with an otherwise normal β-globin gene) in *trans* to the β39 nonsense mutation[303]; one of the affected brothers had a child with β-thalassemia major who inherited the father's β39 nonsense mutation (without the −530 rearrangement) and a structurally normal β-globin gene from an apparently normal mother.

In a study of 100 β-thalassemia genes, Kazazian and coworkers[137,138] identified nine persons in whom the β-globin gene had a normal DNA sequence from a point 600 nucleotides 5′ to the cap site to a point 200 nucleotides 3′ to the end of the gene, as well as a normal DNA sequence of the 400-bp enhancer region located about 0.7 kb 3′ to the gene. These cases appear to represent truly unknown mutations.

Polymorphisms of the Globin Gene Clusters

In contrast to the DNA of exons that shows little or no sequence variability among individuals, the DNA between genes and that of introns can vary significantly in its nucleotide sequence from one person to another; an estimated 1 of every 200 to 400 nucleotides of extragenic DNA may be different in any two persons. Such sequence variability has proved to be informative in a number of genetic studies because it provides a type of marker or fingerprint for a person's genome.

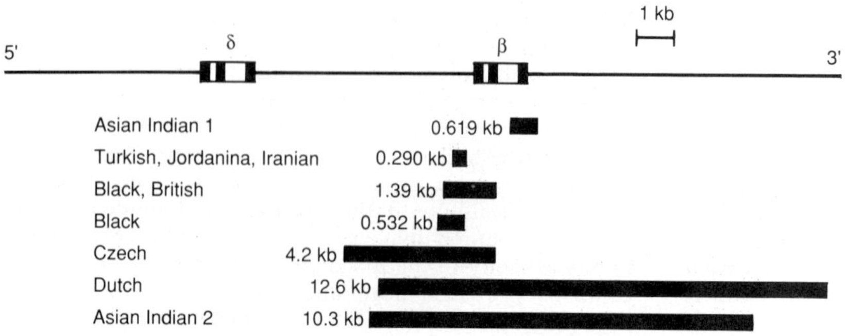

FIGURE 51-14. Deletions of the β-globin gene and flanking DNA associated with β⁰-thalassemia. (After Craig JE, Kelly SJ, Barnetson R, Thein SL. Molecular characterization of a novel 10.3 kb deletion causing β-thalassaemia with unusually high Hb A_2. Br J Haematol 1992;82:735)

Sequence variability is most frequently detected by restriction endonuclease digestion and Southern gel blotting of total cellular DNA, followed by hybridization to a labeled DNA probe from the gene region of interest. The generation of DNA fragments of different sizes in different persons provides evidence for sequence variability in the region of DNA tested; this is called restriction fragment length polymorphism (RFLP). A large number of such polymorphisms have been identified in the β-globin gene cluster. They are found in intergene as well as intervening sequence DNA, and one polymorphism is even present in the coding sequence of the β-globin gene but without causing a change in amino acid sequence. Most of these polymorphisms are common and widely distributed among different racial groups. The location and nature of some of these RFLPs are illustrated in Figure 51-15. These different polymorphisms are not associated with one another in a totally random manner but tend to occur in certain groupings or subsets called *haplotypes*.[304–306]

The nine major haplotypes of the β-gene cluster are illustrated in Figure 51-15. Orkin and coworkers[140] first demonstrated that, in Mediterraneans, different specific β-thalassemia mutations were associated with different haplotypes. The determination of haplotypes by gene mapping therefore provided a relatively simple screening test to identify the most probable mutation in an affected person or to help identify the persons with novel mutations. This strategy was successfully applied to a systematic survey of β-thalassemia mutations in different population groups such as Asian Indians, Chinese, and American blacks.[305,306] Haplotype analysis has also been a useful procedure in prenatal diagnosis of β-thalassemia by analysis of DNA from amniocentesis samples or chorionic villus biopsies (see later section of this chapter on use of restriction fragment length polymorphisms in DNA-based prenatal diagnosis).

RFLPs have also been identified in the α-globin gene cluster and a number of different α cluster haplotypes have been defined.[307–310] As in the β-globin gene cluster, many of these RFLPs are due to single base changes that abolish or create a restriction endonuclease site. A second type of RFLP is also present that is due to the presence of variable numbers of short, tandemly repeated DNA sequences. Such clusters of variable DNA, called hypervariable regions, have been identified at the 3′ end of the cluster, within the introns of the ζ and $\psi\zeta$ genes, between the $\psi\zeta$ and ζ genes, and at a site about 70 kb 5′ of the ζ gene.[308] These polymorphisms have proved useful in the study of the population genetics of α-thalassemia mutations.

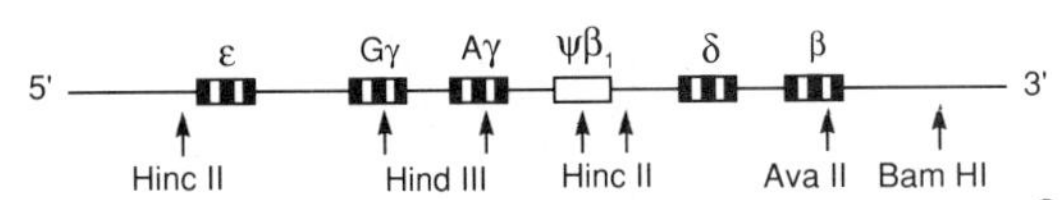

Haplotypes	Hinc II	Hind III	Hind III	Hinc II	Hinc II	Ava II	Bam HI	Overall Frequency
I	+	−	−	−	−	+	+	47%
II	−	+	+	−	+	+	+	17%
III	−	+	−	+	+	+	−	8%
IV	−	+	−	+	+	−	+	1%
V	+	−	−	−	−	+	−	12%
VI	−	+	+	−	−	−	+	6%
VII	+	−	−	−	−	−	+	6%
VIII	−	+	−	+	−	+	−	1%
IX	−	+	−	+	+	+	+	3%

FIGURE 51-15. Different haplotypes of restriction site polymorphisms in the β-gene cluster and their frequency in Mediterranean individuals with β-thalassemia. A plus sign indicates the presence and a minus sign the absence of the particular restriction endonuclease cleavage site. (After Orkin SH, Kazazian HH Jr, Antonarakis SE, et al. Linkage of β-thalassemic mutations and β-globin gene polymorphisms with DNA polymorphisms in the human β-globin gene cluster. Nature 1982;296:627)

Association of RFLP Haplotypes With β-Thalassemia Mutations and Population Genetics of β-Thalassemia and Other β-Chain Hemoglobinopathies

The prevalence of different haplotypes in Mediterranean β-thalassemic patients is shown in Figure 51-15. Follow-up studies of this population using synthetic oligonucleotides (or restriction endonuclease digestion) for direct identification of thalassemic mutations have led to some interesting observations. In general, a given haplotype within this population is usually associated with one specific type of thalassemia. Thus, by haplotype analysis, one can predict with about 90% accuracy the specific mutation causing β-thalassemia in a given person. Exceptions are the following: more than one type of thalassemia mutation can be found within a given haplotype, and a specific type of thalassemia mutation may be associated with two or more different haplotypes in the same population. In haplotype I, which is the most common haplotype in Mediterranean β-thalassemic patients (see Fig. 51-15), about 90% of cases are associated with the mutation at IVS-1 position 110.[311]

Other β-thalassemia mutations are also associated with haplotype I in Mediterraneans: the frameshift mutation at codon 6, Hb Knossos, and even the β codon 39 nonsense mutation. Thus, it cannot be assumed that all Mediterranean β-thalassemic persons with haplotype I have the IVS-1 position 110 mutation. This result is not totally surprising; multiple different independent mutations might be expected to occur on the same chromosomal background if the latter is particularly common in a given normal population, as is haplotype I.

Although a number of examples have been found of the association of a given specific β-thalassemia mutation with more than one different haplotype, the most interesting cases consist of the β-codon 39 nonsense and β^E-globin genes. The β-codon 39 nonsense mutation was shown to be associated with at least nine different chromosomes.[312] In seven of these chromosomes, RFLPs within (or close to) the β-globin gene itself were identical. Thus, one could explain the observation by a single mutation in an ancestral β-globin gene that then spread to other chromosomes by recombination, the crossover site being located between the 5′ side of the β-globin gene and the 3′ side of the polymorphic *HincII* sites around the $\psi\beta1$ gene (see Fig. 51-15). It has been proposed that this region of DNA contains a hot spot for recombination.[304,313]

The β-codon 39 nonsense mutation has also been identified in β-globin genes with different intragenic polymorphic sites or, in the terminology of Orkin and Kazazian,[306] in different *β-globin gene "frameworks."* There are three (or four) basic β-globin gene frameworks that differ by two to five intragenic nucleotide base substitutions.[305,306] The occurrence of the same mutation in two different β-gene frameworks, especially in two frameworks differing by five nucleotides (one in exon 1 and four in IVS-2) implies that the identical mutation must have arisen spontaneously at least twice, once in each framework.

Alternatively, if one holds to the theory of a single ancestral mutation, the findings can be explained only by a rare localized interchromosomal recombination event called gene conversion. Such short discrete recombination or gene conversion events appear to have occurred in the γ-globin genes (in IVS-2) as well as in the histocompatibility and immunoglobulin genes. The Hb E mutation in Asian populations has been identified in two different β-globin gene frameworks, differing by four nucleotides.[314] This finding must also be explained by the occurrence of independent identical mutations or short gene conversion events. A similar phenomenon has also been observed with the Hb S mutation.

The comparison of haplotypes and β-thalassemic mutations in different populations has provided the interesting finding that the same haplotype is generally associated with different forms of β-thalassemia in different populations. In fact, a given β-thalassemia mutation generally appears to be restricted to a particular population, because the same mutation is not usually found in two different racial groups. Of the more than 100 mutations listed in Table 51-2, only 11 have been described in more than one racial group.[137] In such instances, the chromosomal background (haplotype or β-globin gene framework or both) is almost always different in the separate racial groups, indicating that the mutations most likely had independent origins in the different populations.[137]

Molecular Basis of α-Thalassemia

In contrast to β-thalassemia, in which most cases are due to point mutations, the major cause of α-thalassemia consists of deletions that remove one or both α-globin genes from the affected chromosome 16. Nevertheless, a number of nondeletion cases of α-thalassemia have been characterized, and these are generally due to types of point mutations similar to those that cause β-thalassemia.

α-Thalassemia was first intensively studied in Asian populations, where it occurs at a very high incidence. Four main clinical types of α-thalassemia syndromes of progressively increasing severity were defined in this population and were thought to be caused by deletion or inactivating mutation of one, two, three, or four of the α-globin gene loci (Fig. 51-16). The four syndromes were called (1) α-thalassemia-2 or silent carrier state (one inactive α-globin gene); (2) α-thalassemia-1 (two inactive α-globin genes); (3) Hb H disease (three inactive α-globin genes), due to double heterozygosity for α-thalassemia-2 plus α-thalassemia-1; and (4) hydrops fetalis with Hb Bart's (four inactive α-globin genes), due to homozygosity for α-thalassemia-1. An additional common type of α-thalassemia syndrome identified in Asians is associated with the inheritance of Hb Constant Spring (Hb CS), a hemoglobin variant with an elongated α-globin chain due to an α-chain termination mutation (see section on nondeletion forms of α-thalassemia), which interacts with α-thalassemia-1 in the same manner as does α-thalassemia-2 to cause Hb H disease. The hematologic and clinical characteristics of these different conditions are discussed later in this chapter.

On the other hand, the results of genetic analyses in blacks with α-thalassemia did not fit the model proposed for the inheritance of α-thalassemia in Asians. Although the incidence of apparent heterozygous α-thalassemia (α-thalassemia-1 phenotype) was high in blacks, hydrops fetalis was never observed and Hb H disease was rare. It was therefore proposed that the α-thalassemia-1 phenotype in blacks might be associated with the deletion or inactivation of two α-globin genes, but on opposite chromosomes (in *trans*) rather than on the same chromosome (in *cis*), as in Asians (see Fig. 51-16).

The availability of molecular hybridization assays, in particular gene quantitation by DNA–cDNA hybridization assays in solution, led to the first confirmation of some of the genetic theories on the molecular basis of α-thalassemia by demonstrating the actual absence or deletion of the predicted number of α-globin genes in the different α-thalassemia syndromes.[315] The refinement of gene mapping technology (Southern gel blotting) provided additional confirmation of α-globin gene deletions as a cause of α-thalassemia and permitted the characterization of the location and extent of these deletions within the affected α-globin gene cluster. More than 20 different deletions have been identified in the α-globin gene cluster, most of which are illustrated in Figure 51-17. Most result in deletion or inactivation of both α-globin genes on the same chromosome, whereas some are associated with the deletion of only one α-globin gene per chromosome.[308–310]

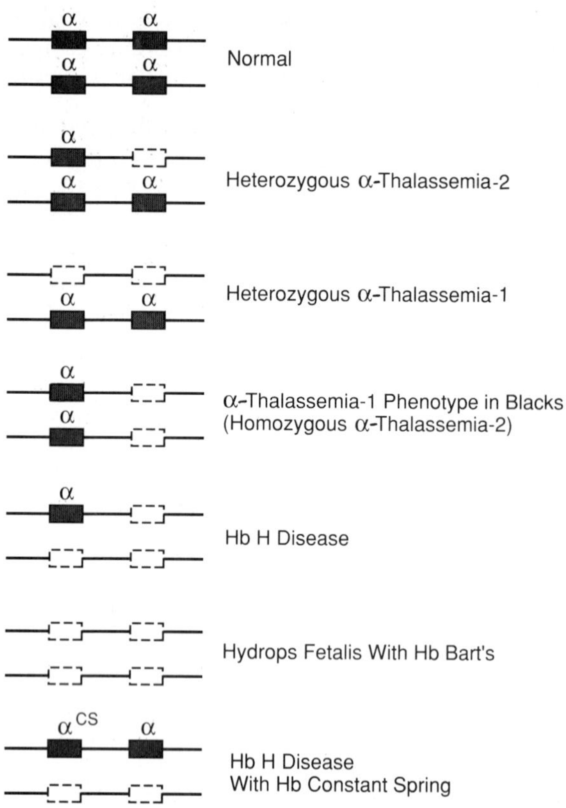

FIGURE 51-16. Model of α-globin gene deletions as the molecular basis for the various α-thalassemia syndromes. Gene deletions are represented by the dashed blocks. (After Bunn HF, Forget BG. Hemoglobin: molecular, genetic and clinical aspects. Philadelphia, WB Saunders, 1986)

Deletion of a Single α-Globin Gene Causing α-Thalassemia-2, or α^+-Thalassemia, Designated $-\alpha$

The heterozygous state for the deletion of a single α-globin gene or silent carrier state can be easily detected by the technique of Southern gel blotting. Normal DNA with two α-globin genes per haploid genome after digestion with the restriction endonuclease *Bam*HI, and hybridization to an α-gene probe yields a single band of about 14 kb. DNA from persons who are obligate carriers for α-thalassemia-2 yields a second shorter band of about 10.5 kb in addition to the normal band.

Detailed restriction endonuclease mapping of the shorter abnormal α-globin gene DNA fragment found in α-thalassemia-2 has established that it contains only one of the two α-globin genes. By using various restriction endonucleases, six different types of (−α) deletions have been defined[137,308–310] (see Fig. 51-17):

1. A deletion of about 3.7 kb (by far the most common) found in Asians, Mediterraneans, and blacks, consistent with a deletion created by nonhomologous crossing over between two α-globin loci, which has been called the rightward deletion and designated $-\alpha^{3.7}$.[316] There are three distinct subtypes of this deletion—

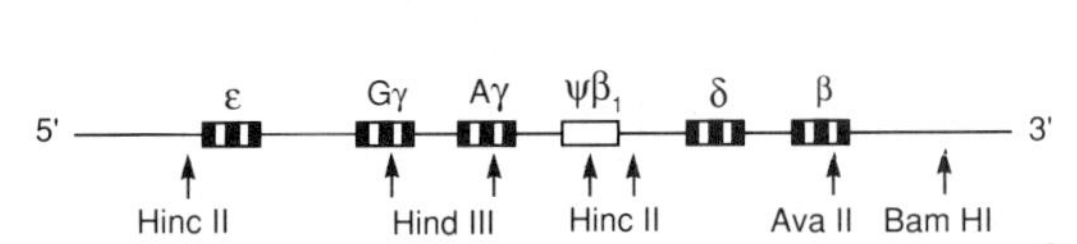

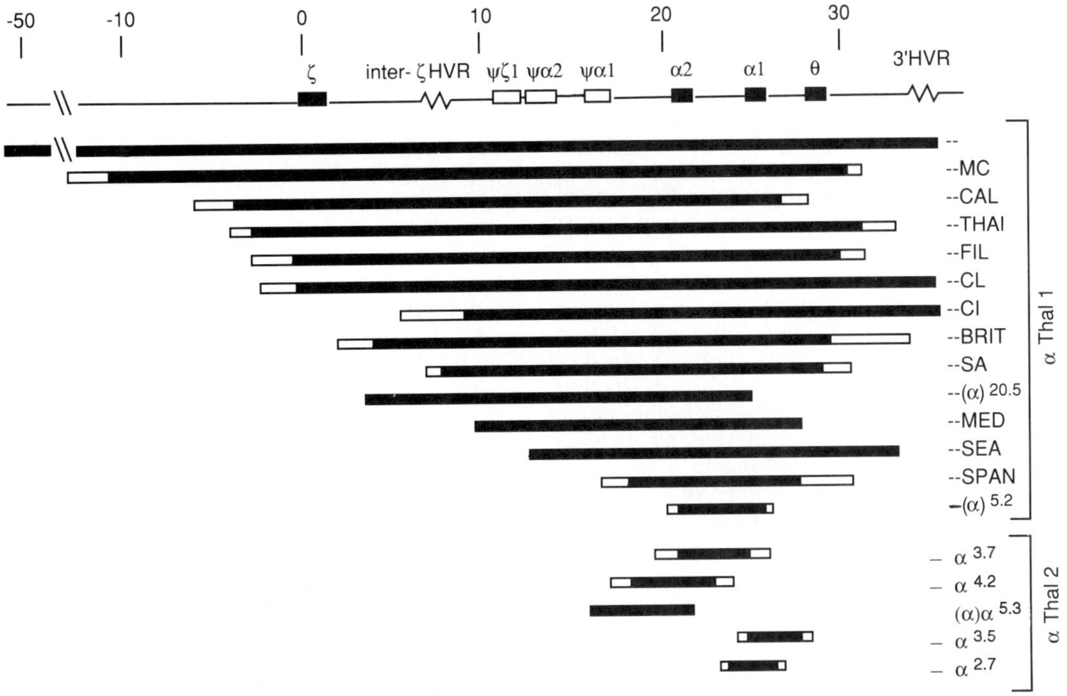

FIGURE 51-17. Extent of various deletions in the α-globin gene cluster associated with α-thalassemia. Reference citations for the individual mutations can be found in the text and elsewhere.[308] (After Higgs DR, Vickers MA, Wilkie AOM, et al. A review of the molecular genetics of the human α-globin gene cluster. Blood 1989;73:1081)

designated types I, II, and III—because of the different sites of crossover between the two α loci.

2. A deletion of about 4.2 kb, found in Southeast Asians and rarely in blacks, consistent with deletion of the 5′ or α2-globin gene, which has been called the leftward deletion and designated $\alpha^{4.2}$.[316]
3. A rare deletion of about 3.5 kb, identified in two Asian Indians, consistent with deletions of the 3′ or α1-globin gene and designated $-\alpha^{3.5}$.[317]
4. A rare deletion of about 2.7 kb in a Chinese family, designated $-\alpha^{2.7}$.[318]
5. A rare deletion of 5.3 kb in an Italian family, designated $(\alpha)\alpha^{5.3}$.[319]
6. A rare deletion of more than 18 kb, involving the α1 and θ1 genes as well as the 3′ hypervariable region of the α cluster, identified in a Czech person[320] (not shown in Fig. 51-17).

Mechanisms of α-Globin Gene Deletion

Structural analysis of the α-globin gene cluster has revealed the presence of homologous stretches of flanking or intergene DNA sequences, which form α-globin gene duplication units of about 4 kb and could serve as foci for nonhomologous crossover or recombination. These homologous duplicated segments are indicated by the boxes labeled X, Y, and Z in Figure 51-18. The two common forms of α-thalassemia-2, $-\alpha^{3.7}$ and $-\alpha^{4.2}$, are thought to result from recombination events involving different segments of this duplication unit. Thus, the common rightward $-\alpha^{3.7}$ deletion would result from mispairing and recombination between the duplicated homologous sequences located in segment Z. The leftward $-\alpha^{4.2}$ deletion would result from misspairing and recombination between the homologous sequences located in segment X (see Fig. 51-18). When recombinant DNA bacteriophage containing the cloned normal human α-globin gene cluster are grown in culture, recombination frequently occurs, generating deletions of a similar nature to those observed in the naturally occurring $-\alpha^{3.7}$ and $-\alpha^{4.2}$ thalassemias. As previously noted, the $-\alpha^{3.7}$ deletion is itself heterogeneous and three different forms have been described—designated $-\alpha^{3.7\text{I}}$, $-\alpha^{3.7\text{II}}$, and $-\alpha^{3.7\text{III}}$—because of crossovers occurring at different points within segment Z.

The unequal crossover mechanism described above predicts the occurrence in some persons of the reciprocal product of such a recombination event, that is, a chromosome bearing three α-globin gene loci. Such is the case,

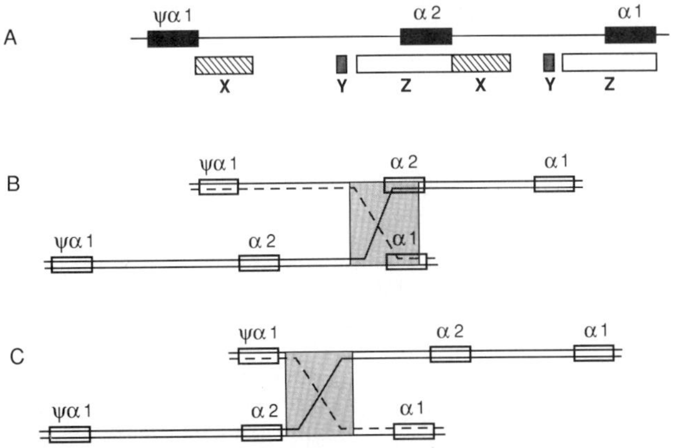

FIGURE 51-18. Model of unequal crossover events in the α-globin gene cluster resulting in α-thalassemia-2 deletions and reciprocal triple α-gene clusters. (**A**) The X, Y, and Z homology blocks in the region of the α-globin genes are shown. (**B**) Mispairings and crossing over in the Z homology block produce a $-\alpha^{3.7}$ chromosome containing a 3.7-kb deletion (*dashed line*). The reciprocal of this event (*solid line*) is a triple α chromosome. (**C**) Mispairing and crossing over in the X homology block produces a single chromosome with a 4.2-kb deletion (*dashed line*). The reciprocal of this event (*solid line*) is also a triple α chromosome. (After Kazazian HH Jr. The thalassemia syndromes: molecular basis and prenatal diagnosis in 1990. Semin Hematol 1990;27:209)

and both possible reciprocal chromosomes, $\alpha\alpha\alpha^{anti\text{-}3.7}$ and $\alpha\alpha\alpha^{anti\text{-}4.2}$, have been found.[308–310] Occasional chromosomes with quadruplicated α-globin genes $\alpha\alpha\alpha\alpha^{anti\text{-}3.7}$ and $\alpha\alpha\alpha\alpha^{anti\text{-}4.2}$ have also been observed, presumably having resulted from subsequent recombination events involving a triplicated locus with a normal locus.[308] The frequency of the ααα-chromosome is unexpectedly high, ranging from 0.01 to 0.08; it has been found in most populations that have been studied, including those in which α-thalassemia is rare.[308]

The possible role of malaria and other selective pressures in causing the high frequency of the ααα chromosome is unknown. Another interesting feature of the ααα locus is that affected homozygotes are hematologically normal even with an excess of α-globin mRNA and α-globin chain synthesis in their erythroid cells.[321] The possibility exists that in some circumstances a mild β-thalassemia phenotype may be conferred by the excess α-globin chain synthesis as a result of the ααα cluster, resulting in a more severe than expected phenotype when one or two ααα chromosomes are coinherited with heterozygous β-thalassemia.[321–323]

The two linked α-globin genes are known to be expressed at different levels: the 5′ or α2-globin gene is expressed at a level about three-fold higher than that of the 3′ or α1-globin gene.[324,325] Therefore, the clinical phenotype of α-thalassemia would be expected to be more severe with deletion or inactivity of the α2 gene. This is generally true in the case of the nondeletion forms of α-thalassemia (see section on nondeletion forms of α-thalassemia). In deletions causing α-thalassemia-2, the situation is more complex, and compensatory mechanisms appear to modify the expected result. Thus, homozygotes for the leftward deletion, who lack both α2 genes, express more α-globin than the expected 25% of normal, and homozygotes for the rightward deletion, who have two hybrid α2/α1 genes express less α-globin than the expected 75% of normal.[326] Nevertheless, the clinical phenotype associated with homozygosity for the $-\alpha^{4.2}$ deletion is more severe than that associated with homozygosity for the $-\alpha^{3.7}$ deletion.[326] It has been estimated that the level of expression of the $-\alpha^{3.7}$ hybrid gene is intermediate between that of a normal α2 and α1 gene,[327] even though the promoter and 5′ flanking DNA of the $-\alpha^{3.7}$ gene is that of the α2 gene and would be expected to direct the synthesis or accumulation of more α-globin mRNA than is actually observed. The precise mechanisms responsible for this phenomenon are unknown.

Homozygosity for α-Thalassemia-2 (−α) as a Cause of the α-Thalassemia-1 Phenotype

When Southern gel blotting was carried out using DNA from blacks with the α-thalassemia-1 phenotype (hematologically apparent α-thalassemia trait), the results were consistent with the genotype −α/−α.[117,328] This observation confirmed earlier theories that black persons with the α-thalassemia-1 phenotype were likely to carry deletions of two α-globin genes *in trans*, −α/−α (homozygosity for α-thalassemia-2), rather than *in cis*, −−/αα, as is the case in Asian subjects heterozygous for α-thalassemia-1 (see Fig. 51-16 and following section). These findings, therefore, provided a definitive explanation for the lack of hydrops fetalis and the rarity of Hb H disease in blacks. Because the α-thalassemia chromosome prevalent in the black population almost always carries one normal α-globin gene (−α), it is virtually impossible for blacks to inherit the genotype found in Asian infants with hydrops fetalis, who lack all four globin genes. The rare cases of Hb H disease in blacks result from inheritance of the prevalent α-thalassemic chromosome together with a much rarer α-thalassemic chromosome in which both α-globin genes are deleted or inactive (see next section).

Another corollary of the above findings is that the heterozygous state for α-thalassemia-2 must be extremely prevalent in the black population. If the prevalence of the α-thalassemia-1 phenotype (homozygous α-thalassemia-2) is 1% to 2% in the black population, then heterozygosity for α-thalassemia-2 must approach 30%. In fact, a survey of a large number of black Americans revealed that 27.5% were heterozygous for the α-thalassemia genotype (−α/αα) and 1.9% were homozygous (−α/−α); the overall frequency of the single α-globin locus was calculated to be 0.16 in this population.[117]

Deletion Causing Lack of Expression of Both α-Globin Genes on One Chromosome: α-Thalassemia-1 or α⁰-Thalassemia

A large number of different deletions have been characterized that inactivate both α-globin genes on the same chromosome (in *cis*) and result in the phenotype of α-thalassemia-1 in heterozygotes. Most of these deletions completely remove both α genes and are designated as −−; two deletions retain portions of one α-globin gene and are designated $-(\alpha)^{5.2}$ and $-(\alpha)^{20.5}$, respectively, according to the total size of the deletion[308,309,329] (see Fig. 51-17). Four different and interesting deletions, designated $(\alpha\alpha)^{RA}$, $(\alpha\alpha)^{MM}$, $(\alpha\alpha)^{TI}$, and $(\alpha\alpha)^{IJ}$, respectively, leave both α-globin genes intact but involve varying amounts of DNA located 5′ to the α cluster (Fig. 51-19). In $(\alpha\alpha)^{RA}$, the approximately 62-kb deletion includes the ζ-globin gene and about 50 kb of upstream DNA.[329,330] In $(\alpha\alpha)^{MM}$, the deletion begins about 7kb 5′ to the ζ gene and extends in the 5′ for at least 105 kb, without involving the telomere.[331] In $(\alpha\alpha)^{TI}$, the deletion begins about 30 kb 5′ to the ζ gene and extends to and includes the telomere (tip) of the short arm of chromosome 16.[332] In $(\alpha\alpha)^{IJ}$, the deletion involves about 35 kb of DNA 5′ to the ζ gene, starting at a point 28 kb 5′ to the gene.[333] The clinical phenotype associated with these unusual deletions is that of α-thalassemia-1, and it is thought that the α-globin

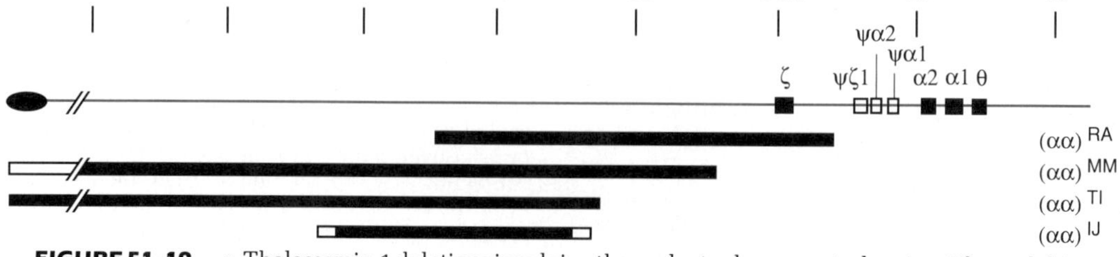

FIGURE 51-19. α-Thalassemia-1 deletions involving the α-cluster locus control region. The α-globin genes are intact but inactive. The telomere of the short arm of chromosome 16 is indicated by the oval at the far left of the α-gene cluster. (After Higgs DR. α-Thalassemias. Bailliere Clin Hematol 1993;6: 117)

genes on the affected chromosomes are totally (or partially) inactive because of the absence in the upstream DNA of an important *cis*-acting element analogous to the β-gene cluster (see section on enhancers and other *cis*-acting sequences and section on γδβ-thalassemia). Functional studies in transgenic mice and in MEL cells after gene transfer, as well as in vivo footprinting studies of erythroleukemia cell lines, have confirmed the existence of LCR-like sequences in the DNA, which is deleted in the (αα)-thalassemia syndromes.[49,334,335]

The most frequently encountered α-thalassemia-1 mutations are the $--^{SEA}$ deletion found in Southeast Asians, the $--^{MED}$ deletion found in Mediterranean persons, and the $--^{FIL}$ deletion found in Filipinos (see Fig. 51-17). The $--^{FIL}$ deletion, which accounts for about 30% of α-thalassemia genes in Filipinos, involves the entire α-globin gene cluster including the functional ζ-globin gene. Homozygosity for this and other deletions involving the ζ gene would not be expected to allow development of the embryo beyond the earliest stages of pregnancy because of total absence of functional embryonic hemoglobin. In contrast, heterozygotes develop normally. The common $--^{SEA}$ deletion, which reaches a gene frequency of 0.1 to 0.2 in certain regions of Southeast Asia, encompasses the θ-globin gene located 3′ to the α1-globin gene. Homozygosity for this deletion clearly allows development beyond the early stages of gestation and there is at least one child with hydrops fetalis due to this deletion who has survived through treatment with blood transfusions and who has apparently developed normally.[336,337] These observations indicate that the presence (or function) of the θ-globin gene is not essential for normal development. Heterozygotes for this and other deletions that preserve the ζ gene express low levels of ζ-globin (less than 1% of total globin) in adult life.[338]

The infrequent cases of Hb H disease in blacks are associated with the inheritance of the following α-thalassemia-1 mutations: $--^{BRIT}$[308,339] (see Fig. 51-17), an incompletely characterized deletion involving the entire α cluster,[340] an approximately 8.5 kb deletion including the α2-, α1-, and θ1-globin genes[341] and mutations, including an initiation codon mutation,[353] a framework mutation in codon 31,[350] and the Hb Evanston missense mutation,[361] affecting the remaining α gene on an -α3.7 α-thalassemia-2 allele.

The mechanism that gave rise to most of the α^0-thalassemia deletions is different from that described for the α^+-thalassemia deletions and, with one exception, consisted of illegitimate recombination events between nonhomologous segments of DNA.[329] In the human genome, a number of different types of repetitive DNA sequences exist, which are primarily located in the intergene DNA and sometimes in introns. One of these families of repetitive DNA sequences is called the *AluI* family because of the usual presence of the recognition site for that particular restriction endonuclease within the repetitive sequence. *AluI* repetitive sequences are about 300 bp in length, occur about 300,000 times within the human genome, and share about 80% homology with one another.[342,343] A number of copies of *AluI* repetitive sequences are found in both the α- and β-globin gene clusters. In some gene systems, recombination between homologous *AluI* repetitive sequences has resulted in gene deletion events. The $(\alpha\alpha)^{RA}$ α-thalassemia deletion appears to have resulted from such a recombination event between two *AluI* repetitive sequences located 62 kb apart.[329]

In other α^0-thalassemia deletions, *AluI* repetitive DNA sequences are frequently found at or near one of the breakpoints, but the significance of this finding is unclear. The 3′ breakpoints of many of the α^0-thalassemia deletions tend to cluster in a 6- to 8-kb region of DNA between the α1-globin gene and a hypervariable region of DNA (3′ HVR in Fig. 51-17) located about 10 kb downstream. Analysis of polymorphisms (RFLPs) in the 5′ flanking DNA of the common $--^{MED}$ and $--^{SEA}$ α^0-thalassemia deletions indicates that these mutations probably arose only once during evolution. Therefore, their high frequency must be attributed to positive selection due to malaria.[308]

Nondeletion Forms of α-Thalassemia

Although rare, a number of different point mutations have been identified as causes of α-thalassemia (Table 51-3). In general, these mutations fall into the same categories or classes of point mutations that have been identified and previously discussed as causes of β-thalassemia (see section on the molecular basis of β-thalassemia): nonfunctional mRNA due to initiation codon mutations, nonsense mutations or frameshifts, splicing defects, polyadenylation signal defects, and unstable globin chains. In fact, nondeletion forms of α-thalassemia provided the first examples of initiator codon[351] and polyadenylation signal[344] mutations. The unstable $\alpha^{Quong\ Sze}$ globin chain is the prototypical example of an extremely unstable globin chain associated

TABLE 51-3. Nondeletion Forms of α-Thalassemia

Mutation	Racial Group	Affected Gene	References
CLEAVAGE/POLYADENYLATION MUTATIONS			
AATAAA → AATAAG	Arab	α2	344, 345
AATAAA → AATGAA	Turkish	α2	346
SPLICING MUTATION			
IVS-1 donor site, 5-bp deletion	Mediterranean	α2	347, 348
MUTATIONS PRODUCING NONFUNCTIONAL mRNAs			
Nonsense mutation			
Codon 116 (G → T)	Black	α2	349
Frameshift mutation			
−2 codon 31 (−AG)	Black	$-\alpha^{3.7}$	350
Initiator codon mutations			
ATG → ACG	Mediterranean	α2	351
ATG → GTG	Mediterranean	α1	352
	Black	$-\alpha^{3.7}$	353
CCACCATG → CC—CATG	North African	$-\alpha^{3.7}$	354
	Mediterranean	$-\alpha^{3.7}$	355
CHAIN TERMINATION MUTATIONS			
Hb Constant Spring (TAA → CAA)	Southeast Asian	α2	356, 357
Hb Icaria (TAA → AAA)	Mediterranean	α2	358
Hb Koya Dora (TAA → TCA)	Asian Indian	α2	359
Hb Seal Rock (TAA → GAA)	Black	α2	360
MISSENSE MUTATIONS PRODUCING UNSTABLE GLOBINS			
Codon 14 (Trp → Arg), Hb Evanston	Black	$-\alpha^{3.7}$	361
Codon 109 (Leu → Arg), Hb Suan Dok	Southeast Asian	α2	362
Codon 110 (Ala → Asp), Hb Petah Tikvah	Middle Eastern	α	363
Codon 125 (Leu → Pro) Hb Quong Sze	Southeast Asian	α2	364

in heterozygotes with a phenotype of typical thalassemia trait without detectable hemolysis or abnormal globin chains, except as a radioactive product in short (5 to 20 minutes) pulse-labeling experiments.[364] One unusual initiator codon mutation involves the adjacent Kozak consensus sequence (deletion of nucleotides −2 and −3) rather than the ATG itself: CCCACCATG → CCCCATG.[354] This mutation illustrates the importance for proper chain initiation of the nucleotides flanking the ATG, particularly the requirement for a purine (usually A) in position −3.[19]

An especially novel form of nondeletion α-thalassemia consists of the chain termination mutants, *Hb Constant Spring* (found not uncommonly in Southeast Asians), *Hb Koya Dora*, *Hb Icaria*, and *Hb Seal Rock*.[356–360] These mutants are due to four different base substitutions in the normal α-chain termination codon, changing it to a codon for one of four different amino acids, respectively, and allowing read-through of the 3′ untranslated sequence of the α mRNA until a new in-phase termination codon is encountered 31 codons later. The striking feature of these four elongated α-chain variants is that they are present in only very low amounts in RBCs of heterozygotes (1% to 2% of the total hemoglobin)—hence the α-thalassemia phenotype.

The precise molecular basis for the uniformly very low level of expression of these chain termination mutants is not clear. It is clear that the low level of Hb Constant Spring is not due primarily to instability of the mutant globin chain itself, because biosynthetic studies reveal that the variant globin chain does not have a high specific activity and is therefore not rapidly turning over in reticulocytes or marrow cells. The rate of globin chain elongation, or translation time, was also measured and found to be the same for α^{CS}-globin chains as for normal α^{A}-globin chains. The mutant α-globin chain is synthesized almost exclusively in bone marrow erythroid cells rather than in peripheral blood, and α^{CS}-globin mRNA is virtually absent in reticulocyte mRNA of affected persons, suggesting the possibility of instability of α^{CS} mRNA as a basis for the low level of synthesis of the mutant globin chain.[325,365]

With one exception, all of the nondeletion α-thalassemia mutations affect the more strongly expressed α2-globin gene. In contrast to the $-\alpha^{4.2}$ deletion of the α2 gene, no compensatory increase occurs in the expression of the linked α1 gene. Therefore, the clinical phenotype associated with these nondeletion mutants is more severe than that of the common −α determinants and more closely resembles that of α-thalassemia-1 rather than α-thalassemia-2. The initiator codon mutation that affects the α1-globin gene is associated with a mild clinical phenotype.[352]

Acquired α-Thalassemia

Two distinct α-thalassemia syndromes are due to acquired or de novo mutations of the α-globin genes: Hb H disease associated with myeloproliferative disorders and Hb H disease associated with mental retardation.

Acquired Hb H Disease Associated With Myeloproliferative Disorders. Hb H disease has occasionally been observed to develop during the course of erythroleukemia or other myeloproliferative disorders, including preleukemic syndromes, such as myelofibrosis and refractory anemia, which eventually progress to acute nonlymphocytic leukemia.[308,310,366] The disorder usually affects elderly males over the age of 60 and is characterized by a dimorphic blood smear containing both normal RBCs and hypochromic RBCs from the leukemic clone that contain numerous inclusion bodies of Hb H after incubation with brilliant cresyl blue. As the disease progresses, the abnormal clone becomes increasingly predominant. The degree of imbalance of globin chain synthesis and of α-globin mRNA deficiency is greater than that observed in the hereditary type of Hb H disease. It is even conceivable that cells of the abnormal leukemic clone synthesize no α-globin chains at all, but this phenomenon is difficult to document in total blood as long as some normal erythroid cells are being produced.

The molecular basis of this fascinating disorder remains obscure. It is clear that the marked deficiency of α-globin chain synthesis is not due to a major deletion or rearrangement in the α-globin gene cluster.[366,367] The defect probably involves the suppression or silencing of all four α-globin genes in affected cells.[367] The results of chromosome transfer experiments suggest that the defect responsible for this disorder may involve the abnormal expression of a *trans*-acting factor—either the absence of a positive regulatory factor required for normal α-globin gene expression or the presence of a negative regulatory factor capable of suppressing α-gene expression.[368]

Hb H Disease in Association With Mental Retardation. A second syndrome that is associated with Hb H as an acquired abnormality is the disorder of mental retardation with Hb H disease.[369] A total of 13 affected persons have been identified.[370,371] In this disorder, those affected have mental retardation (with IQs of 50 to 70), dysmorphic features, and Hb H disease that is inherited in a nontraditional manner. Although one parent may have α-thalassemia-2 by various criteria, the other parent is usually completely normal. In more than 50% of cases, there is the de novo appearance of large deletions involving the entire α-globin gene cluster including the 5′ and 3′ hypervariable regions. In some of these persons, the deletion produces detectable cytogenetic abnormalities of chromosome 16, indicating that a large segment of the chromosome is deleted, sometimes because of unbalanced chromosomal translocations involving the telomeres of the affected chromosomes.[370,372,373] In persons without detectable deletions of the α-globin gene complex, the molecular basis of the disorder remains unknown and may involve the abnormal expression of a *trans*-acting factor, as is presumed in the case of acquired Hb H disease with myeloproliferative disorders (see previous section).[371]

δβ-Thalassemia, γδβ-Thalassemia, Hereditary Persistence of Fetal Hemoglobin, Hemoglobin Lepore, and Related Disorders

A group of β-thalassemia–like disorders is distinguished from the more typical forms of β-thalassemia by the presence of a substantial elevation of Hb F in heterozygotes, as well as in homozygotes and compound heterozygotes. These disorders are usually due to deletions of different sizes involving the β-globin gene cluster, but nondeletion types of disorders have also been identified.[374–376]

Although δβ-thalassemia and HPFH are generally described or referred to as distinct disorders with different phenotypes, they should probably not be considered as unambiguously separate entities but as a group of disorders with a variety of partially overlapping phenotypes that sometimes defy classification as one syndrome or the other. The following are working definitions generally applied to the classification of these disorders. *δβ-Thalassemia* usually refers to a group of disorders associated with a mild but definite thalassemia phenotype of hypochromia and microcytosis together with a modest elevation of Hb F, which, in heterozygotes, is heterogeneously distributed among RBCs. In contrast, *HPFH* refers to a group of disorders with substantially higher levels of Hb F, in which there is usually no associated phenotype of hypochromia and microcytosis. In addition, the increased Hb F in heterozygotes with the typical forms of HPFH is distributed in a relatively uniform (pancellular) fashion among all the RBCs rather than being distributed in a heterogeneous (heterocellular) fashion among a subpopulation of so-called F cells, as in $\delta\beta$-thalassemia.

Homozygotes for both conditions totally lack Hb A and Hb A_2, indicating absence of δ- and β-globin gene expression in *cis* to the $\delta\beta$-thalassemia and HPFH determinants. Although the apparent striking qualitative difference in cellular distribution of Hb F between HPFH and $\delta\beta$-thalassemia may be due in great part to the quantitative differences in Hb F per cell and the sensitivity of the methods used to detect Hb F cytologically, it appears that the increased amount of Hb F in HPFH is caused by a genetically determined failure to suppress γ-globin gene activity postnatally in all erythroid cells, rather than by selective survival of the normally occurring subpopulation of F cells as occurs in sickle cell anemia, β^+-thalassemia, and β^0-thalassemia. In the final analysis, some overlap definitely exists between the two sets of syndromes at the level of their clinical and hematologic phenotypes as well as at the level of their molecular basis.

Deletions Associated With $\delta\beta$-Thalassemia

A large number of different deletions of the β-globin gene cluster have been identified as causes of $\delta\beta$-thalassemia (Fig. 51-20). In almost all patients, partial or total deletions of both the δ- and β-globin genes are the bases for absent δ- and β-globin chain synthesis. The one exception is the so-called Corfu $\delta\beta$-thalassemia, in which the deletion involves only the δ gene, with the defect in β-gene expression being due to a point mutation (G→A) at position 5 of IVS-1 of the linked β-globin gene.[181,182] The $\delta\beta$-thalassemias can be classified into two general categories: $^G\gamma^A\gamma(\delta\beta)^0$-thalassemia, in which both γ genes are intact, and $^G\gamma(^A\gamma\delta\beta)^0$-thalassemia, in which the deletion also involves part or all of the $^A\gamma$ gene and results in increased Hb F that is all of the $^G\gamma$ type. In general, the $\delta\beta$-thalassemia deletions are relatively circumscribed and do not extend far beyond the β-gene cluster. Three $\delta\beta$-thalassemia mutations (Chinese, Spanish, and Japanese deletions) encompass a considerable region of DNA with 3′ endpoints about 75 kb, 100 kb, and more than 100 kb, respectively, to the 3′ side of the β-globin gene. A particularly interesting DNA rearrangement is that causing the Indian $^G\gamma(^A\gamma\delta\beta)^0$-thalassemia, in which there are two deletions involving portions of the $^A\gamma$, δ, and β genes and an inversion of the intergene DNA between the $^A\gamma$ and δ genes.

As indicated by their names, these deletions are usually limited in their geographic distribution. In those cases in which the endpoints have been sequenced, the deletions appear to have arisen by illegitimate recombination events between nonhomologous segments of DNA (see sections on molecular mechanisms associated with the generation of deletions in the β-globin gene cluster).

The cause of the increased Hb F production in $\delta\beta$-thalassemia is poorly understood, and a number of theories have been advanced. One theory proposes that the deletions may lead to disruption of the normal adult chromatin configuration between the fetal and adult domains of the β cluster and thereby allow the γ genes to escape normal repression and be expressed in a subpopulation of adult erythroid cells.[377] Based on observations of possible competition between γ and β promoters for various *cis*- and *trans*-acting factors, such as the LCR[23,46,58–60] (see section on molecular mechanisms and models in section on ontogeny of globin gene expression, another theory proposes that deletion of the δ- and β-gene promoters allows the γ-gene promoters to compete more successfully for the influence of the LCR or other *cis*- and *trans*-acting factors. Finally, as proposed in the case of deletion type HPFH (see section on deletions associated with Hb Kenya and hereditary persistence of fetal hemoglobin), the DNA sequences at the 3′ breakpoint of certain deletions may contain enhancer-like sequences that may activate the γ genes when translocated into their vicinity by the recombination–deletion event.

For example, certain $\delta\beta$-thalassemia deletions, such as the black $^G\gamma(^A\gamma\delta\beta)^0$ and Indian $^G\gamma(^A\gamma\delta\beta)^0$ deletions, leave the 3′ β-gene enhancer intact and result in its translocation closer to the γ-gene promoters. The Chinese, German, and black $^G\gamma(^A\gamma\delta\beta)^0$-thalassemia deletions have 3′ breakpoints similar to those of certain types of deletional $^G\gamma^A\gamma$-HPFH but are presumably associated with a $\delta\beta$-thalassemia rather than an HPFH phenotype because only one γ gene remains functional, whereas in the HPFH deletions both γ genes are functional.

The Hemoglobin Lepore Syndromes

The Hb Lepore syndromes can be considered to be related to the $\delta\beta$-thalassemia syndromes because they are associated with a β-thalassemia phenotype, absence of normal δ- and β-globin gene expression in *cis*, and usually a modest elevation of Hb F. The increase in Hb F is not as striking as that seen in typical cases of $\delta\beta$-thalassemia. Hb Lepore is a structurally abnormal hemoglobin in which the abnormal globin chain is a hybrid or fused globin chain, having the N-terminal amino acid sequence of the normal δ chain and the C-terminal amino acid sequence of the normal β chain.[2] The Lepore gene is almost certainly the result of an unequal crossover event or recombination between the homologous (but nonidentical) δ- and β-globin genes, with the resulting deletion of the 5′ end of the β gene, the 3′ end of the δ gene, and about 7 kb of intergene DNA between the δ and β genes (see Fig. 51-20). Gene mapping studies have in fact confirmed the expected gene deletion.[378,379]

Three different types of Hb Lepore due to crossovers at different positions of the genes have been identified. In the most common form, Hb Lepore Boston or Lepore Washington, the recombination event occurred at the 5′ end of IVS-2 of the β-globin gene.[380–382] The same mutation is found in diverse racial groups and associated with different haplotypes of β-cluster RFLPs.[383] Thus, the mutation appears to have arisen independently on more than one occasion. The Hb Lepore gene behaves as a β-thalassemic gene because of the presence of only a low level of synthesis of its gene product (Lepore $\delta\beta$-globin chain) and absence of normal β-chain production from the affected chromosome; homozygotes produce no Hb A or Hb A_2.

The reasons for the low level of synthesis of Hb Lepore are not known. Synthesis may be decreased because of relative instability of the mRNA for the Lepore chain. Globin chain synthetic studies reveal that synthesis of the Lepore $\delta\beta$ chain, like that of the δ chain of the Hb A_2, occurs primarily in bone marrow cells and is virtually absent or much lower in peripheral blood reticulocytes.[384] In addition, transcription of the Lepore $\delta\beta$ gene is probably reduced because it shares the same 5′ flanking (promoter) sequences as the δ-globin gene, and these sequences, which differ from the corresponding sequences of the β gene, are likely to be responsible (at least partly) for the normally low level of δ-globin gene expression.

Whatever the relative contributions of mRNA instability and decreased gene transcription, Hb Lepore accumulates to a level of about 10% to 15% of the total hemoglobin,

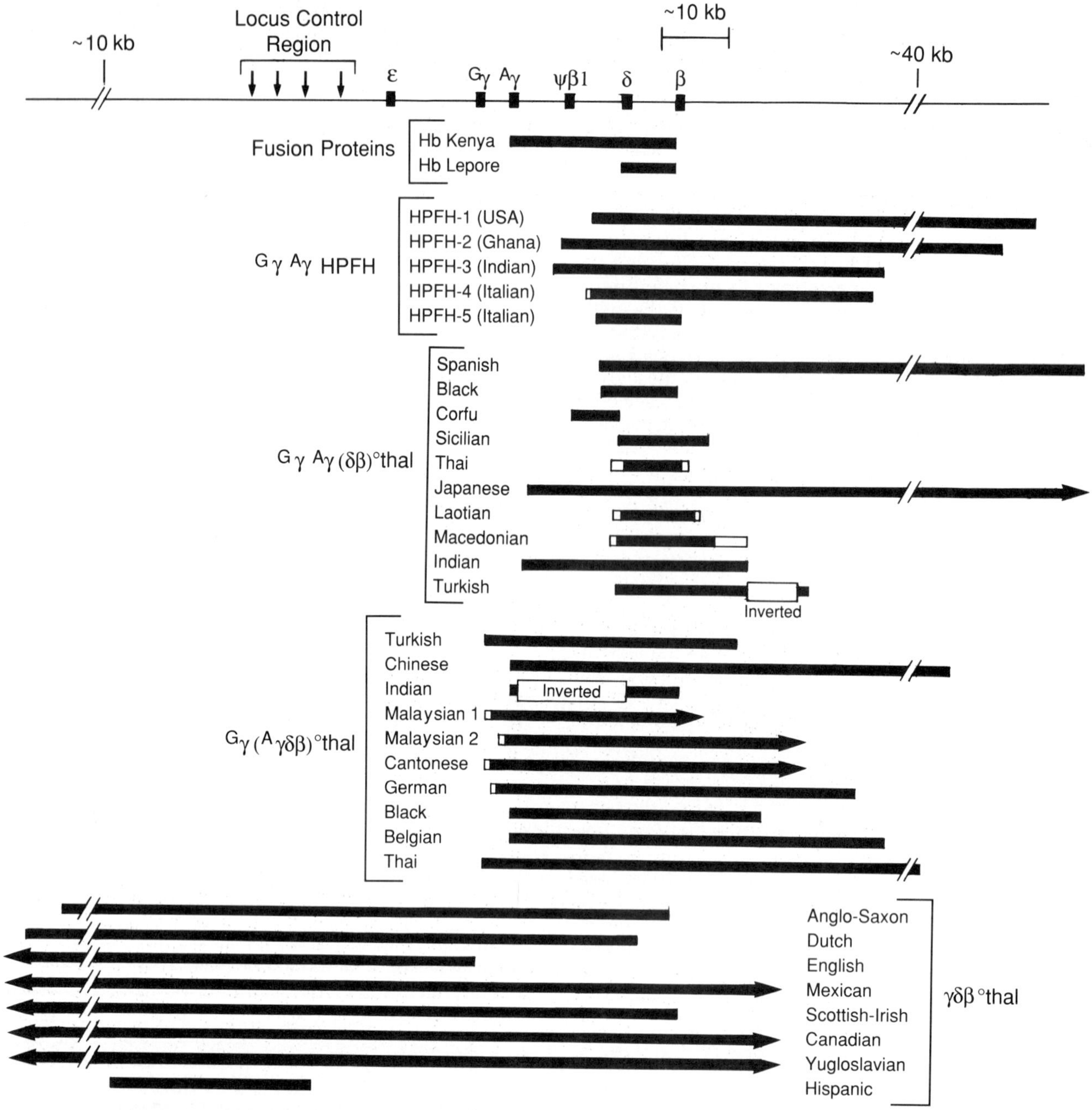

FIGURE 51-20. Deletions involving multiple genes or the locus control region of the β-globin gene cluster associated with fusion proteins, hereditary persistence of fetal hemoglobin, $\delta\beta$-thalassemia, or $\gamma\delta\beta$-thalassemia. The extents of the deletions are indicated by the closed bars, with open bars representing regions where the precise endpoints of the deletions are indeterminate. The open bars in the Indian $^G\gamma(^A\gamma\delta\beta)^0$-thalassemia and Turkish $^G\gamma^A\gamma(\delta\beta)^0$-thalassemia indicate a DNA inversion. The reference citations for the individual mutations are listed elsewhere.[374] (After Bollekens JA, Forget BG. $\delta\beta$ Thalassemia and hereditary persistence of fetal hemoglobin. Hematol Oncol Clin North Am 1991;5:399)

whereas Hb A_2 is rarely increased to levels much greater than 5%. The 5′ flanking DNA adjacent to the δ gene cannot be the only factor influencing the level of expression of the Lepore $\delta\beta$ gene; otherwise, Hb Lepore would be expected to accumulate only to a level similar to that of Hb A_2. It is possible that the enhancer elements in IVS-2, exon 3, and the 3′ flanking DNA of the β-globin gene, now in proximity to the δ promoter because of the recombination event, increase the activity of the δ promoter in the Lepore $\delta\beta$-fusion gene (see previous section on enhancers and other *cis*-acting sequences that influence globin gene expression). Other possible mechanisms to explain the differences between steady-state amounts of Hb Lepore and Hb A_2 are stabilization of the $\delta\beta$ mRNA by 3′ untranslated sequences from the β gene and different affinities of the δ-and $\delta\beta$-globin chains for association with α chains.

The reciprocal product of Lepore type recombination events is the anti-Lepore chromosome, which has been identified for all three types of Lepore crossovers. The anti-Lepore syndromes are not associated with a β-thalassemia phenotype because the affected chromosome carries, in addition to the mutant gene, normal β, and δ genes. Similar to the situation observed in the Hb Lepore syndromes, the synthesis of the anti-Lepore globin chain is almost absent in reticulocytes and is essentially limited to bone marrow cells. This phenomenon has been interpreted as evidence of instability of the anti-Lepore globin mRNA and evidence that both the 5′ and 3′ untranslated sequences of β-globin mRNA are important in maintaining its stability.

Deletions Associated With γδβ-Thalassemia

A number of large deletions are associated with the γδβ-thalassemia (see Fig. 51-20). This syndrome has a distinctive clinical and hematologic phenotype characterized in heterozygous newborns by neonatal hemolysis and normoblastemia, which is self-limited, and in heterozygous adults by the hematologic phenotype of heterozygous β-thalassemia with normal levels of Hb F and Hb A_2. Because of the associated absence of γ-gene expression, homozygosity for this disorder is expected to be lethal early in gestation.

The location and extent of the deletions associated with γδβ-thalassemia are illustrated in Figure 51-20.[385–394] Both endpoints of the deletions have been mapped in only two of the deletions (Anglo-Saxon and Dutch), and in these the total size of the deletion is about 100 kb with the breakpoints staggered by only 3 to 5 kb.[386] Gene mapping studies suggest that in many of the other deletions, the total extent of the deletion probably encompasses even more DNA. For instance, the 5′ breakpoints of five of the deletions are located at an unknown distance 5′ to the breakpoints of the Dutch and the Anglo-Saxon deletions.

The basis for the total absence of γ-, δ-, and β-globin chain synthesis in *cis* to these mutations is clearly understandable in the case of five of the eight deletions shown in Figure 51-20, because the involved genes are either totally or partially deleted. In the case of the three other deletions, the β- or one or both of the γ-globin genes on the affected chromosome are intact but inactive. This surprising finding was initially studied in some detail in the Dutch deletion, in which the β-globin gene with 2.5 kb of its 5′ flanking DNA is intact but appears to be totally inactive. The cloned β-globin gene from this chromosome was shown to be structurally normal and to function normally in gene transfer–expression studies. In fetal liver erythroid cells of an affected fetus, the β-globin gene from the deletion chromosome was found to be hypermethylated, whereas the β gene from the normal chromosome in *trans* was hypomethylated, as is usually found in actively transcribing genes.[395]

The cause of the inactivity and hypermethylation of the β-globin gene on the deletion chromosome was initially poorly understood. Proposed explanations included disruption of chromatin structure preventing normal expression of the β gene or juxtaposition of negative regulatory sequences from the upstream DNA brought into the vicinity of the β gene as a result of the deletion–recombination event. Subsequently, two other families were described, in which the 3′ breakpoint of the deletion was found to be located substantially farther 5′ in the β cluster, leaving considerable amounts of normal β-cluster DNA situated 5′ to the silent β-globin gene. These include the English deletion, in which the 3′ breakpoint is located between the ^{G}γ- and ^{A}γ-globin genes[389] and the Hispanic deletion, in which the entire β cluster is intact and the 3′ breakpoint of the deletion is located about 10 kb 5′ to the ε-globin gene.[393] An explanation for this puzzling inactivity of the structurally normal γ-, δ-, and β-globin genes on these various deletion chromosomes came to light with the discovery of important regulatory sequences located 5′ to the ε-globin gene, the LCR associated with the presence of DNase I hypersensitive or superhypersensitive sites in erythroid cells (see previous section on enhancers and other *cis*-acting sequences that influence globin gene expression).

The most plausible explanation for the inactivity of the β-globin gene (and other nondeleted globin genes) in the Dutch, English, and Hispanic γδβ-thalassemias is the deletion of the LCR region 5′ to the ε gene, which is required for normal activity of the globin genes in the β cluster. The Hispanic γδβ deletion spares hypersensitive site 1 while deleting the other 5′ sites together with about 30 kb of 5′ DNA. These findings suggest that the presence of site 1 alone is not sufficient to allow high levels of activity of the β-gene cluster. In fact, a short deletion involving only site 1 is not associated with a clinical phenotype of γδβ-thalassemia.[396] Studies in transgenic mice and MEL cells suggest that the 5′ hypersensitive sites 2 and 3, which are effectively deleted in the Hispanic γδβ-thalassemia, contain most of the sequences responsible for conferring high levels of globin gene expression.[397,398]

Deletions Associated With Hb Kenya and Hereditary Persistence of Fetal Hemoglobin

Hb Kenya is a structurally abnormal hemoglobin, which, like Hb Lepore, contains a fused β-like globin chain resulting from a nonhomologous crossover event between two globin genes in the β cluster. Whereas the Lepore crossover occurred between the δ- and β-globin genes, the Kenya gene resulted from crossover between the ^{A}γ-and β-globin genes[3] (see Fig. 51-20). The crossover occurred in the second exons of the ^{A}γ and β genes between the codons for amino acids 80 to 87 and resulted in deletion of about 24 kb of DNA from the ^{A}γ to the β gene.[399] Unlike Hb Lepore, which is associated with a β-thalassemic phenotype, Hb Kenya is associated with a phenotype of pancellular ^{G}γ-HPFH. Erythrocytes of affected heterozygotes have normal RBC indices and contain 7% to 23% Hb Kenya as well as about 10% Hb F, all of which is of the ^{G}γ type and is relatively uniformly distributed among the RBCs.

The finding of Hb Kenya was initially thought to provide added support for an early theory that proposed the existence of control elements in the ^{A}γ- to δ-intergene DNA, deletion of which in HPFH (and Hb Kenya) but not in δβ-thalassemia resulted in incomplete postnatal suppression of γ-gene activity in all erythroid cells.[93] The most likely explanation for the HPFH phenotype associated with Hb Kenya is the influence on the ^{G}γ- and Kenya gene promoters of the 3′ β-globin gene enhancer translocated into closer proximity of the γ-globin gene promoters by the crossover–deletion event (see section on enhancers and other *cis*-acting sequences that influence globin gene expression).

Five deletions have been described in the β-globin gene cluster, which are associated with a phenotype of pancellular ^{G}γ^{A}γ-HPFH[377,388,400–410] (see Fig. 51-20). One of these deletions, HPFH-5, recently identified in an Italian family, is relatively short and extends from a point about 3 kb 5′ to the δ gene to a point 0.7 kb 3′ to the β gene, within the proximal portion of its 3′ enhancer.[410] The molecular basis of the HPFH phenotype associated with this deletion is presumably the influence of the translocated 3′ β-gene enhancer on the γ-gene promoters in a manner analogous to that proposed for the basis of the HPFH phenotype of the Hb Kenya syndrome. The other four deletions are considerably more extensive and fall into two different size classes. HPFH-1 and HPFH-2, found in blacks, are the result of extensive deletions of nearly identical sizes, involving about 105 kb of DNA, with breakpoints staggered by only 5 to 6 kb[377,388,400–405] (see Fig. 51-20). The deletions associated with HPFH-3 (in Asian Indians) and HPFH-4 (in Southern Italians) are less extensive, encompassing about 50 kb and 40 kb, respectively. The 3′ breakpoints of these two deletions are separated by only about 2 kb and are located about 30 kb 3′ to the site of the β-globin gene, or about 50 to 60 kb more proximal than the 3′ breakpoints of HPFH-1 and HPFH-2.[406–410]

The 5′ breakpoints of all five HPFH deletions are located between the ψβ and δ genes. The clustering of the 3′ breakpoints of the four largest deletions in two discrete regions has focused attention on the nature of the DNA sequences at these sites and their possible role in the generation of the HPFH phenotype. The DNA sequences at the 3′ breakpoint of HPFH-1 and HPFH-2 have a number of interesting properties: they have gene enhancer activity in various assay systems; they are specifically hypomethylated and contain a DNase I hypersensitive site in erythroid cells; and they contain a large open reading frame.[401,411] All these properties suggest the presence in this DNA of a gene that is active in erythroid cells.

Furthermore, the Spanish type of $^{G}\gamma^{A}\gamma(\delta\beta)^{0}$-thalassemia has a 5′ breakpoint close to that of HPFH-1[412] (see Fig. 51-20), but extends for an additional 6 to 7 kb in the 3′ direction.[401,413] Thus, the deletion of the additional DNA containing the interesting sequences at the 3′ breakpoint of the HPFH-1 and HPFH-2 deletions is associated with a δβ-thalassemia rather than a HPFH phenotype, suggesting a role for these sequences in the generation of the HPFH phenotype in HPFH-1 and HPFH-2. The 3′ breakpoints of HPFH-3 and HPFH-4 are located within a complex array of repetitive DNA sequences,[406] but these DNA sequences have been shown to possess enhancer-like properties in different assay systems, including transgenic mice.[414]

The unifying theory that emerges from the study of the four largest HPFH deletions is that the DNA sequences at the 3′ deletion breakpoints become juxtaposed to the γ genes as a result of the deletion events and may influence γ-gene expression in a manner analogous to the presumed influence of the 3′ β-gene enhancer on γ-gene expression in Hb Kenya and HPFH-5. Mechanisms by which this could occur include the presence of enhancer sequences in the translocated 3′ breakpoint DNA or the presence in this DNA of an active chromatin configuration, which could have a spreading and activating effect on the expression of the neighboring γ-globin genes.

A number of δβ-thalassemia deletions have 3′ breakpoints located near those of the HPFH deletions. These include the Chinese deletion,[415] with a 3′ breakpoint near that of HPFH-2, and the German[416] and Belgian[417] deletions, with 3′ breakpoints near those of HPFH-3 and HPFH-4 (see Fig. 51-20). All these deletions also involve all or part of the $^{A}\gamma$-globin gene and are therefore associated with $^{G}\gamma(^{A}\gamma\delta\beta)^{0}$-thalassemia. It is likely that for a deletion to cause HPFH rather than δβ-thalassemia, two γ or γ-like genes must be intact or functional in *cis* to the deletion. No examples of deletion type HPFH are found in which only one γ gene is intact and functional. In Hb Kenya, the functional $^{A}\gamma\beta$-fusion gene can be considered a γ-like gene.

Molecular Mechanisms Associated With the Generation of Deletions in the β-Globin Gene Cluster

Considerable discussion in the literature has occurred regarding the molecular mechanisms responsible for generating the various deletions observed in the β-globin gene cluster.[405] With the exceptions of Hb Lepore and Hb Kenya, all the deletions in the β-gene cluster are the result of "illegitimate" recombination events in which no significant DNA sequence homology is present at the deletion breakpoints. Sometimes, a simple rejoining of the normal DNA sequences flanking the breakpoints occurs; other times, short segments of foreign DNA are inserted between the breakpoints. In some cases, one of the breakpoints involves a repetitive DNA sequence, either of the *AluI* family or of the L1 family, and some speculation has occurred concerning whether such repetitive DNA sequences serve as hot spots for recombination. Although examples of recombination events between two repetitive DNA sequences of the *AluI* family are found in the α-globin gene cluster and in other gene systems, these are not found in the β-globin gene cluster. It is likely that the finding of repetitive DNA sequences at one or the other breakpoint of a deletion event often occurs by chance alone, given the abundance of such sequences in the β cluster, as in the human genome in general.

A striking feature of the deletions in the β-globin gene locus is the clustering of sets of deletions of about the same size. To explain this phenomenon, Vanin and colleagues[388] proposed a model in which recombination may occur during DNA replication between sequences located at the attachment points of DNA or chromatin to the structure in the cell nucleus (called the nuclear matrix), resulting in loss of an entire chromatin loop. Because chromatin loops are thought to move through the nuclear matrix attachment points during DNA replication like a cable through a reel, different deletions of about the same size, but with different breakpoints, could result from random breakage and joining of DNA at different points in time as they travel through the nuclear matrix.

Nondeletion Forms of δβ-Thalassemia and Hereditary Persistence of Fetal Hemoglobin

δβ-Thalassemia. Although most cases of δβ-thalassemia are due to deletions in the β-globin gene cluster, two distinct syndromes occur in which a δβ-thalassemia phenotype is not associated with a deletion. In these cases, two separate mutations have been found: a point mutation causing β-thalassemia and a second mutation causing increased Hb F production. The form of δβ-thalassemia found in Sardinia is characterized by the synthesis of predominantly $^{A}\gamma$-globin chains of Hb F.[418] The β-globin gene on the affected chromosome carries the common nonsense mutation at codon 39 as the cause of the β-thalassemia phenotype,[419,420] whereas the $^{A}\gamma$-globin gene carries a C→T base substitution at position −196 of the $^{A}\gamma$-gene promoter,[421] which is associated with one form of nondeletion HPFH (see following section).

A Chinese family has also been described in which a δβ-thalassemia phenotype with increased levels of both $^{G}\gamma$- and $^{A}\gamma$-chains of Hb F is not associated with a deletion in the β-globin gene cluster.[422] The β-globin gene on the affected chromosome was found to contain an A → G substitution at position −29 of the β-gene promoter as the cause of the β-thalassemia phenotype,[423] but the mutation responsible for the increased production of Hb F remains unknown.

HPFH. In contrast to the deletional HPFH syndromes in which both linked $^{G}\gamma$ and $^{A}\gamma$ genes are overexpressed, only one or the other γ gene is usually overexpressed in the best characterized nondeletional types of HPFH, although less well-characterized nondeletion forms of $^{G}\gamma^{A}\gamma$-HPFH also exist. Because of the restricted pattern of γ-globin gene expression in the $^{G}\gamma$ and $^{A}\gamma$ forms of nondeletion HPFH, it was assumed that the mutations in these syndromes must be located near the affected gene and molecular studies focused initially on the DNA sequence analysis of the overexpressed γ genes in these disorders.

The results of these structural analyses revealed a number of different point mutations in the promoter region of the overexpressed γ gene in persons with different types of nondeletion HPFH (Table 51-4 and Fig. 51-21). These point mutations have clustered in three distinct regions of the 5′ flanking DNA of the affected γ genes. Five different mutations have been identified in the region located about 200 bp from the cap site or site of transcription initiation of the γ genes, specifically at position −202 (C→G) of the $^{G}\gamma$ gene and positions −202 (C→T), −198 (T→C), −196 (C→T), and −195 (C→G) of the $^{A}\gamma$ gene[424–429] (see Fig. 51-21). This region of DNA, which had not previously been suspected of playing a role in the regulation of γ-gene expression, is very G+C rich, and its sequence bears homology to that of known control elements of other genes, such as the 21-bp repeat of the SV40 virus promoter and the distal element of the thymidine kinase gene of herpes simplex virus.

The G+C-rich sequence of the latter genes is known to be the binding site of a ubiquitous *trans*-acting protein factor called Sp1. Subsequent studies of the γ-gene promoters have demonstrated that the −200 region is also a binding site for Sp1 and at least one other ubiquitous DNA-binding protein.[105,430–433] The −202 (G→C) and −196 mutations are associated with high levels of Hb F (15% to 20%), expressed in a pancellular fashion, whereas the −202 (C→T), −198, and −195 mutations are associated with lower levels of Hb F (3% to 10%), expressed in a heterocellular fashion[1,374,376] (see Table 51-4).

The second region containing a mutation associated with nondeletion HPFH is located at position −175 (see Fig. 51-21). A point mutation (T→C) at this position of either the

TABLE 51-4. Nondeletion Forms of Hereditary Persistence of Fetal Hemoglobin (HPFH) and δβ-Thalassemia

Type and Racial Group	Mutation in Globin Gene	Percentage of Hb F in Heterozygotes	References
PANCELLULAR $^{G}\gamma$ HPFH			
Black	$^{G}\gamma$: −202 (C → G)	15–25	424
Black	$^{G}\gamma$: −175 (T → C)	20–30	434
Sardinian	$^{G}\gamma$: −175 (T → C)	17–21	435
Japanese	$^{G}\gamma$: −114 (C → T)	11–14	443
PANCELLULAR $^{A}\gamma$ HPFH			
Southern Italian	$^{A}\gamma$: −196 (C → T)	12–16	427
Chinese	$^{A}\gamma$: −196 (C → T)	14–21	428
Black	$^{A}\gamma$: −175 (T → C)	36–41*	436
Greek	$^{A}\gamma$: −117 (G → A)	10–20	437, 438
Sardinian	$^{A}\gamma$: −117 (G → A)	12–16	439
Black	$^{A}\gamma$: −117 (G → A)	11–16	440
Black	$^{A}\gamma$: −114 to −102 deleted	30–32	441
PANCELLULAR $^{G}\gamma^{A}\gamma$ HPFH			
Chinese	Unknown	20–25	442
HETEROCELLULAR $^{G}\gamma$ HPFH			
Black (Atlanta)	$^{G}\gamma^{G}\gamma$: −158 (C → T)	2.3–3.8	458, 459
HETEROCELLULAR $^{A}\gamma$ HPFH			
Black	$^{A}\gamma$: −202 (C → T)	1.6–3.9	425
British	$^{A}\gamma$: −198 (T → C)	3.5–10	426
Brazilian	$^{A}\gamma$: −195 (C → G)	4.5–7	429
Black (Georgia)	$^{A}\gamma$: −114 (C → T)	2.6–6	439
HETEROCELLULAR $^{G}\gamma^{A}\gamma$ HPFH			
Swiss	Unknown	1–4	1
Black (Seattle)	Normal γ-gene promoters	3–8	454, 455
$^{A}\gamma$-δβ THALASSEMIA			
Sardinian	$^{A}\gamma$: −196 (C → T)	10–20	418–420
	β: codon 39 (CAG → TAG)		419
$^{G}\gamma^{A}\gamma$-δβ THALASSEMIA			
Chinese	Normal γ-gene promoters β: −29 (A → G)	22.3	422, 423

* The one patient studied was doubly heterozygous for Hb A and Hb C. About 20% of the Hb F (or 8% of the total Hb) was of the $^{G}\gamma$ type, and the $^{G}\gamma$ gene in *cis* to the −175 $^{A}\gamma$ mutation carried the −158 C → T change.

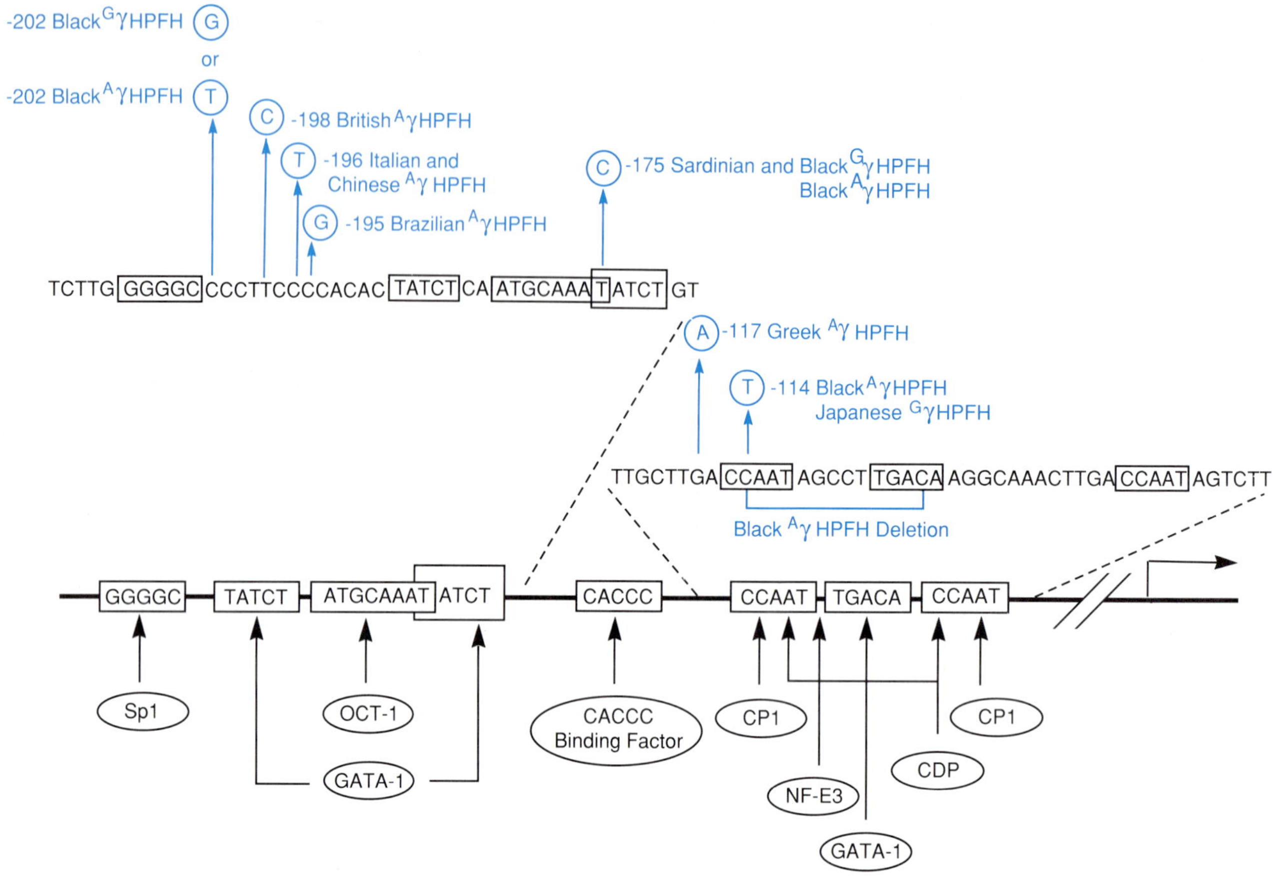

FIGURE 51-21. *Cis*- and *trans*-acting elements of the human γ-globin gene promoters and mutations associated with nondeletion forms of hereditary persistence of fetal hemoglobin (HPFH). (After Bollekens JA, Forget BG. δβ Thalassemia and hereditary persistence of fetal hemoglobin. Hematol Oncol Clin North Am 1991;5:399)

$^G\gamma$- or $^A\gamma$ gene is associated with a phenotype of pancellular HPFH with high levels of Hb F (15% to 25%).[434–436] This region of DNA is noteworthy because it contains an octanucleotide sequence that is present in the promoter region of a number of genes and is the binding site of another ubiquitous *trans*-acting factor called OCT-1. In addition, the octamer consensus sequence of the γ-gene promoters is flanked on either side by a consensus sequence for the erythroid-specific factor GATA-1.[21,24,94–99] The point mutation at position −175 affects the one nucleotide that is present in the partially overlapping binding sites of both OCT-1 and GATA-1.

The third region affected by a point mutation in nondeletion HPFH is the area of a well-known regulatory element of globin and other genes: the CCAAT box sequence. In the γ genes, the CCAAT box is duplicated, and the mutation associated with the Greek ($^A\gamma$) type of nondeletion HPFH is a G→A substitution at position −117, 2 bases upstream of the distal CCAAT box of the $^A\gamma$-globin gene promoter.[437,438] The base change disrupts a pentanucleotide sequence, YYTTGA (Y = pyrimidine), which is highly conserved immediately upstream of the CCAAT sequence in all animal fetal and embryonic genes.[437] Another mutation with a similar phenotype involves the deletion of 13 bp of DNA, from position −102 to −114, encompassing the distal CCAAT box and adjacent 3′ DNA of the $^A\gamma$-globin gene[441] (see Fig. 51-21). The CCAAT box region is known to be the binding site of a number of *trans*-acting factors, including the ubiquitous factors CCAAT binding protein (CP1) and CCAAT displacement factor (CDP), as well as an erythroid-specific factor, NF-E3. A third mutation has also been identified, which consists of a C → T base substitution at position −114 of the $^G\gamma$- or $^A\gamma$-globin gene, within the distal CCAAT consensus sequence.[443,444]

The unifying model by which these various mutations are thought to affect hemoglobin switching proposes that these base changes alter the binding of a number of different *trans*-acting factors to critical regions of the γ-gene promoters and thereby prevent the normal postnatal suppression of γ-gene expression.[376] The mutations could prevent the binding of negative regulatory factors or enhance the binding of positive regulatory factors. Either mechanism could be operative with one mutation or the other.

The following abnormalities of protein–DNA interactions have been observed when nondeletion HPFH γ-globin gene promoter sequences have been compared with normal γ-gene promoter sequences:

1. The point mutation at position −198 clearly results in increased binding affinity of the ubiquitous *trans*-acting factor, Sp1, whereas the mutations at positions −202(C→T) and −196 result in either no change or reduced Sp1 binding.[430–433] The C → G mutation at position −202 gives variable results: increased Sp1 binding in some studies[430,431] but not in others.[432,433] At least one other ubiquitous activity has been identified, the binding of which is decreased by the −202 C → G and −198 mutations.[105,430,433] Finally, the −202 C → G mutation leads to the binding of yet another activity, called −50γ, that usually binds to the −50

region of the γ promoter and may be important for selective γ- over β-globin gene expression during the fetal stage of development.[104,105,433]

2. The T→G mutation at position −175 results in markedly decreased binding of the ubiquitous factor OCT-1,[21,445–447] whereas the binding of the erythroid-specific factor GATA-1 is either unaffected[21,445] or slightly enhanced[446] in different studies. The mutation does alter the DNase I "footprint" pattern of the GATA-1–DNA complex,[21] and the increased functional activity of the mutant promoter in gene transfer–expression studies is dependent on the presence and ability of GATA-1 to bind to the promoter, since additional mutations that abolish GATA-1 binding to the HPFH promoter also abolish its overexpression.[21,99]
3. The G→A mutation at position −117 results in reduced binding of the erythroid-specific factors GATA-1 and NF-E3, and enhanced binding of the ubiquitous factors CP1 and CDP.[445,446,448,449] The 13-bp deletion involving the distal CCAAT box and adjacent 3′ DNA results in the loss of binding of NF-E3, CP1, and CDP, but it leaves GATA-1 binding intact.[449] The C to T mutation at position −114 abolishes binding of CP1 to the distal CCAAT box without affecting the binding of GATA-1.[443]

In addition to the nondeletion forms of HPFH associated with point mutations of the $^G\gamma$ or $^A\gamma$ promoters, there exists another group of related disorders, the molecular basis of which is less well characterized. These disorders include the Swiss, Seattle, and German types of heterocellular HPFH in which the increased Hb F is of both the $^G\gamma$ and $^A\gamma$ types; the Altanta type of heterocellular HPFH in which the elevated Hb F is all of the $^G\gamma$ type; and the Saudi and other related high Hb F determinants with predominance of $^G\gamma$-gene expression.

The Swiss type of the heterocellular HPFH consists of a heterogeneous group of disorders associated with only a slight elevation of Hb F (2% to 3%) in simple heterozygotes but with substantially higher than usual levels of Hb F when coinherited with homozygous sickle cell anemia, homozygous β-thalassemia, or Hb S/β-thalassemia.[1] In some families, the disorder appears to be linked to the β-gene cluster on chromosome 11, but the finding of a small number of crossover events suggests that the locus may be at some distance from the β cluster.[450] In other families, the locus is clearly not linked to the β-gene cluster,[451] and in some of these families an X-chromosome–linked pattern of inheritance of the high Hb F determinant is seen.[452,453]

Heterozygotes with the Seattle type of HPFH have slightly higher levels of Hb F (3% to 8%) than heterozygotes with the Swiss type HPFH.[454] The promoters of the overexpressed $^G\gamma$ and $^A\gamma$ genes have a normal DNA sequence.[455] A cluster of three base substitutions was identified in the 3′ $^A\gamma$-gene enhancer of affected persons,[455] but this was later shown to be a polymorphism also found in persons without HPFH.[456]

The German type of heterocellular HPFH (5% to 8% Hb F) was described in a family in which the mother and daughter were found to have a balanced cyclic translocation involving four chromosomes: 46,XX,t(6;9;11;20), including the portion of chromosome 11 containing the β-gene cluster.[457] The breakpoint of the translocation did not appear to occur within the β cluster itself.

The Atlanta type of $^G\gamma$-HPFH (2.5% to 4% Hb F)[458] is associated with a β-locus that contains two $^G\gamma$ genes, perhaps as the result of a gene conversion event.[459] Both $^G\gamma$ genes have a C→T base substitution at position −158 of the $^G\gamma$ promoter. The possible significance of the −158 C→T base change is discussed below in relation to the high Hb F determinants associated with sickle cell anemia in certain Saudi Arabians and in Africans.

In eastern Saudi Arabia, many patients with homozygous sickle cell anemia or Hb S/β^0-thalassemia have an unusually mild clinical course, associated with consistently high levels of Hb F, in the range of 25% to 40% and with predominance of $^G\gamma$ chains.[460,461] A similar syndrome has also been described in certain Asian Indians with sickle cell anemia.[462,463] In contrast to the situation in blacks of African ancestry with sickle cell anemia and high levels of Hb F, one cannot usually identify in the Saudi or Indian families a parent with slight elevation of Hb F or F-cell numbers consistent with the Swiss type of heterocellular HPFH. The high Hb F genetic determinant appears to be inherited in *cis* to the sickle gene but seems to be expressed only in the presence of erythropoietic stress induced by hemolysis due to the homozygosity for the β^S gene or double heterozygosity for one β^S gene and a β^0-thalassemia gene.

The molecular basis of high Hb F expression in Saudis with sickle cell anemia is poorly understood. Analysis of the cloned genes of affected persons has revealed the presence of the C→T base change at position −158 of the $^G\gamma$-gene promoter and one other probably polymorphic base change (A→G) 29 bp upstream of the initiator codon in the 5′ untranslated sequence of the $^A\gamma$ gene.[464] The C→T base change at position −158 is also found in the $^G\gamma$-gene promoter of African β^S-chromosomes bearing the so-called Senegal haplotype of β-cluster RFLPs.[465] Sickle cell anemia patients with the Senegal haplotype have a predominance of Hb F of the $^G\gamma$ type, but the total elevation of Hb F, although generally higher than that in sickle cell anemia patients with other haplotypes, is not nearly as great as that observed in the Saudi. As in the case of Saudi heterozygotes, heterozygotes for the Senegal haplotype have normal levels of Hb F. The Saudi and Senegal β^S-haplotypes, although similar, differ at the polymorphic *Hinc*II site 5′ to the ε gene. Thus, the β-cluster chromosomal background is not identical in the two populations.

The significance of the −158 C→T base change is not entirely clear. It creates a polymorphism for the enzyme *Xmn*I,[459] which is commonly found in the general population and is associated with high $^G\gamma/^A\gamma$ ratios of Hb F in normal adults. Simple heterozygotes for the −158 C→T base change do not have significantly elevated levels of Hb F and therefore are not classified as having HPFH. When the −158 base change is coinherited with conditions that cause erythroid stress, such as sickle cell anemia, Hb S/β thalassemia, or homozygous β thalassemia, usually a significantly higher than usual synthesis of Hb F occurs, which is predominantly of the $^G\gamma$ type.

The precise role of the −158 base change in the phenomenon of high total levels of Hb F in the presence of erythroid stress remains to be determined. It is conceivable that the base change itself is not directly responsible for the high level of Hb F production but is simply a polymorphism that marks chromosomes with high Hb F genetic determinants, the nature of which is still unknown. Another base change has been identified in the same region of the $^G\gamma$-gene promoter (−161 G→A) in a black family with low levels of Hb F (1% to 2%) and marked predominance of $^G\gamma$ chains.[466]

Isolated δ-Thalassemia and γ-Thalassemia

δ-Thalassemia. Isolated thalassemia affecting the δ-globin gene has been identified in persons who totally lack Hb A_2 and are either homozygous for δ^0-thalassemia or doubly heterozygous for δ^0-thalassemia and $(\delta\beta)^0$-thalassemia. A form of δ^+-thalassemia has also been described in Sardinians in whom partial rather than total suppression of δ-chain synthesis occurs. The clinical significance of heterozygous δ-thalassemia is that if it is coinherited with heterozygous β-thalassemia, the affected person will have a normal level of Hb A_2 and thus the diagnosis of β-thalassemia trait may be missed. In such cases, the δ-thalassemia gene is usually coinherited in *trans* to the β-thalassemia gene. There are two syndromes in which a δ-thalassemia gene is coinherited as a second independent mutation in *cis* to a β-thalassemia gene: δ^0-thalassemia in *cis* to the structurally abnormal $\beta^{Knossos}$ gene (in Mediterraneans, but not blacks of the French West Indies)[467] and δ-thalassemia in *cis* to the β^+-thalassemia caused by a point mutation (C→G) at position 745 of IVS-2.[468]

With one exception (the 7.2-kb Corfu $\delta\beta$-thalassemia deletion without associated β-thalassemia[469]), gene mapping studies have failed to reveal any deletion or rearrangement of the affected δ-globin gene in cases of isolated δ-thalassemia. Gene cloning or PCR analysis and DNA sequence analysis have identified a number of different point mutations in the δ-globin genes of affected persons (Table 51-5).

Many of the molecular defects causing δ-thalassemia are similar in type to those that cause β-thalassemia: premature chain termination due to frameshifts, splicing defects, unstable globin chains, and so on. Two defects are novel and noteworthy, being associated with point mutations in GATA-1 consensus sequences in either the promoter region[477,478] or 3′ flanking DNA of the δ gene[479] with resulting abnormal binding of the transcription factor GATA-1. The promoter mutation at position −77 is associated with decreased GATA-1 binding,[478] whereas the point mutation 69 bp 3′ to the poly (A) addition site is associated with increased binding affinity of GATA-1.[479]

TABLE 51-5. Molecular Defects Causing δ-Thalassemia

Mutation	Phenotype δ^0 or δ^+	Racial Group	References
GENE DELETION			
7.2 kb	0	Sardinian	469
FRAMESHIFT MUTATIONS			
Codon 59 (−A)	0	Greek	470
		Egyptian	471
Codon 91 (+T)	0	Belgian	472
SPLICING DEFECTS			
IVS-1, position 1 (T → C)	0	Italian	473
IVS-2, 3′ end (AG → GG)	0	Greek Cypriot	474
? Codon 30 (G → C)	0	Southern Italian	475
AMINO ACID SUBSTITUTIONS			
Codon 27 (G → T) (Ala → Ser)	+	Sardinian	473
		Greek Cypriot	474
Codon 30 (G → C) (Arg → Thr) (? consensus splice site mutation)	0	Southern Italian	475
Codon 116 (C → T) (Arg → Cys)	+	Greek	474, 476
Codon 141 (T → C) (Leu → Pro)	+	Greek Cypriot	474
GATA-1 CONSENSUS SITE			
−77 (T → C)	0	Japanese	477, 478
Poly(A) addition site + 69 (G → A)	+	Sardinian	479

δ^0-Thalassemia also occurs in nonhuman primates such as the Old World monkeys, who do not synthesize Hb A_2 despite the presence of δ-globin genes in their DNA. A number of different mutations have been identified by cloning and DNA sequence analysis of δ-globin genes from various nonhuman primates, including a frameshift mutation associated with a 1-base insertion at codon 55 in rhesus monkeys and baboons and a 20-bp deletion at the cap site in colobus monkeys.[480,481] It has been postulated that these mutations may be secondary events that occurred by evolutionary drift after a different δ-gene silencing event such as a promoter mutation.[480] The cloned δ-globin genes of colobus and rhesus monkeys have been shown to be transcribed inefficiently, compared with the human δ-globin gene, in a cell-free transcription system. Although the 20-bp deletion could account in part for decreased transcription of the colobus δ gene, the frameshift mutation by itself should not cause decreased transcription of the rhesus δ gene.

The only differences in the promoter sequences of these different δ-globin genes consist of three base substitutions at positions −92, −52, and −23 from the cap site; the base change at position −52 was not found in the baboon.[480] Thus, it has been proposed that one (or both) of the other differences between the human and monkey sequences may be the primary cause of the silencing of the δ gene in all of the Old World monkeys by markedly decreasing the transcriptional activity of the gene.[480]

In an evolutionally more distant prosimian, the brown lemur, a δ-pseudogene has resulted from a crossover between the $\psi\beta1$ gene and the δ gene leading to the formation of a Lepore-like fusion gene having the 5′ end of the nonfunctional $\psi\beta1$ gene and the 3′ end (including IVS-2) of the δ-globin gene.[482]

γ-Thalassemia. Cases of isolated γ-thalassemia have been identified during the course of cord blood screening surveys in infants with unusually high levels of the $^A\gamma$ type of Hb F. Gene mapping studies revealed a deletion of 5 kb consistent with a nonhomologous crossover between $^G\gamma$- and $^A\gamma$-globin genes, creating a single fused γ-globin gene having the 5′ end of the $^G\gamma$ gene and the 3′ end of the $^A\gamma$.[483] Since the homozygous Indian child originally studied synthesized Hb F containing only $^A\gamma^T$ chains with threonine instead of the usual isoleucine at position 75, the crossover in that family must have occurred 5′ to codon 75 in the $^A\gamma$-globin gene, since the γ^T-polymorphism has been identified only in $^A\gamma$-globin chains.

The $(-\gamma)$ thalassemia deletion is analogous to the $(-\alpha)$ deletion causing α-thalassemia-2 and is the reciprocal product of the recombination event leading to chromosomes with triplicated γ-globin genes. Both single and triple γ-gene chromosomes are found in a number of different populations, especially Asian populations.[484–486] The homozygous state for the $(-\gamma)$ deletion is essentially asymptomatic and is characterized by a lower than normal percentage of Hb F in cord blood, all of which is of the $^A\gamma$ type, and by a rapid decrease in the amount of Hb F in the first 2 to 3 months of life. Heterozygotes have an increased proportion of $^A\gamma$ chains in cord blood Hb F; a similar phenotype can result from the inheritance of a chromosome with two $^A\gamma$ genes.[487]

A different deletion has been described that involves 2.5 kb of DNA encompassing the 5′ end of the $^A\gamma$ gene and constitutes a form of isolated $^A\gamma^0$-thalassemia.[488] Cord blood of affected children should have Hb F with disproportionately high levels of $^G\gamma$ chains in heterozygotes and total absence of $^A\gamma$ chains in homozygotes. A similar phenotype can result from inheritance of chromosomes with two $^{G}\gamma$ genes,[487] as observed in the Atlanta type of nondeletion HPFH[459] (see previous section on nondeletion forms of $\delta\beta$-thalassemia and hereditary persistence of fetal hemoglobin).

A 4-bp deletion at positions −222 to −225 of the $^{A}\gamma$-globin gene promoter was found to be associated with unusually low levels of $^{A}\gamma$ chains in a black family[489] and in certain Sardinian β^0-thalassemia (codon 39) patients,[490] and may be the cause of a form of $^{A}\gamma^{+}$-thalassemia. Other studies suggest that this small deletion is a common polymorphism, which does not affect $^{A}\gamma$-globin gene expression.[491]

IMPLICATIONS OF MOLECULAR FINDINGS FOR PRENATAL DIAGNOSIS AND GENE THERAPY

Prenatal Diagnosis

An important step in the prevention of cases of severe homozygous α- or β-thalassemia is the detection of the heterozygous state in adults of reproductive age. Physicians should be aware of the possibility of thalassemia trait occurring in persons with hypochromic anemias that are refractory to iron therapy, and they should perform the necessary diagnostic studies to confirm the diagnosis. In areas where a high incidence of thalassemia trait is present, general population screening is often available. Once identified, affected persons can be educated and counseled with respect to the disease process and its genetics. Two affected heterozygotes contemplating marriage and planning to have a family should be aware of the one-in-four chance of having a severely affected homozygous child. Identification of such couples provides the opportunity for their counseling and education regarding the option of prenatal diagnosis. Nevertheless such information rarely alters the reproductive behavior of couples at risk.

Prenatal diagnosis for hemoglobinopathies has gone through many changes during the past decade because of rapid advances in our understanding of the molecular basis of the thalassemias. Much of this new knowledge has been applied to prenatal diagnosis of thalassemia at the DNA level.[137,138,492]

Fetal Blood Sampling

Before the availability of DNA-based diagnosis, prenatal diagnosis of thalassemia required fetal blood sampling at 18 to 20 weeks' gestation and analysis of globin chain synthesis by isotopic labeling and separation of globin chains to identify the quantitative defect in globin chain synthesis.[493] Although fetal blood sampling has been successfully accomplished by various techniques in many medical centers, the procedure cannot be considered totally safe. In a few cases, fetal loss has occurred because of infection, hemorrhage, premature labor, or undetermined causes. It is estimated from large surveys of the worldwide experience with this procedure that even in the best of hands, there exists a risk of death or serious injury to the fetus in the order of about 5%,[493] which is a much higher risk than that associated with amniocentesis.

With the availability of DNA-based prenatal diagnosis, the demand for prenatal diagnosis by fetal blood sampling and analysis of globin chain synthesis has decreased markedly. Fetal blood sampling is usually limited to cases in which DNA diagnosis is not possible, either because of lack of knowledge of the genotype of the parents or lack of sufficient information concerning linkage of RFLPs, or because the case presents itself too late in the course of the pregnancy to obtain the necessary baseline DNA information from parents and other family members. Such situations are becoming increasingly rare because of the speed and efficiency of DNA-based prenatal diagnosis using the polymerase chain reaction.

DNA-Based Prenatal Diagnosis

The characterization of thalassemia mutations at the DNA level has led to the application of various molecular techniques for the prenatal detection of thalassemia.[137,138] The source of DNA may be amniotic fluid cells obtained by amniocentesis between 14 and 20 weeks of gestation or chorionic villi obtained by ultrasound-guided transcervical or transabdominal sampling (aspiration biopsy) between 8 and 10 weeks of gestation. The latter procedure is increasingly preferred because it allows much earlier diagnosis, counseling, and decision making. Both procedures are considerably safer than fetal blood sampling.

Detection of Globin Gene Deletions

The earliest applications of molecular biology to prenatal detection of thalassemia consisted of molecular hybridization assays in solution or Southern gel blotting assays to detect thalassemia syndromes due to gene deletions such as the common forms of α-thalassemia and $\delta\beta$-thalassemia. Theoretically, any thalassemia defect that is associated with an abnormal globin gene pattern on Southern gel blotting can be detected in this way. However, most of the demand for prenatal diagnosis involves pregnancies at risk for homozygous β-thalassemia in which the molecular defects are mostly the result of point mutations rather than gene deletions.

Use of Restriction Fragment Length Polymorphisms

A widely applied procedure for the prenatal diagnosis of thalassemia in the absence of gene deletion or of a direct assay for the gene mutation was developed after the characterization of RFLPs in the β-globin gene cluster (see previous section on polymorphisms of the globin gene clusters). Thus, it is possible by Southern gel blotting to identify and track, in a given family, linkage of one or more polymorphisms to a β-thalassemic gene that is coinherited with the marker polymorphisms in the family.

Use of this technique for prenatal diagnosis of β-thalassemia is facilitated by the fact that polymorphisms occur at a high frequency at multiple different sites in the β-globin gene cluster and are associated with one another in a nonrandom fashion, forming haplotypes (see Fig. 51-15) that are associated in a given population group with specific molecular forms of thalassemia. Thus, haplotype analysis of RFLPs in fetal DNA became a widely used and precise method to achieve prenatal diagnosis of β-thalassemia.[494]

Although accurate, haplotype analysis remains a labor-intensive procedure requiring analysis of DNA from many family members using a number of different enzymes. Using standard Southern gel blotting, this technique may also require substantial amounts of fetal DNA, which may not always be available. Finally, the test does not provide a definitive answer in about 10% to 15% of cases because of lack of heterozygosity of RFLPs in key family members or lack of sufficient numbers or types of informative family members. For these various reasons, a procedure with 100% applicability would be preferred that can directly rather than indirectly identify mutations in a single assay requiring a small amount of DNA. Such procedures have been devised and are discussed in the following section.

Direct Demonstration of Point Mutations in DNA

The Polymerase Chain Reaction. Point mutations causing β-thalassemia can be detected by Southern gel blotting of total cellular DNA followed by hybridization to allele-specific oligonucleotide (ASO) probes[495–497] (see later section on direct identification of single base substitutions by use of synthetic oligonucleotide probes). The introduction of the polymerase chain reaction (PCR) has greatly facilitated the process of mutation detection.[498,499] The PCR technique uses synthetic oligonucleotides corresponding to sequences flanking a DNA region of interest as primers for the amplification of this DNA segment. This is done in repeated cycles of DNA synthesis in vitro, using a DNA polymerase. The reaction is carried out in an automated apparatus that subjects the sample to repeated cycles of heating to denature the DNA, followed by lowering of the temperature to allow annealing of the primers to the denatured DNA and synthesis of DNA between the two primers by primer extension. A thermostable DNA polymerase is used, which is resistant to inactivation during the heating cycles. After 30 or more cycles, the target sequence is amplified about 1 million-fold over its starting concentration and can be seen as a discrete band after gel electrophoresis. Thus, starting with 1 μg of total cellular DNA in which the β-globin gene is less than 1 part per million, the PCR technique can yield 1 μg of β-globin gene fragment.

The amplified DNA can then be subjected to various analyses, which will be discussed in detail in the following sections: (1) restriction endonuclease digestion and gel electrophoresis to visualize the digestion pattern and (2) blotting of the DNA to filters (dot blots or slot blots) followed by hybridization with normal and mutant ASO probes. The PCR approach is much quicker and simpler than previously used techniques such as Southern gel blotting of total cellular DNA followed by ASO hybridization. An added advantage is that only tiny amounts of DNA are required; thus, the size of the fetal tissue sample is almost never a limiting factor.

Although ^{32}P-labeled oligonucleotide probes are most frequently used, the procedure has been adapted to nonisotopic techniques, thus increasing its access to geographic areas where use of isotopes is not feasible or inconvenient.[500,501] A longer shelf-life of probes can also be achieved by use of ^{35}S- rather than ^{32}P-labeled ATP for end labeling of the oligonucleotide probes.[502] Other modifications of the technique include the use of fluorescence-based color complementation assays[503]; use of specific primers to selectively amplify only a normal or mutant allele[504]; use of immobilized sequence-specific probes in nonisotopic detection assays[505]; and PCR-based mutagenesis to create a restriction endonuclease cleavage site difference between a normal and a mutant allele.[506,507] The PCR technique can also be used to detect RFLPs either singly[508] or in groups using multiplex reactions containing multiple sets of matched primer pairs. Thus, it is possible to carry out haplotyping of β-gene cluster RFLPs using one or two PCR reactions and direct visualization of the PCR products after enzyme digestion and gel electrophoresis and circumventing the need for multiple Southern gel blots and hybridization to multiple different ^{32}P-labeled probes.[509]

Identification of the Mutations in the Couple at Risk. Prenatal diagnosis of β-thalassemia by direct detection of point mutations using PCR or traditional approaches requires prior demonstration of the specific mutations present in the family at risk. In view of the multiplicity of β-thalassemic mutations (see Table 51-2), this may appear at first glance to be a daunting task. However, a given mutation usually occurs only within one racial group, and within a given racial group, five or six specific mutations usually account for about 90% of all cases of β-thalassemia[137,138,492] (Table 51-6). In addition, a given mutation within a given racial group is usually associated with only one particular haplotype of β-gene cluster RFLPs. Thus, when a couple who are at risk present for the first time for prenatal diagnosis of β-thalassemia, it should be relatively easy to establish the nature of the β-thalassemic mutation in each parent (and in any affected offspring) by using PCR-based technology to carry out haplotype analysis and screening for the most likely mutations, based on knowledge of the racial origin and haplotypes of the affected persons. In those cases in which a common mutation is not detected in this initial screening procedure, PCR can be used to amplify and directly sequence the β-globin genes of the undiagnosed parent to identify the nature of the mutation.[149,510]

Another screening procedure to identify the general location of a point mutation is the technique of *denaturing gradient gel electrophoresis.*[511] By initially determining the approximate location of a point mutation in the β-globin gene, the process of specific mutation identification by DNA sequence analysis can be achieved more quickly and efficiently. The technique consists of fractionating DNA fragments, usually PCR products, in a specialized acrylamide gel electrophoresis system that subjects the migrating DNA fragments to a gradient of denaturing forces. Thus, DNA fragments that are identical except for the presence of a single base substitution will denature and acquire altered mobility at different positions in the gel, because different DNA sequences usually require different conditions of denaturation for the two strands to separate or "melt." The differential mobility between mutant and normal fragments can be further enhanced by mixing them together and then subjecting them to denaturation and renaturation, thus allowing the formation of heteroduplexes or hybrid DNA fragments in which one strand is normal

TABLE 51-6. Common β-Thalassemia Mutations in Different Racial Groups

MEDITERRANEAN
IVS-1 position 110 (G → A)
Codon 39, nonsense
IVS-1 position 1 (G → A)
IVS-2 position 745 (C → G)
IVS-1 position 6 (T → C)
IVS-2 position 1 (G → A)
BLACK
−29 (A → G)
−88 (C → T)
Poly (A), (AATAAA → AACAAA)
SOUTHEAST ASIAN
Codons 41/42, frameshift
IVS-2 position 654 (C → T)
Codon 17, nonsense
−28 (A → G)
ASIAN INDIAN
IVS-1 position 5 (G → C)
619-bp deletion
Codons 8/9, frameshift
Codons 41/42, frameshift
IVS-1 position 1 (G → T)

(Data from Kazazian HH Jr, Boehm CD. Molecular basis and prenatal diagnosis of β-thalassemia. Blood 1988; 72:1107)

and the complementary strand contains the base substitution.

The heteroduplexes are substantially more unstable than the parent molecules and thus are more widely separated from the latter after gel electrophoresis. This technique, which was initially applied to the study of cloned globin genes, has also been used successfully to detect single base substitution in thalassemic globin genes by analysis of total cellular DNA digested with appropriate restriction enzymes[512] and, more recently, to efficiently identify β-thalassemic mutations in PCR-generated fragments derived from genomic DNA.[513,514] Computer programs have been derived to facilitate the selection of the location and sequence of PCR primers that are most likely to provide the most efficient detection of mutations by this procedure.[511] This technique constitutes another screening procedure for the identification of those carrying novel or specific mutations in a given region of a globin (or other) gene.

Direct Identification of Mutations by Differences in Restriction Endonuclease Cleavage Pattern Due to the Mutation Itself. A number of the base substitutions (or other subtle mutations) causing α- or β-thalassemia abolish or create cleavage sites for different restriction endonucleases at the precise point of the mutation.[492] They are therefore directly detectable by Southern gel blotting of total cellular DNA or enzymatic digestion and gel electrophoresis of appropriate PCR products. This approach was first used for the successful prenatal diagnosis of Hb O^{Arab} ($\beta^{121\ Glu \rightarrow Lys}$), in which the base substitution abolishes the intragenic *Eco*RI site of the β-globin gene.[515] Widespread use of this approach occurred with the identification of restriction enzymes, such as *Mst*II, having recognition sites, encompassing β-globin gene codon 6, which are abolished by the base substitution causing sickle cell hemoglobin ($\beta^{6\ Glu \rightarrow Val}$). Direct detection of the β^S mutation using PCR followed by digestion of the PCR product with *Mst* II (or other enzymes with similar specificity) constitutes the method of choice for prenatal diagnosis of sickle cell anemia.[516,517]

In β-thalassemia, about 30% to 40% of the mutations, including five of seven common Mediterranean mutations, are directly detectable by restriction endonuclease digestion of DNA.[137,138,492] In some cases, the size of the affected DNA fragments is small, making detection difficult or impossible by traditional Southern gel blotting but not by analysis of PCR products. Nevertheless, some common forms of β-thalassemia, such as the IVS-1 position 110 mutation, do not directly affect restriction endonuclease sites and are therefore not normally detectable by enzymatic digestion and gel analysis. Therefore, a different strategy was initially devised for the direct DNA diagnosis of these thalassemic mutations, as described in the following section.

Direct Identification of Single Base Substitutions by the Use of Synthetic Oligonucleotide Probes. The precedence-setting work of Wallace and colleagues[518,519] established the feasibility of direct detection of single nucleotide base substitutions in globin gene DNA by the use of labeled synthetic oligonucleotide probes about 19 nucleotides long, in which the central nucleotide is either identical with or different from that of the target DNA sequence being analyzed. Hybridization conditions were established that would allow annealing of the synthetic probe to its target only if all 19 nucleotides were perfectly complementary. If the one central nucleotide was different, no hybridization was observed. Thus, it was possible to distinguish with such oligonucleotide probes DNA containing the β^A-globin gene from that containing the β^S-globin gene, initially in cloned DNA samples, then in total cellular DNA. This established the basis for using this procedure in the prenatal detection of β-thalassemic point mutations in fetal DNA samples.

The general strategy for this approach consists of using two ASO probes: one complementary to the normal sequence, the other complementary to the mutant sequence with a single nucleotide substitution. By using the different probes in parallel or sequential hybridization assays, the presence or absence of the normal or the mutant sequence can be detected in the test sample, thereby allowing the detection of heterozygotes as well as homozygotes for the target sequences. Before the introduction of PCR, this procedure was applied to the study of total cellular DNA. Because total cellular DNA contains multiple regions that can hybridize to a given 19-base oligonucleotide, it was not possible to carry out the analysis directly on dots or spots of total unfractioned DNA. If the DNA was first digested with a restriction endonuclease and fractionated by agarose gel electrophoresis, it became possible to separate the specific target DNA fragment containing the β-globin gene away from the nonspecifically hybridizing fragments located elsewhere in the genome.[519]

*Bam*HI is a convenient enzyme for detecting β-thalassemic mutations.[495–497] It yields a 1.8-kb fragment, containing the 5′ end of the β-globin gene, which is well separated from higher molecular weight fragments that hybridize to oligonucleotide probes corresponding to sequences in exon 1, exon 2, or IVS-1 of the β-globin gene, the sites of common point mutations causing β-thalassemia.

With the introduction and availability of PCR, use of ASO hybridization has been made much simpler and quicker. Because of the tremendous amplification of the target sequence, the background hybridization to nonspecific DNA sequences is negligible relative to the authentic hybridization signal. Thus, it is not necessary to fractionate the sample; it can be directly applied to filters and hybridized to the probes. Nevertheless, the specificity of the hybridization and washing conditions must be established for each probe set to ensure accuracy of the assay. Conditions for specificity may vary between different probe sets because of differences in the G+C content of the probes and the nature of the single base-pair mismatch that disrupts hybridization; that is, G to T mismatches are more stable than A to C mismatches.

As previously stated, it is possible to use nonisotopically tagged probes, which have the advantage of having a long shelf-life, thus provide more flexibility to the assay.[500,501] Such probes usually consist of oligonucleotides tagged with horseradish peroxidase or with biotin (or other hapten) and are detected by histochemical assay or enzyme-linked immunoassay. A variation on the nonisotopic detection assay uses reverse dot hybridization, in which the unmodified oligonucleotide probe is immobilized on a filter and the target DNA is amplified using biotinylated primers.[505]

ASO probes are commonly used in the detection of those thalassemia mutations for which there is no detection assay using naturally occurring restriction enzyme sites. Nevertheless, in such cases it is frequently possible to generate by PCR-based mutagenesis restriction enzyme sites, which distinguish the mutant from the normal allele,[506,507] or to use allele-specific primers for the PCR reaction, which will allow the amplification of only the normal or mutant allele.[504]

Summary and Conclusions

Safe, rapid, and accurate procedures are available for the prenatal diagnosis of thalassemia. The method of choice consists of chorionic villus biopsy performed between 8 and 10 weeks of gestation. DNA extracted from the sample is then amplified by using PCR and the amplified DNA analyzed by restriction endonuclease digestion and gel electrophoresis or by hybridization of slot–dot blots with

ASOs. Systematic programs to educate the public and provide comprehensive testing and counseling services in countries and regions where the prevalence of thalassemia is high have resulted in a dramatic decrease in the incidence of new cases of the disease in recent years.[520–522] In the United States, one of the leading centers providing DNA-based prenatal diagnosis of thalassemia, sickle cell anemia and other genetic diseases is in the Division of Genetics, Department of Pediatrics, Johns Hopkins University School of Medicine, under the direction of Dr. Haig H Kazazian, Jr. (Similar diagnostic services are also provided by commercial laboratories such as IG Labs, Inc, Framingham, MA.)

Gene Therapy and Manipulation of Gene Expression

Gene Transfer Approaches

It is clear from the heterogeneity and nature of the molecular defects that cause thalassemia that any practical attempts at gene therapy for thalassemia should be directed at substituting, by various gene transfer technologies, normal globin genes for the defective thalassemic genes, rather than directly correcting the specific defect associated with the mutant gene. A possible exception to this is the potential for correcting the effect of nonsense mutations in thalassemic globin mRNAs by the transfer of suppressor tRNA genes into hematopoietic stem cells, thus providing erythroid cells with a means of translating the mutant globin mRNA into a full-length, functional globin chain. The mutant β-globin mRNA associated with the nonsense mutation at β-globin codon 17 has been successfully translated into normal β-globin chains in frog oocytes after transfer into these cells of genes for an amber suppressor tRNA capable of inserting a lysine at the position of a UAG chain termination codon.[523]

A particular concern regarding gene therapy using amber suppressor tRNA genes resides in the nonspecificity of the approach. In addition to allowing full-length translation of the mutant β-globin mRNAs, the amber suppressor tRNAs allow the readthrough of all normal cellular mRNAs that have a UAG termination codon and therefore lead to the synthesis of many proteins abnormally elongated at their C terminal. The potential harmful effects on hematopoietic cells of such readthrough proteins remains unknown, although in prokaryotic systems, amber suppressor tRNAs do not have a notably harmful or lethal effect. Short-term viability of frog oocytes was not appreciably affected by the presence of amber suppressor tRNA in the experiments resulting in translation of thalassemic globin mRNA containing a nonsense mutation.[523] Nevertheless, although attractive on a theoretical level, this approach is not being actively pursued in practical terms as a possible modality of human gene therapy.

With regard to gene therapy by transfer of normal globin genes into hematopoietic stem cells, a number of obstacles must be overcome: those related to the level of expression of globin genes after transfer into a foreign chromosomal environment and those related to the cell biology of hematopoietic stem cells and the difficulty of introducing genes into the self-renewing or reconstituting hematopoietic stem cell. Great progress has been made in the technical ability to transfer globin gene DNA into a variety of tissue culture cells as well as into primary hematopoietic cells of the bone marrow.[524–530] It has become apparent during the course of these experiments that the transferred globin genes are not usually expressed at high levels in their new chromosomal environment and that the marrow cells successfully transfected are not predominantly self-renewing.

Retroviral Vectors

The most efficient method of transferring genes into cells is by the use of retroviral vectors.[531–533] The gene of interest is inserted into a DNA copy of the virus from which most of the viral genes and control elements have been removed. The DNA is then transfected into a viral packaging cell line that produces all of the necessary components to package RNA copies of the modified retroviral genome into infectious viral particles. After entry of these particles into a target cell, a DNA copy of the viral genome (produced by the reverse transcription of the viral RNA) is integrated randomly into the chromosomal DNA of the host cell. Because the modified retroviral genome lacks essential genes, such as those for viral envelope proteins, no further cycles of viral production can occur. Nevertheless, the integrated viral genome can be transcribed and produce mRNA copies of the gene inserted into it for the purpose of gene therapy. In globin gene transfers, the retrovirus is constructed in such a way that the globin gene is transcribed from its own promoter in an opposite direction from that of viral gene transcription, which occurs from the promoter of the viral long terminal repeat sequence.

One of the earliest successful globin gene transfer experiments in a long-term living animal model system was accomplished by Dzierzak and colleagues.[534] This experiment illustrates some of the practical difficulties of the approach that must be overcome before future applications in humans. The human β-globin gene was successfully transferred by means of a retrovirus into self-renewing hematopoietic stem cells of mice; this was evidenced by the fact that DNA of the transferred globin retrovirus was still detectable in blood cells of the mice 4 to 9 months after transplantation of the virally transduced bone marrow cells. The extent of donor marrow cell engraftment varied between 40% and 98%, whereas the efficiency of infection of the engrafted donor marrow cells ranged between 2% and 100%. The transferred human globin gene was expressed in virtually a tissue-specific manner, globin mRNA being detected in significant amounts essentially only in erythroid cells, although trace amounts were observed in lymphoid cells and macrophages of some of the animals.[534] A disappointing result was the very low level of β-globin mRNA expression that was estimated to correspond to only 0.4% to 4% of the level of the endogenous murine β-globin mRNA when considered on a single copy per genome basis. Similar results were subsequently reported by Bender and colleagues.[535]

Transfers of foreign globin genes by other means such as by microinjection into oocytes to produce transgenic mice or by DNA-mediated gene transfer into MEL cells also generally result in low levels of expression of the transferred globin gene relative to that of endogenous globin genes. The normal chromosomal environment of the endogenous gene is thought to be an important factor contributing to and being necessary for the high level of expression of globin genes. Also, for transferred globin genes to be reproducibly expressed at high levels and in a tissue-specific manner, they may have to become integrated at or near the normal chromosomal site of the endogenous globin gene.

An important feature of the normal chromosomal environment that confers a high level of expression to globin genes is the LCR[46] (see previous section on enhancers and other *cis*-acting elements that influence globin gene expression). It was therefore thought that incorporation of

LCR sequences into the retroviral vectors would overcome the problem of low expression levels. Unfortunately, initial attempts to include LCR sequences in gene transfer vectors has had unexpected deleterious effects on the ability to obtain retroviral stocks of sufficiently high titer to be efficient vehicles for gene transfer into bone marrow hematopoietic stem cells.[536,537] It is nevertheless possible that additional manipulation of these sequences will result in the removal of sequences deleterious for viral production without inhibiting the potentiating effect of the sequences on globin gene expression. The use of LCR-containing retroviral vectors for human β-globin gene transfers into MEL tissue culture cells has resulted in enhanced levels of expression of the transferred gene,[536–539] which, in some cell lines, was equal to or higher than that of the endogenous murine β-globin gene.[536,537] Recently, mice were successfully engrafted with LCR/β-globin retrovirus-transduced hematopoietic stem cells and expressed significantly higher levels of human β globin than in previous studies.[539]

Potential safety problems associated with the use of retroviral vectors as gene transfer vehicles include the following[533]: insertional mutagenesis due to the random nature of the DNA integration event, resulting either in inactivation of an essential gene or inappropriate activation of a nearby latent potentially harmful gene such as a protooncogene, and inadvertent infection of the marrow and therefore the patient, with oncogenic wild type retrovirus, which may contaminate the gene transfer virus stock because of recombination with the viral genome in the packaging cell line. Although these are definite risks, they occur infrequently. In particular, the use of more recently developed disabled viruses has greatly reduced the risk of contaminating wild type retroviruses.[531]

Gene Targeting Approach

An alternative approach to the problem of low expression levels of transferred globin genes is to attempt targeted insertion of the transferred gene into the endogenous globin gene locus by homologous recombination. Although targeted transfer of globin and other genes has been successfully accomplished in tissue culture cells as well as in mouse embryonic stem cells, such homologous recombination events occur very infrequently.[540–542] To be useful in practical terms for gene therapy, this targeting approach requires the ability to carry out selection and subsequent in vitro expansion of the rare cell in which the event has taken place. Unfortunately, in vitro techniques for selection and expansion of self-renewing hematopoietic stem cells are not readily available, although progress along these lines can be anticipated in the near future.

Stem Cell Biology

For effective gene therapy, the gene must be transferred into the self-renewing hematopoietic stem cell. If the gene is transferred only into the more differentiated, non–self-renewing, progenitor or precursor cells, the cell lineage containing the transferred gene will persist only transiently. Unfortunately, gene transfer and integration require cell division, whereas most of the self-renewing stem cells in the bone marrow are usually in the nondividing (G_0) phase of the cell cycle and are therefore relatively refractory to successful gene transfer. Although transfer of globin (and other) genes into the self-renewing hematopoietic stem cell of the mouse has been successfully accomplished,[534] experiments in larger animal species have been generally disappointing, and suggest that gene transfer into self-renewing hematopoietic stem cells of these species occurs at too low a level to achieve any practical therapeutic impact. A promising approach to this problem is the exposure of the bone marrow to various combinations of hematopoietic growth factors—before or during infection with the retroviral vector—to stimulate the self-renewing cell to enter into the cell cycle and divide.

Experiments in the murine model system indicate that a higher proportion of reconstituting or self-renewing stem cells can be infected after prestimulation of the marrow in vitro with hematopoietic growth factors such as interleukin-3 (IL-3) and IL-6.[543,544] The use of stem cell factor (kit ligand) may also be helpful in this regard.[545,546] Prestimulation of cells with hematopoetic growth factors, combined with the use of high-titer viral producer cell lines with or without initial enrichment of stem cells by CD34 antibody selection, has resulted in the successful transfer of a retroviral vector into self-renewing stem cells of the rhesus monkey. Thus far, this has occurred in only about 1% of the reconstituting stem cells.[547–550]

In conclusion, much progress in the successful transfer of globin (and other) genes into hematopoietic cells has been achieved, but more progress is required before gene therapy by globin gene transfer is a reality for the management of thalassemia. If advances in this field continue to occur with the same explosive rapidity as they have, numerous breakthroughs can be anticipated, and perhaps the realization of what has been for many the "impossible dream." Actually, the first practical attempt at gene therapy using a retroviral vector in a human being is underway in two children with immunodeficiency due to adenosine deaminase (ADA) enzyme deficiency.[526] The clinical trial consists of repeated aphereses of the patients' peripheral blood leukocytes followed by stimulation of the lymphoid cells with IL-2, exposure to a retrovirus containing the ADA gene, and reinfusion of the cells into the patient. In this case, the target cells for gene transfer are long-lived T-lymphocytes, not the self-renewing hematopoietic stem cells. Approval by regulatory agencies for similar gene therapy trials using bone marrow or cord blood stem cells of affected newborn infants has been obtained.[526]

Manipulation of Endogenous Globin Gene Expression

Pharmacologic augmentation of γ-globin gene expression is a feasible alternative approach to gene therapy for the control of the pathophysiologic abnormalities in homozygous β-thalassemia as well as in sickle cell anemia. As previously discussed, increased synthesis of Hb F can have a beneficial effect on the severity of homozygous β-thalassemia and sickle cell anemia. Recent studies have demonstrated that it is possible to increase Hb F production in patients with hemoglobinopathies by the administration of various chemotherapeutic agents.

In adult bone marrow cells, the inactive γ-globin genes are in a state of hypermethylation, as is usually the case for inactive genes in animal cells. In contrast, the active γ-globin genes in fetal liver erythroid cells are hypomethylated as expected for any active gene. The importance of DNA methylation in γ-globin gene expression is also illustrated by the finding that permanently methylated γ-globin genes are not expressed normally after gene transfer into tissue culture cells. The chemotherapeutic agent 5-azacytidine prevents the methylation of DNA during DNA replication by inhibiting the enzyme DNA methyltransferase. On the basis of the previously mentioned information, DeSimone and colleagues[551] reasoned that the administration of 5-azacytidine might result in enhanced γ-globin gene expression, and this was the result they obtained after administration of the drug to baboons.

Based on these animal studies, short-term clinical trials of 5-azacytidine therapy were carried out in patients with homozygous β-thalassemia or sickle cell anemia.[552–554] The initial results were encouraging: after administration of the drug, a four- to eight-fold increase occurred in the level of Hb F, and this was accompanied by evidence of decreased hemolysis and decreased ineffective erythropoiesis as well as by a sustained increase in the total hemoglobin for up to 40 days. Studies of DNA methylation showed a decrease in methylation of the γ- and ε-globin genes in bone marrow cells starting as early as 2 days after the drug was given and lasting up to 21 days.

As exciting as these results were, they were greeted with some caution and concern regarding the general applicability and long-term safety of the therapy. The biggest concern was the fact that the drug is probably mutagenic and carcinogenic and that long-term therapy might lead to the development of malignancies. Therefore, the use of 5-azacytidine to stimulate Hb F synthesis in patients with homozygous β-thalassemia is considered highly experimental and, until more information accumulates regarding long-term side effects, limited in its application to patients with advanced disease for whom conventional therapy is not possible. Treatment of a limited number of such patients has resulted in therapeutic benefits.[555,556]

The precise mechanism of action of 5-azacytidine in augmenting Hb F production is not clear and is probably not exclusively or predominantly related to its effects on γ-globin gene demethylation. Administration of a number of other chemotherapeutic agents such as cytosine arabinoside (cytarabine; Ara C) and hydroxyurea also results in enhanced Hb F production, but these agents do not directly influence gene methylation. The current model proposes that these agents influence Hb F production by a combination of cell toxicity and depletion followed by regeneration, resulting in the selective recruitment of erythroid progenitor cells that give rise to precursors with the capacity to produce cells with high levels of Hb F (F cells).[557–560] This is illustrated by the high Hb F pathway of progenitor cell maturation, as shown in Figure 51-8.

It is likely that these chemotherapeutic agents also have a direct effect on globin gene expression in differentiating erythroid precursor cells, perhaps as a result of disruption of the cell cycle. At least in the case of 5-azacytidine, the increased production of Hb F, as evidenced by increased numbers of Hb F-containing reticulocytes, can be observed as early as 2 days after administration of the agents, an interval that is too short to be consistent with the maturation time of newly recruited progenitor cells.[558] This early, apparently direct effect may be due to hypomethylation.

Butyrate is another compound that has been demonstrated to augment Hb F production in various animal model systems (see previous section on ontogeny of globin gene expression). Butyrate is thought to act by altering chromatin configuration. Short-term treatment with butyrate in a limited number of patients resulted in increased levels of γ-globin chain synthesis.[90] Three patients with sickle cell anemia and three patients with β-thalassemia syndromes were treated with short courses (2 to 3 weeks) of continuous intravenous infusions of arginine butyrate. In all six patients γ-globin chain synthesis increased by 6% to 45%. In one patient with homozygous Hb Lepore who was treated for 7 weeks, the hemoglobin level rose from 4.7 to 10.2 g/dL, without significant side effects.[90] Another study examined the effect on F-cell production of an oral agent, sodium 4-phenylacetate, given for therapy of urea-cycle disorders.[89] In 15 nonanemic patients who had received this compound for 5 to 65 months, the mean F-cell level was 12.4% ± 3.1% compared with the level of 3.1% ± 0.2% in normal subjects. Use of this oral agent in four patients with sickle cell anemia has resulted in a significant increase in F-cell levels[561] and, in one patient with β^0-thalassemia, an improvement in α/non-α globin chain synthetic ratio from 0.5 to 1.0.[562] Although no toxic side effects were observed in these short-term trials in humans, the infusion of high doses of butyrate into baboons did result in signifcant neurologic toxicity.[88] Further studies will be required to assess the long-term safety and efficacy of therapy with butyrate.

Because of its relatively low toxicity, hydroxyurea is the chemotherapeutic agent favored for clinical trials in humans.[62,563,565] The combination of hydroxyurea with recombinant hematopoietic growth factors such as erythropoietin is also being tested for possible additional potentiating effects on Hb F production.[566] Clinical trials of hydroxyurea for augmentation of Hb F production are primarily being conducted in patients with sickle cell anemia.[563,564]

CLINICAL ASPECTS OF THE β-THALASSEMIAS

Historical Review

In 1925 and 1927, Cooley and associates described five children with similar clinical radiographic and hematologic abnormalities.[1,567] At that time, many of the severe anemias of infancy and childhood were designated as Von Jach's anemia or pseudoleukemic anemia. Cooley clearly delineated a distinct syndrome from what was a heterogeneous group of disorders. Cooley's patients were severely anemic and had characteristic facies described as "mongoloid." Their skin and sclerae were yellow. Radiographs showed striking enlargement of the marrow spaces of the cranial and facial bones. Splenomegaly was a consistent feature. Their blood smears showed large numbers of normoblasts leading Cooley to designate this condition as "erythroblastic anemia."

Cooley's anemia is known to result from monozygosity for thalassemia genes, which, in the heterozygous state, usually produce β-thalassemia minor (β-thalassemia trait).

Heterozygous β-Thalassemia

Heterozygosity for a β-thalassemia gene usually results in clinical β-thalassemia minor, a mild, nonprogressive, hypochromic microcytic anemia. A partial deficiency of β-chain synthesis can be demonstrated by in vitro globin synthetic studies that show a β-/α-chain ratio of 0.5:0.7.[568] Ferrokinetic studies reveal impaired incorporation of ^{59}Fe into RBC hemoglobin, which is less severe than in homozygous β-thalassemia.[569]

Hematology of β-Thalassemia Minor

The hemoglobin levels of persons affected with β-thalassemia minor average 1 to 2 g/dL less than age- and gender-matched normals. RBCs are hypochromic (mean corpuscular hemoglobin concentration [MCHC] less than 26 pg) and microcytic (mean corpuscular volume [MCV] less than 75 fL, and RBC count is in the high normal range or increased. Osmotic fragility is decreased and a one-tube osmotic fragility test has been used for screening for thalassemia trait.[570]

The blood smear shows varying numbers of target cells but targeting is not as prominent as in the Hb E and Hb C disorders and should not be considered pathognomonic of thalassemia. Poikilocytes, anisocytes, ovalocytes, and basophilic stippling of the RBCs are also usually noted.

Symptomatology of β-Thalassemia Minor

Most persons affected with β-thalassemia minor are asymptomatic, and the blood abnormalities are frequently first noted during routine hematologic examinations. This is especially true when electronic cell counters measuring MCV are used. Some patients complain of increased fatigability. No significant hematologic differences or changes in 2,3-DPG levels or oxygen affinity could be found between a group of β-thalassemia minor women who complained of easy fatigue and a group of β-thalassemia minor women who had no symptoms.[571]

During the last trimester of pregnancy, the hemoglobin level of women with β-thalassemia minor often decreases further and transfusions have sometimes been considered necessary. Because iron deficiency may occur during pregnancy, iron supplements are often used.[572,573]

A small proportion of persons with heterozygous β-thalassemia have more pronounced chronic anemia, splenomegaly, and some bony abnormalities. Splenomegaly, pigmentary gallstones, and leg ulceration may occur in these persons. These patients have been described as having dominant thalassemia trait.[574]

In African and African-American ethnic groups, the prevalence of β-thalassemia trait may be as high as 0.2% to 0.5%. The condition is milder, RBC abnormalities are less marked, and β-/α-globin chain synthetic ratios are higher than those usually observed in whites and Asians.[575] These differences are accounted for by different kinds of thalassemia mutations in blacks.[576]

Differential Diagnosis of Microcytic Anemias

Microcytic anemias have five general causes: iron deficiency; iron malutilization, as in the anemia of chronic infection; thalassemia; lead poisoning; and sideroblastic anemias.

Iron deficiency, either because of inadequate dietary intake or chronic blood loss, is by far the most common cause of microcytic anemia. It is characterized by a hypochromic microcytic anemia of varying degrees of severity and a constellation of biochemical abnormalities that include low serum iron, increased iron binding capacity, low serum ferritin levels, and increased RBC free erythrocyte protoporphyrin (FEP) levels. The anemia responds rapidly and predictably to iron medication.

In contrast, in the anemia of chronic inflammation and infection, serum iron levels are low, but serum iron binding capacity is not increased. Serum ferritin levels are normal or increased. Iron medication does not cause an increase in hemoglobin level.

Lead poisoning is often associated with iron deficiency. Remarkable increases in FEP and elevated levels of blood lead are diagnostic.

The sideroblastic anemias are a heterogeneous group of chronic disorders associated with iron overload. They are rarely confused with β-thalassemia minor.

In a patient with hypochromic microcytic anemia, a diagnosis of β-thalassemia minor can be established by demonstration of increased proportions of Hb A_2 by electrophoresis or column chromatography.

The level of Hb A_2 in β-thalassemia minor is above 3.5% and it averages 5.1% (range 3.5% to 7.1%), which is about twice the normal level. A strong correlation of Hb A_2 levels of affected persons in the same family has been demonstrated.[577,578] Diagnostically elevated Hb A_2 levels are established in affected infants by 4 to 6 months of age, as the postnatal fall in Hb F occurs. In those with β-thalassemia minor who also have severe iron deficiency, Hb A_2 levels are depressed, sometimes in the normal range.[579] If there is any indication of concomitant iron deficiency, Hb A_2 should be determined after a course of iron therapy.

Hb F levels are inconsistently elevated in persons with β-thalassemia minor. The postnatal fall of Hb F is delayed. After an affected infant is about 1 year of age, total Hb F in about 50% of persons is normal (less than 2%). In the remainder, levels of Hb F are moderately elevated (2.1% to 5%). A minor population of RBCs containing increased amounts of Hb F can be demonstrated by acid elution (Kleihauer-Betke technique).[580]

In many instances of hypochromic microcytic anemia, a diagnosis of iron deficiency anemia is entertained and iron therapy is given without significant improvement. A microcytic anemia that does not respond to iron therapy should suggest the possibility of β-thalassemia minor.

Screening for Thalassemia Trait

β-Thalassemia Trait. The purpose of mass screening for thalassemia is to identify persons who are at risk of having a child with a severe disease if they marry another affected person. Mass screening programs are carried out in Italy and Greece, where the incidence of β-thalassemia ia very high. When combined with prenatal diagnosis, the incidence of new cases of β-thalassemia major is being significantly decreased. In high-prevalence areas such as Italy, Greece, and Cyprus with national programs for heterozygote detection and availability of prenatal diagnosis, the birth of homozygote infants has fallen dramatically, in some areas by more than 90%.[581–583] Similar, although less striking, results have been described from London[584] and from Connecticut.[585]

Mass screening may be fraught with difficulties and should be undertaken only with expert professional and laboratory backup. It is essential to ensure voluntary informed participation, confidentiality of results, and meaningful counseling.

The most definitive methods for diagnosis of β-thalassemia are quantitative Hb A_2 determination and globin chain synthesis ratios, as well as direct demonstration of thalassemia mutations in the patient's DNA. These techniques are not applicable to mass screening. Because β-thalassemia minor is almost invariably associated with significant hypochromia (MCHC less than 26 pg) and microcytosis (MCV less than 75 fL), determination of RBC indices by electronic equipment such as the Coulter model S-cell counter has been used as a preliminary indicator of possible thalassemia trait.[586] Microcytosis due to iron deficiency must be excluded. The RBC distribution width is increased in iron deficiency patients but normal in those with β-thalassemia minor.[587] Algorithms have been described for diagnosis of β-thalassemia trait. Stockman and colleagues[588] have suggested the use of FEP measurements in the evaluation of persons with microcytosis. In persons with β-thalassemia trait, FEP levels are normal, whereas FEP levels are elevated in those with iron deficiency and plumbism.

Functions derived from Coulter counter indices have also been suggested for rapid differentiation between the microcytosis of thalassemia and iron deficiency. England and Fraser[589] described a derived function (DF) equal to MCV $-$ RBCs $-$ $(5 \times \text{Hb}) \div 3.4$. DF values higher than 2 were associated with iron deficiency, whereas values less than 2 indicated β-thalassemia trait. Mentzer[590] showed that the ratio of MCV (fL) to RBCs ($\times 10^6$) was also predictive. Values of more than 12 usually indicate iron deficiency, and those less than 11 usually are associated with β-thalassemia trait.

Most screening programs use an initial simple but sensitive screening test such as the MCV determined by electronic cell counters or the osmotic fragility. These screening tests exclude most normal persons but do not differentiate precisely between β-thalassemia trait and iron-deficiency anemia. Microcytic patients with β-thalassemia have elevated Hb A_2 levels. Hb F determinations and hemoglobin electrophoresis are necessary to diagnoses δβ-thalassemia and Hb Lepore traits in those with microcytic RBC. No feasible screening procedures detect the silent carrier of β-thalassemia trait.

α-Thalassemia Trait. α-Thalassemia, which occurs in the same populations as does β-thalassemia, makes screening more complicated. This diagnosis is suggested by a mild, familial hypochromic microcytosis with low or normal levels of Hb A_2 and Hb F and no evidence of iron deficiency. Absolute diagnosis of α-thalassemia requires demonstration of a β/α globin synthetic ratio greater than 1.1, or an enumeration of the number of α-thalassemia genes.[308]

Other Forms of β-Thalassemia

In addition to the common classic β-thalassemia trait characterized by microcytosis and elevated levels of Hb A_2, other variants of thalassemia have been described with different biochemical characteristics.

Silent Carrier

The silent carrier state for a β-thalassemia gene is usually used to describe a parent of a child with homozygous β-thalassemia who is hematologically normal. Although it must be admitted that nonpaternity is a more common explanation, the occurrence of multiple affected children in a given family suggests this condition. Thalassemia-like gene mutations have been demonstrated in some silent carriers. Hb E and unstable hemoglobins may also interact with β-thalassemias to produce a more severe condition in the double heterozygote.[6]

Not all instances of severe disease produced by a mating of a normal person with one with β-thalassemia minor need involve a silent carrier. One instance of a thalassemia mutation in the germ cells of the father of an affected child has been reported.[214]

δβ-Thalassemia (High Hb F Thalassemia)

The hematologic findings are those of a mild hypochromic microcytosis indistinguishable from those of β-thalassemia minor. Hb is elevated from 5% to 15% and is heterogeneously distributed in the RBCs. This condition arises from deletions in (β-globin gene) cluster. The most common deletion is referred to as the Sicilian type. The deletion begins within the δ-globin gene and extends a short distance beyond the β-globin gene (see Fig. 51-20).[591,592] The homozygous state for δβ-thalassemia results in the clinical and hematologic findings of thalassemia intermedia.[1]

Lepore Hemoglobin Syndromes ($\alpha_2[\delta\beta]_2$)

Although usually no qualitatively abnormal hemoglobin species is found in thalassemia, the Lepore hemoglobin syndromes are exceptions.[593] The Lepore hemoglobins contain a unique kind of polypeptide chain, which is a fusion of portions of both δ- and β-chains. The Lepore hemoglobin non-α chains begin with a normal 80 to 100 amino acid sequence of the N-terminal amino δ chain, which is linked to C-terminal sequence of the β chain. Thus, the Lepore hemoglobins are a consequence of unequal crossover between the δ and β loci at meiosis.[594,595] Several different Lepore hemoglobins have been described, resulting from different crossovers.[596] The δ-globin promoter regulates translation, and so Hb Lepore is synthesized at a markedly reduced rate and accounts for only 5% to 15% of the total.

The RBCs in Hb Lepore syndromes have the typical microcytosis and hypochromia of thalassemia. Heterozygosity for the Hb Lepore gene produces β-thalassemia minor, manifested as a mild hypochromic microcytic anemia. The doubly heterozygous state for β-thalassemia and Lepore traits is usually manifested as thalassemia intermedia.[597] Another crossover globin, Hb Kenya, has the normal N-terminal sequence of γ-globin united with the C-terminal sequence of β-globin.[598]

α+β-Thalassemia

Because of the prevalence of both α- and β-thalassemia genes in many populations, a number of various combinations have been observed. α-Thalassemia-1 trait (α−/α−) plus β-thalassemia trait produces a mild microcytic anemia no more severe than either trait alone.[599,600]

β-Thalassemia Intermedia

Five to 10% of patients with apparent homozygous β-thalassemia and others with doubly heterozygous conditions (β-thalassemia, Hb Lepore, and other conditions) have a syndrome of intermediate hematologic severity. Maintenance of a hemoglobin level (6 to 8 g/dL) compatible with reasonably comfortable survival in the absence of regular transfusions are the generally accepted criteria for β-thalassemia intermedia.[601] These patients do not usually have onset of recognized anemia until after 2 years of age. There is a broad range of clinical and hematologic severity. Some of the patients affected with β-thalassemia intermedia have the potential for survival well into adult life with few complications. Some have normal maturation and sexual development. Other patients with β-thalassemia intermedia have significant morbidity including weakness, cardiomegaly, osteoporosis, fractures, and splenomegaly.

All the complications of extramedullary hematopoiesis, especially spinal cord compression, may occur. Disfiguring facial changes may result in a grotesque appearance, causing emotional and psychological distress. Most complications can be prevented by transfusion programs that suppress erythropoiesis by maintaining hemoglobin levels higher than 10 g/dL.

Patients with β-thalassemia intermedia pose a therapeutic dilemma. If transfusions are begun, progressive hemosiderosis will inevitably develop. Failure to institute transfusions may be associated with unacceptable morbidity. A plea is made to consider the patient's total clinical condition, not only the hemoglobin level. Development of effective oral chelation therapy may make this therapeutic decision easier.

Whether or not β-thalassemia intermedia patients are regularly transfused, they may develop iron overload as a result of increased absorption of dietary iron. Chelation therapy with deferoxamine is indicated if patients become significantly iron loaded.

Although there is no specific therapy for patients with β-thalassemia intermedia, therapeutic use of erythropoietin, hydroxyurea, and butyrate is under investigation.[602,603] Prevention of folic acid deficiency by regular supplementation may be important in patients with extreme marrow hyperplasia. Aplastic crises associated with parvovirus infections may also result in life-threatening anemia. Splenectomy is often performed for massive splenomegaly or for the elimination of cytopenias resulting from hypersplenism.

In a 1985 symposium organized by the Thalassemia Program of the New England Regional Genetics Group (NERGG), data were tabulated from 48 patients with β-thalassemia intermedia followed at five northeastern centers (NERGG unpublished data). The mean age of the group was 21.9 years (range 3 to 45). This was distinctly older than a contemporary group of β-thalassemia major patients with a mean age of 14.2 years. Seventy-five percent (36 of 48) of the β-thalassemia intermedia patients had been splenectomized. The mean age at splenectomy was 12.1 years (range 1 to 43). The average hemoglobin of 11 patients who had not been splenectomized was 8.9 g/dL. An increase in hemoglobin level of 1 to 2 g/dL occurred after splenectomy. Facial changes were observed in most patients. These changes were considered severe in 34%, moderate in 40%, mild in 20%, and minimal or none in 6%. Two patients had undergone cosmetic maxillary reconstructive surgery. Twelve of 26 patients (47%) were abnormally short (under the fifth percentile). Forty-three percent were of normal stature. Twenty-one percent of patients had received no blood transfusions; 31% had infrequently received transfusions (1 to 20 transfusions). The remaining 48% had received more than 20 transfusions. Nineteen percent of the patients had been started on regular transfusions.Fifty percent of the patients had serum ferritin levels over 2000 ng/mL. Thirty-eight percent were on chelation therapy, and 12% had declined to initiate chelation therapy. Almost 30% of the patients had fractures, often involving multiple bones. Thirty-five percent had gallstones, and 88% of those had undergone cholecystectomy. Two patients (4%) had cirrhosis, and 5 (10%) had experienced severe bacterial sepsis or meningitis.

Homozygous β-Thalassemia (β-Thalassemia Major)

Modern transfusional therapy has had a major effect on the clinical and laboratory features of β-thalassemia major (homozygous β-thalassemia). The advent of modern hypertransfusion regimens prevents many of the most striking manifestations of the disease.[1,604,605] The deforming skeletal and cosmetic changes, so prevalent in the past, should be, at least in most industrialized countries, of largely historical importance. β-Thalassemia major in its untreated and undertreated form is described first. This description applies to the disease as seen in the United States before about 1965 and is still applicable elsewhere in the world.

Untreated β-Thalassemia

The prognosis for persons with untreated homozygous β-thalassemia is poor. Because of predominant Hb F production, the infant with β-thalassemia major is not significantly anemic at birth, even though decreased β-chain synthesis can be demonstrated at birth and even well before birth.[606,607] Neonatal screening for β-thalassemia has been reported using isoelectric focusing of the globin chains or quantitation of cord blood hemoglobins. Quantitative hemoglobin A determinations of cord blood reveal that thalassemia homozygotes have less than 2% Hb A, heterozygotes have 6.8% to 9.9%, and normals average 20.3%.[608] The absence of Hb A on an ordinary electrophoresis suggests homozygous β-thalassemia. We have seen a patient with homozygous thalassemia who was diagnosed by a state neonatal hemoglobinopathy screening program because his cord blood hemoglobin had only Hb F by electrophoresis.

Clinical manifestations of β-thalassemia major usually become apparent during the second 6 months of life, and the diagnosis is almost always evident by 2 years of age.[609] Pallor, irritability, growth retardation, abdominal swelling due to enlargement of the liver and spleen, and jaundice are the usual presenting clinical features. Baty and colleagues[610] described these symptoms in 13 of 16 patients under 2 years of age. Severe facial and skeletal changes develop later. In early reports, most children died in late infancy or early childhood as a consequence of severe anemia or infection. Silvestroni and Bianco,[611] in a retrospective review from Italy, reported that the average survival of children with untreated β-thalassemia major was less than 4 years and more than 80% died in the first 5 years of life. The length of survival of β-thalassemia major patients without transfusion in developed countries is not known because transfusion is almost universally given. Although life might be extended beyond early childhood, patients would experience considerable morbidity. Such information is unlikely to ever be available.

Conventional Treatment (Low Transfusion)

Transfusions are necessary to prevent early death in β-thalassemia major patients; in 50% of patients transfusion therapy is initiated in the first year of life.[609] Until 15 to 20 years ago, transfusions were given at irregular intervals, often 5 to 10 weeks or more apart. They were often given only when symptoms of severe anemia such as weakness and irritability occurred. The hemoglobin was permitted to fall to 5 to 6 g/dL or even lower, and these children had symptoms caused by severe anemia much of the time. Cardiomegaly, secondary to severe anemia was always present. Levels of serum erythropoietin were very high. Exuberant hypertrophy of erythroid marrow tissue occurred in both medullary and intramedullary sites as a response to the extreme hemolysis and severe anemia.

Transfusions were used sparingly in the 1950s to 1970s because of concerns about transfusion-induced hemosiderosis. Each 200 mL of packed RBCs transfused results in about 200 mg of iron being deposited in the tissues; this iron cannot be eliminated physiologically. After hundreds of transfusions, a massive iron burden occurs, often of more than 40 to 50 g of total body iron. Deposition of the iron and the fibrosis that it evokes cause dysfunction resulting in endocrine abnormalities such as growth retardation, failure of puberty, and diabetes mellitus. Siderofibrosis of the myocardium produces cardiac dysfunction manifested by arrhythmias and congestive heart failure. Before the 1970s, life expectancy of β-thalassemia major patients averaged 15 to 20 years, and survival of transfusion-dependent patients for more than 25 years was distinctly unusual.

Laboratory Findings

The affected child with homozygous β-thalassemia is not usually anemic at birth, but the hemoglobin level decreases progressively during the first months of life. When the child exibits symptoms, the hemoglobin level may be as low as 3 to 4 g/dL. In some patients, anemia develops more slowly, delaying the onset of symptoms until the latter part of the first year of life or later. Increasing splenomegaly is often associated with lower hemoglobin levels. The RBC morphology is strikingly abnormal, with many microcytes, bizarre poikilocytes, and target cells (Fig. 51-22). A characteristic finding is the presence of large, thin, wrinkled, and folded cells containing irregular clumps of hemoglobin.

Fessas[612] described intraerythrocytic inclusions in the peripheral blood cells, especially after splenectomy. These inclusions, best seen with supravital staining with methylene blue or cresyl violet as well as with phase microscopy,

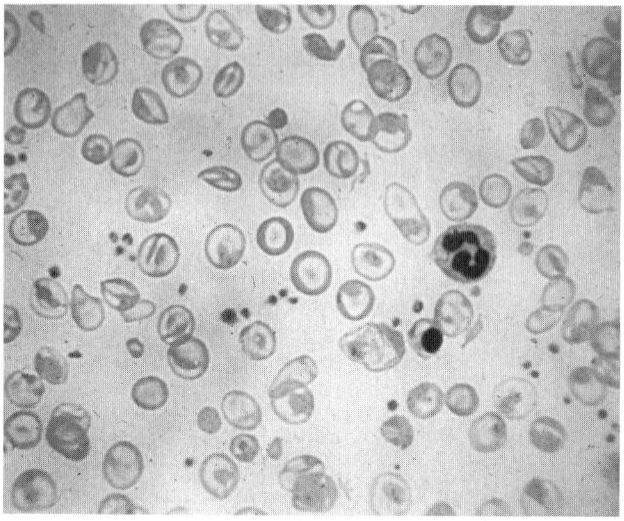

FIGURE 51-22. Peripheral blood of thalassemia major. Marked hypochromia anisocytosis and poikilocytosis and nucleated RBCs are notable. Many of the RBCs contain dense masses of precipitated α-globin chains (inclusion bodies), not visible in the Wright stain.

are aggregates of precipitated, denatured α chains.[613] The so-called Fessas bodies are also found in large numbers within erythroid precursors in the bone marrow and result in intramedullary hemolysis and ineffective erythropoiesis.[614,615] Nucleated RBCs are invariably found, but before splenectomy they may be relatively few in number (1 to 5 per 100 white blood cells [WBCs]). The reticulocyte count is 2% to 8%, which is lower than would be expected considering the degree of marrow erythroid hyperplasia and the degree of hemolysis. The WBC count is moderately elevated because of a polymorphonuclear leukocytosis. The platelet count is usually normal or increased unless considerable splenomegaly has developed, when thrombocytopenia may be seen. The bone marrow is markedly hypercellular as a result of normoblastic erythroid hyperplasia. The RBC precursors also show defective hemoglobinization and reduced amounts of cytoplasm. After splenectomy, a prodigious outpouring of nucleated RBCs into the blood occurs. Striking thrombocytosis (more than 1,000,000/μL) is often noted.

Although rarely used in the diagnostic evaluation of thalassemia, the RBC osmotic fragility is invariably abnormal. The RBCs are resistant to hemolysis in hypotonic sodium chloride solutions and are not entirely hemolyzed even in distilled water. Serum iron is increased, and the iron-binding protein is highly saturated.[616] Serum ferritin levels are elevated in proportion to the number of transfusions the patient has received.

The hemoglobin of the patient with homozygous β-thalassemia is either predominantly Hb F (β^+-thalassemia) or exclusively Hb F (β^0-thalassemia). Cases have been recognized by neonatal hemoglobinopathy screening programs from the fact that no Hb A is present. (Patients with homozygous β^0-thalassemia never produce Hb A.) In the newborn with β^+-thalassemia, more than 90% of hemoglobin is Hb F. With advancing age, this decreases slowly but usually ranges from 20% to 60%. Transfusions with normal Hb A containing RBCs will confound the estimation of the true Hb F level.

Hb A_2 levels tend to parallel the levels of Hb A in β-thalassemia major patients, although at a much lower level. The ratio of A_2 to A_1, which in the normal person is about 1:30, is increased to less than 1:20 in β-thalassemia major patients. Other biochemical abnormalities of the RBC in β-thalassemia major include a postnatal persistence of the i antigen and a decrease of RBC carbonic anhydrase.[617]

The serum is icteric with elevated serum levels of unconjugated bilirubin ranging from 2 to 4 mg/dL. RBC survival in β-thalassemia major patients is variable but usually decreased, with RBC chromium-51 (^{51}Cr) half-life ranging from 6.5 to 19.5 days compared with a normal half-life of 25 to 35 days. Increased plasma iron turnover and poor radioiron utilization indicate ineffective erythropoiesis.[618] Levels of transaminases (SGOT and SGPT) are increased, reflecting hepatic damage secondary to hemosiderosis. Lactic dehydrogenase levels are elevated as a consequence of ineffective erythropoiesis. Serum levels of haptoglobin and hemopexin are usually absent.

Low levels of serum zinc are present, and a relation of this finding to growth failure has been postulated but not established.[619,620] Low levels of serum and leukocyte ascorbic acid are common in thalassemia patients presumably because of increased catabolism of the vitamin in the presence of iron overload.[621] Administration of 100 mg of ascorbic acid per day maintains normal leukocyte levels of ascorbic acid and enhances the effectiveness of deferoxamine.[622] Larger doses of ascorbic acid may induce cardiac compromises.

Biochemical evidence of folic acid deficiency and occasional clinical and hematologic improvement after treatment with this vitamin have been described.[623,624] Although significant changes in hemoglobin levels or transfusions requirements rarely occur after treatment, many treatment centers use daily or biweekly supplementation with 0.5 to 1 mg of folic acid. The rationale for supplementation in well-transfused patients whose erythropoiesis is markedly reduced is unclear.

The large amounts of iron present in these patients' bodies and perhaps a degree of malabsorption secondary to pancreatic and hepatic fibrosis may lead to decreased levels of vitamin E (α-tocopherol), a potent antioxidant. Serum levels of vitamin E are often reduced below 0.5 mg/dL, and evidence of increased RBC membrane lipid peroxidation has been described.[625] Therapy with large doses of vitamin E does not improve survival of transfused RBCs or decrease transfusion requirements.[626]

Patients with β-thalassemia major often have recurrent nosebleeds. Study of the coagulation mechanism reveals abnormalities similar to those found in other patients with liver disease. Lowered levels of factors II, VII, IX, X, XI, and XII are present in older patients. Such coagulation defects are probably not the cause, or at least not the only cause, of nosebleeds because some patients with epistaxis have no significant coagulation defects. A general correlation exists between the coagulation status and the other parameters of hepatic function, both tending to deteriorate in older patients.[627]

Many thalassemia patients have slightly prolonged bleeding times and abnormal platelet aggregation. Although these changes are not usually considered of great clinical significance, some suggest that salicylates should be used with caution in these patients.[628] Other centers routinely administer aspirin because of the thrombocytosis that occurs after splenectomy; increased bleeding has not been observed.

Pathology

The pathologic changes in β-thalassemia major patients reflect chronic, severe hemolytic anemia, the compensatory processes in response to this anemia, the long-term effects of hypoxia, and the consequences of transfusional therapy. Hypertransfusion and chelation therapy can delay or prevent many of these abnormalities.

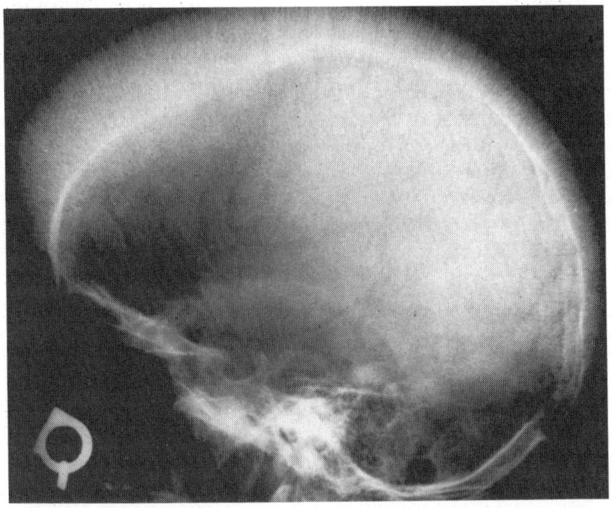

FIGURE 51-23. Lateral roentgenogram of the skull of a patient with thalassemia major. There is marked widening of the diploe of the skull, producing a "hair-on-end" appearance.

Skeletal Changes

Skeletal abnormalities result from hypertrophy and expansion of the erythroid marrow resulting in widening of the marrow space, thinning of the cortex, and osteoporosis.[629–631] They do not result from iron toxicity or vitamin D deficiency or metabolic abnormalities.[632,633]

Striking changes, first described by Cooley, occur in the skull and facial bones. The frontal bones are thickened with prominent frontal bossing. The thickened, membranous bones of the skull do not expand adjacent to the sutures, resulting in a "hot-cross bun" configuration of the skull. Radiographs of the skull show widened diploë with a granular appearance. Perpendicular bone trabeculae ultimately appear, giving the classic "hair-on-end" or crew-cut appearance (Fig. 51-23). Computed tomography scans dramatically demonstrate the bone marrow expansion (Fig. 51-24).

Pneumatization of the maxillary sinusoid is delayed in β-thalassemia major patients, and overgrowth of the maxilla causes malocclusion and jumbling of the upper incisors as well as prominence of the malar eminences. These bone changes produce a mongoloid facies (Fig. 51-25). In the metacarpals, metatarsals, and phalanges, expanded medullary cavities produce rectangular and then convex shapes. Marked enlargement of the nutrient foramina is observed.[634] Osteoporosis and cortical thinning predispose to pathologic fractures of the extremities. Compression fractures of the vertebrae may also occur. Premature fusion of the epiphyses of the long bones, particularly the epiphyses of the proximal humerus results in characteristic shortening of the upper arms.[635,636]

An unusual complication results from expansion of paravertebral (extramedullary) hematopoietic tissue into the spinal canal to cause cord compression.[637,638] Decompressive laminectomy or radiation therapy may be necessary to prevent permanent paralysis.[639]

The bones of β-thalassemia major patients change significantly with age. In older children, bone lesions regress in the arms and legs, correlating with the normal replacement of red marrow by fatty marrow. Radiographic changes become more conspicuous in the skull, spine, and pelvis—sites of active, persistent erythropoiesis.[629]

Liver and Gallbladder

The liver is enlarged in early childhood in a β-thalassemia major patient. This is partly a consequence of extramedullary hematopoiesis, as indicated by reduction of liver size by hypertransfusion.[640] Later, as a consequence of hemosiderosis and sometimes viral hepatitis, it is associated with extensive cirrhosis with nodular aggregates of regen-

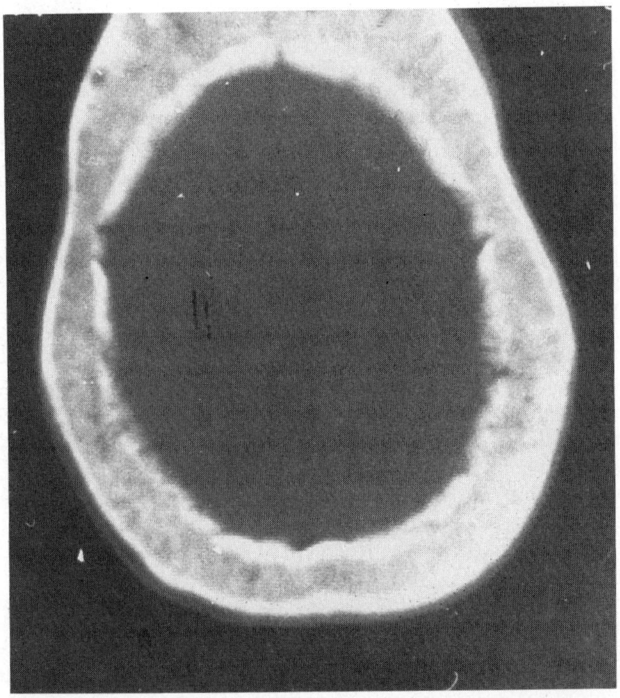

FIGURE 51-24. Computed tomographic scan of the skull of a patient with thalassemia major.

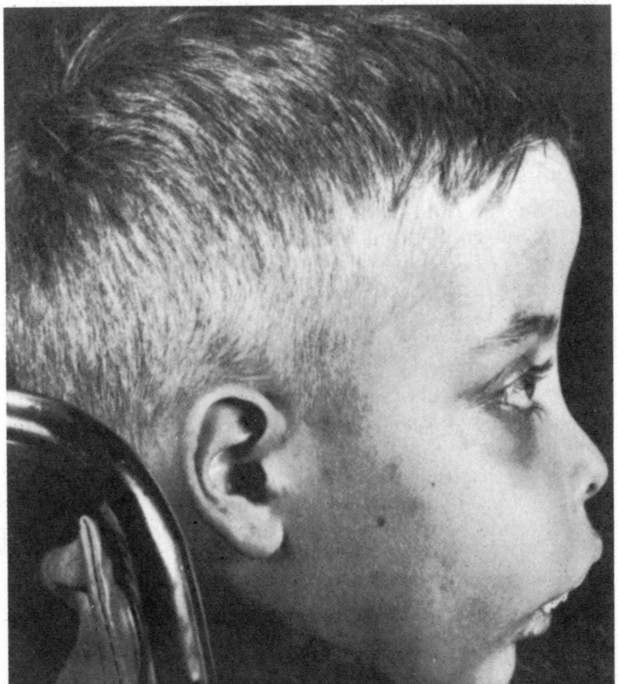

FIGURE 51-25. Profile of a 12-year-old boy with thalassemia major managed by a low transfusion regimen. He demonstrates a classic mongoloid facies. The skull is enlarged, and there is expansion of the maxilla with severe overbite.

erating hepatocytes, separated by broad bands of fibrous tissue.[641] Iron deposition is initially present in Kupffer's cells. With increasing numbers of transfusions, iron deposition ultimately also involves the parenchymal cells, resulting in an appearance indistinguishable from that of idiopathic hemochromatosis.[642,643]

Many of these patients also have hepatitis B and C, which may aggravate liver damage. In Italy, a high incidence of hepatitis B surface markers (HBsAg) and anti-HBc and anti-HBs antibodies were found in a group of 253 children.[644] A high incidence of chronic active hepatitis was observed, and it was postulated that liver iron overload may facilitate persistence of virus-induced progressive liver diseases. In the United States, a much lower incidence of HB infection is seen. In Connecticut, only 1 of 35 thalassemia patients with multitransfusions had serologic evidence of hepatitis B infection.[645] It is common practice to administer hepatitis B vaccine to patients who have had transfusions so that most will have antibodies. Hepatitis C antibodies are also prevalent. In 1990, 60% of Connecticut patients had these antibodies.

Hypergammaglobulinemia, hypoalbuminemia, and moderate decreases in the coagulation factors that are synthesized in the liver are regularly seen. Elevated levels of SGOT and SGPT are found. These correlate with hepatic iron-induced damage and decrease with effective chelation therapy.

Pigmentary gallstones are increasingly more common in patients over 4 years old on a low transfusion program. Two thirds of patients over 15 years have multiple, calcified, bilirubinate calculi. Gallbladder surgery is not usually advocated unless biliary colic or obstructive jaundice has occurred. If gallstones are present at the time of splenectomy, cholecystectomy or stone removal may be considered at that time. Laparoscopic cholecystectomy has been successfully used in several of our patients. The availability of this relatively nontraumatic procedure may lead to reconsideration of intervention in patients with asymptomatic gallstones.

Heart

Cardiac abnormalities cause morbidity and mortality in patients with β-thalassemia major. In children with paucitransfusion, cardiac dilation secondary to anemia is almost always present. During the second decade of life, myocardial siderofibrosis is inevitable, and serious cardiac disorders become common.[646] The first electrocardiographic abnormalities include a prolonged PR interval, first-degree heart block, and premature atrial contractions. The appearance of ST-segment depression and supraventricular ectopic multifocal beats constitute ominous indicators of myocardial damage.[647] Twenty-four-hour Holter electrocardiogram monitoring is a useful technique for determining myocardial irritability.

Echocardiographic estimation of left ventricular function is a reliable, noninvasive indicator of myocardial dysfunction and may reveal abnormalities before other evidence of cardiac disease is found. The left ventricular end systolic pressure-dimension relation (ejection fraction) determined with the echocardiogram is a convenient noninvasive way to assess ventricular contractility. The sensitivity of this technique may be increased by pharmacologic afterloading.[648,649]

Episodes of sterile pericarditis manifested by pain, friction rub, and the presence of a pericardial effusion, best appreciated by echocardiography, occur in about 50% of these patients. Cardiac tamponade has not been observed. Therapy is symptomatic, consisting of bed rest, treatment of any associated infection, and management of superimposed congestive heart failure.[650] When pain and discomfort are present, salicylates or corticosteroid therapy should be used.

Cardiomegaly and left ventricular deterioration progress to chronic refractory congestive heart failure. Therapy at this point consists of careful maintenance of the hemoglobin level above 10 g/dL, judicious use of digitalis and diuretics, dietary control, and salt restriction. Management is difficult because the iron-overloaded myocardium is sensitive to digitalis and has little capacity to improve its performance. Arrhythmias may cause sudden death. Supraventricular tachycardia and atrial fibrillation may necessitate the use of agents such as quinidine and propranolol in conjunction with digitalis to reduce myocardial irritability. These agents further depress ventricular function. These cardiac complications are the usual cause of death in patients with β-thalassemia major in the second or third decade.[646]

Kidneys

The kidneys are enlarged in β-thalassemia major patients. Although this may partly reflect extramedullary hematopoiesis, dilation of the renal tubules has also been described.[651] The urine is dark "coca-cola" brown, especially after splenectomy, because of the excretion of RBC catabolites including dipyrroles and mesobilifuchsins and urobilin, reflecting a severe degree of hemolysis and ineffective erythropoiesis.[652] Large amounts of urates and uric acid are also present in the urine.

Growth and Endocrine Status

In the past, growth retardation was typical even in young children with β-thalassemia. This probably was a consequence of anemia, since hypertransfusion regimens produce relatively normal growth at least during the first decade of life. Under any transfusion program, unless iron overload can be prevented, the adolescent growth spurt is delayed or absent and most patients do not attain normal stature.[653] Assays of growth hormone levels after stimulation vary from low to normal to exaggerated increases.[654,655] Somatomedin levels are low in many patients.[656,657] Treatment with recombinant human growth hormone has not usually produced a satisfactory growth response.

Menarche is frequently delayed. Breast development may be poor, and many girls are oligomenorrheic or amenorrheic. Studies of the hypothalamic pituitary gonadal axis indicate that both pituitary and gonadal damage may be responsible for amenorrhea in thalassemic women.[658,659] The typical management includes small doses of estrogen and progesterone to promote secondary sexual development and cyclic uterine bleeding. A few pregnancies have been reported in patients who were transfusion-dependent from infancy.[660] Other reports appear to describe patients with β-thalassemia intermedia.[660]

Boys are frequently immature, with sparse facial and body hair. Although spermatogenesis may be normal, libido is usually decreased. We have cared for one patient who was sexually active as a young man and fathered a child with β-thalassemia trait at 22 years of age. Physiologic doses of androgens may be used to produce phallic enlargement, a deeper voice, and growth of facial and body hair. The psychological benefits derived from androgen therapy must be weighed against the theoretical risk of inducing hepatic carcinoma.

Evidence of abnormal carbohydrate metabolism, ranging from postprandial hyperglycemia to overt insulin-dependent diabetes mellitus, is common in older patients with β-thalassemia major. One report described only 3 of 22 β-thalassemia patients (3 to 17 years of age), who had normal glucose tolerance tests.[661] Diabetes in these patients is due to iron deposition and associated progressive obliteration of the islets, affecting activity of both α and β cells. In addition, Merkel and associates[662] have reported hyperinsulinemia and a state of insulin resistance that precedes the onset of insulin dependency in many patients. Therapy with oral hypoglycemic agents at least temporarily reversed this hyperinsulinism.[663]

Multiple endocrine abnormalities such as hypothyroidism with low thyroxine and high thyroid-stimulating hormone levels is occasionally seen.[664] Hypoparathyroidism may be symptomatic with hypocalcemia and tetany or may be detected only with provocative tests.[665]

Spleen and Splenectomy

Some β-thalassemia major patients on low transfusion regimens require surgical removal of the spleen because the size of the organ produces mechanical discomfort. Massive splenomegaly is unusual with modern transfusion programs. Although often ascribed to hypersplenism, thrombocytopenia and neutropenia are probably consequences of sequestration of WBCs and platelets in a markedly expanded splenic blood pool in thalassemic patients with splenomegaly. Infection and bleeding are unusual. The usual indication for splenectomy is a progressive shortening of the survival rate of transfused blood cells, as evidenced by an increased transfusional requirement. This makes it difficult to maintain satisfactory hemoglobin levels with a reasonable transfusion interval. Investigators in the United States and England have pointed out that transfusion requirements are considerably less for splenectomized patients than for those whose spleens are still present. A transfusion requirement of more than 200 mL/kg/y of packed RBCs (hematocrit [Hct] 70%) is considered to indicate excessive RBC breakdown. Occasionally, serologic evidence of alloimmunization may be documented with positive Coombs' test results. This may permit selection of compatible donor cells that have normal survival. In most instances, no serologic evidence of RBC incompatibility is found in patients with increased transfusional requirements, and sensitization cannot usually be detected in vitro. RBC survival studies and determination of splenic sequestration by the ^{51}Cr method are of uncertain value for prediction of response after splenectomy. A significant, and especially progressive, increase in transfusional requirement is the most important indication for splenectomy. Splenectomy should be deferred as long as possible, certainly until after the child is 5 or 6 years of age because of the risk of infection in young children.

After splenectomy, usually the requirement for blood transfusions significantly decreases. Thrombocytosis, sometimes very marked (platelet count over $1 \times 10^9/L$), may occur. Because this has not been observed to cause thromboembolic phenomena, antiplatelet aggregation or anticoagulant therapies are probably not indicated. After splenectomy, increased numbers of nucleated RBCs and large numbers of Fessas bodies, precipitated masses of denatured α-globin chains, can be demonstrated in the circulating RBCs. The urine may become considerably darker after splenectomy.

Patients with β-thalassemia major are at significant risk for developing acute, overwhelming, and often fatal postsplenectomy infection.[666] Consistent bacteriologic and clinical features of the postsplenectomy infection include age (infections being most common in young children) and bacterial specificity. The causative organisms are aggressive encapsulated organisms—pneumococcus in two thirds of the cases, and *Haemophilus influenzae* type B and meningococcus in most of the remaining patients. A characteristic clinical pattern is also seen; the disease is fulminant and may proceed from mild fever and headache to hyperpyrexia, prostration, shock, and death within 6 to 12 hours. In the past, as many as 10% to 30% of splenectomized children with β-thalassemia major developed this complication.[667]

The cause of postsplenectomy infection is complex.[668] The macrophage–monocyte tissues of the spleen are unique in their capacity to clear bacteria from the blood in the absence of specific antibody. Also, evidence shows that the spleen actively participates in antibody formation, especially in the early hours of a bloodstream infection. The spleen may also be crucial in the properdin (alternate) pathway, which is so important in opsonization when specific antibody is lacking. High levels of serum iron and saturation of iron-binding protein seen in these patients have also been suggested as predisposing them to infection.

When organisms gain entrance to the bloodstream of nonimmune splenectomized patients, they are not cleared rapidly because most young children lack circulating antibodies to the polysaccharide capsular antigens of pneumococci and *H influenzae* type B organisms. The organisms rapidly proliferate in the circulation, with a doubling time of 20 to 30 minutes. Enormous numbers of bacteria accumulate in a relatively short period of time, and hyperpyrexia, shock, disseminated intravascular coagulation, adrenal hemorrhage, and death may rapidly ensue.[669]

Splenectomy should be deferred as long as possible because humoral immunity to a broad range of bacteria usually develops after the child is 6 years of age, and the risk of postsplenectomy infection decreases markedly after 4 to 5 years of age. Oral penicillin therapy has been advocated as prophylaxis against postsplenectomy infection. The effectiveness of penicillin prophylaxis in preventing pneumococcal bacteremia has been clearly shown in children under 6 years of age with the functional hyposplenism of sickle cell anemia.[670] After splenectomy, parents should be instructed to seek medical attention immediately if the child develops significant fever. Broad-spectrum antibodies (cephalosporin) should be administered to the febrile asplenic child. Polyvalent pneumococcal vaccines are also administered. The duration of immunity and the need for booster injections have not been determined.[671] In addition to postsplenectomy sepsis, severe *Yersinia* and *Vibrio* infections have been noted in splenectomized patients with β-thalassemia major receiving deferoxamine therapy.[672,673]

Treatment for β-Thalassemia

Transfusion

Transfusions are necessary to prevent early death; in 50% of patients with homozygous β-thalassemia (β-thalassemia major), transfusion therapy must be initiated in the first year of life.[674] Before the 1970s, transfusions frequently were given at irregular intervals, often 5 to 10 weeks or more apart. They were given only when symptoms of severe anemia such as fatigue, weakness, and irritability occurred. Because the hemoglobin was permitted to fall to 5 to 6 g/dL or even lower, these children were symptomatic much of the time. Cardiomegaly, a consequence of severe anemia, was universally present. Erythropoiesis was not suppressed and hypertrophy of erythroid marrow tissue occurred in medullary and intramedullary sites as a response to hemolysis and severe anemia.

Transfusions were used sparingly because of fear of the consequences of transfusional hemosiderosis. Each 200 mL of transfused RBCs results in tissue deposition of about 200 mg of iron, which cannot be eliminated by physiologic processes. After years of transfusions, a massive iron burden causes dysfunction of many organ systems and tissues, resulting in endocrine abnormalities, growth retardation, di-

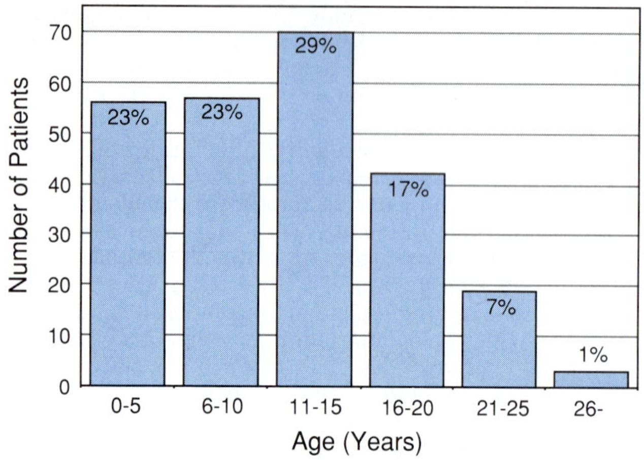

FIGURE 51-26. Age distribution of patients with thalassemia major in 1973, before the advent of effective chelation therapy.

abetes mellitus, and cardiac failure. Before the advent of effective chelation therapy, life expectancy of β-thalassemia major patients averaged only 15 to 20 years[675] (Fig. 51-26).

In 1964, Wolman[676] proposed that transfusions in β-thalassemia major should be viewed as palliative therapy for an inevitably fatal disease. If palliation is defined as the prevention of discomfort and the maintenance of as nearly a normal life as possible, the transfusion programs then in general use were unsatisfactory. The chronic and recurrent symptoms of anemia and the cosmetic consequences of overgrowth of erythropoietic tissue made life unpleasant and uncomfortable for these affected children. Because many of the problems of children with β-thalassemia major treated by infrequent transfusion could be related to anemia per se, several centers initiated transfusion programs designed to ameliorate these symptoms. The hemoglobin levels were maintained above 9 to 10 g/dL. These more vigorous regimens were designated "hypertransfusion," although normotransfusion might be a more descriptive term.[677]

The clinical benefits of hypertransfusion programs were dramatic. The growth of younger children, previously subnormal, returned to normal percentiles for height and weight.[678] Erythropoiesis was effectively suppressed, as evidenced by decreases in numbers of reticulocytes and circulating nucleated RBCs and marked reduction of the level of Hb F. Enlargement of the liver and especially the spleen receded.[679] Changes in facial appearance and osseous abnormalities either did not develop or regressed (Fig. 51-27). Cardiac dilatation decreased, and normal age-appropriate activities were possible.[680,681]

Because hypertransfusion programs require an increase of 25% or more in the amount of blood that must be administered, it was originally feared that this would result in accelerated iron overload, more rapid development of hemosiderotic complications, and death at an earlier age. These concerns were not realized, and life expectancy of children on hypertransfusion programs were not significantly shortened. This may be because the amelioration of severe anemia is associated with a reduction of gastrointestinal iron absorption, which offsets the increased transfusional iron load.

Hypertransfusion has proved to be so clearly clinically superior to older transfusion practices that many treatment centers have adopted this as standard management. The complications of anemia and erythropoietic hypertrophy, so regularly encountered in the past, have become uncommon.[682] Even more vigorous transfusional programs (supertransfusion) aimed at keeping hemoglobin levels at about 12 g/dL have been used to totally suppress erythropoiesis. The blood requirements are said not to be increased by these regimens, and a significant reduction in blood volume can be documented.[683,684] Whether this more aggressive transfusion strategy alters prognosis has not been determined.

To reduce the amount of blood administered, some centers transfuse more frequently (6 to 8 mL/kg RBC every 2 weeks). It was claimed that this results in a 20% decrease in blood requirement but this appears dubious.[685]

Another experimental transfusion program has attempted to reduce transfusion requirements by using a young population of RBCs (neocytes) prepared by differential centrifugation or cell separators.[686] Neocyte preparations have a mean cell age of 30 days compared with the 60 days of unfractionated blood. ^{51}Cr survival (half-life) of transfused neocytes is increased from the 27 days of unfractionated RBCs to 44 days. In one study, the interval between transfusion was increased an average of 2 weeks using neocytes. In another study, only a modest increase in transfusional interval was observed.[687]

Neocyte preparations are much more expensive than ordinary packed or glycerol-frozen RBCs. Whether the modest decrease in transfusion requirements obtained with their use can justify the increased expense remains to be determined. They also entail exposure to twice as many donors and potentially may increase risk of alloimmunization and transfusion-transmitted diseases. A more complicated procedure involving the use of neocyte–gerocyte exchange transfusions has been suggested as a method for further reducing transfusional iron burden, but it appears to be extraordinarily difficult and expensive.[688]

Before the first blood transfusion is given to patients with β-thalassemia major, a complete genotype of the RBCs

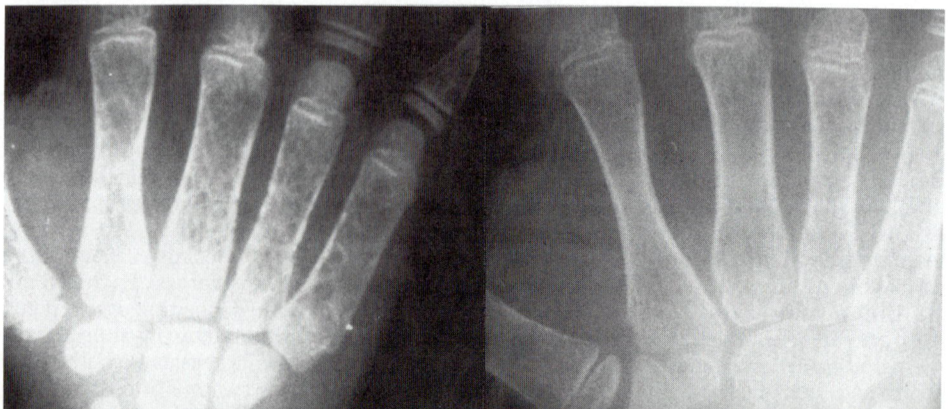

FIGURE 51-27. Effect of hypertransfusion on metacarpal bones of a patient with thalassemia major. The roentgenograms were taken before (*left*) and 1 year after (*right*) institution of hypertransfusion.

should be performed. This information may prove valuable for identifying minor blood group incompatibility if alloimmunization should develop later. Group- and type-specific RBCs that are compatible by the indirect antiglobulin reaction should be used. RBCs are separated from the plasma and buffy coat and concentrated by centrifugation. Ordinary packed RBCs have a hematocrit of 65% to 75%.

Febrile reactions are common in patients who receive multiple transfusions. Because fever associated with transfusions is frequently caused by WBC antibodies, reactions can be minimized by the use of leukocyte-poor RBCs. These can be prepared by repeated centrifugation and washing. Passing blood through special filters can remove 99% of leukocytes. If febrile reactions continue in spite of these precautions, pretransfusion therapy with antihistamines, hydrocortisone (25 to 50 mg), and acetaminophen may reduce their severity. Glycerol-frozen RBC preparations contain few leukocytes, so usually produce few febrile reactions.

Alloimmunization and transfusion reactions may occur even with scrupulous techniques.[689] In an occasional patient, it may be difficult to provide compatible blood. A few instances of what appears to be a superimposed autoimmune hemolytic process with circulating autoantibodies have been described in thalassemia patients.[690,691] A syndrome of posttransfusion hypertension, convulsions, and cerebral hemorrhage, perhaps related to release of vasopressors, has also been reported.[692]

The transmission of viral infections by blood transfusions is a potential problem in thalassemic patients. In the United States, the risk has been dramatically reduced by the use of wholly volunteer donors and appropriate serologic screening of blood before transfusion. In a study from Italy, 25% of patients had serologic evidence of exposure to hepatitis B virus.[693] In contrast, none of 25 patients transfused in Connecticut was positive for hepatitis B antibody.[694] About 15% of thalassemia patients from New York were positive for HIV antibody,[695] but no Connecticut patients had HIV antibody.[694] Hepatitis C remains a transfusion-related risk. We recently found 50% of Connecticut patients to have antibodies for hepatitis C. Serologic screening tests for hepatitis C should reduce the risk in the future.

A single transfusion usually consists of 15 mL/kg of packed RBCs, which raises the patient's hemoglobin level by about 5 g/dL (approximate predicted increase of hemoglobin is mL/kg packed cells divided by 3). In more severely anemic patients, several initial transfusions may be necessary to increase the hemoglobin level to 12 to 14 g/dL, but no more than 15 mL/kg of packed RBCs should be given in a 24-hour period. In patients with cardiac compromise, smaller volumes of RBCs as well as diuretic therapy are necessary.[685] A regular and convenient outpatient schedule can usually be set up for transfusion. When it is well organized, the entire process including cross-matching and transfusion should take 4 to 5 hours.

Iron Chelation Therapy

The accumulation of an excessive and ultimately toxic iron burden is inevitable in transfusion-dependent β-thalassemia major patients. The magnitude of the iron burden is directly proportional to the number of RBC transfusions that the patient has received.[696] The cardiac consequences of transfusional hemosiderosis constitute the major cause of late morbidity and mortality in β-thalassemia major. The daily acquisition of body iron in a child receiving monthly transfusion is about 8 to 16 mg/d from the 250 to 500 mL of RBCs administered every month.[697] Toxic burdens are attained before the child reaches 8 to 10 years of age.

No physiologic mechanisms are available for excretion of excess iron from the body.[698] Phlebotomy, the most effective method for reducing body iron stores, is obviously of no value in a disease that requires regular blood transfusion to sustain life. Pharmacologic approaches to reduce body iron involve the administration of chemical agents (iron chelators), which can combine with body iron and enhance its excretion in urine and stool.

A number of iron chelating agents have been identified and tested in patients with β-thalassemia major. These include penicillamine, ethylenediaminetetraacetic acid (EDTA), diethylenetriaminepentaacetic acid (DPTA), 1,2-dimethyl-3-hydroxypyridin-4-one (L1), deferoxamine B mesylate, and others.[699] Some of these agents lack specificity for iron, some are ineffective, and some have significant toxicities.

Deferoxamine B, a siderophore produced by the bacterium *Streptomyces pilosis*, was introduced three decades ago.[700,701] It has proved to be an effective and nearly specific drug for chelating iron with relatively low toxicity in patients with β-thalassemia major.[702,703] It is the only approved chelating agent for iron overload.

Increased urinary iron excretions after administration of parenteral deferoxamine is proportional to body iron stores.[704] In patients with β-thalassemia major, substantial urinary iron excretion after the administration of 40 mg/kg of deferoxamine does not occur until after 3 to 4 years of regular transfusions. Therefore, deferoxamine chelation therapy is usually begun only after the child is 4 or 5 years of age.[685] By this time, serum ferritin levels usually exceed 2000 ng/mL, and serum transferrin saturation is nearly complete.

In the 1960s, deferoxamine therapy was administered as a daily intramuscular injection of 0.5 to 1 g/d. This was shown to be effective in reducing the rate of hepatic iron accumulation and fibrosis and also in improving cardiac function.[705] Because deferoxamine is rapidly excreted, it was impossible to attain negative iron balance using intermittent deferoxamine injections. Total body iron burden continued to increase because of continuing RBC transfusion. In addition, considerable discomfort was caused by daily intramuscular injections. These factors led to general discontinuation of deferoxamine therapy by most centers after the 1960s.

In 1976, Propper[706,707] demonstrated that the effectiveness of deferoxamine could be markedly increased by prolonged infusion of the drug either intravenously or subcutaneously. Protocols have been developed that can attain negative iron balance in most patients after they reach 5 or 6 years of age. These protocols involve daily extended subcutaneous injections of 1 to 2 g of deferoxamine over extended intervals using portable battery-driven pumps. The pumps impel a syringe containing an aqueous solution of deferoxamine, which is injected subcutaneously through a No. 25 needle placed in the abdomen or thigh. Most patients elect to infuse deferoxamine over 8 to 10 hours at night while sleeping. Regular use of subcutaneous deferoxamine has been shown to improve cardiac function,[708,709] prevent or improve pancreatic dysfunction, improve growth and sexual maturation,[710,711] and extend life.[712,713]

Iron burden can be dramatically reduced as indicated by decreasing levels of serum ferritin (Fig. 51-28). Tachyphylaxis to deferoxamine has not been reported, and the typical reason for apparent lack of effectiveness and increases in serum ferritin levels is noncompliance. The simultaneous use of ascorbic acid, 100 to 200 mg/d, enhances the effectiveness of deferoxamine, presumably by mobilizing iron from tissue store.[714] Larger doses of vitamin C may be associated with cardiac toxicity in iron-overloaded patients and should be avoided.

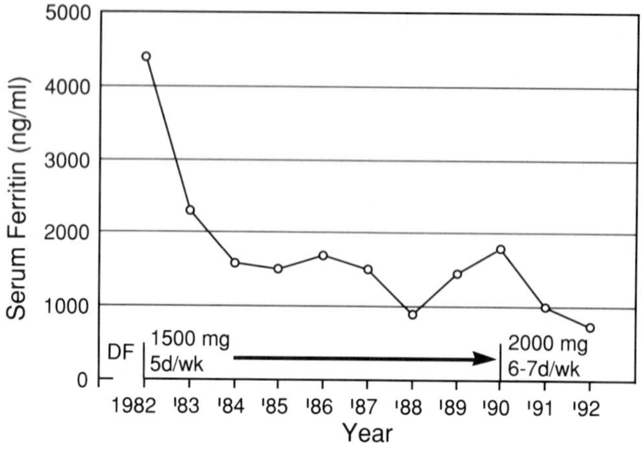

FIGURE 51-28. Serum ferritin levels in a patient with thalassemia major receiving chronic subcutaneous deferoxamine therapy.

Although deferoxamine therapy is almost always well tolerated, uncomfortable side effects as well as other toxicities have been recognized.[715] Hard, painful swellings often occur at the site of injection. These do not appear to be due to hypersensitivity or allergy because they occur only intermittently. Adding small amounts of hydrocortisone to the deferoxamine solution has not proved to be effective in preventing local reactions. Because painful local reactions are a deterrent to use of the medication, placement of permanent venous access devices (such as a Portacath), which permit direct venous infusions are being increasingly used. Other rarer toxicities are visual and auditory neurotoxicity,[716] pulmonary infiltrates,[717] growth failure, and bony changes.[718] Most of these toxicities have been associated with high-dose (over 60 mg/kg/d) therapy.

The combination of a complex, expensive, and uncomfortable drug, the administration protocol, and local toxicities lead to poor compliance of many patients. Although compliance is usually good during early childhood when the medication is administered by a parent, it often becomes poor during later childhood and adolescence. Because no immediate consequences are perceived by the patient when medication is not used regularly, a tangible incentive to continue regular usage is not apparent. Failure to use the drug results in increasing body iron and increases in serum ferritin levels (Fig. 51-29).

The difficulty for most patients to adhere to the chronic subcutaneous deferoxamine regimen has provided a major impetus to the search for alternative—especially oral—iron chelating drugs.[719] Considerable interest is being given to the 3-hydroxypyridin-4-one (L1) family of bidentate iron chelators.[720–722]

L1 increases urinary iron excretion in iron-overloaded animals and patients. Its efficacy in inducing ferriuria is comparable to deferoxamine. L1 does not increase fecal iron excretion, and this may constitute a substantial fraction of total deferoxamine-induced iron excretion.

The effectiveness of L1 in reducing body iron burden and serum ferritin is uncertain. Some studies show unchanged serum ferritin levels after L1 therapy.[723] Other studies showed significant decreases in hepatic iron as well as serum ferritin.[724] Both mild adverse reactions as well as serious side effects—including agranulocytosis—have been reported with L1 therapy.[699] Longer clinical trials with L1 are necessary to determine both efficacy and safety.

A number of other classes of iron chelating drugs are being developed and tested.[699] As of this writing, deferoxamine is the only proven effective iron chelating agent for use in patients with transfusional hemosiderosis.

Bone Marrow Transplantation

Successful use of bone marrow transplantation as curative therapy for β-thalassemia major patients was first accomplished by ED Thomas in 1982. An 18-month-old Italian infant, who had received only a few transfusions, was permanently engrafted with marrow from his histocompatibility complex (HLA)-compatible nonthalassemic sibling.[725] A few additional bone marrow transplantations have been performed in England and the United States, but the largest experience has been reported by Guido Lucarelli and associates[726,727] in Pesaro, Italy. This group has performed more than 450 bone marrow transplantations for β-thalassemia major patients. They have reported that when transplantation is performed early in life, using an HLA-matched donor relative, there is an 80% to 90% probability of cure. Additionally, chronic severe graft-versus-host disease is infrequent in their patients.

These remarkable results have led some authorities to recommend that bone marrow transplantation should be strongly considered in any young β-thalassemia major patient who has a compatible donor.[685,728,729] This opinion is justified on the basis of the high cure rate, great expense of life-long, conventional, transfusion chelation therapy, and the high incidence of noncompliance with chronic deferoxamine chelation therapy.

It should be recognized that current hypertransfusion therapy, combined with vigorous chelation is compatible with a long, healthy life. In addition, because of decreasing family size, HLA-compatible donors are available in only a small percentage of cases. Finally, the development of effective oral iron chelates—which may be imminent—would make compliance with chelation therapy much easier.[699]

At this time, a decision whether to recommend bone marrow transplantation in a young patient with β-thalassemia major who has a suitable donor is controversial. Families should be apprised of the risks and potential benefits of the procedure to helped them make an informed decision. If an HLA-compatible donor is not available, bone marrow transplantation is not usually considered to be an acceptable option.

Bone marrow transplantation has been less extensively attempted in older children and adults, many of whom

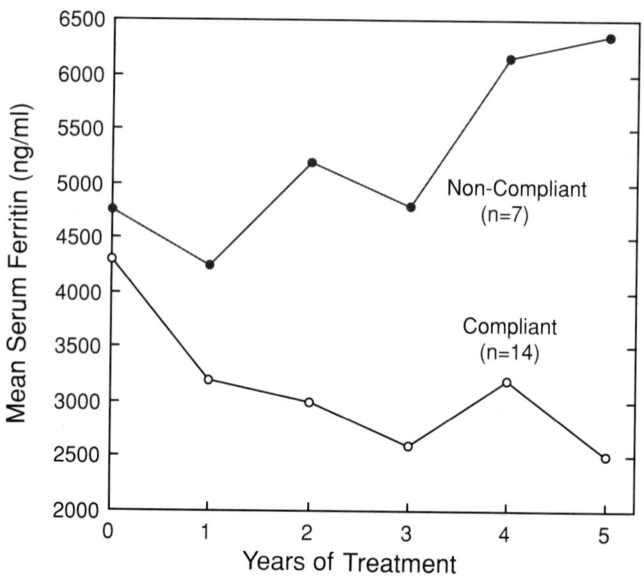

FIGURE 51-29. Serum ferritin levels in groups of patients with thalassemia major who were compliant or noncompliant with subcutaneous deferoxamine therapy.

have significant hepatic hemosiderosis and fibrosis. Lucarelli's early experience with a number of patients over 16 years of age was disappointing, with a high immediate mortality rate and no long-term survivors. More recently, Lucarelli[730] described excellent results of marrow transplantation in older patients who were iron overloaded and had significant hepatic abnormalities. Eighty percent of his adult patients had long-term, disease-free survivals. These results will lead to a reevaluation of the use of bone marrow transplants in older β-thalassemia major patients.

CLINICAL ASPECTS OF THE α-THALASSEMIAS

The α-thalassemias are a group of familial microcytic anemias resulting from decreased synthesis of a α-globin chains. They are difficult to diagnose and identify with certainty because there are no characteristic elevations in Hb A_2 or Hb F. They are more complex and difficult to understand and explain because there are two sets of α genes.

The α-globin genes are duplicated and lie near each other on chromosome 16 (see Fig. 51-2). The classic α-thalassemia syndromes, particularly common in Asian populations, show a strong correlation between the number of genes actually deleted from the chromosome 16 pair and clinical severity. Thus, in α-thalassemia-2 trait (silent carrier state) a single α gene is deleted (−α/αα); in α-thalassemia-1, or classic trait, two α genes are deleted (αα/−−) or (−α/−α), whereas in Hb H disease, three are deleted (−−/−α). Hydrops fetalis is associated with deletion of all four genes (−−/−−; see Fig. 51-16).[1]

α-Thalassemia-1 trait can occur in two ways: two genes can be deleted from the same chromosome 16 (*cis* deletion), or one copy can be deleted from each of the chromosome 16 homologues (*trans* deletion). The *cis* deletion, common in Asia, is the type that is usually associated with hydrops fetalis or Hb H disease. The former usually represents the homozygous state for the *cis* deletion, whereas the latter results from inheritance of the *cis* deletion from one parent and α-thalassemia-2 from the other parent, who is a silent carrier. The *trans* deletion form of α-thalassemia-1 trait (−α/−α) is extremely common in black populations, but the *cis* deletion of both α genes from one chromosome is not encountered. This explains why, despite the high (25% to 30%) incidence of α-gene deletions in blacks, there is a virtual absence of hydrops fetalis or severe Hb H disease.[731]

The α-thalassemias caused by gene deletions are the most common forms encountered (see Fig. 51-17). There are at least 30 α-thalassemia mutations.[1] Nondeletion α-thalassemia alleles are also encountered in 15% to 20% of Mediterranean and Asian patients. These α-thalassemia genes are analogous to common forms of β-thalassemia; that is, the genes are present but rendered hypofunctional or nonfunctional by mutations that disrupt mRNA production.

Structurally abnormal hemoglobins have been found to be associated with α-thalassemia. Hb Quong Sze ($\alpha_2^{125Leu \rightarrow Pro}\beta_2$) has an exceedingly labile α chain that is destroyed so rapidly after its synthesis on ribosomes that no hemoglobin tetramers can be formed.

Silent Carrier (α-Thalassemia-2 Trait) (−α/αα)

α-Thalassemia-2 trait results from deletion of one α gene. No hematologic manifestations occur. The RBCs are not microcytic; Hb A_2 and Hb F are normal. A mild decrease in α-chain synthesis is noted, with β/α ratios slightly exceeding 1. In the newborn period, small amounts (1% to 3%) of Hb Bart's (α_4) may be seen in Asian populations, but have not been regularly seen in black or Mediterranean peoples.[732]

α-Thalassemia Trait (α-Thalassemia-1 Trait) (−α/−α)

α-Thalassemia-1 is a mild, familial, microcytic anemia resulting from deletion of two α genes. It is characterized by levels of Hb A_2 in the low to low normal range (1.5% to 2.5%) and β/α synthetic ratios averaging 1.4. In the newborn period, substantial amounts (5% to 8%) of Hb Bart's are noted, and a relative microcytosis is present in cord blood erythrocytes.[733] When an α-thalassemia-1 gene occurs in persons who are heterozygous for β-chain variant hemoglobins such as Hb S, Hb C, or Hb E, the proportion of the abnormal hemoglobins is lower than that seen in ordinary hemoglobin heterozygotes.[250]

α-Thalassemia-1 is common in Asians and reaches an incidence of 20% in Southeast Asian populations, especially Thais. About 3% to 5% of blacks have this trait and, as mentioned, the deletions are in the *trans* position.[734]

Hb Constant Spring Trait

Hemoglobin polypeptide chain variants are rare in the thalassemias. An exception to this generalization is Hb Lepore. A second class of exceptions are the Hb Constant Spring syndromes.[260,735] These are minor hemoglobins (1% to 2%) found in many Asians and occasionally in whites with α-thalassemia syndromes. There are four different hemoglobins of the Hb Constant Spring type.[736] Each of these has elongated α chains resulting from a single base mutation in the termination codon that normally signals the cessation of mRNA translation after the 141st amino acid is incorporated into the chain. Each of these mutations changes the usual termination codon to a codon that codes for an amino acid. Thus, translation continues beyond the normal stop into the usually untranslated regions of the α-mRNA. Thirty-one additional amino acids are added until the next in-phase termination is encountered. This accounts for the elongated α chain and for the fact that the additional amino acids in all four variants are the same except for the first extra residue at position 142.[261]

The heterozygous state has no hematologic abnormality other than the 1% Hb Constant Spring demonstrated by electrophoresis.[260]

Hb H Disease (−−/−α)

Hb H disease is a moderately severe but variable anemia resulting from combination of an α-thalassemia-1 (−−/) gene and an α-thalassemia-2 (−α/) or Hb Constant Spring (αα CS/).[1] These result in a marked deficiency of α-chain synthesis with β-/α-synthesis ratios of about 5:2. Family studies reveal that one parent is hematologically normal (α-thalassemia-2 trait, silent carrier) and the other has microcytosis and hypochromia (α-thalassemia-1 trait). Hb H disease may resemble β-thalassemia intermedia, with moderately severe anemia, osseous changes, and splenomegaly, or it may be considerably milder. Hb H disease occurs predominantly in Asians, has occasionally been reported in whites, and is rare in blacks.

Hb H (β_4) is unstable and forms precipitates within the RBC that damage the RBC membrane, inducing hemolysis. Hb H can be demonstrated by incubation of RBC in supravital stains, such as 1% brilliant cresyl blue. Multiple small inclusions of precipitated Hb H form in the RBCs. Electrophoresis of freshly prepared hemolysate at alkaline or neutral pH demonstrates a fast-moving component amounting to 10% to 30% of the total hemoglobin. Concomitant iron deficiency may reduce the amount of Hb H in the patient's RBCs.[737] In Hb H disease resulting from interaction of α-thalassemia-1 and Hb Constant Spring traits, the minor slowly migrating Hb Constant Spring band is noted on electrophoresis.[735]

Hydrops Fetalis with Hb Bart's (−−/−−)

Hydrops fetalis, the most severe form of α-thalassemia, is associated with total absence of α-chain synthesis. Affected fetuses are usually born prematurely and either are stillborn or die shortly after birth. Marked anasarca and enlargement of the liver and spleen are present.[738,739] This syndrome has occurred almost exclusively in Southeast Asians, especially in Chinese, Cambodians, Thais, and Filipinos.[740] The influx of these Southeast Asian peoples has made this condition more prevalent in the United States. Several children with hydrops fetalis have been successfully resuscitated and treated with neonatal exchange transfusions. These children have since been maintained on a regular transfusion program because they are obviously totally dependent on RBC transfusion for survival.[741,742]

Severe anemia is usually present in patients with hydrops fetalis, with hemoglobin levels ranging from 3 to 6 g/dL. The RBCs are microcytic and hypochromic, with target cells and large numbers of circulating nucleated RBCs. These RBC morphologic abnormalities and the invariably negative Coombs' test exclude the hemolytic diseases of blood group incompatibility. After incubation with brilliant cresyl blue, intracellular crystals resembling Heinz bodies develop in the RBCs because of precipitation of the unstable Hb Bart's.

Hemoglobin electrophoresis reveals predominantly Hb Bart's (α_4) with a smaller amount of Hb H (β_4). A minor component identified as Hb Portland ($\zeta_2\gamma_2$) migrating in the position of Hb A is also seen. Normal Hb A ($\alpha_2\gamma_2$) and Hb F ($\alpha_2\alpha_2$) are totally absent.[743] Lowered values for alkali-resistant hemoglobin, 35% to 75%, compared with 75% to 90% in infants of comparable gestational age, are explained on the basis of an intermediate degree of alkali resistance of Hb Bart's compared with that of Hb F.

Affected infants have massive enlargement of the liver and spleen. The extreme extramedullary hematopoiesis reflects the profound hemolytic anemia characteristic of this disease. The universal edema of hydrops fetalis is a reflection of severe congestive heart failure in utero. This is partly a consequence of anemia, with hemoglobin levels averaging 6.2 g/dL. The strikingly abnormal oxygen affinity of Hb Bart's also contributes to the pathophysiology. Hb Bart's lacks the normal sigmoid oxygen dissociation curve and is shifted markedly to the left. The shift is so great that oxygen cannot be released to the tissues under conditions of low oxygen tension.[744]

The reason these infants do not die in the earlier trimester of pregnancy is probably because of the presence of Hb Portland ($\zeta_2\gamma_2$). This nontetrameric component has a more favorable oxygen dissociation pattern than Hb Bart's and probably promotes oxygen transport until its concentration decreases in the last trimester.

A high incidence of toxemia of pregnancy has been described in pregnant women carrying severely affected infants.[738,745] This gives increased rationale for prenatal diagnosis of this condition. (See earlier section on prenatal diagnosis.)

CLINICAL ASPECTS OF HEREDITARY PERSISTENCE OF FETAL HEMOGLOBIN

Hereditary persistence of fetal hemoglobin is characterized by high levels of Hb F within the RBCs, which persist after infancy. HPFH results from two kinds of genetic mechanisms (see Figs. 51-20 and 51-21). Large deletions in the region between the γ-globin gene and the δ-globin gene have been described in Africa[377,402] and elsewhere (see Fig. 51-20). In the heterozygous state, 20% to 30% Hb F is present in otherwise normal RBCs. No anemia or microcytosis is found. The RBC distribution of Hb F is pancellular on the Kleihauer-Betke acid elution preparation. Persons who are homozygous for deletional HPFH are healthy. Their RBCs are slightly microcytic and hypochromic and contain 100% Hb F. There is a left shift of the oxygen dissociation curve. Because of the high oxygen affinity of Hb F-containing RBCs, a slight increase in total hemoglobin levels occurs.[744]

The second form of HPFH is caused by nondeletion point mutations usually within the promoter regions of either the $^{G}\gamma$- or $^{A}\gamma$-globin genes (see Fig. 51-21). These mutations are believed to alter the binding of regulatory proteins to the γ promoter.

The levels of Hb F in heterozygotes for nondeletional HPFH are variable, ranging from 3% to 30%. The distribution of Hb F may be pancellular or heterocellular.[746]

Both deletional and nondeletion forms of HPFH can ameliorate the effects of the sickle cell gene. Thus, double heterozygotes for Hb S and HPFH are not anemic and have no intravascular sickling, despite a hemoglobin distribution of 60% to 70% Hb S and 40% to 30% Hb F. This observation has given impetus to the pharmacologic manipulation of therapy in sickle cell anemia patients.

REFERENCES

1. Weatherall DJ, Clegg JB. The thalassemia syndromes, ed 3. Oxford, Blackwell Scientific Publications, 1981.
2. Baglioni C. The fusion of two peptide chains in hemoglobin Lepore and its interpretation as a genetic deletion. Proc Natl Acad Sci USA 1962;48:1880.
3. Kendall AG, Ojwang PJ, Schroeder WA, et al. Hemoglobin Kenya, the product of a γ-β fusion gene: studies of the family. Am J Hum Genet 1973;25:548.
4. Deisseroth A, Nienhuis A, Turner P, et al. Localization of the human α-globin structural gene to chromosome 16 in somatic cell hybrids by molecular hybridization assay. Cell 1977;12:205.
5. Deisseroth A, Nienhuis A, Lawrence J, et al. Chromosomal localization of human β-globin gene on human chromosome 11 in somatic cell hybrids. Proc Natl Acad Sci USA 1978;75:1456.
6. Bunn HF, Forget BG. Hemoglobin: molecular, genetic and clinical aspects. Philadelphia, WB Saunders, 1986.
7. Collins FS, Weissman SM. The molecular genetics of human hemoglobin. Prog Nucleic Acid Res Mol Biol 1984;31:315.
8. Nienhuis AW, Maniatis T. Structure and expression of globin genes in erythroid cells. In: Stamatoyannopoulos G, Nienhuis AW, Leder P, Majerus PW, eds. The molecular basis of blood diseases. Philadelphia, WB Saunders, 1987:28.
9. Hsu S-L, Marks J, Shaw J-P, et al. Structure and expression of the human Θ globin gene. Nature 1988;331:44.
10. Ley TJ, Maloney KA, Gordon JI, et al. Globin gene expression in erythroid human fetal liver cells. J Clin Invest 1988;83:1032.
11. Albitar M, Peschle C, Liebhaber SA. Theta, zeta, and epsilon globin messenger RNAs are expressed in adults. Blood 1989;74:629.
12. Clegg JB. Can the product of the Θ gene be a real globin? Nature 1987;329:465.
13. Padgett RA, Grabowski PJ, Konaroka MM, et al. Splicing of messenger RNA precursors. Annu Rev Biochem 1986;55:1119.
14. Mount SM. A catalogue of splice junction sequences. Nucleic Acids Res 1982;10:459.
15. Smale ST, Baltimore D. The "initiator" as a transcription control element. Cell 1989;57:103.
16. Wickens M. How the messenger got its tail: addition of poly(A) in the nucleus. Trends Biochem Sci 1990;15:277.
17. Wahle E, Keller W. The biochemistry of 3'-end cleavage and polyadenylation of messenger RNA precursors. Annu Rev Biochem 1992;61: 419.
18. Boissel J-P, Kasper TJ, Shah SC, et al. Amino-terminal processing of proteins: hemoglobin South Florida, a variant with retention of initiator methionine and N^{α}-acetylation. Proc Natl Acad Sci USA 1985;82: 8448.
19. Kozak M. The scanning model for translation: an update. J Cell Biol 1989;108:229.
20. Mitchell PJ, Tjian R. Transcriptional regulation in mammalian cells by sequence-specific DNA binding proteins. Science 1989;245:371.

21. Martin D, Tsai S, Orkin S. Increased γ-globin expression in a non-deletion HPFH is mediated by an erythroid-specific DNA-binding factor. Nature 1989;338:435.
22. Tsai S, Martin D, Zon L, et al. Cloning of the cDNA for the major DNA-binding protein of the erythroid lineage through expression in mammalian cells. Nature 1989;339:446.
23. Orkin SH. Globin gene regulation and switching: circa 1990. Cell 1990;63:665.
24. Orkin SH. GATA-binding transcription factors in hematopoietic cells. Blood 1992;80:575.
25. Engel JD, George KM, Ko LJ, et al. Transcription factor regulation of hematopoietic lineage cells. Semin Hematol 1991;28:158.
26. Pevny L, Simon MC, Robertson E, et al. Erythroid differentiatiion in chimaeric mice blocked by a targeted mutatio in the gene for transcription factor GATA-1. Nature 1991;349:257.
27. Simon MC, Pevny L, Wiles MV, et al. Rescue of erythroid development in gene targeted GATA-1 mouse embryonic stem cells. Nature Genetics 1992;1:92.
28. Andrews NC, Erdjument-Bromage H, Davidson MB, et al. Erythroid transcription factor NF-E2 is a haematopoietic-specific basic-leucine zipper protein. Nature 1993;363:722.
29. Khoury G, Gruss P. Enhancer elements. Cell 1983;33:313.
30. Svaren J, Chalkley R. The structure and assembly of active chromatin. Trends Genet 1990;6:52.
31. Lewin B. Commitment and activation at Pol II promoters: a tale of protein-protein interactions. Cell 1990;61:1161.
32. Ptashne M, Gann AAF. Activators and targets. Nature 1990;346:329.
33. Kollias G, Hurst J, DeBoer E, et al. The human β-globin gene contains a downstream developmental specific enhancer. Nucleic Acids Res 1987;15:5739.
34. Trudel M, Magram J, Bruckner L, et al. Upstream Gγ-globin and downstream β-globin sequences required for stage-specific expression in transgenic mice. Mol Cell Biol 1987;7:4024.
35. Behringer RR, Hammer RE, Brinster RL, et al. Two 3′ sequences direct adult erythroid-specific expression of human β-globin genes in transgenic mice. Proc Natl Acad Sci USA 1987;84:7056.
36. Trudel M, Costantini F. A 3′ enhancer contributes to the stage-specific expression of the human β-globin gene. Genes Dev 1987;1:954.
37. Antoniou M, deBoer E, Habets G, et al. The human β-globin gene contains multiple regulatory regions: identification of one promoter and two downstream enhancers. EMBO J 1988;7:377.
38. Wall L, deBoer E, Grosveld F. The human β-globin gene 3′ enhancer contains multiple binding sites for an erythroid-specific protein. Genes Dev 1988;2:1089.
39. Bodine DM, Ley TJ. An enhancer element lies 3′ to the human $^A\gamma$ globin gene. EMBO J 1987;6:2997.
40. Knezetic JA, Felsenfeld G. Identification and characterization of a chicken α-globin enhancer. Mol Cell Biol 1989;9:893.
41. Cao SX, Gitman PD, Dave HPG, et al. Identification of a transcriptional silencer in the 5′-flanking region of the human ε-globin gene. Proc Natl Acad Sci USA 1989;86:5306.
42. Lamb P, Watt P, Proudfoot NJ. Negative regulation of the human embryonic globin genes ζ and ε. In: Stamatoyannopoulos G, Nienhuis AW, eds. Hemoglobin switching: transcriptional regulation, part A. New York, Alan R Liss, 1989:269.
43. Tuan D, Solomon W, Li Q, et al. The "β-like-globin" gene domain in human erythroid cells. Proc Natl Acad Sci USA 1985;82:6384.
44. Forrester WC, Thompson C, Elder JT, et al. A developmentally stable chromatin structure in the human β-globin gene cluster. Proc Natl Acad Sci USA 1986;83:1359.
45. Grosveld F, Blom van Assendelft G, Greaves DR, et al. Position-independent, high-level expression of the human β-globin gene in transgenic mice. Cell 1987;51:975.
46. Townes TM, Behringer RR. Human globin locus activation region (LAR): role in temporal control. Trends Genet 1990;6:219.
47. Forrester WC, Takegawa S, Papayanopoulou T, et al. Evidence for a locus activating region: the formation of developmentally stable hypersensitive sites in globin-expressing hybrids. Nucleic Acids Res 1987;15:10159.
48. Talbot D, Collis P, Antoniou M, et al. A dominant control region from the human β-globin locus conferring integration site–independent gene expression. Nature 1989;338:352.
49. Higgs DR, Wood WG, Jarman AP, et al. A major positive regulatory region located far upstream of the human α-globin gene locus. Genes Dev 1990;4:1588.
50. Moi P, Kan YW. Synergistic enhancement of globin gene expression by activator protein-1-like proteins. Proc Natl Acad Sci USA 1990;87: 9000.
51. Philipsen S, Talbot D, Fraser P, et al. The β-globin dominant control region: hypersensitive site 2. EMBO J 1990;9:2159.
52. Philipsen S, Talbot D, Fraser P, et al. Detailed analysis of the site 3 region of the human β-globin dominant control region. EMBO J 1990;9: 2169.
53. Ikuta T, Kan YW. In vivo protein-DNA interactions at the β-globin gene locus. Proc Natl Acad Sci USA 1991;88:10188.
54. Strauss EC, Orkin SH. In vivo protein-DNA interactions at hypersensitive site 3 of the human β-globin locus control region. Proc Natl Acad Sci USA 1992;89:5809.
55. Ney PA, Sorrentino BP, McDonagh KT, et al. Tandem AP-1-binding sites within the human β-globin dominant control region function as an inducible enhancer in erythroid cells. Genes Dev 1990;4:993.
56. Talbot D, Grosveld F. The 5′HS2 of the globin locus control region enhances transcription through the interaction of a multimeric complex binding at two functionally distinct NF-E2 binding sites. EMBO J 1991;10:1391.
57. Liu D, Chang JC, Moi P, et al. Dissection of the enhancer activity of β-globin 5′ DNaseI-hypersensitive site 2 in transgenic mice. Proc Natl Acad Sci USA 1992;89:3899.
58. Stamatoyannopoulos G. Human hemoglobin switching. Science 1991;252:383.
59. Epner E, Kim CG, Groudine M. What does the locus control region control? Curr Biol 1992;2:262.
60. Dillon N, Grosveld F. Transcriptional regulation of multigene loci: multilevel control. Trends Genet 1993;9:134.
61. Stamatoyannopoulos G, Nienhuis AW. Hemoglobin switching. In: Stamatoyannopoulos G, Nienhuis AW, Majerus PW, Varmus H, eds. The molecular basis of blood diseases, ed 2. Philadelphia, WB Saunders, 1994:107.
62. Ley TJ. The pharmacology of hemoglobin switching: of mice and men. Blood 1991;77:6.
63. Peschle C, Mavilio F, Carè A, et al. Haemoglobin switching in human embryos: asynchrony of $\zeta \rightarrow \alpha$ and $\varepsilon \rightarrow \gamma$-globin switches in primitive and definitive erythropoietic lineage. Nature 1985;313:235.
64. Bard H. Postnatal fetal and adult hemoglobin synthesis in early preterm newborn infants. J Clin Invest 1973;52:1789.
65. Bard H, Prosmanne J. Postnatal fetal and adult hemoglobin synthesis in preterm infants whose birth weight was less than 1,000 grams. J Clin Invest 1982;70:50.
66. Bunch C, Wood WG, Weatherall DJ, et al. Haemoglobin synthesis by foetal erythroid cells in an adult environment. Br J Haematol 1981;49: 325.
67. Wood WG, Bunch C, Kelly S, et al. Control of haemoglobin switching by a developmental clock? Nature 1985;313:320.
68. Delfini C, Saglio G, Mazzo, U, et al. Fetal haemoglobin synthesis following fetal liver transplantation in man. Br J Haematol 1983;55:609.
69. Papayannopoulou T, Nakamoto B, Agostinelli, F, et al. Fetal to adult hemopoietic cell transplantation in man: insights into hemoglobin switching. Blood 1986;67:99.
70. Zanjani ED, Lim G, McGlave PB, et al. Adult haematopoietic cells transplanted to sheep fetuses continue to produce adult globins. Nature 1982;295:244.
71. Papayannopoulou T, Brice M, Stamatoyannopoulos G. Analysis of human globin switching in MEL X human fetal erythroid cell hybrids. Cell 1986;46:469.
72. Wood WG, Weatherall DJ. Haemoglobin synthesis during human foetal development. Nature 1973;244:162.
73. Wood WG, Nash J, Weatherall DJ, et al. The sheep as an animal model for the switch from fetal to adult hemoglobins. In: Stamatoyannopoulos G, Nienhuis AW, eds. Cellular and molecular regulation of hemoglobin switching. New York, Grune & Stratton, 1979:153.
74. Colombo B, Kim B, Perez Atencio R, et al. The pattern of fetal haemoglobin disappearance after birth. Br J Haematol 1976;32:79.
75. Terrenato L, Bertilaccio C, Spinelli P, et al. The switch from Haemoglobin F and A: the time course of qualitative and quantitative variations of haemoglobins after birth. Br J Haematol 1981;47:31.
76. Shepart MK, Weatherall DJ, Conley CL. Semi-quantitative estimation of the distribution of fetal hemoglobin in red cell populations. Bull Johns Hopkins Hosp 1962;110:293.
77. Weinberg RS, Goldberg JD, Schofield JM, et al. Switch from fetal to adult hemoglobin is associated with a change in progenitor cell population. J Clin Invest 1983;71:785.
78. Alter BP, Jackson BT, Lipton JM, et al. Control of the simian fetal hemoglobin switch at the progenitor cell level. J Clin Invest 1981;67: 458.
79. Wood WG, Pearce K, Clegg JB, et al. Switch from foetal to adult haemoglobin synthesis in normal and hypophysectomised sheep. Nature 1977;264:799.
80. Wintour EM, Smith MB, Bell RJ, et al. The role of fetal adrenal hormones in the switch from fetal to adult globin synthesis in the sheep. J Endocrinol 1985;104:165.
81. Perrine SP, Greene MF, Faller, DV. Delay in the fetal globin switch in infants of diabetic mothers. N Engl J Med 1985;312:334.
82. Bard H, Prosmanne J. Relative rates of fetal hemoglobin and adult hemoglobin synthesis in cord blood of infants of insulin-dependent diabetic mothers. Pediatrics 1985;75:1143
83. Perrine SP, Rudolph A, Faller DV, et al. Butyrate infusions in the ovine fetus delay the biologic clock for globin gene switching. Proc Natl Acad Sci USA 1988;85:8540.
84. Burns LJ, Glauber JG, Ginder GD. Butyrate induces selective transcriptional activation of a hypomethylated embryonic globin gene in adult erythroid cells. Blood 1988;72:1536.
85. Constantoulakis P, Papayannopoulou Th, Stamatoyannopoulos G. α-Amino-N-butyric acid stimulates fetal hemoglobin in the adult. Blood 1988;72:1961.
86. Constantoulakis P, Knitter G, Stamatoyannopoulos G. On the induction of fetal hemoglobin by butyrates: in vivo and in vitro studies with sodium butyrate and comparison of combination treatments with 5-AzaC and AraC. Blood 1989;74:1963.

87. Perrine SP, Miller BA, Faller DV, et al. Sodium butyrate enhances fetal globin gene expression in erythroid progenitors of patients with Hb SS and β thalassemia. Blood 1989;74:454.
88. Blau AC, Constantoulakis P, Shaw CM, Stamatoyannopoulos G. Fetal hemoglobin induction with butyric acid: efficacy and toxicity. Blood 1993;81:529.
89. Dover GJ, Brusilow S, Samid D. Increased fetal hemoglobin in patients receiving sodium 4-phenylbutyrate. N Engl J Med 1992;327:569.
90. Perrine SP, Ginder GD, Faller DV, et al. A short-term trial of butyrate to stimulate fetal-globin-gene expression in the β-globin disorders. N Engl J Med 1993;328:81.
91. Boyer SH, Belding TK, Margolet L, et al. Fetal hemoglobin restriction to a few erythrocytes (F cells) in normal human adults. Science 1975;188:361.
92. Wood WG, Stamatoyannopoulos G, Lim G, et al. F-cells in the adult: normal values and levels in individuals with hereditary and acquired elevations of Hb F. Blood 1975;46:671.
93. Huisman THJ, Schroeder WA, Efremov GD, et al. The present status of the heterogeneity of fetal hemoglobin in β-thalassemia: an attempt to unify some observations on thalassemia and related conditions. Ann NY Acad Sci 1974;232:107.
94. Evans T, Felsenfeld G. The erythroid-specific transcription factor Eryfl: a new finger protein. Cell 1989;58:877.
95. Zon LI, Tsai S-F, Burgess S, et al. The major human erythroid DNA-binding protein (GF-1): primary sequence and localization of the gene to the X chromosome. Proc Natl Acad Sci USA 1990;87:668.
96. Trainor CD, Evans T, Felsenfeld G, et al. Structure and evolution of a human erythroid transcription factor. Nature 1990;343:92.
97. Whitelaw E, Tsai S-F, Hogben P., et al. Regulated expression of globin chains and the erythroid transcription factor GATA-1 during erythropoiesis in the developing mouse. Mol Cell Biol 1990;10:6596.
98. Minie ME, Kimura T, Felsenfeld G. The developmental switch in embryonic ρ-globin expression is correlated with erythroid lineage-specific differences in transcription factor levels. Development 1992;115:1149.
99. Nicolis S, Ronchi A, Malgaretti N, et al. Increased erythroid-specific expression of a mutated HPFH γ-globin promoter requires the erythroid factor NFE-1. Nucleic Acids Res 1989;17:5509.
100. Gallarda JL, Foley KP, Yang Z, et al. The β-globin stage selector element factor is erythroid-specific promoter-enhancer binding protein NF-E4. Genes Dev 1989;3:1845.
101. Foley KP, Engel JD. Individual stage selector element mutations lead to reciprocal changes in β- versus ε-globin gene transcription: genetic confirmation of promoter competition during globin gene switching. Genes Dev 1992;6:730.
102. Purucker M, Bodine D, Lin H, et al. Structure and function of the enhancer 3′ to the human $^{A}\gamma$ globin gene. Nucleic Acids Res 1990;18: 7408.
103. Lavelle D, Ducksworth J, Eves E, et al. A homeodomain protein binds to γ-globin gene regulatory sequences. Proc Natl Acad Sci USA 1991;88: 7318.
104. Jane SM, Ney PA, Vanin EF, et al. Identification of a stage selector element in the human γ-globin gene promoter that fosters preferential interaction with the 5′ HS2 enhancer when in competition with the β-promoter. EMBO J 1992;11:2961.
105. Gumucio DL, Heilstedt-Williamson H, Gray TA, et al. Phylogenetic footprinting reveals a nuclear protein which binds to silencer sequences in the human γ and ε globin genes. Mol Cell Biol 1992;12:4919.
106. Raich N, Enver T, Nakamoto B, et al. Autonomous developmental control of human embryonic globin gene switching in transgenic mice. Science 1990;250:1147.
107. Enver T, Ebens AJ, Forrester WC, et al. The human β-globin locus activation region alters the developmental fate of a human fetal globin gene in transgenic mice. Proc Natl Acad Sci USA 1989;86:7033.
108. Behringer RR, Ryan TM, Palmiter RD, et al. Human γ-to β-globin gene switching in transgenic mice. Genes Dev 1990;4:380.
109. Enver T, Raich N, Ebens AJ, et al. Developmental regulation of human fetal-to-adult globin gene switching in transgenic mice. Nature 1990;344:309.
110. Dillon N, Grosveld F. Human γ-globin genes silenced independently of other genes in the β-globin locus. Nature 1991;350:252.
111. Strouboulis J, Dillon N, Grosveld F. Developmental regulation of a complete 70-kb human β-globin locus in transgenic mice. Genes Dev 1992;6:1857.
112. Peterson KR, Clegg CH, Josephson BM, et al. Transgenic mice containing a 248 Kb human β locus YAC display proper developmental control of human globin genes. (Abstract) Clin Res 1993;41:258a.
113. Hanscombe O, Whyatt D, Fraser P, et al. Importance of globin gene order for correct developmental expressions. Genes Dev 1991;5:1387.
114. Pasvol G, Weatherall DJ, Wilson RJM. Effects of foetal haemoglobin on susceptibility of red cells to *Plasmodium falciparum*. Nature 1977;270: 171.
115. Friedman MJ, Traeger W. The biochemistry of resistance to malaria. Sci Am 1981;244:154.
116. Nagel RL, Roth EF, Jr. Malaria and red cell genetic defects. Blood 1989;74:1213.
117. Dozy AM, Kan YW, Embury SH, et al. α-Globin gene organization in blacks precludes the severe form of α-thalassemia. Nature 1979;280: 605.
118. Oppenheimer SJ, Higgs DR, Weatherall DJ, et al. α thalassemia in Papua New Guinea. Lancet 1984;2:424.
119. Rachmilewitz EA, Shinar E, Shalev O, et al. Erythrocyte membrane alterations in beta-thalassemia. Clin Hematol 1985;14:163.
120. Shinar E, Rachmilewitz EA. Oxidative denaturation of red blood cells in thalassemia. Semin Hematol 1990;27:70.
121. Shinar E, Shalev O, Rachmilewitz EA, et al. Erythrocyte membrane skeleton abnormalities in severe beta thalassemia. Blood 1987;70:158.
122. Shinar E, Rachmilewitz EA, Lux SE. Differing erythrocyte membrane skeletal protein defects in alpha and beta thalassemia. J Clin Invest 1989;83:404.
123. Schrier SL, Rachmilewitz E, Mohandas N. Cellular and membrane properties of alpha and beta thalassemic erythrocytes are different: implication for differences in clinical manifestations. Blood 1989;74: 2194.
124. Rouyer-Fessard P, Garel M-C, Domenget C, et al. A study of membrane protein defects and α hemoglobin chains of red blood cells in human β thalassemia. J Biol Chem 1989;264:19092.
125. Sorensen S, Rubin E, Polster H, et al. The role of membrane skeletal-associated α-globin in the pathophysiology of β-thalassemia. Blood 1990;75:1333.
126. Adavani R, Sorenson S, Shinar E, et al. Characterization and comparison of the red blood cell membrane damage in severe human α- and β-thalassemia. Blood 1992;79:1058.
127. Scott MD, Rouyer-Fessard P, Ba MS, et al. α- and β-Haemoglobin chain induced changes in normal erythrocyte deformability: comparison to β thalassemia intermedia and Hb H disease. Br J Haematol 1992;80: 519.
128. Yuan J, Kannan R, Shinar E, et al. Isolation, characterization, and immunoprecipitation studies of immune complexes from membranes of β-thalassemic erythrocytes. Blood 1992;79:3007.
129. Orkin SH, Sexton JP, Cheng T-C, et al. ATA box transcription mutation in β-thalassemia. Nucleic Acids Res 1983;11:4727.
130. Poncz M, Ballantine M, Solowiejczyk D, et al. β-Thalassemia in a Kurdish Jew. J Biol Chem 1983;257:5994.
131. Antonarakis SE, Orkin SH, Cheng T-C, et al. β-Thalassemia in American blacks: novel mutations in the TATA box and IVS-2 acceptor splice site. Proc Natl Acad Sci USA 1984;81:1154.
132. Huang S-Z, Wong C, Antonarakis SE, et al. The same TATA box β-thalassemia mutation in Chinese and US blacks: another example of independent origins of mutation. Hum Genet 1986;74:152.
133. Cai SP, Zhang JZ, Doherty M, Kan YW. A new TATA box mutation mutation detected in prenatal diagnosis. Am J Hum Genet 1989;45: 112.
134. Fei YJ, Stoming TA, Efremov GD, et al. β-Thalassemia due to a T→A mutation within the ATA box. Biochem Biophys Res Commun 1988;153:741.
135. Takihara Y, Nakamura T, Yamada H, et al. A novel mutation in the TATA box in a Japanese patient with β^{+}-thalassemia. Blood 1986;67: 547.
136. Lin L-I, Lin K-S, Lin K-H, Cheng T-Y. A novel −32 (C→A) mutant identified in amplified genomic DNA of a Chinese β-thalassemic patient. Am J Hum Genet 1992;50:237.
137. Kazazian HH Jr. The thalassemia syndromes: molecular basis and prenatal diagnosis in 1990. Semin Hematol 1990;27:209.
138. Kazazian HH Jr, Dowling CE, Boehm CD, et al. Gene defects in β-thalassemia and their prenatal diagnosis. Ann NY Acad Sci 1990;612: 1.
139. Meloni A, Rosatelli MC, Faa V, et al. Promoter mutations producing mild β-thalassemia in the Italian population. Br J Haematol 1992;80: 222.
140. Orkin SH, Kazazian HH Jr, Antonarakis SE, et al. Linkage of β-thalassemic mutations and β-globin gene polymorphisms with DNA polymorphisms in the human β-globin gene cluster. Nature 1982;296: 627.
141. Kulozik AE, Bellan-Koch A, Bail S, et al. Thalassemia intermedia: moderate reduction of β-globin gene transcriptional activity by a novel mutation of the proximal CACCC promoter element. Blood 1991;77: 2054.
142. Efremov DG, Dimovski AJ, Efremov GD. Detection of β-thalassemia mutations by ASO hybridization of PCR amplified DNA with digoxigenin ddUTP labeled oligonucleotides. Hemoglobin 1991;15:525.
143. Coleman MB, Steinberg MH, Harrell AH, et al. The −87 (C→A) β^{+}-thalassemia mutation in a Black family. Hemoglobin 1992;16:399.
144. Rund D, Cohen T, Filon D, et al. Evolution of a genetic disease in an ethnic isolate: β-thalassemia in the Jews of Kurdistan. Proc Natl Acad Sci USA 1991;88:310.
145. Orkin SH, Antonarakis SE, Kazazian HH Jr. Base substitution at position -88 in a β-thalassemic globin gene: further evidence for the role of distal promoter element ACACCC. J Biol Chem 1984;259:8679.
146. Faustino P, Osorio-Almeida L, Barbot J, et al. Novel promoter and splice junction defects add to the genetic, clinical or geographical heterogeneity of β-thalassemia in the Portuguese population. Hum Genet 1992;89:573.
147. Oron V, Filon D, Fearon C, et al. Two novel β-thalassemia mutations in Ashkenazi Jews. (Abstract) Blood 1992;80(Suppl 1):5a.
148. Gonzalez-Redondo JM, Stoming TA, Kutlar A, et al. A C→T substitution at nt -101 in a conserved DNA sequence of the promoter region of the

β-globin gene is associated with "silent" β-thalassemia. Blood 1989;73: 1705.
149. Wong C, Dowling CE, Saiki RK, et al. Characterization of β-thalassemic mutations using direct genomic sequencing of amplified single copy DNA. Nature 1987;330:384.
150. Wong C, Dowling CE, Saiki RK, et al. Characterization of β-thalassaemia mutation using direct genomic sequencing of amplified single copy DNA. Nature 1987;330:384.
151. Orkin SH, Cheng T-C, Antonarakis SE, Kazazian HH Jr. Thalassemia due to a mutation in the cleavage-polyadenylation signal of the human β-globin gene. EMBO J 1985;4:453.
152. Jankovic L, Efremov GD, Petkov G, et al. Two novel polyadenylation mutations leading to β^+-thalassemia. Br J Haematol 1990;75:122.
153. Rund D, Dowling C, Najjar K, et al. Two mutations in the β-globin polyadenylylation signal reveal extended transcripts and new RNA polyadenylylation sites. Proc Natl Acad Sci 1992;89:4324.
154. Huisman THJ. The β- and δ-thalassemia repository. Hemoglobin 1992;16: 237.
155. Kazazian HH Jr, Orkin SH, Antonarakis SE, et al. Molecular characterization of seven β-thalassemia mutations in Asian Indians. EMBO J 1984;3:593.
156. Chibani J, Vidaud M, Duquesnoy P, et al. The peculiar spectrum of β-thalassemia genes in Tunisia. Hum Genet 1988;78:190.
157. Gonzalez-Redondo JM, Stoming TA, Kutlar F, et al. Severe Hb S-β^0-thalassaemia with a T→C substitution in the donor splice site of the first intron of the β-globin gene. Br J Haematol 1989;71:113.
158. Lossi AM, Milland M, Berge-Lefranc JL. A further case of β-thalassemia with an homozygous T→C substitution at the donor splice site of the first intervening sequence of the β-globin gene. Hemoglobin 1989;13: 619.
159. Bouhass R, Aguercif M, Trabuchet G, Godet J. A new mutation at IVS1 nt 2(T→A), in β-thalassemia from Algeria. Blood 1990;76:1054.
160. Gonzalez-Redondo JM, Kattamis C, Huisman, THJ. Characterization of three types of β^0 thalassemia resulting from a partial deletion of the β-globin gene. Hemoglobin 1989;13:377
161. Deidda G, Novelletto A, Hafez M, et al. A new β-thalassemia mutation produced by a single nucleotide substitution in the conserved dinucleotide sequence of the IVS-1 consensus acceptor site (AG→AA). Hemoglobin 1990;14:431.
162. Oner R, Altay C, Gurgey A, et al. β-Thalassemia in Turkey. Hemoglobin 1990;14:1.
163. Yamamoto Ku, Yamamoto Ki, Hattori Y, et al. Two β-thalassemia mutations in Japan: codon 121 (GAA→TAA) and IVS-I-130 (G→C). Hemoglobin 1992;16:295.
164. Orkin SH, Sexton JP, Goff SC, Kazazian HH Jr. Inactivation of an acceptor RNA splice site by a short deletion in β-thalassemia. J Biol Chem 1983;258:7249.
165. Treisman R, Proudfoot NJ, Shander M, Maniatis T. A single base change at a splice site in a β^0-thalassemic gene causes abnormal RNA splicing. Cell 1982;29:903.
166. Wong C, Antonarakis SE, Goff SC, et al. On the origin and spread of β-thalassemia: recurrent observation of four mutations in different ethnic groups. Proc Natl Acad Sci USA 1986;83:6529.
167. Hattori Y, Yamamoto K, Yamashiro Y, et al. Three β-thalassemia mutations in the Japanese: IVS-II-1 (G→A), IVS-II-848 (C→G), and codon 90 (GAG→TAG). Hemoglobin 1992;16:93.
168. Nozari G, Rahbar S, Rahmanzadeh S, Golshairgan A. Splice junction [IVS-II-1 (G→C)] thalassemia: a new mutation detected in an Iranian patient. Hemoglobin 1993;17:279.
169. Atweh GF, Anagnou NP, Forget BG, Kaufman RE. β-Thalassemia resulting from a single nucleotide substitution in an acceptor splice site. Nucleic Acids Res 1985;13:777.
170. Padanilam BJ, Huisman THJ. The β^0-thalassemia in an American Black family is due to a single nucleotide substitution in the acceptor splice junction of the second intervening sequence. Am J Hematol 1986;22: 259.
171. Jankovic L, Dimovski AJ, Sukarova E, et al. A new mutation in the β-globin gene (IVS II-850 G→C) found in a Yugoslavian β-thalassemia heterozygote. Haematologica 1992;77:119.
172. Rosatelli MC, Tuveri T, Scalas MT, et al. Molecular screening and fetal diagnosis of β-thalassemia in the Italian population. Hum Genet 1992;89: 585.
173. Chehab FF, Der Kaloustian V, Khouri FP, et al. The molecular basis of β-thalassemia in Lebanon: application to prenatal diagnosis. Blood 1987;69:1141.
174. Vidaud M, Gattoni R, Stevenin J, et al. A 5′ splice-region G→C mutation in exon 1 of the human β-globin gene inhibits pre-mRNA splicing: a mechanism for β^+-thalassemia. Proc Natl Acad Sci USA 1989;86: 1041.
175. Gonzalez-Redondo JM, Stoming TA, Kutlar F, et al. Hb Monroe or $\alpha_2\beta_2$30(B12)Arg→Thr, a variant associated with β-thalassemia due to a G→C substitution adjacent to the donor splice site of the first intron. Hemoglobin 1989;13:67.
176. Kalaydjieva L, Eigel A, Argiris A, Horst J. The molecular basis of thalassemia in Bulgaria. (Abstract) Third International Conference on Thalassemia and the Hemoglobinopathies, Sardinia, April 1989:43.
177. Cheng T-C, Orkin SH, Antonarakis SE, et al. β-Thalassemia in Chinese: use of in vivo RNA analysis and oligonucleotide hybridization in systematic characterization of molecular defects. Proc Natl Acad Sci USA 1984;81:2821.
178. Hill AVS, Bowden DK, O'Shaughnessy DF, et al. β-Thalassemia in Melanesia: association with malaria and characterization of a common variant (IVS-1 nt 5 G→C). Blood 1988;72:9.
179. Atweh GF, Wong C, Reed R, et al. A new mutation in IVS-1 of the human β globin gene causing β-thalassemia due to abnormal splicing. Blood 1987;70:147.
180. Gonzalez-Redondo JM, Kutlar A, Kutlar F, et al. Molecular characterization of Hb S(C) β-thalassemia in American blacks. Am J Hematol 1991;38:9.
181. Kulozik AE, Yarwood N, Jones RW. The Corfu $\delta\beta^0$ thalassemia: a small deletion acts at a distance to selectively abolish β globin gene expression. Blood 1988;71:457.
182. Kattamis C, Hu H, Cheng G, et al. Molecular characterization of β-thalassaemia in 174 Greek patients with thalassaemia major. Br J Haematol 1990;74:342.
183. Lapoumeroulie C, Pagnier J, Bank A, et al. β-Thalassemia due to a novel mutation in IVS-1 sequence donor site consensus sequence creating a restriction site. Biochem Biophys Res Comm 1986;139:709.
184. Wong C, Antonarakis SE, Goff SC, et al. β-Thalassemia due to two novel nucleotide substitutions in consensus acceptor site sequences of the β-globin gene. Blood 1989;73:914.
185. Chiou SS, Chang TT, Chen PH, et al. Molecular basis and haematological characterization of β-thalassemia major in Taiwan, with a mutation of IVS-1 3′ end TAG→GAG in a Chinese patient. Br J Haematol 1993;83: 112.
186. Gonzalez-Redondo JH, Stoming TA, Lanclos KD, et al. Clinical and genetic/heterogeneity in black patients with homozygous β-thalassemia from the southeastern United States. Blood 1988;72:1007.
187. Murru S, Loudianos G, Deiana M, et al. Molecular characterization of β-thalassemia intermedia in patients of Italian descent and identification of three novel β-thalassemia mutations. Blood 1991;77:1342.
188. Beldjord C, Lapoumeroulie C, Pagnier J, et al. A novel β-thalassemia gene with a single base mutation in the conserved polypyrimidine sequence at the 3′ end of IVS-II. Nucleic Acids Res 1988;16:4927.
189. Varawalla NY, Old JM, Weatherall DJ. Rare β-thalassaemia mutations in Asian Indians. Br J Haematol 1991;79:640.
190. Spritz RA, Jagadeeswaran P, Choudary PV, et al. Base substitution in an intervening sequence of a β^+-thalassemic human globin gene. Proc Natl Acad Sci USA 1981;78:2455.
191. Westaway D, Williamson R. An intron nucleotide sequence variant in a cloned β^+-thalassemia globin gene. Nucleic Acids Res 1981;9: 1777.
192. Metherall JE, Collins FS, Pan J, et al. β^0-Thalassemia caused by a base substitution that creates an alternative splice acceptor site in an intron. EMBO J 1986;5:2551.
193. Dobkin C, Pergolizzi RG, Bahre P, et al. Abnormal splice in a mutant β-globin gene not at the site of a mutation. Proc Natl Acad Sci USA 1983;80:1184.
194. Yang KG, Kutlar F, George E, et al. Molecular characterization of β-globin gene mutations in Malay patients with Hb E-β-thalassaemia and thalassaemia major. Br J Haematol 1989;72:73.
195. Goldsmith ME, Humphries RK, Ley T, et al. Silent substitution in β^+-thalassemia gene activating a cryptic splice site in β-globin RNA coding sequence. Proc Natl Acad Sci USA 1983;80:2318.
196. Hattori Y, Yamane A, Yamashiro Y, et al. Gene analysis of β-thalassemia among Japanese. Hemoglobin 1989;13:657.
197. Orkin SH, Kazazian HH Jr, Antonarakis SE, et al. Abnormal RNA processing due to the exon mutation of the β^E-globin gene. Nature 1982;300: 768.
198. Orkin SH, Antonarakis SE, Loukopoulos D. Abnormal processing of $\beta^{Knossos}$ RNA. Blood 1984;64:311.
199. Ribeiro MLS, Baysal E, Kutlar F, et al. A novel β^0-thalassaemia mutation (codon 15, TGG→TGA) is prevalent in a population of central Portugal. Br J Haematol 1992;80:567.
200. Chang JC, Kan YW. β^0-Thalassemia: a nonsense mutation in man. Proc Natl Acad Sci USA 1979;76:2886.
201. Fucharoen G, Fucharoen S, Jetsrisuparb A, Fukumaki Y. Molecular basis of HbE-β-thalassemia and the origin of HbE in northeast Thailand: identification of one novel mutation using amplified DNA from buffy coat specimens. Biochem Biophys Res Commun 1990;170:698.
202. Fucharoen S, Fucharoen G, Fucharoen P, Fukumaki Y. A novel ochre mutation in the β-thalassemia gene of a Thai. J Biol Chem 1989;264: 7780.
203. Boehm CD, Dowling CD, Waber PG, et al. Use of oligonucleotide hybridization in the characterization of a β^0-thalassemia gene ($\beta^{37\ TGG\rightarrow TGA}$) in a Saudi Arabian family. Blood 1986;67:1185.
204. Trecartin RF, Liebhaber SA, Chang, JC, et al. β^0-Thalassemia in Sardinia is caused by a nonsense mutation. J Clin Invest 1981;68:1012.
205. Moschonas N, deBoer E, Grosveld FG, et al. Structure and expression of a cloned β^0-thalassemic globin gene. Nucleic Acids Res 1981;9:4391.
206. Orkin SH, Goff SC. Nonsense and frameshift mutations in β^0-thalassemia detected in cloned β globin genes. J Biol Chem 1981;256:9782.
207. Pergolizzi R, Spritz RA, Spence S, et al. Two cloned β-thalassemia genes are associated with amber mutations at codon 39. Nucleic Acids Res 1981;9:7065.
208. Jackson IJ, Freund RM, Wasylyk B, et al. The isolation, mapping and

transcription in vitro of a β^0-thalassaemia globin gene. Eur J Biochem 1981;121:27.
209. Gorski J, Fiori M, Mach B. A new nonsense mutation as the molecular basis for β^0-thalassaemia. J Mol Biol 1982;154:537.
210. Chehab FF, Honig GR, Kan YW. Spontaneous mutation in β-thalassemia producing the same nucleotide substitution as that in a common hereditary form. Lancet 1986;1:3.
211. Atweh GF, Brickner HE, Zhu XX, et al. A new amber mutation in a β-thalassemia gene with non-measurable levels of mutant mRNA in vivo. J Clin Invest 1988;82:557.
212. Fucharoen S, Katsube T, Fucharoen G, et al. Molecular heterogeneity of β-thalassaemia in the Japanese: identification of two novel mutations. Br J Haematol 1990;74:101.
213. Divoky V, Gu L-H, Indrak K, et al. A new β^0-thalassaemia nonsense mutation (codon 112, T→A) not associated with a dominant type of thalassaemia in the heterozygote. Br J Haematol 1993;83:523.
214. Kazazian HH Jr, Orkin SH, Boehm CD, et al. Characterization of a spontaneous mutation to a β-thalassemia allele. Am J Hum Genet 1986;38:860.
215. Fei YJ, Stoming TA, Kutlar A, et al. One form of inclusion body β-thalassemia is due to a GAA→TAA mutation at codon 121 of the β chain. Blood 1989;73:1075.
216. Thein SL, Hesketh C, Taylor P, et al. Molecular basis for dominantly inherited inclusion body β-thalassemia. Proc Natl Acad Sci USA 1990;87:3924.
217. Hall GW, Franklin IM, Sura T, Thein SL. A novel mutation (nonsense β127) in exon 3 of the β globin gene produces a variable thalassaemia phenotype. Br J Haematol 1991;79:342.
218. Rosatelli MC, Dozy A, Faa V, et al. Molecular characterization of β-thalassemia in the Sardinian population. Am J Hum Genet 1992;50: 422.
219. Kollia P, Gonzalez-Redondo JM, Stoming TA, et al. Frameshift codon 5 [FSC-5 (-CT)] thalassemia: a novel mutation detected in a Greek patient. Hemoglobin 1989;13:597.
220. Kazazian HH Jr, Orkin SH, Boehm CD, et al. β-Thalassemia due to deletion of the nucleotide which is substituted in sickle cell anemia. Am J Hum Genet 1983;35:1028.
221. Chang JC, Alberti A, Kan YW. A β-thalassemia lesion abolishes the same *MstII* site as the sickle mutation. Nucleic Acids Res 1983;11:7789.
222. Orkin SH, Goff SC. Nonsense and frameshift mutations in β-thalassemia detected in cloned β-globin genes. J Biol Chem 1981;256:9782.
223. Economou EP, Antonarakis SE, Dowling CC, et al. Molecular heterogeneity of β-thalassemia in Mestizo Mexicans. Genomics 1991;11: 474.
224. Chan V, Chan TK, Kan YW, Todd D. A novel β-thalassemia frameshift mutation (codon 14/15) detectable by direct visualization of abnormal restriction fragment in amplified genomic DNA. Blood 1988;72:1420.
225. Deidda G, Novelletto A, Hafez M, et al. A new β-thalassaemia frameshift mutation detected by PCR after selective hybridization to immobilized oligonucleotides. Br J Haematol 1991;79:90.
226. Fattoum S, Guemira F, Öner C, et al. β-Thalassemia, Hb S-β-thalassemia, and sickle cell anemia among Tunisians. Hemoglobin 1991;15:11.
227. Lin L-I, Lin K-S, Lin K-H, Cheng H-C. The spectrum of β-thalassemia mutations in Taiwan: Identification of a novel frameshift mutation. Am J Hum Genet 1991;48:809.
228. Schnee J, Griese EV, Eigel A, Horst J. β-Thalassemia gene analysis in a Turkish family reveals a 7 bp deletion in the coding region. Blood 1989;73:2224.
229. Indrak K, Indrakova J, Kutlar F, et al. Compound heterozygosity for a β^0-thalassemia (frameshift codons 38/39; -C) and a non-deletional Swiss type of HPFH (A→C at nt -110, $^G\gamma$) in a Czechoslovakian family. Ann Hematol 1991;63:111.
230. Fucharoen S, Fucharoen G, Laosombat V, and Fukumaki Y. Double heterozygosity of the β-Malay and a novel β-thalassemia gene in a Thai patient. Am J Hematol 1991;38:142.
231. Kimura A, Matsunaga E, Takihara Y, et al. Structural analysis of a β-thalassemia gene found in Taiwan. J Biol Chem 1983;258:2748.
232. Kinniburgh AJ, Maquat LE, Schedl T, et al. mRNA-deficient β^0-thalassemia results from a single nucleotide deletion. Nucleic Acids Res 1982;10:5421.
233. Losekoot M, Fodde R, van Heeren H, et al. A novel frameshift mutation [FSC 47 (A+)] causing β-thalassemia in a Surinam patient. Hemoglobin 1990;14:467.
234. Fucharoen S, Katsube T, Fucharoen G, et al. Molecular heterogeneity of β-thalassaemia in the Japanese: identification of two novel mutations. Br J Haematol 1990;74:101.
235. Chehab FF, Winterhalter KH, Kan YW. Characterization of a spontaneous mutation in β-thalassemia associated with advanced paternal age. Blood 1989;74:852.
236. Chan V, Chan TK, Todd D. A new codon 71 (+T) mutant resulting in β^0-thalassemia. Blood 1989;74:2304.
237. Basak AN, Özer A, Özcelik H, et al. A novel frameshift mutation: deletion of C in codons 74/75 of the β-globin gene causes β^0-thalassemia in a Turkish patient. Hemoglobin 1992;16:309.
238. DiMarzo R, Dowling CE, Wong C, et al. The spectrum of β-thalassemia mutations in Sicily. Br J Haematol 1988;69:393.
239. Schwartz E, Goltsov AA, Kaboaev OK, et al. A novel frameshift mutation causing β-thalassemia in Azerbaijan. Nucleic Acids Res 1989;17:3997.
240. Indrak K, Brabec V, Indrakova J, et al. Molecular characterization of β-thalassemia in Czechoslovakia. Hum Genet 1992;88:399.
241. Ristaldi MS, Pirastu M, Murru S, et al. A spontaneous mutation produced a novel elongated β-globin chain structural variant (Hb Agnana) with a thalassemia-like phenotype. Blood 1990;75:1378.
242. Kazazian HH Jr, Dowling CE, Hurwitz RL, et al. Dominant thalassemia-like phenotypes associated with mutations in exon 3 of the β-globin gene. Blood 1992;79:3014.
243. Beris PH, Miescher PA, Diaz-Chico JC, et al. Inclusion-body β-thalassemia trait in a Swiss family is caused by an abnormal hemoglobin (Geneva) with an altered and extended β chain carboxy-terminus due to a modification in codon β114. Blood 1988:72:801.
244. Fucharoen S, Kobayashi Y, Gucharoen G, et al. A single nucleotide deletion in codon 123 of the β-globin gene causes an inclusion body β-thalassemia trait: a novel elongated globin chain β^{Makabe}. Br J Haematol 1990, 75:393.
245. Fucharoen G, Fucharoen S, Jetsrisuparb A, et al. Eight-base deletion in exon 3 of the β-globin gene produced a novel variant (β Khon Kaen) with an inclusion body thalassemia trait. Blood 1991;78:537.
246. Fucharoen S, Fucharoen G, Fukumaki Y, et al. Three-base deletion in exon 3 of the β-globin gene produced a novel variant (β^{Gunma}) with a thalassemia-like phenotype. Blood 1990;76:1894.
247. Öner R, Öner C, Wilson JB, et al. Dominant β-thalassaemia trait in a Portuguese family is caused by a deletion of (G)TGGCTGGTGT(G) and an insertion of (G)GCAG(G) in codons 134, 135, 136, and 137 of the β-globin gene. Br J Haematol 1991;79:306.
248. Lam VMS, Xie SS, Tam JWO, et al. A new single nucleotide change at the initiation codon (ATG→AGG) identified in amplified genomic DNA of a Chinese β-thalassemic patient. Blood 1990;75:1207.
249. Koo MS, Kim SI, Cho HI, et al. A β-thalassemia mutation found in Korea. Hemoglobin 1992;16:313.
250. Jankovic L, Efremov GD, Josifovska O, et al. An initiation codon mutation as a cause of a β-thalassemia. Hemoglobin 1990;14:169.
251. Beris P, Darbellay R, Speiser D, Kirchner V, et al. *De novo* initiation codon mutation (ATG→ACG) of the β-globin gene causing β-thalassemia in a Swiss family. Am J Hematol 1993;42:248.
252. Hattori Y, Yamashiro Y, Ohba Y, et al. A new β-thalassemia mutaion (initiation codon ATG→GTG) found in the Japanese population. Hemoglobin 1991;15:317.
253. Rahbar S, Nozari G. A novel β-thalassemia mutation (initiation codon ATG→ATT) with a β-thalassemia intermedia phenotype. (Abstract) Blood 1992;80(Suppl 1):5a.
254. Öner R, Agarwal S, Dimovski AJ, et al. The G→A mutation at position +22 3′ to the cap site of the β-globin gene as a possible cause for a β-thalassemia. Hemoglobin 1991;15:67.
255. Cai S-P, Eng B, Francombe WH, et al. Two novel β-thalassemia mutations mutations in the 5′ and 3′ noncoding regions of the β-globin gene. Blood 1992;79:1342.
256. Huang S-Z, Xu Y-H, Zeng F-Y, et al. A novel β-thalassaemia mutation: deletion of 4 bp (-AAAC) in the 5′ transcriptional sequence. Br J Haematol 1991;78:125.
257. Eng B, Waye JS, Chui DHK. The T→C substitution at nucleotide +1570 of the β-globin gene is a polymorphism. Blood 1992;80:1365.
258. Jankovic L, Dimovski AJ, Kollia P, et al. A C→G mutation at nt position 6 3′ to the terminating codon may be the cause of a silent β-thalassemia. Int J Hematol 1991;54:289.
259. Thein SL, Best S, Sharpe J. Hemoglobin Chesterfield (β28 Leu→Arg) produces the phenotype of inclusion body β thalassemia. Blood 1991;77: 2791.
260. Podda A, Galanello R, Maccioni L, et al. A new unstable hemoglobin variant producing a β-thalassemia–like phenotype. Abstract presented at the Third International Conference on Thalassemia and the Hemoglobinopathies, Sardinia, 1989;51.
261. Coleman MB, Steinberg MH, Adams JG III. Hemoglobin Terre Haute arginine β^{106}: a posthumous correction to the original structure of hemoglobin Indianapolis. J Biol Chem 1991;266:5798.
262. Kobayashi Y, Fukumaki Y, Komatsu N, et al. A novel globin structural mutant, Showa-Yakushiji (β110 Leu-Pro) causing a β-thalassemia phenotype. Blood 1987;70:1688.
263. de Castro CM, Lee M, Fleenor DE, et al. A novel β-globin mutation, β Durham-N.C. [β(114) Leu→Pro], detected by SSCP, produces a dominant thalassemia-like phenotype. (Abstract) Blood 1992;80(Suppl 1): 6a.
264. Treisman R, Orkin SH, Maniatis T. Specific transcription and RNA splicing defects in five cloned β-thalassaemia genes. Nature 1983;302: 591.
265. Busslinger M, Moschonas N, Flavell RA. β^+-Thalassemia: aberrant splicing results from a single point mutation in an intron. Cell 1981;27: 289.
266. Fukumaki Y, Ghosh PK, Benz EJ Jr, et al. Abnormally spliced messenger RNA in erythroid cells from patients with β^+-thalassemia and monkey cells expressing a cloned β^+-thalassemia gene. Cell 1982;28:585.
267. Dobkin C, Bank A. Reversibility of IVS 2 missplicing in a mutant human β-globin gene. J Biol Chem 1985:16332.
268. Fessas P, Loukopoulos D, Loutradi-Anagnostou A, et al. "Silent" β-thalassaemia caused by a "silent" β-chain mutant: the pathogenesis of a syndrome of thalassaemia intermedia. Br J Haematol 1982;51:577.
269. Rouabhi F, Chardin P, Boissel JP, et al. Silent β-thalassemia associated

with Hb Knossos β27 (B9) Ala→Ser in Algeria. Hemoglobin 1983:7: 555.
270. Gonzalez-Redondo JM, Brickner HE, Atweh GF. Abnormal processing of β-Malay globin RNA. Biochem Biophys Res Comm 1989;163:8.
271. Takeshita K, Forget BG, Scarpa A, et al. Intranuclear defect in β globin mRNA accumulation due to a premature translation termination codon. Blood 1984, 64:13.
272. Humphries RK, Ley TJ, Anagnou NP, et al. β^0-Thalassemia gene: a premature termination codon causes β mRNA deficiency without changing cytoplasmic β mRNA stability. Blood 1984;64:23.
273. Baserga SJ, Benz EJ Jr. Nonsense mutations in the human β-globin gene affect mRNA metabolism. Proc Natl Acad Sci USA 1988;85: 2056.
274. Baserga SJ, Benz EJ Jr. β-Globin nonsense mutation: Deficient accumulation of mRNA occurs despite normal cytoplasmic stability. Proc Natl Acad Sci USA 1992;89:2935.
275. Maquat LE, Kinninbergh AJ, Rachmilewitz EA, et al. Unstable β-globin mRNA in mRNA-deficient β^0-thalassemia. Cell 1981;27:543.
276. Maquat LE, Kinninburgh AJ. A β^0-thalassemic β-globin RNA that is labile in bone marrow cells is relatively stable in HeLa cells. Nucleic Acids Res 1985;13:2855.
277. Thein SL. Dominant β thalassemia: molecular basis and pathophysiology. Br J Haematol 1992;80:273.
278. Adams JG III, Boxer LA, Baehner RL, et al. Hemoglobin Indianapolis (β112[G14] arginine): an unstable β-chain variant producing the phenotype of severe β-thalassemia. J Clin Invest 1979;63:931.
279. Adams JG, Coleman MB. Structural hemoglobin variants that produce the phenotype of thalassemia. Semin Hematol 1990;27:229.
280. Padanilam BJ, Felice AE, Huisman THJ. Partial deletions of the 5′ β-globin gene region causes β^0-thalassemia in members of an American black family. Blood 1984;4:941.
281. Anand R, Boehm CD, Kazazian HH, et al. Molecular characterization of a β^0-thalassemia resulting from a 1.4 kilobase deletion. Blood 1988;72: 636.
282. Thein SL, Hesketh C, Brown JM, et al. Molecular characterization of a high A_2 β thalassemia by direct sequencing of single strand enriched amplified genomic DNA. Blood 1989;73:924.
283. Diaz-Chico JC, Yang KG, Kutlar A, et al. An ~ 300 bp deletion involving part of the 5′ β-globin gene region is observed in members of a Turkish family with β-thalassemia. Blood 1987;70:583.
284. Spiegelberg R, Aulehla-Scholz C, Erlich H, et al. A β-thalassemia gene caused by a 290-base pair deletion: analysis by direct sequencing of enzymatically amplified DNA. Blood 1989;73:1695.
285. Gilman J. The 12.6 kilobase DNA deletion in Dutch β-thalassemia. Br Haematol 1987;67:369.
286. Popovich BW, Rosenblatt DS, Kendall AG, et al. Molecular characterization of an atypical β-thalassemia caused by a large deletion in the 5′ β-globin gene region. Am J Hum Genet 1986;39:797.
287. Spritz R, Orkin SH. Duplication followed by deletion accounts for the structure of an Indian deletion β^0-thalassemia gene. Nucleic Acids Res 1982;10:8025.
288. Sanguansermsri T, Pape M, Laig M, et al. β-Thalassemia in a Thai family is caused by a 3.4 kb deletion including the entire β-globin gene. Hemoglobin 1990;14:157.
289. Wayne JS, Cai SP, Eng B, et al. High hemoglobin $A_0^{2\beta}$-thalassemia due to a 532-basepair deletion of the 5′ β-globin gene region. Blood 1991;77: 1100.
290. Thein SL, Old JM, Wainscoat JS, et al. Population and genetic studies suggest a single origin for the Indian deletion β^0 thalassemia. Br J Haematol 1984;57:271.
291. Motum PI, Lindeman R, Hamilton TJ, Trent RJ. Australian β^0-thalassaemia due to a 12 kb deletion commencing 5′ to the β-globin gene. Br J Haematol 1992;82:107.
292. Craig JE, Kelly SJ, Barnetson R, Thein SL. Molecular characterization of a novel 10.3 kb deletion causing β-thalassaemia with unusually high Hb A_2. Br J Haematol 1992;82:735.
293. Motum PI, Kearney A, Hamilton TJ, Trent RJ. Filipino β^0 thalassaemia: a high Hb $A_0^{2\,\beta}$ thalassaemia resulting from a large deletion of the 5′ β globin gene region. J Med Genet 1993;30:240.
294. Codrington JF, Li HW, Kutlar F, et al. Observations on the level of Hb A_2 in patients with different β-thalassemia mutations and a δ chain variant. Blood 1990;76:1246.
295. Schwartz E. The silent carrier of β-thalassemia. N Engl J Med 281: 1327.
296. Semenza GL, Delgrosso K, Poncz M, et al. The silent carrier allele: β thalassemia without a mutation in the β-globin gene or its immediate flanking regions. Cell 1984;39:123.
297. Chebloune Y, Pagnier J, Trabuchet G, et al. Structural analysis of the 5′ flanking region of the β-globin gene in African sickle cell anemia patients: further evidence for three origins of the sickle cell mutation in Africa. Proc Natl Acad Sci USA 85:4431.
298. Wong SC, Stoming TA, Efremov GD, et al. High frequencies of a rearrangement (+ATA; -T) at −530 to the β-globin gene in different populations indicate the absence of a correlation with a silent β-thalassemia determinant. Hemoglobin 1989;13:1.
299. Balanello R, Meloni A, Gasperini D, et al. The repeated sequence $(AT)_X(T)_Y$ upstream to the β-globin gene is a simple polymorphism. Blood 1993;81:1974.
300. Schwartz E, Cohen A, Surrey S. Overview of the β-thalassemias: genetic and clinical aspects. Hemoglobin 1988;12:551.
301. Berg PE, Mittelman M, Elion J, et al. Increased protein binding to a −530 mutation of the human β-globin gene associated with decreased β-globin synthesis. Am J Hematol 1991;36:42.
302. Murru S, Loudianos G, Cao A, et al. A β-thalassemia carrier with normal sequence within the β-globin gene. Blood 1990;76:2164.
303. Murru S, Loudianos G, Porcu S, et al. A β-thalassaemia phenotype not linked to the β-globin cluster in an Italian family. Br J Haematol 1992;81: 283.
304. Antonarakis SE, Boehm CD, Giardina PJ, Kazazian HH Jr., Nonrandom association of polymorphic restriction sites in the β-globin gene cluster. Proc Natl Acad Sci USA 1982;79:137.
305. Antonarakis SE, Kazazian HH Jr., Orkin SH. DNA polymorphism and molecular pathology of the human globin gene clusters. Hum Genet 1985;69:1.
306. Orkin SH, Kazazian HH Jr. The mutation and polymorphism of the human β-globin gene and its surrounding DNA. Annu Rev Genet 1984;18:131.
307. Higgs DR, Wainscoat JS, Flint J, et al. Analysis of the human α-globin gene cluster reveals a highly informative genetic locus. Proc Natl Acad Sci USA 1986;83:5165.
308. Higgs DR, Vickers MA, Wilkie AOM, et al. A review of the molecular genetics of the human α-globin gene cluster. Blood 1989;73:1081.
309. Higgs DR. The molecular genetics of the α globin gene family. Eur J Clin Invest 1990;20:340.
310. Lienhaber SA. α Thalassaemia. Hemoglobin 1989;13:685.
311. Kazazian HH Jr., Orkin SH, Markham AF, et al. Quantification of the close association between DNA haplotypes and specific β-thalassaemia mutations in Mediterraneans. Nature 1984;310:152.
312. Pirastu M, Galanello R, Doherty MA, et al. The same β-globin gene mutation is present on nine different β-thalassemia chromosomes in a Sardinian population. Proc Natl Acad Sci USA 1987;84:2882.
313. Chakravarti A, Buetow KH, Antonarakis SE, et al. Nonuniform recombination within the human β-globin gene cluster. Am J Hum Genet 1984;36:1239.
314. Antonarakis SE, Orkin SH, Kazazian HH Jr., et al. Evidence for multiple origins of the β^E-globin gene in Southeast Asia. Proc Natl Acad Sci USA 1982;79:6608.
315. Kan YW, Dozy AM, Varmus HE, et al. Deletion of α globin genes in haemoglobin H disease demonstrates multiple α globin structural loci. Nature 1975;255:255.
316. Embury SH, Miller JA, Dozy AM, et al. Two different molecular organizations account for the single α-globin gene of the α-thalassemia-2 genotype. J Clin Invest 1980;66:1319.
317. Kulozik AE, Kar BC, Serjeant GR, et al. The molecular basis of α thalassemia in India: its interactions with the sickle cell gene. Blood 1988;71: 467.
318. Zhao J-B, Zhao L, Fei Y-J, et al. A novel α-thalassemia-2 (−2.7 kb) observed in a Chinese patient with Hb H disease. Am J Hematol 1991;38: 248.
319. Lacerra G, Fioretti G, De Angioletti M, et al. $(\alpha)\alpha^{5.3}$: a novel α^+ thalassemia deletion with the breakpoints in the α2-globin gene and in close proximity to an *Alu* family repeat between the $\psi\alpha$2- and $\psi\alpha$1-globin genes. Blood 1991;78:2740.
320. Indrak K, Gu Y-C, Novotny J, Huisman THJ. A new α-thalassemia-2 deletion resulting in microcytosis and hypochromia and *in vitro* chain imbalance in the heterozygote. Am J Hematol 1993;43:144.
321. Camaschella C, Bertero MT, Serra A, et al. A benign form of thalassaemia intermedia may be determined by the interaction of triplicated α locus and heterozygous β-thalassaemia. Br J Haematol 1987;66:103.
322. Galanello R, Ruggeri R, Paglietti E, et al. A family with segregating triplicated alpha globin loci and beta thalassemia. Blood 1983;62:1035.
323. Kulozik AE, Thein SL, Wainscoat JS, et al. Thalassaemia intermedia: interaction of the triple α-globin gene arrangement and heterozygous β-thalassaemia. Br J Haematol 1987;66:109.
324. Orkin SH, Goff SC. The duplicated human α-globin genes: their relative expression as measured by RNA analysis. Cell 1981;24:345.
325. Liebhaber SA, Kan YW. Differentiation of the mRNA transcripts originating from the α1- and α2-globin loci in normals and α-thalassemics. J Clin Invest 1981;68:439.
326. Bowden DK, Hill AVS, Higgs DR, et al. Different hematologic phenotypes are associated with leftward ($-\alpha^{4.2}$) and rightward ($-\alpha^{3.7}$) α^+-thalassemia deletions. J Clin Invest 1987;79:39.
327. Liebhaber SA, Cash FE, Main DM. Compensatory increase in α1-globin gene expression in individual heterozygous for the α thalassemia-2 deletion. J Clin Invest 1985;76:1057.
328. Higgs DR, Old JM, Clegg JB, et al. Negro α-thalassaemia is caused by deletion of a single α-globin gene. Lancet 1979;2:272.
329. Nicholls RD, Fischel-Ghodsian N, Higgs DR. Recombination at the human α-globin gene cluster: sequence features and topological constraints. Cell 1987;49:369.
330. Hatton CSR, Wilkie AOM, Drysdale HC, et al. α-Thalassemia caused by a large (62 kb) deletion upstream of the human α globin gene cluster. Blood 1990;76:221.
331. Romao L, Osorio-Almeida L, Higgs DR, et al. α-Thalassemia resulting from deletion of regulatory sequences far upstream of the α-globin structural genes. Blood 1991;78:1589.

332. Wilkie AOM, Lamb J, Harris PC, et al. A truncated human chromosome 16 associated with α thalassaemia is stabilized by addition of telomeric repeat (TTAGGG). Nature 1990;346:868.
333. Liebhaber SA, Griese E-U, Weiss I, et al. Inactivation of human α-globin gene expression by a de novo deletion located upstream of the α-globin gene cluster. Proc Natl Acad Sci USA 1990;87:9431.
334. Jarman AP, Wood WG, Sharpe JA, Gourdon G. Characterization of the major regulatory element upstream of the human α-globin gene cluster. Mol Cell Biol 1991;11:4679.
335. Strauss EC, Andrews NC, Higgs DR, Orkin SH. *In vivo* footprinting of the human α-globin locus upstream regulatory element by guanine and adenine ligation-mediated polymerase chain reaction. Mol Cell Biol 1992;12:2135.
336. Beaudry MA, Ferguson DJ, Pearse K, et al. Survival of a hydropic infant with homozygous α-thalassemia-1. J Peds 1986;108:713.
337. Bianchi DW, Beyer EC, Stark AR, et al. Normal long-term survival with α-thalassemia. J Peds 1986;108:716.
338. Chui DHK, Wong SC, Chung S-W, et al. Embryonic ζ-globin chains in adults: a marker for α-thalassemia-1 haplotype due to a > 17.5 kb deletion. N Engl J Med 1986;314:76.
339. Steinberg MH, Coleman MB, Adams JH III, et al. A new gene deletion in the α-like globin gene cluster as the molecular basis for the rare α-thalassemia-1 (—/αα) in blacks: Hb disease in sickle cell trait. Blood 1986;67:469.
340. Felice AE, Cleek MP, McKie K, et al. The rare α-thalassemia-1 of blacks is a ζα-thalassemia-1 associated with deletion of all α- and ζ-globin genes. Blood 1984;63:1253.
341. Fei YJ, Liu JC, Walker ELD III, Huisman THJ. A new gene deletion involving the α2-, α1-, and ξ1-globin genes in a black family with Hb H disease. Am J Hematol 1992;39:299.
342. Schmid CW, Jelinek. The Alu family of dispersed repetitive sequences. Science 1982;216:1065.
343. Jelinek WR, Schmid CW. Repetitive sequences in eukaryotic DNA and their expression. Annu Rev Biochem 1982;51:813.
344. Higgs DR, Goodbourn SEY, Lamb J, et al. α-Thalassaemia caused by a polyadenylation signal mutation. Nature 1983;306:398.
345. Thein SL, Wallace RB, Pressley L, et al. The polyadenylation site mutation in the α-globin gene cluster. Blood 1988;71:313.
346. Yüregir GT, Aksoy K, Cürük MA, et al. Hb H disease in a Turkish family resulting from the interaction of a deletional α-thalassaemia-1 and a newly discovered poly A mutation. Br J Haematol 1992;80:527.
347. Orkin SH, Goff SC, Hechtman RL. Mutation in an intervening sequence splice junction in man. Proc Natl Acad Sci USA 1981;78:5041.
348. Felber BK, Orkin SH, Hamer DH. Abnormal RNA splicing causes one form of α-thalassemia. Cell 1982;29:895.
349. Liebhaber SA, Coleman MB, Adams JG III, et al. Molecular basis for non-deletion α-thalassemia in American blacks $\alpha2^{116GAG \rightarrow UAG}$ J Clin Invest 1987;80:154.
350. Safaya S, Rieder RF. Dysfunctional α-globin gene in hemoglobin H disease in blacks. J Biol Chem 1988;263:4328.
351. Pirastu M, Saglio G, Chang JC, et al. Initiation codon mutation as a cause of α-thalassemia. J Biol Chem 1984;259:12315.
352. Moi P, Cash FE, Liebhaber SA, et al. An initiation codon mutation (AUG→GUG) of the human α1-globin gene: structural characterization and evidence for a mild thalassemic phenotype. J Clin Invest 1987;80:1416.
353. Olivieri NF, Chang LS, Poon AO, et al. An α-globin gene initiation codon mutation in a black family with Hb H disease. Blood 1987;70:729.
354. Morle F, Lopez B, Henni T, et al. α-Thalassemia associated with the deletion of two nucleotides at position -2 and -3 preceding the AUG codon. EMBO J 1985;44:1245.
355. Morle F, Starck J, Godet J. α-Thalassemia due to the deletion of nucleotides -2 and -3 preceding the AUG initiation codon affects translation efficiency both in vitro and in vivo. Nucleic Acids Res 1986;14:3279.
356. Milner PF, Clegg JB, Weatherall DJ. Haemoglobin H disease due to a unique haemoglobin variant with an elongated α chain. Lancet 1971;1:729.
357. Clegg JB, Weatherall DJ, Milner PG. Haemoglobin Constant Spring: a chain termination mutant? Nature 1971;234:337.
358. Clegg JB, Weatherall DJ, Contopoulos-Griva I, et al. Haemoglobin Icaria, a new chain termination mutant which causes α-thalassaemia. Nature 1974;251:245.
359. De Jong WW, Khan PM, Bernini LF. Hemoglobin Koya Dora: high frequency of a chain termination mutant. Am J Hum Genet 1975;27:81.
360. Bradley TB, Wohl RC, Smith GJ. Elongation of the α-globin chain in a black family: interaction with Hb G Philadelphia. (Abstract) Clin Res 1975;23:1314.
361. Honig GR, Shamsuddin M, Vida LN, et al. Hemoglobin Evanston (α14 Trp→Arg): an unstable α-chain variant expressed as α-thalassemia. J Clin Invest 1984;73:1740.
362. Sanguansermsri T, Matragoon S, Changloah L, et al. Hemoglobin Suan-Dok ($\alpha_2^{109(G16)LEU \rightarrow ARG}\beta_2$): an unstable variant associated with α-thalassemia. Hemoglobin 1979;3:161.
363. Honig GR, Shamsuddin M, Zaizov R, et al. Hemoglobin Petah Tikvah (α110 Ala→Asp): a new unstable variant with α-thalassemia–like expression. Blood 1981;57:705.
364. Goosens M, Lee KY, Liebhaber SA, Kan YW. Globin structural mutant $\alpha^{125\ Leu \rightarrow Pro}$ is a novel cause of α-thalassaemia. Nature 1982;296:864.
365. Hunt DM, Higgs DR, Winichagoon P, et al. Haemoglobin Constant Spring has an unstable α chain messenger RNA. Br J Haematol 1982;51:405.
366. Higgs DR, Wood WG, Barton C, et al. Clinical features and molecular analysis of acquired Hb H disease. Am J Med 1983;75:181.
367. Anagnou NP, Ley TJ, Chesbro B, et al. Acquired α-thalassemia in preleukemia is due to decreased expression of all four α-globin genes. Proc Natl Acad Sci USA 1983;80:6051.
368. Helder J, Deisseroth A. S1 nuclease analysis of α-globin gene expression in preleukemic patients with acquired hemoglobin H disease after transfer to mouse erythroleukemia cells. Proc Natl Acad Sci USA 1987;84:2387.
369. Weatherall DJ, Higgs DR, Bunch C, et al. Hemoglobin H disease and mental retardation. N Engl J Med 1981;305:607.
370. Wilkie AOM, Buckle VJ, Harris PC, et al. Clinical features and molecular analysis of the α thalassemia/mental retardation syndromes. I. Cases due to deletions involving chromosome band 16p13.3. Am J Hum Genet 1990;46:1112.
371. Wilkie, AOM, Zeitlin HC, Lindenbaum RH, et al. Clinical features and molecular analysis of the α thalassemia/mental retardation syndromes. II. Cases without detectable abnormality of the α globin complex. Am J Hum Genet 1990;46:1127.
372. Lamb J, Harris PC, Lindenbaum RH, et al. Detection of breakpoints in submicroscopic chromosomal translocation, illustrating an important mechanism for genetic disease. Lancet 1989;2:819.
373. Lamb J, Harris PC, Wilkie AOM, et al. *De novo* truncation of chromosome 16p and healing with $(TTAGGG)_n$ in the α-thalassemia/mental retardation syndrome (ATR-16). Am J Hum Genet 1993;52:668.
374. Bollekens JA, Forget BG. δβ Thalassemia and hereditary persistence of fetal hemoglobin. Hematol Oncol Clin North Am 1991;5:399.
375. Poncz M, Henthorn P, Stoeckert C, et al. Globin gene expression in hereditary persistence of fetal hemoglobin and $(\delta\beta)^0$ thalassemia. In: MacLean N, ed. Oxford surveys on eukaryotic genes, vol 5. Oxford, Oxford University Press, 1988:163.
376. Ottolenghi S, Mantovani R, Nicolis S, et al. DNA sequences regulating human globin gene transcription in nondeletional hereditary persistence of fetal hemoglobin. Hemoglobin 1989;13:523.
377. Bernards R, Flavell RA. Physical mapping of the globin gene deletion in hereditary persistence of foetal haemoglobin (HPFH). Nucleic Acids Res 1980;8:1521.
378. Flavell RA, Kooter JM, deBoer E, et al. Analysis of the δ-γ-globin gene loci in normal and Hb Lepore DNA: direct determination of gene linkage and intergene distance. Cell 1978;15:25.
379. Mears JG, Ramirez F, Leibowitz D, et al. Organization of human δ- and β-globin genes in cellular DNA and the presence of intragenic inserts. Cell 1978;15:15.
380. Baird M, Schreiner H, Driscoll C, et al. Localization of the site of recombination in formation of the Lepore Boston globin gene. J Clin Invest 1981;68:560.
381. Mavilio F, Giampaolo A, Care A, et al. The δβ crossover region in Lepore Boston hemoglobinopathy is restricted to a 59 base pairs region around the 5′ splice junction of the large globin gene intervening sequence. Blood 1983;62:230.
382. Chebloune Y, Verdier G. The delta-beta-crossing-over site in the fusion gene of the Lepore-Boston disease might be localized in a preferential recombination region. Acta Haematol 1983;69:294.
383. Lanclos KD, Patterson J, Efremov GD, et al. Characterization of chromosomes with hybrid genes for Hb Lepore-Washington, Hb Lepore-Baltimore, Hb P-Nilotic, and Hb Kenya. Hum Genet 1987;77:40.
384. Wood WG, Old JM, Roberts AVS, et al. Human globin gene expression: control of β, δ and δβ chain production. Cell 1978;15:437.
385. Orkin SH, Goff SC, Nathan DG. Heterogeneity of DNA deletion in γδβ thalassemia. J Clin Invest 1981;67:878.
386. Taramelli R, Kioussis D, Vanin E, et al. γδβ-Thalassemias 1 and 2 are the result of a 100 kbp deletion in the human β-globin cluster. Nucleic Acids Res 1986;14:7017.
387. Van der Ploeg LHT, Konings A, Oort M, et al. γ-β-Thalassemia studies showing that deletion of the γ and δ influences β-globin gene expression in man. Nature 1980;283:637.
388. Vanin EF, Henthorn PS, Kioussis D, et al. Unexpected relationships between four large deletions in the human β-globin gene cluster. Cell 1983;35:701.
389. Curtin P, Pirastu M, Kan YW, et al. A distant gene deletion affects β-globin gene function in an atypical γδβ-thalassemia. J Clin Invest 1985;76:1554.
390. Fearon ER, Kazazian HH, Waber PG, et al. The entire globin cluster is deleted in a form of γδβ-thalassemia. Blood 1983;61:1273.
391. Pirastu M, Kan YW, Lin CC, et al. Hemolytic disease of the newborn caused by a new deletion of the entire β-globin cluster. J Clin Invest 1983;72:602.
392. Trent RJ, Williams BG, Kearney A, et al. Molecular and hematologic characterization of Scottish-Irish type $(\epsilon\gamma\delta\beta)^0$ thalassemia. Blood 1990;76:2132.
393. Driscoll MC, Dobkin CS, Alter BP. γδβ-thalassemia due to a de novo mutation deleting the 5′ β-globin gene activating-region hypersensitive sites. Proc Natl Acad Sci USA 1989;86:7470.

394. Diaz-Chico JC, Huang HJ, Juricic D, et al. Two new large deletions resulting in $\epsilon\gamma\delta\beta$ thalassemia. Acta Haematol 1988;80:79.
395. Kioussis D, Vanin E, deLange T, et al. β-Globin gene inactivation by DNA translocation in $\gamma\beta$-thalassemia. Nature 1983;306:662.
396. Kulozik AE, Bail S, Bellan-Koch A, et al. The proximal element of the β globin locus control region is not functionally required *in vivo*. J Clin Invest 1990;87:2142.
397. Collis P, Antoniou M, Grosveld F. Definition of the minimal requirements within the human β-globin gene and the dominant control region for high level expression. EMBO J 1990;9:223.
398. Ryan TM, Townes TM, Reilly MP, et al. A single erythroid-specific DNAse I superhypersensitive site activates high levels of human β-globin gene expression in transgenic mice. Genes Dev 1989;3:314.
399. Ojwang PJ, Nakatsuji T, Gardiner MB, et al. Gene deletion as the molecular basis for the Kenya -$^G\gamma$-HPFH condition. Hemoglobin 1983;7:115.
400. Collins FS, Cole JL, Lockwood WK, Iannuzzi MC. The deletion in both common types of hereditary persistence of fetal hemoglobin is approximately 105 kilobases. Blood 1987;70:1797.
401. Feingold EA, Forget BG. The breakpoint of a large deletion causing hereditary persistence of fetal hemoglobin occurs within an erythroid DNA domain remote from the β-globin gene cluster. Blood 1989;74:2178.
402. Fritsch EF, Lawn RM, Maniatis T. Characterization of deletions which affect the expression of fetal globin genes in man. Nature 1979;279:598.
403. Tuan D, Feingold E, Newman M, et al. Different 3′-end points of deletions causing $\delta\beta$-thalassemia and hereditary persistence of fetal hemoglobin: implications for the control of γ-globin gene expression in man. Proc Natl Acad Sci USA 1983;80:6937.
404. Tuan D, Murnane MJ, de Riel JK, et al. Heterogeneity in the molecular basis of hereditary persistence of fetal hemoglobin. Nature 1980;285:335.
405. Henthorn PS, Smithies O, Mager DL. Molecular analysis of deletions in the human β-globin cluster: deletion junctions and locations of breakpoints. Genomics 1990;6:226.
406. Henthorn PS, Mager DL, Huisman THJ, et al. A gene deletion ending with a complex array of repeated sequences 3′ to the human β-globin gene cluster. Proc Natl Acad Sci USA 1986;83:5194.
407. Kutlar A, Gardiner MB, Headlee MG, et al. Heterogeneity in the molecular basis of three types of hereditary persistence of fetal hemoglobin and the relative synthesis of the $^G\gamma$ and $^A\gamma$ types of γ chain. Biochem Genet 1984;22:21.
408. Wainscoat JS, Old JM, Wood WG, et al. Characterization of an Indian $(\delta\beta)^0$ thalassemia. Br J Haematol 1984;58:353.
409. Saglio G, Camaschella C, Serra A, et al. Italian type of deletional hereditary persistence of fetal hemoglobin. Blood 1986;68:646.
410. Camaschella C, Serra A, Gottardi E, et al. A new hereditary persistence of fetal hemoglobin deletion has a breakpoint within the 3′ β-globin gene enhancer. Blood 1990;75:1000.
411. Elder JT, Forrester WC, Thompson C, et al. Translocation of an erythroid-specific hypersensitive site in deletion-type hereditary persistence of fetal hemoglobin. Mol Cell Biol 1990;10:1382.
412. Ottolenghi S, Giglioni B. The deletion in a type of $\delta\beta$ thalassemia begins in an inverted Alu I repeat. Nature 1982;300:770.
413. Camaschella C, Serra A, Saglio G, et al. The 3′ end of the deletions of Spanish $(\delta\beta)^0$-thalassemia and Black HPFH 1 and 2 lie within 17 kilobases. Blood 1987;70:593.
414. Anagnou NP, Perez-Stable C, Gelinas R, et al. Sequences located 3′ to the breakpoint of HPFH-3 can modify the developmental expression of the $^A\gamma$ globin gene. (Abstract) Clin Res 1990;38:301A.
415. Mager DL, Henthorn PS, Smithies O. A Chinese $^G\gamma^+(^A\gamma\delta\beta)^0$ thalassemia deletion: comparison to other deletions in the human β globin gene cluster and sequence analysis of the breakpoints. Nucleic Acids Res 1985;13:6559.
416. Anagnou NP, Papayannopoulou T, Nienhuis AW, et al. Molecular characterization of a novel form of $(^A\gamma\delta\beta)^0$-thalassemia deletion with a 3′ breakpoint close to those of HPFH-3 and HPFH-4: insights into a common regulatory mechanism. Nucleic Acids Res 1988;16:6057.
417. Fodde R, Losekoot M, Casula L, et al. Nucleotide sequence of the Belgian $^G\gamma^+(^A\gamma\delta\beta)^0$-thalassemia deletion breakpoint suggests a common mechanism for a number of such recombination events. Genomics 1990;8:732.
418. Cao A, Melis MA, Galanello T, et al. $\delta\beta$(F)-Thalassemia in Sardinia. J Med Genet 1982;19:184.
419. Guida S, Giglioni B, Comi P, et al. The β-globin gene in Sardinian $\delta\beta^0$-thalassemia carries a C→T nonsense mutation at codon 39. EMBO J 1984;3:785.
420. Pirastu M, Kan YW, Galanello R, Cao A. Multiple mutations produce $\delta\beta^0$ thalassemia in Sardinia. Science 1984;223:929.
421. Ottolenghi S, Giglioni B, Pulazzini A, et al. Sardinian $\delta\beta$-thalassemia: a further example of a C to T substitution at position −196 of the $^A\gamma$ globin gene promoter. Blood 1987;69:1058.
422. Atweh GF, Zhu D-E, Forget BG. A novel basis for $\delta\beta$-thalassemia in a Chinese family. Blood 1986;68:1108.
423. Atweh GF, Zhu X-X, Brickner HE, et al. The β-globin gene on the Chinese $\delta\beta$-thalassemia chromosome carries a promoter mutation. Blood 1988;70:1470.
424. Collins FS, Stoeckert CJ Jr, Serjeant GR, et al. $^G\gamma\beta^+$ Hereditary persistence of fetal hemoglobin: cosmid cloning and identification of a specific mutation 5′ to the $^G\gamma$ gene. Proc Natl Acad Sci USA 1984;81:4894.
425. Gilman JG, Mishima N, Wen XJ, et al. Upstream promoter mutation associated with modest elevation of fetal hemoglobin expression in human adults. Blood 1988;72:78.
426. Tate VE, Wood WG, Weatherall DJ. The British form of hereditary persistence of fetal hemoglobin results from a single base pair mutation adjacent to an S1 hypersensitive site 5′ to the $^A\gamma$ globin gene. Blood 1986;68:1389.
427. Giglioni B, Casini C, Mantovani R, et al. A molecular study of a family with Greek hereditary persistence of fetal hemoglobin and β-thalassemia. EMBO J 1984;3:2641.
428. Gelinas R, Bender M, Lotshaw C, et al. Chinese $^A\gamma$ fetal hemoglobin: C to T substitution at position −196 of the $^A\gamma$ gene promoter. Blood 1986;67:1777.
429. Costa FF, Zago MA, Cheng G, et al. The Brazilian type of nondeletional $^A\gamma$-fetal hemoglobin has a C to G substitution at nucleotide-195 of the $^A\gamma$-globin gene. Blood 1990;76:1896.
430. Sykes K, Kaufman R. A naturally occuring gamma globin gene mutation enhances SP1 binding activity. Mol Cell Biol 1989;10:95.
431. Ronchi A, Nicolis S, Santoro C, et al. Increased Sp1 binding mediates erythroid-specific overexpression of a mutated (HPFH) γ-globin promoter. Nucleic Acids Res 1989;24:10231.
432. Fischer K-D, Nowock, J. The T to C substitution at −198 of the $^A\gamma$-globin gene associated with the British form of HPFH generates overlapping recognition sites for two DNA-binding proteins. Nucleic Acids Res 1990;18:5685.
433. Gumucio D, Rood KL, Blanchard-McQuate KL, et al. Interaction of Sp1 with the human γ globin promoter: binding and transactivation of normal and mutant promoters. Blood 1991;78:1853.
434. Surrey S, Delgrosso K, Malladi P, Schwartz E. A single base change at position −175 in the 5′-flanking region of the $^G\gamma$-globin gene from a black with $^G\gamma\beta^+$-HPFH. Blood 1988;71:807.
435. Ottolenghi S, Nicolis S, Taramelli R, et al. Sardinian $^G\gamma$-HPFH: a T→C substitution in a conserved "octamer" sequence in the $^G\gamma$-globin promoter. Blood 1988;71:815.
436. Stoming TA, Stoming GS, Lanclos KD, Nute PE. An $^A\gamma$ type of nondeletional hereditary persistence of fetal hemoglboin with a T→C mutation at position −175 to the cap site of the $^A\gamma$ globin gene. Blood 1989;73:329.
437. Collins FS, Metherall JE, Yamakawa M, et al. A point mutation in the $^A\gamma$-globin gene promoter in Greek hereditary persistence of fetal haemoglobin. Nature 1985;313:325.
438. Gelinas R, Endlich B, Pfeiffer C, et al. G to A substitution in the distal CCAAT box of the $^A\gamma$-globin gene in Greek hereditary persistence of fetal haemoglobin. Nature 313:323.
439. Ottolenghi S, Camaschella C, Comi P, et al. A frequent $^A\gamma$-hereditary persistence of fetal hemoglobin in Northern Sardinia: its molecular basis and haematological phenotype in heterozygotes with β thalassemia. Hum Genet 1988;79:13.
440. Huang HJ, Stoming TA, Harris HF, et al. The Greek $^A\gamma\beta$-HPFH observed in a large black family. Am J Hematol 1987;25:401.
441. Gilman JF, Mishima N, Wen XJ, et al. Distal CCAAT box deletion in the $^A\gamma$ globin gene of two black adolescents with elevated fetal $^A\gamma$ globin. Nucleic Acids Res 1988;16:10635.
442. Zeng Y-T, Huang S-Z, Chen B, et al. Hereditary persistence of fetal hemoglobin or $(\delta\beta)^0$-thalassemia: three types observed in South Chinese families. Blood 1985;66:1430.
443. Fucharoen S, Shimizu K, Fukumaki Y. A novel C-T transition within the distal CCAAT motif of the Gγ-globin gene in the Japanese HPFH: implication of factor binding in elevated fetal globin expression. Nucleic Acids Res 1990;18:5245.
444. Oner R, Kutlar F, Gu L-H, Huisman THJ. The Georgia type of nondeletional hereditary persistence of fetal hemoglboin has a C→T mutation at nucleotide −114 of the $^A\gamma$-globin gene. Blood 1991;77:1124.
445. Gumucio DL, Rood KL, Gray TA, et al. Nuclear proteins that bind to the human γ-globin gene promoter: alterations in binding produced by point mutation associated with hereditary persistence of fetal hemoglobin. Mol Cell Biol 1988;8:5310.
446. Mantovani R, Malgaretti N, Nicolis S, et al. The effects of HPFH mutations in the human γ-globin promoter on binding of ubiquitous and erythroid-specific nuclear factors. Nucleic Acids Res 1988;16:7783.
447. Lloyd JA, Lee RF, Lingrel JB. Mutation in two regions upstream of the $^A\gamma$ globin gene canonical promoter affect gene expression. Nucleic Acids Res 1989;17:4339.
448. Superti-Furga G, Barberis A, Schaffner G, et al. The −117 mutation in Greek HPFH affects the binding of three nuclear factors to the CCAAT region of the γ-globin gene. EMBO J 1988;7:3099.
449. Mantovani R, Superti-Furga G, Gilman J, et al. The deletion of the distal CCAAT-box region of the $^A\gamma$-globin gene in black HPFH abolishes the binding of the erythroid specific protein NFE3 and of the CCAAT displacement protein. Nucleic Acids Res 1989;17:6681.
450. Old JM, Ayyub H, Wood WG, et al. Linkage analysis of non-deletion hereditary persistence of fetal hemoglobin. Science 1982;215:981.
451. Gianni AM, Bregni M, Cappellini MD, et al. A gene controlling fetal hemoglobin expression in adults is not linked to the non-α globin cluster. EMBO J 1983;2:921.

452. Miyoshi K, Kaneto Y, Kawai H, Huisman THJ. X-linked dominant control of F-cells in normal adult life. Blood 1988;72:1854.
453. Dover GJ, Smith KD, Chang YC, et al. Fetal hemoglobin levels in sickle cell disease and normal individuals are partially controlled by an X-linked gene located at Xp22.2. Blood 1992;80:816.
454. Stamatoyannopoulos G, Wood WF, Papayanopoulou T, et al. A new form of hereditary persistence of fetal hemoglobin in blacks and its association with sickle cell trait. Blood 1975;46:683.
455. Gelinas RE, Rixon M, Magis W, Stamatoyannopoulos G. γ Gene promoter and enhancer structure in Seattle variant of hereditary persistence of fetal hemoglobin. Blood 1988;71:1108.
456. Bouhassira EE, Rajagopal K, Ragusa A, et al. The enhancer-like sequence 3′ to the $^{A}\gamma$ gene is polymorphic in human populations. Blood 1989;73:1050.
457. Jensen M, Wirtz A, Walther J-U, et al. Hereditary persistence of fetal haemoglobin (HPFH) in conjunction with a chromosomal translocation involving the haemoglobin β locus. Br J Haematol 1984;56:87.
458. Altay C, Huisman TH, Schroeder WA. Another form of hereditary persistence of fetal hemoglobin (the Atlanta type)? Hemoglobin 1977;1:125.
459. Gilman JG, Huisman THJ. DNA sequence variation associated with elevated fetal $^{G}\gamma$ globin production. Blood 1985;66:783.
460. Pembrey ME, Wood WG, Weatherall DJ, et al. Fetal haemoglobin production and the sickle gene in the oases of eastern Saudi Arabia. Br J Haematol 1978;40:415.
461. Perrine RP, Pembrey ME, John P, et al. Natural history of sickle cell anaemia in Saudi Arabs: a study of 270 subjects. Ann Intern Med 1978;88:1.
462. Kar BC, Satapathy RK, Kulozik RK, et al. Sickle cell disease in Orissa state, India. Lancet 1986;2:1198.
463. Kulozik AE, Kar BC, Satapathy RK, et al. Fetal hemoglobin levels and β^{S} globin haplotypes in an Indian population with sickle cell disease. Blood 1987;69:1742.
464. Miller BA, Olivieri N, Salameh M, et al. Molecular analysis of the high-hemoglobin-F phenotype in Saudi Arabian sickle cell anemia. N Engl J Med 1987;316:244.
465. Nagel RL, Fabry ME, Pagnier J, et al. Hematologically and genetically distinct forms of sickle cell anemia in Africa: the Senegal Type and the Benin Type. N Engl J Med 1985;312:880.
466. Gilman JG, Kutlar F, Johnson ME, Huisman THJ. A G to A nucleotide substitution 161 base pairs 5′ of the $^{G}\gamma$ globin gene cap site (−161) in a high $^{G}\gamma$ non-anemic person. In: Stamatoyannoupoulos G, Nienhuis AW, eds. Developmental control of globin gene expression. New York, Alan R Liss, 1987:383.
467. Galacteros F, Garin DJ, Monplaisir N, et al. Two new cases of heterozygosity for hemoglobin Knossos $\alpha_2\beta_2$ 27 Ala→Ser detected in the French West Indies and Algeria. Hemoglobin 1984;8:215.
468. Oggiano L, Pirastu M, Moi P, Longinotti M, et al. Molecular characterization of a normal Hb A_2 β-thalassaemia determinant in a Sardinian family. Br J Haematol 1987;67:225.
469. Galanello R, Melis MA, Podda A, et al. Deletion δ-thalassemia: the 7.2 Kb deletion of Corfu $\delta\beta$-thalassemia in a non-β-thalassemia chromosome. Blood 1990;75:1747.
470. Loudianos G, Cao A, Pirastu M, et al. Molecular basis of the δ thalassemia in *cis* to hemoglobin Knossos variant. Blood 1991;77:2087.
471. Olds RJ, Sura T, Jackson B, et al. A novel δ^0 mutation in *cis* with Hb Knossos: a study of different genetic interactions in three Egyptian families. Br J Haematol 1991;78:430.
472. Losekoot M, Fodde R, Giordano PC, Bernini LF. A novel δ^0-thalassemia arising from a frameshift insertion, detected by direct sequencing of enzymatically amplified DNA. Hum Genet 1989;83:75.
473. Moi P, Paglietti E, Sanna A, et al. Delineation of the molecular basis of δ- and normal HbA_2 β-thalassemia. Blood 1988;72:530.
474. Trifillis P, Ioannou P, Schwartz E, Surrey S. Identification of four novel δ-globin gene mutations in Greek Cypriots using polymerase chain reation and automated fluorescence-based DNA sequence analysis. Blood 1991;78:3298.
475. Loudianos G, Murru S, Ristaldi MS, et al. A novel δ-thalassemia mutation A G→C substitution at codon 30 of the δ-globin gene in a person of southern Italian origin. Hum Mutat 1992;1:169.
476. Loudianos G, Murru S, Kanavakis E, et al. A new δ chain variant hemoglobin A2-Corfu or $\alpha_2\delta_2$ 116 Arg→Cys (G18), detected by δ-globin gene analysis in a Greek family. Hum Genet 1991;87:237.
477. Nakamura T, Takihara Y, Ohta Y, et al. A δ-globin gene derived from patients with homozygous δ^0-thalassemia functions normally on transient expression in heterologous cells. Blood 1987;70:809.
478. Matsuda M, Sakamoto N, Fukumaki Y. δ-Thalassemia caused by disruption of the site for an erythroid-specific transcription factor, GATA-1, in the δ-globin gene promoter. Blood 1992;80:1347.
479. Moi P, Loudianos G, Lavinha J, et al. δ-Thalassemia due to a mutation in an erythroid-specific binding protein sequence 3′ to the δ-globin gene. Blood 1992;79:512.
480. Martin SL, Vincent KA, Wilson AC. Rise and fall of the delta globin gene. J Mol Biol 1983;164:513.
481. Kimura A, Takagi Y. A frameshift addition causes silencing of the δ-globin gene in an old world monkey, an anubis. Nucleic Acids Res 1983;11:2541.
482. Jeffreys AJ, Barrie PA, Harris S, et al. Isolation and sequence analysis of a hybrid δ-globin pseudogene from the brown lemur. J Mol Biol 1982;156:487.
483. Nakatsuji T, Gardiner MB, Reese Al, et al. Gamma thalassemia resulting from the deletion of a γ-globin gene. Nucleic Acids Res 1983;11:4635.
484. Shimasaki S, Iuchi I. Diversity of human γ-globin gene loci including a quadruplicated arrangement. Blood 1986;67:784.
485. Hill AVS, Bowden DK, Weatherall DJ, Clegg JB. Chromosomes with one, two, three, and four fetal globin genes: molecular and hematologic analysis. Blood 1986;67:1611.
486. Four categories of γ-globin gene triplications: DNA sequence comparison of low $^{G}\gamma$ and high $^{G}\gamma$ triplications. Blood 1988;72:480.
487. Powers PA, Altay C, Huisman THJ, Smithies O. Two novel arrangements of the human fetal globin genes: $^{G}\gamma$-$^{G}\gamma$ and $^{A}\gamma$-$^{A}\gamma$. Nucleic Acids Res 1984;12:7023.
488. Tate VE, Hill AVS, Bowden DK, et al. A silent deletion in the β-globin gene cluster. Nucleic Acids Res 1986;14:4743.
489. Gilman JG, Johnson ME, Mishima N. Four base-pair DNA deletion in human $^{A}\gamma$ globin-gene promoter associated with low $^{A}\gamma$ expression in adults. Br J Haematol 1988;68:455.
490. Manca L, Cocco E, Gallisai D, et al. Diminished $^{A}\gamma^{T}$ fetal globin levels in Sardinian haplotype II β^0-thalassaemia patients are associated with a four base pair deletion in the $^{A}\gamma^{T}$. Br J Haematol 1991;78:105.
491. Coleman MB, Steinberg MN, Adams JG, III. A four-base deletion 5′ to the $^{A}\gamma$ globin gene is a common polymorphism. Blood 1991;78:2473.
492. Kazazian HH Jr, Boehm CD. Molecular basis and prenatal diagnosis of β-thalassemia. Blood 1988;72:1107.
493. Alter BP. Antenatal diagnosis. Ann NY Acad Sci 1990;612:237.
494. Boehm CD, Antonarakis SE, Phillips JA, III, et al. Prenatal diagnosis using DNA polymorphisms: report on 95 pregnancies at risk for sickle-cell disease or β-thalassemia. N Engl J Med 1983;308:1054.
495. Orkin S, Markham AF, Kazazian HH. Direct detection of the common Mediterranean β-thalassemia gene with synthetic DNA probes. J Clin Invest 1983;71:775.
496. Pirastu M, Kan YW, Cao A, et al. Prenatal diagnosis of β-thalassemia: detection of a single nucleotide mutation in DNA. N Engl J Med 1983;309:284.
497. Rosatelli C, Falchi AM, Tuveri T, et al. Prenatal diagnosis of beta-thalassaemia with the synthetic-oligomer technique. Lancet 1985;1:241.
498. Eisenstein BI. The polymerase chain reaction: a new method of using molecular genetics for medical diagnosis. N Engl J Med 1990;322:178.
499. Mullis KB. The unusual origin of the polymerase chain reaction. Scientific American 1990;263:56.
500. Saiki RK, Chang C-A, Levenson CH, et al. Diagnosis of sickle cell anemia and β-thalassemia with enzymatically amplified DNA and nonradioactive allele-specific oligonucleotide probes. N Engl J Med 1988;319:537.
501. Cai S-P, Chang CA, Zhang JZ, et al. Rapid prenatal diagnosis of β thalassemia using DNA amplification and nonradioactive probes. Blood 1989;73:372.
502. Cai S-P, Zhang J-Z, Huang D-H, et al. A simple approach to prenatal diagnosis of β-thalassemia in a geographic area where multiple mutations occur. Blood 1988;71:1357.
503. Chehab FF, Kan YW. Detection of specific DNA sequences by fluorescence amplification: a color complementation assay. Proc Natl Acad Sci USA 1989;86:9178.
504. Wu DY, Ugozzoli L, Pal BK, Wallace RB. Allele-specific enzymatic amplification of β-globin genomic DNA for diagnosis of sickle cell anemia. Proc Natl Acad Sci USA 1989;86:2757.
505. Saiki RK, Walsh SP, Levenson CH, et al. Genetic analysis of amplified DNA with immobilized sequence-specific oligonucleotide probes. Proc Natl Acad Sci USA 1989;86:6230.
506. Lindeman R, Hu SP, Volpato F, Trent RJ. Polymerase chain reaction (PCR) mutagenesis enabling rapid non-radioactive detection of common β-thalassaemia mutations in Mediterraneans. Br J Haematol 1991;78:100.
507. Change J-G, Chen P-H, Chiou S-S, et al. Rapid diagnosis of β-thalassemia mutation in Chinese by naturally and amplified created restriction sites. Blood 1992;80:2092.
508. Sutton M, Bouhassira EE, Nagel RL. Polymerase chain reaction amplification applied to the determination of β-like globin gene cluster haplotypes. Am J Hematol 1989;32:66.
509. Sallee D, Kazazian HH, Jr. Multiplex analysis of β-globin restriction site polymorphisms by PCR: a method for rapid haplotyping and identity exclusion. (Abstract) Am J Hum Genet 1989;45:A216.
510. Engelke DR, Hoener PA, Collins FS. Direct sequencing of enzymatically amplified human genomic DNA. Proc Natl Acad Sci USA 1988;85:544.
511. Myers RM, Maniatis T, Lerman LS. Detection and localization of single base changes by denaturing gradient gel electrophoresis. Methods Enzymol 1987;155:501
512. Myers RM, Lumelsky N, Lerman LS, Maniatis T. Detection of single base substitutions in total genomic DNA. Nature 1985;313:495.
513. Cai S-P, Kan YW. Identification of the multiple β-thalassemia mutations by denaturing gradient gel electrophoresis. J Clin Invest 1990;85:550.
514. Losekoot M, Fodde R, Harteveld CL, et al. Denaturing gradient gel electrophoresis and direct sequencing of PCR amplified genomic DNA: a rapid and reliable diagnostic approach to beta thalassaemia. Br J Haematol 1990;76:269.

515. Phillips JA, III, Scott AF, Kazazian HH, et al. Prenatal diagnosis of hemoglobinopathies by restriction endonuclease analysis: pregnancies at risk for sickle cell anemia and S-O^{Arab} disease. Johns Hopkins Med J 1979;145:57.
516. Embury SH, Scharf SJ, Saiki RK, et al. Rapid prenatal diagnosis of sickle cell anemia by a new method of DNA analysis. N Engl J Med 1987;316:656.
517. Chehab FF, Doherty M, Cai S, et al. Detection of sickle cell anaemia and thalassaemias. Nature 1987;329:293.
518. Wallace RB, Schold M, Johnson MJ, et al. Oligonucleotide directed mutagenesis of the human β-globin gene: a general method for producing specific point mutations in cloned DNA. Nucleic Acids Res 1981;9:3647.
519. Conner BJ, Reys AA, Morin C, et al. Detection of sickle cell β^S-globin allele by hybridization with synthetic oligonucleotides. Proc Natl Acad Sci USA 1983;80:278.
520. Cao A, Rosatelli MC, Leoni GB, et al. Antenatal diagnosis of β-thalassemia in Sardinia. Ann NY Acad Sci 1990;612:215.
521. Loukopoulos D, Hadji A, Papadakis M, et al. Prenatal diagnosis of thalassemia and of the sickle cell syndromes in Greece. Ann NY Acad Sci 1990;612:226.
522. Petrou M, Modell B, Darr A, et al. Antenatal diagnosis: how to deliver a comprehensive service in the United Kingdom. Ann NY Acad Sci 1990;612:251.
523. Temple GF, Dozy AM, Roy KL, Kan YW. Construction of a functional human suppressor tRNA gene: an approach to gene therapy for β-thalassaemia. Nature 1982;296:537.
524. Apperley JF, Williams DA. Gene therapy: current status and future directions. Br J Haematol 1990;75:148.
525. Karlsson S. Treatment of genetic defects in hematopoietic cell function by gene transfer. Blood 1991;78:2481.
526. Anderson WF. Human gene therapy. Science 1992;256:808.
527. Miller AD. Human gene therapy comes of age. Nature 1992;357:455.
528. Verma IM. Gene therapy. Scientific American 1990;263:63.
529. Nienhuis AW, McDonagh KT, Bodine DM. Gene transfer into hematopoietic stem cells. Cancer 1991;67:2700.
530. Mulligan RC. The basic science of gene therapy. Science 260:926.
531. Miller AD. Retrovirus packaging cells. Hum Genet Ther 1990;1:5.
532. Miller AD. Progress toward human gene therapy. Blood 1990;76:271.
533. Cornetta K. Safety aspects of gene therapy. Br J Haematol 1992;80:421.
534. Dzierzak EA, Papayannopoulou T, Mulligan RC. Lineage-specific expression of a human β-globin gene in murine bone marrow transplant recipients reconstitued with retrovirus-transduced stem cells. Nature 1988;331:35.
535. Bender MA, Gelinas RE, Miller AD. A majority of mice show long-term expression of a human β-globin gene after retrovirus transfer into hematopoietic stem cells. Mol Cell Biol 1989;9:1426.
536. Gelinas R, Novak U. Retroviral vectors for the β-globin gene that demonstrate improved titer and expression. Ann NY Acad Sci 1990;612:427.
537. Novak U, Harris EAS, Forrester W, et al. High level β-globin expression after retroviral transfer of locus activation region-containing human β-globin gene derivatives into murine erythroleukemia cells. Proc Natl Acad Sci USA 1990;87:3386.
538. Chang JC, Liu D, Kan YW. A 36-base-pair core sequence of the locus control region enhances retrovirally transferred β-globin gene expression. Proc Natl Acad Sci USA 1992;89:3107.
539. Plavec I, Papayannopoulou T, Maury C, and Meyer F. A human β-globin gene fused to the human β-globin locus control region is expressed at high levels in erythroid cells of mice engrafted with retrovirus-transduced hematopoietic stem cells. Blood 1993;81:1384.
540. Smithies O, Gregg RG, Boggs SS, et al. Insertion of DNA sequences into the human chromosomal β-globin locus by homologous recombination. Nature 1985;317:230.
541. Nandi AK, Roginski RS, Gregg RG, et al. Regulated expression of genes inserted at the human chromosomal β-globin locus by homologous recombination. Proc Natl Acad Sci USA 1988;85:3845.
542. Popovich BW, Kim H-S, Shesely EG, et al. Correction of the human sickle cell gene using targeted gene replacement. In: Stamatoyannopoulos G, Nienhuis AW, eds. The regulation of hemoglobin switching. Baltimore, Johns Hopkins University Press, 1991:526.
543. Bodine DM, Karlsson S, Nienhuis AW. Combination of interleukins 3 and 6 preserves stem cell function in culture and enhances retrovirus-mediated gene transfer into hematopoietic stem cells. Proc Natl Acad Sci USA 1989;86:8897.
544. Bodine DM, Crosier PS, Clark SC. Effects of hematopoietic growth factors on the survival of primitive stem cells in liquid suspension culture. Blood 1991;78:914.
545. Bodine DM, Orlic D, Birkett NC, et al. Stem cell factor increases CFU-S number *in vitro* in synergy with interleukin-6, and *in vivo* as a single factor. Blood 1992;79:913.
546. Toksoz D, Zsebo KM, Smith KA, et al. Support of human hematopoiesis in long-term bone marrow cultures by murine stromal cells selectively expressing the membrane-bound and secreted forms of the human homolog of the steel gene product, stem cell factor. Proc Natl Acad Sci USA 1992;89:7350.
547. Bodine DM, McDonagh KT, Brandt SJ, et al. Development of a high-titer retrovirus producer cell line capable of gene transfer into rhesus monkey hematopoietic stem cells. Proc Natl Acad Sci USA 1990;87:3738.
548. Bodine DM, McDonagh KT, Seidel NE, and Nienhuis AW. Retrovirus mediated gene transfer to pluripotent hematopoietic stem cells. In: Stamatoyannopoulos G, Nienhuis AW, eds. The regulation of hemoglobin switching. Baltimore, Johns Hopkins University Press, 1991;505–525.
549. van Beusechem VW, Kukler A, Heidt PJ, Valerio D. Long-term expression of human adenosine deaminase in rhesus monkeys transplanted with retrovirus-infected bone-marrow cells. Proc Natl Acad Sci USA 1992;89:7640.
550. Moritz T, Luskey B, Kessler S, et al. Expression of the adenosine deaminase (ADA) gene after transduction into rhesus monkey repopulating stem cells. (Abstract) Blood 1992;80(Suppl 1):72a.
551. DeSimone J, Heller P, Hall L, Zwiers D. 5-Azacytidine stimulates fetal hemoglobin synthesis in anemic baboons. Proc Natl Acad Sci USA 1982;79:4418.
552. Ley TJ, DeSimone J, Anagnou NP, et al. 5-Azacytidine selectively increased γ-globin synthesis in a patient with β+ thalassemia. N Engl J Med 1982;307:1469.
553. Charache S, Dover G, Smith K, et al. Treatment of sickle cell anemia with 5-azacytidine results in increased fetal hemoglobin production and is associated with nonrandom hypomethylation of DNA around the $\gamma\delta\beta$-globin gene complex. Proc Natl Acad Sci USA 1983; 80:4842.
554. Ley TJ, DeSimone J, Noguchi CT, et al. 5-Azacytidine increases γ-globin synthesis and reduces the proportion of dense cells in patients with sickle cell anemia. Blood 1976;62:370.
555. Dunbar C, Travis W, Kan YW, Nienhuis A. 5-Azacytidine treatment in a β^0-thalassaemic patient unable to be transfused due to multiple alloantibodies. Br J Haematol 1989;72:467.
556. Lowrey CH, Nienhuis A. Pharmacologic manipulation of globin gene expression with 5-azacytidine has produced long term therapeutic benefits in two patients with β-thalassemia. (Abstract) Blood 1991;78 (Suppl 1):368a.
557. Torrealba-de Ron AT, Papayannopoulou T, Knapp MS, et al. Perturbations in the erythroid marrow progenitor cell pools may play a role in the augmentation of Hb F by 5-azacytidine. Blood 1984;63:201.
558. Humphries RK, Dover G, Young NS, et al. 5-Azacytidine acts directly on both erythroid precursors and progenitors to increase production of fetal hemoglobin. J Clin Invest 1985;75:547.
559. Lavelle D, DeSimone J, Heller P, et al. On the mechanism of Hb F elevations in the baboon by erythropoietic stress and pharmacologic manipulation. Blood 1986;67:1083.
560. Galanello R, Stamatoyannopoulos G, Papayannopoulou T, et al. Mechanism of Hb F stimulation by S-stage compounds. J Clin Invest 1988;81:1209.
561. Dover GJ, Charache SC, Brusilow SW. Sodium phenylbutyrate increases fetal hemoglobin production in patients with sickle cell disease. (Abstract) Blood 1992;80(Suppl 1):73a.
562. Olivieri NF, Costin D, Dover G, et al. γGlobin expression induced by butyrate and an oral derivative can ameliorate a thalassemic phenotype. (Abstract) Blood 1992;80(Suppl 1):343a.
563. Kaufman RE. Hydroxyurea: specific therapy for sickle cell anemia? Blood 1992;79:2503.
564. Rodgers GP, Dover GJ, Uyesaka N, et al. Augmentation by erythropoietin of the fetal-hemoglobin response to hydroxyurea in sickle cell disease. N Engl J Med 1993;328:73.
565. Bunn HF. Reversing ontogeny. N Engl J Med 1993;328:129.
566. Stamatoyannopoulos G, Veith R, Al-Khatti A, Papayannopoulou T. Induction of fetal hemoglobin by cell-cycle–specific drugs and recombinant erythropoietin. Am J Pediatr Hematol Oncol 1990;12:21.
567. Cooley, TB, Witwer ER, Lee P. Anemia in children with splenomegaly and peculiar changes in bones: report of cases. Am J Dis Child 1927;34:347.
568. Nathan DG. Thalassemia. N Engl J Med 1972;286:586.
569. Pearson, HA, McFarland W, King ER. Erythrokinetic studies in thalassemia trait. J Lab Clin Med 1960;56:866.
570. Silvestroni E, Bianco I. A highly cost effective method of mass screening for thalassemia. Br Med J 1983;286:1007.
571. Pearson HA, Motoyama E, Genel M, et al. Intraerythrocytic adaptation (2,3 DPG, P50) in thalassemia minor. Blood 1977;49:463.
572. Hedge UM, Khunda S, Marsh GW, et al. Thalassemia, iron, and pregnancy. Br Med J 1975;3:509.
573. Hocking IW, Ibbotson RN. The effect of beta thalassemia trait on pregnancy with particular reference to its complications and outcome. Med J Aust 1966;2:397.
574. Friedman S, Ozsoylu S, Luddy R, Schwartz E. Heterozygous beta thalassemia of unusual severity. Br J Haematol 1976;32:65.
575. Weatherall DJ. Biochemical phenotypes of thalassemia in the American Negro population. Ann NY Acad Sci 1964;119:450.
576. Kazazian HH Jr. The thalassemia syndromes: molecular basis and prenatal diagnosis in 1990. Semin Hematol 1990;27:209.
577. Gerald PS, Diamond LK. The diagnosis of thalassemia by starch block electrophoresis of the hemoglobin. Blood 1958;13:61.
578. Berman BW, Ritchey AK, Jeckel JF, et al. Hematology of β thalassemia trait: age-related developmental aspects and intra-familial correlations. J Pediatr 1980;97:901.

579. Wasi P, Disthasongchan P, Na-Nakorn S. The effect of iron deficiency on the levels of hemoglobins A_2 and E. J Lab Clin Med 1968;71:85.
580. Shepard MK, Weatherall DJ, Conley CL. Semi-quantitative estimation of the distribution of fetal hemoglobin in red cell populations. Johns Hopkins Med J 1962;110:293.
581. Cao A, Furbetta M, Galanello R, et al. Prevention of homozygous β-thalassemia by carrier screening and prenatal diagnosis in Sardinia. Am J Hum Genet 1981;33:592.
582. Cao A, Rosatelli C, Galanello R, et al. The prevention of thalassemia in Sardinia. Clin Genet 1989;36:277.
583. Alter BP. Antenatal diagnosis of thalassemia: a review. Ann NY Acad Sci 1985;445:393.
584. Modell B, Petrou M, Ward RHT, et al. Effect of fetal diagnostic testing on birth rate of thalassemia major in Britain. Lancet 1984;2:1383.
585. Pearson HA, Guiliotis DK, Rink L, Wells JA. Patient age distribution in thalassemia major: changes from 1973 to 1985. Pediatrics 1987;80:53.
586. Pearson HA, O'Brien RT, McIntosh S. Screening for thalassemia trait by electronic measurement of mean corpuscular volume. N Engl J Med 1973;288:351.
587. Bessman JD, Gilmer PR Jr, Gardner FH. Improved classification of anemias by MCV and RDW. Am J Clin Pathol 1983;80:322.
588. Stockman JA III, Weiner LS, Simon GE, et al. The measurement of free erythrocyte porphyrin (FEP) as a simple means of distinguishing iron deficiency from beta-thalassemia trait in subjects with microcytosis. J Lab Clin Med 1975;85:113.
589. England JM, Fraser PM. Differentiation of iron deficiency from thalassemia trait by routine blood-count. Lancet 1973;1:449.
590. Mentzer WC. Differentiation of iron deficiency from thalassemia trait. Lancet 1973;1:882.
591. Ottolenghi S, Comi P, Giglioni B. δβ-thalassemia is due to a gene deletion. Cell 1976;9:71.
592. Trent RJ, Svirklys L, Jones P. Thai $(\delta\beta)^0$-thalassemia and its interactions with γ-thalassemia. Hemoglobin 1988;12:101.
593. Gerald PS, Efron ML, Diamond LK. A human mutation (the Lepore hemoglobinopathy) possibly involving two "cistrons." Am J Dis Child 1961;102:514.
594. Baglioni C. The fusion of two peptide chains in hemoglobin Lepore and its interpretation as a genetic deletion. Proc Natl Acad Sci USA 1962;48:1880.
595. Baird M, Schreiner H, Driscoll C, Bank A. Localization of the site of recombination in formation of the Lepore Boston globin gene. J Clin Invest 1981;68:560.
596. Duma H, Efremov G, Sadikario A, et al. Study of nine families with hemoglobin-Lepore. Br J Haematol 1968;15:161.
597. Pearson HA, Gerald PS, Diamond LK. Thalassemia intermedia due to interaction of Lepore trait with thalassemia trait. Am J Dis Child 1959;97:464.
598. Kendall AG, Ojwang PJ, Schroeder WA, et al. Hemoglobin Kenya, the product of a gamma-beta fusion gene: studies of the family. Am J Hum Genet 1973;25:548.
599. Pearson HA. Alpha-beta thalassemia disease in a Negro family. N Engl J Med 1966;275:176.
600. Kan YW, Nathan DG. Mild thalassemia: the result of interaction of alpha and beta thalassemia genes. J Clin Invest 1970;49:635.
601. Pearson HA. Thalassemia intermedia: genetic and biochemical considerations. Ann NY Acad Sci 1964;119:390.
602. Rogers GP, Diver G, Uyesaka N, et al. Augmentation by erythropoietin of the fetal hemoglobin response to hydroxyurea in sickle cell disease. N Engl J Med 1993;328:73.
603. Perrine SP, Gorder GD, Faller DV, et al. A short-term trial of butyrate to stimulate fetal-globin-gene expression in the β-globin disordera. N Engl J Med 1993;328:81.
604. Modell B, Bedoukas V. The clinical approach to thalassemia. Orlando, Grune & Stratton, 1984.
605. Fosburg MT, Nathan DG. Treatment of Cooley's anemia. Blood 1990;76:435.
606. Alter BP. Prenatal diagnosis of hemoglobinopathies. Lancet 1981;2:1152.
607. Gaburro D, Valpato, Vigi V. Diagnosis of β thalassemia in the newborn by means of haemoglobin synthesis. Acta Paediatr Scand 1970;59:523.
608. Cossu G, Manca M, Pirastru MG, et al. Neonatal screening of beta-thalassemias by thin layer isoelectric focusing. Am J Hematol 1982;13:149.
609. Logothetis J, Constantoulakis M, Economidou J, et al. Thalassemia major (homozygous beta-thalassemia): a survey of 138 cases with emphasis on neurologic and muscular aspects. Neurology 1972;22:294.
610. Baty JM, Blackfan KD, Diamond LK. Blood studies in infants and children. I. Erythroblastic anemia: a clinical and pathologic study. Am J Dis Child 1932;43:667.
611. Silvestroni E, Bianco I. Screening for microcythemia in Italy: analysis of data collected in the past 30 years. Am J Hum Genet 1975;27:198.
612. Fessas P. Inclusions of hemoglobin in erythroblasts and erythrocytes of thalassemia. Blood 1963;21:21.
613. Fessas P, Loukopoulos D, Kaltsoya A. Peptide analysis of the inclusions of erythroid cells in β-thalassemia. Biochem Biophys Acta 1966;124:430.
614. Nathan DG, Stossel TB, Gunn RB, et al. Influence of hemoglobin precipitation on erythrocyte metabolism in alpha and beta thalassemia. J Clin Invest 1969;48:33.
615. Nathan DG, Gunn RB. Thalassemia: the consequences of unbalanced hemoglobin synthesis. Am J Med 1966;41:815.
616. Smith CH, Sisson TRC, Floyd WH Jr, Siegal S. Serum iron and iron-binding capacity of serum in children with severe Mediterranean (Cooley's) anemia. Pediatrics 1950;5:799.
617. Giblett ER, Crookston MC. Agglutinability of red cells by anti-i in patients with thalassemia major and other haematological disorders. Nature 1964;201:1138.
618. Sturgeon P, Finch CA. Erythrokinetics in Cooley's anemia. Blood 1957;12:64.
619. Arcasoy A, Cavdar AO. Changes of trace metals (serum iron, zinc, copper, and magnesium) in thalassemia. Acta Haematol 1975;53:341.
620. Prasad AS, Diwany M, Gabr M, et al. Biochemical studies in thalassemia. Ann Intern Med 1965;62:87.
621. Cohen A, Cohen IJ, Schwartz E. Scurvy and altered iron stores in thalassemia major. N Eng J Med 1981;304:158.
622. O'Brien RT. Ascorbic acid enhancement of desferrioxamine-induced urinary iron excretion in thalassemia major. Ann NY Acad Sci 1974;232:221.
623. Jandl JH, Greenberg MS. Bone-marrow failue due to relative nutritional deficiency in Cooley's hemolytic anemia: painful "erythropoietic crises" in response to folic acid. N Engl J Med 1959;260:461.
624. Luhby AJ, Cooperman JM, Feldman R, et al. Folic-acid deficiency as a limiting factor in the anemia of thalassemia major. Blood 1961;18:786.
625. Miniero R, Piga A, Luzzatto L, Gabutti V. Vitamin E and β thalassemia. Haematologica 1983;68:562.
626. Hyman CB, Landing B, Alfin-Slater R, et al. D1-α-Tocopherol, iron and lipofuscin in thalassemia. Ann NY Acad Sci 1974;232:211.
627. Hilgartner MW, Smith CH. Coagulation studies as a measure of liver function in Cooley's anemia. Ann NY Acad Sci 1964;119:631.
628. Stuart MJ. Platelet dysfunction in homozygous beta-thalassemia. Pediatr Res 1979;13:1345.
629. Caffey J. Cooley's anemia: a review of the roentgenographic findings in the skeleton. AJR 1957;78:381.
630. Lawson JP, Ablow RC, Pearson HA. The ribs in thalassemia. I. The relationship to therapy. Radiology 1981;140:663.
631. Lawson JP, Ablow RC, Pearson HA. The ribs in thalassemia. II. The pathogenesis of the changes. Radiology 1981;140:673.
632. Dandona P, Menon RK, Houlder S, et al. Serum 1,25 dihydroxy-vitamin D and osteocalcin concentrations in thalassemia. Arch Dis Child 1987;62:474.
633. Rioja L, Girot, R, Garabedian M, Cournot-Witmer G. Bone disease in children with homozygous beta-thalassemia. Bone Miner 1990;8:69.
634. Lawson JP, Ablow RC, Pearson HA. Calvarial and phalangeal vascular impressions in thalassemia. AJR 1984;143:641.
635. Currarino G, Erlandson ME. Premature fusion of epiphyses in Cooley's anemia. Radiology 1964;63:656.
636. Lawson JP, Ablow RC, Pearson HA. Premature fusion of the proximal humeral epiphyses in thalassemia. AJR 1983;140:239.
637. Sorsdahl OS, Taylor PE, Noyes WD. Extramedullary hematopoiesis, mediastinal masses, and spinal cord compression. JAMA 1964;189:343.
638. Editorial. Spinal cord compression in thalassemia. Lancet 1982;1:664.
639. Issaragrisil HC, Piankigagum A, Wasi P. Spinal cord compression in thalassemia: report of 12 cases and recommendations for treatment. Arch Intern Med 1981;141:1033.
640. O'Brien RT, Pearson HA, Spencer RP. Transfusion induced decrease in spleen size in thalassemia major. J Pediatr 1972;81:105.
641. Barry M, Flynn DM, Letsky EA, Risdon RA. Long-term chelation therapy in thalassemia major: effect on iron concentration, liver histology and clincal progress. Br Med J 1974;2:16.
642. Ellis JT, Schulman I, Smith CH. Generalized siderosis with fibrosis of liver and pancreas in Cooley's (Mediterranean) anemia with observations on the pathogenesis of the siderosis and fibrosis. Am J Pathol 1954;30:287.
643. Fink H. Transfusion hemochromatosis in Cooley's anemia. Ann NY Acad Sci 1964;119:680.
644. De Virgelius S, Forelli G, Fargion S, et al. Chronic liver disease in transfusion-dependent thalassemia: hepatitis B virus marker studies. J Clin Pathol 1980;33:949.
645. Pearson HA, Wood C, Andiman W, et al. Low risk of hepatitis B from blood transfusions in thalassemic patients in Connecticut. J Pediatr 1986;108:252.
646. Engle MA. Cardiac involvement in Cooley's anemia. Ann NY Acad Sci 1964;119:694.
647. Engle MA, Erlandson M, Smith CH. Late cardiac complications of chronic, severe, refractory anemia with hemochromatosis. Circulation 1964;30:698.
648. Nienhuis AW, Griffith P, Strawczynski H. Evaluation of cardiac function in patients with thalassemia major. Ann NY Acad Sci 1980;344:384.
649. Leon MB, Borer JS, Bacharach SL. Detection of early cardiac dysfunction in patients with severe beta-thalassemia and chronic iron overload. N Engl J Med 1979;301:1143.
650. Stanfield JB. Acute benign pericarditis in thalassemia major. Proc R Soc Med 1962;55:236.

651. Grossman H, Dische MR, Winchester PH, Canale V. Renal enlargement in thalassemia major. Radiology 1971;100:645.
652. Kreimer-Birnbaum M, Pinkerton PH, Bannerman RM, Hutchison HE. Urinary "dipyrroles": their occurrence and significance in thalassemia and other disorders. Blood 1966;28:993.
653. Johnston FE, Krogman WM. Patterns of growth in children with Cooley's anemia. Ann NY Acad Sci 1964;119:667.
654. Canale VC, Steinherz P, New M, Erlandson M. Endocrine function in thalassemia major. Ann NY Acad Sci 1974;232:333.
655. Pintor C, Cella SG, Manso P, et al. Impaired growth hormone (GH) response to GH-releasing hormone in thalassemia major. J Clin Endocrinol Metab 1986;62:263.
656. Lassman MN, O'Brien RT, Pearson HA, et al. Endocrine function in thalassemia major. Ann NY Acad Sci 1974;232:226.
657. Saenger D, Schwartz E, Markenson AL, et al. Depressed serum somatomedin activity in beta-thalassemia. J Pediatr 1980;96:214.
658. De Sanctis V, Vullo C, Katz M, et al. Hypothalamic-pituitary-gonadal axis in thalassemic patients with secondary amenorrhea. Obstet Gynecol 1988;72:643.
659. Wang C, Tso SC, Todd, D. Hypogonadotropic hypogonadism in severe β thalassemia: effect of chelation and gonadotropin-releasing hormone therapy. J Clin Endocrinol Metab 1989;68:511.
660. Mordel N, Birkenfeld A, Goldfarb AN, Rachmilewitz EA. Successful full-term pregnancy in homozygous β thalassemia major: case report and review of literature. Obstet Gynecol 1989;73:837.
661. Zuppinger K, Molinari B, Hirt A, et al. Increased risk of diabetes mellitus in beta-thalassemia major due to iron overload. Helv Paediatr Acta 1979;34:197.
662. Merkel PA, Simonson DC, Amiel SA, et al. Insulin resistance and hyperinsulinemia in patients with thalassemia major treated by hypertransfusion. N Engl J Med 1988;318:809.
663. Jones TW, Boulware SD, Caprio S, et al. Correction of hyperinsulinemia by glyburide treatment in non-diabetic patients with thalassemia major. Pediatr Res 1993;33:497.
664. Spitz IM, Hirsch HJ, Landau H, et al. TSH secretion in thalassemia. J Endocrinol Invest 1984;7:495.
665. Gertner JM, Broadus AE, Anast CS, et al. Impaired parathyroid response to induced hypocalcemia in thalassemia major. J Pediatr 1979;95:210.
666. Singer DB. Postsplenectomy sepsis. Perspect Pediatr Pathol 1973;1:285.
667. Smith CH, Erlandson ME, Stern G, Hilgartner MW. Postsplenectomy infection in Cooley's anemia: an appraisal of the problem in this and other blood disorders with a consideration of prophylaxis. N Engl J Med 1962;266:737.
668. Pearson HA. The spleen and disturbances of splenic function. In: Nathan DG, Oski FA, eds. Hematology of infancy and childhood. Philadelphia, WB Saunders, 1992.
669. McCracken EH, Dickerman JD. Septicemia and disseminated intravascular coagulation: occurrence in four asplenic children. Am J Dis Child 1969;118:431.
670. Gaston MH, Verter JI, Woods G, et al. Prophylaxis with oral penicillin in children with sickle cell anemia: a randomized trial. N Engl J Med 1986;314:1593.
671. Kafidi KT, Rotschafer JC. Bacterial vaccines for splenectomized patients. Drug Intell Clin Pharmacol 1988;22:192.
672. Roche G, Leheup B, Gerard A, et al. Septicemias a *Yersinia enterocolitica:* revue generale. Rev Med Intern 1982;3:65.
673. Katz BZ. Vibrio vulnificus meningitis in a boy with thalassemia after eating raw oysters. Pediatrics 1988;82:784.
674. Logothetis J, Constantoulakis M, Economidou J, et al. Thalassemia major (homozygous beta thalassemia): a survey of 138 cases with emphasis on neurologic and muscular aspects. Neurology 1972;22:294.
675. Pearson HA, O'Brien RT. The management of thalassemia major. Semin Hematol 1975;12:255.
676. Wolman IJ. Transfusion therapy in Cooley's anemia: growth and health as related to long-range hemoglobin levels: a progress report. Ann NY Acad Sci 1964;119:736.
677. Necheles TF, Chung S, Sabbah R, Whitten D. Intensive transfusion therapy in thalassemia major: an eight-year follow-up. Ann NY Acad Sci 1974;232:179.
678. Kattamis C, Touliatos N, Haidas S, Matsaniotis N. Growth of children with thalassemia: effect of different transfusion regimens. Arch Dis Child 1970;45:502.
679. O'Brien RT, Pearson HA, Spencer RP. Transfusion-induced decrease in spleen size in thalassemia major. J Pediatr 1972;81:105.
680. Piomelli S, Danoff SJ, Becker MH, et al. Prevention of bone malformation and cardiomegaly in Cooley's anemia by early transfusion regimen. Ann NY Acad Sci 1969;165:427.
681. Piomelli S, Karpatkin MH, Arzanian M, et al. Hypertransfusion regimen in patients with Cooley's anemia. Ann NY Acad Sci 1974;232:186.
682. Lawson JP, Ablow RC, Pearson HA. The ribs in thalassemia. I. The relationship to therapy. Radiology 1981;140:663.
683. Gabutti V, Piga A, Nicola P, et al. Hemoglobin levels and blood requirement in thalassemia. Arch Dis Child 1982;57:156.
684. Propper RD, Button LN, Nathan DG. New approaches to the transfusion management of thalassemia. Blood 1980;55:55.
685. Giardina PJ, Hilgartner MW. Update on thalassemia. Pediatr Rev 1992;13:55.
686. Corash L, Klein H, Deisseroth A, et al. Selective isolation of young erythrocytes for transfusion support of thalassemia major patients. Blood 1981;57:599.
687. Cohen AR, Schmidt JM, Martin MB, et al. Clinical trial of young red cell transfusions. J Pediatr 1984;104:865.
688. Propper RD. Neocytes and neocyte gerocyte exchange. Prog Clin Biol Res 1982;88:227.
689. Coles SM, Klein HG, Holland PV. Alloimmunization in two multitransfusion patient populations. Transfusion 1981;21:462.
690. Cividalli G, Sandler SG, Yatziv S, et al. β^0 Thalassemia complicated by autoimmune hemolytic anemia. Globin synthesis during immunosuppressive therapy. Acta Haematol 1980;63:37.
691. Kruatrachue M, Sirisinha S, Pacharee P, et al. An association between thalassemia and autoimmune hemolytic anemia (AIHA). Scand J Haematol 1980;25:259.
692. Constantopoulos A, Matsaniotis N. Hypertension, convulsion, and cerebral hemorrhage in thalassemia patients after multiple blood transfusion. Helv Paediatr Acta 1980;35:269.
693. Moroni GA, Piacentini G, Terzoli S, et al. Hepatitis B and non-A, non-B virus infection in multitransfused thalassemic patients. Arch Dis Child 1984;59:1127.
694. Pearson HA, Wood C, Andiman W, et al. Low risk of hepatitis B from blood transfusion in thalassemia patients in Connecticut. J Pediatr 1986;108:252.
695. Hilgartner MW. Personal communication, 1992.
696. Constantoulakis M, Economidou J, Karagiorga M, et al. Combined long-term treatment of hemosiderosis desferrioxamine and DTPA in homozygous thalassemia. Ann NY Acad Sci 1974;232:193.
697. Modell B, Beck J. Long-term desferrioxamine therapy in thalassemia. Ann NY Acad Sci 1974;232:201.
698. Finch CA, Huebers H. Perspectives in iron metabolism. N Engl J Med 1982;306:1520.
699. Brittenham GM. Development of iron-chelating agents for clinical use. Blood 1992;80:569.
700. Smith RS. Iron excretion in thalassemia major after administration of chelating agents. Br Med J 1962;2:1577.
701. Keberle H. The biochemistry of desferroxamine and its relation to iron metabolism. Ann NY Acad Sci 1964;119:758.
702. Barry M, Flynn DM, Letsky EA, Risdon RA. Long-term chelation therapy in thalassemia major: effect on liver iron concentration, liver histology and clinical progress. Br Med J 1975;2:16.
703. Modell B, Letsky EA, Flynn DM, et al. Survival and desferrioxamine in thalassemia major. Br Med J 1982;2:1081.
704. Giardina PJ, Grady RW, Ehlers JM, et al. Chelation therapy in Cooley's anemia: a decade of experience with subcutaneous desferrioxamine. Ann NY Acad Sci 1990;612:275.
705. Seshadri R, Colebatch JH, Gordon P, Ekert H. Long-term administration of desferrioxamine in thalassemia major. Arch Dis Child 1974;49:621.
706. Propper RD, Shurin SB, Nathan DG. Reassessment of the use of desferrioxamine B in iron overload. N Engl J Med 1976;294:1421.
707. Propper RD, Cooper B, Rufo RR, et al. Continuous subcutaneous administration of desferrioxamine in patients with iron overload. N Engl J Med 1977;297:418.
708. Wolfe L, Olivieri N, Sallan D, et al. Prevention of cardiac disease by subcutaneous deferoxamine in patients with thalassemia major. N Engl J Med 1985;312:1600.
709. Freeman AP, Giles RW, Berdoukas VA, et al. Sustained normalization of cardiac function by chelation therapy in thalassemia major. Clin Lab Haematol 1989;11:299.
710. Borgna-Pignatti C, De Stefano P, Zonta L, et al. Growth and sexual maturation in thalassemia major. J Pediatr 1985;106:150.
711. Bronspiegel-Weintrob N, Olivieri NF, Tyler B, et al. Effect of age at the start of iron chelation therapy on gonadal function in β-thalassemia major. N Engl J Med 1990;323:713.
712. Modell B, Letsky EA, Flynn DM, et al. Survival and desferrioxamine in thalassemia major. Br Med J 1982;284:1081.
713. Zurlo MG, De Stefano P, Borgna-Pignatti C, et al. Survival and causes of death in thalassemia major. Lancet 1989;2:27.
714. O'Brien RT. Ascorbic acid enhancement of desferrioxamine-induced urinary iron excretion in thalassemia major. Ann NY Acad Sci 1974;232: 221.
715. Porter JB, Huehns ER. The toxic effects of desferrioxamine. Baillieres Clin Haematol 1989;2:459.
716. Olivieri NF, Buncie JF, Chew E, et al. Visual and auditory neurotoxicity in patients receiving subcutaneous deferoxamine therapy. N Engl J Med 1986;314:869.
717. Freedman MH, Grisaru D, Olivieri N, et al. Pulmonary syndrome in patients with thalassemia major receiving intravenous desferrioxamine infusions. Am J Dis Child 1990;144:565.
718. Olivieri NF, Koren G, Harris J, et al. Growth failure and bony changes induced by deferoxamine. Am J Pediatr Hematol Oncol 1992;14:48.
719. Third NIH Sponsored Symposium on the Development of Iron Chelation for Clinical Use. University of Florida, Gainesville, May 20–22, 1992.
720. al-Refaie FN, Wonke B, Hoffbrand AV, et al. Efficacy and possible adverse effects of the oral iron chelator 1,2-dimethyl-3-hydroxypyrid-4-one (L1) in thalassemia major. Blood 1992;80:593.
721. Bartlett AN, Hoffbrand AV, Kontoghiorghes GJ. Long-term trial with the oral iron chelator 1,2-dimethyl-3-hydroxypyrid-4-one. Br J Haematol 1990;76:301.

722. Olivieri NF, Koren G, Klein J, et al. Oral iron chelation with 1,2-dimethyl-3-hydroxypyrid-4-one (L1) in thalassemia major (TM): pharmokinetics, safety, and iron excretion. (Abstract) Blood 1990;76(Suppl 1):72a.
723. Kontoghiorghes GJ, Bartlett AN, Hoffbrand AV, et al. Long-term trial with the oral iron chelator 1,2-dimethyl-3-hydroxypyrid-4-one. I. Iron chelation and metabolic studies. Br J Haematol 1990;76:295.
724. Olivieri NF, Koren G, Matsui D, et al. Reduction of tissue iron stores and normalization of serum ferritin during treatment with the oral iron chelator L1 in thalassemia intermedia. Blood 1992;79: 2741.
725. Thomas ED, Buckner CD, Sanders JE, et al. Marrow transplantation for thalassemia. Lancet 1982;2:227.
726. Lucarelli G, Polchi P, Galimberti M, et al. Marrow transplantation for thalassemia following busulphan and cyclophosphamide. Lancet 1985;1:1355.
727. Lucarelli G, Galimberti M, Polchi P, et al. Bone marrow transplantation in patients with thalassemia. N Engl J Med 1990;322:417.
728. Lucarelli G, Weatherall DJ. For debate: (1) Bone marrow transplantation for severe thalassemia; (2) to be or not to be. Br J Haematol 1991;78: 300.
729. Weatherall DJ. Bone marrow transplantation for thalassemia and other inherited disorders of hemoglobin. Blood 1992;80:1379.
730. Lucarelli G, Galimberti M, Polchi P, et al. Bone marrow transplantation in adult thalassemia. Blood 1992;80:1603.
731. Dozy AM, Kan YW, Embury SH, et al. α-Globin gene organization in blacks precludes the severe form of α thalassemia. Nature 1979;280: 605.
732. Kanavakis E, Tzotzos S, Lipaki A, et al. Frequency of alpha thalassemia in Greece. Am J Hematol 1986;22:225.
733. Koenig HM, Vedvick TS. Alpha thalassemia in American born Filipino infants. J Pediatr 1975;87:756.
734. Weatherall DJ. The genetics of thalassemia. Br Med Bull 1969;25:24.
735. Milner PF, Clegg JB, Weatherall DJ. Haemoglobin-H disease due to a unique haemoglobin variant with an elongated α chain. Lancet 1971;1: 729.
736. Benz EJ Jr, Forget BG. The thalassemias: models for the molecular analysis of human disease. Annu Rev Med 1982;33:363.
737. O'Brien RT. The effects of iron deficiency on the expression of hemoglobin H. Blood 1973;41:853.
738. Pearson HA, Shanklin DR, Brodine CR. Alpha-thalassemia as a cause of nonimmunological hydrops. Am J Dis Child 1965;109:168.
739. Kan YW, Allen A, Lowenstein L. Hydrops fetalis with alpha thalassemia. N Engl J Med 1967;276:18.
740. Eng LIL. Alpha-chain thalassemia and hydrops fetalis in Malaya: report of five cases. Blood 1962;20:581.
741. Beaudry MA, Freguson DJ, Pearse K, et al. Survival of a hydropic infant with homozygous alpha-thalassemia-1. J Pediatr 1986;108:713.
742. Bianchi D, Beyer EC, Start AR, et al. Normal long-term survival with alpha-thalassemia. J Pediatr 1986;108:716.
743. Weatherall DJ, Clegg JB, Boon WH. The haemoglobin constitution of infants with haemoglobin Bart's hydrops foetalis syndrome. Br J Haematol 1970;18:357.
744. Benesch RE, Ranney HM, Benesch R, Smith GM. Chemistry of Bohr effect. II. Some properties of hemoglobin H. J Biol Chem 1961;236:2926.
745. Wasi P, Na-Nakorn S. The alpha thalassemias. Clin Haematol 1974;3: 383.
746. Wood WG, Weatherall DJ, Clegg JB. Interaction of heterocellular hereditary persistence of fetal hemoglobin with beta thalassemia and sickle cell anemia. Nature 1976;264:247.

Blood: Principles and Practice of Hematology, edited by Robert I. Handin, Samuel E. Lux, and Thomas P. Stossel. J.B. Lippincott Company, Philadelphia © 1995.

52

Disorders of Hemoglobin Function and Stability

Ronald L. Nagel

This chapter deals with disorders stemming from structural abnormalities (mutations of the coding sequence) that lead to clinical manifestations secondary to alterations of the function (oxygen affinity, electronic state of the heme iron) or stability of the hemoglobin molecule. Not included are disorders resulting from the presence of hemoglobin S (Hb S) or related conditions or the thalassemias.

Hemoglobin disorders can be classified according to the genetic mechanisms involved, the functional abnormalities they engender, or the clinical syndrome with which they are associated. Table 52-1 depicts the classification of these disorders according to the functional abnormality and the clinical syndrome they generate.

The material herein starts with a general introduction on hemoglobin structure and function, followed by a description of the five types of hemoglobinopathies described in Table 52-1.

NORMAL HEMOGLOBIN STRUCTURE AND FUNCTION

Overall Hemoglobin Structure: The Myoglobin Fold

The adult major hemoglobin molecule is a tetramer, since it is formed by four polypeptide chains, two α chains (141 amino acids long), and two β chains (146 amino acids long). The primary structure (amino acid sequence) is illustrated in Table 52-2. Each of these chains is attached to a prosthetic group called *heme*, formed by protoporphyrin IX complexed with an iron molecule. To understand the secondary and tertiary structure, that is, the three-dimensional shape of each of the globin polypeptide chains forming the tetramer, we need to consider (1) the "myoglobin fold," which is the overall architectural strategy that nature has devised for constructing all globin-based oxygen carriers; (2) the peculiarities of the α and β chains that form the major adult human hemoglobin; and (3) the heme and its relation to the protein moiety.

The myoglobin fold is a time-proven structural solution to the secondary and tertiary structure of globin chains. In effect, it has been found to be the structural blueprint of all myoglobin analyzed by x-crystallography, but also of the individual chains of all globin chains so far examined, including vertebrate and mollusk hemoglobins (two dissimilar hemoglobin constructs). Even hemoglobin present in the root nodules of legumes has the same myoglobin fold. This structure clearly was the best solution for heme–globin complexes early in evolution.

Myoglobin, the oxygen-carrying pigment in muscle, is a single polypeptide chain of 153 amino acids and was the first protein in which secondary and tertiary structures were elucidated by x-ray crystallography. John C. Kendrew from Cambridge, England, was awarded a Nobel Prize for his pioneering contribution on this subject[1] (Fig. 52-1).

Myoglobin is a globular and well-packed molecule in which most of the 153 amino acids are arranged in eight (labeled A to H) predominantly α-helical structures: The amide (−CO−NH−) backbone forms a helical structure with 3.6 residues per turn, stabilized by hydrogen bonds between a −C=O with the NH four residues farther down the chain (Fig. 52-2).

All the α helices are right-handed and vary in length between 4 amino acids (minimum number required to construct an α helix) and 28 amino acids. Nevertheless, the terminal portions of the α helices are anomalous since they fit either a 3_{10} helix (four residues per turn) or a π helix (five residues per turn). The remaining amino acids (23 of 153 total) are not arranged in helices, but are participants in two other types of molecular structures: (1) the elbows, hairpin corners of different degrees of sharpness that connect α helices and allow the sequence to wrap itself around the heme; and (2) terminal portions of the sequence (C- and N-terminal portions of the polypeptide chain).

Not all elbows contain residues in nonhelical configuration: the sharp turns between helices A and B, B and C, and D and E do not leave room for them. When there is room for amino acids in the elbows, they are mostly amino acid residues that are not helix makers. For example, proline's side chain introduces strains to the amide plane and, when present in the midst of an α helix, it either results in bending (as in helix E) or interruption (as in C and G helices) of the helix. Other residues, such as glycine are also "α-helix busters."

Another cardinal feature of the myoglobin fold is that different types of amino acid residues tend to occupy the surface of the molecule and the interior portions. The charged amino acids (aspartic, glutamic, lysine, arginine, and histidine) all are present almost exclusively in the exterior of the molecule, in direct contact with the solvent. Also, the uncharged but polar asparagine and glutamine

TABLE 52-1. Classification of Structural Nonsickle Hemoglobinopathies

Functional Abnormalities	Clinical Syndrome
High-affinity hemoglobins	Erythrocytosis
Low-affinity hemoglobins	Cyanosis
Ferric-heme hemoglobins	Pseudocyanosis
Unstable hemoglobins	Heinz body hemolytic anemia
Hemoglobins with abnormal assembly	Dominant thalassemia

tend to be in the exterior of the molecule. The true hydrophobic residues (phenylalanine, leucine, isoleucine, methionine, and valine) are mostly present pointing toward the interior of the molecule away from the solvent, and they stabilize the packing arrangement. Finally, some residues are not strong in either polarity or hydrophobicity because their side chains are too short and have an —OH group or a ring structure (proline, threonine, serine, cysteine, alanine, glycine, tyrosine, tryptophan). These are trump card amino acids; they can be located in the interior or exterior of the molecule. Nevertheless, they play critical roles in the secondary structure, since some of these amino acids can interrupt α helices and others can form structurally and functionally critical hydrogen bonds.

Violations of any of these myoglobin fold rules make the protein unstable in solution, change its functional properties, or both, resulting in the pathologic states to be discussed.

As stated before, the myoglobin fold has been conserved by nature for several millions of years in all globin-based oxygen carriers. The central achievement of this structure is that it solves two fundamental problems: it makes heme water-soluble and it helps maintain the heme iron in the ferrous state. These two physical properties are central and

TABLE 52-2. Primary Structure of Human Globin Subunits*

Helix	α	ζ	Helix	β	δ	γ	ϵ
NA1	1 Val	Ser	NA1	1 Val	Val	Gly	Val
			NA2	2 His	His	His	His
NA2	2 Leu	Leu	NA3	3 Leu	Leu	Phe	Phe
A1	3 Ser	Thr	A1	4 Thr	Thr	Thr	Thr
A2	4 Pro	Lys	A2	5 Pro	Pro	Glu	Ala
A3	5 Ala	Thr	A3	6 Glu	Glu	Glu	Glu
A4	6 Asp	Glu	A4	7 Glu	Glu	Asp	Glu
A5	7 Lys	Arg	A5	8 Lys	Lys	Lys	Lys
A6	8 Thr	Thr	A6	9 Ser	Thr	Ala	Ala
A7	9 Asn	Ile	A7	10 Ala	Ala	Thr	Ala
A8	10 Val	Ile	A8	11 Val	Val	Ile	Val
A9	11 Lys	Val	A9	12 Thr	Asn	Thr	Thr
A10	12 Ala	Ser	A10	13 Ala	Ala	Ser	Ser
A11	13 Ala	Met	A11	14 Leu	Leu	Leu	Leu
A12	14 Trp	Trp	A12	15 Trp	Trp	Trp	Trp
A13	15 Gly	Ala	A13	16 Gly	Gly	Gly	Ser
A14	16 Lys	Lys	A14	17 Lys	Lys	Lys	Lys
A15	17 Val	Ile	A15	18 Val	Val	Val	Met
A16	18 Gly	Ser					
AB1	19 Ala	Thr					
B1	20 His	Gln	B1	19 Asn	Asn	Asn	Asn
B2	21 Ala	Ala	B2	20 Val	Val	Val	Val
B3	22 Gly	Asp	B3	21 Asp	Asp	Glu	Glu
B4	23 Glu	Thr	B4	22 Glu	Ala	Asp	Glu
B5	24 Tyr	Ile	B5	23 Val	Val	Ala	Ala
B6	25 Gly	Gly	B6	24 Gly	Gly	Gly	Gly
B7	26 Ala	Thr	B7	25 Gly	Gly	Gly	Gly
B8	27 Glu	Glu	B8	26 Glu	Glu	Glu	Glu
B9	28 ALa	Thr	B9	27 Ala	Ala	Thr	Ala
B10	29 Leu	Leu	B10	28 Leu	Leu	Leu	Leu
B11	30 Glu	Glu	B11	29 Gly	Gly	Gly	Gly
B12	31 Arg	Arg	B12	30 Arg	Arg	Arg	Arg
B13	32 Met	Leu	B13	31 Leu	Leu	Leu	Leu
B14	33 Phe	Phe	B14	32 Leu	Leu	Leu	Leu
B15	34 Leu	Leu	B15	33 Val	Val	Val	Val
B16	35 Ser	Ser	B16	34 Val	Val	Val	Val
C1	36 Phe	His	C1	35 Tyr	Tyr	Tyr	Tyr
C2	37 Pro	Pro	C2	36 Pro	Pro	Pro	Pro
C3	38 Thr	Gln	C3	37 Trp	Trp	Trp	Trp
C4	39 Thr	Thr	C4	38 Thr	Thr	Thr	Thr
C5	40 Lys	Lys	C5	39 Gln	Gln	Gln	Gln

(continued)

TABLE 52-2. *(Continued)*

Helix	α	ζ	Helix	β	δ	γ	ε
C6	41 Thr	Thr	C6	40 Arg	Arg	Arg	Arg
C7	42 Tyr	Tyr	C7	41 Phe	Phe	Phe	Phe
CE1	43 Phe	Phe	CD1	42 Phe	Phe	Phe	Phe
CE2	44 Pro	Pro	CD2	43 Glu	Glu	Asp	Asp
CE3	45 His	His	CD3	44 Ser	Ser	Ser	Ser
CE4	46 Phe	Phe	CD4	45 Phe	Phe	Phe	Phe
			CD5	46 Gly	Gly	Gly	Gly
CE5	47 Asp	Asp	CD6	47 Asp	Asp	Asn	Asn
CE6	48 Leu	Leu	CD7	48 Leu	Leu	Leu	Leu
CE7	49 Ser	His	CD8	49 Ser	Ser	Ser	Ser
CE8	50 His	Pro	D1	50 Thr	Ser	Ser	Ser
			D2	51 Pro	Pro	Ala	Pro
			D3	52 Asp	Asp	Ser	Ser
			D4	53 Ala	Ala	Ala	Ala
			D5	54 Val	Val	Ile	Ile
			D6	55 Met	Met	Met	Leu
CE9	51 Gly	Gly	D7	56 Gly	Gly	Gly	Gly
E1	52 Ser	Ser	E1	57 Asn	Asn	Asn	Asn
E2	53 Ala	Ala	E2	58 Pro	Pro	Pro	Pro
E3	54 Gln	Gln	E3	59 Lys	Lys	Lys	Lys
E4	55 Val	Leu	E4	60 Val	Val	Val	Val
E5	56 Lys	Arg	E5	61 Lys	Lys	Lys	Lys
E6	57 Gly	Ala	E6	62 Ala	Ala	Ala	Ala
E7	58 His	His	E7	63 His	His	His	His
E8	59 Gly	Gly	E8	64 Gly	Gly	Gly	Gly
E9	60 Lys	Ser	E9	65 Lys	Lys	Lys	Lys
E10	61 Lys	Lys	E10	66 Lys	Lys	Lys	Lys
E11	62 Val	Val	E11	67 Val	Val	Val	Val
E12	63 Ala	Val	E12	68 Leu	Leu	Leu	Leu
E13	64 Asp	Ser	E13	69 Gly	Gly	Thr	Thr
E14	65 Ala	Ala	E14	70 Ala	Ala	Ser	Ser
E15	66 Leu	Val	E15	71 Phe	Phe	Leu	Phe
E16	67 Thr	Gly	E16	72 Ser	Ser	Gly	Gly
E17	68 Asn	Asp	E17	73 Asp	Asp	Asp	Asp
E18	69 Ala	Ala	E18	74 Gly	Gly	Ala	Ala
E19	70 Val	Val	E19	75 Leu	Leu	Ile, Thr	Ile
E20	71 Ala	Lys	E20	76 Ala	Ala	Lys	Lys
EF1	72 His	Ser	EF1	77 His	His	His	Asn
EF2	73 Val	Ile	EF2	78 Leu	Leu	Leu	Met
EF3	74 Asp	Asp	EF3	79 Asp	Asp	Asp	Asp
EF4	75 Asp	Asp	EF4	80 Asn	Asn	Asp	Asn
EF5	76 Met	Ile	EF5	81 Leu	Leu	Leu	Leu
EF6	77 Pro	Gly	EF6	82 Lys	Lys	Lys	Lys
EF7	78 Asn	Gly	EF7	83 Gly	Gly	Gly	Pro
EF8	79 Ala	Ala	EF8	84 Thr	Thr	Thr	Ala
F1	80 Leu	Leu	F1	85 Phe	Phe	Phe	Phe
F2	81 Ser	Ser	F2	86 Ala	Ser	Ala	Ala
F3	82 Ala	Lys	F3	87 Thr	Gln	Gln	Lys
F4	83 Leu	Leu	F4	88 Leu	Leu	Leu	Leu
F5	84 Ser	Ser	F5	89 Ser	Ser	Ser	Ser
F6	85 Asp	Glu	F6	90 Glu	Glu	Glu	Glu
F7	86 Leu	Leu	F7	91 Leu	Leu	Leu	Leu
F8	87 His	His	F8	92 His	His	His	His
F9	88 Ala	Ala	F9	93 Cys	Cys	Cys	Cys
FG1	89 His	Tyr	FG1	94 Asp	Asp	Asp	Asp
FG2	90 Lys	Ile	FG2	95 Lys	Lys	Lys	Lys
FG3	91 Leu	Leu	FG3	96 Leu	Leu	Leu	Leu
FG4	92 Arg	Arg	FG4	97 His	His	His	His
FG5	93 Val	Val	FG5	98 Val	Val	Val	Val
G1	94 Asp	Asp	G1	99 Asp	Asp	Asp	Asp

(continued)

TABLE 52-2. *(Continued)*

Helix	α	ζ	Helix	β	δ	γ	ε
G2	95 Pro	Pro	G2	100 Pro	Pro	Pro	Pro
G3	96 Val	Val	G3	101 Glu	Glu	Glu	Glu
G4	97 Asn	Asn	G4	102 Asn	Asn	Asn	Asn
G5	98 Phe	Phe	G5	103 Phe	Phe	Phe	Phe
G6	99 Lys	Lys	G6	104 Arg	Arg	Lys	Lys
G7	100 Leu	Leu	G7	105 Leu	Leu	Leu	Leu
G8	101 Leu	Leu	G8	106 Leu	Leu	Leu	Leu
G9	102 Ser	Ser	G9	107 Gly	Gly	Gly	Gly
G10	103 His	His	G10	108 Asn	Asn	Asn	Asn
G11	104 Cys	Cys	G11	109 Val	Val	Val	Val
G12	105 Leu	Leu	G12	110 Leu	Leu	Leu	Met
G13	106 Leu	Leu	G13	111 Val	Val	Val	Val
G14	107 Val	Val	G14	112 Cys	Cys	Thr	Ile
G15	108 Thr	Thr	G15	113 Val	Val	Val	Ile
G16	109 Leu	Leu	G16	114 Leu	Leu	Leu	Leu
G17	110 Ala	Ala	G17	115 Ala	Ala	Ala	Ala
G18	111 Ala	Ala	G18	116 His	Arg	Ile	Thr
G19	112 His	Arg	G19	117 His	Asn	His	His
GH1	113 Leu	Phe	Gh1	118 Phe	Phe	Phe	Phe
GH2	114 Pro	Pro	GH2	119 Gly	Gly	Gly	Gly
GH3	115 Ala	Ala	GH3	120 Lys	Lys	Lys	Lys
GH4	116 Glu	Asp	GH4	121 Glu	Glu	Glu	Glu
GH5	117 Phe	Phe	Gh5	122 Phe	Phe	Phe	Phe
H1	118 Thr	Thr	H1	123 Thr	Thr	Thr	Thr
H2	119 Pro	Ala	H2	124 Pro	Pro	Pro	Pro
H3	120 Ala	Glu	H3	125 Pro	Gln	Glu	Glu
H4	121 Val	Ala	H4	126 Val	Met	Val	Val
H5	122 His	His	H5	127 Gln	Gln	Gln	Gln
H6	123 Ala	Ala	H6	128 Ala	Ala	Ala	Ala
H7	124 Ser	Ala	H7	129 Ala	Ala	Ser	Ala
H8	125 Leu	Trp	H8	130 Tyr	Tyr	Trp	Trp
H9	126 Asp	Asp	H9	131 Gln	Gln	Gln	Gln
H10	127 Lys	Lys	H10	132 Lys	Lys	Lys	Lys
H11	128 Phe	Phe	H11	133 Val	Val	Met	Leu
H12	129 Leu	Leu	H12	134 Val	Val	Val	Val
H13	130 Ala	Ser	H13	135 Ala	Ala	Thr	Ser
H14	131 Ser	Val	H14	136 Gly	Gly	Gly, Ala	Ala
H15	132 Val	Val	H15	137 Val	Val	Val	Val
H16	133 Ser	Ser	H16	138 Ala	Ala	Ala	Ala
H17	134 Thr	Ser	H17	139 Asn	Asn	Ser	Ile
H18	135 Val	Val	H18	140 Ala	Ala	Ala	Ala
H19	136 Leu	Leu	H19	141 Leu	Leu	Leu	Leu
H20	137 Thr	Thr	H20	142 Ala	Ala	Ser	Ala
H21	138 Ser	Glu	H21	143 His	His	Ser	His
HC1	139 Lys	Lys	HC1	144 Lys	Lys	Arg	Lys
HC2	140 Tyr	Tyr	HC2	145 Tyr	Tyr	Tyr	Tyr
HC3	141 Arg	Arg	HC3	146 His	His	His	His

* The α and α-related (δ) subunits are shown at the left. The β and β-related (δ, γ, and ε) chains are at the right. The amino acids' relationship to the eight globin helices (A to H) is also shown. Thus, A16 is the 16th amino acid in the A helix. Interhelical elbows are named for the two adjacent helices (eg, AB1 is the first amino acid between helices A and B). The N- and C-terminal residues are labeled NA and HC, respectively. The residues are aligned to maximize the homology between subunits, which causes some gaps.
(Modified from Bunn HF, Forget BG. Hemoglobin: molecular, genetic, and clinical aspects. Philadelphia, WB Saunders, 1986)

indispensable for the oxygen carrying capacity of myoglobin and hemoglobin.

The Heme

The myoglobin fold is wrapped around the heme, which is the combination of a porphyrin ring and an iron molecule. The porphyrin, in turn, is composed of four puerile rings tied together by methenyl (=CH−) bridges. The porphyrin ring in heme is protoporphyrin IX, defined by the type of substitutions found in the carbons not involved in methenyl bridging (Fig. 52-3). All the structural components of heme are arranged in a single plane resulting in a wafer-like structure, hence representing the heme as a flat plate in

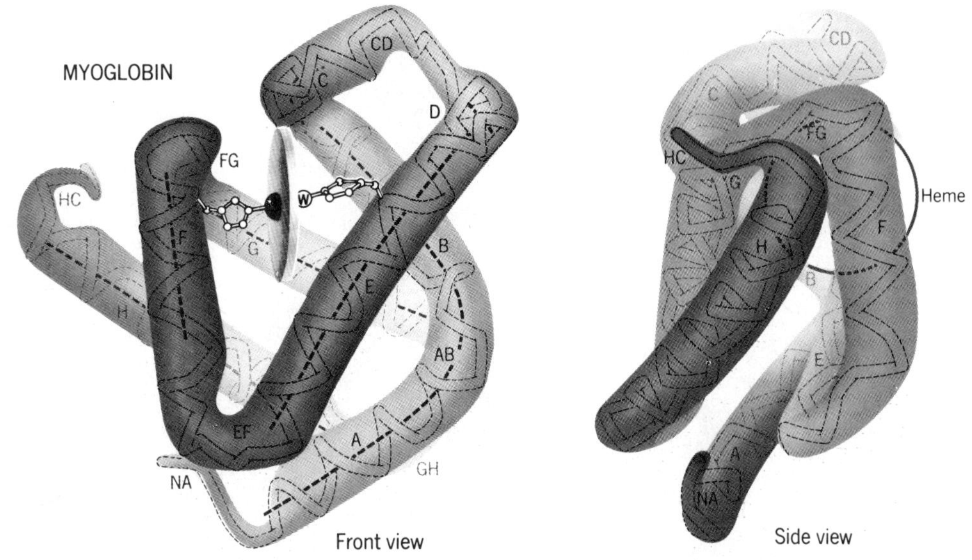

FIGURE 52-1. The myoglobin fold. The myoglobin molecule consists of eight stretches of α helix that surround the heme group forming a pocket. Single letters signify a helix; double letters, a corner or bend (nonhelical regions). The heme pocket is formed by helices E and F. Helices B, G, and H are at the bottom, and the CD corner closes the open end. Histidine side chains interact with the heme from both sides. W depicts the place occupied by the oxygen molecule when it binds to the iron. (Dickerson RE, Geis I. Hemoglobin: structure, function, evolution, and pathology. Menlo Park, CA, Benjamin/Cummings, 1983:26)

the myoglobin model. The centerpiece of the structure is a tetracoordinated iron atom, in which the bonds with puerile rings 4 and 2 are identical, as well as the bonds between the iron and puerile rings 1 and 3. This structure, weighing 616 daltons, contains a large number of alternating double-bond rings and consequently delocalized π electrons.

How Does the Heme Interact With the Globin Portion of Myoglobin? The heme fits snugly in the heme pocket formed by the F and E helices, to which it is tied. It is surrounded by the H, G, and B helices on one side and the C and D helices on the other.

Why is the heme semiburied in the globin heme pocket? Model compound studies suggest that hydrophobic environments are best for the maintenance of the ferrous state of the iron, and the heme pocket is highly hydrophobic and narrow.[2] The heme leaves only the charged propionic side chains significantly exposed to the solvent at the entrance of the niche. The niche is large enough for oxygen to penetrate, although with some slight difficulty, as judged by micropath kinetic measurements. Ligands (molecules capable of binding to the iron) that are significantly larger than oxygen, such as the family of isocyanates, have progressive difficulty in reaching the iron in direct proportion to their bulk.

How Does the Iron of the Heme Interact With the Globin? As mentioned, four valences are consumed by coordination with the four puerile rings. The fifth coordination occurs with a histidine residue in the eighth position of the F helix (His F8), the proximal histidine. The sixth coordination is potentially occupied by an oxygen molecule: in oxymyoglobin, the $-O-O-$ axis is at 59 degrees from the heme plane, whereas this coordination position is occupied in deoxymyoglobin by a water molecule instead. This arrangement renders the favored structure for ferrous or ferric iron, octahedral coordination. Nevertheless, this structure is further complicated by the presence of an interacting histidine, the E7 or distal histidine, on the far site of the oxygen. This residue is too far to coordinate directly with the iron, but the nitrogen in its side chain interacts with the oxygen or the water, further modifying ligand binding.

The fact that the heme–globin arrangement is indispensable for retaining the oxygen-binding iron in the ferrous state becomes abundantly apparent when the class of hemoglobin mutants called M hemoglobins are discussed; these variants result from mutations of the proximal and distal histidines.

α Chains of Hemoglobin

The α chains have the general architecture of the myoglobin fold, but they are shorter chains, involving 141 amino acids rather than 153. This difference comes from the absence of the five residues that form the myoglobin D helix, and six residues from the C-terminal portion (two are the last members of the H helix and four are from the nonhelical tail of myoglobin; Fig. 52-4).

The deletion of the D helix in the α chains has no explanation. The disappearance of the nonhelical C-terminal residues could be related to the important bond between Arg α141 and Tyr α140 and the appropriate receptor, which are important to the conformational changes involved in the oxy-to-deoxy transformation (see later discussion), a central feature of the tetramer structural–functional relation. The N-terminal–added residues in myoglobin might strain these critical molecular distances and make the conformational change impossible.

The differences between α chains and myoglobin could also be derived from the need that α chains have to bind several different β-like chains (γ, δ, ϵ) with varied requirements for the generation of the quaternary structure. Specifically, the generation of a quaternary structure implies changes in the character of the residues involved in subunit contact. That is, residues that are polar in myoglobin (because they are in direct contact with the solvent) might be buried in an intersubunit contact in several of the hemoglobins, and hence have to be replaced by hydrophobic amino acids. Two examples of this are found in residue B15, a lysine in myoglobin that becomes a leucine and residue C1 a histidine in myoglobin, which is a phenylalanine in human α chains.[3]

β Chains of Hemoglobin

The human β chains are also shorter than myoglobin, but less so than α chains, containing 146 residues. The general architecture of the chain, its secondary and tertiary structure, complies closely with the myoglobin fold.[4–6]

Two small structural differences with myoglobin are apparent: the disappearance of two residues from the junction of A and B helices, making the AB elbow sharper, as well as six residues missing from the C-terminal sequence (as in the α chains). The reason for the change in the AB elbow is not understood. The critical bonds involving His β142 and Tyr β145 might be incompatible with the presence of the nonhelical terminal residues found in myoglobin. In

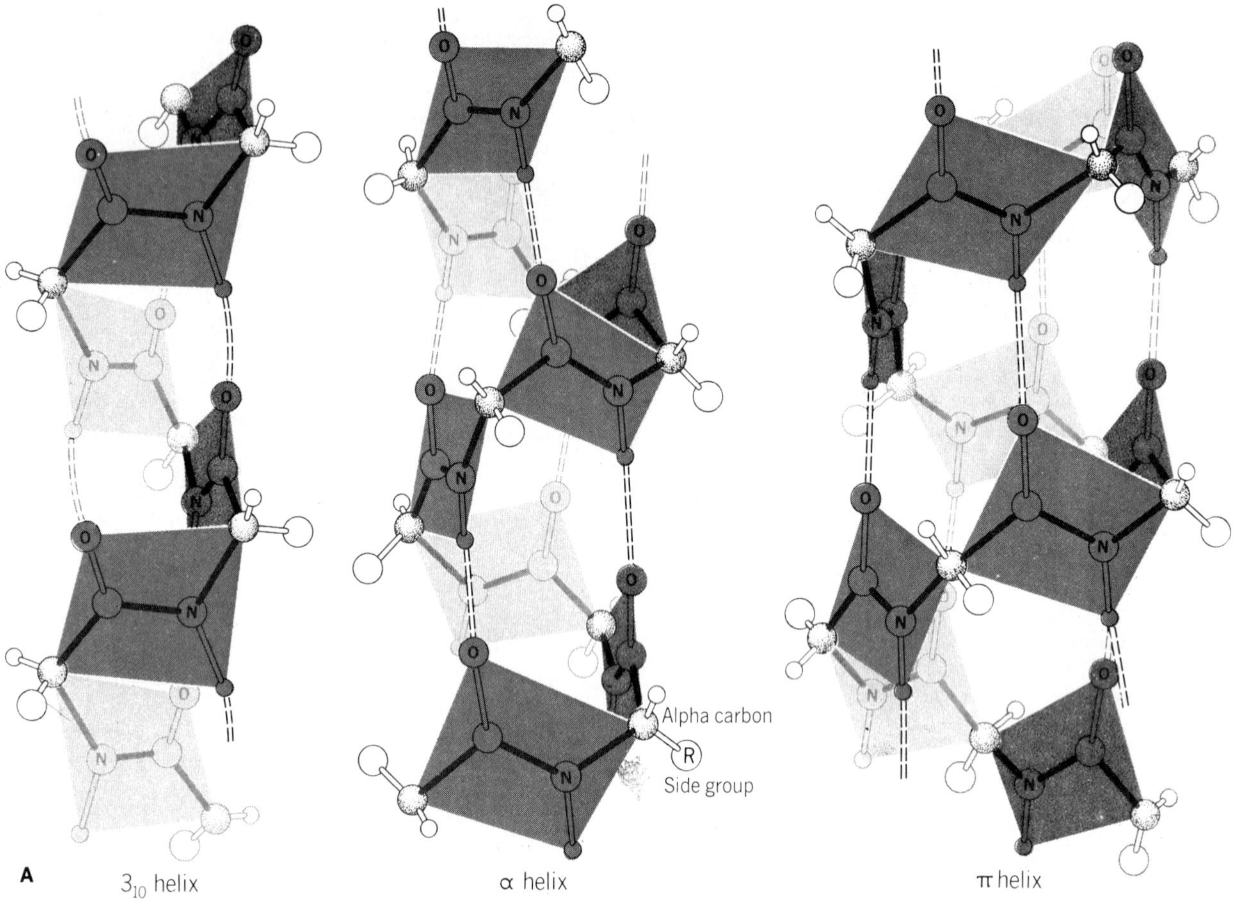

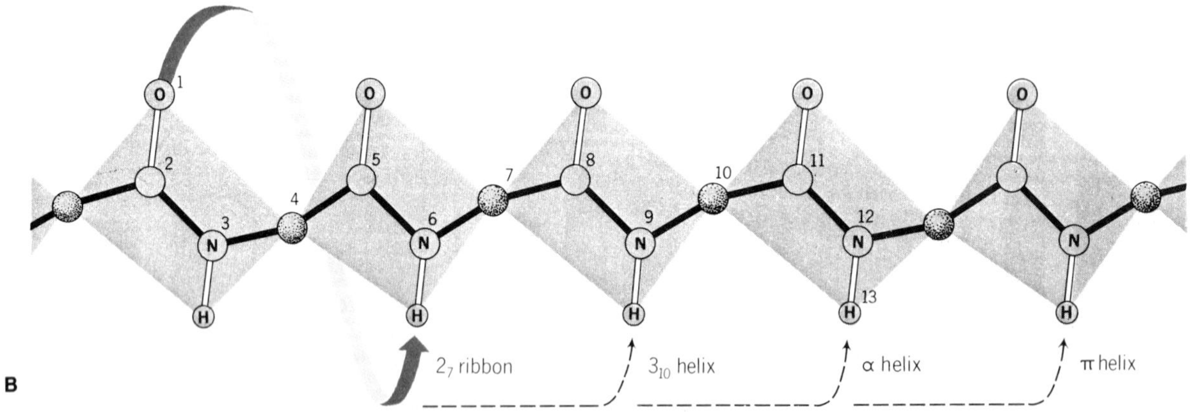

FIGURE 52-2. Coiling of polypeptide chains into helices. (**A**) The 3_{10}, α, and π helices differ in their patterns of hydrogen bonding, shown in **B**. Hydrogen bonds in the α helix are particularly unstrained, making the α helix especially stable. The α carbons are stippled, with small attached spheres for hydrogens and larger spheres for side chains. (**B**) Hydrogen-bonding pattern from one turn of the helix to the next turn for four related helices. Only the α helix is found extensively in proteins; the others are found only occasionally for very short stretches, usually winding down or unwinding the last turn of an α helix. (Dickerson RE, Geis I. Hemoglobin: structure, function, evolution, and pathology. Menlo Park, CA, Benjamin/Cummings, 1983:15)

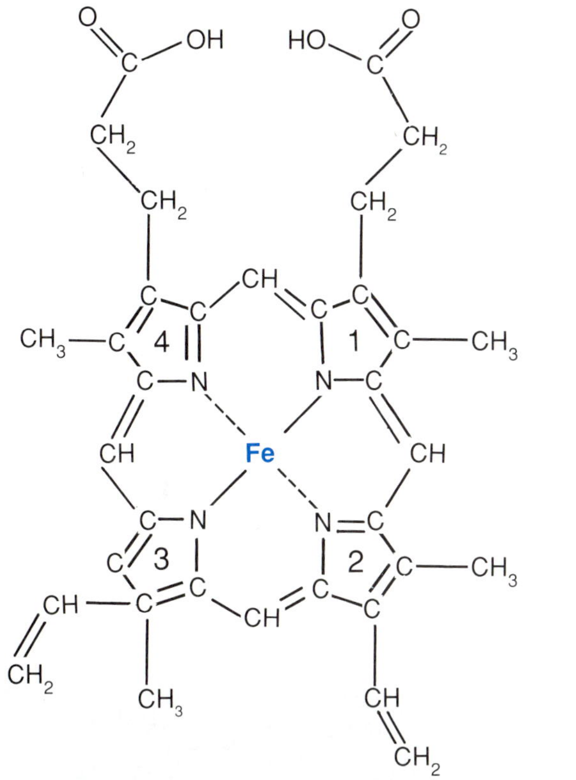

FIGURE 52-3. The protoporphyrin IX heme structure consists of four pyrrole rings with the following side-chain replacements: two methyl and two propionic acids in pyrrole 1 and 4; two methyl and two vinyls in pyrroles 2 and 3. Iron is tetracoordinated by the nitrogens of the pyrrole rings.

the β chains, changes of charged residues to hydrophobic ones can also be observed in the areas of the sequence involved in subunit interaction.

The main secondary and tertiary structural differences between α and β chains are in the D helix, which are absent in the former and present in the latter. The reason for this difference is also not understood.

The Tetramer (Quaternary Structure)

The hemoglobin molecule is a tetramer formed by two α chains and two β chains, with a total molecular weight of 64.5 kd.

How Do the Two Pairs of Chains Arrange Themselves in Space to Generate a Tetramer (Quaternary Structure)? The arrangement of the two types of chains in the tetramer complies with a 222 symmetry. This designation means that the structure can be characterized by three two-fold axes of symmetry, perpendicular to each other, as illustrated in Figure 52-5. To understand this symmetry, consider the upper half (the dark pair of chains) in the vertical axis. If you rotate these two chains by 180 degrees, they will coincide perfectly with the light-colored pair of chains: this is called a *two-fold* or *diad axis of symmetry*; hence, the three twos. Of course, α chains are not identical with β chains. Therefore, in a real hemoglobin molecule this symmetry is only approximate. The homotetramer of β chains (β_4 or Hb H), observed in a severe form of α-thalassemia, exhibits the perfect 222 symmetry in the oxygenated tetramer, since all chains are truly identical.

How Do the Four Chains Interact With Each Other? The tetramer $\alpha_2\beta_2$ exhibits several types of subunit interactions. First, little contact occurs between identical chains, that is, in the $\alpha_1\alpha_2$ or $\beta_1\beta_2$ interfaces. Most of the strong interactions between subunits are in the contacts between the dissimilar pair of chains, that is, in the interfaces $\alpha_1\beta_1$ and or the equivalent $\alpha_2\beta_2$.

The next level of complexity is the contact between these two pairs of unlike chains. The contact occurs in two areas in the surfaces of these dimers: the $\alpha_1\beta_2$ contact (Fig. 52-6) and the equivalent $\alpha_2\beta_1$, which is called the *sliding contact*. Conversely, the $\alpha_2\beta_2$ dimer has areas of interaction between the α and the β chain that are called *packing contacts*.

The packing contacts are strong and can be disrupted only with very high urea concentrations and certain salts, and they remain intact through all the conformational changes of hemoglobin. The sliding contact, on the other hand, is weaker and has strategically located hydrogen bonds and salt bridges that can be broken and reformed elsewhere, allowing the mobility of the two surfaces indispensable for conformational changes (see next section). In conclusion, the interactions between like chains are weak, whereas the interactions between unlike chains are strong; hence, when the tetramer dissociates, $\alpha_1\beta_2$ dimers are generated.

Chothia and colleagues[7] have shown that about 20% of the surface area of the subunits is consumed in subunit–subunit interaction, of which 60% are involved in packing contacts and 35% in sliding contacts.

The Structure–Function Relations for the Binding of Oxygen by Hemoglobin

The primary task of hemoglobin is to carry oxygen from the lungs to the capillaries and carbon dioxide (CO_2) in the reverse direction. In addition, in mammals it has to be able to adapt to sudden changes in oxygenation requirements; therefore, the modulation of its oxygen carrying capacity has to be available. The functions of hemoglobin are summarized as follows:

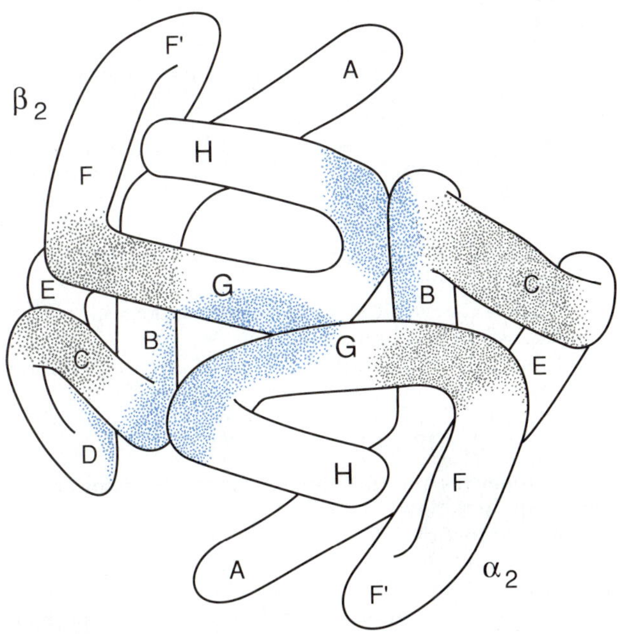

FIGURE 52-4. The $\alpha_2\beta_2$ dimer is seen in a side view. The colored areas depict the packing contacts that hold the dimer together. The sliding contacts with the $\alpha_1\beta_1$ dimer are depicted by areas of gray stippling. (After Dickerson RE, Geis I. Hemoglobin: structure, function, evolution, and pathology. Menlo Park, CA, Benjamin/Cummings, 1983:38)

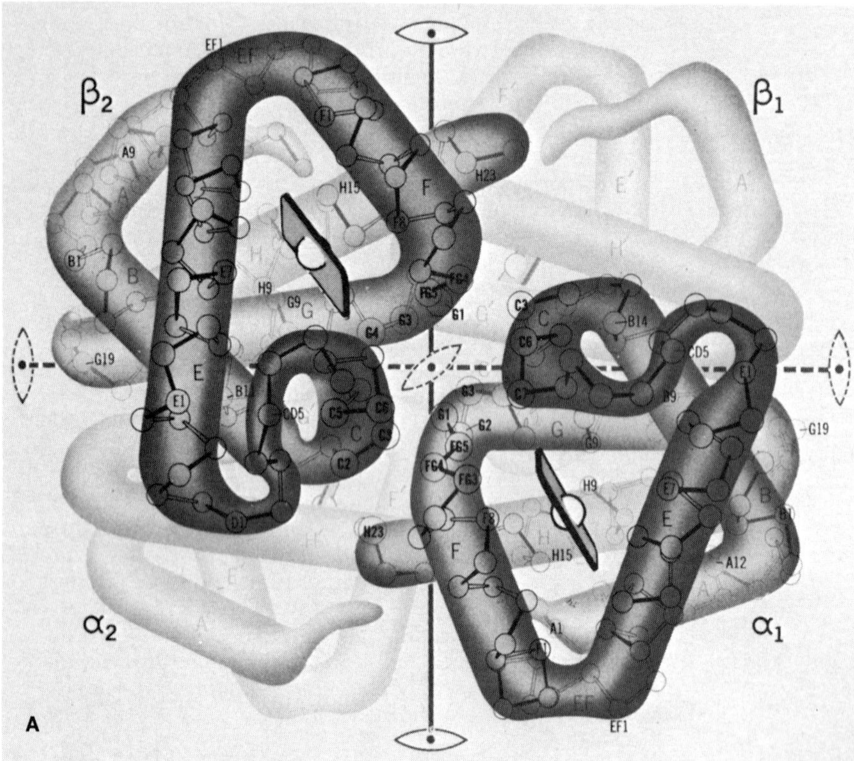

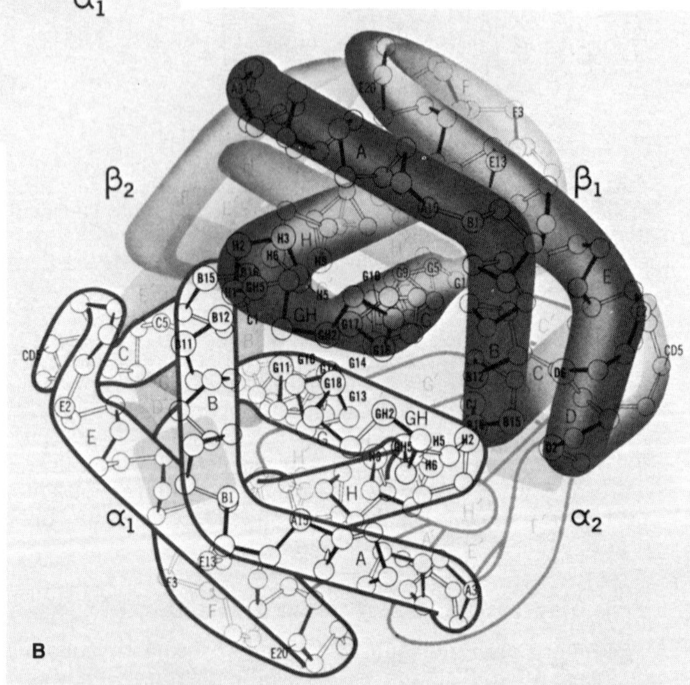

FIGURE 52-5. The four chains of methemoglobin. (**A**) Front view: $\alpha_1\beta_2$ contacts (the $\alpha_2\beta_1$ contacts are identical on the back side of the molecule). (**B**) Right side view: $\alpha_1\beta_1$ contacts (the $\alpha_2\beta_2$ contacts are identical). The two perpendicular pseudoaxes are indicated in **A** by dashes. Only the α carbons of the main chains are shown. Those side chains involved in contacts between subunits are given boldface numbers in large circles. (Dickerson RE, Geis I. Hemoglobin: structure, function, evolution, and pathology. Menlo Park, CA, Benjamin/Cummings, 1983:36)

1. It binds oxygen with a sigmoid curve—that is, allosterically.
2. It binds CO_2 while it is delivering oxygen and releases CO_2 when it is binding oxygen.
3. It binds H^+ efficiently in a low-pH environment and releases it when it encounters high pH (Bohr effect).
4. Oxygen affinity is modulated by allosteric effectors, that is, 2,3-DPG, Cl^-, H^+, and CO_2.

These properties and their molecular mechanisms are described in the following sections.

Hemoglobin Binds Oxygen Allosterically. The myoglobin molecule, being a monomer and having one heme, binds oxygen as predicted by mass law: a plot of the Po_2 versus oxygen saturation can be described by a hyperbole. On the other hand, the hemoglobin tetramer, with four hemes, binds oxygen with a sigmoidal curve (Fig. 52-7). Myoglobin binding of oxygen can be described at equilibrium by the simple relation:

$$y = \frac{K_aPo_2}{1 + K_aPo_2}$$

where
y = fractional saturation of the myoglobin molecule with oxygen
K_a = association constant
Po_2 = partial pressure of oxygen

For the hemoglobin molecule, the binding of oxygen is different, and at equilibrium this reaction can be described by the formula:

$$y = \frac{K_aPo_2{}^n}{1 + K_aPo_2{}^n}$$

The difference is the power of n to which Po_2 is elevated: n is the Hill coefficient, an empiric number that is an index of the sigmoidicity of the curve and a feature of the function that is related to the extent of cooperativity. The Hill coefficient is 2.8 for hemoglobin, whereas it is equal to 1 for myoglobin.

What is Cooperativity? Cooperativity is the reason for the sigmoid shape of the oxygen equilibrium curve of hemoglobin. The initial portion of the curve has a very low

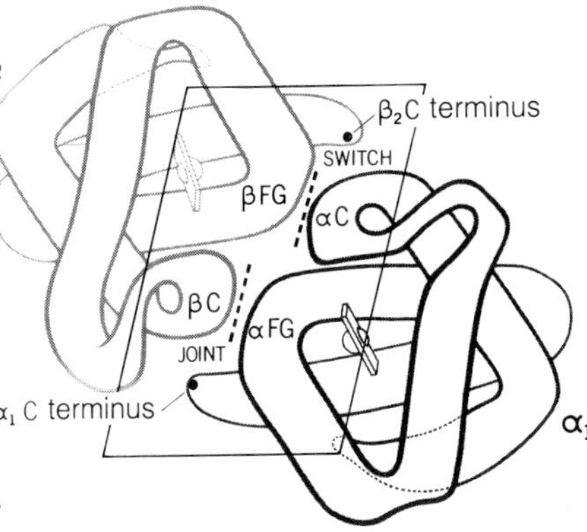

A

FIGURE 52-6. Front view of hemoglobin shows extensive subunit interactions between FG corners and C helices in the $\alpha_1\beta_2$ contacts. The area in **A** is enlarged in **B**. Important interaction regions from top to bottom are the β-chain carboxy terminal, the switch region, the flexible joint, and the α-chain terminal. (Dickerson RE, Geis I. Hemoglobin: structure, function, evolution, and pathology. Menlo Park, CA, Benjamin/Cummings, 1983:43)

Deoxyhemoglobin:

····· H bonds or salt bridges

----- Nonbonded packing contacts

Oxyhemoglobin:

····· H bonds or salt bridges

----- Nonbonded packing contacts

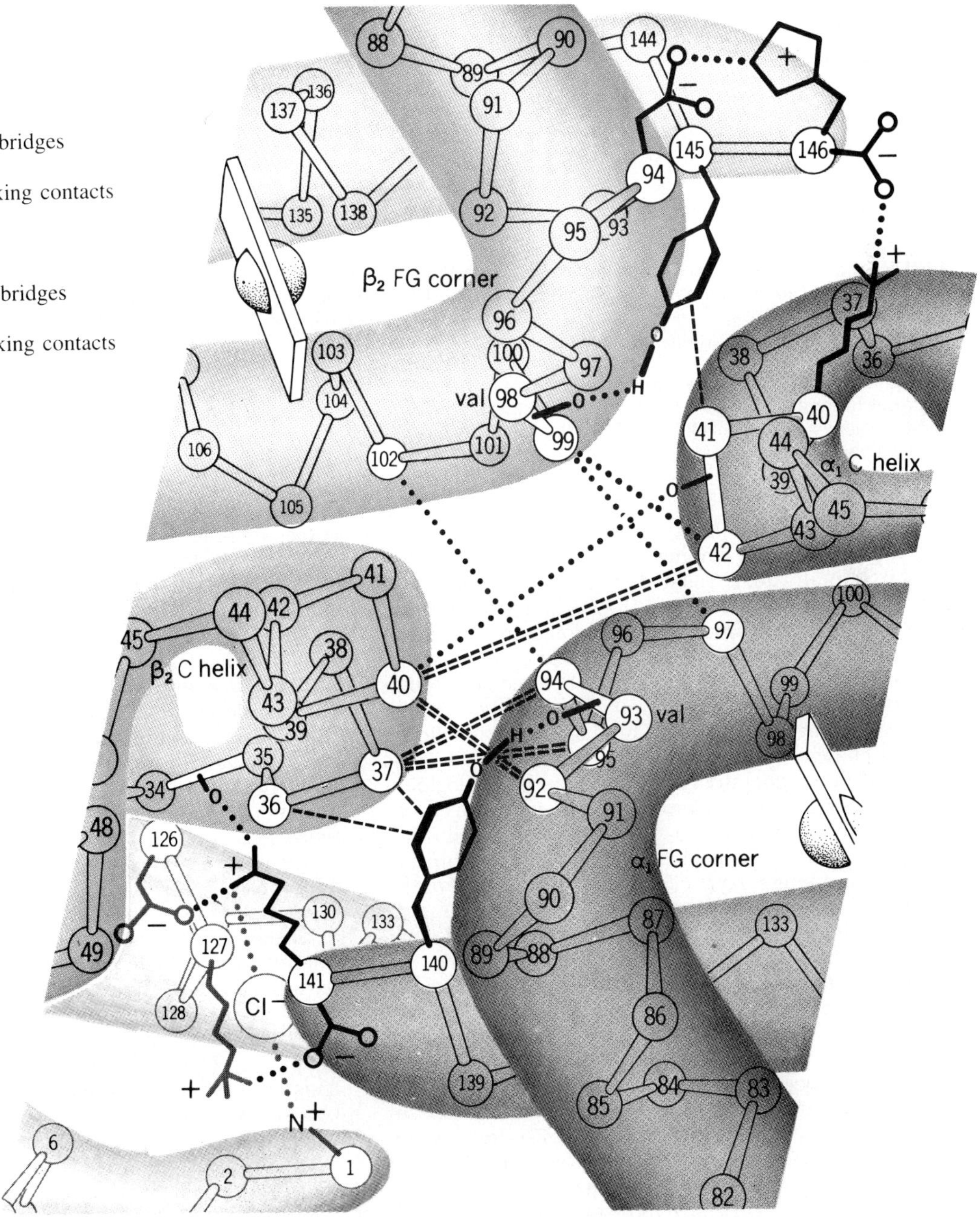

B

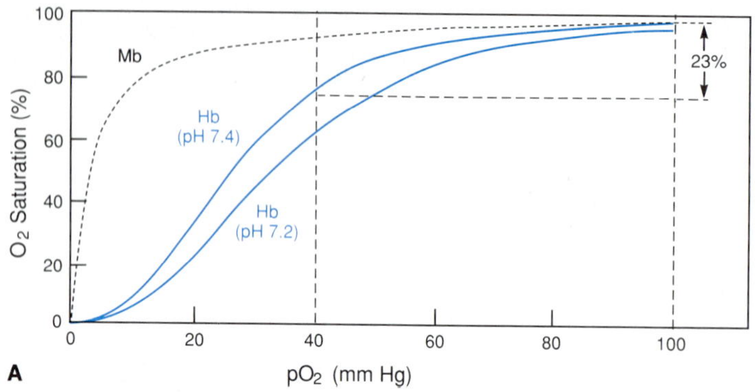

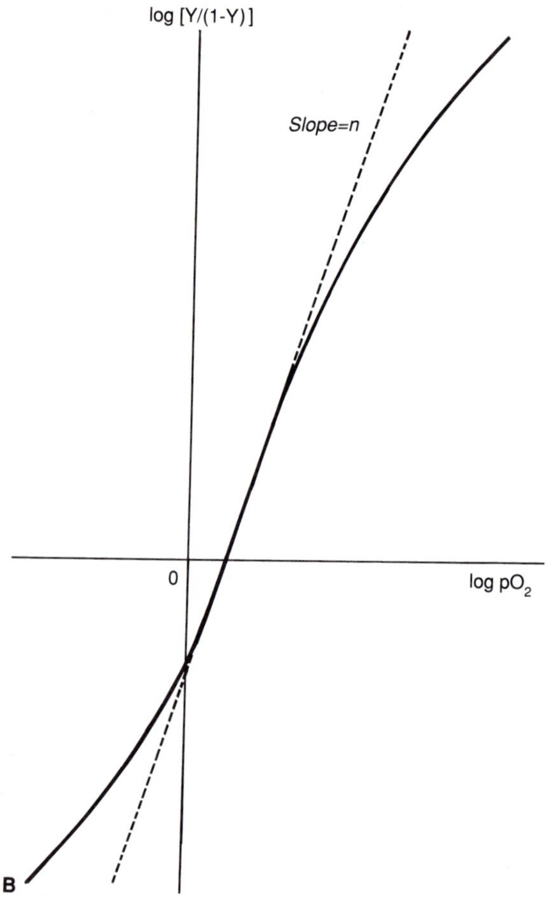

FIGURE 52-7. (**A**) Oxygen equilibrium curves of sperm whale myoglobin (Mb) and hemoglobin (Hb) in human red cells. At pH 7.4 and 37°C, the oxygen saturation of the red cells is 98% at the arterial blood Po_2 (100 mmHg) and 75% at the mixed venous blood Po_2 (40 mmHg) so that oxygen corresponding to 23% saturation difference is transported by circulating RBCs. (**B**) Logarithmic (Hill) plot of oxygen equilibrium curve of human hemoglobin. Y, fractional saturation of hemoglobin with oxygen; n, Hill's coefficient. (After Imai K. Allosteric effects in haemoglobin. Cambridge, Cambridge University Press, 1982)

slope, reflecting a low affinity for oxygen by hemoglobin at the beginning of the loading process. That is, when hemoglobin is totally deoxygenated, it has a rather poor avidity for oxygen (see Fig. 52-7). As the loading proceeds and as the molecule binds more oxygen molecules, the slope of the reaction begins to change rapidly and becomes steep. This means that the affinity for oxygen has becomes much higher despite the sluggish beginnings. In other words, the initial molecules of oxygen that bind a deoxyhemoglobin tetramer change the protein's avidity for oxygen. This property, called cooperativity, ensures that the hemoglobin tetramer, after it begins to accept oxygen, is fully oxygenated promptly. Thus, if we could measure the distribution of oxygen in all the hemoglobin molecules in a solution that contains enough oxygen to oxygenate only half of the hemes available, most molecules would not be oxygenated at all or would be entirely oxygenated, with a small compartment of partially oxygenated hemoglobulins.

How Can Cooperativity Be Explained at the Molecular Level? Formally, there are two overall models. The *sequential* or Koshland-Nemethy-Filmer (KNF) model[8] (Fig. 52-8) involves the change of conformation of each subunit after binding oxygen, combined with a slight modification of the conformation of their neighbors and, as a consequence, progressive increase in their affinity for oxygen. This model predicts a family of conformations between fully deoxygenated and totally oxygenated molecules, each one exhibiting slightly higher overall affinity for the ligand.

The *two-state* (or *concerted*) model of Monod, Wyman, and Changeaux[7] (MWC model) contains two fundamentally different conformations, one for oxygenated hemoglobin, another for the deoxygenated molecule. In its strictest form, this model does not accept meaningful intermediate conformations, only two extreme ones. It predicts that the molecule of hemoglobin will bind two or three molecules of oxygen at low affinity (deoxy conformation) and then, suddenly, the molecule will flip to the oxygenated conformation, drastically increasing the oxygen affinity of the molecule as a whole. Max Perutz and colleagues[9] have applied this model with great success to hemoglobin.

The two-state model was originally developed to explain the function of enzymes, particularly the role of effectors; these effectors, although not binding at the active site, were nevertheless able to modify the activity of protein. The conceptual breakthrough came with the realization that the effector induces a change in conformation of the molecule as a whole producing, from a distance, a significant change in the conformation and function of the active site. This process was called *allostery* or *allosteric changes*, meaning different shapes.

Formally, the two-state model can be defined by two quantities: c, which represents the difference in activity between the two enzyme states, but in the special case of hemoglobin, corresponds to the ratio in oxygen affinity constants between the two conformation states (K_a oxy/K_a deoxy = c). The second quantity, L, defines the equilibrium constant for the conformational change itself between the two states: T for tense, the nonaccepting or low-affinity state (the deoxygenated conformer in the case of hemoglobin) and the R for relaxed, the accepting or high-affinity state (the oxygenated conformer in the case of hemoglobin). For the fully unliganded state, $(T_o)/(R_o) = L = 10{,}000$, under physiologic conditions. That is, when molecules of hemoglobin are fully deoxygenated, 10,000 molecules are in the T state and 1 molecule in the R state. We will see later in the text the influence of effectors (2,3-diphosphoglycerate [2,3-DPG], H^+, CO_2 and Cl^-) on these parameters.

As soon as the first molecule of oxygen is added, the ratio

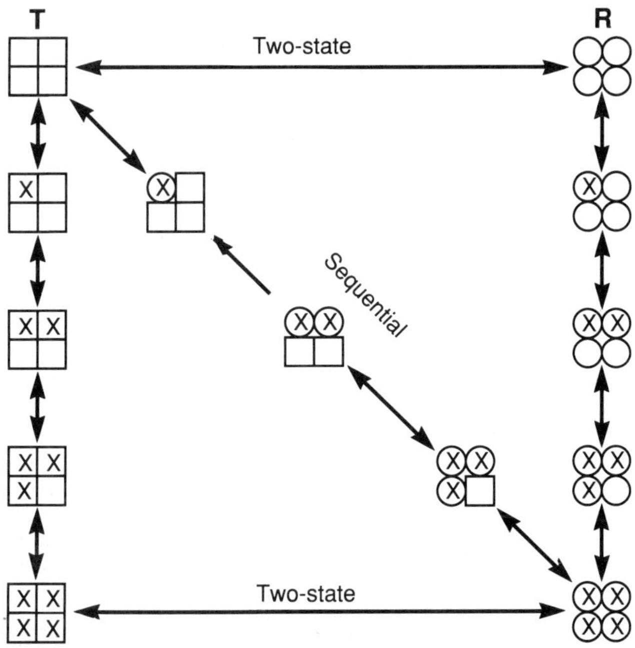

FIGURE 52-8. Contrasting ways of generating cooperativity according to the two-state (Monod-Wyman-Changeaux) and sequential (Koshland-Nemethy-Filmer) models. Each subunit has two distinct tertiary conformations, one with higher ligand affinity for ligand X than the other. In the two-state model, the oligomeric molecule is postulated to exist in only two global conformations, T and R. In quaternary T, all subunits have the low-affinity tertiary conformation t (*squares*); in quaternary R, they all have the high-affinity conformation r (*circles*). The fully unligated oligomer favors T, whereas the R form predominates in fully ligated molecules. Changes in conformation of individual subunits occur in a concerted or all-or-none fashion so that the oligomer is always symmetric. The sequential model is indicated by the diagonal, where species proceed through a sequence of intermediate conformations. Ligand binding induces a change to the high-affinity conformation (r) in each ligated subunit, whereas the unligated subunits retain their low-affinity conformations (t). Altered pairwise contacts of each ligated subunit with its neighbors influence the neighboring subunit's tendency to bind the next ligand and to switch to the high-affinity form. The sequential model can account for both positive and negative cooperativity (binding a ligand diminishes the affinity for subsequent binding), whereas the two-state model can accommodate only positive cooperativity. (After Komiyama N, Shih DT, Looker D, et al. Was the loss of the D helix in alpha globin a functional neutral mutation? Nature 1991;352:349)

of the two conformers will be defined by: $(T_1)/(R_1) = Lc$. Baldwin and Chothia's[10] number for c is around 0.01; therefore, the ratio will be 10 to 1. When two molecules of oxygen are added, the ratio will be $(T_2)/(R_2) = Lc_2 = 1$; hence, the same number of T molecules and R molecules will be present. When three molecules are bound, the ratio becomes $(T_3)/(R_3) = Lc_3 = -100$, which means that 100 molecules are in the R form and 1 in the T form. Finally, when all four sites are saturated, $(T_4)/(R_4) = Lc_4 = -10{,}000$. There are 10,000 molecules in the R form for every T hemoglobin molecule. Thus, the significant switch of conformation must occur in hemoglobin somewhere in between the binding of two and three molecules of oxygen.

In contrast, the sequential (KNF) model has progressive subunit conformation changes that are stepwise but not necessarily equal. The first subunit oxygenated will change conformation from t_1 to r_1 and so progressively, until $t_4 \rightarrow R_4$. This produces stepwise but nonequal increments in affinity for the successive subunits liganded.

The question is which of these two models better explains the data available on hemoglobin ligand binding. Crystallography has defined two extreme conformations of hemoglobin, one oxy and one deoxy, both of which are different, but this result does not decide the issue, since the two models proposed have different "initial" and "final" conformers. The present state of evidence suggests that, in general, the two-state model explains most of the experimental data accumulated for the functional properties of the hemoglobin molecule. The broad categories of evidence are the following:

1. In the cyanomethemoglobin–oxyhemoglobin hybrids of the type of $\alpha_2\beta_2$CMet and α_2CMetβ_2,[11] two hemes are frozen in the liganded oxygenated-like state (cyanomethemoglobin) and they can be interrogated (by nuclear magnetic resonance [NMR] spectroscopy) as to their R or T state, when the other two hemes are deoxygenated or oxygenated. The experiment demonstrates that the cyanomet hemes do not change when the ferrous hemes are either oxygenated or deoxygenated. In other words, they are fixed in the R (oxy) conformer. Nevertheless, if the R conformer is forced into the T state by a powerful allosteric inhibitor (such as inositolhexaphosphate [IHP]), the spectrum of the cyanomet hemes changes to the T state. Therefore, the environment of the hemes is sensitive to protein conformational changes and not to the individual state of the subunits.
2. Hybrid hemoglobin molecules constructed with nitrous oxide–bound hemoglobins have been examined by spectral methods.[12,13] They can also be driven to the deoxy conformer, even when fully liganded, by the superallosteric inhibitor, IHP. Iron–histidine interactions can be observed to go from the R to the T state in spite of the liganded state of the molecule. Again, these results are a strong argument for the two-state model.
3. The properties of hemoglobin mutants are largely concordant with the two-state model.[14,15]

Nevertheless, detailed thermodynamic descriptions of the hemoglobin molecule by Gary Ackers and colleagues[16] and other data by Ho and Russu,[15] indicate that the two-state model must be relaxed to accept some amount of stepwise conformational change. As usual, nature refuses the straitjacket of simple theoretical modeling. Miura and colleagues[17] find NMR evidence of tertiary conformational changes that are incompatible with the strict two-state model system. Ackers and colleagues[16] find thermodynamic evidence of a "third allosteric structure." Perella and associates,[18] using low temperature isoelectric focusing techniques, find that the distribution of intermediate ligand states is compatible with a third allosteric structure, which in effect brings features of the KNF sequential model to the MWC two-state model. Nevertheless, the extent of departure from the MWC model is well settled: the use of mixed-state hybrids for defining some of the evidence overstates the KNF feature of heme–heme interaction. In other words, the big picture remains the overall T-to-R transition of the whole hemoglobin molecule (two-state model), but the small (but significant) picture is the T-to-R transitions in each subunit.

An important area that has not been fully defined is subunit specificity. Does oxygen (or other ligands) bind differently to α and β chains? Are the two chains equally likely to bind the first molecule of ligand? Are the pathways that lead to conformational changes identical if the first ligand bound attaches to the α or the β chains? Some of these questions have been answered for bulky ligands that fit differently in the heme slits of the α and β chains, but they have not been conclusively answered for smaller, physiologically relevant ligands, such as oxygen and carbon monoxide.

What are the Precise Structural Events Underlying Cooperativity? We will examine the conformational restraints characterizing the T and R state, the triggering mechanism at the heme, and the micropath that leads from the iron to the switching of conformers.

The critical differences between R and T conformers are confined to the areas of contact between the $\alpha_1\beta_2$ and $\alpha_2\beta_1$ dimers. The $\alpha_1\beta_1$ and $\alpha_2\beta_2$ areas of contact are essentially immobile during the conformational change, since these dimers move as a unit. These events are pictured in Figure 52-9.

Three regions of the molecule sustain the major changes during the R to T conformational change, which is a 15-degree rotation of the $\alpha_1\beta_1$ dimer with respect to the $\alpha_2\beta_1$

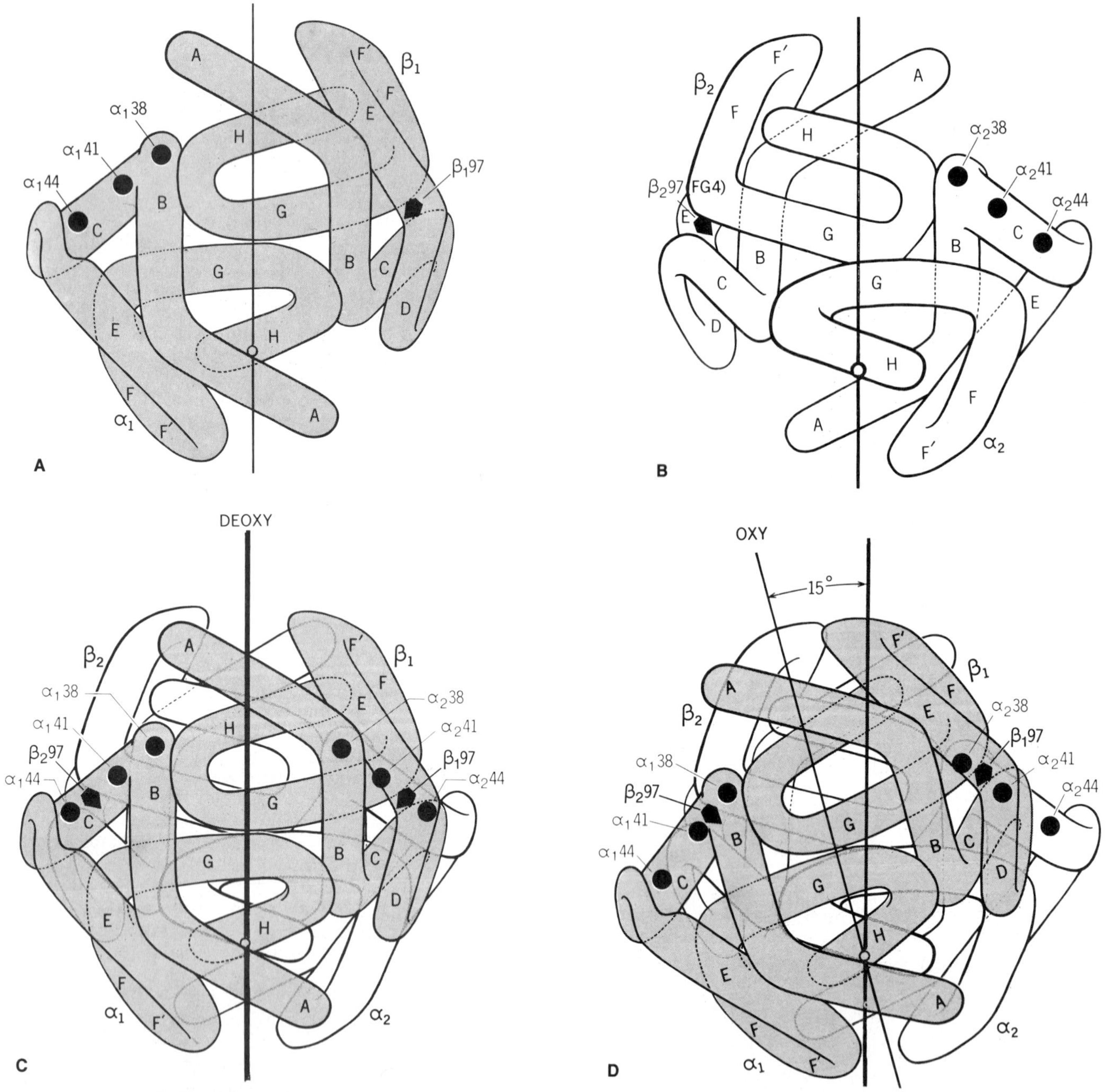

FIGURE 52-9. Subunit motion in hemoglobin. Side views of the separated $\alpha_1\beta_1$ and $\alpha_2\beta_2$ dimers and their combination into deoxyhemoglobin and oxyhemoglobin. (**A**) The $\alpha_1\beta_1$ dimer is seen from outside the molecule, and the four critical residues appear on the undersides of the helices as seen here. (**B**) The $\alpha_2\beta_2$ dimer is seen from inside the molecule. These two dimers are superimposed in **C** and **D**. Critical α-chain residues in the switch region are noted. (**C**) The complete tetramer is shown in its deoxyhemoglobin conformation. Note the position of β97 relative to α41 and α44. (**D**) In oxyhemoglobin, the $\alpha_1\beta_1$ is rotated 15 degrees relative to $\alpha_2\beta_2$. The new position of β97 is between α41 and α38. (Dickerson RE, Geis I. Hemoglobin: structure, function, evolution, and pathology. Menlo Park, CA, Benjamin/Cummings, 1983:39)

dimer around a pivot passing through the terminal portions of the H helix in both chains. The asymmetry of the pivot results in great changes (7Å translation) in the way the two β chains are deployed with respect to each other and in considerably smaller changes between the two α chains. The movements involve exclusively the residues that touch each other in the $\alpha_1\beta_2$ areas of contact. These are of two types: one between the FG corner of the β chains and the C helix of the α chains, and the other involving the FG corner of the α chains contacting the C helix of the β chains. In the pivotal sliding of the two dimers with respect to each other, the contact involving the β FG corner is farther away from the pivotal axis; therefore, the translation is farther. Baldwin and Chothia[10] have called this contact point the *switch region* (see Fig. 52-6A). The other contact is less affected, because the α FG corner is much closer to the pivotal axis. The same authors have called this area the *flexible joint*. The third important change is in the set of salt bridges between the H helix (C-terminal portion of the β chain) and the C helix of the α chain and between the C-terminal portion of the α chains and the C helix of the β chain. These contact points have no particular name, but they are referred to here as the *C-terminal changes*. Detailed residue interactions are depicted in Figure 52-9.

All these H bonds and salt bridges are broken in the oxy conformer, providing one of the most important sources of the difference in free energy between the T and R states in hemoglobin.

What Is the Triggering Mechanism at the Level of the Heme for the Conformational Change? The iron in deoxyhemoglobin is slightly out of the plane of the heme (domed configuration) because the puerile rings are also slightly pyramidal (Fig. 52-10). The angle between the heme plane and the iron is 8 degrees in the α heme and 7 degrees in the β heme. The His F8 axis is 8 degrees off center, and the Val FG5 is in contact with vinyl side chain of pyrrole 3 (Fig. 52-11). When the ligand binds the sixth coordinating position of the iron, significant stearic stresses are introduced, particularly between the heme and the proximal histidine, the ligand and the heme, and the heme and the Val FG5. To relieve this strain, the histidine moves 8 degrees to become perpendicular to the heme, significantly decreasing the doming of the iron (the angle between iron and the heme falls to 4 degrees). Also, displacement of FG5 is present in the direction of His F8. The configuration around the heme has now changed to the oxygenated or R state, and a chain of events involving the critical interactions in the $\alpha_1\beta_2$ area of contact follows.

What is the Micropath Followed by Conformational Change Extending From the Heme to the Globin? The best interpretation of the available data is the following. In the α chain, the displacement of the His F8 to straighten up its 8-degree tilt in the liganded heme requires that the F helix move with it. This displacement of the F helix along its axis is accompanied by a shift downward, which moves closer to the heme. The heme shifts toward the interior of the heme pocket. The changes in the F helix are propagated along the E and G helices, but leave the rest of the α chain unchanged. In the β subunit, the changes are similar, except that the heme also tilts around a puerile 2–4 axis. In both heme niches, the Val FG5 moves closer to the vinyl side chains; this Van der Waals contact breaks the critical H bonds between Val 98 and Tyr 145 in the β chain and between Val 98 and Tyr 140 in the α chain. The rest of the H bonds and salt bridges described before for the C terminals become weakened to the point of breakage, releasing the molecule from the T state (closed and low affinity) to the R state (open and high affinity).

The general features of this micropath for the confor-

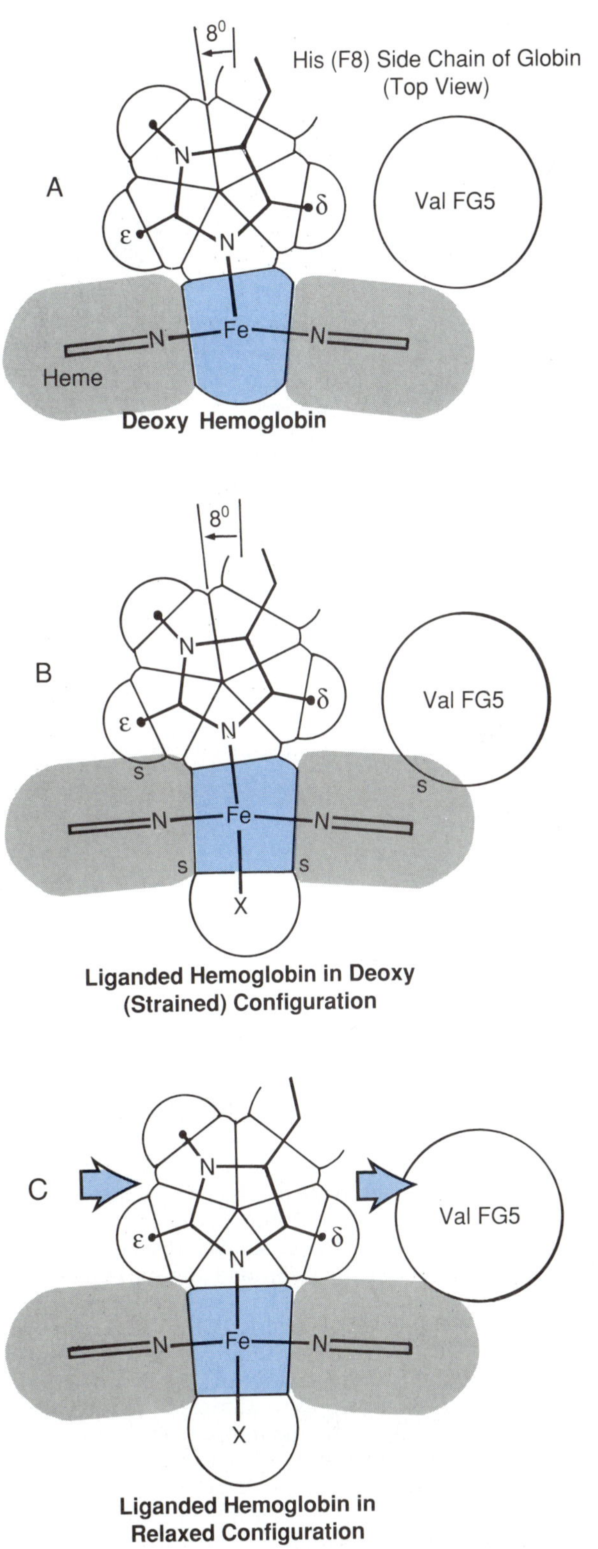

FIGURE 52-10. Ligation and strain in the heme environment. (**A**) Unliganded heme in deoxyhemoglobin, with the histidine tilted, the iron out of plane, and the heme in contact with the Val FG5 side chain. (**B**) Liganded heme held in its deoxy configuration before the T-to-R subunit transition. Steric strain (marked s) among heme, histidine, ligand (X), and valine can be relieved only after this transition. (**C**) Relaxed, unstrained liganded heme after the T-to-R shift. Both His F8 and Val FG5 have shifted to the right, and the histidine now is perpendicular to the heme plane. The heme is largely undomed. (After Dickerson RE, Geis I. Hemoglobin: structure, function, evolution, and pathology. Menlo Park, CA, Benjamin/Cummings, 1983:55)

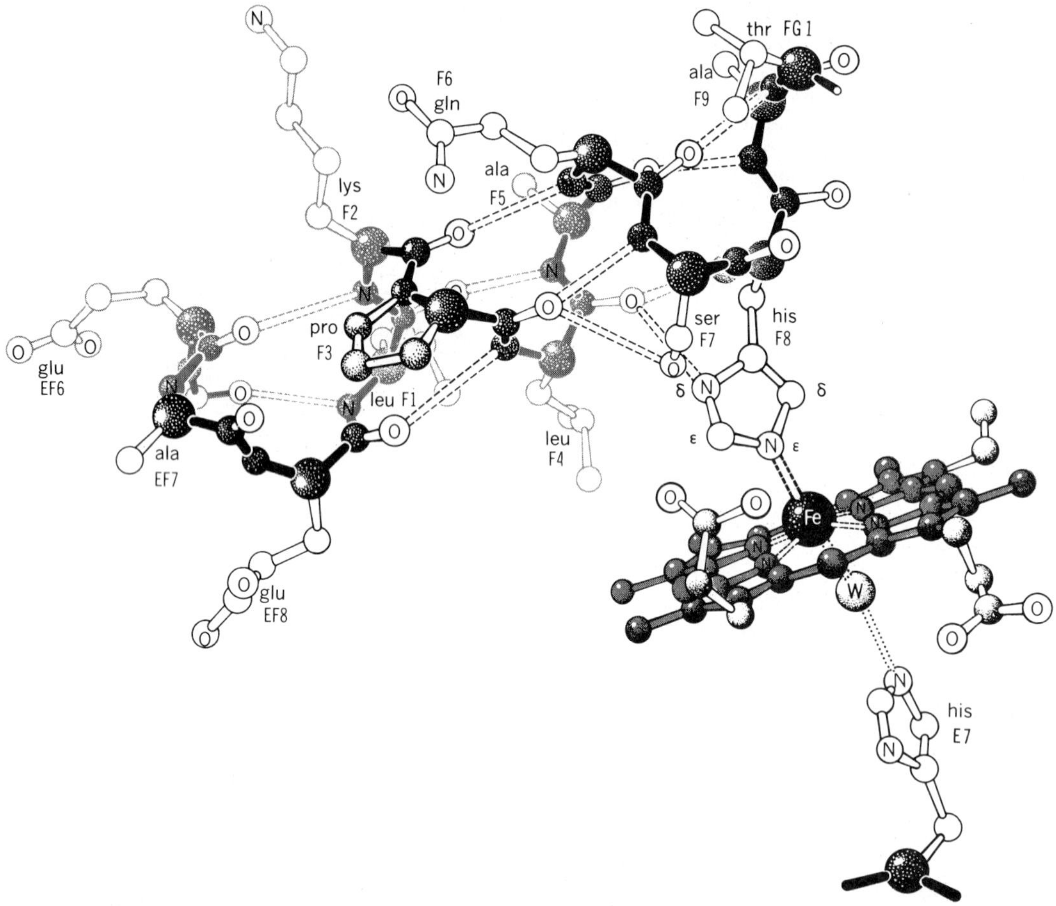

FIGURE 52-11. The F helix. Pro in position F3 interrupts the hydrogen bonding of the F helix. Because prolines lack a free NH, they can appear at the beginning of helices, but not in the middle or at the end. Prolines frequently introduce bends into the polypeptide chain. In the heme environment, octahedral coordination about the iron atom is completed in metmyoglobin by a water molecule at *W*. In deoxymyoglobin, the water molecule is gone, and in oxymyoglobin it is replaced by oxygen. The hydrogen bond between N_δ of the histidine and CO of F4 helps to hold the histidine ring rigidly in place. (Dickerson RE, Geis I. Hemoglobin: structure, function, evolution, and pathology. Menlo Park, CA, Benjamin/Cummings, 1983:27)

mational changes of hemoglobin were proposed early with insufficient evidence.[18] Significant proof had to wait for high-resolution x-ray crystallography, extended x-ray absorption fine structure (EXAFS), and the experiments of Perutz and associates.[19–21]

Hemoglobin Binds CO_2 While It Is Delivering Oxygen and Releases CO_2 When It Is Binding Oxygen. The hemoglobin molecule is designed to bind CO_2 after delivering oxygen to the tissues, helping to dissipate the increase in concentration of CO_2 in the tissues and conveniently delivering this metabolic end product to the alveoli of the lungs. It accomplishes this particular task with ease because CO_2 is an allosteric inhibitor of hemoglobin, decreasing the oxygen affinity of the molecule.

CO_2 binds hemoglobin by forming carbamates with the α amino groups of the α chains. Through this new negative charge, CO_2 can bind Arg 141 in the absence of Cl^- ions. This bond stabilizes the T conformer and decreases the oxygen affinity of the molecule.[22,23] The basic reaction is:

$$Hb-NH_2 + CO_2 \rightarrow Hb-NH-COO^- + H^+$$

Although CO_2 also binds the α amino groups of the β chains, helping to transport more of this metabolic end product, the reaction does not contribute to the allosteric effect. The β-chain carbamate reaction favors the deoxy conformer by the production of H^+, but this effect is counteracted by the reduction of positive charges in the central cavity, an event that favors the R state. Nothing gained, nothing lost.

Hemoglobin Binds H^+ Efficiently in a Low pH Environment and Releases Protons When It Encounters High pH (Bohr Effect). The Bohr effect describes the changes of oxygen affinity secondary to pH changes exhibited by hemoglobin. Within a certain range, the lower the pH the lower the affinity or the higher the p50.[24–27] That is, an increased concentration of protons favors a low-affinity state in hemoglobin. Deoxyhemoglobin binds more protons than the oxy conformer, which means that in the absence of a buffer, a ligand change in hemoglobin can be recorded by a change in the solution pH (Haldane effect).

All the features described in the previous paragraph are the consequence of H^+ ions acting as allosteric inhibitors: H^+ binds more avidly to the deoxy conformer (T state) than the oxy state. The so-called Bohr protons (protons released during oxygenation) originate primarily from the breakage of the C-terminal bonds during ligand binding (Fig. 52-12).

Seventy percent of the Bohr effect is derived from the differences in the pK of the following residues when the molecule changes from the oxy to the deoxy conformation: (1) the two terminal histidines of the β chains (His β146), which Kilmartin[24] has determined account for 40% of the Bohr protons; (2) the α amino groups of the two N-terminal

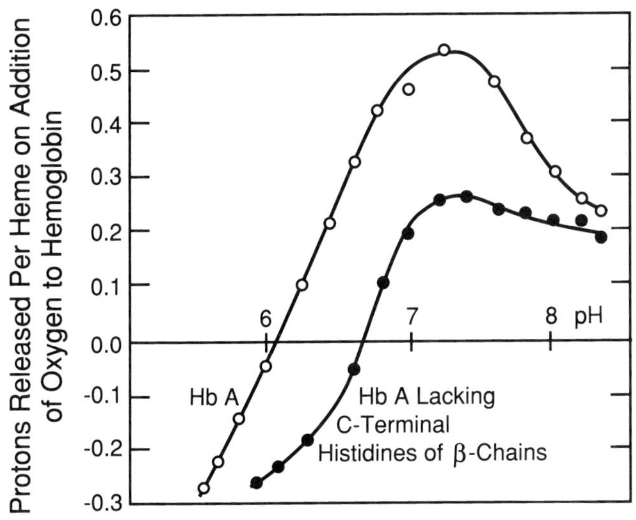

FIGURE 52-12. Discharge of protons on uptake of oxygen (Bohr effect) by normal human hemoglobin A and hemoglobin from which the C-terminal histidines of the β chains have been cleaved with carboxypeptidase B (des His 146β hemoglobin). Note the reversal of the alkaline Bohr effect at pH 6.0 in Hb A and at the pH 6.7 in des His hemoglobin and the halving of the alkaline Bohr effect in the latter. (After Kilmartin JV, Wootton JF. Inhibition of Bohr effect after removal of C-terminal histidines from haemoglobin β chains. Nature 1970;228:766)

residues (Val 1) of the α chains (25%); and (3) His α122, which Nishikura has found contributes 10% of the Bohr protons (although no rationale for this effect has been found). The remaining 25% is probably derived from several residues, including His β143, Lys β144, and other surface histidines.

The Oxygen Affinity of Hemoglobin is Modulated by Other Allosteric Effectors, Such as 2,3-DPG and Cl^-. In addition to H^+ and CO_2, other intraerythrocytic components also act as allosteric effectors. The Beneshes[28] discovered the effects of 2,3-DPG on the function of hemoglobin when they noticed, while examining tabular data in preparation for a lecture to medical students, that this intraerythrocytic organic phosphate was almost equimolar to hemoglobin. Oxygen equilibrium measurements in the presence and absence of 2,3-DPG rapidly demonstrated that this effector drastically displaces the p50 of hemoglobin (partial pressure of oxygen at which hemoglobin is half saturated) to the right, making the hemoglobin less avid for the ligand.

Independently and simultaneously, Chanutin and Curnish,[29] who were close to retirement after many years of studying organic polyphosphates, realized that these substances have an important biologic effect on the red blood cell. These discoveries were followed by the finding that inositol hexaphosphate, a higher-level polyphosphate than 2,3-DPG, and a more powerful effector, has the same function as 2,3-DPG, but at lower concentrations, in the red cells of birds. Finally, in some fish, red cell adenosine triphosphate (ATP) or guanosine triphosphate seem to be the physiologic oxygen modulators.

In an allosteric model, the effector must bind differentially to each one of the conformational states. For an effector to be an inhibitor (a molecule that decreases the activity of the molecule—in this case the oxygen affinity), it must bind more strongly to the T form. Crystallographic evidence of Arnone[30] has demonstrated that 2,3-DPG binds to the central cavity of hemoglobin, that is, the space surrounding the true diad axis of symmetry between the two β chains (Fig. 52-13). The displacement of the β chains away from each other by 7Å in deoxyhemoglobin makes this single site in the tetramer capable of accommodating the highly negatively charged 2,3-DPG molecule, whereas the tighter $\beta\beta$ interaction in oxyhemoglobin does not allow the effector to penetrate the central cavity. The five negative charges of 2,3-DPG find proper positive charges to form salt bridges just under the edge of the central cavity between the β chains. The globin residues involved in the binding are the two amino terminals of the α and β chains, the two β143 histidines, and one of the two β82 lysines.

This site in the central cavity is the only binding site for 2,3-DPG in hemoglobin; therefore, one 2,3-DPG molecule binds per tetramer of hemoglobin. This is unusual, since in hemoglobin, because of its 222 symmetry, most binding sites have an equivalent counterpart on the other side of the molecule. The central cavity is the exception, reinforcing that this molecule does not have perfect 222 symmetry due to the nonidentity of the α and β chains. The other end of the central cavity, surrounded by α chains, does not move apart much during deoxygenation, as previously discussed, and does not form a proper binding site for 2,3-DPG.

The purpose of this effector is to modulate the oxygen equilibrium curve according to physiologic requirements. For example, in anemia the synthesis of 2,3-DPG increases, favoring the release of oxygen and partially coping with the decrease in the number of oxygen carriers.

Chloride (Cl^-) is another allosteric inhibitor of hemoglobin. It also decreases the oxygen affinity of the molecule. Two mechanisms are involved. Cl^- binds preferentially to the deoxy conformer, the classic mechanism by which allosteric inhibitors work in hemoglobin. As noted earlier, Arg α141, among its many interactions, forms a salt bridge with the amino terminals of the opposite α chain across the $\alpha_1\beta_1$ area of contact through a Cl^- ion (Fig. 52-14). These bonds are broken in the oxy conformer and the binding of Cl^- is no longer possible. The other type of Cl^- binding to hemoglobin is less clear. Bonaventura and colleagues[31] have found that anions, including Cl^-, in the absence of 2,3-DPG can bind the positive charges available in the central cavity. This binding might not affect the oxygen affinity of hemoglobin through the T-to-R conversion, since the same effect is observed in isolated chains. The physical basis of this effect remains unresolved.

Oxygen Transport by the Red Cell

Oxygen-Binding Properties of the Red Cell

The oxygen equilibrium of red cells depends on (1) the intrinsic oxygen affinity of the hemoglobin molecule (determined in solutions stripped of phosphate), (2) intraerythrocytic pH, (3) the intraerythrocytic concentration of 2,3-DPG, (4) temperature, and (5) pCO_2.

Intraerythrocytic pH. The Bohr effect of whole blood is remarkably similar to hemoglobin in solution. For normal blood (37°C and 40 mmHg of CO_2), the log p50/pH is close to 0.5. Intracellular pH is 0.2 units below the extracellular pH, determined by the concentration of permeant ions H^+, OH^-, Cl^-, and bicarbonate and the the major impermeant ions, hemoglobin itself and 2,3-DPG.

The concentrations of solutes inside and outside the red cell follow the Gibbs–Donnan relation that requires electroneutrality and due consideration to activity coefficient differences in the two compartments. As hemoglobin and 2,3-DPG, which are negatively charged at pH 7.4, are trapped inside the red cell, erythrocyte Cl^- concentration has to be decreased; thus, the ratio of 0.7 between intracellular and extracellular Cl^-. Calculation of the Gibbs–Donnan equilibrium predicts the observed 0.2 pH unit difference between the inside and outside of the red cell, sug-

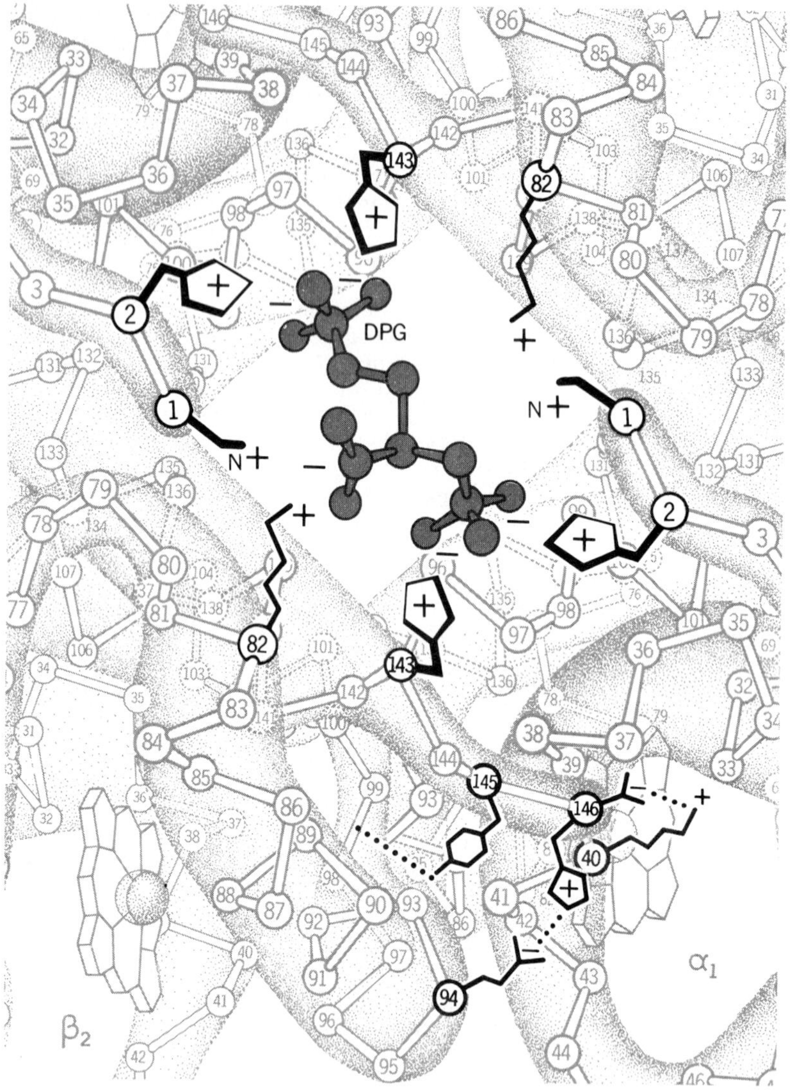

FIGURE 52-13. Amino acid side chains around the 2,3-diphosphoglycerate (2,3-DPG) binding site. This top view of the central cavity in human deoxyhemoglobin shows the positive charges lining the DPG site: two each from the amino terminal (Val β1), from His β2, from Lys β82, and from His β143. The DPG molecule with its five negative charges sits in the middle of this ring of positive charges. The fetal γ chain loses two of its eight positive charges by substituting Ser for His at β143, decreasing the affinity for DPG. Also shown are the salt bridges and the hydrogen-bonding pattern around the carboxyl terminus of the β chain (*lower part of figure*), which emphasizes their contribution to the Bohr effect. (Dickerson RE, Geis I. Hemoglobin: structure, function, evolution, and pathology. Menlo Park, CA, Benjamin/Cummings, 1983:44)

gesting that no significant participant is missing in this phenomenon.

2,3-DPG. The normal level of red cell 2,3-DPG is 12.8 (μmol/g hemoglobin) for males and 13.8 (μmol/g hemoglobin) for females for the Sigma kit that is based on the method of Rose.[32] Children younger than 5 years of age and elderly patients have increased and decreased levels of 2,3-DPG, respectively.[33,34] This amount makes the organic phosphate almost equimolar with hemoglobin in red cells, whereas in other cells it exists in very small concentrations.

Metabolically, 2,3-DPG is generated by the Rapoport–Luebering shunt from 1,3-DPG by DPG synthase or mutase. Its level depends on the rates of synthesis and hydrolysis. The rate of synthesis is complex and depends on the amount of the substrate 1,3-DPG generated by glycolysis, which in turn increases directly with pH, and the amount of 1,3-DPG entering the Rapoport–Luebering shunt. The alternative pathway for 1,3-DPG, and the most energetic, is to be converted into 3-phosphoglycerate and generate an ATP molecule. This alternative is probably greatly affected by the activity of the synthase, which is stimulated in direct proportion to the red cell pH and is under end-product inhibition by the concentration of 2,3-DPG.

Hypoxia has a tremendous impact on these relations, and Duhm has put together a scheme that clarifies the consequence of acidosis and alkalosis (Fig. 52-15), an event of significant clinical implications.

Temperature. The p50 of blood is almost doubled by an increase of 10°C (between 20° and 30°C). This seems appropriate to deal with hypothermia and hyperthermia. Cold decreases metabolic requirements and reduces the need for oxygen. During fever, metabolism is increased dramatically, and an increase in the delivery of oxygen is required. The basis for this phenomenon is primarily the temperature-induced changes on the hemoglobin molecule.

Oxygen Transport to the Tissues

The fundamental relation that describes the delivery of oxygen to the tissues is the Fick equation:

$$V_{O_2} = 0.139(Q)(Hb)(Sa_{O_2} - SV_{O_2})$$

which says that the amount of oxygen delivered to the tissues (V_{O_2}) in liters per minute is the product of three independent variables: (1) the blood flow (Q); (2) the amount of O_2 carried by that flow, which is the product of 0.139 and the grams of hemoglobin (1.39 is the amount of oxygen, in millimeters of mercury, that a fully saturated gram of hemoglobin is capable of carrying); and (3) the extraction of oxygen at the level of the tissues, which is the difference

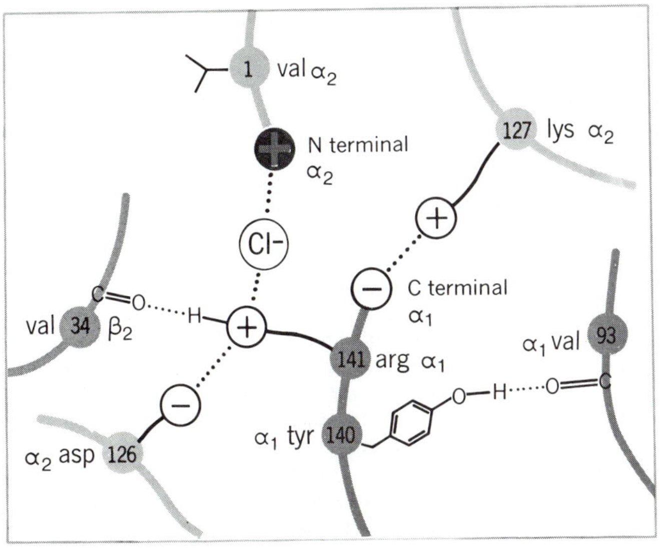

FIGURE 52-14. Salt bridges and hydrogen bonds (the distinction is often unclear from radiographic analyses) between other groups and the N-terminal and C-terminal residues in the α chains of deoxyhemoglobin. All these bonds are ruptured in oxyhemoglobin. A shift to the oxy configuration brings the α carboxy terminals closer together. The side chain of Arg $\alpha_1$141(HC3) is squeezed out, rupturing all the bonds shown. One of the two groups that contribute to the Bohr effect by becoming partially deprotonated in the oxy configuration is shown by a black-encircled plus sign. (Dickerson RE, Geis I. Hemoglobin: structure, function, evolution, and pathology. Menlo Park, CA, Benjamin/Cummings, 1983:45)

between the saturations of the arterial blood and the mixed venous blood.

The consequence of this analysis is that when regulation of oxygen release is desired, it is best done in the following areas:

Blood flow (Q): This is in turn affected by cardiac output and by microcirculatory size and distribution

Hemoglobin concentration (Hb): The red cell mass is the balance between erythropoiesis and red cell destruction and is actively regulated by erythropoietin. This hormone responds to hypoxia detected in the postarterial side of the renal circulation by a detection system that has not been defined.

Oxygen extraction by the tissues ($S_aO_2 - S_vO_2$): This parameter depends on the shape of the oxygen equilibrium curve, as discussed previously, and on tissue PO_2. The determinants of tissue PO_2 and its regulation are poorly understood.

MOLECULAR PATHOLOGY AND THE PATHOPHYSIOLOGY OF HEMOGLOBIN ABNORMALITIES

High Ligand Affinity Hemoglobins: Erythrocytosis

Structural Defects

Mutations resulting in changes in the primary structure of the α or β chains can lead to changes in the affinity toward ligand of these hemoglobin variants. Increases in the oxygen affinity of hemoglobin can come about by various mechanisms. In most instances, the changes in oxygen affinity are in concordance with our understanding of the structural–functional relations in hemoglobin. In a few instances, the known alterations of the primary structure are not sufficient to explain the observed effect, given the state of our knowledge.

The mutations that generate high-affinity hemoglobins can arise from single-point substitutions, double-point substitutions (although some of these could be crossover events between two mutated chains), deletions, additions, frameshift mutations, and fusion genes.

The molecular mechanisms of ligand high-affinity hemoglobin mutants are summarized here and described in the following sections (for some high-affinity hemoglobins, there is no explanation for their functional behavior):

- Alteration of the switch region, the flexible joint, or the C terminals in the $\alpha_1\beta_2$ area of contact that favor

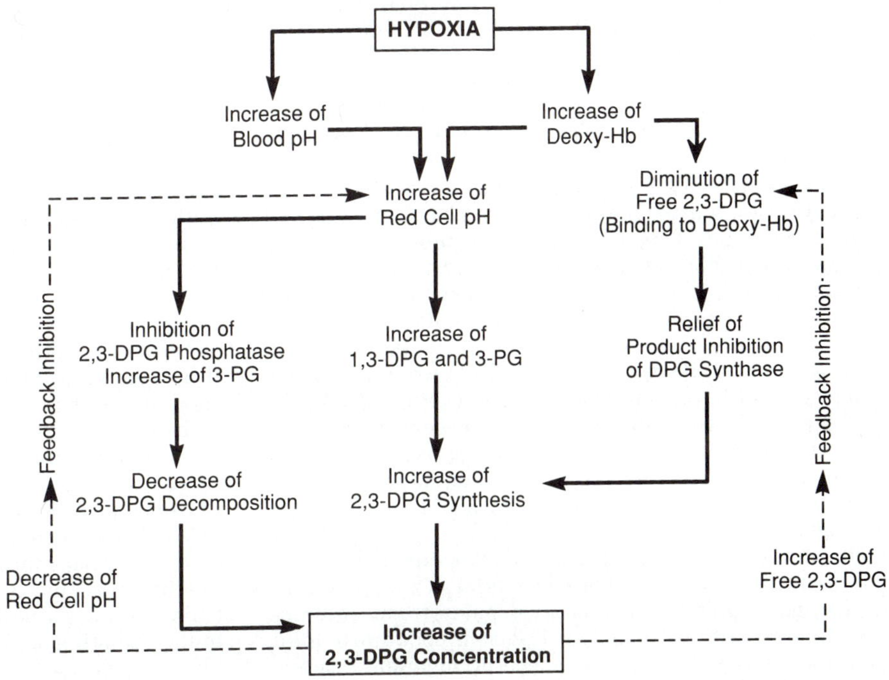

FIGURE 52-15. Effect of hypoxia on red cell pH and 2,3-diphosphoglycerate (DPG). (After Bunn HF, Forget BG. Hemoglobin: molecular, genetic, and clinical aspects. Philadelphia, WB Saunders, 1986)

the R state, either by stabilizing this conformer or by destabilizing the T state

- Alteration of the $\alpha_1\beta_1$ area of contact with disruption of the overall architecture of hemoglobin that favors the R state
- Mutations that decrease the affinity of hemoglobin for 2,3-DPG
- Reducing heme interaction by restraining the quaternary conformation through polymerization
- Elengation of the globin chain, disrupting the quaternary structure

Alterations of the Switch Region, Flexible Joint, or C Terminals in the $\alpha_1\beta_2$ Area of Contact. These alterations favor the R state, either by stabilizing this conformer or by destabilizing the T state. *Hb Poissy* (β56 (D7)Gly → Arg and 86(F2) Ala → Pro)[35] is a double-site mutation; one mutation (at the β56 site Arg) had been described previously as *Hb Hamadan, exhibiting* no functional abnormalities. When a second case was found in 1982 in France, the patient exhibited erythrocytosis and red cells with a high affinity for oxygen. A discrepancy that needed explanation was apparent. Recent reexamination of the structure of the mutation by high-performance liquid chromatography (HPLC) methods revealed that the French propositus carries a β chain with two mutations, one identical with Hb Hamadan and the other an electrophoretically silent mutation in the same β chain but at position 86, in which an alanine has been substituted by a proline. This new hemoglobin has a three-fold increase in oxygen affinity, with a low n (Hill) coefficient and a diminished Bohr effect. It also shows a biphasic curve in the autoxidation rate, suggesting a great inequivalency in the propensity for methemoglobin formation (conversion of heme iron from ferrous to ferric) of the α and β hemes. NMR studies in this mutant suggest that the helix-breaking proline residue displaces the F helix toward the heme, destabilizing this helix toward the critical FG corner. This interferes with the $\alpha_1\beta_2$ contact area, favors the R state, and modifies the environment of the hemes.

Hb Chesapeake (α92(FG4) Arg → Leu)[37–39] was the first high-affinity mutant described in a classic paper by Charache and colleagues.[38] At pH 8.61, it is a fast-moving electrophoretic variant, representing about 20% of the hemolysate. It has a moderately high oxygen affinity (whole blood Po_2: 19 mmHg) and normal Bohr and 2,3-DPG effects, and it produces moderate erythrocytosis. It involves a substitution of an invariant residue (a residue in most α chains analyzed regardless of species). The molecular mechanism is the stabilization of the R state at the level of the $\alpha_1\beta_2$ area of contact.

Hb J Capetown (α92(FG4) Arg → Gln) occurs at the same site as Hb Chesapeake and has similar characteristics, although the stabilization of the R state is probably less significant. The initial report that this abnormal hemoglobin had a very low n value, proved to be incorrect.[40] The observation was based on total hemolysate data that corresponded to the addition of two curves with a very displaced p50, but a not so different n value.[41] The copresence of two hemoglobins (the patient was a heterozygote)—Hb A and Hb Capetown—generates a flattened oxygen equilibrium curve since Hb Capetown begins loading oxygen first because of its high affinity. From this combination curve, a reliable n value cannot be calculated for each individual hemoglobin.

Hb Nunobiki (α141(HC3) Arg → Cys) is one of four mutations at the same site, all of which exhibit a high affinity for oxygen, significantly decreased heterotropic interactions (effect of H^+, Cl^-, and 2,3-DPG), and moderate to mild erythrocytosis.[42] The mutation affects an invariant residue. Hb Nunobiki merits special mention. At pH 8.6, Hb Nunobiki is an electrophoretically fast-moving abnormal hemoglobin, expressed at a low level (13%). Most α-chain abnormalities represent 20% to 25% of the hemolysate, since they are produced by one of four α genes.

The consequences of the presence of the cysteine residue in position α141 are varied. First, during storage the hemoglobin changes mobility (becomes faster), presumably through the oxidation of the cysteine residue to a negatively charged sulfoxide ($-SO^-$) or sulfitic acid ($-SOO^-$). Second, Hb Nunobiki is more resistant to autoxidation, probably because of two circumstances: the protection toward oxidants rendered by its high-affinity status and the addition of a new site (cysteine residue) for the consumption of the oxidants. Third, the low percentage of the α mutant is explained by the fact that it is a mutant of the α_1 gene (closest to the 3′ region of the cluster), which Orkin has shown to be expressed one third to two thirds less than the α_2 gene. Finally, as with other mutations of the N-terminal end of the α chains, Hb Nunobiki produces little erythrocytosis in spite of its high affinity, because of the low percentage that is present in the red cells. The high ligand affinity is due to the breaking of the C-terminal-to-C-terminal salt bridge indispensable for the stabilization of the T state. Hence, the R state is greatly favored.

There are six known mutations of the β99(Gl) site: *Hb Kempsey* (Asp → Asn) (β99)[43]; *Hb Yakima* (Asp → His)[36,44]; *Hb Radcliffe* (Asp → Ala)[45]; *Hb Ypsilanti* (Asp → Tyr)[46]; *Hb Hotel-Dieu* (Asp → Gly)[47]; and *Hb Chemilly* (Asp → Val).[48] These five electrophoretically apparent mutations constitute about 40% to 50% of the hemolysate, exhibit moderately high oxygen affinity, show a 25% to 60% decrease in the Bohr effect, exhibit clinically apparent erythrocytosis, and are the molecular consequence of disturbances in the $\alpha_1\beta_2$ area of contact. In Hb Yakima, as determined by x-ray crystallography of the deoxy form, the intersubunit deoxy bonds between β99(Gl) and αC7 and αG4 are broken, a situation that favors the R or oxy conformation. More recently, crystallography of CO Hb Ypsilanti, another mutation of β99, has disclosed an important characteristic of this mutant. At a 3-Å resolution, it appears that CO Hb Ypsilanti has a feature never before observed in abnormal hemoglobins: a different and stable quaternary structure along the $\alpha_1\beta_1$ area of contact. The two stable dimers in the liganded form of carboxyhemoglobin (CO Hb) Ypsilanti rotate beyond the limit observed in the R/T difference. The consequence of this rotation is that many of the salt bridges stabilizing the R structure are lost, but the H bonding between Asp β94 and β102 is retained and new bonds are formed by the mutated Tyr β99 with Asn α97 and Thr α38. This new quaternary conformation, baptized as Y by authors to differentiate it from the R and T conformers, could be a transient conformation attained during the normal RT transition that is stabilized by the mutation.

The response to 2,3-DPG is moderately decreased in Hb Kempsey and Hb Radcliffe and is slightly decreased in Hb Hotel Dieu. In other mutations, it has not been measured. It is interesting that Hb Ypsilanti and Hb Radcliffe form stable hybrids in the hemolysates in which the abnormal β chains coexist with normal β chains.

Three mutations are described for site β146 (HC3): *Hb Hiroshima* (His → Asp)[49,50]; *Hb York* (His → Pro); and *Hb Cowtown* (His → Leu). These hemoglobins are detectable by electrophoresis, and Hb Hiroshima also by cellulose acetate. They have moderately increased oxygen affinity and a Bohr effect that is half-normal (Fig. 52-16). In addition, Hb Cowtown has a decreased 2,3-DPG effect. All of these mutants disrupt a T-state salt bridge and eliminate the residue originating 50% of the Bohr protons. The decrease of

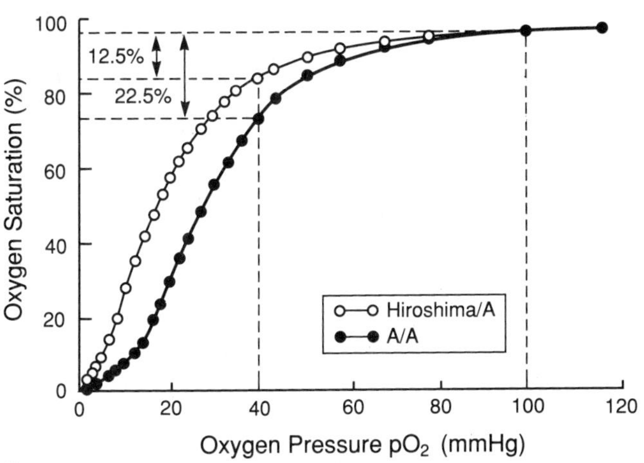

FIGURE 52-16. Oxygen equilibrium curves of red cells from a healthy person (A/A) and that of an Hb Hiroshima heterozygote (Hiroshima/A). Oxygen pressure is plotted against oxygen saturation. Vertical dotted lines mark the typical PO_2 of the lungs (100 mmHg) and of the tissues (40 mmHg). Horizontal dotted lines mark the oxygen extraction (lungs − tissues) for normal red cells (22.5%) and the reduction observed for the high-affinity red cells (12%).

the 2,3-DPG binding might be secondary to the reduction of positive charges in the central cavity or to the destabilization of the T state.

Alteration of the $\alpha_1\beta_1$ Area of Contact With Disruption of the Overall Architecture of Hemoglobin That Favors the R State. *Hb San Diego* (β109[Gll] Val → Met) is an electrophoretically silent mutation with moderately high oxygen affinity, a normal Bohr effect and clinically apparent erythrocytosis.[51] The molecular mechanism probably involves a stearic hindrance, induced by the larger bulk of methionine, compared with valine in the $\alpha_1\beta_1$ contact, particularly in the deoxy configuration. This biases the molecule toward the R state.

Mutations That Decrease the Affinity of Hemoglobin for 2,3-DPG. Three mutations of β82(EF6) have been described: *Hb Rahere* (Lys → Thr)[52]; *Hb Helsinki* (Lys → Met)[53]; and *Hb Providence* (Lys → Asn → Asp).[54,55] All these mutants have moderately high oxygen affinity and moderate erythrocytosis. Hb Helsinki, in addition, has a mild decrease in the Bohr effect. In Hb Providence, the new Asn suffers deamination in vivo, generating an Asp (electrophoretically detectable). All these mutants have drastically reduced 2,3-DPG binding due to the elimination of one of the normal binding sites for this allosteric effect. This position in the β chains involves an invariant residue, suggesting the importance that nature places on the binding of polyphosphates.

Reduction of Heme Interaction by Restraining the Quaternary Conformation Through Polymerization. *Hb Porto Alegre* (β9[A6] Ser → Cys) is an extremely interesting mutant with higher than normal oxygen affinity and a tendency to aggregate.[56,57] No erythrocytosis is apparent in the carriers. The polymerization of Hb Porto Alegre is based on the formation of −S−S− bonds in oxygenated samples, and thus is different from Hb S. The polymerization of this mutant diminishes heme–heme interaction and increases the oxygen affinity. This is a unique molecular mechanism.

Hb Olympia (β20[B2] Val → Met) is a hard to detect silent mutation (not detectable by isoelectric focusing) that produces moderate erythrocytosis because of a moderately increased oxygen affinity with a normal Bohr effect.[58,59] Difficulties in isolation impaired the study of this mutation. It is particularly intriguing because the mutation affects an exterior residue that is not involved in any of the areas of contact associated with quaternary conformational changes. However, the mystery has been solved. Using a case of β-thalassemia associated with Hb Olympia in a Greek person (thus an almost pure solution of Hb Olympia hemolysate), Edelstein and colleagues[59] confirmed its high affinity, low *n* value, and normal heterotropic interactions with 2,3-DPG and Cl^-. In addition, detailed analysis of the oxygen equilibrium curve showed a pH dependency of the *n* value, suggesting that the tetramer molecules self-aggregate in the deoxy state at a high pH. This was confirmed with centrifugation studies in the liganded and unliganded states. Small-angle diffraction studies need to be done to determine the actual size of the aggregate.[59]

Elongation of the Globin Chain Disrupting the Quaternary Structure. *Hb Tak* is an abnormal hemoglobin that corresponds to an elongation of the β chains by 11 residues (157 residues total) probably due to unequal crossing-over.[60–62] The abnormal hemoglobin constitutes 40% of the hemolysate, has a high oxygen affinity with no cooperativity (n = 0), and no allosteric effects with pH or 2,3-DPG. This is not surprising since the C terminal of the β chain is actively involved in the conformational changes of the hemoglobin molecule by stabilizing the T state. Hence, Hb Tak, by having these stabilizing interactions disrupted, is totally frozen in the R state. It is also slightly unstable. In spite of these severe functional abnormalities, the heterozygous patient exhibited no erythrocytosis. This puzzling situation could be explained by the extraordinarily biphasic oxygen affinity curve observed with mixtures of Hb Tak and Hb A, suggesting that no hybrid formation is present. The top portion of the oxygen equilibrium curve of the mixture is normal and begins to be abnormal only below 40% saturation. As physiologic oxygen exchange occurs (most frequently above that level of saturation), the tissues might not be aware of the presence of the abnormal hemoglobin.

Hb Saverne corresponds to an elongation of the β chains, probably because of a frameshift mutation involving a deletion of the second base of the triplet coding for His143.[63,64] New residues are added for a total of 156. This abnormal hemoglobin is 30% of the hemolysate, has a slightly faster electrophoretic mobility than Hb A, has a high oxygen affinity, lacks cooperativity, and has a low Bohr effect. Again, the disruption of the C terminals due to the excess residues also disrupts the stabilization of the T conformer, favoring the R state. The patient has a compensated hemolytic anemia that could be the consequence of the conflicting effects of high affinity and instability.

Another extended chain has been described, *Hb Thionville*, which has intrinsically high affinity due to changes in the $\alpha_1\beta_1$ contact surface, but because it is an α-chain abnormality, it is expressed only at a 21% level and does not reach functional importance or cause clinical consequences. Nevertheless, this abnormality illuminates another feature of hemoglobin synthesis. In humans, globin translation is initiated by a methionine residue that is cleaved after the chain has reached about 30 amino acids by the enzyme methionine aminopeptidase. If a charged amino acid is introduced as in α Thionville, the cleavage does not take place and there is one amino acid extension at the N terminal. In the β chain, this same phenomenon has been described in *Hb Doha*. In another case, the β_1 valine is replaced by methionine (*Hb South Florida*). The posttranslation modification continues because a globin chain with an N-terminal methionine is acetylated when the chain reaches about 50 residues in length. As discussed below, N-terminal valine strongly inhibits acetylation, as demonstrated in normal α and β chains, whereas Met–Glu

(text continues on page 1611)

TABLE 52-3. High-Affinity Hemoglobins

	Mutation	Name	Hb Level and Additional Properties
α SITES			
α 2 (NA2)	Leu → Arg	Chongqing	UN
α6 (A4)	Asp → Ala	Sawara	
	Asp → Asn	Dunn	
	Asp → Val	Ferndown	
	Asp → Tyr	Woodville	
	Asp → Gly	Swan River	
α14 (A12)	Trp → Arg	Evanston	
α16 (A14)	Lys → Met	Harbin	UN
α40 (C5)	Lys → Glu	Kariya	UN
	Lys → Met	Kanagawa	
α44 (CE2)	Pro → Leu	Milledgeville	
	Pro → Arg	Kawachi	
α45 (CE3)	His → Arg	Fort de France	
α84 (F5)	Ser → Arg	Etobioke	
α85 (F6)	Asp → Asn	G-Norfolk	
	Asp → Tyr	Atago	
	Asp → Val	Inksten	
α88 (F9)	Ala → Ser	Loire	
	Ala → Val	Columbia-Missouri	
α90 (FG2)	Lys → Met	Handa Munakate	
α92 (FG5)	Arg → Gln	J Capetown	
	Arg → Ser	Chesapeake	
α95 (G2)	Pro → Ala	Denmark Hill	
	Pro → Ser	Rampa	
	Pro → Arg	St Lukes	
	Pro → Leu	G-Georgia	
α97 (G4)	Asn → His	Dallas	
α126 (H9)	Asp → His	Sassai	
	Asp → Asn	Tarrant	
	Asp → Val	Fukitomi	Hb: 15–19
	Asp → Tyr	Montefiore	
α138 (H21)	Ser → Pro	Attleboro	
α139 (HCl)	Lys → Thr	Tokoname	
	Lys → Glu	Hanamaki	
α140-α141	(Tyr-Arg) → O	Natal	
α141 (HC3)	Arg → His	Suresnes	Hb: 15–19
	Arg → Cys	Nunobiki	
	Arg → leu	Legnano	Hb: 16–20
β2 (NA2)	His → Arg	Deer Lodge	
	His → Gln	Okayama	
β9 (A6)	Ser → Cys	Porto Alegre	Polym
β17-18	(Lys-Val) → O	Lyon	
β20 (B2)	Val → Met	Olympia	
β23 (B5)	Val → O	Freiburg	
	Val → Asp	Strasbourg	
	Val → Phe	Palmerston North	
β27 (B9)	Ala → Val	Grange Blanche	
β34 (B16)	Val → Phe	Pitie-Salpetriere	Hb: 17–20
β36 (C2)z	Pro → Ser	North Chicago	
β37 (C3)	Trp → Ser	Hirose	Dissoc
β40 (C6)	Arg → Lys	Athens-Ga, Waco	Dissoc
	Arg → Ser	Austin	
β51 (D2)	Pro → Arg	Williamette	UN
β68 (E12)	Leu → His	Brisbane, Great Lakes	HB: 15–20; UN

(continued)

TABLE 52-3. *(Continued)*

	Mutation	Name	Hb Level and Additional Properties
β79 (EF3)	Asp → Gly	G-Hsi-Tsou	
β82 (EF6)	Lys → Thr	Rahere	Hb: 19
	Lys → Met	Helsinki	Hb: 14–17
β86 (F2)	Ala → Asp	Olomouc	
β87 (F3)	Thr → O	Tours	
β89 (F5)	Ser → Asn	Creteil	
	Ser → Arg	Vanderbilt	Hb: 19–22
β90 (F6)	Gly → Asp	Pierre Benite	
β93 (F9)	Cys → Arg	Okazaki	
β94 (FG1)	Asp → His	Barcelona	Hb: 18
	Asp → Asn	Bunbury	
β96 (FG3)	Leu → Val	Regina	
β97 (FG4)	His → Gln	Malmo	Hb: 17–21
	His → Leu	Wood	Hb: 17–22
	His → Pro	Nagoya	UN
β99 (G1)	Asp → Asn	Kempsey	Hb: 17–20
	Asp → His	Yakima	Hb: 16–18
	Asp → Ala	Radcliffe	Hb: 17–19
	Asp → Tyr	Ypsilanti	Hb: 15–19
	Asp → Gly	Hotel-Dieu	Hb: 20–24
	Asp → Val	Chemilly	Hb: 19
	Asp → Glu	Cormora	
β100 (G2)	Pro → Leu	Brighham	Hb: 16–18
β101 (G3)	Glu → Lys	British	Hb: 17
	Glu → Gly	Columbia Alberta	Hb: 20
	Glu → Asp	Potomac	Hb: 17–19
β103 (G5)	Phe → Leu	Heathrow	Hb: 16–21
β105 (G7)	Leu → Phe	South Milwaukee	
β109 (G11)	Val → Met	San Dlego	Hb: 16–18
	Val → Leu	Johnston	
β124 (H2)	Pro → Gln	Ty Gard	Hb: 19
β140 (HC2)	(Tyr-Arg) → O	Natal	
β141 (HC3)			
β140 (H18)	Ala → Thr	Saint Jacques	Hb: 19
β142 (H20)	Ala → Asp	Ohio	Hb: 19–20
β143 (H21)	His → Arg	Abruzzo	
	His → Gln	Little Rock	Hb: 20–13
	His → Pro	Syracuse	Hb: 19–24
	His → Asp	Rancho Mirage	
β144 (HCl)	Lys → Asn	Andrew-Minneapolis	Hb:20
	Lys → Glu	Mito	
β145 (HC2)	Tyr → His	Bethesda	Hb: 16–21
	Tyr → Cys	Rainier	Hb:17–21; AKR
	Tyr → Asp	Fort Gordon	Hb: 17–23
	Tyr → Term	Osler, Nancy McKees Rocks	Hb: 18–21
β146 (HC3)	His → Asp	Hiroshima	Hb: 15–17
	His → Pro	York	
	His → Leu	Cowtown	Hb: 18–19
	His → Gln	Kodaira	
INSERTIONS			
144 Lys-Ser-Ile-Thr-150 Lys-Leu-Ala-Phe-Leu-Leu-Ser-Asn 155 Phe-Tyr-COOH		Cranston	

UN, unstable; Hb, hemoglobin in g/dL; Polym, polymerization; Dissoc, tendency to increased dissociation; AKR, alkaline resistance.

is a particularly good combination for complete acetylation. This is the case not only for globin but also for other proteins (such as band 3 protein in the red cell membrane). In *Hb Long Island–Marseille*, the methionine is not acetylated because β_2 is valine.

Finally, Hb Thionville is interesting for two other reasons. Because it is an α-chain abnormality, it identifies the allosteric interactions in which α chains participate. It shows a reduced Bohr effect and reduced Cl^- binding whereas 2,3-DPG binding, which is mainly due to an allosteric interaction of the β chains, is normal. It also illustrates how acetylation of the N terminal interferes with R-to-T transition. This demonstrates the need to keep the N terminal nonacetylated, that is, without methionine, for the conformational changes of hemoglobin to take place.

Some High-Affinity Hemoglobins That Lack an Explanation for Their Functional Behavior. *Hb Heathrow* (β103[G5] Phe → Leu) is an intriguing, electrophoretically silent mutation with moderately high oxygen affinity and clinically apparent erythrocytosis.[65] This mutation affects an invariant residue that guards the entrance of the heme pocket. The molecular mechanism is not known. The smaller side chain at the bottom of the heme pocket might alter ligand micropaths or the electronic environment of the prosthetic group, but this is speculation. We might not know why this mutant has a high oxygen affinity but nature surely does, since the mutated residue is invariant.

Diagnosis of High Oxygen Affinity Hemoglobins

In 1966, Samuel Charache and colleagues[38] described an 81-year-old patient who presented with erythrocytosis, was found to have an abnormal band in his hemoglobin electrophoresis, had an increased oxygen affinity of red cells, and complained of mild angina.

The abnormal hemoglobin proved to be a substitution of leucine for arginine in residue 92 of the α chains. The discovery of the first carrier of Hb Chesapeake opened a new chapter in the study of hemoglobinopathies, since it demonstrated that a variant of this molecule could generate another clinical syndrome. The discovery of this abnormal hemoglobin and others has been useful in the elucidation of the molecular mechanisms underlying the function of normal hemoglobin (Table 52-3).

Because the propositus of the Hb Chesapeake pedigree presented with mild angina, it is legitimate to ask whether this is a characteristic of the carriers of high-affinity hemoglobins. The study of other members of the same pedigree and a large number of carriers of high-affinity hemoglobins have convinced most observers that the presence of these variants is largely without clinical consequences, except for inappropriate iatrogenic interventions when the diagnosis has been ignored or the patients confused with polycythemia vera.

High-affinity hemoglobin patients do not have increased white cell and platelet counts and do not have splenomegaly (except for patients with concomitant β-thalassemia). In addition, sometimes they have a family history of "thick blood." It should be remembered that a significant number of high-affinity hemoglobins have been detected as "fresh mutations," that is, with no abnormal hemoglobin being found among parents or siblings.

The differential diagnosis of a person with erythrocytosis is outlined in Table 52-4. Erythrocytosis should not be confused with polycythemia, in which there is an additional elevation of white cells and platelets and usually no splenomegaly. The diagnosis of the entities in the table requires different methodologic approaches. For example, an increase in erythropoietin can be suspected in the appropriate clinical environment, but can be certified only by measuring blood erythropoietin levels. For this purpose, the best method available is radioimmunoassay, first developed by Sherwood and Goldwasser.[66] This method is available in commercial kits, and the test is also available from commercial laboratories and some academic institutions. Hypoxia of pulmonary or cardiovascular origin can be excluded on the basis of blood gases. Affected patients characteristically have low PO_2 and low O_2 saturations. Patients with red cells that have an altered capacity to transport O_2 have normal PO_2.

TABLE 52-4. Differential Diagnosis of Erythrocytosis (Isolated Increase in Hematocrit and Hemoglobin)

RELATIVE ERYTHROCYTOSIS (NORMAL RED CELL MASS) DUE TO DECREASED PLASMA VOLUME
ABSOLUTE ERYTHROCYTOSIS (INCREASED RED CELL MASS)
Idiopathic familial erythrocytosis
Primary (physiologically inappropriate increase in erythropoietin)
Neoplasms that secrete erythropoietin
Renal lesions that produce erythropoietin
Abnormality in erythropoietin receptor
Secondary (physiologically appropriate increase in erythropoietin)
Arterial hypoxemia
High altitude
Chronic pulmonary disease
Right-to-left cardiac shunts
Massive obesity (pickwickian syndrome)
Hypoxemia secondary to intrinsic red cell changes
High affinity hemoglobin variants
Decreased or absence of 2, 3-DPG mutase
Congenital or acquired methemoglobinemia
Chronic carbon monoxide poisoning (including heavy smoking)

Among the patients with abnormal red cells, the different subtypes can be distinguished by a strategy based on comparing the oxygen affinity of hemolysates (those that contain only hemoglobin at defined conditions of pH and salt) with the oxygen equilibrium of the red cells. The hemolysates identify intrinsic defects in the hemoglobin molecule; study of intact red cells identifies other red cell factors (such as 2,3-DPG) that alter the oxygen affinity of an otherwise normal hemoglobin. Specifically, abnormal hemoglobins have red cells with a high oxygen affinity, a high oxygen affinity hemolysate, and a near normal 2,3-DPG concentration. The enzymatic defects of 2,3-DPG mutase are characterized by high oxygen affinity red cells, normal oxygen affinity of the red cell hemolysate, and a very low 2,3-DPG.[67] All of the above have a normal absorption spectrum of their hemolysates.

Methemoglobin (such as congenital methemoglobinemia) can be identified by the presence of an abnormal peak at 620 nm and carboxy hemoglobin (eg, carbon monoxide poisoning)[68] can be assayed by a three-wavelength calculation, since the spectra of carbon monoxide Hb and oxy Hb differ significantly. Several gas measuring apparatuses are available in hospitals (IL CO-oximeter), which can give an accurate reading of methemoglobinemia and carboxyhemoglobinemia in whole blood.

Finally, patients with familial erythrocytosis have a normal oxygen affinity, whether red cells or hemolysate is used. The disease has a recessive inheritance pattern and is sometimes associated with clubbing.[69]

In terms of the diagnosis of high-affinity hemoglobin variants, the following points should be remembered:

1. Routine hemoglobin electrophoresis is capable of detecting only a fraction of high-affinity mutants. More-sophisticated methods, such as agar electrophoresis or isoelectric focusing, can improve detection, but a group of abnormal hemoglobins with high affinity and neutral substitutions cannot be detected by any electrophoretic methods. Some of these cases apparently can be detected by HPLC. Nevertheless, a normal electrophoresis does *not* exclude the diagnosis of a high-affinity hemoglobin.
2. A p50 value useful for the diagnosis of a high-affinity hemoglobin cannot be a "calculated" p50 from Po_2 data. One has to be able to measure directly the saturation of hemoglobin and the Po_2 to obtain a useful p50. Types of apparatus like the Hem-o-Scan are perfectly adequate for this purpose, but the state of the art equipment is the Imai cell as an attachment to a good recording spectrophotometer.

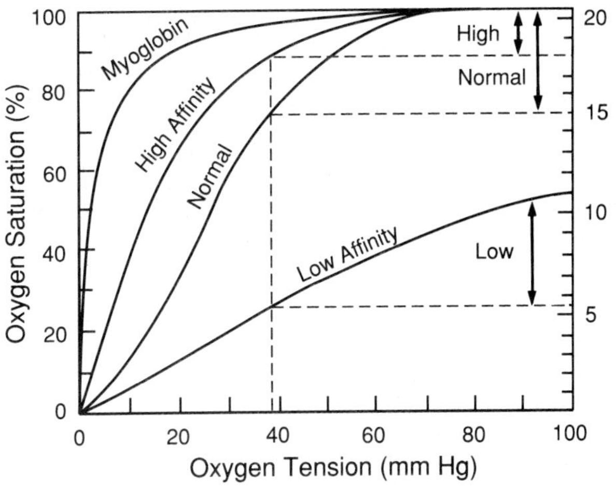

FIGURE 52-17. Oxygen equilibrium curves of myoglobin (no heme–heme interaction, hence n = 1) and of normal hemoglobin red cells, flanked by curves of high-affinity hemoglobin red cells and low-affinity hemoglobin containing red cells. Oxygen tension (Po_2) is plotted against percentage of oxygen saturation and oxygen content in volume percentage. Oxygen content takes into account the amount of hemoglobin present. The oxygen extraction is the difference in oxygen content of red cells at a Po_2 of 100 mmHg in the lungs and a Po_2 of 40 mmHg in the tissues. That subtraction renders about 5 volumes of oxygen for normal hemoglobin. The high-affinity hemoglobin renders 2.5 volumes and causes tissue hypoxia. The very low oxygen affinity hemoglobin (p50 of 85 mmHg as in Hb Beth Israel) results in an extraction of a little over 5 volumes, essentially normal. Nevertheless, any curve between this and the normal will have an increased oxygen extraction, and it is possible the tissues will respond to this increased oxygen delivery with a decrease in the release of erythropoietin and anemia.

Pathophysiologic and Clinical Aspects of High-Affinity Hemoglobins

Most patients with high-affinity hemoglobins and erythrocytosis have a benign clinical course and no apparent complications. Although the first case of a high-affinity hemoglobin was identified in the course of a workup for angina, this circumstance was probably fortuitous.

Patients with *Hb Moke* have been reported to be symptomatic and have benefited from phlebotomy and the transfusion of normal blood, but this is the exception and not the rule.[36] A significant number of these patients are diagnosed in the course of a routine hematologic examination or when the pedigree of a propositus is examined. There are generally no physical findings, except an occasional ruddy complexion. The hemoglobin and hematocrit levels are only moderately increased.

The most pressing reason to diagnose these high-affinity hemoglobins early and accurately is to avoid submitting the patient to unnecessary invasive diagnostic procedures and inappropriate and often dangerous therapeutic interventions. Many of these patients have undergone expensive and unnecessary cardiac catheterization. Others have suffered several courses of radioactive phosphorus (^{32}P) treatment based on a mistaken diagnosis of polycythemia vera. As a rule of thumb, it is reasonable to state that any polycythemia vera patient about to undergo a serious therapeutic intervention should have a whole blood oxygen equilibrium measurement.

The main pending issues that have concerned students of this subject are the following:

Do the carriers of high-affinity hemoglobins have problems in the delivery of oxygen to the tissues?

Patients carrying a physiologically significant high-affinity hemoglobin all their lives are probably reasonably compensated for their abnormality. The reduced delivery of oxygen to the tissues is compensated primarily by increases in erythropoietin-induced red cell mass, probably increases in blood flow, and possibly changes in perfusion patterns in selected regions (Fig. 52-17).

The best evidence of an erythropoietin-mediated increase in red cell mass, responding to hypoxic stimuli, comes from Adamson and colleagues.[71–73] These authors determined that patients with several high-affinity hemoglobins with erythrocytosis had normal urinary erythropoietin levels that dramatically increased when they were phlebotomized to a normal red cell mass. This effect was not observed among patients with idiopathic familial erythrocytosis. Charache and associates[74] have determined that patients with high-affinity hemoglobins have normal oxygen consumption, normal arterial Po_2, slightly reduced mixed venous Po_2 in some cases, and slightly decreased resting cardiac output. More important, these numbers change significantly on phlebotomy or measured exercise, with marked increases in cardiac output and lowering of the mixed venous Po_2. The compensatory mechanisms might include increased perfusion efficiency. For example, patients with Hb Malmo have been shown to have increased myocardial blood flow, and patients with Hb Yakima have increased cerebral flow.

Charache and colleagues[75] have also addressed the issue of the risk involved in pregnancy for mothers with high-affinity hemoglobins. No increase in morbidity or mortality in offsprings or mother is observed, suggesting that compensatory mechanisms other than the differences in oxygen affinity between Hb F and Hb A (the former has lower affinity) must be operative in pregnancies in which the mother's hemoglobin has a higher oxygen affinity than Hb F.

What is the basis of the differences in levels of hemoglobin among carriers of the same high-affinity hemoglobin?

Charache and colleagues[76] observed that carriers of *Hb Osler* had the same oxygen affinity as patients with *Hb McKees Rocks*, but hemoglobin levels were significantly higher (by more than 4 g/dL) in male carriers of the former. When oxygen transport was assessed in these two groups, only a small decrease in mixed venous Po_2 was observed. This could be the consequence of better oxygen extraction by carriers of Hb McKees Rocks, thus not requiring as much of an increase in red cell mass as is needed for those with Hb Osler.

These results imply that epistatic genetic effects might be operating, making the level of increase in red cell mass variable according to a person's genetic makeup. Charache and colleagues[75] have pointed out that adaptation to hypoxia of high altitude is also different in different ethnic groups. Among sherpas of Nepal, a lower hematocrit, no chronic mountain sickness, and a normal oxygen equilibrium curve are found, whereas in the populations adapted to the Andes (Quechuas and Aymaras), a higher hematocrit, chronic mountain sickness, and right-shifted oxygen equilibrium curves are observed. These findings suggest that adaptation might involve choosing among several possible strategies (with potential differences in success) according to the different genetic background.

Should carriers of high-affinity hemoglobins undergo phlebotomy?

The preceding discussion suggests that patients with high-affinity hemoglobins have reached a reasonable compensation of their abnormality with correction of the delivery of oxygen to the tissues in spite of increases in blood viscosity; therefore, no intervention is needed. Butler and associates[76] have done exercise studies before and after phlebotomy in Hb Osler patients and have found no need for phlebotomy. Nevertheless, as mentioned before, reports have been made of individual patients benefiting from the procedure. The possibility arises that in some patients other factors might be interfering with the normal compensation for high-affinity hemoglobin and that the increased viscosity might have become a burden. These are exceptional patients, and prudence dictates that before embarking on a regimen of chronic phlebotomy, one should be conservative and review the case at 6-month intervals during the first few years after diagnosis. In older patients, due vigilance to their coronary status is recommended.

Low ambient P_{O_2} (airplane cabins, living or climbing in mountains) does not represent a risk to patients with these high-affinity hemoglobins. In fact, they are better equipped than the average person to handle such situations, since their hemoglobins bind oxygen avidly. It is interesting that they should be less prone to "the bends" during deep sea diving, since they would release their oxygen with more difficulty during ascension. Nevertheless, this fact should probably not be disclosed to the patient.

Low Oxygen Affinity Hemoglobin Mutants: Cyanosis

Carriers of some low ligand affinity hemoglobin variants are characterized by a slate gray color of the skin and other teguments, secondary to cyanosis. Cyanosis can be present from birth in the α-chain abnormalities and from the middle to the end of the first year of life in the β-chain mutants. This pattern results because α chains are expressed from the second trimester of fetal life, whereas β chains begin to be synthesized in the perinatal period and reach a significant concentration after about 6 months of age. This congenital noncardiopulmonary cyanotic syndrome, secondary to abnormal hemoglobins, has to be distinguished from other causes of cyanosis.

Description and Clinical Features of Low-Affinity Hemoglobins

Many fewer low-affinity hemoglobins are described than high-affinity hemoglobins (Table 52-5). They can be classified as resulting from the following three conditions, which are discussed at length in the section below:

- Alteration of the switch region, the flexible joint, or the C terminals of the $\alpha_1\beta_2$ area of contact that favor the T state, either by stabilizing this conformer or by destabilizing the R state
- Steric hindrance to the heme, resulting in decreased affinity for ligands
- Alteration of the $\alpha_1\beta_1$ area of contact with disruption of the overall architecture of the hemoglobin that favors the T state

Alteration of the Switch Region, Flexible Joint or the C Terminal in the $\alpha_1\beta_2$ Area of Contact That Favor the T State, Either by Stabilizing This Conformer or by Destabilizing the R State. One example is *Hb Titusville* (α94[G1] Asp → Asn),[77] which is the only α-chain mutation with low oxygen affinity described. This mutant has an abnormal electrophoretic mobility in cellulose acetate and makes up 35% of the hemolysate. The propositus had a hemoglobin level of 12.5 g/dL. The mutant hemoglobin has a significant lower oxygen affinity, combined with a reduction of the Bohr effect by over 60% and a clear tendency of the molecule to dimerize. Nevertheless, no apparent cyanosis was detected in this carrier. The molecular defect involves the $\alpha_1\beta_2$ area of contact and the substitution favors the T state of the molecule.

Other examples are the three mutations described for the β102(G4) site: *Hb Kansas* (Asn → Thr),[78,79] *Hb Beth Israel* (Asn → Ser),[80] and *Hb St Mande* (Asn → Tyr).[81] These three abnormal hemoglobins all have low oxygen affinity and produce clinically apparent cyanosis.

Hb Kansas (the first low-affinity hemoglobin described and the most extensively studied) has a very high p50 (about 70 mmHg for whole blood in a heterozygous person compared with 26 mmHg for a normal person), decreased cooperativity, and a normal Bohr effect. The Asn residue at this site is invariant for the β chains; this is not surprising, since the only hydrogen bond across the $\alpha_1\beta_2$ interface in oxyhemoglobin is formed between this Asn and Asp 94. This bond is broken when the molecule assumes the T state. Examination of deoxy Hb Kansas by difference Fourier x-ray diffraction analysis at 5.5 Å resolution has shown that the new Thr residue is incapable of forming this bond. Thus, the low oxygen affinity results from destabilization of the oxy (R) conformer. In addition, other structural changes occur at the $\alpha_1\beta_2$ interface, which accounts for the increased tendency of Hb Kansas to dissociate into $\alpha\beta$ dimers.

Replacement of the same Asn residue by Lys in *Hb Richmond* has not been reported to produce abnormal oxygen-binding properties.[83] With this mutant, Greer[82] has shown that the introduced Lys residue is capable of bridging the $\alpha_1\beta_2$ region by forming a salt bridge with Asp 94 that replaces the original hydrogen bond. Since there are some abnormalities in the $\alpha_1\beta_2$ region on the difference Fourier maps, Greer suggests that detailed analyses of oxygen equilibrium curve might be useful.

Hb Beth Israel was found in a person of Italian descent, but the abnormal hemoglobin was not detected in his parents, and the propositus exhibited clinically apparent cyanosis involving fingers, lips, and nailbeds. He had been severely disciplined in the past for constantly having "dirty hands," and the abnormal skin color was not noticeable to himself or his parent. The cyanosis was detected by a surgeon about to perform a herniorrhaphy. The whole blood p50 was 88 mmHg (normal, 26), and the arterial blood was only 63% saturated despite a normal P_{O_2} of 97 mmHg. The red cell 2,3-DPG was mildly elevated (20 μm/L). The hemolysate showed a low oxygen affinity and a normal Bohr effect. The molecular mechanism involved here is the same as in Hb Kansas, although the defect might be more disruptive locally since serine is shorter than threonine.

Hb St Mande is a mutant making up 38% of the hemolysate that migrates electrophoretically as Hb F. It was found in a person who exhibited labial cyanosis and mod-

TABLE 52-5. Stable Low-Affinity Hemoglobins

	Mutation	Name	Cyanosis	Other Properties
α-CHAIN SITES				
α94 (G1)	Asp → Asn	Titusville	(−)	↑ Dimer
α130 (H13)	Ala → Asp	Yuda	(−)	
β-CHAIN SITES				
β1 (NAI)	Val → AcAla	Raleigh	(−)	↓ Dimer
β11 (A8)	Val → Phe	Washtenaw	(−)	
β21 (B3)	Asp → Gly	Connecticut	(−)	
β37 (C3)	Trp → Arg	Rothschild	(−)	
β41 (C7)	Phe → Ser	Denver	(+)	
β61 (E7)	Lys → Met	Bologna	(−)	
β65 (E9)	Lys → Glu	J Cairo	(−)	↑ Met
β66 (E10)	Lys → Thr	Chico	(−)	
β73 (E17)	Asp → Tyr	Vancouver	(−)	
	Asp → Asn	Korle Bu, G Accra	(−)	
	Asp → Val	Mobile	(−)	
	Asp → Gly	Tilburg	(−)	
β76 (E20)	Ala → Pro	Calais	(−)	↑ Met
β82 (EF6)	Lys → Asn → Asp	Providence	(−)	
β83 (EF7)	Gly → Asp	Pyrgos, Mizunami	(−)	
β90 (F6)	Glu → Lys	Agenogi	(−)	
β102 (G4)	Asn → Thr	Kansas	(+)	↑ Dimer
	Asn → Ser	Beth Israel	(+)	
	Asn → Tyr	Saint Mandé	(+)	
β108 (G11)	Asn → Asp	Yoshisuka	(−)	
	Asn → Lys	Presbyterian	(−)	
β121 (GH4)	Glu → Gln	D Los Angeles, D Punjab	(−)	

Dimer, dissociation into dimers; met, methemoglobin formation.

erate anemia (hemoglobin, 9.6 g/dL). The p50 was 52 mmHg (normal in that laboratory was 28), and the 2,3-DPG concentration was normal. The measured oxygen saturation of arterial blood was 81%. Recent one- and two-dimensional NMR spectroscopy has demonstrated that the quaternary structure of liganded Hb St Mande is different from the R state but also different from the T state.[84] This special ligand quaternary structure also differs from Hb Kansas, which has an NMR spectrum similar to the T state in the liganded molecule. The tertiary conformation around the heme of both chains is altered, suggesting that the β-chain mutations propagate modification to the other subunit, and one of them involving the βLeu141 is long-range interaction.

The intensity of the cyanosis and the extent of the decrease in oxygen affinity are inversely proportional to the length of the substituted side chain at β102. It is maximal when Ser is present, less when Thr is present, and least in Tyr-substituted hemoglobins.

Hb Rothschild (β37[C3] Trp → Arg)[70,85] is a remarkably interesting abnormal hemoglobin that Sharma and coworkers[86] have characterized as alternatively exhibiting low and high affinity, depending on conditions. The overall oxygen affinity curve of this mutant exhibits low affinity.[85] Nevertheless, the situation is far more complicated.[86] This mutant is extensively dissociated into dimers in the liganded state, which explains the low affinity (fully liganded dimers have lower affinity than partially unsaturated dimers). On the other hand, the fully deoxy state of Hb Rothschild has a higher affinity for ligands than the T state of Hb A. This occurrence explains the low/high affinity description of this mutant. This unique set of properties is probably explained by the introduction of an Arg at position 37, which brings this residue in direct conflict with another Arg at position 92(FG4). This clash of positive charges destabilizes the $\alpha_1\beta_2$ subunit contacts and explains the extensive dissociation into αβ dimers. In addition, the T state is less constrained (explaining the higher affinity of the deoxy form) and probably the monoliganded tetramers have increased dissociation, again conspiring against a true T-state behavior. Hb Rothschild has considerable alterations in the intradimer stability and in its capacity to refold.[87] These findings predict small, but potentially significant, changes in the areas of the molecule distal to the substitution.

Stearic Hindrance to the Heme Resulting in Decreased Affinity for Ligands. *Hb Connecticut*, a mutation of β21(B3) Asp → Gly, might be an example of this stearic hindrance to the heme.[88] It is an electrophoretically apparent mutation that amounts to 39% of the hemolysate. It shows a slightly elevated p50 (whole blood p50 was 28.5 compared with a normal of 26 mmHg), a normal Bohr effect, and normal 2,3-DPG interactions. Cyanosis is not apparent clinically, and patients with this mutation are not anemic. Hb Connecticut is of theoretical interest, since it involves a residue that lies outside the areas critical for ligand-dependent conformational changes. Moo-Penn and associates[88] have suggested, on the basis of preliminary radiographic data, that the molecular abnormality probably involves the disruption of the salt bridges between Asp 21 and Lys residues 61 and 65. This event might allow the E helix to come closer to the heme plate, inducing potential stearic hindrance to the binding of ligands.

Hb Bologna (β61[E5] Lys → Met) has an abnormal electrophoretic mobility and accounts for 48% of the hemolysate.[89] The propositus was not anemic or cyanotic. This mutation has also been found in conjunction with β^0-

thalassemia, in which the abnormal hemoglobin makes up 90% of the hemolysate. Remarkably, affected patients had no apparent cyanosis, in spite of a whole blood p50 of 37.6 (normal, 26 mmHg) in the compound heterozygotes and 31 in the simple heterozygotes.

Lys β61 is an external residue, close to the distal heme-linked E7 histidine, and forms a salt bridge with Asp 21 of the same β chain. It is also in contact with β25 of the B helix and two residues in the D helix (β55 and β56). The disruption of any or all of these contacts is likely to alter the oxygen-binding properties of the β heme. Note that the compensatory erythrocytosis observed commonly in thalassemia traits is abolished in the compound heterozygote for β^0-thalassemia and Hb Bologna, demonstrating the increased oxygen delivery secondary to the right shift of the oxygen equilibrium curve.

Hb Chico is a mutation of β66(E10), in which the normal Lys is replaced by Thr. The interesting feature of this variant is the low affinity (p50 about 50% of normal).[90] This feature is not limited to the tetramer, but it is also present in the β Chico isolated chain, suggesting that the mutation creates conditions of decreased affinity for ligands by changes in the heme environment unrelated to the RT transition. The most facile interpretation is that this effect is a consequence of the rupture of the salt bridge that Lys 66 forms with one of the propionate side chains of the β heme. Crystallography shows the hydrogen bonding of the introduced Thr β66 to the distal His β63(E7), Nevertheless, site-directed mutagenesis shows that although distal histidines are important in ligand binding in state α chains, they are not significant in β chains.[91] Hence, the low affinity of Hb Chico must be secondary to direct stearic hindrance.

Alteration of the $\alpha_1\beta_1$ Area of Contact With Disruption of the Overall Architecture of Hemoglobin That Favors the T State. Two mutant hemoglobins have been described for site β108(G10): *Hb Yoshizuka* (Asn → Asp)[92] and *Hb Presbyterian* (Asn → Lys).[93] Hb Yoshizuka is electrophoretically distinct, amounts to 51% of the hemolysate, and has significantly low oxygen affinity and a decreased Bohr effect (by 30%). Affected carriers usually have mild anemia and no cyanosis. Asn 108 lies in the central cavity and is hydrogen-bonded to His 103, a residue located in the $\alpha_1\beta_1$ area of contact. In addition, this residue is linked extensively through hydrogen bonding (by water molecules) to other residues in both the α and β chains. The introduction of the carbonyl group of the Asp residue disrupts this contact severely and changes the electrostatic properties of the central cavity, resulting in destabilization of the oxy conformation.

Hb Presbyterian, in which the mutation introduces a residue with opposite charge than in Yoshizuka (Lys instead of Asp), amounts to 40% of the hemolysate, is an electrophoretically fast component, exhibits significantly low oxygen affinity, and has an abnormally high Bohr effect (increased by 30%) and normal interactions with 2,3-DPG. Heterozygotes are mildly anemic. The molecular mechanism involved here is probably similar to that of Hb Yoshizuka. This hemoglobin does not dissociate normally in the R state, suggesting that it is abnormally biased toward the T state.[93]

The two hemoglobins just discussed teach us that any charge (positive or negative) disrupts drastically the $\alpha_1\beta_1$ area of contact. The difference in Bohr effects can be resolved only after high-resolution crystallography of these hemoglobins.

The three mutations, β73(E17) *Hb Vancouver* (Asp → Tyr),[94] *Hb Korle Bu* (Asp → Asn),[95] and *Hb Mobile* (Asn → Val), belong in the same category as that of the preceding two hemoglobins.[96] These three mutants are similar and account for close to 40% of the hemolysate. Affected patients have no apparent cyanosis. Hb Vancouver has a p50 of 29.5 mmHg for whole blood, but this variant (as well as Hb Mobile) has an *increased* Bohr effect (about 20% higher than normal). The isolated mutants are in the following order of increasing p50: Vancouver > Mobile > Korle Bu > A.[97] The molecular mechanism of these effects is not obvious. Residue β73 is on the surface, and one of its well-known properties is its capacity to interfere with the polymerization of Hb S, as demonstrated by Bookchin and Nagel[98] and confirmed in the crystallographic studies of Wishner and associates.[99] The possibility that bulkier side changes could interfere with the entrance of ligands to the heme and alter the oxygen affinity by stearic hindrance has been suggested.[94] Wajcman and Jones[97] have argued that since the size of asparaginyl and aspartyl residues is almost identical, this theory does not explain the differences in p50 observed. These authors note that the increase in p50 is proportional to the hydrophobicity of the newly introduced residue. Hence, it is likely that the effect is the result of the formation of a hydrophobic bond of increasing strength that perturbs the conformation. A good candidate for the receptor of this interaction is Thr84, located in the EF segment.

Pathophysiologic Considerations

Low-affinity hemoglobins deliver more oxygen to the tissues. Figure 52-17 depicts the amount of oxygen extracted from a curve situated to the right of the normal oxygen equilibrium curve. The oxygen binding at 100 mmHg (lungs) and 40 mmHg (tissues) in a low-affinity curve can be as high as double the difference of a normal oxygen equilibrium curve. Nevertheless, the increase in extraction is not monotonic with the increase in p50 of about 80 mmHg. This analysis predicts that patients with moderately right-shifted red cell oxygen equilibrium curves could be anemic (p50 between 35 and 55 mmHg), but that no anemia should be expected in patients with severely right-shifted curves (p50 around 80 mmHg). The clinical picture observed in patients with Hb Kansas, Hb Beth Israel, Hb Titusville, and Hb Seattle confirm this analysis. Clinically apparent cyanosis is only observed in carriers with red cells with significantly right-shifted curves, that is, over 50 mmHg.

The effect of the right-shifted curve on the level of 2,3-DPG is of interest. In erythrocytes, about 20% of the conversion of 1,3-DPG to 3-phosphoglycerate is done indirectly through the formation of 2,3-DPG. The level of red cell 2,3-DPG is known to rise in many conditions associated with hypoxia, as previously discussed. This effect is probably related to the decrease in oxygen saturation of red cells and is independent of the presence of hypoxia per se; therefore, it applies to the low-affinity hemoglobins despite the absence of tissue hypoxia.

Desaturation increases intraerythrocytic pH as a result of deoxyhemoglobin binding more protons than oxyhemoglobin (Bohr effect). This slight intraerythrocytic alkalosis, in turn, stimulates two enzymes involved in 2,3-DPG synthesis: phosphofructokinase, which controls the overall glycolytic rate, and DPG mutase, which directly controls the rate of 2,3-DPG synthesis. In addition, high pH inhibits 2,3-DPG phosphatase. Hence, high pH simultaneously increases the synthesis of 2,3-DPG and decreases its destruction. Finally, release of end-product inhibition may also be involved. Red cells with low-affinity hemoglobin have an increased proportion of deoxyhemoglobin and will bind more 2,3-DPG, decreasing the free 2,3-DPG and thus inhibiting DPG mutase.[80] Figure 52-18 depicts the oxygen affinity effect of the increased 2,3-DPG in Hb Beth Israel–containing red cells.

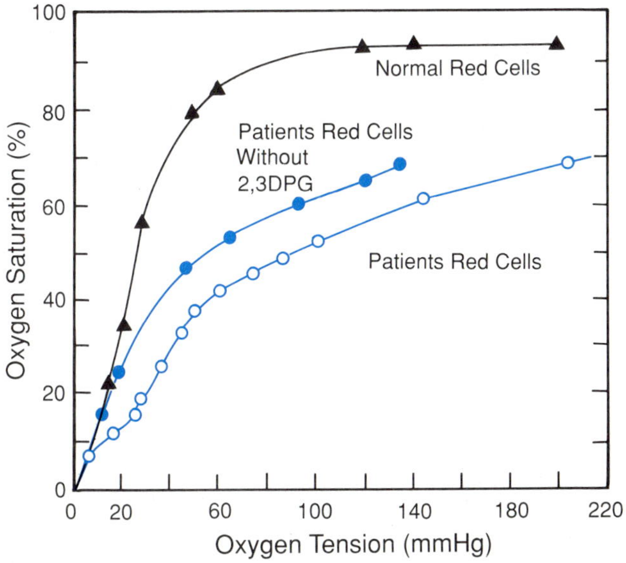

FIGURE 52-18. Oxygen equilibrium curves of normal red cells (*triangles*) and red cells from a patient heterozygous for Hb Beth Israel before (*open circles*) and after (*closed circles*) depletion of 2,3-DPG. The p50 for Hb Beth Israel–containing cells was 88 mmHg (normal, 27 mmHg). Patient's cells depleted of 2,3-DPG had a p50 of 55 mmHg. Normal red cells subjected to the same procedure had a p50 of 16 mmHg. The heterozygous patient's red cells have a biphasic or triphasic curve, composed of the oxygen affinity curves of normal hemoglobin (particularly the bottom portion of the composite patient curve), the abnormal hemoglobin Beth Israel (top of the composite curve), and probably hybrid molecules containing one β Beth Israel chain and one normal β chain (intermediate portion of the curve). (After Nagel RL, Joshua L, Johnson J, et al. Hemoglobin Beth Israel: a mutant causing clinically apparent cyanosis. N Engl J Med 1976;295:125)

Diagnosis of Low-Affinity Hemoglobin Variants

The diagnosis of a low-affinity hemoglobin should always be considered in patients with cyanosis, particularly when cardiopulmonary causes can be ruled out. In patients with cyanosis of unknown origin, it is probably advisable to obtain a hemoglobin electrophoresis and a whole blood p50 before undertaking expensive or risky invasive diagnostic procedures. The search for low-affinity hemoglobins as the explanation for anemia is less compelling, since the yield is probably very low and the tests are not cost-effective. Nevertheless, if other investigations prove to be fruitless, unexplained normocytic anemias deserve to be explored with a hemoglobin electrophoresis and a whole blood p50.

A simple test (even bedside) to distinguish low-affinity hemoglobins and cardiopulmonary cyanosis from methemoglobinemia, M hemoglobins, and sulfhemoglobinemia is to expose blood from the patient to pure oxygen. This will turn the purple-greenish blood of normal persons and that of patients with low-affinity hemoglobins to the bright red color of fully oxygenated blood. In contrast, the blood of patients with methemoglobinemia, sulfhemoglobinemias, or M hemoglobins retains its abnormal color in spite of the exposure to pure oxygen.

M Hemoglobins: Pseudocyanosis

Description and Pathophysiologic Features of the M Hemoglobins

The German physicians Horlein and Weber[100] described a family with congenital cyanosis due to abnormal red cells 1 year before Pauling's discovery of Hb S. These authors determined that the defect was autosomal dominant and was produced by red cells with an abnormal pigment that was similar to methemoglobin. They showed that the genetic defect resided in the globin and not in the heme. This last finding was based on recombination experiments in which the patients' globin was bound to normal heme, and the patients' heme to normal globin. The amino acid substitutions characterizing three of these M hemoglobins were reported by Gerald and Efron.[101] About the same time, Shibata and associates[102] in Japan solved the problem of hereditary nigremia (kuroko or "black child"), which had been observed by clinicians in the Shiden village of the Iwate prefecture for over 160 years. They found a brownish-colored hemoglobin in the hemolysate of a patient of this type, which was later characterized as Hb Iwate.

In the M hemoglobins, each mutated globin chain (α or β) creates an abnormal microenvironment for the heme iron, displacing the equilibrium toward the oxidized or ferric state. The combination of the Fe^{3+} and its abnormal coordination with the substituted amino acid generates an abnormal visible spectrum that resembles but is clearly different from methemoglobin (oxidized heme iron in a normal globin chain). The strength by which the abnormal hemes are locked into this situation differs from one M hemoglobin to another. Figure 52-19 is a diagram of the hemoglobin M mutations.

As shown in Table 52-6, in four of the five known M hemoglobins, the distal or proximal histidine that interacts with the heme iron is replaced by tyrosine, either in the α chains or the β chains. In the fifth, Hb Milwaukee, Val β67 is replaced by a glutamic acid whose longer side chains can reach and perturb the heme iron.

Several molecular abnormalities are associated with the M hemoglobins that are not identical in the five examples. They can be classified into the following categories.

Weak Heme Attachment. The x-ray crystallographic studies on deoxy *Hb M Hyde Park* showed a loss of 20% to 30% of the heme.[103] Others detected a minor component (5%) in the hemolysate of these patients, which migrated between Hb A_2 and Hb A Hyde Park.[104] The α chains of the abnormal component were normal, but only one of the two β^{HP} chains contained heme.

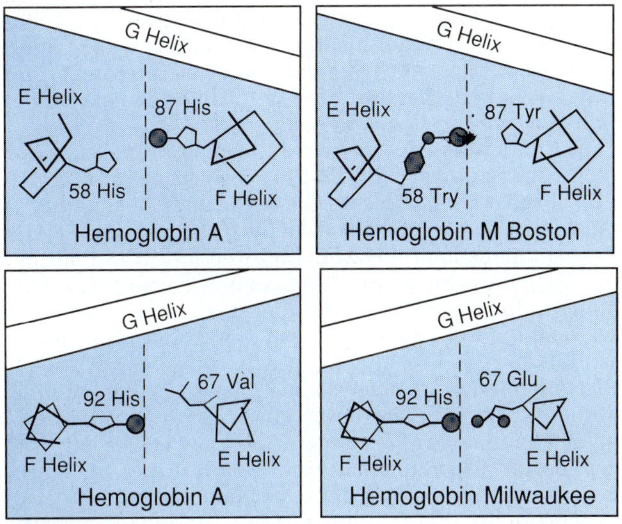

FIGURE 52-19. Schematic depiction of the crystallographic findings in Hb M Boston (**A**; α 58[E7] His → Tyr) and Hb M Milwaukee-1 (**B**; β 67[E11] Val → Glu) compared with normal. (**A** after Pulsinelli PD, Perutz MF, Nagel RL. Structure of hemoglobin M Boston, a variant with a five-coordinated ferric heme. Proc Natl Acad Sci USA 1973;70:3870; **B** after Perutz MF, Pulsinelli PD, Ranney HM. Structure and subunit interaction of haemoglobin M Milwaukee. Nature 1972;237:259)

TABLE 52-6. Human M Hemoglobins

	Hb M Milwaukee	Hb M Boston	Hb M Iwate	Hb M Saskatoon	Hb M Hyde Park	Normal Values
Substitution	β67 (E11) Val → Glu	α58 (E7) His → Tyr	α87 (F8) His → Tyr	β63 (E7) His → Tyr	β92 (F8) His → Tyr	E7: distal histidine F8: proximal histidine
Percentage of total Hb	50	—	19	35	—	—
Hb (g/dL)	14–15	—	17	13–16	10–125	13–16
Reticulocytes (%)	1–2	—	—	0.8–3.2	4–6	1–2
Rate of reduction of Fe^{3+} by dithionite ($T_{1/2}$)	23	260	—	15	55	Too fast to measure
Rate of autooxidation of abnormal chains	13	—	—	26	—	1440 min
p50	Decreased	Decreased	Decreased	Normal	Normal	—
Value in Hill's equation	n = 1.2	n = 1.2	n = 1.1	n = 1.2	n = 1.3	n value for Hb A = 2.7
Bohr effect	Present	Decreased	Decreased	Present	Present	—
Conversion of abnormal subunits to cyanmet with KCN	Fast	Slow	Very slow	Fast	Slow	Very fast

Binding of the Iron to the Remaining Histidine and to the Newly Introduced Tyrosine. The question that has intrigued investigators since beginning the study of the M hemoglobins was the interaction of the mutant tyrosine with the heme iron. The status of proximal histidine (F8) in the β^M chains (Hb Hyde Park) and α^M chains (Hb Iwate) is as follows. Gerald and Efron[101] suggested that in *Hb Hyde Park*, the β heme would move toward the E helix, allowing the iron to be bound by the distal histidine, accommodating the bulkier side chain of the new tyrosine, and generating a phenolic bond to the sixth coordinating position of the iron; this action would stabilize it in the ferric form. Crystallographic studies contradicted this interpretation, demonstrating that the heme was not displaced toward the E helix.[103] Therefore, the Tyr must be accommodated by movements of the F helix, which appears largely destabilized. Independent confirmation was provided by the application of electron nuclear double-resonance spectroscopy.[105] Examination of the N^{14} interactions in Hb M Hyde Park show that none of the high-frequency peaks assigned to the normal proximal histidines indicate that the distal histidines did not take over the role of the proximal histidine. It is likely that that the Tyr in Hb Hyde Park binds the heme iron through a phenolic anion.

The findings on *Hb Iwate* were the opposite. Here, crystallographic studies[103] did find the displacement of the E helix of the α chains toward the heme plate by about 2A, which is the distortion expected if the distal histidine E(7)38 of the α chains had moved to bind the fifth coordinating position in the α-heme iron.[101] To complicate matters, NMR studies indicate that when the abnormal heme is reduced and bound to a ligand the iron now binds the distal histidine.[106,107]

The interactions of the distal histidines (E7) that are substituted by tyrosines in the β^M chain of Hb M Saskatoon and α^M chain in *Hb M Boston* are also known. The data for Hb M Boston are more precise and are illustrated in Figure 52-19. Pulsinelli and colleagues[108] demonstrated by x-ray crystallography that the new residue Tyr 58 (E7) surprisingly fills the fifth coordinating position of the heme iron in spite of the presence of a normal proximal histidine. This bond moves the plane of the heme sufficiently to make the interaction between the proximal histidine and the heme iron impossible. This interpretation has been confirmed by NMR data.[107] No crystallographic data are available on Hb M Saskatoon.

Finally, *Hb M Milwaukee* occupies a particular place in the constellation of the M hemoglobins because it is not a mutation of the proximal or distal histidines, but of a residue nearby (Val 67 [E11]). When substituted by a residue with an appropriate side chain (such as Glu), it perturbs the heme iron and generates an M hemoglobin (defined as a variant having an abnormal methemoglobin-like spectrum). Other mutations of that site, such as Hb Bristol (Asp) or Hb Sidney (Ala), are unstable or have low affinity but do not generate an abnormal ferric state for the heme iron. Perutz and coworkers[109] found by x-ray crystallography that the carboxylic group of the new glutamate occupies the sixth coordination position of the iron, and that the proximal histidine maintains its role as the tenant of the fifth coordinating position. This situation, of course, stabilizes the abnormal ferric state of Hb Milwaukee (see Fig. 52-19).

Oxygen-Binding Properties and R → T Transition of M Hemoglobins. Hb M Milwaukee, Hb M Hyde Park, and Hb M Boston all adopt deoxy or deoxy-like conformation on the deoxygenation of the two normal chains (in spite of the fact that the abnormal chains cannot deoxygenate). This finding helps in understanding the function of normal hemoglobin. It affirms that after two hemes become deoxygenated, the molecule as a whole adopts a deoxy conformation (T state). This is based on crystallography, electron paramagnetic resonance spectroscopy, and NMR spectroscopy,[110] binding of 2,3-DPG,[110] and studies of copolymerization of deoxy Hb C Harlem.[111]

The presence of the Bohr effect and a normal p50 strongly suggest that in Hb M Milwaukee, Hb M Saskatoon, and Hb M Hyde Park the molecule adopts the R state when the two normal chains are oxygenated. NMR studies on Hb M Milwaukee by Linstron and colleagues[112] support the theory that the conformational changes take place when the normal hemes are oxygenated. On the other hand, Hb M Iwate is in the crystallographic T-configuration state when the normal hemes are in the ferric state.[82] This explains its decreased affinity. The molecule does not shift to the R state when the normal hemes are liganded and remains in the low-affinity T state. A similar situation probably exists in Hb M Boston, since the habit of the deoxyhemoglobin crystal remains intact after oxygenation, suggesting that no conformational change has occurred that would necessitate a different crystal structure.[108]

The reason Hb M Saskatoon and Hb M Boston have dif-

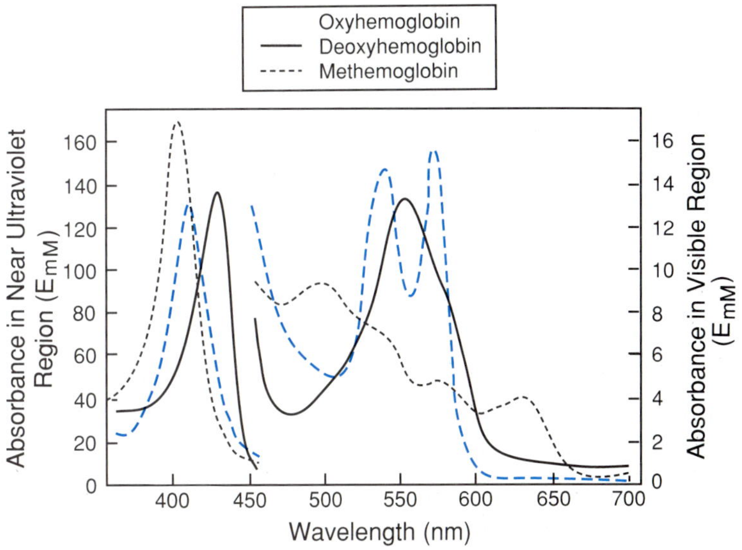

FIGURE 52-20. Light absorption spectra of oxyhemoglobin, deoxyhemoglobin, and methemoglobin in the visible and near ultraviolet regions. E_{mM} is the millimolar extinction coefficient in 0.1 mol/L potassium phosphate buffer (pH 7.4). (After Imai K. Allosteric effects in haemoglobin. Cambridge, Cambridge University Press, 1982)

ferent properties (despite their common substitution of the distal histidine) is that the former does not change conformation when oxygenated and the latter does. Why β chains differ from α chains when their distal histidine is substituted has not been resolved.

Iron Oxidation and Spectral Characteristics. The fundamental characteristic of the M hemoglobins is that their hemes are stabilized in the abnormal ferric state. Hence, they exhibit an abnormal visible spectrum that can be easily distinguished from regular methemoglobins (Figs. 52-20 and 52-21) This characteristic separates these variants from hemoglobin mutants that have a tendency to form normal methemoglobin, such as Hb St Louis,[113] Hb Bicetre,[114] Hb I Toulouse,[115] and Hb Seattle,[116] all of which are unstable (see text that follows) in addition.

The iron atoms in the abnormal subunits of the M hemoglobins exhibit an abnormally low redox potential. Hence, they are oxidized much more rapidly than normally by molecular oxygen,[117] and are resistant to a variable degree to reduction by dithionite. Nagai and colleagues[118] have examined the rate of reduction of the five M hemoglobins with various reductases, including the enzyme active in the normal erythrocyte, NADH–cytochrome b_5 reductase. The surprise is that Hb M Iwate, Hb M Hyde Park, and Hb M Boston are not reduced at all, but Hb M Milwaukee is reduced slowly and Hb M Saskatoon is reduced normally by this reductase. These findings suggest the possibility that in vivo the latter two M hemoglobins might be less oxidized than expected. Full ferric conversion might occur only in vitro, due to the high autoxidation rate of these abnormal hemoglobins. Older red cells might nevertheless have fully oxidized abnormal chains in keeping with the presence of clinically apparent cyanosis.

Column chromatography, which separates the M hemoglobins from hemoglobin A, dramatically demonstrates the differences in the state of the iron in the two hemoglobins.

Clinical Aspects and Diagnosis

The predominant clinical feature associated with Hb M carriers is a condition similar to cyanosis, which can be called *pseudocyanosis*. The coloration of the skin and mucosal membranes may be brownish or slate-colored, more like that seen in methemoglobinemia, but not as blue-purple as in true cyanosis. The distinction is subtle and might not be apparent without contrasting the two conditions simultaneously. The reason for the difference is that the color of the skin is induced by hemoglobin molecules that have an abnormal methemoglobin state, whereas cyanosis is caused by the presence of more than 5 g/dL of deoxyhemoglobin. The cyanosis is present from birth in α-chain abnormalities and from the middle of the

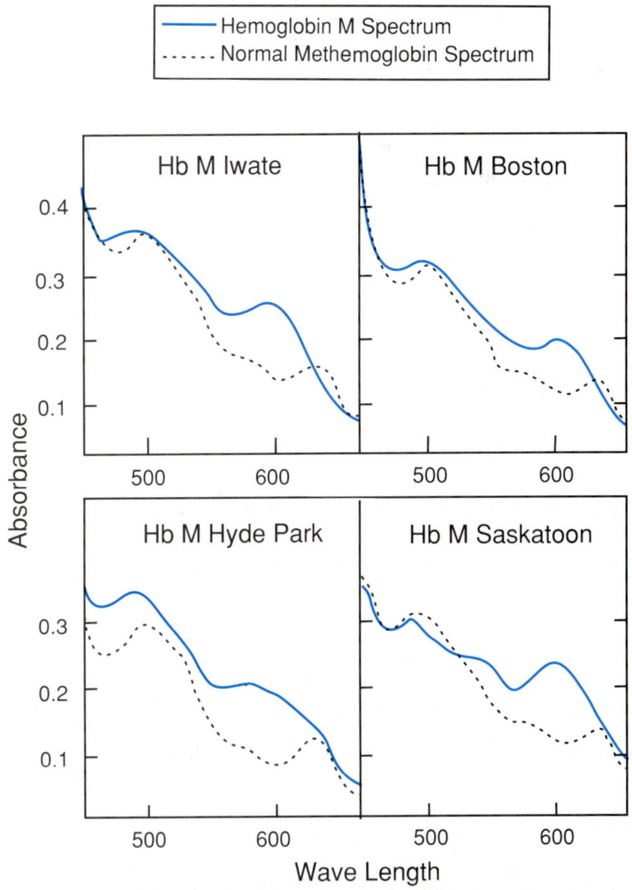

FIGURE 52-21. Spectra between 450 and 650 μm of the oxidized form of four M hemoglobins are compared in each case with the normal methemoglobin spectra. In these spectra, the normal chains are met and the abnormal chains have their own particular spectral properties. (After Shibata S, Miyaji T, Iuchi I. Methemoglobin M's of the Japanese. Bull Yamaguchi Med Sch 1967;14:141)

first year in the β-chain mutants. In addition, a mixture of the abnormal pigment and true cyanosis due to hemoglobin desaturation (of the normal chains) is observed in the low-affinity Hb Ms (Hb M Boston and Hb M Iwate).

Pseudocyanosis is not associated with dyspnea or clubbing, and affected persons apparently have a normal life expectancy. A mild hemolytic anemia (with increased reticulocyte count) has been observed in Hb M Hyde Park and can be explained by the instability of the hemoglobin induced by partial loss of the hemes.

The possibility of Hb M should be considered in all patients with abnormal homogeneous coloration of the skin and mucosa, particularly when pulmonary and cardiac function are normal. The diagnosis can be reinforced by observing an abnormal brown coloration of the blood in a tube. To distinguish this coloration from methemoglobin, the addition of potassium cyanide to the hemolysate is useful. Hemolysates containing methemoglobin turn red; those containing hemoglobin M often change color more slowly. The rate of color conversion varies among the M hemoglobins. A recording spectrophotometer is required for the next step in the diagnosis, although any spectrophotometer can be used for the overall technique that is recommended for the differential diagnosis of cyanotic syndromes (see following section). Figure 52-21 illustrates the differences in the spectra observed with the M hemoglobins, but all clearly differ from the normal methemoglobin spectrum with its maximum at 620 nm.

Electrophoresis is of limited value because the oxy forms are not separable from normal hemoglobin by cellulose acetate. Agar electrophoresis is a little better. Ion exchange chromatography (Biorex 70 equilibrated and developed with 0.196 M $NaPO_4$, pH 6.42) can separate the brown hemoglobin from the normal hemoglobin rendering the diagnosis. Hemoglobin chains can be prepared by blocking the cysteine thiols with p-chloromercuribenzoate and separating the chains electrophoretically or chromatographically. This procedure allows one to determine which chain has an abnormal color.

Perhaps the greatest hazard for carriers of Hb M is misdiagnosis and the risk of expensive and hazardous workups. I am aware of one instance in which a 1-week-old infant was misdiagnosed as having a pseudotruncus arteriosus and underwent surgery with a procedure (Blalock) that did not allow the surgeons to realize the error. When the family study was completed many years later, the father was identified as a carrier of Hb M Boston and the child was also recognized as a carrier of this abnormal hemoglobin.

Differential Diagnosis of Red Cell–Induced Cyanosis (Low-Affinity Hemoglobins) and Pseudocyanosis (M Hemoglobins) From Methemoglobinemia and Sulfhemoglobinemia

In this section, a more general problem is analyzed, the pathophysiologic and diagnostic aspects of the patient with cyanosis not of cardiopulmonary origin.

Although the cardiac and pulmonary systems are major targets in the evaluation of a patient with apparent cyanosis, the differential diagnosis of this clinical sign includes two classes of hemoglobinopathies. First, the presence of an abnormal hemoglobin with a normal visible spectrum but a markedly right-shifted p50 results in significant arterial desaturation.[79,128] Second, in sulfhemoglobin, methemoglobin, and hemoglobin M, the altered visible spectrum of the abnormal pigments is responsible for the gray skin color. The comparative spectral properties of sulfhemoglobin with those of methemoglobin are such that less of the former is needed to produce cyanosis. A patient can be markedly cyanotic with only 12% (1.6 g/dL) sulfhemoglobin.[129,130]

The respiratory status of persons with cyanosis resulting from an abnormal hemoglobin varies with the entity. There is general agreement that clinically apparent dyspnea is not associated with the mutant hemoglobins with right-shifted p50s[79,128] or with the M hemoglobins,[117,131] but can be associated with even relatively mild degrees of methemoglobinemia.[132] For sulfhemoglobinemia, there is no agreement. Most case reports indicate that dyspnea is not a feature, but others state that the symptoms associated with methemoglobinemia and sulfhemoglobinemia are "identical."[132]

Because the altered hemes in Hb M, sulfhemoglobin, and methemoglobin do not transport oxygen, affected persons with all three entities may have normal hemoglobin levels but suffer the physiologic effects of an anemia simply because insufficient functional hemes remain. This effect, in isolation, would be clinically significant only in extreme cases of methemoglobinemia and sulfhemoglobinemia or when the overall hemoglobin level was low. Severe cases of both sulfhemoglobinemia[133] and methemoglobinemia[134] have been reported in which the abundance of nonfunctional hemes was the major concern. In contrast, with hemoglobin M, the proportion of normal to abnormal hemes is genetically determined as greater than 75%, so that the decrease of oxygen binding capacity is a problem only when superimposed on underlying anemia.

The clinical effects of nonfunctional hemes need not be limited to their inability to transport oxygen. Small amounts of nonfunctional hemes can have clinical significance beyond that of comparable degrees of anemia if their presence in partially modified tetramers produces a physiologically dysfunctional shift in the oxygenation curve of neighboring unmodified subunits. This is the molecular basis of the left-shifted oxygenation curve, the impaired oxygen delivery to the periphery, and the resulting respiratory distress seen in relatively mild degrees of methemoglobinemia. This phenomenon, called the *Darling-Roughton effect,* occurs because the oxidized subunits in partially oxidized tetramers are held in an R-like (or liganded) conformation and this increases the oxygen affinity of the remaining subunits in those tetramers.[54,55] Although mixed venous blood is unusually saturated, the abnormal spectrum of the methemoglobin outweighs this effect and the person appears cyanotic. An analogous left shift in the oxygenation curve occurs to a more pronounced degree in carbon monoxide poisoning, and here, too, the impaired oxygen delivery is thought to exacerbate dyspnea.

In the M hemoglobins, the presence of the abnormal nonfunctional hemes in the affected tetramers results in a marked flattening of the oxygen affinity curve. The curve is also right-shifted, especially in the most physiologically relevant P_{O_2} range.[117,135] This leads to normal or even enhanced ability to deliver oxygen to the periphery, which is consistent with the absence of respiratory insufficiency in these syndromes.

The following system has been suggested by Park and Nagel[49] for evaluating the blood of persons with pseudocyanosis with exposure to drugs or chemicals associated with methemoglobinemia or sulfhemoglobinemia.

Procedure: If the visible spectrum of the hemolysate reveals a peak in the 610- to 640-nm range, the following sequence of spectra should be obtained:

- The air-equilibrated sample with and without potassium cyanide
- The sample with dithionite
- The sample with carbon monoxide

Interpretation: If only methemoglobin is present, the abnormal peak will disappear immediately after the addition of dithionite or cyanide. For Hb M, the peak disappears more slowly and can require hours. For sulfhemoglobin, the peak undergoes a slow very decrease as a result of instability.

Differentiation: To distinguish sulfhemoglobin from Hb M, compare the spectra of the air- and CO-equilibrated samples. If CO results in an augmentation and downfield shift of the peak, the sample contains sulfhemoglobin.

Unstable Hemoglobin Variants: Heinz Body Congenital Hemolytic Syndrome

Some hemoglobin mutants have substitutions that alter the solubility of the molecule in the red cell (Table 52-7). The intraerythrocytic precipitated material derived from the unstable abnormal hemoglobin is detectable by a supravital stain as dark globular aggregates called *Heinz bodies*. These intracellular inclusions reduce the life expectancy of the red cell and generate a hemolytic syndrome of varied severity called the *Heinz body hemolytic syndrome*. The word *syndrome* is advisable since this clinical picture is not exclusive to unstable hemoglobins, bu can also be generated by congenital enzyme deficiencies.

Cathie,[137] in 1952, was the first to describe and publish data on a patient with a congenital hemolytic anemia. The baby was diagnosed at 10 months of age when it presented with jaundice, splenomegaly, and pigmenturia. Since this syndrome did not respond to splenectomy, the authors concluded that it was not familial spherocytosis. Eighteen years later, it was identified as a case of Hb Bristol, an unstable variant. In the intervening years, a number of unstable hemoglobins were described and an easy diagnostic test was devised—the heat stability test.

Structural Abnormalities Involved in Unstable Hemoglobins

Substitutions in the primary sequence can lead to alterations in the tertiary or quaternary structure and result in a globin polypeptide chain or a hemoglobin tetramer that is relatively unstable and tends to precipitate inside the red cell (see Table 52-7). The structural alterations leading to this event can be classified as follows:

Mutations That Weaken or Modify the Heme–Globin Interactions. The binding of the heme to the globin is important not only for the oxygen-binding properties of the molecule but also for its stability and solubility. Figure 52-22 depicts several of the mutations involving residues with defined interactions with the heme group. These mutations include the following:

- Substitutions that introduce a charged side chain into the heme pocket where a nonpolar side chain existed previously; examples are Hb Boras, Hb Bristol, Hb Olsted, Hb Himeji, and others
- Deletions involving residues that directly interact with the heme, such as Hb Gun Hill
- The nontyrosine substitutions of the proximal histidine (F8), such as Hb St Etienne (also know as Hb Istanbul), Hb J-Altgeld Gardens, Hb Mozhaisk, Hb Newcastle, Hb Iwata, Hb Redondo (also known as Hb Ishehara)
- Nontyrosine substitutions of the distal histidine (E7), such as Hb Zurich and Hb Bicetre

Hb Zurich is an interesting mutation, which deserves special mention. Caughey's group[138–146] have dissected the molecular pathology associated with this hemoglobin variant. The substitution of an arginine for the distal histidine in the β chains makes the space available for ligand binding around the iron much larger, fundamentally changing some of its interactions with ligands.

Although the extra space in the heme pocket has little effect on the oxygen molecule that binds iron at an angle, a significant difference for carbon monoxide becomes apparent. The biatomic carbon monoxide binds perpendicular to the heme and because of stearic constraints present in the normal heme pocket, its binding to iron is reduced with respect to oxygen. This reduction of the binding constant is a normal adaptation to the endogenous generation of CO (one CO molecule evolves from each heme catabolized) and protects us from excessive accumulation of carboxy hemoglobin (CO Hb). The toxicity of CO stems from the significant reduction in the dissociation constant, compared with oxygen, making CO Hb a particularly stable ligand species.

Carriers of Hb Zurich exhibit an increased affinity for CO due to the increase in binding constant. This molecular pathology is a protective mechanism of sorts. It does not allow the abnormal β chain to become ferric, which would increase its instability. Smokers with Hb Zurich have high levels of CO Hb, but nonsmoking carriers also have abnormal CO Hb levels. Because of the partially protective effect of CO Hb Zurich, Heinz bodies are less common among smokers than nonsmokers with this abnormal hemoglobin.[139]

Hb Zurich carriers have a special susceptibility to hemolytic crises induced by sulfanilamide. The increased aperture of the heme pocket also explains this phenomenon: sulfanilamide is now capable of binding to the heme and producing methemoglobin directly. Again, CO is protective.

Substitutions involving the proximal His βF8 are also interesting. If the substituting residue is Tyr, an M hemoglobin is the result, but if it is another residue, the consequences vary. For example, *Hb Redondo*[140] results from substitution of this residue by Asn (β92[F8] His $\rightarrow$ Asn). The phenotype includes compensated hemolytic anemia, macrocytosis (mean corpuscular volume [MCV] = 111 fL), and the presence of two abnormal hemoglobin bands on electrophoresis (at pH 8.6). The major band migrates in the position of Hb A_2 (10% of total hemoglobin). The minor component (6%) migrates close to the position of Hb S. Both bands lack heme in their β-globin subunits and hence are semihemoglobins. A phenotypic consequence of this phenomenon is that mean corpuscular hemoglobin, mean corpuscular hemoglobin concentration (MCHC), and total hemoglobin are artifactually low, since these parameters are determined by spectrophotometric methods that depend on heme absorption.

The slower electrophoretic band increases during storage, suggesting a posttranslational modification. Adding heme to the hemolysate dramatically decreases the slow-moving band. Amino acid analysis demonstrates that this band has Asp instead of Asn in position β92. Hence, deamination is the posttranslation event generating the second band. Other hemoglobins in which deamination takes place in Asn residues that have been introduced by mutation are *Hb Providence* (β82 Lys $\rightarrow$ Asn) and *Hb Wayne* (frameshift mutation introduces an Asn in position α139). All these mutations comply with the requirements of Robinson[141] that deaminating Asn are usually in α-helix/interhelix interface regions, which increases their flexibility and chances of interaction. In addition, they are usually preceded by Thr, Ser, or Cys and followed by a charged residue. Another interesting hemoglobin is the unstable *Hb La Roche sur Yon* (β81 Leu $\rightarrow$ His). This substitution makes the neighboring Asn at β80 labile, since it becomes partially deaminated. His might have to be added to the list of residues that promote deamination when they preced an Asn residue (assuming the rest of these requirements are met, as in this case).

(text continues on page 1625)

TABLE 52-7. Unstable Hemoglobins

	Mutation	Name	Molecular Mechanism*	Reticulocytes and Additional Abnormalities
α-CHAIN SITE				
α6 (A3)	Asp → O	Boyle Heights		HA
α24 (B5)	Tyr → His	Luxembourg	4	Low
α26 (B7)	Ala → Glu	Shenyang		
α27 (B8)	Glu → Lys	Shuangfeng		Medium
α31 (B12)	Arg → Ser	Prato		
α43 (CE1)	Phe → Val	Torino	1	Medium, LA
	Phe → Leu	Hirosaki		
α47 (CE5)	Asp → Gly	Kokura, Umi, Beilinson	2	Medium, HA
	Asp → His	Hasharon, Sealy, L-Ferrara		Low
	Asp → Asn	Arya		Low
	Asp → Ala	Cordele		Low
α50 (CE8)	His → Arg	Aichi		
α53 (E2)	Ala → Asp	J-Rovigo		Low
α59 (E8)	Gly → Val	Tettori		Medium
α62 (E11)	Val → Met	Evans	1	High
α63 (E12)	Ala → Asp	Pontoise		
α80 (F1)	Leu → Arg	Ann Arbor	2	Medium
α86 (F7)	Leu → Arg	Moabit	1	Medium, LA
α87 (F8)	His → Arg	Iwata		Low, met
α91 (FG3)	Leu → Pro	Port Philip	2	Low
α103 (G10)	His → Arg	Contaldo		Medium
α109 (G16)	Leu → Arg	Suan-Dok	2	
α110 (G17)	Ala → Asp	Petah Tikva		Low
α112 (G19)	His → Asp	Hopkins II	2	Low, HA
α130 (H13)	Ala → Pro	Sun Prairie	2	High, hypo
α131 (H14)	Ser → Pro	Questembert		
α136 (H19)	Leu → Pro	Bibba	2	Medium
	Leu → Arg	Toyama		
β-CHAIN MUTATIONS				
β6 or 7 (A3)	Glu → O	Leiden	3b	Low
β7 (A4)	Glu → Gly	G-San Jose		
β11 (A8)	Val → Asp	Windsor	1	Low, HA
β14 (A11)	Leu → Arg	Sogn		
	Leu → Pro	Saki	2	Low
β15 (A12)	Trp → Arg	Belfast	2	Low, LA
	Trp → Gly	Radwick	3	Low
β22 (B4)	Glu → Lys	E-Saskatoon	3	
β23 (B5)	Val → Gly	Miyashiro		Low, HA
β24 (B6)	Gly → Arg	Riverdale-Bronx	3	Medium, HA
	Gly → Val	Savannah	3	High, HA
	Gly → Asp	Moscva	3	
β26 (B8)	Glu → Lys	E		
	Glu → Val	Mondor		
β27 (B9)	Ala → Asp	Volga, Drenthe	3a	H
β28 (B10)	Leu → Gln	St Louis	1	HA
	Leu → Arg	Chesterfield		Thal
	Leu → Pro	Genova, Hyogo	2	HA
β29 (B11)	Gly → Asp	Lufkin		Medium
β30 (B12)	Arg → Ser	Tacoma	2	Low
β31 (B13)	Leu → Pro	Yokohama	2	Medium
β32 (B14)	Leu → Pro	Perth, Lincoln	2	High
	Leu → Arg	Kobe	3a	High
	Leu → Val	Castilla Muscat		

(continued)

TABLE 52-7. *(Continued)*

	Mutation	Name	Molecular Mechanism*	Reticulocytes and Additional Abnormalities
β33 (B15) or β34 (B16)	Val → O	Korea		
β35 (C1)	Tyr → Phe	Philly	4	Low, HA
β36 (C2)	Pro → Thr	Linkoping		
β38 (C4)	Thr → Pro	Hazebrouck	2	Medium
β39 (C5)	Gln → Glu	Vassa		Low
β41 (C7)/ β42 (CD1)	Phe → O	Bruxelles		
β42 (CD1)	Phe → Ser	Hammersmith		High, LA
	Phe → Leu	Chiba		Medium, LA
	Phe → Val	Louisville, Bucuresti Sendagi, Warsaw		LA
β43 (CD2)	(Phe-Glu-Ser) → O or (Glu-Ser-Phe) → O	Niteroi		LA
β45 (CD4)	Phe → Ser	Cheverly		Low, LA
β48 (CD7)	Leu → Arg	Okaloosa	3a	Low, LA
β49 (CD8)	Phe → Val	Las Palmas		Low
β54 (D5)	Sen → Pro	Jacksonville	3a, 4	High, HA
β55 (D6)	Met → Lys	Matera		
β56 (D7)	Gly-Asn-Pro-Lys) → O	Tochigi		
β57 (E1)	Asn → Lys	G-Ferrara	2	
β60 (E4)	Val → Ala	Collingwood		
	Val → Glu	Cagliari		High, thal
β62 (E6)	Ala → Pro	Duarte	2	Medium, HA
β63 (E7)	His → Pro	Bicetre	2	Medium, met
	His → Arg	Zurich		
β64 (E8)	Gly → Asp	J-Calabria, J Bari		Low, HA
β66 (E10)	Lys → Glu	I-Tolouse	1	Low, met
β67 (E11)	Val → Asp	Bristol	1	High, LA
	Val → Ala	Sydney	1	Medium
β68 (E12)	Leu → Pro	Mizuho	2	
β70 (E14)	Ala → Asp	Seattle	1	Low
β71 (E15)	Phe → Ser	Christchurch	3c	Medium
β74 (E18)	Gly → Val	Bushwick		Low
	Gly → Arg	Aalborg	3a	Low
	Gly → Asp	Shepherds Bush	3	Medium, HA
β74-β75	(Gly-Leu) → O	St Antoine	3b	Medium
β75 (E19)	Leu → Pro	Atlanta	2	
	Leu → Arg	Pasadena		HA
β81 (EF5)	Leu → Arg	Baylor	3a	Low, HA
β83 (EF7)	Gly → Cys	Ta-Li		Polym
β85 (F1)	Phe → Ser	Buenos Aires, Bryn Mawr	1	Medium, HA
β87 (F3)	Thr → O	Tours	2	Medium
β88 (F4)	Leu → Arg	Boros	1	
	Leu → Pro	Santa Ana	2	High
β91 (F7)	Leu → Pro	Sabrine	2	High
	Leu → Arg	Carribean	1	Low, LA
β91–β95 (F7-FG1)	(Leu-His-Cys-Asp-Lys) → O	Gun Hill	3b	Medium
β92 (F8)	His → Gln	St Etienne, Istanbul	1	Low, HA
	His → Asp	J-Altgeld Gardens		Low
	His → Pro	Newcastle	2	Medium, HA
	His → Arg	Mozhaisk		Medium
	His → Asn → Asp	Redondo, Ishehara	1	
β97 (FG4)	His → Pro	Nagoya		
β98 (FG5)	Val → Met	Koln, San Francisco, Ube I	1, 4	Medium, HA
	Val → Gly	Nottingham	1, 3c	High, HA
	Val → Ala	Djelfa	1, 3c	

(continued)

TABLE 52-7. *(Continued)*

	Mutation	Name	Molecular Mechanism*	Reticulocytes and Additional Abnormalities
β101 (G3)	Glu → Gln	Rush		Low
β106 (G8)	Leu → Pro	Southampton, Casper	2	High, HA
	Leu → Gln	Tubingen	1, 3a	High, HA
	Leu → Arg	Terre Haute		
β107 (G9)	Gly → Arg	Burke		Medium, LA
β111 (G13)	Val → Phe	Peterborough	3, 4	Low, LA
	Val → Ala	Stanmore		LA
β112 (G14)	Cys → Arg	Indianapolis	3a, 4	High
β113 (G15)	Val → Glu	New York, Kaohsiung		LA
β115 (G17)	Ala → Pro	Madrid	2	High
β117 (G19)	His → Pro	Saitama	2	High
β119 (GH2)	Gly → Asp	Fannin-Lubbock		
	Gly → Val	Bougardirey-Mali		
β124 (H2)	Pro → Arg	Khartoum	4	
β126 (H4)	Val → Glu	Hofu		
	Val → Gly	Dhonburi, Neapolis	2	M, thal
β127 (H5)	Gln → Lys	Brest	4	High
β128 (H6)	Ala → Asp	J-Guantanamo	4	Low
β129 (H7)	Ala → Pro	Crete		
	Ala → Val	LaDesirade		LA
β130 (H8)	Tyr → Asp	Wien	3a	High
β131 (H9)	Gln → Lys	Shelby	2	
	Gln → Pro	Shanghai		
	Gln → Arg	Sarrebourg		
β134 (H12)	Val → Glu	North Shore	3	Low
β135 (H13)	Ala → Pro	Altdorf	2	Medium
	Ala → Glu	Beckman		
β136 (H14)	Gly → Asp	Hope		
β138 (H16)	Ala → Pro	Brockton	2	Medium
β139 (H17)	Asn → Asp	Geelong		
β140 (H18)	Ala → Asp	Himeji		LA
β141 (H19)	Leu → Arg	Olmsted	3	Low
	Leu → O	Coventry	3b	Medium
β142 (H20)	Ala → Pro	Toyoake	2	Low
δ CHAIN				
δ98 (FG5)	Val → Met	A_2 Wrens		
δ121 (GH4)	Glu → Val	A_2 Manzanares		
$^G\gamma$ CHAIN				
γ130 (H8)	Trp → Gly	F-Poole		
$^A\gamma^T$ CHAIN				
$^A\gamma^T$25 (B7)	Gly → Arg	F-Xin Jiang		
EXTENSION (FRAMESHIFT)				
144 (β) Lys-Ser-Ile-Thr-150 Lys-Leu-Ala-Phe-Leu-Leu-Ser-Asn-155 Phe-Tyr-COOH		Cranston	3	Medium

Low, <5% reticulocytes; medium, 5%–15% reticulocytes; high, 15% reticulocytes; HA, high affinity; LA, low affinity; polym, tendency to polymerize; thal, thalassemia; met, tendency to methemoglobin formation; hypo, hypochromia.

* 1, heme environment; 2, secondary structure; 3, tertiary structure; 3a, change residue in interior; 3b, deletion; 3c, steric hindrance; 4, $\alpha_1 \beta_1$ contact.

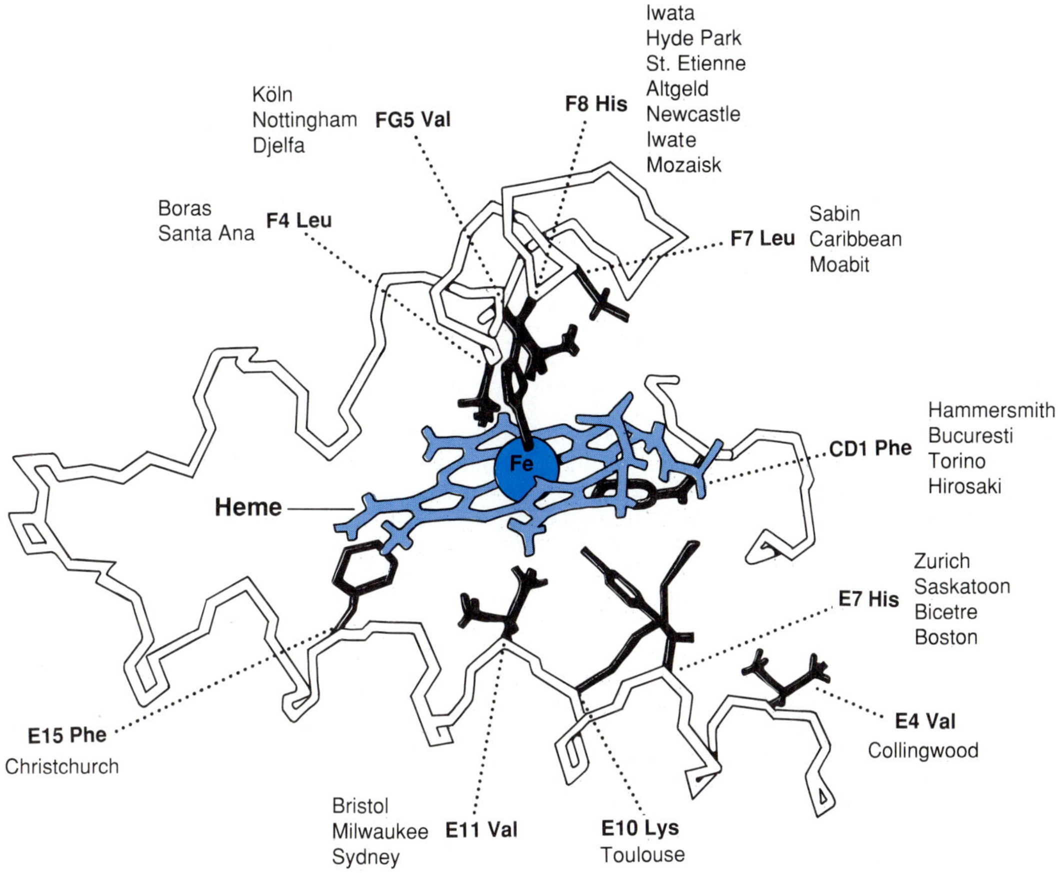

FIGURE 52-22. Diagram of the heme pocket, showing the replacement site of several of the unstable hemoglobins. Valine E4 is at the corner of the pocket, and its side chain does not make contact with the heme but does affect the placement of adjacent amino acid side chains. (After Williamson, et al. Hemoglobin 1983;7:511)

Another fascinating posttranslation modification is illustrated by *Hb Atlanta-Coventry*.[142] In the first report of this hemoglobin, the propositus had a chronic hemolytic anemia and the products of three β-globin genes: 66% of the hemolysate was normal Hb A, 23% was *Hb Atlanta* (β75 Leu → Pro), and 11% was the β Atlanta mutation plus a deletion previously identified in *Hb Coventry* (β141 Leu → O). Elaborate theories were advanced to explain this occurrence, including a β-gene rearrangement generating three β genes due to a Lepore-type unequal crossover involving the β Atlanta gene and the normal neighboring δ genes. Nevertheless, when the genome was examined, no β-gene rearrangement was found and, even more striking, the β141 deletion was not found in the sequence, since the codon for Leu was intact. The authors rechecked the protein to see if they had missed a posttranslation modification and they found by mass spectrometry a 129-da amino acid in the β141 position. The only common amino acid with this weight is glutamic acid, which is impossible, given the charge of the peptide. The likely explanation is the presence in position 141 of *hydroxy*leucine, which fits the weight and other properties of the peptide. The failure to detect this modification by amino acid analysis is probably related to the formation of lactones.

The story does not end here. The Hb Atlanta (β75 Leu → Pro) mutation affects the heme-linked E helix, decreasing the strength of the heme–globin bond. Hb Sidney (β67 Val → Ala) is another unstable hemoglobin with the same mechanism. Hb Coventry was first described in a patient who was also heterozygous for Hb Sidney. Because the peptide mapping of Hb Coventry and Hb Sidney was done from the hemolysate, the authors could not exclude the possibility that the two defects were located in the same chain. The possibility that Hb Sidney could be posttranslationally modified at Leu141 needs to contemplated, particularly since Brennan and associates[143] have identified a mutation in the same site as Hb Sidney, β67 Val → Gly, and found that 5% of the chains had the same 129-dalton residue in position 141.

The question is, therefore, what is it about β141 and mutations in the E helix that make this residue susceptible to hydroxylation? Could *Hb Vicksburg*, which is expressed at an 8% level and is considered a deletion (β75 Leu → O), be another case of hydroxyleucine?

Mutations That Interfere With the Secondary Structure of the Subunits. As previously mentioned, hemoglobin is over 75% α-helical, and any disruption of this secondary structure reduces the solubility of the subunit. Unstable hemoglobin mutants can result from the introduction of proline in the helical structure or the substitution of glycine by a mutation in invariant positions in the bands. Twenty-one of the 139 mutations depicted in Table 52-7 correspond to the introduction of a proline residue.

One special case does not constitute an exception. *Hb Singapore* is an abnormal hemoglobin in which the introduction of a proline is not accompanied by instability. The reason is simple. The substituted residue is the last amino acid of the α chain, Arg 141, and no disruption of an α helix takes place.

Mutations That Interfere With the Tertiary Structure of the Subunits. Hemoglobin is a tight globular protein, which means that the α-helical regions must be folded into a solid sphere. This design introduces enormous constraints to the architecture. Substitutions of the sequence can occur with no change in solubility as long as (1) no charged residues (hydrophilic) are allowed to point inward; (2) no bulky side chains are allowed to substitute for less bulky residues inside the molecule; and (3) the loss of critical nonpolar residues from the surface of the subunit is avoided. A special case is what Fermi and Perutz[146] called the "loss of a nonpolar plug." This is a reference to hydrophobic residues that are located on the surface and serve to prevent water from invading the interior of the molecule. This is a common cause of instability for hemoglobin and about half of the cases correspond to substitution of an Arg for a Leu.

Mutations That Affect Subunit Interactions: Interference With the Quaternary Structure. These mutations involve the introduction of charged residues in the interior or the loss of intersubunit contact hydrogen bonds or salt bridges in the $\alpha_1\beta_1$ area of contact. This contact is critical for stability since it does not dissociate normally, unlike the $\alpha_1\beta_2$ area of contact, which dissociates under conditions found in the red cell, yielding hemoglobin dimers. Because dimerization is a first-order reaction (concentration independent) and tetramerization is a second-order reaction (concentration dependent), the proportion of dimers in the concentrated hemoglobin milieu of the red cell is small. Nevertheless, dissociation is possible and is constantly occurring.

In contrast, the breakdown of $\alpha_1\beta_1$ dimers normally occurs to a vanishingly small extent, but is a great threat to the molecule, since it generates methemoglobin and consequent instability. Dissociation of $\alpha_1\beta_1$ dimers generates monomeric α and β chains, which uncoil, loosening their heme–globin interaction and favoring methemoglobin formation. Several unstable hemoglobin mutations involve residues located in the $\alpha_1\beta_1$ area of contact: Hb Philly,[147] Hb Peterborough,[148] Hb Stanmore,[149] Hb Linkoping,[150] Hb J Guantanamo,[151] and Hb Khartoum.[152]

Hyperunstable Hemoglobins. *Hyperunstable hemoglobins* is a term coined by Ohba[153] to characterize unstable hemoglobins that are either barely detectable or undetectable in hemolysates. These hemoglobins are presumably synthesized normally but are rapidly destroyed, creating a phenotype closer to thalassemia than to the hemolytic anemia normally associated with unstable hemoglobins.

Hb Hirosaki (α43[CE1] Phe → Leu) accounts for 1% of the hemolysate and is clinically silent in some carriers and expressed as a hemolytic anemia in others.[154]

Hb Quong Sze (α125[H8] Leu → Pro) is undetectable in red cells by electrophoresis, chromatography, or biosynthetic studies.[155] It was discovered by sequencing the α_2 gene and confirmed by biosynthesis in a cell-free system.

Hb Toyama (α136[H19] Leu → Arg)[156] corresponds to less than 1% of the hemolysate and is detectable only in biosynthetic studies. Although some of the carriers have severe normocytic hemolytic anemias, others are not anemic but have microcytic red cells.

Presumably, the disappearance of these chains in the cytosol is the consequence of proteases that are particularly effective in digesting the mutated chains. The interesting variability in phenotype strongly suggests the phenomenon of epistasis (the effect of other genes besides the one affected, that is, "epistatic genes," in defining the phenotype). It is possible that persons differ in the level or type of proteases expressed in the red cell cytosol. Carriers have microcytosis and hypochromia if they express effective proteases and have hemolytic anemia if they do not.

Clinical Characteristics of the Congenital Heinz Body Hemolytic Anemias

Anemia is the centerpiece of the syndrome, but its intensity varies widely among patients, depending on the hemoglobin variant.

Unstable hemoglobins are uncommon mutational events generally limited to a single pedigree. The exception is *Hb Köln*, which has been detected in several different pedigrees and geographic locations. The time when anemia appears depends on the chain affected. One of the α-chain mutants, *Hb Hasharon*, which is found predominantly among Ashkenazi Jews, produces significant hemolysis in newborns, but is milder in adults.[157,158] In some carriers, it produces a mild anemia, whereas no hemolysis is observed in other carriers of the same pedigree. Epistatic effects of other nonlinked genes are probably involved here.

Unstable γ-chain variants such as *Hb Poole* have been associated with significant hemolysis in the first semester of life.[22] The condition disappears with the emergence of the β chains as the predominant hemoglobin chain at the end of the first year.

Patients with unstable hemoglobin may have hemolytic crises (abrupt increases in hemolysis over the levels usually found during the steady state) in association with bacterial or viral infections, or with exposure to chemical oxidants. The mechanism of the infection-mediated hemolysis is not clear, but pyrexia and transient acidosis contribute to the phenomenon. Both are capable of increasing hemoglobin denaturation. Drugs, such as sulfonamides, have been directly implicated in the hemolytic crisis of Hb Zurich, as discussed previously, as well as Hb Hasharon, Hb Shepards Bush, Hb Peterborough, and others. The crises are generally self-limited, and stopping all drugs is the prudent course. These patients, like all patients with chronic hemolysis, are susceptible to parvovirus B19-induced aplastic crises.

Patients with unstable hemoglobins can have characteristically dark urine or pigmenturia. The color change is not due to bilirubin, but to the presence of dipyrrole methylenes of the mesobilifuscin group.[160] The origin of these fluorescent compounds is not clear. Their structure—two pyrrole rings still bound to each other by a methenyl bridge—suggests the malfunctioning of the methenyl oxygenase, the enzyme involved in the breaking of the –CH= bridges. Apparently, fluorescent dipyrroles are also present in Heinz bodies.[161]

The absence of pigmenturia does not exclude the diagnosis of unstable hemoglobin, since not all unstable mutants exhibit pigmenturia and the severity of hemolysis is unrelated to pigmenturia. For example, Hb Köln (which induces a severe hemolytic anemia) has in common with Hb Zurich (very little hemolysis) significant pigmenturia.

Congenital Heinz body hemolytic anemias secondary to unstable hemoglobins are generally mild and do not require therapy, except for supportive and preventive measures including administration of folic acid to ensure that the overworked marrow does not become deficient in this nutrient, prevention and prompt treatment of infections, avoidance of pyrexia with aspirin, and avoidance of oxidant drugs, including acetaminophen.

The question of splenectomy arises in the more severe hemolytic cases. No doubt the spleen plays an important pathophysiologic role in the destruction of Heinz body–containing red cells. This fact has to be balanced with the role of the spleen in the susceptibility to pneumococcal infections early in life, and the need to use antipneumococcal vaccines in the case where splenectomy occurs during childhood. According to Koler and colleagues,[162] splenectomy is beneficial, in balance, for the most severe cases of unstable hemoglobinopathies, and partial correction of the anemia has been achieved in some instances. Nevertheless, the patient should be informed that the success of the splenectomy cannot be ensured.

Diagnosis

The elements for the differential diagnosis of unstable hemoglobins are the following:

- Presence of Heinz bodies, spontaneously present in the blood (less frequent) or induced by 24-hour saline incubation of a sterile sample and stained by supravital pigments
- Hemoglobin electrophoresis, only when positive (sometimes a smeared band is observed); negative results are not diagnostically useful
- Positive heat stability test

All these tests are useful and should be pursued because any one of them could be negative. The heat stability test is the least likely to result in a false-negative outcome.

The differential diagnosis of an unstable hemoglobinopathy in the adult is listed with the other causes of congenital Heinz body hemolytic syndrome (for G6PD deficiency, see Chap. 58) and acquired forms of Heinz body hemolytic anemias (acquired methemoglobinemia, chemical and drug oxidants, and other conditions). In rare cases, several of these entities interact with each other to the detriment of the patient.[163]

Because many patients lack Heinz bodies, often the differential diagnosis is with autoimmune hemolytic anemia. In young adults and children, when Heinz bodies are absent, glycolytic enzyme defects, Wilson's disease, and erythropoietic porphyria also have to be considered.

Smear and Heinz Body Preparation. The blood smear is not specific. It reveals anisocytosis, sometimes hypochromia, and often prominent basophilic stippling, Howell-Jolly bodies, and normoblasts. Microspherocytes may be prominent.

Heinz body detection requires the use of methylene blue or crystal violet supravital stains. Heinz bodies appear as pale purple inclusions of 2 μm in diameter or less, singly or a few, and frequently have the appearance of being attached to the membrane. In some cases, Heinz bodies are apparent in fresh blood, but in most cases, incubation for 24 hours (particularly in the absence of glucose but from a sterile tube) is required to elicit them. A normal hemolysate should always be run simultaneously as a control. After splenectomy, Heinz bodies become easier to detect.

Electrophoresis. Hemoglobin electrophoresis can demonstrate an abnormal component, but many times the unstable hemoglobin appears as a diffuse band. This alteration is probably secondary to the partial denaturation of hemoglobin molecules during electrophoresis (because of the heat generated) or during the preelectrophoresis manipulations of the hemolysate. Occasionally, only precipitated material at the origin is observed. Many unstable hemoglobins are not detectable by electrophoresis.

Heat Stability Test. The heat denaturation test, consisting of the incubation of a hemolysate for 1 or 2 hours at 50°C, is a simple and reliable procedure described by Grimes and associates[164,165] 25 years ago. Normal hemolysates are stable under these conditions, and the presence of an unstable hemoglobin is signaled by the appearance of a visible precipitate. Some abnormal hemoglobins, such as Hb Hasharon, precipitate at higher temperatures than 50°C, but if higher temperatures are used controls are indispensable, since normal hemoglobin begins to precipitate at about 55°C.

Other similar laboratory procedures are available. For example, the isopropanol test of Carrell and Kay[166] is used by many laboratories, but it gives false-positive results when the sample contains over 5% Hb F. Zinc acetate precipitation is free from interference with Hb F.[167] The mechanical agitation procedure of Asakura and colleagues[168] has also been shown to be useful in the diagnosis of unstable hemoglobins in several cases.[169]

Pathophysiology of the Heinz Body Hemolytic Syndrome Produced by Unstable Hemoglobins

Thermostability of Hemoglobins. When heat-unstable hemoglobins were related to the presence of a Heinz body hemolytic anemia by Grimes and colleagues,[164,165] the conceptual framework for the understanding of this syndrome was generated. Homeothermic mammals and birds have relatively thermostable hemoglobins. If a hemolysate is incubated for 1 or 2 hours at 50°C, little protein precipitate occurs. This property is observed even among the reptile hemoglobins, although to a lesser degree. Among amphibians and fish, the thermostability of hemoglobin decreases substantially.

At first approximation, these differences may be connected with the environmental mean temperature. Thus, the hemoglobins of heterothermic animals (exposed to low mean temperatures) must have evolved to the hemoglobins of homeothermic animals (exposed to higher mean temperatures) by accumulating mutations in their globin genes (and other genes) that provide thermostable (instead of thermolabile) gene products.[171]

The molecular basis of thermostability is not clear. Perutz[172] has suggested that thermostability of some proteins, including hemoglobin, can be attributed to electrostatic interactions and salt bridge formations, whereas Bigelow[173] contends that hydrophobic interactions are critical. Others claim that both electrostatic and hydrophobic interactions are contributory.[174] Most of this evidence comes from the structural analysis of homologous proteins obtained from thermophilic and mesophilic bacteria[175] or from comparing amino acid sequences in hemoglobins of organisms that prefer different temperatures.[176]

Borgese and colleagues[171] have studied several fish hemoglobins and found that they can be classified into four categories: those stable at all levels of pH (for example, skate hemoglobins); those stable at acid, but unstable at alkaline pH (like the mustelus canis or dogfish hemoglobins); those unstable at acid, but stable at alkaline pH (such as the toad fish hemoglobins); and those unstable at all levels of pH (most fish hemoglobins). Furthermore, the effect of salt (which interferes with electrostatic interactions) and alkylureas (a family of chemicals that interferes with hydrophobic interactions) is revealing: electrostatic interactions are not consistently related to thermostability, whereas all hemoglobins demonstrate increased thermoinstability in the presence of alkylureas. In this model system, hydrophobic interactions are at the heart of the thermostability properties of hemoglobins.

Other contributions to the thermostability come from the strength of the heme–globin bonds. Bunn and Jandl[177] demonstrated that heme exchange between hemoglobin and albumin and between hemoglobins decreases considerably when the methemoglobin heme is ligated with cyanide. Presumably, cyanmethemoglobin has a stronger heme–globin attachment than methemoglobin and is more similar to liganded hemoglobin. Deoxyhemoglobin has the tighter bond.

Autoxidation of Hemoglobin. An old observation is that the generation of methemoglobin increases the thermostability of hemoglobin. Thus, the pathways and events accompanying the conversion of Fe^{2+} to Fe^{3+} in hemoglobin are important in understanding unstable hemoglobins.

When a hemoglobin solution is left on the counter at room temperature, it turns into a brown material that is predominantly methemoglobin. This occurs even more rapidly at 37°C. The chemical basis of autoxidation is probably the generation of superoxide anion (oxygen). This is an infrequent event because most of the time, oxyhemoglobin gives up dimolecular oxygen and converts itself partially into deoxyhemoglobin. The generation of superoxide anion comes from the transfer of a d electron from the heme iron to the unoccupied $\pi 2$ orbital. The loss of this electron converts iron into the low spin ferric state. This reaction is catalyzed by H^+, Cl^-, the superoxide anion itself, and probably by the T state of hemoglobin (generated by 2,3-DPG and other polyphosphates, T-stabilizing mutations, and partial deoxygenation). All of these conditions favor autoxidation. Totally deoxygenated hemoglobin, although in the T state, has no oxygen to contribute to the reaction. Hence, it is more stable with respect to autoxidation.[178]

The decrease in the autoxidation of hemolysates in the presence of EDTA suggests that bivalent cations could play a catalytic role in this process. The best-known effect is that of copper, long known to bind hemoproteins,[179] Cu^{2+} binds specifically to the β chains (and converts the β hemes into methemoglobin) with two high-affinity sites.[180,181] Later work[182,183] confirmed these findings and determined that Cu^{2+} reacts with the β93 cysteine. The mechanism by which the bound Cu^{2+} oxidizes the β hemes is not known.

In contrast, the α chains are a preferred site for autoxidation.[184] Isoelectric focusing is an excellent tool to separate and quantitate the different forms of the autoxidation process.

From the previous discussion, we conclude that the autoxidation of hemoglobin is favored by increased temperature, 2,3-DPG, trace metals, and low pH.

Denaturation of Hemoglobin and Hemichrome Formation. Heinz bodies, one of the hallmarks of the hemolytic syndrome generated by unstable hemoglobins, are the product of hemoglobin denaturation. Initial suggestions were that Heinz bodies are composed by heme-depleted globin chains.[185,186] The pioneering work of Rachmilewitz, in collaboration with Peisach and Blumberg[187–190] allowed the identification of the precipitated material as hemichromes. These are derivatives of the low spin forms of ferric hemoglobin that have the sixth coordination position occupied by a ligand provided by the globin: a hydroxyl group (−OH) or protonated histidyl (reversible hemichromes) or an unprotonated histidyl (irreversible hemichrome)[191] (Fig. 52-23).

Another type of irreversible hemichrome can be generated by having the fifth coordination position occupied by a cysteine and the sixth by an aliphatic amine. All these compounds can be resolved by electron paramagnetic resonance spectroscopy, but not by absorption spectroscopy because their visible spectra are similar. Hemichromes are generated when the heme is dissociated from the heme pocket and rebinds elsewhere in the globin after the α or β chains have suffered some form of uncoiling or denaturation. Irreversible hemichromes seem to be an indispensable stage in the formation of Heinz bodies. Winterbourne and Carrell[192] have found both α and β chains in Heinz bodies. In addition, these authors have worked out a general scheme for the process involved in the generation of Heinz bodies[193] (Fig. 52-24).

From the preceding discussion, it is understandable that any weakening of the heme–globin bond will accelerate hemoglobin denaturation.

Anemia in the Unstable Hemoglobins Generating Heinz Bodies Hemolytic Syndrome. The primary cause of the anemia resides in the reduced life-span of the red cells that contain Heinz bodies. Evidence indicates that Heinz bodies, at least in part, adhere to the cytosolic side of the membrane[194,195] by hydrophobic interactions and not through covalent bonds, as previously suggested.[196,197]

The anion exchanger (AE-1 or band 3: 103 kd) is the most common transmembrane protein in the mature red cell. It spans the membrane with a glycolysated portion on the surface of the red cell, a hydrophobic portion across the lipid bilayer, and a cytosolic domain of about 43 kd (see Chap. 54). The cytosolic domain (N-terminal segment of the protein) has two conformationally independent portions separated by a hinge region. The most N-terminal portion of the cytosolic domain (past the hinge) is highly negatively charged and ends in an acetylated N terminal. The enzymes phosphofructokinase, glyceraldehyde-3-phosphate dehydrogenase, and aldolase bind to this region of band 3 (see Chap. 54). In addition, this is the portion of the molecule to which hemoglobin and hemichromes bind.[198,199]

The negatively charged band 3 sequence threads itself into the positively charged central cavity of hemoglobin, which is why it binds deoxyhemoglobin preferentially and

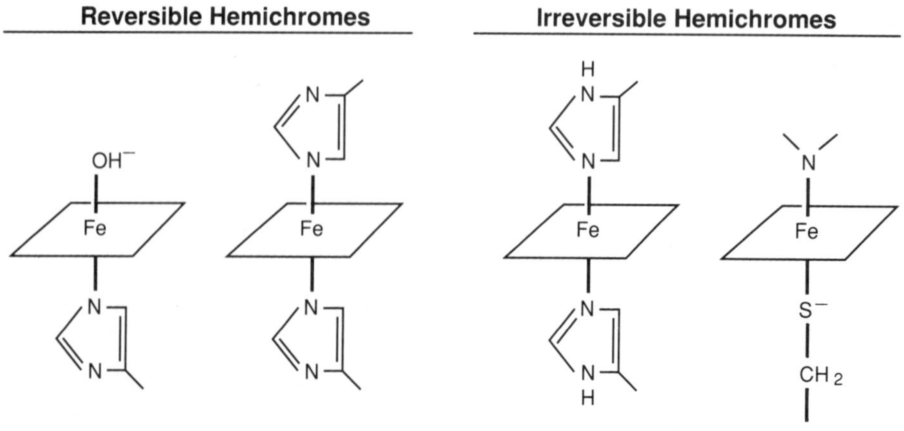

FIGURE 52-23. Diagramatic structure of hemichromes, showing proximal histidine below the plane of the heme and distal histidine above the plane. One or both of the histidines can be substituted. (After Peisach J, Blumberg WE, Rachmilewitz EA. The demonstration of ferrihemochrome intermediates in Heinz body formation following the reduction of oxyhemoglobin A by acetylphenylhydrazine. Biochem Biophys Acta 1975;393:404)

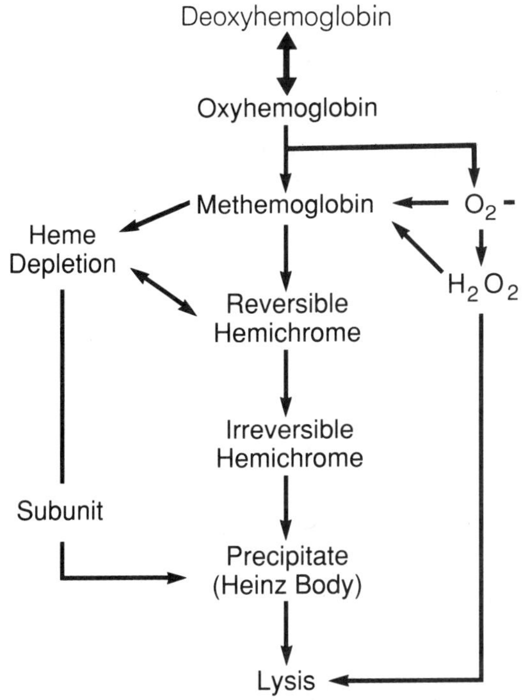

FIGURE 52-24. Scheme of the intraerythrocyte denaturation of unstable hemoglobins as proposed by Winterbourne and Carrell. (After Winterbourne CC, Carrell DW. Studies of hemoglobin denaturation and Heinz body formation in the unstable hemoglobins. J Clin Invest 1974;54:678)

in a reversible way; the higher the positive charge, the higher the affinity. This is why Hb A_2 and Hb C (particularly the latter) attach tenaciously to the membrane. Hb S is intermediate in affinity. Hb C also exhibits reversible binding, and Hb S has an irreversible component, which may be due to hemichrome binding to band 3. Hemichromes bind at the same site as hemoglobin, but the binding seems to be irreversible and causes band 3 molecules (and associated membrane proteins) to aggregate.[198–205]

Unstable hemoglobins generate considerable amounts of hemichromes and some of these bind to band 3. It is not surprising that these red cells exhibit decreased deformability, a characteristic that will condemn them to be preferentially trapped in the red cell quality control organ, the spleen.[206,207] It is possible that Heinz body–containing red cells are pitted initially. The term *pitting* refers to the mechanism by which Heinz bodies and a portion of the overlying plasma membrane are excised from the cell during their passage through the spleen. This manipulation converts red cells progressively into spherocytes through membrane loss, producing a rigid remnant that will be eliminated eventually from the circulation.

Other potential sources of membrane damage come from peroxidation and cross-linking of membrane proteins. These are probably secondary to the presence of free heme and iron and to free radicals generated during methemoglobin formation and hemoglobin denaturation.[208,210] Other evidence of membrane alteration is the presence of abnormal K^+ efflux in some of these cells.[207,211]

Another determinant of the anemia in patients with unstable hemoglobins is the oxygen equilibrium curve. The level of 2,3-DPG is generally normal,[212] but some of the unstable variants have a high or low oxygen affinity. For the reasons discussed before, the high ligand affinity unstable hemoglobins would tend to have less anemia and the low ligand affinity unstable hemoglobins would be characterized by more anemia. Nevertheless, there is considerable overlapping of these abnormal properties.[9]

Unstable hemoglobins with abnormal oxygen affinity include the following:

High oxygen affinity: the β-chain mutant Hb Etobioke and the β-chain mutants (in increasing order of sequence number) St Louis, Genova, Tacoma Philly, Duarte, Zurich, Bicetre, Shepherds Bush, Baylor, Buenos Aires, Boras, Gun Hill, Istanbul, Mozhaisk, Köln, Nottingham, Southampton, Tubingen, Altdorf, Toyoake, and Cranston

Low oxygen affinity: the α-chain mutant Torino and the β-chain mutants Leiden, Hazebrouck, Hammersmith, Louisville, Cheverly, Okaloosa, Bristol, Seattle, Christchurch, Caribbean, Burke

The question of alterations in the synthesis or catabolism of the unstable hemoglobins is also of interest. The extreme case is that in which the hemoglobin is so unstable that none can be detected in the red cell. This is the case for *Hb Quong Sze*, an α-chain mutant that can be identified only by DNA sequencing. Adams and colleagues[214,215] have demonstrated that *Hb Terre Haute* (β106 Leu → Arg), originally incorrectly identified as Hb Indianapolis (β112 Cys → Arg), is an extremely unstable hemoglobin and is expressed as a dominant thalassemic syndrome (see next section), with an α-globin/β-globin synthesis ratio of 0.4:1 (normal, 1:1). In Hb Quong Sze, the abnormal chain is so unstable that it does not have the opportunity to form dimers or tetramers and is destroyed by proteolysis. In Hb Terre Haute, the synthesis of the abnormal hemoglobin is reduced drastically. Other less dramatic instances are represented by unstable hemoglobins with lower than normal synthesis: *Hb Boras*, *Hb Abraham Lincoln*, and *Hb Riverdale-Bronx*. An increase in free heme in erythroblasts (which has been found in unstable hemoglobins with weak heme–globin interactions) may inhibit heme synthesis and significantly reduce δ-aminolevulinic synthetase levels.[216]

Many unstable hemoglobins have a normal rate of synthesis, sometimes unexpectedly, as in *Hb Gun Hill*,[218] which contains a five-residue deletion. With this hemoglobin, Rieder[217] demonstrated that the unstable α chains can exchange with stable α chains from the surplus pool. Hence, very unstable hemoglobins, but those in which the process is not driven by the instability of recently synthesized isolated chains that are incapable of assembly, tend to have, paradoxically, more abnormal hemoglobin, more Heinz bodies, and more severe hemolysis.

Finally, several unstable hemoglobins coexist in the genome with α- or β-thalassemia: the α-chain mutants *Hb Suan-Dok* and *Hb Petah Tikva* coexist in *cis* with α-thalassemia, and the β-chain mutant *Hb Leiden* coexists in *cis* with a β-thalassemia mutation.

Hemoglobin Structural Mutations With Abnormal Assembly: Dominant Thalassemia Syndrome

The dominant thalassemia syndrome includes mutations of the coding region of the globin genes that lead to a significant deficit in synthesis and that present clinically as dominant thalassemia. This definition does not include structural mutations associated with phenotypes resembling β-thalassemia trait. For example, not considered in this group are the δ/β fusion genes (Lepore and anti-Lepore hemoglobins), nor mutations affecting the translation termination codon (Hb Constant Spring, Hb Icaria, Hb Koya Dora, and Hb Seal Rock). We also exclude α- or β-structural mutations that are linked in cis with α- or β-thalassemia, respectively. Finally, neither Hb North Shore-Caracas nor Hb K Woolrich, both of which have a thalassemia syndrome of unknown origin, nor the abnormal mRNA splicing observed in Hb E, Hb Knossos, and Hb Monroe nor proteolytically hypersusceptible Hb Mississippi qualify for this group, since the clinical presentation of the heterozygotes is mild.

Clinical Picture and Diagnosis

The dominant thalassemia syndrome is characterized by significant anemia, often transfusion-dependent, by splenomegaly, and by a blood smear with prominent hypochromia, microcytosis, and basophilic stippling. The reticulocyte count is often high. Inclusion bodies are frequently observed in erythrocyte *precursors* with supravital staining, which is why some authors call this syndrome inclusion body thalassemia. The bone marrow exhibits considerable erythroid hyperplasia, and evidence of ineffective erythropoiesis can be obtained. Finally, the full-fledged thalassemic syndrome is found in members of different generations in the same pedigree, frequently in one of the parents or progeny of the propositus. Although the syndrome is similar to thalassemia intermedia, an astute clinician can exclude this diagnosis when the intensity of the disease in the parents or descendants is equal to that seen in the propositus. Thalassemia intermedia usually results from homozygosity or double heterozygosity for much milder defects; hence, the parents or progeny have a much milder disease. Nevertheless, lack of parental involvement does not exclude the diagnosis since the mutation can be de novo. A thalassemia picture in a patient with an ethnic origin not associated with β-thalassemia should also increase the suspicion of the clinician for this syndrome.

An important point to keep in mind is that electrophoresis might not reveal an abnormal band because the abnormal hemoglobin is either synthesized at an extremely low level, is rapidly catabolized, or both. Specific examples of dominant thalassemia syndrome follow.

Hb Sowa-Yakushiji (β110 Leu → Pro) was found in a Japanese family (β-thalassemia is uncommon in the Japanese). The three affected adults had hemoglobin of 7.6 to 9 g/dL, MCV of about 60, low MCHC, reticulocytes of 2.4 to 4.1, Hb F of 1.2% to 2.0%, Hb A_2 of 5%, hypochromia, a normal hemoglobin electrophoresis (no abnormal bands), and negative heat denaturation and isopropanol tests. Sequence of the β genes and Southern blotting demonstrated a nucleotide mutation affecting codon 110 (CTG → CCG)in all three affected members of the pedigree. HPLC was incapable of detecting the synthesis of the abnormal β chain. The α-chain/β-chain synthesis ratio was 0.7 to 0.8.

Hb Terre Haute (β106 Leu → Arg) was observed in a person of Irish descent. It was originally described as Hb Indianapolis and was incorrectly identified as β112 Cys → Arg. The proband and father had intense anemia (hemoglobin 4.7 to 5.7, MCV 72 to 75, low MCHC, 14% to 15% reticulocytes (some of which could have been inclusion bodies in red cells), hypochromia, nucleated red cells, and basophilic stippling). Hemoglobin electrophoresis was normal, Hb A_2 was normal, and Hb F was 10% to 12%. Labeled amino acids allowed the detection of the β chain of Hb Terre Haute by HPLC. The synthesis ratio of β Terre Haute: β normal was 0.8:1 at 1.25 minutes of incubation during the in vitro synthesis study, but at 20 minutes it had dropped to 0.46:1. Undoubtedly, Hb Terre Haute was rapidly precipitating with subsequent proteolysis.

Most of the residues involved in the packing contact ($\alpha_1\beta_1$ area of contact) correspond to amino acids coded by exon 3, which starts at G6 (β104 and α99) and includes the β106 residue. The pathophysiologic difference with a β-thalassemia trait is the celerity of the precipitation of the abnormal chains and the potential that this process will overwhelm the anti–free radical protecting mechanisms of the red cell and cause oxidative damage.

Hb Manhattan (frameshift −1 [−G]) in codon 109 leads to an elongation of 156 amino acids. This mutation was discovered in a Lithuanian Jew, with life-long hemolytic anemia (hemoglobin 8.5, MCV 67, marked anisocytosis with hypochromia, marked basophilic stippling, reticulocyte count 1.2%, and no spontaneous or incubated Heinz bodies). Synthetic studies did not reveal the abnormal chain, and the α:β ratio was 0.5:1.

Hb Agnana (β94 [+TG] → 156aa) is another frameshift mutation first observed in a Southern Italian child who had a hemoglobin level of 6.6 g/dL at the age of 3 years, hepatosplenomegaly, moderate thalassemia type bone manifestations, large inclusions bodies in cresyl blue-stained smears, normal Hb A_2, 10% level Hb F, and an α-chain/non–α-chain synthetic ratio of 1:5. Electrophoresis and chromatography failed to detect an abnormal hemoglobin. Heat and isopropanol tests were negative. The molecular abnormality was ascertained by direct sequencing of the β gene, in which a TG insertion at codon 94 created a frameshift that elongated the β chain by 10 amino acids. This was a de novo mutation, since both parents were normal. The patient required transfusions every 2 or 3 months, was splenectomized at 14 years, and died at 27 years of hepatic coma.

Pathophysiology

The molecular basis of the dominant thalassemia syndrome is generally of two types: (1) single-point mutations (substitutions or deletions) affecting particularly, but not exclusively, exon 3; and (2) chain-length abnormalities secondary to either a shorter chain (premature termination) or an elongated chain (frameshift mutation leading to an altered stop codon). These mutations also affect exon 3.

The central question of this syndrome is why the phenotype is significantly more intense in severity than β^0-thalassemia trait, in which a similar deficit in the α-globin/β-globin synthetic ratio exists. The answer lies in the notion that in dominant thalassemia the abnormal chain is probably synthesized at a close to normal rate but is rapidly destroyed because it cannot assemble into tetramers. This phenomenon creates inclusions and generates large amounts of free radicals (because of conversion of the heme groups to metheme). The reason for the lack of assembly is that all these mutations affect the residues coded in exon 3 and involved in the $\alpha_1\beta_1$ area of contact, the contact that stabilizes the $\alpha_1\beta_1$ dimer. Without this contact, a tetramer cannot be built. The mutations found in dominant thalassemia affect the $\alpha_1\beta_2$ area of contact, indirectly (as in Hb Chesterfield and Hb Cagliari in which an internal amino acid is replaced by a bulky and charged amino acid or a deletion [Hb Korea]), completely destroying the tertiary structure) or directly as in all the other cases.

Oxidative damage to the red cell membrane has not been studied in these syndromes but is probably severe and may even be the primary basis for the hemolysis.

SULFHEMOGLOBINEMIA

The discussion that follows is largely based on the work of Constance M. Park in collaboration with the author.[129,130]

Sulfhemoglobin, a green pigmented molecule with a sulfur atom incorporated into the porphyrin, has been associated with drug abuse,[219–224] with direct occupational exposure to sulfur compounds,[225] and with environmental exposure to polluted air.[226] Although sulfurated hemoglobin has not been separated until recently[129] from unmodified hemoglobin, it is known that the modified hemes have a drastically right-shifted oxygenation curve that renders them ineffective for oxygen transport.[227] In addition, the fully sulfurated tetramer seems to have no heme–heme interaction (n close to 1).[130] The oxygenation curve shows a right shift in the physiologically relevant Po_2 range. Full saturation of unaltered hemes in the lungs and enhanced oxygen unloading at the tissues would be expected. Since this right shift would ameliorate any decrease in functional hemoglobin mass, sulfuration of hemes may have little physiologic significance as long as sufficient unmodified hemoglobin remains.

For equivalent amounts of abnormal pigment, the patient with sulfhemoglobinemia would be expected to have a bluer appearance than the patient with methemoglobinemia as a result of spectral differences between the pigments, but he or she would be less symptomatic, as a result of the differences in p50 reported here. This is fortunate, since no known treatment is analogous to methemoglobin reduction for reconverting sulfhemoglobin to functional hemoglobin.

An understanding of the molecular basis of the right-shifted oxygenation curve emerges from isoelectric focusing data. In a clinical sample that contains only 12% modified hemes, the distribution of these hemes among partially sulfurated tetramers results in a larger percentage of the tetramers being abnormal.[129] Between 24% and 48% of the hemoglobin tetramers in a clinical sample are abnormal and may contribute to the shift of the oxygenation curve.[130] The actual effect these partially modified molecules have on the oxygenation curve depends on their conformation. Because the half-sulfurated, half-liganded tetramers have an isoelectric point between deoxy and oxyhemoglobin and bind 2,3-DPG under conditions when oxyhemoglobin does not, their conformation must be closer to the T state than is that of oxyhemoglobin.

Whereas in methemoglobinemia some tetramers have subunits frozen in an oxidized R-like state (Darling-Roughton effect), in sulfhemoglobinemia some tetramers have subunits frozen in a T-like state because they remain unliganded at physiologic Po_2.[135] In the former, a left-shifted oxygenation curve and impaired oxygen delivery results; in the latter, a right-shifted curve and enhanced oxygen delivery occur. The slightly high 2,3-DPG in the blood of patients with sulfhemoglobinemia probably reflects increased binding to the T-like sulfurated tetramers rather than an actual increase in free 2,3-DPG.[129]

Sulfhemoglobin and methemoglobin have been reported as coexisting in a number of patients with drug-induced hemoglobinopathy,[133,219–225] and the lists of chemicals and drugs reported to produce these syndromes are overlapping. Acetanilid, usually in the form of Bromo-Seltzer, and phenacetin were found to be the main offenders in 62 cases of sulfhemoglobinemia seen at the Mayo Clinic.[220] The aryl hydroxylamine metabolites of these drugs can serve as reducing agents in a cyclic process capable of generating both sulfhemoglobin[227] and methemoglobin.[228] The origin of the sulfur atom in the former remains unclear, but both H_2S generated by intestinal flora[229] and glutathione[230] have been suggested. It has been noted before that laboratory documentation is often inadequate to distinguish between the various hemoglobin entities, and it is likely that sulfhemoglobin is underdiagnosed.[232] Although acetanilid was removed from Bromo-Seltzer a number of years ago and the Food and Drug Administration removed phenacetin from the US market, sulfhemoglobinemia is not likely to vanish. Sulfonamides, dapsone, and sulfur-containing ointments are reported offenders[225,233,234] and are still widely used. Some drugs reported to produce methemoglobin, including acetaminophen, may also produce sulfhemoglobin when more careful analysis is done.

Furthermore, accidents involving occupational exposure to H_2S are expected to increase[235] and exposure of red cells to H_2S produces sulfhemoglobin within minutes.[236] Although sulfhemoglobin is seldom looked for in this setting, it has been reported and with the increased interest in occupational and environmental pollutants, that the screening of populations at risk may reveal many more subclinical cases.[226,227]

Sulfhemoglobinemia is probably a relatively nontoxic syndrome in persons with hemoglobin A, but it may prove to be suprisingly toxic in those with Hb S, especially compared with methemoglobinemia, which would be expected to ameliorate sickling.[237] The presence of sulfurated subunits shifts the conformation of Hb S tetramers toward the unliganded, polymerizing T form, even in the presence of high Po_2. Microvascular occlusion could be exacerbated by the fact that these tetramers remain in the polymerizing conformation in both the arterial and venous circulation. We have shown that a solution of Hb S that is half-sulfurated does gel at atmospheric Po_2 in concentrations found in red cells.

In summation, the features to remember about sulfhemoglobin are the following. It is a green-pigmented protein that can be accurately identified by spectrophotometric and isoelectric focusing methods (Fig. 52-25). At low concentrations, sulfurated tetramers are shifted toward the deoxy or T form, producing a right shift of the oxygen equilibrium curve. For this reason, dyspnea is absent unless the levels of sulfhemoglobin are extraordinarily high. Mild cases that now go undiagnosed may be revealed in screening studies looking for toxic effects of drugs and environmental pollutants. Even small amounts of sulfhemoglobin may exacerbate sickling disorders. Awareness of this entity and a proper diagnostic approach allow the ascertainment of its true incidence.

METHEMOGLOBINEMIA

Methemoglobinemia is the consequence of the oxidation of the iron (from ferrous to ferric) in the center of the protoporphyrin IX ring that forms the prosthetic group (heme) of hemoglobin. It is a misnomer, as Jaffe[239] has noted, because it is not oxidized hemoglobin circulating in plasma, but oxidized hemoglobin inside the red cells. The more precise name, *methemoglobincythemia*, is too cumbersome. Potentially, methemoglobinemia can induce problems because it renders hemoglobin incapable of binding oxygen (an exclusive property of ferrous heme).

The clinical consequences of methemoglobinemia are generally (but not always) benign, but the change in skin color may be dramatic. Methemoglobinemia belongs in the differential diagnosis of cyanosis. It may be the consequence of genetic abnormalities of the mechanisms involved in maintaining the hemoglobin in the ferrous state and may be capable of binding oxygen (hereditary methemoglobinemia) or may be due to exogenous oxidizing agents that gain access to the interior of red cells (acquired methemoglobinemia).

Hereditary Methemoglobinemia

History and Background

The discovery of methemoglobin brings us back 50 years to a town near Belfast called Banbridge. As Quentin H. Gibson[238] recalls, the whole event can be traced to the practice of Dr. Deeny. Deeny had tried Albert Szent-

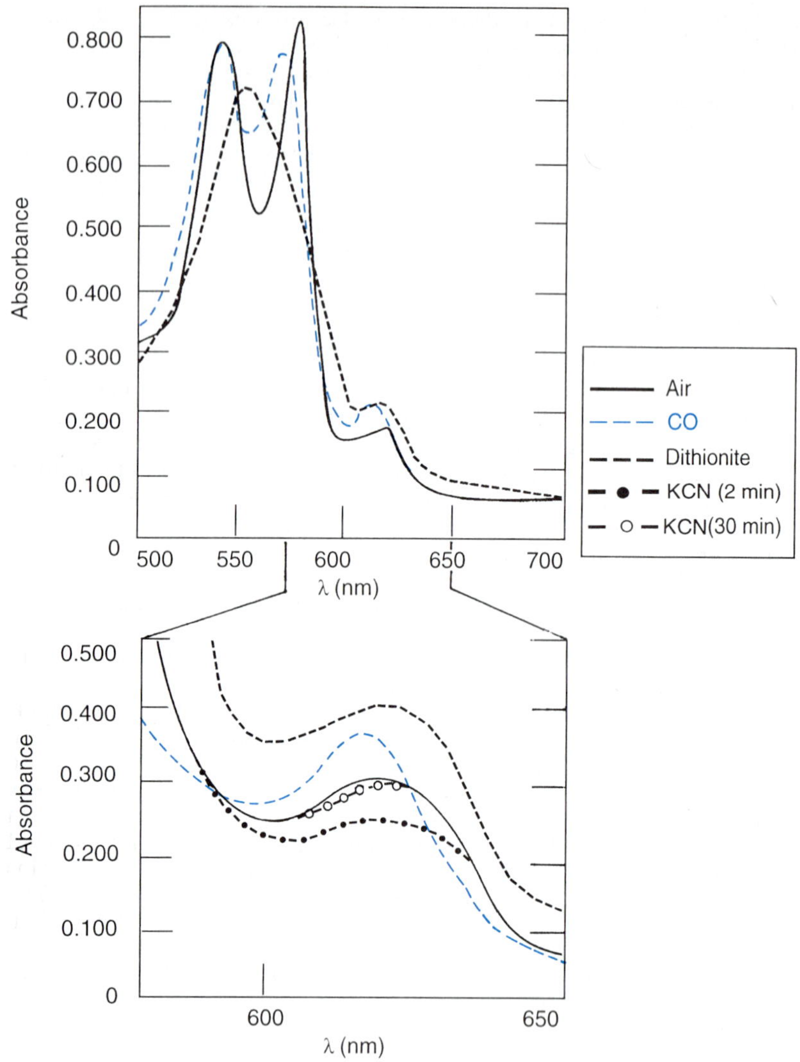

FIGURE 52-25. Visible spectra of the hemolysate of a patient with sulfhemoglobinemia. (**A**) The spectrum of the air-equilibrated sample, the sample after equilibration with carbon monoxide, and the sample treated with the reducing agent dithionite. (**B**) The abnormal peak in the air-equilibrated sample at 2 and 30 minutes after the addition of potassium cyanide (KCN). The augmentation and shift of the peak toward lower wavelength with the addition of carbon monoxide provides the basis for the diagnostic procedure for sulfhemoglobinemia. (After Park CM, Nagel RL. Sulfhemoglobin: clinical and molecular aspects. N Engl J Med 1984;310:1579)

Görgyi's great discovery (ascorbic acid) in a few congestive heart failure patients and was convinced of its efficacy to the reluctance of his colleagues. It is understandable that when he encountered two brothers, Fred and Russell, in the streets of Banbridge who were blue (cyanotic in aspect), he jumped at the opportunity to try ascorbic acid again. He treated one brother and left the other as a control. Sure enough, the treated patient saw his cyanosis disappear fast and dramatically. The untreated brother remained blue. Deeny's skeptical cardiologist colleagues rapidly poked a hole in Deeny's proof: the hearts of Fred and Russell were in excellent and normal condition. One brother was even a member of a field hockey team. Fortunately for all concerned and for hematology, the patients were next studied at the Physiology Laboratory at Belfast, where it was established that their blood contained methemoglobin. The calculated amount of hemoglobin based on gasometry (which depended on the binding of oxygen) was lower than the calculated amount based on colorimetry (which depended on the amount of visible light absorbed by the heme). The diagnosis was clinched by the "observation of the band at 630 nm made with a pocket spectroscope."[238]

Quentin H. Gibson's work in Belfast included using gas manometers to study gas exchange in solutions. Armed with the knowledge that methylene blue speeded up methemoglobin reduction (conversion of ferric to ferrous iron in the heme), he obtained Fred's blood, exposed it to the dye, and observed a burst of oxygen uptake, indicating the reduction of methemoglobin. In addition, by observing that glycolysis was normal in Fred and Russell's red cells and that neither lactate nor glucose, which were known to serve as substrates for the reduction of methemoglobin, were effective in reducing the brother's methemoglobin, Gibson concluded the defect had to be in coenzyme factor I (diaphorase I). He tested this hypothesis, using an enzymatic assay in which fructose diphosphate was converted to triosephosphate by aldolase. This exercise is an example of how an enlightened analysis of a genetic defect can produce powerful insights, even when the only clinical material available is two affected members of a pedigree.

Clinical Aspects

The principle symptom of methemoglobinemia is cyanosis, but the critical question is how much methemoglobin is needed to make cyanosis apparent on examination of the skin and mucosa. Jaffe[239] has calculated that the degree of cyanosis produced by 5 g/dL deoxyhemoglobin (in the ferrous state), is equivalent to 1.5 g/dL of methemoglobin (in the ferric state) or 0.5 g/dL of sulfhemoglobin.

According to Jaffe,[239] hereditary methemoglobinopathies that are the product of an enzyme deficiency (excluding carriers of Hb M) can be classified into four categories:

Type I. Patients affected with this group of methemoglobinopathies are more cyanotic than sick. They have no symptoms except for some fatigue with strenuous exercise in the worst cases. The patients have a normal survival and normal pregnancies. Levels of methemoglobin vary from between 20% and 40% of the total hemoglobin. Despite the mild course, affected patients can develop toxic levels of methemoglobin on exposure to methemoglobin-inducing drugs or chemicals.

Gibson's original patients belonged in this category. The original article describing type I disease contained the solution: the defect was a diaphorase deficiency. Later, Scott[240] confirmed Gibson's findings by demonstrating decreased activity of the red cell–reduced nicotinamide adenine dinucleotide (NADH)-dependent methemoglobin reductase system in Eskimos and American Indians with hereditary methemoglobinemia. NADH was formerly called DNPH or coenzyme I. Methemoglobin reductase is the new name for diaphorase I. Hultquist and Passon[241] made the next major contribution, by demonstrating that NADH-methemoglobin reductase works in conjunction with cytochrome b_5 to reduce methemoglobin. It is interesting that NADH-methemoglobin reductase turns out to have a totally different function in red cell progenitors; it serves as a protease and clips the hydrophobic C-terminal portion of microsomal cytochrome b_5.

Methylene blue works in methemoglobin reductase deficiency because it reduces methemoglobin through a different pathway, using an NADPH (NADH-phosphate)-dependent methemoglobin reductase (diaphorase II), as Gibson had already predicted.

Type II. Hereditary methemoglobinemia type II affects about 10% to 15% of patients. It is a severe and lethal disease, with a strong neurologic component. Although the methemoglobinemia can be treated, the neurologic syndrome is refractory. As Kaplan and colleagues[242–244] have demonstrated, the disease is secondary to a defective NADH-methemoglobin reductase (cytochrome b_5 reductase), in all tissues. The mutation apparently affects the whole molecule.

The defect is autosomal recessive because only the homozygote is affected. The elucidation of this genetic disease involved the finding of Leroux and associates[245] that there are two NADH-methemoglobin reductases in the red cell. One is attached to the membrane and the other is a soluble form, which has been modified by proteolysis so that it no longer assembles itself on the membrane. Because both enzymes are deficient in type II methemoglobinemia patients, Leroux concluded that the primary defect affects the original gene in a way that makes both enzyme forms deficient; hence the symptomatology affects other organs.

Prenatal diagnosis is available for hereditary methemoglobinemia type II but it is generally useful only after the propositus is ascertained, since the disease is recessive.

Type III. Only a few families have been described with type III methemoglobinemia, which is intermediate in severity between types I and II, but closer to type I symptomatically.[246,247] The deficiency of NADH-methemoglobin (cytochrome b_5) reductase is expressed in some nonerythroid cells, including leukocytes, lymphocytes, and platelets. The methemoglobin level is about 25%. The existence of type III methemoglobinemia forces us to be cautious in the use of leukocyte enzyme analyses in the diagnosis of type II.

Type IV. The patient who generated the type IV category of methemoglobinopathy presented with congenital deficiency of cytochrome b_5 (the cofactor, not the enzyme) with a reduction of 23% of the normal level and methemoglobinemia of 12% to 19%.[248] This disorder has no neurologic symptoms and definitely establishes the importance of cytochrome b_5 in the reduction of methemoglobin. The cytochrome b_5 reductase level is normal in red cells.

Pathophysiology

Reduction of Methemoglobin. If normal red cell hemolysates are analyzed for the presence of methemoglobin, less than 0.5% is usually found. Much more is produced, but the red cell has an elaborate mechanism by which the ferric hemes are constantly reduced to the ferrous form (Figs. 52-26 and 52-27). Autoxidation of hemoglobin has been discussed in the section on the M hemoglobins.

Mechanisms capable of reducing methemoglobin include the cytochrome b_5 reductase system, the NADPH–phosphate reductase system, ascorbic acid, and the reduced glutathione.

Cytochrome b_5 Reductase System. This system contains several components.

NADH-DEPENDENT ENZYME: CYTOCHROME b_5 REDUCTASE. This enzyme was purified by Yubisui and Takashita[249] in 1980. It exists in two forms in erythroid cells. It is also known as diaphorase I, NADH-methemoglobin reductase, and NADH-dehydrogenase. It is a soluble enzyme, which reduces methemoglobin, has a molecular weight of about 31,000 without flavine adenine dinucleotide. It contains 275 amino acids and its N terminal is a phenylalanine. The membrane-bound cytochrome b_5 reductase is found in erythroblasts and is probably similar or identical with the liver microsomal enzyme.[250] It contains 300 amino acids, including a membrane-binding domain at the N-terminal end. A 14-carbon fatty acid, myristic acid, is attached to the N-terminal glycine and anchors the enzyme to the membrane. The soluble erythrocyte form is derived from the membrane-bound form by proteolysis of the membrane-binding domain during erythroid maturation. The function of the membrane-bound enzyme in somatic cells is to desaturate and elongate fatty acids in cholesterol biosynthesis and in drug metabolism.

The human gene for this enzyme has been cloned[251] (Fig. 52-28) and consists of nine exons and eight introns (30 kb). Some of the exons and introns are short. For example, the first exon encodes only seven amino acids. The first encoded amino acid is Met. As this is removed, the underlying Gly is spontaneously modified by myristic acid. The cleavage site of the membrane-binding domain lies in the center of the second exon, making it unlikely that the soluble form is generated by alternative splicing. The promoter is of the "housekeeping gene" type, with no TATA box or CAAT box, but several GC boxes.

Some of the mutations that generate NADP-dependent cytochrome b_5 reductase deficiency have been elucidated

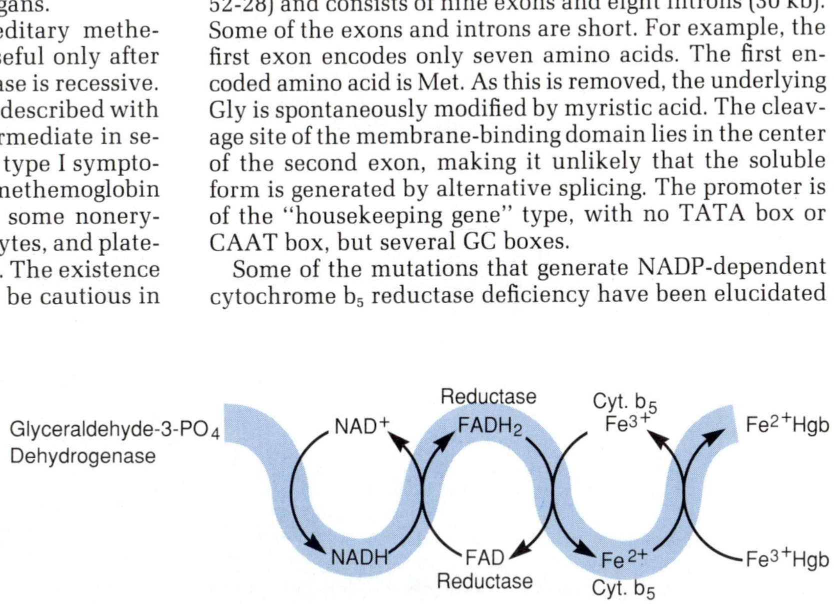

FIGURE 52-26. The absence of methemoglobin-reducing reaction in hemolysates of human erythrocytes suggests the need for a biochemical carrier between NADH and methemoglobin. Because intact erythrocytes contain cytochrome b5 and a flavin-containing cytochrome b5 reductase that is capable of reducing methemoglobin, the sequence shown has been postulated.

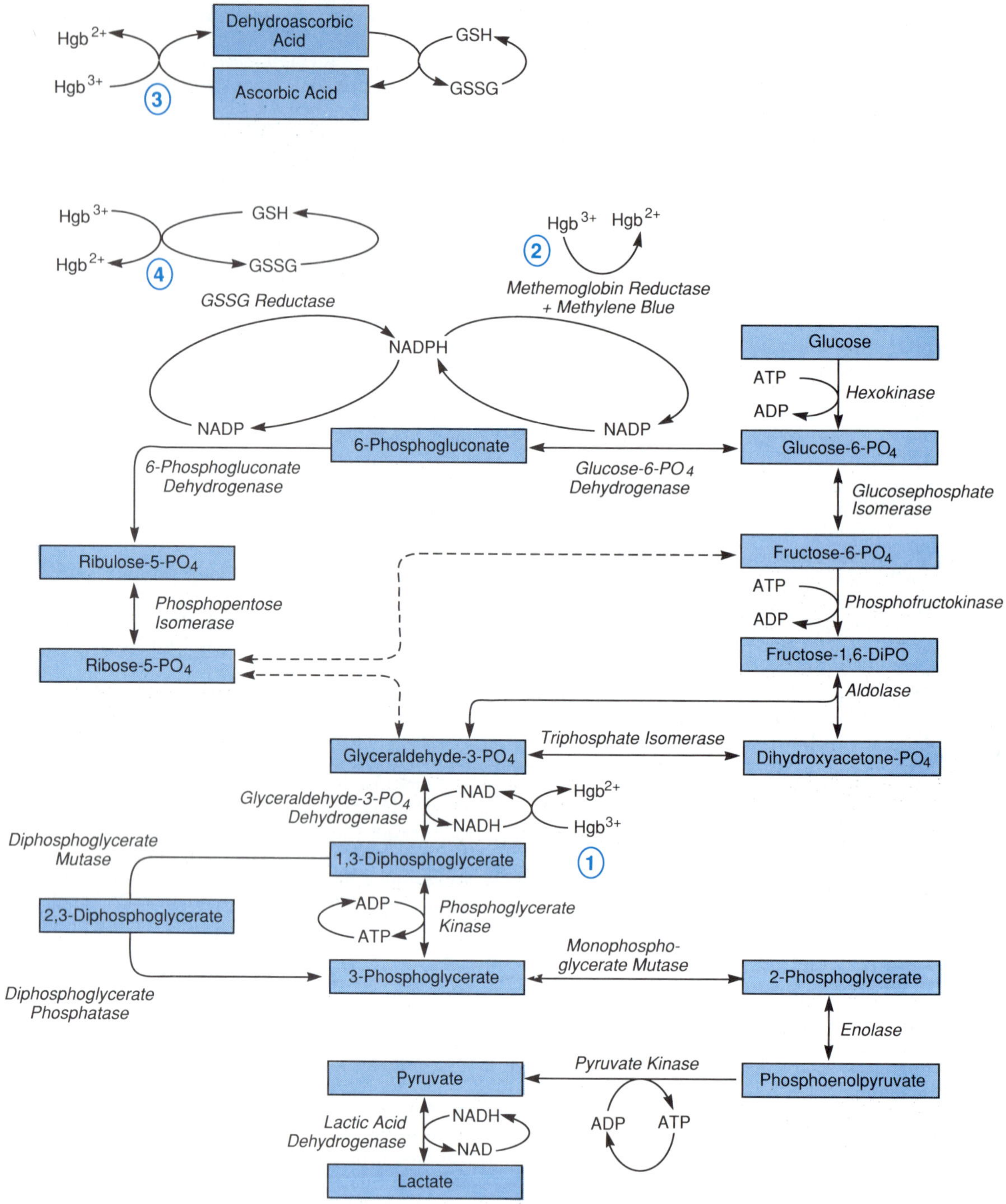

FIGURE 52-27. Pathway for the reduction of methemoglobin.

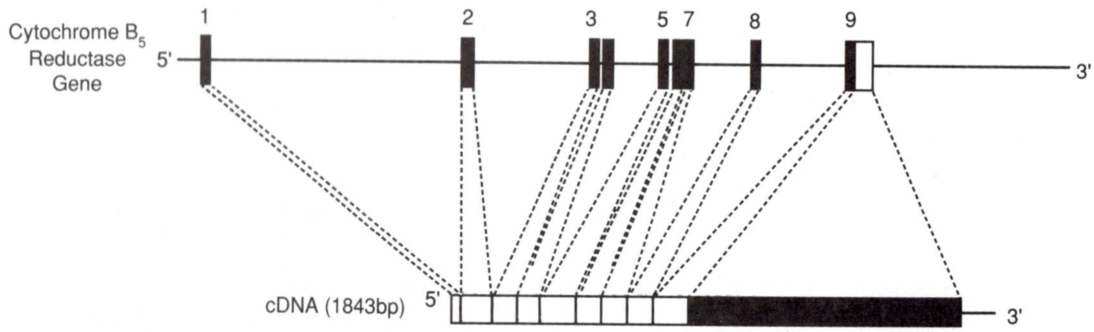

FIGURE 52-28. Organization of the cytochrome b_5 reductase gene and cDNA.

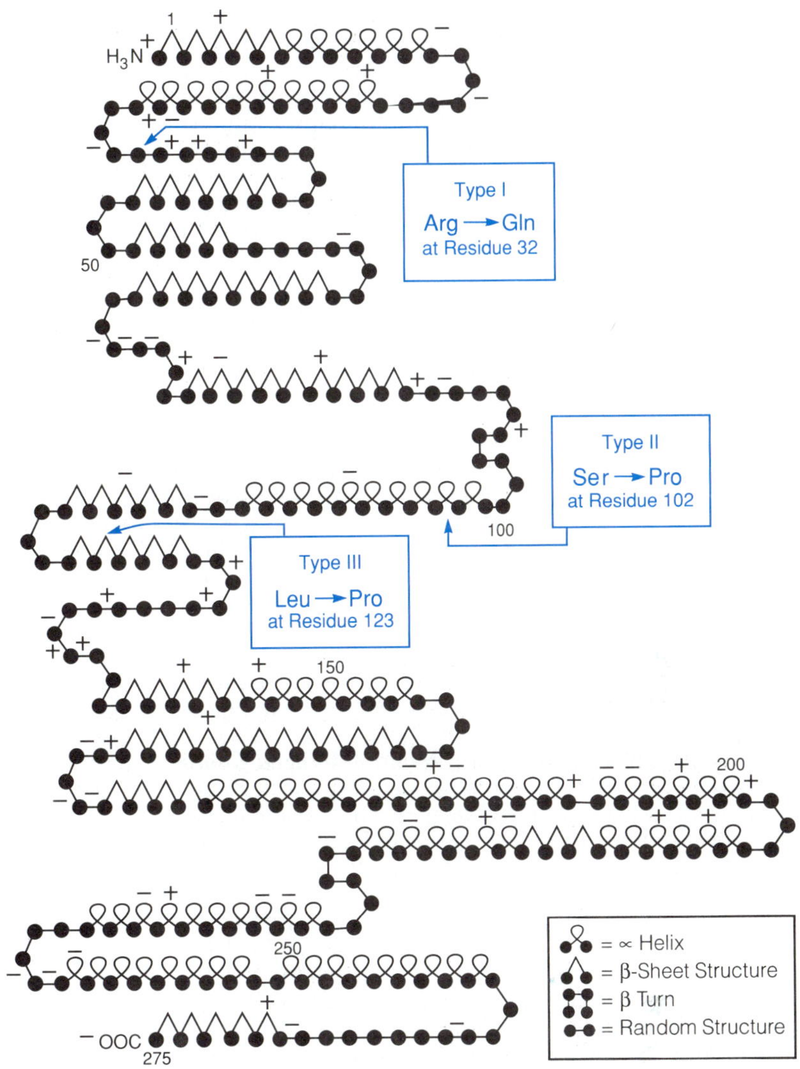

FIGURE 52-29. Location of amino acid substitutions found in cytochrome b_5 reductase (b5R) of homozygotes for hereditary methemoglobinemia types I to III. The secondary structure of the soluble type (erythrocyte type) of b5R is shown. Residue 1 of the soluble type of b5R corresponds to residue 26 of the membrane-bound type. Each substitution is indicated by an arrow. Plus signs indicate positively charged residues, and minus signs negatively charged residues. The variant with Arg–Gln at residue 32 is named b5R Toyoake, that with Ser–Pro at residue 1023 is b5R Hiroshima, and the variant with Leu–Pro at residue 123 is b5R Kurobe. (After Kobayashi Y, Fukumaki Y, Yubisui T, et al. Ser–Pro replacement at residue 127 of NADH–cytochrome b5 reductase causes hereditary methemoglobinemia, generalized type. Blood 1990;75:1408)

(Fig. 52-29). Type I hereditary methemoglobinemia can be the result of a point mutation involving a G → A change in codon 57 of the cytochrome b_5 reductase gene (b_5R-Toyoake). This codon corresponds to residue 32 in the protein. It is normally an arginine and is substituted by a glutamine in the mutated protein.[252] This residue is constant in all enzymes sequenced. The mutation is probably located between an α helix and a β-pleated sheet and might disrupt the conformation of the enzyme.[249,250,254]

Type II hereditary methemoglobinemia is also the result of a single-base mutation in position 102 (b_5R-Hiroshima), in which a serine is replaced by a proline. The substitution is in a region likely to be α-helical. The introduction of a proline in an α helix tends to disrupt the secondary structure and has high probability of inducing significant conformational changes. The mutation is located in exon 5. A mutation associated with type III hereditary methemoglobinemia is located 21 amino acids downstream at position 123: Leu → Pro (b_5R-Kurobe).[255] Again, the introduction of the proline should be disruptive. Why type II is so severe and generalized and why type III is generalized but not severe remain to be elucidated. These mutations, unlike type II, are likely to disrupt the function of the membrane form of the enzyme, particularly its participation in the metabolism of lipids. Fatty acid composition might be altered in patients with type II hereditary methemoglobinemia.[256] Of course, all persons of the same type are unlikely to have the same mutation. This might be true within one ethnic group, but it is less likely as patients from other ethnic backgrounds are examined. Enzymatic differences among patients with type I disease strongly suggest that many other mutations generating this type of methemoglobinemia will be discovered in the future.

NADH. NADH is an indispensable cofactor for cytochrome b_5 reductase. It is generated (reaction 1 in Fig. 52-27) by glyceraldehyde-3-phosphate dehydrogenase, which reduces NADP to NADPH in the process of converting glyceraldehyde-3-phosphate to 1,3 diphosphoglycerate in the glycolytic pathway. Lactic acid dehydrogenase, another enzyme of the glycolytic pathway converts NADPH back into NADP in the process of metabolizing pyruvate to lactic acid. Hence, during steady state there is no net accumulation of NADPH. Nevertheless, when increased methemoglobin levels need to be reduced, pyruvate accumulates because NADH is being consumed in the reduction of methemoglobin.

CYTOCHROME b_5. Cytochrome b_5 is the electron carrier between NADH and methemoglobin. Gacon and colleagues,[257] using an ingenious isoelectric focusing technique, showed that electron transfer between cytochrome b_5 and methemoglobin occurs by means of a complex between the two molecules. The cytochrome binds to four lysines in the heme pocket in both chains. Computer modeling predicts that lysines 56, 60, and 90 interact with cytochrome residues 43 (Glu), 44 (Glu), and 60 (Asp). In addition, an H bond between Lys 61 of the cytochrome serves as a bridge between the two heme propionic side chains of both heme proteins, serving as the micropath for electron transfer. An almost identical interaction occurs in the β chains.

The whole cytochrome b_5 reductase system and the reactions in which this enzyme and its cofactors are involved are depicted in Figure 52-26.

NADPH–Phosphate Reductase System. This reaction (reaction 2 in Fig. 52-27) is probably nonphysiologic since patients with glucose-6-phosphate dehydrogenase (G6PD) deficiency do not have methemoglobinemia. Nevertheless, in the presence of nonphysiologic electron carriers such as methylene blue, this system becomes active. It is the basis for use of methylene blue in the treatment of hereditary methemoglobinemia.

Ascorbic Acid. Ascorbic acid can reduce methemoglobin at a low rate in red cells (reaction 3 in Fig. 52-27). The reduction is combined with oxidation of ascorbic acid to dehydroascorbic acid, which occurs without the help of an enzyme.

Reduced Glutathione (GSH) System. GSH can reduce methemoglobin directly, without enzyme assistance (reaction 4 in Fig. 52-27). The resulting oxidized glutathione (GSSG) is recycled by glutathione reductase.

The four metabolic systems just discussed generate a reducing capacity 250 times greater than that required to reduce physiologically generated red cell methemoglobin.[239]

Protective Mechanisms to Avoid Methemoglobin Formation. Several metabolic processes protect hemoglobin from oxidation to methemoglobin. For example, superoxide dismutase that mops up the toxic superoxide ion, generating hydrogen peroxide. H_2O_2 is also toxic but can be removed by glutathione peroxidase and, less effectively, by the low-affinity enzyme catalase, which intervenes only when peroxides reach an excess. This situation explains why patients with acatalasemia do not have any methemoglobinemia, whereas patients with an inherited deficiency of glutathione peroxidase have low levels of methemoglobin. Glutathione peroxidase is deficient in the red cells of newborns, which might explain their susceptibility to acquired methemoglobinemia.[239]

Acquired Methemoglobinemia

Several chemical agents and drugs can induce methemoglobinemia. Dyes and anilines reduce molecular oxygen and generate methemoglobin, sometimes in cycles, as in the case of phenylhydroxylamine. After reducing oxyhemoglobin, it generates nitrobenzene, which is reduced again to phenylhydroxylamine by red cell enzymes and in turn generates more methemoglobin. Nitrites are common offenders, particularly in children, but the mechanism is less well understood. Recreational use of amyl, butyl or isobutyl nitrites is another cause of acquired methemoglobinemia. In addition, infections might release toxins (including nitrites) that produce methemoglobin.

Differential Diagnosis

The sudden onset of cyanosis, in the absence of cardiopulmonary pathology, suggests acquired methemoglobinemia, although sulfhemoglobin should also be considered. Long-standing cyanosis or the presence of cyanosis in siblings is more compatible with a diagnosis of hereditary methemoglobinemia. Since the latter disorder is recessive, it should not be expected in the parents. The differential diagnosis also includes the M hemoglobins and the low-affinity hemoglobins; since these conditions are dominant, the presence of cyanosis in a parent is diagnostically useful. (Details of the laboratory differential diagnosis are covered in previous sections.) Enzymatic assays or spot tests are available for the methemoglobin reductases, and genetic ascertainment is available for the known mutations. Prenatal diagnosis is available for type II hereditary methemoglobinemia. The efficacy of methylene blue is also diagnostic.

An unusually high incidence of hereditary methemoglobinemia is found among Alaskan Eskimos and Northwest Indians, Navajo Indians, and natives of Yarkusk, Siberia, all of whom may be ethnically connected. The disease has also been observed among Puerto Ricans and in Mediterranean populations.

Treatment of Methemoglobinemia

Acquired methemoglobin is treated first by stopping the offending agent, if it can be identified. Methylene blue, 1 or 2 mg/kg, should be administered intravenously in patients with high levels of methemoglobin (40% to 60%), particularly in those with symptoms. It does not work in patients with coexisting G6PD deficiency. In type I hereditary methemoglobinemia, this intervention is only cosmetic and can be followed by oral methylene blue, 100 to 300 mg/d, to keep the hemoglobin reduced.

In aniline-induced methemoglobinemia, methylene blue can combine with oxyhemoglobin to generate free radicals and produce hemolysis. In these cases, the dye should be limited to two doses.

Patients with methemoglobinemia of over 70% may be at serious risk and should undergo an exchange transfusion.

OTHER NORMAL HEMOGLOBINS AND THEIR MUTATIONS

Hemoglobin F

In 1966, Korber[259] discovered that red cells in newborns are resistant to alkaline denaturation, which was the first suggestion that these cells contain a hemoglobin different from normal adult hemoglobin. Another easily measurable property is found in the ultraviolet spectra of Hb F ($\alpha_2\gamma_2$), which contains a "tryptophan notch" at 252 nm as the result of an extra tryptophan at position γ130 compared with the β chains.[260]

The γ chains are different from the β chains in 39 to 40 positions in the sequence. γ Chains are the product of two genes placed in tandem between the ϵ and pseudo β genes, in the β-like globin cluster on chromosome 11. The only difference between the two γ gene products is the presence of glycine in position γ 136 in the G γ gene, the left gene, and alanine in the same position in the $^A\gamma$ gene, to the right. A common polymorphism is in the $^A\gamma$ gene, in which threonine ($^A\gamma^T$) replaces isoleucine ($^A\gamma^I$).[262] The striking similarities in the protein sequence are reflected at the nucleotide level, where the homology between the two genes is high. Oliver Smithies[263] was the first to point out that this is a consequence of gene conversion, a mutational event in which the sequences upstream replace sequences downstream, particularly in tandem genes, homogenizing them in the process.

That this process is ongoing in this portion of the genome was demonstrated by Bouhassira and colleagues[264] in the Bantu haplotype linked to the β^S gene. They found a subgroup of this haplotype that had undergone an even more recent gene conversion, eliminating several of the few difference in sequence between the two γ genes. One interpretation of this phenomenon is that considerable selective value is placed on the sequence of γ chains and on the structure of Hb F. This is not surprising since Hb F is present throughout most of fetal life (although mostly during the last three trimesters), and abnormalities could easily be fatal.

The functionally important differences between γ and β chains are discussed in the following text:

Sequence Differences

The 39 differences are mostly on the surface of the molecule, exactly 22 of them. Four critical substitutions are in the $\alpha_1\beta_1$ area of contact (the packing contact). This is the strong contact that dissociates only under extreme conditions (very high butyl urea concentration, iodine salts, extreme pH). Nevertheless, two of these substitutions (Thr γ112 and Try γ130) in the $\alpha_1\gamma_1$ contact, could be involved in providing the molecule (Hb F) with its alkaline resistance, as well as its decreased dissociation to monomers. In the β chains, position β112 is a cysteine and β130 is a tyrosine. Both of these residues ionize at alkaline pH, and that could promote dissociation of the dimer into monomers. Threonine and tryptophan are polar but not ionizable. No sequence changes affect the $\alpha_1\beta_2$ area of contact (sliding contact), which is the center of ligand-dependent conformational changes. Other critical sequence differences are discussed with the anomalous functional properties.

Protein Conformation

Crystallographic studies of Hb F at 2.5 A resolution show almost entire isomorphism between Hb A and Hb F.[265] The only difference is in the N-terminal portion. This change increases the distance of 2,3-DPG inserted in the central cavity to the γ2 His, which may contribute to the reduction in the effect 2,3-DPG on Hb F (see following section).

Ligand Binding

Red cells of newborns (containing mostly Hb F) have a higher oxygen affinity than adult red cells (p50 = 29 mmHg compared with 26 mmHg in adults), but the oxygen affinity of neonatal and adult red cell hemolysates are indistinguishable.[266] This suggests that the Hb F and Hb A molecules have identical oxygen-binding properties, but the red cells contain effectors that interact abnormally with Hb F.

2,3-DPG has decreased binding to Hb F.[267] The primary structural basis of this effect is the replacement of β143 His (phosphate binding site in the central cavity) with a serine residue at γ143. This abolishes an important binding site. Secondary effects, as already mentioned, come from displacement of the N-terminal portion of the γ chains, which inhibits the binding of phosphates with γ2 His. Finally, Hb F molecules that are acetylated at the γ-chain N terminal are incapable of binding 2,3-DPG.[268]

The effect of Cl^- is also impaired.[269] This anion also binds in the 2,3-DPG site in the central cavity. At low NaCl concentrations (up to 0.05 mol/L), Hb F has a lower affinity for oxygen than does Hb A. At higher Cl^- concentrations, the differences disappear. This effect is not well understood but might have to do with the diminution of positive charges in the central cavity; therefore, the binding affinity for anions and the destabilizing effect on the T state is reduced. The increased stability of the T state induced by the absence of anion neutralizing positive charges would favor low ligand affinity.

The binding of CO_2 to Hb F is drastically decreased.[270] Fewer carbamates are formed at the N terminal over a wide range of P_{CO_2}. The γ-chain N terminal has a pKa of 8.1, which is considerable higher than the pKa of β chains (pKa 6.6). Under physiologic conditions, 90% of the γ sites are protonated and unable to bind CO_2.

The alkaline Bohr effect (relation between high pH and ligand affinity) is increased by 20% in Hb F–containing red cells.[271] This seems to be a Cl^- effect, since in isolated Hb F at low anion concentrations, hemoglobins A and F have an identical Bohr effect, and the Bohr effect of Hb F increases pari passu with the Cl^- concentration. A plausible explanation is that the binding of Cl^- at low pH to β143 His stabilizes the R state. The absence of this Cl^- site in γ chains would lower the low pH Bohr effect, since it is a situation that favors the T state. As a consequence, the alkaline Bohr effect is favored in Hb F.

Physiology of Hb F–Containing Red Cells

The central question is how the modified properties of Hb F benefit the fetus and the newborn. Perhaps the main feature of fetal circulation, in terms of its differences with postnatal life, is that the oxygen loading is done under more difficult circumstances in the fetus (liquid–liquid interface) than in the neonate (gas–liquid interface). On the plus side, the tissues of the fetus have a high metabolic rate. therefore, the limitation may be on loading sufficient oxygen rather than on delivery of oxygen, since a significant difference between the P_{O_2} of blood and that of tissue is likely to exist in the fetus.

This analysis explains why the oxygen affinity of Hb F–containing red cells is increased, a situation that favors uptake of oxygen in the placenta. It also explains why modulation of delivery of oxygen is less needed, since modulation generally consists in the decrease of the affinity for oxygen in Hb A. Therefore, no 2,3-DPG response is found in Hb F. Moreover, the analysis explains why the Bohr effect is increased, since fetal blood increases its pH when it passes through the intravillous spaces because of release of CO_2. The Bohr effect accounts for 40% of the normal fetal gas exchange.[271] In addition, by having an increased Bohr effect, the fetus can modulate delivery of oxygen to tissues if it is really needed, even in the absence of 2,3-DPG. About 50% of the delivery to tissues is accounted for by the increased Bohr effect. Finally, the increased Bohr effect could also explain the paradox observed by Charache and colleagues,[75] in which mothers with high-affinity hemoglobin variants did not have pregnancy complications or fetal morbidity. The advantage of Hb F is not limited to the p50 difference with Hb A; if the affinity difference is erased, as in Charache's patients, the enhanced Bohr effect can make up at least some of the difference.

Genetic Heterogeneity

As noted earlier, γ chains are synthesized by two sequence-identifiable genes. This genetic heterogeneity is unique among globins. Additional heterogeneity comes from the fact that about 10% to 15% of newborns have a post-translation modification of the N-terminal glycine of the γ chains. Acetylation is common in proteins that have N-terminal alanine, serine, and, to a lesser extent, glycine residues. Hemoglobin needs to have its N terminal free for functional reasons; therefore, it is not surprising that acetylation has been excluded largely by selection. In the case of Hb F, it contributes to the decrease in 2,3-DPG binding, apparently a welcome feature. Acetylation occurs after synthesis, probably early in the process, and involves catalytic transfer of the acetyl moiety from acetyl-CoA to the protein by acetyltransferase.

Hb Raleigh, which involves the replacement of β1 Val by an acetylatable alanine, is 100% acetylated. Cat hemoglobin, in which the β1 residue is serine, is also 100% acetylated (and does not bind 2,3-DPG well).

Laboratory Diagnosis of Hemoglobin F

The best methods for determining the level of Hb F in the hemolysate depend on the concentration. For normal levels, between 0.1% and 1.5% of the total hemoglobin, the immunologic assays are best. Between 1.5% and 40%, alkaline denaturation is accurate. Over 40%, HPLC is probably the best method, although it can also be used at lower concentrations. A method of enriching the Hb F by chromatography or isoelectric focusing, followed by HPLC, allows this technique to be applied to all concentrations of fetal hemoglobins. Disposable columns for the determination of Hb F in hemolysates that contain no Hb A (such as red cells from Hb SS or Hb CC disease patients) are also available and are accurate.

Because Hb F is unevenly distributed among red cells (in normals and in those with most medical conditions except some forms of hereditary persistence of fetal hemoglobin), immunologic techniques that allow the identification of red cells containing Hb F (F cells and F reticulocytes) and measurement of the average amount of Hb F per cell have become powerful tools for the study Hb F expression.[272–275] About 0.5% to 7% of red cells are F cells in normal adults.

Agar electrophoresis at pH 6.4 (available as a kit) offers an interesting method to isolate or identify Hb F. Hemoglobins are subjected to a combination of chromatography and electrophoresis in agar. The agar matrix interacts with the central cavity of hemoglobins,[276] and hemoglobins with abnormalities in that region (such as Hb F) tend to migrate faster (or slower) than their electrophoretic mobility would predict at pH 6.4. Therefore, when a hemoglobin is found in which the electrophoretic mobility in agar is anomalous compared with the mobility under standard conditions (cellulose acetate, pH 8.6), a mutation of the central cavity should be suspected. *Hb Hope* is an example of this phenomenon.

Medical Conditions Outside of Hemoglobinopathies Associated With High Fetal Hemoglobin Expression in Infants and Adults

Newborns have between 65% and 95% Hb F. This amount decreases progressively during the first year of life. The normal adult level is approached by 1 year of age and is achieved by 5 years. Normals have a gender-determining dispersion of their Hb F levels. Miyoshi and colleagues[277] has detected an excess of high normal values in women and have presented evidence that this is inherited as an X-linked characteristic. Identification of an X-linked modulator of Hb F expression is being actively pursued.

Pregnancy is associated with a modest increase in Hb F in the second trimester. Hydatidiform moles are associated with particularly high values. Although maternal pregnancy hormones have been implicated, the mechanism of this elevation is not clear.[278]

Some conditions (besides hemoglobinopathies) retard the down-regulation of Hb F in the first 5 years of life. These conditions include prematurity, trisomy 21, and infants of diabetic mothers.[279] Acceleration of the fall in Hb F is observed in Down's syndrome patients and those with C/D translocations.

Hemolytic anemias, acute bleeding, treatment with hydroxyurea or Ara-C all can be associated with higher than normal values of Hb F, a phenomenon that has been interpreted to mean that under these conditions early progenitors are rushed through development while retaining their fetal hemoglobin program, because the reduction in the number of cells division precluded their down-regulation.

Invariably, juvenile chronic myeloid leukemia and Fanconi's anemia are accompanied by significant elevations of Hb F). Erythroleukemia, paroxysmal nocturnal hemoglobinuria, kala-azar, preleukemia, and recovery from marrow aplasia are also accompanied by variable elevations of Hb F. The highest levels are found in erythroleukemia (Di-Guglielmo's disease). Many other conditions, including solid tumors, exhibit occasionally increased levels of Hb F.[280–282]

Mutations in the $^{G}\gamma$ Genes

Variants of the $^{G}\gamma$ Gene. Thirty-three variants have been described with a single amino acid substitution in the $^{G}\gamma$ gene.[283] Of these, two are unstable: *Hb Poole* (γ 130[H] Trp → Gly), which is significantly unstable and *Hb F Xin Jin* (γ 119[GH] Gly → Arg).[159] A mutation of the same site, but not the same amino acid as Hb Poole, has also been identified in β chains (Hb Wein [β130 Tyr → Asp]).

Also found in Hb F is the equivalent of M hemoglobins in the β chains: *Hb F-M Fort Ripley*, which has a cyanotic phenotype in the newborn and corresponds to the substitution of the proximal histidine γ92(F8) His → Tyr. It is the perfect equivalent to Hb Hyde Park. The other mutation, *Hb F-M Osaka*, involves the distal histidine, γ63(E7) and is equivalent to Hb M Saskatoon. Newborns with α-chain substitutions of the proximal or distal histidines have the same cyanotic phenotype as that of adults, with the cyanosis appearing early in the neonatal period.

Finally, one high-affinity variant has been described: *Hb F Onoda*.

Variants of the $^{A}\gamma$ Gene and the Common Variant $^{A}\gamma^{T}$ (Hb F Sardinia). Twenty variants of the $^{A}\gamma$ gene have been described up until now, but none of them have functional abnormalities. Six variants of the common $^{A}\gamma^{T}$ variant have been described[279] but only Hb F Xinjiang is unstable.

Note that Hb F Texas, Hb F Alexandria, and Hb F Ube have not been assigned to the corresponding γ gene.

Hemoglobin A_2

Hemoglobin A_2 is the product of the combination of α chains with δ chains ($\alpha_2\delta_2$). The δ chains are the product of the δ gene, which transcribes δ message at a low level. Hb A_2 represents about 2.4% of the hemoglobins present in normal hemolysates. The δ gene resides in the cluster of β-like genes between the pseudo-β gene and the β gene.

δ Gene

The δ gene arose from a duplication of the β gene about 40 million years ago (although one cannot exclude the possibility that gene conversion could have erased differences of an older gene). This gene also exists and is expressed at low levels in the new-world primates (1% to 6%). In some old-world primates, the δ gene is present but not expressed. The δ gene is absent in other mammals. In any case, the distribution among animals suggests that this was the last globin gene to emerge in the β-like gene cluster. Its relatively recent appearance (or recent gene conversion) explains why the δ chain exhibits only 10 sequence differences in the β gene.

The low level of transcription might be the consequence of changes in the 5′ flanking region. Of the three CCAAT-like box sequences, none are perfectly conserved. Instability of the δ mRNA may also contribute to the poor expression of the δ gene.

Functional and Structural Aspects

Hb A and Hb A_2 have similar ligand binding curves, although the latter has slightly higher oxygen affinity. The Bohr effect, the cooperativity of ligand binding, and the response to 2,3-DPG are identical.

Among the differences are that Hb A_2 is more thermostable. This is due to a change at $\delta 116$, in which there is an arginine instead of the $\beta 114$ proline. This arginine forms a salt bridge with $\alpha 114$ proline, increasing even further the stability of the $\alpha_1\beta_1$ packing contact. Another difference is that Hb A_2 binds to the red cell membrane better than does Hb A.[289]

The low levels of Hb A_2 and the multiple functionally abnormal mutations found in primate δ-like genes have been quoted as reasons for the lack of functional importance for this minor component and that the δ gene is condemned to the biologic heap of history as a pseudogene. Nevertheless, this analysis presupposes that the only functional role of any hemoglobin is to carry oxygen. If this is so, Hb A_2 is clearly useless. Alternatively, the increased binding of Hb A_2 to the membrane could indicate another role for this hemoglobin. It is necessary to know what proteins in addition to band 3 that this hemoglobin is capable of binding and if this has any functional role. The finding of Hb A_2 at polymorphic frequencies in the Dogon (see following text) stimulates this type of thinking.

Mutational Events Involving the δ Gene

Twenty three single amino acid substitutions, all due to single base changes, have been described in Hb A_2. This might be the tip of the iceberg, since these substitutions are more difficult to detect. Two mutations, *Hb A_2 Wrens* (98[FG5] Val → Met)[290] and *Hb A_2 Manzanares* (δ121[GH4] Glu → Val)[291] are unstable. *Hb A_2 Canada* (δ99 [Asp → Asn])[292] has very high affinity for oxygen, but no erythrocytosis is present.

A common mutation, found mostly among African Americans and Africans is *Hb A_2'*, also called *Hb B_2*. In Africa, it has been described in samples from different geographic locations including Ghana. Hb A_2' has been found at polymorphic frequencies in one of the casts in the Dogon region of the Republic of Mali. Haplotype analysis of the Mali β-like gene cluster demonstrates that all unrelated persons carrying this mutation have the same haplotype. Samples from unrelated African Americans with this mutation also demonstrate haplotype homogeneity. Hence, it is possible that Hb A_2' arose in Africa unicentrically and distributed itself to other regions of Africa by gene flow.

A interesting set of mutational events involve the unequal crossover between the δ gene and the β gene. This generates hemoglobins with portions of δ chains and portions of β chains. They are termed *Lepore-type hemoglobins* after the first family described. The first three examples of this type of event were characterized in heterozygotes by low levels of the Lepore-type hemoglobin (about 20%), electrophoretic migration similar to Hb S, and a thalassemic phenotype (microcytosis, hypochromia, hemolytic anemia). In homozygotes for this condition, severity varies from transfusion dependency to moderate anemia. Populations at risk are principally Italians, Greeks, and Yugoslavians (the latter being the most severe), but examples have been found in Turkish Cypriots, inhabitants of Papua New Guinea, African Americans, Indians, and Romanians.

The Lepore hemoglobins are described in more detail in Chapter 51. Hb Lepore Hollandia, Hb Lepore Baltimore, and Hb Lepore Washington-Boston (the first described) have different lengths of the δ sequence in the N-terminal portion of the hybrid chain and complementary portions of the β chains at the C-terminal end. All have a total of 146 amino acids. The more recently described Lepore-type hemoglobin, Hb Parchman, is a patchwork in which a segment of the β sequence is located in the center of the chain. The location of the crossover is uncertain because, with only 10 amino acid differences between the δ and β chains, there are too few informative sites.

If a Lepore-type unequal crossover occurs, an anti-Lepore hemoglobin molecule is also generated, but finding it depends on its prevalence and on luck. Hb P-Nilotic is the anti-Lepore of Lepore Hollandia. Hb Lincoln Park is probably the same with an added deletion at position δ137. The hemoglobins Miyada and P Congo could be anti-Lepores of Lepore hemoglobins that are yet to be found. Electrophoretically, hemoglobins P Congo, P Nilotic, and Lincoln Park migrate like Hb S, whereas Hb Miyada and Hb Parchman migrate like Hb C.

Variation of Hb A_2 Levels With Other Clinical Conditions

The levels of Hb_2 are elevated in a number of condition; in some instances, this feature is of diagnostic value. The most common clinical instance is β-thalassemia. Hb A_2 is also elevated in sickle trait; SS blood, particularly SS with α-thalassemia; and in acquired conditions such as megaloblastic anemias and hyperthyroidism. Controversial evidence exists that Hb A_2 is elevated in malaria patients. Elevation of Hb A_2 is not due to an increase in the synthesis of δ chains, but is a consequence of the preferential assemblage of δ with α chains, particularly if α chains are in short supply. Decreases of the levels of Hb A_2 are found in α-thalassemia, $\delta\beta$-thalassemia, δ-thalassemia, and hereditary persistence of fetal hemoglobin, either because the δ gene is not present (deletions) or because the α chains are more avid for γ or β chains than for the δ chains.

REFERENCES

1. Kendrew JC, Dickerson RE, Strandberg BE, et al. Structure of myoglobin: a three-dimensional Fourier synthesis at 2 A resolution. Nature 1960;185:422.
2. Tetreau C, Lavalette D, Momenteau M, Lhoste JM. Energy barriers in the binding of CO and O_2 bindings to heme model compounds. Proc Natl Acad Sci USA 1987;84:2267.
3. Komiyama NH, Shih DT, Looker D, et al. Was the loss of the D helix in alpha globin a functionally neutral mutation? Nature 1991;352:349.
4. Perutz MF, Rossman MG, Cullis AF, et al. Structure of haemoglobin: a three-dimensional Fourier synthesis at 5.5 A resolution, obtained by X-ray analysis. Nature 1960;185:416.
5. Baldwin JM. The structure of human carbonmonoxy haemoglobin at 2.7 Å resolution. J Mol Biol 1980;136:103.
6. Fermi G, Perutz MF, Shaanan B, et al. The crystal structure of human deoxyhaemoglobin at 1.7 Å resolution. J Mol Biol 1984;175:159.
7. Chothia C, Wodak S, Janin J. Role of subunit interfaces in the allosteric mechanism of hemoglobin. Proc Natl Acad Sci USA 1976;73:3793.
8. Koshland DE Jr, Nemethy G, Filmer D. Comparison of experimental binding data and theoretical model in proteins containing subunits. Biochemistry 1966;5:365.
9. Monod J, Wyman J, Changeaux JP. On the nature of allosteric transition: a plausible model. J Mol Biol 1967;12:88.
10. Baldwin J, Chothia C. Haemoglobin: the structural changes related to ligand binding and its allosteric mechanism. J Mol Biol 1979;129:175.
11. Perutz MF, Sanders JKM, Chenery DH, et al. Interactions between the quaternary structure of the globin and the spin state of the heme in ferric mixed spin derivatives of hemoglobin. Biochemistry 1978;17:3640.
12. Perutz MF, Kilmartin JV, Nagai K, et al. Influence of globin structures on the state of the heme: ferrous low spin derivatives. Biochemistry 1976;15:378.
13. Maxwell JC, Caughey WS. An infrared study of NO bonding to heme B and hemoglobin A: evidence for inositol hexaphosphate induced cleavage of proximal histidine to iron bonds. Biochemistry 1976;15:388.

14. Perutz MF. Sterochemistry of the cooperative effects in haemoglobin. Nature 1970;288:726.
15. Ho C, Russu IM. Proton nuclear magnetic resonance studies of sickle cell hemoglobin. In: Caughey WS, ed. Biochemical and clinical aspects of hemoglobin abnormalities. New York, Academic Press, 1978:179.
16. Ackers GK, Doyle ML, Myers D, Daugherty MA. Molecular code for cooperativity in hemoglobin. Science 1992;255:54.
17. Miura S, Ikeda-Saito T, Yonetani T, Ho C. Oxygen equilibrium studies of cross-linked asymmetrical cyanomet valency hybrid hemoglobins: models for partially oxygenated species. Biochemistry 1987;26:2149.
18. Perrella M, Colosimo A, Benazzi L, et al. What the intermediate compounds in ligand binding to hemoglobin tell about the mechanism of cooperativity. Biophys Chem 1990;37:211.
19. Nagel RL, Ranney HM, Kucinskies LL. Tyrosine ionization in human CO and deoxyhemoglobin. Biochemistry 1966;5:1934.
20. Ishimor K, Hashimoto M, Imai K, et al. Site-directed mutagenesis in haemoglobin: functional and structural role of the penultimate tyrosine in the alpha subunit. Biochemistry 1994;33:2546.
21. Ackers GK, Hazzard JH. Transduction of binding energy into hemoglobin cooperativity. Trends Biochem Sci 1993:385.
22. Perrella M, Bresciani D, Rossi-Bernardi L. The binding of CO_2 to human hemoglobin. J Biol Chem 1975;250:5413.
23. Perrella M, Kilmartin JV, Fogg J, et al. Identification of the high and low affinity CO_2 binding sites of human haemoglobin. Nature 1975;256:759.
24. Kilmartin JV, Fogg JH, Perutz MF. Role of C-terminal histidine in the alkaline Bohr effect of human hemoglobin. Biochemistry 1980;19:3189.
25. Nishikura K. Identification of histidine-122 α in human haemoglobin as one of the unknown alkaline Bohr groups by hydrogen-tritium exchange. Biochem J 1978;173:651.
26. Russu IM, Ho NT, Ho C. Role of the β 146 histidyl residue in the alkaline Bohr effect of hemoglobin. Biochemistry 1980;19:1043.
27. Perutz MF, Gronenborn AM, Clorc GM, et al. The pKa values of two histidine residues in human haemoglobin, the Bohr effect, and the dipole moments of α-helices. J Mol Biol 1985;183:491.
28. Benesch R, Benesch RE. The effect of organic phosphates from the human erythrocyte on the allosteric properties of hemoglobin. Biochem Biophys Res Commun 1967;26:162.
29. Chanutin A, Curnish RR. Effect of organic and inorganic phosphates on the oxygen equilibrium of human erythrocytes. Arch Biochem Biophys 1967;121:96.
30. Arnone A. X-ray diffraction study of binding of 2,3-diphosphoglycerate to human deoxyhaemoglobin. Nature 1972;237:146.
31. Bonaventura J, Bonaventura C, Amiconi G, et al. Allosteric interactions in non-α chains isolated from normal human hemoglobin, fetal hemoglobin, and hemoglobin Abruzzo [β 143 (H21) His → Arg]. J Biol Chem 1975;250:6278.
32. Rose ZB. The enzymology of 2,3-bisphosphoglycerate. Adv Enzymol 1980;51:211.
33. Card R, Brain M. The "anemia" of childhood. N Engl J Med 1973;288:388.
34. Purcell Y, Brozovic B. Red cell 2,3-diphosphoglycerate concentration in man decreases with age. Nature 1974;251:511.
35. Lacombe C, Craescu CT, Blouquit Y, et al. Structural and functional studies of hemoglobin Poissy $\alpha_2\beta_2$ 56 (D7) Gly → Arg and 86 (F2) Ala → Pro. Eur J Biochem 1985;153:655.
36. Grace RJ, Gover PA, Treacher DF, et al. Venesection in haemoglobin Yakima, a high oxygen affinity haemoglobin. Clin Lab Haematol 1992;14:1995.
37. Clegg JB, Naughton MA, Weatherall DJ. Abnormal human haemoglobins: separation and characterization of the α and β chains by chromatography, and the determination of two new variants, Hb Chesapeake and Hb J (Bangkok). J Mol Biol 1966;19:91.
38. Charache S, Weatherall DJ, Clegg JB. Polycythemia associated with a hemoglobinopathy. J Clin Invest 1966;45:813.
39. Nagel RL, Gibson QH, Charache S. Relation between structure and function in hemoglobin Chesapeake. Biochemistry 1967;6:2395.
40. Lines JG, McIntosh R. Oxygen binding by haemoglobin J Capetown (α2 92 Arg→Gln). Nature 1967;215:297.
41. Nagel RL, Gibson OH, Jenkins T. Ligand binding in the Hb J Capetown. J Mol Biol 1971;58:643.
42. Shimasaki S. A new hemoglobin variant, hemoglobin Nunobiki [α 141 (HC3) Arg→Cys]: notable influence of the carboxy-terminal cysteine upon various physico-chemical characteristics of hemoglobin. J Clin Invest 1985;75:695.
43. Reed CS, Hampson R, Gordon S, et al. Erythrocytosis secondary to increased oxygen affinity of a mutant hemoglobin, hemoglobin Kempsey. Blood 1968;31:623.
44. Jones RT, Osgood EE, Brimhall B, et al. Hemoglobin Yakima. I. Clinical and biochemical studies. J Clin Invest 1967;46:1840.
45. Weatherall DJ, Clegg JB, Callender ST, et al. Haemoglobin Radcliffe ($\alpha_2\beta_2$ 99(GI)Ala): a high oxygen-affinity variant causing familial polycythaemia. Br J Haematol 1977;35:177.
46. Rucknagel DL, Glynn KP, Smith JR. Hemoglobin Ypsilanti characterized by increased oxygen affinity, abnormal polymerization and erythremia. Clin Res 1967;15:270.
47. Blouquit Y, Braconnier F, Galacteros F, et al. Hemoglobin Hotel-Dieu β 99 Asp→Gly (Gl): a new abnormal hemoglobin with high oxygen affinity. Hemoglobin 1981;5:19.
48. Rochette J, Poyart C, Varet B, et al. A new hemoglobin variant altering the $\alpha_2\beta_2$ contact: Hb Chemilly $\alpha_2\beta_2$ 99 (Gl) Asp → Val. FEBS Lett 1984;166:8.
49. Imai K. Oxygen-equilibrium characteristics of abnormal hemoglobin Hiroshima ($\alpha_2\beta_2$ 143 Asp). Arch Biochem Biophys 1968;127:543.
50. Nagel RL, Gibson OH, Hamilton HB. Ligand kinetics in hemoglobin Hiroshima. J Clin Invest 1971;50:1772.
51. Nute PE, Stamatoyannopoulos G, Hermodson MA, et al. Hemoglobinopathic erythrocytosis due to a new electrophoretically silent variant, hemoglobin San Diego (β 109 [Gll] Val → Met). J Clin Invest 1974;53:320.
52. Lorkin PA, Stephens AD, Beard MEJ, et al. Haemoglobin Rahere (β 82 Lys → Thr): a new high affinity haemoglobin associated with decreased 2,3 diphosphoglycerate binding and relative polycythaemia. Br Med J 1975;4:200.
53. Ikkala E, Koskela J, Pikkarainen P, et al. Hb Helsinki: a variant with a high oxygen affinity and a substitution at a 2,3-DPG binding site (β 82 [EF6] Lys → Met). Acta Haematol 1976;56:257.
54. Bonaventura J, Bonaventura C, Sullivan B, et al. Hemoglobin Providence: functional consequences of two alterations of the 2,3-diphosphoglycerate binding site at position β82. J Biol Chem 1976;251:7563.
55. Lorkin PA, Stephens AD, Beard MEJ, et al. Haemoglobin Rahere (β82 Lys→Thr): A new high affinity haemoglobin associated with decreased 2,3-diphosphoglycerate binding and relative polycythaemia. Br Med J 1975;4:200.
56. Bonaventura J, Riggs A. Polymerization of hemoglobins of mouse and man: structural basis. Science 1967;158:800.
57. Tondo CV, Bonaventura J, Bonaventura C, et al. Functional properties of hemoglobin Porto Alegre ($\alpha_2A\beta_2$9 Ser→Cys) and the reactivity of its extra cysteinyl residue. Biochim Biophys Acta 1974;342:15.
58. Stamatoyannopoulos G, Nute PE, Adamson JW, et al. Hemoglobin Olympia (β20 valine → methionine): an electrophoretically silent variant associated with high oxygen affinity and erythrocytosis. J Clin Invest 1973;52:342.
59. Edelstein SJ, Poyart C, Blouquit Y, Kister J. Self-association of haemoglobin Olympia ($\alpha_2\beta_2$ 20 (B2) Val→Met): a human haemoglobin bearing a substitution at the surface of the molecule. J Mol Biol 1986;187:277.
60. Flatz G, Kinderlerer JL, Kilmartin JV, et al. Haemoglobin Tak: a variant with additional residues at the end of the β-chains. Lancet 1971;10:732.
61. Imai K, Lehmann H. The oxygen affinity of haemoglobin Tak, a variant with elongated β chain. Biochim Biophys Acta 1975;412:288.
62. Lehmann H, Casey R, Lang A, et al. Haemoglobin Tak: a β-chain elongation. Br J Haematol 1975;31:119.
63. Delano J, North ML, Arous N, et al. Hb Saverne: a new variant having an elongated β chain. (Abstract) Blood 1984;64(Suppl 1):56a.
64. Delanoe-Garin J, Blouquit Y, Arous N, et al. Hemoglobin Saverne: a new variant with elongated β chains: structural and functional properties. Hemoglobin 1988;12:337.
65. White JM, Szur L, Gillies IDS, et al. Familial polycythaemia caused by a new haemoglobin variant: Hb Heathrow: Hb 103 (G5) phenylalanine → leucine. Br Med J 1973;3:665.
66. Sherwood JB, Goldwasser E. A radioimmunoassay for erythropoietin. Blood 1979;54:885.
67. Rosa R, Prehu MO, Beuzard Y, Rosa J. The first case of a complete deficiency of diphosphoglycerate mutase in human erythrocytes. J Clin Invest 1978;62:907.
68. Kales SN. Carbon monoxide intoxication. Am Fam Physician 1993;48:1100.
69. Adamson JW. Familial polycythemia. Semin Hematol 1975;12:383.
70. Kelly RM, Hui HL, Noble RW. Chloride acts as a novel negative heterotropic effector of hemoglobin Rothschild (beta 37 Trp→Arg) in solution. Biochemistry 1994;33:4363.
71. Adamson JW, Finch CA. Erythropoietin and the polycythemias. Ann NY Acad Sci 1968;149:560.
72. Adamson JW, Hayashi A, Stamatoyannopoulos G, et al. Erythrocyte function and marrow regulation in hemoglobin Bethesda (β 145 Histidine). J Clin Invest 1972;51:2883.
73. Adamson JW, Finch CA. Hemoglobin function, oxygen affinity and erythropoietin. Annu Rev Physiol 1975;37:351.
74. Charache S, Achuff S, Winslow R, et al. Variability of the homeostatic response to altered P(50). Blood 1978;52:1156.
75. Charache S, Catalano P, Burns S, et al. Pregnancy in carriers of high-affinity hemoglobins. Blood 1985;65:713.
76. Butler WM, Spratling L, Kark JA, et al. Hemoglobin Osler: report of a new family with exercise studies before and after phlebotomy. Am J Hematol 1982;13:293.
77. Schneider RG, Atkins RJ, Hosty TS, et al. Haemoglobin Titusville: α94 Asp → Asn, a new haemoglobin with a lowered affinity for oxygen. Biochem Biophys Acta 1975;400:365.
78. Bonaventura J, Riggs A. Hemoglobin Kansas: a human hemoglobin with a neutral amino acid substitution and an abnormal oxygen equilibrium. J Biol Chem 1968;243:980.

79. Reismann KR, Ruth WE, Nomura T. A human hemoglobin with lowered oxygen affinity and impaired heme–heme interactions. J Clin Invest 1961;40:182.
80. Nagel RL, Lynfield J, Johnson J, et al. Hemoglobin Beth Israel: a mutant causing clinically apparent cyanosis. N Engl J Med 1976;295:125.
81. Arous N, Braconnier F, Thillet J, et al. Hemoglobin Saint Mande β102 (G4) Asn → Tyr: a new low oxygen affinity variant. FEBS Lett 1981;126: 114.
82. Greer J. Three dimensional structure of abnormal haemoglobins Kansas and Richmond. J Mol Biol 1971;59:99.
83. Efremov GD, Huisman THJ, Smith LL, et al. Hemoglobin Richmond: a human hemoglobin which forms asymmetric hybrids with other hemoglobins. J Biol Chem 1969;244:6105.
84. Andersen L. J Mol Biol 1975;94:33.
85. Gacon G, Belkhodja O, Wajcman H, Labie D, Najman A. Structural and functional studies of Hb Rothschild β37(C3) Trp→Arg: a new variant of the $\alpha_1\beta_2$ contact. FEBS Lett 1977;82:243.
86. Sharma VS, Newton GL, Ranney HM, et al. Hemoglobin Rothschild (β37(C3) Trp → Arg): a high/low affinity haemoglobin variant. J Mol Biol 1980;144:267.
87. Craik CS, Vallette I, Beychok A, Waks M. Refolding defects in hemoglobin Rothschild. J Biol Chem 1980;255:6219.
88. Moo-Penn WF, McPhedran P, Bobrow S, et al. Hemoglobin Connecticut (β21 (β3) Asp → Gly): a hemoglobin variant with low oxygen affinity. Am J Hematol 1981;11:137.
89. Marinucci M, Giuliani A, Maffi D, et al. Hemoglobin Bologna ($\alpha_2\beta_2$ 61(E5) Lys→Met), an abnormal human hemoglobin with low oxygen affinity. Biochim Biophys Acta 1981;668:209.
90. Bonaventura C, Cashon R, Bonaventura J, et al. Involvement of the distal histidine in the low affinity exhibited by Hb Chico (Lys β66 → Thr) and its isolated β chains. J Biol Chem 1991;266:23033–23040.
91. Olson JS, Mathews AJ, Rohlfs RJ, et al. The role of the distal histidine in myoglobin and hemoglobin. Nature 1988;336:265–266.
92. Imamura T, Fujita S, Ohta Y, et al. Hemoglobin Yoshizuka (G10 (108) β asparagine → aspartic acid): a new variant with a reduced oxygen affinity from a Japanese family. J Clin Invest 1969;48:2341.
93. Moo-Penn WF, Wolff JA, Simon G, et al. Hemoglobin Presbyterian: β108 (G10) asparagine → lysine—a hemoglobin variant with low oxygen affinity. FEBS Lett 1978;92:53.
94. Jones RT, Brimhall B, Pootrakul S, Gray G. Hemoglobin Vancouver [$\alpha_2\beta_2$ 73 (E17) Asp→Tyr]: its structure and function. J Mol Evol 1976;9: 37.
95. Konotey-Ahulu FID, Gallo E, Lehmann H, Ringelhann B. Haemoglobin Korle-Bu (α73 aspartic acid → asparagine) showing one of the two amino acid substitutions of haemoglobin C, Harlem. J Med Genet 1968;5: 107.
96. Schneider RG, Hosty TS, Tomlin G, et al. Hb Mobile ($\alpha_2\beta_2$ 73 (E17) Asp→Val): a new variant. Biochem Genet 1975;13:411.
97. Wajcman H, Jones RT. Propriétés fonctionelles des hémoglobines humaines mutées en position 73. INSERM 1977;70:269.
98. Bookchin RM, Nagel RL. Molecular interactions of sickling hemoglobin. In: Abramson H, Bertles JF, Wethers DC, eds. Sickle cell disease, CV Mosby, St Louis, 1973:140.
99. Wishner BC, Ward KB, Lattman EE, Love WE. Crystal structure of sickle-cell deoxyhemoglobin at 5 A resolution. J Mol Biol 1975;98:179.
100. Horlein H, Weber G. Uber chronisch familiare Methamoglobinanue und eine neue Modifikation des Methamoglobins. Dtsch Med Wochenschr 1948;73:476.
101. Gerald DS, Efron ML. Chemical studies of several varieties of Hb M. Proc Natl Acad Sci USA 1961;47:1758.
102. Shibata S, Tanuira A, Iuchi I. Hemoglobin M_1 demonstration of a new abnormal hemoglobin in hereditary nigremia. Acta Haematol Jpn 1960;23:96.
103. Greer J. Three dimension studies of abnormal human hemoglobins M Hyde Park and M Iwate. J Mol Biol 1971;59:107.
104. Shibata N, Iuchi I. Characterization of a red minor component of abnormal hemoglobin found in HbM of Hyde Park disease. Hemoglobin 1977;1:829.
105. Feher G, Isaacson RA, Scholes CP. Endor studies on normal and abnormal hemoglobins. Ann NY Acad Sci 1973;222:86.
106. Peisach J, Gersonde K. Binding of CO to mutant α chains of HbM Iwate: evidence for distal imidazole ligation. Biochemistry 1977;16:2539.
107. LaMar GR, Nagai K, Jue T, et al. Assignment of proximal histidyl imidozle exchangeable proton NMR resonances to individual subunits in HbA, Boston, Iwate and Milwaukee. Biochem Biophys Res Commun 1980;96:1177.
108. Pulsinelli PD, Perutz MF, Nagel RL. Structure of hemoglobin M Boston, a variant with a five-coordinated ferric heme. Proc Natl Acad Sci USA 1973;70:3870.
109. Perutz MF, Pulsinelli PD, Ranney HM. Structure and subunit interaction of haemoglobin M Milwaukee. Nature 1972;237:259.
110. Raftery MA, Huestis WH. Molecular conformation and cooperativity in hemoglobin. Ann NY Acad Sci 1973;222:40.
111. Caldwell PRB, Nagel RL. The binding of 2,3 diphosphoglycerate as a conformational probe of human hemoglobins. J Mol Biol 1973;74:605.
112. Lindstrom TR, Ho C, Pisciotta AV. Nuclear magnetic resonance studies of haemoglobin M Milwaukee. Nature 1972;237:263.
113. Thillet J, Cohen-Solal M, Seligmann M, Rosa J. Functional and physiochemical studies of hemoglobin St. Louis β 28 (B10) Leu → Gln. J Clin Invest 1976;58:1098.
114. Wajcman H, Krishnamoorthy R, Gacon G, et al. A new hemoglobin variant involving the distal histidine: Hb Bicetre (β63 (E7) His → Pro). J Mol Med 1976;1:187.
115. Rosa J, Labie D, Wajcman H, et al. Haemoglobin I Toulouse: β66 (E10) Lys → Glu: a new abnormal haemoglobin with a mutation localized on the E10 porphyrin surrounding zones. Nature 1969;223:190.
116. Kurachi S, Hermodson M, Hornung S, Stamatoyannopoulos G. Structure of haemoglobin Seattle. Nature 1973;243:275.
117. Bunn HF, Forget BG. Hemoglobin: molecular, genetic and clinical aspects. Philadelphia, WB Saunders, 1986.
118. Nagai M, Yubisui T, Yoneyama Y. Enzymatic reduction of hemoglobin M Milwaukee I and M Saskatoon by NADH: cytochrome b_5 reductase and NADPH flavin reductase purified from human erythrocytes. J Biol Chem 1980;255:4599.
119. Shibata S, Mijaji T, Iuchi I. Methemoglobin M's of the Japanese. Bull Yamaguchi Med Sch 1967;14:141.
120. Shibata S. Hemoglobinopathies in Japan. Hemoglobin 5:509, 1981.
121. Hayashi A, Suzuki T, Shimizu A, Yamamura Y. Properties of hemoglobin M: unequivalent nature of the α and β subunits in the hemoglobin molecule. Biochim Biophys Acta 1968;168:262.
122. Ranney HM, Nagel RL, Heller P, Udem L. Oxygen equilibrium of hemoglobin M(Hyde Park). Biochim Biophys Acta 1968;160:112.
123. Suzuki T, Hayashi A, Shimizu A, Yamamura Y. The oxygen equilibrium of hemoglobin M Saskatoon. Biochim Biophys Acta 1966;127:280.
124. Suzuki T, Hayashi A, Yamamura Y, et al. Functional abnormality of hemoglobin M. Biochem Biophys Res Commun 1965;19:691.
125. Udem L, Ranney HM, Bunn HF, Pisciotta A. Some observations on the properties of hemoglobin $M_{Milwaukee}$. J Mol Biol 1970;48:489.
126. Hayashi A, Suzuki T, Imai K, et al. Properties of hemoglobin M Milwaukee I variant and its unique characteristics. Biochem Biophys Acta 1969;194:6.
127. Nagel RL, Bookchin RM. Human hemoglobin mutants with abnormal oxygen binding. Semin Hematol 1974;11:385.
128. Moo-Penn WF, Bechtel KC, Schmidt RM, et al. Hemoglobin Raleigh (β1 valine → acetylamine). Biochemistry 1977;16:4872.
129. Park CM, Nagel RL. Sulfhemoglobin: clinical and molecular aspects. N Engl J Med 1984;310:1579.
130. Park CM, Nagel RL, Blumberg WE, et al. Sulfhemoglobin: properties of partially sulfurated tetramers. J Biol Chem 1986;261:8805.
131. Beutler E. Hemoglobinopathies producing cyanosis. In: Williams J, Beutler E, Erslev AJ, Lichtman MA, eds. Hematology. New York, McGraw-Hill, 1983.
132. Finch CA. Methemoglobinemia and sulfhemoglobinemia. N Engl J Med 1948;239:470.
133. Pinkas J, Pjaldetti M, Joshua H, et al. Sulfhemoglobinemia and acute hemolytic anemia with Heinz bodies following contact with a fungicide-zinc ethylanol bisthiocarbamate: in a subject with glucose-6-phosphate dehydrogenase deficiency and hypocatalassemia. Blood 1963;21:484.
134. Greenberg HB. Syncope and shock due to methemoglobinemia. Arch Environ Health 1964;9:762.
135. Darling RC, Roughton FJW. The effect of methemoglobin on the equilibrium between oxygen and hemoglobin. Am J Physiol 1942;137:56.
136. Bunn HF, Drysdale JW. The separation of partially oxidized hemoglobins. Biochim Biophys Acta 1971;229:51.
137. Cathie AB. Apparent idiopathic Heinz body anemia. Great Ormond St J 1952;3:3.
138. Asakura T, Adachi K, Shapiro M, et al. Mechanical precipitation of hemoglobin Koln. Biochim Biophys Acta 1975;412:197.
139. Roth EF Jr, Elbaum D, Bookchin RM, Nagel RL. The conformational requirements for the mechanical precipitation of hemoglobin S and other mutants. Blood 1976;48:265.
140. Wajcman H, Vasseur C, Blouquit Y, et al. Hemoglobin Redondo [β92(F8)His → Asn]: an unstable hemoglobin variant associated with heme loss which occurs in two forms. Am J Hematol 1991;38:194.
141. Robinson AB. Evolution and the distribution of glutamyl and asparaginyl residues in proteins. Proc Natl Acad Sci USA 1974;71:885.
142. George PM, Myles Y, Williamson D, et al. A family with haemolytic anaemia and three beta-globins: the deletion in haemoglobin Atlanta-Coventry (beta 75 Leu–Pro, 141 Leu deleted) is not present at the nucleotide level. Br J Haematol 1992;81:93.
143. Brennan SO, Shaw J, Allen J, George PM. Beta 141 Leu is not deleted in the unstable haemoglobin Atlanta-Coventry but is replaced by a novel amino acid of mass 129 daltons. Br J Haematol 1992;81:99.
144. Tucker PW, Phillips SEV, Perutz MF, et al. Structure of hemoglobins Zurich [His E7(63) β → Arg] and Sydney [Val E11(67) → Ala] and role of the distal residues in ligand binding. Proc Natl Acad Sci USA 1978;75: 1076.
145. Virshup DM, Zinkham WH, Sirota RL, Caughey WS. Unique sensitivity of Hb Zurich to oxidative injury by phenazopyridine: reversal of the effects by elevating carboxyhemoglobin in vivo and in vitro. Am J Hematol 1983;14:315.
146. Fermi G, Perutz MF, Williamson D, Stein P, Shih DT. Structure–function relationships in the low-affinity mutant haemoglobin Aalborg (G174 [E18] beta–Arg). J Mol Biol 1992;226:883.

147. Reider RF, Oski FA, Clegg JB. Hemoglobin Philly (β 35 tyrosine → phenylalanine): studies in the molecular pathology of hemoglobin. J Clin Invest 1969;48:1627.
148. King MAR, Wiltshire BG, Lehmann H, Moriomoto H. An unstable haemoglobin with reduced oxygen affinity: haemoglobin Peterborough, β 111 (G13) valine → phenylalanine, its interaction with normal haemoglobin and with haemoglobin Lepore. Br J Haematol 1972;22:125.
149. Como PF, Wylie BR, Trent RJ, et al. A new unstable and low oxygen affinity hemoglobin variant: Hb Stanmore [β111(G13)Val→Ala]. Hemoglobin 1991;15:53.
150. Wada Y, Ikkala E, Imai K, et al. Structure and function of a new hemoglobin variant, Hb Meilahti $\alpha_2\beta_2$ 36(C2)Pro → Thr), characterized by mass spectrometry. Acta Haematol 1987;78:109.
151. Martinez G, Lima F, Colombo B. Haemoglobin J Guantanamo (α_2 β_2 128 (H6) Ala→Asp). A new fast unstable haemoglobin found in a Cuban family. Biochim Biophys Acta 1977;491:1.
152. Clegg JB, Weatherall DJ, Wong Hock Boon, Mustafa D. Two new haemoglobin variants involving proline substitutions. Nature 1969;22:379.
153. Ohba Y. Unstable hemoglobins. Hemoglobin 1990;14:353.
154. Ohba Y, Miyaji T, Matsouka M, et al. Hemoglobin Hirosaki [α43(CE1) Phe→Leu: a new unstable variant. Biochim Biophys Acta 1975;405: 155.
155. Goosens M, Lee KY, Liebhaber SA, Kan YW. Globin structural mutant α125 Leu → Pro is a novel cause of α-thalassemia. Nature 1982;296: 864.
156. Ohba Y, Yamamoto K, Hattori Y, Kawata R, Miyaji T. Hyperunstable hemoglobin Toyama $\alpha_2$136 (H19) Leu → Arg β_2: detection and identification by in vitro biosynthesis with radioactive amino acids. Hemoglobin 1987;11:539.
157. Tatsis B, Dosik H, Rieder R, et al. Hemoblogin Hasharon: severe hemolytic anemia and hypersplenism associated with a mildly unstable hemoglobin. Birth Defects 1972;8:25.
158. Levine RL, Lincoln DR, Buchholz WM, et al. Hemoglobin Hasharon in a premature infant with hemolytic anemia. Pediatr Res 1975;9:7.
159. Lee-Potter JP, Deacon-Smith RA, Simpkiss MJ, et al. A new cause of haemolytic anemia in the newborn: a description of an unstable fetal haemoglobin—F Poole G$\alpha_2\gamma_2$ 130 tryptophan → glycine. J Clin Pathol 1975;28:317.
160. Schmid R, Brecher G, Clemens T. Familial hemolytic anemia with erythrocyte inclusion bodies and a defect in pigment metabolism. Blood 1959;14:991.
161. Eisinger J, Flores J, Tyson JA, Shohet SB. Fluorescent cytoplasm and Heinz bodies of Koln erythrocytes: evidence for intracellular heme catabolism. Blood 1985;65:886.
162. Koler RD, Jones RT, Bigley RH, et al. Hemoglobin Casper: β 106 (G8) Leu → Pro, a contemporary mutation. Am J Med 1973;55:549.
163. Nagel RL, Ranney HM. Drug-induced oxidative denaturation of hemoglobin. Semin Hematol 1973;10:269.
164. Grimes AJ, Meisler A. Possible cause of Heinz bodies in congenital Heinz body anaemia. Nature 1962;194:190.
165. Grimes AJ, Meisler A, Dacie JV. Congenital Heinz-body anaemia: further evidence on the cause of Heinz-body production in red cells. Br Haematol 1964;10:281.
166. Carrell RW, Kay R. A simple method for the detection of unstable hemoglobins. Br J Haematol 1972;23:615.
167. Ohba Y, Hattori Y, Yoshinaka H, et al. Clin Chim Acta 1981;119:179.
168. Asakura T, Adachi K, Shapiro M, et al. Mechanical precipitation of hemoglobin Koln. Biochim Biophys Acta 1975;412:197.
169. Roth EF Jr, Elbaum D, Bookchin RM, Nagel RL. The conformational requirements for the mechanical precipitation of hemoglobin S and other mutants. Blood 1976;48:265.
170. Tondo CV, Mendez HM, Reischl E. Thermostability of hemoglobins in homeothermic and non-homeothermic vertebrates. Comp Biochem Physiol 1980;66B:151.
171. Borgese TA, Harrington J, Borgese JM, Nagel RL. Thermostability of fish hemoglobins. Comp Biochem Physiol 1982;72B:7.
172. Perutz MF. Electrostatic effects in proteins. Science 1978;201:1187.
173. Bigelow C. On the average hydrophobicity of proteins and the relation between it and protein structure. J Theor Biol 1967;16:187.
174. Kauzmann W. Some factors in the interpretation of protein denaturation. Adv Protein Chem 1959;14:1.
175. Argos P, Rossman MG, Grau UM, et al. Thermal stability and protein structure. Biochemistry 1979;18:5698.
176. Perutz MF, Raidt H. Sterochemical bases of heat stability in bacterial ferredoxins and in hemoglobin A_2. Nature 1975;255:256.
177. Bunn FH, Jandl JH. Exchange of heme among hemoglobins and between hemoglobin and albumin. J Biol Chem 1968;243:465.
178. Brooks J. The oxidation of haemoglobin to methaemoglobin by oxygen. II. The relation between the rate of oxidation and the partial pressure of oxygen. Proc R Soc London [B] 1935;118:560.
179. Gurd FRN, Falk KE, Malstrom BG, Vanngard T. The conformational transition of sperm whale ferrimyoglobin in the presence of several equivalents of cupric ion. J Biol Chem 1967;242:5731.
180. Bemski G, Arends T, Blanc G. Electron spin resonance of Cu (II) in copper hemoglobin complexes. Biochem Biophys Res Commun 1969;35: 599.
181. Nagel RL, Bemski G, Pincus P. Some aspects of the binding of Cu (II) to human hemoglobin and its subunits. Arch Biochem Biophys 1970;137:428.
182. Rifkind J. Copper and the autoxidation of hemoglobin. Biochemistry 1974;13:2475.
183. Winterbourne CC, Carrell RW. Oxidation of human hemoglobin by copper. Biochem J 1977;165:141.
184. Mansouri A, Winterhalter KH. Nonequivalence of chains in hemoglobin oxidation. Biochemistry 1973;12:4946.
185. Jacob HS, Winterhalter KH. The role of hemoglobin heme loss in Heinz body formation: studies with a partially heme-deficient hemoglobin and with genetically unstable hemoglobin. J Clin Invest 1970;49:2008.
186. Jacob HS, Winterhalter KH. Unstable hemoglobins: the role of heme loss in Heinz body formation. Proc Natl Acad Sci USA 1970;65:697.
187. Rachmilewitz EA, Peisach J, Blumberg WE. Studies on the stability of oxyhemoglobin A and its constituent chains and their derivatives. J Biol Chem 1971;246:3356.
188. Rachmilewitz EA, Harari E. Intermediate hemichrome formation after oxidation of three unstable hemoglobins (Freiburg, Riverdale-Bronx and Koln). Haematol Bluttransfus 1972;10:241.
189. Rachmilewitz EA, White JM. Haemichrome formation during the in vitro oxidation of haemoglobin Koln. Nature 1973;241:115.
190. Rachmilewitz EA. Denaturation of the normal and abnormal hemoglobin molecule. Semin Hematol 1974;11:441.
191. Peisach J, Blumberg WE, Rachmilewitz EA. The demonstration of ferrihemochrome intermediates in Heinz body formation following the reduction of oxyhemoglobin A by acetylphenylhydrazine. Biochem Biophys Acta 1975;393:404.
192. Winterbourne CC, Carrell RW. Studies of hemoglobin denaturation and Heinz body formation in the unstable hemoglobins. J Clin Invest 1974;54:678.
193. Winterbourne CC, McGrath BM, Carrell RW. Reactions involving superoxide and normal and unstable haemoglobins. Biochem J 1976;155: 503.
194. Rifkind RA. Heinz body anemia: an ultrastructural study. II. Red cell sequestration and destruction. Blood 1965;26:433.
195. Schnitzer B, Rucknagel DL, Spencer HH, Aikawa M. Erythrocytes: pits and vacuoles as seen with transmission and scanning electron microscopy. Science 1971;173:251.
196. Winterbourne CC, Carrell RW. Characterization of Heinz bodies in unstable haemoglobin haemolytic anaemia. Nature 1972;240:150.
197. Chan E, Desforges J. Role of disulfide bonds in Heinz body attachment to membranes. Blood 1974;44:921.
198. Low P. Interaction of native and denatured hemoglobins with Band 3: consequences for erythrocyte structure and function. In: Agre P, Parker JC, eds. Red blood cell membranes. New York, Marcel Dekker, 1989.
199. Low PS, Westfall MA, Allen DP, Appell KC. Characterization of the reversible conformational equilibrium of the cytoplasmic domain of erythrocyte membrane band 3. J Biol Chem 1984;259:13070.
200. Waugh SM, Low PS. Hemichrome binding to band 3: Nucleation of Heinz bodies on the erythrocyte membrane. Biochemistry 1985;24:34.
201. Cho N, Song S, Asher SA. UV resonance Raman and excited-state relaxation rate studies of hemoglobin. Biochemistry 1994;33:5932.
202. Fisher S, Nagel RL, Bookchin RM, et al. The binding of hemoglobin to membranes of normal and sickle erythrocytes. Biochim Biophys Acta 1975;375:422.
203. Shaklai N, Sharma VS, Ranney HM. Interaction of sickle cell hemoglobin with erythrocyte membrane. Proc Natl Acad Sci USA 1981;78: 65.
204. Reiss GH, Ranney HM, Shaklai N. Association of hemoglobin C with erythrocyte ghosts. J Clin Invest 1982;70:946.
205. Walder JA, Chatterjee R, Steck T. et al. The interaction of hemoglobin with the cytoplasmic domain of band 3 of the human erythrocyte membrane. J Biol Chem 1984;259:10238.
206. Jandl JH, Simmons RL, Castle WB. Red cell filtration and the pathogenesis of certain hemolytic anemias. Blood 1961;18:133.
207. Miller DR, Weed RI, Stamatoyannopoulos G, Yoshida A. Hemoglobin Koln disease occurring as a fresh mutation: erythrocyte metabolism and survival. Blood 1971;38:715.
208. Chou AC, Fitch CD. Mechanism of hemolysis induced by ferriprotoporphyrin IX. J Clin Invest 1981;68:672.
209. Allen DW, Burgoyne CF, Groat JD, et al. Comparison of hemoglobin Koln erythrocyte membranes with malondialdehyde-reacted normal erythrocyte membranes. Blood 1984;64:1263.
210. Flynn TP, Allen DW, Johnson GJ, White JG. Oxidant damage of the lipids and proteins of the erythrocyte membranes in unstable hemoglobin disease: evidence for the role of lipid peroxidation. J Clin Invest 1983;71:1215.
211. Jacob HS, Brain MK, Dacie JV. Altered sulfhydryl reactivity of hemoglobins and red blood cell membranes in congenital Heinz body hemolytic anemia. J Clin Invest 1968;47:2664.
212. DeFuria FG, Miller DR. Oxygen affinity in hemoglobin Koln disease. Blood 1972;39:398.
213. Goosens M, Lee KY, Liebhaber SA, Kan YW. Globin structural mutant α 125 Leu → Pro is a novel cause of α-thalassemia. Nature 1982;296: 864.
214. Adams JG III, Boxer LA, Baehner RL, et al. Hemoglobin Indianapolis

(β 112 [G14] arginine): an unstable β-chain variant producing the phenotype of severe β-thalassemia. Nature 1982;296:864.
215. Adams JG, Steinberg MH, Boxer LA, et al. The structure of hemoglobin Indianapolis (β 112 [G14] arginine): an unstable variant detectable only by isotopic labeling. J Biol Chem 1979;254.
216. Kolski GB, Miller DR. Heme synthesis in hereditary hemolytic anemias: decreased δ-amino-levulinic acid synthetase in hemoglobin Koln disease. Pediatr Res 1976;10:702.
217. Rieder RF. Synthesis of hemoglobin Gun Hill: increased synthesis of the heme-free beta^{GH} globin chain and subunit exchange with a free alpha chain pool. J Clin Invest 1971;50:388.
218. Bradley TB, Wohl RC, Rieder RF. Hemoglobin Gun Hill: deletion of five amino acid residues and impaired heme-globin binding. Science 1967;157:1581.
219. Kneezel LD, Kitchens CS. Phenacetin-induced sulfhemoglobinemia: report of a case and review of the literature. Johns Hopkins Med J 1967;139:175.220. Brandenburg RO, Smith HL. Sulfhemoglobinemia: a study of 62 clinical cases. Am Heart J 1951;42:582.
221. Cumming RLC, Pollock A. Drug-induced sulfhaemoglobinemia and Heinz body anemia in pregnancy with involvement of the foetus. Scott Med J 1967;12:320.
222. Reynolds TB, Ware AG. Sulfhemoglobinemia following habitual use of acetanilid. JAMA 1952;149:1538.
223. Evans AS, Enzer N, Eder HA, Finch CA. Hemoglytic anemia with paroxysmal methemoglobinemia and sulfhemoglobinemia. Arch Intern Med 1950;86:22.
224. Lambert M, Sonnet J, Mahien P, Hassoun A. Delayed sulfhemoglobinemia after acute dapsone intoxication. Clin Toxicol 1982;19:45.
225. Ford R, Shkov J, Akman WV, et al. Deaths from asphyxia among fishermen. Morbid Mortal Week Rep 1978;27:309.
226. Medeiros MH, Bechara EJ, Naoum PC, Mourao CA. Oxygen toxicity and hemoglobinemia in subjects from a highly polluted town. Arch Environ Health 1983;38:11.
227. The reversible binding of oxygen to sulfhemoglobin. J Biol Chem 1978;253:7212.
228. Nichol AW, Hendry I, Movell DB, Clezy PS. Mechanism of formation of sulfhemoglobin. Biochim Biophys Acta 1968;156:97.
229. Kiese M. The biochemical production of ferrihemoglobin-forming derivatives from aromatic amines and mechanisms of ferrihemoglobin formation. Pharmacol Rev 1966;18:1091.
230. Gibson GA, Douglas CC. Microbic cyanosis. Lancet 1906;2:72.
231. McCutcheon AD. Sulfhaemoglobinaemia and glutathione. Lancet 1960;2:290.
232. Suzuki T, Hayshi A, Shimizu A, Yamamura Y. The oxygen equilibrium of hemoglobin M Saskatoon. Biochim Biophys Acta 1966;127:280.
233. Basch F. On hydrogen sulfide poisoning from external application of elementary sulfur as an ointment. Arch Exp Pathol Pharmacol 1926;111: 126.
234. Glud TK. Complete recovery from acquired met- and sulfhemoglobinemia following treatment with neomycin and bacitracin. Ugeskr Laeger 1979;141:1410.
235. Burnett E, King EG, Grace M, Hall WF. Hydrogen sulfide poisoning: review of 5 years' experience. Can Med Assoc J 1977;117:1277.
236. Baker CH, Sutton ET, Davis DL. Microvessel mean transit time and blood flow velocity of sulfhemoglobin-RBC. Am J Physiol 1980;238: 745.
237. Beutler E, Milcus BJ. The effect of methemoglobin formation in sickle cell disease. J Clin Invest 1961;40:1856.
238. Gibson QH. The reduction of methaemoglobin in red blood cells and studies on the cause of idiopathic methaemoglobinaemia. Biochem J 1948;42:13–23.
239. Jaffe ER. Methemoglobinemia in the differential diagnosis of cyanosis. Hosp Practice 1985;20:92.
240. Scott EM. The relation of diaphorase of human erythrocytes to inheritance of methemoglobinemia. J Clin Invest 1960;39:1176.
241. Passon PG, Hultquist DE. Soluble cytochrome b5 reductase from human erythrocytes. Biochim Biophys Acta 1972;275:62.
242. Beauvais P, Kaplan JC. La methemoglobinemie congenitale recessive: etude de huit cas avec encephalopathie—nouvelle conception nosologique. J Pediatr 1978;10:145.
243. Kaplan JC, Leroux A, Beauvais P. Formes cliniques et biologiques de déficit en cytochrome b5 reductase. CR Seances Soc Biol 1979;173:368.
244. Kaplan JC, Leroux A, Bakouri S, et al. La lésion enzymatique dans la méthemoglobinemie congénital récessive avec encephalopathie. Nouv Rev Fr Hematol 1974;14:755.
245. Leroux A, Junien C, Kaplan JC, Bamberger J. Generalised deficiency of cytochrome b5 reductase in congenital methaemoglobinaemia with mental retardation. Nature 1975;258:619.
246. Arnold H, Botcher HW, Hufnagel D, Lohr GW. Hereditary methemoglobinemia due to methemoglobin reductase deficiency in erythrocytes and leukocytes without neurological symptoms. Abstracts of the XVII Congress of the International Society of Hematology, Paris, 1978:752.
247. Tanishima K, Tanimoto K, Tomoda A, et al. Hereditary methemoglobinemia due to cytochrome b5 reductase deficiency in blood cells without associated neurologic and mental disorders. Blood 1985;66: 1288.
248. Hegesh E, Avron M. The enzymatic reduction of ferrihemoglobin. II. Purification of a ferrihemoglobin reductase from human erythrocytes. Biochim Biophys Acta 1967;146:397.
249. Yubisui T, Takeshita M. Characterization of the purified NAH-cytochrome b5 reductase of human erythrocytes as a FAD-containing enzyme. J Biol Chem 1980;255:2454.
250. Ozols J, Korza G, Heinemann FS, et al. Complete amino acid sequence of steer liver microsomal NADH-cytochrome b_5 reductase. J Biol Chem 1985;260:11953.
251. Tomatsu S, Kobayashi Y, Fukumaki Y, et al. The organization and the complete nucleotide sequence of the human NADH-cytochrome b5 reductase gene. Gene 1989;80:353.
252. Katsube T, Sakamoto N, Kobayashi Y, et al. Exonic point mutations in NADH-cytochrome B_5 reductase genes of homozygotes for hereditary methemoglobinemia, types I and III: putative mechanisms of tissue-dependent enzyme deficiency. Am J Hum Genet 1991;48:799.
253. Yubisui T, Murakami K, Shirabe K, et al. Structural analysis of NADH-cytochrome B_5 reductase in relation to hereditary methemoglobinemia. In: Brewer GJ, ed. The red cell. New York, Alan R Liss, 1989:107.
254. Zenno S, Hattori M, Misumi Y, et al. Molecular cloning of a cDNA inducting rat NADH cytochrome B_5 reductase and the corresponding gene. Biochem J (Tokyo) 1990;107:810.
255. Kobayashi Y, Fukumaki Y, Yubuisi T, et al. Serine-proline replacement at residue 127 of NADH–cytochrome B_5 reductase causes hereditary methemoglobinemia, generalized type. Blood 1990;75:1408.
256. Hiono H. Lipids of myelin, white matter and gray matter in a case of generalized deficiency of cytochrome B_5 reductase in congenital methemoglobinemia with mental retardation. Lipids 1980;15:272.
257. Gacon G, Lostanlen D, Labie D, Kaplan JC. Interaction between cytochrome B_5 and hemoglobin: involvement of β66(E10) and β95(FG2) lysyl residues of hemoglobin. Proc Natl Acad Sci USA 1980;77:1917.
258. Poulos TL, Mauk AG. Models of the complexes formed between cytochrome β_5 and the subunits of methemoglobin. J Biol Chem 1983;258: 7369.
259. Korber E. Inaugural dissertation: Uber differenzen Blutfarbstoffes: Dorpat, 1866. In: Bischoff H. Z Exp Med 1926;48:472.
260. Jope EM. The ultra-violet spectral absorption of haemoglobin inside and outside the red blood cell. In: Roughton FJW, Kendrew JC, eds. Haemoglobin. London, Butterworths, 1949:205.
261. Schroeder WA, Shelton JR, Shelton JB, et al. The amino acid sequence of the γ-chain of human fetal hemoglobin. Biochemistry 1963;2:992.
262. Schroeder WA, Huisman THJ, Efremov GD, et al. Further studies on the frequency and significance of the $^T\gamma$ chain of human fetal hemoglobin. J Clin Invest 1979;63:268.
263. Slightom JL, Blechl AE, Smithies O. Human fetal $^G\gamma$- and $^A\gamma$-globin genes: complete nucleotide sequences suggest that DNA can be exchanged between these duplicated genes. Cell 1980;21:627.
264. Bouhassira EE, Lachman H, Krishnamoorthy R, Labie D, Nagel RL. A gene conversion located 5′ to the A gamma gene is in linkage disequilibrium with the Bantu haplotype in sickle cell anemia. J Clin Invest 1989;83:2070.
265. Frier JA, Perutz M. Structure of human foetal deoxyhemoglobin. J Mol Biol 1977;112:97.
266. Allen DW, Wyman J, Smith CA. The oxygen equilibrium of foetal and adult human hemoglobin. J Biol Chem 1953;203:81.
267. Tyuma I, Shamizu. Different response to organic phosphates of human fetal and adult hemoglobins. Arch Biochem Biophys 1969;129:404.
268. Schroeder WA, Cua JT, Matsuda G, Fenninger WD. Hemoglobin F_1, an acetyl-containing hemoglobin. Biochem Biophys Acta 1962;63:532.
269. Poyart C, Burseaux E, Guesnon P, Teissiere B. Chloride binding and Bohr effect of human fetal erythrocytes and HbF_{II} solutions. Pfluegers Arch 1978;37:169.
270. Gros G, Bauer C. High pK value of the N-terminal amino group of the gamma chains causes low CO_2 binding of human fetal hemoglobin. Biochem Biophys Res Common 1978;80:56.
271. Burseaux E, Poyart C, Guesnop P, Teissiere B. Comparative effects of CO_2 on the affinity for O_2 of fetal and adult hemoglobins. Pfluegers Arch 1979;378:197.
272. Kleinhauer E, Braun H, Betke K. Demonstration von fetalem Hamoglobin in den Erythrozyten eines Blutausstrichs. Klin Wochenschr 1957;35:637.
273. Dover GJ, Boyer SH, Bell WR. Microscopic method for assaying F cell production: illustrative changes during infancy and in aplastic anemia. Blood 1978;52:664.
274. Dover GJ, Boyer SH, Pembrey ME. F cell production in sickle cell anemia: regulation by genes linked to β-hemoglobin locus. Science 1981;211:1441.
275. Dover GJ, Boyer SH, Charache S, Heintzelman K. Individual variation in the production and survival of F-cells in sickle cell disease. N Engl J Med 1978;299:1428.
276. Winters WP, Seale WR, Yodh J. Interaction of hemoglobin S with anionic polysaccharides. Am J Pediatr Hematol Oncol 1984;6:77.
277. Miyoshi K, Kaneto Y, Kawai H, et al. X-linked dominant control of F-cells in normal adult life: characterization of the Swiss type as hereditary persistence of fetal hemoglobin regulated dominantly by gene(s) on X chromosome. Blood 1988;72:1854.
278. Pembrey ME, Weatherall DJ, Clegg JB. Maternal synthesis of haemoglobin F in pregnancy. Lancet 1973;16:1351.

279. Huehns ER, Hecht F, Keil JV, Motulsky AG. Developmental hemoglobin anomalies in a chromosomal triplication: D_1 trisomy syndrome. Proc Natl Acad Sci USA 1964;51:89.
280. Wood WG, Stamatoyannopoulos G, Lim G, Nute PE. F-cells in the adult: normal values and levels in individuals with hereditary and acquired elevations of Hb F. Blood 1975;46:671.
281. Boyer SH, Belding TK, Margolet L, et al. Variations in the frequency of fetal hemoglobin-bearing erythrocytes (F-cells) in well adults, pregnant women, and adult leukemics. Johns Hopkins Med J 1975;137:105.
282. Newman DR, Pierre RV, Linman JW. Studies on the diagnostic significance of hemoglobin F levels. Mayo Clin Proc 1973;48:199.
283. Huisman T. Abnormal hemoglobin list. Hemoglobin 1992;16:127.
284. Guang W, Ma M, Qian D. Hb F-Xin-Jin or $^{G}\gamma$119(GH2)Gly→Arg: a new unstable fetal hemoglobin variant. Hemoglobin, in press.
285. Priest JR, Watterson J, Jones RT, et al. Mutant fetal hemoglobin causing cyanosis in a newborn. Pediatrics 1989;83:734.
286. Glader BE. Hemoglobin FM-Fort Ripley: another lesson from the neonate. Pediatrics 1989;83:792.
287. Hayashi A, Fujita T, Fujimura M, Titani K. A new fetal hemoglobin, HbF M Osaka (ob2γ^2 63 His → Leu): a mutant with high oxygen affinity and erythrocytosis. Am J Clin Pathol 1979;72:1028.
288. Harano T, Harano K, Doi K, et al. HbF-Onoda or $\alpha^2_G\gamma_2$146(HC3)His → Tyr, a newly discovered fetal hemoglobin variant in a Japanese newborn. Hemoglobin 1990;14:217.
289. Fischer S, Nagel RL, Bookchin RM, et al. The binding of hemoglobin to membranes of normal and sickle erythrocytes. Biochim Biophys Acta 1975;375:422.
290. Codrington JF, Kutlar F, Harris HF, et al. Hb A_2-Wrens or $\alpha_2\delta_2$ 98(FG5) Val→Met, an unstable δ chain variant identified by sequence analysis of amplified DNA. Biochim Biophys Acta 1989;1009:87.
291. Garcia CR, Navarro JL, Lam H, et al. Hb A_2-Manzanares or $\alpha_2\delta_2$ 121(GH4) Glu→Val, an unstable δ chain variant observed in a Spanish family. Hemoglobin 1983;7:435.
292. Salkie ML, Gordon PA, Rigal WM, et al. Hb A_2-Canada or $\alpha_2\delta_2$ 99(G1) Asp→Asn: a newly discovered $\delta\delta$ chain variant with increased oxygen affinity occurring in cis to β-thalassemia. Hemoglobin 1982;6:223.

Blood: Principles and Practice of Hematology,
edited by Robert I. Handin, Samuel E. Lux, and Thomas P. Stossel.
J.B. Lippincott Company, Philadelphia © 1995.

53

The Sickle Syndromes

Orah S. Platt

EPIDEMIOLOGY OF THE SICKLE GENE

World Distribution of the Sickle Mutation

The sickle mutation is a single base change (A to T) in the middle of the triplet that codes for glutamic acid as the sixth amino acid of the hemoglobin β chain (Fig. 53-1). This mutation substitutes valine (Val) for glutamic acid (Glu) and is common among people whose origins are in areas where malaria has been endemic (Fig. 53-2). Nagel and Ranney[1] and Serjeant[2] reviewed the worldwide distribution of the sickle gene and the influence of spontaneous mutation and migration (most often by slave trade). In the various populations of equitorial Africa, the gene frequency ranges from 5% to more than 14%; it is about 4% among Caribbeans, Europeans, and North and South Americans of African descent. The sickle gene is also indigenous to Sicily,[3] Greece,[4] India,[5,6] Saudi Arabia,[7,8] Israel,[9] Turkey,[10] and Iran.[11]

Studies of β-gene cluster polymorphisms from different populations suggest that the sickle mutation arose at least five times, each in the context of a different ancient β haplotype (see Fig. 53-2). In Africa, there are three major sickle haplotypes, each associated with a particular geographic region (see Fig. 53-2): *Senegal* (Atlantic West Africa), *Benin* (Central West Africa), and *Bantu* (also called *CAR*, for Central African Republic).[12] The relative geographic isolation and certain structural features of the 5′-flanking region of these β genes support the hypothesis that they are independent mutations and not recombination events.[13] The Benin type is the most widely dispersed, found not only in Benin but also in Ibadan,[14] Algeria,[12] Sicily,[15] Turkey,[16] Greece,[17] Yemen, and southwest Saudi Arabia.[14] A fourth haplotype is described in a small population found in the Cameroon.[18] Among Jamaican and American sickle cell patients of African heritage, roughly 50% to 70% of chromosomes are Benin, 15% to 30% are Bantu-CAR, and 5% to 15% are Senegal.[19–21] In Africa, the geographic isolation is strong, and virtually all patients are homozygous for a given haplotype. Nagel and coworkers[22,23] document that different homozygotes have different hematologic characteristics. The Bantu-CAR and Senegalese patients have higher levels of fetal hemoglobin and fewer dense cells compared with Beninians. The Senegalese have a high proportion of $^{G}\gamma$ fetal hemoglobin; the Bantu-CAR and Beninians do not. In contrast to what is found among Africans living in Africa, African Americans are mainly heterozygotes. In Los Angeles, 38% of patients are Benin homozygotes (Benin/Benin); 25% are Benin/Bantu-CAR; 13% are Benin/Senegal; 5% are Bantu-CAR homozygotes; and 3% are Bantu-CAR/Senegal.[20] These haplotypes appear to influence overall clinical severity, with the Bantu-CAR being the most and the Senegalese being the least severely affected.[24]

A fifth haplotype is found in India and parts of Saudi Arabia.[14] In Riyadh, Saudi Arabia, all patients with sickle cell anemia are from southwest Saudi Arabia and Yemen and are homozygous Benin. In the eastern oases of Saudi Arabia, the African haplotypes are not seen; an Arab-Indian haplotype is the only one associated with the sickle mutation. This haplotype is also seen in patients from Orissa, India (whether they are of tribal origin or not) and Poona, India. Patients from these regions have long been recognized as having mild disease and elevated levels of fetal hemoglobin.[25–29] The Arab-Indian and Senegalese haplotypes are both associated with elevated fetal hemoglobin, and, as seen in Figure 53-2*A*, are structurally similar in the regions near and in the γ genes.

Malaria and Sickling

Nagel and Roth[30] and Weatherall[31] have reviewed the impact of malaria on the prevalence of genetic red cell disorders and the impact of those disorders on the malaria parasite. Two observations on the epidemiology of malaria in Africa support the concept of *balanced polymorphism:* (1) children with sickle cell trait are less likely to die from *Plasmodium falciparum* than children without trait[32]; and (2) the prevalence of trait increases with age.[33] Balanced polymorphism correctly predicts that because those with sickle trait have a selective advantage, the prevalence of trait rises in endemic areas until it is offset by the early death of patients with homozygous disease.

In humans, *P falciparum* has exoerythrocytic (liver) and intraerythrocytic phases. It is presumably the intraerythrocytic phase that is affected by sickle hemoglobin. Deoxygenated sickle trait red cells containing *P falciparum* are more likely to sickle than unparasitized cells.[34,35] Sickling probably accelerates removal of these cells and their parasites from the circulation. In addition, the loss of potassium, water, or both that accompanies sickling may provide an inhospitable environment for the parasite.[36] In culture, oxygenated trait cells support the growth of *P falciparum*, whereas deoxygenated trait cells do not.[37,38] The parasites may die because they are unable to metabolize polymerized hemoglobin[39] or because they become impaled by it.[40]

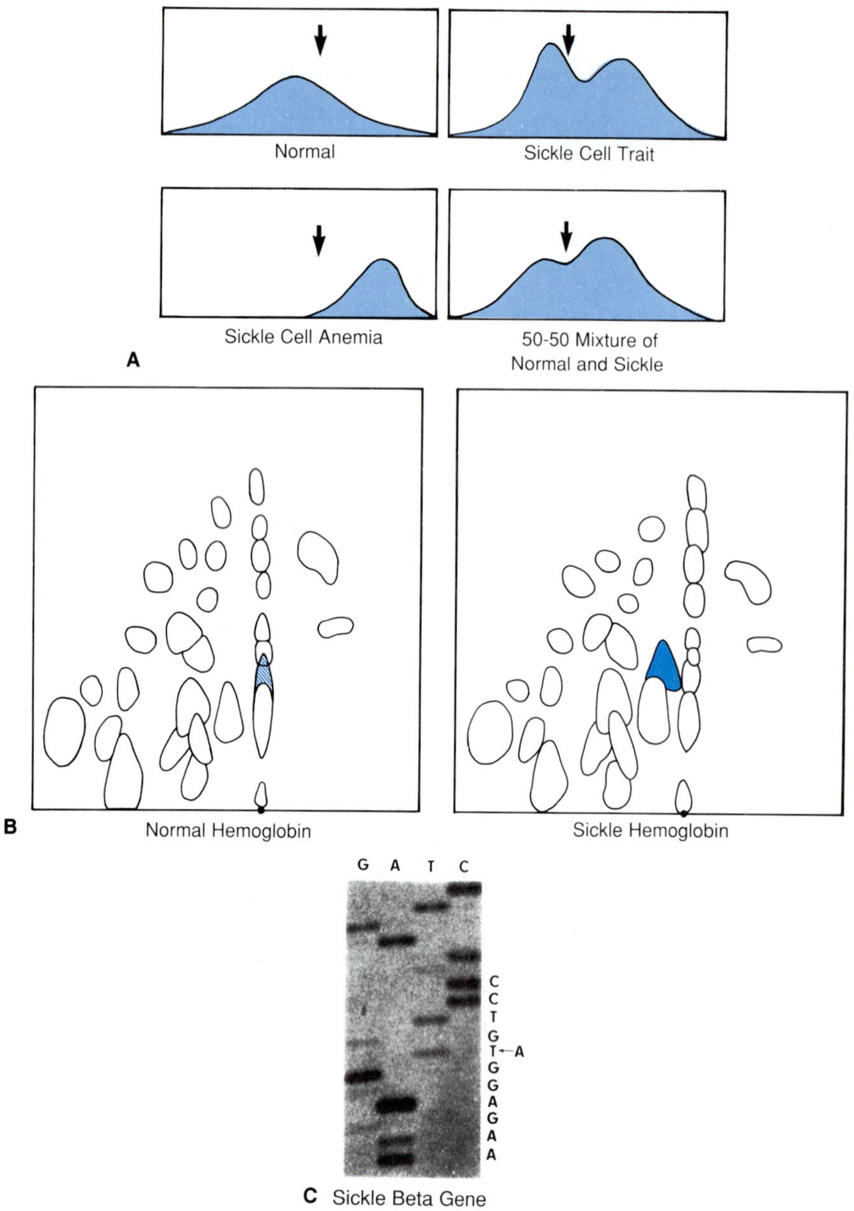

FIGURE 53-1. History of the investigation of the sickle mutation. (**A**) Hemoglobin electrophoresis: the first demonstration of the abnormal electrophoretic mobility of sickle hemoglobin. (**B**) Hemoglobin fingerprinting: the classic globin "fingerprint," demonstrating the specific peptide abnormality (*shaded peptide*) of sickle hemoglobin. (**C**) β-Globin sequencing gel of sickle β globin DNA. (**A** after Pauling L, Itano HA, Singer SJ, Wells IC. Sickle cell anemia: a molecular disease. Science 1949;110:543; **B** after Ingram VM. A specific chemical difference between globins of normal human and sickle cell anaemia hemoglobin. Nature 1956;178:792)

SICKLE HEMOGLOBIN POLYMER

The critical early work of Hahn and Gillespie,[41] Ham and Castle,[42] and Harris[43] contributed to our knowing that deoxygenation causes sickle hemoglobin to polymerize. This fundamental fact remains at the center of our concept of the pathophysiology of the disease. The fascinating history of the early clinical and scientific discoveries in the field are beautifully described by Bunn[44] and Conley.[45] The basic unit of sickle hemoglobin polymerization is the fiber, which is responsible for the viscosity and shape changes characteristic of sickle red cells. Understanding the fine structure of the fiber and the factors that influence its formation is crucial to understanding the clinical manifestations of the disease and to designing rational therapy.

Structure of the Sickle Hemoglobin Fiber

Electron Microscopy

Electron microscopy has proved to be one of the most powerful tools in dissecting the anatomy of the sickle hemoglobin fiber. Electron micrographs of deoxygenated sickle red cells display slender cables of hemoglobin fibers running along the long axis[46–50] (Fig. 53-3). Detailed examination of high-resolution micrographs provides a consistent depiction of the geometry of the fiber.[51–58] It is about 21 nm in diameter and is composed of 14 strands. Cross-sectional analysis shows that the 14 strands are arranged as seven staggered twisted pairs with a repeat of about 300 nm, as shown in Figure 53-4. The double strands are not symmetric since they are staggered by half a tetramer, and each tetramer is tilted slightly off the X-axis of the fiber. This arrangement results in a relative polarity, as illustrated in Figure 53-5.

X-Ray Crystallography

Although electron micrographs provide tremendous insight into the arrangement and orientation of tetramers in sickle hemoglobin fibers, details at the molecular level are available only by x-ray crystallography. This technique requires the use of large crystals of sickle hemoglobin grown in

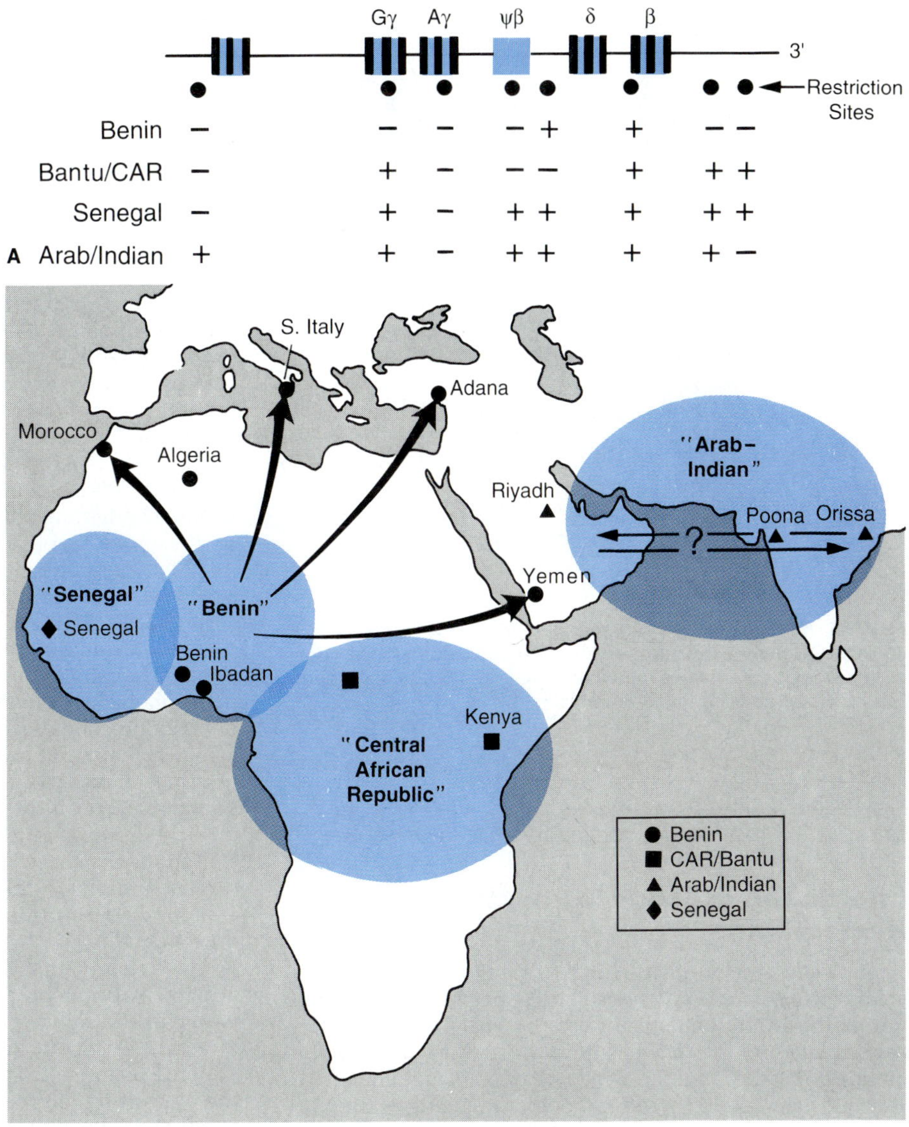

FIGURE 53-2. Worldwide distribution of the sickle haplotypes. (**A**) Each haplotype shown is distinguished by different patterns of restriction enzyme polymorphisms within the β-globin gene cluster on chromosome 11. β^S is associated with each of the different haplotypes shown, indicating it arose independently several times during evolution. (**B**) The distribution and spread of the major sickle haplotypes. (After Ragusa A, Lombardo M, Sortino G, Lombardo T, Nagel RL, Labie D. Beta S gene in Sicily is in linkage disequilibrium with the Benin haplotype: implications for gene flow. Am J Hematol 1988;27:139)

polyethylene glycol. Fortunately, there is considerable evidence that even though the structure of the crystal and the fiber are not identical, many of the important molecular interactions are maintained. In fact, with time[59] or stirring,[60] naturally occurring fibers convert spontaneously to crystals. By x-ray diffraction, the crystal and the fiber are both composed of the same basic structural unit—the double strand.[57,59] The major difference between the fiber and the crystal is that the crystal does not have the twisted 14-stranded arrangement shown in Figure 53-5, but instead has a larger array of evenly matched straight parallel and antiparallel double strands.

The crystal structure was first described at the resolution of 5 Å by Wishner and colleagues[61] and is commonly known as the *Wishner-Love double strand.* Padlan and Love refined the resolution to 3 Å and determined more than 400 atomic-pair interactions in the sickle crystal.[62,63] Most of these are of the van der Waals type, with only rare potential hydrogen bonds and even rarer ionic interactions. Several of these important interactions are shown in Figure 53-6.

In each double strand, there are axial and lateral contacts. *Axial contacts* consist of interactions between α_1 and β_1 chains of one tetramer and the α_2 and β_2 chains of the tetramer directly above or below. Because of the asymmetry of the strand, there are two similar but distinct classes of contacts. Using the standard nomenclature for the domains of the hemoglobin chains (see Chap. 52), in one strand, the dimer below contributes residues from the GH region of the α_1 and residues from the A and G helices and GH regions of the β_1. The tetramer above contributes from the G helix of the β_2 and from the GH regions of both α_2 and β_2. In the other strand, there is an additional contribution from the A helix of the α_2. None of these interactions involves the β-6 valine, so it is not surprising that almost identical interactions are found in crystals of hemoglobins A, F, and C.

Lateral contacts strongly involve the β-6 mutation. Because this mutation is not seen in hemoglobins A, F, or C, crystals of these hemoglobins do not contain the strong interactions that stabilize the double strands. In the sickle crystal, the β-6 valine of the β_2 chain interacts strongly, lying deep within a hydrophobic pocket lined with the Ala 70, Phe 85, and Leu 88 of the adjacent $\beta 1$. This interaction is primarily responsible for the abnormal solubility of deoxy sickle hemoglobin. There is also a probable hydrogen bond between the β_2 Thr 4 and the β_1 Asp 73.

The interactions between double strands largely involve residues from the α chains. Antiparallel pairs are loosely

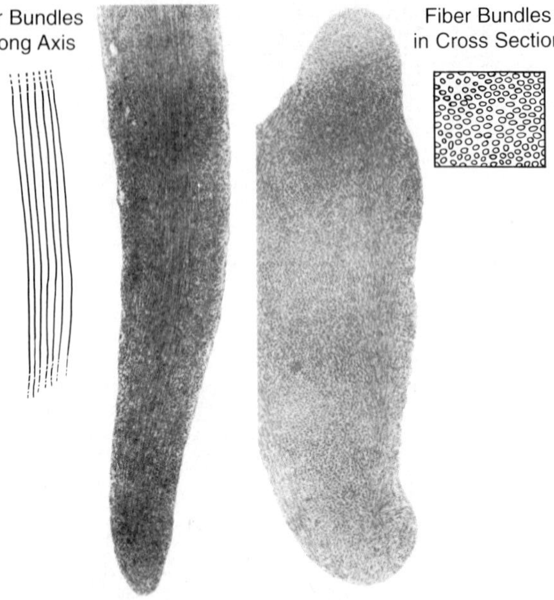

FIGURE 53-3. Electron micrograph of deoxygenated sickle erythrocyte, demonstrating deoxyhemoglobin S fibers. (After Bertles JF, Dobler J. Reversible and irreversible sickling: a distinction by electron microscopy. Blood 1969;33:884)

held, interacting with only a few residues of the α_1 chains. Parallel pairs interact more extensively than antiparallel pairs, with α residues reacting with adjacent β residues.

Interaction of Sickle With Other Hemoglobins

There is a long scientific tradition of studying the properties of mixtures of sickle and nonsickle hemoglobins. Although the methods have changed over the years, these studies continue to provide insight into the structure of the sickle hemoglobin fiber, the clinical behavior of patients with various hemoglobin combinations, and manipulation of hemoglobin as a therapeutic tactic. A summary of the important hemoglobins that affect sickle hemoglobin polymerization is shown in Table 53-1.

Behavior of Hemoglobin Mixtures in Solution

In solution, hemoglobin tetramers continuously dissociate into dimers and reassociate. In the process, tetramers exchange dimers. Consider preparing a solution of equal parts hemoglobins A and S. Initially, there will be two types of tetramer, $\alpha_2\beta_2^S$ (hemoglobin S) and $\alpha_2\beta_2^A$ (hemoglobin A). As the dissociation to dimer and reassociation to tetramer proceeds, hybrid tetramers $\alpha_2\beta^A\beta^S$ are formed. At equilibrium, roughly half of the tetramers will be hybrids, and one fourth will be of pure starting material. Experimentally, the tetramers can be frozen so no hybrid will form. This can be done either by deoxygenating (deoxyhemoglobin does not dissociate) or chemically cross-linking the hemoglobin before mixing. Hybrid formation also takes place in cells. Routine hemoglobin electrophoresis does not reveal the presence of hybrids because electrophoresis conditions favor the formation of dimer.

Sickle Hemoglobin and Hemoglobins With Nonsickle β Chains

Hemoglobin A and numerous β-chain variants affect sickle hemoglobin polymerization (see Table 53-1). In this section, the variants that illustrate the importance of the β-6, β-73, and β-121 positions on the polymerization process are discussed.

β-6 Position

Sickle hemoglobin is a mutation in the β-6 position. Crystallographic data illustrate the critical role this residue plays in the formation of the double strand. Experiments that examine polymerization in solutions containing mixtures of different hemoglobins have strengthened these observations and establish that the lateral contact between the val-6 of the β_2 and the hydrophobic pocket of the β_1 is the primary interaction responsible for the formation of the sickle fiber.

Hemoglobin A. For more than 30 years, we have known that a mixture of sickle and hemoglobin A has a lesser tendency to polymerize than a pure solution of sickle hemoglobin.[64,65] This mixture contains three species: hemoglobin S, hemoglobin A, and the hybrid $\alpha_2\beta^A\beta^S$. The hemoglobin S tetramer can participate in polymerization as usual. The hemoglobin A does not contain the β-6 valine, so it cannot reach into the hydrophobic pocket of the neighboring β chain and participate in the strengthening and growth of the double strand. It can, however, be *incorporated* into the polymer since all the non–β-6 valine contacts are maintained. The hybrid exists in two forms. In one, the β-6 valine is in the correct position to enter the hydrophobic pocket (the β_2 chain) and behaves exactly like hemoglobin S in all its contacts. In the other, the β-6 valine is in the chain that provides the pocket (the β_1 chain). This hybrid behaves exactly like hemoglobin A. The effect of hemoglobin A on the kinetics of polymerization of hemoglobin S is shown in Figure 53-7 and explains the lack of symptoms associated with sickle cell trait.

Hemoglobin C. Like hemoglobin S, hemoglobin C has an amino acid substitution at the β-6 position. In contrast, however, this substitution codes for a hydrophilic lysine (Lys)—a residue that would have difficulty insinuating itself into the hydrophobic pocket that accommodates the mutant valine of the sickle globin. Because the critical lateral interaction between the hydrophobic valine and its hydrophobic pocket cannot take place when the β^C chain is in the β_2 position, one would anticipate that mixtures of hemoglobin S and hemoglobin C would behave exactly like the mixtures of hemoglobin S and hemoglobin A described previously. Early work using a minimal gelling capacity technique suggested, however, that hemoglobin S and C mixtures were *less* soluble than S and A mixtures and were consistent with the fact that individuals heterozygous for hemoglobins S and C (see section on hemoglobin SC disease) are symptomatic, while those heterozygous for hemoglobins A and S (see section on sickle trait) are not.[64,65] Newer studies of the solubility and kinetics of polymerization of these mixtures show little difference between S plus A and S plus C.[66,67] The inconsistency with the earlier results is likely a function of the ionic strength of the experimental conditions.[68] At physiologic salt and hemoglobin concentrations, there is not an important difference in the behavior of these mixtures. The clinical difference between the two syndromes is less a function of the physical interaction of the two hemoglobins and more a reflection of their cellular content and concentration. There is relatively more hemoglobin S in the red cells of patients with SC disease than in those with sickle trait; and the hemoglobin concentration of the SC red cell is higher than the AS red cell.[66,69]

β-73 Position

Hemoglobins C-Harlem and Korle Bu. Hemoglobin C-Harlem is a mutant hemoglobin with two amino acid substitutions: β-6 Glu $\rightarrow$ Val (as in hemoglobin S) and β-73 Asp $\rightarrow$ Asn. This hemoglobin should theoretically polymerize as well as hemoglobin S since it has the criti-

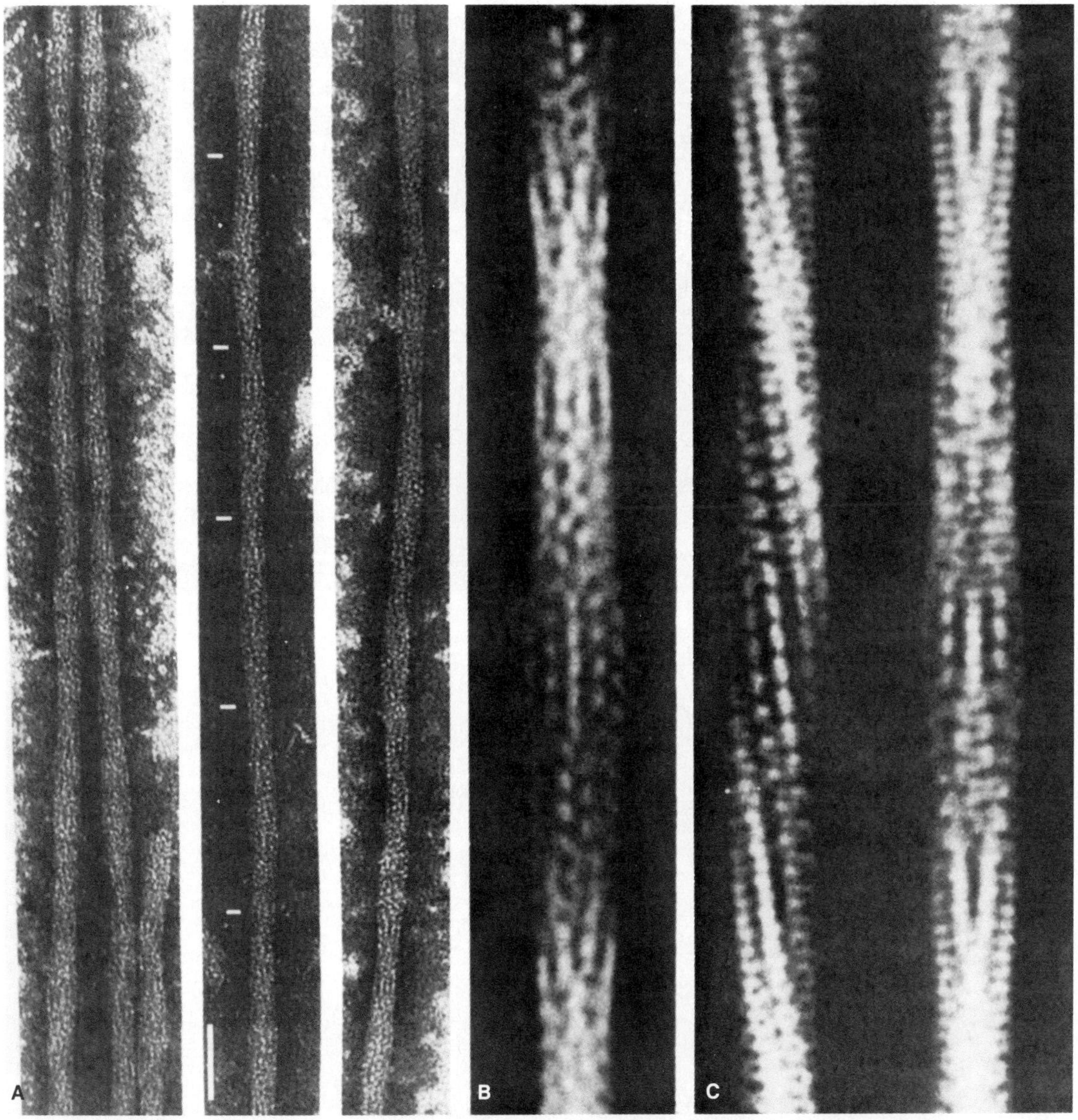

FIGURE 53-4. Structure of the sickle hemoglobin fiber. (**A**) Electron micrographs of negatively stained fibers of deoxyhemoglobin S. (**B**) Fourier transform of the electron microscopic data. (**C**) Electron density models of the fiber, illustrating both the helical projection (*left*) and the surface map (*right*). (After Carragher B, Bluemke DA, et al. Structural analysis of polymers of sickle cell hemoglobin. I. Sickle cell hemoglobin fibers. J Mol Biol 1988;199:315)

cal β-6 valine in every β chain, but it does not.[70,71] Deoxyhemoglobin C-Harlem is three times more soluble than deoxyhemoglobin S, illustrating the importance of having asparagine (Asp) in position 73. Additional studies using the mutant hemoglobin Korle Bu (β-73 Asp → Asn) indicate that this hemoglobin is more effective than hemoglobin A in inhibiting the polymerization of hemoglobin S—convincing evidence that the impact of the β-73 residue is in the trans (β_1) position. This contact is found in the crystal (see Fig. 53-6), where it probably hydrogen-bonds with the β-4 threonine (Thr).[62,63]

β-121 Position

Hemoglobin D. Hemoglobin D (Los Angeles or Punjab) is a mutant with amino acid substitution β-121 Glu → Gln. This hemoglobin is less efficient than hemoglobin A in reducing thepolymerization of hemoglobin S in mixtures,[72] and patients heterozygous for S and D-Los Angeles are symptomatic.[73–75] This suggests that the β-121 residue is important in the formation of the fiber and that a glutamine (Gln) in this position is more favorable for polymerization than glutamic acid (Glu). The crystal structure suggests that this residue is part of an axial contact in which the Glu 121 shares three contacting atoms with the α-16 lysine of the tetramer above[62,63] (see Fig. 53-6). Because this is already a favorable interaction, it is possible that the Gln 121 interacts even more strongly with another residue and enhances the axial contact.

Hemoglobin O Arab. Hemoglobin O-Arab is another mutation at the β-121 position, a substitution of a lysine for glutamic acid. In a minimal gelling capacity assay at high ionic strength, this hemoglobin actually enhanced the polymerization of hemoglobin S.[76] The observation confirms the importance of the β-121 in the formation of the polymer and accurately predicts that patients doubly heterozygous for S and O-Arab are clinically severe.[77]

Sickle and Hemoglobins Without β Chains

Hemoglobin F. In mixing experiments, hemoglobin F is the most efficient hemoglobin for solubilizing hemoglobin S[78–80] (see Fig. 53-7). The effect of hemoglobin F is mediated

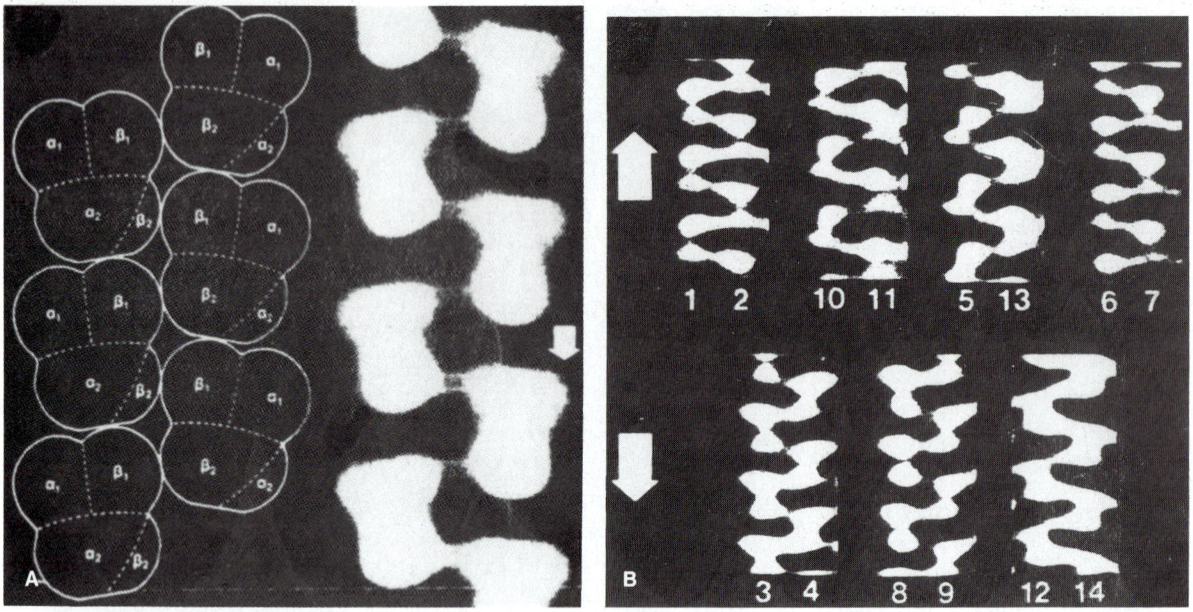

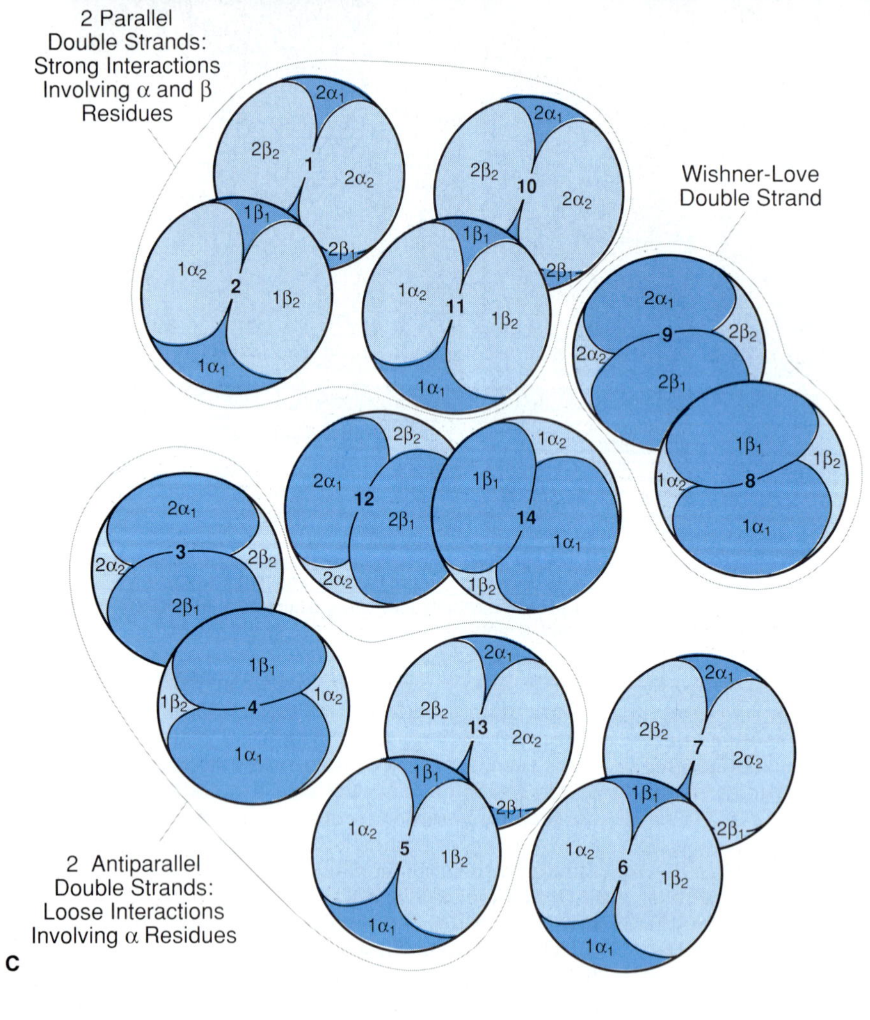

FIGURE 53-5. Polarity of the double strands. (**A**) Diagram of a crystal pair and the corresponding projected electron density. The direction of the heavy arrow indicates polarity. (**B**) Seven reconstructed pairs with the heavy arrows indicating the two opposite polarities. (**C**) Model indicating the arrangement of the double strands to form a fiber, using the conventional numbering system indicated in **B.** Double strands of the same polarity are the same color. (**A** and **B** after Rodgers DW, Crepeau RH, Edelstein SJ. Pairing and polarities of the 14 strands in sickle cell hemoglobin fibers. Proc Natl Acad Sci USA 1987;84:6157; **C** after Dickerson RE, Geis I. Hemoglobin: structure function, evolution and pathology. Menlo Park, CA, Benjamin Cummins, 1983)

through the formation of hybrid tetramers—$\alpha_2\beta^S\gamma$. This hybrid interferes with polymerization *in the solution phase.* Unlike the hybrids formed with hemoglobin A, almost no γ chains are incorporated into the polymer until the amount of hemoglobin F exceeds 30%. The γ loci that are critical in interfering with hemoglobin S polymerization are the γ-80 Asp and γ-87 Gln.[81] In the crystal, the β-87 Thr is an important contact site involved in both lateral interactions and interactions between parallel double strands.[62,63]

Hemoglobin A_2. Hemoglobin A_2 is comparable to hemoglobin F in its ability to interfere with polymerization of hemoglobin S.[81,82] The critical contact residues are the δ-87 Gln and the δ-22 Ala.[81]

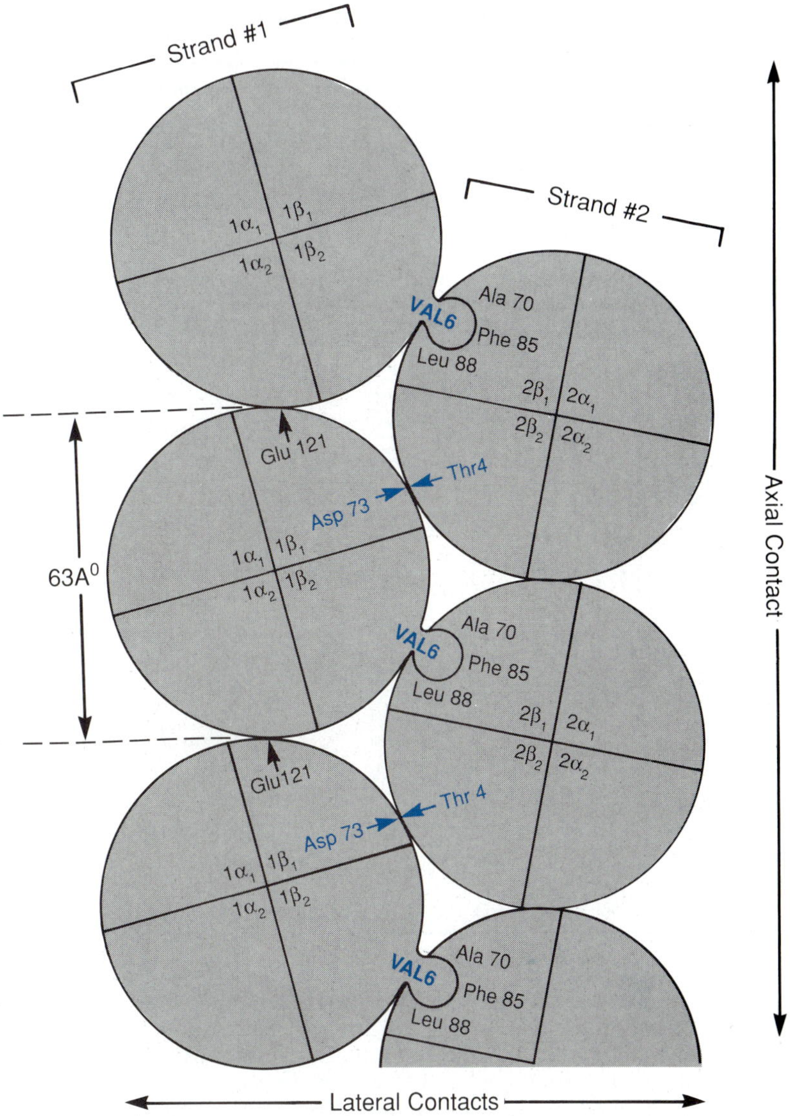

FIGURE 53-6. The Wishner-Love double strand, indicating a number of the key contact residues. (After Wishner BC, Ward KB, Lattman EE, Love WE. Crystal structure of sickle-cell deoxyhemoglobin at 5 A resolution. J Mol Biol 1975;98:179)

Sickle Hemoglobin and α-Chain Variants

Numerous α-chain variants influence hemoglobin S polymerization.[83–88] As can be seen in Table 53-1, effective α mutants generally represent axial or inter–double-strand contacts. Some of the mutants that do not appear as critical contacts in the crystallographic model do appear in the hypothetical model devised to account for the twisting of the double strands that occurs in the fiber and not in the crystal.[89]

Polymerization of Sickle Hemoglobin

Excellent reviews and views of the polymerization of hemoglobin S present different emphases on the relative importance of equilibrium, kinetic, and structural issues in the pathophysiology of disease.[90–93] An overview of the relevant data and some of the areas of controversy are considered in this section.

Polymerization in Solution

Studies at Equilibrium. As seen in Figure 53-8, a sickle hemoglobin gel is a two-phase system with polymer coexisting in equilibrium with tetramers in solution.[94–96] The solubility of sickle hemoglobin can be determined by measuring the concentration of hemoglobin in the supernatant.[95–99] The solubility depends on temperature,[95,96,98] pH,[100,101] and 2,3-diphosphoglycerate (2,3-DPG) concentration.[102,103] The most dramatic environmental influence on the solubility of sickle hemoglobin is oxygen. Complete saturation with oxygen prevents polymer formation, while removal of oxygen promotes polymerization. Between the extremes of a Po_2 of 100 and one of 0, the degree of polymerization of the gel depends on the relative oxygen affinities of the hemoglobin in the polymer phase and the hemoglobin in solution.

As a respiratory pigment, soluble sickle hemoglobin behaves exactly like hemoglobin A. The *solution* oxygen-binding curve (Fig. 53-9) is normal.[104] In contrast, the *polymer*-binding curve is far from normal, exhibiting low affinity and no cooperativity[105–108] (see Fig. 53-9*A*). Knowledge of the solubility as a function of oxygen saturation[106] (see Fig. 53-9*B*) combined with the data on the oxygen binding of solution and polymer phases can be used to construct binding curves and polymerization curves of gels at different hemoglobin concentrations (see Fig. 53-9C and *D*). The more concentrated the solution, the more likely there is to be polymer at a given Po_2, and the more the binding curve deviates away from normal and toward the polymer-

TABLE 53-1. Variant Hemoglobins With Effects on Sickle Hemoglobin Polymerization

Name	Residue	Normal	Mutant
α-CHAIN VARIANTS			
Sawara	α6	Asp	Ala
Anantharaj	α11	Lys	Glu
I	α16	Lys	Glu
Le Lamentin	α20	His	Gln
Memphis	α23	Glu	Gln
Sealy	α47	Asp	His
J-Mexico	α54	Gln	Glu
G-Philadelphia	α69	Asn	Lys
Winnipeg	α75	Asp	Tyr
Stanleyville	α78	Asn	Lys
O-Indonesia	α116	Glu	Lys
β-CHAIN VARIANTS			
C	β6	Glu	Lys
Machida	β6	Glu	Gln
J-Baltimore	β16	Gly	Asp
J-Amiens	β17	Lys	Gln
D-Ouled Rabah	β19	Asn	Lys
I-Toulouse	β66	Lys	Glu
Korle Bu	β73	Asp	Asn
G-Szuhu	β80	Asn	Lys
Pyrgos	β83	Gly	Asp
D-Ibadan	β87	Thr	Lys
Detroit	β95	Lys	Asn
N-Baltimore	β95	Lys	Glu
O-Arab	β121	Glu	Lys
D-Los Angeles	β121	Glu	Gln

binding curve. As is discussed later, this phenomenon, combined with the increased 2,3-DPG, results in the right-shifted oxygen dissociation curve found in patients with sickle cell disease (see Fig. 53-9E). After controlling for 2,3-DPG content and the presence of other hemoglobins (see Fig. 53-9F), these curves accurately predict the behavior of cells with different concentrations of hemoglobin S.

Studies of Kinetics. The binding curves presented in Figure 53-9 are the result of experiments in which hemoglobin solutions were exposed to specific oxygen tensions for relatively long periods of time, allowing polymer to form and reach equilibrium before being analyzed. Understanding the process of polymer *assembly* required an experimental set-up that allowed rapid induction of polymer in a polymer-free solution while continuously monitoring polymer accumulation. Polymer could be induced by temperature jump, and the amount of polymer formed monitored by birefringence,[109–111] viscometry,[112–117] turbidity,[99,105,110,118,119] or nuclear magnetic resonance (NMR).[120–124] Regardless of the detection system used, the results were the same. After the temperature jump, there was a quiet delay period during which there was no apparent polymerization. After the delay, there was a characteristic precipitous and rapid appearance of polymer. These studies illustrated the unprecedented sensitive dependence of the delay on the concentration of sickle hemoglobin. Although most reactions depend on the first or second power of the concentration, this reaction is sensitive to the 30th to 50th power of the hemoglobin S concentration.[125] As is discussed later, this has important therapeutic implications since small changes in hemoglobin S concentration translate into profound changes in the delay time. The temperature jump experiments were informative regarding the kinetics of polymerization for solutions with delay times longer than 100 seconds. To study the process at more realistic physiologic time and hemoglobin concentrations, a technique that could deoxygenate hemoglobin S in milliseconds was devised.[126–128] In these experiments, 10^{-11} mL of solution was saturated with carbon monoxide (carboxyhemoglobin S is soluble at concentrations greater than 45 g/dL[129]), then rapidly dissociated from the carbon monoxide ligand by laser photolysis. The effect of hemoglobin concentration (up to 40 g/dL) on the delay time (down to milliseconds) is shown in Figure 53-10. The reproducibility of delay curves is shown in Figure 53-11. Solutions with long delay times exhibit poor reproducibility and, microscopically, a highly aligned single domain of polymer. In contrast, the solutions with short delay times have highly reproducible curves and, microscopically, multiple small domains of short polymers (see Fig. 53-11). These observations led to the *double-nucleation* hypothesis for the mechanism of hemoglobin S polymerization[130] (Fig. 53-12). This model suggests that two related processes take place in a polymerizing solution: (1) a *homogeneous nucleation* that occurs free in solution, and (2) a *heterogeneous nucleation* that occurs on the surface of polymer. Homogeneous nucleation starts the process. The initial aggregation of monomers in solution is relatively unfavorable until the size of the critical nucleus is reached. At this point, entropy is overcome, and the deposition of more monomers becomes favorable. Heterogeneous nucleation can now proceed on the surface of the already-formed polymer, an autocatalytic process because the surface area available for aggregation is constantly increasing. In slowly polymerizing solutions, homogeneous nucleation is relatively slow and random and is followed by rapid heterogeneous nucleation and polymerization of a single, highly ordered domain. In contrast, rapidly polymerizing solutions contain multiple homogeneous nuclei that ultimately provide polymer surface for the production of multiple small polymer domains by heterogeneous nucleation. What results is a dynamic network of growing and cross-linking fibers.[131]

Polymerization in Cells

Several independent pieces of evidence suggest that polymerization data derived from hemoglobin S solutions apply equally well to intact cells.

^{13}C Nuclear Magnetic Resonance Studies at Equilibrium. Natural abundance ^{13}C NMR spectroscopy has been used to quantitate polymer as a function of oxygen saturation at equilibrium in intact cells in a number of different sickle syndromes and density-separated cells.[132–135] As seen in Figure 53-13, sickle cells of different density (and therefore different hemoglobin concentration) have different polymerization curves. The experimental data are close to theoretical expectations, supporting the hypothesis that hemoglobin S in the cell behaves much like hemoglobin S in a cuvette. The ^{13}C NMR data in Figure 53-13 demonstrate the presence of small amounts of polymer in dense cells even at the relatively high oxygen tensions that are encountered in the *arterial* circulation of some patients with sickle cell disease.[136] This point has been stressed by Noguchi and Schechter and their colleagues[90,137–141] as being of prime importance in understanding the pathophysiology of sickle cell anemia. Two factors powerfully influence the presence of polymer in cells at high oxygen tension: the nonideal behavior of concentrated hemoglobin solutions and the heterogeneous distribution of cell density. *Nonideality* results from the molecular crowding that takes place in concentrated hemoglobin solutions and roughly translates into the observation that "hemoglobin in the red cell behaves chemically as if it were almost 100 times more

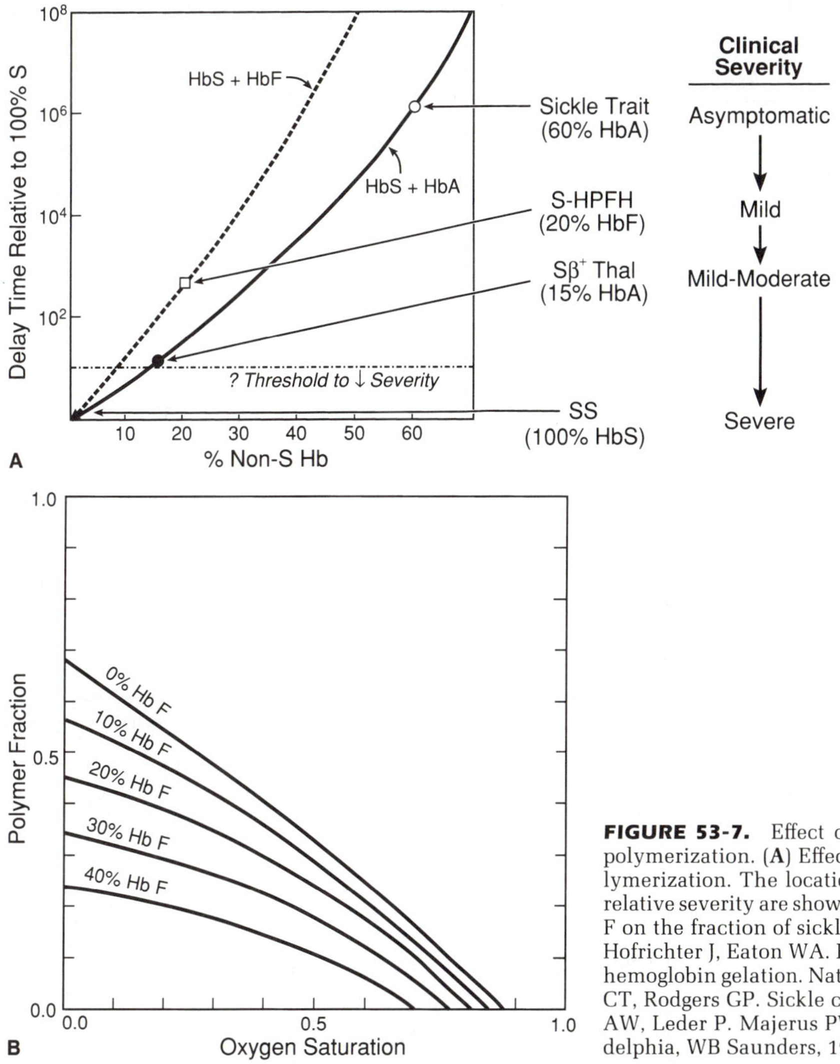

FIGURE 53-7. Effect of nonsickle hemoglobins on sickle hemoglobin polymerization. (**A**) Effect of hemoglobins A and F on the *kinetics* of polymerization. The locations of four common sickle syndromes and their relative severity are shown. (**B**) Effect of different percentages of hemoglobin F on the fraction of sickle polymer at *equilibrium*. (**A** after Sunshine HR, Hofrichter J, Eaton WA. Requirements for therapeutic inhibition of sickle hemoglobin gelation. Nature 1978;275:238; **B** after Schechter AN, Noguchi CT, Rodgers GP. Sickle cell disease. In: Stamatoyannopoulos G, Neinhuis AW, Leder P. Majerus PW, eds. Molecular basis of blood diseases. Philadelphia, WB Saunders, 1987)

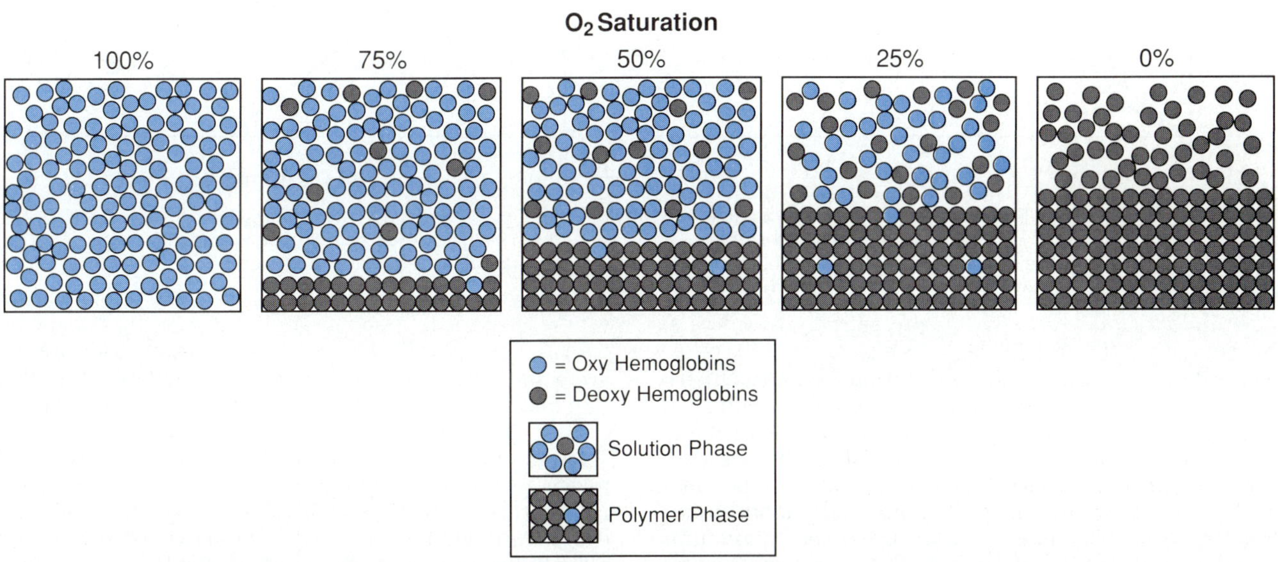

FIGURE 53-8. Sickle hemoglobin at equilibrium at various oxygen saturations. (After Noguchi CT, Schechter AN. Intracellular polymerization of sickle hemoglobin and its relevance to sickle cell disease. Blood 1981;58:1057)

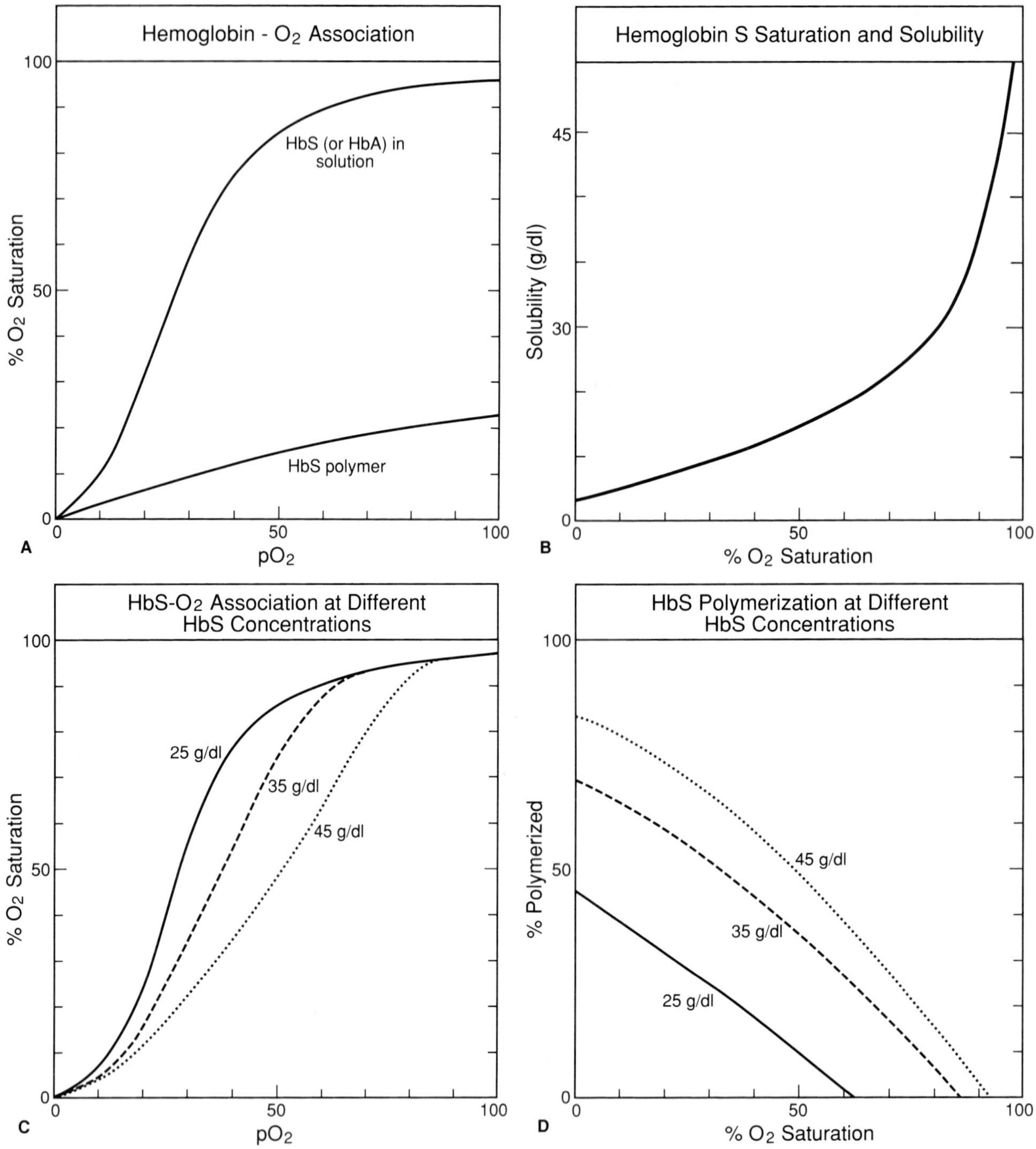

FIGURE 53-9. Relationship between sickle hemoglobin and oxygen. (**A** to **E** after Eaton WA, Hofrichter J. Hemoglobin S gelation and sickle cell disease. Blood 1987;70:1245; **F** after Brittenham GM, Schechter AN, Noguchi CT. Hemoglobin S polymerization: primary determinant of the hemolytic and clinical severity of the sickling syndromes. Blood 1985;65:183)

concentrated than it actually is."[137] Heterogeneous distribution of cell density is a hallmark of the sickle syndromes and results from a complex interplay between sickling and membrane permeability changes. Sickle syndromes with a large number of dense cells have more cells with polymer at high oxygen saturations and are generally more severe (see Fig. 53-9F). The presence of cells with small amounts of polymer on the arterial side of the circulation focuses interest on a part of the vascular tree that, because of its high oxygen tension, has received little attention. Although it remains to be determined which, and to what extent, arteriolar beds are affected in sickle cell disease, these beds are potentially pharmacologically manipulable. Vasodilation may emerge as an important therapy, as suggested in a clinical trial in patients with retinopathy.[142]

Laser Photolysis Studies of Kinetics. The laser photolysis technique that was used to study the kinetics of polymerization of hemoglobin S solutions has been used to study individual red cells.[143] These experiments underscore the concordance between the behavior of hemoglobin S in the test tube and its behavior in the cell. In cells, the distribution of delay times observed correlates with the expected distribution based on cell heterogeneity. In addition, as in solution, the reproducibility of delay time in

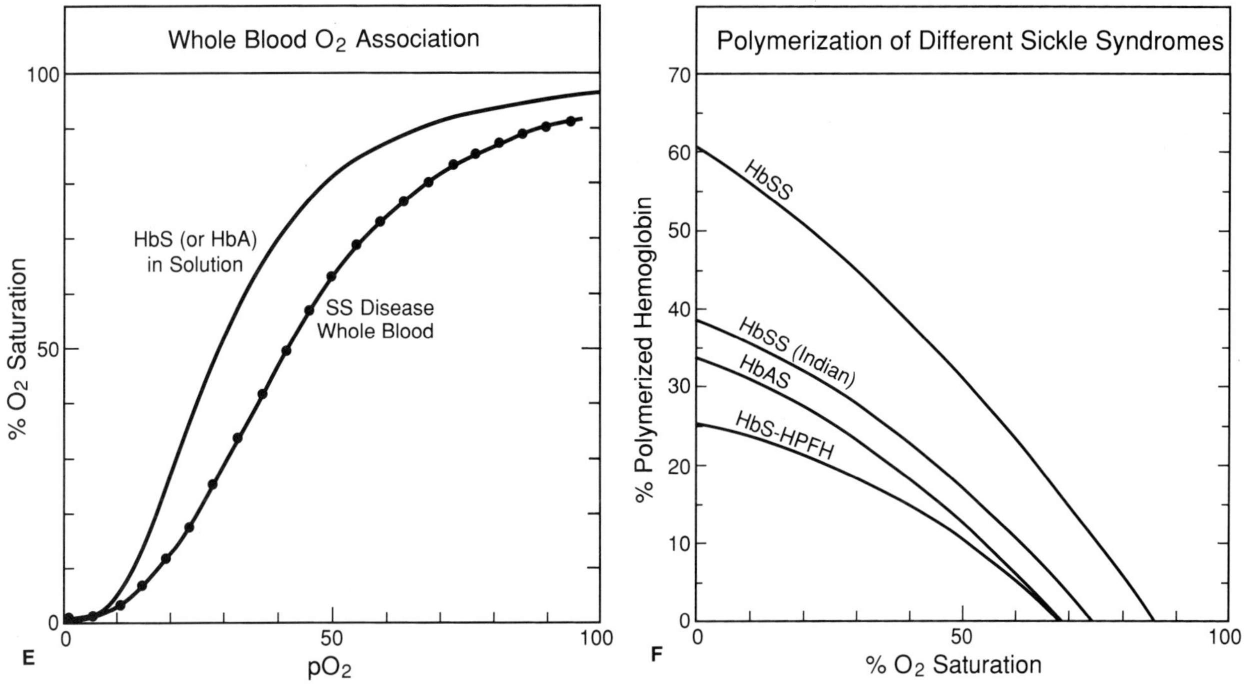

FIGURE 53-9. Continued

cells is best for rapidly polymerizing cells and worst for slowly polymerizing cells. The double-nucleation mechanism (see Fig. 53-12) appears to apply to cells and predicts that dense cells with short delays have multiple small domains of polymer and that light cells have long delays and large single domains (see Fig. 53-11). This view is supported by morphologic studies[144] and may have clinical implications since domains with long fibers are more likely to be rigid and to stretch and potentially damage the membrane than domains with small fibers.[93]

To answer some basic questions as to where, if, and how cells polymerize or sickle in the circulation, a second laser was added to the basic photolysis experiment, allowing cells to be studied at partial desaturation.[145] A critical feature of this work is that as little as 0.05% polymer can be detected in a cell by its marked shortening of the delay time. The loss of delay is always accompanied by cell distortion, while the reacquisition of delay is always accompanied by the restoration of normal morphology. In this experimental setting, as in several rheologic studies,[146–148] morphologic sickling equals polymerization. As seen in Figure 53-14, the curve representing sickling (the loss of delay and normal morphology after a 1-minute exposure to a given saturation) is *not* superimposed on the curve representing unsickling (reappearance of delay and normal morphology after equilibration at a given saturation). This hysteresis occurs because polymer forms after a delay but melts without delay.

Eaton and Hofrichter[91] emphasized the importance of polymerization kinetics in the pathophysiology of sickle cell disease. The relevant time frame for cells in the circulation is roughly 1 second in the alveoli, 3 seconds on the arterial side, 1 second in the capillaries, and 10 seconds in the venous return.[145] Cells with delay times longer than 1 second pass through the microcirculation without sickling. As seen in Figure 53-14, the unsickling curve shows that, *at equilibrium*, about 5% of cells would be sickled at arterial oxygen tensions and 85% at venous tensions. In contrast, the 1-minute sickling curve shows only about 5% sickled at venous tensions. This implies that, under steady-

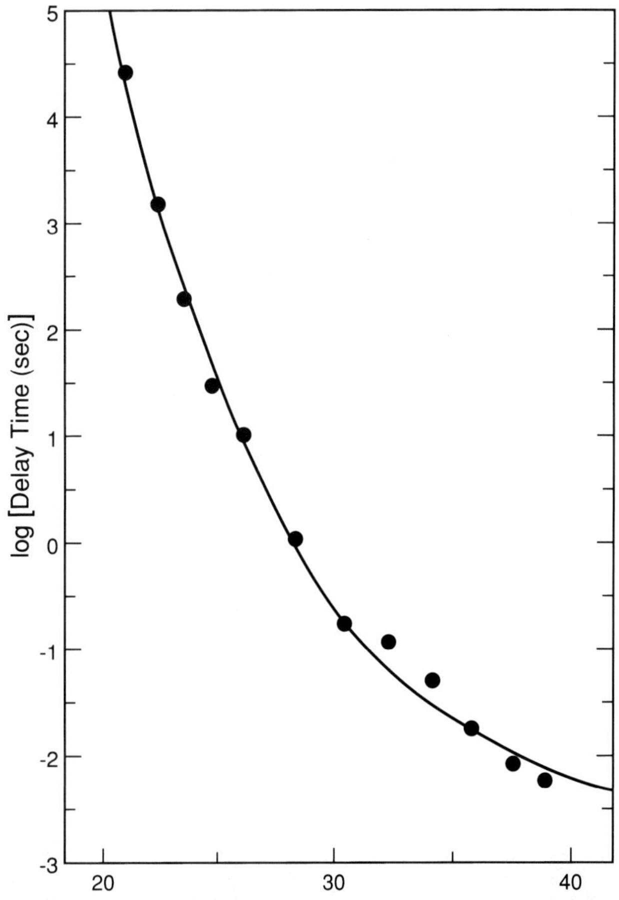

FIGURE 53-10. Effect of hemoglobin concentration on the delay time of polymerization. (After Ferrone FA, Hofrichter J, Eaton WA. Kinetics of sickle hemoglobin polymerization. I. Studies using temperature-jump and laser photolysis techniques. J Mol Biol 1985;183:591)

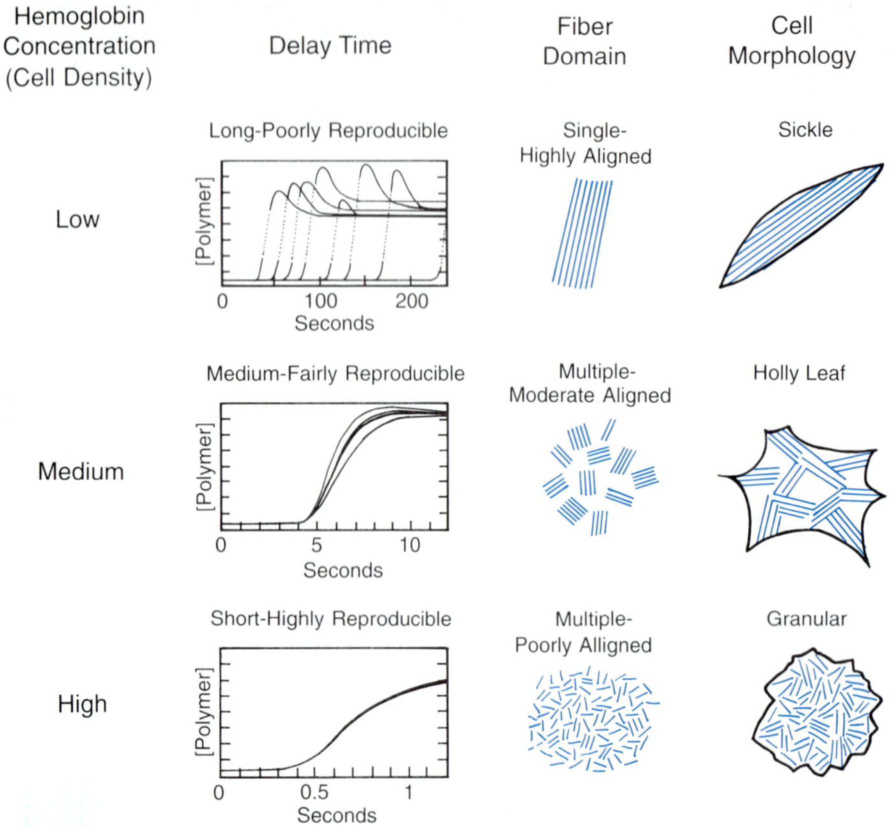

FIGURE 53-11. Illustration of the dependence of delay time, fiber domain, and cell morphology on cell hemoglobin concentration (a measure of cell density). (After Eaton WA, Hofrichter J. Hemoglobin S gelation and sickle cell disease. Blood 1987;70:1245)

state conditions, the delay time is sufficiently long that about 80% of cells are prevented from sickling in the capillaries. This is close to the figure of 10% sickled cells in the arteries and 20% in the veins, compiled from a number of morphologic studies[136,149–151] by Eaton and Hofrichter.[91] Vasoocclusion is favored by factors that either shorten the delay time or increase the transit time.

POLYMERIZATION, RED CELLS, AND THE CIRCULATION

Membrane Damage in Sickle Red Cells

The pathophysiology of sickle cell disease starts with the abnormal gene and its unstable hemoglobin product that polymerizes when deoxygenated. The clinical manifesta-

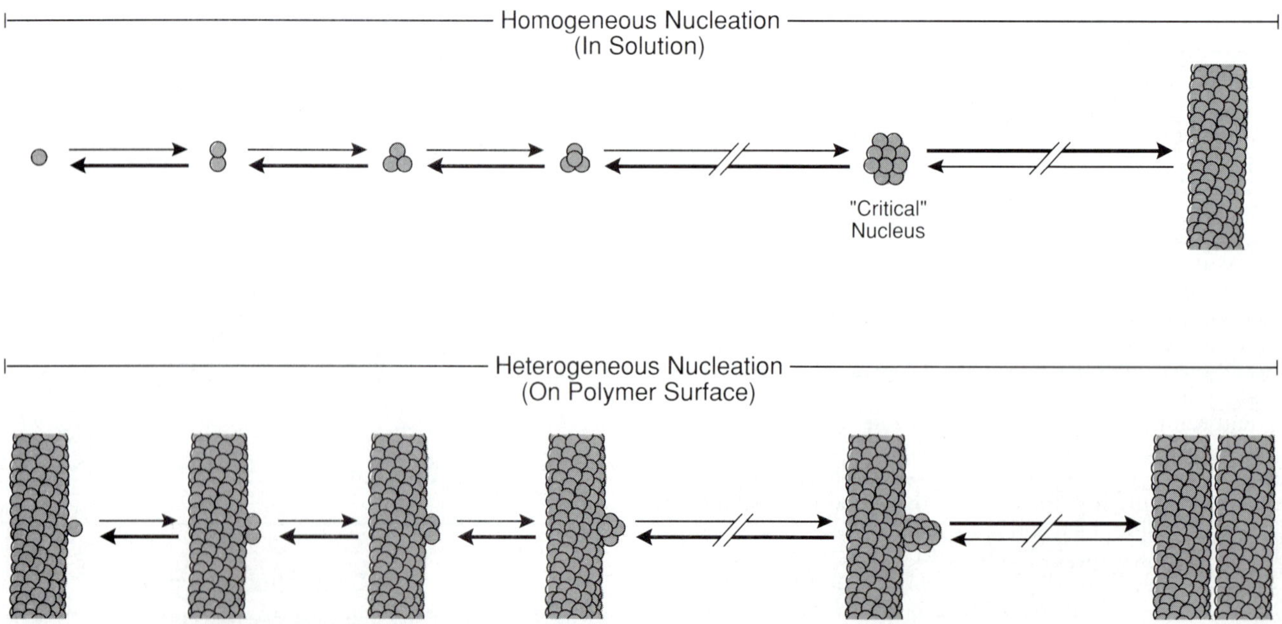

FIGURE 53-12. The double nucleation mechanism of hemoglobin S polymerization hypothesized by Ferrone and colleagues. Gray circles represent molecules of deoxyhemoglobin S. (After Ferrone FA, Hofrichter J, Eaton WA. Kinetics of sickle hemoglobin polymerization. II. A double nucleation mechanism. J Mol Biol 1985;183:611)

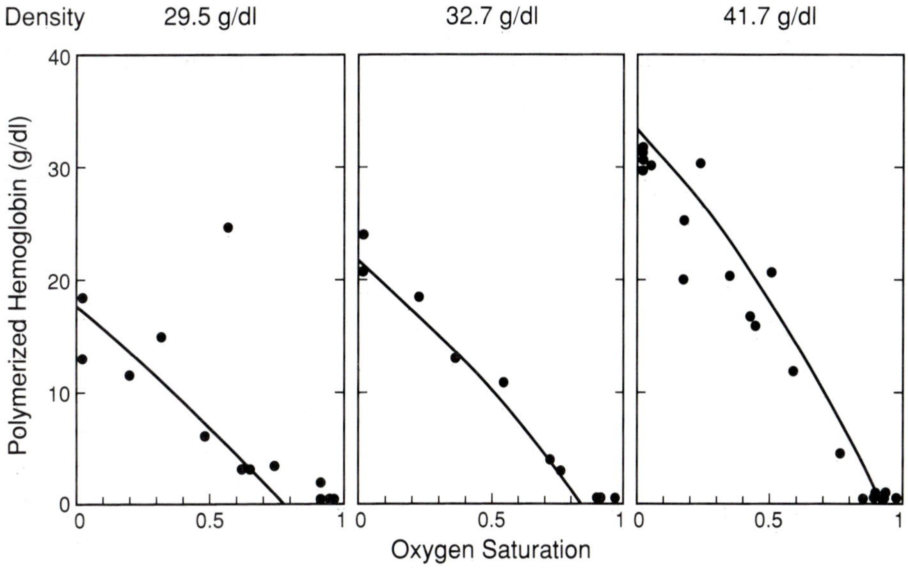

FIGURE 53-13. Relationship between the concentration of polymerized hemoglobin S and oxygen saturation for cells of different density. Density is measured as the mean corpuscular hemoglobin concentration (MCHC). (A fractional oxygen saturation of 1 represents 100% saturation.) (After Noguchi CT, Torchia DA, Schechter AN. Intracellular polymerization of sickle cell hemoglobin: effects of cell heterogeneity. J Clin Invest 1983;72:846)

tions are all secondary phenomena—tissue damage caused by the hemoglobin. Because hemoglobin is packaged as a highly concentrated solution encased by the red cell membrane, the membrane is probably an important modulator of clinical expression. It is the tissue in most intimate contact with the abnormal gene product and is precariously exposed to its noxious by-products and subject to gross physical distortion. The membrane also influences the degree of concentration of the hemoglobin and is the surface that is recognized by proteins and cells in the plasma, by the vascular endothelium, and by reticuloendothelial cells. In this section, the evidence for membrane damage is presented, its cause considered, and its clinical implications discussed. A comprehensive review by Hebbel[152] should be consulted for additional details.

Irreversibly Sickled Cells

Irreversibly sickled cells are the long, slender, pointed cells that persist in well-oxygenated peripheral smears of patients with hemoglobin SS disease (Fig. 53-15). These dense, hemoglobin F–poor cells contain virtually no polymerized hemoglobin when they are fully oxygenated and survive for only a few days.[153,154] Their numbers correlate well with hemolytic rate[155] and spleen size[156] but not with vasoocclusive severity. Experimentally, irreversibly sickled cells can be produced from reversibly sickled cells using a variety of deoxy incubation strategies, including adenosine triphosphate (ATP) depletion,[157] calcium accumulation,[158] ATP maintenance,[159] and oxy–deoxy cycling.[160–163] They provide the most graphic evidence of membrane damage in SS disease. As seen in Figure 53-16, the abnormal shape of an irreversibly sickled cell is maintained by the membrane ghost. Furthermore, when the cell ghost is exposed to a detergent that removes the membrane lipid and integral proteins, the abnormal shape survives in the residual protein skeleton.[164] In normal red cells, the skeleton influences cell shape, permeability, lipid organization, deformability, and movement of intramembranous particles (see Chap. 54). There are abnormalities other than shape in irreversibly sickled cells and other abnormalities in cells with normal shape.

Membrane Control of the Internal Environment

As discussed previously, the red cells in sickle cell anemia are extremely heterogeneous with respect to their hemo-

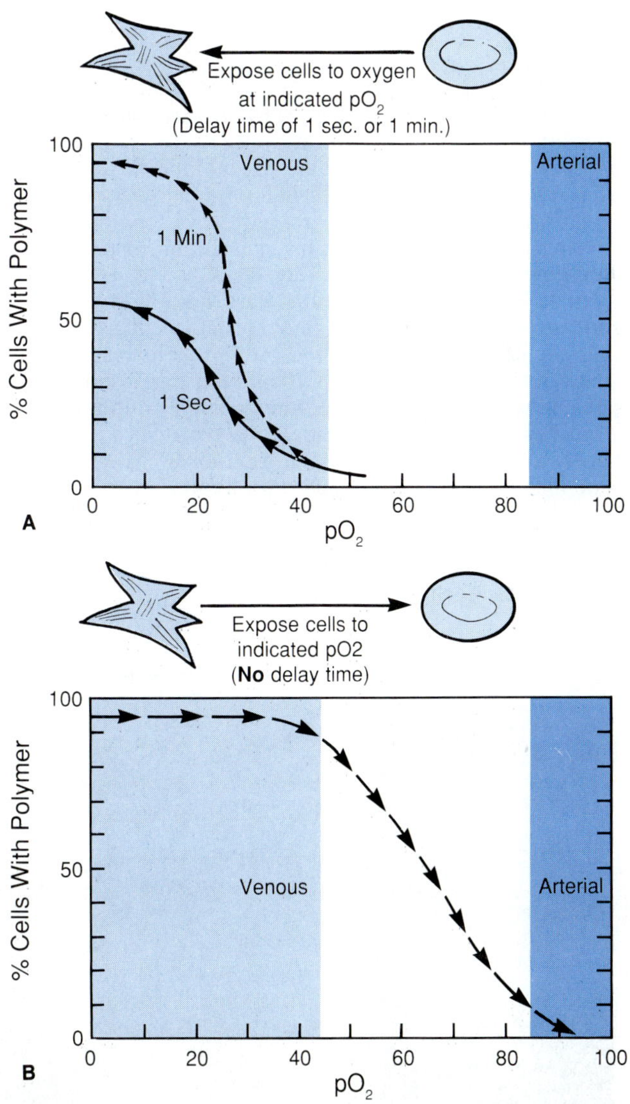

FIGURE 53-14. Sickling **(A)** and unsickling **(B)** curves extrapolated to in vivo conditions. In contrast to the sickling process, there is no delay time for unsickling. The area marked *Venous* extends from a typical venous Po_2 of 40 to 45 mmHg to 0 mmHg, which would not ordinarily occur in vivo.

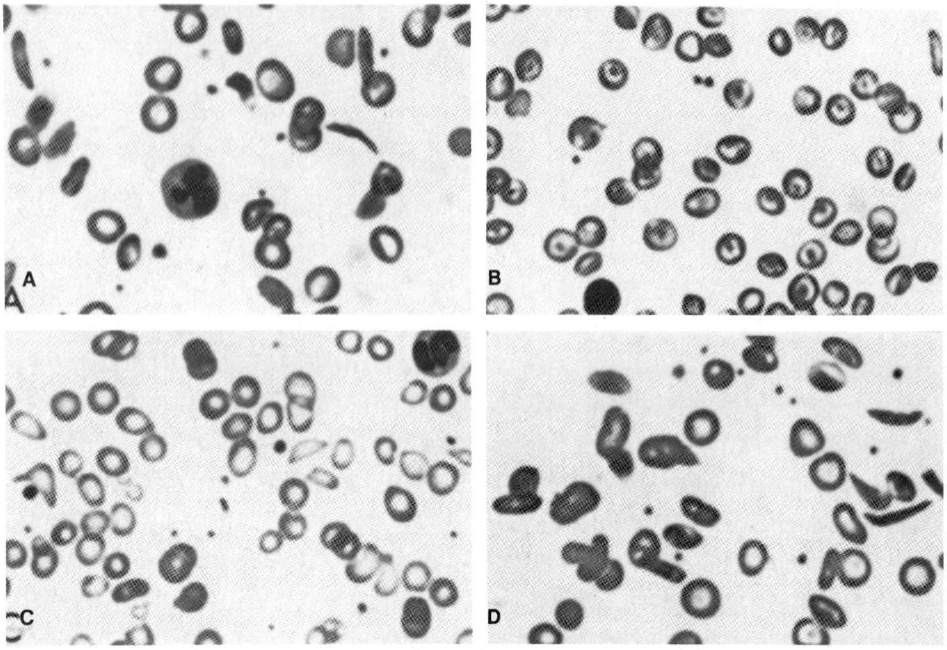

FIGURE 53-15. Peripheral blood smears from persons with sickle cell anemia (**A**), hemoglobin SC disease (**B**), Sβ-thalassemia (**C**), and hemoglobin SD disease (**D**). (After Platt OS, et al. Hematology of infancy and childhood. In: Nathan DG, Oski FA eds. WB Saunders, 1993)

globin concentration. The proportion of dehydrated cells (including irreversibly sickled cells) directly influences the amount of polymer present at a given Po_2. Extreme dehydration, which in itself may cause membrane damage,[165] is a reflection of the abnormal permeability of sickle membranes. Three transport pathways contribute in varying degrees under varying conditions to pathologic dehydration:

Na^+-K^+ Pump. Almost 40 years ago, Tosteson and colleagues[166–168] demonstrated that sickle cells have the unique tendency to lose K^+ and gain Na^+ when deoxygenated. Physical deformation of the membrane is closely associated with the increased permeability,[169,170] and the leak is relatively insensitive to charge but restrictive in size.[171] Because the K^+ lost is balanced by the Na^+ gained, there is no net water movement and no dehydration.[172,173] When the internal Na^+ becomes sufficiently high, however, the Na^+-K^+ pump is stimulated, and the excess Na^+ is expelled. The stoichiometry of the pump is such that for every three Na^+ that are extruded, only two K^+ are imported. This imbalance creates the situation in which the stimulated pump can cause net cation loss and cell dehydration.[174–177]

Ca^{2+}-Activated K Channel. As discussed previously, morphologic sickling is associated with a transient increase in both Na^+ and K^+ permeability. Similarly, Ca^{2+} permeability is increased during sickling, allowing the red cell to accumulate large amounts of calcium.[178–180] Normally, red cells contain 2 to 8 μmol calcium per liter of red cells.[181] In contrast, unfractionated sickle cells contain 40 to 60 μmol calcium, and irreversibly sickled cells contain as much as 200 μmol calcium per liter of red cells.[182–184] In 1956, Gardos[185] showed that red cells with elevated levels of calcium undergo selective K^+ and water loss if they become ATP depleted. The *Gardos phenomenon* has been an attractive hypothesis to explain dehydration in calcium-loaded sickle cells.[172,186–189] However, the excessive Ca^{2+} that is needed to provoke the Gardos phenomenon may not be free in the cytosol[190] but safely sequestered—actively pumped into endocytic vesicles.[191] Compartmentalization may explain why there is no easily measurable Ca^{2+}-

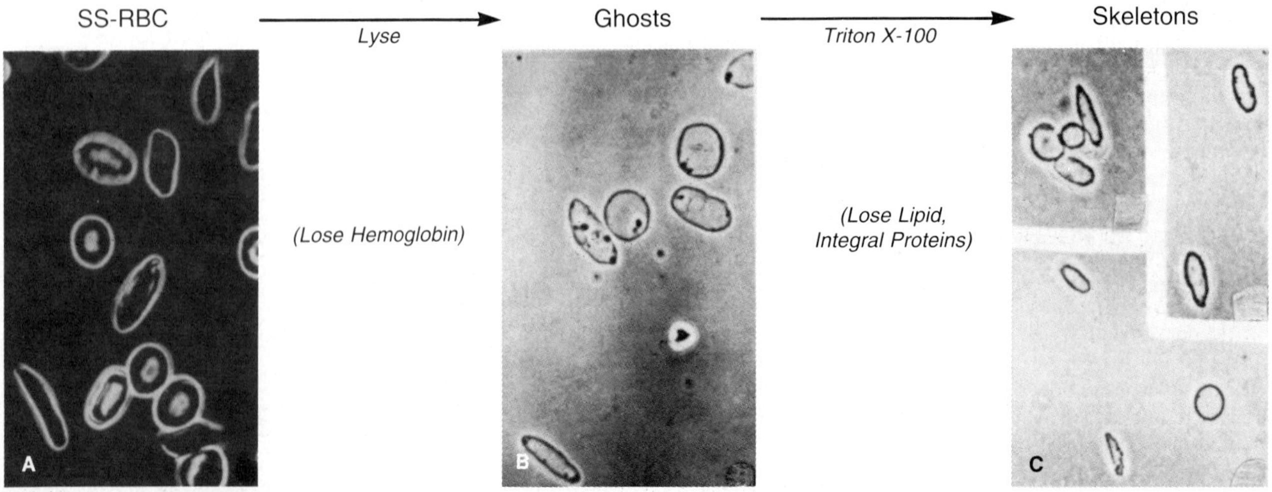

FIGURE 53-16. Demonstration that membrane ghosts and membrane protein skeletons of irreversibly sickled cells maintain the sickle shape. (Lux SE, John KM, et al. Irreversible deformation of the spectrin–actin lattice in irreversibly sickled cells. J Clin Invest 1976;58:955)

dependent K^+ loss in sickle red cells[192,193] but does not exclude the possibility that brief dehydrating pulses of increased cytosolic Ca^{2+} develop during polymerization.

KCl Cotransport System. Attention has focused on what is probably the most important dehydrating transport pathway in RBCs. This system does not require deoxygenation, polymerization, or sickling for its activation—the KCl cotransport system.[194–196] This system is found in normal reticulocytes,[197,198] which may explain its activity in sickle cell anemia. Its presence in cells from patients with hemoglobin C trait[199] and homozygous C disease[200] is not entirely explained by cell age and implies that there may be a functional interaction between positively charged hemoglobin and the membrane. KCl cotransport results in a net loss of water and KCl from the cell and may clarify why cells with hemoglobin C tend to be dehydrated. The pathway is chloride-dependent and is stimulated by acid pH (less than 7.4), cell swelling, and sulfhydryl modification.[201,202] It is inhibited by magnesium.[195,203] Incubation of sickle red cells at low pH suggests that this pathway can lead to cellular dehydration.[196]

Membrane and Outside Surface of the Cell

Abnormal Lipid Orientation. The phospholipids of the red cell bilayer are constantly flipping between the inner and outer leaflets (see Chap. 54). Despite this rapid continuous movement, a degree of asymmetry is maintained, with the amino phospholipids (phosphatidylserine and phosphatidylethanolamine) spending relatively more time in the inner leaflet and the choline-phospholipids (phosphatidylcholine and sphingomyelin) on the external surface. This asymmetry is poorly maintained in sickle cells. Phosphatidylserine and phosphatidylethanolamine partition normally in oxygenated reversibly sickled cells, are more exposed on the surface of deoxygenated reversibly sickled cells, and are permanently externalized in irreversibly sickled cells.[204–208] This anomalous partitioning results in abnormal cell-surface characteristics and reactions. Phosphatidylserine is capable of promoting coagulation, and its exposure on the surface of sickle cells is associated with increased procoagulant activity.[204] It is not known whether such enhanced clotting influences microvascular occlusion. The abnormal surface lipids are also associated with the increased tendency of sickle cells to bind and fuse with lipid vesicles,[209] dehydrate,[210] and adhere to macrophages.[211]

Abnormal Surface Interactions, Topography, and Skeletal Proteins. Surface charge and antigens of red cells are largely carried on the transmembrane protein glycophorin and band 3 (the erythrocyte anion exchange channel; see Chap. 54). The distribution and nature of surface antigen and charge is abnormal in sickle cells, implying an abnormality in the protein structure of the membrane.

Hemoglobin A binds to the membrane[212,213] on the cytoplasmic portion of band 3.[214–218] Sickle hemoglobin binds even more readily than hemoglobin A.[219–223] Denatured hemoglobin, the major constituent of Heinz bodies, binds with extremely high affinity to the cytoplasmic portion of band 3[224] and, in intact cells, causes band 3 to aggregate.[225] Sickle red cells do not contain large classic Heinz bodies but do have small inclusions made of hemichrome—*micro-Heinz bodies.*[226–229] There is a marked redistribution of the membrane proteins of sickle cells near the micro-Heinz bodies. As demonstrated by immunofluorescence microscopy (Fig. 53-17), Heinz bodies underlie (and presumably aggregate) abnormal clusters of band 3, ankyrin, and glycophorins.[230] Band 3 and glycophorin are progressively aggregated in increasingly dehydrated sickle and normal red cells.[230a]

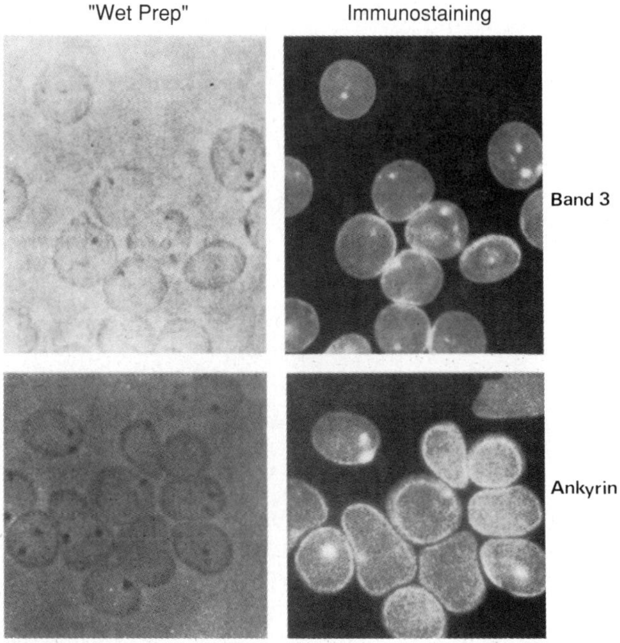

FIGURE 53-17. Demonstration of band 3 and ankyrin clustering at the site of Heinz bodies. All the Heinz bodies, which appear as dark inclusions in the phase contrast ("wet prep") photomicrographs fluoresce when stained by the band 3 antibody, but only a subset stain with an ankyrin antibody. (After Waugh SM, Willardson BM, Kannan R, Labotka R, Low PS. Heinz bodies induce clustering of band 3, glycophorin, and ankyrin in sickle cell erythrocytes. J Clin Invest 1986;78:1155)

Clustered or clusterable band 3 and glycophorins may be responsible for the electron microscopic appearance of uneven clumps of negative charge on the surface of sickle red cells.[231] Such an abnormal surface coincides with the tendency of sickle cells to adhere to endothelial cells.[231] Hebbel's observation that sickle cells adhere to endothelial cells has been confirmed[232] (Fig. 53-18*A*), carefully quantitated,[233] and even demonstrated in a flowing ex vivo vascular system[234,235] (see Fig. 53-18*C*). The endothelial cells may be damaged in the process.[236] The mediators of this unusual adherence are largely unknown, although it appears that at least divalent cations and von Willebrand's factor are involved.[237,238] The synthetic RGDS tetrapeptide reduces the adhesion of sickle cells and supports the role of von Willebrand's factor in the system. The blocking ability of this peptide, however, does not rule out the participation of other adherence proteins, such as fibronectin, which also has an RGDS-binding domain and the ability to bind to sickle cells.[239] When endothelial cells are infected with herpes simplex virus, adherence is enhanced and appears to be mediated through red cell immunoglobulin G (IgG) and the induced Fc receptors on the endothelial cell.[240] Other potentially induced endothelial ligands include a variety of adhesive proteins, such as vascular cell adhesion molecule 1 (VCAM-1).[240a] Such molecules are inducible by cytokines and can be recognized by integrins such as $\alpha_4\beta_1$ on very young sickle reticulocytes. Endothelial adherence has potentially important clinical implications because it is one of the only laboratory measurements that correlates with clinical severity in patients with sickle cell anemia[241,242] (see Fig. 53-18*D*).

Clustering[225,243] and other alterations of band 3[244–246] cause the deposition of specific immunoglobulin[247,248] on the surface of the sickle cell. This pattern of anti–band 3 antibody deposition is related to premature cell senescence and probably contributes to hemolysis.[249] The finding that both

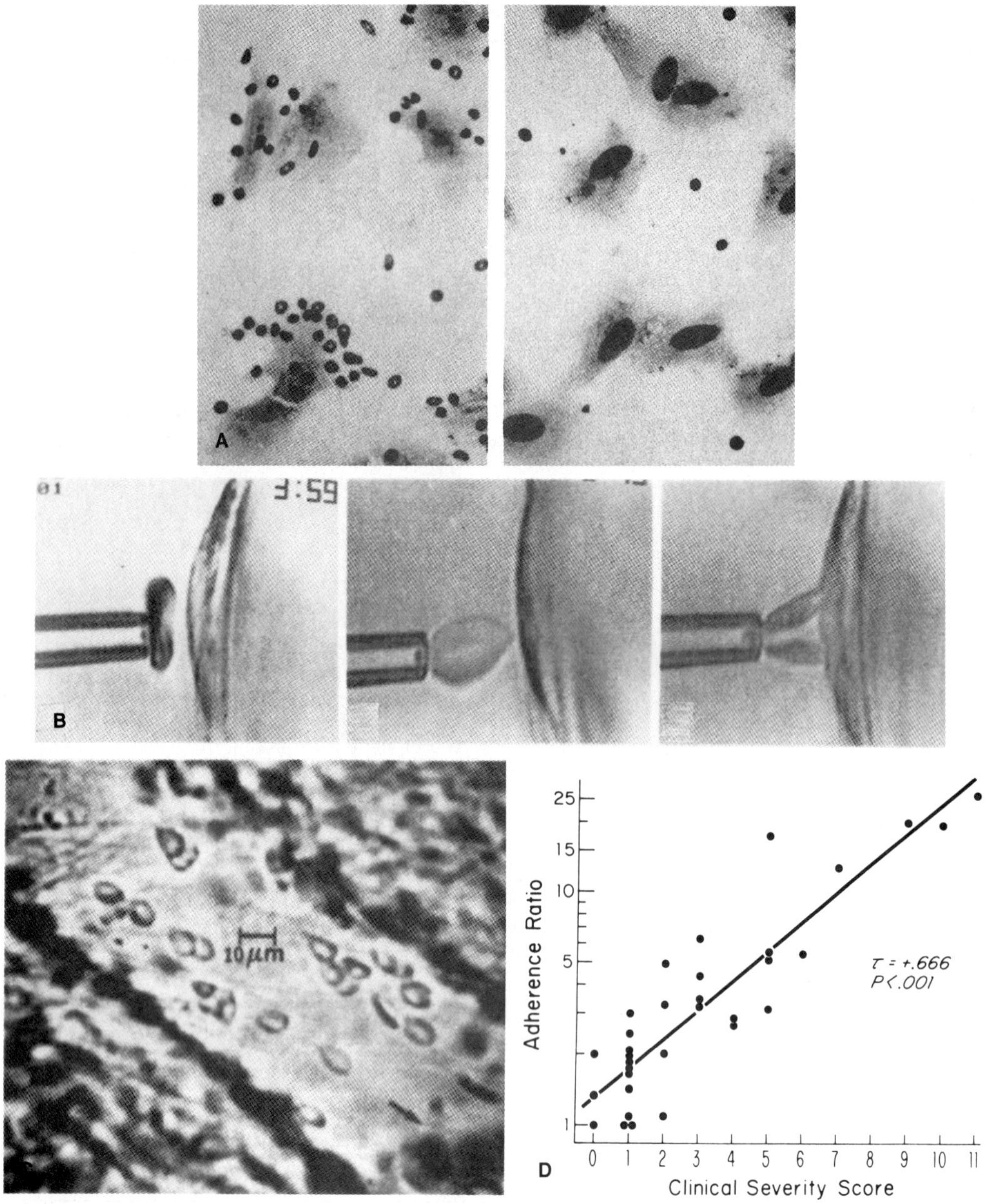

FIGURE 53-18. Sickle erythrocytes and endothelial adherence. Three measures of adherence are shown. (**A**) Increased adherence of sickle (*right*) and normal (*left*) red cells to cultured endothelial cells. The small dark sickle red cells rosette around the much larger endothelial cells (*left*), whereas none of the normal red cells is close to an endothelial cell. (**B**) Increased force of adherence of individual erythrocytes to cultured cells: nonadherent normal cell (*left*), sickle cell with one attachment site (*center*), and sickle cell with multiple attachment sites (*right*). (**C**) Increased adherence of sickle erythrocytes in a flow system (small blood vessels in the rat mesocecum) that mimics in vivo conditions. Transfused sickle cells are adherent to the wall of the blood vessel in the center of the photomicrograph. (**D**) Positive correlation between clinical severity and increased adherence of sickle cells to cultured human venous endothelial cells. (**A** from Hebbel RP, Yamada O, et al. Abnormal adherence of sickle erythrocytes to cultured vascular endothelium: possible mechanism for microvascular occlusion in sickle cell disease. J Clin Invest 1980;65:154; **B** after Mohandas N, Evans E. Sickle erythrocyte adherence to vascular endothelium. J Clin Invest 1985;76:1605; **C** from Kaul DK, Fabry ME, Nagel RL. Microvascular sites and characteristics of sickle cell adhesion to vascular endothelium in shear flow conditions: pathophysiological implications. Proc Natl Acad Sci USA 1989;86:3356; **D** from Hebbel RP, Boogaerts MAB, Eaton JW, Steinberg MH. Erythrocyte adherence to endothelium in sickle-cell anemia: a possible determinant of disease severity. N Engl J Med 1980;302:992)

i and I antigens are increased in sickle cells[250,251] is more likely to be a function of accelerated erythropoiesis than altered skeletal organization.

The skeletal proteins, which interact with and provide structural support for band 3 and the glycophorins, are also affected in sickle cell disease. Long polymers of sickle hemoglobin can physically dissociate the membrane lipid and its associated band 3 from the underlying skeleton.[252] This causes the release of spectrin-free vesicles[253,254] (Fig. 53-19). Chemically, there is good evidence that the thiol redox status of spectrin, ankyrin, and protein 4.1 is abnormal.[255] Sickle protein 4.1 contains 1 to 2 mol% fewer cysteines and about 1 mol% more cysteic acid than the normal protein.[256] The function of sickle ankyrin is abnormal—when exposed on the surface of inside-out vesicles prepared from sickle cells, it binds poorly to spectrin.[257] This functional ankyrin

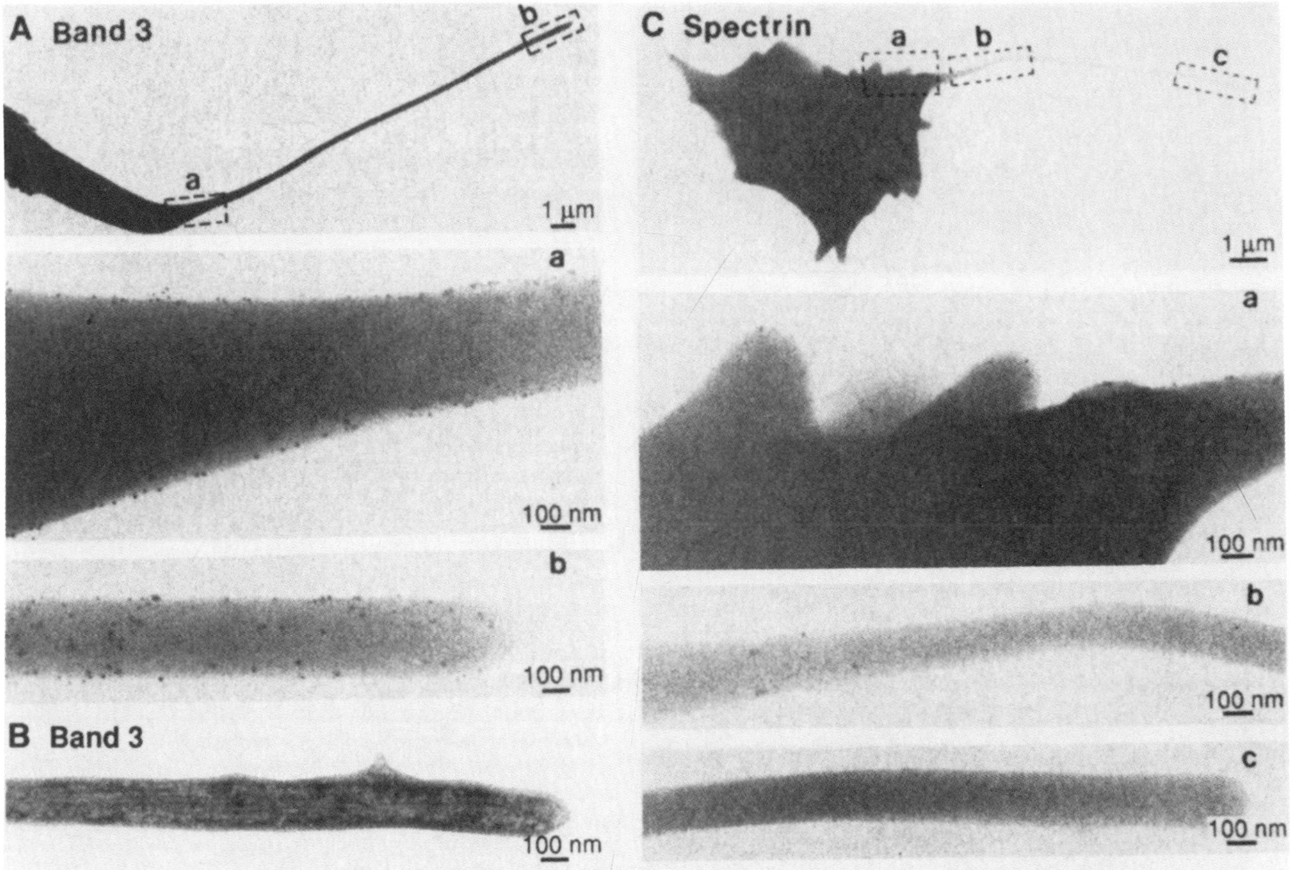

FIGURE 53-19. Transmission electron micrographs of sickled RBCs labeled with antibody-coated gold particles. (**A**) Band 3 labeling of a spicule induced by deoxygenation. The regions marked a and b at the base and tip of the spicule, respectively, are shown in higher magnification below. Band 3 molecules, marked by the gold particles (*small black dots*, 15 nm in diameter), extend to the tip of the spicule. (**B**) Tip of a long spicule negatively stained with uranyl acetate to show that hemoglobin S polymers extend to the end of the spicule. (**C**) Spectrin labeling. High magnifications of regions a, b, and c are also shown. In contrast to band 3, spectrin is absent from the long spicule. The data suggest that hemoglobin polymers pierce the membrane skeleton and extend out from the cell, covered by the lipid bilayer and integral membrane proteins such as band 3, which are detached from the membrane skeleton in the process. (Liu SC, Derick LH, Zhai S, Palek J. Uncoupling of spectrin-based skeleton from the lipid bilayer in sickled red cells. Science 1991;252:574)

abnormality relates to clinical severity of the sickle syndromes (Fig. 53-20). It is also found in other cells with Heinz bodies, such as erythrocytes containing unstable hemoglobins.[258] The pathogenesis of the membrane abnormalities is not known precisely but is likely to be some combination of hemoglobin interaction and oxidation.

Several convincing convergent lines of evidence implicate oxidation as the major contributor to the membrane abnormalities of sickle cells; these are discussed in detail in a review by Hebbel.[259] Sickle red cells generate twice the normal amount of the potent oxidants, superoxide, peroxide, and hydroxyl radical.[260] The inherent tendency of oxyhemoglobin S to autoxidize and form methemoglobin results in the generation of superoxide and the loss of free heme.[261] The liberated heme is capable of damaging the membrane by oxidizing proteins or lipids and also by acting as a structure-perturbing detergent.[262,263] Various components of the sickle membrane contain excessive amounts of free or globin-bound heme, which may cause site-specific damage.[264] For example, free heme may target membrane lipids, while denatured globin-bound heme (hemichrome) may target band 3 and its neighbors, such as ankyrin. Nonheme iron is also found in sickle cells and is enriched in dense cells.[265] Because phospholipase D can liberate free iron from membranes, it is likely that the iron is associated with and can potentially specifically damage aminophospholipids.[265] Many of the abnormal membrane properties of sickle membranes can be circumstantially linked to oxidation. Oxidation of normal cells can result in abnormal cation homeostasis,[266,267] membrane deformability,[268,269] interaction with phagocytes,[270] lipid asymmetry,[271] tendency to form vesicles,[272,273] abnormal binding function of ankyrin,[258] and increased binding of anti–band 3 surface IgG.[274]

Abnormal Red Blood Cell Rheology and Implications for Microvascular Flow

A variety of rheologic techniques demonstrate that even fully oxygenated sickle red cells are less deformable than normal.[275–278] When these cells are fractionated by density and studied, it becomes clear that the major rheologic impairment comes from the very dense cells with high intracellular viscosity.[279–281] When rehydrated to a normal hemoglobin concentration, the rheology of these cells improves but does not normalize. This partial correction implies that there may be a residual abnormal membrane component—perhaps one of the ones described previously, or perhaps related to formation of a complex between spectrin and sickle hemoglobin.[282] Sickle hemoglobin can be experimentally packaged in normal membranes, cre-

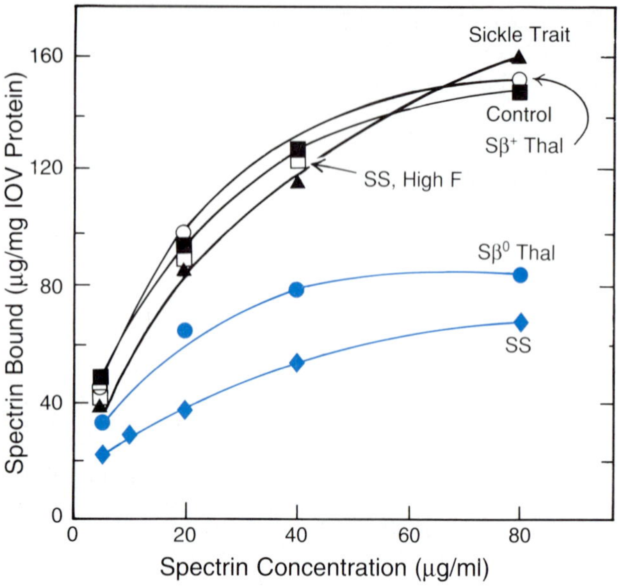

FIGURE 53-20. Binding of normal spectrin to inside-out membrane vesicles (IOV) prepared from erythrocytes from patients with different sickle syndromes. Asymptomatic patients with sickle trait, $S\beta^{+}$-thalassemia, and sickle cell anemia with elevated fetal hemoglobin had normal binding curves. Red cell membranes from the symptomatic persons with sickle cell anemia and $S\beta^{0}$-thalassemia contained decreased spectrin binding sites. (After Platt OS, Falcone JF, Lux SE. Molecular defect in the sickle erythrocyte skeleton: abnormal spectrin binding to sickle inside-out vesicles. J Clin Invest 1985;75:266)

ating a hybrid cell with an abnormal shear modulus. Packaging of hemoglobin A in sickle membranes normalizes the shear modulus.[283] This observation suggests that the interaction of sickle hemoglobin with the membrane causes the abnormal cellular characteristics. In the same series of experiments, however, the abnormal plastic behavior of the very dense sickle cells could not be normalized by exchanging the sickle hemoglobin for hemoglobin A.

Kaul and coworkers[234] showed how the heterogenous sickle red cells behave as they flow through the mesocecal vasculature of the rat. Even when fully oxygenated, flow occasionally ceases as relatively light cells adhere to postcapillary venules and entrap dense cells. Although the dense cells are the least adherent, they do become sequestered in the venules,[284] which may explain why some patients appear to lose their dense cells during vasoocclusion.[285] Precapillary obstruction occurs randomly as dense cells are held up at the arteriole–capillary junction.[286–289] Such periodic plugging of the microvasculature may trigger vasomotor responses and create the periodic flow pattern seen in the skin of patients studied with laser Doppler flow velocimetry.[290]

If oxygenated sickle cells have difficulty traversing the microvasculature, the situation drastically deteriorates when the cells become deoxygenated. As oxygen tension is reduced, so is the deformability of sickle cells.[291–293] Filterability of sickle red cells declines with oxygen tension, and the densest cells appear to be the most sensitive to deoxygenation.[294] Very dense cells become less filterable, even in oxygen tensions found on the arterial side of the circulation.[295] The observation that the rheologic properties of minimally desaturated dense cells correlate with clinical parameters stresses the potential pathophysiologic importance of polymer in the arterial circulation.[296] Ironically, ektacytometric measurements of cell deformability suggest that the cells with the highest hemoglobin concentration require the greatest amount of polymer to be present before deformability is impaired.[297]

STRATEGIES FOR THERAPY

Replace the Defective Gene

Expression of the sickle gene is limited to the erythroid cells of the bone marrow—a tissue that can be transplanted. The first bone marrow transplantation in a patient with sickle cell anemia was done to treat acute myeloblastic leukemia; both conditions were successfully cured.[298] More recently, a child with sickle cell disease and Morquio's syndrome was successfully transplanted.[299] In the United States, there is considerable reluctance to resort to transplantation as primary treatment for any patient with sickle cell disease. The morbidity and mortality associated with transplantation are high compared with the relatively benign course that many patients naturally follow. The gap between transplant morbidity and disease morbidity is particularly wide in young children, who have the fewest symtpoms but who are the best transplantation candidates. A unique approach to this medical dilemma was a formal mock trial complete with barristers, expert witnesses, and a jury.[244a] Although this jury decided not to offer transplantation for all children with symptoms, it is clear that in the coming years, as transplantation technology improves and high-risk sickle cell patients can be identified earlier, transplantation will emerge as an important therapy. In the United States, a prospective clinical trial for selected patients with symptoms is underway, and the European experience is growing rapidly.[300–300b]

More specific *gene therapy* (ie, repairing the sickle gene defect by inserting a normal β gene) is still years away. However, the effectiveness of retroviral gene constructs in inserting functional human β genes (normal and sickle) into transgenic mice is encouraging. Such techniques are well on the way to creating a much-needed mouse model for sickle cell disease.[301,302]

Stimulate Fetal Hemoglobin Production

Because fetal hemoglobin has such a profound inhibitory effect on sickle hemoglobin polymerization, there has been substantial interest in trying to stimulate the dormant γ-globin genes. The first evidence that the chemotherapeutic agent 5-azacytidine could enhance fetal hemoglobin production in anemic primates[303] led to encouraging clinical trials in patients with thalassemia and sickle cell disease.[304–306] The increased production of fetal hemoglobin was thought to be related to the ability of 5-azacytidine to reduce directly methylation and therefore restore transcription of fetal genes. Subsequent trials with other cytotoxic drugs that do not influence DNA methylation, such as cytosine arabinoside and hydroxyurea,[307,308] revealed that "safer" drugs than 5-azacytidine can also stimulate fetal hemoglobin production. Understanding the precise mechanism of this effect continues to be elusive. The simple compounds butyrate and acetate enhance fetal hemoglobin synthesis in sickle red cell progenitors[309,309a] and in vivo.[309b]

Hydroxyurea has been used in several clinical trials.[310–313] Most patients respond with elevated fetal hemoglobin production, but it remains to be seen what factors influence the magnitude of the response and what fraction of patients will ultimately benefit from treatment. Although the anecdotal reports of clinical efficacy are encouraging, further study is necessary before this cytotoxic, teratogenic[314,315] drug can be recommended for general use.

Decrease Concentration of Hemoglobin S

The polymerization of sickle hemoglobin is exquisitely concentration dependent. Any therapy that reduced the mean corpuscular hemoglobin concentration (MCHC) of sickle cells would drastically reduce polymerization. Two approaches to decrease hemoglobin concentration have been tried: (1) lowering plasma osmolarity, and (2) increasing intracellular cation concentrations. The first approach uses desmopressin (DDAVP) and severe dietary salt restriction to decrease the serum sodium to 120 mEq/L. This treatment causes cell swelling, lower MCHC, and fewer painful episodes.[316] Although promising as a strategy, others find this regimen too difficult to maintain, neurologically toxic, and ineffective.[317–319] The second approach relies on a number of compounds that alter the permeability of the red cell membrane and allow sickle cells to become hydrated. The best-studied drug of this group is cetiedil, which is used clinically to treat painful peripheral vascular disease. This drug inhibits morphologic sickling[320,321] and causes cells to gain salt and water.[322] A clinical trial of cetiedil as acute therapy for episodes of pain suggested a modest reduction in the duration of episodes, but there was ultimately no difference in the amount of narcotic required.[323] It is possible that this drug may be useful if given prophylactically, in a better dosing schedule, or in combination with other agents.[324] A potentially promising specific inhibitor of KCl cotransport, [(dihydroindenyl)oxy]alkanoic acid has been described and shown to prevent the dehydration of sickle cells in vitro.[325] The oral antifungal drug clotrimazole can block the Gardos channel and prevent dehydration of sickled red cells in vitro[325a] and in vivo using a mouse model for sickle cell disease.[325b] A clinical trial in humans is underway.

Inhibit Polymerization of Hemoglobin S

Despite the detailed knowledge of the structure of the sickle polymer and the effort that excellent laboratories have expended in designing and demonstrating antisickling compounds, none is used to treat patients. Pragmatic issues of toxicity and red cell membrane permeability are serious problems that may take years to solve. The potentially useful antisickling agents are generally classified as either noncovalent or covalent modifiers of hemoglobin and have a variety of effects on hemoglobin solubility, oxygen affinity, and cell sickling.[326] Urea is the classic noncovalent reagent that disrupts hydrophobic interactions. It is an antisickling agent at molar concentrations in vitro[327] but is ineffective in concentrations that can be achieved clinically.[328] A more specific approach to noncovalent disruption of polymerization is exemplified by the use of *p*-aminobenzoylpolyglutamates with hydrophobic end groups.[329] These relatively potent compounds are designed to interfere with the interaction of the β-6 valine of one strand and the hydrophobic pocket on the adjacent strand.

The covalent modifiers were reviewed by Ueno and colleagues.[330] A variety of effective antisickling agents target a variety of residues. For example, nitrogen mustard reacts with histidine[331]; glyceraldehyde[332] and aspirins[333] react with lysine and cystamine[334]; and glutathione[335] reacts with cysteine. The only agent of this class that has undergone clinical trial is cyanate, a chemical that carbamylates the amino-terminal groups of the α and β chains.[336,337] Despite some initial encouraging clinical experience, serious neurotoxicity[338] and cataract stimulation[339] preclude its use. Extracorporeal carbamylation of blood has been successfully attempted[340] and may eventually become practical enough for large-scale clinical efficacy trials.

Increase Flow in Small Vessels or Decrease Sickle Cell Interactions With Endothelial Cells

Any change in vessel tone that would either facilitate the passage of cells with polymer or speed up the passage of cells about to develop polymer would reduce vascular obstruction. Although it is not known whether clinically important vascular beds affected in sickle cell disease are sensitive to vasodilating agents, a report suggests that retinal and conjunctival flow is improved in patients receiving nifedipine.[142] There is no compelling evidence that the vasodilating calcium-channel blockers have a therapeutic role in sickle cell disease; however, these agents have potential and, like cetiedil (discussed previously), may have the added benefit of preventing cell dehydration by inhibiting cation and water loss.

Therapy aimed at reducing endothelial adherence is also theoretically beneficial and might ultimately involve altering endothelial cell or red cell membrane lipids, surface charge, antigens, receptors, plasma proteins, or the redox status of the cell.[340a]

CLINICAL FEATURES

Nomenclature

In this chapter, the term *sickle cell disease* includes all the symptomatic sickle syndromes (eg, SS disease, S-thalassemias, SC disease) and specifically excludes the asymptomatic carrier state—sickle trait. Table 53-2 lists the shorthand notation for the different sickle syndromes.

Diagnosis

Prenatal Screening

Kazazian and colleagues[341] and Rowley[342] reviewed the history of the development of technology for performing prenatal diagnosis and the North American experience to date. In 1987, 85% of prenatal diagnoses were done using amniotic fluid cells, 13% by chorionic villi, and 2% by examining fetal blood. The sickle gene can be easily detected by Southern blotting using a convenient Mst II,[343–345] Cvn I, or Oxan I site that is specifically obliterated in the β^S gene, or by using a specific oligonucleotide probe.[346] The β^C gene is generally detected by linkage analysis, Hpa I linkage disequilibrium, or a specific oligonucleotide probe.[342] β-Thalassemia is diagnosed by linkage analysis or specific probes. The polymerase chain reaction can be used to amplify the β gene, eliminating considerable analysis time and the need for radiolabeled gene probes.[341,347–349] Using chorionic villus sampling and the polymerase chain reaction, prenatal diagnosis can be made as early as 10 weeks of gestation.

Rowley[342] reviewed the use and outcome of prenatal diagnostic services in the United States. In 1987, the number of pregnancies at risk for SS or SC disease was about 6563, but only 272 prenatal diagnoses were done. It remains to be seen whether the low use rate reflects lack of knowledge and availability of services or informed decision making. In Rochester NY, 47% of a group of informed couples at risk for a hemoglobinopathy requested prenatal diagnosis,[350] suggesting that more couples would seek such services if appropriately informed of their risks. The goal for those seeking prenatal diagnosis was not necessarily to terminate an affected pregnancy; 61% of SS and 77% of SC fetuses were carried to term.[350]

TABLE 53-2. Clinical Features of Sickle Cell Syndromes: Typical Findings

		Complete Blood Cell Count			Morphology		Hemoglobin Electrophoresis						
Syndrome	Abbreviation	Hb (g/dL)	MCV (fL)	Reticulocytes (%)	ISCs	Targets	S	A	F	A_2	Other	Percentage With Splenomegaly	Vasoocclusive Severity (Range)
Sickle cell trait	AS ($\alpha\alpha/\alpha\alpha$)	N	80–90	N	0	0	35–40	50–60	<2	<3.5	—	0	0
Sickle trait (+ α-thalassemia silent carrier)	As ($-\alpha/\alpha\alpha$)	13–14	75–85				30–35	55–65					
Sickle trait (+ α-thalassemia trait)	AS ($-\alpha/-\alpha$)	12–13	70–75				25–30	60–75					
Sickle trait (+ Hb H disease)	AS ($--/-\alpha$)	7–10	50–55				17–25	65–80					
Sickle cell anemia	SS ($\alpha\alpha/\alpha\alpha$)	8	95	>10	4+	3+	80–99	0	2–20	2.8	—	80% in children; ~10% in adults	4+(1+ to 4+)
SS (+ α-thalassemia silent carrier)	SS ($-\alpha/\alpha\alpha$)	8.5	85	~10	3+	3+	80–99	0	2–20	3.3			
SS (+ α-thalassemia trait)	SS ($-\alpha/-\alpha$)	9	75	<10	2+	3+	80–90	0	2–20	3.8			
Sickle C disease	SC	11	80	<10	1+	4+	50	0	<2	<3.5	50% C	60%	2+(1+ to 4+)
Sickle β^+-thalassemia	Sβ^+ thal	10	75	<5	2+	4+	75	15	5	>3.5	—	60%	2+(1+ to 4+)
Sickle β^0-thalassemia	Sβ^0 thal	8	70	~10	3+	4+	90	0	5	>3.5	—	60%	4+(1+ to 4+)

MCV, mean corpuscular volume; ISCs, irreversibly sickled cells; N, normal.

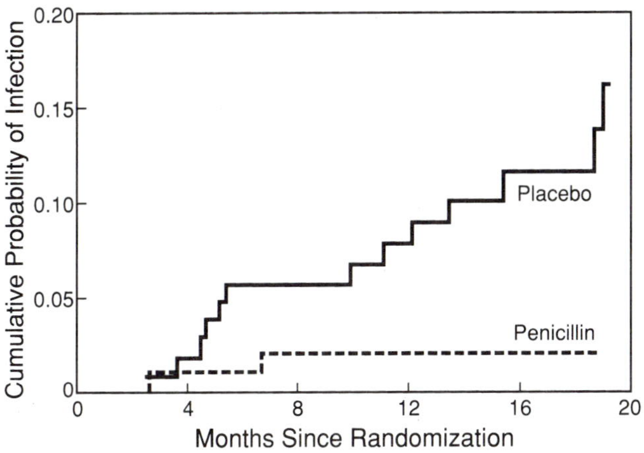

FIGURE 53-21. Effect of prophylactic penicillin on the probability of bacterial sepsis in children with sickle cell anemia under 5 years of age. (After Gaston MH, Verter JI. Prophylaxis with oral penicillin in children with sickle cell anemia: a randomized trial. N Engl J Med 1986;314:1593)

Newborn Screening

The most important therapeutic trial in the sickle cell disease literature is the one by Gaston and coworkers[351] that demonstrated the efficacy of prophylactic penicillin in the prevention of pneumococcal sepsis in young children (Fig. 53-21). This study established that early identification and intervention can have an impact on mortality. As a result, most of the United States has developed procedures to screen newborns for sickle cell disease.[351a] A comprehensive review of the rationale, counseling, follow-up requirements, preliminary data, technical problems, legal issues, ethical issues, and social issues can be found in a recent monograph.[352] Using hemoglobin electrophoresis or chromatography, an experienced laboratory can accurately diagnose sickle cell disease in the newborn. An FA electrophoretic pattern is normal; FAS is sickle trait (or rarely, $S\beta^+$-thalassemia); FS is sickle cell anemia (or rarely, sickle hereditary persistence of fetal hemoglobin, or $S\beta^0$-thalassemia); FSC is SC disease; FAC is C trait; and the presence of Bart's hemoglobin indicates α-thalassemia. The sickle preparation and solubility tests are inaccurate in this age group.[353]

Diagnosing Sickle Syndromes in the Older Child and Adult

Such a wide variation exists in the clinical severity of the sickle syndromes that it is not uncommon to be faced with making a new diagnosis in a relatively asymptomatic adult. This is particularly true for the syndromes that tend to be milder, such as SC disease or $S\beta^+$-thalassemia. As can be seen from Table 53-2, a reliable diagnosis of the major sickle syndromes can be made on the basis of a complete blood count, reticulocyte count, peripheral smear, sickle solubility test, and hemoglobin electrophoresis. For prenatal counseling or research situations, a more specific genetic diagnosis can be assigned at the DNA level, determining α-gene number and β-globin haplotype.

Anemia of Sickle Cell Disease

Chronic Anemia

After the first few months of life, the level of fetal hemoglobin declines (Fig. 53-22), the production of hemoglobin S dominates, and the typical chronic hemolytic pattern of SS disease develops[354,354a] (Fig. 53-23). As seen in Figure 53-15, in SS disease, the peripheral blood has some normal-looking red cells as well as targets, Howell-Jolly bodies, nucleated red cells, fragments, spherocytes, and irreversibly sickled cells. This is a hemolytic anemia with a red cell survival of 10 to 30 days (normal, 120 days) and a rate of heme catabolism (endogenous carbon monoxide production) that is six times normal.[355] The degree of hemolysis is relatively constant for a given patient[356] and is unchanged during uncomplicated vasoocclusive events. The degree of anemia inversely correlates with irreversibly sickled cell count,[357,358] reticulocyte count, and mean corpuscular volume (MCV).[359]

Theoretically, the expanded bone marrow (Fig. 53-24) should be able to compensate for the hemolytic rate of this disease and produce a normal hematocrit. There are several possible explanations for the apparent lack of complete compensation: (1) the amount of erythropoietin is lower than seen in other comparable anemias,[360] possibly because of an altered renal response or to the right-shifted O_2 dissociation curve; (2) the plasma volume is expanded to a greater extent than in other anemias,[357] making the hematocrit appear lower than it really is; and (3) there may be some degree of ineffective erythropoiesis since polymerization and phagocytosis can occur in and to red cell precursors in the marrow[361,362] (Fig. 53-25).

Anemia is probably more of a help than a hindrance in this disease because the increased blood viscosity that accompanies a higher hematocrit may augment sludging and vasoocclusion. This probably explains why patients with SS disease and coexisting α-thalassemia—who have less dense cells, intracellular polymer, and hemolysis—typically have considerable symptoms, with acute pain episodes and avascular necrosis of bones. It also explains why patients with higher hematocrits have a tendency toward more pain crises and episodes of acute chest syndrome. This apparent paradox suggests that phlebotomy might be useful in the treatment of some patients.

Exacerbations of Steady-State Anemia

Iron Deficiency. Florid iron deficiency causing worsening anemia is relatively rare in SS disease, although mild deficiency certainly occurs,[363–366] and the resultant microcytosis can contribute to misdiagnosing $S\beta^0$-thalassemia.[367]

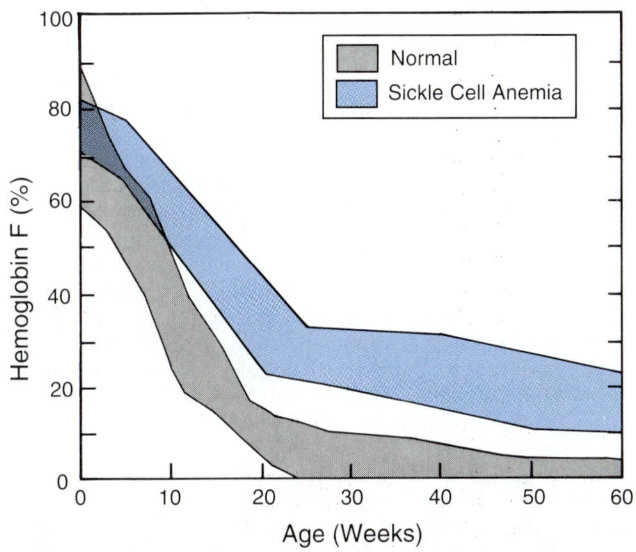

FIGURE 53-22. Age-related changes in fetal hemoglobin in children with sickle cell anemia. (After Platt OS, et al. In: Nathan DG, Oski FA, eds. Hematology of infancy and childhood. WB Saunders, 1993)

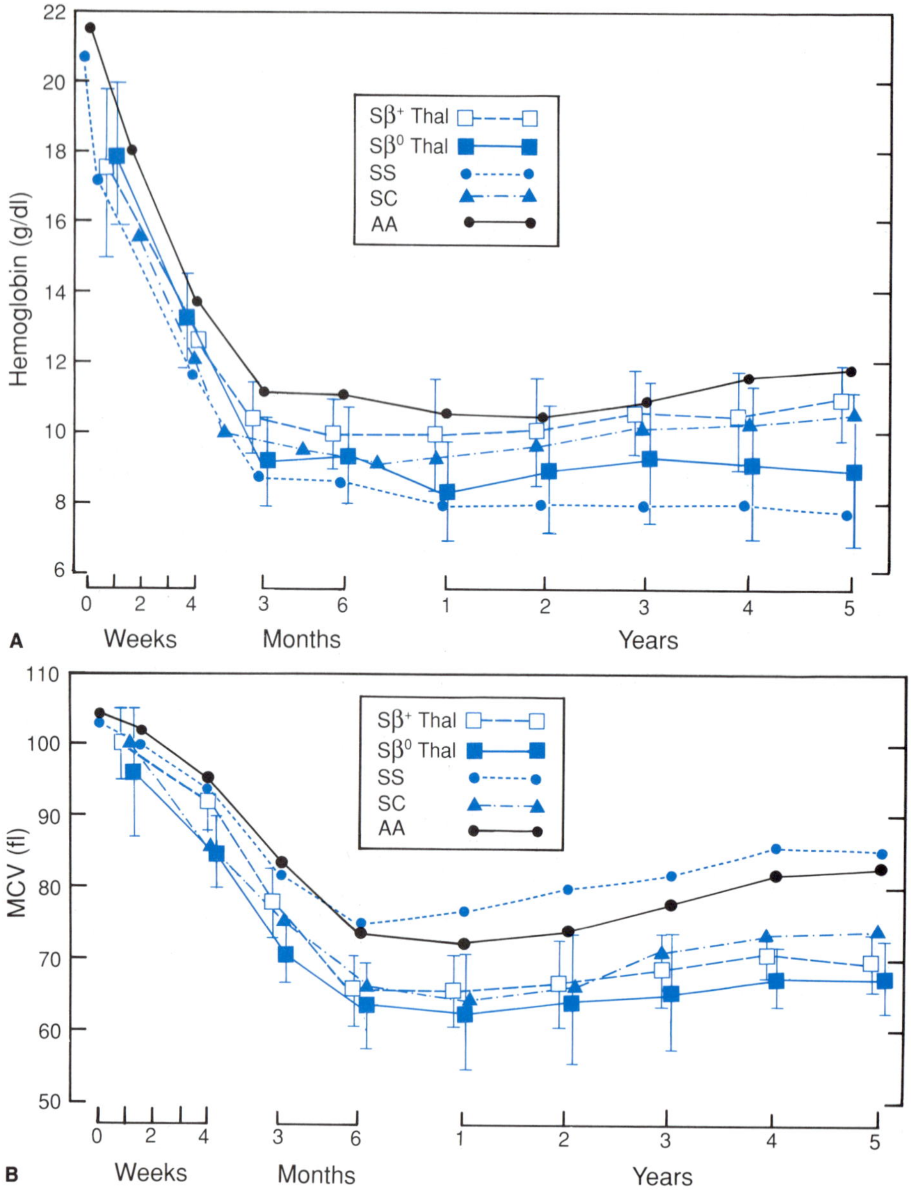

FIGURE 53-23. Early childhood changes in hemoglobin **(A)** and mean corpuscular volume **(B)** in patients with the sickle syndromes (sickle cell anemia, $S\beta^+$-thalassemia, $S\beta^0$-thalassemia, and hemoglobin SC disease). (After Serjeant GR, Ashcroft MT, et al. The clinical features of sickle cell beta thalassemia in Jamaica. Br J Haematol 1973;24:19; and Serjeant GR, Ashcroft MT, et al. The clinical features of haemoglobin SC disease in Jamaica. Br J Haematol 1973;24:491)

Because of the decreased hemoglobin concentration, iron deficiency may result in less hemolysis and fewer painful episodes,[368–370] but withholding iron is not recommended as treatment.

Folic Acid Deficiency. As in all patients with chronic hemolysis, patients with SS disease have increased folic acid requirements. Patients with poor dietary intake of folate may develop a superimposed megaloblastic anemia, particularly if not supplemented during pregnancy or a period of rapid growth. Mild chemical folate deficiency without megaloblastosis is relatively common.[371] It has become general clinical practice to provide prophylactic folate supplementation (1 mg/d), although a controlled trial of placebo versus folate showed a difference of only 4 fL in MCV and no difference in hematocrit or growth in children.[372,373]

Renal Failure. When patients with SS disease develop renal failure, erythropoietin levels fall, and anemia worsens.[374] Many of these patients develop chronic congestive heart failure, become transfusion-dependent, and, like other patients with renal failure, may benefit from high-does exogenous erythropoietin.[374a]

Acute Splenic Sequestration. One of the leading causes of death in children with SS disease is the acute splenic sequestration crisis,[375–380] a complication that has been seen as early as 8 weeks of age.[381] These young children frequently present in hypovolumic shock, having trapped a considerable portion of intravascular volume in a rapidly enlarging spleen. There is often history of dyspnea, left-sided abdominal pain, vomiting, and abdominal distention blossoming over a period of hours. The hemoglobin is at least 2 g/dL lower than usual, with increased reticulocytes, erythroblastosis, and mild to moderate thrombocytopenia. For those who survive the initial episode, about half have a recurrence,[375–377] usually within 6 months.[376,377] In the Jamaican series,[377] the mortality from recurrences reached 14%, although such devastating outcomes are not found in contemporary American series.[382] As used here, the phrase *acute splenic sequestration* refers to a rapidly evolving dramatic event, typically with the spleen palpable below the umbilicus, a hematocrit 40% to 70% of baseline, and fewer than 150,000 platelets. Some patients, who between routine visits may superficially appear to be having acute sequestration and whose hematocrits are falling and

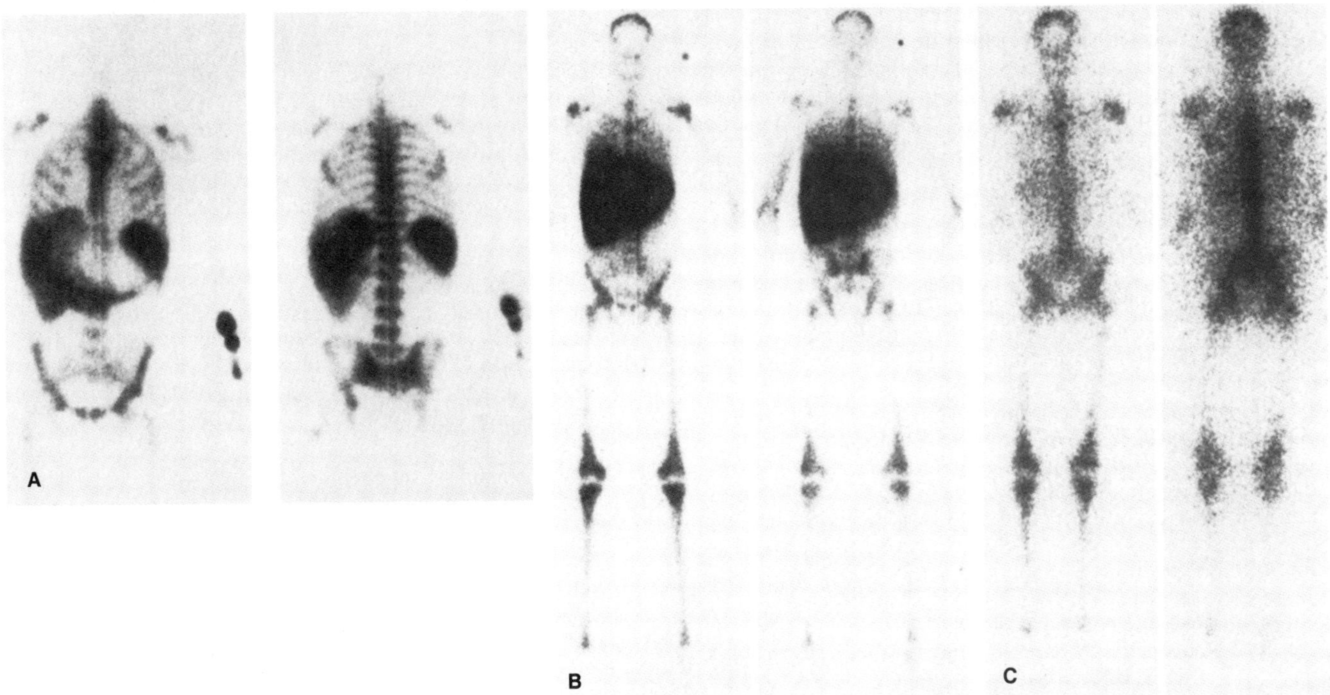

FIGURE 53-24. Bone marrow and reticuloendothelial scans in sickle cell anemia. Three pairs of scans are shown. In each pair the scan on the left is an anterior view and the one on the right is a posterior view. (**A**) Reticuloendothelial (^{99m}Tc-sulfur colloid) scan in a normal adult. Positive areas include the liver, spleen and bone marrow, which is confined to the trunk and pelvis in adults. Reticuloendothelial (RE) scan (**B**) and bone marrow (^{52}Fe) scan (**C**) in an adult with sickle cell disease. The expansion of the bone marrow to the skull and extremities is evident in both scans. The RE scan also shows enlargement of the liver and absence of the spleen. (Fordham EW, Ali A. Radionuclide imaging of bone marrow. Semin Hematol 1981;18:222)

spleens enlarging, are in fact going through the typical hematologic changes of infancy (see Fig. 53-23). Some patients develop mild hypersplenism in association with viral illness, with a larger than usual spleen, and a 20% to 25% drop in hematocrit. At initial presentation, these patients may resemble an early sequestration and should be examined frequently to assess the tempo of the process. It is not known whether these children with a tendency for transient hypersplenism are at high risk for developing fulminant sequestration, but they should be seen frequently and their parents alerted to the possibility.

The acute management of sequestration is straightforward and noncontroversial: immediately restore intravascular volume and oxygen-carrying capacity by transfusion of packed red cells. Once a normal cardiovascular status is restored, the patient usually improves rapidly, and the spleen size and platelet count normalize over days. There is no role for *emergency* splenectomy.

The chronic management is less straightforward and more controversial. The obvious approach to preventing recurrence of splenic sequestration is to remove the spleen. There is understandable reluctance, however, to remove what may be a functional spleen in a very young child, and some have suggested that a maintenance transfusion program be instituted to prevent recurrence.[383] A review of 23 cases of splenic sequestration from Duke University illustrates the problems of transfusion as prevention.[382] In this series, 4 patients underwent prompt splenectomy, 7 were observed carefully without transfusion, and 12 received transfusions (6 to 12 months) and were maintained with a hemoglobin S less than 30%. Of the 7 observed patients, 4 experienced recurrences 3 to 11 months after the initial episode. Of the 12 patients who received transfusions, 2 are still receiving transfusions and are well. Of the remaining 10, 3 experienced recurrences while on transfusion (3 to 9 months after the initial episode), and 4 had recurrences within 3 months of the last transfusion. Only 3 of the patients remain well 11 months to 3.9 years off transfusion therapy. In this series, 14% of children developed red cell antibodies, and one child developed non-A, non-B hepatitis. Eventually, 14 of the 23 patients came to splenectomy. All were immunized against pneumococcus

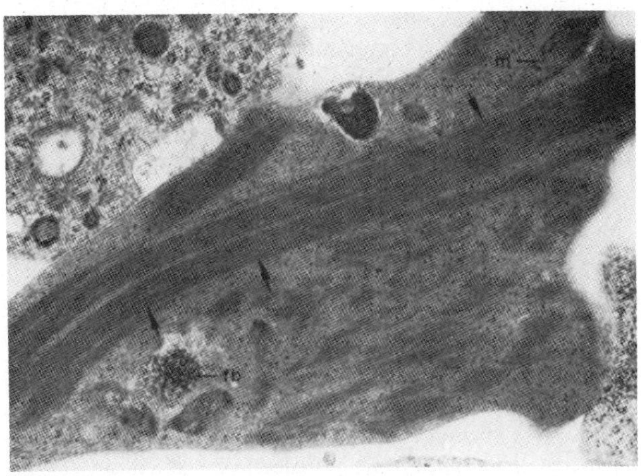

FIGURE 53-25. Sickle hemoglobin polymer (*arrows*) in a bone marrow reticulocyte. (Grasso JA, Sullivan AL, Sullivan LW. Ultrastructural studies of the bone marrow in sickle cell anemia. I. The structure of sickled erythrocytes and reticulocytes and their phagocytic destruction. Br J Haematol 1975;31:135)

and were prescribed prophylactic penicillin. None has experienced a life-threatening infection in a total follow-up period of 65.6 patient-years. Several important lessons can be learned from this series: (1) sequestration can occur while on a transfusion program; (2) sequestration can recur soon after stopping a transfusion program; (3) transfusions are not without risk; (4) immunized and prophylactically treated children can tolerate splenectomy; and (5) sequestration need not be a fatal complication if families are alerted to early signs. Routine care of children should include teaching parents to palpate the child's spleen and to be alert to a rapid inclrease in size. This is a small, uncontrolled, and retrospective study, yet it lends support to those who advocate splenectomy after the first major episode of sequestration.[384]

Splenic sequestration is primarily a disease of young children with SS disease. Occasionally, it occurs in older patients with SC disease and Sβ-thalassemia.[385–387] In adults with these syndromes, acute splenic sequestration is almost never a life-threatening complication and behaves more like a transient episode of hypersplenism, often in the setting of an acute viral illness. One patient with SC disease and hereditary spherocytosis was described who experienced five episodes of sequestration.[388]

Acute Liver Sequestration. Sequestration may also take place in the liver, but because the liver is not as distensible as the spleen, there is rarely associated cardiovascular collapse. These patients experience worsening anemia, an enlarged tender liver, right upper quadrant pain, extreme hyperbilirubinemia (unconjugated bilirubin over 50 mg/dL), elevated transaminases, and increased reticulocytosis.[389] These patients usually recover spontaneously within a week but may be indistinguishable at presentation from those rare patients who go on to die of fulminant hepatic failure.[390,391]

Aplastic Episode. Patients with SS disease are vulnerable to the same life-threatening parvovirus-induced transient cessation of erythropoiesis as are patients with other chronic hemolytic anemias[392] (see Chap. 10). In Jamaica, about 40% of SS and AA children developed parvovirus-specific IgG by age 15 years, although about 20% of these children did not develop aplasia.[392a] Typical patients with aplastic anemia present with various combinations of increased fatigue, headache, gastrointestinal symptoms, pallor, thrombocytopenia, and arthralgia but not the typical rash of fifth disease.[393,394] The short-lived hemoglobin F–poor cells disappear first from the circulation, causing an apparent increase in the percentage of hemoglobin F during these episodes.[395] The hematocrit falls 10% to 15% per day without compensatory reticulocytosis.[396] The virus is *highly* transmissible to medical personnel as well as other close contacts. If one patient in a household becomes aplastic, others are almost certain to follow within a few days.[397] Spontaneous recovery is usually preceded by a sharp increase in peripheral nucleated red cells, then a brisk reticulocytosis, an increase in serum transferrin receptor,[397a] and often hyperbilirubinemia. This recovery phase is probably responsible for many of the cases referred to as *hyperhemolytic episodes*. Spontaneous recovery may not occur before cardiovascular compromise occurs. In the Jamaican experience, 87% of patients required transfusion to tide them over until marrow activity resumed.[393] Recurrence is generally not seen.

Glucose-6-Phosphate Dehydrogenase Deficiency. Glucose-6-phosphate dehydrogenase (G6PD) deficiency (see Chap. 58) is a common genetic variant among people of African heritage. An unexpectedly high prevalence of G6PD deficiency among patients with SS disease originally suggested that the enzyme deficiency confers a protective effect.[398,399] More recent studies suggest that there is no increased prevalence.[400,401] In a study of 801 males with SS disease from the Cooperative Study of Sickle Cell Disease (CSSCD), 4% were G6PD deficient[402] and demonstrated no difference in degree of anemia, MCV, reticulocyte count, bilirubin, serum glutamic-oxaloacetic transaminase, or incidence of painful or acute anemic episodes. Because the sickle red cell is young and the A^- variant of G6PD deficiency typically maintains normal activity in young cells (see Chap. 58), hemolysates from enzyme-deficient SS red cells have normal activity, whereas those from enzyme-sufficient SS red cells have elevated activity.[401] Episodes of accelerated hemolysis in patients with both SS disease and G6PD deficiency have been described.[403] It appears that such accelerated "hyperhemolysis" would be more likely when the average age of the circulating cells is higher, as it is during an aplastic episode.

Growth and Development

Infants with SS disease have normal birthweight[404] but may exhibit growth delay and delayed bone age during childhood.[405–410] In the CSSCD, the 2115 patients studied had normal height and weight until 7 years of age.[411] At this age, growth was delayed compared with normal African American controls (Fig. 53-26). Weight was more affected than height. Patients with SS disease or $S\beta^0$-thalassemia were more delayed than patients with SC disease or $S\beta^+$-thalassemia. In general, by late adolescence, patients caught up with the normal population and attained normal adult height, although weight continued to be low.

Sexual development is also delayed in sickle cell disease[411,412] (Table 53-3). The pattern of sexual delay is similar to that found for growth delay—SS disease and $S\beta^0$-thalassemia patients are more delayed than the SC disease and $S\beta^+$-thalassemia patients. Although there is a delay in sexual maturity, both males and females eventually mature, suggesting that there is no permanent underlying endocrinopathy. This was supported by the careful study of female fertility in Jamaica, which revealed no difference in the interval between sexual exposure and pregnancy between patients and normal controls.[413] Normal thyroid function[412] and hypothalamic–pituitary axis[412,414] have been shown, although some men are infertile and have decreased sperm motility and number.[415] Primary hypogonadism[416,417] and hypothalamic hypogonadism responsive to clomiphene[418] have also been described.

The cause of delayed growth and development among patients with sickle cell disease is not known. The fact that growth is more delayed in SS disease and $S\beta^0$-thalassemia than in SC disease and $S\beta^+$-thalassemia suggests that the degree of anemia or clinical severity may be relevant. Analyses from the CSSCD showed that growth and maturation delays are inversely correlated with hematocrit[419] and do not correlate with the incidence of painful episodes (Espeland M, unpublished data).

Perhaps the hematopoietic and cardiovascular compensation for anemia causes the increased metabolic needs[420] that impair growth if unmet. This is supported by the finding that supplemental nasogastric feeding improves the growth of children with SS disease.[421] In one series, zinc deficiency was also a factor in growth retardation.[422]

Susceptibility to Infection

Despite the fact that sickle cell disease is a disorder of hemoglobin, the single most common cause of death is not polymerization but infection.[423–425] As seen in Table 53-4, the organisms encountered are generally not unusual pathogens, but the infections they cause are more frequent and severe. Characteristically the infections of children are fulminant, without focus, often fatal, and typically

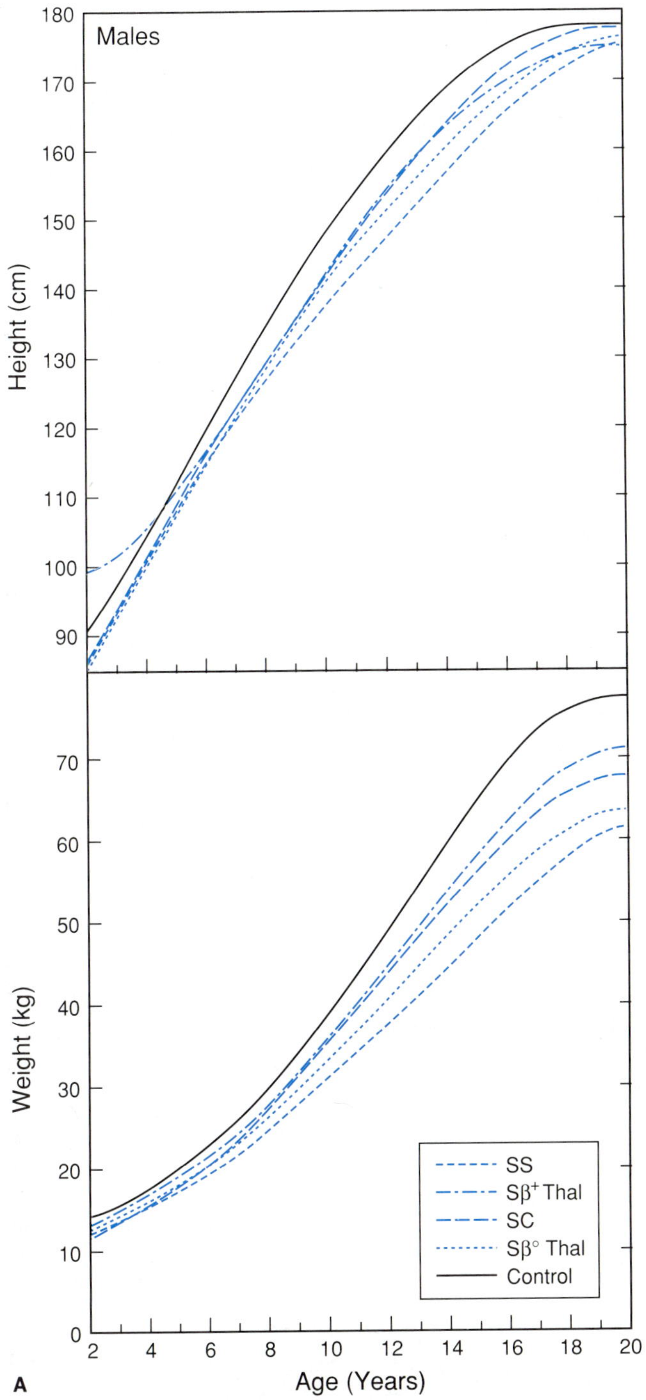

FIGURE 53-26. Height and weight growth curves for patients with sickle cell syndromes. (After Platt OS, Rosenstock W, et al. Influence of sickle hemoglobinopathies on growth and development. N Engl J Med 1984;311:7)

caused by the encapsulated *Streptococcus pneumoniae* and *Haemophilus influenzae*. In adults, death from sepsis is less common, urinary tract and bone foci are more frequent, and *Escherichia coli*, *Salmonella* sp, and *Staphylococcus aureus* are prominent pathogens[426] (Fig. 53-27).

Functional Asplenia and Bacterial Sepsis

The function of the spleen is invariably destroyed in sickle cell disease (see Chap. 46). During the first year of life, most patients with SS disease lose the spleen's ability to clear particulate matter from the blood, referred to as *functional asplenia*.[427,428] This dysfunction is heralded by the appearance of Howell-Jolly bodies and irregular "pocking" of the red cell surface (which can only be seen using a microscope equipped with interference or Nomarski optics).[429] Despite their palpable splenomegaly, these children have no uptake of technetium-99m sulfur colloid (see Fig. 53-24) and are susceptible to the most virulent complication of asplenia: *S pneumoniae* sepsis.[430] Transfusion may temporarily restore splenic function in children under 7 years of age.[431] Bone marrow transplantation may also restore splenic function.[431a]

The timing of the development and the ultimate prevalence of splenic dysfunction varies by genotype[432] (Fig. 53-28). Patients with $S\beta^0$-thalassemia have a spleen pattern

TABLE 53-3. Estimated Median Age at Attainment of Tanner Stages, According to Hemoglobinopathy

	Tanner Stage	Median Age (y) SS	SC	$S\beta^+$	$S\beta^0$
Females					
Breasts	2	11.8	9.8	10.6	11.8
	3	13.5	11.9	12.6	12.8
	4	15.0	13.9	13.8	14.8
	5	17.3	16.0	16.5	17.2
Pubic hair	2	12.0	10.1	10.0	11.5
	3	13.5	11.8	11.2	12.8
	4	15.2	14.0	13.8	14.2
	5	19.2	17.0	17.0	20.8
Males					
Penis	2	12.0	10.4	11.9	12.4
	3	14.2	13.0	13.0	13.2
	4	16.0	14.1	13.5	15.5
	5	17.6	16.6	16.6	18.8
Pubic hair	2	13.2	11.5	12.0	13.2
	3	14.8	13.2	13.0	13.9
	4	16.2	14.2	13.9	16.2
	5	17.9	16.6	17.1	18.5

Platt OS, Rosenstock W, et al. Influence of sickle hemoglobinopathies on growth and development. N Engl J Med 1984;311:7.

virtually identical to that of SS disease; $S\beta^+$-thalassemia has little dysfunction; and SC disease is intermediate. In one series, the risk of a child with SS disease under 5 years of age acquiring S *pneumoniae* sepsis or meningitis was over 15%; the associated mortality was about 30%.[433] It appears that children with SC disease may be at somewhat less risk of bacterial sepsis overall.[434–436] The CSSCD experience showed that the children with SC disease who were younger than 2 years of age had a rate of sepsis indistinguishable from the SS disease group[426] but had a lower mortality rate.

Clinically, the most worrisome organism is S *pneumoniae*. There may be as high as a 400-fold increase in the incidence of S *pneumoniae* sepsis in children with SS disease who are younger than 5 years of age.[437] The course is fulminant and often fatal. In contrast, H *influenzae* sepsis is only two to four times more common in SS disease than in the general population and typically follows a several-day prodrome with low-grade fever, symptoms of upper respiratory tract infection, or otitis media.[437]

Prophylactic Penicillin. Prophylactic penicillin prevents 80% of S *pneumoniae* sepsis in children with SS disease who are less than 3 years of age[438] (see Fig. 53-21). The impact of prophylaxis is tremendous, and newborn screening programs are in place in most of the United States, so that infants with sickle cell disease can be identified early and begun on penicillin. Recommendations for prophylaxis are set forth in the recent National Institutes of Health (NIH) guidelines for management and therapy of sickle cell disease.[439] Our approach is as follows:

1. Give prophylaxis to all children with sickle cell disease (SS, SC, $S\beta$-thalassemia).
2. Start as early as possible, optimally by 3 months of age.
3. Prescribe penicillin, 125 mg orally twice daily, until 3 years of age, then increase to 250 mg orally twice daily until at least 6 years of age (studies are underway to determine the optimal length of prophylaxis).

TABLE 53-4. Infections in Sickle Cell Disease

Infection	Cause	Episodes	Percentage
Pneumonia[501]	No diagnosis	66	65
	Streptococcus pneumoniae	4	4
	Haemophilus influenzae	4	4
	Mycoplasma	16	16
	Virus (confirmed)	8	8
	Other bacterial	4	4
Sepsis[422,425]*	*S pneumoniae*	12	40
	H influenzae	3	11
	Gram-negative enterics	3	11
	Salmonella	3	11
	Anaerobic bacteria	2	8
	Staphylococcus pyogenes	1	4
Meningitis	*S pneumoniae*	35	57
	Partially treated	13	21
	H influenzae	5	8
	Aseptic	4	6
	Others (*Escherichia coli, Staphylococcus aureus, Streptococcus, Neisseria meningiditis*)	4	6
Osteomyelitis[422,425,433]†	*Salmonella*	14	70
	S aureus	3	15
	S pneumonia	3	15
Urinary tract[422,425]*	*E coli*	35	63
	Klebsiella	15	27
	Proteus	2	4
	Others (*S aureus, Herellea vaginicola*, paracoli)	4	8

* Represents 4133 patient-years of observation.
† Represents 7575 patient-years of observation.

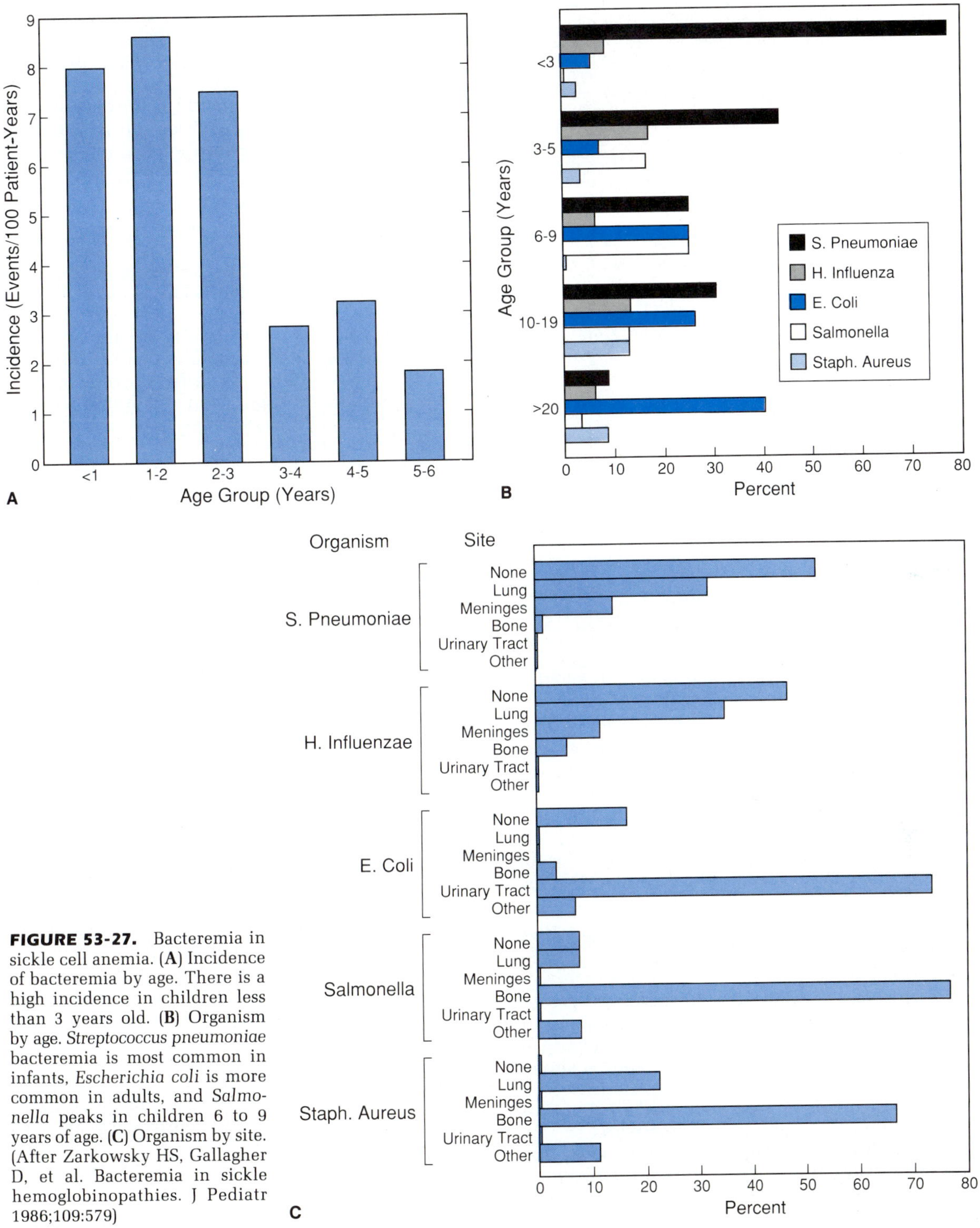

FIGURE 53-27. Bacteremia in sickle cell anemia. (**A**) Incidence of bacteremia by age. There is a high incidence in children less than 3 years old. (**B**) Organism by age. *Streptococcus pneumoniae* bacteremia is most common in infants, *Escherichia coli* is more common in adults, and *Salmonella* peaks in children 6 to 9 years of age. (**C**) Organism by site. (After Zarkowsky HS, Gallagher D, et al. Bacteremia in sickle hemoglobinopathies. J Pediatr 1986;109:579)

4. Prescribe erythromycin for penicillin-allergic children.
5. Do *not* use ampicillin prophylactically—efficacy is unproved, side effects are common, and resistant organisms are likely to emerge.
6. Develop an educational program to encourage compliance and recognition of early signs of infection.

This program does not, and is not intended to, eradicate nasopharyngeal carriage of *S pneumoniae*.[440] The goal is to prevent mortality from bacteremia. The appearance of this organism in the pharynx of a patient does not necessarily indicate poor compliance with penicillin.

Immunization Recommendations. Pneumococcal vaccine has been shown to be efficacious in eliciting a normal antibody response and reducing the incidence of infections with *S pneumoniae* in children older than 2 years of age.[441–444] All children with sickle cell disease should be immunized according to American Academy of Pediatrics recommendations and should receive pneumococcal vaccine in addition (see Chap. 46). Older children and adults may benefit from influenza virus vaccine, and some centers suggest recombinant human hepatitis B vaccine for HBsAb-negative patients.

Empiric Therapy for the Febrile Child

For the child with sickle cell disease, fever may be the only indication of a potentially fatal infection. As a rule, the

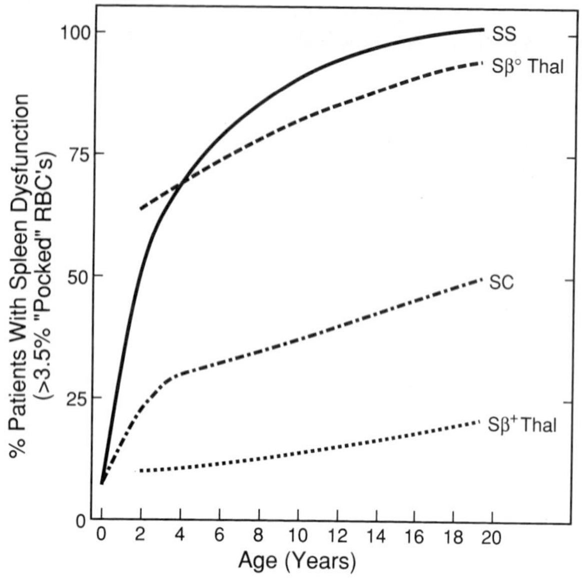

FIGURE 53-28. Splenic function (as measured by peripheral blood "pocked" erythrocytes) by age in the various sickle syndromes. (After Pearson HA, Gallagher D, et al. Developmental pattern of splenic dysfunction in sickle cell disorders. Pediatrics 1985;76:392)

higher the temperature[445] and the higher the erythrocyte sedimentation rate, leukocyte count, and band count,[446] the more likely there is to be a serious bacterial infection. Unfortunately, however, there is no absolutely safe set of numbers that clearly separate febrile children into bacteremic or nonbacteremic groups. This issue is further complicated by the fact that the baseline leukocyte count is typically elevated (presumably because of asplenia) and the sedimentation rate may be lower (because of the anemia and poikilocytosis that disfavor rouleaux formation). The following are guidelines for empiric therapy of febrile children younger than 12years of age who do not have an obvious source[439]:

1. Basic laboratory investigation includes complete blood count, urine analysis, chest radiograph, and cultures of the blood, urine, and throat.
2. Toxic children, or those with temperatures greater than 39.9°C, should be treated with parenteral antibiotics promptly, before radiographs are taken or laboratory results are available. These children should be admitted to the hospital.
3. Lumbar puncture should be performed on toxic children and those with any signs of meningitis.
4. Nontoxic children with temperatures lower than 39.9°C, but with an infiltrate on chest radiograph or with a white blood cell count over 30,000/μL or below 5000/μL should be treated parenterally and admitted to the hospital.
5. Nontoxic children with temperatures lower than 39.9°C, normal chest radiograph, normal leukocyte count, and reliable parents can be treated with a long-acting antibiotic (such as ceftriaxone, 50 mg/kg intravenously) observed over a period of hours, and discharged home for follow-up evaluation and repeated antibiotic dosing the next day.
6. Antibiotics should be selected based on their ability to kill S *pneumoniae* and H *influenzae* and to enter the central nervous system. In areas where β-lactamase–producing H *influenzae* are regularly encountered, β-lactamase–resistant antibiotics should be used.
7. If children do well, and cultures remain negative after 72 hours, antibiotics can be discontinued.
8. Documented sepsis should be treated parenterally for a minimum of 7 days.
9. Bacterial meningitis should be treated for a minimum of 10 days parenterally or for at least 7 days after cerebrospinal fluid sterilization.

Organ System Involvement

Musculoskeletal

Acute Painful Episodes. Acute episodes of bone pain (or *pain crises*—a term that is falling out of favor since it has negative connotations for patients) are such a prominent clinical feature that African tribal names for sickle cell disease are onomatopoetic repetitive descriptions of pain: "chwechweechwa" (Ga tribe), "nwiinii" (Fante tribe), "nucdudui" (Ewe tribe), and "ahotutuo" (Twi tribe). Roughly translated these names mean "beaten up," "body biting," and "body chewing."[447,448] The variation in incidence by age is shown in Figure 53-29.

The patient experiences a deep, gnawing, throbbing pain, usually with little in the way of physical findings. The underlying event appears to be ischemia or infarction of the marrow.[449] In one study, marrow was aspirated serially from a patient with acute sternal pain. The aspirates revealed a pattern that evolved from frank necrosis to purulent neutrophil infiltration and, over a period of weeks, to restored normal marrow.[450] In an informative series by Mankad and colleagues,[451] patients were followed using serial magnetic resonance imaging (MRI) of the long bones. A representative set of studies is shown in Figure 53-30, illustrating the typical mottled appearance of the marrow-infiltrated long bones and how this pattern changes when the patient experiences pain. In one of these patients with acute pain who died, autopsy examination revealed liquefactive necrosis of bone that correlated with local MRI findings of increased T_1 and T_2 signals (Fig. 53-31). The more necrosis present, the more the patient is likely to have local swelling, tenderness, and heat.

It is difficult to distinguish these infarctive changes from bone infection since both processes produce similar physical findings and similar fever, leukocytosis, and acute-phase responses. Even with systemic and local signs, the diagnosis of infarction is statistically more likely. The results of one study suggest that acute long bone infarction is at least 50 times more common than osteomyelitis.[452] Forty-one acute long bone infarcts were examined (38% humerus, 23% tibia, and 19% femur). All patients had local tenderness, with swelling in 85%, joint findings in 68%, and localized warmth in 65%. Fourteen percent of patients

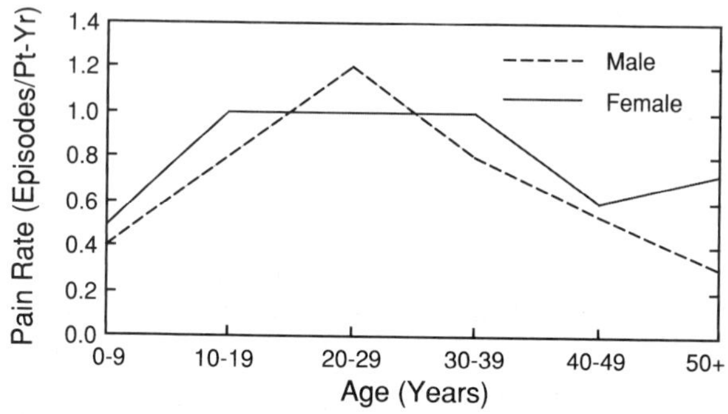

FIGURE 53-29. Pain rate (episodes requiring medical attention per patient-year) by age among patients with sickle cell anemia. (After Platt OS, Thorington BD, et al. Pain in sickle cell disease: rates and risk factors. N Engl J Med 1991;325:11)

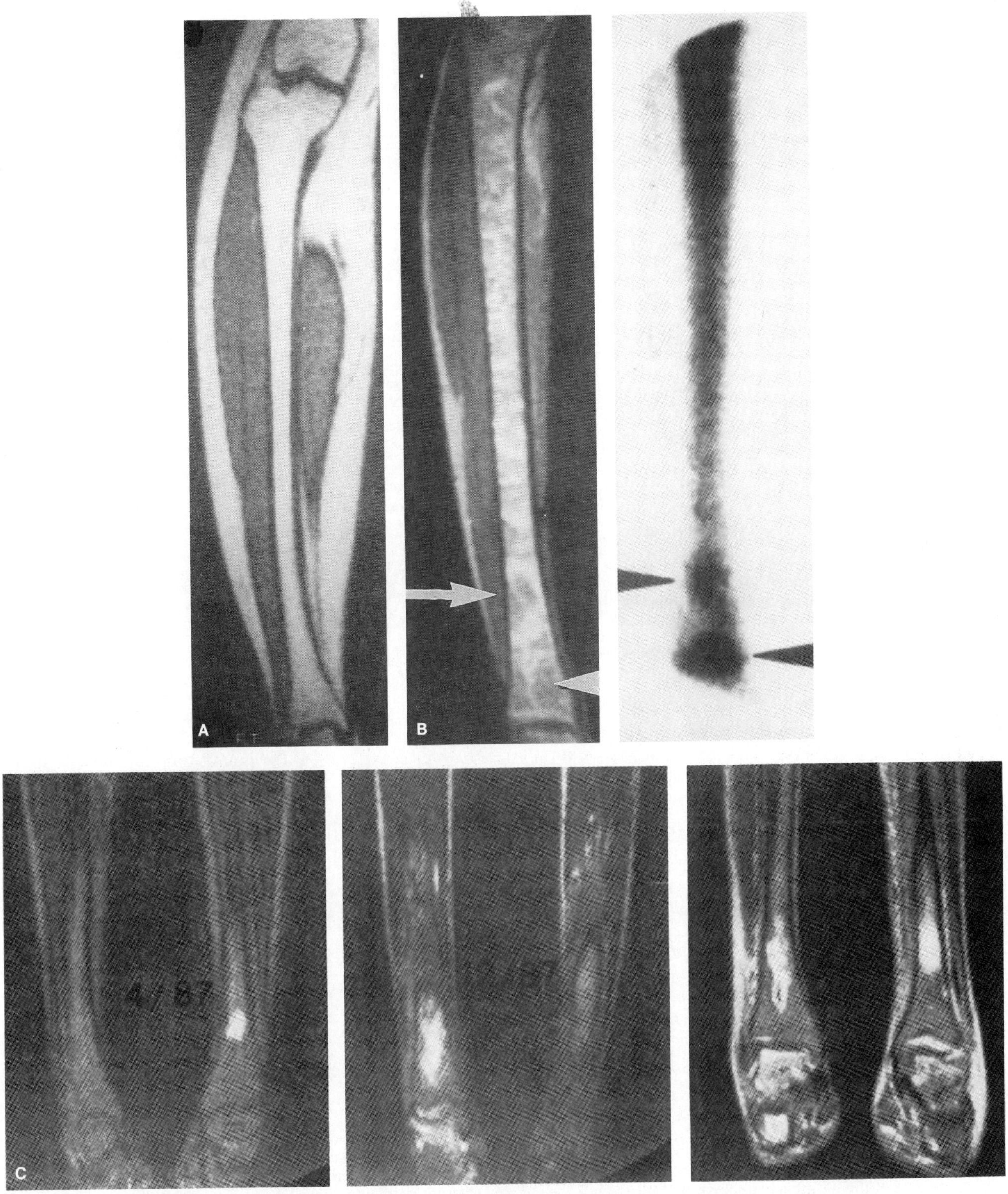

FIGURE 53-30. Magnetic resonance image (MRI) of bones in sickle cell disease. (**A**) MRI of a normal tibia. (**B**) MRI of a tibia (*left*) and the corresponding bone marrow reticuloendothelial (^{99m}Tc-sulfur colloid) scan (*right*) of an *asymptomatic* sickle cell anemia patient. Note the mottled appearance of the bone in the sickle MRI. This is due to areas of bone marrow hyperplasia, which are particularly evident in the two nodules indicated by the arrows. (**C**) Serial studies of an 8-year-old SS patient experiencing pain. In each pair of images, the right leg is on the left and vice versa. (*Left*) In April 1987, a bright lesion can be seen in the asymptomatic left leg at the site of a prior painful episode. (*Middle*) By December 1987, there is resolution of the previous left-sided lesion and the appearance of a new right-sided lesion at the site of a painful vaso-occlusive crisis in the right ankle. (*Right*) In April 1988, a new lesion appeared on the left with another episode of pain. (Mankad VN, Williams JP, Harpen MD, et al. Magnetic resonance imaging of bone marrow in sickle cell disease: clinical, hematological, and pathological correlations. Blood 1990;75:274)

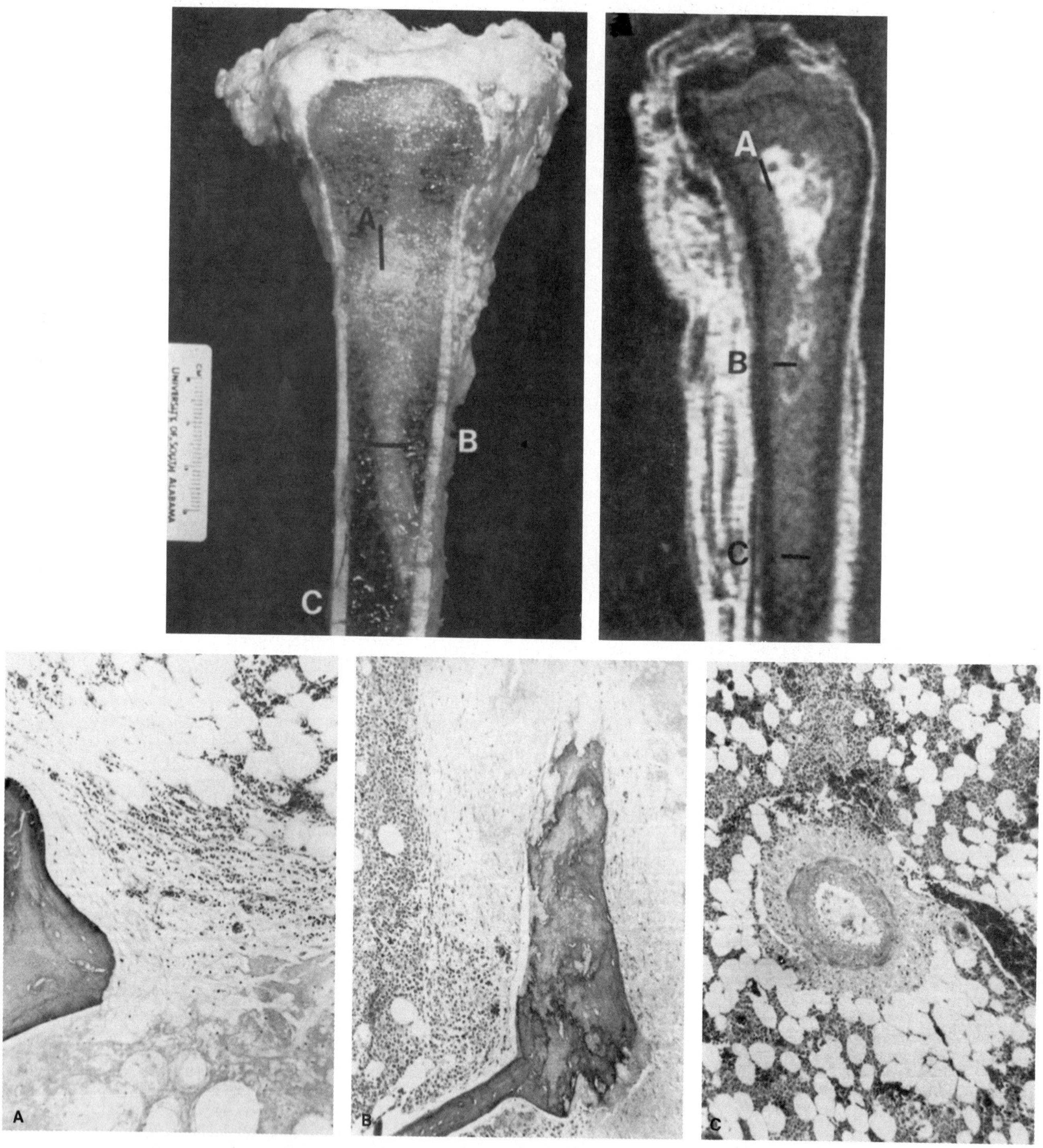

FIGURE 53-31. Pathology of bone pain in a patient with sickle cell anemia. The patient died of pneumococcal pneumonia during a painful episode. Microscopic sections from the corresponding lettered areas in the gross pathology specimen (*top left*) and the magnetic resonance image (*top right*) of the left tibia are shown in **A** through **C** (*below*). (**A**) Current pain site shows liquefactive necrosis and acute inflammatory infiltrate. (**B**) Previous pain site reveals dense fibrosis and regenerative changes. (**C**) Another previous pain site shows hyperplastic erythroid marrow and perivascular fibrosis. (Mankad VN, Williams JP, Harpen MD, et al. Magnetic resonance imaging of bone marrow in sickle cell disease: clinical, hematological, and pathological correlations. Blood 1990;75:274)

appeared toxic; and 21% had a temperature above 39°C. The total leukocyte count varied between 7200 and 43,000/μL (mean, 17,000/μL); absolute band counts ranged from 0 to 2940/μL (mean, 442/μL). Although *most* of the patients did *not* have impressive systemic signs of inflammation, some clearly had classic findings of osteomyelitis. Various radionuclide scans have been reported to be helpful in making the distinction between infarction and infection[453–456]; in this study, however, they did not eliminate osteomyelitis as a possibility.

Most often, patients with acute painful episodes have no local physical findings and only a modest elevation in temperature, heart rate, blood pressure, and leukocyte count. Numerous laboratory changes are observed in patients experiencing painful episodes, including decreased platelets,[457,458] abnormal platelet function,[459–461] normal platelet function,[462,463] evidence of increased fibrinogen turnover,[464–468] elevated myoglobin,[469] elevated α-hydroxybutyrate,[469,470] and a decreased proportion of dense red cells.[471] These findings are interesting from a pathophysiologic point of view, but none is a sufficiently definitive marker of vasoocclusion to warrant its use to identify malingerers. Infections,[447] changes in climate,[472–474] and psychological factors have been suggested as possible precipitating events, although in most cases, no such factors can be identified.

The most frequently involved areas are the knee, lumbosacral spine, elbow, and femur. Less often, the ribs, sternum, clavicles, calcaneus, iliac crest, zygoma, mandible, and maxilla are affected.[447] Involvement of facial bones may result in impressive *facial swelling*,[357] and *rib infection* is commonly associated with the acute chest syndrome.[474a] When the knees or elbows are involved, *joint effusions* (usually noninflammatory) are common. They should be tapped only if the clinical course is strongly suggestive of infection. Sterile purulent effusions can be encountered,[475] so the diagnosis of infection necessarily relies on culture results.

In children younger than 5 years of age, the small bones of the hands and feet may become involved in *dactylitis*, the so-called hand–foot syndrome.[476,477] This is often the first clinical manifestation of the disease.[478] The distressed youngster cries with pain, refuses to use the extremity, and has hot, tender, swollen hands or feet. As in other patients experiencing acute bone involvement, the child may be febrile and have a leukocyte count as high as 60,000/μL. At the onset of soft tissue swelling, usually no bony changes are seen on radiograph. One to 2 weeks later, films demonstrate subperiosteal new bone, irregular areas of radiolucency, and cortical thinning. All these bone changes generally resolve spontaneously over a period of 4 to 8 months. Rarely, permanent shortening of the digits is seen.[479]

No specific treatment is directed toward the underlying pathophysiology of the painful episode. Treatment is supportive. The goals are to alleviate pain and treat underlying problems, especially infection, hypoxia, acidosis, and dehydration. Patients in pain should always be evaluated for possible infection—fever should *not* be assumed to be simply part of the vasoocclusive process. Hypoxia is a serious problem for patients because of the relation between deoxygenation and polymerization. Oxygen therapy is important for *hypoxemic* patients but does little besides causing bone marrow suppression[480] for those who are not. Even *hyperbaric* oxygen is not beneficial in painful crises.[481] Acidosis also potentiates sickling, but empiric use of bicarbonate is not indicated.[482] Dehydrated patients, particularly those with concurrent gastrointestinal fluid losses, need careful restoration of normal volume status. Overhydration (managing fluids at 1.5 or 2 times normal maintenance) must be done with caution since these patients handle rapid infusions poorly and easily develop acute chest syndrome and pulmonary edema—especially when being "run wet" and treated with narcotics at the same time.[483,484] Careful monitoring of weight, electrolytes, and fluid balance is essential.

The careful, consistent, and compassionate use of analgesics in the context of an experienced multidisciplinary team is key to management of painful episodes.[485] The choice, route, and dosage of narcotic agents is a highly charged subject that is unfortunately contaminated by the *misimpression* that the iatrogenic addiction rate is high among sickle cell disease patients. Our approach emphasizes choosing a fixed dose and rate schedule (not as-needed dosing) that is clinically effective for the particular patient. To do this properly requires knowledge of analgesic pharmacokinetics and equianalgesic dosing. This subject is reviewed in detail in an important article by Payne,[486] which should become required reading for caregivers involved with these patients. A summary of basic narcotic charateristis is found in Table 53-5.

Although transfusion (even exchange transfusion) rarely works acutely, a subset of patients with frequent recurrent episodes may benefit from a short course (a few months) of maintenance transfusion. With this approach, these unusual patients (less than 10% of the total) with high pain rates may be kept free of pain for a sufficient period of time to finish a school year or complete an important project.

Osteomyelitis. Definitive diagnosis and appropriate therapy of osteomyelitis requires identification of a specific pathogen. Although blood (and stool in the case of *Salmonella* sp) cultures may be positive, needle aspiration and culturing of suspicious bone lesions is critical. Careful culturing *before* starting antibiotics is essential to avoid unnecessary or inappropriate protracted intravenous therapy. As seen in Table 53-4, in most series, the predominant pathogen is *Salmonella* sp. Pending culture results, empiric antibiotic treatment should cover both *Salmonella* and *Staphylococcus* sp. Fortunately, osteomyelitis is a relatively rare disease. In one study, the New York City Department of Health reviewed its cases of *Salmonella* osteomyelitis between 1964 and 1978[487]; 37 cases were reported, 14 were in patients with sickle cell disease. Only four patients developed chronic osteomyelitis, and *all* these patients had been treated parenterally for less than 1 week. The perfusion of these lesions is severely compromised, and clear-

TABLE 53-5. Characteristics of Commonly Used Narcotic Agents

Agent	Dose (mg) Equianalgesic to 10 mg IM Morphine	Peak Effect (h)	Duration of Effect (h)	Typical Fixed Dose Interval (h)	Comments
Morphine	10 IM 20–60 PO	0.5–1 1.5–2	3–6 4–7	4	Caution with acute lung disease, liver, or renal failure
Hydromorphone (Dilaudid)	1.5 IM 7.5 PO	0.5–1 1–2	3–4 3–4	4	Same precautions as morphine
Meperidine (Demerol)	75 IM 300 PO	0.5–1 1–2	3–4 3–6	4	Normeperidine metabolite is toxic (primarily CNS) and accumulates with dosing, liver disease, renal disease
Methadone	10 IM 20 PO	0.5–1.5	4–6	6	Risk of delayed toxicity because of accumulation

ing these infections requires a more aggressive approach than is generally required in the normal population. A minimum of 6 weeks of treatment with documented efficacious blood levels of antibiotics is recommended.

Aseptic Necrosis. Aseptic necrosis of the femoral head is a serious and often debilitating complication that occurs in young adults with sickle cell disease. This is one of the few complications that is a prominent feature of SC disease, although the incidence is slightly higher among patients with SS disease and is highest among those with SS *and* α-thalassemia.[487a] In the CSSCD, in which patients were screened for the presence of hip disease, 3% of those below 15 years of age had osteonecrosis (all with SS disease, $S\beta^0$-thalassemia, or SC disease). Among those over 45 years of age, 35% of patients with SS disease, 25% with $S\beta^0$-thalassemia, 29% with SC disease, and 40% with $S\beta^+$-thalassemia had osteonecrosis of the hip. Bilateral disease developed in about half of the patients with hip disease, usually by age 25 years. About half of patients had no signs or symptoms at the time of diagnosis, but 21% had signs or symptoms at a later date. The typical radiographic findings[488] of aseptic necrosis are generally not present when the patient first becomes symptomatic, but MRI imaging is useful in documenting subtle early disease.[489,490] Treatment of these lesions is not satisfying. Proscription of weight-bearing for long periods (months) may be helpful in the early stages. For patients who have progressed to severe disease, total hip replacement may be the only way to provide relief of pain and improve mobility. Because the underlying bone is generally of poor quality, hip replacement surgery carries a high complication rate, and early revisions are common.[491,492] The CSSCD experience with hip prosthesis suggests a failure of roughly 10% per year. Experience at the Medical College of Georgia suggests that a relatively simple procedure in which the femoral head is decompressed by removing a small portion of ischemic cancellous *bone–core decompression*[493]—may be a beneficial technique in early lesions (Milner P, personal communication). In the CSSCD, aseptic necrosis of the humeral head followed a genetic pattern similar to that of necrosis of the femoral head.[494] In fact, roughly 75% of SS and SC patients with shoulder disease also had hip disease, although only 20% of them had symptoms from the shoulder disease.

Other Chronic Bone Findings. The chronic hemolytic anemia results in an expanded marrow cavity (see Fig. 53-24) that can be easily seen in radiographs of the skull, which typically show a widened diploic space. Overgrowth of the anterior maxilla may lead to serious orthodontic problems. Vertebrae are usually flattened, with a characteristic biconcave codfish-like shape on radiograph. Older patients may develop chronic back pain as a result of vertebral collapse.

Pulmonary

Acute Chest Syndrome. Episodes of acute chest pain accompanied by radiographic evidence of infiltrate, effusion, or edema are referred to as the *acute chest syndrome.* Johnson and Verdegem[495] reviewed this subject. In the Jamaican series, acute chest syndrome was common and was the leading cause of death among sickle cell disease patients older than 10 years of age.[496,497] In Houston, chest syndrome accounted for 33% of all hospital admissions for sickle cell patients.[498]

As the enigmatic name implies, it is often difficult to be certain of the cause of the acute pulmonary disease. Patients are prone to both infarction and infection, and the two conditions can coexist. The original epidemiology of acute chest syndrome in children suggested that it was predominantly an infection caused by *S pneumoniae.*[499,500] In more recent studies, *S pneumoniae* was not as important a pathogen,[498,501] possibly a reflection of the efficacy of *S pneumoniae* vaccination and the use of prophylactic penicillin. In the Philadelphia study of 102 episodes, 12% were bacterial, 8% were viral, and 16% were mycoplasmal (see Table 53-4). There was a definite seasonal variation in infections. In the autumn, 45% of events were caused by *Mycoplasma* sp; half of the viral pneumonias occurred during January and February. Initial laboratory findings showed decreased hematocrit (down 11% from baseline), increased reticulocyte count (up 15%), increased leukocyte count (up 66%), and decreased platelet count (down 11%). In the Jamaican experience, one third of patients had either a pleural rub or effusion,[502] and in London, *only* 36% of patients had an abnormal chest film on presentation, although all eventually developed abnormal radiographic findings.[503] In children, chest syndrome frequently presents with acute abdominal pain, ileus, hypoxemia, and a normal chest radiograph. Several days may pass before the chest radiograph appears abnormal.

The patient experiencing acute chest syndrome (regardless of the cause) is in a particularly precarious position because hypoxia has such a profound effect on sickling. Most series of acute chest syndrome include a section on autopsy findings. Pulmonary postmortem findings typically include areas of alveolar wall necrosis and focal parenchymal scars.[504,505] In one autopsy, multiple large infarcts, but no accompanying occluded vessels, were found, suggesting that severe vasospasm may play a role in some cases.[506] Pulmonary *emboli of necrotic bone marrow* have been well documented in nine cases: five symptomatic patients with acute chest syndrome (four of whom had accompanying bone pain) died from the bone marrow emboli. Of the four patients with marrow emboli found incidentally at autopsy, one had acute chest syndrome and three had no obvious chest symptoms.[504] Acute chest syndrome often appears in the setting of bone pain. It is possible that the embolization of marrow or fat[507] from ischemic marrow is responsible for these episodes. The unusual physical and laboratory findings associated with *fat embolization* were reviewed by Johnson and Verdegem[495] and should be sought when considering this clinical possibility; they are thrombocytopenia, hypocalcemia, hyperuricemia, lipemia retinalis, upper thoracic and conjunctival petechiae, and lipid droplets in the sputum or urine. A review of the many factors contributing to the pathogenesis of lung disease in hemoglobinopathies can be found in a summary of a National Heart, Lung and Blood Institute workshop.[507a]

Although most patients with acute chest syndrome recover uneventfully, the course is unpredictable, and rapid unexpected deterioration is common. All patients with chest syndrome must be managed in the hospital, in a setting where they can have frequent monitoring of vital signs and arterial blood gasses. A PO_2 of less than 75 mm (or a decrease of 25% from baseline, if the patient is chronically hypoxic) carries a poor prognosis.[508] Because the hemoglobin–oxygen dissociation curve varies among patients, and because the shallow portion of the curve is between a PO_2 of 50 and 100 mmHg, transcutaneous oxygen saturation measurements are *not sufficient* unless there are enough simultaneous direct measurements of arterial PO_2 to detect trends.[508a] This is particularly true for patients with high steady-state hemobglobin concentrations.[508b] In one study, all children with SS disease and acute chest syndrome had transcutaneous saturation measurements below 96%.[508b] Oxygen therapy is of critical importance, and mechanical ventilation is sometimes required. Antibiotics should be used liberally after careful culturing (including stool culture for *Salmonella* sp), keeping in mind the prevalence of

S pneumoniae, H influenzae, and Mycoplasma sp. Transfusion is *critical* for persistently hypoxic patients (Po_2 less than 75 mm, or a decrease of 25% from baseline). Exchange transfusion is indicated if the hematocrit is high and the patient is hypoxic, if the patient is deteriorating rapidly, or if the patient continues to deteriorate after simple red cell transfusion.

Chronic Pulmonary Disease. In one survey, the lung volumes of asymptomatic adolescents with SS disease were normal compared with those of a black control population.[509] In these same patients, resting arterial Po_2 was 65 to 85 mmHg (normal is greater than 87 mmHg). Large alveolar–arterial oxygen Po_2 differences were found in room air (27 to 42 mmHg; normal is less than 16 mmHg) and on 100% O_2 (186 to 246 mmHg; normal is less than 86 mmHg). These values are consistent with increased pulmonary shunting of 12% to 16% (normal is less than 7%). Progressive deterioration in pulmonary function is discussed in detail in a comprehensive review by Powars and colleagues.[510] They identified a group of patients with increasing hypoxia, decreasing lung volumes and flow rates, increasing chest pain, increasing right ventricular dysfunction, and increasing pulmonary artery pressure. These patients had a high mortality rate compared with their matched controls. Half of the identified patients died—some suddenly, with postmortem evidence of myocardial infarction without coronary artery disease and with cor pulmonale. Risk factors for developing chronic lung disease include increased incidence of acute chest syndrome and painful episodes associated with chest pain.

Central Nervous System

Vasoocclusive Stroke. About 7% of patients with SS disease experience acute cerebral infarction.[511,511a] This potential disaster usually occurs spontaneously and without warning, but it also occurs during episodes of pneumonia, aplasia, viral illness, pain, priapism, hyperventilation, and dehydration.[512–514a] Hemiplegia, seizures, speech defects, coma, and visual disturbances are the most common features. The abnormal signs and symptoms may improve slightly or remain constant.[511,515] In untreated patients, the mortality approaches 20%, and about 70% recur within 3 years. Over 70% of the survivors are left with permanent motor disability and deficits in IQ.[511] Angiographic and postmortem examinations usually reveal more vessel involvement than anticipated on clinical grounds. Typically, there are multiple stenoses of internal carotid and anterior and middle cerebral arteries that appear to originate at sites of bifurcations; less frequently, single or no lesions are found.[512,516–518] This is not simple in situ sickling but a definite vasculopathy with intimal, fibroblast, and smooth muscle proliferation[519,520] (Fig. 53-32). Computed tomographic (CT) scanning, MRI, or arteriography is essential to rule out potentially treatable disorders such as subdural hematoma, berry aneurysm, or tuberculous granuloma—all of which have been described in patients with sickle cell disease.[512,521] CT scans are more likely to demonstrate middle cerebral infarcts several days after an acute event and are less sensitive than MRI in demonstrating deep white-matter infarcts in patients with transient ischemic attacks or seizures.[522] The ability to image these "watershed" infarcts by MRI has highlighted the vulnerability of these areas of the brain that are supplied by the distal arteries and that are susceptible to changes in cerebral perfusion.[523] The sensitivity of this technique also creates important clinical conundrums, as exemplified by the finding of *unexpected* infarcts in 11% of patients *without any* history of central nervous system symptoms.[522] Arteriography has been the gold standard for defining the detailed vascular anatomy, a definition that might ultimately prove to have therapeutic implications.[512] Arteriography should *not* be performed until an exchange transfusion has been completed *if hypertonic radiographic dye will be used.* It is likely that noninvasive techniques, such as combined transcranial Doppler and MRI, will ultimately replace arteriography.[524] In fact, promising work from the Medical College of Georgia suggests that transcranial Doppler may be a useful screening tool for identifying children at high risk for stroke.[524a–524c]

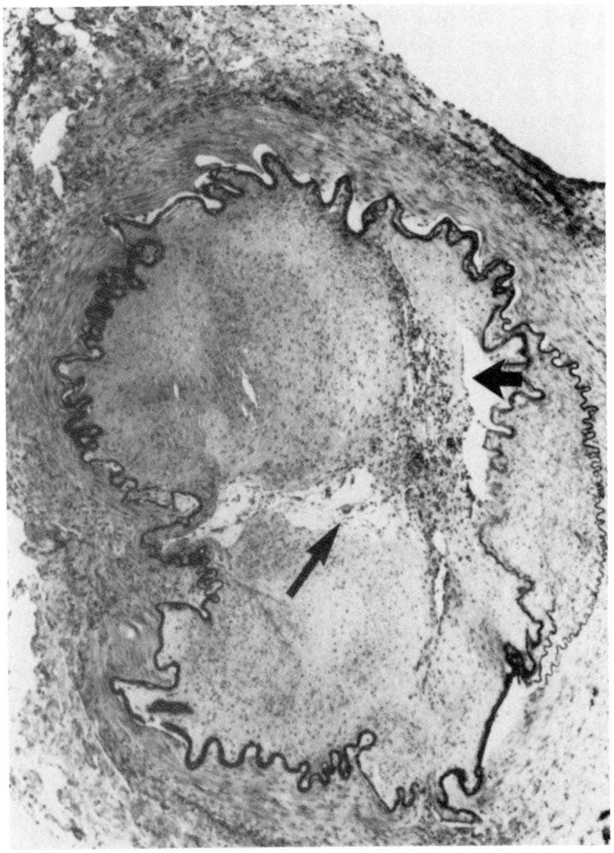

FIGURE 53-32. Cerebral blood vessel pathology in sickle cell anemia patient. Narrowed vessel lumen (*thick arrow*) and marked intimal hyperplasia (*thin arrow*) are visible. (After Koshy M, Thomas C, Goodwon J. Vascular lesions in the central nervous system in sickle cell disease (neuropathology). J Assoc Acad Minority Phys 1990;1:71)

Maintenance transfusion therapy has had a profound influence on the prognosis of patients with stroke.[512,517,525–527] A regular transfusion program designed to keep the hemoglobin S level below 30% lowers the recurrence rate to 10%, although 30% of patients may continue to have residual motor impairment, and 10% develop IQ levels below 70. Transient ischemic attacks *can* occur in patients still on transfusion.[512,528–530] In three such patients,[527] the hemoglobin S levels were 17% to 35%. In patients undergoing transfusion, repeated arteriograms generally show stabilization and smoothing of intimal lesions, whereas patients not receiving transfusions demonstrate progressive vessel damage.[512] Even after improvement of arteriograms, however, patients continue to be at risk of recurrence, as demonstrated by two patients whose arteriograms improved after 1 year of transfusion but who had recurrences after cessation of therapy.[512]

A study of 12 children in Memphis who had been on transfusion therapy for 1 to 2 years revealed a 70% recurrence rate within 5 weeks to 11 months of stopping transfusion.[517] The St Jude's and LeBonheur Children's group reported their updated results on patients who received transfusions for 5 to 12.5 years before discontinuation.[531] All 10 patients had abnormal arteriograms and evidence of encephalomalacia by MRI at the time transfusions were stopped. Five patients had recurrent strokes, and one died suddenly and without explanation (no new stroke at postmortem) 2.5 to 12 months after discontinuation.

Emergency treatment for stroke includes exchange transfusion to limit the extent of the ischemic damage and prepare the patient for possible arteriography (especially if a hypertonic radiographic dye is to be used). Maintenance transfusions may need to be continued indefinitely to prevent recurrence. Although theoretically beneficial, a lifetime of maintenance transfusion carries with it the real risks of infection, red cell antigen sensitization, and iron overload. Despite these hazards, life-long therapy appears to be the only way to prevent recurrent strokes. Follow-up of a group of children from the Children's Hospital of Philadelphia who had undergone 4 years of a transfusion program designed to keep the pretransfusion hemoglobin S level below 30% suggests that the target hemoglobin S level can be safely increased to 50%.[531a]

Intracranial Hemorrhage. Intracranial hemorrhage was reviewed by Van Hoff and colleagues.[532] In adults, hemorrhages are more common than ischemic strokes, although the two frequently coexist.[520] The mean age of occurrence is 25 years, with an overall incidence of about 2%.[511] These bleeds are usually subarachnoid hemorrhages that present as a severe sudden headache, frequently with vomiting, signs of meningismus, and photophobia. They progress rapidly, and the associated overall mortality rate approaches 50% in some series,[511] although others report a more favorable outcome.[533,533a] Not all patients with arteriographically demonstrated bleeds have diagnostic cerebrospinal fluid or CT findings.[533] Because these lesions may be surgically correctable, patients should have angiography after being prepared with exchange transfusion. Bleeding aneurysms probably balloon from damaged intima and fragile collaterals (often resembling moyomoya disease[519]) formed during childhood. This sequence of events is suggested in a series of patients with hemorrhage 4 to 20 or more years after ischemia,[534] although a history of stroke is not invariable.[533] Because the clinical experience with hemorrhage is limited and the mortality high, there is not enough data on survivors to be dogmatic about long-term management. One reasonable approach is to use chronic maintenance transfusion for those who are found to have abnormal vascular anatomy,[532] although three patients are known to have bled while on a transfusion program that maintained their hemoglobin S level lower than 20%.[534]

Cardiac

The chronic anemia of sickle cell disease causes a compensatory increase in cardiac output.[535] As a result, most patients have abnormal cardiac findings.[536–542] On examination, the most common signs are systolic ejection murmur, third heart sound, suprasternal notch thrill, split first heart sound, and diastolic murmur.[541] The cardiac examination may mimic congenital or rheumatic disorders. Cardiomegaly is found in most patients, with electrographic evidence of left ventricular hypertrophy in about half the cases.[542]

Discrete episodes of acute myocardial infarction are relatively rare, considering that this is a disease marked by vasoocclusion and tissue infarction.[542,543] In one review of the postmortem literature, only four classic infarcts were reported among 153 hearts[543]; although 20% of another series of 72 cases had lesions that could be interpreted as ischemic.[544] Despite the high oxygen extraction in the coronary circulation, blood in the coronary sinus has no more sickling than blood in the general circulation,[545] presumably because of the rapid transit time.[535] Atherosclerosis is virtually absent in this population—appearing in none of 100 hearts of patients between 16 and 47 years of age.[543] This is in marked contrast to the findings among those who died on the battlefields of Vietnam, where 45% had atherosclerosis.[546] When injected at autopsy, hearts from patients with SS disease had larger than normal caliber vessels.[547]

Although classic atherosclerosis-related myocardial infarctions are rare, some patients have evidence of tissue damage as measured by various scanning techniques and elevation of cardiac enzymes.[548] It is not known how prevalent these findings are or whether they represent a subtle form of sickle myocardiopathy.[549] Several studies have shown that most patients have normal resting left ventricular function as measured by a variety of noninvasive techniques.[550–553] Several careful studies of a group of patients from Augusta, Georgia, however, demonstrated that one third of children have decreased left ventricular contractility,[554] that 15% develop electrocardiographic evidence of ischemia with exercise,[555] and that those with an ischemic response also have an abnormal ejection fraction in response to exercise.[556] In another study, systemic vascular resistance was significantly reduced, and end-diastolic volume was increased.[557] The authors commented that these abnormal loading conditions, which are common compensatory changes in anemia, may mask left ventricular dysfunction as measured by ejection fraction. As they manipulated the loading conditions, they were able to demonstrate left ventricular dysfunction as a decreased end-systolic stress/end-systolic volume ratio.[557] A study that compared SS disease patients to patients with chronic aortic insufficiency suggested that resting left ventricular function is well preserved, as it is in other chronic high-output states.[558] The authors emphasized that hypertension, a rare finding among SS disease patients,[559] would have extremely deleterious effects on left ventricular function in this high-output state. Although it remains uncertain as to how prevalent or clinically important mild left ventricular dysfunction is under *normal* circumstances, it is well known that, with the stress of volume overload, hypoxemia, hyperthermia, tachycardia, exacerbated anemia, or hypertension, a well-compensated patient can rapidly develop intractable cardiac failure.

Right ventricular dysfunction,[552] pulmonary hypertension, and cor pulmonale can be seen, particularly in patients who have suffered numerous pulmonary infarcts.[560] As discussed in the section on chronic lung disease, patients with cor pulmonale and right ventricular dysfunction have a high mortality rate. Transfusion can increase exercise tolerance and decrease resting heart rate in some patients,[561] and a chronic transfusion program may benefit patients with chronic progressive lung disease.

Arrhythmia appears to be common during painful episodes. In one study, 80% of patients experienced arrhythmia during the first hour of treatment for pain[562]; 67% were atrial, 60% were ventricular, and none was thought to be clinically significant.

Genitourinary

Hyposthenuria and Tubular Defects. Hyposthenuria[563–565] develops during the first 10 years of life and, as with functional asplenia, may be temporarily reversed with transfusion.[566,567] The hypertonic environment of the renal medulla enhances sickling,[568] thereby reducing medullary blood flow and disturbing the countercurrent multiplier system (Fig. 53-33). The abnormal countercurrent multiplier may be the cause of the hyposthenuria, or it may result from diversion of blood flow away from nephrons with long Henle's loops and toward those with short loops.[569] The obligatory water loss results in a tendency toward dehydration and invalidates the use of urine flow or specific gravity as an indicator of the patient's state of hydration. Nocturia and enuresis are common complaints of patients who excrete large volumes of dilute urine.[570] Urinary sodium is rarely high enough to cause hyponatremia.[571] A defect in renal tubular acidification,[572,573] as well as hyporeninemic hypoaldosteronism[574] and impaired potassium excretion,[575,576] have been identified and may result in hyperkalemic acidosis.[577] Mild hyperuricemia is found in patients with impaired secretion of uric acid in the distal tubule.[578] This may rarely lead to urate stones or clinical gout.

Hematuria. About one fourth of patients with SS disease and renal papillary necrosis do not have hematuria[579]; nevertheless, this pathologic entity is thought to be responsible for most of the occasional episodes of hematuria[580] that occur in all the sickle syndromes, including sickle trait. Hematuria is usually mild but can be severe enough to cause significant blood loss.[581–583] Maintenance transfusion may allow bleeding lesions to heal. ε-Aminocaproic acid can be used for refractory bleeding,[584–586] but this must be done cautiously. Patients should be kept on bed rest in the hospital, and a high urine flow should be maintained because of the risk of clotting and obstruction of the ureter or renal pelvis. In patients with long-standing hematuria, iron supplements may be necessary.

Nephrotic Syndrome and Renal Failure. Proteinuria and nephrotic syndrome occur mainly in adults with SS disease.[587] Despite the well-described histology,[588,589] the cause of the glomerular lesion is not known. It may represent a response to iron[590] or immune complex[591,592] deposition. Results from the series of patients observed at Chapel Hill suggest that proteinuria is caused by glomerular capillary hypertension and that it can be reduced by therapy with inhibition of angiotensin-converting enzyme.[592a] Bakir and colleagues[593] reviewed the Chicago experience and reported that 4% of adult SS patients developed nephrotic syndrome; two thirds of these patients went on to develop renal failure, and half of these patients died within 2 years. In the Jamaican experience, 6 of 25 patients older than 40 years of age had diminished creatinine clearance.[594] In Los Angeles, chronic renal failure was found in about 4% of SS patients (median age at onset, 25 years) and in about 2% of SC patients (median age at onset, 50 years). Chronic renal failure contributed little to mortality in patients younger than 10 years but accounted for about 15% of deaths in those older than 10 years.[24] Sickle cell patients with chronic renal failure can be managed remarkably well with peritoneal dialysis, hemodialysis, or transplantation.[595–597]

Priapism. Priapism is a distressing problem that occurs in males of all ages. In a Jamaican questionnaire study of 104 males between 10 and 62 years of age, 42% reported at least one episode of priapism, with a median age of onset of 21 years.[598] The experience of Powars and colleagues[24] in Los Angeles suggests that about 7% of SS and about 2% of SC males develop priapism, with a median age of onset of about 22 years. Because of the relative infrequency with which priapism is an admitting diagnosis in the United States, either there is more priapism in Jamaica or it is usually managed at home in the United States. Four clinical entities are described: *stuttering* priapism, with short (less than 2 to 3 hours), often multiple episodes; *acute prolonged* priapism (more than 24 hours), which can persist for weeks; *chronic* priapism, a painless induration that may last for years; and *acute-on-chronic* priapism, acute painful episodes complicating chronic induration.[439] Sexual dysfunction was reported by 46% of patients with a history of priapism.[598] In general, young patients with brief episodes involving the corpora cavernosa are not likely to become dysfunctional,[599] whereas adults with involvement of the corpora cavernosa and corpus spongiosa tend to have prolonged episodes and a better than 50% chance of becoming impotent.[599a] Urinary retention requring catheterization may complicate the acute episode.[600] These patients are also apparently particularly susceptible to acute severe neurologic complications—even those treated with exchange transfusion.[514a] They should be monitored closely for early neurologic symptoms, especially headache.

The approach to treatment of priapism is not entirely uniform, but a consensus appears in the NIH management and therapy guide[439] and is presented here. Short episodes of acute priapism usually occur on awakening and can be

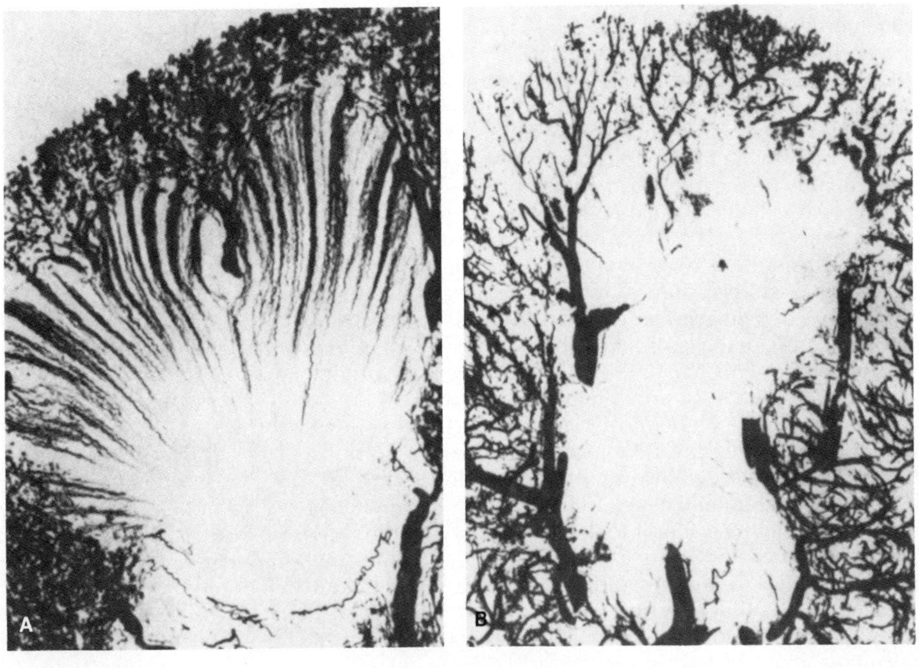

FIGURE 53-33. Vascular anatomy of the kidney in patient with sickle cell disease. Postmortem injection of normal (**A**) and sickle cell (**B**) kidneys. Marked destruction of the vascular anatomy has occurred. (Statius van Eps LW, Schouten H, et al. The influence of red blood cell transfusions on the hyposthenuria and renal hemodynamics of sickle cell anemia. Clin Chim Acta 1967;17:449)

managed at home. Patients should be instructed to urinate frequently, do some vigorous exercise, increase fluid intake, and soak in a warm tub. If the episode does not resolve within 3 hours, the patient should be appear for medical treatment. In adults, treatment of acute priapism that has lasted more than 3 hours should start with prostatic massage (which may induce detumescence) and examination of the prostatic fluid for infection. In all patients, underlying conditions that may predispose to sickling (dehydration, hypoxemia, and infection[601]—particularly prostatitis) should be diagnosed and treated. Patients should receive analgesics (see Table 53-5), and preparations should be made to perform an exchange transfusion. Priapism may respond to simple red cell transfusion,[602] and this may be a reasonable temporizing measure in the first 6 to 8 hours. Some patients begin to improve within hours of an exchange,[603,604] although most do not show signs of detumescence for 24 to 48 hours. Complete detumescence may take weeks to months.

Surgical intervention should be considered only for patients who have *not* shown any signs of detumescence 24 hours after exchange transfusion and should be avoided in patients not receiving transfusions. Although procedures ranging from corporal aspiration and irrigation to saphenocorporal shunts have been advocated in the past,[605–608] there is a high complication rate with subsequent penile deformities and impotence. A first surgical approach is penile aspiration. If this is unsuccessful, Winter's procedure or one of its modifications can be tried, whereby a needle or scalpel is inserted through the glans into one of the corpora and the viscous blood is aspirated. This temporarily allows for drainage of cavernous blood into the systemic circulation and has been successfully used in SS disease patients.[609] Intermittent compression with a blood pressure cuff is critical to limit refilling.

Hepatobiliary

Liver and biliary tract abnormalities are common among SS disease patients[610–612] and typically result from cholelithiasis, hepatic ischemia, and viral hepatitis. Most asymptomatic patients have chronic hyperbilirubinemia (average bilirubin, 3 mg/dL[612]), mild to moderate hepatomegaly (see Fig. 53-24), and moderately elevated transaminases.[613] Chronically elevated levels of alkaline phosphatase are usually of bone origin.[614] A review of the hepatobiliary system in sickle cell disease by Schubert should be consulted for details.[615]

Gallstones. Bilirubin stones are common.[616,617] In one informative series, 226 patients with SS disease had routine sonograms of the gallbladder.[618] Among patients 2 to 4 years of age, the prevalence of stones was 12%. With increasing age, the prevalence increased, reaching 42% in those 15 to 18 years of age. Fourteen patients were noted to have sludge in the gallbladder. They were reexamined up to 2 years later; four had developed stones, six still had sludge, and the sludge had disappeared in four patients. The patients with stones had an average, steady-state total bilirubin (3.8 $\pm$ 0.3 mg/dL) that was higher than that of the patients without stones (2.6 $\pm$ 0.12 mg/dL). Total hemoglobin and reticulocyte counts did not differ significantly between the two groups. Acute cholecystitis presents in these patients with the same signs and symptoms as in other populations, but it is not known what proportion of patients with bilirubin stones eventually develop cholecystitis. Common bile duct stones can be difficult to diagnose solely on the basis of routine laboratory tests and ultrasonography and may require direct examination of the duct.[618a] Convincing evidence suggests that children tolerate *elective* cholecystectomy with little morbidity,[619,620] whereas operating in the setting of acute cholecystitis carries a significant risk of serious complication.[621] Laparoscopic cholecystectomy has been particularly effective in reducing the postoperative hospital stay in children with sickle cell disease.[620a] The NIH management and therapy guide[439] recommends removing the gallbladder electively within 6 weeks of an acute attack to minimize the formation of adhesions, and the guide emphasizes the need for performing an intraoperative cholangiogram to identify intrahepatic or common duct stones. Persistent *Salmonella* bacteremia is also an indication for elective cholecystectomy in a patient with gallstones.

Intrahepatic Sickling and Hepatitis. All episodes of right upper quadrant pain are not cholecystitis.[622] Pain, worsening jaundice, elevations in transaminases, nausea, and low-grade fever are also features of intrahepatic sickling[615,623] and viral hepatitis.[624] Schubert[615] recalls the second reported case of sickle cell disease, described by Washburn in 1911.[625] Despite the fact that 107 gallstones were removed at cholecystectomy, the patient continued to have episodes of right upper quadrant pain postoperatively. Acute intrahepatic sickling usually resolves fairly abruptly, in days to weeks.[615] In contrast, in viral hepatitis, the resolution is more gradual and takes longer.[615] Fulminant hepatic failure with massive cholestasis and rapid progression to hepatic encephalopathy and shock is a rare, often fatal complication that may be amenable to emergency exchange transfusion.[626,627]

A review of postmortem liver pathology among 70 patients from John Hopkins Hospital[628] revealed unexpected hepatic injury. Necrosis, portal fibrosis, regenerative nodules, and cirrhosis were common features thought to be a result of recurrent ischemia and repair.

Skin

Leg ulcers have been described in a number of different anemias, including hereditary spherocytosis, thalassemia, elliptocytosis, and pyruvate kinase deficiency[629]; their presence in sickle cell anemia should therefore not necessarily imply that they represent vasoocclusion. Ulceration may result from increased venous pressure in the legs caused by the expanded blood volume in the hypertrophied bone marrow.[630] A recent review by Koshy and colleagues of the CSSCD experience[631] revealed that there were no ulcers found among 1700 patients younger than 10 years of age. Among older patients with SS disease, the incidence per 100 person-years was as follows: ages 10 to 20, 3; ages 20 to 30, 15; ages 30 to 40, 17; ages 40 to 50, 18; over age 50, 19. For every age group, the presence of α-thalassemia resulted in a lower incidence, for example, 9% in the 20- to 30-year-old group. There were also fewer ulcers among the $S\beta^0$-thalassemia patients, and no ulcers were found in either $S\beta^+$-thalassemia or SC patients. In tropical areas where shoes are not always worn and insect bites are common, leg ulcers are more frequent.[632–634] In Jamaica, leg ulcers typically start in the 10- to 20-year-old group and eventually appear in 75% of adults. Chronic lesions become a major source of morbidity and have a profound negative impact on educational achievement and employment.[635]

Ulcers are usually present over the medial surface of the lower tibia or just posterior to the medial malleolus. They begin as a small depression with central necrosis and, if unattended, may widen to encircle the entire lower leg. In one case, ulcers resulted in chronic osteomyelitis requiring amputation.[631] Initially, the surrounding skin appears healthy, but as the ulcer becomes chronic the skin becomes darker, the follicles and subcutaneous fat are lost, and chronic cellulitis and local adenitis can be severely painful. These ulcers can persist for years.

Treatment of ulcers is a long-term and relatively frustrating process. In the CSSCD, the recurrence rate was high

(25% to 52%) regardless of the treatment program.[631] The NIH management and therapy guide[439] suggests an escalating regimen that starts with local cleaning (several weeks of wet-to-dry dressings every 3 hours) and moves to protection (3 to 4 weeks of weekly changing of Unna boot), transfusion (6 months of maintenance), and eventually skin grafting (split thickness, with continued postoperative maintenance transfusion) for ulcers that have not healed. Logic suggests that early intervention should be beneficial. Patients should be advised to be particularly careful about leg injuries and seek early care for any skin lesions on the legs that do not heal promptly.

Ocular

The review by Cohen and colleagues[636] illustrates the often subtle and always complex nature of the ocular manifestations of sickle cell disease. Before describing the common complications, three important clinical points need to be stressed:

1. Proliferative retinopathy can cause blindness and can be diagnosed reliably only by an ophthalmologist.
2. Eye trauma resulting in blood in the anterior chamber (hyphema) can cause blindness even in patients with sickle cell trait.
3. Retinal surgery should not be done without preoperative transfusion treatment.

Some of the most dramatic and exotic ocular lesions of sickle cell disease are *not* associated with blindness. Saccular comma-shaped dilatations of conjunctival vessels occur in virtually all patients with SS disease, over half of patients with SC disease, and no patients with sickle trait.[637] These benign lesions curiously disappear with the administration of oxygen, with transfusion, or under the heat of the slit lamp[638–640]; appear more prominently with vaso-

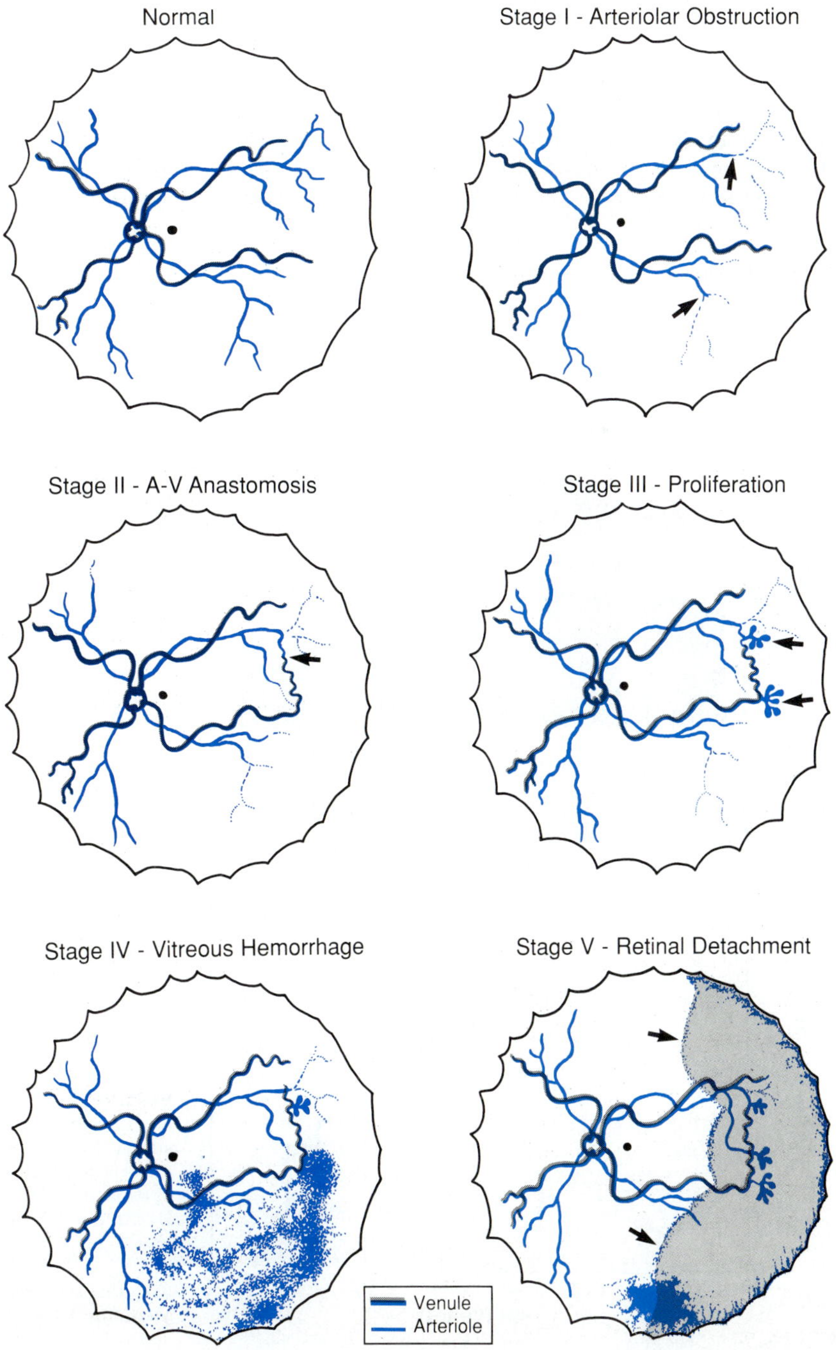

FIGURE 53-34. Goldberg classification of sickle cell retinopathy. (After Goldberg MF. Retinal vaso-occlusion in sickling hemoglobinopthies. Birth Defects 1976;12:475)

constricting eyedrops; and are correlated with the number of circulating irreversibly sickled cells.[641]

Retinopathy is conveniently classified as either proliferative or nonproliferative.[642] Nonproliferative retinopathy generally does not cause blindness and marks localized areas of hemorrhage. Depending on the age, layer, and extent of the bleed, the lesion appears as a salmon patch, schisis cavity, iridescent spot, black sunburst, or mottled brown area.[643–646] In contrast, proliferative retinopathy can ultimately cause blindness by vitreous hemorrhage or retinal detachment. These lesions occur peripherally, out of the of view of nonophthalmologists. The initial insult appears to be cessation of blood flow at the end or bifurcation of an arteriole. Endothelial damage at the site of occlusion is inferred by the abnormal angiographic pattern.[636] Goldberg[647] defined five stages of proliferative retinopathy that progress from discrete peripheral occlusions, through the development of characteristic "sea-fan" neovascularization, and ultimately to retinal hemorrhage and detachment (Fig. 53-34). Although 20% to 60% of patients with sea-fans may cure their own lesions by autoinfarction,[648,649] in well-selected patients with stage III retinopathy, blindness can be prevented by photocoagulation.[650] Surgically amenable lesions typically occur in patients older than 15 years of age and are more common among patients with SC disease. It is reasonable, therefore, that *regular yearly* ophthalmologic examinations begin in the teen-age years. Unfortunately, surgery carries the risk of potentially blinding complications[651,652] and should be undertaken only by retinal specialists.

Rarely, acute painless loss of vision results from central retinal artery occlusion. Although spontaneous restoration of sight may occur, exchange transfusion has been recommended when bilateral disease occurs.[653]

The aqueous humor is an ascorbate-rich fluid that promotes sickling.[636] With even minimal amounts of hyphema, intraocular pressure can be elevated by outflow obstruction. As reviewed by Cohen and colleagues,[636] optimal intraocular pressure for sickle cell patients is less than 25 mmHg. Higher pressure may result in retinal infarction or central retinal artery occlusion. Pressure reduction therapy is complicated because most antiglaucoma medications, at least theoretically, enhance sickling or vasoconstriction (mannitol, acetazolamide, epinephrine). Timolol maleate has been well tolerated in some patients, although if this therapy fails, repeated paracentesis may be required. Hyphema is an *ophthalmologic emergency*, even in patients with sickle *trait*.

Auditory

In patients with SS disease, sensorineural hearing loss can be found at both ends of the auditory spectrum.[654,655] In one study, 12% of children had deficiencies in the high-frequency range.[656] Although there was no excess of meningitis or otitis media in the affected group, five of the six

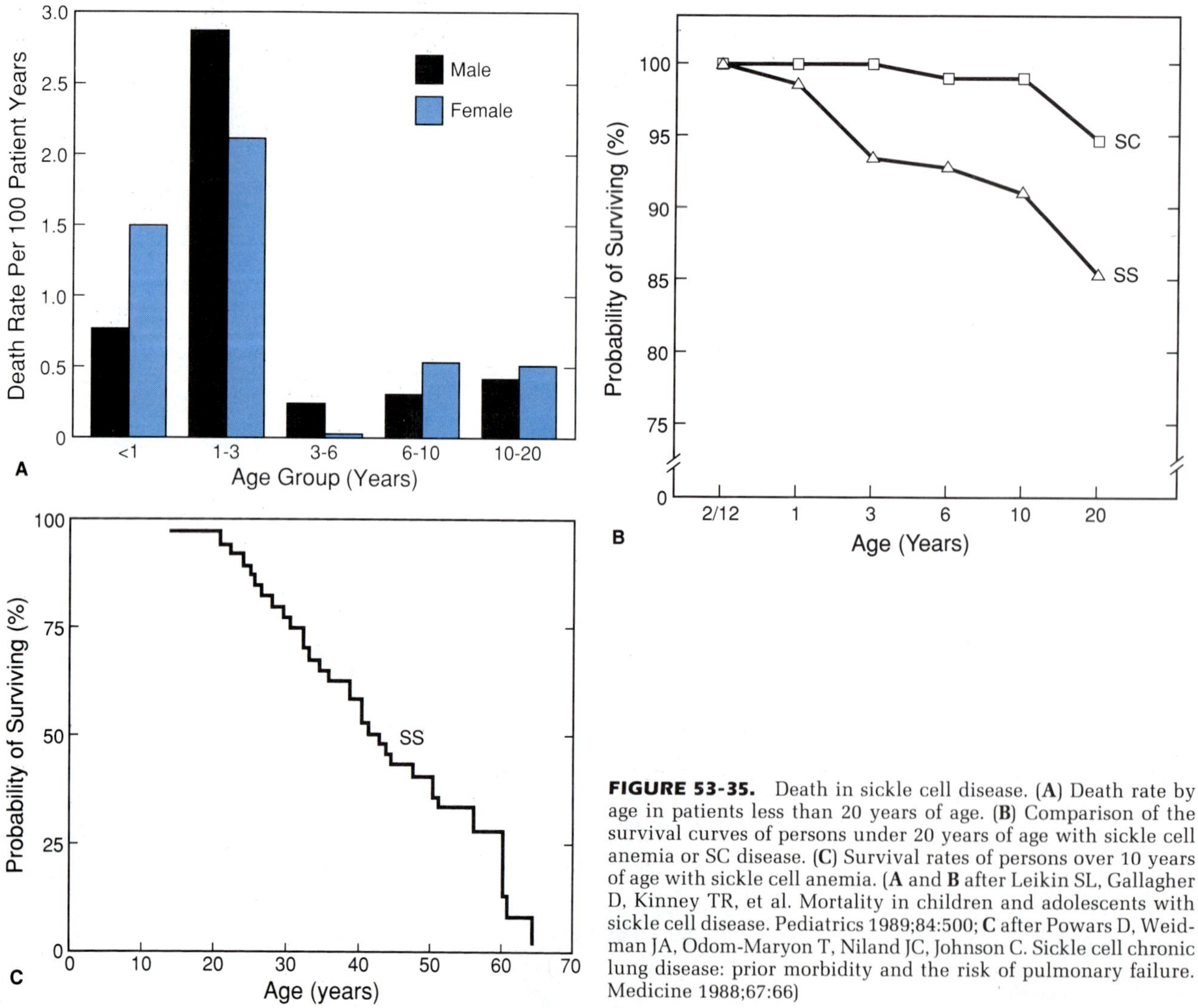

FIGURE 53-35. Death in sickle cell disease. (**A**) Death rate by age in patients less than 20 years of age. (**B**) Comparison of the survival curves of persons under 20 years of age with sickle cell anemia or SC disease. (**C**) Survival rates of persons over 10 years of age with sickle cell anemia. (**A** and **B** after Leikin SL, Gallagher D, Kinney TR, et al. Mortality in children and adolescents with sickle cell disease. Pediatrics 1989;84:500; **C** after Powars D, Weidman JA, Odom-Maryon T, Niland JC, Johnson C. Sickle cell chronic lung disease: prior morbidity and the risk of pulmonary failure. Medicine 1988;67:66)

children with central nervous system disease had abnormal hearing. The underlying pathology appears to be sickling in the cochlear vasculature and loss of hair cells.[657]

Death in Sickle Cell Disease

Both the rate and cause of death varies with age in sickle cell disease. In children, the peak mortality is in the 1- to 3-year-old group, with pneumococcal sepsis, stroke, and splenic sequestration being the most often defined causes of death[658–660] (Fig. 53-35*A*). Older patients die during acute chest syndrome, painful episodes, cerebral vascular accidents, and chronic renal or lung failure.[24,661,662] Leikin and colleagues,[658] from the CSSCD, report that about 85% of SS and 95% of SC patients survive to age 20 (see Fig. 53-35*B*). The work of Powars and colleagues[24] suggests that about half of SS patients survive to their mid-40s, and less than 10% live beyond 60 years of age[24] (see Fig. 53-35C). The widespread use of prophylactic penicillin in young children, aggressive treatment of pulmonary disease and infection, careful selection of patients for transfusion therapy, and thoughtful comprehensive care should further prolong the life expectancy, even before new effective therapies are found.

Management of Patients With Sickle Cell Disease

Routine Health Maintenance

Patients with sickle cell anemia should be followed on a routine basis by a multidisciplinary team of caregivers familiar with the prevention and treatment of the various complications of the disease. The emphasis of the routine visit should be on patient education and anticipation of problems. Patients should be encouraged to participate in self-help groups that are ideally organized and run by patients outside the medical bureaucracy. Routine dental care is critical to avoiding serious oral infections that may lead to osteomyelitis.[663,664] Regular visits with routine laboratory studies when the patient is *well* establish the patient's steady-state normal values and baseline physical findings. These baseline data are extremely helpful in sorting out the problems when the patient is ill. The issues and data

TABLE 53-6. Routine Management of Patients With Sickle Cell Anemia

	Age			
	5 y	5–10 y	10–20 y	20 y+
ISSUES AND EDUCATION				
Penicillin prophylaxis	X			
Splenic sequestration	X			
Fever or infection	X	X	X	X
Coping with pain	X	X	X	X
Dental care	X	X	X	X
Groups for patients	X	X		
Priapism		X	X	X
Smoking		X	X	X
Self-esteem and independence		X	X	X
Education		X	X	X
Recreation		X	X	X
Puberty, birth control, genetics			X	X
Leg ulcers			X	X
Vocational planning, career			X	X
Self-help groups			X	X
Family, planning, fertility				X
Prognosis				X
LABORATORY				
Complete blood cell count	1–3 times a year	1–2 times a year	1–2 times a year	1–2 times a year
Red cell antigen typing	X			
Liver function tests, blood urea nitrogen, creatinine		Every 1–2 y	Every year	Every year
Urinalysis		1–2 times a year	1–2 times a year	1–2 times a year
SPECIAL STUDIES				
Pulmonary function tests		Every 3–5 y	Every 3–5 y	Every 3–5 y
Chest radiographs		Every 3–5 y	Every 2–3 y	Every 2–3 y
Ophthalmologic examination		Every 3–5 y	Every year	Every year
Ultrasound		Every 3–5 y*	Every 3–5 y*	Every 3–5 y*
Magnetic resonance of hips			Every 5 y	Every 5 y
TREATMENT				
Penicillin prophylaxis	X	X?	X?	X?
Folate	X	X	X	X
Pneumococcus, hepatitis B, influenza vaccines	As recommended	As recommended	As recommended	As recommended

* Until positive for stones.

of importance differ with age. Table 53-6 briefly highlights some of the issues and studies that should be considered at each routine visit. This table is not meant to be exhaustive and deals with neither normal routine care nor the management of a patient with a specific chronic problem.

Use and Abuse of Transfusions

Patients with sickle cell disease tolerate (and ironically may benefit from) their anemia. They require transfusion only under unusual situations: acute splenic sequestration, aplastic crisis, central nervous system infarction, acute chest syndrome with hypoxia, prolonged priapism, preparation for some surgery or for diagnostic studies requiring hypertonic dyes, chronic heart failure (especially with the anemia of renal failure), and complicated pregnancy. In particular, there is *no* role for transfusion in managing uncomplicated painful episodes; nor is transfusion indicated to simply improve the baseline hematocrit of otherwise well patients.

Choice of Red Cell Product. In studies of sickle cell disease patients who received blood crossmatched by standard techniques, the rate of sensitization varied between 8% and 50%.[665–670] In the CSSCD series, which looked at 1814 patients receiving transfusions, the overall rate was 18.6%, a rate that increased with increasing number of transfusions.[671] The following antibodies are the most common: anti-E, anti-C, anti-K, anti-Le^a, anti-Fy^a, anti-D, anti-Le^b, anti-Jk^b, anti-S, anti-M, anti-Fy^b, anti-e, and anti-c. It is likely that these antibodies arise as a result of the difference in distribution of antigens between the largely white donor pool and the predominantly black patients.[672] Sensitization (especially multisensitization) can make transfusion difficult or even impossible. In addition, because these antibodies may be transient and therefore not discovered at the time of a subsequent transfusion, they can cause serious delayed transfusion reactions.[673] Sensitization can be successfully reduced by transfusing antigenically matched blood,[669] a worthwhile strategy despite the increased cost.[666] An alternative solution is to increase the pool of black donors. For patients who become sensitized to leukocytes or plasma proteins, filtered or washed cells should be used.

Simple and Exchange Red Cell Transfusions. During episodes of acute splenic sequestration or erythroid aplasia, a standard simple red cell transfusion is the most effective way to restore the abnormally low red cell mass. When the patient is not excessively anemic, however, simple transfusion increases the viscosity of the blood and can potentially lead to *decreased* oxygen delivery.[674] An illustration of the physiology is shown in Figure 53-36. For patients who are not severely anemic, some form of exchange transfusion is recommended to decrease the number of circulating sickle cells while increasing the hematocrit. Partial red cell exchange can be done manually, as described by Charache.[675] A 50-kg adult with a hematocrit of 20% to 27% can have 500 mL of blood removed through a 14- or 16-gauge needle, followed immediately by the infusion of 500 mL of saline. Another 500 mL of blood is removed, and five units of packed cells are then infused promptly. Vital signs and hematocrit must be monitored closely during the procedure. The most rapid and efficient way to perform red cell exchange is by using an automated cell separator.[676–680]

Maintenance Transfusion. Maintenance transfusion programs are designed to suppress erythropoiesis by consistently transfusing to a hematocrit level that is over 35%. The goal is to keep the level of hemoglobin S below 30%. First, a partial exchange is done; then the patient receives a simple transfusion every 3 to 5 weeks. Hemoglobin electrophoresis is monitored at the time of each transfusion to ensure that the transfusion schedule is accomplishing the goal of less than 30% hemoglobin S. Such programs are successful in the long-term management of patients with stroke and may be of use in some patients with recurrent priapism, resistant leg ulcers, unresponsive hematuria, or complicated pregnancy. Iron overload is a serious complication of transfusion therapy[681] and should be treated by chelation (see Chaps. 49 and 51).

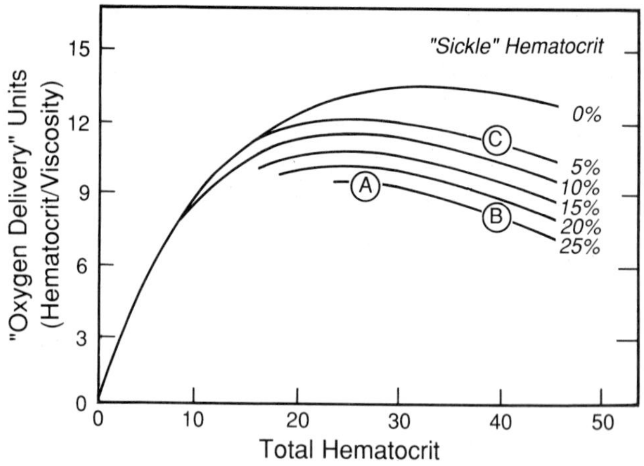

FIGURE 53-36. Effect of transfusion on oxygen delivery in sickle cell anemia. At point A, the patient's total hematocrit = sickle hematocrit = 25%, that is, the patient is untransfused. After a simple transfusion to raise the total hematocrit to 40% (point B), the oxygen delivery is slightly decreased. If an exchange transfusion is performed and the sickle hematocrit is lowered to 5%, while the total hematocrit is increased to 40% (point C), oxygen delivery is markedly improved. The viscosity measurements were made under conditions that approximate those in capillaries: Po_2, 37 mmHg; shear rate, 208 s^{-1}. (After Schmalzer EA, Lee JO, Brown AK, Usami S, Chien S. Viscosity of mixtures of sickle and normal red cells at varying hematocrit levels: implications for transfusion. Transfusion 1987;27:228)

Preparation for Surgery

Patients with sickle cell disease can be operated on safely only when their care is carefully planned and executed by an expert team that includes a surgeon, anesthesiologist, and hematologist. Compulsive attention should be paid to oxygenation, hydration, and acid–base balance during the procedure and in the postoperative period.[682–692] Choice of an anesthetic agent appears not to be as critical as the care with which it is delivered.[691] Burrington and Smith[692] suggest some simple rules: keep the operating room temperature between 26.6° and 29°C (80° and 85°F); ventilate with 100% oxygen before and after extubation or intubation; keep the patient warm in the recovery room; and take special care of intravenous boards, casts, splints, and so forth to ensure good circulation. For procedures that require a bloodless field, tourniquet surgery can be performed safely.[692a]

During and after major surgery, vasoocclusive morbidity and possibly mortality can be minimized by preoperative partial exchange transfusion (30% hemoglobin S or less). Although partial exchange is preferable, surgery can also be done safely with simple transfusion to a hematocrit level of 36%.[693] The risks and benefits of preoperative partial exchange and simple transfusion are being determined in a national collaborative study.[694] For minor procedures that are not associated with prolonged postoperative hypoventilation or atelectasis (eg, tympanostomy tube placement, skin biopsy, first-trimester therapeutic abortion) transfusion may not be necessary[694a] if it is performed with increased monitoring and follow-up in conjunction with an experienced sickle cell team.

Management of Pregnancy

Although women with sickle cell disease usually have successful pregnancies, pregnancy can be associated with serious problems for both mother and fetus.[695] Maternal complications can include increased frequency and severity of painful episodes and chest syndrome, worsening anemia, infections, toxemia, and death.[696] Fetal complications can include spontaneous abortion, prematurity, intrauterine growth retardation, and stillbirth. There has been tremendous improvement in both maternal and fetal outcomes of pregnancy since the mid-1960s.[697–699] With modern obstetric management, regular prenatal care, and better nutrition, maternal mortality has been reduced to less than 1%, and perinatal deaths have declined to less than 15%.[700] Some authors have suggested that pregnancy outcome could be improved further if mothers received transfusions prophylactically.[698,701–705] Results of women treated with transfusion are favorable when compared with historical controls but are not as convincing in contemporary comparisons.[706] Koshy and coworkers[707] carried out a prospective randomized trial of transfusion in pregnancy. Among the 138 women with SS disease, 11% had spontaneous abortions early in pregnancy before randomization. A total of 72 mothers were randomly assigned to receive no prophylactic transfusion or an aggressive transfusion program designed to keep the hemoglobin S level below 35%. The mothers who received prophylactic transfusions had fewer painful episodes, but otherwise, prophylactic transfusion had no impact on maternal morbidity, birthweight, gestational age, fetal distress, or perinatal mortality. All of the 170 placentas studied had evidence of fibrosis of the villi, infarction, and calcification. Fourteen to 18% of the infants had growth retardation, and 5% to 10% were stillborn. No mothers died, but 6% to 17% had urinary tract infections, 3% had nephrotic syndrome, 3% had congestive heart failure, and 6% to 8% had acute chest syndrome. Forty-four percent of the mothers who did not receive prophylactic transfusions developed medical or obstetric indications for transfusion and subsequently underwent transfusion.

Women with sickle cell disease qualify as having high-risk pregnancies and must be followed by the obstetrician and hematologist team. At the initial obstetric visit, complete red cell typing of both mother and father and antibody screening of the mother should be done. Both iron and folate should be prescribed. The early stages of pregnancy should be monitored with serial ultrasonographic studies. Maintenance transfusions should be initiated if the mother becomes increasingly symptomatic with either vasoocclusive or anemia-related problems, or if there is any sign of fetal distress. The newborns should receive standard neonatal care, including screening for sickle cell disease.

Specific Features of Particular Sickle Syndromes

Sickle Cell Trait

Sickle cell trait is a benign condition that occurs in about 8% of African Americans and is *not* associated with increased mortality or morbidity.[708–712] Growth, behavior, and educational development of children with trait is normal,[713,714] and the prevalence of trait among African American players in the National Football League is the same as in the general African American population.[715] There is no increased risk associated with pregnancy,[716] and pulmonary function tests are normal.[717] Although various reports of serious vasoocclusive complications of sickle cell trait appear in the literature,[718] they are extremely rare, and the *causal* link to trait is weak. Finding sickled red cells at autopsy does not mean that sickling took place before or caused death. Under certain *extreme* conditions, however, trait may be associated with sickling and even death; these conditions include pneumonia,[719] unpressurized flying,[720,721] and exercise at high altitudes.[722,723] An alarming retrospective report showed a disturbing discovery of a 30- to 40-fold increase in sudden death during basic training among recruits with sickle trait.[724] Subsequently, a smaller scale prospective study of recruits did *not* reveal any differences in exercise tolerance attributable to sickle trait.[725] It remains to be seen whether or how these findings translate into normal civilian life, but several prominent editorials have emphasized that there is no need to proscribe either military service or vigorous athletics.[726–728] There is no evidence that people with sickle cell trait are at risk during air travel.[729] General anesthesia poses no significant excess risk to patients with sickle cell trait,[730,731] but tourniquet surgery[732] and deep hypothermia should be avoided if possible. The most consistent abnormality found in sickle trait is the inability to produce a highly concentrated urine.[565] Hematuria occurs in 1.5% of the general population and in 2.5% of people with sickle cell trait.[736] This difference in rate is statistically significant but is hardly large enough to attribute any episode of bleeding to trait. In a review of 120,000 people with trait, none had hematuria.[447] There is no associated anemia, no abnormal red cell morphology, and normal red cell survival. Because of a differential in the electrostatic interactions of normal and sickle globin chains (Fig. 53-37), most persons have about 40% hemoglobin S and 60% hemoglobin A. Coexisting α-thalassemia decreases the percentage of hemoglobin S further (see Table 53-2),[733,734] as do iron[735] and folate deficiencies.[736]

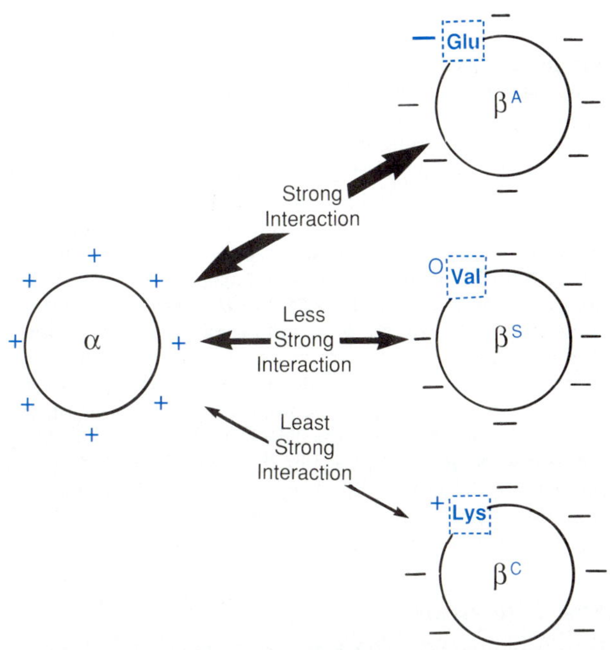

FIGURE 53-37. The relative strength of electrostatic forces between normal α-globin chains, and β-globin variants with different charges. (After Bunn HF, McDonald MJ. Electrostatic interactions in the assembly of haemoglobin. Nature 1983;306:498)

Hemoglobin SS Disease and α-Thalassemia

About 30% of African Americans have three α-globin genes (the silent carrier state of α-thalassemia), and 2% to 3% have only two α-globin genes (α-thalassemia trait).[737] Therefore, the combination of sickle cell anemia and α-thalassemia is common and well-described.[738–757] The crucial diagnostic features include the following:

- Hemoglobin electrophoresis showing no hemoglobin A, high-normal hemoglobin A_2, and predominantly hemoglobin S
- Microcytosis without iron deficiency
- Two parents with sickle trait, one with coexisting α-thalassemia trait (microcytosis and less than 35% hemoglobin S)
- Elevated Bart's hemoglobin in the cord blood
- α-Gene mapping showing two or three α-globin genes

These patients have smaller, lighter cells with a higher hemoglobin level and a lower reticulocyte count. Although the hematologic severity of sickle cell anemia is clearly ameliorated by coexisting α-thalassemia, there is no obvious effect on vasoocclusive severity,[758–761] perhaps because the benefits of a lowered MCHC are offset by the higher hematocrit and higher blood viscosity.[762]

Hemoglobin SS Disease With Elevated Fetal Hemoglobin

As discussed previously, hemoglobin F has a potent inhibitory effect on hemoglobin S polymerization, a feature that has encouraged the development of treatments designed to stimulate hemoglobin F production. Early recognition of the benefit of hemoglobin F came from the observation of Shiite Saudi Arabian patients with elevated levels of hemoglobin F (about 20%, with uneven distribution) and surprisingly mild clinical manifestations.[763–766] The hemoglobin F level in SS is highly variable. This *interperson* variation is in marked contrast to the stability of hemoglobin F levels in *individual* patients.[767] Ultimately, the amount of hemoglobin F in the blood is a function of the number of cells that contain hemoglobin F, the amount they contain, and how well those cells survive compared with cells without hemoglobin F.[768] A considerable proportion of the variation in hemoglobin F production is genetically determined.[769] Three classes of mutations are associated with an increased level of hemoglobin F: (1) large deletions in the β-globin gene cluster; (2) nondeletion or point mutations in the β-globin gene cluster; and (3) mutations *not* linked to the β-globin gene cluster (for details, see Chap. 51). Large deletions are relatively rare among SS disease patients. These virtually asymptomatic (25% to 35% hemoglobin F), mildly microcytic patients are doubly heterozygous for hemoglobin S and either δβ-thalassemia or pancellular hereditary persistence of fetal hemoglobin (HPFH).[770–774] The nondeletion mutations linked to the β-globin gene region are not consistently either heterogeneous or homogeneous in hemoglobin F distribution but are often associated with mild SS disease.[775–778] The Arab-Indian and Senegal haplotypes discussed earlier fall into this category. Hemoglobin F synthesis may also be controlled by genes unassociated with the β-globin gene cluster,[779–781] perhaps even one on the X chromosome.[782]

Sickle β-Thalassemia

Double heterozygotes for hemoglobin S and β-thalassemia have hematologic and clinical severity that correlate with the amount of output from the thalassemia gene.[783–786] Patients with thalassemia genes that produce *no* normal β-globin ($S\beta^0$-thalassemia) are typically of either African or Mediterranean origin. They have mostly hemoglobin S, elevated hemoglobin A_2, variable amounts of hemoglobin F, and *no* hemoglobin A (see Table 53-3). These patients have clinical severity comparable to that seen in SS disease. Features that help distinguish these patients from those with SS disease are their microcytosis and splenomegaly. One parent has sickle trait, and the other has β-thalassemia trait. Red cell morphology is shown in Figure 53-15 and, as in SS disease, has prominent target cells and irreversibly sickled cells. The decreased MCV of $S\beta^0$-thalassemia can be easily missed when examining the peripheral smear because of all the poikilocytosis and anisocytosis.

Patients with thalassemia genes that *do* produce some normal β-globin ($S\beta^+$-thalassemia) tend to have a milder clinical course, comparable to SC disease. These patients can be easily distinguished from those with SS disease by the presence of hemoglobin A in their blood. They also have microcytosis and splenomegaly. The electrophoretic pattern of $S\beta^+$ can be distinguished from sickle trait by the predominance of hemoglobin S over hemoglobin A.

A single base substitution involving the promoter region of a sickle β-globin gene has been reported.[787] In this Moroccan family, the thalassemic sickle gene was associated with a relatively normal hemoglobin level, low MCV (in the 60s), very low hemoglobin S (11%), and high hemoglobin A_2 (6%).[788]

Hemoglobin SC Disease

Patients with hemoglobin SC disease are doubly heterozygous for hemoglobin S ($\alpha_2\beta_2^{6Val}$) and hemoglobin C ($\alpha_2\beta_2^{6Lys}$). The gene originates in the Central West African nation of Burkina Faso, previously called Upper Volta.[1] Among African Americans, the prevalence of C trait is 2% to 3%,[789] and the prevalence of SC is about 0.04%. As seen in Table 53-2, this is a mild chronic hemolytic anemia with variable vasooclusive severity. Adults typically have a hemoglobin between 10 and 13 g/dL and 5% to 10% reticulocytes. The morphology is shown in Figure 53-15 and resembles homozygous hemoglobin C (targets, spherocytes) rather than hemoglobin S (irreversibly sickled cells). Figure 53-23 shows that children with SC disease younger than 5 years of age are characteristically more anemic (hemoglobin, 9 g/dL) and microcytic (MCV, 60 to 70 fL) than adults.[790]

All the major vasoocclusive complications of SS disease, such as recurrent bone pain, abdominal pain, chest syndrome, priapism, and stroke, have been reported in patients with SC disease,[791–794] although the rates are generally lower. Proliferative retinopathy[795–797] appears to be *more* common in SC than in SS disease, while aseptic necrosis of the femoral head[798] and renal papillary necrosis[799] are comparable. Splenomegaly is found in about 60% of patients and may result in splenic infarction[800] and sequestration,[801] especially at high altitudes. As seen in Figure 53-28, loss of splenic function occurs at a later age and is less pervasive in SC than in SS disease. The infection rate in SC disease is also lower than in SS disease,[802] but patients with SC disease have an increased rate of both pneumococcal and *H influenzae* sepsis compared with that found in the general population.[803] Prophylactic penicillin and the bacterial vaccines are recommended for children with SC disease. Previously unvaccinated adults should be vaccinated and instructed to seek immediate medical attention for fever.

SC disease is clinically more severe than sickle trait (AS) using either hematologic or vasoocclusive criteria. It is therefore surprising that mixtures of hemoglobin S and hemoglobin A polymerize almost identically to mixtures of hemoglobin S and hemoglobin C.[804] The polymerization data predict that SC should be clinically as mild as AS.

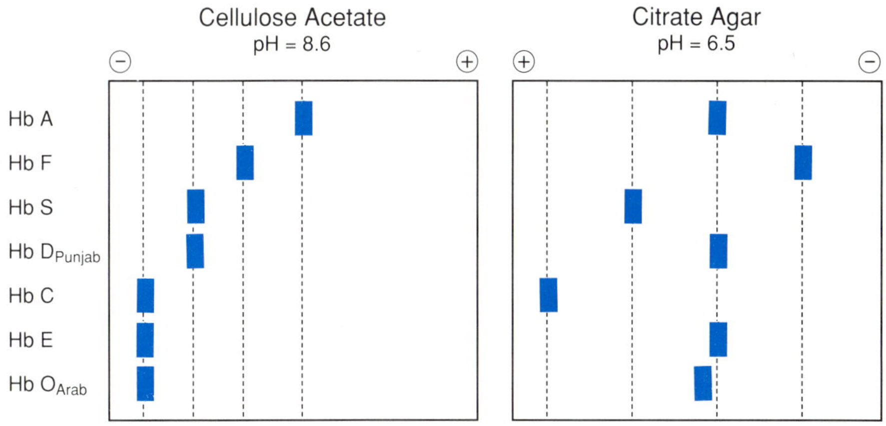

FIGURE 53-38. Electrophoresis of several hemoglobins at pH 8.6 and 6.5. The electrophoresis at pH 6.5 is necessary to distinguish hemoglobin S from hemoglobin D Punjab, and hemoglobin C from hemoglobins E and O Arab.

The apparent dichotomy between the polymerization data and the clinical observations are explained by the relative packaging of these hemoglobins in AS and SC red cells. Two major factors explain why SC cells sickle more readily than AS cells: (1) there is more hemoglobin S in an SC cell, and (2) there is a higher hemoglobin concentration in an SC cell. The higher proportion of hemoglobin S in SC cells is a function of the relative affinities of normal α chains for mutant β chains of different charge. As demonstrated by Bunn and McDonald,[805] electrostatic forces stabilize the $\alpha\beta$ dimer. The relatively positively charged α chain has a high-affinity interaction with the normally slightly negatively charged β chain (see Fig. 53-37). Because of the valine substitution for glutamic acid in the sickle β chain, there is less of a negative charge and therefore less of an affinity for α chains. In a mixture in which normal β^A chains compete with β^S chains, the normal chains have the electrostatic advantage, and a slight predominance of normal over sickle hemoglobin results. In the case of the β^C mutant, whereby a positively charged lysine substitutes for glutamic acid, the interaction is even *less* favorable. This explains the higher proportion of hemoglobin S in SC cells compared with AS cells. This increase results in about a seven-fold increase in the rate of polymerization.[804] When α chains are in short supply, as in α-thalassemia, the competition is enhanced, and the dominance of hemoglobin A over either hemoglobin S or hemoglobin C (or other positive β mutants) is exaggerated (see Table 53-2).

SC cells are also *dehydrated* compared with AS cells.[806] The mechanism involves the KCl cotransport system described earlier. The combination of SC and α-thalassemia trait has been described in a relatively asymptomatic 7-year-old girl with mild anemia (hematocrit, 26%), microcytosis (MCV, 50 to 60 fL), 7% reticulocytes, and about equal amounts of hemoglobin S and hemoglobin C. One parent had 27% hemoglobin S and an MCV of 72 fL; the other had 24% hemoglobin C and an MCV of 57 fL.[807]

Hemoglobinopathies SO_{Arab}, SD, and SE

As shown in Figure 53-38, in the typical screening electrophoresis done at pH 8.6, hemoglobin C is not readily distinguished from hemoglobin O_{Arab}, although the distinction can be made by electrophoresis at pH 6.5. Clinically, patients with SO_{Arab} have a relatively severe disorder with a chronic hemolytic anemia and vasoocclusion.[808,809] Although occasional cases of SC disease may be equally severe, these atypical patients should be evaluated to see whether they are in fact SO_{Arab} heterozygotes.

In contrast, patients who are SE heterozygotes (estimated to be 1 in 100,000 African Americans) have only a mild microcytic anemia (hemoglobin, 13 g/dL; MCV, 70 fL; 35% hemoglobin E; 64% hemoglobin S) and no vasoocclusive symptoms.[810]

SD disease is clinically similar to SS disease. As shown in Figure 53-38, hemoglobin D migrates with hemoglobin S at pH 8.6 but can be distinguished from hemoglobin S at pH 6.5. This distinction may be important when evaluating a child who appears to have SS disease but who has one parent with a negative sickle preparation.

REFERENCES

1. Nagel RL, Ranney HM. Genetic epidemiology of structural mutations of the beta-globin gene. Semin Hematol 1990;27:342.
2. Serjeant GR. Geography and the clinical picture of sickle cell disease. Ann NY Acad Sci 1989;565:109.
3. Schiliro G, Di-Gregorio F, Romeo MA, Russo A. Incidence of hemoglobin S carriers in Sicily. Hemoglobin 1986;10:95.
4. Deliyannis GA, Tavlarakis N. Sickling phenomenon in northern Greece. Br Med J 1955;2:299.
5. Lehmann H, Cutbush M. Sickle-cell trait in southern India. Br Med J 1952;1:404.
6. Negi RS. Sickle cell trait in India: a review of known distribution. Bull Anthropol Surv India 1972;17:439.
7. Lehmann H, Marajian G, Mourant AE. Distribution of sickle-cell hemoglobin in Saudi Arabia. Nature 1963;198:492.
8. Gelpi AP. Glucose-6-phosphate dehydrogenase deficiency, the sickling trait, and malaria in Saudi Arab children. J Pediatr 1967;71:138.
9. Moses WS, Matoth Y, Levin S. Sickle cell disease in Israel: report of 5 cases in an Arab family. Harefuah 1956;51:255.
10. Aksoy M. Sickle-cell trait in south Turkey. Lancet 1955;1:589.
11. Haghshenass M, Ismail-Beigi F, Clegg JB, Weatherall DJ. Mild sickle-cell anaemia in Iran associated with high levels of fetal haemoglobin. J Med Genet 1977;14:168.
12. Pagnier J, Mears JG, Dunda-Belkhodja O, Schaeffer-Rego KE, Beldjord C, Nagel RL, Labie D. Evidence for the multicentric origin of the sickle cell hemoglobin gene in Africa. Proc Nat Acad Sci USA 1984;81:1771.
13. Chebloune Y, Pagnier J, Trabuchet G, et al. Structural analysis of the 5′ flanking region of the beta globin gene in African sickle cell anemia patients: further evidence for three origins of the sickle mutation in Africa. Proc Natl Acad Sci USA 1988;85:4431.
14. Kulozik AE, Haque SK, Hilali AM, et al. Geographical survey of beta S globin gene haplotypes: evidence for an independent Asian origin of the sickle cell mutation. Am J Hum Genet 1986;39:239.
15. Ragusa A, Lombardo M, Sortino G, Lombardo T, Nagel RL, Labie D. Beta S gene in Sicily is in linkage disequilibrium with the Benin haplotype: implications for gene flow. Am J Hematol 1988;27:139.
16. Aluoch HR, Kilinc Y, Aksoy M, et al. Sickle cell anaemia among Eti-Turks: haematological, clinical and genetic observations. Br J Haematol 1986;64:45.
17. Boussio M, Christakis J, Fessas P, Loukopoulos D. The origin of the sickle mutation in Greece: evidence from beta S globin gene cluster polymorphisms. (Abstract) Blood 1987;70:59A.
18. Lapoumeroulie C, Dunda O, Trabuchet G, et al. A novel sickle gene of yet another origin in Africa: the Cameroon type. (Abstract) Blood 1989;74:63A.
19. Antonarakis SE, Boehm CD, Serjeant GR, et al. Origin of the beta S globin gene in blacks: the contribution of recurrent mutation of gene conversion or both. Proc Natl Acad Sci USA 1984;81:853.
20. Schroeder WA, Powars DR, Kay LM, et al. Beta cluster haplotypes,

alpha gene status, and hematological data from SS, SC, and S beta thalassemia patients in southern California. Hemoglobin 13:325, 1989.
21. Hattori Y, Kutlar F, Kutlar A, et al. Haplotypes of β^s chromosomes among patients with sickle cell anemia from Georgia. Hemoglobin 1986;10:623.
22. Nagel RL, Fabry ME, Pagnier J, et al. Hematologically and genetically distinct forms of sickle cell anemia in Africa. N Engl J Med 1985;312: 880.
23. Nagel RL, Rao SK, Dunda-Belkhodja O, et al. The hematological characteristics of sickle cell anemia bearing the Bantu haplotype. Blood 1987;69:1026.
24. Powars, D, Chan L, Schroeder WA. The variable expression of sickle cell disease is genetically determined. Semin Hematol 1990;27:360.
25. Perrine RP, Brown MJ, Clegg JB, Weatherall DJ, May A. Benign sickle-cell anemia. Lancet 1972;2:1163.
26. Pembrey ME, Wood WG, Weatherall DJ, Perrine RP. Fetal haemoglobin production and the sickle gene in the oases of Eastern Saudi Arabia. Br J Haematol 1978;40:415.
27. Perrine RP, Pembrey ME, John P, Perrine S, Shoup F. Natural history of sickle cell anaemia in Saudi Arabs: a study of 270 subjects. Ann Intern Med 1978;88:1.
28. Ali SA. Milder variant of sickle-cell disease in Arabs in Kuwait associated with unusually high level of foetal haemoglobin. Br J Haematol 1970;19:613.
29. Brittenham G, Lozoff B, Harris JW, Mayson SM, Miller A, Huisman THJ. Sickle cell anemia and trait in Southern India: further studies. Am J Hematol 1979;6:107.
30. Nagel RL, Roth EF. Malaria and red cell genetic defects. Blood 1989;74: 1213.
31. Weatherall DJ. Common genetic disorders of the red cell and the "malaria hypothesis." Ann Trop Med Parasitol 1987;81:539.
32. Allison AC. Protection afforded by sickle cell trait against subtertian malarial infection. Br Med J 1954;1:290.
33. Fleming AF, Storey J, Molineaux L, et al. Abnormal haemoglobins in the Sudan savanna of Nigeria. I. Prevalence of haemoglobins and relationships between sickle cell trait, malaria and survival. Ann Trop Med Parasitol 1979;73:161.
34. Luzzatto L, Nwachuku ES, Reddy S. Increased sickling of parasitized erythrocytes is mechanism of resistance against malaria in sickle trait. Lancet 1970;1:319.
35. Roth EF Jr, Friedman M, Ueda Y, Tellez I, Trager W, Nagel RL. Sickling rates of human AS red cells infected in vitro with *Plasmodium falciparum* malaria. Science 1978;202:650.
36. Friedman MJ, Roth EF, Nagel RL, Trager W. *Plasmodium falciparum*: physiological interactions with the human sickle cell. Exp Parasitol 1979;47:73.
37. Friedman MJ. Erythrocytic mechanism of sickle cell resistance to malaria. Proc Natl Acad Sci USA 1978;75:1994.
38. Pasvol G, Weatherall DJ, Wilson RJM. Cellular mechanism for the protective effect of haemoglobin S against *P. falciparum* malaria. Nature 1978;274:701.
39. Eaton WJ, Wood PA. Antimalarial red cells. Prog Clin Biol Res 1983;165:395.
40. Friedman MJ. Ultrastructural damage to the malaria parasite in the sickled cell. J Protozool 1979;26:195.
41. Hahn EV, Gillespie EB. Sickle-cell anemia: report of a case greatly improved by splenectomy. Arch Intern Med 1927;39:233.
42. Ham TH, Castle WB. Relation of increased hypotonic fragility and of erythrostasis to mechanism of hemolysis in certain anemias. Trans Assoc Am Physicians 1940;55:127.
43. Harris JW. Studies on the destruction of red blood cells. VIII. Molecular orientation in sickle-cell hemoglobin solutions. Proc Soc Exp Biol Med 1950;75:197.
44. Bunn HF. Sickle cell disease: molecular and cellular pathogenesis. In: Bunn HF, Forget BG, eds. Hemoglobin: molecular, genetic and clinical aspects. Philadelphia, WB Saunders, 1986:453.
45. Conley CL. Sickle cell anemia: the first molecular disease. In: Wintrobe MM, ed. Blood, pure and eloquent. New York, McGraw-Hill, 1980: 319.
46. Stetson CA Jr. The state of hemoglobin in sickled erythrocytes. J Exp Med 1966;123:341.
47. White JG. The fine structure of sickled hemoglobin in situ. Blood 1968;31:561.
48. Dobler J, Bertles JF. The physical state of hemoglobin in sickle cell anemia erythrocytes in vivo. J Exp Med 1968;127:711.
49. Lessin LS. Helical polymerization of hemoglobin molecules in falciform erythrocytes: A study using unmasking by cold. C R Acad Sci 1968;266:1806.
50. Finch JT, Perutz MF, et al. Structure of sickled erythrocytes and sickle cell hemoglobin fibers. Proc Natl Acad Sci USA 1973;70:718.
51. Dykes G, Crepeau RH, et al. Three-dimensional reconstruction of the fibers of sickle cell hemoglobin. Nature 1978;272:506.
52. Garrell RL, Crepeau RH, et al. Cross-sectional views of hemoglobin S fibers by electron microscopy and computer modeling. Proc Natl Acad Sci USA 1979;76:1140.
53. Dykes G, Crepeau RH, et al. Three dimensional reconstruction of the 14-filament fibers of hemoglobin S. J Mol Biol 1979;130:451.
54. Edelstein SJ. Molecular topology in crystals and fibers of hemoglobin S. J Mol Biol 1981;150:557.
55. Rodgers DW, Crepeau RH, Edelstein SJ. Pairing and polarities of the 14 strands in sickle cell hemoglobin fibers. Proc Natl Acad Sci USA 1987;84:6157.
56. Carragher B, Bluemke DA, et al. Structural analysis of polymers of sickle cell hemoglobin. I. Sickle cell hemoglobin fibers. J Mol Biol 1988;199:315.
57. Bluemke DA, Carragher B, Potel MJ, et al. Structural analysis of polymers of sickle cell hemoglobin. II. Sickle hemoglobin macrofibers. J Mol Biol 1988;199:333.
58. Carragher B, Bluemke DA, Becker M, McDade WA, et al. Structural analysis of polymers of sickle cell hemoglobin. III. Fibers within fascicles. J Mol Biol 1988;199:383.
59. Magdoff-Fairchild B, Chiu CC. X-ray diffraction studies of fibers and crystals of deoxygenated sickle cell hemoglobin. Proc Natl Acad Sci USA 1979;76:223.
60. Pumphrey JG, Steinhardt J. Crystallization of sickle hemoglobin from gently agitated solutions: an alternative to gelation. J Mol Biol 1977;112: 359.
61. Wishner BC, Ward KB, Lattman EE, Love WE. Crystal structure of sickle-cell deoxyhemoglobin at 5 A resolution. J Mol Biol 1975;98: 179.
62. Padlan EA, Love WE. Refined crystal structure of deoxyhemoglobin S. I. Restrained least-squares refinement at 3 A resolution. J Biol Chem 1985;260:8272.
63. Padlan EA, Love WE. Refined crystal structure of deoxyhemoglobin S. II. Molecular interactions in the crystal. J Biol Chem 1985;260: 8280.
64. Singer K, Singer L. The gelling phenomenon of sickle cell hemoglobin: its biological and diagnostic significance. Blood 1953;8:1008.
65. Allison AC. Properties of sickle-cell haemoglobin. Biochem J 1957;65: 212.
66. Bunn HF, Noguchi CT, et al. Molecular and cellular pathogenesis of hemoglobin SC disease. Proc Natl Acad Sci USA 1982;79:7527.
67. Adachi K, Kim J, Travitz R, et al. Effect of amino acid at the beta 6 position on surface hydrophobicity, stability, solubility, and the kinetics of polymerization of hemoglobin: comparisons among Hb A (Glu beta 6), Hb C (Lys beta 6), Hb Machida (Gln beta 6) and Hb S (Val beta 6). J Biol Chem 1987;262:12920.
68. Bookchin RM, Balzas T. Ionic strength dependence of the polymer solubilities of deoxyhemoglobins S + C and S + A mixtures. Blood 1986;67:887.
69. Fabry ME, Kaul DK, et al. SC erythrocytes have an abnormally high intracellular hemoglobin concentration: pathophysiological consequences. J Clin Invest 1982;70:1315.
70. Bookchin RM, Nagel RL, Ranney HM. The effect of $\text{beta}^{73\ \text{Asn}}$ on the interactions of sickling hemoglobins. Biochim Biophys Acta 1970;221: 373.
71. Adachi K, Kim J, Kinney TR, Asakura T. Effect of beta 73 amino acid on the hydrophobicity, solubility, and the kinetics of polymerization of deoxyhemoglobin S. J Biol Chem 1987;262:10470.
72. Adachi K, Kim J, Ballas S, et al. Facilitation of hemoglobin S polymerization by the substitution of Glu for Gln at beta 121. J Biol Chem 1988;263:5607.
73. Sturgeon P, Itano HA, et al. Clinical manifestations of inherited abnormal hemoglobins. I. The interaction of hemoglobin S with hemoglobin D. Blood 1955;10:389.
74. Schneider RG, Veda S, et al. Hemoglobin D Los Angeles in two caucasian families: hemoglobin SD disease and hemoglobin D thalassemia. Blood 1968;32:250.
75. Cawein MJ, Lappat EJ, et al. Hemoglobin SD disease. Ann Intern Med 1966;64:62.
76. Milner PF, Miller C, Grey R, Seakins M, DeJong, WW, Went LN. Hemoglobin O_{Arab} in four negro families and its interaction with hemoglobin S and hemoglobin C. N Engl J Med 1970;283:1417.
77. Charache S, Zinkham WH, et al. Hemoglobin SC, SS/G Philadelphia and SO_{Arab} disease. Am J Med 1977;62:439.
78. Goldberg MA, Husson MA, Bunn HF. The participation of hemoglobins A and F in the polymerization of sickle cell hemoglobin. J Biol Chem 1977;252:3414.
79. Benesch RE, Edalji R, Benesch R, Kwong S. Solubilization of hemoglobin S by other hemoglobins. Proc Natl Acad Sci USA 1980;77:5130.
80. Bookchin RM, Nagel RL, Balazs T. Role of hybrid tetramer formation in gelation of hemoglobin S. Nature 1977;256:667.
81. Nagel RL, Bookchin RM, Johnson J, et al. Structural bases of the inhibitory effects of hemoglobin F and hemoglobin A_2 on the polymerization of hemoglobin S. Proc Natl Acad Sci USA 1979;76:670.
82. Cheetham RC, Huehns ER, Rosemeyer MA. Participation of haemoglobins A, F, A_2, and C in polymerization of haemoglobin S. J Mol Biol 1979;129:45.
83. Benesch RE, Yung S, Benesch R, Mack J, Schneider RG. Alpha-chain contacts in polymerization of sickle haemoglobin. Nature 1976;260: 219.
84. Benesch RE, Kwong S, Benesch R, Edalji R. Location and bond type of intermolecular contacts in the polymerization of haemoglobin S. Nature 1977;269:772.

85. Benesch RE, Kwong S, Edalji R, Benesch R. Alpha-chain mutations with opposite effects on the gelation of hemoglobin S. J Biol Chem 1979;254:8169.
86. Benesch RE, Kwong S, Benesch R. The effect of alpha chain mutations cis and trans to the beta 6 mutation on the polymerization of sickle cell haemoglobin. Nature 1982;299:231.
87. Rhoda MD, Martin J, Bloquit Y, Garel MC, Edelstein SJ, Rosa J. Sickle cell hemoglobin fiber formation strongly inhibited by the Stanleyville-II mutation (beta 78 Asn-Lys). Biochem Biophys Res Commun 1983;111:8.
88. Rhoda MD, Bloquit Y, Caburi-Martin J, et al. Effects of the alpha 20 mutation on the polymerization of Hb S. Biochim Biophys Acta 1984;786:62.
89. Edelstein SJ. Molecular topology in crystals and fibers of hemoglobin S. J Mol Biol 1981;150:557.
90. Noguchi CT, Schechter AN. Sickle hemoglobin polymerization in solution and in cells. Annu Rev Biophys Chem 1985;14:239.
91. Eaton WA, Hofrichter J. Hemoglobin S gelation and sickle cell disease. Blood 1987;70:1245.
92. Schechter AN, Noguchi CT, Rodgers GP. Sickle cell disease. In: Stamatoyannopoulos G, Neinhuis AW, Leder P. Majerus PW, eds. Molecular basis of blood diseases. Philadelphia, WB Saunders, 1987.
93. Ferrone FA. Kinetic models and the pathophysiology of sickle cell disease. Ann NY Acad Sci 1989;565:63.
94. Minton AP. A thermodynamic model for gelation of sickle-cell hemoglobin. J Mol Biol 1974;82:483.
95. Ross PD, Hofrichter J, Eaton WA. Calorimetric and optical characterization of sickle cell hemoglobin gelation. J Mol Biol 1975;96: 239.
96. Ross PD, Hofrichter J, Eaton WA. Thermodynamics of gelation of sickle cell deoxyhemoglobin. J Mol Biol 1977;115:111.
97. Bertles JF, Rabinowitz R, Doebler J. Hemoglobin interaction: modification of solid phase composition in the sickling phenomenon. Science 1970;169:375.
98. Magdoff-Fairchild B, Poillon WN, Li T-I, Bertles JF. Thermodynamic studies of polymerization of deoxygenated sickle cell hemoglobin. Proc Natl Acad Sci USA 1976;73:990.
99. Hofrichter J, Ross PD, Eaton WA. Supersaturation in sickle cell hemoglobin solutions. Proc Natl Acad Sci USA 1976;73:3034.
100. Goldberg MA, Husson MA, Bunn HF. The participation of hemoglobins A and F in the polymerization of sickle hemoglobin. J Biol Chem 1977;252:3414.
101. Briehl RW. Gelation of sickle cell haemoglobin. IV. Phase transitions in hemoglobin S gels: separate measures of aggregation and solution-gel equilibrium. J Mol Biol 1978;123:521.
102. Swerdlow PH, Bryan RA, Bertles JF, Poillon WN, Magdoff-Fairchild B, Milner PF. Effect of 2,3-diphosphoglycerate on the solubility of deoxy sickle hemoglobin. Hemoglobin 1977;1:527.
103. Poillon WN, Kim BC, Walder JA. Deoxygenated sickle hemoglobin: the effects of 2,3-dephosphoglycerate and inositol hexaphosphate on its solubility. In: Beuzard Y, Charache S, eds. Approaches to the therapy of sickle cell anemia. Paris, INSERM, 1986:89.
104. Gill SJ, Benedict RC, Fall L, Spokane R, Wyman J. Oxygen binding to sickle cell hemoglobin. J Mol Biol 1979;130:175.
105. Hofrichter J. Ligand binding and the gelation of sickle cell hemoglobin. J Mol Biol 1979;128:335.
106. Sunshine HR, Hofrichter J, Ferrone FA, Eaton WA. Oxygen binding by sickle cell hemoglobin polymers. J Mol Biol 1982;158:251.
107. Hofrichter J, Eaton WA. Linear dichroism of biological chromophores. Annu Rev Biophys Bioeng 1976;5:511.
108. Eaton WA, Hofrichter J. Polarized absorption and linear dichroism spectroscopy of hemoglobin. Methods Enzymol 1981;76:175.
109. Hofrichter J, Ross PD, Eaton WA. Kinetics and mechanism of deoxyhemoglobin S gelation: a new approach to understanding sickle cell disease. Proc Natl Acad Sci USA 1974;71:4864.
110. Hofrichter J, Ross PD, Eaton WA. A physical description of the gelation of deoxyhemoglobin S. In: Hercules JI, Cottam GL, Waterman MR, Schechter AN, eds. Molecular and cellular aspects of sickle cell disease. Bethesda, DHEW Publication No (NIH) 76-1007, 1976:185.
111. Gill SJ, Spokane R, Benedict RC, Fall L, Wyman J. Ligand-linked phase equilibria of sickle cell hemoglobin. J Mol Biol 1980;140:299.
112. Behe MJ, Englander SW. Mixed gelation theory: kinetics, equilibrium and gel incorporation in sickle hemoglobin mixtures. J Mol Biol 1979;133:137.
113. Wenger GD, Balcerzak SP. Viscometric and spectrophotometric measurements of hemoglobin S polymerization kinetics. Blood 1984;63: 897.
114. Malfa R, Steinhardt J. A temperature-dependent latent period in the aggregation of sickle-cell deoxyhemoglobin. Biochem Biophy Res Commun 1974;59:887.
115. Moffat K, Gibson QH. The rates of polymerization and depolymerization of sickle cell hemoglobin. Biochem Biophys Res Commun 1974;61:237.
116. Harris JW, Bensusan HB. The kinetics of the sol-gel transformation of deoxyhemoglobin S by continuous monitoring of viscosity. J Lab Clin Med 1975;86:564.
117. Danish EH, Harris JW. Viscosity studies of deoxyhemoglobin S: evidence for formation of microaggregates during the lag phase. J Lab Clin Med 1983;101:515.
118. Sunshine HR, Hofrichter J, Eaton WA. Requirements for therapeutic inhibition of sickle hemoglobin gelation. Nature 1978;275:238.
119. Sunshine HR, Hofrichter J, Eaton WA. Gelation of sickle cell hemoglobin in mixtures with normal adult and fetal hemoglobins. J Mol Biol 1979;133:435.
120. Eaton WA, Hofrichter J, Ross PD, Tschudin RG, Becker ED. Comparison of sickle cell hemoglobin gelation kinetics by NMR and optical methods. Biochem Biophys Res Commun 1976;69:538.
121. Waterman MR, Cottam GL. Kinetics of the polymerization of hemoglobin S: studies below normal erythrocyte hemoglobin concentration. Biochem Biophys Res Commun 1976;73:639.
122. Cottam GL, Waterman MR, Thompson BC. Kinetics of polymerization of deoxyhemoglobin S and mixtures of hemoglobin A and hemoglobin S at high concentrations. Arch Biochem Biophys 1977;181:61.
123. Shibata K, Waterman MR, Cottam GL. Alteration of the rate of deoxyhemoglobin S polymerization: effect of pH and percentage of oxygenation. J Biol Chem 1977;252:7468.
124. Waterman MR, Cottam OL, Shibata K. Inhibitory effect of deoxyhemoglobin A_2 on the rate of deoxyhemoglobin S polymerization. J Mol Biol 1979;128:337.
125. San Biagio PL, Hofrichter J, Mozzarelli A, Henry ER, Eaton WA. Current perspectives on the kinetics of hemoglobin S gelation. Ann NY Acad Sci 1989;565:53.
126. Ferrone FA, Hofrichter J, Sunshine HR, Eaton WA. Kinetic studies on photolysis-induced gelation of sickle-cell hemoglobin suggest a new mechanism. Biophys J 1980;32:361.
127. Ferrone FA, Hofrichter J, Eaton WA. Kinetics of sickle hemoglobin polymerization. I. Studies using temperature-jump and laser photolysis techniques. J Mol Biol 1985;183:591.
128. Hofrichter J. Kinetics of sickle hemoglobin polymerization. III. Stochastic fluctuations in polymerization progress curves. J Mol Biol 1986;189:553.
129. Briehl RW, Salhany JM. Gelation of sickle hemoglobin. III. Nitrosyl hemoglobin. J Mol Biol 1975;96:733.
130. Ferrone FA, Hofrichter J, Eaton WA. Kinetics of sickle hemoglobin polymerization. II. A double nucleation mechanism. J Mol Biol 1985;183:611.
131. Samuel RE, Salmon ED, Briehl RW. Nucleation and growth of fibres and gel formation in sickle cell haemoglobin. Nature 1990;345:833.
132. Noguchi CT, Torchia DA, Schechter AN. ^{13}C NMR quantitation of polymer in deoxyhemoglobin S gels. Proc Natl Acad Sci USA 1979;76: 4936.
133. Noguchi CT, Torchia DA, Schechter AN. Determination of deoxyhemoglobin S polymer in sickle erythrocytes upon deoxygenation. Proc Natl Acad Sci USA 1980;77:5487.
134. Noguchi CT, Torchia DA, Schechter AN. Polymerization of hemoglobin in sickle trait erythrocytes and lysates. J Biol Chem 1981;256: 4168.
135. Noguchi CT, Torchia DA, Schechter AN. Intracellular polymerization of sickle cell hemoglobin: effects of cell heterogeneity. J Clin Invest 1983;72:846.
136. Lonsdorfer J, Bogui P, Otayeck A, Bursaux E, Poyart C, Cabannes R. Cardiorespiratory adjustments in chronic sickle cell anemia. Bull Eur Physiopathol Respir 1983;19:339.
137. Noguchi CT, Schechter AN. Intracellular polymerization of sickle hemoglobin and its relevance to sickle cell disease. Blood 1981;58: 1057.
138. Noguchi CT. Polymerization in erythrocytes containing S and non-S hemoglobins. Biophys J 1984;45:1153.
139. Brittenham GM, Schechter AN, Noguchi CT. Hemoglobin S polymerization: primary determinant of the hemolytic and clinical severity of the sickling syndromes. Blood 1985;65:183.
140. Noguchi CT, Rodger GP, Serjeant G, Schechter AN. Levels of fetal hemoglobin necessary for treatment of sickle cell disease. N Engl J Med 1988;318:96.
141. Noguchi CT, Rodgers GP, Schechter AN. Intracellular polymerization: disease severity and therapeutic predictions. Ann NY Acad Sci 1989;565:75.
142. Rodgers GP, Roy MS, Noguchi CT, Schechter AN. Is there a role for selective vasodilation in the management of sickle cell disease? Blood 1988;71:597.
143. Coletta M, Hofrichter J, Ferrone FA, Eaton WA. Kinetics of sickle haemoglobin polymerization in single red cells. Nature 1982;300:194.
144. Askura T, Mayberry J. Relationship between morphologic characteristics of sickle cells and method of deoxygenation. J Lab Clin Med 1984;104:987.
145. Mozzarelli A, Hofrichter J, Eaton WA. Delay time of hemoglobin S polymerization prevents most cells from sickling in vivo. Science 1987;237:500.
146. Nash GB, Johnson CJ, Meiselman HJ. Influence of oxygen tension on the viscoelastic behavior of red blood cells in sickle cell disease. Blood 1986;67:110.
147. Chien S, King RG, Kaperonis AA, Usami S. Viscoelastic properties of sickle cells and hemoglobin. Blood Cells 1982;8:53.
148. Sorette MP, Lavenant MG, Clark MR. Ektacytometric measurement

of sickle cell deformability as a continuous function of oxygen tension. Blood 1987;69:316.
149. Sproule BJ, Halden ER, Miller WF. A study of cardiopulmonary alterations in patients with sickle cell disease and its variants. J Clin Invest 1958;37:486.
150. Jensen WN, Rucknagel DL, Taylor WJ. In vivo study of the sickle cell phenomenon. J Lab Clin Med 1960;56:854.
151. Serjeant GR, Petch MC, Serjeant BE. The in vivo sickle phenomenon: a reappraisal. J Lab Clin Med 1973;81:850.
152. Hebbel RP. Beyond hemoglobin polymerization: the red blood cell membrane and sickle disease pathophysiology. Blood 1991;77:214.
153. Bertles JF, Milner PF. Irreversibly sickled erythrocytes: a consequence of the heterogeneous distribution of hemoglobin types in sickle cell anemia. J Clin Invest 1968;47:1731.
154. Bertles JF, Dobler J. Reversible and irreversible sickling: a distinction by electron microscopy. Blood 1969;33:884.
155. Serjeant GR, Serjeant BE, et al. The irreversibly sickled cell: a determinant of haemolysis in sickle cell anemia. Br J Haematol 1969;17: 527.
156. Serjeant GR. Irreversibly sickled cells and splenomegaly in sickle cell-anemia. Br J Haematol 1970;19:635.
157. Jensen M, Shohet SB, Nathan DG. The role of red cell energy metabolism in the generation of irreversibly sickle cells in vitro. Blood 1973;42:835.
158. Glader BE, Nathan DG. Cation permeability alterations during sickling: relation to cation composition and cellular hydration of irreversibly sickled cells. Blood 1978;51:983.
159. Lessin LS, Kuranstin-Mills J, Walles C, Weems H. Membrane alterations in irreversibly sickled cells: hemoglobin-membrane interaction. J Supramol Struct 1978;9:537.
160. Ohnishi ST, Horiuchi KY, Horiuchi K. The mechanism of in vitro formation of irreversibly sickled cells and modes of action of its inhibitors. Biochim Biophys Acta 1986;886:119.
161. Horiuchi K, Asakura T. Formation of light irreversibly sickled cell. In: Nagel RL, ed. Pathophysiological aspects of sickle vaso-occlusion. Prog Clin Biol Res 1987;240:217.
162. Horiuchi K, Ballas SK, Asakura T. The effect of deoxygenation rate on the formation of irreversibly sickled cells. Blood 1988;71:46.
163. Nash GB, Johnson CS, Meiselman HJ. Rheologic impairment of sickle RBCs induced by repetitive cycles of deoxygenation-reoxygenation. Blood 1988;72:539.
164. Lux SE, John KM, et al. Irreversible deformation of the spectrin-actin lattice in irreversibly sickled cells. J Clin Invest 1976;58:955.
165. Platt O. Exercise-induced hemolysis in sickle cell anemia: shear sensitivity and erythrocyte dehydration. Blood 1982;59:1055.
166. Tosteson DC. The effects of sickling on ion transport. II. The effect of sickling on sodium and cesium transport. J Gen Physiol 1955;39:55.
167. Tosteson DC, Shea E, Darling RC. Potassium and sodium of red blood cells in sickle cell anemia. J Clin Invest 1952;31:406.
168. Tosteson DC, Carlsen E, Dunham ET. The effects of sickling on ion transport. I. Effect of sickling on potassium transport. J Gen Physiol 1955;39:31.
169. Mohandas N, Rossi ME, Clark MR. Association between morphologic distortion of sickle cells and deoxygenation-induced cation permability increase. Blood 1986;68:450.
170. Ney PA, Christopher MM, Hebbel RP. Synergistic effects of oxidation and deformation on erythrocyte monovalent cation leak. Blood 1990;75:1192.
171. Clarke MR, Rossi ME. Permeability characteristics of deoxygenated sickle cells. Blood 1990;76:2139.
172. Glader BE, Nathan DG. Cation permeability alterations during sickling: relation to cation composition and cellular hydration of irreversibly sickled cells. Blood 1978;51:983.
173. Berkowitz LR, Orringer EP. Passive sodium and potassium movements in sickle erythrocytes. Am J Physiol 1985;249:C208.
174. Clark MR, Unger RC, et al. Monovalent cation composition and ATP and lipid content of irreversibly sickled cells. Blood 1978;51:1169.
175. Clark MR, Guatelli JC, White AT, Shohet SB. Study on the dehydrating effect of the red cell Na^+/K^+ pump in nystatin treated cells with varying Na^+ and water contents. Biochim Biophys Acta 1981;646: 422.
176. Joiner CH, Platt OS, Lux SE IV. Cation depletion by the sodium pump in red cells with pathological cation leaks: sickle cells and xerocytes. J Clin Invest 1986;78:1487.
177. Izumo H, Lear S, Williams M, Rosa R, Epstein FH. Sodium-potassium pump, ion fluxes, and cellular dehydration in sickle cell anemia. J Clin Invest 1987;79:1621.
178. Eaton JW, Sketon TD, et al. Elevated erythrocyte calcium in sickle cell disease. Nature 1973;246:105.
179. Palek J. Calcium accumulation during sickling hemoglobin S (HbSS) red cells. Blood 1973;42:988.
180. Palek J, Thomas D, et al. Red cell calcium content and transmembrane calcium movements in sickle cell anemia. J Lab Clin Med 1977;89: 1365.
181. Harrison DG, Long C. The calcium content of human erythrocytes. J Physiol 1968;199:367.
182. May A, Huehns ER. The concentration dependence of oxygen affinity of haemoglobin S. Br J Haematol 1975;30:317.
183. Steinberg MH, Eaton JW, et al. Erythrocyte calcium abnormalities and the clinical severity of sickling disorders. Br J Haematol 1978;40: 533.
184. Bookchin RM, Raventos C, et al. Abnormal vesiculation and calcium transport by "on-step" inside out vesicles from sickle cell anemia: comparisons with transport by intact cells. In: Brewer GJ, ed. The red cell: fifth annual Arbor conference. New York, Alan R. Liss, 1981: 82.
185. Gardos G. The permeability of human erythrocytes to potassium. Acta Physiol Acad Sci Hung 1956;10:185.
186. Jensen M, Shohet SB, Nathan DG. The role of red cell energy metabolism in the generation of irreversibly sickled cells in vitro. Blood
187. Bookchin RM, Ortiz OE, Lew VL. Red cell calcium transport and mechanisms of dehydration in sickle cell anemia. In: Beuzard Y, Charache S, Galacteros F, eds. Approaches to the therapy of sickle cell anemia. Paris, Les Editions INSERM, 1986:291.
188. Ohnishi ST, Horiuchi KY, Horiuchi K. The mechanism of in vitro formation of irreversibly sickled cells and modes of action of its inhibitors. Biochim Biophys Acta 1986;886:119.
189. Horiuchi K, Asakura T. Formation of light irreversibly sickled cells during deoxygenation-oxygenation cycles. J Lab Clin Med 1987;110: 653.
190. Murphy E, Berkowitz LR, Orringer E, Levy L, Gabel SA, London R. Cytosolic free calcium levels in sickle red blood cells. Blood 1987;69: 1469.
191. Lew VL, Hockaday A, Sepulveda M-I, et al. Compartmentalization of sickle cell calcium in endocytic inside-out vesicles. Nature 1985;3315: 586.
192. Lew VL, Bookchin RM. A Ca^{2+}-refractory state of the Ca-sensitive K^+ permeability mechanisms in sickle cell anemia red cells. Biochim Biophys Acta 1980;602:196.
193. Ortiz O, Lew VL, Bookchin RM. Calcium accumulated by sickle cell anemia red cells does not affect their potassium ($^{86}Rb^+$) flux components. Blood 1986;76:710.
194. Brugnara C, Bunn HF, Tosteson DC. Regulation of erythrocyte cation and water content in sickle cell anemia. Science 1986;232:388.
195. Brugnara C, Tosteson DC. Inhibition of K transport by divalent cations in sickle erythrocytes. Blood 1987;70:1810.
196. Brugnara C, Ha TV, Tosteson DC. Acid pH induces formation of dense dells in sickle erythrocytes. Blood 1989;74:487.
197. Brugnara C, Tosteson DC. Cell volume, K transport and cell density in human erythrocytes. Am J Physiol 1987;252:C269.
198. Hall AC, Ellory JC. Evidence for the presence of volume-sensitive KCl cotransport in young human red cells. Biochim Biophys Acta 1986;858:317.
199. Brugnara C, Bunn HF, Tosteson DC. Ion content and transport and the regulation of volume in sickle cells. Ann NY Acad Sci 1989;565: 96.
200. Brugnara C, Kopin AK, Bunn HF, Tosteson DC. Regulation of cation content and cell volume in erythrocytes from patients with homozgous hemoglobin C disease. J Clin Invest 1985;75:1068.
201. Canessa M, Spalvins A, Nagel RL. Volume-dependent and NEM-stimulated K^+, Cl^- transport is elevated in SS, SC and CC human red cells. FEBS Lett 1986;200:197.
202. Canessa M, Fabry ME, Blumenfeld N, Nagel RL. Volume-stimulated, Cl^--dependent K^+ efflux is highly expressed in young human red cells containing normal hemoglobin or HbS. J Membr Biol 1987;97: 97.
203. Canessa M, Fabry ME, Nagel RI. Deoxygenation inhibits the volume-stimulated, Cl^--dependent K^+ efflux in SS and young AA cells: a cytosolic Mg^{2+} modulation. Blood 1987;70:1861.
204. Chiu D, Lubin B, et al. Erythrocyte membrane lipid reorganization during the sickling process. Br J Haematol 1979;41:223.
205. Lubin B, Chiu D, et al. Abnormalities in membrane phospholipid organization in sickled erythrocytes. J Clin Invest 1981;67:1643.
206. Franck P, Chiu D, Op den Kamp JAF, et al. Accelerated transbilayer movement of phosphatidyl choline (PC) in sickled erythrocytes. J Biol Chem 1983;258:8435.
207. Chiu D, Lubin B, et al. Sickled erythrocytes accelerated clotting in vitro: an effect of abnormal membrane lipid asymmetry. Blood 1981;58: 398.
208. Choe HR, Schlegel RA, Rubin E, Williamson P, Westerman MP. Alteration of red cell membrane organization in sickle cell anemia. Br J Haematol 1986;63:761.
209. Schwartz RS, Duzgunes N, et al. Interaction of phosphatidyl serine–phosphatidylcholine liposomes with sickle erythrocytes. J Clin Invest 1982;71:1570.
210. Kuypers FA, Chiu D, et al. The molecular species composition of phosphatidylcholine affects cellular properties in normal and sickle erythrocytes. Blood 1987;70:1111.
211. Schwartz RS, Tanaka Y, Fidler IJ, Chiu DTY, Lubin B, Schroit AJ. Increased adherence of sickled and phosphatidylserine enriched human erythrocytes to cultured human peripheral monocytes. J Clin Invest 1985;75:1965.

212. Shaklai N, Yguerabide J, et al. Interaction of hemoglobin red blood cell membranes as shown by a fluroescent chromophore. Biochemistry 1977;16:5585.
213. Shaklai N, Yguerabide, et al. Classification and localization of hemoglobin binding sites on the red blood cell membrane. Biochemistry 1977;16:5593.
214. Eisinger J, Flores J. Cytosol membrane interface of the human erythrocyte: a resonance energy transfer study. Biophys J 1983;41:367.
215. Eisinger J, Flores J, et al. Association of cytosol hemoglobin with the membrane in intact erythrocytes. Proc Natl Acad Sci USA 1982;79: 408.
216. Cassloy R. Quantitative analysis of the association of human hemoglobin with the cytoplasmic portion of band 3 protein. J Biol Chem 1983;258:3859.
217. Salhany JM, Cordes KA, et al. Light scattering measurements of hemoglobin binding to the erythrocyte membrane: evidence for transmembrane effects related to a disulfic stilbene binding to band 3. Biochemistry 1980;19:447.
218. Sayare M, Schuster TM. Association of hemoglobin A and S with the cytoplasmic surface of the erythroycte membrane. Fed Proc Am Soc Exp Biol 1980;39:1916.
219. Fischer S, Nagel RL, et al. The binding of hemoglobin to membranes of normal and sickle erythrocytes. Biochim Biophys Acta 1975;375: 422.
220. Klipstein FA, Ranney HM. Electrophoretic components of the hemoglobin of red cell membranes. J Clin Invest 1960;39:1894.
221. Bank A, Mears G, et al. Preferential binding of S globin chains associated with stroma in sickle cell disorder. J Clin Invest 1974;54: 805.
222. Shaklai N, Ranney HM. Interaction of sickle cell hemoglobin with erythrocyte membranes. Proc Natl Acad Sci USA 1981;78:65.
223. Fung LWM, Litvin SD, et al. Spin-label detection of sickle hemoglobin-membrane interaction at physiological pH. Biochemistry 1983;22:864.
224. Waugh SM, Low PS. Hemichrome binding to band 3: nucleation of Heinz bodies on the erythrocyte membrane. Biochemistry 1985;24: 34.
225. Low PS, Waugh SM, Zinke K, Drenckhahn D. The role of hemoglobin denaturation and band 3 clustering in red blood cell aging. Science 1985;227:531.
226. Schneider RG, Takeda I, et al. Intraerythrocytic precipitation of haemoglobin S and C. Nature 1972;235:88.
227. Kim HC, Friedman S, et al. Inclusions in red blood cells containg HbS or HbC. Br J Haematol 1980;44:547.
228. Asakura T, Minakata K, et al. Denatured hemoglobin in sickle erythrocytes. J Clin Invest 1977;59:633.
229. Campwala HQ, Desforges JF. Membrane-bound hemichrome in density-separated cohorts of normal (AA) and sickled (SS) cells. J Lab Clin Med 1982;99:25.
230. Waugh SM, Willardson BM, Kannan R, Labotka R, Low PS. Heinz bodies induce clustering of band 3, glycophorin, and ankyrin in sickle cell erythrocytes. J Clin Invest 1986;78:1155.
230a. Corbett JD, Golan DE. Band 3 and glycophorin are progressively aggregated in density-fractionated sickle and normal red blood cells: evidence from rotational and lateral mobility studies. J Clin Invest 1993;91:208
231. Hebbel RP, Yamada O, et al. Abnormal adherence of sickle erythrocytes to cultured vascular endothelium: possible mechanism for microvascular occlusion in sickle cell disease. J Clin Invest 1980;65: 154.
232. Hoover R, Rubin R, Wise G, Warren R. Adhesion of normal and sickle erythrocytes to endothelial monolayer cultures. Blood 1979;54;872.
233. Mohandas N, Evans E. Sickle erythrocyte adherence to vascular endothelium. J Clin Invest 1985;76:1605.
234. Kaul DK, Fabry ME, Nagel RL. Microvascular sites and characteristics of sickle cell adhesion to vascular endothelium in shear flow conditions: pathophysiological implications. Proc Natl Acad Sci USA 1989;86:3356.
235. Kaul DK, ME Fabry, Nagel RL. Erythrocytic and vascular factors influencing the microcirculatory behavior of blood in sickle cell anemia. Ann NY Acad Sci 1989;565:316.
236. Weinstein R, Zhou M, et al. Sickle erythrocytes inhibit human endothelial cell DNA synthesis. Blood 1990;76:2146.
237. Mohandas N, Evans E. Adherence of sickle erythrocytes to vascular endothelial cells: requirement for both cell membrane changes and plasma factors.
238. Mohandas N, Evans E. Rheological and adherence properties of sickle cells. Ann NY Acad Sci 1989;565:327.
239. Patel VP, Ciechanover A, Platt O, Lodish HF. Mammalian reticulocytes lose adhesion to fibronectin during maturation to erythrocytes. Proc Natl Acad Sci USA 1985;82:440.
240. Hebbel RP, Visser MR, Goodman JL, Jacob HS, Vercellotti GM. Potentiated adherence of sickle erythrocytes to endothelium infected by virus. J Clin Invest 1987;60:1503.
240a. Swerlick RA, Eckman JR, Kumar A, et al. Alpha 4 beta 1-integrin expression on sickle reticulocytes: vascular cell adhesion molecule-1–dependent binding to endothelium. Blood 1993;82:1891
241. Hebbel RP, Boogaerts MAB, Eaton JW, Steinberg MH. Erythrocyte adherence to endothelium in sickle-cell anemia: a possible determinant of disease severity. N Engl J Med 1980;302:992.
242. Hebbel RP, Moldow CF, Steinberg MH. Modulation of erythrocyte endothelial interactions and the vasoocclusive severity of sickling disorders. Blood 1981;64:947.
243. Schluter K, Drenckhan D. Co-clustering of denatured hemoglobin with band 3. Proc Natl Acad Sci USA 1986;83:6137.
244. Kay MMB, Sorensen K, Wong P, Bolton P. Antigenicity, storage, and aging: physiologic autoantibodies to cell membrane and serum proteins and the senescent cell antigen. Mol Cell Biochem 1982;49:65.
245. Kay MMB, Goodman SR, Sorensen K, Whitfield CF, Wong P, Zaki L, Rudloff V. Senescent cell antigen is immunologically related to band 3. Proc Natl Acad Sci USA 1983;80:1631.
246. Galili U, Clark MR, et al. Excessive binding of natural anti-alpha-galactosyl immunoglobin G to sickle erythrocytes may contribute to extravascular cell destruction. J Clin Invest 1986;77:27.
247. Green GA, Kalra VK. Sickling-induced binding of immunoglobulin to sickle erythrocytes. Blood 1988;71:636.
248. Petz LO, Yam P, Wilkinson L, Garratty G, Lubin B, Mentzer W. Increased IgG molecules bound to the surface of red blood cells of patients with sickle cell anemia. Blood 1984;64:301.
249. Hebbel RP, Miller WJ. Phagocytosis of sickle erythrocytes: immunologic and oxidative determinants of hemolytic anemia. Blood 1984;64:733.
250. Fukuda M, Fukuda MN, Hakomori S, Papayannopoulou T. Anomalous cell surface structure of sickle cell anemia erythrocytes as demonstrated by cell surface labeling and endo-beta-galactosidase treatment. J Supramol Struct Cell Biochem 1981;17:289.
251. Basu MK, Lee MM, et al. Characteristics of I and P antigen receptors on the membrane of erythrocytes in sickle cell anemia. J Lab Clin Med 1984;103:712.
252. Liu SC, Derick LH, Zhai S, Palek J. Uncoupling of spectrin-based skeleton from the lipid bilayer in sickled red cells. Science 1991;252: 574.
253. Allan D, Limbrick AR, Thomas P, Westerman MP. Microvesicles from sickle erythrocytes and their relation to irreversible sickling. Br J Haematol 1981;47:383.
254. Allan D, Limbrick AR, Thomas P, Westerman MP. Release of spectrin-free vesicles on reoxygentation of sickled erythrocytes. Nature 1982;295:612.
255. Rank B, Carlsson J, Hebbel RP. Abnormal redox status of membrane protein thiols in sickle erythrocytes. J Clin Invest 1985;75:1531.
256. Schwartz RS, Rybicki AC, Heath RH, Lubin BH. Protein 4.1 in sickle erythrocytes: evidence for oxidative damage. J Biol Chem 1987;262: 15666.
257. Platt OS, Falcone JF, Lux SE. Molecular defect in the sickle erythrocyte skeleton: abnormal spectrin binding to sickle inside-out vesicles. J Clin Invest 1985;75:266.
258. Platt OS, Falcone JF. Membrane protein lesions in erythrocytes with Heinz bodies. J Clin Invest 1988;82:1051.
259. Hebbel RP. The sickle erythrocyte in double jeopardy: autoxidation and iron decompartmentalization. Semin Hematol 1990;27:51.
260. Hebbel RP, Eaton JW, Balasingam M, Steinberg MH. Spontaneous oxygen radical generation by sickle erythrocytes. J Clin Invest 1982;70: 1253.
261. Hebbel RP, Morgan WT, Eaton JW, Hedlund BE. Accelerated autoxidation and heme loss due to instability of sickle hemoglobin. Proc Natl Acad Sci USA 1988;85:237.
262. Liu S, Zhai S, Palek J. Detection of hemin release during hemoglobin S denaturation. Blood 1988;71:1755.
263. Jarolim P, Lahav M, Liu SC, Palek J. Effect of hemoglobin oxidation products on the stability of red cell membrane skeletons and the associations of skeletal proteins: correlation with release of hemin. Blood 1990;76:2125.
264. Kuross SA, Rank BH, Hebbel RP. Excess heme in sickle erythrocyte inside-out membranes: possible role in thiol oxidation. Blood 1988;71: 876.
265. Kuross SA, Hebbel RP. Nonheme iron in sickle erythrocyte membranes: association with phospholipids and potential role in lipid peroxidation. Blood 1988;72:1278.
266. Deuticke B, Poser B, Lutkemeier P, Haest CWM. Formation of aqueous pores in the human erythrocyte membrane after oxidative cross-linking of spectrin by diamide. Biochim Biophys Acta 1983;731:196.
267. Hebbel RP, Shalev O, Foker W, Rank BH. Inhibition of erythrocyte Ca^{2+}-ATPase by activated oxygen through thiol- and lipid-dependent mechanisms. Biochim Biophys Acta 1986;862:8.
268. Chasis JA, Mohandas N. Erythrocyte membrane deformability and stability: two distinct membrane properties that are independently regulated by skeletal protein associations. J Cell Biol 1986;103:343.
269. Hebbel RP, Leung A, Mohandas N. Oxidation-induced changes in microrheologic properties of the red blood cell membrane. Blood 1990;76:1015.
270. Hebbel RP, Miller WJ. Phagocytosis of sickle erythrocytes: immunologic and oxidative determinants of hemolytic anemia. Blood 1984;64:733.

271. Franck PFH, Op den Kamp JAF, Roelofsen B, van Deenen LLM. Does dimamide treatment of intact human erythrocytes cause a loss of phospholipid asymmetry? Biochim Biophys Acta 1986;857:127.
272. Smith DK, Palek J. Sulfhydryl reagents induce altered spectrin self-association, skeletal instability, and increased thermal sensitivity of red cells. Blood 1983;62:1190.
273. Rank BH, Moyer NL, Hebbel RP. Vesiculation of sickle erythrocytes during thermal stress. Blood 1988;72:1060.
274. Kay MMB, Bosman GJ, Shapiro SS, Bendich A, Bassel PS. Oxidation as a possible mechanism of cellular aging: vitamin E deficiency causes premature aging and IgG binding to erythrocytes. Proc Natl Acad Sci USA 1986;83:2463.
275. Chien S, Usami S, Bertles JF. Abnormal rheology of oxygenated blood in sickle cell anemia. J Clin Invest 1970;49:623.
276. Messmer MJ, Harris JW. Filtration characteristics of sickle cells. J Lab Clin Med 1970;76:527.
277. Havell TC, Hillman D, Lessin LS. Deformability characteristics of sickle cells by microelastometry. Am J Hematol 1978;4:9.
278. Clark MR. Mean corpuscular hemoglobin concentration and cell deformability. Ann NY Acad Sci 1989;565:284.
279. Clark MR, Mohandas N, Shohet SB. Deformbility of oxygenated irreversibly sickle cells. J Clin Invest 1980;65:189.
280. Gulley ML, Ross DW, Feo C, Orringer EP. The effect of cell hydration on the deformability of normal and sickle erythrocytes. Am J Hematol 1982;13:283.
281. Nash GB, Johnson CS, Meiselman HJ. Mechanical properties of oxygenated red blood cells in sickle cell (HbSS) disease. Blood 1984;63:73.
282. Fortier N, Snyder LM, Garver F, Kiefer C, McKenney J, Mohandas N. The relationship between in vivo generated hemoglobin skeletal protein complex and increased red cell membrane rigidity. Blood 1988;71:1427.
283. Evans EA, Mohandas N. Membrane-associated sickle hemoglobin: a major determinant of sickle erythrocyte rigidity. Blood 1987;70:1443.
284. Kaul DK, Fabry ME, Nagel RL. Vasoocclusion by sickle cells: evidence for selective trapping of dense red cells. Blood 1986;68:1162.
285. Fabry ME, Banjamin L, Lawrence C, Nagel RL. An objective sign in painful crisis in sickle cell anemia: the concomitant reduction of high density red cells. Blood 1984;64:559.
286. Lipowsky HH, Usami S, Chien S. Human SS red cell rheological behavior in the microcirculation of cremaster muscle. Blood Cells 1982;8:113.
287. LaCelle PL. Oxygen delivery to muscle cells during capillary vascular occlusion by sickle erythrocytes. Blood Cells 1977;3:273.
288. Baez S, Kaul DK, Nagel RL. Microvascular determinants of blood flow behavior and Hb SS erythrocyte plugging in microcirculation. Blood Cells 1982;8:127.
289. Klug PP, Lessin LS. Microvascular blood flow of sickled erythrocytes. Blood Cells 1977;3:263.
290. Rodgers GP, Schechter AN, Noguchi CT, Klein HG, Neinhuis A, Bonner RF. Periodic microcirculatory flow in patients with sickle-cell disease. N Engl J Med 1984;311:1534.
291. Klug PP, Lessin LS, Radice P. Rheological aspects of sickle cells as studied by microsieving. Arch Intern Med 1974;133:577.
292. Usami S, Chien S, Scholtz PM, Bertles JF. Effect of deoxygenation on blood rheology in sickle cell disease. Microvasc Res 1975;9:324.
293. Nash GB, Johnson CS, Meiselman HJ. Influence of oxygen tension on the viscoelastic behavior of red blood cells in sickle cell disease. Blood 1986;67:110.
294. Green MA, Noguchi CT, Keidan AJ, Marwah SS, Stuart J. Polymerization of sickle cell hemoglobin at arterial oxygen saturation impairs erythrocyte deformability. J Clin Invest 1988;81:1669.
295. Keidan AJ, Noguchi CT, Player M, Chalder SM, Stuart J. Erythrocyte heterogeneity in sickle cell disease: effect of deoxygenation on intracellular polymer formation and rheology of sub-populations. Br J Haematol 1989;72:254.
296. Keidan AJ, Sowter MC, Johnson CS, et al. Effect of polymerization tendency on haematological, rheological and clinical parameters in sickle cell anaemia. Br J Haematol 1989;71:551.
297. Sorette MP, Lavenant MG, Clark MR. Ektacytometric measurement of sickle cell deformability as a continuous function of oxygen tension. Blood 1987;69:316.
298. Johnson FL, Look AT, et al. Bone marrow transplantation in a patient with sickle cell anemia. N Engl J Med 1984;311:780.
299. Mentzer WC, Packman S, Wara W, Cowan M. Successful bone marrow transplantation in a child with sickle cell anemia and Morquio's disease. Presented at the 15th Annual Meeting of the National Sickle Cell Centers, Oakland, May 1990.
299a. Smith R. Using a mock trial to make a difficult clinical decision. Br Med J 1992;305:1284
300. Vermylen C, Cornu G, Ferster A, et al. Bone marrow transplantation in sickle cell disease: the Belgian experience. Bone Marrow Transplant 1993;12:116.
300a. Giardini C, Galimberti M, Lucarelli G, et al. Bone marrow transplantation in sickle-cell anemia in Pesaro. Bone Marrow Transplant 1993;12:122.
301. Ryan TM, Townes TM, et al. Human sickle hemoglobin in transgenic mice. Science 1990;247:566.
302. Greaves DR, Fraser P, Vidal MA, et al. Transgenic mouse model of sickle cell disorder. Nature 1990;343:183.
303. DeSimone J, Heller P, Hall L, Zwiers D. 5-Azacytidine stimulates fetal hemoglobin synthesis in anemic baboons. Proc Natl Acad Sci USA 1982;79:4428.
304. Ley TJ, DeSimone J, Anagnou NP, et al. 5-Azacytidine selectively increases beta-globin synthesis in a patient with beta$^+$ thalassemia. N Engl J Med 1982;307:1469.
305. Ley TJ, DeSimone J, Noguchi CT, et al. 5-Azacytidine increases alpha-globin synthesis and reduces the proportion of dense cells in patients with sickle cell anemia. Blood 1983;62:370.
306. Charache S, Dover G, Smith K, Talbot CC Jr, Moyet M, Boyer S. Treatment of sickle cell anemia with 5-azacytidine results in increased fetal hemoglobin production and is associated with nonrandom hypomethylation of DNA around the gamma-delta-beta-globin gene complex. Proc Natl Acad Sci USA 1983;80:4842.
307. Platt OS, Orkin SH, Dover G, Beardsley GP, Miller B, Nathan DG. Hydroxyurea enhances fetal hemoglobin production in sickle cell anemia. J Clin Invest 1984;74:652.
308. Veith R, Galanello R, Papayannopoulou T, Stamatoyannopoulos G. Stimulation of F-cell production in sickle-cell anemia treated with cytarabine or hydroxyurea. N Engl J Med 1985;313:1571.
309. Perrine SP, Miller BA, et al. Sodium butyrate enhances fetal globin gene expression in erythroid progenitors of patients with Hb SS and beta thalassemia. Blood 1989;74:454.
309a. Fibach E, Prasanna P, Rodgers GP, et al. Enhanced fetal hemoglobin production by phenylacetate and 4-phenylbutyrate in erythroid precursors derived from normal donors and patients with sickle cell anemia and beta-thalassemia. Blood 1993;82:2203.
309b. Perrine SP, Ginder GD, Faller DV, et al. A short-term trial of butyrate to stimulate fetal-globin-gene expression in the beta-globin disorders. N Engl J Med 1993;328:81
309c. Dover GJ, Brusilow S, Samid D. Increased fetal hemoglobin in patients receiving sodium 4-phenylbutyrate. N Engl J Med 199;327:569.
310. Charache S, Dover GJ, Moyer MA, Moore JW. Hydroxyurea-induced augmentation of fetal hemoglobin production in patients with sickle cell anemia. Blood 1987;69:109.
311. Charache S, Dover GJ, Moore RD, et al. Hydroxyurea: effects on hemoglobin F production in patients with sickle cell anemia. Blood 1992;79:2555.
312. Rodgers GP, Dover GJ, Noguchi CT, Schechter AN, Nienhuis AW. Hematologic responses of patients with sickle cell disease to treatment with hydroxyurea. N Engl J Med 1990;322:1037.
313. Goldberg MA, Brugnara C, Dover GJ, et al. Treatment of sickle cell anemia with hydroxyurea and erythropoietin. N Engl J Med 1990;323:366.
313a. Rodgers GP, Dover GJ, Uyesaka N, et al. Augmentation by erythropoietin of the fetal-hemoglobin response to hydroxyurea in sickle cell disease. N Engl J Med 1993;328:73.
314. Timson J. Hydroxyurea. Mutat Res 1975;32:115.
315. DePass LR, Weaver EV. Comparison of teratogenic effects of aspirin and hydroxyurea in the Fischer 344 and Wistar strains. J Toxicol Environ Health 1982;10:297.
316. Rosa R, Bierer BE, et al. A study of hyponatremia in the prevention and treatment of sickle cell crises. N Engl J Med 1980;303:1138.
317. Leary M, Abramson N. Induced hyponatremia for sickle cell crisis. N Engl J Med 1981;304:844.
318. Charache S, Walker WG. Failure of desmopressin to lower serum sodium or prevent crisis in patients with sickle cell anemia. Blood 1981;58:892.
319. Charache S, Moyer MA, et al. Treatment of acute sickle cell crises with a vasopressin analogue. Am J Hematol 1983;15:315.
320. Benjamin LJ, Kokkini G, Peterson CM. Cetiedil: its potential usefulness in sickle cell disease. Blood 1980;55:265.
321. Asakura T, Ohnishi ST, Adachi K, et al. Effect of ceteidil on erythrocyte sickling: new type of antisickling agent that may affect erythrocyte membranes. Proc Natl Acad Sci USA 1980;77:2955.
322. Schmidt WF, Asakura T, Schwartz, E. Effect of cetiedil on cation and water movements in erythrocytes. J Clin Invest 1982;69:589.
323. Benjamin LJ, Berkowitz LR, Orrigner E, et al. A collaborative double-blind randomized study of cetiedil citrate in sickle cell crisis. Blood 1986;67:1442.
324. Benjamin LJ. Membrane modifiers in sickle cell disease. Ann NY Acad Sci 1989;565:247.
325. Vitoux D, Olivieri O, Garay RP, Cragoe EJ, Galacteros F, Beuzard Y. Inhibition of K^+ efflux and dehydration of sickle cells by [(dihydroindenyl)oxy]alkanoic acid: an inhibitor of the K^+ Cl^- cotransport system. Proc Natl Acad Sci USA 1989;86:4273.
325a. Brugnara C, de Franceshi L, Alper SL. Inhibition of Ca(2+)-dependent K+ transport and cell dehydration in sickle erythrocytes by clotrimazole and other imidazole derivatives. J Clin Invest 1993;92:520.
325b. De Franceschi L, Saadane N, Trudel M, et al. Treatment with oral clotrimazole blocks Ca^{2+}-activated K^+ transport and reverses erthrocyte dehydration in transgenic SAD mice. J Clin Invest 1994;93:1670.

326. Chang H, Ewert SM, et al. Comparative evaluation of fifteen antisickling agents. Blood 1983;61:693.
327. May A, Huens E. The effect of urea on sickling. Br J Haematol 1975;30:21.
328. Cooperative Urea Trials Group. Treatment of sickle cell crisis with urea in invert sugar: a controlled trial. JAMA 1974;228:1125.
329. Benesch RE, Kwong S, Hudson BB, Krumdieck CL. p-Aminobenzoylpolyglutamates with hydrophobic end groups: a new class of inhibitors of hemoglobin S polymerization. J Biol Chem 1988;263:69.
330. Ueno H, Bai Y, Mannin JB. Covalent chemical modifiers of sickle cell hemoglobin. Ann NY Acad Sci 1989;565:239.
331. Roth EF, Nagel RL, Bookchin RM, Grayzel AI. Nitrogen mustard: an in vitro inhibition of erythrocyte sickling. Biochem Biophys Res Commun 1972;48:612.
332. Acharya AS, Manning JM. Reactivity of the amino groups of carbonmonoxy hemoglobin S with glyceraldehyde. J Biol Chem 1980;255:1406.
333. Shansuddin M, Mason RG, Ritchey JM, Honig GR, Klotz IM. Sites of acetylation of sickle cell hemoglobin by aspirin. Proc Natl Acad Sci USA 1974;71:4693.
334. Hassan W, Beuzard Y, Rosa J. Inhibition of erythrocyte sickling by cystamine, a thiol reagent. Proc Natl Acad Sci USA 1976;73:3288.
335. Garel MC, Domenget C, Caburi-Martin J, Prehu C, Galacteros F, Beuzard Y. Covalent binding of glutathione to hemoglobin. I. Inhibition of hemoglobin S polymerization. J Biol Chem 1986;261:14704.
336. Cerami A, Manning JM. Potassium cyanate as an inhibitor of the sickling of erythrocytes in vitro. Proc Natl Acad Sci USA 1971;68:1180.
337. Nigen AM, Njikam N, Lee CK, Manning JM. Studies on the mechanism of the action of cyanate in sickle cell disease. J Biol Chem 1974;249:6611.
338. Peterson CM, Tsairis P, et al. Sodium cyanate-induced polyneuropathy in patients with sickle cell disease. Ann Intern Med 1974;81:152.
339. Charache S, Duffy TR, et al. Toxic-therapeutic ratio of sodium cyanate. Arch Intern Med 1975;135:1043.
340. Diederich DA, Trueworthy RC, et al. Hematologic and clinical responses in patients with sickle cell anemia after chronic extracorporeal red cell carbamylation. J Clin Invest 1976;58:642.
340a. Platt OS. Easing the suffering caused by sickle cell disease. N Engl J Med 1994;330:783.
341. Kazazian HH Jr, Phillips DG, Dowling CE, Boehm CD. Prenatal diagnosis of sickle cell anemia—1988. Ann NY Acad Sci 1989;565:44.
342. Rowley PT. Prenatal diagnosis for sickle cell disease: a survey of the United States and Canada. Ann NY Acad Sci 1989;565:48.
343. Wilson JT, Milner PF, Summer ME, et al. Use of restriction endonucleases for mapping the allele for beta S-globin. Proc Natl Acad Sci USA 1982;79:3628.
344. Orkin SH, Little PFR, Kazazian HH, Boehm CD. Improved detection of the sickle mutation by DNA analysis: application to prenatal diagnosis. N Engl J Med 1982;307:32.
345. Chang JC, Kan YW. A sensitive new prenatal test for sickle-cell anemia. N Engl J Med 1982;307:30.
346. Conner BK, Reyes AA, Morin C, Itakura K, Teplitz RL, Wallace RB. Detection of sickle cell beta-globin allele by hybridization with synthetic oligonucleotides. Proc Natl Acad Sci USA 1983;80:278.
347. Chehab F, Doherty M, Cai S, Kan YW, Cooper S, Rubin E. Detection of sickle cell anemia and thalassemias. Nature 1987;329:293.
348. Embury SH, Scharf SJ, Saiki RK, et al. Rapid diagnosis of sickle cell anemia by a new method of DNA analysis. N Engl J Med 1987;316:656.
349. Kulozik AE, Lyons J, Kohne E, Bartram CR, Kleihauer E. Rapid and non-radioactive prenatal diagnosis of beta thalassaemia and sickle cell disease: application of the polymerase chain reaction (PCR). Br J Haematol 1988;70:455.
350. Rowley PT, Loader S, Sutera CJ, Walden M. Do pregnant women benefit from hemoglobinopathy carrier detection? Ann NY Acad Sci 1989;565:152.
351. Gaston MH, Verter JI, Woods G, et al. Prophylaxis with oral penicillin in children with sickle cell anemia. N Engl J Med 1986;314:1593.
351a. Smith JA, Kinney TR. Sickle cell disease: screening and management in newborns and infants. Am Fam Physician 1993;48:95.
352. Newborn screening for sickle cell disease and other hemoglobinopathies. Pediatrics 1989;83:1.
353. Pearson HA. Neonatal testing for sickle cell diseases: a historical and personal review. Pediatrics 1989;83:815.
354. Serjeant GR, Grandison Y, et al. The development of haematological changes in homozygous sickle cell disease: a cohort study from birth to six years. Br J Haematol 1981;48:533.
354a. Brown A, Sleeper L, Miller S, et al. Reference values and hematologic changes from birth to five years in patients with sickle cell disease. J Dis Child, in press.
355. Bensinger TA, Gillette PN. Hemolysis in sickle cell disease. Arch Intern Med 1974;133:624.
356. Odenheimer DJ, Whitten CF, Rucknagel DA, Sarnaik SA, Sing CF. Stability over time of hematological variables in 197 children with sickle cell anemia. Am J Med Genet 1984;1:461.
357. Serjeant GR. The clinical features of sickle cell disease. New York, Elsevier North-Holland, 1974.
358. Serjeant GR, Serjeant BE, Milner PF. The irreversibly sickled cell: a determinant of hemolysis in sickle cell anemia. Br J Haematol 1969;17:527.
359. Maude GH, Hayes RJ, Serjeant GR. The haematology of steady state homozygous sickle cell disease: interrelationships between haematological indices. Br J Haematol 1987;66:549.
360. Sherwood JB, Goldwasser E, Chilcote R, Carmichael LD, Nagel RL. Sickle cell anemia patients have low erythropoietin levels for their degree of anemia. Blood 1986;67:46.
361. Grasso JA, Sullivan AL, Sullivan LW. Ultrastructural studies of the bone marrow in sickle cell anemia. I. The structure of sickled erythrocytes and reticulocytes and their phagocytic destruction. Br J Haematol 1975;31:135.
362. Grasso JA, Sullivan AL, Sullivan LW. Ultrastructural studies of the bone marrow in sickle cell anemia. II. The morphology of erythropoietic cells and their response to deoxygenation in vitro. Br J Haematol 1975;31:381.
363. Peterson CM, Graziano JH, de Ciutiis A, et al. Iron metabolism, sickle cell disease and response to cyanate. Blood 1975;46:583.
364. Natta C, Weiner MA, Chang H, Wolff JA, Fawaz R. Sickle cell anemia and iron deficiency. JAMA 1982;247:1442.
365. Davies S, Henthorn J, Brozovic M. Iron deficiency in sickle cell anemia. J Clin Pathol 1983;36:1012.
366. Rao KR, Patel AR, McGinnis P, Patel MK. Iron stores in adults with sickle cell anemia. J Lab Clin Med 1984;103:792.
367. Natta C, Weiner MA, Chang H. Sickle cell anemia and iron deficiency: resemblance to sickle thalassemia. JAMA 1982;247:1442.
368. Castro O, Haddy TB. Improved (red cell) survival of iron deficient patients with sickle erythrocytes. N Engl J Med 1983;308:527.
369. Vichinsky E, Klemon K, Embury S. The diagnosis of iron deficiency anemia in sickle cell disease. Blood 1981;58:963.
370. Haddy TB, Castro O. Overt iron deficiency in sickle cell disease. Arch Intern Med 1982;142:1621.
371. Watson-Williams EJ. Folic acid deficiency in sickle cell anemia. East Afr Med J 1962;39:213.
372. Rabb LM, Grandison Y, Mason K, Hayes RJ, Serjeant B, Serjeant GR. A trial of folate supplementation in children with homozygous sickle cell disease. Br J Haematol 1983;54:589.
373. Serjeant GR. Treatment of sickle cell disease in early childhood in Jamaica. Am J Pediatr Hematol Oncol 1985;7:235.
374. Morgan AG, Gruber CA, Serjeant GR. Erythropoietin and renal function in sickle cell disease. Br Med J 1982;285:1686.
374a. Tomson CR, Edmunds ME, Chambers K, et al. Effect of recombinant human erythropoietin on erythropoiesis in homozygous sickle-cell anaemia and renal failure. Nephrol Dialysis Transplant 1992;7:817.
375. Seeler RA. Deaths in children with sickle cell anemia: a clinical analysis of 19 fatal instances in Chicago. Clin Pediatr 1972;11:634.
376. Emond AM, Collis R, Darvill D, et al. Acute splenic sequestration crisis in homozygous sickle cell disease: natural history and management. J Pediatr 1985;107:201.
377. Topley JM, Rogers DW, Stevens MCG, et al. Acute splenic sequestration and hypersplenism in the first five years in homozygous sickle cell disease. Arch Dis Child 1981;56:765.
378. Seeler RA, Shwiaki MZ. Acute splenic sequestration crises (ASSC) in young children with sickle cell anemia. Clin Pediatr 1972;11:701.
379. Thomas AN, Pattison C, Serjeant GR. Causes of death in sickle-cell disease in Jamaica. Br Med J 1985;285:633.
380. Leikin SL, Gallagher D, Kinner TR, et al. Mortality in sickle cell disease. Pediatrics 1989;84:500.
381. Pappo A, Buchanan GR. Acute splenic sequestration in a 2-month-old infant with sickle cell anemia. Pediatrics 1989;84:578.
382. Kinney TR, Ware RE, Schultz WH, Filston HC. Long-term management of splenic sequestration in children with sickle cell disease. J Pediatr 1990;117:194.
383. Rao S, Gooden S. Splenic sequestration in sickle cell disease: role of transfusion therapy. Am J Pediatr Hematol Oncol 1985;7:298.
384. Jenkins ME, Scott RB, et al. Studies in sickle cell anemia. XVI. Sudden death during sickle cell anemia crises in young children. J Pediatr 1960;56:30.
385. Githens JH, Gross GP, Eife RF, et al. Splenic sequestration syndrome at mountain altitudes in sickle/hemoglobin C disease. J Pediatr 1977;90:203.
386. Andrews J, Buchanan GR. Mild splenic sequestration crises in sickle-hemoglobin C disease. Clin Pediatr 1984;23:354.
387. Pearson HA. Hemoglobin S-thalassemia syndrome in Negro children. Ann NY Acad Sci 1969;165:83.
388. Warkentin TE, Barr RD, et al. Recurrent acute splenic sequestration crisis due to interacting gene defects: hemoglobin SC disease and hereditary spherocytosis. Blood 1990;75:266.
389. Buchanan GR, Glader BE. Benign course of extreme hyperbilirubinemia in sickle cell anemia: analysis of six cases. J Pediatr 1977;91:21.
390. Sheehy TW. Sickle cell hepatopathy. South Med J 1977;70:533.

391. Bauer TW, Moore GW, Hutchin GM. The liver in sickle cell disease: a clinicopathologic study of 70 patients. Am J Med 1980;69:833.
392. Serjeant GR, Manson K, et al. Outbreak of aplastic crises in sickle cell anemia associated with parvoviruslike agent. Lancet 1981;1:595.
392a. Serjeant GR, Serjeant BE, Thomas PW, et al. Human parvovirus infection in homozygous sickle cell disease. Lancet 1993;341:1237.
393. Goldstein AR, Anderson MJ, Serjeant GR. Parvovirus associated aplastic crisis in homozygous sickle cell disease. Arch Dis Child 1987;62:585.
394. Saarinen UM, Chorba TL, et al. Human parvovirus B19 induced epidemic of acute red cell aplasia in patients with hereditary hemolytic anemia. Blood 1986;67:1411.
395. MacIver JE, Parker-Williams EJ. Aplastic crisis in sickle-cell anemia. Lancet 1961;1:1086.
396. Singer K, Motulsky AG, et al. Aplastic crisis in sickle cell anemia. J Lab Clin Med 1950;35:721.
397. Leikin SL. The aplastic crisis of sickle cell disease: occurrence in several members of families within a short period of time. Am J Dis Child 1957;93:128.
397a. Sighal A, Cook JD, Skikne BS, et al. The clinical significance of serum transgerrin receptor levels in sickle cell disease. Br J Hematol 1993;84:301.
398. Lewis RA, Kay RW, et al. Sickle cell disease and glucose-6-phosphate dehydrogenase deficiency. J Pediatr 1969;74:544.
399. Piomelli S, Reindorf CA, et al. Interactions of G6PD deficiency and sickle cell anemia. N Engl J Med 1972;287:213.
400. Beutler E, Johnson C, et al. Prevalence of glucose-6-phosphate dehydrogenase deficiency in sickle cell disease. N Engl J Med 1974;290:826.
401. Steinberg MH, Dreiling BJ. Glucose-6-phosphate dehydrogenase deficiency in sickle cell anemia. Ann Intern Med 1974;80:217.
402. Steinberg MH, West MS, Gallagher D, Mentzer W. Effects of glucose-6-phosphate dehydrogenase deficiency upon sickle cell anemia. Blood 1988;71:748.
403. Smits HL, Oski FA, et al. The hemolytic crisis of sickle cell disease: the role of glucose-6-phosphate dehydrogenase deficiency. J Pediatr 1969;74:544.
404. Booker CR, Scott RB, et al. Studies in sickle cell anemia. XXII. Clinical manifestations during the first two years of life. Clin Pediatr 1964;3:111.
405. Whitten C. Growth status of children with sickle cell anemia. Am J Dis Child 1961;102:355.
406. McCormack MK, Dicker L, et al. Growth of children with sickle cell disease. Hum Biol 1976;48:429.
407. Phebus CK, Gloninger MF, et al. Growth patterns by age and sex in children with sickle cell disease. J Pediatr 1984;105:28.
408. Stevens MCC, Maude GH, et al. Prepubertal growth and skeletal maturation in children with sickle cell disease. Pediatrics 1986;78:124.
409. Jiminez CT, Scott RB, et al. Studies in sickle cell anemia. XXII. The effects of homozygous sickle cell disease on onset of menarche, pregnancy, fertility, pubescent changes, and body growth in Negro subjects. Am J Dis Child 1966;111:497.
410. Ashcroft MT, Serjeant GR, Desai P. Heights, weights, skeletal age of Jamaican adolescents with sickle cell anemia. Arch Dis Child 1972;47:519.
411. Platt OS, Rosenstock W, et al. Influence of sickle hemoglobinopathies on growth and development. N Engl J Med 1984;311:7.
412. Luban NLC, Leikin S, August GA. Growth and development in sickle cell anemia. Am J Pediatr Hematol Oncol 1982;4:61.
413. Alleyne SI, Rauseo RD, et al. Sexual development and fertility of Jamaican female patients with homozygous sickle cell disease. Arch Intern Med 1981;141:1295.
414. Oberfield SE, Wethers DL, et al. Growth hormone responses to growth hormone releasing factor in sickle cell disease. Am J Pediatr Oncol 1987;9:331.
415. Osegbe DN, Akinyanju O, et al. Fertility in males with sickle cell disease. Lancet 1981;2:275.
416. Olambiwonnu NO, Penny R, et al. Sexual maturation in subjects with sickle cell anemia: studies of serum gonadotropin concentration, height, weight, and skeletal age. J Pediatr 1975;87:459.
417. Abbasi AA, Prasad AS, et al. Gonadal function abnormalities in sickle cell anemia. Ann Intern Med 1976;85:601.
418. Landerfeld M, Schambelau M, et al. Clomiphine-responsive hypogonadism in sickle cell anemia. Ann Intern Med 1983;99:480.
419. Wethers DL. Delayed growth and sexual maturation in sickle cell disease. Ann NY Acad Sci 1989;565:137.
420. Singhal A, Davies P, Sahota A, et al. Resting metabolic rate in homozygous sickle cell disease. Clin Nutr 1993;57:32.
421. Heymann MB, Vichinsky E, et al. Growth retardation in sickle cell disease treated by nutritional support. Lancet 1985;1:903.
422. Prasad AS. Zinc supplementation and growth in sickle cell disease. Ann Intern Med 1984;100:367.
423. Seeler RA. Deaths in children with sickle cell anemia: a clinical analysis of 19 fatal instances in Chicago. Clin Pediatr 1972;11:634.
424. Barrett-Connor E. Bacterial infection and sickle cell anemia: an analysis of 25 infections in 166 patients and a review of the literature. Medicine 1971;50:97.
425. Robinson MG. Clinical aspects of sickle cell disease. In: Levere RD, ed. Sickle cell anemia and other hemoglobinopathies. New York, Academic Press, 1975.
426. Zarkowsky HS, Gallagher D, et al. Bacteremia in sickle hemoglobinopathies. J Pediatr 1986;109:579.
427. Pearson HA, Spencer RP, et al. Functional asplenia in sickle-cell anemia. N Engl J Med 1969;281:923.
428. O'Brien RT, McIntosh S, et al. Prospective study of sickle cell anemia in infancy. J Pediatr 1976;89:205.
429. Pearson HA, McIntosh S, et al. Interference phase microscopic enumeration of pitted RBC and splenic hypofunction in sickle cell anemia. Pediatr Res 1978;12:471.
430. Seeler RA, Metzger W, et al. *Diplococcus pneumoniae* infections in children with sickle cell anemia. Am J Dis Child 1972;123:8.
431. Pearson HA, Cornelius EA, et al. Transfusion-reversible functional asplenia in young children with sickle cell anemia. N Engl J Med 1970;283:334.
431a. Ferster A, Bujan W, Corazza F, et al. Bone marrow transplantation corrects the splenic reticuloendothelial dysfunction in sickle cell anemia. Blood 1993;891:1102.
432. Pearson HA, Gallagher D, et al. Developmental pattern of splenic dysfunction in sickle cell disorders. Pediatrics 1985;76:392.
433. Overturf GD, Powars D, et al. Bacterial meningitis and septicemia in sickle cell disease. Am J Dis Child 1977;131:784.
434. Buchanan GR, Smith SJ, Holtkamp CA, Fuseler JP. Bacterial infection and splenic reticuloendothelial function in children with hemoglobin SC disease. Pediatrics 1983;72:93.
435. Topley JM, Cupidor L, Vaidya S, Hays RJ, Serjeant GR. Pneumococcal and other infections in children with sickle cell hemoglobin C (SC) disease. J Pediatr 1982;101:176.
436. Powars D, Overturf GD, Wilkins J. Commentary: infections in sickle cell and SC disease. J Pediatr 1983;103:242.
437. Powars D, Overturf G, et al. Is there an increased risk of *Haemophilus influenzae* septicemia in children with sickle cell anemia? Pediatrics 1983;71:927.
438. Gaston MH, Verter JI. Prophylaxis with oral penicillin in children with sickle cell anemia: a randomized trial. N Engl J Med 1986;314:1593.
439. Wilimas JA, Flynn PM, Harris S, et al. A randomized study of outpatient treatment with ceftriaxone for selected febrile children with sickle cell disease. N Engl J Med 1993;329:472.
440. Overturf GC, Field R, Lam C, Lee S, Powars DR. Nasopharyngeal (NP) carriage of S. pneumoniae and relationship to serum antibody in immunized children with sickle cell disease (SCD). Infect Immunol 1980;28:1048.
441. Ammann AJ, Addrego J, et al. Polyvalent pneumococcal-polysaccharide immunization of patients with sickle cell anemia and patients with splenectomy. N Engl J Med 1977;297:897.
442. Overturf GD, Rigau-Perez JG, et al. Pneumococcal polysaccharide immunization of children with sickle cell disease. I. Clinical reactions to immunization and relationship to preimmunization antibody. Am J Pediatr Hematol Oncol 1982;4:19.
443. Chudwin DS, Wara DW, et al. Increases in serum opsonic activity and antibody concentration in patients with sickle cell disease after pneumococcal polysaccharide immunization. J Pediatr 1983;102:51.
444. Buchanan GR, Schiffman G. Antibody responses to polyvalent pneumococcal vaccine in infants with sickle cell anemia. J Pediatr 1980;96:264.
445. McIntosh S, Rooks Y, et al. Fever in young children with sickle cell disease. J Pediatr 1980;96:199.
446. Buchanan GR, Glader BE. Leukocyte counts in children with sickle cell disease. Arch Dis Child 1978;132:396.
447. Konotey-Ahulu FID. The sickle cell diseases. Arch Intern Med 1974;133:611.
448. Baum KF, Dunn DT, et al. The painful crisis of homozygous sickle cell disease: a study of risk factors. Arch Intern Med 1987;147:1231.
449. Milner PF, Brown M, et al. Bone marrow infarction in sickle cell anemia: correlation with hematologic profiles. Blood 1982;60:1411.
450. Charache S, Page DL. Infarction of bone marrow in the sickle cell disorders. Ann Intern Med 1967;67:1195.
451. Mankad VN, Williams JP, Harpen MD, et al. Magnetic resonance imaging of bone marrow in sickle cell disease: clinical, hematological, and pathological correlations. Blood 1990;75:274.
452. Keeley K, Buchanan GR. Acute infarction of long bones in children with sickle cell anemia. J Pediatr 1982;101:170.
453. Sain A, Sham R, et al. Bone scan in sickle cell crisis. Clin Nucl Med 1978;3:85.
454. Alavi A, Schumacher HR, et al. Bone marrow scan evaluation of arthropathy in sickle cell disorders. Arch Intern Med 1976;136:436.
455. Hammel CF, DeNardo SJ, et al. Bone marrow and bone mineral scintigraphic studies in sickle cell disease disease. Br J Haematol 1973;25:593.
456. Lutzker LG, Alavi A. Bone and marrow imaging in sickle cell disease: diagnosis of infarction. Semin Nucl Med 1976;6:83.
457. Gordon PA, Breeze GR, Mann JR, Stuart J. Coagulation fibrinolysis in sickle cell disease. J Clin Pathol 1974;27:485.

458. Freedman ML, Karpatkin S. Elevated platelet count and megathrombocyte number in sickle cell anemia. Blood 1975;46:579.
459. Stuart MJ, Stockman A, Oski FA. Abnormalities of platelet aggregation in the vasoocclusive crisis of sickle cell anemia. J Pediatr 1974;85:629.
460. Leichtman DA, Brewer GJ. A plasma inhibitor of ristocetin-induced platelet aggregation in platelet with sickle hemoglobinopathies. Am J Hematol 1977;2:251.
461. Mehta P, Mehta J. Abnormalities of platelet aggregation in sickle cell disease. J Pediatr 1980;96:209.
462. Buchanan GR, Holtkamp CA. Platelet aggregation, malondialdahyde generation and production time in children with sickle cell anaemia. Thromb Haemost 1981;46:610.
463. Buchanan GR, Hotlkamp CA. Evidence against enhanced platelet activity in sickle cell anaemia. Br J Haematol 1983;54:595.
464. Matti R, Weinger R, Sisc HS. Coagulation, fibrinogen survival and fibrin split products in sickle cell disease. Blood 1973;42:1004.
465. Leslie J, Langler D, Serjeant GR, Serjeant BE, Desai P, Gordon YB. Coagulation changes during the steady state in homozygous sickle cell disease in Jamaica. Br J Haematol 1975;30:159.
466. Ittyerah R, Alkjaersig N, Fletcher A, Chaplin H. Coagulation factor XIII concentration in sickle cell disease. J Lab Clin Med 1976;88:546.
467. Leichtman DA, Brewer GJ. Elevated plasma levels of fibrinopepetide A during sickle cell anemia pain crisis: evidence for intravascular coagulation. Am J Hematol 1978;5:183.
468. Alkjaersig N, Fletcher A, Joist H, Chaplin H Jr. Hemostatic alterations accompanying sickle cell pain crises. J Lab Clin Med 1976;88:440.
469. Roth EF Jr, Bardfeld PA, Goldsmith SJ, Radel E, Williams JC. Sickle cell crisis as evaluated from measurements of hydroxybutyrate dehydrogenase and myoglobin in plasma. Clin Chem 1981;27:314.
470. Karayalcin G, Lanzkowsky P, Kazi AB. Serum alpha-hydroxybutyrate dehydrogenase levels in children with sickle cell disease. Am J Pediatr Hematol Oncol 1981;3:169.
471. Fabry ME, Benjamin L, Lawrence C, Nagel RL. An objective sign in painful crisis in sickle cell anemia: the concomitant reduction of high density red cells. Blood 1984;64:559.
472. Redwood AM, Williams EM. Climate and painful crises of sickle cell disease in Jamaica. Br Med J 1976;1:66.
473. Akinyanju OO. A profile of sickle cell disease in Nigeria. Ann NY Acad Sci 1989;565:126.
474. Ibrahim AS. Relationship between meteorological changes and occurrence of painful sickle cell crises in Kuwait. Trans R Soc Trop Med Hyg 1980;74:159.
474a. Gelfand MJ, Daya SA, Rucknagel DL, et al. Simultaneous occurrence of rib infarction and pulmonary infiltrates in sickle cell disease patients with acute chest syndrome. J Nucl Med 1993;34:614.
475. Diggs LW. Bone and joint lesions in sickle-cell disease. Clin Orthop 1967;51:119.
476. Watson RJ, Burko H, et al. The hand–foot syndrome in sickle-cell disease in young children. Pediatrics 1963;45:975.
477. Worrell VT, Batera V. Sickle cell dactylitis. J Bone Joint Surg 1976;58:1161.
478. Bainbridge R, Higgs DR, Maude GH, Serjeant GR. Clinical presentation of homozygous sickle cell disease. J Pediatr 1985;106:881.
479. Serjeant GR, Ashcroft MT. Shortening of the digits in sickle cell anemia: a sequela of the hand–foot syndrome. Trop Geogr Med 1971;23:341.
480. Embury SH, Garcia JF, et al. Effects of oxygen inhalation on endogenous erythropoietin kinetics, erythropoiesis, and properties of blood cells in sickle cell anemia. N Engl J Med 1984;311:291.
481. Laszlo J, Obenour W, Saltzman HA. Effects of hyperbaric oxygenation on sickle syndromes. South Med J 1969;62:453.
482. Cooperative Urea Trials Group. Clinical trials of therapy for sickle cell vaso-occlusive crises. JAMA 1974;228:1120.
483. Cole TB, Sprinkle RH, Smith SJ, Buchanan GR. Intravenous narcotic therapy for children with severe sickle cell pain crisis. Am J Dis Child 1986;140:1255.
484. Haynes J, Allison R. Pulmonary edema, complication in the management of sickle cell pain crisis. Am J Med 1986;80:833.
485. Vichinsky EP, Johnson R, et al. Multidisciplinary approach to pain management in sickle cell disease. Am J Pediatr Hematol Oncol 1982;4:328.
486. Payne R. Pain management in sickle cell disease, rationale and techniques. Ann NY Acad Sci 1989;565:189.
487. Ortiz-Neu C, Marr JS, et al. Bone and joint infections due to *Salmonella*. J Infect Dis 1978;138:820.
487a. Milner PF, Kraus AP, Sebes JI, et al. Sickle cell disease as a cause of ostenecrosis of the femoral head. N Engl J Med 1991;325:1476.
488. Lee REJ, Golding JSR, Serjeant GR. The radiological features of avascular necrosis of the femoral head in homozygous sickle cell disease. Clin Radiol 1981;32:205.
489. Rao VM, Fishman M, et al. Painful sickle cell crisis: bone marrow patterns observed with MR imaging. Radiology 1986;161:211.
490. Rodgers GP, Noguchi CT, Schechter AN. Non-invasive techniques to evaluate the vaso-occlusive manifestations of sickle cell disease. Am J Pediatr Hematol Oncol 1985;7:245.
491. Bishop AR, Roberson JR, Eckman JR, Fleming LL. Total hip arthroplasty in patients who have sickle-cell hemoglobinopathy. J Bone Joint Surg 1988;70:853.
492. Clarke HJ, Jinnah RH, et al. Total replacement for avascular necrosis in sickle cell disease. J Bone Joint Surg 1989;71:465.
493. Camp JD, Colwell CW Jr. Core decompression of the femoral head for osteonecrosis. J Bone Joint Surg 1986;68A:1313.
494. Milner PF, Kraus AP, Sebes JI, et al. Ostenocrosis of the humeral head in sickle cell disease. Clin Orthop Rel Res 1993;289:136.
495. Johnson CS, Verdegem TD. Pulmonary complications of sickle cell disease. Semin Respir Med 1988;9:287.
496. Thomas AN, Pattison C, et al. Causes of death in sickle cell disease in Jamaica. Br J Med 1982;285:633.
497. DeCeulaer K, McMullen KW, et al. Pneumonia in young children with homozygous sickle cell disease: risk and clinical features. Eur J Pediatr 1985;144:255.
498. Sprinkle RH, Cole T, Smith S, Buchanan GR. Acute chest syndrome in children with sickle cell disease. Am J Pediatr Hematol Oncol 1986;8:105.
499. Barrett-Connor E. Acute pulmonary disease and sickle cell anemia. Am Rev Respir Dis 1971;104:159.
500. Barrett-Connor E. Pneumonia and pulmonary infarction in sickle cell anemia. JAMA 1973;224:997.
501. Poncz M, Kane E, Gill FM. Acute chest syndrome in sickle cell disease: etiology and clinical correlates. J Pediatr 1985;107:861.
502. Petch MC, Serjeant GR. Clinical features of pulmonary lesions in sickle cell anemia. Br Med J 1970;3:31.
503. Davies SC, Luce PJ, et al. Acute chest syndrome in sickle-cell disease. Lancet 1984;1:36.
504. Haupt HM, Moore GW, et al. The lung in sickle cell disease. Chest 1982;81:332.
505. Diggs LW. Pulmonary lesions in sickle cell anemia. Blood 1969;34:734.
506. Athanasou NA, Hatton C, McGee JO, Weatherall DJ. Vascular occlusion and infarction in sickle cell crisis and the sickle chest syndrome. J Clin Pathol 1985;38:659.
507. Hutchinson RM, Merrick MV, White JM. Fat embolism in sickle cell disease. J Clin Pathol 1973;26:620.
507a. Weil JV, Castro O, Malik AB, Rodgers G, et al. NHLBI Workshop summary: pathogenesis of lung disease in sickle hemoglobinopathies. Am Rev Respir Dis 1993;148:249.
508. Charache S, Scott JC, Charache P. Acute chest syndrome in adults with sickle cell anemia: microbiology, treatment, and prevention. Arch Intern Med 1979;139:67.
508a. Pianosi P, Charge TD, Esseltine DW, et al. Pulse oximetry in sickle cell disease. Arch Dis Childhood 1993;68:735.
508b. Rockoff WR, Kunkel N, Silber JH, et al. Pulse oximetry and factors associated with hemoglobin oxygen desaturation in children with sickle cell disease. Blood 1993;81:3422.
509. Wall MA, Platt OS, et al. Lung function in children with sickle cell anemia. Am Rev Respir Dis 1979;120:210.
510. Powars D, Weidman JA, Odom-Maryon T, Niland JC, Johnson C. Sickle cell chronic lung disease: prior morbidity and the risk of pulmonary failure. Medicine 1988;67:66.
511. Powars D, Wilson B, et al. The natural history of stroke in sickle cell disease. Am J Med 1978;65:461.
511a. Balkaran B, Char G, Morris JS, et al. Stroke in a cohort of patients with homozygous sickle cell disease. J Pediatr 1992;120:360.
512. Russell MO, Goldberg HL, et al. Effect of transfusion therapy on arteriographic abnormalities and on recurrence of stroke in sickle cell disease. Blood 1984;63:162.
513. Allen J, Imbus C, Powars D, Haywood LJ. Neurological impairment induced by hyperventilation in children with sickle cell anemia. Pediatrics 1976;58:124.
514. Arnow P, Panwalker A, Garvin J, Rodriguez-Erdmann F. Aspirin hyperventilation and cerebellar infarction in sickle cell disease. Arch Intern Med 1978;138:148.
514a. Rackoff WR, Ohene-Frempong K, Month S, et al. Neurologic events after partial exchange transfusion of priapism in sickle cell disease. J Pediatr 1992;120:882.
515. Portnoy B, Herion JC. Neurological manifestations in sickle cell disease. Ann Intern Med 1972;76:643.
516. Stockman JA, Nigro MA, et al. Occlusion of large cerebral vessels in sickle cell anemia. N Engl J Med 1972;287:846.
517. Wilimas J, Goff JR, et al. Efficacy of tranfusion therapy for one or two years in patients with sickle cell disease and cerebrovascular accidents. J Pediatr 1980;96:205.
518. Boros L, Thomas C, et al. Large cerebral vessel disease in sickle cell anemia. J Neurol Neurosurg Psychiatr 1976;39:1236.
519. Merkel KH, Ginsberg PL, et al. Cerebrovascular disease in sickle cell anemia: a clinical, pathological and radiological correlation. Stroke 1978;9:45.
520. Koshy M, Thomas C, Goodwon J. Vascular lesions in the central nervous system in sickle cell disease (neuropathology). J Assoc Acad Minority Phys 1990;1:71.
521. Hitchock ER, Tsementizis SA, et al. Subarachnoid hemorrhage in sickle cell anemia. Surg Neurol 1983;19:251.

522. Zimmerman RA, Gill F, Goldberg HI, et al. MRI of sickle cell cerebral infarction. Neuroradiology 1987;29:232.
523. Pavlakis SG, Bello J, Prohovnik I, et al. Brain infarction in sickle cell anemia: magnetic resonance imaging correlates. Ann Neurol 1988;23: 125.
524. Adams RJ, Nichols FT, El Gammal T, et al. Noninvasive detection of cerebral vasculopathy using transcranial Doppler and magnetic resonance imaging. Ann NY Acad Sci 1989;565:358.
524a. Adams R. McKie V, Nichols F, et al. The use of transcranial ultrasonography to predict stroke in sickle cell disease. N Engl J Med 1992;326:605.
524b. Adams RL, Nichols FT, Figueroa R, et al. Transcranial Doppler correlation with cerebral angiography in sickle cell disease. Stroke 1992;23:1073
524c. Seibert JJ, Miller SF, Kirby RS, et al. Cerebrovascular disease in symptomatic and asymptomatic patients with sickled cell anemia: screening with duplex transcranial Doppler US—correlation with MR imaging and MR angiography. Radiology 1993;189:457.
525. Russell MO, Goldberg HI, et al. Tranfusion therapy for cerebrovascular abnormalities is sickle cell disease. J Pediatr 1976;88:382.
526. Lusher JM, Haghighat H, et al. A prophylactic transfusion program for children with sickle cell anemia complicated by CNS infarction. Am J Hematol 1976;1:265.
527. Seeler RA, Royal JE. Commentary: sickle cell anemia, stroke, and transfusion. J Pediatr 1980;96:243.
528. Buchanan GR, Bowman WP, et al. Recurrent cerebral ischemia during transfusion therapy in sickle cell anemia. J Pediatr 1983;103:92.
529. Greenbaum BH, Kim HC. Recurrent strokes in two siblings with sickle-cell disease and von Willebrand's disease: implications of the role of platelets. J Pediatr Hematol Oncol 1988;5:239.
530. Miller ST, Rao SP, Jensen D, Brown AK. Is chronic transfusion necessary to prevent recurrent stroke in children with sickle cell disease? Ann NY Acad Sci 1989;565:435.
531. Wang W, Kovnar E, Tonkin I, et al. High risk of recurrent stroke following discontinuation of transfusion in sickle cell patients transfused for 5–20 years. Presented at the 15th Annual Meeting of the National Sickle Cell Centers. Berkeley CA, May, 1990.
531a. Cohen AR, Martin MB, Silber JH, et al. A modified transfusion program for prevention of stroke in sickle cell disease. Blood 1992;79:1657.
532. Van Hoff J, Ritchey AK, Shaywitz BA. Intracranial hemorrhage in children with sickle cell disease. Am J Dis Child 1985;139:1120.
533. Eckman J, Platt A, Oyesiku N. Subarachnoid hemorrhage in patients with sickle cell syndromes: a ten year experience. Presented at 15th Annual Meeting of the National Sickle Cell Centers, Berkeley, CA, May 1990.
533a. Anson JA, Koshy M, Ferguson L, et al. Subarachnoid hemorrhage in sickle cell disease. J Neurosurg 1991;75:552.
534. Powars DR, Adams RJ, Nichols FT, et al. Delayed intracranial hemorrhage following cerebral infarction in sickle cell anemia. J Assoc Acad Minority Phys 1990;1:79.
535. Finch CA. Pathophysiologic aspects of sickle cell anemia. Am J Med 1972;53:1.
536. Lindo CL, Doctor LR. The electrocardiogram in sickle cell anemia. Am Heart J 1955;40:218.
537. Klinefelter HF. The heart in sickle cell anemia. Am J Med Sci 1942;203: 34.
538. Winsor T, Burch GE. The electrocardiogram and cardiac state in active sickle cell anemia. Am Heart J 1944;29:685.
539. Shubin H, Kaufman R, et al. Cardiovascular findings in children with sickle cell anemia. Am J Cardiol 1960;6:875.
540. Sproule BJ, Halden ER, et al. A study of cardiopulmonary alterations in patients with sickle cell disease and its variants. J Clin Invest 1957;37:486.
541. Ng ML, Liebman J, Anslovar J, Gross S. Cardiovascular findings in children with sickle cell anemia. Dis Chest 1967;52:788.
542. Lindsay J, Meshel JC, Patterson RH. The cardivascular manifestations of sickle cell disease. Arch Intern Med 1974;133:643.
543. O'Neill B Jr, Saunders DE Jr, et al. Myocardial infarction in sickle cell anemia. Am J Hematol 1984;16:139.
544. Martin C, Cobb C, Johnson C, Tatter D, Haywood LJ. Cardiovascular pathology in sickle cell disease. J Am Cardiol 1983;1:723.
545. Jensen WN, Rucknagel DL, et al. In vivo study of the sickle cell phenomenon. J Lab Clin Med 1960;56:854.
546. McNamara JJ, Molot MA Jr, et al. Coronary artery disease in combat casualties in Vietnam. JAMA 1971;216:1185.
547. Gerry JL, Buckley MG, et al. Clinicopathologic analysis of cardiac dyfunction in 52 patients with sickle cell anemia. Am J Cardiol 1978;42:211.
548. Haywood LJ, Martin C, Tatter D, Norris S, Johnson CS. Nature of cardiac findings in sickle cell anemia. Ann NY Acad Sci 1989;565: 393.
549. Falk RH, Hood WB Jr. The heart in sickle cell anemia. Arch Intern Med 1982;142:1680.
550. Gerry JL, Baird MG, et al. Evaluation of left ventricular function in patients with sickle cell anemia. Am J Med 1976;60:967.
551. Val-Mejias J, Lee W, et al. Left ventricular performance during and after sickle cell crises. Am Heart J 1979;97:585.
552. Manno BV, Burka ER, et al. Biventricular function in sickle-cell anemia: radionuclide angiographic and thallium-201 scintigraphic evaluation. Am J Cardiol 1983;52:584.
553. Covarrubias EA, Sheikh MU, et al. Left ventricular function in sickle cell anemia: a noninvasive evaluation. South Med J 1980;73:342.
554. Rees AH, Stefadouros MA, et al. Left ventricular performance in children with homozygous sickle cell anaemia. Br Heart J 1978;40:690.
555. Alpert BS, Gilman PA, et al. Hemodynamic and ECG responses to exercise in children with sickle cell anemia: a radionuclide study. Am J Dis Child 1981;135:362.
556. Covits W, Eubig C, et al. Exercise-induced cardiac dysfunction in sickle cell anemia: a radionuclide study. Am J Cardiol 1983;51:570.
557. Denenberg BS, Criner G, et al. Cardiac function in sickle cell anemia. Am J Cardiol 1983;51:1674.
558. Willens HJ, Lawrence C, et al. A noninvasive comparison of left ventricular performance in sickle cell anemia and chronic aortic regurgitation. Clin Cardiol 1983;6:542.
559. Johnson CS, Giorgio AJ. Arterial blood pressure in adults with sickle cell disease. Arch Intern Med 1981;141:891.
560. Moser KM, Shea JC. The relationship between pulmonary infarction, cor pulmonale and the sickle states. Am J Med 1957;22:561.
561. Charache S, Bleecher ER, et al. Effects of blood transfusion on exercise capacity in patients with sickle cell anemia. Am J Med 1983;74:757.
562. Maisel A, Friedman H, et al. Continuous electrocardiographic monitoring in patients with sickle-cell anemia during pain crisis. Clin Cardiol 1983;6:339.
563. Whitten CF, Younes AA, et al. Comparative study of renal concentrating ability in children with sickle cell anemia and in normal children. J Lab Clin Med 1960;55:400.
564. Hatch FE, Culbertson JW, et al. Nature of the renal concentrating defect in sickle cell disease. J Clin Invest 1967;46:336.
565. Schlitt LE, Keital HG. Renal manifestations of sickle cell disease: a review. Am J Med Sci 1960;239:773.
566. Statius van Eps LW, Schouten H, et al. The influence of red blood cell transfusions on the hyposthenuria and renal hemodynamics of sickle cell anemia. Clin Chim Acta 1967;17:449.
567. Statius van Eps LW, Pinedo-Veels C, et al. Nature of concentrating defect in sickle-cell nephropathy. Lancet 1970;1:450.
568. Perillie PE, Epstein FH. Sickling phenomenon produced by hypertonic solutions: a possible explanation for the hyposthenuria of sicklemia. J Clin Invest 1963;42:570.
569. Buckalew VM, Someren A. Renal manifestations of sickle cell disease. Arch Intern Med 1974;133:660.
570. Noll JB, Newman AJ, et al. Enuresis and nocturia in sickle cell disease. J Pediatr 1967;70:965.
571. Radel EG, Kochen JA, et al. Hyponatremia in sickle cell disease: a renal salt losing state. J Pediatr 1976;88:800.
572. Goossens JP, Statius van Eps LW, et al. Incomplete renal tubular acidosis in sickle cell disease. Clin Chim Acta 1972;41:149.
573. Oster JR, Lespier LE, et al. Renal acidification in sickle cell disease. J Lab Clin Med 1976;88:389.
574. Yoshino M, Amerian R, et al. Hyporeninemic hypoaldosteronism in sickle cell disease. Nephrologie 1982;31:242.
575. Oster JR, Lanier DC Jr, et al. Renal response to potassium loading in sickle cell trait. Arch Intern Med 1980;140:534.
576. DeFronzo RA, Taufield PA, Black H, MePhedran P, Cooke CR. Impaired renal tubular potassium secretion in sickle cell disease. Ann Intern Med 1979;90:310.
577. Batille D, Itsarayoungyuen K, Arruda JAL, Kurtzman NA. Hyperkalemic hyperchloremic metabolic acidosis in sickle cell hemoglobinopathies. Am J Med 1982;72:188.
578. Diamond HS, Meisel AD, Holden D. The natural history of urate overproduction in sickle cell anemia. Ann Intern Med 1979;90:752.
579. McCall IW, Moule N, Desai P, Serjeant GR. Urographic findings in homozygous sickle cell disease. Radiology 1978;129:99.
580. Diggs LW. Anatomic lesions in sickle cell disease. In: Abramson H, Bertles JF, eds. Sickle cell disease, diagnosis, management, education and research. St Louis, CV Mosby, 1973.
581. Mostofi FK, Bruegge CFV, et al. Lesions in kidneys removed for unilateral hematuria in sickle cell disease. Arch Pathol 1957;63:336.
582. Lucas WM, Bullock W. Hematuria in sickle cell disease. J Urol 1960;83: 733.
583. Allen TD. Sickle cell disease and hematuria: a report of 29 cases. J Urol 1964;91:177.
584. Bilinsky RT, Kandel GL, et al. Epsilon aminocaproic acid therapy of hematuria due to heterozygous sickle cell diseases. J Urol 1969;102: 93.
585. Black WD, Hatch FE, Acchiardo S. Aminocaproic acid in prolonged hematuria of patients with sicklemia. Arch Intern Med 1976;136:678.
586. McInnes BK. The management of hematuria associated with sickle hemoglobinopathies. J Urol 1980;124:171.
587. Nicholson GD, Amin UF, et al. Proteinuria and the nephrotic syndrome in homozygous sickle cell anaemia. West Ind Med J 1980;29: 239.
588. Bernstein J, Whitten CR. A histologic appraisal of the kidney in sickle cell anemia. Arch Pathol 1960;70:407.

589. Pitcock JA, Muirhead EE, Hatch FE, Johnson JG, Kelly BJ. Early renal changes in sickle cell anemia. Arch Pathol 1970;90:403.
590. McCoy RC. Ultrastructural alterations in the kidney of patients with sickle cell disease and the nephrotic syndrome. Lab Invest 1969;21:85.
591. Pardo V, Strauss J, Kramer H, et al. Nephropathy associated with sickle cell anemia: an autologous immune complex nephritis. II. Am J Med 1975;59:650.
592. Strauss J, Pardo V, Koss MN, Griswold W, McIntosh RM. Nephropathy associated with sickle cell anemia: an autologous immune complex nephritis. I. Am J Med 1975;58:382.
592a. Falk RJ, Scheinman J, Phillips G, et al. Prevalence and pathologic features of sickle cell nephropathy and response to inhibition of angiotensin-converting enzyme. N Engl J Med 1992;326:910.
593. Bakir AA, Hathiwala SC, et al. Prognosis of the nephrotic syndrome in sickle glomerulopathy. Am J Nephrol 1987;7:110.
594. Morgan AG, Serjeant GR. Renal function in patients over 40 with homozygous sickle cell disease. Br Med J 1981;282:1181.
595. Spector D, Zachary JB, et al. Painful crisis following renal transplantation in sickle cell anemia. Am J Med 1978;64:835.
596. Gonzalez-Carrillo M, Rudge CJ, et al. Renal transplantation in sickle cell disease. Clin Nephrol 1982;18:209.
597. Chatterjee SN. National study on natural history of renal allografts in sickle cell disease or trait. Nephrologie 1980;25:199.
598. Emond AM, Holman R, et al. Priapism and impotence in homozygous sickle cell disease. Arch Intern Med 1980;140:1434.
599. Seeler RA. Intensive tranfusion therapy for priapism in boys with sickle cell anemia. J Urol 1973;110:360.
599a. Sharpsteen JR, Powars D, Johnson C, et al. Multisystem damage associated with tricorporal priapism in sickle cell disease. Am J Med 1993;94:289.
600. Grace DA, Winter CC. Priapism: an appraisal of management of twenty-three patients. J Urol 1968;99:301.
601. Karayalcin G, Imran M, et al. Priapism in sickle cell disease: report of five cases. Am J Med Sci 1972;264:289.
602. Seeler RA. Intensive transfusion therapy for priapism in boys with sickle cell anemia. J Urol 1973;110:630.
603. Rifkind S, Waisman J, et al. RBC exchange pheresis for priapism in sickle cell disease. JAMA 1979;242:2317.
604. Walker EM Jr, Mitchum EN, et al. Automated erythrocytopheresis for relief of priapism in sickle cell hemoglobinopathies. J Urol 1983;130:912.
605. Campbell JH, Cummings SD. Priapism in sickle cell anemia. J Urol 1969;101:71.
606. Kinney TR, Harris MB, et al. Priapism in association with sickle hemoglobinopathies in children. J Pediatr 1975;86:241.
607. Howe GE, Prentiss RJ, et al. Priapism: a surgical emergency. J Urol 1969;101:576.
608. Hasen HB, Raines SL. Priapism associated with sickle cell disease. J Urol 1962;88:71.
609. Noe HN, Wilimas J, et al. Surgical management of priapism in children with sickle cell anemia. J Urol 1981;126:770.
610. Alli AF, Lewis EA. The liver in sickle cell disease: pathological aspects based on a report on the pathological study of 77 necropsy and 5 biopsy specimens of liver. Ghana Med J 1969;8:119.
611. Bogosh A, Casselman WGB, et al. Liver disease in sickle cell anemia: a correlation of clinical, biochemical and histochemical observations. Am J Med 1955;19:583.
612. Green TW, Conley CL, et al. Liver in sickle cell anemia. Bull John Hopkins Hosp 1953;92:99.
613. Isichi UP. Liver function and the diagnostic significance of biochemical changes in the blood of African children with sickle cell disease. J Clin Pathol 1980;33:626.
614. Brody JI, Ryan WN, Haider MA. Serum alkaline phosphatase isoenzymes in sickle cell anemia. JAMA 1975;232:738.
615. Schubert TT. Hepatobiliary system in sickle cell disease. Gastroenterol 1986;90:2013.
616. Barrett-Connor E. Cholelithiasis in sickle cell anemia. Am J Med 1968;45:889.
617. Rennels MB, Dunne MG, et al. Cholelithiasis in patients with major sickle hemoglobinopathies. Am J Dis Child 1983;138:66.
618. Sarnaik S, Slovis TL, et al. Incidence of cholelithiasis in sickle cell anemia using the ultrasonic gray-scale technique. J Pediatr 1980;96:1005.
618a. Ware RE, Schultz WH, Filston HC, et al. Diagnosis and management of common bile duct stones in patients with sickle hemoglobinopathies. J Pediatr Surg 1992;27:572.
619. Ware R, Filston HC, Schultz WH, Kinney TR. Elective cholecystectomy in children with sickle hemoglobinopathies: successful outcome using a preoperative transfusion regimen. Ann Surg 1988;208:17.
620. Malone BS, Werlin SL. Cholecystectomy and cholelithiasis in sickle cell anemia. Am J Dis Child 1988;142:799.
620a. Ware RE, Kinney TR, Casey JR, et al. Laparoscopic cholecystectomy in young patients with sickle hemoglobinopathies. J Pediatr 1992;120:58.
621. Stephens CG, Scott RB. Cholelithiasis in sickle cell anemia: surgical or medical management. Arch Intern Med 1980;140:648.
622. Sheehy TW. Sickle cell hepatopathy. South Med J 1977;70:533.
623. Buchanan GR, Glader BE. Benign course of extreme hyperbilirubinemia in sickle cell anemia. Blood 1969;34:734.
624. Barrett-Connor E. Sickle cell disease and viral hepatitis. Ann Intern Med 1968;69:517.
625. Washburn RE. Peculiar elongated and sickle-shaped red blood corpuscles in a case of severe anemia. Va Med 1911;490:1910.
626. Sheehy TW, Law DE, et al. Exchange transfusion for sickle cell intrahepatic cholestasis. Arch Intern Med 1980;140:1364.
627. Klion FM, Weiner MJ, et al. Cholestasis in sickle cell anemia. Am J Med 1964;37:829.
628. Bauer TN, Moore GW, et al. The liver in sickle cell disease: a clinicopathologic study of 70 patients. Am J Med 1980;69:833.
629. Peachy RD. Leg ulceration and haemolytic anaemia: an hypothesis. Br J Dermatol 1978;98:245.
630. Thrall JH, Rucknagel DL. Increased bone marrow blood flow in sickle cell anemia demonstrated by thallium-201 and Tc-99m human albumin microspheres. Radiology 1978;127:817.
631. Koshy M, Entsuah R, Koranda A, et al. Leg ulcers in patients with sickle cell disease. Blood 1989;74:1403.
632. Wolfort FG, Krizek TJ. Skin ulceration in sickle cell anemia. Plast Reconstr Surg 1969;43:71.
633. Serjeant GR. Leg ulceration in sickle cell anemia. Arch Intern Med 1974;133:690.
634. Akinyanju O, Akinsets I. Leg ulceration in sickle cell disease in Nigeria. Trop Geogr Med 1979;31:87.
635. Alleyne S, Wint E, et al. Social effect of leg ulceration in sickle cell anemia. South Med J 1977;70:213.
636. Cohen SB, Fletcher ME, Goldberg MF, Jednock NJ. Diagnosis and management of ocular complications of sickle hemoglobinopathies: parts I-V. Ophthalmic Surg 1986;17:57.
637. Nagpal KC, Asdourian GK, Goldbaum MH, Raichand M, Goldberg MF. The conjunctival sickling sign, hemoglobin S, and irreversibly sickled erythrocytes. Arch Opthalmol 1977;95:808.
638. Paton D. The conjunctival sign of sickle cell disease. Arch Opthalmol 1961;66:90.
639. Fink AI, Funahashi T, Robinson M, Watson RJ. Conjunctival blood flow in sickle-cell disease: preliminary report. Arch Opthalmol 1961;66:824.
640. Paton D. The conjunctival sign of sickle cell disease: further observations. Arch Opthalmol 1962;68:627.
641. Marsh RJ, Ford SM, Rabb MF, Hayes RJ, Serjeant GR. Macular vasculature, visual acuity, and irreversibly sickled cells in homozygous sickle cell disease. Br J Opthalmol 1982;66:155.
642. Nagpal KC, Goldberg MF, Rabb MF. Ocular manifestations of sickle hemoglobinopathies. Surv Ophthalmol 1977;21:391.
643. Goldberg MF. Retinal vaso-occlusion in sickling hemoglobinopthies. Birth Defects 1976;12:475.
644. Welch RB, Goldberg MF. Sickle-cell hemoglobin and its relation to fundus abnormality. Arch Opthalmol 1966;75:353.
645. Romayananda N, Goldberg MF, Green WR. Histopathology of sickle cell retinopathy. Trans Am Acad Opthalmol Otolaryngol 1973;77:652.
646. Asdourian G, Nagpal KC, Goldbaum M, Patrianakos D, Goldberg MF, Rabb M. Evolution of the retinal black sunburst in sickling haemoglobinopathies. Br J Opthalmol 1975;59:710.
647. Goldberg MF. Classification and pathogenesis of proliferative sickle retinopathy. Am J Opthalmol 1971;71:649.
648. Goldberg MF, Jampol LM. Treatment of neovascularization, vitreous hemorrhage, and retinal detachment in sickle cell retinopathy. In: Symposium on medical and surgical diseases of the retina and vitreous: transactions of the New Orleans Academy of Ophthalmology. St Louis, CV Mosby, 1983:53.
649. Condon PI, Serjeant GR. Behaviour of untreated proliferative sickle retinopathy. Br J Ophthalmol 1980;64:404.
650. Goldberg MF. Treatment of proliferative sickle retinopathy. Trans Am Acad Ophthalmol Otolaryngol 1971;75:532.
651. Goldberg MF, Acacio I. Argon laser photocoagulation of proliferative sickle retinopathy. Arch Ophthalmol 1973;90:35.
652. Galinos S, Goldberg MF. Photocoagulation therapy of sickle cell retinopathy. Sight Sav Rev 1972;42:201.
653. Weissman H, Nadel AJ, et al. Simultaneous bilateral retinal arterial occlusions treated by exchange transfusions. Arch Opthalmol 1979;97:2151.
654. Todd GB, Serjeant GR, et al. Sensori-neural hearing loss in Jamaicans with SS disease. Acta Otolaryngol 1973;76:268.
655. Serjeant GR, Norman W, et al. The internal auditory canal and sensorineural hearing loss is homozygous sickle cell disease. J Laryngol Otolarynol 1975;89:453.
656. Friedman EM, Luban NLC, et al. Sickle cell anemia and hearing. Ann Otol Rhinol Laryngol 1980;89:342.
657. Morganstein KM, Manace CD. Temporal bone histopathology in sickle cell disease. Laryngoscope 1969;79:2172.
658. Leikin SL, Gallagher D, Kinney TR, et al. Mortality in children and adolescents with sickle cell disease. Pediatrics 1989;84:500.
659. Seeler RA. Deaths in children with sickle cell anemia: a clinical analysis of 19 fatal instances in Chicago. Clin Pediatr 1972;11:634.

660. Seeler RA, Shwiaki MZ. Acute splenic sequestration crises (ASSC) in young children with sickle cell anemia. Clin Pediatr 1972;11:701.
661. Serjeant GR. Five-year follow-up of Jamaican adults with sickle cell anemia. Br Med J 1975;3:20.
662. Thomas AN, Pattison C, et al. Causes of death in sickle cell disease in Jamaica. Br J Med 1982;285:633.
663. Girasole RV, Lyon ED. Sickle cell osteomyelitis of the mandible: report of three cases. J Oral Surg 1977;35:231.
664. Catena DL. Oral manifestations of the hemoglobinopathies. Dent Clin North Am 1975;19:77.
665. Sarnaik S, Schornack JI, Lusher JM. The incidence of development of irregular red cell antibodies in patients with sickle cell anemia. Transfusion 1986;26:249.
666. Blumberg N, Ross K, Avila E, Peck K. Should chronic transfusion be matched for antigens other than ABO and Rho(D)? Vox Sang 1984;47:205.
667. Orlina AR, Unger PJ, Koshy M. Post-transfusion alloimmunization in patients with sickle cell diseases. Am J Hematol 1978;5:101.
668. Reisner EG, Kostyu DD, Phillips G, Walker C, Dawson DV. Alloantibody responses in multiply transfused sickle cell anemia patients. Tissue Antigens 1987;30:161.
669. Ambruso DR, Githens JH, Alcorn R, et al. Experience with donors matched for minor blood group antigens in patients with sickle cell anemia who are receiving chronic transfusion therapy. Transfusion 1987;27:94.
670. Davies SC, McWillam AC, Hewitt PE, Devenish A. Red cell alloimmunization in sickle cell disease. Br J Haematol 1986;63:241.
671. Rosse WF, Gallagher D, Kinney TR, et al. Transfusion and alloimmunization in sickle cell disease. Blood 1990;76:1431.
672. Vichinsky EP, Earles A, Johnson RA, et al. Alloimmunization in sickle cell anemia and transfusion of racially unmatched blood. N Engl J Med 1990;322:1617.
673. Diamond WJ, Brown FL, Bitterman P, Klein HG, Davey RJ, Winslow RM. Delayed transfusion reaction presenting as sickle-cell crisis. Ann Intern Med 1980;93:231.
674. Schmalzer EA, Lee JO, Brown AK, Usami S, Chien S. Viscosity of mixtures of sickle and normal red cells at varying hematocrit levels: implications for transfusion. Transfusion 1987;27:228.
675. Charache S. Treatment of sickle cell anemia. Annu Rev Med 1981;32:195.
676. Kein HG, Garner RJ, Miller DM, Rosen SL, Statham, Winslow RM. Automated partial exchange transfusion in sickle cell anemia. Transfusion 1980;20:578.
677. Keeling MM, Lavery JP, Clemons AV, Schaefer RL, Bland PD, Hardis EA. Red cell exchange in the pregnancy complication by a major hemoglobinopathy. Am J Obstet Gynecol 1980;138:1.
678. Kernoff LM, Botha MC, Jacobs P. Exchange transfusion in sickle cell disease using a continuous flow blood cell separator. Transfusion 1977;17;269.
679. Key TC, Horger EO, Walker EM, Mitchum EN. Automatic erythrocytophereisis for sickle cell anemia during pregnancy. Ann Obstet Gynecol 1980;138:731.
680. Lenes B, Klein HG, Lakatos E. Selective removal of sickle cells with the IBM 2997 continuous flow blood cell separator. J Clin Apheresis 1983;1:64.
681. Cohen A, Schwartz E. Excretion of iron in response to deferioxamine in sickle cell anemia. J Pediatr 1978;92:659.
682. Searle JF. Anesthesia in sickle states. Anesthesia 1973;28:48.
683. Bentley PG, Howard ER. Surgery in children with homozygous sickle cell anaemia. Ann R Coll Surg Engl 1979;61:55.
684. Browne RA. Anaesthesia in patients with sickle cell anemia. Br J Anaesthesiol 1965;37:181.
685. Gilbertson AA. Anaesthesia in West African patients with sickle cell anaemia. Br J Anaesthesiol 1965;37:614.
686. Howells TH, Huntsman RG. Anaesthesia in sickle cell states. Br Med J 1973;1:174.
687. Spiegelman A, Warden MJ. Surgery in patients with sickle cell disease. Arch Surg 1972;104:761.
688. Chun PK, Flannery EP, et al. Open-heart surgery in patients with hematologic disorders. Am Heart J 1983;105:835.
689. Holzmann L, Finn H, et al. Anesthesia in patients with sickle cell disease: a review of 112 cases. Anesth Analg 1969;48:566.
690. Homi J, Reynolds J, et al. General anesthesia in sickle-cell disease. Br Med J 1979;1:1599.
691. Oduro KA, Searle JF. Anesthesia in sickle cell states: a plea for simplicity. Br Med J 1972;4:596.
692. Burrington JD, Smith MD. Elective and emergency surgery in children with sickle cell disease. Surg Clin North Am 1976;56:55.
692a. Afa-Gyamfi Y, Sankarankutty M, Marwa S. Use of a tourniquet in patients with sickle-cell disease. Can J Anesthesia 1993;40:24.
692b. Griffin RC, Buchanan GR, Elective surgery in children with sickle cell disease without preoperative blood transfusion. J Pediatr Surg 1993;28:681.
693. Janik JS, Seeler RA. Surgical procedures in children with sickle hemoglobinopathy. J Pediatr 1977;91:505.
694. Vichinsky, E. Preoperative transfusion (TX) in sickle cell anemia (SCA). (Abstract) Blood 1989;74:184A.
695. Powars DR, Sandhu M, et al. Pregnancy in sickle cell disease. Obstet Gynecol 1986;67:217.
696. Freeman MG, Ruth GU. SS disease, SC disease and CC disease: obstetric considerations and treatment. Clin Obstet Gynecol 1969;12:134.
697. Milner PF, Jones BR. Outcome of pregnancy in sickle cell anemia and sickle cell-hemoglobin C disease: an analysis of 181 pregnancies in 98 patients, and a review of the literature. Am J Obstet Gynecol 1980;138:239.
698. Pritchard JA. The effects of maternal sickle cell hemoglobinopathies and sickle cell trait on reproductive performance. Am J Obstet Gynecol 1973;117:662.
699. Morrison JC, Fort AT, et al. The modern management of pregnant sickle cell patients. South Med J 1972;65:533.
700. Charache S, Scott J, et al. Management of sickle cell disease in pregnant patients. Obstet Gynecol 1980;55:407.
701. Cunningham FG, Pritchard JA, et al. Pregnancy and sickle cell hemoglobinopathies: results with and without prophylactic transfusions. Obstet Gynecol 1983;62:419.
702. Cunningham FG, Pritchard JA, et al. Prophylactic transfusions of normal red blood cells during pregnancies complicated by sickle cell hemoglobinopathies. Am J Obstet Gynecol 1979;135:994.
703. Morrison JC, Schneider JM, et al. Prophylactic transfusions in pregnant patients with sickle hemoglobinopathies: benefit versus risk. Obstet Gynecol 1980;56:274.
704. Nagey DA, Alawode NA, et al. Isovolumetric partial exchange transfusion in the management of sickle cell disease in pregnancy. II. Simplified ambulatory technique. Am J Obstet Gynecol 1983;147:693.
705. Key TC, Horger EO III, et al. Automated erythrocytopheresis for sickle cell anemia during pregnancy. Am J Obstet Gynecol 1980;138:731.
706. Miller JM Jr, Horger EO Jr, et al. Management of sickle hemoglobinopathies in pregnant patients. Am J Obstet Gynecol 1981;141:237.
707. Koshy M, Burd L, Wallace D, Moawad A, Baron J. Prophylactic red-cell transfusion in pregnant patients with sickle cell disease, a randomized cooperative study. N Engl J Med 1988;319:1447.
708. Boyle E Jr, Thompson C, et al. Prevalence of sickle cell trait in adults of Charleston County. Arch Environ Health 1968;17:891.
709. Ashcroft MR, Miall WE, et al. Comparison between characteristics of Jamaican adults with normal hemoglobin and those with sickle cell trait. Am J Epidemiol 1969;90:236.
710. Ashcroft MT, Desai P. Mortality and morbidity in Jamaican adults with sickle-cell trait and with normal haemoglobin followed up for twelve years. Lancet 1976;2:784.
711. Sears DA. The morbidity of sickle cell trait: a review of the literature. Am J Med 1978;64:1021.
712. Heller P, Best WR, et al. Clinical implications of sickle cell trait and glucose-6-phosphate dehydrogenase deficiency in hospitalized black male patients. N Engl J Med 1979;300:1001.
713. Ashcroft MT, Desai P, et al. Growth, behavior, and educational achievement of Jamaican children with sickle cell trait. Br Med J 1976;1:1371.
714. Kramer MS, Rooks T, et al. Growth and development in children with sickle cell trait. N Engl J Med 1978;299:686.
715. Murphy JR. Sickle cell hemoglobin (Hb AS) in black football players. JAMA 1973;225:981.
716. Blattner P, Dar H, et al. Pregnancy outcome in women with sickle cell trait. JAMA 1977;238:1392.
717. Stinson JM, McPherson GL. Lung volumes and diffusion capacity in sickle cell trait. J Natl Med Assoc 1986;78:505.
718. Harris JW, Kellermeyer RN. The red cell. Cambridge MA: Harvard University Press, 1970:170.
719. Ober WB, Bruno MS, et al. Fatal intravascular sickling in a patient with sickle cell trait. N Engl J Med 1960;263:947.
720. McCormack WF. Abnormal hemoglobins. II. The pathology of sickle cell trait. Am J Med Sci 1961;241:329.
721. Smith EW, Conley CL. Clinical features of the genetic variants of sickle cell disease. Bull Johns Hopkins Hosp 1954;94:289.
722. Jones SR, Binder RA, et al. Sudden death in sickle-cell trait. N Engl J Med 1970;282:323.
723. O'Brien RT, Pearson HA, et al. Splenic infarct and sickle cell trait. N Engl J Med 1972;287:720.
724. Kark JA, Posey DM, Schumacher, Ruehle CJ. Sickle-cell trait as a risk factor for sudden death in physical training. N Engl J Med 1987;317:781.
725. Weissman IM, Zeballos RJ, Martin TW, Johnson BD. Effect of army basic training in sickle-cell trait. Arch Intern Med 1988;148:1140.
726. Charache S. Sudden death in sickle trait. Am J Med 1988;84:459.
727. Sullivan LW. The risk of sickle-cell trait: caution and common sense. N Engl J Med 1987;317:830.
728. Pearson HA. Sickle cell trait and competitive athletics: is there a risk? Pediatrics 1989;83:613.
729. Long ID. Sickle cell trait and aviation. Aviat Space Environ Med 1982;53:1921.
730. Atlas SA. The sickle trait and surgical complications: a matched-pair patient analysis. JAMA 1974;229:1078.
731. Metras D, Quezzin A, et al. Open-heart surgery in sickle-cell haemoglobinopathies: report of 15 cases. Thorax 1982;37:486.

732. Searle JF. Anesthesia and sickle-cell haemoglobin. Br J Anaesthesiol 1972;44:1335.
733. Husiman THJ. Trimodality in the percentages of beta-chain variants in heterozygotes: the effect of the number of active HB structural loci. Hemoglobin 1977;1:349.
734. Steinberg MH, Embury SH. Alpha thalassemia in blacks: genetic and clinical aspects and interactions with the sickle hemoglobin gene. Blood 1986;69:985.
735. Levere RD, Lichtman HS, et al. Effect of iron deficiency anaemia on the metabolism of the heterogenic haemoglobins in sickle cell trait. Nature 1964;202:499.
736. Heller P, Yakulis V, et al. Variation in the amount of hemoglobin S in a patient with sickle cell trait and megaloblastic anemia. Blood 1963;21:479.
737. Milner PF, Garbutt GJ, Nolan-Davis LV, et al. The effect of hemoglobin F and alpha thalassemia on the red cell indices in sickle cell anemia. Am J Hematol 1986;21:383.
738. Serjeant GR, Sommereux AM, et al. Comparison of sickle cell beta° thalassemia in Jamaica. Br J Haematol 1973;24:19.
739. Honig GR, Koshy M, et al. Sickle cell syndromes. II. The sickle cell anemia-alpha thalassemia syndrome. J Pediatr 1978;92:556.
740. Embury SH, Dozy AM, et al. Concurrent sickle cell anemia and alpha-thalassemia: effect on severity of anemia. N Engl J Med 1982;306:270.
741. Higgs DR, Aldridge BE, et al. The interaction of alpha-thalassemia and homozygous sickle cell disease. N Engl J Med 1982;306:270.
742. Higgs DR, Pressley L, et al. The genetics and molecular basis of alpha-thalassemia in association with HbS in Jamaican Negroes. Br J Haematol 1981;47:43.
743. Steinberg MH, Rosenstock W, et al. Effects of thalassemia and microcytosis on the hematological and vasocclusive severity of sickle cell anemia. Blood 1984;63:1353.
744. deCeulaer K, Higgs DR, et al. Alpha-thalassemia reduces the hemolytic rate in homozygous sickle cell disease. N Engl J Med 1983;309:189.
745. Embury SH, Clarke MR, et al. Concurrent sickle cell anemia and alpha-thalassemia. J Clin Invest 1984;74:116.
746. Serjeant BE, Mason KP, et al. Effect of alpha-thalassemia on the rheology of homozygous sickle cell disease. Br J Haematol 1983;55:479.
747. Rodgers GP, Dover GJ, et al. Alpha-thalassemia changes cell density and hemoglobin F in sickle cell disease. Blood 1983;62:60A.
748. Steinberg MH, Embury SH. Alpha thalassemia in blacks: genetic and clinical aspects and interactions with the sickle hemoglobin gene. Blood 1986;68:985.
749. Felice AE, Webber B, Miller A, et al. The association of sickle cell anemia with heterozygous and homozygous alpha-thalassemia-2: in vitro Hb chain synthesis. Am J Hematol 1979;6:91.
750. Altay C, Gravely ME, Joseph BR, Williams DF. Alpha-thalassemia-2 and the variability of hematological values in children with sickle cell anemia. Pediatr Res 1981;15:1093.
751. Fabry ME, Mears JG, Patel P, et al. Dense cells in sickle cell anemia: the effects of gene interaction. Blood 1984;64:1042.
752. Noguchi CT, Dover GJ, Rodgers GP, et al. Alpha thalassemia changes erythrocyte heterogeneity in sickle cell disease. J Clin Invest 1985;75:1632.
753. Embury SH, Clark MR, Monroy G, Mohandas N. Concurrent sickle-cell anemia and alpha-thalassemia: effect on pathological properties of sickle erythrocytes. J Clin Invest 1984;73:116.
754. Serjeant BE, Mason KP, Kenny MW, et al. Effect of alpha thalassemia on the rheology of homozygous sickle cell disease. Br J Haematol 1983;55:479.
755. Embury SH, Backer K, Glader BE. Monovalent cation changes in sickle erythrocytes: a direct reflection of alpha-globin gene number. J Lab Clin Med 1985;106:75.
756. Stevens MCG, Maude GH, Beckford M, et al. Alpha thalassemia and the hematology of homozygous sickle cell diseases in childhood. Blood 1986;67:411.
757. Kulozik AE, Kar BC, Serjeant GR, et al. The molecular basis of alpha thalassemia in India: its interaction with the sickle gene. Blood 1988;71:467.
758. Natta C. Failure of the alpha-thalassemia gene to decrease the severity of sickle cell anemia. Blood 1978;51:1163.
759. Hawker H, Neilson H, Hayes RJ, Serjeant GR. Haematological factors associated with avascular necrosis of the femoral head in homozygous sickle cell disease. Br J Haematol 1982;50:29.
760. Hayes RJ, Condon PI, Serjeant GR. Haematological factors associated with proliferative retinopathy in homozygous sickle cell disease. Br J Opthalmol 1981;65:29.
761. Mears JG, Lachman H, Labie D, Nagel RL. Alpha-thalassemia is related to prolonged survival in sickle cell anemia. Blood 1983;62:286.
762. Serjeant BE, Mason KP, Kenny MW, et al. Effect of alpha thalassemia on the rheology of homozygous sickle cell disease. Br J Haematol 1983;55:479.
763. Perrine RP, Brown MJ, et al. Benign sickle cell anaemia. Lancet 1972: 1:1163.
764. Perrine RP, Pembrey ME, et al. Natural history of sickle cell anemia in Saudi Arabs. Ann Intern Med 1978;88:1.
765. Perrine RP. Cholelithiasis in sickle cell anemia in a Caucasian population. Am J Med 1978;54:327.
766. Pembrey ME, Wood WG, et al. Fetal hemoglobin production in sickle cell anemia in the eastern province of Saudi Arabia is genetically determined. Blood 1986;67:1404.
767. Odenheimer DJ, Whitten CF, Rucknagel DA, et al. Stability over time of hematological variables in 197 children with sickle cell anemia. Am J Med Genet 1984;18:461.
768. Dover GJ, Boyer SH, et al. Individual variation in the production and survival of F cells in sickle-cell disease. N Engl J Med 1978;299:1428.
769. Boyer SH. The emerging complexity of genetic control of persistent fetal hemoglobin biosynthesis in adults. Ann NY Acad Sci 1989;565: 23.
770. Murray N, Serjeant BE, Serjeant GR. Sickle cell-hereditary persistance of fetal haemoglobin and its differentiation from other sickle cell syndromes. Br J Haematol 1988;69:89.
771. Charache S, Conley CL. Hereditary persistence of fetal hemoglobin. Ann NY Acad Sci 1969;165:37.
772. Bradley TB Jr, Brawner JN III, et al. Further observations on an inherited anomaly characterized by persistence of fetal hemoglobin. Bull Johns Hopkins Hosp 1961;108:242.
773. Jacob GR, Raper AB. Hereditary persistence of foetal hemoglobin production and its interaction with sickle cell trait. Br J Haematol 1958;4: 138.
774. Weatherall DJ, Clegg JB. The thalassemia syndromes, ed 2. Oxford UK, Blackwell Scientific, 1972:195.
775. Old JM, Avyub H, et al. Linkage analysis of nondeletion hereditary persistance of fetal hemoglobin. Science 1982;215:981.
776. Milner PF, Leibfarth JD, et al. Increased Hb F in sickle cell anemia is determined by a factor linked to the beta S gene from one parent. Blood 1984;63:64.
777. Stamatoyannopoulos G, Wood WG, et al. A new form of hereditary persistence of fetal hemoglobin in blacks and its association with sickle cell trait. Blood 1975;46:683.
778. Makler MT, Berthrog M, et al. A new variant of sickle cell disease with high levels of foetal haemoglobin homogenously distributed within red cells. Br J Haematol 1974;26:519.
779. Gianni AM, Bregni M, et al. A gene controlling fetal hemoglobin expression in adults is not linked to the non-alpha globin cluster. EMBO J 2:921, 1983.
780. Wood WG, Weatherall DJ, et al. Interaction of heterocellular hereditary persistance of foetal haemoglobin with beta thalassemia and sickle cell anemia. Nature 1976;264:247.
781. Boyer SH, Dover GJ, Serjeant GR, et al. Production of F-cells in sickle cell anemia: regulation by a genetic locus or loci separate from the beta-globin gene cluster. Blood 1984;64:1053.
782. Dover GJ, Smith KD, Chang YC, et al. Fetal hemoglobin levels in sickle cell disease and normal individuals are partially controlled by an X-linked gene located at Xp22.2 Blood 1992;80:816.
783. Weatherall DJ. Biochemical phenotypes of thalassemia in the American Negro population. Ann NY Acad Sci 1964;119:450.
784. Pearson HA. Hemoglobin S-thalassemia syndrome in Negro children. Ann NY Acad Sci 1969;165:83.
785. Weatherall DJ, Clegg JB. The thalassemia syndromes, ed2. Oxford UK, Blackwell Scientific, 1972:252.
786. Serjeant GR, Ashcroft MT, et al. The clinical features of sickle cell beta thalassemia in Jamaica. Br J Haematol 1973;24:19.
787. Baklouti F, Ouazana R, Gonnet C, et al. Beta$^+$ thalassemia in *cis* of a sickle gene: occurrence of a promoter mutation on a beta^S chromosome. Blood 1989;74:1817.
788. Baklouti F, Francina A, Dorleac E, et al. Association in *cis* of beta$^+$ thalassemia and hemoglobin S. Am J Hematol 1987;26:237.
789. Rivers GL, Robbins AB, et al. S-C hemoglobin: a clinical study. Blood 1961;18:385.
790. Stevens MCG, Maude GH, Beckford M, et al. Haematological change in sickle cell-haemoglobin C disease and in sickle-cell-beta thalassaemia: a cohort study from birth. Br J Haematol 1985;60:279.
791. Tuttle AH, Koch B. Clinical and hematological manifestations of hemoglobin C-S disease in children. J Pediatr 1960;56:331.
792. Serjeant GR, Ashcroft MT, et al. The clinical features of haemoglobin SC disease in Jamaica. Br J Haematol 1973;24:491.
793. Rowley PT, Englander D. Hemoglobin S-C disease presenting as acute cor pulmonale. Am Rev Respir Dis 1968;98:494.
794. Fabian RH, Peters BH. Neurological complications of hemoglobin SC disease. Arch Neurol 198;41:289.
795. Goldberg MF. Natural history of untreated proliferative sickle retinopathy. Arch Opthalmol 1971;85:421.
796. Ryan SJ, Goldberg MF. Anterior segment ischemia following scleral buckling in sickle cell hemoglobinopathy. Am J Opthalmol 1971;72: 35.
797. Goldberg MF. Treatment of proliferative sickle retinopathy. Trans Am Acad Opthalmol Otolaryngol 1971;75:532.
798. Barton CJ, Cockshott WP. Bone changes in hemoglobin SC disease. AJR 1962;88:523.
799. Kay CJ. Renal papillary necrosis in hemoglobin SC disease. Radiology 1968;90:897.

800. Yeung KY, Lessin LS. Splenic infarction in sickle cell hemoglobin C disease. Arch Intern Med 1976;1236:905.
801. Githens JH, Gross GP, et al. Splenic sequestration syndrome at mountain attitudes in sickle/hemoglobin C disease. J Pediatr 1977;90:203.
802. Barrett-Connor E. Infection and sickle cell C disease. Am J Med Sci 1971;262:162.
803. Buchanan GR, Smith SJ, et al. Bacterial infection and splenic reticuloendothelial function in children with hemoglobin SC disease. Pediatrics 1983;72:93.
804. Bunn HF, Noguichi CT, Hofrichter J, et al. Molecular and cellular pathogenesis of hemoglobin SC disease. Proc Natl Acad Sci USA 1982;79:7527.
805. Bunn HF, McDonald MJ. Electrostatic interactions in the assembly of haemoglobin. Nature 1983;306:498.
806. Fabry ME, Kaul DK, et al. Sickle cell erythrocytes have an abnormally high intracellular hemoglobin concentration: pathophysiological consequences. J Clin Invest 1982;70:1315.
807. Honig GR, Gunav U, et al. Sickle syndromes. I. Hemoglobin SC-alpha thalassemia. Pediatr Res 1976;10:613.
808. Milner PF, Miller C, et al. Hemoglobin O Arab in 4 Negro famililies and its interaction with hemoglobin S and hemoglobin C. N Engl J Med 1970;283:1417.
809. Charache S, Zinkham WH, et al. Hemoglobin SC, SS/G Philadelphia, and SO_{Arab} disease. Am J Med 1977;62:439.
810. Altay C, Niazi GA, Huisman THJ. The combination of Hb S and Hb E in a black female. Hemoglobin 1976;1:101.

Blood: Principles and Practice of Hematology,
edited by Robert I. Handin, Samuel E. Lux, and Thomas P. Stossel.
J.B. Lippincott Company, Philadelphia © 1995.

54

Disorders of the Red Cell Membrane

Samuel E. Lux
Jiri Palek

The red cell membrane is a small but important structure, less than 0.1% of the cell's thickness and only about 1% of its weight. During erythropoiesis, it responds to erythropoietin and imports the billion or so iron atoms each red cell needs to complete hemoglobin synthesis. The red cell membrane sequesters the reductants required to protect hemoglobin and other cell proteins from corrosion by oxygen; it selectively retains other vital components such as organic phosphates, which are manufactured with precious adenosine triphosphatase (ATP) energy, and lets metabolic detritus escape. Evidence suggests that the red cell membrane may even help regulate metabolism by reversibly binding and inactivating many glycolytic enzymes.[1] In the circulation, it carefully balances cation and water concentrations so that red cells do not shrivel or explode. Simulntaneously, it exchanges tremendous numbers of bicarbonate and chloride anions (about 10 to 30 billion per second per red cell), which aids transfer of carbon dioxide from tissues to lungs.[2] The red cell membrane also maintains a slippery exterior so that red cells do not adhere to endothelial cells or aggregate and clog capillaries. Finally, buttressed by the "membrane skeleton," a protein scaffold that lines the inner membrane surface, the membrane achieves the critical combination of strength and flexibility needed to survive 4 months in the circulation. Failure of any of these or numerous other functions shortens red cell survival, a process termed *hemolysis*. In fact, all hemolysis is ultimately due to membrane failure.

Our modern understanding of membranes began with the deduction by Danielli and Davson[3] nearly six decades ago that membrane lipids are organized into a planar bilayer. Modern views of membrane architecture retain the lipid bilayer as a cornerstone but differ substantially in other ways, especially in regard to the disposition of membrane proteins. These models, which originated in the fluid mosaic model of Singer and Nicolson,[4] emphasize the mobility and asymmetric distribution of the protein and lipid components and present a much more complex and dynamic picture of membrane structure than was originally imagined. The great contribution of the fluid mosaic model was the concept that the lipids were mobile and that some membrane proteins penetrated the lipid bilayer, leading to the classic picture of "protein icebergs floating in a sea of lipid." It is difficult, when the concept of transmembrane proteins seems so natural, to realize how heretical this idea once was.

Our knowledge of red cell membrane proteins has largely been achieved in the past 30 years. Key early discoveries include (1) methods of preparing red cell membranes (or ghosts)[5] and inside-out membrane vesicles[6]; (2) the technique of SDS gel electrophoresis,[7,8] which revealed the complexity of the membrane and provided a simple tool for protein analysis; and (3) the isolation of spectrin[9] and glycophorin,[10] the first purified red cell membrane proteins. Today, we understand the structure of the red cell membrane in considerable detail. All the major proteins have been cloned and sequenced and their interconnections defined. During the past few years, many of the molecular defects responsible for common hereditary disorders of the membrane, such as hereditary spherocytosis (HS) and hereditary elliptocytosis, have been described. In addition, analogues of erythrocyte membrane proteins clearly play prominent structural and functional roles in cell membranes of other tissues.

In this chapter, we will first discuss normal membrane structure, emphasizing aspects that are most involved in the genesis of membrane disease. Later, the focus will be on abnormalities of red cell membranes, particularly HS and hereditary elliptocytosis, the two most common and best understood disorders.

MEMBRANE LIPIDS

Lipid Components of the Bilayer

Lipids make up about 50% of the weight of the red cell membrane (Table 54-1) or about 1.6% of the weight of the hemoglobin. Phospholipids and unesterified (free) cholesterol predominate and are present in nearly equal proportions (cholesterol/phospholipid molar ratio of 0.8).[11–13] Small amounts of glycolipids, principally globoside (73% of the glycosphingolipids) are also present[11] (Fig. 54-1). Thus, the average red cell contains about 250 million phospholipid molecules, 195 million cholesterol molecules, 10 million glycolipid molecules, and 6 million protein molecules in a membrane whose total surface area is about 140 μm^2.[10,14] Phosphatidylcholine (PC), phosphatidylethanolamine (PE), sphingomyelin, and phosphatidylserine (PS) are the predominant phospholipids (see Table 54-1). Their structures are shown in Figure 54-1. Small amounts of phosphatidic acid (PA), phosphatidylinositol (PI), and lysophosphatidylcholine (lyso-PC) are also present. At physiologic pH, PS, PA, and PI have a net negative charge, whereas the other phospholipids are electrically neutral.

TABLE 54-1. Composition of Normal Human Red Cell Membranes

Component	Weight (%)	Grams per Membrane ($\times 10^{-13}$)	Approximate Number of Molecules per Membrane ($\times 10^6$)	Percentage in Outer Half of Bilayer*	Percentage in Inner Half of Bilayer*
PROTEINS AND GLYCOPROTEINS†	**55**	**5.7‡**	**6**		
LIPIDS	**45**	**4.7**	**475**		
Phospholipids§	28	3.0	250‖		
Sphingomyelin (SM)	6.8	0.73	60	80	20
Phosphatidylcholine (PC)	7.0	0.75	65	75	25
Phosphatidylethanolamine (PE)	7.4	0.79	65	20	80
Phosphatidylserine (PS)	4.3	0.46	40	0	100
Phosphatidylinositols (PI)	1.0	0.10	8	0	100
PI	0.34	0.036	3		
PI-4-P	0.22	0.024	2		
PI-4,5-PP	0.39	0.042	3		
Phosphatidic acid (PA)	1.0	0.10	8	Unknown	Unknown
Lysophosphatidylcholine (LPC)	0.3	0.03	3	Unknown	Unknown
Lysophosphatidylethanolamine (LPE)	0.3	0.03	3	Unknown	Unknown
Cholesterol§	13	1.3	195	50	50
Glycolipids¶	3	0.3	10	100	0
Free fatty acids#	1	0.1	20	Unknown	Unknown
	100	**10.4**	**481**		

* Based on data in Blair and Bittman,[87] Low and Finean,[241] and Verkleij et al.[242]
† An average of three reported values in Fairbanks et al.[7]
‡ Calculated from data in Table 54-2.
§ Based on compiled data in Ferrell and Huestis.[243]
‖ Number of phospholipids per ghost based on an average molecular weight of 723 calculated from the average RBC phospholipid polar head group and fatty acid composition.[15]
¶ Based on the data in Sweeley and Dawson.[11]
#An average of two reported values compiled in Cooper.[244]

With the exception of sphingomyelin and lyso-PC, these lipids have two fatty acids attached to a glycerol backbone. These fatty acids are usually in ester linkage, although sometimes, particularly in PE, one of the fatty acids is a vinyl ether (plasmalogen).[15] The lysophospholipids have only one fatty acid and are named for the hemolysis induced by their detergent-like properties.

Asymmetric Organization of Phospholipids in the Bilayer

Membrane phospholipids are arranged with their polar head groups exposed at each membrane surface and their hydrophobic fatty acyl side chains buried in the bilayer core. Small foci of nonbilayer phospholipids may also exist transiently for specific purposes. For example, some theories require the interaction of nonbilayer regions of micellar-like phospholipid during membrane fusion.[16]

Trans Asymmetry

Red cell membrane lipids, like membrane proteins (see discussion under membrane protein structure), are asymmetrically distributed across the bilayer plane.[17–19] This *trans* asymmetry has been established by several different techniques, all of which indicate that choline phospholipids (PC and sphingomyelin) are concentrated in the outer half of the bilayer and that amino phospholipids (PE and PS) and PI are largely confined to the inner half (see Table 54-1). The evidence has been critically reviewed.[20]

The asymmetric distribution of phospholipids reflects a steady state involving a constant exchange (flip-flop) of phospholipids between the two bilayer hemileaflets.[20,21] In pure phospholipid bilayers, this transmembrane diffusion is slow, lasting several hours to days.[21] In contrast, the transmembrane shuttle of phospholipids in biologic membranes is fast. In addition to enzymatic phospholipid translocation described in the next paragraph, phospholipid flip-flop is accelerated by transmembrane proteins, which produce localized discontinuities in the bilayer, or, in the case of neutral phospholipids, by transmembrane pH gradients.[21]

***Trans* Asymmetry is Maintained by a Phospholipid Flippase.** Evidence indicates that phospholipid asymmetry is produced and maintained by an ATP-dependent transport system, called the *aminophospholipid translocase* or *flippase*.[20,22] This enzyme translocates PS and, to a lesser extent, PE from the outer to the inner bilayer.[23–27] The half-lives ($T_{1/2}$) for PS and PE are about 5 and 60 minutes, respectively, at 37°C.[27a] A similar activity exists in all mammalian red cells[28] and in at least some nonerythroid cells and cell organelles.[29] The aminophospholipid translocase requires Mg-ATP at the inner membrane surface[25] and may contain an active site cysteine, since it is inhibited by sulfhydryl-modifying reagents.[30] The flippase is also inhibited by vanadate (50 μmol/L) and free Ca^{2+} (over 0.2 μmol/L).[27] The enzyme has not been isolated. One candidate is a 115- to 130-kd, PS-stimulated, vanadate-inhibited Mg^{2+}-ATPase, of unknown function, which is present in red cell membranes.[31] A more interesting hypothesis is that the flippase may be related to the multidrug resistance (*mdr*) gene product, which is also called the P glycoprotein.[31a] The fact that mice that lack one of the mdr genes (*mdr-2*) are unable to secrete phospholipids into the bile[31b] supports this idea.

A Floppase May Also Be Present. PC and sphingomyelin are not transported inward by the flippase enzyme,[25,27] but red cells are able to transport PC, along with PS and PE from the inner to the outer bilayer.[32] It is

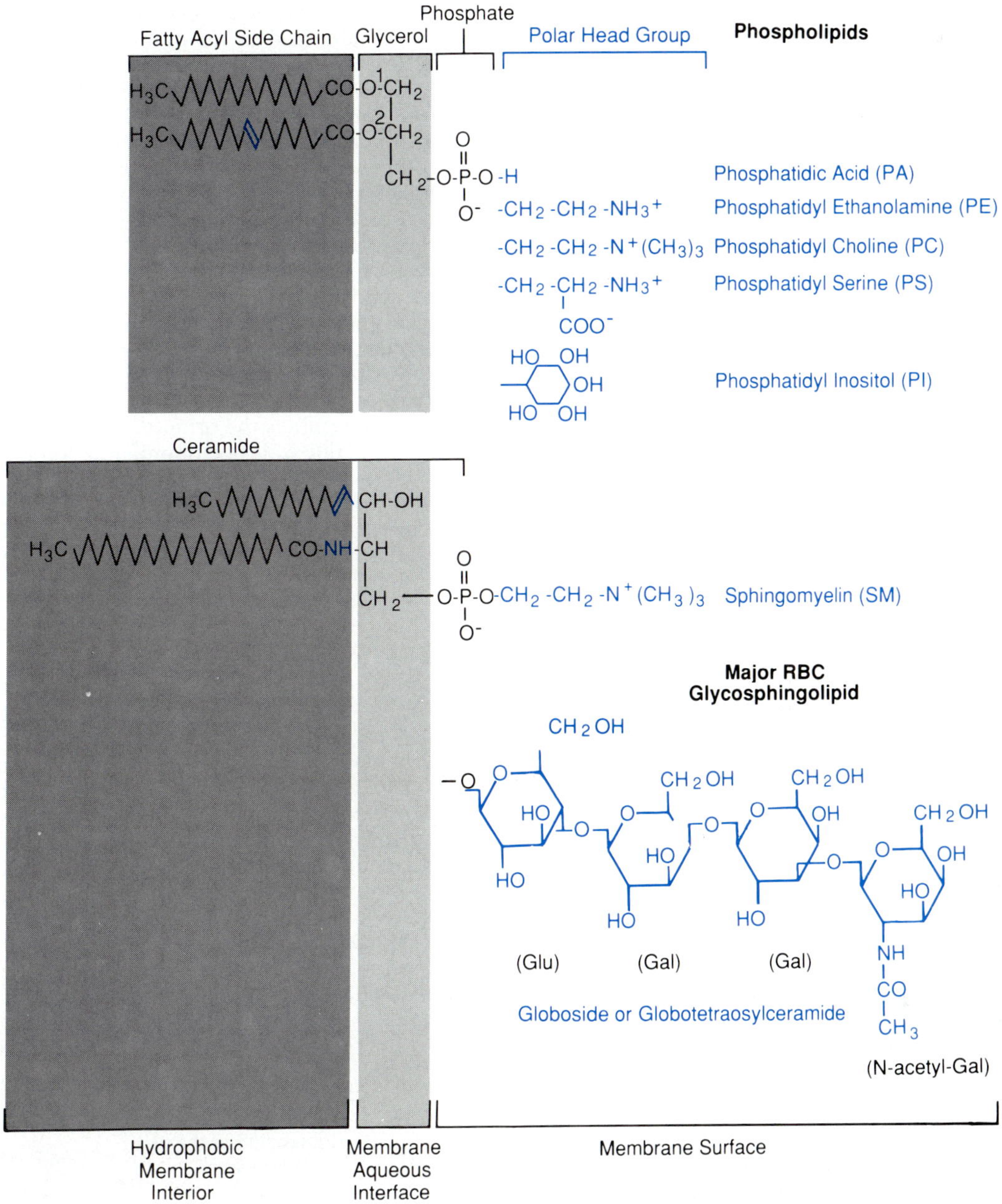

FIGURE 54-1. Structures of the major phospholipids and the predominant glycosphingolipid (globoside) of the red cell membrane. The phospholipid head groups all are attached to similar backbone structures composed of two fatty acyl side chains, a glycerol moiety, and a phosphate. Phosphatidylcholine and sphingomyelin share the same polar group (choline), and sphingomyelin and globoside share the same nonpolar group (ceramide).

not clear whether this floppase activity is a second function of the aminophospholipid (flippase) translocase or whether it is generated by a separate enzyme.[32]

The Flippase Is Not the Rh Protein. For a while, the Rh protein appeared to be the aminophospholipid translocase. A photoactivatable PS analogue that was transported to the inner bilayer by the translocase selectively labeled a 31-kd protein[33] that was precipitated by monoclonal anti-Rh antibodies.[34] The 31-kd protein, which is the same size as Rh proteins,[35] was also labeled by an inhibitor of the translocase.[30] However, the recently cloned Rh proteins[35] do not contain the characteristic nucleotide-binding motif found in ATPases,[36] and Rh_{null} erythrocytes, which lack all Rh antigens (see Chap. 56), have normal translocase activity.[34] Most likely, the Rh proteins are associated with the translocase, perhaps as part of a complex, and are labeled by an "innocent bystander" mechanism.

Spectrin Does Not Help to Maintain Phospholipid Asymmetry. Early experiments suggested that membrane skeletal proteins such as spectrin may help stabilize phospholipid asymmetry through interactions with inner membrane lipids. Spectrin interacts weakly with anionic phospholipids in vitro,[37–40] and phospholipid asymmetry is lost when spectrin is oxidized and cross-linked.[41–44] We now know that the translocase is also sensitive to oxidation[23,27,30] and would have been damaged by the treatments used to oxidize spectrin.[41–44] In addition, heat-treated ghosts, heat-induced vesicles (which are spectrin depleted), and spectrin-deficient hereditary spherocytes are capable of translocating aminophospholipids with the same efficiency as normal ghosts.[45,46] Aminophospholipid translocase appears to be able to maintain phospholipid asymmetry without help from the membrane skeleton, at least under normal conditions.

Calcium Induces a Rapid Phospholipid Scrambling. Increase in intracellular Ca^{2+} leads to activation of a poorly defined lipid translocation pathway in which both PS and PE flip to the outer bilayer leaflet, whereas PC flops inside.[20,47–49] In addition to the inhibitory effect of Ca^{2+} on the aminophospholipid translocase, this rapid phospholipid scrambling may represent another mechanism underlying altered phospholipid asymmetry. The molecular basis of the phenomenon is unknown. Hypothetical possibilities include phospholipase activation leading to formation of diacylglycerol, which may destabilize the lipid bilayer by forming nonbilayer structures, and disruption of lipid bilayer integrity during the plasma membrane fusion that follows Ca^{2+}-induced shedding of membrane microvesicles.[20,49]

Phospholipid Asymmetry Is Lost in Sickle Cells. Phospholipid asymmetry results from the balance of the active translocation of PS and PE and the passive, slow bidirectional flip-flop of phospholipids. Changes in the equilibrium distribution of phospholipids could occur by inhibition of the translocase, acceleration of basal flip-flop rates to a degree that overwhelms the translocase, or both. Phospholipid flip-flop is increased and phospholipid asymmetry is lost in sickle cells,[50–52] in which several forms of skeletal protein damage have been documented[53–55] (see Chap. 53), including decreased phospholipid translocase activity[50] and uncoupling of the lipid bilayer from the underlying skeleton in the sickle cell spicules.[56] Phospholipid asymmetry is also altered in diabetic red cells,[57] which, like sickle cells, tend to adhere to endothelial cells.[57–60]

Externalized PS May Trigger Clotting or Phagocytosis. Red cells, and perhaps other cells,[19] are generally believed to sequester aminophospholipids on the cytoplasmic side of the membrane because the exposed lipids trigger the conversion of prothrombin to thrombin and promote intravascular clotting.[61–63]

In addition, macrophages bind and ingest red cells, or even liposomes, that have PS exposed on their outer surfaces.[64–68] Little is known of the receptor involved, such as whether it is a unique PS receptor or a receptor of known function that also binds PS. It is also unclear whether the PS receptor actually participates in the removal of sickle cells or other damaged cells from the circulation or whether it has other functions such as the scavenging of dead or dying cells that have lost the ability to internalize PS.

Finally, speculation exists that the aminophospholipid translocase might foster endocytosis by "pumping" PS and PE into the inner bilayer.[22] Even a small excess of inner bilayer phospholipids would tend to make the membrane invaginate.

Cis Asymmetry

Macroscopic Domains. Evidence indicates that red cell lipids also exist in different domains within each of the bilayer planes (*cis* asymmetry). Fluorescent phospholipids partition into doughnut-shaped lipid domains up to several microns in diameter within the membrane of red cells or ghosts.[69] These lipid-rich domains are intrinsic structural features of the membrane, not just gel-phase or fluid-phase domains.[69] These domains increase in size when membrane proteins aggregate and they are lacking in large liposomes made solely of membrane lipids, suggesting that proteins play a role in their formation. How and why this occurs is a mystery.

Microscopic Domains. Lipids may also partition on a more microscopic scale within the membrane. Early experiments[70] detected a layer of tightly associated boundary lipids attached to membrane proteins that intruded into the bilayer core. Subsequent work[71] suggested that such lipids were bound only transiently (less than 10^{-7} second) and probably were not distinguishable from other lipids in the bilayer on the time scale of enzyme reactions and other cellular events. Nevertheless, there are probably exceptions to this generalization, because specific lipids are required for the enzymatic functions of some transport proteins, such as the sodium and calcium pumps, and because some membrane proteins, such as glycophorin A (discussed later in this chapter), bind anionic (PS, PI) but not choline (PC, sphingomyelin) phospholipids.[72–75] Positively charged amino acids are concentrated on the cytoplasmic side of the bilayer-spanning domains of glycophorins and other membrane proteins, partly because their position determines the orientation of the protein.[76–78] Although it is not well documented, anionic phospholipids probably cluster near these regions of positive charge. Surface-bound membrane proteins such as spectrin and protein 4.1, which bind preferentially to anionic phospholipids, may also contribute to the nonrandom topography of inner membrane phospholipids.[37–40]

Bilayer Couple Hypothesis

The shape of the lipid bilayer is responsive to slight variations (less than 0.4%) in the surface area of its inner and outer halves.[79,80] This is termed the *bilayer couple effect*.[81] It reflects the tight packing of membrane lipids, the independent motion of lipids in each half of the bilayer, and the extreme thinness of the membrane (less than 0.1% of the diameter of the cell). Processes that expand the outer bilayer (or contract the inner) produce uniform membrane spiculation, called *echinocytosis* (Fig. 54-2). Conversely, relative expansion of the inner bilayer leads to membrane invagination and cup-shaped red cells (stomatocytosis). Strongly charged amphipathic compounds such as phospholipids cause echinocytosis.[80,82] They are trapped in the outer bilayer by their fixed charge. Permeable amphipaths

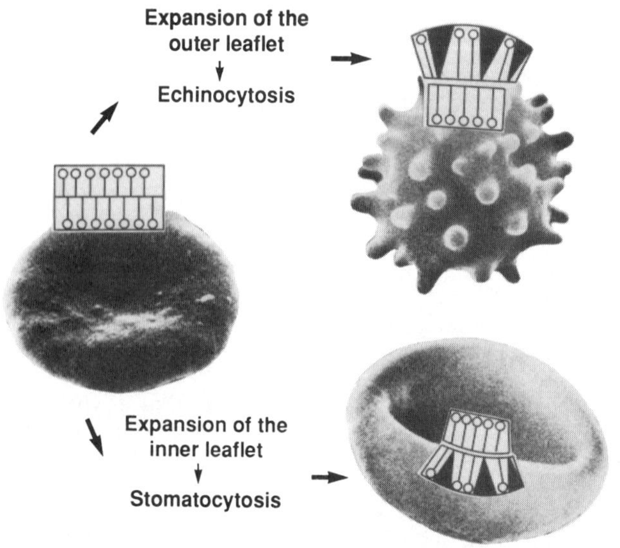

FIGURE 54-2. Bilayer couple hypothesis. Compounds or processes that selectively expand the outer leaflet of the lipid bilayer produce uniform membrane spiculation (echinocytosis). Selective expansion of the inner leaflet of the bilayer leads to membrane invagination and cup-shaped red cells (stomatocytosis). (Palek J, Jarolim P. Clinical expression and laboratory detection or red cell membrane protein mutations. Semin Hematol 1993;30:249)

(eg, weak acids and bases that can cross the membrane in their uncharged form) cause the membrane to extend toward the side of greater accumulation.[83,84] In general, cationic compounds accumulate in the negatively charged inner bilayer, and anionic compounds partition to the neutral outer bilayer. Even subtle effects, such as differences in the cross-sectional area of lipid head groups or fatty acyl tails can lead to changes in membrane curvature.[82]

The bilayer couple hypothesis predicts that shape changes resulting from expansion of one lipid leaflet can be reversed by a commensurate alteration in the other. For example, the intensely spiculated red cells of patients with abetalipoproteinemia can be almost completely converted to biconcave disks by the addition of small amounts (0.1 mmol/L) of chlorpromazine, a cationic amphipath.[85] Unfortunately, this simple test has not been widely applied to pathologic red cells, so it is difficult to estimate how often bilayer couple effects dictate cell shape in vivo.

Glycolipids and Cholesterol

Glycolipids and cholesterol are intercalated between the phospholipids in the bilayer with their long axes perpendicular to the bilayer plane. Red cell glycolipids are located entirely in the external half of the bilayer with their carbohydrate moieties extending into the aqueous phase. They carry several important red cell antigens, including A, B, H, Le^a, Le^b, and P, and may serve other important functions. The P glycolipid, for example, serves as the receptor for B19 parvovirus, the agent responsible for most aplastic crises.[86]

Cholesterol is present in about equal proportions on both sides of the bilayer[87] and equilibrates between them in seconds or less.[88] This facilitates membrane bending, since the movement of cholesterol can offset the difference in surface pressure caused by bending and compressing one of the bilayers relative to the other. At rest, cholesterol appears to have a slightly higher affinity for the outer bilayer. Cholesterol depletion promotes inward curvature of the membrane, whereas cholesterol enrichment favors outward deflection.[89] Cholesterol molecules are relatively buried, because the 3-OH group (the part of the molecule that is closest to the aqueous interface) lies about at the level of the carbonyl group of the phospholipid fatty acids.[90]

Membrane Phosphoinositides

This interesting class of phospholipids includes PI[20] and its phosphorylated forms, PI-4-monophosphate and PI-4,5-bisphosphate (PIP and PIP_2, respectively). In nucleated cells, phosphoinositides are precursors of important intracellular second messengers such as inositol-1,4,5-triphosphate and diacylglycerol.[91,92] In mature erythrocytes, phosphoinositides represent 2% to 5% of the total phospholipids. They reside largely at the inner membrane surface and undergo rapid phosphorylation and dephosphorylation.[92] Phosphoinositides help to regulate Ca^{2+} transport, interact with membrane proteins such as glycophorin C and protein 4.1, and may influence discocyte–echinocyte shape transformation. The subject has been recently reviewed.[92]

Lipid Mobility

Acyl Side Chains

Purified Lipids Exist in Gel or Liquid Crystalline States. Purified phospholipids exhibit discrete, liquid crystalline to gel-phase transitions that are dependent on the length and degree of unsaturation of their acyl side chains. Above the temperature of this transition, the acyl side chains waggle rapidly (10^8 to 10^9 times per second) from side to side, with progressively greater excursions from the glycerol ester linkage to the terminal methyl group.[93,94] The presence of a double bond in the acyl chain increases the disorder and flexibility all along the hydrocarbon chain,[95,96] especially toward the terminal methyl end.[95] Below the temperature of the liquid crystalline to gel transition, acyl chains of purified lipids are extended in stiff, parallel, hexagonally packed arrays, which are more nearly solid than liquid.

Cholesterol Creates an Intermediate State Between Gel and Liquid Lipids. Cholesterol buffers the extremes of the gel and liquid crystalline states. At temperatures above the gel–liquid phase transition, cholesterol partially immobilizes the acyl chains of phospholipids, particularly the proximal 8 to 10 carbons adjacent to the bulky steroid nucleus.[94] Below this transition, cholesterol disrupts the ordering of the acyl chains, in effect preserving membrane fluidity.[97] The net result is that cholesterol tends to abolish the gel to liquid crystalline transition and create a condition of intermediate fluidity in which the proximal ends of the hydrocarbon chains are extended and relatively rigid and the distal ends are disordered and fluid.

The red cell membrane contains relatively large amounts of cholesterol (cholesterol/phospholipid, 0.8 mol/mol) and is relatively less fluid than other plasma membranes.[98] The inner bilayer is more fluid than the outer,[25] probably because it contains more unsaturated fatty acids.[15] The significance of this difference is unknown.

Spectroscopic techniques are available for assessing the motion of various lipid-soluble probes and are widely used to measure lipid fluidity. Decreased red cell lipid fluidity due to membrane cholesterol accumulation has been implicated in the pathogenesis of acanthocytosis associated with abetalipoproteinemia[99] or liver disease (spur cell anemia)[100,101] and with a number of other conditions. It remains to be determined whether the spectroscopic changes observed are due to true alterations in lipid fluidity or to changes in lipid organization that alter the location and properties of the spectroscopic probe.

Lateral Diffusion

Phospholipids move about rapidly within each plane of model lipid bilayers.[98,102,103] From the measured lateral diffusion constants (2 to 5 $\times$ 10^8 cm^2/s), one can calculate that phospholipids exchange places with each other about 10^7 times per second. This rate is slightly damped in the red cell membrane (estimated diffusion constant of 1.4 $\times$ 10^8 cm^2/s),[104] but the difference is about what would be expected, considering the effects of cholesterol on the lateral mobility of phospholipids.[103]

Lipid Renewal Pathways

Mature Erythrocytes Cannot Synthesize Lipids. Mature erythrocytes are unable to synthesize fatty acids, phospholipids, or cholesterol de novo and depend on lipid exchange and fatty acid acylation as mechanisms for phospholipid repair and renewal (Fig. 54-3). Outer bilayer phospholipids (PC, sphingomyelin) exchange slowly (approximate turnover time of 5 days)[105] with the phospholipids of plasma lipoproteins.[106,107] Inner bilayer phospholipids (PS, PE) are unable to participate in this process and are virtually unexchangeable.[105]

Esterification Depletes Red Cell Cholesterol. Fatty acids and lysophosphatides exchange more rapidly. Red cell membrane cholesterol (unesterified) also exchanges readily with the unesterified cholesterol in plasma lipoproteins ($T_{1/2}$ of 7 hours), where it is partially converted to esterified cholesterol by the action of lecithin:cholesterol

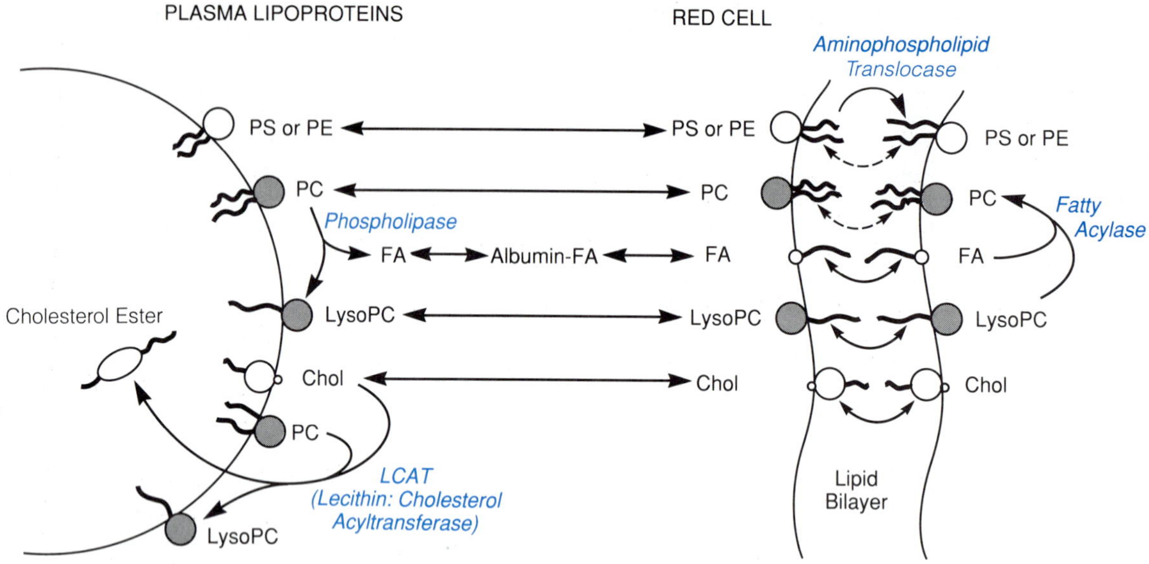

FIGURE 54-3. Pathways for lipid exchange and fatty acid replacement in the red cell membrane. PC, phosphatidylcholine; PS, phosphatidylserine; PE, phosphatidylethanolamine; LysoPC, lysophosphatidylcholine; Chol, cholesterol; FA, fatty acid. (After Becker PS, Lux SE. Disorders of the red cell membrane. In: Nathan DG, Oski FA, eds. Hematology of infancy and childhood, ed 4. Philadelphia, WB Saunders, 1993)

acyltransferase (LCAT). Because the newly formed cholesteryl ester cannot return to the red cell membrane (there is virtually no esterified cholesterol in the membrane), LCAT catalyzes a unidirectional pathway (see Fig. 54-3) that depletes the membrane of cholesterol and decreases its surface area. Conversely, when LCAT is absent or inhibited, excess membrane cholesterol accumulates, expanding the membrane surface area.[108]

Fatty Acid Acylation May Repair Phospholipid Side Chains. The fatty acid acylation pathway is an active metabolic pathway and requires ATP energy. This system combines fatty acids with lysophosphatides (principally lyso-PC) to remake the native phospholipid (see Fig. 54-3).[109–111] The acylase enzyme and its phospholipid products are located in the inner bilayer.[112] In theory, this enzyme should facilitate the renewal of lost or damaged fatty acid side chains and should prevent the accumulation of deleterious lysophosphatides within the membrane; it is not certain whether the phospholipases necessary to remove damaged fatty acids operate in the red cell.

These renewal pathways, although limited, permit a slow replacement of membrane lipid components. About 30 days are required for erythrocyte lipids to reach equilibrium after a change in dietary fatty acids.[113] Theoretically, this could be pathologically significant in persons on unusual diets (eg, infants receiving a high intake of medium-chain triglycerides). To date, no pathologic consequences have been reported.

MEMBRANE PROTEIN STRUCTURE

Composition

The red cell membrane contains 12 major proteins[7] and hundreds of minor ones.[114] The major proteins have been intensively studied and are the subject of many reviews.[113,115–137] Related reviews focus on diseases of the red cell membrane.[138–149] With the exception of a few functionally important proteins, few reviews have emphasized the minor components.[150–152]

Integral and Peripheral Membrane Proteins. The red cell membrane is usually defined by hypotonic hemolysis[5,7] and analyzed by sodium dodecyl sulfate polyacrylamide gel electrophoresis (SDS-PAGE),[7,153,154] which separates the proteins according to molecular weight (Fig. 54-4; Table 54-2). In general, membrane proteins are classified as either

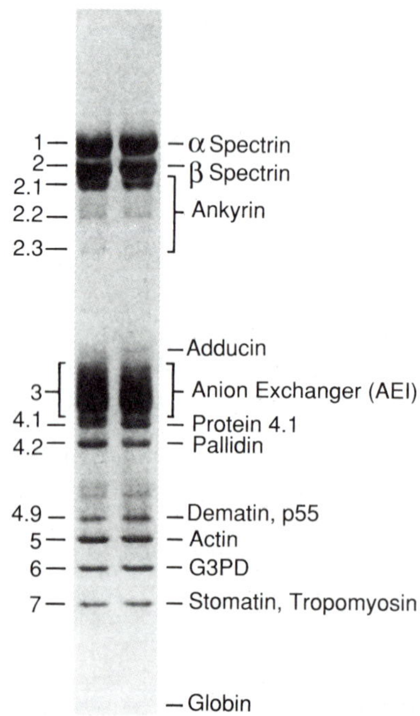

FIGURE 54-4. Major proteins of the red cell membrane. The proteins are separated by SDS gel electrophoresis using the Fairbanks-Agre gel system[7,236] and are stained with Coomassie blue. The glycophorins and the Rh protein bind this dye poorly and are not visible. (After Costa FF, et al. Linkage of dominant hereditary spherocytosis to the gene for the erythrocyte membrane-skeleton protein ankyrin. N Engl J Med 1990;323:1046)

integral or *peripheral*. Integral membrane proteins penetrate or traverse the lipid bilayer and interact with the hydrophobic lipid core. They include transport proteins such as band 3 (AE1), the anion exchange channel, and the glycophorins, which carry membrane receptors and antigens. Peripheral proteins interact with integral proteins or lipids at the membrane surface but do not penetrate into the bilayer core. In the red cell, the major peripheral membrane proteins all are located on the cytoplasmic membrane face and include enzymes such as glyceraldehyde-3-phosphate dehydrogenase (G3PD) and structural proteins such as spectrin and actin.

Intramembranous Particles

Freeze-cleave electron microscopy of erythrocyte membranes reveals randomly distributed intramembranous particles of 80 to 100 Å on both the inner (protoplasmic) and outer (external) bilayer faces. Some studies suggest the more numerous protoplasmic intramembranous particles are primarily band 3 (AE1) dimers and tetramers, and that external intramembranous particles are mostly glycophorins or the glucose transport protein.[155,156]

Band 3

Band 3 (anion exchange protein 1 [AE1]), the erythroid anion exchange protein, is the major integral protein of the red cell. It accounts for 25% to 30% of the membrane protein or about 1.2 million copies per cell. Human band 3 is a single 101,791-dalton polypeptide, containing 911 amino acids.[157,158] It migrates as a diffuse band on SDS gels (see Fig. 54-4) because of heterogenous glycosylation. Human, mouse, chicken, and trout cDNAs of band 3 have been analyzed,[157–161] and most of the mouse gene (20 exons, about 17 kb) has been sequenced.[162] The human gene is located on chromosome 17 (see Table 54-2).

Four to 20 percent[163–165] of different populations are heterozygous for a polymorphic but functionally normal band 3, called *band 3 Memphis*, in which lysine 56 is replaced by glutamic acid.[166–167]

Band 3 is the conduit for the physiologically important chloride–bicarbonate exchange.[168–172] It is also a major binding site for a variety of enzymes and cytoplasmic membrane components. These two functions—transport and binding—are relegated to two structurally independent domains of the molecule[173–174] (Fig. 54-5).

N-Terminal (Cytoplasmic) Domain

N-Terminal Domain Binds Glycolytic Enzymes, Hemoglobin, and Skeletal Proteins. The N-terminal domain is the binding domain. Most of it can be released from the membrane, as a 43-kd fragment, by treatment with chymotrypsin or trypsin.[175] The domain is an elongated, water-soluble, 403–amino acid segment, with a pliant "hinge" near the center (see Fig. 54-5). The first 45 amino acids are highly acidic and probably stretch into the cytoplasm. The remainder of the domain is remarkably mobile. It extends at high pH and contracts at low pH, presumably flexing about the hinge region[174] (Fig. 54-6).

Glycolytic Enzyme Binding Is Regulated by Tyrosine Phosphorylation. The acidic N-terminal sequence contains the binding sites for the glycolytic enzymes G3PD,[176–178] phosphoglycerate kinase (PGK),[179–181] and aldolase.[180,182,183] About 65% of G3PD, 50% of PGK, and 40% of aldolase are bound in the intact red cell.[176,180] Membrane attachment inhibits enzyme activity[177,182,183] and is regulated by substrates, cofactors, and inhibitors of the three enzymes, and by phosphorylation[184] of tyrosine 8. The observations suggest that the protein may be an important regulator of red cell glycolysis. In fact, mild oxidants, which stimulate tyrosine phosphorylation in intact red cells, elevate glycolytic rates.[1]

In Vivo Hemoglobin Is Bound to About Half the Band 3 Molecules. Hemoglobin binds weakly (K_D less than 10^{-4} mol/L) to the acidic N terminal.[185,186] Deoxyhemoglobin binds better than oxyhemoglobin, but 2,3-diphosphoglycerate (2,3-DPG) inhibits deoxyhemoglobin binding.[185] This is understandable from x-ray diffraction studies, which show that the first 5 to 7 amino acids of band 3 insert deeply into the 2,3-DPG–binding cleft of hemoglobin.[186] Nevertheless, because the concentration of hemoglobin is so high, roughly half of the band 3 molecules have hemoglobin attached under physiologic conditions.[185] Hemichromes, a partially denatured form of hemoglobin, bind much better[187,188] and copolymerize with band 3, forming an aggregate.[188–190] This is likely to play a role in red cell senescence.

Ankyrin Binds to the Flexed Conformations of Band 3. Three peripheral membrane proteins, ankyrin,[175,191–195] protein 4.1,[196–197] and pallidin (protein 4.2),[178,198–200] also bind to the cytoplasmic segment of band 3. The ankyrin binding site has been partially characterized and includes sequences from the proximal, medial, and distal portions of the cytoplasmic domain[192,194,201] (see Fig. 54-5). This and other evidence indicate that the domain has a complex folded structure. Ankyrin binds to the flexed conformations of band 3 (see Fig. 54-6), most likely to band 3 tetramers[195] (see section on self-association of band 3). Protein 4.1 binds near the N terminal and competes with ankyrin for attachment.[197] Judging from naturally occurring mutations, pallidin binds in the same region[200] or in the distal part of the domain[202] (see Fig. 54-5).

C-Terminal (Membrane) Domain

Membrane Domain Contains the Anion Exchange Channel. The 52-kd membrane domain (amino acids 404 to 911) contains the anion exchange channel. The 1.2 million channels in each red cell can exchange 10^{10} to 10^{11} HCO_3^- and Cl^- anions per second (calculated from data in Weith and associates[2]). This allows much of the HCO^3 produced in red cells by carbonic anhydrase to be carried in the plasma (Fig. 54-7) and increases CO_2 transport from the tissues to the lungs by about 60%.[2] The H^+ byproduct of the carbonic anhydrase reaction binds to hemoglobin and facilitates O_2 release to the tissues (Bohr effect). All these reactions are reversed in the lungs.

Anion Exchange Occurs by a Ping-Pong Mechanism. It appears that anions move by a "ping-pong" mechanism in which an intracellular anion enters the transport channel and is translocated outward and released, with the channel remaining in the outward conformation until an extracellular anion enters and triggers the reverse cycle.[131,136,203,204] Models have incorporated the concept of a "vestibule,"[136,205] an intermediate structure that is stabilized by the anion and is not accessible to either surface (Fig. 54-8). (This structure has not been directly identified and may not exist.) Whatever the mechanism, it probably involves a fairly large conformational change, since anion transport has a high energy and volume of activation.[206,207] Exchange is extremely rapid ($T_{1/2}$ of 50 msec) for Cl^- and H_3^-, the physiologic anions. The specificity of the channel is broad, and larger anions such as sulfate, phosphate, pyruvate, and superoxide are also transported, although at much slower rates.[131]

A large number of potent and useful anion transport inhibitors are known, especially various stilbene disulfonates such as DIDS (4,4′-diisothiocyanostilbene-2,2′-disulfonate). These bind to two lysine residues, probably Lys 539 and

TABLE 54-2. Major Human Erythrocyte Membrane Proteins

SDS Gel Band[d]	Protein	Mol Wt (Gel) (×10³)	Mol Wt (Calc)[a] (×10³)	Amino Acids	Monomer Copies per Cell[b] (×10³)	Oligomeric State
1	α-Spectrin	240	281	2429	242 ± 20	Heterodimer/tetramer/oligomer
2	β-Spectrin	220	246	2137	242 ± 20	
2.1[g]	Ankyrin[g]	210	206	1880	124 ± 11[g]	Monomer
2.9	α-Adducin	103	81	737	≈30	Heterodimer/tetramer
	β-Adducin	97	80	726	≈30	
3[h]	AE1[f]	90–100[i]	102[j]	911	≈1200	Dimer or tetramer
4.1	Protein 4.1	80 + 78[k]	66[l]	588	≈200	Monomer
4.2	Pallidin	72	77	691	≈250	?Dimer or trimer
4.9[h]	Dematin[n]	48 + 52	43 + 46	383 + ?[n]	≈140	Trimer[n]
	p55	55	53	466	≈80	?Dimer
5[h]	β-Actin	43	42	375	≈500	Oligomer (≈14)
	Tropomodulin	43	41	359	≈30	Monomer
6	G3PD[f]	35	36	335	≈500	Tetramer
7[h]	Stomatin	31	32	288	—	—
	Tropomyosin	27 + 29	28[p]	239[p]	≈70	Heterodimer[p]
8	Protein 8	23	—	—	≈200	—
PAS-1	Glycophorin A[q]	36[r]	14[j]	131	≈1000	Dimer
PAS-2	Glycophorin C[q]	32[r]	14[j]	128	≈200 (C + D)[s]	—
PAS-3	Glycophorin B[q]	20[r]	8[j]	72	≈200	?Dimer
	Glycophorin D[q]	23[r]	11[j]	107	≈200 (C + D)[s]	—
	Glycophorin E[q]	—[t]	6[j]	59	—[t]	—[t]

[a] Calculated from amino acid sequences.
[b] Based on an estimate of 5.7 × 10^{-13} g protein/ghost[7] and on the approximate proportions of each protein, estimated from densitometry of SDS gels. The data for spectrin and ankyrin were measured directly by radioimmunoassay.[245]
[c] Proteins 1 to 8 were estimated from the data in Fairbanks et al,[7] Palek and Jarolim,[149] and Pinder and Gratzer[246] and from unpublished data.[247]
[d] Numbering system of Fairbanks[7] and Steck.[154] Bands 1 to 8 refer to Coomassie blue–stained gels. PAS-1 to PAS-3 refer to periodic acid-Schiff–stained gels.
[e] The GenBank accession number can be used to retrieve the nucleotide and protein sequence from the GenBank database.
[f] HE, hereditary elliptocytosis; HS, hereditary spherocytosis; HPP, hereditary pyropoikilocytosis; HAc, hereditary acanthocytosis; HSt, hereditary stomatocytosis; SAO, Southeast Asian ovalocytosis; AE1, anion exchange protein 1 (erythroid anion exchange protein); G3PD, glyceraldehyde-3-phosphate dehydrogenase.
[g] Protein 2.1 is full-length ankyrin. Other isoforms are evident on SDS gels including band 2.2, 195 kd; band 2.3, 175 kd; and band 2.6, 145 kd. Band 2.2 is produced by alternate splicing. The origin of the other bands is unknown. The data shown are for ankyrin 2.1 except for the number of copies/cell and approximate proportion (wt%), which include all isoforms.
[h] The α- and β-adducins lie in the upper part of SDS gel band 3. Band 4.9 contains both dematin and p55; band 5 contains β-actin and tropomodulin; band 7 contains stomatin and tropomyosin.
[i] The protein runs as a broad band on SDS gels due to heterogeneous glycosylation.

Lys 851, on externally exposed portions of the protein in or near the entrance of the channel.[131,169]

Transport Channel Probably Located at Monomer Interface in Band 3 Dimers. The relation of the transport mechanism and band 3 structure is being investigated. The membrane domain is composed of 12 or 14 transmembrane helices, connected by hydrophilic segments.[136,157] The location and orientation of these structures (which are inside and which are outside) have been intensively studied for many years and recently reviewed.[131,136,157,208,209] The helices must form the transport channel, but how they do so is unknown. Wang and Reithmeier[210] and colleagues have derived a low-resolution structure of band 3 by image analysis of negatively stained two-dimensional crystals of the membrane domain. They find that the membrane domain exists in two different conformations, represented by two crystal structures. Perhaps these are the inward- and outward-facing transporters. The basic structural unit in both is an oblong *band 3 dimer* (about 40 × 110 Å). At the center of the dimer, the two monomers abut and appear to form a channel, presumably the transport channel.[210] There is also a flexible subdomain on the far side of each monomer, which might be formed by one or more of the large cytoplasmic loops between transmembrane helices.

It is unclear whether the apparent morphologic channel is actually one or two functional channels. A variety of studies suggest that each monomer contains a functional anion channel.[211,212] If two channels exist, their location at the interface of band 3 monomers raises the possibility that two anions may be translocated simultaneously in opposite directions or that allosteric interactions between the subunits may regulate transport or both.[213,214]

The Ii Blood Group Antigens Are Carried on Band 3. Band 3 contains a single fatty acid[215] esterified to Cys 843

Approximate Proportion[c] (Wt%)	Peripheral or Integral	GenBank Accession Number[e]	Gene Symbol	Chromosome Location	Gene Size (kb)	Number of Exons	Associated Diseases[f]
14	P	M61877	SPTA1	1q22 → q23	80	52	HE, HPP, HS
13	P	J05500	SPTB	14q23 → q24.2	>100	≈32	HE, HPP, HS
6[q]	P	X16609	ANK1	8p11.2	>120	42	HS
<1	P	X58141	ADDA	4p16.3	—	—	—
<1	P	X58199	ADDB	—	—	—	—
29	I	M27819	EPB3	17q12 → q21	17	20	HS, SAO, HAc
5	P	M14993	EL1	1p33 → p34.2	>250	23	HE
5	P	M30646	ELB42	15q15 → q21	20	13	HS[m]
1	P	—	—	—	—	—	—
	P	M64925	MPP1	Xq28	—	—	—
6	P	X00351	ACTB	7pter → q22	>4	6	—
	P	M77016	TMOD	9q22	—	—	—
5[o]	P	M17851	GAPD	12q13	5	9	—
4	I	M81635	—	—	12	6	?HSt
	P	X04588	TPM3	1q31	—	—	—
1–2	P	—	—	—	—	—	—
1.6	I	X51798	GYPA	4q31	>40	7	None
0.1	I	M36284[s]	GYPC[s]	2q14 → q21	14[s]	4	HE
0.2	I	J02982	GYPB	4q31	>30	5	None
0.02	I	M36284[s]	GYPC[s]	2q14 → q21	14[s]	4	HE
—[t]	I	M29610	GYPE	4q31	>30	4	—

[j] The calculated molecular weight does not include the contribution of the carbohydrate chains.

[k] Protein 4.1 is a doublet (4.1a and 4.1b) on SDS gels. Protein 4.1a is derived from 4.1b by slow deamidation.[248] Its proportion is a measure of RBC age.

[l] Protein 4.1 exists in a very large number of isoforms.[125] The major erythroid isoform is listed here. It is not known why its calculated molecular weight deviates so much from the apparent molecular weight on SDS gels.

[m] Deficiency of pallidin is associated with a variety of morphologies (see text) but spherocytes predominate.[122] An abnormality of a nonerythroid isoform of pallidin is present in the *pallid* mouse mutation.[249]

[n] Only the 48-kd subunit has been cloned.[250] Although dematin is present as a trimer in solution, the 48- and 52-kd subunits have an apparent stoichiometry of 3:1 on SDS gels.

[o] The amount of G3PD (band 6) associated with the membrane varies from person to person (≈3 to 6 wt%).

[p] Tropomyosin is a heterodimer of the 27-kd and 29-kd subunits. There are about 70,000 copies of each chain per RBC. Data for the calculated molecular weight, the number of amino acids and the accession number are for fibroblast tropomyosin. The RBC isoform has not been sequenced.

[q] The glycophorins (GpA to GpD) are visible only on PAS-stained gels.

[r] Molecular weights, including carbohydrate, estimated from mobilities on SDS gels.[251]

[s] Glycophorins C and D are probably synthesized from the same mRNA using different translational start sites.[120] The total number of glycophorin C and D molecules is about 200,000.

[t] Glycophorin E mRNA has been identified but it is not certain that the mRNA is translated.

and a single, complex carbohydrate chain attached to Asn 642[216] (see Fig. 54-5). Removal of the carbohydrate does not affect anion exchange. It is a complex lactosaminoglycan,[217,218] which is variable in length and contains Ii blood group antigens. In fetal cells, it is unbranched and has i specificity.[217,219] In adult red cells, a branched structure with I reactivity is present.[218,219] The rare absence of I antigen in adult cells apparently results from the lack of the branching enzyme.[219]

Self-Association of Band 3. Band 3 forms stable dimers, tetramers, and higher oligomers in solutions of the nonionic detergent $C_{12}E_8$ (octaethylene glycol *n*-dodecyl monoether). These can be separated on sizing columns and quantitated. Normally, 70% is in the dimer form and 30% in tetramers and oligomers. Almost all of the latter is associated with the membrane skeleton,[220] which fits with other evidence that ankyrin binds preferentially to band 3 tetramers.[193,195,221] Since isolated membrane domains only form dimers,[220] tetramers are probably assembled by crosslinking neighboring dimers through the cytoplasmic domain either with ankyrin (the physiologic cross-linker) or by oxidation (disulfide cross-linking),[201] hemichromes,[188–190] or other means.

Association of Band 3 With Glycophorin A. There is increasing evidence that glycophorin A (GPA) and band 3 are associated in the membrane. Two observations stand out: (1) A monoclonal antibody to the Wr^b blood group antigen immunoprecipitates both proteins.[222] (2) The coexpression of GPA in *Xenopus* oocytes enhances expression of band 3, by facilitating transport of band 3 from the endoplasmic reticulum to the cell surface.[223] The purpose of the interaction in vivo is a mystery since red cells that lack GPA are structurally and functionally normal (see text that follows).

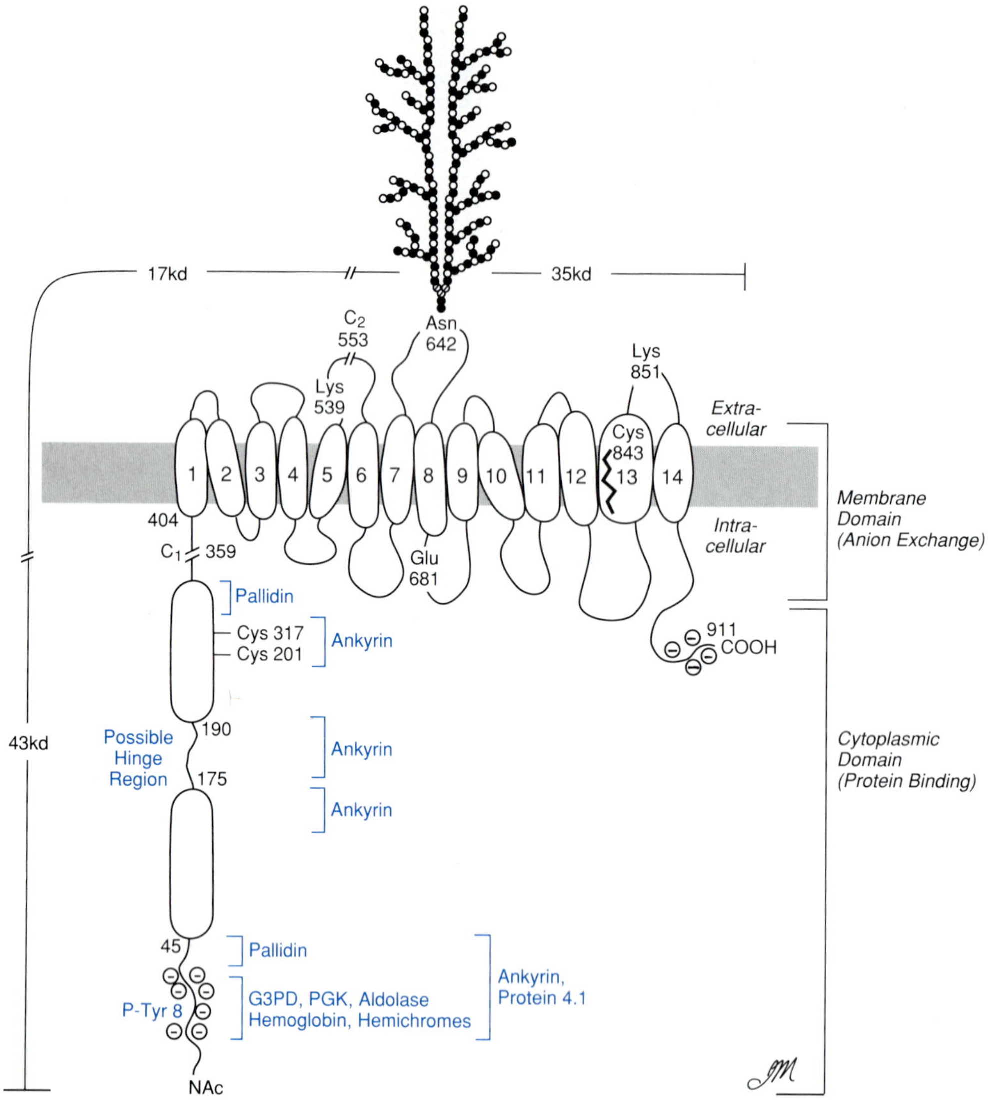

FIGURE 54-5. Organizational model of human erythrocyte anion exchange protein (band 3, AE1). The protein is divided into two structurally and functionally distinct domains: an approximately 43-kd cytoplasmic domain (amino acids 1 to 359), which contains binding sites for several cellular proteins, and an approximately 52-kd (17 kd + 35 kd), transmembrane domain (amino acids 360 to 911), which forms the anion exchange channel. The two regions can be separated by chymotrypsin cleavage at the inner membrane (C1). A second chymotryptic site (C2) is accessible at the external surface.

Cytoplasmic domain: The highly acidic N terminal (amino acids 1 to 45) binds hemoglobin, hemichromes, protein 4.1, and the glycolytic enzymes phosphoglycerate kinase (PGK), aldolase, and glyceraldehyde-3-phosphate dehydrogenase (G3PD). Enzyme attachment is blocked by phosphorylation of tyrosine 8. Ankyrin and probably pallidin (protein 4.2) binding involves several noncontiguous regions scattered throughout the cytoplasmic domain, which suggests that these binding sites are formed by protein folding. A functional hinge exists in the middle of the domain (see Fig. 54-6).

Transmembrane domain: Band 3 may contain as many as 14 transmembrane segments. Their orientation with respect to the inside and outside of the membrane has been extensively studied; almost nothing is known about how they are positioned, relative to each other, to form the anion channel. Lys 539 and Lys 851 are probably the sites where H2-DIDS, a covalent inhibitor of anion transport, attaches to band 3. Lys 851 and Glu 681 (in its protonated form) are candidates for the specific sites involved in monovalent and divalent anion transport, respectively.[136,238,239] A fatty acid, indicated by the zig-zag symbol, is esterified to Cys 843, and a complex carbohydrate structure is attached to Asn 642. Solid circles, N-acetylglucosamine; hatched circles, mannose; open circles, galactose. (After Becker PS, Lux SE. Disorders of the red cell membrane. In: Nathan DG, Oski FA, eds. Hematology of infancy and childhood, ed 4. Philadelphia, WB Saunders, 1993)

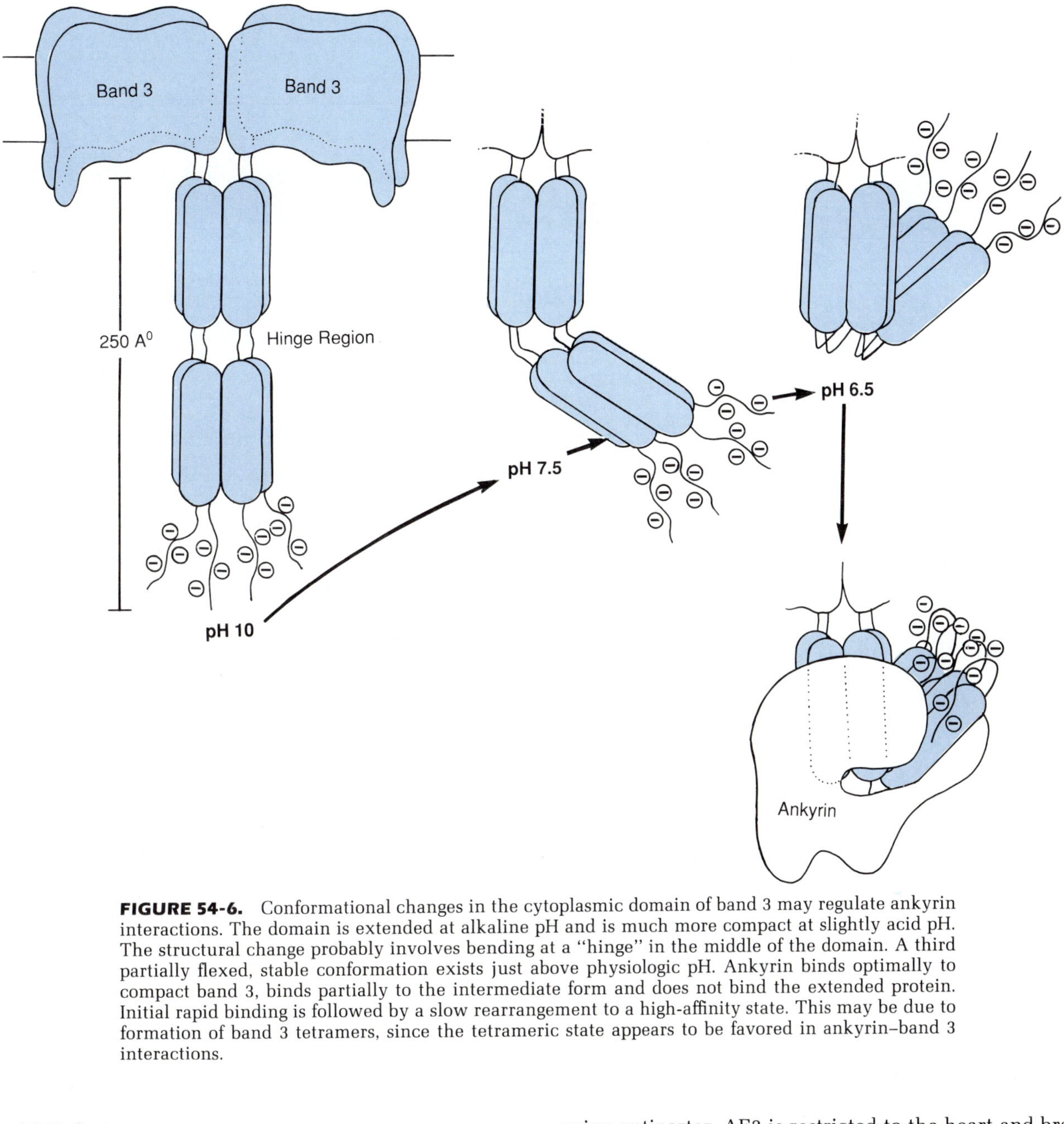

FIGURE 54-6. Conformational changes in the cytoplasmic domain of band 3 may regulate ankyrin interactions. The domain is extended at alkaline pH and is much more compact at slightly acid pH. The structural change probably involves bending at a "hinge" in the middle of the domain. A third partially flexed, stable conformation exists just above physiologic pH. Ankyrin binds optimally to compact band 3, binds partially to the intermediate form and does not bind the extended protein. Initial rapid binding is followed by a slow rearrangement to a high-affinity state. This may be due to formation of band 3 tetramers, since the tetrameric state appears to be favored in ankyrin–band 3 interactions.

Band 3 Defects

Defects of band 3 have been identified in four diseases: (1) HS, due to decreased synthesis, membrane insertion, or stability of band 3, or to mutations in the pallidin binding sites; (2) Southeast Asian ovalocytosis, due to deletion of amino acids 400 to 408; (3) rare forms of inherited acanthocytosis, in which two band 3 variants exhibiting increased anion transport were reported[224–227]; and (4) congenital dyserythropoietic anemia type II (CDA II), in which the lactosaminoglycan side chain is improperly constructed due to lack of the relevant glycosyltransferases. The first three disorders are discussed in later sections. CDA II is covered in Chapter 9.

Anion Exchangers in Nonerythroid Tissues

Two other genes encoding band 3 (AE1)–related anion exchange proteins have been identified: AE2 and AE3[228–230] (reviewed in Alper[115] and Fukuda and associates[219]). AE2 is widely distributed and is probably the general tissue anion antiporter. AE3 is restricted to the heart and brain. Both proteins are larger than AE1 because of addition of about 300 amino acids at the N terminal. All three AEs are strongly conserved, particularly in the membrane domain.[232–234] AE1 is also expressed outside the red cell in the kidney and testis. The kidney transcript lacks the first 66 amino acids and presumably cannot bind glycolytic enzymes and some membrane skeletal proteins[232,233] (see Fig. 54-5).

For interested readers, a number of excellent reviews of band 3 structure and function have appeared.[115,131,133,136,168,174,231,235]

Glycophorins

Glycophorin A. GPA (reviewed by Chasis and Mohandas[121] and Fukuda[126]) is the major sialoglycoprotein of the red cell (about 1 million copies per cell; see Table 54-2). It is also known as PAS 2 or glycoprotein α.[265] The 36-kd protein has a single transmembrane region and is

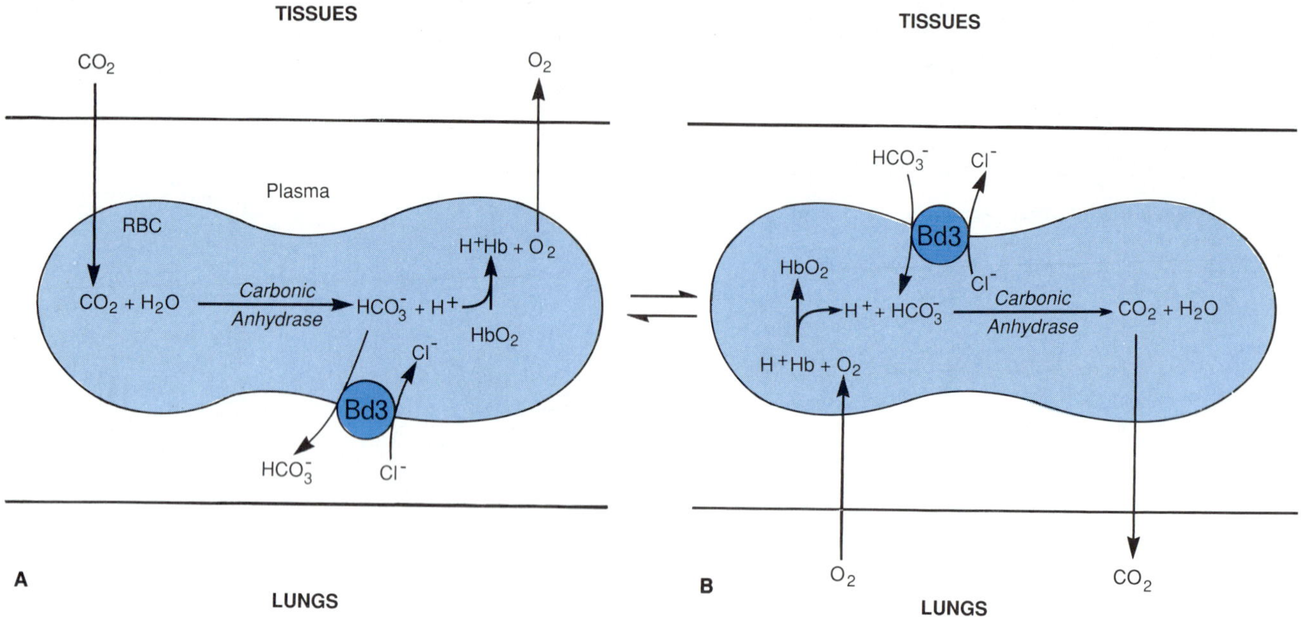

FIGURE 54-7. Function of band 3 in O_2 and CO_2 transport. (**A**) Tissue CO_2 is converted into HCO_3^- and H^+ in the red cell by carbonic anhydrase. Band 3-mediated exchange of the HCO_3^- for Cl^- (Hamburger shift) allows HCO_3^- to be carried in the plasma as well as in the red cell and increases CO_2 transport by 60%. The H^+ binds to hemoglobin and facilitates O_2 release (Bohr effect) and tissue oxygenation. (**B**) These processes are reversed in the lungs, promoting hemoglobin oxygenation and CO_2 release. (After Weith JO et al. Chloride-bicarbonate exchange in red blood cells: physiology of transport and chemical modification of binding sites. Philos Trans R Soy Soc Lond [Biol] 1982;299: 383)

oriented with its N terminal outside[252,289,290] (Fig. 54-9A). The extracellular domain (residues 1 to 61) contains 15 tetrasaccharides that are O-glycosidically linked to serine or threonine residues and one complex oligosaccharide[291] attached to Asn 26. Overall, the carbohydrate accounts for about 60% of the mass of the molecule. This includes much of the sialic acid on the red cell membrane, and the M and N blood group antigens. Amino acid residues 1 and 5 are variable and contribute to the MN blood group antigens, along with sialic acid residues on adjacent O-linked tetrasaccharides.[252] In MM red cells, amino acids 1 and 5 are serine and glycine, respectively; in NN red cells, leucine and glutamic acid are present (Table 54-3).[252]

Little is known about the membrane domain (amino acids 62 to 95), except that it binds negatively charged phospholipids,[72–75] such as PS and PI, and is probably the site of

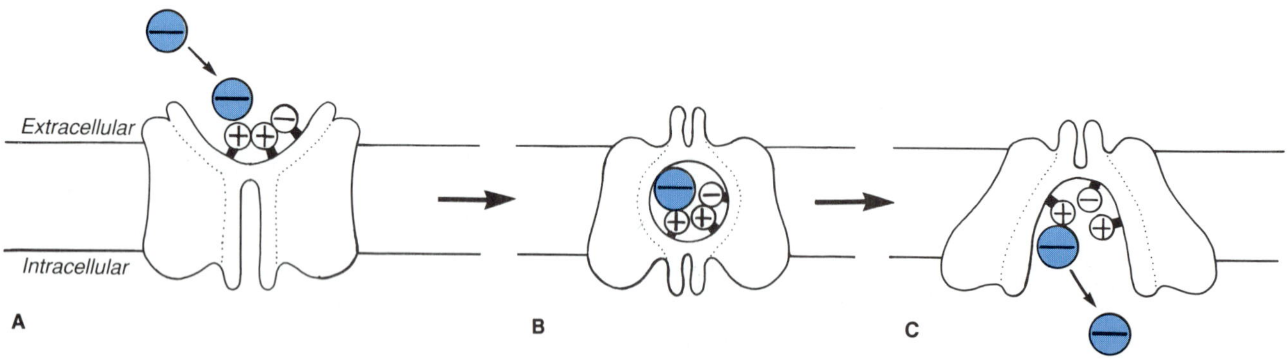

FIGURE 54-8. Model of anion transport. The protein may exist in an outward (**A**) or inward (**C**) facing orientation but may not adopt both of these configurations simultaneously and switches from one to the other only in the absence of an anion rarely (perhaps 1 in 20,000 times). The thin permeability barrier separates funnel-shaped channels that are probably lined with positive charges to exclude cations and guide anions to the critical translocation sites. Lys 851 may be one of the critical sites involved in monovalent anion transport. Glu 681, when protonated, probably serves as the second site needed for transport of divalent anions. In this model, binding of the anion to the translocation sites allows the protein to form a translocation intermediate (**B**), trapping the anion in a protein "vestibule." The hypothesized intermediate is stabilized by chelation of the anion and cannot form without it. Presumably, the protein enclosing the anion must be flexible to accommodate different-sized ions. Dissociation of the transition state moves the anion across the membrane. (After Krupka RM. Role of substrate binding in exchange-only transport systems. II. Implications for the mechanism of the anion exchanger of red cells. J Membr Biol 1989;109:159; Tanner MJA. Molecular and cellular biology of the erythrocyte anion exchanger [AE1]. Semin Hematol 1993;30:34)

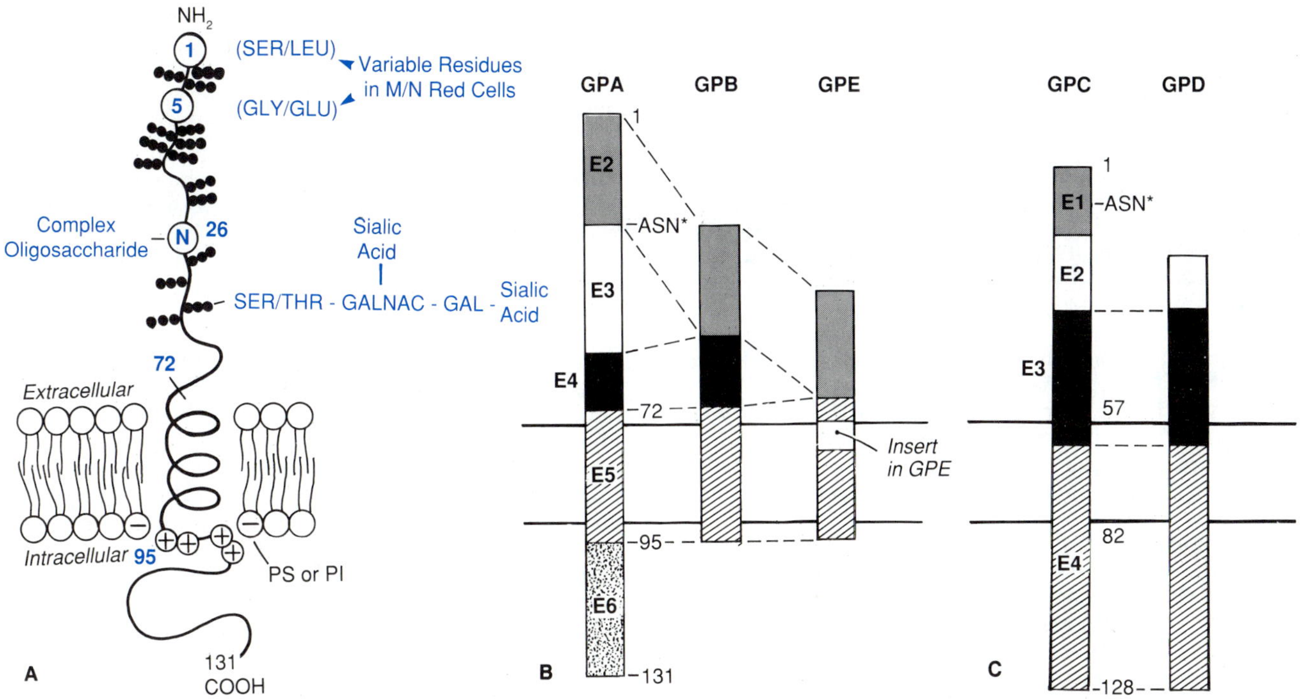

FIGURE 54-9. Structure of red cell glycophorins. (**A**) Organization of glycophorin A (GPA), the major red cell sialoglycoprotein. The external domain has 15 tetrasaccharides attached to serine or threonine residues and one complex oligosaccharide attached to asparagine 26. Residues 1 and 5 are Ser and Gly in M red cells and Leu and Glu in N cells. (**B**) Schematic representation of the domain combinations of GPA, GPB, and GPE. Each box represents the portion of each protein encoded by a specific exon or insertion sequence. (**C**) Schematic representation of the domains contributing to GPC and GPD. (After Becker PS, Lux SE. Disorders of the red cell membrane skeleton: hereditary spherocytosis and hereditary elliptocytosis. In: Scriver CS, Beaudet AL, Sly WS, Valle D, eds. The metabolic basis of inherited disease, ed 7. New York, McGraw-Hill, in press; Fukuda M. Molecular genetics of the glycophorin A gene cluster. Semin Hematol 1993;30:138)

GPA dimerization.[121] The dimeric interaction is strong and difficult to dissociate, even in detergents. Conventional SDS gels contain monomers, dimers, and heterodimers of GPA and similar oligomers of some of the other glycophorins. All these species run anomalously on SDS gels because the large amount of carbohydrate interferes with SDS binding.[292] The carbohydrate also interferes with Coomassie blue staining to the extent that the glycophorins are invisible unless special stains (eg, periodic acid-Schiff) are used. The function of the cytoplasmic domain (residues 96 to 131) is also largely unknown.

A single copy of the gene for GPA is on the long arm of

TABLE 54-3. Variants of Glycophorins A, B, and E

Variant	Defect	References
Amino-terminal	Amino-terminal sequence	
M	Ser-Ser*-Thr*-Thr*-Gly-Val. . .	252, 253
N	Leu-Ser*-Thr*-Thr*-Glu-Val. . .	252, 253
M^c	Ser-Ser*-Thr*-Thr*-Glu-Val. . .	254
M^g	Leu-Ser-Thr-Asn-Glu-Val. . .	255
H^e (Henshaw)	Trp-Ser*-Thr*-Ser*-Gly-Val. . .	256
Other	Structural defects	
En(a−)	Absence of glycophorin A (due to homologous recombination and unequal crossover → partial gene deletions)	126, 252, 257–260
S−s−U−	Absence of glycophorin B (due to homologous recombination and unequal crossover → partial gene deletions)	126, 261–263
M^k	Absence of glycophorins A & B (due to homologous recombination and unequal crossover → partial gene deletions)	126, 264
Mi.I (Miltenberger I), Mi.II, Mi.VII, Mi.VIII	Variants of glycophorin A that differ by one or two amino acids.	265–269
Mi.III, MiJ.L., Mi.V, Mi.VI, Mi.IX, Mi.X, Ph, Pj, Dantu, St^a (types A, B, & C)	Variants due to formation of Lepore-like and anti–Lepore-like hybrids of glycophorins A, B, and E	126, 265, 270–285
Cad	Carbohydrate variant with an abnormal O-linked oligosaccharide containing an extra $\beta(1 \rightarrow 4)$-linked galactosamine on the penultimate galactose residue of both glycophorins A and B	286–288

* O-glycosylation site (see Fig. 54-8).

chromosome 4 (4q31).[285,290] The protein is first detectable in proerythroblasts[121,293] and is a specific marker for erythroid cells.

Glycophorin B. Glycophorin B (GPB; also known as PAS 3 or glycoprotein δ) is almost identical to the N blood group form of GPA for the first 26 amino acid residues except that it lacks the complex oligosaccharide.[252,253] Distally, it lacks a piece of the extracellular domain of GPA corresponding to exon 3 (see Fig. 54-9*B*) and almost all of the cytoplasmic domain. The gene lies just downstream of GPA on chromosome 4 and apparently arose by gene duplication (along with GPE) during primate evolution.[294–297] Besides N-blood group activity, it carries the S, s, and U antigens. The S and s antigens differ by substitutions at residue 29 (S = Met, s = Thr).[253]

Glycophorin E. GlycophorinE (GPE) is the newest glycophorin.[240,298] It lies just beyond GPB, which it resembles in structure (see Fig. 54-9*B*). Nothing is known of its function. In fact, it is not clear whether GPE mRNA is even translated.

Glycophorins C and D. Glycophorins C and D (GPC and GPD, respectively; reviewed by Cartron and colleagues[120] and Chasis and Mohandas[121]) have a general domain structure similar to glycophorins A-B-E, but they are located on a different chromosome (2q14-q21)[299] and their amino acid sequences are unique.[300] GPC (also known as PAS 2′ or glycoprotein β) contains 128 amino acids and bears one N-linked and about 12 O-linked oligosaccharides as well as the Gerbich (Ge:3) blood group antigens (amino acids 41 to 50). Its total molecular weight is about 32 kd. GPD (also known as glycoprotein γ) is a shortened form of GPC, lacking its N-terminal region (see Fig. 54-9*C*). It arises from the same mRNA as GPC by use of an alternate initiation codon.[120,301] Unlike GPA, GPC is not erythroid specific. Low levels of GPC mRNA are detectable in many tissues.[120] In red cells, a desialylated form of GPC is exposed on the surface of early progenitors (BFU-E) and can be a useful marker of early normal or leukemic erythroid differentiation.[302] Normally glycosylated GPC first appears in the CFU-E.[121]

Glycophorin Functions

The functions of the glycophorins are uncertain, except for the obvious function that they provide most of the negative surface charge that red cells require to avoid sticking to each other and to the vascular wall.

The glycophorins have long been considered as possible conduits for transmembrane signaling and bear receptors for *Plasmodium falciparum* (see the section on glycophorins and malaria) and for a number of viruses and bacteria. Studies support this concept in some respects. When wheat germ agglutinin or specific antibodies are attached to the external domain of GPA, the internal domain binds to the underlying membrane skeleton.[303,304] These increased cross-links make the membrane harden dramatically and cause it to acquire irreversible, plastic-like properties on deformation. The effect seems to involve transmembrane communication rather than antibody or lectin cross-linking, since it is also observed with monovalent Fab fragments but is not observed in red cells bearing variant glycophorins that lack a cytoplasmic domain (eg, Miltenberger V [MiV]).[305] The reason why red cells have this interesting property is a mystery. Chasis and Mohandas[121] note that a number of pathogens adhere to red cells and suggest that the consequently stiffened erythrocytes may hasten reticuloendothelial removal of the invaders. This imaginative idea deserves more attention.

GPC binds to protein 4.1 and may help anchor the skeleton to the membrane. This interaction is discussed in the section on protein 4.1 later in this chapter.

Glycophorin Variants

The realization that the MNSs blood group antigens are carried by the glycophorins has led to the discovery of a variety of glycophorin defects in persons with variants of this blood group system (Fig. 54-10; see Table 54-3).

Glycophorin A-B-E Variants. The most dramatic defects result in complete loss of GPA (En(a−) red cells), GPB (S−s− red cells), or both (M^kM^k red cells). These rare defects are often caused by gene deletions from unequal recombination of the neighboring GPA and GPB genes (see Fig. 54-10). The En(a−) red cells are the best studied. They have weak MN blood group antigens and, as expected from the gene defect, lack GPA.[257,260] The red cell compensates for this potentially disastrous loss of surface charge (normally about 60% is from GPA) by increasing the glycosylation of band 3.[257,259,264] As a result the surface charge is only about 20% less than expected.

Recombination events leading to hybrid glycophorin molecules are relatively common among the glycophorin A-B-E variants (see Table 54-3), as would be expected for a cluster of recently duplicated genes.[126,265,271–285] They are believed to result from chromosomal misalignment during meiosis and subsequent nonhomologous cross-over of the chromosomes in the region of GPA and GPB. The mechanism is illustrated at the bottom of Figure 54-10. A similar process is known to be responsible for the Lepore hemoglobins (see Chap. 52). Both Lepore-like and anti–Lepore-like recombinations of the glycophorins occur. In the former, illustrated by the MiV variant,[275,284,285] the normal GPA gene is replaced by a fusion gene containing the N-terminal end of GPA and the C-terminal end of GPB. In the latter, illustrated by the St^a variant,[274,276,279,281] the hybrid protein is reversed (N-terminal GPB, C-terminal GPA) and inserted between the GPA and GPB genes, neither of which is lost.

None of the GPA and GPB variants produces any detectable change in erythropoiesis or in the shape, function, or life-span of the affected red cells. This is true even in those rare persons with complete absence of both GPA and GPB[264] and indicates either that GPA and GPB have no critical basal functions in the erythrocyte or that such functions are duplicated or can be subsumed by some other protein (eg, band 3, GPC).

Glycophorin C-D Variants. Defects in GPC and GPD affect the Gerbich antigen system. Ge− red cells of the Ger, Yus, and Webb phenotypes have mutations in the extracellular domain of GPC. Gerbich-type cells lack exon 2, Yus type cells lack exon 3, and Webb-type cells have a missense mutation of GPC (Asn 8 → Ser).[306] In all three cases, the mutant GPC protein is present although its antigenicity is altered. In the Leach phenotype, on the other hand, GPC protein is absent, due either to a deletion of both exons 3 and 4[307–309] or to a frameshift mutation.[309] The Leach phenotype does not result in significant anemia, but it does cause elliptocytosis,[310,311] as well as a decrease in membrane deformability and mechanical stability.[312,313] In contrast, red cells with the extracellular Ge− mutants and red cells that lack GPA or GPB have normal mechanical properties.[121,314]

Studies suggest that the deficiency of GPC is not directly responsible for the altered mechanical properties. Instead, the mechanical instability appears to be due to a concomitant partial deficiency of protein 4.1. The instability is fully corrected by introducing 4.1 or its spectrin-binding domain (which facilitates spectrin–actin interactions) into GPC-

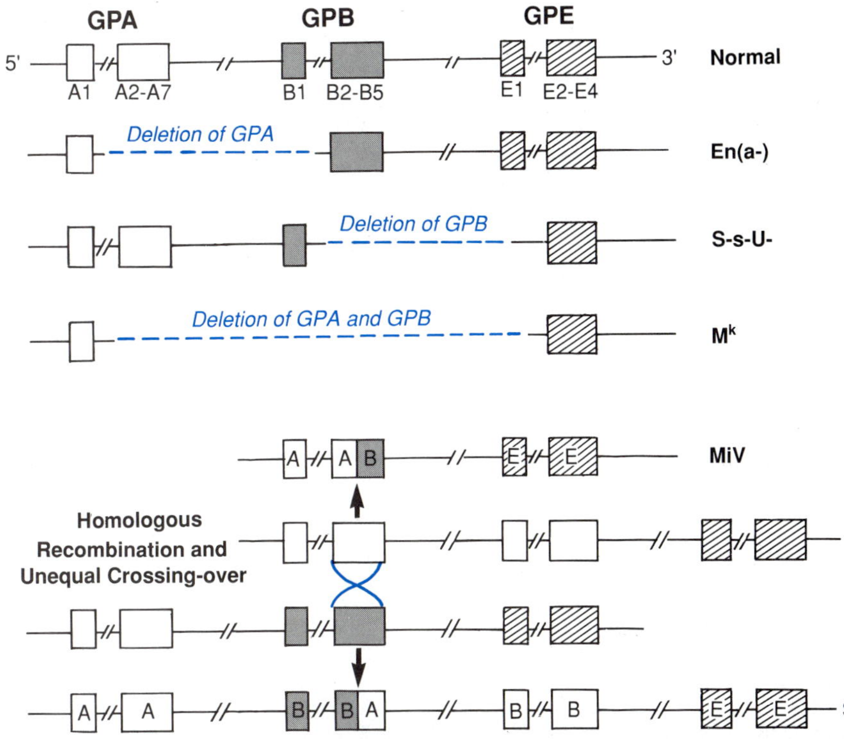

FIGURE 54-10. Glycophorin variants. Organization of the GPA, GPB, and GPE genes on chromosome 4 and probable deletions in the En(a−), S−s−U−, M^k, Miltenberger type V (MiV), and Stones (St^a) variants. The MiV hemoglobins. In MiV red cells, the normal GPB gene is replaced by a fusion gene (Lepore-type recombination). In St^a erythrocytes, the product of the reciprocal exchange is inserted between the GPA and GPB loci, but no normal genes are lost (anti–Lepore-type recombination). (After Vignal A, et al. Promoter sequence and chromosomal organization of the genes encoding glycophorins A, B, and E. Gene 1990;95:289)

deficient red cells.[315] Why protein 4.1 and another recently described protein, p55 (see section on protein p55), are deficient is not completely clear. The cytoplasmic domain of GPC interacts with both proteins and presumably helps bind them to the membrane (see section on protein 4.1).

Glycophorins and Malaria

Research indicates that GPA, and possibly GPB and GPC, are receptors for *P falciparum*. This was first discovered by Perkins[316] and has now been confirmed in many other laboratories (reviewed by Gratzer and Dluzewski[144] and Hermentin and Enders[317]) either by direct competition using the purified sialoglycoproteins or by the inability of *P falciparum* to infect red cells with various glycophorin abnormalities.[318–320] The principal ligand appears to be sialic acid attached through an α2–3 linkage to galactose.[321] It binds to EBA-175, a 175-kd erythrocyte-binding antigen located on the surface of *P falciparum* merozoites,[322] and inhibits parasite invasion.[321]

Other Integral Proteins

The red cell membrane contains a large number of other integral proteins, probably more than 100, which are beyond the scope of this chapter.[114] These include the Rh protein,[150] Kell antigen,[151] glucose transporter, urea transporter, Na^+/K^+-ATPase, Ca^{2+}-ATPase, Mg^{2+}-ATPase, various kinases and phosphatases, acetylcholinesterase, decay accelerating factor, complement proteins (C3b and C4b), and receptors for transferrin, insulin, insulin-like growth factors, thyroid hormone, parathyroid hormone, β-adrenergic agonists, cholinergic agents, diphtheria toxin, ceruloplasmin, and opiates.

MEMBRANE SKELETON

Definition

Operationally, the red cell membrane skeleton is the insoluble proteinaceous residue that remains after extraction of red cells[323] or their ghosts[324] with the nonionic detergent Triton X-100. It makes up 55% to 60% of the membrane protein mass and includes all the spectrin, actin, tropomyosin, tropomodulin, adducin, ankyrin, protein 4.1, dematin (protein 4.9), and a portion of band 3, pallidin (protein 4.2), and the proteins in the band 7 region on SDS gels (see Fig. 54-4). Spectrin, actin, protein 4.1, and dematin (and perhaps tropomodulin and adducin) form the core of the structure, since the skeleton retains its shape when other components are eluted with hypertonic potassium chloride but disintegrates when spectrin or actin are removed.[323] All the major skeletal proteins have been cloned and investigated; their specifications are listed in Table 54-2. They are discussed individually and then considered regarding how they are organized to form the skeleton.

Spectrin

Erythrocyte spectrin is the major skeletal component (reviewed by Gallagher and Forget[127] and Winkelmann and Forget[137]). It is a heterodimer of two enormous polypeptide chains, α-spectrin (2429 amino acids, about 280 kd)[325] and β-spectrin (2137 amino acids, about 246 kd),[326] which are structurally related but functionally distinct. The two chains are aligned side by side in an antiparallel arrangement with respect to their N- and C-terminal ends[327] (Fig. 54-11). Electron microscopy shows spectrin to be a slender, twisted worm-like molecule that extends to a total length of about 100 nm[329,330] (Fig. 54-12). The protein is highly flexible[329,330] and assumes a variety of conformations, an unusual property that may be critical for normal membrane pliancy.

Spectrins Are a Ubiquitous Gene Family. Humans have four spectrin genes: α- and β-spectrin and α- and β-fodrin. Spectrin (also called erythrocyte spectrin, spectrin I, or $spectrin_R$), although it was discovered before fodrin, is the more specialized protein and evolutionarily more recent. α-Spectrin is expressed only in red cells. β-Spectrin is also expressed in an alternatively spliced form in muscle and brain (where it probably pairs with α-fodrin).[137] Fodrin (also called tissue spectrin, brain spectrin, spectrin II, or

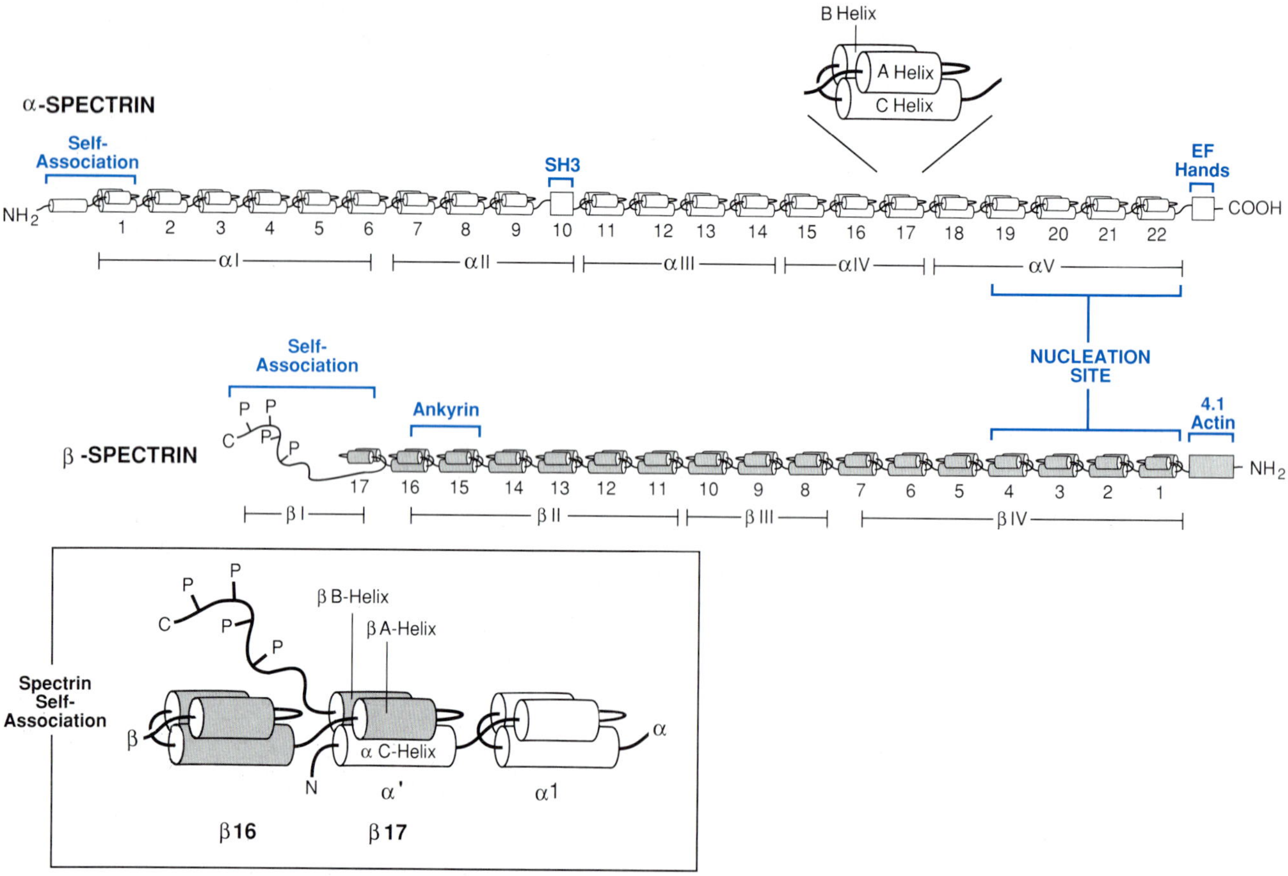

FIGURE 54-11. Spectrin structure. The α and β chains are aligned antiparallel with respect to their N- and C-terminal ends. The approximately 106 amino acid "spectrin repeats" are numbered from the N terminal of each chain. (*Upper right*) In the Speicher Model, each repeat is composed of three α helices (A, B, and C).[328] (*Lower left*) The spectrin self-association site is formed by joining parts of a repeat that are left over at the "head" ends of the two chains. The α chain contributes helix C, the β chain helices A and B. (*Middle*) Some repeats are specialized, such as β15 and part of β16, which form the ankyrin-binding site, and the first four repeats at the "tail" of each chain, which nucleate interchain interactions. Rectangles denote peptide segments that differ from the repeats. They include the actin–protein 4.1 binding sites, a potential Ca^{2+} binding region (EF hands), and an SH3 domain. Each chain can be further divided into large structural domains by gentle proteolysis with trypsin. These domains are marked below each chain. In patients with hereditary elliptocytosis or pyropoikilocytosis, which are due to spectrin defects, the defects lie in the αI (80-kd), αII, and βI domains.

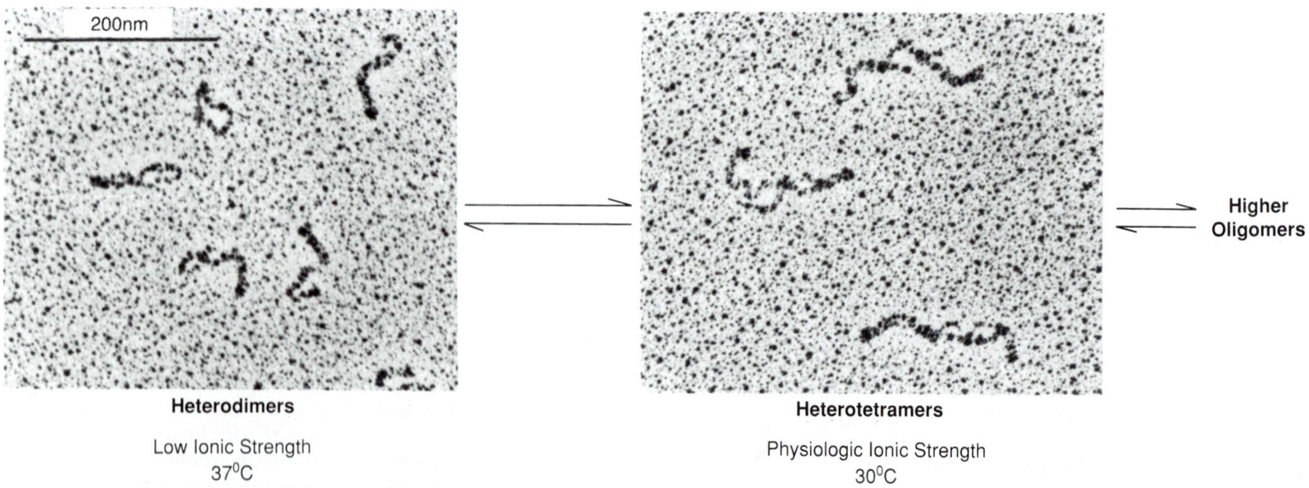

FIGURE 54-12. Electron micrographs (rotary shadowed) of spectrin heterodimers and heterotetramers. The α and β chains of heterodimers are flexible, loosely attached (side to side), and twisted about each other, and heterotetramers are made by end-to-end association of dimers. Factors that favor the dimer or tetramer–oligomer state are listed under the photographs. The dimer–tetramer–oligomer equilibrium is kinetically frozen at 0°C. Spectrin extracted and maintained at 0°C retains the distribution of dimers and tetramers that exists on the membrane.

spectrin$_G$) is expressed in all or almost all cells and tissues except mature red cells (it is found in red cell precursors). It is widely distributed in vertebrates and invertebrates and has been detected in amoebas,[331,332] slime molds,[333] sea urchins,[334,353] flies,[335,335a,336] and plants.[337]

Spectrin and fodrin are similar structurally and functionally and are members of a gene superfamily that includes dystrophin and α-actinin.[338–341] The latter two proteins also contain spectrin/fodrin-like 106–amino acid repeats (see following section) and N-terminal or C-terminal functional regions that are similar to those in spectrin and fodrin.

The α-spectrin gene is located on chromosome 1q22-q23, near the Duffy blood group.[342,342a] β-Spectrin is on chromosome 14q23-q24.2.[343] α-Fodrin and β-fodrin reside on chromosomes 9q34.1 and 2p21, respectively.[344,345]

Spectrin Consists Mostly of Tandem 106–Amino Acid Repeats. Each spectrin chain contains a series of 106–amino acid repeats, hooked end to end like beads on a string.[325,326,346,347] The repeats do not correlate with intron–exon boundaries, which suggests they are ancient.

Each repeat forms a triple helical structure that is about 5 nm long and 2 nm wide and is rotated 60 degrees (right-handed) relative to the neighboring repeats[347] (Fig. 54-13). Expression studies[348] and x-ray crystallography[347] of a repeat from α-fodrin indicate the repeats begin with a straight,

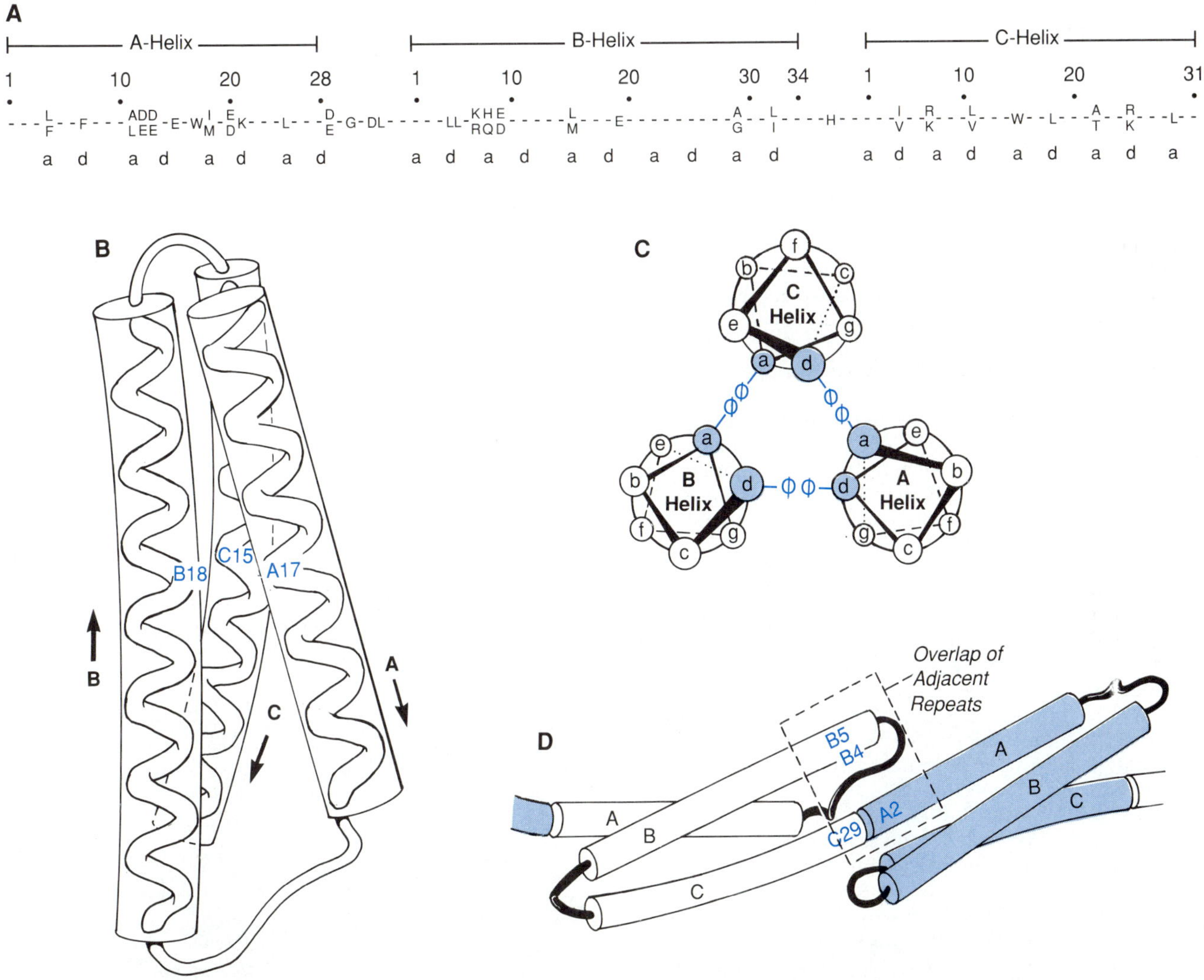

FIGURE 54-13. Structure of spectrin repeats. (**A**) Consensus sequence of human erythrocyte spectrin[127] phased according to crystallographic data,[347] which defines three α helices that encompass the amino acids shown. Less conserved residues are marked with a dash. Residues a and d are the major contact points between helices. They tend to be hydrophobic and are conserved in most spectrins. (**B**) Model of a single repeat based on the crystal structure of *Drosophila* α-fodrin.[347] The positions of the nearly invariant tryptophans at A17 and C15 are shown. They interact with surrounding residues, including B18, at the central junction where the A helix crosses over from B to C. (**C**) Cross-section of a typical repeat. The A, B, and C helices are in a triangular array, and the a and d residues lie on one face of each helix. The side chains of these amino acids are usually hydrophobic (Φ) and interact with each other to stabilize the triple helical configuration. Salt bonds between the typically polar amino acids at positions e and g also help attach the B–C and A–C helices to each other. (**D**) Interconnection of two adjacent repeats. The A and C helices are directly connected, forming one long helix. The distal repeat of each pair is rotated 60 degrees (right-handed). The B helix of the proximal repeat (*black and white*) overlaps the A helix of the following repeat (*colored*). Interactions in the overlap region among conserved hydrophobic residues such as C29, B4, and B5 and the mostly hydrophobic residues at A2 probably stabilize the connection and limit mobility at the repeat junction.

28–amino acid α helix (A helix).* The polypeptide chain then reverses itself and forms a second, long (34 amino acids), α helix (B helix). This is followed by another reverse turn and the C helix (31 amino acids), which bends in the middle. The helices are arranged in a triangular array and held together by both hydrophobic and electrostatic interactions.[347] One face of each helix is lined with mostly hydrophobic amino acids. Since an α helix makes one turn every 3.6 residues, the hydrophobic amino acids are spaced every third or fourth residue at the positions designated a and d in Figure 54-13*A* and *C*.

Additional salt bonds occur between the mostly polar amino acids at positions e and g of the helices (see Fig. 54-13*C*), particularly between helices A–C and B–C.[347] The three helices are tilted away from each other by 10 to 20 degrees so that the C-terminal end of each repeat is wider than the N-terminal end (see Fig. 54-13*B*). This provides room for the following repeat to attach without any adjustment of the structure. The repeats connect to each other through the A and C helices, forming one long α helix.[347] Because of the tight connection, the B helix of the proximal repeat overlaps the A helix of the distal repeat. Interactions between the two helices appear to restrict the mobility of the repeats at the repeat junction and limit the range of motions of the α-fodrin chain. Whether this detail is present in the more flexible erythrocyte spectrin is unknown. Circular dichroism measurements indicate that the spectrin repeats contain 65% to 70% α-helical structure,[349] which is slightly less than the amount (88%) observed in the crystal structure of the fodrin repeat.[347]

α-Spectrin Contains an SH3 Domain. α-Spectrin begins with an isolated, unpaired helix C followed by nine typical 106–amino acid repeats (conformational segments 1 to 9), a small region that lacks homology to the repeats but that is related to SH3 domains (segment 10), and 12 more repeats (segments 11 to 22; see Fig. 54-11). The function of the spectrin SH3 domain is unknown. In other proteins, SH3 domains function as sites for the attachment of various molecules to membranes.[350] This is presumably also true for spectrin, but the ligand or ligands have not been identified. The C terminal of α-spectrin is a unique region that is related to the actin-binding protein, α-actinin. It contains two EF hands: structures that participate in calcium binding and regulate calcium action in other proteins, including α-actinin[351,352] and probably fodrin.[353,354] No evidence exists that spectrin binds calcium or that its interactions with actin and protein 4.1 are regulated by calcium; therefore, the EF hands may be vestigial.

β-Spectrin Contains Binding Sites for Ankyrin, Protein 4.1, and Actin. β-Spectrin contains 17 conformational repeats. The 15th and the first part of the 16th repeats are modified and form the binding site for ankyrin.[355] The N-terminal region (272 residues) contains the actin binding site[356–358] and probably the binding site for protein 4.1.[357,359] It binds actin[358] and is homologous to other actin-binding proteins, including α-actinin, dystrophin, filamin, gelation factor (ABP-120), adducin, and fimbrin (reviewed by Winkelmann and Forget[137]). The actin binding site in gelation factor has been traced to a 27–amino acid sequence within the conserved actin binding domain.[360] Presumably the same site is used by spectrin.

The binding site of protein 4.1 is less well defined. It is probably located just beyond the actin binding site within the N-terminal domain[357,359]: (1) electron micrographs show that protein 4.1 and actin bind at the end of the molecule[356]; (2) photoaffinity labeling of spectrin by protein 4.1 labels the β chain[357]; and (3) a family with HS and a β-spectrin that cannot bind protein 4.1 (to be discussed later in text) has a mutation in the appropriate location (β-spectrin Trp 202 → Arg).[359]

The C-terminal end of β-spectrin contains a 52–amino acid extension that is phosphorylated (3 P-Ser, 1 P-Thr)[361] by a membrane-associated casein kinase I.[362] The function of this region remains a mystery.

Spectrin Tryptic Domains. The spectrin chains can also be divided into reproducible structural domains, each containing several 106–amino acid repeats, by gentle proteolysis[327,363] (Fig. 54-14). There are nine such domains, five on the α-chain (αI [80 kd], αII [46 kd], αIII [52 kd], αIV [52 kd], and αV [41 kd]) and four on the β chain (βI [17 kd], βII [65 kd], βIII [33 kd], and βIV [74 kd]; see Fig. 54-11). As will be shown, many of the molecular defects in hereditary elliptocytosis have been identified as abnormalities in spectrin domain maps after proteolytic digestion.

Spectrin α and β Chains Zip Together. Side-to-side assembly of the spectrin α and β chains occurs in a zipper-like fashion, beginning with a defined *nucleation site* composed of four repeats from each chain, α19 to α22, and β1 to β4.[364] These are located at the tail end of the molecule, the end where actin binds (see Fig. 54-11). Two of the α repeats and one of the β repeats have eight-residue insertions that participate in the interchain interaction.[365] These are located between conformational segments α19 to α20, α20 to α21, and β2 to β3. The model suggests that after the initial tight association of the complementary nucleation sites, a conformational change is propagated, which pro-

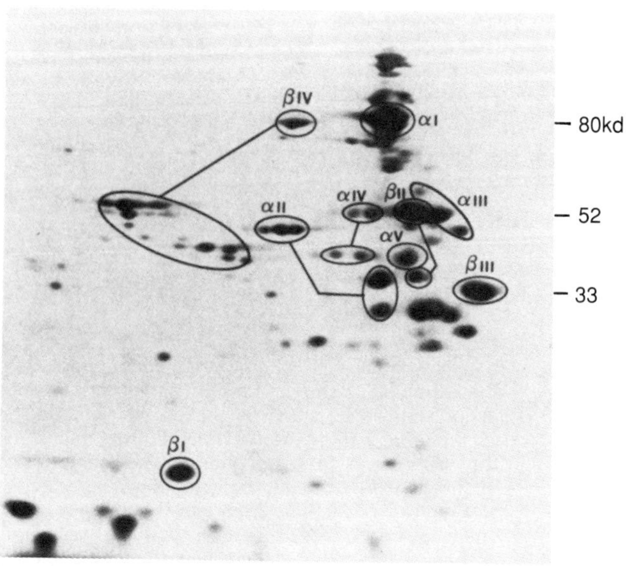

FIGURE 54-14. Tryptic domains of spectrin. The partial tryptic digest is separated by isoelectric focusing, pH 6.5 to 4.5 (*left to right*), followed by SDS gel electrophoresis (*top to bottom*). The major α- and β-chain domain peptides are labeled. (Gallagher PG, Forget BG. Spectrin genes in health and disease. Semin Hematol 1993;30:4)

* Until recently, the spectrin repeat unit was based on the amino acid sequence of the N terminal of the α chain,[346] which begins with an extra, unpaired C helix. Thus, the repeat was defined as the C helix of one folded subunit and the A and B helixes of the next subunit. The newer nomenclature designates a triple helical segment or a conformational repeat that contains all three helices; the sequence of the redefined repeat aligns with its folded structure[328,347] (see Fig. 54-13). The C helix at the beginning of the α chain is now designated α′ (see Fig. 54-11). Thus, helix C of repeat 5 (by the original amino acid sequence designation) is identical with helix C of conformational repeat 4. The amino acid phasing in the consensus sequence in Figure 54-12 and the numbering of repeats in Figure 54-11 and subsequently in the chapter refer to conformational repeats.

motes the pairing of the remaining length of the two chains.[364] In support of this hypothesis is the finding of a common polymorphism, a low-expression allele called α^{LELY} or $\alpha^{V/41}$, which probably interferes with nucleation and effectively decreases synthesis of functionally competent α-spectrin. This important polymorphism is discussed in detail in the section on hereditary elliptocytosis.

Spectrin Molecules Self-Associate to Form Tetramers and Oligomers. Spectrin heterodimers (αβ) associate at the head end of the molecule[329,330] to form heterotetramers ($\alpha_2\beta_2$) and higher oligomers ($\alpha_n\beta_n$)[330,366,367] (see Figs. 54-11 and 54-12). Both tetramers and oligomers exist on the membrane, but tetramers predominate,[330] probably because the association constant for formation of tetramers is substantially higher than for the larger species.[368] At low ionic strength and physiologic temperature (37°C), spectrin dissociates into dimers,[366,367,369] whereas physiologic ionic strength and lower temperatures (25°C) favor the tetramer and oligomer species (see Fig. 54-12). At 0°C, the equilibrium is kinetically frozen.[367] It is possible to extract spectrin from the membrane at such temperatures and examine its association state directly or manipulate it in vitro to produce any desired oligomeric species.[330,366,367,370] Measurements of spectrin eluted from normal ghosts indicate that about 5% of the spectrin is in the dimer form and about 50% is in tetramers.[330] The remainder is divided between higher-order spectrin oligomers and very high molecular weight complexes of spectrin, actin, protein 4.1, and dematin.[330,371] It is also possible to manipulate the dimer–tetramer equilibrium in situ by exposing ghosts to temperatures and salt concentrations that favor or discourage self-association. Ghosts enriched in spectrin dimers are strikingly fragile.[370] The results are compelling testimony to the structural importance of the skeleton for the erythrocyte.

Self-Association Occurs Between the Incomplete Repeats at the Ends of the α and β Chains. The interconversion of spectrin dimers to tetramers involves a reversible opening of the dimer bond and formation of two new αβ attachments. The αβ contact closely resembles the triple helical structure of native spectrin repeats (see Fig. 54-11), except that in the contact site two of the helices are contributed by the C terminal of the β chain (helices A and B) and one (helix C) comes from the N terminal of the α chain.[328] Spectrin dimers exist in open and closed forms, depending on whether the ends of the α and β chains are free (open) or bound to each other (closed). The open and closed states are distinguished by their reactivity and susceptibility to proteases.[328,372,373] Newly assembled spectrin heterodimers are open, and they close by interaction with each other, by forming heterotetramers, or by forming an internal αβ bond. In the latter instance, the longer α chain probably folds back in a hairpin structure to engage the β-subunit.[328] Opening the αβ contact (either the internal bond in closed dimers or the first αβ bond in tetramers) is the rate-limiting step in dimer–tetramer interconversion.[373]

Spectrin Molecules Are Coiled Up In Vivo. Spectrin is thought to function as a kind of spring, such that in vivo the 200-nm tetramers are coiled up with an end-to-end distance of about 76 nm.[374] Measurements suggest that spectrin molecules condense by twisting their α- and β-subunits around a common axis and that the degree of condensation is regulated by varying the pitch and diameter of the twisted double strand. The native molecule would have about 10 turns with a pitch of 7 nm and a diameter of 5.9 nm.[375,376] The coiled spectrin tetramers can extend reversibly when the membrane is stretched but cannot exceed their 200-nm contour length without rupturing.

α-Spectrin Is Synthesized in Excess Relative to β-Spectrin. Spectrin is synthesized early in erythroid development. It is plentiful in pronormoblasts[377] and is detectable in undifferentiated erythroleukemia cells[378] and possibly in mature committed erythroid stem cells (BFU-E and CFU-E).[379]

In chickens, mice, and humans, α-spectrin is synthesized in about threefold excess relative to β-spectrin[380–382] and is degraded by a different, slower pathway.[383] The limited synthesis and more rapid degradation of β-spectrin suggests that its association with the membrane is the rate-limiting step in spectrin assembly.[382,383]

Actin

Red cell actin is structurally and functionally similar to other actins.[384] The β subtype is found in a variety of other nonmuscle cells.[246] Unlike other nonmuscle actins, red cell actin is organized as short double-helical, F-actin protofilaments about 12 to 14 monomers long.[385,386] These short filaments appear to be stabilized by their interactions with spectrin, adducin, protein 4.1, and tropomyosin, and by capping of the slow growing or pointed end of the actin filament by tropomodulin.[387]

Evidence exists that the state of actin polymerization is functionally important to the red cell, since compounds that inhibit actin polymerization increase membrane flexibility and compounds that promote its polymerization make the membrane rigid.[388] Spectrin dimers bind to the side of actin filaments at a site near the tail end of the spectrin molecule[356,358,385,386,389] (see Fig. 54-11). Spectrin tetramers are therefore bivalent and can cross-link actin filaments, but binding is weak (K_D of about 10^{-3} mol/L) and ineffectual in the absence of protein 4.1.[390,391]

Protein 4.1

Protein 4.1 is a core skeletal component that interacts with spectrin and actin and with proteins in the overlying lipid bilayer (reviewed by Conboy and Mohandas[124,125]). The cloned protein is globular (5.7 nm in diameter) and has a molecular weight of 66 kd but migrates as an 80-kd protein on SDS gels. The reason for this unusual discrepancy is unknown. Four structural domains have been defined by proteolysis[392]: NH_2–(30 kd–16 kd–10 kd–22/24 kd)–COOH (Fig. 54-15). Two forms of the intact protein, designated 4.1a (80 kd) and 4.1b (78 kd), are resolved on high-resolution SDS gels.[153] Protein 4.1a is derived from 4.1b by gradual deamidation[248] of Asn 502, within the 22/24-kd domain; therefore 4.1a is more prominent in older erythrocytes.[393]

Protein 4.1 Amplifies Spectrin–Actin Interactions. Protein 4.1 binds tightly (K_D of about 10^{-7} mol/L) to β-spectrin,[357,359,394] very near the actin binding site[356,395] (see Fig. 54-11) and greatly amplifies the otherwise weak spectrin–actin interaction.[389–391] This activity can be traced to the 10-kd domain[396,397] and, at least partly, to a 21–amino acid peptide within the domain.[398,399] Evidence indicates that protein 4.1 also binds directly to F-actin (K_D of about 10^{-7} mol/L).[400] This suggests that it works by bridging spectrin and actin, although other mechanisms have not been excluded.

The interaction of protein 4.1 with spectrin and actin is blocked by protein kinase A phosphorylation, which labels residues in the 16-kd (Ser 331) and 10-kd (Ser 467) domains,[401,402] and by tyrosine kinase phosphorylation, which labels a site (Tyr 418) in the 10-kd domain[403] (see Fig. 54-15). The ternary complex also appears to be regulated by Ca^{2+} and calmodulin.[404–406] Calmodulin binds to protein 4.1 in a Ca^{2+}-independent manner (K_D of about 5×10^{-7}) but, after it is bound, the calmodulin–4.1 complex confers Ca^{2+} sensitivity on the viscosity increase produced by

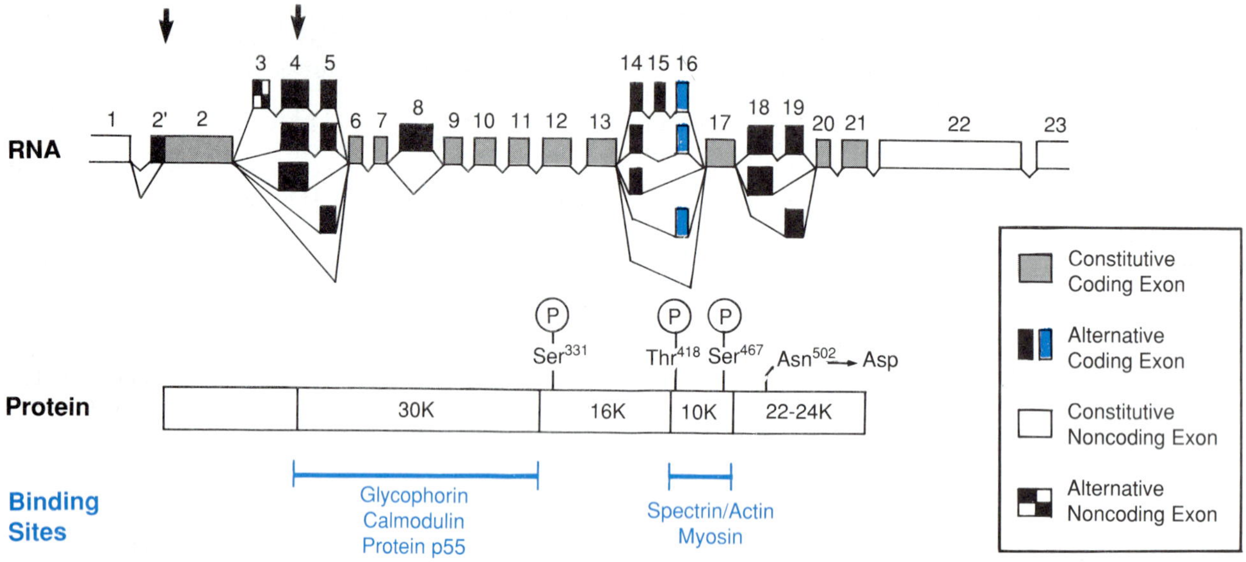

FIGURE 54-15. Protein 4.1. (*Top*) Alternative splicing map of protein 4.1 mRNA. Reticulocyte 4.1 is translated from the downstream AUG (*arrow over exon 4*) and includes a 63-bp (21–amino acid) erythroid-specific sequence (*colored area*) that is critical for spectrin–actin interactions. Many combinations of exons are expressed, although some are observed only in nonerythroid tissues. (*Middle* and *bottom*) Domain map of the 80-kd (erythroid) form of protein 4.1, indicating binding sites, phosphorylation sites, and the location of a C-terminal asparagine that is deamidated in old red cells (After Conboy JG. Structure, function, and molecular genetics of erythroid membrane skeletal protein 4.1 in normal and abnormal red blood cells. Semin Hematol 1993;30:138)

spectrin–actin–4.1 binding.[406] The calmodulin binding site is located within the 30-kd domain.[406]

Protein 4.1 is necessary for normal membrane stability. Patients who lack protein 4.1 have marked hemolysis and fragile membranes,[407] but normal membrane stability is restored when the ghosts are reconstituted with protein 4.1[408] or even with a fusion protein containing only 62 amino acids (21–amino acid spectrin–actin binding site plus the next 41 amino acids).[409]

Protein 4.1 Attaches the Skeleton to GPC and Possibly Other Proteins. Protein 4.1 also binds to the membrane and serves as a secondary attachment site for spectrin. The location of the binding site is controversial. GPA, GPC, and band 3 are the major candidates. The putative interaction with GPA is interesting because it depends on the presence of phosphatidylinositol-4,5-bisphosphate (PI-PP)[410] and therefore could be regulated metabolically or through various signaling pathways. The interaction with band 3 has a high capacity but relatively low affinity.[196] In vitro, band 3 accounts for 60% to 70% of the membrane binding sites. The interaction is blocked by phosphorylation of 4.1 by protein kinase C but not by protein kinase A.[411] The binding sites for GPA, GPC, and band 3 are generally assumed to lie within the 30-kd domain (see Fig. 54-15), based on unpublished preliminary data for GPA.[412] More direct evidence is needed.

The major issue is whether one or all of these interactions occurs in vivo. If *interaction* is defined as being close enough to protein 4.1 to be modified by a radioactive cleavable cross-linker, then all three proteins serve as binding sites.[187] The interaction with GPC is the only one that has been shown to have functional consequences in intact red cells[312,413]: (1) 4.1-deficient red cells are also deficient in GPC but not GPA or band 3[413–415]; (2) the residual GPC is only loosely bound to the skeleton but becomes tightly bound when the deficient cells are reconstituted with protein 4.1[414]; and (3) GPC-deficient red cells are structurally unstable, whereas GPA-deficient cells are mechanically normal.[121,312] In addition, both protein 4.1 and GPC bind p55, which may augment or regulate their interaction (see following section). Preliminary evidence shows that these effects are due to protein 4.1 deficiency rather than 4.1–GPC or 4.1–p55 interactions,[315] since the mechanical weakness of GPC-deficient membranes is fully restored by reconstitution with protein 4.1 or just its spectrin–actin binding domain.[315]

Protein 4.1 also interacts with myosin[416] (see Fig. 54-15), tubulin[417] and PS.[418,419] The interaction with myosin (K_D of 1.4×10^{-7} mol/L) is particularly interesting because the myosin binding site lies within the 10-kd domain that regulates spectrin–actin–4.1 complex formation and because protein 4.1 inhibits the actin-activated Mg^{2+}-ATPase activity of myosin.[416] Finally, protein 4.1 is modified by the addition of the O-linked monosaccharide, *N*-acetylglucosamine to a site in the 22/24-kd domain.[420] The function of this unusual alteration is unknown.

Protein 4.1 Is Expressed in Many Alternatively Spliced Forms. The single gene for protein 4.1 is located on chromosome 1p33-p34.2[421] and is complex. It is more than 90 kb long and contains at least 23 exons, including 10 alternatively spliced exons or motifs.[422] This leads to a remarkably diverse collection of 4.1 isoforms in erythroid and nonerythroid cells[422–425] (reviewed by Conboy[125]). Two are particularly notable. One is a 17-bp motif at the 5′ end of the 4.1 gene that contains an upstream translation initiation sequence. In most tissues, this sequence is spliced in and a downstream 80-bp motif is spliced out. This gives rise to an elongated isoform of protein 4.1 containing an additional 209 amino acids attached to the N terminal of erythroid protein 4.1 (see Fig. 54-15). The other 4.1 isoform is a 63-bp motif within the 10-kd domain that contains the 21–amino acid spectrin–actin binding site. Expression of this motif is linked to terminal erythroid differentiation.[426]

Protein 4.1 is widely expressed in nonerythroid tissues and is part of a superfamily of proteins that includes talin, ezrin, moesin, and radixin.[427,428] They share homology in the N-terminal (30-kd) domain.

Protein p55

Protein p55 is the human homologue of *dlg*, a *Drosophila* tumor suppressor gene.[429] It contains three domains: an N-terminal domain of unknown function that is also present in *dlg*, a central SH3 domain that may be a binding site for other proteins, and a C-terminal guanylate kinase domain.[429–431] There are 80,000 copies of p55 per red cell, probably assembled into dimers.[431] The protein is extensively palmitoylated and tightly bound to the membrane. The p55 gene is located on the long arm of the X chromosome, at Xq28, just beyond the factor VIII gene.[430,432] It is expressed throughout erythroid differentiation and widely expressed in nonerythroid tissues.

Research indicates that p55 interacts with protein 4.1 and GPC, probably bridging between them.[433] Patients who lack either protein also lack p55,[434] and direct binding studies show that p55 binds to the 30-kd domain of protein 4.1 (K_D of about 2×10^{-9} mol/L; see Fig. 54-15) and to the cytoplasmic domain of GPC (K_D about 7×10^{-9} mol/L).[433,435] Considering the wide tissue distribution of all three proteins, this interaction, or interactions of p55 with other members of the 4.1 superfamily, is likely to have a variety of important functions.

Actin-Associated Proteins

Adducin

Adducin is a heterodimer of α (81-kd) and β (80-kd) subunits.[436] The two subunits are homologous[437] and are divided into three domains: a 39-kd N-terminal head domain, which resembles the actin binding regions of proteins in the spectrin superfamily; a 9-kd linking peptide; and a 33-kd protease-sensitive tail. The protein appears at the proerythroblast stage but is not stably incorporated into the membrane skeleton until later in erythroid development.[438] There are 30,000 copies per cell or 1 per actin protofilament.

Adducin is believed to play a role in the early assembly of the spectrin–actin network. The protein binds to actin and, like protein 4.1, increases the binding of spectrin to actin.[436] Unlike protein 4.1, adducin does not interact directly with spectrin in the absence of actin. The adducin–spectrin–actin complex fosters binding of a second spectrin, a reaction that is blocked by calmodulin.[436]

Adducin is present in a variety of nonerythroid tissues and is concentrated at sites of cell-to-cell contact.[439] The protein assembles at these sites in response to extracellular calcium and dissociates after treatment of the cells with phorbol esters,[439] which stimulate phosphorylation of adducin by protein kinase C.[439,440] The protein is also phosphorylated by protein kinase A, but the effect of this kinase is unknown. The data suggest that adducin may allow local regulation of the membrane skeleton by calcium and protein kinase C and attachment of the skeleton to certain parts of the membrane, such as sites of cell contact, which require reinforcement.

Dematin (Protein 4.9)

Human erythrocyte dematin consists of two chains of 48 kd and 52 kd, which are present in a ratio of 3:1 (48 kd:52 kd).[441–443] The native protein is a trimer. It binds to actin and bundles actin filaments into cables.[443] This action is abolished by protein kinase A phosphorylation,[441] but is not affected by protein kinase C. The primary structure of the 48-kd subunit[250] shows that the C-terminal half is similar to villin, an actin-binding protein that induces growth of microvilli and reorganizes actin filaments in brush borders. In contrast to villin, dematin is widely distributed, which raises the possibility that it may substitute for villin and regulate actin organization, under phosphorylation control, in tissues that lack villin. Dematin must also attach to a lipid or integral membrane protein, since it remains associated with the membrane when the other skeletal proteins are extracted; this site has not been identified.

Tropomyosin

Erythrocyte tropomyosin is a heterodimer of 27- and 29-kd subunits that run on SDS gels in the region of band 7.[444] The red cell analogue is similar to other nonmuscle tropomyosins by many criteria,[444,445] except that it polymerizes poorly.[445] This makes sense in the red cell where the double helical actin filaments are short (two chains, each containing six to seven monomers). There is one copy of tropomyosin for each six to eight actin monomers, which is just enough to line both grooves of the actin protofilament.[444] The binding of tropomyosin to actin is not affected by spectrin, but spectrin–actin interactions are inhibited by saturating concentrations of tropomyosin.[445] Possible functions of tropomyosin include stabilizing the short erythroid actin filament and helping determine the sites of spectrin–actin interactions.

Tropomodulin

Tropomodulin is a 41-kd protein that binds to tropomyosin in a 2:1 molar ratio with a K_D of 5×10^{-7} mol/L.[446,447] There are 30,000 copies per red cell, or one per actin protofilament. Tropomodulin associates with the *pointed end* of actin filaments and blocks growth at that end.[387] Whether it binds and caps the filaments directly or binds to one end of tropomyosin[447] and caps actin indirectly is unclear. Tropomyosin binding activity maps to the N-terminal region of the protein.[448] Tropomodulin remains attached to the membrane when spectrin, actin, and tropomyosin are removed. Its binding site has not been identified.

Myosin

Red cells contain a nonmuscle myosin composed of two light chains (19 and 25 kd) associated with a 200-kd heavy chain.[449,450] The protein forms bipolar filaments and has typical ATPase activities.[449,450] There are about 4300 myosins in adult red cells and 2.5 times as many in neonatal erythrocytes,[451] or about one myosin per 50 to 100 actin monomers. This may explain the greater motility of neonatal reticulocytes.

Several reviews focus on the proteins that make up the spectrin–actin junction.[116–118,128]

Ankyrin (Bands 2.1, 2.2, 2.3, and 2.6)

Ankyrin (reviewed by Bennett[119] and Peters and Lux[135]) is a large (206-kd), pyramid-shaped (8.3×10 nm) protein[395] that serves as the high-affinity (K_D of about 10^{-7} mol/L) binding site for the attachment of spectrin to the inner membrane surface.[452–454] Ankyrin binds to spectrin at a site near the end of the molecule involved in dimer–tetramer associations[355,395] (see Fig. 54-11). Judging from its relative abundance (see Table 54-2), each spectrin tetramer binds on the average only one ankyrin molecule, even although two binding sites are available. This is probably because ankyrin binds about 10 times more avidly to spectrin tetramer than to spectrin dimer.[455,456] Ankyrin, in turn, is bound with high affinity (K_D about 10^{-7} to 10^{-8} mol/L) to the cytoplasmic portion of band 3, the true anchor for the membrane skeleton.[175,191,193] Selective disruption of the ankyrin–band 3 interaction in intact red cells, at slightly alkaline pH,[457] markedly decreases membrane stability, emphasizing the importance of the interaction.

N-Terminal Domain Contains a Repeat Motif and the Binding Site for Band 3. Analysis of ankyrin fragments[454,456,458–463] and cDNA clones[464,465] shows that the molecule is divided into three domains (Fig. 54-16). The 89-kd N-terminal domain is almost entirely composed of 24 consecutive 33–amino acid repeats,[464,465] called *SWI/*

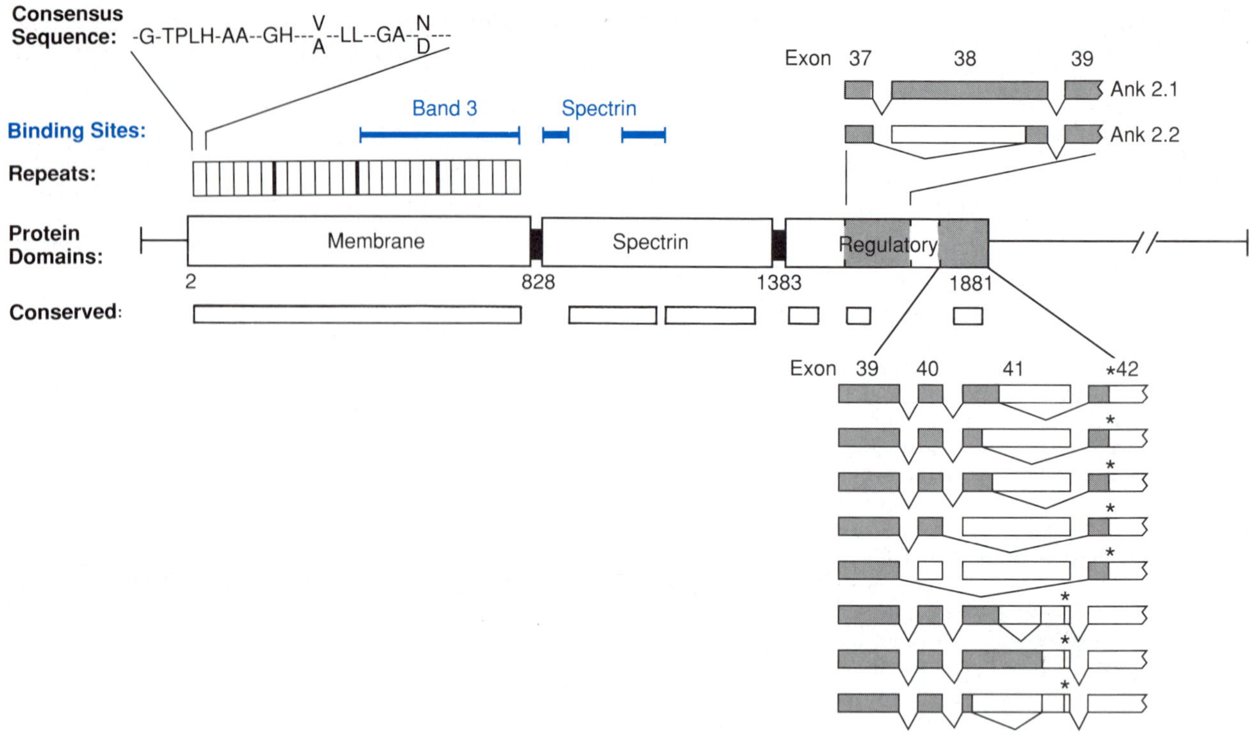

FIGURE 54-16. Structure of erythroid ankyrin (Ank1). The membrane domain (89 kd) contains 24 repeats (33 amino acids each), grouped in folding units of six. Their consensus sequence is shown at the top left in single-letter amino acid code. Dashes indicate less conserved residues. The last 12 repeats form the band 3 binding site, especially repeats 22 and 23. The spectrin domain (62 kd) contains the binding site or sites for spectrin. These two domains are the most conserved. The regulatory domain (55 kd) is thought to modulate the binding functions of the other two domains. In the middle of the domain, a highly acidic inhibitory region in exon 38 is spliced out of full-length ankyrin (Ank2.1) to make Ank2.2. At least eight isoforms of the last three exons exist. The last three isoforms contain a basic sequence (*open area*) that is common in brain Ank1 but rare in the red cell protein. In addition, isoforms lacking exons 38 and 39, 36 through 39, and 36 through 41 have been detected. The asterisk indicates the location of the translation terminator codon.

ANK repeats,[135] which are subdivided into 6-repeat folding units.[462] The repeats are similar to each other and must have formed by repeated duplications of a primordial minigene. Binding sites for band 3[456,459–462] and tubulin,[466,467] especially unpolymerized tubulin,[468] are located in this domain. The band 3 site is formed by the last 12 repeats,[460,462] particularly repeats 22 and 23[461]; the location of the tubulin site has not been further defined.

Similar repeats are found in an enormous variety of proteins in all phyla,[119,135] including bacteria and viruses. These proteins have little in common except the ability to interact with other proteins. The SWI6/ANK repeat must have been an evolutionarily convenient solution to this recurring need.

Spectrin Binds to the Middle Domain. The spectrin binding site is located within a 62-kd globular central domain (previously called the 72-kd domain[452,469]) and appears to involve regions at both the beginning[460] and middle[463] of the domain (see Fig. 54-16). The complementary binding site for ankyrin on spectrin is formed by spectrin repeats 15 and 16[355] (see Fig. 54-11). The intermediate filament proteins vimentin and desmin may also bind to this portion of the molecule.[470,471]

The Alternatively Spliced C-Terminal Domain Contains Regulatory Sequences. The 55-kd C-terminal domain contains regulatory sequences that enhance and diminish the binding of ankyrin to spectrin and the anion exchange protein.[464,468,472,473] Some of these are alternatively spliced, creating ankyrin isoforms of different sizes and functions. For example, ankyrin 2.2 (see band 2.2 in Fig. 54-4) lacks an acidic 162–amino acid sequence from exon 38 that is found in full-sized ankyrin (band 2.1[464]; see Fig. 54-16). The smaller isoform functions like an activated ankyrin, with enhanced binding to band 3, spectrin, and tubulin,[468,473] and the ability to bind to new sites on some other plasma membranes.[472] The 162–amino acid *repressor sequence*, expressed as a separate protein, binds to ankyrin 2.2 and inhibits its interaction with band 3.[468] Eight alternatively spliced isoforms of the three C-terminal exons have been identified.[474,475] In addition, isoforms lacking (1) exons 38 and 39, (2) exons 36 through 39, and (3) exons 36 through 41 have been detected.[476] Some of these shortened RNAs probably form the smallest ankyrin isoforms (bands 2.3, 2.6, and so on; see Fig. 54-4). Together with the 2.1/2.2 isoforms, there are 31 possible combinations, most of which have been observed.[474–477] The C-terminal exons are highly conserved,[478] unlike most of the 55-kd domains, which suggests they also encode regulatory sequences. These may be activating sequences since proteolytic removal of the last 196 amino acids partially deactivates ankyrin, muting its affinity for band 3.[473]

The function of ankyrin is also regulated by phosphorylation.[455,479,480] In vitro, up to seven phosphates are added to ankyrin by the red cell membrane casein kinase I.[479] Unphosphorylated ankyrin binds preferentially to spectrin tetramers and oligomers rather than to spectrin dimers.[455,456,479] This preference is abolished by phosphorylation, which also reduces the capacity of ankyrin to bind band 3.[480] Ankyrin is also phosphorylated by protein kinase A, but the functional effect of the modification has not been studied.

Ankyrin Gene Family. Ankyrin, like spectrin, is a multigene family, and ankyrins are widely expressed,[135] perhaps in all cells. Ank1, the erythrocyte ankyrin, is also found in myocytes,[481–483] endothelial cells,[484] and brain, particularly in Purkinje cells of the cerebellum.[485,486] It is located on the short arm of chromosome 8 near the centromere (8p11.2).[487] Ank2 is an exclusively neural form that is localized to neuronal cell bodies and dendrites.[486,488–490] It resides on chromosome 4 (4q25-q27).[491] Ank3 is the most widely distributed, particularly in epithelia and axons.[492–494] It is also expressed in megakaryocytes, macrophages, myocytes, melanocytes, hepatocytes, and testicular Leydig's cells.[494] Additional ankyrins must exist, but probably not many. Lymphocytes, for example, contain an ankyrin-like protein[495–497] that does not hybridize to sequences from the three known ankyrins.[484]

Nonerythroid Ankyrins Position Integral Proteins in Membranes. Nonerythroid ankyrins bind a variety of integral membrane proteins other than band 3, including Na^+/K^+-ATPase, the voltage-dependent axonal Na channel, the amiloride-sensitive epithelial Na^+ channel, the cardiac Na^+/Ca^{2+} exchanger, CD44, and a group of neurofascin-related brain adhesive proteins.[135] The available data suggest that ankyrins localize these proteins to particular membrane domains, presumably by local interactions with cytoskeletal proteins.[498–503]

Pallidin (Protein 4.2)

Pallidin Binds to Ankyrin and Band 3 and Probably Strengthens Their Interaction. Pallidin is a 77-kd peripheral membrane protein that helps link the skeleton to the lipid bilayer (reviewed by Cohen and associates[122] and Yawata[504]). Pallidin binds to band 3 (AE1) and probably to ankyrin. It certainly binds to ankyrin in solution,[199] but it has been difficult to prove that it binds to ankyrin when ankyrin is attached to band 3. Possibly, the two proteins can bind to different band 3 molecules.[199] In *nb/nb* mice, which lack ankyrin, and in a child with HS and deletion of one ankyrin gene, some reduction in pallidin is also observed.[487,505] In addition, some investigators[506,507] find that ankyrin elutes more easily from the membranes of pallidin-deficient erythrocyte; others have not found this.[508,509]

These observations strongly suggest that pallidin and ankyrin sometimes interact in vivo. Pallidin is also myristylated.[510] The function of this modification is unknown.

Pallidin Is Homologous to Transglutaminases. Pallidin is remarkably homologous to transglutaminases,[511,512] although it possesses no such activity itself because a critical residue in the active site of transglutaminases is not conserved in pallidin.[511] Presumably, some other common property of the two proteins must maintain their homology, but what that may be is a mystery. The pallidin gene is located on chromosome 15q15-q21[513] and resembles transglutaminases in its intron–exon organization.[514] Four isoforms exist caused by alternative splicing of 90-bp and 234-bp exons in the N-terminal end of the protein.[515] The respective proteins are 80 kd (both exons present), 78 kd (small exon absent), 71 kd (large exon absent), and 69 kd (both exons absent). The 78-kd protein is the predominant species (97%) in normal red cells[504]; isoforms lacking the 234-bp exon are rare.

***Pallid* Mice Have a Defect in Pallidin.** In the mouse, pallidin maps to chromosome 2, coincident with the recessive mutation *pallid* (*pa/pa*).[249] The phenotype is characterized by hypopigmentation (abnormal melanosomes), prolonged bleeding time (abnormal platelet dense granules), and increased lysosomal enzyme content in the kidneys (defective lysosomes), which suggests a complex defect in granule/organelle formation.[249] *Pallid* is 1 of 12 genetically independent mouse mutations that map to unique chromosomal loci but have similar phenotypes. They resemble the two human platelet storage pool disease, Hermansky-Pudlak syndrome and Chédiak-Higashi syndrome. In *pallid* mice mRNA transcripts from affected tissues, such as the skin and kidney, are smaller than normal.[249] Transcripts from erythrocytes and other unaffected tissues are normal.

Remarkably, another one of the 12 mutations, *mocha* (*mh/mh*), which is similar to *pallid* phenotypically, may be due to a defect in Ank3.[516] It is hard to believe this is a coincidence. More likely, Ank3 and pallidin interact and are part of a larger structure, such as a granule membrane skeleton, whose individual proteins are candidate genes for the 12 hypopigmentation mutations.

Organization of the Membrane Skeleton

By analogy, the skeleton is sometimes compared with a sweater, which reveals its nodes and individual filaments when stretched but not when collapsed. Stretched skeletons reveal complexes of F-actin (the nodes) cross-linked by molecular filaments of spectrin, when viewed by high-resolution, negative-stained electron microscopy[132,385,386] (Figs. 54-17 and 54-18). Dematin, adducin, and protein 4.1 colocalize with these complexes on immunoelectron microscopy[132] (Fig. 54-19). Most of the complexes are connected by spectrin tetramers (85%) and three-armed hexamers (10%)[386] (see Fig. 54-17). Ankyrin and band 3-containing globular complexes attach to spectrin about 80 nm from its distal end or 20 nm from the site of self-association. The average thickness of the skeletal protein layer has been estimated to be 3 to 6 nm from x-ray diffraction data[517] and 7 to 10 nm from electron micrographs.[518] These dimensions suggest the skeleton is only one or two molecules thick on average, which means it must cover about 25% to 50% of the inner membrane surface area (like a loose-knit sweater). This corresponds reasonably to micrographs of unspread skeletons, where the contracted, collapsed spectrin filaments appear to cover much of the inner membrane surface.

A model of the red cell membrane skeleton based on this and other evidence is shown in Figure 54-20. Similar models have existed, with gradual refinement, since 1979.[519] Spectrin dimers are depicted as twisted, flexible polymers joined head to head to form tetramers and higher order oligomers. Self-association occurs between the N-terminal end of the spectrin α chain and the C-terminal end of the β chain (see Fig. 54-11), as described in detail in the earlier section on spectrin. Spectrin molecules are linked into a two-dimensional network by interactions with a complex of actin protofilaments, protein 4.1, dematin, adducin, and tropomyosin (reviewed by Gilligan and Bennett[128]; see Figs. 54-17 and 54-19). These associations occur at the tail ends of the bifunctional spectrin tetramer. The predicted complexes are morphologically similar to isolated spectrin–actin–4.1 complexes (see Fig. 54-18) and to structures observed in situ in normal ghosts (see Figs. 54-17 and 54-19). They appear to serve as a branch point or "molecular junction" in skeletal construction. On average, six spectrin molecules emanate from each complex, although some variation is found. This is evident in the hexagonal arrangement of spectrin in spread skeletons (see Fig. 54-17). In unperturbed skeletons, most spectrin molecules probably fold up to about one third of their length and do not extensively overlap or intertwine.[375,376]

Individual spectrin tetramers and oligomers are attached to the overlying lipid bilayer through high-affinity interactions with ankyrin and band 3, probably with the assistance of pallidin (protein 4.2). Evidence suggests that band 3 is a mixture of dimers and tetramers in the membrane[220] and that the tetramer probably binds only one molecule of ankyrin.[193,195,221] If so, about 40% of the band 3 molecules are involved in anchoring the membrane skeleton. Although the spectrin tetramer contains two ankyrin binding sites, there is only enough ankyrin to fill one, and generally

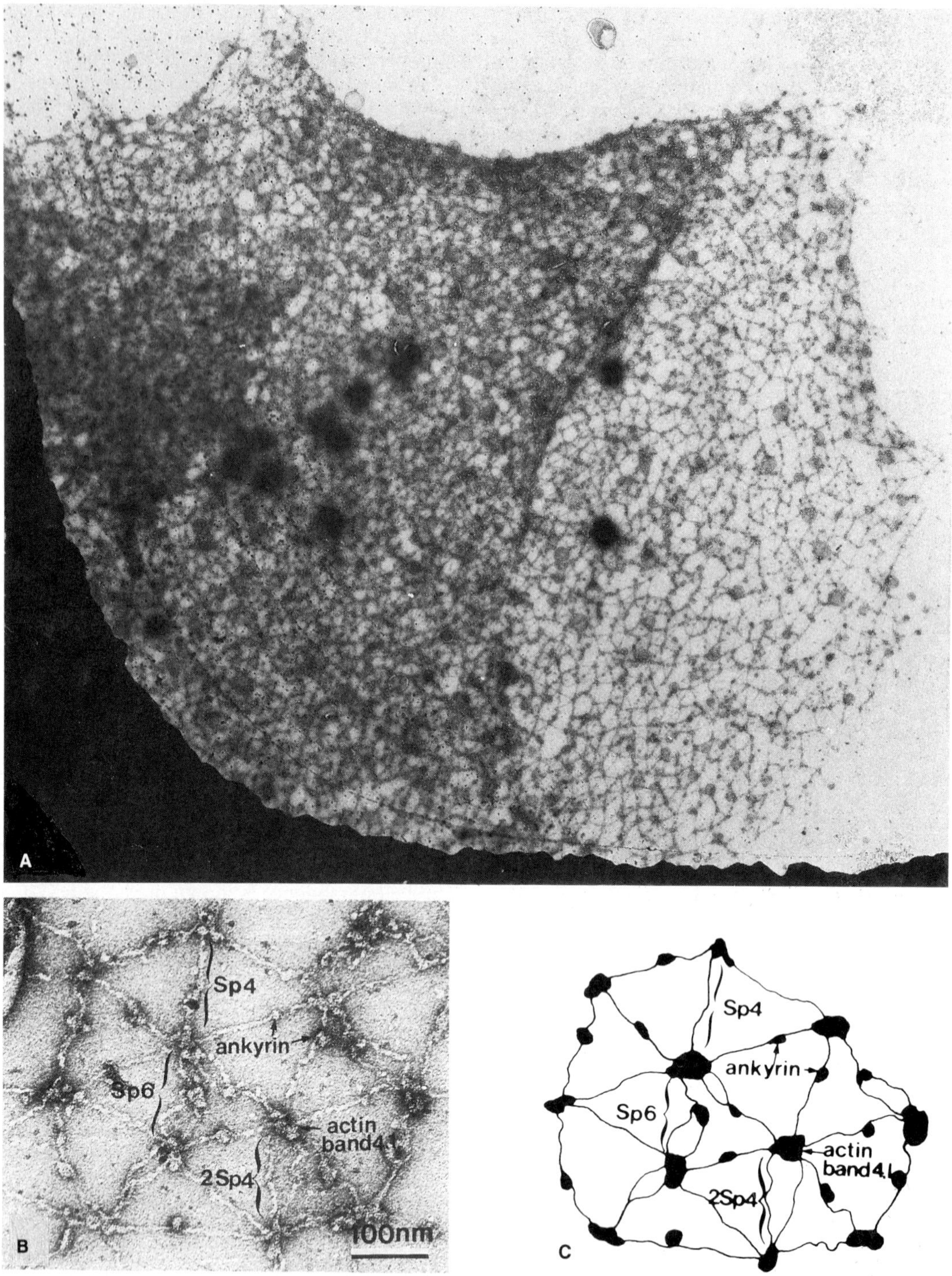

FIGURE 54-17. Electron microscopy of red cell membrane skeletons. The negatively stained skeletons have been artificially expanded to reveal details of their structure. (**A**) Low-magnification view to emphasize the ordered, net-like structure. High-magnification view (**B**) and schematic diagram (**C**) showing the predominantly hexagonal organization of the skeleton. The location of various skeletal elements is shown in C. (Palek J, Sahr KE. Mutations of the red blood cell membrane proteins: from clinical evaluation to detection of the underlying genetic defect. Blood 1992;80:308)

only one is filled in situ (see Fig. 54-17). Interactions among protein 4.1, protein p55, and GPC or between protein 4.1 and band 3 provide secondary sites of attachment.

Modulation of Membrane Skeletal Structure

Red cell membrane proteins are subject to a large number of posttranslational modifications or other regulatory effects: phosphorylation, fatty acid acylation, methylation, glycosylation, deamidation, calpain cleavage, polyphosphoinositide and calmodulin regulation, oxidation, and modification by polyanions (Tables 54-4 and 54-5). Detailed discussion of all these pathways is beyond the scope of this chapter. They have been thoroughly analyzed in a superb review.[92]

Phosphorylation

Almost all the membrane skeletal proteins are phosphorylated by one or more protein kinases (see Table 54-4).

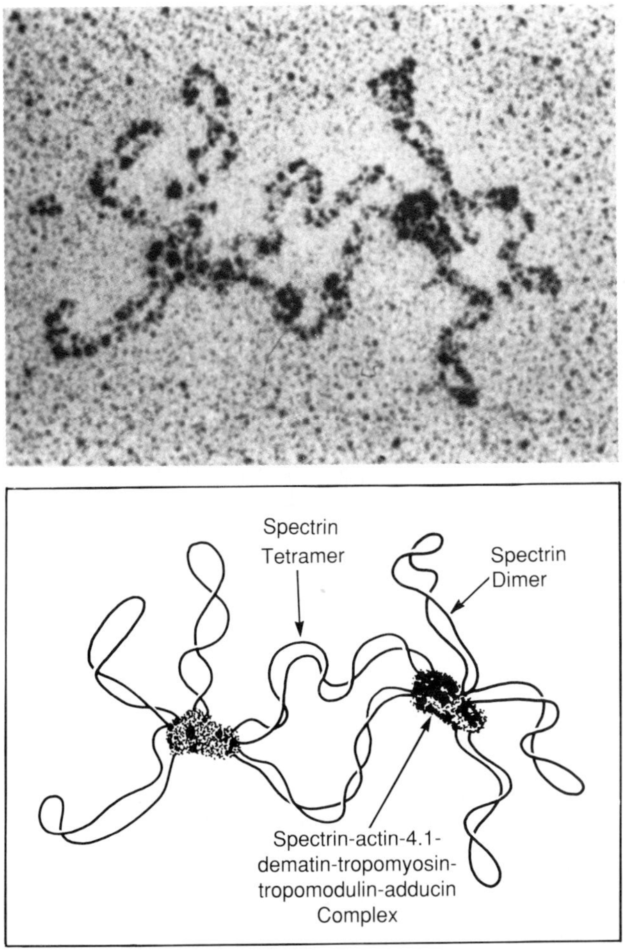

FIGURE 54-18. Two membrane skeletal junction complexes connected by spectrin tetramer strands. (Beaven GH, et al. An examination of the soluble oligomeric complexes extracted from the red cell membrane and their relation to the membrane cytoskeleton. Eur J Cell Biol 1985;35:299)

These include casein kinases (spectrin, ankyrin, band 3, protein 4.1, and dematin); protein kinase A (spectrin, ankyrin, adducin, protein 4.1, and dematin); protein kinase C (adducin, protein 4.1, and dematin); and tyrosine kinases (band 3 and protein 4.1).[92]

In all cases studied, phosphorylation inhibits membrane protein interactions:

1. Ankyrin phosphorylation (casein kinase) abolishes the preference of ankyrin for spectrin tetramer[455,479] and decreases binding to band 3.[480]
2. Phosphorylation of protein 4.1 (several kinases) diminishes its binding to spectrin and its ability to promote spectrin–actin binding[402,403,519a] and decreases its attachment to the membrane.[519b]
3. Phosphorylation by protein kinase C also inhibits binding of protein 4.1 to band 3.[411]
4. Phosphorylation of dematin by PKA prevents actin bundling.[441]
5. Phosphorylation of Tyr 8 at the N terminal of band 3 blocks the binding of glycolytic enzymes[184] and presumably hemoglobin, and results in increased glycolysis.[1]

In contrast, despite extensive study,[367,368,479,520,521] no functional effect of spectrin phosphorylation has been identified.

Polyanions

Physiologic concentrations of organic polyanions such as 2,3-DPG and ATP weaken and dissociate the membrane skeleton[522,523] and increase the lateral mobility of band 3 in ghosts.[524] In vitro, these compounds dramatically inhibit spectrin–actin interactions, even in the presence of protein 4.1.[525] Whether these or other polyanions (eg, polyphosphorylated phosphoinositides) are physiologic mediators in vivo is not clear. Some studies suggest that even supraphysiologic concentrations of 2,3-DPG have little or no effect on intact erythrocytes.[526,527]

Calcium and Calmodulin

Good evidence shows that calmodulin modifies the membrane properties of the red cell.[405] Physiologic concentrations of calmodulin, sealed in red cell ghosts, destabilize membranes in the presence (but not absence) of micromolar concentrations of Ca^{2+}. Studies suggest that the effect may result from interactions of calmodulin with protein 4.1.[406] Submicromolar concentrations of calmodulin, even lower than those that exist in the red cell (3 to 6 μmol/L), block protein 4.1-inducted gelation of actin in the presence of spectrin.[406] The effect is Ca^{2+} dependent. It begins at a Ca^{2+} concentration of 10^{-6} to 10^{-7} mol/L, which is relatively low but still higher than the free Ca^{2+} concentration in the erythrocyte (20 to 40 nmol/L). Ca^{2+}-calmodulin does not block spectrin–actin–4.1 complex formation under these conditions,[406] only the extensive cross-linking needed to cause gelation. Calmodulin also binds to the spectrin β chain in a Ca^{2+}-dependent manner,[404] but the affinity of spectrin for calmodulin is not great and it is unclear whether this effect occurs at the concentrations of calmodulin that exist in erythrocytes.

β-Adducin also binds calmodulin (K_D of 2.3×10^{-7} mol/L).[528] Adducin bound to spectrin and actin fosters the attachment of a second—neighboring—spectrin. This reac-

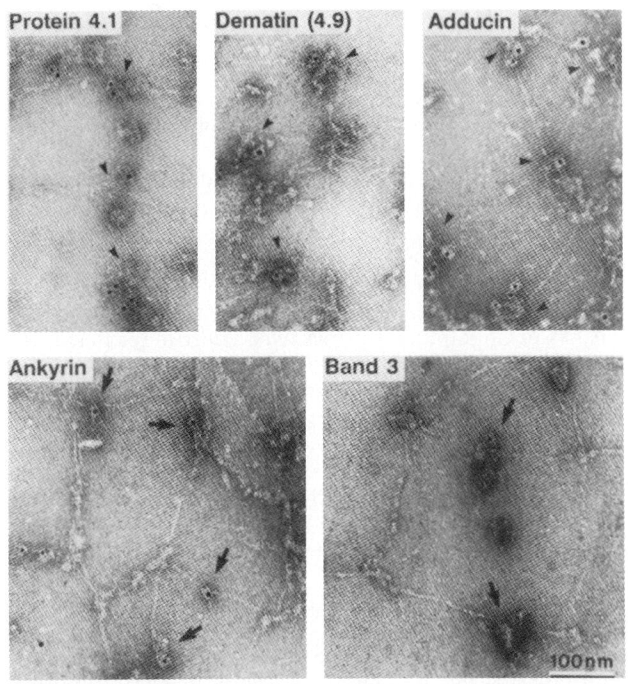

FIGURE 54-19. Immunogold labeling of proteins in red cell membrane skeletons. Expanded membrane skeletons were incubated with affinity-purified antibodies to the membrane skeletal proteins indicated, then washed and stained with 5-nm gold-labeled anti-IgG. Protein 4.1, dematin, and adducin are located in junctional complexes (*arrowheads*), whereas band 3 and ankyrin reside in globular structures (*arrows*) on spectrin filaments, midway between junctional complexes. (Liu S-C, Derick LH. Molecular anatomy of the red blood cell membrane skeleton: structure-function relationships. Semin Hematol 1992;29:231)

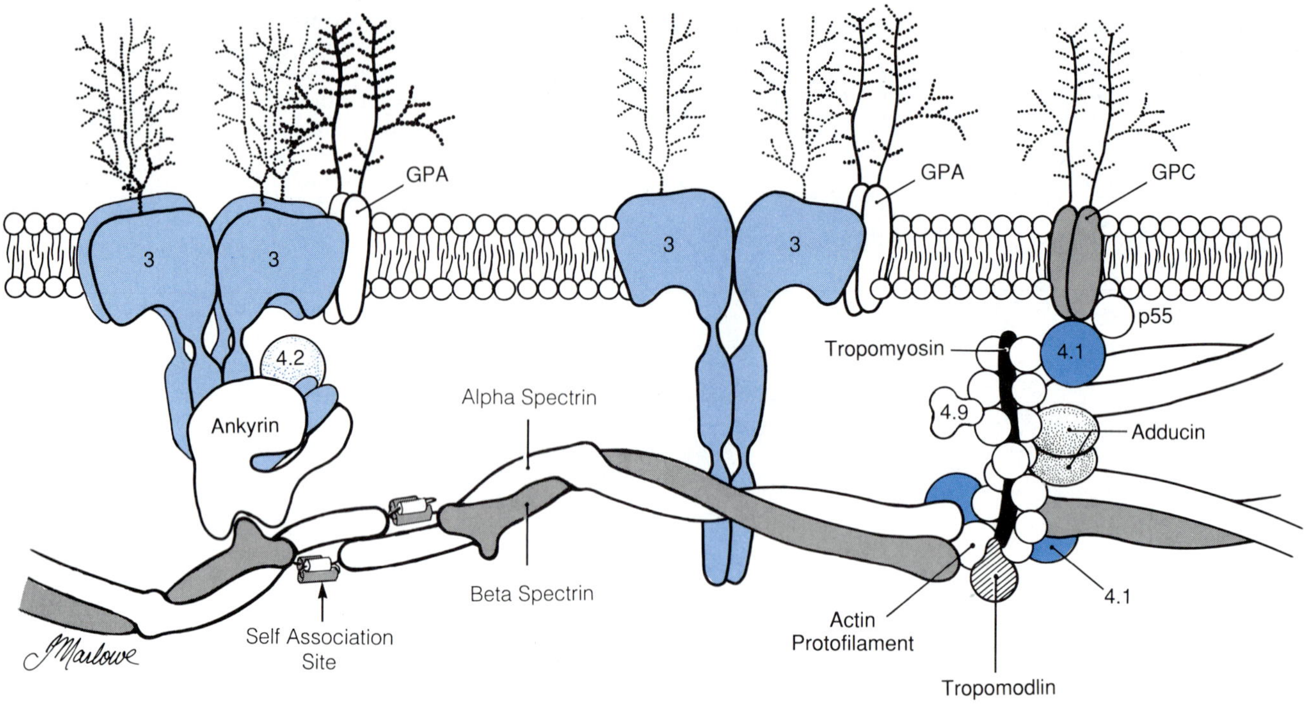

FIGURE 54-20. Schematic model of the red cell membrane. The relative position of the various proteins is correct, but the proteins and lipids are not drawn to scale.

tion is blocked by calmodulin in the presence of Ca^{2+} (over 10^{-7} mol/L).[436,529] The physiologic consequences of this effect are unclear.

Several other Ca^{2+}-dependent events do not require the presence of calmodulin. One event is membrane protein cross-linking, catalyzed by Ca^{2+}-dependent transglutaminase.[530] This cross-linking acts as an endogenous fixative, stabilizing red cell shape.[531,532] The Ca^{2+} concentration required by this reaction is more than 100 times greater than the normal red cell Ca^{2+} concentration, making it unlikely that transglutaminase permanently stabilizes red cell shape in vivo.[531]

A second calmodulin-independent effect of Ca^{2+} is the so-called *Gárdos phenomenon*,[533] a unidirectional K^+ and water loss, producing cellular dehydration. In contrast to transamidative cross-linking, the Ca^{2+} concentration required to trigger the Gárdos channel is low (in the micromolar range) and thus physiologically significant. As discussed in Chapter 53, this pathway contributes to cellular dehydration of sickle red cells.

A third calmodulin-independent Ca^{2+} effect involves calpain, one of a family of Ca^{2+}-stimulated neutral proteases, that are present in a variety of tissues including red cells (reviewed by Cohen and Gascard[92]). Susceptible membrane substrates include ankyrin, protein 4.1, and, to a lesser extent, spectrin and band 3. Finally, Ca^{2+} also induces phospholipid scrambling, as discussed earlier in the chapter.

Thus, increases in intracellular calcium produce a wide range of deleterious effects. Although these phenomena are well studied in vitro, their role in erythrocyte pathology, particularly in acquired disorders associated with abnormal red cell shape, is not well understood.

Biogenesis of the Membrane Skeleton

Synthesis of Band 3 Initiates Assembly of a Stable Membrane Skeleton. Spectrin and ankyrin synthesis is detectable at early stages of erythroid development in avian and mammalian erythroid cells (reviewed by Hanspal and Palek[130] and Lazarides and Woods[534,535]). These proteins turn over rapidly and do not assemble into a permanent network. Synthesis of band 3 (anion exchange protein) and protein 4.1 begins at the proerythroblast stage and increases throughout terminal erythroid maturation, up to the late erythroblast stage. During the same time, the mRNA levels and synthesis of spectrin and ankyrin decline. Even so, the proportion (and actual amounts) of newly assembled spectrin and ankyrin on the membrane progressively increase, and these proteins become more stable, as indicated by their slower turnover. This increased recruitment and stabilization of spectrin and ankyrin, in spite of declining synthesis, are thought to be related to the progressive increase in the synthesis of band 3 and protein 4.1, since these proteins are the principal sites for attachment of the skeleton to the membrane.[130]

Skeletal Proteins Are Synthesized in Excess. The synthesis of membrane skeletal proteins is wasteful. Only a fraction of newly synthesized spectrin, ankyrin, and protein 4.1 is assembled into the permanent skeletal network (Fig. 54-21). The excess proteins are rapidly catabolized.[534,536,537] Furthermore, skeletal protein synthesis is highly asymmetric. This is most striking in spectrin, in which two- to threefold more α-spectrin is produced than β-spectrin (see Fig. 54-21). Yet, the two chains are assembled into the membrane skeleton in equimolar amounts as mixed heterodimers. Because of this high synthetic ratio of α-spectrin to β-spectrin, heterozygotes for a deleted or synthetically inactive α-spectrin allele should be asymptomatic, since sufficient α-spectrin should still be made to pair with all the β-spectrin.

Rate-Limiting Steps of Membrane Skeletal Assembly. As already discussed, the principal rate-limiting step in membrane skeletal assembly is the synthesis of band 3, which contains a high-affinity ankyrin binding site that recruits and stabilizes spectrin and ankyrin on the membrane.[538,539] This view has to be reconciled with observations that some patients with dominantly inherited HS and partial band 3 deficiency, do not have a proportional decrease in the amounts of spectrin and ankyrin in their

TABLE 54-4. Posttranslational Modifications of the Major Red Cell Membrane Proteins

Protein	Modification*	Functional Effect/(Comment)
α-Spectrin	Phosphorylation: PKA	Unknown
β-Spectrin	Phosphorylation: CKI	No effects detected
	Phosphorylation: PKA	Unknown
Ankyrin	Phosphorylation: CKI	Decreased affinity for spectrin tetramers and oligomers
	Phosphorylation: PKA	Unknown
Adducin	Phosphorylation: PKA	Unknown
	Phosphorylation: PKC	Unknown
Band 3	Phosphorylation: CK†	Unknown
	Phosphorylation: TK (Tyr 8)‡	Inhibits binding of glycolytic enzymes → increased glycolysis; may be activated by oxidants
	Glycosylation (Asn 642)	No effects detected
	Palmitoylation (Cys 843)	Unknown
	Methylation	Unknown (low stoichiometry)
Protein 4.1	Phosphorylation: PKA (Ser 331, Ser 467)	Inhibits 4.1-spectrin binding and spectrin–actin–4.1 complex formation
	Phosphorylation: PKC	Inhibits 4.1–spectrin binding, spectrin–actin–4.1 complex formation, and 4.1–band 3 binding
	Phosphorylation: CK	Inhibits 4.1–spectrin binding and binding of 4.1 to membrane
	Phosphorylation: TK (Tyr 418)§	Inhibits spectrin–actin–4.1 complex formation
	Deamidation (Asn 502)	Unknown (converts SDS gel band 4.1b → 4.1a)
	Glycosylation	Unknown (only 20%–40% of protein modified)
Pallidin (4.2)	N-myristoylation (Gly 1)	Unknown
Protein p55	Palmitoylation	Unknown
Dematin (4.9)	Phosphorylation: PKA	Inhibits actin filament bundling
	Phosphorylation: PKC	No effects detected
	Phosphorylation: CK	Unknown

PKA, protein kinase A; PKC, protein kinase C; CK, casein kinase; CKI, casein kinase I; TK, tyrosine kinase.

* Constitutive modifications underlined.

† Several amino acids in the N-terminal region are partially phosphorylated (total incorporated $PO_4 \approx 1$ mol/mol): Ser 29, Thr 39, Thr 42, Thr 48, Thr 49, Ser 50 and Thr 54.

‡ Also some phosphorylation of Tyr 21, Tyr 359 and Tyr 904.

§ May occur only in nonerythroid cells.

(Adapted from Cohen CM, Gascard P. Regulation and post-translational modification of the erythrocyte membrane-skeletal proteins. Semin Hematol 1992;29:244)

TABLE 54-5. Red Cell Membrane Regulatory Pathways

Pathway	Effect	Activation
Ca^{2+}-calmodulin	May regulate membrane mechanical properties by effects on spectrin–actin–4.1 complex or by effects on adducin	Increased intracellular Ca^{2+}
Calpain-mediated proteolysis	Degradation of spectrin, ankyrin, band 3, and protein 4.1	Increased intracellular Ca^{2+}
Deamidation	See Table 54-4	
2,3-Diphosphoglycerate (2,3-DPG)	Decreases membrane mechanical stability, disrupts spectrin–actin–4.1 complexes, inhibits membrane casein kinases	Changes in oxygenation (increased free 2,3-DPG in oxygenated RBCs)
Glycosylation	See Table 54-4	
Methylation	See Table 54-4	
Phosphoinositides	Regulate binding of protein 4.1 to membrane sites (probably glycophorins); may affect casein kinase activity, cation homeostasis, or cell shape	Increased intracellular Ca^{2+} (via activation of phosphoinositidase C), metabolic depletion, PKC activation.
Phosphorylation	See Table 54-4	
Sulfhydryl oxidation	Formation of cross-linked complexes of membrane proteins. Some specific effects: Spectrin: decreased 4.1 binding and ?decreased self-association; Ankyrin: decreased spectrin binding; Band 3: decreased ankyrin binding	Oxidative stress, G6PD deficiency, sickle cell disease, unstable hemoglobinopathies, thalassemias

(Adapted from Cohen CM, Gascard P. Regulation and post-translational modification of erythrocyte membrane-skeletal proteins. Semin Hematol 1992;29:244)

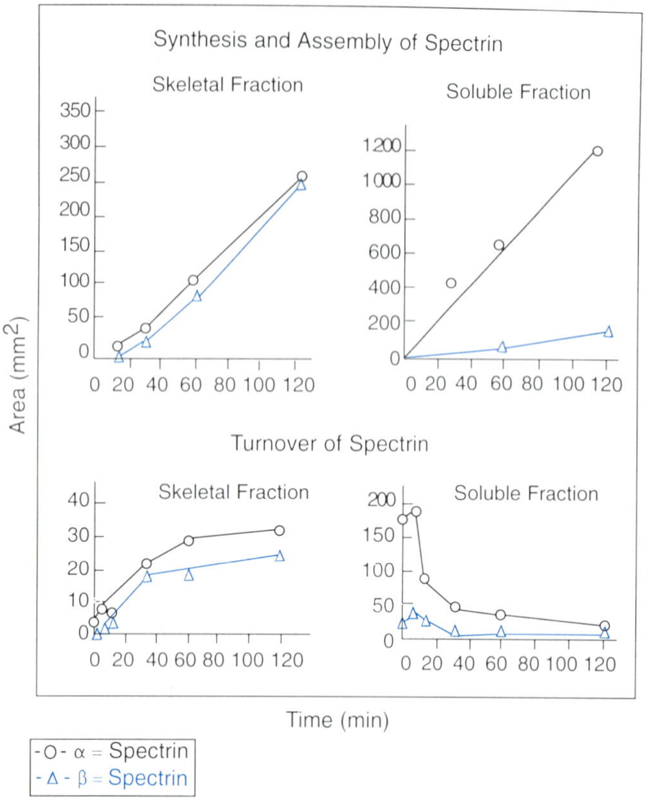

FIGURE 54-21. Synthesis, assembly, and turnover of spectrin in erythroblasts. (*Top*) Synthesis and assembly of α- and β-spectrin. Membrane skeletons and soluble (cytoplasmic) proteins from red cell precursors labeled with a radioactive amino acid were immunoprecipitated with an antispectrin antibody, and the proteins were separated on an SDS gel and autoradiographed. The areas of the scanned autoradiogram peaks are plotted with time. α-Spectrin is synthesized in excess of β-spectrin (*top right*), but both subunits assemble in equivalent amounts on the membrane (*top left*). (*Bottom*) Turnover of spectrin. After a brief period of labeling (pulse), erythroblasts were incubated with nonradioactive amino acids (chase) and the amounts of α- and β-spectrin observed over time. The newly synthesized spectrins are stable if they are incorporated into the membrane skeleton (*bottom left*) but are rapidly degraded if they remain in the cytoplasm (*bottom right*). (After Palek J, Lambert S. Genetics of the red cell membrane. Semin Hematol 1990;27: 290)

membranes.[540,541] The likely explanation is that band 3 is synthesized in excess. About five-fold more band 3 is made than spectrin or ankyrin, but only the tetrameric fraction of band 3 binds ankyrin with high affinity.[195,540] Excess dimeric band 3 is selectively lost in band 3–deficient spherocytes.[540]

The second rate-limiting step is the availability of ankyrin, which provides the high-affinity binding sites for β-spectrin. This is best illustrated by studies of membrane skeletal synthesis in *nb/nb* spherocytic mice[380] and in a severe form of human HS associated with combined deficiency of spectrin and ankyrin.[381] In both disorders, ankyrin synthesis is markedly reduced, which leads to decreased assembly of spectrin and ankyrin on the membrane, in spite of normal spectrin synthesis.[381]

The third rate-limiting step involves synthesis of β-spectrin. Because α- and β-spectrin polypeptides are assembled on the membrane in equimolar amounts and because β-spectrin binds to ankyrin with high affinity, the availability of β-spectrin seems to regulate the amounts of membrane-assembled α/β-spectrin heterodimers. This regulatory role of β-spectrin is illustrated by the effects of erythropoietin on membrane protein assembly. Erythropoietin stimulates the synthesis of β-spectrin and increases assembly of α/β-spectrin heterodimers on the membrane.[542] In contrast, α-spectrin, which is made in excess, does not seem to have a limiting role in the skeletal assembly. α-Spectrin becomes rate limiting only when its synthesis is markedly reduced, as in some patients with recessive HS or hereditary pyropoikilocytosis.

Membrane Remodeling During Enucleation and Reticulocyte Maturation. At the orthochromatic erythroblast stage, when membrane biogenesis is nearly complete, the cell membrane undergoes a series of critical remodeling steps. The cell nucleus is surrounded by an actin ring, which likely participates in the expulsion of the nucleus from the erythroblast. At the same time, the spectrin skeleton segregates into the incipient reticulocyte, whereas some surface receptors cluster in the membrane surrounding the soon-to-be-extruded nucleus.[377] Further membrane remodeling takes place as the young multilobular reticulocyte attains the biconcave shape.[543–546] This involves a loss of lipids and certain surface proteins, including receptors for transferrin and fibronectin.

RED CELL MEMBRANE DEFORMABILITY AND STABILITY

Material Properties

The material properties of the red cell membrane reflect the properties of both the lipid bilayer and the skeleton. During deformation of the red cell membrane, bending is restricted by the incompressibility of the lipid bilayer and is facilitated by rapid translocation of cholesterol from the inner to the outer half of the bilayer.[88] The lipid bilayer cannot expand its surface area more than 3% to 4%. Consequently, when red cells are suspended in hypotonic solutions (such as during osmotic fragility testing (see later in chapter), they swell to a spherical shape and then rupture, discharging their hemoglobin into the supernatant.[546]

The membrane skeleton determines both the solid and semisolid properties of the membrane.[134] The solid properties are exemplified by an elastic extension of the cells, which completely restores their normal shape after the applied force has been removed. An example is a cell that has been deformed when passing through fenestrations of the splenic sinus wall. This elastic recovery of the biconcave shape is facilitated by the unique molecular anatomy of the skeletal lattice. In normal red cells, individual spectrin molecules are arranged in a hexagonal array and are folded in a compact configuration. The junctional complexes are close to each other and are linked by shortened spectrin tetramers, thus allowing large unidirectional extensions without disruption of the lattice (Fig. 54-22). The skeletal connections are unperturbed during such deformations. On the other hand, application of large or prolonged forces allows the skeletal elements to reorganize and make new connections. This produces a permanent plastic deformation (see section on plastic deformation of red cells). When the force is excessive, membrane fragmentation ensues. An example is the poikilocytosis produced in microangiopathic blood vessels where red cells may adhere to damaged endothelium and stretched by the vascular torrent or may be "clotheslined" by fibrin strands.[547] After release, many of the cells are either permanently deformed or fragmented.

Cellular and Molecular Determinants of Red Cell Deformability

The need to undergo large deformations is best exemplified in the wall of the splenic sinus where red cells have to

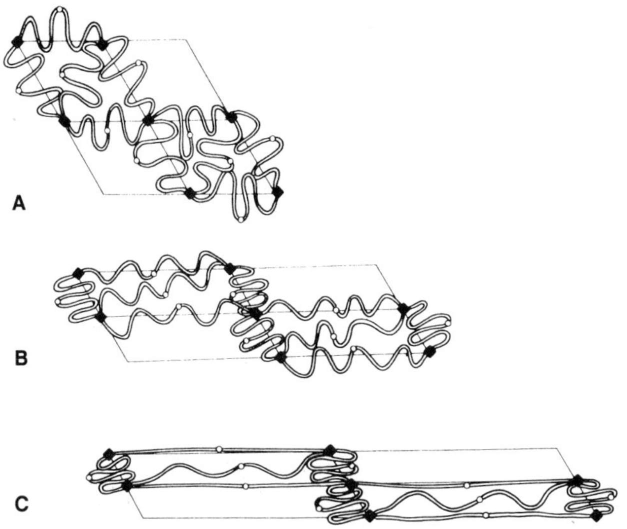

FIGURE 54-22. Model of the effects of deformation on the membrane skeleton. The red cell membrane cannot expand its area. When a force is applied to a section of nondeformed membrane (**A**), extending the lipid bilayer and its attached spectrin molecules (**B**), the bilayer and spectrin molecules in the nonstressed dimension must shrink to maintain a constant area. Eventually, spectrins reach the limit of their length (**C**). Further extension disrupts membrane skeletal interconnections and leads to membrane fragmentation. Spectrin–actin–4.1 junctions (*solid diamonds*), sites of spectrin–spectrin association (*open circles*). (Mohandas N, Chasis JA. Red cell deformability, membrane material properties, and shape: regulation by transmembrane skeletal, and cytosolic proteins and lipids. Semin Hematol 1993;30:171)

squeeze through narrow slits between the endothelial cells that line the splenic sinus wall (see Chaps. 7 and 46 and the later section in this chapter on splenic structure). This whole cell deformability is determined by three factors[134]:

Cell geometry: a large cell surface/volume ratio allows cells to undergo large deformations at a constant volume

Viscosity of the cell contents: determined principally by the properties and the concentration of hemoglobin in the cells

Intrinsic viscoelastic properties of the red cell membrane

Of these factors, the contribution of the surface/volume ratio is the most important, as exemplified by the cellular lesion of hereditary spherocytes, discussed later in this chapter. On the other hand, the intrinsic deformability of the red cell membrane has a relatively small effect on red cell survival. This is best illustrated by the red cell membrane properties of Southeast Asian ovalocytes, which carry a mutant band 3 protein. As will be discussed, both the intact Southeast Asian ovalocyte red cells and their membranes are extremely rigid, but the SAO red cells have a normal survival in vivo.[134,149]

Several molecular alterations increase membrane rigidity. One is accretion of denatured hemoglobin, which may contribute to the membrane rigidity of Heinz body–containing red cells.[548] Others are transamidative or oxidative cross-linking, which make the membrane rigid in vitro.[530–532] Oxidative cross-linking may also be important in vivo, as evidenced by aggregates of oxidant cross-linked proteins in red cells containing unstable hemoglobins.[549] On the other hand, transamidative cross-linking is probably not physiologically significant because the high Ca^{2+} concentrations needed for the reaction are unlikely to be attained in vivo.[531]

Recent studies emphasize the role of integral proteins in regulating membrane deformability. For example, treatment of red cells with antibodies against GPA, including their Fab fragments, leads to reduced deformability via transmembrane signaling. This is exemplified by red cells that lack the cytoplasmic domain of GPA (eg, MiV red cells), which are not influenced by such treatment.[304] Another important factor is the aggregation state of band 3. Membrane rigidity is increased when band 3 molecules are cross-linked with antibodies[550] or, as in Southeast Asian ovalocytosis (see later in text), when mutant band 3s spontaneously stack into linear aggregates.[551,551a] This finding presumably also explains the marked restriction of band 3 mobility in Southeast Asian ovalocyte red cells. Because aggregates of Southeast Asian ovalocyte band 3 contain ankyrin, which attaches the skeleton to the membrane, the decreased mobility of Southeast Asian ovalocyte band 3 may impede skeletal deformation when red cells deform, resulting in a rigid erythrocyte.

Membrane Structural Integrity and Fragmentation

The skeleton is also the principal determinant of membrane stability. As noted earlier, it is possible to manipulate the proportion of spectrin dimers and tetramers in situ by exposing ghosts to temperatures and salt concentrations that favor or discourage self-association. Ghosts enriched in spectrin dimers are strikingly fragile.[370] Similarly, hereditary elliptocytosis and hereditary pyropoikilocytosis are often due to α- or β-spectrin mutations that weaken spectrin self-association. In such cells, the hexagonal skeletal lattice is disrupted,[552] usually in association with red cell fragmentation and poikilocytosis.

Lipid Bilayer Loss and Microvesiculation

The fluid lipid bilayer is stabilized both by the underlying membrane skeleton and the transmembrane proteins. In vitro, the bilayer can be uncoupled from the skeleton at the tips of spiculated red cells by various treatments[553] (Fig. 54-23). The lipids are released in the form of microvesicles, which contain integral proteins but lack skeletal components.[132] Such loss of membrane material may underlie the

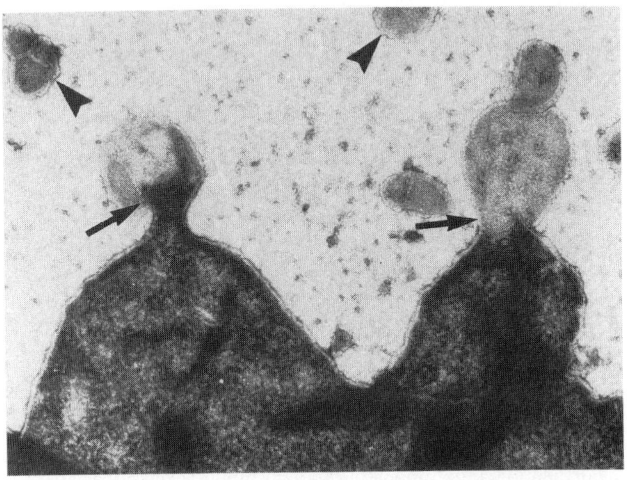

FIGURE 54-23. Microvesiculation. Red cell ghosts treated with hypertonic saline develop spicules. At the end of the spicules, the lipid bilayer often separates from the underlying membrane skeleton. The arrows point to the boundary between the skeleton (*dark areas*) and the unsupported lipids (*light areas*), which are unstable and tend to be released as vesicles (*arrowheads*). A similar process is thought to occur in a variety of disorders associated with spiculation, such as spur cell anemia and possibly hereditary spherocytosis.

surface area deficiency of red cells subjected to prolonged storage[554,555] or of ATP-depleted red cells.[556] Aggregation of the band 3-containing intramembranous particles in the membrane also destabilizes the lipid bilayer.[557] In ghosts, such aggregation can be induced by treatment with Ca^{2+}, Mg^{2+}, polylysine, or basic proteins.[557] The particle-free regions bleb and release lipid microvesicles. As discussed later in this chapter, all these pathways may contribute to the surface deficiency of hereditary spherocytes.

Plastic Deformation of Red Cells

The role of the membrane skeleton in red cell shape is best illustrated by irreversibly sickled cells or hereditary elliptocytes, in which the abnormal shape is retained in the ghosts and membrane skeletons.[558,559] This process is probably an example of plastic deformation, the result of prolonged exposure of red cells to deforming forces, when the proteins of the deformed skeleton undergo active rearrangement that permanently stabilize the cells in the deformed shape[134] (Fig. 54-24). Existing protein–protein contacts disconnect and new associations form. In hereditary elliptocytosis, shape transformations may be facilitated by the weakened skeletal protein interactions.

In addition, both normal and abnormal red cell shapes can be stabilized by intermolecular cross-linking of membrane proteins, either because of a formation of intermolecular disulfide bridges induced by oxidants[531,560] or by transamidative protein cross-linking catalyzed by a Ca^{2+}-activated cytosolic transglutaminase.[531] These protein modifications are like endogenous fixatives and permanently stabilize cell shape in vitro.

Red Cell Surface

The red cell surface is rich in sialic acid residues accounting for the negative surface charge. Ninety percent of these residues reside on GPA; the remainder are shared by other glycophorins, the anion exchange protein, and glycolipids (reviewed by Catron and associates,[120,301] Chasis and Mohandas,[121] Fukuda,[126] and Tanner[136]). Alterations in surface charge distribution are deleterious. For example, surface charge clustering may contribute to adhesion of sickle red cells to the surface of endothelial cells.[561] Several proteins are removed from the surface of reticulocytes that participate in cell–cell and cell–matrix interactions during erythroid differentiation.[545,562,563] One example, $\alpha_4\beta_1$ integrin, interacts with VCAM-1, an endothelial cell adhesion molecule, and may contribute to attachment of sickle cells to the endothelium.[563]

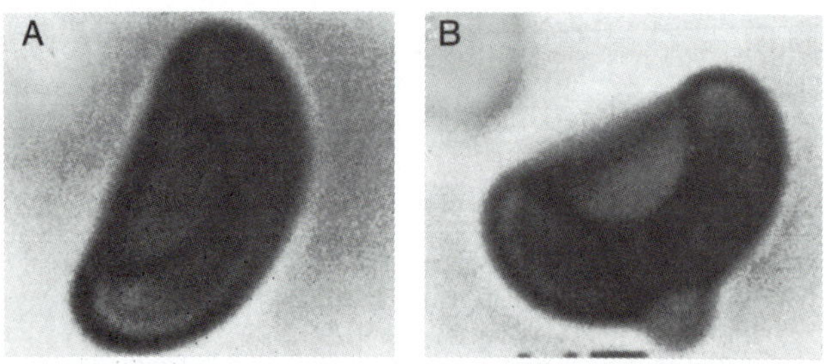

FIGURE 54-24. Plastic deformation. (**A**) Discocytic shape of a red cell at rest in solution. If a nipple of membrane from such a cell is aspirated into a micropipette and immediately released, it snaps back to its original position. If the aspirated membrane is deformed for some time, a permanent nipple forms (**B**) as a result of reorganization of the membrane skeleton in the stressed portion of the membrane. This semisolid behavior is called *plastic deformation* and is believed to be responsible for the irregular shape of poikilocytes, especially in diseases such as hereditary pyropoikilocytosis, in which skeletal reorganization is fostered by genetically weakened skeletal interconnections. (Mohandas N, Chasis JA. Red cell deformability, membrane material properties, and shape: regulation by transmembrane skeletal, and cytosolic proteins and lipids. Semin Hematol 1993;30:171)

The structure and genetic origins of red cell surface antigens, residing either on glycolipids, on externally exposed portions of transmembrane proteins or their carbohydrate side chains, or on the proteins linked via a glycosyl PI anchor, are discussed in Chapter 56. Furthermore, several surface receptors are involved in attachment of malarial parasites to the cells including glycophorins, band 3 protein, and the Duffy blood group antigen (reviewed by Gratzer and Dluzewski,[144] Golan,[564] and Pasvol and associates[565]).

Glycosyl Phosphatidylinositol-Anchored Surface Proteins. To connect externally exposed hydrophilic proteins with the hydrophobic lipid bilayer, nature has devised a hydrophobic glycosyl phosphatidyinositol (GPI) anchor, which is embedded in the outer leaflet of the bilayer. Among the large number of GPI-linked surface proteins, a group of complement-regulatory proteins are clinically the most important[152] (described in detail in Chap. 11). Defective biosynthesis of the GPI anchor precludes attachment of these proteins to the membrane, causing increased susceptibility to hemolysis by complement, as clinically manifested by paroxysmal nocturnal hemoglobinuria. Since this glycolipid anchor is embedded only in the outer leaflet of the bilayer, GPI-anchored surface proteins are not restricted by the membrane skeleton, in contrast to what is found with most transmembrane proteins, and they are much more laterally mobile.[152,564] This high mobility may be important in recruiting complement-regulatory proteins to sites of complement activation. These regulatory proteins are preferentially enriched in the lipid vesicles released from abnormal red cells,[566] such as vesicles derived from spicules of deoxygenated sickle cells. Consequently, GPI-linked proteins are diminished in the densest fraction of sickle cells, rendering them more susceptible to complement-mediated injury.[566]

Lateral Mobility of Transmembrane and Surface Proteins. The mobilities of membrane surface molecules influence the interaction of red cells with the outside environment.[564] For example, cell agglutination requires rapid lateral movements of surface antigens. Their immobilization (eg, by glutaraldehyde) inhibits agglutination.[567]

The lateral mobility of proteins that are anchored exclusively in the outer leaflet of the bilayer (eg, GPI-linked proteins) is fast (see previous section). Conversely, transmembrane proteins, such as band 3, are much less mobile. In band 3, this occurs because of (1) specific binding to ankyrin and the skeleton; (2) steric hindrance by spectrin strands, which entangle the internal portions of band 3; (3) self-association of band 3 into tetramers and higher oligomers; and (4) interaction of band 3 with other transmembrane proteins such as the glycophorins.[564]

MEMBRANE PERMEABILITY

Normally, the red cell membrane is nearly impermeable to monovalent and divalent cations, thereby maintaining a high potassium, low sodium and very low calcium content. In contrast, the red cell is highly permeable to water and anions, which are readily exchanged by the water channel and the anion transport protein, respectively. Glucose is taken up by the glucose transporter,[568,569] whereas larger charged molecules, such as ATP and related compounds, do not cross the normal red cell membrane.

The transport pathways for cations and anions in the human red cell membrane can be divided into five categories (Fig. 54-25).

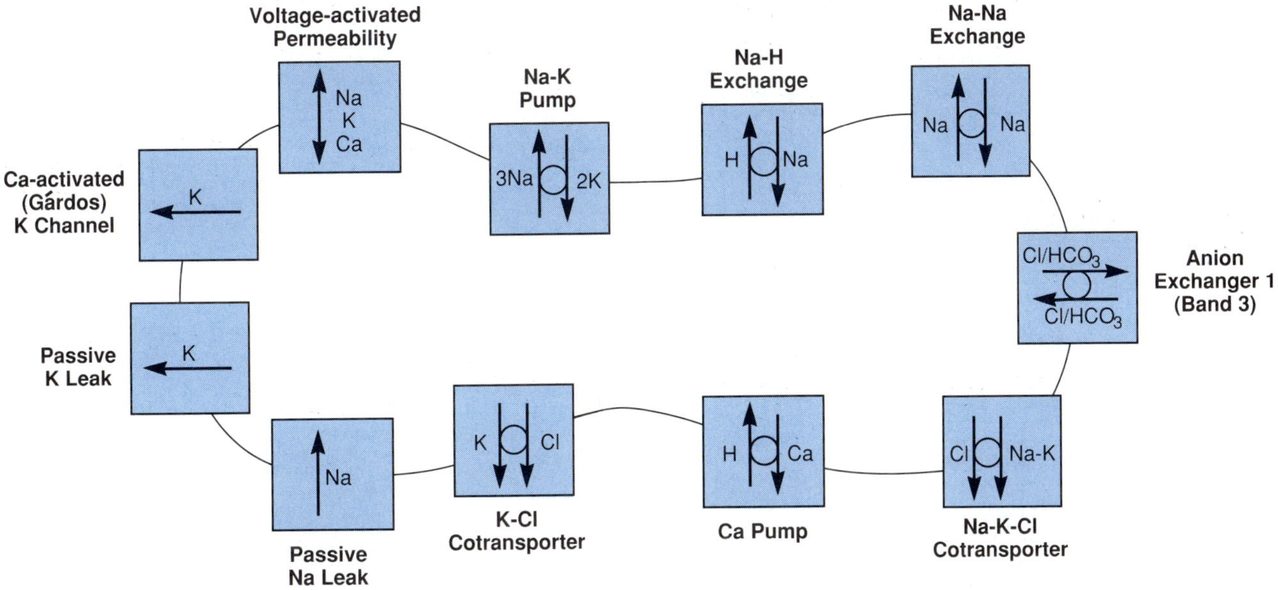

FIGURE 54-25. Red cell membrane ion transport channels, ion exchange channels, and passive permeability pathways.

- Exchangers, such as the Na^+/H^+ exchanger and anion exchanger discussed earlier
- Cotransporters, in which the transmembrane movements of more than one solute are coupled in the same direction (eg, the K^+/Cl^- cotransporter and the $Na^+/K^+/Cl^-$ cotransporter)
- The Ca^{2+}-activated K^+ channel (Gárdos channel) discussed later in chapter
- The cation leak pathways, which allow Na^+ and K^+ to move in the direction of their concentration gradients
- Membrane pumps, such as the ouabain-inhibitable Na^+/K^+ pump and the Ca^{2+} pump, respectively

A detailed review of these pathways is beyond the scope of this chapter. The interested reader is referred to several reviews and monographs.[570–574]

An important feature of the normal red cell is its ability to maintain a constant volume. One of the intriguing, yet unanswered, questions is how cells sense changes in cell volume and activate appropriate volume regulatory pathways. One possibility is that they sense mechanical events, such as membrane stretching.[575] Such a mechanism is unlikely to operate in red cells which, by virtue of their large surface area, can undergo a substantial volume increase without stretching. Another possibility is that cell volume is controlled by the crowding of cytoplasmic macromolecules.[575] According to this theory, cell shrinkage stimulates and swelling inhibits a putative protein kinase, which, in turn, changes the activity of a volume-regulatory cation transporter, such as the K^+/Cl^- cotransporter.[575]

Water Permeability

Water permeability of many cell types is similar to the permeability of pure lipid bilayer membranes, in which water is postulated to enter through small cavities in the bilayer.[576] When phospholipids are in the liquid crystalline state, these cavities are thought to be caused by a noncooperative rotation and kinking around the C-C bonds.[576] In addition, water permeability may be facilitated by lipids with large polar head groups, such as gangliosides and lysophospholipids, which, when dispersed in water, prefer a micellar rather than bilayer configuration. In addition, integral proteins are likely to enhance water diffusion by producing localized discontinuities in the lipid bilayer.[576]

Membranes of red cells and some kidney tubules differ from membranes of most other cells in that they have a high water permeability, being endowed by a molecular water channel protein.[577,578] This protein, designated CHIP 28 (channel-like integral protein of 28 kd) has been cloned and sequenced.[579] The hydropathy analysis indicates six highly hydrophobic membrane segments. Both the N terminal and the C terminal are exposed in the cytoplasm, and two external potential glycosylation sites are present. There are about 200,000 copies of the channel per cell. The suggested function of CHIP 28 is to facilitate rehydration of red cells after their shrinkage in the hypertonic environment of the renal medulla.[580]

Transport Pathways Leading to Cellular Dehydration

Two pathways exert a critical volume regulatory effect (Fig. 54-26). One is the K^+/Cl^- cotransporter, a typical carrier-mediated cotransport pathway, which is particularly active in reticulocytes. It is activated by cell swelling, acidification, depletion of intracellular Mg^{2+}, and thiol oxidation. It is increased in sickle red cells and hemoglobin C erythrocytes, which accounts, in part, for cellular dehydration of these cells.[571–573]

The second transporter is the Gárdos channel, which causes selective loss of K^+ in response to an increase in intracellular ionized calcium[533] (see Fig. 54-26). This channel appears to be regulated by a cytoplasmic protein called calpromotin and by cyclic adenosine monophosphate (cAMP). The channel is inhibited by insect toxins, such as charybdotoxin, and by the Ca^{2+} channel blockers, nitrendipine and nifedipine (reviewed by Bugnara[571] and Joiner[572]). In sickle cells, the combination of the Gárdos pathway and the K^+/Cl^- cotransporter account for the net loss of K^+ and water, leading to cellular dehydration.[572]

Disruption of the Permeability Barrier in Abnormal Red Cells

The effects of breaching the red cell permeability barrier are well illustrated by complement hemolysis. Complement activation on the red cell surface leads to formation of the membrane attack complex, composed of the terminal com-

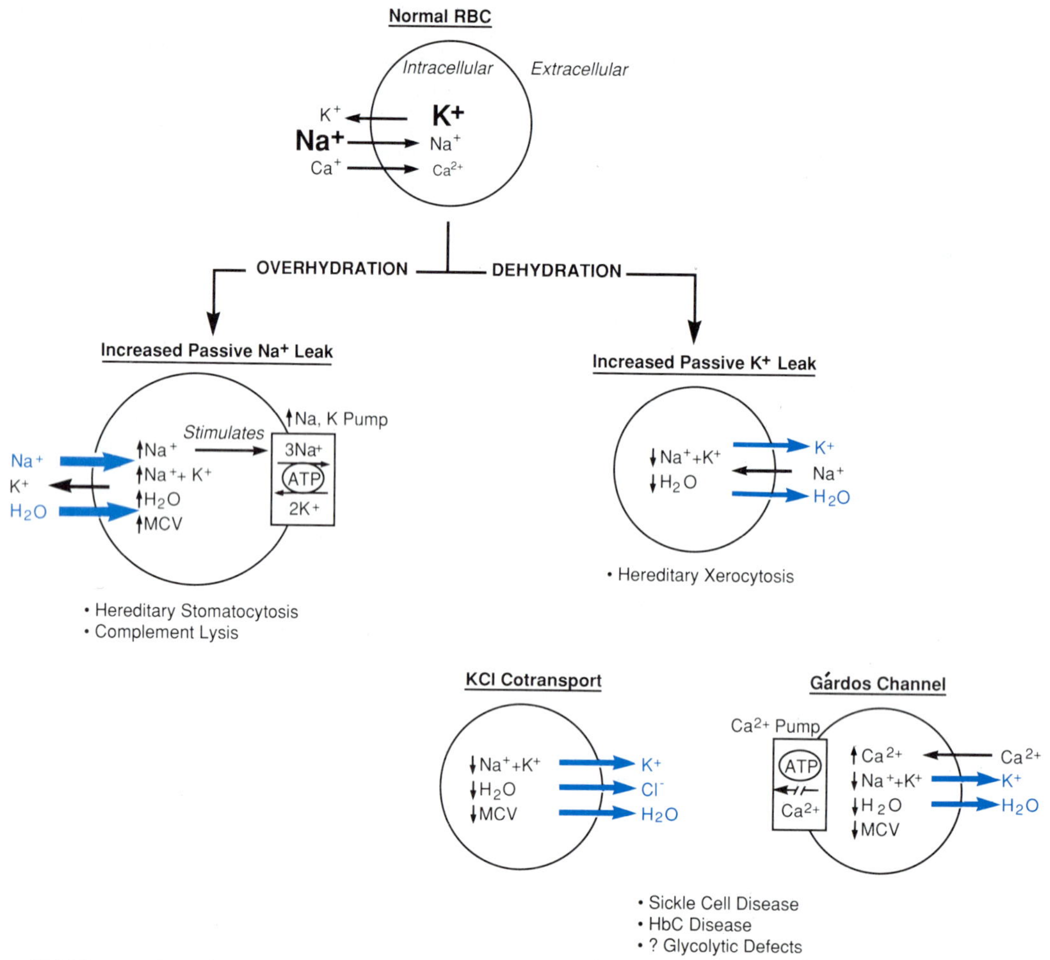

FIGURE 54-26. Cation changes leading to dehydration or overhydration of red cells. (*Left*) Overhydration is caused by a massive unbalanced influx of Na^+, which overwhelms the Na^+/K^+ pump and leads to an increase in total monovalent cations ($Na^+ + K^+$) and cell water. (*Right*) Dehydration is caused by excess, unbalanced K^+ leakage or by activation of K^+ losing channels such as the K^+/Cl^- cotransport channel or the Ca^{2+}-activated Gárdos pathway. Dehydration is associated with a decline in total monovalent cations ($Na^+ + K^+$) and cell water.

plement components embedded in the lipid bilayer (see Chaps. 11 and 16). This multimolecular complex acts as a cation channel, allowing passive movements of sodium, potassium, and calcium across the membrane according to their concentration gradients. Attracted by fixed anions, such as hemoglobin, ATP, and 2,3-DPG, sodium accumulates in the cells in excess of potassium loss and in excess of the compensatory efforts of the Na^+/K^+ pump. The resulting increase in intracellular monovalent cations and water is followed by cell swelling (see Fig. 54-26) and ultimately by colloid osmotic hemolysis.

Another leak pathway has been described in sickle cells. It involves an influx of Na^+ and Ca^{2+} and an efflux of K^+ during deoxygenation and sickling.[571,572] Although the molecular basis of this diffusional pathway is unknown, the magnitude of the Na^+ and K^+ leaks correlates with the degree of morphologic sickling and with lipid bilayer–skeleton uncoupling, suggesting it is caused by mechanical events (reviewed by Joiner[72]). This conclusion is further supported by the observation that Ca^{2+} permeability is increased by mechanical stress.[581] Such permeability pathways may be related to stretch-activated channels, described in various tissues, including endothelial, epithelial, and muscle cells.[582] The mechanism of activation of these channels is unknown, but one of the possibilities involves deformation of the submembrane skeleton.[583,584]

Membrane Pumps

To maintain low intracellular concentrations of sodium and calcium and a high potassium concentration, the membrane is endowed with two cation pumps, both utilizing intracellular ATP as an energy source. The ouabain-inhibitable Na^+/K^+ pump, extrudes sodium and takes up potassium, with a stoichiometry of *three* Na^+ pumped outward for two K^+ pumped inward. This exactly balances the normal passive leaks (Na^+ influx of 1 to 2 mEq per liter of red cells per hour; K^+ efflux of 0.8 to 1.5 mEq per liter of red cells per hour). The enzyme is activated by intracellular Na^+ (K_m of 25 mmol/L) and extracellular K^+ (K_m of 2.5 mmol/L).[585] Because plasma K^+ is high enough to saturate the extracellular K^+ site, Na^+ and K^+ transport is primarily regulated by increases in red cell Na^+ concentration, and cell K^+ losses are rectified only when there is a concomitant Na^+ gain to stimulate active transport. Even then, the ratio between the inward Na^+ leak and outward K^+ leak must not be less than the physiologic ratio of 3:2. At lower ratios, the Na^+/K^+ pump, driven by the Na^+ leak and internal Na^+ concentration will not balance the leaks and will actually exacerbate K^+ loss.[586,587] Consequently, conditions in which K^+ loss approaches or exceeds Na^+ gain lead to irreversible K^+ depletion and cell dehydration.

The calmodulin-activated, Mg^{2+}-dependent Ca^{2+} pump extrudes Ca^{2+} and maintains a low intracellular free Ca^{2+} concentration (20 to 40 nmol/L). It protects red cells from the multiple deleterious effects of Ca^{2+} (echinocytosis, membrane vesiculation, calpain activation, membrane proteolysis, and cell dehydration) described earlier in the chapter. The structure and function of the Na^+/K^+ and Ca^{2+} pumps has been reviewed in detail.[574]

RED CELL MEMBRANE ALTERATIONS OF SENESCENT RED CELLS

Pleiotropic Effects

The removal of senescent red cells from the circulation is a subject of a long-standing interest. As discussed in a comprehensive review of the literature published prior to 1988,[588] the concept of red cell senescence is based on results of radioactive labeling of a cohort of reticulocytes and bone marrow erythroblasts. In many species, including man, the fraction of labeled cells remains constant for a defined time period, followed by a rapid decline of radioactivity, suggesting that the red cells are removed from the circulation in an age-dependent manner. Many techniques have been used to isolate senescent red cells, including methods based on differences in cell density, osmotic fragility, and cell size (reviewed by Clark and Shohet[588,589]). Density separation is most widely used, but the results obtained by this technique must be interpreted with caution. Although red cells exhibit a progressive increase in density as they age in vivo, not all dense red cells are senescent.[588,590,591]

In addition to in vitro separation techniques, various in vivo animal models have been used to study red cell aging.[588] For example, red cells can be labeled with biotin and then removed at defined times with avidin, which complexes tightly to biotin.[592] The senescent cells defined by these techniques exhibit numerous membrane abnormalities, which are summarized in several reviews.[588,590,593,594] Of particular note is the loss of potassium and water, leading to cell dehydration and increased cell density, and the loss of surface area, presumably because of gradual release of membrane microvesicles.[588,589,594,595] The latter phenomenon is probably caused by constant exposure of red cells to the shearing forces of the microcirculation. In addition, red cell membrane proteins and lipids experience oxidative damage, as evidenced by high molecular weight aggregates containing hemoglobin, spectrin, and band 3[596,597] and by adducts of proteins and malonylaldehyde, a product of lipid peroxidation.[598]

Early results suggested that loss of red cell surface charge,[599] due to in vivo loss of sialic acid residues, and exposure of the penultimate β-galactose residues of the carbohydrate side chains were important factors in the recognition and removal of aged erythrocytes.[600] Later studies have revealed that the mild surface charge loss can be entirely explained by the loss of cell surface area[601] and that the surface charge density and the number of sialic acid residues per sialoglycoprotein in senescent red cells is normal.[602,603]

In addition to red cell membrane abnormalities, red cell aging is associated with a decline of many red cell enzyme activities.[604] Red cell ATP concentration is normal.[588] Likewise, no major abnormalities have been detected in Ca^{2+} transport, and no compelling evidence exists that Ca^{2+} accumulates in senescent cells (reviewed by Clark[588]).

Autologous IgG and Destruction by Macrophages

Although some of the above-mentioned alterations may compromise red cell microcirculatory flow, none is likely to destroy old cells. In a creative series of studies begun almost two decades ago, Kay[605] has shown that senescent red cells have small amounts (a few hundred molecules per cell) of autologous IgG on their surface that target the cells for destruction by macrophages. The nature of the "senescent antigen" has been a source of some dispute. Possibilities include band 3 molecules[606–607a] and exposed α-galactosyl residues on membrane glycoproteins.[608,609] The contribution of the latter modification is probably minimal, because the removal of α-galactosyl residues by extensive washing does not affect phagocytosis of senescent erythrocytes.[610] On the other hand, considerable evidence shows that antibodies are bound to band 3 in aged and pathologic red cells.[189,226,227,606–607a,611–613] What is not clear is why.

The most popular view is that antibodies to senescent antigen bind to aggregated or oligomerized band 3.[596,607,612] Band 3 clusters have been visualized by immunofluorescence microscopy and detected by biochemical methods in aged red cells.[596,607,612] Aggregation probably results from cumulative oxidative damage because similar damage, including the binding of autologous IgG, takes place on oxidized red cells or red cells containing Heinz bodies, a product of oxidative denaturation of hemoglobin.[55,189,607,612a,613] The senescent antigen is also exposed on red cells infected with the knobby variant of *P falciparum*.[614]

Intramembranous particles, which are mostly band 3, are not reproducibly clustered in cells that bear senescent IgG.[615] This suggests that other band 3 modifications account for increased binding of autologous IgG. For example, band 3 could be structurally modified by proteolysis or oxidation, or band 3 molecules could be vertically displaced, exposing new antigenic sites or rendering existing sites more accessible to antibodies.

In addition to targeting senescent red cells for macrophage destruction, band 3 antibodies also trigger complement deposition on senescent cells.[594] As noted, this process may be facilitated by loss of GPI-linked complement regulatory proteins from old cells through microvesiculation.

Although the role of autologous IgG in the destruction of senescent erythrocytes is widely accepted, two observations suggest that other mechanisms must be considered. First, blockade of the Fc portion of autologous "senescent" IgG with protein G fails to inhibit red cell phagocytosis.[593] Second, red cell survival is the same in agammaglobulinemic mice as in controls.[593] The latter data may not be applicable to humans, because the removal of mouse red cells from the circulation is random.[588]

Altered phospholipid asymmetry might also contribute to removal of senescent erythrocytes. This could occur from damage to the aminophospholipid translocase by products of lipid peroxidation.[616] Disordered phospholipid asymmetry reportedly activates the alternate complement pathway[617] and targets red cells for destruction by macrophages.[618]

Other alterations of possible pathologic significance include postsynthetic modification of red cell proteins by nonenzymatic glycosylation[619] or carboxymethylation.[620,620a] Glycosylation of membrane proteins, like hemoglobin (to form hemoglobin A_{1c}), occurs gradually over the life of the cell and is proportional to the glucose concentration. Methylation of membrane proteins occurs primarily in older red cells. Ankyrin and protein 4.1 are the principal substrates.

HEREDITARY SPHEROCYTOSIS

Hereditary spherocytosis is a common, inherited hemolytic anemia in which defects of spectrin or the proteins that attach spectrin to the membrane (ankyrin, pallidin, band 3) lead to spheroidal, osmotically fragile cells that are selectively trapped in the spleen and that survive almost normally after splenectomy.

History

In 1871, two Belgian physicians, Vanlair and Masius, in a lengthy report in the Bulletin of the Royal Academy of Medicine of Belgium,[621] described the case of a young woman who suffered from recurrent abdominal pains over her enlarged spleen, associated with prostration, vomiting, jaundice, anemia, aphonia, and marked muscular weakness, The authors noted that during the attack (presumably a hemolytic crisis) most of the woman's red cells were spherical and much smaller than normal, averaging only 4 μm in diameter. The authors named the disease *microcythemia* and depicted the patient's unstained cells, which they called microcytes, in a beautiful lithograph drawn and tinted by Vanlair (Fig. 54-27). The drawing shows numerous spherocytes and some elliptocytes (19% of the evaluable cells), which suggests that iron deficiency or thalassemia may have contributed to the anemia and cell size.

The patient's red cells remained abnormal after her recovery, and her splenomegaly persisted. Vanlair and Masius thought the microcytes were senile red cells (globules atrophiques) and that the spleen assisted in their aging. They argued that when red cells are sequestered in the splenic pulp they lose volume and become dense, spherical, and microcytic. Vanlair and Masius reasoned that an enlarged spleen might produce even more of such cells than a normal spleen and that the liver might complete the work of the spleen by destroying microcytes it received through the splenic vein. They suggested that the large number of microcytes in their patient was due to a combination of splenic enlargement and liver atrophy. Last, the authors noted that the patient's sister had suffered from an identical illness and died during a crisis, and that her mother was also subject to jaundice.

In retrospect, the paper is remarkably prescient. Not only did the authors describe the first example of hereditary hemolytic anemia well before the microscope was in general use in the analysis of blood diseases, but their deductions concerning the pathophysiology of HS, particularly the role of the spleen, predated Ham and Castle's concept of erythrostasis[622] by more than two thirds of a century. Their paper is placed in perspective by the fact that five to seven decades later respected hematologists were still ascribing HS to causes such as hereditary syphilis[623] and splenic hemolysins.[624]

Unfortunately, Vanlair and Masius' report went unnoticed, as did subsequent descriptions of HS in the 1890s by British physicians Wilson and Stanley,[625,626] who clearly recognized the hereditary nature of the disease and were the first to recognize the characteristic pathology of the spleen engorged with red cells. In the German literature, a report by Minkowski[627] in 1900, received wide attention, and many other papers soon appeared,[628,629] including Chauffard's classic description of osmotic fragility[630] and reticulocytosis[631] as hallmarks of the disease. During this time, Widal and associates[632] defined an acquired form of the disease, which we now recognize as warm-antibody immunohemolytic anemia. Because Hayem[633] had previously reported similar cases, the acquired and congenital diseases were soon accorded the Hayem-Widal and Minkowski-Chauffard eponyms.

The use of splenectomy was soon advocated, and in 1911 Micheli[634] removed the spleen from a patient with acquired hemolytic jaundice. The fortunately brilliant result, combined with the subsequent success of splenectomy in the congenital disease,[635] led rapidly to widespread acceptance of the procedure. Actually, the first successful splenectomy for HS was unintentionally performed by Wells in England in 1887,[636] 3 years before Wilson's description of HS in that country. While operating on a jaundiced woman for a supposed uterine fibroid, Wells instead encountered and bravely removed an enormous spleen. The patient recovered and her jaundice disappeared. The events were reconstructed 40 years later by Dawson,[636] who found the characteristic osmotic fragility during an examination of the woman and her son.

Thus, almost all the major clinical feature of HS were defined by the time of Tileston's[637] and Gänsslen's[638] reviews in 1922. The spleen was thought to be involved in red cell destruction, and splenectomy was known to be curative. Nevertheless, except for Vanlair and Masius's farsighted (and still unrecognized) deductions, nothing significant was known about the pathogenesis of the disease.

Readers interested in more details about these and other aspects of the history of HS should consult the chapters by Dacie, Crosby, and Wintrobe in *Blood, Pure and Eloquent*, a captivating account of the history of hematology.[639]

Prevalence and Genetics

Hereditary spherocytosis occurs in all racial and ethnic groups. It is particularly common in Northern European peoples, affecting about 1 in 5000 persons[640]; this is probably an underestimation. Surveys of red cell osmotic fragility, using sensitive assays, suggest that mild forms of HS may be four or five times more common.[641,642] There are no good

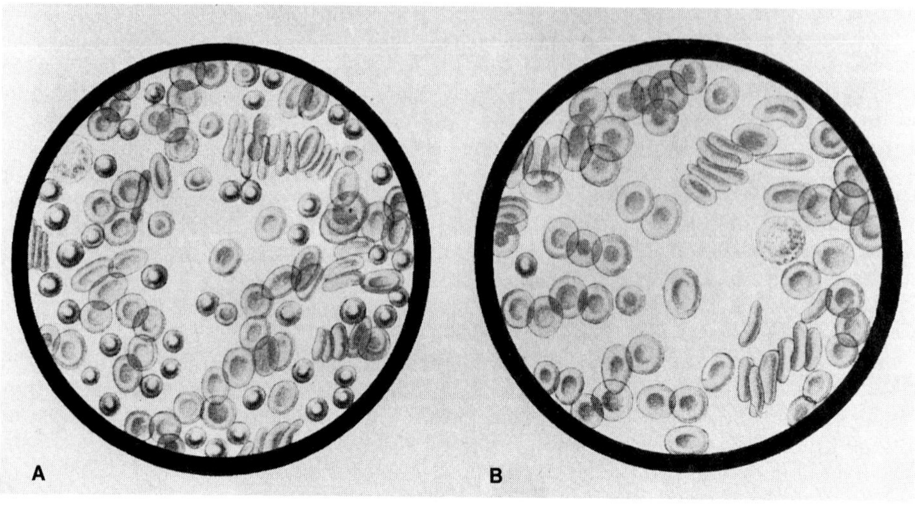

FIGURE 54-27. Lithograph of normal blood cells (**B**) and cells from a patient with "microcythemia" (**A**) described by Vanlair and Masius in 1871. (De la midrocythémie. Bull R Acad Med Belg 1871;5:515)

estimates of the prevalence in other populations, but clinical experience suggests it is less common in African Americans and Southeast Asians.

HS exhibits both dominant and recessive phenotypes. About 75% of families have the autosomal dominant disease.[640,643,644] No definite homozygotes for typical dominant HS have ever been identified, which suggests that homozygosity may be incompatible with life. A report of near-lethal HS (severe intrauterine hydrops fetalis, marked spherocytosis, and extreme spectrin deficiency) in a family in whom one parent has moderate dominant HS and the other has clinically silent disease with only a slightly abnormal osmotic fragility test, supports this supposition.[645] The single exception may be a Portugese family in whom both parents have mild HS and the affected children have moderately severe hemolysis and anemia (Hb 7 to 8 gdL, reticulocytes 7% to 20%).[645a] Two other reports of less severe homozygous HS have appeared,[646,647] but in neither case was homozygosity proved (or likely).

In about 20% to 25% of HS patients, both parents are clinically normal but have subtle laboratory abnormalities that suggest a carrier state[643,648] (see later section on silent carrier state). These patients probably have an autosomal recessive form of the disease,[236,643,648] although it is not always possible to exclude dominant HS with reduced penetrance or dominant HS resulting from a new mutation. For simplicity, the term recessive HS is used in this chapter to identify patients who do not have typical dominant HS. By definition, patients whose parents are completely normal (5% to 10%) are considered to have new mutations.[643]

Etiology: Membrane Protein Defects

The primary molecular defects in HS reside in membrane skeletal proteins, particularly the proteins whose vertical interactions connect the membrane skeleton to the lipid bilayer: spectrin, ankyrin, pallidin (protein 4.2), and band 3 (AE1). All these and other known membrane protein defects are compiled in Table 54-6.

Spectrin

Spectrin Deficiency Is Common in Hereditary Spherocytosis. Red cells from most HS patients are spectrin deficient,[236,643,648,650] including both the dominant and recessive forms. The degree of deficiency correlates well with the spheroidicity of HS erythrocytes,[648,650,795] the severity of hemolysis,[643,648,650] and the response of patients to splenectomy.[648] The spectrin deficiency is evident microscopically (Fig. 54-28). The mechanical properties of the cells, particularly their ability to withstand shear stress, also correlate with their spectrin content[795,796] (Fig. 54-29). Microscopically, HS red cells show fewer spectrin filaments interconnecting spectrin–actin–4.1 junctional complexes,[552] but overall skeletal architecture is preserved, except in the most severe forms of HS.

α-Spectrin: Possible Association With Recessive Hereditary Spherocytosis. The mechanisms of spectrin deficiency are unknown in most HS patients. Initially it seemed probable that recessive and dominant HS would be due to defects in α-spectrin and β-spectrin, respectively. In several species, including humans,[381] α-spectrin exceeds β-spectrin synthesis by about 3 or 4 to 1. Heterozygotes for α-spectrin synthetic defects should still produce enough normal α-subunits to pair with all or nearly all the β chains that are made, so that spectrin deficiency would be evident only in the homozygous state. In fact, this fits with what is observed. Even in the most severe forms of recessive HS, obligate heterozygotes show little or no spectrin deficiency.[236,643,648]

Careful protein mapping and limited sequencing show that a subset (about 55%) of patients with severe recessive HS and marked spectrin deficiency (20% to 40% of normal; Fig. 54-30) have a mutation in the ninth 106–amino acid repeat of α-spectrin (α Ala 969 → Asp, αII domain),[659,660] termed the *spectrin αIIa variant* (see Table 54-6). Studies indicate that that this mutation is an unlikely cause of HS, since it is present in 2%[659,660] to 15%[797] of healthy persons. In addition, in many HS families it is located on a different chromosome and inherited independently from the HS gene.[797] What is not clear is whether it is linked to HS in some families—that is, whether HS is sometimes caused by a defect in α-spectrin. The high incidence of the α Ala 969 → Asp polymorphism in families with severe spectrin-deficient HS[659,660] suggests that this is the case; these studies have been published only in abstract form, so that it is difficult to evaluate the data. In any case, patients with this extremely severe form of recessive HS are rare (less than 2% of all HS patients). Data indicate that defects in ankyrin[723] or pallidin[122] often cause the more typical (milder) recessive disease.

β-Spectrin: Association With Dominant Hereditary Spherocytosis. Deficiency of the scarce β-spectrin chains, on the other hand, should limit formation of spectrin heterodimers and be expressed as a dominant defect. A deficiency of ankyrin should limit spectrin heterodimer formation as well, since spectrin heterodimers are stable only when bound to the membrane[798] and ankyrin, the high-affinity binding site, is normally present in limiting amounts. By the same reasoning, band 3 might also be a culprit, since ankyrin and spectrin do not bind to the membrane until band 3 is expressed[539] and only a fraction of the band 3 molecules are available to bind ankyrin.[193]

Cytogenetic studies support the prediction that some patients with dominant HS have defects in β-spectrin. Kimberling and colleagues[731] detected a loose linkage between polymorphisms of the immunoglobulin heavy chains (IgH) and an HS locus (now called SPH1) by combining observations on 70 patients in 11 informative families. IgH was subsequently localized to chromosome 14q32.3, reasonably close to β-spectrin (14q23-q24.2).[343]

Despite this evidence, defects in β-spectrin have so far been rare. Apparent mutations have been identified in three unrelated dominant HS families, all of whom are heterozygotes for an unstable β-spectrin that lacks the ability to bind protein 4.1 and, as a consequence, binds poorly to actin[719,720] (Fig. 54-31). In one well-studied instance, spectrin Kissimmee,[359,718,720] (see Table 54-6), there is a single amino acid change, β-spectrin Trp 202 → Arg, in a conserved region near the N terminal,[359] which probably forms part of the 4.1 binding site.[395,799]

Ankyrin

A second spherocytosis locus (SPH2) is located on the short arm of chromosome 8. This was first established by showing that HS cosegregated with balanced chromosome translocations in two unrelated families. The translocations involved chromosomes 8 and 12 (t[8;12][p11;p12])[730] and chromosomes 8 and 3 (t[3;8][p21;p11]).[729] Both had breakpoints at 8p11. This locus was confirmed by the subsequent discovery of six patients with a syndrome of psychomotor retardation, short stature, unusual facies, hypogonadism, and moderately severe HS.[487,726–728] Each was heterozygous for an interstitial deletion of chromosome 8 that extended from 8p11,[727] 8p11.1[487,726] or 8p11.22[729] to 8p21.1. The SPH2 locus must lie at the centromeric end of this interval, in 8p11.1 or 8p11.2, since deletions of 8p12 to 8p21[800] and 8p11.2 to 8p21[800a] are associated with psychomotor retar-

(text continues on page 1744)

TABLE 54-6. Hereditary Defects of Membrane Skeletal Proteins

Protein Defects*	Clinical Expression: Heterozygote	Clinical Expression: Homozygote or Compound Heterozygote†	Tryptic Cleavage or Other Studies‡	Primary Structural Defect‡ (Location)§	Prevalence and Other Characteristics	Selected References
SPECTRIN						
Primary Spectrin Deficiency						
Autosomal recessive HS (rHS)	Silent carrier	Moderate to severe HS	Spectrin = 30%–75% of normal	α Ala 969 → Asp (α9 repeat) present in many families with severe recessive HS (probably a linked polymorphism and not the causal defect)	Severe forms of autosomal recessive HS are rare and probably often due to α-spectrin defects; moderate forms of rHS are common ($\approx$25%) and probably due to defects in ankyrin and pallidin as well as α-spectrin	236, 648, 658–660, 797
Defects in α-Spectrin That Impair Spectrin Self-Association						
Sp $\alpha^{I/78}$						
Sp Tunis	Silent carrier to moderately severe HE	?	78-kd peptide cleaved at Lys 16	α Arg 41 → Trp (α': helix C)	Especially in North Africa; single case reports	661, 662
Unnamed mutation				α Arg 45 → Ser (α': helix C)		663
Sp $\alpha^{I/74}$						
Unnamed mutation	Silent carrier to moderately severe HE	Severe HE to HPP†	74-kd peptide cleaved at Lys 48	α Arg 28 → His (α': helix C)	α Arg 28 mutations are relatively common; found in whites, blacks, Arabs, and Melanesians	140, 664–675
Unnamed mutation				α Arg 28 → Cys (α': helix C)		666, 674
Unnamed mutation				α Arg 28 → Leu (α': helix C)		666, 669
Unnamed mutation				α Arg 28 → Ser (α': helix C)		666, 669
Sp Genova				α Arg 34 → Trp (α': helix C)	One report	676
Sp Culoz				α Gly 46 → Val (α': helix C)	One report	677
Unnamed mutation				α Lys 48 → Arg (α': helix C)	One report	669
Sp Lyon			74-kd peptide cleaved at Arg 45	α Leu 49 → Phe (α': helix C)	One report	677
Sp $d^{I/65}$ (Sp $\alpha^{I/68}$)‖						
Unnamed mutation	Silent carrier to mild HE	Moderate to moderately severe HE	65-kd peptide cleaved at Arg 137	α Leu 154 → LeuLeu (α1: helix C)	Common in blacks. Homogenous defect (extra Leu after codon 154)	140, 653, 665, 668, 678–688
Sp Ponte de Sor	Silent carrier	Severe HE		α Gly 151 → Asp (α1: helix C)	One report	689
Sp $\alpha^{I/61}$						
Unnamed mutation	Silent carrier	HPP	61-kd peptide; ?Cleavage site	?	Single report	690
Sp $\alpha^{I/46}$						
Unnamed mutation	Mild HE	HPP	46-kd peptide cleaved at Lys 258	Amino acids 178–226 deleted from α2 repeat (helix A–B link); exon 5 skipped and $\approx$1 kb inserted in intron 5	Single report	691
Sp $\alpha^{I/50a}$ (Sp $\alpha^{I/46}$, Sp $\alpha^{I/46\text{-}50a}$)‖						
Unnamed mutation	Silent carrier to mild HE	HPP	50-kd peptide cleaved at Arg 256 or Lys 258	α Leu 207 → Pro (α2: helix B)	Relatively common in blacks	653, 686, 692
Unnamed mutation				α Leu 260 → Pro (α2: helix C)		653, 686
Unnamed mutation				α Ser 261 → Pro (α2: helix C)		653, 686

Sp $\alpha^{I/43}$						
Unnamed mutation	Mild HE (postsplenectomy)	?	43-kd peptide; ?cleavage site	?	Single report; moderate poikilocytosis	693
Sp $\alpha^{I/36}$						
Sp Sfax	Silent carrier to mild HE	?	36- & 33-kd peptides cleaved from αI domain	Amino acids 363–371 (α3: helix C) deleted due to activation of cryptic splice site in exon 8	Single report	694
Sp $\alpha^{I/50b}$ (Sp $\alpha^{I/46\text{-}50b}$)‖						
Sp Alexandria	Mild to moderately severe HE	?	50-kd peptide cleaved at Arg 468	α His 469 → deleted (α4: helix C)	Single kindred; moderate to marked poikilocytosis	695
Sp Barcelona	Mild to moderately severe HE		50- & 46-kd peptides cleaved Arg 470	α His 469 → Pro (α 4: helix C)	Single Spanish kindred; asymptomatic unless combined with α^{LELY}, then moderately severe	696
Unnamed mutation	Mild HE	?		α His 469 → Arg (α4: helix C)	Probably rare	686, 697
Unnamed mutation	Mild HE			α Glu 471 → Pro (α4: helix C)		653, 686
Sp $\alpha^{II/31}$						
Sp Jendouba	Silent carrier to mild HE	?	Abnormal 31-, 26-, 21-, & 18-kd peptides; cleavage after Lys 788	α Asp 791 → Glu (α7: helix C)	Single report; relatively few, roundish elliptocytes; only slight defect in spectrin self-association	698
Sp $\alpha^{II/21}$						
Sp Oran	Silent carrier	Mild to moderate HE	Abnormal 21- & 16-kd peptides derived from αII domain	Amino acids 822–862 (exon 18) deleted due to A → G (−1) in the acceptor splice site (α8: helix B)	Single report; low expression of mutant allele; normal self-association	699, 700
Sp $\alpha^{II/47}$						
Unnamed mutation	Silent carrier	HPP	?	?	Single report	701
Truncated α-spectrin						
Unnamed mutation	Mild HE	?	235-kd α'-spectrin band on SDS gels	?	Rare. 10%–45% of mutant α-band. ?Mild defect in spectrin self-association	702
Decreased amount of α-spectrin						
Unnamed mutation	Severe hemolytic HE	?	?	?	Single report	703
Defects in β-Spectrin That Impair Spectrin Self-Association						
Sp $\alpha^{I/74}$						
Sp Cagliari	Silent carrier to moderately severe HE	Severe HPP to lethal hydrops fetalis	Increase in the 74-kd fragment cleaved from the αI domain	β Ala 2018 → Gly (β17: helix A)	Single case reports; mutations in β-spectrin that alter cleavage of the neighboring αI domain	704
Sp Providence				β Ser 2019 → Pro (β17: helix A)		705
Sp Mali				β Ala 2053 → Pro (β17: helix B)		656
TRUNCATED β-SPECTRINS						
Sp $\beta^{220/218}$						
Sp Rouen	Moderate HE	?	218-kd β'-chain, reduced phosphorylation	Truncated, G → T (+3) in donor splice site; exon Y skipped → premature termination	Single report; elliptocytes without poikilocytes. GOE = HS pattern;¶ hemolytic crises	706, 707

(continued)

TABLE 54-6. *(Continued)*

Protein Defects*	Clinical Expression: Heterozygote	Clinical Expression: Homozygote or Compound Heterozygote	Tryptic Cleavage or Other Studies‡	Primary Structural Defect‡	Prevalence and Other Characteristics	Selected References
Sp $\beta^{220/216}$						
Sp Nice	Moderate HE	?	216-kd β'-chain; absent phosphorylation	Truncated, AG duplication at codons 2045/2046 → frameshift	Single report; GOE = HS pattern;¶ hemolytic crises	708, 709
Sp Tandil	Moderate HE	?		Truncated, deletion of 7 bp at codon 2041 → frameshift	Single report. GOE = HS pattern¶; Rounded elliptocytes	710
Sp Tokyo	Moderate HE	?		Truncated, deletion of C in codon 2059 → frameshift	Single report	711
Sp $\beta^{220/214}$						
Sp Göttingen	Moderately severe HE	?	214 kd β' chain; absent phosphorylation	Truncated, T → A (+2) in donor splice site of intron following exon X → X skipped → frameshift	Single report; elliptocytes and poikilocytes; MCV 70–90, ↑ OF; hemolytic crises	712, 713
Sp LePuy	Moderate HE	?		Truncated, A → G (+4) in donor splice site of intron following exon X → X skipped → frameshift	Single report; elliptocytes and poikilocytes; OF normal	714, 715
Sp $\beta^{220/210}$						
Sp Yamagata	?	?	210-kd β' chain	?	?	716
ELONGATED β-SPECTRIN						
Sp $\beta^{220/330}$						
Sp Detroit	Silent carrier	?	330-kd spectrin β' chain	?	Single kindred; giant β'-chain only 25% of β-spectrin → probably unstable; not clear that β-spectrin defect impairs self-association since patient also has $\alpha^{I/65}$ defect	717
Defects in β-Spectrin That Impair Binding of Protein 4.1						
Sp Kissimmee	Moderate HS	?	Spectrin low (80% normal)	β Trp 202 → Arg; spontaneous mutation; defect located in N-terminal region, between βIV domain and actin binding site; ? part of 4.1 binding site	Rare; some acanthocytes on blood smear; mutant spectrin unstable, easily oxidized, and binds protein 4.1 very weakly → membrane spectrin content low	359, 718–720
ANKYRIN						
Primary Ankyrin Deficiency						
Dominant HS (dHS)	Mild to moderately severe HS	Severe or ?lethal HS	Spectrin and ankyrin are equally reduced (50%–90% of normal) in most patients	Multiple defects (see below); preliminary data suggest a high frequency of frameshift and nonsense mutations; mostly private mutations	Ankyrin defects are a common cause (est. 20%–50%) of dominant HS mutations	237, 245, 647, 721, 722

Recessive HS (rHS)	Silent carrier	Mild to severe HS	Spectrin and ankyrin are equally reduced (50%–90% of normal) in most patients	Multiple defects (see below); preliminary data suggest a high frequency of mutations in the 5′ untranslated region (exon 1) and putative promoter	Ankyrin defects are also common (est. 40%–70%) in recessive HS	722, 723
5′ UNTRANSLATED REGION/PROMOTER MUTATIONS						
−108 mutation	Silent carrier	?Mild-severe HS	Combined spectrin-ankyrin deficiency	T → C exchange in promoter, 108 bp from translation start site	4 of 31 HS kindreds tested; adjacent to one of the transcription start sites	723
AMINO ACID SUBSTITUTIONS						
Ank Walsrode	Silent carrier	Mild HS	Combined spectrin-ankyrin deficiency	Val 463 → Ile in exon 13 (repeat 14, membrane domain)	1 of 31 HS kindreds tested; patient is combined heterozygote for Ank Walsrode and −108 mutation	723
Ank Düsseldorf	Silent carrier	Severe HS	Near normal spectrin and ankyrin content	Asp 1592 → Asn in exon 38 (regulatory domain)	1 of 31 HS kindreds tested; patient is presumed combined heterozygote for unknown second mutation	723
Ank Bocholt	Silent carrier	Moderate HS	Combined spectrin-ankyrin deficiency	Arg → Trp in alternative isoform of exon 41, 157 bp after start of exon 41 and 16 bp after usual 3′ splice site	1 of 31 HS kindreds tested; patient is combined heterozygote for Ank Bocholt and −108 mutation; alternative exon 41 isoform uncommon in bone marrow RNA, so significance uncertain	762
FRAMESHIFT/NONSENSE MUTATIONS						
Ank Stuttgart	Moderate HS	?	Combined spectrin-ankyrin deficiency	Deletion of GC in codon 329 (exon 10, repeat 10, membrane domain) → premature termination	1 of 31 HS kindreds tested	723
Ank Einbeck	Mild HS	?	Combined spectrin-ankyrin deficiency	Extra C in codon 572 (exon 16, repeat 18, membrane domain) → premature termination	1 of 31 HS kindreds tested	723, 802
Ank Marburg	Moderate-severe HS	?	Combined spectrin-ankyrin deficiency	Four bp deletion in codons 797–798 (exon 22, end of membrane domain) → premature termination	1 of 31 HS kindreds tested	723, 802
Ank Porta Westfalica	Severe HS	?	Combined spectrin-ankyrin deficiency	One bp deletion in codon 1127 (exon 29, spectrin domain) → premature termination	1 of 31 HS kindreds tested	723
Ank Bovenden	Moderate HS	?	Combined spectrin-ankyrin deficiency	Arg 1436 → Stop (TGA) in exon 36 (regulatory domain)	1 of 31 HS kindreds tested	723

(continued)

TABLE 54-6. *(Continued)*

Protein Defects	Clinical Expression: Heterozygote	Clinical Expression: Homozygote or Compound Heterozygote	Tryptic Cleavage or Other Studies‡	Primary Structural Defect‡	Prevalence and Other Characteristics	Selected References
PROBABLE SPLICING DEFECTS						
Ank Prague	HS	?	Deficiency of ankyrin band 2.1. New band at 174 kd (ankyrin 2.2′)	Insertion of 67 aa at splice junction between exons 37 and 38 (Asn 1512 – Gly 1513); abnormal protein cleaved to 174 kd (2.2′) band?	Single family	724, 725
Ank Rakovnik	HS	?	Decrease (25%) in 2.1, increase in band 2.2 (70%)	?	Single family	725
OTHER ANKYRIN DEFECTS						
Ankyrin gene deletions	Severe HS	?	Combined spectrin-ankyrin deficiency. Partial lack of pallidin	Heterozygous interstitial deletions of chromosome 8 from 8p11–8p22.2 (ankyrin located at 8p11.2)	Spontaneous mutations; associated features of growth and developmental retardation and hypogonadism; six kindreds known	484, 487, 726–728, 802
Balanced translocations	HS	?	?	Balanced translocations involving 8p11 (not proven that ankyrin gene involved, though likely)	Typical HS; two kindreds known	729–731
Unstable ankyrin	?	?	Combined spectrin-ankyrin deficiency	Approximately 50% reduction in ankyrin mRNA; unstable ankyrin	Single case; inheritance unclear; severe HS with unsuaul poikilocytosis	381, 732
PROTEIN 4.1						
Primary 4.1 Deficiency						125, 407, 414, 668, 733–744
Unnamed defects	Mild HE	Severe hemolytic HE	Heterozygote = 50% protein 4.1; homozygote = 0% 4.1 and 9% glycophorin C	Deletion (318 bp) encompassing the downstream (erythroid-specific) translation start site in one Algerian kindred.	Heterozygous state relatively common, especially in N Africa (≈33% of HE patients); most studies on one Algerian kindred	125, 407, 408, 733–735, 738
4.1 Madrid	Silent carrier	Severe HE		ATG → AGG in the downstream translation initiation codon	Single report	736
4.1 Mutations Involving the Spectrin–Actin Binding Region#						
$4.1^{68/65}$	Mild HE	?	65- & 68-kd 4.1 isoforms	Deletion of Lys 407-Gly 486 (2 exons)	Single kindred deletion encompasses exon encoding spectrin–actin binding domain; membranes mechanically unstable	125, 741–744
$4.1^{76/78}$	Mild HE	?	76- & 78-kd 4.1 isoforms	Deletion of Lys 407-Glu 427 (1 exon)	Single case in a dog; deletion encompasses exon encoding spectrin-actin binding domain	398
4.1^{95}	Mild HE	?	95-kd 4.1 isoform	Duplication of Lys 407-Gln 529 (3 exons)	Single kindred; duplication of spectrin-actin binding domain; normal membrane stability	125, 741, 742, 744

PALLIDIN (PROTEIN 4.2)						
Primary Pallidin Deficiency						
Pallidin Nippon	Silent carrier	Moderately severe hemolytic anemia	Heterozygote = 50% pallidin; Homozygote <1% pallidin; faint 74/72 kd bands on immunoblots; spectrin = 100%	Ala 142 → Thr in alternatively spliced segment of pallidin → alters RNA processing	Rare in Europeans, relatively common in Japanese; spherocytic elliptocytes, spherocytes and stomatocytes; increased band 3 mobility suggests band 3 detached from skeleton	504, 506–508, 509, 515, 745
Pallidin Tozeur	Silent carrier	Moderate hemolytic anemia	Trace pallidin, slightly ↓ band 3	Arg 310 → Gln	Single consanguinous Tunisian family; mild spherocytosis, slight elliptocytosis; moderate acanthocytosis poikilocytosis	749
Pallidin Lisboa	Silent carrier	Moderate hemolytic anemia	Pallidin completely absent	Deletion of C in codon 88 or 89 → premature termination	Single Portugese family; mild spherocytosis, slight elliptocytosis, moderate acanthocytosis and poikilocytosis	749
GLYCOPHORIN C						
Primary Glycophorin C Deficiency						
Unnamed defect	Silent carrier	Mild HE	Heterozygote = 50% glycophorin C; homozygote = 0% GP C and 30% of normal protein 4.1	Deletion of exons 3 and 4 in glycophorin C gene	Rare; Leach phenotype of Gerbich-negative blood group	307–311, 750–754
Unnamed defect				Deletion of 2 bp in codons 44–45 → premature termination	One patient	309
BAND 3 (ANION EXCHANGER 1, AE1)						
Primary Band 3 Deficiency						
Dominant HS (dHS)	Mild HS	?	Band 3 = 65–85%	Defect unknown in most cases; presumably multiple defects	Probably ≈10–15% of dominant HS; selective loss of band 3 not bound to skeleton → greatest band 3 deficit in old RBCs; normal or near normal RBC spectrin; some mushroom shaped RBCs on blood smears in some families	540, 541, 755–760
Bd3 Prague	HS	?		Duplication of 10 bases following codon 818 → frameshift involving last predicted transmembrane segment		540
Bd3 Coimbra	HS	?Hydrops	Band 3 = 76–82%	Val 488 → Met	Single Portuguese family	761
Bd3 Wilson	HS	?	Band 3 = 72%; normal spectrin	Deletion of G in codons 170–172 → premature termination	Single family; low normal membrane stability in ekacytometer	541, 762
C-terminal Arg mutations	HS	?		Arg 760 → Trp	Single family	758
				Arg 760 → Gln	Two unrelated families	758
				Arg 808 → Cys	Single family	758
				Arg 870 → Trp	Single family	758

(continued)

TABLE 54-6. *(Continued)*

Protein Defects	Clinical Expression: Heterozygote	Clinical Expression: Homozygote or Compound Heterozygote	Tryptic Cleavage or Other Studies‡	Primary Structural Defect‡	Prevalence and Other Characteristics	Selected References
Decreased band 3 and protein 4.1	Compensated hemolysis; normal morphology	Severe hemolysis; elliptocytes & poikilocytes	Band 3 with slightly ↑ mobility on SDS gels; protein 4.1 content ↓ 30%	?	Single family	763
Defects in Band 3 That Impair Pallidin Binding						
Bd3 Tuscaloosa	HS	?	Heterozygote ≈ 70% of normal pallidin	Pro 327 → Arg and a linked polymorphism Lys 56 → Glu (Bd3 Memphis)	Single report; pallidin binding to inside-out RBC membranes (IOVs) ↓ 30%	202
Bd3 Montefiore	?	HS	Homozygote ≈ 12% of normal pallidin; normal amount of spectrin	Glu 40 → Lys	Single patient; pallidin binding to IOVs only ↓ 30%	200
Defects in Band 3 That Reduce Ankyrin Binding						
Band 3 HT	Silent carrier	Acanthocytosis; no hemolysis	Band 3 with slightly ↑ mobility on SDS gels; normal amount of band 3	Pro 868 → Leu	Single report; probably rare; decreased ankyrin binding (50%) and H_2 DIDS labeling; ↑ anion transport	224, 225
Defects in Band 3 That Increase Membrane Rigidity						
Southeast Asian ovalocytosis (SAO)	Stomatocytic elliptocytosis	Probably lethal	Heterozygote ≈ 50% SAO band 3	Deletion of Ala 400 → Ala 408 linked to Bd3 Memphis polymorphism (Lys 56 → Glu); deletion alters signal sequence in first transmembrane helix → misassembly and inability to transport anions; SAO membranes rigid due to ?tendency of SAO band 3 to form linear arrays, ?diminished mobility of cytoplasmic domain → domain entangled in spectrin skeleton, ? ↑ ankyrin binding	Very common (up to 25%) in aborigines of Melanesia and Malaysia; some elliptocytes with characteristic transverse bar; increased ankyrin binding (controversial) and decreased protein 3 mobility → very rigid RBCs that resist invasion by malaria but, remarkably, circulate normally (little or no hemolysis or decreased tissue perfusion)	551, 764–785, 808
SOME ASYMPTOMATIC MEMBRANE PROTEIN POLYMORPHISMS						
Spectrin						
Sp α^{II}	Silent carrier	Silent carrier	Four polymorphic variants identified that differ in pI and molecular weight	Arg 701 → His / Ile 809 → Val / Thr 853 → Arg I: − / − / − II: + / + / − III: + / + / − IV: − / + / +	Common in blacks	786–788

Low Expression Allele						
Sp α^{LELY} (or $\alpha^{V/41}$)	Silent carrier	Silent carrier	Enhanced cleavage of αIV–αV junction after Lys 1920; 41-kd peptide released	Leu 1857 → Val mutation (exon 40) causes the $\alpha^{V/41}$ cleavage defect; a linked 2nd mutation, C → T (−12), in the acceptor splice site of intron 45 → ≈50% in-frame skipping of tiny exon 46 (18 nt); a 3rd linked mutation, G → A (−12, intron 46) may also contribute. Exon 46 lies within the nucleation site that initiates side to side association of α- and β-spectrin chains, α chains lacking exon 46 probably nucleate poorly → increase proportion of α chains from *trans* allele incorporated into spectrin.	Very common: gene frequency ≈30% in Europeans (≈42% heterozygous, ≈8% homozygous); ≈20% in Japanese and African blacks; clinically silent spectrin polymorphism that greatly exacerbates the clinical severity of α-spectrin defects occurring in *trans* and mutes the severity of defects occurring in *cis*	143, 364, 681, 789, 790
Protein 4.1						
4.1 Presles	Silent carrier	Silent carrier	Shortened protein 4.1, migrates with an apparent MW of 73–74 kd	Preferential skipping of one exon (34 amino acids) near the beginning of the 22/24-kd C-terminal domain	Rare	743, 791–794
Band 3						
Bd3 Memphis	Silent carrier	Silent carrier	Bd3 migrates slightly fast on SDS gels	Lys 56 → Glu	Common in blacks, Melanesians	163–167

* The nomenclature for α-spectrin defects includes an abbreviation for spectrin (Sp) followed by a superscript designation of the α-spectrin domain that is altered on tryptic peptide maps (αI to αV) and the size of the largest tryptic peptide that is generated from the mutant domain. Thus, Sp $\alpha^{I/65}$ indicates that the αI domain is affected and that a 65-kd peptide is generated by tryptic cleavage instead of the usual 80-kd peptide. Similarly, the superscript designating β-spectrin mutations reflects the size of the abnormal peptide, which is usually a mixture of normal (220 kd) and abnormal β-spectrin. Thus, the 214-kd Sp LePuy mutation is designated Sp $\beta^{220/214}$. Finally, note that some point mutations of β-spectrin cause abnormal tryptic cleavage of the α-spectrin chain and are therefore included in the Sp $\alpha^{I/74}$ group, the phenotype of their tryptic cleavage.

† Most HPP patients are double heterozygotes for an α-spectrin mutant and a second "silent" defect, usually the common low expression α spectrin allele designated $\alpha^{V/41}$ or α^{LELY} (see Some Asymptomatic Membrane Protein Polymorphisms near end of table). Patients who are double heterozygotes for two different α-spectrin mutants (or homozygous for one) may also exhibit the HPP phenotype.

‡ Note that the numbering of amino acids and codons of α-spectrin is based on the cDNA sequence.[325] which includes six N-terminal amino acids that are not present in the mature protein.[649,650] Other mutations are numbered according to the published cDNA sequences of β-spectrin,[326] ankyrin,[464,465] proteins 4.1[651] and 4.2,[511,512] glycophorin A,[289] glycophorin C,[300] and band 3.[157,158] Exons are numbered using published information for the α-spectrin,[652,653] and glycophorin C[654] genes and unpublished data on ankyrin genomic structure. (Tse WT, Scarpa A, Gallagher PG, Lux SE, Forget BG. Unpublished observations).

§ "(Location)" refers to the repetitive segment (≈106 AA repeats) of α- or β-spectrin and the three antiparallel helices making up the repeats in the revised triple helical models of Speicher,[328,364] Winograd,[348] and Yan.[347] Thus, (α2: helix C) refers to the C helical segment in the second repeat of α-spectrin. The numbering of the repeats and helices is based on their proposed spatial arrangement (see Figs. 54-11 and 54-13) and differs from that originally proposed.[346,649,650,655] The revised model predicts that the triple helical segment at the site of spectrin self-association is composed of repeat 17 of β-spectrin (contributes helices A and B) and the N terminal, α′ repeat of α-spectrin (contributes helix C).[328,656] The first complete repetitive segment of α-spectrin therefore begins with helix A.

‖ The reported differences in molecular weight probably reflect differences in methodology rather than different mutations.

¶ GOE, gradient osmotic ektacytometry[657]; HS pattern, deformability index at isotonicity decreased and maximum deformability index shifted toward hypotonicity.

#The superscript indicates the size (kd) of the elongated (4.1^{95}) or truncated ($4.1^{68/65}$ and $4.1^{76/78}$) 4.1 mutants.

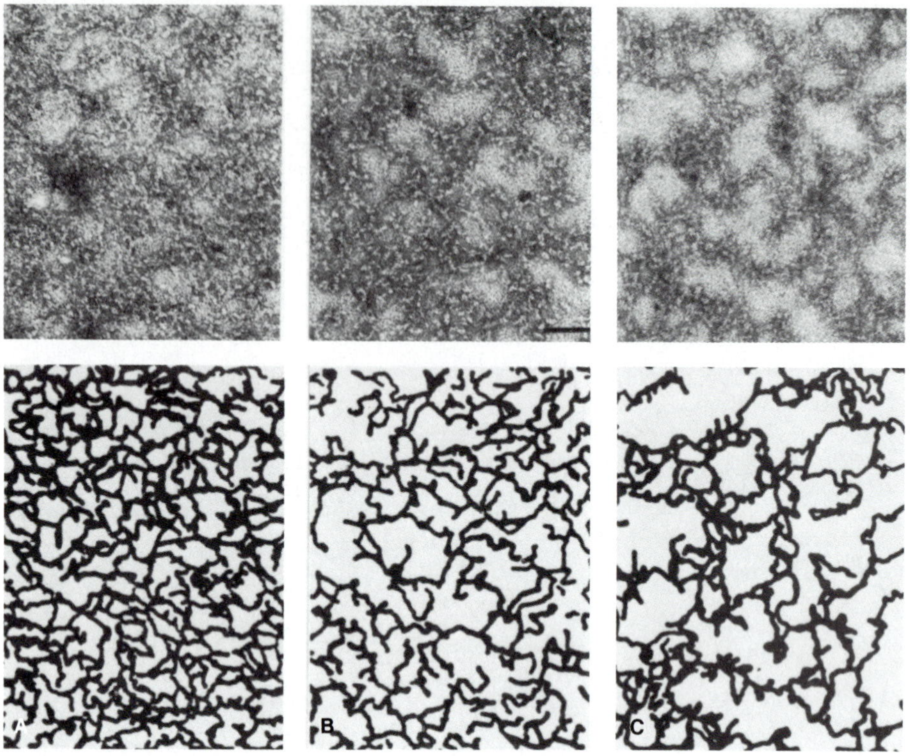

FIGURE 54-28. Density of spectrin on the membrane. Spectrin in situ was visualized by negative stain on electron microscopy (*top row*) in normal ghosts (**A**), 50% spectrin-deficient ghosts from a hereditary spherocytosis patient[732] (**B**), and 70% spectrin-deficient ghosts (**C**), which are partially spectrin-extracted. Tracings of the skeletal network (*bottom row*) indicate the relative change in spectrin density. The bar in **B** indicates 100 nm.

dation, short stature, and hypogonadism, but not HS. Considering how rarely chromosome analyses are performed on HS patients, particularly patients with uncomplicated HS, the existence of these families suggests that mutations at the SPH2 locus are relatively common.

Ank1 has been mapped to 8p11.2 by fluorescent in situ hybridization (FISH)[487] (Fig. 54-32). One copy of the Ank1 gene is missing from DNA of two of the children with HS and heterozygous interstitial deletions of chromosome 8.[487] This was determined visually, using the FISH technique (see Fig. 54-32), and by gene dosage blots. Red cell membranes are deficient in both ankyrin (59% of normal) and spectrin (79%).[487] Pallidin may also be decreased.

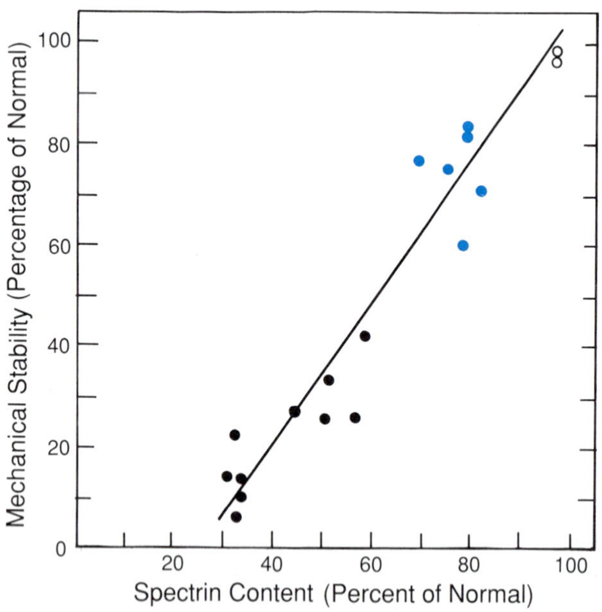

FIGURE 54-29. Relation between membrane mechanical stability, measured with the ektacytometer, and spectrin content in red cells from patients with heterozygous dominant hereditary spherocytosis (HS; *colored circles*), homozygous recessive HS (*solid black circles*), and heterozygous recessive HS (*open black circles*). Membranes from dominant and recessive HS patients fall on the same curve, suggesting that similar mechanisms may be responsible for membrane fragility in the two conditions. (After Chasis JA, et al. Decreased membrane mechanical stability and in vivo loss of surface area reflect spectrin deficiencies in hereditary spherocytosis. J Clin Invest 1988;82:617)

In addition, genetic linkage of HS and ankyrin has been proved, using restriction enzyme polymorphisms, in a single large family with typical dominant HS.[237]

Most Hereditary Spherocytosis Red Cells Are Deficient in Both Spectrin and Ankyrin. Coetzer and coworkers[732] were the first to report combined deficiency of spectrin and ankyrin in two adults, who have an atypical and unusually severe form of HS characterized by bizarre-shaped microspherocytes. Red cell spectrin and ankyrin levels are about 50% normal, apparently as a result of failure of ankyrin synthesis or to synthesis of an unstable molecule.[381] Ankyrin mRNA concentrations are also 50% normal, and pulse chase studies show that newly synthesized ankyrin does not accumulate in the cytoplasm and only reaches half-normal levels on the membrane[381] (Fig. 54-33). In contrast, spectrin mRNA concentrations are normal, although only 50% of the synthesized spectrin attaches to the membrane, presumably because ankyrin sites are decreased.

This work and the studies described earlier showed that ankyrin defects occur in patients with HS; the prevalence of such defects was unclear, particularly in typical dominant HS. Savvides and associates[245] addressed this problem by measuring red cell spectrin and ankyrin levels by radioimmunoassay in 39 patients from 20 typical dominant HS kindreds. The values ranged from 40% to 100% of the normal cellular levels of 242,000 ± 20,500 spectrin heterodimers and 124,500 ± 11,000 ankyrins. Spectrin and ankyrin were both less than the normal range in 75% to 80% of kindreds. Remarkably, *the degree of spectrin and ankyrin deficiency was similar in 19 of the 20 kindreds*[245] (Fig. 54-34). Pekrun and colleagues[722] have obtained similar data in 45 patients.

The combined observations argue strongly that ankyrin deficiency is the primary defect in most patients with dom-

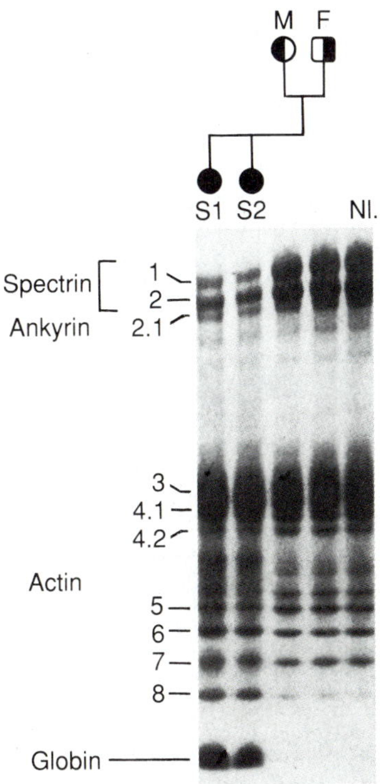

FIGURE 54-30. SDS gel electrophoresis of spectrin-deficient red cell membranes from two sisters (S1 and S2) with severe recessive hereditary spherocytosis. A marked decrease is seen in spectrin α and β chains (bands 1 and 2), but the parents' red cells contain a normal amount of spectrin. (After Agre P, et al. Deficient red-cell spectrin in severe, recessively inherited spherocytosis. N Engl J Med 1982;306:1155)

inant HS and that spectrin deficiency is secondary to the loss of ankyrin attachment sites.

Different Types of Ankyrin Mutations Are Prevalent in Dominant and Recessive Hereditary Spherocytosis. The molecular defects in ankyrin that cause HS are just beginning to be defined. Unfortunately, the easily detected defects, things that change the size of the gene on Southern blots or the size of the protein on Western blots, are not common,[247] although two examples of an altered protein have appeared in preliminary reports.[724,725] In the best-studied case, normal ankyrin (206 kd) is replaced by a 174-kd variant (*ankyrin Prague*), presumably because of abnormal splicing.[724] The variant contains 67 new amino acids inserted at the splice junction between exons 37 and 38 (Asn 1512 → Gly 1513)[725] (Fig. 54-35; see Table 54-6).

More often, the primary defect is a small insertion or deletion, or a missense mutation. Surveys for such defects are in progress[723] and have already identified a number of new mutations (see Fig. 54-35 and Table 54-6). The preliminary results[723] suggest the following:

1. Ankyrin mutations are common, affecting patients with both dominant and recessive HS.
2. Mutations that abolish the normal ankyrin product are prevalent in dominant HS (eg, frameshift mutations or mutations that introduce a stop codon in the coding sequence).
3. Defects upstream of the coding region are common in recessive HS, particularly a T → C exchange in the potential promoter (CC<u>T</u>GG → CC<u>C</u>GG), −108 bp from the translation start site, which is present on one chromosome in 4 of 13 recessive HS families.[723] This defect lies next to one of the several transcriptional start sites of ankyrin.[801] Because this defect is silent in obligate heterozygotes, recessive HS patients must have a second mutation. They have been discovered in two patients: a man with mild HS who carries the −108 mutation and a silent defect in trans, ankyrin Walsrode [Val 463 → Ile (GTC → ATC)]; and a man with moderate HS, the −108 mutation, and Ank Bocholt, an Arg → Trp mutation in an alternatively spliced region near the C terminal.
4. Variations in the clinical severity and red cell ankyrin content of similar mutations indicate that other factors modify the expression of the primary ankyrin defects. For example, ankyrins Marburg and Einbeck are

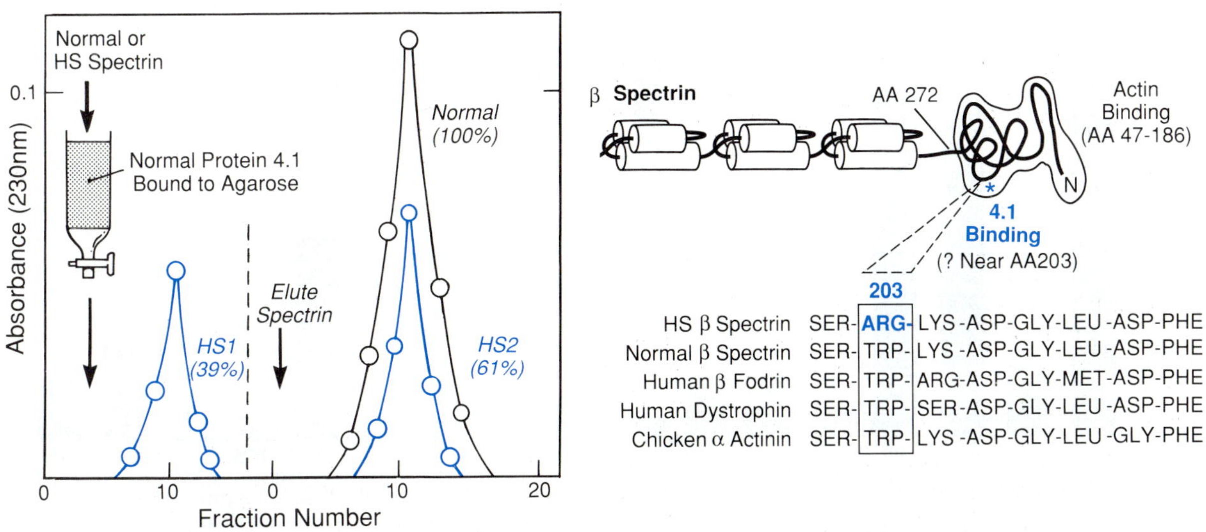

FIGURE 54-31. Defect in binding site for protein 4.1 in β-spectrin Kissimmee. Spectrin from a normal person or a patient with β-spectrin Kissimmee was passed over a column containing immobilized normal protein 4.1. All normal spectrin and 61% of the HS spectrin bound and could be eluted under conditions unfavorable for spectrin–protein 4.1 interactions. Thirty-nine percent of the HS spectrin failed to bind to the column and, in a separate assay, this fraction (Sp Kissimmee) lacked the ability to bind protein 4.1.[720] Recent studies have localized the defect to β-spectrin[718] and defined a mutation in amino acid 202 (Trp → Arg).[359] The mutation is in a conserved region in the N-terminal end of β-spectrin, just beyond the actin-binding domain (amino acids 47 to 186).[358] The region is a likely location for the 4.1 binding site.

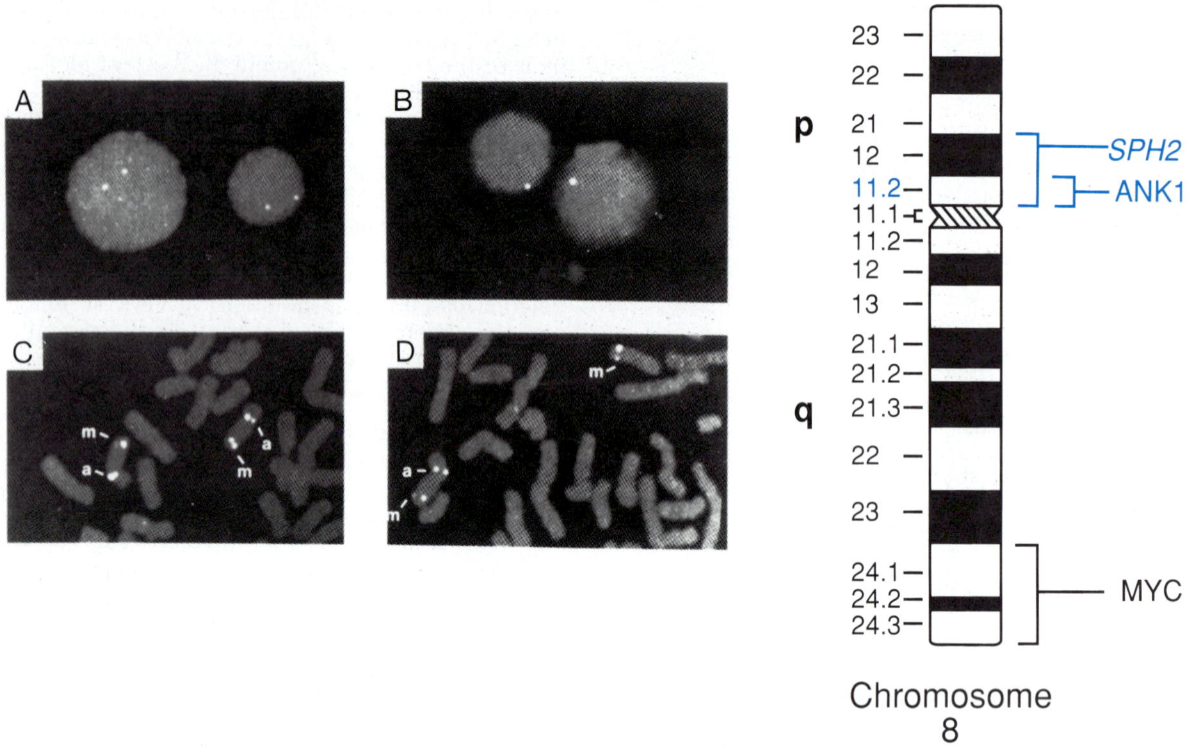

FIGURE 54-32. Demonstration of ANK1 (erythrocyte ankyrin) gene deletion in HS by fluorescence in situ hybridization. (**A** and **B**) Interphase nuclei from a control patient (*left*) and a patient with hereditary spherocytosis and a small, heterozygous deletion (8p11.1-p21.1) of part of the short arm of chromosome 8 that defines the spherocytosis 2 (SPH2) locus (*right*). Two fluorescent spots represent the two normal ankyrin genes in the control patient, but only a single spot is seen in the nuclei of the patient with hereditary spherocytosis. (**C** and **D**) Metaphase spreads of control (*left*) and patient (*right*) cells hybridized with ANK1 (a) and MYC (m) genomic probes. The MYC gene is located at 8q24, near the end of the long arm of chromosome 8. Both normal chromosomes 8 are labeled by both probes, whereas both hereditary spherocytosis chromosomes 8 contain MYC signals, but the one at the top of **D** does not react with the ankyrin probe. (**E**) Map of human chromosome 8 indicating the location of the ANK1 and MYC genes and the SPH2 locus. (After Lux SE, Tse WT, Menninger JC, et al. Hereditary spherocytosis associated with deletion of the human erythrocyte ankyrin gene on chromosome 8. Nature 1990;345:736)

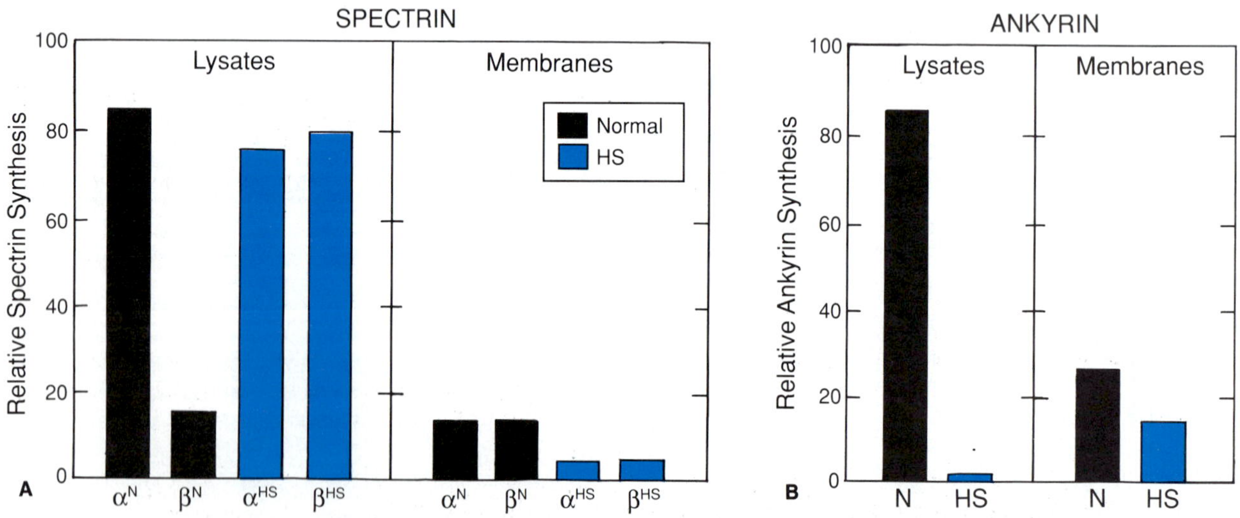

FIGURE 54-33. Synthesis and assembly of spectrin and ankyrin in normal (N) and hereditary spherocytosis (HS) reticulocytes. The HS patient has an unusually severe variant associated with combined spectrin and ankyrin deficiency.[732] (**A**) Newly synthesized α- and β-spectrin in the cytoplasm (lysate) and assembled on the membrane (membrane). Synthesis of α-spectrin exceeds that of β-spectrin by more than 4:1 in normal reticulocytes, but the measurements are about equal in the young reticulocytes from the patient with HS. Only a fraction of the spectrin is assembled into heterodimers and bound to the membrane, and HS spectrin is diminished in this respect. (**B**) Normally ankyrin is also made in excess relative to what is incorporated into the membrane. In this patient with HS, ankyrin is unstable: it fails to accumulate in the cytoplasm and is poorly incorporated into the membrane. (After Hanspal M, Yoon SH, Yu H, et al. Molecular basis of spectrin and ankyrin deficiencies in severy hereditary spherocytosis: evidence implicating a primary defect of ankyrin. Blood 1991;77:165)

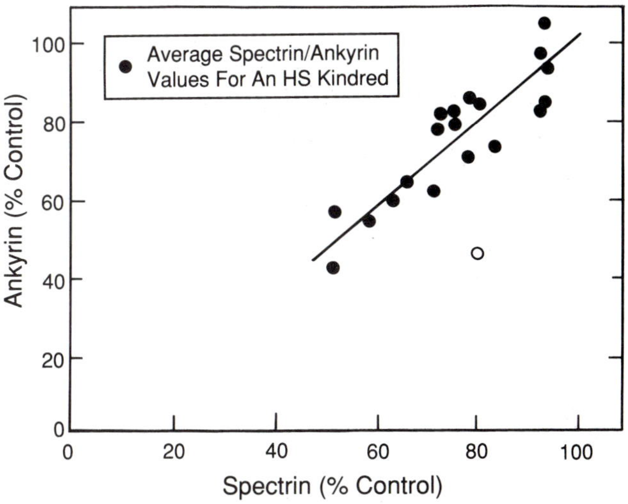

FIGURE 54-34. Correlation of spectrin and ankyrin deficiencies in 20 dominant hereditary spherocytosis kindreds. Each point, expressed as a percentage of the control (taken to be 100%), represents the mean value for a kindred for both red cell spectrin and ankyrin levels. Within experimental error, the degree of spectrin and ankyrin deficiencies is essentially identical in these families with one exception (*open circle*), an otherwise typical family in which red cells are primarily ankyrin deficient. (After Savvides P, Shalev O, John KM, Lux SE. Combined spectrin and ankyrin deficiency is common in autosomal dominant hereditary spherocytosis. Blood 1993;82:2953)

frameshift mutations that occur in the N-terminal (membrane) domain and do not produce a detectable product in mature red cells (see Table 54-6). They would be expected to have a similar phenotype but patients with Ank Marburg have moderate to severe HS and moderate ankyrin deficiency (64% of normal), whereas patients with Ank Einbeck have mild disease and normal ankyrin levels.[723,802] Understanding this and similar variations will be one of the critical problems in HS research in the next few years.

Band 3

Some Hereditary Spherocytosis Patients Have Band 3–Deficient Spherocytes. In about 10% to 20% of patients with dominant HS, the primary protein defect resides in band 3 (AE1).[758] Specific mutations have been identified in several kindreds, and genetic linkage of HS to the band 3 gene (17q21 → qter) has been reported in one family.[759] Affected patients have mild to moderate HS and a 20% to 40% deficiency of band 3,[540,541,755–760,803] which is usually detected as an increase in the spectrin/band 3 ratio on SDS gels.[541,757,804] Where quantitated, red cell spectrin content is normal.[541,803]

In the best-studied case, *band 3 Prague*, 10 nucleotides are duplicated near the C-terminal end of the protein, leading to a shift in the reading frame and an altered C terminal after amino acid 821[540] (70 new amino acids; Fig. 54-36; see Table 54-6). The mutation affects the last transmembrane helix and probably alters insertion of band 3 into the membrane, since the mutant protein is not detectable in mature red cells. The decrease in band 3 content occurs principally in the mobile, dimeric fraction of band 3.[540] Immobilized band 3, which probably includes band 3 bound to ankyrin, is not greatly affected.

Four other band 3 mutations have been identified in dominant HS patients.[758] Curiously, all of them cluster near the C terminal and all replace an arginine with another amino acid (see Fig. 54-36 and Table 54-6). Each of the three affected arginines (Arg 760 [two mutations], Arg 808, and Arg 870) is located at the cytoplasmic end of a predicted transmembrane helix.[157] Arginine residues are located in the same position in most transmembrane proteins and are thought to help orient the membrane-spanning segments.[76–78,805] This suggests that the mutant proteins are not present in the mature red cell because they do not fold and insert into the membrane correctly after synthesis. In addition, some arginines in band 3 appear to be involved in anion transport.[136,806]

Improper membrane insertion of band 3 may not be the only mechanism causing red cell band 3 deficiency. Some patients with dominant HS have a high spectrin/band 3 ratio (band 3 deficiency) in dense, older (reticulocyte-poor) red cells,[756,757,760] but near normal amounts of band 3 in light, young (reticulocyte-rich) cells. This suggests that band 3 is lost as these cells circulate, presumably because of a weakened association with ankyrin. The underlying molecular defect is unknown.

Pallidin (Protein 4.2)

Several investigators have described families with clinically typical recessive HS in which affected patients lack red cell pallidin (protein 4.2; 15q14 → q15).[200,202,504,506,508,509,745–749]

In the most common variant, *pallidin Nippon*, the red cells contain only a small quantity of a 74/72-kd pallidin doublet instead of the usual 72-kd species, because of a

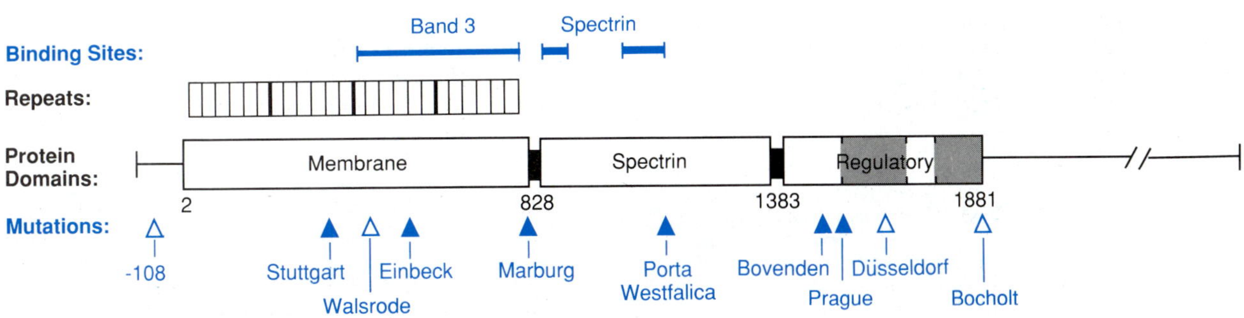

FIGURE 54-35. Ankyrin defects in hereditary spherocytosis (HS). Solid triangles, autosomal dominant mutations; open triangles, autosomal recessive mutations. All the dominant defects are frameshift mutations (Anks Stuttgart, Einbeck, Marburg, Porta Westfalica) or new termination codons (Ank Bovenden) except Ank Prague, a 174-kd variant that results from abnormal splicing. In contrast, in recessive HS, the Ank1 mutations discovered so far include conservative amino acid replacements (Anks Walsrode, Düsseldorf, Bocholt) and a defect adjacent to a transcription start site, −108 bp from the beginning of translation. Ank Bocholt is enclosed in parentheses because the affected amino acid is present only in some isoforms. Solid triangles, autosomal dominant mutations; open triangles, autosomal recessive mutations.

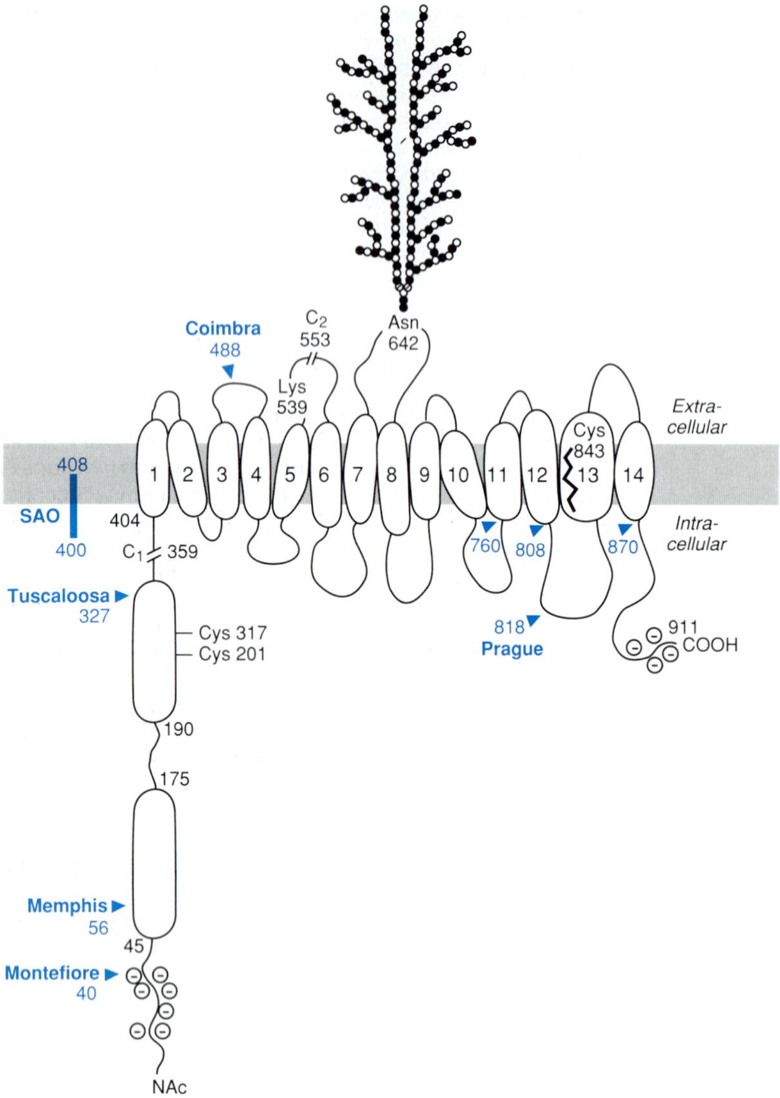

FIGURE 54-36. Band 3 defects and polymorphisms in hereditary spherocytosis (HS) and Southeast Asian ovalocytosis (SAO). In dominant HS with band 3 deficiency, the known mutations cluster near the C terminal. Most involve Arg residues (Arg 760, 808, and 870) at the inside of the membrane that may participate in protein folding. In one case (Bd 3 Prague) an insertion leads to a frameshift. However, conservative substitutions (Bd 3 Coimbra) may also cause band 3 deficiency. In HS associated with pallidin deficiency, mutations exist at residues 40 (Bd 3 Montefiore) and 327 (Bd 3 Tuscaloosa). Presumably, these amino acids lie in or near the pallidin binding site. SAO is caused by a deletion of nine amino acids (residues 400 to 408) and is linked to a common polymorphism (Bd 3 Memphis).

Ala 142 → Thr mutation that affects the processing of pallidin mRNA[515] (Fig. 54-37; see Table 54-6). Pallidin Nippon–deficient membranes lose 70% of their ankyrin with low ionic strength extraction,[506,507] and the ankyrin loss is blocked by preincubation of the membranes with purified pallidin, which suggests pallidin stabilizes ankyrin on the membrane. This hypothesis is supported by the observations that pallidin content is low in ankyrin-deficient *nb/nb* mice (see section on mouse models of HS) and in HS patients who lack one ankyrin gene.[487] In addition, red cells from patients homozygous for pallidin Nippon are fragile and exhibit heat-sensitive skeletons, clumped intramembranous particles (probably band 3 molecules), and increased lateral mobility of band 3.[507] (The latter two findings are puzzling in light of studies in Southeast Asian ovalocytes in which aggregation of intramembranous particles is associated with a decrease in both lateral and rotational mobility[551,807].) Ankyrin lability is not evident in other patients with pallidin deficiency,[508,509] some of whom have normal morphology,[508] acanthopoikilocytosis,[749] or ovalostomatocytosis[747,748] rather than spherocytosis. These differences are presumed to be examples of allelic variation.

Finally, erythrocyte pallidin deficiency has been associated with mutations in the cytoplasmic domain of band

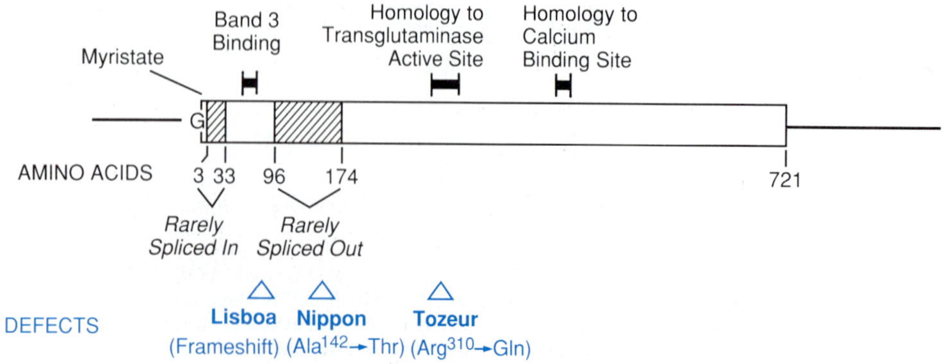

FIGURE 54-37. Pallidin defects in hereditary spherocytosis. The three known mutations are shown relative to the alternatively spliced portions of pallidin and to various functional sites of pallidin (band 3 binding site) and related molecules (active site and calcium binding site of transglutaminases).

3 in two patients. One of the mutations (*band 3 Montefiore*) lies near the N terminal of band 3 (Glu 40 → Lys[200]; see Fig. 54-36); the other (*band 3 Tuscaloosa*) is near the end of the cytoplasmic domain (Pro 327 → Thr).[202] The pallidin binding site probably involves both regions.

Other Membrane Protein Defects of Uncertain Significance

Tight Binding of Spectrin to the Membrane. Inextractable spectrin was first observed some years ago in 2 of 12 HS patients in whom spectrin failed to elute from the membrane after exposure to low ionic strength for 72 hours.[808] These are conditions that generally produce greater than 90% spectrin extraction. A second patient was discovered more recently.[809] The molecular basis of this phenomenon has not been investigated, although the possibility that it is secondary to a defect in ankyrin or β-spectrin is obvious. In addition, some tightly bound spectrin is palmitoylated,[810] and this fraction might be increased.

Increased Membrane Hemoglobin. Hereditary spherocyte membranes contain increased amounts of hemoglobin and catalase.[811] This is a relatively nonspecific finding that is observed in a number of hemolytic anemias. Its molecular basis is not understood.

Enolase Deficiency. Two reports of apparent HS combined with partial enolase deficiency (about 50%) have appeared.[812,813] In the first patient, a French woman, red cell osmotic fragility and autohemolysis tests were typical of HS, although spherocytes were not apparent on the blood smear.[812] Dominant inheritance was suggested by history but could not be established because the affected father was deceased. Dominant inheritance of both HS and partial enolase deficiency was clearly evident in the second family, in whom both diseases could be traced through four generations.[813] In this kindred, the enolase-deficient spherocytes resisted lysis in the acidified glycerol lysis test, another characteristic of typical HS. The similarity of these two cases suggests that they may represent a unique subgroup of HS. In particular, the combination of dominant inheritance and 50% of normal levels of enolase raises the possibility that the primary defect could lie in an enolase-binding membrane protein, assuming that such a protein exists.

Diminished Membrane Protein Phosphorylation. In the late 1970s and early 1980s, the discovery that red cell membrane proteins are phosphorylated was followed by numerous reports that phosphorylation was defective in HS patients. These reports are summarized and analyzed in previous reviews.[814,815] In short, the effects were variable from lab to lab and generally were demonstrable only in ghosts incubated in low ionic strength buffers for relatively long periods. Initial rates of phosphorylation in HS ghosts were normal,[816–818] as was membrane protein phosphorylation of intact spherocytes from persons who had undergone splenectomy.[818] It now appears that the phosphorylation defects were secondary effects.

Defective Phosphorylation-Induced Gelation of Membrane Skeletons. Homogenized suspensions of membrane skeletons from hereditary spherocytes gel poorly or not at all when treated with spectrin kinase, whereas normal skeletons gel firmly under the same conditions.[819] The phenomenon is not understood on a molecular level, but it is specific and reproducibly abnormal in HS.[819,820]

Secondary Defects

A large number of secondary abnormalities have been identified over the years. These are catalogued and discussed in detail in earlier reviews.[814,815]

Membrane Lipids. The principal lipid abnormality of hereditary spherocytes is a symmetric loss of membrane lipids as part of the overall loss of membrane surface, the hallmark of HS pathobiology. The relative proportions of cholesterol and the various phospholipids are normal,[821] and the phospholipids show the usual transmembrane asymmetry, even in severe cases.[46] It has been reported that very long-chain fatty acids are missing from certain classes of phospholipids,[822] but this has not been confirmed.[823] It is unclear whether this difference is due to technical factors or to genetic heterogeneity of the disease. Even if real, it seems likely that the changes in fatty acid composition will be secondary to underlying membrane protein defects.

Cations and Transport. For many years, HS red cells have been known to be intrinsically more leaky to sodium and potassium ions than normal cells.[824–826] A similar defect exists in spectrin-deficient mice.[827] The excessive sodium influx activates Na^+/K^+-ATPase and the monovalent cation pump, and the accelerated pumping in turn increases ATP turnover and glycolysis. At one time, this modest sodium leak was was believed to be responsible for the hemolysis of hereditary spherocytes,[825] particularly those cells trapped in the unfavorable metabolic environment of the spleen, but it now is clear that this is incorrect because the magnitude of the sodium flux does not correlate with the extent of hemolysis in HS.[828] In addition, patients with hereditary stomatocytosis (to be discussed later) and a much greater defect in sodium permeability do not develop microspherocytes and sometimes have little hemolysis.[829] The leak of sodium into red cells in hereditary stomatocytosis is accompanied by the entry of water and cell swelling, a finding that contrasts with the well-established dehydration of hereditary spherocytes.

The dehydration of HS red cells is likely to be inflicted, at least in part, by the adverse environment of the spleen, since spherocytes from surgically removed spleens are the most dehydrated.[830] The pathways causing HS red cell dehydration have not been clearly defined. A likely candidate is increased K^+/Cl^- cotransport, which is activated by acid pH.[573] HS red cells, particularly from subjects who have not undergone splenectomy, have a low intracellular pH,[831] reflecting the low pH of the splenic environment. The K^+/Cl^--cotransport pathway is also activated by oxidation,[832] which is likely to be inflicted by splenic macrophages. Last, hyperactivity of the Na^+/K^+ pump, triggered by increased intracellular Na^+, can dehydrate red cells directly, because three Na^+ ions are extruded in exchange for only two K^+ ions.[586,587] The loss of monovalent cations is accompanied by water.

Glycolysis. In general, glycolysis is mildly accelerated in HS red cells,[825,833,834] mostly to support increased cation pumping,[825] and 2,3-DPG concentrations are slightly depressed,[831,835,836] probably because of activation of 2,3-DPG phosphatase by the acidic intracellular pH of the cell.[836] The latter abnormalities are at least partly due to splenic detention, because the acidosis and DPG deficiency both improve after splenectomy.[831,835]

Phosphoenolpyruvate Transport. An apparently specific decrease in carrier-mediated transport of phosphoenolpyruvate has been noted in red cells of some patients with HS.[837] Unfortunately, only patients who have not had splenectomy were studied, so it is possible that the defect is secondary to the metabolic derangements these cells acquire during their detention in the spleen. More likely, the defect is caused by diminished anion exchange. Band 3 transports pyruvate and probably phosphoenolpyruvate. If so, reduced phosphoenolpyruvate transport would be expected in HS patients with band 3 deficiency. Anion transport is also suppressed (about 30% to 35%) in patients with known ankyrin defects.[802] The molecular explanation is unknown. It is also not known whether pallidin deficiency alters anion transport, but this should be considered because diminished phosphoenolpyruvate transport has been reported only in Japanese patients with HS, a population in which pallidin deficiency is particularly common.

Mouse Models of Hereditary Spherocytosis

Six types of autosomal recessive, spherocytic hereditary hemolytic anemias have been described in the common house mouse, *Mus musculus*. These are designated *ja/ja* (jaundiced), *sph/sph* (spherocytosis), sph^{ha}/sph^{ha} (hemolytic anemia), sph^{2BC}/sph^{2BC}, sph^{2J}/sph^{2J}, and *nb/nb* (normoblastosis).[380,485,838–844] The nomenclature indicates that the six mutants represent three alleles: *ja*, *sph*, and *nb*. The sph^{ha}, sph^{2BC}, and sph^{2J} mutations are allelic variants at the *sph* locus.[839,843] All the mutants have severe hemolysis with marked spherocytosis, bilirubin gallstones, massive hepatosplenomegaly, and reticulocyte counts that approach 100%.[838] Anemia is observed only in the homozygous state and is associated with decreased viability.

All of the *Mus* mutants are spectrin or spectrin–ankyrin deficient (Fig. 54-38) and have extremely fragile red cells.[380,842] Red cells spontaneously vesiculate, and ghosts disintegrate during preparation. The *ja/ja* mutant has a defect in the spectrin β chain (Arg 1160 → Stop)[839] and no detectable spectrin.[380,840] The *sph/sph* variants have α-spectrin mutations.[380,840] They lack α chains, either because of decreased synthesis (*sph*, sph^{2BC}, sph^{2J}) or because of synthesis of an unstable chain (sph^{ha}),[380] but have small amounts of β-spectrin. Knockout of the α-spectrin gene by accidental insertion of a transgene has also been reported.[845] Homozygous animals have a severe spherocytic anemia that is lethal in the first few days of life.

Nb mice have a primary defect in ankyrin. The *nb* mutation maps to the *Ank1* locus on mouse chromosome 8[844] and *nb/nb* animals have only a trace of ankyrin mRNA and protein[380,842,485] (see Fig. 54-38). Interestingly, spectrin levels are relatively preserved in *nb/nb* red cells (50% to 70% of normal). This is in contrast to human ankyrin deficiency (see earlier in text), where ankyrin and spectrin levels are comparably depressed. *Nb/nb* mice also lack ankyrin (Ank1) in cerebellar Purkinje cells.[485,486] This leads to an age-related loss of Purkinje cells during the first 5 to 7 months of life and the emergence of cerebellar ataxia.[485] Spinocerebellar degeneration and related syndromes have also been reported in a few adults with HS,[846–854] although it is not known whether ankyrin is affected.

Fetal *nb/nb* mice have no anemia and normal reticulocyte counts at birth,[855] apparently because of expression of ankyrin-related proteins in utero.[856] Humans may also be protected in utero, at least partially, since hydrops fetalis has not been reported in patients with probable ankyrin defects (combined spectrin–ankyrin deficiency), even those who become transfusion dependent after birth.

Another recessive spherocytic hemolytic anemia has been described in the deer mouse, *Peromyscus maniculatus*.[857] This disorder is less severe and closely resembles the autosomal dominant form of human HS. As in human HS, the spectrin content of the deer mouse erythrocytes is reduced about 20%.[858]

Pathophysiology

Loss of Membrane Surface by Vesiculation

The primary membrane lesions described, all involving "vertical interactions" between the skeleton and the bilayer, fit the prevailing theory that HS is caused by local disconnection of the skeleton and bilayer, followed by vesiculation of the unsupported surface components. This in turn leads to progressive reduction in membrane surface area and to a shape called a *spherocyte*, although it usually ranges between a thickened discocyte and a spherostomatocyte.[859] The phospholipid and cholesterol contents of isolated spherocytes are decreased by 15% to 20%, consistent with the loss of surface area.[860–863]

Despite its popularity, the evidence supporting the vesiculation theory is surprisingly scant. On the plus side, careful biomechanical measurements show that HS membranes are fragile. The force required to fragment the

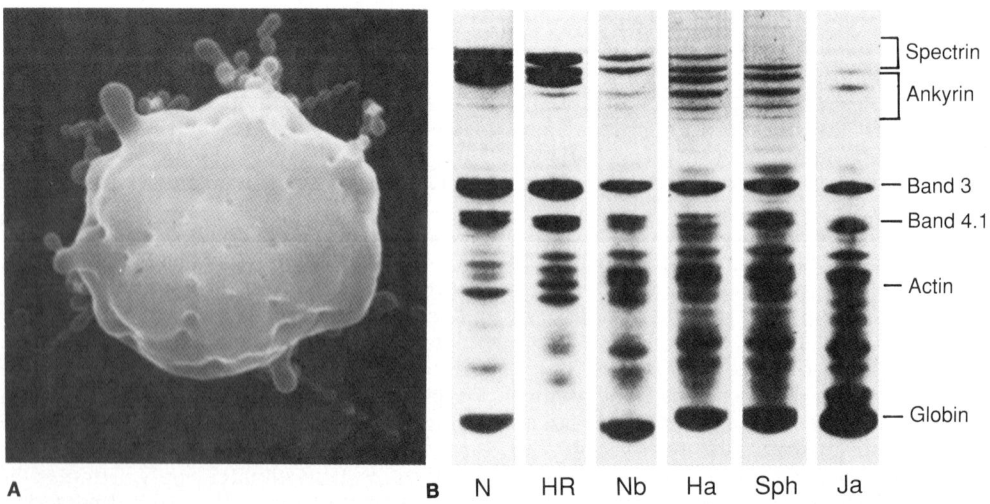

FIGURE 54-38. Hereditary spherocytosis mutants in mice (*Mus musculus*). (**A**) Scanning electron micrograph of sph^{ha}/sph^{ha} red cell. The marked membrane instability and spontaneous vesiculation are evident. (**B**) SDS gels of red cell membrane proteins from normal (N) and high reticulocyte control (HR) mice, and from four Mus mutants: *nb/nb* (Nb), sph^{ha}/sph^{ha} (Ha), *sph/sph* (Sph), and *ja/ja* (Ja). The *ja/ja* and *sph/sph* mutations are defects in synthesis of β- and α-spectrin, respectively. Mice with the sph^{ha}/sph^{ha} mutation synthesize an unstable α-spectrin. The *nb/nb* mice lack ankyrin. (After Lux SE. Spectrin–actin membrane skeleton of normal and abnormal red blood cells. Semin Hematol 1979;16: 21)

membrane is diminished and is proportional to the density of spectrin on the membrane[795,796] (see Figs. 54-28 and 54-29). Membrane elasticity and bending stiffness are also reduced and proportional to spectrin density.[796,864] In addition, HS red cells lose membrane more readily than normal when metabolically deprived[863,865–867] or when their ghosts are subjected to conditions facilitating vesiculation.[868] This has not been shown to occur in metabolically healthy spherocytes, perhaps because it occurs slowly (about 1% to 2% per day) under such conditions.

Because budding red cells are rarely observed in typical HS blood smears, the postulated vesiculation must either involve microscopic vesicles or occur in bywaters of the circulation such as the reticuloendothelial system. Both explanations are probably true. When membrane vesicles are induced in normal red cells, they originate at the tips of spicules, where the lipid bilayer uncouples from the underlying skeleton.[553] The vesicles are small (about 100 nm) and devoid of hemoglobin and skeletal proteins, so that they are invisible during a conventional examination of stained blood films. Tiny (50 to 80 nm) bumps have been detected in preliminary studies with an atomic force microscope, on the surface of HS red cells obtained from patients who are actively hemolyzing[869] (Fig. 54-39). The bumps could be microvesicles, although this needs to be proved using more conventional microscopic techniques. They are less than the length of a spectrin molecule (100 nm) and are not present on red cells from patients who have had splenectomy; this is consistent with the slower rate of surface loss and much longer life-span of HS red cells postsplenectomy.

Is Hereditary Spherocytosis Caused by Spectrin Deficiency or a Lack of Lipid–Band 3 Interactions? The observation that spectrin or spectrin–ankyrin deficiencies are common in HS has led to the suggestion that they are the primary cause of spherocytosis. According to this hypothesis (Fig. 54-40, hypothesis 1), interactions of spectrin with bilayer lipids or proteins are required to stabilize the membrane. Spectrin-deficient areas would tend to bud off, leading to spherocytosis. This conjecture does not explain how spherocytes develop in patients whose red cells are deficient in band 3 or pallidin but have normal amounts of spectrin.[506,541,803]

The alternate hypothesis (see Fig. 54-40, hypothesis 2) argues that the bilayer is stabilized by interactions between lipids and the abundant band 3 molecules. Each band 3 contains about 14 hydrophobic transmembrane helices, many of which must interact with lipids. Such interactions presumably spread beyond the first layer of lipids and influence the mobility of lipids in successive layers. In deficient red cells the area between band 3 molecules would increase, on average, and the stabilizing effect would diminish. Transient fluctuations in the local density of band 3 could aggravate this situation and allow unsupported lipids to be lost, resulting in spherocytosis. Such a hypothesis is supported by earlier microscopic studies of aggregation of intramembranous particles, which leads to intramembranous particle–free domains, as discussed earlier. These domains are unstable, giving rise to surface blebs that are subsequently released from the cells as vesicles.[557] In addition, in a subset of patients with band 3 deficiency, the protein appears to be lost from the cells during their residence in the circulation. The concomitant loss of the "boundary" lipids may contribute to the deficiency of surface area.[757]

Spectrin- and ankyrin-deficient red cells could become spherocytic by a similar mechanism. Since spectrin filaments corral band 3 molecules and limit their lateral movement,[870] a decrease in spectrin would allow band 3s to diffuse and transiently cluster, fostering vesiculation.

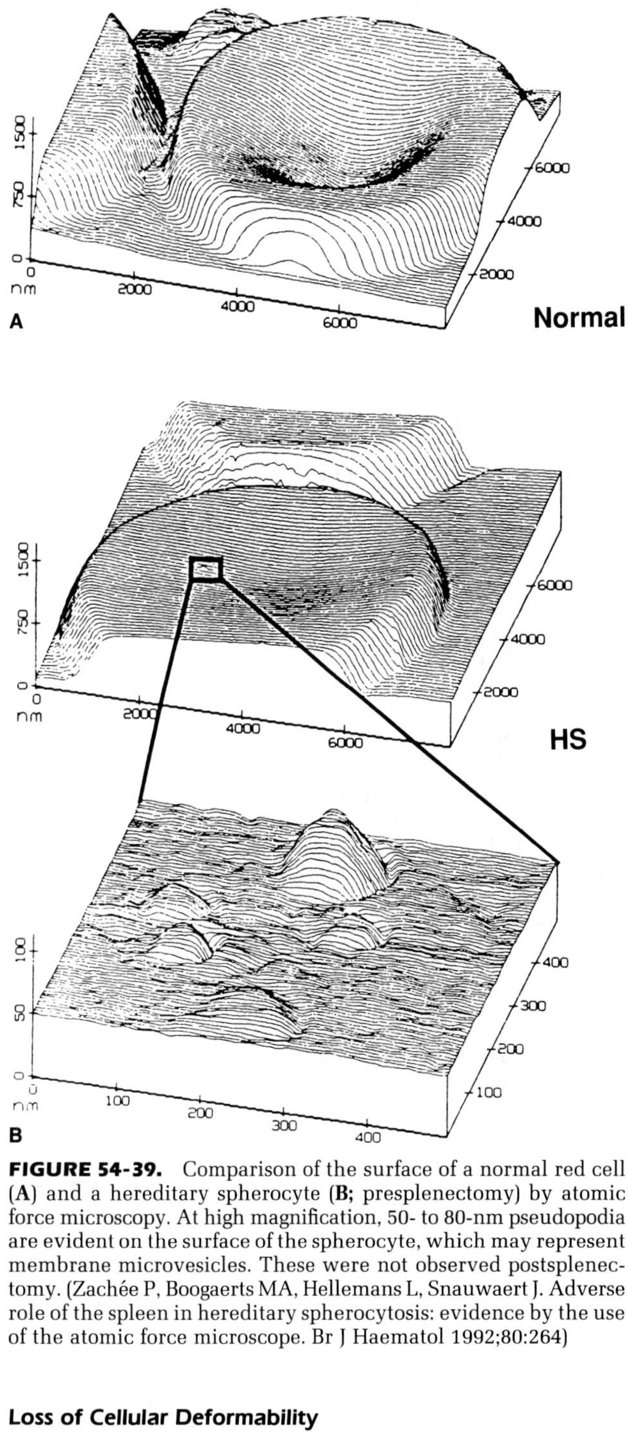

FIGURE 54-39. Comparison of the surface of a normal red cell (**A**) and a hereditary spherocyte (**B**; presplenectomy) by atomic force microscopy. At high magnification, 50- to 80-nm pseudopodia are evident on the surface of the spherocyte, which may represent membrane microvesicles. These were not observed postsplenectomy. (Zachée P, Boogaerts MA, Hellemans L, Snauwaert J. Adverse role of the spleen in hereditary spherocytosis: evidence by the use of the atomic force microscope. Br J Haematol 1992;80:264)

Loss of Cellular Deformability

Hereditary spherocytes hemolyze because of the rheologic consequences of their decreased surface/volume ratio. The red cell membrane is flexible, but it can expand its surface area only about 3% before rupturing.[871] Hence, the cell becomes less and less deformable as surface area is lost. For HS red cells, poor deformability is a hindrance only in the spleen, since the cells have a nearly normal life-span after splenectomy.[872,873]

Sequestration of Hereditary Spherocytes in the Spleen

Spherocytes Are Detained at the Cordal–Sinus Junction. In the spleen, most of the arterial blood empties directly into the splenic cords—a tortuous maze of interconnecting narrow passages formed by reticular cells and lined with phagocytes.[874–879] Histologically, this is an "open" cir-

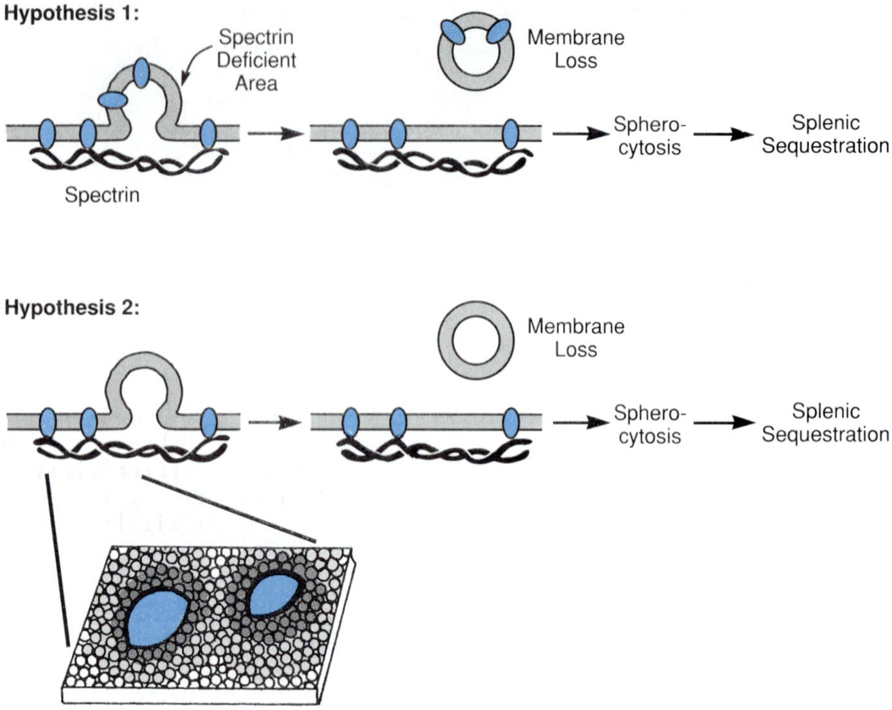

FIGURE 54-40. Two hypotheses concerning the mechanism of membrane loss in hereditary spherocytosis. Hypothesis 1 assumes that the "membrane" (ie, the lipid bilayer and integral membrane proteins) is directly stabilized by interactions with spectrin or other elements of the membrane skeleton. Spectrin-deficient areas, lacking support, bud off, leading to spherocytosis. Hypothesis 2 assumes that the membrane is stabilized by interactions of band 3 with neighboring lipids. The influence of band 3 extends into the lipid milieu because the first layer of immobilized lipids slows the lipids in the next layer, and so on. In band 3–deficient cells, the area between lipid molecules increases and unsupported lipids are lost. Spectrin–ankyrin deficiency allows band 3 molecules to diffuse and transiently cluster, with the same consequences.

culation, but apparently most of the blood that enters the cords normally travels by fairly direct (functionally closed) pathways.[878,879] If passage through these channels is impeded, red cells are diverted deeper into the labyrinthine portions of the cords, where blood flow is slow and the cells may be detained for minutes to hours. Whichever route is taken, to reenter the circulation red cells must squeeze through spaces between the endothelial cells that form the walls of the venous sinuses. Even when maximally distended, these narrow slits are always much smaller than red cells (Fig. 54-41), which are greatly distorted during their passage.[876,878]

Numerous experiments show that spherocytes are selectively sequestered at this juncture.[880–882] As a consequence, spleens from HS patients have massively congested cords and relatively empty sinuses.[874,882a,883,884] In electron micrographs, few spherocytes are seen in transit through the sinus wall[874,883,885] in contrast to that seen in normal spleens, where transiting cells are readily found.[878]

Spherocytes Are "Conditioned" in the Spleen. Evidence is also abundant that HS red cells suffer during detention in the spleen. In HS patients who have not had splenectomy, two populations of spherocytes are detectable: a minor population of hyperchromic "microspherocytes" that form the "tail" of fragile cells in the unincubated osmotic fragility test and a major population that may be only slightly more spheroidal than normal. It was known by 1913 that red cells obtained from the splenic vein were more osmotically fragile than those in the peripheral circulation,[886] and this fact was confirmed by other hematologists of the time.[636,637,887] Its significance was not clear until the classic studies of Emerson and associates[888] and Young and associates[882] in the early 1950s. These investigators showed that osmotically fragile microspherocytes are concentrated in and emanate from the splenic pulp (Fig. 54-42). After splenectomy, spherocytosis persists, but the tail of hyperfragile red cells is no longer evident.[882,888,889] These and other data led to the conclusion that the spleen detains and "conditions" circulating HS red cells in a way that increases their spheroidicity and hastens their demise.[882,888,890] The kinetics of this process were beautifully illustrated in vivo by Griggs and colleagues,[890] who found that a cohort of ^{59}Fe-labeled HS red cells gradually shifted from the major, less fragile population to the more fragile, conditioned population 7 to 11 days after their release into the circulation. Although most conditioned HS red cells that escape the spleen are probably recaptured and destroyed, the damage incurred is sufficient to permit extrasplenic recognition and removal, because conditioned spherocytes, isolated from the spleen and reinfused postoperatively, are rapidly eliminated.[890,891]

Splenic Cords Are Metabolically Inhospitable. The mechanism of splenic conditioning is less certain. It is difficult to obtain accurate information about the cordal environment, but the existing data suggest that it is metabolically inhospitable,[881,888,892,893] although perhaps less so than originally believed.[879] Crowded red cells must compete for limited supplies of glucose[892] in acidic surroundings (pH about 6.6 to 7.2),[879,881,888,893] where glycolysis is inhibited.[894,895] The acidic environment induces chloride and water entry and cell swelling[896] but, as already discussed, it also stimulates the K^+/Cl^- cotransporter, which produces a net loss of potassium and water from the cells. The adverse effects of the cordal environment are further compounded by oxidant producing macrophages. Hence, the spherocyte, detained in the splenic cords because of its surface deficiency, is stressed by erythrostasis in a metabolically threatening environment.

Erythrostasis

As Ham and Castle[622] and Dacie[897] first recognized, the HS red cell is particularly vulnerable to erythrostasis. This is the basis of the well-known autohemolysis test. During prolonged sterile incubation in the absence of supplemental glucose, red cells undergo a series of changes that culminate in hemolysis.[138] The sequence of the changes is the same for HS and normal erythrocytes. Because HS cells are abnormally leaky and bear unstable membranes, their degeneration is accelerated.

HS red cells are initially jeopardized because their membrane permeability to Na is mildly increased.[824,825] Their

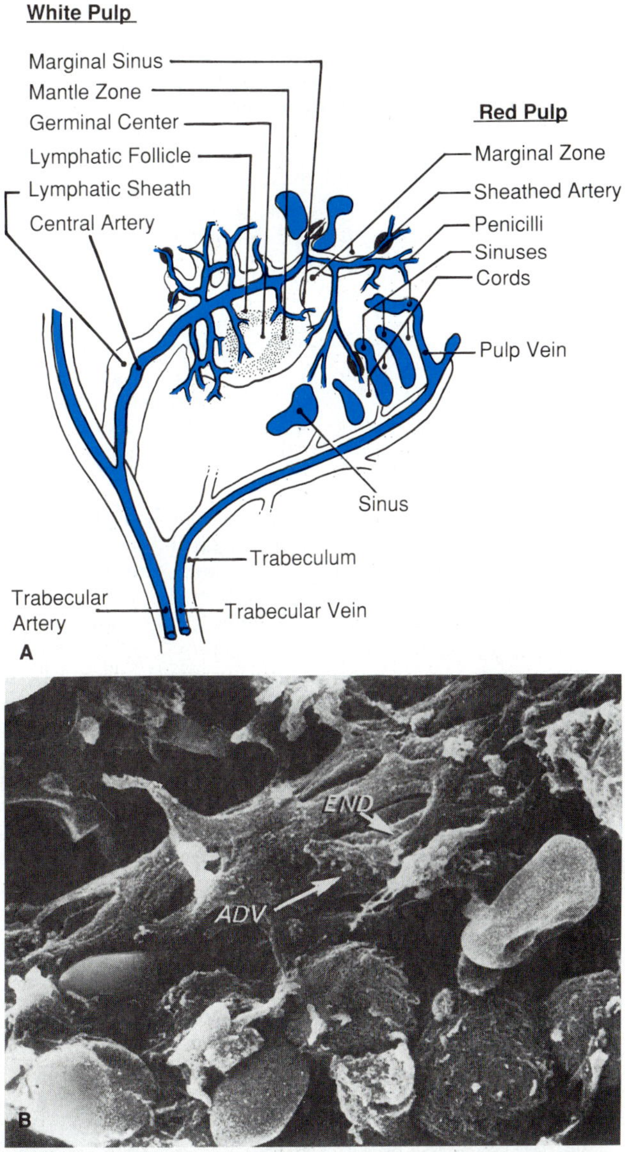

FIGURE 54-41. Splenic anatomy. (**A**) Schematic illustration of the anatomy of the spleen. The components of the white pulp are listed at the left, and of the red pulp are at the right. Blood entering the splenic cords must pass through the walls of the splenic sinuses to reenter the venous circulation. (**B**) Scanning electron micrograph of a splenic sinus viewed from within the splenic cords. The narrow transmural slits between the endothelial cells (END) and adventitial cells (ADV) of the sinus are evident. The edges of these slits probably touch each other in the normal spleen, so the openings are potential structures rather than fixed pores. They are revealed here because of a drying artifact. The adjacent erythrocytes are considerably larger than the slits and hence must be flexible to pass into the splenic sinuses and return to the venous circulation. (After Weiss L. A scanning electron microscopic study of the spleen. Blood 1974;43:665)

propensity to accumulate Na^+ and water is normally balanced by increased Na^+ pumping; the increased dependence on glycolysis is detrimental in erythrostasis where substrate is limited.[825] HS red cells exhaust serum glucose and become ATP depleted more rapidly than normal red cells. As ATP levels fall, ATP-dependent Na^+/K^+ and Ca^{2+} pumps fail, and the cells gain Na^+ and water and swell. Later, when the Ca^{2+}-dependent K^+ (Gárdos) pathway is activated, K^+ loss predominates and the cells lose water and shrink. The Na^+ gain is accelerated in HS red cells but is insufficient by itself to induce hemolysis. HS red cells are doubly jeopardized. As noted earlier, they are inherently unstable and fragment excessively during metabolic depletion.[863,865–867] Membrane lipids (and probably integral membrane proteins) are lost at more than twice the normal rate.[865] At first, this surface loss is balanced by cell dehydration, but eventually (30 to 48 hours) membrane loss predominates, the cells exceed their critical hemolytic volume, and autohemolysis ensues.[138]

Consequences of Splenic Trapping

Calculations[138] indicate the average normal red cell passes through the splenic cords about 14,000 times during its lifetime and has an average transit time of 30 to 40 seconds—close to measured transient times in normal human spleens in vivo.[897a] The calculated residence time of the average HS red cell in the splenic cords is much longer, perhaps as long as 15 to 150 minutes, but still far short of the time required for metabolic depletion to occur.[138]

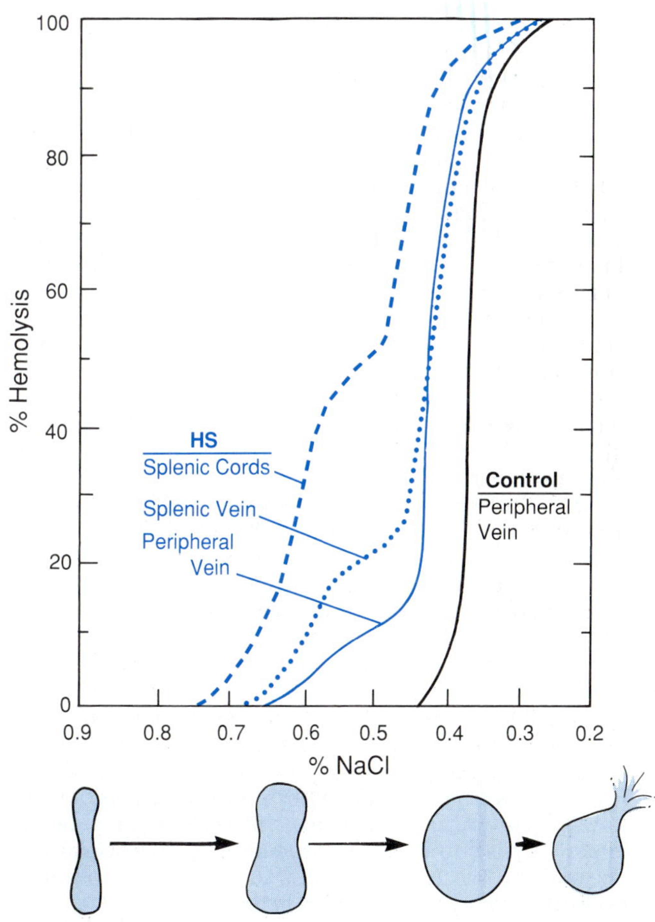

FIGURE 54-42. Osmotic fragility in hereditary spherocytosis. In the osmotic fragility test, red cells are suspended in salt solutions of varying tonicities between isotonic saline (0.9% NaCl; *left*) and distilled water (*right*). Normal red cells swell in hypotonic media and eventually reach a limiting spherical shape, beyond which they hemolyze (*bottom*). Spherocytes, which begin with a lower than normal surface/volume ratio, can swell less before they reach their limiting volume; hence, their osmotic fragility curve is shifted to the left (higher salt concentrations). The spherocytes are said to be osmotically fragile. Before splenectomy, a small proportion of the red cells are extra fragile and produce a tail on the osmotic fragility curve. The cells have been conditioned by the spleen, as shown by their higher concentration in the splenic vein and especially in the splenic cords.

TABLE 54-7. Comparison of Splenic Cordal and Circulating Red Cells in Hereditary Spherocytosis

	Peripheral Red Cells (30% Conditioned)*	Splenic Cordal Red Cells (90% Conditioned)*
Na^+ (mEq/L)	10 ± 2	17 ± 3
K^+ (mEq/L)	78 ± 7	58 ± 12
$Na^+ + K^+$ (mEq/L)	89 ± 9	75 ± 13
ATP (mmol/L)	1.48 ± 0.16	1.46 ± 0.18
ADP (mmol/L)	0.40 ± 0.08	0.85 ± 0.14
2,3-DPG (mmol/L)	4.72 ± 0.35	3.02 ± 0.57
ATP turnover (relative specific activity)	102 ± 9	93 ± 7

* As measured by osmotic fragility tests.
(Data from Mayman D, Zipursky A. Hereditary spherocytosis: the metabolism of erythrocytes in the peripheral blood and in the splenic pulp. Br J Haematol 1974;27:201)

This conclusion is supported by direct analysis of splenic red cells. As shown in Table 54-7, HS red cells obtained from the splenic pulp and containing 80% to 100% conditioned cells are moderately cation depleted and show changes in adenosine diphosphate and 2,3-DPG concentrations consistent with metabolism in an acidic environment, but their ATP levels are *normal*.[830] Others have reported similar findings.[898,899]

Oxidants May Exacerbate Membrane and Water Loss in Hereditary Spherocytosis Red Cells. The data suggest that splenic conditioning is caused by mechanisms other than ATP depletion. For example, potassium loss and membrane instability may be exacerbated by the high concentrations of acids and oxidants that must exist in a spleen filled with activated macrophages lunching on trapped HS red cells. In vitro, oxidants from activated phagocytes can diffuse across the membranes of bystander red cells and damage intracellular proteins within minutes. Red cells moving through the rapid transit pathways in the spleen might escape damage, but those caught in cordal traffic would be vulnerable. Oxidants, even in relatively low concentrations, cause selective K^+ loss by a variety of mechanisms[900–904] and also damage membrane skeletal proteins.[54,597,612a,613,905–907] Finally, there is preliminary evidence that HS red cells may be abnormally sensitive to oxidants.[908] When exposed to peroxides, they undergo remarkable blebbing (and presumably vesiculation)[909] (Fig. 54-43). If a similar process occurs in the spleen, it could be responsible for the excessive surface loss observed in conditioned cells.

Splenic Residence May Activate Membrane Proteases. Residence in the spleen may also activate proteolytic enzymes in the red cell membrane. Membrane proteins of HS red cells from patients with splenomegaly are excessively digested during in vitro incubations, and the degree of proteolysis correlates with splenic size.[910] Whether this occurs in vivo is uncertain, but if so, it could contribute to skeletal weakness and membrane loss.

Macrophages May Directly Condition Hereditary Spherocytes. The possibility that macrophages may directly condition HS red cells must also be considered. It is well known that spherocytosis often results from the interaction of IgG-coated red cells with macrophages, but HS red cells do not have abnormal levels of surface IgG.[911] Macrophages also bear receptors for oxidized lipids (scavenger receptor) and PS, but there is no evidence that HS red cells expose the relevant ligands. The involvement of macrophages is supported by the careful, but frequently ignored, observations of Coleman and Finch,[912] who found that large doses of cortisone markedly ameliorated HS in patients with intact spleens. The effects were similar to those produced by splenectomy. Hemoglobin production, reticulocytosis, and fecal urobilinogen declined; red cell life-span doubled; and hyperspheroidal, conditioned red cells *disappeared* from the circulation. It is well known that similar doses of corticosteroids inhibit splenic processing and destruction of IgG- or C3b-coated red cells in patients with immunohemolytic anemias, probably by suppressing macrophage-induced red cell sphering and phagocytosis.[913,914] Electron microscopy shows that splenic erythrophagocytosis is common in HS patients, particularly in the splenic cords.[883,885,915] In addition, phagocytes expressed from the cords of HS patients contain bits of ghost-like debris,[916] presumably resulting from membrane fragmentation.

Summary of Pathophysiology of HS

In summary, HS red cells are selectively detained by the spleen. This custody is detrimental, leading to a loss of membrane surface that fosters further splenic trapping and

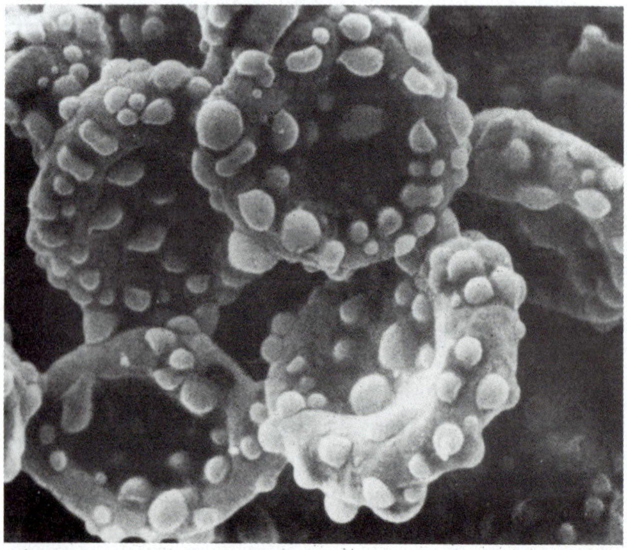

FIGURE 54-43. Blebbing hereditary spherocytosis (HS) red cells exposed to an oxidant (3 mmol/L tert-butyl-hydroperoxide) in vitro. Similar membrane loss could be responsible for splenic conditioning if HS red cells are exposed to sufficient concentrations of phagocyte oxidants during detention in the spleen (an unproven assumption). (Malorni W, Iosi F, Donelli G, et al. A new, striking morphologic feature for the human erythrocyte in hereditary spherocytosis: the blebbing pattern. [Letter] Blood 1993;81:2821)

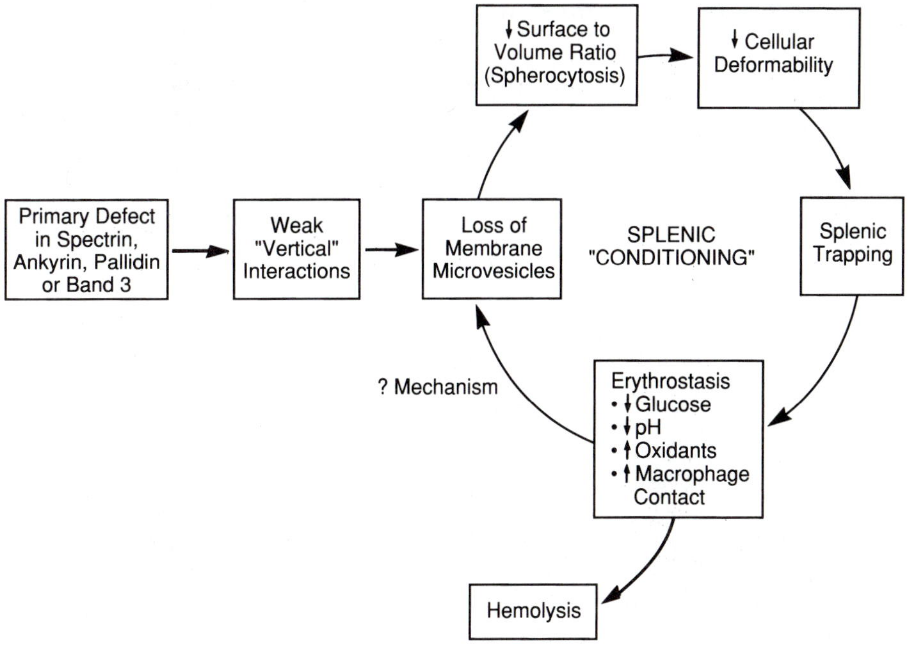

FIGURE 54-44. Pathophysiology of the splenic conditioning and destruction of hereditary spherocytes. (After Becker PS, Lux SE Disorders of the red cell membrane. In: Nathan DG, Oski FA, eds. Hematology of infancy and childhood, ed 4. Philadelphia, WB Saunders, 1993:529)

eventual destruction (Fig. 54-44). It appears that the primary membrane defects involve deficiencies or defects of spectrin, ankyrin, pallidin, or band 3, but much remains to be learned about why these proteins are defective and how this causes surface loss. Obvious membrane budding and fragmentation are rare in HS patients. The speculation is that the HS skeleton (including band 3) may not adequately support all regions of the lipid bilayer, leading to loss of small areas of untethered lipids and integral membrane proteins. As discussed previously, it is not clear whether this is due directly to deficiency of spectrin and ankyrin or whether spectrin–ankyrin deficiency operates indirectly by increasing the lateral mobility of band 3 molecules and decreasing their stabilization of the lipid bilayer (see Fig. 54-40).

The mechanisms of splenic conditioning and red cell destruction are also uncertain. Kinetic considerations make it unlikely that HS red cells are continuously trapped in the cords for the long periods required to induce passive sphering and autohemolysis by metabolic depletion; repetitious accrual of metabolic damage remains a possibility. A special susceptibility of the HS red cell to the acidic, oxidant-rich environment of the spleen[909] and active intervention of macrophages in the processing of erythrostatically damaged spherocytes must also be considered.

Clinical Presentation

Typical HS

The typical clinical picture of HS combines evidence of hemolysis (anemia, jaundice, reticulocytosis, gallstones, and splenomegaly) with spherocytosis (positive osmotic fragility or acidified glycerol lysis tests or both) and a positive family history (Table 54-8). Mild, moderate, and severe forms of HS have been defined according to differences in the hemoglobin and bilirubin concentrations and the reticulocyte count (Table 54-9).[643,722]

Typical HS is associated with both dominant and recessive inheritance. On average, the recessive disease is more severe, but there is considerable overlap.[643,648] Clinical severity and the response to splenectomy roughly parallel the degree of spectrin (or ankyrin) deficiency in patients with defects in either protein.[245,643,648,658,722] Analogous correlations probably exist for patients with mutations in band 3 or pallidin, but this has not been tested.

HS typically manifests in infancy or childhood but may manifest at any age.[917] In children, anemia is the most common presenting complaint (50%), followed by splenomegaly and jaundice with a positive family history (all 10% to 15%).[918] No comparable data exist for adults.

About 60% to 75% of HS patients have incompletely compensated hemolysis and mild to moderate anemia. The

TABLE 54-8. Characteristics of Hereditary Spherocytosis

CLINICAL MANIFESTATIONS
Anemia
Splenomegaly
Intermittent jaundice
From hemolysis
From biliary obstruction
Aplastic crises
Inheritance
Dominant—75%
Nondominant—25%
Rare manifestations
Leg ulcers
Extramedullary hematopoietic tumors
Spinocerebellar ataxia
Myocardiopathy
Excellent response to splenectomy
LABORATORY FEATURES
Reticulocytosis
Spherocytosis
Elevated MCHC
Increased osmotic fragility (especially incubated osmotic fragility test)
Normal Coombs' test
Decreased red cell spectrin, or spectrin and ankyrin, or protein 3, or pallidin (protein 4.2)

TABLE 54-9. Clinical Classification of Hereditary Spherocytosis

	Trait	Mild Spherocytosis	Moderate Spherocytosis	Moderately Severe* Spherocytosis	Severe*§ Spherocytosis
Hemoglobin (g/dL)	Normal	11–15	8–12	6–8	<6
Reticulocytes (%)	1–3	3–8	≥8	≥10	≥10
Bilirubin (mg/dL)	0–1	1–2	≥2	2–3	≥3
Spectrin content (% of normal)†	100	80–100	50–80	40–80‡	20–50
Peripheral smear	Normal	Mild spherocytosis	Spherocytosis	Spherocytosis	Spherocytosis and poikilocytosis
Osmotic fragility					
Fresh blood	Normal	Normal or slightly increased	Distinctly increased	Distinctly increased	Distinctly increased
Incubated blood	Slightly increased	Distinctly increased	Distinctly increased	Distinctly increased	Markedly increased

* Values in untransfused patients.
† Normal (±SD) = 245 ± 27 × 10^5 spectrin dimers per erythrocyte. In most patients ankyrin content is decreased to a comparable degree. A minority of HS patients lack band 3 or protein 4.2 and may have mild to moderate spherocytosis with normal amounts of spectrin and ankyrin.
‡ The spectrin content is variable in this group of patients, presumably reflecting heterogeneity of the underlying pathophysiology.
§ By definition,[643,722] patients with severe spherocytosis are transfusion dependent.
(Adapted from Eber SW, Armbrust R, Shröter W Variable clinical severity of hereditary spherocytosis: relation to erythrocytic spectrin concentration, osmotic fragility and autohemolysis. J Pediatr 1990;177:409 and Pekrun A, Eber SW, Kuhlmey A, Schröter W. Combined ankyrin and spectrin deficiency in hereditary spherocytosis. Ann Hematol 1993;67:89)

anemia is often asymptomatic except for fatigue and mild pallor or, with children, nonspecific parental complaints such as "crabbiness."

Jaundice is seen at some point in about 50% of patients, usually in association with viral infections. It is acholuric, characterized by unconjugated (indirect) hyperbilirubinemia and the *absence* of bilirubinuria.

Palpable splenomegaly is seen in about 50% of infants and 75% to 95% in older children and adults.[918–920] Typically, the spleen is modestly enlarged (2 to 6 cm), but it may be massive.[636,637,921,922] No proven correlation exists between the size of the spleen and the severity of HS, although, given the pathophysiology and the response of the disease to splenectomy, such a correlation probably does exist.

Silent Carrier State

The parents of patients with nondominant HS are clinically asymptomatic and do not have anemia, splenomegaly, hyperbilirubinemia, or spherocytosis on peripheral blood smears.[643,648] Most do have subtle laboratory signs of HS,[643,648] including slight reticulocytosis (average 2.1% ± 0.8%), diminished haptoglobin levels, osmotic fragility, shortened acidified glycerol lysis time,[642] and elevated autohemolysis (see Table 54-9). The incubated osmotic fragility test is probably the most sensitive measure of this condition, particularly the 100% lysis point, which is significantly elevated in carriers (NaCl of 0.43 ± 0.05 g/dL) compared with normal persons (0.23 ± 0.07).[643] No single test is sufficient. Carriers can be detected reliably only by considering the results of a battery of tests.

From the estimated incidence of recessive HS (1 in 20,000—ie, 25% of all HS, which is 1 in 5000 in the United States[640]), one can calculate that 1.4% of the population will be silent carriers. Screens of normal Norwegian[641] or German[642] blood donors with osmotic fragility or acidified glycerol lysis tests show a 0.9% to 1.1% incidence of previously unsuspected very mild HS. Presumably, many of these persons are silent carriers.

Mild Hereditary Spherocytosis

Patients With Mild Hereditary Spherocytosis Have Compensated Hemolysis. Red cell production and destruction are balanced or nearly balanced in about 20% to 30% of HS patients,[919,923] who are said to have "compensated hemolysis." Such patients are not anemic and are usually asymptomatic. Diagnosis may be difficult in some patients because hemolysis, splenomegaly, and spherocytosis are unusually mild. For example, reticulocyte counts are generally less than 6%, and only 60% of patients have significant spherocytosis on peripheral blood smears[643] (see Table 54-9). Red cell spectrin and ankyrin levels are typically more than 80% of normal.[643,762]

Pregnancy, Exercise, and Splenic Enlargement May Exacerbate Mild Hereditary Spherocytosis. Hemolysis may become severe with illnesses that cause splenomegaly, such as infectious mononucleosis.[923a] Hemolysis may also be exacerbated by pregnancy[924,925] or exercise,[926] such that it may impair athletic performance in endurance sports, even in patients with mild disease. Many patients with mild HS are diagnosed during family studies or discovered as adults when splenomegaly or gallstones appear. Although mild HS is usually familial, it develops sporadically in families with more severe disease.[919] This is presumably due to the coinheritance of modifying genes, such as those affecting spectrin or ankyrin synthesis or splenic function.

How Is Compensated Hemolysis Achieved? One of the interesting mysteries about HS is why patients with compensated hemolysis continue to have erythroid hyperplasia when their hemoglobin levels are normal. This phenomenon is difficult to reconcile with the generally accepted theory that erythropoiesis is regulated by tissue hypoxia. One possibility is the concentration of 2,3-DPG, which reportedly is low in hereditary spherocytes prior to splenectomy[831,835] (although the P_{50} of HS blood is normal[835]). Another possibility is that the dehydrated HS red cells are rheologically impaired and do not perfuse the juxtaglomerular renal vessels (where erythropoietin is made) normally, even when the hematocrit is normal. This interesting question deserves to be revisited, especially now that erythropoietin levels can be easily and accurately measured.

Moderately Severe and Severe Hereditary Spherocytosis

A small fraction of HS patients (about 5% to 10%) have moderately severe to severe anemia.[236,643,645,658,726,732,927–929] Patients with moderately severe disease typically have a hemoglobin of 6 to 8 g/dL, reticulocytes 10% or higher, bilirubin 2 to 3 mg/dL, and 40% to 80% of the normal red cell spectrin content (see Table 54-9). This category includes patients with both dominant and recessive HS and a variety of molecular defects.

Patients with severe disease, by definition, have life-threatening anemia and are transfusion dependent. They almost always have recessive HS. Most with severe HS probably have isolated, severe spectrin deficiency (less than 40% of normal),[236,658] which is thought to be due to a defect in α-spectrin.[659,660] Some have ankyrin defects.[723,732] Patients with severe HS are also distinguished by red cell morphology.[236,732] They often have some irregularly contoured or budding spherocytes or bizarre-shaped poikilocytes in addition to typical spherocytes (Fig. 54-45, *panel 4*). Such cells are rare prior to splenectomy in patients with moderately severe disease, although some may be seen postsplenectomy.

In addition to the risks of recurrent transfusions, affected patients often suffer from an aplastic crisis and those with severe HS rarely develop growth retardation,[236,484,921,922] delayed sexual maturation,[921] or aspects of thalassemic facies.[484,921]

Hereditary Spherocytosis in Pregnancy

In general, HS patients who have not had splenectomy have no significant complications during pregnancy except for anemia, which worsens because of plasma volume expansion[930] and sometimes because of increased hemolysis.[924,925] Folic acid deficiency is also a risk.[931,932] One group reported that transfusions were required in 20% of HS pregnancies,[925] but in our experience few HS patients need to receive transfusions.

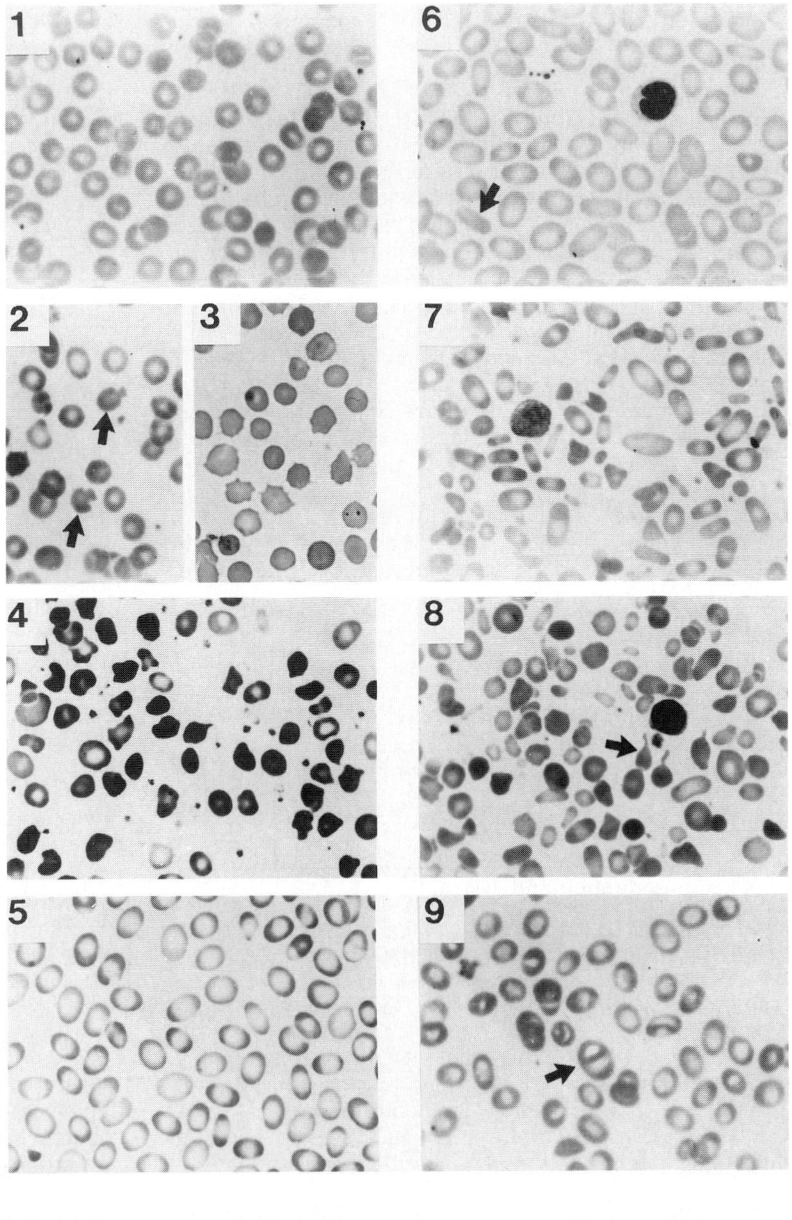

FIGURE 54-45. Red cell morphology in hereditary spherocytosis (HS) and hereditary elliptocytosis (HE). **(1)** Typical HS. Microspherocytes are evident among red cells with some central pallor. **(2)** HS with mushroom-shaped ("pincered") red cells (*arrows*). Pincered cells are found in about 80% of patients with band 3–deficient HS.[929a] **(3)** HS with acanthocytes due to Sp Kissimmee,[359] a variant that lacks the ability to bind protein 4.1. **(4)** Severe HS with spherocytes and bizarre poikilocytes in a patient with combined spectrin–ankyrin deficiency and an unstable ankyrin.[381,732] **(5)** Spherocytic elliptocytosis. Rounded elliptocytes are visible. **(6)** Mild common HE associated with a Sp $\alpha^{I/74}$ mutation. Typical elliptocytes and occasional rod shaped cell are seen (*arrows*). **(7)** "Homozygous" common HE in a patient who is actually a compound heterozygote for Sp $\alpha^{I/74}$ and Sp $\alpha^{I/65}$. A mixture of elliptocytes, fragments, and poikilocytes is shown. **(8)** Hereditary pyropoikilocytosis associated with Sp $\alpha^{I/74}$. Notable are the prominent microspherocytosis and bizarre poikilocytosis, budding (*arrow*), and fragmentation. Also, elliptocytes are sparse. **(9)** Southeast Asian ovalocytosis. A small fraction of the cells show the characteristic transverse bar dividing the central clear space (*arrow*). (Palek J, Lambert S. Genetics of the red cell membrane skeleton. Semin Hematol 1990;27:290)

Hereditary Spherocytosis in the Neonate

Hereditary spherocytosis frequently presents as jaundice in the first few days of life.[933–935] Perhaps as many as 50% of all HS patients have a history of neonatal jaundice,[936] and 91% of infants discovered to have HS in the first week of life are jaundiced (bilirubin more than 10 mg/dL).[934] Hyperbilirubinemia usually appears in the first 2 days of life[933,935,936] and may rise rapidly, driven by the combination of hemolysis and the reduced capacity of the neonatal liver to conjugate bilirubin. Kernicterus is a risk,[933] so that exchange transfusions are sometimes necessary, but in most cases the jaundice is controlled with phototherapy.

Only 43% of neonates with HS are anemic (hemoglobin 15 g/dL or below), and severe anemia is rare.[934] Possibly, human infants with ankyrin defects, like ankyrin-deficient *nb/nb* mice,[855,856] are partially protected in utero by the expression of ankyrin-related proteins in embryonic and fetal erythroblasts. Hydrops fetalis has been reported in an infant with an apparent defect in α-spectrin.[645] Such infants may require intrauterine transfusions.

Diagnosis of Hereditary Spherocytosis Can Be Difficult in Neonates. The diagnosis of HS is often more difficult in the neonatal period than later in life. Splenomegaly is uncommon—at most the spleen tip is palpable[935,936]—and reticulocytosis is variable and usually not severe. Only 35% of affected neonates have a reticulocyte count of 10% or more.[934] In addition, the haptoglobin level is not a reliable indicator of hemolysis during the first few months of life.[937] An even greater problem is that 33% of neonates with HS do not have significant numbers of spherocytes on their peripheral blood smears.[934] Moreover, because fetal red cells are more osmotically resistant than adult cells when fresh, and more osmotically sensitive after incubation at 37°C for 24 hours,[934,938] the osmotic fragility test may give false-positive (incubated osmotic fragility) or false-negative (unincubated osmotic fragility) results unless fetal controls are used. Fortunately, these controls have been published[934] and appear to reliably distinguish neonates with HS, particularly when the incubated osmotic fragility test is used.[934–936]

Some Neonates With Hereditary Spherocytosis Have Transient Sluggish Erythropoiesis. No evidence exists that patients with HS who are symptomatic as neonates have a more severe form of the disease. In fact, most neonates become asymptomatic within the first few weeks of life. Some infants become progressively more anemic and require transfusion. We have found that this usually happens because the marrow response to anemia is more sluggish than normal. The reticulocyte count is relatively low for the degree of anemia. Fortunately, the problem is transient, except in rare patients with severe HS, and usually remits after one or two transfusions. If the child is otherwise well, we allow the hemoglobin to fall to about 5.5 to 6.5 g/dL before giving transfusion to try to stimulate the marrow. We raise the hemoglobin only to 9 to 11 g/dL after transfusion to avoid suppressing the desired marrow response. After the bone marrow "kicks in," the course of the disease depends on the equilibrium between the rates of red cell production and destruction.

Laboratory Features

Many of the laboratory features of HS are common to all hemolytic processes. These include reticulocytosis, erythroid hyperplasia of the bone marrow, unconjugated (indirect) hyperbilirubinemia, and increased fecal urobilinogens.[918,919,939] Plasma hemoglobin is normal[940] and haptoglobin is only variably reduced[941] because most of the hemoglobin released when hereditary spherocytes are destroyed is catabolized at the site of destruction ("extravascular hemolysis").

Peripheral Blood Smear

Spherocytes are the hallmark of HS and are reliably present (97%) in patients with moderate or moderately severe disease.[643] About 25% to 35% of mild HS patients lack the characteristic microspherocytes[643,918,919]; in some, no spherocytes are detectable.[643,919] Actually, hereditary spherocytes are technically misnamed: they range in shape from thickened discocytes to spherostomatocytes.[859]

Generally, spherocytes and microspherocytes are the only abnormal cells in the peripheral smear (other than polychromatophils) in patients with typical mild to moderate HS (see Fig. 54-45, *panel 1*). Patients with band 3-deficient HS may also have a small number of mushroom-shaped red cells or "pincered" cells[148] (see Fig. 54-45, *panel 2*), and some acanthocytes (5% to 10%) are present in patients with spectrin Kissimmee[359,720] (see Fig. 54-45, *panel 3*).

Patients with more severe forms of HS have proportionally more misshapened spherocytes, spiculated red cells, and bizarre-shaped poikilocytes. In the most severe cases, these may dominate the blood smear[236,732] (see Fig. 54-45, *panel 4*). Oblong spherocytes suggest an elliptocytic variant called *spherocytic elliptocytosis* (discussed later in chapter; see Fig. 54-45, *panel 5*).

Because the spherocytic shape is acquired gradually in the circulation, bone marrow erythroblasts are morphologically normal[942] and reticulocytes are only slightly spheroidal.[943] Nucleated red cells are uncommon in HS blood smears[918] except in the most severe forms.[236] Howell-Jolly bodies are also uncommon before splenectomy (4% of patients)[918] and suggest reticuloendothelial blockade.[929]

Red Cell Indices

The mean corpuscular hemoglobin concentration (MCHC) of HS red cells is increased, because of cellular dehydration. Spherocyte Na^+ concentrations are normal or slightly increased, but K^+ concentration and water content are low, particularly in cells harvested from the splenic pulp.[830,943–945] The nature of the permeability defect has not been thoroughly investigated with modern techniques. The average MCHC exceeds the upper limit of normal (36%) in about 50% of HS patients,[919] but all patients have some dehydrated cells. These are best revealed using instruments like the Technicon H1 blood counter (Technicon Corporation, Tarrytown, NY), which measures mean corpuscular volume (MCV) by light scattering and provides a histogram of MCHC[946] that is sufficient, in our experience and others[947,948], to identify all or nearly all HS patients (Fig. 54-46). We find that this simple method is one of the easiest and most accurate ways of diagnosing HS. It is particularly useful when one member of a family is already known to have HS and an inexpensive method of screening other family members is needed.

The MCH and MCV fall within the normal range in HS patients,[919] except in those with severe HS, whose MCV may be slightly low.[236] The MCV is relatively low for the age of the cells (reticulocytes have a high MCV) in all HS patients, reflecting the dehydrated state of HS red cells.

Fragility and Autohemolysis Tests

Osmotic Fragility Test. The state-of-the-art method for demonstrating the low surface/volume ratio of hereditary spherocytes is osmotic gradient ektacytometry.[657] Only a few clinical laboratories are equipped with this instru-

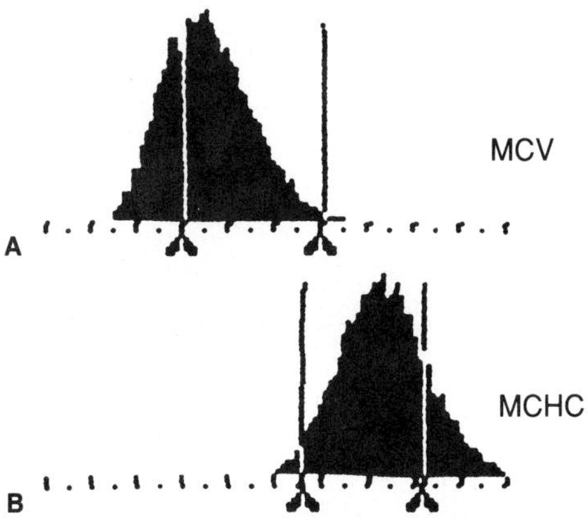

FIGURE 54-46. Histograms of the distribution of MCV (**A**) and MCHC (**B**) in red cells of a patient with hereditary spherocytosis before splenectomy. The vertical lines mark the normal limits of the distributions. The data were collected with a Technicon H1 laser scattering blood counter. The patient has subpopulations of microcytes (low MCV) and dehydrated cells (high MCHC), which presumably represent conditioned microspherocytes. All 21 patients in one study[948] had similar subpopulations. (Pati AR, Patton WN, Harris RI. The use of the Technicon H1 in the diagnosis of hereditary spherocytosis. Clin Lab Haematol 1989;11:27)

mentation. In most, the osmotic fragility test remains the principal diagnostic test.

The osmotic fragility test is performed by suspending red cells in buffered solutions containing various concentrations of sodium chloride.[888,949] In hypotonic solutions, red cells swell until they become spherical and then burst. Cells that begin with a decreased surface/volume ratio, like spherocytes or stomatocytes, reach the spherical limit at a lower salt concentration than normal cells, and are termed *osmotically fragile* (see Fig. 54-42). The method of Parpart and colleagues[949] is recommended with the modified buffers introduced by Godal and associates.[950]

The osmotic fragility test, particularly the *incubated* osmotic fragility, is probably the most sensitive test available for HS. This is surprising since osmotic fragility reflects a secondary property of HS red cells (the loss of surface area) instead of the primary molecular defect. In our experience, direct quantitation of membrane proteins rarely, if ever, detects patients missed by the incubated osmotic fragility test and is a lot more difficult and expensive to perform. The unincubated osmotic fragility test provides useful information on the proportion of conditioned red cells, data that is lost in the incubated test.[882,888,889] Nevertheless, 20% to 25% of HS patients have a normal unincubated osmotic fragility, particularly those with mild HS, who are the most difficult to diagnose.[920,951] The incubated osmotic fragility test is more sensitive[951] and is almost always positive. The test is performed the same way but the whole blood sample is first incubated for 24 hours at 37°C. During this period of time, HS red cells become metabolically depleted and lose membrane fragments more rapidly than normally, which accentuates their spheroidicity and enhances the sensitivity of the test.

Modifications of the osmotic fragility test have been proposed. Some have suggested that addition of 3 μmol/L ouabain during the 24-hour preincubation increases the sensitivity of the incubated osmotic fragility test, particularly for mildly affected subjects.[952,953] Unfortunately, this was not confirmed in a separate study.[954] Another group has used logarithmic transforms of the osmotic fragility curve to simplify calculation of the 50% hemolysis point[955]; this deemphasizes the beginning and endpoints of hemolysis, which can be diagnostically useful in some patients and in silent carriers.[643]

Acidified Glycerol Lysis Test and Pink Test. The glycerol lysis test, in which glycerol is used to retard the osmotic swelling of red cells, was developed as an alternative to the osmotic fragility test. The original test[956] lacked the necessary sensitivity and specificity.[957] An acidified version (acidified glycerol lysis test [AGLT]) was more sensitive,[958] although insufficiently so in some hands,[959] and was not completely specific. For unknown reasons, the accuracy of the standard AGLT is greatly improved when the samples are preincubated at room temperature for 24 hours (incubated AGLT).[960-962] Under these conditions, the sensitivity and specificity of the test approach 100%—similar to that of the incubated osmotic fragility. Eber[642] reinvestigated the buffers used in the test and found that simply increasing the sodium phosphate concentration from 5.3 to 9.3 mmol/L gives 100% sensitivity and specificity without the need for the preincubation step. The modified test is easy to perform and requires little blood. ethylenediaminetetraacetic acid (EDTA) blood (20 μL) is diluted into a saline solution containing 9.3 mmol/L sodium phosphate and 2 mol/L glycerol, pH 6.90, and the fall in absorbance at 625 nm (largely turbidity) is measured as the red cells hemolyze. The $T_{1/2}$ for AGLT lysis is more than 30 minutes for normals and less than 5 minutes for HS samples.[642]

Another adaption of the original glycerol lysis test, called the *Pink test*, is more reproducible and accurate,[963] but also profits from a 1-day preincubation.[964] The test has been adapted for fingerstick blood samples,[964,965] but direct comparisons suggest that it is less specific than the osmotic fragility or incubated AGLT tests.[960,965] Because the modified AGLT test has also been adapted to microsamples,[642] it appears to be the test of choice.

Hypertonic Cryohemolysis Test. This recently described method is based on the fact that HS red cells are particularly sensitive to cooling at 0°C in hypertonic solutions.[966] The authors state that the hypertonic cryohemolysis test is 100% sensitive for HS patients but only 94% specific for normal pesons and 86% for patients with autoimmune hemolytic anemia. The test is independent of the surface/volume ratio of the cells, which is an advantage compared with other diagnostic tests. The use of this test in clinical diagnosis awaits independent verification of its sensitivity and specificity by other laboratories.

Autohemolysis Test. The autohemolysis of HS red cells, incubated in their own plasma in the absence of added glucose, is increased at 48 hours.[897,920,967] In most HS patients, less autohemolysis occurs when supplemental glucose is added.[920,945,967] This is not always true in more severe HS patients,[862] which can cause diagnostic confusion since autohemolysis that is unresponsive to glucose is a feature of some other hemolytic anemias.[967] The test is sensitive and occasionally useful in confirming the diagnosis of HS, but we do not use it routinely.

Membrane Protein Measurements

Membrane protein concentrations are most easily assessed using SDS gels. Individually stained bands are quantified by densitometry or by eluting the dye from an excised band and measuring its concentration spectrophotometrically.[245] This technique is satisfactory for detecting spectrin deficiency (expressed as a spectrin/band 3 ratio),[804] although it is not as accurate as a radioimmunoassay (RIA)[236,245] or ELISA immunoassay,[722] partly because band 3 is lost with other surface components as spherocytes circulate. This is even more true for ankyrin, which is present in smaller amounts and migrates close to β-spectrin on gels. SDS gels do not give reliable results even with a gel system that

TABLE 54-10. Classification of Crises in Hereditary Spherocytosis

Type	Anemia	Reticulocytes	Jaundice	Cause	Comment
Hemolytic	Increased	Increased	Increased	Viral infections → splenomegaly	Frequent, usually mild
Aplastic	Increased	Decreased	Decreased	Parvovirus B19	Occurs once, severe, risk to pregnant contacts
Megaloblastic	Increased	No change or decreased	No change or increased	Relative folic acid deficiency	Rare, preventable

optimizes the spectrin–ankyrin separation[236] (see Fig. 54-4). The popular Laemmli gels are completely unsatisfactory because ankyrin migrates between the spectrin bands in this system. Immunoassays, on the other hand, work well.[245,722] SDS gels are satisfactory for detecting band 3 deficiency (elevated spectrin/band 3 ratio) or pallidin deficiency and are useful in combination with antibody staining (Western blots) for detecting mutant proteins of altered size.

Complications

Crises

Patients with HS, like patients with other hemolytic diseases, are subject to "crises" (Table 54-10).

Hemolytic. Hemolytic crises are probably the most common complications (especially mild hemolytic crises), which usually occur with viral syndromes, particularly in children. They are characterized by a mild transient increase in jaundice, splenomegaly, anemia, and reticulocytosis. No medical intervention is required. Severe hemolytic crises are rare. Characteristic features include jaundice, anemia, vomiting, abdominal pain, and tender splenomegaly.

Aplastic. Aplastic crises are less common but more serious. Severe anemia and death[636,921] can result. These crises are usually caused by parvovirus B19[968] (see Chap. 10), which proliferates in erythropoietic precursors and inhibits their growth.[969,970] In children with HS, the viral infection may present with fever, vomiting, abdominal pain, pallor, extreme lassitude, or other symptoms of anemia.[971,971a] Sometimes multiple family members are affected simultaneously.[971,972] Parvovirus infections are often associated with mild neutropenia or thrombocytopenia, and a few cases of transient pancytopenia have been reported.[973,974]

Parvovirus can also infect susceptible adults and is a particular danger to pregnant women, since it can cause fetal death due to anemia and nonimmune hydrops fetalis.[975–977] The risk of hydrops fetalis for women who become infected during pregnancy is, fortunately, low.[976] Nevertheless, because the virus is highly contagious and easily transmitted to patients and staff[978,979] and because only about 50% of the pregnant population have already acquired protective antibodies, all patients who have or are suspected of having an aplastic crisis should be placed on precautions while hospitalized, and IgG-negative contacts who are pregnant should be tested for evidence of seroconversion. Hydrops fetalis can be detected by ultrasonography and has been successfully treated by intrauterine transfusions.[980]

The sequence of events in an aplastic crisis was best described in the classic article of Owren[971] and is illustrated in Figure 54-47. During the aplastic phase, the hematocrit level and reticulocyte count fall, marrow erythroblasts disappear, and unused iron accumulates in the serum.[971] Giant pronormoblasts often appear and are a hallmark of the cytopathic effects of parvovirus B19.[981] As production of new red cells declines, the remaining cells age, and microspherocytosis and osmotic fragility increase. Bilirubin levels may decrease as the number of abnormal red cells that can be destroyed declines. The return of marrow

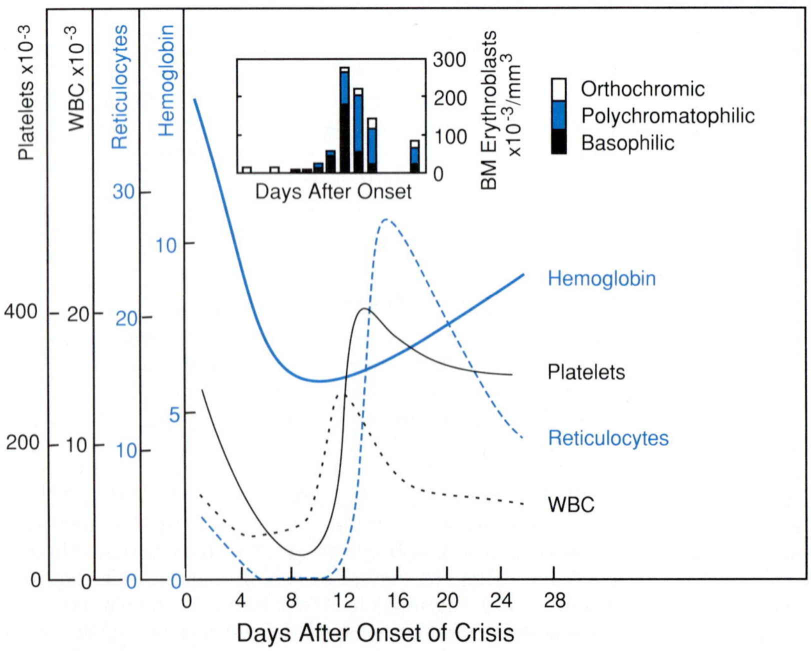

FIGURE 54-47. The temporal sequence of a severe aplastic crisis in a patient with hereditary spherocytosis. Marked reticulocytopenia and mild to moderate leukopenia and thrombocytopenia occurred during the aplastic phase (in this case, the leukopenia and thrombocytopenia were more severe than usual). Reticulocytosis and recovery were heralded by a rise in peripheral blood granulocytes and platelets, and by reappearance of bone marrow normoblasts. (Data from Owren PA. Congenital hemolytic jaundice: the pathogenesis of the hemolytic crisis. Blood 1948;3:231)

function is heralded by a fall in the serum iron concentration and the emergence of granulocytes, platelets, and, finally, reticulocytes (see Fig. 54-47).

It is important to realize that an aplastic crisis may be the first evidence of HS in a patient with compensated hemolysis (mild HS)[982,983] and that the lack of reticulocytes should not eliminate hemolytic anemias from diagnostic consideration. Diagnostic confusion may also arise during reemergence of marrow function, when the physician may mistake an aplastic crisis for a hemolytic crisis.

Because aplastic crises usually last 10 to 14 days[971] (about 50% of the life-span of HS red cells),[897a,984] the hemoglobin value typically falls to about 50% of its usual level before recovery occurs. For this reason, aplastic crises are a serious threat to young children with HS, particularly those with more severe forms of the disease, and these children require careful observation.

Megaloblastic. Megaloblastic crises are rare. They occur when the dietary intake of folic acid is inadequate for the increased needs of the erythroid HS bone marrow. This need is particularly acute during pregnancy[931,932] and during recovery from an aplastic crisis. All patients with HS (or other hemolytic anemias) should routinely receive folic acid supplements (about 1 mg/d) to prevent this complication.

Gallstones

Pigment gallstones have been detected in children with HS as young as 3 years of age[985] but are most common in adolescents and adults. In a retrospective study of 152 consecutive cases of HS conducted prior to the development of ultrasonography, Bates and Brown[986] found gallstones in only 5% of children younger than 10 years of age who were adequately examined, but the incidence rose to 40% to 50% in the second to fifth decades and 55% to 75% thereafter (Fig. 54-48). The rise in incidence of gallstones after age 30 years paralleled the incidence in the general population,[986] which suggests that cholelithiasis due to HS is primarily manifested in the second and third decades.

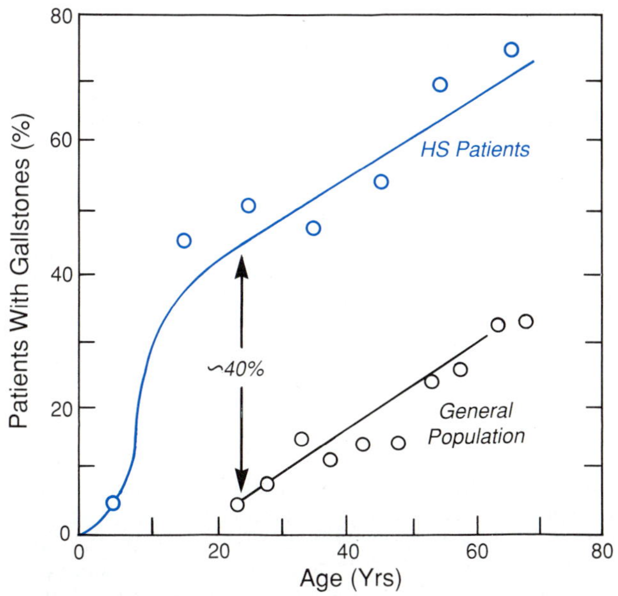

FIGURE 54-48. Proportion of normal and hereditary spherocytosis (HS) patients with gallstones as a function of age. Data are from a study of gallbladder disease in 152 consecutive patients seen at the Cleveland Clinic before 1952.[986] Only patients whose gallbladders were examined at surgery or by cholecystography are included. Data for the general population are from an autopsy series of patients who did not have hemolytic anemia.[987] The prevalence of gallstones rises sharply between the ages of 10 and 30 and parallels that of the general population after 30.

The pigment stones typical of HS and other hemolytic anemias are easily detected by ultrasonography. All HS patients should have ultrasound examinations about every 5 years and before splenectomy. The high incidence of cholelithiasis and the risks of its complications constitute the major impetus for splenectomy in many HS patients. Unfortunately, it is not clear how often patients with pigment gallstones develop *symptomatic* gallbladder disease or biliary obstruction. Anecdotal reports in the old HS literature suggest that 40% to 50% of HS patients with cholelithiasis have symptoms and that a high proportion of stone-containing gallbladders have histologic evidence of cholecystitis.[988] Studies that include large numbers of patients with mild HS show a much lower incidence of symptomatic gallbladder disease.[989] Clearly, more accurate data about the long-term complications of pigment stone disease are needed to assess the risk/benefit ratio of splenectomy in HS patients and the need for cholecystectomy in the asymptomatic patient with stones.

Other Complications

Gout and Leg Ulcers. Rarely, adults with HS develop *gout*,[637,990] *indolent leg ulcers*,[991,992] or a chronic *erythematous dermatitis* on the legs.[993] All three problems are corrected by splenectomy.

Extramedullary Hematopoietic Tumors. Adults with HS may also develop *extramedullary masses of hematopoietic tissue*, particularly alongside the posterior thoracic or lumbar spine[636,990,994–998] or in the hila of the kidneys.[636] The tumors often arise in patients with mild HS, perhaps because they frequently escape splenectomy. The masses gradually enlarge and may be mistaken for neoplasms.[990] Biopsy can lead to extensive bleeding.[990] If necessary, an open biopsy should be performed. Experience suggests that these bone marrow tumors can be diagnosed by magnetic resonance imaging (MRI),[998] which may make biopsies unnecessary. The masses stop growing and undergo fatty metamorphosis after splenectomy but do not shrink in size.[994,996]

Multiple Myeloma. Schafer and colleagues[999] have suggested that untreated HS may predispose patients to a true neoplasm--*multiple myeloma*. Four patients with HS and myeloma have been reported.[999–1001] None had undergone splenectomy, two had gallbladder disease, and one had silicosis. Schafer argues that the association may be due to chronic reticuloendothelial stimulation, since splenic clearance of abnormal red cells induces proliferation of lymphocytes and plasma cells as well as macrophages.[1002] HS patients have a mild, polyclonal hypergammaglobulinemia,[999,1003] and evidence favors the association of myeloma and chronic gallbladder disease.[999,1004]

Hemochromatosis. Untreated HS may also exacerbate *hemochromatosis* in patients who are *heterozygous* for the hereditary disease.[1005–1008] Several patients have subsequently died of liver failure or hepatoma.

Congestive Heart Disease. Untreated HS may also aggravate underlying heart disease and precipitate heart failure. Occasionally, this may be the presenting complaint.[1009]

Angioid Streaks. *Angioid streaks*, which are brownish or gray streaks resembling veins in the optic fundus, have been reported in adult members of several kindreds with HS.[1010,1011] The incidence of this association is unknown. Angioid streaks are relatively common in some other hematologic disorders—notably sickle cell disease and thalassemia[1010]—and may be complicated by retinal vascular proliferation requiring photocoagulation.[1013]

Diagnostic Problems

Other Causes of Spherocytosis

In general, HS is easily diagnosed and differentiated from other causes of spherocytosis (Table 54-11), but there are several situations in which diagnosis can be difficult. In the neonatal period, HS may be hard to differentiate from ABO incompatibility because microspherocytosis is prominent in both conditions and the Coombs' test is sometimes negative in ABO disease. Fortunately, in most affected infants with ABO incompatibility, anti-A (or anti-B) antibodies can be eluted from the red cells, and free anti-A IgG antibodies can be detected in the infant's serum. Occasionally, older patients with immunohemolytic anemias and spherocytosis also have so few antibody molecules attached to their red cells that the Coombs' test is negative and differentiation of the disease from HS is possible only with the use of radioactive antiglobulin reagents.[1014]

Spherocytosis is also seen in Heinz body hemolytic anemias during an acute hemolytic crisis (see Chap. 52). The diagnosis is suggested by the presence of bite cells and blister cells on peripheral blood films and by detecting Heinz bodies in red cells stained with methyl violet.

Aplastic Crisis

Diagnostic difficulties also arise in patients who present during an aplastic crisis. Early in the crisis, the acute nature of the symptoms may suggest an acquired process, and the absence of reticulocytes may divert the physician from a diagnosis of hemolytic anemia. Later, as marrow function returns, physicians may occasionally be misled by the properties of the emerging young HS red cells, which are less spherocytic and osmotically fragile than usual.[943]

Conditions That Camouflage Hereditary Spherocytosis

Hereditary spherocytosis may also be camouflaged by association with disorders that increase the surface/volume ratio of the red cells, such as iron deficiency,[1015] obstructive jaundice,[860] β-thalassemia,[1016] vitamin B_{12} or folate[1017] deficiency, and hemoglobin SC disease.[1018]

Iron deficiency corrects the abnormal shape, fragility, and high MCHC of hereditary spherocytes but does not improve their life-span,[1015] whereas *obstructive jaundice* improves both shape and survival.[860] For example, we have seen a young girl who developed jaundice and symptoms of biliary obstruction at 6 years of age (Fig. 54-49). She had a palpable spleen tip, evidence of mild compensated hemolysis (hemoglobin, 14 g/dL; 3.3% reticulocytes) and a *normal peripheral blood smear and osmotic fragility test* (fresh and incubated). Abdominal x-ray studies showed calcified stones in the gallbladder and common bile duct. After cholecystectomy and relief of the partial biliary obstruction, the child's hemolysis worsened (10.8% reticulocytes), and she developed anemia (hemoglobin, 10.2 g/dL), spherocytosis, and a definitely abnormal incubated osmotic fragility test. She subsequently responded to splenectomy.

The description of a large French family in which HS and *β-thalassemia trait* are independently segregating,[1016] strongly suggests that β-thalassemia ameliorates and partially masks HS. Patients with both traits have signs of both diseases: small, hemoglobin A_2-rich, osmotically fragile cells, and some spherocytes on peripheral blood smears.

Megaloblastic anemia can also mask HS,[1017] at least the morphologic characteristics of the disease. Osmotic fragility is also improved. The masking effect is observed in both vitamin B_{12}[484] and folate[1017] deficiencies and is rapidly reversed after correction of the nutritional deficit.

Coinheritance of HS and *hemoglobin SC disease* may exacerbate the hemoglobinopathy. A 14-year-old boy with both diseases was much more anemic than his SC siblings and had experienced five splenic sequestration crises.[1018] The two diseases may also disguise each other, at least partially. Only a few spherocytes or target cells were evident on the boy's blood smear, and the surface/volume ratio of his red cells (and probably their osmotic fragility) was normal. This is presumably due to the balancing effects of HS (loss of surface area) and hemoglobin SC (loss of cell volume) on red cells. Even *sickle trait* may be worsened by HS. Yang and colleagues[1019] reported two patients with the combination who suffered multiple splenic sequestration crises. On the other hand, spontaneous regression of HS, presumably due to development of a hyposplenic state, has been observed in two family members who had HS and sickle cell trait.[1020]

In these unusual cases, special tools may be needed to confirm the diagnosis of HS, like immunoassays for red cell membrane proteins[236,245,722] or the osmotic gradient ektacytometer (which can independently measure surface area and volume).[657]

TABLE 54-11. Diseases in Which Spherocytosis is the Predominant Morphology

COMMON
Hereditary spherocytosis
Immunohemolytic anemias (warm antibody type)
ABO incompatibility in neonates
UNCOMMON TO RARE
Clostridial sepsis
Hemolytic transfusion reactions
Severe burns and other RBC thermal injuries
Spider, bee, and snake venoms
Severe hypophosphatemia
Hypersplenism*
Acute RBC oxidant injury (G6PD deficiency during hemolytic crisis, favism, oxidant drugs, and chemicals)*

* Hypersplenism and acute red cell oxidant injury are common, but spherocytosis is only rarely the predominant morphology.

Atypical Hereditary Spherocytosis

Zail and coworkers[1021] have described a family with a dominantly inherited disorder characterized by spherocytosis and mild compensated hemolysis in which fresh red cells had a normal or *decreased* osmotic fragility and ^{51}Cr-labeled red cells lacked the characteristic pattern of splenic sequestration that is typical of HS.

HS With Involvement of Nonerythroid Tissues

Two adults with HS and a poorly defined, slowly progressive *spinocerebellar degenerative* syndrome have been described.[847] The existence of similar cases in the older European literature,[846,848–853] and the discoveries that erythrocyte ankyrin[485,492] and β-spectrin[137] are expressed in the cerebellum and spinal cord and that mice with an inherited lack of ankyrin develop delayed cerebellar ataxia because of slow loss of Purkinje's cells,[485] suggest that these patients may have unique spectrin or ankyrin defects.

Similarly, the reports of *hypertrophic cardiomyopathy* segregating with HS in three generations of a Russian family[1022] and of spherocytosis with a *movement disorder*

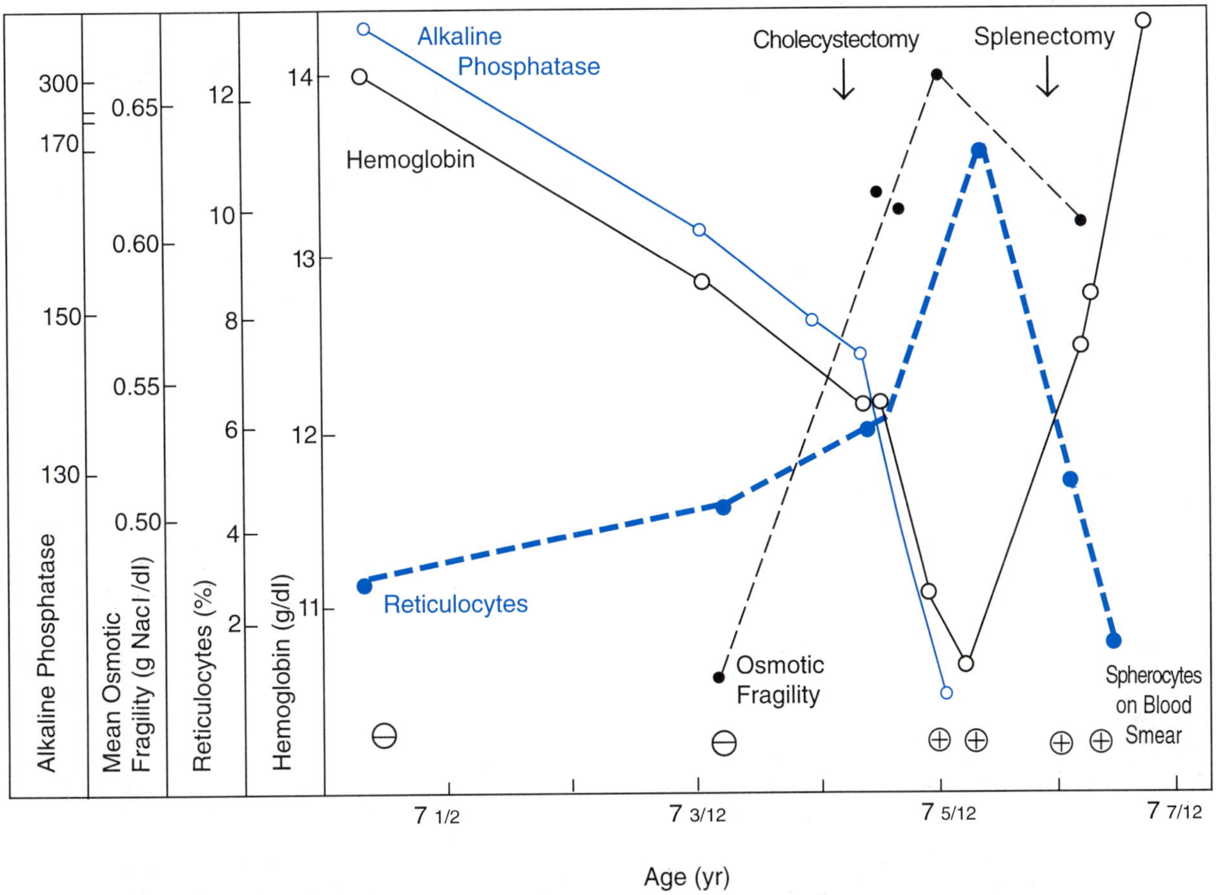

FIGURE 54-49. Hereditary spherocytosis (HS) camouflaged by obstructive jaundice. Patient CD presented at 7 years, 1 month of age with a history of recurrent abdominal pain, vomiting, and jaundice, as well as evidence of biliary obstruction (four gallstones in the common duct). She had a normal hemoglobin measurement, a normal osmotic fragility test, a near-normal reticulocyte count, and normal red cell morphology. After cholecystectomy and relief of obstruction (note fall in alkaline phosphatase), florid HS developed (increased osmotic fragility, reticulocytosis, anemia, and spherocytosis), which improved, as expected, after splenectomy. This patient's course clearly shows that loss of red cell surface area is responsible for hemolysis in HS and that conditions that increase red cell surface area, such as biliary obstruction,[860] can camouflage HS.

and myopathy in two brothers[854] are of interest because erythroid spectrin and ankyrin are also known to be expressed in muscle.[137,247,481,482,1023]

Splenectomy

Splenectomy cures almost all patients with HS, eliminating anemia and reducing the reticulocyte count to near normal levels of 1% to 3%. Patients with the most severe forms of the disease may not achieve a complete remission,[236,648] but will benefit greatly from the procedure.

Risks

Sepsis, Bacterial and Parasitic Infections, and Ischemic Heart Disease. The indications for splenectomy should be weighed carefully, since a small proportion of patients will die from *overwhelming postsplenectomy infections*[1024–1031] (see Chap. 46). Because the risk of postsplenectomy sepsis is high in infancy and early childhood, splenectomy should be delayed until the age of 5 to 9 years, if possible, and until at least 2 or 3 years in all cases, even when chronic transfusions are required in the interim. There is no evidence that further delay is useful—and it may be harmful because the risk of cholelithiasis increases dramatically in children after the age of 10 years[986] (see Fig. 54-48).

It is difficult to estimate the risk of postsplenectomy infections after infancy. The surveys of Green and associates[1026] and Schwartz,[1030] which are the best available, are limited to adults and largely predate immunization for *Streptococcus pneumoniae* and other bacteria. They show an incidence of fulminant sepsis of 0.2 to 0.5 per 100 person-years of follow-up and a death rate of 0.1 per 100 person-years; in addition, other serious bacterial infections (eg, pneumonia, meningitis, peritonitis, bacteremia) are much more common (4.5 per 100 person-years) than normal, particularly in the first few years after the operation. The risk of infection would presumably be lower today, with routine pneumococcal immunization, because 50% to 70% of postsplenectomy sepsis is due to *S pneumoniae* and 80% of pneumococcal disease is due to strains contained in the vaccine. Further risk reductions would be anticipated from the chronic use of prophylactic penicillin. Nevertheless, the risk cannot be reduced to zero. Postsplenectomy infections occur occasionally in successfully immunized patients,[1032–1035] and compliance regarding prophylactic medications is a problem, particularly in teenagers.[1036]

Unfortunately, as discussed in several reviews,[1037–1039] penicillin-resistant pneumococci are increasing rapidly all over the world. In some countries (eg, Hungary), more than half of all isolates are resistant.[1040] In the United States, the prevalence is closer to 5%,[1037,1041] but it is rising. Although most of the pneumococcal strains show some sensitivity to penicillin, some are highly resistant and others are multiply resistant.[1041] The emergence of these strains will greatly complicate the use of antibiotics for pneumococcal prophylaxis during the next decade.

For patients in selected parts of the world, consideration must also be given to the greater risk of red cell parasitic diseases like *P falciparum* malaria and babesiosis[1042–1045] in hosts who have had splenectomy.

The risk of *ischemic heart disease* may also increase after splenectomy. In one careful study, Robinette and Fraumeni[1046] observed that death from ischemic heart disease occurred 1.86 times more often in young men who had undergone splenectomy than in matched controls during a 28-year follow-up period, a significant difference. The cause is unknown, although the chronically higher platelet count postsplenectomy is a good possibility.

The major complication of the operation, other than local infection or bleeding, is *pancreatitis*,[1047] probably due to injury to the tail of the pancreas incurred during removal of the spleen.

Candidates for Splenectomy

All patients with severe spherocytosis should have splenectomy, but without large clinical studies it is difficult to give firm rules regarding splenectomy for patients with mild to moderate HS. We generally defer splenectomy in patients with mild HS and compensated hemolysis. We recommend splenectomy for patients with moderate HS if they suffer from reduced vitality or physical stamina because of anemia, if, later in life, anemia compromises vascular perfusion of vital organs, or if leg ulcers or extramedullary hematopoietic tumors develop. Whether patients with moderate, *asymptomatic* anemia should have a splenectomy remains controversial. The treatment of patients with mild to moderate HS and gallstones is also debatable, particularly since new treatments for gallstones (eg, laparoscopic cholecystectomy, endoscopic sphincterotomy, and extracorporal choletripsy)[1048–1050] lower the risk of this complication. If such patients have *symptomatic* gallstones, we favor a combined cholecystectomy and splenectomy, particularly when acute cholecystitis or biliary obstruction has occurred. In the past, cholecystectomy and splenectomy were sometimes staged but, if both operations are necessary, most surgeons seem willing to do them together.[1051]

Partial Splenectomy and Laparoscopic Splenectomy

Studies of Tchernia and colleagues[1052] suggest that partial splenectomy may be an effective compromise for many HS patients, that is, relieving hemolysis while maintaining some residual splenic phagocytic function (Fig. 54-50). Complications were low and regrowth of the splenic remnant was not observed during a 4-year follow-up period, but more experience and longer follow-ups are needed before the procedure can be recommended. The same can be said of laparoscopic splenectomy, which offers decreased morbidity and more rapid recovery but requires a longer operation.[1052a]

Prophylaxis

All patients who have had a splenectomy must receive polyvalent pneumococcal vaccine, preferably given several weeks preoperatively. Immunization with *Haemophilus influenzae* vaccine and, in some countries, meningococcal vaccines is also recommended, particularly in children. We advocate prophylactic antibiotics after splenectomy, with emphasis on protection against pneumococcal sepsis (penicillin V or equivalent, 125 mg orally twice daily in children younger than 7 years and 250 mg twice daily in older children and adults), at least for the first 5 years after surgery and preferably for life.

Prior to splenectomy, HS patients, like patients with other hemolytic disorders, should take folic acid, 1 mg/d orally, to prevent folate deficiency.

Postsplenectomy Changes

After splenectomy, spherocytosis persists but conditioned microspherocytes disappear, and changes typical of the postsplenectomy state, including Howell-Jolly bodies, target cells, siderocytes, and acanthocytes, become evident in the peripheral blood smear. On average, the MCV and mean red cell surface area increase, and the MCHC and osmotic fragility decrease, but the effects are modest (5% to 10%).[1053] In typical dominant HS, reticulocyte counts fall to normal or near-normal levels,[648] although red cell life-span, if carefully measured, remains slightly shortened (96 ± 13

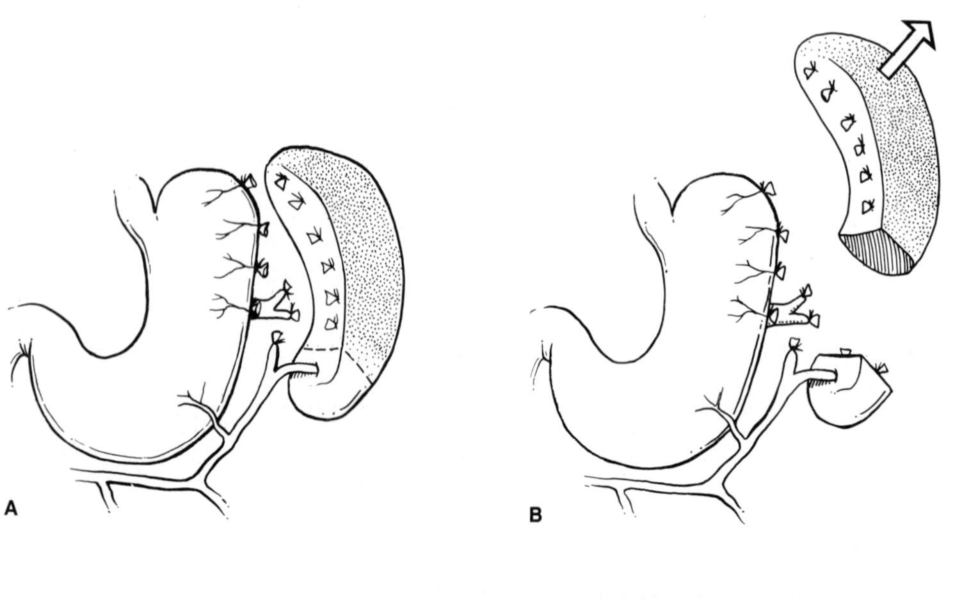

FIGURE 54-50. Surgical technique used for partial (about 80%) splenectomy. (**A**) All vascular pedicles supplying the spleen are divided except those arising from the left gastroepiploic vessels. (**B**) The upper pole of the spleen is removed at the boundary between the well perfused and poorly perfused tissue. (After Tchernia G, Gauthier F, Mielot F, et al. Initial assessment of the beneficial effect of partial splenectomy in hereditary spherocytosis. Blood 1993;81:2014)

days).[873] In all but the most severe cases, anemia and jaundice remit and do not recur.

Splenectomy Failure

The rare splenectomy failure (recurrence of hemolysis) is usually caused by an accessory spleen that was missed during surgery[1054,1055] or by another red cell disorder such as pyruvate kinase deficiency.[1056,1057] *Accessory spleens* occur in 15% to 40% of patients[988,1047,1058] and must always be sought. Recurrence of hemolytic anemia years[1055] or even decades[1054] after splenectomy should raise suspicion of an accessory spleen, particularly when Howell-Jolly bodies are no longer evident on peripheral blood smears. The absence of pitted red cells with crater-like surface indentations (readily seen by interference contrast microscopy) is also a sensitive measure of recrudescent splenic function.[1059,1060] The ectopic splenic tissue can be confirmed by a radiocolloid liver/spleen scan or a scan using ^{51}Cr-labeled, heated red cells.[1054,1061]

HEREDITARY ELLIPTOCYTOSIS

Hereditary elliptocytosis (HE) is a relatively common, clinically and genetically heterogenous disorder characterized by the presence of a large number of elliptically shaped red cells in the peripheral blood. In the more severe forms of the disease, spherocytes or bizarre-shaped poikilocytes are also present and sometimes predominate. Hereditary pyropoikilocytosis (HPP) is an example of the latter situation. Although HPP was previously considered a separate entity, emerging biochemical and genetic information clearly indicates that it is related to HE, so that the two disorders will be considered together.

History

According to Lambrecht,[1062] elliptocytosis was first observed in 1860 by Goltz in Königsburg, Germany, but no written report of this observation is known. The disease was first reported in 1904 by Dresbach,[1063] a physiologist at Ohio State University, in one of his histology students during a laboratory exercise in which the students were examining their own blood. His brief report elicited some controversy since the student died soon thereafter, leading the prominent American physician, Austin Flint, to suggest that he actually had incipient pernicious anemia.[1064] Dresbach replied that the student died of acute rheumatic carditis and took his slides to Germany where famous pathologists such as Ewing, Ehrlich, and Arneth supported his view that the red cell disorder was primary.[1065] This was substantiated during the next two decades by the reports of Bishop,[1066] Sydenstricker[1067] and Huck and Bigelow.[1068] Hunter's demonstration of elliptocytosis in three generations of one family firmly established the hereditary nature of the disease.[1069,1070]

In the 1930s and early 1940s, considerable debate occurred about whether HE was a disease or simply a morphologic curiosity. In retrospect, it is surprising since a number of persons with hemolytic HE were described during this interval,[1062,1071–1075] and some authors had clearly differentiated hemolytic and nonhemolytic forms.[1062,1071,1074] In fact as early as 1928, van den Bergh[1075] even reported that anemia and jaundice cleared up after splenectomy in one patient. Early on, some confusion also existed in differentiating HE from sickle cell anemia and thalassemia and later in differentiating hemolytic HE from HS.[1076] These reports illustrate a point that will be emphasized later—namely, that HE, particularly its hemolytic variants, can sometimes be morphologically deceptive.

For the reader interested in the historical aspects of the disease, the reports of Wyandt and coworkers,[1076] Wolman and Ozge,[1077] and Dacie[1078,1079] are recommended.

Prevalence and Genetics

Hereditary elliptocytosis is clearly heterogenous from a clinical, genetic, and biochemical point of view. This was not appreciated by early investigators, who lumped together all patients with HE. Accordingly, it is difficult to relate much of the available information to the different clinical forms of the disease. The incidence of all forms of HE in the United States is reported to be 1 in 2000 to 4000 persons,[1076,1080] but clinical experience suggests that for whites these early estimates may be too high. Elliptocytic red cells have been observed in all racial and ethnic groups, but the distribution of some of the clinical phenotypes is clearly restricted. Because of a selective pressure exerted by malaria, the prevalence of common HE in equatorial Africa approaches 1%.[1081] In certain ethnic groups of Southeast Asia and Melanesia where malaria is also endemic, the prevalence of Southeast Asian ovalocytosis (a type of HE) is as high as 30%.[764,766,1082] With the exception of HPP, HE is inherited as an autosomal dominant trait with complete penetrance.

Genetic studies show that one of the elliptocytosis genes (El1) is closely linked to the Rh locus on the short arm of chromosome 1 (1p36 to 1p34).[1083–1085] This is the location of the protein 4.1 gene.[651] Another gene (El2) is located on the long arm of chromosome 1, near the Duffy blood group locus (1q24)[1086] in the region where the spectrin α-chain gene is located (1q22 to 1q25).[342] The identification of numerous mutations in both proteins in HE confirms the linkage studies.

Clinical Syndromes

Most reported cases of HE can be classified into one of three clinical categories: common HE, spherocytic HE, or Southeast Asian ovalocytosis (Table 54-12). With the exception of the latter disorder, which is homogenous in molecular genetic terms (see section on Southeast Asian ovalocytosis), these appellations denote clinical phenotypes and not specific molecular etiologies, although correlations between the two exist. Numerous molecular defects in the membrane proteins of HE patients have been identified (see Table 54-6), and HE can also be classified based on these defects.

Common Hereditary Elliptocytosis

Common HE is, by far, the most prevalent form of HE. It is particularly common in African populations. In West Africa, the prevalence approaches 1%.[1081] Almost all of the African mutations involve α-spectrin. Common HE is at least 15 to 25 times less common in Western populations, where in some laboratories about 60% of the cases of HE are due to α-spectrin defects and about 40% are due to defects in protein 4.1.[140,142] Occasional patients with common HE lack GPC or have mutations in β-spectrin that affect the structure of the α chain.[656,704,705] The truncated β-spectrins, which are usually included among mutations causing common HE, are discussed in the section on spherocytic HE later in the chapter.

Heterozygous Common Hereditary Elliptocytosis

The clinical picture of common HE trait varies enormously, from the silent carrier state to moderately severe hemolytic HE. Several clinical patterns can be defined. It is important

TABLE 54-12. Clinical Subtypes of Hereditary Elliptocytosis (HE)

Clinical Manifestations	Laboratory Features
COMMON HE	
Asymptomatic Dominant inheritance: one parent with HE No splenomegaly Variants: Some neonates with moderately severe hemolytic anemia and hereditary pyropoikilocytosis–like smear; converts to typical mild HE by ≈1 y Some patients with mild to moderate chronic hemolysis, due either to coinheritance of low expression α-spectrin variant (α^{LELY}) or to coexistence of chronic disease producing splenomegaly, or to unknown factors	Blood smear: elliptocytes, rod forms, few or no poikilocytes No anemia, little or no hemolysis (reticulocytes = 1–3%) Normal osmotic fragility Usually defect in α-spectrin → decreased spectrin self-association, or to partial deficiency or dysfunction of protein 4.1; rarely due to lack of glycophorin C (which binds 4.1 to the membrane) or to defect in β-spectrin
HOMOZYGOUS COMMON HE AND HEREDITARY PYROPOIKILOCYTOSIS	
Moderate to severe hemolytic anemia Splenomegaly Intermittent jaundice Aplastic crises Recessive inheritance: typically one parent with HE and one with α^{LELY} or both parents with HE Good improvement following splenectomy	Blood smear: bizarre poikilocytes, fragments, ± spherocytes, ± elliptocytes Reticulocytosis; decreased mean corupscular volume due to red cell fragmentation; increased osmotic fragility α-Spectrin defects: Decreased red cell heat stability Marked defect in spectrin self-association In most severe variants, partial spectrin deficiency (indicated by more spherocytes on the blood smear)
SPHEROCYTIC HE	
Mild to moderate hemolytic anemia Splenomegaly Intermittent jaundice Aplastic crises Dominant inheritance pattern Excellent response to splenectomy	Blood smear: rounded elliptocytes, ± spherocytes; may see variable morphology within a kindred; reticulocytosis; increased osmotic fragility; glucose-responsive autohemolysis Primary defect uncertain. Patients with C-terminal tRunctions of β-spectrin have similar clinical picture
SOUTHEAST ASIAN OVALOCYTOSIS	
Asymptomatic Dominant inheritance Lowland aboriginal tribes, especially in Melanesia and Malaysia Very rigid red cells that resist invasion by malarial parasites	Blood smear: rounded elliptocytes, some with a transverse bar that divides the central clear space Little or no anemia or hemolysis Normal osmotic fragility Mutant band 3 that lacks anion exchange function and shows increased interactions with membrane skeleton → rigid membrane

to emphasize that *different members of the same family may exhibit different clinical patterns and even the pattern of same person can vary with time.* The clinical patterns are probably more useful for illustrating the spectrum of common HE than for classifying the disease.

Silent Carrier State. The silent carrier was identified by analyzing asymptomatic members of kindreds with HE or HPP. The affected persons have normal red cell shape and no evidence of hemolysis, but careful measurements show a subtle defect in their membrane skeletons, with decreased red cell thermal stability, decreased mechanical stability of isolated skeletons, an increased fraction of spectrin dimers in 0°C spectrin extracts, abnormal tryptic peptide maps of spectrin, and various combinations of these defects.[656,671,672,1087–1091] (Tests will be discussed in more detail in a later section.) Some patients classified as silent carriers have the same molecular defect as patients with mild common HE.[1088–1091] This underscores the natural variability of these mutations.

More commonly, the silent carrier state is associated with a low-expression α-spectrin allele, α^{LELY} or $\alpha^{V/41}$.[789,790] This common allele contains a mutation within a nucleation site of α-spectrin that diminishes the propensity of Sp α^{LELY} to associate, side by side, with β-spectrin. When present *in trans* with an α-spectrin mutant that causes HE, incorporation of the HE α chain into spectrin αβ heterodimers is favored, leading to an increased proportion of the elliptocytogenic spectrin in the cells and consequently more severe hemolytic disease. The α^{LELY} locus is clinically silent by itself, even when homozygous, but it greatly augments the effects of the *trans* allele and plays a major role in the clinical expression of HE.

Mild Common HE. The most common clinical form of HE is mild common HE.[311,407,661,663,673,678,681,685,737,739,741,1076,1092–1097] Patients are asymptomatic, and HE is often discovered by accident when a blood smear is examined. They have no anemia and no splenomegaly, except for an occasional "spleen tip" (see Table 54-12). Red cell survival may be normal,[1096] but more often there is mild compensated hemolysis with a slight reticulocytosis and a decreased haptoglobin level.[665,678,737,1076,1094,1095] In persons with common HE, the condition is hardly more than a morphologic curiosity.

The peripheral blood smear shows prominent elliptocytosis with little red cell budding or fragmentation and no spherocytosis. Elliptocytes exceed 10% of the red cells by definition and usually exceed 30% (see Fig. 54-45, *panel 6*).[665,1076,1090–1092,1094] In some patients, they reach 100%. In contrast, normal persons have less than 2% to 5% elliptocytes.[665,1090,1091] Slightly higher proportions are seen in patients with anemia, particularly megaloblastic anemias, hypochromic-microcytic anemias, myelodysplastic syndromes,[1098] and myelofibrosis, but even in these persons, elliptocytes do not exceed 35%.[1092]

Common Hereditary Elliptocytosis With Chronic Hemolysis. More severe variants of common HE occur frequently, even within a kindred.[666,670,672,678,685,703] In general, the hemolysis is accompanied by evidence of membrane instability on the peripheral blood smear: budding red cells, fragments, and other bizarre-shaped poikilocytes.

In patients with α-spectrin mutations, significant hemolysis is usually due to coinheritance of the α^{LELY} allele and one of the more deleterious HE alleles[664,681,694,696,789] (see Table 54-12). Of the common mutations (discussed in the later section on α-spectrin defects). Sp $\alpha^{I/74}$ is more severe than Sp $\alpha^{I/46}$ and much more severe than Sp $\alpha^{I/65}$.[142,1099] Patients with $\alpha^{LELY}/\alpha^{I/74}$ have marked hemolysis and elliptopoikilocytosis compared with their $\alpha/\alpha^{I/74}$ siblings, whereas patients with $\alpha^{LELY}/\alpha^{I/65}$ have more elliptocytes than their $\alpha/\alpha^{I/65}$ siblings but no significant hemolysis.[789]

Less often, hemolysis is caused by inheritance of a mutant spectrin that is grossly dysfunctional.[666] This is indicated by dominant transmission of the hemolytic syndrome and by an unusually high fraction of spectrin dimers in 0°C spectrin extracts.

Common Hereditary Elliptocytosis With Sporadic Hemolysis. Patients with common HE may also develop uncompensated hemolysis in response to stimuli that cause hyperplasia of the reticuloendothelial system, particularly when the spleen is involved. Examples include viral hepatitis,[1097] cirrhosis,[1100] infectious mononucleosis,[1095] bacterial infections,[1095] and malaria.[1101,1102] Hemolysis has also been observed with thrombotic thrombocytopenic purpura[1103] and during a renal transplant rejection complicated by DIC,[1103] which suggests that elliptocytes may be especially susceptible to microangiopathic damage. For unknown reasons, pregnancy and vitamin B_{12} deficiency[1104] may also transiently aggravate the disease.[1095]

Neonatal Poikilocytosis. Infants with mild common HE often begin life with moderately severe hemolytic anemia, characterized by marked red cell budding, fragmentation, and poikilocytosis (see Table 54-12) and by neonatal jaundice, which may require an exchange transfusion.[523,663,665,670,685,702,1105–1108] In most cases, enough elliptocytes are present to suggest the diagnosis, but sometimes this is not so and the disorder is mistaken for sepsis, infantile pyknocytosis, or a microangiopathic or oxidant-induced hemolytic anemia.[1105,1106] Neonatal HE can easily be distinguished from these conditions if the parents' smears are examined, since one will have common HE, typically because of a defect in α- or β-spectrin that affects spectrin self-association. It is more difficult to distinguish HE with neonatal poikilocytosis from HPP.

Most α-spectrin variants have been associated with the neonatal poikilocytosis syndrome, but not all neonates are affected.[670,1109] The factors that determine susceptibility are unknown. With time, fragmentation and hemolysis decline, and the clinical picture of mild common HE emerges. This transition requires from 4 months to 2 years. Subsequently, the disease is clinically indistinguishable from typical mild common HE. The prevalence is unknown, but it is not rare.

The fragmenting neonatal red cells are sensitive to heat like hereditary pyropoikilocytes, but, unlike pyropoikilocytes, this sensitivity decreases as the patients mature.[1108] During the conversion, the poikilocytic red cells are dense and rich in hemoglobin F, whereas the smooth elliptocytes are light and enriched in hemoglobin A.[247] This suggests the change in the disease corresponds to the change from fetal to adult erythropoiesis. No variations in the primary α-spectrin defect or its functional effects on spectrin self-association occur during the conversion,[665] so that other skeletal interactions must differ in fetal and adult red cells. Mentzer and colleagues[523] has made the interesting suggestion that 2,3-DPG is the critical agent. Free 2,3-DPG is elevated in fetal red cells, since it is not bound by hemoglobin F. The free anion is known to weaken spectrin–actin–4.1 interactions[522,524,525] and to increase the fragility of isolated ghosts at physiologic concentrations,[523] but it is controversial whether it does so in intact red cells.[526,527] If so, this would certainly aggravate the underlying defect in spectrin self-association.

Common Hereditary Elliptocytosis With Dyserythropoiesis. In a small number of families with otherwise typical common HE, the sporadic occurrence of hemolysis and anemia is at least partially due to the development of dysplastic and ineffective erythropoiesis. All the patients reported with this rare syndrome are from Italy, have less elongated red cells than is typical for common HE, and show the characteristic findings of ineffective erythropoiesis (relatively low reticulocyte counts, indirect hyperbilirubinemia, high serum iron and ferritin, and rapid clearance of ^{59}Fe combined with poor incorporation of ^{59}Fe into new erythrocytes).[1110,1111] Some patients are macrocytic. Others have a few spherocytes, but these probably are an artifact, since osmotic fragility tests are normal.[1111] The patient's bone marrows are hyperplastic, with decreased late erythroblasts and dysplastic features (asynchrony of nuclear cytoplasmic maturation, binuclearity, internuclear bridges, and small numbers of ringed sideroblasts).[1110,1111] Anemia and presumably erythroid dysplasia usually commence during adolescence or early adult life and advance gradually over years. Because dysplasia persists after splenectomy, response to the operation is incomplete.

The available data suggest that dysplasia and elliptocytosis cosegregate, since all persons who were observed to have dysplasia also had elliptocytosis.[1110,1111] If so, these families must represent a unique subtype of common HE. This is supported by the fact that none of the typical HE protein defects were observed in one well-studied family.[1111] Spectrin self-association, spectrin peptide maps, and the concentration of protein 4.1 and other major membrane proteins were normal.

Homozygous Common Hereditary Elliptocytosis

A number of patients who are homozygotes or compound heterozygotes for common HE have been reported.[140,407,665,667,680,690,699,701,736,1076,1099,1112–1118] Some have had a severe or even fatal[1117] transfusion-dependent hemolytic anemia (hemoglobin, 2 to 6 g/dL) with marked fragmentation, poikilocytosis, spherocytosis, and elliptocytosis (see Table 54-11, Fig. 54-45, *panel 7*). In others, hemolysis was less rampant (hemoglobin, 7 to 11 g/dL). These differences appear to reflect variations in the severity of the many α-spectrin mutations that produce common HE[665,668,1099] (see Table 54-6). Clinically, the disease resembles HPP,[665,690] except for the mildest forms. All treated patients have responded dramatically to splenectomy.

Hereditary Pyropoikilocytosis

Hereditary pyropoikilocytosis is an interesting, rare recessive disease, which presents in infancy or early childhood as a severe hemolytic anemia (hemoglobin, 4 to 8 g/dL)[665] characterized by extreme poikilocytosis with budding red cells, fragments, spherocytes, triangulocytes, and other bizarre-shaped cells[1088,1119–1121] and, in some cases, with few or no elliptocytes (see Fig. 54-45, *panel 8*, and Table 54-11). The morphology is similar to that observed in patients with homozygous common HE and common HE with neonatal poikilocytosis. Most cases have occurred in blacks.[668,675,703,1122]

Patients typically present with hyperbilirubinemia in the neonatal period or with anemia in the first few months of life.[1123] The anemia is characterized by splenomegaly, red cell fragmentation, and erythroblastosis.[1123] Complications of severe anemia including growth retardation, frontal bossing, and early gallbladder disease are reported.[1120,1121] Osmotic fragility tests are abnormal, particularly after incubation,[407,680,1119–1121] and autohemolysis is greatly elevated.[1119–1121] The MCV is low (25 to 75 $\mu m)^3$ because of the large number of fragmented red cells.[665,1089–1091,1119,1120] Another characteristic feature of these cells is their remarkable thermal sensitivity. Hereditary pyropoikilocytes fragment at 45° to 46°C (normal is 49°C) after short periods of heating (10 to 15 minutes).[1121] After splenectomy, hemolysis is greatly decreased but not eliminated.[1120,1121] Typically, the hemoglobin after splenectomy is 10 to 14 g/dL with 3% to 10% reticulocytes.[665]

Although HPP was initially considered a separate disease, evidence is convincing that it is related to HE. As already noted, HPP is clinically and morphologically similar to the more severe forms of hemolytic elliptocytosis. In addition, often a parent or sibling has typical mild common HE, and in some of these kindreds an identical molecular defect is observed in siblings with phenotypically different diseases (HPP and common HE). In other families, all the first-degree relatives are phenotypically normal.

Hereditary pyropoikilocyte red cells, but not hereditary elliptocytes, are partially deficient in spectrin, as evidenced by a decreased spectrin/band 3 ratio.[538,665,1124] Typically, one parent of the HPP offspring carries an α-spectrin mutation, whereas the other parent is fully asymptomatic with no detectable biochemical abnormality. Studies of spectrin synthesis and mRNA levels reveal that such asymptomatic parents carry a silent "thalassemia-like" defect of spectrin synthesis.[538] When coinherited with the elliptocytogenic spectrin mutation in the HPP offspring, this thalassemia-like defect enhances the expression of the mutant spectrin in the cells and leads to a superimposed spectrin deficiency. The spectrin deficiency is thought to be responsible for the large number of spherocytes and relative paucity of elliptocytes in some HPP blood smears (see Fig. 54-45, *panel 8*).

Spherocytic Hereditary Elliptocytosis

Spherocytic HE is a dominant disorder, which is a phenotypic hybrid of common HE and HS. Reported only in white families of European descent, it is not linked to the Rh gene and appears to be a unique subtype[1071,1095,1125–1128] (see Table 54- 11). Its prevalence is unknown, but, judging from the number of published reports and our own experience, it is relatively rare, probably accounting for no more than 5% to 10% of HE in patients of European ancestry. Unlike mild common HE, almost all affected patients have some hemolysis. This is usually mild to moderate and often incompletely compensated. The elliptocytes are fewer and plumper than those in mild common HE, and some spherocytes, microspherocytes, and microelliptocytes are usually present (see Fig. 54-45, *panel 5*). Poikilocytes and red cell fragments are uncommon, which distinguishes spherocytic HE from common HE with hemolysis. Red cell morphology may vary, even within the same family. Some family members may have relatively prominent spherocytes and as few as 10% to 20% elliptocytes, whereas others have mostly elliptocytes and very few spherocytes.[484,1071,1125] This may cause diagnostic confusion initially, particularly when the propositus has few elliptocytes. Family studies almost always reveal some members with obvious elliptocytosis.

Like HS red cells, spherocytic elliptocytes are osmotically fragile, particularly after incubation.[484,1125,1127,1128] Excessive mechanical fragility and increased autohemolysis that responds to glucose are also characteristic.[1125,1127,1128] Gallbladder disease is common,[1125,1127] and aplastic crises are a risk. The splenic pathology also mimics that of HS.[1129,1130] Splenic sequestration is evident, red cells are conditioned during splenic passage, and hemolysis abates after splenectomy.[1125,1127,1128,1130]

The molecular pathology of classic spherocytic HE is unknown. Patients with C-terminal truncations of β-spectrin have many of the clinical features of spherocytic HE and perhaps should be recognized as an example of the disorder.[706–710,712–715,1131] Seven such truncations have been identified (see Table 54-6). Affected patients typically have moderate hemolysis and anemia, punctuated by recurrent, severe hemolytic crises.[707,708,712] Blood smears show plump and usually smooth elliptocytes,[707,708,710,1131] although in two patients poikilocytosis was prominent.[712,714] In all but one instance,[707] the hereditary elliptocyte red cells were mildly heat sensitive. All patients with C-terminal truncations of β-spectrin have a positive osmotic fragility test or an osmotic gradient ektacytometry pattern that resembles the pattern in HS, and one patient also had a positive acidified glycerol lysis test.[708] Like HS, the spleen is enlarged and selectively destroys labeled elliptocytes[714] ($T_{1/2}$ of 11 days [normal is 24 to 34 days]), and splenectomy is effective.

Patients who lack GPC (see section on deficiency of glycophorins C and D) also have positive osmotic fragility tests and rounded, smooth elliptocytes.[310,751,752] They should probably also be classified as having a recessive (and unusually mild) variant of spherocytic HE.

Patients who lack protein 4.2 (another recessive condition) sometimes display features of spherocytic HE, such as ovalostomatocytosis.[747,748,504] Protein 4.2 deficiency more often resembles HS, morphologically and pathophysiologically, and is better classified as a variant of that disorder.

Rare patients appear to be compound heterozygotes for HS and HE. One Turkish girl is a particularly good example.[1132] Her mother and father had mild HS and mild common HE (probably), respectively, whereas she suffered from a moderately severe hemolytic anemia (Hb 8.4, reticulocytes 24%, bilirubin 1.6 mg/dL) with frontal bossing, osteoporosis, splenomegaly (10 cm), and a mixture of microspherocytes and rounded elliptocytes.

Etiology

Methods to Define Abnormal Spectrin Structure and Function in Hereditary Elliptocytosis

Thermal Sensitivity of Red Cells and Spectrin. Red cells heated to temperatures approaching 50°C for short periods of time become unstable and fragment spontaneously,[1133–1135] probably owing to denaturation of spectrin.[1136] Normal spectrin denatures at 49°C (10-minute exposure),[559,1136] and normal red cells fragment at the same temperature.[559,778,1121] As noted previously, all patients with HPP (by definition) and some patients with other forms of HE have thermally sensitive red cells. Hereditary pyropoikilocytes and red cells from infants with common HE and neonatal poikilocytosis fragment after 10 minutes at 44° to 46°C.[1108,1121] Red cells from some patients with common HE fragment at 47° to 48°C.[559,1121] As expected, purified spectrin from these red cells is also heat sensitive.[559,1136] This test is limited because we do not understand, in molecular terms, why specific mutations are thermally sensitive. Nevertheless, it remains one of the simplest tests available for assessing HPP in laboratories that do not specialize in membrane protein analysis.

Abnormal Spectrin Oligomerization. Many patients with HE and all patients with HPP are unable to properly convert spectrin dimers to tetramers and higher oligomers in vitro or on the membrane (Fig. 54-51). This important functional property is easily assessed in low temperature spectrin extracts. At 0°C, the equilibrium between spectrin dimer and tetramer is greatly slowed—virtually frozen.[389] When spectrin is extracted from the membrane at 0°C and carefully protected from warming during separation of dimers, tetramers, and oligomers (usually on nondenaturing polyacrylamide gels), the proportion of each spectrin species reflects its relative proportion on the membrane.[330] Patients with defects in spectrin self-association have abnormally high percentages of spectrin dimer in 0°C spectrin extracts (over 10% of total spectrin dimers and tetramers).[672,1137,1138] *The fraction of spectrin dimers is an important functional assessment in patients with α-spectrin defects.* It correlates well with clinical severity[1099] and accurately predicts unusually severe mutations.[666] Conversely, discordance between the degree of hemolysis and the percentage of spectrin dimers may alert the physician to an underlying secondary complication (see previous section on common HE with hemolysis).

Ektacytometry. The ektacytometer can be used to assess red cell membrane deformability and stability in patients with hemolytic disorders.[1139,1140] Isolated red cell ghosts are subjected to a high shear stress in a laser dif-

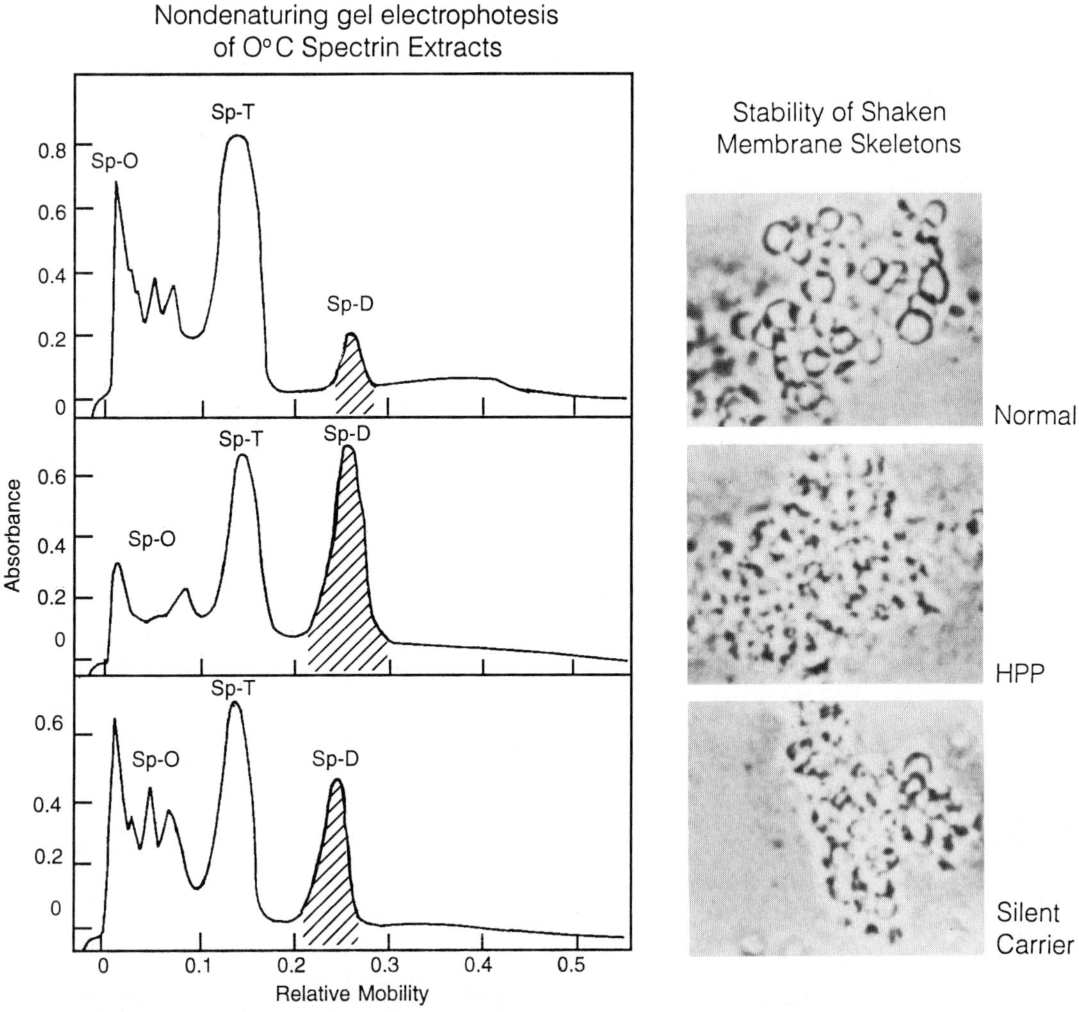

FIGURE 54-51. Increased spectrin dimers and membrane fragility in hereditary elliptocytosis and hereditary pyropoikilocytosis (HPP). (*Left*) Analysis of spectrin dimers (Sp-D), tetramers (Sp-T), and oligomers (Sp-O) by nondenaturing gel electrophoresis in a normal individual, a patient with HPP, and his mother, a silent carrier. The densitometric tracing of the scanned gel is shown. (*Right*) Membrane skeletons from each of the three persons were shaken for 1 hour and examined microscopically. The fraction of spectrin dimers is increased in the HPP patient (about 50%) and his asymptomatic mother (about 30%) compared with normal (8% ± 3%). The membrane skeletons of the patient, and to a lesser extent his mother, are fragile and disintegrate with shaking, whereas normal skeletons remain intact. (After Liu S-C, Palek J, Prchal J, Castlebury RP. Altered spectrin dimer–dimer associations and instability of erythrocyte membrane skeletons in hereditary pyropoikilocytosis. J Clin Invest 1981;68:597)

fraction viscometer, and the *deformability index* (a measure of the average elongation of the sheared ghosts) is recorded as a function of time. Fragile ghosts fragment more quickly than normal, causing their deformability to fall (Fig. 54-52). The technique is a useful screening test, since membrane stability is reduced in almost all membrane skeletal diseases.

In addition, the ektacytometer can be modified to measure cellular deformability at different osmolalities, a technique termed *osmotic gradient ektacytometry*.[657] The resulting curves are dependent on both membrane surface area and cell volume and are a sensitive measure of the surface loss that characterizes many skeletal defects.

Two-Dimensional Spectrin Domain Maps. Spectrin structure is conveniently analyzed by domain mapping[327,363]—limited tryptic digestion, performed at 0°C, followed by one-dimensional (SDS polyacrylamide gel electrophoresis [SDS-PAGE]) or two-dimensional separation (isoelectric focusing, then SDS-PAGE) of the resulting trypsin-resistant domains. A two-dimensional separation of normal spectrin domains is shown in Figure 54-14. The gels are stained with Coomassie blue, and characteristic, reproducible maps are obtained. Among these peptides, the 80-kd αI domain peptide, which contains the self-association site of normal α-spectrin, is the most prominent. Almost all α- or β-spectrin mutations reported are associated with tryptic peptides of abnormal size and mobility that are generated instead of the normal 80-kd peptide. One-dimensional "fingerprints" of domains from patients with various kinds of HE are shown in Figure 54-53. The cleavage sites of the most common abnormal tryptic peptides are located in the third helix of the triple helical spectrin repeats.[143] The reported mutations reside in the vicinity of these cleavage sites either in the same helix or, less commonly, at neighboring sites in helix 1 or 2[143] (Fig. 54-54).

Consequently, tryptic peptide mapping remains a powerful tool to map the approximate sites of the underlying spectrin mutations; the mutations can subsequently be defined by polymerase chain reaction (PCR) amplification and sequencing of the respective region of the cDNA or genomic DNA.

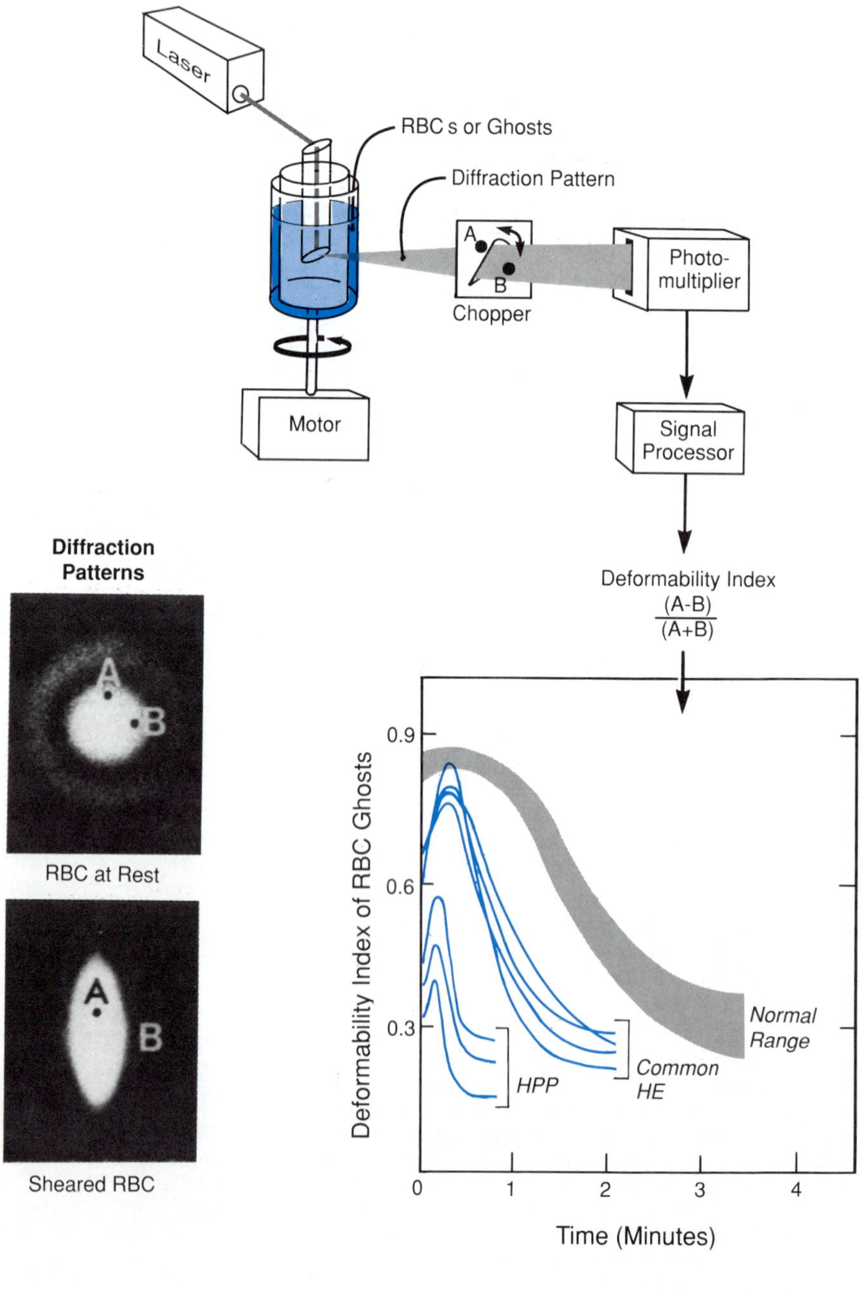

FIGURE 54-52. Membrane fragility of hereditary elliptocytosis (HE) red cells measured with the ektacytometer. The ektacytometer combines a concentric cylinder viscometer with a laser diffractometer. The outer cylinder of the viscometer is spun to produce a uniform shear stress. The laser beam is diffracted by the red cells or ghosts in the sample, and the resulting diffraction patterns are analyzed to give information about the deformation of the sheared cells. In the typical system, the intensity of the laser light is alternately sampled, using a chopper, at two points, A and B, which lie just inside the edge of the resting diffraction pattern. A signal processor converts this information into a *deformability index*, defined as (A − B)/(A + B), which is a measure of the elliptical shape of the sheared cells. To measure membrane stability, ghosts are subjected to a high shear stress (575 dynes/cm^2 in the experiment shown), and the deformability index is determined as a function of time. The deformability index falls as the ghosts fragment, since the fragments have a smaller surface/volume ratio (ie, they are more spheroidal) than the original ghosts. This occurs more rapidly than normally in the fragile HE and hereditary pyropoikilocytosis red cells. In general, ektacytometry is a powerful screening test, since membrane stability is reduced in almost all membrane skeletal disorders. (After Mohandas N, Clark MR, Heath BO, et al. A technique to detect reduced mechanical stability of red cell membranes: relevance to elliptocytic disorders. Blood 1982;59:768; Mohandas N, Clark MR, Jacods MS, Shohet SB. Analysis of factors regulating erythrocyte deformability. J Clin Invest 1980;66:563)

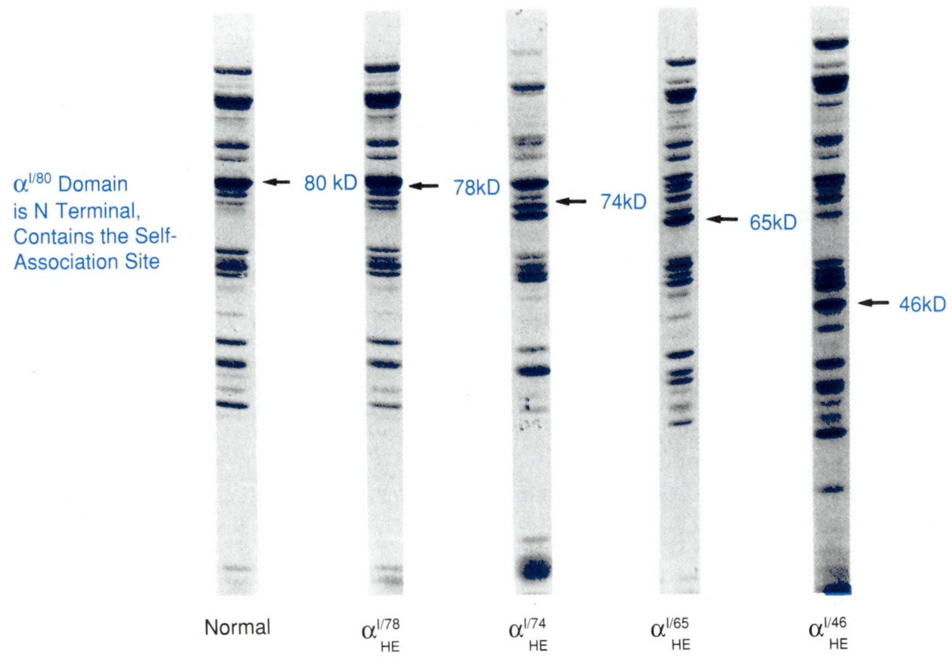

FIGURE 54-53. Spectrin domains in hereditary elliptocytosis. One-dimensional peptide maps of partial tryptic digests of normal spectrin (*left*). The tryptic digestion releases an 80-kd peptide from the N terminal of the normal α chain. In the $\alpha^{I/78}$, $\alpha^{I/74}$, $\alpha^{I/65}$, and $\alpha^{I/46}$ mutant α-spectrins, the 80-kd domain is degraded to smaller peptides (*arrows*) by trypsin because of local conformational changes produced by the mutations. (Delaunay J, Dhermy D. Mutations involving the spectrin heterodimer contact site: clinical expression and alterations in specific function. Semin Hematol 1993;30:21)

DNA Sequencing. Reticulocyte mRNA is first isolated from patients with HE. Reverse transcription and PCR are performed, using specific primers flanking the region suspected to contain the mutation. The cDNA product is subjected to nucleic acid sequencing or other forms of analysis (see Chap. 4). For heterozygotes several independent subclones must be sequenced, since, on average, only 50% will have the mutant allele.

Many individual variations of this technique have been used to identify the mutations described in the following sections. For example, genomic DNA can be substituted for mRNA when intron–exon boundaries are known, and screening techniques can be used to identify the PCR-amplified DNA fragments that should be sequenced. This is particularly advantageous with large proteins, such as spectrin and ankyrin. The SSCP (*Single Strand Conformation Polymorphism*) method[1142,1143] is a simple, sensitive, and appropriately popular example of such a screening test. DNA fragments (200 to 600 bp) are denatured, and the single strands are refolded before running on a nondenaturing gel. Even a single nucleotide change usually alters the folding pattern enough to allow mutant and normal fragments to separate on the gel (about 70% to 90% of mutations). Abnormal fragments are subcloned and sequenced.

α-Spectrin Defects: General Concepts*

Defects in the αI Domain Impair Spectin Self-Association. Defects of spectrin self-association are found in many patients with common HE and in all patients with HPP. Most of the defects lie in the 80-kd αI domain at the

* The nomenclature for α-spectrin defects includes an abbreviation for spectrin (Sp) followed by a superscript designation of the α-spectrin domain that is altered in tryptic peptide maps (α^{I} to α^{V}) and the size of the largest tryptic peptide that is generated from the mutant domain.[1089] Thus, Sp $\alpha^{I/65}$ indicates that the α^{I} domain (80 kd) is affected and that a 65-kd peptide is generated by tryptic cleavage instead of the usual 80-kd peptide.

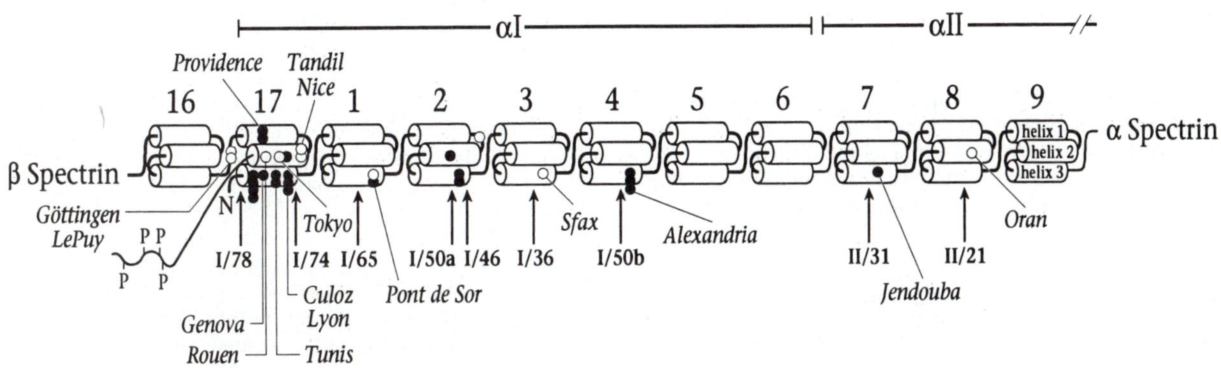

FIGURE 54-54. Spectrin defects in hereditary elliptocytosis. The location of amino acid substitutions (*closed circles*) and insertions, deletions, or truncations (*open circles*) are shown. The tryptic cleavage sites that characterize α-spectrin defects are also indicated. Most defects are close to the site of spectrin self-association. Most α-chain mutations are in helix C (helix 3); less often helix A (helix 1) or helix B (helix 2) are involved. Most β-chain defects are C-terminal truncations. (Becker PS, Lux SE. Disorders of the red cell membrane skeleton: hereditary spherocytosis and hereditary elliptocytosis. In: Scriver CS, Beaudet AL, Sly WS, Valle D, eds. The metabolic basis of inherited disease, ed 7. New York, McGraw-Hill, in press)

N-terminal end of the α-spectrin chain (see Fig. 54-11). Nine tryptic cleavage defects of the αI domain have been identified by peptide mapping (see Table 54-6 and Figs. 54-53 and 54-54). These are characterized by loss of the normal 80-kd αI peptide and the appearance of one of the following:

- A new 78-kd peptide ($\alpha^{I/78}$)
- A new 74-kd peptide ($\alpha^{I/74}$)
- A new 65- or 68-kd peptide ($\alpha^{I/65}$ or $\alpha^{I/68}$)
- A new 61-kd peptide ($\alpha^{I/61}$)
- A new 46-kd peptide ($\alpha^{I/46}$)
- A new 50-kd (or 46-kd) peptide ($\alpha^{I/50a}$ or $\alpha^{I/46-50a}$)
- A new 50-kd peptide with a more basic isoelectric point than $\alpha^{I/50a}$ ($\alpha^{I/50b}$)
- Two new peptides of 43 and 42 kd ($\alpha^{I/43}$)
- Two new peptides of 36 and 33 kd ($\alpha^{I/36}$)

The clinical expression and other characteristics of the variants are shown in Table 54-6.

All αI and αII domain defects produce a similar functional deficit: diminished spectrin self-association, reflected in an increased proportion of spectrin dimers in 0°C low ionic strength extracts of spectrin (see Fig. 54-51), and decreased conversion of spectrin dimers (S_D) to tetramers (S_T) in solution, in ghosts, and on inside-out vesicles. In addition, all patients show decreased red cell thermal stability. The fragile spectrin–spectrin links weaken the membrane skeleton and diminish the resistance of the isolated membrane or skeleton to shear stress[134,523,702,1088,1140] (see Fig. 54-52). This results in a stiff membrane (elevated elastic shear modulus)[1146] rather than a lax one.

More Distant Defects Are Usually Milder. Two defects in the αII domain have also been discovered by peptide mapping, Sp Jendouba ($\alpha^{II/31}$) and Sp Oran ($\alpha^{II/21}$),[698–700] but they have only a feeble effect on the distant self-association process and are mild (see Table 54-6). This illustrates a useful, although inexact, rule: that the severity of a mutation is inversely proportional to its distance from the site of self-association. Two exceptions are notable: Sp $\alpha^{I/65}$ is unusually mild given its relative proximity, and Sp $\alpha^{I/50a}$ and $\alpha^{I/50b}$ are unusually severe.

Most α-Spectrin Defects Occur in Helix C. The precise mutations responsible for HE have been identified in most of these variants. Their positions are shown in Figure 54-54. Curiously, a large number of the mutations occur in helix C of each spectrin repeat, near the C-terminal end of the helix. Why spectrin self-association is particularly sensitive to mutations in this location is a mystery.

Severity of Defect Depends on Amount of Spectrin and Its Effect on Self-Association. In general patients with spectrin defects in the αI or αII domains have common HE (or HPP). The severity of a particular mutation correlates especially with the degree of impairment of spectrin self-association. Electron micrographs of negatively stained red cell membrane skeletons from patients with various α-spectrin mutations corroborate this association[132,552,665] (Fig. 54-55). Severity is also affected by the *amount* of the mutant spectrin, which is strongly influenced by the recently identified Sp α^{LELY} polymorphism.

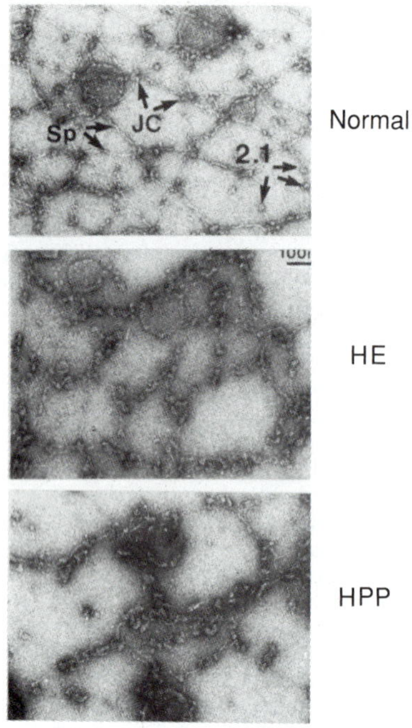

FIGURE 54-55. Electron micrographs of negative-stained membrane skeletons from normal, hereditary elliptocytosis (HE), and hereditary pyropoikilocytosis (HPP) red cells. The regular structure of the normal skeleton is moderately disrupted in the HE skeleton and severely damaged in HPP. JC, junctional complexes; Sp, spectrin tetramers; 2.1, ankyrin molecules. (Liu S-C, Derick LH. Molecular anatomy of the red blood cell membrane skeleton: structure–function relationships. Semin Hematol 1992;29:231)

Spectrin α^{LELY} (or $\alpha^{V/41}$) Polymorphism

Differences in clinical expression are at least partially due to the presence or absence of the Sp α^{LELY} polymorphism on the "normal" spectrin allele, that is, *in trans* to α-spectrin mutations that cause HE.[789] This polymorphism is common, affecting about 30% of the α-spectrin alleles of European whites and 20% of the alleles of Japanese and African blacks.[789,1147] This means that about 42% of the European white population is heterozygous for Sp α^{LELY} and 9% is homozygous. (The comparable figures in Japan and Africa are 32% and 4%.) The exceptional prevalence of the polymorphism suggests it may be experiencing genetic selection. If so, its advantage is unclear.

Recent work shows that Sp α^{LELY} (low-expression allele from Lyon, France) is actually a combination of two linked mutations: one in exon 40 and one in intron 45.[790] The effect of each is shown in Figure 54-56. Exon 40 contributes a point mutation in helix B of α-spectrin repeat 18 that converts Leu 1857 → Val. When folded according to the crystallographic model (see Fig. 54-13), this valine lies next to the tryptic site (Lys 1920) that is cleaved to generate the αIV and αV domains. This results in more rapid cleavage of the αIV to αV junction and an increased concentration of the 41-kd αV domain, the so-called $\alpha^{V/41}$ polymorphism (see Fig. 54-56).

The linked defect is responsible for low expression. It is a C → T substitution at position −12 in the 3′ (acceptor) splice site of intron 45, and it interferes with the splicing of the neighboring exon 46 so that 50% of the resulting RNAs and proteins contain exon 46 and 50% do not[790] (see Fig. 54-56). Exon 46 is small—only six amino acids[652]—so its absence is not evident on SDS gels. It lies in the middle of the site that nucleates assembly of the spectrin α- and β-subunits.[364] Presumably, α chains that lack exon 46 fail to assemble into stable spectrin dimers and are degraded.

The polymorphism is completely silent by itself, even when homozygous, probably because α-spectrin is normally synthesized in a three- or four-fold excess.[536] When Sp α^{LELY} is inherited *in trans* to an α-spectrin mutation, it has the effect of increasing the concentration of the mutant spectrin and the severity of the associated disease[789] (Fig. 54-57). The effect can be dramatic. For example, in one family a patient who was heterozygous for the $\alpha^{I/74}$ mutation ($\alpha^{I/74}/\alpha$) had mild disease and almost no morphologic abnormality, whereas a relative who had also inherited the

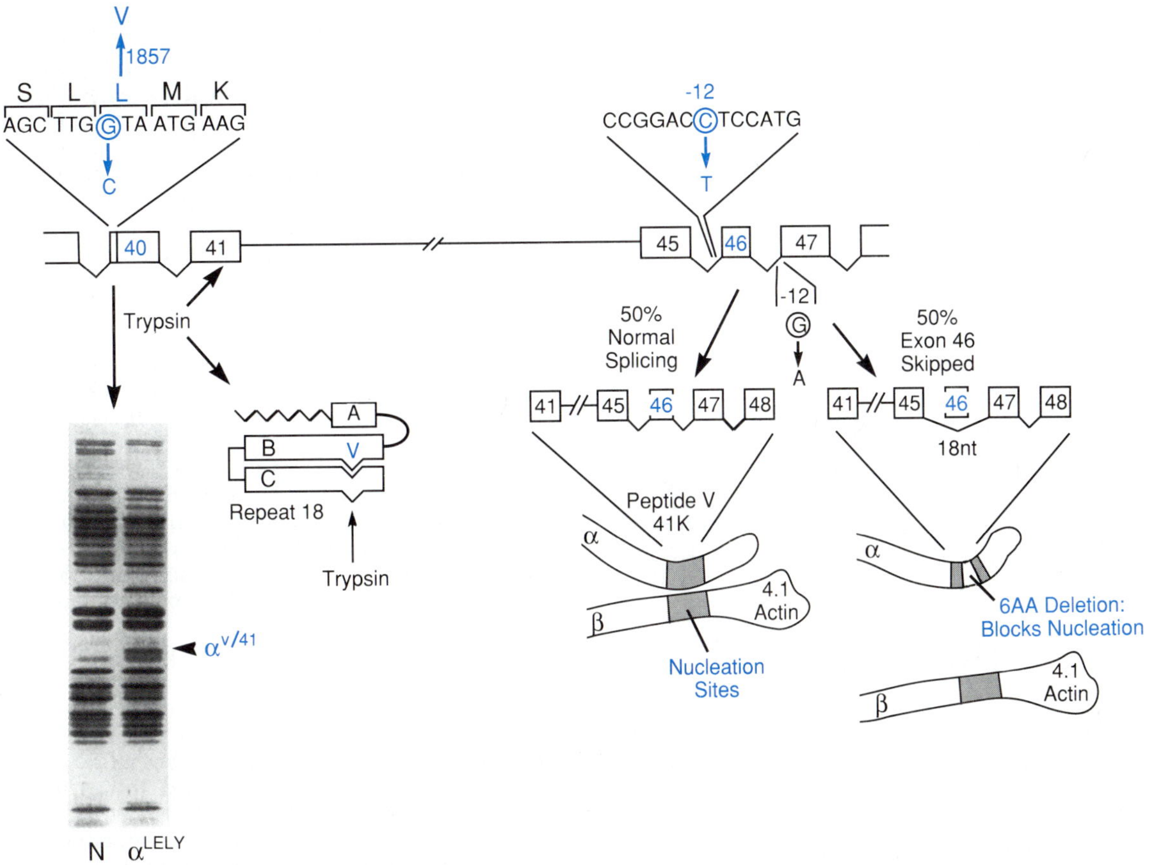

FIGURE 54-56. Nature of the low-expression α^{LELY} allele. The allele contains two linked mutations[790]—a marker mutation, the $\alpha^{V/41}$ defect, and a splicing mutation, the α^{LELY} defect. (*Left*) The $\alpha^{V/41}$ defect is caused by a G → C substitution at the beginning of exon 40, which changes Leu 1857 to Val in helix B of spectrin repeat 18. The valine impinges on the neighboring helix C of the repeat and makes it more trypsin sensitive, leading to a more rapid release of the $\alpha^{V/41}$ peptide from trypsin-treated spectrin derived from the α^{LELY} allele. SDS gels of trypsin-treated normal spectrin and α^{LELY}-containing spectrin are also shown. The $\alpha^{V/41}$ peptide is marked. (*Right*) The linked splicing mutation is a C → T substitution at position −12 in the acceptor splice site of intron 45 (a second linked mutation, G → A, at position −12 of intron 46 may also contribute). This causes exon 46 to be skipped in 50% of α^{LELY} spectrin (*far right*). Exon 46 is very small, only 6 amino acids, but it lies in the center of the nucleation site required for side-to-side association of the spectrin α and β chains. It is likely that the half of α^{LELY} spectrin that lacks exon 46 cannot form spectrin heterodimers and is destroyed. The other 50% of α^{LELY} spectrin contains exon 46 and is functionally normal (although marked by the $\alpha^{V/41}$ tryptic peptide).

α^{LELY} allele ($\alpha^{I/74}/\alpha^{LELY}$) had severe elliptocytosis.[789] Similarly, in another family the α^{LELY} allele increased the proportion of Sp $\alpha^{I/65}$ in heterozygotes from 45% to 65% of the total spectrin.[789] This was associated with an increase in the proportion of elliptocytes from none or only a few to nearly 100%. All α-spectrin mutations seem to be similarly affected.[789] Conversely, when the α^{LELY} allele is on the same chromosome as an α-spectrin mutation, it mutes the elliptocytic phenotype.[1087]

Sp α^{LELY} should be distinguished from the thalassemia-like defect of α-spectrin synthesis which, when coinherited with some of the α-spectrin mutations, produces a phenotype of HPP. The latter defect is characterized by reduced α-spectrin mRNA levels and diminished α-spectrin synthesis.[538] In contrast, α-spectrin mRNA levels are normal in Sp α^{LELY}.

α-Spectrin Defects: Specific Mutations

Spectrin $\alpha^{I/74}$. Sp $\alpha^{I/74}$ makes up a heterogenous collection of defects (see Table 54-6), which result in enhanced tryptic cleavage after Arg 45 or Lys 48 in an extra helical segment (helix C in the crystallographic structure of the repeat[347]) that juts out from the N-terminal end of the α-spectrin chain. This is the end that participates in spectrin self-association (see Fig. 54-11). The corresponding (C-ternminal) end of the β chain also contains extra helices (helices A and B) in repeat 17, followed by a phosphorylated segment. Tse[656] and Speicher[328] and their colleagues have proposed that these three helices pair up, as they do all along the spectrin chain, and that this is the bond responsible for spectrin self-association. Evidence is increasing that this elegant hypothesis is true.

Because the Sp $\alpha^{I/74}$ mutations disrupt one of the three interacting terminal helices, they would be expected to markedly disrupt spectrin self-association. This has been found to be true. Correspondingly, the Sp $\alpha^{I/74}$ mutations are generally considered to be the most severe of the common α-spectrin mutations that cause HE. Rare patients who are homozygous for $\alpha^{I/74}$ usually have life-threatening hemolysis and an HPP-like syndrome.[665,1099] Patients who are compound heterozygotes for Sp $\alpha^{I/74}$ and $\alpha^{I/46}$ or $\alpha^{I/61}$ also have severe hemolysis. In addition, both groups of patients have partial (about 30%) spectrin deficiency,[1124] similar to

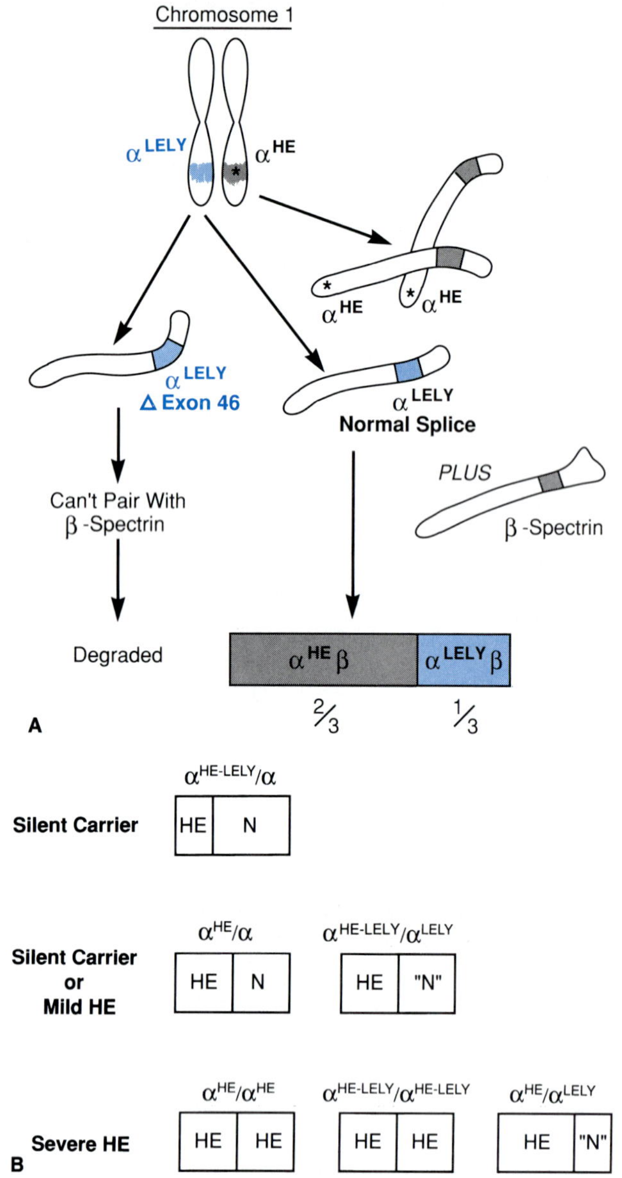

FIGURE 54-57. Effect of α^{LELY} on the proportion of spectrins containing normal and HE α chains. (**A**) When an α^{LELY} allele (*colored*) pairs with an α allele bearing an HE mutation (*asterisk*), the abnormal splicing associated with the α^{LELY} polymorphism decreases the concentration of normal α chains and results in an increased proportion of spectrin containing the HE α chain. (**B**) The consequences of different combinations of normal α chains (α), low expression α chains (α^{LELY}), HE α chains (α^{HE}), and HE mutations developing on an α chain carrying the common α^{LELY} polymorphism ($\alpha^{HE\text{-}LELY}$). The proportions of normal (N) and elliptocytosis (HE) spectrins and the resulting phenotypes are illustrated. (After Delaunay J, Dhermy D. Mutations involving the spectrin heterodimer contact site: clinical expression and alterations in specific function. Semin Hematol 1993;30:21)

that which occurs in HS.[245,658,722] The Sp $\alpha^{I/74}$ patients also have marked microspherocytosis on their blood smears, and sometimes they have so few elliptocytes that the diagnosis of HE is not considered until the parents' smears are examined.

In most cases, the primary defect in Sp $\alpha^{I/74}$ is a single amino acid change near the site of enhanced tryptic cleavage in the α chain (see Table 54-6).[664,666,669,670,674,676,677] Codon 28 is a "hot spot" and has been associated with four different mutations. In three instructive families, the primary defects occur in helix A or B of repeat 17 of β-spectrin[656,704,705] (eg, see Sp Providence in Fig. 54-54). These two helices are adjacent to the $\alpha^{I/74}$ *cleavage site in helix C at the N terminal of the α chain,* if the mechanism of spectrin self-association described above is correct (see Fig. 54-11). In fact, this mutation provides powerful support for the model.

Spectrin $\alpha^{I/50a}$ (or $\alpha^{I/46}$). Sp $\alpha^{I/50a}$ disorder is also heterogenous and variable in severity[140,653,665,668,672,685,686,692,1144,1145] but generally less severe than Sp $\alpha^{I/74}$ and more severe than Sp $\alpha^{I/65}$.[1099] It is particularly common in black populations. Mutations cluster around the site of abnormal tryptic cleavage in helix C of α-spectrin repeat 2, with one informative exception[692], which occurs at an adjacent site in helix B of repeat 2 (see Table 54-6).

Spectrin $\alpha^{I/65}$. This common mutation[140,653,665,668,678–688] is widely distributed in blacks in West Africa (where the prevalence of HE is 0.67%[1081]), in blacks in Central Africa,[147] and in their descendants in the West Indies and North America. It is also seen in Arab populations and is the most common cause of HE in North Africa. This mild disorder causes mild common HE in blacks and is even milder in North Africans, who sometimes have little or no elliptocytosis (silent carriers). Even homozygotes have only mild to moderate hemolysis.

Studies to date indicate that *all patients have the same defect*: insertion of an extra leucine between codons 154 and 155, probably because of duplication of codon 154.[653,686,688,689] The high incidence of Sp $\alpha^{I/65}$ and its homogenous expression strongly suggests that it has experienced genetic selection and that it may provide some protection from malaria or other tropical blood-borne parasites. This has not been systematically tested, although preliminary evidence shows that growth of *P falciparum* is inhibited in $\alpha^{I/65}$ erythrocytes.[1148]

Spectrin $\alpha^{I/78}$. Sp $\alpha^{I/78}$ defect has been observed mostly in North Africans.[661–663] Symptoms are variable, ranging from asymptomatic to moderately severe hemolysis, perhaps related to coinheritance of Sp α^{LELY} (see earlier in chapter), which is common in this population.[789] Primary mutations occur amid those that cause Sp $\alpha^{I/74}$ defects[662,663] (see Table 54-6), but, for unknown reasons, these mutations induce tryptic cleavage at a more proximal site (Lys 16).

Defects of Spectrin Self-Association Involving the β Chain

Two types of β-chain abnormalities have been identified in patients with HE and defective spectrin self-association (see Fig. 54-54): either a truncated β chain[706–716,1131] or, as described earlier, a mutation of the C-terminal end of the β chain that is expressed as Sp $\alpha^{I/74}$.[656,704,705]

As discussed in the section on spherocytic elliptocytosis, truncated β chains have been reported in eight kindreds with HE and chronic hemolysis.[706–716,1131] SDS gels show

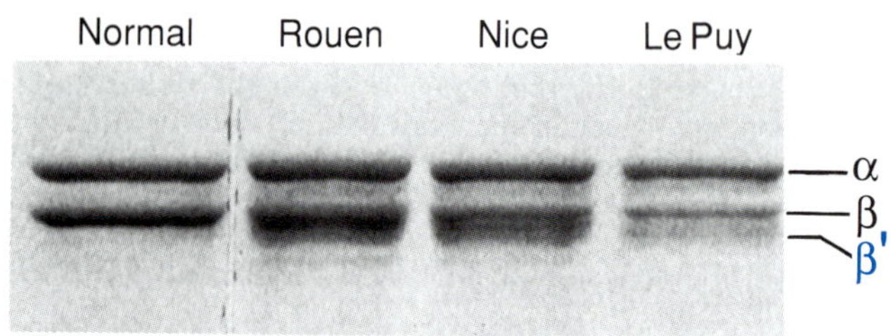

FIGURE 54-58. SDS gel electrophoretic patterns of the α- and β-spectrin subunits and some shortened β' chains due to C-terminal truncations: normal, Sp Rouen ($\beta^{220/218}$), Sp Nice ($\beta^{220/216}$), and Sp Le Puy ($\beta^{220/214}$). (Delaunay J, Dhermy D. Mutations involving the spectrin heterodimer contact site: clinical expression and alterations in specific function. Semin Hematol 1993;30:21)

two β-spectrin bands: β and β′ (Fig. 54-58). The β component comigrates with the normal spectrin β chain (kd), whereas β′ moves faster, consistent with loss of a portion of the peptide chain. The size of the β′ band varies from 210 to 218 kd (see Table 54-6). In most patients, the β′ component is not phosphorylated, which localizes the deletion to the C-terminal end of the β chain. This end of β-spectrin contains four phosphorylation sites within 10 kd of the C terminal.[521] Sp Rouen (218 kd) is an exception; it has the smallest deletion and retains at least one phosphorylation site.[706,707]

The primary molecular defect in β-spectrin has been defined in six of these kindreds. In each case, the coding sequence terminates because of a frameshift. In three instances, a splice site mutation causes the adjacent exon to be skipped (Sp Rouen, Sp Göttingen, and Sp LePuy).[706,707,713,715] In the other three instances, insertions or deletions alter the reading frame (Sp Nice, Sp Tandil, and Sp Tokyo)[709–711] (see Table 54-6).

Functionally, these β-spectrin deletions all result in diminished spectrin self-association. Some of the mutations also foster abnormal tryptic cleavage of the neighboring α chain, similar to that observed in Sp $\alpha^{I/74}$.[708,714] Low-temperature spectrin extracts contain increased spectrin dimer (about 50% of the spectrin dimer plus tetramer pool), and nearly all the mutant β′ spectrin is found in the dimer fraction,[707,714,1131] proving that it is responsible for the functional defect.

Molecular Determinants of the Clinical Severity of Hereditary Elliptocytosis Spectrin Mutations

As already discussed, the severity of hemolysis in common HE often varies, not only among different kindreds but also within a given family. The two principal determinants of severity are the spectrin content of the cells and the percentage of dimeric spectrin in crude spectrin extracts.[147,1099] The fraction of dimeric spectrin, in turn, depends principally on two factors. The first is the dysfunction of the mutant spectrin. Mutations within or near the site of self-association produce a more profound defect of spectrin function and a more severe clinical phenotype than point mutations in more distant triple helical repeats.[143] The second factor is the fraction of the mutant spectrin in the cells. This is determined by the gene dose (simple heterozygote versus homozygote or double heterozygote) and by other genetic defects such as the presence, *in trans*, of a defect leading to reduced α-spectrin synthesis (as described in some subjects with HPP), or the presence, either in *cis* or *in trans*, of Sp α^{LELY}.[143,364,789]

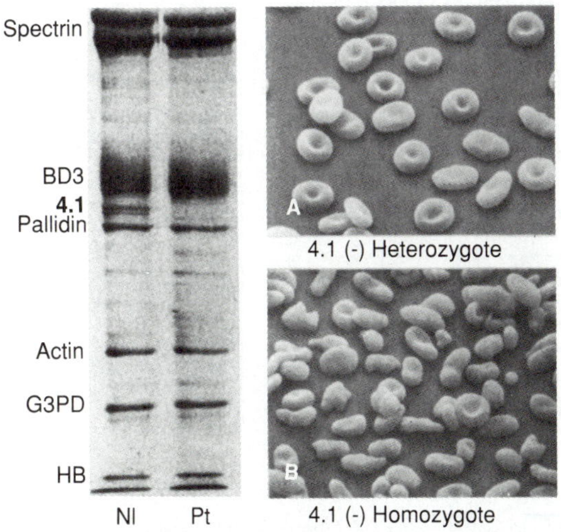

FIGURE 54-59. Deficiency of protein 4.1 in hereditary elliptocytosis (HE). (*Left*) SDS gels (Laemmli system) are of red cell membrane proteins from a normal individual (Nl) and a patient with homozygous HE who lacks protein 4.1 (Pt). (*Right*) Scanning electron micrographs are of red blood cells in protein 4.1–deficient patients. (**A**) Elliptocytes in a patient with heterozygous HE and 50% protein 4.1. (**B**) Elliptocytes, poikilocytes, and fragmented red cells in a patient with homozygous HE and no protein 4.1. (After Tchernia G, Mohandas N, Shohet SB. Deficiency of cytoskeletal membrane protein band 4.1 in homozygous hereditary elliptocytosis: implications for erythrocyte membrane stability. J Clin Invest 1981;68:454)

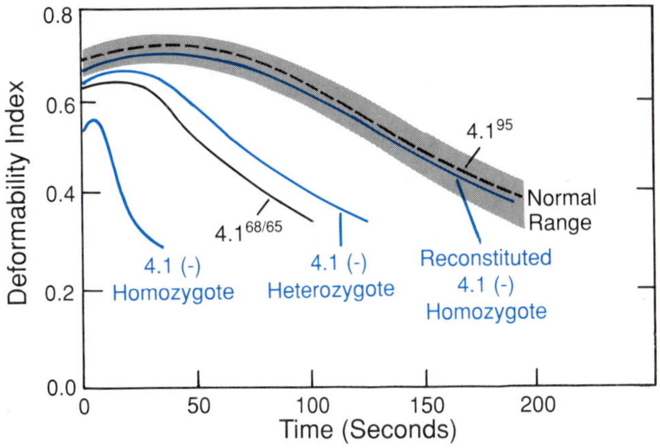

FIGURE 54-60. Red cell membrane stability in defects of protein 4.1. Red cell membranes were subjected to high shear stress in an ektacytometer, and their deformability was measured as a function of time. A fall in deformability occurred as the membranes fragmented. Patients lacking protein 4.1 (4.1 [−] homozygotes) have fragile membranes, and normal fragility can be restored by reconstituting the membranes with normal protein 4.1. (After Mohandas N, Chasis JA. Red cell deformability, membrane material properties, and shape: regulation by transmembrane, skeletal, and cytosolic proteins and lipids. Semin Hematol 1993;30:171)

Deficiency of Protein 4.1

Tchernia[407] and Feo[738] and their colleagues first described the association between HE and protein 4.1 deficiency in a consanguineous Algerian family (Fig. 54-59). Subsequent investigators have shown that protein 4.1 deficiency is a relatively common cause of HE in some Arab and European populations (about 40%).[140,142,668,737,739–741] It is not observed in blacks.[1081]

Clinically, heterozygotes have "classic" mild common HE with a high proportion of elongated, smooth elliptocytes and little or no hemolysis. They have about half the normal amount of protein 4.1. No 4.1 is detectable in homozygotes.

As a consequence, homozygotes have a severe, transfusion-dependent hemolytic anemia with marked osmotic fragility, normal thermal stability, fragmenting elliptocytes, and a good response to splenectomy.[407,736,791] The homozygous red cells fragment much more rapidly than normal at moderate shear stresses, an indication of their intrinsic instability[1140] (Fig. 54-60). Cells from heterozygotes show intermediate stability, similar to other patients with mild common HE. Membrane mechanical stability can be completely restored by reconstituting the deficient red cells with normal protein 4.1[408] or even with a fusion protein containing only 62 amino acids (the 21-amino acid spectrin–actin binding site plus the next 41 amino acids).[409]

In addition to 4.1 deficiency, homozygotes have only about 30% of the normal content of GPC and GPD[414,415,750,736] and lack protein p55.[434,736] This and other evidence[187,312,414] argue persuasively that GPC is one of the membrane attachment sites of protein 4.1, probably with the aid of p55[433,434] (see earlier discussions). Completely 4.1-deficient red cells also manifest other defects. Membrane phospholipid asymmetry is disturbed,[418] and protein 4.9 appears to be missing from isolated membrane skeletons, although not from intact red cell membranes.[407]

In one well-studied Algerian patient,[407] the 4.1(−) mRNA is not translated[734] because of a 318-bp deletion that encompasses the "downstream" translational start site that is used in reticulocytes[125] (Fig. 54-61). Another patient, with 4.1 Madrid, has a point mutation in the same downstream translation start site, with the same consequences.[736] Interestingly (and probably fortunately), expression of protein 4.1 is relatively unimpaired in nonerythroid tissues[424,425] and early erythroblasts[426] because many of the 4.1 isoforms in these tissues initiate translation at an alternatively spliced upstream translation start site.[424,425]

Structural and Functional Defects of Protein 4.1

Two structural defects of protein 4.1 have been identified in patients with HE.

Shortened Protein 4.1 ($4.1^{65/68}$) With Defective Spectrin–Actin Binding. This disorder was discovered in an Italian family with mild common HE (no anemia or reticulocytosis) and mechanically unstable red cells[741,742,744] (see Fig. 54-60). The affected patients are heterozygous for a protein 4.1 variant that has lost two exons (Lys 407 → Gly 486) encoding the spectrin–actin binding region (see Fig. 54-61). The mutant protein runs as a 65- and 68-kd doublet on SDS gels and seems to be present in nearly normal amounts.[741] It is presumed but not proved to be functionally inept.

High-Molecular-Weight Protein 4.1 (4.1^{95} or 4.1 Hurdle-Mills). This variant was discovered in a family of Scotch-Irish ancestry with very mild common HE.[741] The patients are heterozygous for a 95-kd form of protein 4.1, which results from duplication of three exons encoding sequences between Lys 407 and Gln 529[742,744] (see Fig. 54-61). This leads to duplication of the spectrin–actin binding region, but function appears to be preserved, since 4.1^{95} red cell membranes have *normal* mechanical stability[125] (see Fig. 54-60). It is not clear why this functionally normal variant causes HE.

Deficiency of Glycophorins C and D

Deficiency of GPC and GPD, two closely related minor sialoglycoproteins occurs in homozygous 4.1 deficiency and in patients with the rare Leach phenotype of Gerbich-negative (Ge−) red cells. The Gerbich antigen system is carried on both GPC and GPD. Patients with the Leach phenotype of Ge− lack both of these glycophorins.[307,309–311,750–754] Affected patients have very mild common HE[307,310,311,751] with *increased osmotic fragility* (a mild form of spherocytic HE). In some patients, no elliptocytes are observed.[415] In one patient, transient GPC deficiency and elliptocytosis were associated with the development of an autoantibody to GPC.[752] Patients who lack some Ge antigens (so-called Yus and Ge phenotypes) have normal amounts of red cell protein 4.1 and do not have HE. Their red cells contain a hybrid and apparently functionally active glycophorin with features of both GPC and GPD.[120,1149]

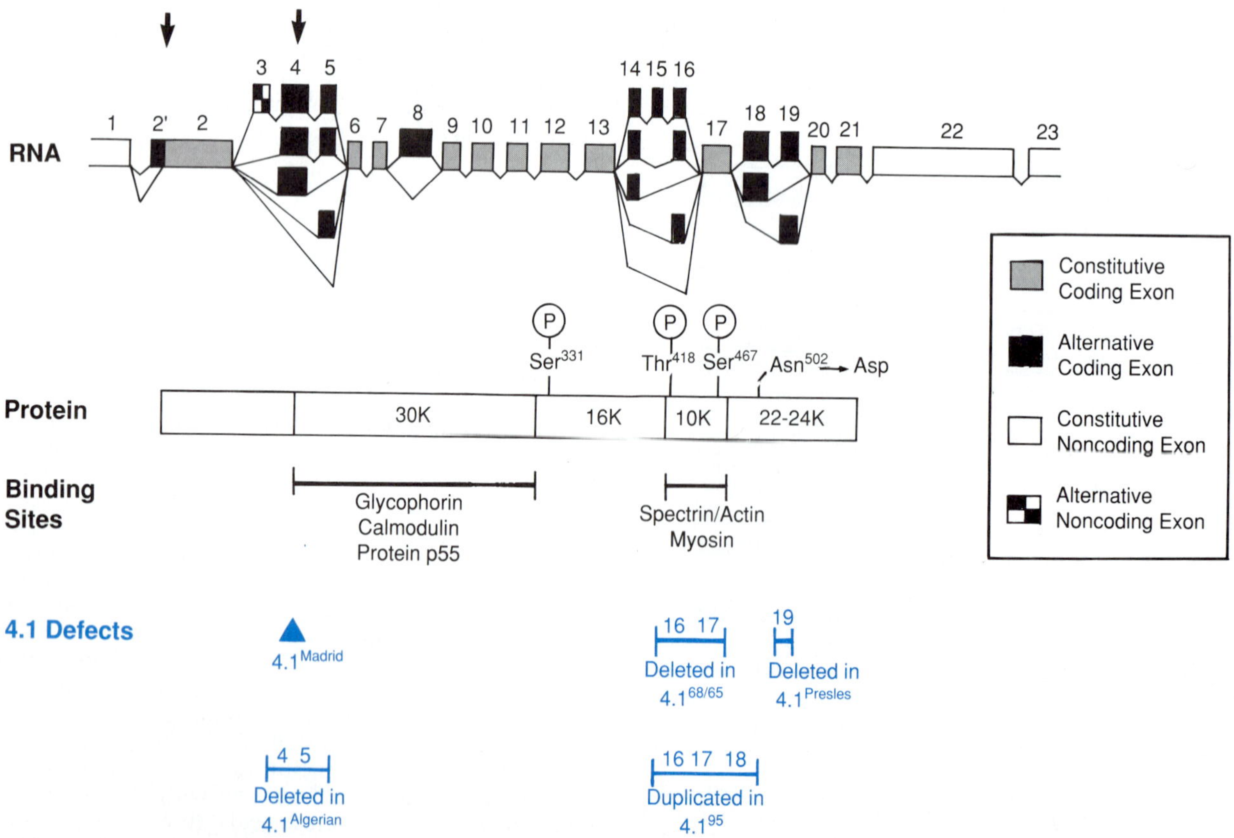

FIGURE 54-61. Defects in protein 4.1. The location of specific defects is shown relative to the structure of 4.1 mRNAs and the protein 4.1 domains. The numbers above the deletions indicate the missing exons. 4.1 Madrid is caused by a mutation in the downstream AUG (arrow in exon 4) that selectively blocks synthesis of red cell 4.1, which begins with the 30K domain.

GPC-deficient red cells lack protein p55,[434] which binds to GPC and protein 4.1.[433] The levels of protein 4.1 are reduced, reflecting a weakened interaction with the membrane. This and other information, discussed earlier, suggest that GPC and protein p55 may create a membrane binding site for protein 4.1. In contrast to that which occurs with GPC deficiency, patients lacking GPA or GPB, or both, are entirely asymptomatic and have normal red cell morphology and mechanical stability.

Pathobiology of the Red Cell Lesion in Common Hereditary Elliptocytosis and Hereditary Pyropoikilocytosis

α-Spectrin Mutations. The principal functional consequence of the elliptocytogenic spectrin mutations is a weakening or even disruption of the spectrin dimer–tetramer contact, and consequently, the two-dimensional integrity of the membrane skeleton.[132] These "horizontal defects" are readily detected by ultrastructural examination of membrane skeletons, which reveals disruption of the normally uniform hexagonal lattice.[552] Consequently, membrane skeletons, cell membranes, and the red cells are mechanically unstable.[132,134] In patients carrying severely dysfunctional spectrin mutations or in those who are homozygous or compound heterozygous for such mutant proteins, this membrane instability is sufficient to cause hemolytic anemia with red cell fragmentation.

How elliptocytes are formed is less clear. In common HE, red cell precursors are round and the cells become progressively more elliptical as they age in vivo.[1076,1092,1150] Red cells distorted by shear stress in vitro or flowing through the microcirculation in vivo have elliptical or parachute-like shapes, respectively.[134,1151] Perhaps elliptocytes and poikilocytes are permanently stabilized in their abnormal shape because the weakened skeletal interactions facilitate skeletal reorganization after prolonged or repetitive cellular deformation. Skeletal reorganization is likely to involve breakage of the unidirectionally stretched protein connections and formation of new contacts that reduce stress on the skeleton and stabilize the deformed shape.[134] This process, first proposed in 1978,[1152] has been shown to account for permanent deformation of irreversibly sickle cells.[1152,1153]

As already noted, HPP red cells have two abnormalities: they contain a mutant spectrin that disrupts spectrin self-association and they are partially deficient in spectrin.[538,1124] This is due either to an elliptocytogenic α-spectrin mutation and a defect involving reduced α-spectrin synthesis or to two elliptocytogenic spectrin alleles. In the latter situation, spectrin deficiency might be a consequence of spectrin instability, which would reduce the amount of spectrin available for membrane assembly. In red cells carrying a lot of unassembled spectrin dimers, the fact that *one* ankyrin is bound per *one* spectrin tetramer (*two* spectrin heterodimers) may also contribute to spectrin deficiency. At best, only about half of the spectrin dimers could succeed in attaching to the available ankyrin binding sites. It would probably be less because unphosphorylated ankyrin binds spectrin dimers about 10 times less avidly than spectrin tetramers.[455,456,479]

The phenotype of HPP, characterized by the presence of fragments and elliptocytes, *together* with evidence of red cell surface area deficiency (microspherocytes), suggests that the membrane dysfunction involves both *vertical* interactions (a consequence of the spectrin deficiency) and *horizontal* interactions (a consequence of the elliptocytogenic spectrin mutations).

Protein 4.1 Mutations. Hereditary elliptocytes that are deficient in protein 4.1 are similar in shape and membrane instability to elliptocytes that result from spectrin mutations.[134] This suggests that 4.1 deficiency principally affects the spectrin–actin contact (a *horizontal* interaction) rather than the skeletal attachment to GPC (a *vertical* interaction).

Permeability of Hereditary Elliptocytosis Red Cells. HE red cells consume more ATP and 2,3-DPG than normal erythrocytes,[1154] probably because of increased transmembrane sodium movements.[1155] As a result of the underlying skeletal defect, HE and HPP red cells are abnormally permeable to Na^+, K^+, and Ca^{2+} ions.[1120,1155] The excessive Ca^{2+} leak was originally thought to be the primary molecular lesion in a patient with a severe microcytic hemolytic anemia and red cell thermal instability,[1120] who was subsequently shown to have a spectrin mutation and probably HPP.[1145]

Common Hereditary Elliptocytosis and Malaria

Epidemiologic studies of the elliptocytogenic mutations of spectrin in central West Africa suggest that their prevalence is considerably greater than would be expected for sporadic mutations. For example, the prevalence of the Sp $\alpha^{I/65}$ mutation approaches 1%[1081] and the mutation is always associated with the same α-spectrin haplotype.[143] Similar findings were reported for two α-spectrin mutations producing the Sp $\alpha^{I/50\text{-}46a}$ phenotype (Leu 207 → Pro and Leu 260 → Pro). These data are interesting in light of in vitro studies, demonstrating diminished malarial parasite entry or growth in red cells that contain some of the elliptocytogenic spectrin mutants or are deficient in protein 4.1.[1148,1156]

Southeast Asian Ovalocytosis

Southeast Asian ovalocytosis (SAO), also known as Melanesian elliptocytosis or stomatocytic elliptocytosis, is inherited in an autosomal dominant pattern.[765–767,775,1157] It is observed in the aboriginal populations of Melanesia and Malaysia and in portions of Indonesia and the Philippines.[764,766,767,769,771,1158] The gene is very common in Melanesia, particularly in lowland tribes where malaria is endemic.[765,781,1157,1158] In these tribes, 5% to 25% of the natives are affected. In vivo evidence shows that SAO provides some protection against all forms of malaria,[765,766,781,1157–1159] particularly heavy infections,[1159] but protection is incomplete. Nevertheless, the prevalence of SAO increases with age in populations challenged by malaria, suggesting that ovalocytic persons have a survival advantage.[1159] In vitro, SAO red cells are resistant to invasion by malarial parasites,[768,774,1160] apparently because the membrane is 10 to 20 times more rigid than normal[776–778,780] (Fig. 54-62*A*). Other membrane characteristics reflect this property. For example, the cells are unusually heat resistant, easily withstanding heating to 49°C, at which temperature normal red cells disintegrate[774]; they do not undergo endocytosis in response to drugs that produce dramatic endocytosis in normal cells[778]; and they strongly resist crenation,[778] even after several days of storage in plasma or buffered salt solutions (see Fig. 54-62*B*). The latter property, combined with the distinctive red cell morphology, provides a simple means of diagnosing SAO.

Most of the SAO cells are rounded elliptocytes, but a few are traversed by one or two transverse bars that divide the central clear space[764,769,771,775,1158] (see Fig. 54-45, *panel 9*). These "elliptical knizocytes" or "stomatocytic elliptocytes" are not seen in any other condition. Hemolysis is apparently mild or absent,[764,766,769,771,780] although extensive hematologic data have not been published. For example, a recently described patient had compensated hemolysis (no anemia), with mild splenomegaly, an absolute reticulocyte count of

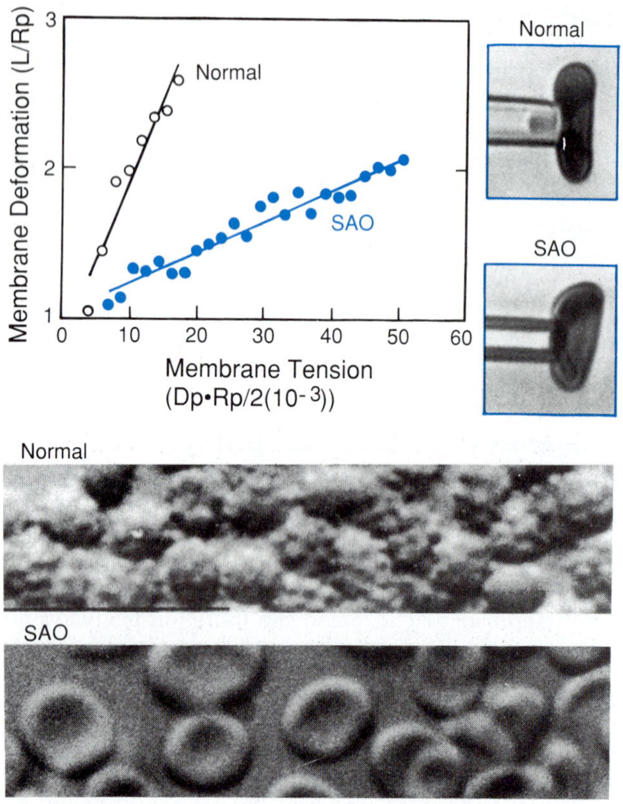

FIGURE 54-62. Membrane stiffness of Southeast Asian ovalocytosis (SAO) red cells as measured by micropipette and lack of crenation. Membrane rigidity of normal and SAO red cells. (*Top right*) Videomicrographs of pipette aspirations of normal and SAO red cells. The SAO cell forms a much smaller tongue of membrane than the normal cell at the same aspiration pressure. (*Top left*) Plots of membrane tension, where Dp = aspiration pressure) versus tongue length (L), both normalized by the pipette radius (Rp). A much higher tension is required to aspirate an equal length of SAO membrane into the pipette (*colored circles*) than normal membrane (*open circles*). (*Bottom*) Failure of SAO red cells to crenate, compared with normal cells, when diluted in saline. This is one of the simplest methods for demonstrating the rigidity of SAO membranes. (Mohandas N, Chasis JA. Red cell deformability, membrane material properties, and shape: regulation by transmembrane, skeletal, and cytosolic proteins and lipids. Semin Hematol 1993;30:171; Saul A, Lamont G, Sawyer WH, et al. Decreased membrane deformability in Melanesian ovalocytes from Papua New Guinea. J Cell Biol 1984;98:1348)

150 to 300 × 10^3 (normal, 40 to 80 × 10^3), mild hyperbilirubinemia, and gallstones.[1160a] This indicates that membrane rigidity is not a major determinant of red cell survival. In another well-studied SAO patient,[771] red cell Na^+ and K^+ permeability was increased, glucose consumption was elevated to compensate for increased cation pumping, autohemolysis was increased, and the cells were osmotically resistant. Curiously, many blood group antigens are poorly expressed on the surface of SAO red cells,[1158] conceivably because the rigid membrane inhibits their clustering and impedes agglutination.

Investigations show that the primary defect in SAO lies in band 3, near the interface of the membrane and cytoplasmic domains (see Fig. 54-36).

Etiology

The finding of tight linkage between an abnormal proteolytic digest of band 3 protein and the SAO phenotype led to detection of the underlying molecular defect.[775] All carriers of the SAO phenotype are heterozygotes. One band 3 allele is normal and the other contains two mutations in *cis*: a deletion of 9 codons encoding amino acids 400 to 408, located at the boundary of the cytoplasmic and membrane domains, and the replacement of Lys 56 by Glu[772,777,780] (see Fig. 54-36). The Lys 56 → Glu substitution is an asymptomatic polymorphism known as band 3 Memphis.[163,166,167] The mutant SAO band 3 exhibits tight binding to ankyrin,[775] increased tyrosine phosphorylation,[1161–1163] inability to transport anions,[779,783] and markedly restricted lateral and rotational mobility in the membrane.[775,777]

Since SAO is caused by deletion of 27 bases from the band 3 gene, amplification of the deleted region in genomic DNA or reticulocyte cDNA is the most specific diagnostic test. This produces a single band in control red cells and a doublet with the second band shorter by 27 bp in SAO cells.[772,777,782]

Molecular Basis of Membrane Rigidity and Malaria Resistance

Southeast Asian ovalocytosis red cells are unique among axially deformed cells in that they are rigid and hyperstable rather than unstable.[776] The SAO band 3 mutation is the first example of a defect of an *integral* membrane protein leading to red cell membrane rigidity, a property that had previously been attributed to the membrane skeleton.[1164]

The molecular mechanism underlying SAO red cell membrane rigidity is not clear. One hypothesis is that conformational changes of the cytoplasmic domain of SAO band 3 preclude lateral movement (extension) of the skeletal network during deformation[777,780] (reviewed by Mohandas and Chasis[134]). A second possibility is that SAO band 3 binds abnormally tightly to ankyrin and thus to the underlying skeleton.[775] In addition, the increased propensity of SAO band 3 to aggregate into higher oligomers may be important, since the oligomers can strengthen band 3 attachment to ankyrin.[551] The tendency of SAO band 3 to form linear arrays[551a] also decreases its mobility within the bilayer. Finally, SAO band 3 may adhere to the skeleton nonspecifically, possibly because of denaturation of the membrane spanning domain.[1165]

The resistance of SAO red cells to malaria is presumably related to the altered properties of SAO band 3. Band 3 serves as one of the malaria receptors, as evidenced by inhibition of in vitro invasion by band 3-containing liposomes.[1166] In normal red cells, parasite invasion is associated with marked membrane remodeling and redistribution of band 3–containing intramembranous particles.[1167] Intramembranous particles cluster at the site of parasite invasion and form a ring around the orifice through which the parasite enters the cell. The invaginated red cell membrane, which surrounds the invading parasite, is free of intramembranous particles. The reduced lateral mobility of band 3 protein in SAO red cells may preclude band 3 receptor clustering and thus prevent attachment or entry of the parasites.[775,777]

Resistance to malaria has also been attributed to diminished anion exchange, caused by the inability of SAO band 3 to transport anions.[779,783] In addition, SAO red cells consume ATP at a higher rate than do normal cells; the ensuing partial depletion of ATP levels in ovalocytes has been proposed to account at least partly for the resistance of these cells to malaria invasion in vitro.[1160] Diminished anion transport and ATP depletion do not appear to play a critical role in malaria resistance of SAO erythrocytes in vivo. This is evidenced by the fact that band 3-deficient HS red cells are considerably less resistant to malaria invasion than are SAO red cells, although both cell types have a similar decrease in anion transport, and by the fact that malaria resistance of SAO red cells is detected in vitro even when red cell ATP levels are maintained.[1168]

OTHER CAUSES OF MEMBRANE INJURY LEADING TO SPHEROCYTOSIS

Relatively few conditions cause "spherocytosis," meaning that spherocytes predominate and are the only significant red cell shape on the peripheral blood smear (see Table 54-11). The definition excludes diseases like HPP, in which spherocytes are common but are clearly only one of many morphologic elements.

Other than HS, immunohemolytic anemias are the most common cause of spherocytosis: AB(H)-related hemolysis in newborns and warm antibody-type autoimmune (or drug-related) hemolytic anemias in older children and adults. These are discussed in Chapters 64 and 55, respectively. Severe hemolytic transfusion reactions (see Chap. 60) are also a form of immunohemolysis and are often marked by spherocytosis but are relatively uncommon.

Patients with acute red cell oxidant injury may also develop spherocytes, although they are rarely the principal morphology. Usually bite cells, blister cells, and dense, irregular contracted cells predominate. Oxidant injury occurs during acute hemolytic episodes in patients with G6PD deficiency (see Chap. 58) and in normal persons exposed to toxic concentrations of oxidant drugs or chemicals. Powerful reducing agents such as arsine (AsH_3) may also cause a spherocytic hemolytic anemia after toxic exposure. Little is known about the specific nature of the membrane injury in any of these conditions.

Other acquired causes of membrane damage and spherocytosis are discussed in the sections that follow.

Thermal Injury

Almost 130 years ago, Schultze[1169] observed that red cells fragment and sphere when heated to temperatures near 50°C for short periods. This phenomenon was further defined by the careful studies of Ham and coworkers[1133,1134] and Kimber and Lander[1135] and is now believed to be due to heat denaturation of spectrin or other membrane proteins.[1136] Essentially identical changes are observed acutely in patients with major cutaneous burns, presumably because of heat exposure of red cells in the skin and subcutaneous tissues. Intravascular hemolysis develops, along with red cell fragmentation and spherocytosis, during the first 24 to 48 hours after the burn.[1170,1171] The severity of the reaction is related to the extent and degree of the burn. Hemolysis is usually evident in patients with third-degree burns involving 15% to 20% or more of the skin.[1170,1172] In severely burned patients, up to 30% of the red cell mass may be destroyed. Acute hemolysis is usually complete by the third postburn day and is followed by the anemia of chronic disease.[1173,1174] A rare variant of this disorder has been reported after infusion of red cells that were inadvertently overheated in a blood warmer.[1175,1176]

Hypophosphatemia

In patients with severe hypophosphatemia (serum phosphorus level 0.1 to 0.3 mg/dL), red cell glucose metabolism is compromised, ATP and 2,3-DPG levels decline, and hemoglobin–oxygen affinity increases.[1177,1178] When red cell ATP falls to low levels (about 10% to 20% of normal), a severe hemolytic anemia characterized by marked microspherocytosis or spheroacanthocytosis results.[1177] Hemolysis remits after phosphate repletion and ATP regeneration.[1177]

Toxins and Venoms

Clostridial Sepsis

Patients With Clostridial Sepsis May Have Spherocytosis and Massive Intravascular Hemolysis. *Clostridium perfringens* septicemia occurs in a variety of clinical situations but must particularly be considered in immunosuppressed patients with gastrointestinal or hematologic malignancies,[1179] in infants with necrotizing enterocolitis,[1180–1183] and in patients with penetrating wounds, septic abortions,[1184] peritonitis after a perforated viscus, and cholecystitis or cholangitis.[1179,1185–1190] Severe, rapidly progressive *intravascular hemolysis* and marked microspherocytosis occur in about 10% of patients with *C perfringens* sepsis,[1179,1188] often in association with shock, disseminated intravascular coagulation, acute renal failure, and a fatal outcome. Hemolysis of the entire red cell mass has been reported[1184,1190–1192] and remarkably is compatible with good tissue oxygenation and survival for hours[1192] despite ineffective transfusion therapy.

The mechanism of red cell damage is disputed and may not be the same for all patients. The bacteria produce several hemolytic toxins, of which α-toxin and Θ-toxin are the best characterized. α-Toxin is a 43-kd protein that has an N-terminal phospholipase C domain and a C-terminal domain that is needed for hemolysis.[1193,1194] Θ-Toxin is a 54-kd, thiol-sensitive, cholesterol-binding protein[1195–1197] that aggregates and forms membranes pores,[1196,1198] leading to colloid osmotic hemolysis.

In addition, *C perfringens* contains a neuraminidase that cleaves terminal sialic acids from red cell membrane glycoproteins in some infected patients.[1199] The underlying galactose residues form the so-called Thomsen-Friedenreich cryptantigen or red cell *T antigen*. The antigen is easily detected because affected red cells are agglutinated by peanut lectin.[1186] Since anti–T antibodies are present in most adult plasma, T activation can cause hemolysis. In septic infants and children who lack T antibodies, hemolysis may follow transfusions.[1180,1181,1183] On the other hand, T activation may precede frank intravascular hemolysis and permit early detection of clostridial sepsis and lifesaving therapeutic intervention.[1186]

Venoms

The venoms of cobras and certain vipers and rattlesnakes may produce severe hemolysis and spherocytosis.[1200–1202] Spherocytic hemolytic anemia may also be seen in persons bitten by the common brown spiders (*Loxosceles reclusus* and *Loxosceles lata*) of the central and southern United States and of South America[1203,1204] and in persons afflicted by massive numbers of honeybee,[1205] wasp,[1206,1207] or yellow jacket[1208] stings. Hemolysis has also been reported in a child stung by a Portuguese man-of-war (jellyfish).[1209]

A full description of the numerous toxins in these venoms and their mechanisms of action is beyond the scope of this chapter. In general, the mechanisms of hemolysis after envenomation are not fully understood. The venoms of snakes and insects often contain phospholipases (particularly phospholipase A_2) and protein toxins that enhance their action. Examples of the latter are the mastoparans of wasp and hornet venoms[1210–1212] and melittin, a polypeptide contained in honeybee (*Apis mellifera*) venom that immobilizes and clusters erythrocyte band 3,[1213–1216] exposing protein-free areas of lipid bilayer to phospholipase attack.[1215]

Brown Spider Bites Sometimes Cause a Coombs'-Positive Hemolytic Anemia. Hemolysis after brown spider bite is characteristically delayed from 1 to 5 days and is caused by a different mechanism.[1204] Affected patients develop a transient, spherocytic, Coombs'-positive hemolytic anemia[1217–1219] with intravascular hemolysis, erythrophagocytosis, and deposition of IgG[1218] and C3[1217] on the red cell surface. In vitro, venom components bind to the red cell membrane[1220] and induce IgG attachment[1218] and activation of complement by the alternative pathway.[1221] The hemolysis usually subsides within a week, but it may be fatal.[1204,1222,1223] The role of complement seems to be critical since C′-deficient guinea pigs are resistant to the venom.[1224] The venom also contains a phospholipase D,[1225] which may contribute to the hemolysis.

With the exception of spider bites, which may be clinically deceptive initially, the potential for a hemolytic catastrophe should be clear in patients who have been bitten or stung.[1204] Sometimes the impending hemolysis is signaled by a rapid rise in the serum potassium level caused by a prelytic leak of this ion from damaged red cells. After hemolysis is established, therapy other than transfusions is usually of little use. Antibiotics and hyperbaric oxygen have occasionally been successful in treating clostridial infections.[1182,1186,1187,1226] In snake bites, localization or drainage of the venom and prompt administration of antivenom can be life-saving.

ECHINOCYTES AND ACANTHOCYTES

The two basic types of spiculated red cells are echinocytes and acanthocytes (Fig. 54-63). Echinocytes have a serrated outline with small uniform projections evenly spread over the circumference of the cell. Acanthocytes have fewer spicules, which vary in size and project irregularly from the red cell surface. These differences are easily appreciated in scanning electron micrographs and can usually be discerned in wet preparations, but they are sometimes hard to distinguish in dried smears. In general, echinocytes have relatively uniform scalloped edges in smears (appearing crenated), whereas acanthocytes are contracted, dense, and irregular. Fortunately, the distinction is not critical. Although echinocytes can appear on their own, acanthocytes are almost always accompanied by echinocytes. From a diagnostic point of view, it is usually best to consider all spiculated red cells as a group and not attempt to include or exclude diseases based on this fine morphologic distinction.

It is important to realize that echinocytes in peripheral blood smears are often artifactual. They are readily produced in vitro by washing red cells in buffers or diluting them in saline,[1227] by contact between red cells and glass surfaces,[1227,1228] and by amphipathic molecules that partition into and expand the outer half of the lipid bilayer (see previous section on the bilayer couple hypothesis).[80–84] High pH values, ATP depletion, and Ca^{2+} accumulation also cause echinocytosis.[1229,1230] Spiculated red cells are consistently present in different parts of a blood smear and on different smears, and it is often useful to examine "wet preps" or red cells fixed with glutaraldehyde (0.5% in phosphate-buffered saline). Wet preps are easily made by diluting a small drop of blood with the plasma from the top of an hematocrit tube and covering the mixture with a coverslip. The cells should be viewed with phase contrast optics or, if necessary, under brightfield conditions with the microscope condenser lowered.

According to Dacie,[1231] normal adults may have up to 3% spiculated red cells in their peripheral blood. In our experience, the limit is less than 1% and probably closer to 0.5%. This percentage is higher in states of functional or actual splenectomy and after the ingestion of certain drugs (eg, salicylates, ethanol, furosemide, and indomethacin).[1232] Postsplenectomy the median number of acanthocytes is 1.7%, with a range of 0% to 8.5%.[1227] In full-term infants, the median number of spiculated red cells is 2% (range, 0% to 6%), whereas in premature babies it is 5.5% (range, 1% to 25%).[1233,1234]

Echinocytes are found in patients with advanced uremia[1235,1236]; in patients with defects of glycolytic metabolism,[1237] especially after splenectomy; in some patients with microangiopathic hemolytic anemias[1238]; and in divers after decompression from pressures of more than 3 to 4 bars[1239] (Table 54-13). They are seen transiently after transfusions with large amounts of stored blood because red cells become echinocytic after a few days of storage.

Acanthocytes and *echinocytes* are common in patients with severe hepatocellular damage,[1240] abetalipoproteinemia,[1241] infantile pyknocytosis,[1242] and the McLeod[1243] and In(Lu)[1244] blood groups (see Table 54-13). Occasionally, they are a predominant (5% to 10% of red cells) morphologic feature in patients with myelodysplasia.[1245,1246] Small numbers of acanthocytes are present in many patients with hypothyroidism[1247] and anorexia nervosa.[1248,1249]

Uremia

Red cell survival is reduced in patients with advanced renal failure.[1250–1252] An extracorporal factor is involved, because red cells from uremic patients survive normally when infused into normal persons, whereas normal red cells survive poorly in uremic patients.[1251] The factor is nondialyz-

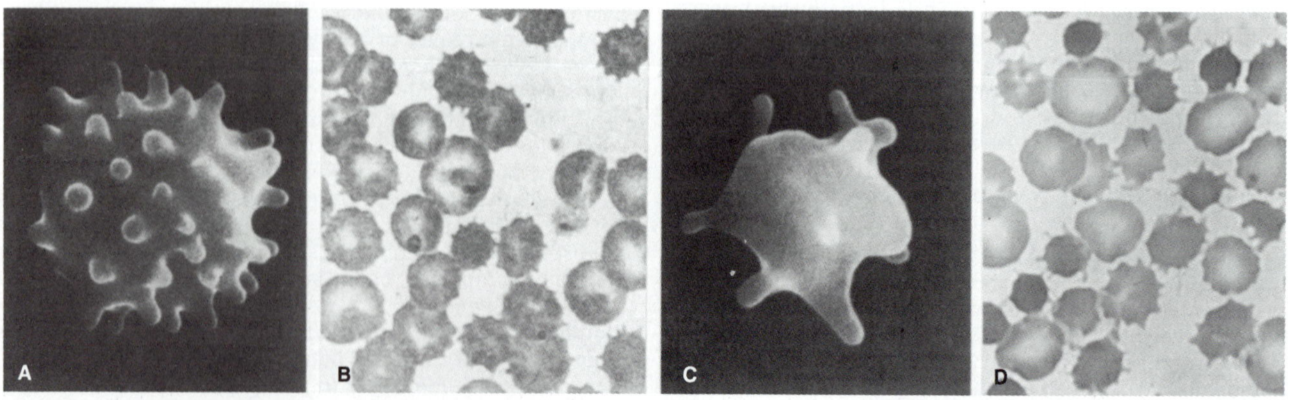

FIGURE 54-63. Morphology of echinocytes and acanthocytes. (**A**) Scanning electron micrograph of a spherical echinocyte. (**B**) Peripheral blood smear of echinocytes in a splenectomized patient with pyruvate kinase deficiency. (**C**) Scanning electron micrograph of an acanthocyte. (**D**) Peripheral smear of acanthocytes in a child with hepatitis and spur cell anemia. (Becker PS, Lux SE. Disorders of the red cell membrane. In: Nathan DG, Oski FA, eds. Hematology of infancy and childhood, ed 4. Philadelphia, WB Saunders, 1993:529)

TABLE 54-13. Conditions Associated with Echinocytosis, Acanthocytosis, or Target Cells

ECHINOCYTES OR ACANTHOCYTES (SPICULATED RED CELLS)
Echinocytes
Premature infants*†
Acute hepatic necrosis (spur cell anemia)
Embden-Myerhof pathway (glycolytic) defects*†
Uremia*
RBC fragmentation syndromes*
Transiently after massive transfusion of stored blood
Divers after decompression*
Heat stroke*
Acanthocytes and Echinocytes
Abetalipoproteinemia
Acanthocytosis with neurologic disease and normal lipoproteins
Choreoacanthocytosis
Hallervorden-Spatz disease
McLeod blood group
In(Lu) blood group
Vitamin E deficiency*†
Infantile pyknocytosis
Anorexia nervosa*†
Hypothyroidism*†
Postsplenectomy*†
Target Cells
Obstructive liver disease
Hypochromic-microcytic anemias
Iron deficiency†
Hemoglobins S, C, D, and E†
Thalassemias
Sideroblastic anemias*†
Hereditary xerocytosis*†
Lecithin:cholesterol acyltransferase deficiency
Fish-eye disease
Postsplenectomy*†

* Disorder sometimes associated with this morphology.
† Indicated morphology usually affects only a small proportion of the red cells.

able and some studies suggest that it is parathyroid hormone (PTH).[1253–1255] PTH is elevated in patients with renal failure as a result of hyperphosphatemia and secondary hyperparathyroidism; PTH levels correlate closely with red cell survival in chronic renal failure patients on dialysis[1255]; and parathyroidectomy abolishes hemolysis in dogs with uremia.[1253] In vitro, relevant levels of PTH or its bioactive N-terminal peptide augment Ca^{2+} entry into red cells via a cAMP-independent pathway and cause the cells to develop filamentous extensions and lose membrane surface (presumably by vesiculation).[1254] These effects are largely blocked by the calcium channel blocker, verapamil.[1254] It is possible that they are responsible for the increased numbers of echinocytes observed in some uremic patients, because increased intracellular Ca^{2+} is markedly echinocytogenic.[1256] This remains to be tested.

Hepatocellular Damage (Spur Cell Anemia)

Anemia in liver disease is complex. Common causes are blood loss, hypersplenism, iron deficiency, folic acid deficiency, and marrow suppression from alcohol, hepatitis virus, and other poorly understood factors.[1257,1258] In addition, in some patients acquired abnormalities of the red cell membrane may contribute to anemia. Two morphologic syndromes are recognized. In one symdrome (to be discussed), target cells predominate. In the other, a syndrome of brisk hemolysis develops in association with acanthocytes or "spur" cells–so-called spur cell anemia.[1240,1259–1269]

Typically, target cells are associated with obstructive liver disease and acanthocytes are associated with hepatocellular disease. In practice, the situation is more complex. It is not uncommon for both morphologies to coexist, and some experimental data suggest they are different stages of the same process. For example, when the bile duct is ligated in a rat, acanthocytes appear within 8 hours, but they convert to target cells when the obstruction persists for 7 days or more.[1270] Nevertheless, acanthocytes (spur cells) and target cells differ in many important respects, and we will consider them separately in this chapter.

Clinical Features

Spur cell anemia is most often observed in patients with alcoholic cirrhosis.[1240,1261–1263,1267,1268] It is also associated with cardiac cirrhosis,[1263] metastatic liver disease,[1266] hemochromatosis,[1265] neonatal hepatitis,[1271] cholestasis,[1259,1260,1269] Wilson's disease,[484] and fulminant hepatitis.[484] Spur cell anemia probably can occur in any disease in which damage to hepatocytes is severe.

Typically, patients have moderately severe hemolysis (hematocrits of 20% to 30%), marked indirect hyperbilirubinemia, splenomegaly, and clinical and laboratory evidence of severe hepatic dysfunction. By definition, over 20% acanthocytes are evident in multiple areas on several peripheral blood smears. Morphologically, the acanthocytes of spur cell anemia are indistinguishable from those seen in patients with abetalipoproteinemia. Echinocytes and target cells are also present in some patients, and spherocytes may develop, presumably from vesiculation (see Fig. 54-23). Occasionally, this may be confusing. In our experience, many of these spherocytes have fine spicules when closely examined (spheroechinocytes), which distinguishes them from true microspherocytes.

The red cell life-span of spur cells is shortened by splenic sequestration[1240,1262,1267,1272] and improves after splenectomy[1272]; nevertheless, spur cell anemia has developed in a patient who has had a splenectomy.[1264] Because splenectomy is a dangerous and often fatal procedure in these very sick patients, it is not generally recommended.[1272] Some success has been reported in treating patients with either phospholipid infusions[1273] or flunarizine[1274]; these approaches are still experimental and their efficacy has not been confirmed.

Etiology and Pathogenesis

The clinical syndrome of spur cell anemia apparently can be produced by at least two different pathogenic mechanisms. In one group—typically patients with alcoholic cirrhosis[1240,1263,1268,1272]—the disorder is due to an acquired abnormality of red cell lipids. The pathophysiology of spurring in these patients has been defined and reviewed by Cooper and associates in a classic series of investigations[99,244,1240,1272,1275–1277] and is illustrated in Figure 54-64. It occurs in two stages: cholesterol loading and splenic remodeling. In the first stage, abnormal, cholesterol-laden, apolipoprotein A-II–deficient lipoproteins, produced by the spur cell patient's diseased liver, transfer their excess cholesterol to circulating erythrocytes and increase erythrocyte membrane cholesterol concentration, the cholesterol/phospholipid ratio, and membrane surface area[1249,1275,1278] (Fig. 54-65; see Fig. 54-64). This is an acquired process and can be mimicked in vitro by incubating normal

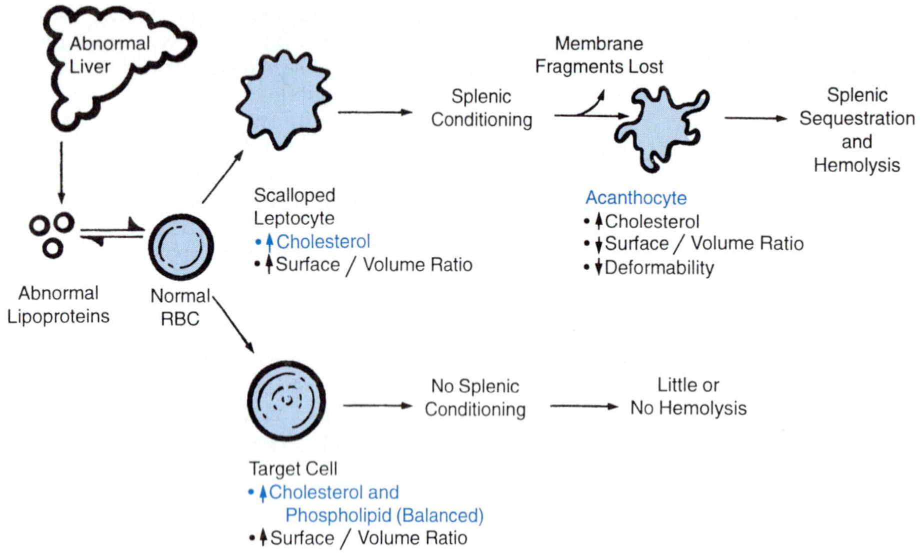

FIGURE 54-64. Pathophysiology of acanthocyte (spur cell) and target cell formation in liver disease. (After Becker PS, Lux SE. Disorders of the red cell membrane. In: Nathan DG, Oski FA, eds. Hematology of infancy and childhood, ed 4. Philadelphia, WB Saunders, 1993:529)

red cells in spur cell plasma[1240,1272] (Fig. 54-66) or in artificial media containing cholesterol-phospholipid dispersions with a cholesterol/phospholipid ratio greater than 1.[1276] It can be reproduced in vivo in dogs[1277] and rabbits[1279] fed a high cholesterol diet. In scanning electron micrographs, these cholesterol-laden cells are flattened and often folded, with an undulating periphery.[1276] They appear scalloped or crenated on dried smears.[1240,1272]

In vivo, the scalloped cells are converted into spur cells by a process involving "splenic conditioning." Over 1 to 7 days, membrane lipids and surface area are lost, cellular rigidity increases (presumably because of a decline in the surface/volume ratio), and the cells become acanthocytes[1240,1272] (see Fig. 54-64). Splenectomy blocks the formation of spur cells and retards their premature destruction but, as noted earlier, it is a high-risk procedure and is seldom indicated.[1272]

Cholesterol-laden incipient spur cells are presumably detained and conditioned by the spleen because they are less deformable than normal cells. How this occurs at a molecular level is not known, but presumably it involves effects of the excess cholesterol on the membrane skeleton or on interconnections between the skeleton and integral membrane proteins. Evidence exists that cholesterol interacts directly with band 3[1280] and possibly with membrane skeleton proteins[1281] and that a slight increase in the cholesterol/phospholipid ratio above normal markedly alters cholesterol organization in the membrane (as measured by accessibility to cholesterol oxidase)[1282] and increases the helical content of one or more of the major membrane proteins.[1283] There is also evidence that membrane proteolytic activity is increased in spur cells and that spur cell plasma can stimulate membrane protein degradation in normal red cells.[1284] These observations are interesting, but more specific information is obviously needed.

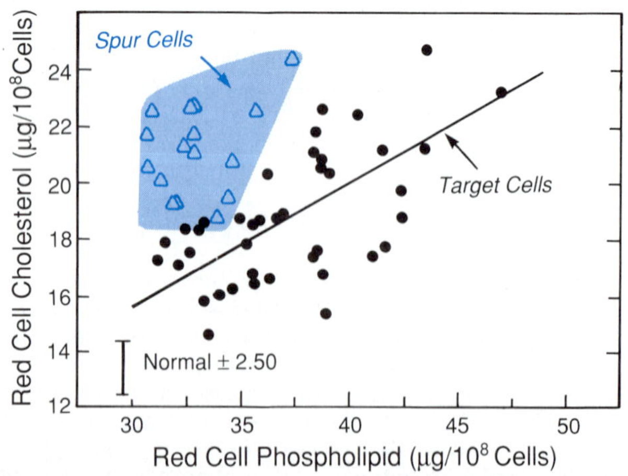

FIGURE 54-65. The cholesterol and phospholipid content of target and spur cells. Target cells (*circles*) tend to have a balanced increase in cholesterol and phospholipid, whereas spur cells (*triangles*) are selectively enriched in cholesterol. (After Cooper RA, Diloy-Puray M, et al. An analysis of lipoproteins, bile acids, and red cell membranes associated with target cells and spur cells in patients with liver disease. J Clin Invest 1972;31:3182)

The second group of patients with liver disease and spur cell anemia differ in that red cell membrane lipids are *normal* and incubation of normal red cells in the patients' plasma does *not* induce spurring.[1262,1266,1267] The pathophysiology of this condition is unknown and largely unstudied. It has been reported in patients with alcoholic cirrhosis[1262,1267] and metastatic liver disease,[1266] and we have observed it in some children with spur cell anemia.

Both alcoholic cirrhosis and metastatic liver disease appear to differ from Zieve's syndrome, a poorly defined syndrome of hyperlipoproteinemia, jaundice, and spherocytic hemolytic anemia, occasionally observed in patients with alcoholic liver disease.[1285]

Abetalipoproteinemia

Abetalipoproteinemia (Bassen-Kornzweig syndrome[1241,1286]) is the paradigm of disorders associated with acanthocytosis. Progressive ataxic neurologic disease, retinitis pigmentosa, fat malabsorption, and the absence of chylomicrons, very low-density lipoproteins (VLDLs, pre-β lipoproteins), and low-density lipoproteins (LDLs; β lipoproteins) are the other major features of this rare autosomal recessive disorder. The disease is caused by failure to synthesize or secrete lipoproteins containing products of the apolipoprotein β (Apo B) gene[1287] due to lack of *microsomal triglyceride transfer protein*,[1288,1289] which catalyzes the transport of triglyceride, cholesteryl ester, and phospholipid between phospholipid surfaces. Microsomal triglyceride transfer protein is a heterodimer of a multifunctional protein called *disulfide isomerase* and a unique 88-kd subunit. It is located in the lumen of the microsomes in liver and intestinal epithelial cells, the sites of lipoprotein synthesis. The 88-kd

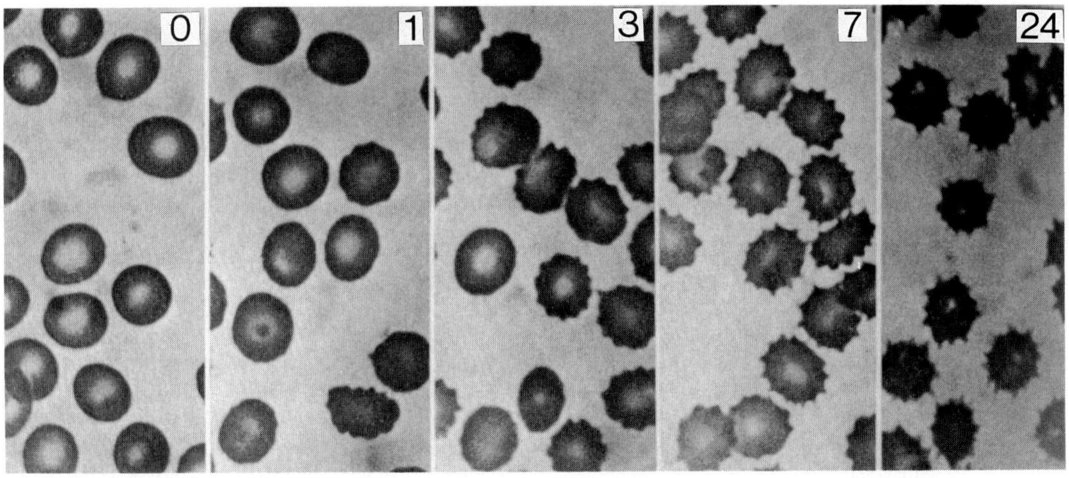

FIGURE 54-66. Production of spur cells in vitro by incubation of *normal* red cells in heated serum from a patient with spur cell anemia. The hours of incubation are shown for each panel. (Cooper RA. Anemia with spur cells: a red cell defect acquired in serum and modified in the circulation. J Clin Invest 1969;48:1820)

subunit is missing in abetalipoproteinemia,[1289] and homozygous null mutations have been demonstrated in the p88 cDNA in two patients.[1288] Apo B is synthesized, but cannot be secreted without its lipid coat.[1290,1291]

Related entities (hypobetalipoproteinemia, normotriglyceridemic abetalipoproteinemia, and chylomicron retention disease) exist that are associated with partial production of Apo β–containing lipoproteins or with secretion of lipoproteins containing truncated forms of Apo β.[1287,1292] Patients with these diseases may also manifest acanthocytosis and neurologic disease, depending on the severity of the lipoprotein defect. Even patients with heterozygous hypobetalipoproteinemia may have acanthocytosis,[1293] although often they do not. An excellent review of the disease is available,[1287] which should be updated this year.[1294]

Characteristically, 50% to 90% of the red cells are acanthocytes.[1287,1295] The shape defect is not evident in nucleated red cells or reticulocytes and worsens as the erythrocytes age.[1287,1295] Membrane protein composition is normal, but membrane lipids are not. PC concentration is decreased by about 20%, and sphingomyelin is correspondingly increased. The cholesterol/phospholipid ratio is normal or mildly elevated.[99,1295–1297] These changes reflect abnormalities in the distribution of plasma phospholipids and a decrease in lecithin:cholesterol acyltransferase activity.[1298] The elevated cholesterol and sphingomyelin decrease lipid fluidity,[99,1296] particularly in the outer half of the bilayer,[1299] and presumably contribute to the acanthocytic shape. They probably do so by expanding the outer bilayer relative to the inner bilayer, since drugs that selectively intercalate into the inner bilayer convert acanthocytes to biconcave disks.[1300] This is almost impossible to prove because the difference in the surface areas of the outer bilayers of an echinocyte or acanthocyte compared with a discocyte is less than 1%.[79]

Because of the fat malabsorption and the absence of LDLs (which transports vitamin E[1301]), the red cells of patients with abetalipoproteinemia are markedly deficient in vitamin E.[1302] Lipid-soluble oxidants such as hydrogen peroxide generate lipid peroxides, damage phospholipids rich in unsaturated fatty acids such as the phospholipids PE and PS, oxidize membrane proteins, and cause hemolysis.[1302] Oxidant sensitivity can be blocked by treatment with a water-soluble form of vitamin E (eg, D-α-tocopherol polyethylene glycol succinate).[1302] Vitamin E deficiency is widely believed to be the primary stimulus for secondary manifestations of the disease, such as neuropathy,[1287] because a similar neuropathy is observed in rare patients with chronic cholestasis[1303–1305] or selective malabsorption of vitamin E.[1306] In the latter defects[1307] and probably in abetalipoproteinemia,[1287,1308] the neurologic symptoms can be delayed or prevented by continuous vitamin E administration.

Despite the increased lipid viscosity and vitamin E deficiency, hemolysis in patients with abetalipoproteinemia is mild.[1287,1295] This contrasts with spur cell anemia, where hemolysis of similarly shaped cells is often severe. Several authors have attributed the difference to the spleen, which is normal in abetalipoproteinemia patients but enlarged and congested by portal hypertension in those with spur cell anemia.[99] Whether this is a sufficient explanation is unknown.

Vitamin E Deficiency

Premature infants (of less than 36 weeks' gestation or weighing less than 2000 g) and children or adults with steatorrhea are susceptible to vitamin E deficiency because of decreased absorption of the vitamin.[1309,1310] The diagnosis has largely disappeared in modern nurseries, partly because of increased breastfeeding and adjustments to the composition of infant formulas, and partly because of the realization that the disease was overdiagnosed[1311] and that overdoses of parenteral vitamin E can be toxic. The experience with patients with disorders of fat malabsorption, such as abetalipoproteinemia (see previous section), and with rare infants with cystic fibrosis who present with hemolysis and edema[1312,1313] that respond to vitamin E, suggest that vitamin E deficiency can be deleterious.

Hemolysis and thrombocytosis are hallmarks of classic vitamin E deficiency[1314–1316]; generalized firm edema is seen in a subset of severely affected infants.[1312,1313,1316] Peripheral blood smears are usually normal but sometimes show variable numbers of irregularly contracted, spiculated cells (acanthocytes or pyknocytes) and small numbers of spherocytes and fragmented red cells.[1313,1315] The mechanism of hemolysis is uncertain. Vitamin E is a lipid-soluble antioxidant, and in its absence lipid peroxidation occurs, with damage to the double bonds of unsaturated fatty acids. Phospholipids rich in unsaturated acyl chains, such as PE, are particularly susceptible[1297,1302,1317]; some evidence shows that damage to membrane protein sulfhydryls may also contribute to hemolysis.[1318]

Vitamin E–deficient rat erythrocytes have many of the characteristics of aged normal red cells,[1319] especially exposure of the so-called senescent antigen[605,606] (see earlier section on red cell membrane alterations of senescent red cells). This cryptic antigen is exposed by incompletely defined modifications of band 3—proteolysis,[606] aggregation,[596,607,612] oxidation[55,189,607,612a,613] or some combination of these perturbations. It is recognized by an IgG autoantibody that initiates removal of the cells by macrophages.[605] Autoantibody attachment is blocked by vitamin E and reversed by thiol-reducing agents in experimental situations[612a], which suggests that membrane lipid oxidation occurs first and leads to the oxidation of band 3 thiols. Similar processes presumably accelerate red cell destruction in vivo in vitamin E deficiency.

Acanthocytosis With Neurologic Disease and Normal Lipoproteins

Amyotrophic Chorea-Acanthocytosis

Amyotrophic chorea-acanthocytosis was first described by Estes and coworkers in 1967[1] and 1968.[1321] Since then, a number of reports have appeared.[1232,1322–1333] More than 30 patients have been described in the Western literature and more than 50 patients in Japan. The disorder is characterized by acanthocytosis, normolipoproteinemia, and progressive neurologic disease beginning in adolescence or adult life (8 to 62 years) and having a variety of manifestations, including orofacial dyskinesia, vocalizations, lip and tongue biting, limb chorea, dysarthria, dysphagia, axonal sensorimotor polyneuropathy, decreased or absent tendon reflexes, muscle hypotonia, distal muscle wasting, and increased creatine phosphokinase. MRI and pathologic examinations show atrophy of the basal ganglia, particularly the caudate and putamen. Mental deterioration is variable,[1328] and little or no hemolysis occurs. In some patients, acanthocytosis precedes neurologic symptoms.[1328] In others, acanthocytosis is not evident in peripheral blood smears but spiculation can be induced in vitro more easily than normally, by echinocytogenic stimuli (eg, saline, contact with glass).[1334]

More than one disorder probably is represented by these reports, because both dominant[1321,1325,1328] and recessive[1322,1327,1331] inheritance is recorded. In addition, variant syndromes with chorea-acanthocytosis and myopathy[1335] and with chorea-acanthocytosis, spherocytosis and hemolysis[854] have been observed.

Other Neurologic Syndromes

Acanthocytosis is also associated with four other unusual neurologic syndromes. One features acanthocytosis and *parkinsonism*, sometimes associated with motor neuron disease[1336] or diurnal dystonia.[1337] The second combines acanthocytosis, *mitochondrial myopathy*, encephalopathy, lactic acidosis, and a stroke-like syndrome.[1336] The third couples acanthocytosis and *Hallervorden-Spatz disease* (progressive dementia, dystonia, spasticity, pallidal degeneration with iron deposition, and often retinal degeneration).[1338–1340] Finally, there is one report uniting acanthocytosis, abnormal lipoproteins, and a Hallervorden-Spatz–like disorder called *HARP syndrome* (hypoprebetalipoproteinemia [decreased VLDLs], acanthocytosis, retinitis pigmentosa, and pallidal degeneration with iron deposition).[1341]

The cause of these disorders is unknown, but evidence is increasing that the red cell membrane is defective, particularly in the typical chorea-acanthocytosis syndrome. The acanthocytic red cells are dense because of excessive K^+ loss[1324] and may[1324] or may not[1332] have an increased proportion of sphingomyelin. In a preliminary report, one research group has observed that cAMP-dependent phosphorylation of red cell dematin (protein 4.9) is impaired in affected patients from two families with "mild spheroacanthocytosis and a choreiform movement disorder or dementia" (probably chorea-acanthocytosis).[1342] Another group notes that ankyrin and proteins 3 and 4.2 self-digest more rapidly than normal in red cells from patients with chorea-acanthocytosis,[1333] which hints at a defect in the vertical connections between the skeleton and the lipid bilayer. In this regard, a specific molecular defect near the C terminal of band 3, Pro 868 → Leu, has been identified[224] in one kindred with chorea-acanthocytosis and mild hemolytic anemia (hematocrit about 34%; reticulocytes about 5%).[225,1343] The affected siblings have 20% to 25% acanthocytes, a slight increase in the apparent molecular weight of band 3 on SDS gels (97 to 99 kd instead of 95 kd), a modest increase in anion transport, and a decrease in ankyrin binding sites.[225] It will be interesting to learn whether similar defects are present in other chorea-acanthocytosis kindreds.

McLeod's Syndrome

McLeod's syndrome is an X-linked anomaly of the Kell blood group system in which red cells or WBCs or both react poorly with Kell antisera but behave normally in other blood group reactions. The affected cells lack Kx, a 37-kd membrane precursor of the Kell antigens.[151,1344,1345] The gene is located on the X chromosome and is referred to as the *Xk* locus.[1346] Male hemizygotes who lack Kx on their red cells have variable echinocytosis or acanthocytosis (8% to 85%), and mild compensated hemolysis (3% to 7% reticulocytes).[1243,1347,1348] Some teardrop erythrocytes and bizarre-shaped poikilocytes are also present. Female heterozygotes have occasional acanthocytes (as expected by the Lyon hypothesis) and mild hemolysis.[1243,1347] The abnormal shape is apparently due to a lack of lipid in the inner bilayer, because it can be corrected by substances like chlorpromazine, which accumulate between inner bilayer lipids.[1349]

Patients with McLeod's syndrome also have a myopathy or neuropathy.[1232,1350–1353] This is first manifested as areflexia and an elevated serum creatine phosphokinase.[1350] Later in adult life, a cardiomyopathy (cardiomegaly) or slowly progressive neuropathy (dystonic or choreiform movements and seizures) may appear. The skeletal muscle myopathy is usually not evident clinically, although myopathic changes may be seen in biopsy specimens.[1232,1352,1353]

The cause of the membrane defect is unknown. The Kx protein is present in small amounts (about 500 copies per red cell)[1345] and has not been cloned. Membrane protein and lipid composition are normal,[1354,1355] but the density of the intramembranous particles is increased.[1354] This suggests that band 3, the major intramembranous particle protein, may be more dissociated in McLeod's red cells than in normal red cells, where it exists primarily as dimers and tetramers.[220] Also present is increased phosphorylation of some lipids and membrane proteins, notably band 3, spectrin, phosphatidic acid, and polyphosphoinositides.[1355] The meaning of these changes is unknown.

The *Xk* gene is less than 500 kb distal to the chronic granulomatous disease locus on the short arm of the X chromosome (Xp21.1).[1356,1357] As a consequence, some males have both chronic granulomatous disease and McLeod's syndrome, caused by deletions that encompass both loci. It is important to recognize patients with McLeod's syndrome because, if they receive transfusions, they may produce antibodies that are compatible only with the Kx-deficient McLeod red cells.[1358,1359]

In(Lu) Gene

The major antigens of the Lutheran blood group system are Lu^a and Lu^b. They are located on two low abundance glycoproteins of 85 and 78 kd.[1360] About 1 person in 3000 to 5000[1244,1361] inherits a *dominantly* acting inhibitor, called *In(Lu)*, which greatly suppresses expression of Lu^a and Lu^b, to the extent that they are not detectable by routine agglutination tests. This is the most common cause of the null Lutheran phenotype, Lu(a−b−). It is interesting for three reasons. First, the *In(Lu)* gene product has broad regulatory powers. It inhibits expression of CD44 (an adhesive protein), MER2 (a common red cell antigen), CR1 (the C3b/C4b complement receptor), AnWj (the erythroid *Haemophilus influenzae* receptor), and the glycolipid antigens P_1 and i, as well as the Lutheran antigens.[1362] Second, although some of these proteins are widely expressed, such as CD44, the action of *In(Lu)* is limited to erythroid cells.[1363] Third, patients with the *In(Lu)* Lu(a−b−) phenotype have abnormally shaped red cells.[1244] The morphology varies from normal or mild poikilocytosis (bumpy, irregular cells) to marked *acanthocytosis.*[1244] No hemolysis or anemia is evident. Osmotic fragility testing of fresh *In(Lu)* Lu(a−b−) red cells produces normal results but, during in vitro incubations, the cells lose K^+ and become osmotically resistant.[1244] The molecular mechanisms responsible for this cation loss and for the regulatory effects of the In(Lu) protein are not known, mostly because the *In(Lu)* gene has not been cloned, but they should be of considerable interest.

Anorexia Nervosa

For unknown reasons, acanthocytosis or echinocytosis is conspicuous in many patients with severe anorexia nervosa.[1248,1249] Patients with undetectable β– and pre-β–lipoproteins (LDLs and VLDLs, respectively) have been reported,[1364] but plasma lipids and LDLs are usually normal or mildly decreased.[1249] In contrast, patients who are heterozygous for congenital hypobetalipoproteinemia typically have normal red cell morphology even when LDL levels are only 10% to 20% of normal.[1287] Severe starvation or malnutrition due to causes other than anorexia nervosa can also produce acanthocytosis[1365–1367] or target cells[1368] and hypobetalipoproteinemia.

Despite the morphologic defect, only a small proportion (about 7%) of anorexia patients are anemic. Mild to moderate leukopenia of neutropenia is common (about 38%), and mild thrombocytopenia is not rare.[1248,1249,1369,1370] The various cytopenias are due to bone marrow hypoplasia,[1249,1369] and their severity correlates with body weight.[1369] The hypoplastic marrow is also deficient in fat, which is replaced by an amorphous ground substance, possibly acid mucopolysaccharide.[1249]

Infantile Pyknocytosis

In 1959, Tuffy and colleagues[1242] described a syndrome of neonatal jaundice and hemolysis associated with variable numbers of distorted, irregularly contracted, spiculated cells, which they called *pyknocytes.* Morphologically, these cells are similar (and possibly identical) to acanthocytes. Normal full-term infants have 0.3% to 1.9% pyknocytes on peripheral blood smears. In premature infants, the normal range is 0.3% to 5.6%.[1242] The affected infants typically present with jaundice and slight hepatosplenomegaly in the first few days of life. Pyknocytosis and hemolytic anemia peak at 3 to 4 weeks of age and then decline spontaneously. Clinical severity is variable, but some infants are severely affected (hemoglobin, 4 to 6 g/dL, 15% to 20% reticulocytes, and 25% to 50% pyknocytes) and some require exchange transfusions.[1242] Transfused erythrocytes become pyknocytic[1242,1371,1372] and survive poorly,[1372] indicating an extracorpuscular defect. Infantile pyknocytosis is seen in both premature and full-term infants. The only consistent chemical abnormality is a mild elevation in serum glutamic oxaloacetic transaminase ([SGOT]; 50 to 250 IU). Parents and siblings are normal.[1342]

The cause of this syndrome has not been clearly defined, and for unknown reasons the diagnosis is seldom made. Infants with severe G6PD deficiency,[1373] neonatal Heinz body hemolytic anemias,[1242,1374] vitamin E deficiency,[1313,1315] glycolytic enzyme deficiencies,[1237] neonatal hepatitis,[1271] HE with neonatal poikilocytosis,[1105,1106] HPP, or microangiopathic hemolytic anemias may present with hemolysis and pyknocytes (or cells resembling pyknocytes) and are sometimes misdiagnosed as having infantile pyknocytosis. In most of the original case reports, evidence is sufficient to exclude those disorders. The transient nature of the disease, its onset after the first week of life, the mild transaminase elevation, morphology, and extracorpuscular etiology constitute a reasonably distinctive combination and imply that infantile pyknocytosis may be a valid entity. The morphology and timing suggest oxidant damage, but other hypotheses are equally tenable.

Hypothyroidism

Patients with hypothyroidism frequently (20% to 65%) have a small number (0.5% to 2%) of acanthocytes in the peripheral blood smears.[1227,1247,1375,1376] Given the high incidence of hypothyroidism, compared with other diseases associated with echinocytosis or acanthocytosis (see Table 54-13), the presence of acanthocytes should prompt physicians to consider testing thyroid function, particularly in adults. Sometimes this will uncover unsuspected cases of hypothyroidism.[1377]

TARGET CELLS

Red cells increase their surface area by an increase in membrane lipids. In dried smears, the excess surface accumulates and bulges outward in the red cell's central clearing, producing the characteristic target cell morphology. In wet preparations, they are bowl-shaped. Target cells also occur when red cell volume is diminished, owing to decreased hemoglobin synthesis (eg, thalassemia, iron deficiency), abnormal hemoglobin charge or aggregation (eg, hemoglobins S, C, D, and E), or decreased cell cations and water. In these cases, a relative increase occurs in the surface/volume ratio. With the exception of dehydrated red cells, an increase in membrane surface, whether relative or absolute, has little effect on red cell deformability or life-span and hence is usually innocuous.

Obstructive Liver Disease

Target cells are particularly characteristic of biliary obstruction,[1378,1379] but also occur in other forms of liver disease. Like spur cells, they form when red cells accumulate excess lipids from abnormal lipoproteins[1275,1379] (see Fig. 54-64). Unlike spur cells, target cells are characterized by a *balanced* increase in both free cholesterol and phospholipids[1275,1380,1381] (see Fig. 54-65). The phospholipid increase is confined to PC.[1275]

The pathogenesis of lipid accumulation in target cells is relatively clear. The process is extracorpuscular, reversible, and caused by an abnormal serum component. Normal cells acquire target cell surface area, morphologic characteristics, and osmotic resistance when transfused into patients with obstructive jaundice or incubated in their serum, whereas target cells from such patients lose their excess lipids and revert to biconcave disks in normal persons or their sera.[1379] Cooper and coworkers[1275] find a close relation between the cholesterol/phospholipid ratios of target cells and serum lipoproteins, particularly LDLs. It is known that in obstructive jaundice a unique, abnormal lipoprotein called LP-X accumulates in the LDL density class.[1382,1383] LP-X contains about equal amounts of free cholesterol and PC, plus small amounts of protein, cholesterol esters, triglycerides, and lithocholic acid.[1382] Normal red cells rapidly acquire excess cholesterol, PC, and surface area when incubated with LP-X in vitro,[1381] and this is the likely source of lipids for membrane expansion and targeting in vivo. Membrane proteins may also be abnormal in these cells. Iida and coworkers[1384] found that pallidin (protein 4.2) was diminished or absent in 11 of 11 Japanese patients with obstructive jaundice and typical lipid-laden target cells. Red cell morphology, membrane lipids, and pallidin content returned to normal in one patient after surgical relief of the biliary obstruction.[1384] To date, this curious observation has never been confirmed or denied and its relevance, if any, to the pathophysiology of targeting remains obscure.

Familial Lecithin:Cholesterol Acyltransferase Deficiency

Familial lecithin:cholesterol acyltransferase (LCAT) deficiency is a rare autosomal recessive disorder characterized by anemia, corneal opacities, hyperlipemia, proteinuria, chronic nephritis, and premature atherosclerosis. An excellent review of the disease has been published[108] and is being updated this year.[1294] LCAT deficiency is relatively asymptomatic during childhood. Proteinuria and corneal opacities are among the earliest manifestations. The latter consist of minute grayish dots that concentrate near the edge of the cornea, resembling arcus senilis.[108] Almost all the patients reported on have had a moderate normochromic anemia (hemoglobin, 8 to 11 g/dL) characterized by prominent target cell formation and decreased osmotic fragility.[108,1385–1387] Hematologic studies suggest that the anemia is due to a combination of moderate hemolysis and decreased erythropoietic compensation, but interpretation of the evidence is complicated by the coexisting renal disease. Other studies have shown that the red cells are abnormally susceptible to peroxidative threat and have mechanically fragile membranes.[1386] There is no obvious explanation for these changes, but they possibly contribute to the shortened red cell life-span.

LCAT deficiency is caused by a variety of mutations of the LCAT gene—mostly missense and frameshift defects.[1388–1391] As expected from the absence of LCAT activity, a pronounced decrease in cholesteryl esters and an increase in free cholesterol and PC in plasma lipoproteins occur.[108] Because LCAT is required for normal lipoprotein formation and catabolism, nascent lipoproteins and abnormal lipoprotein remnants accumulate in the plasma.[108] One of the latter is LP-X.[108,1392] As discussed in the previous section, this lipoprotein is believed to be responsible for target cell formation in patients with the acquired LCAT deficiency of obstructive liver disease[1381] and presumably plays the same role in the familial disease. Free cholesterol and PC levels are markedly elevated in the red cell membranes of LCAT-deficient patients,[1393] but total red cell phospholipid levels are normal because the increase in PC is balanced by a decrease in the phospholipids, PE, and sphingomyelin.[1393] As in liver disease, red cell targeting and lipid abnormalities can be induced by incubation of normal red cells in LCAT-deficient serum and reversed by incubation in normal serum.[1394] Other plasma membranes are probably also affected by the abnormal LCAT-deficient lipoproteins. For example, accumulations of lipid in endothelial membranes may underlie the atherosclerotic and nephritic complications.[108] In addition, phagocytosis of abnormal lipoproteins by reticuloendothelial cells leads to the appearance of foam cells[1385] and sea-blue histiocytes[1395] in the bone marrow, spleen, and other organs. Serum and red cell lipids are improved in vivo when LCAT is supplied by infusions of normal plasma[108]; nevertheless, the short $T_{1/2}$ of this protein (about 4 to 5 d) and the large amounts of plasma required make chronic replacement therapy impractical.

Fish-Eye Disease. Fish-eye disease is caused by partial deficiency of LCAT. It is characterized by corneal opacities (which give the disease its name), hypertriglyceridemia, and very low levels of high-density lipoproteins (HDLs).[108] A report notes increased target cells and decreased osmotic fragility.[1396]

Postsplenectomy

In the first several weeks after splenectomy, target cells gradually increase in number,[1053,1378,1397,1398] eventually (in otherwise normal persons) reaching levels of 2% to 10%.[1397] This change is associated with an increase in osmotic resistance,[1378] membrane lipid content,[860] and mean surface area relative to volume,[1053] indicating expansion of the red cell membrane surface.[1053] By deduction, the spleen must normally remove surplus membrane from such cells–a process referred to as *surface remodeling*. Experimental studies have clearly documented that the stress reticulocytes induced by acute blood loss or hemolysis undergo extensive surface remodeling[1399,1400] and suggest that normal reticulocytes are remodeled to a lesser degree. In addition to membrane lipids, transferrin receptors,[544] fibronectin receptors,[545] and a high molecular weight membrane protein complex[1401] are also removed during the remodeling process. Postsplenectomy blood smears also show increased numbers of acanthocytes,[1227,1402] poikilocytes, and red cells burdened with useless or potentially harmful inclusions (eg, Heinz bodies, Howell-Jolly bodies, siderotic granules, and endocytic vesicles).[1403,1059,1060] The presence of these inclusions attests to the "culling" and "pitting" functions of the spleen.[1403] These and other aspects of splenic function are discussed more fully in Chapter 46.

INHERITED DISORDERS OF RED CELL CATION PERMEABILITY AND VOLUME

Red cell hydration is determined in part by the intracellular concentration of monovalent cations.[1404] A net increase in $[Na^+ + K^+]$ causes water to enter, forming *stomatocytes* or *hydrocytes*, whereas a net loss of monovalent cations produces dehydrated red cells or *xerocytes*.*

In the past 35 years, numerous descriptions of congenital or familial hemolytic anemias associated with abnormal cation permeability and, in some cases, disturbed red cell hydration have appeared.[247,771,829,866,1405–1435] These descriptions range from severe stomatocytosis[1434] to severe

* These cells have also been dubbed *desiccytes*; however, this term, a Latin–Greek chimera, is less desirable.

xerocytosis[1409] and are clinically heterogenous. They can be divided into six provisional categories based on differences of severity, morphology, cation content, lipid and protein composition, genetics, and response to splenectomy (Table 54-14). It is not certain whether these categories are unique entities. None of these apparent disorders is precisely defined in either clinical or molecular terms.

An excellent, but slightly dated, review of these disorders has been published.[1436]

Hereditary Stomatocytosis

Hereditary stomatocytosis (or hereditary hydrocytosis) is a rare syndrome characterized by extraordinary monovalent cation leaks, relative Na^+/K^+-pump failure, and stomatocytic red cell morphology (Fig. 54-67). Ten definite families have been described.[829,1406,1408,1417,1419,1423,1424,1427,1428,1434,1442]

Pathophysiology

Hereditary Stomatocytes Have a Huge Passive Sodium Leak. The major detectable defect in hereditary stomatocytosis is a marked asymmetric increase in passive Na^+ and K^+ permeability (Na^+_{in} greater than K^+_{out}). Permeabilities as great as 15 to 40 times normal are observed.[1427,1434,1442] Because the influx of Na^+ exceeds the loss of K^+, stomatocytic red cells progressively gain cations and water and swell. As a consequence, their average density is less than normal (Fig. 54-68), and the swollen stomatocytes are osmotically fragile. Unlike normal cells, aged stomatocytes are less dense and more stomatocytic than stomatocytic reticulocytes.[829,1406]

Monovalent cation transporters are stimulated by the influx of Na^+, particularly the Na^+/K^+ pump and K^+/Cl^- cotransporter,[1423] but are unable to keep up with the exaggerated cation leaks and are overwhelmed. There is no convincing evidence that Na^+/K^+ pumping is defective: pump kinetics are normal,[829] and the number of pumps is increased several times,[1434,1437] even after correcting for red cell age.[1438] Some authors have observed that Na^+ and K^+ are not transported in the usual ratio (3 Na^+ to 2 K^+)[829,1418,1424] and have argued that the Na^+/K^+ pump is "decoupled"[1424]; other work suggests that this is, at least partly, an artifact of the methods used to measure cation permeability.[1439]

Bifunctional imidoesters, which cross-link proteins, reverse the abnormal shape and permeability of hereditary stomatocytes and normalize their survival in the circulation.[1440–1442] The critical proteins have not been identified because many red cell membrane proteins are cross-linked at the concentrations required to achieve this effect.

Many Patients With Hereditary Stomatocytosis Lack Stomatin (Protein 7.2b). The excess cation permeability is often[1408,1413,1423,1427,1442] but not always[1410,1411] associated with absence of a membrane protein that migrates in the band 7 region on SDS gels (Fig. 54-69). Lande and Mentzer and their colleagues[1413] first observed that one of the four proteins in this region was *absent* in the red cell membranes of a patient with classic hereditary stomatocytosis. Subsequently, the same defect has been found in all eight patients tested from seven other typical stomatocytosis kindreds[1408,1423,1427,1442] and from a patient with cryohydrocytosis[1413] (see following section). The suspect protein (called protein 7.2, or 7.2b, or "stomatin"[1442]) has been isolated and cloned.[1442–1445] It is a 31.5-kd (about 28 kd on SDS gels) basic, phosphorylated (cAMP-dependent kinase), palmitoylated, integral membrane protein with a single transmembrane helix, a small external segment, and a relatively large cytoplasmic domain.[1442,1444,1445] The gene (EPB72) is located on chromosome 9 at 9q34.1.[1446] The protein is widely expressed in nonerythroid tissues and lacks homology with other known proteins. Its function is unknown, but presumably it helps regulate membrane sodium permeability or associates with proteins that do so. The primary structure does not suggest a transport channel, because there is only a single stretch of hydrophobic sequence, but it is possible the protein associates to form a channel.

If stomatin deficiency is the cause of hereditary stomatocytosis, it is necessary to explain why it is *completely absent* in patients with autosomal dominant stomatocytosis. A 50/50 mixture of normal and mutant proteins would be expected. One possibility is that stomatin behaves as a dominant negative mutation. If the protein forms higher-order oligomers, the introduction of even one mutant protomer might destabilize the structure or interfere with its membrane assembly. Alternatively, stomatin might associate with a second protein (the true mutant protein) whose presence could be required to bring stomatin to the membrane, for example, or to modify or stabilize it after it is there. The latter concept is more likely. Three groups have cloned and sequenced cDNAs from stomatocytosis patients with stomatin deficiency,[1447–1449] including the most severe patient yet reported.[1434] All three groups find that the coding sequence of stomatin is *normal*, which is not compatible with a dominant negative mutation.

Stomatocytes are relatively rigid[1420] and expend extraordinary amounts of ATP pumping Na^+ and K^+, attempting to defend the threat of osmotic rupture. They should be uniquely vulnerable to splenic sequestration, and predictably splenectomy has been uniformly beneficial in patients with severe hemolysis.[1406,1420,1423,1424,1428,1434]

Hereditary stomatocytosis is probably more heterogenous than previously suggested. Some patients with severe permeability defects have little or no hemolysis.[829] In addition, studies of 44 Japanese patients with stomatocytosis show that the proportion of stomatocytes and the degree of Na^+ influx do not correlate with each other, and neither correlates with the amount of hemolysis or anemia.[1411] Furthermore, stomatin (protein 7.2b) deficiency was not observed in Japanese patients with the most severe permeability defects and was present to a mild degree in only five of nine patients with more moderate Na^+ leaks. This suggests that hereditary stomatocytosis is either a complex mixture of diseases (a good prospect) or that factors other than Na^+ leak and stomatin content are critical to the demise of the stomatocyte (also likely).

Clinical Features

The diagnostic features of hereditary stomatocytosis include the unique red cell morphology (5% to 50% stomatocytes; see Fig. 54-67), macrocytosis, elevated erythrocyte Na^+ concentration, reduced K^+ concentration, and increased total ($Na^+ + K^+$) content (see Table 54-14). The excess cations elevate cell water (see Fig. 54-26), producing osmotically fragile cells (see Table 54-14). In many patients, hereditary stomatocytes are also moderately deficient in 2,3-DPG.[1420,1434,1437] Perhaps a portion of the 1,3-DPG normally used for 2,3-DPG synthesis is diverted through phosphoglycerate kinase to provide extra ATP for cation transport.[1437] The 2,3-DPG deficiency mildly enhances oxygen affinity[1437] and causes additional water entry and cell swelling. Some patients[1416,1422] and dogs[1450,1451] with hereditary stomatocytosis have an unexplained decrease in red cell glutathione; it is unlikely that this is pathophysiologically significant. As noted, splenectomy reduces the hemolytic rate in patients with severe disease.

TABLE 54-14. Features of Stomatocytosis-Xerocytosis Syndromes*

	Stomatocytosis		Intermediate Syndromes			
	Severe Hemolysis	**Mild Hemolysis**	**Cryohydrocytosis**	**Pseudohyperkalemia**	**Stomatocytic Xerocytosis**	**Xerocytosis***
Hemolysis	Severe	Mild-moderate	Moderate	Mild	Mild	Moderate
Anemia	Severe	Mild-moderate	Mild-moderate	None	None	Mild-moderate
Blood smear	Stomatocytes	Stomatocytes	Stomatocytes or normal	Targets, few stomatocytes	Stomatocytes	Targets; occasional echinocytes, stomatocytes
MCV (80–100 fL)†	110–150	95–130	90–105	83–91	91–98	84–122
MCHC (32%–36%)	24–30	26–29	34–40	34–36	33–39	34–38
Unincubated osmotic fragility	Very increased	Increased	Normal	Normal or slt. decreased	Slightly decreased	Very decreased
RBC Na^+ (5–12)‡	60–100	30–60	40–50	Slt. increased§	10–20	10–30
RBC K^+ (90–103)‡	20–55	40–85	55–65	Slt. decreased §	75–85	60–90
RBC $Na^+ + K^+$ (95–110)‡	110–140	115–145	100–105	Low normal	87–109	75–99
Phosphatidylcholine content	Normal	±Increased	Normal	Normal	Normal	Increased*
Cold autohemolysis (Na^+ leak in)	No	No	Yes	?No	No	No
Cold K^+ leak out	?	?	Yes	Yes	?	No
Stomatin absent	Yes	?	Sometimes	No	?	?No
Effect of splenectomy	Good	Good	Fair	?	?	Poor
Genetics	AD, ?AR	AD	AD	AD	AD	AD
References	1406, 1408, 1415–1417, 1420, 1423, 1427, 1428, 1434	829, 1424	1412, 1421, 1453, 1456	1454, 1455	1422	866, 1407, 1409, 1414, 1425, 1426, 1429, 1430, 1432, 1433, 1435, 1452, 1457

AR, autosomal recessive; AD, autosomal dominant.

* Xerocytosis is very similar, and possibly identical with,[1435] high phosphatidylcholine hemolytic anemia (HPCHA)[1414,1429,1430,1432,1433,1452]; it is not clear whether all patients with xerocytosis have the elevated levels of phosphatidylcholine that characterize HPCHA.

† Normal values are given in parentheses.

‡ Units for RBC cations are milliequivalents per liter of RBCs.

§ Patient RBC Na^+ = 15.7–19.5 mmol/kg cell water (nl, 8.9–12.1); patient RBC K^+ = 126–134 mmol/kg cell water (nl, 133–159).

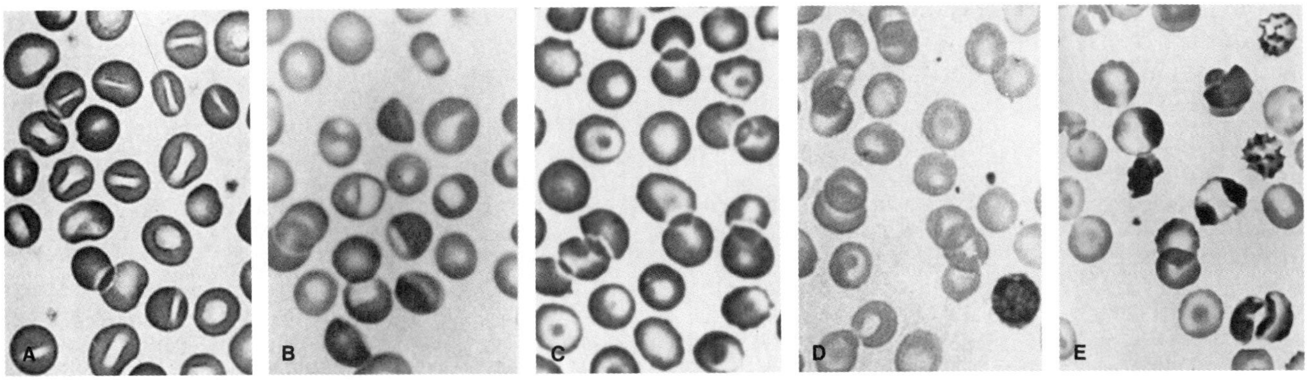

FIGURE 54-67. Peripheral blood morphology in hereditary stomatocytosis and hereditary xerocytosis. (**A**) Stomatocytosis. Many stomatocytes and occasional spherocytes are seen. (**B**) Cryohydrocytosis. Some of the stomatocytes are bowl shaped, some have curvilinear slits, and some have a transverse bar dividing the central clearing. (**C**) Stomatocytic xerocytosis. Moderate numbers of target cells and some crenated cells are present. (**D**) Xerocytosis (mild). Occasional target cells are evident, but most red cells are morphologically unremarkable. (**E**) Xerocytosis (severe). Target cells, echinocytes, and dense crenated cells predominate. In occasional cells, the hemoglobin appears to be puddled in one portion of the cell. (**A** from Turpin F et al[1431]; **B** from Miller G et al[1421]; **C** from Wiley JS et al[1432]; **D** from Jaffé ER, Gottfried EL[1452]; **E** from Glader BE et al[1409])

Hereditary Xerocytosis (High Phosphatidylcholine Hemolytic Anemia)

Several families have been described with a hemolytic anemia in which the red cells are markedly dehydrated, as manifested by an elevated MCHC.[866,1407,1409,1414,1425,1426,1432,1433,1435,1452,1457] Physiologically, the major red cell abnormality in these patients is a change in the relative membrane permeability to potassium. K^+ efflux is increased (two- to four-fold) and approximates Na^+ influx. No metabolic or hemoglobin abnormality accounts for this permeability lesion, and red cell calcium content is not increased. The nature of the permeability defect (the pathways involved) has not been well studied. Monovalent cation pump activity is increased appropriately for the slightly elevated Na^+ content, but the Na^+/K^+ pump cannot compensate for K^+ losses in excess of Na^+ gain. In fact, the action of the pump significantly exacerbates the rate of K^+ loss since three Na^+ ions are pumped out for every two K^+ ions returned.[586,587] As a consequence, xerocytes gradually become cation depleted and lose water in response to decreased intracellular osmolality. This is easily detected by centrifugation on Stractan gradients (see Fig. 54-68).

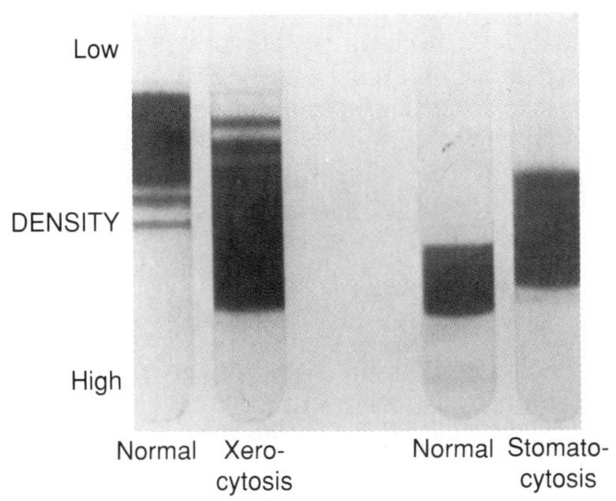

FIGURE 54-68. Separation of hydrocytes and xerocytes by density. (*Left*) Control and hereditary xerocytosis samples. The cells were separated on Stractan density gradients. The xerocytes extend to higher densities than normal red cells. (*Right*) Control and hereditary stomatocytosis samples. Many of the stomatocytes are lighter than the control red cells. (Lande WM, Mentzer WC. Haemolytic anaemia associated with increased cation permeability. Clin Haematol 1985;14:89)

Little is known about the molecular pathology of this rare disease. Where measured, the proportion of red cell membrane PC is increased (12 to 20 fmol/cell; normal, 10 to 12).[1435] The combination of hereditary xerocytosis and high PC is sometimes given the name *high PC hemolytic anemia* (HPCHA),[1414,1429,1433,1435,1452] but there appears to be

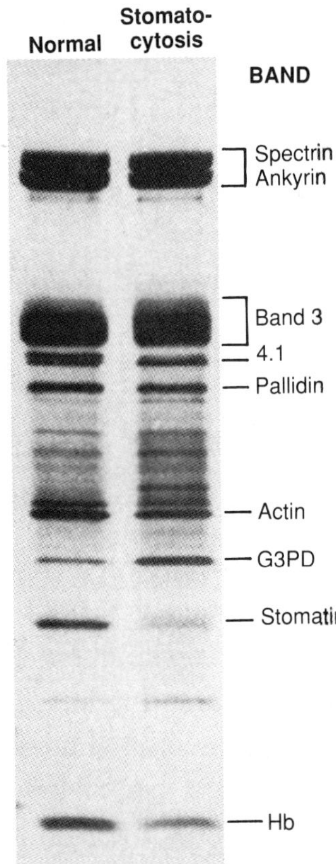

FIGURE 54-69. Stomatin deficiency in hereditary stomatocytosis. SDS gels of normal and stomatocytotic red cells show that the principal (28-kd) band in the band 7 region (band 7.2b, or stomatin) is missing. A similar picture is observed in most European patients with severe hereditary stomatocytosis. Immunoblots confirm that stomatin is absent in these cells. (Rix M, Bjerrum RJ, Wieth JO, Frandsen B. Congenital stomatocytosis with hemolytic anemia: with abnormal cation permeability and defective membrane proteins. Ugeskr Laeger 1991;153:724)

little reason to distinguish HPCHA from hereditary xerocytosis.[1435] Early studies suggested that the excess PC was due to diminished transfer of PC fatty acids to PE,[1429] a pathway that is normally *stimulated* by cellular dehydration.[1457a] It is not clear why this pathway is inhibited in hereditary xerocytosis or how it relates to the underlying membrane leakiness and hemolysis.

Red cells in hereditary xerocytosis are also shear sensitive[1426] and exceptionally prone to membrane fragmentation in response to metabolic stress.[866] This suggests a membrane skeletal defect, but no systematic studies of xerocytotic skeletons have been conducted to date. Conventional analyses of red cell membrane proteins have been normal,[866] except for an increase in the proportion of membrane-associated G3PD in one family.[1458] Quantitatively, all membrane components are increased, because for unknown reasons xerocytes have 15% to 25% more surface area than normal cells.[1459] Xerocytes are relatively rigid cells[1407] and probably develop a dehydration-induced membrane injury.[1426,1460] This poorly defined lesion is also found in irreversibly sickled cells[1460] and presumably is important in the pathophysiology of hemolysis.

Harm, Sauberman, and Snyder and associates[1461–1463] have shown that hereditary xerocytes are unusually sensitive to oxidants. For example, exposure of xerocytes to concentrations of hydrogen peroxide (H_2O_2) that do not affect normal cells causes a rapid loss of intracellular K^+, conversion of hemoglobin to methemoglobin, and cross-linking of hemoglobin to spectrin.[1462,1463] Similar sensitivity occurs in dehydrated *normal* red cells. Conversely, rehydrated xerocytes exhibit a normal reaction to H_2O_2. Native xerocytes contain the abnormal spectrin–globin complex, and the amount correlates with the extent of dehydration in various cellular fractions and with membrane rigidity.[1464] Finally, oxidation of normal erythrocytes with peroxide generates the spectrin–globin complex and rigid membranes.[1465] Complex formation is blocked by carbon monoxide, which prevents hemoglobin oxidation but is not blocked by lipid antioxidants.[1465] This implies a direct role for hemoglobin in cross-linking spectrin.

Clinical Features

In all families with hereditary xerocytosis studied, inheritance appears to be autosomal dominant.[866,1409,1414,1418,1432,1433,1452] Diagnostic red cell features include an increased MCHC and decreased osmotic fragility (resistance to osmotic lysis; see Table 54-14). In the most severely affected patients,[1409] blood smears display contracted and spiculated red cells and red cells in which the hemoglobin appears to be puddled or gelled in one portion of the cell (see Fig. 54-67). Most patients have *nearly normal erythrocyte morphology*, with only a *few target cells* and an occasional echinocyte or stomatocyte.

The characteristic biochemical abnormality is a reduced cell K^+ and total monovalent cation content (see Table 54-14). In older erythrocytes, K^+ approaches half-normal levels.[1435] Red cell 2,3-DPG concentrations are moderately decreased in hereditary xerocytosis,[866,1405,1409,1418,1425] as well as in hereditary hydrocytosis (see earlier section). The reasons for this deficiency are unknown. Because the loss of the polyvalent DPG is compensated by an influx of monovalent chloride ions and water, patients with xerocytosis and unusually low DPG levels have fewer dehydrated red cells than expected for the degree of cation loss, and in rare cases have no dehydration at all.[1405] Patients with low DPG also have increased whole blood oxygen affinity and, consequently, may have little apparent anemia (*relative* polycythemia).[1405] Autohemolysis is increased and responds to glucose,[866,1418,1432,1452] similar to the pattern in HS.

Conventional analyses suggest that hereditary xerocytes are macrocytic, despite their dehydration (see Table 54-14); this is, at least partly, an artifact of cellular stiffness. In Coulter-type electronic counters, the conversion of pulse height (from the resistance of a cell passing through an electric field) to a cellular volume depends on cell shape. Xerocytes do not deform to the same degree as do normal cells, which causes the electronically measured MCV to be about 10% too high.[1459] This also affects the hematocrit, which is calculated from the MCV.

Splenectomy Is Probably Not Beneficial in Hereditary Xerocytosis. In contrast to the situation in hereditary hydrocytosis, in which splenectomy is beneficial, the limited experience available suggests that removing the spleen does not significantly reduce hemolysis in patients with hereditary xerocytosis.[1409,1414] Xerocytes are so functionally compromised that they are easily detected and eliminated in other areas of the reticuloendothelial system. It may even be dangerous: one 46-year-old xerocytosis patient had fatal pulmonary emboli after splenectomy.[1414] Fortunately, most patients are able to maintain a hemoglobin level of at least 9 g/dL, so that splenectomy is not an issue.

Intermediate Syndromes

Hydrocytosis and xerocytosis represent the extremes of a spectrum of red cell permeability defects. A number of families with features of both conditions have been reported. The reported cases seem to fall into three groups whose red cells differ principally in morphology, osmotic fragility, and sensitivity to cold (see Table 54-14).

Cryohydrocytosis

Two unrelated patients have been reported with this disease. The mode of inheritance is not apparent from these cases, but we have seen a third family with 12 affected members in four generations,[1453] which strongly suggests autosomal dominant transmission. The patients have a mild congenital hemolytic anemia characterized by marked autohemolysis *that is greater at 4°C than at 37°C*.[1412,1421,1453,1456] This cold autohemolysis is sensitive to the method of anticoagulation. It is increased in the cold in heparin, EDTA, and defibrinated plasma, but not in acid citrate dextrose.[1412,1421,1453] This may reflect unusual pH sensitivity of the abnormal red cells, because cold hemolysis is accentuated at pH 8 (pH of blood in the first three anticoagulants at 4°C) compared with pH 7.6 (pH of acid citrate dextrose plasma at 4°C).[1412,1421,1422, 1453–1456]

Blood smears show stomatocytes, some of which have an eccentric or curvilinear slit or a transverse bar bisecting the area of central pallor (see Fig. 54-67). Fresh erythrocytes are Na^+ loaded and K^+ depleted (see Table 54-14), but the total concentration of ($Na^+ + K^+$) is normal.[1412,1453] In the cold, Na^+ and K^+ permeabilities are markedly increased. Because Na^+ entry greatly predominates, the red cells rapidly swell and lyse. The primary molecular lesion of this interesting disorder is unknown. Membrane lipids are quantitatively normal,[1412] and with the exception of a mild decrease in red cell glutathione),[1412,1421] no defects in metabolism have been detected. In one patient, stomatin was missing when red cell membrane proteins were analyzed,[1413] but this defect was not observed in our patients.[1453]

Pseudohyperkalemia

Stewart and colleagues[1454,1455] have reported a family with a dominantly inherited disorder characterized by erythrocyte K^+ loss that is exaggerated in the cold. Electrolyte analyses of plasma obtained from blood samples stored for just a few hours at room temperature or lower may falsely suggest that affected persons are hyperkalemic. The disorder resembles cryohydrocytosis except that K^+ loss and dehydration predominate (cryoxerocytosis) instead of Na^+ gain and cryohemolysis. Fortunately, there is little K^+ loss at physiologic temperatures, so that patients have only mildly dehydrated red cells and little or no hemolysis and anemia.[1454,1455]

Stomatocytic Xerocytosis

In 1971, Miller and colleagues[1422] reported 54 patients with dominantly inherited stomatocytosis in a large Swiss-German family. Apparent heterozygotes (51 of 54 patients) had mild hemolysis, 1% to 25% stomatocytes on their peripheral blood smears (see Fig. 54-14), and no anemia. Intracellular potassium and total monovalent cations were mildly decreased, and fresh red cells were osmotically resistant (see Table 54-14). Three probable homozygotes from a consanguineous mating had mild anemia, moderately severe hemolysis, marked stomatocytosis (20% to 35%), and greater cation permeability.[1422,1439] Because net sodium and potassium levels were relatively balanced, cell hydration was not seriously deranged.

Other Stomatocytic Disorders

Acquired Stomatocytosis

In normal people, 3% or less of the red cells on peripheral blood smears are stomatocytic,[1466,1467] although more stomatocytic forms are evident (up to 10%) when sensitive techniques like scanning electron microscopy are used.[1468] Because stomatocytes may occasionally occur as a drying artifact in limited areas of the smear, care must be taken to examine multiple areas on several smears before diagnosing stomatocytosis. In wet preparations, stomatocytes are bowl-shaped (uniconcave). Such preparations are useful in excluding artifactual stomatocytes, but the presence of bowl-shaped cells cannot be used as proof of the presence of stomatocytes because target cells are also bowl-shaped in solution.[1378]

In a prospective study of 4291 peripheral blood smears, Davidson and coworkers[1469] found increased numbers of stomatocytes in 2.3% of the preparations (59% of these smears had 5% to 20% stomatocytes, 35% had 20% to 50% stomatocytes, 6% had greater than 50% stomatocytes). In this and other studies,[1415,1422,1470] a wide variety of drugs and diagnoses were associated with stomatocytosis. Further studies are needed to determine which associations are specific and repeatable.

Two specific associations are alcohol and vinca alkaloids. Acquired stomatocytosis is common in alcoholics, particularly in those with *acute alcoholism*, and may be associated with moderate hemolysis.[1466,1467] Red cell cation measurements have not been reported to date; severe hydrocytosis is unlikely because osmotic fragility tests have been normal.[1466]

Vinca alkaloids (eg, vincristine, vinblastine) frequently induce hemolysis, sometimes with increased membrane Na^+ permeability and stomatocytosis, in the doses used for chemotherapy of leukemias and lymphomas.[1471] This is a particular problem in the rare instances in which these drugs must be given to patients with cancer who also have HS. We have seen two such patients, and in both cases severe hemolysis occurred. The probable explanation is that spherocytes and stomatocytes both have a decreased surface/volume ratio. Imposing a stomatocytic stress on HS red cells will make them even more spheroidal and hasten their demise.

Stomatocytes have also been observed, transiently, on wet preparations of blood from *marathon runners* immediately after a race.[1472] Because some marathon runners develop transient intravascular hemolysis after running (march hemoglobinuria),[1473] the two phenomena may be related. Some years ago, Banga and associates[1474] reported that three of three patients with *march hemoglobinuria* lacked a 29-kd protein (presumably stomatin) in the band 7.2 region of red cell membranes. The defect was similar and probably identical with the defect observed in hereditary stomatocytosis[1408,1413,1423,1442] (see Fig. 54-69), but the patients with march hemoglobinuria did not have any significant hemolysis or abnormal red cell morphology under basal conditions.[1474]

Rh_{null} Disease

The Rh(D) antigen and the other antigens of the Rh group (cCeE) are part of two minor red cell membrane proteins whose structure has been deciphered (see Chap. 56). Patients who lack all Rh antigens (Rh_{null})[1475] have a moderately severe hemolytic anemia (^{51}Cr-labeled red cell $T_{1/2}$ of 10 to 14 days)[1476–1479] characterized by stomatocytosis and spherocytosis. Osmotic fragility is only mildly increased,[1476,1479] but ektacytometry shows a significant loss of membrane surface, particularly in denser (and presumably older) cells.[1476] Red cell membrane K^+ or Rb^+ (a K^+ analogue) permeability is about twice normal, which is compatible with a mild xerocytosis syndrome.[1476,1480] In one patient, most of the Rh_{null} cells were dense and K^+ depleted[1476]; in another patient, cation and water concentrations were normal.[1480]

Stomatocytosis and hemolysis are also features of Rh_{mod} disease, a related anomaly in which the expression of Rh antigens is suppressed but not absent, owing to the influence of a suppressor gene.[1481,1482]

Tangier Disease

Tangier disease is an autosomal recessive condition characterized by splenomegaly, the virtual absence of HDLs, hypertriglyceridemia, mild corneal clouding, peripheral neuropathy, bone marrow foam cells (in 70% of patients), and characteristic orange, cholesteryl ester–laden tonsils.[1483] Cholesteryl esters are greatly elevated in tissue macrophages in Tangier disease because of lack of HDLs, which normally returns cholesteryl esters to the liver. The HDL deficiency is caused by hypercatabolism of the lipoprotein.[1483] Normally, HDL binds to specific receptors on macrophages, is internalized (presumably to load up on cholesteryl esters), and then recycles to the membrane surface. In Tangier disease, for unknown reasons, the protein is misrouted to macrophage lysosomes and destroyed.[1484]

Hematologic examination of one patient with Tangier disease disclosed stomatocytosis, hemolysis (hemoglobin 8.5 g/dL; reticulocytes 6% to 9%), and osmotically sensitive red cells.[1485] Membrane cholesterol was low, the cholesterol/phospholipid ratio was decreased, and phospholipid analysis showed high PC and low sphingomyelin.[1485] Red cell cation concentrations and permeabilities were not investigated. Because hematologic data have rarely been reported in Tangier disease, it is difficult to know whether this patient is exceptional. Previous reports of unexplained hemolysis in three patients suggest that he is not.[1486–1488]

Mediterranean Stomatocytosis

About 25 years ago, several groups independently observed that stomatocytosis was remarkably common among Mediterranean immigrants to Australia.[1470,1489–1491] Norman,[1489] and Jackson and Knight[1490] recorded 41 patients within one small private practice, and Ducrou and Kimber[1470] added an additional 20 patients. The typical stomatocytic morphology was associated with mild to moderate hemolytic anemia, normal red cell cations, and normal osmotic fragility.[1470,1490] Many patients also had macrothrombocytopenia (40,000 to 150,000 platelets, 9 to 120 fL in volume) and slight splenomegaly.

A study of *healthy* Mediterranean immigrants confirmed the increased incidence of stomatocytosis (36% with more than 5% stomatocytes); affected persons were not anemic.[1492] Splenomegaly and macrothrombocytopenia were also common, but they segregated independently of the red cell defect.

The cause of Mediterranean stomatocytosis remains a mystery. It is not even clear whether it still exists, since no further reports have appeared. The general impression is that stomatocytosis is not unusually prevalent in Mediterranean countries or in Mediterranean immigrants in other parts of the world, which suggests an environmental influence, but accurate data concerning the prevalence of stomatocytosis are lacking.

Other Diseases Associated With Stomatocytosis

Stomatocytosis is also observed in at least some patients with the hemolytic anemia that results from adenosine deaminase overproduction.[1493] A preliminary report of mild stomatocytosis and uncompensated hemolysis in a Japanese woman with polyagglutinable red cells and an apparent defect in sialylation of band 3 and glycophorin has also appeared.[1494]

Other Causes of Xerocytosis

ATP Depletion

When red cell ATP concentrations fall below 5% to 15% of normal, the cells leak cations and become rigid and echinocytic.[1495] In plasma or other Ca^{2+}-containing media, a specific K^+ permeability lesion (the Gárdos phenomenon)[533] is superimposed on the unchecked normal leak of Na^+ and K^+ and leads to cation depletion and dehydration. Coincidentally, poorly defined changes occur in membrane skeletal structure.[1496,1497]

These phenomena are presumably involved in the hemolysis that occurs in inherited defects of glycolysis such as pyruvate kinase (PK) deficiency (see Chap. 57). Studies by Nathan,[1498] Mentzer,[1499] and Glader[1500] and their coworkers show that PK-deficient red cells rapidly lose ATP and K^+ and become dehydrated, spiculated, and viscous when incubated in vitro, particularly under conditions in which residual mitochondrial production of ATP is curtailed. In patients who have undergone splenectomy, contracted, crenated red cells are more numerous.[1237,1501] These "deflated echinocytes"[1501] are more rigid than normal[1502] and are relatively scarce in patients who have not had a splenectomy,[1237,1501] which implies that they are premorbid cells given temporary reprieve by removal of the spleen.

Little is known about the status of membrane proteins in red cells with compromised ATP production. Small amounts of disulfide-linked spectrin complexes and marked diminution of spectrin extractability were detected in a patient with glucose phosphate isomerase deficiency,[1503] which suggests that membrane protein damage may be pathologically relevant in these disorders; further experience is required to assess this point accurately.

Irreversibly Sickled Cells

Irreversibly sickled cells are circulating erythrocytes from patients with sickle cell anemia that retain a sickled shape when oxygenated because of an acquired defect in the membrane skeleton.[558] Biochemically, irreversibly sickled cells are deficient in total monovalent cations and water.[1504,1505] The mechanism of their formation and the nature of the acquired membrane defects responsible for their abnormal shape, cation content, and surface topography are detailed in Chapter 53.

OTHER MEMBRANE DISORDERS

Oxidant Hemolysis

Oxidant damage is incurred by the red cell membrane in a variety of inherited disorders involving abnormal hemoglobins or defects in the cells' endogenous system for detoxification of oxidants. These include sickle cell disease (see Chap. 53), thalassemias (see Chap. 51), unstable hemoglobinopathies (see Chap. 52), G6PD deficiency (see Chap. 58), and disorders of glutathione metabolism. A complete description of the membrane lesions associated with these diseases is beyond the scope of this chapter and, in most instances, is covered in the chapters indicated.

Membrane oxidant damage may also result from encounters with exogenous oxidants, one of the most important of these being copper.

Copper Toxicity and Wilson's Disease

Acute Intoxication

Acute copper-induced hemolysis has been reported in humans after accidental or suicidal ingestion, copper sulfate therapy for burns, and copper contamination of hemodialysis units.[1506–1510] It is characterized by flushing, chills, nausea and vomiting, diarrhea, abdominal pain, a metallic taste in the mouth, excessive salivation, headache, weakness, and acute intravascular hemolysis.[1506–1511]

Wilson's Disease

Wilson's disease (hepatolenticular degeneration) is an autosomal recessive disorder of copper metabolism characterized by defective biliary excretion of copper, low plasma ceruloplasmin, and toxic accumulation of copper in liver, erythrocytes, kidneys, corneas, and brain.[1512,1513] The toxic consequences include cirrhosis, hemolysis,[1514–1527] Fanconi's renal tubular syndrome, corneal Kayser-Fleischer rings, and a progressive neurologic syndrome (psychiatric symptoms, loss of coordination, dystonic posturing, involuntary movements, and dysarthria).

The Wilson disease gene is located on chromosome 13 at q14.3 and encodes an integral membrane protein that has the features of a copper-transporting ATPase.[1528–1532] It is predominantly expressed in the liver and kidneys.[1529,1531]

Hemolysis is an early feature of Wilson's disease. It is seen in 20% of patients who present with liver disease[1514] and may be the presenting manifestation.[1515–1521] Because the disease is treatable and because hemolysis may presage fulminant liver disease by days to years,[1512,1517,1520,1521] the clinician must always consider Wilson's disease in children and young adults (4 to 40 years of age) with Coombs'-negative hemolytic anemia. Typically, these previously well patients have chemical evidence of acute hepatocyte damage, mild hepatosplenomegaly, and chemical signs of Wilson's disease (low ceruloplasmin concentration, increased erythrocyte and hepatic copper levels, and increased urinary copper excretion).[1512] Jaundice is common and may be extreme. Hemolysis is at least partially intravascular, and hemoglobin may be detected on urine analysis, but gross hemoglobinuria is uncommon. Peripheral blood smears are usually uncharacteristic, although we have seen one child in whom spur cells and target cells were prominent.

Copper is believed to accumulate in the liver in Wilson's disease patients until it reaches a toxic level. The resulting hepatocellular necrosis releases stored copper into the bloodstream,[1520] where it is rapidly taken up by red cells.[1533] Hemolysis occurs as a consequence of oxidative damage. The oxidative effects of copper are manifold. In vitro, copper inactivates numerous red cell glycolytic and hexose-monophosphate shunt enzymes; directly oxidizes NADPH and glutathione; oxidizes and denatures hemoglobin; damages membrane ATPases, fatty acid acylase, and probably other membrane enzymes; generates lipid peroxides; and cross-links membrane skeletal proteins into disulfide-bonded high molecular weight complexes, increasing membrane permeability and rigidity.[1511,1534] Most of these effects have not been demonstrated at concentrations of copper observed in hemolyzing erythrocytes (150 to 400 μg/100 mL red cells = 2.4×10^{-5} to 6.3×10^{-5} mol/L).[1522,1526] So far, it has not been possible to determine the exact cause of the red cells' demise.

REFERENCES

1. Harrison ML, Rathinavelu P, Arese P, Geahlen RL, Low PS. Role of band 3 tyrosine phosphorylation in the regulation of erythrocyte glycolysis. J Biol Chem 1991;266:4106.
2. Weith JO, Anderson OS, Brahm J, et al. Chloride-bicarbonate exchange in red blood cells: physiology of transport and chemical modification of binding sites. Philos Trans R Soc Lond (Biol) 1982;299:383.
3. Danielli JF, Davson HA. A contribution to the theory of the permeability of thin films. J Cell Comp Physiol 1936;9:89.
4. Singer SJ, Nicolson GL. The fluid-mosaic model of the structure of cell membranes. Science 1972;175:720.
5. Dodge JT, Mitchell C, et al. The preparation and chemical characteristics of hemoglobin-free ghosts of human erythrocytes. Arch Biochem Biophys 1963;100:119.
6. Kant JA, Steck TL. Cation-impermeable inside-out and right-side-out vesicles from human erythrocyte membranes. Nature 1972;240:26.
7. Fairbanks G, Steck TL, Wallach DFH. Electrophoretic analysis of the major polypeptides of the human erythrocyte membrane. Biochemistry 1971;10:2606.
8. Shapiro AL, Vinuela E, Maizel JV. Molecular weight estimation of polypeptide chains by electrophoresis in SDS polyacrylamide gels. Biochem Biophys Res Commun 1967;28:815.
9. Marchesi VT, Steers E Jr. Selective solubilization of a protein component of the red cell membrane. Science 1968;159:203.
10. Marchesi VT, Tillack TW, Jackson RL, Segrest JP, Scott RE. Chemical characterization and surface orientation of the major glycoprotein of the human erythrocyte membrane. Proc Natl Acad Sci USA 1972;69:1445.
11. Sweeley CC, Dawson G. Lipids of the erythrocyte. In: Jamieson GA, Greenwalt TJ, eds. Red cell membrane structure and function. Philadelphia, JB Lippincott, 1969:172.
12. Turner JD, Rouser G. Precise quantitative determination of human blood lipids by thin layer and triethylaminoethyl cellulose column chromatography. Ann Biochem 1970;38:437.
13. Ways P, Hanahan DJ. Characterization and quantification of red cell lipids in normal man. J Lipid Res 1964;5:318.
14. Weinstein RS. The morphology of adult red cells. In: Surgenor DM, ed. The red blood cell, ed 2, vol 1. New York, Academic Press, 1974:214.
15. Van Deenen LLM, De Gier J. Lipids of the red blood cell membrane. In: Surgenor DM, ed. The red blood cell, ed 2, vol 1. New York, Academic Press, 1974:148.
16. Cullis PR, Hope MJ. Effects of fusogenic agents on membrane structure of erythrocyte ghosts and the mechanism of membrane fusion. Nature 1978;271:672.
17. Bergelson LD, Barsukov LI. Topological asymmetry of phospholipids in membranes. Science 1977;197:224.
18. Etemadi AH. Membrane asymmetry: a survey and critical appraisal of the methodology: methods for assessing the unequal distribution of lipids. Biochim Biophys Acta 1980;604:423.
19. Op den Kamp JAF. Lipid asymmetry in membranes. Annu Rev Biochem 1979;48:47.
20. Devaux PF. Protein involvement in transmembrane lipid asymmetry. Annu Rev Biophys Biomol Struct 1992;21:417.
21. Devaux PF. Lipid transmembrane asymmetry and flip-flip in biological membranes and in lipid bilayers. Curr Opin Struct Biol 1993;3:489.
22. Devaux PF. Static and dynamic lipid asymmetry in cell membranes. Biochemistry 1991;30:1163.
23. Connor J, Schroit AJ. Determination of lipid asymmetry in human red cells by resonance energy transfer. Biochemistry 1987;26:5099.
24. Daleke DL, Huestis WH. Incorporation and translocation of aminophospholipids in human erythrocytes. Biochemistry 1985;24:5406.
25. Seigneuret M, Devaux PF. ATP-dependent asymmetric distribution of spin-labeled phospholipids in the erythrocyte membrane: relation to shape changes. Proc Natl Acad Sci USA 1984;81:3751.
26. Tilley L, Cribier S, Roelofsen B, Op den Kamp JAF, Van Deenen LLM. ATP-dependent translocation of amino phospholipids across the human erythrocyte membrane. FEBS Lett 1986;194:21.
27. Zachowski A, Favre E, Cribier S, Hervé P, Devaux PF. Outside-inside translocation of aminophospholipids in the human erythrocyte membrane is mediated by a specific enzyme. Biochemistry 1986;25:2585.
27a. Morrot G, Hervé P, Zachowski A, Fellmann P, Devaux PF. Aminophospholipid translocase of human erythrocytes: phospholipid substrate specificity and effect of cholesterol. Biochemistry 1989;28:3456.
28. Connor J, Schroit AJ. Transbilayer movement of phosphatidylserine in nonhuman erythrocytes: evidence that the aminophospholipid transporter is a ubiquitous membrane protein. Biochemistry 1989;28:9680.
29. Zachowski A, Henry J-P, Devaux PF. Control of transmembrane lipid asymmetry in chromaffin granules by an ATP-dependent protein. Nature 1989;340:75.
30. Connor J, Schroit AJ. Transbilayer movement of phosphatidylserine in erythrocytes: inhibition of transport and preferential labeling of a 31,000-dalton protein by sulfhydryl reactive reagents. Biochemistry 1988;27:848.
30a. Higgins CF, Gottesman MM. Is the multidrug transporter a flippase? Trends Biochem Sci 1972;17:18.
30b. Smit JJ, Schinkel AH, Oude Elferink RP, et al. Homozygous disruption of the murine mdr2 P-glycoprotein gene leads to a complete absence of phospholipid from bile and to liver disease. Cell 1993;75:451.
31. Morrot G, Zachowski A, Devaux PF. Partial purification and characterization of the human erythrocyte Mg-ATPase: a candidate aminophospholipid translocase. FEBS Lett 1990;266:29.
32. Connor J, Pak CH, Zwaal RFA, Schroit AJ. Bidirectional transbilayer movement of phospholipid analogs in human red blood cells: evidence for an ATP-dependent and protein-mediated process. J Biol Chem 1992;267:19412.
33. Schroit AJ, Madsen J, Ruoho AE. Radioiodinated, photoactivatable phosphatidylcholine and phosphatidylserine transfer properties and differential photoreactive interaction with human erythrocyte membrane proteins. Biochemistry 1987;26:1812.
34. Schroit AJ, Bloy C, Connor J, Cartron J-P. Involvement of Rh blood group polypeptides in the maintenance of aminophospholipid asymmetry. Biochemistry 1990;29:10303.
35. Chérif-Zahar B, Bloy C, Le Van Kim C, et al. Molecular cloning and protein structure of a human blood group Rh polypeptide. Proc Natl Acad Sci USA 1990;87:6243.
36. Walker JE, Saraste M, Runswick J, Gay NJ. Distantly related sequences in the alpha and beta subunits of ATP synthase, myosin, kinases, and other ATP-requiring enzymes and a common nucleotide binding fold. EMBO J 1982;8:945.
37. Bonnet D, Begard E. Interaction of anilinonapthyl labelled spectrin with fatty acids and phospholipids: fluorescence study. Biochem Biophys Res Comm 1984;120:344.
38. Cohen AM, Liu S-C, Derick LH, Palek J. Ultrastructural studies of the interaction of spectrin with phosphatidylserine liposomes. Blood 1986;68:920.
39. Maksymiw R, Sui S-F, Gaub H, Sackmann E. Electrostatic coupling of spectrin dimers to phosphatidylserine containing lipid lamellae. Biochemistry 1987;26:2983.
40. Mombers C, De Gier J, Demel RA, Van Deenen LLM. Spectrin-phospholipid interacton: a monolayer study. Biochim Biophys Acta 1980;603:52.
41. Bergmann WL, Dressler V, Haest CW, Deuticke B. Crosslinking of SH groups in the membrane enhances transbilayer orientation of phospholipids: evidence for a limited access of phospholipids to the reorientation sites. Biochim Biophys Acta 1984;769:390.
42. Dressler V, Haest CWM, Plasa G, Deuticke B, Erusalimsky JD. Stabilizing factors of phospholipid asymmetry in the erythrocyte membrane. Biochim Biophys Acta 1984;775:189.
43. Franck PFH, Roelofsen B, Op den Kamp JA. Complete exchange of phosphatidylcholine from intact erythrocytes after protein cross-linking. Biochim Biophys Acta 1982;687:105.
44. Haest CWM, Plasa G, Kamp D, Deuticke B. Spectrin as a stabilizer of the phospholipid asymmetry in the human erythrocyte membrane. Biochim Biophys Acta 1978;509:21.
45. Calvez J-Y, Zachowski A, Herrmann A, Morrot G, Devaux PF. Asymmetric distribution of phospholipids in spectrin-poor erythrocyte vesicles. Biochemistry 1988;27:5666.
46. Kuypers FA, Lubin BH, Yee M, Agre P, Devaux PF, Geldwerth D. The distribution of erythrocyte phospholipids in hereditary spherocytosis demonstrates a minimal role for erythrocyte spectrin on phospholipid diffusion and asymmetry. Blood 1993;81:1051.
47. Verhoven B, Schlegel RA, Williamson P. Rapid loss and restoration

of lipid asymmetry by different pathways in resealed erythrocyte ghosts. Biochim Biophys Acta 1992;1104:15.
48. Williamson P, Kulick A, Zachowski A, Schlegel RA. Devaux PF. Ca^{2+} induces transbilayer redistribution of all major phospholipids in human erythrocytes. Biochemistry 1992;31:6355.
49. Zwaal RFA, Comfurius P, Bevers EM. Mechanism and function of changes in membrane-phospholipid asymmetry in platelets and erythrocytes. Biochem Soc Trans 1993;21:248.
50. Blumenfeld N, Zachowski A, Galacteros F, Beuzard Y, Devaux PF. Transmembrane mobility of phospholipids in sickle erythrocytes: effect of deoxygenation on diffusion and asymmetry. Blood 1991;77:849.
51. Franck PFH, Chiu DT-Y, et al. Accelerated transbilayer movement of phosphatidylcholine in sickled erythrocytes: a reversible process. J Biol Chem 1983;258:8436.
52. Lubin B, Chiu D, et al. Abnormalities in membrane phospholipid organization in sickled erythrocytes. J Clin Invest 1981;67:1643.
53. Platt OS, Falcone JF, Lux SE. Molecular defect in the sickle erythrocyte skeleton: abnormal spectrin binding to sickle inside-out vesicles. J Clin Invest 1985;75:266.
54. Schwartz RS, Rybicki AC, Heath RH, Lubin BH. Protein 4.1 in sickle erythrocytes: evidence for oxidative damage. J Biol Chem 1987;62:15666.
55. Waugh SM, Willardson BM, Kannan R, Labotka RJ, Low PS. Heinz bodies induce clustering of band 3, glycophorin, and ankyrin in sickle cell erythrocytes. J Clin Invest 1986;78:1155.
56. Liu S-C, Derick LH, Zhai S, Palek J. Uncoupling of the spectrin-based skeleton from the lipid bilayer in sickled red cells. Science 1991;252:574.
57. Wautier JL, Paton RC, Wautier MP, et al. Increased adhesion of erythrocytes to endothelial cells in diabetes mellitus and its relationship to vascular complications. N Engl J Med 1981;305:237.
58. Hebbel RP, Yamada O, Moldow CF, Jacob HS, White JG, Eaton JW. Abnormal adherence of sickle erythrocytes to cultured vascular endothelium: possible mechanism for microvascular occlusion in sickle cell disease. J Clin Invest 1980;65:154.
59. Hebbel RP, Boogaerts MA, Eaton JW, Steinberg MH. Erythrocyte adherence to endothelium in sickle-cell anemia: a possible determinant of disease severity. N Engl J Med 1980;302:992.
60. Mohandas N, Evans E. Adherence of sickle erythrocytes to vascular endothelial cells: Requirement for both cell membrane changes and plasma factors. Blood 1984;64:282.
61. Bevers EM, Comfurius P, et al. Generation of prothrombin-converting activity and the exposure of phosphatidyl serine at the outer surface of platelets. Eur J Biochem 1982;122:429.
62. Chiu D, Lubin B, Roelofsen B, Van Deenen LLM. Sickled erythrocytes accelerate clotting in vitro: an effect of abnormal membrane lipid asymmetry. Blood 1981;58:398.
63. Zwaal RFA, Comfurius P, et al. Membrane asymmetry and blood coagulation. Nature 1977;268:358.
64. Allen TM, Williamson P, Schlegel RA. Phosphatidylserine as a determinant of reticuloendothelial recognition of liposome models of the erythrocyte surface. Proc Natl Acad Sci USA 1988;85:8067.
65. McEvoy L, Williamson P, Schlegel RA. Membrane phospholipid asymmetry as a determinant of erythrocyte recognition by macrophages. Proc Natl Acad Sci USA 1986;83:3311.
66. Pradhan D, Williamson PL, Schlegel RA. Phosphatidylserine as a signal for recognition and phagocytosis of erythrocytes by macrophages. (Abstract) Mol Biol Cell 1993;4(Suppl):84.
67. Schwartz RS, Chiu DT, Lubin B. Plasma membrane phospholipid organization in human erythrocytes. (Review) Curr Top Hematol 1985;5:63.
68. Tanaka Y, Schroit AJ. Insertion of fluorescent phosphatidylserine into the plasma membrane of red blood cells: recognition by autologous macrophages. J Biol Chem 1983;258:11335.
69. Rodgers W, Glaser M. Characterization of lipid domains in erythrocyte membranes. Proc Natl Acad Sci USA 1991;88:1364.
70. Jost PC, Nadakavukaren KK, Griffith OH. Phosphatidyl choline exchange between the boundary lipid and bilayer domains in cytochrome oxidase containing membranes. Biochemistry 1977;16:3110.
71. Smith RL, Oldfield E. Dynamic structure of membranes by deuterium NMR. Science 1984;225:280.
72. Armitage IM, Shapiro DL, et al. ^{31}P nuclear magnetic resonance evidence for polyphosphoinositide associated with the hydrophobic segment of glycophorin A. Biochemistry 1977;16:1317.
73. Mendelsohn R, Dluhy RA, Crawford T, Mantsch HH. Interaction of glycophorin with phosphatidylserine: a Fourier transform infrared investigation. Biochemistry 1984;23:1498.
74. Ong RL. ^{31}P and ^{19}F NMR studies of glycophorin-reconstituted membranes: preferential interaction of glycophorin with phosphatidylserine. J Membr Biol 1984;78:1.
75. Yeagle PL, Kelsey D. Phosphorus nuclear magnetic resonance studies of lipid-protein interactions: human erythrocyte glycophorin and phospholipids. Biochemistry 1989;28:2210.
76. Boyd D, Beckwith J. The role of charged amino acids in the localization of secreted and membrane proteins. Cell 1990;62:1031.
77. Parks GD, Lamb RA. Topology of eukaryotic type II membrane proteins: importance of N-terminal positively charged residues flanking the hydrophobic domain. Cell 1991;64:777.
78. Yamane K, Akiyama Y, Ito K, Mizushima S. A positively charged region is a determinant of the orientation of cytoplasmic membrane proteins in *Escherichia coli*. J Biol Chem 1990;265:21166.
79. Beck JS. Relations between membrane monolayers in some red cell shape transformations. J Theor Biol 1978;75:487.
80. Ferrell JE Jr, Lee KJ, Huestis WH. Membrane bilayer balance and erythrocyte shape: a quantitative assessment. Biochemistry 1985;24:2849.
81. Sheetz MP, Singer SJ. Biological membranes as bilayer couples: a molecular mechanism of drug-erythrocyte interactions. Proc Natl Acad Sci USA 1974;71:4457.
82. Christiansson A, Kuypers FA, Roelofsen B, Op den Kamp JAF, Van Deenen LLM. Lipid molecular shape effects erythrocyte morphology: a study involving replacement of native phosphatidylcholine with different species followed by treatment of cells with sphingomyelinase C or phospholipase A. J Cell Biol 1985;101:1455.
83. Isomaa B, Hagerstrand H, Paatero G. Shape transformation induced by amphiphiles in erythrocytes. Biochim Biophys Acta 1987;899:93.
84. Sheetz MP, Painter RG, et al. Biological membranes as bilayer couples. III. Compensatory shape changes induced in membranes. J Cell Biol 1976;70:193.
85. Lange Y, Steck TL. Mechanism of red blood cell acanthocytosis and echinocytosis in vivo. J Membr Biol 1984;77:153.
86. Brown K, Anderson SM, Young NS. Erythrocyte P antigen: cellular receptor for B19 parvovirus. Science 1993;262:114.
87. Blair L, Bittman R. Cholesterol distribution between the two halves of the lipid bilayer of human erythrocyte ghost membranes. J Biol Chem 1978;253:8366.
88. Lange Y, Dolde J, Steck TL. The rate of transmembrane movement of cholesterol in the human erythrocyte. J Biol Chem 1981;256:5321.
89. Lange Y, Slayton JM. Interaction of cholesterol and lysophosphatidylcholine in determining red cell shape. J Lipid Res 1982;23:1121.
90. Huang C-H. A structural model for the cholesterol-phosphatidyl choline complexes in bilayer membranes. Lipids 1977;12:348.
91. Berridge MJ. Inositol trisphosphate and calcium signalling. Nature 1993;361:315.
92. Cohen CM, Gascard P. Regulation and post-translational modification of the erythrocyte membrane and membrane-skeletal proteins. Semin Hematol 1992;29:244.
93. Levine YK, Birdsall NJM, Lee AG, Metcalf JC. ^{13}C nuclear magnetic resonance relaxation measurements of synthetic lecithins and the effect of spin-labeled lipids. Biochemistry 1972;11:1416.
94. McConnell HM, McFarland BG. The flexibility gradient in biological membranes. Ann NY Acad Sci 1972;195:207.
95. Barton PG, Gunstone FD. Hydrocarbon chain packing and molecular motion in phospholipid bilayers formed from unsaturated lecithins. J Biol Chem 1975;250:4470.
96. Seelig A, Seelig J. Effect of a single cis double bond on the structure of a phospholipid bilayer. Biochemistry 1977;16:45.
97. Oldfield E, Chapman D. Effects of cholesterol and cholesterol derivatives on hydrocarbon chain mobility in lipids. Biochem Biophys Res Commun 1971;43:610.
98. Lee AG, Birdsall NJM, et al. Measurement of fast lateral diffusion of lipids in vesicles and in biological membranes by ^{3}H nuclear magnetic resonance. Biochemistry 1973;12:1650.
99. Cooper RA, Durocher JR, Leslie MH. Decreased fluidity of red cell membrane lipid in abetalipoproteinemia. J Clin Invest 1977;60:115.
100. Cooper RA. Abnormalities of cell-membrane fluidity in the pathogenesis of disease. N Engl J Med 1977;297:371.
101. Vanderkooi J, Fischkoff S, et al. Fluorescent probe analysis of the lipid architecture of natural and experimental cholesterol-rich membranes. Biochemistry 1974;13:1589.
102. Devaux P, McConnell HM. Lateral diffusion in spin-labeled phosphatidyl choline multilayers. J Am Chem Soc 1972;94:4475.
103. Wu E-S, Jacobson K, et al. Lateral diffusion in phospholipid multilayers measured by fluorescence recovery after photobleaching. Biochemistry 1977;16:3936.
104. Koppel DE, Sheetz MP, et al. Matrix control of protein diffusion in biological membranes. Proc Natl Acad Sci USA 1981;78:3576.
105. Reed CF. Incorporation of orthophosphate ^{32}P into erythrocyte phospholipids in normal subjects and in patients with hereditary spherocytosis. J Clin Invest 1968;47:2630.
106. Renooij W, Van Golde LMG. The transposition of molecular classes of phosphatidyl choline across the rat erythrocyte membrane and their exchange between the red cell membrane and plasma lipoproteins. Biochim Biophys Acta 1977;470:465.
107. Shohet SB. Release of phospholipid fatty acid from human erythrocytes. J Clin Invest 1970;49:1668.
108. Norum KR, Gjone E, Glomset JA. Familial lecithin:cholesterol acyltransferase deficiency, including fish eye disease. In: Scriver CS, Beaudet AL, Sly, WS, Valle D, eds. The metabolic basis of inherited disease, ed 6. New York, McGraw-Hill, 1989:1181.
109. Mulder E, Van Deenen LLM. Metabolism of red cell lipids. I. Incorporation in vitro of fatty acids into phospholipids from mature erythrocytes. Biochim Biophys Acta 1965;106:106.

110. Oliveria MM, Vaughan M. Incorporation of fatty acids into phospholipids of erythrocyte membranes. J Lipid Res 1964;5:156.
111. Shohet SB, Nathan DG, et al. Stages in the incorporation of fatty acids into red blood cells. J Clin Invest 1968;47:1096.
112. Renooij W, Van Golde LMG, Zwaal RF, Roelofsen B, Van Deenen LL. Preferential incorporation of fatty acids at the inside of human erythrocyte membranes. Biochim Biophys Acta 1974;363:287.
113. Farquhar JW, Ahrens EH Jr. Effects of dietary fats on human erythrocyte fatty acid patterns. J Clin Invest 1963;42:675.
114. Rubin RW, Milikowski C. Over two hundred polypeptides resolved from the human erythrocyte membrane. Biochim Biophys Acta 1978;509:100.
115. Alper SL. The band 3–related anion exchanger (AE) gene family. Annu Rev Physiol 1991;53:549.
116. Bennett V. The spectrin-actin junction of erythrocyte membrane skeletons. Biochim Biophys Acta 1989;988:107.
117. Bennett V. Spectrin-based membrane skeleton: a multipotential adaptor between plasma membrane and cytoskeleton. Physiol Rev 1990;70:1029.
118. Bennett V, Lambert S. The spectrin skeleton from red cells to brain. J Clin Invest 1991;87:1483.
119. Bennett V. Ankyrins: adaptors between diverse plasma membrane proteins and the cytoplasm. J Biol Chem 1992;267:8703.
120. Cartron J-P, Le Van Kim C, Colin Y. Glycophorin C and related glycoproteins: structure, function, and regulation. Semin Hematol 1993;30:152.
121. Chasis JA, Mohandas M. Red blood cell glycophorins. Blood 1992;8:1869.
122. Cohen CM, Dotimas E, Korsgren C. Human erythrocyte membrane protein band 4.2 (pallidin). Semin Hematol 1993;30:119.
123. Coleman TR, Fishkind DJ, Mooseker MS, Morrow JS. Contributions of the beta-subunit to spectrin structure and function. Cell Motil Cytoskeleton 1989;12:248.
124. Conboy JG, Mohandas N. Characterization of the gene coding human erythrocyte protein 4.1: implications for understanding hereditary elliptocytosis. In: Agre P, Parker JC, eds. Red blood cell membranes: structure, function, clinical implications. New York, Marcel Dekker, 1989:167.
125. Conboy JG. Structure, function, and molecular genetics of erythroid membrane skeletal protein 4.1 in normal and abnormal red blood cells. Semin Hematol 1993;30:58.
126. Fukuda M. Molecular genetics of the glycophorin A gene cluster. Semin Hematol 1993;30:138.
127. Gallagher PG, Forget BG. Spectrin genes in health and disease. Semin Hematol 1993;30:4.
128. Gilligan DM, Bennett V. The junctional complex of the membrane skeleton. Semin Hematol 1993;30:74.
129. Goodman SR, Krebs KE, Whitfield CF, Risederer BM, Zagon IS. Spectrin and related molecules. CRC Crit Rev Biochem 1988;23:171.
130. Hanspal M, Palek J. Biogenesis of normal and abnormal red blood cell membrane skeletons. Semin Hematol 1992;29:305.
131. Jennings ML. Structure and function of the red blood cell anion transport protein. Annu Rev Biophys Chem 1989;18:397.
132. Liu S-C, Derick LH. Molecular anatomy of the red blood cell membrane skeleton: structure-function relationships. Semin Hematol 1992;29:231.
133. Low PS, Willardson BM, Thevinin B, et al. The other functions of erythrocyte membrane band 3. In: Hamasaki N, Jennings ML, eds. Anion transport protein of the red blood cell membrane, New York, Elsevier, 1989:103.
134. Mohandas N, Chasis JA. Red cell deformability, membrane material properties, and shape: regulation by transmembrane, skeletal, and cytosolic proteins and lipids. Semin Hematol 1993;30:171.
135. Peters LL, Lux SE. Ankyrins: structure and function in normal cells and hereditary spherocytes. Semin Hematol 1993;30:85.
136. Tanner MJA. Molecular and cellular biology of the erythrocyte anion exchanger (AE1). Semin Hematol 1993;30:34.
137. Winkelmann JC, Forget BG. Erythroid and nonerythroid spectrins. Blood 1993;81:3173.
138. Becker PS, Lux SE. Disorders of the red cell membrane. In: Nathan DG, Oski FA, eds. Hematology of infancy and childhood, ed 4. Philadelphia, WB Saunders, 1993:529.
139. Becker PS, Lux SE. Disorders of the red cell membrane skeleton: hereditary spherocytosis and hereditary elliptocytosis. In: Scriver CS, Beaudet AL, Sly WS, Valle D, eds. The metabolic basis of inherited disease, ed 7. New York, McGraw-Hill, in press.
140. Boivin P, Lecomte MC, Garbarz M, et al. Clinical expression of spectrin alpha I variants. In: Cohen CM, Palek J, eds. Cellular and molecular biology of normal and abnormal erythroid membranes. New York, Wiley-Liss, 1990:235.
141. Davies KA, Lux SE. Hereditary disorders of the red cell membrane skeleton. Trends Genet 1989;5:222.
142. Delaunay J, Alloisio N, Morlé L, Pothier B. The red cell skeleton and its genetic disorders. Mol Aspects Med 1990;11:161.
143. Delaunay J, Dhermy D. Mutations involving the spectrin heterodimer contact site: clinical expression and alterations in specific function. Semin Hematol 1993;30:21.
144. Gratzer WB, Dluzewski AR. The red blood cell and malaria parasite invasion. Semin Hematol 1993;30:232.
145. Lux SE, Becker PS. Disorders of the red cell membrane skeleton: hereditary spherocytosis and hereditary elliptocytosis. In: Scriver CS, Beaudet AL, Sly, WS, Valle D, eds. The metabolic basis of inherited disease, ed 6. New York, McGraw-Hill, 1989:2367.
146. Marchesi SL. The erythrocyte cytoskeleton in hereditary elliptocytosis and spherocytosis. In: Agre P, Parker JC, eds. Red blood cell membranes: structure, function and clinical implications. New York, Marcel Dekker, 1989:77.
147. Palek J, Lambert S. Genetics of the red cell membrane skeleton. Semin Hematol 1990;27:290.
148. Palek J, Sahr KE. Mutations of the red blood cell membrane proteins: from clinical evaluation to detection of the underlying genetic defect. Blood 1992;80:308.
149. Palek J, Jarolim P. Clinical expression and laboratory detection of red cell membrane protein mutations. Semin Hematol 1993;30:249.
150. Cartron J-P, Agre P. Rh blood group antigens: protein and gene structure. Semin Hematol 1993;30:193.
151. Redman CM, Marsh WL. The Kell blood group system and the McLeod phenotype. Semin Hematol 1993;30:209.
152. Rosse WF. The glycolipid anchor of membrane surface proteins. Semin Hematol 1993;30:219.
153. Laemmli UK. Cleavage of structural proteins during the assembly of the head of bacteriophage T4. Nature 1970;227:680.
154. Steck TL. Cross-linking the major proteins of the isolated erythrocyte membrane. J Mol Biol 1972;66:295.
155. Edwards HH, Mueller TJ, et al. Distribution of transmembrane polypeptides in freeze fracture. Science 1979;203:1343.
156. Pinto da Silva P, Torrisi MR. Freeze-fracture cytochemistry: partition of glycophorin in freeze-fractured human erythrocyte membranes. J Cell Biol 1982;93:463.
157. Lux SE, John KM, Kopito RR, Lodish HF. Cloning and characterization of band 3, the human erythrocyte anion exchange protein (AE1). Proc Natl Acad Sci USA 1989;86:9089.
158. Tanner MJA, Martin PG, High S. The complete amino acid sequence of the human erythrocyte membrane anion-transport protein deduced from the cDNA sequence. Biochem J 1988;256:703.
159. Hübner S, Michel F, Rudloff V, Appelhans. Amino acid sequence of band-3 protein from rainbow trout erythrocytes derived from cDNA. Biochem J 1992;285:17.
160. Kim H-RC, Yew NS, Ansorge W, et al. Two different mRNAs are transcribed from a single genomic locus encoding the chicken erythrocyte anion transport proteins (band 3). Mol Cell Biol 1988;8:4416.
161. Kopito RR, Lodish HF. Primary structure and transmembrane orientation of the murine anion exchange protein. Nature 1985;316:234.
162. Kopito RR, Andersson M, Lodish HF. Structure and organization of the murine band 3 gene. J Biol Chem 1987;262:8035.
163. Mueller TJ, Morrison M. Detection of a variant of protein 3, the major transmembrane protein of the human erythrocyte. J Biol Chem 1977;252:6573.
164. Palatnik M, Simoes MLMdS, Alves ZMS, Laranjeira NSM. The 60 and 63 kDa proteolytic peptides of the red cell membrane band-3 protein: their prevalence in human and non-human primates. Hum Genet 1990;86:126.
165. Ranney HM, Rosenberg GH, Morrison M, Mueller TJ. Frequencies of band 3 variants of human red cell membranes in some different populations. Br J Haematol 1990;76:262.
166. Jarolim P, Rubin HL, Zhai S, et al. Band 3 Memphis: a widespread polymorphism with abnormal electrophoretic mobility of erythrocyte band 3 protein caused by the substitution AAG GAG (Lys Glu) in codon 56. Blood 1992;80:1592.
167. Yannoukakos D, Vasseur C, Driancourt C, et al. Human erythrocyte band 3 polymorphism (band 3 Memphis): characterization of the structural modification (Lys56 Glu) by protein chemistry methods. Blood 1991;78:1117.
168. Bar-Noy S, Cabantchik I. Transport domain of the erythrocyte anion exchange protein. J Membr Biol 1990;115:217.
169. Bartel D, Hans H, Passow H. Identification by site-directed mutagenesis of Lys-558 as the covalent attachment site of H_2 DIDS in the mouse erythroid band 3 protein. Biochim Biophys Acta 1989;985:355.
170. Cabantchik ZI, Rothstein A. Membrane proteins related to anion permeability of human red blood cells. I. Localization of disulfonic stilbene binding sites in proteins involved in permeation. J Membr Biol 1974;15:207.
171. Ho MK, Guidotti G. A membrane protein from human erythrocytes involved in anion exchange. J Biol Chem 1975;250:675.
172. Jennings ML. Topography of membrane proteins. Annu Rev Biochem 1989;58:999.
173. Low PS, Westfall MA, Allen DP, Appell KC. Characterization of the reversible conformational equilibrium of the cytoplasmic domain of erythrocyte membrane band 3. J Biol Chem 1984;259:13070.
174. Low PS. Structure and function of the cytoplasmic domain of band

3: center of erythrocyte membrane-peripheral protein interactions. Biochim Biophys Acta 1986;864:145.
175. Bennett V, Stenbuck PJ. Association between ankyrin and the cytoplasmic domain of band 3 isolated from human erythrocyte membrane. J Biol Chem 1980;255:6424.
176. Kliman HJ, Steck TL. Association of glyceraldehyde-3-phosphate dehydrogenase with the human red cell membrane: a kinetic analysis. J Biol Chem 1980;255:6314.
177. Tsai I-H, Prasanna-Murthy SN, Steck TL. Effect of red cell membrane binding on the catalytic activity of glyceraldehyde-3-phosphate dehydrogenase. J Biol Chem 1982;257:1438.
178. Yu J, Steck TL. Associations of band 3, the predominant polypeptide of the human erythrocyte membrane. J Biol Chem 1975;250:9176.
179. De BK, Kirtley ME. Interaction of phosphoglycerate kinase with human erythrocyte membranes. J Biol Chem 1977;252:6715.
180. Jenkins JD, Madden DP, Steck TL. Association of phosphofructokinase and aldolase with the membrane of the intact erythrocyte. J Biol Chem 1984;259:9374.
181. Higashi T, Richards CS, Uyeda K. The interaction of phosphofructokinase with erythrocyte membranes. J Biol Chem 1979;254:9542.
182. Murthy SNP, Liu T, Kaul RK, Kohler H, Steck TL. The aldolase binding site of the human erythrocyte membrane is at the NH_2 terminus of band 3. J Biol Chem 1981;256:11203.
183. Strapazon E, Steck TL. Interaction of the aldolase and the membrane of human erythrocytes. Biochemistry 1977;16:2966.
184. Low PS, Allen DP, Zioncheck TF, et al. Tyrosine phosphorylation of band 3 inhibits peripheral protein binding. J Biol Chem 1987;262: 4592.
185. Chétrite G, Cassoly R. Affinity of hemoglobin for the cytoplasmic fragment of human erythrocyte membrane band 3: equilibrium measurements at physiological pH using matrix-bound proteins: the effects of ionic strength, deoxygenation and of 2,3-diphosphoglycerate. J Mol Biol 185:639–644.
186. Walder JA, Chatterjee R, Steck TL, et al. The interaction of hemoglobin with the cytoplasmic domain of band 3 of the human erythrocyte membrane. J Biol Chem 1984;259:10238.
187. Waugh SM, Low PS. Hemichrome binding to band 3: nucleation of Heinz bodies on the erythrocyte membrane. Biochemistry 1985;24: 34.
188. Waugh SM, Walder JA, Low PS. Partial characterization of the copolymerization reaction of erythrocyte membrane band 3 with hemichromes. Biochemistry 1987;26:1777.
189. Kannan R, Labotka R, Low PS. Isolation and characterization of the hemichrome-stabilized membrane protein aggregates from sickle erythrocytes: major site of autologous antibody binding. J Biol Chem 1988;263:13766.
190. McPherson RA, Sawyer WH, Tilley L. Rotational diffusion of the erythrocyte integral membrane protein band 3: effect of hemichrome binding. Biochemistry 1992;31:512.
191. Bennett V, Stenbuck, PJ. The membrane attachment protein for spectrin is associated with band 3 in human erythrocyte membranes. Nature 1979;280:468.
192. Davis L, Lux SE, Bennett V. Mapping the ankyrin-binding site of the human erythrocyte anion exchanger. J Biol Chem 1989;264:9665.
193. Hargreaves WR, Giedd KN, Verkleij A, Branton D. Reassociation of ankyrin with band 3 in erythrocyte membranes and in lipid vesicles. J Biol Chem 1980;255:11965.
194. Willardson BM, Thevenin BJM, Harrison ML, Kuster WM, Benson MD, Low PS. Localization of the ankyrin binding site on erythrocyte membrane protein, band 3. J Biol Chem 1989;264:15893.
195. Thevenin BJM, Low PS. Kinetics and regulation of the ankyrin-band 3 interaction of the human red blood cell membrane. J Biol Chem 1990;265:16166.
196. Pasternack GR, Anderson RA, Leto TL, Marchesi VT. Interactions between protein 4.1 and band 3: an alternative binding site for an element of the membrane skeleton. J Biol Chem 1985;260:3676.
197. Lombardo CR, Willardson BM, Low PS. Localization of the protein 4.1-binding site on the cytoplasmic domain of erythrocyte membrane band 3. J Biol Chem 1992;267:9540.
198. Korsgren C, Cohen CM. Purification and properties of human erythrocyte band 4.2: association with the cytoplasmic domain of band 3. J Biol Chem 1986;261:5536.
199. Korsgren C, Cohen CM. Associations of human erythrocyte protein 4.2: binding to ankyrin and to the cytoplasmic domain of band 3. J Biol Chem 1988;263:10212.
200. Rybicki AC, Qiu JJH, Musto S, Rosen NL, Nagel RL, Schwartz RS. Human erythrocyte protein 4.2 deficiency associated with hemolytic anemia and a homozygous $_{40}$glutamic acid lysine substitution in the cytoplasmic domain of band 3 (band $3^{Montefiore}$). Blood 1993;81:2155.
201. Thevenin BJM, Willardson BM, Low PS. The redox state of cysteines 201 and 317 of the erythrocyte anion exchanger is critical for ankyrin binding. J Biol Chem 1989;264:15886.
202. Jarolim P, Palek J, Rubin HL, Prchal JT, Korsgren C, Cohen CM. Band 3 Tuscaloosa: Pro^{327} Arg^{327} substitution in the cytoplasmic domain of erythrocyte band 3 protein associated with spherocytic hemolytic anemia and partial deficiency of protein 4.2. Blood 1992;80: 523.
203. Falke JJ, Pace RJ, et al. Direct observation of the transmembrane recruitment of band 3 transport sites by competitive inhibitors: A ^{35}Cl NMR study. J Biol Chem 1984;259:6481.
204. Gunn RB, Fröhlich O. Asymmetry in the mechanism for anion exchange in human red blood cell membranes: evidence for reciprocating sites that react with one transported anion at a time. J Gen Physiol 1979;74:351.
205. Krupka RM. Role of substrate binding in exchange-only transport systems. II. Implications for the mechanism of the anion exchanger of red cells. J Membr Biol 1989;109:159.
206. Canfield VA, Macey RI. Anion exchange in human erythrocytes has a large activation volume. Biochim Biophys Acta 1984;778:378.
207. Dalmark M, Wieth JO. Temperature dependence of chloride, bromide, iodide, thiocyanate and salicylate transport in human red cells. J Physiol 1972;224:583.
208. Cabantchik ZI. The anion transport system of red blood cell membranes. In: JR Harris ed. Blood cell biochemistry, vol 1. New York, Plenum Press, 1990:337.
209. Reithmeier RAF. The erythrocyte anion transporter (band 3). Curr Opin Bacterial Biol 1993;3:515.
210. Wang DN, Kühlbrandt W, Sarabia VE, Reithmeier RAF. Two-dimensional structure of the membrane domain of human band 3, the anion transport protein of the erythrocyte membrane. EMBO J 1993;12:2233.
211. Jennings ML. Topical review: oligomeric structure and the anion transport function of human erythrocyte band 3 protein. J Membr Biol 1984;80:105.
212. Lindenthal S, Schubert D. Monomeric erythrocyte band 3 protein transports anions. Proc Natl Acad Sci USA 1991;88:6540.
213. Salhany JM, Sloan RL, Cordes KA. In situ cross-linking of human erythrocyte band 3 by bis(sulfosuccinimidyl)suberate: evidence for ligand modulation of two alternate quaternary forms: covalent band 3 dimers and noncovalent tetramers formed by the association of two covalent dimers. J Biol Chem 1990;265:17688.
214. Salhany JM, Sloan RL, Cordes KA. Evidence for the development of an intermonomeric asymmetry in the covalent binding of 4,4′-diisothiocyanato-2,2′-disulphonate to human erythrocyte band 3. Biochemistry 1991;30:4097.
215. Okubo K, Hamasaki N, Hara K, Kageura M. Palmitoylation of cysteine 69 from the COOH-terminal of band 3 protein in the human erythrocyte membrane: acylation occurs in the middle of the consensus sequence of F-I-IICLAVL found in band 3 protein and G2 protein of Rift Valley fever virus. J Biol Chem 1991;266:16420.
216. Jay DG. Glycosylation site of band 3, the human erythrocyte anion-exchange protein. Biochemistry 1986;25:554.
217. Fukuda M, Dell A, Fukuda MN. Structure of fetal lactosaminoglycan: the carbohydrate moiety of band 3 isolated from human umbilical cord erythrocytes. J Biol Chem 1984;259:4782.
218. Fukuda M, Dell A, Oates JE, Fukuda MN. Structure of branched lactosaminoglycan, the carbohydrate moiety of band 3 isolated from adult erythrocytes. J Biol Chem 1984;259:8260.
219. Fukuda M, Fukuda MN, et al. Developmental change and genetic defect in the carbohydrate structure of band 3 glycoprotein of human erythrocyte membrane. J Biol Chem 1979;254:3700.
220. Casey JR, Reithmeier RAF. Analysis of the oligomeric state of band 3, the anion transport protein of the human erythrocyte membrane, by size exclusion high performance liquid chromatography. J Biol Chem 1991;266:15726.
221. Mulzer K, Kampmann L, Petrasch P, Schubert D. Complex associations between membrane proteins analyzed by analytical ultracentrifugation: studies on the erythrocyte membrane proteins band 3 and ankyrin. Colloid Polym Sci 1990;268:60.
222. Telen MJ, Chasis JA. Relationship of the human erythrocyte Wr^b antigen to an interaction between glycophorin A and band 3. Blood 1990;76:842.
223. Groves JD, Tanner MJA. Glycophorin A facilitates the expression of human band 3-mediated anion transport in *Xenopus* oocytes. J Biol Chem 1992;267:22163.
224. Bruce LJ, Kay MM, Lawrence C, Tanner MJ. Band 3 HT, a human red-cell variant associated with acanthocytosis and increased anion transport, carries the mutation Pro 868Leu in the membrane domain of band 3. Biochem J 1993;293:317.
225. Kay MMB, Gieljan JC, Bosman GM, Lawrence C. Functional topography of band 3: specific structural alteration linked to functional aberrations in human erythrocytes. Proc Natl Acad Sci USA 1988;85: 492.
226. Kay MMB. Band 3 in aging and neurological disease. Ann NY Acad Sci 1991;621:179.
227. Kay MMB, Marchalonis JJ, Schluter SF, Bosman G. Human erythrocyte aging: cellular and molecular biology. Transfus Med Rev 1991;V:173.
228. Alper SL, Kopito RR, Libresco SM, Lodish HF. Cloning and characterization of a murine band 3-related cDNA from kidney and from a lymphoid cell line. J Biol Chem 1988;263:17092.
229. Demuth DR, Showe LC, Ballantine M, et al. Cloning and structural characterization of a human non-erythroid band 3-like protein. EMBO J 1986;5:1205.

230. Kopito RR, Lee BS, Simmons DM, Lindsey AE, Morgans CW, Schneider K. Regulation of intracellular pH by a neuronal homologue of the erythrocyte anion exchanger. Cell 1989;59:927.
231. Kopito RR. Molecular biology of the anion exchanger gene family. Int Rev Cytol 1990;123:177.
232. Brosius FC 3rd, Alper SL, Garcia AM, Lodish HF. The major kidney band 3 transcript predicts an aminoterminal truncated band 3 polypeptide. J Biol Chem 1989;264:7784.
233. Kudrycki KE, Schull GE. Primary structure of the rat kidney band 3 anion exchange protein deduced from a cDNA. J Biol Chem 1989;264:8185.
234. Kudrycki KE, Newman PR, Schull GE. cDNA cloning and tissue distribution of mRNAs for two proteins that are related to the band 3 chloride-bicarbonate exchanger. J Biol Chem 1990;265:462.
235. Salhany JM. Erythrocyte band 3 protein. Boca Raton, FL, CRC Press, 1990.
236. Agre P, Orringer EP, Bennett V. Deficient red-cell spectrin in severe, recessively inherited spherocytosis. N Engl J Med 1982;306:1155.
237. Costa FF, Agre P, Watkins PC, et al. Linkage of dominant hereditary spherocytosis to the gene for the erythrocyte membrane-skeleton protein ankyrin. N Engl J Med 1990;323:1046.
238. Kawano Y, Okubo K, Tokanaga F, Miyata T, Iwanaga S, Hamasaki N. Localization of the pyridoxal binding site at the COOH-terminal region of the erythrocyte band 3 protein. J Biol Chem 1988;263:8232.
239. Jennings ML, Smith JS. Anion-proton cotransport through the human red blood cell band 3 protein: role of glutamate 681. J Biol Chem 1992;267:13964.
240. Vignal A, London J, Rahuel C et al. Promoter sequence and chromosomal organization of the genes encoding glycophorins A, B, and E. Gene 1990;95:289.
241. Low MG, Finean JB. Modification of erythrocyte membranes by a purified phosphatidylinositol-specific phospholipase C (*Staphylococcus aureus*). Biochem J 1977;162:235.
242. Verkleij AJ, Zwaal RFA, Roelofsen B, Comfurius P, Kastelijn D, Van Deenen LLM. The asymmetric distribution of phospholipids in the human red cell membrane: a combined study using phospholipase and freeze-etch electron microscopy. Biochim Biophys Acta 1973;323:178.
243. Ferrell JE Jr, Huestis WH. Phosphoinositide metabolism and the morphology of human erythrocytes. J Cell Biol 1984;98:1992.
244. Cooper RA. Lipids of human red cell membranes: normal composition and variability in disease. Semin Hematol 1970;7:296.
245. Savvides P, Shalev O, John KM, Lux SE. Combined spectrin and ankyrin deficiency is common in autosomal dominant hereditary spherocytosis. Blood 1993;82:2953.
246. Pinder JC, Gratzer WB. Structural and dynamic states of actin in the erythrocyte. J Cell Biol 1983;96:768.
247. Lux SE, John KM. Unpublished observations.
248. Inaba M, Guptka KC, Kuwabara M Takahashi T, Benz EJ Jr, Maede Y. Deamidation of human erythrocyte membrane protein 4.1: possible role in ageing. Blood 1992;79:3355.
249. White RA, Peters LL, Adkinson LR, Korsgren C, Cohen CM, Lux SE. The murine *pallid* mutation is a platelet storage pool disease associated with the protein 4.2 (pallidin) gene. Nature Genet 1992;2:80.
250. Rana AP, Ruff P, Maalouf GJ, Speicher DW, Chishti AH. Cloning of human erythroid dematin reveals another member of the villin family. Proc Natl Acad Sci USA 1993;90:6651.
251. Blanchard D, Dahr W, Hummel M, et al. Glycophorins B and C from human red cell membrane. J Biol Chem 1987;262:5808.
252. Furthmayr H. Structural comparison of glycophorins and immunochemical analysis of genetic variants. Nature 1978;271:519.
253. Dahr W, Gielen W, et al. Structure of the Ss blood group antigens. I. Isolation of Ss-active glycopeptides and differentiation of the antigens by modification of methionine. Hoppe Seylers Z Physiol Chem 1980;361:145.
254. Dahr W, Kordowicz M, et al. The amino acid sequence of the M^{c}-specific major red cell membrane sialoglycoprotein: an intermediate of the blood group M- and N-active molecules. Hoppe Seylers Z Physiol Chem 1981;362:363.
255. Dahr W, Beyreuther K, et al. Amino acid sequence of the blood group M^{g}-specific major human erythrocyte membrane sialoglycoprotein. Hoppe Seylers Z Physiol Chem 1981;362:81.
256. Dahr W, Kordowicz M, et al. Structural analysis of the Ss sialoglycoprotein specific for Henshaw blood group from human erythrocyte membranes. Eur J Biochem 1984;141:51.
257. Tanner MJA, Anstee DJ. The membrane change in En(a−) human erythrocytes. Biochem J 1976;153:271.
258. Tanner MJA, Jenkins RE, et al. Abnormal carbohydrate composition of the major penetrating membrane protein of En(a−) human erythrocytes. Biochem J 1976;155:701.
259. Gahmberg CG, Myllyla G, et al. Absence of the major sialoglycoprotein in the membrane of human En(a−) erythrocytes and increased glycosylation of Band 3. J Biol Chem 1976;251:6108.
260. Dahr W, Uhlenbruck G, et al. Studies on the membrane glycoprotein defect of En(a−) erythrocytes. I. Biochemical aspects. J Immunogenet 1976;3:329.
261. Tanner MJA, Anstee DJ, et al. A carohydratedeficient membrane glycoprotein in human erythrocytes of phenotype S−s−. Biochem J 1977;165:151.
262. Dahr W, Uhlenbruck G, et al. SDS-polyacrylamide gel electrophoretic analysis of the membrane glycoproteins from S−s−U− erythrocytes. J Immunogenet 1975;2:249.
263. Huang C-H, Johe K, Moulds JJ, Siebert PD, Fukuda M, Blumenfeld OO. δ glycophorin (glycophorin B) gene deletion in two individuals homozygous for the S−s−U− blood group phenotype. Blood 1987;70:1830.
264. Tokunaga E, Sasakawa S, et al. Two apparently healthy Japanese individuals of type M^{k}M^{k} have erythrocytes which lack both blood group MN and Ss-active sialoglycoproteins. J Immunogenet 1979;6:383.
265. Anstee DJ. The blood group MNSs-active sialoglycoproteins. Semin Hematol 1981;15:13.
266. Blanchard D, Asseraf A, et al. Miltenberger class I and II erythrocytes carry a variant of glycophorin A. Biochem J 1983;213:399.
267. Dahr W, Newman RA, Contreras M, et al. Structures of Miltenberger class I and II specific major human erythrocyte membrane sialoglycoproteins. Eur J Biochem 1984;138:259.
268. Dahr W, Beyreuther K, Moulds JJ. Structural analysis of the major human erythrocyte membrane sialoglycoproteins from Miltenberger class VII cells. Eur J Biochem 1987;166:27.
269. Dahr W, Vengelen-Tyler V, Dybkjaer E, Beyreuther K. Structural analysis of glycophorin A from Miltenberger class VIII erythrocytes. Biol Chem Hoppe Seyler 1989;370:855.
270. Johe KK, Smith AJ, Blumenfeld OO. Amino acid sequence of Milll glycophorin: demonstration of δ-α and α-δ junction regions and expression of δ pseudoexon by direct protein sequencing. J Biol Chem 1991;266:7256.
271. Johe KK, Vengelen-Tyler V, Leger R, Blumenfeld OO. Synthetic peptides homologous to human glycophorins of the Miltenberger complex of variants of MNSs blood group system specify the epitopes for Hil, S^{JL}, Hop, and Mur antisera. Blood 1991;78:2456.
272. Mawby WJ, Anstee DJ, et al. Immunochemical evidence for hybrid sialoglycoproteins of human erythrocytes Nature 1981;291:161.
273. Tanner MJ, Anstee DJ, et al. A new human erythrocyte variant (Ph) containing an abnormal membrane sialoglycoprotein. Biochem J 1980;187:493.
274. Johe KK, Smith AJ, Vengelen-Tyler V, Blumenfeld OO. Amino acid sequence of an α-δ glycophorin hybrid: a structure reciprocal to St^{a} δ-α glycophorin hybrid. J Biol Chem 1989;264:17486.
275. Anstee DJ, Mawby WJ, et al. Abnormal blood group Ss-active sialoglycoproteins in the membrane of Miltenberger class III, IV, and V erythrocytes. Biochem J 1979;183:19.
276. Huang C-H, Guizzo ML, Kikuchi M, Blumenfeld OO. Molecular genetic analysis of a hybrid gene encoding St^{a} glycophorin of the human erythrocyte membrane. Blood 1989;74:836.
277. Blumenfeld OO, Smith AJ, Moulds JJ. (1987) Membrane glycophorins of Dantu blood group erythrocytes. J Biol Chem 1987;262:11864.
278. Blanchard D, Cartron JP, et al. Pj variant, a new, hybrid MNSs glycoprotein of the human red cell membrane. Biochem J 1982;203:419.
279. Huang C-H, Blumenfeld OO. Identification of recombination events resulting in three hybrid genes encoding human MiV, MiV(J.L.), and St^{a} glycophorins. Blood 1991;77:1813.
280. Huang C-H, Blumenfeld OO. Molecular genetics of human erythrocyte MiIII and MiVI glycophorins: use of a pseudoexon in construction of two δ-α-δ hybrid genes resulting in antigenic diversification. J Biol Chem 1991;266:7248.
281. Huang C-H, Blumenfeld OO. Multiple origins of the human glycophorin St^{a} gene: identification of hot spots for independent unequal homologous recombinations. J Biol Chem 1991;266:23306.
282. Huang C-H, Kikuchi M, McCreary J, Blumenfeld OO. Gene conversion confined to a direct repeat of the acceptor splice site generates allelic diversity at human glycophorin (*GYP*) locus. J Biol Chem 1992;267:3336.
283. Huang C-H, Skov F, Daniels G, Tippett P, Blumenfeld OO. Molecular analysis of human glycophorin MiIX gene shows a silent segment transfer and untemplated mutation resulting from gene conversion via sequence via sequence repeats. Blood 1992;80:2379.
284. Huang C-H, Blumenfeld OO. Characterization of a genomic hybrid specifying the human erythrocyte antigen Dantu: Dantu gene is duplicated and linked to a δ glycophorin gene deletion. Proc Natl Acad Sci USA 1988;85:9640.
285. Kudo S, Fukuda M. Structural organization of glycophorin A and B genes: glycophorin B gene evolved by homologous recombination at Alu repeat sequences. Proc Natl Acad Sci USA 1989;86:4619.
286. Cartron JP, Blanchard D. Association of human erythrocyte membrane glycoproteins with blood group Cad specificity. Biochem J 1982;207:497.
287. Blanchard D, Cartron JP, et al. Primary structure of the oligosaccharide determinant of blood group Cad specificity. J Biol Chem 1983;258:7691.
288. Herkt F, Parente JP, et al. Structure determination of oligosaccharides isolated from Cad erythrocyte membranes by permethylation anal-

ysis and 500 MHz[1] H-NMR spectroscopy. Eur J Biochem 1985;146: 125.

289. Siebert PD, Fukuda M. Isolation and characterization of human glycophorin A cDNA clones by a synthetic oligonucleotide approach: nucleotide sequence and mRNA structure. Proc Natl Acad Sci USA 1986;83:1665–1669.
290. Rahuel C, London J, d'Auriol L, et al. Characterization of cDNA clones for human glycophorin A: use for gene localization and for analysis of normal of glycophorin-A-deficient (Finnish type) genomic DNA. Eur J Biochem 1988;172:147.
291. Irimura T, Tsuji T, Tagami S, Yamamoto K, Osawa T. Structure of a complex-type sugar chain of human glycophorin A. Biochemistry 1981;20:560.
292. Segrest JP, Jackson RL, et al. Human erythrocyte membrane glycoprotein: a reevaluation of the molecular weight as determined by SDS polyacrylamide gel electrophoresis. Biochem Biophys Res Commun 1971;44:390.
293. Gahmberg CG, Jakinen M, et al. Expression of the major sialoglycoprotein (glycophorin) on erythroid cells in human bone marrow. Blood 1978;52:379.
294. Siebert PD, Fukuda M. Molecular cloning of a human glycophorin B cDNA: nucleotide sequence and genomic relationship to glycophorin A. Proc Natl Acad Sci USA 1987;84:6735.
295. Siebert PD, Fukuda M. Correction. Proc Natl Acad Sci USA 1988;85: 421.
296. Kudo S, Chagnovich D, Rearden A, Mattei M-G, Fukuda M. Molecular analysis of a hybrid gene encoding human glycophorin variant Miltenberger V–like molecule. J Biol Chem 1990;265:13825.
297. Rearden A, Magnet A, Kudo S, Fukuda M. Glycophorin B and glycophorin E genes arose from the glycophorin A ancestral gene via two duplications during primate evolution. J Biol Chem 1993;268: 2260.
298. Kudo S, Fukuda M. Identification of a novel human glycophorin, glycophorin E, by isolation of genomic clones and complementary DNA clones utilizing polymerase chain reaction. J Biol Chem 1990;265:1102.
299. Mattei MG, Colin Y, Le Van Kim C, Mattei JF, Cartron JP. Localization of the gene for human erythrocyte glycophorin C to chromosome 2, q14–q21. Hum Genet 1986;74:420.
300. Colin Y, Rahuel C, London J, et al. Isolation of cDNA clones and complete amino acid sequence of human erythrocyte glycophorin C. J Biol Chem 1986;261:229.
301. Cartron J-P, Rahuel C. Human erythrocyte glycophorins: protein and gene structure analysis. Transfus Med Rev 1992;6:63.
302. Villeval JL, LeVan Kim C, Bettaieb A, et al. Early expression of glycophorin-C during normal and leukemic erythroid differentiation. Cancer Res 1989;49:2626.
303. Chasis JA, Mohandas N, Shohet SB. Erythrocyte membrane rigidity induced by glycophorin A-ligand interaction: evidence for a ligand-induced association between glycophorin A and skeletal proteins. J Clin Invest 1985;75:1919.
304. Chasis JA, Reid ME, Jensen RH, Mohandas N. Signal transduction by glycophorin A: role of extracellular and cytoplasmic domains in a modulatable process. J Cell Biol 1988;107:1351.
305. Chasis JA, Knowles D, Winardi R, George E, Mohandas N. Conformational changes in cytoplasmic domains of band 3 and glycophorin-A affect red cell membrane properties. (Abstract) Blood 1991;78(Suppl 1):252a.
306. Chang S, Reid ME, Conboy J, Kan YW, Mohandas N. Molecular characterization of erythrocyte glycophorin-C variants. Blood 1991;77:644.
307. Anstee DJ, Ridgewell K, Tanner MJ, Daniels GL, Parsons SF. Individuals lacking the Gerbich blood-group antigens have alterations in the human erythrocyte membrane sialoglycoproteins β and τ. Biochem J 1984;221:97.
308. High S, Tanner MJA, MacDonald EB, et al. Rearrangements of the red cell membrane glycophorin C (sialoglycoprotein β) gene: a further study of alterations in the glycophorin C gene. Biochem J. 1989;262: 47.
309. Telen MJ, Le Van Kim C, Chung A, et al. Molecular basis for elliptocytosis associated with glycophorin C and glycophorin deficiency in the Leach phenotype. Blood 1991;78:1603.
310. Anstee DJ, Parsons SF, Ridgewell K, et al. Two individuals with elliptocytic red cells apparently lack three minor sialoglycoproteins. Biochem J 1984;218:615.
311. Daniels GL, Shaw M-A, Judson PA, et al. A family demonstrating inheritance of the Leach phenotype, a Gerbich-negative phenotype associated with elliptocytosis. Vox Sang 1986;50:117.
312. Reid ME, Chasis, Mohandas N. Identification of a functional role for human erythrocyte sialoglycoproteins beta and gamma. Blood 1987;69:1068.
313. Nash GB, Parmar J, Reid ME. Effects of deficiencies of glycophorins C and D on the physical properties of the red cell. Br J Haematol 1990;76:282.
314. Reid ME, Anstee DJ, Jensen RH, Mohandas N. Normal membrane function of abnormal β-related erythrocyte sialoglycoproteins. Br J Haematol 1987;67:467.
315. Discher D, Knowles D, McGee S. Mechanical linkage between red cell skeleton and plasma membrane is *not* a demonstrated function of protein 4.1. (Abstract) Blood 1993;82(Suppl 1):309.
316. Perkins M. Inhibitory effects of erythrocyte membrane proteins on the in vitro invasion of the human malarial parasite (*Plasmodium falciparum*) into its host cell. J Cell Biol 1981;90:563.
317. Hermentin P, Enders B. Erythrocyte invasion by malaria (*Plasmodium falciparum*) merozoites: recent advances in the evaluation of receptor sites. Behring Inst Mitt 1984:121.
318. Pasvol G, Wainscoat JS, et al. Erythrocytes deficient in glycophorin resist invasion by the malarial parasite *Plasmodium falciparum*. Nature 1982;297:64.
319. Cartron JP, Prou O, et al. Susceptibility to invasion by *Plasmodium falciparum* of some human erythrocytes carrying rare blood groups. Br J Haematol 1983;55:639.
320. Hadley TJ, Klotz FW, Pasvol G et al. Falciparum malaria parasites invade erythrocytes that lack glycophorin A and B (M^kM^k):strain differences indicate heterogeneity and two pathways for invasion. J Clin Invest 1988;80:1190.
321. Orlandi PA, Klotz FW, Haynes JD. A malaria invasion receptor, the 175-kilodalton erythrocyte binding antigen of *Plasmodium falciparum* recognizes the terminal neu5A(α2–3)gal-sequences of glycophorin A. J Cell Biol 1992;116:901.
322. Camus D, Hadley TJ. A *Plasmodium falciparum* antigen that binds to host erythrocytes and merozoites. Science 1985;230:553.
323. Sheetz MP. Integral membrane protein interaction with Triton cytoskeletons of erythrocytes. Biochim Biophys Acta 1979;557:122.
324. Yu J, Fischman DA, Steck TL. Selective solubilization of proteins and phospholipids of red blood cell membranes by nonionic detergents. J Supramol Struct 1973;1:233.
325. Sahr KE, Laurila P, Kotula L, et al. The complete cDNA and polypeptide sequences of human erythroid alpha-spectrin. J Biol Chem 1990;265:4434.
326. Winkelmann JC, Chang J-G, Tse WT, Marchesi VT, Forget BG. Full length sequence of the cDNA for human erythroid beta-spectrin. J Biol Chem 1990;265:11827.
327. Speicher DW, Morrow JS, Knowles WJ, Marchesi VT. A structural model of human erythrocyte spectrin: alignment of chemical and functional domains. J Biol Chem 1982;257:9093.
328. Speicher DW, DeSilva TM, Speicher KD, Ursitti JA, Hembach P, Weglarz L. Location of the human red cell spectrin tetramer binding site and detection of a related "closed" hairpin loop dimer using proteolytic footprinting. J Biol Chem 1993;268:4227.
329. Shotton DM, Burke BE, Branton D. The molecular structure of human erythrocyte spectrin: biophysical and electron microscopic studies. J Mol Biol 1979;131:303.
330. Liu S-C, Windisch P, Kim S, Palek J. Oligomeric states of spectrin in normal erythrocyte membranes. Biochemical and electron microscopic studies. Cell 1984;37:587.
331. Pollard TD. Purification of a high molecular weight actin filament gelation protein from *Acanthamoeba* that shares antigenic determinants with vertebrate spectrins. J Cell Biol 1984;99:1970.
332. Choi EY, Jeon KW. Role of spectrin in *Amoeba proteus*, as studied by microinjection of anti-spectrin monoclonal antibodies. Exp Cell Res 1992;199:174.
333. Bennett H, Condeelis J. Isolation of an immunoreactive analogue of brain fodrin that is associated with the cell cortex of *Dictyostelium* amoebae. Cell Motil Cytoskeleton 1988;11:303.
334. Wessel GM, Chen SW. Molecular identification of spectrin in the sea urchin embryo. (Abstract) J Cell Biol 1991;115:464a.
335. Dubreuil R, Byers TJ, Branton D, Goldstein CS, Kiehart DP. Drosophila spectrin. I. Characterization of the purified protein. J Cell Biol 1987;105:2095.
335a. Dubreuil RR, Byers TJ, Sillman AL, Bar-Zvi D, Goldstein LSB, Branton D. The complete sequence of Drosophila alpha-spectrin: conservation of structural domains between alpha-spectrins and alpha-actinin. J Cell Biol 1989;109:2197.
336. Byers TJ, Dubreuil R, Branton D, Kiehart DP, Goldstein LS. Drosophila spectrin. II. Conserved features of the alpha subunit are revealed by analysis of cDNA clones and fusion proteins. J Cell Biol 1975;105: 2103.
337. Michaud D, Guillet G, Rodgers PA, Charest PM. Identification of a 220 kDa membrane-associated plant cell protein immunologically related to human beta-spectrin. FEBS Lett 1991;294:77.
338. Baron MD, Davison MD, Jones P, Critchley DR. The sequence of chick α-actinin reveals homologies to spectrin and calmodulin. J Biol Chem 1987;262:17623.
339. Davison MD, Critchley DR. Alpha-actinins and the DMD protein contain spectrin-like repeats. Cell 1988;52:159.
340. Davison MD, Baron MD, Critchley DR, Wootton JC. Structural analysis of homologous repeated domains in α-actinin and spectrin. Int J Biol Macromol 1989;11:81.
341. Byers TJ, Husain-Chishti A, Dubreuil RR, Branton D, Goldstein LSB. Sequence similarity of the amino-terminal domain of Drosophila beta spectrin to alpha actinin and dystrophin. J Cell Biol 1989;109: 1633.
342. Huebner K, Palumbo AP, Isobe M, et al. The alpha-spectrin gene is

on chromosome 1 in mouse and man. Proc Natl Acad Sci USA 1985;82:3790.
342a. Raeymaekers P, Van Broeckhoven C, Backhovens H, et al. The Duffy blood group is linked to the α-spectrin locus in a large pedigree with autosomal dominant inheritance of Charcot-Marie-Tooth disease type 1. Hum Genet 1988;78:76.
343. Fukushima Y, Byers MG, Watkins PC, Winkelmann JC, Forget BG, Shows TB. Assignment of the gene for β-spectrin (SPTB) to chromosome 14q23q24.2 by in situ hybridization. Cytogenet Cell Genet 1990;53:232.
344. Leto TL, Fortugno-Erickson D, Barton D, et al. Comparison of nonerythroid α-spectrin genes reveals strict homology among diverse species. Mol Cell Biol 1988;8:1.
345. Watkins PC, Eddy RL, Forget BG, et al. Assignment of the gene for non-erythroid β spectrin (SPTBN1) to human chromosome 2p21. (Abstract) Cytogenet Cell Genet 1989;51:1103.
346. Speicher DW, Marchesi VT. Erythrocyte spectrin is comprised of many homologous triple helical segments. Nature 1984;311:177.
347. Yan Y, Winograd E, Viel A, Cronin T, Harrison SC, Branton D. Crystal structure of the repetitive segments of spectrin. Science 1993;262: 2027.
348. Winograd E, Hume D, Branton D. Phasing the conformational unit of spectrin. Proc Natl Acad Sci USA 1991;88:10788.
349. Calvert R, Ungewickell E, Gratzer W. A conformational study of human spectrin. Eur J Biochem 1980;107:363.
350. Koch CA, Anderson D, Moran MF, Ellis C, Pawson T. SH2 and SH3 domains: elements that control interactions of cytoplasmic signaling proteins. Science 1991;252:668.
351. Noegel A, Witke W, Schleicher M. Calcium-sensitive non-muscle α-actinin contains EF-hand structures and highly conserved regions. FEBS Lett 1987;221:391.
352. Waites GT, Graham IR, Jackson P, et al. Mutually exclusive splicing of calcium-binding domain exons in chick α-actinin. J Biol Chem 1992;267:6263.
353. Fishkind DJ, Bonder EM, Begg DA. Isolation and characterization of sea urchin egg spectrin: calcium modulation of the spectrin-actin interaction. Cell Motil Cytoskel 1987;7:304.
354. Wallis CJ, Wenegieme EF, Babitch JA. Characterization of calcium binding to brain spectrin. J Biol Chem 1992;267:4333.
355. Kennedy SP, Warren SL, Forget BG, Morrow JS. Ankyrin binds to the 15th repetitive unit of erythroid and nonerythroid β-spectrin. J Cell Biol 1991;115:267.
356. Cohen CM, Tyler JM, Branton D. Spectrin-actin associations studied by electron microscopy of shadowed preparations. Cell 1980;21:875.
357. Becker PS, Schwartz MA, Morrow JS, Lux SE. Radiolabel-transfer crosslinking demonstrates that protein 4.1 binds to the N-terminal region of beta spectrin and to actin in binary interactions. Eur J Biol Chem 1990;193:827.
358. Karinch AM, Zimmer WE, Goodman SR. The identification and sequence of the actin-binding domain of human red blood cell β-spectrin. J Biol Chem 1990;265:11833.
359. Becker PS, Tse WT, Lux SE, Forget B. β Spectrin Kissimmee: a spectrin variant associated with autosomal dominant hereditary spherocytosis and defective binding to protein 4.1. J Clin Invest 1993;92: 612.
360. Bresnick AR, Janmey PA, Condeelis J. Evidence that a 27-residue sequence is the actin-binding site of ABP-120. J Biol Chem 1991;266: 12989.
361. Harris HW Jr, Lux SE. Structural characterization of the phosphorylation sites of human erythrocyte spectrin. J Biol Chem 1980;255: 11512.
362. Tao M, Conway R, Cheta S. Purification and characterization of a membrane-bound protein kinase from human erythrocytes. J Biol Chem 1980;255:2563.
363. Speicher DW, Morrow JS, Knowles WJ, Marchesi VT. Identification of proteolytically resistant domains of human erythrocyte spectrin. Proc Natl Acad Sci USA 1980;77:5673.
364. Speicher DW, Weglarz L, DeSilva TM. Properties of human red cell spectrin heterodimer (side-to-side) assembly and identification of an essential nucleation site. J Biol Chem 1992;267:14775.
365. Viel A, Branton D. Interchain binding at the tail end of the spectrin dimer from *D. melanogaster*. (Abstract) Mol Biol Cell 1993;4(Suppl): 151a.
366. Morrow JS, Marchesi VT. Self-assembly of spectrin oligomers in vitro: a basis for a dynamic cytoskeleton. J Cell Biol 1981;88:463.
367. Ungewickell E, Gratzer W. Self-association of human spectrin: a thermodynamic and kinetic study. Eur J Biochem 1978;88:379.
368. Shahbakhti F, Gratzer WB. Analysis of the self-association of human red cell spectrin. Biochemistry 1986;25:5969.
369. Ralston G, Dunbar J, White M. The temperature-dependent dissociation of spectrin. Biochim Biophys Acta 1977;491:345.
370. Liu S-C, Palek J. Spectrin tetramer-dimer equilibrium and the stability of erythrocyte membrane skeletons. Nature 1980;285:586.
371. Beaven GH, Jean-Baptiste L, Ungewickell E, et al. An examination of the soluble oligomeric complexes extracted from the red cell membrane and their relation to the membrane cytoskeleton. Eur J Cell Biol 1985;36:299.
372. Morris SA, Eber SW, Gratzer WB. Structural basis for the high activation energy of spectrin self-association. FEBS Lett 1989;244:68.
373. DeSilva TM, Peng K, Speicher KD, Speicher DW. Analysis of human red cell spectrin tetramer (head-to-head) assembly using complementary univalent peptides. Biochemistry 1992;31:10872.
374. Vertessy BG, Steck TL. Elasticity of the human red cell membrane skeleton: effects of temperature and denaturants. Biophys J 1989;55: 255.
375. McGough AM, Josephs R. On the structure of erythrocyte spectrin in partially expanded membrane skeletons. Proc Natl Acad Sci USA 1990;87:5208.
376. Ursitti JA, Pumplin DW, Wade JB, Bloch RJ. Ultrastructure of the human erythrocyte cytoskeleton and its attachment to the membrane. Cell Motil Cytoskel 1991;19:227.
377. Geiduschek JB, Singer SJ. Molecular changes in the membranes of mouse erythroid cells accompanying differentiation. Cell 1979;16: 149.
378. Eisen H, Bach R, Emery R. Induction of spectrin in erythroleukemic cells transformed by Friend virus. Proc Natl Acad Sci USA 1977;74: 3898.
379. Hasthorpe S. Quantification of spectrin-containing erythroid precursor cells in normal and perturbed erythropoiesis. Exp Hematol 1980;8:1001.
380. Bodine DM, Birkenmeier CS, Barker JE. Spectrin deficient inherited hemolytic anemias in the mouse: characterization by spectrin synthesis and mRNA activity in reticulocytes. Cell 1984;37:721.
381. Hanspal M, Yoon SH, Yu H, et al. Molecular basis of spectrin and ankyrin deficiencies in severe hereditary spherocytosis: evidence implicating a primary defect of ankyrin. Blood 1991;77:165.
382. Moon RT, Lazarides E. Beta-spectrin limits alpha-spectrin assembly on membranes following synthesis in a chicken erythroid cell lysate. Nature 1983;305:62.
383. Woods CM, Lazarides E. Degradation of unassembled alpha- and beta-spectrin by distinct intracellular pathways: regulation of spectrin topogenesis by beta-spectrin degradation. Cell 1985;40:959.
384. Tilney LG, Detmers P. Actin in erythrocyte ghosts in its association with spectrin: evidence for a nonfilamentous form of these two molecules in situ. J Cell Biol 1975;66:508.
385. Byers T, Branton D. Visualization of the protein associations in the erythrocyte membrane skeleton. Proc Natl Acad Sci USA 1985;82: 6153.
386. Liu S-C, Derick LH, Palek J. Visualization of the hexagonal lattice in the erythrocyte membrane skeleton. J Cell Biol 1987;104:527.
387. Fowler VM, Sussmann MA, Miller PG, Flucher BE, Daniels MP. Tropomodulin is associated with the free (pointed) ends of the thin filaments in rat skeletal muscle. J Cell Biol 1993;120:411.
388. Nakashima K, Beutler E. Comparison of structure and function of human erythrocyte and human muscle actin. Proc Natl Acad Sci USA 1979;76:935.
389. Ungewickell E, Bennett PM, Calvert R, Ohanian V, Gratzer WB. In vitro formation of a complex between cytoskeletal proteins of the human erythrocyte. Nature 1979;280:811.
390. Cohen CM, Foley SF. The role of band 4.1 in the association of actin with erythrocyte membranes. Biochim Biophys Acta 1982;688:691.
391. Ohanian V, Wolfe LC, John KM, Pinder JC, Lux SE, Gratzer WB. Analysis of the ternary interaction of the red cell membrane skeletal proteins spectrin, actin, and 4.1. Biochemistry 1984;23:4416.
392. Leto TL, Marchesi VT. A structural model of human erythrocyte protein 4.1. J Biol Chem 1984;259:4603.
393. Mueller TJ, Jackson CW, Dockler ME, Morrison M. Membrane skeletal alterations during in vivo mouse red cell aging: increase in the band 4.1a:4.1b ratio. J Clin Invest 1987;79:492.
394. Coleman TR, Harris AS, Mische SM, Mooseker MS, Morrow JS. Beta spectrin bestows protein 4.1 sensitivity on spectrin-actin interactions. J Cell Biol 1987;104:519.
395. Tyler JM, Reinhardt BN, Branton D. Associations of erythrocyte membrane proteins. Binding of purified bands 2.1 and 4.1 to spectrin. J Biol Chem 1980;255:7034.
396. Correas I, Leto TL, Speicher DW, Marchesi VT. Identification of the functional site of erythrocyte protein 4.1 involved in spectrin-actin associations. J Biol Chem 1986;261:3310.
397. Correas I, Speicher DW, Marchesi VT. Structure of the spectrin-actin binding site of erythrocyte protein 4.1. J Biol Chem 1986;261: 13362.
398. Conboy JG, Shitamoto R, Parra M, et al. Hereditary elliptocytosis due to both qualitative and quantitative defects in membrane skeletal protein 4.1. Blood 1991;78:2438.
399. Discher D, Parra M, Conboy JG, Mohandas N. Mechanochemistry of the alternatively spliced spectrin-actin binding domain in membrane skeletal protein 4.1. J Biol Chem 1993;268:7186.
400. Morris MB, Lux SE. Characterization of the binary interaction between human erythrocyte protein 4.1 and actin. Submitted.
401. Horne WC, Prinz WC, Tang EK-Y. Identification of two cAMP-dependent phosphorylation sites on erythrocyte protein 4.1. Biochim Biophys Acta 1990;1055:87.
402. Ling E, Danilov YN, Cohen CM. Modulation of red cell band 4.1

function by cAMP-dependent kinase and protein kinase C phosphorylation. J Biol Chem 1988;263:2209.
403. Subrahmanyam G, Bertics PJ, Anderson RA. Phosphorylation of protein 4.1 on tyrosine-418 modulates its function in vitro. Proc Natl Acad Sci USA 1991;88:5222.
404. Anderson JP, Morrow JS. The interaction of calmodulin with erythrocyte spectrin: inhibition of protein 4.1-stimulated actin binding. J Biol Chem 1987;262:6365.
405. Takakuwa Y, Mohandas N. Modulation of erythrocyte membrane material properties by Ca^{2+} and calmodulin: implications for their role in regulation of skeletal protein interactions. J Clin Invest 1988;78:80.
406. Tanaka T, Kadowaki K, Lazarides E, Sobue K. Ca^{2+}-dependent regulation of the spectrin/actin interaction by calmodulin and protein 4.1. J Biol Chem 1991;266:1134.
407. Tchernia G, Mohandas N, Shohet SB. Deficiency of cytoskeletal membrane protein band 4.1 in homozygous hereditary elliptocytosis: implications for erythrocyte membrane stability. J Clin Invest 1981;68:454.
408. Takakuwa Y, Tchernia G, Rossi M, Benabadji M, Mohandas N. Restoration of normal membrane stability to unstable protein 4.1-deficient erythrocyte membranes by incorporation of purified protein 4.1. J Clin Invest 1986;78:80.
409. Discher D, Parra M, Conboy J, Mohandas N. Identification of the minimal domain of protein 4.1 involved in skeletal interactions. (Abstract) Blood 1993;82(Suppl 1):4a.
410. Anderson RA, Marchesi VT. Regulation of the association of membrane skeletal protein 4.1 with glycophorin by polyphosphoinositide. Nature 1985;318:295.
411. Danilov YN, Fennell R, Ling E, Cohen CM. Selective modulation of band 4.1 binding to erythrocyte membranes by protein kinase C. J Biol Chem 1990;265:2556.
412. Bormann BJ, Knowles WJ, Yang TK, et al. Glycophorin a/protein 4.1 association: molecular map of binding sites. (Abstract) J Cell Biol 107:470.
413. Mueller T, Manson M. Glycoconnectin (PAS2) a membrane attachment site for the human erythrocyte cytoskeleton. In: Kruckeberg W, Eaton J, Greuner G, eds. Erythrocyte membranes 2: recent clinical and experimental advances. New York, Alan R Liss, 1981:95.
414. Reid ME, Takakuwa Y, Conboy JG, Tchernia G, Mohandas N. Glycophorin C content of human erythrocyte membrane is regulated by protein 4.1. Blood 1990;75:2229.
415. Sondag D, Alloisio N, Blanchard D, et al. Gerbich reactivity in 4.1 (−) hereditary elliptocytosis and protein 4.1 level in blood group Gerbich deficiency. Br J Haematol 1987;65:43.
416. Pasternack GR, Racusen RH. Erythrocyte protein 4.1 binds and regulates myosin. Proc Natl Acad Sci USA 1989;86:9712.
417. Correas I, Avila J. Erythrocyte protein 4.1 associates with tubulin. Biochem J 1988;255:217.
418. Rybicki AC, Heath R, Lubin B, Schwartz RS. Human erythrocyte protein 4.1 is a phosphatidylserine binding protein. J Clin Invest 1988;81:255.
419. Sato SB, Ohnishi S. Interaction of a peripheral protein of the erythrocyte membrane, band 4.1, with phosphatidylserine-containing liposomes and erythrocyte inside-out vesicles. Eur J Biochem 1983;130:19.
420. Holt GD, Haltiwanger RS, Torres C-R, Hart GW. Erythrocytes contain cytoplasmic glycoproteins: O-linked GlcNAc on band 4.1. J Biol Chem 1987;262:14847.
421. Tang C-JC, Tang TK. Rapid localization of membrane skeletal protein 4.1 (EL1) to human chromosome 1p33p34.2 by nonradioactive in situ hybridization. Cytogenet Cell Genet 1991;57:119.
422. Huang J-P, Tang C-JC, Kou G-H, Marchesi VT, Benz EJ Jr, Tang TK. Genomic structure of the locus encoding protein 4.1: structural basis for complex combinational patterns of tissue-specific alternative RNA splicing. J Biol Chem 1993;268:3758.
423. Conboy JG, Chan J, Mohandas N, Kan YW. Multiple protein 4.1 isoforms produced by alternative splicing in human erythroid cells. Proc Natl Acad Sci USA 1988;85:9062.
424. Conboy JG, Chan JY, Chasis JA, Kan YW, Mohandas N. Tissue- and development-specific alternative RNA splicing regulates expression of multiple isoforms of erythroid membrane protein 4.1. J Biol Chem 1991;266:8273.
425. Tang TK, Qin Z, Leto T, et al. Heterogeneity of mRNA and protein products arising from the protein 4.1 gene in erythroid and nonerythroid tissues. J Cell Biol 1990;110:617.
426. Chasis JA, Coulombel L, Conboy J, et al. Differentiation-associated switches in protein 4.1 expression: synthesis of multiple structural isoforms during normal human erythropoiesis. J Clin Invest 1993;91:329.
427. Funayama N, Nagafuchi A, Sato N, Tsukita S, Tsukita S. Radixin is a novel member of the band 4.1 family. J Cell Biol 1991;115:1039.
428. Lankes WT, Furthmayr H. Moesin: a member of the protein 4.1-talin-ezrin family of proteins. Proc Natl Acad Sci USA 1991;88:8297.
429. Bryant PJ, Woods DF. A major palmitoylated membrane protein of human erythrocytes shows homology to yeast guanylate kinase and to the product of a Drosophila tumor suppressor gene. (Letter) Cell 1992;68:621–622.
430. Chishti AH, Andrabi KI, Rana A, Keeler M, Maalouf G, Bruns G. Human erythroid p55: homolog of Drosophila tumor suppressor factor is highly conserved X-linked gene product with guanylate kinase activity. (Abstract) Blood 1992;80:149a.
431. Ruff P, Speicher DW, Husain-Chishti A. Molecular identification of a major palmitoylated erythrocyte membrane protein containing the src homology 3 motif. Proc Natl Acad Sci USA 1991;88:6595.
432. Metzenberg AB, Gitschier J. The gene encoding the palmitoylated erythrocyte membrane protein, p55, originates at the CpG island 3′ to the factor VIII gene. Hum Mol Genet 1992;1:97.
433. Marfatia SM, Lue RA, Branton D, Chishti AH. Membrane association of human p55 in a novel complex with protein 4.1 and glycophorin C. (Abstract) Mol Biol Cell 1993;4(Suppl):169a.
434. Alloisio N, Dalla Venezia N, Rana A, et al. Evidence that red blood cell protein p55 may participate in the skeleton-membrane linkage that involves protein 4.1 and glycophorin C. Blood 1993;82:1323.
435. Chishti AH. Personal communication.
436. Gardner K, Bennett V. Modulation of spectrin-actin assembly by erythrocyte adducin. Nature 1987;328:359.
437. Joshi R, Gilligan DM, Otto E, McLaughlin T, Bennett V. Primary structure and domain organization of human alpha and beta adducin. J Cell Biol 1991;115:665.
438. Nehls V, Drenckhahn D, Joshi R, Bennett V. Adducin in erythrocyte precursor cells of rats and humans: expression and compartmentalization. Blood 1991;78:1692.
439. Kaiser HW, O'Keefe E, Bennett V. Adducin: Ca^{++}-dependent association with sites of cell-cell contact. J Cell Biol 1989;109:557.
440. Gardner K, Bennett V. Protein kinase C phosphorylates a recently identified membrane skeleton-associated calmodulin-binding protein in human erythrocytes. J Biol Chem 1986;260:1339.
441. Husain-Chishti A, Levin A, Branton D. Abolition of actin-bundling by phosphorylation of human erythrocyte protein 4.9. Nature 1988;334:718.
442. Husain-Chishti A, Faquin W, Wu C-C, Branton D. Purification of erythrocyte dematin (protein 4.9) reveals an endogenous protein kinase that modulates actin-bundling activity. J Biol Chem 1989;264:8985.
443. Siegel DL, Branton D. Partial purification and characterization of an actin-binding protein, band 4.9, from human erythrocytes. J Cell Biol 1985;100:775.
444. Fowler VM, Bennett V. Erythrocyte membrane tropomyosin. Purification and properties. J Biol Chem 1984;259:5978.
445. Mak AS, Roseborough G, Baker H. Tropomyosin from human erythrocyte membrane polymerizes poorly but binds F-actin effectively in the presence and absence of spectrin. Biochim Biophys Acta 1987;912:157.
446. Fowler VM. Identification and purification of a novel M_r 43,000 tropomyosin-binding protein from human erythrocyte membranes. J Biol Chem 1987;262:12792.
447. Fowler VM. Tropomodulin: a cytoskeletal protein that binds to the end of erythrocyte tropomyosin and inhibits tropomyosin binding to actin. J Cell Biol 1990;111:471.
448. Sung LA, Chien S, Fan Y-S, et al. Human erythrocyte protein 4.2: isoform expression, differential splicing, and chromosomal assignment. Blood 1992;79:2763.
449. Fowler VM, Davis JP, Bennett V. Human erythrocyte myosin: identification and purification. J Cell Biol 1985;100:47.
450. Wong AJ, Kiehart DP, et al. Myosin from human erythrocytes. J Biol Chem 1984;260:46.
451. Colin FC, Schrier SL. Myosin content and distribution in human neonatal erythrocytes are different from adult erythrocytes. Blood 1991;78:3052.
452. Bennett V, Stenbuck PJ. Identification and partial purification of ankyrin, the high affinity membrane attachment site for human erythrocyte spectrin. J Biol Chem 1979;254:2533.
453. Luna EJ, Kidd GH, Branton D. Identification by peptide analysis of the spectrin-binding protein in human erythrocytes. J Biol Chem 1979;254:2526.
454. Yu J, Goodman SR. Syndeins: the spectrin-binding protein(s) of the human erythrocyte membrane. Proc Natl Acad Sci USA 1979;76:2340.
455. Cianci CD, Giorgi M, Morrow JS. Phosphorylation of ankyrin down-regulates its cooperative interaction with spectrin and protein 3. J Cell Biochem 1988;37:301.
456. Weaver DC, Pasternack GR, Marchesi VT. The structural basis of ankyrin function. II. Identification of two functional domains. J Biol Chem 1984;259:6170.
457. Low PS, Willardson BM, Mohandas N, Rossi M, Shohet S. Contribution of the band 3-ankyrin interaction to erythrocyte membrane mechanical stability. Blood 1991;77:1581.
458. Weaver DC, Marchesi VT. The structural basis of ankyrin function. I. Identification of two structural domains. J Biol Chem 1984;259:6165.
459. Wallin R, Culp EN, Coleman DB, Goodman SR. A structural model of human erythrocyte band 2.1: alignment of chemical and functional domains. Proc Natl Acad Sci USA 1984;81:4095.
460. Davis LH, Bennett V. Mapping the binding sites of human erythrocyte

ankyrin for the anion exchanger and spectrin. J Biol Chem 1990;265: 10589.
461. Davis LH, Otto E, Bennett V. Specific 33-residue repeat(s) of erythrocyte ankyrin associate with the anion exchanger. J Biol Chem 1991;266:11163.
462. Michaely P, Bennett V. The membrane-binding domain of ankyrin contains four independently folded subdomains, each comprised of six ankyrin repeats. J Biol Chem 1993;268:22703–22709.
463. Platt OS, Lux SE, Falcone JF. A highly conserved region of human erythrocyte ankyrin contains the capacity to bind spectrin. J Biol Chem 1993;268:24421–24426.
464. Lux SE, John KM, Bennett V. Analysis of cDNA for human erythrocyte ankyrin indicates a repeated structure with homology to tissue-differentiation and cell-cycle control proteins. Nature 1990;344:36.
465. Lambert S, Yu H, Prchal JT, et al. cDNA sequence for human erythrocyte ankyrin. Proc Natl Acad Sci USA 1990;87:1730.
466. Bennett V, Davis J. Erythrocyte ankyrin: immunoreactive analogues are associated with mitotic structures in cultured cells and with microtubules in brain. Proc Natl Acad Sci USA 1981;78:7550.
467. Davis JQ, Bennett V. Brain ankyrin: a membrane-associated protein with binding sites for spectrin, tubulin, and the cytoplasmic domain of the erythrocyte anion channel. J Biol Chem 1984;259:13550.
468. Davis LH, Davis JQ, Bennett V. Ankyrin regulation: an alternatively spliced segment of the regulatory domain functions as an intramolecular modulator. J Biol Chem 1992;267:18966.
469. Bennett V, Stenbuck PJ. Human erythrocyte ankyrin: purification and properties. J Biol Chem 1980;255:2540.
470. Georgatos SD, Marchesi VT. The binding of vimentin to human erythrocyte membranes: a model system for the study of intermediate filament–membrane interactions. J Cell Biol 1985;100:1955.
471. Georgatos SD, Weaver DC, Marchesi VT. Site specificity in vimentin-membrane interactions: intermediate filament subunits associate with the plasma membrane via their head domains. J Cell Biol 1985;100:1962.
472. Davis J, Davis L, Bennett V. Diversity in membrane binding sites of ankyrins: brain ankyrin, erythrocyte ankyrin, and processed erythrocyte ankyrin associate with distinct sites in kidney microsomes. J Biol Chem 1989;264:6417.
473. Hall TG, Bennett V. Regulatory domains of erythrocyte ankyrin. J Biol Chem 1987;262:10537.
474. Gallagher PG, Tse WT, Scarpa AL, Lux SE, Forget BG. Large number of alternatively spliced isoforms of the regulatory region of human erythrocyte ankyrin. Trans Assoc Am Phys 1992;105:268.
475. Jarolim P, Rubin H, Palek J. Multiple alternate splices are detected in reticulocyte mRNA coding for the regulatory domain of human erythroid ankyrin. (Abstract) Blood 1992;80(Suppl 1):144a.
476. Jarolim P. Personal communication.
477. Birkenmeier CS, White RA, Peters LL, Hall EJ, Lux SE, Barker JE. Complex patterns of sequence variation and multiple 5′ and 3′ ends are found among transcripts of the erythroid ankyrin gene. J Biol Chem 1993;268:9533.
478. White RA, Birkenmeier CS, Peters LL, Barker JE, Lux SE. Murine erythrocyte ankyrin cDNA: highly conserved regions of the regulatory domain. Mammal Genome 1992;3:281.
479. Lu P-W, Soong C-J, Tao M. Phosphorylation of ankyrin decreases its affinity for spectrin tetramer. J Biol Chem 1985;260:14958.
480. Soong CJ, Lu PW, Tao M. Analysis of band 3 cytoplasmic domain phosphorylation and association with ankyrin. Arch Biochem Biophys 1987;254:509.
481. Moon RT, Ngai J, Wold BJ, Lazarides E. Tissue-specific expression of distinct spectrin and ankyrin transcripts in erythroid and nonerythroid cells. J Cell Biol 1985;100:152.
482. Nelson WJ, Lazarides E. Goblin (ankyrin) in striated muscle: identification of the potential membrane receptor for erythroid spectrin in muscle cells. Proc Natl Acad Sci USA 1984;81:3292.
483. Lux ML, John KM, Lux SE. Unpublished observations.
484. Lux SE. Unpublished observations.
485. Peters LL, Birkenmeier CS, Bronson RT, et al. Purkinje cell degeneration associated with erythroid ankyrin deficiency in *nb/nb* mice. J Cell Biol 1991;114:1233.
486. Kordeli E, Bennett V. Distinct ankyrin isoforms at neuron cell bodies and nodes of Ranvier resolved using erythrocyte ankyrin-deficient mice. J Cell Biol 1991;114:1243.
487. Lux SE, Tse WT, Menninger JC, et al. Hereditary spherocytosis associated with deletion of the human erythrocyte ankyrin gene on chromosome 8. Nature 1990;345:736.
488. Otto E, Kunimoto M, McLaughlin T, Bennett V. Isolation and characterization of cDNAs encoding human brain ankyrins reveal a family of alternatively spliced genes. J Cell Biol 1991;114:241.
489. Kunimoto M, Otto E, Bennett V. A new 440-kD isoform is the major ankyrin in neonatal rat brain. J Cell Biol 1991;115:1319.
490. Chan W, Kordeli E, Bennett V. 440-kD ankyrinB: structure of the major developmentally regulated domain and selective localization in unmyelinated axons. J Cell Biol 1993;123:1463.
491. Tse WT, Menninger JC, Yang-Feng TL, et al. Isolation and chromosomal localization of a novel non-erythroid ankyrin gene. Genomics 1991;10:858.
492. Kordeli E, Lambert S, Bennett V. Ankyrin$_G$ node: a novel isoform of ankyrin selectively localized to the plasma membrane of axonal initial segments and Nodes of Ranvier in the nervous system. (Abstract) Mol Biol Cell 1993;4(Suppl):99a.
493. Peters LL, Eicher EM, Turtzo LC, Lu FM, Lux SE. Chromosomal location and tissue dependent alternative mRNA processing of murine *Ank-3*, a new member of the ankyrin gene family. (Abstract) Blood 1992;80:272a.
494. Peters LL, Lu FM, John KM, et al. Cloning of a new epithelial-axonal ankyrin gene, *Ank-3*, in the mouse. (Abstract) Mol Biol Cell 1993;4(Suppl):56a.
495. Bourguignon LYW, Walker G, Suchard SJ, Balazovich K. A lymphoma plasma membrane-associated protein with ankyrin-like properties. J Cell Biol 1986;102:2115.
496. Bourguignon LYW, Kalomiris EL, Lokeshwar VB. Acylation of the lymphoma transmembrane glycoprotein, GP85, may be required for GP85-ankyrin interaction. J Biol Chem 1991;266:11761.
497. Gregorio CC, Black JD, Lee JK, Repasky EA. Organization of spectrin and ankyrin in lymphocytes. (Abstract) J Cell Biol 1989;107:26a.
498. Drenckhahn D, Schluter K, Allen DP, Bennett V. Colocalization of band 3 with ankyrin and spectrin at the basal membrane of intercalated cells in the rat kidney. Science 1985;230:1287.
499. Drenckhahn D, Bennett V. Polarized distribution of Mr 210,000 and 190,000 analogs of erythrocyte ankyrin along the plasma membrane of transporting epithelia, neurons and photoreceptors. Eur J Cell Biol 1987;43:479.
500. Kordeli E, Davis J, Trapp B, Bennett V. An isoform of ankyrin is localized at nodes of Ranvier in myelinated axons of central and peripheral nerves. J Cell Biol 1990;110:1341.
501. Li Z, Burke EP, Frank JS, Bennett V, Philipson KD. The cardiac Na^+-Ca^{2+} exchanger binds to the cytoskeletal protein ankyrin. J Biol Chem 1993;268:11489.
502. Nelson WJ, Veshnock PJ. Ankyrin binding to ($Na^+ + K^+$)ATPase and the implications for the organization of membrane domains in polarized cells. Nature 1987;328:533.
503. Srinivasan Y, Elmer L, Davis J, Bennett V, Angelides K. Ankyrin and spectrin associate with voltage-dependent sodium channels in brain. Nature 1988;333:177.
504. Yawata Y. Phenotypic, genetic, and electron microscopic aspects on the red cell membrane protein band 4.2: normal and abnormal. Biochim Biophys Acta (in press).
505. Rybicki AC, Nagel RL, Schwartz RS. Decreased content of protein 4.2 in ankyrin-deficient mouse red cells: evidence for a role of ankyrin in stabilizing the membrane assembly of protein 4.2. (Abstract) Blood 1989;74(Suppl 1):104a.
506. Rybicki AC, Heath R, Wolf JL, Lubin B, Schwartz RS. Deficiency of protein 4.2 in erythrocytes from a patient with a Coombs' negative hemolytic anemia: evidence for a role of protein 4.2 in stabilizing ankyrin on the membrane. J Clin Invest 1988;81:893.
507. Inoue T, Ata K, Yawata A, et al. Electron microscopic and physicobiochemical studies on disorganization of the cytoskeletal network and integral protein (band 3) in red cells of band 4.2 deficiency with a mutation (142 GCT ACT). Submitted.
508. Ghanem A, Pothier B, Maréchal J, et al. A haemolytic syndrome associated with the complete absence of red cell membrane protein 4.2 in two Tunisian siblings. Br J Haematol 1990;75:414.
509. Ideguchi H, Nishimura J, Nawata H, Hamasaki N. A genetic defect of erythrocyte band 4.2 protein associated with hereditary spherocytosis. Br J Haematol 1990;74:347.
510. Risinger M, Dotimas E, Cohen CM. Human erythrocyte protein 4.2, a high copy number membrane protein, is N-myristylated. J Biol Chem 1992;267:5680.
511. Korsgren C, Lawler J, Lambert S, Speicher D, Cohen CM. Complete amino acid sequence and homologies of human erythrocyte membrane protein band 4.2. Proc Natl Acad Sci USA 1990;87:613.
512. Sung LA, Chien S, Chang LS, et al. Molecular cloning of human protein 4.2: a major component of the erythrocyte membrane. Proc Natl Acad Sci USA 1990;87:955.
513. Najfeld V, Ballard SG, Menninger J, et al. The gene for human erythrocyte protein 4.2 maps to chromosome 15q15. Am J Hum Genet 1992;50:71.
514. Korsgren C, Cohen CM. Organization of the gene for human erythrocyte membrane protein 4.2: structural similarities with the gene for the subunit of factor XIII. Proc Natl Acad Sci USA 1991;88:4840.
515. Bouhassira EE, Schwartz RS, Yawata Y, et al. An alanine to threonine substitution in protein 4.2 cDNA is associated with a Japanese form of hereditary hemolytic anemia (protein 4.2^{Nippon}). Blood 1992;79: 1846.
516. Peters LL, Eicher EM, Hoock TC, John KM, Yialamas M, Lux SE. Evidence that the mouse platelet storage pool deficiency mutation mocha is a defect in a new member of the ankyrin gene family, *Ank-3*. (Abstract) Blood 1993;82(Suppl 1):340a.
517. McCaughan L, Krimm S. X-ray and neutron scattering density profiles of the intact human red blood cell membrane. Science 1980;207: 1481.
518. Tsukita S, Tsukita S, Ishikawa H. Cytoskeletal network underlying the human erythrocyte membrane: thin-section electron microscopy. J Cell Biol 1980;85:567.

519. Lux SE. Dissecting the red cell membrane skeleton. Nature 1979;281:426.
519a. Eder PS, Soong CJ, Tao M. Phosphorylation reduces the affinity of protein 4.1 for spectrin. Biochemistry 1986;25:1764.
519b. Chao T-S, Tao M. Modulation of protein 4.1 binding to inside-out membrane vesicles by phosphorylation. Biochemistry 1991;30:10529.
520. Anderson JM, Tyler JM. State of spectrin phosphorylation does not affect erythrocyte shape or spectrin binding to erythrocyte membranes. J Biol Chem 1980;255:1259.
521. Harris HW Jr, Levin N, Lux SE. Comparison of the phosphorylation of human erythrocyte spectrin in the intact red cell and in various cell-free systems. J Biol Chem 1980;255:11521.
522. Sheetz MP, Casaly J. 2,3-Diphosphoglycerate and ATP dissociate erythrocyte membrane skeletons. J Biol Chem 1980;255:9955.
523. Mentzer WC Jr, Iarocci TA, Mohandas N, et al. Modulation of erythrocyte membrane mechanical fragility by 2,3-diphosphoglycerate in the neonatal poikilocytosis/elliptocytosis syndrome. J Clin Invest 1987;79:943.
524. Schindler M, Koppel D, Sheetz MP. Modulation of membrane protein lateral mobility by polyphosphates and polyamines. Proc Natl Acad Sci USA 1980;77:1457.
525. Wolfe LC, Lux SE, Ohanian V. Spectrin-actin binding in vitro: effect of protein 4.1 and polyphosphates. (Abstract) J Supramol Struct Cell Biochem 1981;5(Suppl 5):123.
526. Suzuki Y, Nakajima T, Shiga T, et al. Influence of 2,3-diphosphoglycerate on the deformability of human erythrocytes. Biochim Biophys Acta 1990;1029:85.
527. Waugh RE. Effects of 2,3-diphosphoglycerate on the mechanical properties of erythrocyte membrane. Blood 1986;68:231.
528. Gardner K, Bennett V. A new erythrocyte membrane-associated protein with calmodulin binding activity: identification and purification. J Biol Chem 1986;261:1339.
529. Mische SM, Mooseker MS, Morrow JS. Erythrocyte adducin: a calmodulin-regulated actin-bundling protein that stimulates spectrin-actin binding. J Cell Biol 1987;105:2837.
530. Lorand L, Siefring GE, Jr., Lowe-Krentz L. Enzymatic basis of membrane stiffening in human erythrocytes. Semin Hematol 1979;16:65.
531. Palek J, Liu PA, Liu SC. Polymerisation of red cell membrane protein contributes to spheroechinocyte shape irreversibility. Nature 1978;274:505.
532. Smith BD, La Celle PL, Siefring J, Lowe-Krentz L, Lorand L. Effects of the calcium-mediated enzymatic cross-linking of membrane proteins on cellular deformability. J Membr Biol 1981;61:75.
533. Gárdos G. The role of calcium in the potassium permeability of human erythrocytes. Acta Physiol Acad Sci Hung 1959;15:121.
534. Lazarides E. From genes to structural morphogenesis: the genesis and epigenesis of a red blood cell. Cell 1987;51:345.
535. Lazarides E, Woods C. Biogenesis of the red blood cell membrane-skeleton and the control of erythroid morphogenesis. Annu Rev Cell Biol 1989;5:427.
536. Hanspal M, Palek J. Synthesis and assembly of membrane skeletal proteins in mammalian red cell precursors. J Cell Biol 1987;105:1417.
537. Hanspal M, Hanspal J, Kalraiya R. Asynchronous synthesis of membrane skeletal proteins during terminal maturation of murine erythroblasts. Blood 1992;80:530.
538. Hanspal M, Hanspal JS, Sahr KE, Fibach E, Nachman J, Palek J. Molecular basis of spectrin deficiency in hereditary pyropoikilocytosis. Blood 1993;82:1652.
539. Woods CM, Boyer B, Vogt PK, Lazarides E. Control of erythroid differentiation: Asynchronous expression of the anion transporter and the peripheral components of the membrane skeleton in AEV- and S13-transformed cells. J Cell Biol 1986;103:1789.
540. Jarolim P, Rubin HL, Liu S-C, et al. Duplication of 10 nucleotides in the erythroid band 3 (AE1) gene in a kindred with hereditary spherocytosis and band 3 protein deficiency (Band 3^{PRAGUE}). J Clin Invest 1994;93:121.
541. Lux S, Bedrosian C, Shalev O, et al. Deficiency of band 3 in dominant hereditary spherocytosis with normal spectrin content. (Abstract) Clin Res 1990;38:300a.
542. Hanspal M, Kalraiya R, Hanspal J. Erythropoietin enhances the assembly of α spectrin heterodimers on the murine erythroblast membranes by increasing spectrin synthesis. J Biol Chem 1991;266:15626.
543. Chasis JA, Prenant M, Leung A, Mohandas N. Membrane assembly and remodeling during reticulocyte maturation. Blood 1989;74:1112.
544. Johnstone RM. The transferrin receptor. In: Agre P, Parker JC, eds. Red blood cell membranes: structure, function, and clinical implications. New York, Marcel Dekker, 1989:325.
545. Patel VP, Lodish HF. The fibronectin receptor on mammalian erythroid precursor cells: characterization and developmental regulation. J Cell Biol 1986;102:449.
546. Rand RP, Burton AC. Area and volume changes in hemolysis of single erythrocytes. J Cell Comp Physiol 1963;61:245.
547. Bull BS, Kuhn IN. The production of schistocytes by fibrin strands (a scanning electron microscope study). Blood 1970;35:104.
548. Reinhart WH, Sung LA, Chien S. Quantitative relationship between Heinz body formation and red blood cell deformability. Blood 1986;68:1376.
549. Flynn TP, Allen DW, Johnson GJ, White JG. Oxidant damage of the lipids and proteins of the erythrocyte membranes in unstable hemoglobin disease: evidence for the role of lipid peroxidation. J Clin Invest 1983;71:1215.
550. Chasis JA, McGee S, Anstee D, Mohandas N. Different transmembrane signalling mechanisms mediated by band 3 and glycophorin A. (Abstract) Blood 1993;82(Suppl 1):174a.
551. Liu SC, Nichols PE, Yi SJ, et al. Molecular basis of membrane rigidity in Southeast Asian ovalocytosis: oligomerization of the mutant band 3 protein and its increased association with the membrane skeleton. (Abstract) Blood 1993;82(Suppl 1):308a.
551a. Che A, Cherry RJ, Bannister LH, Dluzewski AR. Aggregation of band 3 in hereditary ovalocytic red blood cell membranes: electron microscopy and protein rotational diffusion studies. J Cell Sci 1993;105:655.
552. Liu S-C, Derick LH, Agre P, Palek J. Alteration of the erythrocyte membrane skeletal ultrastructure in hereditary spherocytosis, hereditary elliptocytosis, and pyropoikilocytosis. Blood 1990;76:198.
553. Liu S-C, Derick LH, Duquette MA, Palek J. Separation of the lipid bilayer from the membrane skeleton during discocyte-echinocyte transformation of human erythrocyte ghosts. Eur J Cell Biol 1989;49:358.
554. Wagner GM, Chiu DT-Y, Qju J-H, Heath RH, Lubin BH. Spectrin oxidation correlates with membrane vesiculation in stored RBC's. Blood 1987;69:1777.
555. Wolfe LC. The membrane and the lesions of storage in preserved red cells. Transfusion 1985;25:185.
556. Lutz HU, Liu S-C, Palek J. Release of spectrin-free vesicles from human erythrocytes during ATP depletion: characterization of spectrin-free vesicles. J Cell Biol 1977;73:548.
557. Elgsaeter A, Shotton DM, Branton D. Intramembrane particle aggregation in erythrocyte ghosts. II. The influence of spectrin aggregation. Biochim Biophys Acta 1976;426:101.
558. Lux SE, John KM, Karnovsky MJ. Irreversible deformation of the spectrin-actin lattice in irreversibly sickled cells. J Clin Invest 1976;58:955.
559. Tomaselli MB, John KM, Lux SE. Elliptical erythrocyte membrane skeletons and heat-sensitive spectrin in hereditary elliptocytosis. Proc Natl Acad Sci USA 1981;78:1911.
560. Haest CWM, Fischer TM, Plasa G, Deuticke B. Stabilization of erythrocyte shape by a chemical increase in membrane shear stiffness. Blood Cells 1980;6:539.
561. Hebbel RP. Beyond hemoglobin polymerization: the red blood cell membrane and sickle cell disease pathophysiology. Blood 1991;77:214.
562. Patel VP, Lodish HF. A fibronectin matrix is required for differentiation of murine erythroleukemia cells into reticulocytes. J Cell Biol 1987;105:3105.
563. Swerlick RA, Eckman JR, Kumar A, Jeitler M, Wick TM. $\alpha_4\beta_1$-Integrin expression on sickle reticulocytes: vascular cell adhesion molecule-1-dependent binding to endothelium. Blood 1993;82:1891.
564. Golan DE. Red blood cell membrane protein and lipid diffusion. In: Agre P, Parker JC, eds. Red blood cell membranes: structure, function, and clinical implications. New York, Marcel Dekker, 1989:367.
565. Pasvol G, Carlsson J, Clough B. The red cell membrane and invasion by malarial parasites. Bailliére's Clini Haematol 1993;6:513.
566. Test ST, Butikofer P, Yee MC, et al. Characterization of the complement sensitivity of calcium-loaded human erythrocytes. Blood 1991;78:3056.
567. Victoria EJ, Muchmore EA, Sudora EJ, Masouredis SP. The role of antigen mobility in anti-Rh(D)-induced agglutination. J Clin Invest 1975;56:292.
568. Chin JJ, Jung EKY, Yung CY. Structural basis of human erythrocyte glucose transporter function in reconstituted vesicles. J Biol Chem 1986;261:7101.
569. Mueckler MM, Caruso C, Baldwin SA, et al. Sequence and structure of a human glucose transporter. Science 1985;229:941.
570. Agre P, Parker JC. Red blood cell membranes: structure, function, clinical implications, New York, Marcel Dekker, 1989.
571. Brugnara C. Membrane transport of Na and K and cell dehydration in sickle erythrocytes. Experientia 1993;49:100.
572. Joiner CH. Cation transport and volume regulation in sickle red blood cells. Am J Physiol 1993;264:C251.
573. Lauf PK, Bauer J, Adragna NC, et al. Erythrocyte K-Cl cotransport: properties and regulation. Am J Physiol 1992;263:C917.
574. Raess BU, Tunnicliff G. The red cell membrane: a model for solute transport. Clifton, NJ, Humana Press, 1989.
575. Parker JC. In defense of cell volume? Am J Physiol 1993;265:1191.
576. De Gier J. Permeability barriers formed by membrane lipids. Bioelectrochem Bioenerg 1992;27:1.
577. Nielsen SB, Smith L, Christensen EI, Knepper M, Agre P. CHIP28 water channels are localized in constitutively water-permeable segments of the nephron. J Cell Biol 1993;120:371.
578. Zeidel ML, Ambudkar SV, Smith BL, Agre P. Reconstitution of functional water channels in liposomes containing purified red cell CHIP28 protein. Biochemistry 1992;31:7436.
579. Preston GM, Agre P. Isolation of the cDNA for erythrocyte integral membrane protein of 28 kilodaltons: member of an ancient channel family. Proc Natl Acad Sci USA 1991;88:11110.

580. Smith BL, Baumgarten R, Nielsen S, Raben D, Zeidel ML, Agre P. Concurrent expression of erythroid and renal aquaporin CHIP and appearance of water channel activity in perinatal rats. J Clin Invest 1993;92:2035.
581. Johnson RM, Gannon SA. Erythrocyte cation permeability induced by mechanical stress: a model for sickle cell cation loss. Am J Physiol 1990;259:C746.
582. Kim Y-K, Dirksen ER, Sanderson MJ. Stretch-activated channels in airway epithelial cells. Am J Physiol 1993;265:1306.
583. Sachs F. Ion channels as mechanical transducers. In: Stein WD, Bronner F, eds. Cell shape: determinants, regulation, and regulatory role. New York, Academic Press, 1989:63.
584. Sachs F. Stretch-sensitive ion channels: an update. In: Corey DP, Roper SD, eds. Sensory transduction. New York, Rockefeller University Press, 1992:242.
585. Garrahan PJ, Glynn IM. Factors affecting the relative magnitude of the sodium:potassium and sodium:sodium exchanges catalyzed by the sodium pump. J Physiol 1967;192:189.
586. Clark MR, Guatelli JC, White AT, Shohet SB. Study of dehydrating effect of the red cell Na^+/K^+ pump in nystatin-treated cells with varying Na^+ and water content. Biochim Biophys Acta 1981;646:422.
587. Joiner CH, Platt OS, Lux SE. Cation depletion by the sodium pump in red cells with pathologic cation leaks. J Clin Invest 1986;78:1487.
588. Clark MR. Senescence of red blood cells: progress and problems. Physiol Rev 1988;68:503.
589. Clark MR, Shohet SB. Red cell senescence. Clin Haematol 1985;14:223.
590. Beutler E. Isolation of the aged. Blood Cells 1988;14:1.
591. Dale GL, Norenberg SL. Density fractionation of erythrocytes by Percoll/hypaque results in only a slight enrichment for aged cells. Biochim Biophys Acta 1990;1036:183.
592. Suzuki T, Dale GL. Senescent erythrocytes: isolation of in vivo aged cells and their biochemical characteristics. Proc Natl Acad Sci USA 1988;85:1647.
593. Gershon H. Is the sequestration of aged erythrocytes mediated by natural autoantibodies? Isr J Med Sci 1992;28:818.
594. Lutz HU. Erythrocyte clearance. In: Harris JR, ed. Blood cell biochemistry, vol 1. New York, Plenum Press, 1990:81.
595. Waugh RE, Mohandas N, Jackson CW, Muller TJ, Suzuki T, Dale GL. Rheologic properties of senescent erythrocytes: loss of surface area and volume with red blood cell age. Blood 1992;79:1351.
596. Jain SK, Hochstein P. Polymerization of membrane components in aging red blood cells. Biochem Biophys Res Commun 1980;92:247.
597. Snyder LM, Fortier NL, Trainor J, et al. Effect of hydrogen peroxide exposure on normal human erythrocyte deformability, morphology, surface characteristics and spectrin hemoglobin crosslinking. J Clin Invest 1985;76:1971.
598. Jain SK. Evidence for membrane lipid peroxidation during the in vivo aging of human erythrocytes. Biochim Biophys Acta 1988;937:205.
599. Danon D, Marikovsky Y. The aging of the red blood cell: a multifactor process. Blood Cells 1988;14:7.
600. Aminoff D, Ghalambor MA, Henrich CJ. GOST, galactose oxidase and sialyl transferase, substrate and receptor sites in erythrocyte senescence. In: Eaton JW, ed. Erythrocyte membranes: recent clinical and experimental advances. New York, Alan R Liss, 1981:269.
601. Gattegno L, Bladier D, Garnier M. Changes in carbohydrate content of surface membranes of human erythrocytes during ageing. Carbohyd Res 1976;52:197.
602. Lutz HU, Fehr J. Total sialic acid content of glycophorins during senescence of human red blood cells. J Biol Chem 1979;254:11177.
603. Seaman GVF, Korok FJ, Nordt FJ. Red cell aging. I. Surface charge density and sialic acid content of density-fractionated human erythrocytes. Blood 1977;50:1001.
604. Beutler E. Biphasic loss of red cell enzyme activity during in vivo aging. Prog Clin Biol Res 1985;95:317.
605. Kay MMB. Mechanism of removal senescent cells by human macrophages in situ. Proc Natl Acad Sci USA 1975;72:3521.
606. Kay MMB. Localization of senescent cell antigen on band 3. Proc Natl Acad Sci USA 1984;81:5753.
607. Schlüter K, Drenckhahn D. Co-clustering of denatured hemoglobin with band 3: its role in binding of autoantibodies against band 3 to abnormal and aged erythrocytes. Proc Natl Acad Sci USA 1986;83:6137.
607a. Lutz HU, Stringaro-Wipf G. Senescent red cell bound IgG is attached to band 3 protein. Biomed Biochim Acta 1983;42:117.
608. Galili U, Macher BA, Buehler J, Shohet SB. Human natural anti-α-galactosyl IgG. II. The specific recognition of α(113)-linked galactose residues. J Exp Med 1985;162:573.
609. Galili U, Flechner I, Knyszynski A, Danon D, Rachmilewitz EA. The natural anti-α-galactosyl IgG on human normal senescent red blood cells. Br J Haematol 1986;62:317.
610. Kay MMB, Bosman GJCGM. Naturally occurring human "antigalactosyl" IgG antibodies are heterophile antibodies recognizing blood-group-related substances. Exp Hematol 1985;13:1103.
611. Kay MMB, Marchalonis JJ, Hughes J, Watanabe K, Schluter SF. Definition of a physiologic aging autoantigen by using synthetic peptides of membrane protein band 3: localization of the active antigenic sites. Proc Natl Acad Sci USA 1990;87:5734.
612. Turrini F, Arese P, Yuan J, Low PS. Clustering of integral membrane proteins of the human erythrocyte membrane stimulates autologous IgG binding, complement deposition, and phagocytosis. J Biol Chem 1991;266:23611.
612a. Beppu M, Mizukami A, Nagoya M, Kikugawa K. Binding of anti-band 3 autoantibody to oxidatively damaged erythrocytes: formation of senescent antigen on erythrocyte surface by an oxidative mechanism. J Biol Chem 1990;265:3226.
613. Lutz HU, Bussolino F, Flepp R, et al. Naturally occurring anti-band-3 antibodies and complement together mediate phagocytosis of oxidatively stressed human erythrocytes. Proc Natl Acad Sci USA 1987;84:7368.
614. Winograd E, Greenan JRT, Sherman IW. Expression of senescent antigen on erythrocytes infected with a knobby variant of the human malaria parasite *Plasmodium falciparum*. Proc Natl Acad Sci USA 1987;84:1931.
615. Lelkes G, Fodor I, Lelkes G, et al. The distribution and aggregatability of intramembrane particles in phenylhydrazine-treated human erythrocytes. Biochim Biophys Acta 1988;945:105.
616. Herrmann A, Devaux PF. Alteration of the aminophospholipid translocase activity during in vivo and artificial aging of human erythrocytes. Biochim Biophys Acta 1990;1027:41.
617. Wang RH, Phillips G Jr, Medof ME, Mold C. Activation of the alternative complement pathway by exposure of phosphatidylethanolamine and phosphatidylserine on erythrocytes from sickle cell disease patients. J Clin Invest 1993;92:1326.
618. Schroit AJ, Madsen JW, Tanaka Y. In vivo recognition and clearance of red blood cells containing phosphatidylserine in their plasma membranes. J Biol Chem 1985;260:5131.
619. Vlassara H, Valinsky J, Brownlee M, Cerami C, Nishimoto S, Cerami A. Advanced glycosylation end products on erythrocyte cell surface induce receptor-mediated phagocytosis by macrophages: a model for turnover of aging cells. J Exp Med 1987;166:539.
620. Barber JR, Clarke S. Membrane protein carboxyl methylation increases with human erythrocyte age. J Biol Chem 1983;258:1189.
620a. Galletti P, Ingrosso D, Nappi A, Gragnaniello V, Iolascon A, Pinto L. Increased methyl esterification of membrane proteins in aged red-blood cells: preferential esterification of ankyrin and band-4.1 cytoskeletal proteins. Eur J Biochem 1983;135:25.
621. Vanlair CF, Masius JB. De la microcythémie. Bull R Acad Med Belg 1871;5:515.
622. Ham TH, Castle WB. Studies on destruction of red blood cells: relation of increased hypotonic fragility and erythrostasis to the mechanism of hemolysis in certain anemias. Proc Am Phil Soc 1940;82:411.
623. Chauffard MA. Pathogénie de l'ictère hémolytique congénitale. Ann Méd 1914;1:3.
624. Dameshek W, Schwartz SO. Hemolysins as the cause of clinical and experimental hemolytic anemias: with particular reference to the nature of spherocytosis and increased fragility. Am J Med Sci 1938;196:769.
625. Wilson C. Some cases showing hereditary enlargement of the spleen. Trans Clin Soc (Lond) 1890;23:162.
626. Wilson C, Stanley D. A sequel to some cases showing hereditary enlargement of the spleen. Trans Clin Soc (Lond) 1893;26:163.
627. Minkowski O. Über eine hereditäre, unter dem Bilde eines chronischen Ikterus mit Urobilinurie, Splenomegalie und Nierensiderosis verlaufende Affektion. Verh Dtsch Kongr Med 1900;18:316.
628. Gilbert A. Castaigne J, Lereboullet P. De l'ictère familial: contribution à l'étude de la diathèse biliaire. Bull Mem Soc Med Hop Paris 1900;17:948.
629. Barlow T, Shaw HB. Inheritance of recurrent attacks of jaundice and of abdominal crises with hepatosplenomegaly. Trans Clin Soc (Lond) 1902;35:155.
630. Chauffard MA. Pathogénie de l'ictère congénital de l'adulte. Semaine Méd (Paris) 1907;27:25.
631. Chauffard MA. Les ictères hémolytiques. Semaine Méd (Paris) 1908;28:49.
632. Widal F, Abrami P, Brulé M. Differentiation de plusieurs types d'ictères hémolytiques par le procédédes hématies déplasmatisées. Presse Med 1907;15:641.
633. Hayem G. Sur une variété particulière d'ictère chronique: ictère infectieux chronique splénomégalique. Presse Méd 1898;6:121.
634. Micheli F. Unmittelbare Effekte der Splenektomie bei einem Fall von erworbenem hämolytischen splenomegalischen Ikterus Typus-Hayem-Widal (Splenohämolytischer Ikterus). Wien Klin Wochenschr 1911;24:1269.
635. Giffin HZ. Haemolytic jaundice: a review of 17 cases. Surg Gynecol Obstet 1917;25:152.
636. Dawson of Penn. The Hume Lectures on haemolytic icterus. Br Med J 1931;1:921.
637. Tileston W. Hemolytic jaundice. Medicine 1922;1:355.
638. Gänsslen M. Über hämolytischen Ikterus. Dtsch Arch Klin Med 1922;140:210.
639. Wintrobe MM. Blood, pure and eloquent. New York, McGraw-Hill 1980.
640. Morton NE, MacKinney AA, Kosower N, Schilling RF, Gray MP. Genetics of spherocytosis. Am J Hum Genet 1962;14:170.

641. Godal HC, Heist H. High prevalence of increased osmotic fragility of red blood cells among Norwegian donors. Scand J Haematol 1981;27:30.
642. Eber SW, Pekrun A, Neufeldt A, Schröter W. Prevalence of increased osmotic fragility of erythrocytes in German blood donors: screening using a modified glycerol lysis test. Ann Hematol 1992;64:88.
643. Eber SW, Armbrust R, Schröter W. Variable clinical severity of hereditary spherocytosis: relation to erythrocytic spectrin concentration, osmotic fragility and autohemolysis. J Pediatr 1990;177:409.
644. Race RR. On the inheritance and linkage relations of acholuric jaundice. Ann Eugenics 1942;11:365.
645. Whitfield CF, Follweiler JB, Lopresti-Morrow L, Miller BA. Deficiency of α-spectrin synthesis in burst-forming units-erythroid in lethal hereditary spherocytosis. Blood 1991;78:3043.
645a. Olim G, Marques S, Saldanha C, Santos D, Barroca P, Silva JME. Red cell abnormalities in a kindred with an uncommon form of hereditary spherocytosis. Acta Méd Portug 1984;6:137.
646. Bernard J, Boiron M, Estager J. Une grand famille hémolytique: treze cas de maladie de Minkowski-Chauffard observés dans la même fratrie. Semaine Hôp Paris 1952;28:3741.
647. Duru F, Gürgey, Öztürk G, Yörükan S, Altay C. Homozygosity for dominant form of hereditary spherocytosis. Br J Haematol 1992;82:596.
648. Agre P, Asimos A, Casella JF, McMillan D. Inheritance pattern and clinical response to splenectomy as a reflection of erythrocyte spectrin deficiency in hereditary spherocytosis. N Engl J Med 1986;315:1579.
649. Speicher DW, Davis G, Yurchenko PD, et al. Structure of human erythrocyte spectrin. I. Isolation of the α-I domain and its cyanogen bromide peptides. J Biol Chem 1983;258:14931.
650. Speicher DW, Davis G, Marchesi VT. Structure of human erythrocyte spectrin. II. The sequence of the alpha-I domain. J Biol Chem 1983;258:14938.
651. Conboy J, Kan YW, Shohet SB, Mohandas N. Molecular cloning of protein 4.1, a major structural element of the human erythrocyte membrane skeleton. Proc Natl Acad Sci USA 1986;83:9512.
652. Kotula L, Laury-Kleintop LD, Showe L, et al. The exon-intron organization of the human erythrocyte α-spectrin gene. Genomics 1991;9:131.
653. Sahr KE, Tobe T, Scarpa A, et al. Sequence and exon-intron organization of the DNA encoding the alpha I domain of human spectrin: application to the study of mutations causing hereditary elliptocytosis. J Clin Invest 1989;84:1243.
654. Colin Y, Le Van Kim C, Tsapis A, et al. Human erythrocyte glycophorin C: gene structure and rearrangement in genetic variants. J Biol Chem 1989;264:3773.
655. Speicher DW. The present status of erythrocyte spectrin structure: the 106-residue repetitive structure is a basic feature of an entire class of proteins. J Cell Biochem 1986;30:245.
656. Tse WT, Lecomte MC, Costa FF, et al. Point mutation in the β-spectrin gene associated with $\alpha^{I/74}$ hereditary elliptocytosis. Implications for the mechanism of spectrin dimer self-association. J Clin Invest 1990;86:909.
657. Clark MR, Mohandas N, Shohet SB. Osmotic gradient ektacytometry: comprehensive characterization of red cell volume and surface maintenance. Blood 1983;61:899.
658. Agre P, Casella JF, Zinkham WH, McMillan C, Bennett V. Partial deficiency of erythrocyte spectrin in hereditary spherocytosis. Nature 1985;314:380.
659. Marchesi SL, Agre PL, Speicher DW, Tse WT, Forget BG. Mutant spectrin α^{II} domain in recessively inherited spherocytosis. (Abstract) Blood 1989;74(Suppl 1):182a.
660. Marchesi SL, Agre PA, Speicher DW. Abnormal spectrin α^{II} domain in recessive spherocytosis. (Abstract) J Cell Biochem Suppl 1989;13B:213.
661. Morlé L, Alloisio N, Ducluzeau MT, et al. Spectrin Tunis ($\alpha^{I/78}$), a new α^{I} variant that causes asymptomatic hereditary elliptocytosis in the heterozygous state. Blood 1988;71:508.
662. Morlé L, Morlé F, Roux AF, et al. Spectrin Tunis (Sp$\alpha^{I/78}$), an elliptocytogenic variant, is due to the CGG TGG codon change (Arg Trp) at position 35 of the α^{I} domain. Blood 1989;75:828.
663. Lecomte MC, Garbarz M, Grandchamp B, et al. Sp $\alpha^{I/78}$: a mutation of the αI spectrin domain in a white kindred with HE and HPP phenotypes. Blood 1989;74:1126.
664. Baklouti F, Maréchal J, Morlé L, et al. Occurrence of the $\alpha^{I\,22ARG\,His\,(CGT\,CAT)}$ spectrin mutation in Tunisia: potential association with severe elliptocytosis. Br J Haematol 1991;78:108.
665. Coetzer T, Lawler J, Prchal JT, et al. Molecular determinants of clinical expression of hereditary elliptocytosis and pyropoikilocytosis. Blood 1987;70:766.
666. Coetzer T, Sahr K, Prchal J, et al. Four different mutations in codon 28 of α spectrin are associated with structurally and functionally abnormal spectrin $\alpha^{I/74}$ in hereditary elliptocytosis. J Clin Invest 1991;88:743.
667. Dhermy D, Lecomte MC, Garbarz M, et al. Molecular defect of spectrin in the family of a child with congenital hemolytic poikilocytic anemia. Pediatr Res 1984;18:1005.
668. Dhermy D, Garbarz M, Lecomte MC, et al. Hereditary elliptocytosis: clinical, morphological, and biochemical studies of 38 cases. Nouv Rev Fr Hématol 1986;28:129.
669. Floyd PB, Gallagher PG, Valentino LA, Davis M, Marchesi SL, Forget BG. Heterogeneity in the molecular basis of hereditary pyropoikilocytosis and hereditary elliptocytosis associated with increased levels of the spectrin $\alpha^{I/74}$-kilodalton tryptic peptide. Blood 1991;78:1364.
670. Garbarz M, Lecomte MC, Féo C, et al. Hereditary pyropoikilocytosis and elliptocytosis in a white French family with the spectrin alpha$^{I/74}$ variant related to a CGT to CAT codon change (Arg to His) at position 22 of the spectrin alpha^{I} domain. Blood 1990;75:1691.
671. Lawler J, Liu S-C, Palek J, Prchal J. Molecular defect of spectrin in hereditary pyropoikilocytosis: alterations in the trypsin resistant domain involved in spectrin self-association. J Clin Invest 1982;70:1019.
672. Lawler J, Liu S-C, Palek J, Prchal J. Molecular defect of spectrin in a subgroup of patients with hereditary elliptocytosis: alteration in the alpha subunit involved in spectrin self association. J Clin Invest 1984;73:1688.
673. Lecomte MC, Dhermy D, Garbarz M, et al. Hereditary elliptocytosis with spectrin molecular defect in a white patient. Acta Haematol (Basel) 1984;71:235.
674. Lorenzo F, Miraglia del Giudice E, Alloisio N, et al. Severe poikilocytosis associated with a de novo alpha 28 Arg Cys mutation in spectrin. Br J Haematol 1993;83:152.
675. Peterson LC, Dampier C, Coetzer T, Lawler J, White J, Palek J. Clinical and laboratory study of two Caucasian families with hereditary pyropoikilocytosis and hereditary elliptocytosis. Am J Clin Pathol 1987;88:58.
676. Miraglia del Giudice E, Perrotta S, Sciarratta G, Cutillo L, Pinto L, Iolascon A. $\alpha^{I/74}$ spectrin Genova: a new elliptocytogenic variant due to Arg Trp substitution at position 34 of α spectrin. (Abstract) Blood 80(Suppl 1):277a.
677. Morlé L, Roux AF, Alloisio N, et al. Two elliptocytogenic $\alpha^{I/74}$ variants of the spectrin α^{I} domain: spectrin Culoz (GGT GTT; α^{I} 40 Gly Val) and spectrin Lyon, (CTT TTT; α^{I} 43 Leu Phe). J Clin Invest 1990;86:548.
678. Alloisio N, Guetorni D, Morlé L, et al. Sp $\alpha^{I/65}$ hereditary elliptocytosis in North Africa. Am J Hematol 1986;23:113.
679. Dhermy D, Garbarz M, Lecomte M-C, et al. Abnormal electrophoretic mobility of spectrin tetramers in hereditary elliptocytosis. Hum Genet 1986;74:363.
680. Garbarz M, Lecomte MC, Dhermy D, et al. Double inheritance of an $\alpha^{I/65}$ spectrin variant in a child with homozygous elliptocytosis. Blood 1986;67:1661.
681. Guetarni D, Roux A-F, Alloisio N, et al. Evidence that expression of Sp $\alpha^{I/65}$ hereditary elliptocytosis is compounded by a genetic factor that is linked to the homologous α-spectrin allele. Hum Genet 1990;85:627.
682. Lawler J, Coetzer TL, Palek J, Jacob HS, Luban N. Sp $\alpha^{I/65}$: a new variant of the alpha subunit of spectrin in hereditary elliptocytosis. Blood 1985;66:706.
683. Lecomte MC, Dhermy D, Garbarz M, et al. Pathologic and nonpathologic variants of the spectrin molecule in two black families with hereditary elliptocytosis. Hum Genet 1985;71:351.
684. Lecomte MC, Dhermy D, Solis C, et al. A new abnormal variant of spectrin black patients with hereditary elliptocytosis. Blood 1985;65:1208.
685. Marchesi SL, Knowles WT, Morrow JS, Bologna M, Marchesi VT. Abnormal spectrin in hereditary elliptocytosis. Blood 1986;67:141.
686. Marchesi SL, Letsinger JT, Speicher DW, et al. Mutant forms of spectrin alpha-subunits in hereditary elliptocytosis. J Clin Invest 1987;80:191.
687. Miraglia del Giudice E, Ducluzeau MT, Alloisio N, et al. $\alpha^{I/65}$ hereditary elliptocytosis in Southern Italy: evidence for an African origin. Hum Genet 1992;89:553–556.
688. Roux AF, Morlé F, Guetarni D, et al. Colonna P, Sahr K, Forget BG, Delaunay J, Godet J. Molecular basis of Sp $\alpha^{I/65}$ hereditary elliptocytosis in North Africa: insertion of a TTG triplet between codons 147 and 149 in the α-spectrin gene from five unrelated families. Blood 1989;73:2196.
689. Dhermy D, Boulanger L, Silva CJ, et al. Spectrin Ponte de Sor (Gly 151 Asp): a mutation of the spectrin α gene associated with Sp $\alpha^{I/65}$ hereditary elliptocytosis. 24th Congress of the International Society of Haematology, (Abstract) 1992: p 143.
690. Lawler J, Coetzer TL, Mankad VN, Moore RB, Prchal JT, Palek J. Spectrin $\alpha^{I/61}$: a new structural variant of α spectrin in a double heterozygous form of hereditary pyropoikilocytosis. Blood 1988;72:1412.
691. Hassoun H, Coetzer TL, Sahr KE, Saad S, Vassiliadis JN, Palek J. An insertion within the α spectrin gene leading to exon skipping in a family with hereditary elliptocytosis (HE) and pyropoikilocytosis (HPP). (Abstract) Blood 80(Suppl 1):276a.
692. Gallagher PG, Tse WT, Coetzer T, et al. A common type of the spectrin α^{I} 46–50a-kD peptide abnormality in hereditary elliptocytosis and hereditary pyropoikilocytosis is associated with a mutation dis-

tant from the proteolytic cleavage site: evidence for the functional importance of the triple helical model of spectrin. J Clin Invest 1992;89:892.
693. Lambert S, Zail S. A new variant of the α subunit of spectrin in hereditary elliptocytosis. Blood 1987;69:473.
694. Baklouti F, Maréchal J, Wilmotte R, et al. Elliptocytogenic $\alpha^{I/36}$ spectrin Sfax lacks nine amino acids in helix 3 of repeat 4: evidence for the activation of a cryptic 5'-splice site in exon 8 of spectrin α-gene. Blood 1992;79:2464.
695. Gallagher PG, Roberts WE, Benoit L, Speicher DW, Marchesi SL, Forget BG. Poikilocytic hereditary elliptocytosis associated with Spectrin Alexandria: an αI/50b kD variant that is caused by a single amino acid deletion. Blood 1993;82:2210.
696. Dalla Venezia N, Alloisio N, Forissier A, et al. Elliptopoikilocytosis associated with the α469 His Pro mutation in Spectrin Barcelona ($\alpha^{I/50-46b}$). Blood 1993;82:1661.
697. Gallagher PG, Marchesi SL, Forget BG. A new point mutation associated with αI/50b kDa hereditary elliptocytosis (HE) and hereditary pyropoikilocytosis (HPP). (Abstract) Clin Res 1991;39:313a.
698. Alloisio N, Wilmotte R, Morlé L, et al. Spectrin Jendouba: an $\alpha^{II/31}$ spectrin variant that is associated with elliptocytosis and carries a mutation distant from the dimer self-association site. Blood 1992;80: 809.
699. Alloisio N, Morlé L, Pothier B, et al. Spectrin Oran ($\alpha^{II/21}$), a new spectrin variant concerning the α^{II} domain and causing severe elliptocytosis in the homozygous state. Blood 1988;71:1039.
700. Alloisio N, Wilmotte R, Maréchal J, et al. A splice site mutation of alpha-spectrin gene causing skipping of exon 18 in hereditary elliptocytosis. Blood 1993;81:2791.
701. Lecomte MC, Féo C, Gautero H, et al. Severe recessive poikilocytic anemia with a new spectrin α chain variant. Br J Haematol 1990;74: 497.
702. Lane PA, Shew RL, Iarocci TA, Mohandas N, Hays T, Mentzer WC. Unique α-spectrin mutant in a kindred with common hereditary elliptocytosis. J Clin Invest 1987;79:989.
703. Lecomte MC, Féo C, Gautero H, et al. Severe hereditary elliptocytosis in two related Caucasian children with a decreased amount of spectrin (Sp) α chain. (Abstract) J Cell Biochem 1989;13B:230.
704. Sahr KE, Coetzer TL, Moy LS, et al. An Ala to Gly substitution in β spectrin associated with spectrin αI/74 in hereditary elliptocytosis (HE) and hereditary pyropoikilocytosis (HPP). (Abstract) Blood (Suppl 1):276a.
705. Gallagher PG, Tse WT, Mohandas N, et al. Spectrin Providence: a defect of erythrocyte beta spectrin ($\beta^{2109\ Ser\text{-}Pro}$) homozygosity for which is associated with fatal hydrops fetalis. (Abstract) Blood 1992;80(Suppl 1):145a.
706. Garbarz M, Tse WT, Gallagher PG, et al. Spectrin Rouen (β220–218), a novel shortened β-chain variant in a kindred with hereditary elliptocytosis: characterization of the molecular defect as exon skipping due to a splice site mutation. J Clin Invest 1991;88:76.
707. Lecomte MC, Gautero H, Bournier O, et al. Elliptocytosis-associated spectrin Rouen ($\beta^{220/218}$) has a truncated but still phosphorylatable beta-chain. Br J Haematol 1992;80:242.
708. Pothier B, Morlé, Alloisio N, et al. Spectrin Nice ($\beta^{220/216}$): a shortened β chain variant associated with an increase of the $\alpha^{I/74}$ fragment in a case of elliptocytosis. Blood 1987;69:1759.
709. Tse WT, Gallagher PG, Pothier B, et al. An insertional frameshift mutation of the beta-spectrin gene associated with elliptocytosis in spectrin Nice ($\beta^{220/216}$). Blood 1991;78:517.
710. Garbarz M, Boulanger L, Pedroni S, et al. Spectrin β^{Tandil}, a novel shortened β-chain variant associated with hereditary elliptocytosis is due to a deletional frameshift mutation in the β-spectrin gene. Blood 1992;80:1066.
711. Kanazaki A, Rabodonirina M, Yawata Y, et al. A deletion frameshift mutation of the β-spectrin gene associated with elliptocytosis in spectrin Tokyo ($\beta^{220/216}$). Blood 1992;80:2115.
712. Eber SW, Morris SA, Schröter W, Gratzer WB. Interactions of spectrin in hereditary elliptocytes containing truncated spectrin β-chains. J Clin Invest 1988;81:523.
713. Yoon SH, Yu H, Eber S, Prchal JT. Molecular defect of truncated β-spectrin associated with hereditary elliptocytosis: β-spectrin Göttingen. J Biol Chem 1991;266:8490.
714. Dhermy D, Lecomte MC, Garbarz M, et al. Spectrin beta-chain variant associated with hereditary elliptocytosis. J Clin Invest 1982;70:707.
715. Gallagher PG, Tse WT, Costa F, et al. A splice site mutation of the β-spectrin gene causing exon skipping in hereditary elliptocytosis associated with a truncated β-spectrin chain. J Biol Chem 1991;266: 15154.
716. Takanashi K, Sugawar T, Sakurai K, et al. A trait of hereditary elliptocytosis with truncated β-spectrin (Spectrin Yamagata $\beta^{220/210}$). Jap J Clin Hematol 1991;32:1365a.
717. Johnson RM, Ravindranath Y, Brohn F, Hussain M. A large erythroid spectrin β-chain variant. Br J Haematol 1992;80:6.
718. Becker PS, Morrow JS, Lux SE. Abnormal oxidant sensitivity and beta-chain structure of spectrin in hereditary spherocytosis associated with defective spectrin-protein 4.1 binding. J Clin Invest 1987;80:557.
719. Goodman SR, Shiffer KA, Casoria LA, Eyster ME. Identification of the molecular defect in the erythrocyte membrane skeleton of some kindreds with hereditary spherocytosis. Blood 1982;60:772.
720. Wolfe LC, John KM, Falcone JC, Byrne AM, Lux SE. A genetic defect in the binding of protein 4.1 to spectrin in a kindred with hereditary spherocytosis. N Engl J Med 1982;307:1367.
721. Iolascon A, Miraglia del Giudice E, Clara C, et al. Ankyrin deficiency in dominant hereditary spherocytosis: report of three cases. Br J Haematol 1991;78:551.
722. Pekrun A, Eber SW, Kuhlmey A, Schröter W. Combined ankyrin and spectrin deficiency in hereditary spherocytosis. Ann Hematol 1993;67:89.
723. Eber SW, Lux ML, Gonzalez JM, et al. Discovery of 8 ankyrin mutations in hereditary spherocytosis (HS) indicates that ankyrin defects are a major cause of dominant and recessive HS. (Abstract) Blood 1993;82(Suppl 1):308a.
724. Jarolim P, Brabec V, Lambert S, Liu S-C, Zhou Z, Palek J. Ankyrin Prague: a dominantly inherited mutation of the regulatory domain of ankyrin associated with hereditary spherocytosis. (Abstract) Blood 1990;76(Suppl 1):37a.
725. Jarolim P, Rubin HL, Brabec V, Palek J. Abnormal alternative splicing of erythroid ankyrin mRNA in two kindred with hereditary spherocytosis (Ankyrin^{Prague} and Ankyrin^{Rakovnik}). (Abstract) Blood 1993;82(Suppl 1):5a.
726. Chilcote RR, Le Beau MM, Dampier C, et al. Association of red cell spherocytosis with deletion of the short arm of chromosome 8. Blood 1987;69:156.
727. Cohen H, Walker H, Delhanty JDA, Lucas SB, Huehns ER. Congenital spherocytosis, B19 parvovirus infection and inherited deletion of the short arm of chromosome 8. Br J Haematol 1991;78:251.
728. Kitatani M, Chiyo H, Ozaki M, Shike S, Miwa S. Localization of the spherocytosis gene to chromosome segment 8p11.22–8p21.1. Hum Genet 1988;78:94.
729. Bass EB, Smith SW Jr, Stevenson RE, Rosse WF. Further evidence for localization of the spherocytosis gene on chromosome 8. Ann Intern Med 1983;99:192.
730. Kimberling WJ, Fulbeck T, Dixon L, Lubs HA. Localization of spherocytosis to chromosome 8 or 12 and report of a family with spherocytosis and a reciprocal translocation. Am J Hum Genet 1975;27: 586.
731. Kimberling WJ, Taylor RA, Chapman RG, Lubs HA. Linkage and gene localization of hereditary spherocytosis (HS). Blood 1978;52: 859.
732. Coetzer TL, Lawler J, Liu S-C, et al. Partial ankyrin and spectrin deficiency in severe, atypical hereditary spherocytosis. N Engl J Med 1988;318:230.
733. Alloisio N, Mark L, Dorléac E, et al. The heterozygous form of 4.1(−) hereditary elliptocytosis [the 4.1(−) trait]. Blood 1985;65:46.
734. Conboy J, Mohandas N, Tchernia G, Kan YW. Molecular basis of hereditary elliptocytosis due to protein 4.1 deficiency. N Engl J Med 1986;315:680.
735. Conboy JG, Chasis JA, Winardi R, Tchernia G, Kan YW, Mohandas N. An isoform-specific mutation in the protein 4.1 gene results in hereditary elliptocytosis and complete deficiency of protein 4.1 in erythrocytes but not in nonerythroid cells. J Clin Invest 1993; 91:77.
736. Dalla Venezia N, Gilsanz F, Alloisio N, Ducluzeau M-T, Benz EJ Jr, Delaunay J. Homozygous 4.1 (−) hereditary elliptocytosis associated with a point mutation in the downstream initiation codon of protein 4.1 gene. J Clin Invest 1992;90:1713.
737. Feddal S, Brunet G, Roda L, et al. Molecular analysis of hereditary elliptocytosis with reduced protein 4.1 in the French Northern Alps. Blood 1991;78:2113.
738. Féo CJ, Fischer S, Piau JP, Grange MJ, Tchernia G. Première observation de l'absence d'une protéine de la membrane érythrocytaire (band-4_1) dans un cas d'anémie elliptocytaire familiale. Nouv Rev Fr Hématol 1981;22:315.
739. Lambert S, Zail S. Partial deficiency of protein 4.1 in hereditary elliptocytosis. Am J Hematol 1987;26:263.
740. Lambert S, Conboy J, Zail S. A molecular study of heterozygous protein 4.1 deficiency in hereditary elliptocytosis. Blood 1988;72: 1926.
741. McGuire M, Smith BL, Agre P. Distinct variants of erythrocyte protein 4.1 inherited in linkage with elliptocytosis and Rh type in three white families. Blood 1988;72:287.
742. Conboy J, Marchesi S, Kim R, Agre P, Kan YW, Mohandas N. Molecular analysis of insertion/deletion mutations in protein 4.1 in elliptocytosis. II. Determination of molecular genetic origins of rearrangements. J Clin Invest 1990;86:524.
743. Garbarz M, Dhermy D, Lecomte MC, et al. A variant of erythrocyte membrane skeletal protein band 4.1 associated with hereditary elliptocytosis. Blood 1984;64:1006.
744. Marchesi S, Conboy J, Agre P, et al. Molecular analysis of insertion/deletion mutations in protein 4.1 in elliptocytosis. I. Biochemical identification of rearrangements in the spectrin/actin binding domain and functional characterizations. J Clin Invest 1990;86:515.
745. Hayashi S, Koomoto R, Yano A, et al. Abnormality in a specific

protein of the erythrocyte membrane in hereditary spherocytosis. Biochem Biophys Res Comm 1974;57:1038.
746. Inoue T, Kanzaki A, Ata K, et al. An unique duplet band 4.2 (72 kD/74 kD) disease of autosomal dominantly inherited stomatocytosis. (Abstract) Blood 1990;76(Suppl 1):9.
747. Yawata Y, Ata K, Kanzaki A, et al. Membrane characteristics of membrane protein band 4.2 deficiency with congenital hemolytic anemia. Blood 1990;76(Suppl 1):21a.
748. Yawata Y. Band 4.2 abnormalities in human red cells. Am J Med Sci (in press).
749. Delaunay J, Hayette S, Cohen C, et al. Hereditary hemolytic anemia associated with the absence of protein 4.2. Molecular Biology of Hematopoiesis, 8th Symposium. (Abstract) Basel, Switzerland, 1993: 65.
750. Alloisio N, Morlé L, Bachir D, Guetarni D, Colonna P, Delaunay J. Red cell membrane sialoglycoprotein beta in homozygous and heterozygous 4.1(−) hereditary elliptocytosis. Biochim Biophys Acta 1985;816:57.
751. Dahr W, Moulds J, Baumeister G, Moulds M, Kiedrowski S. Altered membrane sialoglycoproteins in human erythrocytes lacking the Gerbich blood group antigen. Biol Chem Hoppe Seyler 1985;366: 201.
752. Daniels GL, Reid ME, Anstee DJ, et al. Transient reduction in erythrocyte sialoglycoprotein β associated with the presence of elliptocytes. Br J Haematol 1988;70:477.
753. Reid ME, Matynewycz MA, Walford FE, Crawford MN, Miller LH. Leach type Ge− red cells and elliptocytosis. Transfusion 1987;27: 213.
754. Tanner MJA, High S, Martin PG, et al. Genetic variants of human red cell membrane sialoglycoprotein β: study of the alterations occurring in the sialoglycoprotein β gene. Biochem J 1988;250:407.
755. Floyd P, Bursaux E, Dhermy D, et al. Hereditary spherocytosis associated with defects in the amount and function of erythrocyte band 3. (Abstract) Blood 1992;80(Suppl 1):145.
756. Iolascon A, Miraglia del Giudice E, Perrotta S, et al. Hereditary spherocytosis (HS) due to loss of anion exchange transporter. Haematologica 1992;77:450.
757. Jarolim P, Ruff P, Coetzer TL, et al. A subset of patients with dominantly inherited hereditary spherocytosis has a marked deficiency of the band 3 protein. (Abstract) Blood 1990;76(Suppl 1):37a.
758. Jarolim P, Rubin HL, Brabec V, Chrobak L, Palek J. Clustered arginine substitutions in the membrane domain of erythroid band 3 protein in hereditary spherocytosis with band 3 deficiency. (Abstract) Blood 1993;82(Suppl 1):380a.
759. Prchal JT, Guan Y, Jarolim P, et al. Hereditary spherocytosis in a large family is linked with the band 3 gene and not with α-spectrin, β-spectrin or ankyrin. (Abstract) Blood 78(Suppl 1):81a.
760. Saad STO, Liu S-C, Golan D, et al. Mechanism underlying band 3 deficiency in a subset of patients with hereditary spherocytosis (HS). (Abstract) Blood 1991;78(Suppl 1):81a.
761. Alloisio N, Texier P, Forissier A, et al. Band 3 Coimbra: a variant associated with dominant hereditary spherocytosis and band 3 deficiency. (Abstract) Blood 1993;82(Suppl 1):4a.
762. Eber SW, Lux SE. Unpublished observations.
763. Morlé L, Pothier B, Alloisio N, et al. Red cell membrane alteration involving protein 4.1 and protein 3 in a case of recessively inherited haemolytic anemia. Eur J Haematol 1987;38:447.
764. Amato D, Booth PB. Hereditary ovalocytosis in Melanesians. Papua N Guinea Med J 1977;20:26.
765. Castelino D, Saul A, Myler P, Kidson C, Thomas H, Cooke R. Ovalocytosis in Papua New Guinea: dominantly inherited resistance to malaria. SE Asian J Trop Med Public Health 1981;12:549.
766. Cattani JA, Gibson FD, Alpers MP, Crane GG. Hereditary ovalocytosis and reduced susceptibility to malaria in Papua New Guinea. Trans R Soc Trop Med Hyg 1987;81:705.
767. Fix AG, Baer AS, Lie-Injo LE. The mode of inheritance of ovalocytosis/elliptocytosis in Malaysian Orang Asli families. Hum Genet 1982;61:250.
768. Hadley T, Saul A, Lamont G, Hudson DE, Miller LH, Kidson C. Resistance of Melanesian elliptocytes (ovalocytes) to invasion by *Plasmodium knowlesi* and *Plasmodium falciparum* malaria parasites in vitro. J Clin Invest 1983;71:780.
769. Harrison KL, Collins KA, McKenna HW. Hereditary elliptical stomatocytosis: a case report. Pathology 1976;8:307.
770. Holt M, Hogan PF, Nurse GT. The ovalocytosis polymorphism on the Western border of Papua New Guinea. Hum Biol 1981;53:23.
771. Honig GR, Lacson PS, Maurer HS. A new familial disorder with abnormal erythrocyte morphology and increased permeability of the erythrocytes to sodium and potassium. Pediatr Res 1971; 5:159.
772. Jarolim P, Palek J, Amato D, et al. Deletion in the band 3 gene in malaria resistant Southeast Asian ovalocytosis. Proc Natl Acad Sci USA 1991;88:11022.
773. Sarabia VE, Casey JR, Reithmeier RAF. Molecular characterization of the band 3 protein from Southeast Asian ovalocytes. J Biol Chem 1993;268:10676.
774. Kidson C, Lamont G, Saul A, Nurse G. Ovalocytic erythrocytes from Melanesians are resistant to invasion by malaria parasites in culture. Proc Natl Acad Sci USA 1981;78:5829.
775. Liu S-C, Zhai S, Palek J, et al. Molecular defect of the band 3 protein in Southeast Asian ovalocytosis. N Engl J Med 1990;323:1530.
776. Mohandas N, Lie-Injo LE, Friedman M, Mak JW. Rigid membranes of Malayan ovalocytes: a likely genetic barrier against malaria. Blood 1984;63:1385.
777. Mohandas N, Winardi R, Knowles D, et al. Molecular basis for membrane rigidity of hereditary ovalocytosis: a novel mechanism involving the cytoplasmic domain of band 3. J Clin Invest 1992;89: 686.
778. Saul A, Lamont G, Sawyer WH, Kidson C. Decreased membrane deformability in Melanesian ovalocytes from Papua New Guinea. J Cell Biol 1984;98:1348.
779. Schofield AE, Rearden DM, Tanner MJA. Defective anion transport activity of the abnormal band 3 in hereditary ovalocytic red cells. Nature 1992;335:836.
780. Schofield AE, Tanner MJA, Pinder JC, et al. Basis of unique red cell membrane properties in hereditary ovalocytosis. J Mol Biol 1992;223: 949.
781. Serjeantson S, Bryson K, Amato D, Babona D. Malaria and hereditary ovalocytosis. Hum Genet 1977;37:161.
782. Tanner MJA, Bruce L, Martin PG, Rearden DM, Jones GL. Melanesian hereditary ovalocytes have a deletion in red cell band 3. Blood 1991;78:2785.
783. Tanner MJA, Bruce L, Groves JD, Martin PG, Schofield AE. The defective red cell anion transporter (band 3) in hereditary Southeast Asian ovalocytosis and the role of glycophorin A in the expression of band 3 anion transport activity in *Xenopus oocytes*. Biochem Soc Trans 1992;20:542.
784. Tilley L, Nash GB, Jones GL, Sawyer WH. Decreased rotational diffusion of band 3 in Melanesian ovalocytes from Papua New Guinea. J Membr Biol 1991;121:59.
785. Tilley L, McPherson RA, Jones GL, Sawyer WH. Structural organisation of band 3 in Melanesian ovalocytes. Biochim Biophys Acta 1993;1181:83.
786. Knowles WJ, Bologna ML, et al. Common structural polymorphisms in human erythrocyte spectrin. J Clin Invest 1984;73:973.
787. Gallagher PG, Kotula L, DiPaulo B, Curtis P, Speicher D, Forget BG. Polymorphisms of the αII domain of human α spectrin and of the 3′ untranslated region of α spectrin mRNA. (Abstract) Blood 1991;78(Suppl 1):364a.
788. DiPaolo BR, Speicher KD, Speicher DW. Identification of the amino acid mutations associated with human erythrocyte spectrin αII domain polymorphisms. Blood 1993;82:284.
789. Alloisio N, Morlé L, Maréchal J, et al. Sp$\alpha^{V/41}$: a common spectrin polymorphism at the α^{IV}-α^{V} domain junction: relevance to the expression level of hereditary elliptocytosis due to α-spectrin variants located in *trans*. J Clin Invest 1991;87:2169.
790. Wilmotte R, Maréchal J, Morlé L, et al. Low expression allele a^{LELY} of red cell spectrin is associated with mutations in exon 40 ($\alpha^{V/41}$ polymorphism) and intron 45 and with partial skipping of exon 46. J Clin Invest 1993;91:2091.
791. Alloisio N, Dorléac E, Girot R, Delaunay J. Analysis of the red cell membrane in a family with hereditary elliptocytosis: total or partial absence of protein 4.1. Hum Genet 1981;59:68.
792. Alloisio N, Dorléac E, Delaunay J, et al. A shortened variant of red cell membrane protein 4.1. Blood 1982;60:263.
793. Feddal S, Hayette S, Baklouti F, et al. Prevalent skipping of an individual exon accounts for shortened protein 4.1 Presles. Blood 1992;80:292.
794. Morlé L, Garbarz M, Alloisio N, et al. The characterization of protein 4.1 Presles, a shortened variant of RBC membrane protein 4.1. Blood 1985;65:1511.
795. Chasis JA, Agre PA, Mohandas N. Decreased membrane mechanical stability and in vivo loss of surface area reflect spectrin deficiencies in hereditary spherocytosis. J Clin Invest 1988;82:617.
796. Waugh RE, Agre P. Reductions of erythrocyte membrane viscoelastic coefficients reflect spectrin deficiencies in hereditary spherocytosis. J Clin Invest 1988;81:133.
797. Boivin P, Galand C, Devaux I, et al. Spectrin alpha IIa variant in dominant and non-dominant spherocytosis. Hum Genet 1993;92: 153.
798. Woods CM, Lazarides E. Spectrin assembly in avian erythroid development is determined by competing reactions of subunit homo- and hetero-oligomerization. Nature 1986;321:85.
799. Tyler JM, Hargreaves WR, Branton D. Purification of two spectrin-binding proteins: biochemical and electron microscopical evidence for site specific reassociation between spectrin bands 2.1 and 4.1. Proc Natl Acad Sci USA 1979;76:5192.
800. Beighle C, Karp LE, Hanson JW, Hall JG, Hoehn H. Small structural changes of chromosome 8: two cases with evidence for deletion. Hum Genet 1977;38:113.
800a. Stratton RF, Crudo DF, Varela M, Shapira E. Deletion of the proximal short arm of chromosome 8. Am J Med Genet 1992;42:15.
801. Gallagher PG, Forget BG. Personal communication.
802. Eber SW, Cho M, Brugnara C, et al. Increased band 3 mobility and

decreased anion transport in ankyrin deficient hereditary spherocytes. (Abstract) Blood 1993;82(Suppl 1):175a.
803. Miraglia del Giudice E, Perrotta S, Pinto L, et al. Hereditary spherocytosis characterized by increased spectrin/band 3 ratio. (Letter) Br J Haematol 1990;80:133.
804. Cutillo S, Pinto L, Nobili B, Miraglia del Giudice E, Iolascon A. Spectrin/band 3 ratio as diagnostic tool in hereditary spherocytosis. Eur J Pediatr 1992;151:35.
805. Dalbey RE. Positively charged residues are important determinants of membrane protein topology. Trends Biol Sci 1990;15:253.
806. Julien T, Betakis E, Zaki L. Chemical properties of the anion transport inhibitory binding site of arginine-specific reagents in human red blood cell membranes. Biochim Biophys Acta 1990;1026:43.
807. Liu S-C, Yi SJ, Derick LH, et al. Characterization of the band 3 protein in Southeast Asian ovalocytosis (SAO): interrelationships among band 3 self-association, ankyrin binding, rotational and lateral mobilities. (Abstract) Clin Res 41:135A.
808. Sheehy R, Ralston GB. Abnormal binding of spectrin to the membrane of erythrocytes in some cases of hereditary spherocytosis. Blut 1978;36:145.
809. Price Evans DA, Mackie MJ, Anand R. Diminished extractable spectrin in the erythrocytes of a patient with 'sporadic' hereditary spherocytosis. Acta Haematol 1986;76:136.
810. Mariani M, Maretzki D, Lutz HU. A tightly membrane-associated subpopulation of spectrin is ^{3}H-palmitoylated. J Biol Chem 1993;268:12996.
811. Allen DW, Cadman S, McCann SR, Finkel B. Increased membrane binding of erythrocyte catalase in hereditary spherocytosis and in metabolically stressed normal cells. Blood 1977;49:113.
812. Boulard-Heitzmann P, Boulard M, Tallineau C, et al. Decreased red cell enolase activity in a 40-year-old woman with compensated hemolysis. Scand J Haematol 1984;33:401.
813. Lachant NA, Jennings MA, Tanaka KR. Partial erythrocyte enolase deficiency: a hereditary disorder with variable clinical expression. (Abstract) Blood 1986;68(Suppl 1):55a.
814. Lux SE, Glader BE. Disorders of the red cell membrane. In: Nathan DG, Oski FA, eds. Hematology of infancy and childhood, 2nd ed. Philadelphia, WB Saunders, 1981:456.
815. Lux SE. Disorders of the red cell membrane. In: Nathan DG, Oski FA, eds. Hematology of infancy and childhood, ed 3. Philadelphia, WB Saunders, 1987;444.
816. Beutler E, Guinto E, Johnson C. Human red cell protein kinase in normal subjects and patients with hereditary spherocytosis, sickle cell disease, and autoimmune hemolytic anemia. Blood 1976;48:887.
817. Boivin P, Delaunay J, Galand C. Altered erythrocyte membrane protein phosphorylation in an unusual case of hereditary spherocytosis. Scand J Haematol 1979;23:251.
818. Wolfe LC, Lux SE. Membrane protein phosphorylation of intact normal and hereditary spherocytic erythrocytes. J Biol Chem 1978;253:3336.
819. Pinder JC, Dhermy D, Baines AJ, Lux SE, Gratzer WB. A phenomenological difference between membrane skeletal protein complexes isolated from normal and hereditary spherocytosis erythrocytes. Br J Haematol 1983;55:455.
820. Armbrust R, Eber SW, Schröter W. Absence of phosphorylation-induced gelation of erythrocyte membrane skeletons: a diagnostic tool for hereditary spherocytosis. Ann Hematol 1992;64:93.
821. De Gier J, Van Deenen LLM. Phospholipid and fatty acid characteristics of erythrocytes in some cases of anaemia. Br J Haematol 1964;10:246.
822. Kuiper PJC, Livne A. Differences in fatty acid composition between normal erythrocytes and hereditary spherocytosis affected cells. Biochim Biophys Acta 1972;260:755.
823. Zail SS, Pickering A. Fatty acid composition of erythrocytes in hereditary spherocytosis. Br J Haematol 1979;42:399.
824. Bertles JE. Sodium transport across the surface of red blood cells in hereditary spherocytosis. J Clin Invest 1957;36:816.
825. Jacob HS, Jandl JH. Cell membrane permeability in the pathogenesis of hereditary spherocytosis (HS). J Clin Invest 1964;43:1704.
826. Zipursky A, Israels LG. Significance of erythrocyte sodium flux in the pathophysiology and genetic expression of hereditary spherocytosis. Pediatr Res 1971;5:614.
827. Joiner CH, Barker J, Lux SE. Increased cation permeability in mutant mouse red cells with dysfunctional membrane skeletons. Submitted for publication, 1994.
828. Wiley JS. Red cell survival in hereditary spherocytosis. J Clin Invest 49:666–672.
829. Oski FA, Naiman JL, et al. Congenital hemolytic anemia with high-sodium, low-potassium red cells: studies of three generations of a family with a new variant. N Engl J Med 280:909.
830. Mayman D, Zipursky A. Hereditary spherocytosis: the metabolism of erythrocytes in the peripheral blood and in the splenic pulp. Br J Haematol 1974;27:201.
831. Palek J, Mirevova L, Brabec V. 2,3-Diphosphoglycerate metabolism in hereditary spherocytosis. Br J Haematol 1969;17:59.
832. Olivieri O, Bonollo M, Friso S, Girelli D, Corrocher R, Vettore L. Activation of K^+/Cl^- cotransport in human erythrocytes exposed to oxidative agents. Biochim Biophys Acta 1993;1176:37.
833. Loder PB, Babarczy G, et al. Red cell metabolism in hereditary spherocytosis. Br J Haematol 1967;13:95.
834. Mohler DN. Adenosine triphosphate metabolism in hereditary spherocytosis. J Clin Invest 1965;44:1417.
835. Fernandez LA, Erslev AJ. Oxygen affinity and compensated hemolysis in hereditary spherocytosis. J Lab Clin Med 1972;80:780.
836. Kagimoto T, Hayashi F, et al. Phosphorus^{31} NMR study on nucleotides and intracellular pH of hereditary spherocytes. Experientia 1978;34:1092.
837. Ideguchi H, Hamasaki N, Ikehara Y. Abnormal phosphoenolpyruvate transport in erythrocytes of hereditary spherocytosis. Blood 1981;58:426.
838. Bernstein SE. Hereditary disorders of the rodent erythron. In: Genetics in laboratory medicine, National Academy of Sciences Publication 1679, Washington, DC, 1969:9.
839. Birkenmeier CS, McFarland-Starr EC, Barker JE. Chromosomal location of three spectrin genes: relationship to the inherited hemolytic anemias of mouse and man. Proc Natl Acad Sci USA 1988;85:8121.
840. Bloom ML, Barker JE. A C to T transition in the beta spectrin gene found in the jaundiced mouse DNA. (Abstract) Blood 1993;82(Suppl 1):308a.
841. Greenquist AC, Shohet SB, Bernstein SE. Marked reduction of spectrin in hereditary spherocytosis in the common house mouse. Blood 1978;51:1149.
842. Lux SE. Spectrin-actin membrane skeleton of normal and abnormal red blood cells. Semin Hematol 1979;16:21.
843. Unger AE, Harris MJ, Bernstein SE, Falcone JC, Lux SE. Hemolytic anemia in the mouse: report of a new mutation and clarification of its genetics. J Hered 1983;74:88.
844. White RA, Birkenmeier CS, Lux SE, Barker JE. Ankyrin and the hemolytic anemia mutation, *nb*, map to mouse chromosome 8: presence of the *nb* allele is associated with a truncated erythrocyte ankyrin. Proc Natl Acad Sci USA. 1990;87:3117.
845. Grimber G, Galand C, Garbarz M, et al. Inherited haemolytic anaemia created by insertional inactivation of the alpha-spectrin gene. Transgenic Res 1992;1:268.
846. d'Ermao N, Levi M. Neurological symptoms in anemia, neurological symptoms in blood diseases. Baltimore, University Park Press, 1972:1.
847. McCann SR, Jacob HS. Spinal cord disease in hereditary spherocytosis: report of two cases with a hypothesized common mechanism for neurologic and red cell abnormalities. Blood 1976;48:259.
848. Curshmann H. Über funikuläre Myelose bei hämolytischem Ikterus. Dtsch A Nervenheilk 1931;122:119.
849. Dumolard C, Sarrovy C, Portier A. Ataxie cerebelleuse associée à un syndrome de splénomegalie chronique avec anémie. Bull Soc Med Hop (Paris) 1938;54:71.
850. Lemaire A, Dumolard A, Portici A. Deux cas familiaux de maladie de Friedreich avec maladie hemolytique chez des indigenes algeriens. Bull Soc Med Hop (Paris) 1937;53:1084.
851. Michelazzi AM. Anemia emolitica familiare con sinomatoligia nervosa. Rass Fisiopat Clin Ter 1940;12:145.
852. Percorella F. Sindrome neuroanemica in soggetto con ittero imolitico familiare. Rev Clin Pediatr 1946;44:690.
853. Salmon H. Hämolytischer Ikterus und Degeneration der Hinterstränge. Med Klin 1914;10:312c.
854. Spencer SE, Walker FO, Moore SA. Chorea-amyotrophy with chronic hemolytic anemia: a variant of chorea-amyotrophy with acanthocytosis. Neurology 1987;37:645.
855. Peters LL, White RA, Birkenmeier CS, Bloom ML, Lux SE, Barker JE. Changes in cytoskeletal mRNA expression and protein synthesis during murine erythropoiesis *in vivo*. Proc Natl Acad Sci USA 1992;89:5749.
856. Peters LL, Turtzo C, Birkenmeier CS, Barker JE. Distinct fetal *Ank-1* and *Ank-2* related proteins and mRNAs in normal and *nb/nb* mice. Blood 1993;81:2144.
857. Anderson R, Huestis RR, Motulsky AG. Hereditary spherocytosis in the deer mouse: its similarity to the human disease. Blood 1960;15:491.
858. Falcone J, Lux SE. Unpublished observations.
859. LeBlond PF, De Boisfleury A, Bessis M. La forme des érythrocytes dans la sphérocytose héréditaire: étude au microscope à balayage: rélation avec déformabilité. Nouv Rev Fr Hématol 1973;13:873.
860. Cooper RA, Jandl JH. The role of membrane lipids in the survival of red cells in hereditary spherocytosis. J Clin Invest 1969;48:736.
861. Johnsson R. Red cell membrane proteins and lipids in spherocytosis. Scand J Haematol 1978;20:341.
862. Langley GR, Feldherhof CH. Atypical autohemolysis in hereditary spherocytosis as a reflection of two cell populations: relationship of cell lipids to conditioning by the spleen. Blood 1968;32:569.
863. Reed CF, Swisher SN. Erythrocyte lipid loss in hereditary spherocytosis. J Clin Invest 1966;45:777.
864. Waugh RE. Effects of inherited membrane abnormalities on the viscoelastic properties of erythrocyte membranes. Biophys J 1987;51:363.

865. Cooper RA, Jandl JH. The selective and conjoint loss of red cell lipids. J Clin Invest 1969;48:906.
866. Snyder LM, Lutz HU, Sauberman N, Jacobs J, Fortier NL. Fragmentation and myelin formation in hereditary xerocytosis and other hemolytic anemias. Blood 1978;52:750.
867. Weed RI, Bowdler AJ. Metabolic dependence of the critical hemolytic volume of human erythrocytes: relationship to osmotic fragility and autohemolysis in hereditary spherocytosis and normal red cells. J Clin Invest 1966;45:1137.
868. Liu S-C, Derick LH, Duquette MA. Surface area density of membrane skeleton (MS) in normal red cells and severe hereditary spherocytosis (HS): role in lipid bilayer destabilization. (Abstract) Blood 1988;72(Suppl 1):31a.
869. Zachée P, Boogaerts MA, Hellemans L, Snauwaert J. Adverse role of the spleen in hereditary spherocytosis: evidence by the use of the atomic force microscope. Br J Haematol 1992;80:264.
870. Golan DE, Palek J, Agre PA. Red cell membrane spectrin content regulates band 3 and glycophorin lateral diffusion. (Abstract) Blood 1990;76(Suppl 1):8a.
871. Evans EA, Waugh R, Melnik C. Elastic area compressibility modulus of red cell membranes. Biophys J 1976;16:585.
872. Baird R, McPherson AS, Richmond J. Red blood cell survival after splenectomy in congenital spherocytosis. Lancet 1971;2:1060.
873. Chapman RG. Red cell life span after splenectomy in hereditary spherocytosis. J Clin Invest 1968;47:2263.
874. Barnhart MT, Lusher JM. The human spleen as revealed by scanning electron microscopy. Am J Hematol 1976;1:243.
875. Chen L-T, Weiss L. Electron microscopy of red pulp of human spleen. Am J Anat 1972;134:425.
876. Chen L-T, Weiss L. The role of the sinus wall in the passage of erythrocytes through the spleen. Blood 1973;41:529.
877. Weiss L, Tavassoli M. Anatomical hazards to the passage of erythrocytes through the spleen. Semin Hematol 1970;7:372.
878. Weiss L. A scanning electron microscopic study of the spleen. Blood 1974;43:665.
879. Groom AC. Microcirculation of the spleen: new concepts, new challenges. Microvasc Res 1987;34:269.
880. Johnsson R, Vuopio P. Studies on red cell flexibility in spherocytosis using a polycarbonate membrane filtration method. Acta Haematol 1978;60:329.
881. Murphy JR. The influence of pH and temperature on some physical properties of normal erythrocytes and erythrocytes from patients with hereditary spherocytosis. J Lab Clin Med 1967;69:758.
882. Young LE, Platzer RF, Ervin DM, Izzo MJ. Hereditary spherocytosis. II. Observations on the role of the spleen. Blood 1951;6:1099.
882a. Ferreira JA, Feliu E, Rozman C, et al. Morphologic and morphometric light and electron microscopic studies of the spleen in patients with hereditary spherocytosis and autoimmune haemolytic anaemia. Br J Haematol 1989;72:246.
883. Molnar Z, Rappaport H. Fine structure of the red pulp of the spleen in hereditary spherocytosis. Blood 1972;39:81.
884. Wiland OK, Smith EB. The morphology of the spleen in congenital hemolytic anemia (hereditary spherocytosis). Am J Clin Pathol 1956;26:619.
885. Fujita T, Kashimura M, Adachi K. Scanning electron microscopy (SEM) studies of the spleen-normal and pathological. Scan Electron Microsc Pt 1982;1:435.
886. Banti G. Splenomegalie hemolytique au hemopoietique: le role de la rate dans l'hemolyse. Semin Med 1913;33:313.
887. MacAdam W, Shiskin C. The cholesterol content of the blood in anaemia and its relation to splenic function. Q J Med 1922;16:193.
888. Emerson CP, Jr, Shen SC, Ham TH, et al. Studies on the destruction of red blood cells. IX. Quantitative methods for determining the osmotic and mechanical fragility of red cells in the peripheral blood and splenic pulp: the mechanism of increased hemolysis in hereditary spherocytosis (congenital hemolytic jaundice) as related to the function of the spleen. Arch Intern Med 1956;97:1.
889. Dacie JV. Familial haemolytic anaemia (acholuric jaundice), with particular reference to changes in fragility produced by splenectomy. Q J Med (NS) 1943;12:101.
890. Griggs RC, Weisman R Jr, Harris JW. Alterations in osmotic and mechanical fragility related to in vivo erythrocyte aging and splenic sequestration in hereditary spherocytosis. J Clin Invest 1960;39:89.
891. MacPherson AIS, Richmond J, Donaldson GWK, Muir AR. The role of the spleen in congenital spherocytosis. Am J Med 1971;50:35.
892. Jandl JH, Aster RH. Increased splenic pooling and the pathogenesis of hypersplenism. Am J Med Sci 1967;253:383.
893. LaCelle PL. pH in the mouse spleen and its effect on erythrocyte flow properties. (Abstract) Blood 1974;44:910.
894. Minakami S, Yoshikawa H. Studies on erythrocyte glycolysis. III. The effects of active cation transport, pH and inorganic phosphate concentration on erythrocyte glycolysis. J Biochem (Tokyo) 1966;59:145.
895. Rakitzis ET, Mills GC. Relation of red cell hexokinase activity to extracellular pH. Biochim Biophys Acta 1967;141:439.
896. Parker JC. Ouabain-insensitive effects of metabolism on ion and water content in red blood cells. Am J Physiol 1971;221:338.
897. Dacie JV. Observations on autohemolysis in familial acholuric jaundice. J Pathol Bacteriol 1941;52:331.
897a. Ferrant A, Leners N, Michaux JL, Verwilghen RL, Sokal G. The spleen and haemolysis: evaluation of the intrasplenic transit time. Br J Haematol 1987;65:331.
898. Motulsky AG, Casserd F, Giblett ER, Broun GO Jr, Finch CA. Anemia and the spleen. N Engl J Med 1958;259:1164, 1212.
899. Prankerd TAJ. Studies on the pathogenesis of haemolysis in hereditary spherocytosis. Q J Med (New Series) 1960;24:199.
900. Maridonneau I, Braquet P, et al. Na^+ and K^+ transport damage induced by oxygen free radicals in human red cell membranes. J Biol Chem 1983;258:3107.
901. Orringer EP, Parker JC. Selective increase of potassium permeability in red blood cells exposed to acetylphenylhydrazine. Blood 1977;50:1013.
902. Orringer EP. A further characterization of the selective K movements observed in human red blood cells following acetylphenylhydrazine exposure. Am J Hematol 1984;16:355.
903. Sugihara T, Evans EA, Hebbel RP. Lipid hydroperoxides promote deformation-dependent leak of monovalent cation from erythrocytes. (Abstract) Blood 1990;76(Suppl 1):18a.
904. Wiater LA, Dunham PB. Passive transport of K^+ and Na^+ in human red blood cells: sulfhydryl binding agents and furosemide. Am J Physiol 1983;245:C348.
905. Becker PS, Cohen CM, Lux SE. The effect of mild diamide oxidation on the structure and function of human erythrocyte spectrin. J Biol Chem 1986;261:4620.
906. Johnson GJ, Allen DW, Flynn TP, Finkel B, White JG. Decreased survival in vivo of diamide-incubated dog erythrocytes: a model of oxidant-induced hemolysis. J Clin Invest 1986;66:955.
907. Platt OS, Falcone JF. Membrane protein lesions in erythrocytes with Heinz bodies. J Clin Invest 1988;82:1051.
908. Caprari P, Bozzi A, Ferroni L, Strom R, Salvati AM. Oxidative erythrocyte membrane damage in hereditary spherocytosis. Biochem Int 1982;26:265–274.
909. Malorni W, Iosi F, Donelli G, Caprari P, Salvati AM, Cianciulli P. A new, striking morphologic feature for the human erythrocyte in hereditary spherocytosis: the blebbing pattern. (Letter) Blood 1993;81:2821.
910. De Matteis MC, De Angelis V, Sorrentino F, Bonollo E, Vettore L. Role of spleen in hereditary spherocytosis: evidence for increased in vitro proteolysis of red cell membrane. Br J Haematol 1991;79:108.
911. Szymanski IO, Odgren PR, et al. Red blood cell associated IgG in normal and pathologic states. Blood 1980;55:48.
912. Coleman DH, Finch CA. Effect of adrenal steroids in hereditary spherocytic anemia. J Lab Clin Med 1956;47:602.
913. Atkinson JP, Schreiber AS, et al. Effects of corticosteroids and splenectomy on the immune clearance and destruction of erythrocytes. J Clin Invest 1973;52:1509.
914. Schreiber AD, Parsons J, et al. Effect of corticosteroids on the human monocyte IgG and complement receptors. J Clin Invest 1975;56:1189.
915. Matsumoto N, Ishihara T, Shibata M, Uchino F, Nakashima K, Miwa S. Electron microscopic studies of the spleen and liver in hereditary spherocytosis. Acta Pathol Jpn 1973;23:507.
916. Bowman HS, Oski FA. Splenic macrophage interaction with red cells in pyruvate kinase deficiency and hereditary spherocytosis. Vox Sang 1970;19:168.
917. Friedman EW, Williams JC, Van Hook L. Hereditary spherocytosis in the elderly. Am J Med 1988;84:513.
918. Krueger HC, Burgert EO Jr. Hereditary spherocytosis in 100 children. Mayo Clin Proc 1966;41:821.
919. MacKinney AA Jr, Morton NE, Kosower NS, Schilling RF. Ascertaining genetic carriers of hereditary spherocytosis by statistical analysis of multiple laboratory tests. J Clin Invest 1962;41:554.
920. Young LE, Izzo MJ, Platzer RF. Hereditary spherocytosis. I. Clinical, hematologic and genetic features in 28 cases, with particular reference to the osmotic and mechanical fragility of incubated erythrocytes. Blood 1951;6:1073.
921. Debre R, Lamy M, See G, Schrameck G. Congenital and familial hemolytic disease in children. Am J Dis Child 1938;56:1189.
922. Diamond LK. Indications for splenectomy in childhood: results in fifty-two operated cases. Am J Surg (NS) 1938;39:400.
923. Jensson O, Jonasson JL, et al. Studies on hereditary spherocytosis in Iceland. Acta Med Scand 1977;201:187.
923a. Gehlbach SH, Cooper BA. Haemolytic anaemia in infectious mononucleosis due to inapparent congenital spherocytosis. Scand J Haematol 1970;7:141.
924. Ho-Yen DO. Hereditary spherocytosis presenting in pregnancy. Acta Haematol (Basel) 1984;72:29.
925. Pajor A, Lehoczky D, Szakacs Z. Pregnancy and hereditary spherocytosis: report of 8 patients and a review. Arch Gynecol Obstet 1993;253:37.
926. Godal HC, Refsum HE. Haemolysis in athletes due to hereditary spherocytosis. Scand J Haematol 1979;22:83.
927. Eber SW, Pekrun A, Ahle S, Chaves M, Ungewickell E, Schröter W.

Decreased and increased membrane protein densities in severe recessive spherocytosis. Blood (Abstract) 1991;78(Suppl 1):84.
928. Garwicz S. Atypical spherocytosis: a disease of spleen as well as of red blood cells. Lancet 1975;1:956.
929. Wiley JS, Firkin BG. An unusual variant of hereditary spherocytosis. Am J Med 1970;48:63.
929a. Arnold D, Jarolim P, Palek J. Unpublished observations.
930. Maberry MC, Mason RA, Cunningham FG, Pritchard JA. Pregnancy complicated by hereditary spherocytosis. Obstet Gynecol 1992;79: 735.
931. Delamore IW, Richmond J, Davies SH. Megaloblastic anaemia in congenital spherocytosis. Br Med J 1961;1:543.
932. Kohler HG, Meynell MJ, Cooke WT. Spherocytic anaemia, complicated by megaloblastic anaemia of pregnancy. Br Med J 1960;1:779.
933. Burman D. Congenital spherocytosis in infancy. Arch Dis Child 1985;33:335.
934. Schröter W, Kahsnitz E. Diagnosis of hereditary spherocytosis in newborn infants. J Pediatr 1983;103:460.
935. Trucco JI, Brown AK. Neonatal manifestations of hereditary spherocytosis. Am J Dis Child 1967;113:263.
936. Stamey CC, Diamond LK. Congenital hemolytic anemia in the newborn. Am J Dis Child 1957;94:616.
937. Bergstrand CG, Czar B, et al. Serum haptoglobin in infancy. J Lab Clin Invest 1961;13:576.
938. Erlandson ME, Hilgartner M. Hemolytic disease in the neonatal period and early infancy. J Pediatr 1959;54:566.
939. Watson CJ. Studies of urobilinogen. III. The per diem excretion of urobilinogen in the common forms of jaundice and disease of the liver. Arch Intern Med 1937;59:206.
940. Sears DA, Anderson RP, Foy AL, Williams HL, Crosby WH. Urinary iron excretion and renal metabolism of hemoglobin in hemolytic disease. Blood 1966;28:708.
941. Muller-Eberhard U, Javid J, Liem HH, Hanstein A, Hanna M. Plasma concentrations of hemopexin, haptoglobin and heme in patients with various hemolytic diseases. Blood 1968;32:811.
942. LeBlond PF, LaCelle PL, Weed RI. Rhéologie des érythroblastes et des érythrocytes dans la sphérocytose congénital. Nouv Rev Fr Hématol 1971;11:537.
943. Bell CM, Parker AC, Maddy AH. Abnormal pattern of erythrocyte ageing in hereditary spherocytosis as shown by Percoll density gradient centrifugation. Clin Chim Acta 1984;142:91.
944. Maizels M. The anion and cation content of normal and anaemic bloods. Biochem J 1936;30:821.
945. Selwyn JG, Dacie JV. Autohemolysis and other changes resulting from the incubation in vitro of red cells from patients with congenital hemolytic anemia. Blood 1954;9:414.
946. Mohandas N, Kim YR, Tycko DH, et al. Accurate and independent measurement of volume and hemoglobin concentration of individual red cells by laser light scattering. Blood 1986;68:506.
947. Gilsanz F, Ricard MP, Millan I. Diagnosis of hereditary spherocytosis with dual-angle differential light scattering. Am J Clin Pathol 1993;100:119.
948. Pati AR, Patton WN, Harris RI. The use of the Technicon H1 in the diagnosis of hereditary spherocytosis. Clin Lab Haematol 1989;11: 27.
949. Parpart AK, Lorenz PB, Parpart ER, Gregg JR, Chase AM. The osmotic resistance (fragility) of human red cells. J Clin Invest 1947;26:636.
950. Godal HC, Nyvold N, Russtad A. The osmotic fragility of red blood cells: a re-evaluation of technical conditions. Scand J Haematol 1979;23:55.
951. Young LE. Observations on inheritance and heterogeneity of chronic spherocytosis. Trans Assoc Am Phys 1955;68:141.
952. Jacob HS. Hereditary spherocytosis: a disease of the red cell membrane. Semin Hematol 1965;2:139.
953. Johnsson R, Salminen S. Effect of ouabain on osmotic resistance and monovalent cation transport of red cells in hereditary spherocytosis. Scand J Haematol 1980;29:323.
954. Godal HC, Gjonnes G, et al. Does preincubation of the red blood cells contribute to the capacity of the osmotic fragility test to detect very mild forms of hereditary spherocytosis? Scand J Haematol 1982;29:89.
955. Judkiewicz L, Bartosz G, Oplatowska A, Szczepanek A. Modified osmotic fragility test for the laboratory diagnosis of hereditary spherocytosis. Am J Hematol 1989;31:136.
956. Gottfried EL, Robertson NA. Glycerol lysis time of incubated erythrocytes in the diagnosis of hereditary spherocytosis. J Lab Clin Med 1974;84:746.
957. Zanella A, Milani S, Fagnani G, Mariani M, Sirchia G. Diagnostic value of the glycerol lysis test. J Lab Clin Med 1983;102:743.
958. Zanella A, Izzo C, Rebulla P, Zanuso F, Perroni L, Sirchia G. Acidified glycerol lysis test: a screening test for spherocytosis. Br J Haematol 1980;45:481.
959. Rutherford CJ, Postlewaight BF, Hallowes M. An evaluation of the acidified glycerol lysis test. Br J Haematol 1986;63:119.
960. Bucx MJL, Breed WPM, Hoffman JJML. Comparison of acidified glycerol lysis test, Pink test and osmotic fragility test in hereditary spherocytosis: effect of incubation. Eur J Haematol 1988;40:227.
961. Hoffmann JJ, Swaak-Lammers N, Breed WP, Strengers JL. Diagnostic utility of the pre-incubated acidified glycerol lysis test in haemolytic and non-haemolytic anaemias. Eur J Haematol 1991;47:367.
962. Marik T, Brabec V. Acidified glycerol lysis test in various haemolytic anaemias. Folia Haematol (Leipz) 1990;117:259.
963. Vettore L, Zanella A, et al. A new test for the laboratory diagnosis of spherocytosis. Acta Haematol 1984;72:258.
964. Balari AS, Espinosa JV, Fuertes IF. A new modification of the "Pink test" for the diagnosis of hereditary spherocytosis. Acta Haematol 1989;82:213.
965. Pinto L, Iolascon A, del Giudice EM, Nobili B. A modification of the "Pink test" may improve the diagnosis of hereditary spherocytosis. Acta Haematol 1989;82:53.
966. Streichman S, Gesheidt Y, Tatarsky I. Hypertonic cryohemolysis: a diagnostic test for hereditary spherocytosis. Am J Hematol 1990;35: 104.
967. Young LE, Izzo MJ, Altman KI, Swisher SN. Studies on spontaneous in vitro autohemolysis in hemolytic disorders. Blood 1956;11:977.
968. Young N. Hematologic and hematopoietic consequences of B19 parvovirus infection. Semin Hematol 1988;25:159.
969. Mortimer PP, Humphries RK, et al. A human parvovirus-like virus inhibits haematopoietic colony formation in vitro. Nature 1983;302: 426.
970. Ozawa K, Kurtzman G, Young N. Replication of the B19 parvovirus in human bone marrow cell cultures. Science 1986;233:883.
971. Owren PA. Congenital hemolytic jaundice: the pathogenesis of the hemolytic crisis. Blood 1948;3:231.
971a. Lefrére JJ, Courouce AM, Bertrand Y, et al. Human parvovirus and aplastic crisis in chronic hemolytic anemias: a study of 24 observations. Am J Hematol 1986;23:271.
972. Robins MM. Familial crisis in hereditary spherocytosis: report of six affected siblings. Clin Pediatr 1965;4:210.
973. Hanada T, Koike K, Takeya T, et al. Human parvovirus B19-induced transient pancytopenia in a child with hereditary spherocytosis. Br J Haematol 1988;70:113.
974. Saunders PWG, Reid MM, Cohen BJ. Human parvovirus induced cytopenias: a report of five cases. (Letter) Br J Haematol 1986;53:407.
975. Anand A, Gray ES, Brown T, et al. Human parvovirus infection in pregnancy and hydrops fetalis. N Engl J Med 1987;316:183.
976. Anderson LJ, Hurwitz ES. Human parvovirus B19 and pregnancy. Clin Perinatol 1988;15:273.
977. Leads from the MMWR. Risks associated with human parvovirus B19 infection. JAMA 1989;261:1406.
978. Bell LM, Nasides SJ, Stoffman P, et al. Human parvovirus B19 infection among hospital staff members after contact with infected patients. N Engl J Med 1989;321:485.
979. Shneerson JM, Mortimer PP, Vandervelde EM. Febrile illness due to a parvovirus. Br Med J 1980;280:1580.
980. Schwartz TF, Roggendorf M, Hottentrager B, et al. Human parvovirus B19 infection in pregnancy. (Letter) Lancet 1988;2:566.
981. Ozawa K, Kurtzman G, Young N. Productive infection by B19 parvovirus of human erythroid bone marrow cells in vitro. Blood 1987;70:384.
982. Lefrére JJ, Courouce A-M, Girot R, Bertrand Y, Soulier J-P. Six cases of hereditary spherocytosis revealed by human parvovirus infection. Br J Haematol 1986;62:653.
983. McLellan NJ, Rutter N. Hereditary spherocytosis in sisters unmasked by parvovirus infection. Postgrad Med J 1987;63:49.
984. Stefanelli M, Barosi G, Cazzola M, Orlandi E. Quantitative assessment of erythropoiesis in haemolytic disease. Br J Haematol 1980;45:297.
985. Gairdner D. The association of gall-stones with acholuric jaundice in children. Arch Dis Child 1939;14:109.
986. Bates GC, Brown CH. Incidence of gallbladder disease in chronic hemolytic anemia (spherocytosis). Gastroenterology 1952;21:104.
987. Mentzer SH. Clinical and pathologic study of cholecystitis and cholelithiasis. Surg Gynecol Obstet 1926;42:782.
988. Lawrie GM, Ham JM. The surgical treatment of hereditary spherocytosis. Surg Gynecol Obstet 1974;139:208.
989. MacKinney AA Jr. Hereditary spherocytosis: clinical family studies. Arch Intern Med 1965;116:257.
990. Hanford RB, Schneider GF, MacCarthy JD. Massive thoracic extramedullary hemopoiesis. N Engl J Med 1960;263:120.
991. Lawrence P, Aronson I, Saxe N, Jacobs P. Leg ulcers in hereditary spherocytosis. Clin Exp Dermatol 1991;16:28.
992. Vanscheidt W, Leder O, Vanscheidt E, et al. Leg ulcers in a patient with spherocytosis: a clinicopathological report. Dermatologica 1990;181:56.
993. Beinhauer LG, Gruhn JG. Dermatologic aspects of congenital spherocytic anemia. Arch Dermatol 1957;75:642.
994. Abe T, Yachi A, Ishii Y, et al. Thoracic extramedullary hematopoiesis associated with hereditary spherocytosis. Intern Med 1992;31:1151.
995. Bastion Y, Coiffier B, Felman P, et al. Massive mediastinal extramedullary hematopoiesis in hereditary spherocytosis: a case report. Am J Hematol 1990;35:263.
996. Martin J, Palacio A, Petit J, Martin C. Fatty transformation of thoracic extramedullary hematopoiesis following splenectomy: CT features. J Comput Assist Tomogr 1990;14:477.

997. Pulsoni A, Ferrazza G, Malagnino F, et al. Mediastinal extramedullary hematopoiesis as first manifestation of hereditary spherocytosis (clinical conference). Ann Hematol 1992;65:196.
998. Pietsch B, Sigmund G, Wurtemberger G. Kernspintomographische Befunde der kompensierten chronischen Hamolyse: Fallbericht uber eine hereditare Spharozytose. Aktuelle Radiol 1993;3:266.
999. Schafer AI, Miller JB, Lester EP, Bowers TK, Jacob HS. Monoclonal gammopathy in hereditary spherocytosis: a possible pathogenic relation. Ann Intern Med 1978;88:45.
1000. Fukata S, Tamai H, Nogai K, et al. A patient with hereditary spherocytosis and silicosis who developed an IgA (lambda) monoclonal gammopathy. Jpn J Med 1987;26:81.
1001. Lempert KD. Gammopathy and spherocytosis. Ann Intern Med 1978;89:145.
1002. Jandl JH, Files NM, Barnett SB, MacDonald RA. Proliferative response of the spleen and liver to hemolysis. J Exp Med 1965;122:299.
1003. Schilling RF. Hereditary spherocytosis: a study of splenectomized persons. Semin Hematol 1976;13:169.
1004. Isobe T, Osserman EF. Pathologic conditions associated with plasma cell dyscrasias: a study of 806 cases. Ann NY Acad Sci 1971;190:507.
1005. Blacklock H, Meerkin M. Serum ferritin in patients with hereditary spherocytosis. Br J Haematol 1981;49:117.
1006. Edwards CQ, Skolnick MH, Dadone MM, Kushner JP. Iron overload in hereditary spherocytosis: association with HLA-linked hemochromatosis. Am J Hematol 1982;13:101.
1007. Fargion S, Cappellini MD, Piperno A, Panajotopoulous N, Ronchi G, Fiorelli G. Association of hereditary spherocytosis and idiopathic hemochromatosis: a synergistic effect in determining iron overload. Am J Clin Pathol 1986;86:645.
1008. Mohler DN, Wheby MS. Hemochromatosis heterozygotes may have significant iron overload when they also have hereditary spherocytosis. Am J Med Sci 1986;292: .
1009. Morita M, Hashizume M, Kanematsu T, Sugimachi K, Makizumi K. Hereditary spherocytosis with congestive heart failure: report of a case. Surg Today 1993;23:458.
1010. Clarkson JG, Altman RD. Angioid streaks. Surv Ophthalmol 1982;26:235.
1011. McLane NJ, Grizzard WS, Kousseff BG, Hartmann RC, Sever RJ. Angioid streaks associated with hereditary spherocytosis. Am J Ophthamol 1984;97:444.
1012. Gibson JM, Chaudhuri PR, et al. Angioid streaks in a case of beta thalassemia major. Br J Ophthalmol 1983;67:29.
1013. Deutman AF, Kovacs B. Argon laser treatment in complications of angioid streaks. Am J Ophthalmol 1979;88:12.
1014. Gilliland BC, Baxter E, Evans RS. Red cell antibodies in acquired hemolytic anemia with negative antiglobulin serum tests. N Engl J Med 1971;285:252.
1015. Crosby WH, Conrad ME. Hereditary spherocytosis: observations on hemolytic mechanisms and iron metabolism. Blood 1960;15:662.
1016. Pautard B, Féo C, Dhermy D, Wajcman H, Baudin-Chich V, Delobel J. Occurrence of hereditary spherocytosis and β thalassemia in the same family: globin chain synthesis and visco diffractometric studies. Br J Haematol 1988;70:239.
1017. Blecher TE. What happens to the microspherocytosis of hereditary spherocytosis in folate deficiency? Clin Lab Haematol 1988;10:403.
1018. Warkentin TE, Barr RD, Ali MAM, Mohandas N. Recurrent acute splenic sequestration crisis due to interacting genetic defects: hemoglobin SC disease and hereditary spherocytosis. Blood 1990;75:266.
1019. Yang YM, Donnell C, Wilborn W, et al. Splenic sequestration associated with sickle cell trait and hereditary spherocytosis. Am J Hematol 1992;40:110.
1020. Babiker MA, El Seed FAA. A family with sickle cell trait and hereditary spherocytosis. Scand J Haematol 1984;33:54.
1021. Zail SS, Krawitz P, Viljoen E, Metz J. Atypical hereditary spherocytosis: biochemical studies and sites of erythrocyte destruction. Br J Haematol 1967;13:323.
1022. Moiseyev VS, Korovina EA, Polotskaya EL, Poliyanskaya IS, Yazdovsky VV. Hypertrophic cardiomyopathy associated with hereditary spherocytosis in three generations of one family. (Letter) Lancet 1987;2:853.
1023. Flucher BE, Morton ME, Froehner SC, Daniels MP. Localization of the α_1 and α_2 subunits of the dihydropyridine receptor and ankyrin in skeletal muscle triads. Neuron 1990;5:339.
1024. Heier HE. Splenectomy and serious infection. Scand J Haematol 1980;24:5.
1025. Eraklis AJ, Kevy SV, Diamond LK, Gross RE. Hazard of overwhelming infection after splenectomy in childhood. N Engl J Med 1967;276:1225.
1026. Green JB, Shackford SR, Sise MJ, Fridlund P. Late septic complications in adults following splenectomy for trauma: a prospective analysis in 144 patients. J Trauma 1986;26:999.
1027. Evans DI. Postsplenectomy sepsis 10 years or more after operation. J Clin Pathol 1985;38:309.
1028. Holdsworth RJ, Irving AD, Cuschieri A. Postsplenectomy sepsis and its mortality rate: actual versus perceived risks. Br J Surg 1991;78:1031.
1029. Krivit W. Overwhelming post-splenectomy infection. Am J Hematol 1977;2:193.
1030. Schwartz PE, Sterioff S, Mucha P, Melton LJ, Offord KP. Postsplenectomy sepsis and mortality in adults. JAMA 1982;248:2279.
1031. Singer DB. Postsplenectomy sepsis. In: Rosenberg HS, Bolande RP, eds. Perspectives in pediatric pathology, vol 1. Chicago, Year Book Medical Publishers, 1973:285.
1032. Brivet F, Herer B, Fremaux A, Dormont J, Tchernia G. Fatal post-splenectomy pneumococcal sepsis despite pneumococcal vaccine and penicillin prophylaxis. (Letter) Lancet 1984;1:110.
1033. Buchanan GR, Smith SJ. Pneumococcal septicemia despite pneumococcal vaccine and prescription of penicillin prophylaxis in patients with sickle cell anemia. Am J Dis Child 1986;140:428.
1034. Gonzaga RA. Fatal post-splenectomy pneumococcal sepsis despite prophylaxis. Lancet 1984;2:694.
1035. Wong WY, Overturf GD, Powers DR. Infection caused by *Streptococcus pneumoniae* in children with sickle cell disease: epidemiology, immunologic mechanisms, prophylaxis and vaccination. Clin Infect Dis 1992;14:1124.
1036. Buchanan GR, Siegel JD, Smith SJ, DePasse BM. Oral penicillin prophylaxis in children with impaired splenic function: a study of compliance. Pediatrics 1982;70:906.
1037. Caputo GM, Appelbaum PC, Liu HH. Infections due to penicillin-resistant pneumococci: clinical, epidemiologic, and microbiologic features. Arch Intern Med 1993;153:1301.
1038. Musher DM. Pneumococcal pneumonia including diagnosis and therapy of infection caused by penicillin resistant strains. Infect Dis Clin North Am 1991;5:509.
1039. Chesney PJ. The escalating problem of antimicrobial resistance in *Streptococcus pneumoniae*. Am J Dis Child 1992;146:912.
1040. Marton A, Gulyas M, Munoz R, Tomasz A. Extremely high incidence of antibiotic resistance in clinical isolates of *Streptococcus pneumoniae* in Hungary. J Infect Dis 1991;163:542.
1041. Spika JS, Facklam RR, Plikaytis BD, Oxtoby MJ. Antimicrobial resistance of *Streptococcus pneumoniae* in the United States, 1979–1987. The Pneumococcal Surveillance Working Group. J Infect Dis 1991;163:1273.
1042. Golightly LM, Hirschhorn LR, Weller PF. Infectious disease rounds: fever and headache in a splenectomized woman. Rev Infect Dis 1989;11:629.
1043. Mathewson HO. Self-limited babesiosis in a splenectomized child. Pediatr Infect Dis 1984;3:148.
1044. Rosener F, Zarrabi MH, Benach JL, Habicht GS. Babesiosis in splenectomized adults: review of 22 reported cases. Am J Med 1984;76:696.
1045. Teutsch S, Etkind P, Burwell L, et al. Babesiosis in post-splenectomy hosts. Am J Trop Med Hyg 1980;29:738.
1046. Robinette CD, Fraumeni JF Jr. Splenectomy and subsequent mortality in veterans of the 1939–45 war. Lancet 1977;2:127.
1047. Eraklis AJ, Filler RM. Splenectomy in childhood: a review of 1413 cases. J Pediatr Surg 1972;7:382.
1048. Goekcora JH, Ormeci N, Doekmeci A, Barlas M. Treatment of biliary fistulas and cholelithiasis: is endoscopic sphincterotomy acceptable in the paediatric age groups. Int Surg 1989;74:51.
1049. Holcomb GW 3d, Olsen DO, Sharp KW. Laparoscopic cholecystectomy in the pediatric patient. J Pediatr Surg 1991;26:1186.
1050. Sackmann M, Delius M, Sauerbruch T, et al. Shock wave lithotripsy of gallbladder stones: the first 175 patients. N Engl J Med 1988;318:393.
1051. Pappis CH, Galanakis S, Moussatos G, Keramidas D, Kattamis C. Experience of splenectomy and cholecystectomy in children with chronic haemolytic anaemia. J Pediatr Surg 1989;24:543.
1052. Tchernia G, Gauthier F, Mielot F, et al. Initial assessment of the beneficial effect of partial splenectomy in hereditary spherocytosis. Blood 1993;81:2014.
1052a. Lobe TE, Presbury GJ, Smith BM, Wilimas JA, Wang WC. Laparoscopic splenectomy. Pediatr Ann 1993;22:671.
1053. De Haan LD, Werre JM, Ruben AMTh, Huls HA, De Gier J, Staal GEJ. Alterations in size, shape and osmotic behaviour of red cells after splenectomy: a study of their age dependence. Br J Haematol 1988;69:71.
1054. Bart JB, Appel MF. Recurrent hemolytic anemia secondary to accessory spleens. South Med J 1978;71:608.
1055. MacKenzie FAF, Elliot DH, Eastcott HHG, Hughes-Jones NC, Barkhan P, Mollison PL. Relapse in hereditary spherocytosis with proven splenunculus. Lancet 1962;1:1102.
1056. Brook J, Tanaka KR. Combination of pyruvate kinase (PK) deficiency and hereditary spherocytosis (HS). (Abstract) Clin Res 1970;18:176A.
1057. Valentine WN. Hereditary spherocytosis revisited. West J Med 1978;128:35.
1058. Rutkow IM. Twenty years of splenectomy for hereditary spherocytosis. Arch Surg 1981;116:306.
1059. Buchanan GR, Holtkamp CA. Pocked erythrocyte counts in patients with hereditary spherocytosis before and after splenectomy. Am J Hematol 1987;25:253.

1060. Kvindesdal BB, Jensen MK. Pitted erythrocytes in splenectomized subjects with congenital spherocytosis and in subjects splenectomized for other reasons. Scand J Haematol 1986;37:41.
1061. Satou S, Yokota E, Sugihara J, et al. Relapse of hereditary spherocytosis following splenectomy. Acta Haematol Jpn 1985;48:1337.
1062. Lambrecht K. Die Elliptocytose (Ovalocytose) und ihre klinische Bedeutung. Ergebn Inn Med Kinderheilkd 1938;55:295.
1063. Dresbach M. Elliptical human red corpuscles. Science 1904;19:469.
1064. Flint A. Elliptical human erythrocytes. Science 1904;19:796.
1065. Dresbach M. Elliptical human erythrocytes. Science 1904;21:473.
1066. Bishop FW. Elliptical human erythrocytes. Arch Intern Med 1914;14:388.
1067. Sydenstricker VP. Elliptic human erythrocytes. JAMA 1923;81:113.
1068. Huck JG, Bigelow RM. Poikilocytes in otherwise normal blood (elliptical human erythrocytes). Bull Johns Hopkins Hosp 1923;34:390.
1069. Hunter WC, Adams RB. Hematologic study of three generations of a white family showing elliptical erythrocytes. Ann Intern Med 1923;2:1162.
1070. Hunter WC. Further study of a white family showing elliptical erythrocytes. Ann Intern Med 1932;6:775.
1071. Giffin HZ, Watkins CH. Ovalocytosis with features of hemolytic icterus. Trans Assoc Am Physicians 1939;54:355.
1072. Grzegorzewski H. Über familiäres Vorkommen elliptisher Erythrocyten beim Menschen. Folia Haematol (Leipz) 1933;50:260.
1073. Mason VR. Ovalocytosis (elliptical human erythrocytes). In: Downey H, ed. Handbook of hematology, vol 3. New York, Paul B Hoeber, 1938:2351.
1074. Penfold J, Lipscomb JM. Elliptocytosis in man, associated with hereditary haemorrhagic telangiectasis. Q J Med 1943;12:157.
1075. Van Den Bergh AAH. Elliptische rote Blutköperchen. (Addendum). Dtsch Med Wochenschr 1928;54:1244.
1076. Wyandt H, Bancroft PM, Winship TO. Elliptic erythrocytes in man. Arch Intern Med 1941;68:1043.
1077. Wolman IJ, Ozge A. Studies on elliptocytosis. I. Hereditary elliptocytosis in the pediatric age period: a review of recent literature. Am J Med Sci 1957;234:702.
1078. Dacie JV. The lifespan of the red blood cell and circumstances of its premature death. In: Wintrobe, MM ed. Blood, pure and eloquent. New York, McGraw-Hill, 1980:210.
1079. Dacie JV. Hereditary spherocytosis (HS). In: The haemolytic anaemias, ed 3, vol 1. Edinburgh, Churchill Livingstone, 1985:134.
1080. McCarty SH. Elliptical red blood cells in man: a report of eleven cases. J Lab Clin Med 1934;19:612.
1081. Lecomte MC, Dhermy D, Gautero HY, Bournier O, Galans C, Boivin P. L'elliptocytose hereditaire en Afrique de l'Quest: frequence et repartition des variants de la spectrine. CR Acad Sci Paris 1988;306:43.
1082. Ganesan J, George R, Lie-Injo LE. Abnormal haemoglobins and hereditary ovalocytosis in the Ulu Jempul district of Kuala Pilah, West Malaysia. SE Asian J Trop Med Public Health 1976;7:430.
1083. Morton NE. The detection and estimation of linkage between the genes for elliptocytosis and the Rh blood type. Am J Hum Genet 1956;8:80.
1084. Bannerman RM, Renwick JH. The hereditary elliptocytoses: clinical and linkage data. Ann Hum Genet (London) 1962;26:23.
1085. Cook PJL, Noades JE, Newton MS, De Mey R. On the orientation of the Rh El1, linkage group. Ann Hum Genet (London) 1977;41:157.
1086. Keats BJB. Another elliptocytosis locus on chromosome 1? Hum Genet 1979;50:227.
1087. Dalla Venezia N, Wilmotte R, Morlé L, et al. An α-spectrin mutation responsible for hereditary elliptocytosis associated in *cis* with the $\alpha^{V/41}$ polymorphism. Hum Genet 1993;90:641.
1088. Mentzer WC, Turetsky T, Mohandas N, Schrier S, Wu CS. Identification of the hereditary pyropoikilocytosis carrier state. Blood 1984;63:1439.
1089. Palek J, Lux SE. Red cell membrane skeletal defects in hereditary and acquired hemolytic anemias. Semin Hematol 1983;20:189.
1090. Palek J. Hereditary elliptocytosis and related disorders. Clin Haematol 1985;14:45.
1091. Palek J. Hereditary elliptocytosis:spherocytosis and related disorders: consequences of a deficiency or a mutation of membrane skeletal proteins. Blood Rev 1987;1:147.
1092. Florman AL, Wintrobe MM. Human elliptical red corpuscles. Bull Johns Hopkins Hosp 1938;63:209.
1093. Garrdo-Lacca G, Merino C, Luna G. Hereditary elliptocytosis in a Peruvian family. N Engl J Med 1957;256:311.
1094. Geerdink RA, Helleman PW, Verloop MC. Hereditary elliptocytosis and hyperhaemolysis: a comparative study of 6 families with 145 patients. Acta Med Scand 1966;179:715.
1095. Jensson O, Jonasson TH, Olafsson O. Hereditary elliptocytosis in Iceland. Br J Haematol 1967;13:844.
1096. Motulsky AG, Singer K, Crosby WH, Smith V. The life span of the elliptocyte: hereditary elliptocytosis and its relationship to other familial hemolytic diseases. Blood 1954;9:57.
1097. Pothier B, Alloisio N, Maréchal J, et al. Assignment of spectrin alpha$^{I/74}$ hereditary elliptocytosis to the alpha or beta chain of spectrin through in vitro dimer reconstitution. Blood 1990;75:2061.
1098. Rummens JL, Verfaillie C, Criel A, et al. Elliptocytosis and schistocytosis in myelodysplasia: report of two cases. Acta Haematol 1986;75:174.
1099. Coetzer T, Palek J, Lawler J, et al. Structural and functional heterogeneity of α spectrin mutations involving the spectrin heterodimer self-association site: relationships to hematologic expression of homozygous hereditary elliptocytosis and hereditary pyropoikilocytosis. Blood 1990;75:2235.
1100. Ozer L, Mills GC. Elliptocytosis with haemolytic anaemia. Br J Haematol 1964;10:468.
1101. Kruatrachuo M, Asawapokee N. Hereditary elliptocytosis and *Plasmodium falciparum* malaria. Ann Trop Med Parasitol 1972;66:161.
1102. Nkrumah FK. Hereditary elliptocytosis associated with severe haemolytic anaemia and malaria. Afr J Med Sci 1972;3:131.
1103. Jarolim P, Palek J, Coetzer TL, et al. Severe hemolysis and red cell fragmentation due to a combination of a spectrin mutation with a thrombotic microangiopathy. Am J Hematol 1989;32:50.
1104. Schoomaker EB, Butler WM, et al. Increased heat sensitivity of red blood cells in hereditary elliptocytosis with acquired cobalamin (vitamin B_{12}) deficiency. Blood 1982;59:1213.
1105. Austin RF, Desforges JF. Hereditary elliptocytosis: an unusual presentation of hemolysis in the newborn associated with transient morphologic abnormalities. Pediatrics 1969;44:196.
1106. Carpentieri U, Gustavson LP, Haggard ME. Pyknocytosis in a neonate: an unusual presentation of hereditary elliptocytosis. Clin Pediatr 1977;16:76.
1107. Josephs HW, Avery ME. Hereditary elliptocytosis associated with increased hemolysis. Pediatrics 1965;16:741.
1108. Zarkowsky HS. Heat-induced erythrocyte fragmentation in neonatal elliptocytosis. Br J Haematol 1979;41:515.
1109. Prchal JT, Castleberry RP, Parmley RT, Crist WM, Malluh A. Hereditary pyropoikilocytosis and elliptocytosis: clinical, laboratory, and ultrastructural features in infants and children. Pediatr Res 1982;16:484.
1110. Torlontano G, Fioritoni G, Salvati AM. Hereditary haemolytic ovalocytosis with defective erythropoiesis. Br J Haematol 1979; 43:435.
1111. Jankovic M, Sansone G, Conter V, Iolascon A, Masera G. Atypical hereditary ovalocytosis associated with defective dyserythropoietic anemia. Acta Haematol 1993;89:35.
1112. Evans JPM, Baines AJ, Hann IM, Al-Hakim I, Knowles SM, Hoffbrand AV. Defective spectrin dimer-dimer association in a family with transfusion dependent homozygous hereditary elliptocytosis. Br J Haematol 1983;54:163.
1113. Grech JL, Cachia EA, Calleja F, Pullicino F. Hereditary elliptocytosis in two Maltese families. J Clin Pathol 1961;14:365.
1114. Haddy TB, Rana SR. Homozygous hereditary elliptocytosis with hemolytic anemia. South Med J 1984;77:631.
1115. Iarocci TA, Wagner GM, Mohandas N, Lane PA, Mentzer WC. Hereditary poikilocytic anemia associated with the coinheritance of two α spectrin abnormalities. Blood 1988;71:1390.
1116. Lipton EL. Elliptocytosis with hemolytic anemia: the effects of splenectomy. Pediatrics 1955;15:67.
1117. Nielsen JA, Strunk KW. Homozygous hereditary elliptocytosis as a cause of haemolytic anaemia in infancy. Scand J Haematol 1968;5:486.
1118. Pryor DS, Pitney WR. Hereditary elliptocytosis: a report of two families from New Guinea. Br J Haematol 1967;13:126.
1119. Dacie JV, Mollison PL, Richardson N, Selwyn JG, Shapiro L. Atypical congenital haemolytic anaemia. Q J Med (NS) 1953;22:79.
1120. Wiley JS, Gill FM. Red cell calcium leak in congenital hemolytic anemia with extreme microcytosis. Blood 1976;47:197.
1121. Zarkowsky HS, Mohandas N, Speaker CB, Shohet SB. A congenital haemolytic anaemia with thermal sensitivity of the erythrocyte membrane. Br J Haematol 1975;29:537.
1122. Mallouh A Sadi AR, Ahmad MS, et al. Hereditary pyropoikilocytosis: report of two cases from Saudi Arabia. Am J Med Gen 1984;18:413.
1123. DePalma L, Luban NLC. Hereditary pyropoikilocytosis: clinical and laboratory analysis in eight infants and young children. Am J Dis Child 1993;147:93.
1124. Coetzer T, Palek J. Partial spectrin deficiency in hereditary pyropoikilocytosis. Blood 1986;59:919.
1125. Cutting HO, McHugh, Conrad FG, Marlow AA. Autosomal dominant hemolytic anemia characterized by ovalocytosis: a family study of seven involved members. Am J Med 1965;39:21–34.
1126. Dacie JV. Hereditary elliptocytosis (HE). In: The haemolytic anaemias, ed 3. vol 1. Edinburgh, Churchill Livingstone, 1985:216.
1127. Greenberg LH, Tanaka KR. Hereditary elliptocytosis with hemolytic anemia: a family study of five affected members. Calif Med 1969;110:389.
1128. Weiss HJ. Hereditary elliptocytosis with hemolytic anemia. Am J Med 1963;35:455.
1129. Matsumoto N, Ishihara T, Takahashi M, et al. Fine structure of the spleen in hereditary elliptocytosis. Acta Pathol Jap 1976;26:533.
1130. Wilson HE, Long MJ. Hereditary ovalocytosis (elliptocytosis) with hypersplenism. Arch Intern Med 1955;95:438.
1131. Ohanian V, Evans JP, Gratzer WB. A case of elliptocytosis associated with a truncated spectrin chain. Br J Haematol 1985;61:31.

1132. Aksoy M, Erdem S, Dincol G, Erdogan G, Cilingiroglu K, Dincol K. Combination of hereditary elliptocytosis and hereditary spherocytosis. Clin Genet 1974;6:46.
1133. Ham TH, Shen SC, et al. Studies on the destruction of red blood cells. IV. Thermal injury: action of heat in causing increased spheroidicity, osmotic and mechanical fragilities and hemolysis of erythrocytes: observations on the mechanisms of destruction in such erythrocytes in dogs and in a patient with a fatal thermal burn. Blood 1948;3:373.
1134. Ham TH, Sayre RW, et al. Physical properties of red cells as related to effects in vivo. II. Effect of thermal treatment on rigidity of red cells, stroma and the sickle cell. Blood 1968;32:862.
1135. Kimber RJ, Lander H. The effect of heat on human red cell morphology, fragility and subsequent survival in vivo. J Lab Clin Med 64:922.
1136. Chang K, Williamson JR, Zarkowsky HS. Effect of heat on the circular dichroism of spectrin in hereditary pyropoikilocytosis. J Clin Invest 1979;64:326.
1137. Liu S-C, Palek J, Prchal J, Castlebury RP. Altered spectrin dimer-dimer association and instability of erythrocyte membrane skeletons in hereditary pyropoikilocytosis. J Clin Invest 1981;68:597.
1138. Liu S-C, Palek J, Prchal J. Defective spectrin dimer-dimer association in hereditary elliptocytosis. Proc Natl Acad Sci USA 1982;79:2072.
1139. Chasis JA, Mohandas N. Erythrocyte membrane deformability and stability: two distinct membrane properties that are independently regulated by skeletal protein interactions. J Cell Biol 1986;103:343.
1140. Mohandas N, Clark MR, Health BO, et al. A technique to detect reduced mechanical stability of red cell membranes: relevance to elliptocytic disorders. Blood 1982;59:768.
1141. Mohandas N, Clark MR, Jacobs MS, Shohet SB. Analysis of factors regulating erythrocyte deformability. J Clin Invest 1980;66:563.
1142. Orita M, Iwahana H, Kanazawa H, Hayashi K, Sekiya T. Detection of polymorphisms of human DNA by gel elctrophoresis as single-strand conformation polymorphisms. Proc Natl Acad Sci USA 1989;86:2766.
1143. Sarkar G, Yoon H-S, Sommer SS. Screening for mutations by RNA single-strand conformation polymorphism (rSSCP): comparison with DNA-SSCP. Nucleic Acids Res 1992;20:871.
1145. Lawler J, Palek J, Liu S-C, Prchal J, Butler E. Molecular heterogeneity of a hereditary pyropoikilocytosis: identification of a second variant of the spectrin alpha-subunit. Blood 1983;62:1182.
1146. Chabanel A, Sung K-LP, Rapiejko J, et al. Viscoelastic properties of red cell membranes in hereditary elliptocytosis. Blood 1989;73:592.
1147. Delaunay J. Personal communication
1148. Schulman S, Roth EF Jr, Cheng B, et al. Growth of *Plasmodium falciparum* in human erythrocytes containing abnormal membrane proteins. Proc Natl Acad Sci USA 1990;87:7339.
1149. Le Van Kim C, Colin Y, Blanchard D, Dahr W, London J, Cartron JP. Gerbich blood group of the Ge:-1, -2, -3 types: immunochemical study and genomic analysis with cDNA probes. Eur J Biochem 1987;165:571.
1150. Rebuck JW, van Slyck EJ. An unsuspected ultrastructural fault in human elliptocytes. Am J Clin Pathol 1968;49:19.
1151. Bessis M. Living blood cells and their ultrastructure. New York, Springer-Verlag, 1973:140.
1152. Lux SE, John KM. The role of spectrin and actin in irreversibly sickled cells: unsickling of "irreversibly" sickled ghosts by conditions which interfere with spectrin-actin polymerization. In: Caughey WS, ed. Biochemical and clinical aspects of hemoglobin abnormalities. New York, Academic Press, 1978:335.
1153. Liu S-C, Derick LH, Palek J. Dependence of the permanent deformation of red blood cell membranes on spectrin dimer-tetramer equilibrium: implication for permanent membrane deformation of irreversibly sickled cells. Blood 1993;81:522.
1154. De Gruchy GC, Loder PB, Hennessy IV. Haemolysis and glycolytic metabolism in hereditary elliptocytosis. Br J Haematol 1962;8:168.
1155. Peters JC, Rowland M, Israels LG, Zipursky A. Erythrocyte sodium transport in hereditary elliptocytosis. Can J Physiol Pharmacol 1966;44:817.
1156. Facer CA. Malaria, hereditary elliptocytosis, and pyropoikilocytosis. (Letter) Lancet 1989;1:897.
1157. Baer A, Lie-Injo LE, Welch QB, Lewis AN. Genetic factors and malaria in the Temuan. Am J Hum Genet 1976;28:179.
1158. Booth PB, Serjeantson S, Woodfield DG, Amato D. Selective depression of blood group antigens associated with hereditary ovalocytosis among Melanesians. Vox Sang 1977;32:99–110.
1159. Foo LC, Rekhra JV, Chiang GL, Mak JW. Ovalocytosis protects against severe malaria parasitemia in the Malayan aborigines. Am J Trop Med Hyg 1992;47:271.
1160. Dluzewski AR, Nash GB, Wilson RJ, Reardon DM, Gratzer WB. Invasion of hereditary ovalocytes by *Plasmodium falciparum* in vitro and its relation to intracellular ATP concentration. Mol Biochem Parasitol 1992;55:1.
1160a. Reardon DM, Seymour CA, Cox TM, Pinder JC, Schofield AE, Tanner MJ. Hereditary ovalocytosis with compensated haemolysis. Br J Haematol 1983;85:197.
1161. Jones GL. Red cell membrane proteins in Melanesian ovalocytosis autophosphorylation and proteolysis. (Abstract) Proc Australian Biochem Soc 1984;16:34.
1162. Jones GL, McLemore-Edmundson H, Wesche D, Saul A. Human erythrocyte band 3 has an altered N-terminus in malaria-resistant Melanesian ovalocytosis. Biochem Biophys Acta 1991;1096:33.
1163. Husain-Chishti A, Andrabi K, Palek J, Amato D, Liu SC. Altered tyrosine phosphorylation of the red cell band 3 protein in malaria resistant Southeast Asian ovalocytosis (SAO). (Abstract) Blood 1991;78(Suppl 1):80a.
1164. Mohandas N, Chasis JA, Shohet SB. The influence of membrane skeleton on red cell deformability, membrane material properties, and shape. Semin Hematol 1983;20:225.
1165. Moriyama R, Ideguchi H, Lombardo CR, Van Dort HM, Low PS. Structural and functional characterization of band 3 from Southeast Asian ovalocytes. J Biol Chem 1992;267:25792.
1166. Okoye VCN, Bennett V. Plasmodium falciparum malaria: band 3 as a possible receptor during invasion of human erythrocytes. Science 1985;227:169.
1167. Dluzewski AR, Fryer PR, Griffiths S, Wilson RJM, Gratzer WB. Red cell membrane protein distribution during malarial invasion. J Cell Sci 1989;92:691.
1168. Husain-Chishti A, Jarolim P, Palek J. Unpublished observations.
1169. Schultze M. Ein heizbarer objectisch und seine verwendung bei untersuchungen des blutes. Arch Mikrok Anat 1865;1:1.
1170. Shen SC, Ham TH, et al. Studies on the destruction of red blood cells. III. Mechanism and complication of hemoglobinuria in patients with thermal burns: spherocytosis and increased osmotic fragility of red blood cells. N Engl J Med 1943;229:701.
1171. Topley E. The usefulness of counting "heat-affected" red cells as a guide to the risk of the later disappearance of red cells after burns. J Clin Pathol 1961;14:295.
1172. James GW III, Purnell OJ, et al. The anemia of thermal injury. I. Studies of pigment excretion. J Clin Invest 1951;30:181.
1173. James GW III, Abbott LD, et al. The anemia of thermal injury. III. Erythropoiesis and hemoglobin metabolism studied with N^{15}-glycine in dog and man. J Clin Invest 1954;33:150.
1174. Moore FD, Peacock WC, et al. The anemia of thermal burns. Ann Surg 1946;124:811.
1175. McCollough J, Polesky HF, et al. Iatrogenic hemolysis: a complication of blood warmed by a microwave device. Anesth Analg 1972;51:102.
1176. Staples PJ, Griner PF. Extracorporeal hemolysis of blood in a microwave blood warmer. N Engl J Med 1971;285:317.
1177. Jacob HS, Amsden T. Acute hemolytic anemia with rigid red cells in hypophosphatemia. N Engl J Med 1971;285:1446.
1178. Lichtman MA, Miller DR, et al. Reduced red cell glycolysis, 2,3-diphosphoglycerate and adenosine triphosphate concentration, and increased hemoglobin-oxygen affinity caused by hypophosphatemia. Ann Intern Med 1971;74:562.
1179. Myers G, Ngoi SS, Cennerazzo W, Harris L, DeCosse JJ. Clostridial septicemia in an urban hospital. Surg Gynecol Obstet 1992;174:291.
1180. Mupanemunda RH, Kenyon CF, Inwood MJ, Leigh K. Bacterial-induced activation of erythrocyte T-antigen complicating necrotising enterocolitis: a case report. Eur J Pediatr 1993;152:325.
1181. Placzek MM, Gorst DW. T activation haemolysis and death after blood transfusion. Arch Dis Child 1987;62:743.
1182. Warren S, Schreiber JR, Epstein MF. Necrotizing enterocolitis and hemolysis associated with *Clostridium perfringens*. Am J Dis Child 1984;138:686.
1183. Williams RA, Brown EF, Hurst D, Franklin LC. Transfusion of infants with activation of erythrocyte T antigen. J Pediatr 1989;115:949.
1184. Dean HM, Decker CL, et al. Temporary survival in clostridial hemolysis with absence of circulating red cells. N Engl J Med 1967;277:700.
1185. Ifthikaruddin JJ, Holmes JA. *Clostridium perfringens* septicaemia and massive intravascular haemolysis as a terminal complication of autologous bone marrow transplant. Clin Lab Haematol 1992;14:159.
1186. Batge B, Filejski W, Kurowski V, Kluter H, Djonlagic H. Clostridial sepsis with massive intravascular hemolysis: Rapid diagnosis and successful treatment: intensive Care Med 1992;18:488.
1187. Tsai IK, Yen MY, Ho IC, Yu KW, Liu CY, Cheng DL. *Clostridium perfringens* septicemia with massive hemolysis. Scand J Infect Dis 1989;21:467.
1188. Becker RC, Giuliani M, Savage RA, Weick JK. Massive hemolysis in *Clostridium perfringens* infections. J Surg Oncol 1987;35:13.
1189. Bennett JM, Healey PJM. Spherocytic hemolytic anemia and acute cholecystitis caused by *Clostridium welchii*. N Engl J Med 1963;268:1070.
1190. Mera CL, Freedman MH. Clostridium liver abscess and massive hemolysis: unique demise in Fanconi's aplastic anemia. Clin Pediatr 1984;23:126.
1191. Anonymous. Abdominal pain, total intravascular hemolysis, and death in a 53 year old woman. (Clinical Conference) Am J Med 1992;88:667.
1192. Terebelo HR, McCue RL, Lenneville MS. Implication of plasma free hemoglobin in massive clostridial hemolysis. JAMA 1982;248:2028.
1193. Titball RW, Leslie DL, Harvey S, Kelly D. Hemolytic and sphingo-

myelinase activities of *Clostridium perfringens* alpha toxin are dependent on a domain homologous to that of an enzyme from the human arachidonic acid pathway. Infect Immun 1991;59:1872.
1194. Leslie D, Fairweather N, Pickard D, Dougan G, Kehoe M. Phospholipase C and haemolytic activities of *Clostridium perfringens* alpha toxin cloned in *Escherichia coli*: sequence and homology with a *Bacillus cereus* phospholipase C. Mol Microbiol 1989;3:383.
1195. Iwamoto M, Ohno-Iwashita Y, Ando S. Role of the essential thiol group in the thiol-activated cytolysin from *Clostridium perfringens*. Eur J Biochem 1987;194:25.
1196. Iwamoto M, Ohno-Iwashita Y, Ando S. Effect of isolated C-terminal fragment of theta toxin (perfringolysin O) on toxin assembly and membrane lysis. Eur J Biochem 1990;194:25.
1197. Tweten RK. Cloning and expression in *Escherichia coli* of the perfringolysin O (theta toxin) from *Clostridium perfringens* and characterization of the gene product. Infect Immun 1989;56:3228.
1198. Harriš RW, Sims PJ, Tweten RK. Kinetic aspects of the aggregation of *Clostridium perfringens* theta-toxin on erythrocyte membranes: a fluorescence energy transfer study. J Biol Chem 1991; 266:6936.
1199. Hubl W, Mostbeck B, Hartleb H, Pointner H, Kofler K, Bayer PM. Investigation of the pathogenesis of massive hemolysis in a case of *Clostridium perfringens* septicemia. Ann Hematol 1993;67:145.
1200. Iyaniwura TT. Snake venom constituents: biochemistry and toxicology (part 1). Vet Hum Toxicol 1991;33:468.
1201. Perkash A, Sarup BM. Red cell abnormalities after snake bite. J Trop Med Hyg 1972;75:85.
1202. Reid HA. Cobra-bites. Br Med J 1964;2:540.
1203. Foil LD, Norment BR. Envenomation by *Loxosceles reclusa*. (Review) J Med Entomol 1979;16:18.
1204. Nance WE. Hemolytic anemia of necrotic arachnidism. Am J Med 1961;31:801.
1205. Dacie JV. Haemolytic anemia due to drugs, chemicals and venoms: glucose-6-phosphate dehydrogenase deficiency and favism. In: The haemolytic anaemias, congenital and acquired, ed 2, part 4. New York, Grune & Stratton, 1967:993.
1206. Monzon C, Miles J. Hemolytic anemia following a wasp sting. J Pediatr 1980;96:1039.
1207. Schulte KL, Kochen MM. Haemolytic anemia in an adult after a wasp sting. (Letter) Lancet 1981;2:478.
1208. Bousquet J, Huchard G, et al. Toxic reactions induced by hymenoptera venom. Ann Allergy 1984;52:371.
1209. Guess HA, Saviteer PL, et al. Hemolysis and acute renal failure following a Portuguese man-of-war sting. Pediatrics 1982;70:979.
1210. Argiolas A, Pisano JJ. Facilitation of phospholipase A2 activity by mastoparans, a new class of mast cell degranulation peptides from wasp venom. J Biol Chem 1983;25:13697.
1211. Ho CL, Hwang LL. Structure and biological activities of a new mastoparan isolated from the venom of the hornet *Vespa basalis*. Biochem J 1991;274:453.
1212. Katsu T, Kuroko M, Morikawa T, et al. Interaction of wasp venom mastoparan with biomembranes. Biochim Biophys Acta 1990;1027: 185.
1213. Claque MJ, Cherry RJ. A comparative study of band 3 aggregation in erythrocyte membranes by melittin and other cationic agents. Biochim Biophys Acta 1989;980:93.
1214. Dempsey CE. The actions of melittin on membranes. Biochim Biophys Acta 1990;1031:143–161.
1215. Dufton MJ, Hider RC, Cherry RJ. The influence of melittin on the rotation of band 3 protein in the human erythrocyte membrane. Eur Biophys J 1984;11:17.
1216. Hui SW, Stewart CM, Cherry RJ. Electron microscopic observation of the aggregation of membrane proteins in human erythrocyte by melittin. Biochim Biophys Acta 1990;1023:335.
1217. Eichner ER. Spider bite hemolytic anemia: positive Coombs' test, erythrophagocytosis, and leukoerythroblastic smear. Am J Clin Pathol 1984;81:683.
1218. Hardman JT, Beck ML, et al. Incompatibility associated with the bite of a brown recluse spider *(Loxosceles reclusa)*. Transfusion 1983;23:233.
1219. Madrigal GC, Ercolani RL, Wenzl JE. Toxicity from a bite of the brown spider *(Loxosceles reclusus)*: skin necrosis, hemolytic anemia, and hemoglobinuria in a nine-year-old child. Clin Pediatr 1972;11: 641.
1220. Futrell JM, Morgan PN, et al. Location of brown recluse venom attachment sites on human erythrocytes by the ferritin-labeled antibody technique. Am J Pathol 1979;95:675.
1221. Kurpiewski G, Campbell BJ, Forrester LJ, Barrett JT. Alternate complement pathway activation by recluse spider venom. Int J Tissue React 1981;3:39.
1222. Taylor EH, Denny WF. Hemolysis, renal failure and death, presumed secondary to bite of brown recluse spider. South Med J 1966;59: 1209.
1223. Vorse H, Seccareccio P, Woodruff K, Humphrey GB. Disseminated intravascular coagulopathy following fatal brown spider bite (necrotic arachnidism). J Pediatr 1972;80:1035.
1224. Gebel HM, Finke JH, Elgert KD, Campbell BJ, Barrett JT. Inactivation of complement by *Loxosceles reclusa* spider venom. Am J Trop Med Hyg 1979;28:756.
1225. Bernheimer AW, Campbell BJ, Forrester LJ. Comparative toxinology of *Loxosceles reclusa* and *Corynebacterium pseudotuberculosis*. Science 1985;228:590.
1226. Irvin TT, Moir ERS, et al. Treatment of *Clostridium welchii* infection with hyperbaric oxygen. Surg Gynecol Obstet 1968;127:1058.
1227. Brecher G, Haley JE, Wallerstein RO. Spiculated erythrocytes after splenectomy: acanthocytes or non-specific poikilocytes? Nouv Rev Fr Hématol 1972;12:751.
1228. Furchgott RF. Disk-sphere transformation in mammalian red cells. J Exp Biol 1940;17:30.
1229. Nakao M, Nakao T, et al. Adenosine triphosphate and shape of erythrocytes. J Biochem 1961;45:487.
1230. Palek J, Stewart G, et al. The dependence of shape of human erythrocyte ghosts on calcium, magnesium, and adenosine triphosphate. Blood 1974;44:583.
1231. Dacie JV. The *Haemolytic anaemias*, vol 1. The hereditary haemolytic anaemias, ed 3. Edinburgh, Churchill Livingstone, 1985.
1232. Hardie RJ. Acanthocytosis and neurological impairment: a review. Q J Med 1989;71:291.
1233. Féo CJ, Tchernia G, et al. Observation of echinocytosis in eight patients: a phase contrast and SEM study. Br J Haematol 1978;40:519.
1234. Zipursky A, Brown E, et al. The erythrocyte differential count in newborn infants. Am J Pediatr Hematol 1983;5:45.
1235. Aherne WA. The "burr" red cell and azotaemia. J Clin Pathol 1957;10: 252.
1236. Schwartz SO, Motto SA. The diagnostic significance of "burr" red blood cells. Am J Med Sci 1949;218:513.
1237. Oski FA, Nathan DG, et al. Extreme hemolysis and red cell distortion in erythrocyte pyruvate kinase deficiency. I. Morphology, erythrokinetics and family enzyme studies. N Engl J Med 1964;270:1023.
1238. Dacie JV. Secondary or symptomatic haemolytic anaemias. II. Haemolytic anaemias associated with systemic lupus erythematosus, ulcerative colitis, liver disease, renal disease and vascular disease. In: Haemolytic anaemias, congenital and acquired, ed 2, part 3. New York, Grune & Stratton, 1967;810.
1239. Carlyle RF, Nichols G, et al. Abnormal red cells in blood of men subjected to simulated dives. Lancet 1979;1:1114.
1240. Cooper RA. Anemia with spur cells: a red cell defect acquired in serum and modified in the circulation. J Clin Invest 1969;48:1820.
1241. Bassen FA, Kornzweig AL. Malformation of the erythrocytes in a case of atypical retinitis pigmentosa. Blood 1950;5:381.
1242. Tuffy P, Brown AK, et al. Infantile pyknocytosis: a common erythrocyte abnormality of the first trimester. Am J Dis Child 1959;98: 227.
1243. Symmans WA, Shepard CS, Marsh WL, Oyen R, Shohet SB, Linehan BJ. Hereditary acanthocytosis associated with the McLeod phenotype of the Kell blood group system. Br J Haematol 1979;42:575.
1244. Udden MM, Umeda M, Hirano Y, Marcus DM. New abnormalities in the morphology, cell surface receptors, and electrolyte metabolism of In(Lu) erythrocytes. Blood 1987;69:52.
1245. Doll DC, List AF, et al. Acanthocytosis associated with myelodysplasia. J Clin Oncol 1989;7:1569.
1246. Ohsaka A, Yawata Y, Enomoto Y, et al. Abnormal calcium transport of acanthocytes in acute myelodysplasia with myelofibrosis. Br J Haematol 1989;73:568.
1247. Wardrop C, Hutchison HE. Red-cell shape in hypothyroidism. Lancet 1969;1:1243.
1248. Kay J, Stricker RB. Hematologic and immunologic abnormalities in anorexia nervosa. (Review) South Med J 1983;76:1008.
1249. Mant MJ, Faragher BS. The haematology of anorexia nervosa. Br J Haematol 1972;23:737.
1250. Joske RA, McAlister JM, et al. Isotope investigations of red cell production and destruction in chronic renal disease. Clin Sci (Oxford) 1956;15:511.
1251. Loge JP, Lange RD, et al. Characterization of the anemia associated with chronic renal insufficiency. Am J Med 1958;24:4.
1252. Nathan DG, Schupak E, et al. Erythropoiesis in anephric man. J Clin Invest 1964;43:2158.
1253. Akmal M, Telfer N, et al. Red blood cell survival in chronic renal failure: role of secondary hyperparathyroidism. J Clin Invest 1985;76: 1695.
1254. Bogin E, Massry SG, et al. Effect of parathyroid hormone on osmotic fragility of human erythrocytes. J Clin Invest 1982;69:1017.
1255. Saltissi D, Carter GD. Association of secondary hyperparathyroidism with red cell survival in chronic haemodialysis patients. Clin Sci 1985;68:29.
1256. White JG. Effects of an ionophore A23187 on the surface morphology of normal erythrocytes. Am J Pathol 1974;77:507.
1257. Jandl JH. The anemia of liver disease: observations on its mechanism. J Clin Invest 1955;34:390.
1258. Kimber CD, Deller J, et al. The mechanism of anaemia in chronic liver disease. Q J Med 1965;34:33.
1259. Balistreri WF, Leslie MH, Cooper RA. Increased cholesterol and decreased fluidity of red cell membranes (spur cell anemia) in progressive intrahepatic cholestasis. Pediatrics 1981;67:461.

1260. Cynamon HA, Isenberg JN, Gustavson LP, Gourley WK. Erythrocyte lipid alterations in pediatric cholestatic liver disease: spur cell anemia of infancy. J Pediatr Gastroenterol Nutr 1985;4:542.
1261. Doll DC, Doll NJ. Spur cell anemia. South Med J 1982;75:1205.
1262. Douglass CC, McCall MS, et al. The acanthocyte in cirrhosis with hemolytic anemia. Ann Intern Med 1968;68:390.
1263. Grahn EP, Dietz AA, et al. Burr cells, hemolytic anemia and cirrhosis. Am J Med 1968;45:78.
1264. Greenberg MS, Choi ES. Post-splenectomy spur cell hemolytic anemia. Am J Med Sci 1975;269:277.
1265. Hitchins R, Naughton L, Kerlin P, Cobcroft R. Spur cell anemia (acanthocytosis) complicating idiopathic hemochromatosis. Pathology 1988;20:59.
1266. Keller JW, Majerus PW, et al. An unusual type of spiculated erythrocyte in metastatic liver disease and hemolytic anemia: report of a case. Ann Intern Med 1971;74:732.
1267. Silber R, Amorosi E, et al. Spur-shaped erythrocytes in Laennec's cirrhosis. N Engl J Med 1966;275:639.
1268. Smith JA, Lonergan ET, et al. Spur cell anemia: hemolytic anemia with red cells resembling acanthocytes in alcoholic cirrhosis. N Engl J Med 1964;276:396.
1269. Stillman AE, Giordano GF. Spur cell anemia associated with extrahepatic biliary tract obstruction. Am J Gastroenterol 1983; 78:589.
1270. Taniguchi M, Tanabe F, Ishikawa H, Sakagami T. Experimental biliary obstruction of rat: initial changes in the structure and lipid content of erythrocytes. Biochim Biophys Acta 1983;753:22.
1271. Tchernia G, Navarro J, et al. Anemie hemolytique avec acanthocytose et dyslipidemie au cours de deux hepatites neonatales. Arch Franc Pediatr 1968;25:729.
1272. Cooper RA, Kimball DB, et al. Role of the spleen in membrane conditioning and hemolysis of spur cells in liver disease. N Engl J Med 1974;290:1279.
1273. Salvioli G, Rioli G, Lugli R, Salati R. Membrane lipid composition of red blood cells in liver disease: regression of spur cell anaemia after infusion of polyunsaturated phosphatidylcholine. Gut 1978;19: 844.
1274. Fossaluzza V, Rossi P. Flunarizine treatment for spur cell anaemia. Br J Haematol 1983;55:715.
1275. Cooper RA, Diloy-Puray M, et al. An analysis of lipoproteins, bile acids, and red cell membranes associated with target cells and spur cells in patients with liver disease. J Clin Invest 1972;31:3182.
1276. Cooper RA, Leslie MH, et al. Factors influencing the lipid composition and fluidity of red cell membranes in *vitro*: production of red cells possessing more than two cholesterols per phospholipid. Biochemistry 1978;17:327.
1277. Cooper RA, Leslie MH, Knight D, Detweiler DK. Red cell cholesterol enrichment and spur cell anemia in dogs fed a cholesterolenriched atherogenic diet. J Lipid Res 1980;21:1082.
1278. Duhamel G, Forgez P, et al. Spur cells in patients with alcoholic liver cirrhosis are associated with reduced plasma levels of apo A-II, HDL, and LDL. J Lipid Res 1983;24:1612.
1279. Lichtenstein IH, Zaleski EM, MacGregor RR. Neutrophil dysfunction in the rabbit model of spur cell anemia. J Leuk Biol 1987;42:156.
1280. Schubert D, Boss K. Band 3 protein-cholesterol interactions in erythrocyte membranes: possible role in anion transport and dependency on membrane phospholipid. FEBS Lett 1982;150:4.
1281. Seigneuret M, Favre E, et al. Strong interactions between a spin-labeled cholesterol analog and erythrocyte proteins in the human erythrocyte membrane. Biochim Biophys Acta 1985;813:174.
1282. Lange Y, Cutler HB, et al. The effect of cholesterol and other inter-related amphipaths on the contour and stability of the isolated red cell membrane. J Biol Chem 1980;255:9331.
1283. Rooney MW, Lange Y, et al. Acyl chain organization and protein secondary structure in cholesterol-modified erythrocyte membranes. J Biol Chem 1984;259:8281.
1284. Olivieri O, Guarini P, Negri M, et al. Increased proteolytic activity of erythrocyte membrane in spur cell anaemia. Br J Haematol 1988;70:483.
1285. Zieve L. Jaundice, hyperlipemia and hemolytic anemia: a heretofore unrecognized syndrome associated with alcoholic fatty liver and cirrhosis. Ann Intern Med 1958;48:471.
1286. Salt HB, Wolff OH, Lloyd JK, Fosbrooke AS, Cameron AH, Hubble DV. On having no beta-lipoprotein: a syndrome comprising a-betalipoproteinaemia, acanthocytosis, and steatorrhoea. Lancet 1960;2: 326.
1287. Kane JP, Havel RJ. Disorders of the biogenesis and secretion of lipoproteins containing the B apolipoproteins. In: Scriver CS, Beaudet AL, Sly, WS, Valle D, eds. The metabolic basis of inherited disease, ed 6. New York, McGraw-Hill, 1989:1139.
1288. Sharp D, Blinderman L, Combs KA, et al. Cloning and gene defects in microsomal triglyceride transfer protein associated with abetalipoproteinaemia. Nature 1993;365:65.
1289. Wetterau JR, Aggerbeck LP, Bouma ME, et al. Absence of microsomal triglyceride transfer protein in individuals with abetalipoproteinemia. Science 1992;258:999.
1290. Black DD, Hay RV, Rohwer-Nutter PL, et al. Intestinal and hepatic apolipoprotein B gene expression in abetalipoproteinemia. Gastroenterology 1991;101:520.
1291. Glickman RM, Glickman JN, Magun A, Brin M. Apolipoprotein synthesis in normal and abetalipoproteinemic intestinal mucosa. Gastroenterology 1991;101:749.
1292. Hardman DA, Pullinger CR, Hamilton RL, Kane JP, Malloy MJ. Molecular and metabolic basis for the metabolic disorder normotriglyceridemic abetalipoproteinemia. J Clin Invest 1991;88:1722.
1293. Gheeraert P, DeBuyzere M, Delanghe J, DeScheerder I, Bury J, Rosseneu M. Plasma and erythrocyte lipids in two families with heterozygous hypobetalipoproteinemia. Clin Biochem 1988;21:371.
1294. Scriver CS, Beaudet AL, Sly, WS, Valle D, eds. Metabolic basis of inherited diseases, ed 7. New York, McGraw-Hill, 1994.
1295. Simon ER, Ways P. Incubation hemolysis and red cell metabolism in acanthocytosis. J Clin Invest 1964;43:1311.
1296. Barenholz Y, Yechiel E, et al. Importance of cholesterolphospholipid interaction in determining dynamics of normal and abetalipoproteinemia red blood cell membrane. Cell Biophys 1981;3:115.
1297. Iida H, Takashima Y, et al. Alterations in erythrocyte membrane lipids in abetalipoproteinemia: phospholipid and fatty acyl composition. Biochem Med 1984;32:79.
1298. Cooper RA, Gulbrandsen CL. The relationship between serum lipoproteins and red cell membranes in abetalipoproteinemia: deficiency of lecithin:cholesterol acyltransferase. J Lab Clin Med 1971;78: 323.
1299. Flamm M, Schachter D. Acanthocytosis and cholesterol enrichment decrease lipid fluidity of only the outer human erythrocyte membrane leaflet. Nature 1982;298:290.
1300. Lange Y, Steck TL. Mechanism of red blood cell acanthocytosis and echinocytosis in vivo. J Membr Biol 1984;77:153.
1301. McCormick EC, Cornwell DG, et al. Studies on the distribution of tocopherol in human serum lipoproteins. J Lipid Res 1969;1:211.
1302. Dodge JT, Cohen G, et al. Peroxidative hemolysis of red blood cells from patients with abetalipoproteinemia (acanthocytosis). J Clin Invest 1967;46:357.
1303. Elias E, Muller DPR, Scott J. Association of spinocerebellar disorders with cystic fibrosis or chronic childhood cholestasis and very low serum vitamin E. Lancet 1981;2:1319.
1304. Alvarez F, Landrieu P, Féo C, Lemmonier F, Bernard O, Alagille D. Vitamin E deficiency is responsible for neurologic abnormalities in cholestatic children. J Pediatr 107:422.
1305. Sokol RJ, Guggenheim MA, Heubi JE, et al. Frequency and clinical progression of the vitamin E deficiency neurologic disorder in children with prolonged neonatal cholestasis. Am J Dis Child 1985;139: 1211.
1306. Harding AE, Matthews S, Jones S, Booth IW, Muller DPR. Spinocerebellar degeneration associated with a selective defect of vitamin E absorption. N Engl J Med 1985;313:32.
1307. Sokol RJ, Guggenheim M, Iannaccone ST, et al. Improved neurologic function after long-term correction of vitamin E deficiency in children with chronic cholestasis. N Engl J Med 1985;313:1580.
1308. Muller DPR, Lloyd JK, Bird AC. Long-term management of abetalipoproteinaemia. Arch Dis Child 1977;52:209.
1309. Melhorn DK, Gross S. Vitamin E-dependent anemia in the premature infant. II. Relationships between gestational age and absorption of vitamin E. J Pediatr 1971;79:581.
1310. Ehrenkranz RA. Vitamin E and the neonate. Am J Dis Child 1980;134: 1157.
1311. Zipursky A. Vitamin E deficiency anemia in newborn infants. Clin Perinatol 1984;11:393.
1312. Dolan TF Jr. Hemolytic anemia and edema as the initial signs in infants with cystic fibrosis. Clin Pediatr 1976;15:597.
1313. Monzon CM, Woodruff CW. Anemia and edema as presenting signs in cystic fibrosis: a case report. J Med 1986;17:135.
1314. Melhorn DK, Gross S. Vitamin E-dependent anemia in the premature infant. I. Effects of large doses of medicinal iron. J Pediatr 1971;79: 569.
1315. Oski FA, Barness LA. Vitamin E deficiency: a previously unrecognized cause of hemolytic anemia in the premature infant. J Pediatr 1967;70:211.
1316. Ritchie JH, Fish MB, et al. Edema and hemolytic anemia in premature infants: a vitamin E deficiency syndrome. N Engl J Med 1968;279: 1185.
1317. Jacob HS, Lux SE. Degradation of membrane phospholipids and thiols in peroxide hemolysis: studies in vitamin E deficiency. Blood 1968;32: 549.
1318. Brownlee NR, Huttner JJ, et al. Role of vitamin E in glutathione-induced oxidant stress: methemoglobin, lipid peroxidation, and hemolysis. J Lipid Res 1977;18:635.
1319. Kay MMB, Bosman GJ, et al. Oxidation as a possible mechanism of cellular aging: vitamin E deficiency causes premature aging and IgG binding to erythrocytes. Proc Natl Acad Sci USA 1986;83:2463.
1320. Estes JW, Morley JT, et al. A new hereditary acanthocytosis syndrome. Am J Med 1967;42:868.
1321. Levine IM, Estes JW, et al. Hereditary neurological disease with acanthocytosis. Arch Neurol 1968;19:403.
1322. Alonso ME, Teixeira F, Jimenez G, Escobar A. Chorea-acanthocytosis:

a report of a family and neuropathological study of two cases, Can J Neurol Sci 1989;16:426.
1323. Asano K, Osawa Y, Yanagisawa N, Takahashi Y, Oshima M. Erythrocyte membrane abnormalities in patients with amyotrophic chorea with acanthocytosis. Part 2. Abnormal degradation of membrane proteins. J Neurol Sci 1985;68:161.
1324. Clark MR, Aminoff MJ, Chiu DT, Kuypers FA, Friend DS. Red cell deformability and lipid composition in two forms of acanthocytosis: enrichment of acanthocytic populations by density gradient centrifugation. J Lab Clin Med 1989;113:469.
1325. Critchley EMR, Clark DB, Wikler A. Acanthocytosis and neurological disorder without abetalipoproteinemia. Arch Neurol 1968;18:134.
1326. Faillace RT, Kingston WJ, et al. Cardiomyopathy associated with the syndrome of amyotrophic chorea and acanthocytosis. Ann Intern Med 1982;96:616.
1327. Gross KB, Skrivanek JA, Carlson KC, Kaufman DM. Familial amyotrophic chorea with acanthocytosis: new clinical and laboratory investigations. Arch Neurol 1985;42:753.
1328. Hardie RJ, Pullon HW, Harding AE, et al. Neuroacanthocytosis: a clinical, haematological and pathological study of 19 cases. Brain 1991;114:13.
1329. Sotaniemi KA. Chorea-acanthocytosis: neurological disease with acanthocytosis. Acta Neurol Scand 1983;68:53.
1330. Ueno E, Oguchi K, et al. Morphological abnormalities of erythrocyte membrane in the hereditary neurological disease with chorea, areflexia and acanthocytosis. J Neurol Sci 1982;56:89.
1331. Vance JM, Pericak-Vance MA, Bowman MH, et al. Chorea-acanthocytosis: a report of three new families and implications for genetic counselling. Am J Med Genet 1987;28:403.
1332. Villegas A, Moscat J, Vazquez A, et al. A new family with choreoacanthocytosis. Acta Haematol 1987;77:215.
1333. Vita G, Serra S, Dattola R, et al. Peripheral neuropathy in amyotrophic chorea-acanthocytosis. Ann Neurol 1989;26:583.
1334. Feinberg TE, Cianci CD, Morrow JS, et al. Diagnostic tests for choreoacanthocytosis. Neurology 41:1000.
1335. Lupo I, Aragona F, Fierro B, Savettieri G, Scopa F, Piccoli F. Chorea-acanthocytosis with myopathy: report of a case. Acta Neurol (Napoli) 1987;9:334.
1336. Spitz MC, Jankovic J, Killian JM. Familial tic disorder, parkinsonism, motor neuron disease, and acanthocytosis: a new syndrome. Neurology 1985;35:366.
1337. Peppard RF, Lu CS, Chu NS, Teal P, Martin WR, Calne DB. Parkinsonism with neuroacanthocytosis. Can J Neurol Sci 1990;17:298.
1338. Roth AM, Hepler RS, Mukoyama M, Cancilla PA, Foos RY. Pigmentary retinal dystrophy in Hallervorden-Spatz disease: clinicopathological report of a case. Surv Ophthalmol 1971;16:24.
1339. Swisher CN, Menkes JH, Cancilla PA, Dodge PR. Coexistence of Hallervorden-Spatz disease with acanthocytosis. Trans Am Neurol Assoc 1972;97:212.
1340. Luckenbach MW, Green WR, Miller NR, Moser HW, Clark AW, Tennekoon G. Ocular clinicopathologic correlation of Hallervorden-Spatz syndrome with acanthocytosis and pigmentary retinopathy. Am J Ophthalmol 1983;95:369.
1341. Higgins JJ, Patterson MC, Papadopoulos NM, Brady RO, Pentchev PG, Barton NW. Hypoprebetalipoproteinemia, acanthocytosis, retinitis pigmentosa, and pallidal degeneration (HARP syndrome). Neurology 1992;42:194.
1342. Cianci CD, Mische SM, Morrow JS. Impaired cAMP dependent phosphorylation of erythrocyte protein 4.9 in patients with hereditary spheroechinocytosis and neurodegenerative disease. (Abstract) J Cell Biol 1989;107:469a.
1343. Kay MMB, Goodman J, Lawrence C, Bosman G. Membrane channel protein abnormalities and autoantibodies in neurological disease. Brain Res Bull 1990;24:105.
1344. Redman CM, Marsh WL, Scarborough A, Johnson CL, Rabin BI, Overbeeke M. Biochemical studies on McLeod phenotype red cells and isolation of Kx antigen. Br J Haematol 1988;68:131.
1345. Redman CM, Marsh WL. The Kell antigens and McLeod red cells. In: Agre PC, Cartron J-P, eds. Protein blood group antigens of the human red cell: structure, function and clinical significance. Baltimore, Johns Hopkins University Press, 1992:53.
1346. Marsh WL, Oyen R, Nichols ME, Allen FH. Chronic granulomatous disease and the Kell blood groups. Br J Haematol 1975;29:247.
1347. Taswell HF, Lewis JC, et al. Erythrocyte morphology in genetic defects of the Rh and Kell blood group systems. Mayo Clin Proc 1977;52:157.
1348. Wimmer BM, Marsh WL, Taswell HF, Galey HR. Haematological changes associated with the McLeod phenotype of the Kell blood group system. Br J Haematol 1977;36:219.
1349. Redman CM, Huima T, Robbins E, Lee S, Marsh WL. Effect of phosphatidylserine on the shape of McLeod red cell acanthocytes. Blood 1989;74:1826.
1350. Marsh WL, Marsh NJ, Morore A, Symmans WA, Johnson CL, Redman CM. Elevated serum creatine phosphokinase in subjects with McLeod syndrome. Vox Sang 1981;40:403.
1351. Marsh WL, Redman CM. Recent developments in the Kell blood group system. Transfus Med Rev 1987;1:4.
1352. Swash M, Schwartz MS, Carter ND, Heath R, Leak M, Rogers KL. Benign X-linked myopathy with acanthocytosis (McLeod syndrome): its relationship to X-linked muscular dystrophy. Brain 1983;106:717.
1353. Witt TN Danek A Reiter M Heim MU Dirschinger J Olsen EG. McLeod syndrome: a distinct form of neuroacanthocytosis: report of two cases and literature review with emphasis on neuromuscular manifestations. J Neurol 1992;239:302.
1354. Glaubensklee CS, Evan AP, Galey WR. Structure and biochemical analysis of the McLeod erythrocyte membrane. I. Freeze-fracture and discontinuous polyacrylamide gel electrophoresis analysis. Vox Sang 1982;42:262.
1355. Tang LL, Redman CM, Williams D, Marsh WL. Biochemical studies on McLeod phenotype erythrocytes. Vox Sang 1981;40:17.
1356. Bertelson CJ, Pogo AO, Chadhuri A, et al. Localization of the McLeod locus (XK) within Xp21 by deletion analysis. Am J Hum Genet 1988;42:703.
1357. Francke U, Ochs HD, et al. Minor Xp21 chromosome deletion in a male associated with expression of Duchenne muscular dystrophy, chronic granulomatous disease, retinitis pigmentosa, and McLeod's syndrome. Am J Hum Genet 1985;37:250.
1358. Giblett ER, Klebanoff SJ, et al. Kell phenotypes in chronic granulomatous disease: a potential transfusion hazard. Lancet 1971;1:1235.
1359. Hart MVD, Szaloky A, et al. A "new" antibody associated with the Kell blood group system. Vox Sang 1968;15:456.
1360. Parsons SF, Mallinson G, Judson PA, Anstee DJ, Tanner MJA. Evidence that the Lu^b blood group antigen is located on red cell membrane glycoproteins of 85 and 78 kd. Transfusion 1987;27:61.
1361. Shaw MA, Leak MR, Daniels GL, Tippett P. The rare Lutheran blood group phenotype Lu(a−b−): a genetic study. Ann Hum Genet 1984;48:229.
1362. Telen MJ. The Lutheran antigens and proteins affected by Lutheran regulatory genes. In: Agre PC, Cartron J-P, eds. Protein blood group antigens of the human red cell: structure, function and clinical significance. Baltimore, Johns Hopkins University Press, 1992:70.
1363. Telen MJ, Eisenbarth GS, Haynes BF. Human erythrocyte antigens: regulation of a novel red cell surface antigen by the inhibitor Lutheran *In(Lu)* gene. J Clin Invest 1983;71:1878.
1364. Amrein PC, Friedman R, Kosinski K, Ellman L. Hematologic changes in anorexia nervosa. JAMA 1979;241:2190.
1365. Ero Y, Kitagawa T. Wolman's disease with hypobetalipoproteinemia and acanthocytosis: clinical and biochemical observations. J Pediatr 1970;77:862.
1366. Gracey M, Hilton HB. Acanthocytes and hypobetalipoproteinemia. Lancet 1973;1:679.
1367. Paramathypathy K, Aw SE. Acanthocytosis with beta-lipoprotein deficiency in an Indian girl. Med J Aust 1970;2:1081.
1368. Fondu P, Mozes N, Neve P, Sohet-Robazza, Mandelbaum I. The erythrocyte membrane disturbances in protein-energy malnutrition: nature and mechanisms. Br J Haematol 1980;44:605.
1369. Herpertz-Dahlmann B, Remschmidt H. Blutbildveranderungen bei Anorexia nervosa in Abhangigkeit vom Gewicht. Monatsschr Kinderheilkd 1988;136:739.
1370. Warren MP, Vande Wiele RL. Clinical and metabolic features of anorexia nervosa. Am J Obstet Gynecol 1973;117:435.
1371. Ackerman BD. Infantile pyknocytosis in Mexican-American infants. Am J Dis Child 1969;117:417.
1372. Keimowitz R, Desforges JF. Infantile pyknocytosis. N Engl J Med 1965;273:1152.
1373. Zannos-Mariola L, Kattamis C, et al. Infantile pyknocytosis and glucose-6-phosphate dehydrogenase deficiency. Br J Haematol 1962;8:258.
1374. Allison AC. Acute haemolytic anaemia with distortion and fragmentation of erythrocytes in children. Br J Haematol 1957;3:1.
1375. Horton L, Coburn RJ, England JM, Himsworth RL. The haematology of hypothyroidism. Q J Med 1976;45:101.
1376. Perillie PE, Tembrevilla C. Red-cell changes in hypothyroidism. Lancet 1975;2:1151.
1377. Betticher DC, Pugin P. Hypothyroidie et acanthocytes: importance diagnostique du frottis sanguin. Schweiz Med Wochenschr 1991;121:1127.
1378. Barrett AM. A special form of erythrocyte possessing increased resistance to hypotonic saline. J Pathol Bacteriol 1938;46:603.
1379. Cooper RA, Jandl JH. Bile salts and cholesterol in the pathogenesis of target cells in obstructive jaundice. J Clin Invest 1968;47:809.
1380. Neerhout RC. Abnormalities of erythrocyte stromal lipids in hepatic disease: erythrocyte stromal lipids in hyperlipemic states. J Lab Clin Med 1968;71:438.
1381. Verkleij AJ, Nanta ICD, et al. The fusion of abnormal plasma lipoprotein (LP-X) and the erythrocyte membrane in patients with cholestasis studied by electron microscopy. Biochim Biophys Acta 1976;436:366.
1382. Narayanan S. Biochemistry and clinical relevance of lipoprotein X. (Review) Am Clin Lab Sci 1984;14:371.
1383. Seidel D, Alaupovic P, et al. A lipoprotein characterizing obstructive jaundice. I. Method for quantitative separation and identification of lipoproteins in jaundice subjects. J Clin Invest 48:1211.

1384. Iida H, Hasegawa I, Nozawa Y. Biochemical studies on abnormal membranes: protein abnormality of erythrocyte membrane in biliary obstruction. Biochem Biophys Acta 1976;443:394.
1385. Gjone E, Torsvik H, et al. Familial plasma cholesterol ester deficiency: a study of the erythrocytes. Scand J Clin Lab Invest 1968;21:327.
1386. Jain SK, Mohandas N, et al. Hereditary plasma lecithin-cholesterol acyl transferase deficiency: a heterozygous variant with erythrocyte membrane abnormalities. J Lab Clin Med 1982;99:816.
1387. Murayama N, Asano Y, et al. Decreased sodium influx and abnormal red cell membrane lipids in a patient with familial plasma lecithin: cholesterol acyltransferase deficiency. Am J Hematol 1984;16:129.
1388. Bujo H, Kusunoki J, Ogasawara M, et al. Molecular defect in familial lecithin:cholesterol acyltransferase (LCAT) deficiency: a single nucleotide insertion in LCAT gene causes a complete deficient type of the disease. Biochem Biophys Res Commun 1991;181:933.
1389. Funke H, von Eckardstein A, Pritchard PH, et al. Genetic and phenotypic heterogeneity in familial lecithin:cholesterol acyltransferase (LCAT) deficiency: six newly identified defective alleles further contribute to the structural heterogeneity in this disease. J Clin Invest 1993;91:677.
1390. Klein HG, Lohse P, Duverger N, et al. Two different allelic mutations in the lecithin:cholesterol acyltransferase (LCAT) gene resulting in classic LCAT deficiency: LCAT (tyr 83stop) and LCAT (tyr 156asn). J Lipid Res 1993;34:49.
1391. Maeda E, Naka Y, Matozaki T, et al. Lecithin-cholesterol acyltransferase (LCAT) deficiency with a missense mutation in exon 6 of the LCAT gene. Biochem Biophys Res Commun 1991;178:460.
1392. Gjone E, Javitt N, et al. LP-X and bile acid studies in familial lecithin: cholesterol acyltransferase deficiency. Acta Med Scand 1973;194: 377.
1393. Gjone E, Norum KR, et al. Familial lecithin:cholesterol acyltransferase deficiency. In: Stanbury JB, Wyngaarden JB, et al, eds. The metabolic basis of inherited disease, ed 4. New York, McGraw-Hill, 1978:589.
1394. Norum KR, Gjone E. The influence of plasma from patients with familial lecithin:cholesterol acyltransferase deficiency on the lipid pattern of erythrocytes. Scand J Clin Lab Invest 1968;22:94.
1395. Jacobsen CD, Gjone E, et al. Sea-blue histiocytes in familial lecithin: cholesterol acyltransferase deficiency. Scand J Haematol 1972;9:106.
1396. Frohlich J, Hoag G, McLeod R, et al. Hypoalphalipoproteinemia resembling fish eye disease. Acta Med Scand 1987;221:291.
1397. DeHaan LD, Werre JM, et al. Alterations in size, shape and osmotic behaviour of red cells after splenectomy: a study of their age dependence. Br J Haematol 1988;69:71.
1397. Singer K, Miller EB, et al. Hematologic changes following splenectomy in man, with particular reference to target cells, hemolytic index and lysolecithin. Am J Med Sci 202:171.
1398. Singer K, Weisz L. The life cycle of the erythrocyte after splenectomy and the problems of splenic hemolysis and target cell formation. Am J Med Sci 1945;210:301.
1399. Come SE, Shohet SB, et al. Surface remodeling vs whole-cell hemolysis of reticulocytes produced with erythroid stimulation or iron-deficiency anemia. Blood 1974;44:817.
1400. Shattil SJ, Cooper RA. Maturation of macroreticulocyte membranes *in vivo*. J Lab Clin Med 1972;79:215.
1401. Lux SE, John KM. Isolation and partial characterization of a high molecular weight membrane protein complex normally removed by the spleen. Blood 1977;50:625.
1402. Smith CH, Khakoo Y. Burr cells: classification and effect of splenectomy. J Pediatr 1970;76:99.
1403. Crosby WH. Normal function of the spleen relative to red blood cells: a review. Blood 1959;14:399.
1404. Beilin LJ, Knight GJ, et al. The sodium, potassium, and water contents of red blood cells of healthy human adults. J Clin Invest 1966;45: 1817.
1405. Albala MM, Fortier NL, et al. Physiologic features of hemolysis associated with altered cation and 2,3-diphosphoglycerate content. Blood 1978;52:135.
1406. Bienzle U, Niethammer D, et al. Congenital stomatocytosis and chronic haemolytic anaemia. Scand J Haematol 1975;15:339.
1407. Clark ME, Mohandas N, et al. Effects of abnormal cation transport on deformability of desiccytes. J Supramol Struct 1978;8:521.
1408. Eber SW, Lande WM, Iarocci TA, et al. Hereditary stomatocytosis: consistent association with an integral membrane protein deficiency. Br J Haematol 1989;72:452.
1409. Glader BE, Fortier N, et al. Congenital hemolytic anemia associated with dehydrated erythrocytes and increased potassium loss. N Engl J Med 1974;291:491.
1410. Huppi PS, Ott P, Amato M, Schneider H. Congenital haemolytic anaemia in a low birth weight infant due to congenital stomatocytosis. Eur J Haematol 1991;47:1.
1411. Kanzaki A, Yawata Y. Hereditary stomatocytosis: phenotypical expression of sodium transport and band 7 peptides in 44 cases. Br J Haematol 1992;82:133.
1412. Lande W, Cerrone K, et al. Congenital anemia with abnormal cation permeability and cold hemolysis in vitro. (Abstract) Blood 1979;54(Suppl 1):29a.
1413. Lande WM, Thiemann PV, et al. Missing band 7 membrane protein in two patients with high Na, low K erythrocytes. J Clin Invest 1982;70:1273.
1414. Lane PA, Kuypers FA, Clark MR, 1990; Excess of red cell membrane proteins in hereditary high-phosphatidylcholine hemolytic anemia. Am J Hematol 1990;34:186.
1415. Lo SS, Hitzig WH, et al. Stomatozytose. Schweiz Med Wochenschr 1970;100:1977.
1416. Lo SS, Marti HR, et al. Haemolytic anaemia associated with decreased concentration of reduced glutathione in red cells. Acta Haematol 1971;46:14.
1417. Lock SP, Smith RS, et al. Stomatocytosis: a hereditary red cell anomaly associated with haemolytic anaemia. Br J Haematol 1961;7:303.
1418. McGrath KM. Dehydrated hereditary stomatocytosis: a report of two families and a review of the literature. Pathology 1984;16:146.
1419. Meadow SR. Stomatocytosis. Proc R Soc Med 1967;60:13.
1420. Mentzer WC Jr, Smith WB, et al. Hereditary stomatocytosis membranes and metabolism studies. Blood 1975;46:659.
1421. Miller G, Townes PL, et al. A new congenital hemolytic anemia with deformed erythrocytes (?"stomatocytes") and remarkable susceptibility of erythrocytes to cold hemolysis in vitro. I. Clinical and hematologic studies. Pediatrics 1965;35:906.
1422. Miller DR, Rickles FR, et al. A new variant of hereditary hemolytic anemia with stomatocytosis and erythrocyte cation abnormality. Blood 1971;38:184.
1423. Morlé L, Pothier B, Alloisio N, et al. Reduction of membrane band 7 and activation of volume stimulated (K^+, Cl)-cotransport in a case of congenital stomatocytosis. Br J Haematol 1989;71:141.
1424. Mutoh S, Sasaki R, et al. A family of hereditary stomatocytosis associated with normal level of Na-K-ATPase activity of red blood cells. Am J Hematol 1983;14:113.
1425. Nolan GR. Hereditary xerocytosis: a case history and review of the literature. Pathology 1984;16:151.
1426. Platt OS, Lux SE, et al. Exercise-induced hemolysis in xerocytosis: erythrocyte dehydration and shear sensitivity. J Clin Invest 1981;68: 631.
1427. Rix M, Bjerrum PJ, Wieth JO, Frandsen B. Medfodt stomatocytose med haemolytisk anaemi med abnorm kationpermeabilitet og defekte membranproteiner. (Congenital stomatocytosis with hemolytic anemia: with abnormal cation permeability and defective membrane proteins.) Ugeskr Laeger 1991;153:724.
1428. Schröter W, Ungefehr K, et al. Role of the spleen in congenital stomatocytosis associated with high sodium-low potassium erythrocytes. Klin Wochenschr 1981;59:173.
1429. Shohet SB, Livermore BM, et al. Hereditary hemolytic anemia associated with abnormal membrane lipids: mechanism of accumulation of phosphatidyl choline. Blood 1971;38:445.
1430. Shohet SB, Nathan DG, et al. Hereditary hemolytic anemia associated with abnormal membrane lipids. II. Ion permeability and transport abnormalities. Blood 1973;42:1.
1431. Turpin F, Lortholary P, Lejeune F, Claer R. Un cas d'anémie hémolytique avec stomatocytose. Nouv Rev Franc Hématol 1971;11: 585.
1432. Wiley JS, Ellory JC, et al. Characteristics of the membrane defect in the hereditary stomatocytosis syndrome. Blood 1975;46:337.
1433. Yawata Y, Takemoto Y, Yoshimoto M, et al. The Japanese family of congenital hemolytic anemia with high red cell phosphatidyl choline and increased sodium transport. Acta Haematol Jpn 1982;45:672.
1434. Zarkowsky HS, Oski FA, et al. Congenital hemolytic anemia with high-sodium, low-potassium red cells. I. Studies of membrane permeability. N Engl J Med 1968;278:573.
1435. Clark MR, Shohet SB, Gottfried EL. Hereditary hemolytic disease with increased red blood cell phosphatidylcholine and dehydration: one, two, or many disorders? Am J Hematol 1993;42:25.
1436. Lande WM, Mentzer WC. Haemolytic anaemia associated with increased cation permeability. Clin Haematol 1985;14:89.
1437. Wiley JS, Cooper RA, et al. Hereditary stomatocytosis: association of low 2,3-diphosphoglycerate with increased cation pumping by the red cell. Br J Haematol 1979;41:133.
1438. Wiley JS, Shaller CC. Selective loss of calcium permeability on maturation of reticulocytes. J Clin Invest 1977;59:1113.
1439. Dutcher PO, Segel GB, et al. Cation transport and its altered regulation in human stomatocytic erythrocytes. Pediatr Res 1975;9:924.
1440. Mentzer WC, Lubin BH, et al. Correction of the permeability defect in hereditary stomatocytosis by dimethyl adipimidate. N Engl J Med 294:1200.
1441. Mentzer WC, Lam G, et al. Membrane effects of imidoesters in hereditary stomatocytosis. In: Lux SE, Marchesi VT, et al, eds Normal and abnormal red cell membranes. New York, Alan R Liss, 1979: 265.
1442. Stewart GW, Hepworth-Jones BE, Keen JN, Dash BCJ, Argent AC, Casimir CM. Isolation of cDNA coding for an ubiquitous membrane protein deficient in high Na^+, low K^+ stomatocytic erythrocytes. Blood 1992;79:1593.
1443. Hiebl-Dirschmied CM, Adolf GR, Prohaska R. Isolation and partial characterization of the human erythrocyte band 7 integral membrane protein. Biochim Biophys Acta 1991;1065:195.

1444. Hiebl-Dirschmied C, Entler B, et al. Cloning and nucleotide sequence of cDNA encoding human erythrocyte band 7 integral membrane protein. Biochim Biophys Acta 1991;1090:123.
1445. Wang D, Mentzer WC, Cameron T, Johnson RM. Purification of band 7.2b, a 31-kDa integral membrane phosphoprotein absent in hereditary stomatocytosis. J Biol Chem 1991;266:17826.
1446. Westberg JA, Entler B, Prohaska R, Schröter JP. The gene coding for erythrocyte protein band 7.2b (EPB72) is located in band q34.1 of human chromosome 9. Cytogenet Cell Genet 1993;63:241.
1447. Gallagher PG, Segel G, Marchesi SL, Forget BG. The gene for erythrocyte band 7.2b in hereditary stomatocytosis. (Abstract) Blood 1992;80(Suppl 1):276a.
1448. John KM, Lux SE. Unpublished observations.
1449. Wang D, Turetsky T, Perrine S, Johnson RM, Mentzer WC. Further studies on RBC membrane protein 7.2b deficiency in hereditary stomatocytosis. (Abstract) Blood 80(Suppl 1):275a.
1450. Pinkerton PH, Fletch SM, et al. Hereditary stomatocytosis with hemolytic anemia in the dog. Blood 1974;44:557.
1451. Smith JE, Moore K, et al. Glutathione metabolism in canine hereditary stomatocytosis with mild erythrocyte glutathione deficiency. J Lab Clin Med 1983;101:611.
1452. Jaffé ER, Gottfried EL. Hereditary nonspherocytic hemolytic disease associated with an altered phospholipid composition of the erythrocytes. J Clin Invest 1968;47:1375.
1453. Lux SE, Lanzkowsky P, et al. Unpublished observations.
1454. Stewart GW, Corrall RJM, Fyffe JM, Stockdill G, Strong JA. Familial pseudohyperkalemia. Lancet 1979;2:175.
1455. Stewart GW, Ellory JC. A family with mild hereditary xerocytosis showing high membrane cation permeability at low temperatures. Clin Sci 1985;69:309.
1456. Lande WM, Andrews DL, Thiemann PVM, Mentzer WC. Temperature dependence of RBC passive K efflux in primary permeability disorders: unique finding in a patient with cryohydrocytosis. (Abstract) Blood 1985;66(Suppl 1):34a.
1457. McCormack MK, Geller GR, Krivit W, Krissiep KD, Gantzer ML, Barnett RE. Hemolytic anemia associated with a cation abnormality. (Abstract) J Cell Biol 1975;67:271a.
1457a. Dise CA, Goodman DBP, Rasmussen H. Selective stimulation of erythrocyte membrane phospholipid fatty acid turnover associated with decreased volume. J Biol Chem 1980;255:5201.
1458. Fairbanks G, Dino JE, et al. Membrane alterations in hereditary xerocytosis: elevated binding of glyceraldehyde 3-phosphate dehydrogenase. In: Kruckeberg WC, Eaton JW, et al, eds. Erythrocyte membranes: recent clinical and experimental advances. New York, Alan R Liss, 1978:173.
1459. Sauberman N, Fairbanks G, et al. Altered red blood cell surface area in hereditary xerocytosis. Clin Chim Med 1981;114:149.
1460. Platt OS. Exercise-induced hemolysis in sickle cell anemia: shear-sensitivity and erythrocyte dehydration. Blood 1982;59:1055.
1461. Harm W, Fortier NL, et al. Increased erythrocyte lipid peroxidation in hereditary xerocytosis. Clin Chim Acta 1979;99:121.
1462. Sauberman N, Fortier NL, et al. Spectrin-hemoglobin crosslinkages associated with *in vitro* oxidant hypersensitivity in pathologic and artificially dehydrated red cells. Br J Haematol 1983;54:15.
1463. Snyder LM, Sauberman N, et al. Red cell membrane response to hydrogen peroxide: sensitivity in hereditary xerocytosis and in other abnormal red cells. Br J Haematol 1981;48:435.
1464. Fortier N, Snyder LM, et al. The relationship between in vivo generated hemoglobin skeletal protein complex and increased red cell membrane rigidity. Blood 1988;71:1427
1465. Snyder LM, Fortier NL, et al. Effect of hydrogen peroxide exposure on normal human erythrocyte deformability, morphology, surface characteristics and spectrin hemoglobin crosslinking. J Clin Invest 1985;76:1971.
1466. Douglass CC, Twomey JJ. Transient stomatocytosis with hemolysis: a previously unrecognized complication of alcoholism. Ann Intern Med 1970;72:159.
1467. Wislöff F, Boman D. Acquired stomatocytosis in alcoholic liver disease. Scand J Haematol 1979;23:43.
1468. Simpson LO. Blood from healthy animals and humans contains nondiscocytic erythrocytes. Br J Haematol 1989;73:561.
1469. Davidson RJ, How J, et al. Acquired stomatocytosis: its prevalence and significance in routine haematology. Scand J Haematol 1977;19:47.
1470. Ducrou W, Kimber RJ. Stomatocytes, haemolytic anaemia and abdominal pain in Mediterranean migrants: some examples of a new syndrome? Med J Aust 1969;2:1087.
1471. Ohsaka A, Kano Y, Sakamoto S, et al. A transient hemolytic reaction and stomatocytosis following vinca alkaloid administration. Acta Haematol Jpn 1989;52:7.
1472. Reinhart WH, Chien S. Stomatocytic transformation of red blood cells after marathon running. Am J Hematol 1985;19:201.
1473. Davidson RJL. March or exertional hemoglobinuria. Semin Hematol 1969;6:150.
1474. Banga JP, Pinder JC, et al. An erythrocyte membraneprotein anomaly in march haemoglobinuria. Lancet 1979;2:1048.
1475. Vos GH, Vos D, et al. A sample of blood with no detectable Rh antigens. Lancet 1961;1:14.
1476. Ballas SK, Clark MR, et al. Red cell membrane and cation deficiency in Rh_{null} syndrome. Blood 1984;63:1046.
1477. Seidl S, Spielmann W, et al. Two siblings with Rh_{null} disease. Vox Sang 1972;23:182.
1478. Senhauser DA, Mitchell MW, et al. Another example of phenotype Rh_{null}. Transfusion 1970;10:89.
1479. Sturgeon P. Hematological observations on the anemia associated with blood type Rh_{null}. Blood 1970;36:310.
1480. Lauf PK, Joiner CH. Increased potassium transport and ouabain binding in human Rh_{null} red blood cells. Blood 1976;48:457.
1481. Mallory DM, Rosenfield RE, et al. Rh_{mod}: a second kindred (Craig). Vox Sang 1976;30:430.
1482. Saji H, Hosoi T. A Japanese Rh_{mod} family: serological and haematological observations. Vox Sang 1979;37:296.
1483. Assmann G, Schmitz G, Brewer HB Jr. Familial high density lipoprotein deficiency: Tangier disease. In: Scriver CS, Beaudet AL, Sly WS, Valle D, eds. Metabolic basis of inherited diseases, ed 6. New York, McGraw-Hill, 1989:1267.
1484. Schmitz G, Assmann G, Robenek H, Brennhausen B. Tangier disease: a disorder of intracellular membrane traffic. Proc Natl Acad Sci USA 1985;82:6305.
1485. Reinhart WH, Gössi U, Bütikofer P, et al. Haemolytic anaemia in analpha-lipoproteinaemia (Tangier disease): morphological, biochemical, and biophysical properties of the red blood cell. Br J Haematol 1989;72:272.
1486. Hoffman HN, Fredrickson DS. Tangier disease (familial high density lipoprotein deficiency): clinical and genetic features in two adults. Am J Med 1965;39:582.
1487. Kummer H, Laissue J, et al. Familiäre analphalipoproteinämie (Tangier-Krankheit). Schweiz Med Wochenschr 1968;11:406.
1488. Shaklady MM, Djardjouras EM, Lloyd JK. Red-cell lipids in familial alphalipoprotein deficiency (Tangier disease). Lancet 1968;2:151.
1489. Norman JG. Stomatocytosis in migrants in Mediterranean origin. (Letter) Med J Aust 1969;1:315.
1490. Jackson JM, Knight D. Stomatocytosis in migrants of Mediterranean origin. (Letter) Med J Aust 1969;1:939.
1491. Lander H. More maladies in Mediterranean migrants: stomatocytosis and macrothrombocytopenia. Med J Aust 1971;1:438.
1492. von Behrens WE. Splenomegaly, macrothrombocytopenia and stomatocytosis in healthy Mediterranean subjects (splenomegaly in Mediterranean macrothrombocytopenia). Scand J Haematol 1975;14:258.
1493. Miwa S, Fujii H, et al. A case of red-cell adenosine deaminase overproduction associated with hereditary hemolytic anemia found in Japan. Am J Hematol 1978;5:107.
1494. Wada H, Kanzaki A, Ata K, et al. A new band 3 variant with increased hemolysis, decreased anion transport, glycophorin A anomaly and abnormal rheology. (Abstract) Blood 1990;76(Suppl 1):20a.
1495. Weed RI, LaCelle PL, et al. Metabolic dependence of red cell deformability. J Clin Invest 1969;48:795.
1496. Lux SE, John KM, Ukena TE. Diminished spectrin extraction from ATP-depleted human erythrocytes: evidence relating spectrin to changes in erythrocyte shape and deformability. J Clin Invest 1978;61:815.
1497. Palek J, Liu SC, et al. Metabolic dependence of protein arrangement in human erythrocyte membranes. I. Analysis of spectrin-rich complexes in ATP-depleted red cells. Blood 1978;51:385.
1498. Nathan DG, Oski FA, et al. Extreme hemolysis and red cell distortion in erythrocyte pyruvate kinase deficiency. II. Measurements of erythrocyte glucose consumption, potassium flux and adenosine triphosphate stability. N Engl J Med 1965;272:118.
1499. Mentzer WC, Baehner RL, et al. Selective reticulocyte destruction in erythrocyte pyruvate kinase deficiency. J Clin Invest 1971;50:688.
1500. Glader BE. Salicylate-induced injury of pyruvate kinase-deficient erythrocytes. N Engl J Med 1976;294:916.
1501. Leblond PF, Lyonnais J, et al. Erythrocyte populations in pyruvate kinase deficiency anaemia following splenectomy. I. Cell morphology. Br J Haematol 1978;39:55.
1502. Leblond PF, Coulombe L, et al. Erythrocyte populations in pyruvate kinase deficiency anaemia following splenectomy. II. Cell deformability. Br J Haematol 1978;31:63.
1503. Coetzer T, Zail SS. Erythrocyte membrane proteins in hereditary glucose phosphate isomerase deficiency, J Clin Invest 1979;63:552.
1504. Clark MR, Unger RC, et al. Monovalent cation composition and ATP and lipid content of irreversibly sickled cells. Blood 1978;51:1169.
1505. Glader BE, Lux SE, et al. Energy-reserve and cation composition of irreversibly sickled cells (ISCs) in vivo. Br J Haematol 1978;40:527.
1506. Chuttani HK, Gupta PS, et al. Acute copper sulfate poisoning. Am J Med 39:849.
1507. Fairbanks VF. Copper sulfate induced hemolytic anemia: inhibition of glucose-6-phosphate dehydrogenase and other possible etiologic mechanisms. Arch Intern Med 1967;120:428.
1508. Holtzman NA, Elliot DA, et al. Copper intoxication. N Engl J Med 1966;275:347.

1509. Manzler AD, Schreiner AW. Copper-induced acute hemolytic anemia: a new complication of hemodialysis. Ann Intern Med 1970;73: 409.
1510. Roberts RH. Hemolytic anemia associated with copper sulfate poisoning. Mississippi Doctor 1956;33:292.
1511. Oski FA. Chickee, the copper. (Editorial) Ann Intern Med 1970;73: 485.
1512. Cartwright GE. Diagnosis of treatable Wilson's disease. N Engl J Med 1978;298:1347.
1513. Danks DM. Disorders of copper transport. In: Scriver CS, Beaudet AL, Sly WS, eds. Metabolic basis of inherited diseases, ed 6. New York, McGraw-Hill, 1989:1411.
1514. Walshe JM. Wilson's disease: the presenting symptoms. Arch Dis Child 1962;37:253.
1515. Buchanan GR. Acute hemolytic anemia as a presenting manifestation of Wilson's disease. J Pediatr 1975;86:245.
1516. Forman SJ, Kumar KS, et al. Hemolytic anemia in Wilson disease: clinical findings and biochemical mechanisms. Am J Hematol 1980;9: 269.
1517. Grüter W. Hämolytische Krisen als Frühmanifestation der Wilson'schen Krankheit. Dtsch Z Nervenheilkd 1959;179:401.
1518. Lehr H, Pauschinger M, Pittke E, Kurrle E, Heimpel H. Haemolytic anaemia as initial manifestation of Wilson's disease. Blut 1988;56: 45.
1519. Robitaille GA, Piscatelli RL, Majeski EJ, Gelehrter TD. Hemolytic anemia in Wilson's disease. JAMA 1977;237:2402.
1520. Roche-Sicot J, Benhamou J-P. Acute intravascular hemolysis and acute liver failure associated as a first manifestation of Wilson's disease. Ann Intern Med 1977;86:301.
1521. Willms KG, Blume KG, Löhr GW. Hämolytische Anämie bei Morbus Wilson (Hepatolentikuläre Degeneration). Klin Wochenschr 1972;50: 995.
1522. Deiss A, Lee GR, et al. Hemolytic anemia in Wilson's disease. Ann Intern Med 1970;73:413.
1523. Dobyns WB, Goldstein NP, Gordon H. Clinical spectrum of Wilson's disease (hepatolenticular degeneration). Mayo Clin Proc 1979;54:35.
1524. Hoagland HC, Goldstein NP. Hematologic (cytopenic) manifestations of Wilson's disease. Mayo Clin Proc 1978;53:498.
1525. Iser JH, Stevens BJ, et al. Hemolytic anemia of Wilson's disease. Gastroenterology 1974;67:290.
1526. McIntyre N, Clink HM, et al. Hemolytic anemia in Wilson's disease. N Engl J Med 1967;276:439.
1527. Meyer RJ, Zalusky R. The mechanisms of hemolysis in Wilson's disease: study of a case and review of the literature. Mt Sinai J Med (NY) 1977;44:530.
1528. Petrukhin K, Fischer SG, Pirastu M, et al. Mapping, cloning and genetic characterization of the region containing the Wilson disease gene. Nature Genet 1993;5:338.
1529. Bull PC, Thomas GR, Rommens JM, Forbes JR, Cox DW. The Wilson disease gene is a putative copper transporting P-type ATPase similar to the Menkes gene. Nature Genet 1993;5:327.
1530. Tanzi RE, Petrukhin K, Chernov I, et al. The Wilson disease gene is a copper transporting ATPase with homology to the Menkes disease gene. Nature Genet 1993;5:344.
1531. Yamaguchi Y, Heiny ME, Gitlin JD. Isolation and characterization of a human liver cDNA as a candidate gene for Wilson disease. Biochem Biophys Res Commun 1993;197:271.
1532. Chelly J, Monaco AP. Cloning the Wilson disease gene. Nature Genet 1993;5:317.
1533. Gubler CJ, Labey ME, et al. Studies on copper metabolism. IX. Transportation of copper in blood. J Clin Invest 1953;32:405.
1534. Hochstein P, Kumar KS, et al. Mechanisms of copper toxicity in red cells. In: Brewer GJ, ed. The red cell. New York, Alan R Liss, 1978.

Blood: Principles and Practice of Hematology,
edited by Robert I. Handin, Samuel E. Lux, and Thomas P. Stossel.
J.B. Lippincott Company, Philadelphia © 1995.

55

Autoimmune Hemolytic Anemia

Wendell F. Rosse

Autoimmune immune hemolytic anemias are characterized by the destruction of red blood cells (RBCs) by antibodies produced by the patient. The syndromes of autoimmune hemolytic anemia (AIHA) under this rubric are many and varied; the variety arises from differences in the characteristics of the antibodies involved and the causes of their production.

One of the first syndromes of hemolytic anemia described and clearly differentiated was autoimmune in nature—paroxysmal cold hemoglobinuria, a rare form of AIHA. As early as 1832, physicians in England described "winter hematuria"[1,2] and related the syndrome to secondary and tertiary syphilis. In 1904, Donath and Landsteiner described the serologic reactions that demonstrated the disease was caused by an antibody.[3,4] It has been suggested, however, that both Donath and Landsteiner were not entirely certain what they had discovered.[5]

This discovery was shortly after Ehrlich postulated that such a situation was not possible, that an animal would not make an antibody against its own cells—the famous "horror autotoxicus."[6] It was postulated, perhaps correctly, that the reaction was against antigens on the organism that causes syphilis and that the antibody produced cross-reacted with the cells of the patient.

This syndrome was easily identified because it is characterized by intravascular hemolysis by complement and, for many years, it was thought that this was the only way that RBCs could be destroyed by antibody. Thus, the immunologic nature of the more common form of AIHA, known to be caused by an IgG warm-reacting antibody, was difficult to recognize. Further, this syndrome was confused for many years with congenital hemolytic icterus (hereditary spherocytosis), since both are characterized by the presence of spherocytes in the peripheral blood.[7]

Discovery of the antiglobulin Coombs' test for detection of cell-bound antibody in 1945[11] led to the clear distinction between the two: the test usually was positive in the acquired disease and always negative in the congenital one.[12,13] Within the next few years, the distinction between the positive Coombs' test due to IgG antibody and the non-γ Coombs' test led to the distinction between IgG and IgM antibodies, and the improvement in serologic characterization made more clear the pathophysiology of the disease.[14]

Some antibodies are readily detected by their ability to agglutinate RBCs; this characteristic was used by Landsteiner in demonstrating the alloantibodies to blood groups found in normal serum.[8] Little use was made of this characteristic in identifying antibodies causing hemolytic anemia,[9,10] probably because most antibodies that occur in AIHA agglutinate poorly under physiologic conditions.

In this chapter, we describe the nature of the antibodies that are involved in the syndromes of AIHA and relate their characteristics to the clinical syndromes that result. This builds on the foundation laid by early observations and expanded by the explosion of immunologic knowledge during the past 20 years.

ANTIBODIES

Antibodies encountered in AIHA are of three classes—IgG, IgM, and IgA. These molecules are not known to be different from other immunoglobulin molecules; structurally, they consist of immunoglobulin units containing two light and two heavy chains. The light chains consist of a variable portion and a common portion of equal size. These line up with similarly sized variable and common portions of the heavy chain; these units form the two F(ab) portions of the molecule that bear at their free end the antigen-binding regions composed of the hypervariable portions of a light chain and a heavy chain.

Each heavy chain has two (IgM has three) additional units of the same size that line up with corresponding units of the other heavy chain; these moieties form the Fc portion of the molecule. The Fc portion is separated from the F(ab) portions by a flexible bridge that connects them with the functional regions (on the heavy-chain portion of the molecule) that mediate the effector functions of the molecule.[15,16]

Reaction With Antigen

For antibody molecules to effect lysis of RBCs, they must bind to surface antigens. The binding to antigen depends on a reversible reaction between the antigenic epitope and the antigen-binding pocket of the antibody molecule.[17] Thus, the binding may be more strong or less strong, depending on the biochemical and biophysical characteristics of each.

Antigens that bind the antibodies of AIHA are either protein or polysaccharide in structure. The protein antigens usually are epitopes present on the cells of almost all individuals and are often found on the abundant glycoproteins and lipoproteins of the membrane. Usually, the epitope is not an allomorphic blood group antigen, but occasionally such antigens may be involved in the antigenic structure.

The polysaccharide antigens usually are part of the complex bearing the H, A, and B antigens or the P antigens. These structures may consist of linear or complex, branched arrays of sugars that are attached to lipid (usually sphingolipid) or protein molecules. These structures are present on the RBCs of all individuals, so distinctions of specificity are made on quantitative rather than qualitative bases, or on tests of chemical structure.

The reaction between antigen and antibody may be modified by the temperature at which it takes place. In general, the reaction between a protein antigen and antibody is relatively independent of temperature and can occur at 37°C as well as at lower temperatures. This means that the antibody remains attached to the antigen at the core temperature of the body, which is an important attribute.

Conversely, the reaction of a polysaccharide antigen and its antibody is markedly enhanced at lower temperatures. In most cases, the reaction does not occur to a significant degree at 37°C, indicating that antibody and antigen are not attached to one another at core body temperature. In that case, antigen–antibody interaction can only occur as the blood circulates to the periphery and is cooled sufficiently.

Functional Capacities of Molecules

The means by which antibody molecules mediate destruction of the RBC is determined by their functional capacities—in particular, their capacity to fix complement and their ability to fix to specific receptors that are present on effector cells (eg, phagocytes and "killer" lymphocytes) of the immune system. These capacities differ among isotypes of antibody.

Complement in Destruction of Target Cells

Complement is composed of a group of proteins that effect or augment the destructive reactions of antibodies. When the sequence is completely activated in a series of reactions, a lesion is produced that penetrates the cell membrane and destroys the cell. These reactions are generally so tightly controlled that large amounts of complement must be activated to produce the final destructive event. During activation of the sequence, however, proteins are generated that mediate immune adherence. This may lead to cell-mediated destruction, particularly if an antibody able to mediate immune adherence also is present on the target-cell membrane. The aspects of these reactions relative to immune hemolytic anemia are recounted here.

Fixation of Complement

The ability of an antibody molecule to participate in the fixation of complement depends on specific sequences in the Fc portion of the molecule that interact with the non-collagen portion of the C1q molecule[18,19] (Fig. 55-1); these sequences are present in IgG and IgM molecules but not in IgA molecules. IgA molecules do not fix complement by the classic activation pathway.[20] Two additional conditions must be met before complement can be fixed:

1. The C1q binding site must be accessible to the C1q molecule. This accessibility is impaired in two ways:
   The site may be situated so close to the F(ab) portions of the molecule that these free-swinging "arms" may sterically hinder the fixation of C1q[21] (Fig. 55-2*A*). In IgG_3 and IgG_1 molecules, the C1q-binding site is distant from the F(ab) portion of the molecule because the hinge region between the Fc and the F(ab) domains is long; thus, these two subclasses readily fix C1q if the other conditions are met.[4] Similarly, the binding site in the IgM molecule is distant from the F(ab) domains. The hinge region of IgG_2 and especially IgG_4 molecules is short, however, and the waving F(ab) arms apparently hinder the binding of C1q.[22]
   The site may be hindered by other parts of the molecule. In solution, IgM exists in a planar form; that is, the five monomers are spread out like a cartwheel around the joining J piece. In this conformation, the C1q binding sites of IgM are hidden and not available for binding. When the molecule binds to two epitopes on the same surface, it assumes a conformational configuration that has been likened to a staple or a stool; in this conformation, the C1q binding sites are exposed and binding takes place[23,24] (see Fig. 55-2*B*).
2. For effective binding of C1q to take place, antibody must react with two of the binding regions on the C1q molecule.[25] For two IgG molecules, this means that two molecules must be within about 24 nm to permit the binding of two sites on the C1q molecule[26] (see Fig. 55-2*C*). For IgM molecules, a single molecule is

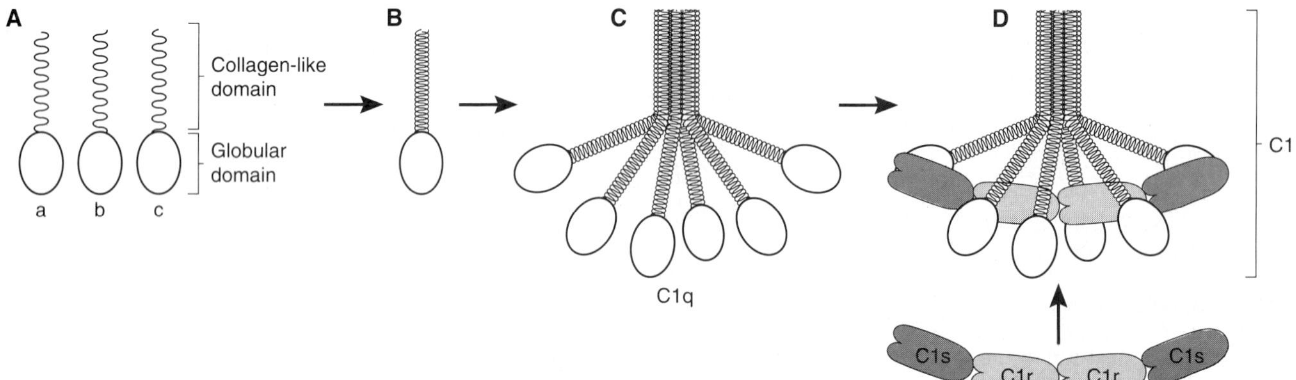

FIGURE 55-1. Structure of the first component of complement. (**A**) Three similar polypeptide chains (a, b, and c) consist of a collagen-like portion (signified by the wavy line) and a globular portion. (**B**) These intertwine to form a heterotrimer; the collagen-like portion becomes rigid and has a bend in it. (**C**) Six of the heterotrimers form a complex structure said to resemble a bunch of flowers held by their lower stems. (**D**) C1r and C1s form a tetramer, which is inserted into the spread ends of the heterotrimers.

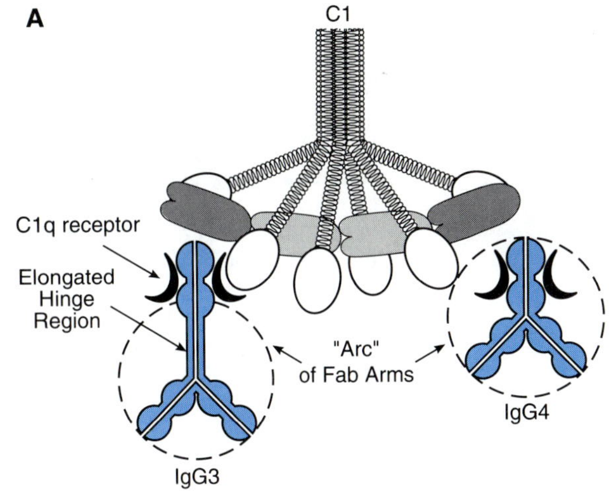

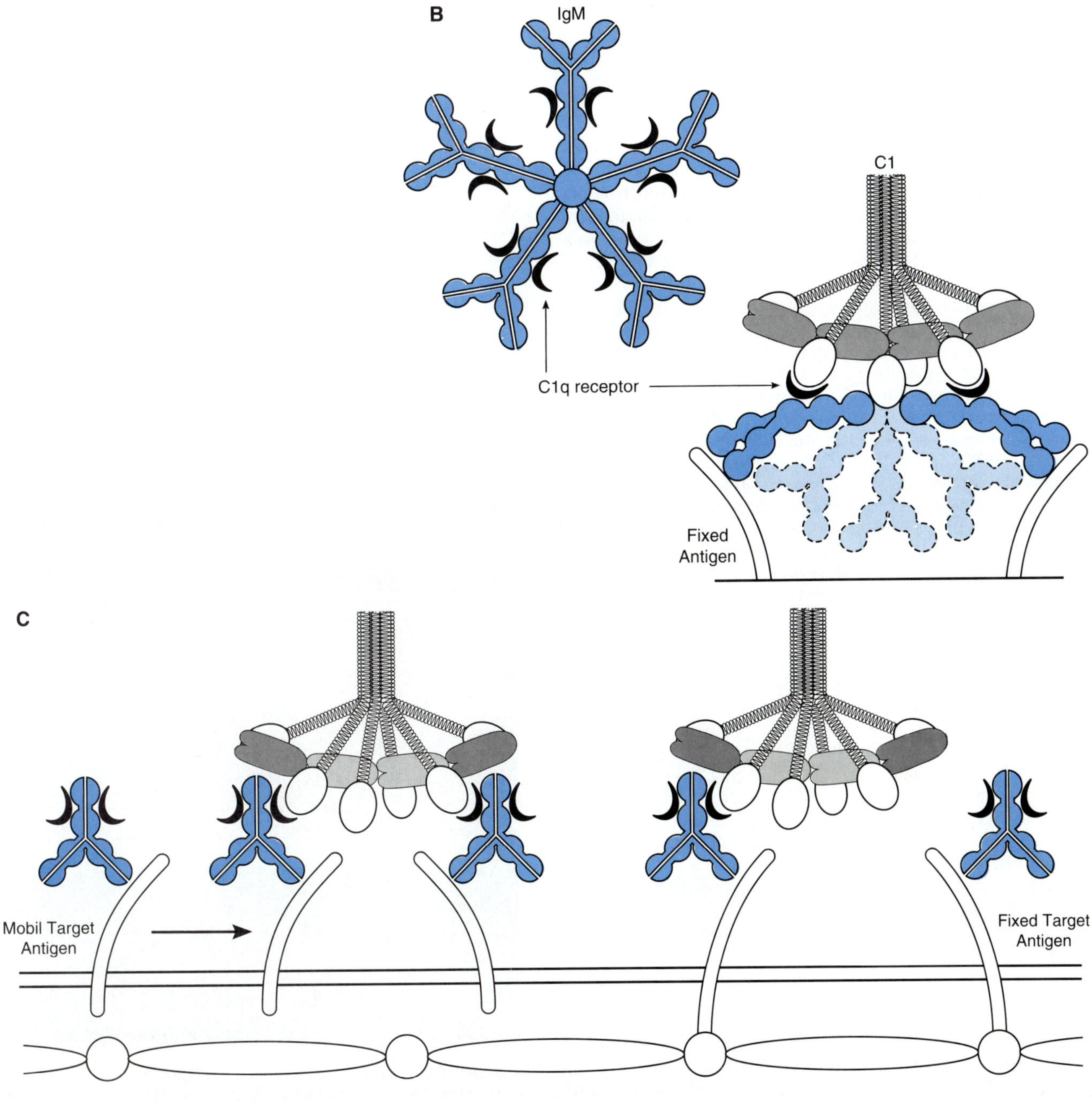

FIGURE 55-2. Binding of C1 to antibodies. (**A**) Binding of C1 to IgG molecules is inhibited by interference from the Fab arms, which is minimized when the hinge region is elongated, as in IgG_3 molecules. (**B**) The C1-binding sites of IgM molecules are not available when the antibody is in the planar form in fluid phase; when two of the monomers are affixed, the molecule assumes an arched form and the C1 binding sites become available for reaction. (**C**) Fixation of C1 by IgG also depends on reaction of two of the receptor binding areas; if this is not possible, as occurs when the antigen-bearing molecule is affixed to the cytoskeleton at relatively great distances, the binding of C1 is too weak to be effective.

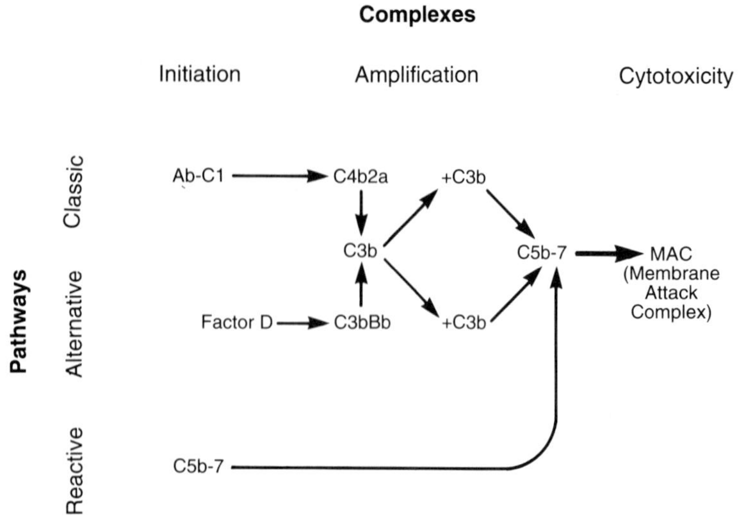

FIGURE 55-3. Activation of complement. Three kinds of complexes are generated: initiation, amplification, and cytotoxicity. These are generated by three different pathways: classic, alternative, and reactive. All result in formation of membrane attack complex.

sufficient, since the C1q-binding areas of two subunits can participate in the reaction; however, the other conditions necessary for C1q binding must be met.

Because of these limitations, complement may not be fixed by all antigen–antibody reactions occurring on the RBC surface.[27] The most common reason for this is the fact that two antigens cannot be sufficiently approximated (to within about 24 nm) to allow antibody molecules affixed to them to bind C1q. In some circumstances, a sparsity of antigenic sites may diminish the chances of two antigens getting together. The usual cause, however, is an inability of the antigen-bearing molecules to move laterally in the membrane. Even sparse antigenic molecules that are able to "patch" or aggregate within the membrane on reaction with antibody are able to fix complement. But if the molecule bearing the antigenic epitope is affixed to the underlying membrane skeleton and thus unable to move laterally in the plane of the membrane, and if the interval at which the molecules are affixed is greater than 24 nm, complement is not fixed, since two C1q-fixing sites cannot be approximated.

Results of Complement Fixation. The activation and control of the complement sequence is complex and involves at least 16 different proteins. The portions that are pertinent to the present discussion are outlined in Figure 55-3.

The fixation of complement by antibody leads to the destruction of the RBC by two major mechanisms. First, the completion of the complement sequence on the surface of the RBC results in the production of a lesion by the terminal components C5 through C9 that breach the lipid bilayer and result in the hemolysis of the cell[28] (Fig. 55-4). Although a single completed lesion is sufficient for the lysis of the cell, the production of a single effective lesion on the normal human RBC by human complement requires a massive activation of complement by antibody, since both the RBC and the serum are endowed with factors that are able to reduce the activation and effectiveness of complement in lysing the cell. Because such massive activation of complement rarely occurs in clinical settings, direct lysis by complement is rarely a major outcome.[29]

In the second mechanism, certain components of complement (C3b and C4b) that are covalently fixed to the membrane of the target cell are able to interact with specific receptors on destructive cells of the immune system, resulting in immune adherence.[30] These receptors are of at least four types, each slightly different in the form of the components to which it binds (Fig. 55-5 and Table 55-1). The immune adherence that results from this binding is frequently not effective in initiating phagocytosis but assists greatly in the destruction of cells to which IgG also is fixed. The effectiveness of this immune adherence is further decreased by degradation of the complement component by specific enzymes, which may release the component from the receptor.[31] For example, the degradation of C3b to iC3b by factor I markedly decreases the adherence to CR1 receptors, and the degradation of iC3b to C3dg by factor I or other serine proteases markedly reduces the adherence to CR3 and CR4 receptors.

Fixation to Antibody-Specific Receptors

There is a second functional attribute of the antibody molecule that mediates destruction of the target cell to which the antibody is affixed—a portion that is able to fix to specific receptors on effector cells reacting with immunoglob-

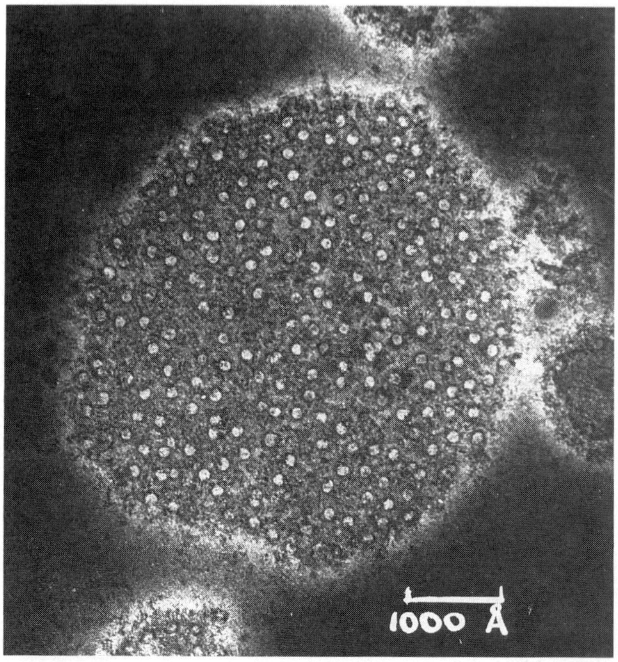

FIGURE 55-4. Electron micrograph of the lesions that appear on the completion of the membrane attack complex of complement. The dark lesions are hydrophilic complexes of protein about 10 nm in diameter in this negatively stained preparation.

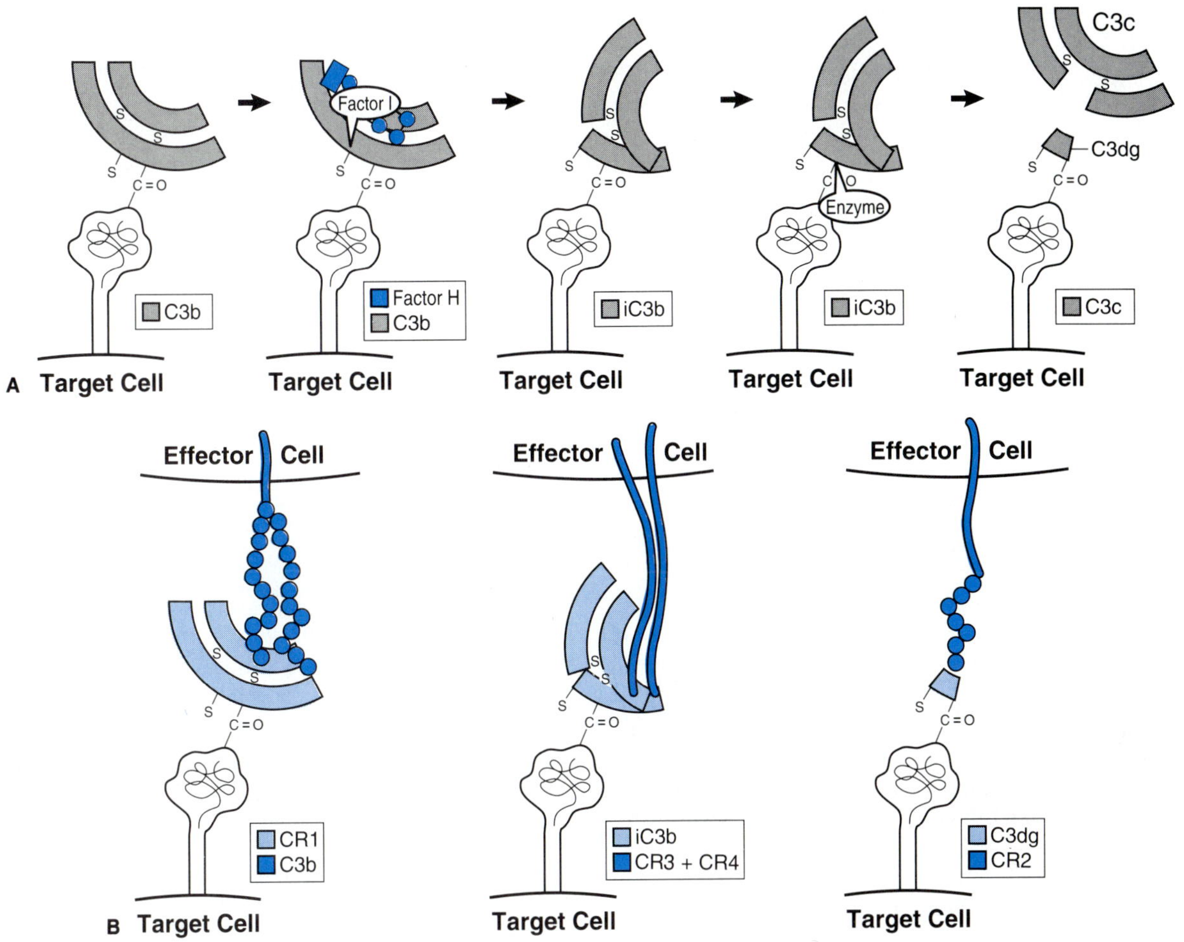

FIGURE 55-5. Degradation of C3b and reaction of the products with specific receptors. (**A**) C3b is cleaved by factor I, which is held in place by factor H, resulting in iC3b; this product is cleaved by a proteolytic enzyme, releasing C3c and leaving C3dg attached to the cell. (**B**) CR1 (a member of the complement regulatory family) reacts preferentially with C3b; CR3 and CR4 (members of the integrin family of proteins) react preferentially with iC3b; CR2 reacts with C3dg.

ulin.[32,33] Such a functional area is present in the Fc portion of IgG and IgA molecules, but it is not present on IgM molecules. Like the C1q-binding area, it may be located within range of the F(ab) arms of the molecule that may impede the binding of IgG_2 and IgG_4 to some of the receptors.

The receptors able to bind to this portion of the immunoglobulin molecule are called Fc receptors. Those reacting with IgG (Fc_γ receptors) are of three distinct molecular types designated I, II, and III, respectively (Table 55-2). These differ in affinity for the Fc portion of the molecule; those with less affinity (II and III) do not bind IgG_2 and IgG_4 well. Specific receptors apparently exist for IgA as well, but they are not well characterized.[34,35]

The effect of immune adherence mediated by Fc receptors is striking. If the effector cell is phagocytic, the cell membrane is stimulated to move in the direction of the attached IgG-coated target.[36] If the membrane of the effector cell is able to engulf the target, it is entirely phagocytosed. If the membrane can engulf only a portion of the target RBC, the cell remnant that is not engulfed becomes spherocytic.

Thus, immune adherence due to the immunoglobulin–Fc-receptor interaction is much more destructive to the RBC than immune adherence due to the C3b (or C4b) and its receptor.[37] The two immune-adherence reactions appear to act in concert. The IgG–Fc receptor reactions are frequently of low affinity, and a number of interactions must accumulate to attain sufficient binding to initiate effective destruction of the cell; therefore, this immune-adherence reaction and its consequences appear to be slow. Reactions

TABLE 55-1. The Biochemistry and Function of Receptors Reacting With Complement Components

Name	Cells	Structure	Ligand
CR1	Erythrocytes, macrophages, monocytes, PMNs, some lymphocytes	Multiple tandem repeats; 205–250 kd	C3b > iC3b
CR2	Lymphocytes	Tandem repeats; 140 kd	C3d
CR3	Macrophages, monocytes, PMNs, some lymphocytes	Integrin family; α = 180 kd; β = 95 kd	iC3b > C3b
CR4	Macrophages	Integrin family; α = 150 kd; β = 95 kd	iC3b (induces phagocytosis)

TABLE 55-2. Summary of the Characteristics of the Fc_{γ} Receptors of Human Cells

Characteristic	FcRI	FcRII	FcRIII
Molecular weight	72 kd	40 kd	50–70 kd
Affinity for IgG monomer	$K_a = 10^8–10^9\ M^{-1}$	Undetectable	Undetectable
Specificity for IgG subclass	1 = 3 > 4; 2 = none	1 = 3 > 2 = 4	3 = 1; 2 and 4 = little or none
Cells			
Monocytes	+	+	−
Macrophages	+	+	+
Neutrophils	−	+	+
Eosinophils	−	+	+
Platelets	−	+	−
Lymphocytes			
B cells	−	+	−
T cells			+
Natural killer cells			+

FcRI, Fc receptor I; FcRII, Fc receptor II; FcRIII, Fc receptor III.

of complement components with their receptors have a higher affinity and do not appear to require accumulated interactions to accomplish effective immune adherence; immune adherence is thus more rapid when mediated by these receptors. When both complement and Fc receptors are present on effector cells, and their ligands are both present on the target RBCs, the reactions of complement and its receptors may rapidly bind the target cells to the effector cells and allow the slower accumulation of effective IgG–Fc receptor interactions to occur.

Methods for Detection of Antibody

Diagnosis of AIHA depends on demonstration of an antibody that is able to interact with the cells of the patient. A number of techniques are available for detecting the antibody on RBCs, in the serum, or both. The fundamental problem of antibody detection is discerning the interaction or the results of an interaction between an immunoglobulin molecule and the cell. The problem is complicated by the characteristics of each.

Agglutination. The simplest reaction that permits detection of the interaction of antibody and erythrocytes is the agglutination reaction: one antigen-binding site on the antibody molecule binds to an antigen on one cell and another antigen-binding site binds to an antigen on another cell. When this occurs multiply, a lattice of cells is formed and agglutination occurs.[38]

For this reaction to occur, the antibody molecule must bridge the charge-related repulsive forces that are associated with the membrane when cells are suspended in saline.[39] These forces maintain cells at a distance of about 24 nm. This distance is easily bridged by IgM molecules, since they possess antigen-binding sites on each of the five monomers (Fig. 55-6*A*), but IgG molecules are too small to do so by a single molecule (see Fig. 55-6*B*) and can bridge the gap only under special circumstances.

To detect IgG molecules by simple agglutination, the distance between the cells must be reduced. This can be done physically by centrifugation, but the forces required are greater than is practical. The addition of anisotropic molecules (eg, albumin, synthetic polymers, or strongly anionic molecules)[40,41] to the medium disperses the ionic cloud and allows approximation of the cells so that a single IgG molecule can affix its antigen-binding sites on different cells (see Fig. 55-6C).

Binding Ligand to Antibody Molecule. The reaction of an antibody with a cell can be detected indirectly by the use of ligands that bind to the antibody molecule. The best known and most useful of these is an antibody to the immunoglobulin molecule, but other ligands—particularly a protein derived from certain strains of *Staphylococcus aureus*, called staphylococcal protein A—that bind to IgG molecules may be used.[42]

Reactions with antiimmunoglobulins made to human serum in rabbits were first used by Coombs in a reaction wherein the endpoint was agglutination of the RBCs.[11] This was possible because one antigen-binding site of the anti-IgG molecule is able to bind to antibody affixed to one cell, and the other antigen-binding site is able to bind to an antibody molecule on another cell. In this way, the distance imposed by mutual repulsion is bridged (see Fig. 55-6*D*). This test has been refined by the use of specific antiimmunoprotein species that allow precise identification of the immunoproteins on the cell surface.[43]

The RBCs must be thoroughly washed to free them of nonspecifically adherent IgG when performing tests using antiglobulins. This is a disadvantage, because this procedure also may remove specifically bound antibody that reacts with low affinity; it may even remove the antigen necessary for antibody binding.

Although useful, the agglutination antiglobulin test is relatively insensitive and difficult to quantitate; the minimum number of molecules that can be detected in the routine test is probably 250 to 500.[44] More-sensitive methods using monoclonal antiglobulin antibodies derived from mouse–human hybridomas have been devised that measure more accurately the amount of antibody on the cells.[45–47] These methods involve labeling the monoclonal antiimmunoglobulin molecule with a radioactive molecule (eg, ^{125}I),[46] an enzyme,[48] or a fluorescent probe.[49] The amount of immunoglobulin affixed is determined by the amount of label affixed when the labeled antiimmunoglobulin molecule is reacted. These techniques detect smaller amounts of affixed antibody (50 to 200 molecules) than the antiglobulin agglutination techniques.

Complement Activation. Complement-fixing antibody in the serum can sometimes be detected by its ability to lyse RBCs by penetration of the lipid bilayer by the membrane attack complex (C5b-9).[50] It is difficult to achieve lysis of human RBCs by human complement, however, because the presence of membrane-bound molecules inhibits the functional activity of homologous complement. Thus, successful completion of the sequence resulting in cell lysis can only occur when complement is massively activated. This usually occurs only when antigen and antibody are

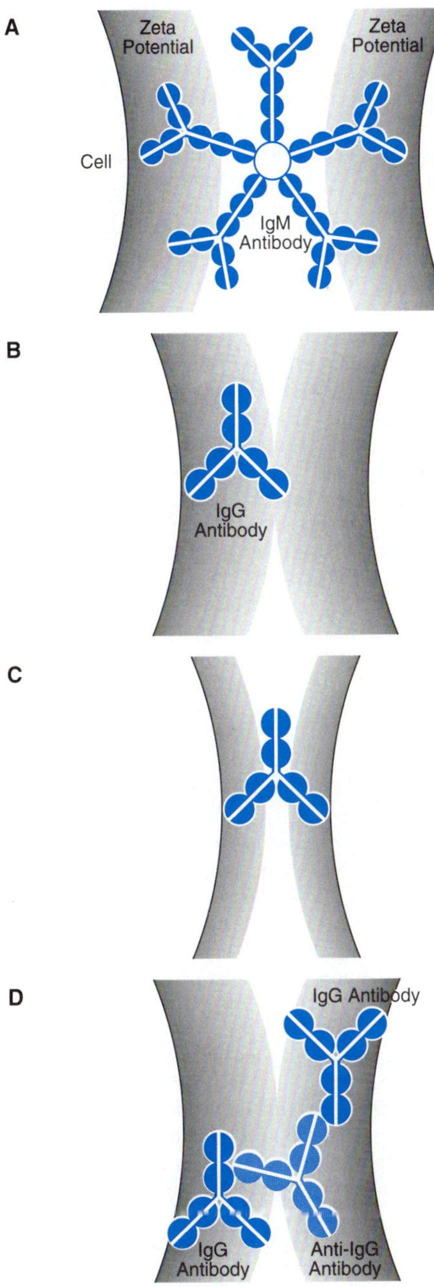

FIGURE 55-6. The conditions that lead to agglutination. (**A**) The large IgM molecule can bridge the repulsive forces of the zeta potential. The smaller IgG molecule cannot bridge (**B**) unless the distance imposed by the zeta potential is reduced (**C**). (**D**) An anti-IgG molecule can bind two bound IgG molecules and bring about agglutination.

both plentiful. For these reasons, tests using hemolysis as an endpoint are insensitive and are more often used to assess the lytic ability of the antibody rather than merely to detect its presence.

The fixation of complement can be detected with greater sensitivity; components C4 and C3 are covalently bound to the membrane during complement activation and may be detected on cells that are attacked by complement but have not lysed. Even when these components are degraded they may be detected on the cell surface by specific antibodies (eg, anti-C3dg and anti-C4d) in both agglutination and ligand-binding assays.[45,47] This testing is of particular importance; if the antibody or the antigen is not stably bound to the membrane, it may provide the only evidence that an immune reaction has occurred on the cell surface.

Detection Tests for Diagnosis of Autoimmune Hemolytic Anemia

Tests on Patient Erythrocytes

The tests outlined may be used in a number of ways to detect antibody in the serum or its effects on cells in the diagnosis of AIHA. The most useful is the detection of antibody, complement, or both on the RBCs of the patient by antibodies to them; in its most commonly used form, it is called the direct antiglobulin test (DAT) or Coombs' test.

Direct Antiglobulin Test. In performing the DAT, the patient's erythrocytes are washed in saline to remove nonspecifically adherent IgG; the washed cells are then incubated with specific antiglobulin antisera. Usually, only anti-IgG (to detect IgG antibodies) and anti-C3d (to detect the presence of complement components) are used in separate reactions. In special tests, other antisera (eg, anti-IgM, anti-IgA) can be used additionally in separate tests. After incubation to allow the antiglobulin molecules to bind, the mixture is gently centrifuged and the cells observed for agglutination. Agglutination indicates that the immunoglobulin or complement component reacting with the antiglobulin is attached to the cell surface.

The amount of antibody or complement may be accurately measured using a monoclonal antibody that is labeled in some way. In this case, the cells are washed thoroughly and incubated with the labeled antibody. The excess antibody is removed either by washing or by sedimenting the cells through immiscible oil by centrifugation. The amount of label fixed to the cells is determined and compared to that fixed to normal RBCs. This technique is useful in detecting small amounts of antibody that are not detectable by the agglutination assay, and in following quantitatively the response of a patient to therapy.

Using anti-IgG and anti-C3dg, four patterns of reaction may be found, depending on whether complement is fixed and whether antibody is detectable (Table 55-3). These are interpreted as follows:

Type 1—antibody alone is fixed. This occurs when the antibody is IgG but is not able to fix complement. The usual reason for this inability is the spacing of the antigens on the cell surface.

Type 2—antibody and complement are fixed. This occurs when the antibody is IgG and the antigen sites are placed so that complement can be fixed. Such antigens

TABLE 55-3. Patterns of Reactions of the Direct Antiglobulin Tests Seen With Specific Antiglobulin Reagents in Patients With Warm Antibody Autoimmune Hemolytic Anemia

Pattern	Reaction With Antiglobulin: Anti-IgG	Anti-C3d	Percentage
I	+	−	35
II	+	+	56
III	−	+	9
IV	−	−	<1

(Data from Issitt PD. Serological diagnosis and characterization of the causative antibodies. In: Chaplin H Jr, ed. Methods in hematology: immune hemolytic anemias. New York, Churchill Livingstone, 1985.)

are either plentiful or are mobile in the plane of the membrane.

Type 3—complement alone is found. When complement components are present but IgG is not, it may be due to one of the following:

The antibody may be IgM or IgA; this can be determined by using specific anti-IgM and anti-IgA in the testing procedure.

The antibody may be IgG, but it is not firmly attached to the antigen and is removed during the washing of the cells. The antibody may be cold reacting (eg, Donath-Landsteiner antibodies) or may be of very low affinity; this can be assessed in tests of patient serum (see later discussion).

The antigen may not be firmly attached to the RBC, causing antigen and antibody to be washed off during cell preparation. This commonly occurs in drug-induced and immune-complex-induced hemolytic anemia.

Type 4—neither IgG nor complement is fixed. If antibody is not IgG, is of low affinity, and is cold reactive, or if it is affixed to an antigen that is not fixed to the membrane *and* complement is not fixed, there may not be evidence that the immune reaction occurred. This occurs in less than 1 in 50 cases.

Tests of Antibody in Serum

Agglutination. The simplest technique for the detection of antibody in patient serum to RBC antigens is direct agglutination, since it involves only the mixing of cells and serum to observe if the cells are agglutinated. It is most useful for the detection of IgM antibodies, which usually are cold reacting and present in the serum in high concentration. The relative concentration of antibody can be estimated by diluting the serum and determining the minimal concentration (usually expressed as the dilution) that effects agglutination. The effect of temperature on agglutination can be easily assessed; the highest temperature at which agglutination can be detected is called the thermal amplitude or thermal maximum. Finally, by using various kinds of cells, the specificity of the antibody can be determined. All of these procedures are important in the characterization of the antibodies in cold agglutinin disease (see later discussion).

The IgG antibodies of warm agglutinin disease are rarely detectable by direct agglutination. Other means—particularly the indirect antiglobulin test (IAT)—usually are sought if such demonstration is needed.

Tests Using Lysis by Complement. Some antibodies in patient serum can be detected and quantitated by their ability to promote complement-mediated lysis. These tests usually are performed by incubating RBCs, patient serum, and normal serum as a source of complement under appropriate temperature conditions. At the end of the reaction, the unlysed cells are sedimented by centrifugation, and the amount of hemoglobin released into the supernatant fluid is assessed.

As noted, such tests for antibody usually are insensitive, since a large amount of complement-fixing antibody is needed to activate sufficient complement to result in the lysis of normal RBCs. The sensitivity of the test can be markedly increased by using the RBCs of patients with paroxysmal nocturnal hemoglobinuria; these cells are characterized by an unusual sensitivity to complement and are lysed by much less antibody. If such cells are not available, normal RBCs can be rendered more sensitive to complement by treatment with aminoethylisothiuonium bromide.[51]

Many of the antibodies for which hemolytic tests are useful are cold reacting and, often, more lysis is obtained if the test is performed in two stages at different temperatures. In the first stage, the RBCs, patient serum, and a source of complement are incubated at a reduced temperature that allows the antibody to bind to the cell but does not promote the activation of complement. The temperature is then raised to 37°C to permit complement activation and lysis of the cells. This test is especially useful in the diagnosis of the IgG cold-reacting antibodies of paroxysmal cold hemoglobinuria (Donath-Landsteiner [D-L] antibody). It is less useful in the demonstration of IgM cold agglutinins because, during the cold phase, the antibody causes too much agglutination, which inhibits the binding of C1.[52] Lysis by these antibodies can sometimes best be demonstrated by incubating RBCs, serum, and complement at an intermediate temperature (eg, 27°C); this is sometimes called a monophasic hemolytic reaction.

Indirect Antiglobulin Test. IgG antibodies in the serum are best detected by the IAT. Normal RBCs in a dilute suspension are incubated for 15 to 30 minutes with the test serum and then washed thoroughly with saline to remove the serum and nonspecifically adherent IgG. Antiglobulin serum or monoclonal antibody against specific immunoproteins (eg, anti-IgG, anti-C3, anti-C4) is then added to the sensitized cells, and the mixture is incubated again. The cells are then centrifuged, and the presence of agglutination is determined. If the cells are agglutinated, they must have acquired antibody, complement, or both from the patient's serum.

A rough estimate of the concentration of antibody in patient serum can be obtained by determining the dilution of serum just sufficient to give a positive reaction. However, the IAT (like the DAT) can be better quantitated using labeled monoclonal antiglobulin antibodies and RBCs from normal donors. After incubation with patient serum, the cells are washed thoroughly and incubated with the labeled monoclonal antibody. The cells are further incubated and washed or sedimented through oil, and the amount of label affixed is determined. This amount is compared to that found on the same normal cells following incubation with normal serum in the first step. Such quantitation is useful in detecting extremely small amounts of affixed antibodies and in following the response to therapy.

The IAT is useful in determining the specificity of the antibody in patient serum. The serum is reacted with a panel of RBCs in which antigenic composition is known; these are selected so that some bear and some lack most of the common antigens of the erythrocyte. After incubation, washing, and reaction with the specific anti-IgG antiserum, some cells may be agglutinated and some may not; this pattern of agglutination is compared to the occurrence of antigens on the cells. If there is congruence between the cells that are agglutinated and the presence of a specific antigen on the agglutinated cells, the specificity of the antibody is determined. Often, the serum of the patient with AIHA reacts with all the cells in the panel; in this case, rare cells lacking antigens that are common in the population (eg, Rh_{null} cells) may be used to try to determine the specificity of the antibody.

The IAT is particularly useful in the detection of drug-related antibodies. In such testing, patient serum is reacted with normal cells with and without the addition of the suspected drug; usually, a source of complement must be included. After incubation, the cells are washed and incubated with anti-IgG and anti-C3, and then centrifuged and observed for agglutination. If the cells incubated with the drug are agglutinated and those not incubated with the drug are not, the assumption is made that antibodies are present in the patient serum that react with the drug in the presence of the cells.

The IAT may be used to detect IgG antibodies of low affinity in patient serum. The affinity of some antibodies can be increased by altering the charge on the RBC by enzymatic digestion or by altering the conditions in which the reaction takes place (eg, reduction in ionic strength or changes in pH). When these altered conditions are used, great care must be taken to be certain that the test has not been rendered so sensitive that the small amount of IgG that is normally adsorbed to the test cells is detected.

The IAT can be used to determine the thermal maximum of the antibody by varying the temperature at which the serum and RBCs are incubated; this is seldom a consideration in the detection or description of autoimmune IgG antibodies, except for those of paroxysmal cold hemoglobinuria. These D-L antibodies may be detected by performing the IAT at 4°C in all the steps. The D-L antibodies fix IgG at 4°C but not at 37°C.

CLINICAL SYNDROMES

The clinical syndromes of AIHA are largely determined by the nature of the antibodies that characterize them, and the two most important attributes of the antibody molecules are isotype and temperature of reaction. Thus, four distinct syndromes can be described:

- The antibody is IgG and warm reacting
- The antibody is IgM and warm reacting
- The antibody is IgM and cold reacting
- The antibody is IgG and cold reacting

Rarely, IgA antibodies are involved, but the clinical syndrome that they cause is little different from that of the IgG or IgM antibodies. When drugs are the cause of immune hemolytic anemia, the clinical syndrome is sufficiently different to merit separate consideration.

Autoimmune Hemolytic Anemia Due to IgG Warm-Reacting Antibody

Clinical Syndrome

Autoimmune hemolytic anemia caused by an IgG warm-reacting antibody can occur at almost any age but is most common in childhood and in young adulthood (ages 25 to 35). Among adults, it is more common in women than men. The clinical syndrome is variable,[53–55] in part depending on age, underlying diseases, and severity.

In children, the onset of anemia may be rapid and profound[56]; not infrequently, hemoglobinuria is present because of the rapidity of the RBC destruction. One third to one half of the patients have histories of a preceding viral infection. Many viruses have been implicated, including those causing exanthems,[57] Epstein-Barr virus (EBV) infection, and cytomegalovirus infection.[58] In these patients, the illness tends to be self-limited, and all evidence of autoantibody production usually disappears within 2 to 4 months.

In the other pediatric patients, the syndrome is not much different than that seen in adults in that it tends to be chronic or relapsing.[56] Many of these patients manifest other evidence of immunologic malfunction, often recognizable as due to an inherited condition.

In adults, the onset of anemia is most frequently moderately rapid, and the patient becomes symptomatic with fatigue and weakness early in the course of the disease. The degree of anemia usually is significant and, in some cases, the oxygen-carrying capacity of the blood may be decreased to dangerous and even fatal levels. There is seldom a history of hemoglobinuria. In elderly patients, particularly those with underlying heart disease, angina pectoris and congestive heart failure may be caused by the strain imposed by the decreased hemoglobin. When the anemia is too severe and not relieved by treatment, cerebral hypoxia leads to coma and death. More than half of patients with this disorder died when no effective treatment was available.

In other patients, the degree of anemia is less severe and the onset of symptoms less abrupt. These patients can sometimes be followed without treatment.

Unless the syndrome is secondary to some other defined illness, the history usually is not helpful. There may be a history of a viral illness 2 to 3 weeks previously; this history is much more common in children and adolescents. Autoimmune hemolytic anemia is much more likely to occur in a patient who has a history, however remote, of AIHA or idiopathic thrombocytopenic purpura. The occurrence of AIHA and autoimmune thrombocytopenia (Evans-Duane syndrome[59]) in the same patient is not unusual. It is estimated that over 30% of patients with AIHA due to IgG antibodies also have IgG antibodies against platelets. These are separable antibodies; those reacting with RBCs do not react with platelets, and vice versa.

No matter what age the patient, physical examination shows little abnormality except for pallor of the skin and mucous membranes. The color of the skin and sclerae may be tinged by jaundice, but if abnormalities of liver function are not present, the degree of jaundice usually is not great. In about 60% of patients, the spleen is enlarged so as to be palpable, but it is rarely greatly so. If the enlargement has been rapid, the spleen may be tender and even may have undergone partial infarction, leading to severe pain in the left upper quadrant, a splenic rub, and a painful spleen on palpation. In such a setting, great care should be taken to be certain that the spleen is not ruptured in the course of examination by palpation.

Laboratory Findings

The hemoglobin and hematocrit are diminished variably. The RBC indices are essentially normal except for some elevation of the mean corpuscular volume (MCV) because of the reticulocytosis; uncommonly, agglutination of the cells may falsely increase the MCV.[60]

The reticulocyte count usually is elevated both relatively and absolutely; in severely anemic patients, it may exceed $500 \times 10^6/L$. On occasion, it may be lower than expected for the degree of anemia; this may have several causes. In some instances, it is suggested that the antibody either suppresses erythropoiesis (as demonstrated by a marrow with erythroid hypoplasia) or destroys the reticulocytes and late precursors (in which case the marrow is often hyperplastic). Aplastic crises may occur any time during the course of the disorder; the most severe of these appear to be due to parvovirus infections.[61] The importance of reticulocytopenia is that it often increases greatly the severity of the anemia, and death is common unless great care is taken.[62]

Cells with the appearance of spherocytes (small dark cells) usually are present on the peripheral blood film (Fig. 55-7*A*); when carefully examined by electron microscopy, these cells are often not truly spherocytic but are concavoconvex[63] (see Fig. 55-7*B*).

The white blood cell count may be elevated during acute hemolysis primarily because of an increase in neutrophils, and counts of 30,000/μm are not uncommon.[64] Monocytes that have ingested RBCs may be found in films prepared from peripheral blood; this usually indicates severe hemolysis. This phenomenon can be more readily reproduced by permitting anticoagulated shed blood to stand.

The platelet count usually is normal unless autoimmune

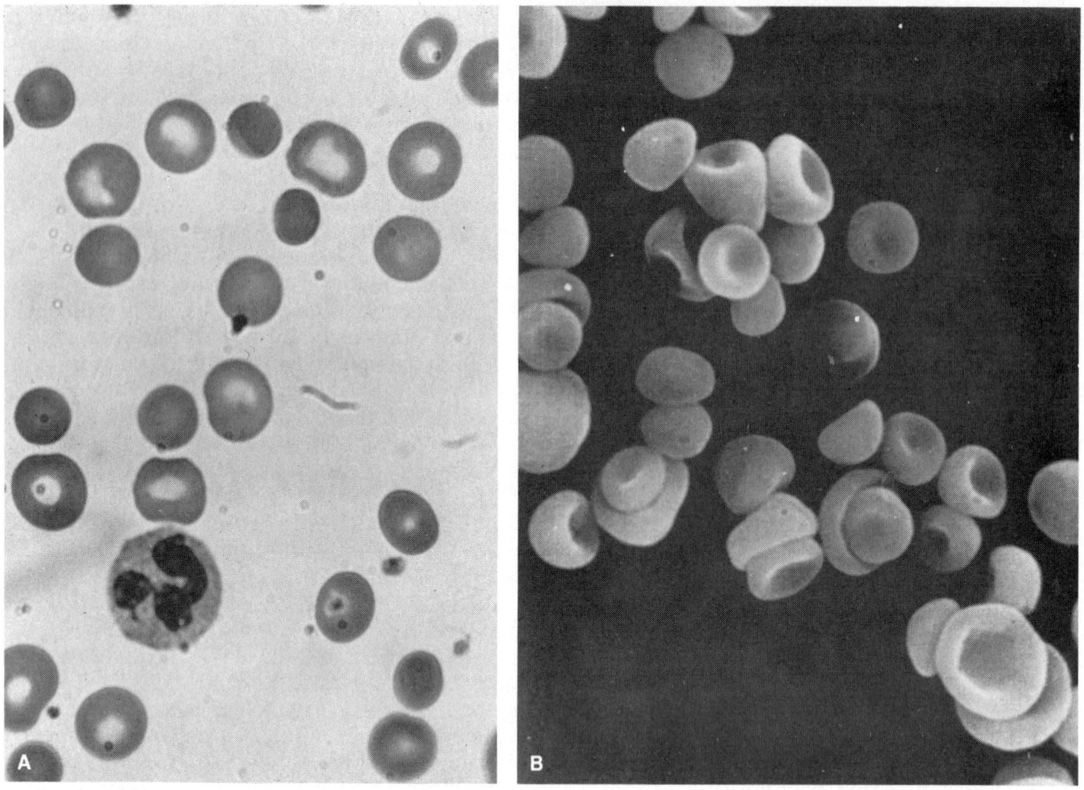

FIGURE 55-7. Spherocytes that appear in hemolytic anemia due to IgG warm-reacting antibodies. (**A**) The appearance on the peripheral film. (**B**) The appearance in scanning electron microscopy.

thrombocytopenia also is present[53]; this occurs in 6% to 13% of patients.[65] Although it is argued that this results in a poorer prognosis,[66] others find this not to be the case.[53] Immune thrombocytopenia may appear at a different time in the patient's life than immune hemolytic anemia.

The bone marrow usually is markedly cellular with a predominance of erythroid precursors. The maturation of the cells usually is normal unless folic acid deficiency is present.[67] A few of the RBC precursors may show dysplastic changes (eg, clefting, "noses," or double nuclei). Rarely, there may be relatively or absolutely decreased numbers of erythrocyte precursors in the marrow.

Diagnostic Tests. In almost all cases of warm-reacting antibody hemolytic anemia due to IgG, the DAT is positive when anti-IgG and anti-C3dg are used as probes in an agglutination assay. Most commonly, both IgG and C3dg are present on the membrane; less commonly, only IgG is present, and uncommonly, IgG is absent but complement is present (see Table 55-3).[68] When complement is not fixed, the antibody often has specificity for the protein or proteins bearing the Rh antigens.

When anti-IgM and anti-IgA antiglobulin antisera are used in the DAT, antibodies of these isotypes may sometimes be identified (Table 55-4). The importance of IgM and IgA warm-reacting antibodies is discussed later.

The DAT can be quantitated by any of several techniques. The simplest is the use of a labeled monoclonal anti-IgG and anti-C3.[46,47] Using these tests, IgG, C3d, or both usually can be detected in small amounts (50 to 200 molecules per cell) on the cells of those patients whose cells do not react with anti-IgG or anti-C3d in the agglutination assay.

Quantitation is useful in following the clinical course of a given patient, since it may show the relative amount of antibody being produced in response to therapy; it is of little value, however, in predicting the rate of hemolysis from patient to patient.[69]

Neither agglutination nor the quantitative DAT measure the amount of antibody on the RBCs in vivo. Cells must be washed during preparation for the DAT, and those antibodies with low affinity are more readily removed in this process than those with a high affinity. Thus, if two patients have antibodies with differing affinity (one low affinity and the other high affinity), the amount of antibody on the cells may be the same in the circulation—perhaps resulting in the same amount of hemolysis—but in the quantitative DAT, much more of the high-affinity antibody remains on the cells after washing than low-affinity antibody.

The IAT is of relatively little value in the diagnosis of AIHA caused by warm-reacting IgG antibody except to distinguish drug-induced immune hemolysis. First, unrelated alloimmune antibodies may be present in patient serum and may be confused with autoantibodies. And second, although the amount of antibody in the serum can be

TABLE 55-4. Incidence of IgG, IgM, and IgA Antibodies in Autoimmune Hemolytic Anemia Due to Warm-Reacting Antibodies

Isotype	Alone (%)	With IgG (%)	With IgM (%)	With IgA (%)	Total* (%)
IgG	72.1	—	4.3	17.2	95.7
IgM	2.1	4.2	—	0	8.4
IgA	4.2	17.2	0	—	23.5

* Two patients had IgG, IgA, and IgM antibodies.
(Courtesy of Petz LD, Garratty G. In: Acquired immune hemolytic anemias. New York, Churchill Livingstone, 1980.)

quantitated, the information is of little value in assessing severity, although it may be used to evaluate response to therapy.

Antibody in the serum or eluted from the RBCs (by heating the cells to 50°C or solubilizing the membrane with organic solvents) may be used to determine its specificity.[70,71] The specificity of the antibody may appear to be for known blood group antigens (eg, anti-e, anti-K) or may be for antigens present on the cells of almost all individuals and only lacking in rare individuals (eg, Rh_{null}, K_o). (Rare cells such as these usually are available at regional transfusion centers such as the American Red Cross, the New York Blood Center, or the Blood Center of Southeastern Wisconsin in Milwaukee.) In the first case, the specificity may be only relative, since in many cases, reaction can be demonstrated by careful techniques with cells lacking the ascribed antigen. For example, many autoimmune anti-e antibodies react with cells of the EE phenotype, even though they react more strongly with cells bearing the e antigen. Such antibodies are called mimicking antibodies.[72]

Many antibodies appear to react with the proteins bearing the Rh antigens. They are classified further by their reactions with cells of rare phenotype (eg, Rh_{null} and D____/D____)[50,73,74]; these cells are available at reference centers specializing in these tests. Some antibodies react with cells bearing the usual allomorphic Rh antigens but do not react with cells partially (D____/D____) or completely (Rh_{null}) missing these antigens. These antibodies presumably react with some nonpolymorphic part of the molecule or molecules bearing the allomorphic Cc and Ee antigens. Other antibodies react with normal cells and partially deleted cells but not with completely deleted cells. The antigen is presumably on some different part of the Rh molecule or molecules than the allomorphic antigens.

Many of the antibodies that do not react with the Rh proteins appear to react with glycophorin molecules, since these antibodies do not bind to cells lacking part or all of these moieties (eg, $En^a(-)$, M^k/M^k cells).[75,76] Using specific enzymes, portions of the glycophorin A molecule may be removed from normal cells, and specificity of autoantibodies for different parts of the molecule may be demonstrated. Many of these antibodies react with the $Wright^b$ (Wr^b) antigen,[77] known to be engendered by a complex of glycophorin A and protein 3 (band 3, AE1).[78] In general, antibodies with these specificities fix complement, since the protein molecules are present in such large numbers that the doublet necessary for C1q fixation is readily generated.

Pathophysiology

The destruction of RBCs by these antibodies is brought about primarily by mechanisms that depend on immune adherence. The IgG molecules are able to adhere to the abundant Fcγ receptors (of which there are at least three kinds),[32] and the adherence is a powerful stimulus to phagocytosis. This adherence is abetted by the simultaneous presence of complement components (C3b and C4b).[79]

The destruction of the cells by the direct lytic action of complement plays a lesser role in the destruction of the RBCs by IgG antibodies in AIHA. Because of the requirement for two molecules of antibody to initiate the reaction, and because of the defense mechanisms of the cells in down-regulating complement, it is uncommon in adults that sufficient activation of complement occurs to result in the completion of a sufficient number of sequences to cause a breaching of the membrane and thus intravascular lysis. In children, in whom the hemolysis tends to be more brisk, hemoglobinuria is more frequent.

The spleen is a primary site of destruction, particularly if complement is not fixed.[80] It is here that the IgG-coated cells are in most intimate contact with the Fc receptor–bearing cells, and the circulation is sufficiently slow that the reaction can occur. Further, partial phagocytosis results in the formation of spherocytes[81] that are less capable of deformation than biconcave discs[82]; they are readily trapped in the cords of Billroth among the phagocytic cells behind the filtering barrier in the spleen, the wall of the splenic sinus[83] (Fig. 55-8). For these reasons, splenectomy is often useful in treatment.

If the amount of antibody affixed to the cell is sufficiently great or if complement if fixed as well, adherence-dependent hemolysis may occur readily in other parts of the reticuloendothelial system. In this case, splenectomy is less effective therapeutically.

The complex relations among the various hemolytic mechanisms are shown in Figure 55-9.

Etiology

Since Ehrlich recognized that the normal immune system did not make antibodies against antigens of self[84] (horror autotoxicus), it has been difficult to understand why this happens in autoimmune diseases. There is little real evidence that explains the phenomenon, but a number of interesting hypotheses are proposed.

When an immune reaction occurs to a foreign antigen, a range of antibodies are first made that vary in their reactivity with the inciting antigen. Those that better fit the antigen are more specific and have a higher affinity; those that fit the antigen less well are less specific (ie, react with different but related structures) and have a lower affinity. Antibodies of the less specific sort may react with self-antigens. In the well-regulated immune system, the clones producing the less-specific antibodies are rapidly suppressed, leaving only the clones producing high-affinity, specific heteroantibodies; this regulation appears to be under the control of antigen-specific suppressor T cells. In the poorly regulated immune system, the production of less-specific antibodies may not be suppressed; if these antibodies cross-react with self-antigens, evidence of autoimmunity is found.

Another theory suggests that autoimmune antibodies arise when mechanisms for the suppression of antibodies against self fail.[85,86] It is known that the immune system makes nonpathogenic antibodies against self-antigens, and that the level of production is normally closely maintained by inhibitory influences—possibly antiidiotype antibodies, possibly specifically programmed suppressor T cells. Autoimmune disease results when such suppression fails and pathogenetic amounts and isotypes of self-reacting antibodies are produced.

The first theory may explain why autoimmune syndromes sometimes follow specific heteroimmune reactions. Such syndromes are frequently seen in childhood, since viral infections are not infrequently followed in 2 to 3 weeks by a bout of AIHA or immune thrombocytopenic purpura. The production of autoantibodies lasts about 3 to 6 weeks but eventually ceases, presumably as the immune system finally regulates itself. It has been suggested but not proven that such patients are more prone to AIHA in later life.

Either theory may account for the AIHA that results from alloimmune reactions. Certain patients, particularly those prone to make alloantibodies, who receive antigenically incompatible transfusions make, in addition to the expected alloantibodies, autoantibodies that are then able to react with their own RBCs.[87] The DAT on the patient's own RBCs is positive (usually only with anti-IgG, since these auto-

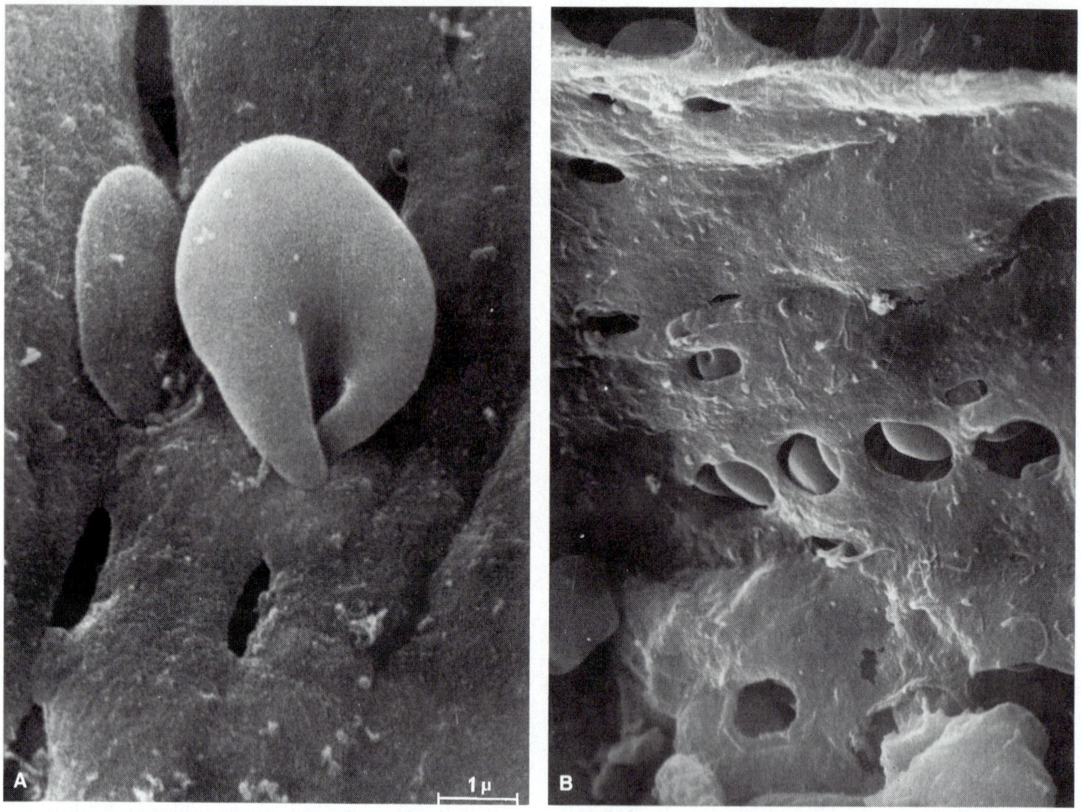

FIGURE 55-8. The wall of the splenic venous sinus as seen in scanning electron microscopy. (**A**) Normal cells can, by deforming, pass the small elliptical apertures to regain the circulation. (**B**) Spherocytes, because they cannot deform, cannot pass the barrier, and are maintained in the cords of Billroth.

antibodies are frequently directed against the nonpolymorphic portions of the Rh proteins) and may be difficult to detect in the presence of alloantibodies reacting with the transfused cells. The amount of hemolysis may be significant, but the production of antibody usually is of short duration, lasting no more than 2 to 3 months. The reaction appears to occur in patients with poorly tuned immune systems that are not able to distinguish self-antigens (since even the alloantigens are not very different from self-antigens) and suppress production of antibodies to them.

Autoimmune hemolytic anemia due to IgG antibody is seen with increased frequency in patients with viral diseases that affect the immune system, particularly human immunodeficiency virus I (HIV-I) infection,[88] infectious mononucleosis,[89] and cytomegalovirus infection.[90] Presumably, the production of antibodies reacting with self-antigens is due to abnormalities of regulation that are induced in the immune cells by the infection.

Association With Other Autoimmune Diseases. Not infrequently, AIHA with warm-reacting IgG antibodies is associated with other evidence of immune dysfunction or other diseases of immune dysfunction (Table 55-5). This is sometimes as minor as alterations in the concentration of immunoglobulins, particularly IgA.[91] In other instances, the abnormalities form a clinical syndrome, such as systemic lupus erythematosus,[92] rheumatoid arthritis[93] or other connective tissue diseases[94–96]; this form of hemolytic anemia is not infrequent in patients with those diseases and, in fact, may precede all other symptoms of the primary disease.

Similarly, patients with congenital disorders of the immune system such as Wiskott-Aldrich syndrome, congenital

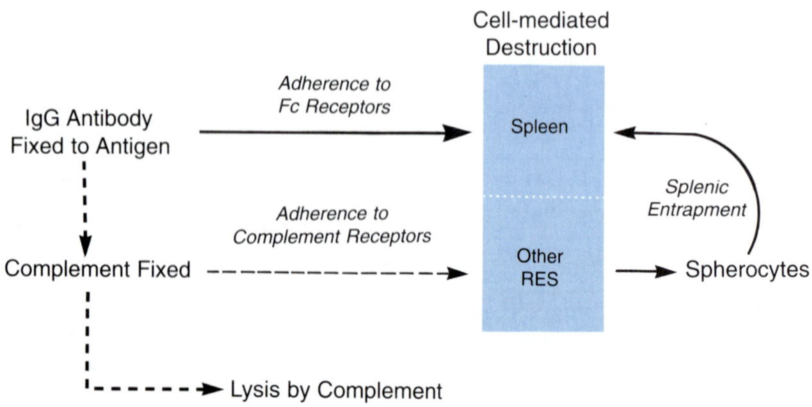

FIGURE 55-9. Mechanisms of lysis in hemolytic anemia due to IgG antibodies.

TABLE 55-5. Diseases in Which Autoimmune Hemolytic Anemia Due to IgG Antibody May Be Seen

INFECTIONS
Postviral autoimmune hemolytic anemia of childhood
Infectious mononucleosis
HIV-1 infection
IMMUNE DEFICIENCY STATES
Hypogammaglobulinemia
Wiskott–Aldrich syndrome
Dysgammaglobulinemia
NEOPLASMS OF THE IMMUNE SYSTEM
Lymphocytic disorders
Chronic lymphocytic leukemia
Non-Hodgkin's lymphoma
Hodgkin's disease
Plasma cell disorders
Waldenstrom's macroglobulinemia
Multiple myeloma
DISEASES OF IMMUNE DYSFUNCTION
Systemic lupus erythematosus
Scleroderma
Rheumatoid arthritis
Sjögren's syndrome
Immune thrombocytopenia (Evans' syndrome)
MISCELLANEOUS DISEASES
Pernicious anemia
Thyroiditis
Ulcerative colitis
Ovarian tumors and cysts
Other tumors

dysgammaglobulinemias, and common variable immunodeficiency may have AIHA due to IgG antibodies.[97–100] The anemia may develop as early as the first year of life and usually is chronic and persistent. It presumably results from the abnormalities of regulation that characterize the primary disease.

Finally, patients with neoplasms of the immune system may have this form of hemolytic anemia. About 20% of patients with chronic lymphocytic leukemia or well-differentiated lymphocytic lymphoma have a positive DAT some time during the course of the disease, even in some instances preceding the lymphocytosis characteristic of the malignant disease.[101,102] The syndrome is reasonably common in Hodgkin's disease[103,104] and thymoma,[105,106] but is perhaps less common in the less differentiated forms of lymphoma.[107,108] The antibody is the result of the underlying or accompanying dysfunction of the immune system and is not the product of the monoclonal malignant lymphocytes; in all cases, multiple isotypes of both light and heavy chains are found among the antibody molecules.[109]

Treatment

The treatment of AIHA of IgG warm antibody type involves the diminution of the concentration of antibody, the reduction in its effectiveness in mediating the destruction of the cells, or both.

Decreasing Antibody Concentration

The concentration of available antibody can most effectively be reduced by diminishing its production. Ideally, one would like to diminish the production of antibody directed only at specific antigen or antigens so that the treatment would not result in general immunosuppression; this is not possible, but the useful treatments reduce the production of autoantibodies more readily than alloantibodies or heteroantibodies.

Prednisone. One of the effects of prednisone is the suppression of the production of IgG antibodies.[110] This effect results only with high doses of the drug, but once suppression has been achieved, it can often be maintained by much lower doses.[106] The production of IgM is not affected; the effect on IgA production is not clear.

In addition to its effects on production, prednisone given in high doses (1 mg/kg/d) also diminishes rapidly the amount of antibody on the circulating RBCs in about two thirds of cases, thus diminishing hemolysis[69]; the reason for this effect is not known. Further, this dose of prednisone appears to interfere with the function of the destructive cells of the immune system, also diminishing hemolysis.[111]

Cytotoxic Drugs. Antibody production can be reduced by the administration of drugs such as alkylating or antimetabolic agents that are cytotoxic to the antibody-producing cells.[112,113] Again, the effect is nonspecific, but the cells actively producing autoantibody appear to be more susceptible to the effects of these drugs than other cells of the immune system. Because the drugs all diminish the production of cells, overdosage results in suppression of the bone marrow, a particularly unfortunate event when greater than normal production of RBCs is necessary.

Cyclophosphamide (Cytoxan) appears to be effective[114] in the treatment of this type of AIHA, resulting in remission is about 40% of cases. Its use is limited by its toxicity; in addition to its immediate toxicity (marrow suppression, bladder irritation, hair loss), cyclophosphamide is significantly leukemogenic.[115]

Azathioprine also has been used in the treatment of AIHA.[116] It is probably a little less likely to induce remission than cyclophosphamide, but its leukemogenic effect is probably lower. Vincristine also has been used as an immunosuppressive agent[117]; the response is often rapid, but short lasting, and its use is limited by neurotoxicity. This treatment is not so effective in this syndrome as it is in immune thrombocytopenic purpura. Vinca-loaded platelets have been used with modest success.[118]

Other cytotoxic regimens, including the use of cyclosporine and radiation, have been suggested but are considered only in cases of desperation.

Plasmapheresis. A reduction in the level of antibody also can be achieved by removing formed antibody from the plasma by plasmapheresis,[119,120] but this procedure is relatively ineffective with IgG antibodies because these molecules are not confined to the intravascular space. Further, since IgG autoantibodies react with antigen at body temperature, they are adsorbed to the RBCs and not removed when plasma is removed. Nevertheless, with persistent daily aphresis, the antibody level can be reduced in some cases, and this may be useful in the case of acute hyperhemolysis.

Reduction in Destruction of Cells

The other approach to the reduction in hemolysis is to diminish the means by which antibody brings about the destruction of cells. This can be accomplished by reducing the interaction of antibody and antigen, reducing the interaction of the antibody-coated cells with the phagocytic cells of the immune system, or removing the site of destruction. Of these, the last is the most effective.

Splenectomy. In this type of AIHA, the spleen is a major site of destruction of RBCs. The removal of the spleen is beneficial in about 65% to 80% of patients and may be all that is necessary in about 50% of these.[121] Splenectomy in children under 5 years of age should be avoided if possible because of the increased incidence of overwhelming sepsis with gram-positive organisms[122]; this complication is much less common in adults. Splenectomy is less likely to be successful if complement is fixed by the antibody since that permits sequestration in other parts of the reticuloendothelial system, particularly the liver. Unfortunately, isotopic studies (usually with ^{51}Cr) localizing the site of sequestration are generally of little value in predicting the success of the operation.[123]

Down-Regulation of Fc Receptors

Intravenous γ-Globulin. The interaction of the IgG molecule and the Fc receptor (responsible for most of the cellular destruction in this form of AIHA) is reversible, and cell-bound IgG can be displaced from the receptor by fluid-phase IgG if it is present in high enough concentration. To this end, purified human γ-globulin given intravenously in large doses (2 g/kg given over 2 or 5 days)[124] has been used to treat autoimmune disease due to IgG antibody. This has met with considerable success in the treatment of idiopathic thrombocytopenic purpura (ITP)[125,126] and with perhaps less[127,128] success in the treatment of AIHA. The effect is transient and the drug is expensive, but it can be used when acute cessation of hemolysis is needed.

Prednisone. One of the effects of prednisone appears to be a down-regulation of the Fc receptors.[112] This effect occurs only with high doses of the drug and may account for some of the rapidity of response when these doses are administered.

Danazol. Certain androgenic steroids also down-regulate Fc receptors and one, danazol, has been used in the treatment of immune destruction of blood cells.[129,130] It appears to be more successful in the treatment of ITP than of AIHA.[131]

Antibodies to Fc Receptors. More recently, monoclonal antibodies to Fc receptors have been used to try to down-regulate their function.[132] This therapy is still under investigation.

Transfusion

Transfusion is frequently necessary in AIHA patients, particularly when the rate of hemolysis is great, as evidenced by a falling or very low hematocrit. In patients over 60 years of age, it is particularly important to be prepared for transfusion of the patient, because these patients are prone to complications such as myocardial infarction and cerebral vascular accident. In general, when a patient is first seen, blood should be made ready for transfusion without waiting for the physiologic consequences of hypoxia to become evident.

Compatibility testing for transfusion of these patients is complicated by the fact that the cells being transfused are nearly always incompatible due to the presence in the serum of autoantibodies. Such antibodies usually do not hemolyze transfused cells at a greater rate than autologous cells. Thus, the transfusion may not be as effective as is normally the case, but it does not cause a massive hemolytic reaction provided alloantibodies are not present.

The detection of alloantibodies is made difficult by the presence of the autoantibody, which must be removed from the serum before one can be sure that no alloantibodies are present. This is often done by repeated adsorption with the patient's own cells that have been heated to 50°C or treated chemically to remove the autoantibody.[133] If this is done thoroughly, any antibody remaining is likely to be an alloantibody that can be identified so that cells lacking its antigen can be found.

These tests are time-consuming, but they should not delay the delivery of a transfusion to the patient in emergent need of blood. In an emergency, type-specific or even O Rh-negative blood may be used. *The patient should not die because of serologic niceties.*

Treatment of Autoimmune Hemolytic Anemia Due to Warm-Reacting IgG Antibodies

The strategy for treatment of AIHA caused by warm-reacting IgG antibodies is dictated by many factors, including the age of the patient, the severity of the hemolysis, and the presence of other medical conditions. Further, it must be flexible to take into account the response or lack of response of the patient (Fig. 55-10).

For most patients, glucocorticoids such as prednisone usually are the first mode of treatment. Prednisone is started at a dose of 1 to 1.5 mg/kg/d; larger relative doses may be used initially in children (2 to 6 mg/kg/d initially, decreasing to 1 to 2 mg/kg/d within a week or so). Unless the patient has particularly severe hemolysis (hemolysis so great that transfusions must be administered every 1 to 2 days), this can be maintained for up to 3 or 4 weeks, or until a response (demonstrated by a reduction in antibody, improved hemoglobin, and reduced reticulocyte count) is seen. Usually, a response is seen within 2 weeks of the initiation of therapy if the regimen is to be successful by itself[134]; if it is not, other treatment is probably needed.

If a response is obtained, the amount of prednisone pre-

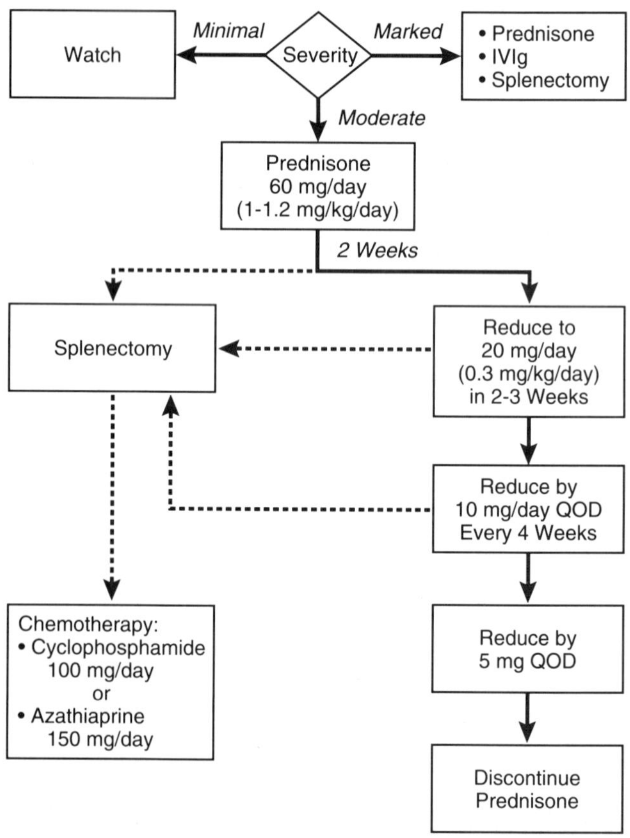

FIGURE 55-10. A schematic diagram for treatment of adult patients with autoimmune hemolytic anemia due to IgG warm-reacting antibodies. Success of the treatment is denoted by a solid arrow to the next step in treatment; lack of success is denoted by an interrupted arrow. Treatment of pediatric patients includes adjustment of the doses of drug for body size (usually relatively larger doses of prednisone) and a greater tendency to avoid therapy, especially splenectomy and chemotherapy.

scribed is reduced, at first fairly rapidly (by 20 mg/d [0.3 mg/kg/d] each week) to a dose of 20 mg/d (0.3 mg/kg/d); this dose is maintained for about one month to determine if the remission continues. The dose is then reduced each month by 10 mg (0.15 mg/kg) on alternate days so that 2 months later, the patient is taking 20 mg (0.3 mg/kg) on alternate days. This dose is then reduced again at monthly intervals until the dose is 10 mg (0.15 mg/kg) on alternate days. If the DAT remains positive, this dose is maintained so long as remission persists.

If, at any point during the course of reduction of dose, exacerbation of hemolysis occurs, the dose is immediately raised to the next level and maintained at that level. If this exceeds a dose tolerable by the patient (certainly no more than 20 mg (0.3 mg/kg) every other day), then other therapy must be contemplated.

Autoimmune Hemolytic Anemia Due to IgM Warm-Reacting Antibodies

IgM autoantibodies are nearly always cold reacting; that is, they do not react with their antigen at body temperature. Rarely, IgM antibodies may react at body temperature, and a particularly severe and difficult syndrome may result.[135,136] The syndrome is like that described for IgG warm-reacting antibodies with some notable exceptions

Often, the amount of hemolysis is great, resulting in severe anemia. In some patients, this may be accompanied by reticulocytopenia, as if the antibody affects the bone marrow. Even in these cases, however, erythroid hyperplasia usually is seen in the bone marrow. Spherocytes are much less prominent or are lacking on the peripheral blood film.

The DAT is negative with anti-IgG and may or may not be positive with anti-C3. Some agglutination may be detected when normal cells are mixed with the serum, but this is rapidly lost on dilution of the serum. The diagnosis is most certainly made by the use of specific anti-IgM antisera in the DAT. The nature of the antigen with which the antibody reacts usually is not known, although serologic specificity has been attributed to the antibody in some cases.

The syndrome may arise without evidence of other disease. It has been seen in patients with malignant lymphocytic neoplasms; it has not been determined in these cases whether the antibody is monoclonal (and therefore presumably the product of the neoplastic cells) or polyclonal (and therefore due to the underlying immunologic abnormalities seen in these diseases).

Treatment of this syndrome is difficult. Prednisone in very high doses (2 mg/kg) has some effect but does not reduce the production of antibody and therefore does not lead to a useful remission. Splenectomy is of no value. Only immunosuppression is successful, and the combination of cyclophosphamide and prednisone has been used.

Autoimmune Hemolytic Anemia Due to IgM Cold-Reacting Antibodies

The second most common syndrome of AIHA is that caused by IgM cold-reacting antibodies.[64,137–141] Because the antibodies occur in the serum in high enough concentration to result in agglutination, the name *cold agglutinin syndrome* is often applied to this symptom complex.

Clinical Syndromes

Three general clinical syndromes may be caused by cold agglutinins. In children and young adults, the syndrome usually is brought on by a viral infection, either infectious mononucleosis or *Mycoplasma pneumoniae* infection. The onset is often abrupt with hemoglobinuria, and the anemia may be severe because of the diminished erythropoiesis caused by the infection. The acute hemolysis usually does not last more than 1 to 3 weeks, and all evidence of cold agglutinins usually are gone within 6 months.

In the chronic cold agglutinin syndrome of adults, the anemia usually is gradual in onset and usually is not severe. Some patients may note initially the onset of acrocyanosis, a purplish to grey discoloration of the fingers, toes, nose, ears, or other peripheral parts on exposure to cold. This is due to the agglutination of the blood as it cools and can often be brought about by immersing the hand in tepid water that is then cooled. The condition is different from Raynaud's phenomenon in that there is no preliminary blanching phase and no reactive red phase once the cyanosis has cleared. Acrocyanosis may be uncomfortable but rarely leads to gangrene.

On physical examination, the patient may exhibit acrocyanosis but usually does not. The spleen is sometimes enlarged, occasionally strikingly so. There usually is no lymph node enlargement unless an accompanying lymphoproliferative disorder is present.[142]

Uncommonly, the syndrome in adults may be acute with severe anemia and marked hemolysis; in some cases, this is due to an antibody that is able to react with its antigen at a temperature approaching 37°C.[143] This syndrome is particularly difficult to treat successfully.

Laboratory Findings

Analysis of the blood is often complicated by the presence of agglutination. Thus, in most automatic counters, the MCV is reported to be remarkably increased unless precautions are taken to warm the blood thoroughly before analysis.[144] Because the hematocrit is calculated from the MCV on such devices, it is also inaccurate under these circumstances.

The agglutination is often visible in the peripheral blood film as aggregates of cells seen even in the thin parts of the preparation (Fig. 55-11). Agglutination also can be distinguished from rouleaux, because the cells are distorted and not simply like stacks of discs.

The reticulocyte count usually is elevated, although the degree of elevation may be suboptimal for the degree of anemia.

The white blood cell count is often somewhat elevated. The lymphocytes usually are normal in appearance unless the patient has a lymphoproliferative disorder. Some of them can be shown to bear the cold agglutinin as surface immunoglobulin. These form rosettes in the cold, with RBCs bearing the antigen.[143]

The bone marrow usually shows erythroid hyperplasia. Careful examination sometimes reveals an increased number of normal-appearing lymphocytes, sometimes in follicles. These lymphocytes exhibit the cold agglutinin as surface immunoglobulin.

The DAT usually is strongly positive with anti-C3dg but not with anti-IgG. Agglutinins are readily demonstrable in the serum. These can sometimes be detected at the bedside, but careful collection of the specimen (maintaining it at 37°C by immersing the tube of blood in warm water until the cells and serum have been separated) and careful analysis are required for reliable diagnosis.

Agglutinin Analysis. Analysis of the agglutinins usually involves three interrelated measures: titer, thermal amplitude or maximum, and specificity. In some instances, the biochemical and immunologic structure of the antibody molecule may be analyzed as well.

Titer. A rough estimate of the concentration of antibody

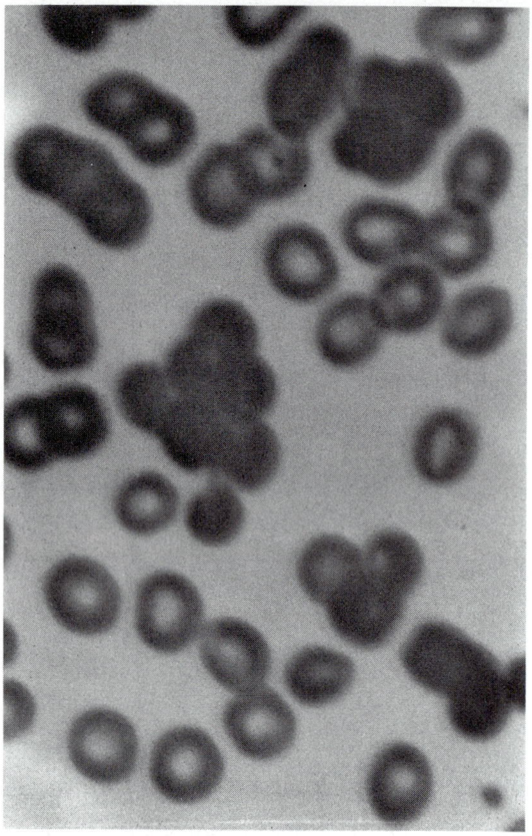

FIGURE 55-11. Appearance of agglutinated red blood cells on the peripheral blood film in a patient with cold agglutinin disease.

in the serum can be made by determining the degree to which the serum can be diluted and yet cause agglutination. A low titer of cold agglutinin (1/10 or so) is present in the serum of most normal donors. Most patients with *M pneumoniae* or EBV infection have a titer between 1/40 and 1/1000. In most cases of symptomatic (hemolytic) cold agglutinin disease, the serum can be diluted more than 1/1000 and often to dilutions exceeding 1/20,000. The titer may vary somewhat when cells of different normal donors are used. For some antibodies, the titer is much greater if albumin is added to the reaction mixture[146]; the significance of this is not clear, since it is not apparent that these antibodies are more hemolytic than those that do not show this difference.[145,147]

Thermal Maximum. The effectiveness of a cold agglutinin in bringing about hemolysis in vivo is determined to a great extent by its thermal maximum; that is, by the highest temperature at which it is able to bind to the antigen on the RBC. The thermal maximum is determined by performing agglutination reactions using the same dilutions of serum and the same RBCs but incubating them at different temperatures. In most cases, there is no agglutination at 37°C. The highest temperature at which agglutination can be distinguished is called the thermal maximum. In rare instances, the thermal maximum may reach 37°C.[143] In these cases, the titer of antibody may be low, but the amount of hemolysis may be great.

Specificity. Cold agglutinins react with polysaccharide antigens that are present on the blood cells of all individuals; thus, specificity cannot be defined, as it is for alloantibodies, by the presence or absence of the antigen on the cells of some but not other individuals in the population. Rather, specificity usually is defined by quantitative relationships of reactions on the cells of different donors, by the effect of various biochemical treatments on the antigen, and by the definition of the structure of the antigen. The latter, while most satisfactory, also is the most difficult.

Most cold agglutinins react with polysaccharide antigens that are part of the complex of molecules bearing the major (ABH) blood group antigens. Two principal types are observed:

- *Anti-I* antibodies agglutinate the cells of normal adult donors in higher titer than the cells of newborn infants or rare (genetic i) adults.[148]
- *Anti-i* antibodies agglutinate the cells of newborn infants in higher titer than the cells of normal adults.[149]
- Other specificities are uncommon and depend on the stability or instability of the antigen on enzymatic treatment of the RBCs[150–152] (Table 55-6).

Structure of Antigens. The biochemistry of these antigens is shown in Figure 55-12. The minimal polysaccharide that can be converted to H, A, or B antigen (the lacto ceramide moiety) consists of four sugars reading from the attachment to the ceramide: glucose–galactose–N-acetylglucosamine–galactose; the immunodeterminant sugars for H, A and B may be attached to the terminal galactose. This backbone can be elongated by the addition of further disaccharide moieties consisting of N-acetylglucosamine—galactose; the resulting entity reacts with anti-i antibodies.[153] After about age 6 months, these disaccharides may be added at two sites on the same galactose molecule, resulting in branching of the structure; the resulting complex polysaccharide reacts with anti-I antibodies.[154]

Some cold agglutinins react better with cells that have or do not have the H, A or B antigens attached to these complexes.[155] They are called by a compound epithet in such a case (eg, anti-AI for such an antibody that reacts

TABLE 55-6. Classification of the Specificities of Cold Agglutinins

Specificity	Adult Versus Fetal RBC	Enzyme Treatment: Proteolytic	Enzyme Treatment: Sialidase	Other Comments
Anti-I	A > F	Enhance	No effect	Structure known
Anti-i	F > A	Enhance	No effect	Structure known
Anti-Pr	A = F	Abolish	Abolish	Has subset variation
Anti-Pr_a	A = F	Abolish	No effect	
Anti-Lud	A > F	Diminish	Abolish	
Anti F1	A > F	No effect	Abolish	Branched polysaccharide complex
Anti-Gd	A = F	No effect	Abolish	On sialic acid bearing ganglioside
Anti-Li	A < F	No effect	Abolish	
Anti-Vo	A < F	No effect	Abolish	Terminally sialylated i antigen

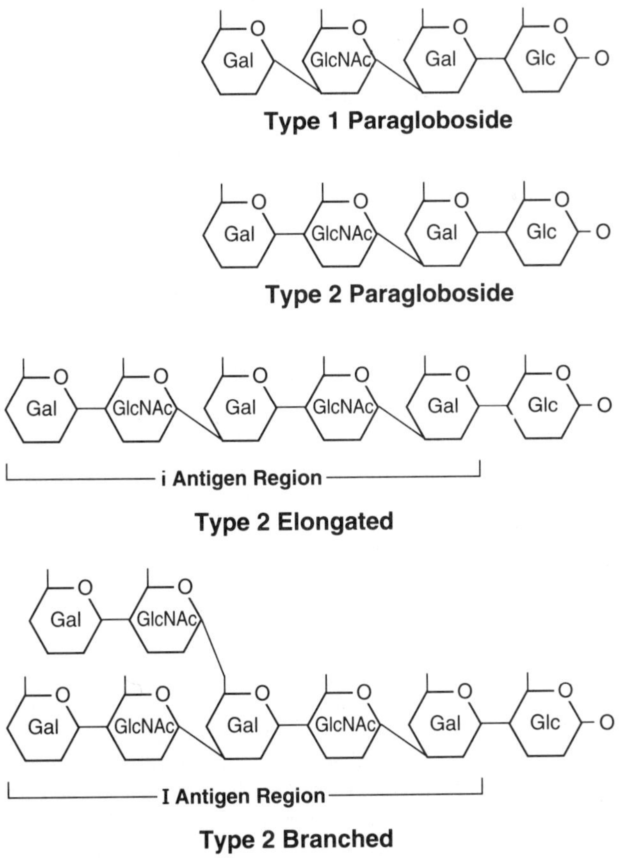

FIGURE 55-12. Structure of the polysaccharide antigens with which cold agglutinins react. The two upper polysaccharides form the basis on which the other members of the group are built. The I and i antigens are the result of further complexity of these molecules. The terminal galactose in all cases can be fucosylated in an α 1 to 2 linkage to make H substance and either can be galactosylated (to make B substance) or N-acetylgalactosylated (to make A substance).

like a cold agglutinin but reacts more strongly with A cells from an adult than with B or O cells).

These antigens are located in the interior of the molecule and therefore do not involve sialic acid, which may terminate a polysaccharide chain. Rarely, the reaction with antibody depends on the presence of this moiety; such antibodies are called anti-Gd,[151] anti-Lud,[152] and so forth. These antibodies do not react with cells that have been treated with sialidase to remove the sialic acid residues.

Rarely, the antigen with which a cold agglutinin reacts is a polysaccharide that is present only on glycoprotein molecules. Such antigens can be removed by proteolytic cleavage of the glycoprotein by, for instance, trypsin. They are called the Pr antigens because they are protein related.[156]

Structure of Antibody Molecule. Cold agglutinins can be easily purified by repeated cycles of adsorption in the cold and elution at 37°C; their structure can then be determined.[157] They are nearly always IgM molecules, although some IgG molecules also may be present[158,159]; rarely, they may have a monomeric rather than the usual pentameric structure.[160] Again rarely, the antibody may be IgA.[161]

The antibody may result from monoclonal or polyclonal production. If polyclonal, the molecules may be similar, but both types of light chain (κ and λ) are present.[162] If monoclonal, all the molecules are identical; this is best seen by showing that a single type of light chain (usually κ) is present.[163]

The monoclonal anti-I antibodies are often similar from patient to patient. The light chain usually is κ, and the framework structure usually is V_{κ}IIIb.[164] The heavy chain usually has the framework structure designated V_HI.[165] Antigens specific for cold agglutinins but common to all of them (idiotopes) usually are expressed in the antigen-combining area of the molecule.[166] These similarities in structure are reflected in similarities in amino acid structure of the molecules.

When the monoclonal cold agglutinin has specificity for antigens other than I, these restrictions on structure may not apply.[167] The light chain is often λ, and the framework structure of the light and heavy chain may be other than noted for anti-I antibodies.

Other Clinically Important Characteristics of Antigen–Antibody Interaction

Inhibition by Bound C3. Some cold agglutinins react less well with cells that have been coated with complement components, particularly C3.[168–170] This presumably is because the affixed C3 molecules cover the antigen sites and sterically hinder the binding of antibody. Because the cells of the patients usually are covered with C3dg, they may be protected in vivo from hemolysis. This property can be tested by determination of agglutination titers with C3-coated cells compared with titers with cells not coated with C3.

Fixation of C1. Because complement plays a dominant role in the pathogenesis of hemolysis by these antibodies, variations in the ability to fix complement may determine the degree of hemolysis in vivo. Some anti-I antibodies appear to affix to the antigen but not to bind complement[138]; thus, they are not highly hemolytic and also may inhibit the binding and hemolysis of other anti-I antibodies.

Pathophysiology

The hemolysis seen in cold agglutinin disease appears to be entirely due to reactions of complement. No Fc receptor for IgM molecules has been reliably reported on phagocytic cells.

Because of the characteristics of antigen–antibody interaction, the fixation of antibody and therefore of complement can occur only as the blood circulates to the periphery and the temperature of the blood drops below the thermal maximum of the antibody. This is more readily attained if the antibody has a high thermal maximum or if the patient is exposed to a colder environment. When this occurs, sufficient antibody is present in the plasma to initiate massively the activation of complement. If sufficient components are affixed to the RBC membrane to overcome the down-regulation of the reactions, lysis of the cell by direct insertion of the membrane attack complex occurs. This results in the intravascular release of hemoglobin,[171] which if sufficiently severe may result in hemoglobinuria and hemosiderinuria.

If the cells survive this attack on the integrity of the membrane, they may then circulate into the central body where the C3b and C4b on their surface may interact with receptors on phagocytic cells of lung, liver, and spleen.[172] The cells bearing these receptors are distributed throughout the reticuloendothelial system, and the circulation of the spleen offers no special advantage in producing cellular destruction. During the circulation, C3b and C4b are enzymatically degraded first to iC3b and iC4b, and further to C3dg and C4d (see Fig. 55-5).[173] As the molecules are degraded, their ability to induce phagocytosis is reduced and the remnants of C3 and C4 (C3dg and C4d) that persist on the membrane probably do not interfere with the longevity of the cells.[136,139]

Etiology

Cold agglutinins may arise from two general causes: reaction to infection or lymphoproliferation. These general causes can be distinguished by the fact that the antibodies that result from infection are polyclonal, whereas those that result from lymphoproliferation are monoclonal; as noted, this distinction can be detected from the isotypic homogeneity or heterogeneity of the light chains.

Cold Agglutinins From Infections. Cold agglutinins are detected frequently during the course of two infections: atypical pneumonia due to *M pneumoniae*,[174] and infectious mononucleosis.[175,176] The presence of the antibody can be of benefit in making the etiologic diagnoses. In both cases, the titer of antibody usually is not markedly elevated (usually less than 1/1200); thus, the amount of hemolysis is not striking.[177,178] The presence of antibody in the serum is limited in time and usually does not last more than 2 to 3 months.

In *M pneumoniae* infections, the antibody usually is anti-I. It appears about 2 weeks after initial symptoms of the infection, like any heteroimmune IgM antibody, and may be a cross-reacting antibody primarily directed at polysaccharide antigens on the organism[179] or at its binding site on the RBC.[180]

A similar antibody may arise in some cases of infection by *Listeria monocytogenes*.[181] The organism has a polysaccharide structure on its surface that closely resembles the antigen reacting with anti-I, and the antibody apparently cross-reacts with the similar structure on the RBC surface.

In infectious mononucleosis due to the EBV virus, cold agglutinins appear in 50% to 80% of cases. The antibody usually is present in relatively low titer (usually less than 1/1200) and is nearly always anti-i. Some of the antibody may be IgG, although IgM antibody usually is present.[126,127] The antibody is thought to be due to the polyclonal stimulation of the B-cell system by this organism; it appears about 2 to 3 weeks after the onset of symptoms and usually is not found 2 to 3 months later. Antibody sufficient to cause clinically significant hemolysis occurs in less than 1 in 1000 cases.[182]

Cold Agglutinins Due to Lymphoproliferative Diseases. Cold agglutinins may result from the monoclonal proliferation of B-cell clones.[111] This proliferation may range in degree of malignancy from benign monoclonal gammopathy (in which the proliferation of the clone is controlled in some degree) to malignant lymphoma.

Chronic cold agglutinin syndrome usually is due to benign monoclonal gammopathy and has many of the characteristics of that syndrome.[107,108] It occurs in older patients; incidence at age less than 50 years is distinctly unusual. It usually is not progressive, and patients may have the syndrome for many years. Occasionally, it may evolve into a more malignant condition.

The cells responsible for the syndrome are benign-appearing plasmacytoid lymphocytes that are rich in discontinuous endoplasmic reticulum and have a small Golgi apparatus. They express the antibody on the surface (see earlier discussion) but also secrete antibody.[113] The antibody is nearly always (90%) anti-I with κ light chains.[131]

The cold agglutinin syndrome rarely occurs in patients with chronic lymphocytic leukemia.[111] The antibody is produced by the malignant clone, and the titer of antibody can be used as a measure of the tumor burden. The antibody usually is anti-I but may have other specificities.

In more malignant lymphomas (particularly diffuse histiocytic lymphoma), cold agglutinin antibody may rarely be produced by the malignant cells.[111] The antibody usually is anti-i and often has λ light chains. The presence of such antibodies may be the first sign of the disease, and the presence of a monoclonal anti-i antibody is nearly pathognomonic of malignant lymphoma.

Rarely, adenocarcinomas may be associated with monoclonal cold agglutinins of anti-I specificity.[183] The relation of the antibody to the underlying disease is not clear, although the young age of the patient and the time of onset of both diseases may sometimes strongly suggest that some causative relation exists.

Treatment

Because of the relatively ineffective mechanisms of cellular destruction initiated by cold agglutinins, the hemolytic anemia is often not severe, and aggressive treatment is often not necessary. This is particularly true of most cases in which the production of antibody is secondary to an infection. When treatment is indicated, it is directed primarily at avoiding the interaction of the antibody with the RBCs or at reducing the production or the serum concentration of antibody. To date, no practical means of reducing the activation or the effectiveness of complement has been devised.

In most cases, the antibody reacts with the RBC only at temperatures less than core body temperature, so avoiding situations where the temperature of the blood is lowered significantly may reduce both the symptoms of cold agglutinin disease and the hemolysis; many patients have a higher hemoglobin in the summer than in the winter. For many patients, the appropriate blood temperature can be maintained by wearing clothing that maintains the peripheral parts of the body at a sufficiently high temperature; such measures include long woolen underwear, down boots, ear muffs, and gloves even in moderate weather. In some cases, removal to a warm climate is necessary.

The necessity for a warm environment sometimes puts patients in peril in particular circumstances. In particular, surgery may be dangerous unless precautions are taken to prevent cooling during the operation.[184,185] Some occupations may not be available to such patients since they involve too much exposure to the cold.

The amount of antibody in the serum can be reduced by plasmapheresis.[139,183,184] This is relatively efficient since the antibody is IgM and is thus confined to the intravascular space. Care must be taken during the procedure to be certain that the blood that is to be returned has not been allowed to become cold—hemolysis may result if this occurs. Unfortunately, the production rate of the antibody is such that the titer rapidly returns to the pretreatment level; this limits this procedure to those instances in which a rapid reduction in antibody titer is needed, since most patients cannot tolerate the amount of plasmapheresis that is required to maintain chronically a low antibody titer.

A reduction in the production of antibody may be difficult to achieve. The production of antibody is not affected by the administration of prednisone, and prednisone usually is not effective in any dose; the exception to this is seen in the unusual patient with an antibody of high thermal amplitude.[143] In these cases, high doses of prednisone may result in amelioration of the hemolysis, probably due to down-regulation of complement receptors rather than a reduction in antibody.

For the reduction in antibody concentration, cytotoxic agents usually are needed. In more benign conditions, daily or intermittent administration of alkylating agents may be used; no clear advantage is known for the agent or for the schedule of treatment.[38,107,188,189] For phenylalanine mustard (Alkeran) the dose is 2 to 4 mg/d or 24 to 30 mg every 3 weeks. For cyclophosphamide, the daily dose is 50 to 100 mg, and the intermittent dose is 500 to 700 mg every 3 weeks. Care must be taken that normal hematopoiesis is not suppressed.

When cold agglutinin disease occurs in the setting of the more malignant lymphoproliferative diseases, the treatment is that of the primary disease. The titer of antibody may indicate the degree of response (Fig. 55-13).

Transfusion. Patients with cold agglutinin syndrome do not often require transfusion. When they do, the presence of the antibody may make blood typing and compatibility testing difficult.

When the cells of patients are tested for the blood group with anti-A and anti-B in the usual way, they are not washed free of the patient's serum. If sufficient serum containing the cold agglutinin is transferred into the tests, the cells agglutinate and appear to be AB in type. The error is readily discovered if the serum is tested for the presence of appropriate alloanti-A or alloanti-B.

As in the case of warm-reacting IgG antibody, the cold agglutinin is likely to react with the cells of all potential donors, and the presence of alloantibodies is difficult to detect. The serum may be absorbed at 4°C with the patient's RBCs; subsequent incubation at 37°C removes the antibody so that the absorption can be repeated. If the antibody is anti-I, it may be removed by rabbit RBC stroma, since these cells bear the I antigen.[181]

Confusion with the cold agglutinin also can be diminished by performing all the reactions of compatibility testing at 37°C; most cold agglutinins do not react at that temperature. Further, the tests using antiglobulin may be done using reagents containing anti-IgG but not anti-C3dg since these detect most significant alloantibodies but do not react with the cold agglutinin autoantibodies.

Hemolytic Anemia Due to Cold-Reacting IgG Antibodies (Paroxysmal Cold Hemoglobinuria)

Paroxysmal cold hemoglobinuria was the first clinical syndrome of AIHA to be definitively described. The primary symptom, hemoglobinuria following exposure to a cold environment—often frightening to the patient and helpful to the physician in making a diagnosis—was first described in England in 1832 in children with congenital lues who

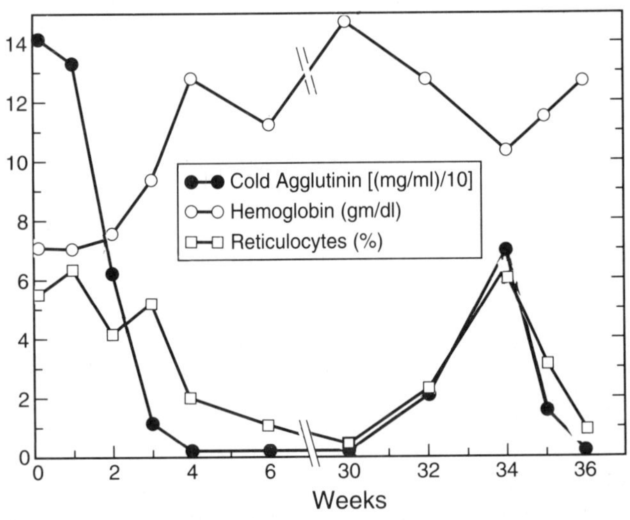

FIGURE 55-13. Cold agglutinin as tumor marker in a patient with undifferentiated lymphocytic lymphoma. The titer, determined by a quantitative hemolysis assay, closely reflects the activity of the disease.

had dark urine when the cold east wind blew.[1] The diagnostic test devised by Donath and Landsteiner was the first to be applied to the diagnosis of AIHA.[3,4]

Clinical Syndrome

Classically, paroxysmal cold hemoglobinuria (PCH) is characterized by the sudden onset of hemoglobinuria after exposure to cold, but many patients may not have this symptom because the concentration of antibody in the serum is insufficient to cause intravascular hemolysis. In other patients, hemoglobinuria may occur without specific exposure to cold if the titer and characteristics of the antibody permit. Thus, the classic symptom is a poor guide to diagnosis in most cases.

Patients with PCH do not exhibit acrocyanosis but may have true Raynaud's phenomenon or other vasomotor phenomena.[190] The reason for this is not clear.

Other symptoms of PCH are those of intermittent hemolysis and include jaundice, weakness, pallor, and, if the anemia is sufficient, cardiac decompensation.

The anemia may range in severity from mild to severe; death may intervene in some cases. The reticulocyte response usually is appropriately high, and leukocytosis may be present during hemolytic episodes. Hemoglobinuria may or may not be seen, but hemosiderinuria is nearly always present.

The DAT, as performed, is either negative or positive only with anticomplement reagents.[191] The IgG antibody usually is washed off during the preparation of the samples at room temperature but may be detected by some of the more sensitive methods. The diagnosis is made by the demonstration of a cold-reacting IgG antibody in the serum. Agglutination in the standard cold agglutination test usually is weak, and titers over 1/100 are rare.

The Donath-Landsteiner bithermic hemolytic test is the classic method of demonstrating the antibodies. In this test, normal RBCs (or, for greater sensitivity, the RBCs of patients with paroxysmal nocturnal hemoglobinuria) are incubated with the patient's serum and a source of complement at 4°C for 30 minutes, then at 37°C for another 30 minutes; if hemolysis occurs in the test sample and does not occur in controls maintained at 37°C for the full time, the test is positive.

The Donath-Landsteiner test is somewhat insensitive, however, and in many patients the cold-reacting IgG antibody can only be demonstrated in the cold indirect Coombs' test in which normal RBCs are mixed with the serum of the patient at 4°C and the binding of IgG antibodies detected by either agglutination by anti-IgG or, preferably, by an assay using a labeled monoclonal anti-IgG.

The determination of the thermal maximum may be important for the same reasons given for its determination for cold agglutinins.[192] This is done by varying the temperature at which the first (cold) phase of the test is conducted.

The antibody usually reacts with the P antigen, a polysaccharide antigen present on the RBCs of nearly all individuals.[193,194] Occasionally, the specificity is for other polysaccharide or polysaccharide-dependent antigens.[195,196] Although there is much discussion about what should be called a D-L antibody, the most logic and pragmatic definition is an IgG antibody that is cold reacting.

Pathophysiology

Hemolysis in PCH is effected for the most part by direct lysis by complement when the circulating blood is exposed to temperature sufficiently decreased to allow interaction of the antibody with the cell and the fixation of complement. Direct intravascular lysis is often more evident in this disorder than in cold agglutinin disease, but the reason is not entirely known. There is some evidence that the fixation of the first component of complement is more efficient since agglutination, which interferes with the binding of this component, does not occur.[52] Since the antibody is IgG, immune adherence by antibody may play a role if the thermal maximum of the antibody is sufficiently high so that some remains on the surface of the RBC when the blood circulates to the warmer interior of the body, where Fc receptors are located.

Etiology

The antibodies characteristic of PCH arise in three clinical settings. They were identified first in patients with advanced syphilis, usually tertiary or congenital. It is thought that, in this infection, the antibody arises in response to P-like antigens on the spirochete and cross-reacts with the P antigen of the RBC. Regardless, the syndrome disappears when the infection is cured.

PCH occurs frequently following a viral illness[197,198] or inoculation[199]; a number of viruses have been implicated, most frequently the childhood exanthems. This reaction occurs most frequently in childhood (usually less than 5 years of age) where it may be the most common form of AIHA.[197] Rarely, the postviral reaction may be seen also in adults. The anemia may be severe, but the syndrome resolves over 3 to 6 weeks even without specific treatment, although multiple blood transfusions are often needed.

PCH can occur also as an autoimmune disease with or without other manifestations of immune dysfunction.[200,201] This form follows the age distribution of other IgG AIHAs. The course usually is chronic, and the degree of anemia is variable; specific treatment is often necessary.

Treatment

The treatment of PCH depends somewhat on its cause. If it is due to syphilis (rarely the case nowadays), that infection should be treated with penicillin. If it is due to viral infections, any treatment is limited in time because of the transient nature of the syndrome.

As in the case of the syndromes due to cold agglutinins, avoidance of the cold can be effective in ameliorating the milder forms of PCH. For many patients, however, this is insufficient and other treatment must be instituted.

The general treatment of PCH is much like that of the syndromes due to warm-reacting IgG (see earlier discussion) with certain exceptions. Prednisone is often effective in reducing the amount of antibody and, if it is unable to do so, cytotoxic agents may be used. Splenectomy and intravenous γ-globulin probably do not have a place in the treatment of PCH unless the antibody has an extremely high thermal maximum.

Transfusion may be necessary and crossmatch may be complicated by the presence of the antibody to a virtually universal antigen; the problem of identifying alloantibodies may be minimized by performing the compatibility testing at 37°C. The rare donors lacking the P antigen may be found, and their blood may be used if it is available.[202] If not, incompatible blood may be given with safety and effectiveness.[203]

Drug-Induced Autoimmune Hemolytic Anemia

Harris and his colleagues[204,205] first recognized that drugs may be able to induce the production of antibodies that are then capable of destroying the circulating RBCs, and since that time, the phenomenon has been ascribed to a bewildering number of drugs[206,207] (Table 55-7).

Two distinct syndromes are described depending on whether the drug is part of the antigen.

Drug as Antigen

Many chemical compounds, including drugs, may act as haptenes; that is, they bind to a carrier and an antibody is formed to the combination. In this case, the drug is an important part of the antigenic configuration. Classically, a haptene is bound securely to the carrier and alone should be able to react with the antibody and inhibit its interaction with the haptene–carrier combination[208]; this may not be true for drugs causing immune hemolytic anemia. It is clear, however, that in most instances, drug-induced immune hemolytic anemia is due to a haptene mechanism.

Clinical Syndrome. For most drugs causing haptene-induced immune hemolytic anemia, the onset of the clinical syndrome usually is fairly abrupt with the rapid onset of anemia.[175] In some instances, hemoglobinemia with resultant hemoglobinuria and hemosiderinuria may be seen; renal failure due to the hemoglobinuria is not uncommon.[209–212] The onset may be so sudden that the reticulocyte count does not have time to rise. The sudden onset may lead to symptoms of hypoxia, especially in older patients, because some of the compensatory mechanisms for the anemia may not have time to occur.

This complication of drug therapy is often seen shortly after the drug is first given to the patient; conversely, it

TABLE 55-7. Drugs Known to Have Caused Immune Hemolytic Anemia

Drug	References
Quinine or Quinidine	194, 232–236
ANTIBIOTICS	
Penicillins	40, 181, 182, 237–239
Cephalothins	240–245
Sulfa drugs	246
p-Aminosalicylic acid (PAS)	177, 247
Rifampicin	186
Stibophen	172, 173, 179, 248
Other	186, 249–251
ANALGESICS AND ANTIRHEUMATICS	
Phenacetin	177, 252
Nonsteroidals	253
NEUROLEPTICS	
Tricyclics	254
Nomifensine	178, 188, 255–257
Phenothiazines	258
Sedatives	259
CARDIOVASCULAR DRUGS	
Thiazides	260, 261
α-Methyldopa	190–193, 262
Procainamide	263
ENDOCRINOLOGIC DRUGS	
Sulfonylureas	184, 264–266
OTHER DRUGS	
Methotrexate	267
Probenecid	268, 269

may occur months to years after the initiation of therapy. Often, only small doses of drug are sufficient to cause the hemolysis, although this varies with the drug.

In other instances, particularly when the drug is penicillin or a drug related to it, the onset usually is less abrupt and the anemia is less severe.[206,213,214] This syndrome usually occurs only when very large doses of penicillin (in excess of 10,000,000 IU/d) are administered; the onset of anemia usually is 5 to 10 days after the initiation of therapy. Hemoglobinuria and renal failure are rare but may occur when complement is fixed (see later discussion).[215]

If the cause is identified, the symptoms usually abate rapidly when the drug is discontinued. In some instances, the antibody appears to be made to an intrinsic structure of the RBC, and hemolysis may last for several weeks in such cases. Nevertheless, the syndrome resolves when the drug is no longer taken.

The antibody usually disappears within a few weeks after the drug is discontinued. If the drug is again administered before this happens, hemolysis may be rapid (within minutes). If the drug is administered after antibody has disappeared, there may be a delay before hemolysis occurs while an anamnestic immune response is mounted. In some instances, reexposure does not cause a recurrence of the syndrome.

Diagnosis. The DAT usually is positive only with anticomplement antisera even though the antibody usually is IgG. This is because the haptene is not sufficiently adherent to the RBC to resist removal during the washing procedure in preparation for the performance of the test. Penicillin and related drugs are exceptional in that they are firmly bound to the membrane of the cell, but the interaction with antibody usually does not fix complement; thus, the DAT usually is positive with anti-IgG, and negative with anti-C3.

The diagnosis of drug-induced immune hemolytic anemia is made by the demonstration that the antibody reacts with RBCs in the presence of the drug but does not react with RBCs in the absence of the drug. Usually, the serum of the patient is mixed with normal RBCs and the drug is added. The occurrence of an interaction is affirmed by agglutination or by the fixation of complement, which either results in lysis of the RBCs or the presence of complement components on the membrane of the test cells. The sensitivity of those tests that are dependent on lysis by complement can be increased by using the cells of patients with paroxysmal nocturnal hemoglobinuria or normal cells that have been treated to be more sensitive to the lytic action of complement.[216] The test is controlled by the omission of the drug; when this is done, the reaction does not occur.

In testing for antibodies to penicillin, normal RBCs are coated with the drug at a high pH[217]; after being washed, they are then reacted with the patient's serum, washed again, and tested with anti-IgG. This procedure affixes the drug to the membrane, and the attachment lasts through several washings.

These tests can be used to determine the fine specificity of the antibody. Congeners of the drug may be used to determine the cross-reactivity of the antibody. Rare cells lacking certain surface proteins (eg, K_o, Lu a[−]b[−]) may not sustain the reaction, indicating that the attachment site of the drug is related to the missing antigenic protein.[184,218–220]

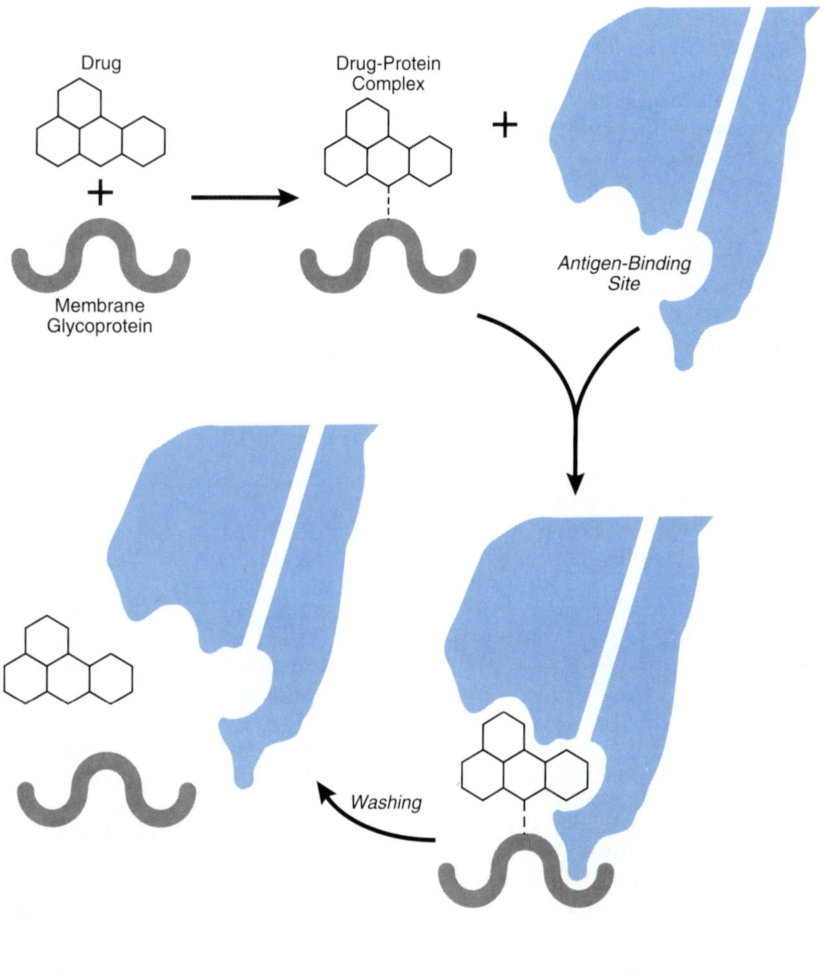

FIGURE 55-14. Binding of antibody to a drug as a haptene. The drug combines with a surface-membrane glycoprotein and is able to stimulate the formation of an antibody. The antibody that is formed reacts with both the drug and, to a lesser extent, the membrane. If the drug is removed, the antibody does not remain bound.

The test may be negative even though the immune hemolytic anemia is drug-related. The antibody may be to a metabolite of the drug; if the metabolites are known, they may be used in the test.[221] If not, the urine of a patient who has ingested the drug may be used to provide the metabolite. The reaction may occur in the absence of the drug even though the drug caused the syndrome (see next section). For these and probably other reasons, a negative test for the specificity of drug-induced immune hemolytic anemia does not mean that the syndrome was not induced by the drug.

When Drug Is Not Antigen

In 1965, Carstairs and associates[222,223] reported that many (about 15%) patients taking the drug α-methyldopa (Aldomet) for hypertension developed a positive DAT; of these, about 10% (1.5% of the total) developed hemolytic anemia. The syndrome occurred more frequently in patients taking high doses (more than 1 g/d) and often did not supervene for several months after the initiation of therapy.

Most patients with positive DATs do not have evidence of hemolysis. With higher titers of antibody (determined by the strength of the DAT or IAT), hemolysis may occur but is seldom severe. Spherocytosis is present in these cases, and the spleen may be enlarged. The reticulocytosis is commensurate with the degree of anemia.

The syndrome usually lasts 4 to 8 weeks after discontinuation of the drug. The degree of hemolysis, when present, gradually diminishes. The DAT gradually weakens and finally disappears.

The DAT is positive with anti-IgG but usually not with anti-C3—unlike the tests in most cases of drug-induced immune hemolytic anemia. Although the drug is clearly implicated in the pathogenesis of the syndrome, the IAT is positive even though the drug is omitted from the reaction. In fact, the antibody in most cases reacts with all RBCs except Rh_{null} cells, suggesting that the antibody reacts with the protein or proteins bearing the Rh antigens[224,225]; this accounts for its inability to fix complement, since antibodies against Rh antigens almost never do so.

Etiology of Drug-Induced Autoimmune Hemolytic Anemia

By definition, the drug is involved in the formation of the antibody. It was first assumed that it acted as a haptene, using some component of the RBC membrane as the carrier, but the reactions did not appear to correspond to those classically described for haptenes. The drug and the antibody in most cases did not appear to be bound to the membrane of the RBC. Further, incubation of the drug and the antibody did not inhibit the ability of the antibody to react with the RBC under appropriate circumstances.[226] For these reasons, it was proposed that the drug reacted with some protein in the plasma, and that the antibody was directed against that complex. This reaction, occurring in the presence of RBCs, resulted in the fixation of complement on the RBC surface. Thus, the RBC was an innocent bystander.

Evidence has accumulated, however, to suggest that the RBC is not so innocent as was thought. In some instances, cells lacking certain membrane proteins or possessing certain blood group antigens do not react with drug and antibody, suggesting that such proteins are necessary for the interaction to occur.[186] Further, in the analogous syndrome, drug-induced immune thrombocytopenia, the drug forms a neoantigen with glycoproteins of the platelet membrane.[227] Both the drug and the glycoprotein are essential for interaction with the antibody, and the reaction stabilizes the drug on the protein. It is probable that the same kinds of reactions take place on RBCs, except that the combination of drug and protein is not stabilized by the interaction, and the drug is washed off readily (Fig. 55-14).

The reaction to α-methlydopa is not explained by this mechanism, since the drug appears to play no part in the structure of the antigen.[190,192] It is hypothesized that the drug in some way alters the immune system so that autoantibodies are produced.[228] It is more likely, however, that the drug alters the structure of the Rh protein or proteins so that cross-reacting antibodies are made[229,230] (Fig. 55-15). These then react with the normal protein and cause hemolytic anemia long after the drug has cleared. A similar mechanism has been postulated for the antibodies produced against nomifensine, a psycholeptic agent introduced in Europe but subsequently withdrawn because of its tendency to cause immune hemolytic anemia.[221]

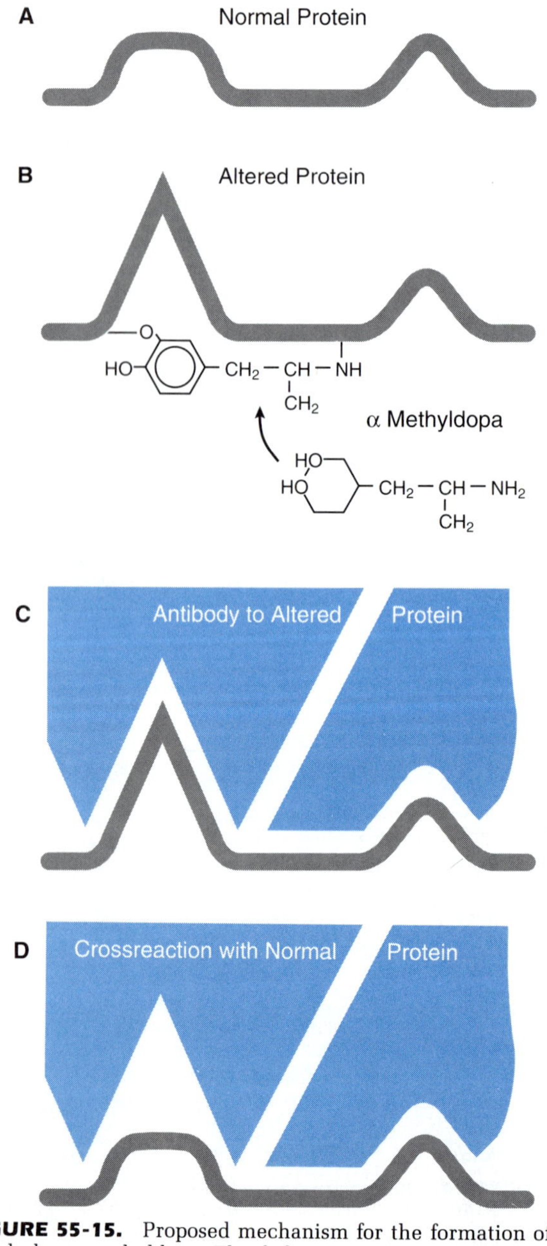

FIGURE 55-15. Proposed mechanism for the formation of antibody by α-methyldopa. This bifunctional agent alters the conformation of the protein so that it appears foreign to the immune system. An antibody is made to the altered protein that cross-reacts with the normal protein.

Therapy

In general, the first thing to be done once drug-induced hemolytic anemia has been identified is to withdraw the drug. In most cases, this results in a fairly rapid resolution of the hemolytic process; the time required depends on the rate of clearance of the drug and the degree to which the antibody reacts with the cell in the absence of the drug. In the latter case, hemolysis persists as long as the antibody is produced, whether or not the drug is present—as occurs with α-methyldopa.

If hemolysis is severe, supportive transfusion may be required. There usually is little problem with the compatibility testing since the drug is not present. This is, of course, not true in cases where the antibody reacts with the membrane in the absence of the drug.

In instances where severe hemolytic anemia occurs after the ingestion of α-methlydopa, further treatment may be necessary. This should consist of the use of prednisone in the manner indicated earlier for warm-reacting IgG antibodies. Such use is not necessary for long periods, since the reaction usually subsides within 3 to 4 months.

The patient should be advised to avoid the causative drug and any analogous drugs that might cross-react. If antibody is still present, a rapid hemolytic reaction may occur. If the antibody has disappeared, an anamnestic reaction may occur and severe hemolysis result.

REFERENCES

1. Elliotson J. Diseases of the heart united with ague. Lancet 1832;1:500.
2. Hassall AH. On intermittent, or winter, haematuria. Lancet 18652:368.
3. Donath J, Landsteiner K. Uber paroxysmale Hameglobinurie. Munch Med Wochenschr 1904;51:1590.
4. Donath J, Landsteiner K. Uber paroxysmale Hamoglobinurie. Z Klin Med 1906;58:173.
5. Goltz D. Das Donath-Landsteiner Hamolysin: die Entstehung eines Mythos in der Medizin des 20 Jahrhunderts. Clio Med 1982;16:193.
6. Ehrlich P, Morgenroth J. Uber Haemolysine: zweite Mittheilung. Berl Klin Wochenschr 1899;36:481.
7. Widal F, Abrami P, Brule M. Les iceteres d'origine hemolytique. Arch Mal Coeur 1908;1:193.
8. Landsteiner K. Uber Agglutilnetionserscheinungen normalen menschlichen Blutes. Wein Klin Wochenschr 1901;14:1132.
9. Widal F, Abrami P, Brule M. Retrocession des symptomes cliniques at des troubles hematiques au cours des icteres hemolytiques acquis. Bull Soc Med Paris 1909;28:73.
10. Dameshek W, Schwartz SO. The presence of hemolysins in acute hemolytic anemia: preliminary note. N Engl J Med 1938;218:75.
11. Coombs RRA, Mourant AE, Race RR. A new test for the detection of weak and 'incomplete' Rh agglutinins. Br J Exp Pathol 1945;26:255.
12. Boorman KE, Dodd BE, Loutit JF. Haemolytic icterus (acholuric jaundice) congenital and acquired. Lancet 1946;1:812.
13. Loutit JF, Mollison PL. Hemolytic icterus (acholuric jaundice), congenital and acquired. J Pathol Bact 1946;58:711.
14. Dacie JV. Acquired hemolytic anemia: with special reference to the antiglobulin (Coombs') reaction. Blood 1953;8:813.
15. Jeske DJ, Capra JD. Immunoglobulins: structure and function. In: Paul WE, ed. Fundamental immunology. New York, Raven Press, 1984:131.
16. Davies DR, Metzger H. Structural basis of antibody function. Annu Rev Immunol 1983;1:87.
17. Wu TT, Kabat EA. An analysis of the sequences of the variable regions of Bence Jones proteins and myeloma light chains and their implications for antibody complementarity. J Exp Med 132:211.1970.
18. Brunhouse R, Cebra JJ. Isotypes of IgG: comparison of the primary structures of three pairs of isotypes which differ in their ability to activate complement. Mol Immunol 1979;16:907.
19. Yasmeen D, Ellerson JR, Dorrington KJ, et al. The structure and function of immunoglobulin domains: IV. the distribution of some effector functions among the $C_{gamma}2$ and $C_{gamma}3$ homology regions of human immunoglobulin G. J Immunol 1976;116:518.
20. Augener W, Grey HM, Cooper N, et al. The reaction of monomeric and aggregated immunoglobulins with C1. Immunochemistry 1971;8:1011.
21. Isenman DE, Dorrington KJ, Painter RH. The structure and function of immunoglobulin domains: II. the importance of interchain disulfide bonds and the possible role of molecular flexibility in the interaction between immunoglobulin G and complement. J Immunol 1975;114:1726.
22. Schumaker VN, Calcott MA, Spiegelberg HL, et al. Ultracentrifuge studies of the binding of IgG of different subclasses to the C1q subunit of the first component of complement. Biochemistry 1978;15:5175.
23. Bubb MO, Conradie JD. The importance of quaternary structure in the expression of the C1-binding site of IgM. Immunology 1976;31:893.
24. Feinstein A, Richardson NE, Gorick BD, et al. Immunoglobulin M conformational change is a signal for complement activation. In: Celada F, Shumaker VN, Sercarz EE, eds. Protein conformation as an immunological signal. New York, Plenum Press, 1983:47.
25. Borsos T, Rapp HJ. Complement fixation of cell surfaces by 19S and 7S antibodies. Science 1965;150:505.
26. Svehag SE, Bloth B. The ultrastructure of human C1q. Acta Pathol Microbiol Scand [B] 1970;78:260.
27. Rosse WF. The fixation of the first component of complement (C'1a) by human antibodies. J Clin Invest 1968;47:2430.
28. Muller-Eberhard HJ. The membrane attack complex. Semin Immunopath 1984;7:93.
29. Rosse WF, Logue GL, Adams J, et al. Mechanisms of immune lysis of the red cells in hereditary erythroblastic multinuclearity with a positive acidified serum test and paroxysmal nocturnal hemoglobinuria. J Clin Invest 1974;53:31.
30. Ross GD, Medof ME. Membrane complement receptors specific for bound fragments of C3. Adv Immunol 1985;37:217.
31. Ross GD, Lambris JD, Cain JA, et al. Generation of three different fragments of bound C3 with purified factor I or serum: I. requirements for factor H vs CR1 cofactor activity. J Immunol 1982;129:2051.
32. Anderson CL, Looney RJ. Human leukocyte IgG Fc receptors. Immunol Today 1986;7:264.
33. Fleit HB, Wright SD, Unkeless JC. Human neutrophil Fcγ receptor distribution and structure. Proc Natl Acad Sci USA 1982;79:3275.
34. Clark DA, Dessypris EN, Jenkins DE jr, et al. Acquired immune hemolytic anemia associated with IgA erythrocyte coating: investigation of hemolytic mechanisms. Blood 1984;64:1000.
35. Gauldie J, Richards C, Lamontagne L. Fc receptors for IgA and other immunoglobulin on resident and activated alveolar macrophages. Mol Immunol 1983;20:1029.
36. Rosse WF, de Boisfleury A, Bessis M. The interaction of phagocytic cells and red cells modified by immune reactions. Blood Cells 1975;1:345.
37. Mantovani B, Rabinovitch M, Nussenzweig V. Phagocytosis of immune complexes by macrophages: different roles of the macrophage receptor sites for complement (C3) and for immunoglobulin (IgG). J Exp Med 1972;135:780.
38. Rosse WF. Detection of antigen-antibody interaction: precipitation, agglutination, and aggregation. In: Clinical hematology: basic concepts and clinical applications. New York, Blackwell, 1990:291.
39. Pollack W, Hager HJ, Recker R, et al. A study of the forces involved in the second stage of hemagglutination. Transfusion 1965;5:158.
40. Bernstein F, Casteneda AR. Alteration in erythrocyte electrical charge associated with mannitol, polyvinylpyrrolidone (PVP), dextrose and various dextran compounds. In: Biophysical mechanisms in vascular homeostasis and intravascular thrombosis. New York, Appleton-Century-Crofts, 1969:103.
41. Jones GE. Intercellular adhesion: modification by dielectric properties of the medium. J Membr Biol 1974;16:297.
42. Goding JW. Use of staphylococcal protein A as an immunological reagent. J Immunol Methods 1978;20:241.
43. Engelfreit CP, von dem Borne AEGKr, Beckers D, et al. Autoimmune haemolytic anaemia: serological and immunological characteristics of the autoantibodies, mechanism of cells destruction. Series Haematol 1974;7:328.
44. Dupuy ME, Elliot M, Masouredis SP. Relationship between red cell bound antibody and agglutination in the antiglobulin reaction. Vox Sang 1964;9:40.
45. Merry AH, Thomson EE, Rawlinson V, et al. The quantification of C3 fragments on normal cells, acquired hemolytic anemia cases and correlation with agglutination of sensitized cells. Clin Lab Haematol 1983;5:387.
46. Merry AH, Thomson EE, Rawlinson VI, et al. A quantitative antiglobulin test for IgG for use in blood transfusion serology. Clin Lab Haematol 1982;4:393.
47. Chaplin H Jr, Monroe MC. Comparisons of pooled polyclonal rabbit anti-human C3d with four monoclonal mouse anti-human C3ds. I. Quantification of RBC-bound C3d and characterization of antiglobulin agglutination reactions against RBCs from 27 patients with autoimmune hemolytic anemia. Vox Sang 1986;50:87.
48. Leikola J, Perkins HA. Enzyme-linked antiglobulin test: an accurate and simple method to quantify red cell antibodies. Transfusion 1980;20:138.
49. Meulen FW van der, de Bruin HG, Goosen PCM, et al. Quantitative aspects of the destruction of red cells sensitized with IgG_1 autoantibodies: an application of flow cytofluorometry. Br J Haematol 1980;46:47.
50. Muller-Eberhard HJ. The membrane attack complex. Semin Immunopath 1984;7:93.

51. Sirchia G, Dacie JV. Immune lysis of AET-treated normal red cells (PNH-like cells). Nature 1967;215:747.
52. Rosse WF, Adams J, Logue G. Hemolysis by complement and cold-reacting antibodies: time and temperature requirements. Am J Hematol 1977;2:259.
53. Allgood JW, Chaplin H Jr. Idiopathic acquired autoimmune hemolytic anemia. Am J Med 1969;43:254.
54. Dacie JV, Worlledge SM. Auto-immune hemolytic anemias. Prog Hematol 1969;6:82.
55. Pirofsky B. Clinical aspects of autoimmune hemolytic anemia. Semin Hematol 1976;13:251.
56. Habibi B, Homberg JC, Schaison G, et al. Autoimmune hemolytic anemia in children: a review of 80 cases. Am J Med 1974;56:61.
57. Zuelzer WW, Mastrangelo R, Stulberg CS. Autoimmune hemolytic anemia: natural history and viral immunologic interactions in childhood. Am J Med 1969;49:80.
58. Horwitz CA, Skradski K, Reece E, et al. Haemolytic anaemia in previously healthy adult patients with CMV infections: report of two cases and an evaluation of subclinical haemolysis in CMV mononucleosis. Scand J Haematol 1984;33:335.
59. Evans RS, Duane RT. Acquired hemolytic anemia: I. the relation of erythrocyte antibody to activity of the disease: II. the significance of thrombocytopenia and leukopenia. Blood 1949;4:1196.
60. Weiss GB, Bessman JD. Spurious automated red cell values in warm autoimmune hemolytic anemia. Am J Hematol 1984;17:433.
61. Young NS, Mortimer PP, Moore JG, et al. Characterization of a virus that causes transient aplastic crisis. J Clin Invest 1984;73:224.
62. Crosby WH, Rappaport H. Reticulocytopenia in autoimmune hemolytic anemia. Blood 1956;11:929.
63. de Boisfleury A. Forme et deformabilite des erythrocytes au cours de l'anemie hemolytique experimentale du rat: etude de leur comportement dans la micro-circulation splenique. (Thesis) d'Univeriste es-Sciences, Faculte des Sciences de Paris, 1977.
64. Dacie JV. The haemolytic anaemias: congenital and acquired. In: The auto-immune haemolytic anaemias, part II. New York, Grune & Stratton, 1962:341.
65. Dausset J, Colombani J. The serology and the prognosis of 128 cases of autoimmune hemolytic anemia. Blood 1959;14:1280.
66. Crosby WH, Rappaport H. Autoimmune hemolytic anemias: I. analysis of hematologic observations with particular reference to their prognostic value: a survey of 57 cases. Blood 1957;12:42.
67. Chanarin I, Dacie JV, Mollin DL. Folic-acid deficiency in haemolytic anaemia. Br J Haematol 1959;5:245.
68. Engelfriet CP, von dem Borne AEGK, Beckers Do, et al. Autoimmune haemolytic anaemia: serological and immunological characteristics of the autoantibodies: mechanisms of cell destruction. Ser Haematol 1974;7:328.
69. Rosse WF. Quantitative immunology of immune hemolytic anemia: II. the relationship of cell-bound antibody to hemolysis and the effect of treatment. J Clin Invest 1971;50:734.
70. Issitt PD. Serological diagnosis and characterization of the causative autoantibodies. In: Chaplin H Jr, ed. Methods in hematology: immune hemolytic aAnemias. New York, Churchill Livingstone, 1985:1.
71. Vos GH, Petz LD, Fudenberg HH. Specificity and immunoglobulin characteristics of autoantibodies in acquired hemolytic anemia. J Immunol 1971;106:1172.
72. Issitt PD. Some messages received from blood group antibodies. In: Red cell antigens and antibodies. American Association of Blood Banks, 1986.
73. Issitt PD, Pavone BG. Critical re-examination of the specificity of auto-anti-Rh antibodies in patients with a positive direct antiglobulin test. Br J Haematol 1978;38:63.
74. Weiner W, Vos GH. Serology of acquired hemolytic anemias. Blood 1963;22:606.
75. Marsh WL, Reid ME, Scott EP. Autoantibodies of U blood group specificity in autoimmune haemolytic anemia. Br J Haematol 1975;29: 247.
76. Issitt PD, Pavone BG, Wagstaff W, et al. The phenotypes En(a−), Wr(a−b−) and En(a+), Wr (a+b−), and further studies on the Wright and En blood groups systems. Transfusion 1976;16:396.
77. Goldfinger D, Zwicker H, Belkin GA, et al. An autoantibody with anti-Wr^b specificity in a patient with warm autoimmune hemolytic anemia. Transfusion 1975;15:351.
78. Telen MJ, Chasis J. Relationship of the human erythrocyte Wr^b antigen to an interaction between glycophorin A and band 3. Blood 1990;76: 842.
79. Kurlander RJ, Rosse WF, Logue GL. Quantitative influence of antibody and complement coating of red cells on monocyte-mediated cell lysis. J Clin Invest 1978;61:1309.
80. Lewis SM, Szur L, Dacie JV. The pattern of erythrocyte destruction in haemolytic anaemia, as studied with radioactive chromium. Br J Haematol 1960;6:122.
81. LoBuglio AF, Cotran RS, Jandl JH. Red cells coated with immunoglobulin G: binding and sphering by mononuclear cells in man. Science 1967;158:1582.
82. Weed RI. The importance of red cell deformability. Am J Med 1966;49: 147.
83. Chen L-T, Weiss L. The role of the sinus wall in the passage of erythrocytes through the spleen. Blood 1973;41:529.
84. Ehrlich P. Collected studies in immunity. In: New York, John Wiley, 1905.
85. Coutinho A. Beyond clonal selection and network. Immunol Rev 1989;110:63.
86. Rossi F, Dietrich G, Kazatchkine MD. Anti-idiotypes against autoantibodies in normal immunoglobulins: evidence for network regulation of human autoimmune responses. Immunol Rev 1989;110:135.
87. Rosse WF. Autoimmune disease due to warm-reacting antibodies: immune hemolytic anemia. In: Clinical hematology: basic concepts and clinical applications. New York, Blackwell, 1990:449.
88. Telen MJ, Roberts KB, Bartlett JA. HIV-associated autoimmune hemolytic anemia: report of a case and review of the literature. J AIDS 1990;3:933.
89. Einzig MJ, Neerhout RC. Hemolytic anemia in infectious mononucleosis. Clin Pediatr 1969;8:171.
90. Horwitz CA, Skradski K, Reece E, et al. Haemolytic anaemia in previously healthy adult patients with CMV infections: report of two cases and an evaluation of subclinical haemolysis in CMV mononucleosis. Scand J Haematol 1984;333:35.
91. Dacie JV, Worlledge SM. Auto-immune hemolytic anemias. Prog Hematol 1969;6:82.
92. Videbaek A. Auto-immune haemolytic anaemia in systemic lupus erythematosus. Acta Med Scand 1962;171:187.
93. MacKenzie MR, Creevy N. Hemolytic anemia with cold detectable IgG antibodies. Blood 1970;36:549.
94. Boling EP, Wen J, Reveille JD, et al. Primary Sjogren's syndrome and autoimmune hemolytic anemia in sisters: a family study. Am J Med 1983;74:1066.
95. Dameshek W, Rosenthal MC. Treatment of acquired hemolytic anemia with a note on the relationship of periarteritis nodosa to hemolytic anemia. Med Clin North Am 1951;35:1423.
96. Jones E, Jones JV, Woodbury JP, et al. Scleroderma and hemolytic anemia in a patient with deficiency of IgA and C4: a hitherto undescribed association. J Rheumatol 1987;14:609.
97. Ashby GH, Evans DI. Cartilage hair hypoplasia with thrombocytopenic purpura, autoimmune haemolytic anaemia and cell-mediated immunodeficiency. J R Soc Med 79:113. 1986.
98. Hinz CF, Boyer JT. Dysgammaglobulilnemia in the adult manifested as autoimmune hemolytic anemia. N Engl J Med 1963;269:1329.
99. Conley ME, Park L, Douglas SD. Childhood common variable immunodeficiency with autoimmune disease. J Pediatr 1986;108:915.
100. Hansen OP, Sorensen CH, Astrup L. Evans' syndrome in IgA deficiency: episodic autoimmune hemolytic anemia and thrombocytopenia during a years observation period. Scand J Haematol 1982;29:265.
101. Kyle RA, Kiely HJM, Stickney JM. Acquired hemolytic anemia in chronic lymphocytic leukemia and the lymphomas: survival and response to therapy in twenty-seven cases. Arch Intern Med 1959;04:61.
102. Dameshek W. Theories of autoimmunity. In: Conceptual advances in immunology and oncology. New York, Hoeber Medical Division, Harper & Row, 1963.
103. Eisner E, Ley MAB, Mayer K. Coombs'-positive hemolytic anemia in Hodgkin's disease. Ann Intern Med 1967;66:258.
104. Weitberg AB, Harmon DC. Autoimmune neutropenia, hemolytic anemia, and reticulocytopenia in Hodgkin's disease. Ann Intern Med 1984;100:702.
105. Halperin IC, Ninogue WF, Komninos ZD. Autoimmune hemolytic anemia and myasthenia gravis associated with thymoma. N Engl J Med 1966;275:663.
106. Mongan ES, Kern WA, Terry R. Hypogammaglobulinemia with thymoma, hemolytic anemia, and disseminated infection with cytomegalovirus. Ann Intern Med 1966;65;548.
107. Freedman J, Cheng LF, Murray D, et al. An unusual autoimmune hemolytic anemia in a patient with immunoblastic sarcoma. Am J Hematol 1983;14:175.
108. White S, Marsden JR, Marks JM, Proctor S. Autoimmune haemolytic anaemia occurring in a patient with mycosis fungoides. Br J Dermatol 1984;110:495.
109. Bakemeier RF, Leddy JP. Heavy:light chain relationships among erythrocyte autoantibodies. J Clin Invest 1967;46:1033.
110. Butler WT. Corticosteroids and immunoglobulin synthesis. Transplant Proc 1975;7:49.
111. Sanders MC, Levinson AI, Schreiber AD. Hormonal modulation of macrophage clearance of IgG-sensitized cells. Trans Assoc Am Physicians 1987;100:268.
112. Worlledge SM, Brain MC, Cooper AC, et al. Immunosuppressive drugs in the treatment of autoimmune haemolytic anaemia. Proc R Soc Med 1968;61:1312.
113. Skinner MD, Schwartz RS. Immunosuppressive therapy. N Engl J Med 1972;287:221.
114. Murphy S, LoBuglio AF. Drug therapy in autoimmune hemolytic anemia. Semin Hematol 1976;13:323.
115. Kyle RA. Second malignancies associated with chemotherapeutic agents. Semin Oncol 1982;9:131.
116. Corley CC. Azothiaprine therapy in autoimmune diseases. Am J Med 1966;41:404.

117. Ahn YS, Harrington WJ, Byrnes JJ, et al. Treatment of autoimmune hemolytic anemia with vinca-loaded platelets. JAMA 1983;249:2189.
118. Gertz MA, Petit RM, Alvaro A, et al. Vinblastine-loaded platelets for autoimmune hemolytic anemia. Ann Intern Med 1981;95:325.
119. Garelli S, Mosconi L, Valbonesi M, et al. Plasma exchange for hemolytic crisis due to autoimmune hemolytic anemia of the IgG warm type. Blut 1980;41:387.
120. Kutti J, Vadenvik H, Safai-Kutti S, et al. Successful treatment of refractory autoimmune haemolytic anaemia by plasmapheresis. Scand J Haematol 1984;32:149.
121. Bowdler AJ. The role of the spleen and splenectomy in autoimmune hemolytic disease. Semin Hematol 1976;13:335.
122. Smith CH, Erlandson M, Schulman I, et al. Hazard of severe infection in splenectomized infants and children. Am J Med 1957;22:390.
123. Parker AC, MacPherson AIS, Richmond J. Value of radiochromium investigation in autoimmune haemolytic anaemia. Br Med J 1977;1: 208.
124. Kurlander RJ, Colman RE, Moore J, et al. Comparison of the efficacy of a two-day and a five-day schedule for infusing intravenous gammaglobulin in the treatment of immune thrombocytopenic purpura in adults. Am J Med 1987;83:17.
125. Imbach P. A multicenter European trial of intravenous immune globulin in immune thrombocytopenic purpura in childhood. Vox Sang 1985;49: 25.
126. Vos JJ, van Aken WG, Engelfriet CP, et al. Intravenous gammaglobulin therapy in idiopathic thrombocytopenic purpura: results with the Netherlands Red Cross immunoglobulin preparation. Vox Sang 1985;49: 92.
127. Macintyre EA, Linch DC, Macey MG, et al. Successful response to intravenous immunoglobulin in autoimmune haemolytic anaemia. Br J Haematol 1985;60:387.
128. Muller-Eckhardt C, Salama A, Mahn I, et al. Lack of efficacy of high-dose intravenous immunoglobulin in autoimmune haemolytic anaemia: a clue to its mechanism. Scand J Haematol 1985;34:394.
129. Ahn YS, Harrington WJ, Simon SR, et al. Danazol for the treatment of idiopathic thrombocytopenic purpura. N Engl J Med 1983;308:1396.
130. Buelli M, Cortelazzo S, Viero P, et al. Danazol for the treatment of idiopathic thrombocytopenic purpura. Acta Haematol 1985;74:97.
131. Ahn YS, Harrington WJ, Mylvaganam R, et al. Danazol therapy for autoimmune hemolytic anemia. Ann Intern Med 1985;102:298.
132. Clarkson SB, Bussel JB, Kimberly RP, et al. Treatment of refractory immune thrombocytopenic purpura with an anti-Fc gamma receptor antibody. N Engl J Med 1986;314:1236.
133. Petz LD. Immunohematology: acquired immune hemolytic anemias. In: Current hematology and oncology, vol 3. New York, John Wiley & Sons, 1984:51.
134. Dameshek W, Komninos ZD. The present status of treatment of autoimmune hemolytic anemia with ACTH and cortisone. Blood 1956;11: 648.
135. Freedman J, Wright J, Lim FC, et al. Hemolytic warm IgM autoagglutinins in autoimmune hemolytic anemia. Transfusion 1987;27:464.
136. Shirey RS, Kickler TS, Bell W, et al. Fatal immune hemolytic anemia and hepatic failure associated with a warm-reacting IgM autoantibody. Vox Sang 1987;52:219.
137. Rosse WF. Autoimmune hemolytic anemia due to cold-reacting antibodies. In: Cold agglutinin disease in clinical immunohematology: basic concepts and clinical applications. Oxford, Blackwell Scientific, 1989.
138. Schubothe H. The cold hemagglutinin disease. Semin Hematol 1966;3: 27.
139. Sokol RJ, Hewitt S, Stamps BK. Autoimmune hemolysis: mixed warm and cold antibody type. Acta Haematol 1983;69:266.
140. Pruzanski W, Shumak KH. Biologic activity of cold reactive autoantibodies. N Engl J Med 1977;297:538.
141. Frank MM, Atkinson JP, Gadek J. Cold agglutinins and cold agglutinin disease. Annu Rev Med 1977;28:291.
142. Crisp D, Pruzanski W. B-cell neoplasms with homogenous cold-reacting antibodies (cold agglutinins). Am J Med 1982;72:915.
143. Schreiber AD, Herskovitz BS, Goldwein M. Low-titer cold-hemagglutinin disease: mechanism of hemolysis and response to corticosteroids. N Engl J Med 1977;296:1490.
144. Bessman JD, Banks D. Spurious macrocytosis, a common clue to erythrocyte cold agglutinins. Am J Clin Pathol 1980;74:797.
145. Feizi R, Werner P, Kunkel, HG, et al. Lymphocytes forming red cell rosettes in the cold in patients with chronic cold agglutinin disease. Blood 1973;42:753.
146. Haynes CR, Chaplin H Jr. An enhancing effect of albumin on the determination of cold hemagglutinins. Vox Sang 1971;20:46.
147. Garratty G, Petz LD, Hoops JK. The correlation of cold agglutinin titrations in saline and albumin with haemolytic anaemia. Br J Haematol 1977;35:587.
148. Wiener AS, Unger LJ, Cohen L, et al. Type-specific auto-antibodies as a cause of acquired hemolytic anemia and hemolytic transfusion reactions: biological test with bovine red cells. Ann Intern Med 1956;44: 221.
149. Marsh WL. Anti-i: a cold antibody defining the I-i relationship in human red blood cells. Br J Haematol 1961;7:200.
150. Roelcke D, Ebert W, Metz J, et al. 1 I-, MN- and Pr_1/Pr-activity of human erythrocyte glycoprotein fractions obtained by ficin treatment. Vox Sang 1971;21:352.
151. Roelcke D. Reaction of anti-Gd, anti-F1 and anti-Sa cold agglutinins with p erythrocytes. Vox Sang 1984;46:161.
152. Roelcke D. The Lud cold agglutinin: a further antibody recognizing N-acetylneuraminic acid-determined antigens not fully expressed at birth. Vox Sang 1981;41:316.
153. Niemann H, Watanabe K, Hakomori SI, et al. Blood groups i and I activities of lacto-N-nor-hexosylceramine and its analogues: the structural requirements for i specificities. Biochem Biophys Res Comm 1978;81:1286.
154. Watanabe K, Hakomori SI, Childs RA, et al. Characterization of a blood group I active ganglioside: structural requirements for the I and i specificities. J Biol Chem 1979;254:3221.
155. Feizi T, Kabat EA. Immunochemical studies on blood groups: LIV. classification of anti-I and anti-i sera into groups based on reactivity patterns with various antigens related to blood group A, B, H, Le^a, Le^b, and precursor substances. J Exp Med 1972;135:1247.
156. Roelcke D. Serological studies on the Pr_1/Pr_2 antigens using dog erythrocytes. Vox Sang 1973;24:354.
157. Fudenberg HH, Kunkel HG. Physical properties of red cell agglutinins in acquired hemolytic anemia. J Exp Med 1957;106:689.
158. Capra JD, Dowling P, Cook S, et al. An incomplete cold-reactive γG antibody with i specificity in infectious mononucleosis. Vox Sang 1969;17:10.
159. Goldberg LS, Barnett EV. Mixed γ G-γ M cold agglutinin. J Immunol 1967;99:803.
160. Spiva DA, George JN, Sears DA. Acute autoimmune hemolytic anemia due to a low molecular weight IgM cold hemolysin associated with episodic lymphoid granulomatous vasculitis. Am J Med 1974;56:417.
161. Angevine CS, Andersen BR, Barnett EV. A cold agglutinin of the IgA class. J Immunol 1966;96:578.
162. Jacobson LB, Longstreth GF, Edgerton TS. Clinical and immunologic features of transient cold agglutinin hemolytic anemia. Am J Med 1973;54:514.
163. Harboe M. Exclusive occurrence of κ chains in isolated cold haemagglutinins. Scand J Haematol 1965;2:259.
164. Feizi T, Lecomte J, Childs R, et al. κ chain (V_kIII) subgroup-related activity in an idiotypic anti-cold agglutinin serum. Scand J Immunol 1976;5:629.
165. Feizi T, Lecomte J, Childs R. An immunoglobulin heavy chain variable region (V_H) marker associated with cross-reactive idiotypes in man. Clin Exp Immunol 1974;30:233.
166. Feizi T, Kunkel HG, Roeleke D. Cross idiotypic specificity among cold agglutinins in relation to combining activity for blood group-related antigens. Clin Exp Immunol 1977;18:283.
167. Feizi T. λ Chains in cold agglutinins. Science 1967;156:1111.
168. Evans RS, Turner E, Bingham M, et al. Chronic hemolytic anemia due to cold agglutinin. II. The role of C′ in red cell destruction. J Clin Invest 1968;47:691.
169. Rosse WF, Sherwood JB. Cold-reacting antibodies: differences in the reaction of anti-I antibodies with adult and cord red blood cells. Blood 1970;36:28.
170. Rosse WF, Adams JP. The variability of hemolysis in the cold agglutinin syndrome. Blood 1980;56:409.
171. Logue, GL, Rosse WF, Gockerman JP. Measurement of the third component of complement bound to red blood cells in patients with cold agglutinin syndrome. J Clin Invest 1973;52:493.
172. Ross GD, Medof ME. Membrane complement receptors specific for bound fragments of C3. Adv Immunol 1985;37:217.
173. Ross GD, Lambris JD, Cain JA, et al. Generation of three different fragments of bound C3 with purified factor I or serum: I. requirements for factor H vs CRa cofactor activity. J Immunol 1982;129:2051.
174. Finland M, Peterson OL, Allen HE, et al. Occurrence of cold isohemagglutinins in various conditions. J Clin Invest 1993;24:451.
175. Jenkins WJ, Koster HG, Marsh WL, et al. Infectious mononucleosis, an unsuspected source of anti-i. Br J Haematol 1965;11:480.
176. Horwitz CA, Moulds J, Henle W, et al. Cold agglutinins in infectious mononucleosis and heterophil-antibody–negative mononucleosis-like syndromes. Blood 1977;50:195.
177. Tanowitz HB, Robbins N, Leidich N. Hemolytic anemia: associated with severe mycoplasma pneumoniae pneumonia. NY State J Med 1979;78:2231.
178. Thurin RH, Bassen F. Infectious mononucleosis and acute hemolytic anemia: report of two cases and review of the literature. Blood 1955;10: 841.
179. Janney FA, Lee LT, Howe C. Cold hemagglutinin cross-reactivity with Mycoplasma pneumoniae. Infect Immun 1978;22:29.
180. Loomes LM, Uemura K, Childs RA, et al. Erythrocyte receptors for Mycoplasma pneumoniae are sialylated oligosaccharides of the Ii antigen type. Nature 1984;307:560.
181. Costea N, Yakulis V, Heller P. Experimental production of cold agglutinins in rabbits. Blood 1965;26:323.
182. Worlledge SM, Dacie JV. Haemolytic and other anaemias in infectious mononucleosis. In: Carter HG, Penman RL, eds. Infectious mononucleosis. Oxford, Blackwell Scientific, 1969.

183. Wortman J, Rosse WF, Logue G. Cold agglutinin hemolytic anemia in nonhematologic malignancies. Am J Hematol 1979;6:275.
184. Landymore R, Isom W, Barlam B. Management of patients with cold agglutinins who require open-heart surgery. Can J Surg 1983;26:79.
185. Blumberg N, Hicks G, Woll J, et al. Successful cardiac bypass surgery in the presence of a potent cold agglutinin without plasma exchange. Transfusion 1983;23:363.
186. Taft EG, Propp RP, Sullivan SA. Plasma exchange for cold agglutinin hemolytic anemia. Transfusion 1977;17:173.
187. Isbister JP, Biggs JC, Penny R. Experience with large volume plasmapheresis in malignant paraproteinaemia and immune disorders. Aust NZ J Med 1978;8:154.
188. Oleson H. Chlorambucil treatment in the cold agglutinin syndrome. Scand J Haematol 1964;1:116.
189. Hippe E, Jensen KB, Olesen H, et al. Chlorambucil treatment of patients with cold agglutinin syndrome. 1970ood 35:68.
190. Dacie JV. The autoimmune haemolytic anaemias IV: paroxysmal cold hemoglobinuria, syphlitic and non-syphlitic. In: The haemolytic anaemias: congenital and acquired. New York, Grune & Stratton, 1962: 545.
191. Petz LD, Garratty G. In: Acquired immune hemolytic anemias. New York, Churchill Livingstone, 1980.
192. Ries CA, Garratty G, Petz LD, et al. Paroxysmal cold hemoglobinuria: report of a case with an exceptionally high thermal range Donath-Landsteiner antibody. Blood 1971;38:491.
193. Worrledge SM, Rousso C. Studies on the serology of paroxysmal cold hemoglobinuria (PCH) with special reference to its relationship with the P blood group system. Vox Sang 1965;10:293.
194. Levine P, Celano MJ, Falkowski F. The specificity of the antibody in paroxysmal cold hemoglobinuria (PCH). Transfusion 1963;3:278.
195. Schwaring GA, Kundu SK, Marcus DM. Reaction of antibodies that cause paroxysmal cold hemoglobinuria (PCH) with globoside and Forssman glycosphingolipids. Blood 1979;53:186.
196. Bell CA, Zwicker H, Rosenbaum DL. Paroxysmal cold hemoglobinuria (PCH) following mycoplasma infection: anti-I specificity of the biphasic hemolysin. Transfusion 1973;13:138.
197. Nordhagen R, Sensvold K, Winsnes A, et al. Paroxysmal cold haemoglobinuria: the most frequent acute autoimmune haemolytic anaemia in children? Acta Paediatr Scand 1984;73:258.
198. O'Neill BJ, Marshall WC. Paroxysmal cold haemoglobinuria and measles. Arch Dis Child 1967;42:183.
199. Bunch C, Schwartz FC, Bird GW. Paroxysmal cold haemoglobinuria following measles immunization. Arch Dis Child 1972;47:299.
200. Bird GW, Wingham J, Martin AJ, et al. Idiopathic non-syphilitic paroxysmal cold haemoglobinuria in children. J Clin Pathol 1976;29:215.
201. Prasad AS, Berman L, Tranchida L, et al. Red cell hypoplasia, cold hemoglobinuria and M-type gamma G serum paraprotein and Bence Jones proteinuria in a patient with lymphoproliferative disorder. Blood 1968;31:151.
202. Rausen AR, LeVine R, Hsu TC, et al. Compatible transfusion therapy for paroxysmal cold hemoglobinuria. Pediatrics 1975;55:275.
203. Wolach B, Heddle N, Barr RD, et al. The variability of hemolysis in the cold agglutinin syndrome. Blood 1981;56:409.
204. Harris JW. Studies on the mechanism of a drug-induced hemolytic anemia. J Lab Clin Med 1954;44:809.
205. Harris JW. Studies on the mechanism of a drug-induced hemolytic anemia. J Lab Clin Med 1956;47:670.
206. Petz LD, Garratty G. In: Acquired immune hemolytic anemia. New York, Churchill Livingstone, 1980.
207. Worlledge SM. Immune drug-induced haemolytic anaemias. Semin Hematol 1969;6:181.
208. Landsteiner K, Jacobs J. Studies on the sensitization of animals with simple chemical compounds. J Exp Med 1936;64:625.
209. MacGibbon H, Loughridge LW, Hourihane DO'B, et al. Autoimmune haemolytic anaemia with acute renal failure due to phenacetin and p-aminosalicylic acid. Lancet 1960;1:7.
210. Bloomfield RJ, Wilson IF. Nomifensine, acute hemolytic anemia, and renal failure. Ann Intern Med 1986;105:807.
211. de Torregrosa MVV, Rosada Rodrigues AL, Montilla E. Hemolytic anemia secondary to stibophen therapy. JAMA 1963;186:598.
212. Lindberg LG, Norden A. Severe hemolytic reaction to chlorpromazine. Acta Med Scand 1961;179:195.
213. Petz LD, Fudenberg HH. Coombs'-positive hemolytic anemia caused by penicillin administration. N Engl J Med 1966;274:171.
214. Swanson MA, Chanmougan D, Schwartz RS. Immunohemolytic anemia due to antipenicillin antibodies. N Engl J Med 1966;274:178.
215. Reis CA, Rosenbaum TJ, Garratty G, et al. Penicillin-induced immune hemolytic anemia. JAMA 1975;233:432.
216. Logue GL, Boyd AE III, Rosse WF. Chlorpropamide-induced immune hemolytic anemia. N Engl J Med 1970;283:900.
217. Spath P, Garratty G, Petz LD. Studies on the immune response to penicillin and cephalothin in humans. II. Immunohematologic reactions to cephalothin administration. J Immunol 1971;107:860.
218. Habibi B, Bretagne Y. Les antigenes de groups sanguins peuvent etre les cibles des conflits immunoallergiques medicamenteux a affinite erythrocytaire. C R Acad Sci 1983;296:693.
219. Habibi B, Basty R, Chodez S, et al. Thiopental-related immune hemolytic anemia and renal failure: specific involvement of red-cell antigen I. N Engl J Med 1985;312:353.
220. Salama A, Mueller-Eckhardt C. Rh blood group-specific antibodies in immune hemolytic anemia induced by nomifensine. Blood 1986;68: 1285.
221. Salama A, Mueller-Eckhardt C. The role of metabolite-specific antibodies in nomifensine-dependent immune hemolytic anemia. N Engl J Med 1985;313:469.
222. Carstairs KC, Worlledge S, Dollery CT, et al. Methyldopa and haemolytic anaemia. Lancet 1966;1:201.
223. Carstairs KC, Breckenridge A, Dollery CT, et al. Incidence of a positive direct Coombs' test in patients on (α)-methyldopa. Lancet 1966;2: 133.
224. LoBuglio AF, Jandl JH. The nature of the alpha-methyl-dopa red-cell antibody. N Engl J Med 1967;276:658.
225. Bakemeier RF, Leddy JP. Erythrocyte autoantibody associated with alpha-methyldopa: heterogeneity of structure and specificity. Blood 1968;32:1.
226. Shulman NR. A mechanism of red cell destruction in individuals sensitized to foreign antigens and its implications in autoimmunity. Ann Intern Med 1964;60:506.
227. Christie DJ, Aster RH. Drug–antibody–platelet interaction in quinine- and quinidine-induced thrombocytopenia. J Clin Invest 1982;70: 989.
228. Kirtland HH, Mohler DN. Chronic stimulation of lymphocyte cyclic AMP: a proposed etiology for methyldopa-induced autoimmunity. Blood 1977;50:295.
229. Green FA, Jung CY, Rampal A, et al. Alpha-methyldopa and the erythrocyte membrane. Clin Exp Immunol 1980;40:554.
230. Green FA, Jung Cy, Hui A. Modulation of alpha-methyldopa binding to the erythrocyte membrane by superoxide dismutase. Biochem Biophys Res Commun 1989;95:1037.
231. Issitt PD. Serological diagnosis and characterization of the causative antibodies. In: Chaplin H Jr, ed. Methods in hematology: immune hemolytic anemias. New York, Churchill Livingston, 1985.
232. Freedman AL, Barr PS, Brody EA. Hemolytic anemia due to quinidine: observations on its mechanism. Am J Med 19596;20:806.
233. Zeigler Z, Shaddock RK, Winkelstein A, et al. Immune hemolytic anemia and thrombocytopenia secondary to quinidine: in vitro studies of the quinidine-dependent red cell and platelet antibodies. Blood 1979;52: 396.
234. Bell CA, Zwicker H, Lee S, et al. Quinidine hemolytic anemia in the absence of thrombocytopenia in a patient with hemoglobin D. Transfusion 1973;13:100.
235. Ballas SK, Caro JF, Miguel O. Quinidine-induced hemolytic anemia: Immunohematological characterization. Transfusion 1978;18:215.
236. Muirhead EE, Halden ER, Groves M. Drug-dependent Coombs' test and anemia. Ann Intern Med 1958;101:87.
237. Strumia PV, Raymond FD. Acquired hemolytic anemia and antipenicillin antibody: case report and review of literature. Arch Intern Med 1962;109:603.
238. Kerr RO, Cardmone J, Dalmasso AP, et al. Two mechanisms of erythrocyte destruction in penicillin-induced hemolytic anemia. N Engl J Med 1972;287:1322.
239. Abraham GN, Petz LD, Fudenberg HH. Immunohaematological cross-allergenicity between penicillin and cephalothin in humans. Clin Exp Immunol 1968;3:543.
240. Gralnick HR, McGinniss MH, Elton W, et al. Hemolytic anemia associated with cephalothin. JAMA 1971;217:1193.
241. Jeannet M, Block A, Dayer JM, et al. Cephalothin-induced immune hemolytic anemia. Acta Haematol 1976;55:109.
242. Forbes CD, Craig JA, Mitchell R, et al. Acute intravascular hemolysis associated with cephalexin therapy. Postgrad Med J 1972;48:186.
243. Gralnick HR, McGinniss MH. Immune cross-reactivity of penicillin and cephalothin. Nature 1967;215:1026.
244. Gralnick HR, Wright LD, McGinniss MH. Coombs' positive reactions associated with sodium cephalothin therapy. JAMA 1967;199:725.
245. Salama A, Gottsche B, Schleiffer T, et al. "Immune complex" mediated intravascular hemolysis due to IgM cephalosporin-dependent antibody. Transfusion 1987;27:460.
246. Tajima H. Clinical studies in hemolytic anemia. Acta Haematol Jpn 1960;23:188.
247. Dausset J, Bergerto-Blondel Y. Etude d'un anticorps allergique actif en presence de para-amino-salicylate de soude (PAS) contre les hematies, les leucocytes et les plaquettes humaines. Vox Sang 1961;6:91.
248. Weiss HJ, Burger RE, Tice AD, et al. Fatal disseminated intravascular coagulation and hemolytic anemia following stibophen therapy. Am J Med Sci 1972;264:375.
249. Wenz G, Klein RL, Lalezari P. Tetracycline-induced immune hemolytic anemia. Transfusion 1974;14:265.
250. Nance SJ, Ladisch S, Williamson TL, et al. Erythromycin-induced immune hemolytic anemia. Vox Sang 1988;55:233.
251. Seldon MR, Bain B, Johnson CA, et al. Ticarcillin-induced immune haemolytic anaemia. Scand J Haematol 1982;28:459.
252. Shinton NK, Wilson C. Autoimmune hemolytic anemia due to phenacetin and p-aminosalicylic acid. Lancet 1960;1:226.
253. Dramer MR, Levene C, Hershko C. Severe reversible autoimmune and

thrombocytopenia with diclofenac therapy. Scand J Haematol 1986;36: 118.
254. Wolf B, Conradty M, Grohmann R, et al. A case of immune complex hemolytic anemia, thrombocytopenia, and acute renal failure associated with doxepin use. J Clin Psychiatry 1989;50:99.
255. Salama A, Mueller-Eckhardt C. Two types of nomifensine-induced immune haemolytic anaemias: drug-dependent sensitization and/or autoimmunization. Br J Haematol 1986;64:613.
256. Salama A, Mueller-Eckhardt C, Kissel K, et al. Ex vivo antigen preparation for the serological detection of drug-dependent antibodies in immune haemolytic anaemias. Br J Haematol 1984;58:525.
257. Fulton JD, Briggs JD, Dominiczak AF, et al. Intravascular haemolysis and acute renal failure induced by nomifensine. Scott Med J 1986;31: 242.
258. Jacobson ES. Immune thrombocytopenia induced by ethchlorvinol. Ann Intern Med 1972;77:73.
259. Habibi B, Basty R, Chodez S, et al. Thiopental-related immune hemolytic anemia and renal failure: specific involvement of red-cell antigen I. N Engl J Med 1985;312:353.
260. Vila JM, Blum L, Dosik H. Thiazide-induced immune hemolytic anemia. JAMA 1978;236:1723.
261. Sirey RS, Bartholomew J, Bell W, et al. Characterization of antibody and selection of alternative drug therapy in hydrochlorothiazide-induced immune hemolytic anemia. Transfusion 1988;28:70.
262. Patten E, Beck CE, Scholl C, et al. Autoimmune hemolytic anemia with anti-Jk[a] specificity in a patient taking Aldomet. Transfusion 1977;17:517.
263. Kleinman S, Nelson R, Smith L, et al. Positive direct antiglobulin tests and immune hemolytic anemia in patients receiving procainamide. N Engl J Med 1984;311:809.
264. Sosler DS, Behzad O, Garratty G, et al. Acute hemolytic anemia associated with a chlorpropamide-induced apparent auto-anti Jk. Transfusion 1984;24:206.
265. Nataas OB, Nesthus I. Immune haemolytic anaemia induced by glibenclamide in selective IgA deficiency. Br Med J 1987;295:366.
266. Kopicky JA, Packman CH. The mechanisms of sulfonylurea-induced immune hemolysis: case report and review of the literature. Am J Hematol 1986;23:283.
267. Woolley PF, Sacher RA, Priego VM, et al. Methotrexate-induced immune haemolytic anaemia. Br J Haematol 1983;54:543.
268. Kickler TS, Buck S, Ness P, et al. Probenecid induced immune hemolytic anemia. J Rheumatol 1986;13:208.
269. Sosler SK, Behzad O, Garratty G, et al. Immune hemolytic anemia associated with probenecid. Am J Clin Pathol 1985;84:391.

Blood: Principles and Practice of Hematology,
edited by Robert I. Handin, Samuel E. Lux, and Thomas P. Stossel.
J.B. Lippincott Company, Philadelphia © 1995.

56

Blood Cell Antigens and Alloimmune Disorders

Peter Agre
Diana Beardsley

BLOOD CELL ANTIGENS

After World War II, blood group serology emerged as a major hospital-based research field, and the contributions of numerous investigators have identified hundreds of different blood antigens of varying clinical and scientific importance. Although a complete analysis of all these antigens is beyond the scope of this chapter, the major antigens, their structural and immunologic features, and their clinical relevance are listed herein. Noted are specialized texts that are available with complete serologic information.[1–3]

The erythrocyte blood group antigens are composed of many families of membrane components. Although each is defined by a specific antibody, the classes of immunoglobulin vary. Some antibodies such as anti-A, and anti-B are immunoglobulins (specifically IgM) and occur naturally. Other antibodies, such as anti-Rh(D), are IgG and result only from transfusion or pregnancy.

Families of related or allelic blood group antigens are called *groups* or *systems*. The genes responsible for antigenic variants within a group are often alleles. The difference between alleles is frequently only a single nucleotide, which leads to a single amino acid substitution in the gene product. Single amino acid substitutions may result in proteins with remarkable immunologic differences or glycosyltransferases with different sugar specificities.

Genes are always written in italics or underlined (eg, *Fy*^{a} and *Fy*^{b}, the major genes of the Duffy system). Allelic genes encode antithetical antigens. Antigens are written without italics or underlining (Fy^a and Fy^b).

The biochemical structures of the different antigen groups are distinct. Members of the ABO antigen system are specific carbohydrate structures attached to glycolipids and several different membrane-spanning proteins by the actions of glycosyltransferases. Members of the MNSs antigen system are specific glycoproteins; the antigenic epitopes contain both carbohydrate and polypeptide. Other antigen systems such as Kell and Kidd are made up of specific polypeptides, and some such as Rh may be complexes of lipid and protein. Although the structural features of some antigens are well understood, the nature of other blood group antigens is only now emerging. The physiologic importance of some antigens is obvious since certain null phenotypes are pathologically affected (such as Rh$_{null}$ or McLeod erythrocytes), whereas other null phenotypes do not result in any detectable hematologic abnormality (such as En[a−]).

A person may become immunized to a specific antigen because of exposure through blood transfusion or pregnancy. The transfusion poses the greater immunologic risk, although pregnancy is obviously a more common event. Other factors influencing the chance of alloimmunization are the abundance and potency of the antigen. The number of antigenic sites varies from about 10^6 A and B antigens per erythrocyte to about 10^3 Le^a sites. Moreover, the frequencies of the different polymorphisms vary among different racial groups for each antigen, which creates additional complexity when matching patient samples.

When various patients who have developed such antibodies are compared, certain antigens are observed as being more immunogenic than others. The D antigen is by far the most immunogenic and accounts for 75% to 85% of all acquired alloantibodies.[4] After the D antigen, other Rh antigens as well as antigens in the Kell, Duffy, and Kidd systems account for most alloimmunization (Table 56-1). In terms of numeric frequency, the D, c, and E antigens more often provoke alloimmunization; when corrected for the likelihood of antigenic mismatch, the Kell antigens are probably even more potent immunogens. Other factors such as history of splenectomy and simultaneous transfusion with multiple foreign antigens may determine whether alloimmunization will occur.

The presence or absence of all antigens is determined by standard serologic methods. Despite the application of automation and the development of manufactured immunologic panels, the basic work of the hospital blood bank laboratory remains the recognition of blood group antigens and antibodies by their ability to produce agglutination, the physical "clump" or "no clump" phenomenon, which is diligently performed countless times each day in every hospital blood bank.

Hemagglutination is well recognized as resulting from the abundance of specific blood group antigens as well as the type of the corresponding antibody. Antibodies of the

TABLE 56-1. Relative Frequencies of Erythrocyte Alloantibodies*

Blood Group System	Relative Frequency of Antibody†	Relative Potency of Antigen (Compared with K)‡
Rh*	0.5	0.3
Kell	0.3	1.0
Duffy	0.15	0.04
Kidd	0.05	0.01
Other	<0.01	Negligible

* Rh(D) excluded.
† Calculated from Grove-Rasmussen and Huggins[4] and Tovey.[7]
‡ Data from Giblett.[5]

IgM class have molecular diameters of 30 nm and directly agglutinate erythrocytes; IgGs have diameters of 12 nm and often fail to agglutinate or can actually block agglutination unless an exogenous source of cross-linking antibody is added (antiglobulin test wherein goat or rabbit antihuman IgG is added to agglutinate the IgG-coated erythrocytes).

Serologists use multiple methods to enhance agglutinability to confirm the presence of antigen or antibody in a patient's blood. Use of low ionic strength buffers and the presence of albumin are often useful. Proteolytic digestion of erythrocytes with papain reduces the electrostatic repulsion between erythrocytes resulting from surface sialoglycoproteins and may also reduce steric restraints to surface antigens, thereby enhancing agglutination. Optimal temperatures of reactivity vary as well and may need to be manipulated to uncover potential reactivity.

EARLY HISTORY OF BLOOD ANTIGENS

The discovery of blood group antigens and the development of transfusion therapy make up a major chapter in the history of medical research. Although investigation of blood transfusions among different species and among humans had been attempted as early as the 17th century, initial efforts were of dubious success and probably provided the first evidence of immune intolerance of transfused blood. Some patients received transfusions repeatedly and were noted to experience feverishness and the passage of dark urine. The effects of these primitive transfusions were sometimes lethal, precipitating the Paris Society of Physicians in 1668 and subsequently the Royal Society of England and the Magistrates of Rome to ban blood transfusions. This prohibition lasted 150 years. The recognition of blood group antigens in the early days of the 20th century made transfusions not only possible, but a major effort of modern hospital laboratory practice.[8]

Karl Landsteiner and the Discovery of the ABO Blood Groups

The discovery of blood group antigens was the direct result of the intense curiosity of Karl Landsteiner (1868 to 1943), whose career was reviewed by his long-term assistant and colleague, Philip Levine (1900 to 1987).[9] Having received his doctorate from the University of Vienna in 1891, Landsteiner postponed his clinical advancement by spending 5 additional years studying chemistry and bacteriology in preparation for a research career. When he finally received a university faculty assistantship, Landsteiner was said to have fulfilled his clinical and teaching duties as rapidly as possible to pursue his experiments.

Although previous investigators had noted that infected patients developed antisera to the invading organisms, Landsteiner had observed that the sera of some of these patients could agglutinate the cells of other patients. Instead of accepting this as the result of the underlying inflammatory disease, Landsteiner made the intuitive leap that this might be unrelated to disease and tested the ability of serum to agglutinate erythrocytes from normal people. The most accessible normal subjects were the investigator's university colleagues. Landsteiner found that the 22 samples fell into three types A, B, and C. Serum from type C (now known as type O) clumped cells from either A or B, but cells from type C were not clumped by serum from A or B. Serum from type A clumped cells from B, and serum from type B clumped cells from A.[10] Moreover, the isoagglutination was due to substances that could be extracted even from dried blood stains, an observation that was to be of great importance in forensic pathology.

The following year, two of Landsteiner's students extended the significance of his report by studying a larger group: 121 patients and 34 healthy people.[11] The relative proportion of the A, B, and C types was the same in patients and in healthy people, thus confirming the lack of disease relation. In addition, they observed four people (now known to be type AB) whose serum failed to agglutinate cells from type A, B, or C, but whose cells were agglutinated by sera from the other groups. Landsteiner recognized that these findings would be essential to the future development of blood transfusions between humans. The importance was not appreciated for several years[12,13] nor was the genetic basis of blood group inheritance.[14] The presence of A, B, and C blood group substances was thereafter recognized in other tissues and secretions. This work, which is the basis from which blood group serology was developed, was appropriately recognized by awarding the 1932 Nobel Prize for Medicine and Physiology to Karl Landsteiner.

INDIVIDUAL BLOOD GROUPS

Polysaccharide Antigens

The polysaccharide antigens make up a class of related structures that result from the actions of several different glycosyltransferases competing for a group of common precursors. These antigens are defined by antibodies with distinct specificity, and the glycosyltransferases are the products of multiple genetic loci. Nevertheless, the core polysaccharides are themselves highly interrelated. The biochemistry and clinical features of the polysaccharide antigens are reviewed in detail elsewhere.[2,15,16]

Biosynthesis

Of the numerous naturally occurring sugars, only a few are immunologically active components of blood group antigens. Because of the restricted geometry of peptide bonds, two amino acids are joined in only two different conformations. In contrast, the glycosidic bonds between two hexose sugars of a disaccharide may take any of dozens of different conformations since there are six positions on each of the two sugars, with either α (below the plane) or β (above the plane) orientation (Fig. 56-1). Therefore, it is not surprising that a host of blood group antigenic structures may be derived by varying assembly of the sugars: D-glucose (Glc), D-galactose (Gal), L-fucose (Fuc), N-acetylglucosamine (GlcNAc), N-acetylgalactosamine (GalNAc), and N-acetylneuraminic acid, only the last being negatively charged at physiologic pH.

The polysaccharide antigens are associated with erythroid and nonerythroid plasma membranes and also exist

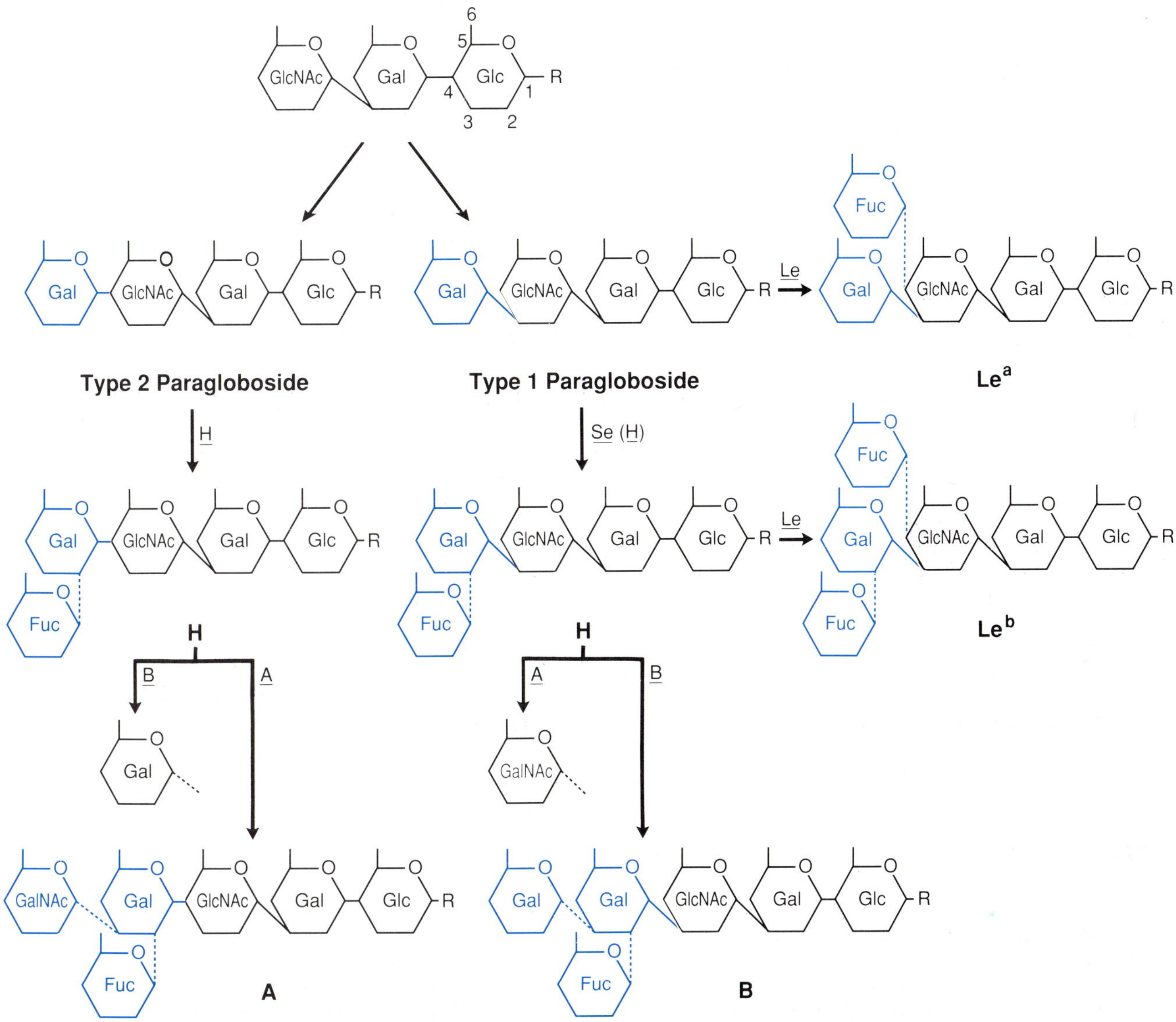

FIGURE 56-1. Diagram of ABH, Lewis, and paragloboside structures. Sugars are denoted as follows: D-glucose (Glc), D-galactose (Gal), L-fucose (Fuc), N-acetylglucosamine (GlcNAc), N-acetylgalactosamine (GalNAc), and N-acetylneuraminic acid (NANA). Glycosidic bonds with α orientation are represented by broken lines, and those with β orientation are represented by solid lines. Genes encoding glycosyl transferases are underlined. R indicates an undesignated polypeptide or lipid. A, B, and H antigens formed on type 2 paraglobosides are expressed on red cell membranes as a result of synthesis in red cells. The A, B, H, and Lewis antigens that are present in the plasma and in secretions are formed on type 1 paraglobosides. Some of the antigens formed on type 1 paraglobosides passively adsorb onto red cell membranes from plasma. The secreted forms of A, B, H, and Lewis antigens have Fuc attached to the position 2 of the terminal Gal on type 1 paragloboside as a result of the action of Se. This figure is a simplification. Only the differing terminal sugars (GalNAc or Gal) are shown on the structures of the B antigen (on type 2 paragloboside) and the A antigen (on type 1 paragloboside). (After Rosse WF, Telen MJ. The biochemistry of the antigens of the red blood cell membrane. In: Agre P, Parker JC, eds. Red blood cell membranes. New York, Marcel Dekker, 1989:299)

as water-soluble complexes in the plasma and in various body secretions. These polysaccharides are conjugated either to specific lipids or proteins. The ABH, Le^a, Le^b, P_1, and P antigens in plasma are glycosphingolipids formed by a glycosidic bond between ceramide and the proximal Glc residue in the polysaccharide moiety (Fig. 56-2; see Fig. 56-1). Certain plasma glycosphingolipids spontaneously partition into the plasma membranes of a variety of cells including erythrocytes, where they make up about 20% of the total membrane-associated polysaccharide antigens.

About 80% of the polysaccharide antigens associated with the erythrocyte membrane are formed by polylactosaminoglycans, complex carbohydrates that are N-linked to asparagine residues in certain membrane proteins, including the anion transporter (band 3, protein 3, AE1), glucose transporter, and probably other integral membrane proteins on erythrocytes and other cells.[18,19]

The polysaccharide antigens in tears, saliva, and other secretions are glycoproteins formed by O linkage between a polysaccharide structure formed from a type 1 paragloboside (see Fig. 56-1) and serine or threonine residues in certain nascent polypeptides that are ultimately secreted as glycoproteins. The presence of the different members of the polysaccharide antigens on erythrocytes, in plasma, or in secretions therefore results from linkages to different proteins and lipids, which is determined by a subtle dif-

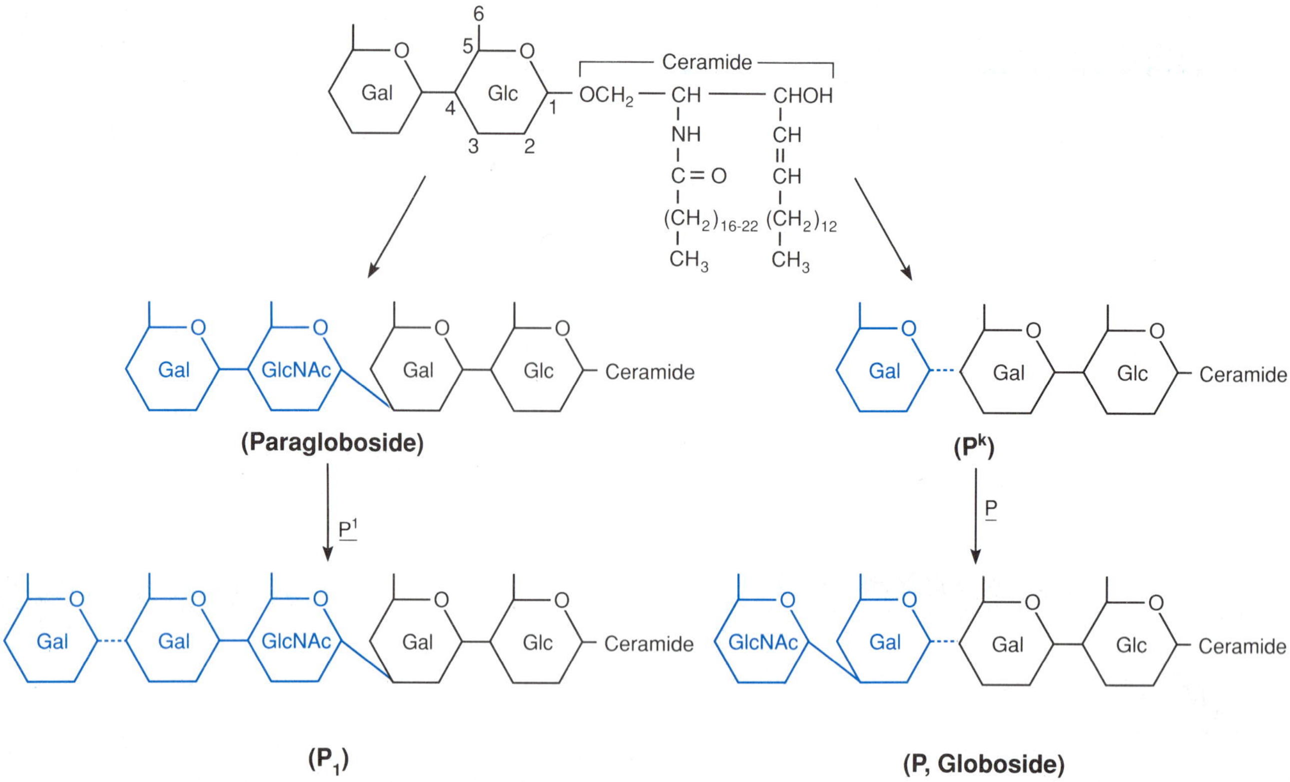

FIGURE 56-2. Diagram of P antigen structures. (After Rosse WF, Telen MJ. The biochemistry of the antigens of the red blood cell membrane. In: Agre P, Parker JC, eds. Red blood cell membranes. New York, Marcel Dekker, 1989:299)

ference in the precursor structures, the type 1 and type 2 paragloboside.

Of all the blood group antigens, the polysaccharide antigens are the most completely understood in terms of primary chemical structure. Nevertheless, the actual three-dimensional organization of these structures in terms of carbohydrate folding and associations between adjacent glycolipids and glycoproteins is poorly understood. Likewise, the biologic importance of these structures remains the subject of speculation.

ABH Antigens

ABH antigens are the most important blood antigens in transfusion medicine, and their discovery heralded the beginning of modern immunohematology (described previously). The ABH substances are formed on the paraglobosides, which are tetrasaccharides created by the addition of galactose to the terminal *N*-acetylglucosamine of a specific trisaccharide attached to lipid (ceramide) or a nascent glycoprotein (see Fig. 56-1). If the addition occurs at position 3, the result is Gal(β1–3)GlcNAc (type 1 paragloboside), whereas addition to position 4 produces Gal(β1–4)GlcNAc (type 2 paragloboside). Although this difference may appear to be subtle, it determines the eventual fate of the mature polysaccharide antigen. The erythrocyte membrane-associated polysaccharide antigens are formed on type 2 paraglobosides, whereas the plasma and secreted antigens are formed on type 1 paraglobosides.

The *H* gene codes for a transferase catalyzing the addition of Fuc to the terminal galactose of type 2 paragloboside, Fuc(α1–2)Gal. A distinct gene *Se* (secretor) catalyzes a similar fucosylation on the type 1 paragloboside. The relation between *H* and *Se* is not altogether clear since they are not alleles. It had been hypothesized that *Se* is a regulator element, although it is currently thought that *H* and *Se* are more likely to be ancestrally related genes, with *H* being expressed in endothelial and erythroid cells, whereas *Se* is expressed in epithelia.[20] The product of *Se* is responsible for ABH blood group substances appearing in saliva, milk, bile, and other secretions.[21] Lack of expression of *Se* is commonly found; about 20% of the general population lacks ABH antigens in their secretions and are referred to as *nonsecretors*, presumably *sese* homozygotes. An extremely rare group of patients (O_h, the Bombay phenotype) lack both *H* and *Se* activities and therefore are devoid of the more mature polysaccharide antigens as well.

Both types of H (formed on type 1 and 2 paraglobosides) can act as acceptors for the transferases encoded by the *A* and *B* alleles, leading to formation of the A and B blood groups, whereas people with group O blood apparently express a nonfunctional transferase.[22] The cDNAs for the A, B, and O transferases have been cloned and sequenced.[23] The differences between A and B cDNAs would change four amino acids, presumably determining specificity for GalNAc or Gal. When compared with A and B, the O cDNA has a single nucleotide deletion resulting in a frame shift and presumably leading to production of an inactive transferase.

The A transferase adds *N*-acetylgalactosamine to the terminal galactose of H substance forming GalNAc(β1–3)Gal, whereas the B transferase adds galactose similarly (see Fig. 56-1). The units formed on type 2 paragloboside appear on the surface of erythrocytes, whereas those from type 1 appear in plasma or secretions. Since both A and B are formed on H substance, it is theoretically possible to convert either to blood group O by elimination of the terminal sugar. This was demonstrated by digestion of B erythrocytes with α-galactosidase, which thereby became group O without affecting in vivo survival.[24]

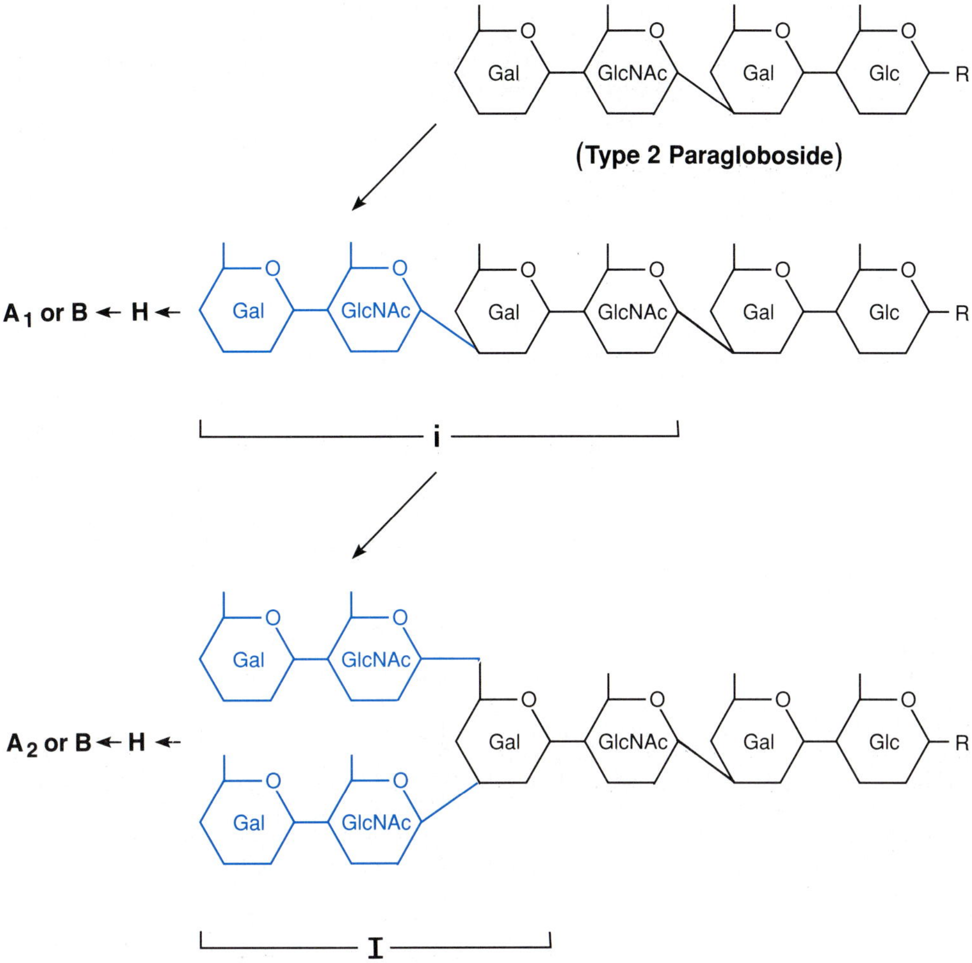

FIGURE 56-3. Diagram of Ii antigen structures. (After Rosse WF, Telen MJ. The biochemistry of the antigens of the red blood cell membrane. In: Agre P, Parker JC, eds. Red blood cell membranes. New York, Marcel Dekker, 1989:299)

Blood type A consists of two subtypes, A_1 and A_2, which differ in the number of A antigens due to the specificity of the two different A transferases. Normal adult A_1 erythrocytes contain about 1 million A sites per cell, four times the number present on A_2 cells.[25] This distinction apparently is due to the action of the A_1 transferase on multiple acceptor sites on branched H structures (Fig. 56-3), thereby increasing the number of A sites per cell. The A_2 variant results from the action of the A_2 transferase acting preferably on the reduced number of sites on the straight chain H structure; this leads to quantitatively less A.[26] Although weakened forms of B are known to exist, no common subtypes have been established.

The discovery of the ABO system resulted from the observation of the naturally occurring antibodies, the isoagglutinins. These agglutinins are of mixed antibody classes, although IgM predominates and is responsible for the direct agglutination. These antibodies can activate complement and are hemolytic. People with type A blood make anti-B, and those with type B make anti-A. People with type O blood make anti-A and anti-B, whereas those with type ABO make neither (Table 56-2). People with the rare Bombay phenotype make anti-A, anti-B, and anti-H. Patients with immune deficiencies such as Wiskott-Aldrich syndrome may have decreased IgM levels and correspondingly reduced titers of anti-A or anti-B. Despite the natural occurrences of these antibodies, immune stimulation due to transfusion of AB-incompatible blood greatly boosts the titers of anti-A and anti-B antibodies of both IgM and IgG classes.

Structures related to the ABH determinants are ubiquitous in biology. A is structurally similar to the Forssman antigen, a glycosphingolipid that can be extracted from a variety of animal tissues and can serve as an immunogen to raise hemolytic antibodies against sheep erythrocytes.[27] Polysaccharide structures similar to ABH have been found on about half of all tested bacterial strains, and the continued exposure to microbial polysaccharide antigens is thought to be responsible for the development of the naturally occurring isoagglutinins.[28] The titers of the naturally occurring antibodies to A and B are low at birth and climb progressively until the child is 5 to 10 years of age, after which they slowly and continuously decline throughout the entire life-span.[29] Experimental animals raised in germ-

TABLE 56-2. ABO System

Group	Erythrocyte Antigens	Serum Antibodies
O	None	Anti-A, anti-B
A (A_1 or A_2)	A	Anti-B
B	B	Anti-A
AB	A and B	None

free environments do not develop isoagglutinins unless they are fed *Escherichia coli*.[30]

The biologic roles of the ABH blood group antigens are not understood. People with all varieties of ABH, Bombay (O_h), and Se are hematologically normal. Nevertheless, the presence of these and related carbohydrate structures are ubiquitous in human and nonhuman populations, suggesting that a natural selection advantage must exist. For example, nonsecretors are phenotypically normal, but they have statistically increased chances of suffering meningococcal or pneumococcal infections, and secreted ABH substances are thought to impede bacterial adherence.[31] Considerable genetic drift has been found among the different human populations, with certain ABH antigens being common in some populations but rare in others (Table 56-3). For example, South American Indians do not have type A or type B red blood cells (RBCs), whereas Australian aboriginals do not have type B RBCs. When compared with types in most Europeans, type B RBCs are much less common among the Basques but are more common among Asians. In countries such as the United States, where cultural mixing is common, relative differences in the prevalence of ABO types are less pronounced but still significant. When compared with Jewish and non-Jewish whites, African American and Asians are more likely to have type B RBCs, whereas Mexican Americans and Native Americans are more likely to have type O RBCs.

Considerable racial variability also exists in the prevalence of most other blood group antigens.[32] Although much has been written about apparent linkage between ABH antigens and a large variety of human diseases and characteristics, these linkages are generally small statistical differences without clear biologic relevance to an individual.[33] Aberrant ABH expression on malignant tissues is well recognized and probably results from loss of specificity of the glycosyltransferases.[34] Expression of A and B antigens is also frequently reduced in acute leukemia patients.

Lewis Antigens

Despite being of large biologic interest, the Lewis antigens are of relatively minor clinical significance in transfusion and pregnancy, although they are important in renal transplantation. *Le* codes for a fucosyltransferase that acts on position 4 of the penultimate GlcNAc on type 1 paragloboside (see Fig. 56-1). This position is already occupied on type 2 paragloboside, which is therefore not an appropriate acceptor. Lewis antigens are glycosphingolipids that are abundant in plasma.[35] The Lewis antigens appear on erythrocytes, platelets, and lymphocytes by adsorption from plasma.[36] Expression of the Lewis antigens is linked to the secretor status since *Se* converts type 1 paragloboside (precursor of Le^a) to H substance (precursor of Le^b); the product of *Le* uses both as substrates. People who express *Se* are typed as Le(a−b+), whereas those who express *sese* are typed as Le(a+b−). Rarely, a person can lack *Le* (that is, *lele*) and is typed as Le(a−b−) but is hematologically normal.

Naturally occurring Lewis antibodies are common in Le(a−b−) people. Lewis antibodies are primarily IgM and are potentially deleterious, but the presence of abundant Lewis antigen in plasma apparently neutralizes the antibodies. Lewis antibodies activate complement but are poor agglutinins. The titer of such antibodies rises during pregnancy, and the presence of Lewis antigens on the maternal cells declines, although this appears to be no hazard to the fetus. Lewis antigens are virtually absent from cord erythrocytes, but their abundance rises within the first few months of life.

TABLE 56-3. Percentages of ABO Groups in Different Populations

	O	A	B	AB
SELECTED NATIVE POPULATIONS				
South American Indian	100	0	0	0
Australian aboriginal	44	56	0	0
Basque	54	43	2	1
Bengali	22	24	38	16
Vietnamese	45	21	29	5
German	43	42	11	4
Italian	46	39	11	4
SELECTED US POPULATIONS				
Native American	89	16	4	<1
Mexican	56	27	13	4
Chinese	40	26	27	7
Black	49	28	19	4
Jewish	38	44	12	6
Non-Jewish white	45	41	11	3

(Adapted from Mourant AE, Kopec AC, Domaniewska-Sobczak K. The distribution of the human blood groups and other biochemical polymorphisms, ed 2. Oxford, Blackwell Scientific Publications, 1976)

Ii Antigens

I and i are not antithetical antigens but are developmentally linked structural variants. The biochemistry of I and i antigens is well understood (see Fig. 56-3). Both I and i are derived from type 2 paragloboside, which may be linked to protein or lipid. The sequential actions of two glycosyltransferases first add N-acetylglucosamine to the paragloboside, GlcNAc(β1–3)Gal, and then add galactose, Gal(β1–4)GlcNAc.[37,38] These enzymes add multiple Gal–GlcNAc units to form a long, straight chain. I resembles i except that the terminal galactose in the paragloboside accepts a second *N*-acetylglucosamine, GlcNAc(β1–6)Gal, which produces a branched structure. The Gal–GlcNAc units may themselves be branched, and as many as five branches may occur in any single polysaccharide unit leading to a highly complex structure. These structures are frequently capped off with ABH antigens, although incomplete polysaccharide units that remain unsubstituted contain exposed I and i structures.

Infants strongly express i, whereas children and adults strongly express I, even though each expresses both antigens.[39] In addition, the appearance of I increases quantitatively during the differentiation of erythroblasts. Normal adult erythrocytes bear about 500,000 I antigens per erythrocyte. The reason for the developmental switch from i to I is not clear, but it may reflect important differences in withstanding exposure to the oxidative atmospheric environment. The lens of the eye shares all the major structural components of the erythrocyte, and persistent expression of i has been linked to a recessive form of cataracts.[22]

Conditions that produce marrow stress, such as severe anemia, frequently lead to enhanced i expression. Increased i is also seen in erythrocytes from patients with rare disorders such as congenital dyserythropoietic anemia, type II, also called hereditary erythroblastic multinuclearity with positive acid serum test (HEMPAS), and is also seen in acute leukemia.[40,41]

Alloantibodies to I and i are not encountered. Cold agglutinin disease is the result of auto–anti-I.[42] For unexplained reasons, patients suffering from infectious mononucleosis or atypical mycoplasmal pneumonia frequently develop auto–anti-I or auto–anti-i antibodies with high titer and high thermal amplitude activity.

P Antigens

The P antigens were first identified by immunization of rabbits with various human erythrocytes.[43] The chemical structure of the P antigens is fundamental to the polysaccharide antigens (see Fig. 56-2). Beginning with the disaccharide, ceramide, different enzymes that are products of nonallelic genes may attach N-acetylglucosamine and galactose to form paragloboside, or, alternatively, galactose may be added directly to form p^k. The p^{1k} gene product subsequently adds a terminal galactose to paragloboside to form P_1 or the P^2 gene product adds N-acetylgalactosamine to p^k to form P globoside.

P^{1k} and P^2 are not allelic. About 75% of people are classed as P_1 and express P, P_1, and P^k, whereas 25% are classed as P_2 and express only P and P^k. Rare P-deficient people with $P_1{}^k$ or $P_2{}^k$ phenotype make P^k but not P, whereas some rare individuals who are *pp* make none of the P antigens and may develop antibodies to P, P_1, and P^k. These people are at increased risk for spontaneous abortions.[44]

The P antigens are plasma glycosphingolipids and are not found in secretions. P is adsorbed to the surface of erythrocytes and other cell types including fibroblasts, lymphocytes, and platelets.[45] The amount of P varies within the population and even varies from cell to cell within a person's blood. Structures similar to the P antigens are ubiquitous in biology, and P antibodies are therefore heterogeneous.[46] Cold reactive antibodies to P_1 may occur naturally but rarely cause transfusion reactions. These antibodies have also been described in P_2 patients suffering from hydatid disease or parasitic flukes. Cold-reactive autoantibodies to P, referred to as the *Donath-Landsteiner antibody*, have been detected in a variety of disease states and may provoke autoimmune hemolysis and paroxysmal cold hemoglobinuria.

The erythrocyte P antigen serves as the cellular receptor for B19 parvovirus,[216a] a virus that invades and destroys erythroblasts and causes aplastic crises in patients with hemolytic anemias. Erythroblasts lacking P antigens are not susceptible to the virus in vitro, and individuals carrying such erythroblasts do not develop antibodies to parvovirus B19.

Glycophorin-Associated Antigens: MN, Ss, and Gerbich

After the discovery of the ABO system, Karl Landsteiner was unable to identify other human blood group isoagglutinins. Nevertheless, he was convinced that additional blood antigens existed. Unfortunately, his investigations were interrupted by World War I and several subsequent years of extreme deprivation. On receiving the sponsorship of Dr. Peyton Rous, he joined the Rockefeller Institute (now University) in 1922. Before his arrival, Landsteiner had confided to Rous that he looked forward to living in a small, inexpensive garden cottage by the sea. Landsteiner had never completely adjusted to apartment living in New York City and even gave up his beloved piano playing to pacify his neighbors.[9]

Encouraged by colleagues at Rockefeller as well as *Drosophila* geneticist T.H. Morgan at Columbia University, Landsteiner and his assistant, Philip Levine, developed a new approach to search for potential membrane-antigenic polymorphisms. They injected rabbits and other nonhuman species with different human erythrocytes in an attempt to raise antisera to yet unrecognized determinants. Using this approach, they discovered a second family of blood group antigens that were not linked to ABO. They named these "M" and "N," since both letters were included in the word *immune* and were located in the alphabet distant from A and B.[43] Subsequent work established that these antigens were associated with the glycophorins.[47,48]

Glycophorins

Glycophorin is a term used to describe the erythrocyte sialoglycoproteins, intensely glycosylated membrane-spanning proteins that carry several blood group antigens including the MN and Ss antigens.[49] Four major species of glycophorins exist and are now known to make up two distinct families, glycophorins A and B, and glycophorins C and D.[50] All four glycophorins share common characteristics: all are membrane proteins with cytoplasmic domains, all contain single hydrophobic transmembrane domains, and all contain extracellular domains with several O-linked oligosaccharides attached to serine or threonine residues (Fig. 56-4).

Glycophorins A and B: MN and Ss Antigens

Glycophorins A and B account for 85% and 10% of the total erythrocyte membrane sialoglycoproteins by weight, existing as about 10^6 and 0.25×10^6 copies per erythrocyte, respectively. Neuraminic acid (sialic acid) is negatively charged at physiologic pH, and the residues in the oligosaccharides attached to glycophorins A and B contribute most of the negative charge associated with the erythrocyte membrane. Glycophorin A contains a single, large, complex asparagine-linked oligosaccharide (polylactosaminoglycan) and 15 O-linked tetrasaccharides.[51] Glycophorin B contains 11 O-linked tetrasaccharides.

The amino acid sequence of glycophorins A and B has been determined by protein sequencing[52] and by analysis of the isolated cDNAs.[53–55] The glycophorin *A* gene and *B* gene were discovered to be derived from the duplication of an ancestral gene.[56] This observation is consistent with the observed close genetic linkage of the MN and Ss antigens, which are expressed on glycophorins A and B, respectively. Also, the close chromosomal location of the glycophorin *A* and *B* genes and unequal crossing-over at meiosis are most likely responsible for the existence of several unusual glycophorin variants that appear to be hybrids of A and B, the Miltenberger and Dantu phenotypes.[57]

The polypeptide backbones of glycophorins A and B contain 131 and 72 amino acids, respectively, of which the first 26 amino acids are nearly identical.[58] A and B have identical bilayer spanning domains, although glycophorin B contains a cytoplasmic domain consisting of only five amino acids. Glycophorins A and B are thought to exist naturally in the membrane as heterodimers or homodimers of α or β subunits, or both.

The M and N antigens are known to result from two amino acid substitutions at the N terminal and fifth residue of the polypeptide (see Fig. 56-4). The M and N antigenic epitopes are determined by these amino acids as well as by the O-linked tetrasaccharides on residues 2, 3, and 4. The N-terminal sequence of glycophorin B is always identical with that of the N antigen variant of glycophorin A, so that all erythrocytes have at least some N expression, but this is not detected by standard serology. The gene frequencies of *M* and *N* are 0.53 and 0.47 among whites, so that appearance of all combinations of M+N−, M+N+, and M−N+ are common. Other rare polymorphisms have also been described such as the M^g phenotype in which asparagine is the fourth amino acid and the surrounding residues lack the usual O-linked oligosaccharides.

The S and s antigens are located only on glycophorin B. These result from a polymorphism at the 29th residue, methionine (S) or threonine (s).[58] The gene frequencies of S and s are 0.33 and 0.67 among whites. S−s− phenotypes have been described in the black population, and most of these patients also test negative for the U antigen, a poorly understood antigen that may be composed of glycophorin B and Rh structural components.[59]

Antibodies to the M and N antigens are often naturally occurring and rarely cause hemolytic transfusion reactions. Anti-S, anti-s, and anti-U are usually naturally occurring and have been implicated in hemolytic transfusion reactions and hemolytic disease of the newborn. Antibodies to N are exceedingly rare, presumably because of the normal presence of N on glycophorin B.

The M, N, S, s, and U antigens are found exclusively on erythrocytes and are totally absent from other blood cells such as platelets, neutrophils, and lymphocytes. Recent work using cDNA probes for glycophorins A and B confirmed the absence of expression of the corresponding mRNAs in nonerythroid cells.[53,60] The physiologic role of these glycophorins is still uncertain. Glycoproteins related

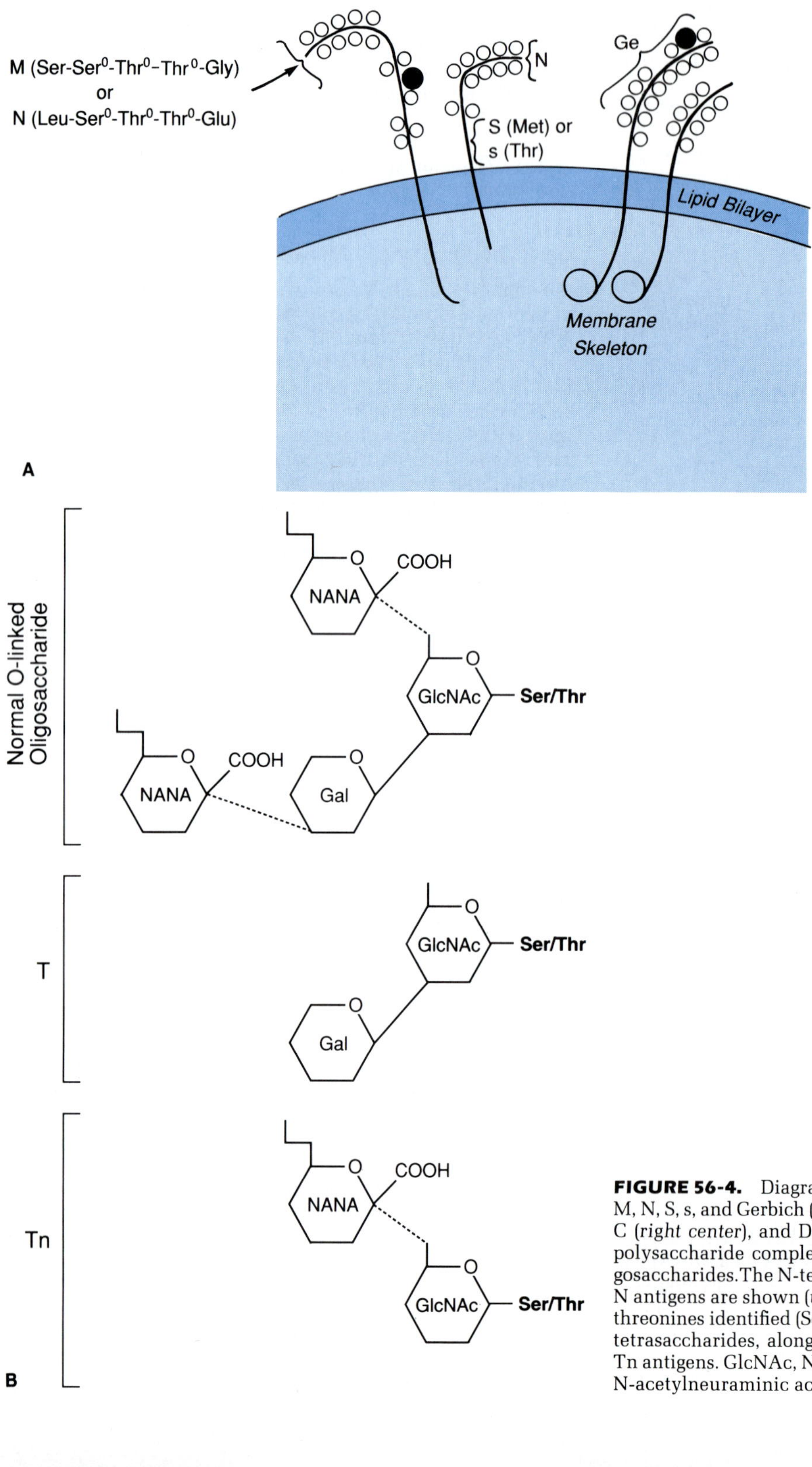

FIGURE 56-4. Diagram of glycophorins and associated antigens M, N, S, s, and Gerbich (Ge). (**A**) Glycophorins A (*left*), B (*left center*), C (*right center*), and D (*right*). Closed circles represent N-linked polysaccharide complexes. Open circles represent O-linked oligosaccharides.The N-terminal amino acid sequences of the M and N antigens are shown (*upper left*) with O-glycosylated serines and threonines identified (Ser^0 and Thr^0). (**B**) Structures of the O-linked tetrasaccharides, along with the structures of the related T and Tn antigens. GlcNAc, N-acetyglucosamine; Gal, galactose; NANA, N-acetylneuraminic acid.

to the glycophorins are found on the surface of nonhuman erythrocytes. Conservation during evolution is highly indicative of a fundamentally significant role for the glycophorins.

Glycophorin A has proved to be a measure of genetic damage resulting from agents such as radiation.[61] Also, despite evolutionary conservation, rare human families have been discovered to totally lack glycophorins A or B or both, and family members suffer no apparent clinical abnormality.[62] The more common of these conditions is the En(a−) phenotype, which totally lacks glycophorin A[63] or bears an abnormal hybrid glycophorin.[64] It is interesting that in these phenotypes, other membrane components are found to have increased amounts of sialic acid.[65] The major role of glycophorins A and B is suggested to be their contribution to overall negative surface charge. Although partial reduction of glycophorin B is known to occur in the Rh_{null} phenotype, the pathologic disorder most likely results from deficiency of the Rh polypeptide, which is needed for membrane stability of glycophorin B.[66]

Glycophorins C and D: Gerbich Antigens

Glycophorins C and D account for only 4% and 1%, respectively, of the total erythrocyte membrane sialoglycoproteins by weight, but they appear to play a more important role in membrane organization. It is clear from protein sequencing and cDNA analysis that glycophorins C and D are highly related to each other and completely unrelated to glycophorins A and B.[67,68] Glycophorin C is a 128 amino acid polypeptide bearing one large N-linked polysaccharide and 12 to 14 O-linked oligosaccharides. Glycophorin D is about 107 amino acids and bears six to eight O-linked structures. Both proteins appear to be encoded by the same gene with an alternate initiation site producing D, a truncated form of C.[69] Unlike glycophorins A and B, which are erythroid specific, glycophorins C and D appear to be transcribed in lymphoid cells and in several tissues, although the glycosylations may reflect significant tissue differences.[68,70]

Glycophorin C contains the high-frequency Gerbich antigens that are of minor clinical importance but have proved to be instructive to our basic understanding of membrane biology. Gerbich-negative patients are rare except among elliptocytosis patients in New Guinea.[71] Extremely rare Europeans with elliptocytosis are Gerbich-negative and lack glycophorins C and D, the Leach phenotype.[72] Other patients lacking Gerbich antigens have glycophorin C molecules with abnormal extracellular domains but normal cytoplasmic domains and normal erythrocyte morphology.[73] Moreover, erythrocytes from elliptocytosis patients who are totally lacking structural protein 4.1 are partially deficient in glycophorin C.[74] Taken together, these and other observations indicate that glycophorin C (and probably D) plays an important role in stabilizing the membrane skeleton by providing a membrane attachment site for protein 4.1[75] (see Fig. 56-4).

Polyagglutination: T Activation and Tn Syndrome

Polyagglutination refers to situations in which the erythrocytes from an individual are agglutinated by the serum of most normal individuals. This most frequently results from antibodies reacting with portions of the O-linked oligosaccharides on the glycophorins. These O-linked oligosaccharides (see Fig. 56-4) are tetrasaccharides composed of two N-acetylneuraminic acid residues linked through galactose and N-acetylgalactosamine to extracellular serine and threonine residues.[76] The underlying structures, referred to as T and Tn antigens, react with naturally occurring antibodies that exist in the plasma of all people except infants. The development of these antibodies is most likely due to exposure to similar antigens within the capsules of gram-negative bacteria. Although anti-T and anti-Tn antibodies exist in the plasma of nearly all adults, the titers are greatly variable among different people.

Exposure of T antigens on the surface of blood cells is referred to as T activation. The phenomenon as first described was an artifact resulting from contamination of blood tubes with microorganisms secreting neuraminidases that removed N-acetylneuraminic acid from O-glycosylated structures on glycophorins and glycolipids, including gangliosides. Authentic T activation is an uncommon clinical disorder resulting from severe infections with a variety of organisms, including pneumococci, streptococci, staphylococci, clostridia, *E coli*, and influenza viruses that secrete neuraminidases and degrade the O-linked oligosaccharides in vivo.

T activation is most often detected because of discrepancies in the determination of ABH antigens on a patient's blood due to the presence of anti-T in the testing sera reacting with T antigens uncovered by the bacterial neuraminidase. Agglutination of T antigens is greater at room temperature than at 37°C. The agglutination is transient and disappears over several weeks after recovery from the infection. Although T agglutination may be demonstrated in vitro, with blood from patients with T activation, usually little or no hemolysis occurs. When present, the hemolysis may actually be the result of other bacterial hemolysins, which may be especially problematic in clostridial infections. In general, the severity of the ongoing infection greatly exceeds the importance of potential hemolysis because of anti-T. Nevertheless, acute presentation of severe hemolytic anemia and hemolytic uremic syndrome has been reported in certain infected patients.[77] This may even be seen in infected infants after transfusion of plasma from adult donors, the source of anti-T antibody.[78]

The Tn syndrome is pathogenically distinct from T activation. The Tn antigen is also deficient in N-acetylneuraminic acid (see Fig. 56-4), but Tn arises from mutations in germ cell lines that affect β3-galactosyltransferase, thereby eliminating the site for addition of a second N-acetylneuraminic acid to the nascent oligosaccharide.[79] Thus, Tn antigens are incompletely formed carbohydrate structures.[80]

Tn syndrome patients usually manifest abnormalities in all blood cell lines and are frequently mosaic for the defect. Microscopic evaluation for agglutination demonstrates mixed-field reactivity, with a subpopulation of erythrocytes (Tn clone) being agglutinated. Overall, the Tn syndrome is more of a laboratory phenomenon than a clinical defect. Although some patients may have mild thrombocytopenia and a subtle degree of anemia, most are clinically normal. The syndrome is generally stable for many years, but emergence of leukemia has been reported in a few Tn patients.[79,81] A related phenomenon has been observed in tumor cells from certain cancer patients. T and Tn antigens are commonly found on the surfaces of nonhematologic malignancies, whereas the surrounding benign tissues lack the T and Tn antigens.[82] Taken together, these observations indicate that the germ cell mutations leading to appearance of Tn may be included in the multistep process from which a malignant transformation emerges.

Glycophorin Antigens and Malaria

Several lines of evidence indicate that the oligosaccharides attached to the glycophorins contribute to the invasion of erythrocytes by malaria merozoites. Unlike the Duffy antigens that are absolutely required for invasion by *P know-*

lesi, the N-acetylneuraminic acid residues attached to glycophorins somehow contribute to invasion by certain strains of *Plasmodium falciparum* but are not absolutely required. Tn erythrocytes partially resist invasion by the Camp strain but not the Thai-Tn strain, and digestion of Tn erythrocytes with trypsin further reduces the degree of invasion.[83,84] Likewise, the Camp strain demonstrates reduced ability to invade M^kM^k erythrocytes that are deficient in glycophorins A and B.[85] Antibodies to glycophorin A inhibit invasion by both *P falciparum* and *P knowlesi*, but this is probably due to changes in membrane skeleton deformability induced by the antibodies.[86]

Proteolipids

A distinct class of blood group antigens behave biochemically as if they were composed of protein and lipid; hence the name proteolipid. The Rh and LW antigens are the most important members of this class.

Discovery of the Rh Antigens

In 1939, Philip Levine, having left Landsteiner's laboratory 7 years earlier, made a report on a patient that led to the recognition of the Rh blood group system. Levine and collaborator, Rufus Stetson, identified a young lady who had just given birth to a stillborn infant who had succumbed to erythroblastosis fetalis. After receiving blood donated by her husband, the patient underwent an immediate and severe transfusion reaction. The investigators noted that the patient's serum agglutinated her husband's erythrocytes even though both were group O. In addition, they found that her serum agglutinated 80 of 104 randomly selected ABO-compatible blood samples.[87] This remarkable observation led to the identification of an antibody as the cause of erythroblastosis fetalis, a common but previously mysterious disease. The key to the observation was that the patient's antibody agglutinated other erythrocytes directly, whereas most Rh-specific antisera were subsequently found to require warming[88] or the addition of a second antibody such as rabbit antihuman globulin.[89]

Rh Genetics

As World War II broke out, researchers on both sides of the Atlantic were actively investigating the newly discovered Rh antigen. The immunologic characteristics of the Rh antigen were soon recognized to be exceedingly complex because of multiple overlapping antigenic variants, and two conflicting genetic theories emerged. Wiener[90] in the United States proposed that Rh antigens are the products of a single complex gene with multiple alleles, referred to as Rh^0, rh', rh'', and so on. Fisher and Race[91] in the United Kingdom proposed that the Rh antigens are products of multiple closely linked genes referred to as *D*, *C*, *E*, and so on. The Fisher-Race theory considers the loci for *DCE* to be so closely spaced that no chromosomal crossing ever takes place during meiosis, and the three genes are inherited en bloc with no recombination between maternal and paternal Rh loci. Recent investigations indicate that alternative splicing of the Rh mRNA or gene duplication are the most likely explanations for multiple distinct antigens encoded by a single locus.[92] The Wiener versus Fisher-Race controversy is therefore likely to end in a draw with both groups partially correct.

TABLE 56-4. Nomenclature for Selected Rh Antigens

Rosenfield	Fisher-Race (CDE)	Wiener (Rh-Hr)
Rh 1	D	Rh_0
2	C	rh'
3	E	rh"
4	c	hr'
5	e	hr"
6	f (ce)	hr
7	Ce	rh_i
12	G	rh^G
25*	LW*	
29	Total Rh	

* The gene that encodes LW is now known to segregate independently from the Rh locus and is no longer assigned to the Rh group system.

TABLE 56-5. Rh Gene Frequencies

		Frequency		
Symbol	**CDE**	**Whites**	**Blacks**	**Asians**
R^1	*CDe*	0.41	0.10	0.55
r	*cde*	0.39	0.15	0.10
R^2	*cDE*	0.14	0.10	0.35
R^0	*cDe*	0.03	0.60	<0.01
r"	*cdE*	All are 0.01 or less		
r'	*CDe*			
R^z	*CDE*			

Rh Nomenclature and Inheritance

The differing genetic viewpoints led to the propagation of different nomenclatures (Table 56-4) proposed by Rosenfield,[93] Fisher and Race,[91] and Wiener,[90] the first being a cataloging system without genetic implications. A system of symbols has evolved for shorthand referral to the antigenic combinations and is commonly used (Table 56-5). The CDE system is also frequently used since it is easily communicated.

The major Rh antigen discovered by Levine and Stetson[87] is referred to as "D." About 85% of Europeans are homozygous or heterozygous for *D* and are referred to as Rh-positive. The remainder of the population do not express *D*, being homozygous for *d* and are referred to as Rh-negative. Although the D antigen is readily detected immunologically, no d antigen has been identified. If there is a *d* gene product, it may be buried in the membrane bilayer. The existence of the C antigen and its antithetical partner c have both been established serologically, and their genes are alleles, C and c. Likewise, E and e are antithetical. The C, c, E, and e antigens are immunologically much less potent and are clinically less important than D. Routine blood typing does not evaluate C, c, E, and e, and Rh-positive indicates the presence of D but does not refer to the presence or absence of C, c, E, or e.

The frequencies of the different Rh genotypes are different among different racial groups (see Table 56-5). Homozygotes for *cde* (r) make up 15% of white, 2% of black, and 1% of Asian populations, whereas homozygotes for *cDe* (R^0) make up 36% of the black population but are rare in whites and Asians.[32] Other than family studies, there is no way to distinguish *DD* people from those with *Dd*. The different Rh antigens occur at different frequencies, so that only probable genotypes may be predicted. For example, people serologically typed as bearing C, c, D, and e antigens may be genetically either *CDe*/*cde* (R^1r) or *CDe*/*cDe* (R^1R^0). The former would be much more likely among whites, and the latter would be much more likely among blacks. The genotype may be better established by studying other relatives, but ambiguities may persist.

D, C, and E Variants and Complexities

The CDE nomenclature is often criticized for being overly simplistic since numerous other Rh-related antigens exist. Table 56-4 lists 10 Rh antigens, but at least 35 others have been identified by specific antisera. In general, those who have difficulties with these variant antigens have been multiply transfused, and no simple method exists for prior recognition. Some of the variant Rh antigens are extremely common, being present in more than 99% of donor samples, whereas others are seen in less than 1% of donor samples.

Variant categories of the D antigen exist, which lack a portion of the D epitope, Rh13, Rh14, Rh15, and Rh16. This phenomenon suggests that the D antigen is a mosaic of several components. Although only rare people lack one of these components, such a person may therefore develop antibodies reacting with the common forms of D but not his or her own.[94] Complex features of the c, C, e, and E antigens have also been identified. Certain Rh antigens such as C^W (Rh8), C^X (Rh9), and Rh39 are related to C, whereas E^W (Rh11) is related to E.

Additional antibodies have added further complexities to our understanding of the Rh antigens. The G antigen may be a portion of Rh structures since it is found on all C-bearing and most D-bearing erythrocytes.[95] Rh29 appears to be a fundamental structural component of all the Rh antigens since it appears to be expressed on all but Rh_{null} erythrocytes.

Antibodies may arise against more than one Rh antigen encoded by the same chromosome. For example, antibodies to Ce (Rh7) react with erythrocytes from people with *Cde/cDE* but not *CDE/cde* genotypes.[96] Likewise, juxtaposition of CE (Rh22) or cE (Rh27) can react with specific antibodies. The molecular explanations for this remain to be established, although the existence of c and E epitopes on the same polypeptide cannot be ruled out.

Rh Antigen Abundance

Unlike the ABH antigens that exist in up to 10^6 copies per erythrocyte, the Rh antigens are exceedingly immunogenic even though far less plentiful. Using ferritin conjugated antibodies to D, it was estimated that *Dd* people express about 9000 to 20,000 D antigens per erythrocyte, whereas *DD* people express 15,000 to 33,000 copies.[97,98] The number of C, c, E, and e antigens is less well agreed on but is in the same range.

Expression of the various Rh antigens is not always comparable and is influenced by other Rh antigens when they are in certain combinations. The molecular explanation for this is unknown, but the effects are well recognized. For example, the expression of D is weakened by the expression of C but increased by the expression of E. For example, cDE/cDE (R_2/R_2) erythrocytes give a stronger reaction with anti-D than do CDe/CDe (R_1/R_1). The existence of D reduces the reactivity of C and E.

The D^u phenotype is sometimes problematic because it behaves immunologically like the D antigen expressed in greatly reduced numbers.[99] Current sensitive methods in blood bank serology can detect most D^u phenotypes. Since the D^u may be immunogenic in Rh-negative patients, D^u donor blood should be treated as Rh-positive, and D^u recipients should be treated as Rh-negative.

Rare people with the phenotype −D− (referred to as *dash D dash*) lack all C, c, E, and e but have an enhanced number of D sites, 100,000 to 200,000 per erythrocyte.[100] The existence of this phenotype is evidence of alternate expression of Rh antigens since they behave as if the people were genotypically *DDD*. Other Rh deletion types have been identified including cD− but not −DE.

Rh Deficiency Phenotypes: Rh_{null} and Rh_{mod} Phenotypes

The most interesting Rh deletions are the Rh_{null} and Rh_{mod} phenotypes.[101] These deletions are extremely rare; only 42 patients with such deletions have been described worldwide. The erythrocytes from Rh_{null} patients are totally devoid of all Rh antigens. Rh_{mod} patients have a similar disorder, but their erythrocytes have barely detectable Rh antigens.[102] The erythrocyte membranes in these phenotypes are structurally defective, and the patients suffer variable degrees of chronic anemia because of the shortened erythrocyte survival.[103] The pathologic nature of these phenotypes is evidence that the Rh polypeptides are essential for normal membrane integrity (see section on biochemistry of Rh antigens).

The peripheral blood of Rh_{null} and Rh_{mod} erythrocytes contains numerous stomatocytes and spherocytes (Fig. 56-5). In some of these cases, the patients have been mistakenly thought to have hereditary spherocytosis at their initial evaluation. The osmotic fragility profile for Rh_{null} cells is different from hereditary spherocytosis. Unincubated Rh_{null} samples are close to the normal range, but after 24 hours of incubation at 37°C, the patient samples undergo a marked shift in the more fragile direction.[101,103] Rh_{null} membranes also have increased cation leak[104,105] and decreased membrane phospholipid organization with increased phosphatidylethanolamine in the outer leaflet of the lipid bilayer.[106]

Clinically, the Rh_{null} and Rh_{mod} syndromes range from virtually normal to moderately anemic.[101] At their basal state, patients in the latter group have increased unconjugated bilirubin, reduced hematocrits, and reticulocytosis of 10% or higher. Chromium-51 RBC survival may be as low as 7 days (normal 25 to 30 days). Splenectomy should be considered for Rh_{null} or Rh_{mod} patients with significant chronic hemolysis. Five Rh_{null} patients with moderately severe anemia have undergone splenectomy, and all experienced great clinical improvement.[101] Like other patients with hemolytic anemia, Rh_{null} patients may suffer periodic hemolytic episodes during viral illnesses and pregnancy.

Since routine blood bank typing tests only for ABO and Rh(D), samples from Rh_{null} patients are therefore read out as Rh-negative since they lack D. Rh_{null} patients who receive blood transfusions or become pregnant may develop antibodies to any Rh antigens in the donor or fetal blood, including Rh29, which likely represents a core component common to all Rh antigens. Although Rh_{mod} patients have barely detectable Rh antigens, they are protected from developing antibodies to Rh antigens that they express.

The Rh_{null} syndrome appears to exist as two types, each expressed recessively. The *amorphic type* appears to be due to a mutation within the Rh gene.[107] Heterozygotes carrying the amorphic Rh_{null} mutation fail to express the Rh antigens carried by the mutant gene. Most Rh_{null} patients and all Rh_{mod} patients have the *regulator type*, which appears to be due to a mutation regulating the expression of Rh antigens. Heterozygotes carrying the regulator Rh_{null} mutation express the Rh antigens carried by the mutant gene at reduced levels. Although the amorphic and regulator types are distinguished by expression of Rh antigens in other family members, it cannot be definitively stated that the mutations are at different loci since they appear to differ only in the level of penetrance and may represent different mutations at the same locus.

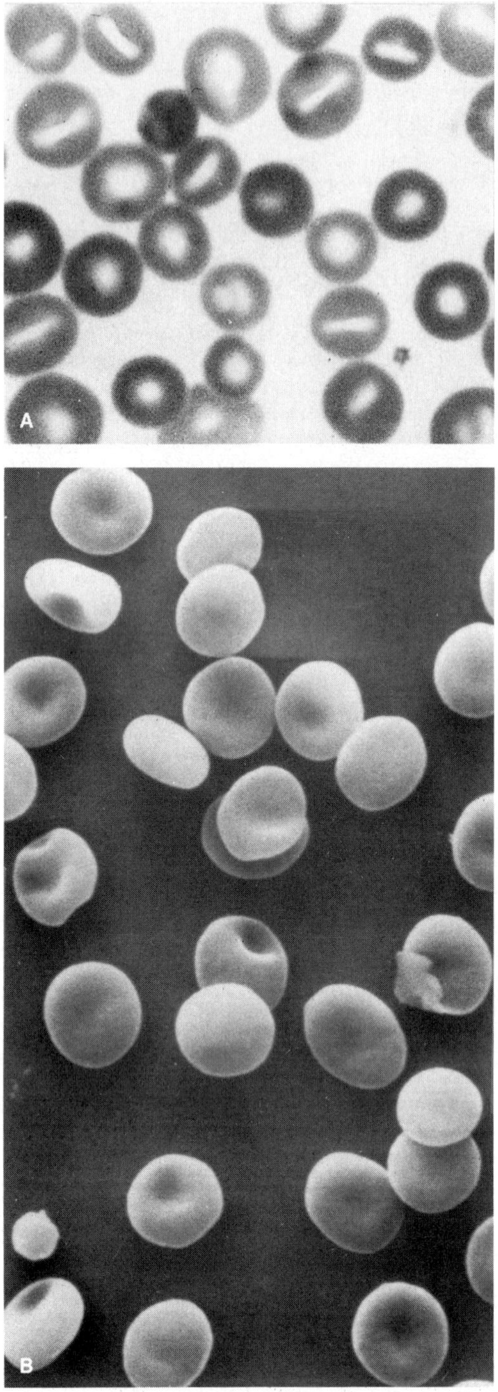

FIGURE 56-5. Wright-stained peripheral blood smear (**A**) and scanning electron micrograph (**B**) of Rh_{null} erythrocytes. (Courtesy of Samir Ballas, Cardeza Foundation, Jefferson Medical College, Philadelphia)

Rh Antibodies

As discussed previously, the Rh antigens are exceedingly immunogenic. Nevertheless, naturally occurring antibodies are rare. Although D is the most immunogenic, antibodies to the other Rh antigens are also found, especially c and E, which are sometimes involved in delayed transfusion reactions (see Chap. 60) and hemolytic disease of the newborn[108] (see Chap. 64). Antibodies to C and e are much less common, and antibodies to C are rarely seen without coexisting antibodies to D. Since the suppression of Rh immunization during pregnancy with passively administered Rh immunoglobulin, the frequencies of anti-D antibodies in Rh-negative women have declined remarkably, and the existence of antibodies specific for c, E, or the combined cE are now relatively more common.

Most Rh antibodies are IgG1 or IgG3 and do not directly agglutinate erythrocytes unless the cells are previously digested with papain to remove surface sialoglycoproteins. Although Rh immunoglobulin is a mixture of antibodies isolated from human serum, monoclonal antibodies with Rh specificity have been developed by using Epstein-Barr virus transformation of human lymphocytes.[109] Commonly, Rh antibodies are confirmed by the antiglobulin test. Rh antibodies fail to activate complement, presumably since the Rh antigens are restricted on the surface of the erythrocyte at distances of 60 to 100 nm, which is beyond the 20-nm span needed for fixation of complement component C1q.

Alloimmunization to D by transfusion and by pregnancy has been thoroughly evaluated and is discussed in detail in Chapter 64. Even small amounts of Rh-positive blood can lead to Rh immunization as assessed by increased clearance of subsequently injected Rh-positive cells[110] or demonstration of circulating antibodies.[111] A minority of Rh-negative people, nonresponders, do not develop antibodies despite repeated injections; the explanation for this is unknown. The existence of other antigenic incompatibilities, such as ABO, is certainly a factor since naturally occurring antibodies to these latter antigens lead to rapid clearance of the injected cells before the patient develops primary Rh immunization.[112] After they are established, Rh-specific antibodies may be detectable in the patient's sera many years after exposure.

Even though the D antigen is found only on erythrocytes, immunization may result from transfusion of platelets or plasma since these may be contaminated with tiny amounts of erythrocytes. Rh immunization has even been reported to result from use of contaminated needles by intravenous drug users.[113] After primary immunization occurs, it cannot be reversed by administration of Rh immunoglobulin.[114]

Biochemistry of Rh Antigens

Despite long-standing interest by numerous investigators, the molecular nature of the Rh antigens remains incompletely resolved. The independent identification of the Rh polypeptide in 1982 by Moore and colleagues[115] in Edinburgh and Gahmberg[116] in Helsinki provided a major advance. The Rh polypeptide is a 32-kd membrane-spanning protein that can be immunoprecipitated with Rh immunoglobulin. Unlike other membrane-spanning proteins, the Rh polypeptide contains no detectable carbohydrate[117] and appears to be associated with the membrane skeleton.[118,119] The Rh polypeptide is missing from Rh_{null} erythrocytes.[120]

Although the purified Rh polypeptide no longer reacts with Rh-specific antibodies, protein polymorphisms have been demonstrated to be linked with specific Rh phenotypes.[92,97,121,122] Immunoprecipitations with monoclonal antibodies specific for D, c, and E permit analysis of the corresponding Rh polypeptides by iodopeptide mapping, a technique that allows estimation of protein homologies based on the two-dimensional "fingerprint" of proteolytic peptide fragments generated from proteins that had all tyrosines radioiodinated. The D, c, and E Rh polypeptides are found to be highly related. The c and E polypeptides are nearly identical, whereas the D polypeptide is less similar.[92] As expected of a fundamental membrane component, proteins related to the Rh polypeptide, but lacking the extracellular antigenic epitope are found in the erythrocyte

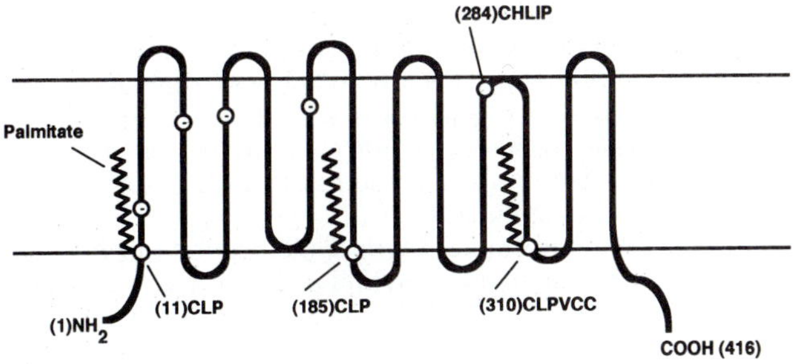

FIGURE 56-6. Diagramatic representation of the membrane organization of a single Rh polypeptide determined from the primary sequence. Carboxy (CCOH) and amino (NH_2) terminals are indicated. Cysteine (C) residues are represented. Probable fatty acid (palmitic acid) acylations are drawn as diagonal jagged lines. Palmitic acids are probably also attached to the two cysteines at positions 314 and 315 (not shown). The circled minus signs indicate negatively charged amino acids within the hydrophobic transmembrane domains. The D and CcEe proteins differ at 36 positions scattered throughout the amino acid sequence. (After Cartron JP, Agre P. Rh antigens: protein and gene structure. Semin Hematol 1993;30:193)

membranes of diverse mammalian species.[121] Determination of the N-terminal amino acid sequence of the Rh polypeptide shows it to be a unique protein.[123–125]

Understanding of Rh structure has greatly advanced in the past several years with the cloning of the two Rh genes[126] and cDNAs;[127,128] the *D* gene and the *CcEe* gene.[129] The genes are located on chromosome 1 (1p34.3-p.36.1).[130] The *D* gene, which encodes the D protein, is missing in Rh(D)-negative erythrocytes.[126] This explains why neither d antigen nor d protein has been found, since there is no *d* gene. The *CcEe* gene encodes the polymorphic C, c, E, and e proteins. These proteins are lacking in rare patients with the –D– phenotype, although the *CcEe* gene is present.[126]

The two genes are highly homologous and presumably evolved by duplication of a common ancestor. The 417–amino acid D and CcEe proteins differ by only 36 amino acids scattered throughout their amino acid sequences.[127,128] Both Rh proteins contain 12 membrane-spanning domains and are thought to be oriented with their amino and carboxy terminals[131,131a] on the inside (Fig. 56-6). They are very hydrophobic and highly palmitoylated[131b,131c]; five of the six cysteines have a palmitic acid attached in a thioester linkage. These cysteines are in the sequence motifs CLP (Cys-Leu-Pro) and CLPVCC (Cys-Leu-Pro-Val-Cys-Cys; see Fig. 56-6). The function of the palmitic acids is unknown.

The Rh protein is thought to exist in a complex with other proteins, including the Rh50 glycoprotein (Rh-related glycoprotein) and perhaps proteins carrying antigens that are absent or markedly diminished in Rh null erythrocytes (eg, LW, Duffy, U, and Duclos).[131d,131e] The Rh50 glycoprotein has recently been cloned.[131f] It contains 409 amino acids and 12 putative transmembrane domains and is ancestrally related to the Rh protein. It is located on chromosome 6 (6p21-qter). The Rh protein and Rh50 glycoprotein resemble transport proteins, with their multiple transmembrane domains, but so far no transport (or other) function has been assigned to either protein.

The amino acid residues responsible for Rh antigenic differences are not clear. In addition to sequence differences, antigenicity may also be modulated by membrane lipid composition, fatty acid acylation of the Rh protein, and the presence or absence of other proteins in the Rh complex.[131a,131b,131g–131i]

LW Antigen

At the time of the Levine and Stetson discovery, Landsteiner and associate, Alexander Wiener[132] (1907 to 1976), were injecting rabbits with erythrocytes from rhesus monkeys. The rabbits developed an antibody to a substance on the surface of the rhesus erythrocytes, and the investigators discovered that the antibody had specificity identical with the antisera of the Levine and Stetson patient. This antigen was therefore referred to as *rhesus* or *Rh*. This observation was unfortunate because it became clear years later that erythrocytes from rhesus monkeys do not contain the Rh antigen but another antigen, which is expressed more abundantly on the surface of Rh-positive human erythrocytes.[133] This antigen is now referred to as LW, named in honor of Landsteiner and Wiener by their colleague, Philip Levine. Although Levine used the opportunity to honor his colleagues, Levine's contributions to immunohematology brought him both the Lasker Award, received jointly with Wiener in 1946, and election to the National Academy of Sciences in 1965.

Unlike Rh, LW is rarely a cause of alloimmunization. It is now clear that Rh and LW are entirely different proteins whose genes are located on different chromosomes. Nevertheless, expression of the two antigens is somehow related since LW is not expressed on Rh_{null} erythrocytes. Unlike the Rh polypeptide, LW is a 40-kd glycosylated membrane protein. Only about 3000 copies are present per erythrocyte.[134] Despite initial speculation, LW is not a glycosylated form of the Rh polypeptide but a unique polypeptide with expression of the antigenic epitope requiring the presence of Mg^{2+}.[135,136]

Other Membrane Glycoproteins

Kell, Kidd, Lutheran, and Duffy are classed together because all are glycoproteins.

Kell System Antigens

After ABO and Rh, the Kell system antigens are the most problematic in terms of alloimmunization. A few weeks after they developed a new antiglobulin test in 1946, Coombs and colleagues[137] detected a novel antibody in the serum of a patient named Mrs. Kell; this explained the hemolytic disease in her newborn. The Kell system antigens are a complex of several sets of autosomal codominant alleles at the Kell locus, of which three sets are of clinical significance (Table 56-6). Unfortunately, Kell terminology is confusing since two different nomenclatures have evolved.[138] K (K1) and k (K2) are also antithetical, with the latter being detected in 98% of whites and more than 99% of blacks. Kp^a (K3) and Kp^b (K4) are antithetical, as are Js^a

TABLE 56-6. Nomenclature and Gene Frequency for Major Kell Antigens

Antigen Symbol		Catalogue Number	Gene Frequencies: Whites	Gene Frequencies: Blacks
Alleles	K	K1	0.05	<0.01
	k	K2	0.95	>0.99
	Kp^a	K3	0.01	<0.01
	Kp^b	K4	0.99	>0.99
	Js^a	K6	<0.01	0.09
	Js^b	K7	>0.99	0.91

(Adapted from Race RR, Sanger R. Blood groups in man, ed 6. Oxford, Blackwell Scientific Publications, 1975)

(K6) and Js^b (K7). Kp^b or Js^b or both are present in more than 99% of random blood samples. Although the gene frequencies may be calculated independently for each Kell antigen, the different sets of alleles are clearly linked.

The expression of Kell system antigens is regulated by an altogether different gene, Kx, which is located on the X chromosome and therefore not genetically linked to the other Kell antigens. The Kx antigen (K15) is of extremely high incidence, and its absence results in the McLeod phenotype.[3]

K_o and McLeod Erythrocytes. Two null phenotypes have been identified, which underline the complexity and biologic importance of the Kell blood group antigens. In rare instances, people with the K_o phenotype lack expression of the Kell system antigens but have hyperexpression of the Kx antigen. K_o erythrocytes are phenotypically normal, and patients suffer no apparent clinical defect. Other rare people with what is referred to as the McLeod phenotype have weak expression of the Kell system antigens and total lack of Kx.[139,140] McLeod patients express abnormal erythrocyte morphology characterized by the existence of acanthocytosis (Fig. 56-7) and chronic hemolysis.[141,142] The peripheral blood of McLeod patients generally shows about 30% of the erythrocytes as having acanthocytic morphology, although this may vary from 10% to 85%.

No reliable morphologic difference is known between McLeod acanthocytes and those in other forms of acanthocytosis. Evaluation of Kell phenotype, serum lipids, liver functions, and family studies permits the distinction. The degree of chronic hemolysis is generally mild and fully compensated. McLeod patients may have had detectable hemolysis when newborns, but as adults they have normal erythrocyte laboratory values with mildly elevated reticulocyte counts (2% to 6%) and reduced serum haptoglobin levels. White blood cell and platelet counts are normal. Female relatives of the McLeod patients who carry the same X chromosome are mosaic for Kell antigens due to lyonization. Their peripheral blood contains 2% to 10% acanthocytes, and microscopic evaluation of agglutination with Kell antisera demonstrates a mixed field of two populations of erythrocytes—aggregated and free.

The McLeod phenotype is sometimes associated either with a subtle form of late-onset muscular dystrophy or with an X-linked form of chronic granulomatous disease.[143] When McLeod patients from multiple kindreds were examined by deletion analysis, it was established that the locus for Kx is on the short arm of the X chromosome between the loci for Duchenne type muscular dystrophy and chronic granulomatous disease, but closer to the latter.[144,145] Moreover, two McLeod patients who were related carried different Kell antigens, confirming that the reduced expression of Kell in the McLeod syndrome results from a mutation in the Kx locus.

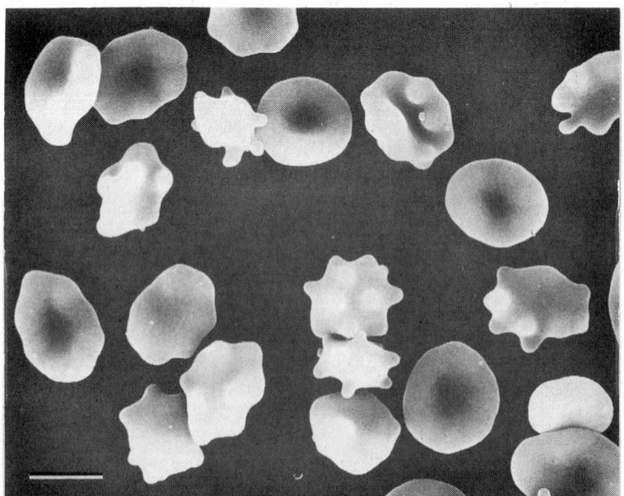

FIGURE 56-7. Scanning electron micrograph of McLeod erythrocytes. (Courtesy of Tellervo Huima, New York Blood Center)

Enhanced membrane bilayer translocation of phosphatidylcholine has been noted in McLeod erythrocytes.[146] This is probably pertinent to the abnormal morphology of the latter since the acanthocytosis can be reversed in vitro by the addition of exogenous lipid to the inner leaflet of the membrane bilayer.[147] Rheologic evaluation of McLeod erythrocyte membranes demonstrates a characteristic rigidity.[148]

Antibodies to Kell Antigens. Kell system antigens are of relatively low abundance on the erythrocyte membrane, existing in about 5000 sites per cell. Despite this, a person lacking a specific Kell system antigen has about a 10% chance of becoming immunized from a single transfusion.[149] Antibodies to Kell system antigens have also been described after certain bacterial infections.[150] Most examples of anti-K1 are IgG1. Kell antibodies may cause large difficulties in obtaining suitable units for blood transfusion since the incidence of several antigens is high. This is especially difficult if K_o or McLeod patients with a history of previous transfusion need subsequent transfusions and possess antibodies to ubiquitous antigens. Severe forms of hemolytic disease of the newborn may result from Kell system antibodies.

Biochemistry of Kell Antigens. Much progress has been made in the definition of Kell system antigens on a molecular level.[151] A 93-kd glycosylated membrane protein has been surface radiolabeled and selectively immunoprecipitated with Kell system antibodies.[152] This protein is distinct from band 3 (anion exchanger) and bears a unique N-terminal amino acid sequence. Indirect evidence indicates that multiple different Kell system antigens reside on this protein. The Kx antigen is located on a different membrane protein of 37 kd.[153] Isolation under nonreducing conditions leads to copurification of several additional membrane proteins, which is compatible with the observation that disulfide bonds are needed for expression of Kell system antigens.[153]

Kidd Antigens

Kidd antigens were first identified because of a novel antibody obtained from the mother of an infant suffering from neonatal hemolysis.[154] Two major alleles have been identified; Jk^a and Jk^b are expressed in nearly identical incidences in the white population, 26% Jk(a+b−), 24% Jk(a−b+), and 50% Jk(a+b+). About 18,000 Kidd system antigens are present per cell.[155]

Antibodies to Jk^a are found more commonly than anti-Jk^b. Most Kidd system antibodies are IgG or mixed IgG and IgM. Kidd antibodies frequently cause delayed transfusion reactions. These antibodies are often difficult to detect since the titer declines rapidly soon thereafter.

Rare people have been identified in Asian and Polynesian populations whose erythrocytes lack Kidd antigens, Jk(a−b−). The erythrocytes from these people resist lysis in 2 mol/L urea.[156] Using resistance to urea lysis as a screening test, 14 of 640,000 Japanese donors were found to be Jk(a−b−), and their erythrocyte membranes contained an abnormal protein of 67 kd.[157] Recent studies demonstrate that Jk(a−b−) erythrocytes are deficient in mediated urea transport.[158] Appearance of these two rare phenotypes led to the hypothesis that Kidd antigens are a component of the urea transporter.

Lutheran Antigens

Lutheran antigens were discovered because of the appearance of a novel antibody in a patient with systemic lupus erythematosus who had received blood from a donor named Lutheran.[160] The Lutheran system is composed of at least three sets of alleles, the most important of which are Lu^a and Lu^b. Clinical difficulties with the Lutheran antigens are uncommon, although delayed transfusion reactions have been described. Anti-Lu^a is usually predominantly IgM. Anti-Lu^b is rare. Relatively little is known about the biochemistry of the Lutheran antigens. About 2000 to 4000 antigens are present in each cell.[161] Lu^b is expressed on 78- and 85-kd membrane proteins that contain N-linked oligosaccharides.[162]

The gene frequency of Lu^a is low, so that only 0.15% of the population are homozygotes and express Lu(a+b−); the remainder of the population express Lu(a+b+) or Lu(a−b+). About 1 person in 3000 has inherited a dominantly acting inhibitor, *In(Lu)*, which partially suppresses the expression of the Lutheran antigens and several other antigens including i, P_1, Au^a, and others.[163] The nature of the *In(Lu)* gene product is uncertain, but it is speculated to be a glycosyltransferase since many of the inhibited antigens contain oligosaccharide.

The *In(Lu)* gene also suppresses expression of an 80-kd membrane glycoprotein normally found on erythrocytes, lymphocytes, and other tissues.[164–167] This protein is referred to as CDw44 and has been characterized in lymphocytes where it is responsible for T-lymphocyte adherence to endothelium.[168] Erythrocyte CD44 is the membrane site for the In^a and In^b antigens.[169,170] The cDNA for CDw44 is homologous to a class of proteins involved in cell interactions with extracellular matrix, the cartilage link proteins, which are hyperexpressed on the surface of carcinomas.[171,172] Recent work shows that CDw44 is also the cell-surface receptor for hyaluronate.[173] *In(Lu)* appears to be lineage specific, and *In(Lu)* patients have suppression of erythrocyte CDw44 but do not appear to have defects in lymphocyte function such as homing.

Duffy Antigens

The Duffy antigens were discovered from an antibody detected in the serum of a patient named Mr. Duffy, a hemophiliac with a need for chronic transfusions.[174] The antigen, Fy^a, was subsequently found in two thirds of whites as Fy(a+b−) or Fy(a+b+), with the remainder expressing Fy(a−b+). Among whites, the gene frequency of Fy^a is 0.43 and of Fy^b is 0.57. In 1955, Sanger and colleagues[175] reported the astonishing observation that two thirds of blacks living in the United States and the United Kingdom and 90% of blacks living in West Africa expressed neither antigen. The existence of Fy(a−b−) was estimated to be 100,000-fold less prevalent among Europeans. This genetic selection was perceived to be the result of malaria (see next section), and the Duffy gene in blacks is referred to as *Fy*.

Additional Duffy antigens have been described and are referred to as Fy3 (anti-Fy3 reacts with all Duffy phenotypes), Fy4, and Fy5 (anti-Fy5 fails to react with Rh_{null} erythrocytes). Duffy was the first blood group antigen for which chromosomal localization was achieved, with the locus existing on the long arm of chromosome 1.[176]

Duffy antigens do not commonly cause alloimmunization but have been implicated in transfusion reactions and hemolytic disease of the newborn. Nevertheless, delayed transfusion reactions have been ascribed to Duffy, which are frequent among blacks with sickle cell disease who require frequent transfusions.[177] Fy(a−b+) whites are multiple vulnerable to immunization than are blacks. Anti-Fy^a is usually IgG1 and is able to activate complement. Antibodies to Fy^b are encountered much more rarely.

The Duffy antigens have been partially characterized biochemically. About 17,000 Duffy antigens are present per erythrocyte.[155] An erythrocyte membrane protein of 35 to 43 kd was found to react specifically on immunoblots with anti-Fy^a.[178] This protein contains at least one asparagine-linked oligosaccharide and migrates as a 26-kd protein after deglycosylation.[179] The Duffy antigens appear to be an oligomeric complex of several additional proteins.[180]

The physiologic role of Duffy antigens is unclear. Nevertheless, structural proteins of the lens of the eye are well known to closely resemble those of the erythrocyte, and an unusual form of cataracts has been found to be inherited in linkage with the Duffy phenotype.[181]

Extensive investigation has implicated a variety of blood group antigens in the invasion of erythrocytes by malarial parasites, but only the role of Duffy antigens has been demonstrated clearly.[182] The invasion of erythrocytes is a complex event that includes merozoite binding to membrane sites, reorientation of the parasite with formation of an electron-dense attachment site, creation of a submembranous vacuole, and insertion of the parasite.[183]

Several lines of evidence indicate that the Duffy antigens are involved in *Plasmodium vivax* invasion, which causes a form of human malaria seen in Asia but not in West Africa where Fy(a−b−) is most common. In the early days of this century when neurosyphilis was treated by malaria-induced fevers, blacks were frequently found to be resistant to therapy.[184] Moreover, among American blacks developing vivax malaria in Vietnam, all were found to bear Fy^a or Fy^b.[185] *P vivax* cannot be cultured and studied directly. Laboratory strains of *P knowlesi*, which causes malaria in monkeys, have been adapted to invade human erythrocytes in vitro. These strains of *P knowlesi* merozoites can bind to human erythrocytes with all Duffy phenotypes, including Fy(a−b−), but can invade only erythrocytes with Fy^a or Fy^b.[186] Addition of antibodies to Fy^a or Fy^b inhibit the invasion of Fy(a+b+) erythrocytes.[187] In addition to Duffy antigens, a second membrane site is believed to be needed for invasion. Additional studies indicate that Duffy antigens are not involved in the invasion of *P falciparum*.

Other Blood Group Antigens

Although numerous other blood group antigens have been described, most are of minor clinical importance and are not understood on a molecular level. The following set of antigens is made up of three groups that are of significant biologic and genetic interest.

Glycosyl Phosphatidylinositol–Linked Antigens

Most of the antigens discussed in this section have a high frequency, one allele existing in most of the population. These antigens are of minor importance to alloimmunization but of great biologic interest because they are members of a new class of membrane proteins that has been discovered to be linked to the lipid bilayer through a glycosylated form of phosphatidylinositol.[188] The glycosyl phosphatidylinositol–linked membrane proteins are diverse with regard to physiologic function and include certain hydrolytic enzymes (such as acetylcholinesterase), cell adhesion molecules (such as neural cell adhesion molecule, N-CAM, and lymphocyte function–associated antigen 3, LFA-3), protozoal coat antigens, and nonerythroid antigens (such as Thy-1, and carcinoembryonic antigen, CEA). They are described in more detail in Chapter 11.

Although some variability is likely, the general structure of glycosyl phosphatidylinositol–linked proteins has been established (Fig. 56-8). The carboxy terminus of the protein is linked by an amide bond to ethanolamine, which is associated by a phosphodiester linkage to mannose within the glycan, a large and complex carbohydrate. At the reducing end of the glycan, the free amino group on N-acetylglucosamine is linked to the head group of phosphatidylinositol, with the fatty acids embedded in the outer leaflet of the lipid bilayer. Glycosyl phosphatidylinositol–linked structures exhibit a characteristic susceptibility to a phosphatidylinositol-specific type of phospholipase C, which cleaves between the phosphate and the first carbon of the glycerol backbone, leading to release of the proteins glycan and diacylglycerol (see arrow in Fig. 56-8).

Erythrocytes from patients with the clonal disorder paroxysmal nocturnal hemoglobinuria (PNH) lack decay-accelerating factor (DAF)[189] and membrane inhibitor of reactive lysis (MIRL).[190] Both DAF and MIRL are involved in restricting complement-induced membrane damage. DAF and MIRL are both anchored to the erythrocyte membrane by glycosyl phosphatidylinositol linkages.[191] The significance of the glycosyl phosphatidylinositol linkage is probably due to enhanced lateral mobility of proteins whose only point of membrane attachment is through a lipid tail. This enhanced mobility is likely to provide DAF and MIRL with greater ability to interact with and inhibit activated membrane complement. Unlike most glycosyl phosphatidylinositol–linked structures, the human erythrocyte forms of these molecules are poor substrates for phosphatidylinositol-specific phospholipase C, presumably due to modification of the inositol head group.

The molecular defect in PNH (see Chap. 11) most likely leads to a failure to make any glycosyl phosphatidylinositol–linked structures on blood cells. Studies on PNH erythrocytes demonstrated that the Cromer-related blood group antigens are deficient in PNH erythrocytes as well as from those of people with the rare *Inab* phenotype, in which only DAF is missing.[192] Thus, although blood cells from PNH patients lack all known glycosyl phosphatidylinositol–linked proteins, the Inab phenotype appears to lack only antigens on the DAF molecule.[193] The functional significance of this is not clear since the PNH erythrocytes have a well-described hemolytic defect, whereas the Inab phenotype expresses no hematologic abnormality (although some patients with Inab phenotype suffer inflammatory protein-losing enteropathy). A recent study shows that several other high-frequency blood group antigens are lacking in PNH erythrocytes, including Cartwright (Yt^a/Yt^b), Holley-Gregory (Hy/Gy^a), John Milton Hagen (JMH), and Dombrock antigens (Do^a/Do^b).[194] These data indicate that the Cromer blood group antigens reside on DAF, and the other high-frequency antigens are likely to reside on other glycosyl phosphatidylinositol–linked structures. The molecular localization of these latter high-frequency antigens is not established.

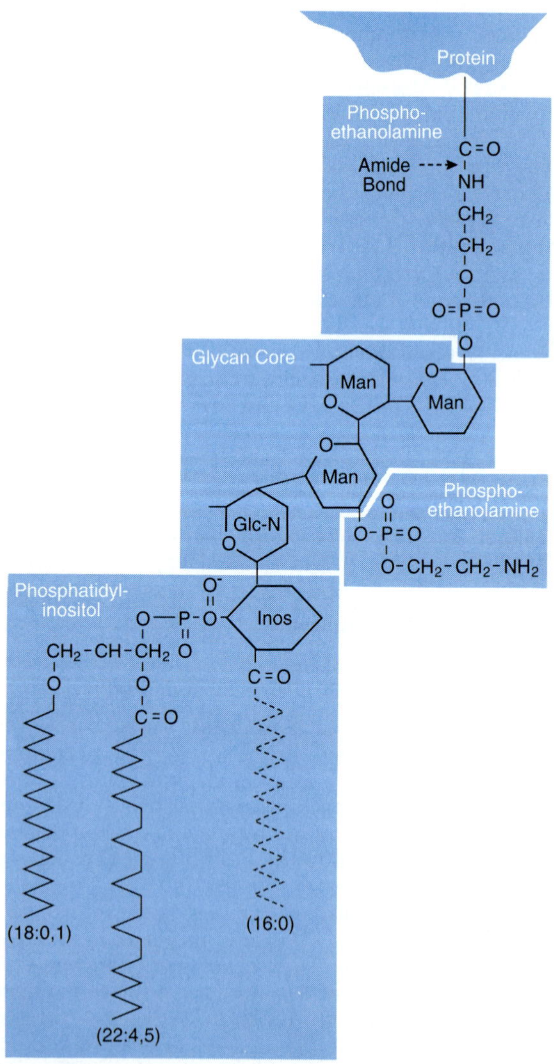

FIGURE 56-8. Diagram of a glycosyl phosphatidylinositol–linked membrane protein. (After Low MG, Saltiel AR. Structural and functional roles of glycosyl-phosphatidylinositol in membranes. Science 1988;239:268)

Chido-Rodgers Antigens

Chido-Rodgers antigens are polymorphic epitopes of the complement component C4d, which may be passively adsorbed to the surface of erythrocytes.[195] Plasma contains abundant complement and effectively neutralizes these antibodies. Neither Chido nor Rodgers is commonly implicated in clinically important alloimmunization. These determinants are enriched on erythrocyte membranes from patients with cold-reacting agglutinins since increased complement deposition occurs.

Xg^a Antigen

The gene Xg^a that encodes the Xg^a antigen has been of great genetic interest since it is carried on the X chromosome.[196] The Xg^a antigen is distinct from Kx, which is also located on the X chromosome and is important in Kell antigen expression (see section on Kell antigen). The allele, *Xg*, is amorphic since no immunologically detectable antigen is expressed. Males therefore either express or fail to express the Xg^a antigen, depending on whether they have inherited Xg^a or *Xg*. The gene frequency for Xg^a is 0.66 in males.[3] Females may be heterozygotes for Xg^a and *Xg*, but due to variable inactivation of the X chromosome (lyonization), one allele may predominate in an individual. Antibodies to Xg^a are rarely of clinical importance.

LEUKOCYTE ANTIGENS

Granulocyte-Specific Antigens

Human leukocytes contain membrane antigens that are important in alloimmunization. These have been reviewed in detail.[197,198] Each line of leukocytes has some antigens expressed only in that lineage, whereas other antigens, such as the HLA antigens, are shared widely among nucleated cells. The shared antigens are not discussed in this chapter because they are covered elsewhere. This section focuses on antigens associated with alloimmune disease, which are restricted to neutrophils, eosinophils, and basophils—the granulocyte-specific antigens. Recent molecular analysis of these antigens has revealed closely related proteins on other cell lineages as well. Several of these leukocyte antigens are likely to be differentiation specific since they are found only after the myelocyte stage of maturation. Disappearance of these antigens has been shown to precede blast crisis of chronic granulocytic leukemia[199] (see Chap. 15).

Because of the pioneering work of Lalezari and others,[203–209] a series of granulocyte antigens is now well characterized (Table 56-7). These antigens were identified because of their involvement in alloimmunization due to pregnancy and transfusions, as well as to autoimmune neutropenias.[198,200,214,215] The granulocyte-specific antigens are less well defined serologically and biochemically than the erythrocyte blood group antigens. This is partly due to technical difficulties in reproducibly measuring granulocyte agglutination, and it is likely that new granulocytic antigens are still to be identified. Rapid progress in the molecular characterizations of granulocyte-specific antigens is now emerging.

NA1 was the first granulocyte-specific antigen to be defined.[203] NA1 is a member of the two-allele NA locus. NA antigens are known to be the surface Fc receptor III,[216] termed CD16 by the International Workshop on Human Leukocyte Differentiation Antigens. In addition to neutrophils, this receptor is also present on macrophages and natural killer cells. The Fc receptor III functions to remove immune complexes from the circulation by phagocytosis. It is linked to the membrane by a glycosyl phosphatidylinositol anchor and, like similarly linked erythrocyte proteins, Fc receptor III is deficient in paroxysmal nocturnal hemoglobinuria.[202,212]

The polymorphisms responsible for the antigenic differences between NA1 and NA2 were recently deduced at the nucleotide level.[210,211] NA1 and NA2 differ by four amino acid residues, of which two are probable sites of N-glycosylation; therefore, NA1 potentially has four N-linked glycans, and NA2 has six. A patient with lupus erythematosus was recently found to lack the neutrophil Fc receptor III despite expressing normal amounts of other Fc and complement receptors.[201] The molecular defect was identified within the Fc receptor III gene. This observation lends support to the speculation that Fc receptor III may be defective in clearing immune complexes in at least some lupus patients.

Initial biochemical characterization of the NB1 antigen demonstrated it to be a 55- to 66-kd glycoprotein found on the plasma membrane and on secondary granules of neutrophils.[213] The antigenic epitope is determined by the structure of the protein core since immunoreactivity is abrogated by reducing agents but not by periodate. The normal biologic role of the NB1-bearing protein is not known.

Other granulocyte antigens have been described for which the basic biologic role is not defined (NC1, ND1, NE1, and the HGA-3 antigens). The gene frequencies at each of these loci is less than 1.0, indicating either that there are alleles that encode amorphic antigens or that antithetical antigens have eluded serologic identification. In addition, autoantibodies with specific reactivity for neutrophils have been identified, and the membrane antigens are likely to be involved in alloimmune disorders also. Autoantibodies reacting with membrane-bound actin and other autoantibodies reacting with the neutrophil cell adhesion complex CD11B/CD18 have both recently been described in patients with autoimmune neutropenia and infections.[217,218]

TABLE 56-7. Human Granulocyte-Specific Antigens

Locus	Antigen	Gene Frequency	References
NA	NA1	0.32	201–205, 208, 210–212, 216
	NA2	0.68	
NB	NB1	0.72	207, 209, 213
	NB2	0.17	
NC	NC1	0.80	206
ND	ND1	0.88	216
NE	NE1	0.12	200
HGA-3	HGA-3a	0.11	214
	HGA-3b	0.13	
	HGA-3c	0.08	
	HGA-3d	0.31	
	HGA-3e	0.09	

Neonatal Alloimmune Neutropenia

Antibodies to granulocyte antigens are involved in at least four disease states: (1) neonatal alloimmune neutropenia, (2) febrile transfusion reactions (see Chap. 60), (3) pulmonary infiltrates after transfusions (see Chap. 60), and (4) autoimmune neutropenia (see Chap. 17). This section will focus on the first disorder since the remaining three are presented elsewhere in the text.

Neonatal alloimmune neutropenia in many ways resembles neonatal hemolytic disease (see Chap. 64). Both result from maternal IgG that crosses the placenta and reacts with antigens on fetal blood cells. Neonatal alloimmune neutropenia is usually recognized because of infections developing in infants soon after birth. This disorder is characterized by severely depressed peripheral neutrophil counts and high titer maternal IgG that reacts with neutrophils of the father and the infant.[204] The N series of granulocyte antigens are frequently involved in this disorder. In a review of neonatal neutropenia in 19 infants from 10 families, 4 mothers had circulating antibodies to NB1, 3 had anti-NA1, 1 had anti-NA2, 1 had anti-NC1, and 1 had an undetermined specificity.[208] Unlike neonatal hemolytic disease, neonatal neutropenia may develop during the first pregnancy, as was found in 4 of the 10 families cited.

The incidence of maternal antibodies to leukocyte antigens is high. In a prospective survey of 200 women analyzed at the end of the first pregnancy or during subsequent pregnancies, 3% were found to have antibodies agglutinating the husband's neutrophils.[219] Despite this risk for isoimmune neutropenia, the actual incidence of the disorder is much lower. Many antibodies detected in multiparous women are probably antibodies to HLA antigens, which usually cause no harm to the fetus since HLA antigens are present in the plasma and on the surface of nearly all fetal cells.

Clinical difficulties due to alloimmune neonatal neutropenia are relatively uncommon but may be severe.[220] The neonatal infections are most frequently staphylococcal skin infections. *E coli* and streptococcal infections are also seen. Although rare, pneumonia and septicemia have been reported. Therapy with corticosteroids is definitely contraindicated because it does nothing to reduce the circulating IgG titer and may harm the infant's own developing immune system. The maternal antibody is gradually cleared by the infant, so that the condition spontaneously resolves 2 to 3 months after birth. Antibiotic therapy specific for the infecting organism should be instituted. In severe cases, the infant may need plasmapheresis followed by infusion of granulocytes harvested from the mother and therefore lacking the involved antigen.

PLATELET ALLOANTIGENS AND ALLOANTIBODIES

Immunization against platelet alloantigens is involved in the pathogenesis of two important hematologic syndromes, neonatal alloimmune thrombocytopenic purpura (NATP) and, posttransfusion purpura (PTP). Infants affected with NATP have platelets containing antigenically different epitopes from their mothers'. An infant's paternally derived antigens elicit formation of maternal IgG alloantibodies, which cross the placenta and destroy fetal platelets. In PTP, the alloimmune response is stimulated after transfusion of blood products. Both of these syndromes can lead to severe thrombocytopenia and life-threatening hemorrhage. Therefore, immediate therapy is important. The platelet alloantigens that have been recognized to date are reviewed here, and these two clinical syndromes of platelet alloimmunization are described. Alloimmunization against platelets can also cause refractoriness to platelet transfusions. This problem is more appropriate to the topic of transfusion medicine and is not discussed in detail in this chapter.

PLATELET ALLOANTIGENS

The platelet-specific alloantigens that have been identified are listed in Table 56-8. Included are the various names used in the literature. The initial descriptions of platelet alloantigens used letters from the surname of the first patient shown to be alloimmunized. This approach yielded multiple names for the same alloantigen (eg, Bak^a = Lek^a, Pen^a = Yuk^b). A systematic nomenclature based on numbered human platelet antigens (HPA) was proposed and has been adopted in much of the literature since 1984.[221] Recently, a nomenclature system has been offered that denotes the parent glycoprotein and the polymorphism responsible for the immunologic allotype.[221] This approach is cumbersome, but it has merit in that it contains precise molecular information; it has not yet been adopted in the literature. Here, we use the HPA terminology for those antigens that have been so named and the family surname terminology for other antigens. Table 56-8 serves as a code for translation between the three systems.

Most of the platelet alloantigens that have been characterized are contained on glycoproteins IIb and IIIa, the complex that binds fibrinogen during platelet aggregation.

TABLE 56-8. Platelet Alloantigens

Human Platelet Antigen Nomenclature	Original Names	Genetic Polymorphism Nomenclature	Gene Frequency (in Whites)
HPA-1a	Pl^{A1}, Zw^a	gpIIIa	0.85
HPA-1b	Pl^{A2}, Zw^b	Pro 33 gpIIIa	0.15
HPA-2a	Ko^b, Sib^b	gpIb	0.93
HPA-2b	Ko^a, Sib^a	Met 145 gpIb	0.07
HPA-3a	Bak^a, Lek^a	gpIIb	0.61
HPA-3b	Bak^b, Lek^b	Ser 843 gpIIb	0.39
HPA-4a	Pen^a, Yuk^b	gpIIIa	0.85
HPA-4b	Pen^b, Yuk^a	Gln 143 gpIIIa	<0.01
HPA-5a	Br^b, Zav^b, Hc^b	gpIa	0.89
HPA-5b	Br^a, Zav^a, Hc^a	Lys 505 gpIa	0.11
HPA-6a	Ca^a, Tu^a	gpIIIa	0.85
HPA-6b	Ca^b, Tu^b	Gln 489 gpIIIa	<0.01

The heterodimer complexes gpIIb/gpIIIa, gpIc/gpIIa and gpIa/gpIIa are members of the integrin superfamily of cytoadhesive receptors. Members of the integrin group occur on a number of different cells, including endothelial cells, fibroblasts, and leukocytes.[223–225] The gpIb/gpIX complex is not a member of this family of cytoadhesions but is a complex including the leucine-rich platelet membrane protein, gpIb.[226–229] All of these non-HLA platelet alloantigens present on platelet glycoproteins are often referred to as "platelet-specific" antigens, although many are also present on the surface glycoproteins of other cell types.[230]

Individual Platelet Specific Alloantigens

HPA-1

The platelet alloantigen system that has been best characterized is the one implicated most frequently in alloimmune diseases, HPA-1a (Pl^{A1} or Zw^a).[231,232] The biallelic HPA-1a and HPA-1b antigens are contained on gpIIIa and depend on the presence of disulfide bonds.[233] The difference between gpIIIa of HPA-1a and HPA-1b platelets is defined by a single amino acid polymorphism (Leu = HPA-1a; Pro = HPA-1b) at residue 33, which is encoded by a single base difference at cDNA position 196.[234] Using site-directed mutagenesis, Goldberger and colleagues[235] documented that this single change accounts for the immunologic differences defined serologically by anti–HPA-1a and anti–HPA-1b antisera. The precise peptide conformation of the HPA epitopes has not yet been elucidated, although a recombinant peptide identical to the 66 amino-terminal residues of gpIIIa was shown to express the HPA-1a antigen.[236] Monoclonal antibodies have been produced that can recognize the difference between denatured HPA-1a and HPA-1b gpIIIa, although they do not recognize the native forms of the protein.[237–239]

The frequency of HPA expression varies among different populations. A small group (2.1%) of whites studied in several series have the HPA-1b phenotype, although HPA-1b is absent in Japanese and other Asian populations studied.[240–243] Although HPA-1 incompatibility accounts for most cases of platelet alloimmune diseases in whites, this situation has not been described in Asians.

HPA-2

The HPA-2 alloantigen system was described independently by alloantibodies found in European[244] and Japanese[245] populations. These antigens are contained on gpIb, a leucine-rich protein component of the platelet membrane.[245–248] The HPA-2a antigen, which is only expressed on the A and B forms of this polymorphic glycoprotein,[248] is located at amino-terminal protion of gpIbα. It is defined by a particular polymorphism at residue 145 (Thr = HPA-2a; Met = HPA-2b).[246,247] Based on the reported cases, this antigen system appears to be most important in refractoriness to platelet transfusions,[244,245] although NATP has been reported.[249]

HPA-3

Glycoprotein IIb contains the polymorphism that defines the HPA-3 antigens (Bak^a and Bak^b or Lek^a and Lek^b).[250–254] The two allelic forms differ by one amino acid near the carboxy terminal of gpIIbα (residue 843; Ser = HPA-3a and Ile = HPA-3b).[255,256] Anti–HPA-3 antibodies have been shown to vary in their dependence on the native conformation and presence of intact carbohydrates on gpIIb.[257] Subsequent studies have found that HPA-3a can be destroyed specifically by removal of O-linked sugars, rather than sialic acid or N-linked carbohydrate[256] and that a single O-linked carbohydrate at residue 847 was responsible for HPA-1a.[257]

Approximately 87.7% of whites have phenotypically HPA-3a platelets (HPA-3a/HPA-3a and HPA-3a/HPA3b); the frequency among Japanese is 78.9%.[240–243] Although maternal–fetal incompatibility for the HPA-3 antigens occurs frequently, only rarely is this situation accompanied by a clinical diagnosis of NATP.[250,259] Studies of fetal platelets in whites suggest that the frequency of this phenotype is significantly lower early in development.[260,261] It is not yet known whether there is a difference in the glycosylation of fetal and adult gpIIb.

HPA-4

Incompatibility of the HPA-4 antigens is the most common cause of alloimmunization among the Japanese population[262] and has been described in rare cases among other ethnic groups.[263–265] This second alloantigen system to be described, which was localized to gpIIIa, is also biallelic.[266–268] The epitopes are determined by an arginine to glutamine polymorphism of gpIIIa at residue 143.[269,270] The binding domain for adhesive macromolecules includes this polymorphic residue; thus, it is not surprising that HPA-4 alloimmunization has been associated with serious hemorrhage in vivo[263] and platelet dysfunction in vitro.[266]

HPA-5

The platelet alloantigen system implicated as the cause of NATP second in frequency after HPA-1 is HPA-5, first named Br, Zav, and Hc.[271–273] The HPA-5a and HPA-5b allelic antigens are contained on the gpIa portion of gpIa/gpIIa, another integrin complex,[271–273] and are determined by a single amino acid polymorphism at residue 505 (Lys in HPA-5a; Glu in HPA-5b).[274] The gpIa/gpIIa complex acts as a collagen receptor, although anti–HPA-5 antibodies do not induce a functional defect in platelets.[274] Although the initial cases of alloimmunization against HPA-5a were NATP, this antigen has also been associated with PTP.[275]

Other Platelet Alloantigens

Another alloantigen system on gpIIIa, Ca, has been reported as a cause of NATP.[276] Designated HPA-6, this antigen is identical to Tu.[277] The precise molecular characterization and genetic specification of these antigens are not yet complete, although the epitope was reported to be in a proximity to the AP3 monoclonal antibody binding site on gpIIIa.[276]

Alloantigens under further investigation include Pl^{T},[278] contained on gpV, Gov,[279] present on a 150-kd platelet protein, and Vis, contained on gpIV.[280] Incompatibility of each of these antigens has been recognized in a single family with NATP. Designation as an HPA allotype awaits confirmation of their characterization. The initial case report of NATP was due to incompatibility of an antigen named Duzo.[281] This antigen was not able to be fully characterized at that time, and the plasma from that case has been depleted.

Several cases of alloimmunization have been reported in which the target antigen is one which occurs with extremely low frequency in the population, usually identified only in the proband case. Such private antigens include Va,[282] Sr,[283] and Mo,[284] which are private epitopes on gpIIIa. The Mo antigen, proposed as HPA-7, is determined by a C → G point mutation on the gpIIIa gene encoding for residue 407 of gpIIIa (proline → alanine).[284]

Antigens Shared With Other Cells

The ABO carbohydrate antigens of erythrocytes are also present platelets.[285–289] These antigens are expressed in variable amounts on platelets from different individuals and can be important in platelet transfusion refractoriness;[289] Rh antigens do not occur on platelets.

The class I antigens of the multiallelic HLA system are present on platelets, although their density is variable. Most cases of platelet transfusion refractoriness on an immune basis are due to anti-HLA antigens. This clinical condition is not discussed further in this chapter. Alloimmunization to HLA has been reported to cause NATP,[290–292] although the coexistence of platelet-specific antibodies may have complicated some of these cases.

Isoantigens

Antibodies produced by individuals who lack a particular platelet glycoprotein on exposure to normal platelets either by pregnancy or transfusion are "isoantibodies." Isoimmunization may have been involved in some of the antibodies that characterized the Pl^{E} antigen on gpIb.[293] The Nak^{a} isoantigen on gpIV was identified in transfusion refractoriness in Japan.[294,295] Isoantibodies can also be formed against gpIIb/gpIIIa by patients with type I Glanzmann's thrombocytopenia who are totally deficient in this glycoprotein complex.[296]

NEONATAL ALLOIMMUNE THROMBOCYTOPENIA

History

Neonatal alloimmune thrombocytopenia was first recognized in 1954[297] in an infant with transient thrombocytopenia whose mother had a normal platelet count. Platelet agglutinins were present in the maternal plasma, and alloimmunity was proposed to be the cause for the infant's thrombocytopenia.[297] The syndrome of NATP due to HPA-1a (Pl^{A1} or Zw^{a}) antigen has been best studied,[231,232] and its clinical features were well characterized in early series.[297a,298] Even in recent series, HPA-1a incompatibility accounts for most of the cases.[299–305] Because the greatest experience has been acquired from cases of HPA-1a incompatibility, current understanding of typical clinical findings and available approaches to diagnosis and management relate primarily to this particular syndrome. In some situations, incompatibility of another antigen is associated with different clinical features; when these have been established, the differences are noted here.

In 1989, the genetic basis defining the HPA-1a and HPA-1b antigens was reported.[234] It is now possible to determine platelet alloantigen genotype directly using amniocytes, chorionic villi, or white cell DNA,[306–309] and these techniques are now being used clinically. It has even been possible to accomplish HPA-1 typing on a single blastomere cell.[310]

Clinical Features

Neonatal alloimmune thrombocytopenia occurs in only 1 of 2000 to 5000 newborns.[311] The hallmark of NATP is severe, isolated thrombocytopenia in an infant who is otherwise healthy. Because the destructive antibodies are produced by the mother, thrombocytopenia is transient. Nevertheless, during the perinatal period, the affected offspring is at risk for serious hemorrhage, which can be fatal or lead to neurologic impairment. The platelet counts in infants who suffer intracranial hemorrhage are usually less than 10,000/μL. It is common for the platelet count to fall immediately after birth before resolution within the first 3 weeks of life.[298] Maternal alloantibody against infant platelets may be present in breast milk, although breast feeding has not been reported to increase the risk of hemorrhage.

The differential diagnosis for an infant with unexpected thrombocytopenia includes maternal autoimmune or drug-dependent thrombocytopenia, preeclampsia, or HELLP syndrome in the mother, as well as neonatal viral or bacterial infection, congential bone marrow hypoplasia, amegakaryocytic thrombcytopenia, osteopetrosis, prematurity, or birth asphyxia in the newborn. Any infant with hepatosplenomegaly or intracranial calcifications should be evaluated for possible congenital viral infection. Isolated thrombocytopenia is typical in NATP even when reported cases are thought to be caused by HLA incompatibility.[290,291]

The analogous alloimmune disorder involving erythrocytes is Rh incomptibility or erythroblastosis fetalis. One significant difference between these two syndromes is that NATP can occur in first pregnancies. In fact, about half the reported cases are in firstborn infants, and the platelet destruction may occur as early as 16 weeks of gestation.[260] Obviously, immunization occurs early in pregnancy, but it is not known whether fetal platelets actually enter the maternal circulation or whether the HPA-1a antigen expressed on tissues of the trophoblast stimulates the maternal immune response.

Bleeding manifestations in the infant affected with NATP range from the skin petechiae and ecchymoses seen in most patients to life-threatening intracranial hemorrhage. In an estimated 10% to 15% of infants with NATP, the outcome is fatal, while neurologic sequelae occur in a similar number.[298,302,303,312] Anti–HPA-1a antibodies have been demonstrated to cause a qualitative platelet defect in vitro.[266,313,314] The HPA-4 epitope is located at the RGD binding region of gpIIIa, and these alloantibodies also interfere with platelet function.[266] Antifunctional effects of antibodies against other alloantigens have not been reported. Not only is there a high risk of serious bleeding in infants with NATP, antenatal hemorrhage can occur, resulting in hydrocephalus, porencephly, seizures, or fetal loss.[263,312,315–322]

Evaluation and Management of the First Affected Infant in a Family

The first infant in a family affected with NATP usually presents with severe isolated thrombocytopenia but no other abnormality. In this circumstance, the diagnosis of NATP is presumptive, based on the clinical presentation. Therapy must be initiated immediately, coincident with the confirmatory immunologic assays, since infants with NATP are at risk for serious CNS hemorrhage.

The laboratory assessment should include tests to determine whether there is a platelet alloantibody detectible in both maternal and fetal plasma or serum. Maternal plasma should be tested against paternal or neonatal platelets as targets. Maternal (antigen-negative) platelets and paternal (antibody-negative) plasma or serum should be used as negative controls. A number of different techniques are used by platelet immunology laboratories for these assays. Most specialists in this field now favor an antigen capture approach for documenting the presence of alloantibodies against a particular glycoprotein complex (eg, the monoclonal antibody immobilization of platelet antigens [MAIPA],[323] immunobead or microtiter well radioimmunoassay,[324] and the antigen capture ELISA or ACE[325] and their modifications). These antibody assays can identify platelet glycoprotein alloantibodies even if anti-HLA antibodies coexist; however, all of these techniques require specification and capture (with a monoclonal antibody) of a particular target platelet glycoprotein complex of interest. Regardless of which alloantigen incompatibility is responsible for NATP, paternal platelets will be obligate antigen-positive targets, while maternal platelets will be negative. The mother's serum often has a higher titer of antibody than does the infant's. A bone marrow aspirate is not included in the evaluation of an infant suspected to have NATP unless hypoproduction is considered to be a possible cause.

It is also necessary to type the mother's and father's platelets for the alloantigens most frequently involved in NATP. Among white populations, HPA-1 and HPA-5 are implicated most frequently,[299–305] whereas for Japanese, HPA-4 (Yuk) is most frequently found.[262] Techniques for the serologic allotyping of platelets include any of the capture assays, FACS, platelet suspension immunofluorescence, radioimmunoassays, immunoblotting, platelet lysis, and complement fixation. All of these serologic approaches require the availability of accurately typed platelets as targets. In recent years, DNA analysis for the specific genotypes of the incompatible platelet antigen has become a possibility for the diagnostic platelet immunology laboratory[306–310]; these techniques are likely to become the standard for platelet allotyping in the near future.

Although NATP may have resolved before completion of a full laboratory evaluation, these studies should be done in a reasonable period of time. It is important to confirm the diagnosis and to identify the specific antigen incompatibility to allow accurate counseling about future pregnancies. Antibody titers peak shortly after birth and then decline, so the investigations should be performed within the first year after delivery, even if the parents are uncertain whether they desire to have more children.

Treatment

Therapeutic management of the affected infant is aimed at increasing the platelet count and reducing the risk of hemorrhage. Modalities that have been used include steroids,[297,298,326,327] exchange transfusion,[298] and transfusion with antigen-negative platelets.[320,327,328] Recently, intravenous immunoglobulin infusion and transfusion of antigen negative platelets have been the mainstays of therapy. Intravenous immunoglobulin, 1 g/kg/d for 1 to 3 days, has been used for the past 10 years.[312,329–332] With intravenous IgG, the platelet count usually rises 10,000 to 20,000/μL/d, reaching 100,000 within 1 week. Transfusion with allocompatible platelets is preferable for the infant with serious hemorrhage, since an immediate correction of thrombocytopenia results.

Random donor platelets have a 98% chance to be HPA-1a. Even if the NATP is caused by HPA-1a incompatibility, a transient improvement in the platelet count may occur.[327,333] Immediate transfusion of random donor platelets is appropriate for the infant with serious hemorrhage. Simultaneously, antigen-negative platelets should be prepared for transfusion. Usually, the only available donor for these platelets is the infant's mother. Transfer of more alloantibody may prolong the NATP; therefore, unnecessary plasma should be removed by concentration or gentle washing of the platelet concentrate.[327,334] Maternal platelets must be irradiated to avoid graft-versus-host disease in the infant if the mother is homozygous for one of the infant's HLA haplotypes. Even maternal platelets should be tested for HIV and hepatitis. Should the mother be HIV-positive, transfusion poses a greater risk of transfer to the infant than would perinatal exposure alone. For the infant with active, life-threatening hemorrhage, abbreviated testing may be necessary.

Management of Future Pregnancies

After one child in a family is affected with NATP, subsequent pregnancies are at high risk for the same syndrome. Although a minority of women make alloantibodies if they are pregnant with a fetus of incompatible platelet type, a woman who has this reaction once is almost certain to do so again. In fact, the severity of both thrombocytopenia and hemorrhage may increase in later pregnancies.[312] The parents should be counseled about the risk of recurrence. It is valuable to know whether the father is homozygous or heterogyzous for the offending allotype. If he is homozygous, a recurrence is virtually certain, whereas the risk is 50% if the father is heterozygous. Management of affected pregnancies should include the expertise of a high-risk perinatal center and a platelet immunology laboratory. Considerable improvements in understanding and outcome of these pregnancies has occurred in recent years. Therefore, recommendations made previously should be reviewed with each subsequent pregnancy.

It is not possible to determine whether a particular fetus is affected based on titers of circulating antiplatelet alloantibody during pregnancy.[298,335] Platelet alloantigens have been demonstrated on platelets as early as 16 weeks of gestational age,[260] and some fetuses have had hemorrhage before this age.[336] By 20 to 24 weeks of gestation, the fetal platelet count and allotype can be determined by percutaneous umbilical blood sampling (PUBS).[312,337] Frequent ultrasound examinations during pregnancy are recommended to observe the clinical status of the fetus. However, antenatal intracranial hemorrhage may not always be obvious on ultrasound.[321]

The period of greatest risk for intracranial hemorrhage in NATP is during labor and delivery. Cesarean section has been recommended for all affected pregnancies,[338,339] unless fetal thrombocytopenia has been corrected.[312,337] Platelet transfusions have been administered to the fetus via PUBS near term to allow a safe, induced vaginal delivery.[335,336] Antigen-negative platelets must be used; they are generally obtained from the mother before the procedure. Most investigators administer platelets to the fetus whenever PUBS is performed to protect against bleeding. The platelets must be irradiated to avoid the possibility of graft-versus-host disease. One group has considered the use of cryopreserved, type-specific platelets for fetal transfusions.[340] Fetal scalp sampling was used at one time during labor to determine the fetal platelet count, but it has been replaced by PUBS at most perinatal centers.[337]

Neither operative delivery nor a perinatal platelet transfusion can affect the risk of antenatal hemorrhage. Recently, investigators have administered intravenous immunoglobulin to the mother to increase the fetal platelet count. Bussel and colleagues[312,341] found an improvement in fetal platelet count in 75% to 80% of pregnancies treated weekly with 1 g/kg of γ-globulin administered intravenously to the mother. They found that treatment with oral steroids was not routinely indicated and may be associated with oligohydramnios. However, other investigators reported a rise in fetal platelet count in only one of seven cases treated with intravenous IgG.[342] For a few pregnancies in families with histories of serious hemorrhage in which maternal intravenous immunoglobulin has not been effective, weekly in utero platelet transfusions have been reported.[336] This heroic approach is not currently recommended for routine management of pregnancies complicated by NATP. In fact, there is no consensus of opinion regarding the management of these pregnancies, as was demonstrated in a recent international forum.[343] Further clinical studies in this area are ongoing.

After birth, the affected infant's platelet count should be monitored closely for the first several days of life. Therapy with intravenous immunoglobulin or transfusion with maternal platelets is indicated if there is bleeding or if the thrombocytopenia is severe. Unless the infant's thrombocytopenia has been corrected, antigen-negative platelets should be available before delivery for immediate administration in the case of serious hemorrhage.

Role of Immune Risk Factors

The syndrome of NATP is diagnosed in only 1 of 2000 to 5000 births,[297,311] although 2% to 3% of pregnant white women are HPA-1b–positive and 85% of their children are HPA-1a–positive. Possible explanations for this marked discrepancy are that HPA-1a is only a weak antigen and that only a minority of the exposed women become immunized and produce IgG anti–HPA-1a antibodies. The second hypothesis has gained much supporting evidence. Reznikoff-Etievant and colleagues[344,345] first reported that mothers of infants with NATP were predominantly of the HLA type B8, DR3 when compared with the general population. The HLA class II superfamily has been confirmed as being of greatest risk for HPA-1a alloimmunization,[346–348] although the precise molecular mechanism has not been elucidated. It is not yet known whether alloimmunization against other platelet specific antigens is affected by immune response restriction, although in one case of NATP due to anti–HPA-1b, the HLA DRw52 was not present.[349]

POSTTRANSFUSION PURPURA

History

The first case reports of the clinical entity now known as posttransfusion purpura (PTP) appeared approximately 30 years ago.[231,232,350] The patients described were women in whom a sudden, severe destructive thrombocytopenia and hemorrhage appeared several days after blood transfusions. One reported patient had potent platelet agglutinins in her serum, but the suspected alloimmune specificity of the antibody could not be determined.[350] Van Loghem and associates[231] defined the platelet specific alloantigen Zw^a (also known as Pl^{A1} and now referred to as HPA-1a), which was present on the platelets of 280 of 287 individuals (97.65%). Since these early reports, numerous other cases with similar clinical features have appeared in the literature; these were tabulated in detail in a comprehensive review[351] and are summarized here. A large European series of PTP cases has subsequently appeared in the literature.[352] The most mysterious aspect of this syndrome is that autologous antigen-negative platelets are destroyed during the development of an alloantibody.

Clinical Presentation

The typical case of PTP occurs in a multiparous woman with HPA-1b platelets who is reimmunized with HPA-1a by blood transfusion and becomes acutely thrombocytopenic about 1 week later. Males have also developed PTP, as have nulliparous females. In these situations, the initial exposure to HPA-1a occurred through a blood transfusion. Most reported patients have been in their 60s and 70s. The history of pregnancy or transfusion and the brief 5- to 10-day period between reexposure and thrombocytopenia suggest that affected patients are undergoing an anamnestic response to the platelet alloantigen. The thrombocytopenia is usually severe, with platelet counts below 10,000/μL; clinical evidence of hemorrhage is common. Petechiae, purpura, and bleeding from puncture sites and surgical wounds often occur, as do hematuria and gastrointestinal hemorrhage. Transfusion of platelets is of no benefit, regardless of their allotype. Examination of the bone marrow reveals active thrombopoiesis, indicating a destructive thrombocytopenia.

The diagnosis of PTP is initially made by excluding other possible causes for thrombocytopenia. The absence of disseminated intravascular coagulation (due to sepsis, hypoxia, tissue necrosis, or erythrocyte transfusion reaction); bone marrow hypoplasia; thrombotic thrombocytopenic purpura; drug-dependent immune thrombocytopenia; autoimmune thrombocytopenia; and other causes for platelet destruction in a previously sensitized individual should suggest the diagnosis of PTP.

Assays for direct and indirect antiplatelet antibodies are usually positive regardless of the method used. The diagnosis is supported by finding an alloantibody in the patient's serum and is further confirmed by documenting that the patient's platelets lack the specific alloantigen target of that antibody. The platelet allotyping may not be feasible until after recovery except by flow cytometric techniques because of very low platelet counts. Most reported cases have been associated with alloimmunization against HPA-1a. The titer of alloantibody usually falls coincident with spontaneous recovery from the thrombocytopenia (within 4 days to 4 months; mean of 27 days).

Although the overall frequency for febrile transfusion reactions among blood product recipients is 1%, as many as 46% of patients diagnosed as having PTP experienced such reactions either with the reimmunizing transfusion or with blood products given later to treat the thrombocytopenia or hemorrhagic complications.[351] Several patients have also suffered hypotension, urticaria, or bronchospasm.

Treatment

At the time the diagnosis of PTP is suspected, any unnecessary medications should be discontinued. In particular, captopril has been reported to enhance the binding of anti–HPA-1a antibodies to platelets by 50%.[354] Numerous treatment modalities have been reported to be beneficial, including corticosteroids, plasmapharesis, exchange transfusion, and intravenous γ-globulin. Some overly aggressive therapies have been attempted without benefit (eg, immunosuppression and splenectomy).[355] High-dose methylprednisolone may be of value,[356] although corticosteroids in the usual doses (1 to 2 mg/kg/d) have not been shown to be beneficial.

Platelet transfusions have not increased the platelet count regardless of whether antigen-positive or antigen-negative platelets were given.[357] Blood transfusions often result in transfusion reactions. Therefore, after the diagnosis is made, blood products should be transfused with careful monitoring for transfusion reaction. Washed red cells may decrease the high risk of febrile transfusion reaction.

Intravenous immunoglobulin therapy is recommended as the treatment of choice.[352,358–365] The recommended doses are those found to be effective in treating autoimmune thrombocytopenia (400 mg to 1 g/kg/d for 2 to 5 days). These recommendations for treatment are based on experience in case reports, since there have been no controlled trials of treatment in this extremely rare syndrome.

Subsequent Transfusion Therapy

After PTP, subsequent transfusions with antigen-incompatible blood products may occur without incident or may initiate thrombocytopenia coincident with another rise in antibody titer.[366,367] Thus, patients with PTP who require blood products again should probably receive autologous or washed red cells or blood products from alloantigen-negative donors.

Role of Immune Risk Factors

The true incidence of PTP is unknown, although it is certainly a rare syndrome, with only about 200 cases reported. Approximately 2% of transfusion recipients of Northern European descent are HPA-1b and many are also multiparious or have received previous transfusions. However, PTP occurs only rarely. Therefore, other factors must be important for the development of this syndrome. Affected patients have high titers of other antibodies, such as anti-HLA.[368] Reznikoff-Etievant and coworkers[344,345] studied HPA-1b–positive mothers of infants with NATP due to anti–HPA-1a antibodies and found an unexpectedly high frequency of the HLA type B3, DR3. Other investigators have confirmed an association with the HLA DRw52 superfamily and PTP.[352,370]

It has been hypothesized that the necessary immunization on reexposure to HPA-1a cannot occur if the anti–HPA-1a titer is very high, since the antigen-positive platelets are cleared rapidly. Thus, a long period (over 10 years) between the two exposures would favor a potent anamnestic response and development of PTP.

In summary, PTP occurs in a HPA-1b–, HLA DRw52–positive woman who has been exposed to HPA-1a many years previously and is then reexposed by a blood transfusion from a HPA-1a–positive donor. The individual at risk may also form potent anti-HLA antibodies. Although no immune risk factors have been associated with PTP when the alloantigenic incompatibility is different from HPA-1a, these cases have not been studied in as much detail.

Mechanism for Destruction of Autologous Platelets

The mechanism for the destruction of autologous, alloantigen-negative platelets during a rise in alloantibody titer is puzzling. A number of hypotheses have been proposed for the destruction of the autologous platelets: (1) immune complex platelet destruction, (2) conversion of antigen-negative platelets by transfer of soluble alloantigen, (3) production of an alloantibody of broad specificity which recognizes both allogeneic (antigen-positive) and autologous (antigen-negative) platelets, and (4) temporary production of a platelet autoantibody.

Shulman and colleagues[368] first recognized that the time course of the thrombocytopenia in PTP coincided with the rise in titer of a complement-fixing, anti–HPA-1a antibody. They suggested that HPA-1a antigen/anti–HPA-1a antibody immune complexes bound to platelets and caused their clearance through an Fc receptor–mediated mechanism. It was proposed that antigen then recirculated and could destroy other platelets.

Other investigators have postulated that soluble HPA-1a material might be adsorbed onto the patients' antigen-negative platelets, with subsequent lysis by anti–HPA-1a.[372] Recent work, however, has shown that soluble antigen does not exist in blood products.[351]

Alternatively, Mueller-Eckhardt[364] proposed that, on stimulation with HPA-1a antigen, some "pseudospecific" antibodies are made that also react with HPA-1b platelets. The binding to HPA-1b platelets may be less avid than to HPA-1a platelets, but it is hypothesized that HPA-1b platelets could still be cleared in the reticuloendothelial system.

A hypothesis first suggested by Morrison and Mollison[373] was that PTP resulted from concurrent production of a platelet autoantibody during a brisk alloimmune response. Two animal models for PTP support this mechanism.[374,375] The autoantibody plus alloantibody mechanism does not explain why eluates prepared from autologous platelets were found to contain potent anti–HPA-1a antibodies.[376] It is known that autoimmune hemolytic anemia can follow erythrocyte alloimmunization[377]; this situation could be explained either by the simultaneous production of autoantibodies or by the formation of pseudospecific antibodies.

SUMMARY

A number of important platelet alloantigens have been identified. Alloimmunization against platelet antigens can lead to severe thrombocytopenia and life-threatening hemorrhage in NATP and PTP. Because effective therapies are now available for both of these rare syndromes, prompt and accurate diagnosis is essential.

REFERENCES

1. Issitt PD. Applied blood group serology, ed 3. Miami, Montgomery Scientific Publications, 1985.
2. Mollison PL, Engelfriet CP, Contreras M. Blood transfusion in clinical medicine, ed 8. Oxford, Blackwell Scientific Publications, 1987.
3. Race RR, Sanger R. Blood groups in man, ed 6. Oxford, Blackwell Scientific Publications, 1975.
4. Grove-Rasmussen M, Huggins CE. Selected types of frozen blood for patients with multiple blood group antibodies. Transfusion 1973;13: 124.
5. Giblett ER. Critique of the theoretical hazard of inter- vs intraracial transfusion. Transfusion 1961;1:233.
6. Grove-Rasmussen M, Huggins CE. Selected types of frozen blood for patients with multiple blood group antibodies. Transfusion 1973;13: 124.
7. Tovey GH. Preventing the incompatible blood transfusion. Haematologia 1974;8:389.
8. Diamond LK. A history of blood transfusion and the story of our blood groups. In: Wintrobe MM, ed. Blood, pure and eloquent. New York, McGraw-Hill, 1980:659.
9. Levine P. A review of Landsteiner's contributions to human blood groups. Transfusion 1961;1:45.
10. Landsteiner D. Uber Agglutinatinserscheinungen normalen menschlichen Blutes. Wien Klin Wochenschr 1901;14:1132.
11. Decastello A von, Sturli A. Uber die Isoagglutinine in Serum gesunder und kranker Menschen. Munchen Med Wochenschr 1901;26:1090.
12. Hektoen L. Isoagglutination of human corpuscles. J Infect Dis 1907;4: 297.
13. Moss WL. Studies of isoagglutinins and isohemolysins. Johns Hopkins Med J 1910;21:63.
14. Dungern E von, Hirszfeld L. Uber gruppenspezifischer Strukturen des Blutes. III. Z Immunitaetsforch 1911;8:526.
15. Hakomori S-i. Blood group ABH and Ii antigens of human erythrocytes. Semin Hematol 1981;18:39.
16. Watkins WM. Blood group substances. Science 1966;152:172.
17. Rosse WF, Telen MJ. The biochemistry of the antigens of the red blood cell membrane. In: Agre P, Parker JC, Red blood cell membranes. New York, Marcel Dekker, 1989:299.
18. Finne J. Identification of the blood-group ABH-active glycoprotein components of human erythrocyte membrane. Eur J Biochem 1980;104:181.
19. Karhi KK, Gahmberg CG. Identification of blood group A-active glycoproteins of the human erythrocyte membrane. Biochem Biophys Acta 1980;622:344.
20. Oriol R, Danilovs H, Hawkins BR. A new genetic model proposing that the *Se* gene is a structural gene closely linked to the *H* gene. Am J Hum Genet 1981;33:421.
21. Hartmann G. Group antigens in human organs. Copenhagen, Munksgaard, 1941.
22. Yoshida A, Yamaguchi YF, Dave V. Immunologic homology of human blood group glycosyltransferases and genetic background of blood group ABO determination. Blood 1979;54:344.
23. Yamamoto F-I, Clausen H, White T, Marken J, Hakomori S-I. Molecular genetic basis of the histo-blood group ABO system. Nature 1990;345: 229.
24. Goldstein J, Siviglia G, Hurst R, Lenny L, Reich L. Group B erythrocytes enzymatically converted to group O survive normally in A, B, and O individuals. Science 1982;215:168.
25. Economidou J, Hughes-Jones N, Gardner B. Quantitative measurements concerning A and B antigen sites. Vox Sang 1967;12:321.
26. Clausen H, Levery SB, Nudelman S, Tsuchiya S, Hakomori S. Repetitive A epitope defined by blood group A_1-specific antibody TH-1. Proc Nat Acad Sci USA 1985;82:1119.
27. Forssman J. Die Herstellung hochwertiger spezifischer Schafhaemolysine ohne Verwendung von Schafblut. Aust Ann Med 1911;15:305.
28. Springer GF, Williamson P, Readler BL. Blood group active gram-negative bacteria and higher plants. Ann NY Acad Sci 1962;182:1341.
29. Thomsen O, Kettel K. Die Staerke der menschlichen Iso-agglutinine und entsprechenden Blutkoerperchenrezeptoren verschiedenen Lebensaltern. Z Immun-Forsh 1929;63:67.
30. Springer GF, Horton RE, Forbes M. Origin of anti-human blood group B agglutinins in white leghorn chicks. J Exp Med 1959;110:221.
31. Blackwell CC, Jondsottir K, Hanson M, et al. Non-secretion of ABO antigens predisposing to infection by *Neisseria meningitidis* and *Streptococcus pneumoniae*. Lancet 1986;2:284.
32. Mourant AE, Kopec AC, Domaniewska-Sobczak K. The distribution of the human blood groups and other biochemical polymorphisms, ed 2. Oxford, Blackwell Scientific Publications, 1976.
33. Marcus DM. The ABO and Lewis blood group system: immunochemistry, genetics, and relation to human disease. N Engl J Med 1969;280: 994.
34. Hakomori S-i. Blood group glycolipid antigens and their modifications as human cancer antigens. Am J Clin Pathol 1984;82:635.
35. Grubb R, Morgan WTJ. The Lewis blood group characters of erythrocytes and body fluids. Br J Exp Pathol 1949;30:198.
36. Sneath JS, Sneath PHA. Transformation of the Lewis groups of human red cells. Nature 1955;176:172.
37. Fukuda M, Fukuda MN, Hakomori S-i. Developmental change and genetic defect in the carbohydrate structure of band 3 glycoprotein of human erythrocyte membrane. J Biol Chem 1979;254:3700.
38. Piller F, Cartron JP. Biosynthesis of i antigenic structures. In: Cartron JP, Rouger P, Salmon C, eds. Red cell membrane glycoconjugates and related genetic. Paris, Lib Arnette, 1983:175.
39. Marsh WL, Jenkins WJ. Anti-i: a new cold antibody. Nature 1960;188: 753.
40. Giblett ER, Crookston MC. Agglutinability of red cells by anti-i in patients with thalassaemia major and other haematological disorders. Nature 1964;201:1138.
41. Hillman RS, Giblett ER. Red cell membrane alteration associated with marrow stress. J Clin Invest 1965;44:1730.
42. Wiener AS. Unger LJ, Cohen L, Feldman J. Type specific cold auto antibodies as a cause of acquired hemolytic anemia and hemolytic transfusion reactions. Ann Intern Med 1956;44:221.
43. Landsteiner K, Levine P. Further observations on individual differences of human blood. Proc Soc Exp Biol NY 1927;24:941.
44. Levine P, Koch E. The rare human isoagglutinin anti-Tj^a and habitual abortion. Science 1954;120:239.
45. Dunstan RA, Simpson MB. Heterogeneous distribution of antigens on human platelets demonstrated by fluorescence flow cytometry. Br J Haematol 1985;61:603.
46. Marcus DM, Kundu SK, Suzuki A. The P blood group system: recent progress in immunochemistry and genetics. Semin Hematol 1981;18: 63.
46a. Brown K, Anderson SM, Young NS. Erythrocyte P antigen: cellular receptor for B19 parvovirus. Science 1993;260:114.
47. Anstee DJ. The blood group MNSs-active sialoglycoproteins. Semin Hematol 1981;18:13.
48. Anstee DJ, Tanner MJA. Structure and function of the red cell membrane sialoglycoproteins. Br J Haematol 1986;64:211.
49. Marchesi VT, Tillack TW, Jackson RL, Segrest JP, Scott RE. Chemical characterization and surface orientation of the major glycoprotein of the human erythrocyte membrane. Proc Natl Acad Sci USA 1972;69: 1445.
50. Furthmayr H. Structural comparison of glycophorins and immunochemical analysis of genetic variants. Nature 1978;271:519.
51. Tomita M, Marchesi VT. Amino-acid sequence and oligosaccharide attachment sites of human erythrocyte glycophorin. Proc Natl Acad Sci USA 1975;72:2964.
52. Tomita M, Furthmayr H, Marchesi VT. Primary structure of human erythrocyte glycophorin A: isolation and characterization of peptides and complete amino acid sequence. Biochemistry 1978;17:4756.
53. Siebert PD, Fukuda M. Isolation and characterization of human glycophorin A cDNA clones by a synthetic oligonucleotide approach: nucleotide sequence and mRNA structure. Proc Natl Acad Sci USA 1986;83:1665.
54. Siebert PD, Fukuda M. Molecular cloning of human glycophorin B cDNA: nucleotide sequence and genomic relationship to glycoprotein A. Proc Natl Acad Sci USA 1987;84:6735.
55. Tate CG, Tanner MJA. Isolation of cDNA clones for human erythrocyte membrane sialoglycoproteins alpha and delta. Biochem J 1988;54: 743.
56. Cartron J-P, Rahuel C. Human erythrocyte glycoproteins: protein and gene structures. Transfus Med Rev 1992;6:63.

57. Anstee DJ, Mawby WJ, Tanner MJA. Abnormal blood-group Ss-active sialoglycoproteins in the membrane of Miltenberger class III, IV and V human erythrocytes. Biochem J 1979;183:193.
58. Dahr W, Beyreuther K, Steinbach H, Gielen W, Kruger J. Structure of the Ss blood group antigens. II. A methionine/threonine polymorphism within the N-terminal sequence of Ss glycoprotein. Hoppe-Seyler's Z Physiol Chem 1980;361:895.
59. Huang CH, Johe K, Moulds JJ, Siebert PP, Fukuda M, Blumenfeld OO. Delta glycoprotein (glycophorin B) gene deletion in two individuals homozygous for the S-s-U-blood group phenotype. Blood 1987;70:1830.
60. Rahuel C, Vignal A, London J, et al. Structure of the 5′ flanking region of the glycophorin A gene and analysis of its multiple transcripts. Gene 1989;85:471.
61. Langlois RG, Bigbee WL, Kyoizumi S, et al. Evidence for increased somatic cell mutations at the glycophorin A locus in atomic bomb survivors. Science 1987;236:445.
62. Darnborough J, Dunsford I, Wallace JA. The En^a antigen and antibody: a genetical modification of human red cells affecting their blood grouping reactions. Vox Sang 1969;17:241.
63. Furuhjelm U, Myllyla G, Nevanlinna HR, et al. The red cell phenotype En(a−) and anti-En^a: serological and physicochemical aspects. Vox Sang 1969;17:256.
64. Langlois RG, Bigbee WL, Jensen RH. Flow cytometric characterization of normal and variant cells with monoclonal antibodies specific for glycophorin A. J Immunol 1985;134:4009.
65. Gahmberg CG, Myllyla G, Leikola J, Pirkola A, Nordling L. Absence of the major sialoglycoprotein in the membrane of human En(a−) erythrocytes and increased glycosylation of band 3. J Biol Chem 1976;251:6108.
66. Schmidt PJ, Vox GH. Multiple phenotypic abnormalities associated with Rh_{null} (. . ./. . .). Vox Sang 1967;13:18.
67. Colin Y, Rahuel C, London J, et al. Isolation of cDNA clones for human erythrocyte glycophorin C. J Biol Chem 1986;261:229.
68. High S, Tanner MJA. Human erythrocyte membrane sialoglycoprotein beta: the cDNA sequence suggests the absence of a cleaved N terminal signal sequence. Biochem J 1987;243:277.
69. El-Maliki B, Blanchard D, Dahr W, Beyreuther K, Cartron JP. Structural homology between glycophorins C and D of human erythrocytes. Eur J Biochem 1989;183:639.
70. Le Van Kim C, Colin Y, Mitjavila MT, et al. Structure of the promoter region and tissue specificity of the human glycophorin C. J Biol Chem 1989;264:20407.
71. Booth PB, McLoughlin K. The Gerbich blood group system, especially in Melanesians. Vox Sang 1972;22:73.
72. Anstee DJ, Parsons SF, Ridgwell K, et al. Two individuals with elliptocytic red cells lack three minor erythrocyte membrane sialoglycoproteins. Biochem J 1984;218:615.
73. Anstee DJ, Ridgwell K, Tanner MJA, Daniels GL, Parsons SF. Individuals lacking the Gerbich blood-group antigen have alterations in the human erythrocyte membrane sialoglycoproteins beta and delta. Biochem J 1984;221:97.
74. Mueller TJ, Morrison M. Glycoconnectin (PAS 2): a membrane attachment site for the human erythrocyte cytoskeleton. In: Kruckenberg WC, Eaton JW, Brewer GJ, eds. Erythrocyte membranes 2: recent clinical and experimental advances, New York, Alan R Liss, 1981:95.
75. Reid EM, Chasis JA, Mohandas N. Identification of a functional role for human erythrocyte sialoglycoproteins beta and gamma. Blood 1987;69:1068.
76. Thomas DB, Winzler RJ. Structural studies on human erythrocyte glycoproteins. J Biol Chem 1969;244:5943.
77. Novak RW, Martin CR. Hemolytic-uremic syndrome and T-cryptantigen exposure by neuraminidase-producing pneumococci: an emerging problem? Pediatr Pathol 1983;1:409.
78. Bird T, Stephenson J. Acute haemolytic anaemia associated with polyagglutinability of red cells. J Clin Pathol 1978;26:868.
79. Bird GWG, Wingham J, Pippard MJ, Hoult JG, Melikian V. Erythrocyte membrane modification in malignant disease of myeloid and lymphoreticular tissues. I. Tn-polyagglutination in acute myelocytic leukaemia. Br J Haematol 1976;33:289.
80. Cartron JP, Andreu G, Cartron J, Bird GWG, Salmon C, Gerbal A. Demonstration of T-transferase deficiency in Tn-polyagglutinable blood samples. Eur J Biochem 1978;92:111.
81. Ness PM, Garratty G, Morel PA, Perkins HA. Tn polyagglutination preceding acute leukemia. Blood 1979;54:30.
82. Springer GF. T and Tn, general carcinoma antigens. Science 1984;224:1198.
83. Cartron JP, Prou O, Leilier M, Soulier JP. Susceptibility to invasion of some human erythrocytes carrying rare blood group antigens. Br J Haematol 1983;55:639.
84. Pasvol G, Jungery M, Weatherall DJ, Parsons SF, Anstee DJ, Tanner MJA. Glycophorin as a possible receptor for *Plasmodium falciparum*. Lancet 1982;2:947.
85. Hadley TJ, Klotz FW, Pasvol G, et al. Falciparum malaria parasites invade erythrocytes that lack glycophorin A and B (M^kM^k). J Clin Invest 1987;80:1190.
86. Pasvol G, Chasis JA, Mohandas N, Anstee DJ, Tanner MJA, Merry A. Inhibition of malarial parasite invasion by monoclonal antibodies against glycophorin A correlates with reduction in red cell membrane deformability. Blood 1989;74:1836.
87. Levine P, Stetson RE. An unusual case of intragroup agglutination. JAMA 1939;113:126.
88. Diamond LK, Abelson N. The demonstration of anti-Rh agglutinins an accurate and rapid slide test. J Lab Clin Med 1945;30:204.
89. Coombs RRA, Mourant AE, Race RR. A new test for the detection of weak and incomplete Rh agglutinins. Br J Exp Pathol 1945;26:255.
90. Wiener AS. The Rh series of allelic genes. Science 1944;100:595.
91. Race RR. An incomplete antibody in human serum. Nature 1944;153:771.
92. Blanchard D, Bloy C, Hermand P, et al. Two-dimensional iodopeptide mapping demonstrates erythrocyte Rh D, c, and E polypeptides are structurally homologous but nonidentical. Blood 1988;72:1424.
93. Rosenfield RE, Allen FH, Rubenstein P. Genetic model for the Rh blood group system Proc Natl Acad Sci USA 1973;70:1303.
94. Sacks MS, Wiener AS, Jahn EF, Spurling CL, Unger LJ. Isosensitization to a new blood factor, Rh^D, with special reference to its clinical importance. Ann Intern Med 1959;51:740.
95. Allen FH Jr, Tippett PA. A new Rh blood type which reveals the Rh antigen G. Vox Sang 1958;3:321.
96. Rosenfield RE, Haber GV. An Rh blood factor, rh_i (Ce), and its relationship to hr (ce). Am J Hum Genet 1958;10:474.
97. Masouredis SP, Sudora EJ, Mahan L, Victoria EJ. Antigen site densities and ultrastructural distribution patterns of red cell Rh antigens. Transfusion 1976;16:94.
98. Rochna E, Hughes-Jones NC. The use of purified ^{125}I-labelled antiglobulin in the determination of the number of D antigen sites on red cells of different phenotypes. Vox Sang 1965;10:675.
99. Masouredis SP. Relationship between Rh_O (D) genotype and quantity of ^{131}I anti-Rh_O (D) bound to red cells. J Clin Invest 1960;39:1450.
100. Race RR, Sanger R, Selwyn JG. A probable deletion in a human Rh chromosome. Nature 1950;166:520.
101. Nash R, Shojania AM. Hematological aspect of Rh deficiency syndrome: a case report and review of the literature. Am J Hematol 1987;24:267.
102. Chown B, Lewis M, Hiroko K, Lowen B. An unlinked modifier of Rh blood groups: effects when heterozygous and when homozygous. Am J Hum Genet 1972;24:623.
103. Sturgeon P. Hematological observations on the anemia associated with blood type Rh_{null}. Blood 1970;36:310.
104. Ballas S, Clark MR, Mohandas N, et al. Red cell membranes and cation deficiency in Rh null syndrome. Blood 1984;63:1046.
105. Lauf PK, Joiner CH. Increased potassium transport and ouabain binding in human Rh null red blood cells. Blood 1976;48:457.
106. Kuyper F, van Linde-Sibenius-Trip M, Roelofsen B, Tanner MJA, Anstee DJ, Op den Kamp JAF. Rh_{null} human erythrocytes have an abnormal membrane phospholipid organization. Biochem J 1984;221:931.
107. Ishimori T, Hasekura H. A Japanese with no detectable Rh blood group antigens due to silent Rh alleles or deleted chromosomes. Transfusion 1967;7:84.
108. Jones AR, Diamond LK, Allen FH Jr. A decade of progress in the Rh blood-group system. N Engl J Med 1954;250:283,324.
109. Goossens D, Champomier G, Rouger P, Salmon C. Human monoclonal antibodies against blood group antigens. J Immunol Methods 1987;101:193.
110. Krevans JR, Woodrow JC, Nosenzo C, Finn R. Patterns of Rh-immunization. Communications at the 10th Congress of the International Society of Haematology, Stokholm, 1964.
111. Woodrow JC, Finn R, Krevans JR. Rapid clearance of Rh positive blood during experimental Rh immunization. Vox Sang 1969;17:349.
112. Murray S, Knox EG, Walker W. Rhesus haemolytic disease of the newborn and the ABO groups. Vox Sang 1965;10:6.
113. Vontver LA. Rh sensitization associated with drug use. JAMA 1973;226:469.
114. Bowman JM, Pollock JM. Reversal of Rh immunization: fact or fancy? Vox Sang 1984;47:209.
115. Moore S, Woodrow CF, McClelland DBL. Isolation of membrane components associated with human red cell antigens Rh_o(D), (c), (E), and Fy^a. Nature 1982;295:529.
116. Gahmberg CG. Molecular identification of the human Rh_o(D) antigen. FEBS Lett 1982;140:93.
117. Gahmberg CG. Molecular characterization of the human red cell Rh_o(D) antigen. EMBO J 1983;2:223.
118. Gahmberg CG, Karhi KK. Association of Rh_o(D) polypeptides with the membrane skeleton in Rh_o(D)-positive human red cells. J Immunol 1984;133:334.
119. Ridgwell K, Tanner MJA, Anstee DJ. The Rhesus (D) polypeptide is linked to the human erythrocyte cytoskeleton. FEBS Lett 1983;174:7.
120. Ridgwell K, Roberts SJ, Tanner MJA, Anstee DJ. Absence of two membrane proteins containing extracellular thiol groups in Rh_{null} human erythrocytes. Biochem J 1983;213:267.
121. Saboori A, Denker BM, Agre P. Isolation of proteins related to the Rh polypeptides from non-human erythrocytes. J Clin Invest 1989;83:187.
122. Suyama K, Goldstein J. Enzymatic evidence for differences in the

placement of Rh antigens within the red cell membrane. Blood 1990;75:255.
123. Avent ND, Ridgwell K, Mawby WJ, Tanner MJA, Anstee DJ, Kumpel B. Protein-sequence studies of Rh-related polypeptides suggest the presence of at least two groups of proteins which associated in the human red-cell membrane. Biochem J 1988;256:1043.
124. Bloy C, Blanchard D, Dahr W, Beyreuther K, Salmon C, Cartron J-P. Determination of the N-terminal sequence of human red cell Rh(D) polypeptide and demonstration that the Rh(D), (c) and (E) antigens are carried by distinct polypeptide chains. Blood 1988;72:661.
125. Saboori AM, Smith BL, Agre P. Polymorphism in the M_r 32,000 Rh protein purified from Rh(D) positive and negative erythrocytes. Proc Natl Acad Sci USA 1988;85:4042.
126. Colin Y, Chérif-Zahar B, Le Van Kim C, et al. Genetic basis of the RhD-positive and RhD-negative blood group polymorphism. Blood 1991;78:2747.
127. Chérif-Zahar B, Bloy C, Le Van Kim C, et al. Molecular cloning and protein structure of a human blood group Rh polypeptide. Proc Natl Acad Sci USA 1990;87:6243.
128. Le Van Kim C, Mouro I, Chérif-Zahar B, et al. Molecular cloning and primary structure of the human blood group RhD polypeptide. Proc Natl Acad Sci USA 1992;89:10925.
129. Cartron JP, Agre P. Rh blood group antigens: protein and gene structure. Semin Hematol 1993;30:193.
130. Chérif-Zahar B, Mattéi MG, Le Van Kim C, et al. Localization of the human Rh blood group gene structure to chromosome 1p34.3-1p36.1 region by in situ hybridization. Hum Genet 1991;86:398.
131. Avent ND, Butcher SK, Liu W, et al. Localization of the C termini of the Rh (rhesus) polypeptides to the cytoplasmic face of the human erythrocyte membrane. J Biol Chem 1992;267:15134.
131a. Hermand P, Mouro I, Huet M, et al. Immunochemical characterization of Rh proteins with antibodies raised against synthetic peptides. Blood (in press).
131b. deVetten MP, Agre P. The Rh polypeptide is a major fatty acid acylated erythrocyte membrane protein. J Biol Chem 1988;263:18193.
131c. Hartel-Schenk S, Agre P. Mammalian red cell membrane Rh polypeptides are selectively palmitoylated subunits of a macromolecular complex. J Biol Chem 1992;267:5569.
131d. Dahr W, Kordowicz M, Moulds J, et al. Characterization of the Ss sialoglycoprotein and its antigen in Rh-null erythrocytes. Blut 1987;54:13.
131e. Tippett P. Regulator genes affecting red cell antigens. Transfus Med Rev 1990;4:56.
131f. Ridgewell K, Spurr NK, Laguda B, et al. Isolation of cDNA clones for a 50 kDa glycoprotein of the erythrocyte membrane associated with Rh (Rhesus) blood-group antigen expression. Biochem J 1992;287:223.
131g. Agre P, Cartron JP. Molecular biology of Rh antigens. Blood 1991;78:551.
131h. Hughes-Jones NC, Gorick BD, Brown D. Differential exposure of epitopes on the human red cell antigen D (Rh). Immunol Lett 1991;27:101.
131i. Shinitzky M, Souroujon M. Passive modulation of blood group antigens. Proc Natl Acad Sci USA 1979;76:4438.
132. Landsteiner K, Wiener AS. An agglutinable factor in human blood recognized by immune sera for rhesus blood. Proc Soc Exp Biol Med 1940;43:223.
133. Levine P, White JA, Stroup M. Seven Ve^a (Vel) negative members in three generations of a family. Transfusion 1961;1:111.
134. Mallinson G, Martin PG, Anstee DJ, et al. Identification and partial characterization of the human erythrocyte membrane component(s) which express the antigens of the LW blood group system. Biochem J 1986;234:649.
135. Bloy C, Hermand P, Cherif-Zahar B, Sonneborn H, Cartron JP. Comparative analysis by two-dimensional iodopeptide mapping of the RhD protein and LW glycoprotein. Blood 1990;75:2245.
136. Bloy C, Hermand P, Blanchard D, Cherif-Zahar B, Goossens D, Cartron J-P. Surface orientation and antigen properties of Rh and LW polypeptides of the human erythrocyte membrane. J Biol Chem 1990;265:21482.
137. Coombs RRA, Mourant AE, Race RR. In vivo isosensitization of red cells in babies with haemolytic disease. Lancet 1946;1:264.
138. Allen FH, Rosenfield RE. Notation for the Kell blood group system. Transfusion 1961;1:305.
139. Giblett E, Klebanoff SJ, Pincus SH, Swanson J, Park BH, McCullough J. Kell phenotypes in chronic granulomatous disease: a potential transfusion hazard. Lancet 1971;1:1235.
140. Marsh WL, Oyen R, Nichols ME, Allen FH. Chronic granulomatous disease and the Kell blood groups. Br J Haematol 1975;29:247.
141. Symmans WA, Shepherd CS, Marsh WL, Oyen R, Shohet SB, Linehan BJ. Hereditary acanthocytosis associated with the McLeod phenotype of the Kell blood group system. Br J Haematol 1979;42:575.
142. Wimer BM, Marsh WL, Taswell HF, Galey WR. Haematological changes associated with the McLeod phenotype of the Kell blood group system. Br J Haematol 1977;36:219.
143. Marsh WL, Redman CM. Recent developments in the Kell blood group system. Trans Med Rev 1987;1:4.
144. Bertelson CJ, Pogo AO, Chaudhuri A, et al. Localization of the McLeod locus (Xk) within XP21 by deletion analysis. Am J Hum Genet 1988;42:703.
145. Frey D, Maechler M, Seger R, Schmid W, Orkin SH. Gene deletion in a patient with chronic granulomatous disease and McLeod syndrome: fine mapping of the Xk gene locus. Blood 1988;71:252.
146. Kuypers FA, van Linde-Sibenius-Trip M, Roelofsen B, Op den Kamp JAF, Tanner MJA, Anstee DJ. The phospholipid organisation in the membranes of McLeod and Leach phenotype erythrocytes. FEBS Lett 1985;184:20.
147. Redman CM, Huima T, Robbins E, Lee S, Marsh WL. Effect of phosphatidylserine on the shape of McLeod red cell acanthocytes. Blood 1989;74:1826.
148. Ballas SK, Bator SM, Aubuchon JP, Marsh WL, Sharp DE, Toy EM. Abnormal membrane physical properties of red cells in McLeod syndrome. Transfusion 1990;30:722.
149. Kornstad L, Heisto H. The frequency of formation of Kell antibodies in recipients of Kell positive blood. Proceedings of the 6th Congress of the European Society of Haematology 1957:754.
150. Marsh WL, Nichols ME, Oyen R, et al. Naturally occurring anti-Kell stimulated by *E coli* enterocolitis in a 20 day old child. Transfusion 1978;18:149.
151. Redman CM, Lee S, Marsh WL. Isolation and partial characterization of Kell blood group antigens. In: Moore SB, ed, Progress in immunohematology. Arlington, VA, American Association of Blood Banks, 1988:141.
152. Redman CM, Avellino G, Pfeffer SR, et al. Kell blood group antigens are part of a 93,000 dalton red cell membrane protein. J Biol Chem 1986;61:9521.
153. Redman CM, Marsh WL, Scarborough A, Johnson CL, Rabin RI, Overbeeke M. Biochemical studies on McLeod phenotype red cells and isolation of Kx antigen. Br J Haematol 1988;42:131.
154. Allen FH, Diamond LK, Niedziela B. A new blood-group antigen. Nature 1951;167:482.
155. Masouredis SP, Sudora E, Mahan L, Victoria EJ. Quantitative immunoferritin microassay of Fy^a, Fy^b, Jk^a, U, and Di^b antigen site numbers on human red cells. Blood 1980;56:969.
156. Heaton DC, McLoughlin K. Jk(a−b−) red blood cells resist urea lysis. Transfusion 1982;22:70.
157. Okubo Y, Yamaguchi H, Nagao N, Tomita T, Seno T, Tanaka M. Heterogeneity of the phenotype Jk(a−b−) found in Japanese. Transfusion 1986;26:237.
158. Frohlich O, Macey RI, Edwards-Moulds J, et al. Urea transport deficiency in Jk (a−b−) erythrocytes. Am J Physiol 1991;260:C778.
160. Callender S, Race RR, Paykoc ZV. Hypersensitivity to transfused blood. Br Med J 1945;2:83.
161. Merry AH, Gardner B, Parsons SF, Anstee DJ. Estimation of the number of binding sites for a murine monoclonal anti-Lu^b on human erythrocytes. Vox Sang 1987;53:57.
162. Parsons SF, Mallinson G, Judson PA, Anstee DJ, Tanner MJA, Daniels GL. Evidence that the Lu^b blood group antigen is located on red cell membrane glycoproteins of 85 and 78 Kd. Transfusion 1987;27:61.
163. Taliano V, Guevin RM, Tippett P. The genetics of a dominant inhibitor of the Lutheran antigens. Vox Sang 1973;24:42.
164. Telen MJ, Eisenbarth GS, Haynes BF. Regulation of expression of a novel erythrocyte surface antigen by the inhibitor Lutheran *In(Lu)* gene. J Clin Invest 1983;71:1878.
165. Telen MJ, Palker TJ, Haynes BF. The *In(Lu)* gene regulates expression of an antigen on an 80 kilodalton protein of human erythrocytes. Blood 1984;64:599.
166. Telen MJ, Shehata H, Haynes BF. Human medullary thymocyte p80 antigen and *In(Lu)*-related p80 antigen reside on the same protein. Hum Immunol 1986;17:311.
167. Telen MJ, Rodgers I, Letarte M. Further characterization of the In(Lu)-related p80 and the defect of In(Lu) Lu(a−b−) erythrocytes. Blood 1987;70:1475.
168. Haynes BF, Telen MJ, Hale LD, Denning SM. CD44 a molecule involved in leukocyte adherence and T cell activation. Immunol Today 1989;10:423.
169. Spring FA, Dalchau R, Daniels GL, et al. The In^a and In^b blood group antigens are located on a glycoprotein of 80,000 MW (the CDw44 glycoprotein) whose expression is influenced by the *In(Lu)* gene. Immunology 1988;64:37.
170. Telen MJ, Ferguson DJ. Relationship of In^b antigen to other antigens on *In(Lu)*-related p80. Vox Sang 1990;58:118.
171. Goldstein LA, Zhou DFH, Picker LJ, et al. A human lymphocyte homing receptor, the Hermes antigen, is related to cartilage proteoglycan core and link proteins. Cell 1989;56:1063.
172. Stamenkovic I, Amiot M, Pesando JM, Seed B. A lymphocyte molecule implicated in lymph node homing is a member of the cartilage link protein family. Cell 1989;56:1057.
173. Aruffo A, Stamenkovic I, Melnick M, Underhill CB, Seed B. CD44 is the principal cell surface receptor for hyaluronate. Cell 1990;61:1303.
174. Cutbush M, Mollison PL, Parkin DM. A new human blood group. Nature 1950;165:188.
175. Sanger R, Race RR, Jack J. The Duffy blood groups of New York Negroes: the phenotype Fy(a−b−). Br J Haematol 1955;1:370.
176. Donahue RP, Bias W, Renwick JH, McKusick VA. Probable assignment

of the Duffy blood group locus to chromosome 1 in man. Proc Natl Acad Sci USA 1968;61:949.
177. Vengelen-Tyler V. Anti-Fy[a] preceding anti-Fy3 or -Fy5: a study of five cases. (Abstract) Transfusion 1985;25:482.
178. Hadley TJ, David P, McGinniss MH, Miller LH. Identification of an erythrocyte component carrying the Duffy blood group Fy[a] antigen. Science 1984;223:587.
179. Tanner MJA, Anstee DJ, Mallinson G, et al. Effect of endoglycosidase F-peptidyl N-glycosidase F preparations on the surface of the human erythrocyte. Carbohydrate Res 1988;15:178.
180. Chaudhuri A, Zbrzezna V, Johnson C, et al. Purification and characterization of an erythrocyte membrane protein complex carrying Duffy blood group antigenicity. J Biol Chem 1989;270:13770.
181. Renwick JH, Lawler SD. Probable linkage between a congenital cataract locus and the Duffy blood group locus. Ann Hum Genet 1963;27: 67.
182. Hadley TJ, McGinniss MH, Klotz F, Miller LH. Blood group antigens and invasion of erythrocytes by malaria parasites. In: Garratty G, ed. Red cell antigens and antibodies, Arlington, VA, American Association of Blood Banks, 1986:17.
183. Dvorak JA, Miller LH, Whitehouse WC, Shiroishi T. Invasion of erythrocytes by malaria merozoites. Science 1975;187:748.
184. Miller LH, Mason SJ, Clyde DF, McGinniss MH. The resistance factor to *Plasmodium vivax* in blacks: the Duffy blood group genotype, FyFy. N Engl J Med 1976;295:302.
185. Miller LG, McGinniss MH, Holland PV, Sigmon P. The Duffy blood group phenotype in American blacks with *Plasmodium vivax* in Vietnam. Am J Trop Med Hyg 1978;27:1069.
186. Miller LH, Mason SJ, Dvorak JA, McGinniss MH, Rothman IK. Erythrocyte receptors for *(Plasmodium knowlesi)* malaria. Science 1975;189: 561.
187. Mason SJ, Miller LH, Shiroishi T, Dvorak JA, McGinniss MH. The Duffy blood group determinants: their role in the susceptibility of human and animal erythrocytes to *Plasmodium knowlesi* malaria. Br J Haematol 1977;36:327.
188. Low MG, Saltiel AR. Structural and functional roles of glycosyl-phosphatidylinositol in membranes. Science 1988;239:268.
189. Nicholson-Weller A, March JP, Rosenfeld SI, Austen KF. Affected erythrocytes of patients with paroxysmal nocturnal hemoglobinuria are deficient in the complement regulatory protein, decay accelerating factor. Proc Natl Acad Sci USA 1983;80:5066.
190. Holguin MH, Fredrick LR, Bernshaw NJ, Wilcox LA, Parker CJ. Isolation and characterization of a membrane protein from normal human erythrocytes that inhibits reactive lysis of the erythrocytes of paroxysmal nocturnal hemoglobinuria. J Clin Invest 1989;84:7.
191. Medof ME, Walter EI, Roberts WL, Haas R, Rosenberry TL. Decay accelerating factor of complement is anchored to cells by a C-terminal glycolipid. Biochemistry 1986;25:6740.
192. Telen MJ, Hall SE, Green AM, Moulds JJ, Rosse WF. Identification of human erythrocyte blood group antigens on decay accelerating factor (DAF) and identification of an erythrocyte phenotype negative for DAF. J Exp Med 1988;167:1993.
193. Daniels GL, Tohoyama H, Uchikawa M. A possible null phenotype in the Cromer-related blood group complex. Transfusion 1982;22: 362.
194. Telen MJ, Rosse WF, Parker CH, Moulds MK, Moulds JJ. Evidence that several high-frequency human blood group antigens reside on phosphatidylinositol-linked erythrocyte membrane proteins. Blood 1990;75:1404.
195. Tilley CA, Romans DG, Crookston MC. Localization of Chido and Rodgers determinants to the C4d fragment of human C4. Nature 1978;276:713.
196. Mann JD, Cahan A, Gelb AG, et al. A sex-linked blood group. Lancet 1962;1:8.
197. Clay ME, Kline WE. Detection of granulocyte antigens and antibodies: current perspectives and approaches. In: Garratty G, ed, Current concepts in transfusion therapy. Arlington, VA, American Association of Blood Banks, 1985:183.
198. McCullough J. Granulocyte antigen systems and antibodies and their clinical significance. Hum Pathol 1983;14:228.
199. Reijden HJ, von dem Borne AEGKr, Verheugt FW, Floor-van Gent AB, Melief J, Engelfriet CP. Granulocyte-specific alloantigen loss in chronic granulocytic leukaemia. Br J Haematol 1979;43:589.
200. Claas FHJ, Langerak J, Sabre LJM, van Rood JJ. A new neutrophil-specific antigen. Tissue Ant 1979;13:129.
201. Clark MR, Liu L, Clarkson SB, Ory PA, Goldstein IM. An abnormality of the gene that encodes neutrophil Fc receptor III in a patient with systemic lupus erythematosus. J Clin Invest 1990;86:341.
202. Huizinga TWJ, Kleijer M, Tetteroo PAT, Roos D, von dem Borne AEGKr. Biallelic neutrophil Na-antigen system is associated with a polymorphism on the phosphoinositol-linked receptor III (CD16). Blood 1990;75:213.
203. Lalezari P, Nussbaum M, Gelman S, Spaet TH. Neonatal neutropenia due to maternal isoimmunization. Blood 1960;15:236.
204. Lalezari P, Bernard GD. A new neutrophile-specific antigen: its role in the pathogenesis of neonatal neutropenia. Fed Proc 1966;25:371.
205. Lalezari P, Bernard JE. An isologous antigen-antibody reaction with human neutrophils related to neonatal neutropenia. J Clin Invest 1966;45:1741.
206. Lalezari P, Thalenfeld B, Weinstein WH. The third neutrophil antigen. In: Terasaki PE, ed. Histocompatibility testing. Baltimore, Williams & Wilkins, 1970:319.
207. Lalezari P, Murphy GB, Allen FH. NB1, a new neutrophil antigen involved in the pathogenesis of neonatal neutropenia. J Clin Invest 1971;50:1108.
208. Lalezari P, Radel E. Neutrophil-specific antigens: immunology and clinical significance. Semin Hematol 1974;11:281.
209. Lalezari P, Petrosova M, Jiang AF, NB2, an allele of NB1 neutrophil specific antigen: relationship to 9a. Transfusion 1982;22:433.
210. Ory PA, Goldstein IM, Kwoh EE, Clarkson SB. Characterization of polymorphic forms of Fc receptor III on human neutrophils. J Clin Invest 1989;83:1676.
211. Ory PA, Clark MR, Kwoh EE, Clarkson SB, Goldstein IM. Sequences of complementary DNAs that encode the NA1 and NA2 forms of Fc receptor III on human neutrophils. J Clin Invest 1989;84:1688.
212. Selvaraj P, Rosse WF, Silber R, Springer TA. The major Fc receptor in blood has a phosphatidylinositol anchor and is deficient in paroxysmal nocturnal hemoglobinuria. Nature 1988;333:565.
213. Stroncek DF, Skubitz KM, McCullough JJ. Biochemical characterization of the neutrophil-specific antigen NB1. Blood 1990;75:744.
214. Thompson JS, Overlin VL, Herbick HM. New granulocyte antigens demonstrated by microgranulocytotoxicity assay. J Clin Invest 1980;65: 143.
215. Verheugt FWA, von dem Borne AEGKr, van Noord-Bokhorst JC, Nijenhuis LE, Engelfriet CP. ND1, a new neutrophil granulocyte antigen. Vox Sang 1978;35:13.
216. Werner G, von dem Borne AEGKr, Bos MJE, et al. Localization of the human NA1 alloantigen on neutrophil Fc receptors. In: Reinherz EL, Haynes BF, Nadler LM, Bernstein ID, eds. Leukocyte typing II: human myeloid and hematopoietic cells, New York, Springer-Verlag, 1986: 109.
217. Hartman KR, Wright DG. Identification of autoantibodies specific for the neutrophil adhesion glycoproteins CD11B/CD18. (Abstract) Blood 1989;74:159.
218. Hartman KR, Mallet MK, Nath J, Wright DG. Antibodies to actin in autoimmune neutropenia. Blood 1990;75:736.
219. Verheugt FWA, van Noord-Bokhorst JC, von dem Borne AEGKr, Engelfriet CP. A family with allo-immune neonatal neutropenia: group specific pathogenicity of maternal antibodies. Vox Sang 1979;36:1.
220. Boxer LA, Yokoyama M. Isoimmune neonatal neutropenia. J Pediatr 1972;80:783.
221. von dem Borne AEGKr. Nomenclature of platelet antigen systems. Br J Haematol 1990;74:239.
222. Newman PJ. Nomenclature of human platelet alloantigens: a problem with the HPA system? Blood 1994;83:1447.
223. Pytela R, Pierschbacher MD, Ginsberg MH, Plow EF, Ruoslahti E. Platelet membrane glycoprotein IIb/IIIa: member of a family of Arg-Gly-Asp-specific adhesion receptors. Science 1986;231:1559.
224. Hynes RO. Integrins: a family of cell surface receptors. Cell 1987;48: 549.
225. Fitzgerald LA, Phillips DR. Structure and function of platelet membrane glycoproteins. In: Kunicki TJ, George JN, eds. Platelet immunobiology: molecular and clinical aspects. Philadelphia, JB Lippincott, 1989:9.
226. Lopez JA, Chung DW, Fujikawa K, et al. Cloning of the alpha chain of human platelet glycoprotein Ib: a transmembrane protein with homology to leucine-rich alpha-2.
227. Titani K, Takio K, Handa M, et al. Amino acid sequence of the von Willebrand factor–binding domain of platelet membrane glycoprotein Ib. Proc Natl Acad Sci USA 1987;84:5610.
228. Du X, Beutler L, Ruan C, Castaldi PA, Berndt MC. Glycoprotein Ib and glycoprotein IX are fully complexed in the intact platelet membrane. Blood 1987;69:1524.
229. Roth GJ. Developing relationships: arterial platelet adhesion, glycoprotein Ib, and leucine-rich glycoproteins. Blood 1991;77:5.
230. Giltay JC, Brinkman HM, von dem Borne AEGK, van Mourik JA. Expression of the alloantigen Zw (or Pl^{A1} on human vascular smooth muscle cells and foreskin fibroblasts: a study on normal individuals and a patient with Glanzmann's thrombasthenia. Blood 1989;73:965.
231. Van Loghem J, Dorfmeijer H, van der Hart M. Serological and genetical studies on a platelet antigen (Zw). Vox Sang 1959;4:161.
232. Shulman NR, Marder V, Hiller M, Collier E. Platelet and leukocyte isoantigens and their antibodies: serologic, physiologic and clinical studies. Prog Hematol 1964;4:222.
233. Kunicki TJ, Aster RH. Isolation and immunologic characterization of the human platelet alloantigen, Pl^{A1}. Mol Immunol 1979;16:353.
234. Newman PJ, Derbes R, Aster RH. The human platelet alloantigens, Pl^{A1} and Pl^{A2}, are associated with a $leucine^{33}/proline^{33}$ amino acid polymorphism in membrane glycoprotein IIIa, and are distinguishable by DNA typing. J Clin Invest 1989;83:1778.
235. Goldberger A, Kolodziej M, Poncz M, Bennett JS, Newman PJ. Effect of single amino acid substitutions on the formation of the PlA and Bak alloantigenic eipitopes. Blood 1991;78:681.
236. Bowditch RD, Tani PH, Halloran CE, Frelinger AL III, McMillan R,

Ginsberg MH. Localization of a Pl^{A1} epitope to the amino terminal 66 residues of platelet glycoprotein IIIa. Blood 1992;79:559.
237. Ryckewaert J-J, Schweizer B, Chapel A. Marguerite G. Production of anti-Pl^{A} monoclonal antibodies. J Lab Clin Med 1992;119:52.
238. Diaz M, Ryckewaert JJ, Masson D, Bensa JC, Marguerie G. Evaluation of monoclonal antibodies with specificity for the human platelet HPA-1 allotypes. Vox Sang 1993;65:219.
239. Liu LX, Nardi M, Flug F, Karpatkin S. Development of a monoclonal antibody capable of differentiating platelet PlA1/PlA1, PlA1/PlA2, and PlA2/PlA2 genotypes. Br J Haematol 1992;81:113.
240. Kunicki T, Aster R. Qualitative and quantitative tests for platelet alloantibodies and drug-dependent antibodies. In: McMillan R, ed. Methods in hematology: immune cytopenias. New York, Churchill Livingstone, 1983:49.
241. Muniz-Diez E, Arilla M, Ibanez M, Bosch MA, Pastoret C, Madoz P. Frequency of platelet alloantigens in the Spanish population. Spanish Sangre 1993;38:289.
242. Santoso S, Santoso S, Kiefel V, Masri R, Mueller-Eckhardt C. Frequency of platelet-specific antigens among Indonesians. Transfusion 1993;33:739.
243. Lin M, Shieh SH, Yang TF. Frequency of platelet-specific antigens among Chinese in Taiwan. Transfusion 1993;33:155.
244. van der Weert C. The platelet agglutination test. In: Histocompatibility Testing, vol 2. Copenhagen, Munksgaard, 1965:161.
245. Saji H, Maruya E, Fujii H, Maekawa T, Akiyama Y, Matsuura T, Hosoi T. New platelet antigen, Sib^{a}, involved in platelet transfusion refractoriness in Japanese man. Vox Sang 1989;56:283.
246. Kuijpers R, Faber NM, Cuypers HThM, Ouwehand WH, von dem Borne AEGKr. Localization of the HPA-2 (Ko) alloantigens on the N-terminal globular fragment of platelet glycoprotein Ibα. Blood 1991;79:283.
247. Murata M, Furihata K, Ishida F, Russell SR, Ware J, Ruggeri ZM. Genetic and structural characterization of an amino acid dimorphism in glycoprotein Ibα involved in platelet transfusion refractoriness. Blood 1992;79:3086.
248. Ishida F, Saji H, Maruya E, Furihata K. Human platelet-specific antigen, Siba, is associated with the molecular weight polymorphism of glycoprotein Ib alpha. Blood 1991;78:1722.
249. Grenet P, Dausset J, Dugas M, Petit D, Badoual J, Tangun Y. Purpura thrombopenique neonatal avec isoimmunization foetomaternelle anti-Ko^{a}. Arch Fr Pediatr 1965;22:177.
250. von dem Borne A, von Riesz E, Verheugt F, et al. Bak^{a}, a new platelet-specific antigen involved in neonatal alloimmune thrombocytopenia. Vox Sang 1980;39:113.
251. Boizard B, Wautier J-L. Lek^{a}, a new platelet antigen absent in Glanzmann's thrombasthenia. Vox Sang 1984;46:47.
252. Von dem Borne A, van der Plas-van Dalen CM. Bak^{a} and Lek^{a} are identical antigens. Br J Haematol 1986;62:404.
253. Keimowitz R, Collins J, Davis K, Aster R. Post-transfusion purpura associated with alloimmunization against the platelet-specific antigen, Bak^{a}. Am J Hematol 1986;21:79.
254. Kieffer N, Boizard B, Didry D, Wautier JL. Nurden AT. Immunochemical characterization of the platelet-specific alloantigen Lek^{a}: a comparative study with the Pl^{A1} alloantigen. Blood 1984;64:1212.
255. Lyman S, Aster RH, Visentin GP, Newman PJ. Polymorphism of human platelet membrane glycoprotein IIb associated with the Bak^{a}/Bak^{b} alloantigen system. Blood 1990;75:2343.
256. Djaffar I, Didier V, Pidard D, Wautier J-L, Rosa J-P. Human Platelet Antigen 3 (HPA-3): localization of the determinant of the alloantibody Leka (HPA-3a) to the c-terminus of platelet glycoprotein IIb heavy chain and contribution of O-linked carbohydrates. Thromb Haemost 1993;69:485.
257. Take H, Tomiyama Y, Shibata Y, et al. Demonstration of the heterogeneity of epitopes of the platelet-specific alloantigen, Baka. Br J Haematol 1990;76:395.
258. Calvete JJ, Muniz-Diaz E. Localization of an O-glycosylation site in the alpha-subunit of the human platelet integrin GPIIb/IIIa involved in Baka (HPA-3a) alloantigen expression. FEBS Lett 1993;328:30.
259. McGrath K, Minchinton R, Cunningham I, Ayberk H. Platelet anti-Bak^{b} antibody associated with neonatal alloimmune thrombocytopenia. Vox Sang 1989;57:182.
260. Gruel Y, Boizard B, Daffos F, et al. Determination of platelet antigens and glycoproteins in the human fetus. Blood 1986;68:488.
261. Hajjar FM, Beardsley DS. Expression of Bak^{a} (Lek^{a}) antigen on fetal and adult platelets. Thromb Haemost 1993;69:1331a.
262. Shibata Y, Miyaji T, Ichikawa Y, Matsuda I. A new platelet antigen system Yuk^{a}/Yuk^{a}. Vox Sang 1986;51:334.
263. Friedman JM, Aster RH. Neonatal alloimmune thrombocytopenic purpura and congenital porencephaly in two siblings associated with a "new" maternal antiplatelet antibody. Blood 1985;65:1412.
264. Morel-Kopp MC, Blanchard B, Kiefel V, Joly C, Mueller-Eckhardt C, Kaplan C. Anti-HPA-4b (anti-Yuka) neonatal alloimmune thrombocytopenia: first report in a caucasian family. Transfus Med 1992;2:273.
265. Puig N, Muniz-Diaz E, Monteagudo E, Ribera A, Montoro JA. A second case of neonatal alloimmune thrombocytopenia by anti-HPA-4b (anti-Yuka) in a caucasian family. Transfus Med 1993;3:164.
266. Furihata K, Nugent DJ, Bissoneet A, Aster RH, Kunicki TJ. On the association of the platelet-specific alloantigen, Pen^{a}, with glycoprotein IIIa: evidence for heterogeneity of glycoprotein IIIa. J Clin Invest 1987;80:1624.
267. Santoso S, Shibata Y, Kiefel V, Mueller-Eckhardt C. Identification of Yuk(b) alloantigen on platelet glycoprotein IIIa. Thromb Haemost 1987;58:197a.
268. Shibata Y, Mori H. A new platelet-specific alloantigen system, Yuk^{a}/Yuk^{b}, is located on platelet membrane glycoprotein IIa. Proc Jpn Acad 1987;63:36.
269. Wang L, Juji T, Shibata Y, Kuwata S, Tokunaga K. Sequence variation of human platelet membrane glycoprotein IIIa associated with the Yuk^{a}/Yuk^{b}, alloantigen system. Proc Jpn Acad 1991;67:102.
270. Wang RG, McFarland J, Furihata K, Friedman K, Newman PJ. An amino acid polymorphism within the RDG binding domain of GPIIIa is associated with the Pen^{a}/Pen^{b} alloantigen system. J Clin Invest 1992;90:2038.
271. Kiefel V, Santoso S, Katzmann B, Mueller-Eckhart C. The Br^{a}/Br^{b} alloantigen system on human platelets. Blood 1989;73:2219.
272. Woods VL, Pischel KD, Avery ED, Bluestein HG. Antigenic polymorphism of human very late activation protein-2 (platelet glycoprotein Ia-IIa). J Clin Invest 1989;83:978.
273. Smith JW, Kelton JG, Horsewood P, et al. Platelet specific alloantigens of the platelet glycoprotein Ia/IIa complex. Br J Haematol 1989;72:534.
274. Santoso S, Kalb R, Walka M, Kiefel V, Mueller-Eckhardt C, Newman PF. The human platelet alloantigens Br(a) and Br(b) are associated with a single amino acid polymorphism on glycoprotein Ia (integrin subunit alpha 2). J Clin Invest 1993;92:2427.
275. Christie DJ, Pulkrabek S, Putnam JL, Slatoff ML, Pischel K. Posttransfusion purpura due to an alloantibody reactive with glycoprotein Ia/IIa (anti-HPA-5b). Blood 1991;77:2785.
276. McFarland JG, Blanchette V, Collins J, Newman PJ, Wang R, Aster RH. Neonatal alloimmune thrombocytopenia due to a new platelet-specific alloantibody. Blood 1993;81:3318.
277. Kekomaki R, Jouhikainen T, Ollikainen J, Westman P, Laes M. A new platelet alloantigen, Tua, on glycoprotein IIIa associated with neonatal alloimmune thrombcytopenia in two families. Br J Haematol 1993;83:306.
278. Ertem M, Moulton T, Ho JS, Beardsley DS. A new platelet alloantigen, Pl^{T}, on glycoprotein V, associated with neonatal alloimmune thrombocytopenia. Pediatr Res 1994;35:160a.
279. Kelton JG, Smith JW, Horsewood P, Humbert JR, Hayward CPM, Warkentin TE. $Gov^{a/b}$ alloantigen system on human platelets. Blood 1990;75:2172.
280. Ertem M, Holtkamp C, Tandon N, Jamieson G, Beardsley DS. "Vis," a new platelet alloantigen on glycoprotein IV associated with neonatal alloimmune thrombocytopenia (NATP). Thromb Haemost 1993;69:997a.
281. Moulinier PJ. Iso-immunization maternelle antiplaquettaire et purpura neonatal. Proceedings of the Sixth Congress of the European Society of Hematology. New York, S Karger, 1958:817.
282. Kekomaki R, Raivio P, Kero P. A new low-frequency platelet alloantigen, Va^{a}, on glycoprotein IIb/IIIa associated with neonatal alloimmune thrombocytopenia. Transfus Med 1992;2:27.
283. Kroll H, Kiefel V, Santoso S, Mueller-Eckhardt C. Sr^{a}, a private platelet antigen on glycoprotein IIIa associated with neonatal alloimmune thrombocytopenia. Blood 1990;76:2296.
284. Kuijpers RWAM, Simsek S, Faber NM, Goldschmeding R, van Wermerkerken RKV, von dem Borne AEGKr. Single point mutation in glycoprotein IIIa is associated with a new platelet-specific allo antigen (Mo) involved in neonatal alloimmune thrombocytopenia. Blood 1993;81:70.
285. Dunstan RA, Simpson MB. Minimal expression of blood group A antigen on human platelets demonstrated by fluorescence flow cytometry. Br J Haematol 1985;61:603.
286. Dunstan RA, Simpson MB, Knowles RW, Rosse WF. The origin of ABH antigens on human platelets. Blood 1985;65:615.
287. Mollicone R, Callard T, Pendu JL, et al. Expression of ABH and X (Le^{a}) antigens on platelets and lymphocytes. Blood 1988;71:1113.
288. Kelton JG, Hamid C, Aker S, Blajchman MA. The amount of blood group A substance on platelets is proportional to the amount in plasma. Blood 1982;59:980.
289. Ogasawara K, Ueki J, Takenaka M, Furihata K. Study on the expression of ABH antigens on platelets. Blood 1993;82:993.
290. Grenet P, Chavelet F, Schaison G, Badonal J. Thrombopenias neonatal par iso-immunization contra des antigens leucoplaquettaires. Nouv Rev Fr Hematol 1967;7:664.
291. Sternbach MS, Malette M, Nadon F, Guevin RM. Severe alloimmune neonatal thrombocytopenia due to specific HLA antibodies. Curr Stud Hematol Blood Transfus 1986;52:97.
292. Lalezari P, Dimitrova A, Diwan A, Einarson M. HLA incompatibility is the most common cause of alloimmune neonatal thrombcytopenia. Blood 1993;82:203a.
293. Furihata K, Hunter J, Aster RH, Koewing GR, Shulman R, Kunicki TJ. Human anti-Pl^{E1} antibody recognizes epitopes associated with the alpha subunit of platelet glycoprotein Ib. Br J Haematol 1988;68:103.

294. Ikeda H, Mitani T, Ohnuma M, Haga H, Ohtzuka S, Nakase T, Sekiguchi S. A new platelet-specific antigen, Nak[a], involved in the refractoriness of HLA-matched platelet transfusion. Vox Sang 1989;57:213.
295. Yamamoto N, Ikeda H, Tandon NN. A platelet membrane glycoprotein (GP) deficiency in healthy blood donors: Nak[a]-platelets lack detectable GPIV (CD36). Blood 1990;76:1698.
296. Nurden AT. Congenital abnormalities of platelet membrane glycoproteins. In Kunicki TJ, George JN, eds. Platelet immunobiology: molecular and clinical aspects. Philadelphia, JB Lippincott, 1989:63.
297. Schulman I, Smith CH, Ando RE. Congenital thrombocytopenic purpura: observation on three infants born to a non-affected mother; demonstration of platelet agglutinins and evidence for platelet isoimmunization. Am J Dis Child 1954;88:784.
297a. Shulman NR, Aster RH, Pearson HA, Hiller MC. Immunoreactions involving platelets. VI. Reactions of maternal isoantibodies responsible for neonatal purpura: differentiation of a second platelet antigen system. J Clin Invest 1962;41:1059.
298. Pearson HA, Shulman NR, Marder VJ, Cone TE. Isoimmune neonatal thrombocytopenic purpura: clinical and therapeutic considerations. Blood 1964;23:154.
299. von dem Borne AE, van Leeuwen EF, von Riesz LE, van Boxtel CJ, Engelfriet CP. Neonatal alloimmune thrombocytopenia: detection and characterization of the responsible antibodies by the platelet immunofluorescence test. Blood 1981;57:649.
300. Taaning E, Antosen H, Peterson S, et al. HLA antigens and maternal antibodies in alloimmune neonatal thrombocytopenia. Tissue Antigens 1983;21:351.
301. Miller WV, Harmon JA. Platelet specific antigen systems and their detection. Prog Clin Biol Res 1984;149:79.
302. Muller JY, Reznikoff-Etievant MF, Patereau C, Dangu C, Chesnel N. Neonatal alloimmune thrombopenia: clinical and biological study of 84 cases. Presse Med 1985;14:83.
303. Muller JY, Patereau C, Reznikoff-Etievant MF, Kaplan C, Simonney N. Neonatal alloimmune thrombopenia. Rev Fr Transfus Immunohematol 1985;28:625.
304. Decary F. Is HLA DR3 a risk factor in PlA1-negative pregnant women? Curr Stud Hematol Blood Transfus 1986;52:78.
305. Mueller-Eckhardt C, Kiefel V, Grubert A, et al. 348 cases of suspected neonatal alloimmune thrombocytopenia. Lancet 1989;1:363.
306. McFarland JG, Aster RH, Bussel JB, Gianopoulos JG, Derbes RS, Newman PJ. Prenatal diagnosis of neonatal alloimmune thrombocytopenia using allele-specific aligonucleotide probes. Blood 1991;78:2276.
307. Metcalfe P, Waters AH. HPA-1 typing by PCR amplification with sequence-specific primers (PCR-SSP): a rapid and simple technique. Br J Haematol 1993;85:227.
308. Anderson BR, Georgsen J, Madsen HO, Taaning E, Grunnet N, Svejgaard A. Human platelet antigen-1 (Zw) typing using PCR-RFLP. Transfus Med 1993;3:153.
309. Williamson LM, Bruce D, Lubenko A, Chana HJ, Ouwehand WH. Molecular biology for platelet alloantigen typing. Transfus Med 1992;2:255.
310. van den Veyver IB, Chong SS, Kristjansson K, Snabes MC, Moise KJ, Hughes MR. Molecular analysis of human platelet antigen system 1 antigen on single cells can be applied to preimplantation genetic diagnosis for prevention of alloimmune thrombocytopenia. Am J Obstet Gynecol 1994;170:807.
311. Blanchette VS, Chen L, Salomon de Friedberg S, Hogan VA, Trudel E, Decary F. Alloimmunization to the Pl[A1] antigen: results of a prospective study. Br J Haematol 1990;74:209.
312. Bussel JB, McFarland JG, Berkowitz R. Antenatal treatment of fetal alloimmune cytopenias. Blut 1989;59:136.
313. Van Leeuwen E, Leeksma O, van Mourik J, Engelfriet C, von dem Borne A. Effect of the binding of anti-Zw[a] antibodies on platelet function. Vox Sang 1984;47:280.
314. Duncan JR, Rosse W. Alloantibody-induced platelet serotonin release is blocked by antibody to the platelet Pl[A1] antigen. Br J Haematol 1986;64:331.
315. Zalneraitis EL, Young RSK, Krishnamoorthy KS. Intracranial hemorrhage in utero as a complication of isoimmune thrombocytopenia. J Pediatr 1979;95:611.
316. Jesurun CA, Levin GS, Sullivan WR, Stevens D. Intracranial hemorrhage in utero re thrombocytopenia. J Pediatr 1980;97:695.
317. Morales WJ, Stroup M. Intracranial hemorrhage in utero due to isoimmune neonatal thrombocytopenia. Obstet Gynecol 1985;65(3 Suppl):208.
318. Naidu S, Messmore H, Caserta V, Fine M. CNS lesions in neonatal isoimmune thrombocytopenia. Arch Neurol 1983;40:552.
319. Chandler D, Daniel SJ. Isoimmune neonatal thrombocytopenia: a case report and a review. Am J Clin Pathol 1985;83:766.
320. Sia CG, Amigo NC, Harper RG, Farahani G, Kochen J. Failure of cesarean section to prevent intracranial hemorrhage in siblings with isoimmune neonatal thrombocytopenia. Am J Obstet Gynecol 1985;153:79.
321. Herman JH, Humbelic MI, Ancona RJ, Kickler TS. In utero cerebral hemorrhage in alloimmune thrombocytopenia. Am J Pediatr Hematol Oncol 1986;8:312.
322. Muhler E, Gurr U, Hornchen H. Intracerebral hemorrhage at 2 different times in neonatal alloimmune thrombocytopenia. Monatsschr Kinderheilkd 1987;135:336.
323. Kiefel V, Santoso S, Weisheit M, Muller-Eckhardt C. Monoclonal antibody-specific immobilization of platelet antigens (MAIPA): a new tool for the identification of platelet-reactive antibodies. Blood 1987;70:1732.
324. McMillan R, Tani P, Millard F, Berchtold P, Renshaw L, Woods VL. Platelet-associated and plasma anti-glycoprotein autoantibodies in chronic ITP. Blood 1987;70:1040.
325. Furihata K, Hunter J, Aster RH, Koewing GR, Shulman R, Kunicki TJ. Human anti-Pl[E1] antibody recognizes epitopes associated with the alpha subunit of platelet glycoprotein Ib. Br J Haematol 1988;68:103.
326. Galea P, Patrick MJ, Goel KM. Isoimmune neonatal thrombocytopenic purpura. Arch Dis Child 1981;56:112.
327. Katz J, Hodder FS, Aster RS, Bennetts GA, Cairo MS. Neonatal isoimmune thrombocytopenia: the natural course and management and the detection of maternal antibody. Clin Pediatr 1984;23:159.
328. Adner MM, Fisch GR, Starobin SG, Aster RH. Use of "compatible" platelet transfusions in treatment of congenital isoimmune thrombocytopenic purpura. N Engl J Med 1969;280:244.
329. McIntosh S, O'Brien RT, Schwartz AD, Pearson HA. Neonatal isoimmune purpura: response to platelet infusions. J Pediatr 1973;82:1020.
329a. Sidiropoulos D, Straume B. The treatment of neonatal isoimmune thrombocytopenia with intravenous immunoglobulin (IgG i.v.). Blut 1984;48:383.
330. Derycke M, Dreyfus M, Ropert JC, Tchernia G. Intravenous immunoglobulins in neonatal isoimmune thrombocytopenia. Arch Dis Child 1985;60:666.
331. Guillois B, Metz C, Guillou MA, Boog G. Treatment of neonatal alloimmune thrombopenia with polyvalent immunoglobulins. Arch Fr Pediatr 1987;44:234.
332. Massey GV, McWilliams NB, Mueller DG, Napolitano A, Maurer HM. Intravenous immunoglobulin in treatment of neonatal isoimmune thrombocytopenia. J Pediatr 1987;111:133.
333. Vain NE, Bedros AA. Treatment of isoimmune thrombocytopenia of the newborn with transfusion of maternal platelets. Pediatrics 1979;63:107.
334. Kalmin ND, Brown DJ. Platelet washing with a blood cell processor. Transfusion 1982;22:125.
335. Kaplan C, Daffos F, Forestier F, et al. Management of alloimmune thrombocytopenia: antenatal diagnosis and in utero transfusion of maternal platelets. Blood 1988;72:340.
336. Waters A, Murphy M, Hambley H, Nicolaides K. Management of alloimmune thrombocytopenia in the fetus and neonate. In: Nance SJ, ed. Clinical and basic science aspects of immunohematology. Arlington, American Association of Blood Banks, 1991:155.
337. Kaplan C, Patereau C, Reznikoff-Etievant MF, et al. Antenatal Pl[A1] typing and detection of GPIIb/IIIa complex. Br J Haematol 1985;60:586.
338. Menutti M, Schwarz RH, Gill F. Obstetric management of isoimmune thrombocytopenia. Am J Obstet Gynecol 1974;118:565.
339. Sitarz AL, Driscoll JM, Wolff JA. Management of isoimmune neonatal thrombocytopenia. Am J Obstet Gynecol 1976;124:39.
340. Richter E, Weigel H, Barz D, Krause KP, Matthes G. Neonatal alloimmune thrombocytopenia: can cryopreserved thrombocytes help? Beitr Infusionsther 1991;28:213.
341. Bussel JB, Berkowitz RL, McFarland JG, Lynch L, Chitbara N. Antenatal treatment of neonatal alloimmune thrombocytopenia. N Engl J Med 1988;319:1374.
342. Kroll H, Giers G, Bald R, et al. Intravenous IgG during pregnancy for (Zw[A]) fetal alloimmune thrombocytopenic purpura? Thromb Haemost 1993;69:997a.
343. Prenatal Management of fetal alloimmune thrombocytopenia. (Editorial) Vox Sang 1993;65:180.
344. Reznikoff-Etievant MF, Lobet R. HLA-B8 antigens and Pl-A1 alloimmunization. Tissue Antigens 1981;18:86.
345. Reznikoff-Etievant MF, Muller JY, Julien F, Patereau C. An immune response gene linked to MHC in man. Tissue Antigens 1983;22:312.
346. Taaning E, Antosen H, Peterson S, et al. HLA antigens and maternal antibodies in alloimmune neonatal thrombocytopenia. Tissue Antigens 1983;21:351.
347. Mueller-Eckhardt C, Mueller-Eckhardt G, Willen-Ohff H, Horz A, et al. Immunogenicity of and immune response to the human platelet antigen Zw[a] is strongly associated with HLA-B8 and DR3. Tissue Antigens 1985;26:71.
348. de Waal LP, van Dalen CM, Engelfriet CP, von dem Borne AEGKr. Alloimmunization against the platelet-specific Zw[a] antigen, resulting in neonatal alloimmune thrombocytopenia or post-transfusion purpura, is associated with the supertypic DRw52 antigen including Dr3. Hum Immunol 1986;17:45.
349. Mueller-Eckhardt C, Becker T, Weisheit M, Witz D, Santoso S. Neonatal alloimmune thrombocytopenia due to fetomaternal Zw[b] incompatibility. Vox Sang 1986;50:94.
350. Zucker MB, Ley AB, Borrelli J, Mayer K, Firmat J. Thrombocytopenia with a circulating platelet agglutinin, platelet lysin, and a clot retraction inhibitor. Vox Sang 1959;4:148.

351. Kunicki TJ and Beardsley DS. The alloimmune thrombocytopenias: neonatal alloimmune thrombocytopenic purpura and post-transfusion purpura. In: Coller B, ed. Progress in thrombosis and hemostasis, vol 9. Philadelphia, WB Saunders, 1989:203.
352. Kroll H, Keifel V, Mueller-Eckhardt C. Post-transfusion purpura: clinical and immunologic studies in 38 patients. Infusionsther Transfusionsmed 1993;20:198.
353. Zucker MB, Ley AB, Borrelli J, Mayer K, Firmat J. Thrombocytopenia with a circulating platelet agglutinin, platelet lysin, and a clot retraction inhibitor. Vox Sang 1959;4:148.
354. Bepler G, Hoffman SE, Thompson BP, Telen MJ, Rosse WF. Captopril-enhanced binding of PlA1 (HPA-1a) antibodies in posttransfusion purpura. Transfusion 1991;31:752.
355. Eden GW, Ostwinkle RJ, Ligorksy RD. Splenectomy in post-transfusion purpura: report of a case. J Am Osteopath Assoc 1985;85:443.
356. Weisberg LJ, Linker CA. Prednisone therapy of posttransfusion purpura. Ann Intern Med 1984;100:76.
357. Gerstner JD, Smith MJ, Davis KD, Cimo PL, Aster RH. Posttransfusion purpura: therapeutic failure of PlA1-negative platelet transfusion. Am J Hematol 1979;6:71.
358. Glud TK, Rosthoj S, Jensen MK, Laursen B, et al. High dose intravenous immunoglobulin for post-transfusion purpura. Scand J Haematol 1983;31:495.
359. Becker T, Panzer S, Maas D, Kiefel V et al. High-dose intravenous immunoglobulin for post-transfusion purpura. Br J Haematol 1985;61:149.
360. Berney SI, Metcalfe P, Wathen NC, Waters AH. Post-transfusion purpura responding to high dose intravenous IgG: further observations on pathogenesis. Br J Haematol 1985;61:627.
361. Taaning E, Morling N, Ovesen H, Svejgaard A. Post-transfusion purpura and anti-Zw^b (-PlA2). Tissue Antigens 1985;26:143.
362. Barre J, Vinsonneau M, Lelarge C, Rendoing J, et al. Post-transfusion thrombopenia treatment with gammaglobulins. Ann Fr Anesth Reanim 1986;5:80.
363. Chong BH, Cade J, Smith JA, Tatoulis J. An unusual case of post-transfusion purpura: a good transient response to high-dose immunoglobulins. Vox Sang 1986;51:182.
364. Mueller-Eckhardt C. Post-transfusion purpura. Br J Haematol 1986;64:419.
365. Mueller-Eckhardt C, Kuenzelen E, Theo-Koerner D, Pralle H. High dose intravenous immunoglobin for post-transfusion purpura. N Engl J Med 1983;398:287.
366. Soulier PJ, Patereau C, Gobert N, Achach P, Muller JY. Post-transfusional immunologic thrombocytopenia: a case report. Vox Sang 1979;37:21.
367. Lau P, Sholtis CM, Aster RH. Post-transfusion purpura: an enigma of alloimmunization. Am J Hematol 1980;9:331.
368. Shulman NR, Aster RH, Lietner A, Hiller MC. Immunoreactions involving platelets. V. Post-transfusion purpura due to a complement-fixing antibody against a genetically controlled platelet antigen: a proposed mechanism for thrombocytopenia and its relevance in "autoimmunity." J Clin Invest 1961;40:1597.
369. Mueller-Eckhardt C, Mueller-Eckhardt G, Willen-Ohff H, Horz A, et al. Immunogenicity of and immune response to the human platelet antigen Zw^a is strongly associated with HLA-B8 and DR3. Tissue Antigens 1985;26:71.
370. de Waal LP, van Dalen CM, Engelfriet CP, von dem Borne AEGKr. Alloimmunization against the platelet-specific Zw^a antigen, resulting in neonatal alloimmune thrombocytopenia or post-transfusion purpura, is associated with the supertypic DRw52 antigen including Dr3. Hum Immunol 1986;17:45.
371. Shulman NR. Platelet immunology. In: Colman RW, Hirsh J, Mauder VJ, Salzman V, eds. Hemostasis and thrombosis: basic principles and clinical practice, ed 2. Philadelphia, JB Lippincott, 1987:342.
372. Kickler TS, Ness PM, Herman JH, Bell WR. Studies on the pathophysiology of post-transfusion purpura. Blood 1986;68:347.
373. Morrison FS, Mollison PL. Post-transfusion purpura. N Engl J Med 1966;243:243.
374. Barnhart DD, Gengozian N. Actively induced thrombocytopenia in the marmoset: a possible autoimmune model. Clin Exp Immunol 1975;21:493.
375. Linklater KA. Post-transfusion purpura in a pig. Res Vet Sci 1977;22:257.
376. Pegels JG, Bruynes EC, Engelfriet CP, von dem Borne AEGKr. Post-transfusion purpura: a serological and immunochemical study. Br J Haematol 1981;49:521.
377. Slichter SJ. Post-transfusion purpura: response to steroids and association with red blood cell and lymphocytotoxic antibodies. Br J Haematol 1982;50:599.

Blood: Principles and Practice of Hematology,
edited by Robert I. Handin, Samuel E. Lux, and Thomas P. Stossel.
J.B. Lippincott Company, Philadelphia © 1995.

57

Disorders of Erythrocyte Glycolysis and Nucleotide Metabolism

Donald E. Paglia

Congenital (or hereditary) nonspherocytic hemolytic anemia is a diagnosis of exclusion. Historically, it has been used to identify a subset of intrinsic erythrocyte defects that could not be ascribed to hemoglobinopathies, thalassemia, paroxysmal nocturnal hemoglobinuria, or hereditary elliptocytosis or spherocytosis. It includes a heterogeneous group of disorders that have in common shortened red blood cell survival times induced by a broad range of metabolic abnormalities. This rather nebulous diagnosis is usually assigned to cases of chronic hemolytic anemia in which hemoglobin abnormalities and antiglobulin reactions are undetectable, microspherocytes are few or essentially absent, and osmotic fragility is normal. In contrast to hereditary spherocytosis, the benefits of splenectomy are generally only partial and inconsistent.

An appreciation of the metabolic basis of these disorders grew from the work of Dacie and colleagues,[1,2] who observed that sterile blood from such patients, when incubated in vitro with various additives, displayed distinctly different hemolytic tendencies. Autohemolysis categorized as type I was only slightly greater than that of normal blood, regardless of the presence of glucose in the incubation medium. Type II autohemolysis was moderately or markedly increased relative to normal controls and was essentially unaffected by glucose supplementation. Defective glycolysis in such cells was further suggested by decreased conversion of glucose to lactate, by accumulation of certain glycolytic intermediates within affected red cells, and by decreased concentrations of erythrocyte adenosine triphosphate (ATP).[3–5]

In 1961, Valentine and colleagues[6,7] demonstrated a common defect, deficiency of pyruvate kinase activity, in several families with chronic hemolytic anemia and type II autohemolysis patterns. This observation, coupled with the demonstration of glucose-6-phosphate dehydrogenase deficiency in primaquine-sensitive erythrocytes,[8] established the metabolic basis of these disorders, which has since been expanded to include a large number of phenotypically diverse enzymopathies of glucose, glutathione, and nucleotide metabolism.[9–17] Additional heterogeneity often exists within a given erythroenzymopathy. A hemolytic syndrome may result not only from insufficient production of normal enzyme protein but also from variant isozymes whose altered primary structures impair substrate or cofactor avidity, alter activation or inhibition characteristics, or decrease stability or specific activity. The common denominator is presumed to be an impairment in energy or antioxidant metabolism that makes the affected cells susceptible to premature hemolysis.[18]

The most common clinical presentations of glycolytic enzymopathies are chronic hemolytic anemia of variable severity and acute hemolytic episodes that are often induced by certain drugs, infections, foods, or the stresses of surgery or pregnancy. Severe cases are manifest in the neonatal period, and some have even been associated with hydrops fetalis. The classic findings of indirect hyperbilirubinemia, with or without icterus, decreased haptoglobin, and compensatory reticulocytosis are usually present along with variable degrees of splenomegaly and erythroid hyperplasia of the marrow. The latter, if sufficiently prominent, may induce skeletal changes by expansion of marrow spaces. A family history of anemia often suggests a hereditary basis for the disorder.

As mentioned previously, the absence of demonstrable antiglobulin reactions or hemoglobin, membrane, or other abnormalities leads to a diagnosis by exclusion. The nonspecific autohemolysis test is essentially obsolete. A precise diagnosis in cases of hereditary nonspherocytic hemolytic anemia requires quantitative enzyme assays to detect a specific enzymopathy. Screening test kits for some of the more common enzyme deficiencies are commercially available, but their qualitative nature makes them particularly susceptible to false-negative results. Several laboratories in the United States, Europe, and Japan have developed the capacity to provide screening services for individual referring physicians and institutions to evaluate suspected cases and to perform detailed biochemical characterization of abnormal enzymes according to internationally standardized criteria. Among these are the laboratories of Drs. Ernest Beutler of the Scripps Clinic and Research Foundation (La Jolla, California), Shiro Miwa of the Okinawa Memorial Institute for Medical Research (Tokyo), Jean and Raymonde Rosa of INSERM Hopital Henri Mondor (Creteil, France), Gerard E.J. Staal of the University Hospital (Utrecht, The Netherlands), Kouichi R. Tanaka of the Harbor–UCLA Medical Center (Torrance, California), and my laboratory at the University of California (UCLA) School of Medicine (Los Angeles).

GLUCOSE METABOLISM IN HUMAN ERYTHROCYTES

The mature erythrocyte represents a highly specialized yet remarkably simplified cell. It consists principally of a plasma membrane enveloping a viscous concentrated (33%) solution of hemoglobin, the latter accounting for about 95% of the cell's dry weight. In the few days required for its reticulocyte precursor to mature, it loses its last vestiges of ribosomal and mitochondrial function, having already dispatched its nucleus by pitting and karyolysis of nuclear remnants. The resultant mature erythrocyte is therefore incapable of oxidative phosphorylation, protein or lipid synthesis, tricarboxylic acid cycling, or most of the diverse and redundant metabolic capacities exhibited by nucleated cells with their complex cytoplasmic organelles.

Although the purpose of gas transport and exchange in the red cell is fulfilled entirely without alteration in energy state, a number of vital cell functions depend on appropriate generation and expenditure of energy. These include (1) initiation and maintenance of glycolysis; (2) cation pumping against electrochemical gradients; (3) synthesis of glutathione and other essential metabolites; (4) nucleotide salvage reactions; (5) maintenance of hemoglobin iron in its functional reduced ferrous state; (6) protection of structural, enzymatic, and hemoglobin proteins from oxidative denaturation; and (7) preservation of membrane phospholipids. These energy needs must be adequately met if the erythrocyte is to survive and function effectively for its expected life-span of 120 days in the peripheral circulation. Inadequate energy production may be reflected by decreased intracellular concentration of ATP, failure of the cation pump, loss of the normal discoid shape and plasticity of the cell envelope, and other membrane alterations that may include Heinz body formation. Such changes may be sufficiently severe to cause intravascular hemolysis or to program the cells for selective removal from the circulation by the reticuloendothelial system.

As summarized in Figure 57-1, energy generation is accomplished almost entirely by glycolysis with storage as high-energy phosphates, particularly ATP, or as reducing energy in the form of glutathione and pyridine nucleotides (NADH and NADPH).

Erythrocyte membranes possess a facilitated transport system for the glucose that is present as an abundant carbon source in the plasma. About 90% of the glucose assimilated by the erythrocyte is normally catabolized by the anaerobic Embden-Meyerhof pathway, providing the cell's principal means of ATP generation. Small and variable amounts of glucose may be diverted through the *hexose monophosphate shunt*, also known as the *pentose phosphate pathway*. Glucose catabolism by this oxidative shunt provides the erythrocyte with a pool of reducing energy to combat ambient oxidative effects on hemoglobin and other proteins. When necessary, glucose shunting through this pathway can increase by more than an order of magnitude.

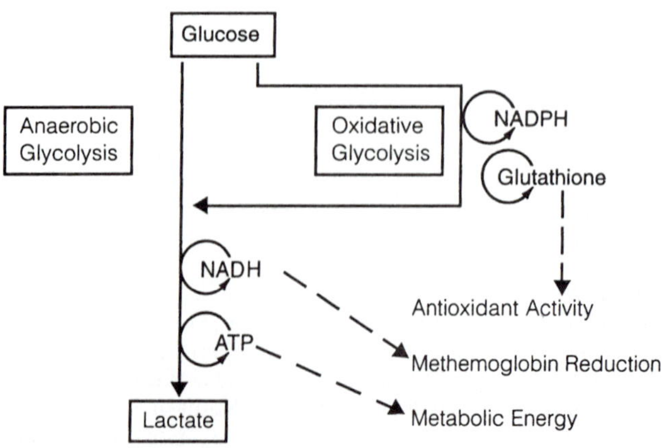

FIGURE 57-1. Energy metabolism of the erythrocyte. Generation of high-energy phosphates and reducing compounds is accomplished principally via glucose catabolism.

Anaerobic Glycolysis

The biochemical pathways available to mature erythrocytes to accommodate their energy needs are shown in greater detail in Figure 57-2. Glucose catabolism is initiated by its phosphorylation to glucose-6-phosphate, a reaction catalyzed by hexokinase. This enzyme has the lowest activity of all the glycolytic enzymes in mature erythrocytes, and its catalytic rate is highly sensitive to pH; to intracellular concentrations of its product, glucose-6-phosphate; and to other metabolites, such as inorganic phosphate, 2,3-diphosphoglycerate, and disulfide compounds. By virtue of these characteristics of hexokinase, the phosphorylation of glucose becomes an important, potentially rate-limiting step in glycolysis.

Isomerization of glucose-6-phosphate to fructose-6-phosphate, catalyzed by glucosephosphate isomerase, provides the substrate for a second major rate-limiting reaction, phosphorylation at the carbon-1 position mediated by phosphofructokinase. Like hexokinase, phosphofructokinase requires magnesium, is optimally active at alkaline pH, and is sensitive to stimulation by inorganic phosphate. It may be under the additional regulatory influences of substrate, product, and other glycolytic metabolite concentrations. The product of this reaction, fructose-1,6-diphosphate, is produced at the cost of two moles of ATP, but its cleavage into dihydroxyacetone phosphate and glyceraldehyde-3-phosphate in the aldolase reaction provides two triose moieties, each of which may then serve as substrate for rephosphorylation of adenosine diphosphate (ADP) by phosphoglycerate kinase and pyruvate kinase. There is thus a net gain of two moles of ATP for every mole of glucose degraded directly to pyruvate or lactate by the Embden-Meyerhof pathway.

Triose degradation begins with glyceraldehyde-3-phosphate formed in the aldolase reaction or by isomerization of dihydroxyacetone phosphate. The latter is catalyzed by triosephosphate isomerase, which has the highest activity of any of the erythrocyte glycolytic enzymes by as much as three orders of magnitude (Table 57-1). Glyceraldehyde-3-phosphate dehydrogenase serves two particularly important functions: it fixes inorganic phosphate into the high-energy compound, 1,3-diphosphoglycerate, and in the process reduces the pyridine cofactor, NAD^+, to NADH, which is the essential cofactor for methemoglobin reductase activity. Two options then ensue: the high-energy phosphate of 1,3-diphosphoglycerate may be transferred to ADP, forming ATP in the phosphoglycerate kinase reaction, or it may be discarded by mutation of the 1,3-phosphodiester to the low-energy intermediate, 2,3-diphosphoglycerate. The intracellular concentration of the latter compound is about 4 mmol/L. It accounts for two thirds or more of the erythrocyte's complement of organic phosphates and has a crucial regulatory influence on hemoglobin oxygen affinity (see Chap. 52).

Mutation of 1,3-diphosphoglycerate to 2,3-diphosphoglycerate constitutes the divergent branch of the Rapoport-Luebering shunt, aptly described by Keitt[19] as the "energy clutch" of ATP generation in erythrocyte metabolism. Triose diverted into the Rapoport-Luebering shunt foregoes the option of ATP generation by phosphoglycerate kinase, yet it provides a large and accessible reservoir of substrate

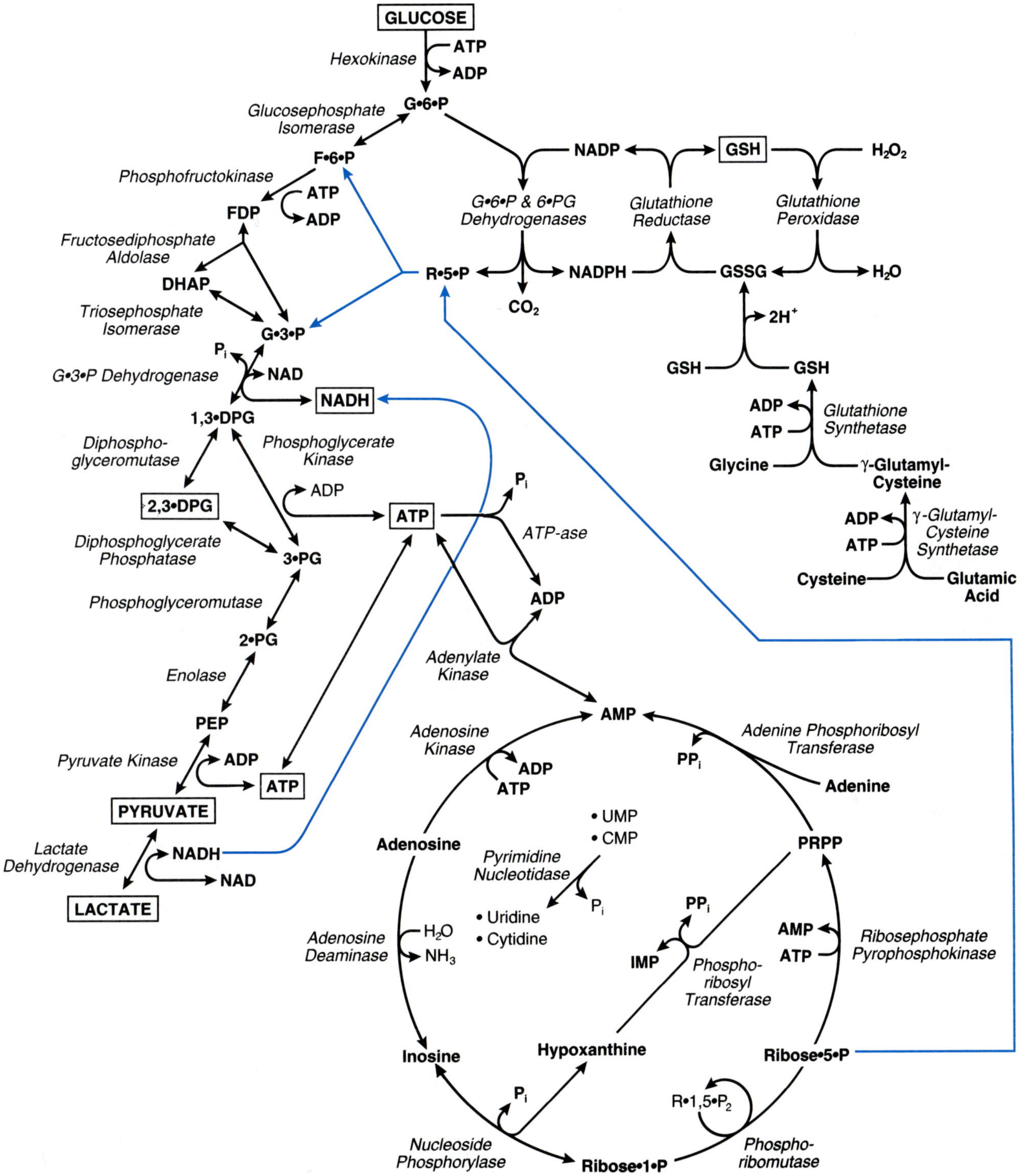

FIGURE 57-2. Biochemical pathways of metabolism in the erythrocyte. Glucose is degraded to lactate anaerobically via the Embden-Meyerhoff pathway (*on the left*) or oxidatively by diversion of glucose-6-phosphate (G-6-P) into the hexose monophosphate shunt (pentose phosphate pathway; *on the right*). Pentose phosphates (R-5-P) generated by this pathway or by nucleoside degradation can be transformed into intermediates of anaerobic glycolysis for further catabolism. NADH serves as cofactor for methemoglobin reductase activity. NADPH is the physiologic cofactor required for maintenance of adequate reduced glutathione (GSH) to combat ambient oxidative stresses. The Rapoport-Luebering shunt shelters an abundant intracellular store of 2,3-diphosphoglycerate (2,3-DPG), which can be degraded to regenerate ATP in response to altered ADP/ATP ratios. (After Scriver CR, Beaudet AL, Sly WS, Valle D, eds. The metabolic basis of inherited disease, ed 6. New York, McGraw Hill, 1989)

TABLE 57-1. Optimal In Vitro Activities of Various Erythrocyte Enzymes

Erythrocyte Enzymes	Relative Activity*
ANAEROBIC GLYCOLYSIS	
Hexokinase	1
Glucosephosphate isomerase	59
Phosphofructokinase	10
Fructosediphosphate aldolase	7
Triosephosphate isomerase	1807
Glyceraldehyde-3-phosphate dehydrogenase	190
Phosphoglycerate kinase	300
Monophosphoglyceromutase	11
Phosphopyruvate hydratase	7
Pyruvate kinase (3 mmol/L PEP)	19
Pyruvate kinase (3 mmol/L PEP + F-1,6-P_2)	20
Pyruvate kinase (0.4 mmol/L PEP)	10
Pyruvate kinase (0.4 mmol/L + F-1,6-P_2)	16
Lactate dehydrogenase	169
HEXOSE MONOPHOSPHATE SHUNT AND GLUTATHIONE CYCLING	
Glucose-6-phosphate dehydrogenase	9
6-Phosphogluconate dehydrogenase	9
Glutathione reductase	6
Glutathione peroxidase	12
Glutathione S-transferase	5
NUCLEOTIDE METABOLISM	
Adenylate kinase	181
Guanylate kinase	9
Cytidylate kinase	10
Uridylate kinase	20
Adenylate deaminase	9
Adenosine kinase	4
Adenosine deaminase	1
Nucleoside phosphorylase	72
Nucleoside diphosphate kinase	9
Ribosephosphate pyrophosphokinase	93
Adenine phosphoribosyltransferase	4
Pyrimidine nucleotidase (uridine monophosphate)	13
Pyrimidine nucleotidase (cytidine monophosphate)	10
Deoxyribonucleotidase (deoxythimidine monophosphate)	20
Deoxyribonucleotidase (deoxyinosine monophosphate)	49
MISCELLANEOUS	
Glutamic oxaloacetic transaminase	4
Malic dehydrogenase	17
Acetylcholinesterase	32
Glyoxalase I	171
Glyoxalase II	63
Triokinase	0.2

PEP, phosphoenolpyruvate.

* Unit relative value corresponds to 0.27 μmol substrate converted per minute by 10^{10} erythrocytes at 37°C or 0.81 μmol substrate per gram of hemoglobin. Values were derived from normal control subjects assayed in the author's laboratory over the preceding 3 years.

to generate ATP by channeling through the pyruvate kinase reaction in terminal glycolysis. The amount of ATP produced per mole of catabolized glucose can thereby be modulated according to the needs of the cell and is governed in large measure by the relative concentrations of ADP and ATP.

The convergent branch of the Rapoport-Luebering shunt is mediated by diphosphoglycerate phosphatase, which irreversibly dephosphorylates 2,3-diphosphoglycerate at the carbon-2 position. Both diphosphoglyceromutase and phosphatase activities are accomplished by the same enzyme protein as it is altered by existent conditions.[20–22] Both activities are inhibited by increasing concentrations of their respective products, and mutation is further inhibited by inorganic phosphate. Mutase activity requires 3-phosphoglycerate as a cofactor and is activated by 2-phosphoglycerate, whereas phosphatase activity is inhibited by the former and unaffected by the latter.

Perhaps the most important modulating influence on activity of the Rapoport-Luebering shunt is provided by intracellular hydrogen ion concentration. Diphosphoglyceromutase is inhibited at acid pH, while diphosphoglycerate phosphatase is simultaneously activated. The effect of acidosis, therefore, is to divert 1,3-diphosphoglycerate through the phosphoglycerate kinase reaction and to mobilize the 2,3-diphosphoglycerate reserve for further degradation, with the consequences of both alternatives being increased generation of ATP by the two distal kinases.

Mutation of 3-phosphoglycerate to the 2-isomer is catalyzed by a monophosphoglyceromutase that requires 2,3-diphosphoglycerate as a cofactor. In actuality, phosphate at the carbon-3 position of the cofactor is transferred to the carbon-2 position of 3-phosphoglycerate, transforming the original substrate into 2,3-diphosphoglycerate and allowing the triose of the original cofactor to continue down the pathway as the substrate of terminal glycolysis. Enolization of 2-phosphoglycerate by phosphopyruvate hydratase produces phospho*enol*pyruvate, the substrate for pyruvate kinase in the last ATP-generating step in glycolysis.

The isozyme of pyruvate kinase normally present in erythrocytes is highly sensitive to allosteric modulation by fructose-1,6-diphosphate. Micromolar concentrations of this glycolytic intermediate markedly increase the affinity of the enzyme for its substrate, phospho*enol*pyruvate, converting its sigmoid kinetic curve into a hyperbole. This provides another point of sensitive control for the overall rate of glycolysis that is additionally influenced by potassium concentrations, which alter affinity for the cofactor, ADP. The product of the pyruvate kinase reaction, pyruvic acid, is diffusible from the cell but also provides a substrate for lactate dehydrogenase activity if the intracellular NAD^+/NADH ratio is appropriate. Conversion of pyruvate to lactate in this reaction regenerates NAD^+ that can be used in the glyceraldehyde-3-phosphate dehydrogenase reaction. NADH provides a reservoir of reducing energy that is essential for maintaining hemoglobin iron in its functional reduced state through the mediation of methemoglobin reductase. Since both pyruvate and lactate are diffusible from the erythrocyte, the direction of the reversible lactate dehydrogenase reaction is governed by the balance between glycolytic use of NAD^+ and oxidation of NADH accompanying methemoglobin reduction.

Phosphorylated compounds generally cannot diffuse across erythrocyte membranes unless assisted by an active transport system. Of the phosphorylated glycolytic intermediates, only phospho*enol*pyruvate appears capable of entering the red cell at low pH through mediation of an anion transport system associated with the band-3 membrane protein.[23,24] After entering the erythrocyte, exogenous phospho*enol*pyruvate is capable of further metabolism to increase intracellular concentrations of both 2,3-diphosphoglycerate and ATP, and this phenomenon has been investigated for its potential to enhance the viability of cells stored for transfusion.[24,25]

Erythrocytes incubated with certain other phosphorylated metabolites or nucleotides may also show significant alterations in intracellular concentrations of glycolytic intermediates and ATP but not by direct incorporation of the exogenous compound. Uniformly labeled fructose-1,6-diphosphate, for example, does not enter the red cell but can increase the intracellular concentration of the same compound by altering membrane cation permeability, effecting an increase in pH that stimulates glycolysis by activation of phosphofructokinase.[26] This can occur in vivo[27] as well as in vitro and may also have potential applications in transfusion medicine or in the treatment of certain erythroid enzyme defects. Similarly, the salutary effect of exogenous ATP on the autohemolysis of incubated erythrocytes appears to be mediated by catabolic degradation and increased glycolysis rather than by direct incorporation of ATP. Regardless of in vitro observations, the physiologic importance of the erythrocyte's capacity to use substrates other than glucose for energy metabolism remains uncertain and controversial.

Aerobic Glycolysis

Oxidative degradation of glucose can occur by diversion of glucose-6-phosphate from the anaerobic Embden-Meyerhof pathway into the hexose monophosphate shunt (the pentose phosphate pathway). Normally, less than 5% to 10% of glucose is catabolized through this pathway, thereby maintaining a pool of reducing energy in the form of NADPH and reduced glutathione. Sudden oxidant challenge, however, can stimulate glucose flow through the shunt by 20- to 30-fold or more.

The ratio of $NADP^+$ and NADPH concentrations provides the principal determinant of hexose monophosphate shunt flow. $NADP^+$ is the obligate pyridine nucleotide cofactor for the two dehydrogenase reactions in the shunt, and NADPH is a potent inhibitor of the initiating enzyme, glucose-6-phosphate dehydrogenase. In these reactions, $NADP^+$ is the hydrogen recipient as glucose-6-phosphate is oxidized at the carbon-1 position, producing carbon dioxide and a phosphorylated pentose, ribulose-5-phosphate. The pentose moiety is subsequently modified and recombined through a series of reactions mediated by a pentose epimerase, isomerase, transketolase, and transaldolase to form two intermediates of the Embden-Meyerhof pathway, glyceraldehyde-3-phosphate and fructose-6-phosphate. The latter may be reversibly isomerized to glucose-6-phosphate and recycled back through the oxidative shunt if the $NADP^+$/NADPH ratio is appropriately compelling.

Under ambient conditions, 1 of 6 mol of glucose traversing the shunt would be lost as carbon dioxide, and the remaining 5 mol would be catabolized to pyruvate-lactate. With shunt stimulation, however, 4 of the 6 mol could be recycled back through the shunt, with only 2 mol committed to triose formation and subsequent anaerobic degradation. This flexibility for diversion of variable amounts of substrate through the hexose monophosphate shunt provides the erythrocyte with its major defense against oxidant damage.

Diversion of glucose from anaerobic to aerobic catabolism is initiated by glucose-6-phosphate dehydrogenase, for which $NADP^+$ is an obligate cofactor. This enzyme is an X-chromosome gene product and exists as a pH-dependent equilibrium of catalytically active homodimers and homotetramers with subunits of about 59 kd. Its activity is strongly influenced by intracellular concentrations of substrate, cofactor, products, hydrogen ions, and metal cations, and its catalytic rate is normally only a small fraction of its potential fully stimulated capacity. NADPH and ATP both serve as inhibitors, competitive with $NADP^+$ and glucose-6-phosphate, respectively. These regulatory properties are physiologically important because they allow appropriate production of NADPH in response to variable oxidative challenges. This pyridine cofactor is crucial to peroxide detoxification by cyclic glutathione peroxidase and reductase activities; additionally, NADPH is avidly bound as a structural component of catalase. The ability of the red cell to survive assaults by ambient oxidants is therefore crucially dependent on effective hexose-monophosphate shunt activity initiated by glucose-6-phosphate dehydrogenase.

The wild enzyme, designated G6PD-B, is common to all cells, but posttranslational modifications may alter its properties slightly from one tissue to another. A normal African isozyme, designated G6PD-A, results from a single amino acid substitution. Its catalytic activity and other biochemical properties are similar or identical to G6PD-B, except for altered electrophoretic migration. An A-minus variant differs by an additional amino acid substitution that significantly decreases its activity, alters other biochemical properties, and has clinical manifestations. The A and A-minus isozymes are common among African Americans (30% and 11%, respectively), and the latter is responsible for an acute hemolytic syndrome associated with administration of certain drugs or other stresses, such as infections, surgery, and perhaps the neonatal period. Glucose-6-phosphate dehydrogenase deficiency and other disorders of the hexose monophosphate shunt are described in detail in Chapter 58, and recent advances have been cogently summarized by Beutler.[27a]

It is curious that a cell whose primary function is to carry molecular oxygen, an explosively reactive oxidant, simultaneously must preserve many of its structural and enzymatic proteins, and even hemoglobin itself, in reduced states to function and survive effectively. This precarious balance is made possible in part by the presence of high concentrations of the cysteine-containing tripeptide, glutathione, which hexose monophosphate shunt activity serves to maintain in the reduced state. Because of its low oxidation potential, this compound readily serves as a sacrificial reductant, protecting less-reactive sulfhydryl groups of cellular proteins from oxidant damage.

Hydrogen peroxide is one such potent oxidant, posing a serious threat because it is constantly generated in small amounts in normal cells and in large amounts by certain drugs, such as primaquine. The selenium metalloenzyme, glutathione peroxidase, catalyzes conversion of hydrogen peroxide to water by coupling it to the oxidative condensation of two molecules of glutathione. The latter can be reduced back to functional tripeptides through disulfide cleavage mediated by the flavin enzyme, glutathione reductase, with NADPH serving as the physiologic hydrogen donor. Oxidants may also induce formation of mixed disulfides between glutathione and other sulfhydryl containing proteins, including hemoglobin, and many of these may also be reduced again through mediation of glutathione reductase. Glutathione itself has a relatively rapid turnover rate in erythrocytes and must be constantly resynthesized from its constituent amino acids, as shown in Figure 57-2.

Many of the deleterious cellular effects of such diverse pathologic processes as inflammation, aging, and radiation and chemical injury are mediated by free radical formation. Sophisticated mechanisms to neutralize free radicals have evolved to protect cell membranes, enzymes, and other cellular components from the destructive structural and functional consequences of lipid peroxidation, altered redox states, and protein denaturation. Human erythrocytes contain a dismutase that inactivates superoxide free radicals by conversion to hydrogen peroxide, which can then be decomposed by catalase or reduced to water by glutathione peroxidase in a coupled oxidation of reduced glutathione. The latter is regenerated by the action of glutathione reductase using NADPH as hydrogen donor.

Defects in any of these enzymes, or in the synthesis and maintenance of glutathione itself, theoretically could compromise antioxidant defenses, potentially rendering such cells susceptible to stress-induced hemolysis. Acatalasemia, however, is not associated with a hemolytic syndrome, and significant deficiencies of superoxide dismutase have not been observed. NADPH is also a tightly bound component of mammalian catalase and is necessary for the enzyme protein's resistance to inactivation by hydrogen peroxide.[28] Contrary to what was implied by earlier studies,[29] it appears that both catalase and glutathione peroxidase are of comparable importance in the physiologic detoxification of peroxidase.[30] A wide range of glutathione peroxidase activities has been observed among certain populations on the basis of heritage[31] or dietary deficiency of selenium,[32,33] an essential enzyme component, but these have not been accompanied by premature hemolysis.

Nucleotide Metabolism

Mature circulating erythrocytes normally contain only trace amounts of nonadenine nucleotides. Because these cells cannot synthesize nucleotides de novo, they have evolved mechanisms that effectively preserve the complement provided them as they emerge from the reticulocyte stage. Some of the known reactions pertinent to erythrocytes are summarized in Figure 57-2.

The adenine nucleotide pool in erythrocytes consists mostly of ATP (85% to 90%), with lesser amounts of ADP (10% to 12%) and adenosine monophosphate (AMP; 1% to 3%), maintained in rapid equilibrium by an active adenylate kinase. Glycolysis generates ATP, but the amount of ATP generated is limited to the ADP available for phosphorylation. The third component, AMP, although present in the smallest concentration, is in a particularly vulnerable position. If it is either deaminated to inosine monophosphate or dephosphorylated to diffusible adenosine, the purine moiety is effectively lost to the cell, and some salvage mechanism must intervene to compensate.

Two potential salvage pathways are apparent in Figure 57-2. Adenine phosphoribosyltransferase in human erythrocytes is sufficient in activity to convert adenine to AMP, but adenine does not appear to be readily available in plasma, and subjects with complete deficiency of the enzyme show no demonstrable alteration in erythrocyte function, longevity, or nucleotide concentrations.[34] By contrast, there is strong evidence to support a physiologic role for adenosine kinase in nucleotide salvage. This pathway accounts for the accumulation of high concentrations of deoxyadenosine phosphates in red cells from some immunodeficient subjects with marked deficiency of the enzyme adenosine deaminase.[35–39] Conversely, patients with hyperactive adenosine deaminase show depletion of their erythrocyte nucleotides.[40–44] Since the kinase and deaminase compete for the same substrate, these observations indicate that nucleotide salvage by adenosine kinase is normally important to maintain the adenine nucleotide pool at constant concentrations.

Except for pyrimidine nucleotidase, none of the other reactions depicted in the nucleotide cycle of Figure 57-2 appears to be physiologically significant for the mature erythrocyte. Deficiencies and hyperactivity states exist for a number of these, including nucleoside phosphorylase, hypoxanthine-guanine phosphoribosyl transferase, and ribosephosphate pyrophosphokinase, and all are apparently devoid of deleterious effects on the red cell.[45] Pyrimidine nucleotidase is physiologically important during reticulocyte maturation. Its substrate specificity allows it to dephosphorylate only the pyrimidine products of RNA degradation, thereby converting them to diffusible nucleosides and clearing them from the cell without simultaneously degrading AMP and affecting the adenine nucleotide pool.[46–48] Red cells also contain a separate deoxyribonucleotidase that may have a corresponding function in DNA catabolism.[49–53]

Erythrocyte Metabolism as a Function of Cell Age

Reticulocytes have a number of metabolic differences compared with mature erythrocytes. Their use of glucose and oxygen is respectively greater by one and two orders of magnitude, largely as a consequence of their transient retention of functional mitochondrial enzymes. Krebs cycle metabolism and oxidative phosphorylation both proceed actively for a short time, as does synthesis of hemoglobin and other proteins.

Additionally, reticulocytes emerge from the marrow with the residua of some glycolytic isoenzymes that are principally present in erythroid precursors but are rapidly inactivated in the postreticulocyte stage. These differences are accentuated in immature macroreticulocytes that may be stimulated to leave the marrow early during the stress erythropoiesis of severe anemia.

All this results in profiles of enzymatic activities and metabolite concentrations that vary considerably between reticulocytes and older erythrocytes. Because the latter can no longer synthesize protein, their enzymes lose activity as the cells progressively age, and each enzyme generally exhibits a characteristic decay rate, depending on its susceptibility to oxidative denaturation, proteolysis, or other processes that result in catalytic inactivation. This phenomenon influences interpretation of analyses for potential enzymatic deficiencies since patients with hemolytic anemia generally have peripheral blood populations inordinately rich in reticulocytes and in metabolically more active, young erythrocytes. These can easily mask a deficiency that might be apparent were older erythrocytes available for analysis. A classic example is the difficulty in establishing a diagnosis of glucose-6-phosphate dehydrogenase deficiency during the period immediately after an acute hemolytic crisis when reticulocytes surge into the peripheral blood to replace the oldest, enzymatically effete erythrocytes that were most susceptible to hemolysis.

The pattern of progressive metabolic depletion as erythrocytes age has been extrapolated to the senescent cell to account for its sharply limited life-span. The traditional view suggests that natural attrition of metabolic capacities eventually leads to a cell that cannot fulfill its energy requirements, and some consequent sequence of events ultimately terminates in cell death. This natural process is presumed to be accelerated by enzymopathies that further restrict energy metabolism in affected erythrocytes, leading to their premature demise.

This hypothesis remains unproved even though abundant supportive data have been generated, particularly by studies related to blood cell preservation for transfusion. Reports in search of the "aging lesion" in erythrocytes continue to expand the literature without resolution of the issue. Decreases in erythrocyte high-energy phosphates and 2,3-diphosphoglycerate concentrations correlate directly with posttransfusion survival,[54] yet studies indicate that the oldest red cell cohorts in vivo actually contain *increased* rather than decreased concentrations of ATP.[55–57] Similarly, the precise event terminating the life of an enzyme-deficient erythrocyte remains uncertain, but the proximal cause-and-effect relation remains unchallenged by more likely hypotheses.

HEMOLYTIC ENZYMOPATHIES OF THE GLYCOLYTIC PATHWAY

Enzyme abnormalities may have perceptible effects on red cell function or survival, depending on the physiologic importance of the affected reactions and on the availability of alternate metabolic pathways. Those enzymopathies that have adverse clinical consequences frequently fall into two patterns. Defects in the hexosemonophosphate shunt and in those reactions normally responsible for generation or maintenance of reduced glutathione generally are associated with periodic hemolytic episodes that are induced by oxidant foods or drugs, the duress of surgery or infections, or other physiologic stresses. By contrast, deficiency states in the Embden-Meyerhof pathway and certain enzymes concerned with nucleotide metabolism are usually expressed by shortened red cell survival and chronic hemolytic anemia. The common denominator among these diverse conditions is an inability to generate sufficient ATP to fulfill cellular energy needs, and this is presumed to be the pathophysiologic basis for premature hemolysis.[18]

Historically, hereditary enzymopathies were first detected as decreases in in vitro activities as measured in optimized assay systems with hemolysates as the source of the enzyme. Observed activities were less than 10% to 20% of those found in normal control hemolysates, and these have come to be termed *quantitative* or *classic* deficiency states. Affected patients were presumed to be homozygotes because intermediate (about 40% to 60%) levels of enzyme activities were often found in parents and relatives, consistent with heterozygous deficiency states. Such inheritance patterns could be explained by the presence of mutant genes that coded for production of an abnormal, catalytically inactive enzyme protein or by null genes that failed to produce appropriate amounts of otherwise normal enzyme protein.

Regardless of the enzyme found to be defective, *no consistent correlation has ever been established between the degree of activity decrements and the severity of their clinical expression.* A number of different abnormalities in biochemical characteristics of affected enzymes can result in functional deficiencies, even though optimal activities observed in vitro may be minimally decreased, normal, or even *increased.* Broad polymorphism in genetic expression has been established for most of the known erythroenzymopathies. Mutant genes may code for production of enzyme proteins that are catalytically impotent; unstable; kinetically aberrant; altered in terms of their response to physiologic activators, inhibitors, cofactors, and allosteric modifiers; or diverse combinations of these characteristics, any of which may be further manifested by altered pH optima, electrophoretic migration rates, and so forth. In the absence of consanguinity, affected patients often represent compound heterozygotes rather than true homozygotes, so mixtures of mutant isozymes are likely to be present in affected cells. A few instances of molecular identity between unrelated mutant variants have been documented. Recent advances in the molecular biology underlying diverse erythroenzymopathies have been reviewed by Beutler[27a] and are summarized in Table 57-2.

Hexokinase

Hexokinase (ATP:D-hexose-6-phosphotranferase, E.C.2.7.1.1) is responsible for priming the glycolytic pump. Because of its crucial importance to the initiation of glycolysis, it was generally assumed that serious hereditary defects in this enzyme would likely be lethal mutations, but a small group of deficient cases with diverse ethnic origins has been detected.[58–73] At least four distinct, tissue-specific isoenzymes of hexokinase are normally identifiable, depending on methods of separation and purification, and these have been designated HK-1 through HK-4.[74] Subtypes of HK-1 are present in erythrocytes,[75–77] including one that predominates in reticulocytes and is presumably responsible for the steep biphasic decay curve observed as reticulocytes mature and erythrocytes age.[78] This complicates diagnosis

TABLE 57-2. Molecular Genetics of Glycolytic Enzymopathies

Enzyme	Main Form in Erythrocytes	Chromosome Locus	Gene Cloned	Mutation Identified
Hexokinase	HK-1	10p11.2	Yes[304]	No
Glucosephosphate isomerase	Same enzyme*	19cen-q13	Yes[334]	Yes[335]
Phosphofructokinase	M, L	1 cen → q32; 21q22.3	Yes[305–307]	Yes[308,336]
Aldolase	A	16q22–q24	Yes[309,310]	Yes[311]
Triosephosphate isomerase	Same enzyme*	12p13	Yes[312]	Yes[313,337]
Phosphoglycerate kinase	PGK-1	Xq13	Yes[314,315]	Yes[153b,153c,316–320]
Diphosphoglycerate mutase	Only in erythrocytes	7q22–q34	Yes[321,322]	Yes[323]
Enolase	α	1pter-p36.13	Yes[324]	No
Pyruvate kinase	L	1q21	Yes[325,338]	Yes[326–331,338]
Lactate dehydrogenase	H	12p12.1–12-2	Yes[332]	Yes[333]

* Same enzyme is present in all cells, including erythrocytes.
(Adapted from Tanaka KR, Paglia DE. Pyruvate kinase and other enzymopathies of the erythrocyte. In: Scriver CR, Beaudet AL, Sly WS, Valle D, eds. The metabolic basis of inherited disease, ed 7. New York, McGraw-Hill, 1994 [in press])

of a deficiency in specimens heavily populated by reticulocytes and young cells. HK-1 is also found in brain but differs from the isozymes found in other blood cells and tissues. Hexokinase is a cytosolic enzyme formed in monomers of about 100 kd. Its governing gene is located on the long arm of chromosome 10,[79] and inheritance of defects conforms to an autosomal recessive mode. Some cases appear to follow a dominant transmission pattern, perhaps with variable penetrance.[68,69]

A wide range of molecular heterogeneity exists among the abnormal HK-1 isozymes that have been reported. Most variants exhibit reduced activities and decreased substrate affinities, but heterogeneity is additionally reflected by alterations in thermostability, electrophoretic migration rates, and variable regulatory responses to glucose-6-phosphate, glucose-1,6-diphosphate, 2,3-diphosphoglycerate, and inorganic phosphate. Decreased production of apparently normal enzyme protein has also been reported.[67] The principal clinical manifestation of severe hexokinase deficiency is confined to erythroid elements as chronic mild to severe hemolytic anemia. Heterozygous deficiency states are without apparent effect on red cell function or longevity, although minor decreases in ATP and some glycolytic intermediates have been observed. In severe cases with heavy transfusion requirements, splenectomy may have some benefits.[58–61,71] Erythrocyte hexokinase deficiency may also occur as one of the multiple abnormalities in Fanconi's anemia.[80]

Glucosephosphate Isomerase

Glucosephosphate isomerase (D-glucose-6-phosphate ketol-isomerase, E.C.5.3.1.9) deficiencies comprise the second most common erythroenzymopathy of anaerobic glycolysis, after those of pyruvate kinase. A single homodimeric enzyme of 134 kd[81–83] is present in humans and is encoded by a gene on chromosome 19.[84] Some slight differences that originally were thought to represent tissue-specific isozymes most likely represent posttranslational modifications rather than distinct isozymes.[85]

Virtually all the mutant gene products reported have been characterized by marked instability. Cells capable of protein synthesis may compensate for this lability by increased enzyme production, but erythrocytes do not share this capacity and consequently die prematurely if glycolysis is sufficiently impaired. Thus, hemolytic anemia may be the only clinical manifestation of this multisystem disorder, although myopathy and mental retardation may sometimes accompany the anemia.[86–88]

In addition to instability, most variant isoenzymes have been characterized by normal substrate affinities, but additional alterations have been observed in catalytic activity, electrophoretic migration rates, pH optima, and varying combinations of these parameters. Stable and kinetically aberrant variants have also been detected.[87–90] Biochemical changes induced by defective enzymes include increased intracellular concentrations of glucose-6-phosphate, decreased concentrations of glycolytic intermediates distal to the point of blockade, altered ATP/ADP concentrations and ratios (both increased and decreased), and severely impaired (less than 1% to 10%) ability to recycle fructose-6-phosphate back through the hexose monophosphate shunt,[91–93] even though shunt activity may increase significantly as glucose-6-phosphate builds up and diversion occurs. Intermediate rates of fructose-6-phosphate recycling have been demonstrated in some heterozygous deficiencies.[92,94] This impairment in hexosemonophosphate shunt recycling may be responsible for the increased susceptibility to oxidant-induced Heinz body formation and glutathione instability that have been observed in some studies of defective glucosephosphate isomerase.

The anemia of glucosephosphate isomerase deficiency varies from mild to severe in homozygotes or compound heterozygotes, and simple heterozygotes are hematologically normal. Severe homozygous deficiency has been documented as a rare cause of hydrops fetalis.[95] Therapeutic attempts to stimulate glycolysis with ascorbic acid, methylene blue, or inorganic phosphate have not been rewarding. Splenectomy in some cases has been followed by variably increased hemoglobin concentrations and decreased transfusion requirements.[96] Prolonged severe anemia that requires frequent transfusions is the principal clinical indication for considering splenectomy, but responses in individual cases remain unpredictable.

Phosphofructokinase

Phosphofructokinase (ATP:D-fructose-6-phosphate 1-phosphotransferase, E.C.2.7.1.11) may be the most important enzyme regulating erythrocyte glycolysis. It occupies a key rate-limiting position in the earliest stage of anaerobic glycolysis, and its activity responds to complex and subtle modulations by a number of metabolites and ions, including ATP, ADP, AMP, 2,3-diphosphoglycerate, and fructose-1,6- and fructose-2,6-diphosphates.[97–102] Additionally, the product of this essentially irreversible reaction, fructose-1,6-diphosphate, is the principal allosteric activator of another crucial rate-limiting enzyme in terminal glycolysis, pyruvate kinase.

Phosphofructokinase is a tetramer composed of three dissimilar subunits, designated L, M, and P (or F) according to their occurrence in liver and leukocytes, muscle, and platelets (or fibroblasts), and ranging in size between 80 and 85 kd.[99–104] Each is encoded by separate genes residing respectively on chromosomes 21, 1, and 10.[105–108] As pointed out by Vora,[109] M subunits tend to predominate in tissues that rely heavily on glycolysis, such as skeletal and cardiac muscle and brain, whereas L subunits appear to be associated with tissue reliance on gluconeogenesis, such as liver and adipose tissue. The red cell contains about equal amounts of L and M subunits arranged in all five possible tetramers: L_4, L_3M_1, L_2M_2, L_1M_3, and M_4.

Deficiencies of phosphofructokinase are multiple and varied, depending on which subunit is affected. Defects of the M subunit, for example, are clinically expressed as myopathies since the skeletal muscle isozyme is the homotetramer M_4. Red cells in such patients must rely completely on the L_4 homotetramer with its decreased activity and substrate affinity. Defects in phosphofructokinase activity due to unstable M subunits may impair red cell glycolysis sufficiently to result in clinically detectable hemolysis without myopathy.[110–113] Cases devoid of either myopathy or hemolysis despite severe reductions in activity have also been observed.

The absence of M subunits in the classic form of phosphofructokinase deficiency (Tarui's disease) reduces erythrocyte phosphofructokinase activities to about half of normal. This results in decreased concentrations of distal glycolytic intermediates, including 2,3-diphosphoglycerate, which can alter the oxygen dissociation curve of hemoglobin sufficiently to induce erythrocytosis. The hemolytic process, therefore, may be well compensated by erythrocytosis, and such patients may be hematologically asymptomatic.[114–116] Tarui's disease is characterized also by glycogen deposition in skeletal muscle (glycogen storage disease type VII), resulting in muscle weakness, cramping, exercise intolerance, and myoglobinuria, sometimes complicated by hyperuricemia and early-onset gout.[114]

Fructosediphosphate Aldolase

Fructosediphosphate aldolase (D-fructose-1,6-bisphosphate D-glyceraldehyde-3-phosphate lyase, E.C.4.1.2.13) reversibly catalyzes the equilibrium between fructose-1,6-diphosphate and its component trioses, dihydroxyacetone phosphate and glyceraldehyde-3-phosphate. It is also a tetrameric enzyme totaling about 158 kd, and three tissue-specific isozymes (A, B, and C) have been described.[117,118] The adolase A gene has been localized to the 16q22-q24 region.[118a] Severe deficiency states have been reported in two unrelated families conforming to an autosomal recessive mode of inheritance. In one case, mild hemolysis with multiple congenital malformations, mental retardation, and glycogen storage disease were present in an uncertain association[119]; in another family, moderately severe chronic hemolysis alone was observed.[120] In the latter, the residual erythrocyte enzyme was unstable and exhibited decreased affinity for its substrate, fructose-1,6-diphosphate. A single amino acid substitution has been demonstrated in one variant.[121]

Triosephosphate Isomerase

Triosephosphate isomerase (D-glyceraldehyde-3-phosphate ketol-isomerase, E.C.5.3.1.1) catalyzes the interconversion of dihydroxyacetone phosphate and glyceraldehyde-3-phosphate. This is a dimeric enzyme molecule totaling 53 kd with identical subunits of 248 amino acids[122] structurally encoded by a single gene on the short arm of chromosome 12.[123,124] All tissues share a common enzyme, and therefore all are affected to some degree by deficiency states. Multiple electrophoretic forms apparently result from posttranslational modifications.[125,126] Null alleles have been detected in a number of subjects who exhibit half of normal activities coupled with comparable amounts of immunologically cross-reacting protein.[127,128]

Clinically, significant deficiencies have been documented in about 30 cases, most of these exhibiting 5% to 20% of the triosephosphate isomerase activity present in normal control erythrocytes.[129–145] Other tissues in which the enzyme has been quantitatively measured also show remarkably reduced enzyme activities. These cases also encompass a broad range of molecular heterogeneity in regard to their residual enzymes, principally manifested as stability, kinetic, and electrophoretic abnormalities. Transmission of the genetic defect follows an autosomal recessive pattern. Clinically affected patients are homozygotes or compound heterozygotes, while simple heterozygotes are devoid of hematologic, neuromuscular, or other abnormalities.

Severe impairment of isomerase activity results in cellular accumulation of potentially toxic dihydroxyacetone phosphate. This triose may be present in affected cells in concentrations as high as 50 times normal.[131,142] The clinical consequences of severe triosephosphate isomerase deficiency are dominated by the severity of neuromuscular abnormalities that invariably accompany this disorder, including tremor, dystonia, pyramidal tract signs, and spinal motor neuron development. These usually become apparent within the first year of life and inexorably progress in severity, with few children surviving to adulthood. A subjective impression of increased susceptibility to infections may reflect leukocyte involvement, but distinct functional abnormalities in phagocytic and bactericidal processes have not been demonstrated. Arrhythmia and sudden death occur presumably as a consequence of cardiac muscle involvement. The hemolytic anemia associated with triosephosphate isomerase deficiency is also moderate to severe and has not been effectively ameliorated by splenectomy.

Phosphoglycerate Kinase

Phosphoglycerate kinase (ATP:3-phospho-D-glycerate 1-phosphotransferase, E.C.2.7.2.3) is the only enzyme of anaerobic glycolysis known to be encoded by a gene on the X chromosome. All tissues except sperm contain the same enzyme (PGK-1),[146,147] which exists as a monomer of 416 amino acids[147] and of about 45 kd.[148] The PGK-2 isoenzyme present in sperm is seperately encoded by an autosomal gene.[148a] Phosphoglycerate kinase catalyzes the first ATP-generating step of glycolysis, transferring the high-energy phosphate of 1,3-diphosphoglycerate to ADP. As shown in Figure 57-2, that substrate may also be converted to a low-energy state and stored as 2,3-diphosphoglycerate by irreversible diversion through the Rapoport-Luebering shunt. The direction of substrate flow is primarily determined by intracellular pH and ATP/ADP ratio. As expected, deficiencies of phosphoglycerate kinase usually show decreased concentrations of ATP and increased concentrations of 2,3-diphosphoglycerate, with a consequent shift in the oxyhemoglobin dissociation curve. Increased intracellular sodium concentrations have also been observed and ascribed to alterations in Na^+-K^+ pump activity secondary to decreased ATP production from this reaction.[149]

Some of the biochemical and clinical heterogeneity in phosphoglycerate kinase deficiency may result from the nature of the specific molecular lesion. The reaction catalyzed by phosphoglycerate kinase is bidirectional. Reverse phosphorylation of 3-phosphoglycerate to 1,3-diphosphoglycerate is a component of gluconeogenesis, a process that is apparently of no consequence to red cell viability. As a matter of technical convenience, in vitro assays often measure this backward reaction, but that may not adequately reflect the effectiveness of the forward, ATP-generating step that is crucial to red cell function and longevity. Some mutations result in gene products that have significantly more catalytic or kinetic impairment in one direction of the reaction relative to the other. This may account for the absence of hemolysis in one variant, such as PGK Creteil, in which the backward reaction is more adversely affected, compared with the overt hemolysis associated with PGK Tokyo, in which the forward reaction is more impaired.

Deficiencies of phosphoglycerate kinase are rare, with 14 variants described, and those that have been documented have shown considerable polymorphism. Seven variants have been sequenced and shown to be due to single amino acid substitutions,[150–153c] occurring in a common region of the enzyme molecule that may adversely affect nucleotide binding.[14,154] Several variants have exhibited abnormal kinetics for substrates or cofactors as well as decreased optimal activities and instability.[150–152,155–164] Although some variants are silent, about half are associated with hemolytic anemia of variable severity and progressive neurologic disturbances in affected males, including mental retardation, emotional lability, behavioral aberrations, dyskinesias, hemiplegia, and aphasia. Affected females exhibit mosaicism with variable populations of normal and enzyme-deficient erythrocytes and hemolytic manifestations that range from moderate to none, and normal neurologic function.

Because a single enzyme form is common to virtually all tissues, they share the enzymopathy that has been demonstrated in skeletal and cardiac muscle, brain, liver, leukocytes, and platelets.[165] Phagocytosis by deficient leukocytes may be ineffective because of impaired bactericidal processes.[166] Patients with isolated myopathy have also been reported,[162,163] as has hemolysis without neuromuscular disease.[164] If severe, the anemia of phosphoglycerate kinase deficiency may improve after splenectomy, but the response rate has been inconsistent. Aplastic crises occasionally occur, but progressive neurologic complications usually dominate the clinical picture.

Pyruvate Kinase

Pyruvate kinase (ATP:pyruvate 2-o-phosphotransferase, E.C.2.7.1.40) is nominally a homotetrameric enzyme composed of about 55- to 60-kd.[167–171] Mammals possess multiple tissue-specific isozymes derived from two principal forms, PK-M and PK-L, dominant in muscle and liver, respectively, which are products of genes on chromosomes 15 and 1 (Fig. 57-3). PK-R isozymes characteristic of red cells are derivative products of the PK-L gene. Close similarities exist between L and R isozymes,[168,172–174] and hepatocytes exhibit decreased pyruvate kinase activity (partially compensated by ongoing synthesis) in many cases of erythrocyte enzyme deficiency.[174–180]

Natural isoenzymes that predominate in adult liver (L), striated muscle and brain (M_1), kidney, leukocytes and platelets (M_2), and erythrocytes (R) all have features in common but are identifiable by distinct biochemical differences.[181–184a] M_2 is the principal form in fetal tissues.[183] Variations in the primary structure of tissue-specific isozymes may be induced by gene rearrangements, alternative RNA splicing, differences in mRNA, or posttranslational proteolytic modifications.[172,173,184–188] Characteristic of the natural isozymes of pyruvate kinase are summarized in Figure 57-3.

Partially purified red cell pyruvate kinase is electrophoretically separable into two bands, homotetrameric R_1 and a heterotetramer, R_2, composed of two paired dissimilar subunits. R_1 and R_2 migrate apart from the L form, even though all three are antigenically identical.[167,176,190] Decreased synthesis of fetal M_2 as erythroid precursors mature[191] allows replacement by R_1 in reticulocytes and young erythrocytes and eventually by R_2, the dominant form in mature erythrocytes.[172,190–194] In some deficiency states, including the animal model in Basenji dogs, R forms may fail to develop properly, and the fetal isozyme persists.[195–197] Persistence of M_2 may also be responsible for certain cases of pyruvate kinase hyperactivity.[198,199]

The R_2 isozyme in mature erythrocytes is more stable than its precursor forms and has greater substrate avidity

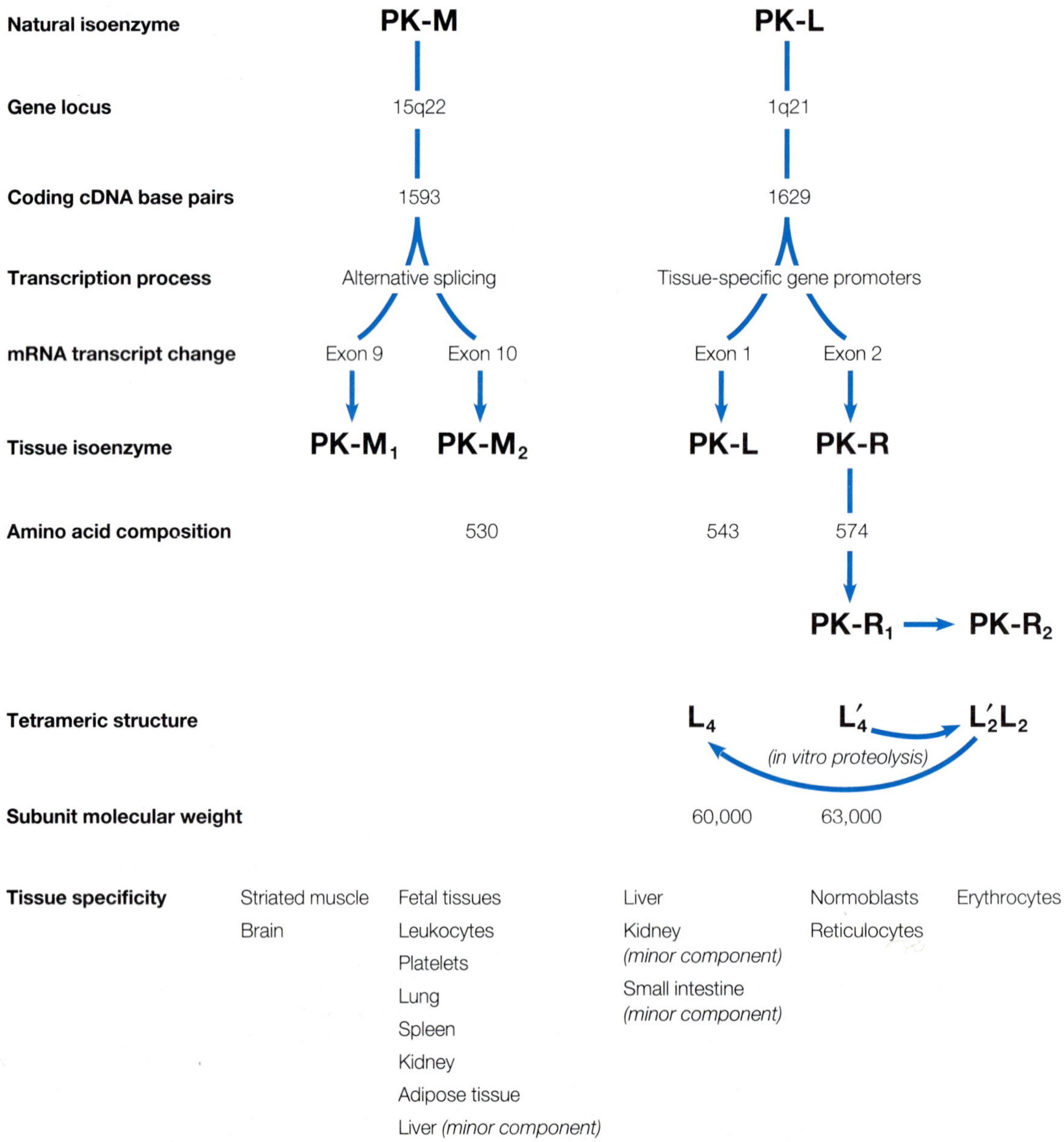

FIGURE 57-3. Characteristics of the natural isoenzymes of human pyruvate kinase.

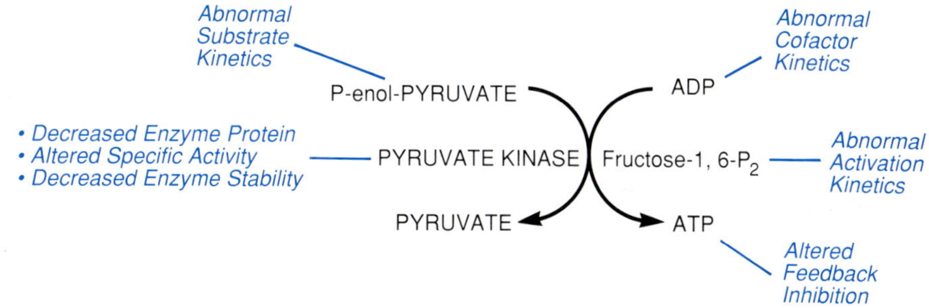

FIGURE 57-4. The pyruvate kinase reaction. The alterations observed in association with various mutant isozymes are indicated.

with more effective regulatory properties.[172,200] Because the R_1 form is the dominant isozyme in reticulocytes, these cells may be particularly vulnerable to further metabolic impairment by mutant variants, perhaps contributing to their selective destruction in some cases of pyruvate kinase deficiency.[201] Although reticulocytes possess the advantage of ATP generation through mitochondrial oxidative phosphorylation, that process is greatly suppressed in the hypoxic and acidic environment of the spleen where these cells may be detained because of their decreased deformability.[202–204] Splenectomy in pyruvate kinase deficiency, therefore, may allow maturation and survival of reticulocytes that otherwise would have perished, accounting for the paradoxical increase in reticulocytosis despite decreased hemolysis that is characteristically observed after splenectomy in this disorder.[205]

Pyruvate kinase catalyzes the second crucial ATP-generative step in glycolysis, which is necessary if there is to be any net gain in ATP. It requires magnesium and potassium for optimal activity, and it is highly sensitive to a number of regulatory influences.[206–208] All the normal tissue-specific isozymes except M_1 are subject to allosteric modulation by substrate or cofactors. The substrate, phospho*enol*pyruvate, and a cofactor product of the phosphofructokinase reaction, fructose-1,6-diphosphate, when combined with the erythrocyte enzyme, increase its substrate avidity, converting a sigmoidal kinetic curve hyperbolic (Michaelis-Menten) kinetics.

Additionally, potassium concentrations influence enzyme affinity for ADP, and increasing concentrations of ATP inhibit activity. These kinetic properties generally follow the R $\leftrightarrow$ T transformation equilibrium model proposed by Monod and colleagues[209] (see Chap. 52). Relaxed (R) conformational changes in the enzyme molecule are induced by attachment of the substrate, phospho*enol*pyruvate, and the allosteric activator, fructose-1,6-diphosphate, which cooperatively increase substrate affinity and catalytic activity. The tight (T) conformation exhibits a sigmoid kinetic curve (Hill's coefficient is about 1.5 to 2), with decreased substrate avidity and low catalytic activities at physiologic concentrations of phospho*enol*pyruvate. The T conformation is also highly sensitive to inhibition by ATP.

These complex qualities reflect a highly ordered, symmetric tertiary protein structure that is common to all the natural pyruvate kinase isozymes and shared by a number of other enzymes possessing helical α/β-barrel configurations.[210] Mutant gene products might exhibit a variety of biochemical abnormalities, dependent on the precise site of the molecular lesion and its consequent effects on tertiary structural conformations. Such is precisely the case with mutant pyruvate kinase isozymes. Alterations affecting various regulatory properties, as well as those that result in significantly decreased stability or catalytic activity (Fig. 57-4), may show identical phenotypic expression as a chronic hemolytic syndrome of variable severity. A number of specific molecular alterations identified among mutant isozymes are summarized in Table 57-3. Baronciani and Beutler[338] have described eight additional mutations.

Pyruvate kinase deficiency was the first enzymopathy of the Embden-Meyerhof pathway to be recognized as a cause of hereditary nonspherocytic hemolytic anemia.[6,7] Along with class I deficiencies of glucose-6-phosphate dehydrogenase, pyruvate kinase defects comprise the most common erythroenzymopathy responsible for chronic hemolysis. Several hundred cases have been identified, and internationally standardized procedures for their evaluation have been adopted.[211] People of Northern European and peri-Mediterranean heritage are most commonly af-

TABLE 57-3. Specific Molecular Lesions Identified in Pyruvate Kinase Deficiency

Variant PK Isoenzyme	Nucleotide		Amino Acid	
	Substitution	Position	Substitution	Position
Beirut[326]				
Tokyo[327]	C → T	1151	Thr → Met	384
Nagasaki[328]				
Linz[326]	C → T	487	Arg → Cys	163
Fukushima[328] Maebashi[328]	C → A	1261	Gln → Lys	421
Sapporo[329]	G → A	1277	Arg → Gln	426
Osaka[330]	G → T	1102	Val → Phe	368
Amish[331]	G → A	1436	Arg → His	479

(Adapted from Tanaka KR, Paglia DE. Pyruvate kinase and other enzymopathies of the erythrocyte. In: Scriver CR, Beaudet AL, Sly WS, Valle D, eds. The metabolic basis of inherited disease, ed 7. New York, McGraw-Hill [in press]) fected, but deficiencies have been observed in a wide range of ethnic and geographic origins.

Genetic transmission follows an autosomal recessive pattern except for rare instances of dominance.[189,212] Homozygosity for the defect results in chronic hemolysis, whereas virtually all heterozygotes are hematologically normal. Because of the broad range of molecular heterogeneity among pyruvate kinase variants and the relative infrequency of consanguinity, most affected patients are not true homozygotes but rather are compound heterozygotes whose red cells contain mixtures of at least two mutant isozymic forms. Because pyruvate kinase is a tetramer, dissimilar subunit assembly could produce as many as five isozymes.[213,214] Although this complicates biochemical characterization, it appears that most clinically significant deficiency states are associated with enzyme variants that have either markedly reduced specific activity, decreased affinity for the substrate phosphoenolpyruvate, reduced stability, or an impaired capacity to respond to allosteric activation by fructose-1,6-diphosphate. Other alterations, such as decreased inhibition by ATP, decreased affinity for the cofactor ADP, increased substrate affinity, and decreased enzyme protein production, have been less commonly observed. Any alteration in the gene product that produces such variable biochemical characteristics may also be reflected in electrophoretic migration patterns, pH optima, and thermal inactivation rates.[185–187,195,213,215–242]

Impairment of glycolysis at the pyruvate kinase step, regardless of the molecular mechanism involved, results in decreased intracellular concentrations of total adenine nucleotides, decreased ATP generation, elevated concentrations of glycolytic intermediates above the blockade (particularly 2,3-diphosphoglycerate and 3-phosphoglycerate), and decreased $NAD^+/NADH$ concentrations with altered ratios. Concentrations of 2,3-diphosphoglycerate may double or triple, shifting the oxyhemoglobin dissociation curve sufficiently to help compensate for the anemia by favoring tissue oxygenation.

The primary clinical consequence of pyruvate kinase deficiency is chronic hemolysis that can vary from completely compensated asymptomatic cases to severe, transfusion-dependent, life-threatening anemias. The latter are often apparent during the neonatal period when exchange transfusions may be required. Severe deficiency may also be manifested by hydrops fetalis. Clinical and laboratory findings are no more distinctive in pyruvate kinase deficiency than in any other chronic hemolytic process. In most cases, peripheral red cell morphology is of little value in diagnosis of pyruvate kinase deficiency, but a number of isolated cases have been distinguished by prominent changes, including acanthocytes, echinocytes, and schistocytes.

Splenomegaly, icterus, indirect hyperbilirubinemia, decreased haptoglobin, bilirubin cholelithiasis, and reticulocytosis with marrow erythroid hyperplasia are commonly observed in direct proportion to the severity of anemia. The stresses of surgery, infections, and pregnancy have all been associated with acute exacerbations of the chronic hemolytic process, and aplastic crises may occur, particularly in association with parvovirus or related infections.[243,244] In severe cases, especially in young children, splenectomy has often resulted in increased erythrocyte and reticulocyte counts and hemoglobin concentrations and has frequently reduced or eliminated transfusion requirements, but there are no reliable criteria by which clinical responses may be reliably predicted. Splenectomy is not advocated for children less than 3 years of age, even if frequent transfusions are required to alleviate symptoms. The risk of iron overload during that period is relatively small compared with the potential hazard of postsplenectomy sepsis.

Erythroenzymopathies Devoid of Premature Hemolysis

Erythroenzymopathies devoid of premature hemolysis have also been documented in a number of instances. Some erythrocyte enzymes exhibit variable electrophoretic migration rates, and others have been found sufficiently defective to result in detectable biochemical alterations but not in hemolytic anemia. Severe deficiency of 2,3-diphosphoglyceromutase, for example, resulted in a virtual absence of intracellular 2,3-diphosphoglycerate. The consequent shift in the oxygen dissociation curve of hemoglobin induced a compensatory erythrocytosis (see Chap. 52) but no evidence of hemolysis or other clinical problems.[245] Similarly, defects in the H subunit of lactate dehydrogenase resulting in severely deficient activities may alter $NAD^+/NADH$ ratios but are unaccompanied by hemolysis.[246–248]

ALTERATIONS IN ERYTHROCYTE NUCLEOTIDE METABOLISM

Defective nucleotide metabolism has been observed in association with hyperactive as well as deficient erythrocyte enzymes. Enzymopathies that may be accompanied by hemolytic processes include overabundance of adenosine deaminase and deficiencies of adenylate kinase and pyrimidine nucleotidase.[45,48,249,250] A number of other deficiency states (eg, those involving adenosine deaminase, purine nucleoside phosphorylase, and the phosphoribosyl transferases acting on adenine, hypoxanthine, and guanine), and hyperactivity of ribosephosphate pyrophosphokinase are apparently unaccompanied by adverse effects on red cells.

Adenylate Kinase

Adenylate kinase (ATP:AMP phosphotransferase, E.C.2.7.4.3) catalyzes the rapidly reversible equilibrium existing among components of the erythrocyte adenine nucleotide pool. Considerable genetic polymorphism exists with at least five identifiable phenotypes.[251–254] Separate loci on chromosome 9 encode AK_1 and AK_3, whereas AK_2 is governed by a gene on the short arm of chromosome 1.[255] The skeletal muscle isozyme is a globular monomer of about 21.5 kd.[256,257]

The erythrocyte isozyme, AK_1, has been found to be variably defective in four kindreds. Among those with moderate to severe hemolytic anemia, residual activities ranged from 44% to less than 10% of normal controls.[258–261] Partial deficiency of glucose-6-phosphate dehydrogenase coexisted in one subject, and psychomotor retardation was present in another in uncertain associations. Genetic transmission appeared consistent with autosomal recessive or dominant inheritance with variable penetrance. Parental adenylate kinase was electrophoretically identical to the common AK_1 phenotype. Heterozygosity was thought to exist in some nonanemic relatives because of half-normal enzyme activities.

In a black American family,[262] however, two siblings displayed widely disparate clinical findings. Both had virtually undetectable adenylate kinase activities; but only one had hemolytic anemia, while the other appeared to be entirely normal. The reason for this disparity remains unexplained. Salvage reactions that generate adenosine monophosphate from adenine or adenosine theoretically require adenylate kinase activity to provide the diphosphates and, ultimately, the triphosphates to maintain the balance of the adenine nucleotide pool. It may be that adenylate kinase activities that are reduced by two or even three orders of magnitude below normal are still adequate to serve that purpose since erythrocyte concentrations of all adenine nucleotides were minimally altered, if at all, in either child.

The importance of adenylate kinase to normal cell function and longevity thus remains unclear. The possibility of compound defects in these cases persists, such as that of glucose-6-phosphate dehydrogenase in one kindred. Alternatively, the association between adenylate kinase deficiency and hemolytic anemia may be fortuitous, placing this erythroenzymopathy into the category of nondiseases described by Beutler.[263]

Adenosine Deaminase

Adenosine deaminase (adenosine aminohydrolase, E.C.3.5.4.4) converts adenosine to inosine, which is not retrievable by mature erythrocytes for reincorporation into the adenine nucleotide pool. Broad genetic polymorphism is expressed by a number of electrophoretic phenotypes,[264,265] and multiple molecular forms predominate in various tissues.[266] Erythrocytes, spleen, and stomach contain a 38-kd monomer. Two monomers may bind to a large dimeric nonenzymatic glycoprotein to form the isozyme characteristic of liver, kidney, and fibroblasts.[267,268] The gene governing adenosine deaminase structure resides on chromosome 20[269,270] and that for the binding protein on chromosome 6.[271] Posttranslational modifications account for additional differences among tissue-specific isozymes.[272,273]

Adenosine deaminase deficiency, such as that underlying certain forms of severe combined immunodeficiency disease,[274] is without apparent effect on erythrocyte function and survival even though the cells may accumulate high concentrations of deoxyadenosine phosphates.[35–39] Marked *elevations* in adenosine deaminase activity, however, have been associated with compensated hemolytic processes in three unrelated families from the United States, Japan, and France.[40–44] This abnormality is transmitted as a genetic *dominant* trait. Catalytic activity measured by standard in vitro assays may be increased by as much as two orders of magnitude over normal controls. The enzyme protein is structurally and biochemically normal.[40–42,275] Even though all tissues share a common catalytic protein component, adenosine deaminase overproduction is apparently isolated to erythroid elements because of a basic defect in mRNA translation.[276,277]

This degree of enzyme hyperactivity is phenotypically expressed as hemolytic anemia that is usually subclinical and well compensated by brisk reticulocytosis. ATP and total adenine nucleotides are about half of normal erythrocyte concentrations. This presumably results from the rapid deamination of plasma adenosine, which reduces or eliminates it as a potential substrate for an essential nucleotide salvage pathway in erythrocytes catalyzed by adenosine kinase.[41,45] The converse situation may be seen in immunodeficiency disease due to severely deficient adenosine deaminase, in which increases in erythrocyte concentrations of adenosine and deoxyadenosine phosphates reflect increased availability of the nucleosides as substrates for phosphorylation by adenosine kinase.

Overproduction of adenosine deaminase is accompanied by prominent elevations in activity of another erythrocyte enzyme, pyrimidine 5′-nucleotidase, but the significance of this linkage is unknown. The nucleotidase appears biochemically normal and does not show any increased ability to dephosphorylate AMP to account for the diminished adenine nucleotide pool.[41,45]

Pyrimidine 5′-Nucleotidase

Pyrimidine 5′-nucleotidase (5′-ribonucleotide phosphohydrolase, E.C.3.1.3.5) is an isoenzyme apparently unique to erythrocytes. Nucleotidases are ubiquitous enzymes that catalyze the hydrolytic dephosphorylation of monophosphate nucleotides to yield the corresponding nucleosides and inorganic phosphate. The isozyme found in erythrocytes, however, is essentially restricted to pyrimidine substrates. During reticulocyte maturation, this permits clearance of pyrimidine products of RNA degradation by dephosphorylation and diffusion while simultaneously protecting adenosine monophosphate from a similar fate.[46,48] A companion isozyme in normal erythrocytes appears to react principally with deoxyribonucleotide substrates and may serve as a complementary system with pyrimidine nucleotidase to clear maturing elements of both DNA and RNA degradation products.[51]

Different gene loci govern production of pyrimidine nucleotidase and deoxyribonucleotidase, but their locations are unknown. In erythrocytes, both are cytosolic enzymes that are easily distinguishable on the basis of substrate specificity, pH optima, sensitivity to heavy-metal inactivation, and other characteristics.[49–53] Deoxyribonucleotidase activity remains unimpaired in cases of severe pyrimidine nucleotidase deficiency.[50,51] Deficiency states for deoxyribonucleotidase have not yet been detected. The erythrocyte protein responsible for pyrimidine nucleotidase activity is about 28 kd.[278] An enzyme with similar characteristics has been detected in rat brain and kidney.[279]

Erythroenzymopathies involving pyrimidine nucleotidase appear to be almost as common as those of pyruvate kinase, particularly among those of peri-Mediterranean, African, and Jewish ancestry.[48,263,280] Hereditary defects are transmitted as autosomal recessive traits, with heterozygotes appearing hematologically and biochemically normal except for intermediate enzyme activities. In the severe deficiency states that characterize homozygosity or compound heterozygosity, residual activities are usually only 5% to 10% of normal, and the hemolytic syndrome that results may be of sufficient severity to require transfusions. Splenectomy has been attempted in some patients with severe hemolysis, but beneficial effects have been inconsistent and unpredictable, occasionally reducing transfusion dependence and elevating hemoglobin and red cell counts. Kinetic, electrophoretic and other abnormalities are sometimes detectable,[281–288] but the common denominator in virtually all cases has been inordinately low catalytic rates.

During reticulocyte maturation, ribonuclease cleavage of RNA into its constituent ribonucleotides provides the in vivo substrates for pyrimidine nucleotidase activity. In severe deficiencies, ineffective hydrolysis of uridine and cytidine monophosphates prevents their clearance from the cell by nucleoside diffusion. This results in accumulation of numerous pyrimidine compounds, most of which are normally undetectable in erythrocytes. This in turn is reflected morphologically by aggregation of undegraded or partially degraded ribosomal nucleoprotein, producing the distinctive basophilic stippling characteristic of this disorder[46,48] (Fig. 57-5).

The principal pyrimidine compounds that accumulate within affected cells are monophosphate, diphosphate, and triphosphate nucleotides, and include phosphodiester conjugates, such as cytidine diphosphate–choline, cytidine diphosphate–ethanolamine, and uridine diphosphate–glucose.[289–292] As much as 80% of the intracellular nucleotides in affected erythrocytes may be pyrimidine compounds, and the absolute concentrations of adenine nucleotides may actually be lower than normal. The presence of pyrimidines provides a simple and useful screening test for detection of the severe deficiency since acid extracts of the cells exhibit ultraviolet absorption spectra in the 265- to 270-nm region that bear no resemblance to the sharp 258-nm adenine absorption peak characteristic of normal erythrocytes.[46,48] (Whole blood is denatured by being rapidly mixed with an equal volume of 1.2 N perchloric acid,

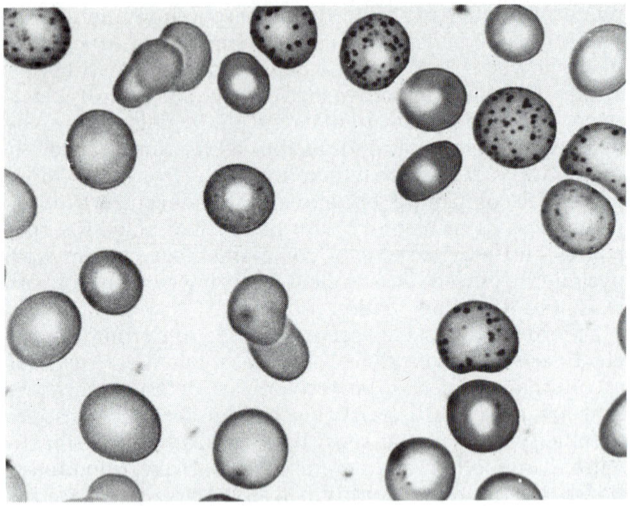

FIGURE 57-5. Coarse basophilic stippling in peripheral erythrocytes characteristic of patients with severe hereditary deficiency of pyrimidine nucleotidase (Wright's stain).

filtered, and its clear supernate diluted 1:10 with 0.1 N hydrochloride. Absorbance is measured in the 220- to 340-nm range.) Several procedures are available for quantitative assay of the enzyme, and recent recommendations for detecting nucleotidase deficiencies have been formulated by an international panel.[293,294]

Glutathione concentrations in erythrocytes with severe nucleotidase deficiency have consistently shown two-fold elevations, and ribosephosphate pyrophosphokinase activities have been reduced to about one fourth of normal. These changes are regarded as epiphenomena without demonstrable roles in the hemolytic process. Their underlying pathogenetic mechanisms remain obscure, but interesting and plausible hypotheses have been proposed.[295–298]

Speculation also continues regarding the pathogenetic mechanisms responsible for premature hemolysis in pyrimidine nucleotidase–deficient red cells. Because the enzyme is not directly involved in energy metabolism and serves no known function beyond the reticulocyte stage, attention has focused on potential effects of the inordinate concentrations of various pyrimidine compounds that accumulate. A suppressive effect on hexose monophosphate shunt activity has been measured and postulated to increase cell susceptibility to oxidant damage.[292] Mentzer and Glader[10] noted the logical possibility of direct physical damage to the cell membrane by particulate remnants of incomplete ribosome degradation, comparable to intracellular Heinz bodies.

Considering the delicate metabolic balance that normally sustains erythrocytes, one that can be disastrously disrupted by any of a variety of enzymopathies, it does not seem too simplistic to suggest that metabolic perturbations might result from competitive displacement of adenine nucleotides by their less effective pyrimidine counterparts.[18,46,48] This might be particularly important to the rate-limiting reactions catalyzed by the three kinases of glycolysis. Such competition has not been readily demonstrable in vitro, so speculation continues, and the precise pathogenetic mechanism remains obscure.

Acquired deficiency of pyrimidine nucleotidase can also be induced by lead toxicity and possibly by other heavy metals to which the enzyme is extraordinarily susceptible to inactivation.[47] Chronic exposure to low levels of lead reduces pyrimidine nucleotidase activities significantly, with negligible effects on glycolytic and many other erythrocyte enzymes.[299–302] At lead concentrations in the regions of 200 μg/dL packed red cells, nucleotidase activities decrease to about those levels seen in severe hereditary deficiencies.[302] At that point, pyrimidine compounds begin to accumulate, the absorption spectra shift, and affected erythrocytes begin to show their characteristic basophilic stippling. In some cases, the complete hereditary deficiency syndrome has been reproduced by lead toxicity, including the epiphenomena involving glutathione and ribosephosphate pyrophosphokinase.[303]

REFERENCES

1. Dacie JV, Mollison PL, Richardson N, Selwyn JG, Shapiro L. Atypical congenital haemolytic anaemia. Q J Med 1953;22:79.
2. Selwyn JG, Dacie JV. Autohemolysis and other changes resulting from the incubation in vitro of red cells from patients with congenital hemolytic anemia. Blood 1954;9:414.
3. de Gruchy GC, Santamaria JN, Parsons IC, Crawford H. Nonspherocytic congenital hemolytic anemia. Blood 1960;16:1371.
4. de Gruchy GC, Crawford H, Morton D. Atypical (nonspherocytic) congenital haemolytic anaemia. Proceedings of the VIIth Congress of the International Society of Hematology, Rome, 1958;2:425.
5. Robinson MA, Loder PB, de Gruchy GC. Red-cell metabolism in non-spherocytic congenital haemolytic anaemia. Br J Haematol 1961;7:327.
6. Valentine WN, Tanaka KR, Miwa S. A specific erythrocyte glycolytic enzyme defect (pyruvate kinase) in three subjects with congenital non-spherocytic hemolytic anemia. Trans Assoc Am Physicians 1961;74:100.
7. Tanaka KR, Valentine WN, Miwa S. Pyruvate kinase (PK) deficiency hereditary non-spherocytic hemolytic anemia. Blood 1962;19:267.
8. Carson PE, Flanagan CL, Ickes CE, Alving AS. Enzymatic deficiency in primaquine-sensitive erythrocytes. Science 1956;24:484.
9. Valentine WN, Tanaka KR, Paglia DE. Pyruvate kinase and other enzyme deficiency disorders of the erythrocyte. In: Scriver CR, Beaudet AL, Sly WS, Valle D, eds. The metabolic basis of inherited disease, ed 6. New York, McGraw-Hill, 1989:2341.
10. Mentzer WC, Glader BE. Disorders of erythrocyte metabolism. In: Mentzer WC, Wagner GM, eds. The hereditary hemolytic anemias. New York, Churchill Livingstone, 1989:267.
11. Dacie J. Hereditary enzyme-deficiency haemolytic anemias. I. Introduction and pyruvate-kinase deficiency. In: Dacie J, ed. The haemolytic anemias. London, Churchill Livingstone, 1985:282.
12. Dacie J. Hereditary enzyme-deficiency haemolytic anaemias. II. Deficiencies of enzymes of the Embden-Myerhoff (EM) pathway other than pyruvate kinase and of enzymes involved in purine and pyrimidine metabolism. In: Dacie J, ed. The haemolytic anemias. London, Churchill Livingstone, 1985:321.
13. Valentine WN, Tanaka KR, Paglia DE. Hemolytic anemias and erythrocyte enzymopathies. Ann Intern Med 1985;103:249.
14. Miwa S, Fujii H. Molecular aspects of erythroenzymopathies associated with hereditary hemolytic anemia. Am J Hematol 1985;19:293.
15. Beutler E. Hemolytic anemia in disorders of red cell metabolism. In: Wintrobe MM, ed. Topics in hematology. New York, Plenum, 1978:199.
16. Sullivan DW, Glader BE. Erythrocyte enzyme disorders in children. Pediatr Clin North Am 1980;27:449.
17. Miwa S. Hereditary disorders of red cell enzymes in the Embden-Meyerhof pathway. Am J Hematol 1983;14:381.
18. Valentine WN, Paglia DE. The primary cause of hemolysis in enzymopathies of anaerobic glycolysis: a viewpoint. Blood Cells 1980;6:819.
19. Keitt AS. Pyruvate kinase deficiency and related disorders of red cell glycolysis. Am J Med 1966;41.
20. Rosa R, Gaillardon J, Rosa J. Diphosphoglycerate mutase and 2,3-diphosphoglycerate phosphatase activities of red cells: comparative electrophoretic study. Biochem Biophys Res Commun 1973;51:536.
21. Rosa R, Audit I, Rosa J. Evidence for three enzymatic activities in one electrophoretic band of 3-phosphoglycerate mutase from red cells. Biochimie 1975;57:1059.
22. Sasaki R, Ikura K, Sugimoto E, Chiba H. Purification of bisphosphoglycerate phosphatase and phosphoglyceromutase from human erythrocytes. Eur J Biochem 1975;50:581.
23. Hamasaki N, Hardjono IS, Minakami S. Transport of phosphoenolpyruvate through the erythrocyte membrane. Biochem J 1978;170:39.
24. Hamasaki N, Kawano Y. Phosphoenolpyruvate transport in the anion transport system of human erythrocyte membranes. Trends Biochem Sci 1987;12:183.
25. Hamasaki N, Hirota-Chigita C. Acid-citrate-dextrose-phosphoenolpyruvate medium as a rejuvenant for blood storage. Transfusion 1983;23:1.
26. Lazzarino G, Cattani L, Costrini R, Mulieri L, Candiani A, Galzigna L. Increase in intraerythrocytic fructose-1,6-diphosphate after incu-

bation of whole human blood with fructose-1,6-diphosphate. Clin Biochem 1984;17:42.

27. Perroni L, Ensoli G, Nunziata A, et al. Comparative study of the effects of fructose-1,6-diphosphate, fructose and physiological saline on the blood levels of glucose and adenosine-triphosphate after oral glucose load. Pharmacol Res Commun 1980;12:147.

27a. Beutler E. Congenital hemolytic anemias related to enzyme defects and acquired hemolytic anemias. Curr Opin Hematol 1993:52.

28. Kirkman HN, Gaetani GF. Catalase: a tetrameric enzyme with four tightly bound molecules of NADPH. Proc Natl Acad Sci USA 1984;81: 4343.

29. Cohen G, Hochstein P. Glutathione peroxidase: the primary agent for the elimination of hydrogen peroxide in erythrocytes. Biochemistry 1963;2:1420.

30. Gaetani GF, Galiano S, Canepa L, Ferraris AM, Kirkman HN. Catalase and glutathione peroxidase are equally active in the detoxification of hydrogen peroxide in human erythrocytes. Blood 1989;73:334.

31. Beutler E, Matsumoto F. Ethnic variation in red cell glutathione peroxidase activity. Blood 1975;46:103.

32. Rea HM, Thomson CD, Campbell DR, Robinson MF. Relation between erythrocyte selenium and glutathione peroxidase (E.C.1.11.1.9) activities of New Zealand residents and visitors to New Zealand. Br J Nutr 1979;42:201.

33. Thomson CD, Rea H, Dolsburg VM, Robinson MF. Selenium concentrations and glutathione peroxidase activities in whole blood of New Zealand residents. Br J Nutr 1977;37:457.

34. Van Acker KJ, Simmonds HA, Potter C, Cameron JS. Complete deficiency of adenine phosphoribosyltransferase: report of a family. N Engl J Med 1977;297:127.

35. Agarwal RP, Crabtree GW, Parks RE Jr, et al. Purine nucleoside metabolism in the erythrocytes of patients with adenosine deaminase deficiency and severe combined immunodeficiency. J Clin Invest 1976;57:1025.

36. Schmalstieg FC, Goldman AS, Mills GC, Monahan TM, Nelson JA, Goldblum RM. Nucleotide metabolism in adenosine deaminase deficiency. Pediatr Res 1976;10:393.

37. Cohen A, Hirschhorn R, Horowitz SD, et al. Deoxyadenosine triphosphate as a potentially toxic metabolite in adenosine deaminase deficiency. Proc Natl Acad Sci USA 1978;75:472.

38. Coleman MS, Donofrio J, Hutton JJ, et al. Identification and quantitation of adenine deoxynucleotides in erythrocytes of a patient with adenosine deaminase deficiency and severe combined immunodeficiency. J Biol Chem 1978;253:1619.

39. Nelson JA, Kuttesch JF, Goldblum RN, Goldman AS, Schmalstieg FC. Analysis of adenosine and adenine nucleotides in severe combined immunodeficiency disease. In: Baer HP, Drummond GI, eds. Physiological and regulatory functions of adenosine and adenine nucleotides. New York, Raven Press, 1979:417.

40. Valentine WN, Paglia DE, Tartaglia AP, Gilsanz F. Hereditary hemolytic anemia with increased red cell adenosine deaminase (45- to 70-fold) and decreased adenosine triphosphate. Science 1977;195:783.

41. Paglia DE, Valentine WN, Tartaglia AP, Gilsanz F, Sparkes RS. Control of red blood cell adenine nucleotide metabolism: studies of adenosine deaminase. In: Brewer GJ, ed. The red cell. New York, Alan R Liss, 1978:319.

42. Fujii H, Miwa S, Suzuki K. Purification and properties of adenosine deaminase in normal and hereditary hemolytic anemia with increased red cell activity. Hemoglobin 1980;4:693.

43. Perignon JL, Hamet M, Buc HA, Cartier P, Derycke M. Biochemical study of a case of hemolytic anemia with increased (85-fold) red cell adenosine deaminase. Clin Chim Acta 1982;124:205.

44. Miwa S, Fujii H, Matsumoto N, et al. A case of red-cell adenosine deaminase overproduction associated with hereditary hemolytic anemia found in Japan. Am J Hematol 1978;5:107.

45. Paglia DE, Valentine WN. Haemolytic anemia associated with disorders of the purine and pyrimidine salvage pathways. Clin Haematol 1981;10:81.

46. Valentine WN, Fink K, Paglia DE, Harris SR, Adams WS. Hereditary hemolytic anemia with human erythrocyte pyrimidine 5′-nucleotidase deficiency. J Clin Invest 1974;54:866.

47. Paglia DE, Valentine WN. Characteristics of a pyrimidine-specific 5′-nucleotidase in human erythrocytes. J Biol Chem 1975;250:7973.

48. Paglia DE, Valentine WM. Hereditary and acquired defects in the pyrimidine nucleotidase of human erythrocytes. Curr Top Hematol 1980;3:75.

49. Swallow DM, Aziz I, Hopkinson DA, Miwa S. Analysis of human erythrocyte 5′-nucleotidases in healthy individuals and a patient deficient in pyrimidine 5′-nucleotidase. Ann Hum Genet 1983;47:19.

50. Paglia DE, Valentine WN, Keitt AS, Brockway RA, Nakatano M. Pyrimidine nucleotidase deficiency with active dephosphorylation of dTMP: evidence of existence of thymidine nucleotidase in human erythrocytes. Blood 1983;61:11:47.

51. DE, Valentine WN, Brockway RA. Identification of thymidine nucleotidase and deoxyribonucleotidase activities among normal isozymes of 5′-nucleotidase in human erythrocytes. Proc Natl Acad Sci USA 1984;81:588.

52. Hirono A, Fujii H, Natori H, Kurokawa I, Miwa S. Chromatographic analysis of human erythrocyte 5′-nucleotidase from five patients with pyrimidine 5′-nucleotidase deficiency Br J Heamatol 1987;65:35.

53. Paglia DE, Valentine WN, Brockway RA, Kanatani M. Substrate specificity and pH sensitivity of deoxyribonucleotidase and pyrimidine nucleotidase activities in human hemolysates. Exp Hematol 1987;15: 1041.

54. Bartlett GR. Red cell metabolism: review highlighting changes during storage. In: Greenwalt TJ, Jamieson GA, eds. The human red cell in vitro. New York, Grune & Stratton, 1974:5

55. Suzuki T, Dale GL. Senescent erythrocytes: isolation of in vivo aged calls and their biochemical characteristics. Proc Natl Acad Sci USA 1988;85:1647.

56. Dale GL, Norenberg SL. Time-dependent loss of adenosine 5′-monophosphate deaminase may explain elevated adenosine 5′triphosphate levels in senescent erythrocytes. Blood 1989;74:2157

57. Paglia DE, Valentive WN, Nakatani M, Brockway RA. AMP deaminase as a cell-age marker in transient erythroblastopenia of childhood and its role in the adenylate economy of erythrocytes. Blood 1989;74: 2161.

58. Valentine WN, Oski FA, Paglia DE, Baughan MA, Schneider AS, Naiman JL. Hereditary Hemolytic anemia with hexokinase deficiency: role of hexokinase in arythrocyte aging. Engl J Med 1967;276:1.

59. Valentine WN, Oski FA, Paglia DE, Baughan MA, Schneider AS, Naiman JL. Erythrocyte hexokinase and hereditary hemolytic anemia. In: Beutler E, ed. Hereditary disorders of erythrocyte metabolism. New York, Grune & Stratton, 1968:288.

60. Keitt AS. Hemolytic anemia with impaired hexokinase activity. J Clin Invest 1969;48:1997.

61. Necheles TF, Rai US, Cameron D. Congenital nonspherocytic hemolytic anemia associated with an unusual erythrocyte hexokinase abnormality. J Lab Clin Med 1970;76:593.

62. Moser K, Ciresa M, Schwarzmeier J. Hexokinasemangel bei hämolytischer Anämie. Med Welt 1970;46:1977.

63. Goebel KM, Gassel WD, Gebel FD, Kafarnik H. Hemolytic anemia and hexokinase deficiency associated with malformations. Klin Wochenschr 1972;50:349.

64. Rijksen G, Staal GEJ. Human erythrocyte hexokinase deficiency: characterization of a mutant enzyme with abnormal regulatory properties. J Clin Invest 1978;62:294.

65. Gilsanz F, Meyer E, Paglia DE, Valentine WN. Congenital hemolytic anemia due to hexokinase deficiency. Am J Dis Child 1978;132: 637.

66. Board PG, Trueworthy R, Smith JE, Moore K. Congenital nonspherocytic hemolytic anemia with an unstable hexokinase variant. Blood 1978;51:111.

67. Beutler E, Dyment PG, Matsumoto F. Hereditary nonspherocytic hemolytic anemia and hexokinase deficiency. Blood 1978;51:935.

68. Siimes MA, Rahiala E-L, Leisti J. Hexokinase deficiency in erythrocytes: a new variant in 5 members of a Finnish family. Scand J Haematol 1979;22:214.

69. Newman P, Muir A, Parker AC. Non-spherocytic haemolytic anemia in mother and son associated with hexokinase deficiency. Br J Haematol 1980;46:537.

70. Paglia DE, Shende A, Lanzkowsky P, Valentine WN. Hexokinase "New Hyde Park": a low activity erythrocyte isozyme in a Chinese kindred. Am J Hematol 1981;10:107.

71. Rijksen G, Akkerman JWN, van den Wall Bake AWL. Generalized hexokinase deficiency in the blood cells of a patient with nonspherocytic hemolytic anemia. Blood 1983;61:12.

72. Magnani M, Stocchi V, Cucchairini L. Hereditary nonspherocytic hemolytic anemia due to a new hexokinase variant with reduced stability. Blood 1985;66:690.

73. Magnani M, Stocchi V, Canestrari F, et al. Human erythrocyte hexokinase deficiency: a new variant with abnormal kinetic properties. Br J Haematol 1985;61:41.

74. Grossbard L, Schimke RT. Multiple hexokinases of rat tissues. Purification and comparisons of soluble forms. J Biol Chem 1966;244: 3546.

75. Holmes EW Jr, Malone JI, Winegrad AI, Oski FA. Hexokinase isoenzymes in human erythrocytes: association of type II with fetal hemoglobin. Science 1967;156:646.

76. Kaplan JC, Beutler E. Hexokinase isoenzymes in human erythrocytes. Science 1968;159:215.

77. Stocchi V, Magnani M, Canestrari F, Dachá M, Fornaini G. Multiple forms of human red blood cell hexokinase. J Biol Chem 1982;257: 2357.

78. Murakami K, Blei F, Tilton W, Seaman C, Piomelli S. An isozyme of hexokinase specific for the human red blood cell (HK_R). Blood 1990;75: 770.

79. Magnani M, Dallapiccola B. Regional mapping of the locus for hexokinase-1 (HK1). Hum Genet 1982;62:181.

80. Löhr GW, Waller HD, Anschutz F, Knoop A. Biochemische Defekte in den Blutzellen bei familiarer Panmyelopathie (Typ Fanconi). Humangenetik 1965;1:383.

81. Caster ND, Yoshida A. Purification and characterization of human phosphoglucose isomerase. Biochim Biophys Acta 1969;181:12.

82. Tilley BE, Gracy RW, Welch SG. A point mutation increasing the

stability of human phosphoglucose isomerase. J Biol Chem 1974;249: 4571.
83. Tsuboi KT, Fukanaga K, Chervenka CH. Phosphoglucose isomerase from human erythrocytes. J Biol Chem 1971;240:7586.
84. McMorris FA, Chen TR, Riciutti F, Tischfield J, Greagan R, Ruddle F. Chromosome assignments in man of the genes for two hexosephosphate isomerases. Science 1973;179:1129.
85. Payne DM, Porter DW, Gracy RW. Evidence against the occurrence of tissue-specific variants and isoenzymes of phosphoglucose isomerase. Arch Biochem Biophys 1972;151:122.
86. Van Biervliet JPGM. Glucosephosphate isomerase deficiency in a Dutch family. Acta Pediatr Scand 1975;64:868.
87. Zanella A, Izzo C, Rebulla P, et al. The first stable variant of erythrocyte glucosephosphate isomerase associated with severe hemolytic anemia. Am J Hematol 1980;9:1.
88. Schröter W, Eber SW, Bardosi A. Generalized glucosephosphate isomerase (GPI) deficiency causing haemolytic anemia, neuromuscular symptoms and impairment of granulocyte function: a new syndrome due to a new stable GPI variant with diminished specific activity (GPI Hamberg). Eur J Pediatr 1985;144:301.
89. Welch SG. Qualitative and quantitative variants of human phosphoglucose isomerase. Hum Hered 1971;21:467.
90. Arnold H, Hasslinger K, Witt I. Glucosephosphate-isomerase type Kayserslautern: a new variant causing congenital nonspherocytic hemolytic anemia. Blut 1983;46:271.
91. Baughan MA, Valentine WN, Paglia DE, Ways PO, Simon ER, DeMarsh QB. Hereditary hemolytic anemia associated with glucosephosphate isomerase (GPI) deficiency: a new enzyme defect of human erythrocytes. Blood 1968;32:236.
92. Paglia DE, Paredes R, Valentine WN, Dorantes S, Konrad PN. Unique phenotypic expression of glucosephosphate isomerase deficiency. Am J Hum Genet 1975;27:62.
93. Oski F, Fuller E. Glucose-phosphate isomerase (GPI) deficiency associated with abnormal osmotic fragility and spherocytes. Clin Res 1971;19:427.
94. Paglia DE, Holland P, Baughan MA, Valentine WN. Occurrence of defective hexosephosphate isomerization in human erythrocytes and leukocytes. N Engl J Med 1969;280:66.
95. Ravindranath Y, Paglia DE, Warrier I, Valentine WN, Nakatani M, Brockway RA. Glucosephosphate isomerase deficiency as a cause of hydrops fetalis. N Engl J Med 1987;316:258.
96. Paglia DE, Valentine WN. Hereditary glucosephosphate isomerase deficiency: a review. Am J Clin Pathol 1974;62:740.
97. Layzer RB, Rowland LP, Bank WJ. Physical and kinetic properties of human phosphofructokinase from skeletal muscle and erythrocytes. J Biol Chem 1969;244:3823.
98. Staal GEJ, Koster JF, Banziger CJM, van Milligen-Boersma L. Human erythrocyte phosphofructokinase: its purification and some properties. Biochim Biophys Acta 1972;276:113.
99. Karadsheh NS, Uyeda K, Oliver RM. Studies on the structure of human erythrocyte phosphofructokinase. J Biol Chem 1977;252:3515.
100. Cottreau D, Levin MJ, Kahn A. Purification and partial characterization of different forms of phosphofructokinase in man. Biochim Biophys Acta 1979;586:183.
101. Kahn A, Meienhofer M-C, Cottreau D, Lagrange J-L, Dreyfus J-C. Phosphofructokinase (PFK) isozymes in man. I. Studies of adult human tissue. Hum Genet 1979;48:93.
102. Meienhofer M-C, Lagrange J-L, Cottreau D, Lenoir G, Dreyfus J-C, Kahn A. Phosphofructokinase in human blood cells. Blood 1979;54: 389.
103. Vora S, Seaman C, Durham S, Piomelli S. Isozymes of human phosphofructokinase: identification and subunit structural characterization of a new system. Proc Natl Acad Sci USA 1980;77:62.
104. Kahn A, Cottreau D, Meienhofer M-C. Purification of F_4 phosphofructokinase from human platelets and comparison with the other phosphofructokinase forms. Biochim Biophys Acta 1980;611:114.
105. Vora S, Durham S, De Martinville B, George DL, Francke U. Assignment of the human gene for muscle-type phosphofructokinase (PFK) to chromosome 1 (region cen→q23) using somatic cell hybrids and monoclonal anti-M antibody. Somatic Cell Mol Genet 1982;8:95.
106. Vora S, Francki U. Assignment of the human gene for liver-type 6-phosphofructokinase isozyme (PFKL) to chromosome 21 by using somatic cell hybrids and monoclonal anti-L antibody. Proc Natl Acad Sci USA 1981;78:3738.
107. Vora S, Miranda A, Hernandez E, Francke U. Regional assignment of the human gene for platelet-type phosphofructokinase (PFKP) to chromosome 10p: novel use of a poly-specific rodent antisera to localize human enzyme genes. Hum Genet 1983;63:374.
108. Van Keuren M, Drabkin H, Hart I, Harker D, Patterson D, Vora S. Regional assignment of human liver-type 6-phosphofructokinase to chromosome 21q 22.3 by using somatic cell hybrids and a monoclonal anti-L antibody. Hum Genet 1986;74:34.
109. Vora S. Isoenzymes of phosphofructokinase. In: Rattazzi MC, Scandalios JG, Whitt GS, eds. Isozymes: current topics in biological and medical research, vol 6. New York, Alan R Liss, 1982:119.
110. Etiemble J, Kahn A, Boivin P, Bernard JF, Goudemand M. Hereditary hemolytic anemia with erythrocyte phosphofructokinase deficiency: studies of some properties of erythrocyte and muscle enzyme. Hum Genet 1976;31:83.
111. Miwa S, Sato T, Murao H, Kozuru M, Ibayashi H. A new type of phosphofructokinase deficiency hereditary nonspherocytic hemolytic anemia. Acta Haematol (Jpn) 1972;35:113.
112. Etiemble J, Picat C, Simeon J, Blatrix C, Boivin P. Inherited erythrocyte phosphofructokinase deficiency: molecular mechanism. Hum Genet 1980;55:383.
113. Waterbury L, Frankel EP. Hereditary nonspherocytic hemolysis with erythrocyte phosphofructokinase deficiency. Blood 1972;39:415.
114. Tarui S, Okuno G, Ikura Y, Tanaka T, Suda M, Nishikawa M. Phosphofructokinase deficiency in skeletal muscle: a new type of glycogenosis. Biochem Biophys Res Commun 1965;19:517.
115. Tarui S, Kono N, Nasu T, Nishikawa M. Enzymatic basis for the coexistence of myopathy and hemolytic disease in inherited muscle phosphofructokinase deficiency. Biochem Biophys Res Commun 1969;34:77.
116. Layzer RB, Rowland LP, Ranney HM. Muscle phosphofructokinase deficiency. Arch Neurol 1967;17:512.
117. Penhoet E, Rajkumar T, Rutter WJ. Multiple forms of fructose diphosphate aldolase in mammalian tissues. Proc Natl Acad Sci USA 1966;56:1275.
118. Lebherz HG, Ruller WJ. Distribution of fructose diphosphate aldolase variants in biological systems. Biochemistry 1969;8:109.
118a. Kukita A, Yoshida MC, Fukushige S, et al. Molecular gene mapping of human adolase A (ALDOA) gene to chromosome 16. Hum Genet 1987;76:20.
119. Beutler E, Scott S, Bishop A, Margolis N, Matsumoto F, Kuhl W. Red cell aldolase deficiency and hemolytic anemia: a new syndrome. Trans Assoc Am Physicians 1974;86:154.
120. Miwa S, Fujii H, Tani K, et al. Two cases of red cell aldolase deficiency associated with hereditary hemolytic anemia in a Japanese family. Am J Hematol 1981;11:425.
121. Kishi H, Mukai T, Hirono A, Fujii H, Miwa S, Hori K. Human aldolase A deficiency associated with a hemolytic anemia: thermolabile aldolase due to a single base mutation. Proc Natl Acad Sci USA 1987;84: 8623.
122. Lu HS, Yuan PM, Gracy RW. Primary structure of human triosephosphate isomerase. J Biol Chem 1984;259:11958.
123. Jongsma APM, Los WRT, Hagemeijer A. Evidence for synteny between the human loci for triosephosphate isomerase, lactate dehydrogenase-B and peptidase-B and the regional mapping of these loci on chromosome 12. Cytogenet Cell Genet 1974;13:106.
124. Decker RS, Mohrenweiser HW. Origin of the triosephosphate isomerase isozymes in humans: genetic evidence for the expression of a single structural locus. Am J Hum Genet 1981;33:683.
125. Eber SW, Krietsch WKG. The isolation and characterization of the multiple forms of human skeletal muscle triosephosphate isomerase. Biochim Biophys Acta 1980;614:173.
126. Yuan PM, Talent JM, Gracy RW. Molecular basis for the accumulation of acidic isozymes of triosephosphate isomerase in aging. Mech Ageing Dev 1981;17:151.
127. Neel JV, Mohrenweiser HW, Meisler MH. Rate of spontaneous mutation at human loci encoding protein structure. Proc Natl Acad Sci USA 1980;77:6037.
128. Gracy RW. Glucosephosphate and triosephosphate isomerases: significance of isozyme structural differences in evolution, physiology, and aging. In: Ratlazzi MC, Scandalios JG, Whitt GS, eds. Isozymes: current topics in biological and medical research, vol 6. New York, Alan R Liss, 1982:183.
129. Schneider AS, Valentine WN, Hattori M, Heins HL Jr. Hereditary hemolytic anemia with triosephosphate isomerase deficiency. N Engl J Med 1965;272:229.
130. Valentine WN, Schneider AS, Baughan MA, Paglia DE, Heins HL Jr. Hereditary hemolytic anemia with triosephosphate isomerase deficiency: studies in kindreds with coexistent sickle cell trait and erythrocyte glucose-6-phosphate dehydrogenase deficiency. Am J Med 1966;41:27.
131. Schneider AS, Valentine WN, Baughan MA, Paglia DE, Shore NA, Heins HL Jr. Triosephosphate isomerase deficiency. A. A multi-system inherited enzyme disorder: clinical and genetic aspects. In: Beutler E, ed. Hereditary disorders of erythrocyte metabolism. New York, Grune & Stratton, 1968:265.
132. Schneider AS, Dunn I, Ibsen KH, Weinstein IM. Triosephosphate isomerase deficiency. B. Inherited triosephosphate isomerase deficiency: erythrocyte carbohydrate metabolism and preliminary studies of the erythrocyte enzyme. In: Beutler E, ed. Hereditary disorders of erythrocyte metabolism. New York, Grune & Stratton, 1968:273.
133. Kaplan JC, Teeple L, Shore NA, Beutler E. Electrophoretic abnormality in triosephosphate isomerase deficiency. Biochem Biophys Res Commun 1968;31:768.
134. Harris SR, Paglia DE, Jaffé ER, Valentine WN, Klein RL. Triosephosphate isomerase deficiency in an adult. Clin Res 1970;18:529.
135. Angelman H, Brain MC, MacIver JE. A case of triosephosphate isomerase deficiency with sudden death. Abstracts from the XIIIth International Congress of Hematology, Munich, 1970:122.
136. Freycon F, Lauras B, Bovier-LaPierre F, Dorche CL, Goddon R. Anemie

hemolytique congenitale par deficit en triosephosphate isomerase. Pediatrie 1975;30:55.
137. Skala H, Dreyfus J-C, Vives-Corrons JL, Matsumoto F, Beutler E. Triosephosphate isomerase deficiency. Biochem Med 1977;18:226.
138. Vives-Corrons J-L, Rubinson-Skala H, Matep M, Estella J, Feliu E, Dreyfus J-C. Triosephosphate isomerase deficiency with hemolytic anemia and severe neuromuscular disease: familial and biochemical studies of a case found in Spain. Hum Genet 1978;42:171.
139. Eber SW, Dunnwald M, Belohradsky BH, et al. Hereditary deficiency of triosephosphate isomerase in four unrelated families. Eur J Clin Invest 1979;9:195.
140. Maquat LE, Chilcote R, Ryan M. Human triosephosphate isomerase cDNA and protein structure: studies of triosephosphate isomerase deficiency in man. J Biol Chem 1985;260:3748.
141. Poll-The BT, Aicardi J, Girot R, Rosa R. Neurological findings in triosephosphate isomerase deficiency. Ann Neurol 1985;17:439.
142. Rosa R, Prehu M-O, Calvin MC, Badoval J, Alix D, Girod R. Hereditary triosephosphate isomerase deficiency: seven new homozygous cases. Hum Genet 1985;71:235.
143. Clark ACL, Szobolotsky MA. Triosephosphate isomerase deficiency: prenatal diagnosis. J Pediatr 1985;106:417.
144. Daar IO, Artymiuk PJ, Phillips DC, Maquat LE. Human triosephosphate isomerase deficiency: a single amino acid substitution results in a thermolabile enzyme. Proc Natl Acad Sci USA 1986;83:7903.
145. Poinsot J, Parent P, Alix D, et al. Un cas d'anemie hemolytique congenitale non spherocytaire par deficit en triose phosphate isomerase diagnostic prenatal. J Genet Hum 1986;34:431.
146. Deys BF, Grzeschick KH, Grzeschick A, Jaffe ER, Siniscalco M. Human phosphoglycerate kinase and inactivation of the X chromosome. Science 1972;175:1002.
147. Michaelson AM, Markham AF, Orkin SH. Isolation and DNA sequence of a full-length cDNA clone for human X chromosome-encoded phosphoglycerate kinase. Proc Natl Acad Sci USA 1983;80:472.
148. Yoshida A, Watanabe S. Human phosphoglycerate kinase. I. Crystallization and characterization of normal enzyme. J Biol Chem 1972;247:440.
148a. McCarrey JR, Thomas K. Human testis-specific PGK gene lacks introns and possesses characteristics of a processed gene. Nature 1987;326:501.
149. Segel GB, et al. Energy metabolism in human erythrocytes: the role of phosphoglycerate kinase in cation transport. Blood 1975;46:271.
150. Yoshida A, Watanabe S, Chem S-H, Giblett ER, Malcolm LA. Human phosphoglycerate kinase. II. Structure of a variant enzyme. J Biol Chem 1972;247:446.
151. Fujii H, Yoshida A. Molecular abnormality of phosphoglycerate kinase–Uppsala associated with chronic nonspherocytic hemolytic anemia. Proc Natl Acad Sci USA 1980;77:5461.
152. Fujii H, Krietsch WKG, Yoshida A. A single amino acid substitution (Asp → Asn) in a phosphoglycerate kinase variant (PGK München) associated with enzyme deficiency. J Biol Chem 1980;255:6421.
153. Fujii H, Chen S-H, Akatsuka J, Miwa S, Yoshida A. Use of cultured lymphoblastoid cells for the study of abnormal enzymes: molecular abnormality of a phosphoglycerate kinase variant associated with hemolytic anemia. Proc Natl Acad Sci USA 1981;78:2587.
153a. Maeda M, Yoshida A. Molecular defect of a phosphoglycerate kinase variant (PGK Matusue) associated with hemolytic anemia: Leu–Pro sustitution caused by a T/A–C/G transition in exam 3. Blood 1991;77:1348.
153b. Maeda M, Bowle EV, Kulkarni R, Beutler E, Yoshida A. Molecular abnormalities of a phosphoglycerate kinase variant generated by spontaneous mutation. Blood 1992;79:2759
153c. Fujii H, Kanno H, Hirono A. Shiomura T, Miwa S. A single amino acid substitution (157 Gly–Val) in a phosphyoglycerate kinase variant (PGK) Shizuoka associated with chronic hemolysis and myoglobinuria. Blood 1992;79:1582
154. Banks RD, Blake CCF, Evans PR, et al. Sequence, structure and activity of phosphoglycerate kinase: a possible hinge-bending enzyme. Nature 1979;279:773.
155. Valentine WN, Hsieh H-S, Paglia DE, et al. Hereditary hemolytic anemia: association with phosphoglycerate kinase deficiency in erthrocytes and leukocytes. Trans Assoc Am Physicians 1968;81:49.
156. Valentine WN, Hsieh H-S, Paglia DE, et al. Hereditary hemolytic anemia associated with phosphoglycerate kinase deficiency in erthrocytes and leukocytes: a probable X-chromosome–linked syndrome. N Engl J Med 1969;280:528.
157. Cartier PP, Habibi B, Leroux JP, Marchad JC. Anemie hemolytique congenitale associee a un deficit en phosphoglycerate kinase dans les globules rouges, les polynucleaires, et les lymphocytes. Nouv Rev Fr Hematol 1971;11:565.
158. Konrad PN, McCarthy DJ, Mauer AM, Valentine WN, Paglia DE. Erythrocyte and leukocyte phosphoglycerate kinase deficiency with neurologic disease. J Pediatr 1973;82:456.
159. Boivin P, Hakim J, Mandereau J, Galand G, Degos F, Schaison G. Deficit en 3-phosphoglycerate kinase erythrocytaire et leucocytaire: étude des propriétés de l'enzyme, de la fonction phagocytaire des polynucleaires et revise de la littertura. Nouv Rev Fr Hematol 1974;14:495.
160. Yoshida A, Miwa S. Characterization of a phosphoglycerate kinase variant associated with hemolytic anemia. Am J Hum Genet 1974;26:378.
161. Dodgson SJ, Lee CS, Holland RAB, O'Sullivan WJ, Vowels MR. Erythrocyte phosphoglycerate kinase deficiency: enzymatic and oxygen binding studies. Aust N Z J Med 1980;10:614.
162. Rosa R, George C, Fardeau M, Calvin M-C, Rapin M, Rosa J. A new case of phosphoglycerate kinase deficiency: PGK Creteil associated with rhabdomyolysis and lacking hemolytic anemia. Blood 1982;60:84.
163. Dimauro S, Dalakas M, Miranda AF. Phosphoglycerate kinase deficiency: another cause of recurrent myoglobinuria. Ann Neurol 1983;13:11.
164. Guis MS, Karadsheh N, Mentzer WC. Phosphoglycerate kinase San Francisco, a new variant associated with hemolytic anemia but not with neuromuscular manifestations. Am J Hematol 1987;25:175.
165. Svirklys LG, O'Sullivan WJ. Tissue levels of glycolytic enzymes in phosphoglycerate kinase deficiency. Clin Chim Acta 1980;108:309.
166. Baehner RL, et al. Metabolic, phagocytic, and bactericidal properties of phosphoglycerate kinase deficient (PGK) polymorphonuclear leukocytes (PMN). Blood 1971;38:833.
167. Ibsen KH, Schiller KW, Taas TA. Interconvertible kinetic and physical forms of human erythrocyte pyruvate kinase. J Biol Chem 1971;246:1233.
168. Marie J, Kahn A, Boivin P. Human erythrocyte pyruvate kinase: total purification and evidence for its antigenic identity with L-type enzyme. Biochim Biophys Acta 1977;481:96.
169. Saheki S, Saheki K, Tanaka T. Peptide structures of pyruvate kinase isozymes. I. Comparison of the four pyruvate kinase isozymes of the rat. Biochim Biophys Acta 1982;704:484.
170. Chern CJ, Kennett R, Engle E, Mellman WJ, Cruce CM. Assignment of the structural genes for the α subunit of hexoseaminidase A, mannose phosphate isomerase, and pyruvate kinase to the region q22-qter of human chromosome 15. Somatic Cell Mol Genet 1977;3:553.
171. Peters J, Nash HR, Eicher EM, Bulfield G. Polymorphism of kidney pyruvate kinase in the mouse is determined by a gene, PK-3, on chromosome 9. Biochem Genet 1981;19:757.
172. Marie J, Garreau H, Kahn A. Evidence for a postsynthetic proteolytic transformation of human erythrocyte pyruvate kinase into L-type enzyme. FEBS Lett 1977;78:91.
173. Marie J, Kahn A. Proteolytic processing of human erythrocyte pyruvate kinase: study of normal and deficient enzyme. Biochem Biophys Res Commun 1979;91:123.
174. Kahn A, Marie J, Boivin P. Pyruvate kinase in man. II. L-type and erythrocyte-type isozymes: electrofocusing and immunologic studies. Hum Genet 1976;33:35.
175. Bigley RH, Koler RD. Liver pyruvate kinase (PK) isozymes in a PK-deficient patient. Ann Hum Genet 1968;31:383.
176. Imamura K, Tanaka T, Nishina T, Nakashima K, Miwa S. Studies on pyruvate kinase (PK) deficiency. II. Electrophoretic, kinetic, and immunological studies on pyruvate kinase of erythrocytes and other tissues. J Biochem 1973;74:1165.
177. Nakashima K, Miwa S, Oda S, Tanaka T, Imamura K, Nishina T. Electrophorectic and kinetic studies of mutant erythrocyte pyruvate kinases. Blood 1974;43:537.
178. Kahn A, Marie J, Galand C, Boivin P. Chronic haemolytic anaemia in two patients heterozygous for erythrocyte pyruvate kinase deficiency: electrofocusing and immunological studies of erythrocyte and liver pyruvate kinase. Scand J Haematol 1976;16:250.
179. Nakashima K, Miwa S, Fujii H, et al. Characterization of pyruvate kinase from the liver of a patient with aberrant erythrocyte pyruvate kinase, PK Nagasaki. J Lab Clin Med 1977;90:1012.
180. Staal GEJ, Rijksen G, Vlug AMC, et al. Extreme deficiency of L-type pyruvate kinase with moderate clinical expression. Clin Chim Acta 1982;118:241.
181. Tanaka T, Harano Y, Sue F, Morimura H. Crystallization, characterization and metabolic regulation of two types of pyruvate kinase isolated from rat tissues. J Biochem 1967;62:71.
182. Bigley RH, Stenzel P, Jones RT, Campos JO, Koler RD. Tissue distribution of human pyruvate kinase isozymes. Enzymol Biol Clin 1968;9:10.
183. Imamura K, Tanaka T. Multimolecular forms of pyruvate kinase from rat and other mammalian tissues. J Biochem 1972;71:1043.
184. Imamura K, Taniuchi K, Tanaka T. Multimolecular forms of pyruvate kinase. II. Purification of M_2-type pyruvate kinase from Yoshida ascites hepatoma 130 cells and comparative studies on the enzymological and immunological properties of the three types of pyruvate kinases, L, M_1, and M_2. J Biochem 1972;72:1001.
184a. Etiemble J, Picat C, Boivin P. A red cell pyruvate kinase mutant with normal L-type PK in the liver. Hum Genet 1982;61:256.
185. Noguchi T, Inque H, Tanaka T. The M_1 and M_2-type isozymes of rat pyruvate kinase are produced from the same gene by alternative RNA splicing. J Biol Chem 1986;261:13807.
186. Marie J, Simon M-P, Dreyfus J-C, Kahn A. One gene, but two messenger RNAs encode liver L and red cell L'pyruvate kinase subunits. Nature 1981;292:70.
187. Noguchi T, Tanaka T. The M_1 and M_2 subunits of rat pyruvate kinase

are encoded by different messenger RNAs. J Biol Chem 1982;257: 1110.

188. Kahn A, Marie J, Garreau H, Sprengers ED. The genetic system of the L-type pyruvate kinase forms in man: subunit structure, interrelation and kinetic characteristics of the pyruvate kinase enzymes from erythrocytes and liver. Biochim Biophys Acta 1978;523:59.
190. Nakashima K. Further evidence of molecular alteration and aberration of erythrocyte pyruvate kinase. Clin Chim Acta 1974;55:245.
191. Max-Audit I, Kechemir D, Mitjavila MT, Vainchenker W, Rotten D, Rosa R. Pyruvate kinase synthesis and degradation by normal and pathologic cells during erythroid maturation. Blood 1988;72:1039.
192. Takegawa S, Fujii H, Miwa S. Change of pyruvate kinase isozymes from M_2 to L type during development of the red cell. Br J Haematol 1983;54:467.
193. Shinohara K, Yamada K, Inoue M, et al. Enzyme activity of cultured erythroblasts. Am J Hematol 1985;20:145.
194. Oda S, Oda E, Tanaka KR. Relationship of density distribution and pyruvate kinase electrophoretic pattern of erythrocytes in sickle cell disease and other disorders. Acta Haematol 1978;60:201.
195. Miwa S, Nakashima K, Ariyoshi K, Shinohara K, Oda E, Tanaka T. Four new pyruvate kinase (PK) variants and a classical type PK deficiency. Br J Haematol 1975;29:135.
196. Takegawa S, Miwa S. Change of pyruvate kinase (PK) isozymes in classical type PK deficiency and other PK deficiency cases during red cell maturation. Am J Hematol 1984;16:53.
197. Black JA, Rittenberg MB, Standerfer RJ, Peterson JS. Hereditary persistence of fetal erythrocyte pyruvate kinase in the Basenji dog. In: Brewer GJ, ed. The red cell: progress in clinical and biological research, vol 21. New York, Alan R Liss, 1978:275.
198. Max-Audit I, Rosa R, Marie J. Pyruvate kinase hyperactivity genetically determined: metabolic consequences and molecular characterization. Blood 1980;56:902.
199. Rosa R, Max-Audit I, Izrael V, Beuzard Y, Thillet J, Rosa J. Hereditary pyruvate kinase abnormalities associated with erythrocytosis. Am J Hematol 1981;10:47.
200. Sprengers ED, Staal GEJ. Functional changes associated with the sequential transformation of L'_4 into L_4 pyruvate kinase. Biochim Biophys Acta 1979;570:259.
201. Mentzer WC Jr, Baehner RL, Schmidt-Schonbein H, Robinson SH, Nathan DG. Selective reticulocyte destruction in erythrocyte pyruvate kinase deficiency. J Clin Invest 1971;50:688.
202. Matsumoto N, Ishihara T, Nakashima K, Miwa S, Uchino F, Kondo M. Sequestration and destruction of reticulocytes in the spleen in pyruvate kinase deficiency hereditary nonspherocytic hemolytic anemia. Acta Haematol (Jpn) 1972;35:525.
203. Leblond PF, Lyonnais J, Delage JM. Erythrocyte populations in pyruvate kinase deficiency anaemia following splenectomy. I. Cell morphology. Br J Haematol 1978;39:55.
204. Leblond PF, Lyonnais J, Delage J-M. Erythrocyte populations in pyruvate kinase deficiency anemia following splenectomy. II. Cell deformability. Br J Haematol 1978;39:63.
205. Bowman HS, Oski FA. Laboratory studies of erythrocytic pyruvate kinase deficiency: pathogenesis of the hemolysis. Am J Clin Pathol 1978;70:259.
206. Koler RD, Vanbellinghen P. The mechanism of precursor modulation of human pyruvate kinase I by fructose diphosphate. Adv Enzyme Regul 1968;6:127.
207. Staal GEJ, Koster JF, Kamp H, van Milligen-Boersma L, Veeger C. Human erythrocyte pyruvate kinase: its purification and some properties. Biochim Biophys Acta 1971;227:86.
208. Black JA, Henderson MH. Activation and inhibition of human erythrocyte pyruvate kinase by organic phosphates, amino acids, dipeptides and anions. Biochim Biophys Acta 1972;284:115.
209. Monod J, Wyman J, Changeux JP. On the nature of allosteric transitions: a plausible model. J Mol Biol 1965;12:88.
210. Muirhead H. Triose phosphate isomerase, pyruvate kinase and other α/β-barrel enzymes. Trends Biochem Sci 1983:326.
211. Miwa S, Boivin P, Blume KG, et al. Recommended methods for the characterization of red cell pyruvate kinase variants: International Committee for Standardization in Haematology. Br J Haematol 1979;43: 275.
212. Etiemble J, Picat C, Dhermy D, Buc HA, Morin M, Boivin P. Erythrocytic pyruvate kinase deficiency and hemolytic anemia inherited as a dominant trait. Am J Hematol 1984;17:251.
213. Valentine WN, Herring WB, Paglia DE, Steuterman MC, Brockway RA, Nakatani M. Pyruvate kinase Greensboro: a four-generation study of a high $K_{0.5s}$ (phosphoenolpyruvate) variant. Blood 1988;72:1054.
214. Valentine WN, Paglia DE. Erythroenzymopathies and hemolytic anemia: the many faces of inherited variant enzymes. J Lab Clin Med 1990;115:12.
215. Paglia DE, Valentine WN, Baughan MA, Miller DR, Reed CF, McIntyre OR. An inherited molecular lesion of erythrocyte pyruvate kinase: identification of a kinetically aberrant isozyme associated with premature hemolysis. J Clin Invest 1968;47:1929.
216. Paglia DE, Valentine WN, Rucknagel DL. Defective erythrocyte pyruvate kinase with impaired kinetics and reduced optimal activity. Br J Haematol 1972;22:651.
217. Miwa S, Nishina T. Studies on pyruvate kinase (PK) deficiency I. Clinical, hematological and erythrocyte enzyme studies. Acta Haematol (Jpn) 1974;37:1.
218. Levinski U, Fajnholc N, Djaldetti M, De Vries A. Hemolytic anemia in pregnancy associated with erythrocyte pyruvate kinase deficiency. Clin Sci 1974;11:43.
219. Kahn A, Marie J, Galand C, Boivin P. Molecular mechanism of erythrocyte pyruvate kinase deficiency. Humangenetik 1975;29:271.
220. Miwa S, Nakashima K, Ariyoshi K, Shinohara K, Oda E, Tanaka T. Four new pyruvate kinase (PK) variants and a classical PK deficiency. Br J Haematol 1975;29:157.
221. Paglia DE, Konrad PN, Wolff JA, Valentine WN. Biphasic reaction kinetics in an anomalous isozyme of erythrocyte pyruvate kinase. Clin Chim Acta 1976;73:395.
222. Shinohara K, Miwa S, Nakashima K, Oda E, Kageoka T, Tsujino G. A new pyruvate kinase variant (PK Osaka) demonstrated by partial purification and condensation. Am J Hum Genet 1976;28:474.
223. Staal GEJ, Ceerdink RP, Vlug AMC, Hamelink ML. Defective erythrocyte pyruvate kinase. Clin Chim Acta 1976;68:11.
224. Paglia DE, Valentine WN, Williams KO, Konrad PN. An isozyme of erythrocyte pyruvate kinase (PK-Los Angeles) with impaired kinetics corrected by fructose-1, 6-diphosphate. Am J Clin Pathol 1977;68: 229.
225. Marie J, Vives-Corrons JL, Kahn A. Hereditary erythrocyte pyruvate kinase deficiency: molecular and functional studies of four mutant PK variants detected in Spain. Clin Chim Acta 1977;81:153.
226. Sprengers ED, Beemer FA, Staal GEJ. A new pyruvate kinase variant: PK-Wouw. J Mol Med 1978;3:271.
227. Zanella A, Rebulla P, Izzo C, Znuso F, Sirchia G. Concomitance of an active and an inactive mutant of red cell pyruvate kinase (PK). Scand J Haematol 1979;22:145.
228. Black JA, Rittenberg MB, Bigley RH, Koler RD. Hemolytic anemia due to pyruvate kinase deficiency: characterization of the enzymatic activity from eight patients. Am J Hum Genet 1979;31:300.
229. Marie J, Zanella A, Vives-Corrons JL, Najman A, Kahn A. Significance of the electrophoretic modifications of defective pyruvate kinase variants: study of six new observations. Clin Chim Acta 1979;93:61.
230. Shinohara K, Tanaka KR. Pyruvate kinase deficiency hemolytic anemia: enzymatic characterization studies in twelve patients. Hemoglobin 1980;4:611.
231. Miwa S, Fujii H, Takegawa S, et al. Seven pyruvate kinase variants characterized by the ICSH recommended methods. Br J Haematol 1980;45:575.
232. Vives-Corrons JL, Marie J, Pujades MA, Kahn A. Hereditary erythrocyte pyruvate-kinase (PK) deficiency and chronic hemolytic anemia: clinical, genetic and molecular studies in six new Spanish patients. Hum Genet 1980;53:401.
233. Vives-Corrons JL, Pujades MA, Aguilar JL, Feliu E, Jou JM. Anemia hemolitica por deficit hereditario de piruvatokinasa eritrocitaria: estudio clinico-familiar y biologico de diez casos. Sangre (Barc) 1980;25: 51.
234. Ishida Y, Miwa S, Fujii H, Fujinami N, Takegawa S, Yamato K. Thirteen cases of pyruvate kinase deficiency found in Japan. Am J Hematol 1981;10:239.
235. Kahn A, Marie J, Vives-Corrons JL, Maigret P, Najman A. Search for relationship between anomalies of the mutant erythrocyte pyruvate kinase variants and their pathological expression. Hum Genet 1981;57: 172.
236. Elder GE, Lappin TRJ, Lawson BE, Bridges JM. Three pyruvate kinase variants with increased affinity for PEP. Br J Haematol 1981;47:371.
237. Paglia DE, Valentine WN. Molecular lesion affecting the ADP-combining site in a mutant isozyme of erythrocyte pyruvate kinase. Proc Natl Acad Sci 1981;78:5175.
238. Dente L, D'Urso M, Di Maio S, Brancaccio B, Luzzatto L. Pyruvate kinase deficiency: characterization of two new genetic variants. Clin Chim Acta 1982;126:143.
239. Schröter W, Lakomek M, Scwarnetzky M, Tillmann W, Winkler H. Pyruvate kinase "Göttingen": congenital hemolytic anemia, evidence of heterozygosity, and lack of enzyme cooperativity. Hum Genet 1982;60:381.
240. Paglia DE, Keitt AS, Valentine WN, Gordon S. Biochemical characterization of three mutant isozymes of erythrocyte pyruvate kinase: PK-"Gainesville," PK-"San Juan," and PK-"Cape Canaveral." Am J Hematol 1983;14:335.
241. Lakomek M, Winkler H, Scharnetzky M, et al. Erythrocyte pyruvate kinase deficiency: characterization of a new variant (PK "Aarau"). Blut 1984;48:123.
242. Muir WA, Beutler E, Wasson C. Erythrocyte pyruvate kinase deficiency in the Ohio Amish: origin and characterization of the mutant enzyme. Am J Hum Genet 1984;36:634.
243. Amankwah KS, Dick BW, Dodge S. Hemolytic anemia and pyruvate kinase deficiency in pregnancy. Obstet Gynecol 1980;55:42S.
244. Duncan JR, Potter CG, Cappellini MD, Kurtz JB, Anderson MJ, Weatherall DJ. Aplastic crisis due to parvovirus infection in pyruvate kinase deficiency. Lancet 1983;2:14.
245. Rosa R, Prehic M-P, Beuzaid Y, Rosa J. The first case of a complete

deficiency of diphosphoglycerate mutase in human erythrocytes. J Clin Invest 1978;62:907.
246. Miwa S, Nishina T, Kakehashi Y, Kitamura M, Hiratsuka A, Shizume K. Studies on erythrocyte metabolism in a case with hereditary deficiency of H-subunit of lactate dehydrogenase. Acta Haematol (Jpn) 1971;34:228.
247. Kitamura M, Iijima N, Hashimoto F, Hiratsuka A. Hereditary deficiency of subunit H of lactate dehydrogenase. Clin Chim Acta 1971;34: 419.
248. Kanno T, Sudo K, Takeuchi I, et al. Hereditary deficiency of lactate dehydrogenase M-subunit. Clin Chim Acta 1980;108:267.
249. Valentine WN, Paglia DE. Erythrocyte disorders of purine and pyrimidine metabolism. Hemoglobin 1980;4:669.
250. Paglia DE, Valentine WN. Hereditary disorders of erythrocyte enzymes in nonglycolytic metabolic pathways. Haematologia 1982;15:381.
251. Fildes RA, Harris H. Nature 1966;209:261.
252. Bowman JE, Frischer H, Ajmar F, Carson PE, Gower MK. Population, family and biochemical investigation of human adenylate kinase polymorphism. Nature 1967;214:1156.
253. Kho JC, Russell PJ Jr. Isoenzymes of adenylate kinase in human tissue. Biochim Biophys Acta 1972;268:98.
254. Russell PJ Jr, Hornstein JM, Goins L, Jones D, Laver M. Adenylate kinase in human tissues. I. Organ specificity of adenylate kinase isoenzymes. J Biol Chem 1974;249:1874.
255. McKusik VA, Ruddle FH. The status of the gene map of the human chromosomes. Science 1977;196:390.
256. Thuma E, Schirmer RH, Schirmer J. Biochim Biophys Acta 1972;268: 81.
257. Von Zabern I, Wittmann-Liebold B, Untucht-Grau R, Schirmer RH, Pai EF. Primary and tertiary structure of the principle human adenylate kinase. Eur J Biochem 1976;68:281.
258. Szeinberg A, Gavendo S, Cahane D. Erythrocyte adenylate-kinase deficiency. Lancet 1969;1:315.
259. Szeinberg A, Kahana D, Gavendo S, Zaidman J, Ben-Ezzer J. Hereditary deficiency of adenylate kinase in red blood cells. Acta Haematol 1969;42:111.
260. Boivin P, Galand C, Hakim J, Simony D, Seligman M. Un nouvelle erythroenzymopathie: anemie hemolytique congenitale non spherocytaire et deficit hereditaire en adenylate-kinase erythrocytaire. La Presse Medicale 1971;79:215.
261. Miwa S, Fujii H, Tani K, Takahashi K, Takizawa T, Igarashi T. Red cell adenylate kinase deficiency associated with hereditary nonspherocytic hemolytic anemia: clinical and biochemical studies. Am J Hematol 1983;14:325.
262. Beutler E, Carson D, Dannawi H, et al. Metabolic compensation for profound erythrocyte adenylate kinase deficiency: a hereditary defect without hemolytic anemia. J Clin Invest 1983;72:648.
263. Beutler E. Red cell enzyme defects as nondiseases and as diseases. Blood 1979;54:1.
264. Spencer N, Hopkinson DA, Harris H. Adenosine deaminase polymorphism in man. Ann Hum Genet 1968;32:9.
265. Hopkinson DA, Cook PJL, Harris H. Further data on the adenosine deaminase (ADA) polymorphism and a report of a new phenotype. Ann Hum Genet 1969;32:361.
266. Edwards YH, Hopkinson DA, Harris H. Adenosine deaminase isozymes in human tissues. Ann Hum Genet 1971;35:207.
267. Daddona PE, Kelley WN. Human adenosine deaminase: purification and subunit structure. J Biol Chem 1977;252:110.
268. Daddona PE, Kelley WN. Human adenosine deaminase binding protein: assay, purification and properties. J Biol Chem 1978;253:4617.
269. Tischfield JA, Creagan RP, Nichols EA, Ruddle FH. Assignment of a gene for adenosine deaminase to human chromosome 20. Hum Hered 1974;24:1.
270. Phillip T, Lenoir G, Rolland MO, et al. Regional assignment of the ADA locus on 20q13.2→qter by gene dosage studies. Cytogenet Cell Genet 1980;27:187.
271. Koch G, Shows TB. A gene on human chromosome 6 functions in assembly of tissue-specific adenosine deaminase isozymes. Proc Natl Acad Sci USA 1978;75:3876.
272. Hirschhorn R, Levytska V, Pollara B, Meuwissen HJ. Evidence for control of several different tissue-specific isozymes of adenosine deaminase by a single genetic locus. Nature New Biol 1973;246:200.
273. Hirschhorn R. Conversion of human erythrocyte-adenosine deaminase activity to different tissue-specific isozymes: evidence for a common catalytic unit. J Clin Invest 1975;55:661.
274. Giblett ER, Anderson JE, Cohen F, Pollara B, Meuwissen HJ. Adenosine deaminase deficiency in two patients with severely impaired cellular immunity. Lancet 1972;2:1067.
275. Fujii H, Miwa S, Tani K, Fujinami N, Asano Y. Overproduction of structurally normal enzyme in man: hereditary haemolytic anaemia with increased red cell adenosine deaminase activity. Br J Haematol 1982;51:427.
276. Chottiner EG, Cloft HJ, Tartaglia AP, Mitchell BS. Elevated adenosine deaminase activity and hereditary hemolytic anemia: evidence for abnormal translational control of protein synthesis. J Clin Invest 1987;79:1001.
277. Chottiner EG, Ginsburg D, Tartaglia AP, Mitchell BS. Erythrocyte adenosine deaminase overproduction in hereditary hemolytic anemia. Blood 1989;74:448.
278. Torrance JD, Whittaker D, Beutler E. Purification and properties of human erythrocyte pyrimidine 5′-nucleotidase. Proc Natl Acad Sci 1977;74:3701.
279. Beutler E, West C. Tissue distribution of pyrimidine 5′-nucleotidase. Biochem Med 1982;27:334.
280. Beutler E, Baranko PV, Feagler J, et al. Hemolytic anemia due to pyrimidine-5′-nucleotidase deficiency: report of eight cases in six families. Blood 1980;56:251.
281. Rosa R, Rochant H, Dreyfus B, Valentin C, Rosa J. Electrophoretic and kinetic studies of human erythrocytes deficient in pyrimidine 5′-nucleotidase. Hum Genet 1977;38:209.
283. Shinohara K, Tanaka KR. Kinetic and electrophoretic studies of human erythrocytes deficient in pyrimidine 5′-nucleotidase. Hum Genet 1979;51:107.
284. Fujii H, Nakashima K, Miwa S, Nomura K. Electrophoretic and kinetic studies of a mutant red cell pyrimidine 5′-nucleotidase. Clin Chim Acta 1979;95:89.
285. Ishida Y, Fujii H, Miwa S. Pyrimidine 5′-nucleotidase deficiency: studies of five cases in two Japanese families. Hemoglobin 1980;4: 683.
286. Ishida Y, Miwa S, Miura Y, Kibe A. Electrophoretic and kinetic studies of human erythrocytes deficient in pyrimidine 5′-nucleotidase. Clin Chim Acta 1980;108:285.
287. Hirono A, Fujii H, Miyajima H, Kawakatsu T, Hiyoshi Y, Miwa S. Three families with hereditary hemolytic anemia and pyrimidine 5′-nucleotidase deficiency: electrophoretic and kinetic studies. Clin Chim Acta 1983;130:189.
288. Hirono A, Fujii H, Natori H, Kurokawa I, Miwa S. Chromatographic analysis of human erythrocyte pyrimidine 5′-nucleotidase from five families with pyrimidine 5′-nucleotidase deficiency. Br J Haematol 1987;65:25.
289. Torrance JD, Whittaker D. Distribution of erythrocyte nucleotides in pyrimidine 5′-nucleotidase deficiency. Br J Haematol 1979;43:423.
290. Swanson MS, Angle CR, Stohs SJ, et al. ^{31}P NMR study of erythrocytes from a patient with hereditary pyrimidine-5′-nucleotidase deficiency. Proc Natl Acad Sci USA 1983;80:169.
291. Swanson MS, Markin RS, Stohs SJ, Angle CR. Identification of cytidine diphosphodiesters in erythrocytes from a patient with pyrimidine nucleotidase deficiency. Blood 1984;63:665.
292. Ericson A, de Verdier C-H, Ruud Hansen TW, Seip M. Erythrocyte nucleotide pattern in two children in a Norwegian family with pyrimidine 5′-nucleotidase deficiency. Clin Chim Acta 1983;134:25.
293. Miwa S, Luzzatto L, Rosa R, et al. Recommended screening test for pyrimidine 5′-nucleotidase deficiency. Clin Lab Haematol 1989;11: 55.
294. Miwa S, Luzzatto L, Rosa R, et al. Recommended methods for an additional red cell enzyme (pyrimidine 5′-nucleotidase assays and the determination of red cell adenosine-5′-triphosphate, 2,3-diphosphoglycerate and reduced glutathione. Clin Lab Haematol 1989;11: 131.
295. Kondo T, Dale GL, Beutler E. Glutathione transport by inside-out vesicles from human erythrocytes. Proc Natl Acad Sci USA 1980;77: 6359.
296. Zerez CR, Lachant NA, Tanaka KR. Pyrimidine nucleotides do not affect the enzymes of glutathione biosynthesis. Enzyme 1985;34:94.
297. Lachant NA, Zerez CR, Tanaka KR. Pyrimidine nucleotides impair phosphoribosylpyrophosphate (PRPP) synthetase subunit aggregation by sequestering magnesium: a mechanism for the decreased PRPP synthetase activity in hereditary erythrocyte pyrimidine 5′-nucleotidase deficiency. Biochim Biophys Acta 1988;994:81.
298. Tomoda A, Noble NA, Lachant NA, Tanaka KR. Hemolytic anemia in hereditary pyrimidine 5′-nucleotidase deficiency: nucleotide inhibition of G6PD and the pentose phosphate shunt. Blood 1982;60: 1212.
299. Paglia DE, Valentine WN, Dahlgren JG. Effects of low-level lead exposure on pyrimidine 5′-nucleotidase and other erythrocyte enzymes: possible role of pyrimidine 5′-nucleotidase in the pathogenesis of lead-induced anemia. J Clin Invest 1975;56:1164.
300. Buc H-A, Kaplan J-C. Red cell pyrimidine 5′-nucleotidase and lead poisoning. Clin Chim Acta 1978;87:49.
301. Angle CR, McIntire MS. Low level lead and inhibition of erythrocyte pyrimidine nucleotidase. Environ Res 1978;17:296.
302. Paglia DE, Valentine WN, Fink K. Lead poisoning: further observations on erythrocyte pyrimidine-nucleotidase deficiency and intracellular accumulation of pyrimidine nucleotides. J Clin Invest 1977;60:1362.
303. Valentine WN, Paglia DE, Fink K, Madokoro G. Lead poisoning: association with hemolytic anemia, basophilic stippling, erythrocyte pyrimidine 5′-nucleotidase deficiency, and intraerythrocytic accumulation of pyrimidines. J Clin Invest 1976;58:926.
304. Nishi S, Seino S, Bell GI. Human hexokinase: sequences of amino- and carboxyl-terminal halves are homologous. Biochem Biophys Res Commun 1988;157:937.
305. Levanon D, Danciger E, Danfni N, Groner Y. Construction of a cDNA clone containing the entire coding region of the human liver-type phosphofructokinase. Biochem Biosphys Res Commun 1987;147:1182.

306. Nakajima H, Noguachi T, Yamasaki T, Kono N, Tanaka T, Tarui S. Cloning of human muscle phosphofructokinase cDNA. FEBS Lett 1987;223:113.
307. Vaisanen PA, Reddy GR, Sharma PM, et al. Cloning and characterization of the human muscle phosphofructokinase gene. DNA Cell Biol 1992;11:461.
308. Nakajima H, Kono N, Yamasaki T, et al. Genetic defect in muscle phosphofructokinase deficiency. J Biol Chem 1990;265:9392.
309. Sakaibara M, Mukai T, Hori K. Nucleotide sequence of a cDNA clone for human aldolase: A messenger RNA in the liver. Biochem Biophys Res Commun 1985;131:413.
310. Maire P, Gautron S, Hakim V, Gregori C, Mennecier R, Kahn A. Characterization of three optional promoters in the 5'region of the human aldolase A gene. J Mol Biol 1987;197:425.
311. Kishi H, Mukai T, Hirono A, Fujii H, Miwa S, Hori K. Human aldolase A deficiency associated with hemolytic anemia: thermolabile aldolase due to a single base mutation. Proc Natl Acad Sci USA 1987;84:8623.
312. Maquat LE, Chilcote R, Ryan PM. Human triosephosphate isomerase cDNA and protein structure: studies of triosephosphate isomerase deficiency in man. J Biol Chem 1985;260:3748.
313. Daar IO, Artymiuk PJ, Phillips DC, Maquat LE. Human triosephosphate isomerase deficiency: a single amino acid substitution results in a thermolabile enzyme. Proc Natl Acad Sci USA 1986;83:7903.
314. Michelson AM, Markham AF, Orkin SH. Isolation and DNA sequence of a full length cDNA clone for human X chromosome–encoded phosphoglycerate kinase. Proc Natl Acad Sci USA 1983;80:472.
315. Singer-Sam J, Simmer RL, Keith DH, et al. Isolation of a cDNA clone for human X-linked 3-phosphoglycerate kinase by use of a mixture of synthetic oligodeoxyribonucleotides as a detection probe. Proc Natl Acad Sci USA 1983;80:802.
316. Fujii K, Kanno H, Hirono A, Shiomura T, Miwa S. A single amino acid Substitution (157 Gly–Val) in a phosphoglyerate kinase variant (PGK Shizuoka) associated and chronic hemolysis and myoglobinuria. Blood 1992;79:1582.
317. Fujii H, Chen S-H, Akasuka J, Miwa S, Yoshida A. Use of cultured lymphoblastoid cells for the study of abnormal enzymes: molecular abnormality of a phosphoglycerate kinase varient associated with hemolytic anemia. Proc Natl Acad Sci USA 1981;78:2587.
318. Fujii H, Krietsch WKG, Yoshida A. A single amino acid substitution (ASP–ASN) in a phosphoglycerate kinase variant (PGK Munchen) associates the enzyme deficiency. J Biol Chem 1980;255:6421.
319. Fujii H, Yoshida A: Molecular abnormality of phosphoglycerate kinase-Uppsala associated with chronic nonspherocytic hemolytic anemia. Proc Natl Acad Sci USA 1980;77:5461.
320. Yoshida A, Watanabe S, Chen S-H, Giblett ER, Malcolm LA: Human phosphoglyverate kinase. II. Structure of variant enzyme. J Biol Chem 1972;247:446.
321. Joulin V, Peduzzi J, Romeo P-H, et al. Molecular cloning and sequencing of the human erythrocyte 2,3-biphosphoglycerate mutase cDNA: revised amino acid sequence. EMBO J 1986;5:2275.
322. Joulin V, Garel M-C, LeBoulch PL, et al. Isolation and characterization of the human 2,3-biphosphoglycerate mutase gene. J Biol Chem 1988;263:15785.
323. Lemarchandel V, Joulin V, Valentin C, et al. Compound heterozygosity in a complete erythocyte bisphosphoglycerate mutase deficiency. Blood 1992;80:2643.
324. Giallongo A, Feo S, Moor R, Croce CM, Showe LC. Molecular cloning and nucleotide sequence of a full-length cDNA for human enolase. Proc Natl Acad Sci USA 1986;83:6741.
325. Tani K, Fujii H, Nagata S, Miwa S. Human liver type pyruvate kinase: complete amino acid sequence and the expression in mammalian cells. Proc Natl Acad Sci USA 1988;85:1792.
326. Neubauer M, Lakomek M, Winkler M, Parke S, Hofferbert S, Schroter W. Point mutations in the L-type pyrate kinase gene of two children with hemolytic anemia caused by pyruvate kinase deficiency. Blood 1991;77:1871.
327. Kanno K, Fujii H, Hirono A, Miwa S. cDNA cloning of human R-type pyruvate kinase and identification of a single amino acid substitution (Thr^{384}–Met) affecting enzymatic stabilility in pyruvate kinase variant (PK Tokyo) associated with hereditary hemolytic anemia. Proc Natl Acad Sci USA 1991;88:8218.
328. Kanno H, Fujii H, Hirono A, Omine M, Miwa S. Identical point mutations of the R-type pyruvate kinase (PK) cDNA found in unrelated PK variants associated with hereditary hemolytic anemia. Blood 1992;79:1347.
329. Kanno H, Fujii H, Miwa S. Low substrate affinity of pyruvate kinase (PK Sapporo) caused by a single amino acid substitution (426 Arg–Gln) associated with hereditary hemolytic anemia. Blood 1993;81: 2439.
330. Kanno H, Fujii H, Tsujino G, Miwa S. Molecular basis of impaired pyruvate kinase isozyme conversation in erythroid cells: a single amino acid substitution near the active site and decreased mRNA content of the R-type PK. Biochem Biophys Res Comm 1993;192:46.
331. Kanno H, Ballas SK, Miwa S, Fujii H, Bowman HS. Molecular abnormality of erythrocyte pyruvate kinase deficiency in the Amish. Blood (in press).
332. Saki I, Shrief FS, Pan Y-CE, Li SS-L. the cDNA and protein sequences of Human lactate dehydrogenase B. Biochem J 1987;248:933.
333. Sudo K, Maekawa, Ikawa S, Machida K, Kitamura M, Li SS. A missense mutation found in human lactate dehydrogenase-B(H) variant gene. Biochem Biophys Res Commun 1990;168:672.
334. Walker JI, Faik P, Morgan MJ. Characterization of the 5' end of the gene for human glucose phosphate isomerase (GPI). Genomics 1990;7: 638.
335. Walker JI, Layton DM, Bellingham AJ, Morgan MJ, Faik P. DNA sequence abnormalities in human glucose 6-phosphate isomerase deficiency. Hum Molec Genet 1993;2:327.
336. Raben N, Sherman J, Miller F, Mena H, Plotz P. A 5' splice junction mutation leading to exon deletion in an Ashkenazic Jewish family with phosphofructokinase deficiency (Tarui disease). J Biol Chem 1993;268:4963.
337. Chang ML, Artymiuk PJ, Wu X, Hollan S, Lammi A, Maquat LE. Human triosephosphate isomerase deficiency resulting from mutation of Phe-240. Am J Hum Genet 1993;52:1260.
338. Baronciani L, Beutler E. Analysis of pyruvate kinase-deficiency mutations that produce nonspherocytic hemolytic anemia. Proc Natl Acad Sci USA 1993;90:4324.

Blood: Principles and Practice of Hematology,
edited by Robert I. Handin, Samuel E. Lux, and Thomas P. Stossel.
J.B. Lippincott Company, Philadelphia © 1995.

58

Glucose-6-Phosphate Dehydrogenase Deficiency and the Pentose Phosphate Pathway

Lucio Luzzatto

HISTORICAL NOTE

The prehistory of glucose-6-phosphate dehydrogenase (G6PD) deficiency begins with an anecdote from the school of Pythagoras (sixth century BC). This great philosopher appears to have admonished his disciples that they should not retreat into a field of fava beans even if their life is at risk (if the anecdote is true, Pythagoras' clinical acumen did not match his mathematic acumen, since adults rarely die of favism). One century later, this notion became enshrined into one of Hippocrates' aphorisms, "*kuamon apecesqe*" ("avoid fava beans"). We do not know whether Lucretius Caro, the Latin poet made famous by his enchanting rendering in verse of natural history, *De Rerum Natura*, had favism in mind when he said that "what is food for some can be harsh poison to others," but the lucid expression of this concept clearly marks him as the founder of pharmacogenetics.

The history of G6PD deficiency began to be recorded, if not by this name, in the Italian medical literature of the 19th century (AD), when "ictero-hemoglobinuric favism" became recognized as a distinct clinical entity. Some astute medical practitioners appreciated that favism "runs in families." In those days, immunology was far more influential than genetics (Paul Ehrlich received a Nobel prize at about the time when Gregor Mendel's work had remained ignored for half a century), and favism was thought to be a manifestation of some kind of allergic reaction.[1,2] In 1923, hemolytic anemia in patients receiving pamaquine for the treatment of malaria was first reported (Table 58-1). "Primaquine sensitivity" came to be perceived as a prominent problem in military medicine during World War II and its aftermath in Korea. The group led by A. S. Alving in Chicago embarked on a systematic study of the syndrome, and in 1956, G6PD deficiency made history when Paul Carson and colleagues[3] discovered that subjects who previously had been identified as primaquine sensitive had a marked deficiency of G6PD activity in their red blood cells. Within a year, similar data appeared from Germany,[4] and in Italy, Sansone and Segni[5] proved that favism was also due to G6PD deficiency. Thus, the problem was solved at the level of biochemical genetics, and G6PD deficiency became a prototype for a variety of disorders due to deficiency in red cells of a specific enzyme, or *enzymopathies*. It took the best part of the next 30 years[6,7]—during which many comprehensive reviews of the subjects have appeared[8–19]—to define the basis of G6PD deficiency at the molecular level.

PENTOSE PHOSPHATE PATHWAY

Glucose-6-phosphate dehydrogenase catalyzes the first reaction of the pentose phosphate pathway (PPP), so named because it brings about the stepwise conversion of G6P to pentose phosphate sugars (Fig. 58-1). These sugars in turn can be recycled by transketolase and transaldolase to F6P and triose phosphate. PPP has thus been regarded as a "shunt" from the classic glycolytic pathway. However, it has long become clear that pentose phosphates, the sugar building blocks of nucleic acids, can be produced directly from F6P, through the concerted action (in reverse) of transketolase and transaldolase, bypassing the first part of the PPP. Thus, the PPP has two main products, namely pentose and NADPH, but the PPP is not indispensable for pentose production. When the cell requires large amounts of pentose, it uses transketolase and transaldolase to bring about a complete conversion of five molecules of F6P (generated from G6P by the glucose phosphate isomerase reaction) to six molecules of R5P through a cycle that, in a strict sense, does not involve the PPP or G6PD. By contrast, the product of the PPP that is *not* produced elsewhere in carbohydrate metabolism is NADPH, and there is every indication that the main role of the PPP, in red cells, is the production of NADPH. At the same time, the role of NADPH is well established as the coenzyme of numerous reductive processes. In fact, one finds one or more NADPH-dependent reactions in most cellular biosynthetic pathways, including fatty acid synthesis, the synthesis of cholesterol and consequently steroid hormones, purine and pyrimidine synthesis, and porphyrin synthesis. We can therefore anticipate that the role of G6PD in any particular cell type will depend on two main considerations: (1) what proportion of NADPH is supplied by G6PD as opposed to other NADPH-generating reactions, and (2) what NADPH-requiring reactions are most important in the physiology of that cell. Two extreme examples can serve to illustrate this point. In the adrenal gland, G6PD is relatively high,[20] and we can presume that its main role is to provide NADPH for steroid hormone

TABLE 58-1. Historical Landmarks in the Study of G6PD Deficiency

		References
19th century	Clinical characterization of favism	1
1923	Hemolytic anemia associated with primaquine sensitivity	209
1932	G6PD activity demonstrated in red cells	210
1956	G6PD deficiency discovered in red cells	3
1960	CNSHA associated with G6PD deficiency	211
1960	G6PD deficiency associated with malaria	118,119
1961	X-linkage of G6PD	212
1962–1963	Somatic cell mosaicism in females heterozygous for G6PD deficiency	88,89
1966	Purification of red cell G6PD to homogeneity	213
1967	Standardization of characterization of G6PD variants	214
1969	Subunit structure of G6PD	37
1981	*Plasmodium falciparum* development is inhibited in G6PD-deficient red cells	135
1986	Cloning and sequence of human G6PD gene	30,67
1988	Molecular basis of G6PD deficiency	106,107

synthesis. In the red cell, G6PD is relatively low, but most of the biosynthetic pathways mentioned have been lost during erythroid cell maturation.[21] Here, the main role of G6PD is unquestionably to maintain a high level of reduced glutathione (GSH; Fig. 58-2). This role is crucial because red cells, being oxygen carriers par excellence, have a literally built-in danger of damage by oxygen radicals, generated continuously in the course of methemoglobin formation.[22]

Control of the Pathway

The first reaction of a metabolic pathway is often rate-limiting, and the PPP is no exception. The first reaction is catalyzed by G6PD,[23,24] and therefore we can expect that control will be exerted here. At the same time, we should consider that the best candidates to regulate physiologically a metabolic reaction are compounds whose concentration will change depending on the needs of the cell. Of the two substrates of G6PD, G6P is not a good candidate because it is always supplied in large amounts through hexokinase, as long as there is glucose in the blood plasma (under most conditions this is a large reservoir). Of the products of G6PD, 6-phosphoglucono-d-lactone is not a good candidate either because it is promptly hydrolyzed to 6-phosphogluconate by a specific lactonase (in fact, the internal ester bond of the lactone is unstable and undergoes hydrolysis even in the absence of the lactonase). Thus, this reaction product is instantly removed and its concentration is uniformly near zero, which makes the G6PD reaction practically irreversible. This leaves the other substrate, NADP, and the other product, NADPH, as possible good candidates for regulation. In fact, there is good evidence that, at least in red cells (where changing the rate of G6PD biosynthesis is not an option), these two compounds are the main agents that control the rate of G6PD activity. This can be understood by considering three important features of the system:

1. The affinity of G6PD for NADP is high: the K_m values measured under different experimental conditions are in the range of 3 to 13 μmol/L.
2. NADPH is an inhibitor with partially competitive kinetics (with respect to NADP) and a K_i of about 16 μmol/L.[25]
3. In normal red cells in the steady state, the concentration of NADP is hardly measurable, whereas NADPH is of the order of 35 μmol/L.[26]

This set of values means that the G6PD reaction is normally almost completely inhibited. Because the total intracellular amount of (NADP + NADPH) is relatively fixed, whenever NADPH is oxidized to NADP, this simultaneously provides substrate for the G6PD reaction and decreases the product inhibition. NADP now is almost quantitatively reduced to NADPH, and the original steady state is restored. In terms of the overall activity of the PPP, it is estimated that, even when it is maximally stimulated, it accounts for less than 10% of the total glucose metabolized by the red cell.[27] In terms of the capacity to generate NADPH, it is remarkable that, because of the low basal activity of G6PD, this can increase by a factor of at least 10 as an instant response to oxidative stress, without any change in the number of G6PD molecules. Detailed analysis of this phenomenon has revealed that, even under maximal stimulation, the activity of G6PD within intact red cells is still about 60 times less than in hemolysates.[28] Thus, the cell appears to have a large reserve potential for NADPH generation.

G6PD Enzyme

Primary Structure

The enzymatically active form of G6PD is either a dimer or a tetramer of a single polypeptide subunit with a molecular mass of 59,096 daltons.[29] The amino acid sequence of the human enzyme has been deduced from the nucleotide sequence of a full-length cDNA clone[30] (Table 58-2).

The rat liver G6PD amino acid sequence, obtained by protein analysis,[31] shows 94% homology to the human sequence and provides evidence that the N-terminal amino acid is N-acetyl-alanine, which must result from post-translational cleavage of the N-terminal methionine followed by acetylation. It is likely that the same is true of the human enzyme.

An understanding of the functional domains of the G6PD molecule is limited by the fact that it has proved difficult to obtain diffracting crystals, and therefore the three-dimensional structure of G6PD is not yet known. However, comparative analysis of G6PD from other organisms has revealed regions of high conservation,[31–34] which may be critical for the function of the enzyme. There is evidence that the G6P-binding site is at or near lysine 205 because this residue can be specifically labeled with pyridoxal 5′-phosphate, and this reaction is prevented by G6P itself.[35] The critical role of this amino acid has been confirmed by showing that its replacement with threonine (produced artificially by site-directed mutagenesis) nearly abolishes catalytic activity.[36] By contrast, there is no conclusive evidence on the location of the NADP-binding site, although the study of variants with altered affinity for NADP has prompted some suggestions in this respect.

Oligomeric Structure

As stated, active G6PD exists either as a dimer or as a tetramer of identical subunits. The dimer–tetramer equilib-

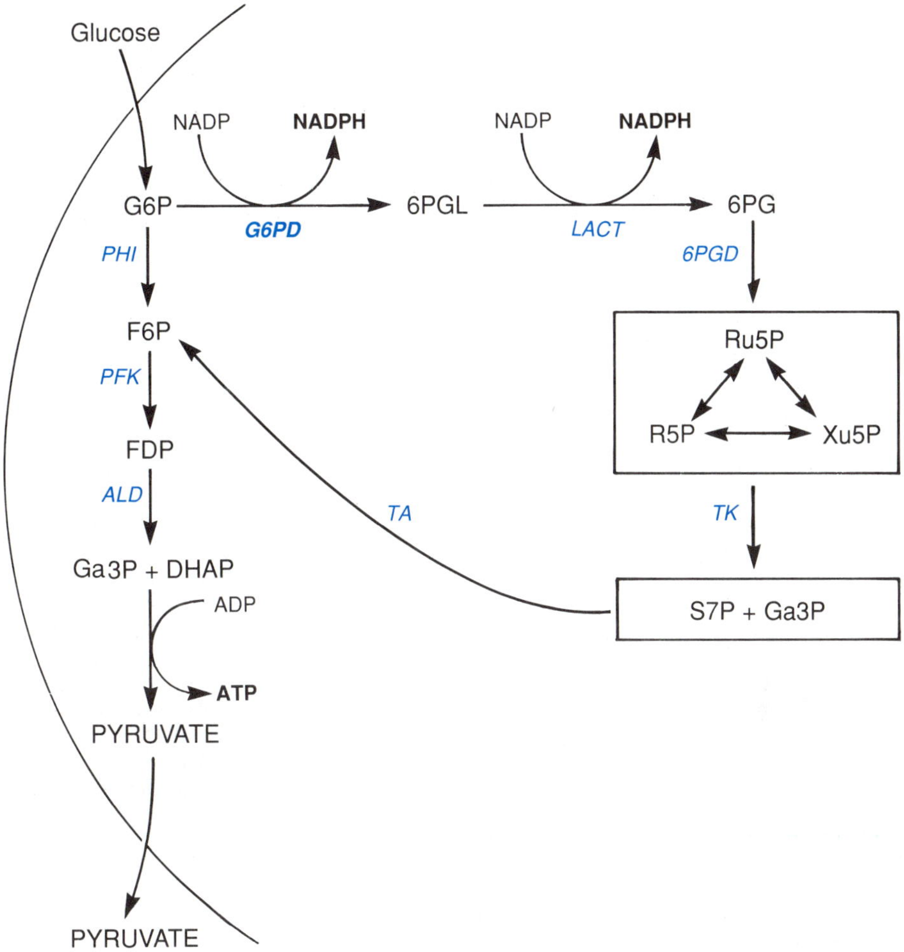

FIGURE 58-1. The pentose phosphate pathway glucose is metabolized anaerobically to pyruvate by way of the Embden-Myerhoff pathway (*left*). The hexose monophosphate shunt, or phosphogluconate pathway (*right*), begins with the dehydrogenation of glucose-6-phosphate (G6P) by glucose-6-phosphate dehydrogenase (G6PD) to yield 6-phosphoglucono-δ-lactone (6PGL). 6PGL is then hydrolyzed to 6-phosphogluconate (6PG) by lactonase (LACT) and decarboxylated by 6-phosphogluconate dehydrogenase (6PGD) to the ketosugar ribulose-5-phosphate (RU5P) and CO_2. Each of these first two steps generates NADPH, which is a critical component of the red cell's glutathione antioxidant system. RU5P is reversibly transformed to xyulose-5-phosphate (Xu5P) by phosphopentose epimerase and into the aldo sugar ribose-5-phosphate (R5P) by phosphopentose isomerase. The thiamine-containing enzyme transketolase (TK) transfers a glycoaldehyde group from Xu5P to R5P, producing sedoheptulose-7-phosphate (S7P) and glyceraldehyde-3-phosphate (Ga3P), which is also an intermediate in the Embden-Myerhoff pathway. Finally, transaldolase (TA) transfers a dihydroxyacetone group from S7P to Ga3P to form fructose-6-phosphate (F6P) and erythrose-4-phosphate (not shown). In addition, TK can convert Xu5P and erythrose-4-phosphate to FDP and Ga3P (not shown). PFK, phosphofructokinase; FDP, fructose-1,6-diphosphate; ALD, aldolase; DHAP, dihydroxyacetone phosphate.

rium is affected by ionic strength and markedly by pH.[37] For instance, at pH 6.0, the enzyme is entirely in tetramer form, whereas at pH 8.0, it is entirely in dimer form. Thus, although the physiologic significance of the interconversion of the two oligomeric forms is unknown, it is interesting that it takes place at around the intracellular pH of red cells. That is, the dimer/tetramer ratio is about 1 at pH 7.2, suggesting that both forms are present in red cells. The specific activity of the enzyme, expressed per mole of subunit, is the same for the dimer and for the tetramer, indicating that it is not affected by the transition from one form of the enzyme to the other. The K_m of G6P is also similar for dimer and tetramer, but around pH 7.2, it has a sharp biphasic pH dependence, which has been attributed to the change in quaternary structure.[38]

Although we are not sure of the significance of the dimer–tetramer interconversion, it is clear that formation of the oligomeric (dimer or tetramer) structure is essential for enzyme activity and that NADP is involved in the process. The evidence for this is as follows:

1. Extensive dialysis in the absence of NADP favors monomer formation and leads to inactivation of G6PD.[39]
2. When G6PD is exposed for short time periods to increasing temperatures, it shows marked stability until

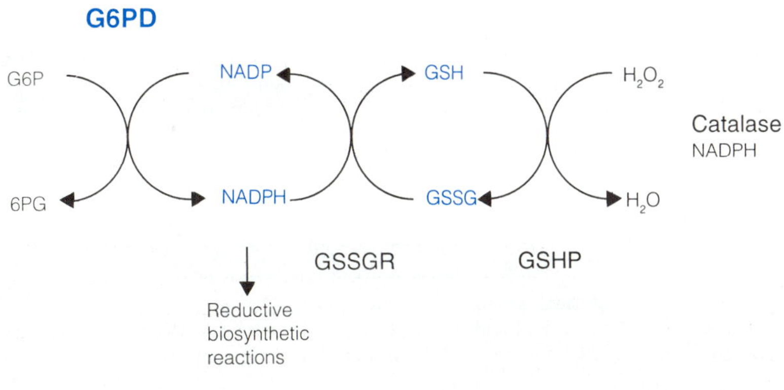

FIGURE 58-2. The principal metabolic role of G6PD in red cells is to protect red cell constituents from oxidants, illustrated here by hydrogen peroxide (H_2O_2). NADPH, a product of the G6PD reaction and the subsequent step in the pentose phosphate pathway, is the hydrogen donor for regeneration of reduced glutathione (GSH) from oxidized glutathione (GSSG), a reaction catalyzed by glutathione reductase (GSSGR). NADPH is also a ligand for catalase, which degrades H_2O_2. G6P, glucose-6-phosphate; 6PG, 6-phosphogluconate; GSHP, glutathione peroxidase.

TABLE 58-2. Numerology of Human G6PD

		References
Number of subunits	2 or 4	37
Number of amino acids	514*	30
Subunit molecular weight (kd)	59, 218	30
Size of mRNA (bp)	2250†	30
Size of genomic gene (kb)	18.5	67
Number of exons	13	67
Specific activity (IU/mg protein)	220	215
K_m of G6P (μmol/L)	72‡	38
K_m of NADP (μmol/L)	16†	25, 216
Activity in red cells (IU/g Hb)	7–10	12

* Without the N-terminal methionine, which has been shown to be absent in rat liver G6PD.[31,217]
† Excluding the poly-A tail.
‡ In trisborate buffer, pH 7.8.

above 50°C, and then it undergoes sharp inactivation, as though the structure collapsed cooperatively.[40] The temperature at which the transition occurs is a function of NADP concentration.

The stabilizing effect of NADP and binding experiments carried out by equilibrium dialysis have led to the notion of the presence of "structural" NADP (1 mol/mol of subunit), which may be distinct from substrate NADP.[41] G6PD preparations may contain inactive monomeric molecules that could not be revealed by conventional analysis based on enzyme activity because as soon as NADP is added to carry out an assay, dimerization would take place, provided the monomer is not irreversibly denatured. On the other hand, there is strong evidence that in vivo there is no significant amount of monomer[42] and that dimerization takes place within milliseconds once NADP is added.[43] Based on the relatively high intracellular concentration of NADP(H), we can presume that subunit association goes on hand in hand with the folding of the polypeptide chain as it is synthesized.

Reaction Mechanism

The kinetics of G6PD have been investigated in considerable detail. NADP became established relatively early in evolution as its coenzyme,[15] and human G6PD has practically no activity with NAD. (Interestingly, the G6PD of *Leuconostoc mesenteroides* has instead a dual specificity: it uses NAD or NADP, depending on the metabolic role of the reaction under different physiologic conditions.[16] Detailed studies of substrate binding[44] and preliminary crystallographic data[45] have been reported for this enzyme.) G6PD is also specific with respect to G6P, and it has relatively low activity on other hexose phosphates (eg, mannose 6-P or galactose 6-P). By contrast, there is significant activity on substrate analogues, such as desamino-NADP and 2-deoxyglucose 6-P. These compounds, although artificial, have been useful in the characterization of variants. The affinity for NADP is about one order of magnitude higher than the affinity for G6P.

Although many natural and nonnatural substances can affect the activity of G6PD, it is not certain which ones may be important physiologically. NADPH, one product of the G6PD reaction, is a potent quasicompetitive inhibitor,[25] and because most of the coenzyme in cells is in the reduced form,[26] we can assume that G6PD is normally under strong inhibition. Because the K_m values for both G6P and NADP are higher than their normal respective intracellular concentrations, it is likely that these two substrates themselves are the main regulators of intracellular G6PD activity, together with NADPH. Any oxidative event that affects the cell alters the NADPH/NADP ratio in favor of NADP. The simultaneous increase in NADP and decrease in NADPH result in an increase in G6PD activity by increasing the substrate drive on the reaction rate and decreasing product inhibition.[46] Under most conditions, this may be the most important short-term regulatory signal, although it is possible that other regulatory effects play a role as well.

GENETICS OF G6PD AND EPIDEMIOLOGY OF G6PD DEFICIENCY

X-Linked Gene for G6PD

The single polypeptide chain of G6PD is encoded in a gene located in the telomeric region of the long arm of the X chromosome[47,48] (band Xq28; Fig. 58-3). (It had been claimed that a portion of the G6PD protein is encoded by an autosomal gene mapped to chromosome 6.[49] However, this latter gene turns out to encode instead guanosine monophosphate

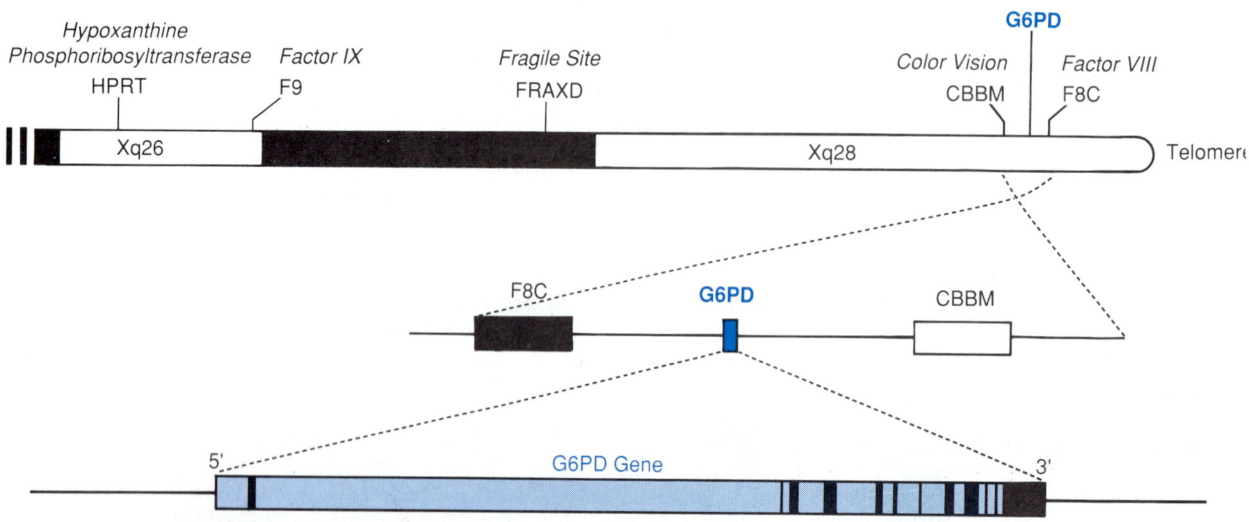

FIGURE 58-3. Arrangement of *G6PD* gene on the long arm of the X chromosome. The gene, with exons depicted in black, is located between the genes for clotting factor VIII (F8C) and color vision (CBBM), near the telomere of the chromosome.

reductase,[50] and the claim has been refuted[51,52] and retracted.[53]) Linkage analysis in appropriate families indicates that the G6PD gene, *Gd*, must lie near the genes for hemophilia A[54] and color blindness.[25] In fact, physical linkage of *Gd* to the genes encoding factor VIII and to those encoding the retinal pigments[55] has been established at the molecular level, and this particular genomic region is one of the best mapped in the entire human genome.[56–64] It also appears to have a high density of genes.[64,66]

At the genomic level, the *Gd* gene consists of 13 exons, the first one of which is noncoding.[67] The total length of the gene, which has been fully sequenced,[68] is of about 18.5 kb, much of which (about 12 kb) consists of intron II. The promoter region is highly GC-rich, as found characteristically in other housekeeping genes analyzed so far.[69] Deletion analysis has revealed that the "essential" portion of the promoter is only about 150 bp long.[70] The significance of the large intron is unknown, but some sequences within introns may be important for efficient transcription.

Since the discovery of G6PD deficiency, it was expected that this condition must result from mutations of the *Gd* gene. In fact, by reference to the best known system in human genetics, namely hemoglobin, it was speculated that there might be two types of mutations. One type, producing qualitative as well as quantitative changes in G6PD, would be analogous to structural hemoglobinopathies and would be expected to be within the coding region. The other type, producing only a reduction in the amount of a qualitatively normal G6PD, would be analogous to thalassemia and might be located in regulatory regions of the gene. Whenever G6PD from G6PD-deficient individuals was subjected to careful biochemical characterization, however, qualitative differences, albeit sometimes only subtle ones, were invariably detected, indicating that in all these cases the mutations were of the first type. Since 1988, identification of individual G6PD mutations at the DNA level has entirely confirmed this indication. All mutations thus far have been structural, and thalassemia-like mutations have not yet been discovered.

Population Genetics

G6PD deficiency is a global feature in the human species. Although it is still often referred to as a problem mainly belonging to Africa and to the Mediterranean, its epidemiology extends instead to all continents.[71] Areas of high prevalence are found in Africa, Southern Europe, the Middle East, South East Asia, and Oceania (Fig. 58-4 and Table 58-3). In the Americas, G6PD deficiency is also prevalent as a result of migrations that have taken place in relatively recent historical times, whereas it is conspicuously absent from the Native American people.

Because the *Gd* gene is X-linked, frequencies of G6PD deficiency in males are identical to gene frequencies. This fact makes it convenient to work out the frequencies of the female genotypes by using the Hardy-Weinberg law (Table 58-4). In contrast to most X-linked conditions, for which it is commonplace to state that males are affected and females are carriers, in many populations the frequency of *Gd*− is sufficiently high to entail the existence of a nonnegligible proportion of *Gd*−/*Gd*− homozygotes.[72] Unfortunately, many studies still report on the *overall* frequency of G6PD deficiency in a mixed group of males and females, which makes it impossible to know the real frequencies of the various genotypes.

X-Chromosome Inactivation

In mammals, the difference between males and females is characteristically associated with having one or two X chromosomes, respectively. Primary sex determination results from a gene[73] located not on the X chromosome but on the Y chromosome, as had been anticipated from the phenotypic difference between XY males and XO females (Turner's syndrome). The presence of one or two X chromosomes, however, constitutes another major difference between the sexes because it imposes the necessity of compensation for gene dosage. It appears reasonable to surmise that X-chromosome inactivation[74,75] has evolved in relation to the necessity to avoid that somatic cells in females would have twice the amount of X-linked gene products compared with males. (Dosage compensation in invertebrates such as *Drosophila* is effected instead by making X-linked genes hyperactive in males[76].) Thus, the level of, for instance, G6PD activity in individual cells of males and females is the same.

X-Chromosome Inactivation Takes Place Early in Embryonic Life. Evidence indicates that, in the fertilized egg, both X chromosomes are active, but soon after implantation (not necessarily at the same time in all tissues throughout the embryo[77]), one of the two X chromosomes is inactivated in each cell of the female embryo. In the extraembryonic

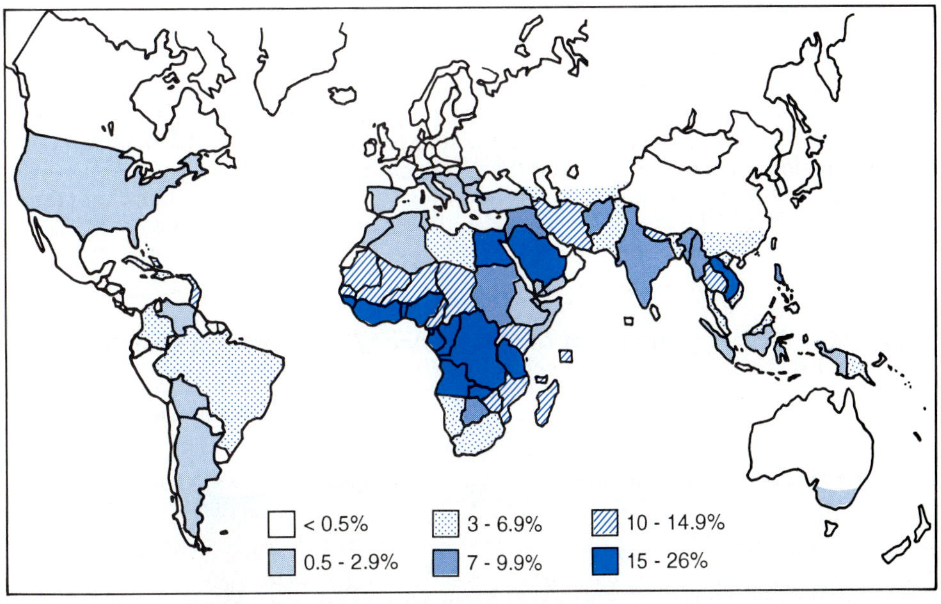

FIGURE 58-4. World distribution of G6PD deficiency. The values shown by the different shadings are frequencies of G6PD-deficient males in the populations of the various countries. These are also gene frequencies because the gene is X-linked. (Luzzato L, Mehta A. In: Scriver CR, Beaudet AL, Sly WS, Valle D, eds. The metabolic basis of inherited disease, ed 6. New York, McGraw-Hill, 1989:2237.

TABLE 58-3. Examples of G6PD Variants

Class	Example	Clinical Features	G6PD Activity (% of normal)	Electrophoretic Mobility	K_m of G6P (μmol/L)	Population Frequency	References
IV	B	None	100	Normal	70	Worldwide	
IV	A	None	110	Fast	70	Polymorphic in Africa	218,219
III	Seattle	Rarely AHA	25	Slow	20	Polymorphic, widespread	108,221,222
III	A^-	AHA, NNJ	110	Fast	70	Polymorphic in Africa, Southern Europe, and Middle East	40,202,223–225
II	Mediterranean	AHA, NNJ	3	Normal	25	Polymorphic in Southern Europe, Middle East, India	106,225,226
I	Santiago de Cuba	CNSHA	2	Slow	45	Rare	106
I	Barcelona	CNSHA and frequent bacterial infection	2	Fast	40	Rare	195

AHA, acute hemolytic anemia; NNJ, neonatal jaundice; CNSHA, chronic nonspherocytic hemolytic anemia.

membranes, the paternal X is preferentially inactivated, but in the embryo itself, X inactivation has two distinctive properties: (1) it occurs at random in each cell, and (2) once it has occurred, it is faithfully maintained in the progeny of each cell.

Genes on the Inactive X Chromosome Are Inactive but Remain Essentially Intact. The process of X chromosome inactivation in vivo appears to be irreversible. In vitro, it is also extremely stable, but occasionally "reactivation" of individual X-linked genes has been observed,[78] and it can be produced artificially by the use of agents such as azacytidine.[79] This finding indicates that individual genes on the inactive X are not lost or disrupted. Although the mechanism of X-chromosome inactivation is not yet completely elucidated, several points are well established:

1. The DNA of an inactive gene on the inactive X is physically modified. This was first formally proved by experiments in which DNA from fibroblast clones from a woman heterozygous for hypoxanthine phosphoribosyltransferase (HPRT) deficiency was transfected into hemizygous HPRT(−) cells. The defect of the recipient cells was correctable by DNA from clones in which the HPRT+ gene was on the active X but not by DNA from clones in which the HPRT+ gene was on the inactive X.[80,81]
2. The physical modification is unlikely to be in the nucleotide sequence because reactivation (as it takes place in gonadal cells) yields a gene with normal expression. By contrast, genes on the inactive X have a different pattern of methylation from those on the active X. For instance, in the case of G6PD, certain C residues are always methylated on both the active and the inactive X, but others are specifically methylated only on the inactive X. The fact that a gene on the inactive X is differently methylated does not by itself prove that this is what makes it inactive, but the ability of 5-azacytidine (a nonmethylatable base analogue) to cause reactivation can be regarded as presumptive evidence in support of this notion.
3. X-chromosome inactivation appears to be a cooperative phenomenon that involves the whole structure of the chromosome, which becomes heterochromatic and late-replicating. Morphologic manifestations of these changes are Barr's bodies in epithelial cells and drumstick appendages in the nuclei of granulocytes.
4. A gene controlling X inactivation has been isolated in both human and mouse. This gene has the unique property of being active only on the inactive X chromosome.[82] Although it is not yet known how this gene exerts its effect, it appears that it plays a key role in causing X inactivation, maintaining it, or both.

Not All Genes on the Inactive X Chromosome Are Inactive. Although the cooperative nature of the X-chromosome inactivation phenomenon is one of its most distinctive features, it has emerged that some X-linked genes are able to escape inactivation. The first well-characterized example was the steroid sulfatase (*STS*) gene, deficiency of which is responsible for metachromatic leukodystrophy.[83] Subsequently, other genes have been proved to escape inactivation.[84,85] In general, they are those that have a homologue on the Y chromosome, and they are clustered on that part of the short arm of the X, which, at the cytogenic level, shows the ability to pair with the Y chromosome (although they may be interspersed with

TABLE 58-4. The Prevalence of G6PD Deficiency in Males and Females Depends on the Overall Gene Frequency in the Population

		Prevalence of G6PD Deficiency (%)			
Gd^- Gene Frequency	Geographic Area (Example)	Male Hemizygotes (All at Risk)	Female Heterozygotes	Female Homozygotes	Females at Risk (%)
Very low: 10^{-4}	Japan	0.01	0.02	0.0001	0.017
Polymorphic, low: 0.02	Southern Italy	2	4	0.04	2.7
Polymorphic, high: 0.65	Kurdish Jews	65	45	42	72

genes subject to inactivation[63]). For these reasons, this region of the X chromosome is referred to as *pseudoautosomal*. The consequence of escape from inactivation is that dosage compensation does not apply—at least not in full—to genes located on this part of the X chromosome. The level of *STS* is higher in normal females than in normal males. The existence of genes such as *STS*, which are active on both the active and the inactive X, provides a good reason for the otherwise intriguing phenomenon that the "inactive" X is not lost through many generations of somatic cell divisions despite its apparent redundancy. It has also been suggested that deficiency of one or more of the genes that escape inactivation may be responsible for the phenotypic features of Turner's syndrome.[86]

X-Chromosome Inactivation Produces Somatic Cell Mosaicism in Females. According to the current estimate of about 100,000 functional genes in the human genome, there must be some 5000 on the X chromosome. We can safely assume that every woman is heterozygous at several of the corresponding genetic loci. A remarkable consequence is that X inactivation produces in each woman two types of somatic cells, which differ from each other in the expression of the respective allelic genes. This situation is referred to as *mosaicism*. Whereas the notion of X chromosome inactivation was first formulated by Mary Lyon from inspection of coat color in mice,[87] the first demonstration of mosaicism at the cellular level was provided by the G6PD system itself, when Beutler and colleagues demonstrated that women heterozygous for G6PD deficiency had two red cell populations, one normal and one deficient.[88] The demonstration that the active and the inactive state of the X were faithfully maintained in somatic cells was also first obtained using G6PD as a marker, when Davidson and colleagues[89] were able to isolate individual fibroblast clones expressing only the A type or the B type of G6PD from a culture of primary diploid fibroblasts of a woman who was genetically a Gd^A/Gd^B heterozygote.

Somatic Cell Mosaicism Sets Heterozygosity for an X-Linked Gene Apart From Heterozygosity for an Autosomal Gene. In most cases, heterozygotes for enzyme deficiencies are asymptomatic because cells with an enzyme level close to half of normal are biochemically normal. By contrast, as a result of X inactivation, the abnormal cells of a woman heterozygous for G6PD deficiency are just as deficient as those of a hemizygous deficient man and therefore just as susceptible to pathology. For this reason, although G6PD deficiency is still often referred to as an X-linked recessive trait, this is a misnomer. A recessive trait is, by definition, not expressed in a heterozygote; instead, G6PD deficiency is expressed in heterozygotes both biochemically and clinically. The expression is decreased, compared with hemizygous males or homozygous females, roughly in proportion to the percentage of G6PD deficient cells in any individual heterozygote. What determines this percentage is not yet completely understood. Because X inactivation is a random phenomenon, it is expected in principle to produce about equal numbers of the two cell types constituting the genetic mosaic of a female organism. Analysis of heterozygotes, however, reveals a normal distribution with a relatively wide variation around the mean. Thus, although most heterozygotes have an intermediate phenotype with respect to their G6PD level, at the extremes of the curve, heterozygotes may have a pseudonormal or a pseudodeficient phenotype. We can envisage at least three (not mutually exclusive) ways by which such extreme phenotypes can arise:

1. Some structural feature of one of the two parental X chromosomes may render its inactivation more likely than that of the other. There is no evidence at the moment for such an occurrence.
2. Because inactivation is a random phenomenon, statistical fluctuation might bring about inactivation to be concordant in most of the cells. For instance, if it occurs in a particular embryo at the eight-cell stage, the probability that the same X chromosome is inactivated in all but one would be $(\frac{1}{2})^7$, or less than 1%. Although this is a small number, this mechanism could apply in an individual case.
3. Once inactivation has taken place, selection might operate on the two types of somatic cells that have emerged (Fig. 58-5, pathway C'). This is especially conspicuous in a heterozygote for a drastically deleterious mutation, such as HPRT deficiency,[90] or in other comparable situations.[91–93]

It is interesting to consider, however, that even an allelic difference that gives a slight growth advantage would see its effect amplified over subsequent rounds of cell division. For instance, if the advantage was 2% (probably undetectable by most available experimental methods), after 10 divisions, the cells with the advantageous gene would exceed the others by a factor of 1.02^{10}, that is, by a factor of nearly 2. After 20 divisions, one population would have practically submerged the other. An interesting feature of this somatic cell selection process is that it could operate at any stage in ontogenesis, and it could operate differently in different tissues because genes conferring a growth advantage in one tissue may not do so in another. Heterozygotes for G6PD mutations causing severe anemia may have an extreme phenotype in red blood cells but not in fibroblasts.[94] Although weights cannot yet be assigned to the role of these three mechanisms, scenario 2 is favored for causing minor deviations from a 1:1 ratio, but scenario 3 is favored for causing marked deviations that produce extreme phenotypes. The frequency of these was estimated at about 1.5% in a study in which G6PD enzyme activity was assayed quantitatively in genetically proved G6PD heterozygotes,[95] but it was much higher in a study in which a methylation-sensitive restriction fragment length polymorphism revealed by the anonymous probe Mb27 was used as marker.[96] In one family, an extremely imbalanced phenotype was observed in every woman heterozygote for two G6PD alleles, and analysis of the data suggested that somatic cell selection was by far the most likely explanation.[97]

Linder and Gartler[98] first pointed out that, because of the mosaic composition of female tissues, any process associated with cellular proliferation would be expected to reflect the mosaic situation, unless it arose from a single cell. Specifically, they showed that each individual uterine leiomyoma from Gd^A/Gd^B heterozygous women express either only G6PD A or only G6PD B. Since then, this approach has been used to test the clonal origin of a variety of solid tumors, leukemias, and related disorders,[99] including polycythemia rubra vera and paroxysmal nocturnal hemoglobinuria.[100] Naturally, this approach is only applicable to women who happen to be heterozygous at the G6PD locus. The electrophoretic A-B polymorphism has been used most commonly because its analysis is easy, but it is confined to women from Africa and of African descent. Subsequently, by taking advantage of the abnormal kinetics of G6PD Mediterranean toward substrate analogues, the same approach has been used in heterozygotes for that gene.[101] More recently, the same concept has been extended to the use as X-linked markers of allelic variation in restriction sites on the X chromosome that are at or near sites characterized by differential methylation on the active versus the inactive X.[22,102,103] With some of these sites, thanks to the presence of variable numbers of tandem repeats, the rate of heterozygosity comes near to 100%, and therefore this approach can be extended to practically all women.[96]

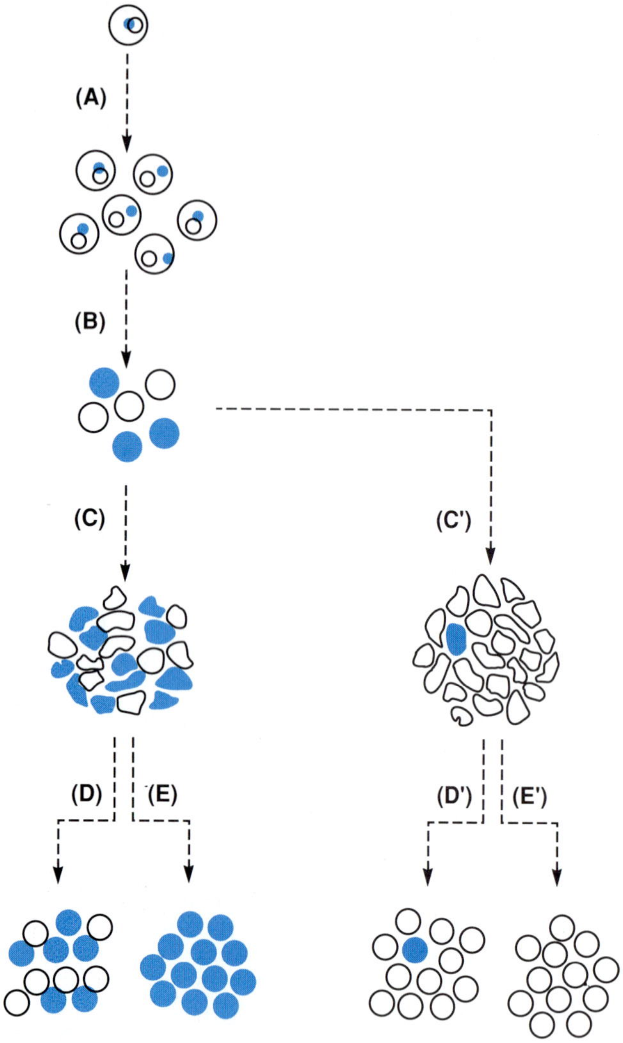

FIGURE 58-5. Use of the G6PD phenotype to obtain information on clonal proliferation and somatic cell selection. (**A**) Embryonic cells before X-chromosome inactivation. The two different colored (blue and white) dots represent expression of two different alleles of G6PD. (**B**) Inactivation of one X chromosome per cell produces two cell populations (blue and white) distinguishable by their G6PD phenotype. (**C**) Proliferation of cells at about even rates produces mosaicism. (**C'**) A differential growth rate of the two cell types resulting from X inactivation (somatic cell selection) may yield a nearly homogeneous population. This could apply to the whole body or to selected tissues because a particular X-linked gene, for which the subject is heterozygous, can only confer a growth advantage in tissues where it is expressed. (**D**) Proliferating tissue, such as an inflammatory process or a healing wound, still produces a mosaic. (**E**) Pathologic proliferation arising from a single ("monoclonal") cell, such as a tumor, produces a homogeneous population. (**D'** and **E'**) If pathologic proliferation arises in a tissue that is already homogeneous, as a result of somatic cell selection, the cell population still is homogeneous (or nearly homogeneous), regardless of whether the proliferative process is monoclonal or polyclonal.

Although this methodology is powerful, it is important to appreciate its limits as well as its potential. The finding of a single X-linked gene expressed in a particular cell population is best described, in phenotypic terms, by saying that the population is homogeneous in that respect. In keeping with the earlier discussion, it may be homogeneous for one of the three following reasons: (1) the population arises from a single cell; (2) the population arises from multiple cells, but selection during growth has favored one cell type over the other; or (3) the population arises from multiple cells in a tissue that already had an extreme phenotype. Only in the first case is the apparently homogeneous population also monoclonal. To safeguard against being misled by the third situation, it is essential to compare the neoplastic population with normal cells of the same lineage. There is no absolute way to eliminate the second possibility. Thus, because mosaicism due to X inactivation precedes pathology, homogeneity for an X-linked marker may be suggestive of monoclonal origin, but it is not as conclusive as the finding of a unique marker such as a chromosomal abnormality or a gene rearrangement. By contrast, the finding that a cell population is not homogeneous with respect to an X-linked marker can be regarded as conclusive evidence that it is *not* monoclonal. This notion has been exploited, for instance, to show that white blood cells of donor origin after bone marrow transplantation arise from a relatively large number (more than 100) of stem cells.[104]

Genetic Heterogeneity of G6PD and of G6PD Deficiency

Analysis of thousands of samples has revealed both qualitative and quantitative changes in the G6PD of human red cells. The parameters most widely used for G6PD characterization are as follows:

- Specific activity in red cells (IU/G Hb)
- Electrophoretic mobility
- Affinity constants (K_m) for the two substrates, G6P and NADP, and for the product inhibitor NADPH (K_i)
- Activity on substrate analogues
- pH Dependence of enzyme activity
- Thermostability

On the grounds of these parameters, some 400 different variants have been reported.[105] From this analysis, G6PD has emerged as the genetic locus in the human genome for which the highest level of heterogeneity is known (Table 58-5). The source of ascertainment of G6PD variants essentially has had two parts. On one hand, variants have been picked up by population screening or by testing clinical samples using methods that measure enzyme activity in a quantitative or semiquantitative way. By this approach, only variants associated with enzyme deficiency are detected. On the other hand, some population studies have been carried out by electrophoretic analysis. By this approach, both deficient variants and variants with charge changes are detected. Thus, it is likely that further heterogeneity has remained hidden thus far because amino acid replacements that do not entail a change in charge remain silent. In addition, many G6PD-deficient samples are not routinely fully characterized.

Classification

To arrange this surplus of variants in relation to features that have biologic and clinical relevance, three main criteria are useful:

Level of residual activity: The variant is normal or deficient with respect to enzyme level.

Clinical manifestations: The variant may be asymptomatic or associated with relatively mild or episodic manifestations, mainly neonatal jaundice and acute hemolytic anemia; or it may be associated with severe manifestations, mainly chronic nonspherocytic hemolytic anemia (CNSHA).

Population frequency: The variant may be only sporadic, or it may have, in one or more populations, a prevalence that qualifies it as polymorphic.

TABLE 58-5. **Summary of G6PD Variants**

Class*	Polymorphic No.	Polymorphic %	Electrophoretic Mobility Fast	Electrophoretic Mobility Normal	Electrophoretic Mobility Slow	Altered Electrophoretic Mobility (%)	Total
I	1	1	24	34	39	64	97
II	37	30	31	37	54	70	122
III	22	21	41	16	46	84	103
IV	12	23	20	3	29	94	52
V	0		2			100	2
TOTAL	72	19	118	90	168	76	376

* Variants are classified on the basis of clinical and biochemical criteria as follows: class I, G6PD deficiency associated with chronic nonspherocytic hemolytic anemia (CNSHA); class II, severely deficient (<10% of normal), but no CNSHA; class III, moderately G6PD deficient (10%–60% of normal); class IV, not significantly deficient (>60% of normal); class V, increased activity.

Population frequency is most useful in indicating whether a particular variant has been subjected to natural selection. The necessary information is not always available, however, because by definition a population study is required for this purpose. Partly for this reason, a classification that has gained wide acceptance and is taxonomically useful is one that uses clinical manifestations and level of residual activity as primary criteria and electrophoretic mobility as a secondary criterion. By reference to a table of variants constructed according to these criteria[105] (Table 58-6), it is relatively easy to work out whether a sample under investigation is likely to correspond to a previously known variant or may be instead a new variant.

Biochemical Versus Molecular Characterization

Since the elucidation of the primary structure of normal G6PD by sequence analysis, it has become possible to determine the basis for G6PD variants by identifying changes at the DNA level. This was carried out initially, in a handful of cases, by constructing genomic libraries from patient DNA, followed by isolation of the appropriate clones by using normal cDNA as a hybridization probe, followed by subcloning in M13 phage and sequencing.[106–109] This laborious procedure was quickly replaced by current methodology, based on use of the polymerase chain reaction technique for amplification of all the G6PD exons, which can then be sequenced with or without prior cloning.[110] Some 40 variants have been analyzed in this way (Fig. 58-6), and a composite pattern is beginning to emerge. First, most variants result from point mutations, that is, single base changes producing single amino acid replacements. The few exceptions are G6PD Sunderland, which has a small deletion of a single codon, and G6PD A− and G6PD Santa Maria, which have two separate point mutations. Second, the mutations are scattered throughout the coding region of G6PD. Third, it is of interest to correlate the molecular information with previous biochemical data. In general, the correlation is good, in the sense that well-characterized biochemical differences have been matched by different underlying mutations. In most cases, the observed electrophoretic mobility matches what could be expected from the amino acid change involved. In several cases, however, samples that had been identified with a particular variant revealed further heterogeneity at the molecular level, for instance, in the cases of G6PD A−[111] and of G6PD Mediterranean.[112,113] This can be easily explained by considering that biochemical differences can be subtle, and whether they are discovered or not depends on how far the analysis is pushed. Conversely, in several cases, variants that had been assigned different names turned out to have the same molecular change, for instance, in the cases of G6PD A−,[111] G6PD Mediterranean,[108] G6PD Walter Reed,[114] G6PD Beverley Hills[114] (the same mutation has been found in G6PD Genova[115]), G6PD Kerala-Kalyan,[116] and others. This finding is more disturbing because it sug-

TABLE 58-6. **Genetic Polymorphism of G6PD**

Class*	Clinical Expression	Residual Activity	No. of Variants (Biochemical)	No. of Variants† (Molecular)	Electrophoretically Normal‡ (%)
I	Severe (CNSHA)	<20	94	27	35
II	Mild	<10	114	13	31
III	Mild	10–60	110	17	15
IV	None	100	52	1	10
V	None	>100	2	0	
TOTAL			372	58	

CNSHA, chronic nonspherocytic hemolytic anemia.

* Defined by a combination of (1) clinical expression (see column 2), and (2) residual activity—a variant is placed in class I if it as associated with CNSHA, regardless of level of residual activity.

† See Table 58-7.

‡ The paucity of electrophoretically normal variants in classes III and IV probably reflects the fact that nondeficient variants are generally detected only if they exhibit an electrophoretic change. By contrast, the fraction of electrophoretically abnormal variants in classes I and II closely approaches the theoretical value of one third (Luzzatto L, Mehta A. Glucose-6-phosphate dehydrogenase deficiency. In: Scriver CR, Beaudet AL, Sly WS, Valle D, eds. The metabolic basis of inherited disease, ed 6. New York, McGraw-Hill, 1989:2237)

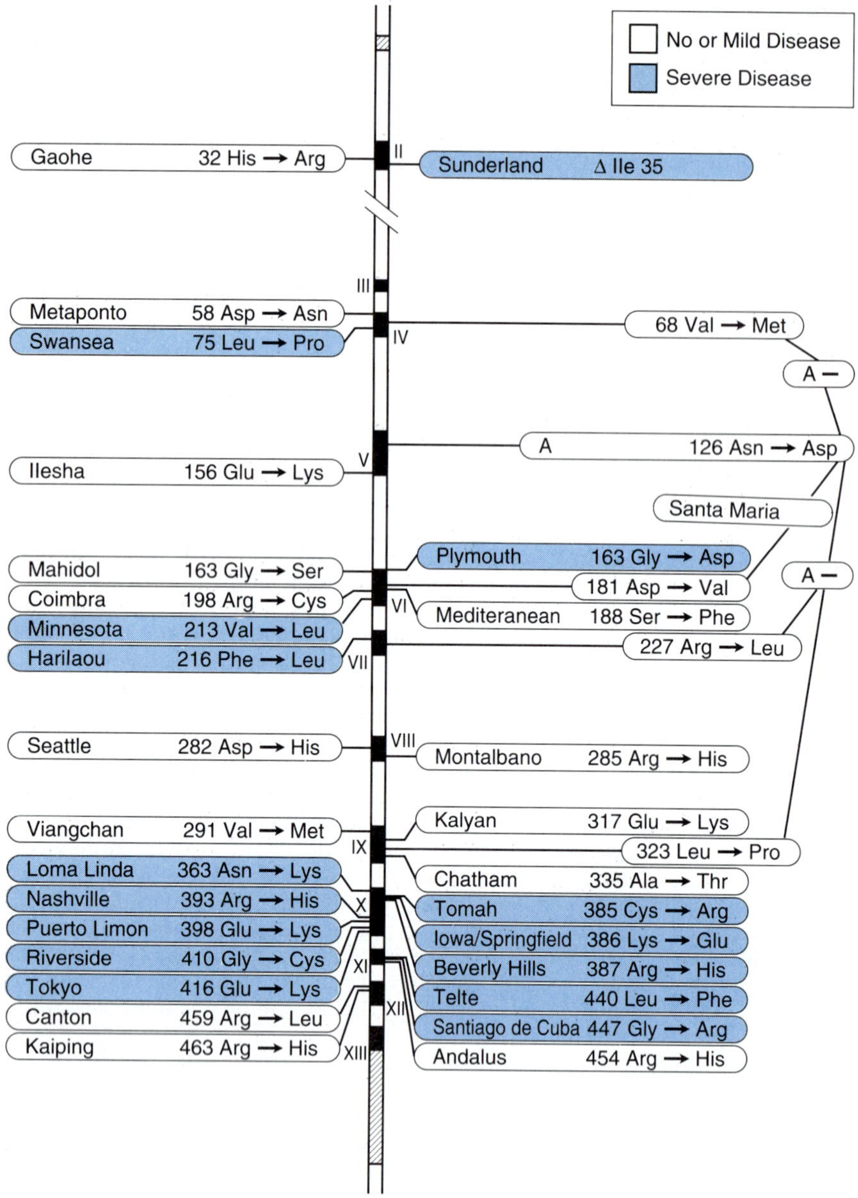

FIGURE 58-6. Molecular basis of G6PD mutations: the human *G6PD* gene and its associated structural mutations. The gene is represented in the center. Exons are in black and are numbered from the 5′ end (*top*). Each boxed entry represents a G6PD variant and the corresponding amino acid replacement. All the variants shown, except G6PD A, are associated with enzyme deficiency. The colored boxes are variants that produce chronic nonspherocytic hemolytic anemia (CNSHA). G6PD A− is heterogeneous. It can result from the combination of the 126 Asn → Asp mutation with any of three additional mutations. In most cases, the second mutation is 68 Val → Met. This figure indicates only some of the variants for which the molecular basis is known. Others are listed in Table 58-7.

gests, at least at first sight, that the biochemical characterization had been inadequate or undermined by poor storage or other artifacts. One might then be tempted to dispense with biochemical characterization altogether, but in this author's view, this would be a mistake for at least two reasons: (1) knowledge of biochemical properties is relevant to the clinical expression of any G6PD variant; and (2) identification of a new molecular lesion in a particular patient, without sufficient knowledge of biochemical properties, would make it impossible to match the new finding with data acquired in the literature before molecular characterization was possible. Certain biochemical properties have proved more useful than others in discriminating among different variants, partly for technical and partly for biologic reasons. For instance, the pH profile has been traditionally recorded as *truncate* or *biphasic*; there are so many variants in each of these two categories that the test is hardly worthwhile from the taxonomic point of view. As another example, the K_m of NADP is difficult to measure and subject to error in unpurified enzyme preparations. By contrast, certain other parameters have proved more reliable and appear to have a higher resolving power.

In summary, a full biochemical characterization, as originally recommended by a WHO Scientific Group, can be regarded as superseded, for classification purposes, by the availability of definitive identification of the underlying mutation from DNA analysis (Table 58-7). On the other hand, for the reasons given earlier, biochemical characterization is still highly recommended[117] and should consist, at a minimum, of the following: residual activity, electrophoretic mobility, K_m of G6P (or activity on substrate analogues), and thermostability. Although it is likely that molecular analysis will become rapidly more widespread, especially in areas where G6PD deficiency is prevalent, relatively few laboratories have retained an interest in biochemical characterization as well as molecular analysis.

Malaria and G6PD Deficiency

Epidemiology

The striking correlation between the worldwide distribution of G6PD deficiency and that of *Plasmodium falciparum* prompted the formulation of the malaria hypothesis some

TABLE 58-7. Genetic Variants of G6PD Characterized at the Molecular Level

Name	Amino Acid Number	Amino Acid Replacement	Class	Electrophoretic Mobility	K_m of G6P (μM)	Population	References
Gaohe	32	His → Arg	III	96	31	Chinese	227
Sunderland	35	Δ Ile	I	95		English	228
Aures	48	Ile → Thr	II	100	59	Algerian	229
Metaponto	58	Asp → Asn	III	90	47	Italian	106,223
A−	68	Val → Met	III	110	60	African	107
	126	Asn → Asp					
Swansea	75	Leu → Pro	I			Welsh	MacDonald et al, unpublished
Ube	81	Arg → Cys	III	108	52	Japanese	230
Lagosanto	81	Arg → His	III			Italian	Ninfali et al, unpublished
Vancouver	106	Ser → Lys	I			Canadian	231
	182	Arg → Trp					
	198	Arg → Cys					
A	126	Asn → Asp	IV	110	60	African	109
Quing-Yan	131	Gly → Val	III	100	56	Chinese	232
Ilesha	156	Glu → Lys	III	75	83	Nigerian	97,106
Mahidol	163	Gly → Ser	II	100	40	Thai, Cambodian	233
Plymouth	163	Gly → Asp	I	103	48	English	Town et al, unpublished
Chinese-3	165	Asn → Asp	II			Chinese	234
Santa Maria	181	Asp → Val	II	98	16	Costa Rican	235
	126	Asn → Asp					
Mediterranean	188	Ser → Phe	II	100	23	Mediterranean, indian	106,236
Coimbra	198	Arg → Cys	II	100	7	Mediterranean	237
Santiago	198	Arg → Pro	I			Chilean	238
Sibari	212	Met → Val	III	100	31	Italian	221
Minnesota	213	Val → Leu	I	95	88	USA—white	239
Harilaou	216	Phe → Leu	I	100		Greek	110
Mexico City	227	Arg → Gln	III	110		Mexican	238
A−	227	Arg → Leu	III	110		USA—black	111
	126	Asn → Asp					
Stonybrook	242–243	Δ Gly, Thr	I				Beutler et al, unpublished
Wayne	257	Arg → Gly	I	107	78		240
Chinese-1	279	Thr → Ser	II			Chinese	241
Seattle	282	Asp → His	III	80	20	European	108
Montalbano	285	Arg → His	III	93	49	Italian	191
Viangchan	291	Val → Met	III	100	105	Laotian	240
Kalyan	317	Glu → Lys	III	75	105	Indian	116
A−	323	Leu → Pro	III	110		USA—black, Spanish	111
	126	Asn → Asp					
Chatham	335	Ala → Thr	III	100	60	Indian	106
Chinese	342	Leu → Phe	III	91	65	Chinese	232
Ierapetra	353	Pro → Ser	II			Greek	238
Loma Linda	363	Asn → Lys	I	98	70	USA—Mexican	239
Tomah	385	Cys → Arg	I				114
Iowa	386	Lys → Glu	I	100	65	USA-white	114
Guadalajara	387	Arg → Cys	I	100	36	Mexican	238
Mount Sinai	387	Arg → Cys	I				Vlachos et al, unpublished
	126	Asn → Asp					
Beverly Hills	387	Arg → His	I	95	41	Italian	114
Nashville	393	Arg → His	I	100	87	USA	239
Alhambra	394	Val → Leu	I	96	55	Finnish, Swedish	238
Puerto Limon	398	Glu → Lys	I	98	32	Costarican	235
Riverside	410	Gly → Cys	I	100	326	German, English	114
Japan	410	Gly → Asp	I			Japanese	239

(continued)

TABLE 58-7. *(Continued)*

Name	Amino Acid Number	Amino Acid Replacement	Class	Electrophoretic Mobility	K_m of G6P (μM)	Population	References
Tokyo	416	Glu → Lys	I	90	65	Japanese	242
Atlanta-I	428	Tyr → Stop	I				Beutler et al, unpublished
Pawnee	439	Arg → Pro	I	103	50	USA—Northern European	238
Telte	440	Leu → Phe	I	100		Italian	Busuttil et al, unpublished
Santiago de Cuba	447	Gly → Arg	I	80	50	Cuban	106
Cassano	449	Gln → His	II	93	14	Italian	221
Maewo	454	Arg → Cys	II	105	8	Polynesian/Filipino	243
Andalus	454	Arg → His	I	100	14	Spanish	112
Canton	459	Arg → Leu	II	105	28	Chinese	244
Cosenza	459	Arg → Pro	II	100	27	Italian	221
Kaiping	463	Arg → His	II	100	40	Chinese	245
Campinas	488	Gly → Val	I			Brazilian	Baronciani et al, unpublished

(Modified from Vulliamy TJ, Beutler E, Luzzato L. Variants of glucose-6-phosphate dehydrogenase are due to missense mutations spread throughout the coding region of the gene. Hum Mutat 1993;2:159)

30 years ago.[118,119] Since then, additional data have consistently corroborated the geographic evidence in the sense that G6PD deficiency has been found at polymorphic frequencies only in populations who are living or have been living for generations in areas where malaria is endemic.

Several apparent discrepancies are easy to explain. In Southern Europe, G6PD deficiency is common, and there is no malaria, but malaria has been eradicated only over the last two to three generations. In North America, there is no malaria, but the prevalence of G6PD deficiency in this continent is entirely accounted for by migrations that have taken place in relatively recent historical times. Conversely, G6PD deficiency is not found at polymorphic frequency in any Native American population. Malaria, which is now endemic in parts of Central and South America, however, is thought to have been imported to those areas in relatively recent times—another scourge of the slave trade.

An overall geographic correlation cannot be regarded by itself as proof of the malaria hypothesis. Additional and compelling evidence has been reviewed elsewhere.[120]

Micromapping. Detailed analysis of the prevalence of G6PD deficiency in relatively narrow geographic areas has consistently shown a good correlation between the frequency of G6PD deficiency and the intensity of malaria transmission, for instance, in East Africa,[119] Papua New Guinea,[121] Sardinia,[122] and Greece.[123] In Sardinia and Greece, the evidence is strengthened by the fact that the population is genetically relatively homogeneous in these areas. Thus, it was possible to use the Wahlund variance of *Gd*− compared with that of other genes as a measure of the likelihood that natural selection intervened.[124]

Convergent Evolution Is Suggested by the Genetic Heterogeneity of Polymorphic G6PD Variants. If G6PD deficiency had spread only by migrations of people and by genetic drift, the same mutant would be found everywhere. Instead, different variants are found to be polymorphic in different parts of the world. This indicates that diverse point mutations must have arisen independently and then spread centrifugally to establish themselves at polymorphic frequencies—a good example of convergent microevolution in the human species. In this respect, the G6PD deficiency polymorphism is more reminiscent of the highly heterogeneous thalassemia system than of the unique mutation of hemoglobin S. In some cases, thanks to the coexistence of silent polymorphisms with mutations causing G6PD deficiency, a true evolutionary history can be outlined.[125,126] At the moment, among the variants most extensively investigated, it appears likely that G6PD A− is relatively recent,[126] whereas G6PD Mediterranean may be ancient. It is widespread[15,60,120,127] and has been found as far East as India[128] and as far West as Portugal.[113]

Clinical Studies

Studies of malaria in the field yield ambiguous data when its prevalence or the rate of parasitemia is compared between normal and G6PD-deficient males or in subjects of both sexes.[129–132] In the single study in which females heterozygous for G6PD deficiency (GdB/GdA−) were rigorously classified (by a combination of a cytochemical test, a quantitative assay, and electrophoretic analysis), a significantly lower *P falciparum* parasitemia was observed.[72,133] This may be crucial for survival because parasitemia is an important determinant of malaria mortality. Thus, any factor that reduces parasitemia may prevent the attainment of high levels that become life-threatening. This finding is consonant with other examples of balanced polymorphism associated with heterozygote advantage, but it *appears* different because the gene concerned is X-linked, and therefore only females can be heterozygous. At the same time, the finding is somewhat paradoxical because it means that having only a proportion of G6PD-deficient red cells (due to X inactivation) is more protective against malaria than having only G6PD-deficient red cells (as in hemizygous males). More field studies need to be carried out in malaria-endemic areas on heterozygotes for G6PD A− and other G6PD-deficient variants because rigorous identification of heterozygotes would be easier using a DNA-based methodology. One study revealed underrepresentation of heterozygotes for G6PD deficiency in a group of children with cerebral malaria in Nigeria.[134]

Mechanism of Protection

The most striking result of a quantitative analysis of malaria parasites in the blood of heterozygotes for G6PD deficiency is the excess of parasites in the normal red cells when compared with the deficient red cells of the mosaic. Because this result is internally controlled (the test cells and the control cells are within the same individual, thanks to mosaicism), it appears that, other things being equal and when given an option, the parasite prefers G6PD-normal red cells. From the in vivo data, however, it was not possible to decide whether this is due to (1) decreased invasion of G6PD-deficient red cells, (2) impaired development of the parasite in these cells, or (3) accelerated removal of parasitized G6PD-deficient red cells. Moreover, the analysis was complicated by the age-dependent nature of G6PD activity, whereby the youngest G6PD-deficient red cells might have been misclassifed as normal.

The Intraerythrocytic Development of *P falciparum* Is Impaired in G6PD-Deficient Red Cells. Once a continuous culture system for *P falciparum* was developed by Trager and Jensen, it became possible to test directly, by controlled in vitro experiments, whether the G6PD genotype of red cells affected their ability to play host to the parasite. Several groups reported that, in G6PD-deficient red cells, invasion by *P falciparum* was normal, but intracellular growth (ie, the process of maturation and schizogony) was impaired.[46,135–138] In some studies, however, the difference was apparent only when the cultures were subjected to oxidative stress.[139] The preferential development of parasites in G6PD-normal as opposed to G6PD-deficient red cells is in keeping with previous evidence obtained in vivo.[140]

***P falciparum* Can Adapt to G6PD-Deficient Red Cells.** The most likely explanation for the inhibition of parasite growth in G6PD-deficient red cells is that the abnormal environment causes oxidative injury to the parasite. Why then are hemizygous or homozygous G6PD-deficient people not protected as well or better than heterozygotes? Further culture experiments have led to the suggestion that the coexistence of two different red cell populations in heterozygotes may be responsible for their relative resistance to malaria.[141–143] Parasites that have survived passage through G6PD-deficient red cells become able to grow normally in this type of host cell after several cycles, explaining why hemizygotes and homozygotes are not protected. This process, which has been described as *adaptation*, is hindered when parasites cycle again through G6PD-normal red cells, offering an explanation for the lower parasitemia in heterozygotes.

***P falciparum* Expresses Its Own G6PD.** Experiments aiming to clarify the mechanism of adaptation revealed the presence, in G6PD-deficient red cells, of a G6PD species distinctly different from red cell G6PD, which must be of parasite origin. This enzyme has been partially purified and characterized,[144] and its presence has been revealed in both G6PD-deficient and G6PD-normal red cells.[145] Thus, the hypothesis that adaptation was mediated by turning on the parasite G6PD gene, which would be turned off in normal cells, does not appear to be supported, and the mechanism of adaptation remains to be elucidated.

The findings summarized previously leave little doubt that the G6PD-deficiency polymorphism is balanced by malaria selection. At the same time, the mechanism of this process is not yet fully explained. The most significant clue is that in vivo protection against malaria is a prerogative of heterozygotes. Mathematic models in which selective advantage is taken to be confined to heterozygous females are consistent with equilibrium frequencies of the *Gd−* gene of the order observed in several human populations.[146]

CLINICAL MANIFESTATIONS OF G6PD DEFICIENCY

G6PD Deficiency–Associated Acute Hemolytic Anemia

The Steady State: Very-Low-Grade Hemolysis

In view of the large number of people who carry a G6PD deficiency gene, it is fortunate that most remain clinically asymptomatic throughout their lifetime. Of those who develop a hemolytic attack, most recover uneventfully. From the clinical point of view, the demarcation between the asymptomatic steady state and the hemolytic attack is sharp. During the steady state, the clinical examination of G6PD-deficient people is entirely negative. Hematologic investigations, including hemoglobin and red cell indices, red cell morphology, reticulocyte count, serum bilirubin, and serum haptoglobin, are also entirely normal. The only way to discover their red cell abnormality, other than a G6PD assay, is to carry out a ^{51}Cr-labeled red cell survival study. Some such studies, carried out in the *absence* of overt hemolysis in G6PD-deficient subjects, have revealed a half-life of 90 to 100 days[147] with some variants, but an entirely normal red cell survival with others (eg, G6PD [A−][148]). In view of the other normal parameters mentioned, the pathophysiologic state of most G6PD-deficient people can best be described as one of very-low-grade, fully compensated hemolysis. Although this must mean that their erythropoietic bone marrow activity is greater than normal, it is not possible to pinpoint any adverse effect of this situation. For instance, unlike other chronic hemolytic disorders, such as sickle cell anemia and hereditary spherocytosis, G6PD-deficient people do not become folate deficient as a result of their presumably increased requirement for folic acid.

Hemolytic Crisis

In most cases, when a G6PD-deficient patient presents with anemia and jaundice, it is possible to identify an exogenous agent that is responsible for the episode.

Inciting Factors. Perhaps because of the historical antecedent whereby primaquine sensitivity was the phrase designating acute hemolytic anemia in people who subsequently turned out to have G6PD deficiency, the general perception is that drugs (Table 58-8) are the most common triggers of hemolysis. In fact, there are three types of triggers: drugs, infections, and fava beans. Large studies on the impact of drugs are lacking, and in many cases, potentially hemolytic drugs are administered in the context of infection. Thus, it is likely that in the past hemolysis was sometimes attributed to drugs used for treating infection when it should have been blamed on the infection itself. Perhaps the best characterized example is lobar pneumonia.[98] It has been suggested that the mechanism by which bacterial infection causes hemolysis may be the release of peroxides during phagocytosis of bacteria by granulocytes.[149] It is more difficult to imagine a mechanism by which viral infection can trigger hemolysis, but this has been documented in the course of viral hepatitis.[150] In areas where fava beans are widely consumed, their ingestion is the most common cause of acute hemolytic anemia associated with G6PD deficiency. Diabetic ketoacidosis is another trigger of hemolysis, but this is rare. A G6PD-deficient homozygous woman (GdA−/GdA−) was studied who also had renal tubular acidosis and evidence of hemolysis, which appeared to correlate with poor control of acidosis.

A question of practical importance is whether the hemolytic risk associated with any particular triggering factor is a function of individual G6PD variants. This presumption

TABLE 58-8. Drugs To Be Avoided in G6PD Deficiency*

ANTIMALARIALS

Primaquine [people with the African A− variant may take it at reduced dosage, 15 mg/d or 45 mg twice weekly under surveillance]

Pamaquine

Chloroquine (may be used under surveillance when required for prophylaxis or treatment of malaria)

SULFONAMIDES AND SULFONES

Sulfanilamide

Sulfapyridine

Sulfadimidine

Sulfacetamide (Albucid)

Sulfafurazone (Gantrisin)

Salicylazosulfapyridine (Salazopyrin)

Dapsone*

Sulfoxone†

Glucosulfone sodium (Promin)

Septrin

OTHER ANTIBACTERIAL COMPOUNDS

Nitrofurans—nitrofurantoin, furazolidone, nitrofurazone

[Nalidixic acid]

Chloramphenicol

p-Aminosalicylic acid

ANALGESICS

Acetylsalicylic acid (aspirin): moderate doses can be used

Acetophenetidin (Phenacetin)

Safe alternative: Paracetamol

ANTHELMINTICS

β-Naphthol

Stibophan

Niridazole

MISCELLANEOUS

Vitamin K analogues (1 mg of menaphthone can be given to babies)

Naphthalene† (moth balls)

Probenecid

Dimercaprol (BAL)

Methylene blue

Arsine†

Phenylhydrazine†

Acetylphenylhydrazine†

Toluidine blue

Mepacrine

* Drugs given in bold print should be avoided by people with all forms of G6PD deficiency; drugs in normal print should be avoided, in addition, by G6PD-deficient people of Mediterranean, Middle Eastern, and Asian origin; items in normal print and within square brackets apply only to people with the African A− variant.

† These drugs or chemicals may cause hemolysis in normal people if given in large doses. Many other drugs may produce hemolysis in particular people.

(WHO Working Group. Glucose-6-phosphate dehydrogenase deficiency. Bull WHO 1989;67:601)

is entirely reasonable in view of the vast genetic heterogeneity of G6PD deficiency. For instance, it is assumed that the risk is generally greater with G6PD Mediterranean than with G6PD A−. Objective evidence, however, for this pharmacogenetic variant-specific heterogeneity is relatively scanty. The best example is probably favism: in the past G6PD A− subjects were thought to be immune, but it is now clear that they are not.[151]

As for drugs, primaquine causes hemolysis regularly, but aspirin causes it only sometimes.[152] It can only be hypothesized that genetic or acquired factors affecting the metabolism of the drug may be responsible.[153,154]

Clinical Features. The course of a drug-induced acute hemolytic attack was well characterized in a series of experiments in the late 1950s on human volunteers. These experiments, although impeccably conducted and fortunately free of long-term consequences, probably would not have obtained Ethics Committee clearance today. When given primaquine at the dose of 30 mg/d, G6PD-deficient (A−) men begin to experience malaise on day 2 or 3; this is sometimes associated with more or less profound weakness and abdominal or lumbar pain. Usually on day 3 or 4, the telltale signs of jaundice and dark urine make their appearance. This is designated as the *acute hemolytic phase;* its intensity and duration depend to some extent on the nature and dosage of the drug and on the type of G6PD variant and, on the average, it lasts about 1 week. In most cases, the hemolytic attack, even if severe, is self-limited and tends to resolve spontaneously.[155] In the absence of additional or preexisting pathology, the bone marrow response is prompt and effective. Depending on the proportion of red cells that are destroyed (reflected in the severity of the anemia), the hemoglobin level may be back to normal in 3 to 6 weeks (recovery phase). The most serious threat in adults is the development of acute renal failure (this is exceedingly rare in children). It is not clear why this should take place only in a small proportion of patients. The most likely explanation is that they have preexisting subclinical renal damage. In such situations, hemodialysis may be required until renal function recovers. After a hemolytic attack, a situation of relative resistance to further drug challenge has been well characterized with G6PD A− (presumably thanks to the considerable proportion in the circulation of red cells that are young and therefore have a higher G6PD level). This is *not* applicable, however, to G6PD Mediterranean,[156] for instance, and it cannot be assumed to apply to others.

Laboratory Findings. Anemia varies from moderate to extremely severe (hemoglobin values of 4 g/dL or less have been recorded). In the absence of other preexisting hematologic abnormalities, the anemia is normocytic and normochromic. The blood smear shows anisocytosis, polychromasia, and other features associated with acute hemolysis, including spherocytes, but it is otherwise unspecific. In severe cases, however, the poikilocytosis is more marked, with bizarre forms and red cells that appear to have an uneven distribution of hemoglobin within them. Although some of these appearances are probably smearing artifacts, electron micrographic evidence suggests that, in some of the cells, opposing surfaces of the membrane have become cross-linked[157] ("blister cells"; Fig. 58-7). The most characteristic poikilocytes are the blister cells, cells in which the cell margin appears dented, as though a portion has been plucked out or bitten away ("bite" cells; see Fig. 58-7). Supravital staining with methyl violet reveals the presence of Heinz bodies consisting of precipitates of denatured hemoglobin (Fig. 58-8) and cells in which, as noted previously, the hemoglobin is excluded from a portion of the cell. It is important to do a methyl violet preparation promptly because Heinz bodies may disappear from the peripheral blood within 24 hours, as they are "pinched off" by the spleen[158] (possibly giving rise to the bite cells). Because many of the red cells thus damaged undergo intravascular hemolysis, haptoglobin is reduced to the point of being undetectable. In severe cases, it is possible to demonstrate free hemoglobin in the plasma (the somewhat incongruous term of *hemoglobinemia* is used to describe this finding in one word). The white blood cell count may be elevated, with predominance of granulocytes. The platelet

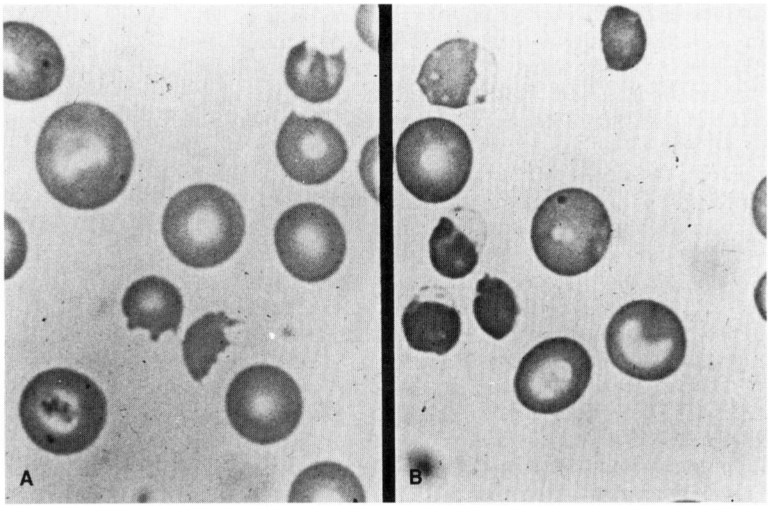

FIGURE 58-7. Peripheral blood smear showing "bite" cells (**A**) and "blister" cells (**B**). A portion of the blister cells is empty of hemoglobin: only a faint outline of the membrane is visible. Bite cells and blister cells appear during severe acute hemolytic crisis in G6PD-deficient people. Between such episodes, the blood smear often appears normal.

count may be normal, increased, or moderately decreased. The unconjugated bilirubin is elevated, but the liver enzymes are usually normal. The dark urine tests strongly positive for blood. It is easy to demonstrate that this is due to hemoglobinuria rather than hematuria because, after centrifugation, the supernatant is as dark as before, and in the sediment, there are few if any red cells.

Favism

Clinical Features. Favism is a dramatic event and, although no age group is spared, it is most often observed in children. A few hours after ingesting fava beans, the child may become fractious and irritable or subdued and even lethargic. Within 24 to 48 hours, fever may develop (up to 38°C), and this may be associated with nausea, abdominal pain, and diarrhea and rarely with vomiting. In striking contrast to these relatively nonspecific symptoms, the patient or relatives observe, within 6 to 24 hours, the telltale and frightening discoloration of the urine. It usually is reported as dark, red, brown, or black or as "passing blood instead of water." At about the same time, jaundice becomes obvious. Physical examination may reveal little more than the signs corresponding to the above symptoms. The child is invariably pale and tachycardiac. In severe cases, there may be evidence of hypovolemic shock or, less likely, of heart failure. The spleen is usually moderately enlarged, and the liver may be also enlarged; either or both may be tender.

The subsequent clinical course depends on the severity of the attack, particularly on what proportion of the patient's red cells have been destroyed. With severe anemia and hypotension, survival may depend on blood transfusion; in milder cases, spontaneous recovery is the rule.

Cause of Hemolysis in Favism. The specificity of favism is extraordinary: the syndrome is caused only in G6PD-deficient people and only by *Vicia faba*. Although there have been claims for acute reactions to peas (*pisismo* in Italian), there are no convincing reports that these were hemolytic attacks. Another recurrent theme in what could be referred to as the favism lore is that it can be triggered by inhalation of the plant flower pollen. I have not obtained satisfactory evidence of a hemolytic attack begun through this port of entry. Thus, although patients must be warned that an attack may recur any time they consume fava beans, they can be reassured that other beans are safe, as are walks in the countryside.

Extensive studies on the components of fava beans responsible for hemolysis have led to the identification of vicine and convicine, two β-glycosides that have as aglycones the substituted pyrimidines divicine and isouramil.[159] These compounds, in the course of their autooxidation, produce free radicals, which in turn oxidize GSH, thus activating the chain reaction of events leading to hemolysis.[160]

Fava beans have been used as staple food for centuries and perhaps millennia precisely in areas where G6PD deficiency is common. A discussion of the possible reasons cannot be given here, but fava beans combine a relatively high nutritional value, a relatively high protein content, and a high level of palatability with a great ease of cultivation because, like other leguminous plants, they require little or no fertilization. From the agricultural point of view, it would be desirable to develop *Vicia faba* mutants that do not have high levels of the dangerous glycosides, but this has not yet been done. These substances may serve as a natural defense of the plant against pests, or they may play a more subtle role in the plant's metabolism.

Fava Bean Ingestion Without Acute Hemolytic Anemia

Role of the Bean. An intriguing feature of favism is its considerably erratic character. It is estimated that, at least in adults, ingestion of fava beans does not trigger acute hemolytic anemia in more than 25% of cases, and even in the same person, favism may occur on one occasion but not on another.[161] Practitioners in endemic areas give ex-

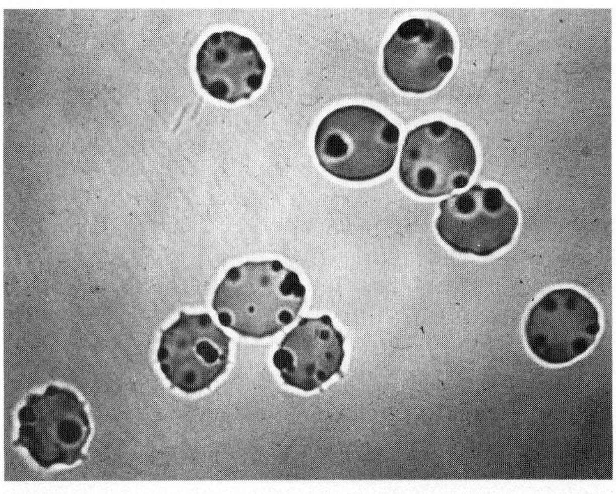

FIGURE 58-8. Heinz bodies in erythrocytes from a G6PD-deficient person. These particles of denatured hemoglobin, which adhere to the red cell membrane and stain with basic dyes, are seen in large numbers after an acute hemolytic crisis.

amples of patients who had their first recognized attacks in their 60s. This feature of favism has practical consequences because, unless it is clearly explained to the public, it may affect the credibility of the physician who advises a patient against recurrence of favism! The reasons for this erratic character are not entirely clear. One obvious factor must be the dosage, that is, the amount of fava beans ingested in relation to body mass, which presumably accounts for the higher rate of favism in children. Another factor must be food processing. Raw fava beans are more likely to cause favism than cooked, frozen, or canned fava beans. A third, and possibly the most important, factor is the maturity of the beans because the young, small beans have higher levels of glucosides. Finally, it is possible that β-glycosidases, present in varying amounts both in the beans and in the intestinal mucosa of the consumer, may play an important role in determining the amount and rate of release of active aglycones.[161]

Role of the* Gd− *Mutation. If factors related to the fava beans are important in determining an attack of favism and its severity, one might expect the type of G6PD-deficient variant in the person ingesting them also to be important. Because early reports on the clinical features of favism and on its epidemiology have come mainly from Southern Italy, Greece, and the Middle East, and because in all these areas, G6PD deficiency has been largely characterized as Mediterranean, this variant has come to be regarded as almost specifically associated with favism. However, favism is common, for instance, in Singapore, where the underlying variants are not always Mediterranean. The occurrence of clinical favism with the African variant A− (which was held as *not* susceptible to favism) was documented.[151] In this respect, it is curious to note that the variant G6PD Betica, originally discovered in patients with favism[127] and previously reported as polymorphic in Spain, turns out to be one and the same as G6PD A−.[111] In a recent carried out in Algeria (D. Nafa, et al, unpublished report), seven different G6PD variants were observed in subjects with G6PD deficiency ascertained because of an attack of favism. Thus, the present evidence suggests that this clinical manifestation can be triggered, under appropriate circumstances, in any G6PD-deficient person. The reason is probably that, whereas subtle kinetic differences among different G6PD variants are important in the steady state, when the rate of operation of the PPP is low, the oxidative action of divicine and isouramil is so drastic that it overrides such differences easily. Once the PPP is maximally stimulated, the only limiting factor for its rate of operation becomes the amount of G6PD activity, which is forced to function at V_{max} level. Thus, it is likely (although not proved) that a G6PD A−–deficient person, with 12% residual activity, needs to eat more fava beans than a G6PD Mediterranean–deficient person, with 3% residual activity. Eventually, the red cell GSH is depleted, and intravascular hemolysis follows.

Diagnosis

The importance of recognizing hemoglobinuria cannot be overemphasized because the presence of this sign restricts considerably the differential diagnosis of hemolytic anemia in general. With a history of fava bean ingestion and the finding of hemoglobinuria (clearly reported or directly observed), the diagnosis is almost always straightforward, and it can be made confidently even before obtaining the final proof that the patient is G6PD deficient. If hemoglobinuria has already subsided, and the history is uncertain, one is faced instead with the much wider differential diagnosis of acute hemolytic anemia. The negative direct antiglobulin test militates against autoimmune hemolytic anemia. In endemic areas, it is important to exclude malaria infection and the much rarer babesiosis. In the hemolytic–uremic syndrome, the red cell morphology is different, and there is evidence of impaired renal function. In all cases, the demonstration of G6PD deficiency is conclusive, and in uncertain cases, it is crucial.

Neonatal Jaundice

Glucose-6-phosphate dehydrogenase activity in the red cells of newborns is somewhat higher than in red cells of adults. Therefore, it may come as a surprise that G6PD deficiency is associated with neonatal jaundice. The word *association* is chosen advisedly because not every G6PD-deficient baby becomes jaundiced after birth: however, numerous studies have shown that the risk of developing neonatal jaundice is much greater in G6PD-deficient than in G6PD-normal newborns.[162–164]

Clinical Features

Neonatal jaundice related to G6PD deficiency differs from the classic Rh-related neonatal jaundice in two main respects: (1) it is rarely present at birth, and the peak incidence of clinical onset is between days 2 and 3[165]; and (2) there is more jaundice than anemia, and the anemia is rarely severe.[166] For this reason, the terms hemolytic disease of the newborn and neonatal jaundice cannot be regarded as interchangeable, at least in the context of G6PD deficiency.

The severity of G6PD-related neonatal jaundice varies enormously from being subclinical to imposing the threat of kernicterus if not treated. Because not *all* G6PD-deficient babies are jaundiced, it is likely that the same factors that cause it to develop may, if more extreme, make it severe. There has been an active search for an additional factor that may cause neonatal jaundice when combined with G6PD deficiency.[167] Marked differences in the incidence of neonatal jaundice have been demonstrated among various Greek islands.[168] Although the study was carried out in the search for an additional genetic factor, thought to be autosomal, it is possible instead that there may be an environmental factor that is different in different islands. In support of the latter possibility, work in Nigeria has revealed that G6PD-deficient babies with neonatal jaundice had a significantly higher rate of exposure to naphthalene (used in their bedding and clothing) than G6PD-deficient control babies.[169]

Pathogenesis

As mentioned earlier, not all G6PD-deficient babies develop jaundice. This erratic character is reminiscent of what applies to acute hemolytic anemia–induced by fava beans or other triggering factors. However, this does not mean that the mechanism is the same. Several studies have addressed the question of which other factor, in addition to G6PD deficiency, is required for the development of neonatal jaundice. One possibility was that, in view of the marked genetic heterogeneity of G6PD deficiency, neonatal jaundice was the prerogative of some babies but not of others. The finding that neonatal jaundice is prevalent in widely remote parts of the world—such as Sardinia,[165] Nigeria,[164] and Malacca[170]—does not support this notion. Alternatively, because fetal red cells differ from those produced after birth in many ways, one might postulate that some newborns have an addition, transient, developmentally related enzyme deficiency that causes neonatal jaundice in G6PD-deficient babies. In this respect, studies have been carried out on glutathione peroxidase, glutathione reductase, and superoxide dismutase, but with negative results.[167]

Partly because of these negative results, attention has been directed away from red cells and toward a hepatic origin of G6PD deficiency–related neonatal jaundice. It is notable that there is a considerable dissociation between hyperbilirubinemia and anemia in G6PD-deficient babies. In one series, there was no difference in the distribution of hematocrit values in the cord blood and on day 3 between jaundiced and nonjaundiced G6PD-deficient babies.[166,171] One wonders therefore whether neonatal hyperbilirubinemia may result from expression of G6PD deficiency in hepatocytes,[172] although a specific biochemical mechanism has not been formulated.

It may be heuristically useful to consider two different types of neonatal jaundice associated with G6PD deficiency: (1) a more common type, best visualized as a marked exaggeration of "physiologic jaundice," that is not greatly influenced by the environment and that may result from G6PD deficiency being expressed in the liver; and (2) a more rare, frankly hemolytic type, which can be visualized as acute hemolytic anemia occurring in a newborn who was exposed to one of the same agents that could cause acute hemolytic anemia even in adults,[173] such as a drug, infection, or some particular local habit (eg, the extensive use of naphthalene [mothballs or camphor balls] in some nurseries).

Management

The management of neonatal jaundice due to G6PD deficiency does not differ from that recommended for other causes. Thus, mild cases do not require treatment; intermediate cases require phototherapy[174]; and severe cases require exchange transfusion treatment, just as in neonatal jaundice due to classic hemolytic disease of the newborn.[175]

G6PD Deficiency and Sickle Cell Anemia

Because the geographic distribution of the β^S globin gene and of the *Gd*− gene overlap extensively, especially in Africa and in people of African descent, one can expect to find the two red cell disorders to coexist frequently. Because the two genes are not genetically linked, the frequency of people having both is the product of the two gene frequencies. For instance, if in a particular population the frequency of hemoglobin AS heterozygotes is 25%, and the frequency of G6PD deficiency in males is 20%, one would predict that one fifth of the AS heterozygotes (ie, 5% of the entire male population) also would be G6PD deficient. Despite some early claims to the contrary,[176] this is found to be the case in a stable population.[177] Because heterozygosity for β^S and heterozygosity for *Gd*− both protect against malaria, it is intriguing to consider whether females with this particular genotypic combination have greater protection than either of the two single heterozygotes. Thus far, such an additive or synergistic effect has not been demonstrated.[133]

A separate question is whether the combination of G6PD deficiency—an asymptomatic condition in the steady state—with *homozygous* sickle cell anemia affects the course of this condition, a serious hemolytic disease even in the steady state. Again, it was claimed that G6PD deficiency ameliorates the course of sickle cell anemia.[176] But a study carried out in Nigeria already in 1975 failed to substantiate this claim.[178] The steady-state hemoglobin level in G6PD-deficient males with sickle cell anemia was slightly lower than in G6PD-normal males with sickle cell anemia. A more recent study from the United States confirmed these findings.[179] We can also ask the reverse question, namely whether sickle cell anemia affects the manifestations of G6PD deficiency. At the biochemical level, the answer is yes because the high reticulocytosis and the globally young red cell population of these patients causes a marked increase in the G6PD activity of G6PD-deficient red cells, especially of those with the A− variant—so much so that these patients are easily misclassified as G6PD normal if an appropriate technique is not used. At the clinical level, one might expect in theory that this relative increase in enzyme level would prevent the development or limit the severity of acute hemolytic anemia consequent to G6PD deficiency. This is difficult to assess in practice because the interaction of infection, drugs, and preexisting anemia is too complex. If the degree of drug-induced hemolysis is less in a patient with sickle cell anemia, however, this is likely to be overridden by the fact that acute intravascular hemolysis would take place on the background of the chronic extravascular hemolysis of sickle cell anemia. Severe exacerbation of anemia has been observed in patients with sickle cell anemia who are also G6PD deficient,[180] it is probably prudent to assume that this combination, if anything, has the potential to increase the clinical load of sickle cell anemia.

Congenital Nonspherocytic Hemolytic Anemia

Clinical Features

In contrast to most G6PD-deficient subjects, who have minimal and subclinical hemolysis in the steady state, a small minority of G6PD-deficient people have a degree of hemolysis that is easily diagnosed by conventional methods and that is sufficiently pronounced to cause them to be anemic. This group of patients is clinically heterogeneous for reasons which are explained later, and therefore it is not possible to describe any level of expression of this condition as being typical.

The patient is almost invariably male and in general presents because of unexplained jaundice. Frequently, the onset is at birth, and a diagnosis is made of neonatal jaundice, which may be severe enough to require exchange transfusion. Unfortunately, anemia recurs, and the jaundice fails to clear completely; this is often the reason for further investigation. In many cases, however, neonatal jaundice may be forgotten, and the patient is only reinvestigated much later in life, for instance, because of gallstones in a child or in a young adult. The severity of anemia ranges in different patients from borderline to transfusion dependent. The anemia is usually normochromic but somewhat macrocytic because a large proportion of reticulocytes (up to 20% or more) cause an increased mean corpuscular volume and a shifted, wider than normal red cell size distribution curve. The red cell morphology is mostly not characteristic, and for this reason, it is referred to in the negative as being *nonspherocytic*. The bone marrow is normoblastic, unless the increased requirement of folic acid associated with the high red cell turnover has caused it to become megaloblastic. There is chronic hyperbilirubinemia, decreased haptoglobin, and increased lactate dehydrogenase. Hemoglobinuria is rare, but hemosiderinuria may be detected sometimes. The spleen is usually moderately enlarged in small children and subsequently may increase in size sufficiently to cause mechanical discomfort, hypersplenism, or both.

Pathophysiology

The clinical picture just described is obviously different from that of G6PD deficiency–related acute hemolytic anemia. It is more reminiscent, instead, of the chronic hemolysis seen in hereditary spherocytosis. Even in severe cases, it is different from thalassemia major because there is no evidence of ineffective erythropoiesis and the destruction is limited to mature circulating red cells. The fact that there is no hemoglobinuria, at least in the steady state, suggests that the hemolysis is mainly extravascular and that its mechanism is different from that of the acute hemolytic variants. Studies of red cell membrane proteins have revealed the presence of high-molecular-weight aggregates,[181] consisting largely of spectrin in CNSHA patients, which have not been found in asymptomatic G6PD-deficient subjects. These findings suggest that the reductive potential of residual G6PD is adequate in the steady state in acute hemolytic variants, whereas in CNSHA, continuous oxidation of sulfydryl groups takes place, followed by irreversible changes in the configuration of membrane proteins. This does not mean that the red cells of patients with severe G6PD deficiency are not vulnerable to acute oxidative damage of hemoglobin as well. The same agents that can cause acute hemolytic anemia in people with the ordinary type of G6PD deficiency can cause severe exacerbations with hemoglobinuria in people with the severe form of G6PD deficiency. The reason that the severity of CNSHA associated with G6PD deficiency is so variable is simply that almost every case is due to a different mutation, and each mutation has a different effect on the stability of the enzyme, its kinetic properties, or both.

Molecular Basis

The course of patients with G6PD deficiency–associated CNSHA is so different from that of most people with G6PD deficiency, who may have the occasional episode of acute hemolytic anemia (no matter how severe), that it appeared highly likely from the phenotype that the underlying genetic basis would be also different. Biochemical studies quickly confirmed this inference. In the early 1960s, characterization of G6PD from rare patients with CNSHA revealed properties that were different from those of the already known polymorphic variants (like G6PD Mediterranean and G6PD A–). Thus, new names, such as G6PD Oklahoma and G6PD Chicago, were coined to designate these new variants. But why would a particular variant cause severe rather than mild hemolysis? In principle, one can visualize two types of reason: *quantitative* and *qualitative*. First, *G6PD deficiency in CNSHA could be simply more extreme*. It stands to reason that if 20% of the normal enzyme activity is adequate for the steady-state requirement of red cell metabolism, 2% may not be adequate. This obvious quantitative consideration plays a role because the G6PD variants associated with CNSHA (class I in Table 58-6) have always represented less than 10% of the normal activity. However, the reverse is not true. Although many of the variants that are *not* associated with CNSHA have more than 10% of normal activity (class III), many others have less (class II), just like CNSHA variants. This clearly indicates that, second, *the molecular properties of individual variants are important determinants of clinical expression*.

Which properties, other than the level of activity, are most important has been keenly debated. Because what we call the *level of enzyme activity* is a V_{max} measurement, the best candidates are properties that influence the activity below V_{max}: the substrate affinities or the effects of natural activators and inhibitors. Because NADP and NADPH are important regulators of G6PD activity in normal cells, one might imagine that mutations causing changes in the K_m of NADP and in the K_i of NADPH would have pronounced pathological effects, and this might be true in some cases. A high K_m of NADP, however, by decreasing the rate of conversion of NADP to NADPH, allows the NADP concentration to rise, thus producing an increase in the rate of the same reaction. The reverse is true if the K_i of NADPH is increased. As a result of this sort of buffering effect, changes in the affinity for these two ligands are to a considerable extent self-defeating. By contrast, an analysis of the K_m values of G6P shows that these are significantly increased in a substantial proportion of class I variants compared with the values in class II and III variants (in which the K_m of G6P is frequently *decreased*). Thus, to a first approximation, it appears that NADP and NADPH have their main role in regulating the physiology of G6PD. The affinity for G6P, instead, has been selected for the pathophysiology of the steady-state activity of the PPP in red cells.

Diagnosis

The diagnosis of G6PD deficiency as such is discussed later, but a special problem in relation to CNSHA is to establish firmly the causal link between the G6PD deficiency and hemolytic anemia. If the patient is, say, of Swedish ancestry or of Japanese ancestry, the link is taken for granted. This is generally justified, given the rarity of G6PD deficiency in these populations. On the other hand, if the patient is from a population in which G6PD deficiency is common, its presence in a patient with CNSHA might be a mere coincidence, and the cause of the CNSHA might be something else altogether. In these cases, it becomes essential to characterize the G6PD of the patient because if it is a common variant, known to be asymptomatic in other subjects, it can be exonerated. If it is a new unique variant, however, it is likely to be the culprit.

PATHOPHYSIOLOGY

When an enzyme is tissue specific, understanding the manifestations of its deficiency is usually rather straightforward. For instance, phenylalanine hydroxylase is mainly expressed in the liver, and this is the basis of phenylketonuria. By contrast, deficiencies of housekeeping enzymes would be expected to affect all tissues of the body, but the clinical manifestations are influenced by where the deficiency causes more damage, although we do not always understand why. For instance, triose phosphate isomerase deficiency and phosphoglycerate kinase deficiency affect all cells, but they cause mainly hemolytic anemia, neuromuscular disease, and brain damage. Because G6PD is also a ubiquitously expressed housekeeping gene, one might expect that G6PD deficiency would be affecting all tissues of the body. Yet, with a few exceptions, G6PD deficiency is essentially a red cell disorder. To some extent, we can now understand why.

G6PD and Red Cell Aging

Compared with most other somatic cells, mature red cells are distinctive in their inability to synthesize protein. In most somatic cells, G6PD is subject to turnover, but in red cells, any G6PD molecule undergoing denaturation or proteolytic breakdown cannot be replaced (this is true of most red cell enzymes).[182] In normal red cells, the decay of G6PD approximates an exponential with a half-life of about 60 days,[183] although it has been claimed to approximate more closely a two-slope curve with a fast breakdown when reticulocytes mature to erythrocytes and a much slower breakdown subsequently.[184] The age dependence of red cell G6PD activity is so characteristic that it almost can be regarded as a marker of red cell age. Normal blood reticulocytes have about five times more activity than the 10%

oldest red cells. Because we know that G6PD is critical to red cell viability, it might be tempting to imagine that aged red cells are removed from the circulation precisely because their G6PD level has become too low. This cannot be so in normal subjects, however, because the level of G6PD even in the oldest cells is higher than the mean level in many G6PD-deficient people. From this analysis, we can infer that there is a threshold level of G6PD activity below which red cells become nonviable. An inevitably approximate estimate may be in the region of 0.1% to 1% of normal[14] if the kinetics of the enzyme are normal—even less if the kinetics of the enzyme are more favorable than normal. Thus, in normal subjects, this threshold is never reached; with common G6PD variants, this threshold is reached only after about 100 days of aging in the circulation. Therefore, the carriers of these variants are hematologically normal in the steady state. With some rare variants of G6PD, this threshold is reached after as few as 10 to 50 days, and therefore they have more or less severe CNSHA.

Mechanism of Hemolytic Crisis

An important and direct pathophysiologic consequence of the marked age dependence of G6PD activity in red cells is that acute hemolytic anemia associated with G6PD-deficiency red cell destruction is an orderly function of red cell age. The oldest red cells with the least G6PD are the first to hemolyze, and the hemolytic process progresses upstream toward the cells with more and more G6PD.[155] As a result, there is a selective enrichment in red cells that, although genetically G6PD deficient, have relatively higher levels of G6PD. This phenomenon can be so marked with certain G6PD variants that patients in the posthemolytic state are found to be relatively refractory to further challenge (the *resistant phase* of the attack). Under these circumstances, ^{51}Cr red cell survival studies show that the half-life is still less than normal, demonstrating that the patient is in a state of compensated hemolysis.[155]

The clinical picture of acute hemolytic anemia associated with G6PD deficiency conveys forcefully the impression that hemolysis results from the action of an exogenous factor on intrinsically abnormal red cells. Hemoglobinemia and hemoglobinuria indicate unambiguously that the hemolysis is at least in part intravascular. To a first approximation, it is easy to visualize the following sequence of events:

1. An oxidative agent causes conversion of GSH to oxidized glutathione.
2. GSH reserve is rapidly depleted due to the limited capacity of G6PD-deficient red cells to regenerate GSH.
3. Once GSH is exhausted, the sulfydryl groups of hemoglobin and probably of other proteins are oxidized to disulfides or sulfoxides.
4. Coarse precipitates of denatured hemoglobin cause irreversible damage to the membrane, and the red cells lyse.

Although GSH depletion is a classic in vitro finding when red cells are challenged, for instance, with acetylphenylhydrazine,[185] not all these steps have been fully documented in vivo. One major difficulty in analyzing the sequential changes that take place in a patient with acute hemolytic anemia from the oxidative attack to the final hemolysis is that red cells sampled from the patient are obviously, at any given stage, those that have not yet hemolyzed. In one careful study, however, it was been demonstrated that in the course of an episode of favism, the first measurable biochemical change is a fall in NADPH, followed by a fall in GSH,[186] in keeping with stages 1 and 2 described earlier. Heinz's bodies are the visible expression of stage 3. Stage 4 is more obscure because we do not know exactly how the membrane is damaged, although studies suggest that binding of hemochromes (arising from hemoglobin denaturation) to band 3 molecules may be one intermediate step.[187,188] Although the diagnostic and pathophysiologic importance of intravascular hemolysis has been emphasized, it is certain that not *all* the hemolysis is intravascular, as witnessed, for instance, by the enlargement of the spleen. It is not difficult to visualize that the most severely damaged red cells hemolyze in the bloodstream without help, whereas less severely damaged red cells are recognized as abnormal by macrophages and undergo extravascular hemolysis in the reticuloendothelial system. This process has been referred to as an example of an "innocent bystander" phenomenon[189] (although the red cells, by virtue of being G6PD deficient, are not that innocent). The role of complement and of of immunoglobulins in extravascular hemolysis of damaged G6PD-deficient red cells mediated by macrophages has been discussed in detail.[161]

Molecular Basis of G6PD Deficiency

In principle, deficiency of G6PD, like that of any other protein, might be due to deletions or to point mutations affecting transcription, processing, or the primary structure. Careful testing of G6PD-deficient cells has uniformly revealed that the enzyme activity, even when severely reduced (sometimes to less than 1% of normal), is never completely absent. This essentially rules out large deletions. Further analysis of enzymic properties of the residual G6PD activity has almost invariably revealed deviations from the properties of the normal enzyme,[14] suggesting that G6PD deficiency is due to structural abnormalities rather than merely to a decrease in number of normal molecules (as would be expected with transcriptional or processing mutants). These predictions have been fully verified because comparison of the DNA sequence of mutant *Gd* genes with the normal gene has revealed, with two exceptions, single point mutations within one of the 12 coding exons.[106,190] It is possible that promoter or splicing mutations exist, but they have not been discovered.

The three exceptions are of considerable interest. The first, G6PD Sunderland, is a 3-base pair deletion, which neatly plucks out one of two neighboring isoleucine codons. Thus, the protein is shortened by a single amino acid. The genesis of the deletion may be related to a short internal repeat. The result is a G6PD variant with marked instability, associated with CNSHA. The other two exceptions are G6PD Santa Maria and G6PD A−. Both are class III variants, and the latter is the common variant in Africa and one of the most common worldwide. These variants have two point mutations: one constant (126 Asn → Asp); the other variable. In G6PD Santa Maria, the second mutation is 181 Asp → Val; in G6PD A−, it is, in at least 90% of cases, 68 Val → Met. Because the first mutation (126 Asn → Asp) is the same found in the nondeficient polymorphic variant G6PD A, one would presume that the second mutation (68 Val → Met) is the one responsible for G6PD deficiency. In fact, this mutation has never been found on its own, suggesting that either it does not exist on its own or that it gives no phenotype. This paradox has been investigated by introducing the two mutations, both separately and in combination, into the normal gene and analyzing their expression in *Escherichia coli*. The results have shown clearly that neither mutation alone causes G6PD deficiency, but the two together do. This is probably the first example in which pathology results from two otherwise harmless mutations that act synergistically when they are in tandem in the same gene.

Changes in the primary structure, that is, substitutions of individual amino acids, can cause G6PD deficiency either by affecting its catalytic function, by decreasing the in vivo stability of the protein, or by both these mechanisms. It is likely that one or the other is the main factor responsible for G6PD deficiency in individual cases. For some variants, an accelerated in vivo breakdown has been demonstrated directly by assaying the activity of G6PD in age-fractionated red cells.[183,191,192] In extreme cases, G6PD deficiency can be visualized simply as resulting from a marked change in the exponential decay constant of the enzyme, where the half-life becomes 10 days or less instead of 50 days. In such cases, the G6PD activity of reticulocytes may be practically normal. In order to demonstrate conclusively a decreased catalytic activity, it is necessary to purify the enzyme to homogeneity, an almost impossible task with severely deficient variants, which are available only in minute quantities from patients' blood samples. In practice, direct measurements of the specific activity of severely deficient variants is only becoming possible now by expression of recombinant human G6PD variants in *E coli*.[51,193]

In summary, and in terms of their biologic significance, we can visualize mutations in the G6PD gene as belonging to three categories:

1. Neutral mutations, like in any other gene. These may or may not become polymorphic, depending on genetic drift and founder effects.
2. Mutations leading to G6PD deficiency that are sufficiently pronounced to cause a problem for *P falciparum*–invading red cells, but not pronounced enough to cause significant hemolysis in the steady state. These have the potential to become polymorphic in a malaria-endemic area.
3. Mutations leading to a qualitatively or quantitatively unacceptably low levels of intracellular activity in the steady state. These cause CNSHA and never become polymorphic.

Mutations of the third group have a further constraint: they must not affect nonerythroid cells too severely, otherwise they would be lethal. Thus, in such mutations, there is probably a strong bias toward unstable ones because they affect red cells much more markedly than other cells. Like other human housekeeping genes we have found so far only those mutations that are compatible with life. An approach to discovering in humans the equivalent of "conditional lethal mutants" in bacteria has not been developed.

Clinical Expression of Different Mutations in the G6PD Gene

The three variants, G6PD A−, G6PD Mediterranean, and G6PD Mahidol are probably the variants for which the clinical manifestations have been best characterized. It is conventionally reported that Mediterranean and Mahidol (class II variants) give more severe manifestations than A− (class III variant). Although this may be true when large series of cases are compared, there is so much overlap among the groups that in an individual case the differences are not relevant with respect to patient management. For instance, whether hemolysis is self-limited depends on the offending agent, on its dose, and on the time course of exposure at least as much as it depends on the G6PD variant involved. Notably, favism has been unambiguously documented with G6PD A− deficiency.[151]

In terms of clinical expression, the demarcation between class I variants and all others is much more clearcut. One of the outstanding questions in the biochemical genetics of G6PD is why a particular variant can cause CNSHA rather than just acute hemolytic anemia. As stated earlier, the level of residual enzyme activity is not the whole answer; this must mean that qualitative differences are important. The most likely way in which a structural change can significantly alter the function of G6PD, *given the same level of deficiency,* is if it affects the binding of one of the main ligands, that is, G6P, NADP, or NADPH. Direct proof of this is still lacking, mainly because we do not have a clear picture of these binding sites. However, there is circumstantial evidence supporting this notion. G6P K_m values are significantly lower in class II and III variants compared with class I variants. Also, three different class I variants have been detected that share marked abnormalities of NADP binding and have point mutations in the three neighboring amino acids: 384 to 386. A mathematic model for predicting the metabolic consequences of altered kinetics of G6PD variants has been proposed[194] and should be tested.

Finally, an obvious but important point to keep in mind, especially in areas of high prevalence of G6PD deficiency, is that the clinical expression may appear to be modified simply because another separate condition coexists in the patient.

G6PD Deficiency in Nonerythroid Cells

As mentioned earlier, because nucleated somatic cells have the capability to synthesize G6PD constitutively, they are less affected than red cells by G6PD deficiency. Specifically, if G6PD deficiency is due to instability of a mutant enzyme, we would not expect nucleated cells to be severely affected. For instance, subjects with G6PD Mediterranean have less than 5% G6PD activity in red cells but about 30% of normal activity in granulocytes; subjects with G6PD A− have about 12% G6PD activity in red cells but near-normal activity in granulocytes. On the other hand, if G6PD deficiency results from a drastic change in catalytic efficiency or in substrate affinity, then deficiency may be more universal. In practice, the only well-documented pathological effect occurs in granulocytes. A few of the class I G6PD variants (eg, G6PD Barcelona[195]) cause granulocyte dysfunction as well as CNSHA. The main effects are impaired phagocytosis and bacterial killing. Patients with these variants have increased susceptibility to bacterial infection, particularly with *Staphylococcus aureus*. G6PD deficiency impairs phagocytosis and killing through a shortage in NADPH supply, similar to that observed in chronic granulomatous disease, in which cytochrome b245 is defective.

Erythrocytes are not the only nonnucleated cells in the body. Another example is in the lens of the eye, and juvenile cataracts have been reported in a number of patients with class I G6PD.[196] In patients with simple G6PD deficiency, an early onset of cataracts has been found in some series[197] but not in others,[198] suggesting that it may be limited to certain variants.

DIAGNOSIS OF G6PD DEFICIENCY

Although the clinical picture of favism and of other forms of acute hemolytic anemia associated with G6PD deficiency is characteristic, the final diagnosis must rely on the direct demonstration of decreased activity of this enzyme in red cells. With neonatal jaundice and CNSHA, the differential diagnosis is much wider, and therefore this test is even more important. The enzyme assay is easy, and numerous screening tests can be used as substitutes if a spectrophotometer is not available. A number of potential snags and sources of error must be understood, however, and the use of commercial kits is not a substitute for such understanding. The following subsections first discuss the value and limitations of the regular quantitative assay and then comment briefly on the use of alternatives.

Tests for G6PD Deficiency

Quantitation

Glucose-6-phosphate dehydrogenase can be assayed by the classic method of Horecker and Smyrniotis,[24] which measures directly the rate of formation of NADPH through its characteristic absorption peak in the near UV at 340 nm. The red cell activity is expressed in international units (micromoles of NADPH produced per minute) per gram of hemoglobin; therefore, it is best to assay the enzyme activity and the hemoglobin concentration in the same hemolysate and work out the ratio. In normal red cells, the range of G6PD activity, measured at 30°C, is 7 to 10 IU/g Hb.

Screening Tests

Several screening tests for G6PD deficiency are useful and reliable provided they are properly run and their limitations are understood. The most popular are the *dye decolorization tests,*[199] the *methemoglobin reduction test,*[200] and the *fluorescence spot test.*[201] All these methods are semiquantitative, and they are meant to classify a sample simply as normal or deficient. The cutoff point can be set by following the appropriate instructions and by trial and error in the individual diagnostic laboratory. One should aim to classify as deficient any sample that less than 30% of the normal activity because above this level, one is unlikely to encounter clinical manifestations. Screening tests are especially useful for testing large numbers of samples. They are also perfectly adequate for diagnostic purposes in patients who are in the steady state, but *not* for patients in the posthemolytic period or with other complications. Also, they cannot be expected to identify all heterozygotes. Finally, an ideal screening test should not give false-negative results (ie, it should not misclassify a G6PD-deficient subject as normal), but it can be allowed to give a few false-positive results (ie, a G6PD-normal subject might be misclassified as G6PD deficient). Ideally, every patient found to be G6PD deficient by screening should be confirmed by the spectrophotometric assay.

A technique that is neglected but that can be useful for some population studies is electrophoresis followed by specific staining for G6PD activity.[72,177] It has the advantage of detecting both electrophoretic variants with normal activity (through displacement of the stained band) and deficient variants (through obvious decrease in staining intensity). The classic starch-gel method,[202] although it may still have the highest resolving power in some cases, has been largely replaced by the use of supporting media that are less laborious to handle, such as cellulose acetate gel[203] and agarose gel.[204]

Cytochemical Tests

G6PD activity can be demonstrated in individual red cells either by the use of a tetrazolium dye,[200,205,206] or by coupling G6PD activity in the intact cell to a methemoglobin elution method.[200] Neither of these techniques has gained wide acceptance in diagnostic laboratories, but they can be useful in special cases and for research purposes.

Practical Problems

The definition of G6PD deficiency is somewhat arbitrary because different genetic variants are associated with different degrees of deficiency. It seems reasonable to choose as the cutoff point a level that can cause clinical manifestations. It can be safely stated that in males there are no hemolytic complications with a red cell G6PD activity greater than 30% of normal. Thus, the demarcation between G6PD-normal and G6PD-deficient males is in principle clearcut. Several problems, however, deserve consideration:

Effect of Red Cell Age

As mentioned earlier, any condition associated with reticulocytosis entails an *increase* in G6PD activity. This means that if the subject is genetically G6PD normal, his red cell G6PD activity is *above* the normal range. This does not affect diagnosis because G6PD deficiency is correctly ruled out. If the subject is genetically G6PD deficient, however, reticulocytosis may raise his red cell G6PD to near or within the normal range, and he may be misclassified as G6PD normal.

Effect of Selective Hemolysis

After a hemolytic attack, two circumstances increase the risk of misdiagnosis: first, if the older red cells have been destroyed selectively; second, if the marrow responds with a sudden outpouring of young cells into the peripheral blood. (A third confusing factor may be admixture of G6PD-normal red cells if the patient had been transfused). Although the reticulocyte count is a good warning to avoid this mistake, it is not a sensitive index of the mean red cell age because reticulocytes turn into morphologically "mature" erythrocytes within 1 to 2 days. In other words, the mean red cell age may be significantly younger than normal even when the reticulocyte count is normal.

There are several ways to circumvent these problems. First, a G6PD level in the low-normal range in the face of reticulocytosis is always suspicious. In general, this finding suggests that the patient is actually G6PD deficient. Second, if the patient is suffering from or is recovering from an acute hemolytic crisis, the suspicion generated from the first finding can be simply kept in store for a few weeks, when the situation will have evolved toward the steady state, and a repeat test will prove whether the patient is G6PD deficient. Third, if either the urgency of some clinical decision or academic curiosity demands a more prompt solution of the problem, the presence of severely G6PD-deficient red cells can be demonstrated either by enzyme assay of the oldest cells (fractionated by sedimentation) or by a cytochemical method.

White Cell Contamination

Because G6PD activity is much higher in leukocytes (particularly in granulocytes) than in erythrocytes, for accurate measurements, it is essential to remove all leukocytes by the Ficoll-Hypaque method, or by filtration through cellulose powder rather than by the cruder approach of sucking off the buffy coat. In most cases, however, this is not necessary just for the purpose of diagnosing G6PD deficiency.

Glucose-6-Phosphate Dehydrogenase Deficiency in Heterozygotes

Heterozygote diagnosis by a quantitative test is not difficult in most cases because the level of G6PD falls between the normal and the deficient male range. In about 10% of cases, however, the G6PD level "trespasses" into either. In addition, the problems outlined for male patients are compounded in the case of heterozygous females, which usually can be overcome by similar methodologies, particularly by the use of a cytochemical test. With good technique, heterozygotes can be detected who have as few as 5% G6PD-deficient red cells. In cases of "extreme phenotypes," sometimes referred to as arising from "imbalanced lyonization," however, no test can demonstrate what is not there. In such cases, one can prove that the female subject is a heterozygote only by pedigree analysis or, if the mutation is known, by DNA analysis. Fortunately, this is not crucial from the clinical point of view. The susceptibility of heterozygotes to develop acute hemolytic anemia, and its severity, are roughly proportional to the percentage of G6PD-deficient red cells. Thus, if this percentage is so low as to be hard to detect, then the patient is most unlikely to have G6PD-related hemolysis.

A special mention should be made of heterozygotes for G6PD variants associated with CNSHA. In the author's experience, the mothers of male patients with this condition are often G6PD normal, either because the variant in the offspring is due to a de novo mutation or because the mother is a heterozygote but is phenotypically normal. In the latter case, somatic selection has favored the hemopoietic progenitor cells with normal G6PD.

TREATMENT OF G6PD DEFICIENCY

Prevention of Clinical Manifestations

Because neonatal jaundice and acute hemolytic anemia are the most common manifestations of G6PD deficiency, it is most important to consider how they can be prevented. The first step is to identify G6PD deficient individuals, and this is where screening is most pertinent. Whether population-wide screening is both desirable and feasible depends primarily on the prevalence of G6PD deficiency in any particular community: this will determine the cost/benefit ratio (the main cost being labor, since the reagents and equipment needed are relatively very cheap). If screening is done at all, it is best done on cord blood, and this is already practiced, for instance, in Sardinia, in Thailand and in Malaysia. Once a subject is known to be G6PD deficient, the two main implications are the risk of neonatal jaundice, and the importance to avoid exposure to agents that can cause acute hemolytic anemia. We cannot prevent neonatal jaundice as yet, but the awareness of G6PD deficiency must entail surveillance for neonatal jaundice until at least day 4, and special recommendations with respect to factors, such as naphthalene, that can cause it or make it worse. By contrast, at least one type of acute hemolytic anemia, namely favism, is totally preventable, if the persons concerned, and their families in the first place, accept the advice to give up eating fava beans. Prevention of infection-induced hemolysis is obviously more difficult. Prevention of drug-induced hemolysis is possible in most cases by choosing alternative drugs, but it may be difficult when there are none. The most common problem is the need to administer primaquine for the eradication of malaria due to *Plasmodium vivax* or to *Plasmodium malariae*: in these cases the administration of a lower dosage for a longer time is the recommended approach, which will still cause hemolysis, but may be of an acceptably mild degree.

A special problem in prevention is what to do about new drugs, the hemolytic potential of which is unknown. Although in vitro methods to test drugs in this respect do exist, such tests are not carried out before drugs are released on the market. This is unfortunate especially when a new drug is introduced in an area where G6PD deficiency is common, and in practice their hemolytic potential will become apparent only from clinical observation.

Treatment of Clinical Manifestations

Management of Acute Hemolytic Anemia and Favism

A patient with acute hemolytic anemia may present a diagnostic problem that, once solved, does not require any specific treatment at all; or the patient may present a medical emergency requiring immediate action. The most urgent question is whether the child needs a blood transfusion. It is difficult to give absolute guidelines, but the following may be useful. If the hemoglobin level is below 7 g/dL, and if there is evidence of continuing hemolysis (especially persisting hemoglobinuria), the child should receive a transfusion as soon as possible.[175] It has been suggested that desferrioxamine could control acute hemolytic anemia in favism,[207] but this has not been confirmed,[208] and withholding a blood transfusion when indicated in this condition should be regarded as dangerous.

The most important complication that may require treatment is acute renal failure, which is exceedingly rare in children. Apart from standard renal failure regimen, hemodialysis may be necessary.

Management of Neonatal Jaundice

This does not differ from management of neonatal jaundice due to causes other than G6PD deficiency. Full details have been given elsewhere.[175]

Management of Chronic Nonspherocytic Hemolytic Anemia

General Care. In general, management does not differ from that of CNSHA due to other causes, such as pyruvate kinase deficiency. If the anemia is not severe, regular folic acid supplements and regular hematologic surveillance suffice. It is important to avoid exposure to potentially hemolytic drugs, and blood transfusion may be indicated when exacerbations occur, mostly with intercurrent infections. In rare patients, the anemia is so severe that it is transfusion dependent. In these cases, blood transfusions usually are needed at about 2-month intervals to keep the hemoglobin in the range of 8 to 10 g/dL. A hypertransfusion regimen aiming to maintain a normal hemoglobin level is not indicated (because there is no ineffective erythropoiesis in the bone marrow). Appropriate iron chelation, however, should be instituted by the age of 2 years and must be continued as long as transfusion treatment is necessary. Sometimes, the transfusion requirement may decrease after puberty.

Splenectomy. A special problem is that of splenectomy. G6PD-deficient red cells are not *selectively* destroyed in the spleen, like in hereditary spherocytosis. The fact that the spleen is usually enlarged, however, suggests that it plays a role in hemolysis. In practice, there are three indications for splenectomy: (1) the spleen becomes a physical encumbrance; (2) there is evidence of hypersplenism; (3) the anemia is severe, even in the absence of the first two indications. Splenectomy may reduce the overall rate of hemolysis just enough to make a transfusion-dependent child become transfusion independent. This is doubly important because it makes it possible to dispense with desferrioxamine. Pneumovax immunization should be given before splenectomy and penicillin prophylaxis after splenectomy.

Genetic Counseling. When a diagnosis of CNSHA is made, the family must be given genetic counseling, and an effort should be made to establish whether the mother is a heterozygote (this may not be easy by conventional techniques). If she is, the chance of recurrence is 1:2 for every subsequent male pregnancy. Prenatal diagnosis can be offered and it can be carried out by a G6PD assay on amniotic fluid cells, although the expression of G6PD deficiency in these cells varies with each G6PD variant. A better alternative probably is to test DNA from chorionic villi with one of the available polymorphic probes that are closely linked to G6PD and for which the mother is heterozygous. Or, if the mutation in the G6PD gene of the boy affected by CNSHA is identified, one can use DNA methods to establish directly whether the mother is heterozygous. Prenatal diagnosis can then be carried out by customized allele-specific oligonucleotide hybridization or by analysis with an appropriate restriction enzyme.

REFERENCES

1. Fermi C, Martinetti P. Studio sul favismo. Ann Igiene Sper 1905;15: 76.
2. Luisada L. Favism: a singular disease affecting chiefly red blood cells. Medicine 1941;20:229.
3. Carson PE, Flanagan CL, Ickes CE, Alving A. Enzymatic deficiency in primaquine-sensitive erythrocytes. Science 1956;124:484–485.
4. Loehr GW, Waller HD. Haemolytische Erythrocytopathie durche Fehlen von Glucose 6-phosphat Dehydrogenase in roten Blutzellen als dominant vererbliche Krankheit. Klin Wochenschr 1958;36:865.
5. Sansone G, Segni G. Prime determinazioni del glutatione (GSH) ematico nel favismo. Boll Soc Ital Biol Sper 1956;32:456.
6. Beutler E. Study of glucose-6-phosphate dehydrogenase: history and molecular biology. Am J Hematol 1993;42:53.
7. Luzzatto L. Glucose 6-phosphate dehydrogenase. Ital J Biochem 1986;35: 375.
8. Beutler E. Glucose-6-phosphate dehydrogenase deficiency. In: Stanbury JB, Wyngaarden JB, Fredrickson DS, Goldstein JL, Brown MS, eds. The metabolic basis of the inherited disease, ed 5. New York, McGraw-Hill, 1983:1629.
9. Piomelli S. G6PD deficiency and related disorders of the pentose pathway. In: Nathan D, Oski F, eds. The pathophysiological basis of pediatric haematology. Philidelphia, WB Saunders, 1974.
10. Yoshida A. Haemolytic anaemia and G6PD deficiency. Science 1973;179: 532.
11. Dacie JV. Hereditary enzyme deficiency haemolytic anaemias. III: Deficiency of glucose-6-phosphate dehydrogenase. In: Dacie JV, ed. Haemolytic anaemias: the Hereditary haemolytic anaemias, ed 3. London, Churchill Livingstone, 1985:364.
12. Beutler E. Haemolytic anaemia in disorders of red cell metabolism (topics in haematology). London, Plenum Medical, 1978.
13. Luzzatto L. Inherited haemolytic states: glucose-6-phosphate dehydrogenase deficiency. Clin Hematol 1975;4:83.
14. Luzzatto L, Testa U. Human erythrocyte G6PD: structure and function in normal and mutant subjects. In: Piomelli S, Yachnin S, eds. Current topics in hematology, vol 1. New York, Alan Liss, 1978:1.
15. Luzzatto L, Battistuzzi G. Glucose 6-phosphate dehydrogenase. Adv Hum Genet 1985;14:217.
16. Levy HR. Glucose 6-phosphate dehydrogenase. In: Meister A, ed. Advances in enzymology, vol. 48. New York, Wiley, 1979:97.
17. Luzzatto L. New developments in glucose-6-phosphate dehydrogenase deficiency. Israel J Med Sci 1973;9:1484.
18. Luzzatto L. Genetic heterogeneity and pathophysiology of G6PD deficiency. Br J Haematol 1974;28:151.
19. Marks PA. Glucose 6-phosphate dehydrogenase. In: Bishop C, ed. The red blood cell, ed 2. New York, Academic Press, 1964.
20. Glock GE, McLean P. Levels of enzymes of the direct oxidative pathway of carbohydrate metabolism in mammalian tissues and tumours. Biochem J 1954;56:171.
21. Marks PA, Johnson AB. Relationship between the age of human erythrocytes and their osmotic resistance: a basis for separating young and old erythrocytes. J Clin Invest 1958;37:1542.
22. Vogelstein B, Fearson ER, Hamilton SR, et al. Clonal analysis using recombinant DNA probes from the X-chromosome. Cancer Res 1987;47: 4806.
23. Warburg O, Christian W. Uber Aktivierung der robinsonschem Hexosemonophosphorsaure in roten Blutzellen und die Gewinnung aktivierender Fermentlosung. Biochem Z 1931;242:206.
24. Horecker BL, Smyrniotis A. Glucose 6-phosphate dehydrogenase. In: Colowick N, Kaplan NO, eds. Methods in enzymology, vol 1. New York, Academic Press, 1955.
25. Luzzatto L. Regulation of the activity of glucose-6-phosphate dehydrogenase by $NADP^+$ and NADPH. Biochim Biophys Acta 1967;146: 18.
26. Kirkman HN, Gaetani GD, Clemons EH, Mareni C. Red cell $NADP^+$ and NADPH in glucose-6-phosphate dehydrogenase deficiency. J Clin Invest 1975;55:875.
27. Brin M, Yonemoto RH. Stimulation of the glucose oxidative pathway in human erythrocytes by methylene blue. J Biol Chem 1958;230:307.
28. Gaetani GF, Parker JC, Kirkman HN. Intracellular restraint: a new basis for the limitation in response to oxidation stress in human erythrocytes containing low activity variants of glucose 6-phosphate dehydrogenase. Proc Natl Acad Sci 1975;71:3584.
29. Cohen P, Rosemeyer MA. Human glucose-6-phosphate dehydrogenase: purification of the erythrocyte enzyme and the influence of ions on its activity. Eur J Biochem 1969;8:1.
30. Persico MG, Viglietto G, Martini G, et al. Isolation of human glucose-6-phosphate dehydrogenase (G6PD) cDNA clones: primary structure of the protein and unusual 5′ non-coding region. Nucleic Acids Res 1986;14:2511.
31. Jeffery J, Soderling-Barros J, Murray LA, et al. Glucose 6-phosphate dehydrogenase: characteristics revealed by the rat liver enzyme. Eur J Biochem 1989;186:551.
32. Bhadbhade MM, Adams MJ, Flynn TG, Levy HR. Sequence identity between a lysine-containing peptide from Leuconostoc mesenteriodes glucose-6-phosphate dehydrogenase and an active site peptide from human erythrocyte glucose-6-phosphate dehydrogenase. FEBS Lett 1987;211:243.
33. Vulliamy T, Mason P, Luzzatto L. The molecular basis of glucose 6-phosphate dehydrogenase deficiency. TIG 1992;8:138.
34. Jeffery J, Persson B, Wood I, Bergman T, Jeffery R, Jörnvall H. Glucose-6-phosphate dehydrogenase: structure function relationships and the *Pichia jadinii* enzyme structure. Eur J Biochem 1993;212:41.
35. Camardella L, Caruso C, Rutigliano B, Romano M, diPrisco G, Descalzi-Cancedda F. Human erythrocyte glucose-6-phosphate dehydrogenase: identification of a reactive lysyl residue labelled with pyridoxal 5′-phosphate. Eur J Biochem 1988;171:485.
36. Mason PJ, Vulliamy TJ, Foulkes NS, Town M, Haidar B, Luzzatto L. The production of normal and variant human glucose-6-phosphate dehydrogenase in cos cells. Eur J Biochem 1988;178:109.
37. Cohen P, Rosemeyer MA. Subunit interactions of human glucose 6-phosphate dehydrogenase from human erythrocytes. Eur J Biochem 1969;8:8.
38. Babalola AOG, Beetlestone JG, Luzzatto L. Genetic variants of human erythrocyte glucose-6-phosphate dehydrogenase: kinetic and thermodynamic parameters of variants A, B and A− in relation to quaternary structure. J Biol Chem 1976;251:2992.
39. DeFlora A, Morelli A, Benatti U, Giuliano F, Molinari MP. Human erythrocyte G6PD: interaction with oxidized and reduced coenzyme. Biochem Biophys Res Commun 1974;60:999.
40. Luzzatto L, Allan NC. Different properties of glucose 6-phosphate dehydrogenase from human erythrocytes with normal and abnormal enzyme levels. Biochem Biophys Res Commun 1965;21:547.
41. DeFlora A, Morelli A, Giuliano F. Human erythrocyte G6PD: content of bound coenzyme. Biochem Biophys Res Commun 1974;59:406.
42. Kahler SG, Kirkman HN. Intracellular glucose 6-phosphate dehydrogenase does not monomerize in human erythrocytes. J Biol Chem 1983;258:717.
43. Cancedda R, Ogunmola GB, Luzzatto L. Genetic variants of human erythrocyte glucose 6-phosphate dehydrogenase: Discrete conformational states stabilized by $NADP^+$ and NADPH. Eur J Biochem 1973;34: 199.
44. Lee WT, Levy HR. Lysine-21 of *Leuconostoc mesenteroides* glucose 6-phosphate dehydrogenase participates in substrate binding through charge-charge interaction. Protein Sci 1992;1:329.
45. Adams MJ, Levy HR, Moffat K. Crystallization of glucose 6-phosphate dehydrogenase from *Leuconostoc mesenteroides*. J Biol Chem 1983;258: 5867.
46. Luzzatto L, Sodeinde O, Martini G. Genetic variation in the host and adaptive phenomena in *Plasmodium falciparum* infection. In: Evered D, Whelan J, eds. Malaria and the red cell: Ciba Foundation Symposium 94. London, Pitman, 1983:159.
47. Pai GS, Sprenkle JA, Do TT, Mareni CE, Migeon BR. Localization of the loci for hypoxanthine phosphoribosyltransferase and glucose-6-phosphate dehydrogenase and biochemical evidence of non-random X chromosome expression from studies of human X-autosome translocation. Proc Natl Acad Sci USA 1980;77:2810.
48. Szabo P, Purrello M, Rocchi M, et al. Cytological mapping of the human glucose-6-phosphate dehydrogenase gene distal to the fragile-X site suggests a high rate of meiotic recombination across this site. Proc Natl Acad Sci USA 1984;81:7855.
49. Kanno H, Huang I-Y, Kan YW, Yoshida A. Two structural genes on different chromosomes are required for encoding the major subunit of human red cell glucose-6-phosphate dehydrogenase. Cell 1989;58: 595.
50. Henikoff S, Smith JM. The human mRNA that provides the N-terminus of chimeric G6PD encodes GMP reductase. Cell 1989;58:1021.
51. Melton DW. HPRT gene organization and expression. In: Maclean M, ed. Oxford surveys on eukaryotic genes, vol 4. Oxford, Oxford University Press, 1987:34.
52. Hollander N, Selvaraj P, Springer TA. Biosynthesis and function of LFA-3 in human mutant cells deficient in phosphatidylinositol-anchored proteins. J Immunol 1988;141:4283.

53. Yoshida A, Kan YW. Origin of "fused" glucose-6-phosphate dehydrogenase. Cell 1990;62:11.
54. Boyer SH, Graham JB. Linkage between the X chromosome loci for glucose 6-phosphate dehydrogenase electrophoretic variation and hemophilia A. Am J Hum Genet 1965;17:320.
55. Patterson M, Schwartz C, Bell M, et al. Physical mapping studies on the human X-chromosome in the region Xq27-Xqter. Genomics 1987;1:297.
56. Schlessinger D, Little RD, Freije D, et al. Yeast artificial chromosome-based genome mapping: some lessons from Xq24-q28. Genomics 1991;11:783.
57. Montanaro V, Casamassimi A, D'Urso M, et al. In situ hybridization to cytogenetic bands of yeast artificial chromosomes covering 50% of human Xq24-Xq28 DNA. Am J Hum Genet 1991;48:183.
58. Kenwrick S, Gitschier J. A contiguous, 3-Mb physical map of Xq28 extending from the colorblindness locus to DXS15. Am J Hum Genet 1989;45:873.
59. Peterlin B, Smahi A, HolvoetVermaut L, Heitz D, Dahl N, HorsCayla MC. An irradiation-reduced hybrid panel for fine-structure mapping of the Xq28 region in the human genome. Cytogenet Cell Genet 1993;62:58.
60. Filosa S, Calabrò V, Lania G, et al. G6PD haplotypes spanning Xq28 from F8C to red/green color vision. Genomics 1993;17:6.
61. Maestrini E, Rivella S, Tribioli C, et al. Identification of novel RFLPs in the vicinity of CpG islands in Xq28: application to the analysis of the pattern of X chromosome inactivation. Am J Hum Genet 1992;50:156.
62. Migeon BR, McGinniss MJ, Antonarakis SE, et al. Severe hemophilia A in a female by cryptic translocation: order and orientation of factor VIII within Xq28. Genomics 1993;16:20.
63. Mandel J-L, Willard HF, Nussbaum RL, Romeo G, Puck JM, Davies KE. Report of the committee on the genetic constitution of the X chromosome. Cytogenet Cell Genet 1989;51:384.
64. Poustka A, Dietrich A, Langenstein G, Toniolo D, Warren ST, Lehrach H. Physical map of human Xq27-qter: localizing the region of the fragile X mutation. Proc Natl Acad Sci 1991;88:8302.
65. Alcalay M, Toniolo D. CpG islands of the X-chromosome are gene associated. Nucleic Acids Res 1988;16:9527.
66. Maestrini E, Tamanini F, Kioschis P, et al. An archipelago of CpG islands in Xq28: identification and fine mapping of 20 new CpG islands of the human X-chromosome. Hum Mol Genet 1992;1:275.
67. Martini G, Toniolo D, Vulliamy TJ, et al. Structural analysis of the X-linked gene encoding human glucose 6-phosphate dehydrogenase. EMBO J 1986;5:1849.
68. Chen EY, Cheng A, Lee A, et al. Sequence of human glucose 6-phosphate dehydrogenase cloned in plasmids and a yeast artificial chromosome. Genomics 1991;10:792.
69. Bird AP. CpG islands as gene markers in the vertebrate nucleus. Trends Genet 1987;3:342.
70. Ursini MV, Scalera L, Martini G. High level of transcription driven by a 400 bp segment of the human G6PD promoter. Biochem Biophys Res Commun 1990;170:1203.
71. WHO Working Group. Glucose-6-phosphate dehydrogenase deficiency. Bull WHO 1989;67:601.
72. Bienzle U, Ayeni O, Lucas AO, Luzzatto L. Glucose-6-phosphate dehydrogenase deficiency and malaria: greater resistance of females heterozygous for enzyme deficiency and of males with non-deficient variant. Lancet 1972;1:107.
73. Sinclair AH, Berta P, Palmer MS, et al. A gene from the human sex-determining region encodes a protein with homology to a conserved DNA-binding motif. Nature 1990;346:240.
74. Monk M. The X chromosome in development in mouse and man. J Inherited Metab Dis 1992;15:499.
75. Lyon MF. Some milestones in the history of X-chromosome inactivation. Ann Rev Genet 1992;26:17.
76. Lucchesi JC. Gene dosage compensation and the evolution of sex chromosomes. Science 1978;202:711.
77. Tan SS, Williams EA, Tam PPL. X-chromosome inactivation occurs at different times in different tissues of the post-implantation mouse embryo. Nature Genet 1993;3:170.
78. Wolf SF, Migeon BR. Studies of X chromosome DNA methylation in normal human cells. Nature 1982;295:667.
79. Gartler SM, Riggs AD. Mammalian X-chromosome inactivation. Ann Rev Genet 1983;17:155.
80. Liskay RM, Evans RJ. Inactive X chromosome DNA-mediated transformation for the hypoxanthine phosphoribosyl transferase gene. Proc Natl Acad Sci 1980;77:4895.
81. Venolia L, Gartler SM. Comparison of transformation efficiency of human active and inactive X-chromosomal DNA. Nature 1983;302:82.
82. Brown CJ, Ballabio A, Rupert JL, et al. A gene from the region of the human X inactivation centre is expressed exclusively from the inactive X chromosome. Nature 1991;349:38.
83. Shapiro LJ. Steroid sulfatase deficiency and X-linked ichthyosis. In: Beaudet AL, Scriver CR, Sly WS, Valle D, eds. The metabolic basis of inherited disorders, ed 6. New York, McGraw-Hill, 1989:1945.
84. Schneider-Gädicke A, Beer-Romero P, Brown LG, Nussbaum R, Page DC. *ZFX* has a gene structure similar to *ZFY*, the putative human sex determinant, and escapes X inactivation. Cell 1989;57:1247.
85. Ellison J, Passage M, Yu LC, Yen P, Mohandas TK, Shapiro L. Directed isolation of human genes that escape X inactivation. Somatic Cell Mol Genet 1992;18:259.
86. Zinn AR, Page DC, Fisher EMC. Turner syndrome: the case of the missing sex chromosome. Trends in Genetics 1993;9:90.
87. Lyon MF. Gene action in the X chromosome in the mouse (*Mus musculus* L.). Nature 1961;190:372.
88. Beutler E, Yeh M, Fairbanks VF. The normal human female as a mosaic of X-chromosome activity: studies using the gene for G6PD deficiency as a marker. Proc Natl Acad Sci USA 1962;48:9.
89. Davidson RG, Nitowsky HM, Childs B. Demonstration of two populations of cells in the human female heterozygous for glucose-6-phosphate dehydrogenase variants. Proc Natl Acad Sci USA 1963;50:481.
90. Nyhan WL, Bakay B, Connors JD, Marks JF, Keele DK. Hemixygous expression of glucose 6-phosphate dehydrogenase deficiency in erythrocytes of heterozygotes for the Lesch-Nyhan syndrome. Proc Natl Acad Sci 1970;65:214.
91. Notarangelo LD, Parolini O, Porta F, et al. Analysis of X-chromosome inactivation and presumptive expression of the Wiskott-Aldrich syndrome (WAS) gene in hematopoietic cell lineages of a thrombocytopenic carrier female of WAS. Hum Genet 1991;88:237.
92. Coleman R, Genet SA, Harper JI, Wilkie AOM. Interaction of incontinentia pigmenti and factor VIII mutations in a female with biased X inactivation, resulting in haemophilia. J Med Genet 1993;30:497.
93. Conley ME, Wang WC, Parolini O, Shapiro DN, Campana D, Siminovitch KA. Atypical Wiskott-Aldrich syndrome in a girl. Blood 1992;80:1264.
94. Town M, Athanasiou Metaxa M, Luzzatto L. Intragenic interspecific complementation of glucose 6-phosphate dehydrogenase in human-hamster cell hybrids. Somatic Cell Mol Genet 1990;16:97.
95. Rinaldi A, Filippi G, Siniscalco M. Variability of red cell phenotypes between and within individuals in an unbiased sample of 77 certain heterozygotes for G6PD deficiency in Sardinians. Am J Hum Genet 1976;28:496.
96. Gale RE, Wheadon H, Linch DC. X-chromosome inactivation patterns using HPRT and PGK polymorphisms in haematologically normal and post-chemotherapy females. Br J Haematol 1991;79:193.
97. Luzzatto L, Usanga EA, Bienzle U, Esan GJF, Fasuan FA. Imbalance in X-chromosome expression: evidence for a human X-linked gene affecting growth of haemopoietic cells. Science 1979;205:1418.
98. Linder D, Gartler SM. Glucose 6-phosphate dehydrogenase mosaicism: utilization as a cell marker in the study of leiomyomas. Science 1965;150:67.
99. Fialkow PJ. Clonal origin of human tumors. Biochim Biophys Acta 1976;458:283.
100. Oni SB, Osunkoya BO, Luzzatto L. Paroxysmal nocturnal hemoglobinuria: evidence for monoclonal origin of abnormal red cells. Blood 1970;36:145.
101. Ferraris AM, Giuntini P, Galiano S, Gaetani GF. 2-Deoxyglucose 6-phosphate utilization in the study of glucose 6-phosphate dehydrogenase mosaicism. Am J Hum Genet 1981;33:307.
102. Gilliland DG, Blanchard KL, Levy J, Perrin S, Bunn HF. Clonality in myeloproliferative disorders: analysis by means of the polymerase chain reaction. Proc Natl Acad Sci 1991;88:6848.
103. Anastasi J, Feng J, Le Beau MM, Larson RA, Rowley JD, Vardiman JW. Cytogenetic clonality in myelodysplastic syndromes studied with fluorescence in situ hybridization: lineage, response to growth factor therapy, and clone expansion. Blood 1993;81:1580.
104. Nash R, Storb R, Neiman P. Polyclonal reconstitution of human marrow after allogeneic bone marrow transplantation. Blood 1988;72:2031.
105. Luzzatto L, Mehta A. Glucose-6-phosphate dehydrogenase deficiency. In: Scriver CR, Beaudet AL, Sly WS, Valle D, eds. The metabolic basis of inherited disease, ed 6. New York, McGraw-Hill, 1989:2237.
106. Vulliamy TJ, D'Urso M, Battistuzzi G, et al. Diverse point mutations in the human glucose-6-phosphate dehydrogenase gene cause enzyme deficiency and mild or severe hemolytic anemia. Proc Natl Acad Sci USA 1988;85:5171.
107. Hirono A, Beutler E. Molecular cloning and nucleotide sequence of cDNA for human glucose-6-phosphate dehydrogenase variant A(−). Proc Natl Acad Sci USA 1988;85:3951.
108. DeVita G, Alcalay M, Sampietro M, Cappellini MD, Fiorelli G, Toniolo D. Two point mutations are responsible for G6PD polymorphism in Sardinia. Am J Hum Genet 1989;44:233.
109. Takizawa T, Yoneyama Y, Miwa S, Yoshida A. A single nucleotide base transition is the basis of the common human glucose-6-phosphate dehydrogenase variant A(+). Genomics 1987;1:228.
110. Poggi V, Town M, Foulkes NS, Luzzatto L. Identification of a single base change in the G6PD gene by PCR amplification of the entire coding region from genomic DNA. Biochem J 1990;271:157.
111. Beutler E, Kuhl W, Vives-Corrons JL, Prchal JT. Molecular heterogeneity of glucose 6-phosphate dehydrogenase A−. Blood 1989;74:2550.
112. Vives-Corrons J-L, Kuhl W, Pujades MA, Beutler E. Molecular genetics

of the glucose-6-phosphate dehydrogenase (G6PD) Mediterranean variant and description of a new G6PD mutant, G6PD Andalus 1361A. Am J Hum Genet 1990;47:575.

113. Corcoran CM, Calabrò V, Tamagnini G, et al. Molecular heterogeneity underlying the G6PD Mediterranean phenotype. Hum Genet 1992;88: 688.

114. Hirono A, Kuhl W, Gelbart T, Forman L, Fairbanks VF, Beutler E. Identification of the binding domain for NADP+ of human glucose-6-phosphate dehydrogenase by sequence analysis of mutants. Proc Natl Acad Sci 1989;86:10015.

115. Gaetani GF, Galiano S, Melani C, et al. A new glucose-6-phosphate dehydrogenase variant with congenital nonspherocytic hemolytic anemia (G6PD Genova): biochemical characterization and mosaicism expression in the heterozygote. Hum Genet 1990;84:337.

116. Ahluwalia A, Corcoran CM, Vulliamy TJ, et al. G6PD Kalyan and G6PD Kerala: two deficient variants in India caused by the same 317Glu → Lys mutation. Hum Mol Genet 1992;1:209.

117. Vulliamy TJ, Beutler E, Luzzatto L. Variants of glucose 6-phosphate dehydrogenase are due to missense mutations spread throughout the coding region of the gene. Human Mutation 1993;2:159.

118. Motulsky AG. Metabolic polymorphisms and the role of infectious diseases in human evolution. Hum Biol 1960;32:28.

119. Allison AC. Glucose 6-phosphate dehydrogenase deficiency in red blood cells of East Africans. Nature 1960;186:531.

120. Luzzatto L. Genetics of red cells and susceptibility to malaria. Blood 1979;54:961.

121. Brabin L, Brabin BJ. Malaria and glucose 6-phosphate dehydrogenase deficiency in populations with high and low spleen rates in Madang, Papua New Guinea. Hum Hered 1990;40:15.

122. Siniscalco M, Bernini L, Filippi G, et al. Population genetics of haemoglobin variants, thalassaemia and glucose-6-phosphate dehydrogenase deficiency, with particular reference to the malaria hypothesis. Bull WHO 1966;34:379.

123. Stamatoyannopoulos G, Panayotopoulos A, Motulsky AG. The distribution of glucose 6-phosphate dehydrogenase deficiency in Greece. Am J Hum Genet 1966;18:296.

124. Piazza A, Mayr WR, Contu L, et al. Genetic and population structure of four Sardinian villages. Ann Hum Genet 1985;49:47.

125. Vulliamy TJ, Othman A, Town M, Nathwani A, Falusi Y, Luzzatto L. Linkage disequilibrium of polymorphic sites in the G6PD gene in African populations and the origin of G6PD A−. Gene Geography 1991;5: 13.

126. Vulliamy TJ, Othman A, Town M, et al. Polymorphic sites in the African population detected by sequence analysis of the glucose 6-phosphate dehydrogenase gene outline the evolution of the variants A and A^-. Proc Natl Acad Sci 1991;88:8568.

127. Vives-Corrons JL, Pujades A. Heterogeneity of "Mediterranean type" glucose 6-phosphate dehydrogenase (G6PD) deficiency in Spain and description of two new variants associated with favism. Hum Genet 1982;60:216.

128. Beutler E, Kuhl W. The NT 1311 polymorphism of G6PD: G6PD Mediterranean mutation may have arisen more than once. Am J Hum Genet 1990;47:1008.

129. Gilles HM, Fletcher KA, Hendrickse RG, Lindner R, Reddy S, Allan NC. Glucose 6-phosphate dehydrogenase, sickling and malaria in African children in South Western Nigeria. Lancet 1967;1:138.

130. Martin SK, Miller LH, Alling D. Severe malaria and glucose 6-phosphate dehydrogenase deficiency: a reappraisal of the malaria/G6PD hypothesis. Lancet 1979;1:524.

131. Segal HE, Noll WW, Thiemanun W. Glucose 6-phosphate dehydrogenase deficiency and falciparum malaria in two Northeast Thai villages. Proc Helminth Soc Wash 1972;39:79.

132. Luzzatto L, Bienzle U. The malaria/G6PD hypothesis. Lancet 1979;1: 1183.

133. Guggenmoos-Holzmann I, Bienzle U, Luzzatto L. *Plasmodium falciparum* malaria and human red cells. II: Red cell genetic traits and resistance against malaria. Int J Epidemiol 1981;10:16.

134. Sodeinde O. Glucose 6-phosphate dehydrogenase deficiency. In: Fleming AF, ed. Epidemiology of haematological disease, part 2. London, Bailliere Tindall, 1992:367.

135. Luzzatto L. Genetics of human red cells and susceptibility to malaria. In: Michal F, ed. Modern genetic concepts and techniques in the study of parasites. Basel, Schwabe, 1981:257.

136. Roth EF Jr, Raventos-Suarez C, Rinaldi A, Nagel RL. Glucose 6-phosphate dehydrogenase deficiency inhibits *in vitro* growth of *Plasmodium falciparum*. Proc Natl Acad Sci 1983;80:298.

137. Golenser J, Miller J, Spira DT, Kosower NS, Vande Waa JA, Jensen JB. Inhibition of the intraerythrocytic development of *Plasmodium falciparum* in glucose 6-phosphate dehydrogenase deficient erythrocytes is enhanced by oxidants and by crisis form factor. Trop Med Parasitol 1988;39:273.

138. Kamchonwongpaisan S, Bunyaratvej A, Wanachiwanawin W, Yuthavong Y. Susceptibility to hydrogen peroxide of *Plasmodium falciparum* infecting glucose-6-phosphate dehydrogenase-deficient erythrocytes. Parasitology 1989;99:2.

139. Marva E, Cohen A, Saltman P, Chevion M, Golenser J. Deleterious synergistic effects of ascorbate and copper on the development of *Plasmodium falciparum*: an *in vitro* study in normal and in G6PD-deficient erythrocytes. Int J Parasitol 1989;19:779.

140. Luzzatto L, Usanga EA, Reddy S. Glucose 6-phosphate dehydrogenase deficient red cells: resistance to infection by malarial parasites. Science 1969;164:839.

141. Usanga EA, Luzzatto L. Adaptation of *Plasmodium falciparum* to glucose 6-phosphate dehydrogenase deficient host red cells by production of parasite-encoded enzyme. Nature 1985;313:793.

142. Luzzatto L, Usanga EA, Modiano G. Genetic resistance to *Plasmodium falciparum*: studies in the field and in cultures *in vitro*. In: Rollinson D, Anderson RM, eds. Ecology and genetics of host-parasite interactions. 1985;11:205.

143. Luzzatto L, O'Brien S, Usanga EA, Wanachiwanawin W. Origin of G6PD polymorphism: malaria and G6PD deficiency. In: Yoshida A, Beutler E, eds. Glucose 6-phosphate dehydrogenase. New York, Academic Press, 1986:181.

144. Ling IT, Wilson RJM. G6PD activity of the malarial parasite *Plasmodium falciparum*. Mol Biochem Parasitol 1988;31:47.

145. Kurdi-Haidar B, Luzzatto L. Expression and characterization of glucose 6-phosphate dehydrogenase of *Plasmodium falciparum*. Mol Biochem Parasitol 1990;41:83.

146. Cavalli-Sforza LL, Bodmer WF. The genetics of human populations. San Francisco, Freeman, 1971.

147. Daley GQ, Van Etten RA, Baltimore D. Induction of chronic myelogenous leukemia in mice by the P210bcr/abl gene of the Philadelphia chromosome. Science 1990;247:824.

148. Lenoir GM, Taub R. Chromosomal translocations and oncogenes in Burkitt's lymphoma. In: Goldman JM, Harnden DG, eds. Genetic rearrangements in leukaemia and lymphoma. London, Churchill Livingstone, 1986:152.

149. Baehner RL, Nathan DG, Castle WB. Oxidant injury of Caucasian glucose-6-phosphate dehydrogenase deficient red blood cells by phagocytosing leukocytes during infection. J Clin Invest 1971;50:2466.

150. Kattamis CA, Tjortjatou F. The hemolytic process of viral hepatitis in children with normal or deficient glucose 6-phosphate dehydrogenase activity. J Pediatr 1970;77:422.

151. Galiano S, Gaetani GF, Barabino A, et al. Favism in the African type of glucose-6-phosphate dehydrogenase deficiency (A−). Br Med J 1990;300:236.

152. Meloni T, Forteleoni G, Ogana A, Francavilla V. Aspirin-induced acute hemolytic anemia in glucose 6-phosphate dehydrogenase deficient children with systemic arthritis. Acta Haematol (Basel) 1989;81:208.

153. Magon AM, Leipzig RM, Zannoni VG, Brewer GJ. Interactions of glucose 6-phosphate dehydrogenase deficiency with drug acetylation and hydroxylation reactions. J Lab Clin Med 1981;97:764.

154. Frischer H, Carson PE. Multiple gene interactions in pharmacogenetics. J Lab Clin Med 1981;97:760.

155. Tarlov AR, Brewer GJ, Carson PE, Alving AS. Primaquine sensitivity: glucose 6-phosphate dehydrogenase deficiency. Arch Intern Med 1962;109:209.

156. Pannacciulli I, Tizianello A, Salvidio E. The course of experimentally-induced hemolytic anemia in a primaquine-sensitive Caucasian. Blood 1965;25:92.

157. Fischer TM, Meloni T, Pescarmona GP, Bosia A, Arese P. Membrane cross bonding in red cells in favic crisis: a missing link in the mechanism of extravascular hemolysis. Br J Haematol 1985;59:159.

158. Rifkind RA. Heinz bodies anaemia: an ultrastructural study. II: Red cell sequestration and destruction. Blood 1965;26:433.

159. Chevion M, Navok T, Glaser G, Mager J. The chemistry of favism-inducing compounds: the properties of isouramil and divicine and their reaction with glutathione. Eur J Biochem 1982;127:405.

160. Winterbourn C, Cowden WB, Sutton HC. Auto-oxidation of dialuric acid, divicine and isouramil: superoxide dependent and independent mechanisms. Biochem Pharmacol 1989;38:611.

161. Arese P, De Flora A. Pathophysiology of hemolysis in glucose 6-phosphate dehydrogenase deficiency. Semin Hematol 1990;27:1.

162. Doxiadis SA, Valaes F. The clinical picture of glucose 6-phosphate dehydrogenase deficiency in early childhood. Arch Dis Child 1964;39: 545.

163. Gibbs WN, Gray R, Lowry M. Glucose 6-phosphate dehydrogenase deficiency and neonatal jaundice in Jamaica. Br J Haematol 1979;43: 263.

164. Bienzle U, Effiong CE, Luzzatto L. Erythrocyte glucose 6-phosphate dehydrogenase deficiency (G6PD type A^-) and neonatal jaundice. Acta Paediatr Scand 1976;65:701.

165. Meloni T, Cutillo S, Testa U, Luzzatto L. Neonatal jaundice and severity of glucose 6-phosphate dehydrogenase deficiency in Sardinian babies. Early Hum Dev 1987;15:317.

166. Meloni T, Cagnazzo G, Dore A, Cutillo S. Phenobarbital for prevention of hyperbilirubinemia in glucose 6-phosphate dehydrogenase-deficient newborn infants. J Pediatr 1973;82:1048.

167. Bienzle U, Effiong CE, Aimaku VE, Luzzatto L. Erythrocyte enzymes in neonatal jaundice. Acta Haematol (Basel) 1976;55:10.

168. Doxiadis SA, Valaes T, Karaklis A, Stavrakakis D. Risk of severe jaundice in glucose 6-phosphate dehydrogenase deficiency of the newborn: differences in population groups. Lancet 1964;2:1210.
169. Owa JA. Relationship between exposure to icterogenic agents, glucose-6-phosphate dehydrogenase deficiency and neonatal jaundice in Nigeria. Acta Paediatr Scand 1989;78:848.
170. Singh A. Glucose 6-phosphate dehydrogenase deficiency: a preventable cause of mental retardation. Br Med J 1986;292:397.
171. Meloni T, Forteleoni G, Dore A, Cutillo S. Neonatal hyperbilirubinaemia in heterozygous glucose-6-phosphate dehydrogenase deficient females. Br J Haematol 1983;53:241.
172. Oluboyede OA, Esan GJF, Francis TI, Luzzatto L. Genetically determined deficiency of glucose 6-phosphate dehydrogenase (type A−) is expressed in the liver. J Lab Clin Med 1979;93:783.
173. Ifekwunigwe AE, Luzzatto L. Kernicterus in G6PD deficiency. Lancet 1966;1:667.
174. Meloni T, Costa S, Dore A, Cutillo S. Phototherapy for neonatal hyperbilirubinemia in mature newborn infants with G6PD deficiency. J Pediatr 1974;85:560.
175. Luzzatto L, Meloni T. Hemolytic anemia due to glucose 6-phosphate dehydrogenase deficiency. In: Brain MC, Carbone PP, eds. Current therapy in hematology–oncology: 1985–1986. Toronto, BC Decker, CV Mosby, 1985:21.
176. Lewis RA, Kay RW, Hathorn M. Sickle cell disease and glucose-6-phosphate dehydrogenase phosphate dehydrogenase. Acta Haematol (Basel) 1966;35:399.
177. Luzzatto L, Allan NC. Relationship between the genes for glucose-6-phosphate dehydrogenase and for haemoglobin in a Nigerian population. Nature 1968;219:1041.
178. Bienzle U, Sodeinde O, Effiong CE, Luzzatto L. G6PD deficiency and sickle cell anemia: frequency and features of the association in an African community. Blood 1975;46:591.
179. Steinberg MH, West MS, Gallagher D, Mentzer W. Effects of glucose-6-phosphate dehydrogenase deficiency upon sickle cell anemia. Blood 1988;71:748.
180. Smits HL, Oski FA, Brody JI. The hemolytic crisis of sickle cell disease: the role of glucose 6-phosphate dehydrogenase deficiency. J Pediatr 1969;74:544.
181. Johnson GJ, Allen DW, Cadman S, et al. Red cell membrane polypeptide aggregates in glucose-6-phosphate dehydrogenase mutants with chronic haemolytic disease: a clue to the mechanism of haemolysis. N Engl J Med 1979;301:522.
182. Adkins B, Leutz A, Graft T. Autocrine growth induced by src-related oncogenes in transformed chicken myeloid cells. Cell 1984;39:439.
183. Piomelli S, Corash LM, Davenport DD, Miraglia J, Amorosi EL. In vivo lability of glucose-6-phosphate dehydrogenase in Gd A and Gd Mediterranean deficiency. J Clin Invest 1968;47:940.
184. Beutler E. The relationship of red cell enzymes to red cell life-span. Blood Cells 1988;14:69.
185. Beutler E, Dern RJ, Alving AS. The hemolytic effect of primaquine. VI: An *in vitro* test for sensitivity of erythrocytes to primaquine. J Lab Clin Med 1955;45:40.
186. Mareni C, Repetto L, Forteleoni G, Meloni T, Gaetani GF. Favism: looking for an autosomal gene associated with glucose-6-phosphate dehydrogenase deficiency. J Med Genet 1984;21:278.
187. Low PS. Structure and function of the cytoplasmic domain of band 3: center of erythrocyte membrane-peripheral protein interactions. Biochim Biophys Acta 1986;864:145.
188. Waugh SM, Walder JA, Low PS. Partial characterization of the copolymerization reaction of erythrocyte membrane band 3 with hemichrome. Biochemistry 1987;26:1777.
189. Kasper ML, Miller WJ, Jacob HS. G6PD deficiency infectious haemolysis: a complement dependent innocent bystander phenomenon. Br J Haematol 1986;63:85.
190. Beutler E. The genetics of glucose-6-phosphate dehydrogenase deficiency. Semin Hematol 1990;27:137.
191. Viglietto G, Montanaro V, Calabrò V, et al. Common glucose 6-phosphate dehydrogenase (G6PD) variants from the Italian Population: biochemical and molecular characterization. Ann Hum Genet 1990;54:1.
192. Morelli A, Benatti U, Gaetani GF, DeFlora A. Biochemical mechanisms of glucose-6-phosphate dehydrogenase deficiency. Proc Natl Acad Sci USA 1978;75:1979.
193. Persico MG, Ciccodicola A, Martini G, Rosner JL. Functional expression of human glucose 6-phosphate dehydrogenase in Escherichia coli. Gene 1989;78:365.
194. Schuster R, Jacobasch G, Holzhutter H-G. Mathematical modelling of metabolic pathways affected by an enzyme deficiency. Eur J Biochem 1989;182:605.
195. Vives-Corrons JL, Feliu E, Pujades MA, et al. Severe glucose-6-phosphate dehydrogenase (G6PD) deficiency associated with chronic haemolytic anaemia, granulocyte dysfunction and increased susceptibility to infections: description of a new molecular variant (G6PD Barcelona). Blood 1982;59:428.
196. Harley JD, Agar NS, Yoshida A. Glucose 6-phosphate dehydrogenase variants: Gd(+) Alexandra associated with neonatal jaundice and Gd(−) Camperdown in a young man with lamellar cataracts. J Lab Clin Med 1978;91:295.
197. Yuregir G, Varinli I, Donma O. Glucose 6-phosphate dehydrogenase deficiency both in red blood cells and lenses of the normal and cataractous native population of Cukurova, the southern part of Turkey: part I. Ophthalmic Res 1989;21:155.
198. Orzalesi M, Fossarello M, Sarcinelli R, Schlich U. The relationship between glucose 6-phosphate dehydrogenase deficiency and cataracts in Sardinia: an epidemiological and biochemical study. Doc Ophthalmol 1984;57:187.
199. Motulsky AG, Campbell-Kraut JM. Population genetics of glucose 6-phosphate dehydrogenase deficiency of the red cell. In: Blumberg BS, ed. Proceedings of conference on genetic polymorphisms and geographic variations in disease. New York, Grune & Stratton, 1961:159.
200. Gall JC, Brewer GJ, Dern RJ. Studies of glucose 6-phosphate dehydrogenase activity of individual erythrocytes: the methemoglobin elution test for the detection of females heterozygous for G6PD deficiency. Am J Hum Genet 1965;17:359.
201. Beutler E. Special modifications for the fluorescent screening test for glucose 6-phosphate dehydrogenase deficiency. Blood 1968;32:816.
202. Boyer SH, Porter IH, Weilbacher RG. Electrophoretic heterogeneity of glucose 6-phosphate dehydrogenase and its relationship to enzyme deficiency in man. Proc Natl Acad Sci 1962;48:1868.
203. Rattazzi MC, Bernini LF, Fiorelli G, Mannucci PM. Electrophoresis of glucose-6-phosphate dehydrogenase: a new technique. Nature 1967;213:79.
204. Forbes J, Steytler JG, van Heerden R. Agarose gel electrophoresis of glucose 6-phosphate dehydrogenase isoenzymes. Clin Chim Acta 1991;199:279.
205. Fairbanks VF, Lampe LT. A tetrazolium-linked cytochemical method for estimation of glucose 6-phosphate dehydrogenase activity in individual erythrocytes: applications in the study of heterozygotes for glucose 6-phosphate dehydrogenase deficiency. Blood 1968;31:589.
206. Jonges GN, Hagen H, Van Noorden CJ, Weening RS, Roos D. Comparison between the chromate inhibition test and a cytochemical method for the determination of glucose-6-phosphate dehydrogenase deficiency in erythrocytes. Clin Chim Acta 1989;181:135.
207. Ekert U, Rawlinson I. Deferoxamine and favism. N Engl J Med 1985;312:1260.
208. Meloni T, Forteleoni G, Gaetani GF. Desferrioxamine and favism. Br J Haematol 1986;63:394.
209. Beutler E. The hemolytic effect of primaquine and related compounds. Blood 1959;14:103.
210. Warburg O, Christian W. Uber ein neues Oxydationserment und sein Absorptionsspektrum. Biochem Z 1932;254:438.
211. Kirkman HN, Riley HD, Crowell BB. Different enzymic expression of human glucose 6-phosphate dehydrogenase. Proc Natl Acad Sci 1960;46:938.
212. Adam A. Linkage between deficiency of glucose 6-phosphate dehydrogenase and colour-blindness. Nature 1961;189:686.
213. Yoshida A. Glucose 6-phosphate dehydrogenase of human erythrocytes: purification and characterization of normal (B^+) enzyme. J Biol Chem 1966;241:4966.
214. Betke K, Brewer GJ, Kirkman HN, et al. Standardization of procedures for the study of glucose-6-phosphate dehydrogenase. WHO Tech Rep Ser 1967;366.
215. Bautista JM, Mason PJ, Luzzatto L. Purification and properties of human glucose-6-phosphate dehydrogenase made in *E. coli*. Biochim Biophys Acta 1991;74:1119.
216. Adediran SA. Sigmoid kinetics of human erythrocyte glucose 6-phosphate dehydrogenase. Arch Biochem Biophys 1988;262:354.
217. Jeffery J, Soderling-Barros J, Murray LA, Hansen RJ, Szepesi B, Jornvall H. Molecular diversity of glucose-6-phosphate dehydrogenase: rat enzyme structure identifies NH2-terminal segment, shows initiation from sites nonequivalent in different organisms and establishes otherwise extensive sequence conservation. Proc Natl Acad Sci USA 1988;85:7840.
218. Kirkman HN, Hendrickson EM. Sex-linked electrophoretic difference in glucose 6-phosphate dehydrogenase. Am J Hum Genet 1963;15:241.
219. Luzzatto L. Studies of polymorphic traits for the characterization of populations: African populations South of the Sahara. Israel J Med Sci 1973;9:1181.
220. Kirkman HN, Simon ER, Pickard BM. Seattle variant of glucose 6-phosphate dehydrogenase. J Lab Clin Med 1965;66:834.
221. Calabrò V, Mason PJ, Civitelli D, et al. Genetic heterogeneity at the glucose 6 phosphate dehydrogenase locus. Am J Hum Genet 1993;52:527.
223. Calabrò V, Giacobbe A, Vallone D, et al. Genetic heterogeneity at the glucose 6-phosphate dehydrogenase locus in southern Italy: a study on a population from the Matera district. Hum Genet 1990;86:49.
224. Town M, Bautista JM, Mason PJ, Luzzatto L. Both mutations in G6PD A− are necessary to produce the G6PD deficient phenotype. Hum Mol Genet 1992;1:171.
225. Kurdi-Haidar B, Mason PJ, Berrebi A, et al. Origin and spread of the glucose 6-phosphate dehydrogenase variant (G6PD Mediterranean) in the Middle East. Am J Hum Genet 1990;47:1013.
226. Kirkman HN, Schettini F, Pickard BM. Mediterranean variant of glucose 6-phosphate dehydrogenase. J Lab Clin Med 1964;63:726.
227. Chao L, Du CS, Louie E, et al. A to G substitution identified in exon 2

of the G6PD gene among G6PD deficient Chinese. Nucleic Acids Res 1991;19:6056.
228. MacDonald D, Town M, Mason PJ, Vulliamy TJ, Luzzatto L, Goff MC. Deficiency in red blood cells. Nature 1991;350:115.
229. Nafa K, Reghis A, Osmani N, et al. G6PD Aures: a new mutation (48 Ile→Thr) causing mild G6PD deficiency is associated with favism. Hum Mol Genet 1993;2:81.
230. Hirono A, Fujii H, Miwa S. Molecular abnormality of G6PD Konan and G6PD Ube. Hum Genet 1993;91:507.
231. Maeda M, Constantoulakis P, Chen CS, Stamatoyannopoulos G, Yoshida A. Molecular abnormalities of a human glucose 6-phosphate dehydrogenase variant associated with undetectable enzyme activity and immunologically cross-reacting material. Am J Hum Genet 1992;51:386.
232. Chiu DTY, Zuo L, Chen E, Louie LT, Lubin BH, Du CS. DNA sequence abnormalities in Chinese glucose 6-phosphate dehydrogenase (G6PD) variants. Blood [Abstract] 1991;78 (Suppl 1):252a.
233. Vulliamy TJ, Wanachiwanawin W, Mason PJ, Luzzatto L. G6PD Mahidol, a common deficient variant in South East Asia is caused by a (163)glycine–serine mutation. Nucleic Acids Res 1989;17:5868.
234. Tang TK, Huamg C-S, Huamg M-J, Tam K-B, Yeh C-H, Tang C-JC. Diverse point mutations result in glucose 6-phosphate dehydrogenase (G6PD) polymorphism in Taiwan. Blood 1992;79:2135.
235. Beutler E, Kuhl W, Saenz GF, Rodriguez W. Mutation analysis of glucose 6-phosphate dehydrogenase (G6PD) variants in Costarica. Hum Genet 87;462:464.
236. Junien C, Kaplan JC, Heienhofer HC, Malgret P, Sender A. G6PD Baudelocque: a new unstable variant characterized in fibroblasts. Enzyme 1974;18:48.
237. Corcoran CM, Calabro V, Tamagnini G, et al. Molecular heterogeneity underlying the G6PD Mediterranean phenotype. Hum Genet 1992;88: 688.
238. Beutler E, Westwood B, Prchal JT, Vaca G, Bartsocas CS, Baronciani L. New glucose 6-phosphate dehydrogenase mutations from various ethnic groups. Blood 1992;80:255.
239. Beutler E, Kuhl W, Gelbart T, Forman M. DNA sequence abnormalities of human glucose 6-phosphate dehydrogenase variants. J Biol Chem 1991;266:4145.
240. Beutler E, Prchal JT, Westwood B, Kuhl W. Definition of the mutations of G6PD Wayne, G6PD Viangchan, G6PD Jammu and G6PD "LeJeune." Acta Haematologica (Basel) 1991;86:179.
241. Beutler E, Westwood B, Kuhl W, Hsia HE. Glucose 6-phosphate dehydrogenase variants in Hawaii. Hum Hered 1992;42:327.
242. Hirono A, Fujii H, Hirono K, Kanno H, Miwa S. Molecular abnormality of a Japanese glucose 6-phosphate dehydrogenase variant (G6PD Tokyo) associated with hereditary nonspherocytic hemolytic anemia. Hum Genet 1992;88:347.
243. Perng L, Chiou S-S, Liu TC, Chang JG. A novel C to T substitution at nucleotide 1360 of cDNA which abolishes a natural HhaI site accounts for a new G6PD deficiency gene in Chinese. Hum Mol Genet 1992;1: 205.
244. Stevens DJ, Wanachiwanawin W, Mason PJ, Vulliamy TJ, Luzzatto L. G6PD Canton: a common deficient variant in South East Asia cause by a 459 Arg→Leu mutation. Nucleic Acids Res 1990;18:7190.
245. Chiu DTY, Zuo L, Chen E, et al. Two commonly occurring nucleotide base substitutions in Chinese G6PD variants. Biochem Biophys Res Commun 1991;180:988.

Blood: Principles and Practice of Hematology,
edited by Robert I. Handin, Samuel E. Lux, and Thomas P. Stossel.
J.B. Lippincott Company, Philadelphia © 1995.

59

Hematologic Aspects of Systemic Disease

Thomas P. Duffy

ANEMIA OF CHRONIC DISEASE

Few alterations in the body's homeostasis are not reflected or expressed in the hematologic system. For example, the renal source of erythropoietin, the hepatic synthesis of coagulation factors, and the leukocyte response to infection demonstrate the fact that pathology in almost any organ system within the body is mirrored in a parallel hematologic response. Systemic disease affects and is affected by changes in hematologic function. These manifestations are so consistent and characteristic that they constitute a major locus for differential diagnosis of systemic disease. Leukocytosis with an increase in band forms is the hallmark of bacterial infection, and eosinophilia has comparable implications for allergic or parasitic diseases. A hematologic abnormality is often the minor detail that defines the focus of the pursuit in establishing the source of pathology elsewhere in the body.

The hematologic aspects of systemic disease are myriad, with some findings diagnostic of a single disorder (such as malaria parasites in red blood cells [RBCs]), whereas others may represent a uniform response to diverse insults. The latter phenomenon assumes its most common guise in the "anemia of chronic disease" (ACD), an anemia that accompanies illnesses as diverse as traumatic, inflammatory, malignant, and infectious states. G.C. Cartwright's prescient recognition of ACD as a unitary pathophysiologic entity[1] stimulated many investigators to explore the cause of this shared response by the body to several different insults. The mechanism is still not completely identified, although the explosion in molecular biology is helping to clarify the pathways involved in the process.[2]

Hypoproliferative Anemia With Low Serum Iron and Transferrin

Persons suffering from infection, malignancy, or inflammation develop within a few weeks of onset of these conditions a characteristic anemia that is independent of any marrow involvement or specific hematologic complication of their disease.[3] A modest shortening of RBC survival is present but not adequately compensated for by the marrow; this reticulocytopenic response suggests that a hypoproliferative defect rather than hemolysis is the major lesion in ACD.[4] The anemia is moderate in degree with the hematocrit usually fixed in the 28% to 32% range; a compensatory erythroid hyperplasia of the marrow or reticulocytosis is not present. The anemia is usually normochromic and normocytic, but a population of hypochromic cells is often evident; 30% to 40% of such patients have a microcytic, hypochromic anemia. Iron studies reveal low serum iron and transferrin levels, contrasting with findings in uncomplicated iron-deficiency anemia in which low iron levels are accompanied by elevated transferrin levels.[5] The transferrin saturation levels in ACD may overlap with those of iron deficiency, contributing to a confusion of these two entities with one another. What distinguishes the two is the abundant stores of reticuloendothelial iron found in those with ACD; the anemia represents, according to Cartwright,[6] a "sideropenic anemia in the face of reticuloendothelial siderosis."

Sequestration of Iron Into Reticuloendothelial Cells

Recycling of iron derived from the breakdown of senescent RBCs and its storage within reticuloendothelial and liver parenchymal cells provide the major source of iron needed for hemoglobin (Hb) synthesis. In progressive iron deficiency, initially no anemia or lowering of serum iron levels is noted until the iron stores within the depots have been exhausted. The body has a reserve of storage iron, which helps guarantee a constant supply of iron for Hb synthesis. In ACD, a low serum iron accompanies iron-deficient anemia, as evidenced by decreased marrow sideroblasts and elevated free erythrocyte protoporphyrins. All these features exist in the presence of abundant reticuloendothelial stores of iron and elevated serum levels of ferritin. The normal mechanism for preferential delivery of iron to support Hb synthesis in developing RBCs is defective on some level in this state. The vector of iron delivery in ACD appears misdirected, and this lesion has been implicated as the source of hypoproliferative ACD.[7]

Several investigators have documented the faulty liberation of iron stores in these states, whereas others question the data or their importance in ACD. Ferrokinetic studies using radiolabeled RBC Hb have demonstrated delayed release of such iron from reticuloendothelial stores.[8] The same delay characterizes the hepatic release of iron derived from free Hb infusions that are taken up by liver parenchymal cells.[9] A similar defect in iron release from intestinal epithelial cells has also been reported.[10] The body appears to closet its iron stores as a feature of ACD, and hypochromic anemia exists in the presence of iron overload.

Restraint of Bacteria or Tumor Growth by Hypoferremia

Cartwright suggested that ACD is part of the body's defense system against various insults; the altered direction of iron flow is purposeful because it creates hypoferremia, a desirable result in the presence of infection or malignancy. All microorganisms require iron for growth and proliferation and many organisms have siderophores, which are iron-complexing molecules that permit successful extraction of iron from plasma.[11] Some malignant cells possess similar devices to ensure their iron requirements for growth.[12–14] A fall in serum iron with ACD deprives the invading cell population of an essential nutrient. The hypoferremia of ACD is a form of nutritional immunity whose advantage to the body in restraining bacterial or tumor cell growth outweighs any associated diversion of iron from erythroid cells. The anemia is the cost of the body's defense against invasion.[15]

Lactoferrin "Iron-Steal" Hypothesis

The cause of hypoferremia in states of infection is not strictly defined. Cartwright and associates[16] showed a rapid fall in serum iron after bacterial challenge of animal models. This phenomenon could be replicated by infusion of *lactoferrin*, an iron transport protein present in the granules of polymorphonuclear cells.[17] Lactoferrin, with an avidity for iron even greater than transferrin, imparts a direction of iron flow away from developing RBCs that do not contain lactoferrin receptors.[18] Any iron scavenged by lactoferrin is rapidly removed from plasma and deposited in reticuloendothelial or hepatic parenchymal cells. Mobilization and activation of polymorphonuclear neutrophils after bacterial infection create a cellular response that is combined with the release of lactoferrin.[19,20] The interposition of this transport protein steals iron from bacterial cells and RBCs alike. This is a teleologic explanation in defense of a positive role for ACD.

The lactoferrin hypothesis may explain ACD as it accompanies infection, but the same leukocytosis and lactoferrin release do not consistently accompany malignancies and their ACD. Lactoferrin does accumulate in several neoplasms and may even be a marker for benign versus malignant tissue.[21] Hypernephroma, a tumor classically associated with anemia, contains significantly increased tissue lactoferrin levels compared with those seen in normal renal tissue. In these circumstances, the vector of iron delivery may favor tumor growth and development, with iron flow more heavily directed to these tissue sites.

Role of Interleukin-1 and Tumor Necrosis Factor

Another possible cause for the hypoferremia of ACD is a disproportionate incorporation of iron into ferritin in storage depots, making the iron less easily mobilizable than the alternate storage form of low molecular weight iron.[22] Since ferritin is an acute phase reactant protein, this shift in iron placement would accompany all the conditions associated with ACD. Neither this mechanism nor lactoferrin's role in host immunity is solidly established as the cause of the hypoproliferative component of ACD. The hypoferremia may be only a part of a more generalized response to infection, malignancy, or inflammation. ACD accompanies other manifestations of systemic disease such as anorexia, weight loss, debilitation, and inflammation.

The signs and symptoms of systemic disease are accompanied by release of acute phase reactants measured in the blood as C-reactive proteins, elevated fibrinogen, haptoglobin, and ceruloplasmin. The presence of these diseases and their activity have traditionally also been monitored by measurement of the erythrocyte sedimentation rate. These seemingly disparate responses to a multitude of bodily insults are now unified in a common pathway of metabolic events initiated by interleukin-1 (IL-1) release from activated macrophages.[23] IL-1 then initiates a cascade of events mediated by the cytokines released from macrophages, lymphocytes, and other numerous cells within the body.[24] Both anabolic and catabolic responses are created with interleukins mediating the host response to infection and inflammation.

An important factor in this network is tumor necrosis factor (TNF), a product of the macrophage with an ability to induce the same spectrum of acute phase changes as IL-1.[25] Injection of TNF reproduces the anorexia, weight loss, and debilitation of chronic disease and likewise inhibits the growth of hematopoietic precursor cells; unifying the entire picture is TNF's induction of hypoferremia as an accompaniment of these chronic disorders.[26]

Cartwright's prescience in recognizing ACD as a single pathophysiologic entity has its explanation in ACD as a participant in the general process of cachexia.[27] ACD, although multifactorial in its causes, has the shared lymphocyte–monocyte reaction to infection, malignancy, and inflammation. RBC survival is abbreviated because of heightened reticuloendothelial activity, the product of activated macrophages, and the effect of fever in shortening the RBC life-span. Hypoferremia is causally related to interleukin–TNF effects on both white blood cell (WBC) and lactoferrin release, with a resultant form of nutritional immunity. A hypoproliferative anemia is created, related to the suppressive effect of the cytokines on progenitor cells.

INFECTIOUS DISEASES

The hematologic aspects of infectious diseases have their historical antecedents in many of the earliest and most important discoveries in the field of hematology. An understanding of pus and its relation to infection and inflammation dates from observations made possible by the staining techniques of Ehrlich, by the recognition of diapedesis and cellular motion by Cornheim, and by phagocytosis by Metchnikoff. These past achievements are complemented by knowledge of the body's humoral and cellular control systems, which modulate the hematologic and immunologic defenses of the body; this interwoven cascade is the means whereby infectious agents are confronted and eliminated and tissue repair occurs.[28] Leukocytosis and a left shift in the WBC differential are the classic accompaniments of bacterial infections.[29] The release of IL-1 after macrophage activation initiates the series of events that mobilizes WBCs from the marrow in response to colony-stimulating factor (CSF) release.[30,31]

The leukocytosis that accompanies bacterial sepsis may be of such magnitude (40,000 to 70,000/μL) that the peripheral blood picture is confused with leukemia, a so-called leukemoid reaction[32] (see Chap. 17). Infections classically associated with a leukemoid blood picture are miliary tuberculosis[33,34] and some bacterial infections such as shigellosis.[35] Other noninfectious causes of leukemoid reactions are corticosteroids, inflammatory states, and nonhematologic malignancies. Corticosteroids create the picture by mobilization of the marginal pool of WBCs into the circulation and inhibition of their emigration into the extravascular space.[36] Tumors may have leukocytosis as a paraneoplastic manifestation, the result of CSF liberation by the neoplasm.[37,38]

Not only is the WBC count increased in bacterial infections, but the morphology of the cells is often a clue to the bacterial origin of a febrile state. These findings include toxic granulations, Döhle bodies, and vacuoles in the polymorphonuclear cells[39,40] (see Chap. 17). Toxic granulations represent nonspecific hypergranulation of the polymorphonuclear leukocytes, whereas Döhle body formation results from aggregation of the endoplasmic reticulum.[41] Vacuolization of polymorphonuclear leukocytes is considered the best of these abnormalities as a clue to the presence of infection, provided that the vacuolization is not artifactually created by WBC ingestion of anticoagulants.[42] Definitive morphologic evidence of bacteria can sometimes be demonstrated, especially in asplenic subjects, by Gram staining a buffy coat preparation of the peripheral blood.[43] In overwhelming sepsis, the organisms are frequently evident in the vacuoles of the polymorphonuclear cells.

The lack of granulocytosis in patients with most viral infections originates in viral induction of an acute phase response that suppresses granulocyte expansion[44,45]; monocytes from virally infected persons do not release IL-1.[46] In addition, the levels of interferon-α, a cause of neutropenia, are elevated in viral states and may inhibit the interleukin–CSF response of bacterial infection.[47] Frequently, lymphocytosis is present with viral infection.[48,49] The specific receptor for viral particles on lymphocytes may be a stimulus for B-lymphocyte proliferation or lymphoid death.[50] T-cell ratios are often reversed in viral infections with increased suppressor T-cell numbers and activation.[51] The atypical lymphocyte or Downey cell of infectious mononucleosis is a stimulated suppressor T cell[52] (see Chap. 22).

Anemia

Common to all chronic infections, and probably playing a role in acute infections as well, is the suppressive effect of the interleukin and TNF on erythropoiesis.[53] In addition, the iron-steal phenomenon deprives microorganisms of iron, which is an essential nutrient for microbial replication, and may be a component of host immunity against infection.[54] Serum levels of iron fall after a bacterial challenge, and the lactoferrin released from stimulated granulocytes is the conduit for this iron to return to reticuloendothelial cells. Many examples of bacterial pathogenicity being dependent on iron availability (*Neisseria gonorrhoeae, Neisseria meningitidis*) support the hypothesis that the anemia of infection is the body's compromise in an attempt to deprive invading microorganisms of iron.[55,56]

The truth of the converse of this situation, that iron overload contributes to increased morbidity and mortality of infection, is controversial.[57] Even critics of the iron overload theory do not seriously question hypoferremia as a host defense mechanism against bacterial infection.

The other erythroid abnormalities seen with infections may involve almost every step in the production and survival of the RBC. Acute viral infection with parvovirus B19, the cause of fifth disease (erythema infectiosum) in children, leads to a direct inhibition of burst-forming unit—erythroid (BFU-E) formation.[58,59] This suppression, which is discussed in detail in Chapter 10, is usually not clinically significant unless the infection occurs in the setting of chronic hemolytic processes such as sickle cell disease or hereditary spherocytosis.[60] In these situations, a life-threatening aplastic crisis may be caused by an otherwise benign viral illness. Epstein-Barr virus has also been incriminated as a cause of RBC aplasia by the mechanism of T-cell suppression of erythroid colony-forming units (CFU-E).[61] Human T-cell lymphocyte virus–III is associated with dysplastic RBC features in the marrow and ineffective erythropoiesis.[62]

Exaggerated and premature RBC destruction accompanies many infections. Heightened reticuloendothelial activity with or without splenomegaly shortens RBC survival in these states. Infections are a leading cause of hemolysis in RBC enzyme deficiency states, but they may also cause excessive hemolysis by direct toxic or immunologic damage to cells.[63] A devastatingly severe form of damage is produced in *Clostridium perfringens* and *Clostridium welchii* sepsis secondary to lecithinase attack on the RBC membrane.[64] The peripheral blood smear findings in this situation are a striking RBC spherocytosis, which is accompanied by elevated levels of free plasma Hb.[65]

Immunologic sensitization may also create membrane damage during infections. *Mycoplasma* and numerous viral infections are associated with the development of cold agglutinins directed against the I or i antigen sites on RBCs. Although these antibodies are commonly detected, they infrequently cause significant hemolytic disease (see Chap. 55). The Donath-Landsteiner antibody, responsible for the bithermal activation of complement and hemolysis in paroxysmal cold hemoglobinuria, is an accompaniment of congenital syphilis and some viral infections, especially mumps.[67] Some bacteria, such as *Haemophilus influenzae*, cause hemolysis via attachment of a capsular polysaccharide to the RBCs, rendering them immunogenic with complement deposition and extravascular hemolysis.[68]

Parasitization of RBCs with resulting hemolysis is the major clinical manifestation of malaria, and the presence of specific malarial forms on the peripheral blood smear contribute the means for identifying the different types of malaria. This parasite and the RBC have an interesting relation dictated by the mechanisms responsible for attachment and entry of the parasite into the cell.[69] The Duffy blood group antigen is necessary for *Plasmodium vivax* attachment to the RBC; its absence prevents *P vivax* infection in vivo[70] (see Chap. 56). The merozoites of *Plasmodium falciparum* probably bind to a glycoprotein constituent of band 3, the site of attachment of the cellular membrane to the ankyrin-linked spectrin.[71] This entryway permits an opening through the cytoskeleton with endocytosis of the parasite. Within the cell, the malaria parasite inserts into the cell membrane a molecular sequence that has striking homology with transferrin; this permits the parasite to obtain iron directly from plasma.[72] The *P falciparum* parasite also can induce knob formation on the RBC membrane. The knobs contain a histidine-rich protein and attach to endothelial cells, which protects the parasites from splenic scrutiny but contributes to the sludging insults of the cerebral, hepatic, and other vessels of the body in *P falciparum* malaria.[73–75] These insults have been reversed by whole blood exchange transfusions.[76]

Other microorganisms may parasitize the RBC with severe hemolysis; *Bartonella bacilliformis*, the bacterial causative agent of bartonellosis (Oroya fever), uses its flagella in drill-like fashion to permit endocytosis of the organism into the cell.[77] The organisms can subsequently be demonstrated inside vacuoles within the RBC. A milder hemolytic anemia is caused by *Babesia microti* microorganisms[78,79]; babesiosis is not life threatening except in asplenic subjects in whom the parasitized RBCs are not contained.[80] Cases of combined babesiosis and Lyme disease are being described, attributable to the shared geographic locale of the tick vectors for these diseases.[81]

Pancytopenia

Splenomegaly, an accompaniment of many chronic infections, may produce a hypersplenic pancytopenic state because of accelerated cell destruction within the hypertrophied organ. A much more severe pancytopenia in the setting of aplastic anemia occurs as an aftermath of bouts of viral hepatitis.[82] The presumptive agent is non-A, non-B hepatitis, because serologic testing for other known hepatitis viruses has been negative. The marrow disorder is not concomitant with the hepatitis but supervenes weeks to months after the hepatic insult. Usually, no relation in severity is found between the preceding hepatitis and the subsequent aplasia of the marrow. Because this form of hepatitis-related aplasia carries a poor prognosis with a rapid and high mortality, these patients are candidates for early marrow transplantation when such an option is available.

Aplastic anemia accompanies hepatitis in an additional setting. A disproportionate number of liver transplantation patients have developed aplastic anemia after transplantation for non-A, non-B hepatitis.[83] The mechanism for the association is not understood, although the hepatitis virus has been demonstrated to be pantropic and probably involves the marrow elements. Several animal and human viruses induce marrow aplasia by direct infection of the marrow.[84] The interval between the initial hepatitis and the subsequent aplasia suggests an immunologic factor in the hepatitis cases followed by aplastic anemia. The relation of hepatitis and aplasia is described in detail in Chapter 10.

Pancytopenia in the context of infection may also occur in association with a benign proliferation of histocytes and a hemophagocytic syndrome that has been confused with malignant histiocytosis[85,86] (see Chap. 32). The marrow is characterized by increased numbers of histiocytes containing ingested platelets, RBCs, and WBCs. Fever, hepatosplenomegaly, lymphadenopathy, and pancytopenia constitute the clinical presentation of both the benign self-limited and the malignant forms of the disease. Viral infections have been most frequently associated with these hemophagocytic syndromes, although bacterial, fungal, and protozoal agents have also been implicated.[87] Some authors have suggested that the morphology of the histiocytes permits a determination of the malignant character of these diseases. The temporal course of the benign form and the presence of a causal organism may be the only means of distinguishing between the two forms.[88]

Bone Marrow Abnormalities

The bone marrow frequently contains clues as to the source of infectious diseases. Histoplasmosis, tuberculosis, kala-azar,[89] and *Candida* all have been identified in marrow macrophages. Marrow granulomas may be a marker of disseminated tuberculosis or histoplasmosis. The liver is more frequently involved than the marrow in miliary tuberculosis, but the marrow biopsy is still important because its findings are complementary to liver biopsy in the search for tuberculosis. Histoplasmosis, like tuberculosis, brucellosis, and *Salmonella*, can be successfully cultured from the marrow aspirate. The organisms are not the only causes of bone marrow granulomas; cytomegalovirus involvement of the marrow creates the same morphologic finding.[90] Bone marrow morphology and culture play an increasingly important role in the identification and isolation of the many organisms (tuberculosis, histoplasmosis, viral infection) that complicate the acquired immunodeficiency state.

Infection is a leading cause of an unusual hematologic lesion, bone marrow necrosis.[91] This complication of sickle cell disease and other hematologic disorders may give rise to marrow embolization and pulmonary damage. Its occurrence in nonsicklers is most frequently in the context of sepsis, with endotoxin considered the toxic etiologic agent. Bone pain may be severe and attributed to other causes.[92] No pathognomonic peripheral blood findings are noted in bone marrow necrosis, although cytopenias and a leukoerythroblastic blood picture are frequently present. The diagnosis requires recognition of necrotic marrow from the involved areas, a frequently overlooked finding. Magnetic resonance imaging may represent a noninvasive means of making the diagnosis.[93]

Hemostatic Involvement With Infectious Diseases

Thrombocytopenia occurs frequently in the setting of a variety of infections. The mechanisms are complex and sometimes unclear since infectious agents may cause many effects on platelet synthesis and destruction. A fall in platelet count is a universal feature of viral infections. The major lesion is attributable to direct viral infection of the megakaryocyte with reduced platelet production.[94] Since platelets possess receptors for viral particles, accelerated platelet destruction may also occur, possibly assisting in containment of the infection.[95–97] An even more significant thrombocytopenia may occur 2 to 3 weeks after the initial viral insult at a time when immunologic mechanisms are most active.[98,99] This complication originates in several possible immunologic reactions. Antibody cross-reactivity as an immunologic overflow phenomenon, immune complex adherence to platelet membranes, and viral hapten deposition all have been implicated in these thrombocytopenic states.[100] These phenomena are discussed in detail in Chapter 34.

Bacterial infections are associated with thrombocytopenia.[101,102] Immune mechanisms play a major role with sensitization of platelets participating in the body's generalized hyperimmune response state.[103] Platelets can function as endotoxin "sponges" and be destroyed as part of the body's containment of endotoxin.[104] Activation of complement in the setting of infection leads to WBC attachment to the pulmonary microvasculature; secondary thrombocytopenia occurs caused by adherence of platelets to the leukocyte-damaged endothelium. This fall in platelet count may be one of the earliest manifestations of impending adult respiratory distress syndromes.[105]

All infectious agents have the potential to initiate a consumption coagulopathy with thrombocytopenia and reduction in several components of the clotting cascade (see Chap. 43).[106] This complication of septicemia is especially prominent when hypotension accompanies the septic state.[107] Bleeding is its most common manifestation, although infection-related disseminated intravascular coagulation (DIC) may infrequently cause the devastating picture of purpura fulminans with thrombosis of the vessels of the extremities and secondary gangrene.[108–110] Sepsis in asplenic persons is sometimes the cause of DIC with adrenal hemorrhage and renal cortical necrosis (Waterhouse-Friderichsen syndrome)[111]; this syndrome has been described most frequently with pneumococcal sepsis,[112,113] but staphylococcal, streptococcal and, meningococcal organisms may create the same picture.[114]

Thrombosis is not a common feature of infection even though IL-1 decreases endothelial cell fibrinolytic activity by increasing the levels of plasminogen activator inhibitors.[115] Thrombophlebitis due to *Campylobacter fetus*, a microaerophilic gram-negative rod, occurs usually in the setting of an underlying medical illness. When phlebitis fails to respond to heparin, this association should be considered.[116] A suppurative thrombophlebitis of the internal jugular vein secondary to an oropharyngeal infection with *Fusobacterium necrophorum* (Lemierre's syndrome) is another example of infection-related thrombosis.[117]

The syndromes of thrombotic thrombocytopenic purpura (TTP) and hemolytic uremic syndrome (HUS) are both characterized by hyaline thrombi, generated throughout the microvasculature of the body in the former and primarily localized to the renal vessels in the latter.[118,119] Although several agents appear to incite these syndromes, a striking correlation exists between HUS and antecedent diarrheal illnesses caused by toxigenic strains of *Shigella* and *Escherichia coli*.[120] These organisms secrete a verotoxin that is damaging to renal cells in culture. This toxin may disrupt the endothelial cell with its stores of von Willebrand factor and result in platelet adhesion to the vessel wall.[121]

MALIGNANT DISEASE

Each step in the body's elegantly modulated system of erythropoiesis alone or in combination may be pathologically altered in the setting of malignancy. The hematologic lesion may originate in sources as diverse as the direct replacement of marrow by the malignancy or, more commonly, as ACD, the anemia that accompanies even extramedullary tumors. The internists' tumor, hypernephroma, has anemia as part of its diagnostic triad with a flank mass and fever.[122,123] Pancreatic carcinoma and other gastrointestinal malignancies so frequently present with anemia that physicians incur a responsibility to examine the gastrointestinal tract in any patient with otherwise unexplained iron-deficiency anemia.[124,125] Erythropoiesis rarely escapes some impairment in the body's altercation with malignancy.

Inhibition of Erythropoiesis by Cancer

Tumor growth in vitro and in vivo is known to be associated with inhibition of normal erythropoiesis.[126,127] What remains controversial is the mechanism or mechanisms that create this impairment. Addition of W-256 cells to erythropoietin stimulated marrow cultures inhibits CFU-E in proportion to the concentration of the cocultured W-256 cells.[128] Cell cytolysis secondary to direct cell interaction with malignant cells has been documented with other tumors, but the effect of W-256 cells is demonstrable even in CFU-E cultures that separate the malignant cells from the population of bone marrow cells. These experiments support earlier observations that marrows from persons with malignancies have decreased responsiveness to erythropoietin stimulation.[129] Linking both observations is the inhibitory effect generated by TNF, which is released in response to tumors.[130,131] This cytokine, part of the body's humoral defenses against tumor invasion, inhibits both CFU-E and BFU-E levels in culture.[132–134] The blunting of the erythropoietin effect in the setting of malignancy becomes part of the body's deployment for containing tumor cell proliferation. The overlapping effect is less surprising with the recognition that hematopoietic elements share many growth receptors with malignant cell populations.[135]

Suppression of erythropoietin effect has not been a universal finding in malignancy-associated anemia. Others have found normal erythropoietin responsiveness in vitro of marrow cells in these diseases.[136] These patients had reduced erythropoietin levels as an explanation for anemia, a finding at variance with other groups.[129] The diversity of findings may be resolved when the complex interlocking of cellular and humoral controls of hematopoiesis is better defined and the different tumor cell contributions to impaired erythropoiesis are identified. The documentation of decreased erythropoietin response accompanying the anemia of cancer[137] and its correction with the administration of erythropoietin indicts erythropoietin deficiency as a major contributor to the anemia of malignancy.[138]

The anemia of malignancy may be moderate in severity when it occurs as a component of the anemia of chronic disease; a more severe anemia is created when pure RBC aplasia supervenes, frequently in the setting of a thymoma or lymphoproliferative disease.[139] About 50% of patients with pure RBC aplasia have a thymoma, and 10% of patients with thymoma have pure RBC aplasia.[140] Krantz and colleagues[141] demonstrated an IgG inhibitor of erythropoiesis in most of these patients. Thymectomy has successfully reversed the aplasia in most patients with thymomas; corticosteroids and cytoxan are also effective in treating this immunologically mediated anemia. Suppressor T-cell inhibition has also been proved to be a cause of pure RBC aplasia with and without associated lymphoproliferative disease.[142–144] Treatment of the underlying disorder with daily cytoxan has reversed this aplasia in some patients. Pure RBC aplasia is also discussed in Chapter 10.

Anemia in the setting of malignancy may be caused by progressive bone marrow infiltration with tumor. Marrow involvement occurs in about 10% of nonhematologic tumors and is frequently heralded by a so-called leukoerythroblastic blood picture.[145] The latter is characterized by the presence in the peripheral blood of nucleated RBC, teardrop RBC, early myeloid forms, and frequently some alteration in platelet size and number. The occurrence of such a constellation in a patient with a malignancy is near-certain evidence of marrow involvement with tumor. Certain tumors such as prostate, breast, and small cell lung carcinomas have a relatively high incidence of marrow metastases, supporting the role of bone scans in establishing the disease stage within these malignancies. A hot spot on bone scan provides an excellent site for marrow biopsy to confirm the presence of tumor, a discovery that may sometimes be the initial documentation of the tumor.

The anemic lesion in malignancy is not confined to marrow suppression or replacement by tumor. Autoimmune hemolytic anemia, which frequently accompanies lymphoproliferative disorders, also occurs with solid tumors, although rarely.[146] This has resulted in the recommendation that a search for occult malignancy be undertaken in elderly persons with otherwise idiopathic autoimmune hemolytic anemia. The variety of tumors discovered has included lung, kidney, testicular, and gastrointestinal malignancies. A more common association of tumors with autoimmune hemolysis is the well-documented linkage of ovarian tumors with corticosteroid- and splenectomy-refractory hemolytic anemia.[147] These are mainly benign tumors such as dermoid cysts, which contain antibodies with Rh specificity. Removal of the tumor reverses the hemolytic process.

Traumatic hemolysis with a microangiopathic blood picture is a feature of metastatic malignancy.[148] This lesion has been attributed to RBC shearing by fibrin strands and pathologically altered small blood vessels[149]; an attendant consumption coagulopathy precipitated by certain tumors was thought to create the fibrin thrombi on which the RBCs were impaled. The documentation that the courses of DIC and microangiopathic hemolytic anemia are not necessarily parallel and that fibrin thrombi are rare at autopsy in such patients has led to alternative hypotheses. Not all patients with tumor-related DIC have evidence of a microangiopathic process; Jacobsen and Jackson[150] found traumatic hemolysis in only 50% of their series. Antman and colleagues[151] relate the RBC lesion to direct contact of the RBC cells with intraluminal embolic tumor cells within the pulmonary vasculature, an involvement they documented in all their cancer patients with microangiopathic hemolytic anemia. The tumor most frequently associated with traumatic hemolysis is a gastric malignancy, highly prone to metastasize to the pulmonary circuit. The horrid prognosis of persons with tumor-related microangiopathy is concordant with widespread metastases as the cause of the lesion.[152]

Erythrocytosis and Malignancy

A classic paraneoplastic manifestation of malignancy is erythrocytosis or secondary polycythemia caused by tumor release of erythropoietin or erythropoietin-like substances.[153,154] An erythropoietin-like substance has been isolated from renal tumors and cerebellar hemangioblastomas; this material is immunologically identical with purified erythropoietin, a finding substantiated in studies of erythropoietin-like activity in secretions of clones of human renal carcinoma cell lines.[155]

The differentiation of this secondary erythrocytosis from polycythemia vera can sometimes be difficult. The panmyeloplasia of polycythemia vera may be mimicked by the leukocytosis and thrombocytosis that frequently accompany malignancy. Radioimmunoassays of erythropoietin may also not detect the erythropoietin-like substances secreted by tumors. The presence of splenomegaly, the bioassay for erythropoietin activity, and in vitro marrow studies may help to differentiate the two entities.[156]

Leukocytosis

Kinetic studies of tumor-induced neutrophilia reveal a major expansion of granulopoietic marrow with a marked increase in marrow neutrophil production and turnover.[157] The leukocytosis associated with some malignancies has been attributed to the necrotic element within the tumors[158]; the WBC elevation constitutes a nonspecific response to inflammation created by the tumor. Knowledge of TNF's effect on the bone marrow, with its release of IL-1 and G-CSF (granulocyte-CSF), updates this relation of tumors with leukocytosis.[159,160] The association of monocytosis with malignancies may also have a similar cause, with macrophage activation by lymphokines and cytokines.[161]

The leukocytosis of malignancy may be of a magnitude to constitute a leukemoid reaction.[162,163] This paraneoplastic phenomenon sometimes has its origin in a pathway analogous to that of erythrocytosis-associated tumors; CSF activity has been isolated from several tumors including sarcomas and carcinomas.[164] An interesting linkage of leukocytosis and humoral hypercalcemia of malignancy with squamous cell tumors and murine mammary cell tumors has been reported.[165] The understanding of these overlapping manifestations is within reach with the availability of cloned interleukins and growth factors. IL-1α–like factor and CSF have both been derived from tumor cells, and transplantation of the tumor into nude mice has resulted in both leukocytosis and hypercalcemia.[166]

Eosinophilia

Eosinophilia is considered a response to malignancy, although the mechanism for its presence remains unclarified.[167,168] Several cases of resolution of eosinophilia after resection of a malignancy have led to the conclusion that some tumors contain an eosinophil chemotactic–stimulatory substance.[169] Reports of isolation of such substances from resected tumors may have anticipated the knowledge of CSF for eosinophils; it is possible that these tumors secrete a particular eosinophil growth factor as a paraneoplastic phenomenon.[170]

Alternatively, tumor-related eosinophilia may relate to the known role of eosinophils in defense against parasites. Eosinophilia may represent a mobilization against tumors, rather than a response directly caused by the tumor.[171] Eosinophil infiltration of tumors occurs and may represent part of the body's defenses against malignancy.[172] The importance of establishing which of these dual roles that eosinophils play in malignancy concerns the practice of reducing eosinophil counts that are considered a threat to the body. The latter appears unwise until a thorough search for malignancy makes a direct attack on the eosinophil appropriate.

Thrombocytosis

Thrombocytosis joins anemia and leukocytosis as common accompaniments of malignancy.[173] Although the platelet elevations are usually moderate, the combination of tumor with infection or bleeding can result in a platelet count elevation that rivals essential thrombocythemia.[174] The two situations can usually be differentiated by the abnormal platelet morphology and prolonged bleeding time seen with primary thrombocythemia. The tumor most frequently associated with thrombocytosis is a bronchogenic carcinoma.[173] Whether thrombocytosis is caused directly by the tumor or is an indirect reaction to disease in the lungs, an important site of megakaryocyte release of platelets, remains to be determined.[175]

Hemostasis and Malignancy

The historical entity of Trousseau's syndrome has been extended by the work of Sacks and colleagues.[176] The original lesion of thrombosis in the setting of malignancy has been amplified to include consumption coagulopathy, arterial and venous thromboses, and marantic endocarditis. The most common associated tumors are mucus-secreting adenocarcinomas. A direct activator of factor V has been isolated from mucin and is considered one of the precipitants of the coagulopathy.[177] Other tumor procoagulants have also been identified, confirming the multiple pathways for activation of the clotting cascade in this condition.[178] Thrombosis is the major component of the syndrome, although some malignancies create a bleeding disorder caused by release of fibrinolysins or rapid consumption of normal clotting factors. Promyelocytic leukemia and prostatic carcinoma are examples of this phenomenon.

The syndrome is not related to the size of the tumor; in fact, the underlying neoplasm often is not obvious and is difficult to find. The problem usually makes itself known when venous thromboses recur while a patient is on coumadin or when thromboses appear in atypical locations. The evidence for DIC may be subtle with normal levels of platelets and fibrinogen representing reductions in the thrombocythemia–hyperfibrinogenemia that accompany malignancies. Elevated fibrin-split products and cryofibrinogens may be further laboratory evidence of the phenomenon.[179,180]

Control of the underlying neoplasm is the primary objective but this is rarely possible because of the refractory nature of the tumor and the presence of metastatic disease. In the presence of the latter, a microangiopathic hemolytic anemia becomes an additional manifestation of the syndrome. Since elimination of the tumor is not possible and coumadin is ineffective in preventing the thromboses, heparin administration becomes the mainstay of symptomatic management. Subcutaneous heparin in amounts to prolong the activated partial thromboplastin time (PTT) 1.5 to 2 times normal control values is usually successful in slightly prolonging life until bleeding or thrombosis, frequently cerebral, results in death. In the late 20th century, Trousseau's syndrome continues with the grim prognosis of its original recognition in the late 19th century.[181]

ANEMIA AND LIVER DISEASE

Anemia in the setting of liver disease is common and multifactorial in its origin.[182] Both acute and chronic liver disease are accompanied by increased portal pressures with the resultant congestive splenomegaly potentially creating any combination of anemia, leukopenia, or thrombocytopenia.[183] The marrow's compensation for such hemolytic insults is frequently dampened or absent because of concomitant vitamin–nutritional deficiencies and the shared toxicity by the liver and bone marrow of the cellular insults imposed by alcohol.[184] Blood loss with the threat of iron deficiency may also contribute to the anemia of liver disease.

Delineation of the causes and even the degree of anemia is difficult in the context of liver disease. Hemodilution occurs secondary to the hyperrenin state of both liver disease and splenomegaly.[185] Increased amounts of atrial natriuretic factor may blunt some of this plasma volume expansion in such patients.[186] Reticulocytosis may represent a marrow's release from alcohol inhibition, the response to replenishment of a missing vitamin or even compensation for gastrointestinal bleeding. Hyperbilirubinemia, elevated lactic dehydrogenase levels and reduced haptoglobin levels may result from liver disease and may not be caused by hemolysis. Since the liver is a storehouse of iron, the serum levels of iron and ferritin are misleadingly elevated with hepatocellular disease.[187] All of these alterations complicate the interpretation of hematologic data in liver disease and enforce the need to recognize the dynamic and multifactorial pathogeneses of anemia in such states.

Liver Disease and the Red Cell Membrane

The RBC membrane is in dynamic equilibrium with the cholesterol–phospholipid components of the surrounding plasma and such membranes undergo remodeling by exchange of molecules with their plasma counterparts.[188] The morphologic abnormalities of RBCs in these conditions are attributable to the alterations in lipids and lipoproteins that accompany liver disease (see Chap. 54). The most common finding is targeting of RBCs secondary to cholesterol accumulation in the RBC membrane leading to an increase in its surface area.[189] These slightly macrocytic cells have a decreased osmotic fragility but experience no shortening of their survival in the absence of congestive splenomegaly. With more severe liver disease, echinocytic transformation of RBC occurs with the formation of scalloped, regularly crenated cell membranes called *spur cells*. An alteration in lipid composition of the membrane is one of the mechanisms for abnormal membrane folding and the loss of membrane fluidity in spur cells.[190] Another contribution to spurring of RBCs is abnormal high-density lipoproteins isolated from jaundiced patients with liver disease. In these patients, the spur cell shape change may be mediated by cell surface receptors for the abnormal HDL molecules.[191]

These primary insults to the RBC membrane are thought to modify the deformability and plasticity of the RBC. The accumulated lipids may alter the steric configuration of membrane proteins or increase calcium permeability, permitting the activation of endogenous proteinases to damage the protein skeleton of the membrane[192]; an increase in intrinsic membrane proteolytic activity has been demonstrated in spur cells, attributed to the lipid alteration in structure.

Acanthocytes, which are irregular, spiculated RBCs, represent the most exaggerated stage of RBC remodeling in liver disease. They may represent a splenic conditioning of the echinocyte stage or the final alteration due to proteinase effects.[193] Whatever the mechanism responsible, these cells have a dramatically shortened RBC survival because of splenic sequestration and destruction of the cells. Unfortunately, splenectomy, which mollifies the hemolysis, is not a recommended intervention because the underlying liver disease makes such a surgical procedure an unacceptable risk. The supervention of spur cell anemia in acute or chronic hepatic disease is usually a manifestation of advanced liver compromise and portends a limited survival.

Alcohol and Hematopoiesis

Significant hematologic damage is incurred by alcoholics because of the combined direct toxicity of alcohol on the marrow and the multiple associated abnormalities in the nutritional and gastrointestinal systems that exist in the alcoholic.[194] Alcohol supplies empty calories for nutrition and is also frequently accompanied by multivitamin deficiencies; alcohol-induced gastritis is threatened with a double jeopardy for bleeding imposed by the combination of thrombocytopenia and a qualitative platelet dysfunction created by the toxin.[195] Congestive splenomegaly, as an accompaniment to both acute alcoholic fatty liver and chronic cirrhosis, may further deplete the RBC pool. These myriad potential pathologic contributions of ethanol to hematopoiesis and its environment readily explain the frequent occurrence of anemia in about 50% of patients hospitalized with acute or chronic alcoholism.[196]

Alcohol and the Red Blood Cell

Heavy alcohol ingestion of over 1 week's duration produces a characteristic vacuolization of the RBC precursors in the marrow, a finding shared with chloramphenicol toxicity, phenylalanine deficiency, and hyperosmolar states.[197] More chronic ingestion of lesser amounts of alcohol results in a mild macrocytosis unaccompanied by any megaloblastic features in the marrow.[198] The vacuolization of normoblasts is short-lived (3 to 5 days) after ethanol withdrawal, whereas the macrocytosis of alcoholism persists for 1 to 2 weeks after abstinence from the toxin.[199] The mechanism for the production of these abnormalities is not established; they occur in the absence of any vitamin deficiency or altered lipid composition of the membrane. Their importance lies in their functioning as suggestive clues for the presence of alcoholism.

Ethanol is also a direct toxin to hematopoietic cells with evidence that ethanol and its breakdown product, acetaldehyde, both inhibit erythroid marrow colony growth in vitro.[200] A further insult to erythropoiesis is produced by a direct antifolate effect of alcohol on the marrow[201]; this compounds an already reduced availability of folate due to alcohol's interference with the normal enterohepatic recirculation of folate and decreased amounts of the active congener of folate, methyl tetrahydrofolate.[202] The sum of these insults to folate metabolism is escalated further by the simultaneous presence of folate deficiency as a result of a poor diet, producing megaloblastic anemia as the most common form of anemia in alcoholics.[203]

The megaloblastic transformation of the marrow due to folate deficiency may not be accompanied by the anticipated striking macrocytosis in the peripheral blood because the condition is often compounded by iron deficiency. This frequently produces a dimorphic RBC picture when there exists competing contributions of both deficiencies to RBC size. Hypersegmentation of the polymorphonuclear cells still remain the marker of megaloblastic hematopoiesis, an important clue when macrocytosis has been blunted by iron lack.[204] Measurement of RBC folate confirms the deficiency, one that may occur in the course of only a few weeks of a folate-deficient diet.

Megaloblastic transformation of the marrow is frequently further complicated by ringed sideroblast formation where iron accumulates in and around altered mitochondria in RBC precursors.[205] This iron fails to be normally incorporated into heme, and the RBC products of this pathway are hypochromic in the face of iron-overloaded mitochondria. The defect originates in alcohol's direct interference in protoporphyrin ring synthesis or in a toxic effect of alcohol on the mitochondria. These insults to normal Hb production and the ineffective hematopoiesis characteristic of megaloblastic lesions alter iron kinetics within the body. Iron measurements are usually falsely elevated in the anemic alcoholic because of the roadblocks that alcohol erects by interfering with erythropoiesis at so many junctures.[206]

After alcohol intake has been discontinued and nutritional supplements provided, the megaloblastic component of the anemia is rapidly reversed. Serum iron levels plummet as normal erythropoiesis supervenes. Sideroblastic features persist for 7 to 10 days, a more prolonged aftermath of alcohol toxicity.[205] The marrow, freed from alcohol's suppressive effect, responds with a reticulocytosis that has frequently been misinterpreted as evidence for hemolysis in the jaundiced, anemic drinker. The finding of reticulocytosis in alcoholics with fatty liver and hypertriglyceridemia became the triad of Zieve syndrome.[207] The original supposition that the triglyceride elevation was causal of the hemolysis has been disproved, and any mild hemolysis is attributed to a hypersplenic insult in these patients. The major component of the reticulocytosis represents the return of a marrow formerly suffering the dual effects of alcohol suppression and vitamin deficiencies.[208]

Alcohol and the White Blood Cell

Leukopenia may be caused by an ethanol effect on the marrow independent of any megaloblastic interference with hematopoiesis. Direct marrow suppression of granulopoiesis by alcohol is accompanied by inhibition of release of CSFs by T lymphocytes.[209,210] This may contribute to the high morbidity and mortality rates associated with pneumococcal sepsis in the alcoholic with leukopenia.[211]

The alcoholic is further handicapped as an infected host because of diminished adherence, chemotaxis, and motility of granulocytes in response to infection.[212] Macrophage function is impaired with decreased motility and phagocytic performance.[213,214] Immune defenses are also diminished. Both lymphopenia and inhibition of lymphocyte transformation are common in alcoholism.[215] The ability to respond with delayed hypersensitivity to new antigens is also compromised.[216] The mechanism of alcohol-related functional defects of WBCs is not established, although a raised intracellular concentration of cyclic adenosine monophosphate in the presence of ethanol has been suggested as the cause.[217]

Alcohol and Platelets

Both platelet number and function are adversely affected by alcohol in the absence of any supplementary contribution of vitamin deficiency or hypersplenism. The thrombocytopenia originates in a modest shortening of platelet survival combined with a more significant impairment of megakaryocytopoiesis.[195] In vivo and in vitro experiments confirm that the number and proliferation of megakarocytes are not altered in the presence of ethanol.[218] The lesion created by the agent appears at the later stages of the megakaryocyte maturation, with inhibition of platelet production. Withdrawal of ethanol is followed within 3 to 5 days by a release of platelets, with levels rebounding to thrombocythemic levels before returning to normal levels in 1 to 3 weeks.[219] Alcohol suppression of thrombopoiesis may be severe enough to result in bleeding, especially when other defects such as gastritis already exist in the patient.

Qualitative platelet abnormalities are also induced by ethanol. With moderate doses (more than 50 g) of ethanol, no direct effect is seen on bleeding time, although this amount of ethanol significantly potentiates prolongation of the bleeding time induced by aspirin and nonsteroidal analgesics. Larger ethanol ingestion results in prolongation of the bleeding time even in the absence of any thrombocytopenia.[221] Defects in platelet aggregation, thromboxane release, and platelet factor 3 availability occur on exposure of platelets to alcohol. These qualitative defects may be secondary to direct toxic effects of ethanol on the platelet membrane in addition to any contribution from an increased plasma osmolality in the presence of ethanol.

THE KIDNEY AND HEMATOPOIESIS

Anemia in Kidney Disease

Anemia, a common effect of acute and chronic renal failure, is often so severe in these conditions that it constitutes the major morbidity of renal disease.[222] It has long been recognized that the anemia, although multifactorial in origin, has erythropoietin deficiency as its primary cause.[223] Progressive renal disease is accompanied by an erythropoietin decline resulting in a hypoproliferative, usually normochromic, normocytic anemia. Transfusion support frequently becomes a necessary intervention, although elevated 2,3-DPG (diphosphoglycerate) levels and a right-shifted oxygen dissociation curve make the RBCs of uremic subjects more effective in the delivery of oxygen than normal RBCs.[224,225] The anemia usually develops when the creatinine clearance falls below 35 to 45 mL/min, although no direct correlation is found between the severity of the anemia and the degree of renal impairment. The Hb level is generally in the 7- to 8-g/dL range in uremic states, with more severe anemia a feature of renoprival states. In the absence of kidneys, the body's limited erythropoiesis has the liver as an extrarenal source of erythropoietin.[226]

It is universally agreed that the anemia of renal disease is an erythropoietin deficiency state.[227] It is still controversial whether serum inhibitors that accumulate in uremic patients contribute to the erythroid hypoplasia.[228,229] Several series have documented improved hematocrits and erythrocyte volumes proportional to the intensity of dialysis treatments, which may remove the inhibitors. Elevated levels of neuraminidase and other proteases have been suggested as inactivators of erythropoietin or its effect on the marrow.[230] The higher Hb levels in uremic patients on chronic ambulatory peritoneal dialysis compared with hemodialysis has been attributed to the greater effectiveness of peritoneal dialysis in removing substances of "middle molecule" range (500 to 5000 daltons).[231] This effect supports the postulated inhibitor role of spermine, a middle molecule substance that accumulates in renal failure and inhibits erythropoiesis in marrow culture.[232,233]

The hypothesis concerning spermine and its precursor, spermidine, has been challenged by further in vitro work demonstrating that the marrow effect of spermidine is nonselective, with a suppression of all marrow elements in culture. Since leukopenia and thrombocytopenia are not usual components of the uremic state, the anemia of renal disease is not thought to be the result of pansuppression by spermidine. The purported role of middle molecule substances has been further questioned by studies demonstrating no difference in RBC mass in chronic ambulatory peritoneal dialysis and hemodialysis patients.[234] The higher Hb levels in the former group are thought to be the result of lower plasma volumes, with hemoconcentration leading to the increase in hematocrit.

Parathyroid hormone has also been indicted as a possible inhibitor of erythropoiesis in uremia, a defect that renal failure states share with primary hyperparathyroidism.[235] The mechanism of this contribution to anemia[236] is probably the one that Fuller Albright postulated more than 50 years ago when he focused on the replacement of the marrow cavity by fibrous tissue in hyperparathyroid states. Removal of hypertrophied parathyroid glands improves the osteitis fibrosa of involved marrows and the anemia that accompanies this abnormality.[237] Treatment with 1,25-dihydroxycalciferol also decreases marrow fibrosis and diminishes the anemia of renal failure.[238,239] The role of parathyroid hormone in these anemias is in remodeling the environment in which hematopoiesis takes place; the more advanced states of bone disease seen in patients with uremia may even lead to splenomegaly secondary to extramedullary hematopoiesis.[240]

The primary role of erythropoietin deficiency in the anemia of renal failure has been incontrovertibly confirmed with the successful trials of recombinant human erythropoietin in both dialyzed and nondialyzed renal failure patients.[241,242] Administration of the hormone has eliminated the need for red cell transfusions or androgens, previously the mainstays in treating the anemia of renal failure.[243,244] The RBC mass is restored to normal, eliminating or overwhelming any contribution of erythropoietin inhibitors to the anemia. The treatment has been remarkably benign with no evidence that antibodies to the erythropoietin develop and weaken the potency of the hormone. Hypertension has sometime worsened, perhaps secondary to the increase in RBC mass, although the plasma volume has not shown a parallel enhancement. The therapeutic success of erythropoietin has brought to a close any doubts concerning the major cause of the anemia of renal failure.

Although erythropoietin treatment reverses the anemia of renal failure, the mild hemolytic component in this condition remains unaffected. It is due to an extracorpuscular factor, since RBCs from affected persons survive normally when transfused into normal subjects.[245] There is significant shortening of RBC survival when blood urea nitrogen (BUN) concentrations are greater than 100 mg/dL; the cause of the abnormality is not strictly defined and may be due to a combination of factors.[246] Abnormal ion transport has been cited as a cause of increased intracellular sodium accumulation.[247] Decreased NADPH (nicotinamide adenine dinucleotide phosphate) generation secondary to defective recycling of glycolytic intermediates through the hexose monophosphate shunt has also been described in RBCs from uremic patients. This abnormality may enhance the sensitivity of such cells to oxidant drug-mediated hemolysis.[248,249] Some hemodialysis baths with their contaminants of copper, nitrate, and chloramine may exaggerate this sensitivity and create a more severe hemolytic picture.[248] The ascorbate–cyanide test identifies subjects as candidates for the development of Heinz body anemias. The extracorpuscular contribution to this RBC insult can be decreased by increasing the number of times dialysis is given, while making certain the dialysate bath is free of contaminants.[249,250]

With moderate degrees of renal failure, the RBCs are normochromic/normocytic with normal osmotic and mechanical fragility. With BUN concentrations greater than 150 mg/dL, the RBC take on a "burr" configuration as a characteristic feature.[251] More dramatic alterations of a microangiopathic nature are a component of traumatic hemolysis in the hemolytic uremic syndrome[252]; the sheared RBCs in this condition are not the effects of renal failure but of the process responsible for the renal failure. A vascular toxin released by several bacterial, enteric pathogens appears to be closely linked to the pathophysiology of hemolytic uremic syndrome.[253,254]

The hemolytic component in uremia-related anemia also may have some contribution from hypersplenism, since splenomegaly may develop in renal failure patients.[255] Extensive exposure to many blood products in hemodialyzed patients frequently results in hepatitis and associated splenomegaly. These patients usually manifest pancytopenia, which responds in part to splenectomy. This complication of hepatitis and splenomegaly with secondary hypersplenism has been described in about 10% of a large series of hemodialyzed patients.

The anemia of renal failure may be worsened in dialyzed patients by the superimposition of iron and folate deficiency. Folate is dialyzable and the already meager stores of this vitamin in these nutritionally marginal patients may become rate limiting. Hypersegmentation of polymorphonuclear neutrophils is described as a feature of uremia alone, but this earliest manifestation of a megaloblastic process is more likely the marker of folate deficiency.[256] Iron lack is another common threat of renal failure because a large blood loss complicates hemodialysis in all patients; about 2 g of iron are lost from the body each year from dialysis alone.[257] This iron deficit is usually more severe because of the occurrence of gastrointestinal blood loss in the setting of uremia-related platelet defects and the structural lesions of angiodysplasia of the bowel that may accompany uremia.[258] Most patients require iron and folate supplementation to compensate for these insults. The administration of erythropoietin may unmask these deficiencies, their presence being signaled by an apparent refractoriness to erythropoietin administration.

Anemia in hemodialyzed patients may be part of the toxicity created by aluminum accumulation[259]; a hypochromic microcytic anemia may occur secondary to this metal's interference with erythropoiesis.[260] Aluminum unloading with desferrioxamine reverses the insult, and dialysis against deionized tap water prevents this complication.[261] Ingestion of aluminum-containing antacids as phosphate binders may also contribute to aluminum accumulation, even in those who are not undergoing dialysis.

Erythrocytosis in Kidney Disease

Although anemia constitutes a major morbidity in renal disease, secondary erythrocytosis is also not an uncommon complication of a wide variety of renal disorders.[262] This increase in RBC mass may originate from erythropoietin release directly from renal carcinoma cells[263,264] or from renal ischemia with conditions such as renal artery stenosis,[265] transplant rejection, and cystic diseases of the kidney.[266] Cystic disease of the kidney may be either a congenital disorder or an acquired cystic disease of end-stage kidney failure on long-term hemodialysis.[267–269] Even diffuse parenchymal renal disease[270] and the nephrotic syndrome[271,272] have been associated with erythrocytosis.

A rare entity, Bartter's syndrome is a hyperrenin state associated with juxtaglomerular apparatus hyperplasia and hypokalemic alkalosis.[273] This disease has been complicated by a high erythropoietin erythrocytosis, initially leading investigators to point to the juxtaglomerular apparatus as the common source for both renin and erythropoietin. The more recent cloning of erythropoietin has allowed its localization within the peritubular cells of the kidney, better explaining the broad range of renal pathology associated with erythrocytosis.[274,275]

ENDOCRINE DISEASE

The multiple hormonal products of the endocrine system of the body have both direct and indirect effects on hematopoiesis. Hypophysectomy creates a normochromic, normocytic anemia in animal models, a lesion that can be corrected with administration of prolactin or growth hormone.[276] Both of these pituitary hormones have a regulatory influence on marrow function at the level of hematopoietic growth factors. Growth hormone has also been demonstrated to stimulate erythropoiesis in vitro.[277]

Hyperthyroidism

Thyroid hormone also has a bimodal effect on erythropoiesis; it directly stimulates human CFU-E formation and indirectly enhances BFU-E proliferation by augmenting the release of soluble burst-promoting factors from accessory cells.[278] Persons with hyperthyroidism frequently have an elevated RBC mass secondary to these effects of excessive thyroid hormone and have an increased requirement for folic acid to accommodate the increased RBC synthesis.[279] A macrocytic anemia may complicate hyperthyroidism in the setting of Graves' disease since pernicious anemia and other immune disorders are linked to Graves' disease.[280] The coagulation and platelet systems are unaffected in hyperthyroidism although these hyperthyroid patients are sensitive to small amounts of coumadin, making regulation of anticoagulation more difficult in this disease.[281]

Hypothyroidism

Hypothyroidism may be complicated by an anemia whose major cause is a reduced RBC mass secondary to the decreased oxygen requirements of the hypothyroid state.[282,283] This anemia is frequently macrocytic, partly because of the cholesterol elevations found in hypothyroidism or to a complicating pernicious anemia. Iron-deficiency anemia also may complicate thyroid hormone deficiency in women because menorrhagia with excessive blood loss is a feature of this hormonal lack.[284] Infrequently, a gelatinous transformation of the marrow may occur with severe hypothyroidism. This marrow myxedema has been accompanied by a severe anemia that was corrected by thyroid hormone replacement.[285]

Hyperparathyroidism

Parathyroid hormone is responsible for remodeling the bony architecture that houses the hematopoietic system. This may explain the 5% to 20% incidence of anemia in patients with hyperparathyroidism in the face of normal renal function.[286,287] The anemia is normocytic and normochromic, and the marrow contains normal precursor elements. When secondary hyperparathyroidism complicates renal disease, the severity of the anemia is best correlated with the bony lesions and myelofibrosis created by the parathyroid hormone excess.[288]

Cushing's Disease and Addison's Disease

The corticosteroid overdrive of Cushing's disease may be accompanied by varying degrees of androgenic excess, which can create a modestly polycythemic picture.[289] The lack of adrenocortical function in Addison's disease is not accompanied by anemia. Lack of salt-retaining hormones in Addison's disease usually results in a hemoconcentrated state with a normal to slightly increased hematocrit.[290] A clue to Addison's disease is the presence of eosinophilia, although this finding is present in only a minority (15%) of such patients.[291]

DIABETES MELLITUS

Red Blood Cells

The major hematologic alterations in diabetes mellitus are not necessarily the direct result of insulin deficiency but probably result from the combined metabolic derangements in carbohydrate and fatty metabolism of the diabetic state.[292] Insulin stimulates human erythroid progenitors in vitro[293,294] and also improves a shortened RBC half-life in poorly controlled diabetes.[295] The major erythroid abnormality in diabetes mellitus is the nonenzymatic, slow, and continuous reaction of plasma glucose with the amino-terminal valine residue of the Hb chain. The resultant glycosylated Hb A_{1C} mirrors the time-averaged concentration of glucose within the RBC over the preceding 6- to 8-week period. Measurements of Hb A_{1C} provide a broader window on the adequacy of glucose control as compared with individual glucose determinations.[296] This glycosylation of Hb interferes with the binding of 2,3-DPG to the Hb molecule, altering the oxygen-binding affinity of affected cells.[297] No measurable differences in the rheologic behavior of cells from diabetics and control subjects are found despite this glycosylation of Hb and cell membrane proteins.[298]

White Blood Cells

Infectious complications punctuate the diabetic state with many defects in leukocyte function incriminated as the causes of this enhanced risk for infection. Decreased leukocyte function in out-of-control diabetes improves with better glucose control[295]; the neutrophil in the diabetic has a decreased rate of glycolysis with reduced phosphofructokinase activity.[299] Defective migration of neutrophils using skin windows is seen in diabetes patients. Defects in leukocyte chemotaxis, phagocytosis, and bacterial killing are also cited in hyperglycemic states.[300]

Platelets

Many alterations in platelet function and the soluble components of the coagulation cascade exist in the patient with diabetes mellitus.[301] Whether these abnormalities are primary or secondary in creating the vascular complications of diabetes mellitus remains controversial.[302] Platelet hyperaggregability with increased ADP-induced activation is a reproducible finding in uncontrolled diabetes and improves with better glucose control.[303] This heightened platelet aggregation is accompanied by high plasma glucose or nonesterified fatty acid inhibition of prostacyclin generation from vessel walls without any comparable effect on thromboxane synthesis.[304] Thrombosis is also favored in diabetes mellitus because of altered antithrombin III activity, because of glycosylation of this molecule at the heparin binding site.[305] Fibrinolysis is also hindered, with elevated euglobulin lysis times and increased activity of plasminogen activator inhibitor.[306]

The clinical relevance of these hemostatic abnormalities remains unsettled. More than suggestive evidence supports a role for glucose and lipid control in helping reverse the hypercoagulable features of diabetes mellitus.

Ketoacidosis

Diabetic ketoacidosis with its severe polyuria is usually complicated by hemoconcentration and falsely elevated hematocrit levels. Acute hemolysis may occur in patients with ketoacidosis if rehydration and glycemic control result in the presence of severe hypophosphatemia.[307] Total body stores of phosphate are usually reduced, even when serum phosphate levels are normal, and may drop to precarious levels as phosphate reenters cells to phosphorylate glucose. An elevation in WBCs commonly accompanies diabetic ketoacidosis[308]; the height of such elevations may result in a leukemoid picture even without any infectious complications.

ANOREXIA NERVOSA

Hematologic abnormalities are common in persons with anorexia nervosa; marrow hypoplasia commonly accompanies this carbohydrate–calorie deficiency state.[309] Pearson's original observation of the marrow accumulation of an acid mucopolysaccharide in persons with anorexia nervosa[310] has been confirmed as a frequent feature of this illness, and its rapid reversibility with clinical improvement in the underlying disease suggests that starvation is the cause.[311]

The peripheral blood findings are variable in anorexia nervosa (see Chap. 54). Most patients have circulating acanthocytes (spur cells), the cause of which is still undetermined.[312] Abetalipoproteinemia is not present, although serum cholesterol levels are reduced in about half of patients.[313] Pancytopenia may supervene when the marrow aplasia is significant; its cause, usually apparent when anorexia nervosa occurs in females, may be perplexing when the more elusive and uncommon illness occurs in men. The unexpected finding of an acid mucopolysaccharide accumulation in the marrows of men with pancytopenia may be the initial clue to the diagnosis of anorexia nervosa.[311]

ANEMIA AND THE ELDERLY

Studies of hematologic parameters in elderly patients have documented an increased incidence of anemia with each successive decade of aging.[314] Hematologic study of healthy, well-nourished elderly populations has not discovered any physiologic anemia of aging.[315]

Animal and human studies have revealed a decreasing marrow reserve as aging proceeds, but the reserve is still adequate to guarantee normal levels throughout the lifetime of the person.[316] Erythropoietin levels do not differ from those in normal, healthy controls.[317] The early stem cell compartments are unperturbed in bone marrows from the elderly; any abnormalities are restricted to defects in the proliferative capacity of more differentiated cell stages.[316]

These observations, plus the fact that many of the changes in hematopoietic function present in elderly subjects are similar to those seen in protein–calorie malnutrition, establish the importance of considering the contribution of an inadequate diet to anemia in the elderly.

Thus, anemia is not the simple accompaniment of aging and should not be attributed to a natural senescence phenomenon. Anemia in the elderly should be considered a sickness index, the sign of a possible malignancy or other systemic disorder.[318]

PREGNANCY

Pregnancy, with a reorientation of the mother's physiology to support the expanding growth of the fetus, is not infrequently complicated by hematologic disorders. Some of these arise from the progressive hypercoagulable state of pregnancy,[319] in preparation for placental separation, whereas other disorders result from pathologic initiation of the clotting cascade secondary to the release of placental, amniotic, or fetal elements.[320] Antecedent hematologic disorders are compounded by the demands of pregnancy and may be exaggerated in severity and impact because of their dual effect on mother and fetus. Leukemia and lymphoma create unique management dilemmas when they are concomitants of pregnancy.[321,322] Other hematologic conditions such as the anticardiolipin syndrome may become problematic only during pregnancy.[323] Management of these conditions must also take into account the effect that any hematologic defects or medications used to reverse these defects may have on the fetus.

Anemia

During the first and second trimesters of pregnancy, a physiologic expansion of the mother's plasma volume occurs, which outdistances a concomitant increase in the RBC mass.[324] This *hydremia of pregnancy* results in a reduction in the normal woman's hematocrit to about 30%, even though the total blood volume is expanded by increases in both the RBC and plasma compartments. This surge in RBC production often outstrips the marginal iron and folate stores of the expectant mother. Laboratory reliance on mean corpuscular volume (MCV) measurements to determine the cause of anemia may be misleading during pregnancy because a combined deficiency may cancel out the extremes of iron (low MCV) and folate (high MCV) deficiency.[325] To avoid the development of anemia secondary to these deficiencies, it is standard practice to supplement all pregnant women with iron and folate. For those women who cannot tolerate iron, monitoring of serum ferritin permits assessment of iron stores and the specific need for iron supplementation.[326]

Other causes of anemia during pregnancy are much rarer. An aplastic anemia that resolves with abortion of the fetus and that has recurred with subsequent pregnancy is thought to have an immunologic basis when it occurs during pregnancy.[327] The devastating anemia secondary to intravascular hemolysis that is associated with clostridial sepsis may be a lethal complication of septic abortions.[328]

Thrombocytopenia

With its potential to exaggerate bleeding during the birth process, thrombocytopenia needs careful assessment and management in the pregnant woman.[329] The incidence of the classic thromboconsumptive processes of idiopathic thrombocytopenic purpura (ITP), thrombotic thrombocytopenic purpura (TTP), and DIC all are increased during pregnancy and are joined by platelet abnormalities as a component of toxemia or eclampsia of pregnancy.[330] Because ITP is most frequently caused by an antibody that crosses the placenta and may create thrombocytopenia in the infant, this condition creates double jeopardy for the mother and fetus.[331]

Idiopathic Thrombocytopenic Purpura

The diagnosis of ITP during pregnancy requires the same constellation of findings as that in the nonpregnant state (see also Chap. 34); the presence or absence of platelet or serum platelet antibodies does not permit any assumptions regarding the fetal platelet count. Percutaneous umbilical blood sampling before labor and scalp vein sampling during delivery are the most common determinants of the optimal route of delivery. A fetal platelet count over 50,000 is usually considered adequate to permit a vaginal delivery.[332] Administration of corticosteroids to the mother in the last 3 weeks before delivery is thought to decrease the severity of the thrombocytopenia in the infant.[333]

Thrombotic Thrombocytopenic Purpura and Eclampsia

Thrombotic thrombocytopenic purpura and eclampsia share the same hematologic features of hemolytic anemia and thrombocytopenia as well as involvement of the kidney and central nervous systems. Because of the rarity of the former and the difficulty of differentiating it from eclampsia, many physicians recommend that TTP during pregnancy be managed as eclampsia, that is, by delivery of the fetus.[334] The mechanism of thrombocytopenia in eclampsia is not certain,[335] although successful reduction of its incidence with acetylsalicylic acid administration to high-risk mothers makes a platelet–endothelial defect most likely.[336,337] The spectrum of toxemia has been extended to include the HELLP syndrome, that is, hemolysis, elevated liver enzymes, and low platelets, which may or may not be accompanied by the more classic evidence of toxemia.[338,339] Management of the hematologic problems of toxemia entails management of the toxemia state, which frequently requires delivery of the infant if the maturity of the fetus allows. Since no transplacental antibody passage occurs in toxemia, this state does not require scalp vein sampling since the infant is not a target for immune thrombocytopenia.[340]

Disseminated Intravascular Coagulation

Because the products of conception can initiate the coagulation cascade when released into the maternal circulation, the course of pregnancy and delivery are not infrequently accompanied by DIC (see also Chap. 43). Fetal death in utero,[341] abruptio placentae,[342,343] and amniotic fluid embolism[344] all are often signaled by bleeding or coagulation abnormalities. Management of these abnormalities requires delivery of the fetus while providing blood component therapy with platelets, fresh frozen plasma, and cryoprecipitate to replace the consumed elements. Amniotic fluid embolism has the specially threatening complication of cardiopulmonary collapse, which requires cardiopulmonary support and corticosteroids in addition to blood product administration.[345] DIC may also accompany the severe hemolytic anemia that occurs when clostridial sepsis follows an abortion.[328]

Sickle Cell Disease and Pregnancy

Exchange transfusion with subsequent maintenance transfusions has been the standard management of the pregnant patient with sickle cell disease because of the documented increase in morbidity and mortality that sickling creates in the mother and child.[346] Improved prenatal and perinatal medical care has led to a reversal of the previous position of transfusing all pregnant sicklers; transfusions are reserved for patients who develop complications during pregnancy (including severe anemia) or for fetal indications[347,348] (see Chap. 53). Management of the pregnant sickle cell patient requires close coordination between the obstetrician and the hematologist because of these concerns.

Pregnancy and Thrombosis

Pregnancy represents a progressive hypercoagulable state during which a marked increase in the incidence of venous thrombosis is seen.[349,350] Because anticoagulation carries a significant risk to the fetus, it is imperative that the indications for initiating this therapy have been established with reasonable certainty. A Doppler ultrasound examination is usually adequate, although venography or a ventilation–perfusion scan with uterine shielding are acceptable tools for diagnosing thrombosis or pulmonary embolism in the pregnant woman.[351] If anticoagulation is indicated on the basis of these tests, heparin is initiated in full therapeutic doses for 7 days and the patient is subsequently maintained on low- to intermediate-dose subcutaneous heparin throughout pregnancy.[352] The drug is discontinued at the time of delivery but reinitiated 24 hours after delivery because of the ongoing risk of thrombosis that persists for 8 to 12 weeks after delivery. *Coumadin is avoided during pregnancy*, especially during the first trimester, because of the risk of a coumadin embryopathy. Heparin escapes this complication because it does not cross the placenta, although it is associated with the threat of bleeding and fetal loss. Either can be used in the postpartum period because neither drug creates problems for the nursing mother or infant.[353,354]

Pregnancy and Inherited Coagulopathies

Neither of the classic hemophilic syndromes complicates pregnancy because of their X-linked mode of inheritance. Von Willebrand's disease (vWD) does require recognition, although the incidence of bleeding secondary to this problem in pregnancy is mitigated by the physiologic increase in factor VIII and von Willebrand's factor (vWF) during pregnancy. Treatment of bleeding due to vWD consists in the use of concentrate or, for short-term control of bleeding, infusions of desmopressin[355] (see Chap. 36). The latter may shorten bleeding times in the various subgroups of vWD, although its use in type IIB vWD may lead to thrombocytopenia due to release of abnormal vWF in this group.[356] Sampling of fetal blood permits prenatal diagnosis of vWD and allows an informed decision regarding any need for cesarean delivery of an infant with vWD.

The universal solution to other coagulation abnormalities consists in administration of fresh frozen plasma in amounts adequate to reverse coagulation test abnormalities. Dysfibrinogenemias and factor XIII deficiency (see Chap. 41) are both associated with spontaneous abortions and abnormal bleeding; plasma infusions throughout pregnancy may be successful in averting complications in these groups.[357]

Hypercoagulable States and Pregnancy

Protein C[358] and antithrombin III[359] deficiency both dramatically increase the risk of thrombotic disease during pregnancy (see also Chap. 44). Anticoagulation with full-dose heparin subcutaneously throughout pregnancy has averted this complication. Preparations of antithrombin III are available and may be infused at the time of delivery.[360]

Essential thrombocythemia (see Chap. 14) may threaten a pregnancy with placental insufficiency secondary to multiple placental infarcts. Antiplatelet therapy with aspirin and dipyridamole as well as platelet pheresis have permitted successful pregnancies in this group.[361] The efficacy of aspirin in essential thrombocytopenia during pregnancy has been questioned by some groups.[362] Paroxysmal nocturnal hemoglobinuria (see Chap. 11) may require low-dose heparinization during pregnancy to avert thrombosis.[363]

COLLAGEN VASCULAR DISEASES

Systemic Lupus Erythematosus

No step in the complicated sequence of hematopoiesis is guaranteed freedom from pathologic involvement with systemic lupus erythematosus (SLE).[364] This threat originates in the interdependence of hematopoiesis and the immune system and the disarray in immune function that characterizes SLE. Antibodies may arise in SLE, which have as their target pluripotent or committed stem cells, creating an aplastic picture that involves all or individual cell lines within the marrow.[365,366] Cellular suppression of marrow cell lines by lymphoid cells may also occur.[367] Immune sensitization of circulating cells can lead to premature destruction of individual cell lines in the peripheral blood.[368] SLE is a leading cause of immune hemolytic anemia and immune thrombocytopenia.[369] The target of the antibody may even be a plasma protein or a phospholipid, producing the so-called lupus anticoagulant with its thrombotic propensity.[370] This immune imbalance with blood elements as a frequent target of the immunologic pathology explains the striking presence of hematologic disorders that characterize SLE.

Anemia

Anemia is the most common finding in patients with SLE, most frequently attributable to ACD. SLE is an inflammatory disorder and the same acute phase reactants of interleukins, TNF, and cachectins are operative in this disorder. In addition, specific interference with marrow production and circulation of RBCs occurs. Although RBC aplasia on a humoral or cellular basis has been identified as a rare occurrence,[371,372] an immune hemolytic anemia is a relatively common complication. It is typically characterized by a serologic pattern of IgG plus component on the red cell surface.[373] Myelofibrosis has also been described in a few patients with SLE; immune complexes have been suggested but not proved to be the cause of this unusual complication of SLE.[374]

Thrombocytopenia

Thrombocytopenia secondary to platelet immune sensitization is the most common immune-mediated hematologic manifestation of SLE.[375] Paralleling the pathophysiology of pure RBC aplasia, immunologic destruction of megakaryocyte precursors by humoral or cellular mechanisms may contribute to the thrombocytopenia.[376–378] Thrombocytopenia may be an initial manifestation of SLE, and serologic investigation for SLE should be a part of any evaluation of ITP in adults, especially in women, and of chronic ITP in children.[379] ITP in this setting has the same therapeutic implication as other immune thrombocytopenias, that is, corticosteroids as a primary intervention with splenectomy reserved for patients who fail corticosteroids. An additional rare cause of thrombocytopenia in SLE patients is platelet consumption in the setting of TTP. Again, this disease syndrome complicating SLE is thought to be due to disordered immune reactivity.[380]

Leukopenia

Leukopenia is a characteristic of SLE, although agranulocytosis is not a common feature of this disease in the absence of a drug reaction.[381] This is an interesting departure from what occurs in rheumatoid arthritis, in which at least two different mechanisms result in absolute leukoneutropenia. Lymphopenia is common in SLE patients along with a reduction in T cells, and B-cell function is hyperactive in this disorder.[364]

Systemic Lupus Erythematosus and the Lupus Anticoagulant–Antiphospholipid Syndrome

Conley and Hartmann's[382] description of a circulating anticoagulant in two SLE patients with a hemorrhagic disorder was the initial piece of a puzzle that is still incomplete. The SLE anticoagulant was first recognized in the laboratory as a prolongation of the PTT and was frequently accompanied by a low titer venereal disease (VDRL) test for syphilis; subsequently it was determined that the antibody–anticoagulant is directed against the phospholipid component of the prothrombin activator complex as well as against the cardiolipin component of the VDRL test.[383] Its pathologic significance is its association with thrombosis, mainly venous, as well as spontaneous abortions thought to be caused by thrombotic occlusions of the placental vasculature.[384] The pathologic spectrum of the SLE anticoagulant has since been amplified to include thrombocytopenia, hemolytic anemia, strokes, livedo reticularis,[385] and even leg ulcers.[386] Its laboratory definition has extended beyond the prolonged PTT to the Russell viper venom test[387] and use of a direct anticardiolipin assay.[388] Although originally considered an SLE anticoagulant, the anticardiolipin antibody is present in rheumatoid disease and even in noncollagen vascular diseases.[389] The primary lesion resides in antibodies directed against phospholipid moieties. Its frequent occurrence in SLE patients (40%) is part of the immunologic overflow in this disease.[390]

The mechanism of thromboses, which occur in about 30% of SLE patients with the anticardiolipin antibody, is not known with certainty. The antibody is an immunoglobulin of an IgG or IgM class; IgG antibodies are more frequently associated with fetal loss, venous thromboses, and thrombocytopenia, whereas IgM antibodies are associated with hemolytic anemia, leg ulcers, and livedo reticularis.[391] Many different deficiencies in coagulation pathways have been linked to the antibody, including prekallikrein inhibition,[392] neutralization of thrombomodulin,[393] inhibition of protein C,[394] and prostacyclin formation.[395] Just as the mechanism by which anticardiolipin antibodies cause thrombosis is controversial,[396] the management of the entity is still not established.[390] Persons with recurrent thrombosis are candidates for anticoagulation, but the appropriate duration (possibly lifelong) of such therapy is not known.[391] Corticosteroid therapy has permitted patients with a history of repeated spontaneous abortions to complete pregnancy, but frequently at the expense of significant corticosteroid side effects such as hypertension and weight gain.[384,397]

Rheumatoid Arthritis

Rheumatoid arthritis represents the classic intersection of ACD and iron-deficiency anemia.[398,399] The latter is a common complication of rheumatoid arthritis because of the gastrointestinal blood loss incurred secondary to longstanding use of aspirin and nonsteroidal analgesics in the symptomatic treatment of this disease.[400] The severe inflammatory nature of the illness also makes it a model for ACD, a sideropenic anemia in the face of reticuloendothelial iron overload (see discussion on ACD at beginning of this chapter). Iron is recognized not only as being closeted in the reticuloendothelial system in rheumatoid arthritis but as accumulating in the involved joints, perhaps playing a role in their destruction.[401] The combined presence in rheumatoid arthritis of two possible lesions that limit iron availability for Hb synthesis makes recognition of a complicating iron-deficiency anemia more difficult in these patients.[402] When iron deficiency does occur, the ferritin level may be as high as 60 to 100 $\mu g/L$.[403] A therapeutic trial of iron results in correction of that part of the anemia attributable to iron deficiency; the hematocrit usually increases to a level of about 30% and stabilizes there even with continued iron replacement therapy.

Other hematologic manifestations of rheumatoid arthritis are a moderately elevated platelet count (7 to $9 \times 10^5/\mu L$)

especially when a prominent vasculitic component is present in the disease.[404] Secondary thrombocythemia is part of the inflammatory response and does not respond to iron replacement. Eosinophilia likewise may be a component of acute rheumatoid disease[405]; the eosinophilia in rheumatoid arthritis may also be an allergic reaction to gold therapy.[406]

Rheumatoid Arthritis and Felty's Syndrome

Severe leukoneutropenia associated with splenomegaly and rheumatoid arthritis constitutes the triad described by Felty in 1924.[407] The syndrome, occurring in 1% of rheumatoid arthritis patients, is complicated by recurrent bacterial infections, leg ulcers, and high serologic titers of rheumatoid factor. The granulocytopenia has had many mechanisms—almost all immune mediated— postulated as its cause.[408,409] Fifty percent of the patients have a "maturation arrest" bone marrow pattern (absence of mature bands and polymorphonuclear cells in the marrow), which is thought to result from immune humoral or cellular mechanisms. The remainder of Felty patients have normal or hypercellular marrows; increased margination and sequestration of neutrophils have been demonstrated in some of these patients.[410]

The role of splenectomy in the management of the neutrophilia-related infection in Felty's syndrome remains controversial.[411,412] Favoring such a surgical intervention is the greater than 50% persistent elevation in neutrophils after splenectomy.[413] Patients who do not respond to splenectomy are cited as evidence that the spleen is not the total explanation of the leukopenia. The parallels to the effect of splenectomy in autoimmune hemolytic anemia suggest that the spleen removes sensitized WBCs from the blood but that the organ may not be the sole scavenger of WBCs in all Felty's patients. Methotrexate treatment of patients with Felty's syndrome is as effective as splenectomy in correcting the neutropenia.[414] This is further evidence that the spleen is a secondary rather than primary contributor to the hematologic picture.

Rheumatoid Arthritis and Large Granular Lymphocytes

A subpopulation of rheumatoid arthritis patients with a clinical picture similar to Felty's syndrome has increased numbers of large granular lymphocytes in the bone marrow or peripheral blood or both.[415] These cells have a characteristic morphology and surface membrane antigen expression, and they infiltrate the red pulp of the spleen, a finding that is not present in patients with Felty's syndrome. The importance of recognizing this variant is that splenectomy is ineffective. Chemotherapy is the treatment of choice.[416]

RED BLOOD CELL THERMAL INJURY

Thermal injury to RBCs creates anemia with the most bizarre and striking alterations in erythrocyte morphology[417] (see Chap. 54). With increasing temperature elevation over a range of 50° to 65°C, increasing RBC fragmentation and microspherocytosis occur, with RBCs of multiple diameters. This phenomenon, accompanied by hemoglobinemia and hemoglobinuria was recognized as a component of extreme body burns as early as 1865. The cells have increased osmotic and mechanical fragility as an aftermath of the membrane burn.[418]

The major late morbidity and mortality in burn patients are secondary to septic complications attributable in major part to neutrophil dysfunction.[419] Leukocytosis and an increase in band forms occur with burns, and these cells demonstrate defective chemotaxis and phagocytic function.[420] Decreased leukotriene generation in granulocytes contributes to this inadequate host response.[421] These cellular defects, combined with abnormalities in cellular and humoral immunity in severely burned patients, often determine the clinical outcome of the impaired burn patient.

Platelets do not escape involvement in burns. An initial thrombocytopenia gives way to thrombocytosis[422]; the latter is probably part of the inflammatory reaction with burns and does not represent a threat to hemostasis.

REFERENCES

1. Cartwright GE. The anemia of chronic disorders. Semin Hematol 1966;3:351.
2. Konijn AM, Hershko C. The anaemia of inflammation and chronic disease. In: DeSouza M, Brock JH, eds. Iron in immunity, cancer and inflammation. Chichester, UK, John Wiley & Sons, 1989:111.
3. Samson D. The anaemia of chronic disorders. Postgrad Med J 1983;59:543.
4. Bentley DP. Anemia of chronic disease. Clin Haematol 1982;11:465.
5. Lee GR. The anemia of chronic disease. Semin Hematol 1983;20:61.
6. Cartwright GE, Lee GR. The anemia of chronic disorders. Br J Haematol 1971;21:147.
7. Fillet G, Beguin Y, Baldelli L. Model of reticuloendothelial iron metabolism in humans: abnormal behavior in idiopathic hemochromatosis and in inflammation. Blood 1989;74:844.
8. Freireich EJ, Miller A, Emerson CP, et al. The effect of inflammation on the utilization of erythrocyte and transferrin bound radio-iron for red cell production. Blood 1957;12:972.
9. Haurani F, Burke W, Martinez E. Defective reutilization of iron in the anemia of inflammation. J Lab Clin Med 1965;65:560.
10. Konijn AM, Hershko C. Ferritin synthesis in inflammation I Pathogenesis of impaired iron release. Br J Haematol 1977;7:37.
11. Cazzola M, Bergamaschi G, Dezza L, et al. Manipulation of cellular iron metabolism for modulating normal and malignant cell proliferation: achievements and prospects. Blood 1990;75:1903.
12. Hann H-WL, Stahlburt MW, Blumberg BS. Iron nutrition and tumor growth: decreased tumor growth in iron-deficient mice. Cancer Res 1988;48:4168.
13. Fernandez-Pol JA. Siderophore-like growth factor synthesized by SV40-transformed cells adapted to picolinic acid stimulates DNA synthesis in cultured cells. FEBS Lett 1978;88:345.
14. Brown J, Woodbury R, Hart C, et al. Quantitative analysis of melanoma-associated antigen in normal and neoplastic tissues. Proc Natl Acad Sci USA 1981;78:539.
15. Weinberg ED. Iron withholding: a defense against infection and neoplasia. Physiol Rev 1984;64:65.
16. Cartwright GE, Launtsen MA, Jones PJ, et al. The anemia of infection. I. Hypoferremia, hypercupremia, and alterations in porphyrin metabolism in patients. J Clin Invest 1946;25:65.
17. Van Swick JC, Masson PC, Heremans JF. The involvement of lactoferrin in the hyposideremia of acute inflammation. J Exp Med 1974;140:1068.
18. Brock JH, Esparza I. Failure of reticulocytes to take up iron from lactoferrin saturated by various methods. Br J Haematol 1979;42:481.
19. Masson PL, Heremans JF, Schowne E. Lactoferrin: an iron binding protein in neutrophilic leukocytes. J Exp Med 1969;130:643.
20. Rado TA, Wei XP, Benz EF Jr. Isolation of lactoferrin cDNA from a human myeloid library and expression of mRNA during normal and leukemic myelopoiesis. Blood 1987;70:989.
21. Loughlin KR, Gittes RF, Partridge D, et al. The relationship of lactoferrin to the anemia of renal cell carcinoma. Cancer 1987;59:566.
22. Roodman GD. Mechanisms of erythroid suppression in the anemia of chronic disease. Blood Cells 1987;13:171.
23. Dinarello CA. Interleukin 1 and the pathogenesis of the acute phase response. N Engl J Med 1984;311:1413.
24. Schooley J, Kullgren B, Allison A. Inhibition by interleuken-1 of the action of erythropoietin on erythroid precursors and its possible role in the pathogenesis of hypoplastic anemias. Br J Haematol 1987;67:11.
25. Tracey KJ, Wei H, Manogue KR, et al. Cachectin/tumor necrosis factor indices cachexia, anemia and inflammation. J Exp Med 1988;167:1211.
26. Means R Jr, Krantz S. Progress in understanding the pathogenesis of the anemia of chronic disease. Blood 1992;80:1639.
27. Beutler B, Cerami A. Cachectin: more than a tumor necrosis factor. N Engl J Med 1987;316:379.
28. Dinarello CA. Interleukin-1. Rev Infect Dis 1984;6:51.
29. Marsh JC, Boggs DR, Cartwright GE, et al. Neutrophil kinetics in acute infection. J Clin Invest 1967;12:1943.

30. Steinbeck M, Roth J. Neutrophil activation by recombinant cytokines. Rev Infect Dis 1989;11:549.
31. Cannistra S, Griffin J. Regulation of the production and function of granulocytes and monocytes. Semin Hematol 1988;25:173.
32. Ramos FJ, Zamora F, Perez-Sicilia M, et al. Chronic granulocytic leukemia versus neutrophilic leukemoid reaction. Am J Med 1990;88: 83.
33. Glasser RM, Walker RJ, Herion JC. The significance of hematologic abnormalities in patients with tuberculosis. Arch Intern Med 1970;125: 691.
34. Twomey JJ, Leavell BS. Leukemoid reaction to tuberculosis. Arch Intern Med 1965;116:21.
35. Halpern Z, Dan M, Gilardi M, et al. Shigellosis in adults: epidemiologic, clinical and laboratory features. Medicine 1989;68:210.
36. Shoenfeld Y, Gurewich Y, Gallant LA, et al. Prednisone-induced leukocytosis: influence of dosage, method and duration of administration on the degree of leukocytosis. Am J Med 1981;71:773.
37. McKee LC Jr. Excess leukocytosis (leukemoid reactions) associated with malignant diseases. South Med J 1985;78:1475.
38. Lee MY, Kaushansky K, Judkins SA, et al. Mechanisms of tumor-induced neutrophilia: constitutive production of colony-stimulating factors and their synergistic actions. Blood 1989;74:115.
39. Liu CH, Lehan C, Speer ME, et al. Degenerative changes in neutrophils: an indicator of bacterial infection. Pediatrics 1984;74:823.
40. Emerson WA, Zieve PD, Krevans JR. Hematologic changes in septicemia. Johns Hopkins Med J 1969;126:69.
41. Easton JA, Fessas C. The incidence of Dohle bodies in various diseases and their association with thrombocytopenia. Br J Haematol 1966;12: 54.
42. Zieve PD, Haghshenass M, Blanks M, et al. Vacuolization of the neutrophil: an aid in the diagnosis of septicemia. Arch Intern Med 1966;118: 356.
43. Brooks GF, Priddle AH, Beaty HN. Early diagnosis of bacteremia by buffy-coat examinations. Arch Intern Med 1973;132:673.
44. Orlic D, Gill R, Feldschuk R, et al. Molecular mechanism for the inhibitory action of interferon on hematopoiesis. Ann NY Acad Sci 1989;554:36.
45. Zoumbos N, Raefsky E, Young N. Lymphokines and hematopoiesis. Prog Hematol 1986;14:201.
46. Helminen M, Vesikari T. Spontaneous and inducible interleukin-1 production from peripheral blood monocytes in bacterial and viral infections in children. Pediatr Infect Dis J 1987;6:1102.
47. Ernstoff M, Galluchio V, Kirkwood J. Analyses of granulocyte-macrophage progenitor cells in patients treated with recombinant interferon alpha-2. Am J Med 1985;79:169.
48. Ackerman Z, Ackerman E, Shouval D. Measles: clinical and laboratory observation in young adults during an epidemic. South Med J 1988;81: 1396.
49. Douglas RG, Alford R, Cate T, et al. The leukocyte response during viral respiratory illness in man. Ann Intern Med 1965;64:521.
50. Blumberg R, Schooley R. Lymphocyte markers and infectious diseases. Semin Hematol 1985;22:81.
51. Tosato G, Magrath I, Koski I, et al. Activation of suppressor T cells during Epstein-Barr-virus–induced infectious mononucleosis. N Engl J Med 1979;301:1133.
52. Wood TA, Frenkel EP. The atypical lymphocyte. Am J Med 1967;42: 923.
53. Johnson RA, Waddelow TA, Caro J, et al. Chronic exposure to tumor necrosis factor in vivo preferentially inhibits erythropoiesis in nude mice. Blood 1989;741:120.
54. Brock JH. Iron and the outcome of infection. Br Med J 1986;293:518.
55. McKenna WR, Mickelsen PA, Sparling PF, et al. Iron uptake from lactoferrin and transferrin by Neisseria gonorrhea. Infect Immun 1988;56: 785.
56. Britigan BE, Cohen MS, Sparling PF. Gonococcal infection: a model of molecular pathogenesis. N Engl J Med 1985;312:1683.
57. Hershko C, Peto TE, Weatherall DJ. Iron and infection. Br Med J 1988;296:660.
58. Young N, Mortimer P. Viruses and bone marrow failure. Blood 1984;63: 729.
59. Rosenfeld SJ, Young NS, Viruses and bone marrow failure. Blood Rev 1991;5:71.
60. Young N. Hematologic and hematopoietic consequences of B19 Parvovirus infection. Semin Hematol 1988;25:159.
61. Socinski MA, Ershler WB, Tosato G, et al. Pure red cell aplasia associated with chronic Epstein-Barr virus infection: evidence for T-cell mediated suppression of erythroid colony forming units. J Lab Clin Med 1984;1041:995.
62. Spivak JL, Bender BS, Quinn TC. Hematologic abnormalities in the acquired immune deficiency syndrome. Am J Med 1984;77:224.
63. Clearfield HR, Brody J, Turner JH. Acute viral hepatitis, glucose-g-phosphate dehydrogenase deficiency and hemolytic anemia. Arch Intern Med 1969;123:689.
64. Bennett JM, Healy PJ. Spherocytic hemolytic anemia and acute cholecystitis caused by *Clostridium welchii*. N Engl J Med 1965;268:1070.
65. Terebelo HR, McCue RL, Leuneville MS. Implications of plasma free hemoglobin in massive clostridial hemolysis. JAMA 1982;248:2028.
66. Murray HW, Masur H, Senterfit LB, et al. The protean manifestations of *Mycoplasma pneumonia* infection in adults. Am J Med 1975;58:229.
67. Nordhagen R, Stensvold K, Winsnes A, et al. Paroxysmal cold hemoglobinuria: the most frequent autoimmune hemolytic anemia in children. Acta Pediatr Scand 1984;73:258.
68. Shurin S, Anderson P, Zollinger J, et al. Pathophysiology of hemolysis in infections with *Hemophilus influenzae* type B. J Clin Invest 1986;77: 1340.
69. Nagel R L, Roth E Jr. Malaria and red cell genetic defects. Blood 1989;74: 1213.
70. Miller LH, Mason SJ, Clyde DF, et al. The resistance factor to *Plasmodium vivax* in blacks: the Duffy blood group genotype FyFy. N Engl J Med 1976;295:302.
71. Okoye V, Bennett V. *Plasmodium falciparum* malaria: band 3 as a possible receptor during invasion of human erythrocytes. Science 1985;227:169.
72. Friedman M, Fukuda M, Lame R. Evidence of a malarial parasite interaction site on the major transmembrane protein of the human erythrocyte. Science 1985;228:75.
73. Allred D, Gruenberg J, Sherman I. Dynamic rearrangements of the erythrocyte membrane internal architecture induced by infection with *Plasmodium falciparum*. J Cell Sci 1986;81:1.
74. MacPherson G, Warrell M, White N, et al. Human cerebral malaria. Am J Pathol 1985;119:385.
75. Aley S, Sherwood J, Howard R. Knob-positive and knob-negative *Plasmodium falciparum* differ in expression of a strain-specific malarial antigen on the surface of infected erythrocytes. J Exp Med 1984;160: 1585.
76. Miller KD, Greenberg AE, Campbell CC. Treatment of severe malaria in the United States with a continuous infusion of quinidine gluconate and exchange transfusion. N Engl Med 1989;321:65.
77. Benson LA, Kar S, McLaughlin G, et al. Entry of *Bartonella bacilliformis* into erythrocytes. Infect Immun 1986;54:347.
78. Auerbach M, Haubenstock A, Soloman G. Systemic babeiosis: another cause of the hemophagocytic syndrome. Am J Med 1986;80:301.
79. Smith RP, Evans AT, Popovsky M, et al. Transfusion-acquired babesiosis and failure of antibiotic treatment. JAMA 1986;256:2726.
80. Golightly L, Hirschhorn L, Weller P. Fever and headache in a splenectomized woman. Rev Infect Dis 1989;11:629.
81. Zaki M. Selected tickborne infections: a review of Lyme disease, Rocky Mountain spotted fever, and babesiosis. NY State Med 1989;89:320.
82. Hagler L, Pastore R, Bergin J. Aplastic anemia following viral hepatitis. Medicine 1975;54:139.
83. Tzakes AG, Arditi M, Whitington PF, et al. Aplastic anemia complicating orthotopic liver transplantation for non-A, non-B hepatitis. N Engl J Med 1988;319:393.
84. Baranski B, Armstrong G, Truman JT, et al. Epstein-Barr virus in the bone marrow of patients with aplastic anemia. Ann Intern Med 1988;109:695.
85. Risdall RJ, McKenna EW, Nesbit ME, et al. Virus-associated hemophagocytic syndrome: a benign histiocytic proliferation distinct from malignant histiocytosis. Cancer 1979;44:993.
86. Dehner L. Morphological findings in the histiocytic sundromes. Semin Oncol 1991;18:8.
87. Reiner A, Spivak J. Hematophagic histiocytosis: a report of 23 new patients and a review of the literature. Medicine 1988;67:369.
88. McKenna RW, Risdall RJ, Brunning RD. Virus associated hemophagocytic syndrome. Human Pathol 1981;12:395.
89. Kitchens CS. Clinical observations of human bone marrow macrophages. Medicine 1977;56:503.
90. Bodem CR, Harmony BH, Taylor HM, et al. Granulomatous bone marrow disease. Medicine 1983;62:372.
91. Kinaly J III, Wheby M. Bone marrow necrosis. Am J Med 1976;60:361.
92. Brown C III. Bone marrow necrosis: a study of seventy cases. J Hopkins Med J 1972;131:189.
93. Weissman D, Negendank W, Ayad A, et al. Bone marrow necrosis in lymphoma studied by magnetic resonance imaging. Am J Hematol 1992;40:42.
94. Oski F, Norman J. Effect of live measles vaccine on the platelet count. N Engl J Med 1966;275:352.
95. Scott S, Reimers H, Chernesky M, et al. Effect of viruses on platelet aggregation and platelet survival in rabbits. Blood 1978;62:47.
96. Terado H, Baldini M, Ebbe S, et al. Interaction of influenza virus with blood platelets. Blood 1966;28:213.
97. Bik T, Sarov I, Livine A. Interaction between vaccinia virus and human blood platelets. Blood 1982;59:482.
98. Ellman L, Carvalito A, Jacobsen B, et al. Platelet autoantibody in a case of infectious mononucleosis presenting as thrombocytopenic purpura. Am J Med 1973;55:723.
99. Cohen JI, Corey GR. Cytomegalovirus infection in the normal host. Medicine 1985;64:100.
100. Wilson J, Neame P, Kelton J. Infection-induced thrombocytopenia. Semin Thromb Hemost 1982;8:217.
101. Goldblum SE, Simon TL, Thilsted JP, et al. Pneumococcus-induced thrombocytopenia in rabbits. J Lab Clin Med 1985;106:298.
102. Oppenheimer L, Hrynuik WM, Bishop AJ. Thrombocytopenia in severe bacterial infections. J Surg Res 1976;20:211.

103. Kelton JG, Neame PB, Gauldie J, et al. Elevated platelet associated IgG in the thrombocytopenia of septicemia. N Engl J Med 1979;300:760.
104. Asprunk DH, Das J. Endotoxin-induced changes in human platelet membranes: morphologic evidence. Blood 1978;51:487.
105. Schneider RC, Zapol WM, Carvalho AC. Platelet consumption and sequestration in severe acute respiratory failure. Am Rev Resp Dis 1980;122:445.
106. Neame P, Kelton J, Walker I, et al. Thrombocytopenia in septicemia: the role of DIC. Blood 1980;56:88.
107. Corrigan JJ Jr, Ray WC, May N. Changes in the blood coagulation system associated with septicemia. N Engl J Med 1968;279:851.
108. Stossel TP, Levy R. Intravascular coagulation associated with pneumococcal bacteremia and symmetrical peripheral gangrene. Arch Intern Med 1970;125:876.
109. Spicer TE, Rau JM. Purpura fulminans. Am J Med 1976;61:566.
110. Beck E, Dejana E. Thrombohemorrhagic phenomena associated with infectious diseases. Semin hematol 1988;25:91.
111. Bisno AL, Freeman JC. The syndrome of asplenia, pneumococcal sepsis and DIC. Ann Intern Med 1970;72:389.
112. Gerjarusak P, Hinthorn D, Liu C. Hyposplenism and DIC in fulminant pneumococcal sepsis. South Med J 1977;70:995.
113. Kingston M, Mackenzie CR. The syndrome of pneumoccemia, DIC and asplenia. Can Med Assoc J 1979;121:57.
114. Ratnoff O, Nebehay W. Multiple coagulative defects in a patient with the Waterhouse-Friderichsen syndrome. Ann Intern Med 1962;56:627.
115. Bevilacqua M, Schleef R, Gimbrone M, et al. Regulation of the fibrinolytic system of cultured human vascular endothelium by interleukin 1. J Clin Invest 1986;78:587.
116. Carbone K, Heinrich M, Quinn T. Thrombophlebitis and cellulitis due to *Campylobacter* sp. fetus. Medicine 1985;64:244.
117. Simave C, Hardy G, Fardy P. The Lemierre syndrome: suppurative thrombophlebitis of the internal jugular vein secondary to oropharyngeal infection. Medicine 1989;68:85.
118. Remuzzi G, Garella S. HUS and TTP: variable expression of a single entity. Kidney Int 1987;32:292.
119. Ridolfi RL, Bell WR. Thrombotic thrombocytopenic purpura: report of 25 cases and review of the literature. Medicine 1981;60:413.
120. Neill MA, Agosti J, Rosen H. Hemorrhagic colitis with *Escherichia coli* 0157:H7 preceding adult hemolytic uremic syndrome. Arch Intern Med 1985;145:2215.
121. Pai CH, Kelly JK. Shiga-like toxin-producing *Escherichia coli*. In: Farthing MJ, Keusch GT, eds. Enteric infection: mechanisms, manifestations, and management. New York, Raven Press, 1989:141.
122. Marshall FF, Walsh PC. Extrarenal manifestations of renal cell carcinoma. J Urol 1977;117:439.
123. Bowman HS, Martinez EJ. Fever, anemia and hyperhaptoglobinemia: an extrarenal triad of hypernephroma. Ann Intern Med 1968;68:613.
124. Beveridge BR, Baumerman RM, Evanson JM, et al. Hypochromic anemia: a retrospective study and follow-up of 378 in-patients. Q J Med 1965;34:145.
125. Rockey DC, Campbell EW Jr. Evaluation of the gastrointestinal tract in patients with iron-deficiency anemia. N Engl J Med 1993;329:1691.
126. Doll D, Weiss R. Neoplasia and the erythron. J Clin Oncol 1985;3:429.
127. Hardy C, Balducci L. Hemopoietic alterations of cancer. Am J Med Sci 1985;290:196.
128. Zucker S, Lysik R, DiSetfano J. Cancer cell inhibition of erythropoiesis. J Lab Clin Med 1980;96:770.
129. Zucker S, Friedman S, Lysik R. Bone marrow erythropoiesis in the anemia of infection, inflammation, and malignancy. J Clin Invest 1974;53:1132.
130. Beutler B, Cerami A. Cachectin, cachexia, and shock. Annu Rev Med 1988;39:75.
131. Balkwill F, Osborne R, Burke F. Evidence for tumour necrosis factor/cachectin production in cancer. Lancet 1987;2:1229.
132. Ulich T, del Castillo J, Guo K, et al. The hematologic effects of chronic administration of the monokines TNF, interleukin-1 and granulocyte-CSF on bone marrow and circulation. Am J Pathol 1987;134:149.
133. Beutler B, Cerami A. Cachectin: more than a tumor necrosis factor. N Engl J Med 1987;316:379.
134. Johnson RA, Waddelow T, Caro, J, et al. Chronic exposure to TNF in vivo preferentially inhibits erythropoiesis in nude mice. Blood 1989;74:130.
135. Berdel WE, Danhauser-Riepl S, Steinhauser G, et al. Various human hematopoietic growth factors (interleukin-3, GM-CSF, G-CSF) stimulate clonal growth of nonhematopoietic tumor cells. Blood 1989;73:80.
136. Dainiak N, Kulkarni V, Howard D, et al. Mechanisms of abnormal erythropoiesis in malignancy. Cancer 1983;51:1101.
137. Miller CB, Jones RJ, Piantadosi S, et al. Decreased erythropoietin response in patients with the anemia of cancer. N Engl J Med 1990;322:1689.
138. Oster W, Herrmann F, Gamm H, et al. Erythropoietin for the treatment of anemia of malignancy associated with neoplastic bone marrow infiltration. J Clin Oncol 1990;8:956.
139. Masaoka A, Hashimoto T, Shibata K, et al. Thymomas associated with pure red cell aplasia: histologic and follow-up studies. Cancer 1989;64:1872.
140. Hirst E, Robertson TI. The syndrome of thymoma and erythroblastopenic anemia. Medicine 1967;46:225.
141. Krantz SB, Kao V. Studies on red cell aplasia. I. Demonstration of a plasma inhibitor to heme synthesis and an antibody to erythroblastic nuclei. Proc Natl Acad Sci USA 1967;58:493.
142. Tetteri A, Windebank KP, Veeder MH, Kiely JM. Steroid-responsive pure red cell aplasia associated with natural killer cell lymphocytosis. Am J Hematol 1989;31:211.
143. Akard LP, Brandt J, Lu L, et al. Chronic T-cell lympholiferative disorder and pure red cell aplasia: further characterization of cell-mediated inhibition of erythropoiesis and clinical response to cytotoxic chemotherapy. Am J Med 1987;83:1069.
144. Mangan KF. T-cell mediated suppression of hematopoiesis. N Engl J Med 1985;312:306.
145. Delsol G, Guiu-Godfrin B, Guiu M, et al. Leukoerythroblastosis and cancer frequency: prognosis and physiopathologic significance. Cancer 1979;44:1009.
146. Spira M, Lynch E. Autoimmune hemolytic anemia and carcinoma: an unusual association. Am J Med 1979;67:753.
147. Bruyere M, Sokal G, Devortille J, et al. Autoimmune haemolytic anaemias and ovarian tumour. Br J Haematol 1971;20:83.
148. Lohrmann HP, Adam W, Heymer B, et al. Microangiopathic hemolytic anemia in metastatic carcinoma: report of eight cases. Ann Intern Med 1973;79:368.
149. Brain MC, Dave J, Hourihane D. Microangiopathic haemolytic anaemia: the possible role of vascular lesions in pathogenesis. Br J Haematol 1962;8:358.
150. Jacobsen RJ, Jackson D. Erythrocyte fragmentation in defibrination syndromes. Ann Intern Med 1974;81:207.
151. Antman KH, Skarm A, Mayer R, et al. Microangiopathic hemolytic anemia and cancer: a review. Medicine 1979;58:377.
152. Murgo AJ. Thrombotic microangiography in the cancer patient including those induced by chemotherapeutic agents. Semin Hematol 1987;24:161.
153. Waldmann, T, Rossi W, Swann R. The erythropoiesis stimulating factors produced by tumors. Ann NY Acad Sci 1968;149:509.
154. Waldmann T, Levin E, Baldwin M. The association of polycythemia with a cerebellar hemangioblastoma: the production of an erythropoiesis stimulating factor by the tumor. Am J Med 1961;31:318.
155. Sytkowski A, Bicknell K, Smith GM, et al. Secretion of erythropoietin-like activity by clones of human renal carcinoma cell line GKA. Cancer Res 1984;44:51.
156. Reid CD, Fidler J, Kirk A. Endogeneous erythroid clones (EEC) in polycythaemia and their relationship to diagnosis and the response to treatment. Br J Haematol 1988;68:395.
157. Lee M, Durch S, Dave D, et al. Kinetics of tumor-induced murine neutrophilia. Blood 1979;53:619.
158. Delmonte L, Liebelt RA. Granulocytosis promoting extract of mouse tumor tissue. Science 1965;148:521.
159. Beutler B, Cerami A. Tumor necrosis, cachexia, shock, and inflammation: a common mediator. Annu Rev Biochem 1988;57:505.
160. Mayer P, Lam C, Obenaus H, et al. Recombinant human GM-CSF induces leukocytosis and activated peripheral blood polymorphonuclear neutrophils in nonhuman primates. Blood 1987;70:206.
161. O'Neill B Jr. Monocytosis in malignant disease. Ann Intern Med 1970;73:991.
162. Ascensao JL, Oken MM, Ewing SL. Leukocytosis and large cell lung cancer: a frequent association. Cancer 1987;60:903.
163. Ramos FJ, Zamora F, Perez-Sicilia M, et al. Chronic granulocytic leukemia versus neutrophilic leukemoid reaction. Am J Med 1990;88:83.
164. Obara TR, Ito Y, Kodama T, Fujimoto Y. A case of gastric carcinoma associated with excessive granulocytosis: production of a colony-stimulating factor by the tumor. Cancer 1985;56:782.
165. Sato K, Mimura H, Han DC. Production of bone-resorbing activity and colony-stimulating activity in vivo and in vitro by a human squamous cell carcinoma associated with hypercalcemia and leukocytosis. J Clin Invest 1986;78:145.
166. Sato K, Fujii Y, Ono M, et al. Production of interleukin 1 α-like factor and colony-stimulating factor by a squamous cell carcinoma of the thyroid (T3M-5) derived from a patient with hypercalcemia and leukocytosis. Cancer Res 1987;47:6474.
167. Beeson P. Cancer and eosinophilia. N Engl J Med 1983;309:792.
168. Weller P. Eosinophilia. J Allergy Clin Immunol 1984;73:1.
169. Lowe D, Jorizzo J, Hutt MSR. Tumor-associated eosinophilia: a review. J Clin Pathol 1981;34:1343.
170. Balducci L, Chapman S, Little D, et al. Paraneoplastic eosinophilia: secretion of eosinophil chemotatic factors. Cancer 1989;64:2250.
171. Silberstein DS, Schoof DD, Rodrick ML, et al. Activation of eosinophils in cancer patients treated with IL-2– and IL-3–generated lymphokine-activated killer cells. J Immunol 1989;142:2162.
172. Isaacson NJ, Rappoport P. Eosinophilia in malignant tumors: its significance. Ann Intern Med 1946;25:893.
173. Levin J, Conley CL. Thrombocytosis associated with malignant disease. Arch Intren Med 1964;114:497.
174. Schafer A. Review: bleeding and thrombosis in the myeloproliferative disorders. Blood 1984;64:1.
175. Bierman HR, Kelly KH, Cordes FL, et al. The release of leukocytes and

platelets from the pulmonary circulation by epinephrine. Blood 1952; 7:683.
176. Sacks G, Levin J, Bell WR. Trousseau's syndrome and other manifestations of chronic disseminated coagulopathy in patients with neoplasms: clinical, pathologic and therapeutic features. Medicine 1977;56:1.
177. Rickles FR, Edwards RL. Activation of blood coagulation in cancer: Trousseau's syndrome revisited. Blood 1983;62:14.
178. Haemostatic abnormalities and malignant disease. (Editorial) Lancet 1986;1:303.
179. Smith SB, Arkin C. Cryofibrinogenemia: incidence, clinical correlations and review of the literature. Am J Clin Pathol 1972;58:524.
180. Moessou MW, Colman RW, Sherry S. Chronic intravascular coagulation syndrome: report of a case with special studies of an associated plasma cryoprecipitate (cryofibrinogen). N Engl J Med 1968;278:815.
181. Bell WR, Starkson NF, Tong S, et al. Trousseau's syndrome: devastating coagulopathy in the absence of heparin. Am J Med 1985;79:423.
182. Jandl JH. The anemia of liver disease: observations on its mechanism. J Clin Invest 1955;34:390.
183. Reynolds TB, Hidemura R, Michel H, et al. Portal hypertension without cirrhosis in alcoholic liver disease. Ann Intern Med 1969;70:497.
184. Eichner ER. The hematologic disorders of alcoholism. Am J Med 1973;54:621.
185. Sheehy JW, Berman A. The anemia of cirrhosis. J Lab Clin Med 1960;56: 72.
186. Kawasaki H, Nemasu J, Maeda N, et al. Plasma levels of atrial natriuretic peptide in patients with chronic liver disease. Am J Gastroenterol 1987;82:727.
187. Lunden L, Aallgren R, Birgegard G, et al. Serum ferritin in alcoholics and the relation to liver damage, iron state and erythropoietin activity. Acta Med Scand 1981;209:327.
188. Reed CF, Murphy M, Roberts G. Phospholipid exchange between plasma and erythrocytes in man and the dog. J Clin Invest 1968;47: 749.
189. Cooper RA, Diloy-Puray M, Lando P, et al. An analysis of lipoproteins, bile acids, and red cell membranes associated with target cells and spur cells in patients with liver disease. J Clin Invest 1972;51:3 182.
190. Cooper RA. Hemolytic syndromes and red cell membrane abnormalities in liver disease. Semin Hematol 1980;17:103.
191. Owen J, Brown D, Harry D, et al. Erythrocyte echinocytosis in liver disease: role of abnormal plasma high density lipoproteins. J Clin Invest 1985;76:2275.
192. Olivieri O, Guarini P, Negri M, et al. Increased proteolytic activity of erythrocyte membrane in spur cell anemia. Br J Haematol 1988;70: 483.
193. Shohet SB. "Acanthocytogenesis"—or how the red cell won its spurs. N Engl J Med 1974;290:1316.
194. Lindenbaum J. Hematologic complications of alcohol abuse. Semin Liver Dis 1987;7:169.
195. Cowan D. Effect of alcoholism on hemostasis. Semin Hematol 1980;17: 137.
196. Eichner ER. The hematologic disorders of alcoholism. Am J Med 1973;54:621.
197. McCurdy P, Rath C. Vacuolated nucleated bone marrow cells in alcoholism. Semin Hematol 1980;17:100.
198. Unger KW, Johnson D. Red blood cell mean corpuscular volume: a potential indicator of alcohol usage in a working population. Am J Med Sci 1974;267:281.
199. Wu A, Chanarin I, Levi AJ. Macrocytosis of chronic alcoholism. Lancet 1974;1:829.
200. Meagher RC, Sieber F, Spivak JL. Suppression of hematopoietic-progenitor-cell proliferation by ethanol and acetaldehyde. N Engl J Med 1982;307:845.
201. Lindenbaum J. Folate and vitamin B-12 deficiencies in alcoholism. Semin Hematol 1980;17:119.
202. Hillman RS, McGuffin R, Campbell C. Alcohol interference with the folate-enterohepatic cycle. Trans Assoc Am Physicians 1977;90:145.
203. Eichner ER, Pierce I, Hillman RS. Folate balance in dietary induced megaloblastic anemia. N Engl J Med 1971;284:933.
204. Spivak JL. Masked megaloblastic anemia. Arch Intern Med 1982;142: 2111.
205. Eichner ER, Hillman RS. The evolution of anemia in alcoholic patients. Am J Med 1971;50:218.
206. Lunden L, Hallgren R, Birgegard G, et al. Serum ferritin in alcoholics and the relation to liver damage, iron state and erythropoietic activity. Acta Med Scand 1981;209:327.
207. Zieve L. Jaundice, hyperlipemia and hemolytic anemia: a heretofore unrecognized syndrome associated with alcoholic fatty liver and cirrhosis. Ann Intern Med 1968;48:471.
208. Tisman G, Herbert V. In vitro myelosuppression and immunosuppression by ethanol. J Clin Invest 1973;52:1410.
209. MacGregor RR. Alcohol and immune defense. JAMA 1986;256:147.
210. Imperia PS, Chikkappa G, Phillips PG. Mechanism of inhibition of granulopoiesis by ethanol. Proc Soc Exp Biol Med 1984;175:219.
211. Perlino C, Rimland D. Alcoholism, leukopenia and pneumococcal sepsis. Am Rev Resp Dis 1985;132:757.
212. Brayton RG, Stokes PE, Schwartz MS, et al. Effect of alcohol and various diseases in leukocyte mobilization, phagocytosis and intracellular bacterial killing. N Engl J Med 1970;282:123.
213. Liu Y. Effects of alcohol on granulocytes and lymphocytes. Semin Hematol 1980;17:130.
214. Liu YK. Phagocytic capacity of reticuloendothlial system in alcoholics. J Reticuloendothel Soc 1979;25:605.
215. Young GP, Weyden MB, Rose IS, et al. Lymphopenia and lymphocyte transformation in alcoholics. Experimentia 1979;35:268.
216. Gluckman SJ, Dvorak VC, MacGregor RR. Host defense during prolonged alcohol consumption in a controlled environment. Arch Intern Med 1977;137:1539.
217. Atkinson JP, Sullivan TJ, Kelly JP, et al. Stimulation by alcohol of cyclic AMP metabolism in human leukocytes: possible role of cyclic AMP in the anti-inflammatory effects of ethanol. J Clin Invest 1977;60: 284.
218. Levine R, Spivak J, Meagher R, et al. Effect of ethanol on thrombopoiesis. Br J Haematol 1986;62:345.
219. Sullivan L, Adams W, Liu Y. Induction of thrombocytopenia by thrombopheresis in man: pattern of recovery in normal subjects during ethanol ingestion and abstinence, Blood 1977;49:197.
220. Deykin D, Jarison P, McMahon L. Ethanol potentiation of aspirin-induced prolongation of the bleeding time. N Engl J Med 1982; 306:852.
221. Mikhailidis DP, Jenkins W, Barradas M, et al. Platelet function defects in chronic alcoholism. Clin Res 1986;293:715.
222. Fried W. Hematologic abnormalities in chronic renal failure. Semin Nephrol 1981;1:176.
223. Jacobson LO, Goldwasser E, Plzak LF, et al. Role of the kidney in erythropoiesis. Nature 1957;129:633.
224. Blumberg A, Marti HA. Adaptation to anemia by decreased oxygen affinity of hemoglobin in patients on dialysis. Kidney Int 1972;1:263.
225. Mitchell T, Pegrum G. The oxygen affinity of hemoglobin in chronic renal failure. Br J Hematol 1971;21:463.
226. Brown S, Caro J, Erslev AJ, et al. Rise in erythropoietin and hematocrit associated with transient liver enzyme abnormalities in anephric hemodialysis patients. Am J Med 1980;62:280.
227. Blumberg A. Pathogenesis of anemia due to kidney disease. Nephron 1989;51(Suppl 1):15.
228. Wallner S, Vantrin R. Evidence that inhibition of erythropoiesis is important in the anemia of chronic renal failure. J Lab Clin Med 1981;97: 170.
229. Caro J, Erslev AJ. Uremic inhibitors of erythropoiesis. Semin Nephrol 1985;5:128.
230. Levinsky H, Gafter U, Levi J, et al. Neuraminidase-like activity in sera of uremic anemic patients. Nephron 1984;37:35.
231. Zappa-Costa A, Caro J, Erslev A. Normalization of hematocrit in patients with end stage renal disease on chronic ambulatory peritoneal dialysis. Am J Med 1982;72:53.
232. Segal G, Stueve T, Adamson J. Spermine and spermidine are non-specific inhibitors of in vitro hematopoiesis. Kidney Int 1987;31:72.
233. Caro J, Ersev A. Uremic inhibitors of erythropoiesis. Semin Nephrol 1985;5:128.
234. Salabindeen A, Hawkins T, Keavy P, et al. Is anemia during continuous ambulatory peritoneal dialysis really better than during haemodialysis? Lancet 1983;2:1046.
235. Klahr S, Slatopolsky E. Toxicity of parathyroid hormone in uremia. Annu Rev Med 1986;37:71.
236. McGonigle R, Wallin J, Husserl F, et al. Potential role of parathyroid hormone as an inhibitor of erythropoiesis in the anemia of renal failure. J Lab Clin Med 1984;104:1016.
237. Barbour G. Effect of parathyroidectomy on anemia in chronic renal failure. Arch Intern Med 1979;139:889.
238. Geary D, Fennell R, Braylan R, et al. Hyperparathyroidism and anemia in chronic renal failure. Eur J Pediatr 1982;139:296.
239. Pitts T, Piramo B, Metro R, et al. Hyperparathyroidism and 1,25-dihydroxy vitamin D deficiency in mild, moderate and severe renal failure. J Clin Endocrinol Metab 1988;67:876.
240. Weinberg S, Lubin A, Weiner S, et al. Myelofibrosis and renal osteodystrophy. Am J Med 1977;63:755.
241. Graber SE, Krantz B. Erythropoietin: biology and clinical use. Hematol Oncol Clin N Am 1989;3:369.
242. Eschbach J, Egue J, Downing M, et al. Correction of the anemia of end-stage renal disease with recombinant erythropoietin. N Engl J Med 1987;316:73.
243. Hendler ED, Goffinet JA, Ross S, et al. Controlled study of androgen therapy in anemia of patients on maintenance hemodialysis. N Engl J Med 1974;291:1046.
244. Neff MS, Goldberg J, Slifkin RF, et al. A comparison of androgens for anemia in patients on hemodialysis. N Engl J Med 1981;304:871.
245. Desforges J. Anemia in uremia. Ann Intern Med 1970;126:808.
246. Adamson J, Eschbach J, Finch CA. The kidney and erythropoiesis. Am J Med 1968;44:725.
247. Welt LG, Sachs JR, McManus TJ. An ion transport defect in erythrocytes from uremic patients. Trans Assoc Am Physicians 1964;77:169.
248. Yawata Y, Howe R, Jacob H. Abnormal red cell metabolism causing hemolysis in uremis. Ann Intern Med 1973;79:362.
249. Yawata Y, Jacob H. Abnormal red cell metabolism in patients with

chronic uremia: nature of the defect and its persistence despite adequate hemodialysis. Blood 1975;45:231.
250. Eaton J, Leida M. Hemolysis in chronic renal failure. Semin Nephrol 1985;5:133.
251. Aherne WA. The "burr" red cell and azotaemia. J Clin Pathol 1957;10: 252.
252. Brain MC, Neame PB. Thrombotic thrombocytopenic purpura and the hemolytic uremic syndrome. Semin Thromb Hemost 1982;8:186.
253. Griffin PM, Olmstead LC, Petras RE. Escherichia coli O157-H7-associated colitis: a clinical and histological study of 11 cases. Gastroenterology 1990;99:142.
254. Martin DL, MacDonald KL, White KE. The epidemiology and clinical aspects of the hemolytic uremic syndrome in Minnesota. N Engl J Med 1990;65:1161.
255. Neiman RS, Bischel MD, Lukes RJ. Hypersplenism in the uremic hemodialyzed patient: pathology and proposed pathophysiologic mechanisms. Am J Clin Pathol 1973;60:502.
256. Hattersley PG, Engels JL. Neutrophilic hypersegmentation without macrocytic anemia. West J Med 1974;121:179.
257. Langnecker RK, Goffnet JA, Handler ED. Blood loss from maintenance hemodialysis. Trans Am Soc Artif Intern Organs 1974;20:135.
258. Navab F, Masters P, Subramani R, et al. Angiodysplasia in patients with renal insufficiency. Am J Gastroenterol 1989;84:1297.
259. Hosokawa S, Oyamaguchi A, Yoshida O. Trace elements and complications in patients undergoing chronic hemodialysis. Nephron 1990;55: 375.
260. Mladenovic J. Aluminum inhibits erythropoiesis in vitro. J Clin Invest 1988;81:1661.
261. Bia M, Cooper K, Schnall S, et al. Aluminum induced anemia: pathogenesis and treatment in patients on chronic hemodialysis. Kidney Int 1989;36:852.
262. Thorling EB. Paraneoplastic erythrocytosis and inappropriate erythropoietin production. Scand J Haematol 1972;(Suppl):17.
263. Okabe T, Urabe A, Kato T, et al. Production of erythropoietin-like activity by human renal and hepatic carcinomas in cell culture. Cancer 1985;55:1918.
264. Da Silva J, Lacombe C, Bruneval P, et al. Tumor cells are the site of erythropoietin synthesis in human renal cancers associated with polycythemia. Blood 1990;75:577.
265. Luke RG, Kennedy AC, Stirling WB. Renal artery stenosis, hypertension and polycythemia. Br Med J 1965;1:164.
266. Rose WF, Waldmann TA, Cohen P. Renal cysts, erythropoietin and polycythemia. Am J Med 1963;34:76.
267. Pollak R, Maddux MS, Cohen J, et al. Erythrocythemia following renal transplantation: influence of diuretic therapy. Clin Nephrol 1988;29: 119.
268. Shalhoub RG, Rajim U, Kim VV. Erythrocytosis in patients on long-term hemodialysis. Ann Intern Med 1982;97:686.
269. Wickre CG, Norman DJ, Bennison A, et al. Postrenal transplant erythrocytosis: a review of fifty-three patients. Kidney Int 1983;23:731.
270. Hoppin EC, Depner T, Yamuchi H, et al. Erythrocytosis associated with diffuse parenchymal lesions of the kidney. Br J Haematol 1976;32: 557.
271. Emanuel DA, Wenzol FJ. Erythrocytosis associated with the nephrotic syndrome. JAMA 1962;181:788.
272. Sonneborn R, Perez GO, Epstein M, et al. Erythrocytosis associated with nephrotic syndrome. Arch Intern Med 1977;137:1068.
273. Erkeleus DW, van Eps LWS. Bartter's syndrome and erythrocytosis. Am J Med 1973;55:711.
274. Lacombe C, DA Silva JL, Bruneval P, et al. Peritubular cells are the site of erythropoietin synthesis in the murine hypoxic kidney. J Clin Invest 1988;81:620.
275. Nissenson A, Nimer S, Wolcott D. Recombinant human erythropoietin and renal anemia: molecular biology, clinical efficacy and nervous system effects. Ann Intern Med 1991;114:402.
276. Nagy E, Berizi I. Pituitary dependence of bone marrow function. Br J Haematol 1989;71:457.
277. Golde DW, Bersch N, Li C. Growth hormone: species specific stimulation of erythropoiesis in vito. Science 1977;196:1112.
278. Dainiak N, Sutter D, Krecztko S. L-Triiodothyronine augments erythropoietin growth factor release from peripheral blood and bone marrow leukocytes. Blood 1986;68:1289.
279. Das KC, Mukkerjee M, Sarkar TK, et al. Erythropoiesis and erythropoietin in hypo- and hyperthyroidism. J Clin Endocrinol Metab 1975;40: 211.
280. Carmel R, Spencer CA. Clinical and subclinical thyroid disorders associated with pernicious anemia. Arch Intern Med 1982;142:1465.
281. Kelle HA, Sawers JS, Boulton FE, et al. Problems of anticoagulation with warfarin in hyperthyroidism. Q J Med 1986;58:43.
282. Horton L, Coburn R. England J, et al. The haematology of hypothyroidism. Q J Med 1985;45:101.
283. Mazzaferri EL. Adult hypothyroidism. Manifestations and clinical presentation. Postgrad Med 1986;29:64.
284. Welansky DC, Greisman B. Early hypothyroidism in patients with menorrhagia. Am J Obstet Gynecol 1989;160:673.
285. Savage RA, Sipple C. Marrow myxedema. Gelatinous transformation of marrow ground substance in a patient with severe hypothyroidism. Arch Pathol Lab Med 1987;111:375.
286. Boxer M, Ellman L, Geller R, et al. Anemia in primary hyperparathyroidism. Arch Intern Med 1977;137:588.
287. Mallette LE, Bilezikian JP, Heath DA, et al. Primary hyperparathyroidism: clinical and biochemical features. Medicine 1974;53:127.
288. Albright F, Aub JC, Bauer W. Hyperparathyroidism. JAMA 1934;102: 1276.
289. Ikkala E, Myllyla G, Pelkneon R, et al. Haemostatic parameters in Cushing's syndrome. Acta Med Scand 1985;217:507.
290. Tudhope GR. Endocrine diseases. Clin Haematol 1972;1:475.
291. Baxter J, Tyrrell JB. The adrenal cortex. In: Felig P, Baxter J, Broadus, et al, eds. Endocrinology and metabolism, ed 2, New York, McGraw-Hill, 1987:551.
292. Jones R, Peterson C. Hematologic alterations in diabetes mellitus. Am J Med 1981;70:339.
293. Bersch N, Groopman JE, Golde DW. Natural and biosynthetic insulin stimulates the growth of human erythroid progenitors in vitro. J Clin Endocrinol Metab 1978;55:1209.
294. Ritchey AK, Tamborlane W, Gertner J. Improved diabetic control enhances erythroid stem cell proliferation in vitro. J Clin Endocrinol Metab 1985;60:1257.
295. Peterson C, Jones R, Koenig R, et al. Reversible hematologic sequelae of diabetes mellitus. Ann Intern Med 1977;86:425.
296. Schwartz JS, Clancy CM. Glycosylated hemoglobin assays in the management and diagnosis of diabetes mellitus. Ann Intern Med 1984;101: 710.
297. Bunn HF, Briehl RW. The interaction of 2,3-diphosphoglycerate with various human hemoglobins. J Clin Invest 1970;49:1088.
298. Williamson JR, Gardner GW, Boylan GL, et al. Microrheologic investigation of erythrocyte deformability in diabetes mellitus. Blood 1985;65: 283.
299. Esmann V. The polymorphonuclear leukocyte in diabetes mellitus. J Clin Chem Clin Biochem 1983;21:561.
300. Mowat AG, Baum J. Chemotaxis of polymorphonuclear leukocytes from patients with diabetes mellitus. N Engl J Med 1971;284:621.
301. Small M, Lowe GD, MacCuish AC, et al. Thrombin and plasmin activity in diabetes mellitus and their association with glycaemic control. Q J Med 1987;65:1025.
302. Mustard J, Packham M. Platelets and diabetes mellitus. N Engl J Med 1984;311:665.
303. Jones DB, Davis T, Brown E, et al. Determinants of ADP-induced platelet aggregation in diabetes mellitus. Diabetologia 1986;29:291.
304. Davi G, Catalano I, Averna M, et al. Thromboxane biosynthesis and platelet function in type II diabetes mellitus. N Engl J Med 1990;322: 1769.
305. Villanueva, Allen N. Demonstration of altered antithrombin III activity due to nonenzymatic glycosylation at glucose concentration expected to be encountered in severely diabetic patients. Diabetes 1988;37:1103.
306. Auwerx J, Bouillon R, Collen D, et al. Tissue-type plasminogen activator antigen and plasminogen activator inhibitor in diabetes mellitus. Arteriosclerosis 1988;8:68.
307. Shilo S, Werner D, Hershko C. Acute hemolytic anemia caused by severe hypophosphatemia in diabetic ketoacidosis. Acta Haematol 1985;73:55.
308. Burris AS. Leukemoid reaction associated with severe diabetic ketoacidosis. South Med J 1986;79:647.
309. Cornbleet PJ, Moir R, Wolf P. A histochemical study of bone marrow hypoplasia in anorexia nervosa. Virchows Arch Pathol Anat Histol 1977;374:239.
310. Pearson H. Marrow hypoplasia in anorexia nervosa. J Pediatr 1967;71: 211.
311. Mant MJ, Faragher PS. The haematology of anorexia nervosa. Br J Haematol 1972;23:737.
312. Smith RR, Spivak JL. Marrow cell necrosis in anorexia nervosa and involuntary starvation. Br J Haematol 1985;60:525.
313. Nestel P. Cholesterol metabolism in anorexia nervosa and hypercholesterolemia. J Clin Endocrinol Metab 1974;38:325.
314. Powers J, Luktenstein M, Collins J, et al. Serum erythropoeitin in healthy older persons. J Am Geriatr Soc 1989;37:388.
315. Lipschitz DA, Udupa KB, Milton KY, et al. Effect of age on hematopoiesis in man. Blood 1984;63:502.
316. Zauber NP, Zauber AC. Hematologic data of healthy very old people. JAMA 1987;257:2181.
317. Lipschitz D, Udupa K. Age and the hematopoietic system. J Am Geriatr Soc 1986;34:448.
318. Baldwin JG. Hematopoeitic function in the elderly. Arch Intern Med 1988;148:2544.
319. Todd M, Thompson JH, Jr, Bowie EJ, et al. Changes in blood coagulation during pregnancy. Mayo Clin Proc 1975;40:370.
320. Weiner CP. The obstetric patient and disseminated intravascular coagulation. Clin Perinatol 1986;13:705.
321. Feliu J, Juarez S, Ordoñez A, Garcia-Paredes ML, et al. Acute leukemia and pregnancy. Cancer 1988;61:580.
322. Caligiuri M, Mayer R. Pregancy and leukemia. Semin Oncol 1989;16: 388.
323. Branch DW, Scott J, Kochenour N, et al. Obstetric complications associated with the lupus anticoagulant. N Engl J Med 1985;313:1322.
324. Hytten F. Blood volume changes in normal pregnancy. Clin Hematol 1985;14:601.

325. Bentley DP. Iron metabolism and anemia in pregnancy. Clin Haematol 1985;14:613.
326. Foulkes J, Goldie DJ. The use of ferritin to assess the need for iron supplements in pregnancy. J Obstet Gynecol 1982;3:11.
327. Suda T, Omine M, Tsuchiya I, et al. Prognostic aspects of aplastic anemia in pregnancy. Blut 1978;36:285.
328. Pritchard J, Whalley PJ. Abortion complicated by *Clostridium perfringens* infection. Am J Obstet Gynecol 1971;111:484.
329. McCrae K, Samuels P, Schriener A. Pregancy-associated thrombocytopenia: pathogenesis and management. Blood 1992;80:2697.
330. Romero R, Duffy TP. Platelet disorders in pregnancy. Clin Perinatol 1980;7:327.
331. O'Reilly RA, Taber BZ. Immunologic thrombocytopenic purpura and pregnancy. Obstet Gynecol 1978;51:590.
332. Nagey DA, Alger LS, Edelman BB, et al. Reacting appropriately to thrombocytopenia in pregnancy. South Med J 1986;79:1385.
333. Karpatkin M, Porges RF, Karpatken S. Platelet counts in infants of women with autoimmune thrombocytopenia: effect of steroid administration to the mother. N Engl J Med 1981;305:936.
334. Schwartz M, Brenner W. The obfuscation of eclampsia by thrombotic thrombocytopenia purpura. Am J Obstet Gynecol 1978;131:18.
335. Redman CW, Platelets and the beginning of preeclampsia. N Engl J Med 1990;323:478.
336. Wallenburg HC, Dekker GA, Makovitz JW, et al. Low dose aspirin prevents pregnancy-induced hypertension and preeclampsia in angiotensin-sensitive primigravida. Lancet 1986;1:1.
337. Sureau C. prevention of perinatal consequences of preeclampsia with low-dose aspirin: results of the Epreda trial. Eur J Obstet Gynecol Reprod Biol 1991;41:71.
338. Baca L, Gibbons R. The HELLP syndrome: a serious complication of pregnancy with hemolysis, elevated levels of liver enzymes, and low platelet count. Am J Med 1988;85:590.
339. Riley CA, Latham PS, Romero R, Duffy TP. Acute fatty liver of pregnancy: a reassessment based on observations in nine patients. Ann Intern Med 1987;106:703.
340. Mimouni F, Miodovinik M. How often does maternal preeclampsia-eclampsia create thrombocytopenia in the fetus? (Letter) Obstet Gynecol 1987;70:811.
341. Romero R, Copel JA, Hobbins JC. Intrauterine fetal demise and hemostatic failure: the fetal death syndrome. Clin Obstet Gynecol 1985;28:24.
342. Sher G. Statland BE. Abruptio placentae with coagulopathy: a rational basis for management. Clin Obstet Gynecol 1985;28:15.
343. Oláh KS, Gee H, Needham PG. The management of severe disseminated intravascular coagulopathy complicating placental abruption in the second trimester of pregnancy. Br J Obstet Gynaecol 1988;95:419.
344. Courtney LD, Allington LM. Effect of amniotic fluid on blood coagulation. Br J Haematol 1972;113:911.
345. Sprung J, Cheng EY, patel S, et al. Understanding and management of amniotic fluid embolism. J Clin Anesth 1992;4:235.
346. Charache S, Niebyl JR. Pregnancy in sickle cell disease. Clin Haematol 1985;14:729.
347. Koshy M, Burd L, Wallace D, et al. Prophylactic red-cell transfusions in pregnant patients with sickle cell disease: a randomized cooperative study. N Engl J Med 1988;319:1447.
348. Wayne A, Kevy S, Nathan D. Transfusion in sickle cell disease. Blood 1993;81:1109.
349. Schaefer AL. The hypercoagulable states. Ann Intern Med 1985;102:814.
350. Rutherford SE, Phelan JP. Thromboembolic disease in pregnancy. Clin Perinatol 1986;13:719.
351. Ginsberg JS, Hirsh J, Rainbow A, Coates G. Risks to the fetus of the radiologic procedures used in the diagnosis of maternal thromboembolic disease. Thromb Haematol 1989;61:189.
352. Letsky E, de Swiet M. Thromboembolism in pregnancy and its management. Br J Haematol 1984;57:543.
353. Ginsberg JS, Hirsh J, Turner D, et al. Risks to the fetus of anticoagulant therapy during pregnancy. Thromb Haemost 1989;61:197.
354. Greer IA, Lowe GD, Walker JJ, et al. Hemorrhagic problems in obstetrics and gynecology in patients with congenital coagulopathies. Br J Obstet Gynaecol 1991;98:909.
355. Chediak JR, Alban GM, Maxey B. von Willebrand's disease and pregnancy: management during delivery and outcome of offspring. Am J Obstet Gynecol 1986;155:618.
356. Rick ME, Williams SB, Sacher RA, et al. Thrombocytopenia associated with pregnancy in a patient with type IIB von Willebrand's disease. Blood 1987;69:786.
357. Caldwell DC, Williamson RA, Goldsmith JC. Hereditary coagulopathies in pregnancy. Clin Obstet Gynecol 1985;28:53.
358. Morrison AE, Walker IO, Black WP. Protein C deficiency and pregnancy: a case report. Obstet Gynecol 1989;73:455.
359. DeStefano V, Leone G, De Carolis S, et al. Management of pregnancy in women with anti-thrombin III congenital defect: report of four cases. Thromb Haemost 1988;59:193.
360. Owen J, Antithrombin III replacement therapy in pregnancy. Semin Hematol 1991;28:46.
361. Jones EC, Mosesson MW, Thomason JL, Jackson TC. Essential thrombocythemia in pregnancy. Obstet Gynecol 1988;71:501.
362. Chow E, Haley L, Vickars L. Essential thrombocytopenia in pregnancy. Am J Hematol 1992;41:249.
363. Solal-Celigney P, Tertian G, Fernandez H, et al. Pregnancy and paroxysmal nocturnal hemoglobinuria. Arch Intern Med 1988;148:593.
364. Budman D, Steinberg A. Hematologic aspects of systemic lupus erythematosus: current concepts. Ann Intern Med 1977;86:220.
365. Bailey F, Lilly M, Bertoli L, Ball G. An antibody that inhibits in vitro bone marrow proliferation in a patient with SLE and aplastic anemia. Arthritis Rheum 1989;32:901.
366. Dainiak N, Hardin J, Floyd V, et al. Humoral suppression of erythropoiesis in SLE and rheumatoid arthritis. Ann Intern Med 1980;69:537.
367. Abdou N, Verdirame J, Amare M, et al. Heterogeneity of pathogenetic mechanism in aplastic anemia. Ann Intern Med 1981;95:43.
368. Alger M, Alarcon-Segovia D, Rivero SJ. Hemolytic anemia and thrombocytopenic purpura: two related subsets of systemic lupus erythematosus. J Rheumatol 1977;4:351.
369. Harvey AM, Shulman LE, Tumulty PA, et al. Systemic lupus erythematosus: review of the literature and clinical analysis of 138 cases. Medicine 1954;33:291.
370. Averbuch M, Korfman B, Levo Y. Lupus anticoagulant, thrombosis and thrombocytopenia in SLE. Am J Med Sci 1987;293:2.
371. Combined pure red cell aplasia and primary hypothyroidism in SLE. Arthritis Rheum 1987;30:839.
372. Cassileth PA, Meyers AR. Erythroid aplasia in systemic lupus erythematosus. Am J Med 1973;55:706.
373. Pirofsky B. Collagen diseases and autoimmune hemolytic anemia. In: Autoimmunization and the autoimmune hemolytic anemias. Baltimore, Williams & Wilkins, 1969:175.
374. Kaelin W, Spivak J. Systemic lupus erythematosus and myelofibrosis. Am J Med 1986;81:935.
375. Karpatkin S, Strick N, Karpatkin MB, et al. Cumulative experience in the detection of antiplatelet antibody in 234 patients with idiopathic thrombocytopenic purpura, systemic lupus erythematosus and other clinical disorders. Am J Med 1972;52:776.
376. Griner P, Hoyer L. Amegakaryocytic thrombocytopenia in SLE. Arch Intern Med 1970;125:328.
377. Stoll DB, Blum S, Pasquale D, et al. Thrombocytopenia with decreased megakarocytes. Ann Intern Med 1981;94:170.
378. Hoffman R, Bruno E, Elwell J, et al. Acquired amegakaryocytic thrombocytopenic purpura: a syndrome of diverse etiologies. Blood 1982;60:1173.
379. Rabinowitz Y, Dameshek W. Systemic lupus erythematosus after "idiopathic" thrombocytopenic purpura: a review. Ann Intern Med 1960;52:1.
380. Dekker A, O'Brien ME, Cammarata RJ. The association of thrombotic thrombocytopenic purpura with systemic lupus erythematosus. Am J Med Sci 1974;267:243.
381. Rustagi P, Currie M, Logue G. Complement-activating antineutrophil antibody in SLE. Am J Med 1985;78:971.
382. Conley CL, Hartmann RC. A hemorrhagic disorder caused by circulating anticoagulant in patients with disseminated lupus erythematosus. J Clin Invest 1952;31:621.
383. Ashershon RA, Kharmashta MA, Hughes GR. Antiphospholipid antibodies and thrombosis. Lancet 1989;2:72.
384. Branch DW, Scott JR, Kochenom NK, et al. Obstetric complications associated with the lupus anticoagulant. N Engl J Med 1985;313:1322.
385. Sneddon JB, Cerebrovascular lesions in livedo reticularis. Br J Dermatol 1965;77:180.
386. Asherson RA, Khamashta MA, Gel A, et al. Cerebrovascular disease and antiphospholipid antibodies in systemic lupus erythematosus, lupus-like disease, and the primary antiphospholipid syndrome. Am J Med 1989;86:391.
387. Thiagarajan P, Pengo V, Shapiro S. The use of the dilute Russell viper venom time for the diagnosis of lupus anticoagulants. Blood 1986;68:869.
388. Petri M, Rhemschmidt M, Whiting-O'Keefe Q, et al. A study of sixty consecutive patients by activated partial thromboplastin time, Russell viper venom time and anticardiolipin antibody level. Ann Intern Med 1987;106:524.
389. Fort J, Cowchock F, Abruzzo J, et al. Anticardiolipid antibodies in patients with rheumatic disease. Arthritis Rheum 1987;30:752.
390. Alarcón-Segovia D, Delezé M, Oria CV, et al. Antiphospholipid antibodies and the antiphospholipid syndrome in SLE. Medicine 1989;68:353.
391. Asherson R, Khamashta M, Ordi-Ros J, et al. The "primary" antiphospholipid syndrome: major clinical and serological features. Medicine 1989;68:366.
392. Sanfellipo MJ, Drayna CJ. Prekallikrein inhibition associated with the "lupus anticoagulant": a mechanism of thrombosis. Am J Clin Pathol 1982;77:275.
393. Freyssinnet JM, Wiesel ML, Gauchy J, et al. An IgM lupus anticoagulant that neutralizes the enhancing effects of phospholipid on purified endothelial thrombomodulin activity: a mechanism for thrombosis. Thromb Haemost 1986;55:309.
394. Cariou R, Tobelem G, Soria J, et al. Inhibition of protein C activation by endothelial cells in the presence of lupus anticoagulant. N Engl J Med 1986;314:1193.

395. Carreras LO, Vermylen JG. "Lupus anticoagulant" and thromboses: possible role of inhibition of prostacyclin formation. Thromb Haemost 1982;48:38.
396. Haselaar P, Derksen R, Blokzijl L, et al. Thrombosis associated with antiphospholipid antibodies cannot be explained by effects on endothelial and platelet prostanoid synthesis. Thromb Haemost 1988;59:80.
397. Feinstein D. Lupus anticoagulant anticardiolipin antibodies, fetal loss, and systemic lupus erythematosus. Blood 1992;80:857.
398. Hochberg M, Arnold CM, Hogan B, et al. Serum immunoreactive erythropoietin in rheumatoid arthritis: impaired response to anemia. Arthritis Rheum 1988;31:1318.
399. Baer AN, Dessypris EN, Goldwasser ER, et al. Blunted erythropoietin response to anaemia in rheumatoid arthritis. Br J Haematol 1987;66:559.
400. Benne JA, Bianchine JR, Johnson PC, et al. Gastrointestinal blood loss caused by tolmetin, aspirin, and indomethacin. Clin Pharmacol Ther 1974;16:821.
401. Munden KD, Senator GB. Iron in the synovial membrane in rheumatoid arthritis and other joint diseases. Ann Rheum Dis 1968;27:38.
402. Baynes RD, Bothwell TH, Bezwoda WR, et al. Hematologic and iron-related measurements in rheumatoid arthritis. Am J Clin Pathol 1987;87:196.
403. Hansen TM, Hansen NE, Birgens HS, et al. Serum ferritin and the assessment of iron deficiency in rheumatoid arthritis. Scand J Rheumatol 1983;12:353.
404. Hutchinson RM, Davis P, Jayson M. Thrombocytosis in rheumatoid arthritis. Ann Rheum Dis 1976;35:138.
405. Panush RS, Franco AE, Schur P. Rheumatoid arthritis associated with eosinophilia. Ann Intern Med 1971;75:199.
406. Davis P, Hughes GR. Significance of eosinophilia during gold therapy. Arthritis Rheum 1974;17:964.
407. Felty AR. Chronic arthritis in the adult associated with splenomegaly and leucopenia: a report of five cases of an unusual clinical syndrome. Johns Hopkins Hosp Bull 1924;35:16.
408. Abdou N, NaPomibejara C, Balentine L, et al. Suppressor cell-mediated neutropenia in Felty's syndrome. J Clin Invest 1978;61:738.
409. Cohen M, Webb J. Antihistone antibodies in rheumatoid arthritis and Felty's syndrome. Arthritis Rheum 1989;32:1319.
410. Campion G, Maddison PJ, Goulding N, et al. The Felty syndrome: a case matched study of clinical manifestations and outcome, serologic features and immunogenetic associations. Medicine 1990;69:69.
411. Breedveld FC, Lafeber GJM, Doeker G, et al. Felty's syndrome: autoimmune neutropenia or immune complex mediated disease? Rheumatol Int 1985;5:253.
412. Breedveld FC, Fibbe WE, Cats A. Neutropenia and infection in Felty's syndrome. Br J Rheumatol 1988;27:191.
413. Moore RA, Brunner CM, Sandusky WR, et al. Felty's syndrome: long-term follow up after splenectomy. Ann Intern Med 1971;75:381.
414. Fiechtner JJ, Miller DR, Starkebaum G. Reversal of neutropenia with methotrexate treatment in patients with Felty's syndrome: correlation of response with neutrophil-reactive IgG. Arthritis Rheum 1989;32:194.
415. Saway PA, Prasthofer E, Barton J. Prevalence of granular lymphocyte proliferation in patients with rheumatoid arthritis and neutropenia. Am J Med 1989;86:303.
416. Linch D, Newland A, Turnbull A, et al. Unusual T cell proliferations and neutropenia in rheumatoid arthritis: comparison with classical Felty's syndrome. Scand J Haematol 1984;33:342.
417. Wallner S, Vautrin R, Katz J, Murphy J. The anemia of thermal injury: partial characterization of an erythroid inhibitory substance. J Trauma 1987;6:639.
418. Ham TH, Shen SC, Fleming E, Castle W. Study on the destruction of red blood cells: IV. Blood 1948;3:373.
419. Felix JC, Davis JM. Neutrophil function in thermally injured patients. In: Gallin JI, Fauci A, eds. Advances in host defense mechanisms, vol 6. New York, Raven Press, 1986:68-.
420. Arturson G. Neutrophil granulocyte functions in severely burned patients. Burns 1985;11:309.
421. Koller M, Konig W, Brom J, et al. Studies on the mechanism of granulocyte dysfunctions in severely burned patients: evidence for altered leukotriene generation. J Trauma 1989;29:435.
422. Eurenuis K, Mortensen R, Meserol P, et al. Platelet and megakaryocyte kinetics following thermal injury. J Lab Clin Med 1972;79:247.

8

Hematologic Therapies

Blood: Principles and Practice of Hematology,
edited by Robert I. Handin, Samuel E. Lux, and Thomas P. Stossel.
J.B. Lippincott Company, Philadelphia © 1995.

60

Transfusion Medicine

Jeffrey McCullough

HISTORY

For centuries, blood has been considered to have mystical properties. During the mid-1600s, a number of major developments led to the beginning of blood transfusion.[1] In 1656, Christopher Wren developed techniques to isolate veins in dogs and carried out many studies of the effects of substances injected into dogs. These culminated in the transfusion of blood from one dog to another. This work was extended by Richard Lower; similar work was done at about the same time in France by Jean Denys. In 1667, Denys carried out what is believed to be the first transfusion of animal (lamb's) blood to a human. The man who received the transfusion complained of "a very great heat along his arm" and a minor nosebleed, but he apparently had no other adverse effects. Soon afterward in England, Lower transfused sheep's blood into a man. In France, Denys continued his animal-to-human transfusions. Some of the most notable transfusions were of calves' blood to a man named Antoine Mauroy. During one transfusion, Mauroy experienced pain in the transfused arm, vomiting, increased pulse, nosebleed, pressure in the chest, and pain over the kidneys; the next day he passed black urine, the now-known classic symptoms of a hemolytic transfusion reaction. After a subsequent transfusion, Mauroy died and Denys was charged with murder. He was exonerated by testimony that the man's wife had given him a liquid, which, when given to a cat, caused death. French physicians determined that transfusion was unsound, the Pope banned the practice, and the English discontinued their transfusion work.

Interest in transfusion was revived during the early 1800s primarily by James Blundell, an obstetrician who believed transfusion would be helpful in treating postpartum hemorrhage. Other work convinced him that transfusions should be between members of the same species, and Blundell is credited with carrying out the first human to human transfusion in 1818.[2] In the United States, transfusions were first used in the mid-1800s, but no record exists of the initial transfusion. Four transfusions were administered during the Civil War.[2] About this time efforts were made, although unsuccessful, to anticoagulate and preserve blood for transfusion. During the last part of the 1800s, the use of animal blood was eliminated, and it was established that the dark urine after transfusion was hemoglobin released from destroyed transfused red blood cells.

The landmark event that opened the way to modern transfusion therapy was the discovery of blood groups by Landsteiner in 1900. In the few years thereafter, the importance of blood typing of donors and recipients, compatibility testing, and donor antibodies were determined. The next major step forward was the development of anticoagulant preservative solutions for blood. Several different citrate solutions were prepared, and citrated blood came into use in treating casualties during World War I. Relatively little progress in transfusion therapy occurred between the two world wars. In 1943, the anticoagulant acid–citrate–dextrose was developed in England. Because this allowed storage of blood for 21 days, transfusion became more practical.

The first blood bank where a stock of blood was maintained apparently was in Barcelona in 1936, although the concept seems to have been developed in Leningrad in 1932.[2] The first blood bank in the United States was established in 1937 at the Cook County Hospital in Chicago.

Transfusion therapy has a broad role in medical care. The availability of an adequate and safe supply of blood and its components is essential for many surgical procedures and the treatment of patients who experience acute or chronic blood loss. Other examples of patients who benefit from transfusion are those with inadequate blood cell production, excessive destruction of their own blood cells, or an inherited defect of red cells or coagulation factors. The discipline within medicine that encompasses expertise in obtaining and preparing blood components, ensuring their appropriate use in patient care, minimizing the complications of transfusion therapy, managing complications when they occur, and dealing with related issues such as the recognition and management of immune destruction of blood cells, transfusion-transmitted diseases, and other approaches to transfusion such as autologous blood donation and intraoperative blood salvage has become known as transfusion medicine.

In the United States, almost all whole blood is collected from nonpaid volunteer donors by either regional community-based or individual hospital-based blood banks. The whole blood is separated into its components shortly after donation, thus allowing each component to be used for the most appropriate specific clinical condition. This approach, called *blood component therapy*, places a responsibility on the clinician to identify the specific blood deficit of the patient and then to choose a specific blood component. For instance, a hemophiliac patient may need only coagulation factor VIII but not red cells or platelets, whereas a patient with anemia of chronic disease may need only red cells.

This chapter describes the approach used to screen potential donors, collect and prepare blood components, and carry out laboratory tests to ensure a compatible transfusion. The situations in which transfusion therapy is used and the recognition and management of the complications of transfusion are discussed.

MEDICAL ASSESSMENT AND SCREENING OF BLOOD DONORS

The collection of blood and preparation of components for transfusion are regulated by the Center for Biologics Evaluation and Research of the Food and Drug Administration (FDA). The FDA considers blood a drug and inspects most blood banks annually much as they inspect facilities that manufacture pharmaceuticals. Although we will not identify each step or procedure that is regulated by the FDA, it can be assumed that almost every procedure that involves the medical assessment of the donor, the collection of blood, and the preparation, storage, and distribution of blood components is regulated.

Whole Blood

Medical History

The first and one of the most important steps in obtaining safe and effective blood components is the medical assessment of the potential donor. Donor medical requirements and many of the questions of the donors are specified by the FDA. In general, the donor medical assessment is designed to ensure that blood donation is not unusually risky for the donor and that the donated blood components are as safe as possible for the recipient. The donor must be in good general health. The specific questions and their rationale are as follows:

1. Have you ever donated blood, platelets, or plasma?

   To avoid iron deficiency, at least 8 weeks must elapse between blood donations. To allow blood volume to reequilibrate, at least 48 hours must elapse after plasmapheresis or cytapheresis.

2. Have you ever been deferred as a blood donor?

   This question helps to evaluate the donor's medical history and may identify health problems that would preclude donation.

3. Are you or have you been pregnant during the last 6 weeks?

   To allow the woman an opportunity to recover from the delivery and to minimize the possibility of iron deficiency, at least 6 weeks must elapse after third-trimester delivery. Potential donors who had a first-trimester abortion can donate whenever their general medical health permits if they meet all other blood donor criteria.

4. Have you had surgery or any major illness in the last 6 months?

   This question helps to evaluate the donor's medical history and may identify health problems that would preclude donation. Donors who have received blood or components during major surgery must be deferred for 6 months, regardless of whether they received blood products. Potential donors who have had minor or uncomplicated surgery are deferred only until the surgical site is healed and the person can resume normal activity. Decisions about which procedures disqualify a donor for 6 months are made at the time of the medical history. Therefore, the distinction between major and minor surgery is not uniformly defined.

5. Have you ever had diseases of the heart, lungs, or liver?

   Potential donors with a history of coronary artery disease and rheumatic heart disease are generally deferred unless it is clear that their cardiac function is good and they can withstand the loss of about 10% of their blood volume in a short period of time. Patients with compromised pulmonary function, active tuberculosis, or other active pulmonary infections should not donate blood. Treated tuberculosis or a positive tuberculin skin test are not reasons for deferral of blood donation. Inflammatory diseases of the liver are almost always cause for deferral. Persons with Gildert's disease may donate blood, although this sometimes causes problems if they have a slightly elevated bilirubin and someone later notices the unusual color of the plasma in the unit of blood.

6. Have you had a recent weight loss?

   This question helps to evaluate the general medical condition of the patient and might indicate the presence of a serious disease. Also, persons on severe diets probably should not donate blood because of possible fluid and electrolyte imbalances.

7. Are you taking any drugs or medications?

   This question also aids in evaluating the general medical condition of the potential donor. Thus, a donor may be deferred not because of the particular medication but because of the condition for which the medication is being taken. Often the medication itself is not a risk for the recipient. In general, the kinds of drugs for which a donor would be deferred because of the significance of the underlying disease are antibiotics, anticonvulsants, anticoagulants, digitalis, insulin, systemic corticosteroids, vasodilators, and antiarrhythmic drugs. Aspirin or aspirin-containing compounds cause abnormal platelet function[3]; thus, donors who will serve as the only source of platelets for a patient should not have ingested aspirin within 2 to 3 days before blood donation. In common practice, this means that donors of whole blood may take aspirin, since their platelets are pooled with those of other donors. When about 20% of the platelets have not been exposed to aspirin, the hemostatic function of the total platelet pool is normal.[3] Thus, the restriction on aspirin ingestion applies primarily to plateletpheresis donors.

   Ingestion of the following commonly used drugs is usually acceptable in most blood banks: tetracyclines or antibiotics taken for acne (acutane disqualifies a donor because it may be a teratogen), topical corticosteroids taken for skin lesions not at the venipuncture site, antihypertensives taken regularly and resulting in an acceptable blood pressure, isoniazid taken because of a positive tuberculin skin test, nonprescription bronchodilators and decongestants, oral hypoglycemic agents in well-controlled diabetics who do not have symptoms of vascular complications, most tranquilizers, hypnotics used at bedtime, oral contraceptives, mild analgesics, vitamins, replacement hormones, weight reduction pills, and marijuana.

8. Have you ever had hepatitis or jaundice?

   This question also usually includes others about previous injections of hepatitis B immunoglobulin, hepatitis vaccine, tattoo, ear piercing, acupuncture, previous transfusions, and the peripheral injection of drugs. The presence of the hepatitis viruses cannot be detected with certainty; thus, potential donors who have a history suggestive of hepatitis or who engage in any activity in which transmission of hepatitis is possible must be deferred. Deferral may be either temporary or permanent, depending on the specific situation.

9. Have you ever had malaria?

   Malaria can be transmitted by blood transfusion.[4] Potential donors who have been in areas in which malaria is endemic and who have not taken antimalaria prophylaxis may donate 6 months after return if they have been symptom free. Potential donors who have had malaria or who have taken prophylaxis while in an endemic malaria area must be symptom free for 3 years after cessation of therapy.

10. Have you ever had a positive test for HIV [human immunodeficiency virus] antibodies? Persons who have AIDS or a positive test for anti-HIV or who are at high risk for acquiring or being infected with HIV should not donate blood.

    Persons who have AIDS or are at high risk for acquiring or being infected with the HIV-1 virus should not donate blood. This includes persons with exposure to an AIDS-infected person or to someone with a positive test for anti–HIV-1, males who have had sex with another male since 1977, present or past intravenous drug abusers, immigrants from Haiti, hemophiliacs, prostitutes, males exposed to prostitutes, or sexual partners of any of the above.

11. Do you have a bleeding tendency?

    Persons with bleeding tendency may have unusual bleeding from the venipuncture site or their plasma may be deficient in coagulation factors, thus preventing effective therapy.

12. Do you have epilepsy, convulsions, or fainting spells?

    Donors who have epilepsy or fainting spells may be more likely to have a reaction or a seizure after blood donation, although this has not been documented.

13. Have you ever had cancer?

    Potential donors who have had leukemia or lymphoma must be deferred. Those who have had minor skin cancer, carcinoma of the cervix, and papillary thyroid carcinoma may donate if the cancer has been adequately treated. Persons with all other forms of cancer must be evaluated by a physician. Although it has not been documented, a theoretical concern exists that cancer can be transmitted by transfusion of malignant cells. Thus, blood banks err on the conservative side by not accepting as donors those with a history of malignancies.

14. Have you been vaccinated or had any shots during the last 12 months?

    In general, recently immunized, symptom-free persons may donate blood. Those who have been vaccinated with live virus vaccines such as measles, rabies, yellow fever, vaccinia, mumps, or oral poliomyelitis should not donate for at least 2 weeks because of the possibility that the virus might be transmitted by blood transfusion. A 1-week waiting period is required for those receiving killed virus, bacterial or rickettsial vaccines, or toxoid. Examples are influenza, diphtheria, tetanus, rabies, and Rocky Mountain spotted fever. Potential donors who have received immune serum globulin should be questioned to determine whether the reason for receiving the immunoglobulin disqualifies them as a donor.

Physical Examination

Potential blood donors undergo a limited physical examination. The donor should have a general appearance of good health and not be under the influence of drugs or alcohol. Donors must weigh at least 110 pounds to enable collection of the standard volume (450 mL) of blood. The risk of adverse reactions is increased in smaller donors.[5] Small donors may be accepted at the discretion of the blood bank physician if some anticoagulant is removed from the blood container and a smaller amount of blood collected. There is no upper limit of weight, but massively obese persons may not be suitable donors because of other aspects of their health status. The potential donor must have a temperature of less than 99.6°F and a pulse of 50 to 100 beats/min. Well-conditioned athletes with pulse rates less than 50 may be accepted. The diastolic and systolic blood pressure must be less than 90 to 180 mmHg. Skin at the venipuncture site must be free of lesions, and the donor's arms are inspected for needle marks suggestive of illicit drug use.

The donor's hemoglobin concentration must be 12.5 g/dL or more. If the hematocrit value is determined, it must be at least 38%. Usually, the hemoglobin concentration is determined using a copper sulfate screening test. A drop of the donor's blood obtained by a fingerstick or ear lobe prick is placed in a copper sulfate solution with a specific gravity of 1.053. If the drop of blood sinks, it contains a sufficient amount of hemoglobin to exceed the minimum requirements. The accuracy, simplicity, and low cost of this screening test have led to its widespread use for many years.

Cytapheresis Donors

Donors undergoing plateletpheresis, leukapheresis, or lymphapheresis must meet all the criteria for donation of whole blood. Because the cytapheresis procedure may have some unique effects on the donor, some additional medical history, physical, or laboratory monitoring criteria are needed. These requirements are described in the following text in relation to each kind of cytapheresis.

Plateletpheresis

Plateletpheresis causes an average decrease in the donor's platelet count of about 30% (75,000/μL), which returns to baseline in 4 days.[6] This is not a risk for healthy normal donors; nevertheless, potential donors should be questioned to ensure that they do not have a bleeding disorder. Plateletpheresis donors should also be questioned carefully to ensure that they are not ingesting drugs such as aspirin, which interferes with platelet function usually by interfering with primary aggregation.[7] Platelets obtained from such donors are not effective clinically. Thus, donors who are going to be the sole source of platelets must not have ingested aspirin for at least 3 days. Plateletpheresis can be done in these donors because, although the platelet lesion is permanent, platelets produced after the drug is no longer circulating are normal. The presence of only 20% normal platelets allows primary aggregation to occur, which in turn causes secondary aggregation of the remaining aspirin-damaged platelets.[3] Although it may be desirable to know the platelet count before donation, this is not required if plateletpheresis is carried out no more often than whole-blood donation is allowed.

Leukapheresis

In addition to the removal of the blood component, donors undergoing leukapheresis receive the blood volume expander, hydroxyethyl starch, a sedimenting agent that improves the granulocyte yield, and corticosteroids to improve the granulocyte yield by increasing the donor's leukocyte count.[8] Thus, these donors must meet all the criteria for whole-blood donation in addition to medical history and physical examination items. Donors are questioned specifically about hypertension, diabetes, peptic ulcers, and bleeding tendency. No additional laboratory tests are necessary before leukapheresis.

Serial Apheresis Donations

In general, if a donor undergoes cytapheresis no more often than is allowable for whole-blood donation (every 8 weeks), no additional laboratory tests or monitoring are necessary. More frequent cytapheresis is sometimes called serial cytapheresis. A donor should not undergo more than 24 plateletpheresis procedures per year, more than 2 procedures in 7 days, nor more than 6 procedures in 1 month. At least 48 hours must elapse between procedures. Serial apheresis donors must be monitored as follows:

1. Red cell loss must average 25 mL or less per week, since the total red cell loss for one calender year must not exceed that allowed for whole-blood donation.
2. The total volume of all blood products retained per plateletpheresis procedure must not exceed 500 to 600 mL, depending on the donor's weight.
3. The total volume of plasma removed must not exceed 15 L/y.
4. The total dose of hydroxyethyl starch must be kept at a minimum.
5. If a donor is to undergo plateletpheresis more often than allowed for whole-blood donation (once every 8 weeks), the predonation platelet count must be known to be greater than 150,000/μL. For logistic reasons, most blood banks obtain a platelet count at the end of the previous donation. If the count is greater than 150,000/μL, it can serve as the predonation count for the subsequent plateletpheresis.

Lymphocyte Depletion in Cytapheresis Donors

Although it appears that some lymphocyte depletion may occur in cytapheresis donors, no adverse effects have been found in association with this.[9–12] Thus, leukocyte or lymphocyte counts are not used to determine the suitability of a potential apheresis donor.

Autologous Blood Donation

Concern about transfusion-transmitted disease in public and health care professionals has led to a large increase in autologous blood donation.[13] Autologous blood can be provided by presurgical donation or by perioperative donation or intraoperative salvage.[14] This section describes the assessment of potential presurgical autologous donors.

Potential autologous blood donors are usually patients with a health problem. Most presurgical patients can be candidates for autologous blood donation. If a patient has special health problems that might increase the risk of blood donation, a knowledgeable physician and good equipment should be available for managing medical emergencies. One absolute contraindication to autologous blood donation is bacteremia, because bacteria can proliferate in stored blood even at 1° to 6°C.[15]

No upper or lower age limit restricts autologous donation. The decision is based on the condition of the donor and in small children on the practical limitation of vascular access and the volume of blood loss the donor can tolerate. There are no specific weight limits, although in donors weighing less than 110 lb (50 kg), proportionally less blood should be withdrawn. The potential donor's hemoglobin concentration must be at least 11 g/dL (hematocrit 34%) to avoid severe iron depletion. As long as the hemoglobin is maintained above 11 g/dL, the patient may donate as often as every 72 hours. This minimum interval is necessary to allow protein mobilization and reequilibration of the donor's blood volume.[16]

Blood from autologous donors who meet all the criteria for allogenic blood donation may be used for other patients if the donor no longer needs the blood. Blood from autologous donors who do not meet all allogenic blood donation criteria must be restricted for use by the donor only. Most autologous blood donors do not meet the FDA criteria for blood donation. This, combined with donation of blood in many situations in which there is a low likelihood of blood use, has resulted in the nonutilization (outdating) of about half of all autologous blood.[13]

Because the patient's ability to donate autologous blood may be limited by his or her iron stores, it is customary to provide iron supplementation. Parenteral administration is not necessary; oral administration is effective. Oral iron, ferrous sulfate, 325 mg three times daily, should be started about 1 week before the first donation and continued after the last donation, depending on the amount of blood donated and the patient's hemoglobin. Erythropoietin can also be used to increase the number of units of blood that can be collected. In many situations, however, it is unclear whether enough additional autologous blood can be obtained to reduce the amount of allogeneic blood used.[18] One group of patients in whom autologous blood donation has great potential but raises questions of safety are those scheduled to undergo cardiac surgery. Most require blood replacement, but they have compromised cardiovascular function. Several studies have shown that under proper medical supervision, autologous blood donation is not an unusual risk for these patients.[19,20]

Autologous blood donation during pregnancy raises additional difficult considerations. The likelihood of transfusion after pregnancy and delivery is less than 3%,[21] and thus autologous donation would seem unnecessary. In addition, the health of two persons (mother and fetus) must be considered in evaluating the possible side effects of blood donation. The effect of blood donation may be difficult to predict because of the large blood volume of the mother and possible hypertension present. Although few data are available, risks of blood donation to the mother during the second[19] and third trimesters[21,22] appear not to be increased. Fetal monitoring revealed no abnormalities due to blood donation during the third trimester in 39 women.[22] Despite these reassuring data in both mothers and their babies, autologous blood donation is not recommended routinely for pregnant patients. It should be limited to situations in which the likelihood of transfusion is increased such as in placenta previa, uterine atony, retained placenta trauma, and abruptio placentae[23] or scheduled cesarean section, eclampsia, or multiple miscarriages.[21]

WHOLE-BLOOD COLLECTION

If the medical assessment indicates that the person meets all the requirements for the particular kind of donation being planned, the donor is then prepared for whole-blood collection or apheresis. The skin at the venipuncture site should be as clean as possible. Several methods of skin preparation are available. In general, these involve scrubbing the area with soap or an iodophor compound, followed by tincture of iodine or iodophor compound, and removal of tincture of iodine with acetone or alcohol. This usually results in an aseptic skin area, although surveillance cultures of the venipuncture site reveal about 1% to 2% incidence of bacterial growth. The bacteria generally do not cause a clinical problem because the most common contaminants do not survive in stored blood and because other contaminants usually occur in small numbers.[24]

The blood containers used today are a series of plastic bags, all sterile, with an integral tubing and needle. The venipuncture is done in the antecubital fossa using the needle (usually 16-gauge) attached to the blood container set.

The standard donation is of about 450 mL (within 10%) of blood collected into 63 mL of citrate phosphate dextrose anticoagulant, resulting in a final volume of 468 to 558 mL. The important steps or issues in blood collection are correct labeling and identification of all bags and specimen tubes, maintaining good blood flow to avoid clotting, and adequate mixing of blood and anticoagulant to avoid clotting or osmotic damage to red cells. The phlebotomy lasts about 7 to 10 minutes; the entire blood donation process including registration, medical assessment, preparation, phlebotomy, and recovery usually takes from 30 to 45 minutes.

Whole blood for transfusion is collected by venipuncture into plastic bags from which it can be separated into its components. After collection of the unit of whole blood, it is usually maintained at room temperature and returned to the blood center, where it is separated into its major components: red cells, platelets, and plasma.

Adverse Reactions to Blood Donation

The donation of 450 mL of whole blood, representing up to 13% of a person's blood volume in about 7 to 10 minutes, is tolerated remarkably well. During and immediately after blood donation, the blood pressure and pulse rate usually remain unchanged, although the central venous pressure may decrease slightly. The blood volume returns to normal in about 72 hours in most donors.[16] A slight increase in reticulocyte count occurs, and the hemoglobin reaches its nadir 1 to 2 weeks after donation.

The overall incidence of adverse reactions observed in most large blood banks is about 1.5% to 2%. Most of these reactions are mild and involve light-headedness, dizziness, pallor, sweating, and nausea. They are caused by hypovolemia. Some, especially first-time donors, may experience a vasovagal reaction. The symptoms are similar to those due to hypovolemia, but the pulse rate slows in a vasovagal reaction. The reaction is not related to the volume of blood lost and may occur before blood is withdrawn. Other adverse effects of blood donation are twitching, muscle spasms, inadvertent puncture of an artery or nerve, hematoma at the venipuncture site, fainting, seizures or serious cardiac events. Such reactions are extremely rare.

Autologous Donors

The techniques of collecting blood from autologous donors are the same as those used to collect blood from homologous donors. It is important that the blood container be labeled at the collection site, preferably at the bedside, to ensure that the correct unit is saved for the donor's later use. If the donor does not meet all the health history and physical criteria for homologous blood donation, this labeling is especially important to minimize the likelihood of the unit's being erroneously transfused to another patient.

Apheresis

Apheresis, meaning to take away, refers to the process of selectively removing one component of whole blood and returning the remainder to the donor. Apheresis can be done on standard units of whole blood with plastic bag systems to isolate platelets (plateletpheresis) or plasma (plasmapheresis). This procedure is time consuming and is no longer widely used. Most apheresis is done using semiautomated instruments sometimes called *blood cell separators*. In the apheresis procedure, blood is pumped from one of the donor's veins into the instrument in which, by centrifugation, it is separated into plasma, platelets, leukocytes, and red cells. The desired component is removed, and the remainder is recombined and returned to the donor. Some variations in the instruments are the use of intermittent versus continuous flow of blood from the donor, the use of one or two donor veins, and the use of one of several different preparations of citrate for anticoagulation while the blood is extracorporeal.

Many different instruments are available for the collection of platelets, granulocytes, lymphocytes, peripheral blood stem cells, or plasma by apheresis (Table 60-1). Instruments available for plateletpheresis were summarized by the FDA. Granulocytes can be collected by at least four instruments. These instruments also can be used to collect lymphocytes. Specific procedures have been described only for collection of peripheral blood stem cells. Pertinent comments about collection of each component are given below. For details of the operation of the instrument and collection procedure, the manufacturer's instructions and references should be consulted.

Platelets

Plateletpheresis usually requires about $1\frac{1}{2}$ hours and involves processing 4000 to 5000 mL of the donor's blood through the instrument. Platelets obtained by plateletpheresis are processed, tested, and labeled in a similar manner to that of whole blood. This includes ABO and Rh typing and testing for all required transfusion-transmitted diseases. The plateletpheresis concentrate may be stored for 24 hours at 20° to 24°C; some newer apheresis instruments allow collection of platelets in a closed system and storage for 5 days. The number of platelets contained in each concentrate is determined, although this information may not necessarily be recorded on the label. Quality control tests must show that at least 75% of the apheresis platelet concentrates produced by each facility contain 3×10^{11} platelets or more. Each platelet concentrate has a volume of about 200 mL and contains few (less than 0.5 mL) red cells so that red cell crossmatching is not necessary. The white blood cell content varies, depending on the instrument and technique used for collection.

Granulocytes

Leukapheresis procedures are usually more complex and lengthy than plateletpheresis. The donor receives up to

TABLE 60-1. Apheresis Instruments

Product	Instrument	Manufacturer	Storage Times
Platelets			
	H-30, H-305	Haemonetics	24h
	V-50 with surge	Haemonetics	24 h/5 d
	Fenwal CS 3000	Baxter	24 h/5 d
	IBM-2997	Cobe/IBM	24 h
	Spectra	Cobe/IBM	5 d
	Didico	Progress	24 h
Granulocytes			
	V-50	Haemonetics	24 h
	Fenwal CS-3000	Baxter	24 h
	IBM-2997	Cobe/IBM	24 h
	Spectra	Cobe/IBM	24 h
Lymphocytes			
	V-50	Haemonetics	18 h
	Fenwal CS-3000	Baxter	18 h
	Spectra	Cobe/IBM	18 h
	IBM-2997	Cobe/IBM	18 h
Peripheral blood stem cells			
	V-50	Haemonetics	2 y
	Spectra	Cobe/IBM	2 y
	CS-3000	Fenwal	2 y
Plasma			
	Fenwal CS-3000	(As a byproduct)	1 y
		Baxter	1 y
	V-50	Haemonetics	1 y
	Autopheresis C	Fenwal	1 y

500 mL of hydroxyethyl starch to improve the efficiency of granulocyte extraction and may receive corticosteroids to increase the yield by elevating the level of circulating granulocytes. Prednisone, 60 mg, can be given orally the evening before or dexamethasone, 4 mg/m^2, can be given intravenously immediately before leukapheresis. The leukapheresis procedure takes 30 to 60 minutes longer than plateletpheresis to process more blood and to improve the granulocyte yield. Usually 6500 to 8000 mL of the donor's blood is processed through the instrument, with removal of about 50% of the granulocyte resulting in a yield of 1 to 2×10^{10} granulocytes in a volume of about 200 mL. Because granulocytes do not completely separate from the red cells, granulocyte concentrates usually contain a substantial amount of red cells (hematocrit 10%, or about 20 mL of red cells); therefore, crossmatching is necessary. Granulocyte concentrates are stored at 20° to 24°C for up to 24 hours, although they should be transfused as soon as possible after collection.[25,26] The granulocyte content of each concentrate is determined but not necessarily indicated on the label. No minimum FDA requirements define the composition of granulocyte concentrates; the American Association of Blood Banks Standards require that 75% of units contain at least 1×10^{10} granulocytes.

Lymphocytes

Lymphocytes are not usually collected as a blood component for transfusion. Lymphocyte collection techniques are used to obtain mononuclear cell concentrates to be used as starting material for the production of cells for adoptive immunotherapy or as a concentrate enriched in peripheral blood stem cells. Lymphocytapheresis also may be done as a therapeutic procedure to treat immune diseases by physical removal of lymphocytes (see the section on therapeutic apheresis).

Peripheral Blood Stem Cells

Hematopoietic stem cells are present not only in the marrow but also in the peripheral circulation as established by cross-circulation and other studies in irradiated animals.[28] There is no uniform agreement that these cells are identical with those in the marrow, and it is not established that peripheral blood stem cells are capable of providing complete hematopoietic reconstitution in humans, although experiments thus far suggest that this is possible.[29] Peripheral blood stem cells have been used successfully for autologous marrow transplantation.[30] These cells are collected by cytapheresis, although the low number of cells in each collection makes it necessary to freeze each peripheral blood stem cell concentrate, collect four to eight, and transfuse all of them at once to provide an adequate dose of cells for successful reconstitution.[31] The techniques used for collection of peripheral blood stem cells are similar to lymphocyte collection procedures. The collection procedure is about 3 hours long; no stimulation of the donor or blood sedimenting agents are used. Usually about 1×10^{10} mononuclear cells are removed and the concentrate obtained has a volume of about 200 mL.

No definitive test exists for the primordial hematopoietic stem cell; therefore, quality control of these peripheral blood stem cell concentrates is difficult. Usually, cell culture techniques are used to determine colony-forming units—granulocyte, monocytic (CFU-C) or colony-forming units—mixed (CFU-MIX) colonies. In practice, the dose for transplantation is usually based on cell counting to obtain at least 3×10^8 mononuclear cells per kilogram of the recipient's body weight. Because the optimal conditions for storage of hematopoietic stem cells are not known,[32] the peripheral blood stem cell concentrates are frozen within a few hours of collection.

Lymphokine-Activated Killer Cells

Lymphokine-activated killer cells are peripheral blood lymphocytes collected by apheresis, then cultured with interleukin-2 and various other additives. The culture techniques produce cells that are cytotoxic to tumor cells but not to nonmalignant cells.[33] Lymphokine-activated killer cells have been used as experimental therapy for several forms of malignancy. Although the ultimate role of this adoptive immunotherapy is not known, the approach of collecting autologous lymphocytes by apheresis and then modifying the lymphocytes in vitro for later autologous use seems likely to undergo extensive clinical investigation during the next few years.

Intraoperative Blood Salvage

One form of autologous blood transfusion is the retrieval of the patient's blood that is shed during surgery and the return of that blood to the patient. Early efforts to salvage and transfuse blood lost during surgery were not successful because of air embolism, coagulopathy, and transfusion of particulate debris. Improved instruments are available, and this process of intraoperative blood salvage or intraoperative autologous transfusion, as it is sometimes called, is being used more often. In intraoperative blood salvage, a suction device is used by the surgeon or assistants to aspirate blood being lost. The blood is immediately anticoagulated, usually with citrate or heparin, then enters a sterile disposable centrifuge bowl where it is washed with saline solution. When the centrifuge bowl is filled with red cells, they are pumped automatically into a bag where they are available for transfusion back to the patient. The centrifuge bowl is now empty and is available to receive more shed blood so that large volumes of blood can be salvaged, washed, and returned to the patient.

Blood that has been salvaged and made ready for transfusion has a hematocrit of about 50%, a supernatant hemoglobin concentration of 100 to 200 mg/dL, and a few leukocytes and platelets, and it may contain some residual heparin. Because the salvaged blood contains no coagulation factors, very few platelets, and possibly at least some heparin, a coagulopathy may develop after transfusion of 1 L or more. Physicians involved with intraoperative blood salvage should be aware of the possible development of a bleeding diathesis and should be prepared to administer fresh frozen plasma or platelet transfusion, if indicated. The red cells obtained by intraoperative blood salvage have a normal intravascular survival[34] and a normal 2,3-diphosphoglycerate (2,3-DPG) level.[35] The normal 2,3-DPG and thus normal oxygen dissociation may give salvaged red cells an advantage over stored homologous red cells, which have a low 2,3-DPG and poor oxygen dissociation.

Intraoperative blood salvage has been used most extensively in cardiac, vascular, urologic, and orthopedic procedures. The amount of homologous blood used can clearly be reduced substantially by intraoperative blood salvage.[36–39] Intraoperative blood salvage is generally not used when there is bacterial contamination of the surgical field. Thus, it is not usually used in patients whose bowel is opened or in trauma. Intraoperative blood salvage also is not used in surgery involving a malignancy. The presence of malignant cells in the peripheral blood raises the possibility of hematogenous spread of the neoplasm. No data support or refute this concern, but in the absence of such data intraoperative blood salvage is unlikely to be used extensively in these patients.

LABORATORY TESTING OF DONATED BLOOD

Before being made available for transfusion, donated blood undergoes several tests involving red cell typing, antibody detection, and screening for transmissible diseases. The use of the tests intended to prevent transfusion-transmitted diseases is discussed more completely in the section on transfusion-transmitted diseases.

ABO and Rh Typing

Red blood cell typing is necessary so that the components can be labeled properly and selected for patients with appropriate ABO and Rh types. Because of their clinical significance, these two blood groups are the only ones that are determined routinely (see section on blood groups).

Red Blood Cell Antibody Detection

Red blood cell antibody detection involves testing the donor's serum against test red cells from two normal subjects whose cells contain the antigens against which most red cell antibodies are directed. Antibodies transfused in the donor plasma can cause hemolysis of the recipient's red cells (intradonor incompatibility).[40] In the past, these problems were avoided by using a minor crossmatch of the donor's serum and the recipient's red cells. Screening for donor antibodies at the time of blood processing has eliminated the need for the minor crossmatch.

Serologic Test for Syphilis

Although syphilis can be transmitted by blood transfusion (see section on transfusion-transmitted disease), this almost never happens in the United States.[41] Most transfusion medicine specialists believe this test is unnecessary. Although the American Association of Blood Banks no longer requires syphilis testing, the FDA and many states do. Thus, all donated blood is tested.

Hepatitis B Surface Antigen

Hepatitis B surface antigen (HBsAg) was the first specific test to detect carrier donors and eliminate a form of posttransfusion hepatitis. The method in widespread use is an enzyme immunoassay using anti-HBs to detect circulating antigen.

Surrogate Tests for Non-A, Non-B Hepatitis

Hepatitis B Core Antibody

As discussed in the section on transfusion-transmitted diseases, a statistical association exists between the occurrence of posttransfusion non-A, non-B hepatitis and transfusion of blood containing hepatitis B core antibody (anti-HBc).[42,43] Thus, although this antibody is directed against a portion of the hepatitis B virus, blood containing anti-HBc is not used for transfusion as a way of reducing posttransfusion non-A, non-B hepatitis. About 1.35% of donated blood is unsuitable for use because it contains anti-HBc. Because it contains hepatitis virus antibodies, plasma from these units of blood can be used to prepare immune serum globulin.

Alanine Aminotransferase

Blood containing elevated alanine aminotransferase (ALT) also has a statistical association with posttransfusion non-

A, non-B hepatitis.[44] Thus, testing for this liver enzyme is also done on all donated blood, and units with ALT levels above a designated cutoff are not used for transfusion in an effort to reduce non-A, non-B hepatitis. A number of non–hepatitis-related factors such as obesity, exercise, and alcohol consumption can elevate the ALT and cause the donor's blood to be unsuitable for transfusion. About 1.2% of donated blood is unsuitable for use because of an elevated ALT.

Human Immunodeficiency Virus

Since 1985, all donated blood is tested for human immunodeficiency virus-1 (for anti–HIV-1). A more complete discussion of transfusion-transmitted HIV is found in the section on transfusion-transmitted diseases. The test used for screening is an enzyme immunoassay. If it is positive, the blood may not be used for transfusion, and a confirmatory test must be done to establish the presence of antibody specificity for HIV-1. About 0.19% of US blood donors are positive for anti–HIV-1, which is only one fortieth to one eightieth of the rate expected from the random population. The significance of the positive screening test in these donors not confirmed by Western blot is not established.

Human T-Cell Lymphotrophic Virus I and II

Human T-cell lymphotrophic virus I (HTLV-I) causes adult T-cell leukemia or tropical spastic paraparesis and can be transmitted by transfusion. Routine testing for anti–HTLV-I was initiated in the United States in 1989. The screening test is an enzyme immunoassaythat detects both anti–HTLV-I and anti–HTLV-II; confirmation of antibody specificity is necessary using a radioimmunoprecipitation assay or a Western blot. The incidence of this virus in US blood donors is low, about 2.5 in 10,000.[46] As with HIV-1, the significance of a positive screening test that is not confirmed by the more specific tests is not known.

Hepatitis C

The hepatitis C virus (HCV) gene has been cloned.[47] Initial trials of an HCV antibody test for blood donor screening revealed an incidence of 0.68% to 2.95%.[48,49] However, only about 25% of these donors' sera could be confirmed to contain specific hepatitis C-RNA.[50] Subsequently, a second-generation anti-HCV test with improved specificity was introduced. However, as many as half of the donors who have a positive screening test cannot be found to harbor HCV-RNA and so probably have false-positive test results. Although all donated blood is now screened for anti-HCV, this has not replaced the use of anti-HBc or ALT as surrogate tests for non-A, non-B hepatitis, because not all donors in whom these tests are abnormal and who transmit non-A, non-B hepatitis have detectable anti-HCV.

Summary

A multifaceted approach is used to attempt to produce the safest possible blood supply. This includes educating donors before donation, obtaining a medical history, increasing the emphasis on determining whether the donor has been involved in AIDS risk behavior, conducting a limited physical examination, laboratory testing of donated blood, determining through a registry whether the donor has been previously deferred or had a positive transmissible disease screening test, and offering to confidentially exclude donor blood from transfusion. The addition of several new viral and related screening tests during the past few years has improved the safety of the blood supply.[51–54] The cost-effectiveness of the steps taken to achieve this is not known. These screening tests result in about 4% of all donated blood being unsuitable for transfusion. Rates of unsuitable blood are much higher in some areas of the United States. Another impact of this increased testing is an increase in the complexity of work and the time involved in making blood available for use after it is collected. This is particularly a problem with products in which the storage period may be short, such as those obtained by apheresis.

PREPARATION, STORAGE, AND CHARACTERISTICS OF BLOOD COMPONENTS

Preparation of Blood Components From Whole Blood

Almost all blood collected in the United States is separated into components: red cells, platelets, and plasma. This allows each component to be stored under conditions that are optimal for that component and avoids the loss of valuable platelets and coagulation factors that would occur if the unit were stored as whole blood at 1° to 6°C. The unit of whole blood is separated into components by centrifugation. Because whole blood is collected in a multiple bag system, the component separation can be accomplished in a closed system avoiding exposure of the blood to the external environment (Fig. 60-1) and the bacterial contamination that might result. A unit of whole blood provides one unit of red cells, one unit of platelet concentrate, one cryoprecipitate, and platelet- and cryoprecipitate-poor plasma. This plasma then undergoes fractionation to provide a variety of blood derivatives (Table 60-2). Other special cellular blood components such as leukocyte-poor or frozen washed red cells are prepared from the unit of red cells after the platelets and plasma have been removed.

Red Blood Cells

After most of the platelets and plasma have been removed, the red cells are resuspended in a solution designed to optimize red cell preservation. The resulting red cell unit has also been called *packed red cells* or *red cell concentrate.* The commonly used red cell preservative solutions contain glucose, adenine, mannitol, and sodium chloride. These preservative solutions allow storage of red cells for 42 days at 1° to 6°C. During storage, some deleterious changes occur in the red cells, such as loss of viability, loss of adenosine triphosphate, increase in cellular rigidity, loss of membrane lipid, change in shape from disk to sphere, formation of microvesicles, loss of 2.3-DPG causing increased affinity of hemoglobin for oxygen, and reduced transmembrane transport of sodium and potassium. Because red cell metabolism continues during storage, metabolites accumulate in stored red cell units and lead to biochemical changes (Table 60-3). Four of these features are discussed more fully: loss of adenosine triphosphate and viability, loss of DPG and function, accumulation of potassium, and hemolysis.

Although a general relation exists between loss of adenosine triphosphate and viability, other factors contribute to this such as loss of membrane lipid and deformability. The red cells with poor viability are removed during the first 24 hours after transfusion, and thereafter the remaining red cells have a normal intravascular half-disappearance time.[40]

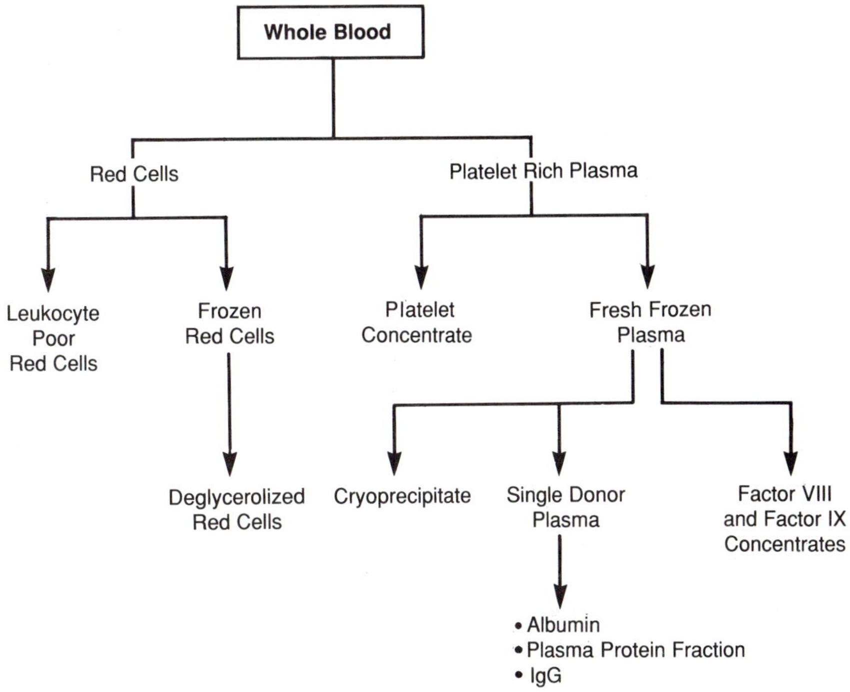

FIGURE 60-1. Preparation of blood components from one unit of whole blood. (After Kennedy MD, ed. Blood transfusion therapy: an audiovisual program, Arlington, VA, American Association of Blood Banks, 1985)

In 1954, Valtis and Kennedy[55] reported that the oxygen dissociation curve was shifted in stored red cells so that the volume of oxygen released to the tissues was reduced. The clinical importance of this observation has been unexpectedly difficult to determine. Studies of animals subjected to hemodilution have shown that hemoglobin concentration (or hematocrit) and avoidance of acidosis were more important than red cell DPG concentration.[40]

Red cell membrane sodium–potassium ATPase is sensitive to decreases in temperature. Thus, during storage at 1° to 6°C, red cells lose potassium into the supernatant (see Table 60-3). Although this is not a problem for most transfusions, older stored red cell units can be a potential problem for neonates (see section on transfusion in special situations).

The cause of the hemolysis that occurs during storage (see Table 60-3) is unknown. Paradoxically, the phthalate plasticizers that leak from the blood bags into the blood during storage seem to have a protective effect and reduce the hemolysis. Thus, the concern that these plasticizers might accumulate in transfusion recipients and cause harm is counterbalanced by their apparent beneficial effect in red cell preservation.

Stored red cells can be rejuvenated by incubating them with adenosine to replenish adenosine triphosphate and with inosine, phosphate, and pyruvate to replenish DPG. This process can produce red cells with good in vivo viability and normal or even above-normal DPG and oxygen transport capability. These techniques have not been adapted for large-scale practical use and are not done as part of routine blood bank operations.

TABLE 60-2. **Blood Derivatives Produced by Fractionation of Plasma**

IMMUNE GLOBULINS
Cytomegalovirus immune globulin*
Hepatitis B immune globulin
Immune globulin intravenous
Immune serum globulin
Rabies immune globulin
Rh(D) immune globulin
Tetanus immune globulin
Varicella zoster immune globulin
COAGULATION PRODUCTS
Activated factor IX complex
Antithrombin III
Coagulation factor IX
Factor VIIA (under development in Europe)
Factor VIII concentrate
Factor IX concentrate-prothrombin complex
Protein C
BLOOD VOLUME EXPANDERS
Albumin
Plasma protein fraction
MISCELLANEOUS
α_1-Antitrypsin
Fibrin glue*

* Not licensed in the United States.

Fresh Frozen Plasma

Fresh frozen plasma is the liquid portion of one unit of blood that has been centrifuged, separated, and frozen solid at −18°C or colder within 6 hours of collection. The unit of whole blood is usually centrifuged using techniques to prepare platelet-rich plasma (see Fig. 60-1). This platelet-rich plasma is then centrifuged and the plasma is removed and frozen giving one unit of fresh frozen plasma and one unit of platelet concentrate. Fresh frozen plasma can be stored for up to 1 year at −18°C or colder. The unit of fresh frozen plasma has a volume of about 185 mL and contains all the constituents of citrated normal plasma. Specifically, this includes the labile and stable coagulation factors, the

TABLE 60-3. Characteristics of Red Cells in As-1 (Adsol) for 42 Days of Storage*

	Days of Storage						
Indices	**0**	**7**	**14**	**21**	**28**	**35**	**42**
ph (37° C)	7.00	6.86	6.69	6.55	—	6.43	6.34
RBC ATP (μmol/gHgb)	4.69	4.97	4.83	4.50	3.75	3.47	3.24
RBC DPG (μmol/gHgb)	10.88	8.16	1.96	0.87	0.65	0.54	0.65
Supernatant sodium (mEq/L)	152	135	131	124	—	126	123
Supernatant potassium (mEq/L)	1.6	17	27	34	—	44	46
Supernatant glucose (mg/dL)	909	780	724	697	660	617	604
Hemolysis (%)	0.02	0.06	0.11	0.14	0.20	0.16	0.24

* As-1 cells: N = 13; volume = 325 ± 29 mL; hematocrit = 58 ± 4%; mean red cell mass = 188 mL; mean supernatant volume = 136 mL; mean total hemoglobin = 19.3 g%.
(Data from Fenwal, Division of Baxter Healthcare, Inc, with permission)

components of the complement and fibrinolytic systems, and the plasma proteins that maintain osmotic pressure and modulate immunity.

For transfusion, fresh frozen plasma is thawed in a 37°C water bath for about 30 minutes. In the past, microwave ovens were not acceptable for thawing fresh frozen plasma because they created hot spots that damaged the plasma proteins. Newer microwave devices may be suitable and thus reduce the time required to make fresh frozen plasma available. After thawing, the plasma should be transfused as soon as possible; it cannot be stored for longer than 24 hours.

Fresh frozen plasma use has increased greatly during the last few years. A National Institutes of Health Consensus Development Conference concluded that this increase was not based on definitive evidence of the effectiveness of fresh frozen plasma but has occurred in the face of evidence of potential risk from its use.[56] The following are indications for use of fresh frozen plasma established by the Consensus Conference:

- Replacement of isolated coagulation factor deficiencies when specific components are not available. Examples include factors V, VIII, IX, X, and XI.
- Reversal of warfarin effect in patients actively bleeding or who require emergency surgery
- Antithrombin III deficiency in patients undergoing surgery or those who require heparin for treatment of thrombosis
- Treatment of thrombotic thrombocytopenic purpura, usually as part of plasma exchange
- Replacement of immunoglobulins in the treatment of immunodeficiency such as in patients with protein-losing enteropathy or in children or adults with immunodeficiency. The availability of intravenous immunoglobulin preparations has almost eliminated this as an indication for fresh frozen plasma.
- Replacement of coagulation factors in massive transfusion. This is a questionable indication. Usually the bleeding diathesis in massive transfusion is due to depletion of platelets rather than coagulation factors. No evidence exists that the empiric use of fresh frozen plasma in some ratio with units of red cells is necessary. Fresh frozen plasma should be used in massive transfusion only when lack of coagulation factors is seen as a major contributor to the bleeding diathesis.
- Replacement of coagulation factors in patients who have depletion of multiple coagulation factors usually due to liver disease and are bleeding or about to undergo surgery

Fresh frozen plasma is not indicated for blood volume replacement or as a nutritional source.

The dose of fresh frozen plasma is difficult to determine because it is usually given to replace multiple plasma proteins and the desired level of each protein may be different. In an average-sized adult, five units of fresh frozen plasma would raise the level of coagulation factors about 30%, a level thought to provide hemostasis. Since this would involve transfusion of about 1000 mL of plasma, the patient's blood volume and cardiovascular status must be considered.

Plasma and Source Plasma

Two other forms of plasma are prepared from whole blood. These are called plasma and liquid plasma. These are the plasma removed from whole blood more than 6 hours and less than 5 days after collection and stored either at −18°C or less (plasma) or at 1° to 6°C (liquid plasma). Source plasma is collected by plasmapheresis and is intended to serve as the raw material for further manufacture into blood derivatives. Several different derivatives are manufactured from human plasma (see Table 60-2).

Cryoprecipitate

Cryoprecipitate is the material that remains insoluble when previously frozen plasma is thawed at 1° to 6°C. Each bag of cryoprecipitate contains about 100 U of factor VIII and 200 mg of fibrinogen and has a volume of about 10 mL. Thus, cryoprecipitate can be used to replace factor VIII or fibrinogen. Cryoprecipitate can be stored for up to 1 year at −18°C or lower.

Cryoprecipitate is thawed in a 37°C water bath and can be stored for up to 6 hours at 1° to 6°C before transfusion. Cryoprecipitate from multiple bags is usually pooled into a single container that is dispensed by the blood bank. To avoid transfusing incompatible ABO antibodies, the ABO type of cryoprecipitate is usually selected to be identical with the patient, although ABO-compatible but nonidentical cryoprecipitate may be used (A cryoprecipitate to O recipient). If there is a shortage of cryoprecipitate, small amounts are ABO-incompatible with the patient can be given. Thus, a patient might receive up to a few hundred milliliters of plasma containing ABO-incompatible antibodies. If the volume of incompatible plasma is limited, usually little risk of hemolysis exists because the volume of plasma from any individual donor who might have a high-titer antibody is only 10 mL. Cryoprecipitate is given without regard to Rh type because it does not contain a sufficient number of red cells to cause immunization.

Random Donor Platelet Concentrates

Preparation

A random donor platelet concentrate is prepared from a standard unit of whole blood. Because cold temperatures damage platelets, the unit of whole blood is maintained at room temperature and platelets are removed within 6 hours of collection. The whole blood is centrifuged and then platelet-rich plasma is passed into a satellite bag (see Fig. 60-1). The bag containing the red cells is detached, the platelet-rich plasma is centrifuged again, and the platelet-poor plasma is passed into another satellite bag leaving the platelet concentrate that is detached. About 50 mL of plasma remains as the suspending medium for the platelets. At least 75% of random donor platelet concentrates contain at least 5.5×10^{10} platelets.[57] This represents recovery of about 20% of the platelets in the original unit of whole blood.

Storage

Random donor platelet concentrates may be stored for up to 5 days at room temperature (20° to 24°C).[57] During storage, platelets lose ability to circulate and to be functionally effective both in vitro and in vivo.[58–61] Many changes that occur during storage have been well described, but the changes crucial to the loss of in vivo effectiveness are not completely understood. During storage, platelets change from disk to spherical shape, have reduced adhesion, aggregation, adenine nucleotides, membrane glycoproteins, and glutathione, and release some α-granule contents into the suspending plasma. The variables known to be important in platelet preservation are temperature, method of agitation, volume of suspending plasma, and type of storage container.[58]

Platelets must be maintained at room temperature. Exposure to cold transforms the platelet from the normal disk to the spherical shape and is associated with abnormal function.[58,59] Also, the pH must be kept above 6.0 to maintain platelet function.[62] This is done by maintaining an adequate volume of plasma, using a container that allows diffusion of oxygen and CO_2, and providing constant mixing of the platelet plasma mixture.

Containers used for red cell and plasma storage are usually made of polyvinyl chloride (PVC) and the plasticizer diethylhexyl-phthalate. Two bags with improved diffusion capacity are available. One is made of polyolefin (PL-732; Fenwal Laboratories, Chicago) instead of PVC and does not contain a plasticizer. The other is made of PVC but uses the plasticizer tri(2-ethyl hexyl)trimellitate (CLX; Cutter Laboratories, Berkeley). The bag is placed on one of several suitable rotating devices for storage. The concentrate can be maintained in this condition for up to 5 days. At the end of the storage period, the intravascular recovery and half-life of the stored platelets are about 51% and 3.1 days.[63] Further evidence of satisfactory function by stored platelets is that they correct the bleeding time in thrombocytopenic patients.[63,64] Actually, satisfactory platelet function can be maintained for up to 7 days,[64,65] but storage longer than 5 days allows bacterial proliferation in some concentrates.[66] This has been associated with transmission of infection.[67,68] Although these complications were infrequent, it was enough of a clinical problem to warrant limiting room temperature platelet storage to 5 days.

Granulocytes

Granulocyte concentrates for transfusion are usually produced by apheresis. The characteristics and storage conditions for these granulocyte concentrates have already been described (see section on blood and component collection). Occasionally, granulocytes may be isolated from fresh units of whole blood. This provides a small number of granulocytes, a dose suitable only for neonatal patients (see section on transfusion in special situations).

TABLE 60-4. Major Red Cell Antigen Systems and General Characteristics of Their Corresponding Antibodies*

Antigen Systems	Number of Antigens	Usual Antibodies	Fix Complement	Optimal Reactivity Temperature	Cause: Transfusion Reactions	Cause: HDN	Cause: Red Cell Immune
ABH	11	IgM/IgG	Yes	Cold	Yes	Yes	No
Lewis	14	IgM	Yes	Cold	No	No	No
I	16	IgM	No	Cold	No	No	No
P	5	IgM	No	Cold	No	No	Yes
Rh	41	IgG	No	Warm	Yes	Yes	Yes
LW	3	IgG	No	Warm	Yes	No†	Yes
Duffy	5	IgG	No	Warm	Yes	Yes	Yes
Kell	21	IgG	No	Warm	Yes	Yes	Yes
Kidd	3	IgG	No	Warm	Yes	Yes	Yes
MN (Ss)	46	IgG/IgM	No	Cold	No	No	No/Yes
Ss	46	IgG/IgM	No	Warm	Yes	Yes	Yes
Lutheran	7	IgM	No	Warm	Yes	Yes	Yes
TOTAL	176						

HDN, hemolytic disease of the newborn.

* The antibody characteristics described are generalizations. Particular antibodies may differ. Reference text should be consulted before decisions are made regarding the identity or clinical significance of an individual serum specimen.

† None reported.

TABLE 60-5. Molecular and Biochemical Characteristics of Some Blood Group Antigens*

Blood Group Antigens	Chromosome of Gene Location	Number of Antigen Sites × 10^3 Red Cell	Molecular Weight of Antigen (kd)	RBC Membrane Components Associated With Antigen Expression	Antigen Composition	cDNA Cloned
AB	9	1000	90–100	Anion transport protein (band 3)	Glycoprotein	Yes
H	19					
Ii	Unknown	500	55	Glucose transport protein (band 4.5)		
		500		Poly-*N*-acetyl lactosaminyl glycolipids	Glycolipid	—
Lewis	19	Unknown	Unknown	Unknown	Glycosphinogolipid	No
P_1	22	Unknown	Unknown	Paragloboside plus a terminal D-galactose	Glycosphinogolipid	No
P	Unknown	Unknown	Unknown	Globoside I	Glycosphinogolipid	No
P^k	Unknown	Unknown	Unknown	Ceramide trihexoside	Glycosphinogolipid	Yes
Rh(D)	1	100–200	30–32	Polypeptides	Lipoprotein	Yes
		100–200	45–100	Polypeptides	Lipoprotein	—
LW	19	3–5	40–47	*N*-glycans	Glycoprotein	Yes
MN	4	200–1000	43*	Glycophorin A	Sialoglycoprotein	Yes
Ss	4	80–250	25*	Glycophorin B	Sialoglycoprotein	Yes
Kell	Unknown	3–6	93*	Disulfide bonding required for antigen activity	Glycoprotein	Yes
K_x	X	Unknown	32	Unknown	Unknown	No
Duffy	1	12	40–50†	*N*-Glycans not required for antigen activity	Glycoprotein	Yes
Lutheran	19	1–4	78–85	*N*-Glycans and disulfide bonding required for antigen activity	Glycoprotein	No
Gerbich	2	60–120	39*	Glycophorin C	Sialoglycoprotein	Yes
		15–20	30*	Glycophorin D	Sialoglycoprotein	Yes
Kidd	18	Unknown	50	Unknown	Unknown	No
Xg	X	Unknown	22–29	Unknown	Unknown	No
Colton	7	Unknown	Unknown	Unknown	Unknown	—
Complement						
Rodgers (C4A)	6	Unknown	96	Unknown	Glycoprotein	Yes
Chido (C4B)	6	Unknown	94	Unknown	Glycoprotein	Yes

* These molecules give anomalous apparent molecular weight on SDS-PAGE. Fy antigen activity is observed over a broad molecular weight range (38–90 kd); the value given corresponds to the region of greatest activity.

(Data from Anstee DJ. Blood group active components of the human cell membrane. In: Garratty G, ed. Red cell antigens and antibodies. Arlington, VA, American Association of Blood Banks, 1986:8; Anstee DJ. Blood group active surface molecules of the human red blood cell. Vox Sang 1990;58:1; and Lewis M, Anstee DJ, Bird GWG, et al. Blood group terminology 1990. Vox Sang 1990;58:142; with permission of the American Association of Blood Banks)

BLOOD GROUPS

Red Blood Cell Blood Groups

New red cell antigen specificities are reported almost weekly. Most of these are variations of the more than 600 red cell antigens that have been identified.[69] These can be categorized in 11 major systems, which account for 172 of the antigens (Table 60-4). Some additional antigens are thought to be part of these systems, but the relation has not been clearly established. Other antigens represent weakly expressed forms of well-defined antigens. Issitt[69] has described 24 additional categories of red cell antigens that are not being called blood groups. In addition, over 200 low-incidence and over 100 high-incidence antigens are thought to be independent of all others. This section describes the red cell antigens and systems most commonly involved in the clinical practice of transfusion medicine. For a more comprehensive description of the hundreds of known red cell antigens, the reader is referred to reference texts.[40,69]

The structure of the red cell membrane and the composition of its major components have been studied extensively. During the past few years, considerable information has been obtained about the composition of antigens of the ABO, Rh, Lewis, P, MN, Kell, Duffy, and Lutheran systems and the relation of these to red cell membrane components.The biochemical composition, molecular weight, and number of antigens per red cell for some antigens has been established (Table 60-5). Blood group antigens are glycoproteins or polypeptides except for ABO antigens, which are also glycolipids. The specificity of several blood group antigens is determined by sugars; thus, the genes responsible for these antigens code for an intermediate molecule, usually an enzyme that creates the antigenic specificity by transferring sugar molecules. The antigens of other blood group systems (Rh and Kell) are proteins and thus directly determined by genes. The size of the antigen-containing molecule ranges from 25 to 100 kd and the number of antigen sites from 1500 to more than 1,000,000 per red cell (see Table 60-5).

ABO System

The ABO system is clinically the most important red cell antigen system because most persons have circulating A and B antibodies that are usually complement-fixing antibodies and cause intravascular hemolysis. The antigenic determinants for A, B, and H are found widely throughout our environment on bacteria, plants, food, and dust. Exposure to these antigens causes the normal development of antibodies against whichever ABH antigens are absent in the individual (Table 60-6).

Composition. The ABH antigen activity is determined by sugars that are linked either to polypeptides (forming a glycoprotein) or to lipids (forming a glycolipid). Because the antigenic activity is determined by sugars and resides in a carbohydrate structure, the antigens are not directly determined by genes. Instead, the ABH genes determine proteins that are sugar-transferring enzymes, collectively called *glycosyltransferases.* The genes for the ABH system are on chromosomes 9 and 19.[70] Each A, B, and H gene codes for a different enzyme (glycosyltransferase), which places a different sugar on the polypeptide or lipid to produce the unique antigen (see Table 60-6). The H gene enables the attachment of L-fucose to the polypeptide or lipid chain. If no A or B gene is present, the H specificity remains and the person is a type O; these red cells do not react with anti-A or B. If an A or B gene or both are present, additional sugars are attached to the L-fucose, giving A, B, or AB specificity.

ABH antigens are widely distributed throughout the body. The ABH antigens present on red cells may be in either the glycoprotein or glycolipid form. ABH glycolipids are also part of most endothelial and epithelial membranes. In addition, the ABH glycolipids are present in a soluble form in plasma. Most other body fluids and secretions contain soluble ABH antigens but in the glycoprotein form. The ability to secrete soluble ABH antigens is controlled by a secretor (Se) gene, which is separate from the ABH system.

The genes for the transferases that determine the red cell ABO type are localized to chromosome 9 q34[71] and have been cloned.[17,71] The A gene is 1062 based pairs long and encodes a 353–amino acid transferase. The O gene is identical to the A gene except that there is a single base deletion at position 258. This causes a frame shift and results in the production of a 115–amino acid transferase that is functionally inactive. Thus, the B gene differs from A by having four consistent base substitutions causing four amino acid substitutions and accounting for the different specificity of the B transferase from the A transferase.[17,81]

Antigen Distribution and Subgroups. In a normal adult, the number of A antigen sites ranges from 1,600,000 (A_1 individual) to 700 (Am individual), the number of B antigen sites is 1,600,000; the number of A,B antigen sites totals 800,000.[40] Normal newborns have about one third the number of antigen sites found in adults. Before the structure and number of A and B antigens were known, it was observed that red cells from some group A persons react more weakly with anti-A sera. These A subgroups were named A_2, A intermediate (A int), A_3, and A_x. It was thought that different forms of the A antigen exist and that sera contained mixtures of antibodies to these different A subgroup antigens. These differences in reactivity appear to be due to variability in the number of antigen sites.[40] Although some persons with these weak A subgroups form anti-A antibodies, this probably does not indicate a qualitative difference in their A antigens but may indicate a quantitative difference.

TABLE 60-6. **Genes and Antigens of the ABH System and ABO Type of Donor Red Cells Suitable for Patients of Different ABO Types**

Gene	Gycosyl Transferase	Antigen-Determining Sugar	ABH Antigen	ABO Type	Antibody Present	Preferable Donor	Other Acceptable Donors*
A	*N*-Acetyl galactosamine transferase	*N*-Acetyl galactosamine	A	A	B	A	O
B	D-Galactosyl transferase	D-Galactose	B	B	A	B	O
H	L-Fucosyl transferase	L-Fucose	H	O	A & B	O	None
A & B			A & B	AB	None	AB	A or B or O

* If blood is used as red blood cells.

The A subgroups are not of major clinical importance. These sera of group A individuals may contain A antibodies. These usually do not react at 37°C and are not considered clinically significant. In rare situations in which the anti-A reacts at 37°C, donors whose red cells are A_2 can be easily identified and a compatible donor can be provided.

Subgroups of B exist but are rare. Persons in this subgroup may also have anti-B in their serum. Since donors with B subgroup red cells are also rare, group O red cells can be used for transfusion.

Bombay Type. The rare Bombay phenotype, first recognized in India, lacks the H gene and is homozygous for its allele h (they are hh). The notation O_h is used for the Bombay type. The lack of an H gene does not allow the attachment of L-fucose to the protein or lipid; thus, these persons have little H antigen. They type as group O, since their red cells do not react with anti-A or anti-B and their serum contains anti-A and anti-B. Their serum also contains anti-H and reacts with group O red cells. Fortunately, such persons are rare because finding compatible red cells is extremely difficult. The only suitable red cells are those from another Bombay person.

Antibodies of the ABH System. ABH antibodies begin to appear during the first few months of life, probably from exposure to ABH antigen-like substances in the environment. Because of this, they are called *naturally occurring antibodies*, but the implication that they form without antigenic stimulation is incorrect. Anti-A or anti-B antibodies are usually combinations of IgM and IgG (see Table 60-4). Because of the IgM content, these sera almost always cause agglutination even at room temperature of red cells containing the corresponding antigen. The IgM composition makes these antibodies effective in fixing complement, and they can be dangerous clinically.

Immunization to A or B antigens can also occur by transfusion of incompatible red cells, inoculation with vaccines containing A or B antigens, transfusion of plasma containing soluble A or B antigens, or pregnancy with an ABO-incompatible fetus. After these kinds of immunizations, the A or B antibody may become more active at 37°C, have a higher IgG component, increase in titer or avidity, and become more strongly hemolytic, and thus even more clinically dangerous.

Anti-H antibodies can occur in persons with little or no H antigen on their red cells. Thus, Bombay type persons (who lack the H gene and do not make H antigens) have an active anti-H, which binds complement and causes hemolysis. A few persons of type A or AB make anti-H probably because almost all their H antigen has been converted to A or B. These anti-H antibodies usually do not react at body temperatures and do not cause hemolysis.

Rh System

The second most important red cell antigen system is the Rh system. This is because a substantial proportion of the population lacks the Rh antigen known as D. The probability of becoming immunized to the D antigen is high and anti-D has serious clinical effects, causing hemolytic disease of the newborn (HDN) or transfusion reactions. In addition to the clinical importance of the Rh system, a lively scholarly debate has been ongoing over the years about the genetics of this system.

Discovery. In 1939, Levine and Stetson[73] reported the case of a woman who delivered a fetus affected by HDN and who, on receiving a transfusion of her husband's blood, experienced a severe transfusion reaction. The researchers hypothesized correctly that the woman had become immunized to a factor that her child had inherited from her husband (the father) but that she lacked. In 1940, Landsteiner and Wiener[74] obtained an antibody from guinea pigs and rabbits immunized with rhesus monkey red cells. This serum had a pattern of reactivity similar to that of Levine and Stetson's patient, and so the blood group system was named Rh for rhesus monkey. Later work established that the animal antirhesus sera and the human antibody did not detect the same antigen, but by that time the nomenclature was established. The pattern of reactivity and the antigen identified by the animal sera has been named *LW* in honor of Landsteiner and Weiner. LW is assigned to a different red cell antigen system from Rh.

Nomenclature and Genetics. The Rh system contains at least 41 different antigens and many other antigenic specificities that may represent weak versions of these antigens or other antigens not yet established as part of Rh system. The antigen detected by the original Levine and Stetson patient's serum is the D antigen. This is present in about 85% of North American whites and is the basis for determining Rh positivity or negativity. That is, persons whose red cells contain the D antigen are Rh-positive and those whose red cells lack the D antigen are Rh-negative.

Four other antigens (C, c, E, and e) were identified that seemed to be inherited in various combinations along with D and became part of the Rh system (Table 60-7). These four antigens along with D account for almost all of the Rh-related transfusion problems encountered in practice. Different nomenclature systems have been used to describe the Rh system (see Table 60-7). The Weiner system supposes that the gene product is a single entity that may have multiple serologic specificities. The Fisher-Race system postulates three closely linked loci, each with its own gene and gene product. The terms that each of these nomenclature systems applies to the different patterns of serologic reactivity are shown in Table 60-7. Rosenfield, and coworkers[77] proposed a third nomenclature in which each Rh antigen is assigned a number and the serologic reactions are used.

Molecular Biology. After almost 50 years of debate about the genetics of the Rh system, molecular biology techniques have provided a considerable amount of information in a few short years. There are three distinct integral membrane proteins (molecular weight, about 32 kd) that carry the Rh antigens. The Rh gene locus is located on chromosome 1 p32-p36 and is composed of two genes.[78] One gene controls expression of the D antigen[79] and one of the CcEe antigens. Thus, Rh-positive (D-positive) persons carry both genes, whereas Rh-negative persons who lack the D antigen carry only the CcEe gene. The two genes are highly homologous and may be the result of duplication of one original ancestral gene.

D Variant or D^u. Many red cell antigens show different degrees of reactivity, but these differences are more of a problem with the D antigen, because all donors and patients are typed for D and because D-negative red cells should be chosen for D-negative patients. Some persons who inherit the D antigen have red cells that react weakly or not at all with certain anti-D reagents. Thus, these persons may appear to be Rh-negative. This situation has been called D variant, D^u, or weak D. The D^u phenomenon can be caused by three different mechanisms. First, when a C gene is on the chromosome opposite from the D gene (*trans* position), the D antigen may be weakened. An example of this is CDe/Cde. This has been called *D^u due to gene interaction*. Second, a D variant or *D^u* can also occur because of a qualitative difference in the D antigen. Rare persons lack a portion of the D antigen molecule and when exposed to the D antigen produce an antibody to that portion of the D antigen that they lack. This has been called *D^u due to D mosaic*. Third, the D gene in some persons codes for an antigen that reacts more weakly. These three forms of D^u

TABLE 60-7. Serologic Reactions and the Wiener and Fisher Race Nomenclature for the Rh System

Reaction With Anti-					Weiner[75]			Fisher Race[76]		
D	**C**	**E**	**c**	**e**	**Most Likely Genotype**	**Phenotype**	**Antigens**	**Most Likely Genotype**	**Phenotype**	**Antigens**
+	+	0	+	+	R^1r	R_1r	Rh_0 rh′ hr′ hr″	CDe/cde	CcDee	CDce
+	+	0	0	+	R^1R^1	R_1R_1	Rh_0 rh′ hr″	CDe/Cde	CCDee	CDe
+	0	+	+	+	R^2r	R_2r	Rh_0 rh″ rh′ hr″	cDE/cde	ccDEe	cDEe
+	0	+	+	0	R^2R^2	R_2R_2	Rh_0 rh″ hr′	cDE/cDE	ccDEE	cDE
+	+	+	+	+	R^1R^2	R_1R_2	Rh_0 rh′ rh″ hr′ hr″	CDe/cDE	CcDEe	CcDEe
+	0	0	+	+	R^0r	R_0r	Rh_0 hr hr	cDe/cde	ccDee	cDe
0	0	0	+	+	rr	rr	hr′ hr″	cde/cde	ccee	ce
0	+	0	+	+	rr	rr	rh′ hr′ hr″	Cde/cde	Ccee	Cce
0	0	+	+	+	r r	r r	rh″ hr′ hr″	cdE/cde	ccEE	cEe
0	+	+	+	+	r r	r r	rh′ rh″ hr′ hr″	Cde/cdE	CcEe	CcEe

occur in about 1% of all Rh-positive persons. The gene interaction and weak D are more common than the D mosaic as causes of *D*^{u}.

These observations are of intellectual interest but have little clinical impact. Persons who are D^u have the D antigen, although some may lack a part of it. Thus, only the rare recipient who is D^u because of a partial absence of D and receives D-positive red cells would make anti-D. Because these patients are rare in practice, it is not necessary to consider this situation. Recipients who are D^u because of gene interaction have all the D antigen and can receive D-positive blood. Thus, it is not necessary to determine whether recipients who appear to be Rh-negative are in fact D^u. They will receive Rh-negative blood.

Rh Null Type. Rarely do persons lack all the Rh antigens. This may be due to the absence of a gene that regulates the expression of Rh antigens or to the presence of an amorphic gene at the Rh locus on chromosome 1. Rh null persons have abnormal red cell morphology and hemolytic anemia, which is usually sufficiently compensated to result in only mild anemia. If exposed to Rh-positive red cells, these persons make an antibody that reacts with all red cells other than Rh null and is considered to be reactive against the entire Rh molecule.

Structure and Composition of the D Antigen. The D antigen is a 28- to 32-kd protein that is associated with the red cell membrane skeleton.[81,82] The protein has an external and intramembranous domain but no cytoplasmic domain. The total amount of D protein per antigen site is about 60,000, indicating that the antigen is probably a dimer or trimer of D proteins,[83] because there are about 30,000 D antigen sites per cell.[84] These cannot move laterally within the membrane but instead are fixed at about 70 nm apart.[85,86] This distance between the D antigen sites probably accounts in part for the lack of complement fixation in D antigen–antibody reactions.

It is surprising that the D protein has been isolated from Rh(D)-negative red cells.[84] Comparison of the protein isolated from Rh-negative cells with the Rh protein isolated from Rh-positive cells reveals slight differences that are probably due to genetic polymorphism.[80] It is postulated that the protein molecule isolated from the Rh-negative cells is a mixture of Rh (c) and (e) proteins. The Rh (c) and (E) proteins have been isolated,[87] and it appears that D, C, and E have regions of identity and regions of diversity.[88] Thus, it appears that C, D, and E are three distinct proteins.[80] These proteins still may be encoded by a single gene so that the controversy between Weiner[75] and Race[76] may end in a draw.[80]

Rh Antibodies. The most common Rh antibody is anti-D. This is almost always an IgG, does not cause agglutination of red cells in vitro, acts at 37°C, and does not bind complement effectively, but causes serious transfusion reactions and red cell destruction by accelerated clearance of cells through the mononuclear phagocyte system.

Kell System

The Kell blood group system includes 24 alloantigens, which can be grouped into four sets of antithetical antigens, two unpaired high-frequency antigens, and 12 related high-frequency antigens. The K gene is autosomal dominant whose frequency differs considerably in different populations. The Kell system is important clinically because the K antigen is next in immunogenicity after D and because antibodies to Kell system antigens (or anti-K) are usually IgG, react at 37°C, and do not bind complement, but can cause severe hemolytic transfusion reactions and HDN. Donors or recipients are not usually typed for Kell unless the recipient has a Kell antibody.

The Kell gene has been cloned and found to be located on the 7 q33 chromosome.[89] The gene produces a 731–amino acid, 93-kd transmembrane glycoprotein. The protein has a 47–amino acid domain within the red cell and a large extracellular C-terminal domain that contains the Kell antigen determinants.[90]

The Kell molecule is a 93-kd glycoprotein[91,92] that apparently is associated with a small (20- to 30-kd), poorly characterized, second protein.[92] Most, if not all, of the Kell antigens are located on this single 93-kd molecule.[93] The antigenicity of Kell antigens is inactivated when the glycoprotein is isolated using reducing conditions that break the disulfide bonds. Thus, the antigen reactivity probably depends on maintenance of the tertiary structure of the surface of the molecule. The Kell molecule glycoprotein molecule is the same size as band 3 of the red cell membrane skeleton; these are different molecules. Another reason that the Kell blood group is interesting is its relation to chronic granulomatous disease (CGD), in which congenital absence of a superoxide-producing cytochrome interferes with the normal oxidative response of neutrophils so that their bactericidal activity is diminished and patients suffer severe, life-threatening infections. The K_x gene locus appears to be on the X chromosome near the CGD locus; thus, about 10% patients have Kell system abnormalities.

In the McLeod phenotype, the red cells express Kell system antigens very weakly and lack K_x, a Kell system precursor substance. Persons with the McLeod phenotype also have bizarre-shaped red cells and a chronic compensated hemolytic anemia. The occurrence of this phenotype in some patients with CGD led to the discovery that the McLeod syndrome involves a spectrum of abnormalities in addition to those involving the Kell system. Other associated abnormalities occur in red cells (acanthocytosis, compensated hemolysis, increased red cell phosphorylation, the nervous system (areflexia, choreiform movements, mild dysarthria, neurogenic myopathy, and muscle wasting), the cardiovascular system (cardiomyopathy), granulocytes (CGD). Other changes such as reduced haptoglobin, elevated creatinine phosphokinase, lactic dehydrogenase, and carbonic anhydrase may be found.

Duffy System

The Duffy system is composed of five antigens that are not present on other blood cells or body tissues. About 13,000 Fy^a or Fy^b antigen sites are on each red cell in persons homozygous for the Fy^a or Fy^b gene.[94] Red cells from persons heterozygous for Fy^a or Fy^b contain about 6000 antigen sites per cell. These red cells often show a weaker agglutination than homozygous cells in serologic tests, a phenomenon called *dosage effect*.

The composition of the Duffy antigens is not completely understood. The molecule containing Fy^a and Fy^b appears to be a glycoprotein with a molecular weight between 40 and 66 kd.[95] The Duffy system is unusual because the antigen frequency varies substantially in different racial groups. In general, the Fy^a gene has a high incidence in Asians, a moderate incidence in whites, and Fy^a and Fy^b have a low incidence in Africans. Both antigens are detectable during fetal development and are present in normal strengths at birth. Duffy was the first blood group locus to be identified on an autosome—chromosome 1. The locus is near the centromere, but it is not clear whether it is on the long or short arm.

Fy^a antibodies may cause severe, even fatal, hemolytic transfusion reactions or severe HDN; transfusion reactions to Fy^a are not common, however, and the HDN is usually mild. Anti-Fy^b is an infrequent cause of transfusion reactions and HDN. Other Duffy system antibodies have not been implicated in clinical problems.

One of the most interesting features of the Duffy system is its association with malaria. Fy^a(a−b−) red cells are resistant to infection by *Plasmodium knowlesi*[96] and probably by *Plasmodium vivax*. The malaria parasites are unable to penetrate red cells lacking the Fy^a or Fy^b antigens because they do not establish a junction site.[97] In West Africa, most blacks are Fy(a−b−) and are resistant to *P vivax* malaria; thus, a natural selection process might have been in effect.

Kidd System

The three antigens of the Kidd system were discovered during the 1950s; no new antigens in this system have been reported since then. Red cells from persons homozygous for Jk^a contain about 11,000 antigen sites[94]; Kidd antigens are not present on other blood cells or tissues. Kidd antigens may be altered by products of bacteria in infected patients. For instance, *Proteus mirabilis* and *Streptococcus faecalis* can cause Jk(b−) cells to become reactive with anti-Jk^b and autohemolysis can occur. The Kidd locus has undergone several different chromosome assignments during the past 15 years. The locus is believed to be a chromosome 18. It is not known whether this genetic locus codes for the Kidd antigens or for a precursor substance or enzyme that determines production of the blood group antigen.

Kidd antibodies are IgG and can cause severe hemolytic transfusion reactions, but they usually cause only mild HDN. In vitro Kidd antibodies may react weakly and cause severe hemolysis despite being IgG. Kidd antibodies usually activate complement. The relatively low number of Kidd antigen sites (11,000) should mean that the distance between antigen sites is too great for complement activation by an IgG molecule; the antigens probably are clustered, thus accounting for weak serologic reactivity, complement activation by IgG, and severe clinical effects.

A unique characteristic of Kidd antibodies is that they often disappear. Thus, they may cause delayed hemolytic transfusion reactions. This occurs when the patient has been immunized previously by pregnancy or transfusion but no longer has circulating antibody so that all the pretransfusion tests are compatible; yet if the patient receives Kidd-positive red cells, the antibody may be resynthesized rapidly, causing hemolysis of the transfused red cells a few hours to days later.

Lutheran System

The Lutheran system has three pairs of antithetical antigens and a seventh antigen that appears to involve one of the pairs of antigens. In addition, six other antigens have Lutheran system nomenclature because they are phenotypically related to the Lutheran system. These para-Lutheran antigens are not genetically related to the Lutheran system.

The structure, composition, and number of Lutheran system antigens per red cell are not well established. Lu^b activity has been found in glycoprotein molecules of 78 to 85 kd, and the number of antigen sites has been reported to be 1000 to 4000 per cell, depending on the zygosity. The antigens are not well developed at birth, and so antigens and antibodies of the Lutheran system cause only mild HDN. Lutheran antibodies may be IgG or IgM or mixtures of these with IgA. The most common Lutheran antibodies are anti-Lu^a and anti-Lu^b.

Anti-Lu^a is usually not active at body temperatures and thus not a problem clinically. It is rarely found because the incidence of Lu(a+) red cells is low; thus, patients are rarely exposed to the antigen. Laboratory test cells often are not Lu(a+), so the antibody is not detected and patients with the antibody would rarely receive a transfusion of Lu(a+) red cells. Anti-Lu^b may cause accelerated destruction of incompatible red cells. This antibody is also rarely found because almost all persons are Lu(b+).

I System

The I blood group system is composed of 16 antigens, the major ones being I and i. One of the unique things about this system is that the presence of the I and i antigens changes with age. At birth, the i antigen is present and I is almost undetectable. During the first 18 months of life, the i antigen declines and is replaced by I. In most adults, little i is detectable, except in rare persons who remain i+ and I−. The other I system antigens are rare forms, transitional forms, or a complex with other antigens. The amount of Ii antigen on red cells varies in different persons, and this also leads to the appearance of different forms of I antigens.

Both anti-I and anti-i are usually autoantibodies that are optimally reactive at cold temperatures and not clinically significant. They do not cause HDN, and only one report is known of an anti-I that caused accelerated destruction of I red cells.[98] The serum of almost all normal adult serum contains anti-I; it is also found in cold agglutinin disease and transiently in *Mycoplasma* pneumonia infection. In cold agglutinin disease, the antibody changes characteristics and is an autologous anti-I that reacts at body temperature, fixes complement, and causes hemolysis. Anti-i is rare but has been associated with infectious mononucleosis.

The i antigen is an oligosaccharide chain attached to a ceramide or protein. I specificity is conferred by the addition of a D-galactose-N-acetyl-D-galactosamine to the i oligosaccharide chain. Thus, it appears that I and i are not alleles but are part of a sequence of steps. The antigen structure is a complex branched chain, and it has been suggested that the variety of antibodies that occurs in the I system is due to formation of antibodies against domains within the antigen molecule.[2]

I and i antigen are present in a soluble form in serum, saliva, breast milk, urine, amniotic fluid, ovarian, and hydatid cyst fluid.

MN System

The M and N antigens were discovered long before Rh by immunizing rabbits with human red cells. The system has five antigens: M and N, which are antithetical; S and s, which are antithetical; and U, which is present in all persons who possess M or N and S or s antigens and in some S−s− persons. The MNU-negative people are usually blacks. Alleles are controlled at the same gene locus. In addition to these five antigens, this system has many variants.

Antibodies to the MN antigens are usually not clinically active. They react below body temperature, have a large IgM component, and thus only rarely cause HDN. Anti-S, anti-s, or anti-U are usually clinically significant. Anti-S occurs infrequently, anti-s is rare, and anti-U is extremely rare. These antibodies may cause a hemolytic transfusion reaction or HDN.

The composition of antigens of this system is well understood. MN antigens are on the sialic acid–rich glycoprotein called *glycophorin A*, and Ss antigens are on the sialic acid–rich glycoprotein called *glycophorin B*. The amino acid sequences of these sialic acid–rich glycoproteins and the location of the antigen activity have been described.[40]

Although anti-M antibodies are often IgG, they are usually not active at body temperatures and do not cause hemolysis, transfusion reactions, or HDN. Unusual examples of anti-M may be active at 37°C and clinically significant. Anti-N is almost always IgM, not reactive at body temperature, and not clinically significant. Anti-S, anti-s, and anti-U are usually IgG warm active antibodies, which may have clinical effects by causing transfusion reactions, hemolysis, or HDN.

The antigens of the MNSs system are located on the red cell membrane sialoglycoproteins.[99] The M and N antigens are on the terminal portion of glycophorin A, of which there are from 200,000 to 1,000,000 copies per red cell. The Ss and probably the U antigens are located on the terminal portion of glycophorin B, of which there are 50,000 to 250,000 copies per red cell.

Glycophorin A has a molecular weight of 43,000 and is composed of 131 amino acids. The MN activity is located in about 70 external amino acids. The remaining amino acids being intramembranous or intracytoplasmic.

P System

The three antigens of the P system define five different P system phenotypes. The antigens are P_1, P, and P^k. All but 1 in 100,000 persons have the P antigen. The two most common phenotypes are P_1 (P_1P) and P_2 (PP); each of these phenotypes has trace amounts of P^k. The amount of P_1 antigen varies greatly among individuals, is not well developed at birth, and does not reach adult levels until the person is about 7 years of age. P-negative (pp) persons are rare.

P system antigens, like the I antigens, seem to be formed in a sequence of steps instead of being antithetical and controlled by allelic genes. They seem to originate from a common precursor and P^k is the precursor of P, but neither P^k nor P are the precursors of P_1.[2] The antigenic determinants are carbohydrates that are linked to glycosphingolipids in the red cell membrane. Genetic control of the P system has been proposed to involve two or three loci. These genes code for enzymes that add the carbohydrates to the lipids in a manner similar to the ABO system genes.

Antigen structures similar to those of the P system are found in animal tissue, pigeons, doves, worms, and *Echinococcus* cyst fluid. Thus, many antibodies of the P system are called *naturally occurring antibodies*, although as with ABO antibodies this is not technically correct. Because some parasites have antigen structures similar to P system antigens, anti-P_1 is sometimes found in patients with parasitic infections.

Antibodies of the P system are common and can range from cold active and clinically insignificant to those that cause severe hemolysis. Anti-P_1 is common, usually cold active, and not clinically significant unless it reacts at body temperatures; anti-PP, P^k made by persons with the rare pp phenotype, anti-P made by persons with the rare P^k phenotype cause hemolysis in vitro and in vivo. A high incidence of miscarriage occurs in women with the pp phenotype, and it has been suggested that anti-PP_k^{1P} may have a pathologic role. Autoanti-P is the specificity of the Donath-Landsteiner antibody found in paroxysmal cold hemoglobinuria. The antibody is often called *biphasic* because it binds to the red cell at cool temperatures, then causes hemolysis at warmer (body) temperature.

Lewis System

The Lewis system is not a blood group system. Lewis antigens are soluble in body fluids, and the antigens present in plasma are adsorbed onto red cells. The Lewis system also differs from most other blood group systems in that the Lewis genes must interact with Hh and secretor genes for Lewis antigens to be produced. There are two antigens in the Lewis system: Le^a and Le^b. The Lewis antigenic specificity is determined by that carbohydrate fucose. The *Le* gene produces a glycosyltransferase, which adds a fucose molecule to a precursor substance (type 1 chain) to produce the Lewis antigen. Thus, Lewis antigens are glycosphingolipids. The exact Lewis antigen produced is determined by the presence or absence of the secretor gene (Se). Se determines the location on the precursor substance (type 1 chain) to which the fucose is added (by the Le gene). Thus, two different antigen specificities are produced, depending on whether the secretor gene is present.

The red cells of newborns lack Lewis antigens, and no Lewis substance is in their plasma, although it is present in their saliva. The adult Le^a antigen phenotype is attained by about 1 year of age but not until about 7 years for Le^b. Lewis antigens are reduced during pregnancy. During pregnancy, an increased lipoprotein to red cell mass results in a shift of glycolipids from red cells to plasma, reducing the Lewis antigen content on the red cells. After transfusion, the transfused donor red cells convert to the Lewis type of the recipient. Thus, Lewis antigen may be acquired or lost through the exchange of glycolipids between the plasma and red cell.

Lewis antibodies are common, usually react below body temperature, are mainly or entirely IgM, and are not clinically significant. These antibodies are usually found in patients who have not received transfusions and are thus sometimes called *natural*, a technically incorrect term since they are probably stimulated by environmental agents. Anti-Le^a is often found in pregnant women, but it is not clear whether the antibody is formed after immunization by fetal red cells. Lewis antibodies do not cause HDN, because they are usually IgM and cannot cross into the fetal circulation. In a few cases, anti-Le^a have caused hemolytic transfusion reactions; usually, the antibodies show reactivity at body temperatures. These reactions can be used as an indication of clinical significance. Lewis antibodies have been implicated in the rejection of transplanted Lewis-positive kidneys.[100] The data on this subject conflict, but Lewis matching of donated kidneys is not done in most transplantation programs.

LW System

The LW antigen is named for Landsteiner and Weiner because it was defined on red cells by the original anti-Rh that the researchers prepared in rhesus monkeys. Only rarely does a person lack LW^a antigen and can make anti-LW^a. Although LW is not genetically part of the Rh system, the expression of LW and Rh is related. Adult D-positive red cells exhibit stronger LW actively than D-negative red cells. Thus, weak examples of anti-LW may appear similar to anti-D because they react with D-positive but not D-negative red cells. Four phenotypes have been observed: LW(a+b−), LW(a+b+), LW(a−b+), LW(a−b−).

LW antibodies are rare. They may cause accelerated destruction of LW-positive red cells; thus, the presence of LW antibodies as an alloantibody should be considered clinically significant. Anti-LW may also occur as a transient autoantibody in persons who temporarily lose LW antigen activity.

Other Blood Group Antigen Systems

Several red cell antigens appear to be related to the HLA system.[100a] HLA class I antigens are present on red cell membranes in variable amounts, 40 to 550 sites. They are attached to the membrane by β_2-microglobulin. These HLA-related red cell antibodies (also known as high-titer, low-affinity [HTLA]) are not considered clinically significant. Chido-Rodgers antigens are C4A plasma components that remain attached to the red cell membrane. Chido-Rodgers antibodies are not considered clinically significant. Several other systems of antigens exist but will not be described in detail here: Wright, Xg, Diego, Cartwright, Scianna, Gerbich, Dombrock, and Colton. They and many other individual or groups of antigens are described in more detail in reference texts.[40]

Antibodies to Red Cell Antigens

Antibodies to red cell antigens vary widely in their characteristics and in vivo significance. Red cell antibodies can be categorized based on their immunoglobulin class, the antigen to which they are directed, the method of stimulation, their optimal temperature of reactions in vitro, whether they fix complement, their action on red cells in vitro, and their in vivo effect such as whether they cause hemolysis, transfusion reactions, or HDN. A summary of the general characteristics of antibodies of the major red cell antigen systems is provided in the preceding section and in Table 60-4; specific antibodies within each system may exhibit different characteristics, so that an appropriate reference text should be consulted before decisions are made regarding the identity or potential clinical effect of a particular antibody. Almost all red cell antibodies are either IgG or IgM. Only rare examples of IgA red cell antibodies are found. Some clinical and laboratory differences between IgM and IgG red cell antibodies exist. The specificities of the most common red cell antibodies found in hospitalized patients, pregnant women, and normal blood donors differ slightly because of the nature of these populations.

The incidence of different antibodies depends on the prevalence of the antigen in the population and the immunogenicity of the antigen. Factors that determine immunogenicity are not fully understood. The combination of the 15% incidence of Rh-negative persons, the 65% likelihood of becoming immunized after exposure to one unit of Rh-positive blood, and the serious clinical effect of anti-D makes the Rh(D) antigen the single most important non-ABO antigen.

The Fab portion of the Ig molecule binds to the antigen-combining site on the red cell surface. The avidity and binding constants for this antigen–antibody reaction vary widely for different red cell antibodies. After binding, the heavy-chain region of the antibody molecule determines the biologic effect of the antibody by activating complement or reacting with receptors in the fixed macrophages of the liver and spleen to cause accelerated red cell clearance.

Platelets

Platelets contain ABH and HLA antigens. Debate exists as to whether the ABO and HLA antigens are integral to the platelet membrane or adsorbed onto the platelet from their soluble form in plasma. Evidence suggests that some ABH antigens are intrinsic to the platelet membrane[101] and some are adsorbed onto the cell surface from the plasma that contains soluble A and B substance. The density of A antigen sites on platelets is only about 5% of that on red cells.[102] In contrast to ABH antigens, HLA antigens are probably integral to the platelet membrane. In addition, there are seven different platelet-specific antigen systems (Table 60-8). Most of these have been localized to particular platelet membrane molecules. Both autoantibodies and alloantibodies occur directed against these alloantigens. These platelet-specific antibodies may cause autoimmune thrombocytopenia or any of several different clinical problems or diseases due to alloimmunization (Table 60-9).

Polymorphonuclear Leukocytes

Granulocytes have been thought to contain ABH antigens on their surface, but recent studies have failed to demonstrate this.[103,104] In addition, granulocytes labeled with indium-111 had normal intravascular recoveries and survivals and migrated normally into skin chambers when injected into subjects who were ABO-incompatible with the granulocyte donors.[105] It is prudent to consider the presence of ABO antigens on granulocytes as unresolved.

HLA-A, HLA-B, and HLA-C (class I) antigens are on the surface of granulocytes,[106] but the antigens are fewer in number than those on lymphocytes.[107] These HLA antigens

TABLE 60-8. Phenotype, Antigen Frequency, and Molecular Association of Platelet-Specific Antigens

Phenotype			
Traditional Nomenclature	International Nomenclature	Antigen Frequency (%)	Platelet Membrane Glycoprotein Association
$P1^{A1}$	HPA-1a	98	IIIa
Pl^{A2}	HPA-1b	27	
Pl^{E1}	NA	>99	Ibα
Pl^{E2}	NA	5	
Bak^{a}	HPA-3a	85	IIb
Bak^{b}	HPA-3b	63	
Pen^{a}	HPA-4a	>99	IIIa
Pen^{b}	HPA-4b		
Ko^{a}	HPA-2a	14	Ib
Ko^{b}	HPA-2b	99	
Pl^{T}		98	V
Br^{a}	HPA-5b	21	Ia
Br^{b}	HPA-5a	81	
Gou^{a}	NA	81	gp175/150
Gou^{b}	NA	64	

NA, not assigned.
(Data primarily from Kickler TS. Management of alloimmunized patients with amegakaryocytic thrombocytopenia. In: Smith DM, Summers SH, eds. Platelets. Arlington, VA, American Association Blood Banks, 1988:115; and von dem Borne, AEGKr, Kuijers RWAM, Goldschmeding R. Platelet antigens in alloimmune thrombocytopenia. In: Nance SJ, ed. Clinical and basic aspects of immunohematology. Arlington, American Association of Blood Banks, 1991:115; with permission of American Association of Blood Banks)

are possibly adsorbed onto the surface of granulocytes[108] rather than being an integral part of the membrane, but this is not established. It appears that HLA-D/DR antigens are not on granulocytes.[104]

Granulocytes also contain several alloantigen systems whose tissue distribution is limited to granulocytes (Table 60-10). These granulocyte-specific antigen–antibody systems are involved in the pathophysiology of several clinical situations (Table 60-11). Both autoantibodies and alloantibodies have been identified, and each may cause severe clinical problems.[109] A situation in which neutrophil-specific antibodies are not important is bone marrow transplantation. We have demonstrated successful marrow engraftment of NA1-positive marrow in a patient with circulating anti-NA1.[110] Stroncek and colleagues[111] reported on a case in which the NB1 granulocyte antibody, present in high titer, apparently caused prolonged neutropenia following transplantation with marrow from an NB1-positive donor. These observations are consistent with evidence that these antigens are not present on promyelocytes, myeloblasts, and earlier uncommitted stem cells but become expressed during myeloid maturation.[112] Thus, the granulocyte-specific antigens can be thought of as differentiation antigens specific for this cell line, which become expressed during maturation of the cell.

Significance of Blood Groups

Red Blood Cells

Red cell blood group antigens have been of interest to blood bankers because of their role in transfusion therapy and

TABLE 60-9. Diseases and Clinical Conditions Due to Platelet-Specific Antibodies

	Most Common Antibody Specificity
Autoantibodies	
Autoimmune thrombocytopenia	$P1^{A1}$
Drug-induced immune thrombocytopenia	?
Alloantibodies	
Alloimmune neonatal thrombocytopenia	$P1^{A1}$
Posttransfusion purpura	$P1^{A1}$
Refractoriness to platelet transfusion	?

TABLE 60-10. Genetic Locus and Antigen Frequency of Granulocyte-Specific Antigens

Locus	Antigen	Phenotype Frequency (%)
NA	NA1	46
	NA2	88
NB	NB1	97
	NB2	32
NC	NC1	91
ND	ND1	98
NE	NE1	23
HGA-3	3a	21
	3b	24
	3c	16
	3d	53
	3e	17

(McCullough J, Clay ME, Press C, Kline W. Granulocyte serology: a clinical and laboratory guide. Chicago, American Society of Clinical Pathologists Press, 1988)

TABLE 60-11. Clinical Situations in Which Granulocyte-Specific Antibody–Antigen Systems Are Causative Agents

Autoantibodies
Autoimmune neutropenia
Drug-induced immune neutropenia
Alloantibodies
Febrile transfusion reactions
Adult respiratory disease syndrome (transfusion-associated acute lung injury)
Alloimmmune neonatal neutropenia
Poor response to granulocyte transfusion

to geneticists because of their ability to serve as a genetic marker. During the past few years, the chromosome location of several blood groups has been established (see Table 60-5). Linkage between some blood groups and diseases are known, and this also helps to localize some blood group genes to certain areas of the chromosomes. Studies of the red cell membrane have also begun to yield information about the structure and composition of red cell (blood group) antigens. Thus, the red cell antigens are no longer of interest only to the serologist–blood banker but are recognized increasingly as parts of important structural or functional components of the cell membrane. Red cell antigens are associated with a variety of conditions ranging from hemolytic anemias to malignancies, stress, and pregnancy (Table 60-12). Some clinical conditions may alter the expression of blood groups, and some rare blood types are associated with abnormal red cell morphology or membrane constituents (Table 60-13).

Platelets

In addition to involvement in several clinical situations (see Table 60-9), some of the platelet-specific antigens are located on molecules that have other important functions. These may be involved in platelet aggregation or platelet adhesion to endothelial cells. It is likely that future studies will demonstrate that abnormalities of these molecules cause alterations in platelet antigens or that altered platelet antigen strength or specificity may affect the structure or function of the cell.

Neutrophils

As with platelets, neutrophil-specific antigens are involved in several important clinical situations. The location of the neutrophil-specific antigen on particular molecules is not as extensively defined as for platelets. The genes for the NA antigens have been cloned,[113,114] and these antigens are part of the Fc receptor molecule,[115] and the NB1 antigen may be part of the receptor for the chemoattractant formyl-methionyl-leucyl-phenylalanine.[116] Thus, it is likely that these neutrophil-specific antigens also will prove to be important in cell membrane structure and function.

LABORATORY DETECTION OF BLOOD GROUPS AND PRETRANSFUSION TESTING

Red Blood Cells

Immunologic Mechanisms of Red Cell Destruction

Because most red cell antibodies are IgM or IgG, red cell destruction involves those two kinds of immunoglobulins either with or without complement. Red cells containing

TABLE 60-12. Clinical Conditions With Red Cell Antigen Alteration

	Red Cell Antigen		
Clinical Condition	**Depressed**	**Increased**	**Antibody**
AIHA	Rh-LW	i	Autoanti-D, LW Anti-Kp^b
Leukemia with monosomy 7	ABH Co^a	IiH	
Myelofibrosis	LW Rh ABH		
Hodgkin's disease			Anti-LW
Paroxysmal nocturnal hemoglobinuria		i	
Paroxysmal cold hemoglobinuria			Autoanti-P
Ovalocytosis	Rh, LW Ss, U Kidd Yt^a, Xg^a	H	
Chronic granulomatous disease	Kell		Anti-KL + K_x
Hereditary hemolytic anemia	Rh Kell Colton		
Sickle cell anemia—stress		i	
Pregnancy	LW Lewis Sd^a		Anti-LW Anti-Lewis
Bacterial infections	Acquired B-antigen T activation		
Chromosomal defects	Rh MN Duffy		

TABLE 60-13. Rare Blood Types Associated With Abnormal Red Cell Morphology or Membrane Constituents

Phenotypes	Biochemical Modification	Morphologic and Functional Abnormality
Rh_{null}	No Rh or LW antigens	Stomatocytes, spherocytes; partially compensated hemolytic anemia
McLeod	Weak expression of normal Kell antigens; K_x absent	Acanthocytes; partially compensated hemolytic anemia
K_0	No normal Kell antigens; K_x present	None observed
p	No normal P antigens; decreased globoside and ceramide trihexoside	None observed
pk	Normal P^1 antigen; CTH increased; globoside decreased	None observed
$P1^{pk}$	Increased GL3 (NAc galactose transferase deficiency)	None observed
Lu(a−b−)	Not studied	Abnormal scanning electron microscopy—wrinkled, furrowed appearance
En(a−)	Glycophorin A absent; depressed MN antigens; enhanced Rho antigen	None observed
S−s−	Glycophorin B absent or abnormal	None observed
M^kM^k	Both glycophorin A and glycophorin B absent	None observed

bound IgG undergo accelerated clearance through the spleen,[2] where Fc receptors of the phagocyte bind to the IgG molecules leading to phagocytosis of the red cell. Although this process does not require complement, binding and phagocytosis are accelerated if the IgG-coated red cell also contains bound complement components.

Complement has one of two roles in the immune destruction of red cells: accelerated clearance by interacting with complement receptors in the fixed macrophage system or causation of membrane damage leading to direct cell lysis. Complement can be activated by either IgG or IgM, although IgM is much more effective, probably because the nature of the IgM molecule places several Fc receptor sites in close proximity. The subclasses of IgG1 and IgG3 are more effective in binding complement than IgG4. The exact mechanisms that determine the ability of different red cell antibodies to activate complement are not known. The situation is more complex than merely the number of Fc sites in close enough proximity to activate C1.[2] For instance, in general, anti-D (an IgG) is not effective in activating complement compared with anti-K or Jk^a (also IgG), which react with antigens that actually have fewer antigen sites than D sites on the red cell.[2]

Activation of C1 begins the complement cascade sequence leading to formation of the membrane attack complex (C5 to C9), which causes lysis of the red cell. The complement system involves several proteins (complement components), the activation of which is influenced by a variety of inhibitors or proteases. Thus, often the process does not proceed to completion of the membrane attack complex and cell lysis. Red cells may be coated with certain complement components that cause accelerated clearance of the red cells by interaction with complement receptors on cells of the fixed macrophage system. The first of these key steps is the activation of C3. After several activation and enzyme cleavage steps, a fragment of C3,C3d remains bound to the red cell membrane antigen–antibody complex. Red cells containing bound C3d undergo accelerated clearance in the liver by interaction with complement receptors in the fixed macrophage system.

Red cell serologic reagents have been developed to detect C3d bound to red cells. These reagents are used for direct antiglobulin testing to determine whether anemia or accelerated red cell destruction may be due to complement activation or complement-binding antibodies or both. For many years, a lively debate took place regarding the value of anti-C3 activity in the reagent antihuman globulin serum used for antibody detection tests and crossmatching. The rationale was that the ability to detect not only IgG but also C3d on the red cell would enhance the likelihood of finding clinically significant antibodies. Many clinically insignificant antibodies active at cold temperatures bind complement. Since these cold antibodies are present normally in many persons, the addition of anti-C3d to antiglobulin serum led to many false-positive tests; this practice has been abandoned.

Although detection of C3d bound to red cells is not helpful for compatibility testing, it is helpful in the evaluation of possible immune hemolytic anemia (see Chap. 55). For instance, some patients with warm antibody type autoimmune hemolytic anemia, cold agglutinin syndrome, and drug-induced immune hemolytic anemias may have red cells that react only with reagents containing anti-C3d activity and not with anti-IgG reagents.

Intravascular Hemolysis. The destruction of red cells by the complement membrane attack complex is called intravascular hemolysis. The red cell membrane is damaged, hemoglobin is released into the circulation, and the classic signs and symptoms of a hemolytic transfusion reaction are seen (see section on complications of transfusion). ABO incompatibility is the best example of red cell antigen–antibody reactions that caused this kind of hemolysis.

Extravascular Hemolysis. Red cell destruction caused by phagocytic cells of the fixed macrophage site is called extravascular hemolysis. This occurs primarily in the spleen and is associated with an increase in bilirubin and its metabolites. In actuality, these distinctions are arbitrary, since complement may be involved in both intravascular and extravascular hemolysis and the degree or severity of hemolysis may be a factor in the symptoms and laboratory findings. For instance, red cells undergoing phagocytosis in the fixed macrophage system may be only partially engulfed and may release some hemoglobin into the intravascular space, thus simulating intravascular hemolysis.

In practice, the red cell serologic tests for compatibility are designed to enhance and speed the cell's reaction to

IgM or IgG antibodies and to detect the reaction by looking for direct cell agglutination or using reagents such as anti-IgG to cause red cell agglutination.

Selection of Blood Types

For routine transfusions, red cells are selected that are identical with the patient's red cells for the ABO and Rh(D) antigens. In some situations, such as massive bleeding or an emergent need for transfusion, red cells that are not ABO and D identical may be used (see also section on transfusions in special situations). When Rh-negative patients experience massive bleeding, it may be necessary to use Rh(D)-positive blood because no Rh-negative red cells are available. This decision should be made by consultation between the blood bank physician and the attending physician. If necessary, Rh-negative red cells can be given to Rh-positive patients. Because Rh-negative red cells lack the D antigen, the Rh-positive patient will experience no unusual adverse effect as long as he or she does not have an anti-D.

It may also be necessary to switch ABO types. When blood of a different ABO type is used, it is used as red cells, not whole blood, to avoid problems due to transfusion of antibodies contained in the plasma. Table 60-6 indicates the ABO types of donor blood that can be used. Despite the small amount of plasma in the red cell unit, hemolysis due to passive transfusion of antibody in these units can occur. This rarely occurs, and the remote possibility of such a problem should not interfere with making red cells available rapidly in urgent situations.

Red Blood Cell Pretransfusion Testing

The crossmatch is only one part of the pretransfusion or compatibility test. The term *pretransfusion testing* refers to all procedures involved in selecting blood products that "will have acceptable survival and will not cause clinically significant destruction of the recipient's own red cells."[57] These procedures include the following:

- Positive identification of recipient and blood sample
- Review of transfusion service records for results of previous testing of samples from the recipient
- ABO and Rh typing. Many clinical conditions and diseases may make interpretation of the results of ABO and Rh typing difficult. Careful attention to detail and to the proper use and interpretation of controls is essential. The ABO and Rh type of the patient is confirmed on each blood sample used for pretransfusion testing to increase the safety of the transfusion by ensuring that the sample is from the correct patient. The ABO and Rh type of the donor blood will have been confirmed when the hospital receives the blood from its regional blood supplier.
- Selection of blood components of appropriate ABO and Rh types
- Antibody detection test (indirect antiglobulin or Coombs' test). In this test, the patient's serum is reacted with red cells usually from two normal persons whose cells contain antigens reactive with all of the common clinically significant antibodies. The cells are usually purchased commercially and subject to FDA requirements for the antigens they contain and their strength of reactivity.

  The conditions of this test usually involve incubation of the patient's serum with test red cells suspended in saline or albumin followed by washing of the red cells, adding antihuman globulin, centrifuging, and looking for agglutination. An extensive literature describes the optimal technique for detecting different antibodies. Some of the methods that may be used are treating the red cells with enzymes, extending the length of incubation, changing the serum cell ratio, altering the incubation temperature, suspending the red cells in low ionic strength solution, and use of chemicals such as polybrene to enhance agglutination. Some of these techniques are used routinely by some blood banks; others are suitable for use only in reference laboratories for investigation of certain antibodies.

  The cornerstone of red cell antibody detection is the use of antihuman globulin. Antihuman globulin is prepared from the serum of rabbits immunized with human IgG (monospecific) or a blend of sera from rabbits immunized with IgG and others immunized with human complement (C3; polyspecific). Antihuman globulin detects IgG (and C3) on the surface of red cells. If the patient's serum contains an IgG antibody that reacts with an antigen on the red cells used in antibody screening tests, it is detected using the antihuman IgG (Fig. 60-2). This test is extremely important since most clinically significant red cell antibodies are IgGs.
- Crossmatch. In the major crossmatch, the recipient's serum is reacted with the intended donor's red cells usually with a technique similar to that used in the antibody detection test. This involves incubation at 37°C and the use of antihuman globulin. Both antiglobulin reagents (polyspecific containing anti-IgG and anti-C3, or monospecific containing anti-IgG only) are in routine use, but the detection of cell-bound C3d may lead to false-positive results and some workers prefer to use the anti-IgG reagent. Various agents or procedural modifications may be used to attempt to enhance or speed antigen–antibody reactions. For patients in whom no antibodies are detected, a complete crossmatch is not necessary.[117] Thus, it is increasingly common to carry out a simplified crossmatch that confirms ABO compatibility if the patient has a negative antibody detection test and has not been pregnant nor received transfusions within the preceding 3 months.[57] This will not prevent an occasional incompatible unit from being transfused, since many blood group antigens of low frequency are not present on the red cells used for antibody screening tests.

  In the minor crossmatch, the donor's serum is reactive with the patient's red cells. This test was intended to detect antibodies in the donor that might cause hemolysis of the patient's red cells. Although a few such cases have been reported, this is rare. The situation is approached by carrying out an antibody detection test on the donor's serum at the time of donor blood processing. If donor antibodies are present, either the unit is not used or the plasma is removed. Thus, the minor crossmatch is not necessary and is no longer used.
- Labeling and issue of the appropriate blood products

Approach to the Patient With an Incompatible Crossmatch

In compatibility testing when there is reactivity in the antibody detection test, serologic studies should be carried out to determine whether a red cell antibody is present. If a clinically significant antibody is identified, donor red cells typed and found to be negative for the corresponding antigen should be compatible when crossmatched. The blood bank staff carries out these procedures and provides compatible blood, although additional time and blood samples may be necessary. For several reasons, the approach of identifying the antibody and selecting known antigen-

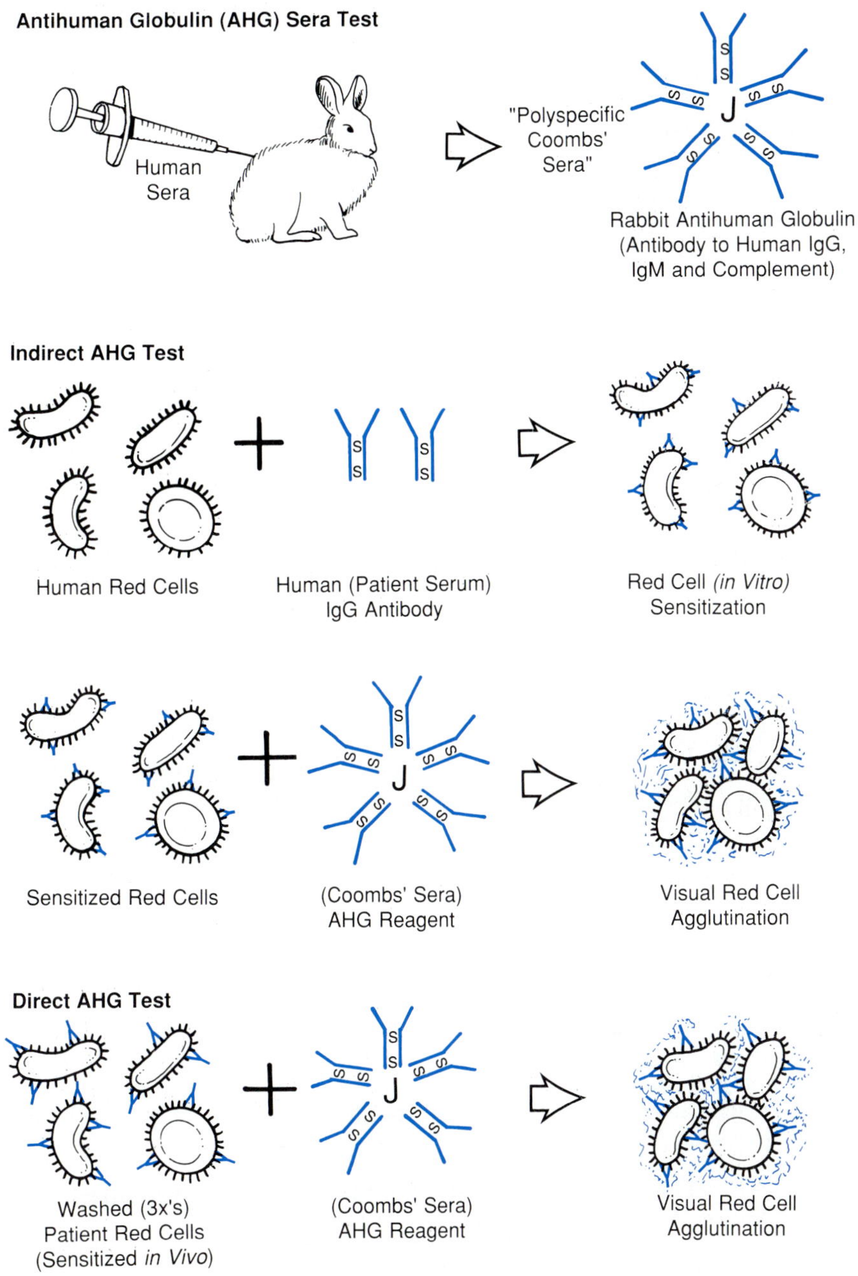

FIGURE 60-2. The antihuman globulin (AHG) test (primary immunization). The AHG reagents currently sold are the products of subsequent immunizations and contain primarily IgG rabbit antibody. (After Harmening D. Modern blood banking and transfusion practices. Philadelphia, FA Davis, 1989)

negative red cells is preferable to merely crossmatching until compatible red cells are found. The panels used for red cell antibody identification do not represent random donors. Thus, the antibody may react with a high proportion of donors making it difficult to obtain compatible red cells; some antibodies react in vitro only with red cells homozygous for the antigen but cause in vivo destruction of heterozygous red cells; and many sera that react in vitro do not signify potential in vivo red cell destruction. Thus, knowledge of the specificity of the red cell antibody and the character of anti–red cell reactivity improves the safety of the transfusion.

Some patients' serum reacts with many or even all of the donors tested. In this situation, it is necessary to determine whether the patient has autoimmune hemolytic anemia. This is usually indicated by a positive direct antiglobulin test. The patient may or may not be anemic. (The selection of blood for patients with autoimmune hemolytic anemia is discussed in the section on transfusion in special situations.) If the patient has a negative direct antiglobulin test and does not have autoimmune hemolytic anemia, but the serum reacts with all donors' red cells tested, it must be determined whether an alloantibody is present against a high-frequency antigen or whether the reactivity is due to other non–red cell blood group factors.

Examples of non–red cell blood group factors are abnormal proteins in the patient's plasma, high titers of normal cold agglutinins, reactivity with test materials such as preservatives or antibiotics used in the test red cell suspension. If it is determined that the patient does have a high-frequency alloantibody, the clinical significance of the antibody determines whether it is preferable to obtain antigen-negative red cells. For instance, this is unnecessary for many antibodies that do not cause transfusion reactions, hemolysis, or accelerated clearance of red cells. If the alloantibody is expected to be clinically significant, most blood banks have local files of rare donors and, if necessary, national rare donor registries of the American Red Cross or American Association of Blood Banks can be contacted. In patients with a clinically significant high-frequency alloantibody, the decision as to whether to delay transfusion to obtain compatible antigen-negative red cells depends on the patient's condition. If the patient's condition does not allow delay, an in vivo crossmatch can be done (see the following section). In situations when no specific antibody has been identified, considerable emphasis has been placed on selecting the least incompatible donor units for transfusion. Although it is unlikely that this is detrimental, no evidence exists to prove that, in these situations, red cells that are less reactive in vitro have better survival in vivo.

In Vivo Compatibility Testing

Occasionally, compatible donor red cells cannot be found either because the patient's serum contains an autoantibody that reacts with all donors' red cells or because the serum contains an alloantibody against an extremely high-frequency antigen and cells lacking the antigen are not available. In these situations, an in vivo crossmatch can be done. This involves labeling with cromium-51 a small volume (usually 5 mL or less) of the red cells to be transfused, injecting them, and determining the percentage that survives 24 hours later.[118] In general, patients do not experience an acute hemolytic reaction if at least 85% of the donor red cells survive 24 hours later.[119] The 85% value should not be used as an arbitrary indication of a safe transfusion. Transfused red cells with lower 24-hour survivals in the in vivo crossmatch may have a better survival when the larger-volume transfusion is given; occasional patients may experience severe hemolysis despite in vivo crossmatch results of greater than 85%.[119] Thus, although an in vivo crossmatch may provide helpful information, it usually does not change the actual management of the patient.

Platelets

Selection of ABO and Rh Type for Platelet Transfusion

ABO antigens are adsorbed onto the surface of the platelet, and the recovery of A_1 platelets transfused into group O patients is decreased.[120] In patients with lymphocytotoxic antibodies against donor cells, the increment in peripheral blood platelet count has been reported to be the same[121] or reduced[122,123] after transfusion of HLA-matched, ABO-incompatible platelets. Although the clinical importance of the ABO effect is not known, it is advisable to transfuse ABO-compatible platelets.[124] If ABO-compatible platelets are not available, ABO-incompatible platelets should be used rather than withholding platelet transfusion.

Incompatibility between the platelet donor plasma and the recipient red cells usually is not clinically important because of the small volume of plasma (50 mL) from each individual platelet concentrate. If large numbers of platelet concentrates are being transfused to an adult or if the patient is a small child, incompatible donor plasma may cause a positive direct antiglobulin test and red cell hemolysis (eg, type O plasma contains anti-A and may react with a type A recipient's red cells). When ABO-compatible platelets are not available, consideration may be given to removing some plasma from the platelet concentrate before transfusion or selecting the platelet ABO type so that ABO-compatible plasma rather than compatible platelets is given. Red cell crossmatching is not necessary before platelet transfusion because the platelet concentrate usually contains about 0.5 mL of red cells.

Rh antigens are not found on platelets. Patients may become immunized to Rh antigens from the red cells contaminating the platelet concentrate. The risk of forming anti-Rh(D) was first reported to be about 8% after 80 to 110 units of platelets.[125] A subsequent study showed no evidence of sensitization in 30 Rh-negative patients after extensive transfusion support with Rh-positive platelets.[126] In a more recent review of 73 Rh-negative oncology patients, 9 (12%) became immunized to the D antigen after receiving a mean of 102 mL of Rh-positive red cells through platelet and granulocyte transfusions.[127] Because of the life-threatening nature of most cases of thrombocytopenia, platelets from Rh-positive donors can be administered to Rh-negative recipients. Rh-negative women of childbearing age with a nonmalignant disease should not receive platelet concentrates from Rh-positive donors because of the possible effect of anti-Rh on future pregnancies. If Rh-positive platelets are given to such a patient, Rh immunization can be prevented by the administration of Rh immune globulin.

Rh-positive platelets have a normal duration of survival in recipients with anti-Rh(D)[128]; thus, the only concern is a possible transfusion reaction to Rh-positive red cells contained in the platelet concentrate. If the platelet concentrates are properly prepared, red cell contamination is 0.5 mL or less per unit, and a significant red cell hemolytic reaction would not be expected even in a recipient with a preformed anti-Rh(D) antibody.

If an Rh-negative patient receives Rh-positive platelets, an attempt to prevent immunization may be desirable. This can be done by giving the patient Rh immune globulin. Since one standard dose (1 mL) of Rh immune globulin prevents immunization from up to 15 mL of Rh-positive red cells, this should cover about 30 units of platelets (25 units $\times$ 0.5 mL = 12.5 mL red cells).[129]

Red Cell Compatibility Testing for Platelet Transfusion

Compatibility testing is not usually done for platelet transfusions because of the small red cell content of the platelet concentrate. Platelets also contain HLA antigens and platelet-specific antigens. Some patients may develop antibodies to these antigens after transfusion, pregnancy, or organ transplantation. When this occurs, transfused platelets may have a decreased recovery and a shortened intravascular survival. These transfused platelets are therefore less effective in controlling hemorrhage. The management of these patients is discussed in the section on transfusion therapy.

Granulocytes

Each granulocyte concentrate contains about 20 mL of red cells, and thus red cell compatibility testing must be done. HLA and granulocyte antibodies can interfere with the ability of transfused granulocytes to circulate and localize at sites of inflammation.[130] This problem could be overcome by carrying out leukocyte compatibility testing. Technical problems make it impractical to do a leukocyte crossmatch of the patient's serum and the donor's cells on the day of transfusion. Donors are usually selected by periodically screening the patient's serum against multiple granulocyte donors. Lack of an effective method of ensuring granulocyte compatibility is a major factor in the limited effectiveness of granulocyte transfusion.

TRANSFUSION THERAPY

Transfusion of Components Containing Red Blood Cells

See also the section on transfusion in special situations.

Clinical Indications

The most common reasons for transfusion are replacement of red cells for oxygen carrying capacity and restoration of blood volume after blood loss. Patients should not receive transfusions based only on their hemoglobin level. In deciding whether a patient requires red cell transfusion, the clinical condition of the patient is of primary importance.

Restoration of Blood Volume. The amount of blood loss that can be tolerated without replacement depends on the condition of the patient. If blood loss has been acute, the patient may have a normal or nearly normal hemoglobin level but may require transfusion for the restoration of blood volume (see section on transfusion in special situations). If blood loss is judged sufficient to require transfusion, it is not necessary to wait until symptoms such as pallor, diaphoresis, tachycardia, and hypotension develop. On the other hand, transfusion should not be initiated too rapidly because it is clear that in most normal patients the loss of about 1 L of blood can be replaced by colloid or crystalloid solutions alone.[131,132]

Improvement of Oxygen-Carrying Capacity. When anemia has developed over a long period of time, the patient adjusts to lower hemoglobin levels and may not require transfusion despite very low hemoglobin levels. No evidence proves that it is necessary to give a transfusion to a patient to reach a normal hemoglobin level before surgery.[133] In addition, there is no specific hemoglobin level above which patients feel better or have better wound healing. In patients with chronic anemia, transfusion should be used only as a last resort, since it may suppress erythropoiesis.

Transfusion in Preparation for Surgery. Most anesthesiologists and surgeons give transfusions to patients when the hemoglobin level is 10 g/dL or less. No scientific or well-described clinical data support this practice. Apparently, many patients would not be at risk if transfusion were withheld until the hemoglobin level was less than 7 g/dL.[133] In baboons subject to normovolemic anemia (exchange transfusion using dextran for replacement of red cells), death occurs at hematocrit levels of about 5%.[133–135] This decline in hemoglobin was accompanied by a linear decrease in mixed venous oxygen tension, an increase in extraction of oxygen from the red cells, and an increase in cardiac output allowing oxygen consumption to remain unchanged until the hematocrit fell to 10% or less.[133] The authors concluded that the normal heart has a remarkable capacity to adjust to acute normovolemic anemia and suggested that most patients should not receive a transfusion unless the hemoglobin level is 7 g/dL or less. Few patients, especially those with normal cardiac function, require transfusions at hemoglobin levels of 10 g/dL. Transfusion to patients with hemoglobin levels of 7 to 10 g/dL should be based on clinical assessment of that particular patient.[134,135]

The few studies that deal with the physiology of blood loss and the indications for red cell transfusion have been done in normal animals or essentially healthy humans. Thus, the indications for transfusion in patients with cardiac disease, coronary atherosclerosis, or other vascular insufficiency are not known. Patients with compromised cardiovascular or cerebrovascular systems may not be able to compensate for anemia effectively. Thus, it has been suggested that the elderly or patients with cardiac or cerebrovascular disease receive transfusions to maintain a hemoglobin of approximately 10 g/dL.[136]

Indications for Specific Red Cell Components

Red Blood Cells. Red cells are the component of choice for any patient with severe anemia. Most patients who require red cell replacement do not also need intravascular volume replacement. In patients who do need intravascular volume and red cell replacement, crystalloid or colloid solutions, not human plasma, are the preferred solutions for intravascular volume replacement. The latter solutions have few, if any, adverse effects, and their use allows the plasma from the original unit of whole blood to be used for the production of coagulation factor concentrate. Thus, almost all transfusions given for red cell replacement are red cells.

Whole Blood. Whole blood is rarely used for transfusion. Instead, whole blood can be replaced with mixtures of separate components such as red cells and crystalloid or colloid solutions.

Leukocyte-Poor Red Blood Cells. Patients who receive multiple transfusion and multiparous women may develop antibodies to leukocytes and platelets. When patients with leukocyte antibodies receive blood containing incompatible leukocytes, febrile transfusion reactions may occur.[109] These leukocyte reactions do not cause red cell hemolysis but can be extremely uncomfortable for the patient and are potentially fatal. Symptoms such as chills, fever, headache, malaise, nausea, vomiting, and chest or back pain may persist for up to 8 hours and seem to be caused by immune damage to donor granulocytes. The incidence and severity of leukocyte transfusion reactions are directly related to the number of incompatible leukocytes transfused.[137] Therefore, leukocyte-poor blood is indicated for patients who have repeated febrile transfusions reactions. Because febrile reactions occur sporadically, patients should not be switched to leukocyte-poor red cells after a single reaction.

Leukocyte-poor red cells can be prepared by centrifuging, washing, or freezing an ordinary unit of red cells, or by filtering them (see Table 60-14). Filters have become available that remove about 99% of leukocytes, do not require priming, and allow flow rates of about 50 mL/min. These filters are effective in preventing febrile transfusion reactions,[138] and the use of leukocyte-poor red cells for patients receiving multiple transfusions may reduce the likelihood of platelet refractoriness.[139–141] Although this simple bedside method of providing leukocyte-poor red cells is becoming widely used, these filters are expensive and should not be used indiscriminately.[138]

Washed Red Blood Cells. Washed red cells are composed of red cells suspended in an electrolyte solution (Table 60-14); most plasma, platelets, and leukocytes have been removed, although leukocyte removal is not as complete as with frozen deglycerolized red cells. After washing, the storage period is 24 hours. Washed red cells are indicated for patients who have reactions caused by plasma. For instance, patients with IgA deficiency can have severe, often fatal, anaphylactic reactions when exposed to plasma containing IgA.[40] Although washed red cells have been used to prevent febrile reactions due to transfused leukocytes, the availability of filters for leukocyte removal should eliminate this indication.

Frozen Deglycerolized Red Blood Cells. Frozen deglycerolized red cells are composed of essentially pure red cells suspended in an electrolyte solution (Table 60-14). Most of the plasma, platelets, and leukocytes have been removed. The main advantage of frozen red cells is that they can be stored for years, thus allowing development of a depot of red cells of rare types or storage of autologous red cells. This is the most important value of frozen red cells. They have been used in the past as a leukocyte-poor blood product or in place of washed red cells. These uses are not recommended. Leukocyte-poor red cells can be prepared more quickly and less expensively by filtration, and frozen red cells have no advantage over washed red cells for patients who have reactions to plasma.

Because of the extensive washing, it has been speculated that frozen deglycerolized red cells may carry no risk of transmitting viruses such as hepatitis, HIV, and cytomegalovirus (CMV). One study indicates that this may be true.[142] It would be preferable to see data confirming that

TABLE 60-14. General Comparison of Methods of Preparing Leukocyte-Depleted Red Cells for Transfusion

Method	White Cells Removed (%)	Approximate No. WBCs Remaining	Original Red Cells Remaining (%)	Comment
Centrifugation	85	1×10^9	80	Product may contain dextran or hydroxyethyl starch, 24-h storage
Sedimentaion (dextran)	95	0.9×10^9	90	24-h storage; product may contain dextran or hydroxyethyl starch
Freezing deglycerolizing	98	0.1×10^9	90	24-h storage
Washing	85	0.1×10^9	85	24-h storage
Spin cool filter	90	0.3×10^9	90	24-h storage
Nylon filter	65	1.5×10^9	88	Heparin required; 24-h storage
New generation filters*	99	5×10^7	95	Bedside use

* Refers to general results from several different manufacturers' filters that have become available during the late 1980s.

frozen deglycerolized red cells have no risk of CMV transmission before accepting this as established fact.

Effects of Red Blood Cell Transfusion

Circulation. When a unit of red cells or whole blood is transfused rapidly (30 to 60 minutes) to a patient with a normal blood volume, the blood volume is increased by the volume of the component. The blood volume returns to its pretransfusion level by about 24 hours. If plasma alone is transfused, the blood volume may readjust more rapidly. Some patients, such as those with chronic renal disease, may require prolonged periods to readjust their blood volume.

Hemoglobin Concentration. The effects of red cell transfusion on the recipient's hemoglobin level and hematocrit are affected by the recipient's blood volume, pretransfusion hemoglobin level, the patient's clinical condition (stable, bleeding, and so on), and the hemoglobin content of the donor unit. For instance, a hypothetical patient with a blood volume of 5000 mL and hemoglobin concentration of 8 g/dL has a total of 400 g of hemoglobin. If a unit of red cells is transfused, the blood volume becomes 5300 mL, the total hemoglobin 460 g, and the hemoglobin concentration 8.7 g/dL. If the patient is able to readjust the blood volume to baseline levels within 24 hours, the result will be 5000 mL blood volume, 460 g hemoglobin, and a hemoglobin concentration of 9.2 g/dL.

Red Blood Cell Production. Transfusion of red cells may result in a decrease in the recipient's red cell production rate due to suppression of erythropoietin. Thus, many patients with a stable chronic anemia may receive less than expected benefit from red cell transfusion, since their hemoglobin levels may fall to pretransfusion levels because of diminished production of their own red cells and the clearance of the transfused cells.

Survival of Transfused Red Blood Cells. The normal red cell has a life-span of about 120 days. This is reflected after transfusion in that about 1% of the donor cells are lost each day.[40] Each unit of blood contains red cells of all ages between 1 and 120 days. As the unit of blood is stored, the red cells continue to age; these senescent red cells are removed from the circulation within 24 hours after transfusion. Thus, when stored blood is transfused, a slight decrease occurs in the proportion of red cells surviving 24 hours after transfusion, depending on the length of time that the blood has been stored. For instance, about 80% of red cells stored in the anticoagulant AS-1 (Adsol) for 42 days survive after transfusion. These red cells then survive normally and are destroyed linearly with a mean half-life of 50 to 60 days.[40] The survival of transfused red cells is also affected by the recipient's health and may be decreased in patients with active bleeding (and iatrogenic blood loss), hemolytic anemia due to defects extrinsic to the red cells (autoantibodies, hypersplenism), and chronic renal or liver failure.

Transfusion of Products Containing Coagulation Factors

The components that can be used to replace coagulation factors are fresh frozen plasma, cryoprecipitate, factor VIII concentrates, and factor IX concentrates. In considering the use of coagulation components, it is convenient to separate situations requiring replacement of multiple factors from those requiring an isolated component.

Deficiency of Multiple Coagulation Factors

The most common combination deficiency of coagulation factors involves those dependent on vitamin K for synthesis. This type of coagulation disorder is best managed by treating the underlying condition with or without vitamin K administration. The coagulation factors can be replaced using plasma of any age since these coagulation factors do not deteriorate during storage of whole blood at 1° to 6°C. Commercial concentrates containing factor IX (II, VII, IX, X complex) should not be used to replace an acquired deficiency of multiple factors because of the high hepatitis risk of these concentrates.[143]

Deficiency of Factor VIII

Deficiencies of coagulation factors may exist as isolated or combined deficiencies and may be acquired or inherited. Isolated inherited deficiencies of each of the coagulation factors have been described, although the most common is hemophilia A or factor VIII deficiency. Opinions differ regarding the level of factor VIII that is desirable to attain in the management or prevention of bleeding episodes (see Chap. 39).

Factor VIII can be replaced with cryoprecipitate, fresh frozen plasma, or a number of factor VIII concentrates. These concentrates are assayed for factor VIII activity and can be stored at 4°C for extended periods. As mentioned, each bag of cryoprecipitate contains about 100 U of factor VIII (see section on preparation, storage, and characteristics of blood components). Factor VIII concentrates are reproduced by several manufacturers. These are available usually as lyophilized material containing anywhere from 200 to 1500 U of factor VIII in a volume of about 30 mL after reconstitution. Factor VIII concentrate prepared using recombinant DNA techniques is now available from the manufacturers.

One unit of factor VIII equals the factor VIII activity of 1 mL of fresh normal pooled plasma. Factor VIII levels are usually reported as a percentage of normal. The intravascular recovery of factor VIII is close to 100% so the amount of factor VIII required to achieve a specified factor VIII level can be estimated as follows:

$$\text{Weight (kg)} \times 70 \text{ mL/kg} = \text{blood volume (mL; adults)}$$

$$\text{Blood volume (mL)} \times (1 - \text{hematocrit}) = \text{plasma volume (mL)}$$

$$\text{Plasma volume (mL)} \times (\text{desired factor VIII level [\%]} - \text{initial factor VIII [\%]}) = \text{units of factor VIII required}$$

Example: To raise the factor VIII level to 50% in a 70-kg patient with a hematocrit of 40% and a factor VIII level of 0%:

$$70 \text{ kg} \times 70 \text{ mL/kg} = 4900 \text{ mL}$$

$$4900 \text{ mL} \times (1 - 0.4) = 2940 \text{ mL}$$

$$2940 \text{ mL} \times (0.5 - 0) = 1470 \text{ U}$$

Because each bag of cryoprecipitate contains about 100 U of factor VIII, 15 bags of cryoprecipitate are required.

When the initial factor VIII level is not known, it can be assumed to be 0% in a patient with severe classic hemophilia A. The half-life of factor VIII after transfusion is 8 to 12 hours; therefore, it is usually necessary to repeat the factor VIII transfusion at 8- to 12-hour intervals to maintain hemostatic levels. Some hemophiliacs may have an inhibitor that causes a shortened half-life of factor VIII after transfusion. The calculations just described provide an estimate of the factor VIII level attained immediately after transfusion, and the dosage should be adjusted so that the minimum desired level is reached before the next transfusion.

Example: If the desired minimum factor VIII level is 30% and the half-life of factor VIII is 12 hours, it is necessary to elevate the patient's initial factor VIII to 60% so that the level just before the next dose will be 30%. Patient's plasma volume = 2940 mL (from preceding example). Required: 2940 mL × (60 − 0) or 1764 U to elevate factor VIII to 60%. Twelve hours later, half of the factor VIII remains; thus, the factor VIII level is 30%. For the next dose of factor VIII, 2940 × (0.6 − 0.3) or only 882 U is required to elevate factor VIII to 60%.

After the dose of factor VIII is determined, the necessary amount of cryoprecipitate or factor VIII concentrate can be calculated easily. The duration of treatment with factor VIII depends on the type and location of the hemorrhage and on the clinical response of the patient.

Deficiency of Factor IX

Isolated inherited deficiency of factor IX is called *hemophilia B* and is clinically similar to hemophilia A. Factor IX is stable in plasma when stored at 4° or −20°C. Thus, stored blood, liquid plasma, or fresh frozen plasma can be used to replace factor IX. It is difficult to replace large amounts of factor IX because of the volume of these components. Within the last few years, commercial preparations containing concentrated factor IX (II, VII, IX, X complex) have become available and can be used when large amounts of factor IX must be administered. Hepatitis is a major risk in transfusion of factor IX concentrates.[143] A purified factor IX concentrate is now available, and this is replacing factor IX complex for the treatment of hemophilia B.

Hypofibrinogenemia

Hypofibrinogenemia may occur as an isolated inherited deficiency or may be acquired secondary to obstetric complications, disseminated intravascular coagulation (DIC), and some forms of cancer. In acquired hypofibrinogenemia, treatment should be directed toward the underlying cause of the disease rather than toward replacement of fibrinogen. Many physicians provide fibrinogen replacement during correction of the underlying disorder. Usually, a fibrinogen level of 50 mg/dL prevents spontaneous hemorrhage, and 100 mg/dL allows adequate hemostasis after trauma or surgery.[144] Cryoprecipitate is usually used as the source of fibrinogen for replacement therapy.[145] The dose of fibrinogen can be determined by either of the following: 100 mg fibrinogen per kg of body weight raises the fibrinogen to more than 100 mg/dL[144]; or, one bag of cryoprecipitate per 100 mL plasma volume increases the fibrinogen to 200 mg/dL. Since each bag of cryoprecipitate from a single donor contains about 200 mg of fibrinogen, the dose of fibrinogen for an adult is 6000 to 8000 mg, although this varies according to the patient's fibrinogen level. Thus, usually about 30 bags of cryoprecipitate are used. If cryoprecipitate is used as a source of fibrinogen, a quality control program should be established by the blood bank so that its fibrinogen content will be known.

Transfusion Techniques and Blood Group Compatibility of Components Used to Replace Coagulation Factors

In the transfusion of plasma components, procedures of patient and blood component identification, venipuncture, infusion solutions, and the use of filters are the same as described for red cell transfusion. Since serious reactions may occur during the transfusion of plasma components, the attendant should obtain the patient's vital signs before initiating transfusion. The patient should be reevaluated about 15 minutes later to ensure that the transfusion is proceeding uneventfully and evaluated at the end of the transfusion to determine whether any adverse reaction has occurred. The rate of administration should be as rapid as possible, but it depends on the patient's ability to tolerate the volume being transfused. Usually, one unit of plasma with a volume of about 200 mL can be given in 30 minutes. Fresh frozen plasma need not be ABO-identical but should be compatible with the recipient's red cells (see Table 60-6) and can be given without regard to Rh type. Red cell compatibility testing is not necessary.

Cryoprecipitate should also be administered as ABO-compatible whenever possible. Although the volume of each unit is small, most therapy involves many units; thus, the total volume of plasma may be large. Cryoprecipitate can be administered without regard to Rh type. While compatibility testing is not necessary, ABO-incompatible cryoprecipitate and commercial concentrated preparations of factor VIII contain anti-A and anti-B, which may cause a positive direct antiglobulin test or a hemolytic anemia if massive doses are administered.[146] In addition, the recipient's fibrinogen may become elevated by the fibrinogen contained in cryoprecipitate if many units are given.

Transfusion of Platelets

Indications for Platelet Transfusion

Platelets may be transfused either to prevent bleeding (prophylactic) or to treat active bleeding. The decision whether to transfuse platelets depends on the clinical condition of the patient, the cause of the thrombocytopenia, the platelet count, and the functional ability of the patient's own platelets. Patients with transient thrombocytopenia due to chemotherapy for malignancy including bone marrow transplantation form the largest group of patients receiving platelet transfusions.[147] Most of the transfusions to these patients are for prophylaxis of bleeding (Table 60-15). Hemorrhage is the major cause of death in patients with bone marrow failure.[148] Little risk of spontaneous hemorrhage is present when the platelet concentration is more than 20,000/μL, but the risk increases with lower platelet concentrations.[149] Because of ethical concerns, there are few controlled studies of prophylactic platelet transfusion. The available studies support the use of prophylactic transfusions, and many physicians use platelet transfusions to prevent serious bleeding when the platelet concentration is lower than 20,000/μL.[150–152] Others, however, withhold prophylactic platelet transfusions or use them only when the platelet count is considerably lower.[153,154] The typical dose of platelets in a prophylactic platelet transfusion is one unit per 10 kg body weight per day. No evidence shows that large prophylactic doses of platelets are necessary to maintain the platelet concentrations at higher levels. Some patients with stable but low platelet counts such as those with aplastic anemia or autoimmune thrombocytopenia have little evidence of bleeding and do not require prophylactic platelet transfusions.[155]

When considering platelet transfusion in a bleeding patient, data relating the bleeding time to the platelet count are helpful. Platelet transfusions are not necessary for bleeding patients with a platelet concentration over 100,000/μL because these patients have a normal bleeding time.[156] With platelet concentrations below 100,000/μL, the bleeding time is increasingly prolonged, although it is only slightly prolonged when the platelet concentration is above 75,000/mL. The optimal platelet level to achieve in a bleeding patient is not known. In one study of patients with platelet concentrations less than 100,000/μL who were undergoing surgery, prophylactic platelet transfusions were given to those whose platelet concentration was less than 50,000/μL.[157] Bleeding was similar in patients with less than 50,000/μL who received platelet transfusion compared with those whose platelet concentration was greater than 50,000/μL but did not receive platelet transfusion. The bleeding did not relate to the platelet concentration but to the severity of the surgical procedure. Thus, in actively bleeding patients, platelet transfusion should be considered in patients with a platelet concentration of less about 75,000/μL. An attempt to achieve a level greater than 50,000/μL is recommended. If the patient's platelets are dysfunctional, as from drugs, the bleeding time may be much longer than would be expected based on the degree of thrombocytopenia. In those situations, the decision to give a platelet transfusion is made on clinical grounds alone.

In patients with autoimmune thrombocytopenic purpura, the bleeding time also is prolonged when the platelet concentration is less than 100,000/μL.[156] Spontaneous bleeding is uncommon despite the level of thrombocytopenia, possibly because the few platelets circulating are young and provide a shorter bleeding time than would be expected for that degree of thrombocytopenia.[156] These patients have platelet autoantibodies; thus, transfused platelets usually have a short survival and limited effectiveness. Platelet transfusion may be effective in controlling serious active bleeding (as in surgery) but is not recommended for prevention of bleeding.

In patients with drug-induced immune thrombocytopenia, the offending drug should be discontinued and the patient closely observed. Because transfused platelets have shortened survival, they are recommended in these patients only for treatment of severe thrombocytopenia with active hemorrhage.

TABLE 60-15. Situations in Which Platelet Transfusion May Be Necessary

DECREASED PRODUCTION
Chemotherapy
Aplastic anemia
Irradiation
INCREASED DESTRUCTION
Disseminated intravascular coagulation
Thrombotic thrombocytopenia purpura
Cavernous hemangioma
Autoimmune thrombocytopenia
Drug-induced immune thrombocytopenia
Neonatal alloimmune thrombocytopenia
DILUTION
Massive transfusion
PLATELET DYSFUNCTION
Exposure to certain drugs
Congenital platelet defects (name)
Damage due to extracorporeal devices
Extracorporeal membrane oxygenator
Cardiopulmonary bypass instruments
Metabolic effects
Uremia

Outcome of Platelet Transfusion

A dose–response effect is seen from platelet transfusion. One to 3 hours after transfusion, the platelet concentration increases about 10,000/μL when 1×10^{11} platelets are transfused into a 70-kg patient.[158] A platelet concentrate usually contains about 0.7×10^{11} platelets, which should cause a platelet concentration increase of 5000 to 10,000/μL in an average-sized adult. Thus, in an adult with 1.8 m^2 body surface area, if it is desired to elevate the platelet concentration from 5000 to 40,000/μL, seven units of platelet concentrate would be required: (40,000 ÷ 5000) 5000 = 7. Another simpler way to determine the dose of platelets is to give one unit of platelet concentrate per 10 kg of body weight. This should increase the platelet concentration about 40,000/μL. The 1-hour posttransfusion platelet concentration is an excellent predictor of an effective platelet transfusion.[159]

Lack of Response to Platelet Transfusion (Refractoriness)

Many patients do not attain the expected posttransfusion increment in platelet concentration because platelet survival can be affected by many clinical factors in the patient. If splenomegaly exists, many of the transfused platelets are sequestered in the spleen and do not remain in the circulation.[160] In patients who have platelet antibodies, such as those with autoimmune thrombocytopenic purpura or those who are immunized to antigens of the HLA system, survival of circulating platelets is extremely brief, sometimes only a matter of minutes. In a careful study of 941 platelet transfusions to 133 patients, Bishop and colleagues[161] found the following factors to be associated with a reduced response to transfusion: DIC, amphotericin administration, palpable spleen, presence of HLA antibody, presence of platelet antibody, and status after marrow transplantation and fever. Active bleeding previously thought to be associated with a reduced response to platelet transfusion was not found to be so in this study. Thus, patients can be refractory as a result of alloimmunization (HLA or platelet antibodies) or nonimmune factors.

The exact percentage of patients whose refractoriness is caused by alloimmunization compared with that caused by nonimmune factors is not known. In one study, about 38% of patients who received multiple platelet transfusions, such as those with acute leukemia or undergoing bone marrow transplantation, become refractory to platelets.[162] This occurred after about nine transfusions involving 61 units of platelets. It appears that patients who become refractory do so after relatively few transfusions and that some patients do not become refractory, regardless of the number of transfusions.[162] In some studies, refractoriness is associated with the presence of HLA antibodies,[159,163] although no generally accepted laboratory test is available that defines with high precision refractoriness due to alloimmunization. Many of these refractory patients also have one or more clinical factors that could account at least partly for the refractoriness. Because of the difficulty in managing patients who are refractory to platelet transfusion, considerable interest exists in preventing alloimmunization. This has been attempted using single-donor platelets,[164] leukocyte-poor blood components,[165] and ultraviolet irradiation.[166]

Lack of response to platelet transfusion is often associated with bleeding. Patients are usually ill with problems such as fever, sepsis, DIC, or viral infections. Whether patients with similar clinical problems who are responsive to platelets have fewer bleeding problems has not been established. Because refractoriness is often associated with bleeding and a poor outcome, it is important to define the steps that can be taken to improve the response to transfusion in these patients.

Management of the Patient Refractory to Platelet Transfusion

Clinical factors such as infection that might cause refractoriness should be sought and, if present, appropriate treatment should be initiated to correct them. Other simple steps that may be helpful are the use of ABO-compatible platelets or platelets less than 24 hours old and review of the techniques for platelet transfusion to ensure that platelets are not being damaged or lost because of improper handling after leaving the blood bank. Because ABO incompatibility appears to result in a reduced posttransfusion recovery,[67,122,167] posttransfusion response may be improved by giving ABO-incompatible platelets. Platelets stored for several days may also give reduced increments[168]; thus, a transfusion of fresher platelets should be attempted.

If these measures fail, efforts should be made to use platelets that are matched to the recipient. Refractoriness due to alloimmunization is primarily caused by HLA- and platelet-specific antibodies. Thus, an improved response may be obtained by selecting a platelet donor whose HLA type matches that of the recipient.[121,169,170] If the patient has an HLA-identical sibling, those platelets may be effective.[171] Many blood banks also have large files of HLA-typed volunteer donors so that HLA-matched platelets can be located for most patients. Most HLA-matched platelets obtained from unrelated donors have some antigens mismatched with the patient. Although the average response to these partially matched transfusions is similar to that from fully matched HLA-identical transfusions, about 30% of HLA-matched transfusions do not provide a satisfactory response.[121,169,170] Also, since these patients require frequent platelet transfusions, many donors who are matched to the patient must be available to sustain the patient for days or a few weeks.[172]

Another approach that should be effective is crossmatching the patient's serum and the potential donor's cells. Many studies of the value of platelet crossmatching have been done, but it is difficult to draw conclusions broad enough to determine appropriate transfusion practice.[67] Although it appears that in most patients HLA antibodies are responsible for refractoriness, platelet-specific antibodies may sometimes be involved. Thus, the optimal in vitro method that should be used for platelet crossmatching is not known. The positive predictive value of platelet crossmatching ranged from 73 to 100% and the negative predictive value 52% to 92% in 10 studies summarized by Heal and coworkers.[67] Thus, in patients with no complicating clinical factors other than apparent alloimmunization, substantial numbers of patients experienced a successful transfusion despite an incompatible crossmatch or an unsuccessful transfusion despite a compatible crossmatch. Platelet crossmatching is performed in some centers and generally appears about as effective as HLA matching.[173] A practical suggested strategy for dealing with patients who are refractory to platelet transfusion is as follows:

1. Treat any correctable clinical factors present that may cause platelet refractoriness. Until these factors are eliminated, recognize that any of the following steps may not be effective.
2. Ensure that the patient is receiving the correct dose of platelets.
3. Give at least one test transfusion of platelets that are not more than 48 hours old and preferably less than 24 hours old.
4. Ensure that platelets being transfused are ABO-compatible.
5. If these steps have failed, give at least one and preferably two or three transfusions of HLA-matched platelets.
6. Determine whether the patient has HLA- or platelet-specific (or both) antibodies. If so and if HLA-matched platelets are unsuccessful, give a transfusion of crossmatch-compatible platelets.

Other strategies that have not generally been effective are use of cyclosporine, plasma exchange, and intravenous immunoglobulin.

Granulocyte Transfusion

An inverse relation exists between the granulocyte count and the presence of infection. As the granulocyte count falls below 1000/mL, risk of infection increases,[174] which is further increased by the duration of granulocytopenia.[175] The increasingly common and aggressive treatment of patients with hematologic malignancies and aplastic anemia has made granulocytopenia common. During the early 1970s, almost 80% of deaths in patients with bone marrow failure were due to infection.[148,174] Because of the success of platelet transfusion in the management of hemorrhage due to thrombocytopenia, considerable interest existed in transfusion of granulocytes for the management of infection in granulocytopenic patients. Because of the small number of granulocytes in the peripheral blood of normal humans, collection of cells for transfusion has been difficult. During the late 1960s and early 1970s, several blood cell separators were devised to allow collection of about 1×10^{10} granulocytes from a normal donor.[8] These cells function normally in vitro and have normal in vivo survival and migration to sites of infection.[8,176]

A variety of patients have been involved in clinical studies of granulocyte transfusions, including those with acute leukemia, chronic leukemias, aplastic anemia, Hodgkin's disease, lymphoma, and solid tumors. Patients with fever of unknown origin do not experience improvement as a result of granulocyte transfusion.[177] Most clinical trials of granulocyte transfusion involve patients with gram-negative bacteremia,[178] and little information is available regarding other organisms. Also, little information is available that collates the site of infection other than bacteremia with response to granulocyte transfusion.[178] A series of studies in the 1970s established that granulocyte transfusion provided improved survival in patients with documented gram-negative sepsis who remained granulocytopenic for at least 10 days.[179,180] Some additional data indicated that granulocytes may be helpful in patients with other kinds of documented infections (either gram-positive or gram-negative) and with granulocytopenia of more than 10 days' duration.[180]

Most patients can be expected to respond to antibiotics, and granulocyte transfusion is rarely used for bacterial infections. Granulocyte transfusion should not be initiated for at least 96 hours after the onset of clinical signs or symptoms of an infection. This allows transfusions to be given only to patients who do not respond to antibiotics. Many patients who do not respond have severe (less than 100/μL) and prolonged neutropenia. The fever may be due to documented or assumed fungal infection, which requires amphotericin therapy.[181,182] When signs and symptoms of infection persist in these patients, granulocyte transfusions are often used. No clinical trials have documented the effectiveness of granulocyte transfusion for fungal infections, although animal[183] and clinical[184] studies support their use and granulocytes kill fungi in vitro.

The minimum dose of granulocytes required for clinical efficacy has not been established. Results have been encouraging from the use of about 5×10^9 granulocytes/m^2/d[179]; this represents less than 5% of the total daily granulocyte production by normal humans. Thus, most investigators believe it is necessary to transfuse at least 1×10^{10} granulocytes each day. The minimum number of transfusions necessary for improvement differs depending on the patient's clinical status. Granulocyte transfusion should be used as a course of treatment similar to that of antibiotics. Monitoring clinical symptoms such as temperature elevation as a means of deciding daily whether to use granulocyte transfusions can be misleading and creates logistical problems with procurement of granulocytes. Since antibiotics would not be discontinued on the basis of brief clinical improvement, after granulocyte transfusions have been initiated they should be continued daily until the patient's general condition has stabilized and improved. In general, it is advisable to consider a course of granulocyte transfusion therapy for at least 7 days.

Most experience with granulocyte transfusion involves treatment of existing infection. At one time, considerable interest existed in the use of granulocytes to prevent infection in granulocytopenia patients. Prophylactic granulocyte transfusions are not helpful in this regard for newly diagnosed patients with acute myelogenous leukemia.[185]

Blood Derivatives

With the use of large-scale separation and manufacturing techniques, several proteins can be isolated from plasma and prepared for therapeutic use. These proteins are called blood derivatives and include a large number of blood proteins (see Table 60-2).

Procedures for the fractionation of plasma became available during the 1940s. The process involves processing a large pool of plasma, usually 10,000 L (50,000 donor units) using cold ethanol fractionation. Different plasma proteins have different solubilities that allow their separation. This process has for over 40 years provided the blood derivatives, albumin, immune serum, γ-globulin, and, during the past 20 years, coagulation factor VIII concentrate and, more recently, factor IX complex concentrate. Until the past few years, techniques were not available to sterilize some blood derivatives after manufacture. Thus, because of the large number of units of donor plasma in each pool, the probability of contamination of the pool with viruses (hepatitis, HIV, and others) was high, and the risk of disease transmission from these nonsterilized blood derivatives was high.[143,186] This risk was accentuated because much of the plasma that serves as the raw material for the manufacture of blood derivatives was obtained from paid donors; a group known to provide blood with an increased likelihood of transmitting disease.[187] Until recently, only albumin and immune globulin carried no risk of disease transmission: albumin because it was sterilized by heating and immune globulin because none of the known infectious agents were contained in that fraction prepared from the plasma or the procedure renders them noninfectious. Because of the recognition of the high risk of disease transmission by coagulation factor concentrates, methods were developed to sterilize them.[188] About 1989, factor VIII concentrates that are prepared using monoclonal antibody technology became available. These also can be treated to prevent transmission of lipid-enveloped viruses such as hepatitis B and HIV.[189] However, these methods do not inactivate viruses that lack a lipid envelope, such as hepatitis A and parvovirus. A risk of transmission of these agents remains.

Coagulation Factor VIII and IX Concentrates

See Chapters 39 and 40 for a more detailed discussion.

Immune Serum Globulins

The γ-globulin (immune globulin]) prepared by the traditional plasma fractionation technique contained aggregated or oligomeric molecules of immune globulin, which, when injected intravenously, activated complement and resulted in severe reactions.[190] Administration of γ-globulin intramuscularly has been effective in preventing bacterial infections in patients with agammaglobulinemia and in preventing certain viral infections in immunologically normal persons (Table 60-16). Several important limitations were created by the necessity of intramuscular administration (Table 60-17). Immune globulin suitable for intravenous administration became available in the United States in about 1985. Four brands are available (Table 60-18). These are prepared from the plasma of normal donors and can be expected to have an antibody content reflective of normal healthy persons in a large population. Some differences are found in the IgA content, the relative proportions of IgG subclasses, and in vitro activity against some

TABLE 60-16. Clinical Uses of Intramuscular Immune Serum Globulin

Disease	Ig Preparation
Hepatitis A	ISG
Hepatitis B	HBIG
Measles	ISG
Chickenpox	VZIG
Rabies	RIG
Humoral immunodeficiency	ISG

TABLE 60-17. **Comparison in IMIg and IVIg**

Issues	IMIg	IVIg
Cost	Low	High
Bioavailability	60% dose degraded at injection site	100% of dose bioavailable
Patient tolerance	Injection painful	Injection minimally painful
Allergic reactions	Few, minor	More likely; may be systematic and severe
Plasma IgG	Difficult to maintain	Easy to maintain
Dose	Limited	High dose possible
Indications	Replacement therapy Viral prophylaxis	Replacement therapy; viral prophylaxis immunomodulation

(Adpated from Sacher RA. Intravenous gammaglobulin products: development, pharmacology, and precautions. In: Garner RJ, Sacher RA, eds. Intravenous gammaglobulin therapy. Arlington, VA, American Association of Blood Banks, 1988:1)

viruses. The differences in IgA content are clinically important, since the brands that contain much IgA may cause a reaction if given to an IgA-deficient patient with anti-IgA. The clinical significance of other differences among the brands has not been established.

Intravenous immune globulin is approved for use by the FDA for treatment of persons with impaired humoral immunity, specifically for primary (congenital) immune deficiency, and for (idiopathic) autoimmune thrombocytopenia. The value of intravenous immune globulin in other immune deficiency states such as in AIDS has not been established.

As with immune globulin preparations used intramuscularly, intravenous immune globulin with especially high activity against a particular virus can be prepared from plasma that has a high level of antibody to that virus. Such preparations of intravenous CMV immune globulin have shown promise in clinical trials, but these are not yet widely available.[191,192]

The availability of intravenous immune globulin makes it possible to maintain the serum IgG level at near normal in immune-deficient patients. The amount required varies with the size of the patient and the indication. Usually, 100 to 200 mg/kg/mo is used as a starting dose for patients with primary immune deficiencies. Larger doses are usually used for patients with autoimmune thrombocytopenic purpura. The half-life of the intravenous immune globulin is 21 to 25 days, which is similar to native IgG.

Adverse reactions to intravenous immunoglobulin occur in 2% to 10% of patients' injections. Reactions are local, such as erythema, pain, phlebitis, and eczema. Systemic symptoms include fever, chills, myalgias, back pain, nausea, and vomiting. Some reactions in some patients are dose related and can be reduced or eliminated by slowing the rate of infusion. The nature and incidence of adverse reactions may differ among the different products, but is not clear and is beyond the scope of this chapter.

Because intravenous immune globulin is made from large pools of human plasma, it contains a variety of antibodies, including those against blood groups and possibly anti-HB_s, anti-HB_c, anti-CMV, and others. Donor screening should eliminate some of these (anti-HIV), but patients may have transiently positive tests for certain antibodies that are passively acquired from intravenous immune globulin. For instance, marrow transplantation patients being treated with intravenous immune globulin had a 49% incidence of positive direct antiglobulin test and 25% incidence of positive red cell antibody detection.[193] Transient hemolysis has been reported in autoimmune thrombocytopenic purpura patients being treated with intravenous immune globulin.[193] Thus, although hemolysis is unusual, a larger proportion of patients receiving intravenous immune globulin develop circulating or cell-bound blood group antibodies. This possibility should be considered if unexplained hemolysis occurs in patients being treated with intravenous immune globulin.

Cytomegalovirus-Negative Blood Components

Cytomegalovirus can be transmitted by blood transfusion with a severe, even fatal result (see section on transfusion-transmitted diseases). Transfusion-transmitted CMV can be prevented by using CMV antibody-negative blood components. This section describes the indications for CMV-negative blood components in different situations.

Neonates

Landmark studies by Yaeger and colleagues[194] established that neonates weighing less than 1200 g born to CMV-negative mothers were at substantial risk of developing CMV disease if they received blood from CMV antibody-positive donors. Serious disease or death occurred in 50% of infected neonates. These observations have been supported by some studies but not by others. This is not surprising because of the large variation in the rate of occurrence of CMV in blood donors in different parts of the United States. It has been suggested that at least some of the differences in the studies just described could be accounted for by a changing incidence of transfusion-transmitted CMV infection due to differences in techniques of CMV testing of donated blood, less frequent use of fresh blood components, greater use of plasma containing CMV antibodies, and a changing donor population due to HIV and non-A, non-B hepatitis screening practices. Because the magnitude of this problem varies considerably, the incidence of CMV disease in neonates should be established locally to determine whether CMV antibody-negative blood components should be provided. In practice, most neonatologists have elected to use CMV-negative blood components routinely for patients weighing less than 1200 g.

Pregnant Women

Cytomegalovirus infection of the fetus is a severe clinical problem causing growth or mental retardation or both, hepatitis, deafness, intracranial calcifications, and bleeding diathesis. Congenital CMV infections due to primary infection in the mother are usually more serious than those due to recurrent maternal CMV infection.[195] Thus, it is prudent to avoid primary CMV infection in pregnant

TABLE 60-18. General Comparison of Intravenous Immune Globulin Products

Category	Gammagard	Sandoglobulin	Gamimune-N	American Red Cross
Manufacturer	Hyland	Sandoz	Cutter	Baxter (Hyland) Health Care
Method of preparation	Cohn-Oncley ion-exchange ultrafiltration	Cohn-Oncley ph 4 + pepsin	Cohn-Oncley pH 4.25 + low salt	Cohn-Oncley ion-exchange ultrafiltration
Indication	Primary immunodeficiencies + ITP	Primary immunodeficiencies + ITP	Primary immunodeficiencies + ITP	Primary Immunodeficiencies + ITP
Contraindication	None‡	IgA deficiency with antibodies to IgA	IgA deficiency with antibodies to IgA	None†
IgA content	1.6 U/mL	720 U/mL	270 U/mL	10 μg/mL or less
Adverse reactions	<6%	2.5%	2.6% systemic 11.6% local 43.8% (local/adult ITP)	<6%
pH (after reconstitution)	6.8	6.6	4.25	6.8
Donors in pool	4000–5000	8000	2000	65,000
Half-life	24 d	23 d	21 d	24 d
Gamma-globulin	>90%	96%	98%	>90%
Monomers	95%	92%	95%	93%
IgG subclass*				
IgG1	67%	55%	67%	65%†
IgG2	25%	36%	27%	23%†
IgG3	7%	6%	5%	8%†
IgG4	<1%	3%	<1%	4%†
Shelf life	27 mo	36 mo	24 mo	24 mo
Reconstitution time	5 min	5 min	In solution	5 min
Administration	Filter required	No filter	No filter	Filter required
Storage	Room temperature	Room temperature	Refrigerate	Room temperature

* ITP, idiopathic thrombocytopenic purpura.
† Based on information from American Red Cross.
‡ Caution with IgA deficiency.
(Adapted from Skvaril F, Gardi A. Differences among available immunoglobulin preparations for intravenous use. Pediatr Infect Dis J 1988;7:S-43.)

women. Although no specific clinical studies of this situation have been reported, it is advisable to provide CMV antibody-negative blood to pregnant women or for intrauterine transfusion of the fetus.[196]

Kidney Transplantation

Cytomegalovirus disease is common in renal transplant recipients, occurring in 60% to 90% of patients. Because CMV can be serious, causing graft rejection or even death, its prevention is important. The cause of CMV disease in these patients may be reactivation of latent previous CMV infection; acquisition of CMV from the donor organ; or acquisition of CMV from blood transfusion. CMV incidence ranges from 30% to 70% in the blood donor population, and most renal transplantation patients have received previous transfusions, further increasing the proportion of those who have previous CMV infection.[197] Thus, reactivation of a previous infection is by far the most common cause of CMV disease in these patients.[198,199]

About 77% of CMV antibody-negative patients who receive a kidney from a CMV antibody-positive donor develop CMV infection compared with 8% to 20% in similar patients who receive a kidney from a CMV antibody-negative donor but receive CMV antibody-positive blood transfusions.[198,199] If CMV antibody-negative patients receive a kidney from a CMV antibody-negative donor and then receive CMV antibody-negative blood components, the possibility of developing CMV infection is almost zero.[199] Thus, it is advisable to provide CMV antibody-negative blood components for the latter patients.

Renal transplantation patients with anti-CMV may develop CMV disease from acquisition of a second strain of the virus from the donor organ.[200] Acquisition of a second strain of CMV by blood transfusion has not been reported. Thus, providing CMV antibody-negative blood components for CMV antibody-positive patients to avoid acquiring a new CMV strain is not recommended until and unless this is shown to be a larger clinical problem than it appears.

Bone Marrow Transplantation

A major complication of marrow transplantation, CMV is more common and more severe in these patients because they are more severely immunosuppressed than solid organ recipients. CMV disease occurs in 40% to 50% of patients undergoing allogeneic marrow transplantation and is an important source of posttransplantation mortality.[201] As with renal transplantation, most CMV disease in marrow transplantation patients occurs in patients with CMV antibody and is probably due to reactivation of virus from a previrus infection, not to acquisition of a new strain.[202] In CMV antibody-negative patients who receive marrow from a CMV antibody-negative donor, the risk of developing CMV infection is about 40%.[202] The likelihood of these patients acquiring CMV infection is almost eliminated by the use of CMV antibody-negative blood components.[202,203] Thus, it is customary to provide CMV antibody-negative blood components to CMV antibody-negative marrow transplantation patients whose marrow donor is CMV antibody-negative. Providing CMV antibody-negative blood components for marrow transplantation patients may be difficult in areas with a large marrow transplantation program and a high CMV incidence in the donor population. Other approaches under study for the prevention of CMV infection are the use of CMV intravenous immunoglobulin,[191,192] ordinary intravenous immunoglobulin,[204] or leukocyte-poor blood components.[205,206]

The intravenous immunoglobulin is extremely expensive and the availability of CMV intravenous immunoglobulin is limited. Since most CMV disease occurs in marrow transplantation patients who are CMV antibody-positive, extension of the use of CMV antibody-negative blood components to potential marrow transplantation patients who are CMV antibody-negative has been suggested. Thus, they would not become infected with CMV as a result of transfusions received earlier in their disease and before entering a marrow transplantation program. This would create major, if not impossible, logistic problems for blood banks to attempt to provide these products for many patients with leukemia, other hematologic malignancies, aplastic anemia, and inherited metabolic disease. This practice has not been shown to be necessary or cost-effective and is not recommended.

Heart, Heart–Lung, Liver, and Pancreas Transplantation

Few data are available describing CMV infections in patients with heart, heart–lung, liver, and pancreas transplantation. One small study of heart transplantation patients demonstrated that CMV infection was transmitted by either the donor heart or blood components.[207] When both the donor organ and all blood components were CMV antibody-negative, CMV infection was prevented in heart[207] as well as liver[208] transplant recipients. A more recent study of heart transplantations showed a low (1.5%) incidence of CMV infection.[209] Although the data are not extensive and are conflicting for these transplantation situations, the patients are immune-suppressed and CMV infection is a clinical problem that can be prevented by the use of CMV antibody-negative blood components. This practice is advisable in CMV antibody-negative patients who receive an organ from a CMV antibody-negative donor. CMV infections in CMV antibody-positive heart transplantation patients are due to reactivation of latent virus[210]; therefore, the use of CMV antibody-negative blood components is not indicated for these patients.

Acquired Immunodeficiency Syndrome

Patients with acquired immunodeficiency syndrome (AIDS) have severely impaired immune function, and CMV infections are an important clinical problem for them. Thus, use of CMV antibody-negative blood components is indicated for CMV antibody-negative AIDS patients, although no clinical trials have been carried out to form the basis for this practice. The same potential extension of the use of CMV antibody-negative blood components mentioned for potential marrow transplantation patients also applies to persons infected with HIV-1. That is, use of CMV antibody-negative blood components for CMV antibody-negative patients infected with the HIV virus but who are asymptomatic. This practice would prevent the development of latent CMV infection in these patients that could reactivate later when AIDS develops. The cost-effectiveness and practicality of this approach have not been established, and use of CMV antibody-negative components for these patients is not recommended.

Severe Combined Immunodeficiency

No specific studies or data are available regarding prevention of CMV infection by the use of CMV antibody-negative components in patients with severe combined immunodeficiency. Because these patients are severely immunocompromised, provision of CMV antibody-negative blood components is the typical transfusion practice.

Patients Receiving Extensive Chemotherapy

As more varied chemotherapy regimens are used, patients are experiencing greater drug-induced immunosuppression. In general, CMV infection has not been an important clinical problem in patients receiving extensive chemotherapy. Since there is no good way of determining the level of immune function at which patients become increasingly susceptible to CMV infection, the use of CMV antibody-negative blood components is not recommended in these patients.

Irradiated Blood Components

Viable lymphocytes contained in blood components can cause fatal graft-versus-host disease (GVHD) in susceptible patients.[211] To prevent transfusion-induced GVHD, blood components are subjected to γ-radiation that interferes with the ability of lymphocytes to proliferate. Irradiation with 1500 to 5000 rad reduces the incorporation of thymidine-14C into mitogen-stimulated lymphocytes by 85% to 98.5%.[212] Lymphocyte response to allogeneic lymphocytes may be a more physiologic indicator of the ability of cells to cause GVHD. A much lower dose of radiation interferes with lymphocyte response to allogeneic cells. Only 500 rad is necessary to abolish lymphocyte proliferation in mixed lymphocyte culture.[213,214]

Doses of up to 5000 rad do not have an adverse effect on red cells, platelets, or granulocytes.[212,215] Red cell survival in vivo and certain in vitro assays are normal after up to 10,000 rad.[215] Granulocyte chemotaxis may be slightly reduced by even 500 rad, but this does not become significant until greater than 10,000 rad.[214] High doses of radiation such as 40,000 rad are required to interfere with phagocytosis and microbial killing.[214–216]

More disagreement exists about the effect of irradiation on platelets. In vitro platelet function studies have generally been normal after up to 5000 rad.[212] One study showed normal in vivo survival,[217] and one showed a 33% reduction in vivo recovery and diminished correction of the bleeding time by irradiated platelets.[215] Since Button and coworkers[215] did not observe a difference in the platelet increment after transfusion of irradiated platelets compared with that of unirradiated platelets, they concluded that 5000 rad was a clinically acceptable dose.

In almost all studies of irradiation on blood components, the cells were studied shortly after irradiation. As the use of irradiated blood components has increased, interest has developed in irradiating the components after collection and storing them for use days or weeks later. Doses of 2000 or 3000 rad to units of red cells resulted in potassium levels two and three times higher than normal after storage for 4 to 5 days.[218,219] This suggests that leakage of potassium from the red cells occurred during postirradiation storage, which indicates radiation damage to the red cell membrane or the sodium–potassium pump. Based on these studies and the lack of data establishing safety, storage of components after irradiation is not recommended.

Because it is difficult to quantitate cellular immunity, no in vitro assays are available which define the degree of immunodeficiency that makes a patient susceptible to transfusion-associated GVHD. Even if better assays were available, these assays probably would not be helpful because the degree of HLA matching between patient and blood donor may be a factor in the likelihood of the occurrence of GVHD. In the following situations, patients are so severely immunocompromised that transfusion-associated GVHD is likely unless blood components are irradiated:

Fetuses. Fatal GVHD can occur from viable lymphocytes in blood used for intrauterine or exchange transfusion.[220] All blood components used for these indications should be irradiated.

Neonates. Although neonates do not have adult levels of immune competence, few reports exist of transfusion-associated GVHD in neonates.[220,221] No evidence has been found that newborns who do not have a congenital immunodeficiency are at increased risk of developing transfusion-associated GVHD. Routine irradiation of blood components for all neonates is not recommended.

Persons with congenital immunodeficiency. Patients with severe combined immunodeficiency syndrome or Wiskott-Aldrich syndrome have severe defects in immunity. These patients have a high probability of developing transfusion-associated GVHD, even from one unit of fresh plasma and should receive irradiated blood components.[220,222]

Persons undergoing allogeneic bone marrow transplantation. These patients are severely immunocompromised by the radiation with or without chemotherapy, which was given to prepare them for the transplantation and in many situations to eradicate residual disease. The GVHD that commonly follows allogeneic bone marrow transplantation is due to viable lymphocytes in the donor marrow.[211] Irradiation of all blood components became routine, but, as a result, no data are available that describe the risk of development of transfusion-associated GVHD in allogeneic bone marrow transplant recipients. The risk can be presumed to be extremely high, and so irradiated blood components are used routinely.[211] Unless the allogeneic bone marrow transplantation patient has a disease that necessitates the use of irradiated blood products, these products are not necessary until the transplantation preparation regimen is begun. Before that time, the blood components should be selected based on the patient's underlying disease.

Persons undergoing autologous bone marrow transplantation. Although there are some differences in the irradiation and chemotherapy preparation for patients undergoing autologous and those undergoing allogeneic bone marrow transplantation, generally patients undergoing autologous bone marrow transplantation are severely immunocompromised. Because the use of irradiated blood components was an established a custom in allogeneic bone marrow transplantation, this practice has been adopted for autologous bone marrow transplantation without clinical or laboratory study.

Several other clinical situations are noted in which isolated cases of transfusion-associated GVHD have been reported and for which a few medical centers use irradiated blood components. There is no consensus on recommended practice.

Hematologic malignancies. Some patients with acute leukemia, lymphoma, or Hodgkin's disease who are receiving chemotherapy often along with radiation have developed transfusion-associated GVHD.[223–227] The risk of transfusion-associated GVHD in these patients has been estimated at 0.1% to 1.0%, but this risk is difficult to determine because of the lack of comprehensive follow-up studies.[228] The data are insufficient to establish whether blood components for these patients should be routinely irradiated.

Aplastic anemia. Patients with aplastic anemia usually do not have defective cellular immunity. No cases of transfusion-associated GVHD due to transfusion of normal cells have been documented. Thus, use of irradiated blood components is not necessary.

Solid tumors. One patient with neuroblastoma and one with glioblastoma have developed transfusion-associated GVHD.[226,229] Some treatment protocols for these patients result in rather severe immune compromise; the data are not adequate to recommend irradiation of blood products for these patients except in therapy involving severe immunodeficiency.

AIDS. Despite the fact that AIDS patients have severely impaired immune function, no cases of transfusion-associated GVHD have been reported. This may be because these patients receive irradiated blood components in some centers. The risk of developing transfusion-associated GVHD is not known for AIDS patients.

Transfusion-associated GVHD and granulocyte transfusions. During the 1970s, there was concern that granulocyte transfusion posed a greater risk of transfusion-associated GVHD than other cellular blood components.[230] This risk was probably due to the increased risk of transfusion-associated GVHD from transfused chronic myelogenous leukemia cells,[231] not from normal donor cells. Thus, routine irradiation of granulocyte concentrates obtained from normal donors is not necessary. The decision to irradiate granulocytes should be based on the patient's underlying condition. Chronic myelogenous leukemia cells are rarely used for transfusions but, if so, they should be irradiated.

Irradiation of noncellular blood components. Transfusion-associated GVHD has occurred in patients with congenital immunodeficiency after transfusion of fresh liquid plasma,[222,232,233] but has not been reported to be caused by previously frozen components, fresh frozen plasma, or cryoprecipitate. These components contain fragments of leukocytes but few, if any, viable lymphocytes. They would not be expected to cause transfusion-associated GVHD. Although irradiation of fresh frozen plasma and cryoprecipitate is probably not necessary, many blood banks irradiate these components to avoid clerical errors in which a cellular blood component might not be irradiated when necessary.

Transfusion-associated GVHD from partially HLA-matched, related, or unrelated donors. Several years ago, some cases of transfusion-associated GVHD occurred after transfusion from relatives who were partially HLA-matched with the patient[222,226,233] or from unrelated but partially HLA-matched donors.[223,234] This raised the concern that transfusion-associated GVHD might develop in patients not severely immunocompromised if there was partial HLA matching between the patient and the blood donor. Because most of the patients involved in these reports were severely immunocompromised, this remained a theoretical concern until 1989. After that, several reports suggested that this situation might be more common than previously believed. Thaler and colleagues[235] reported transfusion-associated GVHD apparently due to fresh blood donated by children in two immunocompetent patients who underwent cardiac surgery. In each case, one of the blood donors was homozygous for an HLA class I antigen haplotype shared with the recipient. Thus, the recipient would not have recognized the HLA class I antigens as foreign. Additional reports of transfusion-associated GVHD were seen in Japan in patients who received fresh blood after cardiac surgery, in a woman who received a transfusion after delivery,[236] in a cardiac surgery patient in New York,[237] and in a Japanese woman who received transfusion after cholecystectomy.[238] The apparent high incidence of this situation in Japan may be due to the rather high incidence of certain HLA antigens in the Japanese, with the likelihood that a random unrelated donor may be partially HLA-matched with the recipient. The incidence of transfusion-associated GVHD in immunocompetent patients in the United States is not know. No evidence shows that this is a problem when unrelated donors are used; the increasing use of directed donors who are related to the patient may increase the likelihood of transfusion-associated GVHD. The problem can be prevented by irradiating the blood components donated by first-degree relatives of the patient.

Neocytes

Many patients, especially those with hemoglobinopathies, require chronic transfusion therapy and may become iron overloaded. Iron chelation and removal or supertransfusion strategies have been used in these patients. Another approach is the transfusion of red cell units enriched with younger cells (neocytes) so that the transfusion requirements would be reduced. These neocyte units have increased the interval between transfusion by about 13 days (range, 30 to 43 days)[239] and have provided a 41% increase in intravascular survival.[240] Neocyte units are usually prepared by cytapheresis using blood cell separators and thus are expensive. It is not clear whether the advantages of neocytes will be sufficient to warrant their broad use in the therapy of patients requiring chronic transfusions.

Fibrin Glue

Fibrin glue refers to the use of fibrinogen in some form along with thrombin as a topical adhesive to control bleeding.[241] Fibrin glue is used predominantly by surgeons to deal with microvascular bleeding in cardiovascular surgery to reduce mediastinal drainage, to seal synthetic vascular grafts, to seal bleeding surfaces of the liver or spleen, to seal dura, for use in maxillofacial surgery, and for peripheral nerve repair.

No one specifically defined fibrin glue product is used. Cryoprecipitate dispensed in syringes can be used along with thrombin, or a more pure form of fibrinogen sometimes produced with chemical additives can be used.[241] Since fibrin glue is made from human plasma, transmission of diseases can occur. The probability of this is not known[241]; in the absence of definitive data, fibrin glue should be considered to have the same risk of disease transmission as other blood components.

Potential Role of Hematopoietic Growth Factors in Transfusion Therapy

The coming availability of hematopoietic growth factors opens a new era in transfusion medicine. The first of these, erythropoietin, can eliminate the need for red cell transfusions in most patients with end-stage renal failure.[242] Nationally, the use of erythropoietin has been estimated to eliminate as many as 50,000 transfusions.[243] These units of red cells would then be available for other patients and would allow renal failure patients to maintain higher hemoglobin levels, have an improved quality of life,[243,244] and avoid the complications of transfusions. Erythropoietin is likely to be used and may be of some value in patients with other forms of anemia, even those not due to erythropoietin deficiency. Thus, the potential exists for managing many anemic patients with erythropoietin alone or some combined strategy of erythropoietin plus red cell replacement in which the red cell transfusion requirement is substantially reduced. Erythropoietin is also being studied for its potential value in increasing autologous blood donation and in reducing the homologous blood requirements of patients undergoing elective surgery. It seems clear that this exciting new drug has the potential to drastically alter red cell transfusion practices.

Clinical trials of granulocyte-macrophage colony-stimulating factor (GM-CSF) suggest that the period of chemotherapy-induced leukopenia may be reduced in patients with malignancy or those undergoing bone marrow transplantation. Although this may have a major impact on the morbidity and mortality of these procedures, it probably will not greatly alter transfusion therapy in the near future since leukocyte replacement is not widely practiced. Reducing the incidence or severity of infection could modify transfusion therapy if sepsis and DIC are avoided, with the resulting decline in use of platelets and fresh frozen plasma.

The long-sought thrombopoietin may have been isolated recently.[244a,244b] If so, development and use of a platelet growth factor should have a major impact on transfusion medicine. The incidence of platelet transfusions has increased more rapidly than that of other blood components.[147] These tranfusions constitute a large part of the activity of most large blood banks. The ability to shorten the duration of thrombocytopenia, reduce the risk of hemorrhage, and reduce the need for platelet transfusion has a great potential benefit and would affect many patients with chemotherapy-induced thrombocytopenia. The effect of a platelet growth factor and GM-CSF in shortening the period of cytopenia with resultant reduction in the need for blood components could be counterbalanced by an overall increase in the number of patients being treated or by escalation in the extent of therapy given. Thus, the effect on the overall need for blood products is difficult to predict.

TRANSFUSION IN SPECIAL SITUATIONS

Acute Blood Loss

Physiology and Therapy

When patients experience acute massive blood loss, the need for volume replacement is urgent. The manifestations are due to blood volume depletion, not to depletion of red cell mass. Thus, blood loss can be replaced initially with electrolyte solutions, normal serum albumin or synthetic volume expanders such as Dextran or Volex (hydroxyethyl starch). Several compensatory mechanisms act to maintain blood flow to and oxygenation of the brain and heart. These mechanisms include adrenergic nervous system stimulation, release of vasoactive substance, hyperventilation, shift of fluid from intracellular space to extracellular space, shift of fluid from the interstitial to the intravascular space, and renal conservation of water and electrolytes. A detailed discussion of this situation is beyond the scope of this chapter.

Two major points deserve emphasis: (1) Because the manifestations of acute blood loss are due to hypovolemia, early and aggressive replacement of intravascular volume is essential. (2) Unless the patient has a very low initial hemoglobin or has severely impaired cardiovascular function, red cell replacement is not necessary during initial therapy of acute blood loss. If blood loss continues, the situation becomes one of massive transfusion and thus additional therapeutic considerations.

Blood Bank Procedures

A blood specimen should be obtained and sent to the blood bank for emergency typing and crossmatching. An ABO and Rh type can be performed quickly, and blood of the same type as the patient is selected. This blood can be released under an emergency crossmatching procedure that requires about 15 minutes. Thus, partially crossmatched blood of the patient's type can be available quickly.

Blood released using an emergency crossmatch procedure involves shortening the incubation period of patient's serum and donor's red cells. Usually, this is done in a way to detect only ABO incompatibility, since this usually provokes the most disastrous kind of transfusion reaction. Alternatively, blood may be released without a crossmatch. If the blood bank has a sample of the patient's blood, the ABO type can be determined quickly and ABO type-specific blood released without a crossmatch. Generally, Rh-positive blood is chosen, but Rh-negative blood may be used, depending on the hospital's inventory and the age and sex of the patient. When the patient's ABO type is not known, group O red cells are used. This has led to the designation of the donor of group O Rh-negative blood as a universal donor, since these red cells would not be hemolyzed by either anti-A, anti-B, or any Rh(D) antibody present, and would not immunize recipients to the D antigen. Group O Rh-negative (universal donor) red cells do not avoid the risk that the recipient may have another red cell antibody or an red cell autoantibody; therefore, hemolysis or transfusion reactions can occur. Stocking O Rh-negative red cells routinely in emergency departments is inappropriate. The red cells may not be stored properly, and there may not be a system of checks for release the units—practices that can lead to serious problems. Techniques of fluid management and resuscitation are so highly developed that patients can be maintained for the few minutes required to obtain red cells from the blood bank.

Blood bank personnel are well aware that situations may develop in which there is an urgent need for blood; thus, each blood bank should have a procedure for the rapid release of red cells.[57] In these situations, clear, concise, and informative communication from the physician to the blood bank and from the blood bank to the physician is essential. To avoid frivolous release of incompletely or uncrossmatched red cells, the blood bank personnel usually ask questions about the patient situation. The physician must take responsibility and clearly indicate the urgent nature of the patient's situation to the blood bank personnel. After the emergency has passed, the physician is expected to sign a form taking responsibility for the emergency release of the blood.

Massive Transfusion

Massive transfusion is transfusion equivalent to the patient's blood volume during a 24-hour interval. The effects of massive transfusion on the recipient are listed in Table 60-19 and are due to the biochemical (see Table 60-3) and functional characteristics of stored blood. The following

TABLE 60-19. Potential Complications of Massive Transfusion

Altered hemoglobin function
Dilution thrombocytopenia
Dilutional decrease in factor V or VIII or both
Acid–base imbalance
Citrate toxicity
Hypothermia
Microembolization
Infusion of plasticizers
Infusion of vasoactive substances
Electrolyte imbalance

(Collins JA. Problems associated with the massive transfusion of stored blood. Surgery 1974;75:274)

three changes in stored blood are of particular concern in massive transfusion:

- Decline in the number and function of platelets
- Decline in the levels of coagulation factors V and VIII
- Shift in the oxygen saturation curve of hemoglobin to make oxygen less readily released to the tissues

Several clinical studies substantiate that thrombocytopenia is the most common coagulation abnormality in patients receiving a massive transfusion.[245,246] The platelet count is usually inversely proportional to the number of units of blood transfused.[245] Well-defined coagulation disorders can be identified in one half to two thirds of patients, and these disorders are usually caused by dilutional thrombocytopenia. Transfusion of large amounts of blood depleted of platelets and factors V and VIII may create deficiencies in the recipient because of dilution of the recipient's blood with this depleted stored blood. In addition, the hemostatic process that occurs in the bleeding patient consumes the patient's own platelets and coagulation factors and compounds the depletion state. Usually, factor VIII is rapidly replaced by the patient, and factor V levels do not fall below levels needed for hemostasis. Measurement of fibrinogen, which is not depleted in stored blood, is also often helpful as an aid in diagnosing DIC,[245,246] but the prothrombin time (PT), partial thromboplastin time (PTT), and bleeding time generally are not helpful in elucidating the cause of abnormal bleeding.[245,247]

Predetermined standard schemes for transfusion of platelets[248] or fresh frozen plasma[249] or both[246] are not effective clinically. Patients undergoing massive transfusions should be followed closely with PT, PTT, fibrinogen, and platelet count. If coagulation abnormalities or thrombocytopenia develop, these deficiencies should be replaced with the appropriate blood components based on the degree of abnormality observed.

During storage, red cell DPG levels decline. This is associated with a shift in the oxygen dissociation curve of hemoglobin to increased oxygen binding and decreased ability to release oxygen to the tissues. Although DPG levels are regenerated and oxygen dissociation returns to nearly normal about 24 hours after transfusion,[250] there has been concern that massive transfusion of DPG-depleted red cells might result in poor oxygen delivery. The clinical importance of this has been more difficult to determine than expected. Studies have shown that animals can compensate well for DPG-depleted red cells if the hematocrit and blood volume were maintained.[251] Thus, it appears that in humans moderate depletion of DPG is tolerated in most patients. In patients with anemia or compromised cardiopulmonary function, low DPG levels may be detrimental but there is little evidence supporting this.

The likelihood of development of hypocalcemia from the infusion of large amounts of citrate during massive transfusion has been overemphasized.[252] Routine administration of calcium during massive transfusion is probably not necessary.

If large amounts of cold blood are transfused rapidly, cardiac arrhythmia may occur, oxygen and energy requirements are increased, metabolism of citrate and lactate are impaired, potassium is released from the intracellular space, and the affinity of hemoglobin for oxygen is increased.[253] Thus, in massive transfusion, warming of blood to about 37°C is necessary. Stored blood contains an acid load primarily the result of citric acid and lactic acid. This may be an exaggerated problem because patients undergoing massive transfusion may have a metabolic acidosis. Often, worsening acidosis is related to the inability to control hemorrhage and shock. Routine administration of alkalinizing agents in these patients gives an additional sodium load and might shift the oxygen dissociation curve to impair the release of oxygen from red cells. Thus, use of alkalinizing agents should be based on specific results of monitoring the patient rather than predetermined arbitrary schedules.

Infusion of microemboli, plasticizers, and vasoactive substances are theoretical concerns, which have not been demonstrated to cause clinical problems. Potassium, ammonia, and phosphate levels are elevated in stored blood, but this does not cause clinical problems except in the transfusion to neonates of stored blood with high potassium levels.

Occasionally, it may be necessary to change to a different blood group in massive transfusion. The patient's history and clinical situation should be considered as well as the potential blood supply. It is sometimes more desirable to switch Rh types (such as from Rh-negative to Rh-positive) than to switch ABO group.

Cardiovascular Surgery

Patients undergoing cardiopulmonary bypass often develop thrombocytopenia and platelet function abnormalities.[254] Most patients do not experience unusual bleeding, and the extent of bleeding is not associated with these hemostatic abnormalities.[254] Thus, the routine transfusion of platelets after cardiopulmonary bypass is not indicated. Patients who develop excessive bleeding should be managed like any other surgical patients; that is, transfusion is indicated if the platelet count is less than 50,000/μL or a severe platelet function defect is present.

Patients undergoing cardiopulmonary bypass do not have abnormalities of the plasma coagulation system except from heparin administered as part of the bypass procedure. Thus, fresh frozen plasma or cryoprecipitate is not necessary. The use of DDAVP (deamino D-arginine vasopressin) may reduce blood loss in patients undergoing complex cardiovascular procedures.[255]

The volume of blood lost by patients undergoing cardiopulmonary bypass is relatively small, usually two to six units. This can be replaced using routine red cell components according to usual blood bank practices. Because the red cells may undergo some trauma in the bypass instrument, it is advisable that not all units of red cells be near the end of their storage period. The practice of using units that have been stored for different periods is standard blood bank practice.

Bone Marrow Transplantation

Patients who are candidates for or are undergoing bone marrow transplantation have unique transfusion requirements. This is because of the severe immunosuppression these patients undergo, their temporary inability to produce blood cells, and the fact that their blood type may change and they may become a temporary or permanent chimera. Since transfusion therapy may differ before and after transplantation, these situations will be considered separately.

Pretransplantation

Before transplantation, bone marrow transplantation patients are not immunosuppressed and thus may become immunized after transfusion. The presence of HLA antibodies is associated with marrow graft rejection[256] and pretransplantation transfusions are associated with decreased patient[257] or graft survival.[258] Thus, patients with aplastic anemia should be evaluated quickly and marrow transplantation, if indicated, done as quickly as possible. The indications for transfusion of the various blood components are the same as indications for other relatively stable anemic, thrombocytopenic, or leukopenic patients. Because of the potentially serious adverse effect of transfusion on marrow engraftment and survival in these patients, transfusion should be given only after careful consideration of the patient's condition. In fact, Storb and Weiden[259] have recommended that prophylactic platelets be given only when the platelet count is less than 5000/μL. For patients who require red cell or platelet transfusions before transplantation, recommendations are as follows:

1. Red cells should be depleted of leukocytes. This can be done by filtration, washing, or freezing and deglycerolizing.
2. Platelet concentrates should be depleted of leukocytes. This can be done by centrifugation, filtration, or certain apheresis collection procedures (see section on preparation, storage, and characteristics of blood components).
3. The use of single-donor instead of pooled random-donor platelet concentrates should be considered. Although it is not firmly established, the use of single-donor platelets may delay alloimmunization (see section on transfusion therapy).
4. Family members should not be used as blood or component donors because of the risk of alloimmunization and an unsuccessful marrow graft.[259]

Patients with inborn errors of metabolism or other nonmalignant diseases rarely require transfusion before marrow transplantation. If transfusion is necessary, these patients should be managed similarly to patients with aplastic anemia. Patients with malignancies who are going to undergo bone marrow transplantation usually have received multiple transfusions during the initial chemotherapy of their underlying disease. The effects of these transfusions on subsequent marrow engraftment are not as severe as for aplastic anemia patients because the chemotherapy is extremely immunosuppressive. Thus, transfusion therapy for these patients can be that necessitated by their chemotherapy. No modifications are necessary because they may become bone marrow transplantation candidates in the future. Transfusions from family members should be avoided.[259] These patients usually have no transfusion requirements in the immediate pretransplantation period because they are in hematologic remission.

Posttransplantation

Because of the severe immunosuppression caused by the pretransplantation preparative regimen, fatal GVHD can occur because of transfusion of viable lymphocytes in blood components.[211] Transfusion-related GVHD can be prevented by irradiating all blood components with at least 1500 rad (see section on transfusion therapy).

About 20 to 30 days elapse between transplantation and marrow engraftment. The return of production of different cell lines varies so that although the duration of transfusion therapy is usually 4 to 6 weeks, the need for different components may vary for each patient (Table 60-20). Almost all patients require platelet and red cell transfusions, but since marrow transplantation does not usually interfere with the production of coagulation factors, transfusion of fresh frozen plasma and cryoprecipitate are necessary only if complications such as DIC develop. Although marrow transplantation patients are severely neutropenic, granulocyte transfusions are not usually necessary.

The indications for the transfusion of blood components are the same as those for other kinds of patients (see section on transfusion therapy). One unique consideration is the source of platelets. Either random or single-donor (apheresis) platelets can be used. Many marrow transplantation physicians prefer to use single-donor platelets in hopes of delaying alloimmunization and refractoriness; it is not established whether this practice has any overall benefit to the patient.

If patients become refractory to platelet transfusion, HLA-matched unrelated or family donor platelets can be used. This and other approaches to the management of patients

TABLE 60-20. Blood Components for 25 Consecutive Patients Undergoing Allogeneic and Autologous Bone Marrow Transplantation at the University of Minnesota, 1989

	Patients Transfused (%)	Units		
		Median	Range	Average
ALLOGENEIC				
Red blood cells	96	16	2–62	19.5
Fresh frozen plasma	20	0	1–59	5.2
Cryoprecipitate	12	0	1–15	0.8
Random platelet concentrates	96	60	6–566	159.8
Apheresis platelet concentrates	88	21	3–95	26.3
Granulocyte concentrates	4	0	0–14	0.6
Cytomegalovirus-negative products	68	2	1–71	6.3
AUTOLOGOUS				
Red blood cells	100	11	1–25	12.7
Fresh frozen plasma	16	0	2–66	3.3
Cryoprecipitate	4	0	0–5	0.2
Random platelet concentrates	96	39	2–172	59.6
Apheresis platelet concentrates	84	7	1–56	13.0
Granulocyte concentrates	4	0	0–5	0.2
Cytomegalovirus-negative products	44	0	1–43	3.6

refractory to platelet transfusion are described in more detail in the section on transfusion therapy. Another unique feature of bone marrow transplantation patients is that the marrow donor is available as a potential platelet donor. Platelets are occasionally obtained from the marrow donor if the patient is refractory and experiencing serious bleeding problems, but this decision requires considerable thought because of ethical considerations regarding the donor.

ABO- and Rh-Incompatible Transplantation

Marrow transplantation can be accomplished successfully between ABO-incompatible persons[260–263] because it appears that hematopoietic stem cells lack ABH antigens.[262] ABO-incompatible transplantation may involve patient antibody directed against donor cells (major incompatibility, that is, patient O, donor A) or donor antibody directed against the patient's red cells (minor incompatibility, that is, patient A, donor O). Blood components given near the time of bone marrow transplantation should be compatible with both the donor and the recipient to minimize the chance of red cell hemolysis. Therefore, it may be necessary to use components of different ABO types at different times during the patient's course (Fig. 60-3). For instance, in major ABO incompatibility, transfusion of small amounts of donor type red cells before transplantation might stimulate production of a high titer of ABO antibodies. Transfusion of plasma containing antibodies against the donor's red cells might cause some hemolysis of red cells in the marrow being transplanted. In minor ABO incompatibility, it is desirable to transfuse red cells of the donor's type to reduce the number of recipient type red cells that might be hemolyzed by donor antibodies developing posttransplantation. The choice of blood components for these and other blood group-incompatible situations is shown in Figure 60-3.

Rh-mismatched transplantations are also successful, even when Rh-positive marrow is transplanted to patients with anti-D.[264] When an Rh-positive patient receives Rh-negative marrow, some original-patient Rh-positive red cells circulate for weeks after transplantation. Some of these patients have developed anti-D.[263] It is not known whether avoidance of Rh-positive blood components in the posttransplantation period would prevent this. We suggest converting to the use of Rh-negative red cells at the time of transplantation. When an Rh-negative patient receives Rh-positive marrow, no cases of Rh immunization have been reported. These patients can receive Rh-positive blood products after transplantation.

Intravenous Immune Globulin

Because patients are severely immunodeficient after bone marrow transplantation, infections with opportunistic organisms are a major problem. Intravenous immune globulin provides a new approach to the prevention or treatment of some of these infections. Varicella zoster immune globulin has been shown to prevent varicella infections in other immunosuppressed patients.[265] CMV intravenous immune globulin[191,192] or ordinary intravenous immune globulin[204] may prevent CMV infections in bone marrow transplantation patients. Studies are underway to establish the role of these immune globulins in bone marrow transplantation patients.

Solid Organ Transplantation

Of patients receiving solid organ transplants, kidney recipients often require transfusion before transplantation because of the anemia associated with end-stage renal disease. During the 1960s and early 1970s, transfusions were minimized to reduce the probability of alloimmunization to HLA antigens and resulting difficulty obtaining a kidney transplant. In 1973, a landmark study showed that kidney graft survival was better in patients who received transfusions compared with those who did not.[266] Separate studies showed that in patients receiving a living related donor kidney, pretransplantation transfusions from the intended kidney donor were associated with improved graft survival.[266,267] Both of these observations led to the change in practice to intentionally give transfusions to patients before transplantation. Despite a large number of studies, the biologic mechanism that accounts for the transfusion effect has not been defined.

Transfusion practice changed again during the mid-1980s. The use of cyclosporine for immunosuppression and other improvements in patient care increased patient and graft survival rates to a level at which a beneficial effect of blood transfusion was no longer apparent. In addition, the growing concern about transfusion-transmitted diseases caused elimination of intentional pretransplantation transfusions and in most centers a reversion to a more conservative use of transfusions. The use of erythropoietin in patients with end-stage renal disease has greatly reduced the need for transfusion. When transfusion is necessary for patients with end-stage renal disease awaiting transplantation, it usually involves only red cells to maintain hemoglobin levels.

Usually the hemoglobin is maintained at about 6.5 to 7 g/dL, although transfusion should be individualized for

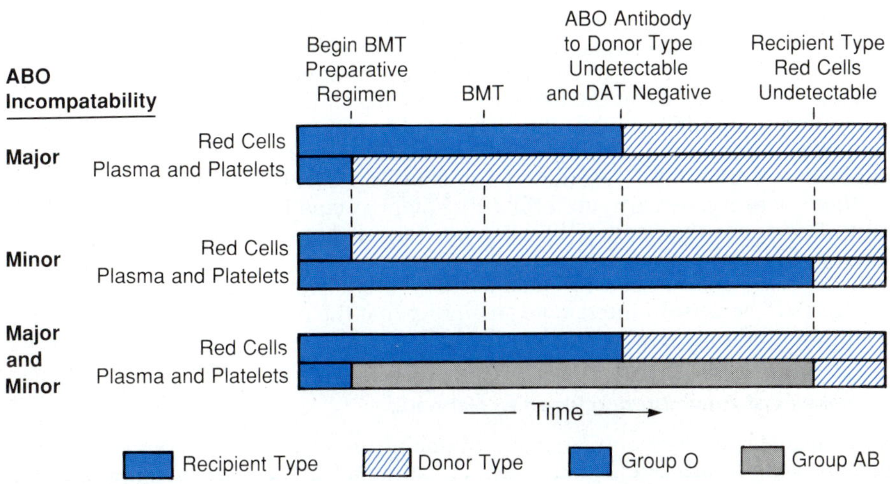

FIGURE 60-3. Recommended ABO type of blood components for use in ABO-incompatible bone marrow transplants. (After McCullough J, Lasky LC, Warkentin PI. Role of the blood bank in bone marrow transplantation. In: McCullough J, Sandler SG, eds. Advances in immunobiology blood cell antigens and bone marrow transplantations, vol 149. New York, Alan R Liss, 1984:379)

each patient's needs. Leukocyte-poor red cells are usually used to reduce the likelihood of HLA alloimmunization, which can result in difficulty in obtaining a compatible kidney for transplantation. During the perioperative and postoperative period, red cell transfusions may be necessary to replace operative blood loss or maintain the hemoglobin. If complications develop involving bleeding, sepsis, and so on, transfusion of other blood components can be given based on the specific needs of the patient. The use of CMV-negative blood for renal transplantation patients is discussed in the section on transfusion therapy.

There are no special transfusion requirements for other patients undergoing solid organ transplantations except for the use of CMV-negative components for patients who are CMV antibody-negative and receive an organ from a CMV antibody-negative donor.

Neonates

Transfusion of very small patients presents some unique considerations.[268] The smaller the neonate, the more likely he or she will receive a transfusion. Neonates may require any of the blood components that are available for adults.

Red Blood Cell Transfusions

Neonates may require red cell transfusions or exchange transfusion for hyperbilirubinemia, correction of symptomatic neonatal anemia, or acute or chronic blood loss. Blood drawn for laboratory tests is a common reason for red cell transfusion. These replacement transfusions are not recommended routinely but instead should be based on the neonate's hemoglobin value and clinical condition. Sacher and colleagues[268] recommend replacement transfusion when more than 5% of the neonate's blood volume has been removed in less than 10 days or when a 10% reduction has occurred in the infant's blood volume and the infant's initial hematocrit was 50% or greater. Red cell transfusions for neonates can be given as packed red cells. Usually, red cells less than 7 days old are used to avoid transfusing supernatant containing high levels of potassium and lactic acid. Red cells, as produced by most blood banks, are suspended in a medium containing glucose, sodium, adenine, mannitol, citrate, and phosphate. Although no reports have been made of complications caused by transfusing these materials to neonates, little data are available on this subject. There is no specific indication for routine use of frozen, thawed, or washed red cells.

Pretransfusion Testing

Because the neonate's immune system is not fully functional, any blood group antibodies in the neonate are those of the mother. Thus, a blood sample is usually obtained from both the mother and the newborn. The ABO and Rh types of both are determined, and the mother's serum is tested for the presence of unexpected (non-ABO) red cell antibodies. If a clinically significant antibody is present, mother's serum is usually used for subsequent compatibility testing for the neonate because her serum should have higher levels of antibody. If no unexpected red cell antibodies are present, no additional compatibility testing is required[57] because of the remote possibility that the neonate would form a new red cell antibody.[269]

Techniques of Administering Blood to Neonates

Most neonates require only a small volume of the component being transfused (usually less than 20 mL). Thus, the tubing sets, and other devices designed for adults, cause waste of a large proportion of the components. This problem has been minimized by use of small tubing sets and infusion pumps to control the transfusion of small volumes. Standard units of blood have a much greater volume than any one neonate requires (unless blood loss is occurring). Blood banks have devised several ways to provide small-volume blood components while not wasting the remainder of the original donor unit. These techniques may involve the use of multiple-bag systems, dispensing of components in syringes, or the use of specially collected small units. Walking donor programs are not recommended because they are associated with serious problems.[270]

Cytomegalovirus-Negative Blood Components

Neonates of less than 1500 g birthweight are at increased risk of CMV infection from blood transfusions.[194] Thus, it is common to provide CMV-negative cellular blood components for such patients. The American Association of Blood Banks Standards[57] recommend this only when local data indicate that transfusion-transmitted CMV disease is a problem. For a more detailed discussion, see section on transfusion therapy.

Irradiated Blood Components

Because neonates do not have a fully developed immune response, physicians have been concerned that transfused blood components could cause GVHD in neonates. Some physicians have recommended the routine use of irradiated blood components to prevent GVHD in neonates. Many thousands of neonates have received transfusions of unirradiated blood components without developing GVHD. No evidence proves that this is a clinical problem; thus, irradiation of blood components for all routine transfusions to neonates is not necessary.

Platelet Transfusions

Neonates may require platelet transfusions for most of the same reasons as those of adults and for additional reasons such as neonatal alloimmune thrombocytopenia, infection-related thrombocytopenia, thrombocytopenia due to maternal problems (idiopathic thrombocytopenic purpura or systemic lupus erythematosus), respiratory distress syndrome, phototherapy, polycythemia, necrotizing enterocolitis, and certain congenital diseases such as Wiskott-Aldrich syndrome. Neonates can receive platelet transfusions in a volume and dose based on the size and platelet count of the patient. The recommended dose is one unit of platelets per 10 kg body weight or four units per square meter of body surface area. Thus, neonates usually require less than one unit. If a higher than usual posttransfusion count is desired, the platelet unit can be centrifuged and concentrated to provide a larger dose of platelets in the volume desired for transfusion. Platelets should be ABO- and Rh-identical with the patient.

Granulocyte Transfusions

Neonatal sepsis has a high mortality rate. Granulocyte transfusions have been reported to be helpful in those patients who are neutropenic (fewer than 3000/μL) and have an inadequate marrow response.[271] Since it is often impractical to do a bone marrow examination to determine marrow reserve, some have suggested that marrow reserves are depleted if more than 70% of circulating neutrophils are immature forms[271] and that this be used as an indication for granulocyte transfusion in these patients. A major practical problem is that granulocyte transfusions to neonates are usually needed urgently, but lack of good preservation techniques make them difficult to obtain. Granulocytes either obtained by leukapheresis or separated from whole blood have been used, but the logistic problems have never been satisfactorily solved and granulocyte transfusions are not widely used for neonates.

Exchange Transfusion of the Neonate

The indications for exchange transfusion in the neonate are hyperbilirubinemia, sepsis, DIC, polycythemia, respiratory distress syndrome, hyperammonemia, anemia, toxin removal, thrombocytopenia, and sickle cell disease. The exchange transfusion can be done through the umbilical vein or a peripheral vein using a continuous or discontinuous procedure. The effectiveness of these two procedures is similar (Fig. 60-4). A one-blood volume exchange should remove about 65% of the original intravascular constituent and a two-blood volume exchange about 85%. In a discontinuous exchange of a stable infant, aliquots of 10 to 20 mL may be done, but the aliquot should not exceed 10% of the patient's blood volume.

Exchange transfusion is usually done with red cells that are only a few days old. Red cells are usually suspended in additive solutions containing glucose and adenine (see section on techniques of blood transfusion). The hematocrit of the blood used for exchange can be adjusted to elevate the hemoglobin in anemic patients. If necessary, because of coagulopathy, fresh frozen plasma can be used along with the red cells to provide coagulation factors during the exchange transfusion. The potential complications of exchange transfusion are infection, rebound hypoglycemia, hypocalcemia (due to citrate anticoagulant in the exchange blood), hyperkalemia (if older red cells are used), late-onset alkalosis, volume overload, hemolysis, thrombocytopenia, neutropenia, coagulopathy, GVHD, and hypothermia. These can be avoided or minimized by careful technique and good general patient care; on the other hand, since many of these patients are ill and unstable, exchange transfusion can be a risky procedure.

Pediatric Patients

Pediatric patients may require transfusion of any of the blood components for most of the reasons described for adults. Because of the size of neonates, the techniques of transfusion and the doses of components may be different from those of adults. In addition, because the volumes of blood components being transfused to neonates and pediatric patients may be considerably smaller than for adults, the equipment for transfusion may be different. For adults, it is recommended that needles for transfusion be no smaller than 21 gauge. Hemolysis can occur from high or very low flow rates and occur in smaller needles, especially when older stored blood is used.[272] Citrated blood stored about 24 hours has been administered through 27-gauge needles with no hemolysis. Thus, the use of butterfly or angiographic catheter needles of 22 to 27 gauge is acceptable.

In patients who will receive many transfusions during a course of therapy (as in bone marrow transplantation and chemotherapy), indwelling catheters such as Broviac or Hickman may be used for transfusion.[273] All blood products should be filtered, and filters with small internal volumes are available. For small patients receiving small volumes of blood, it is customary to control the rate of transfusion by using a constant infusion or syringe pump. In general, these devices work well for this purpose, but the particular brand of device should be tested to ensure accuracy and lack of hemolysis.[272] Guidelines regarding solutions for use in transfusing blood components are similar to those used for transfusion of adults.

Transfusion of red cell products may be necessary for red cell mass replacement to maintain oxygen delivery to the tissues. The typical dose of red cells is 3 to 5 mL/kg, which should elevate the hemoglobin 1 g/L. The typical dose of fresh frozen plasma is 10 to 15 μL/kg.[144] This dose should be adequate to control bleeding in most situations unless DIC is occurring. Cryoprecipitate can be used to replace fibrinogen or factor VIII. The typical dose is one donor unit (bag) per 3 to 5 kg. Another approach is one bag of cryoprecipitate per 100 mL plasma volume.[144] This should raise the fibrinogen level to 200 μg/dL, which provides adequate hemostasis for trauma or surgery. A random donor platelet concentrate should increase the platelet count 8000 to 10,000/μL in a 70-kg adult with about 1.7 m^2 body surface area.[158] Thus, the expected response to platelet transfusion can be calculated using the formula described in the section on platelet transfusion. Another approach for determining the dose of platelets is that one unit of random donor platelet concentrate per 10 kg of recipient body weight should elevate the platelet count about 40,000/μL.

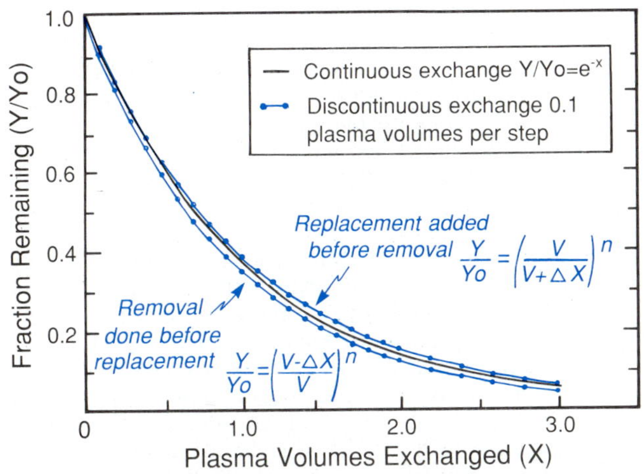

FIGURE 60-4. Calculated fraction of material remaining during exchange assuming an isolated, well-mixed box. Discontinuous exchange calculations assume 0.1 plasma volumes per step. (After Chopek M, McCullough J. Protein and biochemical changes during plasma exchange. In: Therapeutic hemapheresis. Arlington, VA, American Association of Blood Banks, 1980:13)

Hemophilia Patients

The use of blood components and derivatives containing factor VIII is described in the section on transfusion therapy.

Autoimmune Hemolytic Anemia

The causes and pathophysiology of autoimmune hemolytic anemia are described in Chapter 55. The general approach is described here for identifying the antibodies, selecting red cells for transfusion, and carrying out compatibility testing. The decision to give a transfusion to a patient with autoimmune hemolytic anemia should be based on the severity of the anemia, whether the anemia is rapidly progressive, and the associated clinical findings.[2] In patients with newly diagnosed autoimmune hemolytic anemia, the hemoglobin should be measured frequently to determine whether the anemia is stable or progressing. Transfusion is not recommended unless the hemoglobin is in the 5- to 8-g/dL range. Many of these patients compensate for their anemia, especially when on bed rest in the hospital, and transfusion is not necessary. When anemia becomes severe, cardiovascular or neurologic symptoms are usually seen.

These may involve angina, cardiac failure, mental confusion, weakness, or obtundation. Transfusion is indicated for such patients.

Although autoimmune hemolytic anemia patients are experiencing hemolysis, they usually do not experience symptoms of an acute hemolytic transfusion reaction.[2] Transfusion in patients with autoimmune hematolytic anemia involves risks in addition to those usually associated with transfusion.

The unique potential complications of transfusion in autoimmune hemolytic anemia patients are increased hemolysis and congestive heart failure. The increased hemolysis can occur because red cell destruction is a mass action phenomenon so that the number of red cells (red cell mass) destroyed increases as the total body red cell mass is increased by transfusion. Transfusion may also cause congestive heart failure as a result of circulatory overload if the patient has poor cardiac reserve.

If transfusion is indicated, the two goals of compatibility testing are to select red cells that will survive at least as long as the patient's own cells and to avoid transfusing red cells that are incompatible with any clinically significant alloantibodies that the patient may have.

In the serologic investigation of autoimmune hemolytic anemia patients, ABO and Rh typing are usually done without difficulty, although proper controls must be used especially with the Rh typing to ensure that the results are not obscured by spontaneous agglutination caused by the autoantibody. If the patient has not received a transfusion in the recent past, it is advisable to type the red cells for other clinically significant antigens to aid in identifying any alloantibodies that may be present.

Selecting the red cell units that will have optimal survival may be difficult. The patient's serum will react with red cells from all donors because the autoantibodies have a broad spectrum of reactivity. Thus, the autoantibody may obscure alloantibodies in the patient's serum. It is usually not possible to obtain red cells for transfusion that are compatible (negative crossmatch). The patient's serum is studied to determine whether the autoantibody has any blood group specificity and whether any alloantibodies are present. If the autoantibody has blood group specificity, selection of donor red cells lacking the corresponding antigen may provide cells that survive better than the patient's cells,[2] although the data to support this practice are not convincing. It is not advisable to give Rh-positive red cells to an Rh-negative patient solely to avoid an apparent autoantibody specificity. For instance, if the autoantibody has anti-E specificity, it will be difficult to locate Rh-negative red cells that lack E (cdE/cdE) because this is an unusual Rh phenotype. If such a patient is Rh-negative, cde/cde with the common phenotype can be used.

Several serologic techniques are also available to detect alloantibodies that may be present from previous transfusions or pregnancy. These techniques use two approaches: (1) removing the autoantibody from the patient's red cells to determine which antigens the patient lacks and might be immunized against, and (2) absorbing the patient's serum using autologous red cells or those known to possess certain combinations of antigens to try to identify an underlying alloantibody. If any clinically significant alloantibodies are present, red cells selected for transfusion should lack the corresponding antigen.

Because of the autoantibodies, red cells from all donors have a shortened survival. Despite this, patients with autoimmune hemolytic anemia do not require unusual or special red cell components. The usual packed red cells are satisfactory. Choose units that are not close to the end of their storage life to obtain the maximum benefit from the transfusion by avoiding loss of senescent red cells. It may also be advisable to use leukocyte-poor red cells to avoid a possible febrile transfusion reaction that might be confused with a hemolytic reaction and at least might temporarily interrupt the transfusion. No reason is found to use frozen deglycerolized red cells for autoimmune hematolytic anemia patients.

Pregnant Women

Anemia is common during pregnancy; in the rare situations in which pregnant patients require transfusion, it is usually because of another complicating factor. If transfusions are necessary, the choice of blood components should be based on the specific reason for the transfusion (eg, acute blood loss). It is recommended that pregnant patients receive CMV-negative blood components (see section on transfusion therapy).

Autoimmune Thrombocytopenia

Most patients with autoimmune thrombocytopenia do not require platelet transfusion despite low platelet counts. It has been suggested that these patients have a population of young platelets that provide better hemostasis than would be expected based on their platelet count.[156] For instance, when autoimmune thrombocytopenic patients undergo splenectomy, platelet transfusions are rarely required.[274] This is fortunate because autoimmune thrombocytopenic patients have platelet autoantibodies that severely shorten the intravascular survival of transfused platelets. When autoimmune thrombocytopenic patients do experience serious hemorrhage, platelet transfusions should be given. The transfused platelets may survive for only a few minutes or hours, and a beneficial effect may not be obtained.[160]

Neonatal Alloimmune Thrombocytopenia

Neonatal alloimmune thrombocytopenia is estimated to occur in 1 of 5000 live births. It is the platelet analogue of HDN. In neonatal alloimmune thrombocytopenia, the mother becomes immunized to an antigen that she lacks but that the fetus has inherited from the father. Maternal IgG antiplatelet antibodies then cross the placenta and cause thrombocytopenia in the fetus. Mortality rates of about 15% have been reported, primarily as a result of intracranial hemorrhage either before birth or during vaginal delivery.[275] Testing of sera of pregnant women at risk of delivering a baby with neonatal alloimmune thrombocytopenia is helpful if an antibody is detected but failure to find platelet antibody does not ensure that the baby's platelet count will be normal.[276]

The management of neonatal alloimmune thrombocytopenia involves transfusion of platelets that lack the offending antigen or exchange transfusion to remove the offending antibody. Platelets lacking the antigen can be obtained from the mother, although the plasma containing the antibody should be removed before transfusion and the platelets resuspended in saline or AB plasma. It may be difficult for the mother to donate a unit of blood because of postpartum anemia or for logistic reasons when the infant has been transferred to another hospital. The antibody most frequently responsible for neonatal alloimmune thrombocytopenia is anti-Pl^{A1}. Most large blood banks have a few Pl^{A1}-negative donors available to provide compatible platelets when laboratory facilities are available to quickly determine the serologic specificity of the antibody. The half-life of IgG is about 21 days; therefore, more than one platelet transfusion may be necessary in severely affected infants. Alternatively, exchange transfusion can be done using techniques similar to those recommended for HDN. Because it is impossible to remove all of the antibody, management using platelet transfusions is preferable to exchange transfusion.

Neonatal Alloimmune Neutropenia

Neonatal alloimmune neutropenia is the neutrophil analogue of HDN and neonatal alloimmune thrombocytopenia. It is extremely rare; only a few cases have been reported in the literature and there are no estimates of its incidence. Patients usually are discovered because they develop infection at a circumcision site or in the perineal area. Cases due to several different neutrophil-specific antibodies have been reported.[277] Although these infants can be given granulocytes obtained from a whole-blood donation by the mother, the short half-life of granulocytes limits the effectiveness of this approach. Thus, exchange transfusion is the recommended approach for these patients.

Rare Blood Types

There is no universal definition of a rare blood type. For clinical transfusion purposes, it usually refers to the blood of a person who lacks a blood group antigen that is present in very high incidence in the normal population. This means that the person will almost certainly be exposed to the antigen if pregnant or receiving a transfusion. Almost all of these patients have circulating antibody against the antigen, which is what brings them to the attention of the blood bank. Thus, the first question is whether the antibody is clinically significant and likely to cause accelerated destruction of red cells. In general, antibodies that react in vitro at body temperature (37°C) may be clinically significant, although many such antibodies are not significant. Reference texts should be consulted in making the decision. Use of an in vivo crossmatch may be helpful (see section on laboratory detection of blood groups and pretransfusion testing). If the antibody is clinically significant, efforts should be made to obtain red cells that lack the antigen. If such compatible donors are not available through the local blood supplier, donors can be sought from the American Association of Blood Banks and the American National Red Cross, who maintain national registries of rare blood donors.

Considerable planning may be necessary to obtain the red cells, especially when the donors live in other cities. If the transfusion is to replace blood loss during elective surgery, it may be necessary to plan the surgery around the availability of blood. Red cells from some rare donors may be available only in the frozen state, which may create additional problems when the transfusion is for anticipated but uncertain blood loss. To avoid wasting rare red cells and also to avoid giving the patient unnecessary transfusion, close communication between the blood bank and the clinician is essential.

If the need for transfusion is urgent, it is helpful to consider in greater detail the likely clinical effect of the antibody. If the antibody can be expected to cause a shortened red cell survival but little or no acute hemolysis or symptoms, the decision might be made to use incompatible red cells, at least to maintain the patient until antigen-negative compatible red cells can be located.

Patients with rare blood types who do not have an antibody occasionally become known to the blood bank. For those patients, it is not customary to provide red cells negative for the rare antigen of concern. The decision to use antigen-negative blood should be based on the clinical significance of the antibody they might produce, the antigenicity of the antigen, the patient's present medical condition, and the likelihood of the patient requiring transfusion or becoming pregnant.

TECHNIQUES OF BLOOD TRANSFUSION

Blood transfusions must be administered according to clearly defined procedures that are well understood and carried out by qualified personnel. Many complications of transfusion are caused by improper handling or administration of blood products or the administration of the incorrect product to the patient. Each hospital should have its own specific blood administration procedures and should designate persons to be authorized to administer blood components. Blood components are prescription drugs and thus can be administered only on the written order of a physician. The physician's order should include the blood component to be administered, any special requirements, the rate of administration, and any other instructions for care of the patient during the transfusion.

Obtaining Consent for Transfusion

After blood transfusion has been determined to be necessary, the procedure should be explained to the patient to minimize apprehension and to obtain consent. Increased awareness of the risk of transfusion on the part of physicians and patients has drawn attention to the manner in which consent for transfusion is obtained.[278] This is done in a variety of ways. Although a single approach cannot be defined, clearly physicians will be expected to ensure that patients understand the risks of transfusion and any alternatives to homologous donor blood that might be available.

Obtaining the Blood Sample for Compatibility Testing

One of the most common errors that leads to administration of incompatible red cells is mislabeling the blood sample to be used for compatibility testing. Each hospital should have a specific written procedure for this, and persons collecting blood samples for compatibility testing should be familiar with and follow that procedure. One of the most crucial steps is that the label should be applied to the blood specimen at the patient's bedside, and the label should indicate the patient's full name and hospital number. The blood sample should not be obtained from an arm being used for infusion of intravenous fluids because these may alter the blood specimen and invalidate the crossmatch. If the blood sample is being obtained from an indwelling catheter, the catheter must be properly irrigated to clear it of any solutions being infused before the blood sample for compatibility testing is collected.

Blood Administration Sets and Filters

Red blood cells, platelets, granulocytes, fresh frozen plasma, and cryoprecipitate are administered through a filter because fibrin clots and other particulate debris may be present. Traditional blood administration sets have contained filters with a pore size of about 170 mm. The blood filter, intravenous tubing, and other special drip chambers, if used, must be discarded immediately after the blood component has been transfused. When consecutive units of blood or components are given, the filter and intravenous tubing should be discarded periodically and a new filter and tubing used after about 2 units of red cells or components.

During the mid-1970s, it was suggested that the syndrome of acute respiratory distress, which often accompanied massive transfusion, was caused by the lodging of blood microemboli in the pulmonary microcirculation. As a result, several commercial microaggregate filters were developed, and their use was advocated routinely in patients receiving a massive transfusion. These filters were more expensive, and at least some had lower maximum flow rates than standard blood filters. Considerable debate exists as to the role of microaggregates in acute respiratory distress syndrome and the optimal uses for these microaggregate filters. Factors such as shock and complement activation were thought to be important. Clinical laboratory studies have never established the effectiveness of these microaggregate filters in preventing acute respiratory distress syndrome.[138] Several new filters have been developed, which remove up to 99.9% of leukocytes as well as microaggregates in stored blood. Because these filters are costly, indiscriminate use is to be avoided. Febrile transfusion reactions can be prevented by less expensive filters. Leukocyte depletion may delay or prevent alloimmunization and platelet refractoriness in some patients[139–141,165]; the optimal cost-effective strategy and patient population are not known.[138] Leukocyte depletion also may prevent transmission of some cell-associated viruses such as CMV,[205,206] but more data are necessary to establish this as an indication for blood filtration.

Venipuncture

Blood components are administered intravenously. A vein should be selected that is large enough to accommodate the needle but is comfortable for the patient. Veins in the antecubital fossa are most accessible and widely used. Transfusion in these veins limits the patient's ability to flex the elbow during the transfusion. Veins in the forearm or hand are equally suitable, although venipuncture in these areas may be more difficult or painful for the patient.

The venipuncture should be started before or at the time that the blood component is being obtained from the blood bank so that the component can be transfused immediately after it arrives at the patient care unit, thus minimizing the chance of improper storage after leaving the blood bank.

Air should be cleared from the administration set before venipuncture. Venipuncture can be performed with a needle attached to a syringe or attached directly to the blood administration set. Red cells should be administered with a needle of 19 gauge or larger. Other blood components such as platelets, cryoprecipitate, fresh frozen plasma, and blood derivatives can be administered through smaller needles. The transfusion of blood components through a central line used to measure central venous pressure is not recommended. If blood or components are administered through this line, the manometer should be discontinued, and the intravenous tubing cleared of the blood components before obtaining the central venous pressure reading.

Starting the Transfusion

Blood components, except platelets and thawed cryoprecipitate, should be stored in a regulated blood bank refrigerator until immediately before transfusion. Do not place blood components in the ward refrigerator or near a window, since freezing and thawing or overheating from sunshine may cause red cell hemolysis. Red cells must be stored between 1° and 6°C. Because it is impossible to monitor the temperature of the blood while it is outside the blood bank, it is customary for the blood bank to establish a time limit within which the blood may be out of the control of the blood bank and still be suitable for use. This time limit is established by each hospital, but usually is 30 to 60 minutes. Thus, if the transfusion cannot be started within 30 minutes after the blood arrives at the patient care unit, the blood should be returned to the blood bank for further storage.

Infusion Solutions

Sodium chloride injection (normal saline) is the only suitable solution for use in the transfusion of blood components containing red cells, platelets, or leukocytes. In vivo hemolysis of red cells exposed to various intravenous solutions seems to depend primarily on the amount of red cell swelling that occurs in vitro.[279] Five percent dextrose in water is not satisfactory for filling or flushing blood administration sets because red cell clumping and swelling with subsequent hemolysis may occur.[280] Lactated Ringer's solutions may cause clot formation because they contain calcium that recalcifies the anticoagulated blood. Great care must be taken to ensure that drugs that are toxic to blood components are not infused through the same administration set as the blood component.

Medications are never added directly to the blood component or infused simultaneously through the same intravenous line. The blood component must be clamped off, and the intravenous line cleared with saline before administering intravenous medications.

Identification of the Patient and Blood Component

Before beginning the transfusion, it is extremely important to identify correctly the patient and the blood component. Failure to do this is one of the most common errors that are made, which result in fatal transfusion reactions.[173] It is ideal for two persons to carry out the steps involved in cross-checking the information.

Rate of Transfusion

The rate of transfusion depends on the clinical condition of the patient and the component being transfused. Most patients who are not in congestive heart failure or in danger of fluid overload tolerate the transfusion of one unit of red cells in 1 to 2 hours. The transfusion should be completed in less than 4 hours because of the dangers of bacterial proliferation, which may occur as blood warms to room temperature.[15,281]

Warming of Blood

Blood does not need to be warmed before transfusion except in unusual circumstances such as in massive transfusions or when the administration rate is greater than 50 mL/min, in exchange transfusion of a newborn, or in patients with potent cold agglutinins. If blood must be warmed before transfusion, it should be done with a blood warmer device designed specifically for blood transfusion. These devices usually maintain the temperature at about 35°C but always at less than 38°C. Hemolysis may occur when blood is subjected to temperatures higher than 40°C. Blood should never be warmed by placing it near a radiator, heater, or stove. Microwave instruments have not been satisfactory for warming red cells because they cause focal overheating and red cell hemolysis.

Nursing Care of Patients Receiving a Transfusion

Proper nursing care is important for patients receiving transfusions of all blood components including platelets, plasma products, cryoprecipitate, and albumin, in addition to red cells. During the first 15 minutes, the rate of transfusion should be slow—about 2 mL/min. This minimizes the volume transfused if the patient experiences an immediate reaction. The nurse should observe the patient during at least the first 5 minutes of the transfusion, then return after 15 minutes to ensure that the transfusion is proceeding uneventfully. If so, the rate of flow can be increased to the rate ordered by the physician. Baseline values for temperature, pulse, respirations, and blood pressures should be obtained before beginning the transfusion and determined every hour until 1 hour after transfusion. At the completion of the transfusion, the nurse should record whether any adverse reactions have occurred.

COMPLICATIONS OF TRANSFUSION: RECOGNITION AND MANAGEMENT

Despite its lifesaving role, risks are associated with blood transfusion. The complications of transfusion can be categorized as immunologic or nonimmunologic. The immunologic complications involve various forms of what are usually thought of as transfusion reactions. Nonimmunologic complications are usually due to the physical effects of the blood component or to transmission of disease.

It is difficult to determine a single value for the overall risk from a transfusion. Adverse effects during or shortly after completion of the transfusion occur after about 1% to 3% of transfusions. The incidence of long-term or later adverse effects of transfusion are more variable because many of these are due to disease transmission, the likelihood of which depends on the prevalence of the diseases in the donor population. Almost 20% of transfusions have been estimated to result in some kind of adverse effect[282] (Table 60-21), and the fatality rate is about 0.5 to 1 per 100,000 patients who receive a transfusion.[283] This amounts to about 35 transfusion-related deaths per year in the United States.

TABLE 60-21. Complications of Transfusion

Complication	Cause or Impact
Immunization	May cause future problems
Febrile reaction	White blood cells in component
Urticarial reaction	Plasma proteins in component
Pulmonary reaction (ARDS)	PMN antibodies in patient
Anaphylactic reaction	Plasma proteins (IgA) in component
Hemolytic reaction	Red blood cell antibodies in patient or component
Iron overload	Caused by chronic transfusions
Circulatory overload	Caused by whole blood
Massive transfusion	
Citrate toxicity	Caused by citrate anticoagulant
Cold blood	May cause arrhythmia
Acidosis–alkalosis	Caused by citric acid; lactic acid
Microemboli	May cause ARDS
Hyperkalemia	May cause arrhythmia
Graft-versus-host disease	Caused by viable lymphocytes
Posttransfusion purpura	Caused by platelet antibody
Transfusion-transmitted diseases	Caused by virus, spirochete, parasite
Bacterial sepsis	Caused by contaminated component

ARDS, adult respiratory distress syndrome; PMN, polymorphonuclear neutrophil.

Transfusion Reactions

Many kinds of transfusion reactions can occur (see Table 60-21). These can be categorized generally as hemolytic, febrile, allergic, and pulmonary.

Hemolytic Transfusion Reactions

Several kinds of problems can lead to red cell hemolysis in transfusion recipients (Table 60-22). Probably the most dangerous immunologic complication of transfusion is an ABO-incompatible hemolytic transfusion reaction. About 41% of transfusion fatalities reported to the FDA are due to ABO-incompatible transfusions.[283] This means that 16 patients die each year, making the apparent incidence of fatal ABO-incompatible transfusion 1 in 200,000 patients.

The severity of hemolytic transfusion reactions due to ABO incompatibility is probably because the patient has preformed ABO antibodies, which often are IgM and bind complement, causing activation of the complement system with the sequelae of red cell lysis and other symptoms. The nature and severity of the symptoms do not correlate with the severity or ultimate outcome of a hemolytic transfusion reaction. Some patients may experience a severe reaction after receiving only 20 mL of ABO-incompatible red cells,[284,285] whereas others may tolerate an entire unit with no unusual signs or symptoms. The reaction may begin almost immediately on beginning the transfusion or up to several hours after transfusion. The symptoms that may accompany a hemolytic transfusion reaction include fever, chills, flushing, low back pain, hypotension, dyspnea, abdominal pain, vomiting, diarrhea, chest pain, and unexpected bleeding. In one study of 47 patients with hemolytic reactions, the most common symptoms were fever with or without chills (40%), chest pain (12%), and hypotension (12%).[284]

Most symptoms of a hemolytic transfusion reaction are due to complement activation. Several activated components of the complement system, especially C3a and C5a, are vasoactive and cause the release of serotonin and histamine from mast cells, possibly accounting for the hypotension that often occurs.

The coagulation system may be activated in several ways: antigen–antibody complexes activate Hageman factor (XII), which in turn activates the coagulation system; red cell stroma contain thromboplastic substances that activate the coagulation system; activation of platelets releases platelet factor 3, which activates the coagulation system; hypotension leads to tissue hypoxia causing release of tissue factors, which in turn activates the coagulation system. Thus, through one or more of these mechanisms, patients with a severe hemolytic transfusion reaction may develop a coagulopathy or disseminated intravascular coagulation.

Hemolytic transfusion reactions also may cause oliguria

TABLE 60-22. Causes of Red Cell Hemolysis Associated WIth Red Cell Transufsions

Red cell antibody in recipient
Red cell antibody in transfused plasma
Large volumes of aged red cells
Addition of drugs or intravenous solutions to donor unit
Bacterial contamination of red cell unit
Red cell enzyme deficiency in the donor
Excessive warming of donor unit
Erroneous freezing of donor unit
Trauma to red cells from extracorporeal instruments

and renal failure. The specific cause of this is not known, but several mechanisms may be involved. These are that activated Hageman factor (XII) promotes the release of bradykinin that causes vasoconstriction and hypotension and that DIC causes the formation of microthrombi. These events in combination cause a reduced renal blood flow and renal damage.

A classic pattern of alteration is found in laboratory tests in a hemolytic transfusion reaction (Fig. 60-5). In any series, the incidence of abnormalities in different tests cannot be easily related to this pattern because patients are studied at different periods after the onset of hemolysis. Nevertheless, one study illustrates the kind of laboratory abnormalities seen in practice. Pineda and colleagues[284] found the following percentages of test abnormalities in 47 patients who experienced an acute hemolytic transfusion reaction: hemoglobinemia or hemoglobinuria, 87%; urine hemosiderin, 42%; reduced serum haptoglobin, 87%; elevated bilirubin, 80%; positive direct antiglobulin, 87%; unexpected red cell antibody, 85%. Thus, laboratory testing generally should be helpful in diagnosing hemolysis, and the red cell serologic studies have a high sensitivity in detecting the antibody involved.

Febrile Reactions

Febrile reactions occur in association with about 0.5% to 1.0% of transfusions. They are caused by leukocyte antibodies in patients, which react with leukocytes in the transfused components.[109,286] The severity of the reaction is directly related to the number of leukocytes in the blood component.[137] These febrile/leukocyte reactions can be prevented by removing leukocytes from the blood components.[286,287] This can be done in several different ways (see Table 60-14). Many reactions can be prevented by the administration of antipyretics such as acetaminophen. Neither of these strategies is recommended routinely because there is only a 12% likelihood that a patient will experience a reaction to the following transfusions.[287] Thus, the use of antipyretics or leukocyte-poor red cells should be reserved for patients who have experienced two or more reactions.

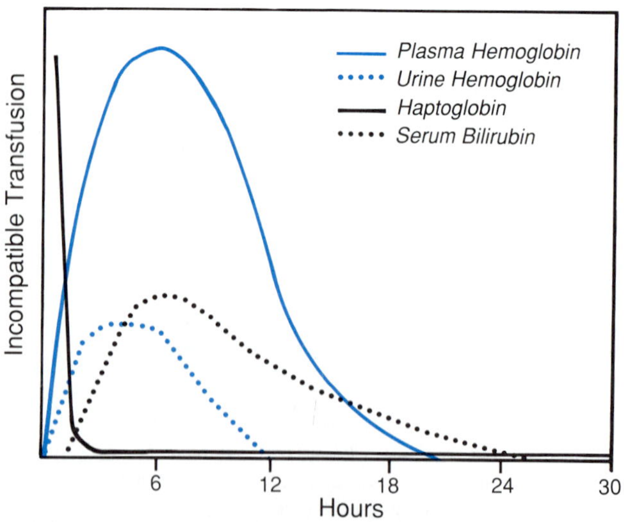

FIGURE 60-5. Time relation of pigmentary changes in serum after hemolytic transfusion reaction (not drawn to scale). (After Huestis DW, Bove JR, Case J. Complications of transfusion. In: Practical blood transfusion, ed 4. Boston, Little, Brown, 1988:251)

Allergic Reactions

Allergic reaction is probably the most common kind of reaction, which occurs after 1% to 2% of transfusions. Allergic reactions involve hives only with no other symptoms. In this situation, the patient can be given an antihistamine, and after 15 to 30 minutes the transfusion can be restarted. This is the only situation in which transfusion may be restarted.

Pulmonary Reactions

The most severe form of a leukocyte reaction is the acute, sometimes fatal, pulmonary reaction. The reaction is uncommon—only about 25 cases have been reported[109]—but they are probably more common than this suggests.[288] Most of these reactions seem to involve transfusion of leukocyte antibodies in the donor unit that react with the patient's leukocytes. Pulmonary reaction was first described in 1957 when Brittingham[286] reported that transfusion of 50 mL of whole blood containing a leukoagglutinating antibody caused fever, vomiting, diarrhea, chills, dyspnea, tachycardia, hypotension, cyanosis, pulmonary infiltrates, and leukopenia. Although the pathophysiology of these reactions is not completely understood, it is thought that transfused leukocyte antibody may react with leukocytes activating complement, causing adherence of granulocytes to pulmonary endothelium with release of proteolytic enzymes and toxic oxygen metabolites that cause further endothelial damage. It has been suggested that plasma from multiparous donors not be used for transfusion, although this practice has not been implemented. Thus, prompt recognition and treatment of these reactions are essential.

Anaphylactic Reactions

Patients who are IgA deficient and have anti-IgA antibodies may experience an anaphylactic reaction when they receive blood components containing anti-A.[289] These reactions may be dramatic and rapidly fatal. The treatment is the same as for any anaphylactic reaction. The reactions can be prevented by using red cells or platelet concentrates washed to remove plasma IgA and using plasma components prepared from IgA-deficient donors. Although such donors are not readily available, most blood banks have access to blood components from IgA-deficient donors through rare donor registries.

Reactions to Platelets

Patients with platelet or HLA antibodies may have febrile nonhemolytic reactions, probably as a result of leukocytes contained in the platelet concentrates. In addition, platelets may be trapped in the pulmonary capillaries causing dyspnea and pulmonary edema. This is particularly likely if aggregates of platelets are transfused. If the platelets are properly prepared, they contain few aggregates. Allergic reactions may also occur with platelet transfusions.

Signs, Symptoms, and Management of a Transfusion Reaction

The most common symptoms of transfusion reaction are chills, fever, and urticaria. It is not possible to predict the cause or ultimate severity of a transfusion reaction from the presenting symptoms. Therefore, all patients who exhibit signs or symptoms during or within several hours after transfusion should be managed initially as if a transfusion reaction were occurring. The monitoring and nursing care that should be provided to patients receiving a transfusion are described in the section on techniques of blood transfusion. Because the symptoms of different kinds of transfusion reactions vary widely, it is difficult to accurately define the type of reaction occurring. Nevertheless, it is necessary to manage the specific clinical problems present. The following symptoms are more likely to relate to different kinds of transfusion reactions:

Acute hemolytic reaction—restlessness, anxiety, severe chills, rapid temperature increase, headache, pleuritic pain, lumbar or thigh pain, hemoglobinuria, nausea, vomiting, pulse rate increase, blood pressure increase, oliguria, and feeling of impending doom

Febrile (leukocyte reaction)—chills, temperature increase greater than 1°C, nausea, and muscle aching

Allergic reaction—rash, hives, facial swelling, and respiratory distress

Cardiac overload or acute respiratory distress syndrome—sudden dyspnea, cyanosis, cough, frothy sputum, blood pressure increase, distended neck veins, and central venous pressure increase

Steps to Take When a Transfusion Reaction Occurs

When a transfusion reaction is suspected, the following steps should be taken:

1. Stop the transfusion immediately.
2. Leave the needle in the vein and begin infusing normal saline while vital signs are obtained.
3. Carry out a brief physical examination.
4. Obtain temperature, pulse, respiratory rate, and blood pressure readings.
5. Auscultate the lungs and heart.
6. Inspect the skin for hives.
7. Inspect the patient for signs of abnormal bleeding.
8. Obtain a new blood sample for repeat red cell compatibility testing and inspection of the plasma for evidence of hemolysis.
9. Obtain a urine sample if the patient can void.
10. Obtain a chest radiograph if pulmonary symptoms are prominent.
11. Make a preliminary assessment of the situation.

Initial Treatment of a Transfusion Reaction

Respiratory problems may require epinephrine, nasal oxygen, or incubation. Hypotension should be treated with infusions of crystalloid. Red or pink plasma or serum suggesting hemolysis necessitates accurate monitoring of urine flow. If necessary, the patient should be catheterized. If evidence of oliguria is present, mannitol should be added to maintain urine volume at about 100 mL/h. If the patient demonstrates only hives, he or she can be given diphenhydramine, 50 mg intramuscularly, and the transfusion can be restarted slowly after about 15 minutes.

Graft-Versus-Host Disease

Transfusion-associated GVHD is caused by viable lymphocytes contained in blood components. In patients who are severely immunocompromised, transfused lymphocytes proliferate causing a syndrome characterized by fever, liver dysfunction, skin rash, diarrhea, and marrow hypoplasia. The syndrome begins less than 30 days after transfusion and is fatal in about 90% of patients.[212] The cellular mechanisms involved in transfusion-associated GVHD are assumed to be similar to those in GVHD due to allogeneic bone marrow.[212] Transfusion-associated GVHD can be prevented by irradiating the blood components before transfusion (see section on transfusion therapy).

Other Complications of Blood Transfusion

Immunization to Blood Group Antigens

As a result of exposure to blood, patients may form antibodies to red cells; lymphocyte, granulocyte, or platelet surface antigens; or plasma proteins. The likelihood of antibody formation depends on the immunogenicity of the antigen and the ability of the patient to mount an antibody response. Each kind of antibody can cause a particular clinical problem later if the patient requires subsequent transfusions, organ, or tissue grafts or becomes pregnant (Table 60-23).

Iron Overload

Patients who receive chronic transfusion therapy may become overloaded with iron and develop iatrogenic hemochromatosis. Iron chelators, supertransfusion, and neocytes have been used but this problem remains as a serious potential complication.

Other

Citrate toxicity, hypocalcemia, acidosis, alkalosis, cold blood, microemboli, and hyperkalemia all are potential complications of massive transfusions. These are discussed more completely in the section on transfusion in special situations.

TRANSFUSION-TRANSMITTED DISEASES

The AIDS epidemic has focused an enormous amount of attention on transfusion-transmitted diseases. Despite the fact that blood is probably safer than it has ever been, the AIDS epidemic and the growing awareness of posttransfusion hepatitis have heightened the public's fears of blood transfusion. Some beneficial effects of this phenomenon are that physicians have become more conservative in their use of blood components, and the process of informing patients and obtaining their consent for transfusion has been strengthened.

TABLE 60-23. Kinds of Clinical Problems Caused by Immunization After Blood Transfusion

Antibody Target	Possible Clinical Problem
Red cells	Hemolytic reactions; difficulty locating compatible blood if transfusion needed; hemolytic disease of the newborn
Lymphocytes (HLA)	Febrile reaction; difficulty locating compatible organ if transplant needed; poor response to platelet transfusion
Granulocytes	Febrile reaction; acute pulmonary reaction; poor response to granulocyte transfusions; alloimmune neonatal neutropenia
Platelets	Poor response to platelet transfusions; alloimmune neonatal thrombocytopenia; posttransfusion purpura
Plasma proteins	Allergic reaction; anaphylactic reaction (IgA)

Posttransfusion Hepatitis

Posttransfusion hepatitis can be caused by hepatitis A, hepatitis B, hepatitis C, CMV, or Epstein-Barr virus, or it may be defined as non-A, non-B hepatitis, which means hepatitis due to none of the agents listed above. Posttransfusion hepatitis is the most common disease transmitted by blood transfusion. Estimates of the incidence of posttransfusion hepatitis are complicated, because figures depend on the blood donor population and on when the studies were done. Prospective studies involving the period of 1974 to 1981 showed rates of posttransfusion hepatitis ranging from 5.9% to 21%.[2,290] Some of these studies involved patients who received many units of blood, and most studies defined hepatitis as abnormal liver function without regard to clinical symptoms. Posttransfusion hepatitis is a major health problem because, based on the estimated number of persons who receive transfusions in the United States annually and the proportion of those who survive the illness that necessitated the transfusion, an estimated 120,000 cases of posttransfusion hepatitis occur annually.[291] The current estimate of the incidence of posttransfusion hepatitis is one case per 3300 units of blood transfused.[52]

Hepatitis A

Hepatitis A usually produces a short period of viremia, which occurs for about 7 days before onset of acute symptoms. Although about 10% of patients may have a relapsing course for up to 1 year, hepatitis A generally does not involve a carrier state, and thus no chronic viremia is present. Although posttransfusion hepatitis A is rare, it can occur if a person is unaware of the hepatitis A exposure and donates blood during the few days of viremia before symptoms develop.[292,293] Because of the absence of hepatitis A antibodies at the time of viremia and the rarity of posttransfusion hepatitis A, laboratory testing of blood donors for hepatitis A is not done. Thus, in evaluating a patient with suspected posttransfusion hepatitis, hepatitis A should be considered but only as a remote possibility.

Hepatitis B

Until a few years ago, blood transfusion was an important method of spread of hepatitis B, and hepatitis B was a major complication of transfusion. This is also because of the biology of hepatitis B infection. The most common response to infection with the hepatitis B virus is asymptomatic. If the person does develop symptoms, viremia and HBsAg positivity occur 2 to 6 weeks before onset of symptoms; thus, an infectious but apparently healthy person may meet all the donor medical history and laboratory testing criteria and donate a unit of infectious blood. Persons who develop symptomatic hepatitis B virus infection would be screened from subsequent blood donations on the basis of their medical history. About 90% of acute hepatitis B virus infections clinically resolve, the virus disappears, and the person becomes HBsAg-negative. Antibody to the hepatitis B virus (anti-HBs) develops in almost all (80% to 90%) of these persons. In about 10% of patients, chronic hepatitis B infection develops, the virus persists, and the person remains HBsAg-positive. If any of these persons have experienced a subclinical (asymptomatic) initial infection, he or she would pass the medical history, but the blood would be found to be infectious by the HBsAg testing done before release of blood for transfusion.

In the past, hepatitis B was an important complication of blood transfusion.[294,295] The adoption of routine screening of blood donors for HBsAg reduced the incidence of posttransfusion hepatitis B. Data defining the extent of reduction are not available because studies were not done throughout the introduction of routine hepatitis B testing and because the donor population has also changed. More recently, hepatitis B has represented only about 10% of all posttransfusion hepatitis. The reasons for this continued small number are not understood. In 1987, routine screening of blood donor's antibody to the hepatitis B core antigen (anti-HBc) was introduced in an effort to reduce the transmission of non-A, non-B hepatitis. An additional benefit of this screening is the possible further reduction or virtual elimination of the remaining cases of transfusion-transmitted hepatitis B.[42,43,296]

Non-A, Non-B Hepatitis

Non-A, non-B hepatitis has been a diagnosis of exclusion, referring to hepatitis not due to the agents described above. The disease does have some general characteristics. There are two forms: one form is similar to hepatitis A in that it has an epidemic person to person spread, and the other form resembles hepatitis B in that it is sporadic and is usually related to parenteral exposure.

Considerable debate has occurred as to whether non-A, non-B hepatitis has a major long-term health impact. Of patients with posttransfusion hepatitis, 50% to 70% had liver function abnormalities for 1 to 3 years.[291,297] Of those who underwent liver biopsy, 90% had either chronic active or chronic persistent hepatitis or cirrhosis. Non-A, non-B hepatitis appears to lead to cirrhosis or chronic hepatitis.[298]

In 1986, blood banks in the United States instituted routine testing of donors for ALT and anti-HBc as a way of reducing posttransfusion non-A, non-B hepatitis. The use of the tests that are not specific for non-A, non-B hepatitis had been controversial. In 1981, data from the transfusion-transmitted virus study showed that an association existed between elevated ALT and posttransfusion non-A, non-B hepatitis[295] and that excluding blood with an elevated ALT would reduce posttransfusion non-A, non-B hepatitis by 30%. A similar study at the National Institutes of Health gave a similar result.[44] Neither study was randomized and blood with elevated ALT was not excluded from use; thus, the effect on reduction in posttransfusion non-A, non-B hepatitis was a calculated projected one not actually observed. ALT as a screening test for blood donors is helpful in only a general way because eliminating blood with an elevated ALT would not eliminate about 70% of posttransfusion hepatitis; also, about 70% of donors with elevated ALT are not implicated in posttransfusion hepatitis. No study has ever documented the actual reduction in posttransfusion due to ALT testing of donated blood.

Later, the transfusion-transmitted virus study data were analyzed to determine whether an association between anti-HBc and posttransfusion non-A, non-B hepatitis existed.[42] This and the National Institutes of Health data[43] showed that posttransfusion non-A, non-B hepatitis was more than twice as common in recipients of anti-HBc–positive blood compared with anti-HBc–negative blood. It was projected that eliminating blood that was anti-HBc–positive would eliminate about 40% of posttransfusion hepatitis. As with ALT, no study has been carried out to establish in practice the impact of anti-HBc testing.

The two tests have little overlap in the persons who are positive for either test and so seem to identify two different groups.

Hepatitis C

A virus has been identified that appears to account for most posttransfusion non-A, non-B hepatitis. Termed *hepatitis C* (HCV), the virus is an RNA virus similar in classification to a *Togavirus*.[47] Anti-HCV was found in six of seven human sera that caused non-A, non-B hepatitis in chimpanzees and in donor units from 9 of 10 patients with posttransfusion non-A, non-B hepatitis.[47] About 80% of patients with posttransfusion non-A, non-B hepatitis in Italy and Japan and 15 of 15 patients in the United States had anti-HCV.[299] Anti-HCV has been found in 0.68% of French,[48] 0.87% of Italian,[49] and 0.5% of US blood donors.[50] Unfortunately, only 54% of persons with antibodies to HCV were also anti-HBc–positive and 33% had an elevated ALT. Thus, although the long-awaited screening test for the non-A, non-B (HCV) virus has become available, it is necessary to continue to test donors for ALT and anti-HBc. The ability to detect HCV and to screen donors for its antibody has made it possible to determine the effect of efforts to reduce the risk of posttransfusion non-A, non-B hepatitis. The introduction of ALT and anti-HBc as surrogate tests resulted in a 57% decrease in the risk of infection per unit of blood transfused, and the addition of anti-HCV testing caused a further decrease of 36%.[51] Thus, overall, there has been about a 94% decrease in the risk of infection per unit of blood, and the remaining risk is about one case of hepatitis C per 3000 units of blood transfused.[51]

HIV Infection and AIDS

The possibility of transfusion-transmitted AIDS first arose in 1982 with the report of hemophiliacs with *Pneumocystis carinii* pneumonia and an apparently new syndrome similar to that occurring in homosexual men.[300] Later that year, the occurrence of the syndrome in a child who had received a transfusion from a donor who later developed AIDS further linked transfusion to AIDS.[301] First, epidemiologic evidence, then more clear and extensive clinical and laboratory evidence established that AIDS is caused by the HIV-1 retrovirus and can be transmitted by blood transfusion.[302]

A number of studies have shown that HIV-1 infection can be transmitted by blood transfusion.[302–307] In 1983, blood banks altered their medical screening practices to defer potential donors from AIDS risk groups such as sexually active homosexual males and Haitian immigrants. Intravenous drug abusers, another AIDS high-risk group, were already not acceptable donors. In late 1984, the HIV-1 virus was shown to be the cause of AIDS, and in May 1985, routine testing of all donated blood for anti–HIV-1 was begun. These steps were extrememly effective in reducing the infectivity of blood.[54]

HIV-1 is a retrovirus, and the proviral DNA is integrated into the host DNA, thus conferring permanent infection. Development of antibodies does not result in eradication of the virus but signifies previous infection and probable present infectivity. Although rare exceptions have been reported,[308,309] once they are present, anti-HIV persists until the person exhibits symptoms.[310] The specific practices used by blood banks in the medical history and laboratory testing of donors are described earlier in this chapter (see sections on medical assessment and screening of blood donors and laboratory testing of donated blood). Thus, the test for HIV-1 antibody is used to detect infectious donated blood.

HIV-1 Antibody Tests

The HIV-1 antibody test is an excellent test. The specificity of a test is the probability that the test will be negative when the infection is not present. In a study of more than 67,000 blood donors in Atlanta, the HIV-1 antibody test had a test specificity of 99.82%.[311] In a separate study,[312] 630,190 units of blood from an estimated 290,110 donors were tested for HIV-1 antibody. No false-positive results were obtained and, with a 95% confidence interval, no more than four false-positive tests would have been expected in this low-risk population of Minnesota blood donors. In this study, the estimated test specificity was 99.9994%. In widespread clinical use, the HIV antibody test has generally been shown to detect HIV antibody in 98% to 100% of AIDS patients and to give a negative test result in about 99.8% of persons who have not been infected with HIV. Although the specificity and sensitivity of the HIV antibody tests is excellent, the predictive value of a positive HIV antibody test in blood donors is low because of the low incidence of HIV infection in that population.

In a population with a known prevalence of the virus for a test with a known sensitivity and specificity, the positive, predictive value varies with the prevalence of the virus in the population. Thus, the predictive value of the HIV-1 antibody test is slightly different in different parts of the United States where the incidence of HIV in blood donors is different.

When a blood donor is found to be anti-HIV–positive on initial testing, the test is repeated in duplicate. If at least one of the repeat tests is also positive, the donor unit is said to be repeatedly reactive and that unit is discarded. Units that are not positive on the repeat test (thus not repeatable reactive) are suitable for transfusion. The blood sample from all repeatable reactive donors is then tested using the Western blot, which identifies antibodies directed against the individual structural polypeptides of HIV.[313] There is no uniform standard, national interpretation of what represents a positive Western blot test. In general, the serum must have antibodies to the p24 gag protein, the p31 pol protein, and the gp41 and/or gp120/160 env glycoproteins. Some other criteria may be used by some laboratories for the definition of a positive Western blot.

A number of other patterns of reactivity with different bands may be observed. These are usually classified as indeterminate. The implication of these indeterminate Western blot results for the significance of infection by HIV or for the person's future health is not known. Little is known about the incidence of loss of antibody, but this is probably rare in asymptomatic persons.[308,309] Some persons with an indeterminate pattern of reactivity on the Western blot may show conversion to a clearly positive pattern in blood samples obtained a few weeks later. Many other persons do not show any change in the pattern of reactivity of their serum, and the implication of this regarding the presence of HIV infection and the person's future health is not known.

Risk of Acquiring HIV Infection From Transfusion of Anti-HIV–Positive Blood

The risk of acquiring HIV infection after transfusion with anti–HIV-1–positive blood has been estimated to be as high as 70% to 91%.[314,315] Before the introduction of HIV-1 antibody testing in May 1985, an estimated 12,000 patients were infected with HIV-1 by transfusion.[316,317] The incubation period between transmission-transmitted HIV-1 infection and the development of AIDS is difficult to determine but may be 4.5 to 14.2 years.[318]

Risk of Acquiring HIV by Transfusion of Anti-HIV–Negative Blood

Acquiring HIV from anti-HIV transfusion could occur from blood donated during the interval between the acquisition of the virus and the development of the antibody (window phase) or by asymptomatic persons who carry the virus but who have lost the antibody. It has been thought that the window interval between infection and antibody appearance was about 6 to 12 weeks. Two reports describe a disturbingly long window period of 31 and 35 months,[319,320] and in other reports HIV was recovered from the lymphocytes of high-risk persons who did not have anti-HIV.[309,321] It is likely that HIV-1 infection could be transmitted by anti–HIV-1–negative donors in this window period, which is estimated to be about 45 days.[52] The incidence of this occurring is difficult to determine. The present risk of acquiring HIV infection through blood transfusion is extremely low. The risk depends on the prevalence of HIV infection in the community and thus on the donor population from which the unit of blood was obtained. Thus, it is difficult to apply a single risk figure to the entire United States. Estimates of the risk of acquiring HIV from a unit of blood that has been tested and found to be negative for HIV antibody range from 1 in 33,000 units,[322] to 1 in 40,000 units,[323] to 1 in 60,000 units,[324] to 1 in 68,000 units[325] to 1 in 200,000 units.[317,326] The last estimate would cause 72 to 90 persons to become infected with HIV annually by transfusion of donated blood that was negative for HIV antibodies, although worst-case estimates are as high as 460.[327] An estimate of the risk of all transfusion-transmitted diseases is shown in Table 60-24.

Approaches to Reducing the Window Phase

Since the virus should be present during the window phase before the development of antibody and since HIV antigen has been detected in some patients before their becoming HIV antibody-positive, it has been suggested that HIV antigen screening of blood donors may be an effective way of reducing or eliminating transmission of infection by blood donated during the window phase. Two large studies, each involving about 500,000 blood donors, did not reveal a single case of a blood donor's serum containong HIV antigen but no HIV antibody. Thus, HIV antigen testing does not appear to be helpful and it seems unlikely that this will be adopted for routine blood donor screening.

Other approaches for reducing the window phase include the use of tests in which the antigens used in the test are produced by recombinant DNA techniques and the use of the polymerase chain reaction to amplify DNA sequences, thus making it possible to detect minute amounts of proviral DNA. None of these laboratory approaches seem likely to be effective in the near future. Continued emphasis must be placed on the medical history process used to identify blood donors who might be at risk of transmitting HIV infection. In addition, public education and education of potential blood donors continue to be essential to encourage high-risk persons not to donate blood.

Malaria

Transmission of malaria by transfusion is possible but so rare in North America that few physicians have seen a case. All four species of *Plasmodium* can survive in refrigerated blood and have caused transfusion-transmitted malaria, although most cases involve *P malariae*.[4] Malaria has been transmitted by platelet transfusion as well as by red cells, and malarial parasites have been found in platelets of infected persons. Thus, periodic spiking fever in a patient who has recently received a transfusion could be due to malaria, but this would be unlikely.

Donors who might transmit malaria are screened out by medical history. *P falciparum* and *P vivax* produce symptoms within 6 months of infection. Thus, travelers returning from malaria areas are deferred for 6 months unless they have taken antimalaria prophylaxis in which case they are deferred for 3 years. *P malariae* infection may produce no symptoms for years, and so the present screening procedures would not defer such donors. The risk is extremely small and adjustment of present donor criteria is not warranted. Laboratory testing of donors for malaria is not practical or cost-effective in the United States.

TABLE 60-24. Risk of Transfusion-Transmitted Infections per Unit of Blood Transfused

Infection	1 in
HIV	225,000
HTLV-I or II	50,000
Hepatitis B	200,000
Hepatitis C	3300
Syphilis	Extremely rare if at all

Syphilis

Transmission of syphilis by blood transfusion was common in the early days of blood transfusion but is now extremely rare. The treponema survives in refrigerated blood for 48 hours.[328] Thus, syphilis can be transmitted from components stored only a few days or from platelet concentrates stored at room temperature.[41] All blood donors are tested for syphilis; this is not an effective method of preventing transfusion-transmitted syphilis in the United States. Serologic tests for syphilis are negative in 25% to 50% of persons at the time of spirochetemia during primary syphilis. With the present general concern regarding the safety of the blood supply, it is unlikely that the requirement for routine syphilis testing will be eliminated.

Cytomegalovirus

Cytomegalovirus is a herpesvirus that is common in the general population. In healthy persons, infection with CMV usually causes few or no symptoms. CMV can be transmitted by blood transfusion to both immunocompetent and immune-deficient patients. The earliest indication that CMV could be transmitted by blood transfusion was the observation of a mononucleosis-like syndrome that occurred several weeks after open heart surgery in immunocompetent patients. This became known as *postperfusion* or *postpump syndrome*. The heterophile-negative cases were shown to be due to CMV[329] and the heterophile-positive cases to Epstein-Barr virus.[329,330] Most of the immunocompetent patients who acquired transfusion-transmitted CMV were asymptomatic; in contrast, CMV can be a serious viral pathogen in patients with either congenital or acquired immunodeficiency. Thus, posttransfusion CMV infection can range from asymptomatic with development of CMV antibody (in patients who are immunocompetent) to an infectious mononucleosis-like syndrome to severe even fatal generalized CMV infection.

The incidence of CMV antibodies in blood donors ranges from 30% to 80%. Healthy persons who pass all the medical screening requirements for blood donation may harbor CMV and transmit the virus through their donated blood components to susceptible patients. The CMV remains latent in the leukocytes of many infected, healthy persons but efforts to isolate the virus have been unsuccessful.[331] Thus, no practical laboratory test is available to determine which patients previously infected with CMV but healthy enough to donate blood may transmit the virus. Most previously infected persons have CMV antibodies and this is used as a screening test, but only 2% to 12% of these persons blood may be capable of transmitting the virus.[332] A suggestion that persons with IgM anti-CMV are more likely to transmit the virus than those with IgG anti-CMV has not been substantiated. Since the virus resides in the leukocytes, blood components depleted of leukocytes may have a reduced or even absent risk of transmitting CMV infection.[205,206] Plasma components (fresh frozen plasma, liquid plasma, cryoprecipitate) contain few leukocytes, and it does not appear that these components transmit CMV infection. Frozen deglycerolized red cells contain only about 1% to 5% of the original leukocytes and do not appear to transmit CMV infection,[142] although washed red cells may transmit CMV.[333]

In summation, the approaches that have been used to prevent transfusion-transmitted CMV infection include the use of CMV antibody-negative blood products, the use of leukocyte-depleted blood products, the administration of acyclovir prophylactically,[334] the administration of CMV immune globulin,[191,192] and the administration of intravenous immunoglobulin.[204] The effectiveness of preventing transfusion-transmitted CMV in the specific situations in which CMV infection is a clinical problem is described in the section on transfusion therapy.

Human T-Cell Lymphotrophic Virus I

Human T-cell lymphotrophic virus I (HTLV-I), the first human retrovirus identified, causes adult T-cell leukemia and tropical spastic paraparesis. The virus is endemic in parts of Japan and the Caribbean but has a low incidence in the United States. No cases of transfusion-transmitted adult T-cell leukemia or tropical spastic paresis have been identified. Transmission of the virus by blood transfusion does occur.[335] About 60% of seronegative recipients developed anti–HTLV-I after transfusion of cellular blood products containing anti–HTLV-I.[335] In the United States, anti–HTLV-I is found almost exclusively in intravenous drug abusers or persons from areas endemic for HTLV-I. The incidence of anti–HTLV-I in blood donors is 0.025%.[46] Because of the potential for disease transmission, routine testing of all donated blood for anti–HTLV-I was initiated in the United States in December 1988. The screening test currently in use also detects antibodies to the HTLV-II virus. Confirmatory tests are used to distinguish these. No disease association is known for HTLV-II. Guidelines are now available for counseling donors found to test positive for anti–HTLV-I or II.[336] It is hoped that these donor-screening steps will avoid the potential problem of transfusion-transmitted adult T-cell leukemia or total serum protein.

Chagas' Disease

The parasite, *Trypanosoma cruzi*, is endemic in many parts of Central and South America. This organism causes Chagas' disease in which patients may develop megacolon, megaesophagus, and possibly heart failure. The organism can survive in refrigerated blood and can be transmitted by transfusion.[337] Many patients with chronic *T cruzi* may be asymptomatic and thus can pass the blood donor medical questions. Cases of transfusion-transmitted Chagas' disease are extremely rare in the United States. No laboratory tests or screening procedures are used in the United States to detect carriers of *T cruzi*. In some endemic areas of Central and South America, donated blood is screened for *T cruzi*.

Babesiosis

Babesia microti and *B bovi* are protozoa that occasionally infect humans by tick bites. The protozoan causes an acute illness of fever, malaise, and sometimes hemolytic anemia; many infected persons are asymptomatic. Thus, *B microti* can be transmitted by blood donated by asymptomatic infected donors.[338] The ticks are prevalent in the northeast, mid-Atlantic, and upper midwest. No suitable laboratory screening test is available. Some blood banks defer persons from heavily tick-infested areas during the summer months.

Lyme Disease

Borrelia burgdorferi, a spirochete transmitted by ticks to humans, causes an acute illness of fever, malaise, and an erythematous annular spreading skin lesion followed by a chronic phase characterized by neurologic or cardiac symptoms or both with or without arthritis. In up to 40% of persons, the infection is asymptomatic.[339] The spirochetes survive in stored blood for up to 45 days.[340] Thus, transmission of *B burgdorferi* by transfusion is theoretically possible but has not been reported. Although a serologic test is available, it is not a suitable laboratory test for donor screening and the widespread prevalence of the tick makes it impractical to defer donors from endemic areas.[339]

Parvovirus

The parvovirus B19 has been implicated as a cause of aplastic anemia.[341] This virus has been transmitted by transfusion of coagulation factor concentrates but not by cellular blood components.[342] Parvovirus is a common infection in children. Infected persons may be asymptomatic or have a mild febrile illness. Infections apparently are uncommon in adults. This, combined with the brief period of viremia, makes transmission of parvovirus by blood transfusion unlikely, even rare. No laboratory screening of donated blood is done for parvovirus.

Other Diseases

Theoretically, any disease in which microbes circulate in the blood and survive for a few days in stored blood components could be transmitted by transfusion. The diseases of most concern have been discussed. A few other diseases that almost never occur owing to transfusions in the United States are toxoplasmosis, leishmaniasis, microfilaria, and African trypanosomiasis.

THERAPEUTIC APHERESIS

The pathophysiology and symptoms of some diseases are due to the excessive accumulation of blood cells or plasma constituents. In these situations, blood cell separators ordinarily used to collect blood components by apheresis from normal donors can also be used therapeutically. Plasma, granulocytes, lymphocytes, platelets, or red cells can be removed selectively from patients.

Plasma Exchange

Clinical Uses

Plasma exchange is the most common form of therapeutic apheresis and is used in a variety of diseases to remove IgG antibodies, IgM antibodies, immune complexes, or excess accumulation of normal substances, or to replace normal constituents (Table 60-25). Plasma exchange as a therapy has suffered from the general problem that it is used in many diseases in which the pathophysiology is poorly understood. Often, no specific laboratory measurements are available of a known pathologic agent that can be correlated with improvement in laboratory values and the patient's clinical condition after plasma exchange. As a result, no careful controlled trials of plasma exchange in many of these diseases have been reported. Since many of these

TABLE 60-25. Indications for Therapeutic Apheresis Generally Accepted for Reimbursement by Third-Party Payors

PLASMA EXCHANGE	
IgG	
	Myasthenia gravis
	Eaton-Lambert syndrome
	Goodpastures syndrome
	Myeloma with renal failure
	Guillain-Barré syndrome
	Hemophilia with factor VIII inhibitor
	Chronic inflammatory demyelinating polyradiculopathy
IgM	
	Waldenström's macroglobulinemia
	Cryoglobulinemia
	Hyperviscosity
Immune complex	
	Glomerulonephritis, rapidly progressive
	Rheumatoid vasculitis
Metabolic	
	Refsum's disease
	Hyperlipoproteinemia, familial
	Cholestasis—intractable pruritus
Unknown	
	Thrombotic thrombocytopenic purpura
	Thyroid storm
	Scleroderma, refractory
	Polymyositis, refractory
CYTAPHERESIS	
Acute leukemia—debulking	
Hairy-cell leukemia—maintenance	
Thrombocytosis, symptomatic	
Chronic myelogenous leukemia, acute symptoms	
RED CELL EXCHANGE	
Sickle cell disease	

patients experience fluctuations or spontaneous improvements, the exact benefits of plasma exchange are difficult to document. The effectiveness and role of plasma exchange in the management of specific diseases are generally outlined in Table 60-25. Multiple sclerosis is not listed because although one controlled trial showed a benefit from plasma exchange, this has not been confirmed and the data are not adequate to establish the value of plasma exchange in this disease.[343]

Plasma Exchange Techniques

In plasma exchange using blood cell separators, the whole blood enters the instrument in which most of the red cells, leukocytes, and platelets are separated from the cell-poor plasma. This plasma is replaced with one or more of several available solutions. These include fresh frozen plasma, albumin, and saline. Vascular access for plasma exchange may be by peripheral veins (preferable) or by venous catheters. If catheters are used, they must have sufficient rigidity so they do not collapse when negative pressure for blood removal is applied. Also, it is not advisable to position the return catheter near the right atrium endocardium because of the possibility that the replacement solution might create an irritable focus and result in cardiac arrhythmia.

Usually, plasma exchange therapy involves several exchanges over a period of days or weeks. How frequently the exchange is carried out depends on the situation. For instance, in myasthenia gravis patients, we often use a course of six plasma exchanges over 2 weeks, possibly adding one or two more procedures, if indicated. In contrast, treatment of a patient with a factor VIII inhibitor might involve plasma exchange daily for several days.

The volume of plasma to be exchanged is usually based on the estimated plasma volume of the patient. Because there is continuous mixing in the patient of replacement solution and patient's plasma, the relation between the fraction of the unwanted compound remaining and the proportion of the patient's plasma volume exchanged is an exponential one (see Fig. 60-4). After exchange equal to the patient's plasma volume, the unwanted component is reduced to about 35% of the initial value. Exchanging two times the patient's plasma volume further reduces the unwanted component only to about 15% of the initial value. Because of this diminishing effectiveness, we usually try to exchange about 1.5 times the patient's plasma volume. Depending on the size of the patient, this procedure may last 4 to 6 hours.

Usually, albumin alone or albumin plus saline are used as replacement solutions. This avoids the possibility of disease transmission and allergic reactions from fresh frozen plasma. As discussed later, the loss of coagulation or other proteins is not so extreme that replacement with fresh frozen plasma is necessary in otherwise stable patients. Fresh frozen plasma should be used only when replacement of coagulation factors is necessary or of other unknown but essential constituents such as in the therapy of thrombotic thrombocytopenic purpura.

Removal of such a large volume of plasma has several biochemical effects.[344] Because some platelets are in the plasma being removed, about a 30% decrease in the platelet count takes about 3 days to return to baseline. The changes in the proteins IgG, IgM, IgA, factor V, ferritin, transferrin, lactic dehydrogenase, serum glutamic oxaloacetic transaminase, and alkaline phosphatase follow closely the decrease expected, based on the volume of plasma removed. When no fresh frozen plasma is used for replacement, coagulation test results are abnormal at the end of the plasma exchange. For instance, the PT is usually 20 seconds or more, the PTT more than 180 seconds, and the fibrinogen decreased by about 70%.[344] These test values return to baseline in about 24 hours except for fibrinogen, which normalizes in 72 hours.

Complement components C_3, C_4 and CH_{50} can be depleted when albumin is used as the replacement fluid. Because of its rapid synthetic rate, complement is not depleted unless plasma exchange is carried out daily for several days.[345]

No clinically important changes in electrolytes result from plasma exchange. If fresh frozen plasma is used for replacement, the citrate anticoagulant may cause reduced ionized calcium and symptoms of paresthesia and muscle cramping. Although some reduction in ionized calcium levels may be found, even when albumin is used as the replacement solution,[344] routine supplementation with calcium during plasma exchange is not recommended.

Complications

Apheresis of normal donors for the production of blood components is well tolerated with few side effects and only rare serious complications. As Huestis and colleagues[346] pointed out, "a patient sick enough to require removal of plasma and its substitution with another fluid cannot be expected to react the same as a healthy donor." The nature and incidence of complications probably depend on the condition of the patient before plasma exchange. For instance, a stable patient with myasthenia gravis might have fewer complications than an actively bleeding hemophilia patient with a factor VIII inhibitor. Complications can be categorized as those related to vascular access, replacement solutions, or the procedure itself. In the category of replacement solution complications, seen are citrate-induced hypocalcemia, coagulation factor depletion, depletion of other functional proteins, electrolyte abnormalities, and reactions or disease transmission when plasma is used. Procedure-related complications refers to hypotension or hypertension due to fluid imbalance or to problems related to the blood cell separator instrument. In the most comprehensive report of complications of plasma exchange, side effects occurred during 12% of procedures and involved 40% of patients.[347] The incidence of severe complications was 0.5%. In general, plasma exchange is a safe procedure, which should be used only in "appropriate clinical circumstances with careful observation of the patient."[346]

Therapeutic Cytapheresis

In some patients with hematologic proliferative disorders, symptoms and severe complications can occur because of the high levels of circulating cells. In one study, leukemic cellular aggregates were the cause of death in 24% of patients with acute myelogenous leukemia and 60% of patients with chronic myelogenous leukemia.[348] All patients who died with leukocyte counts greater than 200,000/μL and 50% of those who died with leukocyte counts between 50,000 and 200,000/μL had prominent cellular aggregates and thrombi in their tissues.

Symptomatic vascular slugging due to high levels of circulating leukemia cells can be a medical emergency. Central nervous system leukostasis can lead to cerebral vascular neurosis with intracranial hemorrhage or thrombosis,[349] pulmonary insufficiency,[350] or coronary artery occlusion.[351] Thus, rapid medical intervention may be necessary.

Blood cell separators can be used to accomplish this by removing abnormal accumulations of leukocytes, platelets, or red cells (see Table 60-24). In therapeutic cytapheresis, the blood cell separator instrument is operated similar to that in collection of the particular blood component from a normal donor. The procedure is usually lengthened to process more blood and thus remove a large number of cells. The number of cells removed depends on the initial level but can be 10^{11} or even 10^{12}. The peripheral leukocyte or platelet count may be reduced by 20% to 80%, depending on the initial level.[352]

Fewer complications generally occurred from cytapheresis than plasma exchange, because in cytapheresis the small volume of cells removed is replaced by saline or anticoagulant. Patients undergoing therapeutic cytapheresis are often seriously ill, and the cytapheresis procedure may be risky because of other factors such as bleeding or central nervous system problems.

As in therapeutic plasma exchange, few controlled trials have been carried out. No doubt, cytapheresis can be used to lower rapidly the elevated cell levels in acute or chronic leukemia and thrombocytosis. Sometimes the procedure is done to prevent potential problems such as central nervous system vascular slugging in patients with chronic myelogenous leukemia, reduction of metabolic problems due to cell lysis during chemotherapy of acute myelogenous leukemia, or thrombotic episodes in patients with thrombocytosis. In other situations, cytapheresis is done to treat existing problems such as central nervous system symptoms in acute or chronic myelogenous leukemia patients with high leukocyte counts.

The medical literature is helpful in establishing the general indications for these procedures, but it is often difficult to decide for specific patients whether cytapheresis is necessary and, when done, whether it was helpful. The following is a summary of the value of therapeutic cytapheresis in specific situations:

Chronic myelogenous leukemia. Symptoms of leukostasis may develop when the leukocyte count exceeds 100,000/μL. If the clinical condition warrants, one or two cytapheresis procedures can be used to rapidly lower the leukocyte level. Chemotherapy should also be started because cytapheresis is not effective maintenance therapy.

Chronic lymphocytic leukemia. It is unclear whether high leukocyte levels in affected patients create problems. Although the count can be lowered rapidly by cytapheresis, this is not recommended unless the patient has symptoms that result from high levels of circulating lymphocytes.

Acute myelogenous leukemia. Patients who present with leukocyte counts greater than 100,000/μL (usually mostly myeloblasts) may have serious problems during the first few days of chemotherapy. These problems that include leukostasis, hyperuricemia, renal failure, and DIC are thought to be due partly to the lysis of a large number of leukemia cells. The problems may be reduced or prevented by lowering the leukocyte count by cytapheresis. Usually, one or two cytapheresis procedures suffice.

Thrombocytosis. Thrombocytosis that occurs as part of myeloproliferative diseases can lead to hemorrhage or thrombosis, especially in the central nervous system. Platelet counts of 1,000,000/μL or more may occur. Cytapheresis can be used to lower the platelet count rapidly with the expectation that complications of thrombocytosis would be prevented.[352]

Sickle cell disease. Red cell exchange is done when removal of a large proportion of the patient's circulating red cells is desired. Use of a blood cell separator makes it possible to rapidly remove patient red cells and replace them with normal donor cells while maintaining hemostasis and fluid balance. This approach has been used to prevent a sickle cell crisis in patients with sickle cell disease. The overall experience with red cell exchange in the management of sickle cell crisis is insufficient to allow a conclusion about its benefit.

BLOOD SUBSTITUTES

The functions of blood can be grouped generally as maintenance of intravascular volume, oxygen delivery to tissues, provision of coagulation factors, provision of some defense mechanisms, and transport of metabolic waste products. A blood substitute, or artificial blood, substitutes only for the oxygen delivery function. Thus, more appropriate terms are hemoglobin or red cell substitute.

For years, considerable interest has existed in the use of a red cell substitute that would effectively transport oxygen from the lungs to the tissues. The ideal acellular red cell substitute would not require crossmatching or blood typing, could be stored preferably at room temperature for a long period, have a reasonable intravascular life-span and thereafter be excited promptly, and be free of toxicity or disease transmission. The two compounds that have undergone the most study are hemoglobin and perfluorocarbons. Hemoglobin chemically binds oxygen, whereas perfluorocarbons have a solubility for oxygen 20 times greater than that of water. The physiologic benefit of this high solubility for oxygen has been demonstrated dramatically by the survival of mice completely immersed in a solution of well-oxygenated perfluorocarbons. During the 1980s, a specific perfluorocarbon product underwent clinical trials in patients who required urgent medical care and who refused to receive blood components. The amount of oxygen that can be delivered is based on the oxygen content of inspired air. At ambient oxygen tension, the perfluorocarbon product was not effective but when patients breathed 100% oxygen, perfluorocarbon provided increased oxygen consumption, an increased mixed venous oxygen tension, and an increased mixed venous hemoglobin saturation.[353]

A study of 186 patients revealed no important adverse effects of the perfluorocarbon on hemodynamics, blood gases, hematologic parameters, coagulation tests, electrolytes, renal function, and liver enzymes.[354] The perfluorocarbon product was toxic to macrophages[355] and in some patients caused bronchospasm, leukopenia, thrombocytopenia, and complement activation.[356] In a careful study, eight severely anemic patients (hemoglobin, 1.2 to 4.5 g/dL) who received the perfluorocarbon product were compared with 15 who did not.[357] All patients refused blood transfusion. The amount of perfluorocarbon that could be given to patients and the oxygen tension, even when 100% oxygen was inspired, were such that the perfluorocarbon contributed only about 50% of the oxygen carrying capacity of the patient's plasma. The amount of oxygen delivered by the perfluorocarbon was not clinically significant, and the patients did not benefit. The major observation in this study was the ability of all the patients to tolerate remarkably low hemoglobin levels, and the lack of need for increased arterial oxygen content in the 15 control patients who had hemoglobin levels of about 7 g/dL.

Work with hemoglobin solutions has progressed steadily. Hemoglobin can be prepared in solution by lysis of red cells. If the remaining cell stroma is removed, the stroma-free hemoglobin is relatively nontoxic and nonantigenic. Stroma-free hemoglobin in solution has a short intravascular life-span and a low P50 (point at which 50% is saturated). Thus, research has focused on modifying the structure of the hemoglobin molecule or binding hemoglobin to other molecules to overcome these two problems. Much of this work is proprietary; thus, little information is available in the scientific literature. At least one stroma-free hemoglobin product has undergone extensive in vitro, and animal trials and will be used experimentally in humans soon.[358] It is likely that in the not-too-distant future a hemoglobin substitute will become available.

Hemoglobin substitutes are likely to supplement, not replace, most red cell transfusions. Because the intravascular life-span of the hemoglobin substitutes probably would be a few days, the major use is expected to be in the treatment of acute blood loss. Because blood typing and crossmatching would not be necessary, hemoglobin substitutes might be stocked in ambulances and used by paramedics outside of health care facilities. Other potential uses of hemoglobin substitutes are for organ perfusion and preservation before transplantation and for improvement of oxygen delivery to tissues that have an impaired blood supply. If the use of hemoglobin solutions follows this course, the need for donated blood may increase rather than decline, as might have been expected.

REFERENCES

1. Myhre BA. The first recorded blood transfusions: 1656 to 1668. Transfusion 1990;30:358.
2. Petz LD, Swisher SN, eds. Clinical practice of transfusion medicine, ed 2. New York, Churchill Livingstone, 1989.
3. Stuart MJ, Murphy S, Oski FA, et al. Platelet function in recipients of platelets from donors ingesting aspirin. N Engl J Med 1972;287:1105.
4. Bruce-Chwatt LJ. Transfusion-associated parasitic infections. In: Dodd RY, Barker LF, eds. Infection, immunity and blood transfusion. New York, Alan R Liss, 1985:101.
5. McVay PA, Andrews A, Kaplan EB, et al. Donation reactions among autologous donors. Transfusion 1990;30:249.
6. Lasky LC, Lin A, Kahn RA, McCullough J. Donor platelet response and product quality assurance in plateletpheresis. Transfusion 1981;21:247.
7. O'Brien JR, Finch W, Clark E. A comparison of an effect of different anti-inflammatory drugs on human platelets. J Clin Pathol 1970;23:522.
8. McCullough J. Leukapheresis and granulocyte transfusion. CRC Crit Rev Clin Lab Sci 1979;10:275.
9. Senhauser DA, Westphal RG, Bohman JE, Neff JC. Immune system changes in cytapheresis donors. Transfusion 1982;22:302.
10. Heal JM, Horan PK, Schmitt TC, Bailey G, Nusbacher J. Long-term follow-up of donors cytapheresed more than 50 times. Vox Sang 1983;45:14.
11. Koepke JA, Parks WM, Goeken JA, et al. The safety of weekly plateletapheresis: effect on the donors' lymphocyte population. Transfusion 1981;21:59.
12. Matsui Y, Martin-Alosco S, Doenges E, et al. Effects of frequent and sustained plateletapheresis on peripheral blood mononuclear cell populations and lymphocyte functions of normal volunteer donors. Transfusion 1986;26:446.
13. Wallace EL, Surgenor DM, Hao HS, An J, Chapman RH, Churchill WH. Collection and transfusion of blood and blood components in the United States, 1989. Transfusion 1993;33:139.
14. Members of the National Blood Resource Education Program Expert Panel on the Use of Autologous Blood. The use of autologous blood: The national blood resource education program expert panel. JAMA 1990;263:414.
15. Braude AI, Carey FJ, Siemienski J. Studies of bacterial transfusion reactions from refrigerated blood: the properties of cold growing bacteria. J Clin Invest 1955;34:311.
16. Adamson J, Hillman RS. Blood volume and plasma protein replacement following acute blood loss in normal man. JAMA 1968;205:609.
17. Yamamoto F, Marken J, Tsuji T, White T, Clausen H, Hakomori S. Cloning and characterization of DNA complementary to human UDP-GalNAc:Fucα1→2Galα1→3GalNAc transferase (histo-blood group A transferase) mRNA. J Biol Chem 1990;265:1146.
18. Goodnough LT, Rudnick S, Price, TH, et al. Increased preoperative collection of autologous blood with recombinant human erythropoietin therapy. N Engl J Med 1989;321:1163.
19. Mann M, Sacks HJ, Goldfinger D. Safety of autologous blood donation prior to elective surgery for a variety of potentially "high-risk" patients. Transfusion 1983;23:229.
20. Owings DV, Kruskall MS, Thurer RL, Donovan LM. Autologous blood donations prior to elective cardiac surgery. JAMA 1989;262:1963.
21. Kruskall MS. Controversies in transfusion medicine: the safety and utility of autologous donations by pregnant patients—pro. Transfusion 1990;30:168.
22. Kruskall MS, Leonard S, Klapholz H. Autologous blood donation during pregnancy: analysis of safety and blood use. Obstet Gynecol 1987;70:938.
23. Kamani AA, McMorland GH, Wadsworth LD. Utilization of red blood cell transfusion in an obstetric setting. Am J Obstet Gynecol 1988;159:1177.
24. Hamil TR. The 30-minute rule for reissuing blood: are we needlessly discarding units? Transfusion 1990.
25. McCullough J, Weiblen BJ, Fine D. Effects of storage of granulocytes on their fate in vivo. Transfusion 1983;23:20.
26. McCullough J. Granulocyte function during short-term liquid storage. Exp Hematol 1983;5:95.
27. Spangrude GJ, Heimfeld S, Weissman IL. Purification and characterization of mouse hematopoietic stem cells. Science 1988;241:58.
28. Storb R, Graham TC, Epstein RB, Sale GE, Thomas ED. Demonstration of hematopoietic stem cells in the peripheral blood of baboons by cross circulation. Blood 1977;50:537.
29. Lasky LC. Hematopoietic reconstitution using progenitors recovered from blood. Transfusion 1989;29:552.
30. Kessinger A, Armitage JO, Landmark JD, et al. Autologous peripheral hematopoietic stem cell transplantation restores hematopoietic function following marrow ablative therapy. Blood 1988;71:723.
31. Lasky LC, Smith JA, McCullough J, Zanjani ED. Three hour collection of committed and multipotent hematopoietic progenitors by apheresis. Transfusion 1987;27:276.
32. Lasky LC, McCullough J, Zanjani ED. Liquid storage of unseparated human bone marrow: evaluation of hematopoietic progenitors by clonal assay. Transfusion 1986;26:331.
33. Klein HG, Leitman SF. Adoptive immunotherapy in the treatment of malignant disease. Transfusion 29:170, 1989.
34. Ray JM, Flynn JC, Bierman AH. Erythrocyte survival following intraoperative autotransfusion in spinal surgery: an in vivo comparative study and 5-year update. Spine 1986;11:879.
35. McShane AJ, Power C, Jackson JF, et al. Autotransfusion: quality of blood prepared with a red cell processing device. Br J Anaesth 1987;59:1035.

36. McCarthy PM, Popovsky, MA, Schaff HV, et al. Effect of blood conservation efforts in cardiac operations at the Mayo Clinic. Mayo Clin Proc 1988;63:225.
37. Tawes RL, Scribner RG, Duval TB, et al. The cell-saver and autologous transfusion: an underutilized resource in vascular surgery. Am J Surg 1986;152:105.
38. Popovsky MA, Devine PA, Taswell HF. Intraoperative autologous transfusion. Mayo Clin Proc 1985;60:125.
39. Hallet JW, Popovsky MA, Ilstrup MS. Minimizing blood transfusions during abdominal aortic surgery: recent advances in rapid autotransfusion. J Vasc Surg 1987;5:601.
40. Mollison PL, Engelfriet CP, Contreras M. Blood transfusion. In: Clinical medicine, ed 8. Great Britain, Alden Press, 1987:613.
41. Chambers RW, Foley HT, Schmidt PJ. Transmission of syphilis by fresh blood components. Transfusion 1969;9:32.
42. Stevens CE, Aach RD, Hollinger FB. Hepatitis B virus antibody in blood donors and the occurrence of non-A, non-B hepatitis in transfusion recipients: an analysis of the transfusion-transmitted viruses study. Ann Intern Med 1984;101:733.
43. Koziol DE, Holland PV, Alling DW, et al. Antibody to hepatitis B core antigen as a paradoxical marker for non-A, non-B hepatitis agents in donated blood. Ann Intern Med 1986;104:488.
44. Alter HJ, Purcell RH, Holland PV, Alling DW, Koziol DE. Donor transaminase and recipient hepatitis: impact on blood transfusion services. JAMA 1981;246:630.
45. Dodd RY. The risk of transfusion-transmitted infection. (Editorial) N Engl J Med 1992;327:419.
46. Williams AE, Fang CT, Slamon DJ, et al. Seroprevalence and epidemiologic correlates of HTLV-1 infection in U.S. blood donors. Science 1988;240:643.
47. Choo QL, Kuo G, Weiner AJ, et al. Isolation of a cDNA derived from a blood-borne non-A, non-B viral hepatitis genome. Science 1989;244:359.
48. Janot C, Courouce AM, Maniez M. Antibodies to hepatitis C virus in French blood donors. Lancet 1989;2:796.
49. Sirchia G, Bellobuono A, Giovanetti A, Marconi M. Antibodies to hepatitis C virus in Italian blood donors. Lancet 1989;2:797.
50. Kleinman S, Alter H, Busch M, et al. Increased detection of hepatitis C virus (HCV)–infected blood donors by a multiple-antigen HCV enzyme immunoassay. Transfusion 1992;32:805.
51. Donahue JG, Munoz A, Ness PM, et al. The declining risk of posttransfusion hepatitis C virus infection. N Engl J Med 1992;327:369.
52. Dodd RY. The risk of transfusion-transmitted infection. (Editorial) N Engl J Med 1992;327:419.
53. McCullough J. The nation's changing blood supply system. JAMA 1993;269:2239.
54. Busch MP, Young MJ, Samson SJ, et al. Risk of human immunodeficiency virus (HIV) transmission by blood transfusions before the implementation of HIV-1 antibody screening. Transfusion 1991;31:4.
55. Valtis DJ, Kennedy AC. Defective gas-transport function of stored red blood-cells. Lancet 1954;1:119.
56. National Institutes of Health Consensus Conference. Fresh frozen plasma: indications and risks. JAMA 1985;253:546.
57. Standards for blood banks and transfusion services, ed 15. Arlington, VA, American Association of Blood Banks, 1989.
58. Slichter SJ, Harker LA. Preparation and storage of platelet concentrates. II. Storage and variables influence platelet viability and function. Br J Haematol 1976;34:403.
59. Filip DJ, Aster RH. Relative hemostatic effectiveness of human platelets stored at 4°C and 22°C. J Lab Clin Med 1978;91:618.
60. Kunicki TJ, Tuccelli M, Becker GA, Aster RH. A study of variables affecting the quality of platelets stored at "room temperature." Transfusion 1975;15:414.
61. Holme S, Vaidja K, Murphy S. Platelet storage at 22°C: effect of type of agitation on morphology, viability and function in vitro. Blood 1978;52:425.
62. Murphy S, Sayer SN, Garner FH. Storage of platelet concentrates at 22°C. Blood 1970;35:549.
63. Murphy S, Kahn RA, Holme S, et al. Improved storage of platelets for transfusion in a new container. Blood 1982;60:194.
64. Hogge DE, Thompson BW, Schiffer CA. Platelet storage for 7 days in second-generation blood banks. Transfusion 1986;26:131.
65. Simon TL, Nelson EJ, Murphy S. Extension of platelet concentrate storage to 7 days in second-generation bags. Transfusion 1987;27:6.
66. Heal JM, Singal S, Sardisco E, Mayer T. Bacterial proliferation in platelet concentrates. Transfusion 1986;26:388.
67. Heal JM, Blumberg N, Masel D. An evaluation of crossmatching, HLA, and ABO matching for platelet transfusions to refractory patients. Blood 1987;70:23.
68. Braine HG, Kickler TS, Charache P, et al. Bacterial sepsis secondary to platelet transfusion: an adverse effect of extended storage at room temperature. Transfusion 1986;26:391.
69. Issitt PD. Applied blood group serology, ed 3. Miami, FL, Montgomery Scientific Publications, 1985.
70. Cook PJL, Roboon EB, Buckton KE, et al. Segregation of ABO, AK1 and ACONS in families with abnormalities of chromosome 9. Ann Hum Genet 1978;41:365.
71. Ferguson-Smith M, Aitken D, Turleau C, de Grouchy J. Localization of the human ABO:Np1:AK-1 linkage group by regional assignment of AK-1 to 9q34. Hum Genet 1976;34:35.
72. Yamamoto F, Clausen H, White T, Marken J, Hakomori S. Molecular genetic basis of the histo-blood group ABO system. Nature 1990;345:229.
73. Levine P, Stetson R. An unusual case of intragroup agglutination. JAMA 1939;113:126.
74. Landsteiner K, Wiener AS. An agglutinable factor in human blood recognizable by immune sera phoresis blood. Proc Soc Exp Biol Med 1940;43:223.
75. Wiener AS. Genetic theory of the Rh blood types. Proc Soc Exp Bio Med 1943;54:316.
76. Race RR. An "incomplete" antibody in human serum. Nature 1944;153:771.
77. Rosenfield RE, Allen FH Jr, Swisher SN, Kochwa S. A review of Rh serology and presentation of a new terminology. Transfusion 1962;2:287.
78. Cherif-Zahar B, Mattei MG, Le Van Kim C, Bailly P, Cartron JP, Colin Y. Localization of the human Rh blood group gene structure to chromosome 1p34.3-1p36.1 region by in situ hybridization. Hum Genet 1991;86:98.
79. Le Van Kim C, Mouro I, Cherif-Zahar B, et al. Molecular cloning and primary structure of the human blood group RhD polypeptide. Proc Natl Acad Sci USA 1992;89:10925.
80. Smith BL, Agre P. The erythrocyte membrane skeleton: site of the molecular defects of congenital anemias and the Rh antigens. In: Moore SB, ed. Progress in immunohematology. Arlington, VA, American Association of Blood Banks, 1988:119.
81. Moore S, Woodrow CF, McClelland DB. Isolation of membrane components associated with human red cell antigens Rho(D), (c), (E), and Fy^a. Nature 1982;295:529.
82. Gahmberg CG. Molecular identification of the human Rho(D) antigen. FEBS Lett 1982;140:93.
83. Saboori AM, Smith BL, Agre P. Polymorphism in the M_r 32,000 Rh protein purified from Rh(D) positive and negative erythrocytes. Proc Natl Acad Sci (USA) 1988;85:4042.
84. Masouredis SP, Sudora EJ, Mahan L, Victoria EJ. Antigen site densitities and ultrastructural distribution patterns of red cell Rh antigens. Transfusion 1976;16:94.
85. Nicolson GL, Masouredis SP, Singer SJ. Quantitative two-dimensional ultrastructural distribution of Rho(D) antigenic sites on human erythrocyte membranes. Proc Natl Acad Sci USA 1971;68:1416.
86. James NT, James V. Nearest neighbor analyses on the distribution of Rh antigens on erythrocyte membranes. Br J Haematol 1978;40:657.
87. Moore S, Green C. The identification of specific Rhesus polypeptide blood group ABH active glycoprotein complexes in the human red cell membrane. Biochem J 1987;244:735.
88. Bloy C, Blanchard D, Dahr W, et al. N-terminal sequence of blood group Rh(D) polypeptide and demonstration that the Rh(D), (c), and (E) antigens are carried by distinct polypeptide chains. Blood.
89. Lee S, Zambas ED, Marsh WL, Redman CM. The human kell blood group gene maps to chromosome 7q33 and its expression is restricted to erythroid cells. Blood 1993;81:2804.
90. Lee S, Zambas ED, Marsh WL, Redman CM. Molecular cloning and primary structure of Kell blood group protein. Proc Natl Acad Sci USA 1991;88:6353.
91. Redman CM, Marsh WL, Mueller KA, et al. Isolation of Kell-active protein from the red cell membrane. Transfusion 1984;294:176.
92. Redman CM, Avellino G, Pfeffer SR, et al. Kell blood group antigens are part of a 93,000 dalton red cell membrane protein. J Biol Chem 1986;261:9521.
93. Redman CM, Lee S, Marsh WL. Isolation and partial characterization of Kell blood group protein. In: Moore, SB, ed. Progress in immunohematology. Arlington, VA, American Association of Blood Banks, 1988:141.
94. Masouredis SP, Sudora E, Mahan L, Victoria EJ. Quantitative immunoferritin microscopy of Fy^a, Fy^b, Jk^a, U, and Di^b antigen site numbers of human red cells. Blood 1980;56:969.
95. Hadley TJ, David PH, McGinniss MH, Miller LH. Identification of an erythrocyte component carrying the Duffy blood group Fy^a antigen. Science 1984;223:597.
96. Miller LH, Mason SJ, Devorak JA, et al. Erythrocyte receptors for plasmodium knowlesi malaria, Duffy blood group determinants. Science 1975;189:561.
97. Miller LH, Aikawa M, Johnson JG, Shiroishi T. Interaction between cytochalasin B-treated malarial parasites and erythrocytes: attachment and junction formation. J Exp Med 1979;149:172.
98. Chaplin H, Hunter VL, Malech AC, Kilzer P, Rosche ME. Clinically significant allo-anti-I in an I-negative patient with massive hemorrhage. Transfusion 1986;25:57.
99. Dahr W, Uhlenbruck G, Bird GW. Further characterization of some heterophile agglutinins reacting with alkali-labile carbohydrate chains of human erythrocyte glycoproteins. Vox Sang 1978;28:133.
100. Oriol R, Cartron J, Yvart J, et al. The Lewis system: new histocompatiblity antigens in renal transplantation. Lancet 1978;1:574.
100a. Swanson J. Laboratory problems associated with leukocyte antibodies. Recent Adv Immunohematol 1973:121.

101. Dunstan RA, Simpson MB, Knowles RW, Rosse WF. The origin of ABO antigens on human platelets. Blood 1985;65:615.
102. Kools A, Collins J, Aster RH. Studies of the ABO antigens of human platelets. (Abstract) Transfusion 1981;21:615.
103. Clay ME, Kline WE. Detection of granulocyte antigens and antibodies: current proposectives and approaches. In: Garratty G, ed. Current concepts in transfusion therapy. Arlington, VA, American Association of Blood Banks, 1985:229.
104. Dunstan RA, Simpson MB, Sanfilippo FP. Absence of specific HLA-DR antigens on human platelets and neutrophils. (Abstract) Blood 1984;64:85a.
105. McCullough J, Clay M, Loken M, Hurd D. Effect of ABO incompatibility on fate in vivo of ^{111}Indium granulocytes. Transfusion 1988;28:358.
106. Clay ME, Kline WE, McCullough J. Granulocyte antigens and antibodies: current concepts of detection and histocompatibility testing. In: Dutcher J, ed. Modern transfusion therapy. Boca Raton, FL, CRC Press 1990:182.
107. Thompson JS. Antileukocyte capillary agglutinating antibody in pre- and post-transplantation sera. In: Rose NR, Friedman H, eds. Manual of clinical immunology. Washington, DC, American Society of Microbiology, 1976:868.
108. Minchinton RM, Waters AH, Malpas JS, et al. Platelet- and granulocyte-specific antibodies after allogeneic and autologous bone marrow grafts. Vox Sang 1984;46:125.
109. McCullough J, Clay ME, Press C, Kline W. Granulocyte serology: a clinical and laboratory guide. Chicago, ASPC Press, 1988:83–112.
110. Warkentin PI, Clay ME, Kersey JH, et al. Successful engraftment of NA1 positive bone marrow in a patient with a neutrophil antibody, anti-NA1. Hum Immunol 1981;2:173.
111. Stroncek DF, Shapiro RS, Filipovich AH, Plachta LB, Clay ME. Prolonged neutropenia resulting from antibodies to neutrophil-specific antigen NB1 following marrow transplantation. Transfusion 1993;33:158.
112. Boxer LA, Yokoyama M, Lalezari P. Isoimmune neonatal neutropenia. J Pediatr 1972;80:783.
113. Trounstine ML, Peitz GA, Yssel H, et al. Reactivity of cloned, expressed human FcRIII isoforms with monoclonal antibodies which distinguish cell type specific and allelic forms of Fc-gamma-RIII. Int Immunol 1990;2:303.
114. Ory PA, Clark MR, Kwoh EE, Clarkson SB, Goldstein IM. Sequences of complementary DNAs that encode the NA1 and NA2 forms of Fc receptor III on human neutrohpils. J Clin Invest 1989;84:1688.
115. Huizinga TWS, Kleijer M, Tetteroo PAT, Roos D, von dem Born AEGKr. Bialletic neutrophil Na-antigen system is associated with a polymorphism on the phospho-inositol-linked Fc receptor III (CD16) Blood 1990;75:213.
116. Richards KL, McCullough J. Chemotactic and chemokinetic responsiveness of fresh and stored human granulocytes. Annual meeting of the American Society for Cell Biology. (Abstract) J Cell Biol 1982;95:324a.
117. Shulman IA, Nelson JM, Saxena S, et al. Experience with routine use of an abbreviated crossmatch. Am J Clin Pathol 1984;82:178.
118. International Committee for Standardization in Hematology: recommended method for radioisotope red cell survival studies. Br J Hematol 1980;45:659.
119. Silvergleid AJ, Wells RP, Hafleigh EB, et al. Compatibility test using 51Cr-labeled red blood cells in crossmatched positive patients. Transfusion 1978;18:8.
120. Aster R. Effect of anticoagulant and ABO incompatibility on recovery of transfused human platelets. Blood 1965;26:732.
121. Lohrman HP, Bull MI, Decter JA, et al. Platelet transfusions from HLA compatible unrelated donors to alloimmunized patients. Ann Intern Med 1974;80:9.
122. Duquesnoy RJ, Anderson AJ, Tomasulo PA, Aster RH. ABO compatibility and platelet transfusions of alloimmunized thrombocytopenic patients. Blood 1979;54:595.
123. Heal JM, Jones ME, Forey J, et al. Fatal salmonella septicemia after platelet transfusion. Transfusion 1987;27:2.
124. Murphy S. ABO blood groups and platelet transfusion. Transfusion 1988;28:401.
125. Goldfinger D. McGinnis MH. Rh incompatible platelet transfusions-risks and consequences of sensitizing immunosuppressed patients. N Engl J Med 1971;284:942.
126. Lichtiger B, Surgeon J, Rhorer S. Rh-incompatible platelet transfusion therapy in cancer patients. Vox Sang 1983;45:139.
127. Baldwin ML, Ness PM, Scott, D, et al. Alloimmunization to D antigen and HLA in D-negative immunosuppressed oncology patients. Transfusion 1988;28:330.
128. Pfisterer H, Thierfelder S, Kottusch H. Untersuchung menschlicher thrombocyten auf rhesus-antigen durch abbaustudien in vivo nach 51Cr-markierung. Klin Wochenschr 1967;45:519.
129. Pollack W, Ascari WQ, Kochesky RJ, et al. Studies on Rh prophylaxis. I. Relationship between doses of anti-Rh and size of antigenic stimulus. Transfusion 1971;11:333.
130. McCullough J, Clay M, Hurd D, Richards K, Ludvigsen C, Forstrom L. Effect of leukocyte antibodies and HLA matching on the intravascular recovery, survival and tissue localization of 111-indium granulocytes. Blood 1986;67:522.
131. Gollub S, Svigals R, Bailey CP, et al. Electrolyte solutions in surgical patients refusing transfusion. JAMA 1971;215:2077.
132. Rigor B, Bosomworth P, Ruth BF, Jr. Replacement of operative blood loss of more than 1 liter with Hartmann's solution. JAMA 1968;203:111.
133. Office of Medical Applications of Research, National Institutes of Health. Perioperative red cell transfusion. JAMA 1988;260:2700.
134. Welch HG, Meehan KR, Goodnough LT. Prudent strategies for elective red blood cell transfusion. Ann Intern Med 1992;116:393.
135. American College of Physicians. Practice strategies for elective red blood cell transfusion. Ann Intern Med 1992;115:403.
136. Faust RJ. Perioperative indications for red blood cell transfusion: has the pendulum swung too far? Mayo Clin Proc 1993;68:512.
137. Perkins HA, Payne R, Ferguson J, et al. Nonhemolytic febrile transfusion reactions: quantitative effects of blood components with emphasis on isoantigenic incompatibility of leukocytes. Vox Sang 1966;11:578.
138. Snyder EL. Clinical use of white cell-poor blood components. Transfusion 1989;29:568.
139. Class FHJ, Smeenk RJT, Schmidt R, et al. Alloimmunization against the MHC antigens after platelet transfusions is due to contaminating leukocytes in the platelet suspension. Exp Hematol 1981;9:84.
140. Eernisse JG, Brand A. Prevention of platelet refractoriness due to HLA antibodies by administration of leukocyte-poor blood components. Exp Hematol 1981;9:77.
141. Schiffer CA, Dutcher JP, Aisner J, et al. A randomized trial of leukocyte depleted platelet transfusion to modify alloimmunization in patients with leukemia. (Abstract) Blood 1980;56:182a.
142. Brady MT, Milam JD, Anderson DC, et al. Use of deglycerolized red blood cells to prevent posttransfusion infection with cytomegalovirus in neonates. J Infect Dis 1984;150:334.
143. Factor IX complex and hepatitis. Food Drug Admin Drug Bull 1976;6:22.
144. Corrigan, JJ. Hemorrhagic and thrombotic disease in childhood and adolescence. New York, Churchill Livingstone, 1985.
145. Ness PM, Perkins HA. Cryoprecipitate as a reliable source of fibrinogen replacement. JAMA 1979;241:1690.
146. Rosati LA, Barnes B, Oberman H, Penner J. Hemolytic anemia due to anti-A in concentrated hemophilic factor preparations. Transfusion 1970;10:139.
147. McCullough J, Steeper TA, Connelly DP, Jackson B, Huntington S, Scott EP. Platelet utilization in a university hospital. JAMA 1988;259:2414.
148. Hersch EM, Bodey GP, Nies BA, Freireich EJ. Causes of death in acute leukemia: a ten year study of 414 patients from 1954–1963. JAMA 1965;193:105.
149. Gaydos LA, Freireich EJ, Mantel N. The quantitative relation between platelet count and hemorrhage in patients with acute leukemia. N Engl J Med 1962;266:905.
150. Roy AJ, Jaffe N, Djerassi I. Prophylactic platelet transfusions in children with acute leukemia: a dose-response study. Transfusion 1973;13:283.
151. Higby DJ, Cohen E, Holland JF, Sinks L. The prophylactic treatment of thrombocytopenic leukemia patients with platelets: a double blind study. Transfusion 1974;14:440.
152. Soloman J, Bokefkamp T, Fahey JL, et al. Platelet prophylaxis in acute non-lymphocytic leukemia. Lancet 1978;1:267.
153. Baer MR, Bloomfield CD. Controversies in transfusion medicine. Prophylactic platelet transfusion therapy: pro. Transfusion 1992;32:377.
154. Patten E. Controversies in transfusion medicine. Prophylactic platelet transfusion revisited after 25 years: con. Transfusion 1992;32:381.
155. Slichter S, Harker LA. Thrombocytopenia: mechanisms and management of defects in platelet production. Clin Haematol 1978;7:523.
156. Harker LA, Slichter SJ. The bleeding time as a screening test for evaluation of platelet function. N Engl J Med 1972;287:155.
157. Bishop JF, Schiffer CA, Aisner J, Matthews JP, Wiernik PH. Surgery in acute leukemia: a review of 167 operations in thrombocytopenic patients. Am J Hematol 1987;26:147.
158. Freireich EJ, Kliman A, Gaydos LA, et al. Response to repeated platelet transfusion from the same donor. Ann Intern Med 1963;50:277.
159. Daly PA, Schiffer CA, Aisner J, Wiernik PH. Platelet transfusion therapy: one-hour posttransfusion increments are valuable in predicting the need for HLA-matched preparations. JAMA 1980;243:435.
160. Aster RH, Jandl JH. Platelet sequestration in man. II. Immunological and clinical studies. J Clin Invest 1964;43:856.
161. Bishop JF, McGrath K, Wolf MM, et al. Clinical factors influencing the efficacy of pooled platelet transfusions. Blood 1988;71:383.
162. Dutcher JP, Schiffer CA, Aisner J, Wiernik PH. Alloimmunization following platelet transfusion: the absence of a dose-response relationship. Blood 1981;57:395.
163. Dutcher JP, Schiffer CA, Aisner J, Wiernik PH. Long-term follow-up of patients with leukemia receiving platelet transfusions: identification of a large group of patients who do not become alloimmunized. Blood 1981;58:1007.
164. Gmur J, von Felten A, Osterwalder B, et al. Delayed alloimmunization using random single donor platelet transfusions: a prospective study in thrombocytopenic patients with acute leukemia. Blood 1983;62:473.

165. Sniecinski I, O'Donnell MR, Nowicki B, Hill LR. Prevention of refractoriness and HLA-alloimmunization using filtered blood products. Blood 1988;71:1402.
166. Deeg HJ. Transfusions with a tan: prevention of allosensitization by ultraviolet irradiation. Transfusion 1989;29:450.
167. Lee EJ, Schiffer CA. ABO compatibility can influence the results of platelet transfusion: results of a randomized trial. Transfusion 1989;29:384.
168. Lazarus HM, Herzig RH, Warm SE, Fishman DJ. Transfusion experience with platelet concentrates stored for 24 to 72 hours at 22°C. Transfusion 1982;22:39.
169. Duquesnoy RJ, Filip DJ, Rodey GE, et al. Successful transfusion of platelets "mismatched" for HLA antigens to alloimmunized thrombocytopenic patients. Am J Hematol 1977;2:219.
170. Duquesnoy RJ, Vieira J, Aster RH. Donor availability for platelet transfusion support of alloimmunized thrombocytopenic patients. Transplant Proc 1977;9:519.
171. Yankee RA, Grumet FC, Rogentine GN. Platelet transfusion therapy: the selection of compatible platelet donors for refractory patients by lymphocyte HLA typing. N Engl J Med 1969;281:1208.
172. Bolgiano DC, Larson EB, Slichter SJ. A model to determine required pool size for HLA-typed community donor apheresis programs. Transfusion 1989;29:306.
173. Moroff G, Garratty G, Heal JM, et al. Selection of platelets for refractory patients by HLA matching and prospective crossmatching. Transfusion 1992;32:633.
174. Bodey GP, Buckley M, Sath YS, Freireich EJ, Quantitative relationships between circulating leukocytes and infection in patients with acute leukemia. Ann Intern Med 1966;64:328.
175. Gurwith MJ, Brunton JL, Lank BA, et al. Granulocytopenia in hospitalized patients. I. Prognostic factors and etiology of fever. Am J Med 1978;61:121.
176. Freireich EJ, Levin RH, Wang J. The function and gate of transfused leukocytes from donors with chronic myelocytic leukemia in leukopenic recipients. Ann NY Acad Sci 1965;113:1081.
177. Alavi JB, Roat RK, Djerassi I, et al. A randomized clinical trial of granulocyte transfusions for infection of acute leukemia. N Engl J Med 1977;296:706.
178. Strauss RG. Therapeutic neutrophil transfusions: are controlled studies no longer appropriate? Am J Med 1978;65:1001.
179. Graw RH Jr, Herzig G, Perry S, Henderson ES. Normal granulocyte transfusion therapy. Treatment of septicemia due to gram-negative bacteria. N Engl J Med 1972;287:367.
180. Herzig GP, Graw RG Jr. Granulocyte transfusions for bacterial infections. In: Brown EB, ed. Progress in hematology, vol 9. New York, Grune & Stratton, 1975:207.
181. Degregorio MW, Lee WMF, Linker CA, et al. Fungal infections in patients with acute leukemia. Am J Med 1982;73:543.
182. Young LS. Nosocomial infections in the immunocompromised adult. Am J Med 1981;70:398.
183. Ruthe RC, Ansersen BR, Cunningham BL, Epstein RB. Efficacy of granulocyte transfusions in the control of systemic candidiasis in leukopenic host. Blood 1978;52:493.
184. Raubitschek AA, Levin AS, Stites DP, et al. Normal granulocyte infusion therapy for aspergillosis in chronic granulomatous disease. Pediatrics 1973;51:230.
185. Strauss RG, Connett JE, Gale RP, et al. A controlled trial of prophylactic granulocyte transfusion during initial induction. N Engl J Med 1981;305:597.
186. Evatt B, Gompaerts E, McDougal J, Ramsey R. Coincidental appearance of LAV/HTLV antibodies in hemophiliacs and the onset of the AIDS epidemic. N Engl J Med 1985;312:483.
187. Walsh JH, Purcell RH, Morrow AG, et al. Post-transfusion hepatitis after open-heart operations: incidence after administration of blood from commercial and volunteer donor populations. JAMA 1970;211:261.
188. Prince AM, Horowitz B, Brotman B. Sterilization of hepatitis and HTLV-III viruses by exposure to try (n-butyl) phosphate and sodium cholate. Lancet 1986;1:706.
189. Aronson, DL. The development of the technology and capacity for the production of factor VIII for the treatment of hemophilia A. Transfusion 1990;30:748.
190. Barundun S, Kistler P, Jeunet F, et al. Intravenous administration of human gamma globulin. Vox Sang 1962;7:157.
191. Condie RM, O'Reilly RJ. Prevention of cytomegalovirus infection by prophylaxis with an intravenous, hyperimmune, native, unmodified cytomegalovirus globulin. Am J Med 1984;76:134.
192. Meyers JD, Leszczynski J, Zaia JA, et al. Prevention of cytomegalovirus infection by cytomegalovirus immune globulin after marrow transplantation. Ann Intern Med 1983;98:442.
193. Sacher RA. Intravenous gammaglobulin products: development, pharmacology, and precautions. In: Garner RJ, Sacher RA, eds. Intravenous gammaglobulin therapy. Arlington, VA, American Association of Blood Banks, 1988:1.
194. Yaeger AS, Grumet FC, Hafleigh EB, et al. Prevention of transfusion-acquired cytomegalovirus infections in newborn infants. J Pediatr 1981;98:281.
195. Stagno S, Pass RF, Dworsky ME, et al. Congenital cytomegalovirus infection: the relative importance of primary and recurrent maternal infection. N Engl J Med 1982;306:945.
196. Adler SP. Neonatal cytomegalovirus infections due to blood. CRC Crit Rev Clin Lab Sci 1985;23:1.
197. Tegtmeier GE. Cytomegalovirus and blood transfusion. In: Dodd RY, Barker LF, eds. Infection, immunity, and blood transfusion, vol 182. New York, Alan R Liss, 1985:175.
198. Glenn J. Cytomegalovirus infection following renal transplantation. Rev Infect Dis 1981;3:1151.
199. Rubin RH, Tolkoff-Rubin NE, Oliver D, et al. Multicenter seroepidemiologic study of the impact of cytomegalovirus infection on renal transplantation. Transplantation 1985;40:243.
200. Chou S. Acquisition of donor strains of cytomegalovirus by renal-transplant recipients. N Engl J Med 1986;314:1418.
201. Miller W, Flynn P, McCullough J, et al. Cytomegalovirus infection after bone marrow transplantation: an association with acute graft-vs-host disease. Blood 1986;67:1162.
202. Bowden RA, Sayers M, Flournoy N, et al. Cytomegalovirus immune globulin and seronegative blood products prevent primary cytomegalovirus infection after marrow transplantation. N Engl J Med 1986;314:1006.
203. Miller WJ, McCullough J, Balfour HH, et al. Prevention of CMV infection following bone marrow transplantation: a randomized trial of blood product screening. Bone Marrow Transplant.
204. Winston DJ, Ho WG, Lin C, et al. Intravenous immunoglobulin for modification of cytomegalovirus infections associated with bone marrow transplantation. Am J Med 1984;76:128.
205. Gilbert GL, Hudson IL, Hayes JJ. Prevention of transfusion-acquired cytomegalovirus infection in infants by blood filtration to remove leucocytes. Lancet 1989;1:1228.
206. Murphy MF, Grint PCA, Hardiman AE, Lister TA, Waters AH. Use of leukocyte-poor blood components to prevent primary cytomegalovirus (CMV) infection in patients with acute leukemia. Br J Haematol 1988;70:253.
207. Preiksaitis JK, Rosno S, Grumet C, Merigan TC. Infections due to herpesviruses in cardiac transplant recipients: role of the donor heart and immunosuppressive therapy. J Infect Dis 1983;147:1974.
208. Rakela J, Wiesner RH, Taswell HF, et al. Incidence of cytomegalovirus infection and its relationship to donor-recipient serologic status in liver transplantation. Transplant Proc 1987;19:2399.
209. Preiksaitis JK, Grumet FC, Smith WK, Merigan TC. Transfusion-acquired cytomegalovirus infections in cardiac surgery patients. J Med Virol 1985;15:283.
210. Adler SP, Baggett J, McVoy M. Transfusion-associated cytomegalovirus infections in seropositive cardiac surgery patients. Lancet 1985;743.
211. Thomas ED, Storb R, Clift RA, et al. Bone-marrow transplantation. N Engl J Med 1975;292:832.
212. Leitman SF, Holland PV. Irradiation of blood products: indications and guidelines. Transfusion 1985;25:293.
213. Sprent J, Anderson RE, Miller JFAP. Radiosensitivity of T and B lymphocytes. II. Effect of irradiation on response of T cells to alloantigens. Eur J Immunol 1974;4:204.
214. Valerius NH, Johansen KS, Nielsen OS, et al. Effect of in vitro x-irradiation on lymphocyte and granulocyte function. Scand J Hematol 1981;27:9.
215. Button LN, DeWolf WC, Newburger PE, Jacobson MS, Kevy SV. The effects of irradiation on blood components. Transfusion 1981;21:419.
216. Holley TR, Van Epps DE, Harvey RL, et al. Effect of high doses of radiation on human neutrophil chemotaxis, phagocytosis, and morphology. Am J Pathol 1974;75:61.
217. Greenberg ML, Chanana AD, Cronkite, et al. Extracorporeal irradiation of blood in man: radiation resistance of circulating platelets. Radiat Res 1968;35:147.
218. Ramirez AM, Woodfield DG, Scott R, McLachlan J. High potassium levels in stored irradiated blood. (Letter) Transfusion 1987;27:444.
219. Rivet C, Baxter A, Rock G. Potassium levels in irradiated blood. (Letter) Transfusion 1989;29:185.
220. Parkman R, Mosier D, Umansky I, et al. Graft-versus-host disease after intrauterine and exchange transfusions for hemolytic disease of the newborn. N Engl J Med 1974;290:359.
221. Bohm N, Kleine W, Enzel U. Graft-versus-host disease in two newborns after repeated blood transfusions because of Rhesus incompatibility. Beitr Pathol 1977;160:381.
222. Douglas SD, Fudenberg HH. Graft versus host reaction in Wiskott-Aldrich syndrome: antemortem diagnosis of human GVH in an immunologic deficiency disease. Vox Sang 1969;16:172.
223. Weiden PL, Zuckerman N, Hansen JA, et al. Fatal graft-versus-host disease in a patient with lymphoblastic leukemia following normal granulocyte transfusions. Blood 1981;57:328.
224. Siimes MA, Koskimies S. Chronic graft-versus-host disease after blood transfusions confirmed by incompatible HLA antigens in bone marrow. Lancet 1982;1:42.
225. Lowenthal RM, Menon C, Challis DR. Graft-versus-host disease in consecutive patients with acute myeloid leukemia treated with blood cells from normal donors. Aust NZ J Med 1981;11:179.
226. Schmidmeier W, Feil W, Gebhart W, et al. Fatal graft-versus host reaction following granulocyte transfusions. Blut 1982;45:115.
227. Cohen D, Weinstein H, Mihm M, Yankee R. Nonfatal graft-versus-

host disease occuring after transfusion with leukocytes and platelets obtained from normal donors. Blood 1979;53:1053.
228. von Fliedner V, Higby DJ, Kim U. Graft-versus-host reaction following blood transfusion. Am J Med 1982;72:951.
229. Woods WG, Lubin BH. Fatal graft versus host disease following a blood transfusion in a child with neuroblastoma. Pediatrics 1981;67: 217.
230. Ford JM, Lucey JJ, Cullen MH, et al. Fatal graft-versus-host disease following transfusion of granulocytes from normal donors. Lancet 1976;2:1167.
231. Schwarzenberg L, Mathe G, Amiel JL, et al. Study of factors determining the usefulness and complications of leukocyte transfusions. Am J Med 1967;43:206.
232. Hathaway WE, Githens JH, Blackburn WR, et al. Aplastic anemia, histiocytosis and erythrodermia in immunologically deficient children: probable human runt disease. N Engl J Med 1965;271:953.
233. Park BH, Good RA, Gate J, et al. Fatal graft-versus-host reaction following transfusion of allogeneic blood and plasma in infants with combined immunodeficiency disease. Transplant Proc 1974;6:385.
234. Dinsmore RE, Straus DJ, Pollack MS, et al. Fatal graft-versus-host disease following blood transfusion in Hodgkin's disease documented by HLA typing. Blood 1980;55:831.
235. Thaler M, Shamiss A, Orgad S, et al. The role of blood from HLA-homozygous donors in fatal transfusion-associated graft-versus-host disease after open-heart surgery. N Engl J Med 1989;321:25.
236. Sheehan T, McLaren KM, Brettle R, Parker AC. Transfusion-induced graft-versus-host disease in pregnancy. Clin Lab Haematol 1987;9: 205.
237. Arsura EL, Bertelle A, Minkowitz S, Cunningham JN, Crob D. Transfusion-associated graft-versus-host disease in a presumed immunocompetent patient. Arch Intern Med 1988;148:1941
238. Otsuka S, Kunieda K, Hirose M, et al. Fatal erythroderma (suspected graft-versus-host disease) after cholecystectomy. Transfusion 1989;29: 544.
239. Propper RD, Button LN, Nathan DG. New approaches to the transfusion management of thalassemia. Blood 1980;55:55.
240. Bracey AW, Klein HG, Chambers S, Corash L. Ex vivo selective isolation of young red blood cells using the IBM-2991 cell washer. Blood 1983;61:1068.
241. Gibble JW, Ness PM. Fibrin glue, the perfect operative sealant? Transfusion 1990.
242. Eschbach JW, Egrie JC, Downing MR, Browne JK, Adamson JW. Correction of the anemia of end-stage renal disease with recombinant human erythropoietin. N Engl J Med 1987;316:73.
243. Eschbach JW, Abdulhadi MH, Browne JK, et al. Recombinant human erythropoietin in anemic patients with end-stage renal disease: results of a phase III multicenter clinical trial. Ann Intern Med 1989;111: 992.
244. Lundin AP. Quality of life: subjective and objective improvements with recombinant human erythropoietin therapy. Semin Nephrol 1989;9:22.
244a. Lok S, Kaushansky K, Holly RD, et al. Cloning and expression of murine thrombopoietin cDNA and stimulation of platelet production in vivo. Nature 1994;369:565.
244b. de Sauvage FJ, Hass PE, Spencer SD. Stimulation of megakaryocytopoiesis and thrombopoiesis by the c-Mpl ligand. Nature 1994;369: 533.
245. Counts RB, Haisch C, Simon TL, Maxwell NG, Heimbach DM, Carrico CJ. Hemostasis in massively transfused trauma patients. Ann Surg 1979;190:91.
246. Mannucci PM, Federici AB, Sirchia G. Hemostasis testing during massive blood replacement: a study of 172 cases. Vox Sang 1982;42: 113.
247. Wilson RF, Dulchavsky SA, Soullier G, Beckman B. Problems with 20 or more blood transfusions in 24 hours. Am Surg 1987;53:410.
248. Reed RL, Ciavarella D, Heimbach, DM, et al. Prophylactic platelet administration during massive transfusion. Ann Surg 1986;203:40.
249. Martin DJ, Lucas CE, Ledgerwood AM, et al. Fresh frozen plasma supplement to massive red blood cell transfusion. Ann Surg 1985;202: 505.
250. Beutler E, Wood L. The in vivo regeneration of red cell 2,3 diphosphoglyceric acid (DPG) after transfusion of stored blood. J Lab Clin Med 1969;74:300.
251. Collins JA. Abnormal hemoglobin-oxygen affinity and surgical hemotherapy. In: Collins JA, Lundsgaard-Hansen P, eds. Surgical hemotherapy. Bibl Hematol 1980:46.
252. Perkins HA, Snyder M, Thagher C, Rolfs MR. Calcium ion activity during rapid exchange transfusion with citrated blood. Transfusion 1971;11:204.
253. Collins JA. Problems associated with the massive transfusion of stored blood. Surgery 1974;75:274.
254. Bick RL. Hemostasis defects associated with cardiac surgery, prosthetic devices, and other extracorporeal circuits. Semin Thromb Hemost 1980;11:249.
255. Salzman EW, Weinstein MJ, Weintraub RM, et al. Treatment with desmopressin acetate to reduce blood loss after cardiac surgery. N Engl J Med 1986;314:1402.
256. Storb R, Prentice RL, Thomas ED. Marrow transplantation for treatment of aplastic anemia: an analysis of factors associated with graft rejection. N Engl J Med 1977;296:61.
257. Storb R, Thomas ED, Buckner CD, et al. Marrow transplantation in 30 "untransfused" patients with severe aplastic anemia. Ann Intern Med 1980;92:30.
258. Champlin RE, Horowitz MM, van Bekkum DW, et al. Graft failure following bone marrow transplantation for severe aplastic anemia: risk factors and treatment results. Blood 1989;73:606.
259. Storb R, Wieden PL. Transfusion problems associated with transplantation. Semin Hematol 1981;18:163.
260. Gale RP, Feig S, Ho W, et al. ABO blood group system and bone marrow transplantation. Blood 1977;50:184.
261. Buckner CP, Clift RA, Sanders JE, Thomas ED. The role of a protective environment and prophylactic granulocyte transfusion in marrow transplantation. Transplant Proc 1978;10:255.
262. Hershko C, Gale RP, Ho W, Fitchen J. ABH antigens and bone marrow transplantation. Br J Haematol 1980;44:65.
263. Lasky L, Warkentin P, Ramsay N, Kersey J, McGlave P, McCullough J. Hemotherapy in patients undergoing blood group incompatible bone marrow transfusion. Transfusion 1983;23:277–285.
264. Berkman EM, Caplan SN. Engraftment of Rh positive marrow in a recipient with Rh antibody. Transplant Proc 1977;9:215.
265. Gershon AA, Steinberg S, Brunell PA. Zoster immune globulin: a further assessment. N Engl J Med 1974;290:243.
266. Opelz G, Sengar DPS, Mickey MR, et al. Effect of blood transfusions on subsequent kidney transplants. Transplant Proc 1973;5:253.
267. Opelz G, Terasaki PI. Improvement of kidney-graft survival with increased numbers of blood transfusions. N Engl J Med 1978;299:799.
268. Sacher RA, Luban NLC, Strauss RG. Current practice and guidelines for the transfusion of cellular blood components in the newborn. Transfusion Med Rev 1989;3:39.
269. Ludvigsen CW, Swanson JL, Thompson TR, McCullough JJ. The failure of neonates to form red blood cell alloantibodies in response to multiple transfusions. Am J Clin Pathol 1987;2:250.
270. Oberman HA. Transfusion of the neonatal patient. Transfusion 1974;14:183.
271. Christensen RD, Rothstein G, Anstall HB, et al. Granulocyte transfusions in neonates with bacterial infection, neutropenia, and depletion of mature marrow neutrophils. Pediatrics 1982;70:1.
272. Butch SH, Coltre MA. Techniques of transfusion. In: Kasprisin DO, Luban NLC, eds. Pediatric transfusion medicine, vol 1. Boca Raton, FL, CRC Press, 1987:91.
273. Warkentin PI. Transfusion therapy for the pediatric oncology patient. In: Kasprisin DO, Luban NLC, eds. Pediatric transfusion medicine, vol 2. Boca Raton, FL, CRC Press, 1987:19.
274. Schwartz SI, Bernard RP, Adams JT, Bauman AW. Splenectomy for hematologic disorders. Arch Surg 1970;101:338.
275. Pearson HA, Shulman NR, Marder VJ, Cone TE. Isoimmune neonatal thrombocytopenia purpura: clinical and therapeutic considerations. Blood 1964;23:154.
276. McFarland JG, Frenzke M, Aster RH. Testing of maternal sera in pregnancies at risk for neonatal alloimmune thrombocytopenia. Transfusion 1989;29:128.
277. Lalezari P. Alloimmune neonatal neutropenia. In: Engelfriet CP, von Loghem JJ, von dem Borne AEGKr, eds. Immunohematology. Amsterdam, Elsevier Science Publishers, 1984:178.
278. Widmann FK. Informed consent for blood transfusion: brief historical survey and summary of a conference. Transfusion 1990;30:460
279. DeCesare WR, Bove JR, Ebaugh FG, Jr. The mechanism of the effect of iso- and hyperosmolar dextrose-saline solutions on in vivo survival of human erythrocytes. Transfusion 1964;4:237.
280. Ryden SE, Oberman HA. Compatibility of common intravenous solutions with CPD blood. Transfusion 1975;15:250.
281. Braude AI. Transfusion reactions from contaminated blood: their recognition and treatment. N Engl J Med 1958;258:1289.
282. Walker RH. Special report: transfusion risks. Am J Clin Pathol 1987;88: 374.
283. Sazama K. 355 reports of transfusion-associated deaths. Transfusion 1990;30:583.
284. Pineda AA, Brzica SM, Taswell HF. Hemolytic transfusion reaction: recent experience in a large blood bank. Mayo Clin Proc 1978;53: 378.
285. Honing CL, Bove JR. Transfusion-associated fatalities: review of burea of biologics reports, 1976–1978. Transfusion 1980;20:653.
286. Brittingham TE, Chaplin H. Febrile transfusion reactions caused by sensitivity to donor leukocytes and platelets. JAMA 1957;165:819.
287. Menitove JE, McElligott MC, Aster RH. Febrile transfusion reaction: what blood component should be given next. Vox Sang 1982;42:318.
288. Popovsky MA, Chaplin HC, Moore SB. Transfusion-related acute lung injury: a neglected, serious complication of hemotherapy. Transfusion 1992;32:589.
289. Vyas GN, Holmdahl L, Perkins HA, Fudenberg HH. Serologic speci-

ficity of human anti-IgA and its significance in transfusion. Blood 1969;34:573.
290. Bove JR. Transfusion-associated hepatitis and AIDS: what is the risk? N Engl J Med 1987;317:242.
291. Alter HJ. You'll wonder where the yellow went: a 15-year retrospective of posttransfusion hepatitis. In: Moore SB, ed. Transfusion-transmitted viral diseases. Arlington, VA, American Association of Blood Banks, 1987:53.
292. Hollinger FB, Khan NC, Oefinger PA, et al. Posttransfusion hepatitis type A. JAMA 1983;250:2313.
293. Noble RC, Kane MA, Reeves SA, Roeckel I. Posttransfusion hepatitis A in a neonatal intensive care unit. JAMA 1984;252:2711.
294. Alter HJ, Holland PV, Purcell RH, et al. Posttransfusion hepatitis after exclusion of commercial and hepatitis-B antigen-positive donors. Ann Intern Med 1972;77:691.
295. Aach RD, Szmuness W, Mosley JW. Serum alanine aminotransferase of donors in relation to the risk of non-A, non-B hepatitis in recipients. N Engl J Med 1981;304:989.
296. Stevens CE, Taylor PE, Liu P. Hepatitis B virus infection: epidemiology and immunoprophylaxis. In: Moore SB, ed. Transfusion-transmitted viral diseases. Arlington, VA, American Association of Blood Banks, 1987:1.
297. Dienstag JL. Non-A, non-B hepatitis: I. Recognition, epidemiology, and clinical features. Gastroenterology 1983;85:439.
298. Koretz RL, Abbey H, Coleman E, Gitnick G. Non-A, non-B posttransfusion hepatitis. Ann Intern Med 1993;119:110.
299. Alter HJ, Purcell RH, Shih JW, et al. Detection of antibody to hepatitis C virus in prospectively followed transfusion recipients with acute and chronic non-A, non-B hepatitis. N Engl J Med 1989;321:1494.
300. Centers for Disease Control (CDC): Pneumocystis carinii pneumonia among persons with hemophilia A. MMWR 1982;31:365.
301. Centers for Disease Control (CDC). Possible transfusion-associated acquired immune deficiency syndrome (AIDS): California. MMWR 1982;31:652.
302. Curran JW, Lawrence DN, Jaffe HW, et al. Acquired immunodeficiency syndrome (AIDS) associated with transfusions. N Engl J Med 1984;310: 69.
303. Peterman TA, Jaffe HW, Feorino PM, et al. Transfusion-associated acquired immunodeficiency syndrome in the United States. JAMA 1985;254:2913.
304. Jaffe HW, Sarngadharan MG, DeVico AL, et al. Infection with HTLV-III/LAV and transfusion-associated acquired immunodeficiency syndrome: serologic evidence of an association. JAMA 1985;254:770.
305. Feorino PM, Kalyanaraman VS, Haverkos HW, et al. Lymphadenopathy associated virus infection of a blood donor-recipient pair with acquired immunodeficiency syndrome. Science 1984;225:69.
306. Feorino PM, Jaffe HW, Palmer E, et al. Transfusion-associated acquired immunodeficiency syndrome: evidence for persistent infection in blood donors. N Engl J Med 1985;312:1293.
307. Lange JMA, van den Berg H, Dooren LJ, et al. HTLV-III/LAV infection in nine children infected by a single plasma donor: clinical outcome and recognition patterns of viral proteins. J Infect Dis 1986;154:171.
308. Farzadegan H, Polis MA, Wolinsky SM, et al. Loss of human immunodeficiency virus type 1 (HIV-1) antibodies with evidence of viral infection in asymptomatic homosexual men. Ann Intern Med 1988;108:785.
309. Salahuddin SZ, Markham PD, Redfield RR, et al. HTLV-III in symptom-free seronegative persons. Lancet 1984;2:1418.
310. Roy MJ, Damato JJ, Burke DS. Absence of true seroreversion of HIV-1 antibody in seroreactive individuals. JAMA 1993;269:2876.
311. Ward JW, Grindon AJ, Feorino PM, et al. Laboratory and epidemiologic evaluation of an enzyme immunoassay for antibodies to HTLV-III. JAMA 1986;256:357.
312. MacDonald KL, Jackson JB, Bowman RJ, et al. Performance characteristics of serologic tests for human immunodeficiency virus type 1 (HIV-1) antibody among Minnesota blood donors. Ann Intern Med 1989;110:617.
313. The Consortium for Retrovirus Serology Standardization. Serological diagnosis of human immunodeficiency virus infection by Western blot testing. JAMA 1988;260:674.
314. Menitove JE. Status of recipients of blood from donors subsequently found to have an antibody to HIV. N Engl J Med 1986;315:1095.
315. Donegan E and the Transfusion Safety Study Group. Serum antibody positivity in recipients of anti-HIV positive blood. Transfusion 1986;26: 576.
316. Centers for Disease Control (CDC). Human immunodeficiency virus infection in transfusion recipients and their family members. MMWR 1987;36:137.
317. Peterman TA, Lui KJ, Lawrence DN, Allen JR. Estimating the risks of transfusions-associated acquired immune deficiency syndrome and human immunodeficiency virus infection. Transfusion 1987;27:371.
318. Lui KJ, Lawrence DN, Morgan WM, et al. A model-based approach for estimating the mean incubation period of transfusion-associated acquired immunodeficiency syndrome. Proc Natl Aca Sci 1986;83: 3051.
319. Ranki A, Valle SL, Krohm M, et al. Long latency precedes overt seroconverstion in sexually transmitted human-immunodeficiency-virus infection. Lancet 1987;2:589.
320. Imagawa DT, Lee MH, Wolinsky SM, et al. Human immunodeficiency virus type 1 infection in homosexual men who remain seronegative for prolonged periods. N Engl J Med 1989;320:1458.
321. Mayer KH, Stoddard AM, McCusker J, et al. Human T-lymphotropic virus type III in high-risk, antibody-negative homosexual men. Ann Intern Med 1986;104:194.
322. Cohen ND, Munoz A, Reitz BA, et al. Transmission of retroviruses by transfusion of screened blood in patients undergoing cardiac surgery. N Engl J Med 1989;320:1172.
323. Busch MP, Bernard EE, Khayam-Bashi H, et al. Evaluation of screened blood donation from human immunodeficiency virus type I infection by culture and DNA amplification of pooled cells. N Engl J Med 1991;325:1.
324. Donahue JG, Nelson KE, Munoz A, et al. Transmission of HIV by transfusion of screened blood. N Engl J Med 1990;323:1709.
325. Kleinman S, Secord K. Risk of human immunodeficiency virus (HIV) transmission by anti-HIV negative blood: estimates using the lookback methodology. Transfusion 1988;28:499.
326. Bove JR. Transfusion-associated hepatitis and AIDS: what is the risk? N Engl J Med 1987;317:242.
327. Ward JW, Holmberg SD, Allen JR, et al. Transfusion of human immunodeficiency virus (HIV) by blood transfusions screened as negative for HIV antibody. N Engl J Med 1988;318:473.
328. Turner TB, Diseker TH. Duration of infectivity of Treponema pallidum in citrated blood stored under conditions obtaining in blood banks. Bull Johns Hopkins Hosp 1941;68:269.
329. Tegtmeier GE. Transfusion-transmitted cytomegalovirus infections: significance and control. Vox Sang 1986;51:22.
330. Gerber P, Walsh JH, Rosenblum EN. Association of EB-virus infection with the post-perfusion syndrome. Lancet 1969;1:593.
331. Jackson JB, Orr HT, McCullough JJ, Jordan MC. Failure to detect human cytomegalovirus DNA in IgM-seropositive blood donors by spot hybridization. J Infect Dis 1987;156:1013.
332. Adler SP. Transfusion-associated cytomegalovirus infections. Rev Infect Dis 1983;5:977.
333. Luban NLC, Williams AE, MacDonald MG, et al. Low incidence of acquired cytomegalovirus infection in neonates transfused with washed red blood cells. Am J Dis Child 1987;141:4161.
334. Meyers JD, Reed EC, Shepp DH, et al.. Acyclovir for prevention of cytomegalovirus infection and disease after allogeneic marrow transplantation. N Engl J Med 1988;38:70.
335. Okochi K, Sato H. Adult T-cell leukemia virus, blood donors and transfusion: experience in Japan. Prog Clin Biol Res 1985;182:245.
336. Centers for Disease Control and Prevention and the U.S.P.H.S. Working Group. Guidelines for counseling persons infected with human T-lymphotropic virus type I (HTLV-I) and type II (HTLV-II). Ann Intern Med 1993;1888:448.
337. Schmunis GA. Chagas' disease and blood transfusion. In: Dodd RY, Barker LF, eds. Infection, immunity and blood transfusion. New York, Alan R Liss, 1985:127.
338. Smith RP, Evans AT, Popovsky M, et al. Transfusion-acquired babesiosis and failure of antibiotic treatment. JAMA 1986;256:2726.
339. Aoki SK, Holland PV. Lyme disease: another transfusion risk? Transfusion 1989;29:646.
340. Badon SJ, Fister RD, Cable RG. Survival of Borrelia burgdorferi in blood products. Transfusion 1989;29:581.
341. Serjeant GR, Mason K, Topley JM, et al. Outbreak of aplastic crisis in sickle cell anemia associated with parvovirus-like agent. Lancet 1981;2:595.
342. Mortimer PP, Luban NL, Kelleher JF, Cohen BJ. Transmission of serum parvovirus-like agent by clotting factor concentrates. Lancet 1983;2: 482.
343. Consensus Conference. The utility of therapeutic plasmapheresis for neurological disorders. JAMA 1986;256:1333.
344. Chopek M, McCullough J. Protein and biochemical changes during plasma exchange. In: Therapeutic hemapheresis. Arlington, VA, American Association of Blood Banks, 1980:13.
345. Keller AJ, Urbaniak SJ. Intensive plasma exchange on the cell separator: effects on serum immunoglobulins and complement components. Br J Haematol 1978;38:531.
346. Huestis DW, Bove, JR, Case J. Complications of transfusion: practical blood transfusion, ed 4. Boston, Little, Brown, 1988:251.
347. Sutton DMC, Nair RC, Rock NG, Canadian Apheresis Study Group. Complications of plasma exchange. Transfusion 1989;29:124.
348. McKee LC, Collins RD. Intravascular leukocyte thrombi and aggregates as a cause of morbidity and mortality in leukemia. Medicine 1974;53: 463.
349. Freireich EJ, Thomas LB, Frei E, Fritz RD, Forkner CE. A distinctive type of intracerebral hemorrhage associated with "blastic crisis" in patients with leukemia. Cancer 1960;13:146.
350. Lokich JJ, Moloney WC. Fatal pulmonary leukostasis following treat-

ment of acute myelogenous leukemia. Arch Intern Med 1972;130: 759.

351. Roberts WC, Bodey GP, Wertlake PT. The heart in acute leukemia: a study of 420 autopsy cases. Am J Cardiol 1968;21:388.

352. Steeper TA, Smith JA, McCullough J. Therapeutic cytapheresis using the Fenwal CS-3000 blood cell separator. Vox Sang 1985;48:193.

353. Tremper KK, Friedman AE, Levine EM. The preoperative treatment of severely anemic patients with a perfluorochemical oxygen-transport fluid, fluosol-DA. N Engl J Med 1982;307:277.

354. Mitsuno T, Ohyanagi H, Naito R. Clinical studies of A perfluorochemical whole blood substitute (Fluosol-DA). Ann Surg 1982;195: 60.

355. Bucala R. Cytotoxicity of a perfluorocarbon blood substitute to macrophages in vitro. Science 1983;220:965.

356. Vercellotti GM, Hammerschmidt DE, Craddock PR, Jacob HS. Activation of plasma complement by perfluorocarbon artificial blood: probable mechanism of adverse pulmonary reactions in treated patients and rationale for corticosteroid prophylaxis. Blood 1982; 59:1299.

357. Gould SA, Rosen AL, Sehgal R, et al. Fluosol-DA as a red-cell substitute in acute anemia. N Engl J Med 1986;314:1653.

358. Winslow RM. Blood substitutes: current status. Transfusion 1989;29: 753.

Blood: Principles and Practice of Hematology,
edited by Robert I. Handin, Samuel E. Lux, and Thomas P. Stossel.
J.B. Lippincott Company, Philadelphia © 1995.

61

Medical Therapy of Hematologic Malignancies

Nathan A. Berger
Hillard M. Lazarus

HISTORICAL PERSPECTIVE

The modern age of cancer chemotherapy can be considered to have begun around the turn of the century with the synthesis and use of sulfur mustard for its vesicant properties in chemical warfare.[1] It was soon noted that victims of mustard gas attacks showed leukopenia, bone marrow aplasia, and lysis of lymphoid tissues.[2–4] By the time of World War II, new chemical analogues were synthesized, and biologic investigations demonstrated that nitrogen mustard could cause regression of animal tumors without killing the host.[5,6] In subsequent studies, nitrogen mustard was shown to cause regression of human tumors along with severe bone marrow depression; in particular, it was shown to be useful for control of Hodgkin's disease and chronic myelogenous leukemia (CML).[5,7,8] This initial success of systemic chemotherapy led to the synthesis of numerous nitrogen mustard analogues with different pharmacologic properties and improved efficacy in a variety of neoplastic disorders.

Several other classes of chemotherapeutic agents were discovered during the 1940s. Studies of the structure and function of the vitamin folic acid led to the synthesis of antagonists such as aminopterin and methotrexate, which were initially found to cause leukopenia and subsequently shown to be useful in the treatment of leukemia.[9,10] Also during the 1940s, Hitchings, Elion and colleagues,[11,12] and others began to synthesize purine and pyrimidine analogues to be used for the investigation of nucleic acid metabolism. In 1952, they reported the synthesis of 6-mercaptopurine and its ability to interfere with nucleic acid synthesis.[12] It was soon shown to cause leukopenia and to be effective in the treatment of acute lymphoblastic leukemia (ALL).[13]

In his 1943 description of Cushing's syndrome, Albright[14] noted the association of lymph node atrophy with overproduction of adrenal corticosteroids, and by 1950, Pearson and Eliel[15,16] had shown the efficacy of cortisone in the treatment of patients with lymphoid neoplasms. Thus, by the early 1950s, several different classes of drugs were in use for the treatment of hematologic malignancies, and the tools for developing combination chemotherapy regimens were in hand. These drugs led the way for the synthesis of many new agents that now enable us to cure some malignancies and to control many others. In this regard, it is interesting to read, in the second edition of the *Pharmacologic Basis of Therapeutics* by Goodman and Gilman, published in 1960, the following statement: "It should be stated at the outset that no chemical compound has yet been found which is capable of curing any form of cancer."[17] Over thirty years later, with a great expansion in the number of chemotherapeutic agents and the development of many new ways to use them, we control many types of malignancies and, more important, achieve cures in several others. In fact, we can cure some of the most fulminant hematologic malignancies. Now, we frequently hear that despite the excitement and availability of biologic response modifiers, they have not yet been successfully used to cure cancer. Hopefully, our therapeutic trials should soon bring us to the point where we will be able to look back on these statements with the same perspective that we now view the 1960 statement regarding chemotherapy.

Although specific regimens for treating each of the hematologic malignancies are contained in the relevant chapters, it is useful to consider the treatment of ALL from a historical viewpoint to illustrate many of the principles involved in treating hematologic malignancies. Our ability to eradicate leukemic cells and allow the regrowth of normal hematopoietic precursors is documented in the remarkable step-by-step success story associated with the treatment of ALL. In 1960, a child with ALL had only a 10% chance of long-term survival. Now, a child with ALL has about a 70% chance of long-term survival, and almost all children with certain subsets of ALL can be cured of their disease.[18,19] Initial progress against this disease came with the demonstration that so-called remissions could be induced by administration of the folate antagonist aminopterin[10] or by administration of a corticosteroid hormone.[15,16] These remissions, however, were temporary, and relapses were almost inevitable.[20,21] The use of chemotherapeutic agents in combination to treat ALL made it clear that this approach could result in disappearance of all clinical and laboratory evidence of disease.[18,19,22] If chemotherapy was stopped after induction of this so-called complete remission, the disease usually recurred, indicating the persistence of undetectable tumor cells that later proliferate to sufficient numbers and produce clinically apparent relapse. Subsequent trials showed that additional courses of intensive chemotherapy could prolong remission durations, suggesting that these second courses of induction therapy served to further reduce the malignant cell mass, that is, consolidate the remission induction.[23] Additional trials showed that continuation of chemotherapy for extended periods beyond those needed to induce remission resulted in long-term disease-free intervals and ultimately, in some cases, to long, unmaintained remissions and apparent cures.[12,19,24–26]

Subsequent experience with ALL showed that the blood–brain barrier made the central nervous system (CNS) a unique sanctuary where leukemic cells could escape the effects of systemic chemotherapy and later proliferate to cause a CNS relapse and subsequently cause systemic disease recurrence.[27,28] Treatment of these sanctuary sites with intrathecal chemotherapy, craniospinal irradiation, or both led to improved long-term remissions and improved the cure rate for ALL.[29–32] Studies are directed at defining the optimal regimen for CNS prophylaxis in ALL since some patients are at low risk for CNS relapse, and significant long-term CNS effects (eg, learning disabilities or more severe dysfunction) may occur as a sequelae of CNS treatment.[32–35]

Addition of maintenance therapy regimens consisting of daily 6-mercaptopurine and weekly methotrexate to the treatment of patients with ALL produced prolonged disease-free survival in at least 40% to 50% of those who entered complete remission.[36–38] Further studies suggested that a more intensive approach to remission maintenance by employing a three-drug induction regimen, early intensification with multiple agents, and four-drug maintenance therapy may result in improved disease-free survival.[36,39]

Some patients in relapse were shown to be cured by bone marrow transplantation, and this procedure has been applied efficiently in second remissions, producing 25% to 30% disease-free survival.[40] Because some high-risk patients can be identified prospectively by age or cytogenetic abnormalities, such as the Philadelphia chromosome t[9;22] or the t[4;11] translocation, or by markedly elevated leukocyte counts at diagnosis and other factors such as slow attainment of complete remission, many transplantation centers have begun to offer bone marrow transplantations in first remission for such patients.[40,41]

Although dramatic strides have been made in the treatment of childhood leukemia, less favorable results are attained in adult ALL.[42–44] Hence, bone marrow transplantation is advocated for adult ALL patients who relapse and are induced into second remission as well as for some children and adults in first remission, as noted previously.[40,41,45] Up to half of these patients may achieve long-term disease-free survivals after allogeneic bone marrow transplantation. Complications such as graft-versus-host disease, interstitial pneumonitis, chemotherapy-induced nonmyeloid organ toxicity, and opportunistic infections seriously limit the success of this approach. In addition, only one third of patients have a suitably matched sibling donor, in part because of the relatively small size of US families.[46,47] These limitations have led to a number of promising trials using autologous bone marrow transplantation in which residual leukemic cells are purged ex vivo, from the marrow, by pharmacologic or immunologic techniques.[48–50] In addition, the use of unrelated matched or haploidentical sibling donor marrow transplants has shown promise when used in first or second remissions.[51]

THERAPEUTIC GOALS

The hematologic malignancies are a diverse group of disorders characterized by different clinical syndromes and disease durations that vary with the affected cell lines and their associated biologic properties. Disease manifestations and clinical courses are also influenced by the acute or chronic nature of the malignant process, the age of the patient, and a variety of other factors. Knowledge of these differences and their relation to normal hematopoietic cell biology and biochemistry are essential to understanding the different rationales and strategic approaches employed in the treatment of hematologic malignancies. Thus, a major goal of systemic therapy in all the hematologic malignancies is reduction of the malignant cell mass; however, this goal is approached with varying degrees of intensity, depending on the disease and the associated clinical syndrome. For example, the acute leukemias usually are characterized by a rapid and fulminant course associated with expansion of immature cells such as lymphoblasts or myeloblasts, with organ invasion and suppression of normal blood-forming elements that results in systemic manifestations of anemia, thrombocytopenia, and granulocytopenia. The approach to the acute leukemias is to treat them aggressively with curative intent to eradicate the malignant cell clone. In contrast, the indolent phase of CML, which usually lasts for several years, is characterized by an expanded production of granulocytes, which maintain most of their functional capacity; whereas in the accelerated phase or blast crisis, this disease resembles acute leukemia. Thus, the chronic phase is frequently treated to produce symptomatic control of the granulocyte mass and associated organomegaly, whereas blast crisis is treated more like acute leukemia. In recent years, however, more aggressive approaches employing bone marrow transplantation using sibling-matched or unrelated-matched allogenic marrow, or autologous bone marrow have been initiated that can effectively eradicate the malignant cell clones and cure CML in its various stages.[52–55]

An entirely different clinical course is shown by polycythemia vera, which is characterized in its initial stages by the expansion of normal-functioning erythrocytes frequently accompanied by leukocytosis and thrombocytosis. The pathophysiology of this disease is associated with an overexpanded red blood cell (RBC) mass rather than with any functional abnormality of the erythrocytes. Thus, this disease may be controlled for long periods using phlebotomy to maintain RBC mass within normal levels.[56] Similarly, chronic lymphocytic leukemia (CLL) usually is treated to control excessive production and expansion of the malignant cell population.[57,58] Attempts at eradication or cure are usually not made since effective therapies for this purpose have not been developed (with the exception of a few patients who have undergone allogeneic or autologous bone marrow transplantation[58a]). Another situation exists with multiple myeloma in which the expansion of a malignant clone of plasma cells and their by-products results in lytic bone lesions, abnormal immunoglobulin and electrolyte metabolism, and suppression of normal hematopoietic elements. In this disease, therapy needs to be directed at control of the malignant cell mass and of the effects of the abnormal immunoglobulin metabolism and bone resorption.

THERAPEUTIC STRATEGIES AND TERMINOLOGY

The operational approach to therapy of the hematologic malignancies involves several distinct stages. *Induction therapy* is the initial use of one or more courses of chemotherapy to reduce or eradicate malignant cells or tumor masses. In the chronic leukemias, induction therapy is used to achieve gradual cytoreduction and control of the malignant cell mass. In the acute leukemias, induction therapy is used to achieve rapid cytoreduction and eradication of the malignant cell mass. *Complete response or remission* indicates that all clinical evidence of malignancy has been eliminated and, in the case of hematologic malignancies, that normal bone marrow cellularity and function have been restored.[59] Because of the therapeutic approaches outlined previously, complete response is usually the goal of therapy in acute leukemia, whereas control is the goal of therapy in chronic leukemia. Complete response, however, is not to be equated with cure since subclinical disease persists and will become clinically apparent if therapy is discontinued. Hence, as described later, consolidation and possibly maintenance therapy are used after complete response is attained.

When a complete response has been achieved and disease signs and symptoms have disappeared for at least 1 month, the patient is considered to be in *complete remission*. *Partial response* and *partial remission* indicate that the malignant cell mass has been significantly reduced (eg, by 50% or more) from its original presentation but that clinical signs of disease may persist. *Stable disease* indicates that the malignant cell mass has neither decreased nor increased appreciably, and *progressive disease* indicates that the malignant cell mass has increased beyond that noted at the start of therapy.[59]

Relapse is the recurrence of laboratory or clinical signs of disease at some time after complete remission has been achieved, and *remission duration* is the time from the achievement of complete remission to the time of relapse. Although apparent complete responses may sometimes be obtained with a single intensive course of chemotherapy, the rapid reoccurrence of disease in acute leukemia indicates the persistence of leukemic cells.[60] Such relapses underscore the importance of recognizing that the term complete remission is an operational term used to describe the clinical situation in which there are no overt signs of disease; however, subclinical disease is usually present under these conditions.[61]

At diagnosis, the bone marrow in most cases of acute leukemia is largely replaced by leukemic blast cells, although in some cases, the bone marrow may be hypoplastic.[62] Expansion of the leukemic cell population suppresses most normal marrow elements. Nonleukemic hematopoietic stem cells, however, appear to remain present in the marrow in sufficient numbers to totally repopulate the marrow with normal blood elements if permitted to do so.[63,64] The ability to cure acute leukemia depends on eradicating the malignant cells while leaving the normal hematopoietic stem cells to later undergo differentiation and repopulation of the marrow.[63,64]

From a cytokinetic viewpoint, patients whose bone marrow is mostly replaced by leukemic cells harbor between 10^{11} and 10^{12} malignant cells in their body.[65] When effective treatment is used to reduce the cell number by several orders of magnitude or logs to 10^9 cells, it is relatively impossible, by morphologic or histochemical techniques, to detect leukemic cells in the bone marrow. Leukemic cells, however, frequently contain nonrandom chromosomal translocations such as the *bcl-2* or t[14;18] translocation in lymphoid malignancies and the Philadelphia chromosome t[9;22] or *bcr/abl* translocation in CML.[61,66] B-cell malignancies also may contain molecular rearrangements in the immunoglobulin genes, such as *CDR3*, the complementarity-determining region III of the immunoglobulin heavy chain that can serve as unique clonal markers.[61] Molecular rearrangements of the T-cell receptor may be used as unique clonal markers of the latter cell type. When leukemic cells have such known markers, Southern blot hybridization can be used to detect residual leukemic cells at a frequency as low as 1% of the total number of cells.[61,66] Use of the polymerase chain reaction, in which rare sequences of DNA or RNA can be amplified and detected, has made it possible to detect these characteristic chromosomal translocations to reveal the presence of residual leukemic cells with a much greater sensitivity, approaching 1 in 1,000,000 cells.[67–70] Thus, some patients in complete remission may still harbor 10^8 to 10^9 leukemic cells in their bone marrow, and without further treatment, proliferation of these cells may lead to relapse within a short period.[60,61,68] When a group of acute myelogenous leukemia (AML) patients achieving complete remission were randomized to continue treatment versus no further postremission therapy, all patients who received no additional therapy relapsed within 9 months, with a median remission duration of 4 months.[60] The patients who received additional therapy had a median remission duration of 8 months, and several were still disease-free after 2 years.[60]

The high relapse rate after remission-induction therapy and the achievement of apparent complete remission, coupled with the understanding that as many as 10^9 leukemic cells could remain in the body but escape routine detection, led to the concept of consolidation therapy. *Consolidation therapy* is administered after remission induction and is aimed at further reducing the malignant cell mass by the use of additional intensive courses of chemotherapy. Patients receiving consolidation therapy given as a repeat course of induction therapy or other intensive therapy have an improved remission duration and are more likely to be disease-free after 2 years.[23] In some cases, however, it is clear that even consolidation therapy does not sufficiently reduce malignant cells to offer long-term remissions or cures and that patients may relapse shortly after induction and consolidation therapy. Therefore, patients with ALL are usually treated with *maintenance therapy*, composed of repeated courses of less intense chemotherapy given over long periods to further eliminate or suppress malignant cells.[24–26] In acute myeloblastic leukemia, however, maintenance therapy has been largely abandoned since such therapy was associated with toxicity but added no additional antitumor or survival benefit.

An alternative approach developed to eliminate residual malignant cells is *intensification therapy*. This strategy employs an intensive course of cytotoxic therapy given at a late time after remission induction or after a period of maintenance therapy. It is theoretically used to protect against the gradual expansion of malignant cells. The use of high-dose chemotherapy and bone marrow transplantation while a patient is in remission may be considered a form of intensification therapy.[41,42]

CHEMOTHERAPEUTIC AGENTS USED IN THE THERAPY OF HEMATOLOGIC MALIGNANCIES

The hematologic malignancies are systemic diseases that in general require a systemic approach to therapy. Thus, chemotherapy with cytotoxic agents is the major approach to treatment of these disorders, and many of the chemotherapeutic agents in use for cancer chemotherapy have been developed for their antileukemic potential. Biologic response modifiers and immunotoxins constitute a more recent approach to systemic therapy, with great promise. Surgery is rarely used in the treatment of hematologic malignancies, while radiation therapy is used for controlling specific and localized problems such as the prophylaxis or treatment of leukemic meningitis.

Chemotherapeutic agents can be classified chemically according to their structure, biochemically according to their mechanisms of actions, or biologically according to their ability to affect cancer cells at various phases of the cell division cycle. These agents also can be classified biologically according to their ability to kill replicating or resting cells. These distinctions are based on laboratory experiments and are critically important in understanding how various agents may be used alone or in combination to kill cancer cells.

Phase-specific agents act on proliferating cells during distinct phases of the cell growth cycle. In some cases, these agents kill proliferating cells during specific phases of the growth cycle; in other cases, the agents prevent progression through the proliferation cycle by arresting growth in specific phases.[71,72]

To fully appreciate the phase-specific effects of selected agents, it is necessary to understand the different biologic and biochemical components of the cell cycle.

The cell generation cycle is divided into four phases: G_1, S, G_2, and M.[65,73] G_1 begins immediately after mitosis; it is the period when the cell carries out its usual nonmitotic functions, and it lasts until the beginning of S phase, which is the synthetic period during which DNA synthesis takes place and the genome is replicated. G_2 is the period between the end of DNA synthesis and the beginning of cell division. M is the mitotic phase, during which chromosomal condensation occurs, the mitotic spindle appears, sister chromatids separate, and the process of cell division occurs with the production of two daughter cells. G_0 cells are those that have left the cycling pool, either temporarily or permanently. Cells that are temporarily in G_0 retain clonogenic potential and can be recruited back into the proliferative cycle by appropriate stimuli or growth factors.[73,74] A fraction of hematopoietic stem cells are characteristically in the G_0 phase, so that they are not severely affected by cycle-specific agents and can be recruited back into the cell cycle. Alternatively, some G_0 cells may be terminally differentiated and cannot be recruited back into the cell cycle. Examples of the latter include mature granulocytes and normoblasts.

Figure 61-1 provides an illustration of the cell cycle and some agents that act at specific phases. Examples include the DNA synthesis inhibitor cytosine arabinoside, which

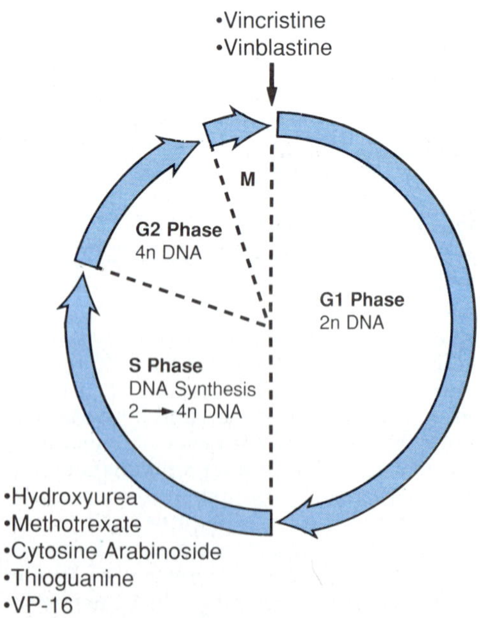

FIGURE 61-1. Phases of the cell cycle in which some antitumor agents have their major toxic effects. The designations 2n and 4n refer to the DNA content of the cell relative to the 1n DNA content, which represents a single copy of the genome found in gamete cells after meiotic division.

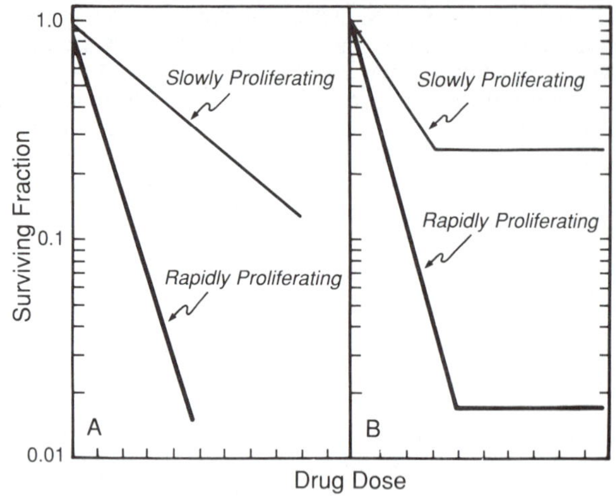

FIGURE 61-2. Theoretic cell survival curves for slowly and rapidly proliferating cells. (**A**) Effect of cycle-independent agents. (**B**) Effect of cycle-specific agents.

blocks cells in the S phase or DNA synthetic phase, and the mitotic spindle inhibitor vincristine, which interferes with cells progressing through the division or mitotic phase of the cell cycle.

Cycle-dependent agents kill both cycling and resting cells but are more active against cycling cells. Methotrexate, 5-fluorouracil, doxorubicin, and daunorubicin are examples of cycle-dependent agents that are S-phase selective. In contrast, cycle-independent agents are equally toxic to proliferating and resting cells. Cyclophosphamide is an example of a cycle-dependent agent that is not phase specific, whereas BCNU (carmustine) is an example of a cycle-independent agent. An important difference between cycle-dependent and cycle-independent agents is the characteristic cytotoxicity or survival curves. Figure 61-2 shows that agents that are cell cycle–specific kill all cells in a specific phase of the cell cycle during a given time of exposure. Once that fraction of the population is killed, the survival curve reaches a plateau. If the entire population proliferates more rapidly, more cells pass through any particular phase of the cell cycle and a greater number of cells are exposed to the agent during their vulnerable phase and consequently killed. Cycle-independent agents, such as many alkylating agents, produce a continuous exponential decrease in cell survival because they affect all cells in the population regardless of their phase in the cell cycle. Nonetheless, these agents may also be more active in rapidly proliferating cells, probably because the cells lack the time to repair damage before completing the cell cycle.[72–75]

The considerations just outlined are important in determining the potential usefulness of an agent for different types of malignancies as well as for inclusion in combination chemotherapy regimens. For example, phase-specific agents are most useful for malignancies with a high level of proliferating cells. In contrast, phase-specific agents are less effective against tumors with low proliferation rates, such as in most carcinomas. Furthermore, when used in the latter situation, phase-specific agents are more likely to cause toxic side effects. Many normal tissues, including epithelium, such as skin and gastrointestinal mucosa, have proliferation rates higher than the tumor and may therefore show increased sensitivity to these agents. Cycle-independent agents such as alkylating agents are useful for tumors with low proliferation rates. Of the hematologic malignancies, CLL, a disease of long-lived B lymphocytes, probably has one of the lowest proliferation rates.[57,58] This disease is often effectively treated with chlorambucil, which is a cycle-independent nitrogen mustard analogue.

The agents commonly used for the treatment of hematologic malignancies are listed in Table 61-1. They are classified into groups that reflect their mechanisms of actions and chemical structures.

Antimetabolites

The antimetabolites are a diverse series of agents. They are often analogues of natural metabolites, and they usually interfere with essential metabolic processes, thereby leading to cell death. The antimetabolites most frequently used in therapy of hematologic malignancies include methotrexate, cytosine arabinoside, thiopurines, and hydroxyurea. Recent additions to this group of agents include deoxycoformycin, chlorodeoxyadenosine, and fludarabine phosphate.

Methotrexate

Methotrexate is a synthetic analogue of folic acid that acts as a competitive inhibitor of dihydrofolate reductase[76,77] (Fig. 61-3). It prevents the conversion of dihydrofolate to tetrahydrofolate, resulting in the rapid depletion of reduced folate pools.[76,77] The latter are required for one-carbon transfer in purine and thymidilate synthesis. By interfering with thymidine and purine availability, methotrexate inhibits DNA synthesis. It acts as an S-phase selective agent and is most active against rapidly proliferating cells. Methotrexate may be administered orally or intravenously. It is also one of the major drugs given by intrathecal administration for the treatment of CNS leukemia.[31,32] Methotrexate is highly useful in the treatment of ALL but must be administered in adequate concentrations. Children exposed to relatively low concentrations of drug because of rapid clearance are more likely to relapse during maintenance therapy.[78] Methotrexate is predominantly toxic to rapidly proliferating tissues such as the bone marrow, skin, and gastrointestinal epithelium. The drug also may be associated with renal damage after high-dose therapy, where it is especially likely to precipitate in acid urine.[79] Methotrexate is also associated with hepatic damage after prolonged administration, as may occur with its use in maintenance regimens. The intrathecal administration of methotrexate, which involves direct instillation into the cerebrospinal fluid, has been associated with acute meningeal irritation as well as with more chronic necrotizing leukoencephalopathy. Many studies correlated serum methotrexate concentrations with the risk of toxicity,[79,80] which includes renal failure, stomatitis, mucositis, bone fractures in pediatric patients, rash, hepatitis, megaloblastic anemia, and pulmonary infiltrates with eosinophilia.[81–84] Alterations in levels of dihydrofolate reductase or binding affinity of the enzyme for methotrexate contribute to methotrexate resistance.[85,86] Methotrexate resistance also is associated with alterations in cellular transport mechanisms.[86]

Cytosine Arabinoside

Cytosine arabinoside is a nucleoside analogue useful in the treatment of acute myelogenous leukemia, acute lymphocytic leukemia, and lymphoma.[87–89] It contains arabinose as the sugar moiety instead of ribose or deoxyribose (Fig. 61-4). Cytosine arabinoside is metabolized by the cell as if it were a DNA building block. The agent requires intracellular metabolism for conversion to its active form, cytosine arabinoside triphosphate. As a nucleoside triphosphate analogue, it acts as an S-phase–specific agent to inhibit DNA synthesis by inhibiting DNA polymerase.[90] It also can be incorporated into nascent DNA chains, where, because of the alteration in the sugar moiety, it distorts DNA structure and acts as a chain terminator.[91] In addition, cytosine arabinoside has been shown to have an effect on sugar nucleotide and phospholipid metabolism, which may contribute to its cytotoxicity.[92] Cytosine arabinoside resistance is associated with low levels of the activating enzyme deoxycytidine kinase, which is required for phosphorylation of cytosine arabinoside, or with high levels of the enzyme cytidine deaminase, which converts cytosine arabinoside monophosphate to uracil arabinoside monophosphate.[93,94] This nucleoside is poorly absorbed from the gastrointestinal tract and is administered by the intravenous route. Fever is a common side effect,[95] but its major toxicity is to rapidly proliferating tissues, resulting in rash and diarrhea.[84,95,96] Because of its CNS penetration, systemic administration of cytosine arabinoside during high-dose therapy may eradicate CNS leukemia.[97] In high doses, however, cytosine arabinoside has been associated with neurologic, ophthalmologic, and hepatic abnormalities[98–100] as well as severe skin, gastrointestinal, and lung dysfunction.[101–104] These effects may be seen, in part, because cytosine arabinoside in high dose produces metabolites that interfere with inactivation (excretion) of active drug.[105]

Thiopurines

The thiopurines are purine analogues with a sulfur substituted for the keto group at the 6 position of the purine ring (Fig. 61-5). These drugs are the result of a program in nucleic acid analogue design, were synthesized in the early 1950s, and have been used as antileukemic agents ever since.[11,13] Their development was the basis for awarding the Nobel Prize in 1988 to George Hitchings and Gertrude Elion. Substitution of sulfur at the 6 position of hypoxanthine results in creation of the drug 6-mercaptopurine, which is useful in the treatment of ALL; and substitution at the 6 position of guanine gives 6-thioguanine, which is used in the treatment of AML.[13] The drugs are metabolized by the intracellular enzyme hypoxanthine guanine phosphoribosyl transferase (HGPRT) to their nucleoside monophosphates and subsequently converted to deoxynucleoside triphosphates, which are incorporated into DNA, where they alter macromolecular stability and function.[106–108] As the monophosphates, the nucleoside analogues interfere with de novo purine synthesis, leading to depletion of purine pools. These agents are S-phase–active drugs. 6-Thioguanine shows considerable synergy with cytosine arabinoside when given in an appropriate schedule. The thiopurines are toxic to rapidly proliferating cells, resulting in bone marrow and gastrointestinal toxicity. They also are associated with hepatic toxicity. Resistance to thioguanine in rodent cells is commonly associated with low levels or absence of the enzyme HGPRT, but in human leukemic cells, it is more commonly associated with increased catabolism of the thiopurine nucleotides to nucleosides.[108] The thiopurines are variably absorbed from the gastrointestinal tract, but 6-mercaptopurine is routinely administered orally as part of maintenance therapy regimens. Decreased absorption is associated with relapses in children, and the serum concentrations should be monitored for efficacy.[109,110]

Hydroxyurea

Hydroxyurea is an S-phase–specific agent that inhibits ribonucleotide reductase, a key regulatory enzyme responsible for conversion of ribonucleotides to deoxy-

TABLE 61-1. Agents Commonly Used in the Chemotherapy of Hematologic Malignancies

Agents and Class	Target and Mechanism of Antileukemic Effect	Nonhematologic Toxicities	Route of Administration
ANTIMETABOLITES			
Methotrexate	Synthetic folic acid analogue; inhibits dihydrofolate reductase; interferes with one-carbon metabolism; interferes with thymidine and purine synthesis, resulting in limitation of DNA synthesis	Mucositis, hepatic fibrosis, renal failure	IV, PO
Cytosine arabinoside	Pyrimidine nucleoside analogue; inhibits DNA polymerase; incorporates into DNA as chain terminator	Mucositis, hepatotoxicity, neurotoxicity	IV
6-Mercaptopurine, 6-thioguanine	Purine analogues; inhibit PRPP aminotransferase and purine synthesis, resulting in limitation of DNA synthesis; incorporates into DNA, producing delayed DNA damage and toxicity	Hepatotoxicity	PO
Hydroxyurea	Chelator; inhibits ribonucleotide reductase, limiting production of deoxyribonucleotides and thereby interfering with DNA synthesis	Stomatitis	PO
Deoxycoformycin	Purine nucleoside analogue; inhibits adenosine deaminase, leading to accumulation of adenosine nucleotides, DNA strand breaks, and depletion of NAD	Gastrointestinal disturbances, neurotoxicity	IV
Chlorodeoxyadenosine	Purine nucleoside analogue; activates pathway, leading to DNA strand breaks and depletion of NAD		IV
Fludarabine phosphate	Purine nucleoside analogue; resistant to adenosine deaminase; inhibits ribonucleotide reductase, DNA polymerase, and DNA synthesis	Neurotoxicity, multifocal demyelination	IV
ALKYLATING AGENTS			
Chlorambucil	Benzene butanoic acid derivative of nitrogen mustard; causes DNA alkylation and cross-link formation	Gastrointestinal disturbances	PO
Melphalan	Phenylalanine derivative of nitrogen mustard; preferentially localized in tumors using glutamine or leucine transport systems; causes DNA alkylation and cross-link formation	Gastrointestinal disturbances	PO, IV
Cyclophosphamide	Nitrogen mustard analogue, metabolized to phosphoramide mustard; causes DNA alkylation damage	Hemorrhagic cystitis, gastrointestinal disturbances	PO, IV
Busulfan	Alkyl sulfonate derivative; causes DNA alkylation damage and cross-link formation	Pulmonary fibrosis, hyperpigmentation	PO
BCNU	Nitrosourea; causes DNA alkylation and cross-link formation	Pulmonary fibrosis	IV
ANTITUMOR ANTIBIOTICS			
Daunorubicin, doxorubicin	Anthracyclines; intercalate DNA, causing DNA damage and free radical generation; stabilize topoisomerase II–cross-linked DNA strand breaks	Cardiomyopathies	IV
Mitoxantrone, idarubicin, epirubicin	Semisynthetic anthraquinone; DNA intercalator; stabilizes topoisomerase II–cross-linked DNA strand breaks; activates pathways, leading to cell death		IV
PLANT ALKALOIDS			
Vincristine, vinblastine	Tubulin-binding agents; inhibitors of microtubule formation; cause disruption of mitotic spindle and mitotic arrest	Neuropathies, mucositis	IV
Etoposide (VP-16); teniposide (VM-26)	Semisynthetic podophyllotoxin; stabilize topoisomerase II–cross-linked DNA strand breaks; activate pathway, leading to cell death, which probably involves major deletion of essential genetic material	Gastrointestinal disturbance, hypotension	IV, PO

(continued)

TABLE 61-1. *(Continued)*

Agents and Class	Target and Mechanism of Antileukemic Effect	Nonhematologic Toxicities	Route of Administration
m-AMSA	Synthetic acridine derivative; DNA intercalator; stabilizes topoisomerase II–cross-linked DNA strand breaks; activates pathway, leading to cell death	Gastrointestinal disturbances	IV
MISCELLANEOUS			
L-Asparginase	Bacterial enzyme; degrades L-asparagine, thereby removing an essential amino acid, resulting in limitation of protein synthesis	Hypersensitivity reactions, anaphylaxis, decreased hepatic protein synthesis, cerebral dysfunction, pancreatitis	IV, IM
Prednisone	Corticosteroid; immediate target is steroid-binding receptor, which translocates to nucleus and induces nuclear apoptosis (probably through induction of endonuclease)	GI bleeding, diabetes, electrolyte disorders, Cushing's syndrome, osteoporosis	IV, PO
Interferon-α	Biologic response modifier; reduces malignant cells in hairy-cell leukemia and chronic myelogenous leukemia	Fever, malaise	IV, SC
All-*trans*-retinoic acid	Vitamin A derivative; action mediated through retinoic acid receptor; induces differentiation	Dry skin or mucous membranes; retinoic acid syndrome	

PRPP, phosphoribosylpyrophosphate.

ribonucleotides[112,113] (Fig. 61-6). By restricting the availability of deoxyribonucleotides, hydroxyurea indirectly inhibits DNA synthesis. This mechanism of interfering with DNA synthesis by reducing precursors differs from the inhibition of DNA synthesis caused by alkylating agents, which is mediated through the primary induction of DNA damage. Because hydroxyurea does not directly cause DNA damage, it is much less likely than alkylating agents to act as a potent mutagen. In addition, its effects are rapidly reversible within days of stopping therapy, which is in contrast to the effects of alkylating agents, from which it may take weeks to months to recover. Because of its low mutagenic potential, good absorption after oral administration, short half-life, and rapid reversibility, many physicians prefer hydroxyurea as the agent of choice for symptomatic treatment of patients with CML in chronic phase.[114]

Deoxycoformycin

2′-Deoxycoformycin is a natural product derived from cultures of *Streptomyces antibioticus*.[115] It is a purine nucleoside analogue that functions as an inhibitor of adenosine deaminase, a key enzyme in purine salvage metabolism responsible for conversion of adenosine to inosine (Fig. 61-7). Inhibition of this enzyme results in an accumulation of adenine nucleotide pools. Elevated levels of deoxyadenosine triphosphate (dATP) in these pools appear to be associated with the development of DNA strand breaks, and alterations of nicotinamide adenine dinucleotide (NAD) metabolism ultimately leading to cell death.[116,117] The accumulation of DNA strand breaks activates the nuclear enzyme poly(ADP-ribose) polymerase and stimulates the synthesis of poly(ADP-ribose) from NAD.[117,118] NAD pools are subsequently consumed in proportion to activation of the polymerase. Since NAD is required for glycolysis and generation of ATP, the consumption of NAD leads to an inability to synthesize ATP, and cells die from failure to maintain energy-dependent processes.[117–119] This pathway of cell death involves damage to DNA but does not require cell replication. Thus, it is cell cycle independent. Accumulation of deoxyadenosine also interferes with S-adenosyl homocystine hydrolase, leading to accumulation of S-adenosyl homocysteine, which is toxic to lymphocytes.[120] Cytotoxicity of deoxycoformycin correlates with accumulation of dATP, and certain lymphoid cells are particularly sensitive to killing by this compound.[121] Deoxycoformycin is unusual as an antimetabolite in that it shows marked toxicity to noncycling cells and is therefore useful for treating tumors with low growth fractions. This agent is intensely lymphocytoxic, and its use can lead to an in-

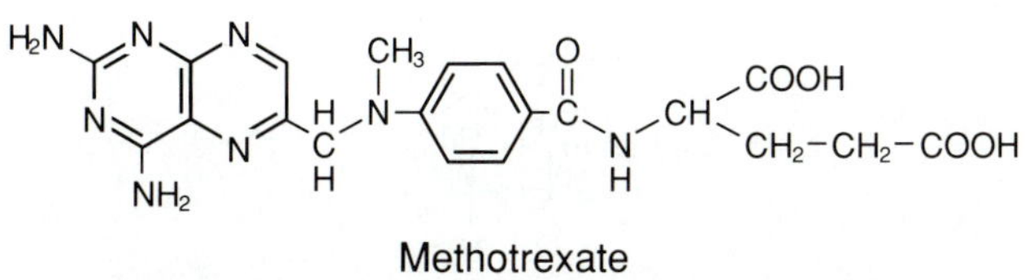

FIGURE 61-3. Chemical structure of methotrexate.

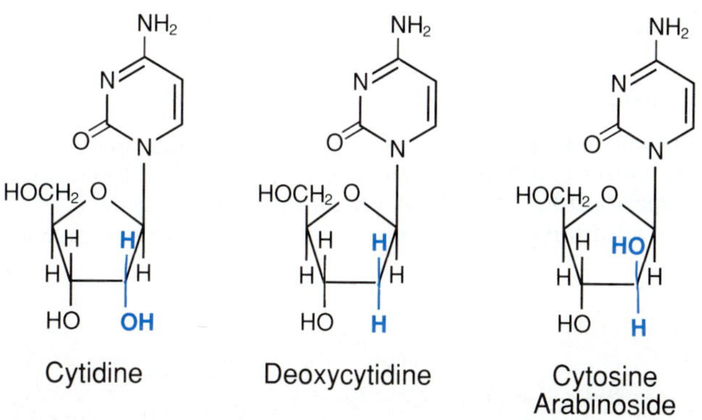

FIGURE 61-4. Chemical structures of cytosine arabinoside and normal ribonucleoside and deoxynucleoside analogues cytidine and deoxycytidine.

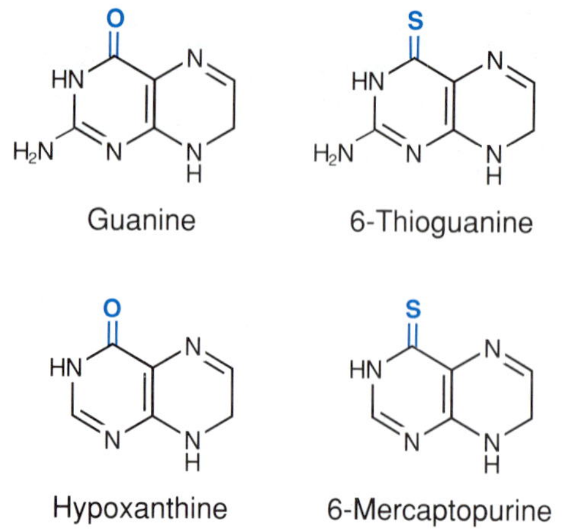

FIGURE 61-5. Chemical structures of the natural purines guanine and hypoxanthine and the chemotherapeutically useful analogues 6-thioguanine and 6-mercaptopurine.

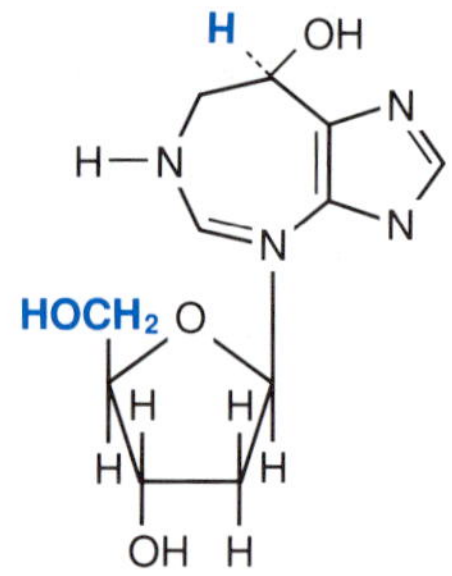

FIGURE 61-7. Chemical structure of deoxycoformycin.

crease in infection. It is particularly useful in treating hairy-cell leukemia and shows promise in CLL and some B-cell lymphomas.[122–127b] When used in intensive treatment regimens, deoxycoformycin was severely toxic to the CNS (lethargy, seizures), liver, and kidney, but use of lower doses in patients who were not acutely ill gave much more favorable results.[122,127–130] Toxicities include mild myelosuppression, fever, keratoconjunctivitis, diarrhea, mild nausea, vomiting, and reversible hepatitis.

Chlorodeoxyadenosine

2′-Chlorodeoxyadenosine is an adenosine analogue resistant to adenosine deaminase[131,132] (Fig. 61-8). It is phosphorylated intracellularly by deoxycytidine kinase, then converted to the 5′-triphosphate derivative, which accumulates in cells and is incorporated into DNA. Its activity is independent of cell proliferation, and it is highly toxic to resting and slowly dividing lymphocytes. Unlike deoxycoformycin, it is not an inhibitor of adenosine deaminase.[132] Its exact mechanism of action is unknown, but it activates a similar pathway to that initiated by deoxycoformycin in terms of the accumulation of DNA strand breaks, activation of poly(ADP-ribose) polymerase, and depletion of NAD leading to cell death.[115,119] Chlorodeoxyadenosine is toxic to human lymphoblasts in the nanomolar range and appears to be effective in the treatment of lymphoid malignancies such as CLL and hairy-cell leukemia.[133–134c] In clinical trials, 2′-chlorodeoxyadenosine has shown the remarkable ability to induce long-term remissions of several years' duration in patients with hairy-cell leukemia after a single 7-day infusion.[134,134d,134e]

Fludarabine Phosphate

Fludarabine phosphate is the 2-fluoro,5′-monophosphate derivative of adenine arabinoside[135] (Fig. 61-9). Fludarabine is resistant to deamination by adenosine deaminase.[136–138] The addition of the 5′-monophosphate derivative increases the aqueous solubility of the nucleoside analogue.[138] In vivo, the monophosphate derivative is dephosphorylated before cellular uptake. It is then rephosphorylated intracellularly and converted to its active form of fluoroadenine arabinoside triphosphate.[135,137] Cells that lack the ability to phosphorylate this agent are resistant to fludarabine.[138,139] Because of its resistance to deamination by adenosine deaminase, fludarabine derivatives are able to accumulate in cells to higher levels than nonfluorinated derivatives. The triphosphate analogue may accumulate in cells in concentrations as high as 500 μmol/L, which is significantly greater than can be achieved by adenine arabinoside triphosphate.[135] The activity of the nucleotide analogue is similar to cytosine arabinoside triphosphate or adenine arabinoside triphosphate in that it interferes with DNA synthesis, DNA polymerase, and ribonucleotide reductase.[136,137] It may also act to interfere with DNA chain elongation.[138] Fludarabine phosphate has recently become available for clinical use; it shows great promise for treatment of CLL refractory to conventional therapy.[140–143] Fludarabine phosphate in higher doses causes neurotoxicity, including optic neuritis progressing to blindness and altered mental status progressing to lethargy and frank coma.[144] The neurotoxicity frequently shows a delayed onset, is progressive, and may be associated with multifocal myelin degeneration.[145] Fludarabine phosphate has been shown to cause a fulminant tumor lysis syndrome in patients with high-volume lymphoid malignancies.[146]

Alkylating Agents

The essential properties of alkylating agents that make them useful in chemotherapy is their ability to form cytotoxic adducts with DNA. The alkylating agents form positively charged, electrophilic groups that react with the negatively charged, electron-rich, nucleophilic groups in macromolecules such as DNA, RNA, and protein[147] (Fig. 61-10). Alkylating agents also react with low-molecular-weight compounds such as glutathione. Because

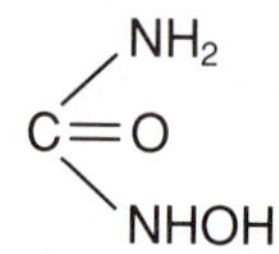

FIGURE 61-6. Chemical structure of hydroxyurea.

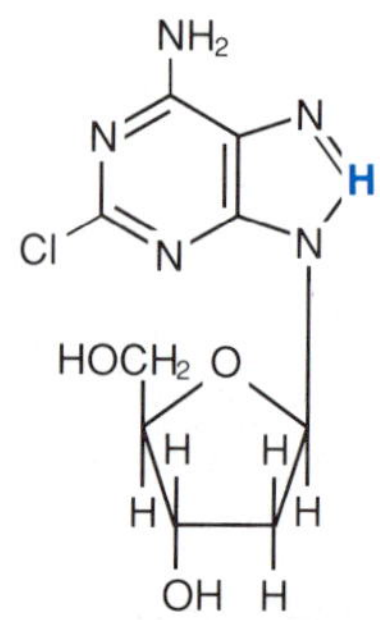

FIGURE 61-8. Chemical structure of 2′-chlorodeoxyadenosine.

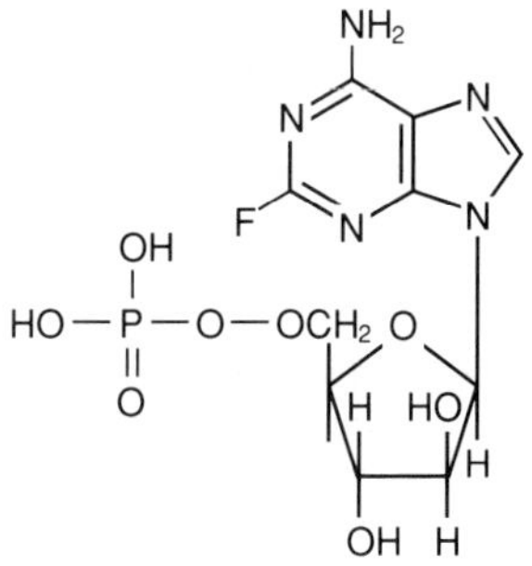

FIGURE 61-9. Chemical structure of fludarabine phosphate.

the latter reactions inactivate the alkylating agents, they may contribute to the development of drug-resistance mechanisms. From a chemotherapeutic viewpoint, reactions with DNA are of critical importance and are responsible for the pharmacologic usefulness of the alkylating agents. By attacking the different nucleophilic nitrogen, oxygen, and phosphate groups in DNA, alkylating agents alter DNA structure and function leading to cell death. A variety of DNA lesions occur in response to the DNA adducts induced by alkylating agents. These include ring openings, base deletions, and strand scissions. Many of the DNA lesions are further acted on by DNA repair enzymes. These reactions can result in complete repair or, when they are only partially completed, can result in additional DNA damage such as the creation of abasic sites or DNA strand breaks. In addition, bifunctional alkylating agents, such as melphalan, chlorambucil, or BCNU, with the capacity to generate two electrophilic groups and form two adducts with DNA, are capable of forming DNA cross-links.[148] The latter interfere with replication, repair, and transcription processes. Because of their primary effect on DNA, these agents not only kill cells but also are highly mutagenic. All the alkylating agents are potential carcinogens; their use sometimes results in the induction of secondary leukemias in patients receiving alkylating agents for lymphomas and nonhematologic malignancies.[149–152] Induction of solid tumors has not been commonly associated with alkylating agent therapy. Most of the alkylating agents interfere with gonadal function, impair fertility, and are teratogenic.[153,154]

Several alkylating agents are useful in the treatment of hematologic malignancies. Many, including chlorambucil, melphalan, and cyclophosphamide, are nitrogen mustard derivatives with chloroethyl functional groups. Busulfan is an alkylsulfonate derivative useful in treating CML, and BCNU is a nitrosourea derivative useful in treating multiple myeloma. All these agents possess the ability to cross-link DNA, and patterns of sensitivity and resistance to these agents have been shown to correlate with cross-link formation and repair.[153–155] Although similar in mechanism of action, these agents do not exhibit cross-resistance in clinical situations.[156]

Chlorambucil

Chlorambucil (Fig. 61-11) is a benzene butanoic acid derivative of nitrogen mustard. It is a bifunctional alkylating agent, stable in aqueous solution. It is completely absorbed from the gastrointestinal tract and reaches peak plasma levels within 1 hour of an oral dose.[157] Because of its convenience, ease of administration, and predictable myelotoxicity, it is the alkylating agent of choice for treatment of CLL. It is usually administered on a daily basis for prolonged periods, with dose adjustments to maintain control of the malignant cell mass without severely suppressing normal blood elements. It is also effective when given in high doses on an intermittent basis, but its usefulness is limited because of its effects on platelets (causing an unpredictable thrombocytopenia as well as pulmonary disease out of proportion to dose with prolonged use) and its association with the development of acute leukemia.[158,159]

Melphalan

Melphalan (see Fig. 61-11), the phenylalanine derivative of nitrogen mustard, is actively transported into cells by their glutamine and leucine transport system.[160] The phenylalanine moiety was originally joined to nitrogen mustard with the expectation that this would increase its uptake into malignant melanoma cells, which use tyrosine for the formation of melanin.[161] Absorption from the gastrointestinal tract is variable, but it is usually administered orally, and its subsequent half-life is about 3 hours or less.[162,163] Among the hematologic malignancies, melphalan, in conventional doses, is primarily used for the treatment of myeloma.[164] A parenteral preparation is used in high-dose regimens, with or without marrow transplantation in the treatment of AML[165,166] and multiple myeloma.[167,168]

Cyclophosphamide

Cyclophosphamide (see Fig. 61-11) differs from the two previously noted alkylating agents in that it requires a multistep activation process before it can function as an antitumor alkylating agent[153,169] (Fig. 61-12). The hepatic

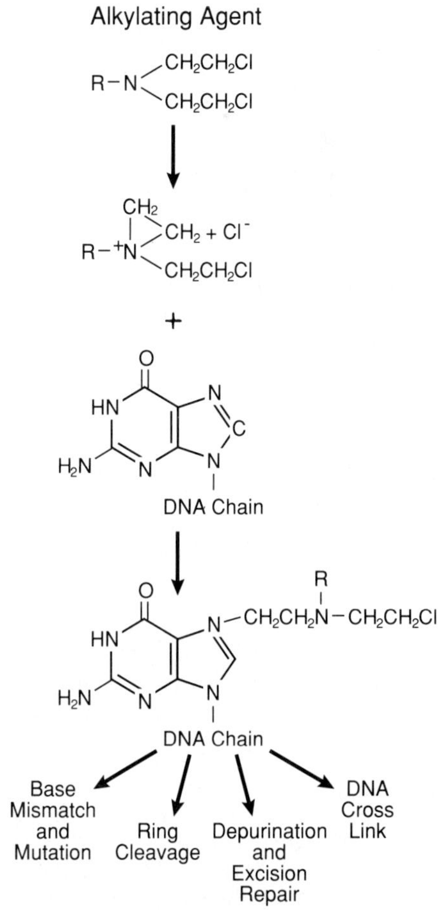

FIGURE 61-10. Example of an alkylating agent reaction and its consequences.

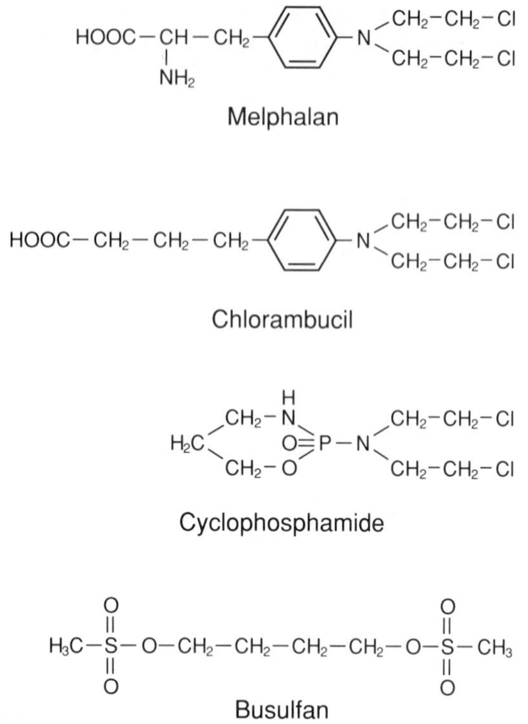

FIGURE 61-11. Chemical structures of alkylating agents used in hematologic malignancies.

microsomal oxidase system converts the original compound to 4-hydroxycyclophosphamide, which undergoes spontaneous tautomerism to aldophosphamide. The latter compound is taken up by cells, where it is converted intracellularly to the cytotoxic agent phosphoramide mustard, which is then available to react with nucleophilic groups in DNA. Cyclophosphamide has been used in various combinations for the treatment of lymphoid and myeloid leukemias. It also has an important use in allogeneic bone marrow transplantations, where its immunosuppressive effects help prevent graft rejection.[153,170]

Cyclophosphamide is well absorbed after oral administration and is used both orally and intravenously. Cyclophosphamide results in significant myelosuppression and immunosuppression. Excretion of active metabolites in the urine can lead to hemorrhagic cystitis in as many as 10% of patients.[171] Drug-induced hemorrhagic cystitis may be avoided by encouraging adequate hydration with 3 to 4 L of fluid per day and encouraging frequent urination for 24 hours after administration of cyclophosphamide. Other approaches to prevent this problem include the use of N-acetylcysteine.[172,173] A syndrome of inappropriate secretion of antidiuretic hormone can occur with cyclophosphamide, which necessitates close monitoring of serum and urine electrolytes and patient intake and output, and acute cardiac injury temporally associated with very-high-dose cyclophosphamide has been described.[174–176]

A cyclophosphamide derivative, 4-hydroperoxycyclophosphamide, which can be directly activated by tumor cells, is used in bone marrow purging procedures in association with high-dose chemotherapy programs and autologous bone marrow rescue.[177,178] In these programs, patients are treated systemically with high-dose chemotherapy to eliminate leukemic cells. Portions of bone marrow are removed before the high-dose therapy and treated with the chemotherapeutic agent 4-hydroperoxycyclophosphamide, ex vivo, with the goal of removing residual leukemic cells.[177,178] The purged autologous marrow, presumably free of occult leukemic cells, is then reinfused to rescue the host from the side effects of the severe chemotherapy-induced marrow aplasia.

Busulfan

Busulfan (see Fig. 61-11) is a bifunctional alkylating agent whose activity is mediated by two methane sulfonate groups. Hydrolysis of the methane sulfonates leads to the formation of carbonium ions, which bind to nucleophilic sites on DNA and result in DNA cross-links.[179,180] The drug also binds extensively to sulfhydryl groups in proteins, but the DNA adducts formed by busulfan account for its major antitumor effect. The drug is well absorbed from the gastrointestinal tract and is commonly used in the treatment of chronic-phase CML.[181,182] It is also an important component of the busulfan and cyclophosphamide regimen for allogeneic and autologous bone marrow transplantations.[183,184] Busulfan administration can result in increased pigmentation, especially over bony prominences and, in high doses, in the axilla and groin.[183,185] Busulfan can cause pulmonary fibrosis resembling that seen after pulmonary irradiation, and it may also cause testicular atrophy and hepatocellular dysfunction.[186–188] Busulfan given in high-dose transplantation regimens can cause hepatic venooc-

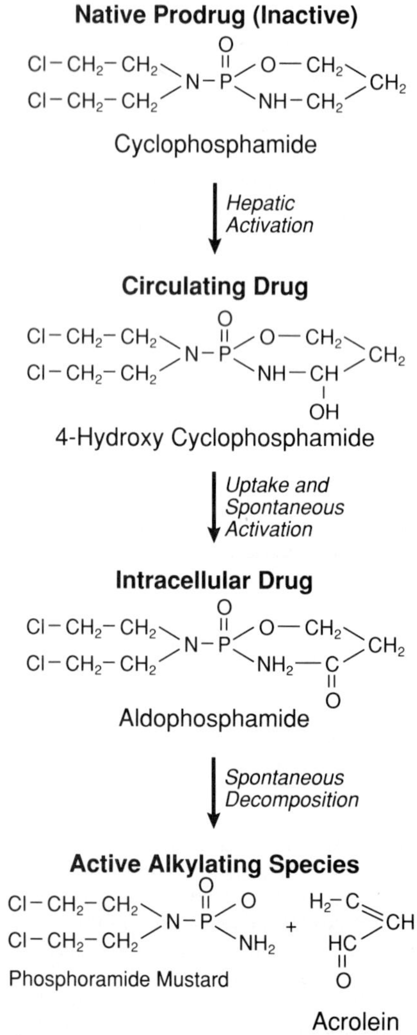

FIGURE 61-12. Cyclophosphamide activation process.

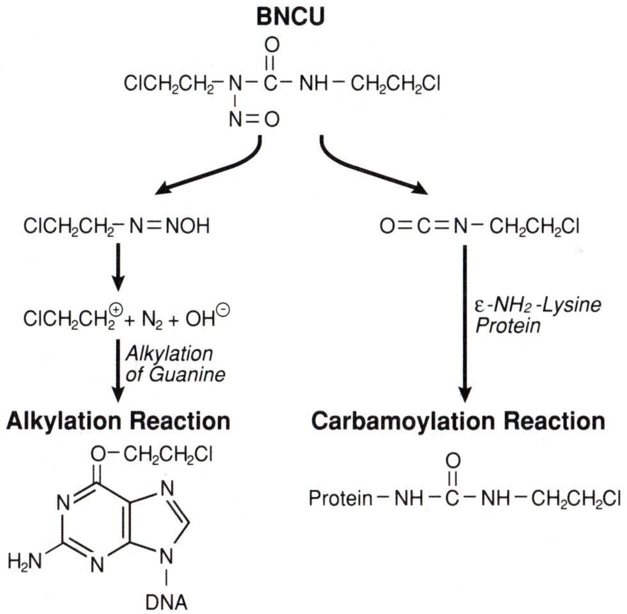

FIGURE 61-13. Chemical structure and metabolism of BCNU.

clusive disease, mucositis, hemorrhagic cystitis, seizures, rash, pneumonitis, and diarrhea.[189–193]

BCNU

BCNU (Fig. 61-13), sometimes used in the treatment of myeloma and AML, is the only nitrosourea commonly employed in treating the hematologic malignancies. It is highly lipid-soluble, and its functional activity resides in its ability to generate a reactive chloroethyl carbonium ion that alkylates DNA and leads to strand breakage and cross-link formation.[194,195] It also dissociates to form an isocyanate group that has the capacity to react with amine groups in a carbamoylation reaction.[196] The carbamoylation of protein, however, has not been shown to significantly potentiate the antitumor effects of BCNU, which are primarily mediated through the alkylation of DNA. The drug is absorbed after oral administration; however, it is usually given intravenously because of lack of stability and rapid decomposition. The plasma half-life of BCNU after intravenous administration is about 30 minutes.[197,198] BCNU is highly toxic to hematopoietic skin cells and may show cumulative toxicity to bone marrow. BCNU administration may also cause pulmonary fibrosis in up to 30% of patients, and this may occur years after treatment.[199–203a] In high doses, BCNU may produce hepatic dysfunction and dementia.[202,204,205]

Antitumor Antibiotics

Anthracyclines

Anthracyclines are a series of natural products that perturb cell membranes, mitochondria, nuclear structure, and function.[206–211] Their major chemotherapeutic action appears to be associated with their nuclear effects, where they have been shown to bind DNA by intercalation, cause consequent DNA unwinding, cause direct single- and double-stranded DNA breaks, and interfere with function cf several nuclear enzymes.[210–212] In particular, interference with topoisomerase II and stabilization of a topoisomerase II–DNA complex appear to be important mechanisms of anthracycline toxicity.[213] Topoisomerase II is responsible for the unwinding and rewinding of DNA required during replication, repair, transcription, and many other processes. Thus, interference with topoisomerase II activity interferes with all these other functions. Anthracyclines may also lead to the formation of DNA deletions, which could contribute to drug-induced cytotoxicity and mutagenicity. Daunorubicin (Fig. 61-14) is the anthracycline most commonly used in the treatment of hematologic malignancies. In combination with cytosine arabinoside, it has had a major impact on remission-induction therapy for AML.[214] It is also used in treatment of ALL.[215] Regimens employing doxorubicin, vinca alkaloids, and dexamethasone have been shown to be effective in treating refractory myeloma and CLL.[216] Newer anthracyclines, such as idarubicin, show great promise for being even more effective in the treatment of the acute leukemias as well as the potential for being less toxic.[217–219] Anthracycline-induced myocardial damage represents a major dose-limiting toxicity of this class of agents.[221–223] This is further discussed in the section on cardiac complications of chemotherapy.

Mitoxantrone

Mitoxantrone is a synthetic anthraquinone resembling the anthracyclines in structure and function (Fig. 61-15). It is a DNA intercalating agent whose cytotoxicity is associated with its ability to form DNA–topoisomerase II complexes.[213,224] Its effects are similar to those described later for etoposide or amsacrine, and it can be used in combination with these agents. It shows some but not complete cross-resistance with the anthracyclines. In preclinical studies, it was found to be highly synergistic with cytosine arabinoside. Mitoxantrone has been used in second-line therapy for AML and ALL and is being evaluated as first-line therapy. Because of the lack of complete cross-resistance with anthracyclines, it is useful for treatment of patients refractory to the latter.[225,226] Dose-limiting toxicity is myelosuppression and mucositis, and other toxicities include gastrointestinal and cardiac effects. As described in the section on cardiac abnormalities, mitoxantrone can lead to the development of cardiomyopathy, and it has cumulative effects with anthracyclines. Gastrointestinal toxicity is less severe and less frequent than with other anthracycline anticancer drugs.[227] Also, alopecia is milder than seen with doxorubicin, and injury after extravasation is considerably less than with doxorubicin or mitomycin C.[227] Absorption after oral administration is poor, and the drug must be administered intravenously.

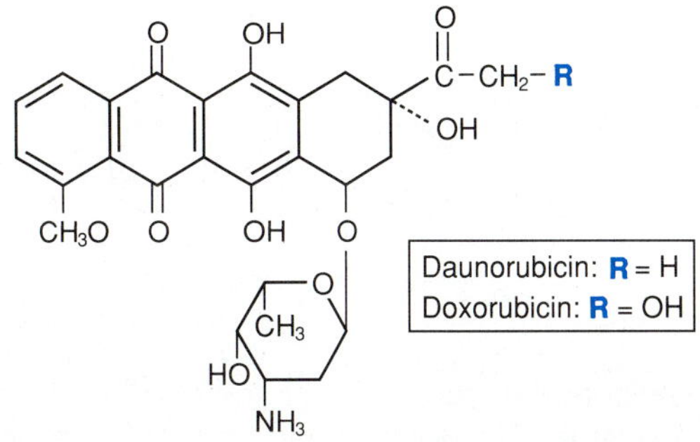

FIGURE 61-14. Chemical structures of daunorubicin and doxorubicin.

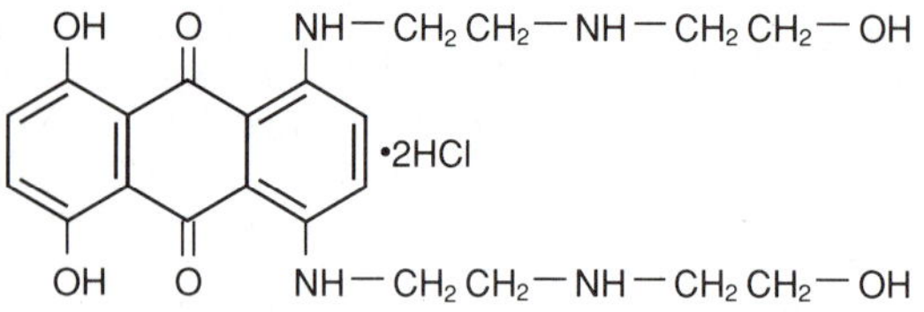

FIGURE 61-15. Chemical structure of mitoxantrone hydrochloride.

Plant Alkaloids

Vinca Alkaloids

Vincristine and vinblastine (Fig. 61-16) are alkaloids extracted from the periwinkle plant. Their antitumor mechanism of action involves binding and inactivation of tubulin with consequent inhibition of microtubule assembly and prevention of mitotic spindle formation.[228,229] By virtue of their action on mitotic spindle formation, the vinca alkaloids are phase-specific agents. They interfere with proliferation in the mitotic phase of the cell cycle.[71,230] Binding to tubulin also interferes with microtubule function in axoplasmic transport and accounts for the neurotoxicity associated with these agents.[231] Adverse neurologic effects constitute the most troublesome and dose-limiting toxicities of vincristine.[232,233] Peripheral neuropathies, including paresthesias of the fingertips and toes and loss of deep tendon reflexes, are among the earliest signs to be detected. Motor neuropathies, including foot drop, ataxia, and weakness progressing to paralysis, may occur with continued administration. Autonomic neuropathies, including constipation, ileus, atony of the bladder, and orthostatic hypotension, may also occur. Individual doses often are limited to a maximum of 2 mg to reduce the incidence of severe neurotoxicity. Early signs of neurotoxicity, such as paresthesia and loss of deep tendon reflexes, are reversible with drug cessation. In contrast to vincristine, vinblastine does not commonly cause neurotoxicity. Its dose-limiting toxicity is myelosuppression. These agents are primarily used in the treatment of acute lymphocytic leukemia.

Podophyllotoxins

Etoposide (VP-16) and teniposide (VM-26) are semisynthetic derivatives of podophyllotoxin extracted from the mandrake plant[234,235] (Fig. 61-17). These agents act as inhibitors of topoisomerase II leading to stabilization of DNA–topoisomerase II complexes, thereby interfering with replication and transcription processes.[236,237] Formation of the DNA–topoisomerase II complex results in the formation of protein–cross-linked DNA strand breaks and DNA recombination events, leading to an increased incidence of sister chromatid exchanges and chromosomal abnormalities.[238,239] These events ultimately lead to cell death by a pathway that may include genetic recombination and deletion of major segments of essential genetic material. Resistance mechanisms are associated with alterations in topoisomerase II that result in loss of the drug's ability to induce formation of the DNA–topoisomerase II complexes.[239,240] Resistance has also been associated with the pleiotropic resistance pathway, discussed in the section on drug-resistance mechanisms.[241]

VP-16 and VM-26 are cycle-active agents that have their major effect when cells are exposed during S phase.[242,243] The drug can be administered orally or intravenously. About half of the oral dose is absorbed, requiring that the oral dose be doubled to achieve the same drug level as obtained by intravenous administration.[244] VP-16 and VM-26 are useful in the treatment of acute leukemia, and the major toxic effect is myelosuppression.[245] VP-16 is also used in combination with fractionated total-body irradiation as a potent treatment of ALL and AML in the setting of allogeneic bone marrow transplantation.[245,247] In high dose, VP-16 may cause transient metabolic acidosis, liver dysfunction, and hemorrhagic cystitis as a result of urinary excretion of native drug.[246] Other toxicities of VP-16 include severe myelosuppression, esophagitis, mucositis, fever, chills, hepatocellular injury, peripheral neuropathy, rash, hypotension, nausea, vomiting, alopecia, and radiation-recall reactions.[248]

Amsacrine

Amsacrine (m-AMSA) is an acridine derivative (Fig. 61-18). It functions as a DNA-intercalating agent that serves to inhibit and stabilize DNA–topoisomerase II complexes.[249,250] This is in contrast to VP-16 and VM-26, which stabilize the DNA-topoisomerase II complex but are not DNA intercalators. Nevertheless, the consequences of stabilizing the DNA–topoisomerase II complex are similar for all these drugs, leading to protein–cross-linked DNA strand breaks, increased DNA recombinational events, chromosomal aberrations, and cell death. The cytotoxic effects of m-AMSA are greatest during S phase when topoisomerase II levels increase.[242] m-AMSA is administered intravenously, and its primary toxicity is dose-related myelosuppression and gastrointestinal toxicity. Cardiac arrhythmia

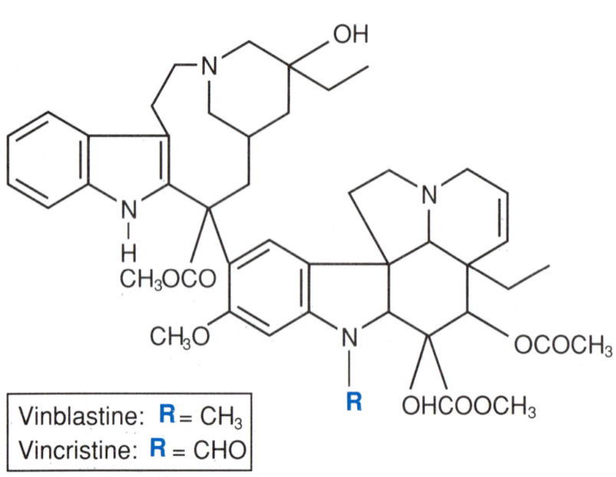

FIGURE 61-16. Chemical structure of vinca alkaloids.

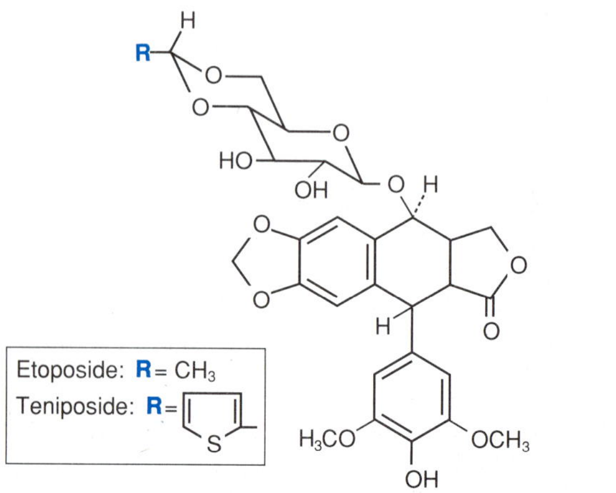

FIGURE 61-17. Chemical structures of etoposide and teniposide.

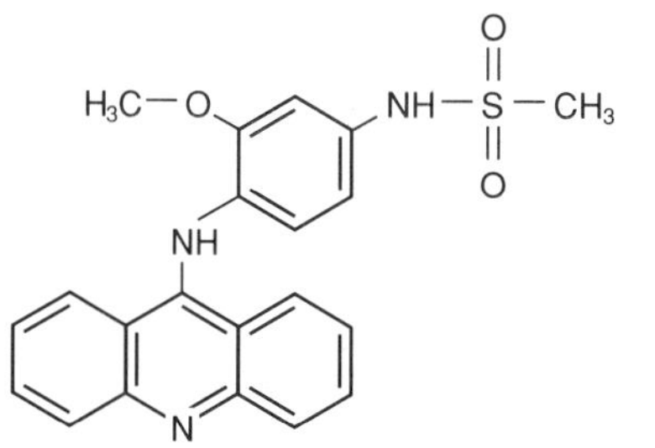

FIGURE 61-18. Chemical structure of m-AMSA.

(especially in hypokalemic patients), congestive heart failure, liver dysfunction (hyperbilirubinemia and transaminase elevation), and CNS abnormalities (seizures and neuropathy) are not uncommon.[251] Other toxic effects include rash, skin discoloration, nausea, vomiting, mucositis, and alopecia. It is effective in the treatment of AML and ALL.[225,252] Cells show some degree of cross-resistance between m-AMSA, VP-16, and VM-26[236]; however, cells resistant to one agent may still retain sensitivity to the others. Resistance mechanisms for m-AMSA involve the multidrug-resistance pathway as well as alterations in topoisomerase II.[241]

Miscellaneous Agents

L-Asparaginase

L-Asparaginase, an enzyme with a molecular weight of 133,000, purified from bacterial sources, represents a unique approach to chemotherapy.[253] The enzyme is administered intravenously or intramuscularly to degrade circulating pools of L-asparagine. This amino acid is required as an essential nutrient by some tumor cells, especially the lymphoblasts in ALL.[254,255] The consequent lack of asparagine results in direct restriction of protein synthesis and secondary inhibition of nucleic acid synthesis. Since it affects protein synthesis based on the cell's requirements for asparagine, rather than depending on any aspect of proliferative capacity, L-asparaginase is unique among chemotherapeutic agents in that it does not affect other rapidly proliferating tissues, such as the gastrointestinal mucosa. Thus, L-asparaginase is highly useful in combination chemotherapy regimens in which the tumor cells require asparagine as an essential nutrient. Based on the requirement of lymphoblasts for exogenous asparagine, L-asparaginase is an important component of therapy for acute lymphocytic leukemia.[256,257] In addition, because of its unique mechanism of action, it may not contribute to the toxic effects of many other chemotherapeutic agents, which affect all rapidly dividing cells. The use of the sequential combinations of high-dose cytosine arabinoside plus L-asparaginase and high-dose methotrexate plus L-asparaginase have been particularly effective since the L-asparaginase rescues normal tissues and provides antitumor effect.[258,259] L-Asparaginase causes systemic toxicity by altering the synthesis of other proteins, such as albumin, insulin, and coagulation factors XI and IX as well as antithrombin III, protein C, and protein S.[260] Hypersensitivity reactions occur in up to 10% of patients.[261] These reactions may vary from rashes, urticaria, and arthralgia to serious problems, including respiratory distress, anaphylaxis, and death.[261–263] Several reports suggest that the frequency of these side effects can be decreased without a loss of efficacy with a change from intravenous to intramuscular administration.[264,265] The allergic reactions may occur even with the first dose of L-asparaginase.[263] Because of these side effects, it is recommended by the manufacturer that all patients who are receiving L-asparaginase for the first time or after an interval of 1 week or more receive an intradermal skin test of 2 IU.[261] The skin test site is observed for allergic reactions, including wheal or erythema formation, for 1 hour. In patients with positive skin tests, the benefit of using the agent must be weighed against the risks of developing severe and potentially fatal allergic reactions. If the drug is to be administered despite a positive skin test, it should be given according to the manufacturer's directions to desensitize the patient with potential allergic reactions. Even if the skin test is negative, severe allergic reactions may still occur, and the physician must be prepared to treat severe allergic reactions, including anaphylaxis. L-Asparaginase obtained from *Erwinia carotovora* is less likely to be associated with this problem than enzyme from an *Escherichia coli* source.[266] Hyperamylasemia progressing to hemorrhagic pancreatitis may also occur as an effect of L-asparaginase therapy.[267] Thrombosis is a major complication of L-asparaginase therapy; with an incidence ranging from 1% to 12% in different series.[268,269] Hemorrhage complicating L-asparaginase therapy occurs only rarely.

Glucocorticosteroids

The glucocorticosteroids are analogues of normal corticosteroids. They have a lympholytic action and are useful in therapy of acute and chronic lymphocytic leukemia and in the lymphoid variety of CML blast crisis.[15,16,20,21] Their mechanism of action requires that the steroid first bind to a cytoplasmic receptor, which then undergoes conformational change. The complex subsequently translocates to the nucleus, where it binds to chromatin and activates a predetermined program of gene expression.[270] In lymphoid cells, the glucocorticoid-induced program includes the increased activity of one or a series of proteins that cause cell lysis.[270] One of these proteins, whose activity increases in response to corticosteroids, appears to be an endonuclease that results in DNA degradation and so-called apoptosis or nuclear disintegration in susceptible target cells. Toxic effects of corticosteroid therapy are similar to the effects of hyperadrenocorticosteroidism and include weight gain, fluid retention, cushingoid appearance, glucose intolerance, immunosuppression, and the development of upper gastrointestinal ulcer disease.[14]

Interferons

Interferons represent an exciting new series of regulatory proteins that have been introduced into the chemotherapeutic armamentarium as biologic response modifiers.[271] These agents are produced naturally in the body in small quantities. As a result of recombinant DNA technology, they are available in pure form in sufficient quantities for clinical study and therapeutic use. Interferon was first recognized for its ability to interfere with the growth of influenza virus.[272] Interferons have been shown to suppress hematopoiesis in vivo and in vitro, and they are thought to be mediators of immune cell suppression of hematopoiesis in vivo.[273–275] Interferons occur in three major types: α, derived primarily from leukocytes; β, from fibroblasts; and γ, from lymphocytes.[276,277] Interferon-α, made by recombinant DNA technology, is approved and available for clinical use. It is a protein with an approximate molecular weight of 19 kd. Although its exact growth regulatory mechanism of action has not been defined, interferon clearly acts as a suppressor of cell growth.[278,279] It has rapidly become a mainstay in the treatment of hairy-cell leukemia[122,280] and shows promise for treatment of CML and multiple myeloma.[281–283b]

All-*Trans*-Retinoic Acid

Recent attempts to treat a variety of malignancies with differentiating agents have been particularly successful using all-*trans*-retinoic acid for patients with acute promyelocytic leukemia.[283c–283f] In vitro, retinoic acid, a derivative of vitamin A, has been shown to induce differentiation in hepatoma cell lines, teratocarcinoma cell lines, and the HL-60 promyelocytic leukemia cell line.[283g,283h] Treatment of bone marrow suspensions from patients with a variety of leukemic subtypes shows that retinoic acid most successfully induces differentiation in cells from patients with acute promyelocytic leukemia. During the past 10 years, there have been anecdotal reports of beneficial-differentiating effects of retinoic acid in patients with myelodysplastic syndrome and AML. Recent clinical trials have demonstrated that treatment with all-*trans*-retinoic acid results in high rates of remission induction in patients with acute promyelocytic leukemia, particularly those with the characteristic t(15;17) translocation.[283c–283f] This translocation results in a fusion protein involving the α-retinoic acid receptor.[283i–283l] In contrast to the usual results that occur when this disease is treated with intensive cytotoxic therapy, patients treated with all-*trans*-retinoic acid experience dry skin and mucous membranes, hyperleukocytosis rather than leukopenia, and normalization of laboratory values relative to the disseminated intravascular coagulation usually associated with acute promyelocytic leukemia.[283c–283f] In these patients, remissions apparently occurred by differentiation and maturation of leukemic leukocytes rather than by their eradication. As many as 25% of patients treated with all-*trans*-retinoic acid may experience retinoic acid syndrome, consisting of fever, hypotension, dyspnea, pleuropericardial effusions, and pulmonary infiltrates.[283e] Transfusion requirements were reduced. Remission durations were in the range of 3 to 12 months. Thus, differentiation therapy with all-*trans*-retinoic acid appears to be superior to cytotoxic therapy for remission induction in acute promyelocytic leukemia; however, remissions are not durable. Cytotoxic chemotherapy is still required for disease eradication.

STRATEGIES FOR COMBINATION CHEMOTHERAPY

As noted previously, chemotherapeutic agents were initially used individually with some success in producing disease control. Although some agents are still used independently, especially for control of chronic leukemias, the most dramatic results in the treatment of hematologic malignancies have been associated with the use of combinations of agents with curative intent. The successful use of combination chemotherapy to treat ALL made it clear that this approach could result in the eradication of all clinical and laboratory evidence of disease.[27–30] In fact, the use of combination chemotherapy for ALL was one of the first demonstrations in humans that systemic malignancies could be cured by chemotherapy.[27]

The major goal of combination chemotherapy is to combine two or more agents to produce additive or synergistic antitumor effects, preferably without compounding toxicity. The principles underlying combination chemotherapy are based on sophisticated studies undertaken in both the in vitro and preclinical situations and ultimately corroborated in the clinical realm. It is estimated that the spontaneous rate of mutation of a malignant cell to a resistant phenotype for a single drug is 1 in 10^6 to 1 in 10^7 cancer cells. The likelihood of spontaneous mutations in patients with clinically apparent tumors is high since such patients have body tumor burdens of 10^{11} cells or higher.[65] Since patients are likely to have cells resistant to any particular single agent, the idea of using a series of different drugs is theoretically attractive.

Several bases are used for selecting the drugs in a combination chemotherapy regimen. These include, but are not limited to, an empiric approach, a cell cycle rationale, or a tumor kinetic approach. In the empiric approach, agents are combined that act individually against a tumor but have differing mechanisms of action and are not cross-resistant. This is an effective means of attacking the tumor as well as decreasing the emergence of drug resistance. Agents generally are selected that have different dose-limiting toxicities, with the expectation that combinations of such agents will result in subadditive toxicity. This is clearly demonstrated by the VAMP regimen shown in Table 61-2, which was successfully employed more than two decades ago to treat childhood ALL.[284]

Another empiric basis for developing chemotherapy regimens is to combine antimetabolites or other cycle-specific agents with cycle-nonspecific agents such as corticosteroids or alkylating agents. Such a design incorporates agents that are not schedule-dependent to kill resting cancer cells (eg, corticosteroids or alkylators) with the phase-specific agents (antimetabolites, vinca alkaloids) that are effective against malignant cells in cell cycle. Some tumors are composed of various-sized populations of resting and actively proliferating cells, requiring therapy with agents directed at each type of population. An additional benefit of this approach to therapy is that as the tumor burden is lowered, more cells enter cell cycle and become more susceptible to killing by all agents employed. Damage to normal tissues in this

TABLE 61-2. VAMP: Combination Chemotherapy Regimen for Acute Lymphoblastic Leukemia

Agent	Mechanism of Action	Toxicity
Vincristine	Binds microtubules and interferes with mitotic spindle formation	Neurotoxicity
Amethopterin	Folic acid analogue; inhibits dihydrofolate reductase, with subsequent interference with thymidine and DNA synthesis	Mucositis
Mercaptopurine	Functions as purine analogue to inhibit purine synthesis and damage DNA	Hepatotoxicity
Prednisone	Corticosteroid; effects are mediated by first binding to steroid receptor, causing lymphocytolysis	Cushing's syndrome

pattern would not be overlapping—the usefulness of alkylators is limited by bone marrow suppression—while damage to other organs would be more selective (eg, peripheral nervous system damage by vinca alkaloids).

This concept has been modified because of a greater understanding of pharmacokinetics and tumor biology. Alkylating agents were initially thought to have similar mechanisms of action and possess cross-resistance. It has subsequently been shown that alkylating agents are not generally cross-resistant, and in some cases, they exhibit considerable synergy with other alkylators, antimetabolites, and antitumor antibiotics.[156] Thus, it is not unusual for combination chemotherapy regimens to contain multiple agents with somewhat similar mechanisms of action, such as the use of BCNU, melphalan, and cyclophosphamide in the treatment of multiple myeloma. The dose-limiting toxicity (eg, myelosuppression) associated with the use of multiple alkylating agents can be overcome by bone marrow or hematopoietic stem cell infusions, and bone marrow transplantation can be successfully undertaken.[184] Thus, given the appropriate supportive care circumstances, even combinations of agents with similar toxicities can be highly effective.

When combination chemotherapy is based on cell cycle considerations, agents are combined that act at different phases of the cell cycle, such as the use of cytosine arabinoside (which is effective during S phase) in combination with vincristine (which is effective during mitosis). The successful use of these agents is highly schedule-dependent.[285] Administration of the two agents together can result in an antagonistic or less than additive effect, whereas administration of the agents at appropriately spaced intervals to take advantage of cells cycling through mitosis and then through S phase provides synergistic cell killing.[285] Similar considerations pertain to the combination of cytosine arabinoside and mercaptopurine. Both agents are active in S phase. As shown in Figure 61-19, the combination is less than additive when the agents are given together. When they are scheduled at appropriate intervals, however, so that each agent is exposed independently to a cohort of cells traversing S phase, their effects become synergistic.[286] Thus, optimal tumor cell kill is achieved when the mercaptopurine is administered 16 hours before or after the cytosine arabinoside. Such results have been easy to demonstrate with transplantable tumors in animal systems. Because of the difficulty of performing these studies in patients, however, this combination has not been extensively applied in the clinical setting.[287]

Selection of drugs for single-agent or combination chemotherapy is frequently based on tumor kinetics. Understanding tumor kinetics requires a measurement of growth fraction or fraction of tumor cells that are in cell cycle at any time. It can be determined experimentally in vivo or in vitro by labeling cells in DNA synthesis with tritiated thymidine and then using autoradiographic techniques for detection.[65] Techniques using bromodeoxyuridine incorporation and its detection with fluorescent-labeled monoclonal antibodies and flow cytometry have been developed to assess growth fractions.[288] Flow cytometry is also useful to identify cells in specific phases of the cell cycle.[65]

When combination chemotherapy is based on tumor kinetics, an attempt is usually made to recruit noncycling cells into the cell cycle, where they show greater susceptibility to cycle-specific agents. This approach is useful for tumors with a large cell mass when there is a small growth fraction. Although many of the hematologic malignancies are rapidly progressive, fulminant diseases, they frequently have small growth fractions.[289] The first agent employed in this type of therapy is usually cycle-independent and

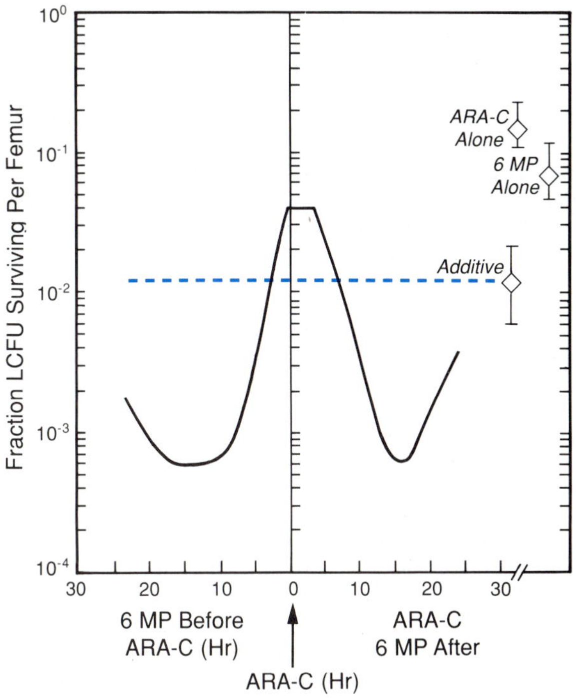

FIGURE 61-19. Survival of leukemia colony-forming units (LCFU) as a function of sequence and interval between the administrations of cytosine arabinoside (ARA-C) and 6-mercaptopurine (6-MP). (Valeriote F, Vietti T, Edelstein M. The combined effect of 1-β-D-arabinofluransylcytosine and thiopurines. Cancer Chemother Rep 1976;60:1925)

used to produce sufficient tumor cell kill to stimulate the remaining tumor cells to proliferate. This renders them more susceptible to a phase-specific agent, which is most effective in killing proliferating cells. This approach underlies the successful combination of anthracyclines with cytosine arabinoside for treatment of acute leukemia.[290]

DRUG-RESISTANCE MECHANISMS

Drug resistance in the hematologic malignancies is multifactorial. Malignant cells may escape the cytotoxic effects of chemotherapy by intrinsic mechanisms. In addition, malignant cells may reside in sanctuaries, which are sites where the cells are protected from chemotherapeutic exposure. An example of such a sanctuary is the CNS, where infiltrated leukemic cells are protected from the effects of systemically administered drugs by the blood–brain barrier. Cells can proliferate in this protected environment and cause CNS leukemia.[28,29] They can also reside there in a resting state for prolonged periods before beginning to proliferate, causing delayed CNS relapse and progression to systemic disease. This is a common problem in acute lymphocytic leukemia, and as many as half of patients with this disease may develop CNS relapses. Effective prophylaxis regimens, however, have been devised for eradicating CNS disease.[291–294] The sanctuary effect can be overcome with agents such as methotrexate or cytosine arabinoside administered intrathecally to mechanically circumvent the barrier.[291,292] Other approaches to overcome the barrier include giving high doses of systemic chemotherapy with the expectation that high drug levels in the blood will establish sufficient concentration gradients to provide cytotoxic drug levels in the cerebrospinal fluid.[293,294] High-dose cytosine arabinoside given intravenously has been shown to eradicate CNS leukemia and lymphoma and has the potential to provide effective prophylaxis.[293,294] Since it is not affected by the blood–brain barrier, radiation therapy also serves as an important approach to treat CNS leukemia.[295] The most effective approach to the treatment of CNS leukemia in ALL has been the use of cranial irradiation in combination with intrathecal methotrexate.[29,31] This approach may result in late sequelae, however, and trials are directed at identifying effective regimens devoid of these complications.[296] The testes provide another sanctuary that serves as a common site for recurrence of ALL.[297–299]

Intrinsic mechanisms of resistance are commonly associated with enzymatic alterations, a variety of which can render hematopoietic cells resistant to commonly used chemotherapeutic agents. These mechanisms have been shown to contribute to resistance in experimental systems and may also contribute to clinical resistance. Methotrexate resistance is associated with quantitative and qualitative alterations of the target enzyme, dihydrofolate reductase.[300,301] Quantitative increases in this enzyme have been shown to be associated with increased copies of the gene for dihydrofolate reductase, and cells with amplification of this gene and its enzyme product can be selected for by progressive exposure to increasing concentrations of methotrexate. Amplification of gene copies and increased levels of the enzyme dihydrofolate reductase have been shown to be associated with a morphologic increase in chromosome fragments, referred to as *double minute chromosomes*.[302]

Resistance to cytosine arabinoside is associated with decreased levels of deoxycytidine kinase or with increased levels of cytidine deaminase.[93,94] Low levels of the former enzyme result in failure of cytosine arabinoside to be converted to its activated phosphorylated form. Elevated levels of the latter enzyme result in conversion of cytosine to uridine nucleotides, which have negligible toxic effects. Biochemical regimens have been devised to protect cytosine arabinoside against deamination to uridine derivatives, but these have not effectively altered resistance or sensitivity patterns.

Alterations in topoisomerase II are associated with resistance to epipodophyllotoxin, daunorubicin, and m-AMSA.[239,240] Resistance to nitrosoureas can be associated with alterations in concentration of the DNA repair protein O^6alkylguanine-DNA alkyltransferase.[303] The latter enzyme directly removes alkylation lesions from the O^6 position of guanine residues in DNA.[304] This is the initial lesion formed in the development of BCNU-induced DNA cross-links, and the alkyltransferase can effectively prevent development of these cytotoxic lesions.

An unusual pleiotropic drug-resistance pattern, termed *multidrug resistance*, has been found to be associated with the presence of increased levels of a membrane glycoprotein that prevents the accumulation of cytotoxic agents in malignant cells.[241,305,306] The term multidrug resistance refers to the situation in which a tumor exposed to one chemotherapeutic agent becomes simultaneously resistant to a series of agents that share little structural similarity.[241,306] The agents to which this resistance pattern commonly develops include anthracyclines, vinca alkaloids, epipodophyllotoxin, actinomycin, and mithramycin.[241,306] All these agents are natural or semisynthetic products. They are hydrophobic molecules with complex ring structures and contain a positively charged nitrogen residue. The mechanism of resistance frequently involves amplification of the multidrug-resistance (*mdr*) gene[306,307] and the overproduction of a 170-kd membrane glycoprotein termed p170 or *P glycoprotein*.[241,306,308] This protein functions as an ATP-dependent membrane pump that probably serves under normal conditions to rid cells of natural toxins.[309] It confers resistance to tumor cells by preventing intracellular accumulation of anticancer drugs. Increased P glycoprotein is clearly associated with acquired drug resistance in ALL, CML, and multiple myeloma.[310–313] The effect of the P glycoprotein can be overcome by phenothiazine and calcium-channel blockers, and clinical trials are underway to determine whether agents such as trifluoperazine, cyclosporine, and verapamil will successfully reverse multidrug resistance in vivo.[314–316b]

BONE MARROW TRANSPLANTATION

In many cases, tumor cell resistance to cytotoxic drugs may be dose-dependent. This resistance may be difficult to overcome, even with increased doses of cytotoxic drugs due, in part, to the fact that the normal hematopoietic tissues may be irreversibly damaged by the dose required to eradicate tumor cells. Bone marrow transplantation with high-dose chemotherapy has been successfully used for over 20 years to bypass this problem and defeat drug-resistance mechanisms.[317–323] Doses of radiation and chemotherapy can be given in greatly increased concentrations since the marrow injury is obviated or attenuated by the later infusion of bone marrow containing sufficient hematopoietic stem cells to reconstitute normal marrow function. Such an approach takes advantage of the steep dose–response effect usually observed in hematopoietic malignancies and sometimes in solid tumors,[324–326] and this modality can lead to long-term disease-free survival or cure in a variety of malignancies.[319,320,322,323]

A number of bone marrow transplantation regimens are available, and their use depends, in part, on the source of bone marrow. The source of the hematopoietic stem cells can be syngeneic, derived from an identical twin; allogeneic, generally derived from an HLA-identical sibling; or autologous, derived from the patient.[327] Hematopoietic stem cells can also be obtained from the peripheral blood using a series of leukapheresis to obtain sufficient stem cells to reconstitute the bone marrow.[328] The most successful results of bone marrow transplantation are in those patients that have a low tumor burden, such as those that are in clinical remission at the time of transplantation or in whom the therapy is begun early in the disease course before resistance mechanisms result in an otherwise relatively refractory disease state.[319,320,322] Further details regarding the use of bone marrow transplantation for hematologic malignancies are contained in the relevant chapters.

CLINICAL TRIALS AND COOPERATIVE GROUPS

The approach to the patient with a hematologic malignancy requires the input and interaction of a variety of specialized professionals. As detailed here, the formulation and execution of an effective management plan requires the active participation of one or more medical oncologists or hematologists, oncology nurses, surgical subspecialists, blood bankers with a state-of-the-art blood bank, experienced laboratory and clinical pathologists, and medical subspecialists (eg, ancillary support services, including a sophisticated staff and consultants in diagnostic radiology, radiation therapy, and microbiology, to name a few). Despite the combined experiences of such personnel and disciplines, it is not always clear in which direction the management of an individual patient should be directed. In addition, although many diseases are responsive to modern therapeutic approaches, a great deal still needs to be learned before hematologic malignancies are treated optimally. In particular, the wealth of experience from in vitro and preclinical scientific investigations needs to be brought to the bedside.

The forum for this approach is the area of clinical trials. Promising new agents can be administered to patients and evaluated in a scientific manner. In general, clinical trials are designed using a protocol format. Such a document is painstakingly written, with input from many of the personnel who are engaged in the care of patients with hematologic malignancies. In addition, other people, such as a biostatistician, clinical pharmacologist, and protocol coordinator or data manager, provide input. These people help determine the sample size and duration of time likely required to answer the questions of such a trial as well as the means to collect and analyze data regarding toxicity and efficacy.

Clinical trials are performed in three classes or phases.[329,330] Phase I trials examine progressively higher doses and differing dose schedules of promising new agents in cohorts of patients. The intent of such an investigation is to establish the toxicities of a drug when given as a single agent and to establish the maximal tolerable dose and side effects at that dose. Small numbers of patients are enrolled at a time, and these individuals are observed closely since the effects of the new agent may be different in humans than those observed in trials conducted in animals. This type of trial typically enrolls no more than 20 to 30 patients. Candidates for phase I studies are patients whose tumors are resistant to all known forms of therapy or those who have tumor types for which there are no known forms of effective therapy available. Both hematologic malignancy and solid tumor malignancy patients are eligible for such trials. On successful completion of a phase I trial, the maximal dose and dosing schedule of a heretofore unknown agent is established.

Subsequently, this single agent is examined in phase II clinical trials. Here, the agent is tested against a broad group of neoplastic diseases to examine the antitumor effect of that agent at a dose and schedule determined in the phase I trial. This phase II study customarily enrolls 15 to 25 patients for each tumor subtype. Using a sample size of this magnitude provides for determining approximate response rate of that agent, but the confidence interval for the value may be large. In addition, such trials may be conducted at a single institution. Hence, to better appreciate the toxicity and efficacy of the agent in question, confirmatory phase II trials enrolling larger patient sample sizes and involving other centers for corroboration frequently are undertaken. Many agents may be tested in the context of phase II trials, but only those few agents that appear to have a high therapeutic ratio and are reasonably efficacious are tested further in phase III clinical trials.

The next step in drug development is that of a phase III trial. In this situation, a new agent alone or in combination with another modality or agent is tested prospectively, head to head against the most effective available regimen for a particular disease stage or type. Patients who show specific disease characteristics and meet specific criteria for inclusion and exclusion are assigned in a randomized fashion to the different therapeutic trial regimens. The most effective of the regimens being evaluated becomes the new approach to therapy and the standard for future comparisons.

This process of therapeutic development is arduous and time-consuming and requires the participation of many willing patients and clinical investigators. To ensure that scientific principles are sound and that resources are used in an efficient manner, specific groups have been designated to conduct such trials. These groups may be composed of a number of investigators at a single institution. Alternatively, investigators from many institutions have banded together to accomplish this task in a more expeditious fashion. These groups are referred to as cooperative groups, and in the United States, they include the Eastern Cooperative Oncology Group, the Southwest Oncology Group, Cancer and Acute Leukemia Group B, the Pediatric Oncology Group, the Children's Cancer Study Group, and the Northeast Central Oncology Group, to name a few. The National Institutes of Health through the National Cancer Institute and their Cancer Therapy Evaluation Program provides funding for these cooperative groups and, with the Food and Drug Administration, monitor the work of these investigators. Detailed and updated print-outs of all the active studies being conducted by these groups, as well as state-of-the-art therapeutic regimens, are available through a National Cancer Institute–maintained information network known as Physician's Data Query (PDQ). PDQ also provides the names, addresses, and telephone numbers of physicians, institutions, and cooperative groups using these protocols. PDQ is available from the National Library of Medicine's MEDLARS computer system. It can be accessed from most medical libraries or through several commercial database vendors by any personal computer equipped with an 80-character-wide display line and a modem.

Many agents under study are referred to as investigational agents. These drugs have not been released for commercial use and require the use of an investigational new drug license. In general, clinical trials of this nature are scrutinized closely. On successful completion of these studies and corroboration of the findings, the results are presented in the medical literature and various scientific forums and are adopted by the medical community as the accepted approach to treating patients with neoplastic disorders.

MANAGEMENT AND COMPLICATIONS OF PATIENTS DURING THERAPY FOR HEMATOLOGIC MALIGNANCIES

Venous Access

Remission-induction and intensification therapy in hematologic malignancies frequently require vigorous support with antibiotics, blood products, antiemetics, parenteral alimentation, and other intravenous medications. Easy venous access should be established before the institution of therapy by inserting cutaneous venous catheter devices. About half of all hospitalized patients in the United States undergo insertion of an intravenous vascular-access device.[331] Many of these devices are inserted in central veins, and their use has greatly facilitated the delivery of health care, especially in cancer patients. Central venous catheters allow greater ease in the administration of intravenous fluids and medications, decrease the risk of infiltration from caustic agents (eg, anthracycline chemotherapy, parenteral alimentation), and allow greater delivery of blood component transfusions, intravenous antibiotics, and chemotherapeutic drugs. These devices are essential for patients who have seriously impaired peripheral venous access due to obesity or previous cytotoxic therapy. Central venous catheters may be used in lieu of peripheral venipuncture blood sampling, significantly improving the quality of life in patients who have a great fear of recurrent needle punctures, such as children.[332]

A number of different types of catheters are commercially available, including totally implantable systems that allow for subcutaneous access (eg, MediPort, Port-o-Cath) and external Silastic catheters (eg, Broviac, Hickman, Groshong, Raaf). These devices are available in multilumen models, which allow for various types of infusions to occur simultaneously. In the past, central venous catheter placement required direct visualization of a branch of a great vessel through the deltopectoral groove, but a direct cannulation technique has since been developed that reduces the degree of tissue injury and allows safe insertion into a large vein, such as the subclavian, even in the severely neutropenic and thrombocytopenic patient.[333] In patients who are unable to undergo placement of this prosthesis in the upper torso, a femoral placement has been successfully used.[334] Large-bore catheters also have been safely inserted into the lumbar area.[335]

Complications can occur with central venous catheters, infectious or thrombotic being the most common. It is critical that the catheter be cared for using strict aseptic technique to flush and prevent thrombosis, while avoiding the introduction of infection. External catheters are usually flushed with a dilute heparin-containing solution (10 IU/mL) twice daily.[336] Despite flushing with heparin, clotting still can occur.[337] The exit site usually is cleaned with hydrogen peroxide and dressed with a povidine-iodine ointment and sterile gauze every other day. Implantable devices generally are filled monthly with a heparin solution (100 IU/mL) and do not require any direct skin care or dressing.

About 1% of patients with central venous catheters experience sepsis, and 10% to 20% of such experiences may be fatal.[331,338] Cancer patients are particularly prone to infection because of the use of immunosuppressive therapy. Some groups have estimated infectious complications as high as 30%.[339–345] Infectious complications may be local (exit site or tunnel infection) or disseminated (bacteremia or fungemia). Rarely, septic thrombophlebitis and endocarditis can occur.

Exit site infections, noncatheter site infections, and bacteremias of unknown origin can be eradicated in most instances without removal of the catheter.[339,340,345] Other infectious situations, such as combined local tract and persistent disseminated infection, may require device removal.[346] Therefore, it is important to determine the specific type of infection. In the febrile patient, two sets of blood cultures should be drawn from all lumens of the central venous catheter as well as from a peripheral vein.[347] Patients who have a positive microbiologic result from blood obtained by central venous catheter but a negative peripheral venipuncture can be assumed to have an infected catheter. Patients who fail to clear subsequent blood cultures on appropriate antibiotics should have the catheter removed. If both sites of blood sampling contain microorganisms while receiving appropriate antibiotics, efforts should be directed to discovering other sites of infection to avoid needless removal of the catheter.

Staphylococcus epidermidis infections are the most common type of bacterial infection affecting the central venous catheter, although other opportunistic organisms can occur (eg, *Pseudomonas* sp, *Candida* sp).[340,344,345,348] One group has recommended that staphylococcal infections of the venous access device may be prevented using a heparin-vancomycin catheter flush.[349] Clotted catheters may have a significantly higher risk for infection caused by colonization by bacteria.[350] Restoring the patency of the catheter using urokinase solutions locally or systemically may be indicated.[351–354]

The incidence of thrombosis varies with the catheter used. Depending on the definition of thrombosis and type of catheter used, the incidence ranges from 5.7%[355] to 65%.[335] These episodes include formation of fibrin sheaths,[337,356–358] superior vena cava syndrome,[346,359,360] septic thrombophlebitis,[361] pulmonary embolism,[362] and infection as a result of thrombosis.[340]

Catheters usually can be removed using local anesthesia without difficulty. Occasionally, thromboembolism may occur during removal in a patient with a preexisting clot.[363] Thus, it is recommended to lyse the clot in this population before proceeding with catheter removal. This can be accomplished by infusion of urokinase directly through the catheter.[351]

Hematologic Problems

Most antineoplastic agents are associated with injury to tissues that rapidly proliferate, such as the gastrointestinal tract, integument, and lymphohematopoietic tissues. Although chemotherapeutic agents have effects on many other tissues, especially with more prolonged administration, the more immediate effects are reflected as toxicity to these organs. Cytotoxic drug exposure causes marrow injury, resulting in anemia, thrombocytopenia, and neutropenia. Pancytopenia requires that the patient receive vigorous supportive care in the form of blood component transfusions as well as prophylaxis and treatment for infectious disease.

Anemia may develop as a result of a hematologic malignancy or in the course of its treatment. Anemia can also occur as a result of hemorrhagic or hemolytic processes. Symptoms of anemia generally occur over a period of time but may develop suddenly. Packed RBC transfusions should be administered routinely to maintain the hematocrit above 25% in stable patients or at a higher level in patients with cardiovascular or cerebrovascular disease. Transfusion reactions of a minor or major nature can occur as a result of blood infusions. Minor transfusion reactions, including fever and chills, are usually due to the infusion of small numbers of contaminating leukocytes in the packed RBC unit, which can be prevented by using RBCs that have been washed free of leukocytes or by using highly efficient filters to remove these cells.[364] Premedication of the patient with antipyretics and antihistamines may also help avoid these reactions.

Major transfusion reactions are less common and include pain at the injection site, chest or back pain, hypotension, cyanosis, shortness of breath, and blood in the urine. In addition, noncardiogenic pulmonary edema may develop,[365–367] in some cases as a result of leukoagglutination from passive transfer of antileukocyte antibodies.[367] Such reactions may be more common in the patient who has received numerous blood transfusions. If a major transfusion reaction develops, the transfusion should be discontinued immediately and the patient should receive intravenous fluids, diphenhydramine, and glucocorticoid therapy.[368]

Thrombocytopenia

Thrombocytopenia remains a major life-threatening sign in the patient receiving cytotoxic drug therapy. In recent years, the widespread availability of platelet transfusions has reduced dramatically the morbidity and mortality due to thrombocytopenia. In most situations, the thrombocytopenia develops as a result of damage to bone marrow and decreased megakaryocyte production, but in some patients (such as those with acute progranulocytic leukemia or infection), either disseminated intravascular coagulation or immune-mediated thrombocytopenia may be involved.[369] In others, the occurrence of splenomegaly and sequestration may result in thrombocytopenia.

Severe thrombocytopenia due to marrow replacement, failure, or cytotoxic damage is a medical emergency and requires that platelet transfusion therapy be instituted immediately. Traditionally, the threshold for platelet transfusion has been a platelet count lower than 20,000/μL. More recent data suggest, however, that a platelet count of 5000/μL may be a more appropriate threshold for transfusions and 10,000/μL as a threshold if fever or minor hemorrhagic manifestations are present.[369,369a] Manifestations of visceral bleeding or mucosal bleeding may be readily apparent in the form of petechiae, or blood can be detected in the stool. Patients should receive 4 units of platelets per square meter or 1 unit per 10 kg. The effect of a transfusion should be judged by the clinical result and the platelet count obtained 1 hour later.[370–372] Practically, this translates to about 6 to 10 units per transfusion. The platelets for transfusion can be obtained from combinations of many donors (random-donor platelets) or from one donor (single-donor platelets). In the former situation, the platelets in each unit of whole blood are pooled or mixed; in the latter situation, a single donor's blood volume can be processed many times using sophisticated pheresis instruments, so that blood is continuously circulated through an apparatus that returns the RBCs to the donor and allows the platelets to be harvested. Transfusions of platelet concentrates can be arranged readily through the blood bank. In the stable, afebrile, nonalloimmunized patient, an increase in platelet count of about 30,000 to 15,000 platelets/μL can be expected 1 hour and 20 hours, respectively, after the transfusion. Platelet count increases (corrected for body surface area and number of units transfused) that are less than 10,000 and 5000 platelets/μL/m^2 after 1 hour and 20 hours, respectively, are unacceptably low, warranting further evaluation.[373] Transfused platelets typically survive only 2 or 3 days in the stable thrombocytopenic patient. Thus, daily or alternate-day platelet transfusions must be given to keep the platelet count at a sufficient level to ensure prevention of hemorrhage in a stable patient, and transfusions should be given more frequently (ie, twice daily or more) in a bleeding patient. In the patient who has fever, disseminated intravascular coagulation, sepsis, or splenomegaly or who is receiving drugs that interfere with platelet function (such as amphotericin B), increments in platelet count after transfusion may not be noted. Such a patient should continue to receive platelet transfusions, but consultation with a transfusion specialist should be undertaken. Failure to increment counts after platelet transfusion may reflect alloimmunization, and specific strategies must be enlisted to deal with this problem. Because of storage at room temperature, platelet transfusions can, on rare occasions, become contaminated and lead to infection.[374] Improvements in transfusion medicine, including development of in vitro testing methods to better define host status, should provide a more compatible blood product. These advances include HLA matching of donor platelets with the patient and actually performing a platelet crossmatch assay. New filters are available that remove significant numbers of the contaminating leukocytes, and their use can prevent platelet transfusion reactions and transmission of agents such as cytomegalovirus.[375,376]

Leukopenia and Granulocytopenia

Patients with hematologic disorders are at significant risk for infection due to predisposing factors, including defects in humoral and cellular immunity, disruption of integumental or mucosal surfaces, status of hyposplenism or asplenism, and use of prosthetic devices.[377] Cytotoxic drug treatments may result in failure of the marrow to produce adequate numbers of neutrophils, further predisposing these patients to serious, life-threatening infection. The incidence and severity of infection rises substantially as a result of granulocytopenia, especially when the neutrophil count is less than 100/μL[378]; on the other hand, infections can occur in patients in whom the neutrophil count is normal or nearly normal.[379] Infections due to neutropenia are a major cause of morbidity and mortality in patients with hematologic malignancies.[380,381] Infections with gram-positive organisms such as *Streptococcus* sp or *Staphylococcus* sp, as well as the enteric gram-negative pathogens such as *Klebsiella* sp, *E coli*, and *Pseudomonas* sp, have been recognized for a long time.[382–387] After a prolonged duration of neutropenia, other opportunistic infections may develop, including infections with *Candida* sp, *Aspergillus* sp, and other fungi.[388–391] These pathogens, usually colonizing the host, may gain access to the bloodstream and result in local or widespread infection.

The occurrence of neutropenia and fever in patients with hematologic malignancies is a medical emergency. It should never be disregarded as being tumor related. The practice of empirically beginning antibacterial agent therapy in the neutropenic patient has markedly reduced the morbidity and mortality of febrile granulocytopenic patients.[380,382,392] Thorough clinical assessment to direct the clinician to the source of the infection must be undertaken immediately and completed rapidly. This examination helps direct the clinician to the likely source of the infection, but in patients with a blunted immune response and lowered granulocyte pool, the usual clinical findings of infection may be masked. It is of crucial importance that the blood, urine, sputum, and other body fluids, such as stool, pleural, or peritoneal specimens, if available, be obtained for culture and Gram stain. In addition, specific attention should be directed to abnormal findings, and specimens should be submitted for routine culture as well as cultured for pathogens of an unusual nature. At this point, empiric antibacterial agent therapy should be instituted. Many regimens have been devised and range from monotherapy treatment with single-agent ceftazidime to triple therapy, using an aminoglycoside and an extended spectrum penicillin as initial therapy.[394–397a] In the intensively treated host, such as the bone marrow transplant recipient, such initial treatment with a single agent may be inadequate, and combination regimens may be preferred.[398] One suggested approach to management of the febrile neutropenic patient is shown in Figure 61-20. This regimen has been effectively used at the Ireland Cancer Center, University Hospitals of Cleveland, and Case Western Reserve University. It may serve as a guide for providing effective therapy against infection in a patient with hematologic malignancies.

Disseminated fungal infections are common in patients who are granulocytopenic and are also subject to treatment with broad-spectrum antibiotics. The longer the period of neutropenia, the greater is the chance for fungal infection to occur.[392] Amphotericin B therapy is commonly used in an empiric fashion when fevers persist after 3 to 5 days of antibacterial agent therapy.[399–401] In one prospective randomized trial,[399] patients benefited significantly from the early empiric use of amphotericin B. Antifungal treatment with amphotericin B is clearly indicated when a fungal infection is documented, and in the case of aspergillosis, higher doses should be used.[402] Other indications for starting amphotericin B are listed in Table 61-3.

Granulocyte transfusions rarely are used because of excessive morbidity, including transfusion reactions, pulmonary infiltrates, alloimmunization, cytomegalovirus infection, and inadequate cell number.[403] Granulocyte transfusions usually are reserved for neutropenic patients with persistent gram-negative bacteremia or a progressive local infection despite an adequate trial of appropriate an-

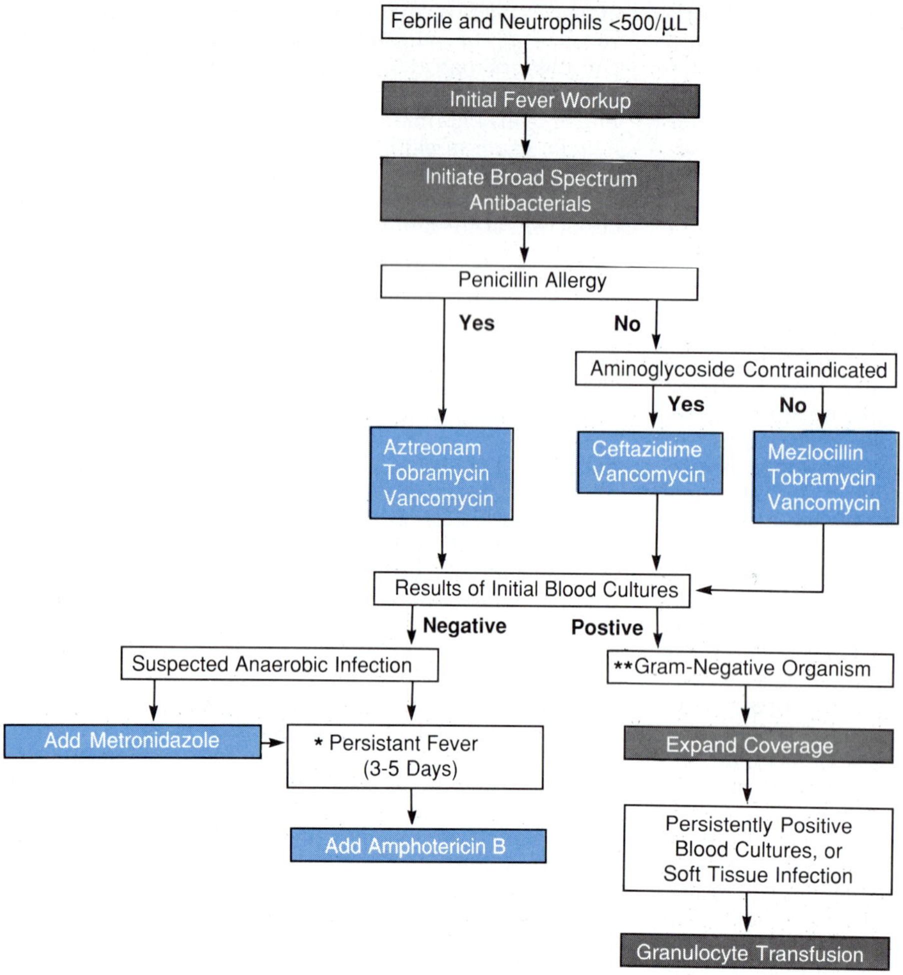

FIGURE 61-20. The Ireland Cancer Center approach to the febrile neutropenic patient. The single asterisk refers to the need to continue to perform serial reevaluation using history, physical, microbiologic culture, and routine radiographic studies. Double asterisks refer to the need to include two antibacterial agents, which bacteria are sensitive to in vitro, and to continue other antimicrobial therapy. (After Lazarus HM, Creger RJ, Gerson SL. Infectious emergencies in oncology patients. Semin Oncol 1989;16:543)

tibiotics.[377] Granulocyte transfusions generally are ineffective against fungal infections.

Gastrointestinal Tract Disorders

Cells lining the gastrointestinal tract exhibit rapid turnover, and drugs used to treat hematologic malignancies may induce serious injury to the intestinal mucosa, leading to a series of problems in the host. Many agents are associated with significant nausea and vomiting. Later, diarrhea, stomatitis, and esophagitis may occur. A syndrome referred to as *neutropenic enterocolitis* also may develop.[404–411] In this syndrome, which generally affects acute leukemia patients who are pancytopenic and receiving broad-spectrum antibiotics as well as corticosteroids, chemotherapy may induce damage to the mucosa.[412] Fever, abdominal pain and tenderness, watery diarrhea, and bleeding may result.[407] Serious electrolyte abnormalities and elevation in serum bilirubin may ensue, and mortality due to sepsis, bowel perforation, or obstruction may occur. About one third of patients who develop this syndrome manifest fungemia or gram-negative bacteremia.[413] Vigorous supportive care, including the possibility of surgical intervention, may be necessary. Patients may develop severe malnutrition, requiring the institution of parenteral alimentation.

Perirectal infections are common in neutropenic patients, especially in those with a history of hemorrhoidal problems.[414] They also may result from aggressive rectal examination or rectal temperature probe or suppository use, all of which should be avoided or approached with caution. A general surgeon should be consulted when perirectal problems occur. Treatment consists of supportive care measures, such as stool softeners and sitz baths. Antibiotic therapy, sometimes with incision and drainage of the infected site, constitutes the cornerstones of management.[415,416]

TABLE 61-3. Indications for the Initiation of Amphotericin B Therapy

Blood culture growing fungus
Diagnostic biopsy or culture showing fungus from skin, lung, sinuses, or esophagus
Endophthalmitis
New or persistent fever despite broad-spectrum antibacterial agents
New or persistent infiltrate on chest radiograph or sinus films
Previous invasive fungal infection
Abrupt clinical deterioration, such as change in mental status, despite broad-spectrum antibacterial agent therapy

(Lazarus HM, Creger RJ, Gerson SL. Infectious emergencies in oncology patients. Semin Oncol 1989;16:543)

Metabolic Problems

Patients with a hematologic malignancy may experience significant metabolic derangements as a result of the disease or its treatment. Tumor lysis syndrome is a well-recognized complication that may occur spontaneously or shortly after institution of cytotoxic drug therapy, radiation, corticosteroids, and interferon.[417–425] The syndrome, in part because of the lysis of tumor cells and the liberation of intracellular constituents in quantities that exceed excretory capacity of the kidneys, is associated with hyperkalemia, hyperphosphatemia, hypocalcemia, and sometimes lactic acidosis. The potential for developing this syndrome should be recognized, and patients with large tumor cell burdens who are undergoing intensive chemotherapy should receive intravenous hydration with fluids containing bicarbonate. Uric acid may also be generated and lead to acute renal failure as a result of uric acid nephropathy. Uric acid is more soluble at elevated pH conditions, and hydration and alkalinization of the urine helps prevent this problem. Despite the administration of allopurinol, during massive tumor lysis, urinary excretion of serum uric acid may still increase. If renal insufficiency develops, allopurinol should be discontinued immediately since hepatotoxicity may result from increased blood levels of the major metabolite oxypurinol.[426,427] Allopurinol blocks the conversion of uric acid to xanthine and hypoxanthine, and since xanthine is less soluble in alkaline urine, xanthine nephropathy can occur.[428,429] In addition, prophylactic use of high doses of allopurinol, 600 $mg/m^2/d$ in divided doses beginning shortly before institution of cytotoxic therapy and continuing for several days during therapy, may prevent this problem. In patients with high tumor cell burdens, attempts should be made to initially use therapeutic modalities that can control the tumor load without contributing to abrupt metabolic derangements. Notably, patients with hyperleukocytosis and leukostasis should undergo either therapeutic leukapheresis or gentle cytoreduction with agents such as hydroxyurea, 2 to 6 g/d, in conjunction with hydration and allopurinol to prevent hyperuricemia.

Other metabolic consequences that result from cytotoxic drug exposure include the development of a glucose intolerance or diabetic-like state from the use of corticosteroids.[14] Cushing's syndrome and pancreatitis may also develop as a result of the use of these agents. Pancreatitis also has been recognized to occur with the agent L-asparaginase.

Skin Injury

A number of cytotoxic drugs have been associated with damage to the integument. Rashes due to cytosine arabinoside, methotrexate, hydroxyurea, or radiation therapy have been well described.[430–432] Radiation recall, in which erythema arises in a preexisting radiation therapy port, and radiation enhancement (increased radiation-induced erythema) have been well documented to occur after treatment with methotrexate, doxorubicin (Adriamycin), BCNU, and actinomycin D.[433–438]

Liver Disease

Hepatocellular dysfunction after exposure to a variety of agents is well described. Agents such as methotrexate, cytosine arabinoside, 6-thioguanine, 6-mercaptopurine, and others in conventional dose have been associated with hepatocellular dysfunction and rarely with hepatic venoocclusive disease.[439–444] BCNU and busulfan have been reported to cause this problem when used in high doses.[189,193,444] Cyclophosphamide has been reported to cause this problem only when used in high doses. The likelihood of developing hepatocellular dysfunction may increase with prolonged exposure to cytotoxic agents or may be noted with use of these agents in high doses. Hepatic venoocclusive disease occurs at a higher rate in patients receiving high-dose chemotherapy in the context of bone marrow transplantation, especially in patients with elevated transaminase before transplantation.[189,445,446] In this syndrome, the agents may cause direct injury to the intima of the central hepatic vein, resulting in thrombosis and worsening of hepatocellular dysfunction. The clinical syndrome presents with right upper quadrant pain, unexplained weight gain, and edema.[445,447] It may have a fulminant or chronic course or may resolve over time.[445,447,448]

Hepatocellular dysfunction may occur during the course of therapy as a result of exposure to antibacterial (trimethoprim-sulfamethoxazole, piperacillin), antifungal (ketoconazole), or antiviral (acyclovir, ganciclovir) agents. Use of parenteral alimentation also may result in hepatocellular dysfunction (asymptomatic mild elevation of transaminases and rarely cholestasis). The most common cause of hepatocellular dysfunction during treatment for cancer is transmission of infection, notably viral infectious agents. Hepatitis B and C viruses clearly are the most common offending agents, although it has become clear that cytomegalovirus and occasionally human immunodeficiency virus may result in hepatocellular injury.[449]

Genitourinary Tract Abnormalities

Damage to the genitourinary tract can occur after exposure to a variety of agents or as a result of the response to therapy. Urate nephropathy and other metabolic problems may lead to direct damage to the genitourinary tract. Certain drugs, such as etoposide and cyclophosphamide, may be excreted as native compounds or active metabolites that injure the uroepithelium, leading to hemorrhage and subsequent fibrosis.[172,245] These problems can generally be avoided by use of vigorous hydration and frequent voiding during the period of treatment or by use of urinary tract protective agents.[450,451]

Cardiac Abnormalities

Anthracycline antibiotics, such as daunorubicin and doxorubicin, as well as the newer agents mitoxantrone, idarubicin, and epirubicin, have been associated with cumulative cardiac damage.[220–223,452–461] Most of the newer agents were developed on the theoretic grounds that they were less likely to cause cardiac damage.[454,458] Administration of anthracyclines may cause acute abnormalities seen on electrocardiogram within hours or days after administration that resolve as the injury is repaired.[452] With repeated drug administration, cumulative endomyocardial damage ensues, eventually resulting in cardiomyopathy. Half of patients show some functional cardiac impairment by the time they receive a cumulative dose of doxorubicin of 500 mg/m^2, and as many as 10% of patients who receive 550 mg/m^2 develop clinically significant cardiomyopathy and congestive heart failure.[220,452,464] The latter is generally unresponsive to medical management. Anthracycline-induced cardiomyopathy may be characterized by electrocardiogram abnormalities, especially reduction in voltage of QRS complex and prolongation of systolic intervals, as well as functional cardiac abnormalities, including reduction in ejection fraction as measured by radionuclide-gated cardiac blood pool scans.[459–462] These clinical findings generally parallel changes noted on endomyocardial biopsy.[459,460] Thus, administration of doxorubicin and daunorubicin is frequently stopped at doses above 450 and 550 mg/m^2, respectively. Conversely, young patients and those without a history of cardiac dysfunction may continue with therapy if they are closely monitored using functional cardiac testing, such as the gated-pool radionuclide scan.[459,461] In one recent study,[458] however, noninvasive cardiac monitoring did not predict the development of cardiomyopathy until it became apparent clinically. When higher anthracycline cumulative doses are reached, the physician must evaluate the potential benefit versus the risk of developing irreversible congestive heart failure. For similar reasons, mitoxantrone is usually stopped at a cumulative dose of 165 mg/m^2, or at 100 mg/m^2 if given after other anthracycline therapy. The myocardial toxicity of anthracyclines is more likely to occur in elderly patients, especially those with preexisting heart disease, such as coronary artery disease or cardiomyopathy, and in patients who received other injurious treatment, such as radiation therapy to the mediastinum.[464,465]

Pulmonary Abnormalities

The lung is a target organ for a variety of cytotoxic agents. Classically, the syndrome of fleeting pulmonary infiltrates and pleural effusion in association with eosinophilia has been described after exposure to methotrexate.[83] This may represent a form of hypersensitivity reaction since rechallenge with methotrexate is not usually associated with this problem. On the other hand, exposure to any of the alkylating agents used to treat hematologic malignancies, including melphalan, cyclophosphamide, nitrogen mustard, BCNU, and other drugs may result in progressive pulmonary fibrosis.[466–468] Chronic alkylating agent exposure may result in the occurrence of pulmonary dysfunction even after cessation of the therapy, even many months later. In some patients, a syndrome of pneumonitis may occur earlier. The effect of this injury may respond to a brief course of corticosteroids.[202,469] In some patients, however, corticosteroids are ineffectual, and a more protracted and relentless pulmonary fibrosis picture may develop.

Neurologic Injury

Neurologic injury has been well appreciated after exposure to a variety of agents.[232] Vincristine is associated with cumulative peripheral neuropathy,[232] and cytosine arabinoside in conventional doses also can cause peripheral neuropathy.[470] High-dose cytosine arabinoside is associated with penetration of the CNS and the development of either global cerebral dysfunction or acute cerebellar injury.[97,471,472] Patients older than 50 years of age, those with a history of neurologic dysfunction, and those with renal or hepatic dysfunction are predisposed to develop high-dose cytarabine CNS toxicity.[473,474] Other agents used in high doses may also cause neurologic syndromes not generally appreciated at conventional doses, including nitrogen mustard and BCNU.[475–478] In other situations, a multifocal coagulative necrosis of the white matter of the brain has been noted after successful combination treatment of CNS leukemia, especially with methotrexate and irradiation.[33,34,479,480] Fludarabine phosphate has been associated with delayed and progressive neurologic problems, including optic neuritis, blindness, lethargy, and coma.[141,142]

REFERENCES

1. Meyer V. Physiologische wirkung der Gechlorten Schwefeträthyle. Berichte 1887;20:1729.
2. Krumbhaar EB, Krumbhaar HD. The blood and bone marrow in yellow cross gas (mustard gas) poisoning: changes produced in the bone marrow of fatal cases. J Med Res 1919;40:497.
3. Lynch V, Smith HW, Marshall EK Jr. On dichloroethylsulphide (mustard gas). I. The systemic effects and mechanism of action. J Pharmacol Exper Ther 1918;12:265.
4. Marshall EK Jr. Mustard gas. JAMA 1919;73:684.
5. Goodman LS, Wintrobe MM, Dameshek W, et al. Nitrogen mustard therapy: use of methylbis (B-chlorethyl) amino hydrochloride for Hodgkin's disease, lymphosarcoma, leukemia and certain allied and miscellaneous disorders. JAMA 1946;132:126.
6. Graef I, Karnofsky DA, Jager VB, et al. The clinical and pathological effects of nitrogen and sulphur mustards in laboratory animals. Am J Pathol 1948;24:1.
7. Jacobson LO, Spurr CL, Barron ESG, et al. Nitrogen mustard therapy: studies on the effect of methyl-bis(betachloroethyl) amine hydrochloride on neoplastic diseases and allied disorders of the hemopoietic system. JAMA 1946;132:263.
8. Rhoads CP. Nitrogen mustards in the treatment of neoplastic disease. JAMA 1946;131:656.
9. Franklin AL, Stokstad ELR, Jukes TH. Acceleration of pteroylglutamic acid in mice and chicks by chemical antagonist. Proc Soc Exp Biol Med 1947;65:368.
10. Farber S, Diamond LD, Mercer RD, et al. Temporary remissions in acute leukemia in children produced by folic acid antagonist, 4-aminopteroylglutamic acid (aminopterin). N Engl J Med 1948;238:787.
11. Hitchings GH, Elion GB, Falco EA, et al. Studies on analogs of purines and pyrimidines. Ann NY Acad Sci 1950;52:1318.
12. Elion GB, Burge E, Hitchings GH. Studies on condensed pyrimidine systems. IX. The synthesis of 6-substituted purines. J Am Chem Soc 1952;74:411.
13. Burchenal JH, Murphy ML, Ellison RR, et al. Clinical evaluation of a new antimetabolite, 6-mercaptopurine in the treatment of leukemia and allied diseases. Blood 1953;8:965.
14. Albright F. Cushing's syndrome: its pathological physiology, its relationship to the adreno-genital syndrome, and its connection with the problem of the reaction of the body to injurious agents ("alarm reaction" of Selye). Harvey Lect 1942–43;38:123.
15. Pearson OH, Eliel LP, Rawson RW, et al. ACTH- and cortisone-induced regression of lymphoid tumors in man: a preliminary report. Cancer 1949;2:943.
16. Pearson OH, Eliel LP. Use of pituitary adrenocorticotropic hormone (ACTH) and cortisone in lymphomas and leukemias. JAMA 1950;143:1349.
17. Goodman LS, Gilman A. The pharmacological basis of therapeutics, ed 2. New York, Macmillan, 1960:1414.
18. Niemeyer CM, Hitchcock-Bryan S, Sallan SE. Comparative analysis of treatment programs for childhood acute lymphoblastic leukemia. Semin Oncol 1985;12:122.
19. Gaynon PS. Primary treatment of childhood acute lymphoblastic leukemia of non-T cell lineages (including infants). Hematol Oncol Clin North Am 1990;4:915.
20. Vietti TJ, Sullivan MP, Berry DH, et al. The response of acute childhood leukemia to an initial and a second course of prednisone. J Pediatr 1965;66:18.
21. Wolff JA, Brubaker CA, Murphy ML, et al. Prednisone therapy of acute childhood leukemia: prognosis and duration of response in 300 treated patients. J Pediatr 1967;70:626.
22. Aur RJA, Simone J, Hustu HO, et al. Central nervous system therapy and combination chemotherapy of childhood lymphocytic leukemia. Blood 1971;37:272.
23. Van Eys J, Berry D, Crist W, et al. A comparison of two regimens for high-risk acute lymphocytic leukemia in childhood. Cancer 1989;63:23.
24. Simone JV, Aur RJA, Hustu HO, et al. Three to ten years after cessation of therapy in children with leukemia. Cancer 1978;42:839.
25. George SL, Aur RJA, Mauer AM, et al. A reappraisal of the results of stopping therapy in childhood leukemia. N Engl J Med 1979;330:269.
26. Land VJ, Berry DH, Herson J, et al. Long-term survival in childhood acute leukemia: "late relapses." Med Pediatr Oncol 1979;7:19.
27. Frei E III, Karon M, Levin RH, et al. The effectiveness of combinations of antileukemia agents in inducing and maintaining remission in children with acute leukemia. Blood 1965;26:642.
28. Hustu HO, Aur RJA. Extramedullary leukemia. Clin Haematol 1978;7:313.
29. Aur RJA, Simone JV, Hustu HO, Verzosa MS. A comparative study of central nervous system irradiation and intensive chemotherapy early in remission of childhood acute lymphocytic leukemia. Cancer 1972;29:381.
30. Haghbin M, Murphy ML, Tan CC, et al. A long-term clinical follow-up of children with acute lymphoblastic leukemia treated with intensive chemotherapy regimens. Cancer 1980;46:241.
31. Inati A, Sallan SE, Cassady JR, et al. Efficacy and morbidity of central nervous system "prophylaxis" in childhood acute lymphoblastic leukemia: eight years' experience with cranial irradiation and intrathecal methotrexate. Blood 1983;61:297.
32. Sullivan MP, Chen T, Dyment PG, et al. Equivalence of intrathecal chemotherapy and radiotherapy as central nervous system prophylaxis in children with acute lymphocytic leukemia: a Pediatric Oncology Group Study. Blood 1982;60:948.
33. Rubenstein LJ, Herman MM, Long TF, Wilbur JR. Disseminated necrotizing leukoencephalopathy: a complication of treated central nervous system leukemia and lymphoma. Cancer 1975;35:291.
34. Price RA, Jamieson PA. The central nervous system in childhood leukemia. II. Subacute leukoencephalopathy. Cancer 1975;35:306.
35. Peylan-Ramu N, Poplack DG, Pizzo PA, et al. Abnormal CT scans of the brain in asymptomatic children with acute lymphocytic leukemia after prophylactic treatment of the central nervous system with radiation and intrathecal chemotherapy. N Engl J Med 1978;298:815.

36. Riehm H, Feikert H-J, Lampert F. Acute lymphoblastic leukaemia. In: Voute PA, Barrett A, Bloom HJG, et al, eds. Cancer in children: clinical management. Heidelberg, Springer-Verlag, 1986:101.
37. Freireich EJ, Gehan E, Frei E III, et al. The effect of 6-mercaptopurine on the duration of steroid-induced remission in acute leukemia: a model for evaluation of other potentially useful therapy. Blood 1963;21:699.
38. Aur RFA, Simone JV, Verzosa MS, et al. Childhood acute lymphocytic leukemia. Cancer 1978;42:2123.
39. Clavell LA, Gelber RD, Cohen HJ, et al. Four-agent induction and intensive asparaginase therapy for treatment of childhood acute lymphoblastic leukemia. N Engl J Med 1986;315:657.
40. Chao NJ, Blume KG. Bone marrow transplantation: what is the question? Ann Intern Med 1990;113:340.
41. Blume KG, Forman SJ, Snyder DS, et al. Allogeneic bone marrow transplantation for acute lymphoblastic leukemia during first complete remission. Transplantation 1987;43:389.
42. Jacobs AD, Gale RP. Recent advances in the biology and treatment of acute lymphoblastic leukemia in adults. N Engl J Med 1984;311:1219.
43. Hoelzer D, Gale RP. Acute lymphoblastic leukemia in adults: recent progress, future directions. Semin Hematol 1987;24:27.
44. Linker CA, Levitt LJ, O'Donnell M, et al. Improved results of treatment of adult acute lymphoblastic leukemia. Blood 1987;69:1242.
45. Champlin R, Gale RP. Acute lymphoblastic leukemia: recent advances in biology and therapy. Blood 1989;73:2051.
46. Beatty PG, Dahlberg S, Mickelson EM, et al. Probability of finding HLA-matched unrelated marrow donors. Transplantation 1988;45:714.
47. Westoff CF. Fertility in the United States. Science 1986;234:544.
48. Ramsay NKC, Kersey JH. Perspective: indications for marrow transplantation in acute lymphoblastic leukemia. Blood 1990;75:815.
49. Kersey JH, Weisdorf D, Nesbit ME, et al. Comparison of autologous and allogeneic bone marrow transplantation for treatment of high risk refractory acute lymphoblastic leukemia. N Engl J Med 1987;317:461.
50. Ritz J, Sallan SE, Bast RC, et al. Autologous bone marrow transplantation in CALLA positive acute lymphoblastic leukemia after in vitro treatment with J5 monoclonal antibody and complement. Lancet 1982;2:60.
51. Kernan NA, Brtsch G, Ash RC, et al. Analysis of 462 transplantations from unrelated donors facilitated by the National Marrow Donor Program. N Engl J Med 1993;328:593.
52. Thomas ED, Clift RA, Fefer A, et al. Marrow transplantation for the treatment of chronic myelogenous leukemia. Ann Intern Med 1986;104:155.
53. Goldman JM, Apperley JF, Jones L, et al. Bone marrow transplantation for patients with chronic myelogenous leukemia. N Engl J Med 1986;314:202.
54. Barnett MJ, Eaves CJ, Phillips GL, et al. Successful autografting in chronic myeloid leukaemia after maintenance of marrow in culture. Bone Marrow Transplant 1989;4:345.
55. McGlave PB, Arthur D, Miller WJ, et al. Autologous transplantation for CML using marrow treated ex vivo with recombinant human interferon gamma. Bone Marrow Transplant 1990;6:115.
56. Berk PD, Goldberg JD, Donovan PB, et al. Therapeutic recommendations in polycythemia vera based on polycythemia vera study group protocols. Semin Hematol 1986;23:132.
57. Gale RP, Foon KA. Chronic lymphocytic leukemia, recent advances in biology and treatment. Ann Intern Med 1985;103:101.
58. Cheson BD. Current approaches to the chemotherapy of B-cell chronic lymphocytic leukemia: at review. Am J Hematol 1989;32:72.
58a. Khouri IF, Keating MJ, Vriesendorp HM, et al. Autologous and allogeneic bone marrow transplantation for chronic lymphocytic leukemia: preliminary results. J Clin Oncol 1994;12:748.
59. Oken MM, Creech RH, Tormey DC, et al. Toxicity and response criteria of the Eastern Cooperative Oncology Group. Am J Clin Oncol 1982;5:649.
60. Cassileth PA, Harrington DP, Hines JD, et al. Maintenance chemotherapy prolongs remission duration in adult acute nonlymphocytic leukemia. J Clin Oncol 1988;6:583.
61. Yamada M, Hudson S, Tournay O, et al. Detection of minimal disease in hematopoietic malignancies of the B-cell lineage by using third-complementarity-determining region (CDR-III)–specific probes. Proc Natl Acad Sci USA 1989;86:5123.
62. Needleman SW, Burns CP, Dick FR, Armitage JO. Hypoplastic acute leukemia. Cancer 1981;48:1410.
63. Duttera MJ, Bull JM, Northrop JD, et al. Serial in vitro bone marrow culture in acute lymphocytic leukemia. Blood 1973;42:687.
64. Mangalik A, Robinson WA, Holton CP, et al. Granulopoietic studies in acute lymphocytic leukemia of children. Blut 1977;34:77.
65. Arlin ZA, Fried J, Clarkson BD. Therapeutic role of cell kinetics in acute leukemia. Clin Haematol 1978;7:339.
66. Cleary ML, Chao J, Warnke R, Sklar J. Immunoglobulin gene rearrangement as a diagnostic criterion of B-cell lymphoma. Proc Natl Acad Sci USA 1984;81:593.
67. Roth MS, Antin JH, Bingham EL, Ginsburg D. Detection of Philadelphia chromosome-positive cells by the polymerase chain reaction following bone marrow transplant for chronic myelogenous leukemia. Blood 1989;74:882.
68. Yamada M, Wasserman R, Lange B, et al. Minimal residual disease in childhood B-lineage lymphoblastic leukemia. N Engl J Med 1990;323:448.
69. Eisenstein BI. The polymerase chain reaction: a new method for using molecular genetics for medical diagnosis. N Engl J Med 1990;322:178.
70. Morgan GJ, Hughes T, Janssen JW, et al. Polymerase chain reaction for detection of residual leukemia. Lancet 1989;1:928.
71. Tannock IF. Cell kinetics and chemotherapy: a critical review. Cancer Treat Rep 1978;62:1117.
72. Madoc-James H, Mauro F. Site of action of cytotoxic agents: in the cell life cycle in antineoplastic and immunosuppressive agents. Heidelberg, Springer-Verlag, 1974:205.
73. Hill BT. Cancer chemotherapy: the relevance of certain concepts of cell cycle kinetics. Biochim Biophys Acta 1978;516:389.
74. Baserga R. Multiplication and division in mammalian cells. New York, Marcel Dekker, 1976:53.
75. Salmon SE, Hamburger AW, Soehnlen B, et al. Quantitatition of differential sensitivity of human-tumor stem cells to anticancer drugs. N Engl J Med 1978;298:1321.
76. Jolivet J, Cowan KH, Curt GA, et al. The pharmacology and clinical use of methotrexate. N Engl J Med 1983;309:1094.
77. Bleyer WA. The clinical pharmacology of methotrexate: new applications of an old drug. Cancer 1978;41:36.
78. Evans WE, Crom WR, Abramowitch M, et al. Clinical pharmacodynamics of high-dose methotrexate in acute lymphocytic leukemia: identification of a relation between concentration and effect. N Engl J Med 1986;314:471.
79. Pitman SW, Frei E III. Weekly methotrexate-calcium leucovorin rescue. Effect of alkalinization on nephrotoxicity: pharmacokinetics in the CNS; and use in CNS non-Hodgkin's lymphoma. Cancer Treat Rep 1977;61:695.
80. Bleyer WA. Methotrexate: clinical pharmacology, current status, and guidelines. Cancer Treat Rev 1977;4:87.
81. Abelson HT, Fasburg MT, Beardsley GP, et al. Methotrexate-induced renal impairment: clinical studies and rescue from systemic toxicity with high-dose leucovorin and thymidine. J Clin Oncol 1983;1:208.
82. Weinstein GD. Methotrexate. Ann Intern Med 1977;86:199.
83. Sostman HD, Matthay RA, Putman CE, et al. Methotrexate-induced pneumonitis. Medicine 1976;55:371.
84. Bronner AK, Hood AF. Cutaneous complications of chemotherapeutic agents. J Am Acad Dermatol 1983;9:645.
85. Bertino JR, Cashmore A, Fruk M, et al. The induction of leukocyte and erythrocyte dihydrofolate reductase by methotrextate. Clin Pharmacol Ther 1965;6:763.
86. Jolivet J, Cowan KH, Crut GA, et al. The pharmacology and clinical use of methotrexate. N Engl J Med 1983;309:1094.
87. Rai KR, Holland JF, Glidewell OJ, et al. Treatment of acute myelocytic leukemia: a study by Cancer and Leukemia Group B. Blood 1981;58:1203.
88. Yates J, Glidewell O, Wiernik P, et al. Cytosine arabinoside with daunorubicin or Adriamycin for therapy of acute myelocytic leukemia: a CALGB study. Blood 1982;60:454.
89. Morra E, Lazzarino M, Alessandrino P, et al. VP16213 and cytosine arabinoside combination chemotherapy for refractory acute lymphoblastic leukemia in adults. Eur J Cancer Clin Oncol 1984;20:1471.
90. Cohen SS. The lethality of ara nucleotides. Med Biol 1979;54:299.
91. Fridland A. Inhibition of DNA chain initiation by 1-β-D-arabinofuranosyl cytosine (ara C) in human fibroblasts. J Supramol Struct 1978;771:331.
92. Lauzon GJ, Paterson ARP, Belch AW. Formation of 1-β-D-arabinofuranosylcytosine diphosphate choline in neoplastic and normal cells. Cancer Res 1978;38:1730.
93. Tattersall MNH, Ganeshaguar K, Hoffbrand AV. Mechanisms of resistance of human acute leukaemia cells to cytosine arabinoside. Br J Haematol 1974;27:29.
94. Steuart CD, Burke PJ. Cytidine deaminase and the development of resistance to arabinosyl cytosine. Nature 1971;233:109.
95. Bensinger TA, Fahey JL, Kellon DB, et al. Febrile response to cytarabine. JAMA 1974;229:1578.
96. Salavin RE, Dias MA, Saral R. Cytosine arabinoside induced gastrointestinal toxic alterations in sequential chemotherapeutic protocols. Cancer 1978;42:1747.
97. Morra E, Lazzarino M, Inverardi D, et al. Systemic high-dose Ara-C for the treatment of meningeal leukemia in adult lymphoblastic leukemia and non-Hodgkin's lymphoma. J Clin Oncol 1986;4:1207.
98. Lazarus HM, Herzig RH, Herzig GP, et al. Central nervous system toxicity of high-dose cytosine arabinoside. Cancer 1981;48:2577.
99. Herzig RH, Wolff SN, Lazarus HM, et al. High-dose cytosine arabinoside therapy for refractory leukemia. Blood 1983;62:361.
100. Lass JH, Lazarus HM, Reed MD, et al. Topical corticosteroid therapy for corneal toxicity from systemically administered cytarabine. Am J Ophthalmol 1983;94:617.
101. Burgdorf WHC, Gilmore WA, Ganick RG. Peculiar acral erythema

secondary to high-dose chemotherapy for acute myelogenous leukemia. Ann Intern Med 1982;97:61.
102. Haupt H, Hutchins G, Moore G. Ara-C lung: noncardiogenic pulmonary edema complicating cytosine arabinoside therapy of leukemia. Am J Med 1981;70:250.
103. Johnson H, Smith T, Desforges J. Cytosine-arabinoside-induced colitis and peritonitis: nonoperative management. J Clin Oncol 1985;3:607.
104. Pizzuto J, Aviles A, Ramos E, et al. Cytosine arabinoside induced liver damage: histopathologic demonstration. Med Pediatr Oncol 1983;11:287.
105. Capizzi RL, Yang JL, Chen E, et al. Alterations of the pharmacokinetics of high-dose Ara-C by its metabolite, Ara-U, in patients with acute leukemia. J Clin Oncol 1983;1:763.
106. Elion GB, Callahan S, Rundles RW, Hitchings GH. Relationship between metabolic fates and antitumor activities of thiopurines. Cancer Res 1963;23:1207.
107. Rosman M, Williams HE. Leucocyte purine phosphoribosyltransferases in human leukemias sensitive and resistant to 6-thiopurines. Cancer Res 1973;33:1202.
108. Christie NT, Drake S, Meya RE, et al. 6-thioguanine-induced DNA damage as a determinant of cytotoxicity in cultured Chinese hamster ovary cells. Cancer Res 1984;44:3665.
109. Rosman M, Lee MH, Creasey WA, Sartorelli AC. Mechanisms of resistance to 6-thiopurines in human leukemias. Cancer Res 1974;34:1952.
110. Zimm S, Collins JM, Riccardi R, et al. Variability bioavailability of oral mercatopurine: is maintenance chemotherapy in acute lymphoblastic leukemia being optimally delivered? N Engl J Med 1983;308:1005.
111. Koren G, Ferrazini G, Sulh H, et al. Systemic exposure to mercaptopurine as a prognostic factor in acute lymphocytic leukemia in children. N Engl J Med 1990;323:17.
112. Young CW, Hodas S. Hydroxyurea: inhibitory effect on DNA metabolism. Science 1964;146:1172.
113. Yeh Y-Ch, Tessman I. Differential effect of hydroxyurea on a ribonucleotide reductase system. J Biol Chem 1978;253:1323.
114. Kennedy BJ. Hydroxyurea therapy in chronic myelogenous leukemia. Cancer 1972;29:1052.
115. Agarwall RP. Inhibitors of adenosine deaminase. Pharmacol Ther 1982;17:399.
116. Seto Sh, Carrera CJ, Kubota M, et al. Mechanism of deoxyadenosine and 2-chlorodeoxyadenosine toxicity to nondividing human lymphocytes. J Clin Invest 1985;75:377.
117. Berger NA. Poly(ADP-ribose) in the cellular response to DNA damage. Radiat Res 1985;101:4.
118. Sims JL, Berger SJ, Berger NA. Poly(ADP-ribose) polymerase inhibitors preserve NAD^+ and ATP pools in DNA-damaged cells: mechanism of stimulation of unscheduled DNA synthesis. Biochemistry 1983;22:5188.
119. Berger SJ, Sudar DC, Berger NA. DNA damage induced alterations in glucose metabolism by activation of poly(ADP-ribose) polymerase. Biochem Biophys Res Commun 1986;134:227.
120. Hershfield MS, Kredich NM, Ownby DR, et al. In vivo inactivation of 5-adenosyl homocysteine hydrolase by 2'deoxyadenosine in adenosine deaminase-deficient patients. J Clin Invest 1979;63:807.
121. Mitchell BS, Koller CA, Heyn R. Inhibition of adenosine deaminase activity results in cytotoxicity to T lymphoblasts in vivo. Blood 1980;56:556.
122. Spiers ASD, Moore D, Cassileth PA, et al. Remissions in hairy cell leukemia with pentostatin (2'-deoxycoformycin). N Engl J Med 1987;316:825.
123. Spiers ASD, Ruckdeschel JC, Horton J. Effectiveness of pentostatin (2'-deoxycoformycin) in refractory lymphoid neoplasms. Scand J Haematol 1984;32:130.
124. O'Dwyer PJ, Wagner B, Leyland-Jones B, et al. 2'-Deoxycoformycin (pentostatin) for lymphoid malignancies: rational development of an active new drug. Ann Intern Med 1988;108:733.
125. Grever MR, Leiby JM, Kraut EH, et al. Low-dose deoxycoformycin lymphoid malignancy. J Clin Oncol 1985;3:1196.
126. Smyth JF, Prentice HG, Proctor S, et al. Deoxycoformycin in the treatment of leukemias and lymphomas. Ann NY Acad Sci 1985;451:123.
127. Grever MR, Siaw MFE, Jacob WF, et al. The biochemical and clinical consequences of 2'-deoxycoformycin in refractory lymphoproliferative malignancy. Blood 1981;57:406.
127a. Ho AD, Thaler J, Stryckmans P, et al. Pentostatin in resistant chronic lymphocytic leukemia: a phase II trial of the European Organization for Research and Treatment of Cancer. J Natl Cancer Inst 1990;82:1416.
127b. Cassileth PA, Chevuart D, Spiers ASD, et al. Pentostatin induces durable remission in hairy cell leukemia. J Clin Oncol 1991;9:243.
128. Poplack DG, Sallan SE, Rivera G, et al. Phase I study of 2'-deoxycoformycin in acute lymphoblastic leukemia. Cancer Res 1981;41:3343.
129. O'Dwyer PJ, Spiers ASD, Marsoni S, et al. Association of severe and fatal infections and treatment with pentostatin. Cancer Treat Rep 1986;70:1117.
130. Prentice HG, Russell NH, Lee N, et al. Therapeutic selectivity of and prediction of response to 2'-deoxycoformycin in acute leukemia. Lancet 1981;2:1250.
131. Carson DA, Wasson DB, Taetle R, Yu A. Specific toxicity of 2-chlorodeoxyadenosine toward resting and proliferating human lymphocytes. Blood 1983;62:737.
132. Carson DA, Wasson DB, Beutler E. Antileukemic and immunosuppressive activity of 2-chloro-2'-deoxyadenosine. Proc Natl Acad Sci USA 1984;81:2232.
133. Piro LD, Carrera CJ, Beutler E, Carson DA. 2-chlorodeoxyadenosine: an effective new agent for the treatment of chronic lymphocytic leukemia. Blood 1988;72:1069.
134. Piro LD, Carrera CJ, Carson DA, Beutler D. Lasting remissions in hairy-cell leukemia induced by a single infusion of 2-chlorodeoxyadenosine. N Engl J Med 1990;322:1117.
134a. Estey EH, Kurzrock R, Kantarjian HM, et al. Treatment of hairy cell leukemia with 2-chlorodeoxyadenosine (2-CdA). Blood 1992;79:882.
134b. Piro LD, Carrera CJ, Carson DA, et al. Lasting remissions in hairy cell leukemia induced by a single fusion of 2-chlorodeoxyadenosine. N Engl J Med 1990;322:1117.
134c. Saven A, Carrera CJ, Carson DA, et al. 2-Chlorodeoxyadenosine treatment in refractory chronic lymphocytic leukemia. Leukemia Lymphoma 1991;5(Suppl):133.
134d. Saven A, Piro LD. Newer purine analogues for the treatment of hairy-cell leukemia. Drug Ther 1993;330:691.
134e. Saven A, Piro LD. 2-Chlorodeoxyadenosine: a newer purine analog active in the treatment of indolent lymphoid malignancies. Ann Intern Med 1994;120:784.
135. Plunkett W, Chubb S, Alexander L, Montgomery JA. Comparison of the toxicity and metabolism of 9-β-D-arabinofuranosyl-2-fluoroadenine and 9-β-D-arabinofuranosyladenine in human lymphoblastoid cells. Cancer Res 1980;40:2349.
136. Brockman RW, Schabel FM, Montgomery JA. Biologic activity of 9-β-D-arabinofluransyl-2-fluoroadenine, a metabolically stable analog of 9-β-D-arabinofuranosyladenine. Biochem Pharmacol 1977;26:2193.
137. White EL, Shaddix SC, Brockman RW, Bennett LL Jr. Comparison of the actions of 9-β-D-arabinofuranosyl-2-fluoroadenine and 9-β-D-arabinofuranosyladenine on target enzymes from mouse tumor cells. Cancer Res 1982;42:2260.
138. Plunkett W, Huang P, Gandhi V. Metabolism and action of fludarabine phosphate. Semin Oncol 1990;17:3.
139. Brockman RW, Cheng Y-C, Schabel FM Jr, et al. Metabolism and chemotherapeutic activity of 9-β-D-arabinofuranosyl-2-fluoroadenine against murine leukemia L1210 and evidence for its phosphorylation by deoxycytidine kinase. Cancer Res 1980;40:3610.
140. LePage GA, Naik SR, Katakkan SB, et al. 9-β-D-arabinofuranosyladenine 5'-phosphate metabolism and excretion in humans. Cancer Res 1975;35:3036.
141. Grever MR, Kopecky KJ, Coltman CA, et al. Fludarabine monophosphate: a potentially useful agent in chronic lymphocytic leukemia. Nouv Rev Fr Hematol 1988;30:457.
142. Keating MJ, Kantarjian H, O'Brien S, et al. Fludarabine: a new agent with marked cytoreductive activity in untreated chronic lymphocytic leukemia. J Clin Oncol 1991;9:44.
143. Keating MJ. Fludarabine phosphate in the treatment of chronic lymphocytic leukemia. Semin Oncol 1990;17:49.
144. Warrell RP Jr, Berman E. Phase I and II study of fludarabine phosphate in leukemia: therapeutic efficacy with delayed central nervous system toxicity. J Clin Oncol 1986;4:74.
145. Chun HG, Leyland-Jones BB, Caryk SM, Hoth DF. Central nervous system toxicity of fludarabine phosphate. Cancer Treat Rep 1986;70:1225.
146. Chun HG, Leyland-Jones B, Cheson BD. Fludarabine phosphate: a synthetic purine antimetabolite with significant activity against lymphoid malignancies. J Clin Oncol 1991;9:175.
147. Ludlum DB. Alkylating agents and the nitrosoureas. In: Becker FF, ed. Cancer: a comprehensive Treatise, vol. 5. New York, Plenum, 1977:285.
148. Kohn KW. Interstrand cross-linked of DNA by 1,3-bis(2-chlorethyl)-1-nitrosourea and other 1-(2-haloethyl)-1-nitrosoureas. Cancer Res 1977;37:1450.
149. Casciato DA, Scott JL. Acute leukemia following prolonged cytotoxic agent therapy. Medicine 1979;58:32.
150. Coltman CA Jr, Dixon DO. Second malignancies complicating Hodgkin's disease: a Southwest Oncology Group 10-year followup. Cancer Treat Res 1982;66:1023.
151. Aisenberg AC. Acute nonlymphocytic leukemia after treatment for Hodgkin's disease. Am J Med 1983;75:449.
152. Pedersen-Bjergaard J, Larsen SO. Incidence of acute nonlymphocytic leukemia, preleukemia, and acute myeloproliferative syndrome up to 10 years after treatment of Hodgkin's disease. N Engl J Med 1982;207:965.
153. Colvin M. The alkylating agents. In: Chabner BA, ed. Pharmacologic principles of cancer treatment. Philadelphia, WB Saunders, 1982:276.
154. Calabresi P, Parks RE Jr. Antiproliferation agents and drugs used for immunosuppression. In: Gilman AG, Goodman LS, Rall TW, Murad

F, eds. The pharmacological basis of therapeutics, ed 7. New York, Macmillan, 1985:1247.
155. Hemminki K, Ludlum DB. Covalent modification of DNA by antineoplastic agents. JNCI 1984;73:1021.
156. Bergsagel DE. Treatment of plasma cell myeloma with cytotoxic agents. Arch Intern Med 1975;135:172.
157. Alberts DS, Chang SY, Chen HS, et al. Pharmacokinetics and metabolism of chlorambucil in man: a preliminary report. Cancer Treat Rep 1979;6:9.
158. Cole SR, Myers TJ, Klatsky AU. Pulmonary disease with chlorambucil therapy. Cancer 1978;41:455.
159. Berk PD, Goldberg JD, Silverstein MN, et al. Increased incidence of acute leukemia in polycythemia vera associated with chlorambucil therapy. N Engl J Med 1981;304:441.
160. Vistica DT. Cytotoxicity as an indicator for transport mechanism: evidence that melphalan is transported by two leucine-preferring carrier systems in the L1210 murine leukemia cell. Biochim Biophys Acta 1979;550:309.
161. Bergel F, Stock JA. Cytotoxic alpha amino acids and endopeptides. Br Emp Cancer Camp Annu Rep 1953;31:6.
162. Alberts DS, Chang SY, Chen HSG, et al. Oral melphalan kinetics. Clin Pharmacol Ther 1979;26:737.
163. Tattersall MHN, Jarman M, Newlands ES, et al. Pharmaco-kinetics of melphalan following oral or intravenous administration in patients with malignant disease. Eur J Cancer 1978;14:507.
164. Waldenström J. Melphalan therapy in myelomatasis. Br Med J 1964;1: 859.
165. Dale BM, Sage RE, Norman JE, et al. Bone marrow transplantation following treatment with high dose melphalan. Transplant Proc 1985;17:1711.
166. Maraninchi D, Pico JL, Hartmann O, et al. High dose melphalan with or without marrow transplantation: a study of dose-effect in patients with refractory and/or relapsed acute leukemias. Cancer Treat Rep 1986;70:445.
167. Selby P, McElwain TJ, Nandi AC, et al. Multiple myeloma treated with high dose intravenous melphalan. Br J Haematol 1987;66:55.
168. Barlogie B, Alexanian R, Dicke KA, et al. High-dose chemoradiotherapy and autologous bone marrow transplantation for resistant multiple myeloma. Blood 1987;70:869.
169. Takamizawa A, Matsumoto S, Iwata T, et al. Studies on cyclophosphamide metabolites and their related compounds. II. Preparation of an active species of cyclophosphamide and some related compounds. J Am Chem Soc 1973;95:985.
170. Santos GW, Sensenbrenner LL, Burke PJ, et al. The use of cyclophosphamide for clinical marrow transplantation. Transplant Proc 1972;4:559.
171. Droller MJ, Saral R, Santos G. Prevention of cyclophosphamide-induced hemorrhagic cystitis. Urology 1982;20:256.
172. Brock N, Pohl J. Prevention of urotoxic side effects by regional detoxification with increased selectivity of oxazophosphorine cytostatics. IARC Sci Publ 1986;78:269.
173. Blacklock H, Ball L, Knight C, et al. Experience with mesna in patients receiving allogeneic bone marrow transplants for poor prognostic leukemia. Cancer Treat Rev 1983;10:45.
174. Appelbaum FR, Strauchen JA, Graw RG, et al. Acute lethal carditis caused by high-dose combination chemotherapy: a unique clinical and pathological entity. Lancet 1976;1:58.
175. Mills BA, Roberts RW. Cyclophosphamide-induced cardiomyopathy: a report of two cases and review of the English literature. Cancer 1979;43:2223.
176. DeFronzo RA, Braine H, Colvin OM, et al. Water intoxication in man after cyclophosphamide therapy. Ann Intern Med 1973;78:861.
177. Cassileth PA, Andersen J, Lazarus HM, et al. Autologous bone marrow transplant in acute myeloid leukemia in first remission. J Clin Oncol 1993;11:314.
178. Yeager AM, Kaizer H, Santos GW, et al. Autologous bone marrow transplantation in patients with acute nonlymphocytic leukemia using ex vivo marrow treatment with 4-hydroperoxycyclophosphamide. N Engl J Med 1986;315:141.
179. Nadkarni MV, Trams EG, Smith PK. Preliminary studies on the distribution and fate of TBM, TEPA and myleran in the human. Cancer Res 1959;19:713.
180. Warwick GP. The mechanism of action of alkylating agents. Cancer Res 1963;23:1315.
181. Cannellos GP. The treatment of chronic granulocytic leukemia. Clin Haematol 1977;6:113.
182. Koefler HP, Golde DW. Chronic myelogenous leukemia: new concepts. N Engl J Med 1981;304:1201.
183. Biggs JC, Szer J, Crilley P, et al. Treatment of chronic myelogenous leukemia with allogeneic bone marrow transplantation after preparation with Bu CY 2. Blood 1992;89:1352.
184. Santos GW, Tutschka PJ, Brookmeyer R, et al. Marrow transplantation for acute nonlymphocytic leukemia after treatment with busulfan and cyclophosphamide. N Engl J Med 1983;309:1347.
185. Kyle RA, Schwartz RS, Oliner HL, Dameshek W. A syndrome resembling adrenal contical insufficiency associated with long term busulfan (myleran) therapy. Blood 1961;18:497.
186. Burns WA, McFarland W, Mathews MJ. Busulfan induced pulmonary disease. Am Rev Respir Dis 1970;101:408.
187. Boyles PW. Interstitial pulmonary fibrosis after long term busulfan therapy. Clin Med 1971;76:11.
188. Leake E, Smith WB, Woodluff JH. Diffuse interstitial pulmonary fibrosis after busulphan therapy. Lancet 1963;2:432.
189. Jones RJ, Lee KSK, Beschorner WE, et al. Venoocclusive disease of the liver following bone marrow transplantation. Transplantation 1987;44:778.
190. Ehrsson H, Hassan M, Ehrnebo M, et al. Busulfan kinetics. Clin Pharmacol Ther 1983;34:86.
191. Beschorner WE, Pino J, Boitnott JK, et al. Pathology of the liver with bone marrow transplantation: effects of busulfan, carmustine, acute graft-versus-host disease, and cytomegalovirus infection. Am J Pathol 1980;99:369.
192. Peters WP, Henner WD, Grochow LB, et al. Clinical and pharmacologic effects of high dose single agent busulfan with autologous bone marrow support in the treatment of solid tumors. Cancer Res 1987;47:6402.
193. Atkinson K, Biggs J, Noble G, et al. Preparative regimens for marrow transplantation containing busulphan are associated with haemorrhagic cystitis and hepatic veno-occlusive disease but a short duration of leucopenia and little oro-pharyngeal mucositis. Bone Marrow Transplant 1987;2:385.
194. Ewig RAG, Kohn KW. DNA damage and repair in mouse leukemia L1210 cells treated with nitrogen mustard, 1,3-bis(2-chloroethyl)-1-nitrosourea, and other nitrosoureas. Cancer Res 1977;37:2114.
195. Ewig RAG, Kohn DW. DNA-protein cross-linking and DNA interstrand cross-linking by haloethylnitrosoureas in L1210 cells. Cancer Res 1978;38:3197.
196. Kahn HE Jr. Comparison of biochemical and biological effects of four nitrosoureas with differing carbamoylating activities. Cancer Res 1978;38:2363.
197. Henner WD, Peters WP, Eder JP, et al. Pharmacokinetics and immediate effects of high-dose carmustine in man. Cancer Treat Rep 1986;70:877.
198. Levin VA, Hoffman W, Weinkam RJ. Pharmacokinetics of BCNU in man: a preliminary study of 20 patients. Cancer Treat Rep 1978;62: 1305.
199. O'Driscol BR, Hasleton PS, Taylor PM, et al. Active lung fibrosis up to 17 years after chemotherapy with carmustine (BCNU) in childhood. N Engl J Med 1990;323:378.
200. Holoye PY, Jenkins DE, Greenberg SD. Pulmonary toxicity in long-term administration of BCNU. Cancer Treat Rep 1976;60:1691.
201. Weiss RB, Poster DS, Penta JS. The nitrosoureas and pulmonary toxicity. Cancer Treat Rev 1981;8:111.
202. Phillips GL, Fay JW, Herzig GP, et al. Intensive 1,3 bis(2-chloroethyl)-1-nitrosourea (BCNU), NSC#-436650 and cryopreserved autologous marrow transplantation for refractory cancer: a phase I–II study. Cancer 1980;52:1792.
203. Durant JR, Norgard MJ, Murad TM, et al. Pulmonary toxicity associated with bischloroethylnitrosourea (BCNU). Ann Intern Med 1979;90:191.
203a. Jones RB, Matthes S, Shpall EJ, et al. Acute lung injury following treatment with high-dose cyclophosphamide, cisplatin, and carmustine: pharmacodynamic evaluation of carmustine. J Natl Cancer Inst 1993;75:640.
204. Takvorian T, Parker LM, Hochberg FH, et al. Autologous bone marrow transplantation: host effects of high-dose BCNU. J Clin Oncol 1983;1: 610.
205. Peters WP, Eder J, Henner W, et al. Novel toxicities associated with high-dose combination alkylating agents with autologous bone marrow support (ABMS 11). Proc Am Soc Clin Oncol (Abstract) 1985;4: 139.
206. Friedmann CA. Structure-activity relationships of anthraquinones in some pathological conditions. Pharmacology 1980;20:113.
207. Pigram WJ, Fuller W, Hamilton LDH. Stereochemistry of intercalation: interaction of daunomycin with DNA. Nature 1972;235:17.
208. Murphree SA, Cunningham LS, Hwang KM, Sartorelli AC. Effects of Adriamycin on surface properties of sarcoma 180 ascites cells. Biochem Pharmacol 1976;25:1227.
209. Mikkelsen RB, Lin PS, Wallach DF. Interaction of Adriamycin with human red blood cells: a biochemical and morphologic study. J Mol Med 1977;2:33.
210. Crooke ST, DuVernay VH, Galvan L, Prestayko AW. Structure-activity relationships of anthracyclines relative to effects on macromolecular synthesis. Mol Pharmacol 1978;14:290.
211. Lown JM, Sim S, Majumdar KC, Chung R. Strand scission of DNA by bound Adriamycin and daunomycin in the presence of reducing agents. Biochem Biophys Res Commun 1977;79:705.
212. Goldenberg GJ, Wang H, Blaair GW. Resistance to Adriamycin: relationship of cytotoxicity to drug uptake and DNA single- and double-strand breakage in cloned cell lines of Adriamycin-sensitive and -resistant P388 leukemia. Cancer Res 1986;46:2978.
213. Tewey KM, Rowe TC, Yang L, et al. Adriamycin-induced DNA damage is mediated by mammalian DNA topoisomerase II. Science 1984;226:466.

214. Yates J, Glidewell O, Wiernik P, et al. Cytosine arabinoside with daunorubicin or Adriamycin for therapy of acute myelocytic leukemia: a CALGB study. Blood 1982;60:454.
215. Sallan SE, Camitta BM, Cassady JR, et al. Intermittent combination chemotherapy with Adriamycin for childhood acute lymphoblastic leukemia: clinical results. Blood 1978;51:425.
216. Barlogie B, Smith L, Alexanian R. Effective treatment of advanced multiple myeloma refractory to alkylating agents. N Engl J Med 1984;310:1353.
217. Vogler WR, Velez-Garcia E, Omura G, Raney M. A phase-three trial comparing daunorubicin or idarubicin combined with cytosine arabinoside in acute myelogenous leukemia. Semin Oncol 1989;16:21.
218. Wiernik PH, Case DC Jr, Periman PO, et al. A multicenter trial of cytarabine plus idarubicin or daunorubicin as induction therapy for adult acute nonlymphocytic leukemia. Semin Oncol 1989;16:25.
219. Berman E, Heller G, Sautorsa J, et al. Results of a randomized trial comparing idarubicin and cytosine arabinoside with daunorubicin and cytosine arabinoside in adult patients with newly diagnosed acute myelogenous leukemia. Blood 1991;77:1666.
220. Praga C, Beretta C, Vigo PL, et al. Adriamycin cardiotoxicity: a survey of 1273 patients. Cancer Treat Rep 1979;63:827.
221. Gottdiener JS, Mathisen DJ, Borer JS, Bonow RO, Green MV, Rosenberg SA. Doxorubicin cardiotoxicity: assessment of the left ventrical dysfunction by radionuclide cineangiography. Ann Intern Med 1981;94:430.
222. Buzdar AU, Marcus C, Smith TL, Blumenschein GR. Early and delayed clinical cardiotoxicity of doxorubicin. Cancer 1985;55:2761.
223. Olson RD, Mushlin PS. Doxorubicin cardiotoxicity: analysis of prevailing hypotheses. FASEB J 1990;4:3076.
224. Durr FE. Biologic and biochemical effects of mitoxantrone. Semin Oncol 1984;11:3.
225. Hiddeman W, Kreutzman H, Straif K, et al. High dose arabinoside and mitoxantrone: a highly effective regimen in refractory acute myeloid leukemia. Blood 1987;69:744.
226. Ho AD, Lipp T, Ehninger G, et al. Combination of mitoxantrone and etoposide in refractory acute myelogenous leukemia: an active and well-tolerated regimen. J Clin Oncol 1988;6:213.
227. Shenkenberg TD, Von Hoff DD. Mitoxantrone: a new anticancer drug with significant clinical activity. Ann Intern Med 1986;105:67.
228. Owellen RJ, Owens AH, Donigian DW. The binding of vincristine, vinblastine and colchicine to tubulin. Biochem Biophys Res Commun 1972;47:685.
229. Owellen RJ, Hartke CA, Dickerson RM, Hains FO. Inhibition of tubulin-microtubule polymerization by drugs of the vinca alkaloid class. Cancer Res 1976;36:1499.
230. Madoc-Jones H, Mauro F. Interphase action of vinblastine and vincristine: differences in their lethal action through the mitotic cycle of cultured mammalian cells. J Cell Physiol 1968;72:185.
231. Igbal Z, Oohs S. Uptake of vinca alkaloids into mammalian nerve and its subcellular components. J Neurochem 1980;34:59.
232. Weiss HD, Walker MD, Wiernik PH. Neurotoxicity of commonly used antineoplastic agents. N Engl J Med 1974;291:127.
233. Robertson GL, Bhoopalam N, Zelkowitz LJ. Vincristine neurotoxicity and abnormal secretion of antidiuretic hormone. Arch Intern Med 1973;132:717.
234. Vogelzang NJ, Raghavan D, Kennedy BJ. VP-16-213 (etoposide): the mandrake root from Issyk-Kul. Am J Med 1982;72:136.
235. Issel BF. The podophyllotoxin derivatives VP16-213 and VM26. Cancer Chemother Pharmacol 1982;7:73.
236. Ross W, Rowe T, Glisson B, et al. Role of topoisomerase II in mediating epipodophyllotoxin-induced DNA cleavage. Cancer Res 1984;44:5857.
237. Chen GL, Yang L, Rowe TC, et al. Nonintercalative antitumor drugs interfere with the breakage-reunion reaction of mammalian DNA topoisomerase II. J Biol Chem 1984;259:13560.
238. Long BH, Musial ST, Brattain MG. Comparison of cytotoxicity and DNA breakage activity of congeners of podophyllotoxin including VP16-213 and VM26: a quantitative structure-activity relationship. Biochemistry 1984;23:1183.
239. Spiridonidis CA, Chatterjee S, Petzold SJ, Berger NA. Topoisomerase II: dependent and independent mechanisms of etoposide resistance in Chinese hamster cell lines. Cancer Res 1989;49:644.
240. Sinha BK, Haim N, Dusre L, et al. DNA strand breaks produced by etoposide (VP-16, 213) in sensitive and resistant breast tumor cells: implications for the mechanism of action. Cancer Res 1988;48:5096.
241. Endicott JA, Ling V. The biochemistry of P-glycoprotein-mediated multidrug resistance. Annu Rev Biochem 1989;58:137.
242. Chow K-C, Ross WE. Topoisomerase-specific drug sensitivity in relation to cell cycle progression. Mol Cell Biol 1987;7:3119.
243. Sullivan DM, Latham MD, Ross WE. Proliferation-dependent topoisomerase II content as a determinant of antineoplastic drug action in human, mouse, and Chinese hamster ovary cells. Cancer Res 1987;47:3973.
244. Hainsworth J, Johnson DH, Frazier SR, Greco FA. Chronic daily administration of oral etoposide in a phase I trial. J Clin Oncol 1989;7: 396.
245. Björkholm M. Etoposide and teniposide in the treatment of acute leukemia. Med Oncol Tumor Pharmacother 1990;7:3.
246. Blume KG, Forman SJ, O'Donnell MR, et al. Total body irradiation and high-dose etoposide: a new preparative regimen for bone marrow transplantation in patients with advanced hematologic malignancies. Blood 1987;69:1015.
247. Stadtmauer EA, Cassileth PA, Gale RP. Etoposide in leukemia, lymphoma, and bone marrow transplantation. Leuk Res 1989;13:639.
248. O'Dwyer PJ, Leyland-Jones B, Alonso MT, et al. Etoposide (VP-16-213): current status of an active anticancer drug. N Engl J Med 1985;312:692.
249. Nelson EM, Tewey KM, Lui LF. Mechanism of antitumor drug action: poisoning of mammalian DNA topoisomerase II on DNA by 4′-(9-acridinylamino)-methanesulfon-*m*-anisidide. Proc Natl Acad Sci USA 1984;81:1361.
250. Estey EH, Silberman L, Beran M, et al. The interaction between nuclear topoisomerase II activity from human leukemia cells, exogenous DNA, and 4′-(9-acridinylamino) methanesulfon-*m*-anisidide (*m*-AMSA) or 4-(4,6-*O*-ethylidene-β-D-glucopyranoside) (VP-16) indicates the sensitivity of the cells to the drug. Biochem Biophys Res Commun 1987;144:787.
251. Louie AC, Issel BF. Amsacrine (AMSA): a critical review. J Clin Oncol 1985;3:562.
252. Arlin ZA, Feldman E, Kempin S, et al. Amsacrine with high dose cytarabine is highly effective therapy for refractory and relapsed acute lymphoblastic leukemia in adults. Blood 1988;72:433.
253. Jackson RC, Handschumacher RE. *Escherichia coli* L-asparginase: catalytic activity and subunit nature. Biochemistry 1970;9:3585.
254. Haley EE, Fischer GA, Welch AD. The requirement for L-asparagine of mouse leukemia cells L5178Y in culture. Cancer Res 1961;21:532.
255. Haw T, Ohnuma T. L-aspriginase: *in vitro* inhibition of blastogenesis by enzyme from *Erwinia carotovora*. Nature 1972;239:50.
256. Jones B, Holland JF, Glidewell O, et al. Optimal use of L-asparaginase (NSC-109229) in acute lymphocytic leukemia. Med Pediatr Oncol 1977;3:387.
257. Sallan SE, Hitchcock-Bryan S, Gelber R, et al. Influence of intensive asparaginase in the treatment of childhood non-T-cell acute lymphoblastic leukemia. Cancer Res 1983;43:5601.
258. Capizzi RL. Schedule dependent synergism and antagonism between methotrexate and asparaginase. Biochem Pharmacol 1974;23:151.
259. Capizzi RL, Davis R, Powell B, et al. Synergy between high-dose cytarabine and asparaginase in the treatment of adults with refractory and relapsed acute myelogenous leukemia: a Cancer and Leukemia Group B study. J Clin Oncol 1988;6:499.
260. Oettegen HF, Stephenson PA, Schwartz MK, et al. Toxicity of E. coli L-asparaginase in man. Cancer 1970;25:253.
261. Cairo MS. Adverse reactions of L-asparaginase. Am J Pediatr Hematol Oncol 1982;4:335.
262. Ohnuma T, Holland JF, Sinks LF. Biochemical and pharmacological studies with L-asparaginase in man. Cancer Res 1970;30:2297.
263. Wiemann MC, Calabresi P. Pharmacology of antineoplastic agents. In: Calabresi P, Schein PS, Rosenberg SA, eds. Medical oncology. New York, Macmillan, 1985:292.
264. Nesbit M, Chard R, Evans A, et al. Evaluation of intramuscular versus intravenous administration of L-asparaginase in childhood leukemia. Am J Pediatr Hematol Oncol 1979;1:9.
265. Ortega JA, Nesbit ME, Donaldson MH, et al. L-asparaginase, vincristine, and prednisone for induction of first remission in acute lymphoblastic leukemia. Cancer Res 1977;37:535.
266. Ohnama T, Holland JR, Meyer P. *Erwinia carotovora* asparaginase in patients with prior anaphylaxis to asparaginase from *E. coli*. Cancer 1972;30:376.
267. Capizzi RL, Bertino JR, Handschumacher RE. L-asparaginase. Annu Rev Med 1970;21:433.
268. Priest JR, Ramsay NKC, Bennett AJ. The effect of L-asparaginase on antithrombin III, plasminogen, and plasma coagulation during therapy for acute lymphoblastic leukemia. J Pediatr 1982;100:990.
269. Kucuk O, Kwaan HC, Gunnar W, et al. Thromboembolic complications with L-asparaginase therapy. Cancer 1985;55:702.
270. Distelhorst CW. Recent insight into the structure and function of the glucocorticoid receptor. J Lab Clin Med 1989;113:404.
271. Krown SE. Interferons and interferon inducers in cancer treatment. Semin Oncol 1986;13:207.
272. Isaacs A, Lindenman: I. Virus interference. I. The interferon. Proc R Soc Lond (Biol) 1957;147:258.
273. Zoumbos NC, Djeu JY, Young NS. Inteferon is the suppressor of hematopoiesis generated by stimulated lymphocytes in vitro. J Immunol 1984;133:769.
274. Neumann HA, Fauser AA. Effect of interferon on pluripotent hemapoietic progenitors (CFU-GEMM) derived from human bone marrow. Exp Hematol 1982;10:587.
275. Broxmeyer HE, Lu L, Platzer E, et al. Comparative analysis of the influences of human gamma, alpha and beta interferons on human multipotential (CFU-GEMM), erythroid (BFU-E) and granulocyte-marcophage (CFU-GM) progenitor cells. J Immunol 1983;131:1300.
276. Stewart WE II, Blalack JE, Bruke DC, et al. Interferon nomenclature. J Immunol 1980;125:2353.
277. Trotta PP. Preclinical biology of alpha interferons. Semin Oncol 1986;13:3.
278. Broxmeyer HE, Lu L, Platzer E, et al. Comparative analysis of the influences of human gamma, alpha and beta interferons on human

multipotential (CFU-GEMM), erythroid (BFU-E) and granulocyte-macrophage (CFU-GM) progenitor cells. J Immunol 1983;131:1300.
279. Borden EC, Hogan TF, Voelkel JC. The comparative antiproliferative activity in vitro of natural interferons α and β for diploid and transformed human cells. Cancer Res 1982;42:4948.
280. Quesada JR, Reuben JA, Mannint JT, et al. Alpha interferon for induction of remission in hairy cell leukemia. N Engl J Med 1984;310:15.
281. Talpaz M, Kantarjian HM, McCredie K, et al. Hematologic remission and cytogenetic improvement induced by recombinant human interferon alpha A in chronic myelogenous leukemia. N Engl J Med 1986;314:1065.
282. Cooper MR. Interferon in the treatment of multiple myeloma. Semin Oncol 1986;13:13.
283. Mandelli F, Auvisati G, Amadosi S, et al. Maintenance treatment with recombinant interferon alpha-2b in patients with multiple myeloma responding to conventional induction chemotherapy. N Engl J Med 1990;322:1430.
283a. Talpaz M, Kantarjian H, Kurzrock R, et al. Interferon-alpha produces sustained cytogenetic responses in chronic myelogenous leukemia. Ann Intern Med 1991;114:532.
283b. Mandelli R, Avvisati G, Amadori S, et al. Maintenance treatment with recombinant interferon alfa-2b in patients with multiple myeloma responding to conventional induction chemotherapy. N Engl J Med 1990;322:1430.
283c. Huang ME, Ye YC, Chen SR, et al. Use of all-*trans* retinoic acid in the treatment of acute promyelocytic leukemia. Blood 1988;72:567.
283d. Castaigne S, Chomienne C, Daniel MT, et al. All-*trans* retinoic acid as a differentiation therapy for acute promyelocytic leukemia. I. Clinical result. Blood 1990;76:1704.
283e. Warrell RP Jr, de Thé H, Wang Z-Y, et al. Acute progranulocytic leukemia. N Engl J Med 1993;329:177.
283f. Grignani F, Fagioli M, Alcalay M, et al. Acute promyelocytic leukemia: From genetics to treatment. Blood 1994;83:10.
283g. Brietman TR, Selonick SE, Collins SJ. Induction of differentiation of the human promyelocytic leukemia cell lines (HL-60) by retinoic acid. Proc Natl Acad Sci USA 1980;77:2936.
283h. Collins SJ, Robertson KA, Mueller L. Retinoic acid-induced granulocytic differentiation of HL-60 myeloid leukemia cells is mediated directly through the retinoic acid receptor (RAR-alpha). Mol Cell Biol 1990;10:2154.
283i. Gallagher RE, Said F, Pua I, et al. Expression of retinoic acid receptor alpha mRNA in human leukemia cells with variable responsiveness to retinoic acid. Leukemia 1989;3:789.
283j. Lemons RS, Eilender D, Waldmann RA, et al. Cloning and characterization of the t(15;17) translocation breakpoint region in acute promyelocytic leukemia. Gene Chromosome Cancer 1990;2:79.
283k. Miller WH Jr, Moy D, Li A, et al. Retinoic acid induces down-regulation of several growth factors and proto-oncogenes in a human embryonal cancer cell line. Oncogene 1990;5:511.
283l. de Thé H, Chomienne C, Lanotte M, et al. The t(15;17) translocation of acute promyelocytic leukemia fuses the retinoic acid receptor alpha gene to a novel transcribed locus. Nature 1990;347:558.
283m. Chomienne C, Ballerini P, Balistrand N, et al. All trans retinoic acid in acute promyelocytic leukemias. II. In vitro studies: structure–function relationship. Blood 1990;76:1710.
284. Henderson ES. Combination chemotherapy of acute lymphocytic leukemia of childhood. Cancer Res 1967;27:2570.
285. Vadlamudi S, Goldin A. Influence of mitotic cycle inhibitors on the antileukemic activity of cytosine arabinoside (NSC-63878) in mice bearing leukemia L1210. Cancer Chemother Rep 1971;5:547.
286. Valeriote F, Vietti T, Edelstein M. The combined effect of 1-β-D-arabinofluransylcytosine and thiopurines. Cancer Chemother Rep 1976;60:1925.
287. Valeriote F, Edelstein M. The role of cell kinetics in cancer chemotherapy. Semin Oncol 1977;4:217.
288. Begg AC, McNally NJ, Schrieve DC, et al. A method to measure the duration of DNA synthesis and the potential doubling time from a single sample. Cytometry 1985;6:620.
289. Preisler HD, Azarnia N, Raza A, et al. Relationship between the percent of marrow cells in S phase and the outcome of remission-induction therapy for acute nonlymphocytic leukaemia. Br J Haematol 1984;56:399.
290. Vaughan WP, Karp JE, Burke PJ. Two-cycle timed-sequential chemotherapy for adult acute nonlymphocytic leukemia. Blood 1984;64:975.
291. Sullivan MP, Vietti TJ, Fernbach DJ, et al. Clinical investigations in the treatment of meningeal leukemia: radiation therapy regimen vs. conventional intrathecal methotrexate. Blood 1969;34:301.
292. Green DM, West CR, Brecher ML, et al. The use of subcutaneous cerebrospinal fluid reservoirs for the prevention and treatment of meningeal relapse of acute lymphoblastic leukemia. Am J Pediatr Hematol Oncol 1982;4:147.
293. Balis FM, Savitch JL, Bleyer WA, et al. Remission induction of meningeal leukemia with high-dose intravenous methotrexate. J Clin Oncol 1985;3:485.
294. Frick J, Ritch PS, Hansen RM. Successful treatment of meningeal leukemia using systemic high dose cytosine arabinoside. J Clin Oncol 1984;2:365.
295. Kun LE, Camitta BM, Mulhern RK. Treatment of meningeal relapse in childhood acute lymphoblastic leukemia. I. Results of craniospinal irradiation. J Clin Oncol 1984;2:359.
296. Pizzo PA, Poplack DG, Bleyer WA. Neurotoxicities of current leukemia therapy. Am J Pediatr Hematol Oncol 1979;1:127.
297. Medical Research Council's Working Party on Leukaemia in Childhood. Testicular disease in acute lymphoblastic leukaemia in childhood. Br Med J 1978;1:334.
298. Nesbit ME, Robinson LL, Ortega JA, et al. Testicular relapse in childhood acute lymphoblastic leukemia: association with pretreatment patient characteristics and treatment. Cancer 1980;45:2009.
299. Bowman WP, Aur RJA, Hustu HO, et al. Isolated testicular relapse in acute lymphocytic leukemia of childhood: categories and influence on survival. J Clin Oncol 1984;2:924.
300. Dedhar S, Hartley D, Goldie JH. Increased dihydrofolate reductase activity in methotrexate-resistant human promyelocytic-leukaemia (HL-60) cells. Biochem J 1985;225:609.
301. Meltzer PS, Cheng YC, Trent JM. Analysis of dihydrofolate reductase gene amplification in a methotrexate-resistant human tumor cell line. Cancer Genet Cytogenet 1985;17:289.
302. Curt GA, Carney DN, Cown KH, et al. Unstable methotrexate resistance in human small-cell carcinoma associated with double-minute chromosomes. N Engl J Med 1983;308:199.
303. Gerson SL, Trey JE. Modulation of nitrosourea resistance in myeloid leukemias. Blood 1988;71:1487.
304. Gerson SL, Trey ME, Miller K. Potentiation of nitrosourea cytotoxicity in human leukemic cells by inactivation of O^6alkylguanine-DNA alkyltransferase. Cancer Res 1988;48:1521.
305. Riordan JR, Denchars K, Kartner N, et al. Amplification of P-glycoprotein genes in multidrug-resistant mammalian cell lines. Nature 1985;316:817.
306. Pastan I, Gottesman M. Multiple-drug resistance in human cancer. N Engl J Med 1987;316:1388.
307. Roninson IB, Chin JE, Choi K, et al. Isolation of human mdr DNA sequences amplified in multidrug-resistant KB carcinoma cells. Proc Natl Acad Sci USA 1986;83:4358.
308. Akiyama S, Fojo A, Hanover JA, et al. Isolation and genetic characterization of human KB cell lines resistant to multiple drugs. Somatic Cell Mol Genet 1985;11:117.
309. Willingham MC, Cornwell MM, Cardarelli CO, et al. Single cell analysis of daunomycin uptake and efflux in multidrug-resistant and sensitive KB cells: effects of verapamil and other drugs. Cancer Res 1986;46:5941.
310. Pirker R, Goldstein LJ, Ludwig H, et al. Expression of a multidrug resistance gene in blast crisis of chronic myelogenous leukemia. Cancer Commun 1989;1:141.
311. Ma DD, Davey RA, Harman DH, et al. Detection of a multidrug resistant phenotype in acute non-lymphoblastic leukaemia. Lancet 1987;135.
312. Dalton WS, Grogan TM, Meltzer PS, et al. Drug-resistance in multiple myeloma and non-Hodgkin's lymphoma: detection of P-glycoprotein and potential circumvention by addition of verapamil to chemotherapy. J Clin Oncol 1989;7:415.
313. Rothenberg ML, Mickley LA, Cole DE, et al. Expression of the mdr-1/P-170 gene in patients with acute lymphoblastic leukemia. Blood 1989;74:1388.
314. Pastan IH, Gottesman MM. Molecular biology in multidrug resistance in human cells. In: DeVita VT Jr, Hellman S, Rosenberg SA, eds. Important advances in oncology. Philadelphia, JB Lippincott, 1988:3.
315. Cornwell MM, Pastan I, Gottesmann MM. Certain calcium channel blockers bind specifically to multidrug resistant human KB carcinoma membrane vesicles and inhibit drug binding to P-glycoprotein. J Biol Chem 1987;262:2166.
316. Ozols R, Cunnion RE, Klecker RW, et al. Verapamil and Adriamycin in the treatment of drug resistant ovarian cancer patients. J Clin Oncol 1987;5:641.
316a. List AF, Spier C, Greer J, et al. Phase I/II trial of cyclosporine as a chemotherapy-resistance modifier in acute leukemia. J Clin Oncol 1993;11:1652.
316b. Sikic BI. Modulation of multidrug resistance: at the threshold. J Clin Oncol 1993;11:1629.
317. Santos GW. History of bone marrow transplantation. Clin Haematol 1983;12:611.
318. Frei E III, Canellos GP. Dose: a critical factor in cancer chemotherapy. Am J Med 1980;69:585.
319. O'Reilly RJ. Allogeneic bone marrow transplantation: current status and future directions. (Review) Blood 1983;62:941.
320. Cheson BD, Lacerna L, Leyland-Jones B, et al. Autologous bone marrow transplantation: current status and future directions. Ann Intern Med 1989;110:51.
321. Thomas ED, Storb R, Clift RA, et al. Bone marrow transplantation. N Engl J Med 1975;292:832.
322. Thomas ED. Marrow transplantation for malignant diseases (Karnofsky Memorial Lecture). J Clin Oncol 1983;1:517.

323. Frei E III, Antman K, Teicher B, et al. Bone marrow autotransplantation for solid tumors: prospects. J Clin Oncol 1989;7:515.
324. Appelbaum FR. Marrow transplantation for hematologic malignancies: a brief review of current status and future prospects. Semin Hematol 1988;25:16.
325. Appelbaum FR, Thomas ED. Crossing the bridge from hematologic malignancies to solid tumors. J Clin Oncol 1986;4:2.
326. Appelbaum FR. Hammering away at solid tumors. Cancer Treat Rep 1987;71:115.
327. Champlin RE, Gale RP. Role of bone marrow transplantation in the treatment of hematologic malignancies and solid tumors: critical review of syngeneic, autologous, and allogeneic transplants. Cancer Treat Rep 1984;68:145.
328. Kessinger A, Armitage JO, Landmark JD, et al. Autologous peripheral hematopoietic stem cell transplantation restores hematopoietic function following marrow ablative therapy. Blood 1988;71:723.
329. Leventhal BG. An overview of clinical trials in oncology. Semin Oncol 1988;15:414.
330. Piatadosi S. Principles of clinical trial design. Semin Oncol 1988;15: 423.
331. Hampton AA, Sheretz RJ. Vascular-access infections in hospitalized patients. Surg Clin North Am 1988;68:57.
332. Gilman FA, Palmer TF, Hrabovsky EE. The use of right atrial catheters in pediatric cancer patients. W Va Med J 1986;J82:37.
333. Stellato TA, Gauderer MWL, Lazarus HM, et al. Percutaneous silastic catheter insertion in patients with thrombocytopenia. Cancer 1985;56: 2691.
334. Lazarus HM, Creger RJ, Bloom AD, Shenk R. Percutaneous placement of femoral central venous catheter in patients undergoing transplantation of bone marrow. Surg Gynecol Obstet 1990;170:403.
335. Haire WD, Lieberman RP, Lund GB, Wieczorek BM, Armitage JO, Kessinger A. Translumbar inferior vena cava catheters: safety and efficacy in peripheral blood stem cell transplantation. Transfusion 1990;30:511.
336. Haire WD, Edney JA, Landmark JD, Kessinger A. Thrombotic complications of subclavian apheresis catheters in cancer patients: prevention with heparin infusion. J Clin Apheresis (Abstract) 1989;5: 41A.
337. Anderson AJ, Krasnow SH, Boyer MW, et al. Hickman catheter clots: a common occurence despite daily heparin flushing. Cancer Treat Rep 1987;71:651.
338. Corona ML, Peters SG, Narr BJ, Thompson RL. Infections related to central venous catheters. Mayo Clin Proc 1990;65:979.
339. Raaf JH. Results from use of 826 vascular access devices in cancer patients. Cancer 1985;55:1312.
340. Press OW, Ramsey PG, Larson EB, Fefer A, Hickman RO. Hickman catheter infections in patients with malignancies. Medicine 1984;63: 189.
341. Larson EB, Wooding M, Hickman RO. Infectious complications of right atrial catheters used for venous access in patients receiving intensive chemotherapy. Surg Gynecol Obstet 1981;153:369.
342. Lowder JN, Lazarus HM, Herzig RH. Bacteremias and fungemias in oncologic patients with central venous catheters: changing spectrum of infection. Arch Intern Med 1982;142:1456.
343. Quinn JP, Counts GW, Meyers JD. Intracardiac infections due to coagulase-negative *Staphylococcus* associated with Hickman catheter. Cancer 1986;57:1079.
344. Krog MPM, Ekbom A, Nystrom-Rosander C, Rudberg CR, Simonssen NOB. Central venous catheters in acute blood malignancies. Cancer 1987;59:358.
345. Harvey MP, Trent RJ, Joshua DE, Ramsey-Stewart G, Storey DW, Kronenberg H. Complications associated with indwelling venous Hickman catheters in patients with hematologic disorders. Aust NZ J Med 1986;16:211.
346. Lazarus HM, Lowder JN, Herzig RH. Occlusion and infection in Broviac catheters during intensive cancer therapy. Cancer 1983;52:2342.
347. Wing EJ, Norden CW, Shadduck RK, et al. Use of quantitative bacteriologic techniques to diagnose catheter-related sepsis. Arch Intern Med 1979;139:482.
348. Schuman ES, Winters V, Gross GF, Hayes JF. Management of Hickman catheter sepsis. Am J Surg 1985;149:627.
349. Schwartz C, Hendrickson K, Powell K. Prevention of intraluminal catheter infections by vancomycin. Proc Am Soc Clin Oncol 1989;8: 329.
350. Reed WP, Newman KA, De Jonge C, et al. Prolonged venous access for chemotherapy by means of the Hickman catheter. Cancer 1983;52: 185.
351. Fraschini G, Jadeja J, Lawson M, et al. Local infusion of urokinase for the lysis of thrombosis associated with permanent central venous catheters in cancer patients. J Clin Oncol 1987;5:672.
352. Glynn M, Langer B, Jeejeebhoy KN. Therapy for thrombotic occlusion of long-term intravenous alimentation catheters. JPEN 1980;4: 387.
353. Hurtubise MR, Bottino JC, Lawson M, et al. Restoring patency of occluded central venous catheters. Arch Surg 1980;115:212.
354. Lawson M, Bottino JC, Hurtubise MR, McCredie K. The use of urokinase to restore the patency of occluded central venous catheters. Am J IV Ther Clin Nutr 1982;9:29.
355. Williams BM, Sanders JE, Clift RA, et al. Use of arteriovenous shunts and right atrial catheters for daily granulocyte collection. J Clin Apheresis 1987;3:171.
356. Wagman LD, Kirkemo A, Johnston MR. Venous access: a prospective, randomized study of the Hickman catheter. Surgery 1984;95:303.
357. Caruana RJ, Raja RM, Zeit RM, Goldstein SJ, Kramer MS. Thrombotic complications of indwelling central venous catheters used for chronic hemodialysis. Am J Kidney Dis 1987;9:497.
358. Tchekmedyian NS, Newman K, Moody MR, et al. Case report: special studies of the Hickman catheter of a patient with recurrent bacteremia and candidemia. Am J Med Sci 1986;291:419.
359. Pessa ME, Howard RJ. Complications of Hickman-Broviac catheters. Surg Gynecol Obstet 1985;161:257.
360. Jacobs MB, Yeager M. Thrombotic and infectious complications of Hickman-Broviac catheters. Arch Intern Med 1984;144:1597.
361. Topiel MS, Bryan RT, Kessler CM, Simon GL. Case report: treatment of Silastic catheter-induced central vein septic thrombophlebitis. Am J Med Sci 1986;291:425.
362. Leiby JM, Purcell H, De Maria JJ, Kraut EH, Sagone AL, Metz EN. Pulmonary embolism as a result of Hickman catheter-related thrombosis. Am J Med 1989;86:228.
363. Brismar B, Hardstedt C, Jacobson S. Diagnosis of thrombosis by catheter phlebography after prolonged central venous catheterization. Ann Surg 1981;194:779.
364. Meryman HT, Hornblower M. The preparation of red cells depleted of leukocytes: review and evaluation. Transfusion 1986;26:101.
365. Levy GJ, Shabot MM, Hart ME, et al. Transfusion-associated noncardiogenic pulmonary edema: report of a case and a warning regarding treatment. Transfusion 1986;26:278.
366. Hammerschmidt DE, Jacob HS. Adverse pulmonary reactions to transfusion. Adv Intern Med 1982;27:511.
367. Popovsky MA, Abel MD, Moore SB. Transfusion-related acute lung injury associated with passive transfer of antileukocyte antibodies. Am Rev Respir Dis 1983;128:185.
368. Smith DM. Management of transfusion reactions. In: Judd WJ, Barnes A, eds. Clinical and serological aspects of transfusion reactions. American Association of Blood Banks 1982:121.
369. Beutler E. Platelet transfusions: the 20,000/μL trigger. Blood 1993;81: 1411.
369a. Gmür J, Burger J, Schauz U, et al. Safety of stringent prophylactic platelet transfusion policy for patients with acute leukemia. Lancet 1991;338:1223.
370. Dutcher JP, Schiffer CA, Aisner J, et al. Long-term follow-up of patients with leukemia receiving platelet transfusions: identification of a large group of patients who do not become alloimmunized. Blood 1981;58:1007.
371. Daly PA, Schiffer CA, Aisner J, et al. Platelet transfusion therapy: one-hour post-transfusion increments are valuable in predicting the need for HLA matched preparations. JAMA 1980;243:435.
372. Consensus Conference. Platelet transfusion therapy. JAMA 1987;257: 1777.
373. Schiffer CA, Wade JC. Supportive care: issues in the use of blood products and treatment of infection. Semin Oncol 1987;14:454.
374. Morrow JF, Braine HG, Kickler TS et al. Septic reactions to platelet transfusions: a persistent problem. JAMA 1991;266:555.
375. Patten E, Patten S. Preparation of leukocyte-poor platelet concentrates. Transfusion 1989;29:562.
376. Hillyer CD, Snydman DR, Berkman EM. The risk of cytomegalovirus infection in solid organ and bone marrow transplant recipients: transfusion of blood products. Transfusion 1990;30:659.
377. Lazarus HM, Creger RJ, Gerson SL. Infectious emergencies in oncology patients. Semin Oncol 1989;16:543.
378. Bodey GP, Buckley M, Sathe YS, et al. Quantitative relationships between circulating leukocytes and infection in patients with acute leukemia. Ann Intern Med 1966;64:328.
379. Whimbey E, Kiehn TE, Brannon P, et al. Bacteremia and fungemia in patients with neoplastic disease. Am J Med 1987;82:723.
380. Pizzo PA, Robichaud KJ, Wesley R, et al. Fever in pediatric and young adult patients with cancer: a prospective study of 1001 episodes. Medicine 1982;61:153.
381. Pizzo PA, Commers J, Cotton D, et al. Approaching the contraversies in antibacterial agent management of cancer patients. Am J Med 1984;76:436.
382. European Organization for the Research and Treatment of Cancer International Antimicrobial Therapy Project Group. Three antibiotic regimens in the treatment of infection in febrile granulocytopenic patients with cancer. J Infect Dis 1978;137:14.
383. Schimpff SC, Young VM, Greene WH, et al. Origin of infection in acute nonlymphocytic leukemia: significance of hospital acquisition of potential pathogens. Ann Intern Med 1972;77:707.
384. Schimpff SC, Satterlee W, Young VM, et al. Empiric therapy with carbenicillin and gentamicin for febrile patients with cancer and granulocytopenia. N Engl J Med 1971;284:1061.
385. Reed E, Arneson M, Vaughn W, et al. Streptococcus viridans (SV): a significant cause of neutropenic fever (NF) that caused death in some patients not empirically treated for gram positive (GP) bacteria. (Abstract) Proc Am Soc Clin Oncol 1990;9:321.
386. Rubin M, Hathorn JW, Marshall D, et al. Gram-positive infections

and the use of vancomycin in 550 episodes of fever and neutropenia. Ann Intern Med 1988;108:30.
387. Martin MA, Pfaller MA, Wenzel RP. Coagulase-negative staphylococcal bacteremia: mortality and hospital stay. Ann Intern Med 1989;110:9.
388. Wingard JR, Santos GW, Saral R. Differences between first and subsequent fevers during prolonged neutropenia. Cancer 1987;59:844.
389. Gold JWM. Opportunistic fungal infections in patients with neoplastic disease. Am J Med 1984;76:458.
390. Maksymiuk AW, Thongprasert S, Hopfer R, et al. Systemic candidiasis in cancer patients. Am J Med 1984;77:20.
391. Gerson SL, Talbot GH, Hurwitz S, et al. Prolonged granulocytopenia: the major risk factor for invasive pulmonary aspergillosis in patients with acute leukemia. Ann Intern Med 1984;100:345.
392. Joshi JH, Schimpff SC. Therapy of infection in granulocytopenic patients with cancer. Clin Oncol 1983;2:611.
393. Bodey GP, Jadeja L, Elting L. *Pseudomonas* bacteremia: retrospective analysis of 410 episodes. Arch Intern Med 1985;145:1621.
394. Wade JC, Johnson DW, Bustamante CL. Monotherapy for empiric treatment of fever in granulocytopenic cancer patients. Am J Med 1986;80:85.
395. Pizzo PA, Hathorn JW, Hiemenz J, et al. A randomized trial comparing ceftazidime alone with combination antibiotic therapy in cancer patients with fever and neutropenia. N Engl J Med 1986;315:552.
396. Reilly JT, Brada M, Bellingham AJ, et al. Ceftazidime compared to tobramycin and ticarcillin in immunocompromised haematological patients. J Antimicrob Chemother 1989;12:89.
397. Fainstein V, Bodey GP, Elting L, et al. A randomized study of ceftazidime compared to ceftazidime and tobramycin for the treatment of infections in cancer patients. J Antimicrob Chemother 1989;12:101.
397a. De Pauw BE, Deresinski SC, Feld R, et al. Ceftazidime compared with piperacillin and tobramycin for the empiric treatment of fever in neutropenic patients with cancer. Ann Intern Med 1994;120:834.
398. Klastersky J. Concept of empiric therapy with antibiotic combinations: indications and limits. Am J Med 1986;80:2.
399. European Organization for the Research and Treatment of Cancer International Antimicrobial Therapy Cooperative Group. Empiric antifungal therapy in febrile granulocytopenic patients. Am J Med 1989;86:668.
400. DeGregorio MW, Lee WMF, Linker CA, et al. Fungal infections in patients with acute leukemia. Am J Med 1982;73:543.
401. Holleran WM, Wilbur JR, DeGregorio MW. Empiric amphotericin B therapy in patients with acute leukemia. Rev Infect Dis 1985;7:619.
402. Burch PA, Karp JE, Merz WG, et al. Favorable outcome of invasive aspergillosis in patients with acute leukemia. J Clin Oncol 1987;5:1985.
403. Lazarus HM. Granulocyte transfusions: have we learned anything? J Lab Clin Med 1990;115:271.
404. Dosik GM, Luna M, Valdivieso M, et al. Necrotizing colitis in patients with cancer. Am J Med 1979;67:645.
405. Varki AP, Armitage JO, Feagler JR. Typhilitis in acute leukemia: successful treatment by early surgical intervention. Cancer 1979;43:695.
406. Mower WJ, Hawkins JA, Nelson EW. Neutropenic enterocolitis in adults with acute leukemia. Arch Surg 1986;121:571.
407. Shamberger RC, Weinstein HJ, Delorey MJ, et al. The medical and surgical management of typhlitis in children with acute nonlymphocytic (myelogenous) leukemia. Cancer 1986;57:603.
408. Skibber JM, Matter GJ, Pizzo PA, et al. Right lower quadrant pain in young patients with leukemia. Ann Surg 1987;206:711.
409. Gandy W, Greenberg BR. Successful medical management of neutropenic enterocolitis. Cancer 1983;51:1551.
410. Alt B, Glass NR, Sollinger H. Neutropenic enterocolitis in adults: review of the literature and assessment of surgical intervention. Am J Surg 1985;149:405.
411. Kunkel JM, Rosenthal D. Management of the ileocecal syndrome: neutropenic enterocolitis. Dis Colon Rectum 1986;29:196.
412. Lea JW Jr, Masys DR, Shackford SR. Typhlitis: a treatable complication of acute leukemia therapy. Cancer Clin Trials 1980;3:355.
413. Sternberg D, Gold J, Brodin A. Necrotizing entercolitis in leukemia. Arch Intern Med 1973;131:538.
414. Schimpff SC, Wiernik PH, Block JB. Rectal abscesses in cancer patients. Lancet 1972;2:844.
415. Barnes SG, Sattler FR, Ballard JO. Perirectal infections in acute leukemia: improved survival after incision and débridement. Ann Intern Med 1984;100:515.
416. Villar HV, Warneke JA, Peck MD, et al. Role of surgical treatment in the management of complications of the gastrointestinal tract in patients with leukemia. Surg Gynecol Obstet 1987;165:217.
417. Cohen LF, Balow JE, Magrath IT. Acute tumor lysis syndrome: a review of 37 patients with Burkitt's lymphoma. Am J Med 1980;68:486.
418. O'Regan S, Carson S, Chesney RW, et al. Electrolyte and acid-base disturbances in the management of leukemia. Blood 1977;49:345.
419. Stapleton FB, Strother DR, Roy S III, et al. Acute renal failure at onset of therapy for advanced stage Burkitt lymphoma and B cell acute lymphoblastic lymphoma. Pediatrics 1988;82:863.
420. Fer MF, Bottino GC, Sherwin SA, et al. Atypical tumor lysis syndrome in a patient with T cell lymphoma treated with recombinant leukocyte interferon. Am J Med 1984;77:953.
421. Vogler WR, Morris JG Jr, Winton EF. Acute tumor lysis in T-cell leukemia induced by amsacrine. Arch Intern Med 1983;143:165.
422. Gomez GA, Han T. Acute tumor lysis syndrome in prolymphocytic leukemia. Arch Intern Med 1987;147:375.
423. Smith T. Tumor lysis syndrome after steroid therapy for anaphylaxis. South Med J 1988;81:415.
424. Dhingra K, Newcom SR. Acute tumor lysis syndrome in non-Hodgkin's lymphoma induced by dexamethasone. Am J Hematol 1988;29:115.
425. Zusman J, Brown DM, Nesbit ME. Hyperphosphatemia, hyperphosphaturia, and hypocalcemia in acute lymphoblastic leukemia. N Engl J Med 1973;289:1335.
426. Elion GV, Benezra FM, Beardmore TD, et al. Studies with allopurinol in patients with impaired renal function. Adv Exp Med Biol 1980;122:263.
427. Al-Kawas FH, Seeff LB, Berendson RA, et al. Allopurinol hepatotoxicity: report of two cases and review of the literature. Ann Intern Med 1981;95:588.
428. Hande KR, Hixson CV, Chabner BA. Postchemotherapy purine excretion in lymphoma patients receiving allopurinol. Cancer Res 1981;41:2273.
429. Spector T. Inhibition of urate production by allopurinol. Biochem Pharmacol 1977;26:355.
430. Doyle LA, Berg C, Bottino G, et al. Erythema and desquamation after high-dose methotrexate therapy. Ann Intern Med 1983;98:611.
431. Levine LE, Medenica MM, Lorincz AL, et al. Distinctive acral erythema occuring during therapy for severe myelogenous leukemia. Arch Dermatol 1985;121:102.
432. Kennedy BJ, Smith LR, Goltz RW. Skin changes secondary to hydroxyurea therapy. Arch Dermatol 1975;111:183.
433. D'Angio GJ, Farber S, Maddock CL. Potentiation of x-ray effects by actinomycin D. Radiology 1959;73:175.
434. Greco FA, Brereton HD, Kent H, et al. Adriamycin and enhanced radiation reaction in normal esophagus and skin. Ann Intern Med 1976;85:294.
435. Phillips TL, Fu KK. Acute and late effects of multimodal therapy on normal tissues. Cancer 1977;40:489.
436. Kim YH, Aye MS, Fayos JV. Radiation necrosis of the scalp: a complication of cranial irradiation and methotrexate. Radiology 1977;124:813.
437. Donaldson SS, Glick JM, Wilbur JR. Adriamycin activating a recall phenomenon after radiation therapy. Ann Intern Med 1974;81:407.
438. Solberg LA, Wick MR, Bruckman JE. Doxorubicin-enhanced skin reaction. Mayo Clin Proc 1980;55:711.
439. Clark PA, Hsia YE, Huntsman RG. Toxic complications of treatment with 6-mercaptopurine: two cases with hepatic necrosis and intestinal ulceration. Br Med J 1960;1:393.
440. Satti MB, Weinbren K, Gordon-Smith EC. 6-Thioguanine as a cause of toxic veno-occlusive disease of the liver. J Clin Pathol 1982;35:1086.
441. Gill RA, Onstad GR, Cardamone JM, et al. Hepatic veno-occlusive disease caused by 6-thioguanine. Ann Intern Med 1982;96:58.
442. Griner PF, Elbadawi A, Packman CH. Veno-occlusive disease of the liver after chemotherapy of acute leukemia: report of two cases. Ann Intern Med 1976;85:578.
443. Woolley PV. Hepatic and pancreatic damage produced by cytotoxic drugs. Cancer Treat Rev 1983;10:117.
444. McIntyre RE, Magidson JC, Austin GE, et al. Fatal veno-occlusive disease of the liver following high-dose 1,3 bis(2-chloroethyl)-1-nitrosourea (BCNU) and autologous bone marrow transplantation. Am J Clin Pathol 1981;75:614.
445. Rollins BJ. Hepatic veno-occlusive disease. Am J Med 1986;81:297.
446. McDonald GB, Sharma P, Matthews DE, et al. Veno-occlusive disease of the liver after bone marrow transplantation: diagnosis, incidence and predisposing factors. Hepatology 1984;4:116.
447. Lazarus HM, Gottfried MR, Herzig RH, et al. Veno-occlusive disease of the liver after high-dose mitomycin-C therapy and autologous bone marrow transplantation. Cancer 1982;49:1789.
448. Ayash LJ, Hunt M, Antman K, et al. Hepatic venoocclusive disease in autologous bone marrow transplantation of solid tumors and lymphomas. J Clin Oncol 1990;8:1699.
449. Wong KK, Hirsch MS. Herpes virus infections in patients with neoplastic disease; diagnosis and therapy. Am J Med 1984;76:464.
450. Burket H. Clinical overview of mesna. Cancer Treat Rev 1983;10:175.
451. Garrick CL, Cronin SM, Sensenbrenner LL. Effect of mesna on cyclophosphamide. DICP 1989;23:798.
452. Young RC, Ozols RF, Myers CE. The anthracycline antineoplastic drugs. N Engl J Med 1981;305:139.
453. Lenaz L, Page JA. Cardiotoxicity of Adriamycin and related anthracyclines. Cancer Treat Rev 1976;3:111.
454. Schell F, Yap HY, Blumenschein GR, et al. Potential cardiotoxicity with mitoxantrone. Cancer Treat Rep 1983;66:1641.
455. Mathe G, Bayssas M, Gouveia J, et al. Preliminary results of a phase II trial of aclacinomycin in acute leukaemia and lymphosarcoma:

an oncostatic anthracyclin that rarely is cardiotoxic and induces no alopecia. Cancer Chemother Pharmacol 1978;1:259.

456. Daghestani AN, Arlin ZA, Leyland-Jones B, et al. Phase I and II clinical and pharmacological study of 4-demethoxydaunorubicin. Cancer Res 1985;45:1408.

457. Jain KK, Casper ES, Geller NL, et al. A prospective randomized comparison of epirubicin and doxorubicin in patients with advanced breast cancer. J Clin Oncol 1985;3:818.

458. Nielsen D, Jansen JB, Dombernowsky P, et al. Epirubicin cardiotoxicity: a study of 135 patients with advanced breast cancer. J Clin Oncol 1990;8:1806.

459. Bristow MR, Mason JW, Billingham ME, et al. Doxorubicin cardiomyopathy: evaluation by phonocardiography, endomyocardial biopsy, and cardiac catheterization. Ann Intern Med 1978;88:168.

460. Alexander J, Dainiak N, Berger JH, et al. Serial assessment of doxorubicin cardiotoxicity with quantitative radionuclide angiography. N Engl J Med 1979;300:278.

461. Torti FM, Bristow MM, Lum BL, et al. Cardiotoxicity of epirubicin and doxorubicin: assessment by endomyocardial biopsy. Cancer Res 1986;46:3722.

462. Morgan GW, McIlveen BM, Freedman A, et al. Radionuclide ejection fraction in doxorubicin cardiotoxicity. Cancer Treat Rep 1981;65: 629.

463. Billingham ME, Mason JW, Bristow MR, Daniel JR. Anthracycline cardiomyopathy monitored by morphologic changes. Cancer Treat Rep 1978;62:865.

464. Von Hoff D, Layard M, Basa P, et al. Risk factors for doxorubicin-induced congestive heart failure. Ann Intern Med 1979;91:710.

465. Minow RA, Benjamin RS, Lee ET, et al. Adriamycin cardiomyopathy: risk factors. Cancer 1977;39:1397.

466. Ginsberg SJ, Comis RL. The pulmonary toxicity of antineoplastic agents. Semin Oncol 1982;9:34.

467. Cooper J, White DA, Matthay RA. Drug induced pulmonary disease. I. Cytotoxic drugs. Am Rev Respir Dis 1986;133:321.

468. Simasoto Y, Baba K, Watanabe S. Pulmonary lesions produced by antitumor drugs: studies on autopsy cases. Jpn J Cancer Clin 1971;17: 21.

469. Antman K, Eder JP, Elias A, et al. High-dose combination alkylating agent preparative regimen with autologous bone marrow support: the Dana-Farber Cancer Institute/Beth Israel Hospital experience. Cancer Treat Rep 1987;71:119.

470. Russell JA, Powles RL. Neuropathy due to cytosine arabinoside. Br Med J 1974;4:652.

471. Dworkin LA, Goldman RD, Zivin LS, et al. Cerebellar toxicity following high-dose cytosine arabinoside. J Clin Oncol 1985;3:613.

472. Grossman L, Baker MA, Sutton DMC, et al. Central nervous system toxicity of high dose cytosine arabinoside. Med Pediatr Oncol 1983;11: 246.

473. Damon LE, Mass R, Linker CA. The association between high-dose cytarabine neurotoxicity and renal insufficiency. J Clin 1989;7:1563.

474. Nand S, Messmore HL Jr, Patel R, et al. Neurotoxicity associated with systemic high-dose cytosine arabinoside. J Clin Oncol 1986;4: 571.

475. Bethlenfalvay NC, Bergin JJ. Severe cerebral toxicity after intravenous nitrogen mustard therapy. Cancer 1972;29:366.

476. Sullivan KM, Storb R, Shulman HM, et al. Immediate and delayed neurotoxicity after mechlorethamine preparation for bone marrow transplantation. Ann Intern Med 1982;97:182.

477. Burger PC, Kamenar E, Schold SC, et al. Encephalomyelopathy following high-dose BCNU therapy. Cancer 1981;48:1318.

478. Weiss GB, Weiden PL, Thomas ED. Central nervous system disturbances after combined administration of procarbazine and mechlorethamine. Cancer Treat Rep 1977;61:1713.

479. Gangi D, Reaman GH, Cohen SR, et al. Leukoencephalopathy and elevated levels of myelin basic protein in the cerebrospinal fluid of patients with acute lymphoblastic leukemia. N Engl J Med 1980;303: 19.

480. Rubenstein LJ, Herman MM, Long TF, Wilbur JR. Disseminated necrotizing leukoencephalopathy: a complication of treated central nervous system leukemia and lymphoma. Cancer 1975;35:291.

Blood: Principles and Practice of Hematology,
edited by Robert I. Handin, Samuel E. Lux, and Thomas P. Stossel.
J.B. Lippincott Company, Philadelphia © 1995.

62

Radiation Therapy in the Treatment of Hematologic Malignancies

Peter M. Mauch
C. Norman Coleman

The history of radiation therapy began nearly 100 years ago with the discoveries of x-rays by Roentgen in 1895 and radium by the Curies shortly thereafter. Radiation therapy consisted of primitive equipment, crude dosimetry, and little knowledge of normal tissue or tumor radiation biology for the next 30 years. By 1930, the development of reliable orthovoltage equipment enabled treatment of deeper tumors than had been possible previously. Fractionated radiation treatments were developed by Coutard in Paris in the 1930s. Modern high-energy megavoltage equipment was first available in the 1950s with cobalt-60 (^{60}Co).[1] The linear accelerator, designed from microwave technology developed for radar in World War II, was first used in the United States by Kaplan and his group at Stanford University in the late 1950s. Radiation therapy as a medical subspecialty began to flourish in the 1960s, and while remaining part of the American College of Radiology, it is independent of diagnostic radiology, with a separate training curriculum and board examinations.

Advances in radiation biology paralleled these technical developments. The importance of oxygen in tumor sensitivity to radiation was noted as early as 1910[2]; however, its possible role in clinical treatment was not suggested by Thomlinson and Gray until 1955.[3] In 1956, Puck and Marcus published the first survival curve for mammalian cells.[4] This demonstrated the relation of fractional cell survival to dose of radiation and marked the beginning of modern radiation biology. Modern radiation biology evolved from these initial in vivo cell survival assays for tumor and normal tissues[5] to our current understanding of the cellular, molecular, and genetic effects of radiation.

The development of radiation oncology and biology has interacted closely with knowledge of normal and malignant tissues. Much of the early work in mice and other mammals centered around the blood and lymphatic system. The mouse provided an important means to measure early bone marrow stem cell damage. A number of normal and malignant tissue cell lines were derived from hematologic and lymphatic tissues from mice and other animals. These studies of radiation effects on the bone marrow stem cells and on specific normal and malignant tissues provided guidelines for the development of treatment plans. The early success of radiation therapy in the treatment of lymphomas and Hodgkin's disease provided encouragement for treatment of other tumors. These developments in radiation therapy are detailed in the next sections.

RADIATION PHYSICS

Types of Radiation

The ionizing radiation (photons) used in clinical treatment is part of the electromagnetic spectrum. The energy of radiation is equal to the frequency (υ) times Planck's constant ($E = h\upsilon$). The frequency equals the speed of light (c) divided by the wavelength (λ) of the radiation ($\upsilon = c/\lambda$). Therefore, the energy of an electromagnetic wave is related inversely to its wavelength $E = hc/\lambda$; the shorter the wavelength of photons, the greater is their energy.[6] X-rays have wavelengths below 10 nm, putting them below the ultraviolet spectrum. Diagnostic x-rays are in the 0.1- to 10-nm range (Fig. 62-1). Photons produced from a linear accelerator have wavelengths of 10^{-3} to 10^{-4} nm. The energy is described in terms of electron volts (eV). Orthovoltage or kilovoltage radiation is in the thousands of electron volts (keV); megavoltage radiation is in the millions of electron volts (MeV).

The energy of the x-rays chosen for therapy is such that they eject an electron from the target tissue, thus the term *ionizing radiation*. The precise interaction with matter depends on the energy of the irradiation. Relatively low-energy x-rays (orthovoltage) interact by the photoelectric effect, whereby the energy of the incoming photon is transferred to an orbital electron, usually the one closest to the nucleus. The probability of interaction is proportional to Z^3 (Z is the atomic number). Orthovoltage x-rays are preferentially absorbed in tissues such as bone that have a much higher Z than soft tissues. The Compton effect is the dominant process by which radiation is absorbed in the energy range of most clinical linear accelerators (1 to 15 MeV). It depends on electron density rather than the atomic number of the material. Lower-electron-density tissues absorb less irradiation than higher-electron-density soft tissues. Corrections for differences in electron density are being incorporated into computerized treatment planning systems. As the energy of the x-ray increases above 20 MeV, absorption is by pair production. This process is proportional to Z^2. Machines that produce photons with energies in the pair-production range are not commonly used in radiation therapy.[6]

High-energy radiation is produced by linear accelerators or from radioactive decay. The photons produced from radioactive decay are called *gamma rays*. They are identical to the x-rays produced by accelerators. Radioactive isotopes can be produced that emit gamma rays at sufficient energy

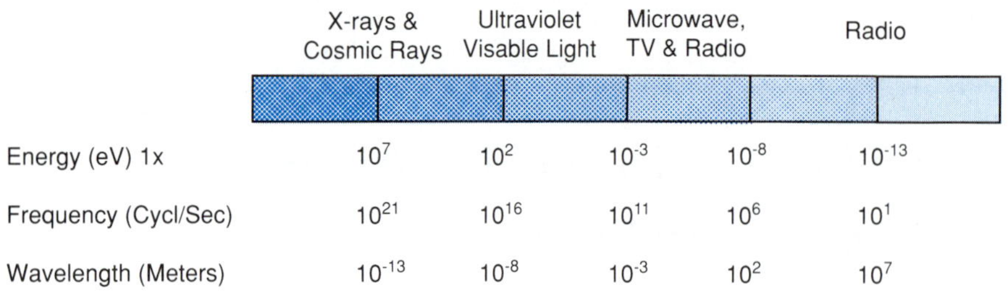

FIGURE 62-1. Relative positions of commonly used regions of the electromagnetic spectrum. (After Purdy JA, Lightfoot DA, Glasgow GP. Principles of radiologic physics, dosimetry and treatment planning. In: Perez CA, Brady LW, eds. Principles and practice of radiation oncology. Philadelphia, JB Lippincott, 1987:129)

and dose rates to be used in clinical external-beam therapy. The most common isotope for external-beam irradiation is ^{60}Co (half-life, 5.26 years). This isotope was in use before the availability of linear accelerators and is still widely used. The decay of ^{60}Co to nickel produces two gamma rays of energy that are 1.17 and 1.33 MeV (average, 1.25 MeV). This is similar to the average energy produced by a 4-MeV linear accelerator. Linear accelerators are more difficult to maintain and require highly trained personnel to service them. Their major advantage over cobalt is that they emit radiation from a smaller source and, as a result, have a much sharper beam edge.

For interstitial or intracavitary implants (brachytherapy), other isotopes are used. The more common ones are cesium-137 (^{137}Cs) for intracavitary gynecologic placements (average photon energy, 0.662 MeV; half-life, 30 years); iridium-192 (^{192}Ir) for removable interstitial implants to gynecologic, head and neck, breast, and other tumors (average photon energy, 0.38 MeV; half-life, 74.2 days); iodine-125 (^{125}I) for permanent prostate cancer implantation or as a high-dose-rate, removable source for brain tumors (average photon energy, 0.028 MeV; half-life, 60 days); gold-198 (^{198}Au) for permanent implants (average photon energy, 0.416 MeV; half-life, 2.7 days); and phosphorus-32 (^{32}P), administered as a colloidal solution for treating the pleural or peritoneal space or as a suspension for treating patients with myeloproliferative disorders (average electron energy, 1.71 MeV; no photons; half-life, 14.3 days). The most widely known isotope, radium, was historically used for both intracavitary insertions and interstitial implants. Radium's high photon energies, long half-life (1622 years), and production of radioactive radon gas as a decay product make it less useful than ^{137}Cs, the isotope that has replaced it.[6–8]

Electrons are used for cancer therapy in addition to photons. These can be generated from radioactive isotopes (^{32}P) or alternatively from the linear accelerator. Linear accelerators bombard a target with electrons to produce photons. The photons are a by-product of this bombardment, but electrons can be used directly with the proper extraction techniques. Most high-energy accelerators have electrons for patient treatment. Neutrons, protons, helium and carbon ions, and pi-mesons are other particles used for experimental radiation therapy. Neutrons have the advantage of a lower dependence on oxygen for cell killing; otherwise, their depth-dose characteristics are similar to photons. Because of their mass and charge, the other particles can be sharply localized in tissue (Bragg's peak). They are, therefore, useful for precise localization, usually of relatively small lesions, such as ocular melanoma, pituitary tumors, arteriovenous malformations, or chordomas. These are not discussed further in this chapter since their use is limited and they are available only to a few centers.

Most external-beam treatment is delivered by linear accelerators. Many of the new-generation accelerators produce photon beams with two different energies and electrons with five or six different energies. The therapist can select the energy that best fits the location and depth of the tumor.

Physical Interaction of Radiation With Tissues

The photon beam produced by linear accelerators is in the megavoltage range and has three important properties: it gives a relatively low dose to the superficial tissue (skin-sparing effect), it is penetrating, and it has sharp edges (the exception being ^{60}Co). The curves in Figure 62-2 represent the percentage depth dose of radiation beams of different energies for depth in water. The point along the path of the beam that has the highest dose is called d_{max} and is defined as the 100% dose point. For photon beams, the d_{max} increases with increasing energy, the precise location depending on machine design as well as energy.[6] It ranges from about 1 cm for a 4-MeV beam to 3 to 4 cm for a 25-MeV beam.[6] Although this skin-sparing effect is useful for avoiding skin reactions, it may lead to underdosing superficial tumors, such as inflammatory breast cancer or the superficial nodes in lymphoma or head and neck cancers. Therefore, photon energies above 8 MeV that have a d_{max} greater than 2 cm should be used with caution. Similarly, the 50% depth dose increases with energy, from 13.8 cm for a 4-MeV beam to over 22 cm for a 22-MeV beam.[6] Most accelerators have their photon energy in the 6- to 10-MeV range. The higher energy beams, with their deeper penetration, are particularly useful for large patients with deep-seated tumors. The dose delivered to tissue is described in units named *Grays* (1 Gy = 1 joule/kg). This unit has replaced the past terminology unit, the rad. The interconversion between rad and Gray is simple: 1 cGy = 1 rad, or

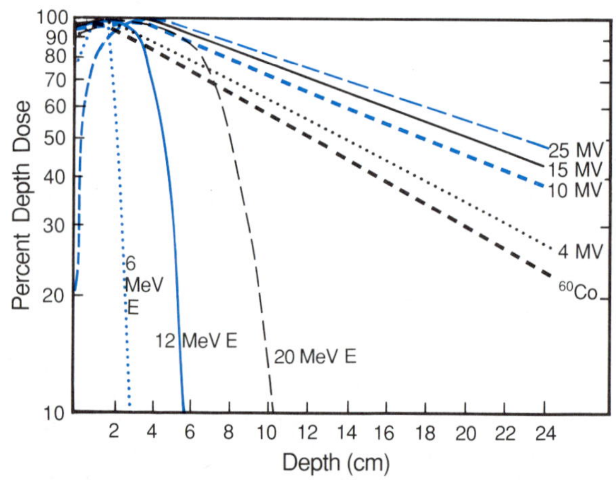

FIGURE 62-2. Percentage depth dose of radiation in tissue for x-ray beams of varying energy. As described in the text, the highest dose along the path of a beam is defined as the 100% point, or d_{max}. Therefore, d_{max} is the depth at which the maximal dose is achieved. For megavoltage x-rays, d_{max} does not occur on the skin because of the dose build-up characteristics of x-rays in tissue. As the depth in tissue increases, the energy deposited in the tissue decreases. For example, at a depth of 10 cm, the percentage depth dose (relative to d_{max}) is 70% for cobalt and 85% for a 15-MV beam. Electron beams produce dose only in the more superficial tissues, with a sharp decline toward zero.

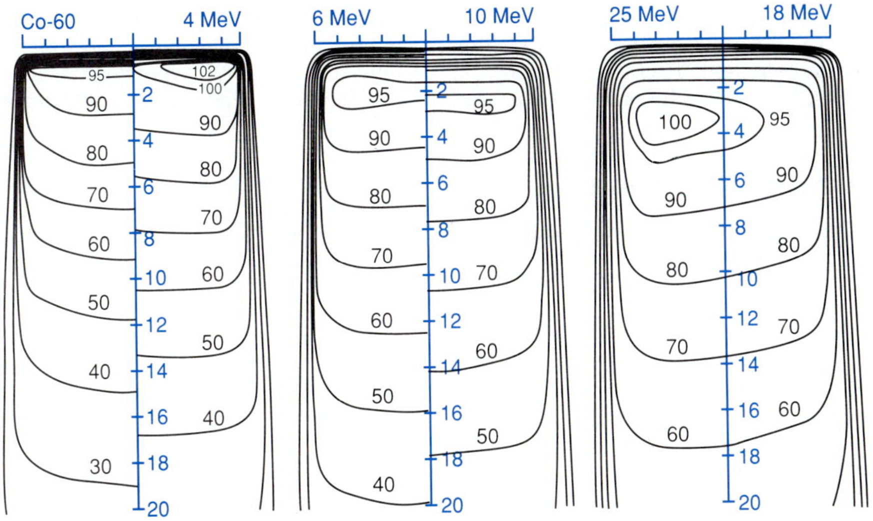

FIGURE 62-3. Beam profiles for photon beams of increasing energy. Each beam width is 10 cm (half of each beam from the central axis is illustrated). The lines shown are isodose lines, which are points along the beam that all have the same dose. (Isodose lines are analogous to the topographic contour maps, where the lines represent a given altitude, and to weather maps, where the contour lines represent equal temperatures.) The dose on the individual isodose lines is the percentage depth relative to 100% (the 100% point occurs at the depth defined as d_{max}). The isodose beams are relatively flat across the beam due to the design of the treatment machines. The higher energy beams are more penetrating; that is, at a given dose, the isodose line is higher for the higher-energy beams. The beam edges are sharp for the linear accelerator fields, with little scatter dose given beyond the edges. See text for further description. (After Glasgow GP, Sampiere VA, Purdy JA. External beam dosimetry and treatment planning. In: Perez CA, Brady LW, eds. Principles and practice of radiation oncology. Philadelphia, JB Lippincott, 1987:159)

1 Gy = 100 rad. The dose to be delivered depends on knowledge of tumor and normal tissue biology and on clinical experience of the radiation oncologist.

The profile for 10 × 10 cm beams of different energies is shown in Figure 62-3. The isodose lines denote all points that will receive the same dose.[9] They are normalized against the d_{max}, the point at which the dose is 100%. Thus, if 200 cGy is given to d_{max}, tissues at the 50% line will receive 100 cGy. Conversely, to give 100 cGy to a tumor at a depth of 13 cm with the 4-MeV beam (this is at the 50% isodose line), the tissue at d_{max} will receive 200 cGy. In practice, a single beam is rarely used; radiation therapy is usually delivered as opposed pairs (anteroposterior, two laterals, or an oblique pair) or as more than two fields to produce a desired dose distribution.[9]

As illustrated in Figure 62-3, the isodose curves are relatively flat. The target and flattening filter in the accelerator are designed to achieve this. There are times when a slanted edge is desirable, however, as with tangential fields for breast cancer. The shape of the isodose curves can be altered by a wedge, a device that can be placed in the head of the machine to absorb graded amounts of radiation across the treatment field. The wedge angle can vary, thereby producing the desired isodose curves (Fig. 62-4). To adjust treatment to the patient's surface irregularities, a compensator can be used as an alternative to the wedge. Compen-

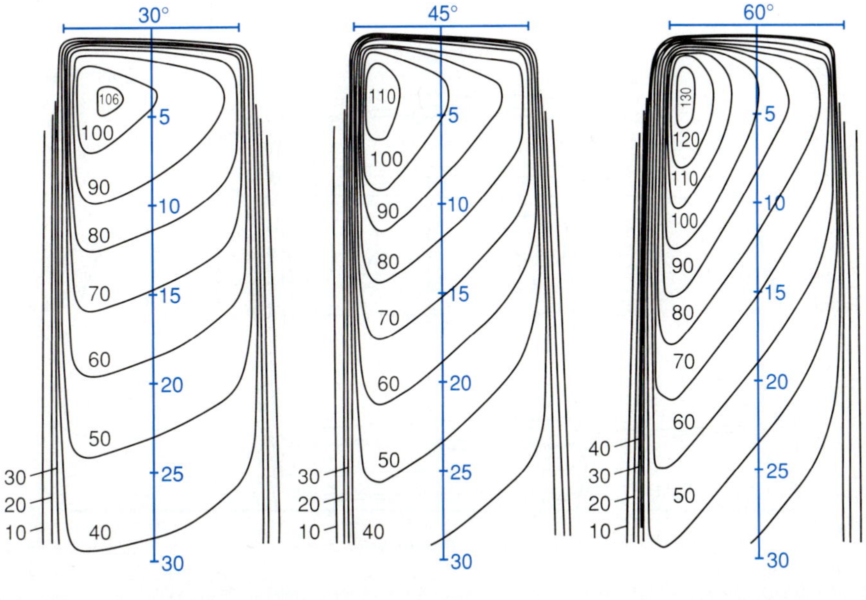

FIGURE 62-4. Effect of wedges placed in the accelerator on the beam profile. Rather than being perpendicular to the beam as in Figure 62-3, the isodose curves angle across the central axis. The angle depends on the wedge chosen—30, 45, or 60 degrees. Such an angled profile is necessary for treating curved surfaces. (After Purdy JA, Lightfoot DA, Glasgow GP. Principles of radiologic physics, dosimetry and treatment planning. In: Perez CA, Brady LW, eds. Principles and practice of radiation oncology. Philadelphia, JB Lippincott, 1987:129)

sators more precisely adjust the radiation to patient contour changes than the wedge, but they are harder to fashion and must be made for each patient. Their use is important for large irregular areas, such as in the treatment of head and neck cancers.

Simulation and Treatment Planning

Radiation treatment requires a precise knowledge of normal anatomy and a detailed knowledge of growth patterns of tumors. Both computed tomographic (CT) and magnetic resonance imaging (MRI) scanning can define the anatomic location of tumors and closely approximated normal tissues. Such images, however, may have inherent distortions that need to be accounted for when planning patient treatment.

Patient treatment plans are developed at a simulator before commencement of radiation therapy. The simulator contains a diagnostic x-ray tube, usually with fluoroscopic capabilities, but otherwise it has geometry identical to that of the treatment unit. Complicated tumor volumes can be defined from a CT scan with the patient in the treatment position. In complicated cases, the data are entered on a computer, the tumor volume is defined three-dimensionally, and simulated beams are created. A plan is then designed with the aid of sophisticated computing to optimize tumor dose with minimal normal tissue doses. Plans may have fields at varying angles, some wedged or intermittently wedged; the beams may be a combination of photon beams and electron beams. For routine cases, often larger fields are used initially to treat areas of potential microscopic involvement, followed by a smaller cone-down field to deliver a higher dose to the area of gross tumor involvement. There may be two or more cone-down fields for head and neck cancers. Since the probability of error increases with complex, multifaceted plans, easier and simpler plans should always be considered in designing treatment.

Figure 62-5 illustrates two treatment plans: a pair of opposed tangential fields for breast cancer and a four-field technique for a pelvic tumor. With the treatment of thoracic or abdominal tumors, both the location of normal tissues of particular concern (kidney, spinal cord) and the tumor location are drawn on the plan, and doses are specified to each area. Once treatments have begun, port films are taken weekly with the accelerator to verify patient and field position. Most departments have a weekly review of treatment plans and verification films. Additional chart review by a physicist or dosimetrist is done to verify the dose calculations. This peer review and quality control system help optimize treatment delivery while maintaining safety.

RADIATION BIOLOGY

Interaction of Photons With Tissues

Photons deposit energy in irradiated tissue by ejection of electrons; this causes ionization of the effected molecule. The energy is deposited at random. The density of ioniza-

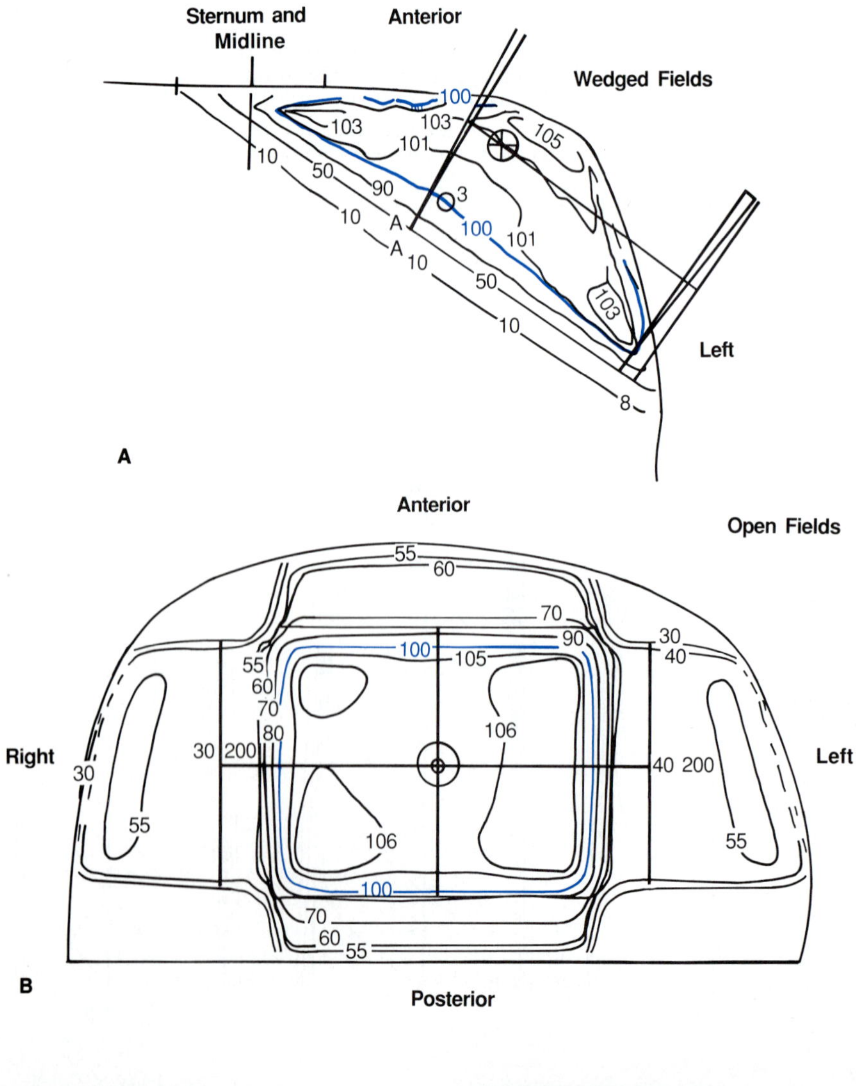

FIGURE 62-5. Treatment plans for breast and chest wall cancer and for a pelvic tumor. (**A**) For breast cancer, two tangential fields are used: one entering across midline and the other laterally. Both are wedged, yielding a homogenous dose within the treatment volume. The tumor dose is 100% (4500 cGy); only a few small regions receive a dose as high as 105% (4725 cGy). (**B**) For treating deep-seated pelvic tumors, such as prostate tumors, the bladder and back part of the rectum are excluded, and the tumors are treated with only the anterior and posterior fields. Similarly, the femoral heads are excluded from the anterior and posterior fields, lessening their dose.

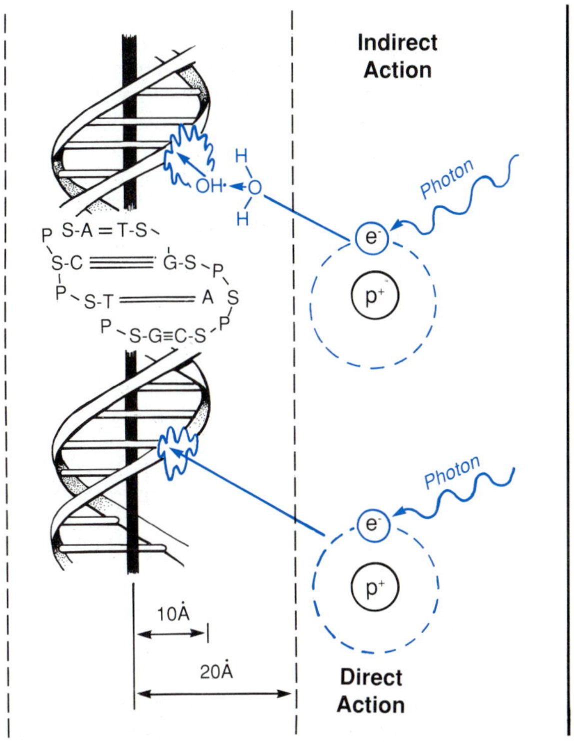

FIGURE 62-6. Schematic depiction of the direct and indirect effects of radiation on DNA. Radiation can directly damage DNA or can produce ionization in nearby water molecules that can lead to DNA damage. (After Hall EJ. The oxygen effect and reoxygenation. In: Radiobiology for the radiologist, ed 4. Philadelphia, JB Lippincott, 1994:137)

tions along the path of radiation is defined by the term *linear energy transfer* (LET) measured in keV/μm of path length.[2] The LET for different types of energy are: photons, 0.3; neutrons, 12; heavy charged particles, 100 or more. As the LET increases, dependence on oxygen for cell killing decreases. This is one of the potential advantages of neutron or particle therapy in patients with large poorly oxygenated tumors. For x-ray therapy, the final deposition of energy is produced by the secondary electrons resulting from the initial interaction between the photon and the irradiated tissue. These electron energies vary. The energy deposition of the relatively high energy electrons (1 to 10 MeV) is low; however, as the electron slows down, it can produce areas called *blobs, spurs*, and *short tracks* that are densely ionized. Thus, there is a high LET component to low LET radiation.

Although the exact mechanism is not known, it is believed that the DNA double-strand breaks are critical for cell death.[10] Radiation can deposit its energy directly in the DNA or in water near the DNA, a process called the *indirect effect* (Fig. 62-6). The latter produces free-radical intermediates, the most reactive of which is the hydroxyl radical. The double-strand break could be caused by direct ionization, probably in a blob or spur of energy from the secondary electron. Alternatively, it could be produced as a result of locally, multiple damaged sites, as described by Ward.[11] It is not known whether the critical lesions are produced randomly along the DNA or at a susceptible site, such as the DNA associated with the nuclear matrix, or the replication fork. With sufficient DNA damage, cell death occurs. Given the redundancy of cellular macromolecules, radiation-induced damage to cellular components is not thought to be as important in causing cell death as is DNA damage.

Cell Survival Curves

A typical cell survival curve for mammalian cells, relating the log of the surviving fraction with dose of radiation, is shown in Figure 62-7. It is characterized by an initial shoulder region and a terminal exponential portion. When sufficient dose is given that the shoulder region is passed, cell survival declines exponentially as the dose is increased. The relation between dose and cell killing is not exponential in the shoulder region, that is, some of the dose is wasted. A simple model to envision such an interaction is the multitarget model in which a minimal number of targets must be hit before cell death occurs. If only four or five critical targets are hit, the cell has accumulated the radiation dose necessary to hit the four targets; since all the necessary sites were not hit, the cell will survive. This is defined as *sublethal injury*. Once the exponential portion is reached, all cells will have had four targets hit; thus, each additional hit will result in cell death.

As time passes after the dose of radiation, these four targets may be repaired. If a second treatment is given at a sufficiently later time, it will again require five hits (not just one) to kill the cell. In other words, the shoulder has reappeared. The reappearance of the shoulder indicates that a repair process has gone on. Since the injury in the shoulder is defined as sublethal injury, its repair is called *sublethal injury repair*. The precise nature of the lesions and the biochemical repair processes involved are not clearly defined.

The clinical daily dose of 200 cGy is on the shoulder region.[2] By altering the timing between fractions, the time required for the reappearance of the shoulder region is about 6 hours. Thus, most multifraction regimens, such as twice-daily radiation therapy, allow 6 hours between treatments so that there is no unsuspected increase in nor-

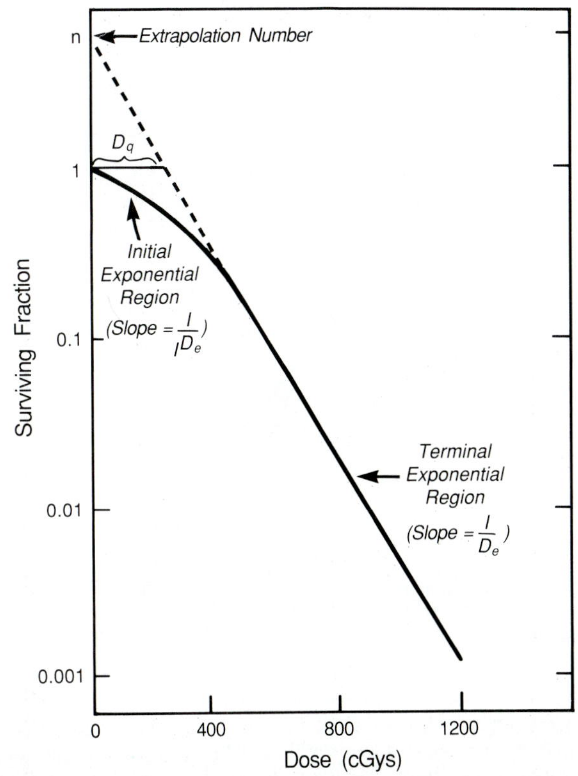

FIGURE 62-7. Cell survival curve. (After Withers HR. Biologic basis of radiation therapy. In: Perez CA, Brady LW, eds. Principles and practice of radiation oncology, ed 2. Philadelphia, JB Lippincott, 1992:72)

mal tissue injury, which might occur if treatments are given too closely together.

The precise mathematic shape of the cell survival curve has been the subject for much debate. The model in use is the linear-quadratic model, in which the surviving fraction = $-_e(\alpha D + \beta D^2)$. Cell survival depends on both single-hit and multihit phenomena. The single-hit cell killing is proportional to the radiation dose, D. The multihit killing is proportional to the radiation dose squared, D^2. For a given cell line, the relative efficacy of single-hit killing is defined by α, and for the multihit killing, by β. The term used to describe the relative proportion of cell killing by the two components is the α/β ratio. A high ratio implies a greater α component, which tends to produce a straighter curve.

Survival curves are important in clinical radiation therapy. In general, survival curves are similar among tumors and normal tissues. Although for many reasons, a direct correlation between in vitro cell survival and tumor curability cannot be made, tumors that have a higher surviving fraction, or less steep slope on the survival curve, are generally less curable.[12,13] The shape of the survival curve may be different for tumors and acute reactions than for late-responding tissues. Acute and late reactions define normal tissue toxicity. Acute reactions occur at the time of treatment and, if sufficiently severe, may cause a treatment break. These include skin and mucosal reactions. Acute reactions almost always heal. Late reactions occur months to years after radiation therapy and are defined in terms of organ dysfunction, necrosis, fibrosis, failure, and so forth. These are generally not reversible, although some may be remediable, such as bowel obstruction, and many are tolerable, such as a slightly dry mouth or diminished bladder capacity.

The shape of the survival curves for the production of acute verses late injury has important implications for radiation therapy because the size of the dose per fraction can affect the relation between tumor control and late radiation injury.[5] Figure 62-8 illustrates the theoretic relation

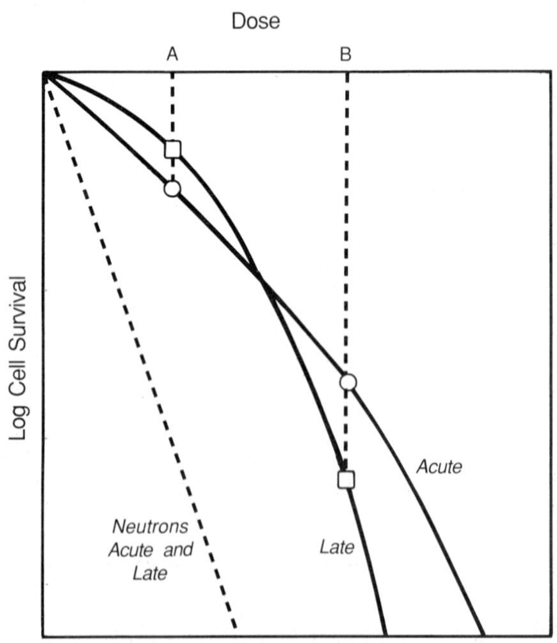

FIGURE 62-8. Cell survival for acute reactions and tumors compared with late-responding tissues. The curves are fit using the relation, surviving fraction = e − (aD + bD^2). Cell survival depends on a single hit. (After Withers HR. Biologic basis of radiation therapy. In: Perez CA, Brady LW, eds. Principles and practice of radiation oncology, ed 2. Philadelphia, JB Lippincott, 1992:79)

between early- and late-responding tissues, the former representing tumor. The α/β ratio is higher for tumors than for late-responding tissues, thereby giving the late-responding tissues a survival curve that is curvier in the clinical dose range. At a lower dose per fraction (A), there is more damage to the tumor than to the normal tissues; whereas at B, the converse is true. Although the relations between absolute total dose and effect (eg, toxicity or local control) differ for the various tissues, this observation is part of the rationale for some of the new fractionation regimens.

Four R's of Radiation Biology

The laboratory and clinical findings of classic radiation biology have been defined in terms of the four R's: repair, redistribution, repopulation, and reoxygenation. Two basic types of repair have been defined operationally. It is likely that similar biochemical mechanisms are involved to some extent for both. Sublethal damage repair was described previously. The reappearance of the shoulder between two doses of radiation is due in part to sublethal damage repair. The second type of repair is called *potentially lethal damage repair*. Cells treated in plateau phase produce a given level of survival immediately after treatment. If the cells remain in situ for a number of hours after treatment, the proportion of surviving cells will increase. The increase in survival over time after a single treatment is defined as potentially lethal damage repair. The importance to clinical outcome of each of these repair processes is not completely understood.

Redistribution refers to the synchronization of the cell cycle that occurs after a single dose of radiation.[2] Cells have decreasing radiosensitivity as from M/G2 to G1 to early S to late S phase. The relative radioresistance of S phase has prompted the combined use of radiation with S-phase–specific drugs. Unfortunately, the clinical use of radiation to synchronize cells for subsequent chemotherapy has not been successful. The potential interaction of radiation and chemotherapy is extremely complex, and many theoretically designed combinations have either not worked or not added selectively to tumor cell killing over that of normal tissue. Nevertheless, a few studies have shown some clinical advantage to the use of radiation and the cycle active agents 5-fluorouracil for anal cancer or hydroxyurea for cervical cancer.

Tumors and normal tissues *repopulate* during a course of irradiation. Normal tissue repopulation is observable with the healing of mucosal and skin reactions that takes place despite continuing the radiation. The repopulation of tumors has been inferred from split-course radiation regimens in which there are a few weeks of no treatment between treatment segments. In settings in which the total dose was the same, local control was worse for split-course than for continuous treatment. Split-course regimens are used increasingly in combined modality regimens. In this situation, however, the chemotherapy is administered between the radiation segments, which theoretically prevents significant repopulation.

Hypoxic cells are relatively radioresistant. For the same portion of cell killing, hypoxic cells require two to three times the dose as the same cells treated in normoxic conditions.[2] Most rodent tumors contain hypoxic cells. Given the relative radioresistance of these cells, it would be expected that the proportion of hypoxic cells would increase rapidly after a few treatments as the more sensitive oxygenated cells are killed. In general, however, this is not the case. A process called *reoxygenation* takes place that maintains the proportion of hypoxic cells at a relatively constant number. The exact mechanism of reoxygenation is not known but likely involves shifts in blood flow.[14] Without reoxygenation, radiation therapy probably would not cure many solid tumors.

Fractionation and Dose

The standard treatment for radiation therapy is 180 to 200 cGy per day, 5 days per week. The total dose depends on the clinical setting and type of tumor. The approximate dose needed for a probability of more than 95% local control of non-Hodgkin's lymphoma (NHL) is 3600 to 4000 cGy for low-grade and 4000 to 5000 cGy for intermediate-grade histologies. For epithelial tumors, the required dose is 5000 to 6000 cGy for microscopic disease, 6000 to 6600 cGy for tumors 2 cm in diameter or smaller, 6500 cGy for postoperative high-risk head and neck cancer or sarcomas, 7000 cGy for epithelial tumors 4 cm in diameter, and 7000 cGy or more for tumors larger than 6 cm. As the required dose increases, it becomes difficult to treat with external beam alone because of the high risk of toxicity to surrounding normal tissues. In such cases, brachytherapy is used, which can deliver a high dose to a small volume. It is critical for clinicians to be aware that although the probability of local control is below 95%, large tumors can be controlled with radiation. Using the criteria of complete or partial response, there are few instances in which the response to irradiation is less than 50%.

Altered fractionation is used more frequently. High doses per fraction (hypofractionation) are useful for palliative regimens. Relatively large doses are given one to four times per week, resulting in a large total weekly dose, such as 3000 cGy in 10 fractions over 2 weeks. An alternative method is to use accelerated fractionation, which keeps the same total dose but decreases the time over which it is given. Such a regimen might be used for a rapidly growing tumor, such as Burkitt's lymphoma. The schedule would be 200 cGy twice daily for a total of 2000 cGy per week. The fractions should be separated by 4 to 6 hours to allow time for sublethal damage repair. Bone marrow transplantation regimens often consist of 175 to 200 cGy twice daily for 3 to 4 days (total dose, 1200 to 1400 cGy).

Hyperfractionation uses a small single dose given 2 to 3 times per day. The total time is about the same as with standard fractionation, but the total dose must be higher to obtain the same effect.[5] The rationale for hyperfractionation is derived from Figure 62-8; the lower dose per fraction spares late-responding tissues relative to tumor. An example of such a regimen is 110 cGy given twice daily (1100 cGy per week, 10 fractions per week) to a total dose of about 8000 cGy. The long-term normal tissue effects of head and neck treatment with such a schedule are similar to those of 200 cGy fractions given once per day to a total dose of about 7000 cGy. Hyperfractionation is being evaluated in clinical trials to determine the maximal safe total dose that can be delivered and whether or not this approach improves the therapeutic index. At times, hybrid regimens are used, such as 160 cGy given twice daily. This is referred to as an *accelerated hyperfractionation regimen*. Therefore, when considering a total dose received by a patient, it is imperative to consider the dose per fraction, the number of doses per week, the total dose, the total treatment time, and, when considering retreatment, the time elapsed since completion of the previous course of therapy.

NEW RADIATION MODALITIES

A number of novel approaches are being used to enhance the local efficacy of radiation therapy. Oxygen-mimetic, electron-affinic radiation sensitizers are used to sensitize the hypoxic cells.[2] The agent under investigation in the United States is SR 2508 (etanidazole). The thiol compound, WR-2721, is being investigated as a protector of normal tissues. This compound is a scavenger of free radicals and prevents cellular and DNA damage. Both the sensitizers and protectors are being investigated as modifiers of chemotherapy.[15]

Hyperthermia involves the heating of tissues with microwaves or ultrasound to achieve target temperatures of 43°C. The precise mechanism of radiation enhancement by hyperthermia is not known. In practice, it is difficult to obtain a sustained minimal tumor temperature of 43°C, but newer technical devices are being developed that may improve this. The use of trimodality therapy—heat, radiation, and chemotherapeutic agents—is also being explored.[16]

Both radiation therapy and chemotherapy are used in many clinical settings. A number of different strategies are used, including adjuvant chemotherapy, toxicity independence (additivity), and sensitization. The dose and schedule of both the chemotherapeutic agents and irradiation are often altered to accommodate their use in a combined modality regimen.[17]

TOXICITY OF IRRADIATION

Whole-Body Irradiation

The toxicity of whole-body irradiation depends on total dose. Very high doses, about 10,000 cGy, produce the cerebrovascular syndrome of confusion and collapse, with death occurring within hours. Doses of 500 to 1200 cGy cause death in a week or less from the gastrointestinal syndrome. The gastrointestinal tract is denuded with associated diarrhea and massive fluid loss, and often, infection occurs. The hematopoietic syndrome occurs after total-body doses of 250 to 500 cGy. This is characterized by pancytopenia with bleeding and infection. The ensuing peak time to death due to failure of the hematopoietic system is about 30 days. The mean lethal whole-body dose is about 400 cGy, but the outcome depends on therapeutic interventions, including supportive care and, possibly, bone marrow transplantation.[2]

Clinical Radiation Tolerance

The extent and frequency of injury to normal tissues depend on both radiation dose and volume treated. The risk can be enhanced by surgery and chemotherapy. Precise organ tolerances are not known, but estimates can be derived from published case reports and small series.

If a relatively large single dose is given to the whole brain, a syndrome of headache, nausea, and vomiting may be seen. With small fractionated doses, the postirradiation somnolence syndrome, seen most frequently in children, occurs 6 to 8 weeks after treatment. This is not due to brain necrosis but most likely is a result of demyelination. Brain tolerance is about 5500 to 6000 cGy, but small volumes can tolerate higher doses. Focal brain necrosis, which may require surgical resection, can occur with high local doses.[18]

About 1 to 3 months after irradiation to a modest length of spinal cord, as is used in patients treated for Hodgkin's disease, patients may develop Lhermitte's syndrome, which can persist for a few months to several years.[19] Lhermitte's syndrome is an electric shock-like feeling in the arms, legs, and back brought on with flexion of the neck. This is self-limiting and is not a harbinger of late injury. At doses in excess of 5000 cGy, radiation myelitis may occur. The use of certain cytotoxic agents, such as doxorubicin, when combined with radiation may increase the risk of spinal cord injury. The clinical syndrome depends on the total-dose fractionation scheme, and length of cord irradiated and can vary from only minimal symptoms to, at its worst, a complete functional cord transection.[18] Radiation injury to the peripheral nervous system is uncommon unless fields have been overlapped or more than one course of treatment given. Brachial neuritis, however, can be seen after conventional doses of irradiation and may be viral.[20] Complete resolution may require 1 year or longer.

Radiation injury to the heart may involve a number of different cardiac tissues. Cardiac injury is rare unless the entire heart is treated to more than 4000 cGy or unless doses of 5000 to 6000 cGy are given to a large portion of the heart. An early finding is asymptomatic pericardial effusion that may resolve or ultimately progress to constrictive pericarditis, requiring pericardiectomy. Myocardial damage may lead to heart failure. Valvular thickening and dysfunction may also occur. Accelerated coronary artery disease can produce a myocardial infarction. Vessels in any radiation field may be injured, but this is relatively uncommon. Anthracyclines enhance the risk of myocardial injury, and symptomatic problems can occur at lower radiation doses than would otherwise be expected. This risk is dependent on the cumulative dose of anthracyclines received.[18] A more detailed discussion of cardiac and pulmonary injury is provided in the section on Hodgkin's disease.

The lungs are particularly sensitive to irradiation injury. Acute injury, as well as long-term fibrosis and loss of pulmonary function, can occur. Fractionated doses as low as 2000 cGy or single doses as low as 800 cGy can cause radiation pneumonitis. Acute radiation pneumonitis can occur up to 6 months after treatment and is characterized by a dry cough, dyspnea, low-grade fever, and radiographic changes within the radiation fields. Treatment for symptomatic relief may require corticosteroids, but if possible, these should be avoided. If used, they must be tapered slowly. Patients who had prior lung irradiation can later develop radiation pneumonitis if steroids administered for other reasons are rapidly tapered.[21] For example, this can occur in patients with Hodgkin's disease treated with mantle-field irradiation followed by the administration of prednisone in the MOPP chemotherapy regimen. Once the radiation pneumonitis resolves, long-term fibrosis and pulmonary dysfunction are usually not seen.

The amount of lung that can be permanently damaged without producing symptoms depends on the presence of underlying lung pathology. In general, a mantle field produces little or no symptoms even though 10% to 15% of the lung receives high doses of irradiation. The use of chemotherapeutic agents, in particular bleomycin, may lower the threshold for clinical radiation lung injury.[18] A relatively rare picture of the adult respiratory distress syndrome may occur soon after limited thoracic irradiation. It involves the entire lung and is not limited to the radiation field.[22]

Kidney tolerance is similar to that of lung. A portion of the kidney that receives a total dose in excess of 2000 cGy will permanently lose function. The development of late hypertension or renal failure depends on the volume of kidney irradiated. Even if a portion of one kidney is treated to a high dose, it is rare to see any clinical signs or symptoms. If cisplatin is administered after kidney irradiation, the toxicity of the platinum may be increased.[18]

The irradiation of a large segment of liver to a dose in excess of 3000 cGy produces a clinical syndrome of hepatomegaly, ascites, and elevated liver function tests. Radiation injury is similar to that of venoocclusive disease, a syndrome that occurs with the high-dose alkylating agent regimens used in some marrow transplantation programs. If not fatal, radiation hepatopathy completely resolves. After paraaortic irradiation, the serum alkaline phosphatase level can be mildly elevated for up to 1 year or longer from the portion of the level in the radiation field. This elevation should not be misinterpreted as recurrent tumor, but elevations greater than three to four times normal should arouse suspicion.[18]

The gastrointestinal tract is modestly sensitive to irradiation, with small bowel tolerance lower than that of esophagus or large bowel. During radiation therapy, patients receiving large abdominal or pelvic fields get some degree of bowel irritation. This can be minimized by using a bland diet to decrease bowel activity. Permanent gastrointestinal injury can occur at doses above 4500 cGy. Prior surgery, with resultant loss of small bowel mobility, greatly increases the risk of injury. Bowel injury usually occurs months to years after treatment and can present as diarrhea, perforation, or obstruction. Late injury may require surgical excision of the damaged bowel segment, but this should be done only after a trial of conservative management.[18]

Virtually all organs are susceptible to injury. The following are the lower limits for permanent injury for some other organs: bone marrow stroma, 4000 cGy; spleen with functional asplenia, 4000 cGy; ovary, 2000 cGy; skin, 5500 cGy; salivary and endocrine glands, 4500 cGy; bladder, 6000 cGy; peripheral nerve, bone, and muscle, 6000 cGy; oral cavity mucosa, 6000 cGy. Acute reactions (eg, bowel, skin, mucosa, hair loss, blood count depression) occur 2 to 3 weeks after the start of treatment. These systems may recover despite an early decrease in function and the continuation of therapy. Conservative management helps a patient get through treatment with a minimum of treatment breaks.[18] As a rule, the presence or extent of an acute reaction does not predict the likelihood of a late reaction.

A major concern after treatment with radiation or chemotherapy is the development of secondary malignancies.[18,23] The risks for second tumor development include predisposition, as with retinoblastoma; underlying illness; altered immunity from the disease itself or its treatment; age of patient and other environmental factors, such as smoking; extent of irradiation; and type, dose, and duration of chemotherapeutic agents. Figure 62-9 illustrates the actuarial risk for developing a secondary malignancy after treatment for Hodgkin's disease.[23] Given the immunologic abnormalities associated with Hodgkin's disease, it is not known if these risks would be seen in patients with other conditions. The risk of leukemia appears to be related primarily to the use of alkylating agents. The solid tumors appear later than the secondary leukemias. Most are probably associated with radiation, but some occur from other causes; examples include secondary melanoma in patients

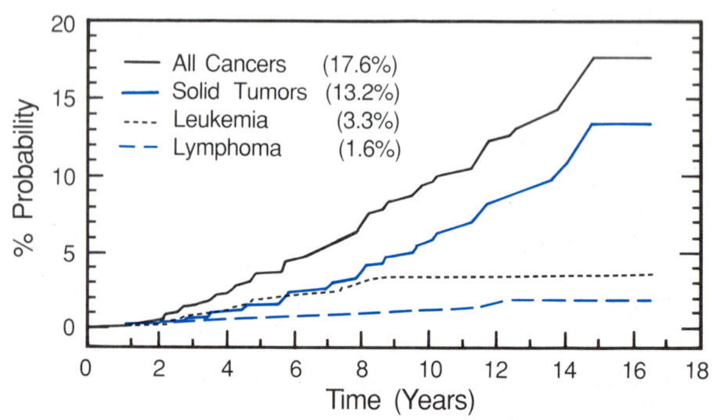

FIGURE 62-9. Probability of secondary neoplasms in patients treated for Hodgkin's disease. (After Tucker MA, Coleman CN, Cox RS, et al. Risk of second cancer after treatment for Hodgkin's disease. N Engl J Med 1988;318:76)

with dysplastic nevus syndrome, in which the risk for melanoma is associated with immunosuppression and ultraviolet radiation, not ionizing radiation; and secondary lung cancers, most of which occur in smokers. Curative treatment should not be compromised to avoid secondary malignancies, but it should be modified to decrease this risk if possible. Careful, lifelong surveillance is required since many secondary malignancies occur beyond 5 or even 10 years after treatment, and about half are curable if diagnosed early.

SPECIFIC USES OF RADIATION THERAPY FOR TREATMENT OF HEMATOLOGIC AND LYMPHOID MALIGNANCY

It is beyond the scope of this chapter to discuss in detail the pros and cons of irradiation for many of the hematologic and lymphoid malignancies. For Hodgkin's disease and NHL, there is considerable debate as to the relative roles of surgery, chemotherapy, and radiation therapy. We discuss some of the details of treatment and the issues regarding treatment selection for these diseases in the following sections.

Early-Stage Hodgkin's Disease

Radiation therapy remains the standard treatment for most patients with early-stage Hodgkin's disease. Routine staging laparotomy for most patients with clinical stage (CS) IA-IIA, IB-IIB, and IIIA disease has provided for the precise localization of disease and the use of radiation therapy alone if disease is limited to sites above the diaphragm.[24–27] Such an approach has resulted in fewer patients requiring combination chemotherapy for cure.

The freedom from first relapse (FFR) and overall survival rates for patients with pathologic stage (PS) IA-IIA Hodgkin's disease are excellent after treatment with radiation therapy alone. In one study, patients treated with radiation therapy alone had a 10-year actuarial FFR of 77% with treatments that varied from involved-field to total lymphoid irradiation (TLI).[25] Treatment with mantle followed by paraaortic and splenic pedicle irradiation resulted in a 14-year actuarial FFR of 82% and survival of 90% in another study.[26] These results are similar to those seen with the use of TLI.

PS IB-IIB Hodgkin's disease patients treated with radiation therapy alone have relapse-free and overall survival rates similar to those of stage IA-IIA patients.[27] Treatment of PS IB-IIB patients with combined radiation therapy and chemotherapy (CMT) does not improve the FFR or survival rates as compared with radiation therapy alone.[27,28] Results with mantle and paraaortic irradiation in the treatment of PS IB-IIB Hodgkin's disease patients appear similar to those with TLI.

For all PS I-II Hodgkin's disease patients, FFR and survival rates appear equivalent either with radiation therapy alone or initial CMT.[25] This suggests that stage I-II patients seen at experienced centers can be effectively treated with radiation therapy alone, with combination chemotherapy reserved for relapse. Excellent results of this treatment, however, depend on the precise anatomic location of disease obtained at staging laparotomy and splenectomy.

The successful treatment of early-stage supradiaphragmatic Hodgkin's disease with radiation therapy alone depends on knowledge of the anatomic location of disease in the thorax, careful treatment planning to minimize the volume and dose of radiation to normal tissues, and daily attention to treatment administration. Hodgkin's disease patients treated with radiation therapy alone at medical centers where large numbers of such patients are routinely seen appear to have a lower risk of relapse than patients treated at institutions that see only small numbers of patients.[29] Thus, treatment of Hodgkin's with radiation demands a level of care and expertise that appears to benefit from a large prior clinical experience.

Three separate radiation fields are employed in the treatment of Hodgkin's disease: mantle, paraaortic and splenic pedicle (splenic), and pelvic.

Mantle Irradiation

The mantle field treats the submandibular, cervical, supraclavicular, infraclavicular, axillary, mediastinal, and hilar lymph nodes. Patients should not be treated in centers that do not have a simulator (described previously) available for treatment planning. A 4- to 8-MeV linear accelerator is ideal for delivery of the mantle irradiation. Higher-energy machines should be avoided because they allow too much skin-sparing and underdose superficial nodes. Treatment with ^{60}Co should also be avoided because the lower energy results in greater inhomogeneity of dose and the penumbra results in more radiation to normal tissues at the field edges.

The superior border of the mantle field should be 1 to 2 cm above the angle of the jaw to allow for treatment of the submandibular and subdigastric nodes. In the presence of high neck nodes, the ipsilateral preauricular nodes are included. The head should be extended so that the edge of the field passes along the lower border of the external auditory meatus. The fields should include both axillae. The position of the axillary nodes changes with the arms up as compared with treatment with the arms akimbo. Thus, lung block adjustments must be made based on arm position. Children without palpable axillary adenopathy should have blocks placed to protect the humeral epiphyses. The inferior border of the mantle field generally is placed at the bottom of T8 or T9 unless there is involvement of the subcarinal or cardiac nodes or pericardial involvement, in which case the field must be extended lower. The T8 and T9 inferior border allows the spleen or splenic pedicle to be included in the paraaortic field.

Individual contoured divergent blocks should be fashioned to protect normal heart and lung. These are made with a special device, then mounted on a tray and placed into the head of the linear accelerator to protect the desired areas from the radiation beam.[30,31] At a minimum, weekly portal films are obtained while the patient is on treatment to make sure that the proper areas are being protected. Figures 62-10 and 62-11 show examples, respectively, of a simulator planning film and of a verification portal film with the lung and cardiac blocks in place. These blocks are shaped around hilar and mediastinal nodes. Mantle patients are often treated at extended machine-to-patient distances (source-to-skin distance, 110 cm or greater) to allow for better tissue homogeneity and to permit treatment of the large fields often needed to cover the nodes above the diaphragm. Equally weighted anterior and posterior fields should be used, with both fields treated daily. Patients with large mediastinal adenopathy may be treated initially with small blocks for 1500 to 2000 cGy. Then, after a 1- to 2-week treatment break to allow for tumor shrinkage, larger blocks can be fashioned to protect additional heart and lung now free of lymph node involvement. Some recommend prophylactic low-dose whole-lung irradiation in patients with hilar or large mediastinal adenopathy to reduce the risk of pulmonary relapse. One technique includes the use of a transmission block, which allows the lungs to receive a fraction of the total daily radiation dose during the mantle treatments.[19] As an alternative, the entire mantle

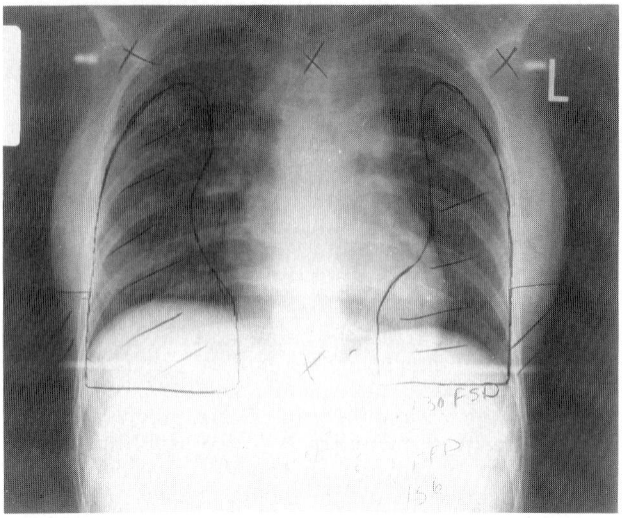

FIGURE 62-10. Simulator film of a mantle field in a patient with early-stage Hodgkin's disease. Areas blocked to protect the heart and lungs are indicated.

(and lungs) receive 150 cGy/d for 10 fractions before adding full-thickness lung blocks.[32] Regardless of the technique, the utility of prophylactic lung irradiation is controversial.[33] Other technical details should include the addition of a small anterior larynx block after 2000 cGy, a posterior cervical spine block after 3000 cGy, and a subcarinal block covering the low heart after 3000 to 3400 cGy. Differences in tissue separation result in the cervical spinal cord receiving about 8% to 10% more radiation than the thoracic cord. The posterior cervical spinal block is used to compensate for this difference.

Patients should receive doses of 3600 to 4000 cGy to the mantle field with an additional cone-down dose, for a total of 4000 to 4400 cGy to areas of bulk disease. If patients are also receiving chemotherapy, it may be possible to reduce the total dose of radiation used, but specific guidelines are not available. All patients receiving mantle irradiation should have separate dose calculations for the inferior portion of the heart, the axilla, and the neck. The precise details regarding blocks and dose vary among other excellent institutions.

Acute side effects seen during mantle irradiation include mild pharyngitis, low posterior scalp epilation, loss or change in taste, mouth dryness and thickening of saliva, mild skin erythema on the shoulders and neck, generalized fatigue, and occasionally nausea. It is common for patients to lose 5 to 10 pounds during treatment mainly as a result of salivary and taste changes. Mouth dryness and taste changes occur 1 to 2 weeks into treatment, and the pharyngitis and epilation occur after 2 to 3 weeks, with resolution after placement of the larynx block. The acute symptoms are transitory. The pharyngitis lasts 1 to 2 weeks. The taste gradually returns after 1 to 2 months, and hair starts to regrow after 3 months; the fatigue and weight loss usually reverse within 2 to 4 weeks. In younger patients (15 to 40 years old), saliva is back to normal usually by 6 months. In patients older than 40 years of age, recovery may be slower, and mild xerostomia can last up to a year or more. Patients should brush daily with fluoride gel during and after radiation to prevent an increase in dental cavities, which is often encountered from the radiation-induced changes in salivary pH. Fluoride applications are continued at least until the patient's salivary function returns to normal and preferably for 2 years after the end of treatment.

Pulmonary Complications. Severe pulmonary complications are rarely seen in the standard treatment for Hodgkin's disease. In early-stage patients treated with radiation therapy alone, the risk of pneumonitis, previously described in this chapter, is 5%, with about one third of affected patients requiring corticosteroids for symptomatic relief.[26] The risk of pneumonitis is greater if whole-lung irradiation or chemotherapy is part of the initial treatment. In patients with large mediastinal adenopathy, the transverse mediastinal size is often exaggerated when the patient is prone or supine, increasing the amount of heart or lung in the treatment field. Techniques to reduce this increase in size and to allow larger lung and cardiac blocks include radiation therapy machine gating to respiration[34] and treatment in the sitting-up position.[35] Pneumonitis is radiographically diagnosed by the appearance of infiltrates usually confined to the original radiation fields, but superimposed bacterial or fungal infections must also be considered. If the patient has been on chemotherapy or prednisone, both radiation pneumonitis and *Pneumocystis carinii* pneumonia can occur. If infiltrates are seen outside the radiation field or do not conform to the entire radiation portal, the diagnosis of infection is more likely than radiation pneumonitis. Radiation pneumonitis can also mimic recurrent Hodgkin's disease, and thoracic CT scanning can often help determine the correct diagnosis (Fig. 62-12). With severe radiation pneumonitis, prednisone, 60 to 80 mg/d, may be helpful for symptomatic improvement and clearing of infiltrates.[19] If patients fail to improve on prednisone, radiation pneumonitis with a superimposed infection is more likely the diagnosis.

Mild perihilar, perimediastinal, and apical pulmonary fibrosis occurs in all patients after mantle irradiation and is seen as soon as 6 months after treatment. Symptomatic changes in pulmonary function are rare. Several studies have measured changes in pulmonary function after irra-

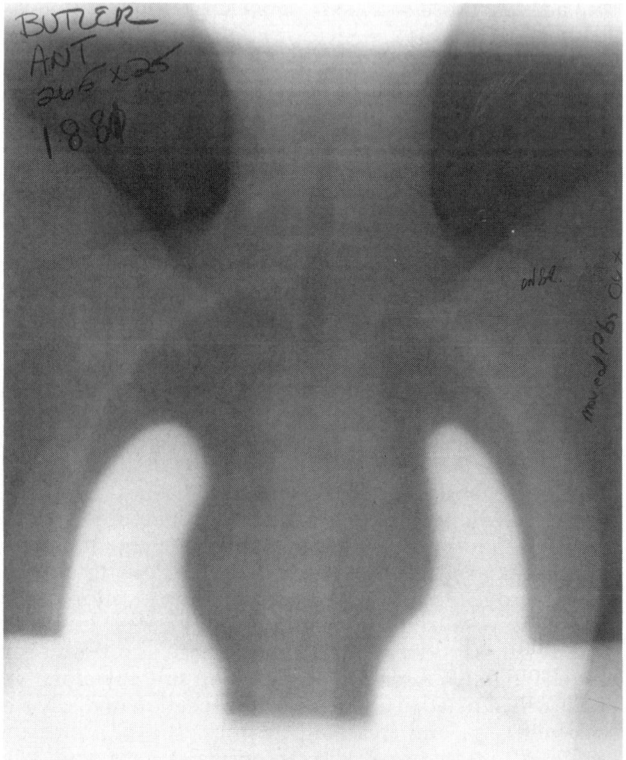

FIGURE 62-11. Simulator film of a paraaortic field. Note the treatment of the splenic pedicle region.

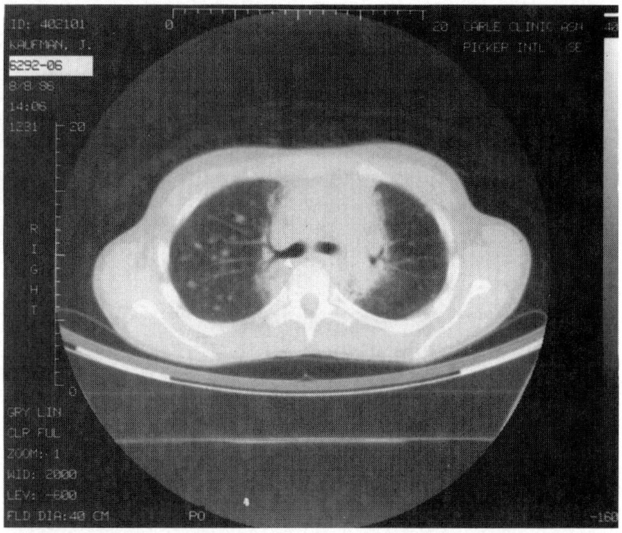

FIGURE 62-12. Representative film of a thoracic computed axial tomographic scan of a patient who had central radiation pneumonitis as well as evidence of recurrent Hodgkin's disease (multiple pulmonary nodules).

diation. One report demonstrated no effect of mantle-field irradiation in arterial blood gas tensions.[36] Another study noted changes in the peak oxygen consumption, but these were minimal. The largest changes were seen in patients with extensive intrathoracic disease; yet even in this group, the mean peak oxygen consumption was only 15% below that predicted.[37]

Cardiac Complications. The general effects of radiation on the heart were described previously. Radiation-related cardiac disease is dose dependent. The radiation technique used, the size of the left ventricular block, and the fraction size when equally weighted anterior and posterior fields are administered are important factors to consider. Doses of greater than 4500 cGy to the anterior heart, even when a ventricular block is in place, have been associated with severe complications, including constrictive pericarditis with tamponade and severe vascular, valvular, and myocardial dysfunction. Early studies using a short focus to skin distance and anterior weighted fields resulted in doses of 4500 to 6000 cGy to the anterior heart. With modern radiation therapy, symptomatic radiation-induced heart disease as a late manifestation of mantle irradiation is rare. Asymptomatic changes are more common and include mild pericardial thickening, valvular thickening or effusion, and a decrease in the left ventricular ejection fraction.[38,39] The frequency of these changes varies and is dose-related. The most common symptomatic effect is radiation pericarditis. In a review of 590 patients receiving mantle irradiation, pericarditis occurred in only 13 patients (2.2%), and all patients recovered with conservative management.[33] Myocarditis associated with congestive heart failure can also be seen, may be virus-induced, but is extremely rare (less than 1% of patients).

Cardiac irradiation may also potentiate accelerated coronary artery disease and early myocardial infarctions. Coronary artery disease has been described for high doses of radiation.[40,41] There is less evidence that it is increased with conventional doses, but several studies have reported a mild increased risk.[33,42] Further studies with concomitant analysis of other risk factors must be done to determine which group of patients is at highest risk.

Thyroid Complications. Thyroid dysfunction after radiation therapy is common.[33,43–46] Except for the small amount of midline shielding that is achieved with the anterior larynx and posterior spine blocks, it is not possible to shield the thyroid during mantle irradiation. Clinical hypothyroidism used to occur in nearly 20% of patients but is now less common because of frequent testing of serum thyroxine and thyroid-stimulating hormone levels and placement of patients on thyroid supplementation for laboratory evidence of mild thyroid dysfunction.[33] In one report, the 15-year actuarial risk of developing a thyroid abnormality was 29% for adults and 64% for children 16 years of age or younger.[33] Thyroid abnormalities may occur late, and long-term surveillance is important. Patients should be tested every 6 to 12 months for thyroid function, and if the thyroid-stimulating hormone level is significantly elevated on repeat testing, thyroid replacement should be initiated.

Although radiation-induced hypothyroidism is thought to be a result of direct cellular injury from ionizing radiation, the presence of thyroiditis in some patients suggests that thyroid injury may also develop from autoantibodies. Although rare, some patients develop palpable thyroid nodules, lymphocytic infiltration, and Hürthle cell nodules.[47,48] Graves' disease with exophthalmos has also been described as a result of high-dose thyroid irradiation.[49,50]

Thyroid cancer after irradiation for Hodgkin's disease appears to be rare.[47,48] High-dose irradiation is presumed to cause sufficient damage to the thyroid follicular cells to prevent subsequent cell division and mutagenesis, therefore resulting in less risk of cancer induction than is seen with lower radiation doses.

Matching of Mantle and Paraaortic Fields. An extremely important part of the radiation therapy management of patients with early-stage Hodgkin's disease is the matching of the divergent mantle and paraaortic fields. Tragic consequences of lower-extremity weakness progressing to paraplegia can result from an excessively high dose to the spinal cord at the level of the match between the mantle and paraaortic field due to a field overlap. Sophisticated treatment planning is needed to deliver an adequate dose of irradiation to the lymph nodes anterior to the vertebral body at the match point while preventing a high dose to the spinal cord. The use of a treatment simulator is mandatory when matching mantle with paraaortic and splenic pedicle fields. In centers with careful treatment planning, radiation myelitis resulting from field overlap should never occur. Radiation-induced transverse myelitis usually occurs 9 months to several years after irradiation. Patients notice lower-extremity weakness, which progresses to loss of bowel and bladder function and flaccid paralysis. When such neurologic symptoms occur, patients should be evaluated to rule out trauma with vertebral body damage, recurrent Hodgkin's disease with extradural involvement, and paraneoplastic or demyelinization syndromes. MRI or CT scanning analysis of cerebrospinal fluid protein, glucose cellular analysis, and a bone scan should be obtained. In addition, the previous radiation fields should be reviewed and the spinal cord dose estimated. Radiation myelitis is extremely rare when less than 5000 cGy is delivered in conventional fractions (180 to 200 cGy/d).[51] The potential for radiation myelitis may increase when long segments of the cord are irradiated or when there is initial tumor involvement of the cord.

A number of different matching techniques exist, but all use several basic principles. A calculated skin gap based on the source-to-skin distance to allow for field divergence is used to match the upper border of the paraaortic field with the lower border of the mantle field at midplane.[52,53] Permanent tattoos marking the bottom of the mantle and top of the paraaortic fields should be used. Special films to carefully visualize the vertebral bodies should be obtained at the time of filming for the mantle and paraaortic treatments. These should show the divergent edge of both fields. As an added safety precaution, we recommend placement of half-value layer blocks on the posterior mantle and posterior paraaortic fields to block the lower and upper 1 cm of the spinal cord within the two fields, respectively. Another technique uses match-line wedges to optimize dose homogeneity in this region.[54]

Paraaortic Irradiation

Laterally, the paraaortic field should cover most of the transverse processes of the vertebral bodies. The upper border is determined by the match with the mantle field. This is planned so that the splenic pedicle region can be included in the paraaortic field. If a staging laparotomy has been done, the splenic hilar region (marked at laparotomy by clips) should also be treated (Fig. 62-13). If the patient has not had a staging laparotomy and splenectomy, the entire spleen must be treated. Splenic volumes can be obtained either from the liver and spleen scan or from a CT scan of the abdomen. The left kidney volume should be identified at planning (by an intravenous pyelogram or from the CT scan) and as much of the kidney protected as possible. The lower border of the paraaortic field should be placed at the bottom of L4. In patients with subcarinal disease, the lower border of the mantle field must be placed lower, often at T10 to T12. In this situation, the upper border of the spleen is higher than the spinal cord match, and those areas that were previously treated in the mantle field must be blocked. This is a difficult technique if splenic treatment is required in the presence of extensive subcarinal disease. Splenectomy should be considered in this circumstance even if not indicated as part of staging.

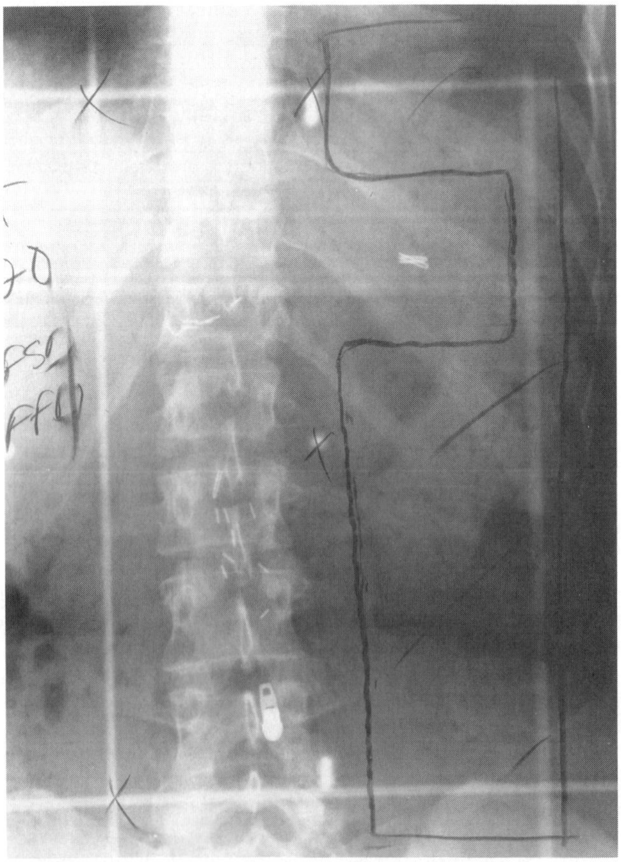

FIGURE 62-13. Portal (verification) film of a mantle field. This film is taken on the treatment unit and should match the simulator film shown in Figure 62-10.

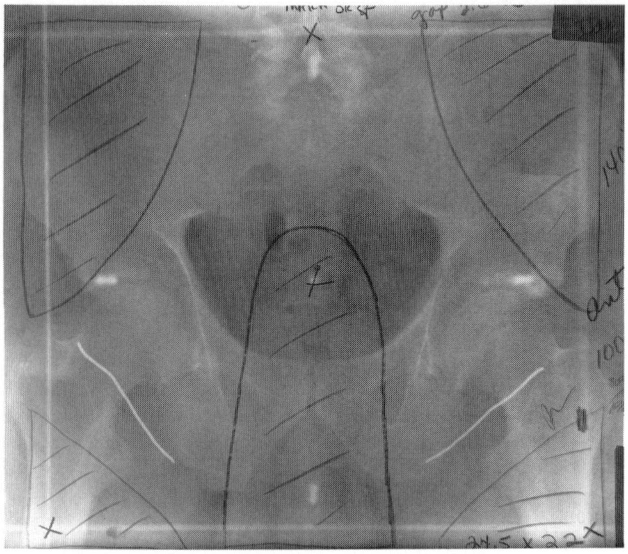

FIGURE 62-14. Simulator films of a pelvic field. Areas blocked to protect the iliac crest marrow and bladder are indicated.

Treatment of the paraaortic nodes should be associated with few or no complications. Acute side effects include nausea and vomiting associated with treating a portion of the stomach. They are more likely to occur when the entire spleen is treated. The doses needed to cure Hodgkin's disease are greater than normal kidney tolerance. None of the right kidney and only a small portion of the left upper kidney should be in the standard paraaortic and splenic pedicle field. When the intact spleen is treated, sometimes a greater portion of the left kidney is necessarily included in the field, and it is important to determine that adequate right renal function is present. It is extremely rare to see long-term clinical or laboratory evidence of renal impairment after paraaortic irradiation for Hodgkin's disease.[55] Nonetheless, when the spleen anatomically covers a substantial portion of the left kidney, splenectomy should be considered as an alternative to splenic irradiation.

Long-term bowel difficulties and chronic, intermittent colicky pain, diarrhea, or malabsorption are extremely rare after paraaortic irradiation. Small bowel obstruction is also unusual but is seen in some patients. In the absence of pathologic or radiologic evidence for focal radiation enteritis, it is most likely the sequela of surgical staging or a combination of both the staging and the irradiation. Small bowel obstruction requiring surgical intervention occurs in fewer than 1% of patients.[26]

Pelvic Irradiation

The use of pelvic irradiation is limited to patients with infradiaphragmatic presentations, stage III1A patients receiving TLI, and stage III patients with extensive paraaortic and pelvic disease receiving CMT. The pelvic field treats the common iliac, hypogastric, external iliac, and inguinal nodes (Fig. 62-14). When there is gross pelvic nodal involvement, the femoral nodes should also be treated. The upper border of the pelvic field can be matched to the low paraaortic field border, with the gap technique described previously.[53] Sometimes, the pelvic and paraaortic nodes can be treated in one large inverted-Y field. This is most common in pediatric patients or in patients with extensive abdominal involvement in whom the match between the mantle and paraaortic fields would include known nodal involvement. The pelvic field technique includes a central block to protect the bladder and the ovaries in women who have undergone oophoropexy.

The acute effects of pelvic irradiation include transient diarrhea and urinary frequency. Chronic effects are potential long-term bone marrow suppression and sterility. With total nodal irradiation, a large portion of the bone marrow is in the pelvic field, and delivering adequate chemotherapy for relapse may be difficult after such treatment. Irradiation of the ovaries to 3500 cGy causes sterility and amenorrhea in all women. Oophoropexy is a procedure designed to move the ovaries with their vascular pedicles to the midline, suturing one ovary anteriorly and one posteriorly low on the uterus.[56] Metallic clips are placed at the suture sites to aid in localizing the ovaries during simulation. A double midline pelvic block is added to further reduce the dose to the ovary. With this technique, the ovarian dose can usually be kept to less than 250 cGy. As a result, 60% of patients retain menstrual function, and normal pregnancies have been reported.[57]

Radiation injury to the testes in Hodgkin's disease results primarily from external and internal scatter from the pelvic nodal irradiation. The risk of sterility to men varies and depends on the field size, field shape, and distance from the field edge to the testes. The position of the lower border is important. If the femoral nodes are treated, the risk of sterility is greater. Although a small amount of scatter occurs from the mantle and paraaortic fields,[58] there is no evidence that sterility results from the scatter from these two fields.[59] The estimated testicular dose from the pelvic field ranges from 140 to 300 cGy.[60] A scrotal shield of two half-value layers should be used to reduce external scatter. When the pelvic field is treated with scrotal shielding, the total testicular dose can be kept under 100 cGy in some patients.[61] A single dose of 100 cGy to the testes would allow recovery of sperm counts within 1 to 2 years,[62] but when the dose is given in low amounts over the entire course of radiation, as is the case with scatter, the risk of sterility may be higher.[60]

Early-Stage Non-Hodgkin's Lymphoma

Hodgkin's disease and NHL present with different distribution and staging patterns. As few as 10% of all NHL patients appear to have true stage I disease.[63,64] An analysis of stage distribution from the tumor registry at the Harvard Joint Center for Radiation Therapy (JCRT) demonstrated that about 15% of patients with NHL had stage I-II disease, in contrast to 60% of patients presenting with Hodgkin's disease. Localized extralymphatic involvement is more common in NHL than in Hodgkin's disease and can often occur as an isolated site of involvement (stage IE) or with adjacent nodes (stage IIE). There appears to be no difference in prognosis between stage I-II NHL patients with localized extralymphatic involvement and those who have only nodal involvement.[65,66]

The standard staging system employed for NHL is the same as that proposed for Hodgkin's disease at the Ann Arbor Conference in 1971.[67] A number of prognostic factors predict survival differences among subgroups of patients with NHL that are not included in the Ann Arbor staging system. Patients with stage I disease or stage II disease with two contiguous sites appear to have similar prognoses, which are superior to that of patients with more advanced stage II, III, or IV disease.[68,69] Other factors that predict for a worse prognosis include the presence of bulky nodal diseases (10 cm or larger), multiple extranodal sites, age (60 years or older), high lactate dehydrogenase level, and the presence of systemic symptoms.[69–73] Incorporation of these factors into a standard staging system for NHL patients would allow for more accurate prediction of outcome and better standardization of treatment.

Staging laparotomy and splenectomy results have enhanced our understanding of the distribution patterns of NHL. This procedure should not be performed in general practice, however, because it is morbid and rarely influences treatment. Most NHL patients have CS III-IV disease. These patients are treated with chemotherapy in most centers, and thus, routine staging laparotomy is not indicated for them. Staging laparotomy could be considered for about 20% of patients who remain CS I or II after sequential staging tests, but only if they are to be treated subsequently with radiation therapy alone rather than with systemic treatment.[74] Even in this setting, staging laparotomy is not generally needed for patients with small cell lymphomas when regional radiation therapy fields are being used. Such treatment has little morbidity, and if relapse occurs, there is no evidence that salvage treatment is compromised. The use of chemotherapy for most patients with stage I-II diffuse large cell lymphomas also obviates the use of staging laparotomies for these patients.[69,75,76]

Dose, Field Size, and Recurrence Patterns

Modern radiotherapeutic techniques for the treatment of NHL include the use of opposed or multiple field arrangements, treatment simulation, and contoured divergent blocks to protect normal tissue. Considerable local control data per radiation dose exists to aid in formulation of treatment plans for patients receiving radiation therapy alone.[77,78] The data are retrospective and are not controlled for tumor bulk or disease response, but they provide useful guidelines. For small cell and mixed lymphomas, 3500 to 4000 cGy in fractionated doses given over 4 to 5 weeks appears sufficient to achieve local control in most patients. Higher doses may occasionally be needed in patients with bulky adenopathy. For most patients with diffuse large cell lymphomas, at least 4500 to 5000 cGy in fractionated doses is needed.

The local control frequency after radiation therapy for patients at the JCRT by disease size and histology is shown in Table 62-1. Local control was worse for patients with bulky disease (10 cm or larger). Increased local recurrence has also been reported by Bush and Gospodarowicz[70] for patients with nodes larger than 5 cm. Initial chemotherapy and radiation therapy appears to reduce the frequency of recurrence and to improve the probability for local control of disease in patients with diffuse large cell lymphomas.[69] If both chemotherapy and radiation therapy are used, it may be possible to reduce the total dose of radiation therapy administered, but specific guidelines are not available.

Recommendations for radiation field size vary greatly for patients with stage I-II NHL. Even within individual reports, field sizes vary, and comparison of results is difficult

TABLE 62-1. Local Control After Radiation Therapy for Stage I and II Non-Hodgkin's Lymphoma

Disease Extent	Small Cell Histology*	Large Cell Histology*
<10 cm	34/34 (100%)	17/17 (100%)
≥10 cm	7/12 (57%)	6/11 (55%)

* Fractions represent number of patients with initial site of disease controlled over total number of patients. The median dose was 5000 cGy for large cell lymphomas, 3800 cGy for nodular lymphomas, and 4100 cGy for diffuse small cell lyphomas.
(Data from the Harvard Joint Center for Radiation Therapy)

because no corrections were made for tumor bulk or number of sites involved. There is no evidence, however, that large extended or total nodal irradiation fields add substantially to the freedom from relapse in stage I-II patients, as compared with involved or limited fields.[79] An analysis of recurrence patterns in patients treated with involved or limited fields has helped provide additional information (Table 62-2). Involved-field recurrences were seen only in patients with bulky (10 cm or larger) abdominal or mediastinal disease. Extranodal recurrences occurred 25% of the time. Transdiaphragmatic sites were the most common location for nodal recurrences and made up 40% of all relapses. Only 10% of relapses were contiguous. Fuks and colleagues[79] reported that the primary site of failure for patients treated with limited irradiation for NHL was in nonirradiated lymph node regions; noncontiguous lymph nodes were sites for recurrence more frequently than contiguous lymph node regions. Chen and colleagues[66] reported that contiguous nodal recurrences made up only 11% of all relapses in their study. Thus, contiguous relapses in NHL patients after treatment with involved-field or regional radiation therapy are rare, and even using larger fields (less than TLI) often does not cover potential nodal sites of relapse.

Influence of Histology

Low-grade lymphomas (diffuse lymphocytic, well-differentiated; nodular mixed; nodular lymphocytic, poorly differentiated). Patients with stage I-II nodular small cell lymphomas have an excellent probability of surviving 10 years after local-regional radiation therapy alone.[65,66] There is some debate about whether these patients are curable. In support of curative treatment, two studies demonstrate flattening of the relapse-free survival curve 4 to 5 years after local-regional radiation therapy. Of 130 stage IA-IIA nodular NHL patients treated with radiation therapy alone, over 70% were alive and 50% were free from first relapse at 10 years.[78] There were no relapses more than 6 years after treatment. Similar results for patients with low-grade stage I-II NHL are reported by Paryani and colleagues.[80] Patients younger than 40 years of age had a significantly better rate of survival than older patients, and a flat FFR curve was seen for this younger subset of patients. Patients with low-grade stage I-II NHL should be treated with local-regional radiation therapy.

Intermediate-grade lymphomas (diffuse lymphocytic, poorly differentiated; diffuse mixed; nodular histiocytic, excluding diffuse histiocytic). Information regarding FFR and survival after local-regional radiation therapy alone for stage I-II patients with intermediate-prognosis lymphomas is sparse, and the 5-year survival is not as good as that seen for the nodular lymphoma patients.[65,66] For patients with nonbulky stage I or limited stage II disease, the FFR and survival at 6 years after local-regional radiation therapy was greater than 80% in one study.[69] Similarly, another study reported a 70% 10-year FFR for stage I-II patients younger than 60 years of age who did not have bulky disease.[70] In contrast, patients older than 60 years of age or with bulky disease had a substantially worse prognosis with radiation therapy alone.[69,70]

Intermediate- to high-grade lymphomas (diffuse histiocytic; diffuse immunoblastic). The diffuse, large cell (cleaved or noncleaved) lymphomas are classified as intermediate-grade lymphomas by the working formulation. These have been combined, however, with the diffuse large cell immunoblastic (high-grade) lymphomas for this discussion because treatment recommendations and prognosis are similar for these histologic groups.

A number of trials have demonstrated that radiation therapy followed by combination chemotherapy improves the disease-free and overall survival compared with treatment with radiation therapy alone for stage I-II large cell lymphoma patients.[75,76,81,82] Results from a retrospective analysis of stage I-II patients with diffuse large cell or diffuse undifferentiated histology treated at the JCRT are shown in Table 62-3. Patients with stage I-II nonbulky disease (smaller than 10 cm, two sites or less) had a significantly better FFR and survival than patients with stage I-II extended disease (more than two sites or disease extent 10 cm or larger). Within each subgroup, the use of combination chemotherapy significantly improved the FFR and survival rates as compared with radiation therapy alone with chemotherapy reserved for relapse. All these results suggest that chemotherapy may not be as effective at the time of relapse as when used initially for patients with early-stage high-grade lymphomas.

The efficacy of combination chemotherapy alone in the treatment of patients with advanced diffuse large cell lymphomas[83–86] has led to its proposed use in stage I-II patients.[87] In this setting, the role for adjuvant involved-field irradiation after chemotherapy continues to be evaluated. Some studies favor its selected use,[69] argue against its use,[87] or present excellent results with chemotherapy and involved-field irradiation without studying the role of each.[88] A potential advantage of involved-field irradiation may include the ability to reduce the number of cycles of chemotherapy; this needs further study.

Little data are available to recommend specific chemotherapy combinations for stage I-II diffuse large cell lym-

TABLE 62-2. Number and Sites of Relapse in 74 Stage I and II Patients Treated With Radiation Therapy Alone

Site of Relapse	Disease Size <10 cm	Disease Size ≥10 cm	Total No. of Relapses (% by Site)
Initial site	0	10	10 (25)
Contiguous site	4	0	4 (10)
Transdiaphragmatic nodal	10	6	16 (40)
Extranodal	6	4	10 (25)
Recurrences/patients treated*	20/51	20/23	40/74

* Contiguous, nodal recurrence in a lymph node group adjacent to the radiation field.
(Mauch R, Leonard R, Skarin A, et al. Improved survival following combined radiation therapy and chemotherapy for unfavorable prognosis stage I–II non-Hodgkin's lymphomas. J Clin Oncol 1985;3:1301)

TABLE 62-3. Stage I and II Diffuse Large Cell or Undifferentiated Non-Burkitt's, Non-Hodgkin's Lymphoma

Treatment Modality	Disease Size <10 cm (No. of Patients)	Disease Size ≥10 cm (No. of Patients)
FREEDOM FROM FIRST RELAPSE (at 6 y)		
CT or CMT	81% (23)	44% (23)
RT	52% (17)	9% (11)
P	0.3	0.001
SURVIVAL (at 6 y)		
CT or CMT	96%	56%
RT	61%	18%
P	0.03	0.003

CT, chemotherapy alone; CMT, chemotherapy and local field treatment; RT, radiation therapy alone; *P*, probability.
(Mauch R, Leonard R, Skarin A, et al. Improved survival following combined radiation therapy and chemotherapy for unfavorable prognosis stage I–II non-Hodgkin's lymphomas. J Clin Oncol 1985;3:1301)

phoma patients. One series reported an advantage to the BACOP combination chemotherapy regimen (bleomycin, Adriamycin [doxorubicin], cyclophosphamide, Oncovin [vincristine], and prednisone) plus radiation therapy as compared with the CVP combination chemotherapy regimen (cyclophosphamide, vincristine, and prednisone) plus radiation therapy.[89] No other comparative studies of different combination chemotherapy regimens are available for early-stage patients. Until further information is available, the type of combination chemotherapy recommended should reflect that routinely used for stage III-IV disease.

Extranodal Lymphomas

Few guidelines have been developed for the treatment of early-stage NHL arising in specific extranodal sites in spite of a large number of reported studies. Since involvement of each specific site is rare, these studies are often faulted for small numbers of patients, a variable treatment policy extending over a long period of time, and a mix of histologic subtypes, the distribution of which may vary from site to site. It has been reported that early-stage patients with lymphomatous involvement of certain specific sites may have a better prognosis than those with such involvement of other sites. For example, patients with primary lymphoma of the thyroid or stomach have been reported to have an especially favorable disease course. It appears, however, that once variations in histology and bulk are accounted for, with few exceptions, patients with early-stage disease have similar prognoses regardless of initial site of involvement. Several large series support this. In a retrospective study of stage I-II patients with primary gastrointestinal lymphomas, separate analysis by histologic subtype using the Rappaport, Lukes-Collins, or Kiel classifications revealed marked differences in prognosis by subtype.[90] Similar differences in prognosis based on histology have been reported for cutaneous malignant lymphomas.[91] In an analysis of 111 patients with stage I-II diffuse NHL (over 80% were diffuse histiocytic), specific survival analysis by site of presentation revealed no differences in 5-year survivals.[92] Thus, once patients were stratified by histology, prognostic differences were not seen.

The general treatment philosophy for patients with extranodal NHL should be similar to that for patients with nodal presentations. For example, if early-stage diffuse large cell nodal lymphomas are treated with chemotherapy and adjuvant radiation therapy, then a similar plan should be used for patients with extranodal presentations. Within each specific extranodal site, however, treatment refinements or alterations may be needed. Some limited examples of this are illustrated next. Patients with primary testicular lymphomas when treated with local-regional radiation therapy have a high risk of recurrence in nodal sites above the diaphragm[89] and in the retroperitoneum, lung, and central nervous system (CNS).[93] Thus, local-regional radiation therapy is probably not sufficient treatment for these patients regardless of histology. Resection of gastric lymphomas by subtotal gastrectomy often reduces the risk of perforation, improves local control, and may reduce the need for adjacent radiation therapy.[94] Different sites may have distinctly different prognostic features. For example, gastric lymphomas extending through the wall or involving nodes have a worse prognosis. Diffuse large cell lymphomas with a pattern of diffuse sclerosis that involves bulky mediastinal or retroperitoneal nodes appear in some studies to have a worse prognosis than tumors without sclerosis.[95–97] Patients with paranasal sinus lymphomas may have a high percentage of CNS recurrence, and some have recommended prophylactic CNS irradiation for these patients.[98]

Lymphomas can involve the orbit, conjunctiva, or the eye itself and respond to local-regional radiation therapy with similar success as other lymphoma sites.[99] Local-regional radiation therapy should be used alone for low- and intermediate-grade lymphomas of the orbit or conjunctiva. Large cell patients have a high risk of developing a CNS relapse. These patients should receive orbital plus CNS treatment.[100]

Primary lymphoma of the brain has a poor prognosis, and patients have a high risk of local recurrence in most series. Although the numbers are small, better survival has been seen with initial tumor resection and with higher radiation doses. It is difficult to demonstrate an advantage for whole-brain irradiation over local tumor irradiation, but most series use large fields initially. Even with high doses (5000 cGy or more) and large fields, however, the local failure rate is significant. Some preliminary observations with high-dose methotrexate followed by cranial irradiation have yielded promising results.[101] This is an area that needs continued investigation.

Low-Grade Disease

Wide-field irradiation played a major role in the treatment of patients with stage III-IV nodular small cell lymphomas in the past. The use of this approach in the current management of NHL is limited because of the availability of effective chemotherapy, bone marrow transplantation as an alternative for patients with advanced lymphomas, and a better appreciation of the long-term toxicities of large-field irradiation. The results of treatment with low-dose total-body irradiation (TBI) and high-dose total-node irradiation are briefly summarized next.

Medinger and Craver[102] first reported an improvement in the median survival rates of patients with advanced-stage low-grade lymphomas treated with low-dose TBI, as compared with involved-field radiation therapy alone. Subsequently, a number of studies evaluated the effectiveness of TBI administered at 15 cGy twice weekly for 5 weeks to a total of 150 cGy,[103] or 10 cGy administered three times a week to a total of 100 to 150 cGy, with a second course given 8 weeks later if needed.[104] Areas of bulk disease were often boosted with involved-field radiation therapy. Thrombocytopenia (fewer than 40,000 platelets/μL) was seen in 40% of patients. Previously untreated patients had a 69% to 80% complete remission rate and a 3-year survival similar to that seen with the CVP combination chemotherapy regimen. Patients with intermediate- or high-grade tumors did considerably worse.[103,105,106] Although a few patients with tumors of low-grade histology remain disease free after 10 years, there is no convincing evidence that low-dose TBI provides curative treatment.[105] The treatment is easily administered but toxic to the marrow and rarely used.

High-dose wide-field radiation therapy alone has also been used for treatment of stage III nodular lymphomas.[107,108] Treatment has included TLI along with irradiation of the spleen, mesenteric nodes, and Waldeyer's ring. Even with such extensive treatment, there is no evidence for a flattening of the disease-free survival curve, and survival is no better than with less intensive regimens. One study identified a group of stage IIIA follicular lymphoma patients with less than five sites of involvement and disease extent smaller than 10 cm that appeared to have a flattening of the FFR curve.[109] This presentation is unusual, however, and the group of patients small. The use of routine wide-field irradiation alone for patients with low-grade stage III NHL is no longer optimal because of the high relapse rates, the high rate of histologic conversion, and the inability to give intensive treatment at relapse due to prior marrow toxicity.

As an alternative approach, some have proposed the use of both intensive radiation therapy and chemotherapy for stage III follicular lymphoma patients. Results with the CHOP-Bleo combination chemotherapy regimen (cyclophosphamide, doxorubicin, vincristine, prednisone, and bleomycin) and wide-field irradiation have been reported. Longer follow-up is needed, but there is no convincing evidence that this regimen is curative.[110]

The standard recommended treatment for patients with low-grade stage III-IV NHL is careful observation for asymptomatic patients with minimal disease and mild cytotoxic therapy for symptomatic patients.[111,112] More intensive combination chemotherapy or high-dose cyclophosphamide and TBI followed by bone marrow transplantation should be reserved for patients with more aggressive disease, with histologic conversion to a higher grade, or in clinical trials. This initial treatment approach could change if evidence for cure is demonstrated in investigational studies. In the meantime, this conservative approach reduces toxicity and appears not to compromise subsequent therapeutic options. High-dose TBI for recipient preparation for autologous bone marrow transplantation for advanced or relapsed lymphoma patients is covered elsewhere in this book.

Leukemia and Myeloma

The primary treatment for the leukemias and multiple myeloma is systemic therapy. The overall management of these disease entities is described elsewhere in this book. The role of radiation therapy in the overall management of these patients is complex and depends on the overall treatment plan. Therefore, only a few of the principles of radiation therapy are included here.

Acute Lymphoblastic Leukemia and Lymphoma

The predominant role for radiation therapy is for CNS prophylaxis.[113–117] Having been employed routinely in the past, the delayed toxicity of CNS dysfunction has led to a reconsideration of the routine use of radiation therapy. Whether the dysfunction is due to the radiation, the intrathecal therapy, or some combination of the two remains to be firmly established. Nevertheless, it is becoming clear that low-risk patients (3 to 6 years of age, leukocyte count less than 10,000/μL) can be adequately treated with intrathecal therapy alone.[114] Radiation therapy is occasionally used for palliation or for salvage for CNS[117] or testicular relapse.[118] In general, with the current intensive induction regimens, most patients with relapse in these sites soon experience a systemic relapse as well. Thus, although the irradiation may offer prolonged control of these sites, most of these patients require additional systemic treatment. In a recent study, cranial irradiation in the treatment of hyperleukocytosis at the time of diagnosis was not shown to be of benefit.[119]

Chronic Leukemias

Radiation is primarily used for local palliation for chronic myelogenous leukemia and chronic lymphocytic leukemia. The site most frequently palliated is the spleen. In general, radiation is administered cautiously to avoid serious blood count depression. Usually, a dose of 25 to 50 cGy is administered three to five times a week. Symptomatic pain relief occurs in most patients, but spleen-related anemia or thrombocytopenia is rarely corrected.[120,121] There is no clear dose–response relation, so the treatment and total dose often are titrated until symptoms are relieved or until the blood counts no longer permit additional treatment. When other sites are palliated, the local disease can be surprisingly resistant. This is commonly seen in patients who have circulating malignant cells. Often, the combination of systemic therapy plus local treatment provides the best local palliation.

Solitary Plasmacytoma and Multiple Myeloma

Solitary plasmacytomas may occur in bone or in soft tissue. Although most series contain a small number of patients, it appears that the patients with osseous plasmacytomas are more likely to develop multifocal plasmacytomas or multiple myeloma than are patients with soft tissue disease.[122–126] Radiation therapy produces long-term control in more than 80% of irradiated sites. The precise dose needed has been debated, but at least 4000 to 5500 cGy should be administered.[124–126]

Radiation is often used as palliation for patients with bony lesions from multiple myeloma. A typical palliative regimen might be 3000 cGy every 2 weeks. The dose and fractionation must be tailored to the clinical setting. A patient with newly diagnosed multiple myeloma who is expected to live many years should be treated with a higher total dose and a lower dose per fraction. Lesions near the spine cord should be treated with a dose equivalent to 4000 cGy because a local failure would be hard to retreat. Occasionally, hemi-body irradiation may be used to palliate patients with involvement of multiple bony sites.

Large-field irradiation has been attempted as a means of consolidating initial chemotherapy for patients with multiple myeloma. McIntyre and colleagues[127] reported that total bone marrow irradiation of 1500 cGy did not benefit the few patients who were able to complete treatment. In this trial of 20 patients, 6 did not respond to melphalan, and an additional 8 were not able to complete the prescribed dose. Although only limited data are available, it appears that this approach is unlikely to be of major clinical benefit.

REFERENCES

1. Perez CA, Brady LW. Introduction. In: Principles and practice of radiation oncology. Philadelphia, JB Lippincott, 1987:1.
2. Hall EJ. Radiobiology for the radiologist, ed 4. Philadelphia, JB Lippincott, 1994.
3. Thomlinson RH, Gray LH. The histological structure of some human

lung cancers and possible implications for radiotherapy. Br J Cancer 1955;9:539.
4. Puck TT, Marcus PT. Action of x-rays on mammalian cells. J Exp Med 1956;103:653.
5. Withers HR. Biologic basis of radiation therapy. In: Perez CA, Brady LW, eds. Principles and practice of radiation oncology. Philadelphia, JB Lippincott, 1987:67.
6. Purdy JA, Lightfoot DA, Glasgow GP. Principles of radiologic physics, dosimetry and treatment planning. In: Perez CA, Brady LW, eds. Principles and practice of radiation oncology. Philadelphia, JB Lippincott, 1987:129.
7. Kahn FM. In: The physics of radiation therapy. Baltimore, Williams & Wilkins, 1984:354.
8. Glasgow GP, Perez CA. Physics of brachytherapy. In: Perez CA, Brady LW, eds. Principles and practice of radiation oncology. Philadelphia, JB Lippincott, 1987:213.
9. Glasgow GP, Sampiere VA, Purdy JA. External beam dosimetry and treatment planning. In: Perez CA, Brady LW, eds. Principles and practice of radiation oncology. Philadelphia, JB Lippincott, 1987:159.
10. Elkind MM. DNA damage and cell killing: cause and effect? Cancer 1985;56:2351.
11. Ward JF. Mechanisms of DNA repair and their potential modification for radiotherapy. Int J Radiat Oncol Biol Phys 1986;12:1027.
12. Fertil B, Malaise EP. Intrinsic radiosensitivity of human cell lines is correlated with radioresponsiveness of human tumors: analysis of 101 published survival curves. Int J Radiat Oncol Biol Phys 1985;11:1699.
13. Weichelbaum RR, Dahlberg W, Little JB. Inherently radioresistant cells exist in some human tumors. Proc Natl Acad Sci USA 1985;82:4732.
14. Coleman CN. Hypoxia in tumors: a paradigm for the approach to biochemical and physiologic heterogeneity. JNCI 1988;80:310.
15. Coleman CN, Bump EA, Kramer RA. Chemical modifiers of cancer treatment. J Clin Oncol 1988;6:709.
16. Herman TS, Teicher BA. Sequencing of trimodality therapy [cis-diamminedichloroplatinum(II)/hyperthermia/radiation] as determined by tumor growth delay and tumor cell survival in the FSaIIc fibrosarcoma. Cancer Res 1988;48:2693.
17. Steel GG. The search for therapeutic gain in the combination of radiotherapy and chemotherapy. Radiother Oncol 1988;11:31.
18. Coleman CN, Howes AE. Overall principles of cancer management. In: Massachusetts American Cancer Society manual. Boston, American Cancer Society, 1990:57.
19. Carmel RJ, Kaplan HS. Mantle irradiation in Hodgkin's disease: an analysis of technique, tumor eradication, and complications. Cancer 1976;37:2813.
20. Salner AL, Botnick LE, Herzog AG, et al. Reversible brachial plexopathy following primary radiation therapy for breast cancer. Cancer Treat Rep 1981;65:797.
21. Castellino RA, Glatstein E, Turbow MM, et al. Latent radiation injury of lungs or heart activated by steriod withdrawal. Ann Intern Med 1974;80:593.
22. Byhardt RW, Abrams R, Almagro U. The association of adult respiratory distress syndrome (ARDS) with thoracic irradiation (RT). Int J Radiat Oncol Biol Phys 1988;15:1441.
23. Tucker MA, Coleman CN, Cox RS, et al. Risk of second cancer after treatment for Hodgkin's disease. N Engl J Med 1988;318:76.
24. Mauch P, Silver B, Yeap B, Larson D, Osteen R, Hellman S. Factor analysis in predicting for positive surgical staging in Hodgkin's disease (HD). Proc Am Soc Clin Oncol 1988;7:224.
25. Hoppe RT, Coleman CN, Cox RS, et al. The management of stage I-II Hodgkin's disease with irradiation alone or combined modality therapy: the Stanford experience. Blood 1982;59:455.
26. Mauch P, Tarbell N, Weinstein H, et al. Stage IA-IIA supradiaphragmatic Hodgkin's disease: prognostic factors in surgically staged patients treated with mantle and para-aortic irradiation. J Clin Oncol 1988;6:1576.
27. Crnkovich MJ, Leopold K, Hoppe RT, Mauch PM. Stage I to IIB Hodgkin's disease: the combined experience at Stanford University and the Joint Center for Radiation Therapy. J Clin Oncol 1987;5:1041.
28. Rosenberg SA, Kaplan HS. The evolution and summary results of the Stanford randomized clinical trials of the management of Hodgkin's disease. Int J Radiat Oncol Biol Phys 1985;11:5.
29. Hanks GE, Kinzie J, White RL, et al. Patterns of care outcome studies: results of the national practice in Hodgkin's disease. Cancer 1983;51:569.
30. Paliwal BR, Asp L. A technique to evaluate styrofoam cutouts used in irregular field shaping. Int J Radiat Oncol Biol Phys 1976;1:791.
31. Powers WE, Kinzie JJ, Demidecki AJ, et al. A new system of field shaping for external beam radiation therapy. Radiology 1973;108:407.
32. Mauch P, Goodman R, Hellman S. The significance of mediastinal involvement in early stage Hodgkin's disease. Cancer 1978;42:1039.
33. Tarbell NJ, Thompson L, Mauch P. Thoracic irradiation in Hodgkin's disease: disease control and long-term complications. Int J Radiat Oncol Biol Phys 1990;18:275.
34. Willett CG, Linggood RM, Stracher MA, et al. The effect of the respiratory cycle on mediastinal and lung dimensions in Hodgkin's disease. Cancer 1987;60:1232.
35. Chayt KJ, Svensson G, Rhodes LP, Mauch PM. Treatment of Hodgkin's disease patients with bulky mediastinal nodes in the upright position. Int J Radiat Oncol Biol Phys 1989;17:139.
36. Host H, Vale JR. Lung function after mantle field irradiation in Hodgkin's disease. Cancer 1973;32:328.
37. Watchie J, Coleman CN, Raffin TA, et al. Minimal long-term cardiopulmonary dysfunction following treatment for Hodgkin's disease. Int J Radiat Oncol Biol Phys 1987;13:517.
38. Gomez GA, Park JJ, Panahon AM, et al. Heart size and function after radiation therapy to the mediastinum in patients with Hodgkin's disease. Cancer Treat Rep 1983;67:1099.
39. Perrault DJ, Levy M, Herman JD, et al. Echocardiographic abnormalities following cardiac radiation. J Clin Oncol 1985;3:546.
40. Brosius FC, Waller BF, Roberts WC. Radiation and heart disease: analysis of 16 young (aged 15 to 33 years) necropsy patients who received over 3,500 rads to the heart. Am J Med 1981;70:519.
41. McReynolds RA, Gold GL, Roberts WC. Coronary heart disease after mediastinal irradiation for Hodgkin's disease. Am J Med 1976;60:39.
42. Boivin JF, Hutchison GB. Coronary heart disease mortality after irradiation for Hodgkin's disease. Cancer 1982;49:2470.
43. Fuks Z, Glatstein E, Marsa GW, et al. Long-term effects of external radiation on the pituitary and thyroid glands. Cancer 1976;37:1152.
44. Glatstein E, McHardy-Young S, Brast N, et al. Alterations in serum thyrotropin (TSH) and thyroid function following radiotherapy in patients with malignant lymphoma. J Clin Endocrinol Metab 1971;32:833.
45. Mauch PM, Weinstein H, Botnick L, et al. An evaluation on long-term survival and treatment complications in children with Hodgkin's disease. Cancer 1983;51:925.
46. Nelson DF, Reddy KV, O'Mara RE, et al. Thyroid abnormalities following neck irradiation for Hodgkin's disease. Cancer 1978;42:2553.
47. McDougall IR, Coleman CN, Burke JS, et al. Thyroid carcinoma after high-dose external radiotherapy for Hodgkin's disease: report of three cases. Cancer 1980;45:2056.
48. Pretorius HT, Katikineni M, Kinsella TJ, et al. Thyroid nodules after high-dose external radiotherapy. JAMA 1982;247:3217.
49. Loeffler JS, Tarbell NT, Garber JR, Mauch PM. The development of Graves disease following radiation therapy for Hodgkin's disease. Int J Radiat Oncol Biol Phys 1988;14:175.
50. Wasnich RD, Grumet FC, Payne RO, et al. Graves ophthalmopathy following external neck irradiation for non-thyroidal neoplastic disease. J Clin Endocrinol Metab 1973;37:703.
51. Wara WM, Phillips TL, Sheline GE, et al. Radiation tolerance of the spinal cord. Cancer 1975;35:1558.
52. Page V, Gardner A, Karzmark CJ. Physical and dosimetric aspects of radiotherapy of malignant lymphomas. II. The inverted-Y technique. Radiology 1970;96:619.
53. Lutz W, Larsen RD. Technique to match mantle and paraaortic fields. Int J Radiat Oncol Biol Phys 1979;2:149.
54. Fraass BA, Tepper JE, Glatstein E, et al. Clinical use of a match-line wedge for adjacent megavoltage radiation field matching. Int J Radiat Oncol Biol Phys 1983;9:209.
55. Birkhead BM, Dobbs CE, Beard MF, et al. Assessment of renal function following irradiation of the intact spleen for Hodgkin's disease. Radiology 1979;130:473.
56. Ray GR, Trueblood HW, Enright LP, et al. Oophoropexy: a means of preserving ovarian function following pelvic megavoltage radiotherapy for Hodgkin's disease. Radiology 1970;96:175.
57. Horning SJ. Female reproductive potential after treatment for Hodgkin's disease. N Engl J Med 1981;304:1377.
58. Kinsella TJ, Fraass BA, Glatstein E. Late effects of radiation therapy in the treatment of Hodgkin's disease. Cancer Treat Rep 1982;66:991.
59. Cunningham J, Mauch P, Rosenthal DS, et al. Long-term complications of MOPP chemotherapy in patients with Hodgkin's disease. Cancer Treat Rep 1982;66:1015.
60. Speiser B, Rubin P, Casarett G. Aspermia following lower truncal irradiation in Hodgkin's disease. Cancer 1973;32:692.
61. Jackson HL, Hass AC, Sooby D, et al. The gonadal exposure of boys and young men treated with inverted "Y" fields: its reduction and genetic significance. Radiology 1970;96:181.
62. Rowley MJ, Leach DR, Warner GA, et al. Effect of graded doses of ionizing radiation on the human testis. Radiat Res 1974;59:665.
63. Chabner BA, Johnson RE, Young RC, et al. Sequential non-surgical and surgical staging of non-Hodgkin's lymphoma. Ann Intern Med 1976;85:149.
64. Anderson T, Chabner BA, Young RC, et al. Malignant lymphoma. I. The histology and staging of 473 patients at the National Cancer Institute. Cancer 1982;50:2699.
65. Reddy S, Saxena VS, Pellettiere EV, et al. Early nodal and extra nodal non-Hodgkin's lymphomas. Cancer 1977;40:98.
66. Chen MG, Prosnitz LR, Gonzalez-Serva A, et al. Results of radiotherapy in control of stage I and II non-Hodgkin's lymphoma. Cancer 1979;43:1245.
67. Carbone PP, Kaplan HS, Musshoff K, et al. Report of the Committee on Hodgkin's disease staging classification. Cancer Res 1971;31:1860.
68. Rosenberg SA. Validity of the Ann Arbor staging classification for the non-Hodgkin's lymphoma. Cancer Treat Rep 1977;61:1023.
69. Mauch P, Leonard R, Skarin A, et al. Improved survival following combined radiation therapy and chemotherapy for unfavorable prognosis stage I-II non-Hodgkin's lymphomas. J Clin Oncol 1985;3:1301.
70. Bush RS, Gospodarowicz M. The place of radiation therapy in the

management of patients with localized non-Hodgkin's lymphoma. In: Rosenberg SA, Kaplan HS, eds. Malignant lymphomas. Cambridge, MA, Academic Press, 1982:485.
71. Rudders RA, Kaddis M, DeLellis RA, et al. Nodular non-Hodgkin's lymphoma: factors influencing prognosis and indications for aggressive treatment. Cancer 1979;43:1643.
72. Ciampi A, Bush RS, Gospodarowicz M, et al. An approach to classifying prognostic factors related to survival experience for non-Hodgkin's lymphoma patients—based on a series of 982 patients: 1967–1975. Cancer 1981;47:621.
73. Shipp MA, Harrington DP, Klatt MM et al. Identification of major prognostic subgroups of patients with large-cell lymphoma treated with M-BACOD or M-BACOD. Ann Intern Med 1986;104:757.
74. Vokes EE, Ultmann JE, Golomb HM, et al. Long-term survival of patients with localized diffuse histiocytic lymphoma. J Clin Oncol 1985;3:1309.
75. Monfardini S, Banfi A, Bonadonna G, et al. Improved five year survival after combined radiotherapy-chemotherapy for stage I-II non-Hodgkin's lymphoma. Int J Radiat Oncol Biol Phys 1986;6:125.
76. Nissen NI, Ersbll J, Hansen HS, et al. A randomized study of radiotherapy versus radiotherapy plus chemotherapy in stage I-II non-Hodgkin's lymphomas. Cancer 1983;52:1.
77. Fuks Z, Kaplan HS. Recurrence rates following radiation therapy of nodular and diffuse malignant lymphomas. Radiology 1973;108:675.
78. Bush RS, Gospodarowicz M, Sturgeon J, et al. Radiation therapy of localized non-Hodgkin's lymphoma. Cancer Treat Rep 1977;61:1129.
79. Fuks Z, Glatstein E, Kaplan HS. Patterns of presentation and relapse in the non-Hodgkin's lymphomata. Br J Cancer 1975;31:286.
80. Paryani SB, Hoppe RT, Cox RS, et al. Analysis of non-Hodgkin's lymphomas with nodular and favorable histologies, stages I and II. Cancer 1983;52:2300.
81. Landberg TG, Hakansson LG, Moller TR, et al. CVP remission maintenance in stage I or II non-Hodgkin's lymphomas. Cancer 1979;44:831.
82. Carde P, Burgers JMV, von Glabbekem, et al. Combined radiotherapy–chemotherapy for early stage non-Hodgkin's lymphoma: the 1975–1980 EORTC controlled lymphoma trial. Radiother Oncol 1984;2:301.
83. Laurence J, Coleman M, Allen SL, et al. Combination chemotherapy of advanced diffuse histocytic lymphoma with the six-drug COP-BLAM regimen. Ann Intern Med 1982;97:190.
84. Skarin AT, Canellos GP, Rosenthal DS, et al. Improved prognosis of diffuse histiocytic and undifferentiated lymphoma by use of high dose methotrexate alternating with standard agents (M-BACOD). J Clin Oncol 1983;1:91.
85. Fisher RI, DeVita VT Jr, Hubbard SM, et al. Diffuse aggressive lymphomas: increased survival after alternating flexible sequences of Promace and MOPP chemotherapy. Ann Intern Med 1983;98:304.
86. Klimo P, Connors JM. MACOP-B chemotherapy for the treatment of diffuse large cell lymphoma. Ann Intern Med 1985;102:596.
87. Miller TP, Jones SE. Initial chemotherapy for clinically localized lymphomas of unfavorable histology. Blood 1983;62:413.
88. Longo DL, Glatstein E, Duffey PL, et al. Treatment of localized aggressive lymphomas with combination chemotherapy followed by involved-field radiation therapy. J Clin Oncol 1989;7:1295.
89. Bonnadonna G, Bajetta E, Lattuada A, et al. CVP Versus BACOP chemotherapy sequentially combined with irradiation in stage I-II diffuse non-Hodgkin's lymphomas. In: Jones SE, Salman SE, eds. Adjuvant therapy of cancer, ed 4. New York, Grune & Stratton, 1984:661.
90. Weingrad DN, DeCosse JJ, Sherlock P, et al. Primary gastrointestinal lymphoma: a 30 year review. Cancer 1986;49:1258.
91. Burke JS, Hoppe RT, Cibull ML, et al. Cutaneous malignant lymphoma: a pathologic study of 50 cases with clinical analysis of 37. Cancer 1981;37:300.
92. Paryani S, Hoppe RT, Burke JS, et al. Extralymphatic involvement in diffuse non-Hodgkin's lymphoma. J Clin Oncol 1983;1:682.
93. Paladugu RR, Bearman RM, Rappaport H. Malignant lymphoma with primary manifestation in the gonad: a clinicopathologic study of 38 patients. Cancer 1980;45:561.
94. Paulson S, Sheehan RG, Stone MJ, et al. Large cell lymphomas of the stomach: improved prognosis with complete resection of all intrinsic gastrointestinal disease. J Clin Oncol 1983;1:263.
95. Ree HJ, Leone LA, Crowley JP. Sclerosis in diffuse histocytic lymphoma. Cancer 1982;49:1636.
96. Miller JB, Variakojis D, Bitran JD, et al. Diffuse histiocytic lymphoma with sclerosis: a clinicopathologic entity frequently causing superior venacaval obstruction. Cancer 1981;47:748.
97. Trump DL, Mann RB. Diffuse large cell and undifferentiated lymphomas with prominent mediastinal involvement: a poor prognostic subset of patients with non-Hodgkin's lymphoma. Cancer 1982;50:277.
98. Jacobs C, Hoppe RT. Non-Hodgkin's lymphomas of head and neck extranodal sites. Int J Radiat Oncol Biol Phys 1985;11:357.
99. Kim YH, Fayos JV. Primary orbital lymphoma: a radiotherapeutic experience. Int J Radiat Oncol Biol Phys 1976;1:1099.
100. Margolis L, Fraser R, Lichter A, et al. The role of radiation therapy in the management of ocular reticulum cell sarcoma. Cancer 1980;45: 688.
101. Loeffler JS, Ervin TJ, Mauch P, et al. Primary lymphomas of the central nervous system: patterns of failure and factors that influence survival. J Clin Oncol 1985;3:490.
102. Medinger FG, Craver LF. Total body irradiation. AJR 1942;48:651.
103. Chaffey JT, Rosenthal DS, Maloney WC, et al. Total body irradiation as treatment for lymphosarcoma. Int J Radiat Oncol Biol Phys 1976;1: 399.
104. Johnson RE. Total body irradiation (TBI) as primary therapy for advanced lymphosarcoma. Cancer 1975;35:242.
105. Thar TL, Million RR, Noyes WD. Total body irradiation in non-Hodgkin's lymphoma. Int J Radiat Oncol Biol Phys 1979;5:171.
106. Lybeert ML, Meerwaldt JH, Deneve W. Long-term results of low dose total body irradiation for advanced non-Hodgkin's lymphoma. Int J Radiat Oncol Biol Phys 1987;13:1167.
107. Glatstein E, Fuks Z, Goffinet DR, et al. Non-Hodgkin's lymphomas of stage III extent: is total lymphoid irradiation appropriate treatment? Cancer 1976;37:2806.
108. Cox JD, Komaki R, Kun LE, et al. Stage III nodular lymphoreticular tumors (non-Hodgkin's lymphoma): results of central lymphatic irradiation. Cancer 1981;47:2247.
109. Paryani SB, Hoppe RT, Cox RS, et al. The role of radiation therapy in the management of stage III follicular lymphomas. J Clin Oncol 1984;2: 841.
110. McLaughlin P, Fuller LM, Velasquez WS, et al. Stage III follicular lymphoma: durable remissions with a combined chemotherapy radiotherapy regimen. J Clin Oncol 1987;5:867.
111. Rosenberg SA. The low grade non-Hodgkin's lymphomas: challenges and opportunities. J Clin Oncol 1985;3:299.
112. Ezdinli EZ, Anderson JR, Melvin F, et al. Moderate versus aggressive chemotherapy of nodular lymphocytic poorly differentiated lymphoma. J Clin Oncol 1985;3:769.
113. Ortega JA, Nesbit ME, Sather HN, et al. Long-term evaluation of a CNS prophylaxis trial-treatment comparisons and outcome after CNS relapse in childhood ALL: a report from the Children's Cancer Study Group. J Clin Oncol 1987;5:1646.
114. Littman P, Coccia P, Bleyer WA, et al. Central nervous system (CNS) prophylaxis in children with low risk acute lymphoblastic leukemia (ALL). Int J Radiat Oncol Biol Phys 1987;13:1443.
115. Clavell LA, Gelber RD, Cohen HJ, et al. Four-agent induction and intensive asparaginase therapy for treatment of childhood acute lymphoblastic leukemia. N Engl J Med 1986;315:657.
116. Coleman CN, Picozzi VJ, Cox RS, et al. Treatment of lymphoblastic lymphoma in adults. J Clin Oncol 1986;4:1628.
117. Kim TH, Ramsay NK, Steeves RA, et al. Intermittent central nervous system irradiation and chemotherapy for central nervous system leukemia in children. Int J Radiat Oncol Biol Phys 1987;13:1451.
118. Kim TH, Hargreaves HK, Chan WC, et al. Sequential testicular biopsies in childhood acute lymphocytic leukemia. Cancer 1986;57:1038.
119. Maurer HS, Steinherz PG, Gaynon PS, et al. The effect of initial management of hyperleukocytosis on early complications and outcome of children with acute lymphoblastic leukemia. J Clin Oncol 1988;6:1425.
120. Wagner H, McKeough PG, Desforges J, et al. Splenic irradiation in the treatment of patients with chronic myelogenous leukemia or myelofibrosis with myeloid metaplasia: results of daily and intermittent fractionation with and without concomitant hydroxyurea. Cancer 1986;58:1204.
121. Guiney MJ, Liew KH, Quong GG, et al. A study of splenic irradiation in chronic lymphocytic leukemia. Int J Radiat Oncol Biol Phys 1989;16: 225.
122. Meis JM, Butler JJ, Osborne BM, et al. Solitary plasmacytomas of bone and extremedullary plasmacytomas: a clinicopathologic and immunohistochemical study. Cancer 1987;59:1475.
123. Knowling MA, Harwood AR, Bergsagel DE. Comparison of extramedullary plasmacytomas with solitary and multiple plasma cell tumors of bone. J Clin Oncol 1983;1:255.
124. Mendenhall CM, Thar TL, Million RR. Solitary plasmacytoma of bone and soft tissue. Int J Radiat Oncol Biol Phys 1980;6:1497.
125. Mill WB, Griffith R. The role of radiation therapy in the management of plasma cell tumors. Cancer 1980;45:647.
126. Mill WB, Wasserman TH. Multiple myeloma and plasmacytomas. In: Perez CA, Brady LW, eds. Principles and practice of radiation oncology. Philadelphia, JB Lippincott, 1987:1086.
127. McIntyre OR, Tefft M, Propert K, et al. Melphalan and prednisone plus total bone marrow irradiation as initial treatment for multiple myeloma. Int J Radiat Oncol Biol Phys 1988;15:1007.

Blood: Principles and Practice of Hematology,
edited by Robert I. Handin, Samuel E. Lux, and Thomas P. Stossel.
J.B. Lippincott Company, Philadelphia © 1995.

63

Bone Marrow Transplantation

Joseph H. Antin
Brian R. Smith

Since the late 1950s, when the first tentative steps in marrow transplantation were undertaken, bone marrow transplantation has developed into a major therapeutic endeavor practiced at more than 200 transplant centers worldwide. The reasons for this widespread adoption of a complex, expensive, and difficult form of therapy are diverse; however, the primary motivation has been the ability to offer curative therapy to patients with previously incurable illnesses. The unique opportunity afforded by marrow grafting to observe the regeneration of the immune and hematopoietic systems, as well as the therapeutic value of the procedure, has stimulated the development of some form of marrow transplantation in many medical centers. As in many medical endeavors, however, the resolution of some problems has uncovered questions and dilemmas that are likely to keep experimental transplant units busy for years.

Although several intrepid clinicians attempted the therapeutic use of bone marrow before the development of immunosuppression,[1–3] the successful use of marrow transplantation awaited an understanding of immunosuppression and histocompatibility. The first indication that marrow grafting was possible was based on early studies in mice demonstrating that lethally irradiated rodents could be saved by shielding the spleen[4,5] or by the infusion of bone marrow.[6] Additional studies by a variety of investigators[1] demonstrated that the infused bone marrow could reestablish hematopoiesis in the irradiated host animal. Survival was poor in some of the animals,[7] but the reason was unclear until Billingham and Brent[8] first described diarrhea, sparse fur, skin lesions, an odd gait, and retarded growth in mice with transplants. They called this syndrome *runt disease*. The phenomenon was rapidly confirmed, and their observations were expanded by several groups. It was later realized that this secondary disease, or runt disease, was actually a graft-versus-host reaction (GVHR).[9,10–12] Billingham[10] summarized the available knowledge about GVHR and formulated the principle that GVHR occurs when immunologically competent cells are infused into an antigenically distinct recipient who is incapable of rejecting them. These immunologically active cells were soon demonstrated to be T lymphocytes.[13] The recognition of histocompatibility antigens in mice and humans led to strategies for the immunologic matching of host and recipient to facilitate engraftment and to prevent GVHR.[1,14,15] The stage was set for the application of marrow transplantation to human diseases.

The first modern attempts to use marrow transplantation clinically were undertaken by Thomas and colleagues in 1957.[16] They used unmatched marrow in an effort to treat malignancies in six patients. Although two patients had temporary signs of donor hematopoiesis, none of the patients survived. A radiation accident in Belgrade provided Mathé and coworkers[17] an opportunity to perform marrow transplantation in five patients using marrow from unrelated volunteers. Although temporary grafts were observed (based on red cell phenotyping), all the patients had recovery of endogenous hematopoiesis, and four survived. Indeed, the temporary support of hematopoiesis until autologous recovery was Mathé's goal. These encouraging studies led to another 154 reported marrow transplantations between 1959 and 1962.[18] Transplants were performed, using a variety of conditioning regimens, for aplastic anemia, leukemia, lymphoma, solid tumors, and immunodeficiencies; but because of the poor results, the number of marrow transplantations declined until 1968, when several investigators were successful in treating immunodeficiencies with marrow grafting.[19–21] Since then, the development of effective antibiotics, improvements in blood product support, and refinements in the understanding of immunosuppression, graft-versus-host disease (GVHD), and conditioning regimen toxicity have allowed the successful application of marrow transplantation to thousands of patients with marrow failure, immune defects, and malignancies.[22–24]

RATIONALE

The observation that hematopoietic stem cells obtained from bone marrow grow and mature indefinitely when infused into a suitable host led to the development of strategies for the use of this resource in overcoming the problems inherent in the treatment of diseases of hematopoietic origin. There are three primary uses for marrow transplantation: (1) to replace a missing hematopoietic or lymphoid component in disorders such as aplastic anemia or severe combined immunodeficiency syndrome (SCIDS); (2) to protect the recipient from dose-limiting myelotoxicity of intensive antineoplastic therapy for leukemia, lymphoma, and perhaps other malignancies; or (3) to allow the destruction of abnormal hematopoiesis (eg, thalassemia) and its replacement with normal stem cells. In some cases, there may also be a secondary benefit from the recognition and destruction or inhibition of residual host malignant

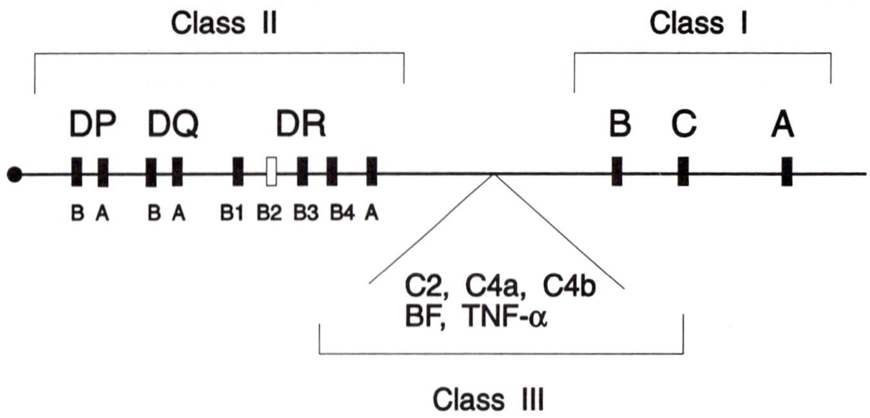

FIGURE 63-1. An example of a simplified schematic representation of the MHC locus on chromosome 6. The black circle indicates the relative position of the centromere. The solid bars are genes, and the open bar signifies a pseudogene.

cells by infused lymphocytes in a form of adoptive immunotherapy called the *graft-versus-leukemia (GVL) reaction.*

HLA CONSIDERATIONS

The human major histocompatibility complex (MHC) locus is a highly polymorphic area on the short arm of chromosome 6 that codes for the cell surface proteins that compose the HLA-A, B, and C antigens (class I MHC); those that constitute the HLA-DR, DP, and DQ antigens (class III MHC), and some additional proteins, such as glyoxalase and complement components C4A, C4B, factor B, and C2[14,15,25,26] (Fig. 63-1). The complement components (class II MHC) are polymorphic, and specific alleles can be detected and grouped into complotypes.[14] Besides DR, the class II MHC antigens are actually composed of at least two proteins, DP and DQ, which may also be important in determining compatibility, although less is known about the role of these antigens in bone marrow transplantation.[26] The class I histocompatibility gene complex proteins are expressed on nearly all nucleated cells, and the products of parental haplotypes are codominantly expressed (Fig. 63-2). Class II antigens are inducible on many cells, but they are constitutively expressed on some cells, such as B cells. HLA molecules are intrinsic to the function of the immune response since many foreign antigens must be recognized in association with host HLA proteins, and HLA antigens are crucial components of the interactions between T lymphocytes, macrophages, and other accessory cells. In an MHC-incompatible bone marrow transplantation, the recipient's MHC can be recognized as foreign by donor lymphocytes that do not share the same determinants, giving rise to GVHD. Similarly, host lymphocytes that persist after the pretransplantation conditioning regimen can recognize donor hematopoietic cells and reject the graft. In addition, the MHC mediates communication between T cells and accessory cells such as endothelial cells. This function is crucial for the recovery of the immune response of the patient, and failure of this communication may result in immunoincompetence despite successful engraftment.

The source of the marrow and the genetic relation of the donor and host determines the type of transplantation. In autologous bone marrow transplantation (ABMT), marrow or peripheral blood stem cells are removed from the patient and cryopreserved before the administration of cytotoxic therapy. After a suitable time for the drugs and metabolites to be excreted, the marrow is thawed and infused. It is not a marrow transplant per se, and it might be more accurately termed *autologous marrow, stem cell,* or *progenitor cell infusion.* If the donor is an identical twin, the transplant is termed *syngeneic.* Transplants performed using the bone marrow of donors other than identical twins are called *allogeneic.* Allogeneic transplants are either MHC matched, if all the MHC loci are shared, or MHC mismatched, if there are any histocompatibility differences. In Figure 63-2, sibling 1 and sibling 3 are HLA-identical, or fully matched—they received the same parental chromosomes. Siblings 2 and 4 are completely mismatched, while sibling 2 is haploidentical to siblings 1 and 3—they share a single chromosome. It is important to consider the genotype of the family as well as the phenotype. Sibling 1 differs from the mother by a single HLA-A antigen; even though the offspring share only one chromosome with the parent (they are haploidentical by genotype), they are considered partially matched. If the phenotype of one of the parents were homozygous, it would be difficult to tell whether two sib-

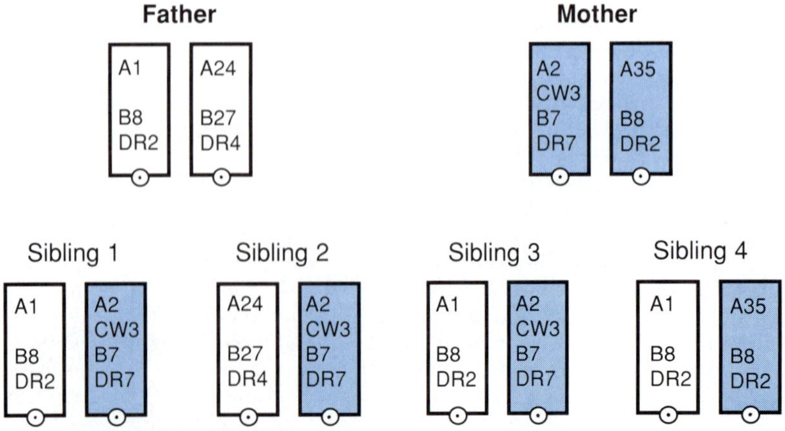

FIGURE 63-2. The chromosome on the left is from the father, and the one on the right is from the mother. The set of HLA antigens on a single chromosome is called a *haplotype.* Four combinations of haplotypes are possible, and each child has a 25% chance of receiving any one of them.

lings who appeared HLA-identical were matched because they received the same chromosomes (genotype match) or different chromosomes (phenotype match by genotype mismatch). Occasionally by chance a parent is HLA-compatible with an offspring—they are phenotypically matched, but unless there is extensive inbreeding, they are genetically haploidentical. The importance of these distinctions is that there may be important antigenic differences that are not measured with routine HLA typing. As reagents for studying the MHC have improved, many apparently discrete HLA antigens have been subdivided into two discrete antigens. These are referred to as *splits*. Thus, the A28 antigen has been split into Aw68 and Aw69. Molecular analysis of the MHC has revealed further heterogeneity.

Another level of complexity is introduced by the mixed lymphocyte culture (MLC). Some class II MHC antigens historically had been difficult to identify with typing sera, but lymphocytes respond to differences in class II MHC antigens by proliferating. Thus, patients who differ at class II MHC loci can be identified using MLC.

If the stimulator is a homozygous typing cell, MLC can be used to determine the HLA-D phenotype. (DR stands for D-related and is determined serologically; although the D and DR are similar, they are not identical.) HLA-D typing using homozygous typing cells is rarely done, and MLC is becoming a less important criterion of compatibility as molecular genetic approaches are more widely used. The results of MLC are indicated as reactive or nonreactive. Nonreactive MLC results are required to consider a donor–recipient pair to be matched. In practice, problems commonly arise in obtaining usable MLC results. It may not be possible to obtain an adequate number of reactive lymphocytes from an infant with SCIDS to perform a satisfactory MLC. Furthermore, the patient's T cells may proliferate poorly. Patients with chronic myelogenous leukemia (CML) may have high background counts because of proliferation of malignant myeloid cells, and it may be impossible to obtain adequate stimulator B cells (that constitutively express class II MHC antigens) to perform an MLC. It may be useful in these settings to examine complotypes. The complement components that share chromosome 6 are polymorphic, and because of linkage disequilibrium, this set of proteins tends to be inherited as a group with HLA antigens. Thus, if the complotype is informative, it may support class II MHC identity indirectly.[27]

The advent of the polymerase chain reaction (PCR) and other improvements in molecule biology have allowed further refinements in HLA typing. Two additional techniques deserve mention. Restriction fragment-length polymorphism (RFLP) analysis detects length differences in HLA alleles after digestion of DNA with restiction enzymes and hybridization with specific cDNA probes. RFLP studies have been helpful in assigning class II typing in some patients in whom serologic typing was unreliable. It is being supplanted by a more direct technique in which sequence-specific oligonucleotide probes recognizing specific DNA sequences in the hypervariable regions of the class II genes are amplified using PCR technology. A large panel of probes can be studied rapidly on very small amounts of DNA. This technique is proving extremely useful in defining previously unrecognized heterogeneity in the class II genes, and many of the serologically defined alleles can now be subtyped.[28,29] These developments have led to an alteration in nomenclature to distinguish serologically obtained typing from molecular genetic typing (Table 63-1). In the new nomenclature, B1 refers to the DRB1 gene (see Fig. 63-1). An asterisk indicates that the type was derived using molecular techniques. The first two numbers (eg, *04*01) refer to the old serologic specificity, and the last two numbers (eg, 04*01*)

TABLE 63-1. Nomenclature of DR4 Alleles

HLA Allele (SSOP)	HLA-DR Type (Serologic)	HLA-D-Associated Specificity (T-Cell Defined)
DRB1*0401	DR4	Dw4
DRB1*0402	DR4	Dw10
DRB1*0403	DR4	Dw13
DRB1*0404	DR4	Dw14
DRB1*0405	DR4	Dw15
DRB1*0406	DR4	Dw'KT2'
DRB1*0407	DR4	Dw13
DRB1*0408	DR4	Dw14
DRB1*0409	DR4	
DRB1*0410	DR4	
DRB1*0411	DR4	

(Adapted from Bodmer JG, Marsh SEG, Albert ED, et al. Nomenclature for factors of the HLA system, 1990. Hum Immunol 1991;31:186)

are the new specificity. The increase in heterogeneity is apparent. This new information may be particularly important in the selection of unrelated donors and in some families with homozygosity in the class II locus.

GVHD and graft rejection occur in substantial numbers of patients who received apparently fully matched allografts. Thus, it is likely that there are additional antigens that are important in determining compatibility. X-ray crystallography has been crucial in the understanding of the function of the MHC molecules.[30–32] These molecules have a peptide-binding cleft where the bulk of the polymorphism in these molecules is concentrated. This cleft binds either self or nonself (eg, viral) peptides and presents them to T lymphocytes.[33–36] These observations provide a framework for understanding why GVHD and graft rejection occur in patients who are otherwise MHC-compatible. Although the MHC is located on chromosome 6, it is likely that the other (self) peptides are coded elsewhere in the genome and are probably not identical, even in siblings. In MHC-matched, unrelated patients, differences are are even more likely, contributing to the high incidence of acute GVHD in these patients.[37] Furthermore, there are very minor sequence differences in the MHC proteins that may be detected by the donor lymphocytes. The subtlety of the immune system's ability to recognize small differences in HLA molecules was recently demonstrated when marrow graft rejection could be attributed to a single amino acid difference in HLA-B44.[38] Standard HLA typing and MLC cannot detect these differences; however, Vogelsang and colleagues[39] developed a skin explant model that allows the prediction of GVHD in HLA-compatible, MLC-nonreactive pairs. The general applicability of this test is unclear, but it was the first indication that alloreactivity based on minor histocompatibility antigens or factors other than MHC can be identified. Subsequent studies have suggested that limiting-dilution analysis of donor interleukin-2 secreting T-cell precursors may be another way of detecting reactivity to minor histocompatibility antigens.[40]

Occasionally, a crossover occurs in meiosis that results in transfer of DNA between parental chromosomes. In the example shown in Figure 63-2, the paternal somatic phenotype would be as shown, but some gametes might be A1, B8, DR4. Offspring from sperm with this genotype would not be HLA-identical to any of the siblings but would be single-antigen mismatches with siblings 1 and 3. Crossovers occur more rarely between HLA-A and HLA-B and sometimes occur between HLA-DR and HLA-D. If a crossover occurs in the class II MHC regions between HLA-DR and

HLA-D, the donor–recipient pair may be HLA-identical but MLC-reactive. This situation would also be considered a single-antigen mismatch, but the siblings are not genotypically haploidentical since some of the genetic material from the rearranged chromosome 6 is common to both.

The final data required are the results of a crossmatch. A crossmatch detects serum antibodies directed against the donor cell HLA antigens, and donors against whom antibodies are made are generally avoided.[41]

The determination of degree of mismatch requires one additional consideration, the direction or vector of the mismatch. If the recipient identifies the donor as foreign, the vector is said to be in the graft rejection direction; that is, if an allogeneic response occurs, the result is graft rejection. If the donor identifies foreign antigens on host cells, the vector is said to be in the GVHD direction. In Figure 63-3, if the father were to donate marrow for his offspring, paternal lymphocytes would only recognize the A2 antigens as foreign since the father's cells already express A1, B8, and DR2. This is a single-antigen mismatch in the graft-versus-host vector. The recipient's lymphocytes, however, recognize both B7 and DR4 as foreign; therefore, it is a two-antigen mismatch in the graft rejection vector. The mother and offspring are single-antigen mismatches in both directions, and thus, everything else being equal, the mother is the preferred donor. The same approach applies to MLC.

Calculations based on the average family size in the United States and Western Europe indicate that only 30% to 40% of people have HLA- and MLC-compatible siblings. Thus, most people with diseases that are susceptible to marrow grafting do not have compatible sibling donors. Several strategies may be considered to increase the pool of potential marrow donors, including ABMT; MHC-mismatched family members; fetal hematopoietic tissues (fully MHC-mismatched); and HLA compatible, unrelated donors. Except for autologous marrow, all these alternative sources of hematopoietic stem cells are considered MHC-mismatched. Fetal liver transplants are rarely performed.

The national Marrow Donor Program was developed to provide unrelated donor bone marrow for patients without histocompatible siblings. Because of the tremendous heterogeneity of the HLA system, it is unlikely that a patient is HLA and MLC identical to a stranger. Because of linkage disequilibrium, however, some HLA types are more common than others, particularly within ethnic or racial groups. Extensive calculations on the probability of finding unrelated donors have been performed by Beatty and colleagues[42] and are summarized next. The size of the donor pool is important in determining the likelihood of finding a compatible donor. If an HLA-A, B, or DR identical donor is sought, the average probability of finding at least one compatible person with hypothetical registries of 10,000 and 100,000 donors is 43% and 75%, respectively. If one also considers MLC and HLA-D compatibility, however, the likelihood decreases to 14% and 32%, respectively. The effects of linkage disequilibrium on these probabilities is profound. For example, a patient with common haplotypes, such as A1, A3, B7, B8, DR2, DR3, has a 69% chance of finding an MLC-nonreactive donor in a 1000-donor registry, while a patient with rare haplotypes, such as A1, A24, B35, Bw50, DR5, DR7, has a 21% chance of finding an MLC-nonreactive donor in a 100,000-donor registry. Similar calculations led to the conclusion that with a registry of 50,000 participants, 17% of patients have common haplotypes and a more than 90% chance of finding a donor; 48% of patients have uncommon haplotypes and a less than 10% chance of finding a donor; and the remainder of patients have a less than 50% chance of finding a compatible donor. Nevertheless, this form of marrow transplantation is being performed with increasing frequency.[43–46]

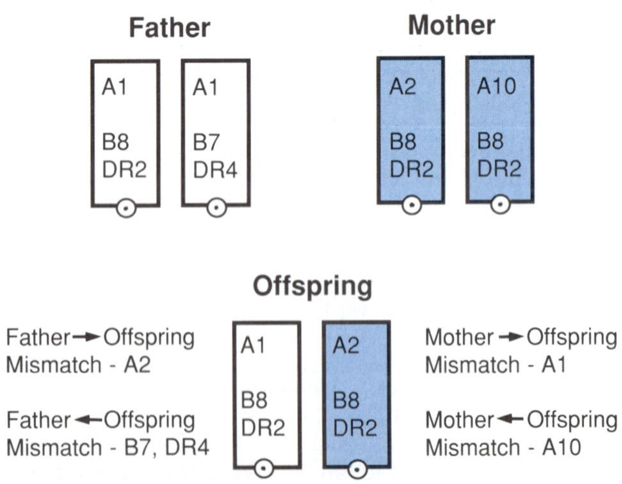

FIGURE 63-3. Schematic representation of the HLA complex demonstrating that the degree of mismatch in donor–recipient pairs depends on the vector. →, graft-versus-host vector; ←, graft rejection vector.

PRETRANSPLANTATION EVALUATION

Donor Selection

In a given family, there is a 25% probability that two siblings are a complete match, so the likelihood of finding a compatible donor depends on the family size. In some large families, there is more than one available sibling donor, and in some genetically restricted communities, there may be extended family members who match the patient. If only one donor is available, the decision about donor selection is simplified. This decision is based on determining that the donation of marrow does not entail significant risk to the donor and that the donor does not have a disease that can be transmitted to the recipient. The disease for which marrow grafting is being considered plays a major role in this determination. For example, patients with aplastic anemia can alternatively be treated with antithymocyte globulin (ATG) therapy, with about a 50% response rate. Thus, if the only acceptable marrow donor were pregnant, it would be preferable to treat the patient with ATG and consider marrow transplantation later, if the ATG were unsuccessful. In contrast, a patient with second- or subsequent-remission acute lymphocytic leukemia or CML in accelerated phase has few alternatives, and after appropriate consideration of the anesthesia risks, it might be reasonable to use a pregnant donor.

Donor Evaluation

Once one or more HLA- and MLC-compatible relatives have been identified, the donors must be evaluated for their own health and to determine the most appropriate donor if more than one is available. The procurement of marrow from small children is feasible but requires special care.[47] The components of a useful evaluation are listed in Table 63-2. The history has always been an important part of the evaluation of potential marrow donors. Prior experience with general or regional anesthesia may be important in assessing the risk of a procedure that has no physical benefit for the donor and that can occasionally be harmful.[48,49] Furthermore, if a donor is considered to be well and the conditioning regimen is initiated, but the donor is subsequently found to be ill or unable to be anesthetized (eg, malignant hyperthermia), then both the well donor and

TABLE 63-2. Transplant Donor and Recipient Evaluation Guidelines

DONOR EVALUATION

Complete history, especially of allergies or other indications of surgical or anesthetic risk, hepatitis, drug use, and sexual history

Physical examination

Complete blood count and differential

Chemistry profile

Viral serologies: herpes simplex, hepatitis C, hepatitis B surface antigen and antibody, Epstein-Barr virus, cytomegalovirus, human immunodeficiency virus, HTLV-I, HTLV-II

Red cell phenotyping: extended panel, including as many of the minor antigens as possible, such as Kell, Duffy, M, and N; leukocyte isoenzymes?; immunoglobulin isotypes?; restriction fragment length polymorphisms

Electrocardiogram

Chest radiograph

Urinalysis

Human chorionic gonadotropin

RECIPIENT EVALUATION

All of the above

Toxoplasmosis and varicella titers

Radionuclide ventriculogram or echocardiogram

Pulmonary function tests

Ophthalmologic evaluation

the irreversibly pancytopenic patient are at risk of death or serious morbidity. In recent years, the specter of human immunodeficiency virus (HIV) infection has become a major concern. Any potential donor must be screened for HIV antibodies; however, a small proportion of patients are viremic in the absence of antibody. The determination of the current and past sexual habits of potential donors and a review of possible risk factors is crucial. Unfortunately, although this aspect of donor evaluation should be simple, family members who have engaged in high-risk activities that may result in HIV infection may keep silent to avoid familial disapproval, and some may not realize they are engaged in high-risk behavior. It is important to have a separate interview with the potential donor to be sure that the history is accurate and, if necessary, to provide the HIV-seropositive or high-risk donor with a reasonable excuse for being unable to donate marrow. Screening for HTLV-1 and HTLV-2 is also important.

The need for physical examination, complete blood counts, urinalysis, and chemistry profile do not require further discussion, except to emphasize that these tests must be undertaken sufficiently in advance of the transplant that abnormalities are recognized before the start of the conditioning regimen. Viral serologies can provide useful information on which to base a decision to chose one available donor over another. For instance, cytomegalovirus (CMV) infection is one of the major hurdles encountered by patients with transplants. If the recipient has not been exposed to CMV, the use of marrow and blood products from CMV-negative donors dramatically reduces the risk of symptomatic CMV disease, while marrow and blood products from CMV-positive donors increase the risk of fatal CMV infection.[50] On the other hand, if the recipient is seropositive for CMV, the status of the donor is probably irrelevant since, in that setting, most clinical CMV disease is due to reactivation of endogenous virus.[51] The value of HIV testing is self-evident; there is no benefit in substituting one fatal disease for another.

Hepatitis B, hepatitis C, and Epstein-Barr virus (EBV) exposures are bigger problems. Clinical hepatitis B is to be expected if the donor has circulating HBsAg (presumably in association with active Dane's particles). The effects of hepatitis B acquired in this fashion in transplantation patients are variable.[52–54] Obviously, it is preferable to select a donor who has surface antibody or no exposure, but the presence of HBsAg should be considered in the context of the disease being treated. For newly diagnosed aplastic anemia, the use of ATG is preferable; if the patient failed to respond to immunosuppression, a transplant from a HBsAg-positive donor might be considered. Similarly, a patient with acute myelogenous leukemia would not receive a transplant in first remission in this setting but rather in relapse or subsequent remission. Similar considerations apply for hepatitis C. The clinical relevance of EBV infection is even less well understood. It is unlikely that an acute infectious mononucleosis-like syndrome would be detected in a patient who received a conditioning regimen since a large part of the syndrome of infectious mononucleosis is due to the reactive expansion of T lymphocytes. Furthermore, EBV exposure in the community is widespread, and clinical problems with acute EBV infection after marrow grafting are uncommon.[55–57] This relative lack of sequelae is surprising since the primary means of controlling the virus, T lymphocytes, are absent or dysfunctional. One would expect the uncontrolled proliferation of donor or residual host B lymphocytes in this milieu. Indeed, in HLA-mismatched transplants, a proportion of patients die from lymphoproliferative disorders in which EBV has been implicated.[58,59]

It may be useful to obtain blood samples for extended red cell typing,[60] leukocyte isoenzymes,[61] immunoglobulin (Ig) isotypes,[62] or RFLP[63] at the time of donor evaluation. These tests are particularly valuable in determining, with some degree of confidence, that twins are monozygotic. One can never be sure of monozygosity, but the more polymorphic determinants that are the same, the lower is the probability that they are dizygotic. Although the presence of informative polymorphisms is not ordinarily a factor in donor selection for nontwin siblings, if two donors are otherwise equivalent, it is preferable to use the donor with the more useful polymorphisms. This facilitates the determination of engraftment, the presence of mixed chimerism, and perhaps the occasional development of leukemia in donor cells.

Other factors that must be considered include the age and sex of the donors. Data indicate that the use of donors of the opposite sex (particularly female donors for male recipient) doubles the risk of GVHD.[64,65] Situations in which parous females donate to male recipients carry the highest risk. There is probably also an influence of donor age on the risk of GVHD, and it is generally believed that younger donors are preferable. The data on donor age are difficult to assess since siblings tend to be of similar ages and the risk may be largely confined to the age of the recipient. In inbred families or populations with limited genetic heterogeneity, there occasionally may be a potential donor who is not a sibling. In that case, the sibling is usually still considered the preferred donor, since non-HLA phenotypic differences are likely to play a role in graft rejection and GVHD. Other considerations, however, such as viral exposure or pregnancy, might make the extended family member the preferred donor.

Patient Evaluation

The primary concern in evaluating a patient for marrow grafting is the determination that the results of the procedure warrant the risks of the transplant. An accurate assessment of the risk requires a knowledge of the general health of the subject, that is, the subject's ability to withstand the rigors of the conditioning regimen, the risk of GVHD, the risk of relapse, and the risk of long-term morbidity related to immunosuppression.

Relatively few pretransplantation evaluations can accurately predict the risk of death or serious morbidity. Most of the poor prognostic features constitute relative rather than absolute contraindications to the procedure. It is important to provide the patient with an accurate estimate of risks, however, so that he or she may judge the merits of pursuing an expensive, uncomfortable, and potentially lethal procedure.

All conditioning regimens function on the borders of nonhematopoietic organ tolerance (discussed later). Consequently, organs that are compromised before the procedure are more likely to be injured during the conditioning regimen. The basic evaluation outlined in Table 63-2 can be used to assess risk in a general way. Electrocardiography, echocardiography or radionuclide scan, and chest radiography may detect the presence of anthracycline cardiotoxicity. If reduction in cardiac reserve is apparent, it would not be wise to subject the patient to high doses of known cardiac toxins such as cyclophosphamide. If marrow transplantation is to be undertaken, it might be more easily accomplished with etoposide and total-body irradiation (TBI)[66] or arabinosylcytosine and TBI.[67] Patients with normal hearts who have not had prior anthracyclines sometimes develop heart failure[68]; thus, the presence of clinical or subclinical cardiac dysfunction is likely to predict further reductions in cardiac performance. Conditioning regimens that rely on BCNU, busulfan, or TBI commonly result in progressive respiratory failure because of interstitial pneumonia. Studies have demonstrated that the presence of small degrees of airways obstruction before the transplantation predicts late (1 year or more) declines in forced expiratory volume and forced vital capacity.[69] Patients who previously received bleomycin or busulfan may be at further risk for progressive lung failure. Bleomycin-induced lung disease is best detected by measuring the carbon monoxide diffusing capacity.[70–73]

Liver injury due to venoocclusive disease can be predicted by the presence of abnormal liver function tests within the year preceding the marrow transplantation.[74] Because the mortality of venoocclusive disease is high, it is important to establish the presence of this risk factor in advance.

Hypertension may be exacerbated by the use of cyclosporine or steroids. Steroids and hyperalimentation may also worsen glucose intolerance. Any reduction in creatinine clearance may affect the ability to use nephrotoxins, such as cyclosporine, aminoglycosides, and amphotericin B. Conditioning regimens used for the treatment of solid tumors such as neuroblastomas often include nephrotoxins such as cisplatin or high-dose melphalan, and conditioning regimens that do not include classic nephrotoxins may also result in renal insufficiency after marrow transplantation,[75] possibly by causing or exacerbating radiation nephritis. Prior bladder injury in a patient who has received cyclophosphamide or ifosfamide may predispose to more severe injury after transplantation conditioning. In such patients, one should consider the use of urothelial protective agents, such as 2-mercaptoethanesulfonate (mesna; discussed later), or a regimen that does not include cyclophosphamide.

Ophthalmologic evaluation is often useful to detect evidence of prior CMV or toxoplasmosis. In addition, conditioning regimens and corticosteroids can cause cataracts, and it is valuable to have a baseline slit-lamp evaluation.[76,77]

As for donors, an evaluation of viral exposure is helpful before undertaking a marrow transplantation. The only absolute contraindication to marrow transplantation is HIV infection. Transplantation has been performed in patients who are infected with HIV,[78,79] but there has been no alteration in the presence of the virus. The virus infects nonhematopoietic cells, such as central nervous system neurons, that act as a reservoir for HIV and cause progressive neurologic dysfunction. The infection of these cells is not affected by the transplantation. Prior exposure to CMV denotes a high but not inevitable likelihood of CMV dissemination. As in the examples given previously, a CMV-positive patient with first-remission acute nonlymphocytic leukemia (ANLL) might be better served by waiting until relapse or subsequent remission. It is also helpful to know whether the patient has been exposed to varicella and herpes simplex viruses since prophylactic acyclovir can substantially reduce morbidity in patients harboring these infections. Toxoplasmosis can flare as a complication of immunosuppression, and prior knowledge of infection can assist in the differential diagnosis of problems that develop later. Hepatitis B antigenemia is another condition that probably predisposes to venoocclusive disease and that is likely to persist through the transplantation. Fulminant hepatitis B reactivation has been reported,[54] but the risk of transplantation does not appear to be excessive.[80] Recognition of this virus is important not only to properly evaluate the patient but also to protect staff against accidental exposures.

Thus, a complete medical evaluation allows the transplantation team to estimate the risks of the procedure and to minimize those risks. As noted previously, the presence of mild or in some cases moderate organ dysfunction may not be an absolute contraindication to marrow grafting but may affect the timing of transplantation and may significantly affect the assessment of the value of the procedure as it is presented to the patient.

BONE MARROW PROCUREMENT

Bone marrow is distributed throughout the axial skeleton, but anatomic constraints limit the reasonable sites for marrow procurement to the pelvis and sternum. Bone marrow is obtained from the donor under general or regional anesthesia by multiple needle aspirates of the iliac crests using large-gauge marrow aspirate needles, and the marrow is added to a heparinized electrolyte solution. Most groups attempt to obtain 1 to 4 $\times$ 10^8 nucleated cells per kilogram of recipient weight—in practice, this amounts to about 10 mL of marrow per kilogram of recipient weight. This volume of marrow amounts to 1% to 5% of the donor's total marrow volume, and its removal causes no cytopenia other than anemia proportionate to the blood loss. If the marrow is to be manipulated to remove T lymphocytes or malignant cells, there are substantial nonspecific losses, and 15 to 20 mL/kg is often obtained. Older donors may have less-cellular marrows, and relatively larger volumes may be required.[49] The marrow sample contains a substantial amount of particulate matter, including blood clots, bone particles, and fat, and is usually filtered through mesh before infusion into the patient. The stress placed on the donor is proportional to the size of the recipient. Often, if the donor is small, and a large amount of marrow is to be obtained, it is wise to phlebotomize the marrow donor 2 to 4 weeks in advance for autologous transfusion. This blood partially restores the donor's hematocrit after the marrow harvest.

The risk to the donor is small. Bortin and Buckner[48] reviewed 3290 marrow harvests and found a life-threatening complication rate of 0.27% and no deaths or permanent injuries. Cardiopulmonary events, cerebrovascular accidents, and infectious complications do occur, however, and donors need to be counseled appropriately. Pain persists for several days but sometimes longer. Occasional donors develop local neuropathies as a result of injury to the lateral femoral cutaneous nerve.

CONDITIONING REGIMENS

The treatment that precedes a marrow transplantation is generally referred to as the *conditioning regimen*. For a successful marrow graft to take place, a conditioning regimen must be established that satisfies the following criteria:

1. It must have the capacity to eradicate malignant (eg, leukemic) or abnormal (eg, thalassemic) cells when administered once over a brief period, while respecting the sensitivity of normal, nonhematopoietic tissues.
2. It must suppress the immune response of the recipient to prevent marrow rejection.
3. It may need to provide for the creation of space in the marrow for the newly infused bone marrow cells.[81]

Examples of conditioning regimens are shown in Figure 63-4.

Eradication of Abnormal Cells

Chemotherapy and radiation therapy kill malignant cells by first-order kinetics—they kill a fixed *proportion* of cancer cells. Thus, if a patient has a large leukemic cell burden,

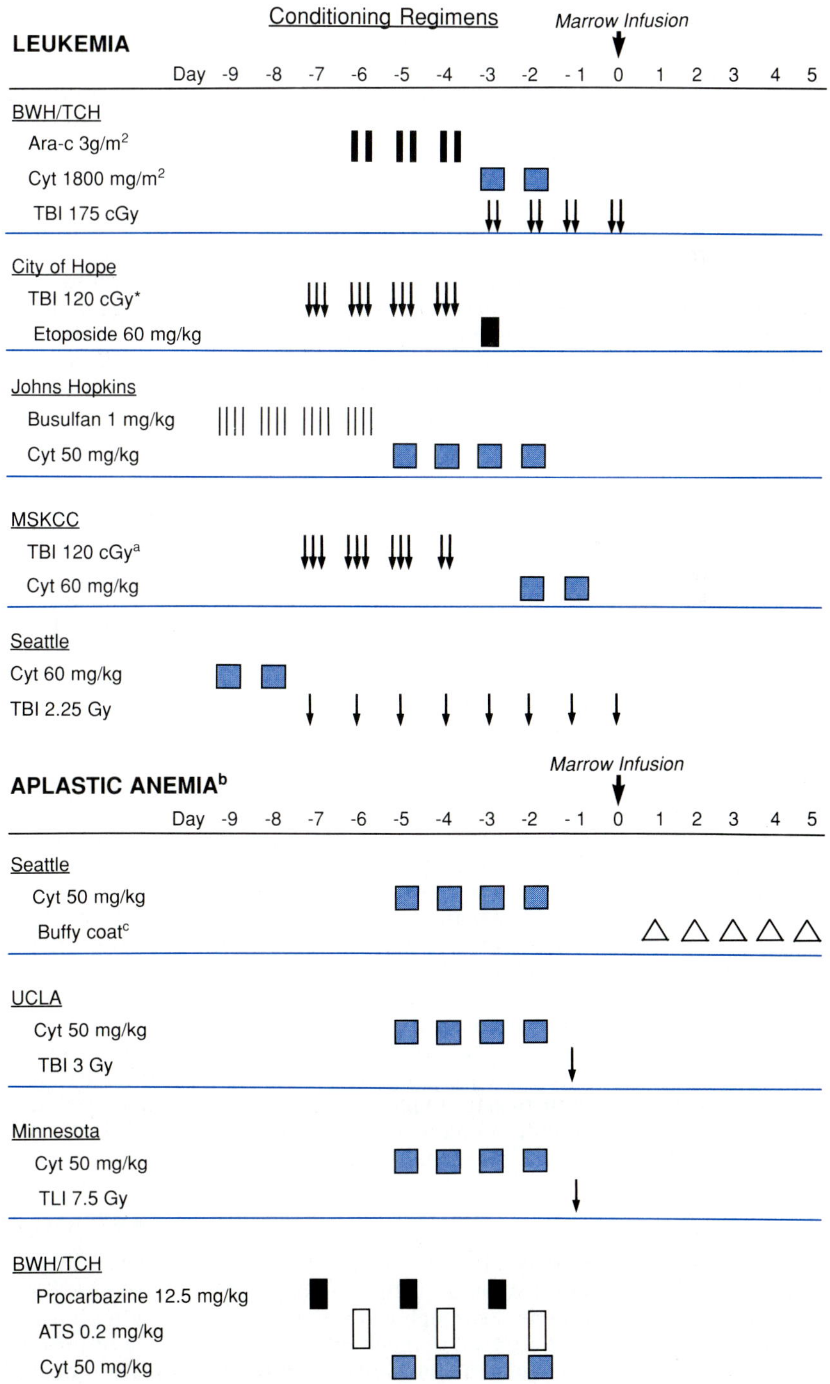

FIGURE 63-4. Conditioning regimens. [a]Data also include electron-beam radiation to the chest wall and to the testes for acute lymphoblastic leukemia. [b]Transfused patients. [c]Derived by leukapheresis of the donor and administered intravenously on days 1 to 3 or 1 to 5. (Data from references 66, 85, 90, 93, 457, 546, 548, 758, 759)

the efficacy of the conditioning regimen is determined by the balance between the number of leukemic cells destroyed and the number of these residual blasts with clonogenic capacity. Transplantation conditioning regimens attempt to exploit the steep dose–response relations that chemotherapy-sensitive tumors often demonstrate.[82] In contrast to standard nontransplantation therapy, in which moderate doses are administered repetitively over a long period, a single high dose is administered. Because sensitivity to drugs or drugs plus radiation is crucial to the success of this brief exposure to therapy, any effective therapy is more likely to cure the neoplasm if the number of cells treated is low and if the dose–response curve for the therapy is steep. Thus, eradication of the malignancy is easier when the malignant cell burden is minimal and the cells are not likely to have acquired a high degree of resistance. As a rule, this means that transplantation in early stages of disease is more likely to cure the neoplasm than if the procedure is undertaken after extensive, unsuccessful prior therapy. Nevertheless, it is likely that in some cases, the administration of very high doses of drugs or radiation can overcome even established, resistant cells.

The advantage of transplant conditioning regimens over standard chemotherapy is the ability to escalate the dose up a steep dose–response curve since myelotoxicity, which is the chief dose-limiting toxicity of most regimens, is not limiting. A steep dose–response curve is apparent with the use of radiation therapy and alkylating agents.[82,83] Early attempts to perform transplantations with single agents were unsuccessful.[22,84] Most transplantations for malignancies are based on a combination of cyclophosphamide and TBI or cyclophosphamide and busulfan. Variations in agent, dose rate and fractionation of TBI, and timing are common; examples are shown in Figure 63-4, but there is little evidence to suggest that one regimen is preferable to another. Higher doses may result in fewer relapses, but toxicity tends to increase.[85] TBI can be given either as a single fraction or fractionated into multiple doses in an attempt to reduce nonhematopoietic toxicity. Children clear busulfan twice as fast as adults do, and appropriate alterations in dosing are critical.[86]

Immunosuppression

If a transplantation is undertaken without the use of immunosuppression, it is usually unsuccessful. The failure is due to the recognition of donor cells as foreign by recipient T cells and perhaps to some extent by recipient natural killer (NK) cells. In general, the therapies employed for the eradication of leukemic cells are highly immunosuppressive. Combinations of cyclophosphamide and TBI or cyclophosphamide and busulfan result in graft rejection rates of 5% or less in histocompatible patients if transplantation is performed without depletion of T lymphocytes. This low rejection rate is observed regardless of the transfusion history of the patient and may be attributable to the immunosuppressive nature of the antileukemic therapy and the effectiveness of TBI and cyclophosphamide as immunosuppressants.

In contrast, patients with aplastic anemia are at high risk of graft rejection. If no conditioning regimen is used, half of transplants between identical twins are rejected,[87] and this graft failure rate can be abrogated with cyclophosphamide.[88] In previously transfused patients who receive transplants from nonidentical siblings, the use of cyclophosphamide alone is associated with a 30% to 60% rejection rate.[89,90] The risk of rejection is related to the degree of sensitization of the recipient's lymphocytes to alloantigens and the dose of bone marrow administered.[91] The single most important prognostic variable in determining the likelihood of engraftment in severe aplastic anemia is the administration of transfusions before transplantation.[92] In contrast to the observations in kidney allograft recipients, any blood products administered more than 48 hours before transplantation increase the likelihood of rejection, and the administration of blood products from family members results in the worst engraftment problems. Because it is often difficult to avoid transfusion in severely pancytopenic patients while awaiting HLA testing and the availability of a transplant bed, most patients with aplastic anemia receive blood products before transplantation. If they are given during the conditioning regimen or within 48 hours of starting, they are less immunogenic. The total number of blood products received appears to be less relevant than the timing of the transfusions. Most transfusions cannot be restricted according to the transplant team's convenience, and intensive immunosuppressive regimens were devised to overcome sensitization. There are no malignant clones to eradicate, and most conditioning regimens for aplastic anemia do not take advantage of the immunosuppression afforded by TBI; those that do use a relatively low dose.[93] The Minnesota group successfully employed total lymphoid irradiation.[94] The immunologic reactivity of most patients with aplastic anemia is normal, and they are capable of responding to minor histocompatibility antigens expressed on the donor marrow. Thus, the introduction of more intensive immunosuppression has reduced rejection rates in transfused patients to the level of 5% to 15%. The main caveat to the use of TBI in aplastic anemia is that the risk of secondary malignancy appears to be higher.[95]

The risk of graft failure in leukemic patients may increase to almost the rate observed in aplastic patients if donor T cells are removed from the marrow before infusion. The rate of graft failure may increase to as much as 30% after T-cell depletion. If there are histocompatibility differences between recipient and donor, the likelihood of graft failure or rejection is even higher—50% in some series.[96–98] This difference is likely to be related to the persistence of residual host T cells that survive the conditioning regimen.[99,100] Donor T cells included in the marrow infusion may provide a further increment of immunosuppression by inhibiting or destroying these residual host elements. This can be considered a form of GVHR. If T cells are not present, recipient T cells that recognize donor antigens on stem cells may prevent the establishment of a functioning graft. Indirect evidence for the importance of an early GVHR was provided by the Seattle group.[91] Buffy coat cells (which are predominantly T cells) administered after transplantation reduce the rejection rate substantially,[101] presumably by inhibiting or killing the residual host T cells; although the stimulation of hematopoiesis by T-cell–derived growth factors cannot be excluded, nor can the addition of peripheral blood stem cells. Indeed, several investigators have demonstrated the expansion of recipient T cells, which are capable of inhibiting marrow growth in vitro.[99,102] Increasing immunosuppression with high-dose arabinosylcytosine[96] or possibly by leaving a small number of T cells in the donor marrow may abrogate some of this difficulty, but at the cost of increased immunosuppression, increased drug-related toxicity, and perhaps increased GVHD. Thus, new approaches are needed to provide further immunosuppression if donor T cells are removed.

Creation of Space

The need for space or a niche for engrafted marrow is a concept that is difficult to demonstrate in clinical transplantation. In murine models, if no conditioning regimen is administered, *parabiosis*, or marrow grafting between histocompatible pairs that can be distinguished with a marker, results in only small numbers of engrafted cells.[103] These animals are immunologically identical, and although they have graft failure, they do not have graft rejection. Infusion of histocompatible bone marrow to infants with SCIDS without destruction of the residual host hematopoietic environment results in mixed lymphohematopoietic chimerism, in which the lymphocytes are derived from the donor and the hematopoietic elements are derived from the host.[63,104] This probably results from selective colonization of the empty thymus by donor-derived cells. Thus, the space exists in advance and is not created by the conditioning regimen. Transplantation for diseases other than SCIDS requires immunosuppression, myelosuppression, or both. It is presumed that only immunosuppression need be administered to patients with aplastic anemia since they already have an empty niche but that both immunosuppression and space need to be established in patients with malignancies or congenital disorders of hematopoiesis or metabolism.

The distinction between graft failure and graft rejection is important. *Graft rejection* implies the recognition and suppression or destruction of hematopoietic stem cells by the recipient's T cells or NK cells and that the defect can be overcome by further suppression of host immunity. *Graft failure* is a more general term that is applied when the reason the graft has not taken is unclear, but nonimmunologic etiologies are considered. Reasons for graft failure might include an insufficient viable stem cell dose, microenvironment abnormality, or immunologic rejection. Regimens that are complicated by graft failure may not be improved by increasing the degree of host immunosuppression. This distinction is particularly important when the donor marrow is manipulated, for instance, treated with monoclonal antibodies or pharmacologic agents. If the lack of hematopoietic recovery is due to iatrogenic stem cell injury, increasing immunosuppression only increases the morbidity of the procedure. If the problem is that the T-cell depletion has abrogated a necessary degree of GVHR, then increased immunosuppression is warranted. In practice, the distinction is rarely clear.

In clinical bone marrow transplantation, the failure to provide space usually goes hand in hand with insufficient immunosuppression, and the cause of graft failure is difficult to ascribe to lack of a hematopoietic niche. Credence must be given to the concept that the hematopoietic microenvironment may be abnormal in some patients. It is most apparent in patients with myelofibrosis, in whom normal hematopoiesis is not restored until the fibrous tissue is removed from the marrow. This remodeling of the microenvironment can be observed in repeated marrow biopsies of patients with myelofibrosis or osteopetrosis.[105–107] In disorders in which a microenvironment injury is likely, engraftment may be slow, and the patient may succumb before the establishment of normal lymphohematopoiesis.[108] A particularly interesting question involves the possibility of microenvironment abnormalities in patients with aplastic anemia. Occasional patients with aplastic anemia may also fall into this category.[1,109,110] It is not clear whether marrow transplantation is possible in these patients (who are impossible to identify in advance) since there is no evidence that stromal elements are transplanted.[111]

Assessment of Engraftment

To confirm the success of the transplantation procedure, it is necessary to establish that the patient's marrow and lymphoid elements are derived from the donor and not the result of autologous recovery. When engraftment is successful, the patient is said to be chimeric; that is, the patient has a mixture of recipient tissues (liver, muscle) and donor tissues (blood, lymphoid cells). If all the transplanted elements are derived from the donor, the chimerism is complete; if there are both host and donor elements discernible in the marrow or blood, the patient is said to be a mixed or incomplete chimera. As noted previously, in SCIDS, the establishment of mixed lymphohematopoietic chimerism is expected. It is likely that when marrow transplantation is used to treat inherited disorders of metabolism, such as Gaucher's disease, stable mixed chimerism would also be acceptable; if the transplanted macrophages could dispose of the excessive glucocerebroside that characterizes Gaucher's disease, there would be no need to transplant granulocytes, erythrocytes, and so forth. Furthermore, the reestablishment of normal hematopoiesis in patients with aplastic anemia can occasionally be observed to be due to recovery of predominantly host hematopoiesis, an observation that contributed to the suggestion that many cases of aplastic anemia are immunologically mediated. Since the chemotherapeutic conditioning regimens commonly used for aplastic anemia are not likely to be irreversibly toxic to stem cells, many aplastic patients do exhibit some degree of mixed chimerism.

The importance of establishing the degree of chimerism is most apparent in patients receiving transplants for leukemia and in the interpretation of the incidence of GVHD. The presence of residual host elements in the blood or marrow of a patient with leukemia generally indicates that the malignancy will relapse, although the predictive value of this type of analysis has not been established.[60,100,112,113] In the evaluation of experimental therapies to prevent GVHD, it is also important to establish the presence of mixed chimerism. The prevention of GVHD per se may increase the rate of mixed chimerism since GVHD is probably an important mechanism for immunosuppression after marrow grafting.[99] Because mixed chimerism may be associated with a lower risk of GVHD,[114] its presence is an important variable in the analysis of GVHD prophylaxis trials. In addition, relapse of leukemia has been occasionally observed in donor rather than recipient cells.[115–117] The detection of this fascinating phenomenon requires the ability to differentiate unequivocally host from donor cells.

Determination of the origin of the various elements of the marrow and immune system depends on the ability to identify the cells of interest, isolate them in pure form, and probe them for differences that were identified between the recipient and donor at the time of pretransplantation evaluation. Methods used to differentiate host and donor include erythrocyte antigen testing,[60,118,119] HLA typing, leukocyte isoenzymes,[61,118] Ig isotype analysis,[62] Barr's body analysis and karyotyping, and DNA sequence polymorphism or RFLP analysis.[60,63,120,121] The most commonly available technique is karyotyping. Less than half of all marrow transplantations are between patients of different sexes, however, and special karyotypic differences, such as the presence of satellites and variability of quinacrine banding, are useful only in experienced centers. Furthermore, karyotype analysis is only applicable to cells that are dividing or can be made to divide. Erythrocyte antigen testing and Ig isotype analysis take advantage of the polymorphic nature of red cell-surface proteins and Ig isotypes, respectively. Because erythrocyte transfusions and γ-globulin infusions are often administered in the course of marrow transplantation, these techniques are primarily useful in the late stages of marrow grafting when residual transfused blood products are no longer present. Patients who undergo MHC-compatible allogeneic marrow grafting do not have HLA differences between host and donor since histocompatibility is one of the primary criteria for the selection of donors. Therefore, the extreme polymorphism of the HLA locus can be exploited only in MHC-mismatched patients. In practice, several of these techniques are used simultaneously, but RFLP analysis is the most useful test for evaluating nucleated cells.

TOXICITY AND COMPLICATIONS

Application of the principles outlined previously has resulted in the establishment of conditioning regimens that function on the borders of tissue tolerance for several nonhematopoietic tissues, including mucous membranes, gastrointestinal tract, lungs, liver, bladder, and heart.[122–124]

The mucous membranes are generally the first nonhematopoietic organs to demonstrate toxicity. Ulceration of the buccal mucosa, often extending into the pharynx and esophagus, is extremely uncomfortable and interferes with oral nutrition and speech. Commonly, herpes simplex virus reactivates during this period, worsening the oral injury; and oral fungi, primarily *Candida* sp, are frequently associated pathogens. It is often necessary to resort to parenteral narcotic infusions to control the pain; topical anesthetics must be used cautiously to avoid blunting the gag reflex and predisposing the patient to aspiration. It is exceedingly important that careful dental care, including filling of caries, cleaning of the teeth and gums, extraction of unsalvageable teeth, and eradication of infections and loci capable of supporting infection, be undertaken before transplantation. Close attention to oral hygiene dramatically reduces oral complications during this stage of marrow grafting. Prophylactic administration of acyclovir and nystatin, fluconazole, or clotrimazole, combined with aggressive débridement, is variably effective in controlling the mucositis. Ordinarily, the mucositis is self-limited, but it can occasionally lead to life-threatening bleeding or require intubation or tracheostomy to maintain a patent airway. Once the mucositis resolves, xerostomia is a frequent problem and may persist for weeks or months. It is due in part to damage to salivary glands in the buccal mucosa as well as the parotid and submaxillary glands. Artificial saliva is sometimes helpful.

The injury to oral mucous membranes may be reflected from one end of the gastrointestinal tract to the other. Severe diarrhea is a frequent complication of conditioning therapy, and it must be distinguished from other common causes of diarrhea, including viral, protozoal, or bacterial gastroenteritis; pseudomembranous enterocolitis; giardiasis; or acute GVHD. There may be altered absorption of nutrients and medications because of the severe mucosal injury. Nausea and vomiting or simply anorexia contribute to poor nutrition, and patients often require total parenteral nutrition to maintain an adequate caloric intake. Abdominal pain can be a major problem, since narcotics may reduce gut motility and predispose to the development of ileus and consequent fluid and electrolyte disorders. Pancreatitis occasionally complicates the picture, although it is rarely severe. Gastrointestinal bleeding is commonplace and may be severe. Often, there are multiple ulcerations of the mucosa extending the length of the gastrointestinal tract, and the residual mucosa is friable and easily injured. The bleeding is compounded by thrombocytopenia. As a rule, injury to the gut begins to resolve with the recovery of granulocytes in the blood if GVHD does not supervene.[74]

The liver is a major site for both detoxification and activation of chemotherapeutic agents. In addition to the usual viral insults resulting from multiple blood transfusions, the liver has to contend with the toxic effects of chemotherapeutic agents, irradiation, and a variety of other hepatotoxins, such as antibiotics and hyperalimentation. It is not surprising, therefore, that hepatotoxicity is a major problem in some patients. In addition to the usually mild and reversible hepatic injury that is often observed in severely ill patients on multiple supportive therapies, the liver is subject to venoocclusive disease.[74,125–128] This condition results in centrilobular necrosis and reticulin deposition around central veins and may occur in as many as one fourth of transplant recipients. It must be distinguished from other hepatic insults, such as viruses, GVHD, acalculous cholecystitis, and gallstones. Liver biopsy and diagnostic procedures such as endoscopic retrograde cholangiopancreatogram are often difficult to perform in thrombocytopenic patients. There is no specific therapy for venoocclusive disease, and it may be fatal in half of patients who develop it. Supportive management includes careful attention to volume status and avoidance of hepatic and renal toxins.

A form of hemorrhagic cardiomyopathy that occurs in small numbers of transplant recipients can be directly attributed to cyclophosphamide.[129] Although the prior use of anthracyclines appears to predispose to cardiotoxicity, that relation has not been established clearly.[130–132] The sudden development of congestive heart failure, with pericardial effusion, cardiomegaly, and loss of electrocardiogram voltage occurring 1 to 10 days after the administration of cyclophosphamide, is a characteristic clinical picture. If the pericardial effusion is large, it may require drainage. Cyclophosphamide cardiotoxicity is often refractory to therapy with diuretics and inotropic agents, and as many as half of patients who develop the clinically apparent form die. Another cardiovascular complication seen after marrow grafting is hypertension. Cyclosporine appears to be the predominant risk factor, but glucocorticoids contribute.[133] Although usually not detected clinically, nonbacterial thrombotic endocarditis is often discovered at autopsy.[134] This possibility should be kept in mind if embolic disease is suspected.

The lungs are another major site for conditioning regimen toxicity. Idiopathic interstitial pneumonitis occurs in 10% to 25% of recipients and differs from the other forms of conditioning regimen toxicity in that it is usually delayed and usually occurs 30 to 100 days after transplantation. Patients generally develop tachypnea, arterial hemoglobin desaturation, and dyspnea, and often they require mechanical ventilation. The main entities from which it must be distinguished are CMV, *Pneumocystis carinii*, diffuse alveolar hemorrhage,[135] and other nonbacterial pneumonias. The pneumonitis occurs after autologous as well as allogeneic marrow transplantation, but the incidence is lower in the autologous group.[136] That observation, coupled with GVHD as an important risk factor, suggests that idiopathic interstitial pneumonia may be a manifestation of GVHD or of the immunosuppression associated with GVHD in some patients. Multivariate analysis suggests that the use of methotrexate rather than cyclosporine as GVHD prophylaxis is also associated with greater risk.[73] The diagnosis can be made confidently only after open lung biopsy. The mortality from this form of pneumonitis is more than 90%.[69,71–73,137,138] Even without clinically apparent pneumonitis, many patients develop obstructive and restrictive respiratory abnormalities.[69]

A severe form of obstructive airway disease due to bronchiolitis obliterans has been described in 5% to 10% of recipients of allogeneic transplants, primarily with the development of chronic GVHD.[139,140] This lung pathology does not appear to occur after ABMT, and it is not associated with methotrexate or other GVHD prophylaxis. A similar picture is observed in patients after lung or heart–lung transplantations,[141] in some autoimmune disorders, and after some viral infections.[142] It is unknown whether this disorder is due to reactivity of donor T lymphocytes against bronchial epithelium in a GVHR or whether the profound immunoincompetence associated with GVHD predisposes to viral injury. If it is progressive, bronchiolitis obliterans has a high mortality,[139] but occasional patients respond to high-dose steroids.

Metabolites of cyclophosphamide are primarily excreted in the urine. Acrolein is the major offending agent and is toxic to the urothelial lining of the entire collecting system. Diffuse mucosal ulceration may occur with severe hemorrhage, dysuria, urethral obstruction with clots, and eventual interstitial cystitis, which can result in a shrunken, fibrotic bladder and may require excision or reconstructive surgery. The hemorrhage is often substantial, and its control may strain the creativity of the transplantation team. Thrombocytopenia often contributes to the bleeding, but even if the platelet count can be maintained above 50,000/μL, bleeding is often difficult to abort. Intravesical alum or formaldehyde is toxic and should be avoided. There are two approaches to avoid hemorrhagic cystitis: (1) saline diuresis is established with or without a bladder lavage through an indwelling catheter to reduce the concentration of acrolein in the urine and to reduce the contact time with the lining of the collecting system; (2) mesna, a sulfhydryl-containing uroprotective agent, is given intravenously. It binds acrolein in the urine and prevents its toxic effects, apparently without limiting the effectiveness of the cyclophosphamide.[143] Predisposing factors include prior bladder irradiation and possibly prior therapy with busulfan.[144,145] Hemorrhagic cystitis may occur in children as well as adults. Although it has been reported to be associated with adenovirus and BK viruria, other studies have not detected virus.[144,146–148]

Several other toxicities related to conditioning regimens deserve mention. Cataracts are a common delayed complication of marrow transplantation, usually occurring more than 2 years after therapy.[76,77] Extensive studies of growth and endocrinologic function in children and adolescents have documented abnormalities in pituitary, thyroid, gonadal, and adrenal function.[149–153] It is clear that growth is reduced and sexual maturation is delayed in many prepubertal children who undergo marrow transplants.[149,154] The probability of becoming infertile depends on the conditioning regimen used. Many younger patients who receive regimens that do not include TBI for aplastic anemia maintain their fertility[151,155,156]; however, TBI usually results in sterility for both males and females.[149] Patients need to be made aware of this complication, and sperm banking or appropriate counseling can be arranged in advance. Hypothyroidism may develop insidiously months to years after the transplantation.[149,157]

Central nervous system complications are uncommon. The exceptions include busulfan-containing regimens, which may cause seizures, and nitrogen mustard, which causes a toxic encephalopathy.[158] Patients with acute lymphoblastic leukemia (ALL) who had prior central nervous system prophylaxis or therapy may be at higher risk of delayed leukoencephalopathy.[159,160] Reversible neurologic abnormalities may be associated with parenteral acyclovir use.[161]

Renal disease generally has not been considered a major late complication of marrow transplantation. However, a hemolytic-uremic syndrome has been recognized in both children and adults.[162,163] This problem occurs 3 to 11 months after transplantation, and renal biopsy is consistent with radiation nephritis. Although congestive heart failure, hypertension, anemia, and thrombocytopenia may be severe, the syndrome has a tendency to resolve spontaneously with supportive care.

Toxicity may be related in part to the extent of prior therapy. Although little objective data exist, many transplant physicians agree that for similar conditioning regimens, patients with the least prior therapy have the fewest difficulties.

SECOND MALIGNANCIES

Radiation, alkylating agents, and immunosuppressants are well known to be associated with the development of therapy-induced malignancies. Thus, a major concern is the long-term effect of conditioning regimens on increasing numbers of transplantation survivors. Secondary malignancies appear to fall into three groups that are not mutually exclusive: lymphoproliferative disorders in donor or recipient cells, solid tumors, and leukemia in donor cells.

Lymphoproliferative disorders are probably due to the severe immunoincompetence that is associated with GVHD, mismatched transplants, and immunosuppressive therapy with steroids, cyclosporine, or monoclonal antibodies.[58,59,164] They are primarily large cell, B-cell immunoblastic lymphomas, and many are associated with EBV.[58,59,165–168] They can occur in cells of host or donor origin and may progress from a polyclonal to an oligoclonal then monoclonal proliferation. The time to the development of the lymphoproliferation is short—30 to 1400 days from transplantation. It is probable that immunoincompetence related to the transplantation or immunosuppressive therapy result in uncontrolled proliferation of either EBV-infected recipient B cells or nasopharyngeal cells that have survived the conditioning regimen or to donor B cells that were infused with the marrow.[57] EBV, however, may also be transmitted by means of blood transfusion. Prophylactic acyclovir was reported to reduce the incidence of EBV-related lymphomas,[169] but other data show no benefit.[58,59] The mortality of this complication is extremely high; most patients die unless immunosuppression can be reduced.

Solid tumors have been reported in patients who have undergone marrow grafting.[123,170,171] Because of the infrequency of the reports, accurate assessment of risk is difficult.

The development of new leukemias in donor cells is particularly intriguing. ANLL[172,173] and ALL[115,116,174–179] have both been reported. The pathogenesis of these malignancies is unclear, but consideration must be given to microenvironmental abnormalities, viral or chemical agent, or a familial predisposition.

ABO CONSIDERATIONS

Compatibility for the HLA antigens does not guarantee ABO compatibility. In general, ABO incompatibility is not a major problem in selecting a marrow donor and performing transplantation. Marrow stem cells do not express ABO antigens, although they can be detected on committed progenitors[180]; consequently, graft failure from ABO incompatibility is not a concern. ABO incompatibility causes three problems: (1) immediate transfusion reactions related to the infusion of large numbers of erythrocytes with the marrow stem cells, (2) late autoimmune hemolytic anemias that develop if residual isohemagglutinin-producing B lymphocytes survive the conditioning regimen, and (3) hemolytic anemia due to the infusion of mature isohemagglutinin-producing donor B lymphocytes with the marrow. Although some authors have found ABO incompatibility to be a risk factor for GVHD,[181] that finding is disputed.[182]

Immediate Isohemagglutinin Reactions

Erythrocytes of type O donors are not recognized by recipient isohemagglutinins. Thus, marrow containing type O red blood cells can usually be infused directly into an ABO-mismatched patient without difficulty. Rarely, a type O donor has high enough titers of isohemagglutinin in the plasma component of the marrow to cause self-limited hemolysis in the recipient. A more common problem occurs when the recipient has isohemagglutinin against the donor (eg, type A marrow into a type O recipient or type B marrow into a type A recipient). If the marrow is infused directly, without either reduction of the isohemagglutinin titers or removal of marrow erythrocytes, a major ABO-mismatched transfusion reaction may occur, and the consequences can be devastating. Three techniques allow the infusion of ABO-mismatched marrow. Isohemagglutinin titers should be checked well in advance of transplantation. If the recipient's isohemagglutinin titers are low, after the conditioning regimen has started, small amounts of packed red blood cells of donor type can be infused *slowly*.[183,184] This infusion serves to adsorb isohemagglutinins present at the time of transplantation. As long as the conditioning regimen has begun, there appears to be little chance that the infusion will stimulate an anamnestic response. All subsequent transfusions should be of the same blood type as the donor to ensure that any remaining isohemagglutinin that is produced will be adsorbed, and platelet transfusions should be ABO compatible, if possible, to prevent the infusion of additional isohemagglutinins contained in the platelet-rich plasma. In general, this approach is reasonable if the isohemagglutinin titer is less than 1/32. For patients who have high isohemagglutinin titers, it is preferable to use plasmapheresis to decrease the titer before converting the blood type. Since the antibodies of concern are primarily IgM, two to four whole-plasma-volume plasmaphereses generally reduce the titer to a manageable level, and some investigators have combined plasmapheresis with immunoadsorption of residual erythrocytes.[185] Transient hemoglobinuria is common. If plasmapheresis is not available or practical, the problem can be avoided by removing the erythrocytes from the marrow before infusion. Dextran or hydroxyethyl starch sedimentation,[186,187] or density gradient centrifugation,[188,189] removes most of the red blood cells and reduces the risk of an immediate reaction. When red blood cells are removed from the marrow, but no effort is made to reduce the isohemagglutinin titer of the recipient, high titers persist, and there may be slow recovery of erythrocyte production by the marrow since erythroid progenitors may be lysed in situ. This intramedullary hemolysis results in delayed reticulocytosis and prolongs the need for red cell transfusion therapy.[186,190] Once the marrow appears to have engrafted by virtue of leukocyte and platelet recovery, a rapid reticulocytosis may result from plasmapheresis.[191–193] If more than one MHC-compatible donor is available, donor selection should include consideration of ABO type.

Delayed Isohemagglutinin Reactions

The B lymphocytes infused with the marrow stem cells may include isohemagglutinin-producing cells. These cells become a problem primarily when the donor is type O and the recipient is not. With this type of ABO mismatch, mature isohemagglutinin-producing cells are stimulated by exposure to large amounts of ABO substance. They then divide and within 1 to 6 weeks produce enough antibody to generate severe hemolysis.[194–196] This severe reaction usually occurs in patients receiving cyclosporine or who received T-cell–depleted marrow; presumably the absence of functional suppressor T lymphocytes allows the reaction to occur unabated. The direct antiglobulin test becomes positive for C3, IgG, and IgM. The hemolysis can be severe enough to be life-threatening, and it requires prompt therapy with packed red blood cells that are type O or the ABO type of the donor. Immunosuppression with prednisone or plasmapheresis may also be of value. Similar reactions have occurred when large numbers of lymphocytes were passively transferred into an ABO-mismatched recipient of a liver transplant.[197] This reaction needs to be distinguished from microangiopathic hemolytic anemia with renal insufficiency, which is not immunologically mediated, and appears to reflect a form of radiation nephritis.[75] Although many allogeneic transplants involve donor–recipient pairs that are mismatched for other erythrocyte antigens (eg, Rh, Kell, Duffy, MN), hemolysis on this basis is rare.

HEMATOPOIETIC AND IMMUNOLOGIC RECONSTITUTION

The nature and tempo of hematopoietic and immune recovery after marrow grafting varies with the source of donor cells, the state of the recipient hematopoietic organs, posttransplantation drug therapy, and clinical status of the patient. Higher marrow infusate doses may lead to more rapid recovery[198]; cryopreservation and purging of autologous marrow before reinfusion may sometimes lead to delayed reconstitution, especially in platelet recovery[199,200]; significant myelofibrosis or splenomegaly, before transplantation, may delay reconstitution[108,201]; GVHD prophylaxis with methotrexate postpones recovery compared with cyclosporine prophylaxis[202,203]; and viral infection (especially of the herpesvirus group) may also lead to a delay in reappearance of normal blood counts.[204] A schematic representation of hematopoietic and immune reconstitution in relation to infectious complications and time after transplantation is shown in Figure 63-5.

In experimental animals, hematopoietic reconstitution may occur from a restricted number of clones. Lemischka and colleagues,[205] using retrovirus-mediated gene transfer to mark stem cells, were able to demonstrate that only one to two stem cell clones are sufficient to give rise to most hematopoietic elements after injection into lethally irradiated mice. Although polyclonal models have been proposed for human transplantation,[206] there is preliminary evidence that monoclonal stem cell reconstitution occurs in some patients.[207] Thus, it remains uncertain as to how many donor stem cells in humans give rise to the eventual fully reconstituted hematopoietic and immune systems.

Hematopoiesis reflects a progressive expansion, maturation, and differentiation of cells. The most primitive pluripotent stem cells are the ultimate source of all mature blood elements. They are characterized by their capacity for self-renewal, and they are capable of sustaining a lifetime of hematopoiesis. If a transplant were performed with a pure population of stem cells, hematopoietic recovery would be slow, because the stem cells need to mature over the course of weeks into fully differentiated blood cells. Once expansion and differentiation begin, the cells are called *progenitors*. Hematopoietic progenitors divide and increase in numbers, but they do not self-renew. Therefore, a transplant composed entirely of progenitors will engraft more rapidly; the rapidity depends on the relative proportion of early versus late progenitors. Early progenitors require more time to differentiate and expand so engraftment would be slower, whereas late progenitors may need only to go through a few divisions to produce mature cells, and mature cells would appear in the blood much sooner. On the other hand, a transplant composed entirely of committed progenitors will ultimately fail. The lack of self-renewal will result in late marrow failure. Most strategies to accelerate hematopoietic recovery provide for the transfusion of an adequate number of stem cells but are focused primarily on stimulating the late progenitors with hematopoietic growth factors. When hematopoietic growth factors are used to accelerate neutrophil recovery after mar-

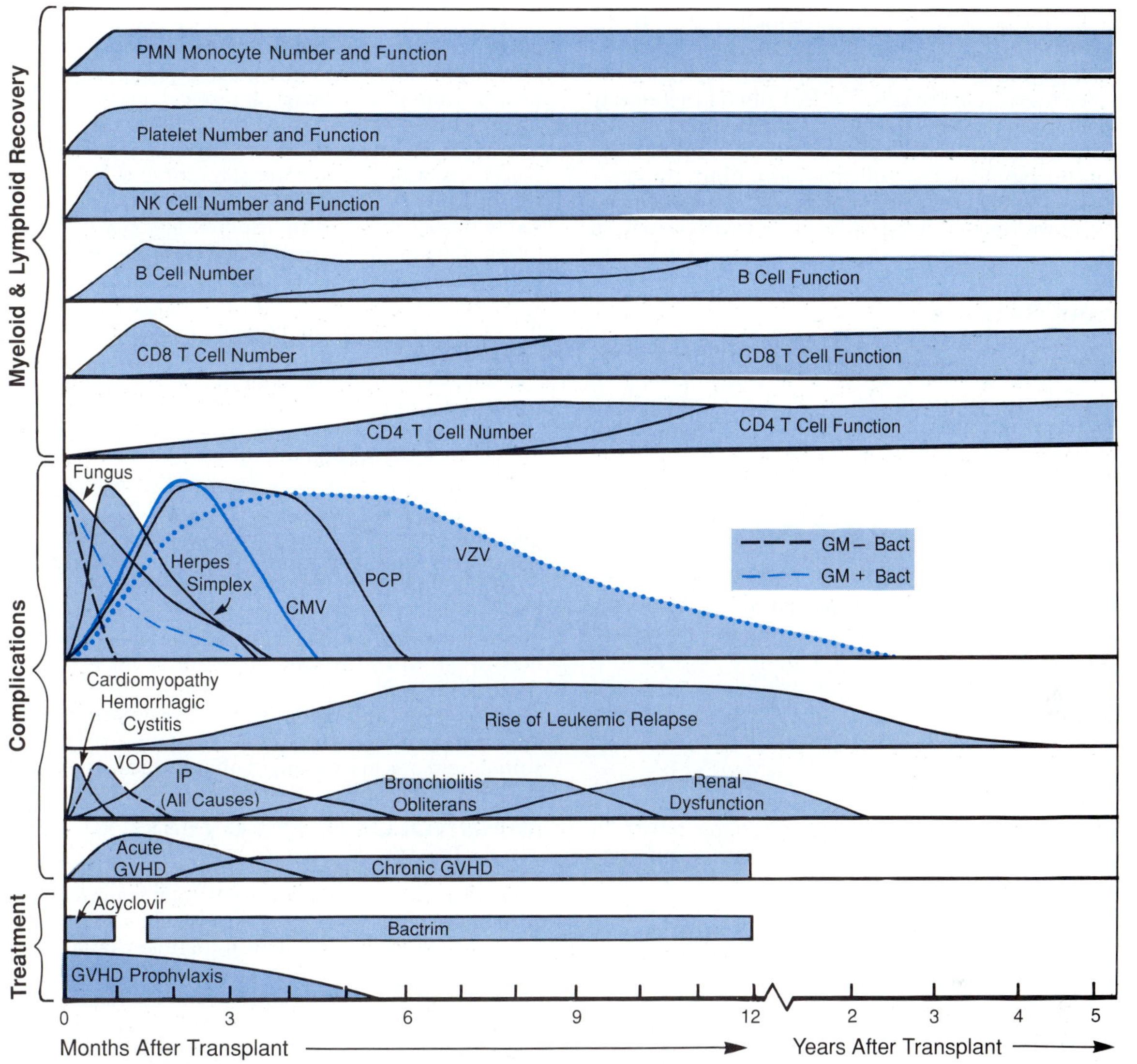

FIGURE 63-5. Schematic representation of the recovery of important classes of lymphocytes and hematopoietic cells and the relation of immune and hematopoietic recovery to infectious, immunologic, and neoplastic risks after transplantation. If graft-versus-host disease occurs, immunologic recovery is shifted to the right—it takes longer to establish normal numbers of functionally competent lymphocytes. Hematopoietic recovery is generally not affected. VOD, venoocclusive disease.

row grafting, the time to first appearance of neutrophils is not usually improved, but once they appear the rate of increase is faster.[208] If the growth factor is stopped, the rate of neutrophil increase returns to baseline. This probably reflects transient stimulation of a relatively limited number of progenitors. One strategy to increase the number of committed progenitors infused is to stimulate the marrow to release large numbers of peripheral blood progenitors either using growth factors or by performing leukapheresis during the recovery from a cycle of chemotherapy when progenitor numbers are known to increase. These progenitors are then used alone or to supplement marrow. After progenitor and stem cell infusion, hematopoietic growth factors are generally administered again. This technique has resulted in a shorter period until neutrophils recover.[209–215]

Granulocyte and Monocyte Recovery

When donor cells are infused into a patient with a marrow and spleen that are morphologically normal before the transplantation conditioning, careful inspection of the blood demonstrates the appearance of nucleated red blood cells and early myeloid forms within 7 to 10 days after infusion. It has been postulated that these early cells result from the presence in the marrow inoculum of relatively mature progenitors that undergo rapid terminal differentiation,[216] rather than from progeny derived from more primitive stem cells. During this initial 2 weeks, the bone marrow is hypocellular, but the spleen may show evidence of colony-like hematopoietic activity, reminiscent of the appearance of colony-forming unit–spleen (CFU-S) in rodent models of transplantation.[109,110]

About 14 to 28 days after transplantation, blood mononuclear cells (some with an atypical lymphocyte morphology) and granulocytes appear. The granulocyte count generally reaches greater than 500/μL within 10 to 21 days after infusion. The earliest recovering granulocytes have normal phagocytic, oxidative burst, and cytolytic capacity.[217] Similarly, quantitative monocyte recovery to normal levels is usually complete by 3 to 4 weeks. These early monocytes also demonstrate normal phagocytic function and usually normal antigen-presentation function, although some studies have noted a variable loss of this latter ability in the monocytes derived from patients 3 to 4 months after transplantation.[218,219] By contrast, the fixed tissue accessory cell populations, including alveolar macrophages[220] and Langerhans cells in the skin,[221,222] are often functionally impaired after the pretransplantation conditioning regimen for weeks to months. These cells remain of residual host derivation for months after transplantation but are gradually replaced with cells of donor origin.[223,224] It is believed that these new donor-derived cells subsequently function normally.

Erythroid Recovery

Reticulocytes are detected 1 to 2 weeks after the commencement of lymphoid and monocyte engraftment and generally peak at 4 to 6 weeks after grafting. Donor-derived red cells in the early recovery period after transplantation often show fetal-like attributes, including macrocytosis, increased i antigen expression, a fetal program of globin synthesis, and increased fetal hemoglobin levels.[225–228] The marrow red cell precursors may be mildly dysplastic.[229] This pattern is reminiscent of that seen with severe stress erythropoiesis, although in the case of marrow transplantation, these characteristics may persist for up to a year after the procedure. Erythropoietin levels are depressed after both autologous and allogeneic marrow transplantation,[230,231] and data are accumulating that the use of recombinant human erythropoietin may accelerate red cell recovery.[232,233]

Platelet Recovery

Platelet recovery usually occurs last, after the return to normal levels of most other blood elements except lymphocytes. Although platelet counts of greater than 20,000/μL are often obtained by 3 to 4 weeks, some patients remain transfusion-dependent for months. Isolated thrombocytopenia in the presence of normal myelopoiesis and erythropoiesis after allogeneic transplantation has been described in up to one third of patients.[234] In some patients, this thrombocytopenia is transient; after an initial platelet rise to greater than 100,000/μL within the first month after transplantation, the platelet count falls to the less than 10,000 to 45,000/μL range, usually with recovery by the third posttransplantation month. This event is often drug-associated (especially trimethoprim-sulfamethoxazole) or virus-associated but has also been reported to occur as an apparent autoimmune phenomenon.[235,236] Chronic persistent thrombocytopenia appears to be a more ominous event. It is frequently, although not exclusively, associated with severe acute or chronic GVHD and often portends a poor survival. Some ABMT regimens have also been associated with prolonged severe thrombocytopenia, and as outlined earlier, splenomegaly or severe marrow fibrosis may also lead to persistent thrombocytopenia after transplantation.

Functional Bone Marrow Recovery

Full morphologic recovery of normal bone marrow cellularity usually takes from 2 to 3 months after transplantation. In patients receiving transplants for aplastic anemia who demonstrate failure to engraft or graft rejection, increased mast cells have been observed in the bone marrow,[237] but the relation of this observation to the engraftment process, if any, remains unknown. Although it would appear logical that the rapidity of bone marrow and blood cell recovery after transplantation should be predictable by quantification of donor marrow CFUs, experimental results have been in conflict in this regard, with some studies noting a correlation,[238–240] while others do not.[241,242] Measurement of progenitors by a variety of CFU assays in posttransplantation marrows has generally shown slow but steady recovery over several months. Examination of serial plasma samples for hematopoietic growth-promoting activity has demonstrated markedly depressed support for burst-forming unit–erythroid and CFU-GEMM (granulocyte, erythroblast, monocyte, megakaryocyte) for prolonged periods of time after transplantation, while support for CFU-GM (granulocyte-macrophage) and CFU-Meg (megakaryocyte) is high within the first 30 days after transplantation.[243] Clinical studies of ABMT, and, to a limited extent, allogeneic transplantation, using the recombinant growth factors granulocyte-macrophage colony-stimulating factor (GM-CSF) and granulocyte colony-stimulating factor (G-CSF) after marrow infusion have demonstrated more rapid recovery of counts and reduction in the incidence of posttransplantation complications.[244,245]

The regeneration of the stromal component of the human marrow microenvironment after transplantation is an important concomitant of normal hematopoiesis. Most experimental data suggest that stromal cells are derived from different progenitors than hematopoietic elements. In patients with leukemia, conflicting data have been reported regarding the involvement of stromal elements in the malignant clone.[246,247] Similarly, conflicting data have been presented regarding the posttransplantation donor versus host origin of the stromal elements.[248,249] It is likely that these issues will remain unresolved until improved methods of isolating and defining the marrow stroma in humans are developed, but it is generally believed that the marrow stroma remains of host origin after marrow transplantation.

IMMUNOLOGIC RECOVERY

Most clinical problems in marrow transplantation result from disruption of an ordered immune system and the variable establishment of new, donor-derived but host-tolerant lymphopoiesis. These include the failure of new marrow to engraft (host-versus-graft disease or graft rejection), the attack of new marrow on the host (GVHD), and the failure of adequate immune reconstitution after transplantation, resulting in infectious complications. Although the recovery of myeloid hematopoiesis in uncomplicated transplantations is usually complete by the third month after transplantation, the recovery of lymphocyte numbers and function often requires 6 months to 2 years to reach a stable state.[250,251] Even more than in the case of myeloid recovery, a myriad of clinical variables affects the reconstitution of the immune system: patient age, GVHD prophylaxis, cryopreservation of donor marrow (with or without chemotherapeutic or antibody purging), and herpesvirus infections, especially CMV.[252,253] In addition, study of the recovery of the immune system may be further complicated by the effects of other concomitant clinical events, including frequent blood transfusions.[254] The following broad outline of recovery holds in most cases, however.

Natural Killer Cell Recovery

In the initial 2 months after transplantation, cells of NK and B-lymphocyte surface phenotype are the first to return to normal numbers in the circulation. NK cells, defined by the expression of CD11 or CD56 and the simultaneous absence of CD3 on the membrane, reach normal or supranormal levels usually by the fourth week in syngeneic, autologous, and allogeneic transplants.[255–258] These cells demonstrate normal cytolytic function at the same time they reach normal numbers. They have many of the characteristics of activated killer cells.[259] Patients with CMV infection may show increased number and cytolytic activity of these cells. The effect of GVHD on the recovery of this population is probably small and is difficult to determine.

B-Lymphocyte Recovery

Cells of B-lymphocyte surface phenotype (CD19+, CD20+, SIg+) likewise reach normal levels early after transplantation in patients undergoing relatively uncomplicated MHC-compatible allogeneic or syngeneic transplants. Recovery of circulating phenotypic B cells may be delayed in some patients with GVHD and in patients receiving MHC-incompatible transplants[260] as well as in some patients receiving autologous grafts for non-Hodgkin's lymphoma, perhaps related to treatment of the marrow with anti–B-cell monoclonal antibodies.[261]

In contrast to the rapid quantitative recovery of circulating B cells in many patients, functional recovery assessed by in vitro assays of cellular proliferation and Ig secretion may be extremely slow in both allogeneic and autologous transplant recipients.[262–269] The pathogenesis of this dysfunction is probably multifactorial, involving intrinsic B-cell defects as well as T-lymphocyte immunoregulatory defects and the decreased production of relevant cytokines.[270,271]

The in vitro abnormalities observed are reflected at least in part in in vivo dysfunction. For example, while most patients after allogeneic transplantation recover normal serum IgM levels within the first 2 months, some patients (most prominently, although not exclusively, those with chronic GVHD) have clinically significant decreased serum IgG levels[272] that may be associated with recurrent infections and possibly bronchiolitis obliterans.[273–275] Moreover, it has been suggested that there is also a subgroup of patients whose total serum IgG returns to normal levels but who remain deficient in specific IgG subclasses, usually IgG-2 and IgG-4. These patients appear to be at increased risk for bacterial infections.[276] Conversely, some patients with acute GVHD develop polyclonal hypergammaglobulinemia.[277] Almost three fourths of patients demonstrate low serum IgA levels for a year or more after transplantation, although the clinical consequences of that immunodeficiency are uncertain. Finally, serum IgE levels are frequently markedly elevated after transplantation.[278,279] Although there is a temporal association of this latter phenomenon with acute GVHD, it is also observed in identical-twin transplants, and its pathogenesis remains unknown.

In the first 2 to 3 weeks after transplantation, serum γ-globulin represents residual host-derived antibody, which decreases with a variable half-life dependent on the presence or absence of concomitant infection and complications such as protein-losing enteropathy. Most evidence suggests a conversion to donor-derived antibody by day 100 in most patients.[280] Some studies have suggested transfer of donor antigen-specific immunity at the B- and T-cell level to marrow transplant recipients.[281,282]

Finally, the appearance of monoclonal and oligoclonal Ig banding on serum protein electrophoresis appears to be a common phenomenon in the early months after transplantation.[283–286] Whether this represents a reflection of normal immune ontogeny or oligoclonal regeneration of the B-cell repertoire or is a consequence of the immune dysregulation posttransplantation is unknown, but the M components generally resolve without clinical sequelae.

T-Lymphocyte Recovery

T-lymphocyte reconstitution after transplantation is slowest of all the hematopoietic-derived elements.[287–292] Among the T-cell subtypes, the CD3+ CD8+ subset recovers most rapidly in patients undergoing all types of transplantation, often reaching normal levels in the uncomplicated situation by 6 to 10 weeks after grafting. The CD3+ CD4+ subset, in contrast, usually requires 6 months or more to reach normal levels. Patients with GVHD tend to have a more rapid and greater rise in CD3+ CD8+ cells and a markedly slower recovery in CD3+ CD4+ cells. Thus, while most marrow transplant recipients retain an inverted CD3+ CD4+/CD3+ CD8+ ratio for months to perhaps years after transplantation, the severity of that inversion is increased in those patients with GVHD. This abnormality of T-cell–subset distribution is also exacerbated by CMV infection.[293,294] It is observed in recipients of autologous as well as allogeneic transplants, but generally to a much lesser extent in the autologous transplant recipient.[295]

As in the case of B lymphocytes, functional recovery of T cells after transplantation is even slower than phenotypic recovery. Simple in vitro measures of T-cell function, such as their ability to proliferate in response to stimulation by lectins, mitogens, or anti-CD3 antibody, their ability to perform a cytolytic effector function, and their ability to secrete cytokines, remain markedly depressed for up to a year or more after transplantation.[296] Similarly, in vivo tests of cellular immunity, such as skin testing either to neoantigens or recall antigens, remains markedly impaired for years in many patients.[297] Even when bulk in vitro assays of T-lymphocyte function normalize, limiting dilution culture methods continue to reveal abnormal T-cell proliferative function as well as diminished cytokine secretion and cytolytic function.[298] Again, GVHD affects the rate of recovery of normal T-cell immunity,[299] probably as a result of the GVHD as well as the treatment regimens employed. There is no clear difference in T-cell recovery observed between patients who receive cyclosporine and those who receive methotrexate for posttransplantation immunoprophylaxis.[300] Patients with chronic GVHD remain the most immunosuppressed for the longest periods in virtually all studies. T-cell depletion of donor marrow (to prevent GVHD; discussed later) exacerbates the cellular immune defect for at least the first 6 months after transplantation.[301]

The pathogenesis of these cellular immunologic lesions is probably multifactorial. In addition to defects in signal transduction mechanisms necessary for the activation of the T cell, defects in interleukin-2[302,303] and interferon-γ[304] production have been noted, although the latter observation is disputed.[305] Active suppression by nonspecific suppressor cells, especially in patients with chronic GVHD, has been delineated,[306–308] as has an inhibitory influence of prostaglandin E_2.[309] The fact that these defects persist at the single cell level,[298] however, confirms that the defects observed are not solely the result of dysregulation but must also represent intrinsic abnormalities of the T cell. As in the case of posttransplantation B-lymphocyte recovery, several phenotypically unusual T-cell subsets have been defined, including cells of CD3+, CD4−, CD8−, and CD3+, CD5− subtypes.[256,310] Whether unique functional aspects of such cells will help to further define the immune abnormalities of these patients remains to be seen.

Partial Chimerism

Patients receiving transplants after a conditioning regimen including TBI or high-dose busulfan are expected to eventually become permanent full chimeras. All their hematopoietic-derived cells should become exclusively of donor origin, although transient persistence of slowly dividing host elements might be expected. For example, it is known that the turnover of fixed tissue macrophages from host to donor origin may require 6 or more months,[311] while circulating monocytes are usually solely of donor origin as soon as they are measurable. Full chimerism, however, does not always occur. In particular, patients receiving bone marrow from which mature T cells have been depleted ex vivo (discussed later) are sometimes found to have persistent host elements capable of undergoing successful cell division.[312,313] Such partial chimerism has been reported to occur in as many as two thirds of patients receiving ex vivo manipulated marrow allografts.[314] Moreover, patients undergoing transplantation with preparatory regimens that are less rigorous (eg, for aplastic anemia) may also develop permanent partial chimerism in the absence of donor marrow manipulation. Some patients who received ablative conditioning also were reported to be mixed chimeras. The incidence of this occurrence in non–T-cell–depleted transplants is probably 5% to 25%.[60,114,315,316] Whether the detection of such chimerism increases the likelihood of leukemic relapse remains controversial.

Finally, there are some clinical situations in which permanent host-origin myeloid and accessory cell elements coresiding with permanent donor-origin lymphocytes is routinely expected. This form of mixed chimerism occurs in the transplantation of patients with SCIDS. About half of children with SCIDS have B cells at the time of transplantation. After transplantation, the T cells are of donor origin, while the B cells remain of donor origin. As more and more transplants are carried out between allogeneic donor–recipient pairs who are not genotypically identical at the MHC loci, MHC disparity between antigen-presenting cells and helper T lymphocytes may be a clinically important factor in determining long-term immune function.[317,318]

Infections After Marrow Transplantation: Clinical Correlates of Immune Reconstitution

The major infectious risk periods after transplantation are predictable from the pattern of immune reconstitution. Before engraftment, major risk is from bacterial and fungal infection due to profound granulocytopenia and damage to the integument secondary to both preparatory chemoradiation therapy and GVHD prophylaxis with agents such as methotrexate. As for all granulocytopenic patients, most of these infections result from endogenously carried organisms that seed the bloodstream from gut or skin. In addition, since these patients virtually always have one or more surgically implanted intravenous lines, *Staphylococcus epidermidis* and *S aureus* and *Candida* sp should be considered early in the differential diagnosis of fever.

During the later part of this period and extending into the immediate posttransplantation period, viral infections become common. Herpes simplex reactivation generally occurs earliest. Although oral lesions are common, profound mucositis can sometimes obscure the classic vesicular eruption. A number of studies have documented the value of routine acyclovir prophylaxis in recipients of allogeneic marrow transplants[319–323] in delaying or preventing reactivation of herpes simplex and, in some cases, accelerating engraftment in patients receiving methotrexate GVHD prophylaxis. Furthermore, additional evidence suggests that prophylactic acyclovir may also help prevent or delay reactivation of herpes zoster and perhaps CMV infection (discussed later).[324,325]

After engraftment, bacterial infections due to endogenous organisms are infrequent. If patients are hypogammaglobulinemic, however, particularly in the setting of chronic GVHD, they are susceptible to infections with encapsulated organisms such as *Haemophilus influenzae* and *Streptococcus pneumoniae*. Moreover, herpes zoster reactivation may occur, CMV infection is common, and, in the absence of prophylactic therapy, *Pneumocystis carinii* infections are observed. The latter is generally avoided with prophylactic trimethoprim-sulfamethoxazole.[326] Recent experience with aerosolized pentamidine or dapsone in patients with acquired immunodeficiency syndrome suggests that transplant recipients who cannot tolerate trimethoprim-sulfamethoxazole may be able to receive *Pneumocystis* prophylaxis.[327] This approach has not been well studied. Varicella zoster infections occur in at least half of transplant recipients at risk for reactivation of this pathogen within the first year.[328,329] Of these three pathogens, however, CMV infection is the most common cause of serious morbidity and mortality after marrow grafting, occurring in about 15% to 20% of all allogeneic marrow transplant recipients. Indeed, CMV is the most common infectious cause of death in these patients.[330,331]

In patients who are seropositive for CMV at the time of transplantation, infection is most often the result of reactivation of latent virus.[332] In patients who are seronegative, the disease is acquired either from donor marrow or from blood products. Although many CMV infections are asymptomatic, some patients develop fever, leukopenia, hepatitis, enteritis, esophagitis, retinitis, or pneumonia. Pneumonia is the most ominous clinical syndrome developing in CMV-infected patients; about one third of patients with CMV infection progress to pneumonia on the average of 60 or more days after transplantation, and mortality in that group is historically estimated at 85% or more. This represents the incidence of CMV pneumonia in allogeneic transplantation. In syngeneic and autologous transplants, the overall incidence of serious CMV disease is far less.[333] In fact, in a survey of 100 recipients of syngeneic marrow, no patient developed CMV pneumonia, even though the rate of infection remained high.[334] Thus, GVHD, even when subclinical, appears to lead to a high risk of progression of CMV infection to lethal pneumonias.[335] Other risk factors for the development of fatal CMV infection include older age, receipt of granulocyte transfusions, TBI, and perhaps increased transplant immunosuppression.[336] One report suggests that immune donors may protect seronegative recipients, but these data require confirmation.[337] Based on these clinical observations and on murine experimentation, it has been postulated that CMV pneumonia is an immunopathologic disease,[338–340] that is, that the pulmonary damage occurs secondary to the attack of cytolytic T cells directed against viral antigens expressed on lung tissue.

Prophylaxis against CMV pneumonia is obviously crucial in the management of postallogeneic transplant recipients. Since seronegative transplant recipients who have seronegative bone marrow donors contract the disease only through administration of CMV-positive blood products, administration of only CMV-negative blood to these patients markedly reduces the incidence of this complication. Because CMV is transmitted with the leukocytes, filtered or deglycerolized packed red blood cells and filtered platelets may reduce the risk of infection if CMV-seronegative blood products are not available.[341–343] Granulocyte transfusions are strongly associated with CMV infection.[344] Administration of either commercial γ-globulin or CMV Ig was associated with a reduction in CMV infection and pneumonia in some series[345,346] and had little or no effect in others.[347] Some studies of γ-globulin infusion demonstrated a reduction in acute GVHD and other infectious complications.[345,346,348] The mechanism for these improvements is uncertain.

For patients who are seropositive, neither the use of seronegative blood products nor the use of routine posttransplantation intravenous γ-globulin decreased the risk of CMV infection.[336] Although vidarabine and interferon were of no benefit,[349,350] the administration of prophylactic acyclovir significantly decreased both CMV infection and disease.[351] The incidence of invasive disease was reduced from 38% to 22% by the administration of intravenous acyclovir, 500 mg/m^2 every 8 hours from 5 days before to 30 days after transplantation, without significant toxicity. In this particular study, overall patient survival for the first 100 days after transplantation was also improved by the administration of acyclovir.

The most significant advance in the reduction of morbidity and mortality from CMV disease was the introduction of prophylactic ganciclovir. Several different regimens have been shown to be effective, but regimens that are associated with ganciclovir-induced neutropenia may be complicated by bacterial infections.[352–354] An effective regimen that does not appear to be excessively myelosuppressive is ganciclovir, 5 mg/kg twice daily for 2 weeks then 5 times a week for 100 to 120 days. Additional therapy with intravenous γ-globulin, 500 mg/kg/wk, may also be beneficial if given through 100 days after transplantation. One caveat in the use of prophylactic ganciclovir is that when CMV infection does occur, it may manifest as declining granulocyte count, often with abnormal liver function tests and fever. There is a tendency to attribute this syndrome to ganciclovir and to stop administering the drug, when it may actually reflect CMV infection, requiring an increase in ganciclovir to full therapeutic dose.

CMV pneumonia occurs at a similar time after transplantation as idiopathic interstitial pneumonia. The distinction is important, since ganciclovir and foscarnet are useful in treating the infection. Open lung biopsy has been the primary diagnostic procedure used to establish the cause of diffuse interstitial pulmonary infiltrates. The morbidity of this procedure is substantial; bronchoalveolar lavage with centrifugation cultures is a highly sensitive and specific technique that can rapidly detect pulmonary CMV and may largely supplant open lung biopsy.[355]

Once CMV pneumonia develops, it is generally treated with ganciclovir and intravenous Ig.[356,357] For patients that do not respond to ganciclovir, foscarnet appears to be an effective alternative.[358]

FAILURE TO ENGRAFT

Two major mechanisms can account for failure to engraft: (1) failure of self-renewing donor stem cells to establish residence in the host, or (2) active rejection of transplanted cells by the host immune system. In practice, it may be difficult to distinguish between these two problems. Primary failure to engraft can occur in autologous, syngeneic, or allogeneic transplantation and may be due to an inadequate stem cell inoculum, the destruction of stem cells by an exogenous agent, or an inhospitable bone marrow microenvironment. Remarkably, relatively few drugs interfere with long-term engraftment,[359] although prudence has dictated the judicious use of agents that cause marrow hypoplasia or cytopenia. Similarly, although CMV, HSV and other infections may slow engraftment, complete failure to engraft is not well documented.[360] Finally, although there remains much discussion about the role of the microenvironment in engraftment, and there is convincing animal data,[361] it is difficult to document graft failure from a defective microenvironment in humans, except in myelofibrosis and osteopetrosis.

In animal models of transplantation, two major cell types have been implicated as mediators of active immunologic graft rejection: NK cells[362–365] and cytolytic T lymphocytes.[366,367] Because it is unusual for patients receiving transplants for leukemic disorders using ablative conditioning regimens and unmanipulated MHC-compatible sibling donor marrow to demonstrate a failure to engraft (incidence estimated at less than 1%), evidence for an active immunologic process in graft rejection in humans comes from two major clinical experiences: transplantation for aplastic anemia and the use of T-cell–depleted donor marrows to reduce the incidence and severity of GVHD in allogeneic transplantation. In transplants performed for aplastic anemia, almost all patients demonstrate an initial rise in blood counts in the first 14 to 28 days after grafting. Some patients subsequently undergo a sudden drop in counts, with loss of all donor cells.[368–370] This is in sharp clinical contrast to a primary failure of the counts to rise. It is well established that patients with aplastic anemia who did not undergo transfusion before marrow grafting have an extremely low incidence of this type of graft rejection, even when conditioned for their transplant with cyclophosphamide alone.[371] By contrast, patients who have undergone multiple transfusions have a rejection rate approaching 50% when given this type of conditioning; and those who have received family-member transfusions have an even greater rejection rate. Thus, pretransplantation sensitization of the host immune system to donor cell antigens appears to lead to an increased risk of active graft rejection. Even aplastic patients who receive a syngeneic transplant in which no difference in antigens should be possible may demonstrate graft failure.[372,373] In one such well-studied case, NK cells were implicated as the cause.[374]

Depletion of mature T cells from donor marrow to abrogate GVHD (discussed later) has led to significant insights into the immunology of human marrow graft rejection. T-lymphocyte–depleted marrow increases the rate of graft rejection.[375] In patients with transplants for leukemia, the rejection rate may change from less than 3% to as high as 15%. It has been possible in some cases to examine the circulating lymphoid cells in these patients that appear during the rejection. Both NK cells and cytolytic T cells have been observed to suppress hematopoietic progenitor cells.[376–378] Such data have been used to support the idea that donor buffy coat cells reduce the incidence of graft rejection in aplastic anemia patients by providing donor T lymphocytes that suppress or lyse residual host-derived lymphocytes that have survived the conditioning regimen and that could mediate rejection. It is also possible that graft failures in patients given T-cell–depleted marrows results from a lack of necessary growth factor production by infused marrow cells. This explanation is somewhat less tenable since increased pretransplantation immunosuppression alone increases the engraftment rate in these patients.[96,379]

Finally, the more recent transplantation experience in patients with hematologic malignancies receiving donor marrow from family members who were not MHC-identical confirms that HLA incompatibility and prior alloimmunization are the most important clinical factors associated with engraftment failure in this patient group. Incompatibility at HLA-B and D and a positive crossmatch for donor lymphocytotoxic antibodies were independent risk factors that led to a 12.3% incidence of graft rejection for recipients of MHC-incompatible marrow, as compared with a 2% graft rejection incidence for matched sibling donor marrow.[41] Moreover, residual host lymphocytes were detected in most patients who failed to engraft, further suggesting the importance of an immune mechanism.

GRAFT-VERSUS-HOST DISEASE

In solid organ transplantation, the major immunologic obstacle to a successful procedure is graft rejection, that is, a failure of the host immune system to develop tolerance for the transplanted organ (host-versus-graft disease). In allogeneic marrow transplantation, however, the conditioning regimens effectively eliminate the host immune system. Therefore, the major immunologic impediment to be faced is the establishment of tolerance of the donor marrow for the host. The failure to induce such tolerance leads to GVHD. As noted earlier, the GVHD reaction was first reported in experimental animals—described as secondary disease or runting—in the late 1950s and subsequently recognized as a clinical syndrome in humans.[1,9] Billingham[10] succinctly described the essential elements of GVHD:

1. The graft must contain immunologically competent cells.
2. The host must possess important transplantation isoantigens that are lacking in the graft donor, so that the host appears foreign to it, and is, therefore, capable of stimulating it antigenically.
3. The host itself must be incapable of mounting an effective immunologic reaction against the graft, at least for sufficient time for the latter to manifest its immunologic capabilities, that is, it must have security of tenure.

Two points are clear from this description. First, only patients receiving allogeneic (either MHC-matched or mismatched) grafts should be capable of developing GVHD (but see later discussion). Second, occasional experiments of nature can also result in GVHD. Thus, children born with severe congenital immunodeficiency can have transplacental passage of maternal lymphocytes, which may result in clinical GVHD in the untransfused newborn. Such a syndrome was first described in the mid-1960s, with demonstration of maternal lymphocytes in the child in at least one case.[380,381]

Two syndromes can be delineated: acute and chronic GVHD. For the sake of definition in clinical trials, 100 days after transplantation is often taken as an arbitrary dividing line between acute GVHD and chronic GVHD. The clinical syndrome of chronic GVHD, however, as described below, can commence before such an arbitrary cut-off, and some patients may demonstrate aspects of both syndromes simultaneously.

Acute Graft-Versus-Host Disease

Description and Diagnosis

Acute GVHD usually begins within the first 4 weeks after transplantation but can occur any time within the first 4 months. It is characterized by a clinicopathologic syndrome involving the skin, liver, and gastrointestinal tract. A maculopapular, erythematous exanthem appears, frequently involving palms and soles. In its mildest manifestation, it may involve less than one fourth of the body surface, but in its severest form, it can progress to total-body erythema, gross bullae formation, and sloughing of skin. The loss of the integument leads to a markedly increased risk of infection, especially with normal skin flora such as *S aureus* and *S epidermidis*. Liver function abnormalities of both inflammatory and obstructive chemistries are seen. Again, mild cases may demonstrate only a three- to four-fold rise in the ALT (alanine aminotransferase) and AST (aspartate aminotransferase), while the most severely affected patients have serum bilirubin levels higher than 10 mg/dL and loss of liver synthetic function. Involvement of the gut is manifest by anorexia, crampy pain and watery, secretory diarrhea, which can progress to bloody diarrhea and frank ileus. In severe cases, a major protein-losing enteropathy results, with hypoalbuminemia. This problem may be exacerbated by severe hepatic dysfunction. The combination of major insensible fluid losses through a damaged integument, decreased hepatic synthetic function, and massive diarrhea make frequent evaluation of blood, urine, and stool electrolytes and careful input and output measurements a necessity.

Often, all three organ systems are involved to about the same severity. Isolated intestinal disease may be common. Gastric GVHD is a frequent cause of otherwise unexplained nausea and vomiting after transplantation.[382] Routine endoscopic evaluation of patients with otherwise apparent clinical GVHD has demonstrated pathologic evidence of intestinal GVHD in about 13% of patients.[383] Gastroscopy and biopsy can confirm this diagnosis and distinguish it from candidiasis, HSV, CMV, or peptic gastritis. Isolated skin involvement is relatively easy to assess with a skin biopsy, but the liver is much more difficult to assess, since thrombocytopenia usually precludes liver biopsy. because the liver is subject to many potential toxins and infections, the diagnosis of isolated hepatic GVHD must be made cautiously. Clinical grading is usually carried out using a modification of the Seattle criteria,[22] as outlined in Tables 63-3 and 63-4. As described in detail later, clinical grade correlates with overall survival. Patients who die from acute GVHD generally do so from concomitant infection, pneumonitis, or, more rarely, overwhelming hepatic failure.

The histology of acute GVHD in the involved organs generally involves evidence of single cell death accompanied by cellular atypia, edema, and a sparse lymphocytic infiltrate. In the skin, this is manifested by epidermal and basal cell vacuolar degeneration, disorganization of epidermal cell maturation, eosinophilic body formation, and melanocyte incontinence.[384] In the liver, bile duct atypia, cellular degeneration, and cholestasis are seen; in the gut, the colon is more frequently involved than the ileum and shows histologic evidence of crypt cell necrosis and dropout and flattening of the villous architecture[385] (Fig. 63-6 and 63-7). The dermatopathologic changes of mild acute GVHD can be indistinguishable from the cytotoxic effect of conditioning regimens or drug eruptions.[386] Radiologic ex-

TABLE 63-3. Staging of Acute Graft-Versus-Host Disease

Stage	Skin	Liver	Intestine
1	Maculopapular rash on <25% of body surface	Bilirubin, 2–3 mg/dL	Diarrhea, >10 mL/kg/d
2	Maculopapular rash on 25%–50% of body surface	Bilirubin, 3–6 mg/dL	Diarrhea, >20 mL/kg/d
3	Generalized erythroderma	Bilirubin, 6–15 mg/dL	Diarrhea, >30 mL/kg/d
4	Generalized erythroderma; bulla formation; desquamation	Bilirubin, >15 mg/dL	Severe diarrhea, abdominal pain, with or without ileus

TABLE 63-4. Grading of Acute Graft-Versus-Host Disease

	Organ Stage		
Grade	**Skin**	**Intestine**	**Liver**
I	1–2	0	0
II	0	1	0–1
	0	0–1	1
	1–3	1	0–1
	1–3	0–1	1
	3	0	0
III	0–3	0–2	2–3
	0–3	2–3	0–3
	0–3	0–3	4*
IV	0–3	4	0–4
	4	0–4	0–4

* If Karnovsky performance status is ≤30%, then grade 4.
(Adapted by the Multicenter FK506 Study Group, sponsored by Fujisawa)

amination of the gut usually demonstrates nonspecific changes that are consistent with the histology of the reaction.

The differential diagnosis of acute GVHD can be extensive and difficult. Skin rashes after transplantation are often due to drug eruptions. These include delayed reactions to conditioning regimen agents; reactions to antibiotics; allergic reactions to topical agents; and manifestations of transfusion reactions. Gastrointestinal dysfunction is expected after TBI. Viral infection, especially CMV and herpes; parasitic infection; pseudomembranous colitis; stress gastritis; and drug reactions can all mimic GVHD of the gut. The potential causes of liver dysfunction include hyperalimentation, venoocclusive disease, viral hepatitis, and drug-induced hepatitis (including cyclosporine, methotrexate, and estrogens that may be administered to prevent breakthrough vaginal bleeding). It is important, therefore, to recognize that acute GVHD is most often a clinical diagnosis. The changes of mild to moderate acute GVHD, especially in skin in the first month after transplantation, are mimicked by the effects of the cytotoxic chemotherapy and radiation therapy conditioning regimens and drug therapy.[387] Moreover, even the signs of more severe acute GVHD, such as a significant epidermal mononuclear cell infiltrate, can be modified by procedures such as T-cell depletion of donor marrow.[388] GVHD lesions in other organs, particularly the gut, can also be imitated by infectious processes, such as CMV and other herpesviruses, although classic viral inclusions are not seen in GVHD.[389] This is not to denigrate the value of biopsy examination since it often is helpful in distinguishing this diagnosis from those clinical syndromes that may mimic GVHD, such as venoocclusive disease of the liver.[390] Finally, it may be impossible to discriminate between these lesions since there is a high association of GVHD with herpesvirus infection (CMV, herpes simplex, and possibly EBV)[391–394] as well as an association between the development of GVHD and venoocclusive disease of the liver.

Whether GVHD can actually affect organs other than the classic triad remains an incompletely resolved issue. The most likely other candidate is the lung. Pneumonitis may occur in 20% to 60% of allogeneic transplant recipients but in many fewer autologous transplant recipients. Causes include CMV infection; other viral infections, such as adenovirus, herpesvirus, and parainfluenza; bacterial, fungal, or protozoan infection; and treatment-induced injury due to radiation, conditioning chemotherapy, or methotrexate. The incidence, severity, and mortality of pneumonia increases with the severity of GVHD, but this association does not necessarily imply that the GVHD, as opposed to the concomitant immunosuppression and treatment, is causative. A particular histopathologic syndrome of lymphocytic bronchitis has been attributed directly to GVHD,[395] although this has not been universally accepted.[396] In addition, other chronic posttransplantation pulmonary syndromes, especially bronchiolitis obliterans, may represent a manifestation of chronic GVHD (discussed later).

Similarly, although renal[397] and urinary tract[398,399] symptoms occur after transplantation, they are attributable to either drug-related or infection-related complications, with no supportive evidence for a role of GVHD. Neurologic complications are likewise not infrequent[400,401] but cannot be ascribed to GVHD.

Pathophysiology

In animal models of marrow transplantation, the initiation of the acute GVHR is dependent on the presence of mature T lymphocytes in the marrow inoculum as a necessary (but not sufficient) condition.[402,403] The severity of the reaction is further dependent on two major factors: the number of T cells in the inoculum and the number and type of major and minor histocompatibility antigen disparities between donor and recipient. Donor and recipient differences at either the MHC class I or class II antigen loci can lead to fatal GVHD.[404,405] In GVHD initiated by minor histocompatibility differences, the number and relative strength of those differences is important. During the GVHD reaction, cytolytic T lymphocytes directed against host cells can be readily identified,[406] although it is possible that other cell types, such as NK cells, may also participate in the effector phase of the GVHD response.[407] The particular subtype of T lymphocyte responsible for initiating the reaction remains somewhat controversial, and unresolved in humans. In full H-2 mismatched murine models, where donor and host differ at both MHC class I and class II loci, the CD4+ lymphocyte subset is the predominant (but not exclusive) effector.[408,409] The same T-cell subset is the effector in MHC class II–mismatched, class I–identical transplant combinations, while the CD8+ lymphocyte subset may control the initiation of GVHD in class I–mismatched transplants. In the case of minor histocompatibility antigen differences, the CD8+ T-cell subset is primarily responsible for GVHD. As in humans, the immunodeficiency resulting from GVHD may be multifactorial and include the development of natural suppressor cell activity.[410]

The primary role of T lymphocytes in initiating GVHD in humans has been confirmed in experimental clinical trials in which these cells were depleted from donor marrow ex vivo (discussed later). Studies have also confirmed that GVHD depends on the quantity of T cells infused into the recipient.[411] The issue of what cell types may participate in the effector phase of the response in humans remains unsettled, despite immunopathologic studies of involved organs.[412]

Data are accumulating that mechanisms other than direct T-cell mediated tissue damage are important in the pathogenesis of GVHD. One poorly explained feature of GVHD is the relative limitation of manifestations to the skin, gut, liver and perhaps lung. These organs share an exposure to bacteria, particularly gram-negative rods. Animals raised in germ-free environments do not develop GVHD after marrow grafting, but fatal GVHD supervenes when they are recontaminated.[413] Furthermore, several other observations link GVHD and the consequences of infection: (1) GVHD tends to flare with a variety of infections; (2) laminar air flow rooms and gut decontamination reduce

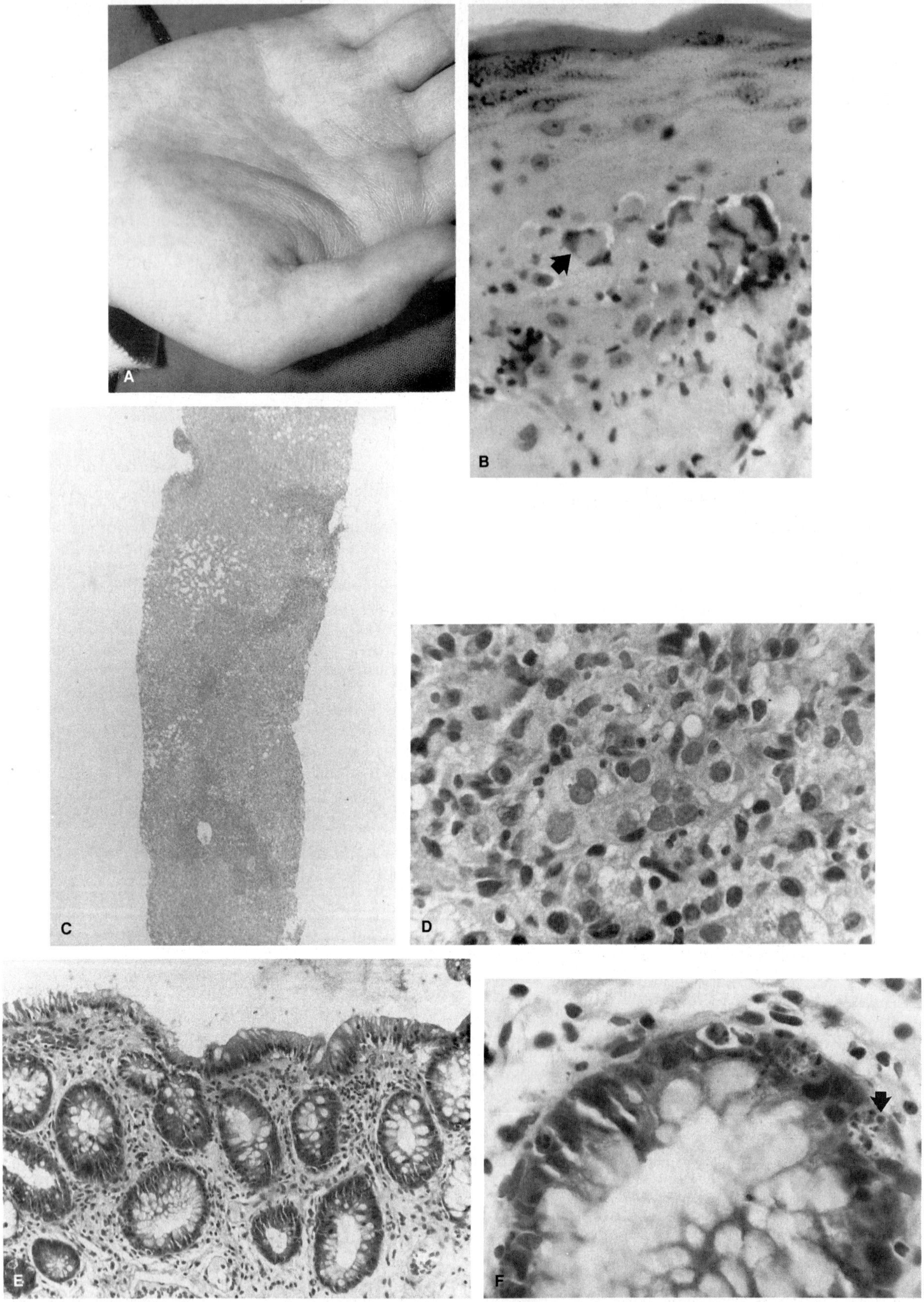

FIGURE 63-6. Acute graft-versus-host disease (GVHD). (**A**) Maculopapular rash with palmar involvement. This is a characteristic appearance of acute cutaneous GVHD and is easily confused with drug eruptions. (**B**) Skin biopsy demonstrates disorganization of epidermal cell maturation, epidermal basal cell vacuolar degeneration, and eosinophilic bodies (*arrow*), which represent dead epidermal cells. There is a mild mononuclear cell infiltrate (×400). Liver biopsy specimens show portal triaditis (**C**; ×25) and bile duct degeneration with mononuclear cell infiltrate (**D**; ×400). (**E**) Colonic mucosal biopsy shows epithelial atrophy (×200). (**F**) High-power view of the same colonic biopsy demonstrates necrosis of epidermal cells (*arrow*; ×400). (See Color Figure 63-6.) (Courtesy of Dr. James Crawford, Pathology Department, Brigham and Women's Hospital, Boston)

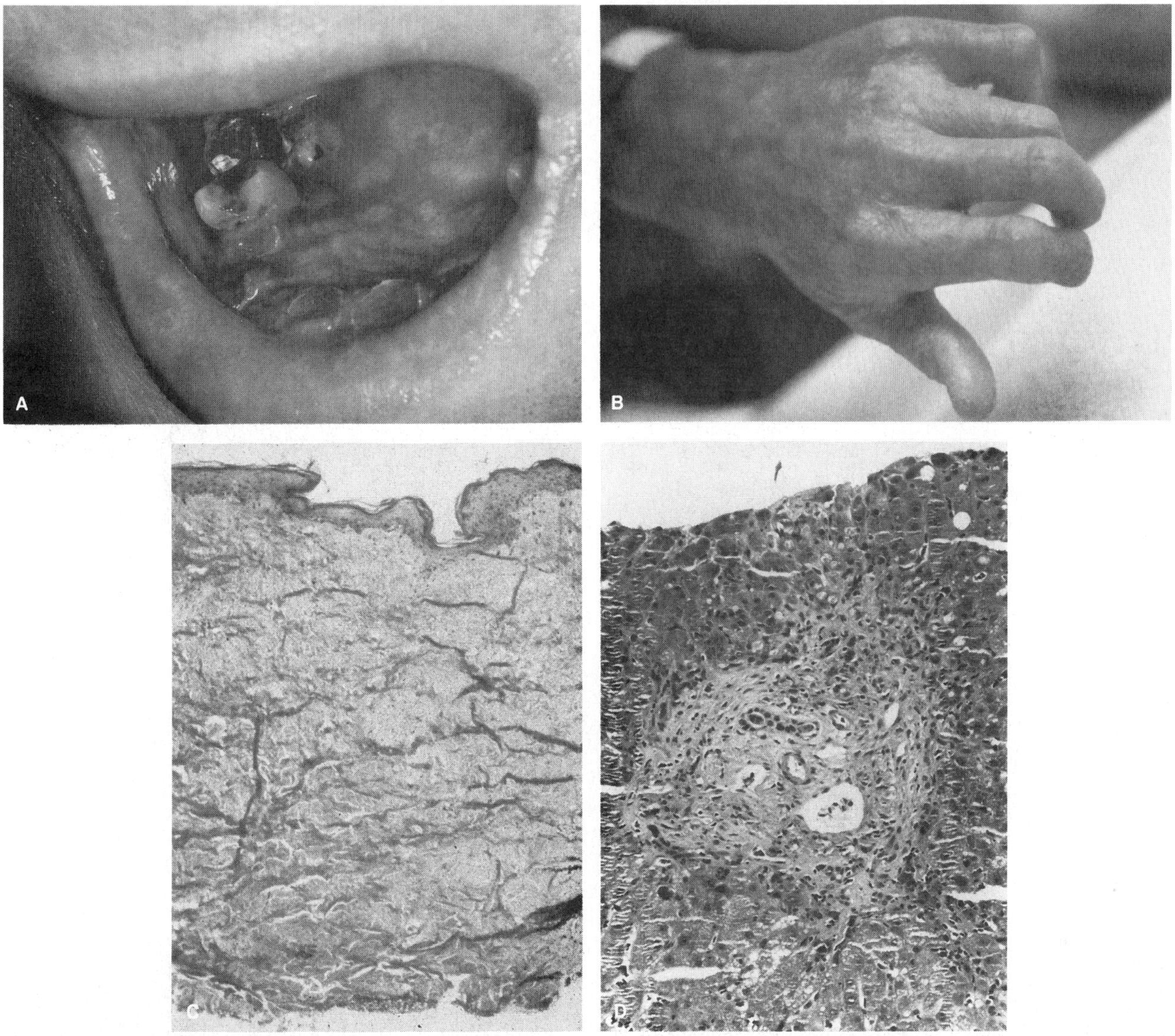

FIGURE 63-7. (A) Oral mucosa with lacy, white plaques that are similar to lichen planus. Caries are due to xerostomia, steroid-induced diabetes mellitus, and chronic grinding of the teeth. (B) Severe atrophy of the skin with flexion contractures. (C) Skin biopsy specimen shows epidermal atrophy with loss of rete pegs and dermal fibrosis. (D) Liver biopsy demonstrates bile duct damage, fibrosis in portal areas, and chronic cholestasis. (See Color Figure 63-7.)

acute GVHD in transplantations performed for aplastic anemia; and (3) high doses of intravenous Ig ameliorate GVHD.[414–419] One explanation for these associations is the possibility that cytokines produced by exposure to bacterial products such as endotoxin result in increased inflammation, increased expression of class II antigens on cell surfaces, increased nitric oxide production, and the production of additional cytokines, such as interleukin-1, tumor necrosis factor-α, and interferon-γ, in a disordered fashion. Direct experimental support for the role of cytokines in GVHD is starting to accumulate.

Risk Factors and Prognosis

The greatest risk factor for the development of GVHD in humans is the MHC compatibility of the donor and recipient. Transplants using methotrexate or cyclosporine as GVHD prophylaxis, undertaken between related patients who differ at more than a single MHC locus, result in a near 100% incidence of GVHD, with most patients developing severe (grade III or IV) disease.[420,421] This observation has resulted in most allogeneic transplantation in the past 20 years that were carried out in patients who had a family member donor identical at all phenotypically measurable MHC loci or, at most, who differed at a single locus. Even in related, MHC-matched transplantations, the incidence of acute GVHD is 25% to 70%. The mortality rate from the disorder varies with severity. Since there may be some beneficial effect of GVHD in patients with malignant disorders, the association of GVHD with morbidity and mortality is probably best observed in patients with transplants for aplastic anemia.[422]

Although a final consensus has not been reached, additional risk factors for the development of acute GVHD include older age of recipient, older age of donor, prior donor transfusions, disease stage, conditioning regimen, and sex mismatching of donor and recipient.[423,424–427] Sex mismatching appears to have its greatest effect when parous females donate to males. There may be a hierarchy with female donors and male recipients at worst risk, followed by female donors and female recipients, then male donors and female recipients, and finally male donors and male recipients. Postulated, and somewhat controversial, risk factors include certain HLA types,[423,428] presence or absence of splenectomy,[420] and ABO mismatching.[181] All observers agree that increasing severity of GVHD results in decreasing patient survival.

Why age, sex mismatching, and the other clinical variables mentioned change the risk of development of GVHD remains speculative. Normal T-lymphocyte differentiation, and, in particular, the elimination of autoreactive clones and the education of immature T cells in the recognition of self MHC, normally occurs in the thymus. Although data suggest that extrathymic differentiation is possible, the prevention of rampant autoimmune disease and the establishment of immunocyte communication in early life are predominantly thymic functions. By puberty, the human thymus has involuted significantly. Moreover, treatment with radiation and chemotherapy can further damage the thymic epithelium on which the T-cell education process takes place. Therefore, the recapitulation of the immune system after marrow transplantation may be aberrant, especially in older patients; and this immune imbalance might lead to a GVHD reaction. Sex mismatching may lead to increased GVHD either by presensitization of donor T cells to foreign antigens, as in parous women, or by reaction to a minor histocompatibility difference between donor and recipient.

An association also exists between infection with members of the herpesvirus family, especially CMV, and GVHD, although the cause-and-effect relation remains unclear.[429,430]

Finally, in vitro predictive tests for GVHD have been described.[431,432] In one case, recipient skin explants were incubated with donor lymphocytes and examined for histopathologic signs of GVHD. In another, a mixed epidermal cell lymphocyte reaction was used. A more sensitive test of donor-recipient recognition involves a limiting-dilution analysis of donor IL-2–secreting T-cell precursors. High levels of IL-2–secreting precursors are associated with a high risk of developing acute GVHD, whereas low precursor numbers seem to identify patient–donor pairs at reduced risk of GVHD. All these tests probably detect donors that are capable of reacting to recipient minor histocompatibility antigens.[433] If these tests continue to prove useful, they will be a helpful adjunct to the clinician in designing new posttransplantation protocols since eliminating the need for GVHD prophylaxis in a subset of patients would likely lead to more rapid immune reconstitution and possibly improved overall survival.

Prophylaxis

Because patient survival is reduced by the development of severe acute GVHD, it is logical that prevention of this disorder might lead to improved clinical results in transplantation. A number of preventive regimens have been used that employ both single-agent and multiagent posttransplantation immunosuppression.[434] Some commonly used regimens are shown in Figure 63-8.[435–437]

Randomized trials have consistently shown that combination therapy is more effective than single-agent prophylaxis. It is reasonable to expect an overall rate of grade II to IV GVHD of 25% to 40%. Ramsay and colleagues[438] randomly assigned patients to a regimen of either 100-day methotrexate alone or methotrexate, ATG (seven doses), and prednisone (days 8 to 20) and noted a 48% incidence of acute GVHD in the methotrexate-alone group as opposed to 21% in the combination regimen. In this study, as has been seen in a variety of trials, increasing rigor of posttransplantation immunosuppression led to a decreased incidence of clinically diagnosed acute GVHD but failed to show a patient survival advantage. The failure to clearly improve survival, especially of patients with transplants for leukemia, while decreasing morbidity and mortality directly attributable to GVHD in some trials may be due to an increase in the incidence of late infectious complications and leukemic relapse in the face of increased immunosuppression (see section on graft-versus-leukemia). Some authors have suggested that reducing the amount of routine posttransplantation immunosuppression and then treating GVHD when it occurs might be an alternate strategy,[439] although others have reported a syndrome of hyperacute GVHD if no prophylaxis is used.[440]

The regimen of cyclosporine plus methotrexate has been reported to improved control of GVHD and increase survival in several studies. In patients with transplants for aplastic anemia,[441] 18% of those receiving cyclosporine plus methotrexate developed significant acute GVHD, compared with 53% in the group receiving methotrexate alone, with respective actuarial 2-year survival rates of 82% and 60%. No difference in the incidence of chronic GVHD was observed (9 of 19 versus 6 of 14, respectively). As noted, reduction of GVHD is most likely to benefit patients receiving transplants for nonmalignant disorders since there is no postulated benefit from adoptive immunotherapy (ie, GVL) in that group. What, then, is the result of the improved combination regimen in patients with transplants for leukemia? In the initial study of patients receiving transplants for ANLL,[202] 33% of those receiving cyclosporine and methotrexate developed GVHD, compared with 54% in the cyclosporine-only group (P = .014); the actuarial survival rate at 1.5 years was 80% versus 55%, respectively (P = .042). Similar improvement was shown for patients receiving transplants for CML. Unfortunately, with longer follow-up, subsequent studies have shown a loss of the survival advantage in most patient groups.[442] With a 3- to 4.5-year follow-up, the survival rate for the ANLL patients is identical (41% in each group), with only a trend toward a survival advantage in CML (73% versus 54%, P = .09). The loss of survival advantage was due to an increase in leukemic relapse. As for other studies, reduction in the incidence of acute GVHD led to no change in the overall incidence of chronic GVHD (about 25% in both groups). Similar results were reported in a large-scale retrospective analysis by the IBMTR.[443] Thus, although the combination regimen has benefits in early posttransplantation management, pharmacologic approaches to GVHD remain suboptimal.

As noted, the intensity of the conditioning regimen influences the incidence of GVHD. In part, this effect may be related to increased tissue injury and inflammatory cytokine production, but the more severe mucositis may also prevent the administration of the full dose of methotrexate.[444–446] Some regimens use prednisone, but its addition to cyclosporine and methotrexate has not improved survival.[447] Unfortunately, the drugs available for GVHD prophylaxis are incompletely effective and have substantial toxicity. Methotrexate often worsens mucositis induced by the conditioning regimen, and it can increase the risk of interstitial pneumonia. Cyclosporine is hepatotoxic and nephrotoxic, and it is often difficult to attain the necessary degree of GVHD control without drug-induced toxicity.

Because acute GVHD can be completely abrogated in animal models by depleting mature T lymphocytes from donor marrow, trials of ex vivo marrow T-cell depletion in humans were begun in the early 1980s.[448–451] A multitude of techniques may be used to accomplish this purpose: sheep erythrocyte rosetting with or without soybean lectin separation,[452,453] monoclonal antibody plus a source of complement,[454,455] immunotoxin conjugates,[456,457] and counterflow elutriation.[458,459] When antibodies are used,

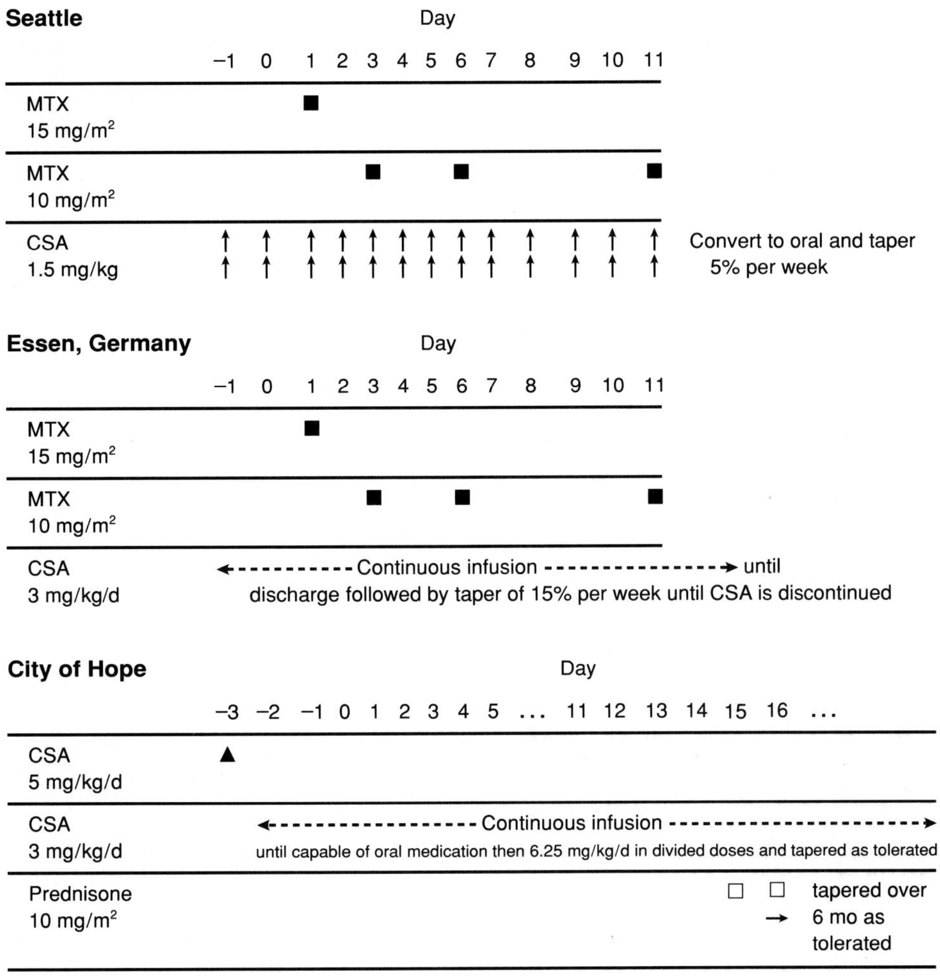

FIGURE 63-8. Three examples of prophylactic regimens for acute graft-versus-host disease. CSA, cyclosporine; MTX, methotrexate. (Data from references 435 to 437)

they may be directed against any of a number of pan-T surface markers (eg, CD3, CD5, CD2), or an attempt may be made to deplete only a particular subset of T lymphocytes.[460] All these variations introduce significant variation in the final result. In some cases, such as the soybean lectin and rosette technique, B cells are depleted along with T cells. Some T-cell antigens modulate rapidly (eg, CD3). If the procedure depends on complement for lysis, there may be inadequate time of exposure, and depletion of the T cells may be relatively inefficient. On the other hand, if an antibody is linked to an immunotoxin that must be internalized to be effective, then modulation may be preferable to optimize death of the target cells. Additional variables include incomplete T-cell depletion with some monoclonal antibodies (such as anti-CD8 or anti-CD5) and sparing of NK cells. Leaving some functionally competent cells may retain the antileukemic effect or may enhance engraftment.

A randomized trial of T-cell depletion versus standard pharmacologic prophylaxis demonstrated the following instructive findings.[461] Although the incidence and severity of acute GVHD was significantly reduced by this procedure, overall survival remained the same. This occurred because of an increased incidence of graft rejection and of leukemic relapse. These same trends have been seen in most other series and in a large retrospective study of the IBMTR.[462] In addition, most series also demonstrate a reduction in overall incidence of chronic GVHD. It is postulated, as mentioned earlier, that the increased risk of graft rejection occurs because of the loss of donor immunologic attack on residual host elements (NK or T cells) that are capable of mounting the rejection reaction. Moreover, additional studies have demonstrated delayed immunologic reconstitution, a possible increased risk of late infections[463] in the HLA-incompatible setting, and a possible increased risk of posttransplantation lymphoproliferative syndrome.[168,457,464,465] These results are reminiscent of early trials of pharmacologic immunosuppression for GVHD. There appears to be a fine line between adequate immunosuppression to prevent (or ameliorate) GVHD and excess immunosuppression that leads to immunologic complications.

Is there a potential future for the T-cell depletion approach? Trials are exploring several options. First, the increased incidence of graft rejection can be reduced by increasing pretransplantation immunosuppressive conditioning. This may be possible to a limited degree since toxicity from methotrexate and cyclosporine would be avoided. Furthermore, improvement in conditioning regimens may also reduce leukemic relapses. Second, the use of cytokines after transplantation might be capable of partially reversing the more severe immunologic defect, although the fear of increasing GVHD remains. Third, based on murine studies, it might be possible to deplete only the particular subset of T cells that is the primary mediator of the GVHD reaction and leave intact the remainder of the T-lymphocyte system. Ultimately, one would want to eliminate only those preformed T cells that are host-specific from the donor marrow. Finally, T-cell depletion might be used to prevent acute, transplant-related toxicity. Subsequently, limited numbers of T cells could be infused to establish a GVL reaction.[466]

Treatment

Once acute GVHD develops, despite prophylaxis, several agents are available for treatment:

- Corticosteroids (generally methylprednisolone): either in doses of 2 to 5 mg/kg/d or in high-dose pulses of 500 mg/m^2 for 10 days[467]
- Cyclosporine: doses similar to those used in prophylaxis regimens
- ATG[468]

Large retrospective studies of the treatment of GVHD have demonstrated that most potent immunosuppressive agents are useful to some extent, with the notable exception of azathioprine, and that patients with complete responses to therapy generally do well.[469] Unfortunately, a substantial proportion of patients do not respond to treatment or experience relapse. The complete response rate for initial therapy was only 20% (complete and partial responses occurred in 44%), and an additional 20% to 40% of patients responded to secondary therapy.[470,471] These patients have a poor overall survival because of both to direct complications of GVHD and opportunistic infections related to prolonged immunosuppression. Acute GVHD developing after unrelated donor transplant seems to be particularly difficult to treat successfully.[472]

Occurrence After Syngeneic and Autologous Transplantations

With an identical-twin donor or an autologous transplant, there are, by definition, no discernible antigenic differences between donor and host. Therefore, based on the pathophysiology outlined previously, it should be impossible to generate a GVHD reaction. Nonetheless, in 1979, a syndrome indistinguishable from acute cutaneous GVHD was reported in three recipients of syngeneic marrow transplants.[473] Two of the patients had normal postconditioning regimen skin biopsies with subsequent development of histologic changes consistent with acute GVHD. No evidence of other organ involvement was found, and none of the patients developed chronic GVHD. Subsequent reports have also supported the existence of this phenomenon,[474–476] including several patients with concomitant liver and gastrointestinal manifestations. A similar syndrome has been observed in recipients of autologous transplants.[474,475,477]

The mechanism by which a GVHD-like reaction could occur in the syngeneic or autologous transplantation setting remains uncertain. Several trivial explanations are possible: the GVHD might actually result from nonirradiated blood products accidentally given to the patient. Alternatively, the reaction might be a drug or radiation effect or a viral infection (such as CMV). Both animal models and clinical observations suggest that an immunologic explanation is also possible. An interesting rodent model has been developed in which rats receiving syngeneic or autologous transplants are treated with cyclosporine after transplantation.[478–480] On cessation of the drug, classic GVHD develops. Injury to the thymus and the presence of cyclosporine during T-cell differentiation have been shown to inhibit the differentiation of thymocytes into mature T cells, specifically interfering with the normal deletion of T-cell clones whose antigen receptors react with self.[481–483] Thus, it is possible that ablative pretransplantation conditioning in humans leads to sufficient thymic damage to induce an autoimmune GVHD-like syndrome. Supporting such a hypothesis is the fact that only one patient has been reported in the literature who developed syngeneic GVHD who did not have ablative conditioning.

Finally, clinicopathologic syndromes similar to GVHD have been observed in patients treated with interleukin-2 or interleukin-2–activated killer lymphocytes,[484] suggesting that nonspecific effects of released cytokines may provide a unifying hypothesis for the GVHD-like appearance of some viral syndromes as well as these syngeneic and autologous transplantation syndromes.

Chronic Graft-Versus-Host Disease

Description and Diagnosis

Chronic GVHD may develop from 2 months to 2 years after allogeneic marrow transplantation. It is the most insidious of transplantation complications and, in some respects, the most difficult to handle. In about one third of the patients who develop the disease, it evolves in an uninterrupted progression from prior acute GVHD (progressive chronic GVHD). In another third of patients, it arises after complete or near complete resolution of acute GVHD (so-called quiescent cGVHD), while in the final third of patients, the disorder appears de novo with no previous evidence of clinically apparent acute GVHD. It may occur in a limited form with relatively localized skin involvement or mild hepatic dysfunction or in a generalized form with extensive involvement of multiple organs[485–487] (Table 63-5). The latter syndrome presents earlier after transplantation, on average, than the former. In its most severe form, it is characterized by scleroderma, erythematous skin changes with scarring and ulcer formation, patchy hyper- and hypopigmentation, lichen planus, alopecia, malar erythema, photosensitivity, xerostomia, severe keratoconjunctivitis sicca,[488] myositis, synovitis, tendonitis, joint contractures, desquamative esophagitis with stricture formation, and abnormal (usually cholestatic) liver function tests. Mucositis can be severe and debilitating. The disease is accompanied by persistent severe immunodeficiency and failure to reconstitute both the humoral and cellular arms of the immune response. This immune failure, coupled with the integumentary loss and cholestasis, heightens the risk of severe infection in these patients and includes a marked increase in gram-positive infections.[489] Flares of chronic GVHD often occur during tapering of cyclosporine or prednisone, but they

TABLE 63-5. Chronic Graft-Versus-Host Disease Classification

LIMITED CHRONIC GRAFT-VERSUS-HOST DISEASE
Localized skin involvement with or without:
Hepatic dysfunction due to chronic graft-versus-host disease
Normal platelet count (>100,000/μL)
EXTENSIVE CHRONIC GRAFT-VERSUS-HOST DISEASE
Generalized skin involvement; or
Localized skin involvement and/or hepatic dysfunction due to chronic graft-versus-host disease, plus any of the following:
Liver histology showing chronic aggressive hepatitis, bridging necrosis, or cirrhosis
Involvement of the eye: Schirmer's test with <5 mm of wetting
Involvement of minor salivary glands or oral mucosa demonstrated on labial biopsy
Involvement of any other target organ
Chronic thrombocytopenia (platelets <100,000/μL) continuously despite normal granulocyte and reticulocyte counts

also appear to be induced by solar exposure and infections. The use of sunscreen, hats, and long-sleeved clothing is important to prevent such exacerbations. Infections such as shingles may be followed by localized chronic GVHD in the area of viral infection or in a generalized worsening of skin disease.

The histology of chronic GVHD in involved organs resembles chronic inflammation and fibrosis (see Fig. 63-6). In the skin, epidermal hypertrophy and lichen planus–like reaction progress to epidermal fibrosis and atrophy.[490] In the localized variant, dense dermal fibrosis may be seen without an inflammatory reaction. Gingival biopsies demonstrate mucositis and squamous cell necrosis similar, but not identical, to that seen in Sjögren's syndrome.[491] Liver biopsies demonstrate chronic active hepatitis with bridging necrosis and cirrhosis in the more severe cases that may go on to cirrhosis.

Although the diagnosis of severe cases of GVHD is not difficult on clinical grounds alone, definitive recognition of the disease in early stages may be made on the basis of skin biopsy, gingival biopsy, and Schirmer's test. Some authorities advocate the routine use of such studies at day 100 after transplantation in all patients so that subclinical disease can be recognized early and therapy begun.

Chronic GVHD is more of a multisystem disease than acute GVHD. Some patients have features of both conditions throughout a prolonged transition period. Aside from the organs discussed previously, what other organs are involved by the disease? Again, it may be difficult to distinguish organ involvement by the condition from organ damage due to secondary infection. Nonetheless, the only other organ suspected of involvement is the lung. After transplantation, many patients develop pulmonary impairment, usually of a combined restrictive and obstructive nature. Bronchiolitis obliterans, a progressive condition in many cases, may develop 6 or more months after transplantation and may be a direct result of chronic GVHD. It is usually associated with hypogammaglobulinemia.[142,492–494] This condition may also be found in patients in the absence of chronic GVHD. Whether that implies that the pathophysiology is of single-organ GVHD in those cases or that the link between these conditions is not one-to-one is unknown. It is likely that bronchiolitis obliterans is triggered by infection.

Pathophysiology

It remains an open question both in experimental animal models and in humans whether chronic GVHD is yet another manifestation of the same pathophysiology responsible for acute GVHD or whether it is, at least sometimes, an intrinsically different disorder. Conceptually, chronic GVHD could represent either a continued attack of committed, mature T cells infused with donor marrow against the host with a failure to develop adequate suppression of these elements. Alternatively, it could represent the manifestations of an autoimmune process, that is, a failure of uncommitted T cells, newly maturing from the lymphoid stem cell, to become host tolerant because of an inadequate thymic or extrathymic environment in which to differentiate. The question is not simply an academic one, since if the latter mechanism is correct, one must predict that even total depletion of all committed T cells from donor marrow in humans will not eliminate chronic GVHD. Indeed, the latter mechanism would suggest that to eliminate chronic GVHD, one needs to supply the newly maturing marrow with an adequate environment for differentiation.

In animal models, evidence for both mechanisms has been proposed.[495,496] In humans, most trials of ex vivo T-cell depletion of donor marrow that have successfully reduced the incidence and severity of acute GVHD have not clearly reduced the incidence of chronic GVHD. However, pharmacologic manipulations that significantly reduce the incidence of acute GVHD (such as cyclosporine plus methotrexate) have not clearly reduced the incidence of chronic GVHD. Trials of thymic transplantation to prevent chronic GVHD have not been successful.[497]

Risk Factors and Prognosis

The most significant risk factors for the development of chronic GVHD are the presence of prior acute GVHD and increasing age of the patient.[498,499] In addition, patients who received the Seattle aplastic anemia conditioning regimen that included the infusion of donor buffy coat cells were at increased risk for the development of chronic GVHD, and some authors find a higher incidence in patients who previously had CMV infection.[500] As for acute GVHD, the exact pathophysiologic mechanism by which these characteristics increase the risk of developing chronic GVHD is uncertain. Since donor buffy coat contains large numbers of nonirradiated, immunocompetent lymphocytes, it is believed that this procedure increases risk by increasing total T-cell dose.

Because of the legion manifestations of the disease and the uneven involvement of different organ systems in different patients, a simple prognostic grading system such as that used for acute GVHD is not in common use. Karnofsky's index or other indices of overall patient performance are probably most useful, but patients who have thrombocytopenia associated with their disease have a particularly grim prognosis.[234] This does not relate to morbidity due to bleeding complications; rather, it presumably serves as an index of overall disease activity since the cause of death in these patients is generally an infection.

Treatment

Treatment of chronic GVHD involves immunosuppressive agents. The Seattle group[501] carried out a randomized trial of prednisone alone, 1 mg/kg every other day, versus a combination of prednisone and azathioprine, 1.5 mg/kg/d, in all patients with extensive chronic GVHD who also had a platelet count of at least 100,000/μL. All patients also received trimethoprim-sulfamethoxazole, one double-strength tablet twice daily, and received a median of 2 years of therapy. Complications included diabetes (5%), aseptic necrosis (5%), and infection. Recurrent malignancy occurred equally in the two groups, but nonrelapse mortality was only 21% in the steroid-only group compared with 40% in the prednisone plus azathioprine group. Moreover, the incidence of disseminated varicella, bacteremia, and interstitial pneumonitis in the steroid versus two-drug group was 11% versus 24%, 6% versus 11%, and 5% versus 14%, respectively. Thus, treatment with alternate-day steroids alone gave significantly better results in these patients. In the same study, patients with platelet counts of less than 100,000/μL were uniformly treated with steroids alone. As expected, these patients had a significantly worse overall prognosis (58% nonrelapse mortality) and higher incidence of disseminated varicella (34%), bacteremia (34%), and interstitial pneumonitis (18%).

Patients with thrombocytopenia and extensive chronic GVHD have been treated with prednisone, 1 mg/kg every other day, alternating with cyclosporine, 6 mg/kg every 12 hours every other day, and continuous trimethoprim-sulfamethoxazole prophylaxis. Complete response rates of 33% were observed, and improvements in survival rates to over 50% were seen even in patients who did not respond to prior therapy.[502] In summary, for patients with mild chronic GVHD, alternate-day steroids appears to be sufficient therapy, while patients with severe chronic GVHD may benefit from the addition of cyclosporine.

Supportive therapy of patients with chronic GVHD is crucial. Prophylaxis with trimethoprim-sulfamethoxazole, use of artificial tears, and avoidance of solar exposure should be combined with a program of psychological support and physical and occupational therapy. Many of these patients are subject to recurrent infections, especially from encapsulated organisms. This results from their combination immunodeficiency: decreased total IgG, inability to mount a new antibody immune response, functional asplenia, and poor integument. Patients with severe disease and those with recurrent infections likely benefit from penicillin prophylaxis, and replacement γ-globulin must also be considered.

Graft-Versus-Leukemia Reaction

The ability of the immune system to destroy allogeneic and syngeneic tumor cells has been amply demonstrated in both animal models and in humans.[503,504] Indeed, the concept of adoptive immunotherapy for acute leukemia dates back to the 1960s.[505] In some experimental systems, a GVL reaction can be detected that is separable from the GVHR[506,507]; while in other models, the two appear to go hand in hand.[508] In human allogeneic marrow transplantation, a GVL effect can also be demonstrated, empirically, to accompany the GVHR[509–512]; and in selected subsets of patients, chronic GVHD, presumably accompanied by the GVL effect, may even contribute to increased overall patient survival as a result of a decrease in disease recurrence. As noted earlier, one of the most effective means of reducing GVHD is donor marrow T-cell depletion. Unfortunately, accompanying that decrease in GVHD is an increase in leukemic relapse.[513] In an analysis of 208 CML patients from eight transplantation centers, 17 of 102 patients who received T-cell–depleted marrow relapsed, and only 2 or 106 patients receiving unmanipulated marrows had recurrent disease.[514] It is not known whether improvements in conditioning regimens or earlier transplantation offset the loss of GVL.

Because clinical data suggest that further improvements in transplantation conditioning regimen effectiveness are likely to be accompanied by further increases in toxicity,[124] it is attractive to consider using the GVL reaction in a controlled fashion. The Seattle group attempted just such a manipulation.[515] By randomly assigning patients to receive three different GVHD prophylaxis regimens, they were able to vary the incidence of grade II to IV acute GVHD from 25% (long-course methotrexate) to 59% (short-course methotrexate) to 82% (methotrexate plus donor buffy coat). Nonetheless, as was discussed earlier, the incidence of chronic GVHD was identical in the three groups (33%, 51%, 44%, respectively). Overall disease-free survival rates with median follow-up of about 5 years were 41%, 30%, and 24% in the three groups, respectively. There was no difference in 5-year probability of recurrent malignancy, although nonrelapse mortality did differ at the extremes (34% versus 45% versus 64%). Thus, in this study, it was not possible to harness GVHD to obtain an adjustable beneficial clinical effect. In part, their failure to observe an improvement in survival may reflect the poor underlying prognosis of the selected patients or insensitivity of their illnesses to GVL. However, another possibility is that increasing acute GVHD in the peritransplant period increases GVHD-related mortality disproportionately to that caused by GVL. Subsequent studies using infusions of peripheral blood leukocytes obtained by leukapheresis have shown an impressive antileukemic effect with surprisingly mild GVHD.[516,517] These new data emphasize the importance of the GVL reaction in the outcome of marrow transplantation, particularly in CML.

Transfusion-Associated Graft-Versus-Host Disease

In addition to marrow transplant recipients and neonatal immunodeficient children, clinical GVHD may also occur in immunosuppressed patients receiving nonirradiated cellular blood products. This has been described in patients with Hodgkin's disease, ANLL, ALL, SCIDS, Wiskott-Aldrich syndrome, neonatal or intrauterine exchange transfusion, liver transplantations, and other disorders,[518–524] although the overall incidence in all these conditions remains low. It is most commonly observed in young (small) children. This is presumed to reflect the relatively high dose of lymphocytes per kilogram of host body weight that occurs in such a child. The minimal dose of lymphocytes necessary to initiate the reaction has been estimated at 10^7/kg. In these circumstances, only the T lymphocytes engraft. Typically, 2 to 4 weeks after a transfusion, the patient develops characteristic rash, liver function abnormalities, diarrhea, and subsequently pancytopenia and perhaps respiratory failure. In contrast to GVHD developing after marrow grafting, pancytopenia is prominent because of suppression of the host's hematopoiesis by the transfused T cells. Both because of this profound cytopenia and because of the host's marked immunodeficiency, fatalities are high in this variant of GVHD when it occurs in an obviously recognizable presentation (estimated at 75% to 90% mortality). Whether the disorder may occur in a mild forme fruste in other postchemotherapy patients is unknown but occasionally suspected. Irradiation of blood products with 1500 to 3000 cGy virtually eliminates the risk of developing GVHD from blood products.

One possible exception to the rule that the development of GVHD only occurs in patients who are profoundly immunosuppressed, and therefore incapable of rejecting the donor lymphocytes, has been described.[525] In two patients who were fully immunocompetent, a fatal syndrome clinically and pathologically identical to transfusion-associated GVHD developed after receiving family blood products during cardiac surgery. The family donor in this case was HLA homozygous for one of the recipient's MHC haplotypes. In this circumstance, it is postulated that the host was incapable of recognizing the donated blood as foreign since the donor expresses only HLA antigens identical to the host. Nonetheless, since the host expresses an HLA haplotype different from the donor, a GVHD reaction may occur.

APLASTIC ANEMIA

Before the application of marrow transplantation, the outlook for patients with severe aplastic anemia was grim[526,527]. Early studies by Thomas and colleagues,[528] however, demonstrated the feasibility of replacing missing or defective hematopoietic stem cells with normal donor cells. In addition to important therapeutic progress, marrow transplantation led to further understanding of the pathogenesis of idiopathic aplastic anemia. In reports of 21 syngeneic transplants performed without the use of immunosuppression, 12 patients failed to engraft, and 8 subsequently successfully engrafted after receiving second transplants conditioned with cyclophosphamide.[529] Subsequent studies also demonstrated a substantial rate of autologous recovery of hematopoiesis after cyclophosphamide-conditioned transplants.[530–534] These data suggested that some patients with aplastic anemia had cellular or humoral inhibition of hematopoiesis rather than deficient numbers of stem cells. The response of patients with aplastic anemia to intensive immunosuppression further supports this view.[535] Another category of aplastic anemia has been inferred by observations of lymphoid chimerism without myeloid chimerism after marrow grafting. These observations suggest that a small proportion of cases of aplastic anemia are due to the inability of the bone marrow microenvironment to support hematopoiesis.[1,109,110]

Soon after the application of marrow grafting to severe aplastic anemia, it was recognized that, in addition to GVHD,[536] graft rejection was a major problem. Typically, the rejection rate was 30% to 45%, and the mortality in patients without sustained grafts was 80%.[537–539] Although several risk factors for graft rejection were suggested by different groups,[539,540] the primary determinant of the likelihood of rejection in HLA-compatible transplantation is prior blood transfusion. Patients who remain untransfused 72 hours before receiving the beginning of the conditioning regimen have a graft failure rate of 10% and an actuarial 10-year survival rate of 82%.[541] It is thought that the rejection rate rises after blood transfusion because of transfusion-induced sensitization to minor histocompatibility antigens.[542,543] Transfusions from family members are the most likely to sensitize the patient to minor histocompatibility determinants and should be avoided. Many patients with aplastic anemia require transfusions before the ascertainment of a HLA-compatible donor and the initiation of transplantation. It is inappropriate to withhold blood products from pancytopenic patients who require them. It appears that the risk of rejection, however, is a function of the number of transfusions received.[540] Consequently, new strategies were directed at reducing the relapse rate. TBI in doses commonly used to treat leukemia was successful at reducing the graft failure rate to low levels—but at the expense of increased mortality due to interstitial pneumonia and GVHD.[538–540,544] Less intensive radiotherapeutic regimens (see Fig. 63-4) that rely on cyclophosphamide and low-dose TBI,[545] total lymphoid irradiation,[546] or thoracoabdominal irradiation[547] resulted in rejection rates of 5% to 10% and overall survival rates of 62% to 78%. Some data indicate that total lymphoid irradiation is preferable to TBI since it is associated with similar graft failure rates but better overall survival.[315,540] However, concern has been raised about the risk of secondary malignancies. Similar results (rejection rate, 10%; 5-year actuarial survival rate, 61%) were achieved with cyclophosphamide-procarbazine-ATG serum.[548] The Seattle group observed that the number of marrow cells infused was an important determinant of engraftment,[549,550,551] and they infused donor-derived buffy coat cells for 1 to 3 or 1 to 5 days after the marrow infusion. This tactic led to a similar decline in graft rejection and a 67% actuarial 10-year survival rate, but at the expense of increased chronic GVHD.[91,101] The reason that buffy coat is effective may be due to the addition of stem cells, but it may also relate to the ability of infused T cells or NK cells to inhibit or destroy residual host lymphocytes that would mediate graft rejection, or to the addition of lymphokine-producing cells. Cyclosporine is a potent immunosuppressive agent that can reduce the graft rejection rate to about 8%, but the risk of late (4 to 7.5 months) graft failure increases to about 9% when cyclosporine is withdrawn.[530] Second transplants can be performed, and 40% of patients may be long-term survivors.[540,552]

The use of mismatched or matched, unrelated donors in the treatment of aplastic anemia is less successful. The graft rejection rate is high, and there appears to be a higher incidence of GVHD.[45,553,554] The use of these alternate donors, however, may prove life-saving for occasional patients with refractory aplastic anemia.

Prospective trials have been undertaken to compare allogeneic marrow transplantation to conventional therapy for aplastic anemia. The International Aplastic Anemia Study Group published a prospective study of androgens or marrow transplantation in 110 patients with aplastic anemia.[555] They concluded that marrow transplantation was superior therapy to androgens and that marrow grafting was the treatment of choice for patients with compatible donors. Improvements in the immunosuppressive therapy of aplastic anemia and improvements in transplantation results have made the choice of marrow transplantation less straightforward. The UCLA group prospectively compared ATG to marrow transplantation in patients younger than 25 years of age and found a 2-year actuarial survival rate of 72% in the transplant group compared with 45% in the ATG group. This difference, however, did not reach statistical significance. The patients with transplants had better blood counts and performance status.[556] A prospective European study treating patients 40 years of age or younger showed a survival advantage in an antilymphocyte globulin–treated group (75%) compared with a transplantation-treated group (46%),[557] but the group with transplants did not fare as well as most centers report. Although not a comparative, prospective study, Sanders and colleagues[558] also reported a high survival rate (70%) in children receiving transplants for aplastic anemia, supporting a recommendation to transplant all young people who have compatible donors.[559] These recommendations were confirmed in a large retrospective analysis of European data, which indicated a significant advantage for marrow transplantation for patients 20 years or age or younger (64% versus 38%), but more equivalent results in older patients.[560] ATG can result in long-term survival rates of 30% to 70%, but often with incomplete recovery and a tendency to relapse.[531] Furthermore, the development of clonal disorders, such as paroxysmal nocturnal hemoglobinuria (PNH) and myelodysplasia, are increasingly recognized in long-term survivors of immunosuppressive therapy.[561,562]

Advantages and disadvantages to each approach are as follows: marrow transplantation offers a high likelihood of cure but is more expensive, has more acute toxicity, and may result in chronic GVHD. Immunosuppression with ATG is also effective, but often does not cure the aplastic anemia. It requires prolonged supportive care, but has fewer side effects. A reasonable recommendation is to transplant all patients who have identical twin donors. In patients who are 30 to 40 years of age or younger, allogeneic transplantation is the treatment of choice if there is a compatible donor. If there are risks for either the patient or marrow donor, such as pregnancy, recent hepatitis, and so forth, the balance is in favor of immunosuppression. For patients more than 40 years of age, ATG should be administered and marrow grafting reserved for those who fail to respond or who relapse. If no compatible donor is known, ATG is the treatment of choice, and marrow grafting from a mismatched or matched, unrelated donor is reserved for patients in whom immunosuppressive therapy is unsuccessful.[553,554]

The cause of the aplastic anemia does not appear to be an important consideration. Successful transplantation has been reported for aplastic anemia due to pregnancy, gold, drugs, and hepatitis.[91,315,529,530,563–566]

PAROXYSMAL NOCTURNAL HEMOGLOBINURIA

Paroxysmal nocturnal hemoglobinuria is an acquired disorder of hematopoiesis that can result in aplastic anemia. Even in the absence of marrow failure, the thrombotic and hemolytic complications of PNH can be lethal. Because PNH is a clonal disorder that can result in acute leukemia, it is important to establish that a conditioning regimen designed primarily for immunosuppression in aplastic anemia is adequate to eliminate the PNH clone. If the marrow is extremely hypocellular (10% or more), immunosuppression appears to be adequate to prevent mixed chimerism.[119,567–569] Mixed hematopoietic chimerism, however, may be common in aplastic anemia. The Seattle group[114] noted a 58% incidence of temporary mixed chimerism in 96 patients with transplants for aplastic anemia. Recovery of endogenous hematopoiesis after marrow grafting for aplastic anemia was been discussed previously. Because cyclophosphamide does not necessarily ablate stems cells, these observations suggest that patients receiving transplants after primarily immunosuppressive conditioning regimens, when the marrow is not severely hypocellular, may have a high incidence of relapse of PNH. TBI and busulfan have both been used in an effort to destroy the PNH clone, but both patients treated with TBI died of interstitial pneumonia.[119,570] For patients with cellular marrows, combination busulfan and cyclophosphamide appears to be an effective regimen.[110]

CHRONIC MYELOGENOUS LEUKEMIA

Chronic myelogenous leukemia is a stem cell disorder that has stubbornly resisted curative therapy with conventional doses of chemotherapy or irradiation. It can be controlled with relatively nontoxic therapy, like hydroxyurea or α-interferon, but it relentlessly progresses to an aggressive phase that is ultimately fatal. In contrast to the acute leukemias, in which long-term disease-free survival may be achieved with standard chemotherapy, CML is only cured by bone marrow transplantation.

Timing of Bone Marrow Transplantation

The likelihood of eradicating the leukemic population is largely dependent on the timing of transplantation. Several large studies indicate that transplantation in chronic (stable) phase is associated with a long-term disease-free survival rate of 55% to 87%, depending on age, the presence of GVHD, and the compatibility of the donor. In contrast, once accelerated phase supervenes, the survival rate drops substantially to 18% to 30%. If the transplantation is undertaken in blast crisis, the results are the worst, with a 10% to 15% long-term survival rate.[513,571–577] Patients in accelerated phase, who have donors, should receive transplants as soon as possible. Patients who achieve a second stable phase after chemotherapy for blast transformation do about as well as patients undergoing transplants in accelerated phase.[572,573] Given the poor overall results in transplantation for blast crisis, if the blast crisis is lymphoid, attempts at establishing a second stable phase with intensive chemotherapy are warranted.

The high transplantation-related mortality requires circumspection when recommending the procedure to patients in chronic phase, particularly if the patient falls into a good prognostic category.[578,579] The Seattle group has suggested that performing the transplantation as soon as possible in chronic phase results in improved survival. Patients undergoing transplantation less than 1 year from diagnosis had about an 80% actuarial survival rate at 4 years, compared with about 40% if the transplantation occurred 1 to 3 years from diagnosis, and about 20% if it occurred more than 3 years after diagnosis.[572] A recent analysis of the Seattle data suggests that early transplantation can result in survival rates in excess of 90% in selected patients.[580] The relation between early transplantation and survival was also noted in other studies.[581,582]

Age younger than 20 to 30 years has been a consistently good prognostic finding.[513,572,573] This advantage stems in part from the age-related increase in GVHD that contributes to mortality in older patients. Recommendation for marrow transplantation must be weighed carefully against the risk of early death. The development of accelerated phase is often unpredictable, however, and transplantation is appropriate for patients younger than 60 years of age early in chronic phase.

Unrelated donor transplantation has been applied to patients with CML without family member donors, and the actuarial survival rate ranges from 30% to 45% in published series.[583–586] The relapse rate appears to lower after unrelated donor marrow transplantation, providing further evidence of a GVL effect. Unfortunately, the risk of severe acute GVHD (about 65%) and chronic GVHD (about 55%) is high when unrelated donor marrow is used.

Role of Splenectomy or Splenic Irradiation

Splenic enlargement is characteristic in CML, and the spleen is engorged with leukemic cells. The large spleen may sequester cells and make transfusion support difficult. Consequently, splenectomy has been proposed as a means of debulking the leukemia and to facilitate platelet transfusion.[587] Engraftment occurs somewhat faster in the absence of the spleen, and transfusion support is easier, but there is a tendency for more acute GVHD.[572,588–590] Retrospective and prospective studies show no significant survival or disease-free survival benefit for splenectomy or splenic irradiation.[588,591]

Prior Therapy

Therapy of stable-phase CML is generally decided by the primary hematologist rather than the transplantation center, but there are no firm guidelines on which to base a recommendation. There may be more interstitial pneumonia in patients who received busulfan before transplantation.[572,582] It was not possible to establish an unequivocal correlation between prior therapy and survival, but it is prudent to avoid busulfan if possible and use hydroxyurea or α-interferon.

Relapse

The recognition that some patients have persistence or recurrence of Philadelphia (Ph) chromosome–positive cells that may not go on to clinical disease has led to a distinction between cytogenic and clinical relapses.[513,514,572,592–594] The presence of Ph metaphases in the marrow up to 2 years after transplantation does not necessarily indicate that clinical relapse is forthcoming.[593] More sensitive molecular genetic techniques may be useful in assessing the frequency and significance of residual Ph-positive cells.[595–597] Risk of relapse after transplantation varies according to several risk factors. The primary concern is stage of disease; relapse rates vary from 9% to 30% for transplants performed in stable phase to 25% to 30% for transplants performed in accelerated phase CML, and up to 80% for transplants done in blast crisis. The only other risk factors for relapse appear to be the presence or absence of GVHD and T-lymphocyte depletion. In retrospective studies, patients with acute GVHD had a relative risk of relapse of 0.7; chronic GVHD was associated with a relative risk of 0.4; and both acute and chronic GVHD was associated with the lowest risk, 0.2.[513,514,598] This reduction in relapse rate is not achieved without cost—GVHD is associated with a higher mortality. T-lymphocyte depletion of the marrow appears to reduce the GVL effect regardless of the presence of GVHD,[513,514,599] but the reduction in mortality from GVHD offsets the increased relapse rate, and the overall survival rates are similar. In one study, relapse was associated with slow return of blood counts, and the authors suggested that the absence of donor T cells in the marrow allowed residual recipient T cells to inhibit donor hematopoiesis and allow leukemic cell proliferation. This mechanism might function in addition to the abrogation of GVL, but it might be amenable to more intensive immunosuppression.[599] Further studies are required to determine if GVL and GVHD can be dissociated, perhaps by selective T-cell depletion, or if improvements in conditioning regimens will allow the use of effective means to reduce GVHD but prevent graft failure and relapse.

Autologous Transplantation

Efforts to prolong stable phase by performing ABMTs with either marrow or peripheral blood stem cells were undertaken by several investigators.[600–602] There was rapid recovery of stable-phase CML in many patients, but death due to blastic transformation was inevitable, and this therapy is used only experimentally, since there is no evidence that it cures CML.

ACUTE LEUKEMIA

Acute Nonlymphocytic Leukemia

Bone marrow transplantation is the preferred treatment for patients with advanced ANLL. The initial studies of marrow grafting in ANLL were undertaken on patients with refractory disease, and 10% to 30% disease-free survival rates[603–605] encouraged the use of allogeneic marrow grafting for patients in remission. It was hoped that transplantation before the development of multidrug resistance would improve the results of therapy. This expectation was confirmed by the 20% to 35% disease-free survival rates of patients receiving transplants in second or subsequent remission.[606,607] Long-term survival is rare after leukemic relapse, and marrow grafting offers the only chance of obtaining a prolonged remission. The application of marrow transplantation even earlier in the course of the disease, after first remission, results in improved antileukemic effects with long-term disease-free survival rates of 40% to 60% and relapse rates of 0% to 25% (Table 63-6).

Most investigators agree that marrow transplantation is a better antileukemic therapy than conventional chemotherapy. Deaths from the conditioning regimen and from subsequent GVHD, however, negate some of the advantages of transplantation. Thus, controversy has arisen regarding the best approach to patients in first remission who have compatible donors and who are younger than 45 to 50 years of age. Indeed, there is probably less controversy about patients 25 years of age or younger than about 25- to 45-year-old patients. The prospective, controlled study with the longest follow-up was performed by Appelbaum and colleagues in Seattle.[608,609] These authors found a significantly better disease-free survival rate in the marrow transplantation group. Reiffers and colleagues[610] performed a prospective study comparing allogeneic transplantation, ABMT, and chemotherapy. They also found a statistically significant benefit to early allogeneic marrow grafting

TABLE 63-6. Marrow Transplantation for Treatment of Acute Nonlymphocytic Leukemia in First Remission

Group	Treatment	No.	Actuarial Disease-Free Survival Rate (%)		Relapse Rate (%)	
COMPARATIVE STUDIES						
Seattle[608,609]	Combination chemotherapy	43	21	$P < .009$	79	
	Cyt/FTBI	33*	48		17	
Reiffers et al[610]	Combination chemotherapy	20	16 (95% CI ± 15)	$P < .002$	83	$P < .00005$
	Cyt/FTBI	20	66 (95% CI ± 21)		18	
UCLA[615]	Combination chemotherapy	44	27 (95% CI ± 14)	$P > .4$	71 (95% CI ± 14)	$P < .01$
	Cyt/TBI	23	40 (95% CI ± 21)		40 (95% CI ± 25)	
Begg et al[614] (metaanalysis)	ECOG trial	84	16 (95% CI ± 8)	$P < .05$		
	BMT (two centers)	94	53 (95% CI ± 13)			
Marsden[611,612]	Combination chemotherapy	39	16	$P < .005$		
	Cyt/TBI	98	51			
NONCOMPARATIVE STUDIES						
Seattle[616]	Cyt/SFTBI or FTBI	231	43 (95% CI ± 7)		25 (95% CI ± 7)	
Minnesota[617]	Cyt/SFTBI or FTBI	73	60 (95% CI ± 12)		13 (95% CI ± 10)	
Hopkins[618]	Busulfan/cyt	49	45 (SE ± 7)		~13	
MSKCC[619]	HFTBI/cyt	30	55 (SE ± 5.2)		10	
Duarte[620]	Ara-c/cyt/SFTBI or cyt/FTBI	69	51 (SE ± 6)		24 (SE ± 6)	
EGBMT[606]	Varied	578	~50			
IBMTR[626]	Varied	704	48 (95% CI ± 5)		20 (CI ± 4)	
CHILDREN						
Seattle[621]	Cyt/SFTBI or FBTBI	38	64 (95% CI ± 16)		~18%	
Minnesota[617,622]	Cyt/SFTBI or FTBI	41	61 (95% CI ± 16)		15 (95% CI ± 14)	

Ara-c, arabinosylcytosine; BMT, bone marrow transplantation; cyt, cyclophosphamide; ECOG, Eastern Cooperative Oncology Group; EGBMT, European Group for Bone Marrow Transplantation; IBMTR, International Bone Marrow Transplant Registry; MSKCC, Memorial Sloan-Kettering Cancer Center; TBI, total-body irradiation; (F, fractionated; HF, hyperfractionated; SF, single fraction).

* Includes 10 patients who had a match but refused transplantation. If those patients are excluded, $P < .004$.

compared with chemotherapy when either actual treatment or designated treatment was considered. An additional nonprospective study by the Royal Marsden group,[611,612] a small prospective study by Conde and colleagues,[613] and a metaanalysis[614] support the view that marrow grafting in first remission results in a better disease-free survival rate than chemotherapy alone. Another prospective study by the UCLA group[615] confirmed a lower relapse rate but could not demonstrate longer disease-free survival.

Although marrow transplantation is probably beneficial, it is important to remember that the data collected apply only to young patients with histocompatible siblings. Because the median age of patients with ANLL is about 50 years and most patients do not have an HLA- and MLC-compatible donor, marrow grafting benefits only a minority of patients.

If marrow transplantation is not performed in first complete remission, consideration must also be given to the fate of patients who have compatible donors but relapse. Transplants performed in resistant relapse usually have a poor outcome—10% to 15% disease-free survival rate. Of patients who experience relapse, only about 30% to 40% achieve a second remission, and marrow transplantation in second remission benefits about 20% to 30% of those patients. Thus, less than 20% of patients who require reinduction are cured by transplants. Deaths during reinduction, anthracycline cardiomyopathy, infections, bleeding, or other complications exclude additional patients. It appears, however, that marrow grafting in early relapse, before any attempt at second remission induction, is associated with a 20% to 30% disease-free survival.[607,616] Twenty to 30% of patients in whom marrow transplantation is delayed until relapse never require transplantation, and an additional 20% to 30% are cured with marrow grafting. The projected number of cured patients is similar to results with patients receiving transplants while in first remission. Larger prospective trials are required to establish the best approach. One problem with this more conservative approach is that it assumes prior HLA typing and immediate access to marrow transplantation. In practice, delays occur, and many patients require induction chemotherapy before consideration of marrow grafting. As control of GVHD improves and less toxic conditioning regimens are established, transplantation in first remission may be preferred. If the patient does not have an HLA- and MLC-compatible donor, transplantation with a partially matched family member or a matched, unrelated donor should not be undertaken in first remission unless warranted by other factors, such as cytogenetic abnormalities.

Prognostic Factors

Most studies identified only age and remission status as significant prognostic factors in determining disease-free survival,, although one collaborative study found that female sex, larger proportion of circulating blasts, absence of hepatitis, and shorter duration of symptoms were beneficial.[623] Other studies identified leukocyte count lower than 10,000[608] or 20,000/μL,[624] French-American-British (FAB) class M4 to M5[624,625] or M4 to M6,[608] and extramedullary disease at diagnosis[625] as poor prognostic factors. The largest analysis of risk factors for disease-free survival in ANLL in first remission was carried out by the IBMTR. They found age 25 years or younger, leukocyte count lower than 75,000/μL, and absence of other organ impairment to be independent favorable prognostic factors. FAB classification correlated only to the extent that M4 to M5 ANLL tended to have higher leukocyte counts.[626] It would be valuable to have detailed data regarding immunologic markers, cytogenic abnormalities, and type of induction therapy since it appears likely that factors, which are important in remission duration for chemotherapy, also apply to some extent to marrow transplantation.

Relapse

As noted, the risk of relapse is related to the stage at which transplantation occurs. Although efforts generally are made to avoid acute and chronic GVHD, GVHD appears to exert an antileukemic effect.[509,511,512] Evidence from the IBMTR indicates that T-cell depletion or transplantation from an identical twin results in higher relapse rates, although the effect on overall survival is not known.[598] This is further indirect evidence of a GVL effect. A similar increased relapse rate may occur after pharmacologic GVHD prophylaxis with the combination of methotrexate and cyclosporine.[627,628] Efforts to harness GVL as a form of adoptive immunotherapy have been unsuccessful.[515]

Secondary Myelogenous Leukemia and Myelodysplasia

These hematopoietic diseases share the common feature of refractoriness to standard therapy. Although patients with myelodysplastic syndromes may have long survivals, these diseases are ultimately fatal. Myelodysplasia and leukemia that arise from prior irradiation or chemotherapy are particularly difficult to treat, and long-term survival is rare. Marrow transplantation has been successfully applied to patients with primary and secondary myelodysplasia and secondary leukemia in both adults and children.[629–633] Disease-free survivals are generally better in primary myelodysplasia and are similar to the results expected in de novo ANLL. The primary adverse prognostic factor is marrow fibrosis. Although marrow grafting can result in resolution of fibrosis, severe fibrosis is associated with a high risk of graft failure.[108]

Acute Lymphoblastic Leukemia

The use of marrow grafting in ALL is tempered by the excellent long-term disease-free survivals routinely achieved in this disease, especially in children. As with ANLL, however, marrow grafting is the preferred therapy for advanced ALL. Although recent intensive regimens have improved remission durations in patients who have relapsed, most centers have poor long-term survival of patients who are no longer in first remission. Furthermore, certain high-risk subgroups of patients with ALL, such as those who have a Ph chromosome, do poorly with routine therapy and are candidates for marrow grafting in first remission. Studies of marrow transplantation in first remission have been carried out in patients considered to be at high risk of relapse—those older than 20 to 30 years of age; with leukocyte counts higher than 10,000 to 25,000/μL; and with the Ph chromosome, t(4;11), or a mediastinal mass. Actuarial disease-free survival rates of 42% to 89% and actuarial relapse rates of 0% to 31% have been reported[634–641] (Table 63-7), but there have been no prospective studies comparing marrow grafting to chemotherapy in these patients. Patients in second or subsequent remission are much more likely to die of their disease, and marrow grafting has been intensively applied to this group of patients. Many different conditioning regimens have been used, and patients have been treated at different times in the course of their disease, so the results of marrow transplantation reflect this heterogeneity. Disease-free survival rates of 22% to 62% have been reported, with relapse rates of 13% to 62%.[638,639,641–645]

TABLE 63-7. Marrow Transplantation for Treatment of Acute Lymphoblastic Leukemia in Remission

Study	Remission Status	Treatment	No.	Actuarial Disease-Free Survival Rate (%)	Relapse Rate (%)
MSKCC[639]	First	HFTBI/cyt	31	64 (SE ± 9)	13 (SE ± 7)
	Second		12	42 (SE ± 14)	25 (SE ± 13)
	Third or relapse		16	23 (SE ± 11)	64 (SE ± 16)
Duarte[634]	First	Ara-c/cyt/SFTBI or FTBI/cyt	39	63 (SE ± 9)	16 (SE ± 8)
IBMTR[641]	First	Varied	299	42 (95% CI ± 9)	29 (95% CI ± 9)
	Second		391	26 (95% CI ± 6)	52 (95% CI ± 8)
GEGMO[635]	First	Varied	27	59 (SE ± 18)	14 (SE ± 15)
EGBMT[636]	First	Varied	57	~60	6
	Second		96	~40	34
	Third or more		39	~12	73
Seattle[644]	Second	Cyt/SFTBI or Cyt/FTBI	57	40	42
Cleveland[645]	Second or third	Ara-c/FTBI	20	58	17

Ara-c, arabinosylcytosine; cyt, cyclophosphamide; IBMTR, International Bone Marrow Transplant Registry; EGBMT, European Group for Bone Marrow Transplantation; GEGMO, Groupe d'Etudes de la Greffe de Moelle Osseuse; MSKCC, Memorial Sloan-Kettering Cancer Center; TBI, total-body irradiation (F, fractionated; HF, hyperfractionated; SF, single fraction).

There have been few prospective studies comparing chemotherapy to marrow transplantation in this setting, and the results are at odds.[646,647] Not all groups are convinced that marrow transplantation affects survival in ALL.[646,648,649] Furthermore, a prospective study performed in Minnesota suggested that ABMT may result in survivals equivalent to allogeneic marrow grafting.[650] Survival rates of patients treated in relapse parallel the results observed in relapsed ANLL or CML in blast crisis—10% to 15%.[604,642] Data for several published studies on patients in remission are summarized in Table 63-7.

Prognostic Factors

If transplantation is undertaken in first remission, the factors of non–T-cell phenotype, leukocyte count at diagnosis of 50,000/μL or higher, male donor to female recipient, and GVHD may be associated with a reduction in leukemia-free survival, while use of corticosteroids appears to increase leukemia-free survival.[641] It has been difficult to identify prognostic factors that predict relapse after marrow transplantation in second or subsequent remission,[104,644] although the Westminster group found standard prognostic factors in ALL to apply to marrow transplantation.[651] A recent analysis by the IBMTR identified age 16 years or older, relapse while on therapy, GVHD prophylaxis without methotrexate, and absence of GVHD as factors that predict for a poor outcome.[641] This difficulty may arise in part from the high relapse rates observed in these patients and the heterogeneity of pretransplantation chemotherapy regimens as well as transplantation-conditioning regimens.

Relapse

Graft-versus-leukemia appears to be an important mechanism for control of residual ALL. Several studies indicate substantially reduced relapse rates in patients with GVHD, as compared with patients without GVHD or patients who received autologous transplants.[509,511,512,643,650] An unexpected finding was the reduction in relapse rate from 71% to 19% associated with the prophylactic use of partially purified human leukocyte interferon. This benefit occurred independent of GVHD. Survival was no different between the groups, perhaps owing to increased leukoencephalopathy in the interferon-treated group.[652] Methotrexate used for GVHD prophylaxis may have antileukemic activity,[641] but attempts to exploit antimetabolites as maintenance therapy have been unsuccessful.[643] There is a substantial risk of central nervous system relapse (actuarial relapse rate is about 38%) that can be largely abrogated by the use of intrathecal methotrexate after transplantation (actuarial relapse rate of 7%), but with a dose-related increased risk of leukoencephalopathy in patients who received prior CNS therapy.[653] Occasional patients who relapse after marrow grafting for ALL can sometimes achieve a complete remission with standard antileukemia therapy, although they relapse eventually.[654]

Autologous Marrow Transplantation

The success of allogeneic marrow grafting and the recognition that lack of a suitable donor, patient age, and GVHD-related toxicity limit its application in patients with leukemia spurred the investigation of ABMT as a form of rescue after high-dose chemotherapy. Limitations to its use include concerns about infusing viable, clonogenic leukemic cells and a limited ability to detect minimal residual disease, but several important considerations affect the use of autografting. First, it appears unlikely that the results of ABMT in a given situation will be better than the results of syngeneic marrow grafting. Thus, for similar conditioning regimens, the relapse rate after syngeneic transplantation probably reflects the best that can be achieved with ABMT. Second, because substantial numbers of patients who receive allogeneic or syngeneic transplants relapse, conditioning regimens are not completely effective in eradicating residual leukemia. Finally, concern about unidentified leukemia in the harvested marrow and the need to remove those cells should be commensurate with the risk of leukemic relapse from disease that persists after the conditioning regimen. There is no point in purging the harvested marrow of leukemic cells if there is a high likelihood that there will be equal or greater numbers of viable leukemic cells in the patient after the conditioning regimen.

It is unlikely that marrow harvested in second or subsequent remission will not contain leukemic cells; however, the ability of these cells to reestablish clinical leukemia is unknown. Investigators who are concerned about these cells have attempted to reduce the numbers of malignant cells by treating the harvested marrow ex vivo with monoclonal antibodies,[655–657] in vitro marrow culture,[658] or the addition of pharmacologic agents.[199,659] On the other hand, calculations based on animal models suggest that leukemic blasts have low clonogenicity and survive cryopreservation poorly and that conditioning regimens may alter the marrow microenvironment in a way that favors normal progenitors.[660,661] If one further estimates that the harvested marrow contains only a small proportion of the total-body leukemic burden, the contribution of these cells to relapse may be small. For instance, if there were 10^7 to 10^8 residual leukemic cells in the patient's marrow at harvest, and 1% to 5% of the marrow was removed, then about 10^5 to 10^6 leukemic cells would have been harvested. As few as 1% of the leukemic cells may be clonogenic, and these must survive cryopreservation and grow in a suboptimal microenvironment. If calculations based on rodent models apply, these additional factors may reduce the effective leukemic dose by an additional 1 to 2 logs.[660–662] Thus, some investigators are performing ABMTs for leukemia in first or subsequent remission without marrow purging.[663,664] Since no controlled comparative studies have been reported, the value of purging remains an open question. Retrospective analysis of registry data is equivocal,[664,665] and assessing the value of purging requires a large, multicenter trial.

In analyzing the results of ABMT in leukemia, it is important to assess the duration of the preceding remissions. Patients with long remissions from chemotherapy tend to have long remissions after ABMT; thus, unless the follow-up is as long as the chemotherapy-induced remissions, the benefit of ABMT is exaggerated. Furthermore, how soon it is performed after remission is also important, since the subset of patients who can maintain long remissions before ABMT may have more favorable prognoses. Because it reduces the number of harvested leukemic cells and the number of leukemic cells that have to be destroyed by the conditioning regimen, consolidation therapy before ABMT is likely to be advantageous. Finally, patients with ALL who experienced relapses while on therapy had a shorter survival compared with patients who had relapses after completing maintenance treatments in some series[666] but not in others.[650] Patients with Ph-positive ALL are also unlikely to do well with ABMT.

ABMT is an effective therapy for both ANLL and ALL. A disease-free survival rate of 50% to 70% at 2 to 4 years can be achieved in both ANLL and ALL in first remission.[663–665] Transplantations performed in second or subsequent remission have been reported to produce long-term survival rates that vary from 0% to 50%.[199,655,663–666] The Minnesota group demonstrated that in patients with high-risk ALL, allogeneic and purged ABMTs have similar outcomes. As noted in previous studies, the relapse rate was lower in the allogeneic patients with GVHD, but the toxicity related to the procedure was greater, and the overall disease-free survival rates were not statistically different (20% autologous versus 27% allogeneic).[650]

One problem observed during autografting for acute leukemia was delayed recovery of hematopoiesis. This delay probably results from a deficiency of harvested progenitors and toxicity of the marrow purging agents. In an effort to overcome this problem and to hasten hematopoietic recovery, administration of hematopoietic growth factors after transplantation have been examined, with mixed results.[667,668] The use of myeloid CSFs should be undertaken with caution in myeloid leukemias.

HODGKIN'S DISEASE AND NON-HODGKIN'S LYMPHOMA

Hodgkin's Disease

Advances in the treatment of Hodgkin's disease have resulted in the cure of a substantial proportion of patients. Even patients who relapse after primary treatment may respond to additional chemotherapy or radiation therapy. Primary resistance to therapy, relapse early after the completion of chemotherapy, or relapse after a second chemotherapeutic regimen, however, is followed by disease progression and, ultimately, death. Because Hodgkin's disease is sensitive to both chemotherapy and radiation therapy, it was logical to increase the dose of these modalities and use allogeneic and autologous marrow grafting to reconstitute the marrow.

Allogeneic transplantation is the least studied approach to the therapy of Hodgkin's disease.[669] Its potential advantage is the applicability to patients in whom pelvic irradiation has made ABMT difficult and to patients with therapy-induced stem cell damage. Theoretic benefits include eventual restoration of normal immunity, infusion of disease-free marrow, and avoidance of alkylating-agent treated marrow, which may develop myelodysplasia or secondary leukemia. On the other hand, the risks of GVHD are substantial, and many patients cannot receive TBI safely because of the striking increase in interstitial pneumonia in patients who had prior mantle irradiation.[670,671] Recurrence rates after local irradiation suggest that the dose of TBI that can be safely administered may not be curative in most patients.[672,673]

ABMT appears to be an effective way of intensifying therapy and obtaining long disease-free survivals in patients with Hodgkin's disease. Because of concern about radiation therapy, most conditioning regimens have avoided TBI and concentrated on high-dose chemotherapy. As noted previously, treatment with autologous marrow is precluded by the prior use of pelvic irradiation, and some investigators have used autologous peripheral blood stem cells instead.[674] In general, patients are considered candidates for ABMT if the disease is resistant to primary therapy or if they relapse after conventional salvage regimens. The likelihood of obtaining a complete remission varies with the conditioning regimen used and the responsiveness of the disease. Because of heterogeneity of patients and treatment protocols, only broad conclusions can be drawn. Examples of reported conditioning regimens and responses are shown in Table 63-8. Substantial heterogeneity in dose and entrance criteria are found in the various studies, so the response rates are not strictly comparable, and the optimal dose and regimen have not been established. It is clear that complete response rates of more than 45% are achievable with intensive therapy and that many of these remissions translate into long-term survivals. Most relapses occur in sites of previous disease rather than as diffuse parenchymal seeding, supporting the contention that marrow purging is not necessary in this disease. The primary causes of treatment-related death are interstitial pneumonia and sepsis related to myelosuppression. The interstitial pneumonia appears to be more severe with higher doses of BCNU.

Multivariate analysis has led to the identification of groups of patients with different outcomes after ABMT for Hodgkin's disease. Poor performance status, failure of more than two prior chemotherapy regimens,[675] and large tumor

TABLE 63-8. **High-Dose Therapy and Autologous Marrow Infusion for Treatment of Hodgkin's Disease**

Center	Conditioning Regimen	No.	Complete Response (%)	Treatment-Related Deaths (%)	Actuarial Disease-Free Survival Rate (%)
London[676]	BEAM	44	50 (at 6 mo)	5	~65*
Vancouver[677]	CBV	55	80 (95% CI 75–84)	20	66 (95% CI 53–79)†
MD Anderson/Nebraska[675]	CBV	61	46	7	38
Boston[678]	CBV	30	44	17	~48
Genoa[679]	CBV	50	48	4	~45

BEAM, BCNU, etoposide, arabinosylcytosine; melphalan; CBV, cyclophosphamide, BCNU, etoposide (VP-16).
* Overall survival.
† Overall survival. Freedom from progression was 77% (95% CI 64–90).

size[676] have been identified as adverse prognostic factors. Thus, if ABMT is to be considered, it is most likely to be successful if applied soon after relapse or recognition that primary therapy is unsuccessful and after therapy to reduce the bulk of the disease.

Of concern in evaluation of the data are the relative indolence of Hodgkin's disease in many patients and the persistence of radiographic abnormalities in the absence of disease. Thus, long-term follow-up is necessary to establish cure rates in this disease.

Non-Hodgkin's Lymphoma

The use of marrow transplantation in non-Hodgkin's lymphoma was a natural outgrowth of the observations of long-term disease-free survivals in relapsed leukemia. Proper understanding of the role of marrow transplantation in these disorders requires a clear understanding of their heterogeneity. High- and intermediate-grade lymphomas often have excellent responses to conventional chemotherapy, and long disease-free survivals are common. Low-grade and some intermediate-grade lymphomas are extremely sensitive to chemotherapy or radiation therapy; however, that sensitivity has not translated into cures. A corollary of these observations is that the more aggressive lymphomas that are not cured are unlikely to have enduring responses to additional chemotherapy, whereas subsequent therapy is often useful in low-grade lymphomas. Furthermore, the duration of follow-up required to demonstrate a benefit from intensive therapy is much shorter for relapsed, aggressive lymphomas. Apparent benefits from intensive therapy in indolent lymphomas require confirmation over many years. Consequently, most of the literature on the management of non-Hodgkin's lymphoma with bone marrow transplantation deals with high- or intermediate-grade disease in which beneficial effects can be evaluated within a relatively brief period.

The results of transplantation for relapsed or resistant lymphoma parallel the treatment results of the resistant, relapsed leukemias. Therapy of bulky, resistant disease is generally much less effective than the treatment of a low volume of sensitive disease. The excellent results of conventional therapy require the selection of patients who are likely to do poorly, if marrow transplantation is to be applied early in the course of therapy of non-Hodgkin's lymphoma.

Allogeneic transplantation has been applied to small numbers of patients, in large part because of the relative success of ABMT. Nevertheless, in patients who have a compatible donor and in whom marrow harvesting is not feasible by virtue of pelvic irradiation, myelodysplasia, or marrow involvement with lymphoma, marrow grafting is a valuable approach. Long-term disease-free survival rates of 10% to 56% have been reported in this group of refractory patients.[670,680–682] A graft-versus-lymphoma effect has also been detected.[683] Because TBI was a principal component of therapy, prior chest irradiation and perhaps the prior use of drugs such as bleomycin contributed to a high incidence of fatal interstitial pneumonia.

ABMT could be applied to larger numbers of patients than allogeneic transplantation, and thus, attracted more attention. Early reports by Appelbaum and colleagues[684,685] of successful high-dose therapy of Burkitt's lymphoma resulted in the initiation of large numbers of subsequent trials of ABMT in all categories of non-Hodgkin's lymphoma.[686–688] Some of these results are summarized in Table 63-9. As with Hodgkin's disease, many of the regimens rely on high doses of chemotherapeutic agents to take advantage of steep dose–response relations, to avoid pulmonary toxicity in previously irradiated patients, and because the maximal safe dose of TBI may not be curative in many patients with aggressive lymphomas.

In properly selected patients, it appears that regimens based on chemotherapy or TBI are effective, although it is likely that TBI-containing regimens are most effective in patients with minimal disease.[689–691] In addition, chemotherapy regimens may allow the subsequent use of local radiation therapy for sites of resistant disease.

Prognostic Factors

The extreme heterogeneity of the disease and the importance of treatment-related characteristics of the tumor, such as complete response to initial therapy, continued sensitivity to chemotherapy, and bulk of disease, make comparisons between groups difficult. It is not surprising that using ABMT early in the course of the disease is more effective than waiting until bulky, resistant disease has developed.[689] Investigators who wish to apply ABMT early in the course of the illness have attempted to identify prognostic factors at diagnosis that predict a poor response to primary therapy. These factors include slow response to primary therapy, high lactate dehydrogenase levels, large mass (more than 10 cm), and two or more extranodal sites of disease.[686,689,694]

Purging

Non-Hodgkin's lymphomas have a well-described propensity to circulate in the blood and invade the bone marrow.[695,696] Often, the level of involvement may not be clinically apparent.[697,698] Several investigators have attempted to purge the marrow of clinically detectable and undetectable lymphoma cells with either immunologic or phar-

TABLE 63-9. High-Dose Therapy and Autologous Marrow Infusion for Treatment of Non-Hodgkin's Lymphoma

Study	Conditioning Regimen	Stage	No.	Marrow Purging	Actuarial Disease-Free Survival at 2–4 Years (%)
Philip et al[692]	BACT; BEAM	Initial partial remission	17	None	75†
Verdonck et al[691]	Cyt/SFTBI	Complete remission	10	None	70†
MSKCC[689]	HFTBI/cyt	Initial remission (complete and partial)	14	4-HC (4)	79
		Relapsed, resistant	17	4-HC (10)	20
DFCI[690]	cyt/FTBI	Sensitive relapse*	49	Anti-B1	65
Wheeler et al[678]	CBV	Relapsed, resistant	28	None	46‡
Philip et al[693]	Variable	Sensitive relapse	25	None	36
		Resistant relapse	22	None	14
		Primarily resistant	39	None	0

BACT, BCNU, arabinosylcytosine, cyclophosphamide, thioguanine; BEAM, BCNU, etoposide, arabinosylcytosine, melphalan; CBV, cyclophosphamide, BCNU, etoposide (VP-16); cyt, cyclophosphamide; TBI, total-body irradiation (SF, single fraction; F, fractionated; HF, hyperfractionated.

* Includes six low-grade lymphomas.

† Overall survival.

‡ Freedom from progression.

macologic techniques.[689,690,699] Immunologic purging has the disadvantage that the cell-surface phenotype of lymphomas is heterogeneous, so a single antibody may not treat all lymphomas. Furthermore, heterogeneity of cell-surface antigen expression within the lymphoma may be a problem. Finally, the cell type damaged by the antibody may not be the lymphomatous stem cell.[686,700–702] PCR technology has been used to detect residual lymphoma cells after purging to determine both the efficacy of purging and whether detectable lymphoma has an effect on outcome. In ABMT for low- and intermediate-grade lymphomas with t(14;18), the prescence of detectable *bcl*-2 gene rearrangements was associated with a high relapse rate, suggesting that the purging may have been of use. On the other hand, the ability to detect residual disease after purging may also simply select patients with better prognoses.[703] In practice, whether or not the marrow has been treated, relapse occurs most often at sites of previous disease rather than as diffuse seeding of parenchymal organs with nodules of similar age. As noted in the discussion of acute leukemia, until the conditioning regimens are capable of eradicating residual disease more effectively, it may be impossible to determine whether purging has a role in ABMT for lymphoma. This assessment requires a large, randomized trial.

Peripheral Blood Progenitor Transplants

It has become evident that the mononuclear cell fraction of blood contains a sufficient quantity of hematopoietic progenitors to perform an ABMT if large numbers of cells are collected.[210,704] Peripheral blood progenitors (and probably stem cells) are collected by leukapheresis and cryopreserved until 6 to 8 $\times 10^9$ nucleated cells/kg are obtained. The proportion of hematopoietic progenitors in the blood increases substantially in the recovery phase after high-dose chemotherapy and in the presence of infusions of hematopoietic growth factors such as sargramostim and filgrastim.[211–215] These cells can then be used alone in patients with marrow involvement or histories of pelvic irradiation, or they can be used in conjunction with bone marrow in an effort to accelerate blood count recovery. The durability of engraftment in patients receiving only peripheral blood progenitors and the optimal schedules for chemotherapy and growth factor administration remain to be determined.

Another source of peripheral blood stem cells that has been gaining attention is umbilical cord blood.[705,706] The proportion of stem cells in cord blood is higher than is found in blood from mature donors. Furthermore, T-cell numbers and function are depressed in cord blood, making it an attractive source of stem cells for allogeneic transplantation. Substantial logistical problems will need to be overcome before umbilical cord blood becomes a practical resource.

OTHER MALIGNANCIES

Any disorder of lymphoid or hematopoietic tissue is a potential target of marrow transplantation. The primary criteria for success are the responsiveness of the disease to the conditioning regimen and the age and physical status of the patient. Both allogeneic and autologous transplantation have been shown, in small studies, to have some palliative benefit in multiple myeloma,[707–709] chronic lymphocytic leukemia,[710] and histiocytosis X.[711] Some chemotherapy-responsive solid tumors, such as breast cancer and neuroblastoma, may also respond to marrow transplantation. A discussion of those diseases is beyond the scope of this chapter.

GENETIC DISORDERS

Conceptually, any congenital disorder whose only clinical manifestation is in cells of hematopoietic origin (eg, thalassemia, sickle cell anemia, SCIDS, Wiskott-Aldrich syndrome) can be permanently corrected by allogeneic bone marrow transplantation from an unaffected donor.

In addition, a number of congenital enzyme deficiencies, although manifest in many parts of the body, can be clinically corrected if a source of the enzyme is distributed to all relevant areas by a cell of bone marrow origin, such as the monocyte-macrophage (eg, Gaucher's disease, mucopolysaccharidoses).[712]

Immunodeficiency Disorders

Many congenital immunodeficiencies that represent a failure of T-cell, B-cell, NK-cell, or phagocyte function have been delineated. Some of these, such as selective IgA deficiency, are relatively common and also generally benign in their clinical manifestations. Others are uniformly fatal. The two major such disorders for which marrow transplantation has been applied are SCIDS and Wiskott-Aldrich syndrome.

Severe Combined Immunodeficiency

Severe combined immunodeficiency syndrome represents a pathophysiologically diverse group of diseases, all characterized by a profound deficiency of cellular immunity that results in recurrent infections and death at an early age.[713,714] Some kindreds demonstrate an autosomal recessive and others an X-linked mode of inheritance. Although, in most cases, the basic lesion is undefined, two well-defined enzyme deficiencies are associated with SCIDS: adenosine deaminase and purine nucleoside phosphorylase deficiency. Regardless of cause, however, marrow transplantation represents the treatment of choice for this otherwise uniformly fatal disorder.

The profound deficiency in T-cell immunity in this disorder is illustrated by the fact that about one fourth of SCIDS neonates are engrafted with maternal cells in utero. The extent of that graft varies, as does the presence or absence of concomitant GVHD after birth, because of the obligatory haploidentical graft.[715,716] Indeed, GVHD may be the presenting manifestation of SCIDS in an infant.

When an MHC-compatible sibling donor is available, pretransplantation conditioning is usually not necessary since the recipient, by definition, lacks an immune system capable of rejecting the infused marrow, and a physiologic niche for the lymphoid stem cell appears to be present in most cases. Historically, many patients have been deliberately given lower doses of nucleated cells than the typical transplantation patient (often 0.5×10^8 cells) in an attempt to reduce the risk of acute GVHD. Failure to engraft, even with these lower doses, has been unusual.[717–720] In addition, many patients have received transplants without post-transplantation prophylactic immunosuppression for GVHD. Even with the lack of prophylactic therapy, acute GVHD in these patients has generally been relatively mild, and chronic GVHD is rare. Whether this is due to the young age of the patient and donor, the low dose of marrow used, the lack of pretransplantation conditioning, the partial mixed chimerism obtained, or some aspect of the underlying disease is unknown.

After transplantation, these patients become partial mixed chimeras with T lymphocytes uniformly of donor origin but myeloid and erythroid cells of host origin.[721] B lymphocytes are of donor origin about half the time, a result consistent with the fact that some SCIDS patients have normal numbers of B cells at the time of transplantation and thus may lack a niche for the B-lymphocyte stem cell. Successful transplantation results in return of measurable T-lymphocyte numbers and function. About 15% of patients who receive MHC-compatible sibling donor marrows fail to develop normal B-cell function after transplantation and may therefore require continued replacement γ-globulin. The overall long-term success rate of MHC-compatible transplantation is over 65%.

For patients without a histocompatible donor, the use of a haploidentical parent as donor, combined with ex vivo T-cell depletion of the donor marrow, has been remarkably successful. Before the development of adequate T-cell depletion techniques, at least 35 patients underwent transplantation with unmanipulated histoincompatible marrow.[719] None survived long. With the use of haploidentical, T-cell–depleted marrow, however, long-term success rates of 50% to 75% have been achieved.[722–726] In many cases, several grafts may be necessary, and pretransplantation conditioning may also be required. Late complications include an occasional failure to achieve complete immune reconstitution and, rarely, the development of a B-cell–derived fatal lymphoproliferative disease.[168]

Wiskott-Aldrich Syndrome

This X-linked disorder is characterized by eczema, thrombocytopenia, small platelets, and severe depression of T-cell immunity with resultant recurrent infections. It is associated with a specific defective surface membrane sialoglycoprotein on lymphocytes.[727] Unlike patients with SCIDS, successful transplantation of patients with Wiskott-Aldrich syndrome requires an ablative conditioning regimen.[728] Wiskott-Aldrich syndrome patients also differ from patients with SCIDS in that they may develop both fatal acute and chronic GVHD. Nevertheless, long-term successful results are reported in over 70% of patients receiving histocompatible marrow grafts.[729,730]

Hemoglobinopathies

Marrow transplantation has been carried out to cure patients with thalassemia.[731–735] Initially, patients with advanced disease fared poorly after transplantation when given irradiation as part of the conditioning regimen. This poor outcome discouraged more frequent application of this therapy. More recent series, however, in which patients were conditioned with high-dose chemotherapy (busulfan and cyclophosphamide), achieved more encouraging results. In 222 patients less than 16 years of age with β-thalassemia, the actuarial survival rate at 2 years was 82%, with a disease-free survival rate of 75%. In this group of patients receiving multiple transfusions, the graft failure rate was about 5%. Deaths were due to graft rejection, pneumonitis, and septicemia, with either acute or chronic GVHD as contributing factors in about half the fatalities. The primary determinants of outcome were related to extent of prior chelation therapy, presence of portal fibrosis, and presence of hepatomegaly. When these factors were organized into three risk groups based on severity, the probability of event-free survival ranged from 94% in class 1, to 77% in class 2, and to 53% in class 3. Although studies in leukemic patient populations have documented a significantly increased risk of serious venoocclusive disease in patients with abnormal hepatic function before transplantation, there was little liver disease after transplantation in the thalassemic population, even though most patients had biopsy-proven hepatic dysfunction due to iron overload and transfusion-associated hepatitis before transplantation. In experimental models, iron overload is reversed by marrow transplantation[736]; whether this occurs in humans is unknown but expected. Thus, marrow grafting (at least from MHC-identical sibling donors) is a viable therapeutic option for patients with thalassemia. It appears that this approach is preferable to a program of vigorous transfusion and iron chelation therapy.

For patients with sickle cell anemia, marrow transplantation remains an experimentally possible treatment approach, but its ultimate role in the management of this disease remains undetermined. Patient selection is critical given the variable natural history of sickle cell disease. As expected, this therapy can eliminate sickle hemoglobin production.[737,738] Transplantation is associated with a high mortality from GVHD, infections, and conditioning regimen toxicity, however, and it is difficult to identify the patients who will be most disabled and in whom the transplantation-related morbidity and mortality is justified. However, children with strokes have a poor prognosis with conventional therapy and would be good transplant candidates if donors are available.

Osteopetrosis

Infantile malignant osteopetrosis (marble bone disease) is an autosomal recessive disorder characterized by absent or dysfunctional osteoclasts. Since experimental work demonstrated the origin of the osteoclast from a bone marrow–derived cell, specifically the monocyte-macrophage, it is logical to postulate that marrow transplantation of a normal hematopoietic stem cell could be the reverse of this disease. It has been demonstrated that after transplantation, the posttransplantation osteoblasts are of recipient origin, the posttransplantation osteoclasts are of donor origin, and bone remodeling can be expected.[739–741]

Storage Diseases

Congenital deficiencies of enzymes that result in disease by virtue of the accumulation of toxic products are potentially treatable by a variety of replacement techniques.[742] Infusion of the enzyme or a modified form of the enzyme is possible in some experimental circumstances, for example, in the treatment of non–storage disorders, such as adenosine deaminase deficiency[743] or α_1-antitrypsin deficiency.[744] An alternative is to transplant a tissue that contains cells of normal enzymatic function that can act by replacing the tissue-specific abnormal cells of the host and also as a source of enzyme to correct the systemic disorder. Two major such tissues have been so used: the liver[745] and the bone marrow. Whether the systemic disorder is in fact corrected by such an approach obviously depends on a variety of kinetic and distribution considerations. In some storage diseases, such as Gaucher's disease, much of the morbidity is caused by macrophages that are engorged, cause mass effects, and injure normal organ parenchyma. Replacement of these macrophages with cells that have the proper enzymatic pathways should alleviate much of the pathology.

Lysosomal storage diseases that have been treated with allogeneic marrow transplantation include Gaucher's disease,[311] the mucopolysaccharidoses[746] (including Hurler's disease,[747] Hunter's disease, Sanfilippo's syndrome type B, Morquio's disease, and Maroteaux-Lamy syndrome[748]), and metachromatic leukodystrophy. In general, the systemic enzymatic defect has been well corrected by the allograft in these patients. One of the critical issues in the application of this technique to some of these disorders is the question of whether neurologic disease can be corrected by marrow transplantation. Some experimental evidence has suggested that pluripotent hematopoietic progenitors may exist in the central nervous system and that microglial cells may be of bone marrow origin.[749,750] In addition, it may be possible for toxic substrates to be transported across the blood–brain barrier and enzymatically degraded in the systemic circulation with beneficial result. In the twitcher mouse (an animal model of the sphingolipidosis, Krabbe's disease), however, marrow grafting from unaffected donors leads to improvement in peripheral neuropathy, but central nervous system disease progresses unabated.[751] Data on humans remain incomplete, and the issue is unresolved; successful marrow grafting is more likely to prevent organ damage than to reverse established injury. Thus, transplantation needs to be undertaken in infancy or even in utero.

Other Red Cell, Granulocyte, and Platelet Disorders

Other genetic diseases manifested primarily in the marrow are susceptible to transplantation. Diseases for which marrow grafting has proved successful include: Kostmann's syndrome,[752] chronic granulomatous disease,[753] neutrophil-actin dysfunction,[754] Chédiak-Higashi syndrome,[755] and Diamond-Blackfan anemia.[756,757]

REFERENCES

1. Santos GE. The history of bone marrow transplantation. Clin Haematol 1983;12:611.
2. Morrison M, Samwick AA. Intramedullary (sternal) transfusion of human bone marrow. JAMA 1940;115:1708.
3. Osgood EE, Riddle MC, Mathews TJ. Aplastic anemia treated with daily transfusions and intravenous marrow. Ann Intern Med 1939;13:357.
4. Jacobsen LO, Simmons EL, Marks EL, et al. The role of the spleen in radiation injury and recovery. J Lab Clin Med 1950;35:746.
5. Barnes DWH, Loutit JF. Spleen protection: the cellular hypothesis. In: Bacq ZM, Alexander P, eds. Radiobiology symposium 1954. New York, Academic Press, 1955:134.
6. Lorenz E, Uphoff D, Reid TR, et al. Modification of irradiation injury in mice and guinea pigs by bone marrow injections. JNCI 1951;12:197.
7. Barnes DWH, Loutit JF. Immunological and histological response following spleen treatment in irradiated mice. In: Mitchel JS, Holmes BE, Smith CL, eds. Progress in radiobiology. Edinburgh, Oliver & Boyd, 1956:291.
8. Billingham RE, Brent L. A simple method for inducing tolerance of skin homografts in mice. Transplant Bull 1957;4:67.
9. Van Bekkum DW, De Vries MJ. Radiation chimeras. New York, Academic Press, 1967:79.
10. Billingham RE. The biology of graft-versus-host reactions. Harvey Lect 1966–1967;62:21.
11. Simonsen M. Graft versus host reactions: their natural history and applicability as tools of research. Prog Allergy 1971;6:349.
12. Elkins WL. Cellular immunology and pathogenesis of graft-versus-host reaction. Prog Allergy 1971;15:78.
13. Grebe SC, Streilein JW. Graft-versus-host reactions: a review. Adv Immunol 1976;22:120.
14. Yunis EJ, Awdeh Z, Raum D, Alper CA. The MHC in human bone marrow transplantation. Clin Haematol 1983;12:641.
15. Bach FH, Sachs DH. Current concepts: immunology. Transplantation immunology. N Engl J Med 1987;317:489.
16. Thomas ED, Lochte HL, Lu WC, Ferrebee JW. Intravenous infusion of bone marrow in patients receiving radiation and chemotherapy. N Engl J Med 1957;257:491.
17. Mathé G, Jammet H, Pendic B, et al. Transfusions et greffes do moelle osseuse homologue chez des humans irradiés a haute dose accidentellement. Rev Franç Etudes Clin et Biol 1959;4:226.
18. Bortin MM. A compendium of reported human bone marrow transplants. Transplantation 1970;9:571.
19. Gatti RA, Meuwissen HJ, Allen HD, Hong R, Good RA. Immunological reconstitution of sex-linked lymphopenic immunological deficiency. Lancet 1968;2:1366.
20. Bach FH, Albertini RJ, Joo P, Anderson JL, Bortin MM. Bone marrow transplantation in a patient with Wiskott-Aldrich syndrome. Lancet 1968;2:1364.
21. De Koning J, Dooren LJ, van Bekkum DW, Dicke KA, Radl J. Transplantation of bone-marrow cells and fetal thymus in an infant with lymphopenic immunological deficiency. Lancet 1969;1:1223.
22. Thomas ED, Storb R, Clift RA, et al. Bone marrow transplantation. N Engl J Med 1975;292:832.
23. O'Reilly RJ. Allogeneic bone marrow transplantation: current status and future directions. Blood 1983;62:941.
24. Nathan DG, ed. Bone marrow transplantation. Clin Haematol 1983;12:611.
25. Bach FH, van Rood JJ. The major histocompatibility complex: genetics and biology. N Engl J Med 1976;295:806.
26. Solheim BG, MØller E, Ferrone S, eds. HLA class II antigens: a comprehensive review of structure and function. New York, Springer Verlag, 1986.

27. Dorak MT, Chalmers EA, Sproul AM, et al. MHC class III polymorphisms in selection of donors for BMT. Bone Marrow Transplant 1993;11:37.
28. Bodmer JG, Marsh SEG, Albert ED, et al. Nomenclature of factors of the HLA system, 1990. Hum Immunol 1991;31:186.
29. Hansen JA, Choo SY, Geraghty DE, Mickelson E. The HLA system in clinical marrow transplantation. Hematol Oncol Clin North Am 1990;4: 507.
30. Bjorkman PJ, Saper MA, Samaoui M, et al. The foreign antigen binding site and T cell recognition regions of class I histocompatibility antigens. Nature 1987;329:506.
31. Bjorkman PJ, Saper MA, Samaoui B, et al. Structure of the human class I histocompatibility antigen HLA-A2. Nature 1987;329:512.
32. Garrett TPJ, Saper MA, Bjorkman PJ, et al. Specificity pockets for the side chains of peptide antigens in HLA-Aw68. Nature 1989;342:692.
33. Wallny HJ, Rammensee HG. Identification of classical minor histocompatibility antigen cell-derived peptide. Nature 1990;343:275.
34. Germain RN. Immunology: the ins and outs of antigen presentation and processing. Nature 1986;322:687.
35. Bevan MJ. Antigen recognition: class discrimination in the world of immunology. Nature 1987;325:192.
36. Adorini L, Appella E, Doria E, et al. Competition for antigen presentation in living cells involves exchange of peptides bound by class II MHC molecules. Nature 1989;342:800.
37. Martin PJ. Increased disparity for minor histocompatibility antigens as a potential cause of increased GVHD risk in marrow transplantation from unrelated donors compared with related donors. Bone Marrow Transplant 1991;8:217.
38. Fleischauer K, Kernan NA, O'Reilly RJ, Dupont B, Tang SY. Bone marrow-allograft rejection by T lymphocytes recognizing a single amino acid difference on HLA-B44. N Engl J Med 1990;323:1818.
39. Vogelsang GB, Hess AD, Berkman AW, et al. An in vitro predictive test for graft versus host disease in patients with genotypic HLA-identical bone marrow transplants. N Engl J Med 1985;313:645.
40. Theobald M, Nierle T, Bunjes D, Arnold R, Heimpel H. Host-specific interleukin-2-secreting donor T-cell precursors as predictors of acute graft-versus-host disease in bone marrow transplantation between HLA-identical siblings. N Engl J Med 1992;327:1613.
41. Anasetti C, Amos D, Beatty PG, et al. Effect of HLA compatibility on engraftment of bone marrow transplants in patients with leukemia or lymphoma. N Engl J Med 1989;320:197.
42. Beatty PG, Dahlberg S, Mickelson EM, et al. Probability of finding HLA-matched unrelated marrow donors. Transplantation 1988;45:714.
43. Kernan NA, Bartsch G, Ash RC, et al. Analysis of 462 transplantations from unrelated donors facilitated by the National Marrow Donor Program. N Engl J Med 1993;328:593.
44. McGlave P, Bartsch G, Anasetti C, et al. Unrelated donor marrow transplantation therpay for chronic myelogenous leukemia:initial experience of the National Marrow Donor Program. Blood 1993;81:543.
45. Beatty PG, Anasetti C, Hansen JA, et al. Marrow transplantation from unrelated donors for treatment of hematologic malignancies: effect of mismatching for one HLA locus. Blood 1993;81:249.
46. Ash RC, Casper JT, Chitambar CR, et al. Successful allogeneic transplantation of T-cell–depleted bone marrow from closely HLA-matched unrelated donors. N Engl J Med 1990;322:485.
47. Sanders J, Buckner CD, Bensinger WI, et al. Experience with marrow harvesting from donors less than two years of age. Bone Marrow Transplant 1987;2:45.
48. Bortin MM, Buckner CD. Major complications of marrow harvesting for transplantation. Exp Hematol 1983;11:916.
49. Buckner CD, Clift RA, Sanders JE, et al. Marrow harvesting from normal donors. Blood 1984;64:630.
50. Bowden RA, Sayers M, Flournoy N, et al. Cytomegalovirus immune globulin and seronegative blood products to prevent primary cytomegalovirus infection after marrow transplantation. N Engl J Med 1986;314:1006.
51. Winston DJ, Eng-Shang H, Miller MJ, et al. Molecular epidemiology of cytomegalovirus infections associated with bone marrow transplantation. Ann Intern Med 1985;102:16.
52. Falk PM, Feig SA, Gitnick GL, Wilkinson RW, Gale RP. Transplantation of hepatitis B surface antigen positive bone marrow. Transfusion 1978;18:242.
53. Beard ME, Heaton DC, Hamer JW, et al. Bone marrow transplantation for acute leukemia and severe marrow aplasia: an analysis of five patients. NZ Med J 1981;94:249.
54. Pariente EA, Goudeau A, Dubois F, et al. Fulminant hepatitis due to reactivation of chronic hepatitis B virus infection after allogeneic bone marrow transplantation. Dig Dis Sci 1988;33:1185.
55. Lange B, Henle W, Meyers JD, et al. Epstein-Barr virus–related serology in marrow transplant recipients. Int J Cancer 1980;26:151.
56. Sullivan JL, Wallen WC, Johnson FL. Epstein-Barr virus infection following bone-marrow transplantation. Int J Cancer 1978;22:132.
57. Hanto DW, Frizzera G, Gajl-Peczalska KJ, Simmons RL. Epstein-Barr virus, immunodeficiency, and B cell lymphoproliferation. Transplantation 1985;39:461.
58. Shapiro RS, McClain K, Frizzera G, et al. Epstein-Barr virus associated B cell lymphoproliferative disorders following bone marrow transplantation. Blood 1988;71:1234.
59. Zutter MM, Martin PJ, Sale GE, et al. Epstein-Barr virus lymphoproliferation after bone marrow transplantation. Blood 1988;72:520.
60. Petz LD, Yam P, Wallace RB, et al. Mixed hematopoietic chimerism following bone marrow transplantation for hematologic malignancies. Blood 1987;70:1331.
61. Blume KG, Beutler E, Bross KJ, et al. Genetic markers in human bone marrow transplantation. Am J Hum Genet 1980;32:414.
62. Witherspoon WP, Schanfield MS, Storb R, Thomas ED, Giblett ER. Immunoglobulin production of donor origin after marrow transplantation for acute leukemia or aplastic anemia. Transplantation 1978;26: 407.
63. Ginsburg D, Antin JH, Smith BR, et al. Origin of cell populations after bone marrow transplantation: analysis using DNA sequence polymorphisms. J Clin Invest 1985;75:596.
64. Gale RP, Bortin MM, van Bekkum DW, et al. Risk factors for graft-versus-host disease. Br J Haematol 1987;67:397.
65. Atkinson K, Farrell C, Chapman G, et al. Female marrow donors increase the risk of acute graft-versus-host disease: effect of donor age and parity and analysis of cell subpopulations in the donor marrow inoculum. Br J Haematol 1986;63:231.
66. Blume KG, Forman SJ, O'Donnell MR, et al. Total body irradiation and high-dose etoposide: a new preparatory regimen for bone marrow transplantation is patients with advanced hematologic malignancies. Blood 1987;69:1015.
67. Coccia PF, Strandjord SE, Warkentin PI, et al. High-dose cytosine arabinoside and fractionated total-body irradiation of children with acute lymphoblastic leukemia in remission. Blood 1988;71:888.
68. Goldberg MA, Antin JH, Guinan EC, Rappeport JM. Cyclophosphamide cardiotoxicity: analysis of dosing as a risk factor. Blood 1986;68:1114.
69. Clark JG, Schwartz DA, Flournoy N, et al. Risk factors for airflow obstruction in recipients of bone marrow transplants. Ann Intern Med 1987;107:648.
70. Thomas ED, Clift RA, Fefer A, et al. Marrow transplantation for the treatment of chronic myelogenous leukemia. Ann Intern Med 1986;104: 155.
71. Wingard JR, Mellits Ed, Sostrin MB, et al. Interstitial pneumonitis after allogeneic bone marrow transplantation. Nine-year experience at a single institution. Medicine 1988;67:175.
72. Valteau D, Hartmann O, Benhamou E, et al. Nonbacterial nonfungal interstitial pneumonitis following autologous bone marrow transplantation in children treated with high-dose chemotherapy without total-body irradiation. Transplantation 1988;45:737.
73. Weiner RS, Bortin MM, Gale RP, et al. Interstitial pneumonitis after bone marrow transplantation. Ann Intern Med 1986;104:168.
74. McDonald GB, Shulman HM, Sullivan KM, Spencer GD. Intestinal and hepatic complications of human bone marrow transplantation: part I. Gastroenterology 1986;90:460.
75. Guinan EC, Tarbell NJ, Niemeyer CM, et al. Intravascular hemolysis and renal insufficiency after bone marrow transplantation. Blood 1988;72:451.
76. Deeg HJ, for the Seattle Marrow Transplant Team. Acute and delayed toxicities of total body irradiation. Int J Radiat Oncol Biol Phys 1984;10: 957.
77. Deeg HJ, Flournoy N, Sullivan KM, et al. Cataracts after total body irradiation and marrow transplantation: a sparing effect of dose fractionation. Int J Radiat Oncol Biol Phys 1984;10:957.
78. Vilmer E, Rhodes-Feuillette A, Rabian C, et al. Clinical and immunological restoration in patients with AIDS after marrow transplantation, using lymphocyte transfusions from the marrow donor. Transplantation 1987;44:25.
79. Verdonck LF, de Gast GC, Lange JM, et al. Syngeneic leukocytes together with suramin failed to improve immunodeficiency in a case of transfusion-associated AIDS after syngeneic bone marrow transplantation. Blood 1988;71:666.
80. Reed EC, Myerson D, Corey L, Meyers JD. Allogeneic marrow transplantation in patients positive for hepatitis B surface antigen. Blood 1991;77:195.
81. Van Bekkum, DW. Conditioning regimens for marrow grafting. Semin Hematol 1984;21:81.
82. Frei EJ, Canellos GP. Dose, a critical factor in cancer chemotherapy. Am J Med 1980;69:585.
83. Skipper HE, Schabel FM Jr, Wilcox WS. Experimental evaluation of potential anticancer agents. XII. On the criteria and kinetics associated with "curability" of experimental leukemia. Cancer Chemother Rep 1964;35:1.
84. Santos GW, Sensenbrenner LW, Burk PJ, et al. Marrow transplantation in man following cyclophosphamide. Transplant Proc 1971;3:400.
85. Clift RA, Buckner CD, Applebaum FR, et al. Allogeneic marrow transplantation in patients with acute myeloid leukemia in first remission: a randomized trial of two irradiation regimens. Blood 1990;76:1867.
86. Grochow LB, Krivit W, Whitley CB, Blazar B. Busulfan disposition in children. Blood 1990;75:1723.
87. Champlin RE, Feig SA, Sparkes RS, Gale RP. Bone marrow transplantation from identical twins in the treatment of aplastic anemia: implications for the pathogenesis of the disease. Br J Haematol 1984;56: 455.
88. Appelbaum FR, Fefer A, Cheever MA, et al. Treatment of aplastic

anemia by bone marrow transplantation in identical twins. Blood 1980;55:1033.
89. Bortin MM, Gale RP, Rimm A. Advisory Committee of the Marrow Transplant Registry: allogeneic bone marrow transplantation for 144 patients with severe aplastic anemia. JAMA 1981:245:1132.
90. Storb R, Thomas ED, Buckner ED, et al. Marrow transplantation for aplastic anemia. Semin Hematol 1984;21:27.
91. Deeg HJ, Self S, Storb R, et al. Decreased incidence of marrow graft rejection in patients with severe aplastic anemia: changing impact of risk factors. Blood 1986;68:1363.
92. Champlin RE, Horowitz MM, van Bekkum DW, et al. Graft failure following bone marrow transplantation for severe aplastic anemia: risk factors and treatment results. Blood 1989;73:606.
93. UCLA Bone Marrow Transplant Team. Prevention of graft rejection following bone marrow transplantation. Blood 1981;57:9.
94. Ramsey NKC, Kim T, Nesbit ME, et al. Total lymphoid irradiation and cyclophosphamide as preparation for bone marrow transplantation in severe aplastic anemia. Blood 1988;55:344.
95. Deeg HJ, Witherspoon RP. Risk factors for the development of secondary malignancies after marrow transplantation. Hematol Oncol Clin North Am 1993;7:417.
96. Bozdech MJ, Sondel PM, Trigg ME, et al. Transplantation of HLA-haploidentical T-cell depleted marrow for leukemia: addition of cytosine arabinoside to the pretransplant conditioning regimen prevents rejection. Exp Hematol 1985;13:1201.
97. Gale RP. T cells, bone marrow transplantation, and immunotherapy: use of monoclonal antibodies. In: Fahey JL, moderator. Immune interventions in disease. Ann Intern Med 1987;106:257.
98. Butturini A, Gale RP. T cell depletion in bone marrow transplantation for leukemia: current results and future directions. Bone Marrow Transplant 1988;3:185.
99. Butturini A, Seeger RC, Gale RP. Recipient immune-competent T lymphocytes can survive intensive conditioning for bone marrow transplantation. Blood 1986;68:954.
100. Bretagne S, Vivaud M, Kuentz M, et al. Mixed blood chimerism in T-cell–depleted bone marrow transplant recipients: evaluation using DNA polymorphisms. Blood 1987;70:1692.
101. Anasetti C, Storb R, Longton G, et al. Donor buffy coat cell infusion after marrow transplantation for aplastic anemia. (Letter) Blood 1988;72: 1099.
102. Kernan NA, Flomenberg N, Dupont B, O'Reilly R. Graft rejection in recipients of T-cell–depleted HLA-nonidentical marrow transplants for leukemia: identification of host-derived antidonor allocytotoxic T lymphocytes. Transplantation 1987;43:842.
103. Ford CE. Traffic of lymphoid cells in the body. In: Wolstenhome GEW, Porter R, eds. The thymus: experimental and clinical studies. Boston, Little, Brown, 1966:131.
104. Rappeport JM, Smith BR, Parkman R, Rosen FS. Application of bone marrow transplantation in genetic diseases. Clin Haematol 1983;12: 755.
105. Smith JW, Shulman HM, Thomas ED, et al. Bone marrow transplantation for acute myelosclerosis. Cancer 1981;48:2198.
106. Dokal I, Jones L, Deenamode M, et al. Allogeneic bone marrow transplantation for primary myelofibrosis. Br J Haematol 1989;71:158.
107. Coccia PF, Krivit W, Cervenka J, et al. Successful bone marrow transplantation for infantile malignant osteopetrosis. N Engl J Med 1980;302: 701.
108. Rajantie J, Sale GE, Deeg HJ, et al. Adverse effect of severe marrow fibrosis on hematologic recovery after chemoradiotherapy and allogeneic bone marrow transplantation. Blood 1986;67:1693.
109. Antin JH, Weinberg DS, Rappeport JM. Evidence that pluripotential stem cells for splenic colonies in humans after marrow transplantation. Transplantation 1985;39:102.
110. Gale RP, Falk P, Feig SA, Cline MJ. Failure of recovery following syngeneic marrow grafting in aplastic anemia. Exp Hematol 1977;5:103A.
111. Laver J, Jhanwar SC, O'Reilly RJ, Castro-Malaspina H. Host origin of the human hematopoietic microenvironment following allogeneic bone marrow transplantation. Blood 1987;70:166.
112. Schmitz N, Gödde-Salz E, Löffler H. Cytogenetic studies on recipients of allogeneic bone marrow transplants after fractionated total body irradiation. Br J Haematol 1985;60:239.
113. Walker H, Singer CRJ, Patterson J, et al. The significance of host haematopoietic cells detected by cytogenetic analysis of bone marrow from recipients of bone marrow transplants. Br J Haematol 1986;62: 385.
114. Hill RS, Peterson FB, Storb R, et al. Mixed hematologic chimerism after allogeneic marrow transplantation for severe aplastic anemia is associated with a higher risk of graft rejection and a lessened incidence of acute graft-versus-host disease. Blood 1986;67:811.
115. Schmitz N, Johannsen W, Schmidt G, et al. Recurrence of acute lymphoblastic leukemia in donor cells after allogeneic marrow transplantation associated with a deletion of the long arm of chromosome 6. Blood 1987;70:1099.
116. Marmont A, Frassoni F, Bacigalupo A, et al. Recurrence of Ph^1-positive leukemia in donor cells after marrow transplantation for chronic granulocytic leukemia. N Engl J Med 1984;310:903.
117. Boyd CN, Ranberg R, Thomas ED. The incidence of recurrence of leukemia in donor cells after allogeneic bone marrow transplantation. Leuk Res 1982;6:833.
118. Sparkes MC, Crist ML, Sparkes RS, et al. Gene markers in human bone marrow transplantation. Vox Sang 1977;33:202.
119. Antin JH, Ginsburg D, Smith BR, et al. Bone marrow transplantation of paroxysmal nocturnal hemoglobinuria: eradication of the PNH clone and documentation of complete lymphohematopoietic engraftment. Blood 1985;66:1247.
120. Weitzel JN, Hows JM, Jefferys AJ, et al. Use of a hypervariable minisatellite DNA probe (33.15) for evaluating engraftment two or more years after bone marrow transplantation for aplastic anemia. Br J Haematol 1988;70:91.
121. Blazar BR, Orr HT, Arthur DC, et al. Restriction fragment length polymorphisms as markers of engraftment in allogeneic bone marrow transplantation. Blood 1985;66:1436.
122. Champlin RE, Gale RP. The early complications of bone marrow transplantation. Semin Hematol 1984;21:101.
123. Sullivan KM, Deeg HJ, Sanders JE, et al. Late complications after marrow transplantation. Semin Hematol 1984;21:53.
124. Bearman SI, Appelbaum FR, Buckner CD, et al. Regimen-related toxicity in patients undergoing bone marrow transplantation. J Clin Oncol 1988;6:1562.
125. McDonald GB, Hinds MS, Fisher LD, et al. Veno-occlusive disease of the liver and multiorgan failure after bone marrow transplantation: a cohort study of 355 patients. Ann Intern Med 1993;118:255.
126. Shulman HM, Hinterberger W. Hepatic veno-occlusive disease—liver toxicity syndrome after bone marrow transplantation. Bone Marrow Transplant 1992;10:197.
127. McDonald GB, Sharma P, Matthews DE, et al. The clinical course of 53 patients with venocclusive disease of the liver after marrow transplantation. Transplantation 1985;39:603.
128. Jones RJ, Lee KSK, Beschorner WE, et al. Venoocclusive disease of the liver following bone marrow transplantation. Transplantation 1987;44: 778.
129. Braverman AC, Antin JH, Plappert MT, Cook EF, Lee RT. Cyclophosphamide cardiotoxicity in bone marrow transplantation: a prospective evaluation of new dosing regimens. J Clin Oncol 1991;9:1215.
130. Steinherz LJ, Steinherz PG, Mangiacasale D, et al. Cardiac changes with cyclophosphamide. Med Pediatr Oncol 1981;9:417.
131. Gottdiener JS, Appelbaum FR, Ferrans VJ, et al. Cardiomyopathy associated with high dose cyclophosphamide therapy. Arch Intern Med 1981;141:768.
132. Goldberg MA, Antin JH, Guinan EC, Rappeport JM. Cyclophosphamide cardiotoxicity: an analysis of dosing as a risk factor. Blood 1986;68: 1114.
133. Loughran TP, Deeg HJ, Dahlberg S, et al. Incidence of hypertension among 112 patients randomized to either cyclosporine or methotrexate as graft-versus-host disease prophylaxis. Br J Haematol 1985;59:547.
134. Patchell RA, White CL, Clark AW, et al. Nonbacterial thrombotic endocarditis in bone marrow transplant patients. Cancer 1985;55:631.
135. Chao NJ, Duncan SR, Long GD, Horning SJ, Blume KG. Corticosteroid therapy for diffuse alveolar hemorrhage in autologous bone marrow transplant recipients. Ann Intern Med 1991;114:146.
136. Wingard JR, Sostrin MB, Vriesendorp HM, et al. Interstitial pneumonitis following autologous bone marrow transplantation. Transplantation 1988;46:61.
137. Cordonnier C, Bernaudin JF, Bierling P, et al. Pulmonary complications after allogeneic bone marrow transplantation: a study of 130 consecutive transplanted patients. Cancer 1987;58:1047.
138. Meyers JD, Flournoy N, Thomas ED, et al. Non-bacterial pneumonia after allogeneic marrow transplantation: a review of ten years' experience. Rev Infect Dis 1982;4:1119.
139. Holland KH, Wingard JR, Beschorner WE, et al. Bronchiolitis obliterans and its relationship to chronic graft-vs-host disease and low serum IgG. Blood 1988;72:621.
140. Ralph DD, Springmeyer SC, Sullivan DM, et al. Rapidly progressive air-flow obstruction in marrow transplant recipients. Am Rev Respir Dis 1984;129:641.
141. Burke CM, Theodore J, Dawkins KD, et al. Post-transplant obliterative bronchiolitis and other late lung sequelae in human heart–lung transplantation. Chest 1984;824.
142. Epler GR, Colby TV, McLoud TC, et al. Bronchiolitis obliterans organizing pneumonia. N Engl J Med 1985;312:152.
143. Hows JM, Mehta A, Ward L, et al. Comparison of mesna with forced diuresis to prevent cyclophosphamide induced haemorrhagic cystitis in marrow transplantation: a prospective randomized study. Br J Cancer 1984;50:753.
144. Brugieres L, Hartmann O, Travagli JP, et al. Hemorrhagic cystitis following high-dose cyclophosphamide and bone marrow transplantation in children with malignancies: incidence, clinical course, and outcome. J Clin Oncol 1989;7:194.
145. Thomas AE, Patterson J, Prentice HG, et al. Haemorrhagic cystitis in bone marrow transplantation patients: possible increased risk associated with prior busulfan therapy. Bone Marrow Transplant 1987;1:347.
146. Arthur RR, Shah KV, Baust SJ, et al. Association of BK viruria with hemorrhagic cystitis in recipients of bone marrow transplants. N Engl J Med 1986;315:230.

147. Rice SJ, Bishop JA, Apperley J. BK virus as cause of haemorrhagic cystitis after bone marrow transplantation. Lancet 1985;2:844.
148. Ambinder RF, Burns W, Forman M, et al. Hemorrhagic cystitis associated with adenovirus infection in bone marrow transplantation. Arch Intern Med 1986;146:1400.
149. Sanders JE, Pritchard S, Mahoney P, et al. Growth and development following marrow transplantation for leukemia. Blood 1986;68:1129.
150. Sanders JE, Buckner CD, Leonard JM, et al. Late effects on gonadal function of cyclophosphamide, total body irradiation and marrow transplantation. Transplantation 1983;36:252.
151. Sanders JE, Buckner CD, Amos D, et al. Ovarian function following marrow transplantation for aplastic anemia or leukemia. J Clin Oncol 1988;6:813.
152. Lieper AD, Stanhope R, Lau T, et al. The effect of total body irradiation and bone marrow transplantation during childhood and adolescence on growth and endocrine function. Br J Haematol 1987;67:419.
153. Lio S, Arcese W, Papa G, Darmiento M. Thyroid and pituitary function following bone marrow transplantation. Arch Intern Med 1988;148: 1066.
154. Sklar CA, Kim TH, Ramsay NK. Testicular function following bone marrow transplantation during or after puberty. Cancer 1984;53:1498.
155. Schmidt H, Ehninger G, Dopfer R, Waller HD. Pregnancy after bone marrow transplantation for severe aplastic anemia. Bone Marrow Transplant 1987;2:329.
156. Deeg HJ, Kennedy MS, Sanders JE, et al. Successful pregnancy after marrow transplantation for severe aplastic anemia and immunosuppression with cyclosporine. JAMA 1983;250:647.
157. Sklar CA, Kim TH, Ramsay NKC. Thyroid dysfunction among long-term survivors of bone marrow transplant. Am J Med 1982;73:688.
158. Sullivan KM, Storb R, Shulman H, et al. Immediate and delayed neurotoxicity after meclorethamine preparation for bone marrow transplantation. Ann Intern Med 1982;97:182.
159. Thompson CB, Sanders JE, Flournoy N, et al. The risks of central nervous system relapse and leukoencephalopathy in patients receiving marrow transplants for acute leukemia. Blood 1986;67:195.
160. Atkinson K, Clink H, Lawler S, et al. Encephalopathy following bone marrow transplantation. Eur J Cancer 1977;13:623.
161. Wade JC, Meyers JD. Neurologic symptoms associated with parenteral acyclovir treatment after marrow transplantation. Ann Intern Med 1983;98:921.
162. Guinan EC, Tarbell NJ, Niemeyer CM, Sallan SE, Weinstein HJ. Intravascular hemolysis and renal insufficiency after bone marrow transplantation. Blood 1988;72:451.
163. Rabinowe SN, Soiffer RJ, Tarbell NJ, et al. Hemolytic-uremic syndrome following bone marrow transplantation in adults for hematologic malignancies. Blood 1991;77:1837.
164. Gossett TC, Gale RP, Fleischman H, et al. Immunoblastic sarcoma in donor cells after bone-marrow transplantation. N Engl J Med 1979;300: 904.
165. Schubach WH, Hackman R, Neiman PE, et al. A monoclonal immunoblastic sarcoma in donor cells bearing Epstein-Barr virus genomes following allogeneic marrow grafting for acute lymphoblastic leukemia. Blood 1982;60:180.
166. Martin P, Schulman H, Schubach W, et al. Fatal Epstein-Barr virus associated proliferation of donor B-cells after treatment of acute graft-versus-host disease with a murine anti-T-cell antibody. Ann Intern Med 1984;101:310.
167. Schubach W, Miller G, Thomas ED. Epstein-Barr virus genomes are restricted to secondary neoplastic cells following bone marrow transplantation. Blood 1985;65:535.
168. Shearer WT, Ritz J, Finegold M, et al. Epstein-Barr virus-associated B-cell proliferation of diverse clonal origins after bone marrow transplantation in a 12-year-old patient with severe combined immunodeficiency. N Engl J Med 1985;312:1151.
169. Trigg ME, Finlay JL, Sondel PM. Prophylactic acyclovir in patients receiving bone marrow transplants. N Engl J Med 1985;312:1708.
170. Deeg HJ, Sanders J, Martin P, et al. Secondary malignancies after marrow transplantation. Exp Hematol 1984;12:660.
171. Deeg HJ, Witherspoon RP. Risk factors for the development of secondary malignancies after marrow transplantation. Hematol/Oncol Clin N Am 1993;7:417.
172. Witherspoon RP, Schubach W, Neiman P, et al. Donor cell leukemia developing six years after marrow grafting for acute leukemia. Blood 1985;65:1172.
173. Elfenbein GJ, Brogaonkar DS, Bias WB, et al. Cytogenetic evidence for recurrence of acute myelogenous leukemia after allogeneic bone marrow transplantation in donor hematopoietic cells. Blood 1978;52:627.
174. Thomas ED, Bryant JL, Buckner CD, et al. Leukaemic transformation of engrafted human marrow cells in vivo. Lancet 1972;1:1310.
175. Newburger PE, Latt SA, Pesando JM, et al. Leukemia relapse in donor cells after allogeneic bone-marrow transplantation. N Engl J Med 1981;304:712.
176. Smith JL, Heerema NA, Provisor AJ. Leukaemic transformation of engrafted bone marrow cells. Br J Haematol 1985;60:415.
177. Fialkow PJ, Thomas ED, Bryant JI, Neiman PE. Leukaemic transformation of engrafted human marrow cells in vivo. Lancet 1971;1:251.
178. Goh K, Klemperer MR. In vivo leukemic transformation: cytogenetic evidence of in vivo leukemic transformation of engrafted marrow cells. Am J Hematol 1977;2:283.
179. Feig SA, Dreazen O, Simon M, et al. B cell acute lymphoblastic leukemia (ALL) in donor cells following bone marrow transplantation for T cell ALL. Bone Marrow Transplant 1988;3:331.
180. Blacklock HA, Katz F, Michalevicz R, et al. A and B blood group antigen expression on mixed colony cells and erythroid precursors: relevance for human allogeneic bone marrow transplantation. Br J Haematol 1984;58:267.
181. Bacigalupo A, Van Lint NT, Occhini D, et al. ABO compatibility and acute graft versus-host-disease following allogeneic bone marrow transplantation. Transplantation 1988;45:1091.
182. Hershko G, Gale RP, Ho W. ABH antigens and bone marrow transplantation. Br J Haematol 1980;44:65.
183. Tichelli A, Gratwohl A, Wenger A, et al. ABO-incompatible bone marrow transplantation: in vivo adsorption, an old forgotten method. Transplant Proc 1987;19:4632.
184. Gale RP, Feig S, Ho W, et al. ABO blood group system and bone marrow transplantation. Blood 1977;50:185.
185. Buckner CD, Clift RA, Sanders JE, et al. ABO-incompatible marrow transplants. Transplantation 1978;26:233.
186. Braine HG, Sensenbrenner LL, Wright SK, et al. Bone marrow transplantation with major ABO blood group incompatibility using erythrocyte depletion of marrow prior to infusion. Blood 1982;60:420.
187. Dinsmore RE, Reich LM, Kapoor N, et al. ABH incompatible bone marrow transplantation: removal of erythrocytes by starch sedimentation. Br J Haematol 1983;54:441.
188. Jin NR, Hill R, Segal G, et al. Preparation of red-blood-cell–depleted marrow for ABO-incompatible marrow transplantation by density-gradient separation using the IBM 2991 blood cell processor. Exp Hematol 1987;15:93.
189. Gilmore ML, Prentice HG, Blacklock HA, et al. A technique for rapid isolation of bone marrow mononuclear cells using Ficoll-metrizoate and the IBM 2991 blood cell processor. Br J Haematol 1982;50:619.
190. Hows JM, Chipping PM, Palmer S, Gordon-Smith EC. Regeneration of peripheral blood cells following ABO incompatible allogeneic bone marrow transplantation for severe aplastic anemia. Br J Haematol 1983;53:145.
191. Bensinger WI, Buckner CD, Thomas ED, Clift RA. ABO-incompatible marrow transplants. Transplantation 1982;33:427.
192. Warkentin PI, Yomtovian R, Hurd D, et al. Severe delayed hemolytic transfusion reaction complicating an ABO-incompatible bone marrow transplantation. Vox Sang 1983;45:40.
193. Ockleford PA, Hill RS, Nelson R, et al. Serological complications of a major ABO incompatible bone marrow transplantation in a Polynesian with aplastic anemia. Transfusion 1982;22:62.
194. Sniecinski IJ, Oien L, Petz LD, Blume KG. Immunohematologic consequences of major ABO-mismatched bone marrow transplantation. Transplantation 1988;45:530.
195. Hows JM, Beddow K, Gordon-Smith E, et al. Donor derived red blood cell antibodies and immune hemolysis after allogeneic bone marrow transplantation. Blood 1986;67:177.
196. Hazlehurst GR, Brenner MK, Wimperis JZ, Knowles SM, Prentice HG. Haemolysis after T-cell depleted bone marrow transplantation involving minor ABO incompatibility. Scand J Haematol 1986;37:1.
197. Ransey G, Nusbacher J, Starzl TE, Lindsay GD. Isohemagglutinins of graft origin after ABO-unmatched liver transplantation. N Engl J Med 1984;311:1167.
198. Niederwieser D, Pepe M, Storb R, et al. Improvement in rejection, engraftment rate, and survival without increase in graft-versus-host disease by high marrow cell dose in patients transplanted for aplastic anemia. Br J Haematol 1988;69:23.
199. Yeager AM, Kaizer H, Santos GW, et al. Autologous bone marrow transplantation in patients with acute nonlymphocytic leukemia using ex vivo marrow treatment with 4-hydroperoxycyclophosphamide. N Engl J Med 1986;315:141.
200. Harada M, Yoshida T, Ishino C, et al. Hematologic recovery following autologous and allogeneic bone marrow transplantation. Exp Hematol 1983;11:841.
201. Banaji M, Bearman SI, Buckner CD, et al. The effects of splenectomy on engraftment and platelet transfusion requirements in patients with chronic myelogenous leukemia undergoing marrow transplantation. Am J Hematol 1986;22:275.
202. Storb R, Deeg HJ, Whitehead J, et al. Methotrexate and cyclosporine compared with cyclosporine alone for prophylaxis of acute graft versus host disease after marrow transplantation for leukemia. N Engl J Med 1986;314:729.
203. Hows JM, Kaffaf S, Palmer S, et al. Regeneration of peripheral blood cells following allogeneic bone marrow transplantation for severe aplastic anemia. Br J Haematol 1982;52:551.
204. Verdonck LF, van Heugten H, de Gast GC. Delay in platelet recovery after bone marrow transplantation: impact of cytomegalovirus infection. Blood 1985;66:921.
205. Lemischka I, Raulet DH, Mulligan RG. Developmental potential and dynamic behaviour of hematopoietic stem cells. Cell 1986;45:917.
206. Nash R, Storb R, Neiman P. Polyclonal reconstitution of human marrow after allogeneic bone marrow transplantation. Blood 1988;72:2031.

207. Turhan AG, Humphries RK, Phillips GL, et al. Clonal hematopoiesis demonstrated by X-linked DNA polymorphisms after allogeneic bone marrow transplantation. N Engl J Med 1989;320:1655.
208. Brandt SJ, Peters WP, Atwater SK, et al. Effect of recombinant human granulocyte-macrophage colony-stimulating factor on hematopoietic reconstitution after high-dose chemotherapy and autologous bone marrow transplantation. N Engl J Med 1988;318:869.
209. Kessinger A, Armitage JO, Smith DM, et al. High-dose therapy and autologous peripheral blood stem cell transplantation for patients with lymphoma. Blood 1989;74:1260.
210. Kessinger A, Bierman PJ, Vose JM, Armitage JO. High-dose cyclophosphamide, carmustine, and etoposide followed by autologous peripheral stem cell transplantation for patients with relapsed Hodgkin's disease. Blood 1991;77:2322.
211. Gianni AM, Siena S, Bregni M, et al. Granulocyte-macrophage colony-stimulating factor to harvest circulating haemopoietic stem cells for autotransplantation. Lancet 1989;2:580.
212. Sheridan WP, Begley CG, Juttner Ca, et al. Effect of peripheral-blood progenitor cells mobilised by filgrastim (G-CSF) on platelet recovery after high dose chemotherapy. Lancet 1992;339:640.
213. Haas R, Ho AD, Bredthauer U, et al. Successful autologous transplantation of blood stem cells mobilized with recombinant human granulocyte-macrophage colony-stimulating facor. Exp Hematol 1990;18:94.
214. Elias AD, Ayash L, Anderson KC, et al. Mobilization of peripheral blood progenitor cells by chemotherapy and granulocyte-macrophage colony-stimulating factor for hematologic support after high-dose intensification for breast cancer. Blood 1992;79:3036.
215. Huan SD, Hester J, Spitzer G, et al. Influence of mobilized peripheral blood cells on the hematopoietic recovery by autologous marrow and recombinant human granulocyte-macrophage colony-stimulating factor after high dose cyclophosphamide, etoposide and cisplatin. Blood 1992;79:3388.
216. Burakoff SJ, Lipton JM, Nathan DG. Recapitulation of the immune response and haematopoietic system in bone marrow transplantation. Clin Haematol 1983;12:695.
217. Rappeport JM, Newburger PE, Goldblum RM, et al. Allogeneic bone marrow transplantation for chronic granulomatous disease. J Pediatr 1982;101:952.
218. Tsoi M-S, Dobbs S, Brkic S, et al. Cellular interactions in marrow-grafted patients. II. Normal monocyte antigen-presenting and defective T-cell proliferative functions early after grafting and during chronic graft versus host disease. Transplantation 1984;37:556.
219. Reittie JE, Poulter LW, Prentice HG, et al. Differential recovery of phenotypically and functionally distinct circulating antigen-presenting cells after allogeneic marrow transplantation. Transplantation 1988;45:1084.
220. Winston DJ, Territo MC, Ho WG, et al. Alveolar macrophage dysfunction in human bone marrow transplant recipients. Am J Med 1982;73:859.
221. Perreault C, Pelletier M, Landry D, Gyger M. Study of Langerhans cells after allogeneic bone marrow transplantation. Blood 1984;63:807.
222. Murphy GF, Merot Y, Tong AKF, et al. Depletion and repopulation of epidermal dendritic cells after allogeneic bone marrow transplantation in humans. J Invest Dermatol 1985;84:210.
223. Thomas ED, Ramberg RF, Sale GE, et al. Direct evidence for a bone marrow origin of the alveolar macrophage in man. Science 1976;192:1016.
224. Gale RP, Sparkes RS, Golde DW. Bone marrow origin of hepatic macrophages (Kupffer cells) in humans. Science 1978;201:937.
225. Alter BP, Rappeport JM, Huisman THJ, Schroeder WA. Fetal erythropoiesis following bone marrow transplantation. Blood 1976;48:843.
226. Papayannopoulou Th, Chen P, Maniatis A, Stamatoyannopoulos G. Simultaneous assessment of i-antigenic expression and fetal hemoglobin in single red cells by immunofluorescence. Blood 1980;55:221.
227. Papayannopoulou T, Nakamoto B, Agostinelli F, et al. Fetal to adult hemopoietic cell transplantation in humans: insights into hemoglobin switching. Blood 1986;67:99.
228. Winkler KJ, Rea CD, Rahbar S, et al. Heterogeneous ontogeny of erythropoiesis after bone marrow ablation and allogeneic bone marrow grafting. Blood 1983;61:167.
229. Rozman C, Feliu E, Granena A, et al. Transient dyserythropoiesis in repopulated human bone marrow following transplantation: an ultrastructural study. Br J Haematol 1982;50:63.
230. Schapira L, Antin JH, Ransil BJ, et al. Serum erythropoietin levels in patients receiving intensive chemotherapy and radiotherapy. Blood 1990;76:2354.
231. Miller CB, Jones RJ, Zahurak ML, et al. Impaired erythropoietin response to anemia after bone marrow transplantation. Blood 1992;80:2677.
232. Stefmann JL, López J, Otero MJ, et al. Erythropoietin treatment in allogeneic BMT accelerates erythroid reconstitution: results of a prospective randomized trial. Bone Marrow Transplant 1992;10:541.
233. Mitus AJ, Antin JH, Rutherford CJ, McGarigle C, Churchill WH, Goldberg MA. Significant reduction in homologous red cell transfusion requirements with the use of recombinant human erythropoietin in allogeneic bone marrow transplantation. Blood 1992;80(Suppl 1):330a.
234. First L, Smith BR, Lipton J, Nathan DG, Parkman RP, Rappeport JM. Isolated thrombocytopenia following allogeneic bone marrow transplantation: existence of transient and chronic thrombocytopenia syndromes. Blood 1985;65:368.
235. Minchinton RM, Waters AH, Malpas JH, et al. Selective thrombocytopenia and neutropenia occurring after bone marrow transplantation: evidence of an autoimmune basis. Clin Lab Haematol 1984;6:157.
236. Anasetti C, Rybka W, Sullivan KM, et al. Graft versus host disease is associated with autoimmune like thrombocytopenia. Blood 1989;73:1054.
237. Naeim F, Smith GS, Gale RP. Morphologic aspects of bone marrow transplantation in patients with aplastic anemia. Hum Pathol 1978;9:295.
238. Faile A, Maraninchi D, Gluckman E, et al. Granulocyte progenitor compartments after allogeneic bone marrow grafts. Scand J Haematol 1981;26:202.
239. Arnold R, Schmeiser T, Heit W, et al. Hemopoietic reconstitution after bone marrow transplantation. Exp Hematol 1986;14:271.
240. Rowley SD, Zuehlsdorf M, Braine HG, et al. CFU-GM content of bone marrow graft correlates with time to hematologic reconstitution following autologous bone marrow transplantation with 4-hydroperoxycyclophosphamide purged bone marrow. Blood 1987;70:271.
241. Atkinson K, Norrie S, Chan P, et al. Lack of correlation between nucleated bone marrow cell dose, marrow CFU-GM dose, or marrow CFU-E dose and the rate of HLA-identical sibling marrow engraftment. Br J Haematol 1985;60:245.
242. Torres A, Alonso MC, Gomez C, et al. No influence of number of donor CFU-GM on granulocyte recovery in bone marrow transplantation for acute leukemia. Blut 1985;50:89.
243. Yamasaki K, Solberg LA Jr, Jamal N, et al. Hemopoietic colony growth promoting activities in the plasma of bone marrow transplant recipients. J Clin Invest 1988;82:255.
244. Nemunaitis J, Singer JW, Buckner CD, et al. Use of recombinant human granulocyte-macrophage colony-stimulating factor in autologous marrow transplantation for lymphoid malignancies. Blood 1988;72:834.
245. Taylor KM, Jagannath S, Spitzer G, et al. Recombinant human granulocyte colony-stimulating factor hastens granulocyte recovery after high-dose chemotherapy and autologous bone marrow transplantation in Hodgkin's disease. J Clin Oncol 1989;7:1791.
246. Golde DW, Hocking WG, Quan SG, et al. Origin of human bone marrow fibroblasts. Br J Haematol 1980;44:183.
247. Singer JW, Keating A, Cuttner J, et al. Evidence for a stem cell common to hematopoiesis and its in vitro microenvironment: studies of patients with clonal hematopoietic neoplasia. Leuk Res 1984;8:545.
248. Keating A, Singer JW, Killen PD, et al. Donor origin of the in vitro haematopoietic microenvironment after marrow transplantation in man. Nature 1982;298:280.
249. Laver J, Jhanwar SC, O'Reilly RJ, Castro-Malaspina H. Host origin of the human hematopoietic microenvironment following allogeneic bone marrow transplantation. Blood 1987;70:1966.
250. Lum LG. The kinetics of immune reconstitution after human marrow transplantation. Blood 1987;69:369.
251. Paulin T, Ringden O, Nilsson B. Immunological recovery after bone marrow transplantation: role of age, graft versus host disease, prednisolone treatment and infections. Bone Marrow Transplant 1987;1:317.
252. Verdonk LF, de Gast GC. Is cytomegalovirus infection a major cause of T cell alterations after (autologous) bone marrow transplantation? Lancet 1984;1:932.
253. Gratama JW, Naipal AMIH, Oosterveer MAP, et al. Effects of herpes virus carrier status on peripheral T lymphocyte subsets. Blood 1987;70:516.
254. Gascon P, Zoumbos NC, Young NS. Immunological abnormalities in patients receiving multiple blood transfusions. Ann Intern Med 1984;100:173.
255. Ault KA, Antin JH, Ginsburg D, et al. Phenotype of recovering lymphoid cell populations following marrow transplantation. J Exp Med 1985;161:1483.
256. Smith BR, Rappeport JM, Burakoff SJ, Ault KA. Clinical correlates of unusual circulating lymphocytes appearing post marrow transplantation. In: Gale RP, Champlin R, eds. Progress in bone marrow transplantation, vol 53. New York, Alan R Liss, 1987:659.
257. Hokland M, Jacobsen N, Ellegaard J, Hokland P. Natural killer function following allogeneic bone marrow transplantation. Transplantation 1988;45:1080.
258. Hercend T, Takvorian T, Nowill A, et al. Characterization of natural killer cells with antileukemic activity following allogeneic bone marrow transplantation. Blood 1986;67:722.
259. Reittie JE, Gottlieb D, Heslop HE, et al. Endogenously generated activated killer cells circulate after autologous and allogeneic marrow transplantation but not after chemotherapy. Blood 1989;73:1351.
260. Antin JH, Ault KA, Rappeport JM, Smith BR. B lymphocyte reconstitution after human bone marrow transplantation: the Leu-1 antigen defines a functionally distinct population of B lymphocytes. J Clin Invest 1987;80:325.
261. Anderson KC, Ritz J, Takvorian T, et al. Hematologic engraftment and immune reconstitution posttransplantation with anti-B1 purged autologous bone marrow. Blood 1987;69:597.
262. Ringden O, Witherspoon R, Storb R, et al. B cell function in human

marrow transplant recipients assessed by direct and indirect hemolysis in gel assays. J Immunol 1979;123:2729.
263. Pahwa S, Friedrich W, Evans R, et al. Humoral immune response in vitro after bone marrow transplantation. Pediatr Res 1981;15:601.
264. Kiesel S, Pezzutto A, Moldenhauer G, et al. B cell proliferative and differentiation responses after autologous peripheral blood stem cell or bone marrow transplantation. Blood 1988;72:672.
265. Witherspoon RP, Storb R, Ochs D, et al. Recovery of antibody production in human allogeneic marrow graft recipients: influences of time post-transplantation, the presence or absence of chronic graft-versus-host disease, and antithymocyte globulin treatment. Blood 1981;58:360.
266. Lum LG, Seigneuret MC, Storb R, et al. In vitro regulation of immunoglobulin synthesis after marrow transplantation. I. T and B cell deficiencies in patients with and without chronic graft versus host disease. Blood 1981;58:431.
267. Witherspoon RP, Lum LG, Storb R. Immunologic reconstitution after human marrow grafting. Semin Hematol 1984;21:2.
268. Shiobara S, Witherspoon RP, Lum LG, Storb R. Immunoglobulin synthesis after HLA identical marrow grafting. V. The role of peripheral blood monocytes in the regulation of in vitro immunoglobulin secretion stimulated by pokeweed mitogen. J Immunol 1984;132:2850.
269. Korsmeyer SJ, Elfenbein GJ, Goldman CK, et al. B cell, helper T cell, and suppressor T cell abnormalities contribute to disordered immunoglobulin synthesis in patients following bone marrow transplantation. Transplantation 1982;33:184.
270. Matsue K, Lum LG, Witherspoon RP, Storb R. Proliferative and differential responses of B cells from human marrow graft recipients to T-cell derived factors. Blood 1987;69:308.
271. Storek J, Saxon A. Reconstitution of B cell immunity following bone marrow transplantation. Bone Marrow Transplant 1992;9:395.
272. Noel DR, Witherspoon RP, Storb R, et al. Does graft versus host disease influence the tempo of immunological recovery after allogeneic human marrow transplantation? Blood 1978;51:1087.
273. Witherspoon RP, Storb R, Ochs HD, et al. Recovery of antibody production in human allogeneic marrow graft recipients: influence of time post transplant, the presence or absence of chronic graft versus host disease, and anti-thymocyte globulin treatment. Blood 1981;58:360.
274. Holland HK, Wingard JR, Beschorner WE, et al. Bronchiolitis obliterans in bone marrow transplantation and its relationship to chronic graft versus host disease and low serum IgG. Blood 1988;72:621.
275. Perreault C, Glasson M, Gyger M, et al. Serum immunoglobulin levels following allogeneic bone marrow transplantation. Blut 1985;51:137.
276. Smith BR, Schur PH, Rappeport JM. Prolonged selective IgG4 deficiency post bone marrow transplantation. Blood 1987;70:113A.
277. Ringden O, Sundberg B, Markling L, Tollemar J. Polyclonal antibody secretion during acute graft versus host disease. Scand J Immunol 1987;26:469.
278. Saryan F, Rappeport J, Leung DYM, et al. Regulation of human IgE synthesis in acute graft versus host disease. J Clin Invest 1983;71:556.
279. Heyd J, Donnenberg AD, Burns WH, et al. Immunoglobulin E levels following allogeneic, autologous, and syngeneic bone marrow transplantation. Blood 1988;72:442.
280. Witherspoon RP, Schanfield MS, Storb R, et al. Immunoglobulin production of donor origin after marrow transplantation for acute leukemia or aplastic anemia. Transplantation 1978;26:407.
281. Lum LG, Seigneuret MC, Storb R. The transfer of antigen specific immunity from marrow donors to marrow recipients. J Clin Immunol 1986;6:1.
282. Lum LG, Munn NA, Schanfield MS, Storb R. The detection of specific antibody formation to recall antigens after human bone marrow transplantation. Blood 1986;67:582.
283. Hammarstrom L, Smith CIE. Frequent occurrence of monoclonal gammopathies with an unbalanced light chain ratio following bone marrow transplantation. Transplantation 1987;43:449.
284. Pruzanski W, Cowan DH, Merrett RA, Freedman NH. IgG1 kappa M component after bone marrow transplantation. Clin Immunol Immunopathol 1973;1:311.
285. Vossen JM, Holl RA, Asma GEM, et al. Reconstitution of the B cell system following allogeneic bone marrow transplantation: an accelerated recapitulation of ontogenic development. In: Eibl M, Rosen S, eds. Primary immunodeficiency diseases. Amsterdam, Elsevier, 1986: 309.
286. Mitus AJ, Stein R, Rappeport JM, et al. Monoclonal and oligoclonal gammopathy following bone marrow transplantation. Blood 1989;74: 2764.
287. Friedrick W, O'Reilly RJ, Koziner B, et al. T lymphocyte reconstitution in recipients of bone marrow transplants with and without GVHD: imbalances of T cell subpopulations having unique regulatory and cognitive function. Blood 1982;59:696.
288. Gratama JW, Naipal A, Oljans P, et al. T lymphocyte repopulation and differentiation after bone marrow transplantation: early shifts in the ratio between T4+ and T8+ T lymphocytes correlate with the occurrence of graft versus host disease. Blood 1984;63:1416.
289. Anderson KC, Ritz J, Takvorian T, et al. Hematologic engraftment and immune reconstitution posttransplantation with anti-B1 purged autologous bone marrow. Blood 1987;69:597.
290. Velardi A, Terenzi A, Cucciaioni S, et al. Imbalances within the peripheral blood T-helper (CD4+) and T-suppressor (CD8+) cell populations in the reconstitution phase after human bone marrow transplantation. Blood 1988;71:1196.
291. Witherspoon RP, Kopecky K, Storb R, et al. Immunologic recovery in 48 patients following syngeneic marrow transplant for hematologic malignancy. Transplantation 1982;33:143.
292. Linch DC, Knott LJ, Thomas RM, et al. T cell regeneration after allogeneic and autologous bone marrow transplantation. Br J Haematol 1983;53:451.
293. de Gast GC, Verdonck LF, Middeldorp JM, et al. Recovery of T cell subsets after autologous bone marrow transplantation is mainly due to proliferation of mature T cells in the graft. Blood 1985;66:428.
294. Schroff RW, Gale RP, Fahey JL. Regeneration of T cell subpopulations after bone marrow transplantation: cytomegalovirus infection and lymphoid subset imbalance. J Immunol 1982;129:1926.
295. Ueda M, Harada M, Shiobara S, et al. T lymphocyte reconstitution in long-term survivors after allogeneic and autologous marrow transplantation. Transplantation 1984;37:552.
296. Rappeport JM, Dunn MJ, Parkman R. Immature T lymphocytes in the peripheral blood of bone marrow transplant recipients. Transplantation 1983;36:674.
297. Witherspoon RP, Matthews D, Storb R, et al. Recovery of in vivo cellular immunity after human marrow grafting. Transplantation 1984;37:145.
298. Rozans M, Smith BR, Burakoff SJ, Miller RA. Long lasting deficit of functional T cell precursors in human bone marrow transplant recipients revealed by limiting dilution methods. J Immunol 1986;136:4040.
299. Noel DR, Witherspoon RP, Storb R, et al. Does graft versus host disease influence the tempo of immunologic recovery after allogeneic human marrow transplantation? An observation on 56 long term survivors. Blood 1978;51:1087.
300. Witherspoon RP, Deeg HJ, Lum LG, et al. Immunological recovery in human marrow graft recipients given cyclosporine or methotrexate for the prevention of graft versus host disease. Transplantation 1984;37: 456.
301. Daley JP, Rozans MK, Smith BR, et al. Retarded recovery of functional T cell frequencies in T cell depleted bone marrow transplant recipients. Blood 1987;70:960.
302. Welte K, Ciobanu N, Moore MAS, et al. Defective interleukin 2 production in patients after bone marrow transplantation and in vitro restoration of defective T lymphocyte proliferation by highly purified interleukin 2. Blood 1984;64:380.
303. Azogui O, Gluckman E, Fradelizi D. Inhibition of IL2 production after human allogeneic bone marrow transplantation. J Immunol 1983;131: 1205.
304. Mizuno S-I, Morishima Y, Kodera Y, et al. Gamma interferon production capacity and T lymphocyte subpopulation after allogeneic bone marrow transplantation. Transplantation 1986;41:311.
305. Cooley MA. Cytokine activity after human bone marrow transplantation. J Immunol 1987;138:3742.
306. Tsoi MS, Storb R, Dobbs S, et al. Non-specific suppressor cells in patients with chronic graft versus host disease after marrow grafting. J Immunol 1979;123:1970.
307. Harada M, Ueda M, Nakao S, et al. Nonspecific suppressor T cells cause decreased mixed lymphocyte culture reactivity in bone marrow transplant patients. J Immunol 1986;137:428.
308. Lum LG. The kinetics of immune reconstitution after human marrow transplantation. Blood 1987;69:369.
309. Klingemann H-G, Tsoi M-S, Storb R. Inhibition of prostaglandin E2 restores defective lymphocyte proliferation and cell mediated lympholysis in recipients after allogeneic marrow grafting. Blood 1986;68: 102.
310. Bierer BE, Burakoff SJ, Smith BR. A large proportion of T lymphocytes lack CD5 expression after bone marrow transplantation. Blood 1989;73: 1359.
311. Rappeport JM, Ginn EI. Bone-marrow transplantation for severe Gaucher's disease. N Engl J Med 1984;311:84.
312. Bertheas MF, Maraninchi D, Lafage M, et al. Partial chimerism after T cell depleted allogeneic bone marrow transplantation in leukemic HLA-matched patients: a cytogenetic documentation. Blood 1988;72: 89.
313. Bretagne S, Vidaud M, Kuentz M, et al. Mixed blood chimerism in T cell depleted bone marrow transplant recipients: evaluation using DNA polymorphism. Blood 1987;70:1962.
314. Schattenberg A, De Witte T, Salden M, et al. Mixed hematopoietic chimerism after allogeneic transplantation with lymphocyte depleted bone marrow is not associated with a higher incidence of relapse. Blood 1989;73:1367.
315. Shank B, Brochstein JA, Castro-Malaspina H, et al. Immunosuppression prior to marrow transplantation for sensitized aplastic anemia patients: comparison of TLI with TBI. Int J Radiat Oncol Biol Phys 1988;14:1133.
316. Lawler SD, Baker MC, Harris H, et al. Cytogenetic studies on recipients of allogeneic bone marrow using the sex chromosomes as markers of cellular origin. Br J Haematol 1984;56:431.
317. Chu E, Umetsu D, Rosen F, Geha RS. Major histocompatibility restriction of antigen recognition by T cells in a recipient of haplotype mismatched human bone marrow transplantation. J Clin Invest 1983;72: 1124.

318. Roncarolo MG, Touraine J-L, Banchereau J. Cooperation between major histocompatibility complex mismatched mononuclear cells from a human chimera in the production of antigen specific antibody. J Clin Invest 1986;77:673.
319. Shepp DH, Newton BA, Dandliker PS, et al. Oral acyclovir therapy for mucocutaneous herpes simplex virus reactivation after marrow transplantation. Ann Intern Med 1985;102:703.
320. Wade JC, Newton B, Flournoy N, Meyers JD. Oral acyclovir for prevention of herpes simplex virus reactivation after marrow transplantation. Ann Intern Med 1984;100:823.
321. Lundgren G, Wilczek H, Lonnqvist B, et al. Acyclovir prophylaxis in bone marrow transplant recipients. Scand J Infect Dis 1985;47:137.
322. Shepp DH, Dandliker PS, Flournoy N, Meyers JD. Sequential intravenous and twice daily oral acyclovir for extended prophylaxis of herpes simplex virus infection in marrow transplant patients. Transplantation 1987;43:654.
323. Saral R, Burns WH, Laskin OL, et al. Acyclovir prophylaxis of herpes-simplex-virus infections: a randomized, double-blind, controlled trial in bone-marrow-transplant recipients. N Engl J Med 1981;305:63.
324. Dorsky DI, Crumpacker CS. Drugs five years later: acyclovir. Ann Intern Med 1987;107:859.
325. Meyers JD, Reed EC, Shepp DH, et al. Acyclovir for prevention of cytomegalovirus infection and disease after allogeneic marrow transplantation. N Engl J Med 1988;318:70.
326. Hughes WT, McNobb PC, Makres TD, et al. Efficacy of trimethoprim and sulfamethoxazole in the prevention and treatment of Pneumocystis carinii pneumonitis. J Infect Dis 1973;128:607.
327. Bernard EM, Pagel L, Schmitt HJ, et al. Clinical trial with aerosol pentamidine for prevention of *Pneumocystis carinii* pneumonia. Clin Res 1987;35:468a.
328. Atkinson K, Meyers JD, Storb R, et al. Varicella-zoster virus infection after marrow transplantation for aplastic anemia or leukemia. Transplantation 1980;29:47.
329. Sullivan KM, Deeg HJ, Sanders JE, et al. Late complications after marrow transplantation. Semin Hematol 1984;21:53.
330. Meyers JD, Flournoy N, Thomas ED. Risk factors for cytomegalovirus after human marrow transplantation. J Infect Dis 1986;153:478.
331. Weiner RS, Bortin MM, Gale RP, et al. Interstitial pneumonitis after bone marrow transplantation: assessment of risk factors. Ann Intern Med 1986;104:168.
332. Winston DJ, Huang ES, Miller MJ, et al. Molecular epidemiology of cytomegalovirus infections associated with bone marrow transplantation. Ann Intern Med 1985;102:16.
333. Wingard JR, Chen DYH, Burns WH, et al. Cytomegalovirus infection after autologous bone marrow transplantation with comparison to infection after allogeneic bone marrow transplantation. Blood 1988;71: 1432.
334. Miller W, Flynn P, McCullough J, et al. Cytomegalovirus infection after bone marrow transplantation: an association with graft versus host disease. Blood 1986;67:1162.
335. Miller W, Flynn P, McCullough J, et al. Cytomegalovirus infection after bone marrow transplantation: an association with acute graft-v-host disease. Blood 1986;67:1162.
336. Meyers JD. Prevention and treatment of cytomegalovirus infection after marrow transplantation. Bone Marrow Transplant 1988;3:95.
337. Grob JP, Grundy JE, Prentice HG, et al. Immune donors can protect marrow-transplant recipients from severe cytomegalovirus infections. Lancet 1987;1:774.
338. Frank I, Friedman HM. Progress in the treatment of cytomegalovirus pneumonia. Ann Intern Med 1988;109:769.
339. Grundy JE, Shanley JD, Griffiths PD. Is cytomegalovirus interstitial pneumonitis in transplant patients an immunopathological condition? Lancet 1987;2:996.
340. Ruutu P, Ruutu T, Volin L, et al. Cytomegalovirus is frequently isolated in bronchoalveolar lavage fluid of bone marrow transplant recipients without pneumonia. Ann Intern Med 1990;112:913.
341. Verdonck LF, de Graan-Hentzen YCE, Dekker AW, et al. Cytomegalovirus seronegative platelets and leukocyte-poor red blood cells from random donors can prevent primary cytomegalovirus infection after bone marrow transplantation. Bone Marrow Transplant 1987;2:73.
342. Yeager AS, Grumet FC, Hafleigh EB, et al. Prevention of transfusion-acquired cytomegalovirus infections in newborn infants. J Pediatr 1981;98:218.
343. Bowden RA, Slichter SJ, Sayers MH, Mori M, Cays MJ, Meyers JD. Use of leukocyte-depleted platelets and cytomegalovirus-seronegative red blood cells for prevention of primary cytomegalovirus infection after marrow transplantation. Blood 1991;76:246.
344. Hersman J, Meyers JD, Thomas ED, et al. The effect of granulocyte transfusions on the incidence of cytomegalovirus infection after allogeneic marrow transplantation. Ann Intern Med 1982;96:149.
345. O'Reilly RJ, Reich L, Gold J, et al. A randomized trial of intravenous hyperimmune globulin for the prevention of cytomegalovirus (CMV) infections following marrow transplantation: preliminary results. Transplant Proc 1983;15:1405.
346. Winston DJ, Ho WG, Lin C-H, et al. Intravenous immune globulin for prevention of cytomegalovirus infection and interstitial pneumonia after bone marrow transplantation. Ann Intern Med 1987;106:12.
347. Bowden RA, Sayers M, Flournoy N, et al. Cytomegalovirus immune globulin and seronegative blood products to prevent primary cytomegalovirus infection after marrow transplantation. N Engl J Med 1986;314:1006.
348. Kubanek B, Ernst P, Ostendorf P, et al. Preliminary data of controlled trial of intravenous hyperimmune globulin in the prevention of cytomegalovirus infection in bone marrow transplant recipients. Transplant Proc 1985;17:468.
349. Kraemer KG, Neiman PE, Reeves WC, Thomas ED. Prophylactic adenine arabinoside following marrow transplantation. Transplant Proc 1978;10:237.
350. Meyers JD, Flournoy NE, Sanders JE, et al. Prophylactic human leukocyte interferon after allogeneic bone marrow transplantation. Ann Intern Med 1987;107:809.
351. Meyers JD, Reed EC, Shepp DH, et al. Acyclovir for prevention of cytomegalovirus infection and disease after allogeneic marrow transplantation. N Engl J Med 1988;318:70.
352. Schmidt GM, Horak DA, Niland JC, et al. A randomized, controlled trial of prophylactic ganciclovir for cytomegalovirus pulmonary infection in recipients of allogeneic marrow transplants. N Engl J Med 1991;324:1005.
353. Goodrich JM, Bowden RA, Fisher L, Keller C, Schoch G, Meyers JD. Ganciclovir prophylaxis to prevent cytomegalovirus disease after allogeneic marrow transplant. Ann Intern Med 1993;118:173.
354. Winston DJ, Ho WG, Bartoni K, et al. Ganciclovir prophylaxis of cytomegalovirus infection and disease in allogeneic bone marrow transplant recipients: results of a placebo-controlled, double-blind trial. Ann Intern Med 1993;118:179.
355. Crawford SW, Bowden RA, Hackman RC, et al. Rapid detection of cytomegalovirus pulmonary infection by bronchoalveolar lavage and centrifugation culture. Ann Intern Med 1988;108:180.
356. Emanuel D, Cunningham I, Jules-Elysee K, et al. Cytomegalovirus pneumonia after bone marrow transplantation successfully treated with the combination of ganciclovir and high dose intravenous gamma globulin. Ann Intern Med 1988;109:777.
357. Reed EC, Bowden RA, Dandliker PS, et al. Treatment of cytomegalovirus pneumonia with ganciclovir and intravenous cytomegalovirus immunoglobulin in patients with bone marrow transplants. Ann Intern Med 1988;109:783.
358. Drobyski WR, Knox KK, Carrigan DR, Ash RC. Foscarnet therapy of ganciclovir-resistant cytomegalovirus in marrow transplantation. Transplantation 1991;52:155.
359. Agura ED, Vila E, Petersen FB, et al. The use of raniditine in bone marrow transplantation: a review of 223 cases. Transplantation 1988;46: 53.
360. Ballen KK, Donadio D, Bouloux C, McCarthy P, Weinstein H, Antin JH. Herpes simplex virus and neutropenia following bone marrow transplantation. Transplantation 1992;54:553.
361. McCullough EA, Siminovitch L, Till JE, et al. The cellular basis of the genotypically determined hemopoietic defect in anemic mice of genotype Sl/Sld. Blood 1965;26:399.
362. Waterfall M, Rayfield LS, Brent L. Abrogation of resistance to bone marrow transplantation by induction of specific tolerance in natural killer cells. Nature 1984;311:663.
363. Kiessling R, Hochman PS, Haller O, et al. Evidence for a similar or common mechanism for natural killer cell activity and resistance to hemopoietic grafts. Eur J Immunol 1977;7:655.
364. Warner JF, Dennert G. Bone marrow graft rejection as a function of antibody-directed natural killer cell. J Exp Med 1985;161:563.
365. Raff RF, Deeg HJ, Loughran JP, et al. Characterization of host cells involved in resistance to marrow grafts in dogs transplanted from unrelated DLA-nonidentical donors. Blood 1986;68:861.
366. Schwartz E, Lapidot T, Gozes D, et al. Abrogation of bone marrow allograft resistance in mice by increased total body irradiation correlates with eradication of host clonable T cells. J Immunol 1987;138:460.
367. Reisner Y, Ben-Bassat I, Dover D, et al. Demonstration of clonable alloreactive host T cells in a primate model of bone marrow transplantation. Proc Natl Acad Sci USA 1986;83:4012.
368. Deeg HJ, Self S, Storb R, et al. Decreased incidence of marrow graft rejection in patients with severe aplastic anemia: changing impact of risk factors. Blood 1986;68:1363.
369. Elfenbein GJ, Mellitus ED, Santos GW. Engraftment and survival after allogeneic bone marrow transplantation for severe aplastic anemia. Transplant Proc 1983;15:1412.
370. Champlin RE, Horowitz MM, van Bekkum DW, et al. Graft failure following bone marrow transplantation for severe aplastic anemia: risk factors and treatment results. Blood 1989;73:606.
371. Storb R, Thomas ED, Buckner CD, et al. Marrow transplantation in thirty "untransfused" patients with severe aplastic anemia. Ann Intern Med 1980;92:30.
372. Champlin RE, Feig SA, Sparkes RS, Gale RP. Bone marrow transplantation from identical twins in the treatment of aplastic anemia: implication for the pathogenesis of the disease. Br J Haematol 1984;56: 455.
373. Applebaum FR, Cheever MA, Fefer A, et al. Recurrence of aplastic anemia following cyclophosphamide and syngeneic bone marrow transplantation: evidence for two mechanisms of graft failure. Blood 1985;65:533.
374. Goss GD, Wittwer MA, Bezwoda WR. Effect of natural killer cells on

syngeneic bone marrow: in vitro and in vivo studies demonstrating graft failure due to NK cells in an identical twin treated by bone marrow transplantation. Blood 1985;66:1043.

375. Martin PJ, Hansen JA, Storb R, Thomas ED. Human marrow transplantation: an immunological perspective. Adv Immunol 1987;40:379.
376. Kernan NA, Flomenberg N, Dupont B, O'Reilly RJ. Graft rejection in recipients of T cell depleted HLA-nonidentical marrow transplants for leukemia. Transplantation 1987;43:842.
377. Bunjes D, Heit W, Arnold R, et al. Evidence for the involvement of host derived OKT8-positive T cells in the rejection of T-depleted, HLA-identical bone marrow grafts. Transplantation 1987;43:501.
378. Bierer BE, Emerson SG, Antin J, et al. Regulation of cytotoxic T lymphocyte mediated graft rejection following bone marrow transplantation. Transplantation 1988;46:835.
379. Soderling CCB, Song CW, Blazar BR, Vallera DA. A correlation between conditioning and engraftment in recipients of MHC mismatched T cell depleted bone marrow transplants. J Immunol 1985;135:941.
380. Kadowaki JI, Zuelzer WW, Brough AJ, et al. Lymphoid chimaerism in congenital immunological deficiency syndrome with thymic alymphoplasia. Lancet 1965;2:1152.
381. Hathaway WE, Brangle RW, Nelson TL, Roeckel IE. Aplastic anemia and alymphocytosis in an infant with hypogammaglobulinemia: graft versus host reaction? J Pediatr 1966;68:713.
382. Spencer GD, Hackman RC, McDonald GB, et al. A prospective study of unexplained nausea and vomiting after marrow transplantation. Transplantation 1986;42:602
383. Weisdorf DJ, Snover DC, Haake R, et al. Acute upper gastrointestinal graft-versus-host disease: clinical significance and response to immunosuppressive therapy. Blood 1990;76:624.
384. Lerner KG, Kao GF, Storb R, et al. Histopathology of graft versus host reaction (GvHR) in human recipients of marrow from HL-A matched sibling donors. Transplant Proc 1974;6:367.
385. Sale GE, Shulman HM, McDonald GB, Thomas ED. Gastrointestinal graft versus host disease in man: a clinicopathological study of the rectal biopsy. Am J Surg Pathol 1979;3:291.
386. Sale GE, Lerner KG, Barker EA, et al. The skin biopsy in the diagnosis of acute graft versus host disease in man. Am J Pathol 1977;89:621.
387. Sviland L, Pearson AD, Eastham EJ, et al. Histological features of skin and rectal biopsy specimens after autologous and allogeneic bone marrow transplantation. J Clin Pathol 1988;41:148.
388. Elliott CJ, Sloane JP, Sanderson KV, et al. The histological diagnosis of cutaneous graft versus host disease: relationship of skin changes to marrow purging and other clinical variables. Histopathology 1987;11: 145.
389. Snover DC. Mucosal damage simulating acute graft versus host reaction in cytomegalovirus colitis. Transplantation 1985;39:669.
390. Shulman HM, McDonald GB, Matthews D, et al. An analysis of hepatic veno-occlusive disease and centrilobular hepatic degeneration following bone marrow transplantation. Gastroenterology 1980;79:1178.
391. Gleichmann E, Gleichmann H. Essential similarity between graft versus host disease and viral infections. Transplantation 1976;22:399.
392. Gratama JW, Sinnige LGF, Weijers TF, et al. Marrow donor immunity to herpes simplex virus: association with acute graft versus host disease. Exp Hematol 1987;15:735.
393. Gratama JW, Stijnen T, Weiland HT, et al. Herpes virus immunity and acute graft versus host disease. Lancet 1987;1:471.
394. de Gast GC, Gratama JW, Ringden O, Gluckman E. The multifactorial etiology of graft-versus-host disease. Immunol Today 1987;8:209.
395. Beschorner WE, Saral R, Hutchins GM, et al. Lymphocytic bronchitis associated with graft versus host disease in recipients of bone marrow transplants. N Engl J Med 1978;299:1030.
396. O'Brien KD, Hackman RC, Sale GE, et al. Lymphocytic bronchitis unrelated to acute graft versus host disease in canine marrow graft recipients. Transplantation 1984;37:233.
397. Bergstein J, Andreoli SP, Provisor AJ, Yum M. Radiation nephritis following total body irradiation and cyclophosphamide in preparation for bone marrow transplantation. Transplantation 1986;41:63.
398. Droller MJ, Saral R, Santos G. Prevention of cyclophosphamide induced hemorrhagic cystitis. Urology 1982;20:256.
399. Arthur RR, Shah KV, Baust SJ, et al. Association of BK viruria with hemorrhagic cystitis in recipients of bone marrow transplants. N Engl J Med 1986;315:230.
400. Patchell R. Neurological complications of bone marrow transplantation. Neurology 1985;35:300.
401. Wiznitzer M. Neurologic complications of bone marrow transplantation in childhood. Ann Neurol 1984;16:569.
402. Korngold R, Sprent J. Lethal graft versus host disease following bone marrow transplantation across minor histocompatibility barriers in mice: prevention by removing mature T cells from marrow. J Exp Med 1978;148:1687.
403. Korngold R, Sprent J. Lethal GVHD across minor histocompatibility barriers: nature of the effector cells and role of the H-2 complex. Immunol Rev 1983;71:5.
404. Klein J. H-2 mutations: their genetics and effect on immune function. Adv Immunol 1978;26:55.
405. Klein J, Park JM. Graft versus host reaction across different regions of the H-2 complex of the mouse. J Exp Med 1973;137:1213.
406. Hamilton BL, Brevan MJ, Parkman R. Anti-recipient cytotoxic T lymphocyte precursors are present in the spleen of mice with acute graft versus host disease due to minor histocompatibility differences. J Immunol 1981;126:621.
407. Charley MR, Mikhael A, Bennett M, et al. Prevention of lethal, minor determinant graft-host disease in mice by the in vivo administration of anti-asialo GM1. J Immunol 1983;131:2101.
408. Vallera DA, Soderling CCB, Kersey JH. Bone marrow transplantation across major histocompatibility barriers in mice. J Immunol 1982;128: 871.
409. Korngold R, Sprent J. Surface markers of T cells causing lethal graft vs host disease to class I vs class II H-2 differences. J Immunol 1985;135: 3004.
410. Maier T, Holda JH, Claman HN. Graft versus host reactions across minor murine histocompatibility barriers. II. Development of natural suppressor cell activity. J Immunol 1985;135:1644.
411. Kernan NA, Collins NH, Julano L, et al. Clonable T lymphocytes in T cell depleted bone marrow transplants correlate with the development of graft versus host disease. Blood 1986;68:770.
412. Volc-Platzer B, Rappersberger K, Mosberger I, et al. Sequential immunohistologic analysis of the skin following bone marrow transplantation. J Invest Dermatol 1988;91:162.
413. Van Bekkum DW, Roodenburg J, Heidt PJ, van der Waaij D. Migration of secondary disease of allogeneic mouse radiation chimeras by modification of the intestinal microflora. J Natl Cancer Inst 1974; 52:401.
414. Gratama JW, Stijinen T, Weiland HT, et al. Herpes-virus immunity and acute graft-versus-host disease. Lancet 1987;1:471.
415. Beelen DW, Haralambie E, Brandt H, et al. Evidence that sustained growth suppression of intestinal anaerobic bacteria reduces the risk of acute graft-versus-host disease after sibling marrow transplanatation. Blood 1992;80:2668.
416. Storb R, Prentice RL, Buckner CD, et al. Graft-versus-host disease and survival in patients with aplastic anemia treated by marrow grafts from HLA-identical siblings: beneficial effects of a protective environment. N Engl J Med 1983;308:302.
417. Sullivan KM, Kopecky KJ, Jocom J, et al. Immunomodulatory and antimicrobial efficacy of intravenous immunoglobulin in bone marrow transplantation. N Engl J Med 1990;323:705.
418. Ferrara JLM, Deeg HJ. Graft-versus-host-disease. N Engl J Med 1991;324: 667.
419. Antin JH, Ferrara JLM. Cytokine dysregulation and acute graft-versus-host disease. Blood 1992;80:2964.
420. Ringden O, Nilsson B. Death by graft versus host disease associated with HLA mismatch, high recipient age, low marrow cell dose, and splenectomy. Transplantation 1985;40:39.
421. Powles RL, Kay HEM, Clink HM, et al. Mismatched family donors for bone marrow transplantation as treatment for acute leukemia. Lancet 1983;1:612.
422. Storb R, Prentice RL, Buckner CD, et al. Graft versus host disease and survival in patients with aplastic anemia treated with marrow grafts from HLA-identical siblings: benefits of a protective environment. N Engl J Med 1983;308:302.
423. Bross DS, Tutschka PJ, Farmer ER, et al. Predictive factors for acute graft versus host disease in patients transplanted with HLA-identical bone marrow. Blood 1984;63:1265.
424. Storb R, Prentice RL. Treatment of aplastic anemia by marrow transplantation from HLA identical siblings: prognostic factors associated with graft versus host disease and survival. J Clin Invest 1977;59:625.
425. Gale RC, Bortin MM, van Bekkum DW, et al. Risk factors for acute graft-versus-host disease. Br J Haematol 1987;67:397.
426. Weisdorf DJ, Haake R, Blazar B, et al. Risk factors for acute graft-versus-host disease in histocompatible donor bone marrow transplantations. Transplantation 1991;51:1197.
427. Nash RA, Pepe MS, Storb R, et al. Acute graft-versus-host-disease: analysis of risk factors after allogeneic marrow transplantation and prophylaxis with cyclosporine and methotrexate. Blood 1992;80:1838.
428. Storb R, Hansen JA, Prentice RL, Thomas ED. Association between HLA-B antigens and acute graft versus host disease. Lancet 1983;2: 816.
429. Vimer E, Mazeron MC, Rabian C, et al. Clinical significance of cytomegalovirus viremia in bone marrow transplantation. Transplantation 1985;40:30.
430. Gratama JW, Stijnen T, Weiland HT, et al. Herpes virus immunity and acute graft versus host disease. Lancet 1987;1:471.
431. Vogelsang GB, Hess AD, Berkman AW, et al. An in vitro predictive test for graft versus host disease in patients with genotypic HLA-identical bone marrow transplants. N Engl J Med 1985;313:645.
432. Bagot M, Cordonnier C, Tilkin A-F, et al. A possible predictive test for graft versus host disease in bone marrow graft recipients: the mixed epidermal cell-lymphocyte reaction. Transplantation 1986;41:316.
433. Theobald M, Nierle T, Bunjes D, Arnold R, Heimpel H. Host-specific interleukin-2-secreting donor T-cell precursors as predictors of acute graft-versus-host disease in bone marrow transplantation between HLA-identical siblings. N Engl J Med 1992;327:1613.
434. Vogelsang GB, Hess AD, Santos GD. Acute graft-versus-host disease: clinical characteristics in the cyclosporine era. Medicine 1988;67:163.
435. Storb R, Deeg HJ, Pepe M, et al. Methotrexate and cyclosporine versus cyclosporine alone for prophylaxis of graft-versus-host disease in pa-

tients given HLA-identical marrow grafts for leukemia: long-term follow-up of a controlled trial. Blood 1989;73:1729.
436. Beelen DW, Quabeck K, Kaiser B, et al. Six weeks of continuous intravenous cyclosporine and short-course methotrexate as prophylaxis for acute graft-versus-host disease after allogeneic bone marrow transplantation. Transplantation 1990;50:421.
437. Forman SJ, Blume KG, Krance RA, et al. A prospective randomized study of acute graft-versus-host disease in 107 patients with leukemia: methotrexate/prednisone v cyclosporine A/prednisone. Transplant Proc 1987;19:2605.
438. Ramsay NKC, Kersey JH, Robison LL, et al. A randomized study of the prevention of acute graft versus host disease. N Engl J Med 1982;306:392.
439. Lazarus HM, Coccia PF, Herzig R, et al. Incidence of acute graft versus host disease with and without methotrexate prophylaxis in allogeneic bone marrow transplant patients. Blood 1984;64:215.
440. Sullivan KM, Deeg HJ, Sanders J, et al. Hyperacute graft versus host disease in patients not given immunosuppression after allogeneic marrow transplantation. Blood 1986;67:1172.
441. Storb R, Deeg HJ, Farewell V, et al. Marrow transplantation for severe aplastic anemia: methotrexate alone compared with a combination of methotrexate and cyclosporine for prevention of acute graft versus host disease. Blood 1986;68:119.
442. Storb R, Deeg HJ, Pepe M, et al. Methotrexate and cyclosporine versus cyclosporine alone for prophylaxis of graft versus host disease in patients given HLA-identical marrow grafts for leukemia: long term followup of a controlled trial. Blood 1989;73:1729.
443. Ringdén O, Horowitz MM, Sondel P, et al. Methotrexate, cyclosporine, or both to prevent graft-versus-host disease after HLA-identical sibling bone marrow transplants for early leukemia? Blood 1993;81:1094.
444. Nash RA, Pepe MS, Storb R, et al. Acute graft-versus-host disease: analysis of risk factors after allogeneic marrow transplantation and prophylaxis with cyclosporine and methotrexate. Blood 1992;80:1838.
445. Clift RA, Buckner CD, Applebaum FR, et al. Allogeneic marrow transplantation in patients with acute myeloid leukemia in first remission: a randomized trial of two irradiation regimens. Blood 1990;76:1867.
446. Clift RA, Buckner CD, Applebaum FR, et al. Allogeneic marrow transplantation in patients with chronic myelogenous leukemia in the chronic phase: a randomized trial of two irradiation regimens. Blood 1991;76:1660.
447. Storb R, Pepe M, Anasetti C, et al. What role for prednisone in prevention of acute graft-versus-host disease in patients undergoing marrow transplant. Blood 1990;76:1037.
448. Reisner Y, Kapoor N, Kirkpatrick D, et al. Transplantation for acute leukemia with HLA-A and B nonidentical parental marrow cells fractionated with soybean agglutinin and sheep red blood cells. Lancet 1981;2:327.
449. Reinherz EL, Geha R, Rappeport JM, et al. Reconstitution after transplantation with T lymphocyte depleted HLA haplo mismatched bone marrow for severe immunodeficiency. Proc Natl Acad Sci USA 1982;79:6047.
450. Prentice HG, Blacklock HA, Janossy G, et al. Use of anti-T-cell monoclonal antibody OKT3 to prevent acute graft versus host disease in allogeneic bone marrow transplantation for acute leukemia. Lancet 1982;1:700.
451. Filipovich AH, McGlave PB, Ramsay NKC, et al. Pretreatment of donor bone marrow with monoclonal antibody OKT3 for prevention of acute graft versus host disease in allogeneic histocompatible bone marrow transplantation. Lancet 1982;1:1266.
452. O'Reilly R, Collins NH, Kernan N, et al. Transplantation of marrow-depleted T cells by soybean lectin agglutination and E-rosette depletion: major histocompatibility complex-related graft resistance in leukemic transplant patients. Transplant Proc 1985;17:455.
453. Reisner Y. A shorter procedure for preparing E-rosette–depleted bone marrow for transplantation. Transplantation 1986;42:312.
454. Racadot E, Hervé P, Beaujean F, et al. Prevention of graft-versus-host disease in HLA-matched bone marrow transplantation for malignant diseases: a multicentric study of 62 patients using 3-pan-T monoclonal antibodies and rabbit complement. J Clin Oncol 1987;5:426.
455. Hale G, Cobbold S, Waldman H, for Campath-1 Users. T cell depletion with campath-1 in allogeneic bone marrow transplantation. Transplantation 1988;45:753.
456. Filipovich AH, Vallera DA, Youle RJ, et al. Graft-versus-host disease prevention in allogeneic bone marrow transplantation from histocompatible siblings. Transplantation 1987;44:62.
457. Antin JH, Bierer BE, Smith BR, et al. Selective depletion of bone marrow T lymphocytes with anti-CD5 monoclonal antibodies: effective prophylaxis for graft-versus-host disease in patients with hematologic malignancies. Blood 1991;78:2139.
458. Wagner JE, Donnenberg AD, Noga SJ, et al. Lymphocyte depletion of donor bone marrow by counterflow centrifugal elutriation: results of a phase I clinical trial. Blood 1988;72:1168.
459. De Witte T, Hoogenhout J, de Pauw B, et al. Depletion of donor lymphocytes by counterflow centrifugation successfully prevents acute graft-versus-host disease in matched allogeneic marrow transplantation. Blood 1986;67:1302.
460. Champlin R, Ho W, Gajewski J, et al. Selective depletion of CD8+ T lymphocytes for prevention of graft-versus-host disease after allogeneic bone marrow transplantation. Blood 1990;76:418.
461. Mitsuyasu RT, Champlin RE, Gale RP, et al. Treatment of donor bone marrow with monoclonal anti-T-cell antibody and complement for the prevention of graft versus host disease. Ann Intern Med 1986;105:20.
462. Marmont AM, Horowitz MM, Gale RP, et al. T-cell depletion of HLA-identical transplants in leukemia. Blood 1991;78:2120.
463. Pirsch JD, Maki DG. Infectious complications in adults with bone marrow transplantation and T-cell depletion of donor marrow. Ann Intern Med 1986;104:619.
464. Smith BR, Burakoff SJ, Weinstein H, et al. Differential outcome of histocompatible versus histoincompatible Leu-1 depleted bone marrow transplants. Blood 1986;68:292A.
465. Martin PJ, Shulman HM, Schulaach WH, et al. Fatal Epstein-Barr virus associated proliferation of donor B cells after treatment of acute graft versus host disease with a murine anti-T cell antibody. Ann Intern Med 1984;101:310.
466. Slavin S, Ackerstein A, Weiss L, et al. Immunotherapy of minimal residual disease by immunocompetent lymphocytes and their activation by cytokines. Cancer Invest 1992;10:221.
467. Kanojia MD, Anagnostou AA, Zander AR. High dose methylprednisolone treatment for acute graft versus host disease after bone marrow transplantation in adults. Transplantation 1984;37:246.
468. Storb R, Gluckman E, Thomas ED. Treatment of established human graft versus host disease by anti-thymocyte globulin. Blood 1974;44:57.
469. Weisdorf D, Haake R, Blazar B, et al. Treatment of moderate/severe acute graft-versus-host disease after allogeneic bone marrow transplantation: an analysis of clinical risk features and outcome. Blood 1990;75:1024.
470. Martin PJ, Schoch G, Fisher L, et al. A retrospective analysis of therapy for acute graft-versus-host disease: initial treatment. Blood 1990;76:1464.
471. Martin PJ, Schoch G, Fisher L, et al. A retrospective analysis of therapy for acute graft-versus-host disease: secondary treatment. Blood 1991;77:1821.
472. Roy J, McGlave PB, Filipovich AH, et al. Acute graft-versus-host disease following unrelated donor marrow transplantation: failure of conventional therapy. Bone Marrow Transplant 1992;10:77.
473. Rappeport JM, Mihm M, Reinherz EL, et al. Acute graft versus host disease in recipients of bone marrow transplants from identical twin donors. Lancet 1979;2:717.
474. Gluckman E, Devbergie A, Sohier J, Saurat JH. Graft versus host disease in recipients of syngeneic bone marrow. Lancet 1980;1:253.
475. Hood AF, Vogelsang GB, Black LP, et al. Acute graft versus host disease: development following autologous and syngeneic bone marrow transplantation. Arch Dermatol 1987;123:745.
476. Einsele H, Ehninger G, Schneider EM, et al. High frequency of graft versus host like syndromes following syngeneic bone marrow transplantation. Transplantation 1988;45:579.
477. Thein SL, Goldman JM, Galton DAG. Acute "graft versus host disease" after autografting for chronic granulocytic leukemia in transformation. Ann Intern Med 1981;94:210.
478. Hess AH, Horwitz L, Beschorner WE, Santos GW. Development of graft versus host disease like syndrome in cyclosporine treated rats after syngeneic bone marrow transplantation. J Exp Med 1985;161:718.
479. Glazier A, Tutschka PJ, Farmer ER, Santos GW. Graft versus host disease in cyclosporine treated rats after syngeneic and autologous bone marrow reconstitution. J Exp Med 1983;158:1.
480. Beschorner WE, Hess AD, Shinn CA, Santos GW. Transfer of cyclosporine associated syngeneic graft versus host disease by thymocytes. Transplantation 1988;45:209.
481. Jenkins MK, Schwartz RH, Pardoll DM. Effect of cyclosporine on T cell development and clonal deletion. Science 1988;241:1655.
482. Fischer AC, Laulis MK, Horwitz L, et al. Host resistance to cyclosporine induced syngeneic graft versus host disease. J Immunol 1989;143:827.
483. Shi Y, Sahai BM, Green DR. Cyclosporin A inhibits activation induced cell death in T cell hybridomas and thymocytes. Nature 1989;339:625.
484. Gaspari AA, Lotze MT, Rosenberg SA, et al. Dermatologic changes associated with interleukin-2 administration. JAMA 1987;258:1624.
485. Shulman HM, Sullivan KM, Weiden PL, et al. Chronic graft versus host disease syndrome in man: a long term clinicopathological study of 20 Seattle patients. Am J Med 1980;69:204.
486. Graze PR, Gale RP. Chronic graft versus host disease: a syndrome of disordered immunity. Am J Med 1979;66:611.
487. Sullivan KM, Shulman HM, Storb R, et al. Chronic graft versus host disease in 52 patients: adverse natural course and successful treatment with combination immunosuppression. Blood 1981;57:267.
488. Izutsu KT, Sullivan KM, Schubert MM, et al. Disordered salivary immunoglobulin secretion and sodium transport in human chronic graft versus host disease. Transplantation 1983;35:441.
489. Atkinson K, Storb R, Prentice RL, et al. Analysis of late infections in 89 long term survivors of bone marrow transplantation. Blood 1979;53:720.
490. Shulman HM, Sale GE, Lerner KG, et al. Chronic cutaneous graft versus host disease in man. Am J Pathol 1978;91:545.

491. Sale GE, Shulman HM, Schubert MM, et al. Oral and ophthalmic pathology of graft versus host disease in man: predictive value of the lip biopsy. Hum Pathol 1981;12:1022.
492. Kurzrock R, Zander A, Kanojia M, et al. Obstructive lung disease after allogeneic bone marrow transplantation. Transplantation 1984;37:156.
493. Weiner RS, Bortin MM, Gale RP, et al. Interstitial pneumonitis after bone marrow transplantation. Ann Intern Med 1986;104:168.
494. Wingard JR, Santos GW, Saral R. Late onset interstitial pneumonia following allogeneic bone marrow transplantation. Transplantation 1985;39:21.
495. Parkman R. Clonal analysis of murine graft versus host disease. J Immunol 1986;136:3543.
496. Korngold R, Sprent J. T cell subsets and graft versus host disease. Transplantation 1987;44:335.
497. Atkinson K, Storb R, Ochs HD, et al. Thymus transplantation after allogeneic bone marrow graft to prevent chronic graft versus host disease in humans. Transplantation 1982;33:168.
498. Storb R, Prentice RL, Sullivan KM, et al. Predictive factors in chronic graft versus host disease in patients with aplastic anemia treated by marrow transplantation from HLA-identical siblings. Ann Intern Med 1983;98:461.
499. Ringden O, Paulin T, Lonnqvist B, Nilsson B. An analysis of factors predisposing to chronic graft versus host disease. Exp Hematol 1985;13: 1062.
500. Lonnqvist B, Ringden O, Wahren B, et al. Cytomegalovirus infection associated with and preceding chronic graft versus host disease. Transplantation 1984;38:465.
501. Sullivan KM, Witherspoon RP, Storb R, et al. Prednisone and azathioprine compared with prednisone and placebo for treatment of chronic graft versus host disease: prognostic influence of prolonged thrombocytopenia after allogeneic transplantation. Blood 1988;72:546.
502. Sullivan KM, Witherspoon RP, Storb R, et al. Alternating-day cyclosporine and prednisone for treatment of high-risk graft-v-host disease. Blood 1988;72:555.
503. Barnes DWH, Corp MJ, Loutit JF, Neal FE. Treatment of murine leukaemia with x-rays and homologous bone marrow. Br Med J 1956;2: 626.
504. Horowitz MM, Gale RP, Sondel PM, et al. Graft-versus-leukemia reactions after bone marrow transplantation. Blood 1990;75:555.
505. Mathe G, Amiel JL, Schwarzenberg L, et al. Adoptive immunotherapy of acute leukemia: experimental and clinical results. Cancer Res 1965;25:1525.
506. Bortin MM, Truitt RL, Rimm AA, Bach FH. Graft versus leukemia reactivity induced by alloimmunization without augmentation of graft versus host reactivity. Nature 1979;281:490.
507. Moscovitch M, Slavin S. Anti tumor effects of allogeneic bone marrow transplantation in (NZB x NZW) F1 hybrids with spontaneous lymphosarcoma. J Immunol 1984;132:997.
508. Tutschka PH, Berkowitz SD, Tuttle S, Klein J. Graft versus leukemia in the rat: the antileukemic effect of syngeneic and allogeneic graft versus host disease. Transplant Proc 1987;19:2668.
509. Weiden PL, Flournoy N, Thomas ED, et al. Antileukemic effect of graft versus host disease in human recipients of allogeneic marrow grafts. N Engl J Med 1979;300:1068.
510. Weisdorf DJ, Nesbit ME, Ramsay NKC, et al. Allogeneic bone marrow transplantation for acute lymphoblastic leukemia in remission: prolonged survival associated with acute graft versus host disease. J Clin Oncol 1987;5:1348.
511. Weiden PL, Sullivan KM, Flournoy N, et al. Antileukemic effect of chronic graft versus host disease. Contribution to improved survival after allogeneic marrow transplantation. N Engl J Med 1981;304:1529.
512. Sullivan KM, Weiden PL, Storb R, et al. Influence of acute and chronic graft-versus-host disease on relapse and survival after bone marrow transplantation from HLA-identical siblings as treatment of acute and chronic leukemia. Blood 1989;73:1720.
513. Goldman JM, Gale RP, Horowitz MM, et al. Bone marrow transplantation for chronic myelogenous leukemia in chronic phase: increased risk for relapse associated with T cell depletion. Ann Intern Med 1988;108:806.
514. Apperley JF, Mauro FR, Goldman JM, et al. Bone marrow transplantation for chronic myeloid leukaemia in first chronic phase: importance of a graft versus leukaemia effect. Br J Haematol 1988;69:239.
515. Sullivan KM, Storb R, Buckner CD, et al. Graft versus host disease as adoptive immunotherapy in patients with advanced hematologic malignancies: a randomized study of short course methotrexate versus standard methotrexate versus standard methotrexate plus buffy coat cells following allogeneic marrow transplantation. N Engl J Med 1989;320:828.
516. Kolb HJ, Mittermüller J, Clemm C, et al. Donor leukocyte transfusions for treatment of recurrent chronic myelogenous leukemia in marrow transplant patients. Blood 1990;76:2462.
517. Porter D, Roth M, McGarigle C, Ferrara J, Antin J. Adoptive immunotherapy induces molecular remission in relapsed CML following allogeneic bone marrow transplantation (BMT). Proc Am Soc Clin Oncol 1993;12:303.
518. Von Fliedner V, Higby DJ, Kim U. Graft-versus-host reaction following blood product transfusion. Am J Med 1982;72:951.
519. Brubaker BB. Human post-transfusion graft versus host disease. Vox Sang 1983;45:401.
520. Weiden P. Graft versus host disease following blood transfusions. Arch Intern Med 1984;144:1557.
521. Dinsmore RE, Straus DJ, Pollack MS, et al. Fatal graft versus host disease following blood transfusion in Hodgkin's disease documented by HLA typing. Blood 1980;55:831.
522. Parkman R, Mosier D, Umansky I, et al. Graft versus host disease after intrauterine and exchange transfusions for hemolytic disease of the newborn. N Engl J Med 1974;290:359.
523. Burdick JF, Vogelsang G, Smith WJ, et al. Severe graft-versus-host disease in a liver-transplant recipient. N Engl J Med 1988;318:689.
524. Anderson KC, Weinstein HJ. Transfusion-associated graft-versus-host disease. N Engl J Med 1990;323:515.
525. Thaler M, Shamiss A, Orgad S, et al. The role of blood from HLA homozygous donors in fatal transfusion-associated graft versus host disease after open-heart surgery. N Engl J Med 1989;321:25.
526. Lewis SM. Course and prognosis in aplastic anemia. Br Med J 1965;1: 1027.
527. Camitta BM, Thomas ED, Nathan DG, et al. A prospective study of androgens and bone marrow transplantation for treatment of severe aplastic anemia. Blood 1979;53:504.
528. Thomas ED, Buckner CD, Storb R, et al. Aplastic anemia treated by marrow transplantation. Lancet 1972;1:284.
529. Champlin RE, Feig SA, Sparkes RS, Gale RP. Bone marrow transplantation from identical twins in the treatment of aplastic anemia: implication for the pathogenesis of the disease. Br J Haematol 1984;56: 455.
530. Hows JM, Palmer S, Gordon-Smith EC. Cyclosporine and graft failure following bone marrow transplantation for severe aplastic anemia. Transplantation 1985;60:611.
531. Gluckman E, Barrett AJ, Arcese W, et al. Bone marrow transplantation in severe aplastic anemia: a survey of the European Group for Bone Marrow Transplant (EGBMT). Br J Haematol 1981;49:165.
532. Sensenbrenner LL, Steele AA, Santos GW. Recovery of hematologic competence without engraftment following attempted bone marrow transplantation for aplastic anemia: report of a case with diffusion chamber studies. Exp Hematol 1977;5:51.
533. Territo MC, for the UCLA Bone Marrow Transplant Team. Autologous bone marrow repopulation following high dose cyclophosphamide and allogeneic marrow transplantation in aplastic anemia. Br J Haematol 1977;36:305.
534. Thomas ED, Storb R, Giblett ER, et al. Recovery from aplastic anemia following attempted marrow transplantation. Exp Hematol 1976;4:97.
535. Gluckman E, Marmont A, Speck B, Gordon-Smith EC, for the Working Party on Severe Aplastic Anemia of the European Group for Bone Marrow Transplantation. Immunosuppressive treatment of aplastic anemia as an alternative treatment for bone marrow transplantation. Semin Hematol 1984;21:11.
536. Storb R, Prentice RL, Buckner CD, et al. Graft-versus-host disease and survival in patients with aplastic anemia treated by marrow grafts from HLA-identical siblings: beneficial effects of a protective environment. N Engl J Med 1983;308:302.
537. Advisory Committee of the Bone Marrow Transplant Registry. Bone marrow transplantation from histocompatible, allogeneic donors for aplastic anemia: a report from the ACS/NIH Bone Marrow Transplant Registry. JAMA 1976;236:1131.
538. Bortin MM, Gale RP, Rimm AA, for the Advisory Committee of the International Bone Marrow Transplant Registry. Allogeneic bone marrow transplantation for 144 patients with severe aplastic anemia. JAMA 1981;245:1132.
539. Storb R, Thomas ED, Buckner CD, et al. Marrow transplantation for aplastic anemia. Semin Hematol 1984;21:27.
540. Champlin RE, Horowitz MM, van Bekkum DW, et al. Graft failure following bone marrow transplantation for severe aplastic anemia. Blood 1989;73:606.
541. Anasetti C, Doney KC, Storb R, et al. Marrow transplantation for severe aplastic anemia: long term outcome in fifty "untransfused" patients. Ann Intern Med 1986;104:461.
542. Santos GW, Sensenbrenner LL. A sensitive and quantitative assay for non H-2 histocompatibility antigens. Exp Hematol 1971;21:19.
543. Storb R, Epstein RB, Rudolph RH, Thomas ED. The effect of prior transfusions on marrow grafts between histocompatible canine siblings. J Immunol 1970;105:627.
544. Gluckman E, Horowitz MM, Champlin RE, et al. Bone marrow transplantation for severe aplastic anemia: influence of conditioning and graft-versus-host disease prophylaxis regimens on outcome. Blood 1992;79:269.
545. Feig SA, Champlin R, Arenson E, et al. Improved survival following bone marrow transplantation for aplastic anemia. Br J Haematol 1983;54:509.
546. McGlave PB, Haake R, Miller W, et al. Therapy of severe aplastic anemia in young adults and children with allogeneic bone marrow transplantation. Blood 1987;70:1325.
547. Gluckman E, Socie G, Devergie E, Bourdeau-Esperou H, Traineau R, Cosset JM. Bone marrow transplantation in 107 patients with severe

aplastic anemia using cyclophosphamide and thoracoabdominal irradiation for conditioning: long-term follow-up. Blood 1991;78:2451.
548. Smith BR, Guinan EC, Parkman R, et al. Efficacy of a cyclophosphamide-procarbazine-antithymocyte serum regimen for prevention of graft rejection following bone marrow transplantation for transfused patients with aplastic anemia. Transplantation 1985;39:671.
549. Storb R, Doney KC, Thomas ED, et al. Marrow transplantation with or without donor buffy coat cells for 65 transfused aplastic anemia patients. Blood 1982;59:236.
550. Niederwieser D, Pepe M, Storb L, et al. Improvement in rejection, engraftment rate and survival without increased graft-versus-host disease by high marrow cell dose in patients transplanted for aplastic anemia. Br J Haematol 1988;69:23.
551. Deeg HJ, Self S, Storb R, et al. Decreased incidence of marrow graft rejection in patients with severe aplastic anemia: changing impact of risk factors. Blood 1986;68:1363.
552. Storb R, Weiden PL, Sullivan KM, et al. Second marrow transplants in patients with aplastic anemia rejecting the first graft: use of a conditioning regimen including cyclophosphamide and antithymocyte globulin. Blood 1987;70;116.
553. Ash RC, Casper J, Menitove, et al. Successful allogeneic marrow transplantation utilizing closely matched unrelated donors. Blood 1988;72: 378A.
554. Hows JM, Yin JL, Marsh J, et al. Histocompatible unrelated volunteer donors compared with HLA nonidentical family donors in marrow transplantation for aplastic anemia and leukemia. Blood 1986;68:1322.
555. Camitta BM, Thomas ED, Nathan DG, et al. A prospective study of androgens and bone marrow transplantation for treatment of severe aplastic anemia. Blood 1979;53:504.
556. Bayever E, Champlin R, Ho W, et al. Comparison between bone marrow transplantation and antithymocyte globulin in treatment of young patients with severe aplastic anemia. J Pediatr 1984;105:920.
557. Speck B, Gratwohl A, Nissen C, et al. Treatment of severe aplastic anemia. Exp Hematol 1986;14:126.
558. Sanders JE, Whitehead J, Storb R, et al. Bone marrow transplantation experience for children with aplastic anemia. Pediatrics 1986;77:179.
559. Thomas ED, Storb R. Acquired severe aplastic anemia: progress and perplexity. Blood 1984;64:325.
560. Bacigalupo A, Hows J, Gluckman E, et al. Bone marrow transplantation (BMT) versus immunosuppression for the treatment of severe aplastic anemia (SAA): a report of the EBMT SAA Working Party. Br J Haematol 1988;70:177.
561. Tichelli A, Gratwohl A, Würsch A, Nissen C, Speck B. Late haematological complications in severe aplastic anemia. Br J Haematol 1988;69: 413.
562. De Planque MM, Klein-Nelemans JC, van Krieken HJM, et al. Evolution of acquired severe aplastic anaemia to myelodysplasia and subsequent leukaemia in adults. Br J Haematol 1988;70:55.
563. Kojima S, Matsuyama K, Kodera Y. Bone marrow transplantation for hepatitis-associated aplastic anemia. Acta Haematol 1988;79:7.
564. Doney K, Storb R, Buckner CD, et al. Marrow transplantation for treatment of pregnancy-associated aplastic anemia. Exp Hematol 1985;13: 1080.
565. Baldwin JL, Storb R, Thomas ED, Mannik M. Bone marrow transplantation in patients with gold-induced marrow aplasia. Arthritis Rheum 1977;20:1043.
566. Witherspoon RP, Storb R, Shulman H, et al. Marrow transplantation in hepatitis-associated aplastic anemia. Am J Hematol 1984;17:269.
567. Szer J, Deeg HJ, Witherspoon RP, et al. Long-term survival after marrow transplantation for paroxysmal nocturnal hemoglobinuria with aplastic anemia. Ann Intern Med 1984;101:193.
568. Hershko C, Gale RP, Ho WG, Cline MJ. Cure of aplastic anemia in paroxysmal nocturnal hemoglobinuria by marrow infusion from identical twin: failure of peripheral-leucocyte transfusion to correct marrow aplasia. Lancet 1979;1:945.
569. Hows JM, Palmer S, Gordon-Smith EC. Use of cyclosporin A in allogeneic bone marrow transplantation for severe aplastic anemia. Transplantation 1982;33:382.
570. Gluckman E, Devergie A, Dutreix A, et al. Bone marrow grafting in aplastic anemia after conditioning with cyclophosphamide and total body irradiation with lung shielding. In: Thierfelder S, Rodt H, Kolb HJ, eds. Immunobiology of bone marrow transplantation. Berlin, Springer Verlag, 1980:339.
571. Speck B, Bortin MM, Champlin R, et al. Allogeneic bone-marrow transplantation for chronic myelogenous leukemia. Lancet 1984;1:665.
572. Thomas ED, Clift RA, Fefer A, et al. Marrow transplantation for the treatment of chronic myelogenous leukemia. Ann Intern Med 1986;104: 155.
573. McGlave P, Arthur D, Haake R, et al. Therapy of chronic myelogenous leukemia with allogeneic bone marrow transplantation. J Clin Oncol 1987;5:1033.
574. Martin P, Clift RA, Fisher LD, et al. HLA-identical marrow transplantation during accelerated-phase chronic myelogenous leukemia: analysis of survival and remission duration. Blood 1988;72:1978.
575. Marmont A. Allogeneic bone marrow transplantation for chronic granulocytic leukemia: progress and controversies. Acta Haematol 1987;78:181.
576. McGlave PB, Arthur DC, Weisdorf D, et al. Allogeneic bone marrow transplantation as treatment for accelerating chronic myelogenous leukemia. Blood 1984;63:219.
577. Wagner JE, Zahurak M, Piantadosi S, et al. Bone marrow transplantation of chronic myelogenous leukemia in chronic phase: evaluation of risks and benefits. J Clin Oncol 1992;10:779.
578. Sokal JE, Baccarani M, Tura S, et al. Prognostic discrimination among younger patients with chronic granulocytic leukemia: relevance to bone marrow transplantation. Blood 1985;66:1352.
579. Segel GB, Simon W, Lichtman MA. Variables influencing the timing of marrow transplantation in patients with chronic myelogenous leukemia. Blood 1986;68:1055.
580. Thomas ED, Clift RA. Indications for bone marrow transplantation in chronic myelogenous leukemia. Blood 1989;73:861.
581. Bacigalupo A, Frassoni F, Lint MT, et al. Bone marrow transplantation for chronic granulocytic leukemia. Cancer 1986;58:2307.
582. Biggs JC, Szer J, Criley P, et al. Treatment of chronic myeloid leukemia with allogeneic bone marrow transplantation after preparation with BuCy2. Blood 1992;80:1352.
583. McGlave P, Beatty P, Ash R, Hows JM. Therapy for chronic myelogenous leukemia with unrelated donor bone marrow transplantation: results in 102 cases. Blood 1990;75:1728.
584. McGlave P, Bartsch G, Anasetti C, et al. Unrelated donor bone marrow transplantation therapy for chronic myelogenous leukemia: intial experience of the National Marrow Donor Program. Blood 1993;81:543.
585. Ash RC, Casper JT, Chitambar CR, et al. Successful allogeneic transplantation of T-cell–depleted bone marrow from closely HLA matched unrelated donors. N Engl J Med 1990;322:485.
586. Kernan NA, Bartsch G, Ash RC, et al. Analysis of 462 transplantations from unrelated donors facilitated by the National Marrow Donor Program. N Engl J Med 1993;328:693.
587. Gluckman E, Devergie A, Bernheim A, Berger R. Splenectomy and bone marrow transplantation in chronic granulocytic leukaemia. Lancet 1983;1:1392.
588. Gratwohl A, Goldman J, Gluckman E, Zwaan F. Effect of splenectomy on survival in chronic granulocytic leukemia. Lancet 1985;2:1290.
589. Baughan AS, Worsley M, McCarthy DM, et al. Hematological reconstitution and severity of graft-versus-host disease after bone marrow transplantation for chronic granulocytic leukemia: the influence of previous splenectomy. Br J Haematol 1984;56:455.
590. Ringdén O, Nilsson B. Death by graft-versus-host disease with HLA mismatch, high recipient age, low marrow cell dose, and splenectomy. Transplantation 1985;40:39.
591. Gratwohl A, Hermans J, Biezen AV, et al. No advantage for patients who receive splenic irradiation before bone marrow transplantation for chronic myelogenous leukemia: results of a prospective randomized study. Bone Marrow Transplant 1992;10:147.
592. Zaccaria A, Rosti G, Testoni N, et al. Chromosome studies in patients with Philadelphia chromosome-positive chronic myeloid leukemia submitted to bone marrow transplantation: results of a European Cooperative Study. Cancer Genet Cytogenet 1987;26:5.
593. Arthur CK, Apperley JF, Guo AP, et al. Cytogenetic events after bone marrow transplantation for chronic myeloid leukemia in chronic phase. Blood 1988;71:1179.
594. Cooperative Study Group on Chromosomes in Transplanted Patients. Cytogenetic follow-up of 100 patients submitted to bone marrow transplantation for Philadelphia chromosome positive chronic myeloid leukemia. Eur J Haematol 1988;40:50.
595. Roth MS, Antin JH, Bingham EL, Ginsburg D. Detection of Philadelphia chromosome positive cells by the polymerase chain reaction following bone marrow transplant for chronic myelogenous leukemia. Blood 1989;74:882.
596. Miyamura K, Tahara T, Tanimoto M, et al. Long persistent bcr-abl positive transcript detected by polymerase chain reaction after marrow transplant for chronic myelogenous leukemia without clinical relapse: a study of 64 patients. Blood 1993;81:1089.
597. Hughes TP, Morgan GJ, Martiat P, Goldman JM. Detection of residual leukemia after bone marrow transplant for chronic myeloid leukemia: role of polymerase chain reaction in predicting relapse. Blood 1991;77: 874.
598. Horowitz MM, for the Advisory Committee of the International Bone Marrow Transplant Registry. Evidence for a graft versus leukemia effect in clinical bone marrow transplantation. Exp Hematol 1988;16:547.
599. Hale G, Cobbold S, Waldmann H, for CAMPATH-1 Users. T cell depletion with CAMPATH-1 in allogeneic bone marrow transplantation. Transplantation 1988;45:753.
600. Buckner CD, Stewart D, Clift RA, et al. Treatment of blastic transformation of chronic granulocytic leukemia by chemotherapy, total-body irradiation and infusion of cryopreserved autologous marrow. Exp Hematol 1978;6:96.
601. Preisler HD, Raza A, Higby D, et al. Treatment of myeloid crisis of chronic myelogenous leukemia. Cancer Treat Rep 1984;68:1351.
602. Marcus RE, Goldman JM. Autografting in chronic granulocytic leukaemia. Clin Haematol 1986;15:235.
603. Thomas ED, Buckner CD, Banaji M, et al. One hundred patients with acute leukemia treated by chemotherapy, total body irradiation, and allogeneic marrow transplantation. Blood 1977;49.

604. Badger C, Buckner CD, Thomas ED, et al. Allogeneic marrow transplantation for acute leukemia in relapse. Leuk Res 1982;6:383.
605. Fefer A, Cheever MA, Thomas ED, et al. Bone marrow transplantation for refractory acute leukemia in 34 patients with identical twins. Blood 1981;57:421.
606. Report from the Working Party on Leukaemia, European Group for Bone Marrow Transplantation. Allogeneic bone marrow transplantation for leukaemia in Europe. Lancet 1988;1:1379.
607. Clift RA, Buckner CD, Appelbaum FR, et al. Allogeneic marrow transplantation during untreated first relapse of acute myeloid leukemia. J Clin Oncol 1992;10:1723.
608. Appelbaum FR, Dahlberg S, Thomas ED, et al. Bone marrow transplantation or chemotherapy after remission induction for adults with acute nonlymphocytic leukemia. Ann Intern Med 1984;101:581.
609. Appelbaum FR, Fisher LD, Thomas ED, and the Seattle Marrow Transplant Team. Chemotherapy v marrow transplantation for adults with nonlymphocytic leukemia: a five-year follow-up. Blood 1988;72:179.
610. Reiffers J, Gaspard MH, Maraninchi D, et al. Comparison of allogeneic or autologous bone marrow transplantation and chemotherapy in patients with acute myeloid leukaemia in first remission: a prospective controlled trial. Br J Haematol 1989;72:57.
611. Powles RL, Morgenstein G, Clink HM, et al. The place of bone-marrow transplantation in acute myelogenous leukaemia. Lancet 1980;1:1047.
612. Lakhani AK, Helenglass G, Powles RL, et al. Allogeneic bone marrow transplantation in first remission acute myeloid leukemia: a study of 98 patients with long follow-up. Bone Marrow Transplant 1987;2:27.
613. Conde E, Iriondo A, Rayon C, et al. Allogeneic bone marrow transplantation versus intensification chemotherapy for acute myelogenous leukaemia in first remission: a prospective controlled trial. Br J Haematol 1988;68:219.
614. Begg CB, McGlave PB, Bennett JM, et al. A critical comparison of allogeneic bone marrow transplantation and conventional chemotherapy as treatment for acute nonlymphocytic leukemia. J Clin Oncol 1984;2:369.
615. Champlin RE, Ho WG, Gale RP, et al. Treatment of acute myelogenous leukemia: a prospective controlled trial of bone marrow transplantation versus consolidation chemotherapy. Ann Intern Med 1985;102:285.
616. Clift RA, Buckner CD, Thomas ED, et al. The treatment of acute nonlymphocytic leukemia by allogeneic bone marrow transplantation. Bone Marrow Transplant 1987;2:243.
617. McGlave PB, Haake RJ, Bostrom BC, et al. Allogeneic bone marrow transplantation for acute nonlymphocytic leukemia in first remission. Blood 1988;72:1512.
618. Geller RB, Saral R, Piantadosi S, et al. Allogeneic bone marrow transplantation after high-dose busulfan and cyclophosphamide in patients with acute nonlymphocytic leukemia. Blood 1989;73:2209.
619. Dinsmore R, Kirkpatrick D, Flomenberg N, et al. Allogeneic bone marrow transplantation for patients with acute nonlymphocytic leukemia. Blood 1984;63:649.
620. Forman SJ, Krance RA, O'Donnell MR, et al. Bone marrow transplantation for acute nonlymphoblastic leukemia during first complete remission. Transplantation 1987;43:650.
621. Sanders JE, Thomas ED, Buckner CD, et al. Marrow transplantation for children in first remission of acute nonlymphoblastic leukemia. Blood 1985;66:460.
622. Weisdorf DJ, McGlave PB, Ramsay NKC, et al. Allogeneic bone marrow transplantation for acute leukaemia: comparative outcomes for adults and children. Br J Haematol 1988;69:351.
623. Tallman S, Kopecky KJ, Amos D, et al. Analysis of prognostic factors for the outcome of marrow transplantation or further chemotherapy for patients with acute nonlymphocytic leukemia in first remission. J Clin Oncol 1989;7:326.
624. Bostrom B, Brunning RD, McGlave PB, et al. Bone marrow transplantation for acute nonlymphocytic leukemia in first remission: analysis of prognostic factors. Blood 1985;65:1191.
625. Zwaan FE, Hermans J, Lyklema A. Factors influencing long-term leukemia-free survival after allogeneic bone marrow transplantation for acute leukemia. In: Hagenbeek A, Lowenberg B, eds. Minimal residual disease in acute leukemia. Amsterdam, Martinus Nijhoff, 1986: 295.
626. International Bone Marrow Transplant Registry. Transplant or chemotherapy in acute myelogenous leukaemia. Lancet 1989;1:1119.
627. Buckner CD, Clift RA, Storb R, et al. Pre- and post-marrow transplant regimens in patients with acute nonlymphoblastic leukemia in first remission. Exp Hematol 1988;16:546.
628. Storb R, Deeg HJ, Pepe M, et al. Methotrexate and cyclosporine versus cyclosporine alone for prophylaxis of graft-versus-host disease in patients given HLA-identical marrow grafts for leukemia: long term follow-up of a controlled trial. Blood 1989;73:1729.
629. Longmore G, Guinan EC, Weinstein HJ, Gelber RD, Rappeport JM, Antin JH. Bone marrow transplantation for myelodysplasia and secondary acute non-lymphoblastic leukemia. J Clin Oncol 1990;8:1707.
630. O'Donnell MR, Nademanee AP, Snyder DS, et al. Bone marrow transplantation for myelodysplastic and myeloproliferative syndromes. J Clin Oncol 1987;5:1822.
631. Appelbaum FR, Storb R, Ramberg RE, et al. Treatment of preleukemic syndromes with marrow transplantation. Blood 1987;69:92.
632. Geller RB, Vogelsang GB, Wingard JR, et al. Successful marrow transplantation for acute myelocytic leukemia following therapy for Hodgkin's disease. J Clin Oncol 1988;6:1558.
633. Sargur M, Buckner CD, Appelbaum FR, et al. Marrow transplantation for acute nonlymphocytic leukemia following therapy for Hodgkin's disease. J Clin Oncol 1987;5:731.
634. Blume KG, Forman SJ, Snyder DS, et al. Allogeneic bone marrow transplantation for acute lymphoblastic leukemia during first complete remission. Transplantation 1987;43:389.
635. Vernant JP, Marit G, Maraninchi D, et al. Allogeneic bone marrow transplantation in adults with acute lymphoblastic leukemia in first complete remission. J Clin Oncol 1988;6:227.
636. Zwaan FE, Hermans J, Barrett AJ, Speck B. Bone marrow transplantation for acute lymphoblastic leukaemia: a survey of the European Group for Bone Marrow Transplantation (E.G.B.M.T.). Br J Haematol 1984;58: 33.
637. Forman SJ, O'Donnell MR, Nademanee AP, et al. Bone marrow transplantation for patients with Philadelphia chromosome-positive acute lymphoblastic leukemia. Blood 1987;70:587.
638. Herzig RH, Bortin MM, Barrett AJ, et al. Bone-marrow transplantation in high-risk acute lymphoblastic leukaemia in first and second remission. Lancet 1987;1:786.
639. Brochstein JA, Kernan NA, Groshen S, et al. Allogeneic bone marrow transplantation after hyperfractionated total-body irradiation and cyclophosphamide in children with acute leukemia. N Engl J Med 1987;317:1618.
640. McCarthy DM, Barrett AJ, MacDonald D, et al. Bone marrow transplantation for adults and children with poor risk acute lymphoblastic leukemia in first complete remission. Bone Marrow Transplant 1988;3: 331.
641. Barrett, Horowitz MM, Gale RP, et al. Marrow transplantation for acute lymphoblastic leukemia: factors affecting relapse and survival. Blood 1989;74:862.
642. Buckner CD, Clift RA. Marrow transplantation for acute lymphoblastic leukemia. Semin Hematol 1984;21:43.
643. Weisdorf DJ, Nesbit ME, Ramsay NKC, et al. Allogeneic bone marrow transplantation for acute lymphoblastic leukemia in remission: prolonged survival associated with acute graft-versus-host disease. J Clin Oncol 1987;5:1348.
644. Sanders JE, Thomas ED, Buckner CD, Doney K. Marrow transplantation for children with acute lymphoblastic leukemia in second remission. Blood 1987;70:324.
645. Coccia PF, Strandjord SE, Warkentin PI, et al. High-dose cytosine arabinoside and fractionated total-body irradiation: an improved preparative regimen for bone marrow transplantation of children with acute lymphoblastic leukemia in remission. Blood 1988;71:888.
646. Buchanan GR, Boyett JM, Rivera GK. Intensive combination chemotherapy for patients with acute lymphoblastic leukemia (ALL) in second marrow remission: a Pediatric Oncology Group study. Proc Am Soc Clin Oncol 1988;7:188.
647. Johnson FL, Thomas ED, Clark BS, et al. A comparison of marrow transplantation with chemotherapy for children with acute lymphoblastic leukemia in second and subsequent remission. N Engl J Med 1981;305:846.
648. Pinkel D. Allogeneic bone marrow transplantation in children with acute leukemia: a practice whose time has gone. Leukemia 1989;3: 242.
649. Chessells, Rogers DW, Leiper AD, et al. Bone-marrow transplantation has a limited role in prolonging second marrow remission in childhood lymphoblastic leukemia. Lancet 1986;1:1239.
650. Kersey JH, Weisdorf D, Nesbit ME, et al. Comparison of autologous and allogeneic bone marrow transplantation for treatment of high risk refractory acute lymphoblastic leukemia. N Engl J Med 1987;317:461.
651. Barrett AJ, Joshi R, Kendra JR, et al. Prediction and prevention of relapse of acute lymphoblastic leukaemia after bone marrow transplantation. Br J Haematol 1986;64:179.
652. Meyers JD, Flournoy N, Sanders JE, et al. Prophylactic use of human leukocyte interferon after allogeneic marrow transplantation. Ann Intern Med 1987;107:809.
653. Thompson CB, Sanders JE, Flournoy N, et al. The risks of central nervous system relapse and leukoencephalopathy in patients receiving marrow transplants for acute leukemia. Blood 1986;67:195.
654. Bostrom B, Woods WG, Nesbit ME, et al. Successful reinduction of patients with acute lymphoblastic leukemia who relapse following bone marrow transplantation. J Clin Oncol 1987;5:376.
655. Ramsay N, LeBien T, Nesbit M, et al. Autologous bone marrow transplantation for patients with acute lymphoblastic leukemia in second or subsequent remission: results of bone marrow treated with monoclonal antibodies BA-1, BA-2 and BA-3 plus complement. Blood 1985;66: 508.
656. Ball ED, Mills LE, Coughlin CT, et al. Autologous marrow transplantation in acute myelogenous leukemia: in vitro treatment with myeloid cell–specific monoclonal antibodies. Blood 1986;68:1311.
657. Ritz J. Use of monoclonal antibodies in autologous and allogeneic bone marrow transplantation. Clin Haematol 1983;12:813.
658. Chang J, Coutinho L, Morgenstern G, et al. Reconstitution of haematopoietic system with autologous marrow taken during relapse of acute

myeloblastic leukaemia and grown in long-term culture. Lancet 1986;1: 294.
659. Gorin NC, Douay L, Laporte JP, et al. Autologous bone marrow transplantation using marrow incubated with Asta Z 7557 in adult acute leukemia. Blood 1986;67:1367.
660. Hagenbeek A, Marten ACM. Reinfusion of leukemic cells with the autologous marrow graft: preclinical studies on lodging and regrowth of leukemia. Leuk Res 1985;9:1389.
661. Hagenbeek A, Marten ACM. The efficacy of high-dose cyclophosphamide in combination with total body irradiation in the treatment of acute myelocytic leukemia: studies in a relevant rat model (BNML). Cancer Res 1983;43:408.
662. Hagenbeek A, Martens ACM, Schultz FW. Residual leukemic cells in autologous marrow grafts do not significantly contribute to leukemia relapse after bone marrow transplantation. Exp Hematol 1988;16:492.
663. Burnett AK, McKinnon S. Autologous bone marrow transplantation in first remission AML using nonpurged marrow: update. In: Hagenbeek A, Lowenberg B, eds. Minimal residual disease in acute leukemia. Dordrecht, The Netherlands, Martinus Nijhoff, 1986:211.
664. Gorin NC, Herve P, Aegerter P, et al. Autologous bone marrow transplantation for acute leukaemia in remission. Br J Haematol 1986;64: 385.
665. Gorin NC, Aegerter P. Autologous bone marrow transplantation for acute leukemia in remission: third European survey—March, 1986. Bone Marrow Transplant 1986;1:255.
666. Billett A, Ritz J, Niemeyer C, Gelber R, Sallan S. Antibody-purged autologous bone marrow transplantation (TP) for relapsed non-T-cell acute lymphoblastic leukemia (ALL) in childhood. Blood 1988;72:380A.
667. Nemunitis J, Rabinowe SN, Singer JW, et al. Recombinant granulocyte-macrophage colony-stimulating factor after autologous bone marrow transplantation for lymphoid cancer. N Engl J Med 1991;324:1773.
668. Blazar BR, Kersey JH, McGlave PB, et al. In vivo administration of recombinant human granulocyte/macrophage colony-stimulating factor in acute lymphoblastic leukemia receiving purged autografts. Blood 1989;73:849.
669. Appelbaum FR, Sullivan KM, Thomas ED, et al. Allogeneic marrow transplantation in the treatment of MOPP-resistant Hodgkin's disease. J Clin Oncol 1985;3:1490.
670. Appelbaum FR, Sullivan KM, Buckner CD, et al. Treatment of malignant lymphoma in 100 patients with chemotherapy, total body irradiation, and marrow transplantation. J Clin Oncol 1987;5:1340.
671. Phillips GL, Wolff S, Herzig G, et al. Local radiotherapy followed by cyclophosphamide, fractionated total body irradiation and autologous marrow transplantation for refractory malignant lymphoma. Blood 1983;62:228A.
672. Kaplan HS. Evidence for a tumoricidal dose level in the radiotherapy of Hodgkin's disease. Cancer Res 1966;26:1250.
673. Kaplan HS. Hodgkin's disease. Cambridge, MA, Harvard University Press, 1980:366.
674. Kessinger A, Armitage JO, Landmark JD, et al. Autologous peripheral hematopoietic stem cell transplantation restores hematopoietic function following marrow ablative therapy. Blood 1988;71:723.
675. Jagannath S, Armitage JO, Dicke KA, et al. Prognostic factors for response and survival after high-dose cyclophosphamide, carmustine, and etoposide with autologous bone marrow transplantation for relapsed Hodgkin's disease. J Clin Oncol 1989;7:179.
676. Gribben JG, Linch DC, Singer CRJ, et al. Successful treatment of refractory Hodgkin's disease by high-dose combination chemotherapy and autologous bone marrow transplantation. Blood 1989;73:340.
677. Reece D, Connors J, Fay J, et al. Augmented cyclophosphamide (C), BCNU (B), and etoposide (V) = CBV and autologous bone marrow transplantation for progressive Hodgkin's disease (HD). Blood 1988;72: 402A.
678. Wheeler C, Antin JH, Churchill WH, et al. Cyclophosphamide, carmustine and etoposide with autologous bone marrow transplantation in refractory Hodgkin's disease and non-Hodgkin's lymphoma: a dose finding study. J Clin Oncol 1990;8:648.
679. Carella AM, Congiu AM, Gaozza et al. High-dose chemotherapy with autologous bone marrow transplantation in 50 advanced resistant Hodgkin's disease patients: an Italian study group report. J Clin Oncol 1988;6:1411.
680. Phillips GL, Herzig RH, Lazarus HM, et al. High-dose chemotherapy, fractionated total-body irradiation, and allogeneic marrow transplantation for malignant lymphoma. J Clin Oncol 1986;4:480.
681. Tannir NM, Spitzer G, Zander AR, et al. High-dose chemoradiotherapy and bone marrow transplantation in patients with refractory lymphoma. Eur J Cancer Clin Oncol 1983;19:1091.
682. O'Leary M, Ransay NKC, Nesbit ME, et al. Bone marrow transplantation for non-Hodgkin's lymphoma in children and young adults. Am J Med 1983;74:497.
683. Jones RJ, Ambinder RF, Piantadosi S, Santos GW. Evidence of graft-versus-lymphoma effect associated with allogeneic bone marrow transplantation. Blood 1991;77:649.
684. Appelbaum FR, Deisseroth AB, Graw RG, et al. Prolonged complete remission following high dose chemotherapy of Burkitt's lymphoma in relapse. Cancer 1978;41:1059.
685. Appelbaum FR, Herzig GP, Ziegler JL, et al. Successful engraftment of cyropreserved autologus bone marrow in patients with malignant lymphoma. Blood 1978;52:85.
686. Singer CRJ, Goldstone AH. Clinical studies of ABMT in non-Hodgkin's lymphoma. Clin Haematol 1986;15:105.
687. Philip T, Pinkerton R, Hartmann O, et al. The role of massive therapy with autologous bone marrow transplantation in Burkitt's lymphoma. Clin Haematol 1986;15:205.
688. Canellos GP, Nadler GP, Takavorian T. Autologous bone marrow transplantation in the treatment of malignant lymphoma and Hodgkin's disease. Semin Hematol 1988;25:58.
689. Gulati SC, Shank B, Black P, et al. Autologous bone marrow transplantation for patients with poor-prognosis lymphoma. J Clin Oncol 1988;6:1303.
690. Takvorian T, Canellos GP, Ritz J, et al. Prolonged disease-free survival after autologous bone marrow transplantation in patients with non-Hodgkin's lymphoma with a poor prognosis. N Engl J Med 1987;316: 1499.
691. Verdonck LF, Dekker AW, Vendrik PJ, et al. Intensive cytoreductive therapy followed by autologous bone marrow transplantation for patients with hematologic malignancies or solid tumors. Cancer 1987;60: 289.
692. Philip T, Hartmann O, Biron P, et al. High-dose therapy and autologous bone marrow transplantation in partial remission after first-line induction therapy for diffuse non-Hodgkin's lymphoma. J Clin Oncol 1988;6:1118.
693. Philip T, Armitage JO, Spitzer G, et al. High-dose therapy and autologous bone marrow transplantation after failure of conventional chemotherapy in adults with intermediate-grade or high-grade non-Hodgkin's lymphoma. N Engl J Med 1987;316:1499.
694. Shipp MA, Harrington DP, Klatt MM, et al. Identification of major prognostic subgroups of patients with large-cell lymphoma treated with m-BACOD or M-BACOD. Ann Intern Med 1986;104:757.
695. Bennett JM, Cain KC, Glick JH, et al. The significance of bone marrow involvement in non-Hodgkin's lymphoma: the Eastern Cooperative Oncology Group experience. J Clin Oncol 1986;4:1462.
696. Tweeddale ME, Lim B, Jamal N, et al. The presence of clonogenic cells in high-grade malignant lymphomas: a prognostic factor. Blood 1987;69: 1307.
697. Smith BR, Weinberg DS, Robert NJ, et al. Circulating monoclonal B lymphocytes in non-Hodgkin's lymphoma. N Engl J Med 1984;311: 1476.
698. Benjamin D, Magrath IT, Douglas EC, Corash LM. Derivation of lymphoma cell lines from microscopically normal bone marrow in patients with undifferentiated lymphomas: evidence of occult bone marrow involvement. Blood 1983;61:1017.
699. Braine HG, Santos GW, Kaizer H, et al. Treatment of poor prognosis non-Hodgkin's lymphoma using cyclophosphamide and total body irradiation regimens with autologous bone marrow rescue. Bone Marrow Transplant 1987;2:7.
700. Freedman AS, Boyd AW, Anderson KC, et al. Immunologic heterogeneity of diffuse large cell lymphoma 1985;65:630.
701. Sklar J, Cleary ML, Thielemans K, et al. Biclonal B cell lymphoma. N Engl J Med 1984;311:20.
702. Siegelman MH, Cleary ML, Warake R, Sklar J. Frequent biclonality and Ig gene alteration among B cell lymphomas that show multiple histologic forms. J Exp Med 1985;161:850.
703. Gribben JG, Freedman AS, Neuberg D, et al. Immunologic purging of marrow assessed by PCR before autologous marrow transplantation for B-cell lymphoma. N Engl J Med 1991;325:1525.
704. Kessinger A, Armitage JO, Smith DM, et al. High-dose therapy and autologous peripheral blood stem cell transplantation for patients with lymphoma. Blood 1989;74:1260.
705. Gluckman E, Broxmeyer HE, Auerbach AD, et al. Hematopoietic reconstitution in patients with Fanconi's anemia by means of umbilical-cord blood from and HLA-identical sibling. N Engl J Med 1989;321: 1174.
706. Broxmeyer HE, Douglas GW, Hangoc, et al. Human umbilical cord blood as a potential source of transplantable hematopoietic stem/progenitor cells. Proc Natl Acad Sci USA 1989;86:3828.
707. Bartologie B, Hall R, Zander A, et al. High-dose melphalan with autologous bone marrow transplantation for multiple myeloma. Blood 1986;67:1298.
708. Gahrton G, Tura S, Flesch M, et al. Bone marrow transplantation in multiple myeloma: report from the European Cooperative Group for Bone Marrow Transplantation. Blood 1987;69:1262.
709. Gahrton G, Tura S, Ljungman P, et al. Allogeneic bone marrow transplantation in multiple myeloma. N Engl J Med 1991;325:1267.
710. Michallet M, Corront B, Hollard D, et al. Allogeneic bone marrow transplantation in chronic lymphocytic leukemia: 8 cases. Blood 1988;72:396A.
711. Ringdén O, Ahström L, Lönnqvist B, et al. Allogeneic bone marrow transplantation in a patient with chemotherapy-resistant progressive histiocytosis X. N Engl J Med 1987;316:733.
712. Parkman R. The application of bone marrow transplantation to the treatment of genetic diseases. Science 1986;232:1373.
713. Rosen FS, Wedgwood RJ, Aiuti F, et al. Primary immunodeficiency diseases. Clin Immunol Immunopathol 1983;28:450.

714. Gelfand EW, Dosch HM. Diagnosis and classification of severe combined immunodeficiency disease. Birth Defects Original Article Series 1983;19:65.
715. Pollack MS, Kirkpatrick D, Kapoor N, et al. Identification by HLA typing of intrauterine derived maternal T cells in four patients with severe combined immunodeficiency. N Engl J Med 1982;397:662.
716. Thompson LF, O'Connor RD, Bastian JF. Phenotype and function of engrafted maternal T cells in patients with severe combined immunodeficiency. J Immunol 1984;133:2513.
717. Gatti RA, Meuwissen HJ, Allen HD, et al. Immunological reconstitution of sex-linked lymphopenic immunological deficiency. Lancet 1968;2:1366.
718. Bortin MM, Rimm AA. Severe combined immunodeficiency disease: characterization of the disease and results of transplantation. JAMA 1977;238:591.
719. Kenny AB, Hitzig WH. Bone marrow transplantation for severe combined immunodeficiency syndrome. Eur J Pediatr 1979;131:155.
720. Rappeport JM, Smith BR, Parkman RP, Rosen FS. Bone marrow transplantation in genetic diseases. Clin Haematol 1983;12:755.
721. Parkman RP, Gelfand EW, Rosen FS, et al. Severe combined immunodeficiency and adenosine deaminase deficiency. N Engl J Med 1975;292:714.
722. Reisner Y, Kapoor N, Kirkpatrick D, et al. Transplantation for severe combined immunodeficiency with HLA, A, B, D, DR incompatible parental marrow cells fractionated by soybean agglutinin and sheep red blood cells. Blood 1983;61:341.
723. Friedrich W, Goldmann SF, Vetter U, et al. Immunoreconstitution in severe combined immunodeficiency after transplantation of HLA-haploidentical, T cell depleted bone marrow. Lancet 1984;1:761.
724. Reinherz EL, Geha R, Rappeport JM, et al. Reconstitution after transplantation with T-lymphocyte depleted HLA haplotype-mismatched bone marrow for severe combined immunodeficiency. Proc Natl Acad Sci USA 1982;79:6047.
725. Fischer A, Durandy A, de Villartay J-P, et al. HLA haploidentical bone marrow transplantation for severe combined immunodeficiency using E rosette fractionation and cyclosporine. Blood 1986;67:444.
726. Buckley R, Schiff SE, Sampson HA, et al. Development of immunity in human severe primary T cell deficiency following haploidentical bone marrow stem cell transplantation. J Immunol 1986;136:2398.
727. Remold-O'Donnell E, Kenny DM, Parkman R, Cairns L, Savage B, Rosen FS. Characterization of a human lymphocyte surface sialoglycoprotein that is defective in Wiskott-Aldrich syndrome. J Exp Med 1984;159:1705.
728. Parkman R, Rappeport JM, Geha R, et al. Complete correction of the Wiskott-Aldrich syndrome by allogeneic bone marrow transplantation. N Engl J Med 1978;298:921.
729. Kapoor N, Kirkpatrick D, Blaese RM, et al. Reconstitution of normal megakaryopoiesis and immunological functions in Wiskott Aldrich syndrome by marrow transplantation following myeloablation and immunosuppression with busulfan and cyclophosphamide. Blood 1981;57:692.
730. Ochs HD, Lum LF, Johnson LF, et al. Bone marrow transplantation in the Wiskott-Aldrich syndrome. Transplantation 1982;34:284.
731. Lucarelli G, Galimberti M, Polchi P, et al. Bone marrow transplantation in patients with thalassemia. N Engl J Med 1990;322:417.
732. Lucarelli G, Galimberti M, Polchi P, et al. Bone marrow transplantation in patients with adult thalassemia. N Engl J Med 1992;80:1603.
733. Weatherall D. Bone marrow transplantation for thalassemia and other inherited disorders of hemoglobin. Blood 1992;80:1379.
734. Lin KH, Lin KS, Feig SA. Marrow transplantation for thalassemia. Bone Marrow Transplant 1986;1:115.
735. Lucarelli G, Galimberti M, Polchi P et al. Marrow transplantation in patients with advanced thalassemia. N Engl J Med 1987;316:1050.
736. Weiden PL, Hackman RC, Deeg HJ, et al. Long term survival and reversal of iron overload after marrow transplantation in dogs with congenital hemolytic anemia. Blood 1981;57:66.
737. Johnson FL, Look AT, Gockerman J, et al. Bone marrow transplantation in a patient with sickle cell anemia. N Engl J Med 1984;311:780.
738. Vermylen C, Robles EF, Ninane J, Cornu G. Bone marrow transplantation in five children with sickle cell anaemia. Lancet 1988;1:1427.
739. Coccia PF, Krivit W, Cervenka J, et al. Successful bone marrow transplantation for infantile malignant osteopetrosis. N Engl J Med 1980;302:701.
740. Ballet JJ, Griscelli C, Courtris C, et al. Bone marrow transplantation in osteopetrosis. Lancet 1977;2:1137.
741. Sorbell M, Kapoor N, Kirkpatrick D, et al. Marrow transplantation for juvenile osteopetrosis. Am J Med 1981;70:1280.
742. Hirschhorn R. Therapy of genetic disorders. N Engl J Med 1987;316:624.
743. Hershfield MS, Buckley RH, Greenberg ML, et al. Treatment of adenosine deaminase deficiency with polyethylene glycol modified adenosine deaminase. N Engl J Med 1987;316:589.
744. Wewers MD, Casolaro A, Sellers SE, et al. Replacement therapy for alpha-1 antitrypsin deficiency associated with emphysema. N Engl J Med 1987;316:1055.
745. Groth CG, Ringdén O. Transplantation in relation to the treatment of inherited disease. Transplantation 1984;38:319.
746. Hobbs JR. Displacement bone marrow transplantation for some inborn errors. J Inherit Metabol Dis 1990;13:1572.
747. Hobbs JR, Hugh-Jones K, Barrett AJ, et al. Reversal of clinical features of Hurler's disease and biochemical improvement after treatment by bone marrow transplantation. Lancet 1981;2:709.
748. Krivit W, Pierpont ME, Ayaz K, et al. Bone marrow transplantation in the Maroteaux-Lamy syndrome (mucopolysaccharidosis type VI). N Engl J Med 1984;311:1606.
749. Bartlett PF. Pluripotential hematopoietic stem cells in adult mouse brain. Proc Natl Acad Sci USA 1982;79:2722.
750. Konigsmark BW, Sidman RL. Origin of brain macrophages in the mouse. J Neuropathol Exp Neurol 1963;22:643.
751. Yeager AM, Brennan S, Tiffany C, et al. Prolonged survival and remyelination after hematopoietic cell transplantation in the twitcher mouse. Science 1984;225:1052.
752. Rappeport JM, Parkman R, Newburger P, et al. Correction of infantile agranulocytosis (Kostman's syndrome) by allogeneic bone marrow transplantation. Am J Med 1980;68:605.
753. Rappeport JM, Newburger PE, Goldblum RM, et al. Allogeneic bone marrow transplantation for chronic granulomatous disease. J Pediatr 1982;101:952.
754. Camitta BM, Quesenberry PJ, Parkman R, et al. Bone marrow transplantation for an infant with neutrophil dysfunction. Exp Hematol 1977;5:109.
755. Elin RJ, Reynolds HY, Durbin WA, et al. Chediak-Higashi syndrome: reversal of increased susceptibility to infection by bone marrow transplantation. Blood 1976;47:555.
756. Iriondo A, Garijo J, Baro J, et al. Complete recovery of hemopoiesis following bone marrow transplant in a patient with unresponsive congenital hypoplastic anemia. Blood 1984;64:348.
757. Lenarsky C, Weinberg K, Guinan E, et al. Bone marrow transplantation for constitutional pure red cell aplasia. Blood 1988;71:226.
758. Santos GW, Tutschka PJ, Brookmeyer, et al. Marrow transplantation for acute nonlymphocytic leukemia after treatment with busulfan and cyclophorphamide. N Engl J Med 1983;309:1347.
759. Shank B, Hopfan S, Kim JH, et al. Hyperfractionated total body irradiation for bone marrow transplantation. I. Early results in leukemia patients. Int J Radiat Biol Phys 1981;7:1109.

Blood: Principles and Practice of Hematology,
edited by Robert I. Handin, Samuel E. Lux, and Thomas P. Stossel.
J.B. Lippincott Company, Philadelphia © 1995.

64

Neonatal Anemia

Lawrence C. Wolfe

Neonatal, and perhaps fetal, hematology has opened doors of investigation to many important principles of hematology and immunology. The pathophysiology of neonatal blood disorders often seems more finite than that of older children or adults, but in reality it is more dynamic and often more complicated. The neonate can be afflicted with quantitative and qualitative defects in red blood cells, white blood cells, and platelets in a similar manner to the way in which older children and adults are afflicted. Most of the hematologic illnesses unique to the neonate are related to the immediate presentation of primary conditions (such as congenital spherocytosis), illnesses acquired through the maternal–fetal connection (such as hemolytic diseases of the newborn and maternal-to-fetal viral illness), or the delayed appearance of conditions associated with developmental changes (such as β-thalassemia) or maturation (such as anemia of prematurity).

NORMAL HEMATOLOGIC VALUES IN NEONATES

One of the most difficult concepts in neonatal hematology is that values given as normal for the neonate simply refer to the observed measurement of any parameter at a given gestational age or chronologic age. This should not be mistaken for a normal function of that given parameter. For example, Table 64-1 presents some normally observed red cell[1–4] and coagulation values[5,6] in neonates of various age groups. The low hemoglobin levels that are regularly observed in almost all infants several weeks after birth may be reported as within the normal range for age. Nevertheless, these values correspond to decreased oxygen-carrying capacity, which may lead to the symptoms, signs, and complications of tissue hypoxia. Premature infants with lower hemoglobins are obviously at greater risk. Analogously, the clinical significance of the prolonged partial thromboplastin time seen in most neonates, that is, a proclivity toward bleeding with less trauma, is still present. Lower levels of antithrombin III, protein C, and protein S create higher risks for thrombosis as well. Thus, as we present normal data, these laboratory values must be interpreted in light of the functional health status of the infant involved.

GESTATIONAL PHYSIOLOGY

The onset of hemopoiesis is in the broad islands of the embryonic sac. There, cells seem destined to become both vascular endothelium and stem cells for hemopoiesis. The earliest red cell precursors appear to be ready to enter the bloodstream in the third week of development, remarkably about the time when the blood is set in motion by the developing heart.[7] Embryonic stem cells then follow along the creation of endothelial channels and reticuloendothelial supporting tissue to temporarily take up residence in the liver and, to a lesser extent, in the spleen. By 8 weeks of gestation, differentiated cells of the erythroid series and the myeloid series are being created in the liver and slowly begin to move to the bone marrow.[8] Megakaryocytes are primarily seen in the bone marrow after the erythroid and myeloid series have arrived.[9] Extramedullary hematopoiesis ebbs compared with bone marrow at about 30 weeks of gestation (Fig. 64-1). The embryology of erythroid hematopoiesis does not end with the birth of the child, since postbirth developmental changes continue. This is demonstrated most dramatically in postbirth red cell changes. The switch from fetal to adult hemoglobin and fetal to adult red cells is not complete in some situations up to 1 year after birth.[9]

Figure 64-1 demonstrates the appearance of globin chain produced from the onset of erythroid hematopoiesis in the neonate. Early in gestation, the embryonic hemoglobins predominate. Animal models such as the mouse suggest that these embryonic globins have a very high oxygen affinity consistent with the very low oxygen tensions to which the embryo is subjected.[10] At birth, fetal hemoglobin (Hb F) predominates, but synthesis of Hb F diminishes rapidly after birth replaced by β-chain synthesis.[9] Figure 64-1 enables the clinician to understand the appearance of embryonic globin pairs, globin tetramers, and β-globin structural mutants. When specific globins are not synthesized appropriately (thalassemias), early embryonic globin parings may persist and tetramers of single globins without complementary chains are observed.

In homozygous α-thalassemia, Hb Gower 1 ($\zeta_2\epsilon_2$), Hb Portland ($\zeta_2\gamma_2$) and Hb Bart's (γ_4) are the only globin species observed in the stillborn hydropic infant. If only three α genes are deficient, the infant survives and the fetal switch of globins leads to a diminishment in the amount of Hb Bart's (γ_4), the production of some normal Hb F ($\alpha_2\gamma_2$) and Hb A ($\alpha_2\beta_2$), and a postbirth excess of β chains producing Hb H (β_4). Deficiency of β-chain synthesis would prevent or limit the postbirth production of Hb A ($\alpha_2\beta_2$), but since excess α chains do not associate into stable tetramers, no unusual hemoglobin species are observed in these postbirth cells on hemoglobin electropoiesis. Rather, α-chain association with alternate non–α chains (δ:Hb A_2; γ:Hb F) is seen.

TABLE 64-1. Selected Mean Red Cell and Coagulation Reference Values for Healthy Full-Term Infants (HFT) and Healthy Premature Infants (HP)

	Day 1		Day 5		Day 30		
	HFT	HP	HFT	HP	HFT	HP	Adult
Hb (g/dL)	19.0	19.4	17.6	17.8	14.2	10.0	15.0
MCV (μ^3)	119	115	114	112	105	101	87
PT (sec)	13.0	13.0	12.4	12.5	11.8	11.8	12.4
PTT (sec)	42.9	53.6	42.6	50.5	40.4	44.7	33.5
Factor VII (U/mL)	0.66	0.67	0.89	0.84	0.90	0.83	1.05
Factor IX (U/mL)	0.53	0.35	0.53	0.42	0.51	0.44	1.09
Protein S (U/mL)	0.36	0.26	0.50	0.37	0.63	0.56	0.92
Protein C (U/mL)	0.35	0.28	0.42	0.31	0.43	0.37	0.96
AT III (U/mL)	0.63	0.38	0.67	0.56	0.78	0.59	1.05

PT, prothrombin time; PTT, partial thromboplastin time; MCV, mean corpuscular volume.

Pathophysiology of Hemoglobin Function at Birth

While all this response to genetic programming is underway, physiologic adaptations occur to accomplish the change from prenatal to postnatal life. The predominance of Hb F with its left-shifted oxygen dissociation curve is beneficial to the fetus, who suffers no tissue oxygen debt as a result of the increased oxygen uptake by hemoglobin in the placental circulation at the intrauterine Po_2 of 30 mmHg[9,11] (Fig. 64-2). This left shift of Hb F relates primarily to the decreased interaction of Hb F with 2,3-DPG (diphosphoglycerate). In the past, it was perceived as logical for neonates with respiratory compromise to receive adult blood which, because of its relatively right-shifted hemoglobin oxygen dissociation curve, rapidly unloads oxygen to anoxic tissues. It has been possible to support neonates for prolonged periods with profoundly low arterial Po_2 levels. Neonates cared for with this level of oxygenation usually have the syndrome of persistent fetal circulation or severe cyanotic congenital heart disease. Theoretically, the use of Hb A blood in this group of neonates could lead to a relative decrease in the oxygen content of blood as a result of the right shift of adult hemoglobin and to a concurrent decrease in oxygen loading in the lungs.

Calculations of theoretical arteriovenous oxygen saturation differences show a breakpoint in the value of adult hemoglobin to deliver oxygen to tissues. When venous Po_2 falls below 10 mmHg, more oxygen is theoretically delivered to tissues by a left-shifted (fetal-like) hemoglobin curve[12] (see Fig. 64-2). This would occur most commonly when arterial Po_2 is less than 50 mmHg. Transfusion of fetal blood is largely impractical, but attempts at conserving fetal blood (avoiding phlebotomy) as well as use of adult blood with maximal 2,3-DPG levels for transfusion is warranted in this special group of infants. Conversely, neonates without severe respiratory disease are not put at physiologic risk by the presence of transfused Hb A.

Developmental Changes in Red Cell Structure

In addition to the issues of hemoglobin structure, function, and production, red cells in fetal life are clearly different in their architecture as well. A large body of descriptive discussion outlines differences between fetal and adult red cells. Tables 64-2 and 64-3 summarize these differences. The clinician should be aware of those differences that relate to certain pathophysiologies. First, as a general characteristic, fetal red cells are less osmotically fragile.[13] Hence, an attempt to diagnose congenital spherocytosis using the osmotic fragility test in the immediate neonatal period can lead to false-normal results. Fortunately, this happens only rarely.

The most clinically apparent red cell membrane difference between adult and neonatal red cells is in the expression of red cell antigens. Although it is not well understood, a decrease in the number of recognizable blood group A

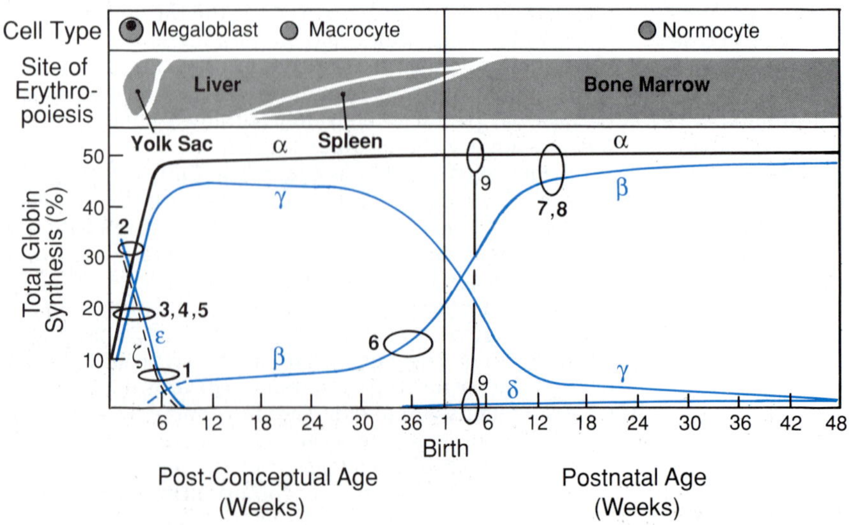

FIGURE 64-1. Developmental sequence of location of hematopoiesis and hemoglobin synthesis. The lassos connect globins that associate under normal and abnormal circumstances:

1. Pre-α: ϵ_4, $\zeta_2\epsilon_2$ (Gower 1)
2. Early α: $\alpha_2\epsilon_2$, (Gower 2)
3. Decreased or absent α: $\zeta_2\gamma_2$ (Portland)
4. Decreased or absent α: γ_4 (Bart's)
5. α Present: $\alpha_2\gamma_2$ (normal Hgb F)
6. Decreased or absent α (late): β_4 (Hgb H)
7. Postbirth normal: $\alpha_2\beta_2$ (Hgb A)
8. β Variants of Hgb A (eg $\alpha_2\beta_2$: Hgb S)
9. Normal: $\alpha_4\delta_2$ (Hgb A2)

(After Brown MS. Fetal and neonatal erythropoiesis in developmental and neonatal hematology. New York, Raven Press, 1988)

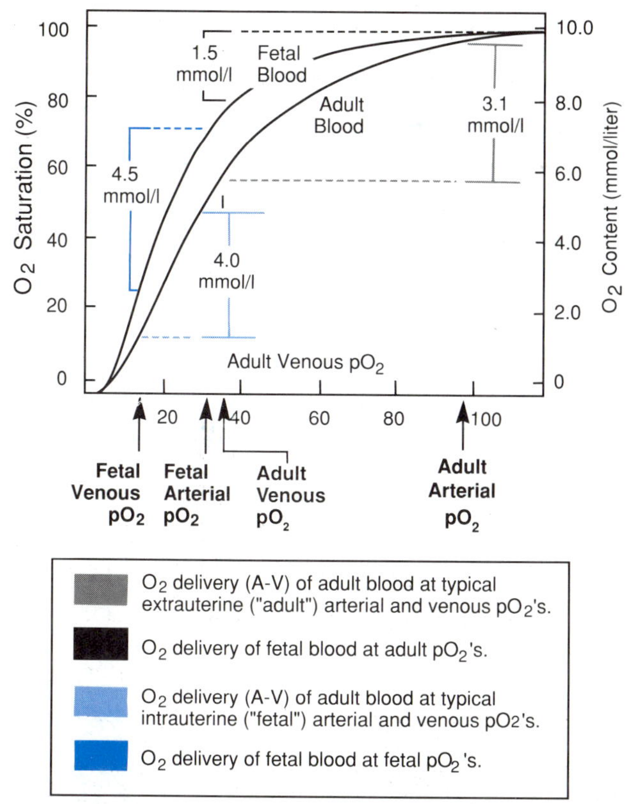

FIGURE 64-2. Difference in the hemoglobin—oxygen dissociation curve between newborns and adults. The left shift of the newborn curve enhances the amount of oxygen that can be delivered at lower oxygen tensions. For example, comparing the difference in oxygen content of blood at fetal arterial and venous PO_2s, fetal blood delivers 4.9 mmol/L, whereas adult blood delivers only 4 mmol/L. In contrast, at typical adult arterial and venous PO_2s, adult blood delivers more oxygen (3.1 mmol/L) than fetal blood (1.5 mmol/L). After Stockman JA. Fetal hematology. In: Eden RD, Boehm FH, eds. Assessment and care of the fetus. Norwalk, CT, Appleton & Lange, 1989:124)

and B antigens occurs on neonatal red cells.[14] Therefore, the neonate could have hemolytic disease based on the acquisition of anti-A or anti-B hemolysins from the mother across the placenta and mysteriously have a negative Coombs' test. This phenomenon probably also explains the less severe clinical picture of ABO incompatibility when compared with Rh blood group incompatibility.[15]

Functional differences may also be important in the membrane skeletons of fetal red cells. A number of observations suggest that membrane skeletons of normal adult red cells are loosened by elevated concentrations of 2,3-DPG.[16,17] Fetal red cells have a very large concentration of free 2,3-DPG by virtue of the diminished binding of 2,3-DPG by Hb F. This may be one of the reasons for shortened fetal red cell survival. In addition, this relation of 2,3-DPG to membrane skeletal components, as well as an enhanced tendency of Hb F to denature and damage the membrane, may exaggerate the anemia seen in other congenital hemolytic anemias, especially the unusual syndromes of hereditary elliptocytosis with neonatal poikilocytosis[18] (see Chap. 54).

Although no clinical syndromes are recognized specific to the alterations of the glycolytic pathways seen in fetal cells, it is likely that the decreased phosphate uptake into both adenosine triphosphate and 2,3-DPG has physiologic and pathophysiologic effects. The latter may contribute to the shortened red cell life-span of fetal red cells.

Fetal red cells appear to be more oxidant sensitive than their adult counterparts.[7] Table 64-3 lists those differences and the differences in enzyme systems important in protecting normal fetal and adult red cells from oxygen injury. The actual oxidant sensitivity probably results from a combination of factors. Term neonates, and especially premature infants, have lower serum vitamin E concentrations, which can last until they are up to 10 weeks of age.[19] This change in oxidant susceptibility can have acute and chronic effects, depending on the oxidant challenge. Acute oxidant stress from chemicals or infection can lead to rapid hemolysis associated with jaundice, reticulocytosis, and the appearance of bite cells and blister cells in the peripheral smear. Chronic effects include an exaggeration of the physiologic nadir of anemia.

TABLE 64-2. Some Structural Characteristics of Fetal Cells Compared With Adult Red Cells

MEMBRANE STRUCTURE AND FUNCTION
Less osmotically fragile[13]
Differences in surface antigen expression
A and B antigens diminished[14]
Lewis system diminished[15]
I antigen very diminished (or absent); i antigen present[15]
Possible decreased structural stability secondary to increased levels of unbound 2,3-DPG[16–18]
Membranes less deformable
Red cells of different shapes with a greater predominance of stomatocytes (bowl-shaped cells) than adult cells[20]
Disc:stomatocyte ratios—adult 78:18; term newborn 43:40, premature 40:29. Increased variability of the smear with multiple morphologic changes.
Red cell membrane pocks (secondary to decreased splenic function)[21]

Fetal Red Blood Cell Morphology

The classic study of Zipursky and associates[20] demonstrated the remarkable variety of red cell morphology observed in

TABLE 64-3. Some Metabolic Characteristics of Fetal Red Cells Compared With Adult Red Cells

ENERGY-RELATED METABOLISM
Glucose consumption increased
Decreased activity of phosphofructokinase
Decreased phosphate uptake with slower incorporation into ATP
Accelerated decline of ATP during short incubations
2,3-DPG METABOLISM
Decreased phosphate incorporation in 2,3-DPG
Accelerated decline of 2,3-DPG levels during brief in vitro incubations
PROTECTION AGAINST HEMOGLOBIN AND MEMBRANE OXIDATION
Decreased activity of: NADP-dependent methemoglobin reductase, catalase, glutathione peroxidase, and glutathione synthetase
Increased methemoglobin content
Increased tendency for Heinz body formation in presence of oxidant compounds
Decreased membrane sulfhydryl groups
Decreased fetal plasma antioxidant activity

ATP, adenosine triphosphate.

(After Oski F. Hematology: the erythrocyte and its disorders. In: Nathan DA, Oski FA, eds. Hematology of infancy and childhood, ed 4. Philadelphia, WB Saunders, 1993:25)

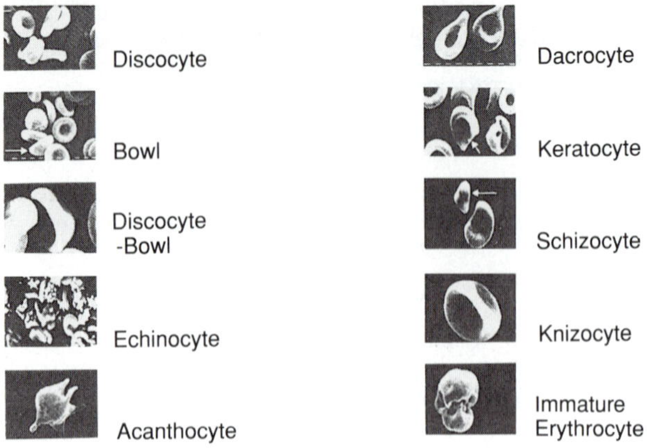

The Erythrocyte Differential Count
Median (5% to 95% Range)

Cell Type	Premature Infant	Term Infant	Normal Adult
Discocyte	39.5 (18-57)	43 (18-62)	78 (42-94)
Bowl	29.0 (13-53)	40 (14-58)	18 (4-50)
Discocyte-Bowl	3.0 (0-10)	2 (0-5)	2 (0-4)
Spherocyte	0.0 (0-3)	0 (0-1)	0 (0-0)
Echinocyte	5.5 (1-23)	1 (0-4)	0 (0-3)
Acanthocyte	0.0 (0-2)	1 (0-2)	0 (0-1)
Dacrocyte	1.0 (0-5)	1 (0-3)	0 (0-1)
Keratocyte	3.0 (0-7)	2 (0-5)	0 (0-1)
Schizocyte	2.0 (0-5)	0 (0-2)	0 (0-1)
Knizocyte	3.0 (0-11)	3 (0-8)	1 (0-5)
Immature Erythrocyte	1.0 (0-6)	0 (0-2)	0 (0-0)

FIGURE 64-3. Varied morphology associated with neonatal smears. (Zipursky A, Brown E, Palko J, Brown EJ. The erythrocyte differential count in newborn infants. Am J Pediatr Hematol Oncol 1983;5:45)

the premature and term infant compared with that of a normal adult (Fig. 64-3). Many of these differences are associated with the absence of splenic function seen in the neonatal period. This inhibition in splenic function is also manifested by the appearance of pits or pocks on the surface of the red cells[21] (see also Chap. 46). Compared with adult normal red cells (2.6% of red cells have pits), 24.3% of red cells from term infants and 47.2% of red cells from premature infants are pitted. The number of pitted cells usually decreases to adult values in term infants at 2 months of age; premature infants may require several more weeks.

In addition to being suggestive of the fetus's increased risk for overwhelming sepsis because of hyposplenism, the presence of this varied morphology may also be a record of turbulence in the neonatal circulation and the residue of fetal circulation (flow through the foramen ovale and the patent ductus arteriosus). Perusal of a smear of the neonate in the context of working up neonatal anemia or of attempting to find clues to systemic illness is complicated by this built-in variability. Hence, the morphologist should be careful not to react simply to the presence of poikilocytosis ("hemolytic" morphology) because this is the norm in neonatal smears. Rather, the approach should be to observe the predominant morphology.

Fetal and Neonatal Red Cell Life-Span

A large body of evidence suggests that the fetal red cell, identified by the presence of Hb F and i antigen on its surface, has a shortened red cell survival. Many of the studies have used chromium-51 (^{51}Cr)–labeled neonatal red cells for survival studies in adults.[22] Table 64-4 presents a summary of collected ^{51}Cr isotope survival data. Agreement using multiple techniques makes it clear that neonatal red cells, particularly from premature infants, have a shorter survival than adult erythrocytes.[7] No clear understanding of why neonatal red cells have a shortened survival is available. In terms of their basic membrane protein and lipid structure, neonatal and adult red cell membranes are qualitatively and quantitatively similar. The metabolism of neonatal red cells does not differ markedly from adult red cells; nevertheless, a few differences deserve discussion.

As mentioned previously, neonatal cells do not tolerate in vitro metabolic stress, demonstrating rapid shape changes and decreased deformability. The reason for this susceptibility is unknown. In addition, normal red cell membranes exposed to free 2,3-DPG undergo a loss of integrity as a result of the diminished interaction between red cell spectrin and actin in the presence of elevated concentrations of 2,3-DPG.[16–18] Because of the decreased interaction of 2,3-DPG with deoxyhemoglobin F, the amount of free 2,3-DPG at any level of hemoglobin oxygen saturation is higher in fetal and neonatal red cells. Premature infants, who have relatively low concentrations of Hb A, have higher free 2,3-DPG levels. In addition, factors that shift the hemoglobin oxygen dissociation curve to the right, such as hypoxia in the tissues, further increase the amount of free 2,3-DPG. This might create a paradoxical shortening of red cell life-span in the face of increased tissue oxygen needs.

APPROACH TO NEONATAL ANEMIA AND THE ANEMIA OF PREMATURITY

Creation of a data base of normal hematologic data from small, difficult to access neonates has always been a challenge. Analysis of a given value must be based on an understanding that many dynamic changes are ongoing with each postnatal day of life. Alterations in values during the first 8 weeks of life are perhaps the most dramatic changes seen in normal hematologic data. Thus, one must take into account the prenatal gestational age of the infant, the infant's functional health status, the presence of cardiac or pulmonary pathology, and the postnatal age of the infant. In addition, the acute changes related to the conduct of labor, the presence or absence of umbilical vessel transfusion, and the exact nature of the blood sampling methodology must be considered as well. When the effects of these variables are learned, their actions on the known pattern of postnatal changes in red cell mass and function can be predicted. Figure 64-4 is a developmental approach to the appearance of various causes of anemia. This chapter presents discussions of these illnesses in the order in which a clinician needs to detect the problem and to suggest therapy to protect the child.

TABLE 64-4. Survival Studies of Neonatal Red Cells*

	Adults	Term Infants	Premature Infants
^{51}Cr half-life (d)	25–30	23.3	16.6
Calculated survival (d)	120	60–70	35–50

* Mean of six studies in term infants (51 subjects) and four studies in premature infants (31 subjects).

(Data from Pearson HA. Life-span of the fetal red blood cell. J Pediatr 1967;70:166)

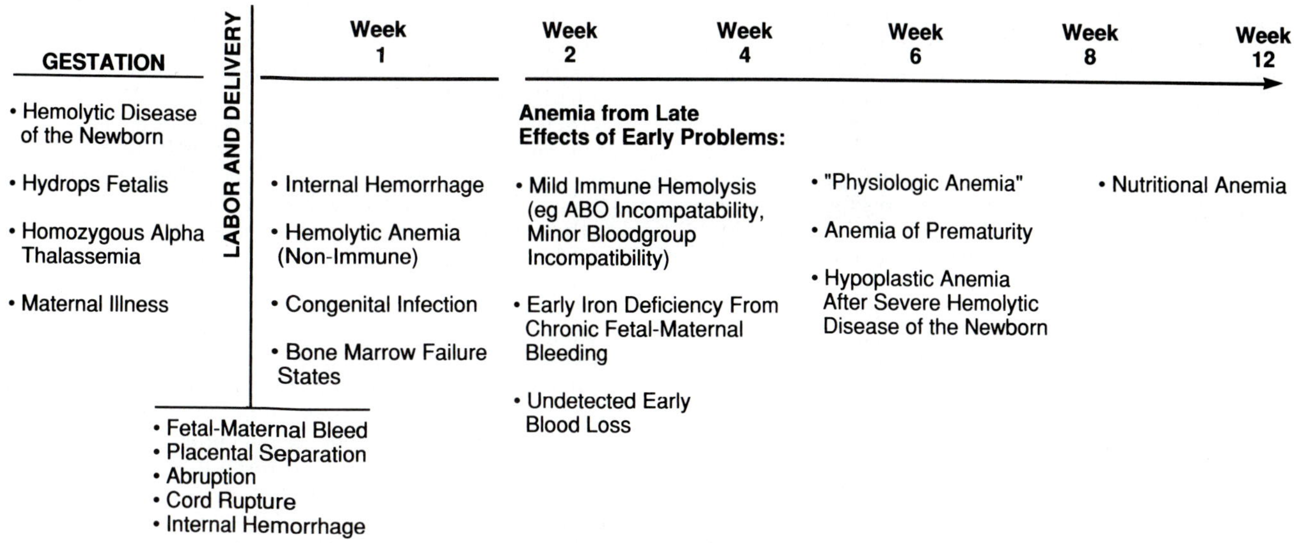

FIGURE 64-4. Developmental differential diagnosis of neonatal anemia.

PRENATAL ANEMIA

The major causes of prenatal anemia, which are important to detect, are homozygous α-thalassemia and hemolytic disease of the newborn (HDN; erythroblastosis fetalis). (Homozygous α-thalassemia will be discussed in the section on hemoglobinopathies.) Because the classic case of severe HDN begins in gestation, we will discuss it in this section.

HEMOLYTIC DISEASE OF THE NEWBORN

The immunologic fortress between mother and child during pregnancy can be breached by sensitization to fetal red cell antigens occurring as a result of micro or macro fetal–maternal hemorrhage. The humoral response of the mother's immune system to the appearance of these fetal antigens, if they differ from her own genotype, can pass across the placenta and bind to the fetal red cells, leading to extravascular hemolysis in the affected infant. This is hemolytic disease of hte newborn.

As depicted in Figure 64-5, several discrete events must come together for the fetal red cell to be at risk for hemolysis. First, the mother must have had prior sensitization by a fetal antigen that she does not have. In most cases, an amnestic response of the immune system is required to create specific immunoglobulin G (IgG) in large enough quantities to pass through the placenta and lead to fetal red cell hemolysis. This prior sensitization can occur in many ways, but the most common way is through prior pregnancy, because of the small amounts of fetal–maternal hemorrhage that occur in most pregnancies.[23] The capacity

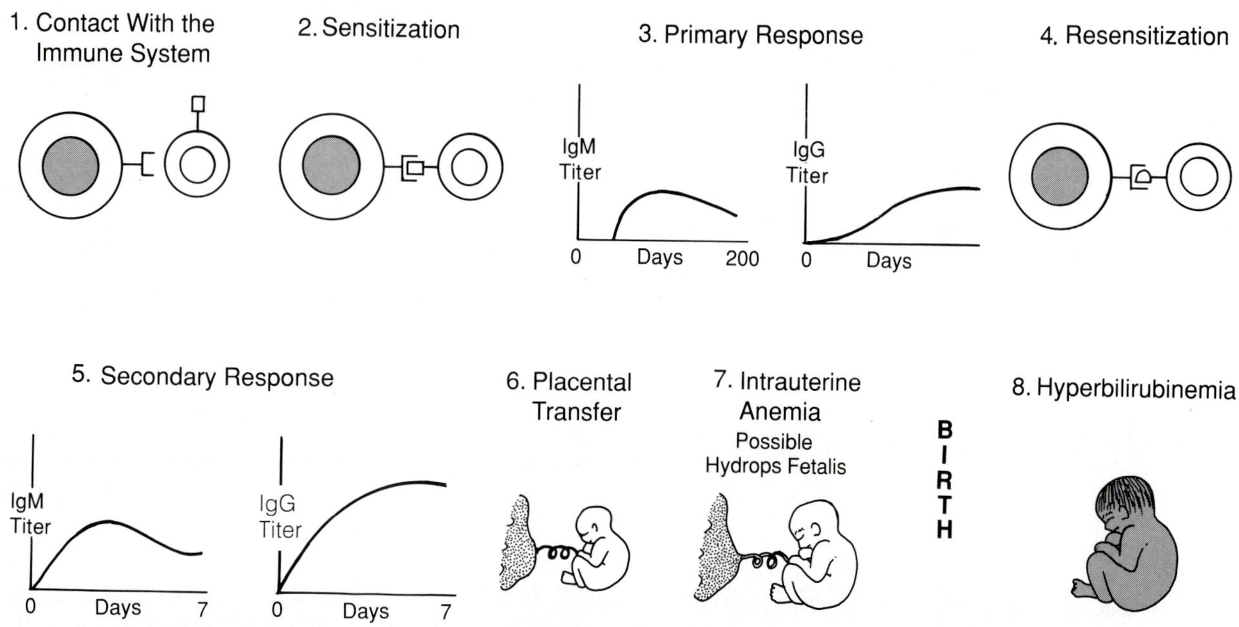

FIGURE 64-5. Necessary steps in the evolution of hemolytic disease of the newborn. Although the figure depicts the Rh(D) antigen, this sequence occurs in all prenatal sensitization, regardless of the red cell antigen involved.

of red cell antigens to induce sensitization varies, so it is important to understand the amount of red cells and the number of exposures to a particular antigen required to elicit a significant maternal immune response.[24]

The next step is the actual maternal response to immunization. The primary response to immunization usually leads to the production of a small amount of IgM and IgG directed toward the antigen. A second exposure often leads to an explosive increase in both IgG and IgM activities with the IgM activity falling after a month's time, and the IgG level rising and remaining elevated as long as antigenic stimulation is present.[25] After the antibody toward a fetal antigen is created in the mother, it must cross the placenta. Because placental transfer of antibodies depends on the Fc portion of the IgG molecule, IgM antibodies do not penetrate the fetal circulation. As the amount of IgG antibody directed against a fetal antigen increases, more may cross the placenta into the fetal circulation. In general, the time course of IgG passage is slow, with a half-life of about 3 weeks.[25] Hence, the effect of the rising titer in the maternal circulation is blunted by the delay in the movement of antibody across the placenta. It is not surprising, then, that investigators have considered the rise in maternal titer to a given antigen to be a strong indicator of fetal outcome.[26]

Next, the clinician must assess the effect of having the antibody and the fetal red cells that contain the targeted antigen together in vivo. For reasons that have not been elucidated, antibodies of a given class or subclass may have different interactions, depending on the antigen to which they are directed. Table 64-5 demonstrates some of the more common antigens and whether they produce HDN.

TABLE 64-5. **Relative Strength of Antigens on Cord Cells and Antigens Implicated in Hemolytic Disease of the Newborn (HDN)**

Antigen Strength	Blood Group System or Antigen	Caused HDN
I. Well-developed at birth	MNSsU	Yes*
	Rh	Yes
	Kell	Yes
	Duffy	Yes
	Kidd	Yes
	Diego	Yes
	Dombrock	Yes (mild)
	Scianna	
	Gerbich	Yes (mild)
	En^a	
	Yt^b	
II. Present at birth—weaker than adult	ABH	Yes
	P	Not
	Lutheran	Yes
III. Very weak or absent at birth	Yt^a	
	Vel	
	Lewis	
	I	No
	Sd^a	No

* Anti-M is rarely a cause of HDN.
† Anti-Tj^a (Anti-PP1P^k) has caused HDN.
(Kline W. Chemistry of blood group antigens and antibodies in hemolytic disease of the newborn. In: Bell C, ed. A seminar on perinatal blood banking. Washington, DC, American Association of Blood Banks, 1978:21)

In general, the *antigen strength* (the amount of agglutination seen with incubation of red cells with a given concentration of specific antibody) relates to the severity of disease seen in HDN. If an IgG hemolysin is present and an antigen is strong enough to lead to the binding of this antibody to the red cell, removal of the red cell with extravascular hemolysis will occur. This can be quantitatively described by analyzing red cell survival after the coating of red cells with more and more antigen-directed IgG.[27]

The final step, the entrapment of coated red cells by the spleen and reticuloendothelial system, may also be affected by gestational or neonatal age and well-being. Nonetheless, when all these antigen–antibody variables fall into place, hemolysis does not appear to be significantly curtailed by the known hyposplenism of the neonate. In vivo, anemia is the cost of this red cell antibody interaction sometimes leading to fetal death before intrauterine transfusion or direct fetal intravascular transfusion.

Clinically, HDN carries with it other potential sequelae beyond the effects of anemia in the neonatal period. Hyperbilirubinemia and its toxicities are also challenges for the neonate with hemolysis. This depends on the rate of entrapment of red cells by the neonatal reticuloendothelial system and the production of bilirubin from the grams of hemoglobin processed in the reticuloendothelial system. Using this model, the effect of various red cell incompatibilities can be examined and understood.

RH(D) DISEASE

Because Rh(D) disease is the most serious form of HDN, we will critically examine the effect of Rh(D) incompatibility within the pattern described in the previous section. (For a description of the Rh blood group system antigen, see Chapter 56.) The first step in assessing the intensity of HDN involving Rh(D) antigen is a consideration of how the mother first becomes sensitized to the antigen and how consistent sensitization is. How often will an Rh(D)-negative mother encounter an Rh(D)-positive fetus? The risk of this setup obviously is related to the prevalence of Rh(D)-positive and Rh(D)-negative persons. Among white populations, the incidence of the Rh(D)-negative genotype ranges between 11% and 21%. American blacks have an incidence of 5.5%. Virtually no Rh(D)-negative persons are found among Japanese, Chinese, and most American Indian groups. Therefore, the combination of an Rh(D)-negative mother and an Rh(D)-positive fetus is much greater in the white population.[25,28]

An Rh(D)-negative woman can be exposed to Rh(D)-positive cells either through transfusion or as a result of intermittent fetal–maternal transfusion. The percentage of sensitization under these circumstances is not 100%.[25] Previous studies have demonstrated that exposure to either fetal or adult Rh(D)-positive erythrocytes can lead to Rh(D) immunization in Rh(D)-negative persons. As expected, the incidence of sensitization from a single injection of Rh(D)-positive erythrocytes increases as the volume of Rh(D)-positive cells is increased.[25,29] Usually, the Rh(D)-negative mother becomes sensitized as a result of multiple small exposures to fetal blood across the placenta throughout the pregnancy. Evidence for this comes from studies that examine the effect of repeated injections of small infusions of fetal or adult Rh(D)-positive erythrocytes in normal Rh(D)-negative volunteers.[25,29–32] Although this is a highly effective way to achieve the formation of anti-Rh(D) in the Rh(D)-negative person, not all Rh(D)-negative persons are sensitized by even extreme exposures. Twenty to 40% of Rh(D)-negative persons exposed even multiple times to red cells expressing the Rh(D) antigen do not become sensitized.[7]

As an experimental extension of this idea, Zipursky and colleagues[29] analyzed the risk of formal sensitization in relation to the calculated volume of fetal red cells found in the maternal circulation postpartum by the Kleihauer-Betke test. Of those women who had 0.1 mL or less of fetal red cells in their circulation, only 3% were sensitized. Five of 35 mothers (14.3%) who had more than 0.1 mL of fetal cells detected postpartum were sensitized. These data strongly support prevention strategies designed to diminish the amount of exposure of an Rh(D)-negative mother to fetal Rh(D)-positive red cells by clearing them rapidly with passively administered anti-Rh(D) antibody.

When an Rh(D)-negative mother is exposed to Rh(D)-positive cells and is destined to be a responder, a primary immunization occurs. This involves the appearance of small amounts of IgM or IgG anti-Rh(D) that is detectable in maternal serum. In mothers who encounter a large volume of Rh(D)-positive fetal red cells, such as in toxemia of pregnancy or placental injury (such as abruption), the clinician is more likely to subsequently discover obvious anti-Rh(D) in the serum. In most cases, the primary immunization is not detectable using standard serologic methods. In both situations, an amnestic response occurs during the next pregnancy of an Rh(D)-positive fetus. Based on approximations of the number of women exposed to a given volume of red cells and the percentage of responders, Zipursky has calculated that of 1000 women sensitized in a first pregnancy to Rh(D), significant titers of anti-Rh(D) will occur in 160 subsequent pregnancies with an Rh(D)-positive fetus.[25]

From these maternal titers, a slow transference of antibodies, especially of the IgG class, will cross the placenta and begin binding to Rh(D)-positive red cells in the fetal circulation.[23] Rh(D) antigen is well established on fetal red cells, and the amount of antibody–antigen binding is directly proportional to the rate of red cell removal, and hence to the survival of the sensitized fetal red cells. Higher titers of maternal anti-Rh(D) may lead to higher titers of fetal anti-Rh(D), a shorter red cell survival, more severe anemia, and more problems with hyperbilirubinemia. Figure 64-6 represents the data of Mollison and colleagues[27] examining red cell survival as it relates to how densely coated red cells are with anti-Rh(D) antibody. The amount of anti-Rh(D) on each red cell is obviously a strong determinant of survival. It is logical, then, that the maternal titer of anti-Rh(D) has long been used to guide concerns about fetal status during pregnancy.

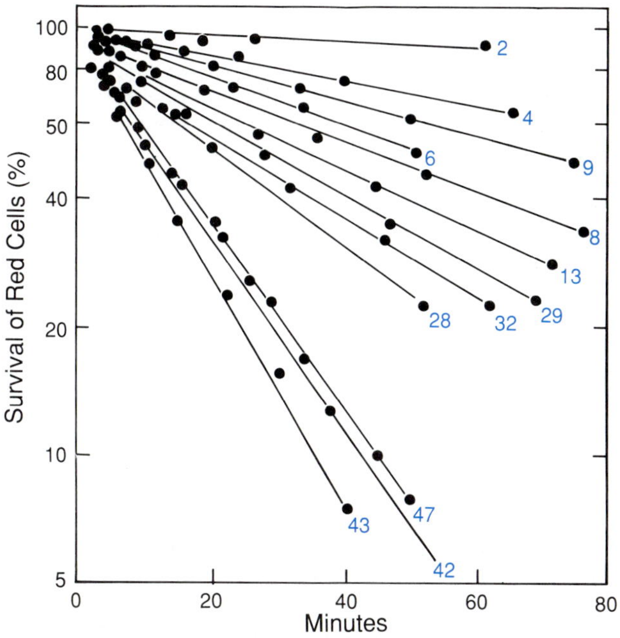

FIGURE 64-6. In vivo survival of Rh-D positive red cells coated with anti-Rh(D) antibody. The numbers next to each line represent the amount (micrograms per milliliter of red cells) of anti-Rh(D) antibody on the red cells. The greater the amount of antibody on the red cell, the shorter the red cell survival (After Mollison PL, Crome P, et al. Rate of removable from the circulation of the red cells sensitized with different amounts of antibody. Br J Hematol 1965;11:461)

Prevention Strategies for Anti-Rh(D) Immunization

In the discussion of Rh(D) HDN, the best strategy is prevention of sensitization. Thus, before considering therapy for the disease, we will discuss its prevention using RhoGAM (anti-Rh[D]). The discovery that passively administered anti-Rh(D) could prevent maternal immunization by fetal Rh(D)-positive cells led to a rapid fall in the incidence of anti-Rh(D) HDN.[33] The use of RhoGAM has reduced the immunization rate (in ABO-compatible pregnancies) from about 15% to about 1.5%.[34–37]

Effect of ABO Incompatibility on Rh(D) Sensitization

In addition to our previous discussion about limiting the volume of fetal blood that would expose an Rh(D)-negative mother to Rh(D)-positive fetal red cells, another important experimental observation gave great optimism for the success of such an approach. Examination of Rh immunization in Rh(D)-negative women producing Rh(D)-positive fetuses revealed a striking lack of sensitization when the infant's ABO blood type was A or B and the mother's was O. Rh(D)-positive fetal cells that might sensitize the Rh(D) mother were thought to be removed from the circulation by maternal anti-A or anti-B, preventing the maternal immune system from being presented with the Rh(D) antigen.[38] Further experiments by Stern and associates[39] revealed that ABO-incompatible Rh(D)-positive red cells did not sensitize Rh(D)-negative persons in experimental models in both animals and humans. Of importance is the fact that this ABO protection did not protect an ABO-incompatible Rh(D)-positive fetus from sensitizing the mother if the mother had a prior sensitization from an Rh(D)-positive ABO-compatible donor. These studies, along with the theoretical value of simply removing Rh(D)-positive cells from the circulation by anti-Rh(D), led to the institution of Rh immunoprophylaxis.[40]

Treatment With Anti-Rh(D)

In its beginnings, 300 μg of anti-Rh(D) (RhoGAM) were administered intramuscularly at the time of delivery of an Rh(D)-positive fetus to an Rh(D)-negative mother under circumstances in which an episode of fetal–maternal bleeding was considered possible, such as in amniocentesis, and in therapeutic or spontaneous abortions in which the neonate's blood type remained unknown. The dose of 300 μg is estimated to be protective for fetal–maternal bleeding episodes up to 15 mL of packed red cells, which accounts for 99.7% of all pregnancies.[33,41] Nonetheless, even when scrupulously adhered to, the current regimens of anti-Rh(D) prophylaxis lead to a 1.5% immunization rate for Rh(D)-negative mothers. Reasons for this failure rate are largely theoretical. One theory supposes that an Rh(D)-negative mother is sensitized as a fetus by maternal–fetal bleeding from her Rh(D)-positive mother (grandmother theory).[33,42,43]

Another theory suggests that the effectiveness of anti-Rh(D) by the intramuscular route of administration may suffer as a result of individual variations in absorption of the antibody, leaving a small group of patients who are inadequately protected. An experimental intravenous preparation is available, but this has not come into wide use in America.[44] Large fetal–maternal bleeding episodes might also account for immunoglobulin failure, although few pregnancies have fetal–maternal bleeds greater than 15 mL of packed red cells.

Most popular is the theory that antepartum immunization occurs. Studies have demonstrated that as pregnancy progresses, a greater number of fetal–maternal bleeds take place, even though the size of the fetal–maternal hemorrhage is less than 0.1 mL. Nonetheless, investigators have found fetal cells in the maternal circulation during the third trimester from 10% to 30% of the time.[45] This has led to considerable interest in the use of Rh immunoprophylaxis at 28 weeks of gestation in all previously unsensitized Rh(D)-negative mothers. Studies have shown that the administration of another 300-μg dose of anti-Rh(D) at 28 weeks does achieve its theoretical increment of protection of an additional 60% to 90%, lowering the sensitization rate from 1.5% to somewhere between 0.8% and 0.15%.[25,37]

Clearly, the best way to treat a disease is to prevent its occurrence. Anti-Rh(D) has proved to be virtually nontoxic. Rh(D)-positive infants are not born with significant hemolytic anemia as the result of the small passive transfer of Rh(D) antibody into the infant. Physicians involved with the treatment of neonates are well aware of the phenomenon of a positive Coombs' test seen in an Rh(D)-positive fetus born to a mother who has received antenatal anti-Rh(D).[33] Experienced clinicians realize that this is a temporary artifact not leading to any major clinical symptomatology. It can be a source of confusion if other reasons for anemia in the neonatal period are occurring simultaneously. One way to analyze the amount of Rh(D) antibody in a neonate whose mother has received antepartum anti-Rh(D) is to look at the ability of maternal serum to agglutinate Rh(D)-positive red cells and at the strength of the direct antiglobulin test of the Rh(D)-positive neonate. If the maternal indirect Coombs' test is weak and directed against Rh(D), it is usually due to the passively administered anti-Rh(D), and the direct Coombs' test results of the infant will be weak as well.

Although the practice is controversial, most centers consider administering antenatal anti-Rh(D) for all nonimmunized Rh(D)-negative mothers to further decrease the potential for development of severe erythroblastosis fetalis from Rh(D) disease.

Typical Clinical Issues

The basic pattern of HDN is set by individual variations of the fetal–maternal unit in the steps outlined previously. Although ABO incompatibility occurs most frequently, the clinical picture of moderate to severe erythroblastosis fetalis, which is the most severe form of HDN, is primarily seen in association with anti-Rh(D) antibody. We will discuss the clinical picture of HDN in reference to the latter illness. In the clinical syndrome of HDN, the clinician must distinguish three separate periods of illness:

1. The in utero threat to the child is one of anemia, hydrops fetalis, and stillbirth. Problems of hyperbilirubinemia are handled during this time by the detoxification systems of the mother. Hence, hyperbilirubinemia causes no threat to the child in utero.
2. At birth, the child undertakes the task of detoxifying the increasing amounts of bilirubin formed as the result of ongoing hemolysis. The second period is devoted primarily to strategies to prevent central nervous system injury as the result of hyperbilirubinemia. This period begins shortly after birth. Complicating medical problems and the stresses and risks of exchange transfusion also ensue during this time.
3. Finally, the issues surrounding prevention of anemia in the womb and detoxification of hyperbilirubinemia after birth usually lead to an exaggeration of physiologic anemia with a chronic hypoproductive anemia that can go on for over 3 months.

Each of these zones of illness is considered individually and discussed in reference to Rh(D) disease.

A cycle of red cell destruction and ineffective red cell production is set up by immune hemolytic anemia occurring in the infant as a result of the passage of Rh(D) antibodies from the mother to an Rh(D)-positive fetus. Red cells sensitized by maternal antibody are destroyed in the reticuloendothelial system of the fetus. Fetal red cells have a relatively short life-span to begin with (see Table 64-4), and the life of the antibody-coated Rh(D)-positive fetal red cell is further shortened. The relative deficiency of oxygen-carrying capacity in the fetus leads to enhanced erythropoietin production, increased bone marrow erythroid production, and hepatosplenomegaly with extramedullary hematopoiesis as the fetus makes a vain attempt to keep up with the hemolytic rate.[46] Uninterrupted, this cycle may lead to an enlarging mass of erythroid-producing tissue in the placenta and throughout the reticuloendothelial system of the fetus. it may also cause an increase in plasma volume, high-output congestive heart failure secondary to anemia, the appearance of hydrops fetalis, and, ultimately, tissue hypoxia, acidosis, and death.

The severity of the anemia is directly related to the balance between red cell destruction and red cell production and is the key determinant of the severity of the illness of the infant. Individual variations in maternal antibody production and fetal red cell destruction determine whether an infant is born with a mild hemolytic anemia and mild hyperbilirubinemia or is a stillborn succumbing to chronic severe hemolytic anemia and hydrops fetalis.[25,27]

Somewhere in the downward spiral of hemolytic disease of the newborn, the syndrome of hydrops fetalis occurs. Hydrops fetalis can be seen when any pathophysiology leads to severe chronic fetal anemia. The syndrome is characterized by massive edema and anasarca with pleural effusions and ascites.[25] The edema is easily demonstrable by ultrasonography.[47,48] Before the use of anti-Rh(D), the cause of hydrops fetalis in most infants was Rh(D) erythroblastosis fetalis. The combination of prevention strategies and the treatment of affected fetuses with intrauterine peritoneal transfusion or intrauterine direct intravascular transfusion has fortunately led to a much decreased incidence of this syndrome as the result of Rh(D) disease.[33]

Theoretically, this severe edematous disorder would be a direct outgrowth of severe anemia and congestive heart failure. However, hydrops has occurred in fetuses without significant anemia, and there have been severely anemic fetuses who have not had hydrops fetalis.[49] Other factors are likely to be involved. One candidate is the degree of tissue hypoxia, since that would be subject to a variety of factors, including maternal health, the integrity of the placental unit, and individual variations in infant cardiac function, as well as the degree of anemia.[50] Increases in tissue hypoxia are known to lead to elevated central venous and arterial pressures, which cause further stress to a fetal heart trying to keep up with anemia.

Treatment of Rh(D) Erythroblastosis Fetalis

Intrauterine Transfusions

All Rh(D)-positive neonates growing in an Rh(D)-negative sensitized mother are at risk for intrauterine death. The treatment of severe Rh(D) HDN was the first example of direct fetal therapy. Although intrauterine transfusion into the peritoneum of the infant was a remarkable step forward, with fetal death rates as high as 6% it should considered a risky procedure.[51] Hence, a number of studies have been done to find criteria to target intrauterine transfusion therapy to the infant at the greatest risk. Because of the ability to accelerate the maturation of fetal lungs in utero with corticosteroids, the risk of early delivery of a child also has to be taken into consideration, a risk that is probably less than 2% in fetuses older than than 33 weeks.[52]

The following are the current criteria that the clinician should use in deciding whether an intrauterine transfusion should be performed.

- History of previous infant with severe Rh(D) anti-hemolytic disease
- Rising maternal titer of Rh anti-Rh(D)
- Ultrasonography: presence of placental enlargement, ascites, effusions, anasarca
- Amniotic fluid bilirubin

The history of a previous stillbirth and the rate of rise of maternal anti-Rh(D) titer are best used as discriminators for deciding which mothers should receive amniocentesis. Monitoring the infant by ultrasonography should be added to this list, since disturbances of fetal growth and the presence of edema, pleural effusions, or ascites are more quantitative findings and suggest a move to amniocentesis.[47]

Nonetheless, the gold standard for deciding which infants require intrauterine, intraperitoneal, or intravascular transfusions is the spectrophotometric profile of amniotic fluid bilirubin levels. Figure 64-7 shows the classic profile, scanning the wavelength between 350 and 700 nm and looking at optical density (absorbance) at 450 mm compared with baseline. The amount of bilirubin in the amniotic fluid is an indicator of the degree of hemolysis occurring in the neonate. Intensity of hemolysis is related to the severity of the anemia. Accordingly, the amount of bilirubin in the amniotic fluid can be correlated to the incidence of severe anemia and stillbirth. When amniocentesis is performed (usually at 20 to 21 weeks) to assess fetal risks for stillbirth, measurement of the amniotic fluid bilirubin is made. The level of bilirubin is low in infants without HDN (0.04 mg/dL). When the optical density at 450 nm rises above 0.1, the diagnosis of a sensitized pregnancy becomes definitive.[53] When a value above 0.1 is seen, the obstetrician may elect sampling at 1- or 2-week intervals, depending on other parameters that suggest the urgency of the situation (rising maternal titer, ultrasonographic changes). If a rising trend is seen within zone 2 or from zone 2 to zone 3, fetal anemia is likely to be life-threatening.[54]

Intrauterine intraperitoneal transfusion was the only option for severely afflicted infants until the technique of intrauterine direct intravascular transfusion became available. Intrauterine intraperitoneal transfusion carries with it a 5% or 6% mortality rate to the treated infants, although maternal morbidity is low.[51] In the technique, donor blood with a hematocrit level of 80% to 90% is instilled into the fetal peritoneal cavity by direct injection. Most of the cells are eventually absorbed, but the amount of donor blood is limited by fetal age because of pressure created within the fetal abdomen.[54,55]

During the past several years, intrauterine intravascular transfusion has begun to replace the intraperitoneal transfusion technique.[56,57] In intravascular transfusion, a needle is guided directly into the fetal circulation. In this method, more of the infused hemoglobin gains immediate access to the infant's circulation with far less risk. Intraperitoneally administered red cells require fetal breathing movements to coerce red cells into the circulation, and thus the effect of transfusion is much less in a sick, inert neonate. Intravascular transfusion leads to immediate improvement. Therefore, infants discovered late in their disease or infants with hydrops fetalis respond much better to the intravascular technique.[56] Harman and colleagues[56] attempted a case control comparison of intraperitoneal with intravascular intrauterine transfusion. Not unexpectedly, they found a significantly lower incidence of fetal mortality (8 of 44 intraperitoneal, 1 of 44 intravascular), decreased risks of procedural complication (39 of 104 intraperitoneal, 17 of 173 intravascular), fewer infants born with Apgar scores less than 7 at 5 minutes (13 of 34 intraperitoneal, 6 of 42 intravascular), and fewer days in the intensive care nursery (8.25 intraperitoneal, 6.1 intravascular). With time, the intravascular approach will probably completely supplant the use of intraperitoneal transfusion.

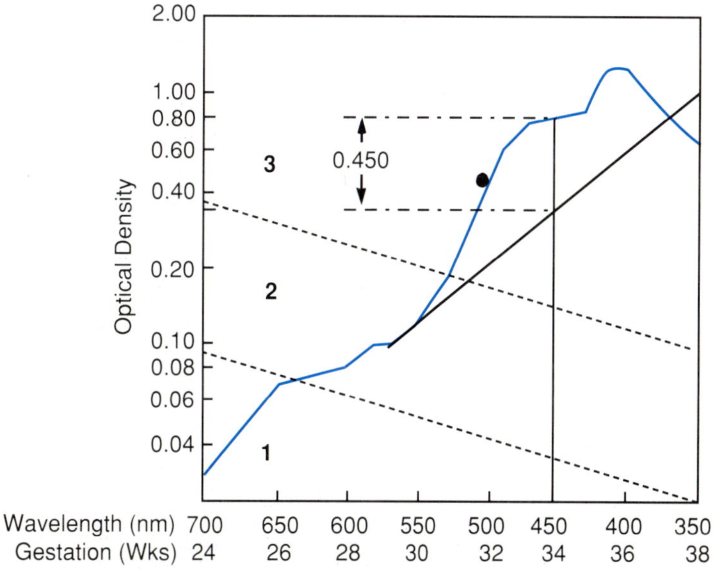

FIGURE 64-7. Amniotic fluid spectrophotometric measurement of bilirubin. The optical density is measured from 350 to 700 nm. The optical density at 450 nm contributed by bilirubin is measured by the increase in optical density at that wavelength above the projected baseline (*straight line*). The corrected optical density 450 in this case is 0.45. This value is then replotted on the same graph, using the optical density scale on the Y axis and the gestational age scale on the X axis, and its position relative to zones 1, 2, and 3 (defined by the slanted lines) is noted. In this case (32.5 weeks of gestation), the resultant point (*dot*) lies in zone 3, a region that indicated severe disease with impending fetal death. Zone 2 represents less severe disease, and zone 1 indicates very mild disease or an Rh-negative fetus. (After Bowman JM, Pollock JM. Amniotic fluid spectrophotometry and early delivery in the management of erythroblastosis fetalis. Pediatrics 1965;35:815)

Patients successfully receiving intrauterine transfusion can be safely delivered after 33 weeks if the lecithin/sphingomyelin ratio of the amniotic fluid is mature (over 1.5).[25] Such maturity can be hastened by the use of maternal corticosteroids, if indicated. As mentioned previously, infants with little evidence of severe hemolysis or severe anemia can be delivered at this time to avoid future intrauterine risks. Those requiring intrauterine transfusion, especially when treated by the intravascular route, may be induced for delivery later, since they would clearly not be suffering from as severe an anemia.

At birth, many infants given intravascular transfusion require exchange transfusion, despite the fact that Rh(D)-positive erythrocytes are not seen in cord blood and the reticulocyte count appears low. This is most likely caused by the continuing presence of maternal anti-Rh(D) in the plasma of the neonate, hemolyzing the reticulocytes and some late erythroid precursors. This has special significance in the consideration of late anemia.

Hyperbilirubinemia

At birth, even infants with severe HDN may not be jaundiced because the placenta clears bilirubin using maternal liver function.[23] In infants with severe HDN, a cord bilirubin should be performed, because this is often a useful determinant and may be elevated even in the absence of clinical jaundice.[58] In most HDN patients, jaundice is seen within the first day of life and continues to rise until either the rate of hemolysis falls or the maturing fetal liver is better able to handle the hyperbilirubinemia. In utero, bilirubin is bound to fetal albumin and probably crosses the chorionic membrane, attaches to maternal albumin, and is detoxified. Small amounts of bilirubin enter the amniotic fluid. This relatively small pool turns over slowly but is important as an indicator of the rate of hemolysis in the fetus.[59] The neonate faces continued hemolysis, even after multiple intrauterine intraperitoneal or vascular transfusions, because of continued production of Rh(D)-positive red cells. Given that 1 g of hemoglobin leads to the formation of 35 mg of bilirubin, the neonate's diminished ability to clear bilirubin is often no match for the accelerated bilirubin production.

This deficient metabolism appears to be caused by impairment of at least two major steps in the detoxification of bilirubin. First, a deficiency of the hepatocyte bilirubin-binding proteins decreases the amount of bilirubin held in the cell and prepared for the action of enzymatic metabolism.[60] In addition, the enzyme responsible for the metabolism of bilirubin (glucuronyltransferase) is remarkably deficient, leading to decreased formation of bilirubin glucuronide, the major form of bilirubin excreted in the bile.[61] Finally, the relative hypomotility of the bowel of the sick neonate leads to enhanced enterohepatic circulation, with return of bilirubin into the blood.

Hyperbilirubinemia in the neonate can clearly cause brain damage, resulting in severe neurologic damage (deafness, ataxia, cerebral palsy) and rarely in death (see Chap. 50). Evidence that brain damage is a result of bilirubin includes yellow staining of the basal ganglia and cerebellum, kernicterus,[25] studies in hyperbilirubinemic rats demonstrating injury to brain cell mitochondria,[62] and the known distribution of bilirubin in the brains of hyperbilirubinemic rats.[63]

Although the exact mechanisms of the damage to brain tissue by bilirubin is not known, much work has been done in an attempt to identify a level of hyperbilirubinemia at which brain injury might occur. The data suggest that conjugated bilirubin and albumin-bound unconjugated bilirubin do not enter the central nervous system and do not cause toxicity.[64] Therefore, approaches examining at what level bilirubin causes central nervous system toxicity attempt to measure how much bilirubin is unconjugated and unbound to albumin (free unconjugated bilirubin). Many different techniques have been used to make this analysis. Recent techniques can determine free bilirubin levels directly. These levels range from 0.1 to 1 mg/dL.[65] None of the sophisticated bilirubin assays can be applied practically at the present time, and none are backed by enough clinical data to justify their widespread use in determining the need for exchange transfusion.

An understanding of the factors that regulate the unconjugated free bilirubin pool will help guide clinical decisions regarding the treatment of hyperbilirubinemia. Free unconjugated bilirubin produced during the processing of hemolyzed red cells binds primarily to albumin. Albumin contains two major binding sites: a primary higher affinity site and a secondary lower affinity site.[61] Free heme can compete with unconjugated bilirubin for binding at the primary binding site, so in situations in which a large amount of intravascular hemolysis (such as oxidative hemolytic anemia) is present, less bilirubin may be bound to the high-affinity site, increasing the level of free bilirubin.[66] The secondary binding site, with its lower affinity, permits the dangerous displacement of bilirubin as a result of acidosis, drugs,[67] or an increase in fatty acid levels. Table 64-6 lists situations that theoretically render an infant more susceptible to the toxic effects of hyperbilirubinemia.

Treatment

Three approaches are commonly used to treat neonatal hyperbilirubinemia (see Chap. 50).

Phototherapy. In situations in which the risk of a free bilirubin level is small and the clinician wishes to blunt the rate of rise of serum bilirubin, phototherapy is widely used. This method can be successful, thus making exchange transfusion unnecessary. It is critical to observe the hemoglobin of the child simultaneously, since ongoing hemolysis may necessitate transfusion to increase oxygen-carrying capacity, but go unnoticed because bilirubin levels and clinical jaundice seem to be under control.

Drug Therapy. The use of phenobarbital, which stimulates the hepatic metabolism of bilirubin, and synthetic metallaoporphyrins, which inhibit the formation of bilirubin by blocking heme oxygenase, is under scrutiny. These approaches are especially important in units caring for neonates with severe hyperbilirubinemia who

TABLE 64-6. Risk Factors for Injury During Neonatal Hyperbilirubinemia

FACTORS LEADING TO AN INCREASE IN FREE SERUM UNCONJUGATED BILIRUBIN
Hypoalbuminemia
Intravascular hemolysis
Acidosis
Free fatty acids (starvation, dehydration)
Drugs
Antibiotics: sulfonimides, oxacillin, gentamicin
Antiinflammatories: salicylate, hydrocortisone
Central-acting agents: caffeine
DIRECT EFFECTS ON THE NEONATAL BRAIN THAT MAY CONTRIBUTE TO BILIRUBIN TOXICITY
Prematurity
Hypoxia
Hypoglycemia

have scant resources for phototherapy and exchange transfusion.[68]

Exchange Transfusion. The most definitive treatment for hyperbilirubinemia related to HDN is exchange transfusion. This procedure is not without risk, especially in the low birth weight infant. Accordingly, clinicians have attempted to devise guidelines that balance the risk of central nervous system damage with the risk of exchange transfusion and the possibility of less toxic approaches, such as phototherapy, succeeding. In most cases, the decision for exchange transfusion is based on the observation of the rate of rise of bilirubin in the immediate neonatal period. Severely affected infants, especially those who have not had intrauterine transfusions and hence continue to have a large percentage of circulating Rh(D)-positive red cells, may be considered for immediate exchange transfusion.

Investigators have come up with varying criteria for immediate exchange. Cord hemoglobins of 10.5[69] to 13[58] g/dL, and cord bilirubin levels above 4[58] to 4.5[69] mg/dL have been suggested. Oski recommends that immediate exchange be reserved for the asphyxiated, severely anemic neonate, with frequent bilirubin determinations after birth to detect the infant who may be at future risk of bilirubin toxicity.[70] The guidelines for exchange transfusion due to anemia are based on older studies and do not reflect the changing nature of the red cell population in the severely affected neonate who has been rescued from severe intrauterine anemia by direct intravascular transfusion of Rh(D)-negative red cells. In the case of such infants, although the hematocrit may not approach an expected hematocrit at birth, the amount of hemolysis and bilirubin formation are significantly less, since a large percentage of the cells are Rh(D)-negative.

The rate of rise of indirect bilirubin in the neonate after birth still continues to be the major determinant for exchange transfusion in those infants whose cord bilirubin does not exceed 4 mg/dL, but who continue at risk for hyperbilirubinemia because of ongoing hemolysis. Most neonatologists perform exchange transfusion in full-term infants with levels of indirect bilirubin greater than 20 mg/dL within the first 72 hours of life. In those centers with access to assays of free indirect bilirubin, any evidence of free unconjugated bilirubin should also prompt exchange transfusion, even if the total indirect bilirubin is less than 20 mg/dL.[25] One investigator has suggested that exchange transfusion should be considered in any infant whose serum bilirubin concentration (in mg/dL) exceeds his or her age in hours.[58] A rate of rise of indirect bilirubin greater than 0.17 mg/dL/h during the first 12 hours after birth has also been suggested.[70]

Figure 64-8 demonstrates one of the standard graphic approaches also used in the literature to aid in deciding when to exchange. All agree that the presence of the accelerators of bilirubin toxicity (see Table 64-6) should encourage earlier exchange transfusion than might be considered from the rate of rise of bilirubin alone.

Only the clinician at the bedside with a knowledge of the risks and benefits of exchange transfusion and an understanding of how the functional health status of the affected neonate contributes to his or her sensitivity to bilirubin damage can decide how to interpret the various guideposts in the literature in reference to the individual child.

Practical Issues in Neonatal Exchange Transfusion. Exchange transfusion may benefit the neonate with severe HDN in three ways: by reversing anemia, by washing out bilirubin, and by removing Rh(D)-positive red cells and replacing them with Rh(D)-negative cells, thus removing the source of continued bilirubin production.

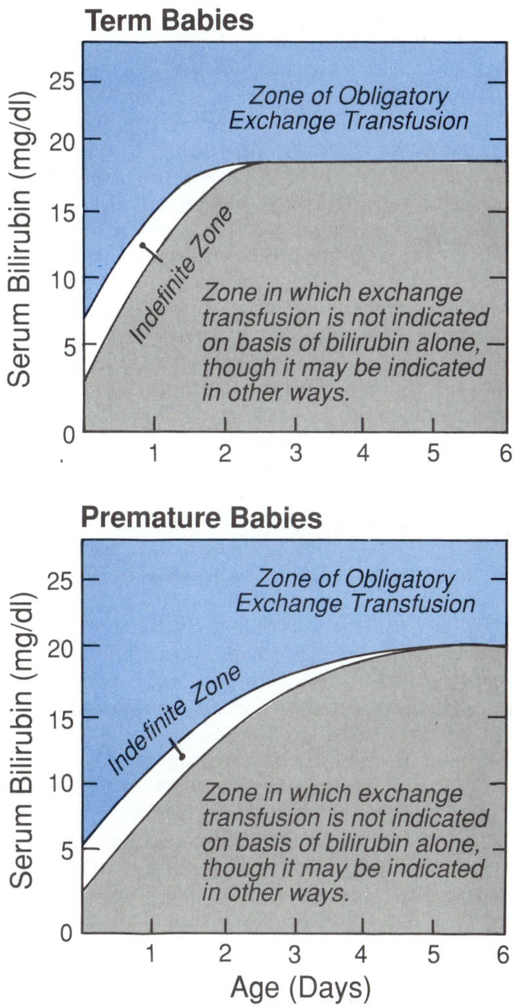

FIGURE 64-8. Graphical guidelines for exchange transfusion in term and premature infants. (After Oski FA, Naiman JL. Hematologic problems of the newborn. Philadelphia, WB Saunders 1982:302)

The procedure of exchange transfusion is simple. The blood of the neonate containing bilirubin (bound and free) and sensitized red cells available for hemolysis is removed and replaced with blood containing fresh albumin for bilirubin adsorption (to decrease free unconjugated bilirubin levels) and new adult red cells of a blood group that will not hemolyze. The exchange procedure always represents a risk to the neonate. In general, the greater the need of the infant for exchange transfusion, the more likely are increased risk factors (eg, prematurity, acidosis, hypoglycemia). Several aspects of the exchange require careful consideration: the blood product used, the desired volume of exchange, and toxic side effects of the exchange.

Most sources recommend using ABO-compatible, Rh(D)-negative fresh whole blood (less than 5 days old) or other appropriate antigen-negative blood (for HDN caused by antigens other than Rh[D]), on the basis that this will preserve 2,3-DPG levels (preventing tissue hypoxia) and diminish hyperkalemia. (Potassium levels rise in the supernatant of red cells throughout storage.[25]) Modern blood bank programs store primarily blood components, with red cells stored in adenine-containing storage solutions. Thus, blood for exchange transfusion is prepared by reconstituting the freshest compatible packed red cell units with fresh frozen plasma. Most hospitals follow their own consistent program based on their resources and the availability of fresh donor blood. Both patterns of transfusion (fresh whole blood 6 to 90 hours old or reconstituted units) have been successfully used.[71]

The desired volume of exchange also varies among practitioners. Early exchange to remove sensitized red cells and prospectively decrease bilirubin production can be very successful. Seventy-five percent of recipient red cells are removed after a single volume exchange, 90% after a double volume exchange.

Removal of total body bilirubin is more difficult.[71] Unconjugated bilirubin is bound to albumin in the intravascular and extravascular spaces. Double volume exchange transfusion removes 90% of intravascular albumin and 150% of the preexchange amount of intravascular bilirubin.[72] Hence, bilirubin must be rapidly moving from extravascular sites to the new albumin being infused. Because the serum bilirubin falls much less than would be expected from these numbers (an average 55% of the preexchange value), there must be a large extravascular bilirubin compartment.[25] Often, serum bilirubin levels paradoxically rise after exchange transfusion, since more bilirubin is attracted from the extravascular space by fresh albumin.

Figure 64-9 shows that the efficiency of exchange transfusion begins to drop at 1 volume of exchange. This suggests that after the sensitized red cells of the infant have been effectively removed (first 2-volume exchange), more efficiency in bilirubin removed would be obtained by doing two separate 1-volume exchanges, allowing time for bilirubin movement into the extravascular space for exchange removal.[71] Some investigators have recommended extra infusion of albumin before or at the time of exchange transfusion to create a larger intravascular albumin pool to expand the amount of extravascular bilirubin attracted to the intravascular space. More bilirubin can be removed in this way, but care must be taken to avoid volume overload or hematocrit dilution in these sick newborns.[25]

In addition to the usual problems associated with transfusion (see Chap. 60), exchange transfusion in neonates requires special attention to some specific problems.[70] Because most exchange transfusions are now done with reconstituted components, excess potassium may be infused during exchange. Although this usually does not cause symptoms, close monitoring is required. In neonates with concomitant renal failure, red cells may be washed before reconstitution. The slow hepatic metabolism of citrate also contributes to hypocalcemia. Most neonatal centers have protocols involving the prophylactic infusion of calcium during exchange transfusion or careful monitoring of ionized calcium.[2] Acidosis may occur secondary to an acid load from the exchange unit; but once again, this rarely requires specific therapy.[69] Blood sugar should also be monitored since these infants can have ongoing hyperinsulinemia or, conversely, poor glucose tolerance from illness or infection. Finally, postexchange thrombocytopenia is expected in exchanges using blood over a few hours old and may require platelet transfusion.

Graft-versus-host disease has been observed when unirradiated blood has been used for intrauterine transfusion or for exchange transfusion after birth. Most centers have a protocol for irradiating units before use.[71] The sudden appearance of conjugated hyperbilirubinemia, skin rash, eosinophilia, and changes in stool pattern should lead to an investigation of whether unirradiated blood was used in error.

Exchange transfusions continue until bilirubin levels either stabilize consistently below the toxic ranges or a decrease in the rate of bilirubin rise permits control of the hyperbilirubinemia by less invasive modalities.

Although the clinician has improved anemia and is helping to prevent bilirubin toxicity, several attendant syndromes may be encountered. First, severe hypoglycemia has been observed in erythroblastosis, associated with hypertrophy and hyperplasia of the pancreatic islets of Langerhans.[73,74] Hypoglycemia can occur shortly after birth but is usually encountered within the first 24 hours of birth.

Inspissated Bile Syndrome and Other Complications of Erythroblastosis Fetalis

Ironically, conjugated hyperbilirubinemia (occasionally surpassing 20 mg/dL) sometimes can be seen from the moment of birth.[75] This can create confusion and lead clinicians toward the diagnosis of hepatitis, other viral illness, or sepsis, if red cell sensitization is not known to exist before

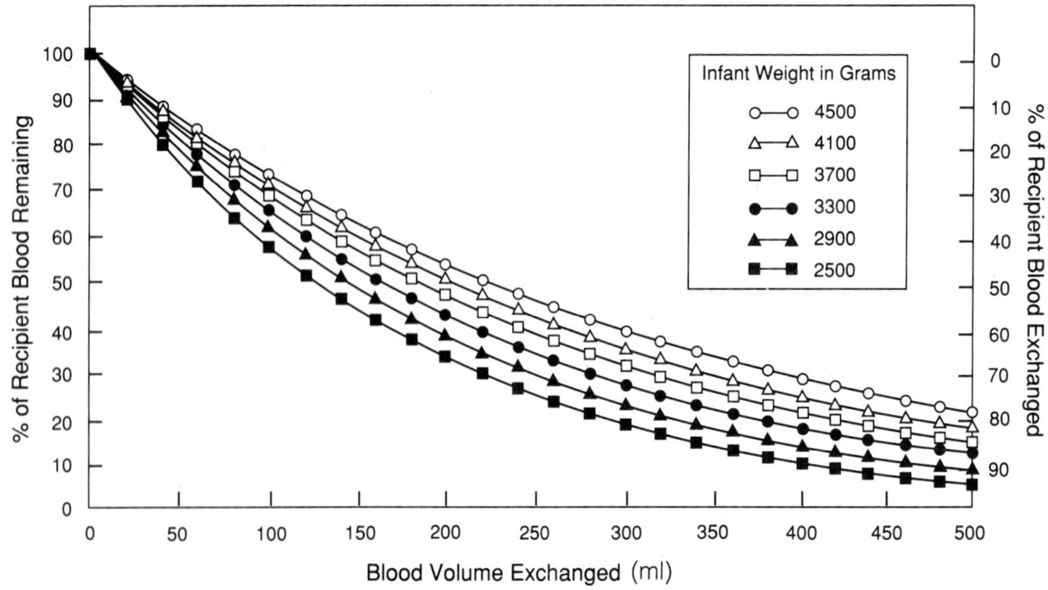

FIGURE 64-9. Predicted efficiency of exchange transfusion in neonates of various birthweights. The curve flattens beyond 250 mL of blood exchanged (about one blood volume for a 3000-g infant), indicating decreased efficiency of neonatal blood removal. (After Buchholz DH. Blood transfusion: merits of component therapy. I. The clinical use of red cells, platelets, and granulocytes. J Pediatr 1974;84:1)

delivery. The cause of inspissated bile syndrome is unknown, but as the hemolysis abates and the general health of the infant improves, the hyperbilirubinemia regresses without sequelae. Table 64-7 compares the clinical features of erythroblastosis fetalis with nonimmune hemolysis and the various congenital viral syndromes that often appear in the differential diagnosis.

Finally, the additive effects of postexchange thrombocytopenia and disseminated intravascular coagulation (either from asphyxia or a separate illness) can place these infants at risk for spontaneous hemorrhagic complications such as intraventricular or intrapulmonary hemorrhage.[25]

Patients with severe erythroblastosis fetalis may develop prolonged chronic hyporegenerative anemia, beginning days to weeks after birth.[76] This will be discussed later in the chapter along with the anemia of prematurity, which it resembles.

ABO INCOMPATIBILITY

ABO incompatibility between mother and fetus is more common and less severe than Rh(D) incompatibility. Hemolytic disease is seen almost exclusively when the mother is blood type O and the infant is type A or B. This happens in about 15% of pregnancies and creates an opportunity for ABO incompatibility to occur.[25] HDN due to ABO incompatibility occurs in far less than 15% of pregnancies.[15] Hence, as in Rh disease, the setup is seen more frequently than the actual disease.

ABO incompatibility is different in mechanism as well as severity from Rh(D) incompatibility. The type O mother has preformed anti-A and anti-B in her serum. Primary immunization to A and B antigens and development of anti-A and anti-B antibodies occurs early in the mother's life, ostensibly from exposure to bacterial and food antigens. Hence, inoculation of the mother with type A or B fetal red cells may cause an anamnestic response during the first sensitizing pregnancy, which usually is not seen until the second sensitizing pregnancy in Rh(D) disease. The frequent lack of hemolysis (HDN) in ABO-mismatched infants may be due to the high proportion of anti-A or anti-B IgM in the maternal circulation, which can lyse sensitizing fetal red cells before they activate the immune system. The process is analogous to the blunting of Rh(D) sensitization in mothers who are ABO incompatible with their infants.[77]

Also unique to the maternal part of ABO incompatibility is the fact that preformed IgG and IgM antibodies against A and B antigens exist in the mother of an ABO-incompatible child. The response to sensitization may lead to an increase in IgM, IgG, or both, and leads to particularly high titers of IgG antibody in only a small proportion of the maternal population.[15] HDN secondary to ABO incompatibility usually occurs in infants of mothers with high IgG titers. Unlike in Rh(D) disease, in which an isolated anamnestic response occurs to a selected antigen that is independent of other ABO antigens, in ABO incompatibility it is very difficult to measure a rising titer since the IgM and IgG anti-A and anti-B antibodies must first be separated. This is not routinely done.[25] In addition, ABO incompatibility rarely if ever leads to stillbirth, making the determination of the severity of the disease during pregnancy of little clinical value.

In mothers with high titers of IgG anti-A or anti-B, which penetrates the serum of the type A or B fetus, the degree of hemolysis is consistently less than that seen in Rh(D) disease. The common, speculative explanation for this is that adult red cells have 26,000 reactive A antigens (or B in type B mothers) on their surface, whereas fetal red cells can have as few as 7500. This diminishes the efficiency of red cell removal by keeping the density of IgG lower on

TABLE 64-7. Diagnostic Features of Some Transplacentally Acquired Infections Compared With Erythroblastosis Fetalis

Finding	Congenital Syphilis	Toxoplasmosis (Generalized Form)	Cytomegalic Inclusion Disease	Rubella Syndrome	Erythroblastosis Fetalis	Nonimmune Hemolytic Anemia
Anemia	++++	+++	++	++	+++	++
Jaundice	+++	+++	+++	+	+++	++
Thrombocytopenia	++	+	+++	+++	+	0
Hepatomegaly	++++	+++	++++	++	++	+
Splenomegaly	++++	++++	++++	++	++	+
Purpura	++	+	+++	+++	+	0
Skin rash	+	+	0	+	0	0
Chorioretinitis	+	+++	+	+	0	0
Intracranial calcifications	0	+	+++	?	0	0
Generalized edema	++	+	+	?	+	0
ADDITIONAL FINDINGS						
	Mucocutaneous lesions Periostitis Snuffles Postive serology	Convulsions Microcephaly Hydrocephaly Positive dye test Lymphadenopathy	Pneumonia Cytomegalic inclusion cells in urine	Cataract Glaucoma Heart defects Deafness Microcephaly Hydrocephaly Bone lesion Rubella virus recoverable	Positive Coombs' test Evidence of blood group incompatiblity between mother and child	Morphology usually helpful

0, not described; +, present in about 1–25% of cases; ++, present in about 26–50% of cases; +++, present in about 51–75% of cases; ++++, present in about 76–100% of cases.
(Adapted from Oski F, Naiman J. The hematologic aspects of the maternal–fetal relationship. In: Hematologic problems of the newborn. (Philadelphia, WB Saunders, 1982:36)

the surface of the red cell. This lack of efficiency is also seen when performing the direct Coombs' (antiglobulin) test on neonatal red cells to determine whether anti-A or anti-B antibodies are attached.[78] In ABO incompatibility, the direct Coombs' test may be negative, is usually weakly positive, and is rarely strongly positive.[15] The clinician is usually attracted to these infants by neonatal hyperbilirubinemia.

To confirm ABO incompatibility as the cause of neonatal jaundice in a given child, several factors should be taken into account:

1. The clinician should examine the mother's and the infant's blood type. Type O mothers and type A and B neonates are the usual setup for ABO incompatibility.
2. The direct antiglobulin test may be positive, but as mentioned, the lack of a positive Coombs' test does not rule out ABO incompatibility as a source of hemolysis.
3. Examination of the smear of the infant usually reveals a predominance of spherocytes. In this circumstance, the distinction between ABO incompatibility and hereditary spherocytosis requires further thought. Additional serologic evidence of ABO incompatibility may lead the clinician in that direction. Of greater immediate value is the fact that 75% of infants born with hereditary spherocytosis have a parent with the disease. Only 25% of hereditary spherocytosis results from spontaneous mutations or nondominant variants.
4. In the absence of a positive Coombs' test, but with hemolysis, jaundice, or spherocytosis being present, the serologic observation of free anti-A or anti-B in the neonate's serum can often be the important clue in distinguishing ABO incompatibility, other types of HDN, and hereditary spherocytosis.

The diagnostic clues just mentioned, in addition to the mild to moderate immediate hemolysis and hyperbilirubinemia usually seen, often lead directly to the diagnosis of ABO incompatibility. Criteria are the same for the treatment of hyperbilirubinemia and for exchange transfusion as in other types of HDN. Although acute anemia is rare in ABO incompatibility, it is not uncommon to see a rapid fall in hematocrit levels toward the physiologic nadir, followed by a prolonged hyporegenerative anemia similar to that seen in Rh(D) incompatibility (but usually less severe). Nonetheless, the neonatologist or pediatrician following up on the infant should be aware of the possibility of more severe and more long-lasting anemia in these infants.

MINOR BLOOD GROUP INCOMPATIBILITIES

As Rh(D) sensitization has become less common as a result of passive immunization with anti-Rh(D) and with the recognition that ABO incompatibility rarely causes severe hemolysis, clinical attention has focused on HDN caused by minor blood group antibodies. Table 64-8 gives general guidance for the flow of work in the blood bank to identify these antigens.[50,63] The common antigens can be identified in most blood banks capable of running red cell antigen panels. Reference laboratories may be required for the more infrequently seen antigens. Under these circumstances, a positive Coombs' test is usually found, and affected children can be treated for hyperbilirubinemia in the same manner as in any other case of HDN. The importance of the ultimate identification of the antibody relates to the choice of red cells for transfusion and to problems with subsequent pregnancies. The choice of red cells for transfusion on an urgent basis is indicated in Table 64-8. Although these minor blood group antigens usually do not cause disease as

TABLE 64-8. Chart for Detection of Neonatal Hemolytic Antibodies Against Minor Blood Group Antigens

Maternal or Neonatal Serum Reactions With Antibody Screening Cells	Results of Testing Reagent Red Cell Panel (Including Maternal Cells)	Further Investigation	Antigens Involved	Approach to Transfusion
POSITIVE				
	Antibodies identified (eg, anti-K, anti-c, anti-e)		Common non-Rh(D) antigens: Kell, Duffy, Kidd, c, C, E, e, Lutheran, M, N, S, s, Dombrock	Compatible blood
	All cells of panel positive except maternal cells	Rare cells tested Antibody to high-frequency antigen discovered	High-frequency antigens: P, Cartwright Colton, Diego	Look for donor among mother's siblings In emergency, use mother's red cells
	All cells positive, including maternal cells	Check for maternal autoantibody	Panagglutinin	Use least-incompatible transfusion (nonmaternal) in emergency
NEGATIVE				
	Father's cells positive; mother's cells negative	Rare cells tested Antibody to low-frequency antigen detected	Low-frequency antigens: variants of MNSS, variants of Kell, variants of Rh	Blood without low-frequency antigens Readily available
	Father's cells negative; mother's cells negative or positive	Review history for possibility of drug-sensitized red cells	Antipenicillin Anticephalosporin	Compatible blood unsensitized by drugs

(Modified from Sabo BH. A seminar in perinatal blood banking. 1978:36)

severe as Rh(D) erythroblastosis fetalis, subsequent pregnancies should be monitored for the signs of intrauterine hemolysis and the mother and infant should be treated using the same criteria as for Rh(D) disease.

ANEMIA AT THE TIME OF BIRTH

Central Versus Capillary Blood Sampling

A note of caution must be made when discussing neonatal anemias. An assumption exists that the measured value for the hemoglobin or hematocrit can be compared with known standards to determine the need for further evaluation in the newborn. However, these values show wide variations in the newborn. In cases in which cord blood is used or a central access is available (umbilical artery or vein catheterization), values reflect the central hemoglobin and hematocrit and are generally reliable. Capillary blood measurements are subject to variability and tend to overestimate the actual central hematocrit. The capillary/central or capillary/peripheral venous hematocrit ratios can be as high as 1.2:1, especially in those infants in whom an accurate value is most important, such as those who are premature, acidotic, hypotensive, or severely anemic.[7,79]

Placental Transfusions

The relation of the infant and the umbilical cord to the placenta in the period immediately after birth affects the infant's blood volume and placental separation and the possibility of fetal–maternal hemorrhage. For infants of any gestational age, the gravitational effect of positioning the infant below the level of the placenta allows blood to pass through the umbilical vein into the infant by passive gravitational flow. In concert, flow from the infant to the mother is prevented as a result of arteriospasm and constriction of the umbilical arteries immediately after birth.[7]

The effects of this placental transfusion may be dramatic, since the placental vessels contain up to one third of the fetal blood volume. If the infant is held below the level of the placenta (about 40 cm below the mother's introitus), the placental transfusion will be complete within 30 seconds.[80] Holding the infant above the level of the placenta leads to an opposite effect, causing fetal blood to flow passively back toward the placenta and the maternal–placental unit. Hence, it is possible for an infant to be born with a 10% to 20% loss of blood volume on the basis of positioning of the child at birth in relation to the placenta. This fact is well accepted, and it is standard obstetric practice to include a period with the neonate still in touch with placental circulation in a position below the introitus. This positioning is of less concern in normal term infants and of greater concern in infants delivered by cesarean section.

Although there may be concerns regarding control of neonatal temperature if the premature neonate is held below the perineum for any length of time, premature infants or those with severe respiratory compromise may benefit the most from the placental transfusion of fetal red cells.[81] The extra volume of fetal blood maintains oxygen-carrying capacity and a left-shifted hemoglobin oxygen saturation curve in the premature infant or the infant born under conditions in which hypoxia is present at birth. The only exception to this practice is when placental transfusion needs to be avoided in patients with known red cell sensitization (such as erythroblastosis fetalis) or who are immediately expected to need transfusion or exchange transfusion for other reasons. In HDN patients, leaving behind sensitized red cells in the placental circulation may be viewed as the beginning of an exchange transfusion.

Under the typical conditions of placenta to neonate transfusion, the blood volume associated with the maternal–fetal transfusion may increase the neonatal blood volume up to 10 mL/kg. Because much of the plasma associated with this blood volume is absorbed quickly into the fetal circulation and the extra volume is subsequently excreted, the major change that occurs is a change in the red cell mass, which is much higher in the group of neonates who receive transfusions (49 mL/kg red cells at 72 hours of age) compared with neonates whose cords are clamped immediately (31 mL/kg red cells).[82] The placental transfusion can lead to an increase in hemoglobin at 1 to 3 days of age by as much as 3 to 7 g/dL.[7,83–84] The difference in red cell mass that occurs without placental transfusion may adversely affect infants under stress around the time of delivery, such as infants delivered by cesarean section, those with respiratory distress syndrome or transient tachypnea of the newborn, premature infants, infants with cyanotic congenital heart disease, asphyxiated infants, infants with meconium aspiration, and infants with persistent fetal circulation.

Despite these differences, which have been confirmed by other investigators, by the time the infant is 3 months of age, no differences in hemoglobin or hematocrit levels are found as a result of the initial transfusion.[84] Therefore, it is interesting to note that an ultimately reduced red cell mass is frequently observed in patients with respiratory distress syndrome and in newborns delivered with a tight nuchal cord who may have perinatal asphyxia.[85] In patients with chronic asphyxia within the intrauterine environment, an increase in red cell mass, probably compensatory, is a response to chronic hypoxia. If the placental transfusion is lost in such infants, the appropriate adaptation is lost.

Fetal–Maternal Hemorrhage

The structure of the fetal–placental unit sets up a large pressure gradient from umbilical artery to intervillous space. The separation and the boundary of the maternal intervillous space from the fetal pulsatile blood circulation are thin (two layers of cells), and there is constant possibility for the rupture of the trophoblastic–endothelial juncture and the contamination of the maternal intervillous space with fetal blood[86] (Fig. 64-10*A*) Given this fragile mechanical relation, it is surprising that fetal–maternal hemorrhage does not happen more often. Although it is clear that fetal red cells also enter the maternal circulation before the third trimester (see Fig. 64-11*B*), most fetal–maternal hemorrhage occurs during labor and childbirth (see Fig. 64-11*C*).

Fetal red cells can be detected in the maternal circulation in a number of ways. Using agglutination procedures, one can detect red cells bearing nonmaternal blood group antigens in the maternal circulation, which subsequently can be shown to be those of the newborn infant.[7] The most clinically useful tests are the postpartum elevation of Hb F in the maternal circulation and the microscopic demonstration of fetal red cells in the mother using the Kleihauer-Betke staining procedure.[87] In this method, Hb A is denatured and eluted from smears of adult red cells with an acid solution, leaving behind largely empty red cell membranes. Hb F resists denaturation and elution, so fetal cells stain darkly. Simple observation of the acid-treated maternal blood smear can give a qualitative picture, but one can estimate the actual amount of fetal blood lost using the following formula: 2400 $\times$ the ratio of fetal to maternal cells = one milliliter of fetal blood. Using this equation, Mollison[88] has observed that most deliveries result in less than 3 mL of fetal blood in the maternal circulation, and only 0.3% have a fetal–maternal transfusion of 10 mL or more. Obviously, conditions that elevate ma-

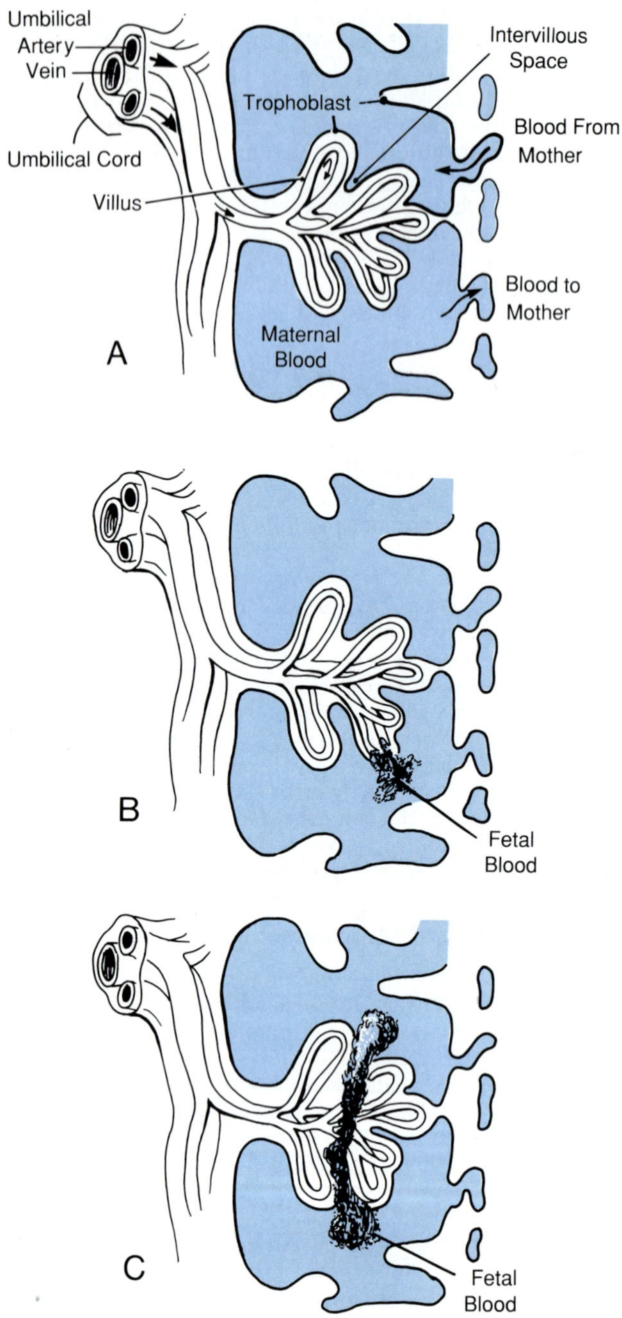

FIGURE 64-10. Anatomic issues in fetomaternal hemorrhage. (**A**) Resting state: fragile capillary networks are present. (**B**) Minor small bleed, known to occur in almost all pregnancies. (**C**) Major possibility of significant exchange of fetal and maternal blood as a result of abruption (more severe) or normal childbirth.

ternal Hb F production confuse this analysis (thalassemia minor, sickle cell disease, hereditary persistence of Hb F, and pregnancy-induced maternal Hb F production).

Fetal–maternal hemorrhage can produce a number of clinical pictures, depending on the amount of bleeding and when it occurs during pregnancy, labor, or delivery. Table 64-9 lists the most helpful discriminators in distinguishing the type and severity of hemorrhage or pallor at birth. At the time of birth, the anemia observed can vary from 3 to 12 g/dL with survival.[7]

A clinician should be especially aware of the clinical picture of acute hemorrhage at the time of delivery, since the hemoglobin level may not have fallen dramatically enough to immediately suggest that the ensuing hypovolemic shock requires whole blood or red cell transfusion rather than simple volume replacement. Small hemorrhages before delivery present as anemia with no sign of hypovolemic shock. If enough time has elapsed, this anemia may be accompanied by reticulocytosis and may be initially confused with a hemolytic process. Under these circumstances, perusal of the neonate's smear reveals mild macrocytosis and polychromasia, but no predominant morphology suggestive of a hemolytic process. The absence of jaundice and a negative Coombs' test also lead one to suspect fetal–maternal hemorrhage rather than hemolysis. If the loss of blood is significant but spaced over weeks before delivery, the child may be normovolemic but pale at birth and have evidence of an iron-deficient hypochromic-microcytic anemia.

When the diagnosis of acute or chronic fetal hemorrhage is made, therapy is dictated by the clinical condition of the child. If the infant is in shock with tachycardia, pallor, and a low central venous pressure, rapid blood transfusion with whole blood or red cells is indicated. In patients born without hypovolemia, but with pallor and signs of subacute or chronic hemorrhage, packed red cell transfusion may be necessary if cardiopulmonary compromise is present. All neonates in this scenario require supplemental iron to replenish the iron lost by bleeding.

Umbilical Cord Hemorrhage

The umbilical cord can rupture from traction during a difficult delivery, or it can be weakened by arteriovenous malformation or velamentous insertion. One in 10,000 pregnancies is associated with umbilical cord bleeding or rupture. Affected neonates are at high risk for shock and death.[89] The worst scenario is acute hemorrhage at the time of birth. Similar serious perinatal bleeding can occur as a result of placenta previa or abruptio placentae.

Twin–Twin Hemorrhage

Another form of perinatal hemorrhage occurs in the bleeding from one monozygotic twin to another within a monochorionic placenta. Most monozygotic twins are born with a monochorionic placenta (up to 70%).[90] Up to 30% of such pregnancies are associated with twin to twin transfusion.[91] The clinical picture depends on the degree of hemorrhage of one twin to another and the timing of the hemorrhage. In twin–twin transfusion, one twin bleeds into the other, leaving the donor twin anemic and the recipient twin polycythemic. Both twins may be sick; the anemic donor twin may develop congestive heart failure and the plethoric recipient twin may require treatment for hyperviscosity syndrome, hyperbilirubinemia, and rarely disseminated intravascular coagulation.[92] In twin–twin transfusion, in which the donor twin has been chronically oozing blood into the recipient, the clinician observes the classic presentation of a small anemic infant with a reticulocytosis from chronic bleeding and a larger plethoric infant whose weight is at least 20% higher. In more acute transfusions, occurring closer to the time of delivery, the difference in weight of the infants does not exceed 20%, and an equal chance exists of either twin being the red cell donor.[93]

Internal Hemorrhage

In addition to fetal–maternal hemorrhage and the effects of placental separation, neonates can also experience internal bleeding with symptoms of mild to severe acute blood loss. These internal hemorrhages are not necessarily manifested at the time of delivery. They may appear on

TABLE 64-9. Differential Diagnosis of Pallor at Birth

Feature	Asphyxia	Acute Blood Loss	Chronic Blood Loss	Hemolytic Disease
Respiratious	Retractions, cyanosis	Rapid without effort	Little distress unless congestive heart failure	Rapid if congestive heart failure
Arterial blood pressure	May be elevated or decreased	May be elevated or decreased	Usually normal	Usually normal
Central venous pressure	Normal or elevated	Low	Normal or elevated	Usually normal
Hepatosplenomegaly	Organs may be pushed down by lungs	None	Hepatomegaly if congestive heart failure	Hepatosplenomegaly
Jaundice	Perhaps	If loss of blood into tissues (eg, scalp)	Usually not	Yes
Hemoglobin	Normal	Normal initially, drops after 24 hours	Low at birth	Low at birth
Red cell morphology	Normal	Normal/macrocytic	May be hypochromic microcytic	May have hemolytic morphology
Other	Responds to O_2 intrauterine	Weak pulses	—	May have positive direct Coombs' test or positive family history

(Adapted from Oski F. Hematology: the erythrocyte and its disorders. In: Nathan DA, Oski FA, eds. Hematology of infancy and childhood, ed 4. Philadelphia, WB Saunders, 1993:34)

physical examination shortly after birth or present as sudden hypotension and pallor at 1 to 2 days of life. The site of the bleeding often can be specified by individual characteristics[7] (Table 64-10).

Bleeding beneath the scalp can be limited (cephalohematoma) or global (subgaleal bleeding across sutures under scalp), and the associated blood loss may be mild to severe and life-threatening. The sequestration of large amounts of blood can lead to hyperbilirubinemia requiring therapy. The presence of extensive subgaleal bleeding should prompt a search for coagulopathy in the child, either endogenous (such as hemophilia, vitamin K deficiency) or exogenous (such as maternal aspirin ingestion).[7,94]

Rupture of the liver and bleeding into the retroperitoneal space may occur in normal infants after difficult deliveries.[19] The clinician can be faced at birth or during the next 48 hours with an infant showing the signs of shock from sudden hypovolemia. Abdominal distention may be diffuse (abdominal and scrotal swelling) or associated with an abdominal mass (subcapsular hepatic hematoma), and there may be evidence of shifting dullness if free blood is in the peritoneal space. After the hypovolemia is stabilized, abdominal ultrasonography may point to the site of the hemorrhage as well as confirm the presence of fluid in the abdomen. These situations may be life-threatening, and surgical intervention may be necessary. When adrenal gland hemorrhage occurs, it may be bilateral and the syndrome of addisonian crisis may occur.

TABLE 64-10. Sites of Internal Neonatal Hemorrhage

Site	Comment
Cephalohematoma	Swelling confined by sutures
Subgaleal bleed	Swelling over the entire calvarium
Retroperitoneal	Associated with difficult delivery
Kidney	Hematuria and hypertension may be present
Spleen	More likely to occur in association with other causes of splenomegaly (erythroblastosis fetalis)
Adrenal	Can lead to collapse associated with adrenocorticoid insufficiency
Liver	Can be devastating and lead to stillbirth; usually presents 1–2 days after birth with sudden collapse, if not apparent at birth; subcapsular 50% of the time (may feel mass)
Intracranial bleed	Low-birthweight or very premature infant or coagulopathy
Gastrointestinal	Blood in stool; can distinguish from swallowed maternal blood using the Apt test

Intracranial bleeding is unfortunately common in very premature or low birth weight infants. It can cause symptoms of acute blood loss along with changes in central nervous system function, but anemia rarely is the only finding associated with the intraventricular hemorrhage.[19,95]

It follows that whenever an infant experiences a difficult delivery or there are concerns about the potential for neonatal hemorrhage, a hematocrit value should be recorded at birth. This should be repeated at 12 to 24 hours to examine whether equilibration has occurred, revealing neonatal blood loss.

ANEMIA IN THE FIRST WEEKS OF LIFE

Many factors affect the hemoglobin level in the first 8 weeks of life (see Fig. 64-4), including the following:

- Normally functioning bone marrow
- The thermostat-like response of the bone marrow to decreased erythropoietin associated with the increased Po_2 observed after birth in the newborn circulation
- The gestational age of the infant at birth
- Nutritional influences
- The presence of intrinsic (such as congenital red cell membrane or metabolic anomalies) or extrinsic (such as sensitization by antibodies and drugs) factors that shorten red cell life-span

Tables 64-11 and 64-12 document the expected red cell values at birth, depending on gestational age and the changes in red cell parameters over the first 12 weeks of life for the term infant.

TABLE 64-11. **Red Cell Values on First Postnatal Days**

	Gestational Age (Wk)							
	24–25 (7)*	26–27 (11)	28–29 (7)	30–31 (25)	32–33 (23)	34–35 (23)	36–37 (20)	Term (19)
RBC × 10^6	4.65 ± 0.43†	4.73 ± 0.45	4.62 ± 0.75	4.79 ± 0.74	5.0 ± 0.76	5.09 ± 0.5	5.27 ± 0.68	5.14 ± 0.7
Hb (g/dL)	19.4 ± 1.5	19.0 ± 2.5	19.3 ± 1.8	19.1 ± 2.2	18.5 ± 2.0	19.6 ± 2.1	19.2 ± 1.7	19.3 ± 2.2
Hematocrit (%)	63 ± 4	62 ± 8	60 ± 7	60 ± 8	60 ± 8	61 ± 7	64 ± 7	61 ± 7.4
MCV (μ^3)	135 ± 0.2	132 ± 14.4	131 ± 13.5	127 ± 12.7	123 ± 15.7	122 ± 10.0	121 ± 12.5	119 ± 9.4
Reticulocytes (%)	6.0 ± 0.5	9.6 ± 3.2	7.5 ± 2.5	5.8 ± 2.0	5.0 ± 1.9	3.9 ± 1.6	4.2 ± 1.8	3.2 ± 1.4
Weight (g)	725 ± 185	993 ± 194	1174 ± 128	1450 ± 232	1816 ± 192	1957 ± 291	2245 ± 213	

MCV, mean corpuscular volume.
* Number in parentheses indicates number of infants.
† Mean values ± SD.
(From Zaizov R, Matoth Y. Red cell values on the first postnatal day during the last 16 weeks of gestation. Am J Hematol 1976;1:276)

The diagnosis of anemia in the newborn can be made using these tables. The cardiorespiratory status and gestational age of the infant should be noted before deciding whether a given hemoglobin level provides enough oxygen-carrying capacity for the infant's needs. The neonate with hypoxia, as in respiratory distress syndrome, cyanotic congenital heart disease, and persistent fetal circulation, requires a higher level of oxygen-carrying capacity than the neonate with normal lungs. Therefore, when comparing a hematocrit level with given red cell standards, the value requiring clinical action must be continually put into the perspective of the cardiopulmonary needs of the patient.

Hemolytic Anemias

In addition to bleeding, hemolytic processes, especially immunohemolytic processes, are common causes of anemia in the first week of life. Table 64-13 lists hemolytic processes in the neonatal period. Immune causes have been discussed in detail. Specific congenital hemolytic anemias have been discussed in detail in previous chapters. A few points may be made about neonatal hemolytic syndromes.

Congenital infections often lead to a picture of hemolytic anemia. This can be confusing in the setting in which no apparent immune setup or genetic history of hemoglobinopathy or membrane disorder is present. Table 64-7 represents an attempt at differential diagnosis among these disorders.

In an infant with hyperbilirubinemia (indirect), a negative Coombs' test, and reticulocytosis, the most likely causes are bleeding into an enclosed space (see earlier discussion of internal hemorrhage) and hemolytic anemia of a nonimmune type. Examination of the smear and analysis of the predominant morphology (see Chap. 47) often lead to a definitive diagnosis.

TABLE 64-12. **Normal Red Cell Values During the First 12 Weeks of Life in the Term Infant**

Age	N	Hb (g/dL) ± 1SD	Hct (%) ± 1SD	MCV (μm^3) ± 1SD	Reticulocytes ± 1SD
DAYS					
1	19	19.0 ± 2.2	61 ± 7.4	119 ± 9.4	3.2 ± 1.4
2	19	19.0 ± 1.9	60 ± 6.4	115 ± 7.0	3.2 ± 1.3
3	19	18.7 ± 3.4	62 ± 9.3	116 ± 5.3	2.8 ± 1.7
4	10	18.6 ± 2.1	57 ± 8.1	114 ± 7.5	1.8 ± 1.1
5	12	17.6 ± 1.1	57 ± 7.3	114 ± 8.9	1.2 ± 0.2
6	15	17.4 ± 2.2	54 ± 7.2	113 ± 10.0	0.6 ± 0.2
7	12	17.9 ± 2.5	56 ± 9.4	118 ± 11.2	0.5 ± 0.4
WEEKS					
1–2	3	17.3 ± 2.3	54 ± 8.3	112 ± 19.0	0.5 ± 0.3
2–3	11	15.6 ± 2.6	46 ± 7.3	111 ± 8.2	0.8 ± 0.6
3–4	17	14.2 ± 2.1	43 ± 5.7	105 ± 7.5	0.6 ± 0.3
4–5	15	12.7 ± 1.6	36 ± 4.8	101 ± 8.1	0.9 ± 0.8
5–6	10	11.9 ± 1.5	36 ± 6.2	102 ± 10.2	1.0 ± 0.7
6–7	10	12.0 ± 1.5	36 ± 4.8	105 ± 12.0	1.2 ± 0.7
7–8	17	11.1 ± 1.1	33 ± 3.7	100 ± 13.0	1.5 ± 0.7
8–9	13	10.7 ± 0.9	31 ± 2.5	93 ± 12.0	1.8 ± 1.0
9–10	12	11.2 ± 0.9	32 ± 2.7	91 ± 9.3	1.2 ± 0.6
10–11	11	11.4 ± 0.9	34 ± 2.1	91 ± 7.7	1.2 ± 0.7
11–12	13	11.3 ± 0.9	33 ± 3.3	88 ± 7.9	0.7 ± 0.3

MCV, mean corpuscular volume.
(Matoth Y, Zaizov R, Varsano I. Postnatal changes in some red cell parameters. Acta Paediatr Scand 1971;60:317).

TABLE 64-13. Causes of a Hemolytic Process in the Neonatal Period

Immune
Rh incompatibility
ABO incompatiblity
Minor blood group incompatibility
Maternal autoimmune hemolytic anemia
Drug-induced hemolytic anemia
Infection
Bacterial sepsis
Congenital infections:
Syphilis
Malaria
Cytomegalovirus
Rubella
Toxoplasmosis
Disseminated herpes
Disseminated intravascular coagulation
Macroangiopathic and microangiopathic hemolytic anemias
Cavernous hemangioma
Large vessel thrombi
Renal artery stenosis
Severe coarctation of the aorta
Galactosemia
Prolonged or recurrent acidosis of a metabolic or respiratory nature
Hereditary disorders of the red cell membrane
Hereditary spherocytosis
Hereditary elliptocytosis
Hereditary stomatocytosis
Other rate membrane disorders
Pyknocytosis
Red cell enzyme deficiencies
Most common are glucose-6-phosphate dehydrogenase deficiency, pyruvate kinase deficiency, pyridine-5′-nucleotidase deficiency, and glucose phosphate isomerase deficiency
α-Thalassemia syndromes
α-Globin structural abnormalities
γ-Thalassemia syndromes
γ-Globin structural abnormalities

(Oski F, Naiman J. The erythrocyte and its disorders. In: Nathan DG, Oski F, eds. Hematology of infancy and childhood, ed 4. Philadelphia, WB Saunders, 1993:34)

Oxidant Hemolysis

Oxidant hemolysis in the newborn is common and is not always associated with a known enzymopathy (see Chap. 58) or with chronic Heinz body hemolytic anemia[96] (see Chap. 52). It is an acute hemolytic event, presumably related to the oxidant sensitivity of neonatal red cells (see Table 64-3). Infants 2 or 3 days old have sudden indirect hyperbilirubinemia, a drop in hematocrit, and the appearance of "bite" cells, "blister" cells, spherocytes, and some dense, contracted, irregularly shaped red cells on the peripheral blood smear. Such infants should be carefully monitored, and a small phlebotomy should be performed for enzyme screening and a Heinz body test. Usually, no obvious source for the presumed oxidant stress is found and the episode is over within a few days. Transfusion is rarely required, in which case, infants usually respond well without further hemolysis. In infants who continue to have hemolysis, a more aggressive search for the cause is warranted (such as analysis for an unstable hemoglobin or enzymopathy). This should include an attempt to identify unstable hemoglobins, especially the unstable γ hemoglobins, whose fleeting nature precludes diagnosis if the opportunity to find them is lost (as by a middle-of-the-night transfusion).

Drugs. Theoretically, drugs known to create oxidant-induced hemolysis in G6PD-deficient individuals should be avoided in premature or term babies. Happily, most of these medications (sulfonamides, nitrofurans, antimalarials, analgesics such as acetylsalicylic acid, anthelmintics, and dyes such as methylene blue and toluidine blue) are rarely indicated in neonates. Ironically, methylene blue does have an indication to treat methemoglobinemia in certain at-risk infants. No oxidant hemolysis has been observed under these circumstances.

Vitamin E Deficiency. Vitamin E deficiency in infants leads to a hemolytic anemia characterized by spherocytes, occasional condensed spiked cells (pyknocytes) and other fragments. In addition, some babies have edema of the lower extremities and thrombocytosis.[97] Vitamin E supplementation eliminates all these findings.[97] Currently, provision of vitamin E in infant formulas and total parenteral nutrition has virtually eliminated this syndrome.

Hereditary Elliptocytosis

Infantile hemolytic elliptocytosis, termed *hereditary elliptocytosis* (hereditary elliptocytosis with neonatal poikilocytosis; see Chap. 54), is a disorder that resembles hereditary pyropoikilocytosis in clinical appearance. The disease is more common in patients of African American and Hispanic descent but also occurs in other racial groups. Patients have severe hemolysis and may require exchange transfusion for hyperbilirubinemia. They usually do not require transfusion for anemia. During the first year of life, the hemolysis improves and the patient is left with typical, mild hereditary elliptocytosis. Sometimes the evolution in the only way to distinguish hereditary elliptocytosis with neonatal poikilocytosis from hereditary pyropoikilocytosis. It has been proposed that the elevated 2,3-DPG levels caused by Hb F in the infant's cells may destabilize a structural unit of the membrane skeleton. As the infant ages and Hb F levels fall, free 2,3-DPG levels fall as well and membrane function improves.

Infantile Pyknocytosis

Infantile pyknocytosis (see Chap. 54) is a hemolytic anemia characterized by condensed spiked red cells and spherocytes. It is rarely diagnosed today, and one wonders whether improvement in neonatal care (nutritional supplementation with vitamin E and other cofactors) has eliminated this illness. It was always more common in premature infants and reflected an exaggeration of the normal numbers of echinocytes and acanthocytes seen in neonatal smears (normal patients have up to 5.5% spiculated red cells; patients with pyknocytosis have up to 50%). The illness was self-limited and usually ended in the second or third month of life. If new cases of pyknocytosis occur, they will undoubtedly be probed with all the new tools of the red cell physiologist.

Hemoglobinopathies

The presentation of hemoglobinopathies in the neonate is often in flux, since certain anomalies that cause hemolysis may resolve within the neonatal period (γ-chain defects), whereas the most common postnatal hemoglobin synthesis defect, β-thalassemia, is usually not clinically evident until the fetal switch has occurred.

α-Globin Defects. Because α-chain synthesis does not vary between neonatal and adult life, the α-chain variants do not usually cause any new clinical syndromes not recognized at birth. One interesting exception, the structural mutant *Hb Hasharon*, is a mild unstable hemoglobin when the abnormal α is paired with γ chains, but it is no longer unstable when paired with β chains. As might be expected, this hemoglobin produces a mild hemolytic anemia that reverses to normal as the fetal-to-adult hemoglobin switch occurs.[98]

α-Thalassemia. Homozygous α-thalassemia leads to the death of the affected fetus in utero from severe hemolytic anemia. In this case, the only hemoglobin usually seen in the stillborn is Hb Bart's (γ_4), although a small amount of Hb Portsmouth (ζ_2, γ_2) may be present (see Fig. 64-1). The neonate is born with the full-blown syndrome of hydrops fetalis. In the rare situation in which the child is born alive, death from cardiopulmonary collapse occurs within minutes. A report has been made of a patient with hydrops fetalis surviving into childhood as the result of vigorous resuscitation and transfusion in the immediate neonatal period after premature delivery.[99] Many centers are screening now for α-thalassemia within the southeast Asian population, where *cis-α* gene deletions are common. In a known genetic setup, prenatal diagnosis of an affected child may be performed to allow consideration of early abortion for these largely doomed children and for maternal safety.

The infant with three functionless α genes (Hb H disease) produces a small amount of functioning normal hemoglobin from the one functional gene. At birth, hemoglobin electrophoresis demonstrates normal hemoglobin concentration (Hb A), Hb Bart's (made up of γ-chain tetramers left over from the fetal switch) and Hb H (composed of β-chain tetramers unable to find an α globin. The last gives this α-thalassemia syndrome its name—*Hb H disease*. Infants with Hb H disease are born with significant anemia as well as microcytosis. Targeting is prominent, and the broad, thin cells look somewhat larger on blood smears than they actually are (as documented by the mean corpuscular volume). The anemia is sufficient to sustain life without transfusion, although neonatal hyperbilirubinemia can be a problem. The appearance of microcytosis and significant anemia first suggest chronic fetal–maternal hemorrhage. If the reticulocyte count is elevated and the patient is in an ethnic group that is likely to have α- thalassemia trait (such as Southeast Asian), Hb H disease should be suspected.

Microcytosis alone without anemia is suggestive of mild chronic fetal–maternal hemorrhage, but it can also mean early α-thalassemia trait. In this case, the microcytosis associated with α-thalassemia trait creates a red cell that is significantly smaller than normal for age but that might be overlooked because normal fetal red cells are considerably larger than adult red cells (normal, 106 $\pm$ 5.7 fL; α-thalassemia trait, 94 fL.)[7] In this case, family studies confirm the diagnosis; occasionally, Hb H can be detected as well, and in the neonatal period, small amounts of Hb Bart's are present.

γ-Globin Structural Defects. γ-Chain structural defects, such as Hb F Poole, have led to Heinz body hemolytic anemia in the neonatal period.[100] As might be expected, this syndrome disappears as the fetal switch occurs.

γ-Thalassemias. To my knowledge, no infant with γ-thalassemia has been born alive. However, one full-term infant has been reported with a hemolytic hypochronic anemia at birth, which transformed as the child matured into the father's β-thalassemia trait.[101] It could be assumed that a γ-thalassemia trait would lead to birth with mild to moderate anemia and microcytosis, but this has not been observed.

β-Chain Structural Defects: Hb S. β-Chain structural variants do not begin to show problems until β globin is well represented as a percentage of the neonate's hemoglobin. Oski[7] points out that the amount of Hb A is usually less than 30% of the normal hemoglobin at birth, but that chronic red cell destruction from hemolytic anemia can accelerate the γ-to-β chain switch, causing earlier expression of β variants.

Of the structural β mutants, the recognition of Hb S in the neonatal period is perhaps the most important. Although Hb S is likely to be a small fraction of the globin at birth, after birth the amount of Hb S rises rapidly. In the immediate neonatal period, an increased incidence of jaundice requiring phototherapy is found. Typical clinical complications of sickle cell disease such as infant dactylitis do not usually occur before an infant is 2 months of age. Nonetheless, at least one case report of sudden infant death was found to be associated with a widespread neonatal vasoocclusion.[102] On this basis, Oski[7] recommends that exchange transfusion be considered in any neonate demonstrating symptoms of sickle cell crisis in the first several days of life.

β-Thalassemia. The expression of β-thalassemia is usually not apparent in the first days of life. Unlike α-thalassemia trait, the cells are not microcytic and anemia is not present, because γ globin is still the dominant gene at this time. As the percentage of Hb F falls during the first 2 to 3 months of life, the stigmata of β-thalassemia trait first appear, leading to microcytosis and mild anemia as the child's bone marrow awakens from the physiologic nadir. If a severe β-thalassemia syndrome has been inherited by the child, the syndrome of microcytic hypochromic hemolytic anemia appears shortly after birth, leading over a short period of time to a transfusion requirement.

Bone Marrow Failure Syndromes

Bone marrow failure states can be seen as early as the first few days of life. As an example, at birth infants with Blackfan-Diamond anemia may manifest depressed hemoglobin values as low as 9.4 g/dL.[103] (See a detailed discussion in Chapter 9.) Most patients present later, within the first 6 months of life. In the neonatal period, few clues suggest the presence of Blackfan-Diamond anemia except for poor red cell production. Alternatively, affected patients may have physical anomalies, particularly unusual thumb changes (deformed thumb, triphalangeal thumb, duplication of a thumb, and bifid thumb). Less specific anomalies that can be associated with pure red cell aplasia and congenital pure red cell aplasia include microcephaly, cleft palate, and webbed neck.[7]

Thrombocytopenia and bone marrow failure can also present within the first few days of life as a result of a congenital infection such as rubella. As previously noted, congenital infections can also present as hemolytic anemia (see Table 64-7). Rare diseases such as congenital leukemia (see Chap. 18) and osteopetrosis (see Chap. 9) also produce anemia during the early days of life. Both these illnesses are manifested by the appearance of leukoerythroblastosis in the peripheral blood and usually present with pancytopenia rather than a pure anemia.

ANEMIA AFTER THE FIRST WEEKS OF LIFE

Physiologic Anemia of Prematurity

The revolutionary changes affecting the transition from life in the womb to life apart from the mother create dramatic changes in the relation of erythroid production and the changing cardiopulmonary circuits. Immediately after birth, the hemoglobin levels begin to fall in neonates who do not have severe chronic hypoxia despite treatment, hemolytic disorders, or bone marrow failure. Figure 64-11 demonstrates the rate of fall in normal neonates. Eventually, a signal is sent to the erythroid marrow to begin to produce red cells again, and over a period of weeks the

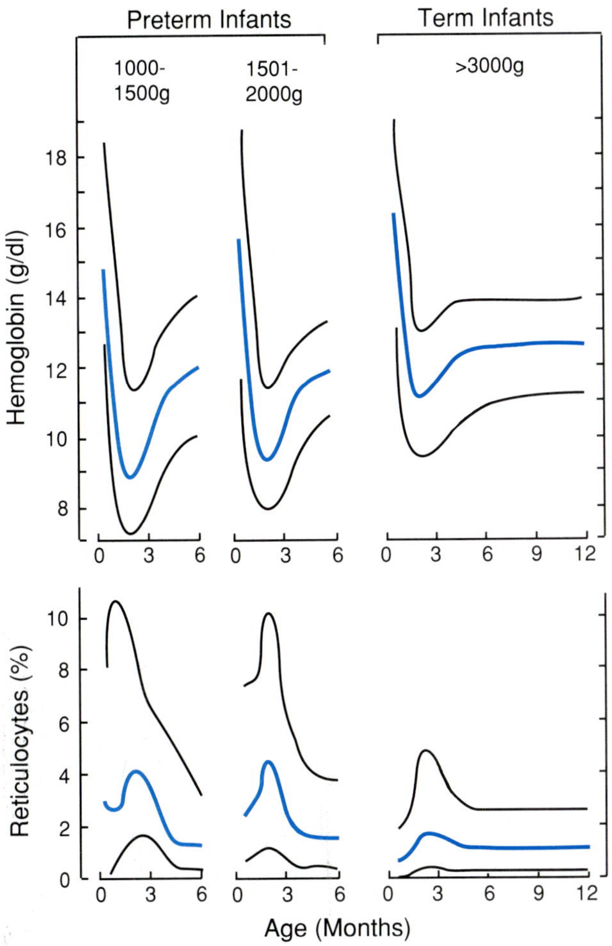

FIGURE 64-11. The mean (*colored*) and range (*black*) of normal hemoglobin and reticulocyte values for healthy and preterm infants. Premature infants become more anemic sooner after birth and return their hemoglobin toward normal later. (After Dallman PR. Anemia of prematurity. Annu Rev Med 1981;32:143)

hemoglobin rises toward the normal level, usually beginning at 2 to 3 months of age. The phenomenon of lowered hemoglobin in these infants is often termed the *physiologic anemia of prematurity*. This should not be taken to mean that it is normal for a neonate to be anemic at this time. As we shall see later, any permutation of this pattern can lead to anemic symptomatology in neonates. This physiologic anemia can vary because of concomitant conditions in the rate of initial fall of the hematocrit, the lowest hematocrit achieved (nadir), and the amount of time hemoglobin levels remain depressed. A basic understanding of the shape of this curve is necessary before the clinician can begin to deal with variations from normal and design appropriate therapy.

As a result of the sudden increase in hemoglobin saturation seen as the infant moves from maternal oxygenation to environmental oxygenation, the degree of tissue hypoxia changes dramatically and erythropoietin levels fall. Hence, red cell production begins to decrease. Fetal red cells have a shortened life-span for a number of reasons. Hence, the initial fall in hemoglobin is the combined result of decreased production and increased destruction of red cells. If neonatal factors that decrease red cell survival or further compromise erythropoiesis (TORCH infections, drugs, and so on) are present, the infant's hemoglobin falls faster toward the nadir.

At some point, the loss of oxygen-carrying capacity manifested by the drop in hemoglobin turns on erythropoietin production, stimulating erythroid activity and new red cell production. The set point at which this occurs is the result of a balance of many factors. Just like the regulation of a thermostat, there also seems to be a sluggishness to respond that may be clinically important if the infant's needs for oxygen-carrying capacity are high. Ample evidence suggests that erythropoietin concentration governs erythropoiesis in the neonate.[7] It is elevated in the cord blood of neonates with hemolytic anemia and persists in the circulation in patients with acute or chronic hypoxia.[104] In most situations, the degree of tissue hypoxia correlates with the production of erythropoietin. Hence, an understanding of the oxygen needs of the infant (well or sick) enables the clinician to determine whether an appropriate erythroid response is present.

Shortly after birth, as the infant's hemoglobin levels fall, the hemoglobin oxygen saturation curve shifts more and more to the right. When the amount of oxygen-carrying capacity does not meet the tissue needs of the infant in a more protective fashion, or as venous oxygen saturation begins to diminish, erythropoietin activity increases and the normal term infant begins to make red cells. Because erythropoietin levels have been virtually undetectable for several weeks, a delay always is seen between the time of increased erythropoietin concentration and the appearance of reticulocytosis, because of the need to revive red cell precursors. During this time, the oxygen requirements of the neonate are only marginally covered, and the physiology of the child is required to make other adaptations for short periods of time. Some of these adaptations may be recognized as symptomatology by the clinician caring for the child.

Symptoms such as increased heart rate, increased respiratory rate, fatigue during feeding, and poor feeding can occur as the "thermostat" is set in motion. In term infants who begin life with a normal hematocrit and normal bone marrow function, the response at the time of the physiologic nadir of anemia leads to no symptoms because the adaptation is made easily. Infants compromised by prematurity, poor nutrition, and low birthweight may experience symptoms before the appropriate bone marrow response occurs. Thus, in situations in which the hematocrit falls sooner to the levels at which oxygen-carrying capacity is diminished, but there is otherwise normal red cell production and survival, the nadir occurs earlier, but the healthy term neonate responds to the earlier appearance of this low oxygen-carrying capacity, with an early appearance of erythropoietin and revival of red cell production.

In the preterm infant, the low-birthweight infant, and neonates who have been sick and received multiple transfusions, the erythropoietin response to a given degree of tissue hypoxemia is less than that seen in term infants[105,106] (Fig. 64-12). This is expressed by an increased sluggishness of the oxygen sensor to tissue hypoxia. Therefore, these infants are more likely to suffer symptoms of tissue hypoxia and may require transfusion.

Vitamin E Deficiency

Nutritional factors also contribute to the fall in hemoglobin after birth. All neonates are relatively deficient in vitamin E at birth. The amount of vitamin E required by the growing infant depends on the degree of deficiency and the amount of polyunsaturated fatty acids in the diet.[19] Breast milk provides an appropriate ratio of these factors, but earlier prepared formulas had too much polyunsaturated fats and not enough vitamin E. Formulas on the market now have corrected ratios of vitamin E and fatty acids. Vitamin E deficiency appears to cause hemolysis and seems important in improving the parameters of the physiologic nadir.[97]

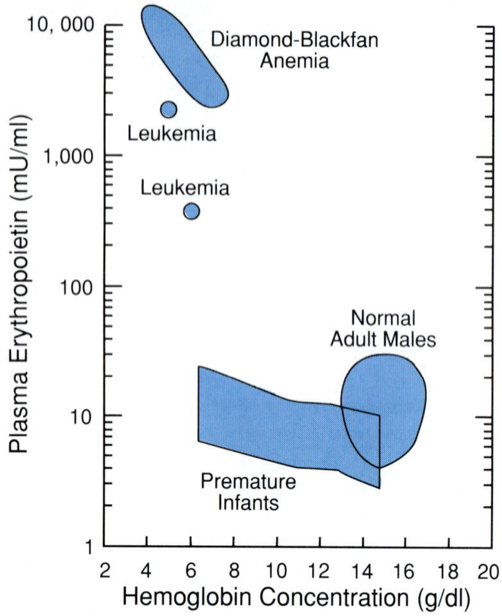

FIGURE 64-12. Relationships between hemoglobin concentration and plasma erythropoietin concentration in 21 premature infants, 7 patients with Diamond-Blackfan anemia, and 2 patients with acute lymphocytic leukemia. (After Stockman JA III, Graeber JE, Clark DA, McClellan K, Garcia JF, Kavey RE. Anemia of prematurity: determinants of the erythropoietin response. J Pediatr 1984;105:786)

Perhaps most important was the need to counter the oxidant effects of exogenously administered iron given to prevent iron deficiency.[4,107]

Iron Deficiency

Iron deficiency occurred frequently in infants at 2 to 3 months of age before the beginning of widespread iron supplementation.[3] Breastfed infants appear to have an appropriate amount of nutrient available, but premature or formula-fed infants are at risk. The chance of iron deficiency is theoretically inversely proportional to the cord blood hematocrit and blood volume (red cell mass). Premature infants who do not receive supplementation almost always become anemic and iron deficient.[108]

It is generally aggreed that with an appropriate ratio of vitamin E to polyunsaturated fatty acid and with iron supplementation of premature infants (commencing no later than 2 months) and term infants (commencing between 4 and 6 months), nutritional influences on erythropoiesis are minimized.[109]

TRANSFUSION AND ERYTHROPOIETIN TREATMENT IN THE PRETERM INFANT

When symptoms of anemia ensue during adaptation to physiologic anemia, the clinician is often faced with issues regarding transfusion. This is a controversial area and final decisions are ultimately based on clinical judgments. A few findings may help to guide clinical decision making. First, hemoglobin concentration alone may be a poor indicator of adequacy of oxygen delivery. Table 64-14 shows how the composition of hemoglobins (Hb F and Hb A), and the intactness of cardiopulmonary function (as manifested by arterial oxygen saturation) dramatically affect the neonatal hemoglobin level to maintain theoretical oxygen requirements. Although another carefully watched parameter, heart rate, has been associated with low central venous oxygen tensions, it has been discredited as a single factor governing the decision to transfuse. In general, final considerations should be based on a number of factors:

Symptoms—the infant's weight gain and fatigue during feeding
Signs—tachypnea, tachycardia, congestive hepatomegaly, and rarely râles
Laboratory values—hemoglobin and hematocrit, reticulocyte count, and the presence or absence of nucleated red cells on the peripheral smear (heralds of reticulocytosis)

After transfusion, the failure of an appropriate erythropoietin response in this group of patients often brings the clinician to the brink of transfusion in a cyclic fashion over weeks to months. The cycle occurs as the result of the inhibiting effect of transfusion on erythropoietin synthesis. As the oxygen-carrying capacity is restored to the neonate during transfusion, the call from the tissues for erythropoietin formation stops. Hence, bone marrow preparation for erythroid activity ceases, and the cycle occurs again as the transfused red cell oxygen-carrying capacity diminishes over time.

This vicious cycle of transfusion followed by symptoms requiring transfusion has led many investigators to consider the use of synthetically produced pure erythropoietin.[110–116] This would theoretically lead to increased erythroid activity from endogenous production with the creation of a proliferative erythroid mass in the infant. The cycle would ostensibly be broken for two reasons. First, the maturation of the tissue hypoxia sensor leading to more appropriate erythropoietin response might occur while endogenous erythropoietin is given, leaving behind an appropriate system to respond to anemia when exogenous erythropoietin is withdrawn. Second, the creation of an active erythroid mass would decrease the delay time associated with the rise of endogenous erythropoietin from the infant.

Use of erythropoietin for the anemia prematurity is under intense investigation. The appropriate timing and dose are to be worked out. In most studies that have been performed up to this point, the number of transfusions has been diminished but not stopped entirely.[112,113] In addition, a loss of neutrophil reserve has been demonstrated. This has led to severe neutropenia in at least one study[112] and significant neutropenia in other studies.[110–112] One recent study suggests that newer dose schedules may be more successful, but cost–benefit issues remain to be evaluated.[117]

TABLE 64-14. Theoretical Hemoglobin Levels (g/dL) Required in Low Birth Weight Infants to Maintain a Central Venous Oxygen Tension of 30 mmHg*

	Arterial Oxygen Saturation (%)†			
P_{50} (mmHg)	95	90	85	80
20‡	10.0	13.0	20.0	>25.0
23	7.3	9.0	11.0	15.5
25	6.2	7.3	8.8	11.0
27§	5.3	6.3	7.3	8.9

* Assumes a cardiac output of 250 mL/kg/min and an oxygen consumption of 6.5 mL/kg/min.
† The lower the arterial oxygen saturation, the less resting pulmonary function (eg, bronchopulmonary dysplasia).
‡ P_{50} of Hb F.
§ P_{50} of Hb A.
(Adapted from Oski FA. Hematology: the erythrocyte and its disorders. In: Nathan DA, Oski FA, eds. Hematology of infancy and childhood, ed 4. Philadelphia, WB Saunders, 1993:40)

At the same time, some significant improvements in the transfusion of neonates have occurred. Global blood bank regulations have significantly decreased the transmission of disease through transfusion. This has occurred not only because of accelerated screening of blood, but also because of the development of multiple "pedipacks," enabling the segregation of a single donor's blood into multiple small units for several of a given neonate's transfusions. This limits donor exposure significantly. A comparison of the current practice of transfusing the neonate when significant hypoxia begins to cause symptoms, rather than the prophylactic use of recombinant erythropoietin, requires a sophisticated analysis of the cost, benefit, and risk of the two modalities.

The clinician needs to realize that in otherwise healthy term infants it can be useful to tolerate some symptoms of tissue hypoxia rather than transfuse early and prevent endogenous erythropoietin formation. This practice is best reserved for infants beyond 40 weeks of gestational age. Before this time, appropriate endogenous erythropoietin production may not be available.

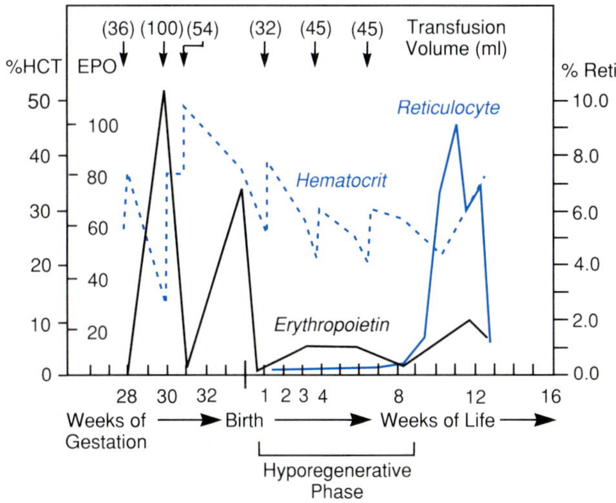

FIGURE 64-13. Hemoglobin, erythropoietin (in mU/mL), and reticulocyte levels during hyporegenerative anemia after intravascular transfusion for Rh hemolytic disease of the newborn. Arrows depict intravascular prebirth and postbirth transfusion. There is a prolonged postbirth decrease in erythropoietin levels. (After Thorp J, O'Connor T, Callenbach J, et al. Hyporegenerative anemia associated with intrauterine transfusion in rhesus hemolytic disease. Am J Obstet Gynecol 1991;165:79)

LATE ANEMIA IN HEMOLYTIC DISEASE OF THE NEWBORN

A state of mild to moderate chronic anemia usually ensues in treated neonates with HDN, as hyperbilirubinemia begins to abate. This occurs for a number of reasons. First, these infants are usually premature. Second, they have the expected normal response to the sudden increase in oxygen available in the outside world. This leads to a suppression of erythropoietin formation as tissue hypoxia disappears. In addition, multiple intrauterine transfusions and any exchanges or packed red cell transfusions that occur around the time of the birth lead to further suppression of erythropoiesis. When this occurs and few of the infant's antigen laden cells are being released from the bone marrow, less bilirubin is generated, the amount of treatment necessary for hyperbilirubinemia is lessened, and, usually between 3 and 5 days of age, the need for an exchange transfusion is gone.

Figure 64-13, which is from the data of Thorp and associates,[118] shows the hematocrit of an infant who suffered from maternal Rh sensitization. This child had severe Rh disease and required three intrauterine–intravascular transfusions and early delivery at 34 weeks of gestation. At the time of birth, the child's hematocrit was 36 and the blood contained 100% type O, Rh-negative adult donor red cells. Immediately after birth, erythropoietin levels fell almost to zero, and no reticulocytes could be demonstrated. By the ninth day, the infant had a symptomatic anemia with a hematocrit of 25% and therefore received a transfusion. This pattern repeated itself several times until 12 weeks of life when erythropoietin levels appeared to rise and reticulocytosis signaled the ability of the neonate to maintain its own hematocrit. This infant suffered the usual lack of erythropoietin formation observed in physiologic anemia of term and premature infants. In addition, the continuing presence of maternal antibody directed against the production of the neonate's own red cells prevented effective reticulocytosis in response to even small amounts of erythropoietin and hence forced the transfusion of Rh-negative cells to remove symptoms. After transfusion occurred, the stimulus to form erythropoietin was lost. This created a circle of transfusions and erythropoietin suppression leading to more transfusions that was harder to break than the similar types of situations that evolve with the anemia of prematurity.

This same cycle of transfusion suppressing erythropoietin and slowing bone marrow recovery from the anemia is also observed when exchange transfusion is used for nonimmune congenital hemolytic anemias, such as hereditary spherocytosis. Unlike the immune hemolytic anemias, these patients may have a small amount of bone marrow red cell production (reticulocyte counts of 1% to 3%), but they still occasionally require rescue by transfusion from the symptoms of anemia.

As with the anemia of prematurity, at some point, transfusions are stopped and some symptoms are tolerated to stimulate expression of increasing levels of erythropoietin. At what point this can be done depends on the general health and nutrition of the infant. As in this case, it usually happens at 8 to 12 weeks after birth. Attempts have been made to provide exogenous erythropoietin for the treatment of anemia related to Rh hemolytic disease.[119] Obviously in the presence of a significant titer of maternal anti-Rh(D) antibody, erythropoietin in these infants serves no purpose, for as soon as a red cell is produced, it is removed from the circulation secondary to interaction with the antibody. Hence, in most cases exogenous erythropoietin should be given when the infant has cleared most of the maternal antibody and might be able to tolerate anemia longer and recover his or her own erythropoietin concentration. It is likely that the use of erythropoietin for the treatment of this anemia will ultimately follow the same recommendation of balancing risk and toxicity that will come out of the study of the use of erythropoietin in the anemia of prematurity.

GENERAL APPROACH TO THE ANEMIC NEWBORN

This chapter has detailed many of the specific conditions involved in the appearance of anemia in the neonate. The emphasis has been on the physiology and pathophysiology of anemia as it relates to the developmental sequence that occurs during the transition from fetal to neonatal life and from neonatal to infant life. Figure 64-14 is a flow chart of the author's approach to the diagnosis of anemia in the

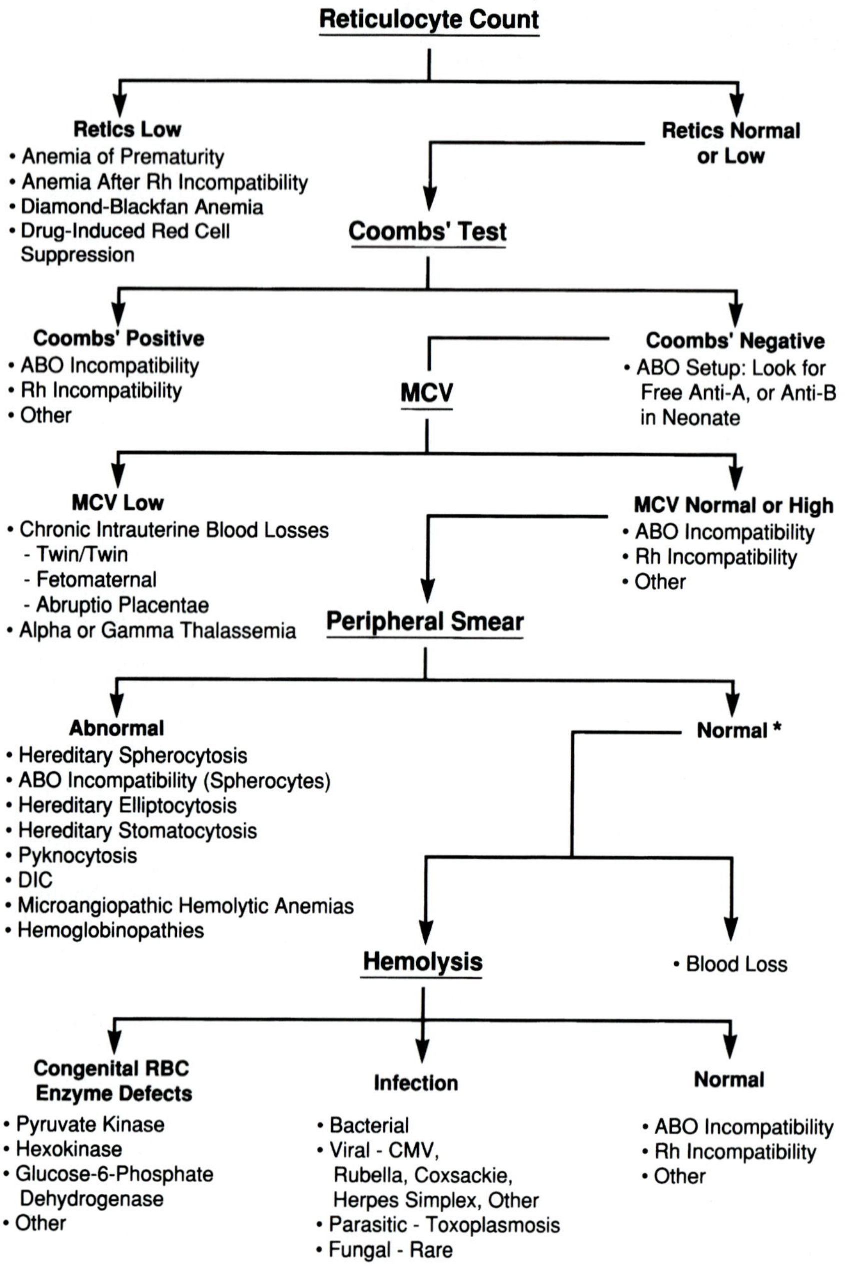

FIGURE 64-14. An approach to neonatal anemia. Asterisk indicates a smear with no predominant morphology (see Table 47-4). (After Oski F. Hematology: the erythrocyte and its disorders. In: Nathan DA, Oski FA, eds. Hematology of infancy and childhood, ed 4. Philadelphia, WB Saunders, 1993:38)

neonate and reflects much of the information and discussion within the chapter. Many neonatal anemias disappear spontaneously as a result of the Hb F switch, changes in the relation of the red cell to its milieu (eg, mild HDN), changes in neonatal erythrocyte membrane physiology (eg, hereditary elliptocytosis with neonatal poikilocytosis), or increasing red cell resistance to oxidant threats (such as Heinz body hemolytic anemia). In the many situations in which hyperbilirubinemia is not serious enough to require intense investigation and in which anemia is mild, it may be prudent to reserve intensive investigation with phlebotomy until the infant is older, when intravenous access is easier and the child can better tolerate the blood loss.

REFERENCES

1. Matoth Y, Zaizov R, Varsano I. Postnatal changes in some red cell parameters. Acta Paediatr Scand 1971;60:317.
2. Stockman JA. Anemia of prematurity. Clin Perinatol 1977;4:239.
3. Zaizov R, Matoth Y. Red cell values on the first postnatal day during the last 16 weeks of gestation. Am J Hematol 1976;1:275.
4. Melhorn DK, Gross S, Childers G. Vitamin E dependent anemia in the premature infant. I. Effect of large doses of medicinal iron. J Pediatr 1971;79:569.
5. Andrew M, Paes B, Milner R, et al. Development of the human coagulation system in the full-term infant. Blood 1987;70:165.
6. Andrew M, Paes B, Milner R, et al. Development of the human coagulation system in the healthy premature infant. Blood 1980;72:1651.
7. Oski F. Hematology: the erythrocyte and its disorders. In: Nathan DA, Oski FA, eds. Hematology of infancy and childhood, ed 4. Philadelphia, WB Saunders, 1993:18.
8. Thomas DB. Yoffey JM. Human foetal haematopoiesis. II. Hepatic haematopoiesis in the human foetus. Br J Haematol 1964;10:193.
9. Pearson H. Disorders of hemoglobin synthesis and metabolism. In: Oski F, Naiman JL, eds. Hematologic problems in the newborn, ed 3. Philadelphia, WB Saunders, 1972:245.
10. Wells RMG. Haemoglobin-oxygen affinity in developing embryonic erythroid cells of the mouse. J Comp Physiol 1979;129:333.
11. Stockman JA III. Fetal hematology. In: Eden RD, Boehm FH, eds. Assessment and care of the fetus. Norwalk, CT, Appleton & Lange, 1990: 113.
12. Wimberley PD. A review of oxygen delivery in the neonate. Scand J Clin Lab Invest 1982;42(Suppl 160):1.
13. Sjolin S. The resistance of red cells in vitro: a study of the osmotic properties, mechanical resistance and the storage behavior of red cells of fetuses, children, and adults. Acta Paediatr Scand 1954;43:1.
14. Voak D, Williams MA. An explanation of the failure of the direct antiglobulin test to detect erythrocyte sensitization in ABO haemolytic

disease of the newborn and observations on pinocytosis of IgG anti-A antibodies by infant (cord) red cells. Br J Hematol 1971;20:9.
15. Mollison PL. Blood transfusion in clinical medicine, ed 4. Oxford, Blackwell Scientific, 1967:275.
16. Sheetz MP, Casaly J. 2,3 diphosphoglycerate and ATP dissociate erythrocyte membrane skeletons. J Biol Chem 1980;255:9955.
17. Wolfe LC, Lux SE, Ohanian V. Regulation of spectrin-actin binding by protein 4.1 and polyphosphates. J Cell Biol 1980;87:203a, Abstract.
18. Advani R, Mentzer W, Andrews D, Schrier S. Oxidation of Hemoglobin F is associated with the aging process of prenatal red blood cells. Pediatr Res 1992;32:165.
19. Oski FA. Anemia in the neonatal period. In: Oski FA, Naiman JL, eds. Hematologic problems in the newborn, ed 3. Philadelphia, WB Saunders, 1982:56.
20. Zipursky A, Brown E, Polk J, Brown EJ. The erythrocyte differential count in newborn infants. Am J Pediatr Hematol Oncol 1983;5:45.
21. Holroyde CP, Oski FA, Gardner FH. The pocked erythrocyte. N Engl J Med 1969;281:516.
22. Pearson HA. Life-span of the fetal red blood cell. J Pediatr 1967;70: 166.
23. Hemolytic disease of the newborn. Raritan, NJ, Ortho Diagnostics, 1968:5.
24. Kline W. Chemistry of blood group antigens and antibodies in hemolytic disease of the newborn. In: Bell C, ed. Seminar on perinatal blood banking. Washington, DC, American Association of Blood Banks, 1978:1.
25. Zipursky A. Isoimmune hemolytic diseases. In: Nathan DG, Oski FA, eds. Hematology of infancy and childhood, ed 4. Philadelphia, WB Saunders, 1993:44.
26. Werth A. Prenatal evaluation of hemolytic disease of the fetus. In: Bell C, ed. Seminar on perinatal blood banking. Washington, DC, American Association of Blood Banks, 1978:55.
27. Mollison PL, Crane P, Jones HJ, Rochna E. Rate of removal from the circulation of red cells sensitized with different amounts of antibody. Br J Haematol 1965;11:461.
28. Prokop O, Uhlenbruck G. Human blood and serum groups. New York, Wiley Interscience, 1969:218.
29. Zipursky A, Pollock J, Neelands P, et al. The transplacental passage of foetal red blood cells and the pathogenesis of Rh immunization during pregnancy. Lancet 1963;2:489.
30. Cook I. Primary rhesus immunization of male volunteers. Br J Haematol 1971;20:369.
31. Weiner AS. Further observations on isosensitization to the Rh factor. Proc Soc Exp Biol Med 1949;70:576.
32. Clarke CA, Donohoe WTA, McConnell RB, et al. Further experimental studies on the prevention of Rh haemolytic disease. Br Med J 1963;1: 979.
33. Nusbacher J. Evaluation and management of the nonimmunized patient. In: Tregallas WM, Wallas CH, eds. Prenatal and perinatal immunohematology. Washington, DC, American Association of Blood Banks, 1981:17.
34. Bowman JM. Rh erythroblastosis fetalis 1975. Semin Hematol 1975;12: 189.
35. White CA, Visscher RD, Visscher HC, Wade MI. Rh (D) immune globulin prophylaxis: a double blind cooperative study. Obstet Gynecol 1976;36: 341.
36. Freda VJ, Gorman JG, Polloch W, Bave E. Prevention of Rh hemolytic disease: ten years' clinical experience with the Rhogam immune globulin in Rh antibody mediated immunosuppression. Raritan, NJ, Ortho Diagnostics, 1975:71.
37. Davey MG, Zipursky A. McMaster Conference on the Prevention of Rh immunization. Vox Sang 1979;36:50.
38. Levine P. Serological factors as possible cause of spontaneous abortion. J Hered 1943;34:71.
39. Stern K, Davidson I, Masiatis L. Experimental studies on Rh immunization. Am J Clin Pathol 1956;26:833.
40. Zipursky A. Rh hemolytic disease of the newborn: the disease eradicated by immunology. Clin Obstet Gynecol 1977;20:759.
41. Polloch W, Ascari WQ, Kochesky RJ, et al. Studies on Rh prophylaxis. I. Relationship between doses of anti-Rh and size of antigenic stimulus. Transfusion 1971;44:333.
42. Taylor JF. Sensitization of Rh negative daughters by their Rh-positive mothers. N Engl J Med 1967;276:547.
43. Bowen FW, Renfield M. The detection of anti–D in Rh D–negative infants born of Rh D–positive mothers. Pediatr Res 1976;20:213.
44. Hoppe HH, Mester T, Hennig W, Krebs HJ. Prevention of Rh immunization: modified production of IgG anti-Rh for intravenous application by ion exchange chromatography. Vox Sang 1973;25:308.
45. Cohen F, Zuelzer WF, Gustafson DC, Evan MM. Mechanisms of isoimmunization. I. The transplacental passage of fetal erythrocytes in homospecific pregnancies. Blood 1964;23:621.
46. Gilmore JR. Erythroblastosis foetalis. Arch Dis Child 1944;19:1.
47. Harman CR. Specialized applications of obstetric ultrasound: management of the alloimmunized pregnancy. Semin Perinatol 1985;9:184.
48. Harmon CR. Fetal monitoring in the alloimmunized pregnancy. Clin Perinatol 1989;26:691.
49. Parkin J, Walker W. Peritoneal dialysis in severe hydrops fetalis. Lancet 1968;2:283.
50. Phibbs RH, Johnson P. Circulatory changes in newborns with erythroblostosis fetalis. Pediatr Res 1967;1:321.
51. Bowman JM, Friesen RF, Bowman WD, et al. Fetal transfusion in severe Rh isoimmunization. JAMA 1969;207:1101.
52. Boggs TR. Proper place of intrauterine transfusions in management of fetuses with Rh hemolytic disease. Clin Pediatr 1970;9:636.
53. Watson D, Mackay EV, Trevella W. Amniotic fluid analysis and foetal erythroblastosis. Clin Chim Acta 1965;23:500.
54. Bowman J. Clinical management of the immunized patient. In: Tregellas WM, Wallas CH, eds. Prenatal and perinatal immunohematology. Washington, DC, American Association of Blood Banks, 1981:61.
55. Frigoletto FD Jr, Umansky I. Intrauterine transfusion in 365 fetuses during fifteen years. J Obstet Gynecol 1981;139:781.
56. Harman CR, Bowman JM, Manning FA, Menticglou SM. Intrauterine transfusion: intraperitoneal versus intravascular approach: a case-control comparison. Am J Obstet Gynecol 1990;102:1053.
57. Ronkin S, Benjamin C, Wapner R, et al. Intravascular exchange and bolus transfusion in the severely isoimmunized fetus. Am J Obstet Gynecol 1989;160:407.
58. Walker W. Hemolytic disease of the newborn. In: Gairdner D, Hull D, eds. Recent advances in pediatrics, ed 4. London, JA Churchill, 1971: 119.
59. Cherry SH, Rosenfield RE, Kochwa S. Mechanism of accumulation of amniotic fluid pigment in erythroblastosis fetalis. Am J Obstet Gynecol 1970;106:297.
60. Levi AJ, Gatmaitan Z, Arias IM. Deficiency of hepatic organic anion-binding protein, impaired organic anion uptake by liver and "physiologic" jaundice in newborn monkeys. N Engl J Med 1970;283:1136.
61. Thaler MM. Perinatal bilirubin metabolism. Adv Pediatr 1972;19:215.
62. Schutta HS, Johnson L, Neville HE. Mitochondrial abnormalities in bilirubin encephalopathy. J Neuropath Exp Neurol 1970;29:296.
63. Diamond L, Schmid R. Experimental bilirubin encephalopathy: the mode of entry of bilirubin 14C into the central nervous system. J Clin Invest 1966;45:678.
64. Chan G, Schiff D. Competitive binding of free fatty acids and bilirubin to albumin differences in HBABA dye versus Sephadex G-25 interpretation of results. Clin Biochem 1971;4:208.
65. Zamet P, Chung F. Separation by gel filtration and micro-determination of unbound bilirubin. Acta Paediatr Scand 1971;60:33.
66. Odell GB, Cohen SN, Kelly PC. Studies in kernicterus. II. The determination of the saturation of serum albumin with bilirubin. J Pediatr 1969;74:214.
67. Stern L. Drug interactions. II. Drugs, the newborn infant, and the binding of bilirubin to albumin. Pediatrics 1972;49:916.
68. Valaes TN, Harvey-Wilkes K. Pharmacologic approaches to the prevention and treatment of neonatal hyperbilirubinemia. Clin Perinatol 1990;17:245.
69. Bowman J, Friesen R. Hemolytic disease of the newborn. In: Gellis S, Kagan B, eds. Current pediatric therapy, ed 3. Philadelphia, WB Saunders, 1968:367.
70. Naiman JL. Erythroblastosis fetalis. In: Oski FA, Namain JL, eds. Hematologic problems in the newborn, ed 3. Philadelphia, WB Saunders, 1982:283.
71. Luban N. Blood groups and blood component transfusion. In: Miller D, Baehner R, McMillan C, eds. Blood diseases of infancy and childhood, ed 5. St Louis, CV Mosby, 1984:46.
72. Valaes T. Bilirubin distribution and dynamics of bilirubin removal by exchange transfusion. Acta Paediatr 1963;(Suppl 1):149.
73. Driscoll BG, Steinke J. Pancreatic insulin content in severe erythroblastosis fetalis. Pediatrics 1967;39:54.
74. Price HV. Hypoglycaemia complicating haemolytic disease of the newborn. Arch Dis Child 1969;44:248.
75. Dunn PM. Obstructive jaundice and haemolytic disease of the newborn. Arch Dis Child 1963;38:54.
76. Thorp J, O'Connor T, Callenbach J, et al. Hyporegenerative anemia associated with intrauterine transfusion in rhesus hemolytic disease. Am J Obstet Gynecol 1991;165:79.
77. Klemper M. Hemolytic anemias: immune defects. In: Miller D, Baehner R, McMillar C, eds. Blood diseases of infancy and childhood, ed 5. St Louis, CV Mosby, 1984:231.
78. Voak D, Williams MA. An explanation of the failure of the direct antiglobulin test to detect erythrocyte sensitization in ABO haemolytic disease of the newborn and observations on pinocytosis of IgG anti-A antibodies by infant (cord) red cells. Br J Haematol 1971;20:9.
79. Linderhamp O, Vesmold HT, Strohhacker I, et al. Capillary-venous hematocrit differences in newborn infants. I. Relationship to blood volume, peripheral blood flow, and acid base parameters. Eur J Pediatr 1977;127:9.
80. Colozzi AE. Clamping of the umbilical cord: its effect on the placental transfusion. N Engl J Med 1954;250:629.
81. Yao AO, Lind J, Tiisala R, Michelsson K. Placental transfusion in the premature infant with observation on clinical course and outcome. Acta Paediatr Scand 1969;58:561.
82. Usher R, Shephard M, Lind J. The blood volume of the newborn infant and placental transfusion. Acta Paediatr 1963;52:497.

83. Demarsh QB, Alt HL, Windle WF. Factors in influencing blood picture of newborn. Am J Dis Child 1948;75:860.
84. Lanzkowsky P. Effects of early and late clamping of umbilical cord on infant's hemoglobin level. Br Med J 1980;2:1777.
85. Faxelius G, Raye J, Gutberlet R, et al. Red cell volume measurements and acute blood loss in high-risk newborn infants. J Pediatr 1977;90: 273.
86. McIntosh S, Pearson H. Origin and development of blood cells and coagulation factors: maternal–fetal interactions. In: Miller D, Baehner R, McMillan C, eds. Blood diseases of infancy and childhood, ed 5. St Louis, CV Mosby, 1984:3.
87. Kleihauer E, Braun H, Betke K. Demonstration von fetalem Hamoglobin in den Erythrocyten eines Blütausstrichs (Demonstration of fetal hemoglobin in erythrocytes of a blood smear). Klin Wochenschr 1957;35: 637.
88. Mollison PL. Quantitation of the extent of transplacental hemorrhage. Br Med J 1972;3:31.
89. Kirkman HN, Riley HD Jr. Post-hemorrhagic anemia and shock in the newborn due to hemorrhage during delivery: report of 8 cases. Pediatrics 1959;24:92.
90. Benirschke K. Accurate recording of twin placentation. Obstet Gynecol 1961;18:334.
91. Strong SJ, Corney G. The placenta in twin pregnancy. New York, Pergamon Press, 1967.
92. Pochedly C, Musker S. Twin-to-twin transfusion syndrome. Postgrad Med 1970;47:172.
93. Tan KL, Tan R, Tan SH, Tan AM. The twin transfusion syndrome: clinical observations on 35 affected pairs. Clin Pediatr 1979;18:111.
94. Pachman DJ. Massive hemorrhage in the scalp of the newborn infant. Pediatrics 1962;29:907.
95. Papila LA, Burstein J, Burstein R, Koffler H. Incidence and evolution of subependymal and intraventricular hemorrhage. J Pediatr 1978;92: 529.
96. Oski F. Disorders of red cell metabolism. In: Oski F, Naiman JL, eds. Hematologic problems in the newborn, ed 3. Philadelphia, WB Saunders, 1982:97.
97. Oski FA, Barness LA. Vitamin E deficiency: a previously unrecognized cause of hemolytic anemia in the premature infant. J Pediatr 1967;70: 211.
98. Levine RL, Lincoln DR, Buchholz WM, et al. Hemoglobin Hasharon in a premature infant with hemolytic anemia. Pediatr Res 1975;9:7.
99. Bianch D, Beyer E, Staru A, et al. Normal long-term survival with α-thalassemia. J Pediatr 1986;108:716.
100. Lee-Potter JP, Deacon-Smith RA, Simpkiss MJ, et al. A new cause of haemolytic anaemia in the newborn. J Clin Pathol 1975;28:317.
101. Kan YW, Forget G, et al. Gamma-beta thalassemia: a cause of hemolytic anemia in the newborn. N Engl J Med 1972;286:129.
102. Hegyi T, Delphin ES, Bank A, et al. Sickle cell anemia in the newborn. Pediatrics 1977;60:213.
103. Diamond LK, Allen DM, Magill FB. Congenital (erythroid) hypoplastic anemia. Am J Dis Child 1961;102:403.
104. Halvorsen S, Finne PH. Erythropoietin production in the human fetus and newborn. Ann NY Acad Sci 1968;149:576.
105. Stockman JA III, Graeber JE, Clark OA. Anemia of prematurity: determinants of the erythropoietin response. J Pediatr 1984;105:786.
106. Stockman JA III. Erythropoietin: off again, on again. J Pediatr 1988;1112: 906.
107. Williams ME, Shott RJ, Oski FA. Role of dietary iron and fat on vitamin E deficiency anemia of infancy. N Engl J Med 1975;292:887.
108. Lundstrom U, Siimes MA, Dallman PR. At what age does iron supplementation become necessary in low-birth-weight infants? J Pediatr 1977;91:878.
109. Forbes G, Woodruff C, eds. Pediatric nutrition handbook. Elle Grove Village, IL, American Academy of Pediatrics, 1989:216.
110. Halperin OS, Wacher P, Lacourt G, et al. Effects of recombinant human erythropoietin in infants with anemia of prematurity: a pilot study. J Pediatr 1990;116:779.
111. Shannon K, Mantzer W, Abels R, et al. Recombinant human erythropoietin in the anemia of prematurity: results of a placebo-controlled pilot study. J Pediatr 1991;118:949.
112. Ohis R, Christensen RD. Recombinant erythropoietin compared with erythrocyte transfusion in the treatment of anemia of prematurity. J Pediatr 1991;119:781.
113. Shannon K, Mentzer W, Abels R, et al. Enhancement of erythropoiesis by recombinant human erythropoietin in low birth weight infants: a pilot study. J Pediatr 1992;120:586.
114. Herger P, Bechensteen A, Halvorsen S. Erythropoietin treatment of protein and iron supplemented premature SGA infants. (Abstract) Pediatr Res 1992;31:267A.
115. Messer J, Donato L, Matis J, Haddad J. Prevention of anemia of prematurity with human recombinant erythropoietin. (Abstract) Pediatr Res 1992;31:269A.
116. Kling P, Widness J, Guillery E, Veng-Pederson P. Lack of erythropoietin efficacy associated with developmental differences in erythropoietin pharmacokinetics. (Abstract) Pediatr Res 1992;31:268A.
117. Maier RF, Obladen M, Sciggalla P, et al. The effect of epoetin beta (recombinant human erythropoietin) on the need for transfusion in very low birth weight infants: European Multicentre Study Group. N Engl J Med 1994;330:1173.
118. Thorp J, O'Connor T, Callenbach J, et al. Hyporegenerative anemia associated with intrauterine transfusion in Rhesus hemolytic disease. Am J Obstet Gynecol 1991;165:79.
119. Bussel JB, Inglis SR, Chervenak FA. Erythropoietin (EPO) treatment for anemia in Rh disease. (Abstract) Pediatr Res 1992;31:265A.

Appendix

Data of Importance in Hematology

Blood: Principles and Practice of Hematology,
edited by Robert I. Handin, Samuel E. Lux, and Thomas P. Stossel.
J.B. Lippincott Company, Philadelphia © 1995.

Normal Blood Values

APPENDIX 1

Normal Leukocyte Counts*

	Total Leukocytes		Neutrophils			Lymphocytes			Monocytes		Eosinophils	
Age	**Mean**	**Range**	**Mean**	**Range**	**%**	**Mean**	**Range**	**%**	**Mean**	**%**	**Mean**	**%**
Birth	18.1	9.0–30.0	11.0	6.0–26.0	61	5.5	2.0–11.0	31	1.1	6	0.4	2
12 h	22.8	13.0–38.0	15.5	6.0–28.0	68	5.5	2.0–11.0	24	1.2	5	0.5	2
24 h	18.9	9.4–34.0	11.5	5.0–21.0	61	5.8	2.0–11.5	31	1.1	6	0.5	2
1 wk	12.2	5.0–21.0	5.5	1.5–10.0	45	5.0	2.0–17.0	41	1.1	9	0.5	4
2 wk	11.4	5.0–20.0	4.5	1.0–9.5	40	5.5	2.0–17.0	48	1.0	9	0.4	3
1 mo	10.8	5.0–19.5	3.8	1.0–9.0	35	6.0	2.5–16.5	56	0.7	7	0.3	3
6 mo	11.9	6.0–17.5	3.8	1.0–8.5	32	7.3	4.0–13.5	61	0.6	5	0.3	3
1 y	11.4	6.0–17.5	3.5	1.5–8.5	31	7.0	4.0–10.5	61	0.6	5	0.3	3
2 y	10.6	6.0–17.0	3.5	1.5–8.5	33	6.3	3.0–9.5	59	0.5	5	0.3	3
4 y	9.1	5.5–15.5	3.8	1.5–8.5	42	4.5	2.0–8.0	50	0.5	5	0.3	3
6 y	8.5	5.0–14.5	4.3	1.5–8.0	51	3.5	1.5–7.0	42	0.4	5	0.2	3
8 y	8.3	4.5–13.5	4.4	1.5–8.0	53	3.3	1.5–6.8	39	0.4	4	0.2	2
10 y	8.1	4.5–13.5	4.4	1.8–8.0	54	3.1	1.5–6.5	38	0.4	4	0.2	2
16 y	7.8	4.5–13.0	4.4	1.8–8.0	57	2.8	1.2–5.2	35	0.4	5	0.2	3
21 y	7.4	4.5–11.0	4.4	1.8–7.7	59	2.5	1.0–4.8	34	0.3	4	0.2	3

* Numbers of leukocytes are in thousands per μL; ranges are estimates of 95% confidence limits; and percentages refer to differential counts. Neutrophils include band cells at all ages and a small number of metamyelocytes and myelocytes in the first few days of life.

(Dallman PR. In: Rudolph AM, ed. Pediatrics, ed 16. New York, Appleton-Century-Crofts, 1977:1178)

APPENDIX 2

Absolute Blood Phagocyte Concentrations

	Concentration (cells/μL; 95% range [mean])			
Population	**Band Forms**	**Segmented Forms**	**Band and Segmented Forms**	**Monocytes**
AMERICAN ADULTS*				
White subjects	200–2150 (600)	1500–6050 (3000)		220–950 (460)
Black subjects	60–1650 (300)	1100–6700 (2700)		210–1050 (470)
EUROPEAN ADULTS†				
White subjects			3487–9206	221–843
AMERICAN INFANTS AND CHILDREN‡				
Birth			6000–26000 (11000)	400–3100 (1050)
7 d			1500–10000 (5500)	300–2700 (1100)
4 y			1500–8500 (3800)	0–800 (450)
10 y			1800–8000 (4400)	0–800 (350)

* Orfanakis NG, Ostlund RE, Bishop CR, Athens JW. Normal blood leukocyte concentration values. Am J Clin Pathol 1970;53:647.

† England JM, Bain BJ. Total and differential leukocyte count. Br J Haematol 1976;33:1.

‡ Altman PL, Katz DD. Human health and disease. In: FASEB biology handbooks II. Washington, DC, FASEB, 1977:161.

APPENDIX 3

Leukocytes: Absolute and Relative Values for a Normal Population*

	Absolute Number (Cells × 10^9/L From Log Plots)		Relative Number (%)	
	Median	95% Range	Mean	95% Range
Total leukocytes	7.0	4.3–10.0		
Neutrophils—bands	0.52	0.1–2.1	9.5	0–21.5
Neutrophils—segmented	3.0	1.1–6.05	43.5	24.8–62.3
Neutrophils—total	3.65	1.83–7.25	53.0	34.6–71.4
Eosinophils	0.15	0–0.7	3.2	0–7.8
Basophils	0.03	0–0.15	0.6	0–1.8
Lymphocytes	2.5	1.5–4.0	36.1	19.6–52.7
Monocytes	0.43	0.2–0.95	7.1	2.4–11.8

* 291 adults in Salt Lake City.
(Orfanakis NG, Ostlund RE, Bishop CR, Athens JW. Normal blood leukocyte concentration. Am J Clin Pathol 1970;53:647)

APPENDIX 4

Leukocyte Alkaline Phosphatase Scores in Normal Subjects

Group	Number	Mean	95% Limits
Male	51	73	22–124
Female	50	92	33–149
Total	101	82	25–139

(Cartwright GE. Diagnostic Laboratory hematology, ed 4. New York, Grune & Stratton, 1968)

APPENDIX 5

Bone Marrow Cell Populations of Normal Infants*

	Month						
Cell Type	**0 (n = 57)**	**1 (n = 71)**	**2 (n = 48)**	**4 (n = 19)**	**6 (n = 22)**	**12 (n = 18)**	**18 (n = 19)**
Small lymphocytes	14.42 ± 5.54	47.05 ± 9.24	42.68 ± 7.90	47.06 ± 8.77	47.55 ± 7.88	47.11 ± 11.32	43.55 ± 8.56
Transitional cells	1.18 ± 1.13	1.95 ± 0.94	2.38 ± 1.35	1.64 ± 1.01	2.31 ± 1.16	2.32 ± 1.90	1.99 ± 1.00
Proerythroblasts	0.02 ± 0.06	0.10 ± 0.14	0.13 ± 0.19	0.05 ± 0.10	0.09 ± 0.12	0.02 ± 0.04	0.08 ± 0.13
Basophilic erythroblasts	0.24 ± 0.25	0.34 ± 0.33	0.57 ± 0.41	0.24 ± 0.24	0.32 ± 0.24	0.30 ± 0.25	0.50 ± 0.34
Early erythroblasts	0.27 ± 0.26	0.44 ± 0.42	0.71 ± 0.51	0.28 ± 0.30	0.41 ± 0.30	0.39 ± 0.27	0.59 ± 0.34
Polychromatic erythroblasts	13.06 ± 6.78	6.90 ± 4.45	13.06 ± 3.48	6.84 ± 2.58	7.30 ± 3.60	6.83 ± 3.75	6.97 ± 3.56
Orthochromatic erythroblasts	0.69 ± 0.73	0.54 ± 1.88	0.66 ± 0.82	0.34 ± 0.30	0.38 ± 0.56	0.37 ± 0.51	0.44 ± 0.49
Extruded nuclei	0.47 ± 0.46	0.16 ± 0.17	0.26 ± 0.22	0.16 ± 0.17	0.16 ± 0.22	0.23 ± 0.25	0.21 ± 0.19
Late erythroblasts	14.22 ± 7.14	7.60 ± 4.84	13.99 ± 3.82	7.34 ± 2.54	7.85 ± 4.11	7.42 ± 4.11	7.62 ± 3.63
Early/late erythroblasts ratio	1:50	1:15	1:18	1:23	1:17	1:17	1:10
Fetal erythroblasts	14.48 ± 7.24	8.04 ± 5.00	14.70 ± 3.86	7.62 ± 2.56	8.25 ± 4.31	7.81 ± 4.26	8.21 ± 37.1
Blood reticulocytes	4.18 ± 1.46	1.06 ± 1.13	3.39 ± 1.22	1.65 ± 0.73	1.74 ± 0.80	1.79 ± 0.79	1.84 ± 0.46
Neutrophils							
Promyelocytes	0.79 ± 0.91	0.76 ± 0.65	0.78 ± 0.68	0.59 ± 0.51	0.67 ± 0.66	0.69 ± 0.71	0.64 ± 0.59
Myelocytes	3.95 ± 2.93	2.50 ± 1.48	2.03 ± 1.14	2.32 ± 1.59	2.22 ± 1.25	2.32 ± 1.14	2.49 ± 1.39
Early neutrophils	4.74 ± 3.43	3.27 ± 1.94	2.81 ± 1.62	2.91 ± 2.01	2.89 ± 1.71	3.02 ± 1.52	3.14 ± 1.75
Metamyelocytes	19.37 ± 4.84	11.34 ± 3.59	11.27 ± 3.38	6.04 ± 3.63	11.02 ± 3.12	11.10 ± 3.82	12.42 ± 4.15
Bands	28.89 ± 7.56	14.10 ± 4.63	13.15 ± 4.71	13.93 ± 6.13	14.00 ± 4.58	14.02 ± 4.88	14.20 ± 5.23
Mature neutrophils	7.37 ± 4.64	3.64 ± 2.97	3.07 ± 2.45	4.27 ± 2.69	4.85 ± 2.69	5.65 ± 3.92	6.31 ± 3.91
Late neutrophils	55.63 ± 7.98	29.08 ± 6.79	27.50 ± 6.88	31.30 ± 7.80	29.86 ± 6.74	30.77 ± 8.69	32.93 ± 7.01
Early/late neutrophil ratio	1:12	1:9	1:9	1:11	1:10	1:10	1:10
Total neutrophils	60.37 ± 8.66	32.35 ± 7.68	30.31 ± 7.27	34.21 ± 8.61	32.75 ± 7.03	33.79 ± 8.76	36.06 ± 7.40
Total eosinophils	2.70 ± 1.27	2.61 ± 1.40	2.50 ± 1.22	2.37 ± 4.13	2.08 ± 1.16	1.92 ± 1.09	2.70 ± 2.16
Total basophils	0.12 ± 0.20	0.07 ± 0.16	0.08 ± 0.10	0.11 ± 0.14	0.10 ± 0.13	0.13 ± 0.15	0.10 ± 0.12
Total myeloid cells	63.19 ± 9.10	35.03 ± 8.09	32.90 ± 7.85	36.69 ± 8.91	34.93 ± 7.52	35.83 ± 8.84	38.86 ± 7.92
Monocytes	0.88 ± 0.85	1.01 ± 0.89	0.91 ± 0.83	0.75 ± 0.75	1.21 ± 1.01	1.46 ± 1.52	2.12 ± 1.59
Miscellaneous							
Megakaryocytes	0.06 ± 0.15	0.05 ± 0.09	0.10 ± 0.13	0.06 ± 0.06	0.04 ± 0.07	0.05 ± 0.08	0.07 ± 0.12
Plasma cells	0.00 ± 0.02	0.02 ± 0.06	0.02 ± 0.05	0.01 ± 0.03	0.03 ± 0.07	0.03 ± 0.07	0.06 ± 0.08
Unknown blasts	0.31 ± 0.31	0.62 ± 0.50	0.58 ± 0.50	0.56 ± 0.53	0.56 ± 0.48	0.37 ± 0.33	0.43 ± 0.45
Unknown cells	0.22 ± 0.34	0.21 ± 0.25	0.16 ± 0.24	0.23 ± 0.25	0.10 ± 0.15	0.11 ± 0.14	0.20 ± 0.23
Damaged cells	5.79 ± 2.78	5.50 ± 2.46	5.09 ± 1.78	4.80 ± 2.29	5.04 ± 1.08	5.34 ± 2.19	5.05 ± 2.15
Total	6.38 ± 2.84	6.39 ± 2.63	5.94 ± 1.94	5.66 ± 2.30	5.78 ± 1.16	5.90 ± 2.03	5.81 ± 2.16

n, number of infants studied at each age.

* Percentages of cell types (means ± SD) in tibial bone marrow of infants from birth to 18 months of age. Based on differential counts of 1000 cells classified on stained smears on each of 10 serial marrow samples from normal American infants of European, African, and Asian origin, aspirated from the same population of infants.

(Rosse C, Kraemer MJ, Dillon TL, McFarland R, Smith NJ. Bone marrow cell populations of normal infants: the predominance of lymphocytes. J Lab Clin Med 1977;89:1228)

Blood: Principles and Practice of Hematology,
edited by Robert I. Handin, Samuel E. Lux, and Thomas P. Stossel.
J.B. Lippincott Company, Philadelphia © 1995.

Leukocytes

APPENDIX 6

Differential Counts of Bone Marrow Aspirates From 12 Heathy Men

	Mean (%)	Observed Range (%)	95% Confidence Limits (%)
Neutrophilic series (total)	53.6	49.2–65.0	33.6–73.6
Myeloblasts	0.9	0.2–1.5	0.1–1.7
Promyelocytes	3.3	2.1–4.1	1.9–4.7
Myelocytes	12.7	8.2–15.7	8.5–16.9
Metamyelocytes	15.9	9.6–24.6	7.1–24.7
Band	12.4	9.5–15.3	9.4–15.4
Segmented	7.4	6.0–12.0	3.8–11.0
Eosinophilic series (total)	3.1	1.2–5.3	1.1–5.2
Myelocytes	0.8	0.2–1.3	0.2–1.4
Metamyelocytes	1.2	0.4–2.2	0.2–2.2
Band	0.9	0.2–2.4	0–2.7
Segmented	0.5	0–1.3	0–1.1
Basophilic and mast cells	0.1	0–0.2	
Erythrocytic series (total)	25.6	18.4–33.8	15.0–36.2
Pronormoblasts	0.6	0.2–1.3	0.1–1.1
Basophilic	1.4	0.5–2.4	0.4–2.4
Polychromatophilic	21.6	17.9–29.2	13.1–30.1
Orthochromatic	2.0	0.4–4.6	0.3–3.7
Lymphocytes	16.2	11.1–23.2	8.6–23.8
Plasma cells	1.3	0.4–3.9	0–3.5
Monocytes	0.3	0–0.8	0–0.6
Megakaryocytes	0.1	0–0.4	
Reticulum cells	0.3	0–0.9	0–0.8
M/E ratio	2.3	1.5–3.3	1.1–3.5

(Wintrobe MM, Lee GR, Boggs DR, et al, eds. Clinical hematology, ed 7. Philadelphia, Lea & Febiger, 1974:1796)

APPENDIX 7

Lymphoid Cell Differentiation

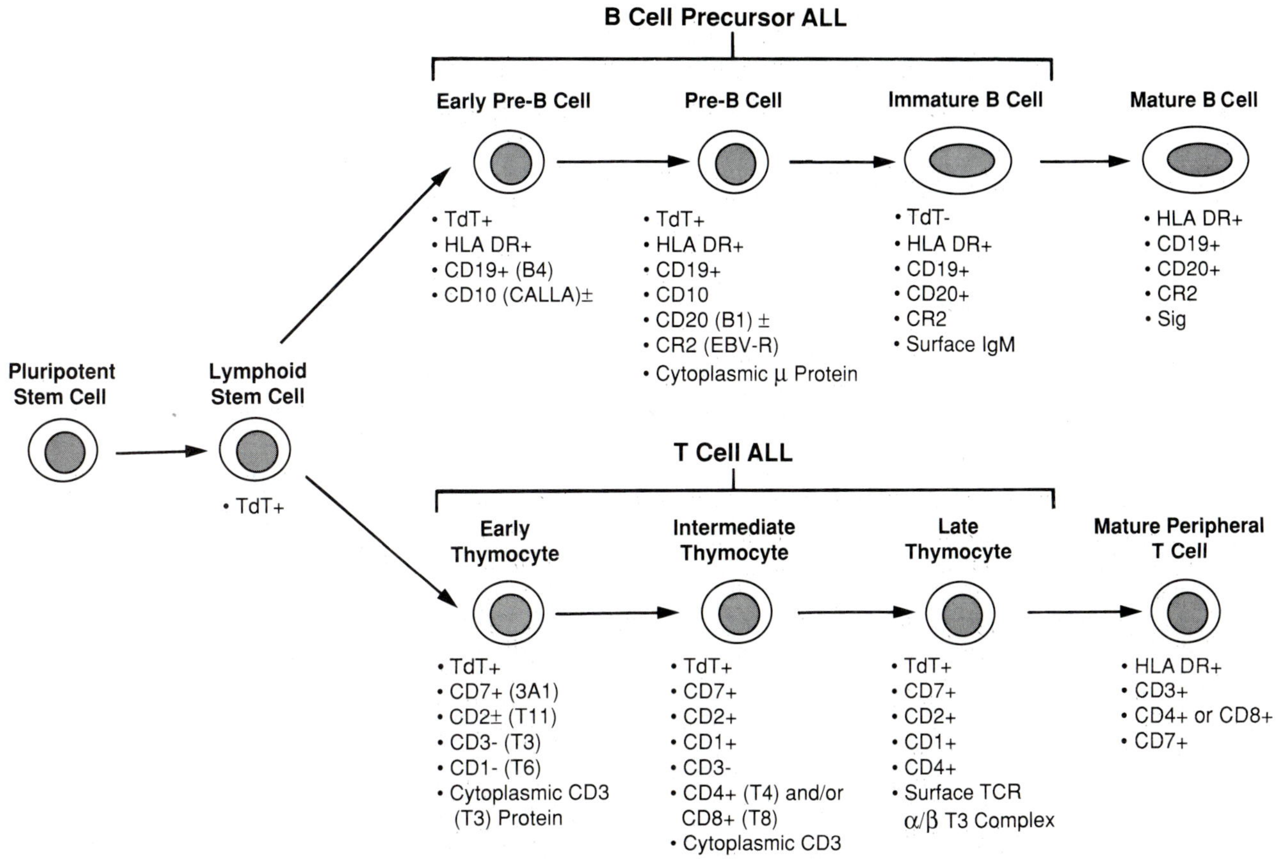

Model showing stages of cellular development based on terminal deoxynucleotide transferase (TdT) activity, binding to commonly used monoclonal antibodies, T-cell receptor gene rearrangement, and the presence of immunoglobulin molecules. CD, cluster differentiation antigens (see Appendix 8).

APPENDIX 8

Cluster Differentiation (CD) Antigens

CD	Other Names or Defining Antibodies	MW Reduced (kd)	Expression	Comments
CD1	T6, Leu-6	43–49	Thy, DC, B(s)	MHC class I–like structure; ? presentation function
CD2	T11, Leu-2, LFA-2	45–58	T, NK	CD58 (LFA-3) receptor, sheep RBC receptor
CD3	T3, Leu-4	γ25–28 δ20 ε20 ζ16 η22	T	Complex of 5 peptides; associates with T-cell receptor. Involved in T-cell activation
CD4	T4, Leu-3	55	T(s), Mo, Mac	Accessory molecule in MHC class II antigen recognition; HIV receptor; involved in T-cell activation;
CD5	T1, Leu-1, Ly-1	67	T, B(s)	CD72 receptor, T-cell activation; marker of IL10-producing autoimmune B cells
CD6	T12	100–130	T, brain	?Role in signal transduction
CD7	Leu-9, gp40	40	T, Thy	Earliest T lineage marker; prothymocyte
CD8	T8, Leu-2	α32–34 β32–34	T(s)	MHC class I receptor
CD9	—	22–27	P, early B, Eo, Bo, T(act)	Platelet activation and aggregation; binds to gpIIb/IIIa (CD41/CD61)
CD10	CALLA, J5, neutral endopeptidase, enkephalinase	100	LP, G(s), BM stroma	Zn metalloprotease
CD11a	LFA-1, LeuCAMa, α_L integrin	180	L, G, Mo, Mac, T (memory)	Integrin α chains; associate with CD18 CD11a/CD18 is ICAM-1/ICAM-2/ICAM-3 receptor
11b	CR3, LeuCAMb, MAC-1, Mo-1, α_M integrin	170	M, NK	CD11b/CD18 is iC3b receptor; it also binds factor X, ICAM-1, and fibrinogen
11c	LeuCAMc, α_X integrin	150	M, Mac	CD11c/CD18 binds fibrinogen and ?iC3b; marker for hairy cell leukemia.
CDw12	—	90–120	Mo, G, P	Function unknown
CD13	Aminopeptidase N	150–170	G, Mo, Bo, Eo, Oc, Ep, F, brain	Zn metalloprotease
CD14	—	53–55 (Mo) 64 (B)	MO, Mac, G(s), B	Receptor for complex of lipopolysaccharide (LPS) and LPS-binding protein; induces TNFα synthesis
CD15	Lewis x (Le^x) 3-fucosyl-N-acetyl-lactosamine	<1	G, Eo, Mo	Pentasaccharide; sialylated derivative (CD15s, sLe^x) is ligand for CD62 and ELAM-1
CD16	FcγRIII	50–80	G, NK, Mac	Low-affinity receptor for aggregated IgG; mediates phagocytosis and ADCC
CDw17	Lactosylceramide	—	G, Mo, P	Glycosphingolipid
CD18	Integrin β_2	95	Leukocytes	Adhesion molecule (see CD11)
CD19	B4, Leu-12	95	B, DC	Regulates B-cell proliferation
CD20	B1, Leu-16, Bp35	33–37	B	?Calcium channel
CD21	—	145	B, DC, Ep, Thy(s)	C3d (CR2) receptor; EBV receptor; ?interferon-α receptor
CD22	BL-CAM	130/140 (heterodimer)	B(s)	Adhesion protein, CD22α binds to Mo and RBC; CD22β binds B and T cells
CD23	FcεRII, Blast-2	45	Mo, Mac, Eo, P, DC, B(s)	Low-affinity IgE receptor
CD24	—	35–45	B, G	GPI-anchored; function unknown
CD25	Tac, IL-2Rα	α55	T(act), B(act), Mo(act), BMP, Thy(s), glia	IL2 receptor α chain (β chain is CD122); activation/proliferation of T, Thy, NK, B, Mac
CD26	—	110	EC, Ep	Dipeptidyl peptidase IV; cell-surface protease
CD27	—	50–55	T	Function unknown
CD28	Tp44	44	T, PC	Binds B7 B-cell ligand
CD29	Integrin β_1	130	Leukocytes	Forms integrin with CD49
CD30	Ki-1, Ber-H2 antigen	105–120	B(act), T(act)	Function unknown
CD31	PECAM-1	130–140	P, EC, Mo, G, L(s)	Function unknown
CD32	Fc γRII	40	Mo, B, G, P, EC, placenta	Low-affinity receptor for aggregated IgG; activates G, Mo; inhibits B cells; ? role in placental IgG transport
CD33	—	67	G/Mac precursors	Function unknown
CD34	—	105–120	BMP, EC	Earliest marker for BM progenitors

(continued)

APPENDIX 8 *(Continued)*

CD	Other Names or Defining Antibodies	MW Reduced (kd)	Expression	Comments
CD35	Complement receptor 1 (CR1)	250	E, B. T(s), G, Mo, DC, Mac	C3b/C4b receptor; mediates phagocytosis
CD36	OKM5, gpIV	88	P, EC, Mo	Platelet glycoprotein IV; *Plasmodium falciparum* receptor; may bind collagen, thrombospondin
CD37	—	40–52	B	Function unknown
CD38	T10	45	Early/activated B & T	Function unknown
CD39	—	78	NK(act), T(s), Mac, DC, LC	Function unknown
CD40	—	50	B	Function unknown
CD41	gpIIb, α_{IIb} integrin	125, 22	P	Associates with gpIIIa (CD61) → fibrinogen, von Willebrand factor (vWF), thrombospondin, fibronectin, vitronectin receptor; defective in thrombasthenia
CD42a	gpIX	23	P	vWF receptor; defective in Bernard-Soulier syndrome
42b	gpIBα	135, 23		
42c	gpIBβ	22		
42d	gpV	85		Thrombin receptor
CD43	Sialophorin, leukosialin	115–135 (G, P) 95–115 (T)	Leukocytes, P, Thy, BMP	Mucin-like protein; major sialoglycoprotein of T cells; binds ICAM-1 (CD54); enhances T-cell activation; decreased in Wiskott-Aldrich syndrome
CD44	Phagocytic glycoprotein 1 (Pgp-1), Hermes antigen In(Lu)-related p80	80–95, 130	Leukocytes, Thy, E, Ep, F, Msk, brain	Adhesion protein; hyaluronic acid receptor; binds leukocytes to high venular endothelium; binds ankyrin; part of RBC Lutheran antigen
CD45	Leukocyte common antigen (L-CA), B220, T200, Ly-5	180–240	Leukocytes, P	T-cell receptor signaling; binds CD22 in B cells
CD46	Membrane cofactor protein (MCP)	51–58, 59–68	Leukocytes, P, EC, Ep, F, Placenta	Involved in degradation of C3b/C4b by factor I
CD47	—	47–52	Leukocytes, P, E, Ec, Ep, F	Function unknown; not expressed in Rh_{null} RBC
CD48	Blast-1, HuLy-m3, BCM1 antigen	40–57	B, T, Thy, Eo, Ep	GPI-anchored; function unknown
CD49	Integrins α_{1-6}, very late antigen (VLA) α chains 1–6. CD49a-CD49f are α chains of VLA1–VLA6.	a, 210 b, 160 c, 125 d, 150, 80, 70 e, 135, 25 f, 120, 25	Leukocytes, P, Ep	Complex family of adhesion proteins; various CD49/CD29 complexes bind collagen, laminin, fibronectin, VCAM-1, and high endothelial cells in venules
CD50	ICAM-3	124	Leukocytes	Adhesion protein
CD51	α_V integrin	125, 24	P(weak)	Binds RGD proteins
CD52	Campath-1	21–28	B, T, G(s)	Function unknown
CD53	—	35–42	Leukocytes, P, Ob, Oc	Function unknown
CD54	ICAM-1	85–110	Wide distribution	Adhesion protein; binds CD11a/CD18 and CD11b/CD18 integrins; Also binds CD43 and *Plasmodium falciparum*–infected RBC; rhinovirus receptor
CD55	Decay accelerating factor (DAF)	64–73	Wide distribution	GPI-anchored; prevents assembly of C3 convertase; absence contributes to pathophysiology of PNH
CD56	N-CAM isoform, Leu-19, NKH-1	175–185	NK, non–MHC-restricted L	Cell adhesion, ?Including NK:target cell adhesion
CD57	Leu-7, HNK-1	—	NK, B, T(s), Mo(s)	Function unknown
CD58	LFA-3	55–70	Wide distribution including L, EC, Mac	Adhesion protein; binds CD2; role in T-cell activation and monocyte IL-1 release
CD59	MIRL, Protectin, HRF20, MACIF, P-18, H19	19	Leukocytes, EC, Ep, placenta	GPI-anchored; blocks complement C8/C9 membrane attack complex; absence contributes to pathophysiology of PNH
CDw60	UM4D4	—	T(s), Mo, P	T-cell stimulation; augments CD3 signaling
CD61	gpIIIa, integrin β_2, vitronectin receptor	105	P, Mac	CD41/CD61 is gpIIb/gpIIIa complex involved in platelet adhesion/aggregation; CD51/CD61 is vitronectin receptor ($\alpha_V\beta_3$ integrin).

(continued)

APPENDIX 8 *(Continued)*

CD	Other Names or Defining Antibodies	MW Reduced (kd)	Expression	Comments
CCD62E	E-selectin, ELAM-1	115	EC	Adhesion of phagocytes to endothelial cells; binds sLe^x
62L	L-selectin, LAM-1 LECAM-1	75–80	Leukocytes	Adhesion of lymphocytes to high endothelial venules and neutrophils to endothelium; binds sLe^x and mucin
62P	P-selectin, PADGEM, GMP-140	150	P, EC	Adhesion protein; located in secretory granules → membrane on activation; mediates platelet–neutrophil interactions; Binds sLe^x (sCD15) and sulfated galactosylceramides
CD63	ME491, MLA1, PTLGP40	53	P, Mo, Mac	Lysosomal membrane protein → plasma membrane on activation; involved in neutrophil–endothelial and other cellular interactions
CD64	FcγRI	72	Mac, Mo, N (γIFN-induced)	γ-IFN-induced, high-affinity IgG receptor; binds monomeric IgG; role in ADCC and clearance of immune complexes
CDw65	—	—	G, Mo(s)	Marker of myeloid lineage; function unknown
CD66a	BGP-1	180–200	N, BMP, Ep(s)	Function unknown
66b	CD67, p100, CGM6	95–100	G	Function unknown
66c	NCA	90–95	—	—
66d	CGM1	30	—	—
66e	CEA	180–200	—	Carcinoembryonic antigen
CD67	Now called CD66b	—	—	—
CD68	—	110	Mac, Mo, N, Bo, L(s), Liver, Ep(s),	Present in lysosomes as well as membrane; function unknown
CD69	AIM, EA 1, MLR-3. Leu-23	28, 32	L(act), P, Thy	Function uncertain
CD70	—	55, 75, 95, 110, 170	B(act), T(act)(s)	CD27 ligand; function unknown
CD71	T9	90–95	Proliferating cells	Transferrin receptor; iron transport
CD72	—	42	B	CD5 ligand; ?Role in B-cell proliferation
CD73	—	69	L(s), EC(s), Ep(s)	GPI-anchored ecto-5′-nucleotidase; dephosphorylates nucleoside monophosphates → uptake
CD74	MHC class II; associated invariant chain (Ii or Iγ)	43, 41, 35, 33	MHC II–positive cells; B, Mo, T(s), Ep(s)	Mostly intracellular; associates with α and β chains of MHC class II molecule. ?Prevents binding of endogenous peptides to class II
CDw75	—	53, 87	B, Ep, E precursors	?Mediates B-cell interactions as CD22 receptor
CDw76	—	85, 67	B, T(s), EC(s), Ep	Function unknown
CD77	Globotriaosylceramide, P^k blood group antigen	—	B(s), DC, EC, Ep(s)	Marker for Burkitt's lymphoma, function unknown
CDw78	Ba antigen, Leu-21	—	B(act), Mac, Ep	Function unclear
CD79a	mb-1, Igα	33, 40	—	—
79b	B29, Igβ	33, 40	—	—
CD80	B7, BB1	60	—	—
CD81	TAPA-1	22	Wide distribution	?Antiproliferative function
CD82	R2, IA4, 4F9	50–53	L(act)	Function uncertain
CD83	HB15	43	—	—
CDw84	—	73	—	—
CD85	VMP-55, GH1/75	120, 83	—	—
CD86	FUN-1, BU63	80	—	—
CD87	UPA-R	50–65	—	—
CD88	C5aR	42	N, Mac, Mast, Msm	C5a receptor; role in chemotaxis; stimulates respiratory burst and degranulation of N, mast
CD89	FcαR	55–75	Mo, G, Mac, T(s), B(s)	IgA receptor
CDw90	Thy-1	25–35	Early Thy	Prothymocytes, GPI-anchored; function unknown
CD91	α_2M-R	600	—	—
CDw92	—	70	—	—
CD93	—	120	—	—
CD94	KP43	43	—	—
CD95	APO-1, FAS	42	—	—
CD96	TACTILE	160	—	—

(continued)

APPENDIX 8 *(Continued)*

CD	Other Names or Defining Antibodies	MW Reduced (kd)	Expression	Comments
CD97	—	74, 80, 89	—	—
CD98	4F2, 2F3	80, 40	Mo, L(act), NK(act), Mc, K	Function uncertain
CD99	E2, MIC2	32	—	—
CD100	BB18, A8	150	—	—
CDw101	BB27, BA27	140	—	—
CD102	ICAM-2	60	EC, L, Mo, liver, kidney	Adhesion protein; ligand for LFA-1 integrin (CS11a/CD18); ?facilitates recirculation of memory T cells
CD103	HML-1	150, 25	—	—
CD104	β_4 integrin chain	220	—	—
CD105	endoglin	95	EC, BM(s), Mac(act)	Function unknown
CD106	VCAM-1, INCAM-110	100, 110	EC, Mac, DC, kidney, F, myoblasts	Receptor for VLA4 (CD49d/CD29)
CD107a	LAMP-1	110	—	Lysosomal membrane glycoprotein
107b	LAMP-2	120	—	Lysosomal membrane glycoprotein
CDw108	—	80	—	—
CDW109	8A3, 7D1	170/150	—	—
CD115	CSF-1R, M-CSFR c-fms protooncogene	150	Mo, Mac, BMP, placenta	Stimulates proliferation and differentiation of Mo/Mac and their progenitors
CDw116	HGM-CSFR, GM-CSFR	75–85	Mo, N, Eo, F, EC, BMP, Ob	Stimulates proliferation and differentiation of N, Eo, Mo, and their progenitors, and RBC progenitors
CD117	SCFR, cKIT	145	—	c-*kit* receptor
CDw119	IFNγR	90	—	γ-Interferon receptor
CD120a	TNFR, 55kd	55	Ep, wide distribution	Receptor for TNFα and TNFβ
120b	TNFR, 75kd	75	M, wide distribution	Receptor for TNFα and TNFβ
CDw121a	IL-1R; type1	80	T, Thy, F, C, EC, K, synovial cells, liver	IL-1 receptor; T/Thy activation, fibroblast proliferation, acute phase reaction
121b	IL-1R; type 2	68	B, Mo, Mac	
CD122	IL-2Rβ	75	B(act), Mo(act), NK, T(act)	IL-2 receptor β chain, activation/proliferation of T, Thy, NK, B, Mac
CDw124	IL-4R	140	B, T, BMP, F, Ep, Ec	IL-4 receptor; stimulates B/T-cell growth IgG_1/IgE production, MHC class II expression, and Mac activation
CD126	IL-6R	80	B(act), PC	IL-6 receptor; stimulates B/T/PC growth, proliferation/differentiation of BM progenitors, and hepatic acute phase response
CDw127	IL-7R	75	LP, proB, T, Thy, Mo	IL-7 receptor; stimulates growth of proB/preB/Thy/T cells and activation of Mo
CDw128	IL-8R	58–67	N, Bo, T(s), Mo, K	IL-8 receptor, chemotaxis of N/Bo/T; activates N/Bo, increases N/Mo adhesion to EC
CDw130	IL-GR-gp130SIG	130	—	—

(act), activated cells of the type indicated; B, B lymphocytes; Bo, basophils; BM, bone marrow; BMP, bone marrow progenitors; C, chondrocytes; DC, dendritic cells; E, erythrocytes; EC, endothelial cells; Eo, eosinophils; Ep, epithelial cells; F, fibroblasts; G, granulocytes; K, keratinocytes; L, lymphocytes; LC, Langerhans' cells; LP, lymphoid progenitors; M, myeloid cells; Mac, macrophages; Mast, mast cells; Mc, cardiac muscle; Mo, monocytes; Msk, skeletal muscle; Msm, smooth muscle; N, neutrophils; NK, natural killer cells; Ob, osteoblasts; Oc, osteoclasts; P, platelets; PC, plasma cells; (s), protein expressed on a subset of indicated cells; T, T lymphocytes; Thy, thymocytes.

(Compiled from Barclay AN, Birkeland ML, Brown MH, et al (eds). The leucocyte antigen facts book. London, Academic Press, 1993; Knapp W. Rieber P, Dörken B, et al. Toward a better definition of human leukocyte surface molecules, Immunol Today 1989;10:254; and Schlossman SF, Boumsell L, Gilks W, et al. CD antigens 1993. Blood 1994;83:879)

APPENDIX 9

Adhesion Proteins

Receptor	Other Names	Size (kd)	Distribution	Ligands	Functions
INTEGRINS					
LPAM-1	$\alpha_4\beta_7$	160, 130	L	VCAM-1, fibronectin, ligand on HEV	Lymphocyte–EC adhesion
VLA-4	LPAM-2, CD49d/CD29, $\alpha_4\beta_1$	160, 130	WBC, melanoma	VCAM-1	Lymphocyte–EC adhesion; tumor–EC adhesion
CD11/CD18					
CD11a	LFA-1, $\alpha_L\beta_2$	180, 95	WBC	ICAM-1, ICAM-2, ICAM-3	Leukocyte–leukocyte adhesion; leukocyte–EC adhesion
CD11b	Mac-1, Mo-1, CR3, $\alpha_M\beta_2$	170, 95	N, Mo, NK fibrinogen	iC3b, ICAM-1, X	Cell–cell adhesion, phagocytosis, complement binding
CD11c	$\alpha_X\beta_2$	150, 95	G, Mo, Mac	Fibrinogen, ?iC3b	Cell–cell adhesion
SELECTION FAMILY					
E-selectin	ELAM-1, CD62E	115	EC(act)	Sialyated, fucosylated molecules (e.g., sLe^x)	Adhesion of WBC to EC activated by LPS, IL-1, or TNF; EC–EC binding in angiogenesis
L-selectin	LAM-1, CD62L, LECAM-1, Leu-8	75 (L) 90–100 (N, Mo)	L, N, Mo	sLe^x, mucin	Initial adhesion of N to EC in areas of inflammation; adhesion of L to HEV
P-selectin	PADGEM, GMP-140, CD62P	150	P, Meg, EC	sLe^x, sulfated galactosylceramide	Adhesion of activated platelets to N and Mo; adhesion of N and Mo to activated EC
IgG SUPERFAMILY					
ICAM-1	CD54	95	Many cells; induced by inflammation	CD11a/CD18 (LFA-1); CD11b/CD18 (Mac-1), CD43 (sialophorin), *P falciparum*–infected RBC	Leukocyte adhesion; rhinovirus receptor
ICAM-2	CD102	60	EC, Mo, DC, L(s), liver, kidney	CD11a/CD18 (LFA-1)	?Lymphocyte recirculation; cell–cell adhesion
ICAM-3		124	L	CD11a/CD18 (LFA-1), CD11b/CD18 (Mac-1)	Unknown
VCAM-1		110	EC(act), Mac, DC, Mb, F, Ep	CD49d/CD29 (VLA-4, α_4, β_1)	Adhesion of WBC to EC activated by IL-1 or TNF; other cell–cell adhesion
VCAM-1(alt)		90	EC	CD49d/CD29 (VLA-4, α_4,β_1)	Unknown
LFA-2	CD2	45–58	T, NK	LFA-3 (CD58)	T-cell adhesion
LFA-3	CD58	55–70	Wide distribution	LFA-2 (CD2)	T-cell adhesion
PECAM-1	CD31, endoCAM	130	EC, P, T, Mo, G	?PECAM-1	Initiation of EC–EC adhesion; platelet–Mo–EC adhesion
Ca^{2+}-independent CAMs					
N-CAM	D2, BSP-2	180, 140, 120	Brain, heart, muscle, kidney	Homophilic cell–cell binding	
Ng-CAM	L1, NILE	200	Neural and glial cells	Homophilic (neural–neural) and heterophilic (neural–glial) interactions	
CADHERINS					
Ca^{2+}-dependent CAMs					
N-Cadherin	A-CAM, N-Cal-CAM	135	Brain, muscle, lens		

(continued)

APPENDIX 9 *(Continued)*

Receptor	Other Names	Size (kd)	Distribution	Ligands	Functions
E-Cadherin	L-CAM, Uvomorulin, Arc-1, cell CAM, 120/80	120–125	Epithelium		
P-Cadherin			Placenta, epithelium, mesothelium		
CARTILAGE-LINK PROTEINS					
CD44	H-CAM, Pgp-1, Hermes antigen, In(Lu)-related p80	80–95, 130	WBC, Thy, E, Ep, F, muscle, brain	Hyaluronic acid, ligand on HEV	Cell–matrix interaction; homing of lymphocytes to HEV
OTHER PROTEINS					
CD36	gpIV	88	P, EC, Mo	Thrombospondin, ?collagen	Platelet–monocyte adhesion

(act), activated cells of the type indicated; B, B lymphocytes; DC, dendritic cells; E, erythrocytes; EC, endothelial cells; Ep, epithelial cells; F, fibroblasts; HEV, high endothelium venules; iC3b, inactive fragment of complement protein C3b; L, lymphocytes; Mac, macrophages; Mb, myoblasts or myocytes; Meg, megakaryocytes; Mo, monocytes; N, neutrophils; NK, natural killer cells; P, platelets; (s), protein expressed on a subset of indicated cells; sLe^x, sialylated Lewis x antigen; T, T lymphocytes; Thy, thymocytes; VCAM-1, vascular cell adhesion molecule 1; WBC, white blood cells, leukocytes; X, factor X.

(Adapted from Albelda SM, Buck CA. Integrins and other cell adhesion molecules. FASEB J 1990;4:2868)

APPENDIX 10

Integrin Family

Integrin $\alpha\beta$ Heterodimer	β Subunit	Other Names	α Subunit	Other Names	Ligands of the Integrin Heterodimer
VLA FAMILY					
VLA-1	β_1	VLAβ, gpIIa	α_1	CD44a	L, C
VLA-2, gpIa/IIa		CD29	α_2	CD44b, gpIa	C, L
VLA-3			α_3	CD44c	Fn, L, C
VLA-4			α_4	CD44d	VCAM-1, Fn
VLA-5, fibronectin receptor			α_5	CD44e, gpIc	Fn
VLA-6, laminin receptor			α_6	CD44f, gpIc	L
β_1, α_7			α_7		L
β_1, α_8			α_8		—
β_1, α_V			α_V	CD51	Fn, Vn
LEUCAM FAMILY					
LFA-1	β_2	CD18	α_L	CD11a	ICAM-1, ICAM-2, ICAM-3
Mac-1, CR3			α_M	CD11b	iC3b, ICAM-1, Fb, factor X
p150, 95			α_X	CD11c	Fb, ?iC3b
CYTOADHESION FAMILY					
CD41a, gpIIb/IIIa	β_3	CD61, gpIIIa	α_{IIb}	CD41, gpIIb	Fb, Fn, Vn, vWF, Ts
Vitronectin receptor			α_V	CD51	Vn, Fb, vWF, C, Ts, Fn, L, Op
β_4, α_6	β_4		α_6	CD49f	L
β_6, α_V	β_5	β_X, β_s	α_V	CD51	Vn, Fn
β_6, α_V	β_6		α_V	CD51	Fn
β_7, α_4, LPAM-1	β_7	β_P	α_4	CD49d	Fn, VCAM-1, ligand on HEV
β_8, α_V	β_8		α_V	CD51	Unknown

C, collagen; Fb, fibrinogen; Fn, fibronectin; HEV, high endothelium venules; iC3b, inactive fragment of complement protein C3b; ICAM-1, Intercellular adhesion molecule 1; L, lamin; Op, osteopontin; Ts, thrombospondin; VCAM-1, vascular cell adhesion molecule 1; Vn, vitronectin; vWF, von Willebrand factor.

Blood: Principles and Practice of Hematology,
edited by Robert I. Handin, Samuel E. Lux, and Thomas P. Stossel.
J.B. Lippincott Company, Philadelphia © 1995.

Plasma Proteins

APPENDIX 11

Relation of Serum Protein Levels to Age

	Total Proteins (g/dL)		Albumin (g/dL)		Alpha-1	
	Mean	Range	Mean	Range	Mean	Range
Cord blood	6.22 ± 1.21	4.78–8.04	3.23 ± 0.82	2.17–4.04	0.41 ± 0.10	0.25–0.66
1–3 mo	5.64 ± 1.04	3.64–7.38	3.41 ± 0.72	2.05–4.46	0.24 ± 0.09	0.08–0.43
4–6 mo	5.43 ± 0.84	4.29–6.10	3.46 ± 0.36	3.17–3.88	0.17 ± 0.04	0.12–0.25
7–12 mo	6.54 ± 0.76	5.10–7.31	3.62 ± 0.60	3.22–4.31	0.35 ± 0.15	0.15–0.55
13–24 mo	6.66 ± 0.93	3.69–7.50	3.63 ± 0.80	1.89–5.03	0.31 ± 0.15	0.09–0.58
25–36 mo	6.98 ± 0.66	6.38–8.06	4.11 ± 0.78	3.57–5.50	0.23 ± 0.09	0.19–0.26
3–5 y	6.65 ± 0.85	4.88–8.06	3.95 ± 0.57	2.93–5.21	0.21 ± 0.08	0.08–0.40
6–8 y	6.95 ± 0.55	5.97–7.94	4.03 ± 0.45	3.26–4.95	0.22 ± 0.09	0.09–0.45
9–11 y	7.43 ± 0.84	6.32–9.00	4.24 ± 0.79	3.16–4.97	0.30 ± 0.07	0.12–0.38
12–16 y	7.25 ± 0.85	6.25–8.75	4.26 ± 0.64	3.19–5.13	0.19 ± 0.07	0.09–0.32
Adult	7.41 ± 0.96	6.44–8.32	4.31 ± 0.59	3.46–4.78	0.23 ± 0.06	0.16–0.30

	Alpha-2 (g/dL)		Beta (g/dL)		Gamma (g/dL)	
	Mean	Range	Mean	Range	Mean	Range
Cord blood	0.68 ± 0.14	0.44–0.94	0.74 ± 0.30	0.42–1.56	1.28 ± 0.23	0.81–1.16
1–3 mo	0.74 ± 0.24	0.40–1.13	0.59 ± 0.20	0.39–1.14	0.66 ± 0.24	0.25–1.05
4–6 mo	0.67 ± 0.11	0.52–0.84	0.61 ± 0.14	0.44–0.76	0.61 ± 0.26	0.24–0.90
7–12 mo	0.99 ± 0.30	0.78–1.46	0.79 ± 0.16	0.63–0.91	0.84 ± 0.36	0.32–1.18
13–24 mo	0.88 ± 0.42	0.41–1.36	0.77 ± 0.31	0.36–1.41	1.09 ± 0.32	0.36–1.62
25–36 mo	0.89 ± 0.14	0.68–1.09	0.67 ± 0.14	0.47–0.91	1.08 ± 0.28	0.73–1.46
3–5 y	0.70 ± 0.15	0.43–0.99	0.67 ± 0.11	0.47–1.01	1.13 ± 0.31	0.54–1.66
6–8 y	0.67 ± 0.10	0.50–0.83	0.72 ± 0.11	0.45–0.93	1.21 ± 0.32	0.70–1.95
9–11 y	0.75 ± 0.27	0.67–0.87	0.84 ± 0.16	0.63–1.02	1.46 ± 0.41	0.79–2.03
12–16 y	0.71 ± 0.15	0.50–0.97	0.68 ± 0.15	0.48–0.88	1.40 ± 0.31	1.08–1.96
Adult	0.61 ± 0.14	0.51–0.86	0.81 ± 0.22	0.59–1.06	1.45 ± 0.46	0.68–2.11

(Park BH, Ellis EF. In: Johnson TR, Moore WM, eds. Children are different: developmental physiology, ed 2, Columbus, OH, Ross Laboratories, 1978:188)

APPENDIX 12

Normal Values for 14 Human Serum Proteins*

	Mean (mg/dL)	Range (mg/dL)
Albumin	4000	3200–5500
α_1-Antitrypsin	240	160–360
α_1-Acid glycoprotein (orosomucoid)	100	40–150
C1 inhibitor	18	11–26
Ceruloplasmin	32	18–45
α_2-Macroglobulin	550 (pediatric)	200–700†
	300 (female, adult)	120–540†
	240 (male, adult)	90–400†
Haptoglobin	108	25–180‡
Transferrin	280	200–350
Low-density lipoprotein	105	40–140§
C3	165	90–220‖
C4	30	10–40
IgA	240	60–360¶
IgM	105	25–170¶
IgG	1100	700–1500#

* Values derived from a large northern New England white population
† Varies markedly during and about the time of puberty.
‡ Varies from 0 to normal adult levels during first 2 weeks of life
§ Varies from 10% of normal to normal adult levels during first year of life.
‖ Varies from 50% of normal to normal adult levels during the first month of life.
¶ Varies from 0 to normal adult levels during first year of life
#Varies from adult normal levels at birth to 25% of normal at about 3 months, returning to adult normal during next several years.
(Ritchie RF. Automated immunoprecipitation analysis of serum proteins. In: Putnam FW, ed. The plasma proteins, ed 2, vol 2. San Diego, Academic Press, 1975:376)

APPENDIX 13

Serum Immunoglobulin Levels in Normal Individuals*

Subjects		IgG		IgA		IgM	
Age	No.	mg/dL	% of Adult Level	mg/dL	% of Adult Level	mg/dL	% of Adult Level
Newborn	20	1004 (598–1672)	95	<5 (0–<5)	<2	9 (6–15)	12
1–3 mo	10	365 (218–610)	34	32 (20–53)	12	24 (11–51)	32
4–6 mo	12	381 (228–636)	36	44 (27–72)	17	38 (25–60)	50
7–9 mo	10	488 (292–816)	46	44 (27–73)	17	47 (18–124)	62
10–18 mo	13	640 (383–1070)	60	67 (27–169)	25	56 (28–113)	74
2 y	8	708 (423–1184)	67	89 (35–222)	33	65 (32–131)	86
3 y	6	798 (477–1334)	75	100 (40–251)	38	57 (28–116)	75
4 y	8	906 (542–1515)	85	120 (48–301)	45	41 (20–82)	54
5 y	5	901 (539–1506)	85	134 (53–336)	50	52 (26–106)	68
6y	11	954 (571–1597)	90	131 (52–329)	49	57 (28–115)	75
7 y	11	1066 (638–1783)	100	223 (89–559)	84	48 (24–98)	63
8 y	8	976 (583–1631)	92	213 (85–535)	80	55 (27–112)	72
9 y	7	1006 (599–1673)	95	230 (92–578)	86	56 (28–113)	74
10 y	7	991 (593–1657)	93	188 (75–472)	71	60 (29–120)	79
11 y	7	989 (586–1637)	93	257 (102–644)	97	56 (28–113)	74
12 y	7	855 (511–1430)	81	232 (92–581)	87	55 (27–111)	72
13 y	13	961 (575–1607)	91	235 (94–588)	88	52 (26–105)	68
14 y	8	940 (562–1571)	89	217 (86–544)	82	67 (33–135)	88
Adult	30	106 (635–177)	100	266 (106–668)	100	76 (37–154)	100

* Geometric means are presented for each immunoglobulin at every age. The bounds, given in parentheses, are obtained by taking the mean logarithm ± twice the pooled standard deviations of the mean logarithms, and then taking the antilogs of the results. In the case of IgA, the first four age groups have a pooled standard deviation separate from the other ages. In the case of IgM, the bounds of the first four age groups are ± twice the individual group standard deviations.
(Buckley RH, Dees SC, O'Fallon WM. Pediatrics 1968;41:600)

APPENDIX 14

Metabolic Parameters of Human Immunoglobulins

	IgG					IgA			
	IgG1	**IgG2**	**IgG3**	**IgG4**	**IgM**	**IgA1**	**IgA2**	**IgE**	**IgD**
Serum concentration (mg/dL)									
Adult	600–1500				75–150	200–300		0.02–0.06	0.01–3
Range	1200				97	250		0.04	2.2
Mean	840	240	80	40	—	220	30	—	—
Fetus (6 months; mean)	300				20	ND		0.003	0.05
Newborn	1200 (all maternal)				30	ND		0.003	0.1
6-month-old	400				40	25		0.006	0.1
1-year-old	800				60	60		0.01	0.3
Fraction of total serum immunoglobulin (%)	75–80				10	10–15		<0.01	<1
Fraction of total serum IgG (%)	70	18	8	4	—	—		—	—
Fraction of body pool intravascular (%)	45				80	42		50	75
Time (days)	23				5.1	5.8		2.5	2.6
	23	23	9	23	—	—		—	—
Fractional catabolic rate (plasma pool catabolized/d)	6.7				25	18		91	37
Metabolic rate (mg/kg/d)	33				6.9	24		0.003	0.4

ND, not determined.

Blood: Principles and Practice of Hematology,
edited by Robert I. Handin, Samuel E. Lux, and Thomas P. Stossel.
J.B. Lippincott Company, Philadelphia © 1995.

Malignancy

APPENDIX 15

The French–American–British (FAB) Classification System of Acute Nonlymphocytic Leukemia

FAB Type	Definition	Blasts ANC	Blasts NEC	Nucleated Erythroblasts	Morphology	Cytochemistry
M1	AML without maturation	>30	>90	<50	Undifferentiated; <10% promyelocytes or monocytes; acute myeloblastic leukemia	>3% POX or SBB+
M2	AML with maturation	>30	30–89	<50	>10% promyelocytes, myelocytes; <20% monocytic cells; AML with partial differentiation	POX+, SBB+, PAS–
M3	Acute promyelocytic leukemia	>30	30–89	<50	>20% abnormal hypergranular promyelocytes; Auer rods common; acute promyelocytic leukemia	POX+, SBB+, PAS–
M3v	Microgranular variant	>30	30–89	<50	Microgranular variant, may have folded nucleus	POX+, SBB+, PAS–
M4	Acute myelomonocytic leukemia	>30	30–79	<50	>20% promonocytes and monocytes; >20% granulocytic component; blood monocytes $>5 \times 10^9$/L or lysozyme more than three times normal	POX+, NASDA+
M4Eo	M4 with eosinophilia	>30	30–79	<50	>5% eosinophils with abnormal eosinophil and basophilic granules	POX+, NASDA+, eosinophils are PAS+
M5a	Acute monocytic leukemia, poorly differentiated		>80*	<50	>80% of monocytic cells are monoblasts; acute monoblastic leukemia	POX, NASDA+ (inhibited by NaF)
M5b	Acute monocytic leukemia, differentiated		>80*	<50	<80% of monocytic cells are monoblasts, rest are promonocytes and monocytes	Same as M5a
M6	Acute erythroleukemia		>30	>50	Megaloblastoid, erythroid, and myeloid blasts; multinucleated; erythroleukemia	PAS+, ringed sideroblasts with iron stain
M7	Acute megakaryoblastic leukemia	>30		<50	Large polymorphic blasts, cytoplasmic blebs; gpIb or IIb/IIIa+; myelofibrosis; acute megakaryoblastic leukemia	POX–, SBB–, NASDA+; platelet POX+ on electron microscopoe
MDS	Myelodysplastic syndrome	<30	<30		Megaloblastoid; nuclear and cytoplasmic dysynchrony; nuclear anomalies; myelodysplastic syndromes	

AML, acute myelogenic leukemia; ANC, all nucleated cells; MDS, myelodysplastic syndrome; NASDA, napthol-ASD chloroacetate esterase; NEC, nonerythroid cells; PAS, periodic acid–Schiff stain; POX, myeloperoxidase, SBB, Sudan black B stain.
* Includes monoblasts, promonocytes, and monocytes.

APPENDIX 16

Immunophenotype Analysis of Acute Myelogenic Leukemia

CD	Antibodies	M1/M2	M3	M4/M5	M6	M7	B-ALL	T-ALL
MYELOID LINEAGE								
CD11b	Anti-Mo1		+	++	−	−	−	−
CD13	Anti-MY7	+	+	++	+	+	−	−
CD14	Anti-Mo2, MY4	−	−	++	−	−		−
CD15	Anti-MY1	+	++	++	−	−	−	−
CD33	Anti-MY9	++	++	++	++	++	−	−
CD34	Anti-MY10	++	+	+	+	+	+	+
T LINEAGE								
CD2	Anti-T11	−	−	−	−	−	−	++
CD3	Anti-T3	−	−	−	−	−	−	+
CD5	Anti-T1	−	−	−	−	−	−	++
CD7	3A1	+	+	+	+	+	+	++
B LINEAGE								
CD10	Anti-CALLA	−	−	−	−	−	+	−
CD19	Anti-B4	−	−	−	−	−	+	−
CD20	Anti-B1	−	−	−	−	−	+	−
ERYTHROID LINEAGE								
	Anti-glycophorin A	−	−	−	++	−	−	−
MEGAKARYOCYTE LINEAGE								
CD41	Anti-gpIIb/IIIa	−	−	−	−	++	−	−
CD42	Anti-gbIb	−	−	−	−	++	−	−

CALLA, common acute lymphoblastic leukemia antigen; CD, cluster differentiation; B-ALL, B-lineage acute lymphobastic leukemia; T-ALL, T-lineage acute lymphoblastic leukemia; +++, expressed by over 20% of blasts in more than 50% of cases; ++, expressed by over 20% of blasts in 20% to 50% of cases; +, expressed by over 20% of blasts in 5% to 20% of cases; −, expressed by less than 5% of cases.

APPENDIX 17

Chromosomal Abnormalities and Genes in Hematopoietic Disorders

Hematopoietic Disorders	Chromosomal Abnormality	Genes Involved	
Chronic myeloid leukemia			
	t(9;22)(q34;q11)	*ABL1*	*BCR*
Acute myeloid leukemia			
	t(6;9)(p23;q34)	*DEK*	*CAN*
	t(8;21)(q22;q22)	*ETO/CDR*	*AML1*
	t(9;11)(p22;q23)		*ALL1/MLL/TRX1*
	t(9;22)(q34;q11)	*ABL1*	*BCR*
	t(15;17)(q22;q11-21)	*PML*	*RARA*
	inv(16)(p13q22) or t(16;16)(p13;q22)	*MYH11*	*CBFB*
B-cell leukemias and lymphomas			
	t(1;19)(q23;p13)	*PBX1*	*E2A*
	t(2;8)(p12;q24)	*IGK*	*MYC, PVT1*
	t(2;14)(p13;q32)		*IGH*
			IGHG2
	t(4;11)(q21;q23)	*AF4*	*ALL1/MLL/TRX1*
	t(5;14)(q31;q32)	*IL3*	*IGH*
	t(8;12)(q24;q22)	*MYC*	*BTG1*
	t(8;14)(q24;q32)	*MYC*	*IGH*

(continued)

APPENDIX 17 *(Continued)*

Hematopoietic Disorders	Chromosomal Abnormality	Genes Involved	
	t(8;22)(q24;q11)	*MYC, PVT1*	*IGL*
	t(9;14)(p11;q32)		*IGHA*
	t(9;14)(p13;q32)		*IGHA*
	t(9:22)(q34;q11)	*ABL1*	*BCR*
	t(10;14)(q24;q32)	*LYT10*	*IGHA1*
	t(11;14)(q13;q32)	*BCL1/PRAD1*	*IGH*
	t(11;14)(q23;q32)	*RCK*	*IGH*
	t(11;19)(q23;p13)	*ALL1/MLL/TRX1*	
	t(14;18)(q32;q21)	*IGH*	*BCL2*
	t(14;19)(q32;p13)	*IGH*	*BCL3*
	t(17;19)(q22;p13)	*HLF*	*E2A*
T-cell leukemias and lymphomas			
	t(1;3)(p34;p21)	*TAL1*	
	t(1;7)(p32;q35)	*TAL1*	*TCRB*
	t(1:7)(p34;q34)	*LCK*	*TCRB*
	t(1;14)(p32;q11)	*TAL1*	*TCRD*
	ins(2;2)(p13;p11-14)	*REL*	
	t(4;16)(q26;p13)	*IL2*	*BCMA*
	inv(7)(p15q35)	*TCRG*	*TCRB*
	t(7;9)(q35;q32)	*TCRB*	*TAL2*
	t(7;9)(q35;q34.3)	*TCRB*	*TAN1*
	t(7;10)(q35;q24)	*TCRB*	*HOX11*
	t(7;11)(q35;p13)	*TCRB*	*RBTNL1*
	t(7;14)(q35;q32)	*TCRB*	
	t(7;19)(q35;p13)	*TCRB*	*LYL1*
	t(8;14)(q24;q11)	*MYC*	*TCRA*
		PVT1	*TCRD*
	t(10;14)(q24;q11)	*HOX11*	*TCRD*
	t(11;14)(p13;q11)	*RBTNL1*	*TCRD*
	t(11;14)(p15;q11)	*RBTN1*	*TCRD*
	inv(14)(q11q32.1)	*TCRA*	*IGH*
	t(14;14)(q11;q32)	*TCRA*	

ABL1, Abelson murine leukemia viral (v-*abl*) oncogene homologue 1; *AF4,* AF4 (or FEL) putative transcription factor; *ALL1,* acute lymphocytic leukemia oncogene 1, homologous to *Drosophila trithorax* developmental regulator; *AML1,* acute myeloid leukemia 1 oncogene, transcription factor homologous to *Drosophila runt* segmentation gene; *BCL1,* B-cell CLL/lymphoma oncogene 1; *BCL2,* B-cell CLL/lymphoma oncogene 2; *BCL3,* B-cell CLL/lymphoma oncogene 3: *BCMA,* B-cell maturation gene; *BCR,* breakpoint cluster region tyrosine kinase; *BTG1,* BTG1 antiproliferative gene, homologous to murine *PC3* gene; *can,* Cain gene, acute myeloid leukemia 220-kd chromosome 9q34 breakpoint; *CBFB, CBF-β* (or PEBP2-β) transcription factor; *CDR,* cyclin D–related gene; *DEK,* acute myeloid leukemia 43-kd chromosome 6p23 breakpoint; *E2A.* E2A transcription factor; *ETO,* ETO (eight twenty-one) transcription factor; *HLF,* hepatic leukemia factor; *HOX11,* homeobox region 11, spleen developmental regulator (T-cell lymphoma 3–associated breakpoint); *IGH,* immunoglobulin heavy chain gene cluster; *IGHA,* immunoglobulin heavy chain, α; *IGHA1,* immunoglobulin heavy chain, α_1; *IGHG2,* immunoglobulin heavy chain, γ_2 (Gm marker); *IGK,* immunoglobulin light chain, κ gene cluster; *IGL,* immunoglobulin light chain, λ gene cluster; *IL2,* interleukin 2; *IL3,* interleukin 3; *LCK,* lymphocyte-specific protein kinase; *LYL1,* lymphoblastic leukemia derived sequence 1; *LYT10,* B-cell lymphoma–associated oncogene, NF-κB p50 transcription factor homologue; *MLL,* myeloid/lymphoid or mixed-lineage leukemia gene, homologous to *Drosophila trithorax* developmental regulator; *MYC,* avian myelocytomatosis viral (v-*myc*) oncogene homologue; *MYH11,* myosin, heavy polypeptide 11, smooth muscle; *PBX1,* pre–B-cell transcription factor 1; *PML,* promyelocytic leukemia; *PRAD1,* parathyroid adenomatosis 1; *PVT1*; *pvt*-1 (murine) oncogene homologue, MYC activator; *RARA,* retinoic acid receptor, α; *RBTN1,* rhombotin 1; *RBTNL1,* rhombotin-like 1; *RCK,* RC-K8 B-lymphoma cell line breakpoint, putative RNA helicase; *REL,* avian reticuloendotheliosis viral (v-*rel*) oncogene homologue; *TAL1,* T-cell acute lymphocytic leukemia 1; *TAL2,* T-cell acute lymphocytic leukemia 2; *TAN1,* translocation-associated *Drosophila notch* homologue 1; *TCRA,* T-cell receptor, α; *TCRB,* T-cell receptor, β; *TCRD,* T-cell receptor, δ; *TCRG,* T-cell receptor, γ; *TRX1,* human trithorax gene 1 (HTRX-1), transcription factor.

Blood: Principles and Practice of Hematology,
edited by Robert I. Handin, Samuel E. Lux, and Thomas P. Stossel.
J.B. Lippincott Company, Philadelphia © 1995.

Coagulation

APPENDIX 18

Normal Values for Tests of Hemostasis and Blood Coagulation

Test	Normal Range [±2 SD]
Platelet count	140–440 × 10^9/L
Bleeding time	
Ivy	1–9 min*
Duke	1–4 min
Partial thromboplastin time	
Standard	68–82 s†
Activated	32–46 s†
Plasma prothrombin time	11–15 s‡
Coagulation time (glass tubes)	8–18 min
Plasma thrombin time	13–17 s
Fibrinogen assay	160–415 mg/dL
Euglobulin clot lysis time	>2 h†
Fibrin degradation products	8 μg/dL†

* Confidence limits determined by logarithmic plot.
† Minor variations depend on exact technique used.
‡ Significant variations depend on thromboplastin used.

APPENDIX 19

Reference Values for Coagulation Tests in Healthy Full-Term Infants During the First 6 Months of Life Compared With Values for Adults*

Coagulation Test	Day 1		Day 5		Day 30		Day 90		Day 180		Adults	
	Mean	95% Range	Mean	95% Range	Mean	95% Range	Mean	95% Range	Mean	95% Range	Mean	95% Range
PT (s)	13.0	10.1–15.9†	12.4	10.0–15.3	11.8	10.0–14.3†	11.9	10.0–14.2†	12.3	10.7–13.9†	12.4	10.8–13.9
INR	1.0	0.53–1.62	0.89	0.53–1.48	0.79	0.53–1.26	0.81	0.53–1.26	0.88	0.61–1.27	0.89	0.64–1.17
APTT (s)	42.9	31.3–54.5	42.6	25.4–59.8	40.4	32.0–55.2	37.1	29.0–50.1†	35.5	28.1–42.9†	33.5	26.6–40.3
TCT (s)	23.5	19.0–28.3†	23.1	18.0–29.2	24.3	19.4–29.2†	25.1	20.5–29.7†	25.5	19.8–31.2†	25.0	19.7–30.3
Fibrinogen (g/L)	2.83	1.67–3.99†	3.12	1.62–4.26†	2.70	1.62–3.78†	2.43	1.50–3.79†	2.51	1.50–3.87†	2.78	1.56–4.00
II (U/mL)	0.48	0.26–0.70	0.63	0.33–0.93	0.68	0.34–1.02	0.75	0.45–1.05	0.88	0.60–1.16	1.08	0.70–1.46
V(U/mL)	0.72	0.34–1.08	0.95	0.45–1.45	0.98	0.62–1.34	0.90	0.48–1.32	0.91	0.55–1.27	1.06	0.62–1.50
VII (U/mL)	0.66	0.28–1.04	0.89	0.35–1.43	0.90	0.42–1.38	0.91	0.39–1.43	0.87	0.47–1.27	1.05	0.67–1.43
VIII (U/mL)	1.00	0.50–1.78†	0.88	0.50–1.54†	0.91	0.50–1.57*	0.79	0.50–1.25†	0.73	0.50–1.09	0.99	0.50–1.49
vWF (U/mL)	1.53	0.50–2.87	1.40	0.50–2.54	1.28	0.50–2.46	1.18	0.50–2.06	1.07	0.50–1.97	0.92	0.50–1.58
IX (U/mL)	0.53	0.15–0.91	0.53	0.15–0.91	0.51	0.21–0.81	0.67	0.21–1.13	0.86	0.36–1.36	1.09	0.55–1.63
X (U/mL)	0.40	0.12–0.68	0.49	0.19–0.79	0.59	0.31–0.87	0.71	0.35–1.07	0.78	0.38–1.18	1.06	0.70–1.52
XI (U/mL)	0.38	0.10–0.66	0.55	0.23–0.87	0.53	0.27–0.79	0.69	0.41–0.97	0.86	0.49–1.34	0.97	0.67–1.27
XII (U/mL)	0.53	0.13–0.93	0.47	0.11–0.83	0.49	0.17–0.81	0.67	0.25–1.09	0.77	0.39–1.15	1.08	0.52–1.64
PK (U/mL)	0.37	0.18–0.69	0.48	0.20–0.76	0.57	0.23–0.91	0.73	0.41–1.05	0.86	0.56–1.16	1.12	0.62–1.62
HMWK (U/mL)	0.54	0.06–1.02	0.74	0.16–1.32	0.77	0.33–1.21	0.82	0.30–1.46†	0.82	0.36–1.28†	0.92	0.50–1.36
XII_a (U/mL)	0.79	0.27–1.31	0.94	0.44–1.44†	0.93	0.39–1.47†	1.04	0.36–1.72†	1.04	0.46–1.62†	1.05	0.55–1.55
XIII_b (U/mL)	0.76	0.30–1.22	1.06	0.32–1.80†	1.11	0.39–1.73†	1.16	0.48–1.84†	1.10	0.50–1.70†	0.97	0.57–1.37

PT, prothrombin time; APTT, activated partial thromboplastin time; TCT, thrombin clotting time; VIII, factor VIII procoagulant; vWF, von Willebrand factor, prekallikrein; HMWK, high-molecular-weight kininogen.

* All factors, except fibrinogen, are expressed as units per milliliter (U/mL), where pooled plasma contains 1 U/mL. All values are expressed as the mean, followed by the lower and upper boundary encompassing 95% of the population. Between 40 and 77 samples were assayed for each value for the newborn. Some measurements were skewed because of a disproportionate number of high values. The lower limit, which excludes the lowest 2.5% of the population, has been given.

† Values that are indistinguishable from those of the adult.

(Andrews M, Paes B, et al. Development of the hemostatic system in the neonate and young infant. Am J Pediatr Hematol Oncol 1990;12:95)

APPENDIX 20

Reference Values for Coagulation Tests in the Healthy Premature Infant (30–36 Weeks' Gestation) During the First 6 Months of Life*

	Day 1		Day 5		Day 30		Day 90		Day 180		Adult	
	Mean	95% Range	Mean	95% Range	Mean	95% Range	Mean	95% Range	Mean	95% Range	Mean	95% Range
PT (sec)	13.0	10.6–16.2†	12.5	10.0–15.3†	11.8	10.0–13.6†	12.3	10.0–14.6†	12.5	10.0–15.0†	12.4	10.8–13.9
INR	1.0	0.61–1.7	0.91	0.53–1.48	0.79	0.53–1.11	0.88	0.53–1.32	0.91	0.53–1.48	0.89	0.64–1.17
aPTT (sec)	53.6	27.5–79.4‡	50.5	26.9–74.1	44.7	26.9–62.5	39.5	28.3–50.7	37.5	27.1–53.3†	33.5	26.6–40.3
TCT (sec)	24.8	19.2–30.4†	24.1	18.8–29.4†	24.4	18.8–29.9†	25.1	19.4–30.8†	25.2	18.9–31.5†	25.0	19.7–30.3
Fibrinogen (g/L)	2.43	1.50–3.73†‡	2.80	1.60–4.18†‡	2.54	1.50–4.14†	2.46	1.50–3.52†	2.28	1.50–3.60	2.78	1.56–4.00
II (U/mL)	0.45	0.20–0.77	0.57	0.29–0.85‡	0.57	0.36–0.95‡	0.68	0.30–1.06	0.87	0.51–1.23	1.08	0.70–1.46
V (U/mL)	0.88	0.41–1.44†‡	1.00	0.46–1.54†	1.02	0.48–1.56†	0.99	0.59–1.39†	1.02	0.58–1.46†	10.6	0.62–1.50
VII (U/mL)	0.67	0.21–1.13	0.84	0.30–1.38	0.83	0.21–1.45	0.87	0.31–1.43	0.99	0.47–1.51†	1.05	0.67–1.43
VIII (U/mL)	1.11	0.50–2.13	1.15	0.53–2.05†‡	1.11	0.50–1.99†‡	1.06	0.58–1.88†‡	0.99	0.50–1.87†‡	0.99	0.50–1.49
vWF (U/mL)	1.36	0.78–2.10	1.33	0.72–2.19	1.36	0.66–2.16	1.12	0.75–1.84†	0.98	0.54–1.58†	0.92	0.50–1.58
IX (U/mL)	0.35	0.19–0.65‡	0.42	0.14–0.74‡	0.44	0.13–0.80	0.59	0.25–0.93	0.81	0.50–1.20	1.09	0.55–1.63
X (U/mL)	0.41	0.11–0.71	0.51	0.19–0.83	0.56	0.20–0.92	0.67	0.35–0.99	0.77	0.35–1.19	1.06	0.70–1.52
XI (U/mL)	0.30	0.08–0.52‡	0.41	0.13–0.69‡	0.43	0.15–0.71‡	0.59	0.25–0.93‡	0.78	0.46–1.10	0.97	0.67–1.27
XII (U/mL)	0.38	0.10–0.66‡	0.39	0.09–0.69‡	0.43	0.11–0.75	0.61	0.15–1.07	0.82	0.22–1.42	1.08	0.52–1.64
PK (U/mL)	0.33	0.09–0.57	0.45	0.25–0.75	0.59	0.31–0.87	0.79	0.37–1.21	0.78	0.40–1.16	1.12	0.62–1.62
HMWK (U/mL)	0.49	0.09–0.89	0.62	0.24–1.00‡	0.64	0.16–1.12‡	0.78	0.32–1.24	0.83	0.41–1.25†	0.92	0.50–1.36
XIIIa (U/mL)	0.70	0.32–1.08	1.01	0.57–1.45†	0.99	0.51–1.47†	1.13	0.71–1.55†	1.13	0.65–1.61†	1.05	0.55–1.55
XIIb (U/mL)	0.81	0.35–1.27	1.10	0.68–1.58†	1.07	0.57–1.57†	1.21	0.75–1.67	1.15	0.67–1.63	0.97	0.57–1.37

PT, prothrombin time; APTT, activated partial thromboplastin time; TCT, thrombin clotting time; VIII, factor VIII procoagulant; vWF, von Willebrand factor; PK, prekallikrein; HMWK, high-molecular-weight kininogen; INR, International Normalized Ratio.

* All factors except fibrinogen are expressed as units per milliliter (U/mL), where pooled plasma contains 1.0 U/mL. All values are given as mean followed by the lower and upper boundaries encompassing 95% of the population. Between 40 and 96 samples were assayed for each value for the newborn. Some measurements were skewed because of a disproportionate number of high values. The lower limit, which excludes the lower 2.5% of the population, has been given.

† Values are indistinguishable from those of adults.

‡ Values different from those of the full-term infants.

(Andrew M, Paes B, Johnston M. Developent of the hemostatic system in the neonate and young infant. Am J Pediatr Hematol Oncol 1990;12:95)

APPENDIX 21

Reference Values for the Inhibitors of Coagulation in Healthy Full-Term Infants During the First 6 Months of Life Compared With Those in Adults*

Coagulation Inhibitors	Day 1		Day 5		Day 30		Day 90		Day 180		Adults	
	Mean	95% Range	Mean	95% Range	Mean	95% Range	Mean	95% Range	Mean	95% Range	Mean	95% Range
ATIII (U/mL)	0.63	0.39–0.87	0.67	0.41–0.93	0.78	0.48–1.08	0.97	0.73–1.21†	1.04	0.84–1.24†	1.05	0.79–1.31
α_2-M (U/mL)	1.39	0.95–1.83	1.48	0.98–1.98	1.50	1.06–1.94	1.76	1.26–2.26	1.91	1.49–2.33	0.86	0.52–1.20
C_1E-INH (U/mL)	0.72	0.36–1.08	0.90	0.60–1.20†	0.89	0.47–1.31	1.15	0.71–1.59	1.41	0.89–1.93	1.01	0.71–1.31
α_1-AT (U/mL)	0.93	0.49–1.37†	0.89	0.49–1.29†	0.62	0.36–0.88	0.72	0.42–1.02	0.77	0.47–1.07	0.93	0.55–1.31
HCII (U/mL)	0.43	0.10–0.93	0.48	0.10–0.96	0.47	0.10–0.87	0.72	0.10–1.46	1.20	0.50–1.90	0.96	0.66–1.26
Proteins C (U/mL)	0.35	0.17–0.53	0.42	0.20–0.64	0.43	0.21–0.65	0.54	0.28–0.80	0.59	0.37–0.81	0.96	0.64–1.28
Protein S (U/mL)	0.36	0.12–0.60	0.50	0.22–0.78	0.63	0.33–0.93	0.86	0.54–1.18†	0.87	0.55–1.19†	0.92	0.60–1.24

ATIII, antithrombin III; α_2-M, α_2-macroglobulin; C_1E-INH, C_1-esterase inhibitor; α_1-AT, α_1-antitrypsin; HCII, heparin cofactor II.

* All values are expressed in units per milliliter (U/mL), where pooled plasma contains 1 U/mL. All values are given as a mean, followed by the lower and upper boundary encompassing 95% of the population. Between 40 and 75 samples were assayed for each value for the newborn. Some measurements were skewed because of a disproportionate number of high values. The lower limits, which excludes the lowest 2.5% of the population, have been given.

† Values are indistinguishable from those of adults.

(Andrew M, Paes B, Johnston M. Development of the hemostatic system in the neonate and young infant. Am J Pediatr Hematol Oncol 1990;12:95)

APPENDIX 22

Replacement Therapy for Congenital Coagulation Disorders

Coagulation Factor	Factor Source (Concentration)	Recovery in the Circulation (%)	Biologic Half-Life	Desired Level for Hemostasis During Surgery	Estimated Therapeutic Dose (per kg body weight)	
					Initial	Maintenance
Factor I (fibrinogen)	Cryoprecipitate (200–300 mg/bag)	About 60	80 h	100 mg/dL	2–3 bags/10 kg	1 bag/15 kg daily
Factor II (prothrombin)	Fresh frozen plasma* Factor IX concentrate†	50	72 h	25%–30%	15–20 mL/kg 20 U/kg	3mL/kg every 12–24 h 10–20 U/kg every 12 h
Factor V	Fresh frozen plasma*	75	12–36 h	25%	15–20 mL/kg	3–6 mL/kg daily
Factor VII	Fresh frozen plasma* Factor IX concentrate†	100	3–6 h	15%–25%	10–20 mL/kg 20–50 U/kg	3–6 mL/kg every 8–12 h
Factor VIII	Fresh frozen plasma* Cryoprecipitate (100 U/bag) Factor VIII concentrate†	90–100	8–12 h	25%–80% (depends on type and extent of surgery or bleed and interval from surgery)	15–50 U/kg 1 bag/2 kg 15–50 U/kg	Every 8–12 h
Factor IX	Plasma* Factor IX concentrate†	25–50	18–24 h	25%–50% (depends on type and extent of surgery or bleed and interval from surgery)	25–50 U/kg (plasma can be given only for mild deficiency)	Every 12–24 h
Factor X	Fresh frozen plasma* Factor IX concentrate†	Varies: 50–90	25–40 h	10%–25%	15–20 mL/kg	3–6 mL/kg every 24 h
Factor XI	Fresh frozen plasma*	90	48–72 h	20%–25%	15–20 mL/kg	3–6 mL/kg every 12 h
Factor XIII	Fresh frozen plasma* Cryoprecipitate (50–100 U/bag)	Varies: 50–100	8–12 d	5%	500 mL 4–6 bags	Every 21 days Every 21 days

* One milliliter of plasma containing approximately 1 unit of factor activity.
† Factor activity variable and stated on label of product.
(Hilgartner M. Transfusion principles for congenital coagulation disorders. In: Hoffman R, Benz EJ Jr, Shattil SJ, Furie B, Cohen HJ, eds. Hematology: basic principles and practice. New York, Churchill Livingstone, 1991;1633)

APPENDIX 23

Red Blood Cell Values at Various Ages: Mean and Lower Limit of Normal (−2D)*

	Hemoglobin (g/dL)		Hematocrit (%)		RBC Count (10^{12}/L)		MCV (fL)		MCH (pg)		MCHC (g/dL)	
Age	**Mean**	**−2 SD**	**Mean**	**−2 SD**	**Mean**	**−2 SD**	**Mean**	**−2 SD**	**Mean**	**−2 SD**	**Mean**	**−2 SD**
Birth (cord blood)	16.5	13.5	51	42	4.7	3.9	108	98	34	31	33	30
1–3 d (capillary)	18.5	14.5	56	45	5.3	4.0	108	95	34	31	33	29
1 wk	17.5	13.5	54	42	5.1	3.9	107	88	34	28	33	28
2 wk	16.5	12.5	51	39	4.9	3.6	105	86	34	28	33	28
1 mo	14.0	10.0	43	31	4.2	3.0	104	85	34	28	33	29
2 mo	11.5	9.0	35	28	3.8	2.7	96	77	30	26	33	29
3–6 mo	11.5	9.5	35	29	3.8	3.1	91	74	30	25	33	30
0.5–2 y	12.0	10.5	36	33	4.5	3.7	78	70	27	23	33	30
2–6 y	12.5	11.5	37	34	4.6	3.9	81	75	27	24	34	31
6–12 y	13.5	11.5	40	35	4.6	4.0	86	77	29	25	34	31
12–18 y												
Female	14.0	12.0	41	36	4.6	4.1	90	78	30	25	34	31
Male	14.5	13.0	43	37	4.9	4.5	88	78	30	25	34	31
18–49 y												
Female	14.0	12.0	41	36	4.6	4.0	90	80	30	26	34	31
Male	15.5	13.5	47	41	5.2	4.5	90	80	30	26	34	31

MCV, mean corpuscular volume; MCH, mean corpuscular hemoglobin; MCHC, mean corpuscular hemoglobin concentration.

* These data have been compiled from several sources. Emphasis is given to recent studies employing electronic counters and to the selection of populations that are likely to exclude individuals with iron deficiency. The mean ± 2 SD can be expected to include 95% of the observations in a normal population.

(Dallman PR. In: Rudolph A, ed. Pediatrics, ed 16. New York, Appleton-Century-Crofts, 1977:1111)

Blood: Principles and Practice of Hematology,
edited by Robert I. Handin, Samuel E. Lux, and Thomas P. Stossel.
J.B. Lippincott Company, Philadelphia © 1995.

Erythrocytes

APPENDIX 24

Normal Hematologic Values During the First 2 Weeks of Life in the Term Infant

Value	Cord Blood	Day 1	Day 3	Day 7	Day 14
Hb (g/dL)	16.8	18.4	17.8	17.0	16.8
Hematocrit (%)	53.0	58.0	55.0	54.0	52.0
Red cells (/μL)	5.25	5.8	5.6	5.2	5.1
MCV (fL)	107	108	99.0	98.0	96.0
MCH (pg)	34	35	33	32.5	31.5
MCHC (g/dL)	31.7	32.5	33	33	33
Reticulocytes (%)	3–7	3–7	1–3	0–1	0–1
Nucleated RBCs (/μL)	500	200	0–5	0	0
Platelets (1000/μL)	290	192	213	248	252

* Hb, hemoglobin; MCV, mean corpuscular volume; MCH, mean corpuscular hemoglobin; MCHC, mean corpuscular hemoglobin concentration.
(Oski FA, Nalman JL. Hematologic problems in the newborn, ed 2. Philadelphia, WB Saunders,1972: 13)

APPENDIX 25

Hemoglobin Concentrations (g/dL) for Iron-Sufficient Preterm Infants*

Age	Birthweight 1000–1500 g	Birthweight 1501–2000 g
2 wk	16.3 (11.7–18.4)	14.8 (11.8–19.6)
1 mo	10.9 (8.7–15.2)	11.5 (8.2–15.0)
2 mo	8.8 (7.1–11.5)	9.4 (8.0–11.4)
3 mo	9.8 (8.9–11.2)	10.2 (9.3–11.8)
4 mo	11.3 (9.1–13.1)	11.3 (9.1–13.1)
5 mo	11.6 (10.2–14.3)	11.8 (10.4–13.0)
6 mo	12.0 (9.4–13.8)	11.8 (10.7–12.6)

* Serum ferritin ≥10 ng/mL.
(Lundstrom U, Siimes MA, Dallman PR. At what age does iron supplementation become necessary in low birth weight infants? J Pediatr 1977;91:878)

APPENDIX 26

Hemoglobin and Mean Corpuscular Volume Percentile Curves for Children

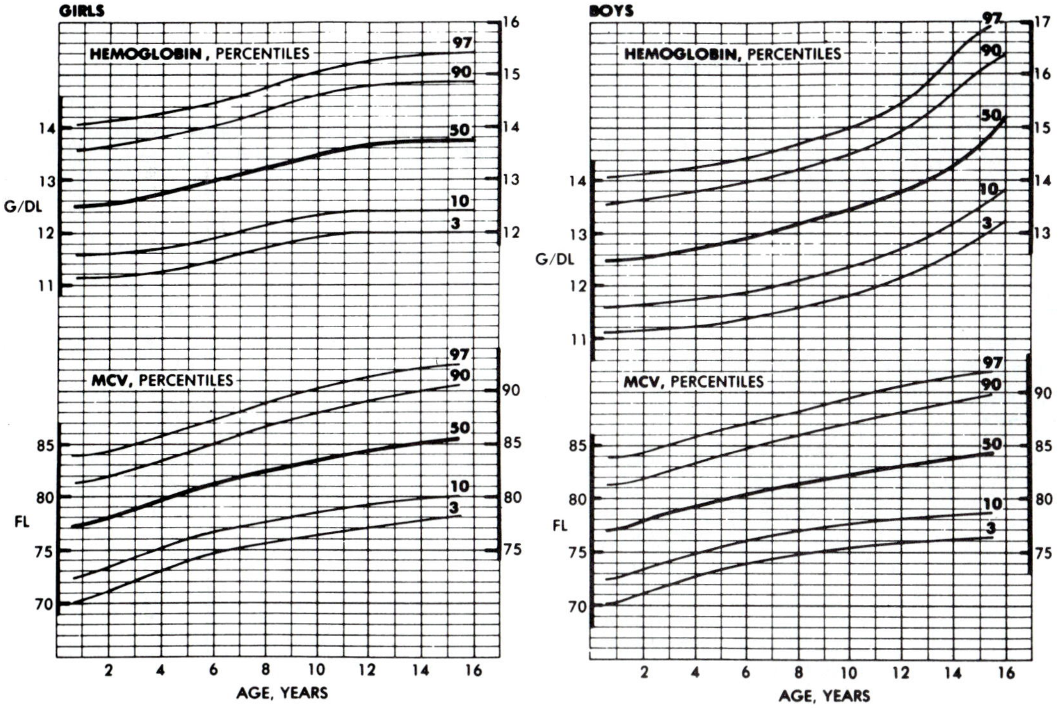

These figures were obtained from populations of nonindigent white US or Finnish children who did not have laboratory evidence of iron deficiency, thalassemia minor, or hemoglobinopathy. (Dallman PR, Siimes MA. Percentile curves for hemoglobin and red cell volume in infancy and childhood. J Pediatr 1979;94:26)

APPENDIX 27

Effect of Pregnancy, With and WIthout Iron Supplementation, on Hematocrit and Hemoglobin Values*

Time	Hematocrit (Mean; %)			Hemoglobin (Mean; g/dL)		
	No Supplement	Intramuscular Supplement†	Oral Supplement‡	No Supplement	Intramuscular Supplement†	Oral Supplement‡
WEEKS OF GESTATION						
0	42.0	—	—	13.4	—	—
12	38.3	40.6	35.7	12.5	13.1	11.4
16	39.5	37.9	36.3	12.4	12.1	11.4
20	36.4	37.0	37.1	11.7	11.8	11.8
24	35.6	36.3	37.1	11.4	11.8	11.8
28	34.6	36.9	36.8	11.0	11.8	11.8
32	34.1	37.2	37.0	10.6	12.1	11.8
36	34.3	37.5	37.5	10.7	12.1	12.0
40	34.9	38.5	38.7	10.9	12.7	12.4
DAYS POSTPARTUM						
2	33.6	37.1	37.3	10.4	12.2	11.9
6	34.9	38.9	40.1	10.7	12.4	12.8
21	38.1	42.0	41.1	11.6	13.6	13.0
42	39.1	41.5	39.8	11.9	13.1	12.6
180	39.2	40.1	40.8	12.1	12.4	12.9

* About 20 persons were in each group.
† 1000 mg iron as iron dextran.
‡ 39 mg elemental iron twice daily.
(de Leeuw NKM, Lowenstein L, Hsieh YS. Iron deficiency and hydremia in normal pregnancy. Medicine 1966;45:291)

APPENDIX 28

Red Cell Kinetic Parameters in Normal Subjects

Parameter	Value	Unit
Red cell mass	Males: 28.7 ± 3.8	mL/kg
	Females: 25.3 ± 2.6	
Plasma volume	Males: 36.9 ± 4.2	
	Females: 41.9 ± 4.4	
^{51}Cr disappearance half-time	Range: 28–35	Days
	Males: 30.1 ± 4.0	
	Females: 29.4 ± 2.1	
Rate of ^{51}Cr label elution	Range: 0.68–1.31	% per day
Plasma iron disappearance half-time	85 ± 5	Minutes
Incorporation of ^{59}Fe into erythrocytes	82 ± 1	
	Range: 79–89	% at 14 days
Plasma iron turnover	0.75 ± 0.02	mg/100 mL whole blood/d
	121 ± 17	μM/L whole blood/d
Erythroid iron turnover	0.56	mg/100 mL whole blood/d
	86 ± 10	μmol/L whole blood/d

APPENDIX 29

Estimated Blood Volumes

			Total Blood Volume (mL/kg)	
Age	Plasma Volume (mL/kg)	Red Cell Mass (mL/kg)	From Plasma Volume	From Red Cell Mass
Newborn	41.3	43.1	82.1	86.1
	46			84.7
			78	
1–7 d	51–54		82–86	
		37.9		77.8
1–12 mo	46.1		78.1	
		25.5		72.8
1–3 y	44.4		73.8	
	47.2		81.8	
		24.9		69.1
4–6 y	48.5		80.0	
	49.6		85.6	
		25.5		67.5
7–9 y	52.2		87.6	
	49.0		86.1	
		24.3		67.5
10–12 y	51.9		87.6	
	46.2		83.2	
		26.3		67.4
13–15 y	51.2		88.3	
16–18 y	50.1		90.2	
Adults	39–44	25–30	68–88	55–75

(Price DC, Ries C. In: Handmaker H, Lowenstein JM, eds. Nuclear medicine in clinical pediatrics. New York, Society of Nuclear Medicine, 1975:279)

APPENDIX 30

Estimation of Red Cell, Plasma, and Total Blood Volume in Adult Men and Women*

	Men			Women		
Volume	a	b	SD (mL)	a	b	SD (mL)
Red cell volume	490	21.4	200	409	18.3	139
Plasma volume	1050	19.6	260	455	28.9	213
Total blood volume	1530	41.0	400	864	47.2	319

* For a subject of given weight (w; in kg) in a normal mean red cell, plasma, or total blood volume (V; in mL) can be calculated from the formula, $V = a + bw$. Example: In a 70-kg man, the mean red cell volume is $490 \pm (21.4 \times 70) = 1988$ mL ± 2 SD; range = 1988 ± 400; or 1588 to 2388 mL. The expected normal range can be calculated from the formula, range = mean ± 2 SD.

Calculations are based on red cell volume measured by ^{51}Cr method and on plasma and blood volumes calculated from the volume and volume of packed red cells without correction for trapped plasma or "body hematocrit" differences.

(After Brown E, et al. Red cell, plasma and blood volume in healthy women measured by radiochromium cell labeling and hematocrit. J Clin Invest 1962;41:2182; and Wennesland R, et al. Red cell, plasma, and blood volume in healthy men measured by radiochromium cell tagging and hematocrit. J Clin Invest 1959;38:1065)

APPENDIX 31

Values of Serum Iron, Iron-Binding Capacity, and Transferrin Saturation From Infants During the First Year of Life*

			Age (mo)						
			0.5	1	2	4	6	9	12
Serum Iron	Median	(μg/dL)	120	125	87	84	77	84	78
	95% range		63–201	58–172	15–159	18–164	28–135	34–135	35–155
Iron-Binding Capacity	Mean ± SD	(μg/dL)	191 ± 43	199 ± 43	246 ± 55	300 ± 39	321 ± 51	341 ± 42	358 ± 38
% Saturation	Median		68	63	34	27	23	25	23
	95% range		30–99	35–94	21–63	7–53	10–43	10–39	10–47

* The data were collected from healthy full-term Finish infants whose formula and cereal were supplemented with iron throughout the first year. Infants with a hemoglobin < 11 g/dL, MCV < 71 fL, or serum ferritin < 10/ng/mL were excluded.

(Saarinen UM, Siimes MA. Developmental changes in serum iron, total iron-binding capacity, and transferrin saturation in infancy. J Pediatr 1977;91;875–877)

APPENDIX 32

Serum and Transferrin Saturation

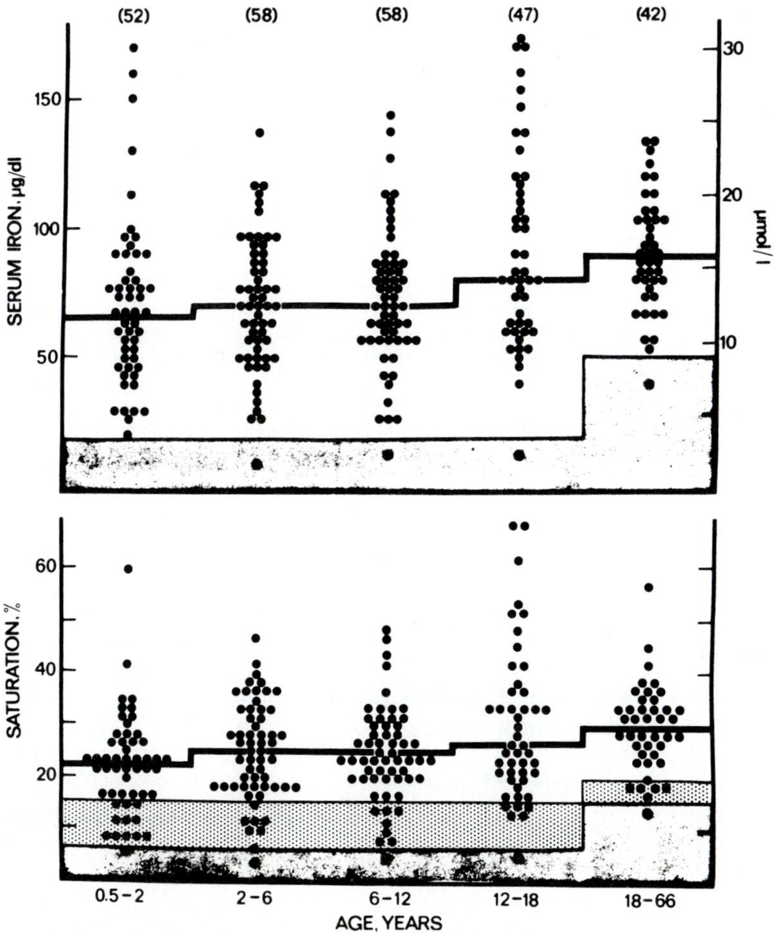

Values in subjects with values for hemoglobin, mean corpuscular volume, free erythrocyte protoporphyrin, and serum ferritin. (Koerper MA, Dallman P. Serum iron concentration and transferrin saturation in the diagnosis of iron deficiency in children: normal developmental changes. J Pediatr 1977;91:870)

APPENDIX 33

Normal Ranges for Folate Assays and FIGLU Test*

	Range	Mean
SERUM FOLATE		
Adults	6.0–18.6	9.7
Children 1 y	3.0–35	9.3
Children 1–6 y	4.1–21.2	11.4
Children 1–10 y	6.5–16.5	10.3
RED CELL FOLATE		
Adults	160–640	316
Infants <1 y	74–995	277
Children 1–11 y	96–364	215
WHOLE BLOOD FOLATE		
Adults	50–140	89
Adults	60–400	195
Infants <1 y	20–160	87
Infants 1 y	31–400	86
Infants 2–24 mo	35–160	96†
Children up to 11 y	52–164	97

	Histidine Load	Collection Period	Total FIGLU
FIGLU EXCRETION			
Adults	15 g	0–8 h	Up to 17 mg
Infants	100–300 mg/kg	0–6 h	Up to 6 mg
Children	0.12 g/lb	0–24 h	Up to 30 mg

* Serum folate levels (fasting) below 3.0, red cell folate below 100, or whole blood folate below 60 can be regarded as abnormal.
† Derived after correction for a packed cell volume of 45%.
(Willoughby MLN. Pediatric haematology. New York, Churchill Livingstone, 1977:17)

APPENDIX 34

Normal Serum Folic Acid Levels (ng/mL)

Age	Range	Mean ± SD
NORMAL PREMATURE INFANTS		
1–4 days	7.17–52.00	29.54 ± 0.98
2–3 weeks	4.12–15.62	8.61 ± 0.55
1–2 months	2.81–11.25	5.84 ± 0.35
2–3 months	3.56–11.82	6.95 ± 0.50
3–5 months	3.85–16.50	8.92 ± 0.86
5–7 months	6.00–12.25	9.02 ± 0.74
NORMAL CHILDREN		
1–6 years	4.12–21.15	11.37 ± 0.82
NORMAL ADULTS		
20–45 years	4.50–28.00	10.29 ± 1.14

(Shojania A, Gross S. Folic acid deficiency and prematurity. J Pediatr 1964;64:323)

APPENDIX 35

Erythropoietin Titers

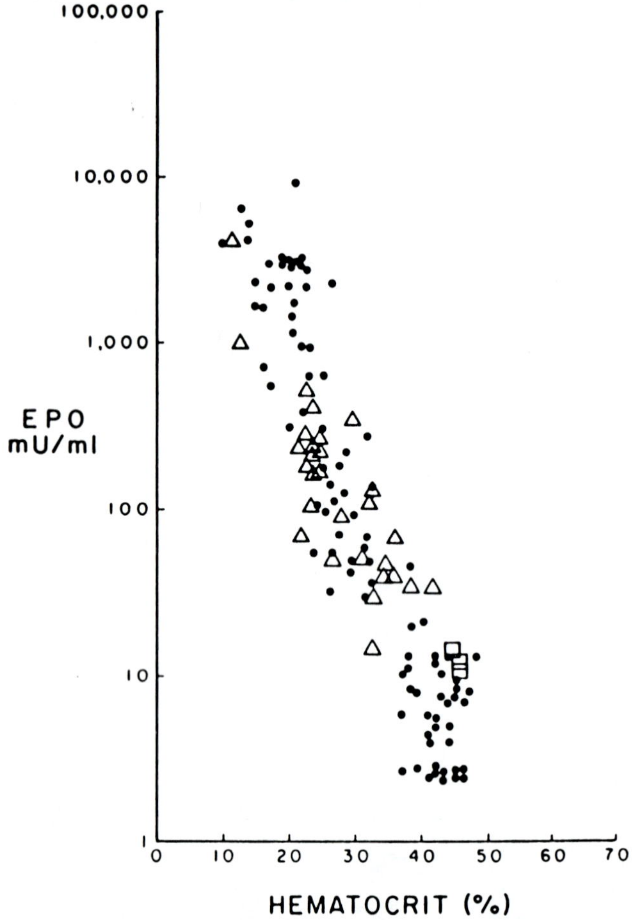

Titers were measured with biologic (BA) and radioimmune (RIA) assays in normal subjects and in patients with anemia caused by renal or chronic diseases. Circles, anemic and normal subjects (BA); squares, normal subjects (RIA); triangles, anemic patients (RIA). (Ersler AJ, Wilson J, Caro J. Erythropoietin titers in anemic, nonuremic patients. J Lab Clin Med 1987;109:429)

APPENDIX 36

Effect of Altitude on Hematocrit in Normal Males

Altitude ft	Altitude m	n	Hematocrit* (%)
0	0	721	47
4400	1340	744	49.5
7457	2280	100	51
12,240	3740	40	54
14,900	4540	32	61
17,800	5430	10	69

* Mean values in males.
(Cartwright GE. Diagnostic laboratory hematology, ed 4. New York, Grune & Stratton, 1968)

APPENDIX 37

Differentiation of Hemoglobins by Cellulose Acetate and Citrate–Agar Gel Electrophoresis

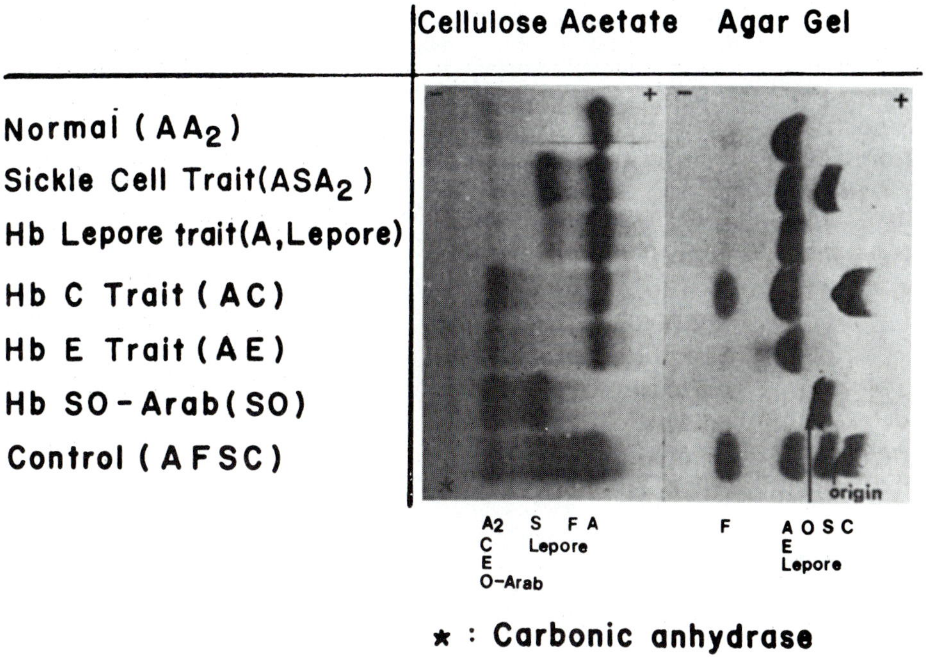

Origin is at the left border of the photograph of the cellulose acetate strip. (Kim HC. Inherited hemoglobinopathies in children. Clin Pediatr 1981;20:161)

APPENDIX 38

Electrophoretic Relative Mobilities of Hemoglobin Variants Under Different Conditions

Supporting Medium, Buffer, and pH	Relative Migration Rates of Various Hemoglobins*															
Starch gel, paper, starch block, agarose; barbital, pH 8.6; tris-EDTA-borate buffer, pH 8.8			⋮			C	E O A_2 1		S DL 5G P		A FMK			J 46N3 2	H I	+
Cellulose acetate; tris-EDTA-borate buffer, pH 8.6†	⋮			C A_2 7		S D		A	J		H					+
Starch gel, paper, starch block; phosphate buffer, pH 6.8		C O A_2			L		S DGPF 5E		A JN K	I		2	⋮	H		+
Agar gel; phosphate or citrate buffer, pH 6.2		F				A D E A_2 G ‡		S O7	HL Q	⋮	C					+

1, Alexander; 2, Barts; 3, Hopkins I; 4, Hopkins II; 5, Lepore; 6, Norfolk; 7, C_{Harlem}.

* Dotted lines indicate origin.

† With a discontinuous buffer system, migration is to the cathodal side, possibly because of a greater electroendosmotic flow.

‡ Also I, J, P, 1, 2, 3, 4, 5.

(Kim HC, Adachi K, Schwartz E. Separation of hemoglobins. In: Williams WJ, Beutler E, Erslev AJ, Lichtman MA. Hematology, ed 4. New York, McGraw-Hill, 1990:1712)

APPENDIX 39

Percentage of Hemoglobins F and A2 in Newborns and Adults*

	HbF (%) (Gα/Aα Ratio)	Hb A2 (%)
Newborn	60–90 (3:1)	<1.0
Adult	<1.0 (2:3)	1.6–3.5

* The α chains of fetal hemoglobin contain either a glycyl residue or an alanyl residue at position 136. The Gα/Aα ratio in the newborn undergoes a considerable change between the third and fourth month of life, at which time it approximates that of the HB F of adults.[16]

(Charache S. In: Altman PL, Dittmer DS, eds. Human health and disease. Bethesda, Federation of American Societies for Experimental Biology, 1977:159)

APPENDIX 40

Time Course of the Relative Hb F Concentration in Blood From Normal Infants

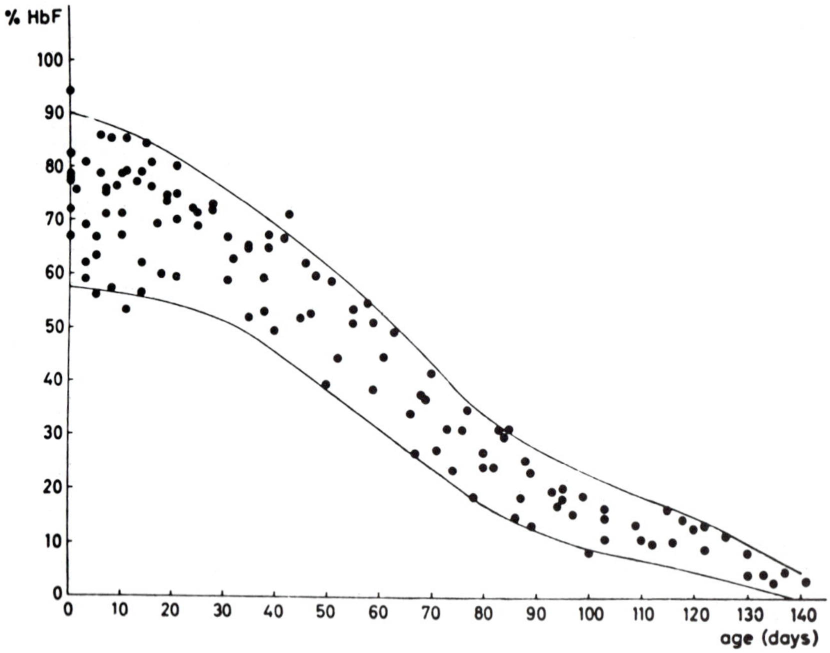

(After Garby I, Sjölin S. Development of erythropoiesis. Acta Paediatr [Stockh] 1962;51: 245)

APPENDIX 41

Methemoglobin Levels in Normal Subjects*

	No. Cases	Methemoglobin (g/dL)			Methemoglobin as Percentage of Total Hemoglobin		
		Mean	Range	SD	Mean	Range	SD
Prematures	50	0.38	(0.02–0.83)	±0.10	2.2	(0.08–4.7)	±1.10
Newborns (1–10 d)	39	0.22	(0.00–0.58)	±0.17	1.5	(0.00–2.8)	±0.81
Infants (1 mo–1 y)	8	0.14	(0.02–0.29)	±0.09	1.2	(0.17–2.4)	±0.78
Children (1–14 y)	35	0.11	(0.00–0.33)	±0.09	0.79	(0.00–2.4)	±0.62
Adults (14–78 y)	30	0.11	(0.00–0.28)	±0.09	0.82	(0.00–1.9)	±0.63

* Apparently well individuals without cyanosis or respiratory disease. The nitrate level in the milk and water ingested by the infants was less than 0.027 ppm. The premature infants were treated with oral vitamin C.

(Kravitz H, Elegant LD, et al. Methemoglobin values in premature and mature infants and children. Am J Dis Child 1956;91:2–5)

APPENDIX 42

Normal Values for Osmotic Fragility

Sodium Chloride Conc. in g/dL	Percentage of Hemolysis: Before Incubation	Percentage of Hemolysis: After Incubation
0.85	0	0
0.75	0	0–2
0.65	0	0–19
0.60	0	0–40
0.55	0	5–70
0.50	0–5	36–88
0.45	0–45	54–96
0.40	50–90	65–100
0.35	90–99	72–100
0.30	97–100	80–100
0.20	100	91–100
0.10	100	100

(Cartwright GE. Diagnostic laboratory hematology, ed 4. New York, Grune & Stratton, 1968)

APPENDIX 43

Plasma Concentration of Hemopexin and Haptoglobin in Term and Premature Infants on the First Day of Life

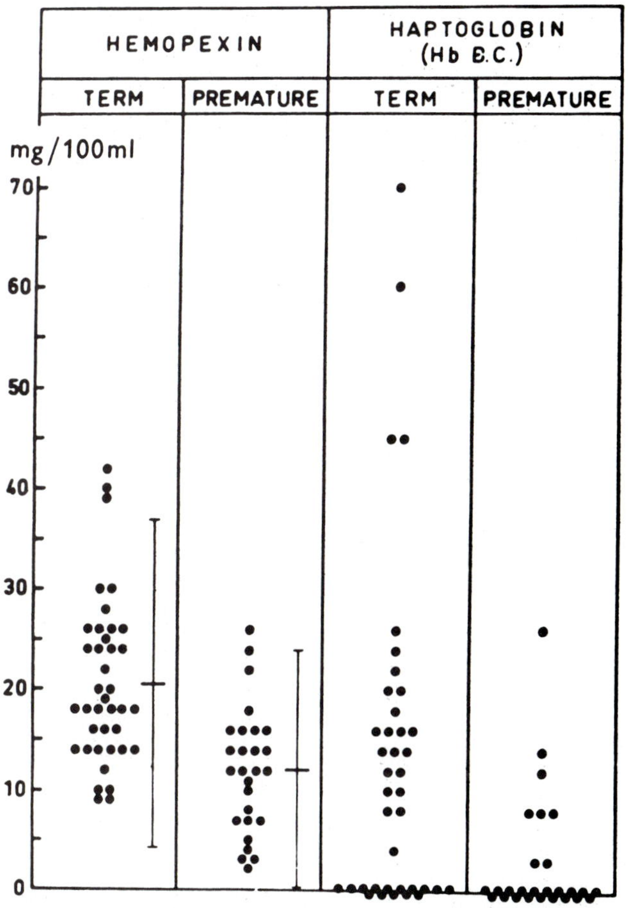

The means ± are indicated to the right of the hemopexin results.
(Lundh B, Oski FA, et al. Plasma hemopexin and haptoglobin in hemolytic diseases of the newborn. Acta Paediatr Scand 1970;59:121)

APPENDIX 44

Activities of Red Cell Enzymes in Normal Adults

Enzyme	Activity at 37°C (mean ± SD)
Acetylcholinesterase	36.93 ± 3.83
Adenosine deaminase	1.11 ± 0.23
Adenylate kinase	258 ± 29.3
Aldolase	3.19 ± 0.86
Bisphosphoglyceromutase (2,3-diphosphoglyceromutase)	4.78 ± 0.65
Catalase	15.3 ± 2.4 × 10^4
Enolase	5.39 ± 0.83
Epimerase	0.23 ± 0.06
Galactokinase	0.029 ± 0.004
Galactose-1-phosphate uridyl transferase	28.4 ± 6.94
Glucose phosphate isomerase	60.8 ± 11.0
Glucose-6-phosphate dehydrogenase	8.34 ± 1.59
WHO method	12.1 ± 2.09
γ-Glutamyl-cysteine synthetase	0.43 ± 0.04
Glutathione peroxidase*	30.82 ± 4.65
Glutathione reductase without FAD	7.18 ± 1.09
Glutathione reductase with FAD	10.4 ± 1.50
Glutathione-S-transferase	6.66 ± 1.81
Glyceraldehyde phosphate dehydrogenase	226 ± 41.9
Glutamic oxaloacetic transaminase without PLP	3.02 ± 0.67
Glutamic oxaloacetic transaminase with PLP	5.04 ± 0.90
Hexokinase	1.78 ± 0.38
Hypoxanthine phosphoribosyl-transferase	1.72 ± 0.30
Lactate dehydrogenase	200 ± 26.5
Methemoglobin reductase	2.60 ± 0.71
Monophosphoglyceromutase	37.71 ± 5.56
NADH-methemoglobin reductase	19.2 ± 3.85 (30°)
NADPH diaphorase	2.26 ± 0.16
Phosphofructokinase	11.01 ± 2.33
Phosphoglucomutase	5.50 ± 0.62
Phosphoglycerate kinase	320 ± 36.1
Phosphoglycolate phosphatase	1.23 ± 0.10
Pyrimidine 5′ nucleotidase	0.11 ± 0.03
Pyruvate kinase	15.0 ± 1.99
6-Phosphogluconate dehydrogenase	8.78 ± 0.78
Triose phosphate isomerase	2111 ± 397

(Beutler E, Blum KG. In: Altman PL, Dittmer DS, eds. Human health and disease. Bethesda, Federation of American Societies for Experimental Biology, 1977:156; and Beutler E. Red cell metabolism: a manual of biochemical methods, ed 3. Orlando, Grune & Stratton, 1984)

APPENDIX 45

Level of Intermediates in Red Cells of Normal Adults

Intermediate	Abbreviation	Concentration (mean ± 1 SD)		
		nmol/g Hb	nmol/mL Red Cells	μmol/L in Whole Blood
Adenosine-5′-diphosphate	ADP	6635 ± 105	216 ± 36	—
Adenosine-5′-monophosphate	AMP	62 ± 10	21.1 ± 3.4	—
Adenosine-5′-triphosphate	ATP	4230 ± 290 (whites)	1438 ± 99	—
		3530 ± 301 (blacks)	1200 ± 102	—
2,3-Diphosphoglycerate	2,3-DPG	1227 ± 1870	4171 ± 636	—
Glutathione	GSH	6570 ± 1040	2234 ± 354	—
Glutathione (oxidized)	GSSG	12.3 ± 4.5	4.2 ± 1.53	—
Glucose-6-phosphate	G6P	82 ± 22	27.8 ± 7.5	—
Fructose-6-phosphate	F6P	27 ± 5.8	9.3 ± 2.0	—
Fructose-6-diphosphate	FDP	5.6 ± 1.8	1.9 ± 0.6	—
Dihydroxyacetone phosphate	DHAP	27.6 ± 8.2	9.4 ± 2.8	—
3-Phosphoglyceric acid	3-PGA	132 ± 15.0	44.9 ± 5.1	—
2-Phosphoglyceric acid	2-PGA	21.5 ± 7.35	7.3 ± 2.5	—
Phosphoenolpyruvate	PEP	35.9 ± 6.47	12.2 ± 2.2	—
Creatine	—	1310 ± 310 (male)	445 ± 105	—
	—	1500 ± 250 (female)	510 ± 85	—
Lactate	—	—	—	932 ± 211
Pyruvate	—	—	—	53.3 ± 21.5

(Beutler E. Red cell metabolism: a manual of biochemical methods, ed 3. Orlando, Grune & Stratton, 1984)

APPENDIX 46

Relative Frequencies of Erythrocyte Alloantibodies

Blood Group System	Relative Frequency of Antibody	Relative Potency of Antigen (Compared With K)
Rh*	0.5	0.3
Kell	0.3	1.0
Duffy	0.15	0.04
Kidd	0.05	0.01
Other	<0.01	Negligible

* Rh(D) excluded.

Blood: Principles and Practice of Hematology,
edited by Robert I. Handin, Samuel E. Lux, and Thomas P. Stossel.
J.B. Lippincott Company, Philadelphia © 1995.

APPENDIX 47

The Genetic Code

1st position (5′ end) ↓	2nd position U	2nd position C	2nd position A	2nd position G	3rd position (3′ end) ↓
U	Phe	Ser	Tyr	Cys	**U**
	Phe	Ser	Tyr	Cys	**C**
	Leu	Ser	STOP	STOP	**A**
	Leu	Ser	STOP	Trp	**G**
C	Leu	Pro	His	Arg	**U**
	Leu	Pro	His	Arg	**C**
	Leu	Pro	Gln	Arg	**A**
	Leu	Pro	Gln	Arg	**G**
A	Ile	Thr	Asn	Ser	**U**
	Ile	Thr	Asn	Ser	**C**
	Ile	Thr	Lys	Arg	**A**
	Met	Thr	Lys	Arg	**G**
G	Val	Ala	Asp	Gly	**U**
	Val	Ala	Asp	Gly	**C**
	Val	Ala	Glu	Gly	**A**
	Val	Ala	Glu	Gly	**G**

APPENDIX 48

Amino Acids

Amino Acid	Three-Letter Abbreviation	One-Letter Symbol
BASIC (+)		
Arginine	Arg	R
Histidine	His	H
Lysine	Lys	K
ACIDIC (−)		
Aspartic acid	Asp	D
Glutamic acid	Glu	E
POLAR		
Asparagine	Asp	N
Cysteine	Cys	C
Glutamine	Glu	Q
Glycine	Gly	G
Serine	Ser	S
Threonine	Thr	T
Tyrosine	Tyr	Y
NONPOLAR		
Alanine	Ala	A
Isoleucine	Ile	I
Leucine	Leu	L
Methionine	Met	M
Phenylalanine	Phe	F
Proline	Pro	P
Tryptophan	Trp	W
Valine	Val	V

APPENDIX 49

SI Unit Conversion Table

Constituent	Traditional Units	Multiplication Factor*	SI Units
δ-Aminolevulinic acid (U)	mg/d	7.63	μmol/d
Bilirubin			
Direct (S)	mg/dL	17.1	μmol/L
Total (S)	mg/dL	17.1	μmol/L
Calcium (S)	mg/dL	0.25	mmol/L
Coproporphyrin (U)	μg/d	1.5	nmol/d
Erythrocyte count (B)	number per μL	10^6	number per L
Fibrinogen† (factor I) (P)	mg/dL	0.01	g/L
	mg/dL	0.029	μmol/L
Folic acid (S)	ng/mL	1.0	μg/L
	ng/mL	2.27	nmol/L
Haptoglobin (S)	mg/dL	0.01	g/L
Hematocrit (B)	%	0.01	ratio
Hemoglobin‡ (B)	g/dL	1.0	g/dL
Iron (S)	μg/dL	0.179	μmol/L
Iron-binding capacity (S)	μg/dL	0.179	μmol/L
Leukocyte count (B)	number per μL	10^6	number per L
Mean corpuscular hemoglobin	pg	1.0	pg
Mean corpuscular hemoglobin concentration	%	1.0	g/dL
Mean corpuscular volume	μm^3	1.0	fL
Packed cell volume (B)	%	0.01	ratio
Phosphorus (S)	mg/dL	0.323	mmol/L
Platelet count (B)	number per μL	10^6	number per L
Prophobilinogen (U)	mg/d	4.42	μmol/D
Protoporphyrin (erythrocyte)	μg/dL	0.018	μmol/L
Reticulocyte count (B)	%	0.01	ratio
	number per μL	10^6	number per l
Transferrin (S)	mg/dL	0.01	g per l
Urea nitrogen (B)	mg/dL	0.36	mmol/L
Uric acid (S)	mg/dL	0.0595	mmol/L
Uroporphyrin (U)	μg/d	1.2	nmol/d
Vitamin B_{12} (S)	pg/mL	1.0	ng/L
	pg/mL	0.738	pmol/L

B, blood; S, serum; P, plasma; U, urine.
* Conventional units multiplied by this factor yield SI units.
† The molar concentration is calculated assuming a molecular weight of 340,000.
‡ Hemoglobin is not usually expressed in molar terms because of uncertainty regarding the polymeric state of the molecule. If the unit (globin chain) molecular weight is assumed to be 16,000, the multiplication factor is 0.62 to convert g/dL to mmol/L. If a molecular weight of 64,500 is assumed (hemoglobin molecule, $\alpha_2\beta_2$ tetramer), the conversion factor is 0.155.
(Data from Baron DN, Broughton PMG, Cohen M, Lansley TS, Lewis SM, Shinton NK. The use of SI units in reporting results obtained in hospital laboratories. J Clin Pathol 1974;27:590; Young DS. "Normal laboratory values" [case records of the Massachusetts General Hospital] in SI units. N Engl J Med 1975;292:795; Lehmann HP. Metrication of clinical laboratory data in SI units. Am J Clin Pathol 1976;65:2)
(Williams WJ, Beutler E, Ersler AJ, Lictman MA. Hematology, ed 4. New York, McGraw-Hill, 1990: 1784)

Blood: Principles and Practice of Hematology,
edited by Robert I. Handin, Samuel E. Lux, and Thomas P. Stossel.
J.B. Lippincott Company, Philadelphia © 1995.

Index

Page numbers in italic type indicate figures, numbers preceded by CF refer to color figures, and numbers followed by *t* indicate tables.

A

B

C

D

E

H

J

K

L

M

O

Q

R

T

U

V

W

X

Y

Z